COLOR ATLASES

I. ATLAS OF CARDIOLOGY

I-1A Exercise sestamibi study **I-1B** Exercise sestamibi study **I-2** Transesophageal echocardiographic view **I-3** Transesophageal echocardiographic view

II. ATLAS OF DERMATOLOGY

A. Common Skin Diseases and Lesions
IIA-1 Acne vulgaris **IIA-2** Acne rosacea **IIA-3** Psoriasis **IIA-4** Atopic dermatitis **IIA-5** Dyshidrotic eczema **IIA-6** Seborrheic dermatitis **IIA-7** Stasis dermatitis **IIA-8A** Allergic contact dermatitis **IIA-8B** Allergic contact dermatitis **IIA-9** Lichen planus **IIA-10** Seborrheic keratoses **IIA-11** Vitiligo **IIA-12** Alopecia areata **IIA-13** Pityriasis rosea **IIA-14A** Urticaria **IIA-14B** Dermatographism **IIA-15** Epidermoid cysts **IIA-16** Keloids **IIA-17** Cherry hemangiomas **IIA-18** Frostbite **IIA-19** Frostbite

B. Cutaneous Neoplasms
IIB-20 Kaposi's sarcoma **IIB-21** Non-Hodgkin's lymphoma **IIB-22** Basal cell carcinoma **IIB-23** Mycosis fungoides **IIB-24** Metastatic carcinoma **IIB-25** Keratoacanthoma **IIB-26** Squamous cell carcinoma **IIB-27** Actinic keratoses

C. Pigmented Lesions—Benign and Malignant
IIC-28 Nevus **IIC-29** Dysplastic nevi **IIC-30** Superficial spreading melanoma **IIC-31** Lentigo maligna melanoma **IIC-32** Nodular melanoma **IIC-33** Acral lentiginous melanoma

D. Infectious Disease and the Skin
IID-34 Erysipelas **IID-35** Spread of herpes zoster with chemotherapy **IID-36** Varicella **IID-37** Herpes zoster **IID-38** Impetigo contagiosa **IID-39** Tender vesicles and erosions **IID-40** Lacy reticular rash of erythema infectiosum **IID-41** Molluscum contagiosum **IID-42** Oral hairy leukoplakia **IID-43** Pseudomembranous oral candidiasis **IID-44** Fulminant meningococcemia **IID-45** Rocky Mountain spotted fever **IID-46** Erythema chronicum migrans **IID-47** Primary syphilis **IID-48** Secondary syphilis **IID-49** Condylomata lata **IID-50** Secondary syphilis **IID-51** Tinea corporis **IID-52** Scabies **IID-53** Skin lesions **IID-54** Chancroid **IID-55** Condylomata acuminata **IID-56** A patient with features of polar lepromatous leprosy **IID-57** Skin lesions of neutropenic patients **IID-58** Septic emboli **IID-59** Vegetations **IID-60** Disseminated gonococcemia

E. Immunologically Mediated Skin Disease
IIE-61A Systematic lupus erythematosus **IIE-61B** Acute LE **IIE-62** Discoid lupus erythematous **IIE-63** Dermatomyositis **IIE-64** Scleroderma **IIE-65** Dermatomyositis **IIE-66** Scleroderma **IIE-67** Erythema multiforme **IIE-68** Dermatitis herpetiformis **IIE-69A** Pemphigus vulgaris **IIE-69B** Pemphigus vulgaris **IIE-70** Erythema nodosum **IIE-71** Vasculitis **IIE-72** Bullous pemphigoid

F. Skin Manifestations of Internal Disease
IIF-73 Acanthosis nigricans **IIF-74** Pretibial myxedema **IIF-75** Plaque of Sweet's syndrome **IIF-76** Bilateral rheumatoid nodules **IIF-77** Neurofibromatosis **IIF-78** Coumarin **IIF-79A** Sarcoid **IIF-79B** Sarcoid **IIF-80** Pyoderma gangrenosum

III. ATLAS OF ENDOSCOPIC FINDINGS

III-1 Normal esophagus **III-2** Peptic regurgitant esophagitis **III-3** Ulcerated squamous cell carcinoma **III-4** Moniliasis of the esophagus **III-5** Barrett's metaplasia of the esophagus **III-6** Normal body of the stomach **III-7** Large, benign, lesser curve gastric ulcer **III-8** Gastric polyp **III-9** Arteriovenous malformation **III-10** Normal pylorus **III-11** Normal duodenal bulb **III-12** Duodenal ulcer **III-13** Normal papilla of Vater **III-14** Periampullary carcinoma **III-15** Endoscopic papillotomy **III-16** Normal colon **III-17** Colonic adenomatous polyp **III-18** Colonic adenomatous polyps **III-19** Colon adenocarcinoma **III-20** Crohn's colitis **III-21** Severe ulcerative colitis **III-22** Kaposi's sarcoma **III-23** Colonic varices **III-24** Ileal pouch

IV. ATLAS OF FUNDUSCOPIC FINDINGS

IV-1 Retinal vasculitis, uveitis, and hemorrhage **IV-2** Cytomegalovirus **IV-3** Hollenhorst plaque **IV-4** Central retinal artery occlusion **IV-5** Hypertensive retinopathy **IV-6** Central retinal vein occlusion **IV-7** Anterior ischemic optic neuropathy **IV-8** Retrobulbar optic neuritis **IV-9** Optic atrophy **IV-10** Papilledema **IV-11** Optic disc drusen **IV-12** Retinal detachment **IV-13** Glaucoma **IV-14** Age-related macular degeneration **IV-15** Diabetic retinopathy **IV-16** Retinitis pigmentosa **IV-17** Melanoma of the choroid **IV-18** Kayser-Fleischer ring

V. ATLAS OF HEMATOLOGY

V-1 Normal blood smear **V-2** β-Thalassemia intermedia **V-3** Uremia **V-4** Burkitt's lymphoma **V-5** Marrow iron stores **V-6** Multiple myeloma (marrow) **V-7** Reactive lymphocytes (infectious mononucleosis) **V-8** Immunohemolytic anemia **V-9** Leukoerythroblastic smear **V-10A** Normal granulocyte **V-10B** Normal monocyte and lymphocyte **V-11** Normal granulocyte precursors in marrow **V-12** Leukemic cell in acute promyelocytic leukemia **V-13** Aplastic anemia **V-14** Normal bone marrow biopsy **V-15** Erythroid hyperplasia **V-16** Iron-deficiency anemia **V-17** Chronic lymphocytic leukemia **V-18** Hodgkin's disease, mixed cellularity **V-19** Marrow fibrosis **V-20** Acute myelocytic leukemia **V-21** Liver disease **V-22** Diffuse large B cell lymphoma **V-23** Neutrophils with toxic granulation **V-24** Megaloblastic anemia **V-25** Leukemic cells in acute lymphoblastic leukemia **V-26** Hereditary spherocytosis **V-27** Spur cell anemia **V-28** Traumatic hemolysis **V-29** Granulocytic hyperplasia **V-30** Follicular lymphoma **V-31** Auer rod **V-32A** Normal eosinophil **V-32B** Basophil **V-33** Megaloblastic erythropoiesis **V-34A** Chédiak-Higashi anomaly **V-34B** Pelger-Hüet anomaly **V-35** Band with Döhle body **V-36** Chronic granulocytic leukemia **V-37** Ringed sideroblast **V-38** Hypersegmentation **V-39** Sickle cell anemia **V-40** Adult T cell leukemia/lymphoma

VI. ATLAS OF DIAGNOSTIC MICROBIOLOGY

VI-1 Gram-stained sputum **VI-2** *Streptococcus pneumoniae*
P. falciparum—thin film: **VI-3 to VI-8**
P. vivax—thin film: **VI-9 to VI-13**
P. ovale—thin film: **VI-14 to VI-17**
P. malariae—thin film: **VI-18 to VI-21**
Babesia—thin film: **VI-22**
P. falciparum—thick film: **VI-23, VI-24**
P. vivax—thick film: **VI-25 to VI-27**
P. ovale—thick film: **VI-28 to VI-30**
P. malariae—thick film: **VI-31 to VI-33**

HARRISON'S 15TH EDITION

PRINCIPLES OF
INTERNAL
MEDICINE

EDITORS OF PREVIOUS EDITIONS

T. R. HARRISON
Editor-in-Chief, Editions 1, 2, 3, 4, 5

W. R. RESNICK
Editor, Editions 1, 2, 3, 4, 5

M. M. WINTROBE
Editor, Editions 1, 2, 3, 4, 5
Editor-in-Chief, Editions 6, 7

G. W. THORN
Editor, Editions 1, 2, 3, 4, 5, 6, 7
Editor-in-Chief, Edition 8

R. D. ADAMS
Editor, Editions 2, 3, 4, 5, 6, 7, 8, 9, 10

P. B. BEESON
Editor, Editions 1, 2

I. L. BENNETT, JR.
Editor, Editions 3, 4, 5, 6

E. BRAUNWALD
Editor, Editions 6, 7, 8, 9, 10, 12, 13, 14
Editor-in-Chief, Edition 11

K. J. ISSELBACHER
Editor, Editions 6, 7, 8, 10, 11, 12, 14
Editor-in-Chief, Editions 9, 13

R. G. PETERSDORF
Editor, Editions 6, 7, 8, 9, 11, 12, 13
Editor-in-Chief, Edition 10

J. D. WILSON
Editor, Editions 9, 10, 11, 13, 14
Editor-in-Chief, Edition 12

J. B. MARTIN
Editor, Editions 10, 11, 12, 13, 14

A. S. FAUCI
Editor, Editions 11, 12, 13
Editor-in-Chief, Edition 14

R. ROOT
Editor, Edition 12

D. L. KASPER
Editor, Editions 13, 14

S. L. HAUSER
Editor, Edition 14

D. L. LONGO
Editor, Edition 14

HARRISON'S 15TH EDITION

PRINCIPLES OF INTERNAL MEDICINE

EDITORS

EUGENE BRAUNWALD, MD, MD(Hon), ScD(Hon)

Distinguished Hersey Professor of Medicine,
Faculty Dean for Academic Programs at Brigham and
Women's Hospital and Massachusetts General Hospital,
Harvard Medical School; Vice-President for Academic
Programs, Partners HealthCare Systems, Boston

ANTHONY S. FAUCI, MD, ScD(Hon)

Chief, Laboratory of Immunoregulation; Director,
National Institute of Allergy and Infectious Diseases,
National Institutes of Health, Bethesda

DENNIS L. KASPER, MD, MA(Hon)

William Ellery Channing Professor of Medicine,
Professor of Microbiology and Molecular Genetics,
Executive Dean for Academic Programs, Harvard
Medical School; Director, Channing Laboratory,
Department of Medicine, Brigham and Women's
Hospital, Boston

STEPHEN L. HAUSER, MD

Betty Anker Fife Professor and Chairman,
Department of Neurology,
University of California San Francisco,
San Francisco

DAN L. LONGO, MD

Scientific Director, National Institute on Aging,
National Institutes of Health,
Bethesda and Baltimore

J. LARRY JAMESON, MD, PhD

Irving S. Cutter Professor and Chairman,
Department of Medicine,
Northwestern University Medical School;
Physician-in-Chief, Northwestern
Memorial Hospital, Chicago

McGraw-Hill
MEDICAL PUBLISHING DIVISION

New York   San Francisco   Washington, DC   Auckland   Bogotá   Caracas   Lisbon   London
Madrid   Mexico City   Milan   Montreal   New Delhi   San Juan   Singapore   Sydney   Tokyo   Toronto

McGraw-Hill
A Division of The **McGraw·Hill** *Companies*

Note: Dr. Fauci and Dr. Longo's works as editors and authors were performed outside the scope of their employment as U.S. government employees. These works represent their personal and professional views and not necessarily those of the U.S. government.

Harrison's
PRINCIPLES OF INTERNAL MEDICINE
Fifteenth Edition

1234567890 DOWDOW 0987654321
ISBN 0-07-007272-8 (Combo)
0-07-007273-6 (Vol. 1)
0-07-007274-4 (Vol. 2)
0-07-913686-9 (Set)

FOREIGN LANGUAGE EDITIONS
Arabic (Thirteenth Edition)—McGraw-Hill Libri Italia srl (est. 1996)
Chinese (Twelfth Edition)—McGraw-Hill Book Company—Singapore © 1994
Croatian (Thirteenth Edition)—Placebo, Split, Croatia
French (Fourteenth Edition)—McGraw-Hill Publishing Co., Maidenhead, UK © 1999
German (Fourteenth Edition)—McGraw-Hill Publishing Co., Maidenhead, UK © 1999
Greek (Fourteenth Edition)—Parissianos, Athens, Greece © 2000
Italian (Fourteenth Edition)—McGraw-Hill Libri Italia srl, Milan © 1999
Japanese (Eleventh Edition)—Hirokawa © 1991
Polish (Fourteenth Edition)—Czelej Publishing Company, Lubin, Poland (est. 2000)
Portuguese (Fourteenth Edition)—McGraw-Hill Interamericana do Brasil Ltda © 1998
Romania (Fourteenth Edition)—Teora Publishers, Bucharest, Romania (est. 2000)
Spanish (Fourteenth Edition)—McGraw-Hill Interamericana de Espana, Madrid © 1998
Turkish (Thirteenth Edition)—McGraw-Hill Libri Italia srl (est. 1996)

This book was set in Times Roman by Progressive Information Technologies. The editors were Martin Wonsiewicz and Mariapaz Ramos Englis. The production director was Robert Laffler. The index was prepared by Irving C. Tullar. The text and cover designer was Marsha Cohen/Parallelogram Graphics.

R. R. Donnelley and Sons, Inc. was the printer and binder.

Library of Congress Cataloging-in-Publication Data

Harrison's principles of internal medicine—15th ed./editors, Eugene Braunwald . . . [et al.].   p. cm.
  Includes bibliographical references and index.
  ISBN 0-07-913686-9 (set)—ISBN 0-07-007273-6 (v. 1)—ISBN 0-07-0072744-4 (v. 2)
    1. Internal medicine. I. Braunwald, Eugene, date
RC46.H333 2001
616—dc21
                                                                          00-063809

DEDICATION

KURT J. ISSELBACHER

With this edition, the editors acknowledge the many contributions of our colleague Kurt J. Isselbacher, who served as an editor of *Harrison's* for nine editions, the sixth through the fourteenth, including Editor-in-Chief of the ninth and thirteenth editions. For more than three decades Dr. Isselbacher played a decisive role in ensuring that *Harrison's* epitomized the state of the art and science of internal medicine and the essence of accuracy and clarity. His indelible contributions to *Harrison's* are felt in the fifteenth edition and will endure into the future.

Dr. Isselbacher is a graduate of Harvard College and of the Harvard Medical School. His further training included a residency in medicine at the Massachusetts General Hospital and a research fellowship at the National Institutes of Health. Chosen to lead the Gastrointestinal Unit of the MGH at the remarkable age of 31, over the ensuing 30 years as Chief of that Unit, he was a leader in advancing both the clinical specialty of gastroenterology and the basic understanding of gastrointestinal disease. Under his leadership, the MGH Gastrointestinal Unit became renowned for its training program in academic gastroenterology as well as for being one of the world's leading centers for clinical and research activities in gastroenterology. In 1987, Dr. Isselbacher undertook new challenges as the first Director of the Cancer Center at the MGH, bringing his characteristic insight and leadership to this new task. In a relatively short time, the MGH Cancer Center has emerged as a premier cancer research institute. Dr. Isselbacher holds the Mallinckrodt Distinguished Professorship of Medicine at Harvard Medical School, and he has been a powerful force for excellence in scholarship at this institution since his graduation. For almost 30 years he served as Chairman of the Executive Committee of Harvard's Departments of Medicine and played a pivotal role in the departments' growth and quest for excellence.

Dr. Isselbacher combines the attributes of an excellent scientist with those of a superb clinician and teacher. He has trained generations of physicians and investigators, including many who are now leaders in academic medicine. As the author of more than 400 scientific articles in leading journals, his research contributions include definition of enzymatic defects in absorptive disorders, and delineation of biochemical mechanisms of absorption, malabsorption, protein synthesis, derangements of metabolism, and immunologic aspects of hepatic gastrointestinal disease. Kurt Isselbacher has been a recipient of many well-earned honors, including the Distinguished Achievement Award and the Friedenwald Medal of the American Gastroenterological Association, the John Phillips Memorial Award for distinguished contributions to clinical medicine from the American College of Physicians, as well as the Kober Medal of the Association of American Physicians. He is a member of the National Academy of Sciences and of its Institute of Medicine and has served as President of the American Gastroenterological Association, the American Association for the Study of Liver Disease, and the Association of American Physicians.

Kurt Isselbacher exemplifies the highest values of medicine. A caring, empathic physician, he consistently combines compassion with incisive analysis in the care of patients. With contributions as a clinician, teacher, scientist, and editor, he has advanced the care of patients with gastrointestinal disorders and cancer while educating generations of physicians.

DEDICATION

JEAN DONALD WILSON

Jean Wilson served as editor of the ninth through the fourteenth editions of *Harrison's Principles of Internal Medicine* from 1978 to 1998; he was Editor-in-Chief of the twelfth edition. A native of Texas, Jean Wilson attended the University of Texas at Austin and the University of Texas Southwestern Medical School in Dallas. He trained as a resident in internal medicine and as a fellow in endocrinology and metabolism at Parkland Hospital. With the exception of 2 years of research in biochemistry in the intramural program of the National Institutes of Health, Dr. Wilson spent his entire career at the University of Texas Southwestern Medical School, where he now holds the Charles Cameron Sprague Distinguished Chair in Biomedical Science.

Dr. Wilson is one of America's most distinguished biomedical scientists and is largely responsible for working out the mechanism of action and physiology of the male sex hormones from the embryo to the normal and diseased adult. Among his many important discoveries has been the 5α-reductase reaction, whereby male target tissues convert testosterone to the more active androgen, dihydrotestosterone. He has been honored many times for his research, having received the Ernst Oppenheimer Memorial Award of the Endocrine Society, the Amory Prize of the American Academy of Arts and Sciences, the Lita Annenberg Hazen Award for Excellence in Clinical Research, the Henry Dale Medal of the Society for Endocrinology, the Gregory Pincus Award of the Worcester Foundation for Experimental Biology, the Fred Conrad Koch Award of the Endocrine Society, and the Kober Medal of the Association of American Physicians.

Amongst his memberships are the National Academy of Sciences, the Institute of Medicine of the National Academy of Sciences, and the American Academy of Arts and Sciences. He is a Fellow of the Royal College of Physicians. He has served as President of the American Society for Clinical Investigation, the Association of American Physicians, and the Endocrine Society. For two decades, Dr. Wilson directed the enormously successful MD/PhD program and for 8 years, the highly esteemed Endocrine-Metabolism Division at Southwestern.

Perhaps the finest thing that can be said of Jean Wilson is that he is a professor of internal medicine in the complete sense. He is, and always has been, a superb teacher and exemplary clinician while constantly maintaining a sterling career in research. Perhaps nothing describes him better than the enduring image of this renowned academic physician trimming callouses and ulcers in the Diabetic Foot Care Clinic at Parkland Memorial Hospital, his teaching hospital, where the patients are the medically indigent of Dallas.

Dr. Wilson is a man of diverse interests, a true intellectual. One of his great gifts and loves is scientific and medical editing. He served as Editor-in-Chief of the *Journal of Clinical Investigation* and of *Williams Textbook of Endocrinology*. As an editor of *Harrison's* for two decades, Dr. Wilson made ample use of his conspicuous strengths as clinician, teacher, and scientist. His meticulous scholarship and high standards have had an enormous impact, not only on the Endocrinology, Metabolism, and Genetics sections, for which he had primary responsibility, but on the entire book.

DEDICATION

JOSEPH B. MARTIN

The editors wish to acknowledge the enormous contributions made by Joseph B. Martin, who edited the Neurology section of *Harrison's* from the tenth to the fourteenth editions. Dr. Martin followed Dr. Raymond D. Adams as editor of the Neurology section. In retrospect, the choice of Joseph Martin to replace Adams was prescient. It foresaw the transformation of neurology in the 1980s and 1990s from a largely descriptive discipline to one of the most dynamic and rapidly evolving areas of internal medicine. With his appointment as editor, the textbook had secured the foremost leader in the new field of molecular neurology to its ranks. Beginning with the tenth edition, Martin built upon the powerful didactic structure of the "syndromic approach" to neurology created by Adams and emphasized advances in molecular genetics and cell biology that reclassify neurologic diseases, clarify disease mechanisms, and offer new insights into clinical diagnosis and therapy. During his tenure, the neurology section of *Harrison's* became the best resource of its kind for the exposition of new discoveries in neurology and contributed substantially to the growing overall success of the textbook.

Born in Bassano, Alberta, Canada, Dr. Martin received his premedical and medical education at the University of Alberta, Edmonton, trained in neurology at Case Western University, and received the PhD from the University of Rochester. His career in academic medicine began in 1971 at McGill University in Montreal, where he established an independent laboratory focused on hypothalamic regulation of pituitary hormone secretion, and where he quickly rose to become Chair of the Department of Neurology and Neurosurgery. In 1978, he joined the faculty at Harvard Medical School as Bullard (later Julianne Dorn) Professor of Neurology and Chief of the Neurology Service at Massachusetts General Hospital. While at Harvard,

he established the Huntington's Disease Center Without Walls, which in 1983 reported the spectacular finding of a genetic marker linked to Huntington's disease, thereby inaugurating the modern era of molecular neurogenetics. In 1989 Dr. Martin joined the University of California, San Francisco, initially serving as Dean of the School of Medicine and subsequently as Chancellor. Among his many achievements at UCSF was the conception of a major new research campus in San Francisco, which is fast becoming a reality. In July 1997, he returned to Harvard as the Caroline Shields Walker Professor of Neurobiology and Clinical Neuroscience and Dean of the Faculty of Medicine. A wonderful teacher and physician, Joe Martin has inspired a generation of housestaff, students, and colleagues at Harvard and UCSF.

Dr. Martin has received many honors, including honorary degrees from five distinguished universities and the Abraham Flexner Award of the Association of American Medical Colleges. He serves or has served on the editorial boards of nineteen medical and neurology journals. He is a member of the Institute of Medicine of the National Academy of Sciences and has served as President of the American Neurological Association.

Dr. Martin's many contributions to this textbook were enhanced by his extraordinary organizational skills and by a clear and direct style of writing and editing that permitted him to distill complex concepts into easily readable prose accessible to a general medical readership. As an example, his chapter on neurogenetics has become an instant classic and a highlight of each new edition of the book. The editors greatly value their friendship with this remarkable man whose integrity and intellectual strengths have served *Harrison's* so well during the past two decades.

CONTENTS

SECTION 2
DISORDERS OF HEMATOPOIESIS

SECTION 3
DISORDERS OF HEMOSTASIS

Part Seven

INFECTIOUS DISEASES

SECTION 1
BASIC CONSIDERATIONS IN INFECTIOUS DISEASES

SECTION 2
CLINICAL SYNDROMES: COMMUNITY-ACQUIRED
INFECTIONS

Part Ten

DISORDERS OF THE KIDNEY AND URINARY TRACT

Part Eleven

DISORDERS OF THE GASTROINTESTINAL SYSTEM

SECTION 1
DISORDERS OF THE ALIMENTARY TRACT

SECTION 2
LIVER AND BILIARY TRACT DISEASE

Part Fourteen
NEUROLOGIC DISORDERS

SECTION 1
DIAGNOSIS OF NEUROLOGIC DISORDERS

SECTION 2
DISEASES OF THE CENTRAL NERVOUS SYSTEM

SECTION 3
DISORDERS OF NERVE AND MUSCLES

SECTION 4
CHRONIC FATIGUE SYNDROME

SECTION 5
PSYCHIATRIC DISORDERS

SECTION 6
ALCOHOLISM AND DRUG DEPENDENCY

Part Fifteen

ENVIRONMENTAL AND OCCUPATIONAL HAZARDS

SECTION 1
SPECIFIC ENVIRONMENTAL AND OCCUPATIONAL HAZARDS

SECTION 2
ILLNESSES DUE TO POISONS, DRUG OVERDOSAGE, AND ENVENOMATION

APPENDICES

CONTRIBUTORS

Numbers in brackets refer to chapters written or co-written by the contributor.

ELIAS ABRUTYN, MD
Professor of Medicine and Public Health; Associate Provost and Associate Dean for Faculty Affairs, Department of Medicine, Division of Infectious Diseases, MCP Hahnemann University School of Medicine, Philadelphia [143, 144]

JOHN W. ADAMSON, MD
Director, Blood Research Institute, Blood Center of Southeastern Wisconsin, Milwaukee [61, 105]

DAVID A. AHLQUIST, MD
Professor of Medicine, Mayo Medical School; Consultant in Gastroenterology, Mayo Clinic and Foundation, Rochester [42]

LEENA ALA-KOKKO, MD
Collagen Research Unit, Biocenter Oulu and Department of Medical Biochemistry, University of Oulu, Finland [351]

MUHAMMAD T. AL-LOZI, MBBS
Assistant Professor of Neurology, Washington University, St. Louis [101]

MICHAEL J. AMINOFF, MD
Professor of Neurology, University of California San Francisco, San Francisco [22, 357, 363]

KENNETH C. ANDERSON, MD
Associate Professor of Medicine, Harvard Medical School; Medical Director, Blood Component Laboratory, Dana-Farber Cancer Institute, Boston [114]

ELLIOTT M. ANTMAN, MD
Associate Professor of Medicine, Harvard Medical School; Director, Samuel A. Levine Cardiac Unit, Brigham and Women's Hospital, Boston [243]

FREDERICK R. APPELBAUM, MD
Member and Director, Clinical Research Division Fred Hutchinson Cancer Research Center; Professor and Head, Division of Medical Oncology, University of Washington School of Medicine, Seattle [115]

GORDON L. ARCHER, MD
Chairman, Division of Infectious Diseases, Department of Internal Medicine; Professor of Medicine and Microbiology/Immunology, Medical College of Virginia, Campus of Virginia Commonwealth University, Richmond [137]

JAMES O. ARMITAGE, MD
Dean, College of Medicine, and Professor of Internal Medicine, Section of Oncology/Hematology, University of Nebraska, Omaha [112]

ARTHUR K. ASBURY, MD
Van Meter Professor of Neurology Emeritus, University of Pennsylvania School of Medicine, Philadelphia [23, 377, 378]

JOHN R. ASPLIN, MD
Assistant Professor of Medicine, Section of Nephrology, University of Chicago, Pritzker School of Medicine, Chicago [276, 279]

JOHN C. ATHERTON, MRCP
Lecturer, Department of Medicine, Division of Gastroenterology and Institute of Infections and Immunity, University of Nottingham, Nottingham, England [154]

PAUL S. AUERBACH, MD
Clinical Professor of Surgery, Division of Emergency Medicine, Stanford University School of Medicine, Los Altos [397]

K. FRANK AUSTEN, MD
Theodore Bevier Bayles Professor of Medicine, Harvard Medical School; Director, Inflammation and Allergic Diseases Research Section, Division of Rheumatology, Immunology and Allergy, Brigham and Women's Hospital, Boston [310]

BERNARD M. BABIOR, MD, PhD
Head, Division of Biochemistry, Department of Molecular and Experimental Medicine, The Scripps Research Institute; Professor and Staff Physician, Division of Hematology and Oncology, Department of Medicine, Scripps Clinic and Research Foundation, La Jolla [107]

KAMAL F. BADR, MD
Professor and Chair, Department of Internal Medicine, American University of Beirut (Lebanon); Attending Physician, American University of Beirut Medical Center, Beirut, Lebanon [278]

DONALD S. BAIM, MD
Professor of Medicine, Harvard Medical School; Director, Center for Minimally Invasive Therapy, Brigham and Women's Hospital, Boston [228, 245]

ROBERT L. BARBIERI, MD
Kate Macy Ladd Professor Obstetrics, Gynecology and Reproductive Biology, Harvard Medical School; Chairman, Department of Obstetrics and Gynecology, Brigham and Women's Hospital, Boston [7]

TAMAR F. BARLAM, MD
Assistant Professor of Medicine, Harvard Medical School; Senior Associate Physician, Beth Israel Deaconess Medical Center, Boston; Director, Project on Antibiotic Resistance, Center for Science in the Public Interest, Washington, D.C. [19, 150]

KENNETH J. BART, MD, MPH, MSHPM
Director, Graduate School of Public Health, San Diego State University, San Diego [122]

M. FLINT BEAL, MD
Anne Parrish Titzel Professor and Chairman of Neurology, Weill Medical College; Neurologist-in-Chief, New York Presbyterian Hospital, New York [367, 376]

ROBERT S. BENJAMIN, MD
Internist and Professor of Medicine, Chairman, Department of Melanoma/Sarcoma Medical Oncology; Medical Director, Multidisciplinary Sarcoma Center, The University of Texas M.D. Anderson Cancer Center, Houston [98]

JOHN E. BENNETT, MD
Head, Clinical Mycology Section, Laboratory of Clinical Investigation, National Institute of Allergy and Infectious Diseases, National Institutes of Health, Potomac [200, 201, 202, 203, 204, 205, 206, 207, 208]

EDWARD J. BENZ, JR., MD
Richard and Susan Smith Professor of Medicine, Professor of Pediatrics and Pathology, Harvard Medical School; President, Dana-Farber Cancer Institute, Boston [106]

PAUL D. BERK, MD
Department of Medicine, Division of Liver Disease, Mount Sinai School of Medicine, New York [294]

DAVID R. BICKERS, MD
Carl Truman Nelson Professor and Chairman, Department of Dermatology, Columbia University, New York [60]

HENRY J. BINDER, MD
Professor of Medicine, Section of Digestive Diseases, Yale University, New Haven [286]

THOMAS D. BIRD, MD
Professor of Neurology, University of Washington; Chief of Neurology, Veterans Affairs Medical Center, Seattle [26, 362, 379]

NEIL R. BLACKLOW, MD
Richard M. Haidack Distinguished Professor of Medicine, Molecular Genetics and Microbiology, University of Massachusetts Medical School, Worcester [187]

MARTIN J. BLASER, MD
Frederick J. King Professor of Internal Medicine, Chairman, Department of Medicine, and Professor of Microbiology, New York University School of Medicine, New York [154, 158]

CLARA D. BLOOMFIELD, MD
Director, The Ohio State University Comprehensive Cancer Center; Deputy Director, The Arthur G. James Cancer Hospital and Richard J. Solove Research Institute; William G. Pace III Endowed Chair in Cancer Research; Director and Professor, Division of Hematology and Oncology, Department of Internal Medicine, College of Medicine and Public Health, The Ohio State University, Columbus [111]

RICHARD S. BLUMBERG, MD
Associate Professor of Medicine, Harvard Medical School; Chief, Division of Gastroenterology, Department of Medicine, Brigham and Women's Hospital, Boston [287]

JEAN L. BOLOGNIA, MD
Professor of Dermatology, Yale University School of Medicine, New Haven [57]

GEORGE J. BOSL, MD
Chairman, Department of Medicine, Memorial Sloan-Kettering Cancer Center; Professor of Medicine, Cornell University Medical College, New York [96]

PATRICK BOSQUE, MD
Assistant Professor of Neurology, Institute for Neurodegenerative Diseases, University of California San Francisco, San Francisco [375]

RICHARD C. BOUCHER, MD
William Rand Kenan Professor of Medicine, University of North Carolina at Chapel Hill; Director, Cystic Fibrosis/Pulmonary Research & Treatment Center, Chapel Hill [257]

KAREN D. BRADSHAW, MD
Associate Professor of Obstetrics and Gynecology, The University of Texas Southwestern Medical Center, Dallas [52, 336]

HUGH R. BRADY, MD, PhD
Professor of Medicine and Therapeutics, University College Dublin; Mater Misericordiae Hospital, Dublin, Ireland [269, 273, 274, 275]

KENNETH D. BRANDT, MD
Professor of Medicine and Head, Rheumatology Division, Indiana University School of Medicine; Director, Indiana University Multipurpose Arthritis and Musculoskeletal Disease Center, Indianapolis [321]

EUGENE BRAUNWALD, MD, MD(Hon), ScD(Hon)
Distinguished Hersey Professor of Medicine; Faculty Dean for Academic Programs at Brigham and Women's Hospital and Massachusetts General Hospital, Harvard Medical School; Vice-President for Academic Programs, Partners HealthCare System, Boston [32, 33, 34, 36, 37, 224, 225, 231, 232, 236, 237, 238, 239, 243, 244]

IRWIN M. BRAVERMAN, MD
Professor of Dermatology, Yale University School of Medicine, New Haven [57]

OTIS W. BRAWLEY, MD
Assistant Director, Office of Special Populations Research, Office of the Director, National Cancer Institute, National Institutes of Health, Bethesda [80]

JOEL G. BREMAN, MD, DTPH
Deputy Director, Division of International Training and Research, Fogarty International Center, National Institutes of Health, Bethesda [214]

BARRY M. BRENNER, MD, DSc(Hon), DMSc(Hon)
Samuel A. Levine Professor of Medicine, Harvard Medical School; Director, Renal Division, Brigham and Women's Hospital, Boston [47, 49, 268, 269, 270, 271, 273, 274, 275, 277, 278, 281]

ROBERT M. BRENNER, MD
Associate Medical Director, Clinical Research, Amgen Inc., Thousand Oaks, California [268]

CHARLES G. D. BROOK, MA, MD
Emeritus Professor of Pediatric Endocrinology, University College London, London, UK [8]

CLAIRE V. BROOME, MD
Senior Advisor to the Director, Integrated Health Information Systems, Centers for Disease Control and Prevention, Atlanta [142]

ROBERT H. BROWN, JR., DPhil, MD
Associate Neurologist, Massachusetts General Hospital; Professor of Neurology, Harvard Medical School, Boston [365, 383]

ROBERT C. BRUNHAM, MD
Professor of Medicine; Director and Medical Director, University of British Columbia Centre for Disease Control, Vancouver, BC, Canada [133]

H. FRANKLIN BUNN, MD
Professor of Medicine, Harvard Medical School; Physician, Brigham and Women's Hospital, Boston [107, 108]

DAVID M. BURNS, MD
Professor of Medicine, University of California San Diego, San Diego [390]

MICHAEL J. BURNS, MD
Instructor of Medicine, Harvard Medical School; Department of Emergency Medicine, Division of Toxicology, Beth Israel Deaconess Medical Center, Boston [396]

JOAN R. BUTTERTON, MD
Assistant Professor of Medicine, Harvard Medical School; Assistant in Medicine, Infectious Disease Division, Massachusetts General Hospital, Boston [131]

JOHN C. BYRD, MD
Director of Clinical Research, Hematology-Oncology Service, Department of Medicine, Walter Reed Army Medical Center, Washington, D.C. [111]

STEPHEN B. CALDERWOOD, MD
Chief, Division of Infectious Diseases, Massachusetts General Hospital; Associate Professor of Medicine (Microbiology and Molecular Genetics), Harvard Medical School, Boston [131]

MICHAEL CAMILLERI, MD
Professor of Medicine and Physiology, Mayo Medical School; Consultant in Gastroenterology, Physiology and Biophysics, Mayo Clinic and Mayo Foundation, Rochester [42]

GRANT L. CAMPBELL, MD, PhD
Division of Vector-Borne Infectious Diseases, National Center for Infectious Diseases, Centers for Disease Control and Prevention, Fort Collins [162, 175]

MARK D. CARLSON, MD
Vice Chair, Department of Medicine, University Hospitals of Cleveland; Associate Professor of Medicine, Case Western Reserve University School of Medicine, Cleveland [21]

CHARLES B. CARPENTER, MD
Professor of Medicine, Harvard Medical School; Senior Physician, Brigham and Women's Hospital, Boston [272]

BRUCE R. CARR, MD
Professor and Director, Division of Reproductive Endocrinology, and Holder, Paul C. MacDonald Distinguished Chair in Obstetrics and Gynecology, The University of Texas Southwestern Medical Center, Dallas [52, 336]

AGUSTIN CASTELLANOS, MD
Professor of Medicine and Director, Clinical Electrophysiology, University of Miami School of Medicine, Miami [39]

PHILLIP F. CHANCE, MD
Professor of Pediatrics and Neurology, University of Washington School of Medicine; Chief, Division of Genetics and Development, Children's Hospital and Regional Medical Center, Seattle [379]

FENG-YEE CHANG, MD, DSc
Associate Professor of Medicine, National Defense Medical Center; Chief, Division of Infectious Diseases, Tri-Service General Hospital, Taipei, Taiwan [151]

YUAN-TSONG CHEN, MD, PhD
Professor of Pediatrics and Genetics, and Chief, Division of Medical Genetics, Duke University Medical Center, Durham [350]

JOHN S. CHILD, MD
Professor of Medicine, University of California, Los Angeles; Co-Chief, Cardiology and Co-Director, Ahmanson/UCLA Adult Congenital Heart Disease Center, UCLA Medical Center, Los Angeles [234]

OLIVIER M. CHOSIDOW, MD
Department of Internal Medicine, Pitie-Salpêtrière Hospital, Paris, France [59]

RAYMOND T. CHUNG, MD
Medical Director, Liver Transplant Program; Director, Liver Service, Gastrointestinal Unit, Massachusetts General Hospital; Assistant Professor of Medicine, Harvard Medical School, Boston [299]

FREDRIC L. COE, MD
Professor of Medicine and Physiology and Director, Clinical Research Training Program, University of Chicago Pritzker School of Medicine, Chicago [276, 279]

ALAN S. COHEN, MD
Distinguished Professor of Medicine in Rheumatology, Emeritus, and Conrad Wesselhoeft Professor of Medicine, Emeritus, Boston University School of Medicine; Chief of Medicine and Director, Emeritus, Thorndike Memorial Laboratory, Boston City Hospital, Boston [319]

JEFFREY I. COHEN, MD
Head, Medical Virology Section, Laboratory of Clinical Investigation, National Institute of Allergy and Infectious Diseases, National Institutes of Health, Bethesda [184, 193]

FRANCIS S. COLLINS, MD, PhD
Director, National Human Genome Research Institute, National Institutes of Health, Bethesda [81]

WILSON S. COLUCCI, MD
Professor of Medicine, and Chief, Cardiovascular Medicine, Boston University School of Medicine, Boston [240]

GERALD A. COLVIN, DO
Assistant Professor of Medicine and Medical Research Scientist, University of Massachusetts Memorial Medical Center, Worcester [104]

MAUREEN T. CONNELLY, MD, MPH
Instructor in Medicine, Harvard Medical School; Harvard Pilgrim Health Care, Boston [10]

MAX D. COOPER, MD
Professor of Medicine, Pediatrics and Howard Hughes Medical Institute Investigator, University of Alabama at Birmingham, Birmingham [308]

LAWRENCE COREY, MD
Professor, Medicine and Laboratory Medicine, and Head, Virology Division, University of Washington; Head, Program in Infectious Diseases, Fred Hutchinson Cancer Research Center, Seattle [182, 197]

FELICIA COSMAN, MD
Associate Professor of Clinical Medicine, Columbia University; Medical Director, Clinical Research Center, Helen Hayes Hospital, West Haverstraw [342]

MARK A. CREAGER, MD
Associate Professor of Medicine, Harvard Medical School; Director, Vascular Center, Brigham and Women's Hospital, Boston [247, 248]

PHILIP E. CRYER, MD
Irene E. and Michael M. Karl Professor of Endocrinology and Metabolism, and Director, Division of Endocrinology, Diabetes and Metabolism, Washington University School of Medicine, St. Louis [334]

RONALD G. CRYSTAL, MD
Bruce Webster Professor of Medicine, Director, Institute of Geriatric Medicine, and Director, The Arthur and Rochelle Belfer Gene Therapy Care Facility, Weill Medical College of Cornell University, New York [318]

JOHN J. CUSH, MD
Medical Director, Arthritis Center, Presbyterian Hospital of Dallas, Dallas [320]

CHARLES A. CZEISLER, MD, PhD
Professor of Medicine, Harvard Medical School; Director, Sleep Disorders and Circadian Medicine, Brigham and Women's Hospital, Boston [27]

MARINOS C. DALAKAS, JR., MD
Chief, Neuromuscular Diseases Section, National Institute of Neurological Disorders and Stroke, National Institutes of Health, Bethesda [382]

DANIEL F. DANZL, MD
Professor and Chair, Department of Emergency Medicine, University of Louisville School of Medicine, Floyd Knobs, IN [20]

ROBERT B. DAROFF, MD
Chief of Staff and Senior Vice President for Academic Affairs, University Hospitals of Cleveland; Professor of Neurology and Associate Dean, Case Western Reserve University School of Medicine, Cleveland [21]

MEHUL T. DATTANI, MD
Senior Lecturer/Honorary Consultant in Pediatric Endocrinology, Institute of Child Health and Great Ormond Street Children's Hospital, London, UK [8]

CHARLES E. DAVIS, MD
Professor of Pathology and Medicine, University of California - San Diego School of Medicine; Director Emeritus, Microbiology Laboratory, UCSD Medical Center, San Diego [211]

JOHN DEL VALLE, MD
Professor of Medicine, Division of Gastroenterology, Department of Medicine, University of Michigan School of Medicine, Ann Arbor [285]

BRADLEY M. DENKER, MD
Assistant Professor of Medicine, Harvard Medical School; Associate Physician, Brigham and Women's Hospital, Boston [47]

DAVID T. DENNIS, MD, MPH
Chief, Bacterial Zoonoses Branch, Centers for Disease Control and Prevention, Fort Collins [162, 175]

ROBERT L. DERESIEWICZ, MD
Assistant Professor of Medicine, Harvard Medical School, Boston [139]

ROBERT J. DESNICK, PhD, MD
Professor and Chairman, Department of Human Genetics, Mount Sinai School of Medicine, New York [346]

BETTY DIAMOND, MD
Chief, Division of Rheumatology, Department of Microbiology and Immunology, Albert Einstein College of Medicine, New York [307]

JULES L. DIENSTAG, MD
Associate Professor of Medicine, Harvard Medical School; Physician, Massachusetts General Hospital, Boston [91, 295, 296, 297, 301]

WILLIAM P. DILLON, MD
Professor of Radiology, Neurology and Neurosurgery; Chief, Diagnostic Neuroradiology, University of California San Francisco, San Francisco [358]

CHARLES A. DINARELLO, MD
Professor of Medicine, University of Colorado Health Sciences Center, Denver [17]

ROBERT G. DLUHY, MD
Professor of Medicine, Harvard Medical School, Brigham and Women's Hospital, Boston [331]

RAPHAEL DOLIN, MD
Maxwell Finland Professor of Medicine, and Dean for Clinical Programs, Harvard Medical School, Boston [181, 189, 190]

DANIEL B. DRACHMAN, MD
Professor of Neurology and Neurosciences; Director, Neuromuscular Unit, The Johns Hopkins University School of Medicine, Baltimore [380]

JEFFREY M. DRAZEN, MD
Professor of Medicine, Harvard Medical School; Senior Physician, Brigham and Women's Hospital, Boston [249, 250, 251, 266]

THOMAS D. DUBOSE, JR., MD
Peter T. Bohan Professor and Chairman, Department of Internal Medicine; Professor of Molecular and Integrative Physiology, University of Kansas School of Medicine, Kansas City [50]

J. STEPHEN DUMLER, MD
Associate Professor and Associate Director, Division of Medical Microbiology, Department of Pathology, The Johns Hopkins Medical Institutions, Baltimore [177]

ANDREA E. DUNAIF, MD
Associate Professor of Medicine, Director, Center of Excellence in Women's Health, Harvard Medical School; Chief, Division of Women's Health and Senior Physician, Brigham and Women's Hospital, Boston [6]

MARLENE DURAND, MD
Assistant Professor of Medicine, Harvard Medical School, Boston [30]

JANICE DUTCHER, MD
Professor of Medicine, New York Medical College; Associate Director for Clinical Affairs, Our Lady of Mercy Comprehensive Cancer Center, New York [102]

JOHANNA DWYER, MD
Professor of Medicine and Community Health, Tufts University School of Medicine; Professor, Tufts University School of Nutrition Science and Policy; Senior Scientist, Jean Mayer USDA Human Nutrition Research Center at Tufts University, Boston [73]

VICTOR J. DZAU, MD
Hersey Professor of the Theory and Practice of Physic (Medicine), Harvard Medical School; Chairman, Department of Medicine, and Director of Research, Brigham and Women's Hospital, Boston [247, 248]

JEFFERY S. DZIECZKOWSKI, MD
Assistant Professor, Departments of Pathology and Internal Medicine, Wayne State University School of Medicine, Detroit [114]

J. DONALD EASTON, MD
Professor and Chair, Department of Clinical Neurosciences, Brown University School of Medicine; Neurologist-in-Chief, Rhode Island Hospital, Providence [361]

DAVID A. EHRMANN, MD
Associate Professor, Section of Endocrinology, Department of Medicine, University of Chicago, Chicago [53]

JOHN W. ENGSTROM, MD
Associate Professor of Neurology, and Vice Chairman, Department of Neurology, University of California San Francisco, San Francisco [16, 366]

ALAN EPSTEIN, MD
Assistant Professor of Medicine, Brown University School of Medicine, Providence [289]

ANTHONY S. FAUCI, MD
Chief, Laboratory of Immunoregulation; Director, National Institute of Allergy and Infectious Diseases, National Institutes of Health, Bethesda [191, 305, 309, 317]

MURRAY J. FAVUS, MD
Professor of Medicine, University of Chicago Pritzker School of Medicine; Director, General Clinical Research Center; Director, Bone Program, Chicago [279]

ROBERT G. FENTON, MD, PhD
Associate Professor of Medicine, University of Maryland Greenebaum Cancer Center, Baltimore [82]

HOWARD L. FIELDS, MD, PhD
Professor of Neurology and Physiology, University of California San Francisco, San Francisco [12]

GREGORY A. FILICE, MD
Associate Professor of Medicine, University of Minnesota; Chief, Infectious Disease Section, Veterans Affairs Medical Center, Minneapolis [165]

ROBERT FINBERG, MD
Professor of Medicine, and Chair Department of Medicine, University of Massachusetts Medical School, Worcester [85, 136]

JOYCE D. FINGEROTH, MD
Assistant Professor of Medicine, Harvard Medical School; Physician, Beth Israel Deaconess Medical Center, Boston [136]

JEFFREY S. FLIER, MD
George C. Reisman Professor of Medicine, Harvard Medical School; Vice-Chair for Research, and Chief, Division of Endocrinology, Department of Medicine, Beth Israel Deaconess Medical Center, Boston [77]

JUDAH FOLKMAN, MD
Surgeon-in-Chief, Emeritus, Director, Surgical Research Laboratory, Children's Hospital; Andrus Professor of Pediatric Surgery, Professor of Cell Biology, Department of Surgery, Harvard Medical School, Boston [83]

SONIA FRIEDMAN, MD
Instructor in Medicine, Harvard Medical School; Associate Physician in Medicine, Brigham and Women's Hospital, Boston [287]

WILLIAM F. FRIEDMAN, MD
J.H. Nicholson Professor of Pediatrics (Cardiology); Associate Dean for Academic Affairs, University of California, Los Angeles School of Medicine and UCLA Medical Center, Los Angeles [234]

ADRIANE FUGH-BERMAN, MD
Assistant Clinical Professor, Department of Health Care Sciences, George Washington University School of Medicine, Washington, D.C. [11]

ROBERT F. GAGEL, MD
Chairman, Department of Internal Medicine Specialties, and Chief, Section of Endocrine Neoplasia and Hormonal Disorders, University of Texas M.D. Anderson Cancer Center, Houston [339]

JOHN I. GALLIN, MD
Director, NIH Warren Grant G. Magnuson Clinical Center; NIH Associate Director for Clinical Research; Chief Laboratory of Host Defenses, National Institute of Allergy and Infectious Diseases, National Institutes of Health, Bethesda [64]

ABHIMANYU GARG, MD
Professor, Department of Internal Medicine, Center for Human Nutrition, University of Texas Southwestern Medical Center at Dallas; Director, Diabetes Clinic, Department of Veterans Affairs Medical Center, Dallas [354]

ROBERT H. GELBER, MD
Clinical Professor of Medicine and Dermatology, University of California San Francisco, San Anselmo [170]

JEFFREY A. GELFAND, MD
Visiting Professor of Medicine, Harvard Medical School; Distinguished Professor of Medicine, Tufts University School of Medicine; Attending Physician in Infectious Diseases, Massachusetts General Hospital, Boston [17, 125]

ANNE A. GERSHON, MD
Professor of Pediatrics, and Director of Division of Pediatric Infectious Diseases, Columbia University College of Physicians and Surgeons, New York [194, 195, 196]

MARC GHANY, MD
Medical Staff Fellow, Liver Diseases Section, Digestive Diseases Branch, National Institute of Diabetes and Digestive and Kidney Diseases, National Institutes of Health, Bethesda [292]

RAYMOND J. GIBBONS, MD
Arthur M. and Glady D. Gray Professor of Medicine, Mayo Medical School, Rochester [227]

BRUCE C. GILLILAND, MD
Professor of Medicine and Laboratory Medicine, University of Washington School of Medicine, Seattle [313, 325, 326]

HENRY N. GINSBERG, MD
Irving Professor of Medicine, Columbia University College of Physicians and Surgeons, New York [344]

ELI GLATSTEIN, MD
Vice-Chairman and Clinical Director, Radiation Oncology, University of Pennsylvania Medical Center, Philadelphia [394]

ROBERT M. GLICKMAN, MD
Professor of Medicine and Dean, New York University School of Medicine, New York [46]

IRA J. GOLDBERG, MD
Professor of Medicine, Division of Preventive Medicine and Nutrition, Columbia University College of Physicians and Surgeons, New York [344]

ARY L. GOLDBERGER, MD
Associate Professor of Medicine, Harvard Medical School; Director, Margret and H.A. Rey Laboratory for Nonlinear Dynamics in Medicine, Beth Israel Deaconess Medical Center, Boston [226]

SAMUEL Z. GOLDHABER, MD
Associate Professor of Medicine, Harvard Medical School; Director, Venous Thromboembolism Research Group; Director, Cardiac Center's Anticoagulation Service, Brigham and Women's Hospital, Boston [261]

DONALD E. GOODKIN, MD
San Rafael, California [371]

RAJ K. GOYAL, MD
Associate Chief of Staff for Research and Development, VA Medical Center; Mallinckrodt Professor of Medicine, Harvard Medical School, West Roxbury [40, 284]

GREGORY A. GRABOWSKI, MD
Professor of Pediatrics; Director, Division and Program in Human Genetics, Children's Hospital Research Foundation, Cincinnati [349]

JACOB GREEN, MD
Associate Professor of Medicine, Department of Nephrology, Technion Faculty of Medicine, Haifa, Israel [270]

HARRY B. GREENBERG, MD
Senior Associate Dean for Research, Professor of Medicine, Microbiology and Immunology, and ACOS for Research VAPAHCS, Stanford University, Stanford [192]

NORTON J. GREENBERGER, MD
Professor of Medicine, and Senior Associate Dean for Medical Education, University of Kansas School of Medicine, Kansas City [302, 303, 304]

JOHN S. GREENSPAN, BDS, PhD
Professor and Chair, Department of Stomatology and Director, Oral AIDS Center, School of Dentistry; Professor, Department of Pathology, and Director, AIDS Clinical Research Center, School of Medicine, University of California San Francisco, San Francisco [31]

DARYL R. GRESS, MD
Associate Professor of Neurology and Neurosurgery; Director, Neurovascular Service, University of California San Francisco, San Francisco [376]

JAMES E. GRIFFIN, MD
Diana and Richard C. Strauss Professor in Biomedical Research, and Professor of Internal Medicine, University of Texas Southwestern Medical Center, Dallas [335, 338]

WILLIAM GROSSMAN, MD
Myer Friedman Distinguished Professor of Medicine, University of California San Francisco; Chief of Cardiology, University of California San Francisco Medical Center, San Francisco [228]

RASIM GUCALP, MD
Associate Professor of Medicine, Department of Oncology, Montefiore Medical Center, Albert Einstein College of Medicine, New York [102]

BEVRA HANNAHS HAHN, MD
Professor of Medicine, Chief of Rheumatology, and Vice-Chair, Department of Medicine, University of California, Los Angeles, Los Angeles [311]

STEPHEN M. HAHN, MD
Assistant Professor of Medicine, Department of Radiation Oncology, University of Pennsylvania Medical Center, Philadelphia [394]

JANET E. HALL, MD
Associate Professor of Medicine, Harvard Medical School; Assistant Chief, Reproductive Endocrine Unit, Massachusetts General Hospital, Boston [54]

SCOTT A. HALPERIN, MD
Professor of Pediatrics, and Associate Professor of Microbiology and Immunology, Dalhousie University; Head, Pediatric Infectious Diseases, IWK-Grace Health Center, Halifax, Nova Scotia, Canada [152]

CHARLES H. HALSTED, MD
Professor of Internal Medicine, Division of Clinical Nutrition and Metabolism, University of California-Davis School of Medicine, Davis [74]

ROBERT I. HANDIN, MD
Professor of Medicine, Harvard Medical School; Co-Director, Hematology Division, and Executive Vice Chairman, Department of Medicine, Brigham and Women's Hospital, Boston [62, 116, 117, 118]

GAVIN HART, MD, MPH
Director, STD Services, Royal Adelaide Hospital; Clinical Associate Professor, School of Medicine, Flinders University, Adelaide South Australia, Australia [164]

WILLIAM L. HASLER, MD
Associate Professor of Internal Medicine, Division of Gastroenterology, University of Michigan Medical Center, Ann Arbor [41]

TERRY HASSOLD, PhD
Professor, Department of Genetics, Case Western Reserve University and the Center for Human Genetics, University Hospitals of Cleveland, Cleveland [66]

STEPHEN L. HAUSER, MD
Betty Anker Fife Professor and Chairman, Department of Neurology, University of California San Francisco, San Francisco [355, 356, 361, 367, 368, 371, 378]

BARTON F. HAYNES, MD
Frederic M. Hanes Professor of Medicine, and Chair, Department of Medicine, Duke University Medical Center, Durham [305]

J. CLAUDE HEMPHILL III, MD
Assistant Professor of Neurology, University of California San Francisco; Director, Neurovascular and Neurocritical Care Program, San Francisco General Hospital, San Francisco [376]

PATRICK H. HENRY, MD
Chairman, Department of Medicine, St. John's Mercy Medical Center, St. Louis [63]

BARBARA L. HERWALDT, MD, MPH
Medical Epidemiologist, Division of Parasitic Diseases, Centers for Disease Control Prevention, Atlanta [215]

MARTIN S. HIRSCH, MD
Professor of Medicine, Harvard Medical School; Director, AIDS Clinical Research, Massachusetts General Hospital, Boston [185]

BERNARD HIRSCHEL, MD
Associate Professor of Medicine; Head, HIV/AIDS Section, Division of Infectious Diseases, University Hospital, Geneva [171]

MICHAEL F. HOLICK, MD, PhD
Professor of Medicine, Department of Endocrinology, Diabetes and Metabolism, Boston University School of Medicine, Boston [340]

STEVEN M. HOLLAND, MD
Senior Investigator and Head, Immunopathogenesis Unit, Clinical Pathophysiology Section, Laboratory of Host Defenses, National Institute of Allergy and Infectious Diseases, National Institute of Health, Bethesda [64]

KING K. HOLMES, MD, PhD
Professor of Medicine, and Director, Center for AIDS and Sexually Transmitted Diseases, University of Washington; Head, Infectious Diseases, Harborview Medical Center, Seattle [132, 133]

RANDALL K. HOLMES, MD, PhD
Professor and Chair, Department of Microbiology, University of Colorado School of Medicine, Denver [141]

ERIC G. HONIG, MD
Professor of Medicine, Emory University School of Medicine, Atlanta [258]

JAY H. HOOFNAGLE, MD
Director, Division of Digestive Diseases and Nutrition, National Institute of Diabetes and Digestive and Kidney Diseases, National Institutes of Health, Bethesda [292]

JONATHAN C. HORTON, MD, PhD
Associate Professor of Ophthalmology, Neurology, and Physiology, University of California San Francisco, San Francisco [28]

LYN HOWARD, MB
Professor of Medicine, Associate Professor of Pediatrics, and Head-Division of Clinical Nutrition in Department of Medicine, Albany Medical College, Albany [76]

HOWARD HU, MD, DPH
Associate Professor of Occupational Medicine, Harvard School of Public Health; Assistant Professor of Medicine, Harvard Medical School; Associate Physician, Channing Laboratory, Brigham and Women's Hospital, Boston [5, 391, 395]

GARY W. HUNNINGHAKE, MD
Professor, Department of Internal Medicine, and Director, Division of Pulmonary, Critical Care, and Occupational Medicine, University of Iowa College of Medicine, Iowa City [253]

EDWARD P. INGENITO, MD
Assistant Professor of Medicine, Harvard Medical School; Director, Pulmonary Function Laboratory, Brigham and Women's Hospital, Boston [266]

ROLAND H. INGRAM, JR., MD
Martha West Looney Professor Emeritus, Emory University School of Medicine, Atlanta [32, 258, 265]

THOMAS S. INUI, ScM, MD
President and CEO, The Fetzer Institute, Kalamazoo, Michigan [10]

MARK A. ISRAEL, MD
Professor, Departments of Neurological Surgery and Pediatrics; Director, Preuss Laboratory of Molecular Neuro-Oncology, University of California San Francisco, San Francisco [370]

KURT J. ISSELBACHER, MD
Distinguished Mallinckrodt Professor of Medicine, Harvard Medical School; Physician and Director, Massachusetts General Hospital Cancer Center, Boston [91, 282, 289, 295, 296, 297, 345]

RICHARD F. JACOBS, MD, FAAP
Horace C. Cabe Professor of Pediatrics, University of Arkansas for Medical Sciences; Chief, Pediatric Infectious Diseases, Arkansas Children's Hospital, Little Rock [161]

J. LARRY JAMESON, MD, PhD
Irving S. Cutter Professor and Chairman, Department of Medicine, Northwestern University Medical School; Physician-in-Chief, Northwestern Memorial Hospital, Chicago [65, 68, 327, 330]

ROBERT T. JENSEN, MD
Digestive Diseases Branch, National Institute of Diabetes and Digestive and Kidney Diseases, National Institutes of Health, Bethesda [93]

DONALD R. JOHNS, MD
Associate Professor of Neurology and Ophthalmology; Harvard Medical School; Director, Division of Neuromuscular Disease, Beth Israel Deaconess Medical Center, Boston [67]

BRUCE E. JOHNSON, MD
Associate Professor of Medicine, Brigham and Women's Hospital and Harvard Medical School; Program Director, Lowe Center for Thoracic Oncology, Dana-Farber Cancer Institute, Boston [100]

MICHAEL JOSEPH, MD
Physician, Weber Medical Clinic, Ltd., Olney, Illinois [30]

MARK E. JOSEPHSON, MD
Professor of Medicine, Harvard Medical School; Director of the Harvard Thorndike Electrophysiology Institute and Arrhythmia Services, Beth Israel Deaconess Medical Center, Boston [229, 230]

EDWARD L. KAPLAN, MD
Professor of Pediatrics, Department of Pediatrics, University of Minnesota Medical School, Minneapolis [235]

MARSHALL M. KAPLAN, MD
Professor of Medicine, Tufts University School of Medicine; Chief, Gastroenterology Department, New England Medical Center, Boston [45, 293]

ADOLF W. KARCHMER, MD
Chief, Division of Infectious Diseases, Beth Israel Deaconess Medical Center; Professor of Medicine, Harvard Medical School, Boston [126]

DENNIS L. KASPER, MD, MA (Hon)
William Ellery Channing Professor of Medicine, Professor of Microbiology and Molecular Genetics, Executive Dean for Academic Programs, Harvard Medical School; Director, Channing Laboratory, Department of Medicine, Brigham and Women's Hospital, Boston [19, 119, 130, 145, 150, 160, 167]

LLOYD H. KASPER, MD
Professor of Medicine (Neurology) and Microbiology, Dartmouth Medical School, Hanover [217]

MARK A. KAY, MD, PhD
Director, Program in Human Gene Therapy, and Associate Professor, Departments of Pediatrics and Genetics, Stanford University School of Medicine, Stanford [69]

ELAINE T. KAYE, MD
Clinical Instructor in Dermatology, Harvard Medical School; Assistant in Medicine, Department of Medicine, Children's Hospital Medical Center, Weston [18]

KENNETH M. KAYE, MD
Assistant Professor of Medicine, Harvard Medical School; Associate Physician, Division of Infectious Diseases, Brigham and Women's Hospital, Boston [18]

GERALD T. KEUSCH, MD
Associate Director for International Research; Director, Fogarty International Center, National Institutes of Health; Professor of Medicine, Tufts University School of Medicine; New England Medical Center, Bethesda [122, 157, 159]

J. S. KEYSTONE, MD
Professor of Medicine, University of Toronto; Centre for Travel and Tropical Medicine, Division of Infectious Disease, Toronto General Hospital, Toronto, Ontario, Canada [123]

ELLIOTT KIEFF, MD, PhD
Albee Professor of Medicine and Microbiology and Molecular Genetics, Harvard Medical School, Boston [180]

TALMADGE E. KING, JR., MD
Constance B. Wofsy Distinguished Professor and Vice Chairman, Department of Medicine, University of California San Francisco; Chief, Medical Services, San Francisco General Hospital, San Francisco [259]

LOUIS V. KIRCHHOFF, MD, MPH
Professor, Department of Internal Medicine, University of Iowa; Staff Physician, Department of Veterans Affairs Medical Center, Iowa City [216]

JOEL N. KLINE, MD
Assistant Professor, University of Iowa College of Medicine, Iowa City [253]

HOWARD K. KOH, MD, PhD
Professor of Dermatology, Medicine and Public Health, Boston University Schools of Medicine and Public Health; Co-Director, Skin Oncology Program, Director, Cancer Prevention and Control Center, Boston [86]

ANTHONY L. KOMAROFF, MD
Professor of Medicine, Harvard Medical School; Senior Physician, Brigham and Women's Hospital, Boston [6]

PETER KOPP, MD
Assistant Professor of Medicine, Division of Endocrinology, Metabolism and Molecular Medicine, Northwestern University, Chicago [65]

WALTER J. KOROSHETZ, MD
Associate Professor of Neurology and Medicine; Associate Director, Stroke and Clinical Neurology Services, Massachusetts General Hospital, Harvard Medical School, Boston [374]

P. E. KOZARSKY, MD
Associate Professor of Medicine, Emory University School of Medicine; Adjunct Assistant Professor of Medicine, Emory University School of Public Health, Atlanta [123]

BARNETT S. KRAMER, MD, MPH
Director, Office of Medical Applications of Research, National Institutes of Health, Bethesda [80]

STEPHEN M. KRANE, MD
Persis, Cyrus and Marlow B. Harrison Professor of Medicine, Harvard Medical School; Physician and Chief, Arthritis Unit, Massachusetts General Hospital, Boston [340, 343]

HELENA KUIVANIEMI, MD, PhD
Associate Professor, Wayne State University School of Medicine, Detroit [351]

LOREN LAINE, MD
Professor of Medicine, University of Southern California School of Medicine, Los Angeles [44]

ANIL K. LALWANI, MD
Associate Professor, Department of Otolaryngology- Head and Neck Surgery, University of California San Francisco, San Francisco [29]

LEWIS LANDSBERG, MD
Professor of Medicine, Vice-President for Medical Affairs, and Dean, Northwestern University Medical School, Chicago [72, 332]

H. CLIFFORD LANE, MD
Head, Clinical and Molecular Retrovirology Section, Laboratory of Immunoregulation; Clinical Director, National Institute of Allergy and Infectious Diseases, National Institutes of Health, Bethesda [309]

THOMAS J. LAWLEY, MD
Professor, Department of Dermatology, and Dean, Emory University School of Medicine, Atlanta [55, 56, 58]

RAPHAEL C. LEE, MBME, MD, ScD, PhD(Hon)
Professor of Surgery (Plastic), Professor of Organismal Biology and Anatomy (Biomechanics) and, Director, Electrical Injury Research Program, University of Chicago; Attending Surgeon, Ancilla / St. Mary's Burn Center, Chicago [393]

THOMAS H. LEE, MD, MSc
Associate Professor, Harvard Medical School; Medical Director, Partners Community Health Care, Inc., Boston [13]

CAMMIE F. LESSER, MD, PhD
Infectious Disease Fellow, University of Washington, Seattle [156]

MATTHEW E. LEVISON, MD
Professor of Medicine and Public Health, and Chief, Division of Infectious Diseases, Allegheny University of the Health Sciences, Philadelphia [255]

PETER LIBBY, MD
Mallinckrodt Professor of Medicine, Harvard Medical School; Chief, Cardiovascular Medicine, Brigham and Women's Hospital, Boston [241, 242]

RICHARD W. LIGHT, MD
Professor of Medicine, Vanderbilt University; Director, Pulmonary Diseases, Saint Thomas Hospital, Nashville [262]

CHRISTOPHER H. LINDEN, MD
Associate Professor, Department of Emergency Medicine, University of Massachusetts Medical School, Worcester [396]

ROBERT LINDSAY, MBChB, PhD
Professor of Clinical Medicine, Columbia University College of Physicians and Surgeons; Chief, Internal Medicine, Helen Hayes Hospital, West Haverstraw, New York [342]

MARC E. LIPPMAN, MD
John G. Searle Professor and Chairman, Department of Internal Medicine, University of Michigan Health Science System, Ann Arbor [89]

PETER E. LIPSKY, MD
Scientific Director, National Institute of Arthritis and Musculoskeletal and Skin Diseases, National Institutes of Health, Bethesda [307, 312, 315, 320]

LEO X. LIU, MD, DTMH
Assistant Professor of Medicine, Harvard Medical School; Division of Infectious Diseases, Department of Medicine, Beth Israel Deaconess Medical Center, Boston [219]

BERNARD LO, MD
Professor of Medicine and Director, Program in Medical Ethics, University of California San Francisco, San Francisco [2]

DAN L. LONGO, MD
Scientific Director, National Institute on Aging, National Institutes of Health, Bethesda and Baltimore [61, 63, 79, 82, 84, 103, 112, 113, 191]

FRANK M. LONGO, MD, PhD
Professor of Neurology, University of California San Francisco; Chief of Neurology, Veterans Affairs Medical Center, Department of Neurology, San Francisco [359]

NICOLA LONGO, MD, PhD
Associate Professor, Division of Medical Genetics, Department of Pediatrics, Emory University School of Medicine Atlanta [352, 353]

DANIEL H. LOWENSTEIN, MD
Carl W. Walter Professor of Neurology and Dean for Medical Education, Harvard Medical School, Boston [360]

SHEILA A. LUKEHART, PhD
Research Professor of Medicine, Division of Allergy and Infectious Diseases, University of Washington School of Medicine, Seattle [172, 173]

M. MONIR MADKOUR, DM
Military Hospital, Riyadh, Saudi Arabia; Faculty of Medicine, Ain Shams University, Cairo, Egypt, Riyadh, Saudi Arabia [160]

LAWRENCE C. MADOFF, MD
Assistant Professor of Medicine, Harvard Medical School; Associate Physician, Channing Laboratory and Division of Infectious Diseases, Brigham and Women's Hospital, Boston [119, 127]

JAMES H. MAGUIRE, MD
Associate Professor of Medicine, Harvard Medical School; Department of Immunology and Infectious Diseases, Harvard School of Public Health, Boston [129, 323, 398]

ADEL A.F. MAHMOUD, MD, PhD
President, Merck Vaccines, Merck & Co., Inc., Whitehouse Station, New Jersey [222]

RONALD V. MAIER, MD
Professor and Vice Chairman of Surgery, University of Washington; Surgeon in Chief, Harborview Medical Center, Seattle [38]

MARK E. MAILLIARD, MD
Associate Professor of Medicine, Division of Gastroenterology and Hepatology, University of Nebraska Medical Center, Omaha [298]

DANIEL B. MARK, MD, MPH
Professor of Medicine, Duke University Medical Center; Director, Outcomes Research and Assessment Group, Durham [3, 4]

THOMAS MARRIE, MD
Professor and Chair, Department of Medicine, University of Alberta, Edmonton, Alberta, Canada [177]

JOSEPH B. MARTIN, MD, PhD, MA (Hon)
Dean of the Faculty of Medicine; Caroline Shields Walker Professor of Neurobiology and Clinical Neuroscience, Harvard Medical School, Boston [12, 356, 359, 366]

JANET R. MAURER, MD
Head, Section of Advanced Lung Disease and Lung Transplantation, Division of Pulmonary and Critical Care Medicine, and Medical Director, Transplant Center, The Cleveland Clinic Foundation, Cleveland [267]

ROBERT J. MAYER, MD
Professor of Medicine, Harvard Medical School; Vice-Chair for Academic Affairs, Department of Adult Oncology, Dana-Farber Cancer Institute, Boston [90, 92]

JOHN D. MCCONNELL, MD
Professor and Chairman, Department of Urology, The University of Texas Southwestern Medical Center, Dallas [48]

WILLIAM M. MCCORMACK, MD
Professor of Medicine and of Obstetrics and Gynecology, and Chief, Division of Infectious Diseases, State University of New York, New York [178]

E. REGIS MCFADDEN, JR., MD
Argyl J. Beams Professor of Medicine, Director, Division of Pulmonary and Critical Care Medicine, University Hospitals of Cleveland, Cleveland [252]

KEVIN T. MCVARY, MD
Associate Professor, Department of Urology, Northwestern University Medical School, Chicago [51]

NANCY K. MELLO, PhD
Professor of Psychology (Neuroscience), Harvard Medical School; Alcohol and Drug Abuse Research Center, McLean Hospital, Belmont [389]

SHLOMO MELMED, MD
Professor and Director, Cedars Sinai Research Institute, University of California Los Angeles School of Medicine, Los Angeles [328]

JERRY R. MENDELL, MD
Chairman and Professor of Neurology; Director, Neuromuscular Disease Center, The Ohio State University, Columbus [381, 383]

JACK H. MENDELSON, MD
Professor of Psychiatry (Neuroscience), Harvard Medical School; Alcohol and Drug Abuse Research Center, McLean Hospital, Belmont [389]

ROBERT O. MESSING, MD
Associate Professor of Neurology, and Associate Director, Ernest Gallo Clinic and Research Center, University of California San Francisco, San Francisco [386]

M. -MARSEL MESULAM, MD
Ruth and Evelyn Dunbar Professor of Neurology and Psychiatry; Director, Center for Behavioral and Cognitive Neurology; Director, Alzheimer's Program, Northwestern University Medical School, Chicago [25]

SUSAN MIESFELDT, MD
Assistant Professor of Medicine, Division of Hematology and Oncology, University of Virginia Health System, Charlottesville [68]

EDGAR L. MILFORD, MD
Associate Professor of Medicine, Harvard Medical School; Director of Renal Transplantation, Brigham and Women's Hospital, Boston [272]

SAMUEL I. MILLER, MD
Professor of Medicine and Microbiology, University of Washington, Seattle [156]

JOHN D. MINNA, MD
Professor, Internal Medicine and Pharmacology; Director, Hamon Center for Therapeutic Oncology Research, University of Texas Southwestern Medical Center, Dallas [88]

JEROME H. MODELL, MD
Associate Vice President for Health Affairs, and Professor of Anesthesiology, College of Medicine, University of Florida, Gainesville [392]

THOMAS A. MOORE, MD
Clinical Assistant Professor, Department of Internal Medicine, University of Kansas School of Medicine, Wichita [212]

MARC MOSS, MD
Assistant Professor of Medicine, Emory University School of Medicine; Director, Medical Intensive Care Unit, Grady Memorial Hospital, Atlanta [265]

ROBERT J. MOTZER, MD
Associate Attending Physician, Division of Solid Tumor Oncology, Department of Medicine, Memorial Sloan-Kettering Cancer Center; Associate Professor of Medicine, Cornell University Medical College, New York [94, 96]

HARALAMPOS M. MOUTSOPOULOS, MD
Professor and Director, Department of Pathophysiology, National University School of Medicine; President of the National Organization for Medicines, Athens, Greece [314, 316]

ROBERT S. MUNFORD, MD
Jan and Henri Bromberg Professor of Internal Medicine, and Professor of Microbiology, University of Texas Southwestern Medical Center, Dallas [124, 146]

TIMOTHY F. MURPHY, MD
Professor of Medicine and Microbiology, and Chief, Division of Infectious Diseases, State University of New York at Buffalo, Buffalo [149]

DANIEL M. MUSHER, MD
Professor of Medicine, and Professor of Molecular Virology, Baylor College of Medicine; Chief, Infectious Diseases, Veterans Affairs Medical Center, Houston [138, 148]

ROBERT J. MYERBURG, MD
Professor of Medicine and Physiology; Director, Division of Cardiology, University of Miami School of Medicine, Miami [39]

GERALD T. NEPOM, MD, PhD
Professor, Department of Immunology, University of Washington School of Medicine; Director, Virginia Mason Research Center, Seattle [306]

RICHARD A. NISHIMURA, MD
Professor of Medicine, Mayo Medical School, Rochester [227]

ROBERT L. NORRIS, MD
Associate Professor of Surgery, Department of Surgery; Chief, Division of Emergency Medicine, Stanford University, Stanford [397]

THOMAS B. NUTMAN, MD
Head, Helminth Immunology Section, Laboratory of Parasitic Diseases, National Institute of Allergy and Infectious Diseases, National Institutes of Health, Bethesda [220, 221]

JOHN A. OATES, MD
The Thomas F. Frist, Sr. Professor of Medicine, and Professor of Pharmacology, Vanderbilt University School of Medicine, Nashville [70]

RICHARD J. O'BRIEN, MD
Chief, Research and Evaluation Branch Division of Tuberculosis Elimination, Centers for Diseases Control and Prevention, Atlanta [169]

PATRICK T. O'GARA, MD
Associate Professor of Medicine, Harvard Medical School; Director, Clinical Cardiology, Brigham & Women's Hospital, Boston [34]

CHRISTOPHER A. OHL, MD
Assistant Professor of Medicine, Section on Infectious Diseases, Wake Forest University School of Medicine; Director, Center for Antimicrobial Utilization, Stewardship and Epidemiology, Baptist Medical Center, Winston-Salem [155]

RICHARD K. OLNEY, MD
Professor of Neurology, University of California San Francisco, San Francisco [22]

YVONNE M. O'MEARA, MD, FRCPI
Senior Lecturer in Medicine, University College Dublin; Consultant Nephrologist, Mater Misericordiae Hospital, Dublin, Ireland [274, 275]

ANDREW B. ONDERDONK, PhD
Professor of Pathology, Harvard Medical School; Director of Clinical Microbiology, Brigham and Women's Hospital, Boston [121]

ROBERT A. O'ROURKE, MD
Charles Conrad Brown Distinguished Professor of Cardiovascular Science, University of Texas Health Science Center at San Antonio, San Antonio [225]

CHUNG OWYANG, MD
Professor of Internal Medicine, H. Marvin Pollard Collegiate Professor and Chief, Division of Gastroenterology, Department of Internal Medicine, University of Michigan Medical Center, Ann Arbor [288]

JEFFREY PARSONNET, MD
Associate Professor of Medicine and of Microbiology, Dartmouth Medical School; Staff Physician, Infectious Diseases Section, Dartmouth-Hitchcock Medical Center, Lebanon [139]

SHREYASKUMAR R. PATEL, MD
Associate Professor of Medicine, Department of Melanoma/Sarcoma, Medical Oncology, University of Texas, MD Anderson Cancer Center, Houston [98]

GUSTAV PAUMGARTNER, MD
Professor of Medicine, Ludwig Maximiliam University of Munich, Durchwal, Germany [302]

STEPHEN J. PEROUTKA, MD
Burlingame, California [15]

MICHAEL C. PERRY, MD, MS
Professor of Internal Medicine; Director, Division of Hematology/Oncology, Nellie B. Smith Professor of Oncology, University of Missouri/Ellis Fischel Cancer Center; Consultant, Harry S. Truman VA Hospital, Columbia [103]

ALAN PESTRONK, MD
Professor of Neurology, Washington University, St. Louis [101]

CLARENCE J. PETERS, MD
Chief, Special Pathogens Branch, Centers for Disease Control and Prevention; Adjunct Professor of Microbiology and Immunology, Emory University, Atlanta [198, 199]

ELIOT A. PHILLIPSON, MD
Sir John and Lady Eaton Professor and Chair, Department of Medicine, University of Toronto, Toronto, Ontario, Canada [263, 264]

GERALD B. PIER, PhD
Professor of Medicine (Microbiology and Molecular Genetics), Harvard Medical School; Microbiologist, Brigham and Women's Hospital, Boston [120]

DANIEL K. PODOLSKY, MD
Mallinckrodt Professor of Medicine, Harvard Medical School; Chief of Gastrointestinal Unit; Director, Center for the Study of Inflammatory Bowel Disease, Massachusetts General Hospital, Boston [282, 299, 300]

RONALD E. POLK, Pharm. D.
Professor, Pharmacy and Medicine, School of Pharmacy Medical College of Virginia Campus, Virginia Commonwealth University, Richmond [137]

MATTHEW POLLACK, MD
Professor of Medicine, Uniformed Services University; F. Edward He'bert School of Medicine; Attending Staff Physician, Internal Medicine and Infectious Diseases, National Naval Medical Center, Bethesda [155]

JOHN T. POTTS, JR., MD
Distinguished Jackson Professor of Clinical Medicine, Harvard Medical School; Director of Research, Massachusetts General Hospital, Boston [341]

LAWRIE W. POWELL, MD, PhD
Professor of Medicine, The University of Queensland and Royal Brisbane Hospital, Brisbane, Queensland, Australia [345]

ALVIN C. POWERS, MD
Associate Professor of Medicine, Molecular Physiology and Biophysics, Vanderbilt University School of Medicine; Chief, Section of Endocrinology and Diabetes, VA Medical Center, Nashville [333]

DANIEL S. PRATT, MD
Assistant Professor of Medicine, Tufts University School of Medicine; Medical Director of Liver Transplantation, New England Medical Center, Boston [45, 293]

DARWIN J. PROCKOP, MD, PhD
Professor and Director, Center for Gene Therapy, Philadelphia [351]

DANIEL T. PRICE, MD
Assistant Professor of Medicine, Boston University School of Medicine; Staff Physician, Boston Veterans Affairs Medical Center, West Roxbury [240]

STANLEY B. PRUSINER, MD
Director, Institute for Neurodegenerative Diseases; Professor, Departments of Neurology, Biochemistry and Biophysics, University of California San Francisco, San Francisco [375]

PETER J. QUESENBERRY, MD
Professor of Medicine, University of Massachusetts School of Medicine, Worcester [104]

SANJAY RAM, MD
Assistant Professor of Medicine, Section of Infectious Diseases, Boston University School of Medicine and Boston Medical Center, Boston [147]

DIDIER RAOULT, MD
Professor of Medicine, Unité des Rickettsies, School of Medicine, University of Aux-Marseille, Marseille, France [177]

NEIL H. RASKIN, MD
Professor of Neurology, University of California San Francisco, San Francisco [15]

MARIO RAVIGLIONE, MD
TB Coordinator, Communicable Disease Programme, World Health Organization, Geneva, Switzerland [169]

SHARON L. REED, MD
Professor of Pathology and Medicine, and Director, Microbiology and Virology Laboratories, University of California, San Diego Medical Center, San Diego [213]

ANTONIO J. REGINATO, MD
Professor of Medicine, and Head, Division of Rheumatology, Cooper University Medical Center, Robert Wood Johnson Medical School at Camden, Camden [322]

RICHARD C. REICHMAN, MD
Professor of Medicine, Microbiology and Immunology, Head Infectious Diseases Unit, Senior Associate Dean for Clinical Research, University of Rochester School of Medicine and Dentistry, Rochester [188]

CAROL M. REIFE, MD
Clinical Assistant Professor of Medicine, Jefferson Medical College, Thomas Jefferson University, Philadelphia [43]

JOHN T. REPKE, MD
Chris J. and Marie A. Olson Professor of Obstetrics and Gynecology, and Chairman, Department of Obstetrics and Gynecology, University of Nebraska Medical Center, Omaha [7]

NEIL M. RESNICK, MD
Professor of Medicine, University of Pittsburgh School of Medicine; Chief, Division of Gerontology and Geriatric Medicine, University of Pittsburgh Healthcare System, Pittsburgh [9]

VICTOR I. REUS, MD
Professor of Psychiatry, University of California San Francisco; Medical Director, Langley Porter Hospital, San Francisco [385]

PETER A. RICE, MD
Professor of Medicine and Chief, Section of Infectious Diseases, Boston University School of Medicine and Boston Medical Center, Boston [147]

STUART RICH, MD
Professor of Medicine, Rush Medical College; Director, Rush Heart Institute Center for Pulmonary Heart Disease, Chicago [260]

GARY S. RICHARDSON, MD
Assistant Professor of Psychiatry, Case Western Reserve University; Senior Research Scientist, Sleep Disorders and Research Center, Henry Ford Hospital, Cleveland [27]

CELESTE ROBB-NICHOLSON, MD
Assistant Professor of Medicine, Harvard Medical School; Assistant Physician, Massachusetts General Hospital, Boston [6]

GARY L. ROBERTSON, MD
Professor of Medicine and Neurology, Northwestern University Medical School, Chicago [329]

DAN M. RODEN, MD
Professor of Medicine and Pharmacology; Director, Division of Clinical Pharmacology, Vanderbilt University School of Medicine, Nashville [70]

KAREN L. ROOS, MD
Professor of Neurology, Indiana University School of Medicine, Indianapolis [372]

ALLAN H. ROPPER, MD
Professor and Chairman of Neurology, Tufts University School of Medicine; Chief, Division of Neurology, St. Elizabeth's Medical Center, Boston [24, 369]

ROGER N. ROSENBERG, MD
Zale Distinguished Chair in Neurology; Professor of Neurology and Physiology, University of Texas Southwestern Medical Center; Attending Neurologist, Parkland Hospital and Zale-Lipsky University Hospital, Dallas [364]

WENDELL ROSSE, MD
Florence Reynaud McAlister Professor of Medicine and Medical Research, Department of Medicine, Duke University Medical School, Durham [108]

DAVID W. RUSSELL, MD, PhD
Associate Professor of Medicine, Division of Hematology University of Washington School of Medicine, Seattle [69]

ROBERT M. RUSSELL, MD
Professor of Medicine and Nutrition, Tufts University; Associate Director, USDA Human Nutrition Research Center, Tufts University, Boston [75]

THOMAS A. RUSSO, MD, CM
Assistant Professor of Medicine, Division of Infectious Diseases, Department of Medicine, State University of New York at Buffalo, Buffalo [153, 166]

STEPHEN M. SAGAR, MD
Professor of Neurology, Case Western Reserve School of Medicine, Cleveland [370]

EDWARD A. SAUSVILLE, MD, PhD
Associate Director, Developmental Therapeutics Program, Division of Cancer Treatment and Diagnosis, National Cancer Institute, Bethesda [84]

MOHAMED H. SAYEGH, MD
Associate Professor of Medicine, Harvard Medical School; Research Director, Laboratory of Immunogenetics and Transplantation, Brigham and Women's Hospital, Boston [272]

I. HERBERT SCHEINBERG, MD
Senior Lecturer in Medicine, College of Physicians and Surgeons, Columbia University, New York [348]

HOWARD I. SCHER, MD
Attending Physician, Chief, Genitourinary Oncology Service, Division of Solid Tumor Oncology, Department of Medicine, Memorial Sloan-Kettering Cancer Center; Professor of Medicine, Department of Medicine, Weill Medical College, New York [94, 95]

ALAN L. SCHILLER, MD
Irene Heinz Given and John LaPorte Given Professor and Chairman of Pathology, Mount Sinai School of Medicine; Chairman of Pathology, The Mount Sinai Hospital, New York [343]

HARRY W. SCHROEDER, JR., MD, PhD
Professor of Medicine and Microbiology, University of Alabama at Birmingham, Birmingham [308]

JOHN S. SCHROEDER, MD
Professor of Medicine, Cardiovascular Medicine, Stanford University School of Medicine, Stanford [233]

ANNE SCHUCHAT, MD
Chief, Respiratory Diseases Branch, Division of Bacterial and Mycotic Diseases, National Center for Infectious Diseases, Centers for Disease Control and Prevention, Atlanta [142]

MARC A. SCHUCKIT, MD
Professor of Psychiatry, University of California San Diego, and Veterans Affairs Medical Center, San Diego [387, 388]

PETER H. SCHUR, MD
Professor of Medicine, Harvard Medical School; Physician, Brigham and Women's Hospital, Boston [324]

STUART SCHWARTZ, PhD
Professor, Department of Genetics, Case Western Reserve University and the Center for Human Genetics, University Hospitals of Cleveland, Cleveland [66]

DAVID S. SEGAL, PhD
Professor of Psychiatry, University of California San Diego, La Jolla [388]

JULIAN L. SEIFTER, MD
Associate Professor of Medicine, Harvard Medical School; Physician, Brigham and Women's Hospital, Boston [281]

ANDREW P. SELWYN, MA, MD
Professor of Medicine, Harvard Medical School, Boston [244]

STEVEN I. SHERMAN, MD
Associate Professor, Section of Endocrine Neoplasia and Hormonal Disorders, University of Texas M.D. Anderson Cancer Center, Houston [339]

KARL SKORECKI, MD
Annie Chutick Professor of Medicine, Bruce Rappaport Faculty of Medicine, Technion-Israel Institute of Technology; Director, Department of Nephrology and Molecular Medicine, Rambam Medical Center, Haifa, Israel [270]

WILLIAM SILEN, MD
Johnson and Johnson Distinguished Professor of Surgery, and Dean for Faculty Development and Diversity, Harvard Medical School; Physician, Brigham and Women's Hospital, Boston [14, 290, 291]

GARY G. SINGER, MD
Assistant Professor of Medicine, Washington University School of Medicine; Associate Director, Transplant Nephrology, Barnes Jewish Hospital, St. Louis [49]

AJAY K. SINGH, MD
Associate Professor of Medicine, Harvard Medical School; Director of Clinical Nephrology, Brigham and Women's Hospital, Boston [271]

JEAN D. SIPE, PhD
Scientific Review Administrator, Center for Scientific Review, National Institutes of Health; Adjunct Professor, Department of Biochemistry, Boston University School of Medicine, Bethesda [319]

WADE S. SMITH, MD, PhD
Assistant Professor of Neurology; Director, Stroke Service, University of California San Francisco, San Francisco [361]

JAMES B. SNOW, JR., MD
Professor Emeritus, Department of Otorhinolaryngology, University of Pennsylvania; former Director, National Institute on Deafness and Other Communication Disorders, National Institutes of Health, Bethesda [29]

ARTHUR J. SOBER, MD
Associate Professor of Dermatology, Harvard Medical School; Associate Chief of Dermatology, Massachusetts General Hospital, Boston [86]

MICHAEL F. SORRELL, MD
Robert L. Grissom Professor of Medicine; Medical Director, Liver Transplant Program, University of Nebraska Medical Center, Omaha [298]

PETER SPEELMAN, MD
Division of Infectious Diseases, Tropical Medicine and AIDS, Department of Internal Medicine, Academic Medical Center, University of Amsterdam, Amsterdam, The Netherlands [174]

FRANK E. SPEIZER, MD
Edward H. Kass Professor of Medicine, Harvard Medical School; Co-Director, Channing Laboratory, Brigham and Women's Hospital, Boston [5, 254, 391]

ANDREW SPIELMAN, ScD
Professor of Tropical Public Health, Harvard School of Public Health, Boston [398]

JERRY L. SPIVAK, MD
Professor of Medicine and Oncology, The Johns Hopkins University School of Medicine, Baltimore [110]

WALTER E. STAMM, MD
Professor of Medicine and Head, Division of Allergy and Infectious Diseases, University of Washington School of Medicine, Seattle [179, 280]

ALLEN C. STEERE, MD
Zucker Professor of Medicine, Tufts University School of Medicine; Chief, Rheumatology/Immunology, New England Medical Center, Boston [176]

ROBERT S. STERN, MD
Carl J. Herzog Professor of Dermatology, Harvard Medical School; Dermatologist-in-Chief, Beth Israel Deaconess Medical Center, Boston [59]

DENNIS L. STEVENS, MD, PhD
Professor of Medicine, University of Washington School of Medicine, Seattle; Chief, Infectious Diseases, VA Medical Center, Boise [128]

RICHARD M. STONE, MD
Associate Professor of Medicine, Harvard Medical School; Clinical Director, Adult Leukemia Program, Dana-Farber Cancer Institute, Brigham and Women's Hospital, Boston [99]

STEPHEN E. STRAUS, MD
Chief, Laboratory of Clinical Investigation, National Institute of Allergy and Infectious Diseases, National Institutes of Health, Bethesda [384]

MORTON N. SWARTZ, MD
Professor, Department of Medicine, Harvard Medical School; Chief, James Jackson Firm Medical Services, Massachusetts General Hospital, Boston [374]

ROBERT A. SWERLICK, MD
Associate Professor, Department of Dermatology, Emory University School of Medicine, Atlanta [56]

A. JAMIL TAJIK, MD
Thomas J. Walker Jr. Professor of Medicine and Pediatrics, Mayo Medical School; Chair, Division of Cardiovascular Diseases, Mayo Clinic, Rochester [227]

JOEL D. TAUROG, MD
Professor of Internal Medicine, and William M. and Gay Burnett Professor for Arthritis Research, University of Texas Southwestern Medical Center; Interim Chief, Division of Rheumatic Diseases and Interim Director, Harold C. Simmons Arthritis Research Center, Dallas [306, 315]

SCOTT J. THALER, MD
Director, Clinical Monitor, Clinical Research, Vaccines, Merck Research Laboratories, Merck & Co., Inc., Blue Bell [323]

LUCY STUART TOMPKINS, MD, PhD
Professor of Medicine (Infectious Diseases and Geographic Medicine), Professor of Microbiology, Immunology and Pathology, Stanford University School of Medicine, Stanford [163]

MARK TOPAZIAN, MD
Associate Professor of Medicine, Yale University School of Medicine; Assistant Director, Gastrointestinal Procedure Center, Yale New Haven Hospital, New Haven [283]

PHILLIP P. TOSKES, MD
Professor of Medicine and Director, Division of Gastroenterology, Hepatology and Nutrition; Associate Chairman for Clinical Affairs, Department of Medicine, University of Florida, Gainesville [303, 304]

JEFFREY M. TRENT, PhD
Chief, Laboratory of Cancer Genetics; Director, Division of Intramural Research, National Human Genome Research Institute, National Institutes of Health, Bethesda [81]

GERARD TROMP, PhD
Assistant Professor, Wayne State University School of Medicine, Detroit [351]

KENNETH L. TYLER, MD
Vice Chairman and Professor of Neurology, Professor of Medicine, Microbiology and Immunology, University of Colorado Health Sciences Center; Chief, Neurology Service, Denver VA Medical Center, Denver [372, 373]

EVERETT E. VOKES, MD
Duchossois Professor, Departments of Medicine and Radiation Oncology; Director, Section of Hematology/Oncology, University of Chicago Medical Center, Chicago [87]

MATTHEW K. WALDOR, MD
Assistant Professor of Medicine, New England Medical Center, Tufts University School of Medicine, Boston [159]

DAVID WALKER, MD
Professor and Chairman, Department of Pathology, University of Texas Medical Branch, Galveston [177]

RICHARD J. WALLACE, JR., MD
Professor and Chairman, Department of Microbiology and Research, University of Texas Health Center at Tyler, Tyler [168]

B. TIMOTHY WALSH, MD
William and Joy Ruane Professor of Pediatric Psychopharmacology, Department of Psychiatry, College of Physicians and Surgeons, Columbia University; Director, Eating Disorders Research Unit, New York State Psychiatric Institute, New York [78]

PETER D. WALZER, MD
Professor of Medicine, University of Cincinnati College of Medicine; Chief, Infectious Diseases, VA Medical Center, Cincinnati [209]

FREDERICK C.S. WANG, MD
Associate Professor of Medicine, Harvard Medical School; Physician, Brigham and Women's Hospital, Boston [180, 186]

CARL V. WASHINGTON, JR., MD
Assistant Professor of Dermatology, Emory University School of Medicine; Director, Mohs Surgery Unit, The Emory Clinic, Atlanta [86]

ANTHONY P. WEETMAN, MD, DSC
Professor of Medicine and Dean, University of Sheffield Medical School; Consultant Physician, Northern General Hospital, Sheffield, UK [330]

STEVEN E. WEINBERGER, MD
Professor of Medicine, Harvard Medical School; Vice-Chairman, Department of Medicine, Beth Israel Deaconess Medical Center, Boston [33, 249, 250, 251, 256]

ROBERT A. WEINSTEIN, MD
Professor of Medicine, Rush Medical College; Chairman of Infectious Diseases, Cook County Hospital, Chicago [134]

PETER F. WELLER, MD
Professor of Medicine, Harvard Medical School; Co-Chief, Division of Infectious Diseases, Chief, Division of Allergy and Inflammation, Department of Medicine, Beth Israel Deaconess Medical Center, Boston [210, 218, 219, 220, 221, 223]

MICHAEL R. WESSELS, MD
Associate Professor of Pediatrics and Medicine, Harvard Medical School; Chief, Division of Infectious Diseases, Children's Hospital; Channing Laboratory, Brigham and Women's Hospital, Boston [140]

MEIR WETZLER, MD
Assistant Professor of Medicine, State University of New York at Buffalo, Buffalo [111]

A. CLINTON WHITE, JR., MD
Associate Professor of Medicine, Department of Medicine, Microbiology and Immunology, Baylor College of Medicine, Houston [223]

NICHOLAS J. WHITE, DSC, MD
Professor of Tropical Medicine, Mahidol University, Thailand and Oxford University, UK, Bangkok, Thailand [214]

RICHARD J. WHITLEY, MD
Loeb Eminent Scholar Chair in Pediatrics, Professor of Pediatrics, Microbiology and Medicine, University of Alabama at Birmingham, Birmingham [183]

GRANT R. WILKINSON, PhD
Professor of Pharmacology, Vanderbilt University School of Medicine, Nashville [70]

GORDON H. WILLIAMS, MD
Professor of Medicine, Harvard Medical School; Chief, Endocrine-Hypertension Division, Brigham & Women's Hospital, Boston [35, 246, 331]

JEAN D. WILSON, MD
Charles Cameron Sprague Distinguished Chair and Clinical Professor of Internal Medicine, The University of Texas Southwestern Medical Center, Dallas [335, 337, 338]

JOHN W. WINKELMAN, MD, PhD
Assistant Professor of Psychiatry, Harvard Medical School; Medical Director, Sleep Health Center, Brigham and Women's Hospital, Boston [27]

BRUCE U. WINTROUB, MD
Associate Dean, Professor and Chair of Dermatology, University of California at San Francisco, San Francisco [59]

GREGORY P. WITTENBERG, MD
Rapid City Medical Center, LLP, Rapid City [86]

ALLAN W. WOLKOFF, MD
Department of Medicine and Marion Bessin Liver Center, Albert Einstein College of Medicine, New York [294]

ALASTAIR J.J. WOOD, MB, ChB
Assistant Vice Chancellor, Professor of Medicine, Professor of Pharmacology, Vanderbilt University, School of Medicine, Nashville [71]

ROBERT L. WORTMANN, MD
Professor and Chairman, Department of Internal Medicine, University of Oklahoma College of Medicine, Tulsa [347]

PAUL W. WRIGHT, MD
Director of Predoctoral Education and Professor of Family Practice, University of Texas Health Center, Tyler [168]

JOSHUA WYNNE, MD, MBA
Professor of Internal Medicine, Wayne State University, Detroit [238]

KIM B. YANCEY, MD
Senior Investigator, Dermatology Branch, Division of Clinical Sciences, National Cancer Institute, National Institutes of Health; Adjunct Professor, Department of Dermatology, Uniformed Services University of the Health Sciences, Bethesda [55, 58]

JAMES B. YOUNG, MD
Professor of Medicine, Northwestern University Medical School; Attending Physician, Northwestern Memorial Hospital, Chicago [72, 332]

NEAL S. YOUNG, MD
Chief, Hematology Branch, National Heart, Lung and Blood Institute, National Institutes of Health, Bethesda [109]

ROBERT C. YOUNG, MD
President, Fox Chase Cancer Center, Philadelphia [97]

ALAN S.L. YU, MB, BChir
Assistant Professor of Medicine, Harvard Medical School; Associate Physician, Renal Division, Brigham and Women's Hospital, Boston [277]

VICTOR L. YU, MD
Professor of Medicine, University of Pittsburgh; Chief, Infectious Disease Section, VA Medical Center, Pittsburgh [151]

DORI F. ZALEZNIK, MD
Assistant Professor of Medicine, Harvard Medical School; Senior Physician, Beth Israel Deaconess Medical Center, Wellesley, Boston [130, 135, 145]

PETER ZIMETBAUM, MD
Instructor in Medicine, Harvard Medical School; Cardiovascular Division, Beth Israel Deaconess Medical Center, Boston [229, 230]

PHILIPPE E. ZIMMERN, MD
Associate Professor of Urology, The University of Texas Southwestern Medical School, Dallas [48]

The first edition of *Harrison's Principles of Internal Medicine* was published in the middle of the twentieth century, more than 50 years ago. In this fifteenth edition, the first of the new century, the text has undergone major revision to reflect further understanding of the biology and pathophysiology of disease and at the same time to retain those facts that, while not new, remain clinically useful and important. Virtually every chapter in this new edition has been completely or substantially rewritten, and a record 86 are new or have new authors. In this preface, we cannot describe all of these changes; however, we would like to call to the reader's attention those that are particularly noteworthy.

Part One, "Introduction to Clinical Medicine," contains new chapters dealing with decision making and cost awareness in clinical medicine. A growing number of patients are turning to alternative therapies, and these are discussed in a new chapter. New authors describe contemporary approaches to medical problems associated with pregnancy and the peripartum period. The chapters on medical ethics and on segments of the population that often present special problems—adolescents, women, and the elderly—have been revised and updated.

Part Two, "Cardinal Manifestations and Presentation of Disease," serves as a comprehensive introduction to clinical medicine, examining current concepts of the pathophysiology and differential diagnosis to be considered in patients with these manifestations. Major symptoms are reviewed and correlated with specific disease states, and clinical approaches to patients presenting with these symptoms are summarized. New chapters have been prepared on chest discomfort, headache, hypothermia, shock, and disorders of smell, taste, and hearing. A new chapter succinctly outlines a rational approach to the febrile patient presenting to the emergency department. The sections on alterations in gastrointestinal and sexual function are almost entirely new.

Given the explosive advances in human genetics, including the completion of a working draft of the sequence of the entire human genome and its growing relevance to clinical practice, Part Three, "Genetics and Disease," has been expanded and completely rewritten with new chapters on human genetics, chromosomal genetics, genetic defects, mitochondrial dysfunction, genetic screening and counseling, as well as gene therapy.

Part Four, "Clinical Pharmacology," provides a sound theoretical basis for pharmacotherapy, so critical to every aspect of medical practice.

Part Five, "Nutrition," has been extensively revised, with five new authors contributing chapters. This section covers nutritional considerations related to clinical medicine, including nutritional requirements, assessment of nutritional status, protein-energy malnutrition, and enteral and parenteral nutrition. It contains a new chapter on obesity, which incorporates the results of rapidly developing basic research in this important field.

The core of *Harrison's* encompasses the disorders of the organ systems and is contained in Parts Six through Fifteen. These sections include succinct accounts of the pathophysiology of the diseases involving the major organ systems and emphasize clinical manifestations, diagnostic procedures, differential diagnosis, and treatment strategies. The treatment sections of virtually every chapter have been amplified and updated. They are supplemented by the liberal use of algorithms, and are clearly highlighted. Guidelines for disease management prepared by specialty societies are included for the first time.

Part Six, "Oncology and Hematology," includes twelve chapters with new authors, including a new chapter by Judah Folkman on angiogenesis. In addition, a new chapter has been added on the medical problems that can arise in patients cured of cancer, including disease-related and treatment-related sequelae. The chapters on myeloid and lymphoid neoplasms include the new World Health Organization classification schemes. A conscientious effort has been made to provide specific, up-to-date treatment recommendations. Where appropriate, diagnostic and management algorithms have been incorporated.

Changes in Part Seven, "Infectious Diseases," include the latest information on the pathology, genetics, and epidemiology of infectious diseases while focusing sharply on the needs of clinicians who must accurately diagnose and treat infections in their patients. Specific recommendations are offered for therapeutic regimens, including the drug of choice, dose, duration, and alternatives. Current figures and trends in antimicrobial resistance are presented and considered in light of their impact on therapeutic choices. New authors cover the latest advances in the management of diseases such as infective endocarditis, meningococcal and gonococcal infections, and schistosomiasis. The overview of pathogenesis from earlier editions has been expanded to encompass viruses, fungi, and parasites as well as bacteria. The Atlas of Hematology includes a complete diagnostic set of spectacular color plates showing malaria-infected red blood cells.

In Part Eight, "Disorders of the Cardiovascular System," a new chapter on the prevention of atherosclerosis focuses not only on the importance of the traditional risk factors but also on the novel risk factors that influence plaque stability. Global risk assessment and management are described. Both primary and secondary prevention of atherosclerosis are discussed. Myocardial imaging by means of ultrasound or radionuclide techniques, at rest and during stress, plays an ever more critical role in assessment of patients with ischemic heart disease, and a new chapter focuses on the clinical use of these important technologies.

Despite major advances in its diagnosis and therapy, acute myocardial infarction remains the most common cause of death in industrialized nations. The chapter on acute myocardial infarction provides important new information on myocardial reperfusion therapy, thrombolysis, and primary coronary angioplasty and summarizes guidelines for acute coronary care and for risk stratification in the postinfarct patient. Unstable angina and congestive heart failure have emerged as two of the most common conditions leading to hospital admission in Western nations. Important advances in pathophysiology and therapy of these two very important conditions are included.

Enormous strides have been made in the use of lung transplantation for selected patients with end-stage, irreversible, pulmonary parenchymal and vascular disease, and Part Nine, "Disorders of the Respiratory System," provides a chapter that focuses on patient selection for this therapy. New chapters on interstitial and granulomatous lung diseases as well as on sleep apnea provide contemporary views of these conditions at the interface between basic science and clinical pulmonology.

In Part Ten, "Disorders of the Kidney and Urinary Tract," there has been considerable revision, with a new chapter on dialysis, incorporating the most recent advances.

In Part Eleven, "Disorders of the Gastrointestinal System," several new authors have contributed to the section on liver and biliary tract disease, and all chapters have been extensively revised. The section is pivoted by a new chapter on "Approach to the Patient with Liver Disease." Recent advances in the therapy of hepatitis B and C have been highlighted. New authors have contributed chapters on endoscopy, peptic ulcer disease, disorders of absorption, inflammatory bowel disease, and irritable bowel syndrome. Our new contributors include the leaders in gastroenterology and hepatology.

In Part Twelve, "Disorders of the Immune System, Connective Tissue, and Joints," the updating focuses on therapy. The chapter on

"Introduction to the Immune System" has been completely rewritten and provides a comprehensive review of the human immune system, using the modern designations of innate versus adaptive immunity. The chapter on HIV disease and AIDS is comprehensive and up-to-date and includes coverage of the natural history, epidemiology, and immunopathogenic mechanisms of HIV disease. In addition, the chapter contains both an organ system by organ system approach and a delineation of the major complications of HIV disease. The sections on therapy include a state-of-the-art discussion of the striking treatment advances of HIV infection with combinations of antiretroviral agents as well as the complications of such therapy.

Profound changes can be found in Part Thirteen, "Endocrinology and Metabolism." Many new authors have been recruited, and all chapters have been extensively revised under the direction of our new editor, Dr. J. Larry Jameson. Nine of these chapters are completely new, including those on the pituitary, thyroid, diabetes mellitus, and osteoporosis. These clinically demanding topics retain a traditional pathophysiologic approach that characterizes the field of endocrinology. In addition, new insights from genetics permeate this section, and the results of evidence-based medicine provide a firm foundation for medical decision making and treatment.

Part Fourteen, "Neurologic Disorders," has been thoroughly updated and expanded. The theme of genetics is emphasized throughout the section, and new chapters highlight the remarkable progress made during the "decade of the brain" in the 1990s that has elucidated the molecular basis of many neurologic and psychiatric diseases. One of the new chapters, written by 1997 Nobel Laureate Stanley B. Prusiner, summarizes the unique biology of prions and the clinical features of human prion disorders, including "mad cow disease."

The very latest information can be found on treatment of epilepsy, Parkinson's disease, and Alzheimer's disease. Coverage of immune-mediated disorders of the nervous system has been greatly expanded to include the many new insights into pathogenesis and treatment that have appeared since the fourteenth edition. The chapter on cerebrovascular diseases offers state-of-the-art information on prevention and treatment of stroke, the third leading killer in the developed world; this chapter is a mini-textbook of stroke and stroke therapy. Another feature of the fifteenth edition is a discussion of the acute neurologic disorders encountered in the setting of critical illness; this chapter should be of value to all physicians who care for hospitalized patients.

Throughout the book, there is an emphasis on the use of neuroimaging figures to illustrate the various disorders discussed. *Harrison's* exceptional collection of high-quality neuroimaging photographs sets a new standard for textbooks of medicine.

Finally, Part Fifteen, "Environmental and Occupational Hazards," has been expanded and reorganized.

In view of the requirements for continuing education for licensure and relicensure, as well as the emphasis on certification and recertification, a revision of the Pre-Test Self-Assessment and Review will again be published with this edition. It consists of several hundred questions based on *Harrison's*, along with answers and explanations for the answers. The *Companion Handbook* that was pioneered as a supplement to the eleventh edition of *Harrison's* has been updated and will appear shortly after the publication of this edition. A CD-ROM version of *Harrison's* has been available since the thirteenth edition. An expanded CD-ROM version of the fifteenth edition will be available and will be regularly updated. In 1998, *Harrison's* went online to provide a "living" textbook of internal medicine. In addition to providing full search capabilities of the text, *Harrison's Online* offers daily updating, reports of clinical trials, practice guidelines, and concise reviews of timely topics, as well as new references with links to MEDLINE abstracts.

The fifteenth edition of *Harrison's* welcomes a new editor, Dr. J. Larry Jameson, who has taken on principal responsibility for the sections on Nutrition, Genetics, Endocrinology, and Metabolism and whose impact on this edition is already clear. Dr. Kurt J. Isselbacher, Dr. Jean D. Wilson, and Dr. Joseph B. Martin have left the editorial group. Their enormous contributions to *Harrison's* are cited elsewhere. Special thanks go to Dr. Robert F. Schrier who has prepared biographies of Nobel Prize Laureates in Physiology or Medicine. These brief essays remind us how deeply our current knowledge and practice of medicine depends on seminal contributions to biomedical science and informs about the lives of some of the most outstanding contributors.

We wish to express our appreciation to our many associates and colleagues, who, as experts in their fields, have helped us with constructive criticism and helpful suggestions. We acknowledge especially the contributions of:

Donna Ambrosino, Peter Banks, Richard Blumberg, Douglas Brust, Myron Cohen, Jonathan Edlow, Christopher Fanta, Mary Gillam, Douglas Golenbach, Fred Gorelick, Charles Halsted, Lee Kaplan, Peter Kopp, Bruce Levy, Leo Liu, William Lowe, Lawrence Madoff, Josh Meeks, Mark Molitch, Chung Owyang, Eugene Pergament, Alice Pau, Gerald Pier, Peter Rice, Paul Sax, Tom Schnitzer, Julian Seifter, Anushua Sinha, Steven Weinberger, Michael Wessels, and Lee Wetzler.

This book could not have been edited without the dedicated help of our co-workers in the editorial offices of the individual editors. We are especially indebted to Scott Cromer, Pat Duffey, Sarah Anne Matero, Julie McCoy, Elizabeth Robbins, Kathryn Saxon, Marie Scurti, and Julieta Tayco.

Finally, we continue to be indebted to two outstanding members of the McGraw-Hill organization: Mariapaz Ramos Englis, Senior Managing Editor, and Martin J. Wonsiewicz, Publisher. They are an effective team who have given the editors constant encouragement and sage advice and have been of enormous help in bringing this edition to fruition in a timely manner.

The Editors

PART ONE

INTRODUCTION TO CLINICAL MEDICINE

The Editors

THE PRACTICE OF MEDICINE

WHAT IS EXPECTED OF THE PHYSICIAN The practice of medicine combines both science and art. The role of *science in medicine* is clear. Science-based technology and deductive reasoning form the foundation for the solution to many clinical problems; the spectacular advances in genetics, biochemistry, and imaging techniques allow access to the innermost parts of the cell and the most remote recesses of the body. Highly advanced therapeutic maneuvers are increasingly a major part of medical practice. Yet skill in the most sophisticated application of laboratory technology and in the use of the latest therapeutic modality alone does not make a good physician. One must be able to identify the crucial elements in a complex history and physical examination and extract the key laboratory results from the crowded computer printouts of laboratory data in order to determine in a difficult case whether to "treat" or to "watch." Deciding when a clinical clue is worth pursuing, or when it should be dismissed as a "red herring," and estimating in any given patient whether a proposed treatment entails a greater risk than the disease are essential to the decision-making process that the skilled clinician must exercise many times each day. This combination of medical knowledge, intuition, and judgment defines the *art of medicine*, which is as necessary to the practice of medicine as is a sound scientific base.

The editors of the first edition of this book articulated what is expected of the physician in words that, although they reflect the gender bias of that era, still ring true as a universal principle:

No greater opportunity, responsibility, or obligation can fall to the lot of a human being than to become a physician. In the care of the suffering he needs technical skill, scientific knowledge, and human understanding. He who uses these with courage, with humility, and with wisdom will provide a unique service for his fellow man, and will build an enduring edifice of character within himself. The physician should ask of his destiny no more than this; he should be content with no less.

Tact, sympathy and understanding are expected of the physician, for the patient is no mere collection of symptoms, signs, disordered functions, damaged organs, and disturbed emotions. He is human, fearful, and hopeful, seeking relief, help and reassurance.

THE PATIENT-PHYSICIAN RELATIONSHIP It may seem trite to emphasize that physicians need to approach patients not as "cases" or "diseases" but as individuals whose problems all too often transcend their physical complaints. Most patients are anxious and frightened. Physicians should instill confidence and reassurance, overtly and in their demeanor, but without an air of arrogance. A professional attitude, coupled with warmth and openness, can do much to alleviate the patients' anxiety and to encourage them to share parts of their history that may be embarrassing. Some patients "use" illness to gain attention or to serve as a crutch to extricate themselves from a stressful situation; some even feign physical illness; others may be openly hostile. Whatever the patient's attitude, the physician needs to consider the setting in which an illness occurs—in terms not only of the patients themselves but also of their families and social and cultural backgrounds. The ideal patient-physician relationship is based on thorough knowledge of the patient, on mutual trust, and on the ability to communicate with one another.

The direct, one-to-one patient-physician relationship, which has traditionally characterized the practice of medicine, is increasingly in jeopardy because of the increasing complexity of medicine and change in health care delivery systems. Often the management of the individual patient is a team effort involving a number of several different physicians and professional personnel. The patient can benefit greatly from such collaboration, but *it is the duty of the patient's principal physician to guide them through an illness*. To carry out this difficult task, this physician must be familiar with the techniques, skills, and objectives of specialist physicians and of colleagues in the fields allied to medicine. In giving the patient an opportunity to benefit from scientific advances, the primary physician must, in the last analysis, retain responsibility for the major decisions concerning diagnosis and treatment.

Patients are increasingly cared for by groups of physicians in clinics, hospitals, integrated health care delivery systems, and health maintenance organizations (HMOs). Whatever the potential advantages of such organized medical groups, there are also drawbacks, chiefly the loss of the clear identification of the physician who is primarily and continuously responsible for the patient. Even under these circumstances, it is essential for each patient to have a physician who has an overview of the problems and who is familiar with the patient's reaction to the illness, to the drugs given, and to the challenges that the patient faces.

The practice of medicine in a "managed care" setting puts additional stress on the classic paradigm of the patient-physician relationship. Many physicians must deal with a patient within a restricted time frame, with limited access to specialists, and under organizational guidelines that may compromise their ability to exercise their individual clinical judgment. As difficult as these restrictions may be, it is the ultimate responsibility of the physician to determine what is best for the patient. This responsibility cannot be relinquished in the name of compliance with organizational guidelines.

The physician must also bear in mind that the modern hospital constitutes an intimidating environment for most patients. Lying in a bed surrounded by air jets, buttons, and lights; invaded by tubes and wires; beset by the numerous members of the health care team—nurses, nurses' aides, physicians' assistants, social workers, technologists, physical therapists, medical students, house officers, attending and consulting physicians, and many others; sharing rooms with other patients who have their own problems, visitors, and physicians; transported to special laboratories and imaging facilities replete with blinking lights, strange sounds, and unfamiliar personnel—it is little wonder that patients may lose their sense of reality. In fact, the physician is often the only tenuous link between the patient and the real world, and a strong personal relationship with the physician helps to sustain the patient in such a stressful situation.

Many trends in contemporary society tend to make medical care impersonal. Some of these have been mentioned already and include (1) vigorous efforts to reduce the escalating costs of health care; (2) the growing number of managed care programs, which are intended to reduce costs but in which the patient may have little choice in selecting a physician; (3) increasing reliance on technologic advances and computerization for many aspects of diagnosis and treatment; (4) increased geographic mobility of both patients and physicians; (5) the need for numerous physicians to be involved in the care of most patients who are seriously ill; and (6) an increasing tendency on the part of patients to express their frustrations with the health care system by legal means (i.e., by malpractice litigation). Given these changes in the medical care system, it is a major challenge for physicians to maintain the *humane* aspects of medical care. The American Board of Internal Medicine has defined humanistic qualities as encompassing integrity, respect, and compassion. Availability, the expression of sincere concern, the willingness to take the time to explain all aspects of the illness, and a nonjudgmental attitude when dealing with patients whose cultures, lifestyles, attitudes, and values differ from those of the physician are just a few of the characteristics of the humane physician. Every physician will, at times, be challenged by patients who evoke strongly negative (or strongly positive) emotional responses. Physicians should be alert to their own reactions to such patients and situations and should consciously monitor and control their behavior so that the patients' best interests remain the principal motivation for their actions at all times.

An important aspect of patient care involves an appreciation of the "quality of life," a subjective assessment of what each patient values most. Such an assessment requires detailed, sometimes intimate knowledge of the patient, which can usually be obtained only through deliberate, unhurried, and often repeated conversations. It is in these situations that the time constraints of a managed care setting may prove problematic.

The famous statement of Dr. Francis Peabody is even more relevant today than when delivered more than three-quarters of a century ago:

The significance of the intimate personal relationship between physician and patient cannot be too strongly emphasized, for in an extraordinarily large number of cases both the diagnosis and treatment are directly dependent on it. One of the essential qualities of the clinician is interest in humanity, **for the secret of the care of the patient is in caring for the patient.**

CLINICAL SKILLS   History Taking   The written history of an illness should embody all the facts of medical significance in the life of the patient. Recent events should be given the most attention. The patient should, at some point, have the opportunity to tell his or her own story of the illness without frequent interruption and, when appropriate, receive expressions of interest, encouragement, and empathy from the physician. The physician must be alert to the possibility that any event related by the patient, however trivial or apparently remote, may be the key to the solution of the medical problem.

An informative history is more than an orderly listing of symptoms; something is always gained by listening to patients and noting the way in which they describe their symptoms. Inflections of voice, facial expression, gestures, and attitude may reveal important clues to the meaning of the symptoms to the patient. Taking history often involves much data gathering. Patients vary in their medical sophistication and ability to recall facts. Medical history should therefore be corroborated whenever possible. The family and social history can also provide important insights into the types of diseases that should be considered. In listening to the history, the physician discovers not only something about the disease but also something about the patient. The process of history taking provides an opportunity to observe the patient's behavior and to watch for features to be pursued more thoroughly during the physical examination.

The very act of eliciting the history provides the physician with the opportunity to establish or enhance the unique bond that is the basis for the ideal patient-physician relationship. It is helpful to develop an appreciation of the patient's perception of the illness, the patient's expectations of the physician and the medical care system, and the financial and social implications of the illness to the patient. The confidentiality of the patient-physician relationship should be emphasized, and the patient should be given the opportunity to identify any aspects of the history that should not be disclosed.

Physical Examination   Physical signs are objective indications of disease whose significance is enhanced when they confirm a functional or structural change already suggested by the patient's history. At times, however, the physical signs may be the only evidence of disease.

The physical examination should be performed methodically and thoroughly, with consideration for the patient's comfort and modesty. Although attention is often directed by the history to the diseased organ or part of the body, the examination of a new patient must extend from head to toe in an objective search for abnormalities. Unless the physical examination is systematic, important segments may be omitted. The results of the examination, like the details of the history, should be recorded at the time they are elicited, not hours later when they are subject to the distortions of memory. Skill in physical diagnosis is acquired with experience, but it is not merely technique that determines success in eliciting signs. The detection of a few scattered petechiae, a faint diastolic murmur, or a small mass in the abdomen is not a question of keener eyes and ears or more sensitive fingers but of a mind alert to these findings. Since physical findings are subject to changes, the physical examination should be repeated as frequently as the clinical situation warrants.

Laboratory Tests   The availability of a wide array of laboratory tests has increased our reliance on these studies for the solution of clinical problems. The accumulation of laboratory data does not relieve the physician from the responsibility of careful observation, examination, and study of the patient. It is also essential to bear in mind the limitations of such tests. By virtue of their impersonal quality, complexity, and apparent precision, they often gain an aura of authority regardless of the fallibility of the tests themselves, the instruments used in the tests, and the individuals performing or interpreting them. Physicians must weigh the expense involved in the laboratory procedures they order relative to the value of the information they are likely to provide.

Single laboratory tests are rarely ordered. Rather, they are generally obtained as "batteries" of multiple tests, which are often useful. For example, abnormalities of hepatic function may provide the clue to such nonspecific symptoms as generalized weakness and increased fatigability, suggesting the diagnosis of chronic liver disease. Sometimes a single abnormality, such as an elevated serum calcium level, points to particular diseases, such as hyperparathyroidism or underlying malignancy.

The thoughtful use of screening tests should not be confused with indiscriminate laboratory testing. The use of screening tests is based on the fact that a group of laboratory determinations can be carried out conveniently on a single specimen of blood at relatively low cost. Screening tests are most useful when they are directed towards common diseases or disorders in which the result directs other useful tests or interventions that would otherwise be costly to perform. Biochemical measurements, together with simple laboratory examinations such as blood count, urinalysis, and sedimentation rate, often provide the major clue to the presence of a pathologic process. At the same time, the physician must learn to evaluate occasional abnormalities among the screening tests that may not necessarily connote significant disease. An in-depth workup following a report of an isolated laboratory abnormality in a person who is otherwise well is almost invariably wasteful and unproductive. Among the more than 40 tests that are routinely performed on patients, one or two are often slightly abnormal. If there is no suspicion of an underlying illness, these tests are ordinarily repeated to ensure that the abnormality does not represent a laboratory error. If an abnormality is confirmed, it is important to consider its potential significance in the context of the patient's condition and other test results.

Imaging Techniques   The availability of ultrasonography, a variety of scans that employ isotopes to visualize organs heretofore inaccessible, computed tomography, and magnetic resonance imaging has opened new diagnostic vistas and has benefited patients because these new techniques have largely supplanted more invasive ones. While the enthusiasm for noninvasive technology is understandable, the expense entailed in performing these tests is often substantial and should be considered when assessing the potential benefits of the information provided.

PRINCIPLES OF PATIENT CARE   Medical Decision-Making   Both during and in particular after the physician has taken the history, performed the physical examination, and reviewed the laboratory and imaging data, the challenging process of the differential diagnosis and medical decision-making begins. Formulating a differential diagnosis requires not only a broad knowledge base but also the ability to assess the relative probabilities of various diseases and to understand the significance of missing diagnoses that may be less likely. Arriving at a diagnosis requires the application of the scientific method. Hypotheses are formed, data are collected, and objective conclusions are reached concerning whether to accept or reject a particular diagnosis. Analysis of the differential diagnosis is an iterative process. As new information or test results are acquired, the group of disease processes being considered can be contracted or expanded appropriately. Medical decision-making occurs throughout the diagnostic and treatment process. It involves the ordering of additional tests, requests for consults, and decisions regarding prognosis and treatment. This process requires an in-depth understanding of the natural history and pathophysiology of disease, explaining why these features are strongly emphasized in this textbook. As described below, medical decision-making should be evidence-based, thereby ensuring that patients derive the full benefit of the scientific knowledge available to physicians.

Evidence-Based Medicine   Sackett has defined evidence-based medicine as "the conscientious, explicit and judicious use of current best evidence in making decisions about the care of individual patients." Rigorously obtained evidence is contrasted with anecdotal experience, which is often biased. Even the most experienced physicians can be influenced by recent experiences with selected patients, unless they are attuned to the importance of using larger, more objective studies for making decisions. The prospectively designed, double-blind, randomized clinical trial represents the "gold standard" for providing evidence regarding therapeutic decisions, but it is not the only source. Valuable evidence about the natural history of disease and prognosis can come from prospective cohort studies and analytic surveys. Persuasive evidence on the accuracy of diagnostic tests can be derived from cross-sectional studies of patients in whom a specific disorder is suspected. Evidence is strengthened immensely when it has been confirmed by multiple investigations, which can be compared with one another and presented in a meta-analysis or systemic overview.

In failing to apply the best and most current evidence, the physician places the patient at unnecessary risk. However, a knowledge of or rapid access to the best available evidence is not sufficient for optimal care. The physician must know whether the evidence is relevant to the patient in question and, when it is, the consequences of applying it in any particular situation. The skills and judgment required to apply sound evidence represent an increasing challenge. Indeed, one might redefine a "good doctor" as one who uses the ever-growing body of rigorously obtained evidence (the science of medicine) in a sensible, compassionate manner (the art of medicine).

While an understanding of biologic and physiologic mechanisms forms the basis of contemporary medicine, when a therapeutic modality is selected, the highest priority must often be placed on improving *clinical outcome* rather than interrupting what is believed to be the underlying process. For example, for decades patients who had suffered myocardial infarction were treated intuitively with drugs that suppress frequent ventricular extrasystoles, since these were believed to be harbingers of ventricular fibrillation and sudden death. Clinical trials, however, have provided firm evidence that the antiarrhythmic agents actually increase the risk of death in such patients. This finding suggests that the extrasystoles are *markers* of high risk rather than the *cause* of fatal events.

Practice Guidelines   Physicians are faced with a large, increasing, and often bewildering body of evidence pointing to potentially useful diagnostic techniques and therapeutic choices. The intelligent and cost-effective practice of medicine consists of making selections most appropriate to a particular patient and clinical situation. Professional organizations and government agencies are developing formal clinical practice guidelines in an effort to aid physicians and other caregivers in this endeavor. When guidelines are current and properly applied, they can provide a useful framework for managing patients with particular diagnoses or symptoms. They can protect patients—

particularly those with inadequate health care benefits—from receiving substandard care. Guidelines can also protect conscientious caregivers from inappropriate charges of malpractice and society from the excessive costs associated with the overuse of medical resources. On the other hand, clinical guidelines tend to oversimplify the complexities of medicine. Different groups with differing perspectives may develop divergent recommendations regarding issues as basic as the need for periodic sigmoidoscopy in middle-aged persons. Furthermore, guidelines do not—and cannot be expected to—take into account the uniqueness of each individual and of his or her illness. The challenge for the physician is to integrate into clinical practice the useful recommendations offered by the experts who prepare clinical practice guidelines without accepting them blindly or being inappropriately constrained by them.

Assessing the Outcome of Treatment   Clinicians generally use *objective* and readily measurable parameters to judge the outcome of a therapeutic intervention. For example, findings on physical or laboratory examination—such as the level of blood pressure, the patency of a coronary artery on an angiogram, or the size of a mass on a radiologic examination—can provide information of critical importance. However, patients usually seek medical attention for *subjective* reasons; they wish to obtain relief from pain, to preserve or regain function, and to enjoy life. The components of a patient's health status or quality of life can include bodily comfort, capacity for physical activity, personal and professional function, sexual function, cognitive function, and overall perception of health. Each of these important areas can be assessed by means of structured interviews or specially designed questionnaires. Such assessments also provide useful parameters by which the physician can judge the patient's subjective view of his or her disability and the response to treatment, particularly in chronic illness. The practice of medicine requires consideration and integration of both objective and subjective outcomes.

Care of the Elderly   Over the next several decades, the practice of medicine will be greatly influenced by the health care needs of the growing elderly population. In the United States the population over age 65 will almost triple over the next 30 years. It is essential that we understand and appreciate the physiologic processes associated with aging; the different responses of the elderly to common diseases; and disorders that occur commonly with aging, such as depression, dementia, frailty, urinary incontinence, and fractures. The elderly have more adverse reactions to drugs, in large part due to altered pharmacokinetics and pharmacodynamics. Commonly used medications such as digoxin and aminoglycosides have prolonged half-lives in the elderly, and tissues such as the central nervous system are more sensitive to certain drugs, such as the benzodiazepines and narcotics. The large number of drugs used by the elderly increases the risk of unwanted interactions, especially when care is provided by several physicians in an uncoordinated manner.

Diseases in Women versus Men   In the past, many epidemiologic studies and clinical trials focused on men. It is now appreciated that there are significant gender differences in diseases that afflict both men and women. Mortality rates are substantially higher in women than in men under the age of 50 suffering acute myocardial infarction. Hypertension is more prevalent in African-American women than in their male counterparts (and in African-American than in white males); osteoporosis is more common in women, reflecting the menopausal loss of estrogen; diseases involving the immune system, such as lupus erythematosus, multiple sclerosis, and primary biliary cirrhosis, occur more frequently in women; and the average life expectancy of women is greater than that of men. Recently, considerable attention has been paid to women's health issues, a subject that regrettably did not receive sufficient attention in the past. Ongoing study should enhance our understanding of the mechanisms of gender differences in the course and outcome of certain diseases.

Iatrogenic Disorders   In an *iatrogenic disorder*, the deleterious effects of a therapeutic or diagnostic maneuver cause pathology independent of the condition for which the intervention was performed. Adverse drug reactions occur in at least 5% of hospitalized patients, and the incidence increases with use of a large number of drugs. No matter what the clinical situation, it is the responsibility of the physician to use powerful therapeutic measures wisely, with due regard for their beneficial action, potential dangers, and cost. Every medical procedure, whether diagnostic or therapeutic, has the potential for harm, but it would be impossible to provide the benefits of modern scientific medicine if reasonable steps in diagnosis and therapy were withheld because of possible risks. *Reasonable* implies that the physician has weighed the pros and cons of a procedure and has concluded, on the basis of objective evidence whenever possible, that it is necessary for establishing a diagnosis, for the relief of discomfort, or for the cure of disease. However, the harm that a physician can do is not limited to the imprudent use of medication or procedures. Equally important are ill-considered or unjustified remarks. Many a patient has developed a cardiac neurosis because the physician ventured a grave prognosis on the basis of a misinterpreted finding of a heart murmur. Not only the diagnostic procedure or the treatment but the physician's words and behavior are capable of causing injury.

Informed Consent   Patients often require diagnostic and therapeutic procedures that are painful and that pose some risk. For many such procedures, patients are required to sign a consent form. The patient must understand clearly the risks entailed in these procedures; this is the definition of *informed consent*. It is incumbent on the physician to explain the procedures in a clear and understandable manner and to ascertain that the patient comprehends both the nature of the procedure and the attendant risks. The dread of the unknown that is inherent in hospitalization can be mitigated by such explanations.

Incurability and Death   No problem is more distressing than that presented by the patient with an incurable disease, particularly when premature death is inevitable. What should the patient and family be told, what measures should be taken to maintain life, what can be done to maintain the quality of life, and how is death to be defined?

The concept of incurable illness and terminal care often evokes examples of cancer. However, patients with many other end-stage diseases including chronic obstructive pulmonary disease, congestive heart failure, renal or hepatic failure, and overwhelming infection face similar issues. The same principles of terminal care should be applied in each of these cases. Doing seemingly small things, focused on the needs of the patient, can do much to restore comfort or dignity during a person's final weeks or days. In the same way that pain should be attentively managed with analgesia, every effort should be made to alleviate shortness of breath and to provide good skin care.

Although some would argue otherwise, there is no ironclad rule that the patient must immediately be told "everything," even if the patient is an adult with substantial family responsibilities. How much is told should depend on the individual's ability to deal with the possibility of imminent death; often this capacity grows with time, and whenever possible, gradual rather than abrupt disclosure is the best strategy. A wise and insightful physician is often guided by an understanding of what a patient wants to know and when he or she wants to know it. The patient's religious beliefs may also be taken into consideration. The patient must be given an opportunity to talk with the physician and ask questions. Patients may find it easier to share their feelings about death with their physician, who is likely to be more objective and less emotional, than with family members. As William Osler wrote:

> One thing is certain; it is not for you to don the black cap and, assuming the judicial function, take hope away from any patient . . . hope that comes to us all.

Even when the patient directly inquires, "Am I dying?" the physician must attempt to determine whether this is a request for information or a demand for reassurance. Only open communication between the patient and the physician can resolve this question and guide the physician in what to say and how to say it.

The physician should provide or arrange for emotional, physical, and spiritual support and must be compassionate, unhurried, and open. There is much to be gained by the laying on of hands. Pain should be adequately controlled, human dignity maintained, and isolation from the family avoided. These aspects of care tend to be overlooked in hospitals, where the intrusion of life-sustaining apparatus can so easily detract from attention to the whole person and encourage concentration instead on the life-threatening disease, against which the battle will ultimately be lost in any case. In the face of terminal illness, the goal of medicine must shift from *cure* to *care*, in the broadest sense of the term. In offering care to the dying patient, the physician must be prepared to provide information to family members and to deal with their guilt and grief. It is important for the doctor to assure the family that everything possible has been done.

"Do Not Resuscitate" Orders and Cessation of Therapy   When carried out in a timely and expert manner, cardiopulmonary resuscitation is often useful in the prevention of sudden, unexpected death. However, unless there are reasons to the contrary, this procedure should not be used merely to prolong the life of a patient with terminal, incurable disease. The decision whether or not to resuscitate or even to treat an incurably and terminally ill patient must be reviewed frequently and must take into consideration any unexpected changes in the patient's condition. In this context, the administration of fluids or food is considered therapy that may be withdrawn or withheld. These decisions must also take into account both the underlying medical condition, especially its reversibility, and the wishes of the patient, especially if these have been expressed in a living will or advance directive. If the patient's wishes cannot be ascertained directly, a close relative or another surrogate who can be relied on to transmit the patient's wishes and to be guided by the patient's best interests should be consulted. The patient's autonomy—whether the choice is to continue or discontinue treatment or to be resuscitated or not in the event of a cardiopulmonary arrest—must be paramount. The courts have ruled that competent patients may refuse therapy and that an incompetent patient's previously stated wishes regarding life support should therefore be respected. The issues involving death and dying are among the most difficult in medicine. In approaching them rationally and consistently, the physician must combine both the science and the art of medicine.

THE EXPANDING ROLE OF THE PHYSICIAN   Genetics and Medicine   The genomic era is likely to lead to a revolution in the practice of medicine. Obtaining the DNA sequence of the entire human genome may help to elucidate the genetic components of common chronic diseases—hypertension, diabetes, atherosclerosis, many cancers, dementias, and behavioral and autoimmune disorders. This information should make it possible to determine individual susceptibility to these conditions early in life and to implement individualized prevention programs. Subclassification of many diseases on a genetic basis may allow the selection of appropriate therapy for each patient. As the response to drugs becomes more predictable, pharmacotherapy should become more rational. In short, the completion of the Human Genome Project is likely to lead to a substantial increase in physicians' ability to influence their patient's health and well-being.

Patients will be best served if physicians play an active role in applying this powerful, sensitive new information rather than being passive bystanders who are intimidated by the new technology. This is a rapidly evolving field, and physicians and other health care professionals must remain updated to apply this new knowledge. Genetic testing requires wise counsel based on an understanding of the value and limitations of the tests as well as the implications of their results for specific individuals.

Medicine on the Internet   The explosion in use of the Internet through personal computers is having an important impact on many practicing physicians. The Internet makes a wide range of information available to physicians almost instantaneously at any time of the day or night and from anywhere in the world. This medium holds enormous potential for delivering up-to-date information, practice guidelines, state-of-the-art conferences, journal contents, textbooks (including this text), and direct communications with other physicians and specialists, thereby expanding the depth and breadth of information available to the physician about the diagnosis and care of patients. Most medical journals are now accessible on-line, providing rapid and comprehensive sources of information. Patients, too, are turning to the Internet in increasing numbers to derive information about their illnesses and therapies and to join Internet-based support groups. Physicians are increasingly challenged by dealing with patients who are becoming more sophisticated in their understanding of illness. At this time, there is one critically important caveat. Virtually anything can be published on the Internet, thus circumventing the peer-review process that is an essential feature of quality publications. Physicians or patients who search the Internet for medical information must be aware of this danger. Notwithstanding this limitation, appropriate use of the Internet is revolutionizing information access for physicians and is a positive force in the practice of medicine.

Delivering Cost-Effective Medical Care   As the cost of medical care has risen, it has become necessary to establish priorities in the expenditure of resources. In some instances, preventive measures offer the greatest return for the expenditure; outstanding examples include vaccination, improved sanitation, reduction in accidents and occupational hazards, and biochemical- and DNA-based screening of newborns. For example, the detection of phenylketonuria by newborn screening may result in a net saving of many thousands of dollars.

As resources become increasingly constrained, the physician must weigh the possible benefits of performing costly procedures that provide only a limited life expectancy against the pressing need for more primary care for those persons who do not have adequate access to medical services. For the individual patient, it is important to reduce costly hospital admissions as much as possible if total health care is to be provided at a cost that most can afford. This policy, of course, implies and depends on close cooperation among patients, their physicians, employers, payers, and government. It is equally important for physicians to know the cost of the diagnostic procedures they order and the drugs and other therapies they prescribe and to monitor both costs and effectiveness. The medical profession should provide leadership and guidance to the public in matters of cost control, and physicians must take this responsibility seriously without being or seeming to be self-serving. However, the economic aspects of health care delivery must not interfere with the welfare of patients. The patient must be able to rely on the individual physician as his or her principal advocate in matters of health care.

Accountability   Medicine is a satisfying but demanding profession. Physicians must understand the characteristics of the populations they serve, and they must appreciate their patients' social and cultural attitudes to health, disease, and death. As the public has become more educated and more sophisticated regarding health matters, their expectations of the health system in general and of their physicians in particular have risen. Physicians are expected to maintain mastery of their rapidly advancing fields (the *science* of medicine) while considering their patient's unique needs (the *art* of medicine). Thus, physicians are held accountable not only for the technical aspects of the care that they provide but also for their patient's satisfaction with the delivery and costs of care.

In the United States, there are increasing demands for physicians to account for the way in which they practice medicine by meeting certain standards prescribed by federal and state governments. The hospitalization of patients whose health care costs are reimbursed by the government and other third parties is subjected to utilization review. Thus the physician must defend the cause for and duration of a patient's hospitalization if it falls outside certain "average" standards. Authorization for reimbursement is increasingly based on documentation of the nature and complexity of an illness, as reflected by recorded elements of the history and physical examination. The purpose of these regulations is both to improve standards of health care and to contain spiraling health care costs. This type of review is being extended to all phases of medical practice and is profoundly altering the practice of medicine. Physicians are also expected to give evidence of

their continuing competence through mandatory continuing education, patient-record audits, recertification by examination, or relicensing.

Continued Learning   The conscientious physician must be a perpetual student because the body of medical knowledge is constantly expanding and being refined. The profession of medicine should be inherently linked to a career-long thirst for new knowledge that can be used for the good of the patient. It is the responsibility of a physician to pursue continually the acquisition of new knowledge by reading, attending conferences and courses, and consulting colleagues and the Internet. This is often a difficult task for a busy practitioner; however, such a commitment to continued learning is an integral part of being a physician and must be given the highest priority.

Research and Teaching   The title *doctor* is derived from the Latin *docere*, "to teach," and physicians should share information and medical knowledge with colleagues, with students of medicine and related professions, and with their patients. The practice of medicine is dependent on the sum total of medical knowledge, which in turn is based on an unending chain of scientific discovery, clinical observation, analysis, and interpretation. Advances in medicine depend on the acquisition of new information, i.e., on research, which often involves patients; improved medical care requires the transmission of this information. As part of broader societal responsibilities, the physician should encourage patients to participate in ethical and properly approved clinical investigations if they do not impose undue hazard, discomfort, or inconvenience. To quote Osler once more:

To wrest from nature the secrets which have perplexed philosophers in all ages, to track to their sources the causes of disease, to correlate the vast stores of knowledge, that they may be quickly available for the prevention and cure of disease—these are our ambitions.

BIBLIOGRAPHY

COLLINS FS: Shattuck Lecture: Medical and Societal Consequences of the Human Genome Project. N Engl J Med 341:28, 1999

COUNCIL ON GRADUATE MEDICAL EDUCATION: *Thirteenth Report: Physician Education for a Changing Health Care Environment.* US Department of Health and Human Services, March 1999

SACKETT DL et al: *Evidence Based Medicine: How to Practise and Teach EBM.* London. Churchill Livingstone, 1997

TAUBES G: Looking for the evidence in medicine. Science 272:22, 1996

2   *Bernard Lo*

ETHICAL ISSUES IN CLINICAL MEDICINE

Physicians frequently confront ethical issues in clinical practice that are perplexing, time-consuming, and emotionally draining. Experience, common sense, and simply being a good person do not guarantee that physicians can identify or resolve ethical dilemmas. Knowledge about common ethical dilemmas is also essential.

FUNDAMENTAL ETHICAL GUIDELINES

Physicians should follow two fundamental but frequently conflicting ethical guidelines: respecting patient autonomy and acting in the patient's best interests.

RESPECTING PATIENT AUTONOMY   Competent, informed patients may refuse recommended interventions and choose among reasonable alternatives.

Informed Consent   Informed consent requires physicians to discuss with patients the nature of the proposed care, the alternatives, the risks and benefits of each, the likely consequences, and to obtain the patient's agreement to care. Informed consent involves more than obtaining signatures on consent forms. Physicians need to educate patients, answer questions, make recommendations, and help them deliberate. Patients can be overwhelmed with medical jargon, needlessly complicated explanations, or too much information at once.

Nondisclosure of Information   Physicians may consider withholding a serious diagnosis, misrepresenting it, or limiting discussions of prognosis or risks because they fear that a patient will develop severe anxiety or depression or refuse needed care. Patients should not be forced to receive information against their will. Most people, however, want to know their diagnosis and prognosis, even if they are terminally ill. Generally, physicians should provide relevant information, offer empathy and hope, and help patients cope with bad news.

Emergency Care   Informed consent is not required when patients cannot give consent and when delay of treatment would place their life or health in peril. People are presumed to want such emergency care, unless they have previously indicated otherwise.

Futile Interventions   Autonomy does not entitle patients to insist on whatever care they want. Physicians are not obligated to provide futile interventions that have no physiologic rationale or have already failed. For example, cardiopulmonary resuscitation would be futile in a patient with progressive hypotension despite maximal therapy. But physicians should be wary of using the term "futile" in looser senses to justify unilateral decisions to forego interventions when they believe that the probability of success is too low, no worthwhile goals can be achieved, the patient's quality of life is unacceptable, or the costs are too high. Such looser usages of the term are problematic because they may be inconsistent and mask value judgments.

ACTING IN THE BEST INTERESTS OF PATIENTS
The guideline of *beneficence* requires physicians to act for the patient's benefit. Laypeople do not possess medical expertise and may be vulnerable because of their illness. They justifiably rely on physicians to provide sound advice and to promote their well-being. Physicians encourage such trust. Hence, physicians have a fiduciary duty to act in the best interests of their patients. The interests of the patient should prevail over physicians' self-interest or the interests of third parties, such as hospitals or insurers. These fiduciary obligations of physicians contrast sharply with business relationships, which are characterized by "let the buyer beware," not by trust and reliance. The guideline of "*do no harm*" forbids physicians from providing ineffective interventions or acting without due care. This precept, while often cited, provides only limited guidance, because many beneficial interventions also have serious risks.

CONFLICTS BETWEEN BENEFICENCE AND AUTONOMY   Patients' refusals of care may thwart their own goals or cause them serious harm. For example, a young man with asthma may refuse mechanical ventilation for reversible respiratory failure. Simply to accept such refusals, in the name of respecting autonomy, seems morally constricted. Physicians can elicit patients' expectations and concerns, correct misunderstandings, and try to persuade them to accept beneficial therapies. If disagreements persist after discussions, the patient's informed choices and view of his or her best interests should prevail. While refusing recommended care does not render a patient incompetent, it may lead the physician to probe further to ensure that the patient is able to make informed decisions.

PATIENTS WHO LACK DECISION-MAKING CAPACITY

Patients may not be able to make informed decisions because of unconsciousness, dementia, delirium, or other conditions. Physicians should ask two questions regarding such patients: Who is the appropriate surrogate? What would the patient want done?

ASSESSING CAPACITY TO MAKE MEDICAL DECISIONS   All adults are considered legally competent unless declared incompetent by a court. In practice, physicians usually determine that patients lack the capacity to make health care decisions and arrange for surrogates to make them, without involving the courts. By definition, competent patients can express a choice and appreciate the medical situation, the nature of the proposed care, the alternatives, and the risks, benefits, and consequences of each. Their choices should be consistent with their values and should not result from delusions or hallucinations. Psychiatrists may help in difficult cases because they are skilled at interviewing mentally impaired patients and can identify treatable depression or psychosis. When impairments are fluctuating or reversible, decisions should be postponed if possible until the patient recovers decision-making capacity.

CHOICE OF SURROGATE   If a patient lacks decision-making capacity, physicians routinely ask family members to serve as surrogates. Most patients want their family members to be surrogates, and family members generally know the patient's preferences and have the patient's best interests at heart. Patients may designate a particular individual to serve as proxy; such choices should be respected. Some states have established a prioritized list of which relative may serve as surrogate if the patient has not designated a proxy.

STANDARDS FOR SURROGATE DECISION MAKING
Advance Directives   These are statements by competent patients to direct care if they lose decision-making capacity. They may indicate (1) what interventions they would refuse or accept or (2) who should serve as surrogate. Following the patient's advance directives, surrogate respects patients' autonomy.

Oral conversations are the most frequent form of advance directives. While such conversations are customarily followed in clinical practice, casual or vague comments may not be trustworthy.

Living wills direct physicians to forego or provide life-sustaining interventions if the patient develops a terminal condition or persistent vegetative state. Generally patients may refuse only interventions that "merely prolong the process of dying."

A health care proxy is someone appointed by the patient to make health care decisions if he or she loses decision-making capacity. It is more flexible and comprehensive than the living will, applying whenever the patient is unable to make decisions.

Physicians can encourage patients to provide advance directives, to indicate both what they would want and who should be surrogate, and to discuss their preferences with surrogates. In discussions with patients, physicians can ensure that advance directives are informed, up-to-date, and address likely clinical scenarios. Such discussions are best carried out in the ambulatory setting. The federal Patient Self-Determination Act requires hospitals and health maintenance organizations to inform patients of their right to make health care decisions and to provide advance directives.

Substituted Judgment   In the absence of clear advance directives, surrogates and physicians should try to decide as the patient would under the circumstances, using all information that they know about the patient. While such substituted judgments try to respect the patient's values, they may be speculative or inaccurate. A surrogate may be mistaken about the patient's preferences, particularly when they have not been discussed explicitly.

Best Interests   When the patient's preferences are unclear or unknown, decisions should be based on the patient's best interests. Patients generally take into account the quality of life as well as the duration of life when making decisions for themselves. It is understandable that surrogates would also consider quality of life of patients who lack decision-making capacity. Judgments about quality of life are appropriate if they reflect the patient's own values. Bias or discrimination may occur, however, if others project their values onto the patient or weigh the perceived social worth of the patient. Most patients with chronic illness rate their quality of life higher than their family members and physicians do.

Legal Issues   Physicians need to know pertinent state laws regarding patients who lack decision-making capacity. A few state courts allow doctors to forego life-sustaining interventions only if patients have provided written advance directives or very specific oral ones.

Disagreements Disagreements may occur among potential surrogates or between the physician and surrogate. Physicians can remind everyone to base decisions on what the patient would want, not what they would want for themselves. Consultation with the hospital ethics committee or with another physician often helps resolve disputes. Such consultation is also helpful when patients have no surrogate and no advance directives. The courts should be used only as a last resort when disagreements cannot be resolved in the clinical setting.

DECISIONS ABOUT LIFE-SUSTAINING INTERVENTIONS

Although medical technology can save lives, it can also prolong the process of dying. Competent, informed patients may refuse life-sustaining interventions. Such interventions may also be withheld from patients who lack decision-making capacity on the basis of advance directives or decisions by appropriate surrogates. Courts have ruled that foregoing life-sustaining interventions is neither suicide nor murder.

MISLEADING DISTINCTIONS People commonly draw distinctions that are intuitively plausible but prove untenable on closer analysis.

Extraordinary and Ordinary Care Some physicians are willing to forego "extraordinary" or "heroic" interventions, such as surgery, mechanical ventilation, or renal dialysis, but insist on providing "ordinary" ones, such as antibiotics, intravenous fluids, or feeding tubes. However, this distinction is not logical because all medical interventions have both risks and benefits. Any intervention may be withheld, if the burdens for the individual patient outweigh the benefits.

Withdrawing and Withholding Interventions Many health care providers find it more difficult to discontinue interventions than to withhold them in the first place. Although such emotions need to be acknowledged, there is no logical distinction between the two acts. Justifications for withholding interventions, such as refusal by patients or surrogates, are also justifications for withdrawing them. In addition, an intervention may prove unsuccessful or new information about the patient's preferences or condition may become available after the intervention is started. If interventions could not be discontinued, patients and surrogates might not even attempt treatments that might prove beneficial.

DO NOT RESUSCITATE (DNR) ORDERS When a patient suffers a cardiopulmonary arrest, cardiopulmonary resuscitation (CPR) is initiated unless a DNR order has been made. Although CPR can restore people to vigorous health, it can also disrupt a peaceful death. After CPR is attempted on a general hospital service, only 14% of patients survive to discharge, and even fewer in certain subgroups. DNR orders are appropriate if the patient or surrogate requests them or if CPR would be futile. To prevent misunderstandings, physicians should write DNR orders and the reasons for them in the medical record. "Slow" or "show" codes that merely appear to provide CPR are deceptive and therefore unacceptable. Although a DNR order signifies only that CPR will be withheld, the reasons that justify DNR orders may lead to a reconsideration of other plans for care.

ASSISTED SUICIDE AND ACTIVE EUTHANASIA Proponents of these controversial acts believe that competent, terminally ill patients should have control over the end of life and that physicians should relieve refractory suffering. Opponents assert that such actions violate the sanctity of life, that suffering can generally be relieved, that abuses are inevitable, and that such actions are outside the physician's proper role. These actions are illegal throughout the United States, except that physician-assisted suicide is legal in Oregon under certain circumstances. Whatever their personal views, physicians should respond to patients' inquiries with compassion and concern. Physicians should elicit and address any underlying problems, such as physical symptoms, loss of control, or depression. Often, additional efforts to relieve distress are successful, and after this is done patients generally withdraw their requests for these acts.

CARE OF DYING PATIENTS Patients often suffer unrelieved pain and other symptoms during their final days of life. Physicians may hesitate to order high doses of narcotics and sedatives, fearing they will hasten death. Relieving pain in terminal illness and alleviating dyspnea when patients forego mechanical ventilation enhances patient comfort and dignity. If lower doses of narcotics and sedatives have failed to relieve suffering, increasing the dose to levels that may suppress respiratory drive is ethically appropriate because the physician's intention is to relieve suffering, not hasten death. Physicians can also relieve suffering by spending time with dying patients, listening to them, and attending to their psychological distress.

CONFLICTS OF INTEREST

Acting in the patient's best interests may conflict with the physician's self-interest or the interests of third parties such as insurers or hospitals. The ethical ideal is to keep the patient's interests paramount. Even the appearance of a conflict of interest may undermine trust in the profession.

FINANCIAL INCENTIVES In managed care systems, physicians may serve as gatekeepers or bear financial risk for expenditures. Although such incentives are intended to reduce inefficiency and waste, there is concern that physicians may withhold beneficial care in order to control costs. In contrast, physicians have incentives to provide more care than indicated when they receive fee-for-service reimbursement or when they refer patients to medical facilities in which they have invested. Regardless of financial incentives, physicians should recommend available care that is in the patient's best interests—no more and no less.

DENIALS OF COVERAGE Utilization review programs designed to reduce unnecessary services may also deny coverage for care that the physician believes will benefit the patient. Physicians should inform patients when a plan is not covering standard care and act as patient advocates by appealing such denials of coverage. Patients may ask physicians to misrepresent their condition to help them obtain insurance coverage or disability. While physicians understandably want to help patients, such misrepresentation undermines physicians' credibility and violates their integrity.

GIFTS FROM PHARMACEUTICAL COMPANIES Physicians may be offered gifts ranging from pens and notepads to lavish entertainment. Critics worry that any gift from drug companies may impair objectivity, increase the cost of health care, and give the appearance of conflict of interest. A helpful rule of thumb is to consider whether patients would approve if they knew physicians had accepted such gifts.

OCCUPATIONAL RISKS Some health care workers, fearing fatal occupational infections, refuse to care for persons with HIV infection or multidrug-resistant tuberculosis. Such fears about personal safety need to be acknowledged, and institutions should reduce occupational risk by providing proper training, equipment, and supervision. Physicians should provide appropriate care within their clinical expertise, despite personal risk.

MISTAKES Mistakes are inevitable in clinical medicine. They may cause serious harm to patients or result in substantial changes in management. Physicians and students may fear that disclosing such mistakes could damage their careers. Without disclosure, however, patients cannot understand their clinical situation or make informed choices about subsequent care. Similarly, unless attending physicians are informed of trainees' mistakes, they cannot provide optimal care and help trainees learn from mistakes.

LEARNING CLINICAL SKILLS Learning clinical medicine, particularly learning to perform invasive procedures, may present inconvenience or risk to patients. To ensure patient cooperation, students may be introduced as physicians, or patients may not be told that trainees will be performing procedures. Such misrepresentation undermines trust, may lead to more elaborate deception, and makes it difficult for patients to make informed choices about their care. Patients should be told who is providing care, what benefits and burdens can be attributed to trainees, and how trainees are supervised. Most patients, when informed, allow trainees to play an active role in their care.

IMPAIRED PHYSICIANS   Physicians may hesitate to intervene when colleagues impaired by alcohol abuse, drug abuse, or psychiatric or medical illness place patients at risk. However, society relies on physicians to regulate themselves. If colleagues of an impaired physician do not take steps to protect patients, no one else may be in a position to do so.

CONFLICTS FOR TRAINEES   Medical students and residents may fear that they will receive poor grades or evaluations if they act on the patient's behalf by disclosing mistakes, avoiding misrepresentation of their role, and reporting impaired colleagues. Discussing such dilemmas with more senior physicians can help trainees check their interpretation of the situation and obtain advice and assistance.

ADDITIONAL ETHICAL ISSUES

MAINTAINING CONFIDENTIALITY   Maintaining the confidentiality of medical information respects patients' autonomy and privacy, encourages them to seek treatment and to discuss their problems candidly, and prevents discrimination. Physicians need to guard against inadvertent breaches of confidentiality, as when talking about patients in elevators. Maintaining confidentiality is not an absolute rule. The law may require physicians to override confidentiality in order to protect third parties, for example, reporting to government officials persons with specified infectious conditions, such as tuberculosis and syphilis; persons with gunshot wounds; and victims of elder abuse and domestic violence. Computerized medical records raise additional concerns because breaches of confidentiality may affect many patients.

ALLOCATING RESOURCES JUSTLY   Allocation of limited health care resources is problematic. Ideally, allocation decisions should be made as public policy, with physician input. At the bedside, physicians generally should act as patient advocates within constraints set by society, reasonable insurance coverage, and sound practice. *Ad hoc* rationing by the individual physician at the bedside may be inconsistent, discriminatory, and ineffective. In some cases, however, two patients may compete for the same limited resources, such as physician time or a bed in intensive care. When this occurs, physicians should ration their time and resources according to patients' medical needs and the probability of benefit.

ASSISTANCE WITH ETHICAL ISSUES   Discussing perplexing ethical issues with other members of the health care team, colleagues, or the hospital ethics committee often clarifies issues and suggests ways to improve communication and to deal with strong emotions. When struggling with difficult ethical issues, physicians may need to reevaluate their basic convictions, tolerate uncertainty, and maintain their integrity while respecting the opinions of others.

BIBLIOGRAPHY

ALPERS A, LO B: When is CPR futile? JAMA 273:156, 1995

AMERICAN COLLEGE OF PHYSICIANS: *American College of Physicians Ethics Manual.* Ann Intern Med, 128:576, 1998

BEAUCHAMP TL, CHILDRESS JF: *Principles of Biomedical Ethics*, 5th ed. New York, Oxford University Press, 2000

EMANUEL EJ et al: The practice of euthanasia and physician-assisted suicide in the United States: Adherence to proposed safeguards and effects on physicians. JAMA 280:507, 1998

GRISSO T, APPELBAUM P: *Assessing Competence to Consent to Treatment: A Guide for Physicians and Other Health Professionals.* New York, Oxford University Press, 1998

KASSIRER JP: Managed care and the morality of the marketplace. N Engl J Med 333:50, 1995

LO B: *Resolving Ethical Dilemmas: A Guide for Clinicians*, 2d ed. Philadelphia, Lippincott Williams & Wilkins, 2000

MEISEL A: *The Right to Die*, 2d ed. New York, Wiley, 1995

QUILL TE et al: Palliative options of last resort: A comparison of voluntarily stopping eating and drinking, terminal sedation, physician-assisted suicide, and voluntary active euthanasia. JAMA 278:2099, 1997

TULSKY JA et al: Opening the black box: How do physicians communicate about advance directives. Ann Intern Med 129:441, 1998

---

3   *Daniel B. Mark*

DECISION-MAKING IN CLINICAL MEDICINE

To the medical student who requires 2 h to collect a patient's history and perform a physical examination, and several additional hours to organize them into a coherent presentation, the experienced clinician's ability to reach a diagnosis and decide on a management plan in a fraction of the time seems extraordinary. While medical knowledge and experience play a significant role in the senior clinician's ability to arrive at a differential diagnosis and plan quickly, much of the process involves skill in clinical decision-making. The first goal of this chapter is to provide an introduction to the study of clinical reasoning.

Equally bewildering to the student are the proper use of diagnostic tests and the integration of the results into the clinical assessment. The novice medical practitioner typically uses a "shotgun" approach to testing, hoping to a hit a target without knowing exactly what that target is. The expert, on the other hand, usually has a specific target in mind and efficiently adjusts the testing strategy to it. The second goal of this chapter is to review briefly some of the crucial basic statistical concepts that govern the proper interpretation and use of diagnostic tests; quantitative tools available to assist in clinical decision-making will also be discussed.

CLINICAL DECISION-MAKING

CLINICAL REASONING   The most important clinical actions are not procedures or prescriptions but the judgments from which all other aspects of clinical medicine flow. In the modern era of large randomized trials, it is easy to overlook the importance of this elusive mental activity and focus instead on the algorithmic practice guidelines constructed to improve care. One reason for this apparent neglect is that much more research has been done on how doctors *should* make decisions (e.g., using a Bayesian model discussed below) than on how they actually *do*. Thus, much of what we know about clinical reasoning comes from empirical studies of nonmedical problem-solving behavior.

Despite the great technological advances of the twentieth century, uncertainty still plays a pivotal role in all aspects of medical decision-making. We may know that a patient does not have long to live, but we cannot be certain how long. We may prescribe a potent new receptor blocker to reverse the course of a patient's illness, but we cannot be certain that the therapy will do so without side effects. Uncertainty in medical outcomes creates the need for probabilities and other mathematical/statistical tools to help guide decision-making. (These tools are reviewed later in the chapter.)

Uncertainty is compounded by the information overload that characterizes modern medicine. Today's experienced clinician needs close to 2 million pieces of information to practice medicine. Doctors subscribe to an average of 7 journals, representing over 2500 new articles each year. Computers offer the obvious solution both for management of information and for better quantitation and management of the daily uncertainties of medical care. While the technology to computerize medical practice is available, many practical problems remain to be solved before patient information can be standardized and integrated with medical evidence on a single electronic platform.

The following three examples introduce the subject of clinical reasoning:

- A 46-year-old man presents to his internist with a chief complaint of hemoptysis. The physician knows that the differential diagnosis of hemoptysis includes over 100 different conditions, including cancer and tuberculosis (Chap. 33). The examination begins with some general background questions, and the patient is asked to describe his symptoms and their chronology. By the time the examination is completed, and even before any tests are run, the physician has formulated a working diagnostic hypothesis and planned a series of steps to test it. In an otherwise healthy and nonsmoking patient recovering from a viral bronchitis, the doctor's hypothesis would be that the acute bronchitis is responsible for the small amount of blood-streaked sputum the patient observed. In this case, a chest x-ray and purified protein derivative (PPD) skin test may be sufficient.
- A second 46-year-old patient with the same chief complaint who has a 100-pack-year smoking history, a productive morning cough, and episodes of blood-streaked sputum may generate the principal diagnostic hypothesis of carcinoma of the lung. Consequently, along with the chest x-ray and PPD skin test, the physician refers this patient for bronchoscopy.
- A third 46-year-old patient with hemoptysis who is from a developing country is evaluated with an echocardiogram as well, because the physician thinks she hears a soft diastolic rumble at the apex on cardiac auscultation, suggesting rheumatic mitral stenosis.

These three vignettes illustrate two aspects of expert clinical reasoning: (1) the use of cognitive shortcuts, or *heuristics*, as a way to organize the complex unstructured material that is collected in the clinical evaluation; and (2) the use of diagnostic hypotheses to consolidate the information and indicate appropriate management steps.

THE USE OF COGNITIVE SHORTCUTS Heuristics reduce the complexity of a problem to a manageable level. Psychologists have found that people rely on three basic types of heuristics. For example, when assessing a patient, clinicians often weigh the probability that this patient's clinical features match those of the class of patients with the leading diagnostic hypotheses being considered. In other words, the clinician is searching for the diagnosis for which the patient appears to be a representative example; this cognitive shortcut is called the *representativeness heuristic*. It may take only a few characteristics from the history for an expert clinician using the representativeness heuristic to arrive at a sound diagnostic hypothesis. For example, an elderly patient with new-onset fever, cough productive of copious sputum, unilateral pleuritic chest pain, and dyspnea is readily identified as fitting the pattern for acute pneumonia, probably of bacterial origin. Evidence of focal pulmonary consolidation on the physical examination will increase the clinician's confidence in the diagnosis because it fits the expected pattern of acute bacterial pneumonia. Knowing this allows the experienced clinician to conduct an efficient, directed, and therapeutically productive patient evaluation although there may be little else in the history or physical examination of direct relevance. The inexperienced medical student or resident, who has not yet learned the patterns most prevalent in clinical medicine, must work much harder to achieve the same result and is often at risk of missing the important clinical problem in a sea of compulsively collected but unhelpful data.

However, physicians using the representativeness heuristic can reach erroneous conclusions if they fail to consider the underlying prevalence of two competing diagnoses. Consider a patient with pleuritic chest pain, dyspnea, and a low-grade fever. A clinician might consider acute pneumonia and acute pulmonary embolism to be the two leading diagnostic alternatives. Clinicians using the representativeness heuristic might judge both diagnostic candidates to be equally likely, although to do so would be wrong if pneumonia was much more prevalent in the underlying population. Mistakes may also result from a failure to consider that a pattern based on a small number of prior observations will likely be less reliable than one based on larger samples.

A second commonly used cognitive shortcut, the *availability heuristic*, involves judgments made on the basis of how easily prior similar cases or outcomes can be brought to mind. For example, the experienced clinician may recall 20 elderly patients seen over the past few years who presented with painless dyspnea of acute onset and were found to have acute myocardial infarction. The novice clinician may spend valuable time seeking a pulmonary cause for the symptoms before considering and discovering the cardiac diagnosis. In this situation, the patient's clinical pattern does not fit the expected pattern of acute myocardial infarction, but experience with this atypical presentation, and the ability to recall it, can help direct the physician to the diagnosis.

Errors with the availability heuristic can come from several sources of recall bias. For example, rare catastrophes are likely to be remembered with a clarity and force out of proportion to their value, and recent experience is, of course, easier to recall and therefore more influential on clinical judgments.

The third commonly used cognitive shortcut, the *anchoring heuristic*, involves estimating a probability by starting from a familiar point (the anchor) and adjusting to the new case from there. For example, a clinician may judge the probability of colorectal cancer to be extremely high after an elevated screening carcinoembryonic antigen (CEA) result because the prediction of colorectal cancer is anchored to the test result. Yet, as discussed below, this prediction would be inaccurate if the clinical picture of the patient being tested indicates a low probability of disease (for example, a 30-year-old woman with no risk factors). Anchoring can be a powerful tool for diagnosis but is often used incorrectly (see "Measures of Disease Probability and Bayes' Theorem," below).

DIAGNOSTIC HYPOTHESIS GENERATION Cognitive scientists studying the thought processes of expert clinicians have observed that clinicians group data into packets or "chunks," which are stored in their memories and manipulated to generate diagnostic hypotheses. Because short-term memory can typically hold only 7 to 10 items at a time, the number of packets that can be actively integrated into hypothesis-generating activities is similarly limited. The cognitive shortcuts discussed above play a key role in the generation of diagnostic hypotheses, many of which are discarded as rapidly as they are formed.

A diagnostic hypothesis sets a context for diagnostic steps to follow and provides testable predictions. For example, if the enlarged and quite tender liver felt on physical examination is due to acute hepatitis (the hypothesis), certain specific liver function tests should be markedly elevated (the prediction). If the tests come back normal, the hypothesis may need to be discarded or substantially modified.

One of the factors that makes teaching diagnostic reasoning so difficult is that expert clinicians do not follow a fixed pattern in patient examinations. From the outset, they are generating, refining, and discarding diagnostic hypotheses. The questions they ask in the history are driven by the hypotheses they are working with at the moment. Even the physical examination is driven by specific questions rather than a preordained checklist. While the student is palpating the abdomen of the alcoholic patient, waiting for a finding to strike him, the expert clinician is on a focused search mission. Is the spleen enlarged? How big is the liver? Is it tender? Are there any palpable masses or nodules? Each question focuses the attention of the examiner to the exclusion of all other inputs until answered, allowing the examiner to move on to the next specific question.

Negative findings are often as important as positive ones in establishing and refining diagnostic hypotheses. Chest discomfort that is not provoked or worsened by exertion in an active patient reduces the likelihood that chronic ischemic heart disease is the underlying cause. The absence of a resting tachycardia and thyroid gland enlargement reduces the likelihood of hyperthyroidism in a patient with paroxysmal atrial fibrillation.

While the representativeness and availability heuristics may play the major roles in shaping early diagnostic hypotheses, the acuity of a patient's illness can also be very influential. For example, clinicians are taught to consider aortic dissection routinely as a possible cause of acute severe chest discomfort along with myocardial infarction, even though the typical history of dissection is different from myocardial infarction and dissection is far less prevalent (Chap. 247). This recommendation is based on the recognition that a relatively rare but catastrophic diagnosis like aortic dissection is very difficult to make unless it is explicitly considered. If the clinician fails to elicit any of the characteristic features of dissection by history and finds equivalent blood pressures in both arms and no pulse deficits, he or she may feel comfortable in discarding the aortic dissection hypothesis. If, however, the chest x-ray shows a widened mediastinum, the hypothesis may be reinstated and a diagnostic test ordered [e.g., thoracic computed tomography (CT) scan, transesophageal echocardiogram] to evaluate it more fully. In noncritical situations, the prevalence of potential alternative diagnoses should play a much more prominent role in diagnostic hypothesis generation. The value of conducting a rapid systematic clinical survey of symptoms and organ systems to avoid missing important but inapparent clues cannot be overstated.

Because the generation and evaluation of appropriate diagnostic hypotheses is a skill that not all clinicians possess to an equal degree, errors in this process can occur, and in the patient with serious acute illness these may lead to tragic consequences. Consider the following hypothetical example. A 45-year-old male patient with a 3-week history of a "flulike" upper respiratory infection (URI) presented to his physician with symptoms of dyspnea and a productive cough. Based on the presenting complaint, the clinician pulled out a "URI Assessment Form" to improve quality and efficiency of care. The physician quickly completed the examination components outlined on this structured form, noting in particular the absence of fever and a clear chest examination. He then prescribed an antibiotic for presumed bronchitis, showed the patient how to breathe into a paper bag to relieve his "hyperventilation," and sent him home with the reassurance that his illness was not serious. After a sleepless night with significant dyspnea unrelieved by rebreathing into a bag, the patient developed nausea and vomiting and collapsed. He was brought into the Emergency Department in cardiac arrest and could not be resuscitated. Autopsy showed a posterior wall myocardial infarction and a fresh thrombus in an atherosclerotic right coronary artery. What went wrong? The clinician decided, even before starting the history, that the patient's complaints were not serious. He therefore felt confident that he could perform an abbreviated and focused examination using the URI assessment protocol rather than considering the full range of possibilities and performing appropriate tests to confirm or refute his initial hypotheses. In particular, by concentrating on the "URI," the clinician failed to elicit the full dyspnea history, which would have suggested a far more serious disorder, and did not even search for other symptoms that could have directed him to the correct diagnosis.

This example illustrates how patients can diverge from textbook symptoms and the potential consequences of being unable to adapt the diagnostic process to real-world challenges. The expert, while recognizing that common things occur commonly, approaches each evaluation on high alert for clues that the initial diagnosis may be wrong. Patients often provide information that "does not fit" with any of the leading diagnostic hypotheses being considered. Distinguishing real clues from false trails can only be achieved by practice and experience. A less experienced clinician who tries to be too efficient (as in the above example) can make serious judgment errors.

MAJOR INFLUENCES ON CLINICAL DECISION-MAKING

More than a decade of research on variations in clinician practice patterns has shed much light on forces that shape clinical decisions. The use of heuristic "shortcuts," as detailed above, provides a partial explanation, but several other key factors play an important role in shaping diagnostic hypotheses and management decisions. These factors can be grouped conceptually into three overlapping categories: (1) factors related to physician personal characteristics and practice style, (2) factors related to the practice setting, and (3) economic incentive factors.

Practice Style Factors   One of the key roles of the physician in medical care is to serve as the patient's agent to ensure that necessary care is provided at a high level of quality. Factors that influence this role include the physician's knowledge, training, and experience. It is obvious that physicians cannot practice evidence-based medicine if they are unfamiliar with the evidence. As would be expected, specialists generally know the evidence in their field better than do generalists. Surgeons may be more enthusiastic about recommending surgery than medical doctors because their belief in the beneficial effects of surgery is stronger. For the same reason, invasive cardiologists are much more likely to refer chest pain patients for diagnostic catheterization than are noninvasive cardiologists or generalists. The physician beliefs that drive these different practice styles are based on personal experience, recollection, and interpretation of the available medical evidence. For example, heart failure specialists are much more likely than generalists to achieve target angiotensin-converting enzyme (ACE) inhibitor therapy in their heart failure patients because they are more familiar with what the targets are (as defined by large clinical trials), have more familiarity with the specific drugs (including dosages and side effects), and are less likely to overreact to foreseeable problems in therapy such as a rise in creatinine levels or symptomatic hypotension. Other intriguing research has shown a wide distribution of acceptance times of antibiotic therapy for peptic ulcer disease following widespread dissemination of the "evidence" in the medical literature. Some gastroenterologists accepted this new therapy before the evidence was clear (reflecting, perhaps, an aggressive practice style), and some gastroenterologists lagged behind (a conservative practice style, associated in this case with older physicians). As a group, internists lagged several years behind gastroenterologists.

The opinion of influential leaders can also have an important effect on practice patterns. Such influence can occur at both the national level (e.g., expert physicians teaching at national meetings) and the local level (e.g., local educational programs, "curbside consultants"). Opinion leaders do not have to be physicians. When conducting rounds with clinical pharmacists, physicians are less likely to make medication errors and more likely to use target levels of evidence-based therapies.

The patient's welfare is not the only concern that drives clinical decisions. The physician's perception about the risk of a malpractice suit resulting from either an erroneous decision or a bad outcome creates a style of practice referred to as *defensive medicine*. This practice involves using tests and therapies with very small marginal returns to preclude future criticism in the event of an adverse outcome. For example, a 40-year-old woman who presents with a long-standing history of intermittent headache and a new severe headache along with a normal neurologic examination has a very low likelihood of structural intracranial pathology. Performance of a head CT or magnetic resonance imaging (MRI) scan in this situation would constitute defensive medicine. On the other hand, the results of the test could provide reassurance to an anxious patient.

Practice Setting Factors   Factors in this category relate to the physical resources available to the physician's practice and the practice environment. *Physician-induced demand* is a term that refers to the repeated observation that physicians have a remarkable ability to accommodate to and employ the medical facilities available to them. A classic early study in this area showed that physicians in Boston had an almost 50% higher hospital admission rate than did physicians in New Haven, despite there being no obvious differences in the health of the cities' inhabitants. The physicians in New Haven were not aware of using fewer hospital beds for their patients, nor were the Boston physicians aware of using less stringent criteria to admit patients.

Other environmental factors that can influence decision-making include the local availability of specialists for consultations and procedures, "high tech" facilities such as angiography suites, a heart surgery program, and MRI machines.

Economic Incentives   Economic incentives are closely related to the other two categories of practice-modifying factors. Financial issues can exert both stimulatory and inhibitory influences on clinical practice. In general, physicians are paid on a fee-for-service, capitation, or salary basis (Chap. 4). In fee-for-service, the more the physician does, the more the physician gets paid. The incentive in this case is to do more. When fees are reduced (discounted fee-for-service), doctors tend to increase the number of services billed for. Capitation, in contrast, provides a fixed payment per patient per year, encouraging physicians to take on more patients but to provide each patient with fewer services. Expensive services are more likely to be affected by this type of incentive than inexpensive preventive services. Salary compensation plans pay physicians the same regardless of the amount of clinical work performed. The incentive here is to see fewer patients. Recognizing these powerful shapers of physician behavior, managed care plans have begun to explore combinations of the three reimbursement types with the goal of improving individual physician productivity while restraining their use of expensive tests and therapies.

In summary, expert clinical decision-making can be appreciated as a complex interplay between cognitive devices used to simplify large amounts of complex information interacting with physician biases reflecting education, training, and experience, all of which are shaped by powerful, sometimes perverse, external forces. In the next section, we will review a set of statistical tools and concepts that can assist in making clinical decisions under uncertainty.

QUANTITATIVE METHODS TO AID CLINICAL DECISION-MAKING

The process of medical decision-making can be divided into two parts: (1) defining the available courses of action and estimating the likely outcomes with each, and (2) assessing the desirability of the outcomes. The former task involves integrating key information about the patient along with relevant evidence from the medical literature to create the structure of a decision problem. The remainder of this chapter will present some quantitative tools to assist the clinician in these activities. These tools can be divided into those that assist the clinician in making better outcome predictions, which are then used to make decisions, and those that support the decision process directly. While these tools are not yet used routinely in daily clinical practice, the computerization of medicine is creating the required substrate for their future widespread dissemination.

QUANTITATIVE MEDICAL PREDICTIONS   Diagnostic Testing   The purpose of performing a test on a patient is to reduce uncertainty about the patient's diagnosis or prognosis and to aid the clinician in making management decisions. Although diagnostic tests are commonly thought of as laboratory tests (e.g., measurement of serum amylase level) or procedures (e.g., colonoscopy or bronchoscopy), any technology that changes our understanding of the patient's problem qualifies as a diagnostic test. Thus, even the history and physical examination can be considered a form of diagnostic test. In clinical medicine, it is common to reduce the results of a test to a dichotomous outcome, such as positive or negative, normal or abnormal. In many cases, this simplification results in the waste of useful information. However, such simplification makes it easier to demonstrate some of the quantitative ways in which test data can be used.

To characterize the accuracy of diagnostic tests, four terms are routinely used (Table 3-1). The *true-positive rate*, i.e., the sensitivity, provides a measure of how well the test correctly identifies patients with disease. The *false-negative rate* is calculated as (1 − sensitivity). The *true-negative rate*, i.e., the specificity, reflects how well the test correctly identifies patients without disease. The *false-positive rate* is

Table 3-1   Measures of Diagnostic Test Accuracy

Test Result	Disease Status	
	Present	Absent
Positive	True-positive (*TP*)	False-positive (*FP*)
Negative	False-negative (*FN*)	True-negative (*TN*)

IDENTIFICATION OF PATIENTS WITH DISEASE

True-positive rate (sensitivity) = $TP/(TP + FN)$
False-negative rate = $FN/(TP + FN)$
True-positive rate = $1 -$ false-negative rate

IDENTIFICATION OF PATIENTS WITHOUT DISEASE

True-negative rate (specificity) = $TN/(TN + FP)$
False-positive rate = $FP/(TN + FP)$
True-negative rate = $1 -$ false-positive rate

(1 − specificity). A perfect test would have a sensitivity of 100% and a specificity of 100% and would completely separate patients with disease from those without it.

Calculating sensitivity and specificity require selection of a cutpoint value for the test to separate "normal" from "diseased" subjects. As the cutpoint is moved to improve sensitivity, specificity typically falls and vice versa. This dynamic tradeoff between more accurate identification of subjects with versus those without disease is often displayed graphically as a receiver operating characteristic (ROC) curve. An ROC curve plots sensitivity (y-axis) versus 1 − specificity (x-axis). Each point on the curve represents a potential cutpoint with an associated sensitivity and specificity value. The area under the ROC curve is often used as a quantitative measure of the information content of a test. Values range from 0.5 (no diagnostic information at all, test is equivalent to flipping a coin) to 1.0 (perfect test).

In the diagnostic testing literature, ROC areas are often used to compare alternative tests. The test with the highest area (i.e., closest to 1.0) is presumed to be the most accurate. However, ROC curves are not a panacea for evaluation of diagnostic test utility. Like Bayes' theorem, they are typically focused on only one possible test parameter (e.g., ST segment response in a treadmill exercise test) to the exclusion of other potentially relevant data. In addition, ROC area comparisons do not simulate the way test information is actually used in clinical practice. Finally, biases in the underlying population used to generate the ROC curves (e.g., related to an unrepresentative test sample) can bias the ROC area and the validity of a comparison among tests.

Measures of Disease Probability and Bayes' Theorem   Unfortunately, there are no perfect tests; after every test is completed the true disease state of the patient remains uncertain. Quantitating this residual uncertainty can be done with Bayes' theorem. This theorem provides a simple mathematical way to calculate the posttest probability of disease from three parameters: the pretest probability of disease, the test sensitivity, and the test specificity (Table 3-2). The pretest probability is a quantitative expression of the confidence in a diagnosis before the test is performed. In the absence of more relevant information it is usually estimated from the prevalence of the disease in the underlying population. For some common conditions, such as coronary artery disease (CAD), nomograms and statistical models have been created to generate better estimates of pretest probability from elements of the history and physical examination. The posttest probability, then, is a revised statement of the confidence in the diagnosis, taking into account both what was known before and after the test.

To understand how Bayes' theorem creates this revised confidence statement, it is useful to examine a nomogram version of Bayes' theorem that uses the same three parameters to predict the posttest probability of disease (Fig. 3-1). In this nomogram, the accuracy of the diagnostic test in question is summarized by the likelihood ratio for a

Table 3-2   Measures of Disease Probability

Pretest probability of disease = probability of disease before test is done; may use population prevalence of disease or more patient-specific data to generate this probability estimate.

Posttest probability of disease = probability of disease accounting for both pretest probability and test results; also called predictive value of the test.

Bayes' theorem
    Computational version:

$$\text{Posttest probability} = \frac{\text{Pretest probability} \times \text{test sensitivity}}{\begin{array}{c}\text{Pretest probability} \times \text{test sensitivity} + \\ (1 - \text{disease prevalence}) \times \text{test false-positive rate}\end{array}}$$

    Example [with a pretest probability of 0.50 and a "positive" diagnostic test result (test sensitivity = 0.90, test specificity = 0.90)]:

$$\text{Posttest probability} = \frac{(0.50)(0.90)}{(0.50)(0.90) + (0.50)(0.10)}$$
$$= 0.90$$

positive test, which is the ratio of the true-positive rate to the false-positive rate [or sensitivity/(1 − specificity)]. For example, a test with a sensitivity of 0.90 and a specificity of 0.90 has a likelihood ratio of 0.90/(1 − 0.90), or 9. Thus, for this hypothetical test, a "positive"

FIGURE 3-1 Nomogram version of Bayes' theorem used to predict the post-test probability of disease (left-hand scale) using the pretest probability of disease (right-hand scale) and the likelihood ratio for a positive test (middle scale). The likelihood ratio is calculated as the sensitivity/(1 − specificity). To use, place a straight edge connecting the pretest probability and the likelihood ratio, and read off the posttest probability. This figure illustrates the value of a positive exercise treadmill test (likelihood ratio 4) and a positive exercise thallium SPECT study (likelihood ratio 9) in the patient with a pretest probability of coronary artery disease of 50%. Treadmill results shown in solid line; thallium results in dashed line. (*Adapted from Fagan TJ: N Engl J Med 293:257, 1975.*)

result is 9 times more likely in a patient with the disease than in a patient without it. The more accurate the test, the higher the likelihood ratio. However, if sensitivity is excellent but specificity is less so, the likelihood ratio will be substantially reduced (e.g., with a 90% sensitivity but a 60% specificity, the likelihood ratio is 2.25). Most tests in medicine have likelihood ratios for a positive result between 1.5 and 20.

Consider two tests commonly used in the diagnosis of CAD, an exercise treadmill and an exercise thallium-201 single photon emission CT (SPECT) test (Chap. 244). Meta-analysis has shown the treadmill to have an average sensitivity of 66% and an average specificity of 84%, yielding a likelihood ratio of 4.1 [0.66/(1 − 0.84)]. If we use this test on a patient with a pretest probability of CAD of 10%, the posttest probability of disease following a positive result rises only to about 30%. If a patient with a pretest probability of CAD of 80% has a positive test result, the posttest probability of disease is about 95%.

The exercise thallium SPECT test is a more accurate test for the diagnosis of CAD. For our purposes, assume that it has both a sensitivity and specificity of 90%, yielding a likelihood ratio of 9.0 [0.90/(1 − 0.90)]. If we again test our low pretest probability patient and he has a positive test, using Fig. 3-1 we can demonstrate that the posttest probability of CAD rises from 10 to 50%. However, from a decision-making point of view, the more accurate test has not been able to improve diagnostic confidence enough to change management. In fact, the test has moved us from being fairly certain that the patient did not have CAD to being completely undecided (a 50:50 chance of disease). In a patient with a pretest probability of 80%, using the more accurate thallium SPECT test raises the posttest probability to 97% (compared with 95% for the exercise treadmill). Again, the more accurate test does not provide enough improvement in posttest confidence to alter management, and neither test has improved much upon what was known from clinical data alone.

If the pretest probability is low (e.g., ≤20%), even a positive result on a very accurate test will not move the posttest probability to a range high enough to rule in disease (e.g., ≥80%). Conversely, with a high pretest probability, a negative test will not adequately rule out disease. Thus, the largest gain in diagnostic confidence from a test occurs when the clinician is most uncertain before performing it (e.g., pretest probability between 30 and 70%). For example, if a patient has a pretest probability for CAD of 50%, a positive exercise treadmill test will move the posttest probability to 80% and a positive exercise thallium SPECT test will move it to 90% (Fig. 3-1).

Bayes' theorem, as presented above, employs a number of important simplifications that should be considered. First, few tests have only two useful outcomes, positive or negative, and many tests provide numerous pieces of data about the patient. Even if these can be integrated into a summary result, multiple levels of useful information may be present (e.g., strongly positive, positive, indeterminate, negative, strongly negative). While Bayes' theorem can be adapted to this more detailed test result format, it is computationally complex to do so. Second, Bayes' theorem assumes that the information from the test is completely unique and nonoverlapping with information used to estimate the pretest probability. This independence assumption, however, is often wrong. In many cases, test results are correlated with patient characteristics. For example, the findings of cardiomegaly and pulmonary edema on chest x-ray are correlated with the historic features of heart failure and with the physical findings of a displaced left ventricular apical impulse, an S_3 gallop, and rales. The unique predictive information contributed by the test in this case (the chest x-ray) is only a fraction of its total information because much had already been learned about the probability of heart failure before the test was done.

Finally, it has long been thought that sensitivity and specificity are prevalence-independent parameters of test accuracy, and many texts still make this assertion. This statistically useful assumption, however, is clinically wrong. For example, a treadmill exercise test has a sensitivity in a population of patients with one-vessel CAD of around 30%, whereas the sensitivity in severe three-vessel CAD approaches

80%. Thus, the best estimate of sensitivity to use in a particular decision will often vary depending on the distribution of disease stages present in the tested population. A hospitalized population typically has a higher prevalence of disease and in particular a higher prevalence of more advanced disease stages than an outpatient population. As a consequence, test sensitivity will tend to be higher in hospitalized patients, whereas test specificity will be higher in outpatients.

Statistical Prediction Models Bayes' theorem, as presented above, deals with a clinical prediction problem that is unrealistically simple relative to most problems a clinician faces. Prediction models, based on multivariable statistical models, can handle much more complex problems and substantially enhance predictive accuracy for specific situations. Their particular advantage is the ability to take into account many overlapping pieces of information and assign a relative weight to each based on its unique contribution to the prediction in question. For example, a logistic regression model to predict the probability of CAD takes into account all of the relevant independent factors from the clinical examination and diagnostic testing instead of the small handful of data that clinicians can manage in their heads or with Bayes' theorem. However, despite this strength, the models are too complex computationally to use without a calculator or computer (although this limit may be overcome when medicine is practiced from a fully computerized platform.) To date, only a handful of prediction models have been developed and properly validated. The importance of independent validation in a population separate from the one used to develop the model cannot be overstated. Unfortunately, most published models have not been properly validated, making their utility in clinical practice uncertain at best.

When statistical models have been compared directly with expert clinicians, they have been found to be more consistent, as would be expected, but not significantly more accurate. Their biggest promise, then, would seem to be to make less-experienced clinicians more accurate predictors of outcome.

DECISION SUPPORT TOOLS

DECISION SUPPORT SYSTEMS Over the past 30 years, many attempts have been made to develop computer systems to help clinicians make decisions and manage patients. Conceptually, computers offer a very attractive way to handle the vast information load that today's physicians face. The computer can help by making accurate predictions of outcome, simulating the whole decision process, or providing algorithmic guidance. Computer-based predictions using Bayesian or statistical regression models inform a clinical decision but do not actually reach a "conclusion" or "recommendation." Artificial intelligence systems attempt to simulate or replace human reasoning with a computer-based analogue. To date, such approaches have achieved only limited success. Reminder or protocol-directed systems do not make predictions but use existing algorithms, such as practice guidelines, to guide clinical practice. In general, however, decision

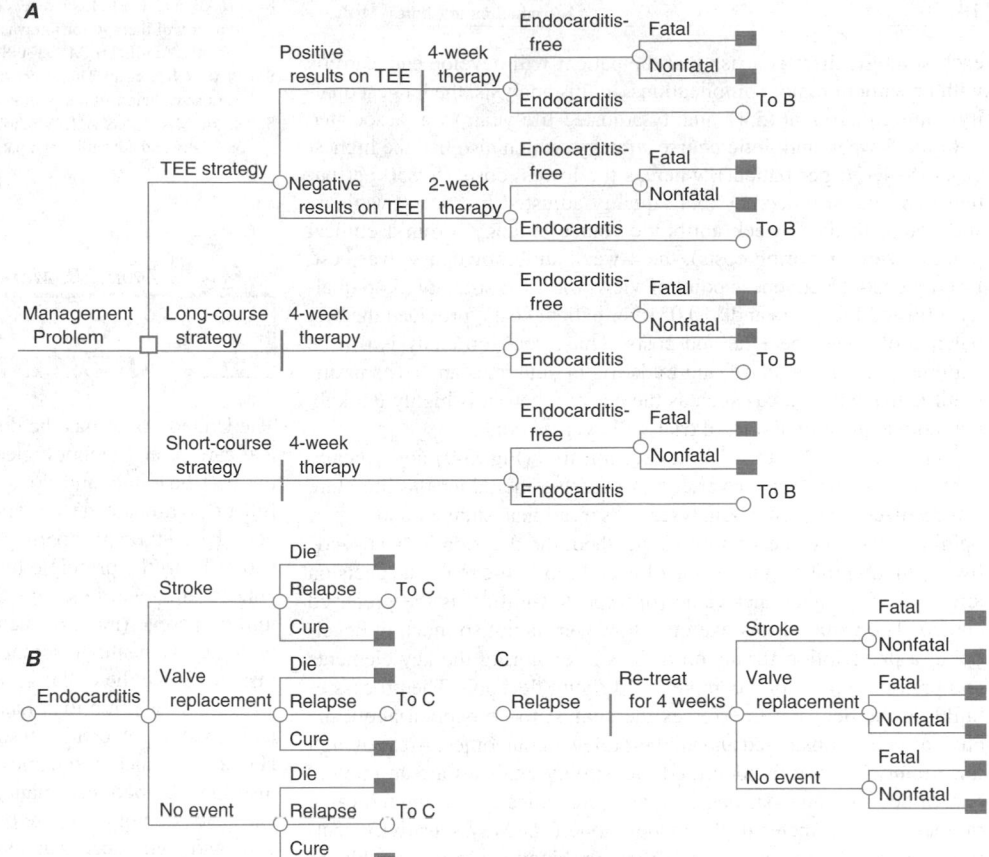

FIGURE 3-2 Decision model used to evaluate strategies for management of the risk of infective endocarditis after catheter-associated *Staphylococcus aureus* bacteremia. The square node indicates a decision between possible management strategies, round nodes represent chance events, and rectangular (or terminal) nodes indicate the outcomes of interest. All nonterminal chance nodes in the main tree (structure *A*) enter substructure *B*. All nonterminal chance nodes in substructure *B* enter substructure *C*. TEE, transesophageal echocardiography. *(From Rosen et al.)*

support systems have shown little impact on practice. Reminder systems, although not yet in widespread use, have shown the most promise, particularly in correcting drug dosing and in promoting guideline adherence. The full potential of these approaches will only be achieved when computers are fully integrated into medical practice.

DECISION ANALYSIS Compared with the methods discussed above, decision analysis represents a completely different approach to decision support. Its principal application is in decision problems that are complex and involve a substantial risk, a high degree of uncertainty in some key area, or an idiosyncratic feature that does not "fit" the available evidence. Three general steps are involved. First, the decision problem must be clearly defined. Second, the elements of the decision must be made explicit. This involves specifying the alternatives being considered, their relevant outcomes, the probabilities attached to each outcome, and the relative desirability (called "utility") of each outcome. Cost can also be assigned to each branch of the decision tree, allowing calculation of cost-effectiveness (Chap. 4).

An example of a decision tree used to evaluate strategies for management of the risk of infective endocarditis after catheter-associated *Staphylococcus aureus* bacteremia is shown in Fig. 3-2. Approximately 35,000 cases of *S. aureus* bacteremia occur each year in the United States. The development of complicating endocarditis, which occurs in about 6% of cases, is associated with high morbidity (31% mortality, 21% stroke rate) and medical costs. The three choices for management of the bacteremia are (1) transesophageal echocardiography (TEE), (2) a 4-week course of intravenous antibiotics (long-course), or (3) a 2-week course of intravenous antibiotics (short-course). In the TEE strategy, a 4-week course of antibiotics is given if endocarditis is evident and a 2-week course is given if it is not. With each strategy, there is a risk that the patient will develop endocarditis with or without major complications. In this analysis, the longest quality-adjusted survival (5.47 quality-adjusted life-years) was associated with the 4-week antibiotic course strategy, which also had the highest costs ($14,136 per patient), whereas the lowest costs ($9830 per patient) and worst outcomes (5.42 quality-adjusted life-years) were associated with the 2-week antibiotic course strategy. From a clinical point of view (ignoring costs), the 4-week antibiotic course was best. From a cost-effectiveness point of view, the TEE strategy (5.46 quality-adjusted life-years and $10,051 per patient costs) provided the best balance of added benefits and costs. Thus, decision analysis can be extremely helpful in clarifying tradeoffs in outcomes and costs in difficult management areas such as the above where it is highly unlikely that an adequate randomized trial will ever be done.

The data needed to fill in a decision tree (Fig. 3-2) are typically cobbled together from a variety of sources, including the literature (randomized trials, meta-analyses, observational studies) and expert opinion. Once the decision tree is finished, the decision is "analyzed" by calculating the average value of each limb of the tree. The decision arm with the highest net value (or expected utility) is the preferred choice. The value of this exercise, however, is not so much in developing a prescription for action as it is in exploring the key elements and pressure points of a complex or difficult decision. The process of building the decision tree forces the analyst to be explicit about the choices being considered and all their relevant outcomes. Areas of high uncertainty are readily identified. Sensitivity analyses are an integral part of decision analysis and involve systematically varying the value of each key parameter in the model alone (one-way sensitivity analysis,) in pairs (two-way), or in higher combinations (multivariable) to assess the impact on choice of preferred management strategy. In the above example, varying the incidence of endocarditis resulting from *S. aureus* bacteremia from 3% to over 50% had no impact on the choice of TEE as the preferred strategy.

User friendly personal computer–based software packages now make the creation and analysis of decision trees much more straightforward than in the past. However, the process is still too cumbersome and time-consuming to be used on a routine basis. When medicine is practiced from a fully computerized platform, a library of prestructured decision trees with user modifiable values can be made available to support practitioners working with individual patients.

CONCLUSIONS

In this era of evidence-based medicine, it is tempting to think that all the difficult decisions practitioners face have been or soon will be solved and digested into practice guidelines and computerized reminders. For the foreseeable future, however, such is not the case. Meta-analyses cannot generate evidence where there are no adequate randomized trials, and most of what clinicians face will never be thoroughly tested in a randomized trial. Excellent clinical reasoning skills and experience supplemented by well-designed quantitative tools and a keen appreciation for individual patient preferences will continue to be of paramount importance in the professional life of medical practitioners for years to come.

BIBLIOGRAPHY

AYANIAN JZ et al: Knowledge and practices of generalist and specialist physicians regarding drug therapy for acute myocardial infarction. N Engl J Med 331:1136, 1994

EDDY DM: Anatomy of a decision. JAMA 263:441, 1990

HIRTH RA et al: Specialist and generalist physicians' adoption of antibiotic therapy to eradicate *Helicobacter pylori* infection. Med Care 34:1199, 1996

KASSIRER JP, KOPELMAN RI: *Learning Clinical Reasoning.* Baltimore, Williams & Wilkins, 1991

NAYLOR CD: Gray zones of clinical practice: Some limits to evidence-based medicine. Lancet 345:840, 1995

ROSEN AB et al: Cost-effectiveness of transesophageal echocardiography to determine the duration of therapy for intravascular catheter-associated *Staphylococcus aureus* bacteremia. Ann Intern Med 130:810, 1999

SCHULMAN KA et al: The effect of race and sex on physicians' recommendations for cardiac catheterization. N Engl J Med 340:618, 1999

SEKKARIE MA, MOSS AH: Withholding and withdrawing dialysis: The role of physician specialty and education and patient functional status. Am J Kidney Dis 31:464, 1998

4   *Daniel B. Mark*

ECONOMIC ISSUES IN CLINICAL MEDICINE

The United States has the distinction of having some of the best medical care of any technologically advanced country. We have many of the best hospitals and doctors in the world. The research pipeline is full of significant new therapeutic advances, with revolutionary genetic-based therapies perhaps only a decade away. Our citizens largely subscribe to the principle that excellent medical care should be available to all, regardless of ability to pay. Yet we also have over 43 million people (most of them employed and earning minimal wages) without any health insurance and many more who are inadequately insured. Since the collapse of the Clinton health care reform efforts in 1994, U.S. health policy has been directed by marketplace forces that have created powerful and sometimes perverse incentives in medicine: Health insurance companies that use every available means to avoid insuring sick people; "managed care" programs that really only manage costs; doctors who are provided incentives to provide less medical care; and pharmaceutical companies that develop powerful and expensive new drugs priced beyond the reach of many of the elderly and chronically ill who need them most.

Facing such powerful and chaotic forces, physicians tend to focus narrowly on what they are most comfortable with, taking care of individual patients and conducting academic investigations. Many doctors consider economics too arcane for them to grasp and therefore do not even try. Consequently, when presented with economic arguments and evidence they are often unable to discriminate the legitimate from the fallacious. More importantly, they are ill equipped to defend their patients' interests in the crucible of cost containment that characterizes the modern managed care era.

This chapter has two goals: first, to provide a brief introduction to some of the larger economic forces that shape modern medical practices, and second, to introduce the economic tools that are used for assessing the value of medical practices, including cost effectiveness analysis.

HEALTH CARE SPENDING AND FINANCING

HOW MUCH IS SPENT ON HEALTH CARE? In 1997, the United States spent $1.1 trillion on its health care system, representing 13.5% of the gross domestic product (GDP) (a crude measure of national income). Most of this ($969 billion) was spent on personal health care: 34% went to hospitals, 20% to physicians, 7% to nursing homes, and 8% to outpatient pharmaceuticals. In comparison, Canada and Western European countries spend a substantially smaller portion (6 to 10%) of their national income on health care but their citizens appear to be equally healthy, at least by crude metrics such as life expectancy and infant mortality rates. Economists and politicians have for years used such data to argue that the United States spends too much on health care. The issue of how much to spend is an inherently political one, however, and the discipline of economics has little to say about it.

WHO PAYS FOR HEALTH CARE? Two major factors are continually driving up the costs of medical care: introduction into medical practice of new medical technologies (drugs, devices, procedures) that have a high price tag, and the aging of the U.S. population (since older people require more medical care than younger ones). These costs are distributed unevenly across society. In 1997, the government paid about 47% of the total national health care bill (75% federal, 25% states), private insurance paid about 32%, and individuals paid 17%. The government, of course, gets its money from taxpayers and uses the health care segment of its budget to pay for the Medicare and Medicaid programs (discussed below). To respond to rising medical costs, the government can increase taxes or redistribute funds from other programs such as defense and education. Neither of these options are politically attractive. Alternatively, because of its size in the medical marketplace, the government can impose lower prices on providers to make the available funds go farther (see "Cost-Containment Strategies," below). Much of the private insurance bill is subsidized by employers through their employee benefits packages. As medical costs go up, health insurance costs also rise and businesses must either pass on higher premium and copayment costs to their employees, raise their prices (potentially impairing their competitive position in the marketplace), or reduce their profit margin (a very unpopular move with stockholders). Like the government, businesses may also negotiate lower prices with health care providers and/or health insurance plans.

PUBLIC FINANCING OF HEALTH CARE The public sector (i.e., government as an agent for society) finances the Medicare and Medicaid programs as well as the Veteran's Administration Hospital system, the Department of Defense military care system, the Public Health Service, and the Indian Health Service. Of these, Medicare is by far the largest and most influential, with 39 million people receiving health insurance at a total cost in 1997 of $214.6 billion (20% of total national health expenditures). The Medicare program was enacted in 1965 by Congress as an amendment to the Social Security Act of 1935 and was envisioned by President Lyndon B. Johnson as a first step toward universal health insurance in the United States, a key part of his "great society" plan. Its impact on the evolution of the U.S. health care system has been profound. The original congressional act provided health care insurance for the elderly (defined as those 65 and older) who were eligible for social security (i.e., retired workers who had paid into the system during their working years and their dependents). Amendments in 1972 extended coverage to the disabled of all ages (currently numbering around 5 million) and to patients with chronic renal failure (who currently number about 284,000).

Medicare consists of two related insurance programs. The Medicare Hospital Insurance Trust Fund (also known as Part A) covers hospital care and skilled nursing home care and is funded by compulsory federal payroll taxes on employers and employees. Medicare Part B, the Medical Supplementary Insurance Program, covers physician fees as well as laboratory and other diagnostic tests and is funded by general federal tax revenues and patient premiums. Both programs have substantial gaps in coverage, necessitating supplemental insurance (so-called Medigap policies) for those who can afford them. Because of its compulsory income redistribution feature, taking tax money from current workers to pay for health care for elderly citizens (many of whom are on fixed income close to the poverty level), Medicare is both a health insurance program and a social welfare program designed to combat poverty in the disabled and elderly. In exchange for their tax money, the 150 million workers funding the program are promised the same type of social security when they become elderly (paid for by future generations of workers).

Medicaid is a social insurance program for the poor that is jointly run by the federal and state governments. The federal government gives each state a grant of money for the program based on that state's per capita income (in 1997, this amount totaled $95 billion), and the states pay for the rest ($65 billion in 1997). The program, like Medicare, was enacted by Congress in 1965 as a part of President Johnson's "great society" program. It is larger than Medicare in terms of eligible beneficiaries (41 million people) but smaller in terms of budget ($160 billion, or 12% of the total national health expenditures). Because the requirements to qualify for Medicaid are stringent, many low-income individuals under age 65 (especially the working poor) do not qualify. Eligibility criteria are set by each state within general federal guide-lines, and the income and asset tests individuals must meet to qualify vary widely among states. Many of the dollars in the Medicaid program actually pay for care for elderly and disabled Medicare beneficiaries who also qualify for Medicaid on the basis of poverty.

PRIVATE FINANCING OF HEALTH CARE Approximately 70% of the non-elderly U.S. population is covered by some form of private medical insurance. The feasibility of group insurance for medical care was initially demonstrated in the 1930s by Blue Cross, a franchise of nonprofit groups providing hospitalization insurance in order to help prop up the financially strapped U.S. hospital industry. Blue Shield, a separate organization modeled after Blue Cross, started providing insurance for in-hospital physician services in 1939. During World War II, employee wages were frozen by the government and to entice workers, who were in short supply, some employers started offering health insurance as a fringe benefit. With the feasibility of employer-sponsored group health insurance demonstrated by the experience of the "Blues," commercial insurers began to enter the market. To win the support of doctors and hospitals, insurers agreed to pay "reasonable and customary charges" and to defer all medical management decisions to doctors. This "fee-for-service" reimbursement system, created in the post-World War II era, sowed the seeds of the tremendous inflation observed in the U.S. medical system during the 1970s and 1980s.

The original focus of indemnity insurance plans was to cover individuals against catastrophic financial losses from high medical care bills. Insurance is a contract for protection against specific hazards that are unpredictable for individuals but can be defined with confidence for large groups. "Major medical" health insurance was designed to provide coverage for catastrophic illness, a relatively rare event in most populations. Group coverage is less expensive than individual coverage because it allows the insurance company to diffuse the risk of a large payout among a big pool of individuals who will pay premiums but make no claims. When coverage is shifted from a focus on rare catastrophes to routine maintenance medical care (comprehensive insurance policies), health insurance becomes a means for payment of expected rather than unexpected care. The consequence is higher health insurance premiums. The early appeal of health maintenance organizations (HMOs) was that they appeared to offer an economically efficient way to provide routine preventive care and to manage the occasional catastrophic illness.

MANAGED CARE Managed care is a generic term that embraces a wide spectrum of systems for integrating the financing and delivery of health care. Managed care organizations (MCOs) contract with doctors and hospitals to provide comprehensive care to enrolled members for a fixed, prospectively set, premium. HMOs are a form of managed care originally organized between the 1940s and 1960s as an alternative to the prevailing fee-for-service–based private insurance. With the advent of serious medical inflation in the 1970s, the HMO model was promoted by the federal government as a way to control the growth in medical spending. Early enthusiasm for this initiative was limited; in 1984, only 5% of individuals with employer-based health insurance were in an HMO. However, by 1998 that figure had risen to 85%. The exponential growth of managed care started in the 1990s in part as an employer-driven response to the uncontrolled medical inflation of the previous two decades.

The massive increase in demand for managed care by employers and by the Medicare program produced a rapid, and sometimes bewildering, evolution in the managed care industry. One important trend has been the growth of for-profit (i.e., investor owned) managed care companies. Over half of HMO members now belong to a for-profit plan. Investment dollars from Wall Street have made it easier for these plans to respond quickly to increased employer demand for managed care options. However, compared with their not-for-profit counterparts, for-profit HMOs spend a smaller proportion of each premium dollar paying for health care for members (the paradoxically named "medical loss ratio"), since stockholders also have to be paid. As a result, for-profit HMOs are less successful than not-for-profit plans in providing preventive care (a presumed strength of managed care).

Another prevalent trend of the 1990s was the move from traditional HMO models to virtual HMOs, built from contractual relationships with community physicians and hospitals. The three HMO models are the staff model, the group model, and the Independent Practice Association (IPA). The staff model HMO is a vertically integrated organization. That is, it owns its own hospitals, employs all its physicians full time for a set salary, and is focused in a particular geographic area. The group model HMO, exemplified by Group Health Cooperative of Puget Sound, contracts with one or more large multispecialty group practices to care for its patients for a preset capitated reimbursement. These physicians do not care for non-HMO patients. In the IPA model, the HMO contracts with an association of self-employed physicians who maintain their own offices and see both HMO and non-HMO patients. The network model refers to a hybrid of the other three forms of HMO. IPA and network model HMOs now have the majority of HMO membership in the United States.

The other portion of the managed care industry is represented by point of service (POS) plans and preferred provider organizations (PPOs). POS plans incorporate key features of both HMOs and traditional fee-for-service plans. A patient may choose care from a provider network or go outside the network. Care within network requires only a minimal copayment, while care outside the network requires a deductible and a large (e.g., 30%) copayment. The goal of the plan is to offer patients a choice but to provide major financial incentives to stay within the HMO portion of the plan. PPOs use a defined provider network (physicians, hospitals) that has agreed to accept discounted fee-for-service to care for enrolled members. PPOs may incorporate various managed care features, such as physician gatekeepers and utilization review.

THE UNINSURED AND UNDERINSURED   Data from the U.S. Census Bureau indicate that 43.4 million people had no health insurance for all of 1997 and 71.5 million people were without insurance for at least part of the year. The great majority of uninsured individuals either work for small employers who do not offer a health insurance benefit or, more commonly, cannot afford the premiums of the plan(s) that are offered. Underinsurance also has a significant impact on the working poor by requiring them to pay an excessive proportion of their family's income for health insurance premiums and out-of-pocket medical costs (deductibles, copayments, and uninsured care). Outpatient prescription medications are a major source of underinsurance. Prescription drug costs are now the fastest growing segment of the national medical budget and the least likely segment to be covered by insurance. The elderly are particularly affected, since Medicare does not currently cover outpatient prescriptions and even Medigap policies have limited coverage.

Some states have experimented with expanded coverage through their Medicaid programs to help the uninsured poor (such as the Oregon Medicaid program). For the forseeable future, however, it does not appear that the federal government will address this problem comprehensively.

COST-CONTAINMENT STRATEGIES   Current projections from the federal government's Health Care Finance Administration (HCFA) are that health care expenditures will double (to $2.2 trillion, or 16.2% of the GDP) by 2008. Over the past 30 years, the U.S. health care system has experimented with a vast array of cost-containment approaches. Conceptually, there are four major ways to control medical spending: (1) control prices, (2) control volume of care provided, (3) control the total budget available to pay for care, and (4) shift costs to another payer.

Two of the most important price control initiatives in medicine have been the Medicare Hospital Prospective Payment System and the Medicare Fee Schedule for physicians. In 1983, Medicare replaced its retrospective cost-based hospital reimbursement system with a pro-

spective payment system. In this system, all hospitalizations are classified into one of approximately 500 Diagnosis Related Groups (DRGs) based on the principal discharge diagnosis for the hospitalization and a few selected additional factors such as age, the performance of surgery, and the presence of complications. Each DRG is assigned an average reimbursement (adjusted annually). If the hospital can provide care for less than this amount, they make a profit. If they spend more than this amount, they lose money. The DRG system was designed to promote efficiency and cost containment in hospital-based care. While it has helped to control Medicare costs, it has not reduced overall U.S. health care costs, probably because of substantial cost-shifting by hospitals to the private insurance sector.

Between 1975 and 1987, Medicare payments to physicians increased at an annual rate of 18%, well above the rate of inflation. While total spending for physician services accounts for less than 25% of the Medicare budget, physicians have control over aspects of care (use of procedures, length of stay, hospital admission) that extend their direct influence to over 75% of the Medicare budget. Recognizing the importance of physicians in cost containment, Congress directed the development of a new physician payment system based on the use of a resource-based relative value scale (RBRVS). The Medicare Fee Schedule, which was first used in 1992, has three components: (1) a measure of the total work (time and complexity) involved in each physician service and standardized across all specialties, (2) a practice expense to cover the cost of running an office, and (3) an amount to cover malpractice insurance costs. The Medicare Fee Schedule classifies all physician services using the American Medical Association's Current Procedural Terminology (CPT) codes. Each CPT code has an associated relative value units (RVUs) weight. The RVU weights are multiplied by a national conversion factor to generate the actual physician fee associated with the service in question.

Price controls are attractive for cost containment because they are less expensive administratively than volume controls and don't involve micromanagement of clinical care. Price controls alone, however, don't generally achieve control of costs because of compensatory responses of providers. For example, under Medicare prospective payment, hospitals have shifted much care to the outpatient setting, where DRGs are not used. Physicians have responded to lower fees by an increased volume and intensity of service.

Volume controls include various programs to limit the diffusion of expensive technologies (such as heart surgery) or extra hospital beds. Limits can be operationalized using either a regulatory approach [such as certificate of need (CON) programs] or a budgetary approach. Utilization review approaches attempt to discern which expensive care items are medically necessary and which are not.

Budgetary controls are simpler than either price or volume control approaches. In Canada, for example, hospitals have global annual budgets. How the money is spent is decided by each hospital. If the budget is exceeded, there are no guarantees that the shortfall will be covered.

Finally, payers can control their costs by cost-shifting to other willing payers. For example, as health insurance premiums rise, employers can choose to pass these costs on to employees. Hospitals and doctors who lose money caring for Medicare patients can try to make up their losses by charging more to private insurance patients. Insurance companies can choose to offer limited or no coverage for outpatient pharmaceuticals, shifting the full cost of expensive new medicines directly to patients.

MEDICAL ECONOMIC CONCEPTS AND TOOLS

MEDICAL COST CONCEPTS   Medical cost analysis is a field that borrows heavily from both economics and accounting. Economics provides the theoretical structure that defines the key questions to be addressed, and accounting provides many of the measurement tools. Traditional economics has as one of its major axioms that societal resources are finite. For this reason, society must choose from among the many ways that resources can be used and not all of society's goals can be fulfilled. Economics has devised a theoretical framework and a set of tools (including cost-effectiveness analysis) to help define the major competing goals for societal resources and to assist in selecting from among the ones that most efficiently fulfill societal needs. "Cost" in economics refers not so much to money but rather to the lost opportunities that occur when the limited societal resources are expended in a particular way. For example, if our medical armamentarium is enhanced over the next decade by discovery of powerful but expensive therapies and these are incorporated into standard clinical practice, the ability of the country to invest in education, defense, or transportation may be compromised. This notion of cost as a lost opportunity to use resources in alternative ways is referred to as *opportunity cost*. While representing the purest economic notion of cost, there is no practical way to measure it.

Accountants, who are much more concerned with issues of measurement, have proposed a "gold standard" of cost measurement, *true accounting cost*, that involves enumerating all the individual resources consumed in the production of a particular medical good or service and assigning market prices for each of them. The total cost is then the sum of the dollar costs for all the component resources. Even this calculation, however, may be prohibitively difficult in "real world" applications, for several reasons. First, all medical care requires not only the easily identifiable components of personnel time and disposable supplies but also the infrastructure components such as the rent on the office building where the care is provided, the cost of utilities, and the expense of an office staff. Second, even if all the components can be identified, enumeration of exactly what is used may be prohibitively expensive. Finally, medicine does not have publicly available "market prices" that can be readily obtained for a medical cost analysis, the way one can obtain prices for automobiles or refrigerators. The reasons for this relate to the lack of a true competitive free market in medicine along with the severe price distortion created in medical charges by cost-shifting practices.

KEY COST TERMS   Several key sets of cost terms are used in medicine. As the volume of health care produced is increased or decreased, costs may exhibit either variable or fixed "behavior." *Variable costs* change with each unit shift in production volume (up or down). For example, each vaccination administered to a group of children increases costs (related to the dose of vaccine and the disposable syringe) in a predictable linear fashion. *Fixed costs* do not shift with short-term changes in the volume of care provided. For example, the rent on the clinical building and the cost of heating, lighting, and so forth do not change according to the number of individuals vaccinated per day. Some types of costs display hybrid features of both variable and fixed components. For example, clinic personnel costs (e.g., nurses, secretaries) may be fixed if these personnel are paid a salary regardless of clinic volume. If the clinic volume goes up so much that evening hours must be added, either new personnel must be hired or existing personnel must work overtime. Either of these changes would graft a variable component onto the fixed personnel costs.

Marginal cost is a concept often used by economists to refer to the cost of producing one more unit of a given health care good or service. For example, the costs of doing one more or one less diagnostic cardiac catheterization would be its marginal cost. For all practical purposes, this is the same as its variable costs (since fixed costs do not change with small changes in volume). While the concept of unit changes in volume is theoretically interesting, a more pragmatic issue is the cost effect of changing a group of patients from one strategy to another. Many experts use the term *incremental costs* to refer to this type of shift (although some use marginal and incremental synonymously). Incremental analysis is a key component of cost-effectiveness analysis (see below).

Another set of cost terms relates to the traceability of costs to the production of health care goods and services. *Direct costs*, such as nursing and physician personnel and disposable supplies, can be clearly linked to the health care provided and are under the control of the health care providers. *Indirect costs*, sometimes known as *overhead*, cannot. For example, the utility, laundry, maintenance, and administration costs of a hospital cannot be linked with the care of an individual patient and are generally not under the control of the physicians and nurses providing the medical care. The distinction of direct versus indirect is useful in cost-containment efforts, where the first step is to identify all major cost components and decide how they are to be controlled.

One common error in the evaluation of medical costs is to focus on the cost of a test or therapy in isolation. Virtually every major medical management decision creates downstream consequences. For example, if physicians order a screening diagnostic test and the result is abnormal, they will need to do a confirmatory or more definitive test. If they order a potent new antibiotic and a fraction of patients develop liver failure as an unexpected toxicity, the total cost of that course of antibiotic includes not only the cost of the drug itself but also the costs of treating the liver failure in the fraction of patients who develop it. Extra costs added as a consequence of some diagnostic or therapeutic decision are referred to as *induced costs*. Similarly, if a management decision produces downstream savings, these would be referred to as *induced savings*. For example, administration of HMG CoA reductase inhibitors to patients with hypercholesterolemia can prevent future myocardial infarctions and revascularization procedures, both of which entail expensive hospitalizations.

One final important cost concept relates to the societal costs of lost productivity (primarily lost time from work) due to illness. While economists often refer to these as indirect costs, confusion with the accounting concept of indirect costs (overhead) has led many to prefer the alternative term, *productivity costs*.

COST MEASUREMENT   Using varying degrees of simplification, medical costs can be measured using either bottom-up or top-down approaches. Bottom-up approaches build from component resources to calculate total cost for an episode or type of care. Microcosting is the gold standard approach. It involves careful enumeration of all resources consumed and detailed cost-accounting estimation of the costs for each component resource. A number of medical centers have now installed computer-based cost-accounting systems that perform a modified type of microcosting analysis. For difficult-to-obtain resource use data (such as time required for a particular type of care by a given type of personnel), these systems use expert opinion in place of empirical data. The other extreme of the bottom-up category of approaches involves enumeration and costing for only the "big ticket" or expensive items, such as hospitalization episodes and costly tests and procedures.

The top-down methods of medical cost estimation calculate a cost estimate from aggregated data. One such approach uses hospital billing charge data and charge-to-cost conversion ratios (which each hospital produces annually in its Medicare Cost Report) to estimate hospital costs. Despite the approximations involved, this approach, which can be used for most nonfederal U.S. hospitals, has provided good agreement with bottom-up estimates in the few instances where formal comparisons have been made. The other top-down approach is the use of DRG assignments and reimbursement rates to provide standard cost weights for hospitalization episodes.

COST-EFFECTIVENESS ANALYSIS   Given a finite budget (for health care overall or for a particular health system), how can we use the available money to provide the most health benefits for our patients? For the clinician, who is less concerned with such policy issues, a prevalent question is whether a new treatment is economically attractive. The analysis method used to address this question is dependent on how the effectiveness and costs of the new therapy compare with those of "standard care" (Fig. 4-1). *Cost-effectiveness analysis* is used when effectiveness of the new treatment is greater and its costs are higher. This analysis calculates the ratio of added (or incremental)

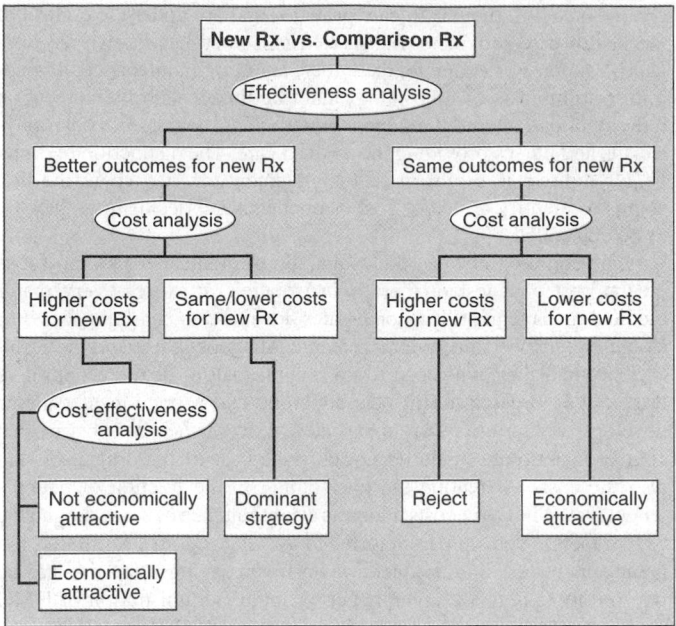

FIGURE 4-1 Schematic representation of patterns of outcome and cost differences that may result when a new therapy or strategy is compared with an existing standard. Effectiveness is always considered first because if the new therapy is less effective, its cost is rarely of concern. If effectiveness is better, or at least equivalent, then costs are prepared. If the outcomes are better but the net costs are higher, cost effectiveness analysis is then performed. If the costs are equivalent or lower, the therapy is said to be *dominant* (i.e., it becomes the preferred option). If outcomes are equivalent, cost analysis is used to select the more efficient, less costly option. This form of cost analysis is sometimes referred to as *cost minimization* or *cost-efficiency analysis.*

health benefits to added costs produced by a new therapy or strategy relative to some reference standard. The general formula is:

$$\text{Cost-effectiveness ratio} = \frac{C_{\text{new}} - C_{\text{usual care}}}{E_{\text{new}} - E_{\text{usual care}}}$$

where C = costs and E = effectiveness.

The cost-effectiveness ratio provides a quantitative statement of the amount of money required to produce a single extra unit of benefit with the new therapy relative to usual care or some other relevant reference standard. The benefit can be calculated in any meaningful clinical unit, such as added survivors or extra patients with a correct diagnosis. However, the vast majority of cost-effectiveness analyses use the epidemiologic concept of life-years to express incremental benefit. Virtually all benchmarks for cost effectiveness relate to this endpoint. Because some therapies affect quality of life but not quantity, a more generally relevant effectiveness measure combines qualify of life and life expectancy into a single composite metric, the quality-adjusted life year (QALY). Calculation of incremental dollars required to add an extra QALY is called *cost-utility analysis.* The QALY is a useful concept, but many details regarding measurement and interpretation remain controversial. The third form of economic efficiency analysis, *cost-benefit analysis*, requires conversion of health benefits into monetary equivalents. Because such conversions are controversial, this form of analysis is rarely used in medicine. In theory, the time horizon of a cost-effectiveness analysis should be long enough to capture all important cost and health consequences of the therapy or strategy being evaluated. Most often, analysts use a lifetime time frame. Because very few empirical studies are long enough to observe lifetime outcomes (especially when chronic diseases are being studied), models are required to extrapolate from available data.

A cost-effectiveness analysis can be done from a variety of perspectives, but the most widely applicable perspective is societal. Other perspectives are often much narrower and may include unattractive qualities. For example, a managed care organization may be interested only in short-term costs and outcomes, knowing that patients tend to change their health insurance every few years.

The benchmarks for cost-effectiveness ratios are determined by comparison with other well-accepted therapies in widespread medical use. A useful benchmark is hemodialysis for chronic renal failure, since the federal government has paid for all renal failure patients to get dialysis since 1973 through the End Stage Renal Disease Program. Recent estimates are that it costs this Medicare program about $50,000 to add 1 life-year to a chronic renal failure patient. Partly for this reason, many analysts use a cost-effectiveness ratio of <$50,000 per added life-year to identify therapies that are economically attractive (i.e., have a favorable balance of extra costs to extra benefits), while therapies with ratios >$100,000 per added life-year are deemed economically unattractive and therapies between $50,000 and $100,000 per added life-year are in the economic "gray zone."

Several caveats about cost-effectiveness analysis should be noted. First, cost-effectiveness analysis is descriptive, not prescriptive. It measures value that could be produced with available health care dollars but does not mandate how these dollars are to be used. If an expensive new therapy is introduced and is found to be very economically attractive by the above benchmarks, it will still not get used if there is no money in the budget to pay for it. Second, a cost-effectiveness ratio is only as good as the data that were used to calculate it. High-quality results can be obtained if economic analysis is prospectively incorporated into the design of large-scale multicenter randomized trials. Third, although cost-effectiveness ratios are often presented as deterministic (i.e., no variability), they often incorporate large amounts of uncertainty. This should be examined either with sensitivity analyses (varying each key parameter through a plausible range to see if the results are materially changed) or calculation of confidence limits.

MEDICAL ECONOMICS AND CLINICAL PRACTICE
In evaluating new therapies, three issues must be addressed: (1) is the new therapy significantly better than what is currently available? (2) how much does it cost and is it economically attractive? and (3) how many patients will need this therapy and is it affordable? The clinician should be primarily concerned with the answer to the first question. Although cost issues are now a reality of daily clinical life and cost-containment pressures are often substantial, decisions by clinicians that are based primarily on economic rather than clinical considerations put the physician in the role of the double agent (i.e., acting on behalf of both the patient and the payer) and compromise our fiduciary obligation to patients. The second question addresses cost effectiveness and, if favorable, can be used to support an argument by clinicians for adoption of the therapy. In the ideal world, at least, therapies that have a large database of evidence demonstrating effectiveness and economic attractiveness should be given preference over therapies that do not have such supporting data. The final question is of primary concern to payers and health policy analysts. An effective therapy that is too expensive to use is of little more value than a therapy that has yet to be discovered.

BIBLIOGRAPHY

AZIMA NA, WELCH HG: The effectiveness of cost effectiveness analysis in containing costs. J Gen Intern Med 13:664, 1998

BODENHEIMER T: The American health care system: Physicians and the changing medical marketplace. N Engl J Med 340:584, 1999

CANTOR SB, GANIATS TG: Incremental cost effectiveness analysis: The optimal strategy depends on the strategy set. J Clin Epidemiol 52:517, 1999

GRANATA AV, HILLMAN AL: Competing practice guidelines: Using cost effectiveness analysis to make optimal decisions. Ann Intern Med 128:56, 1998

HLATKY MA et al: for the BARI Investigators: Medical care costs and quality of life after randomization to coronary angioplasty or coronary bypass surgery. N Engl J Med 336:92, 1997

KUTTNER R: The American health care system: Health insurance coverage. N Engl J Med 340:163, 1999

MARK DB et al: Cost effectiveness of thrombolytic therapy with tissue plasminogen activator as compared with streptokinase for acute myocardial infarction. N Engl J Med 332:1418, 1995

5

Howard Hu, Frank E. Speizer

INFLUENCE OF ENVIRONMENTAL AND OCCUPATIONAL HAZARDS ON DISEASE

Exposures to hazardous materials and processes in the home, the workplace, and the community can cause or exacerbate a multitude of diseases. Physicians commonly treat the sequelae of such diseases in the practice of medicine; however, unless the underlying connection with hazardous exposures is identified and mitigated, treatment of manifestations rather than the cause at best only ameliorates the condition. At worst, the neglect of hazardous exposures may lead to both failure of treatment and failure to recognize a public health problem with wide significance.

No existing surveillance or reporting system can estimate the total contribution of hazardous exposures to morbidity and mortality. However, careful histories have identified occupational factors as etiologic in more than 10% of all admissions to general internal medicine wards in hospitals, with even higher percentages when the primary illness is either respiratory or musculoskeletal. Estimates of the number of new cases of disease due to work in the United States range from 125,000 to 350,000 per year; these cases do not include 5.3 million work-related injuries.

Environmental exposures are increasingly associated with decrements in measures of health whose outcomes range from subclinical to clinically catastrophic. For example, exposure to lead at levels that are common in the general population has been associated with increased blood pressure and decreased creatinine clearance. Ambient air pollution with respect to levels of ozone and fine-particulate matter has been related to increased rates of hospital admission for respiratory and cardiovascular diseases and to increased mortality rates, respectively. Indoor exposure to radon and passive indoor exposure to environmental tobacco smoke have been linked with an increased risk of lung cancer. There is pressure on clinicians to be aware of and act on this type of information, which is suggestive but not necessarily conclusive with respect to causation.

Patients are becoming increasingly concerned about hazardous exposures. More than 15% of patients seen in one study conducted in a primary care clinic expressed the opinion that their health problems were work-related, and 75% of this subgroup of patients reported exposure to one or more recognized toxic agents. Patients often want answers to very specific questions, such as: Is the water in our town safe to drink? Could my breathing problem be related to the new roofing sealant used in my building at work? Physicians are consulted because they are the most trusted sources of information on health risks, including chemical risks. Unfortunately, few physicians have more than rudimentary training in environmental and occupational medicine. Therefore, it becomes important for primary care physicians to be able to recognize symptoms precipitated by exposure to environmental or occupational hazards and either to manage these cases or to make appropriate referrals.

Many manifestations of exposure-related illnesses are nonspecific (e.g., dizziness, headache) or are commonly encountered in general internal medicine (e.g., myocardial infarction, cancer). The establishment of a connection with an environmental or occupational hazard requires a high index of suspicion and the application of fundamental concepts of environmental/occupational medicine. Furthermore, early recognition by physicians of unusual patterns of illness or of evidence of asymptomatic exposure to toxins with low-level effects (e.g., an elevated blood lead level) can alert health officials to the need for control measures. Case reports either sent to local authorities or published in the literature often prompt follow-up studies that can lead to the identification of new hazards. In many states and countries, the reporting by physicians of occupational/environmental diseases is mandatory. For instance, beginning in 1992, physicians in Massachusetts were required to report cases of pneumoconiosis, occupational asthma, carpal tunnel syndrome, and carbon monoxide poisoning, among other conditions. Identification of an environmental/occupational etiology of an illness may have important economic ramifications for the patient (e.g., the awarding of worker's compensation, which covers medical bills as well as lost wages). Finally, physicians are frequently asked to provide expert medical testimony during litigation on the causal relationship between toxic exposures and diseases. In this setting, the more knowledgeable the physician is about potential hazardous exposures, the better prepared he or she is to serve the patient.

THE ENVIRONMENTAL/OCCUPATIONAL HISTORY

For a physician, the most critical steps toward recognizing these disorders are remembering to consider them in the differential diagnosis and taking an appropriate environmental/occupational history as part of the medical workup. The level of detail that is called for depends on the clinical situation. *Information should always be obtained on current and major past occupations, and patients should be asked whether they think their health problem is related to their work or to any particular environment or exposure.* In the review of systems, patients should be asked if they have been exposed to dusts, fumes, chemicals, radiation, or loud noise. When patient and physician are confronted with an illness of uncertain etiology, these factors should be explored in more detail, with the environmental/occupational history as the point of departure. (A brief outline of a sample history is shown in Table 5-1.)

The identification of specific chemical exposures can be difficult. Household products must list chemical ingredients on their labels, and this information may prove useful. For workplace exposures, the U.S. Occupational Safety and Health Administration (OSHA) requires chemical suppliers to provide material safety data sheets with their products and requires employers to retain these sheets and make them available to employees. The data sheets can be obtained by the physician or employee by a telephoned or written request; failure of an

Table 5-1 Initial Clinical Approach to the Recognition of Illness Caused by Environmental or Occupational Hazards

1. Screening questions
   a. Chief symptom and history of present illness
      • What kind of work do you do?
      • Do you think your health problems are related to your work, home, or any other particular environment or exposure?
      • Does the timing of your symptoms have any relation to being at work or at home or to any other particular exposures or activities?
   b. Review of systems
      • Are you now or have you previously been exposed to dusts, fumes, chemicals, radiation, or loud noise?
2. Detailed questioning based on initial suspicion
   • Chronology of jobs: Job title, type of industry, dates of work, description of job, a typical day, potentially hazardous exposures, protective equipment used
   • Chronology of residences: Description of potentially hazardous exposures (e.g., furnaces, pesticide application, home hobbies involving chemicals)
   • Identification of other employees or household members who have similar health problems
   • Exploration in detail of the temporal link between potential exposures and chief symptoms
   • Clinical clues (suspicious scenarios; see text)

SOURCE: Adapted from Newman, 1995.

employer to provide them within 30 days of such a request is a violation of OSHA regulations and is punishable by fines. In addition to providing information on chemical ingredients and percent composition, the material safety data sheets provide basic information on toxicity. This information is seldom adequate from a clinical perspective but may indicate the general type of toxicity to be anticipated.

EVALUATION OF POSSIBLE CHEMICAL OR ENVIRONMENTAL HAZARDS   Given the wide variety of toxic exposures that may be uncovered during a workup, a clinician should routinely consult additional reference material to evaluate whether particular hazards may be associated with the illness at hand. Many sources of information exist. OSHA and some regional poison-control centers have extensive information on hazards and brief summary documents that can be transmitted over the Internet or by telephone or facsimile. Depending on the area, other resources may include county and state health departments; regional offices of the National Institute for Occupational Safety and Health and the Environmental Protection Agency; the Consumer Products Safety Commission in Washington, DC; academic institutions; websites of these institutions; and individual toxicologists, occupational/environmental medicine specialists, or industrial hygienists. Sophisticated computerized databases are also available, including detailed listings on CD-ROM information systems. MEDLARS, the electronic database maintained by the National Library of Medicine, is accessible by modem or the Internet and is familiar to many physicians. Files other than MEDLINE, such as the Hazardous Substances Databank, provide specific toxicity information on chemicals and include toxicologic references not covered by MEDLINE. Many of these databases can also be accessed through the Internet.

As with any other illness, laboratory investigation may be crucial. For example, tests of carboxyhemoglobin level to document carbon monoxide exposure or of serum anticholinesterase level to document organophosphate pesticide absorption should be performed within hours of exposure. As in cases of acute drug overdose, it is useful to freeze samples of urine and serum from any patient suspected of having had an acute chemical exposure; such specimens can be analyzed at a later date by sensitive methods of detection. Use of other tests must rely on knowledge of the specific hazard or illness in question.

SUSPICIOUS SCENARIOS   Some medical problems or clinical scenarios demand a particularly high degree of suspicion of occupational or environmental factors as causative or contributing agents.

Respiratory Disease   The contribution of occupational/environmental factors to respiratory disease is generally underrecognized, particularly among patients who smoke and among the elderly (Chap. 254). For instance, asthma related to chemical exposure may be treated without regard to cause or may be erroneously diagnosed as acute tracheobronchitis. A study of new-onset asthma among HMO members in Massachusetts found that 21% of these individuals met criteria for clinically significant asthma attributable to occupational exposures. The types of exposures and jobs in these cases varied widely; examples include exposure to smoke in a firefighter, to welding fumes in a technical school student, to cleaning compounds in a bartender, and to epoxy in an archery repairman. No single type of job or exposure predominated. Other examples of etiologic errors include shortness of breath from asbestosis that is attributed to chronic obstructive pulmonary disease and chemical pneumonitis that is misdiagnosed as a bacterial infection.

Cancer   Many cancers are thought to be causally related to occupational and environmental factors in addition to tobacco. Some are particularly likely to have a chemical etiology or another environmental cause, including cancers of the skin (solar radiation, arsenic, coal tar, soot); lung (asbestos, arsenic, nickel, radon); pleura (almost exclusively asbestos); nasal cavity and sinuses (chromium, nickel, wood

and leather dusts); liver (arsenic, vinyl chloride); bone marrow (benzene, ionizing radiation); and bladder (aromatic amines).

Coronary Disease and Hypertension   Carbon monoxide exposure is common, particularly in homes with malfunctioning furnaces or in workplaces close to motor vehicle exhaust. By reducing oxygen transport by hemoglobin and inhibiting mitochondrial metabolism, carbon monoxide can aggravate coronary disease. Methylene chloride, a solvent used in paint stripping, is converted to carbon monoxide and thus poses the same risk. Exposure to carbon disulfide, a chemical used in the production of rayon, accelerates the rate of atherosclerotic plaque formation. Chronic lead exposure, even at modest levels, is a risk factor for the development of hypertension as well as abnormalities of cardiac conduction.

Hepatitis/Chronic Liver Disease   In the absence of evidence that a viral infection, alcohol ingestion, or drug use is the main cause of hepatitis (Chaps. 295, 296, and 297), the involvement of a toxin must be considered. Toxin-induced hepatic injury may be cytotoxic, cholestatic, or both. The list of hepatotoxic agents is long, including organic synthetic compounds such as carbon tetrachloride (used in solvents and cleaning fluids) and methylene diamine (a resin hardener); pesticides such as chlordecone (Kepone); metals, particularly arsenic (used in pesticides and paints and found in well water); and natural toxins such as the pyrrolidizine alkaloids.

Kidney Disease   Many chemical and environmental factors can cause renal injury (Chap. 269). The etiology of much chronic kidney disease, however, remains unknown. An increasing body of evidence now links chronic renal failure with hypertension to lead exposure. One study demonstrated that chelation therapy with EDTA slowed the progression of renal insufficiency in patients with a mildly elevated body lead burden. Some studies suggest that chronic exposure to hydrocarbons (e.g., gasoline, paints, solvents) may lead to various types of glomerulonephritis, including Goodpasture's syndrome. Environmental cadmium exposure has been found to promote calcium loss via urinary excretion, which results in skeletal demineralization and thus in an increased risk of fractures.

Peripheral Neuropathy   Organic solvents such as *n*-hexane, heavy metals such as lead and arsenic, and some organophosphate compounds can damage the axons of peripheral nerves. Dimethylaminopropionitrile, an industrial catalyst, causes bladder neuropathy. Nerve entrapment syndromes of the upper extremity, such as carpal tunnel syndrome, may be caused by jobs that involve repetitive motion, especially those requiring the maintenance of awkward positions.

Central Nervous System Disorders   Fatigue, memory loss, difficulty in concentration, and emotional lability have been linked to chronic exposure to solvents such as toluene and perchloroethylene. Painters, metal degreasers, plastics workers, and cleaners are commonly exposed to solvents and develop these symptoms at a high rate. Among the features that distinguish these patients are characteristic patterns on formal neurobehavioral testing and stabilization of symptoms with gradual improvement after discontinuation of the exposure. Other substances associated with neurobehavioral dysfunction include metals, particularly lead, mercury, arsenic, and manganese; pesticides, such as organophosphates and organochlorines; polychlorinated biphenyls (PCBs); and gases such as carbon monoxide.

Environmental factors are also suspected of contributing to other neurologic diseases, such as degenerative disorders, motor neuron diseases, and extrapyramidal disorders. For example, a study in monozygotic and dizygotic twin pairs found a similarity in concordance indicating that environmental (as opposed to genetic) factors play a major etiologic role in cases of typical Parkinson's disease beginning after the age of 50 years.

Teratogenesis and Reproductive Problems   Toxins can impair successful reproduction at a variety of levels. Examples include insecticides and herbicides, PCBs and polybrominated biphenyls (PBBs), ethylene oxide (a sterilizing gas used in hospitals), metals (lead, arsenic, cadmium, mercury), and solvents. Dibromochloropropane, a nematocide, suppresses spermatogenesis. Some toxins, such as PCBs,

PBBs, and chlorinated pesticides, are concentrated in milk. Concern has arisen over the ability of specific organic pollutants, particularly pesticides, to persist in the environment and accumulate in human tissues. Some of these chemicals may disrupt endocrine function, and these effects may be related to phenomena such as the observed increases in the incidences of testicular cancer, breast cancer, and hypospadias.

Immunosuppression, Autoimmunity, and Hypersensitivity Evidence is increasing that exposures to some chemical agents can compromise the immune system, thereby leading to a generalized increase in the incidence of tumors (e.g., exposure to PBBs) or infections (e.g., respiratory infections after exposure to common air pollutants). Mercury, dieldrin, and methylcholanthrene are known to elicit autoimmune responses. Some chemicals are potent allergic sensitizers that cause dermal and respiratory problems (Chaps. 60 and 254).

BIOLOGICAL MARKERS An increasing number of methods are available for measuring and interpreting toxic exposure, including (1) the internal dose of specific toxins and (2) markers of the biologic effects of toxins. Internal-dose markers are relevant for toxins that are sequestered in the human body, such as lead (in blood), arsenic (in hair), and other metals (Chap. 395), and for halogenated compounds (such as PCBs). Examples of markers of the biologic effects of toxins include depressed levels of acetylcholinesterase in serum after exposure to organophosphate pesticides, sister chromatid exchanges in peripheral lymphocytes after exposure to the carcinogen ethylene oxide, and DNA adducts after exposure to tobacco smoke carcinogens.

MANAGING A HAZARD-RELATED ILLNESS Once a chemical or another environmental hazard has been identified as an important contributor to an illness, the next step is to prevent further exposure. Although for chronic diseases such as cancer this step may be irrelevant for the patient in question, prevention of further exposure may still be critical for other persons who have been similarly exposed. When prevention of further exposure is important, *the physician must be willing to become an active advocate for the patient.* This advocacy may involve writing a letter stating that the patient should no longer be exposed to a hazard or should remain out of work. Alternatively, it may involve contacting appropriate officials in government, industry, or labor or other advocates who can deal with a hazardous exposure. Treatment is dependent on the specific hazard.

In few areas of medicine does a physician deal with more scientific uncertainty. Comprehensive information on toxicants is available for only a small percentage of chemicals. In general, the physician should take a conservative approach (i.e., advise the patient to avoid a hazard likely to have contributed to illness) and should use common sense and up-to-date information to evaluate causal relationships.

LOW-LEVEL EXPOSURES AND THEIR EFFECTS The subclinical effects of toxins that are widespread in our environment and our workplaces are of increasing concern. Given the absence of any demonstrable effect threshold, low-level exposure to carcinogens should be avoided; not only carcinogenic but also noncarcinogenic effects of chronic low-level exposure to these substances are important.

Perhaps lead provides the most important example of low-level noncarcinogenic effects that constitute a major public health problem. Multiple pathways of exposure, including the combustion of leaded gasoline, the use of lead-based paints and solder, and the presence of lead in cans containing food, have contributed to exposure of the entire population. Such low-level exposures can impair neurobehavioral development in infants and children and can raise blood pressure in adults. Furthermore, absorbed lead is stored in the skeleton and may reenter the circulation at times of heightened bone turnover (e.g., pregnancy, lactation, osteoporosis, hyperthyroidism). Subclinical toxic effects can be prevented if chronic low-level exposure is detected early and curtailed. In the case of lead, such exposure is detected by tests of blood lead level, which should be performed regularly in young children living in old housing and as a precautionary measure in adults with a history of lead exposure.

BIBLIOGRAPHY

DeRosa C et al: Environmental exposures that affect the endocrine system: Public health implications. J Toxicol Environ Health B Crit Rev 1:3, 1998

Dockery DW et al: An association between air pollution and mortality in six U.S. cities. N Engl J Med 329:1753, 1993

Gennart J-P et al: Importance of accurate employment histories of patients admitted to units of internal medicine. Scand J Work Environ Health 17:386, 1991

Institutes of Medicine: *Role of the Primary Care Physician in Occupational and Environmental Medicine.* Washington, DC, National Academy Press, 1988

Lin JL et al: Chelation therapy for patients with elevated body lead burden and progressive renal insufficiency. A randomized, controlled trial. Ann Intern Med 5:7, 1999

Milton DK et al: Risk and incidence of asthma attributable to occupational exposure among HMO members. Am J Ind Med 33:1, 1998

Newman LS: Current concepts: Occupational illness. N Engl J Med 333:1128, 1995

Paul M (ed): *Occupational/Environmental Hazards and Reproductive Health: A Guide for Clinicians.* Baltimore, Williams & Wilkins, 1992

Rom WN: *Environmental and Occupational Medicine.* Philadelphia, Lippincott-Raven, 1998

Staessen JA et al: Environmental exposure to cadmium, forearm bone density, and risk of fractures: Prospective population study. Lancet 353:1140, 1999

Tanner CM et al: Parkinson disease in twins. An etiologic study. JAMA 281:341, 1999

 6

Anthony L. Komaroff, Celeste Robb-Nicholson, Andrea E. Dunaif

WOMEN'S HEALTH

In recent years, the medical problems and health care of women have received increasing attention. There are poorly understood differences between men and women, both in morbidity and mortality and in the expression of diseases. Many research studies of disease prevention and pathophysiology have included only male subjects; most illnesses that can affect both sexes have not been as well studied in women. It also appears that women receive different care than men for certain common health problems. Finally, an increasing number of women are seeking health care in multidisciplinary women's health units that combine the expertise of gynecology, psychiatry, and internal medicine or family medicine.

MORBIDITY AND MORTALITY IN WOMEN **Morbidity** Past studies have found that women experience more days of restricted activity than men at all ages, over and above the restricted activity caused by obstetric and gynecologic conditions. However, a study in 1998 concluded differently. Women make more visits to physicians, particularly for acute self-limited illnesses.

Mortality In the developed nations, women live longer than men. In the United States, as of 1996, the projected average life expectancy from birth is 79.1 years for females, and 73.1 years for males. Although there are more male fetuses conceived than female fetuses, females have a survival advantage when compared to males, in all age groups. The longer life expectancy of women versus men in developed countries is due in large part to the difference in mortality caused by ischemic heart disease (IHD).

As shown in Table 6-1, the leading causes of death among young women in the United States are accidents, homicide, and suicide. During the middle years, breast cancer is a slightly more common cause of death than IHD and lung cancer. In women between ages 65 and 74, IHD, lung cancer, and cerebrovascular disease supercede breast cancer as the leading causes of death. Among women of all ages, IHD is the leading cause of death by a substantial margin, with a mortality rate five to sixfold higher than the rate for either lung or breast cancer. Nevertheless, polls find that U.S. women believe breast cancer poses the greatest threat to their lives.

Table 6-1   Death Rates (per 100,000) for the Leading Causes of Death in U.S. Women, 1996

Ages 25–34 Total: 74.7	Ages 45–54 Total: 323.3	Ages 65–74 Total: 1,979.0	All Ages Total: 806.5
1. Motor vehicle accidents (10.7)	1. Breast cancer (38.8)	1. Ischemic heart disease (452.6)	1. Ischemic heart disease (172.8)
2. HIV infection (8.5)	2. Ischemic heart disease (30.2)	2. Lung cancer[a] (209.0)	2. Cerebrovascular disease (71.9)
3. Homicide (5.5)	3. Lung cancer[a] (29.0)	3. GI cancer[b] (147.1)	3. Lung cancer[a] (45.6)
4. Non-motor vehicle accidents (5.0)	4. GI cancer[b] (20.2)	4. COPD[c] (136.7)	4. GI cancer[b] (20.2)
5. Suicide (5.0)	5. Cancer of the genital organs (16.4)	5. Cerebrovascular disease (120.1)	5. COPD[c] (38.0)

[a] Cancer of respiratory and intrathoracic organs, predominantly lung cancer.
[b] Cancer of digestive organs and peritoneum.
[c] Chronic obstructive pulmonary disease, including asthma, and allied conditions.
SOURCE: Adapted from National Center for Health Statistics Web site, Vital Statistics of the United States, 1996, general mortality table GMWK290. URL: www.cdc.gov/nchswww/data/gm290.pdf

Social Factors Influencing Morbidity and Mortality   Gender differences in morbidity and mortality may be explained in part by psychosocial factors such as socially-defined gender roles, poverty, participation in the work force, health insurance, and lifestyle.

In the past 30 years in the United States, there has been a "feminization of poverty." One-third of families headed by women currently live in poverty, and the fraction is greater than one-half for African-American and Latino women. Almost a fifth of women over age 65 live below the poverty level. People of lower socioeconomic status experience poorer health and a higher mortality rate than those in higher income groups. The poor are more likely to smoke and less likely to have recommended preventive measures, including cancer screening. Lack of adequate health insurance is a major problem for many women; in general, they are more likely than men to have low-paying, part-time, non-union jobs that do not provide health insurance. Women who are divorced or widowed may also lose health insurance that they had through their husbands.

PREVENTION (See also Chap. 10)   Primary prevention and screening are crucial elements in improving the health of women. Based upon available literature and the consensus of experts, various authoritative organizations have published guidelines on preventive practices in women.

Most physicians believe that a baseline history and physical examination is useful to set the stage for preventive measures appropriate to each patient. In general, authorities recommend that blood pressure be measured every other year throughout life. Counseling on diet, smoking cessation, exercise, and use of seatbelts are of demonstrated value in the primary prevention of diseases and accidents. Counseling about safe sexual practices, alcohol abuse, and violence are also recommended.

Screening for glaucoma is recommended for African-American women over age 40 and for Caucasian women over age 50. Yearly examinations to test visual acuity are recommended for women over age 70.

Regular screening for breast, cervical, and colorectal cancer is recommended, but how often tests should be performed and which tools to use are still being debated. Most authorities recommend annual clinical breast examination in all women beginning at age 35 to 40. There is strong evidence to support the efficacy of annual mammography in women age 50 to 59. For women age 60 or older, the evidence for screening is less strong. The benefits of screening for women between the ages of 40 and 49 are still being debated.

Most authorities recommend Pap smear screening beginning at age 18 or when a woman becomes sexually active. After two or three consecutive normal Pap smears, most groups recommend Pap smear testing every three years. If Pap smears have been normal for 10 years, they can be discontinued in women after age 65.

Recommendations for colorectal cancer screening vary. For patients over 50, the American Cancer Society recommends yearly fecal occult blood testing and rectal examination combined with flexible sigmoidoscopy every 5 years, colonoscopy every 10 years, or double-contrast barium enema every 5 to 10 years.

Bone mineral testing has gained rapid acceptance as a screening tool for detecting osteoporosis, as well as for predicting the likelihood of the condition in the future. With the advent of multiple preventive and therapeutic strategies for osteoporosis, many authorities now recommend bone mineral testing to screen for the condition. A bone mineral density test is recomended for all women over age 65 as well as for all postmenopausal women who are at increased risk for developing osteoporosis (Chap. 342).

Cigarette smoking, a major risk factor for cardiovascular diseases and cancers in women, has been well studied (Chap. 390). Over the past 60 years there has been a sharp decline in smoking among men, but not among women; teenage women smoke at higher rates than their male counterparts. "Low-yield" cigarettes are marketed heavily to women. The Nurses' Health Study showed that one-third of the excess risk of ischemic heart disease was eliminated two years after smoking cessation, and that all of the excess risk was eliminated by 10 to 14 years after smoking cessation.

The National Cholesterol Education Program recommends that total cholesterol and high-density lipoprotein (HDL) levels be measured once. If both are normal, a repeat test after 5 years is recommended. A meta-analysis of several small studies of women showed an increased risk of IHD in women with serum cholesterol greater than 265, a ratio of total cholesterol to HDL cholesterol greater than 4, or an elevated fasting triglyceride.

In various case-control and observational studies, postmenopausal estrogen therapy is associated with a 40 to 50% reduction in deaths due to IHD, but its value in a prospective, randomized trial has not yet been documented.

Calcium and estrogen, as well as alendronate and the selective estrogen receptor modulators, tamoxifen and raloxifene, slow the development of osteoporosis and reduce the frequency of hip and vertebral fracture in postmenopausal women. In randomized clinical trials, both tamoxifen and raloxifene have been shown to reduce the risk of breast cancer in postmenopausal women.

Considerable research indicates that a relatively high dietary intake of various antioxidants (including vitamins E and C) is associated with lower rates of vascular disease and malignancies. Randomized trials of supplemental antioxidants are under way. Preliminary research indicates that regular aspirin use is associated with reduced rates of IHD and colorectal carcinoma.

GENDER DIFFERENCES IN DISEASE   Obviously, some diseases and conditions occur exclusively (or nearly exclusively) in women—e.g., menopause and various breast and gynecological disorders. These are discussed elsewhere in this book (Chaps. 52, 89, 336, 337). In this chapter, we seek to highlight some gender differences in diseases that occur in both women and men.

Ischemic Heart Disease (See also Chap. 244)   Many persons think of IHD as a primary problem for men rather than women, perhaps because men have more than twice the total incidence of cardiovascular morbidity and mortality between the ages of 35 and 84. However, as stated earlier, in the United States IHD is among the leading causes of death among women as well as men (Table 6-1). The curve for the IHD mortality rate in women lags behind that for men by about a decade. Nevertheless, nearly 250,000 women die annually from IHD; after age 40, one in three women will die from heart disease. Although IHD mortality has been falling in men in the United States over the past 30 years, it has been increasing in women.

Why are IHD rates lower in women? They have a more favorable risk profile in some respects: higher HDL cholesterol levels, lower triglyceride levels, and less upper-body obesity than men. But women also have a less favorable risk profile in other respects: more obesity, higher blood pressure, higher plasma cholesterol levels, higher fibrinogen levels, and more diabetes. The simplest explanation for the sex differential in IHD is the "cardioprotective" effect of estrogen, which can be due to improvement of the lipid profile, a direct vasodilatory effect, and perhaps other factors. HDL cholesterol levels appear to be a particularly important risk factor for IHD in women. HDL levels are higher in all age groups in women compared to men, and are higher in premenopausal and estrogen-treated postmenopausal women. Smoking is the most important risk factor for IHD in women.

IHD presents differently in men and women. In the Framingham study, angina was the most frequent initial symptom of IHD in females, occurring in 47% of women, whereas myocardial infarction was the most frequent initial symptom in males, occurring in 46% of men. The exercise electrocardiogram has a substantial false positive as well as false negative rate for women, compared to men.

Women, particularly African-American women, have a higher risk of morbidity and mortality than men following a myocardial infarction. Compared to men, women who obtain coronary artery bypass graft surgery have more advanced disease, a higher perioperative mortality rate, less relief of angina, and less graft patency; however, 5- and 10-year survival rates are similar. Women undergoing percutaneous transluminal coronary angioplasty have lower rates of clinical and angiographic success than men, but also a lower rate of restenosis and a better long-term outcome. Women may benefit less and have more frequent serious bleeding complications from thrombolytic therapy than do men. Factors such as older age, more comorbid conditions, and more severe IHD in women at the time of events or procedures appear to account for at least part of the gender differences observed. Women with IHD benefit at least as much as men, and perhaps more, from reductions in cholesterol level.

The incidence of IHD increases markedly at menopause, consistent with the hypothesis that estrogens are cardioprotective. A number of observational studies have supported this hypothesis by demonstrating significant decreases in IHD in women on hormone replacement therapy (HRT), both estrogen alone and estrogen-progestin combination therapy. However, the HERS, a recent clinical trial of HRT for the *secondary* prevention of IHD, showed no significant difference in cardiovascular events between therapy with combined continuous conjugated equine estrogen (0.625 mg qd) and that with medroxyprogesterone acetate (2.5 mg qd), compared to placebo over four years. Indeed, in the HRT group, there was about a 50% increase in cardiovascular events in the first year of the trial. The Women's Health Initiative is investigating directly the impact of various HRT modalities as a *primary* prevention of IHD risk. Until further data are available, caution should be exercised in prescribing HRT to women with a history of IHD, or for cardioprotection alone.

Hypertension (See also Chap. 246)   Hypertension is more common in U.S. women than men, largely owing to the high prevalence of hypertension in older age groups and the longer survival rate for women. Both the effectiveness and the adverse effects of various antihypertensive drugs appear to be comparable in women and men. Benefits of treatment for severe hypertension have been dramatic in both women and men. However, in clinical trials of the treatment of mild to moderate hypertension, women have had a smaller decrease in morbidity and mortality than men, perhaps because women have a lower risk of myocardial infarction and stroke than men to begin with. Older women benefit at least as much as men from treatment, as demonstrated by the Systolic Hypertension in Elderly study. The incidence of hypertension (above 140/90) appears to be low (less than 5%) with the current low-dose oral contraceptives. Postmenopausal estrogen therapy is not associated with increases in blood pressure.

Immunologically Mediated Diseases   Several immunologically mediated diseases—e.g., rheumatoid arthritis, systemic lupus erythematosus, multiple sclerosis, Graves' disease, and thyroiditis—oc-cur much more frequently in women than in men. In animal models of rheumatoid arthritis—lupus and multiple sclerosis, for example—it is the females of the species that are predominantly affected. On the other hand, animal studies indicate that females are less susceptible to infection.

In short, female animals appear to have more vigorous immune responses, with both beneficial and adverse consequences. Increasing evidence indicates that estrogens upregulate both cellular and humoral immunity. Also, some immunocytes contain estrogen, progestin and androgen receptors, and the uterus produces a variety of cytokines, suggesting a complex interaction between the reproductive and immune systems.

Osteoporosis (See also Chap. 342)   This condition is much more prevalent in postmenopausal women than in men of similar age. Osteoporotic hip fractures are a major cause of morbidity in elderly women. Men accumulate more bone mass and lose bone more slowly than women. Gender differences in bone mass are found as early as infancy. Calcium intake, vitamin D and estrogen all play important roles in osteoporosis; calcium intake is an important determinant of peak bone mass, particularly during adolescence. Vitamin D deficiency is surprisingly common in elderly women. Receptors for estrogens and androgens have been identified in bone. The aromatase enzyme system, which converts androgens to estrogens, is also present in bone.

Therapy with HRT, or with calcium and vitamin D, has been shown to reduce the risk of osteoporotic fractures. Newer modalities, such as bisphosphonates (alendronate), calcitonin, and raloxifene, a selective estrogen receptor modulator, prevent bone loss and reduce the risk of osteoporotic fractures.

Alzheimer's Disease (See also Chap. 362)   Alzheimer's disease (AD) affects approximately twice as many women as men, in part because women live longer. Several observational studies suggest that HRT may decrease the risk of AD and improve cognitive function in older women. These benefits are seen in both current as well as past HRT users. In a few experimental studies, estrogen replacement has been shown to be associated with improved memory compared to placebo treatment. Estrogens enhance neuronal growth and activity, providing a biologic basis for these putative cognitive effects of HRT. Prospective clinical trials, including the Women's Health Initiative, are underway to pursue these intriguing observations.

Diabetes Mellitus (See also Chap. 333)   Estrogens enhance insulin sensitivity in women but not in men. Despite this, the prevalence of type 2 diabetes mellitus (DM) is higher in women, which is related in part to the higher prevalence of female obesity. Premenopausal women with DM lose the cardioprotective effect of female gender and have identical rates of IHD to those in males. This is partially explained by the presence of several IHD risk factors in women with DM: obesity, hypertension and dysplipidemia. Recent evidence suggests that vascular responses differ in women with DM, as compared to normal women. Polycystic ovary syndrome and gestational diabetes mellitus—common conditions in premenopausal women—are associated with a significantly increased risk for type 2 DM.

Psychological Disorders (See also Chap. 385)   Depression, anxiety panic disorder and eating disorders (bulimia and anorexia nervosa) occur more often in women than in men. Epidemiologic studies from both developed and developing nations consistently find major depression to be twice as common in women as in men, with the gender disparity becoming evident in early adolescence. Depression occurs in 10% of women during pregnancy and in 10 to 15% of women during the first several months of the postpartum period. The incidence of major depression diminishes after age 45, and does not increase with the onset of menopause. Depression in women also appears to have a worse prognosis than in men; episodes of depression last longer and there is a lower rate of spontaneous remission.

Social factors may account for the greater prevalence of some disorders in women; the traditionally subordinate role of women in society may generate feelings of helplessness and frustration which contribute to psychiatric illness. In addition, it is likely that biological factors, including hormonally influenced neurochemical changes, also play a role. The limbic system and hypothalamus—areas of the brain thought to subserve appetite, satiety and emotion—contain estradiol and testosterone receptors.

Alcohol and Drug Abuse (See also Chap. 387)   One-third of Americans who suffer from alcoholism are women. Women alcoholics are less likely to be diagnosed than men; a greater proportion of men than women seek help for alcohol and drug abuse. Men are more likely to go to an alcohol or drug treatment facility, while women tend to approach a primary care physician or mental health professional for help under the guise of a psychosocial problem. Late-life alcoholism is more common in women than men. In 1997, an epidemiologic survey reported that, among women over age 59, an estimated 1.8 million were addicted to or abused alcohol, and over 2.8 million were addicted to or abused psychoactive or mood-altering prescription drugs.

On average, alcoholic women drink less than alcoholic men, but exhibit the same degree of impairment. Blood alcohol levels are higher in women than in men after drinking equivalent amounts of alcohol, adjusted for body weight. This greater bioavailability of alcohol in women is probably due to the higher proportion of body fat and lower total body water. Women also have a lower gastric "first-pass metabolism" of alcohol, associated with lower activity of gastric alcohol dehydrogenase. In addition, alcoholic women are more likely than alcoholic men to abuse tranquilizers, sedatives, and amphetamines. Women alcoholics have a higher mortality rate than do nonalcoholic women and alcoholic men. Compared to men, women also appear to develop alcoholic liver disease and other alcohol-related diseases with shorter drinking histories and lower levels of alcohol consumption. Alcohol abuse also poses special risks to women who are or wish to become pregnant, adversely affecting fertility and the health of the baby (fetal alcohol syndrome).

Finally, there is growing evidence that for several illicit drugs, women proceed more rapidly to drug dependence than do men.

Human Immunodeficiency Virus Infection (See also Chap. 309) As of September 1998, the Centers for Disease Control and Prevention estimate that between 120,000 and 160,000 adolescent and adult women in the United States were living with HIV infection, including those with AIDS (Table 6-1). Between 1985 and 1998, the proportion of all U.S. AIDS cases reported among women more than tripled, from 7 to 23%. HIV infection was the fourth leading cause of death among U.S. women age 25 to 44 in 1997, and the second leading cause of death among African-American women in this age group. The CDC estimates that 30% of the approximately 40,000 new HIV infections in the United States each year are among women.

Between 1996 and 1997 the incidence of new AIDS cases in the United States decreased by 18% and that of AIDS-related deaths by 42%, largely because of advances in HIV therapies. The decline continued between 1997 and 1998, albeit at a slower rate. AIDS incidence and AIDS-related mortality fell by 11 and 20%, respectively. However, AIDS incidence and deaths are not decreasing as rapidly among women as among men. HIV and AIDS continue to affect women in racial/ethnic minorities and lower socioeconomic classes disproportionately. CDC estimates that 64% of new HIV infections in 1998 occured among African-American women, 18% among Hispanic women, and 18% among white women. Of the new HIV infections among women in the United States in 1998, CDC estimates that 75% of women were infected through heterosexual sex and 25% of women through injection drug use.

Violence Against Women   Violence against women in the United States is an enormous problem. Incidents of both rape and domestic violence are vastly underreported. Sexual assault is one of the most common crimes against women. One in five adult women in the United States reports having experienced sexual assault during her lifetime. Adult women are much more likely to be raped by a spouse, ex-spouse, or acquaintance than by a stranger.

Domestic violence is defined in the American Medical Association guidelines as "an ongoing, debilitating experience of physical, psychologic, and/or sexual abuse in the home, associated with increasing isolation from the outside world and limited personal freedom and accessibility to resources." It affects women of all ages, ethnic orientations, and socioeconomic groups. Based upon national crime statistics, every year an estimated 2 million women in the United States are severely injured and more than 1000 are killed by their current or former male partner. Domestic violence is the most common cause of physical injury in women, exceeding the combined incidence of all other types of injury (such as from rape, mugging, and auto accidents). Women who are young, single, pregnant, recently separated or divorced, or who have a history of substance abuse or mental illness, or a partner with substance abuse or mental illness, are at increased risk of domestic violence.

Domestic violence and sexual assault are associated with increased rates of physical and psychologic symptoms, medical office visits, and hospitalizations. Given this indirect presentation of the consequences of violence, and the high prevalence of unreported violence, clinicians should have a low threshold for pursuing the possibility of violence in female patients, particularly those with vague symptoms and psychological disorders.

The immediate treatment of rape and domestic violence focuses on assessing and treating physical injuries; providing emotional support; assessing and dealing with the risks of sexually transmitted infection and pregnancy; evaluating the safety of the patient and other family members; and documenting the patient's history and physical examination findings. In addition to dealing with the medical and psychological issues, appropriate care includes providing information about legal services, shelters and safe houses, hotlines, support groups, and counseling services.

RESEARCH IN WOMEN'S HEALTH   The growing recognition of the importance of women's health has spawned a number of research efforts, including large observational studies and clinical trials. The U.S. National Institutes of Health has introduced guidelines to mandate the inclusion of women in clinical studies, and the reporting of gender-specific data.

Studies of Prevention   Large observational studies of men and women, such as the Rancho Bernardo Study and the Framingham Study, designed to analyze data specific to women have been on the increase. The Nurses' Health Study has been following more than 200,000 women, many for more than 20 years, prospectively collecting data to study the impact of smoking, diet, physical activity, medications, prevention and screening behaviors, and some psychosocial factors on the risk of various medical disorders, including breast cancer, IHD, stroke, diabetes, and fracture, as well as causes of mortality.

These studies have set the stage for clinical trials such as the Postmenopausal Estrogens/Progestins Intervention (PEPI) Trial, the first multicenter, randomized, double-blind, placebo-control trial of the effects of three estrogen/progestin regimens on risk factors for cardiovascular disease, bone mineral density, and endometrial hyperplasia. The study found that estrogen, alone or in combination with progestin, increased serum levels of HDL and decreased low-density lipoprotein (LDL) and fibrinogen levels. While unopposed estrogen (without progestins) resulted in the most beneficial effects on lipids, it was also associated with an increased risk of endometrial hyperplasia.

In 1992, the NIH funded the Women's Health Initiative (WHI), a study of the health of postmenopausal women. The WHI, the largest research study ever funded by the NIH, involves over 160,000 postmenopausal women participating at 45 clinical centers across the United States through the year 2002. The WHI study includes both a prospective observational study and an interventional randomized trial involving over 63,000 women, which is designed to test the effects of a low-fat diet, hormone replacement therapy, and calcium and vitamin

D supplementation on the risks for cardiovascular disease, breast cancer, and osteoporotic fractures.

Many other studies currently in progress promise new insights into the health of women within the next decade.

Pharmacologic Studies   Historically, women have been underrepresented in drug trials, even though the majority of pharmaceuticals sold in the United States each year are used by women. However, this has been rapidly changing. The FDA requires information on the safety and effectiveness of experimental drugs in women, on the effects of the menstrual cycle and menopause on a drug's pharmacokinetics, and on a drug's influence on the effectiveness of oral contraceptives. The increased emphasis on entering women into drug trials is likely to yield important information. Studies that have included women indicate that there are clinically significant differences in the way women respond to a number of frequently prescribed pharmaceuticals, including sedative-hypnotics, antidepressants, antipsychotics, anticonvulsants, and β-adrenergic blocking agents. The 1992 FDA Adverse Experience Report found that women have a higher frequency of adverse drug reactions than men. Other studies suggest that the efficacy of many drugs may be different in women compared to men. For example, women require lower doses of neuroleptics to control schizophrenia than men do. Women awaken from anesthesia faster than do men who are given the same doses of anesthetics, and they have a more powerful response to certain classes of analgesics than men. The reasons for these differences are not clear. However, these observations have spurred researchers to consider separating out the effects of gender in future clinical research in an effort to define "gender-based" biologic processes.

CONCLUSION   At the same time that the health of women is undergoing more rigorous study and women's clinics are becoming increasingly common and popular, a growing fraction of health professionals are women. The number of women physicians has increased by 300% between 1970 and 1990, and more than 40% of all U.S. medical students now are women. This infusion of women into the physician work force is likely to lead to a still greater recognition of the unique aspects of health and disease in women.

BIBLIOGRAPHY

CDC FACT SHEET, September 99. HIV/AIDS among U.S. women: Minority and young women at continuing risk. www.cdc.gov/nchstp/hiv_aids/pubs/facts/women.htm

COLDITZ GA: The Nurses' Health Study: A cohort of U.S. women followed since 1976. J Am Med Women's Assoc 50:40, 1995

COUNCIL ON SCIENTIFIC AFFAIRS, AMERICAN MEDICAL ASSOCIATION: Violence against women. Relevance for medical practitioners. JAMA 267:3184, 1992

GIJSBERS VAN WIJK CMT et al: Symptom sensitivity and sex differences in physical morbidity: A review of health surveys in the United States and the Netherlands. Women Health 17:91, 1991

HULLY S et al: Randomized trial of estrogen plus progestin for secondary prevention of coronary heart disease in postmenopausal women. Heart and Estrogen/Progestin Replacement Study (HERS) Research Group. JAMA 280: 605, 1998

KAPLAN NM: The treatment of hypertension in women. Arch Intern Med 185:563, 1995

MINKOFF HL, DEHOVITZ JA: Care of women infected with the human immunodeficiency virus. JAMA 266:2253, 1991

MURABITO JM: Women and cardiovascular disease: Contributions from the Framingham Heart Study. J Am Med Women's Assoc 50:35, 1995

MUSTARD CA et al: Sex differences in the use of health care services. N Engl J Med 338: 1678, 1998

RICH-EDWARDS JW et al: The primary prevention of coronary heart disease in women. N Engl J Med 332:1758, 1995

RODIN J, ICKOVICS JR: Women's health. Review and research agenda as we approach the 21st century. Am Psychol 45:1018, 1990

SHAYWITZ SE et al: Effects of estrogen on brain activation patterns in postmenopausal women during working memory tasks. JAMA 281:1197, 1999

VERBRUGGE LM, WINGARD DL: Sex differentials in health and mortality. Women Health 12:103, 1987

WEISSMAN MM, OLFSON M: Depression in women: Implications for health care research. Science 269:799, 1995

WINKLEBY MA et al: Ethnic and socioeconomic differences in cardiovascular disease risk factors: findings for women from the Third National Health and Nutrition Examination Survey, 1988–1994. JAMA 280:356, 1998

WRITING GROUP FOR THE PEPI TRIAL: Effects of estrogen or estrogen/progestin regimens on heart disease risk factors in postmenopausal women: The Postmenopausal Estrogen/Progestin Interventions Trial. JAMA 273:199, 1995

Robert L. Barbieri, John T. Repke

7 MEDICAL DISORDERS DURING PREGNANCY

Approximately 4 million births occur in the United States each year. A significant proportion of these are complicated by one or more medical disorders. Two decades ago, many medical disorders were contraindications to pregnancy. Advances in obstetrics, neonatology, obstetric anesthesiology, and medicine have increased the expectation that pregnancy will result in an excellent outcome for both mother and fetus despite most of these conditions. Successful pregnancy requires important physiologic adaptations, such as a marked increase in cardiac output. Medical problems that interfere with the physiologic adaptations of pregnancy increase the risk for poor pregnancy outcome; conversely, in some instances pregnancy may adversely impact an underlying medical disorder.

HYPERTENSION (See also Chap. 246)

In pregnancy, cardiac output increases by 40%, most of which is due to an increase in stroke volume. Heart rate increases by approximately 10 beats per minute during the third trimester. In the second trimester of pregnancy, systemic vascular resistance decreases and this is associated with a fall in blood pressure. During pregnancy, a blood pressure of 140/90 mmHg is considered to be abnormally elevated and is associated with a marked increase in perinatal morbidity and mortality. In all pregnant women, the measurement of blood pressure should be performed in the sitting position, because for many the lateral recumbent position is associated with a blood pressure lower than that recorded in the sitting position. The diagnosis of hypertension requires the measurement of two elevated blood pressures, at least 6 h apart. Hypertension during pregnancy is usually caused by preeclampsia, chronic hypertension, gestational hypertension, or renal disease.

PREECLAMPSIA   Approximately 5 to 7% of all pregnant women develop *preeclampsia*, the new onset of hypertension (blood pressure > 140/90 mmHg), proteinuria (>300 mg per 24 h), and pathologic edema. Although the precise placental factors that cause preeclampsia are unknown, the end result is vasospasm and endothelial injury in multiple organs. Preeclampsia is associated with abnormalities of cerebral circulatory autoregulation, which increase the risk of stroke at near-normal blood pressures. Risk factors for the development of preeclampsia include nulliparity, diabetes mellitus, a history of renal disease or chronic hypertension, a prior history of preeclampsia, extremes of maternal age (>35 years or <15 years), obesity, factor V Leiden mutation, angiotensinogen gene T235, antiphospholipid antibody syndrome, and multiple gestation.

There are no well-established strategies for the prevention of preeclampsia. Clinical trials have demonstrated that low-dose aspirin treatment does *not* prevent preeclampsia in either low- or high-risk women. Two meta-analyses reported that dietary calcium supplementation appeared to be effective in reducing the risk of developing preeclampsia. Subsequently, however, a large randomized clinical trial in low-risk women did not demonstrate a protective effect of calcium supplementation. Therefore, calcium supplementation may be considered in women at high risk for preeclampsia (see above). The observation that dietary intervention may reduce the risk of hypertension in men and nonpregnant women raises the possibility that dietary manipulations will be discovered that reduce the risk of preeclampsia.

Severe preeclampsia is the presence of new-onset hypertension and proteinuria accompanied by central nervous system dysfunction (headaches, blurred vision, seizures, coma), marked elevations of blood pressure (>160/110 mmHg), severe proteinuria (>5 g per 24 h), oliguria or renal failure, pulmonary edema, hepatocellular injury (ALT > 2× the upper limits of normal), thrombocytopenia (platelet count < 100,000/μL), or disseminated intravascular coagulation. Women with *mild preeclampsia* are those with the diagnosis of new-onset hypertension, proteinuria, and edema without evidence of severe pre-eclampsia. The *HELLP* (*h*emolysis, *e*levated *l*iver enzymes, *l*ow *p*latelets) syndrome is a special subgroup of severe preeclampsia and is a major cause of morbidity and mortality in this disease. The presence of platelet dysfunction and coagulation disorders further increases the risk of stroke.

℞ **TREATMENT**   Preeclampsia resolves within a few weeks after delivery. For pregnant women with preeclampsia prior to 37 weeks' gestation, delivery reduces the mother's morbidity but exposes the fetus to the risk of premature delivery. The management of pre-eclampsia is challenging because it requires the clinician to balance the health of both mother and fetus simultaneously and to make management decisions that afford both the best opportunities for infant survival. In general, prior to term, women with *mild* preeclampsia can be managed conservatively with bed rest, close monitoring of blood pressure and renal function, and careful fetal surveillance. For women with *severe* preeclampsia, delivery is recommended after 32 weeks' gestation. This reduces maternal morbidity and slightly increases the risks associated with prematurity for the newborn. Prior to 32 weeks' gestation, the risks of prematurity for the fetus are great, and some authorities recommend conservative management to allow for continued fetal maturation. Expectant management of severe preeclampsia remote from term affords some benefits for the fetus with significant risks for the mother. Such management should be restricted to tertiary care centers where maternal-fetal medicine, neonatal medicine, and critical care medicine expertise are available.

The definitive treatment of preeclampsia is delivery of the fetus and placenta. For women with severe preeclampsia, aggressive management of blood pressures > 160/110 mmHg reduces the risk of cerebrovascular accidents.

Intravenous labetalol or hydralazine are the drugs most commonly used to manage preeclampsia. Alternative agents such as calcium channel blockers may be used. Elevated arterial pressure should be reduced slowly to avoid hypotension and a decrease in blood flow to the fetus. *Angiotensin-converting enzyme (ACE) inhibitors as well as angiotensin-receptor blockers should be avoided in the second and third trimesters of pregnancy because of their adverse effects on fetal development.* Pregnant women treated with ACE inhibitors often develop oligohydramnios, which may be caused by decreased fetal renal function.

Magnesium sulfate is the treatment of choice for the prevention and treatment of eclamptic seizures. Two large randomized clinical trials have demonstrated the superiority of magnesium sulfate over phenytoin and diazepam. Magnesium may prevent seizures by interacting with *N*-methyl-D-asparate (NMDA) receptors in the central nervous system. Given the difficulty of predicting eclamptic seizures on the basis of disease severity, it is recommended that once the decision to proceed with delivery is made, all patients carrying a diagnosis of preeclampsia be treated with magnesium sulfate (see Guideline).

CHRONIC ESSENTIAL HYPERTENSION   Pregnancy complicated by chronic essential hypertension is associated with intrauterine growth restriction and increased perinatal mortality. Pregnant women with chronic hypertension are at increased risk for superimposed preeclampsia and abruptio placenta. Women with chronic hypertension should have a thorough prepregnancy evaluation, both to identify remediable causes of hypertension and to ensure that the

Regimens for the Administration of Magnesium Sulfate for Seizure Prophylaxis in Women in Labor with Preeclampsia

Intramuscular	Intravenous
10 g (5 g IM deep in each buttock)[a]	6-g bolus over 15 min
5 g IM deep q4h, alternating sides	1–3 g/h by continuous infusion pump
	May be mixed in 100 mL crystalloid; if given by intravenous push, make up as 20% solution; push at maximum rate of 1g/min
	40-g $MgSO_4 \cdot 7H_2O$ in 1000 mL Ringers lactate; run at 25–75 mL/h (1–3 g/h)[a]

[a] Made up as 50% solution

prescribed antihypertensive agents are not associated with adverse pregnancy outcome (e.g., ACE inhibitors, angiotensin-receptor blockers). α-Methyldopa and labetalol are the most commonly used medications for the treatment of chronic hypertension in pregnancy. Baseline evaluation of renal function is necessary to help differentiate the effects of chronic hypertension versus superimposed preeclampsia should the hypertension worsen during pregnancy. There are no convincing data that demonstrate that treatment of mild chronic hypertension improves perinatal outcome.

GESTATIONAL HYPERTENSION   This is the development of elevated blood pressure during pregnancy or in the first 24 h post partum in the absence of preexisting chronic hypertension and other signs of preeclampsia. Uncomplicated gestational hypertension that does not progress to preeclampsia has not been associated with adverse pregnancy outcome or adverse long-term prognosis.

RENAL DISEASE (See also Chap. 268)

Normal pregnancy is characterized by an increase in glomerular filtration rate and creatinine clearance. This occurs secondary to a rise in renal plasma flow and increase glomerular filtration pressures. Patients with underlying renal disease and hypertension may expect a worsening of hypertension during pregnancy. If superimposed preeclampsia develops, the additional endothelial injury results in a capillary leak syndrome that may make the management of these patients challenging. In general, patients with underlying renal disease and hypertension benefit from more aggressive management of blood pressure than do those with gestational hypertension. Preconception counseling is also essential for these patients so that accurate risk assessment can occur prior to the establishment of pregnancy and important medication changes and adjustments be made. In general, a prepregnancy serum creatinine level <133 μmol/L (<1.5 mg/dL) is associated with a favorable prognosis. When renal disease worsens during pregnancy, close collaboration between the nephrologist and the maternal-fetal medicine specialist is essential so that decisions regarding delivery can be weighed in the context of sequelae of prematurity for the neonate versus long-term sequelae for the mother with respect to future renal function.

Successful pregnancy after renal transplantation has been reported increasingly. Predictors for success include a normal-functioning transplanted kidney, absence of rejection for at least 2 years prior to the pregnancy, absence of hypertension, and preferably minimal doses of immunosuppressant medications. Pregnancies in women using cyclosporine are more likely to be complicated by renal insufficiency and/or the development of hypertension. Such patients require very careful maternal and fetal surveillance. Nearly half of these pregnancies deliver preterm, and 20% of neonates are small for their gestational age. Rejection occurs in approximately 10% of pregnancies, and approximately 15% of patients will have deterioration in their renal function that persists after delivery. While pregnancy is generally well tolerated in renal transplant recipients, controversy remains as to whether or not deterioration of graft function is accelerated by pregnancy. More aggressive management of blood pressure has been suggested in this group of patients in an effort to protect the grafted kidney.

Another subset of patients with chronic renal disease and hypertension are those patients whose pregnancies are complicated by systemic lupus erythematosus (SLE) (Chap. 311). In the past, SLE was considered to be a contraindication to pregnancy. With improved understanding of the effects of SLE on pregnancy, and vice versa, and with improved pharmacologic methods for managing SLE, successful pregnancy outcome is likely. Good prognostic factors for establishment of pregnancy in the presence of SLE are as follows:

1. Disease quiescence > 6 months
2. Normal blood pressure (with or without medication)
3. Normal renal function [creatinine < 133 μmol/L (< 1.5 mg/dL)]
4. Absence of antiphospholipid antibodies
5. Minimal or no need for immunosuppressive drugs
6. Absence of prior adverse reproductive outcome

Previously a point of controversy, there is now increasing consensus that pregnancy and the postpartum period are times of increased lupus activity. In severe flares early in gestation, pregnancy termination is often recommended. If pregnancy termination is not an option, then medical therapy to manage the lupus flare should not be influenced by the pregnancy, provided informed consent for treatment is obtained from the patient. Pulsed glucocorticoid therapy, azathioprine, hydroxychloroquine, and cyclophosphamide have all been used successfully in pregnancy.

CARDIAC DISEASE

VALVULAR HEART DISEASE (See also Chap. 236) This is the most common cardiac problem complicating pregnancy.

Mitral Stenosis This is the valvular disease most likely to cause death during pregnancy. The pregnancy-induced increase in blood volume and cardiac output can cause pulmonary edema in women with mitral stenosis. Pregnancy associated with long-standing mitral stenosis may result in pulmonary hypertension. Sudden death has been reported when hypovolemia has been allowed to occur in this condition. Careful control of heart rate, especially during labor and delivery, minimizes the impact of tachycardia and reduced ventricular filling times on cardiac function. Pregnant women with mitral stenosis are at increased risk for the development of atrial fibrillation and other tachyarrhythmias. Medical management of severe mitral stenosis and atrial fibrillation with digoxin and beta blockers is recommended. Balloon valvulotomy can be carried out during pregnancy.

Mitral Regurgitation and Aortic Regurgitation These are both generally well tolerated during pregnancy. The pregnancy-induced decrease in systemic vascular resistance reduces the risk of cardiac failure with these conditions. As a rule, mitral valve prolapse does not present problems for the pregnant patient and aortic stenosis, unless very severe, is also well tolerated. In the most severe cases of aortic stenosis, limitation of activity or balloon valvuloplasty may be indicated.

For women with artificial valves contemplating pregnancy, it is important that warfarin be stopped and heparin initiated prior to conception. Warfarin therapy during the first trimester of pregnancy has been associated with fetal chondrodysplasia punctata. In the second and third trimester of pregnancy, warfarin may cause fetal optic atrophy and mental retardation.

CONGENITAL HEART DISEASE (See also Chap. 234) The presence of a congenital cardiac lesion in the mother increases the risk of congenital cardiac disease in the newborn. Prenatal screening of the fetus for congenital cardiac disease with ultrasound is recommended. Atrial or ventricular septal defect is usually well tolerated during pregnancy in the absence of pulmonary hypertension, provided that the woman's prepregnancy cardiac status is favorable. Use of air filters on intravenous sets during labor and delivery in patients with intracardiac shunts is generally recommended.

OTHER CARDIAC DISORDERS Supraventricular tachycardia (Chap. 230) is a common cardiac complication of pregnancy. Treatment is the same as in the nonpregnant patient, and fetal tolerance of medications such as adenosine and calcium channel blockers is acceptable. When necessary, electrocardioversion may be performed and is generally well tolerated by mother and fetus.

Peripartum cardiomyopathy (Chap. 238) is a rare disorder of pregnancy associated with myocarditis, and its etiology remains unknown. Treatment is directed toward symptomatic relief and improvement of cardiac function. Many patients recover completely; others are left with a progressive dilated cardiomyopathy. Recurrence in a subsequent pregnancy has been reported, and women should be counseled to avoid pregnancy after a diagnosis of peripartum cardiomyopathy.

SPECIFIC HIGH RISK CARDIAC LESIONS **Marfan Syndrome** (See also Chap. 351) This is an autosomal dominant disease, associated with a high risk of maternal morbidity. Approximately 15% of pregnant women with Marfan syndrome develop a major cardiovascular manifestation during pregnancy, with almost all women surviving. An aortic root diameter <40 mm is considered to be associated with a favorable outcome of pregnancy. Prophylactic therapy with beta blockers has been advocated, although large-scale clinical trials in pregnancy have not been performed.

Pulmonary Hypertension (See also Chap. 260) Maternal mortality in the setting of severe pulmonary hypertension is high, and primary pulmonary hypertension is a contraindication to pregnancy. Termination of pregnancy may be advisable in these circumstances to preserve the life of the mother. In the Eisenmenger syndrome, i.e., the combination of pulmonary hypertension with right-to-left shunting due to congenital abnormalities (Chap. 234), maternal and fetal death occur frequently. Systemic hypotension may occur after blood loss, prolonged Valsalva maneuver, or regional anesthesia; sudden death secondary to hypotension is a dreaded complication. Management of these patients is challenging, and invasive hemodynamic monitoring during labor and delivery is generally recommended.

In patients with pulmonary hypertension, vaginal delivery is less stressful hemodynamically than Cesarean section, which should be reserved for accepted obstetric indications.

DEEP VENOUS THROMBOSIS AND PULMONARY EMBOLISM
(See also Chaps. 248 and 261)

A hypercoagulable state is characteristic of pregnancy, and deep venous thrombosis (DVT) is a common complication. Indeed, pulmonary embolism is the most common cause of maternal death in the United States. Activated protein C resistance caused by the factor V Leiden mutation increases the risk for DVT and pulmonary embolism during pregnancy. Approximately 25% of women with DVT during pregnancy carry the factor V Leiden allele. The presence of the factor V Leiden mutation also increases the risk for severe preeclampsia. If the fetus carries a factor V Leiden mutation, the risk of extensive placental infarction is very high. Additional genetic mutations associated with DVT during pregnancy include the prothrombin G20210A mutation (heterozygotes and homozygotes) and the methylenetetrahydrofolate reductase C677T mutation (homozygotes).

℞ **TREATMENT** Aggressive diagnosis and management of DVT and suspected pulmonary embolism optimize the outcome for mother and fetus. In general, all diagnostic and therapeutic modalities afforded the nonpregnant patient should be utilized in pregnancy. Anticoagulant therapy with heparin is indicated in pregnant women with DVT. Warfarin therapy is contraindicated in the first trimester due to its association with fetal chondrodysplasia punctata. In the second and third trimesters, warfarin may cause fetal optic atrophy and mental retardation. In the initial treatment of DVT, heparin, which does not cross the placenta, may be administered as an intravenous bolus of approximately 100 IU per kilogram of body weight. Continuous heparin infusion is generally initiated at 1000 IU/h and then titrated to achieve a target activated partial thromboplastin time of 50 to 80 s. After initial intravenous anticoagulation, intermittent subcutaneous heparin therapy with 10,000 IU two or three times daily may be employed. When deep venous thromboembolism occurs in the postpartum period, heparin therapy for 7 to 10 days may be followed by warfarin therapy for 3 to 6 months. Warfarin is not contraindicated in breast-feeding women.

Low-molecular-weight heparins are of sufficient size and charge that they do not cross the placenta and may be substituted for unfractionated heparin in the pregnant patient. Recent concerns about low-molecular-weight heparin use and epidural hematoma suggest that caution be used in the anesthetic management of patients who had been receiving low-molecular-weight heparin near the onset of labor.

ENDOCRINE DISORDERS

DIABETES MELLITUS (See also Chap. 333)   In pregnancy, the fetoplacental unit induces major metabolic changes, the purpose of which is to shunt glucose and amino acids to the fetus while the mother uses ketones and triglycerides to fuel her metabolic needs. These metabolic changes are accompanied by maternal insulin resistance, caused in part by placental production of steroids, a growth hormone variant, and placental lactogen. Although pregnancy has been referred to as a state of accelerated starvation, it is better characterized as accelerated ketosis. In pregnancy, after an overnight fast, plasma glucose is lower by 0.8 to 1.1 mmol/L (15 to 20 mg/dL) than in the nonpregnant state. This is due to the use of glucose by the fetus. In early pregnancy, fasting may result in circulating glucose concentrations in the range of 2.2 mmol/L (40 mg/dL) and may be associated with symptoms of hypoglycemia. In contrast to the decrease in maternal glucose concentration, plasma hydroxybutyrate and acetoacetate levels rise to two to four times normal after a fast.

℞ **TREATMENT**   Pregnancy complicated by diabetes mellitus is associated with higher maternal and perinatal morbidity and mortality rates. Preconception counseling and treatment are important for the diabetic patient contemplating pregnancy. Optimizing preconception glucose control and attention to other dietary needs such as appropriate levels of folate can significantly reduce the risk of congenital fetal malformations. Folate supplementation reduces the incidence of fetal neural tube defects, which occur with greater frequency in fetuses of diabetic mothers. In addition, optimizing glucose control during key periods of organogenesis reduces other congenital anomalies including sacral agenesis, caudal dysplasia, renal agenesis, and ventricular septal defect.

Once pregnancy is established, glucose control should be managed more aggressively than in the nonpregnant state. In addition to dietary changes, this requires more frequent blood glucose monitoring and often involves additional injections of insulin or conversion to an insulin pump. Fasting blood glucose levels should be maintained at <5.8 mmol/L (<105 mg/dL) with no values exceeding 7.8 mmol/L (140 mg/dL). Commencing in the third trimester, regular surveillance of maternal glucose control as well as assessment of fetal growth (obstetric sonography) and fetoplacental oxygenation (fetal heart rate monitoring or biophysical profile) optimize pregnancy outcome. Pregnant diabetic patients without vascular disease are at greater risk for delivering a macrosomic fetus, and attention to fetal growth via clinical and ultrasound examinations is important. Fetal macrosomia is associated with an increased risk of maternal and fetal birth trauma. Pregnant women with diabetes have an increased risk of developing preeclampsia, and those with vascular disease are at greater risk for developing intrauterine growth restriction, which is associated with an increased risk of fetal and neonatal death. Excellent pregnancy outcomes in patients with diabetic nephropathy and proliferative retinopathy have been reported with aggressive glucose control and intensive maternal and fetal surveillance.

Glycemic control may become more difficult to achieve as pregnancy progresses. Because of delayed pulmonary maturation of the fetuses of diabetic mothers, early delivery should be avoided unless there is biochemical evidence of fetal lung maturity. In general, efforts to control glucose and maintain the pregnancy until the estimated date of delivery result in the best overall outcome for both mother and newborn.

GESTATIONAL DIABETES   All pregnant women should be screened for gestational diabetes unless they are in a low-risk group. Women at low risk for gestational diabetes are those <25 years of age; those with a body mass index < 25 kg/m², no maternal history of macrosomia or gestational diabetes, and no diabetes in a first-degree relative; and those not members of a high-risk ethnic group (African American, Hispanic, Native American). A typical two-step strategy for establishing the diagnosis of gestational diabetes involves administration of a 50-g oral glucose challenge with a single serum glucose measurement at 60 min. If the serum glucose is < 7.8 mmol/L (<140 mg/dL), the test is considered normal. Serum glucose > 7.8 mmol/L (>140 mg/dL) warrants administration of a 100-g oral glucose challenge with serum glucose measurements obtained in the fasting state, and at 1, 2, and 3 h. Normal values are serum glucose concentrations <5.8 mmol/L (<105 mg/dL), 10.5 mmol/L (190 mg/dL), 9.1 mmol/L (165 mg/dL), and 8.0 mmol/L (145 mg/dL), respectively.

Pregnant women with gestational diabetes are at increased risk of preeclampsia, delivering infants who are large for their gestational age, and birth lacerations. Their fetuses are at risk of hypoglycemia and birth trauma (brachial plexus) injury.

℞ **TREATMENT**   Gestational diabetes is first treated with dietary measures. Inability to maintain fasting glucose concentrations <5.8 mmol/L (<105 mg/dL) or 2-h postprandial glucose concentrations <6.7 mmol/L (<120 mg/dL) should prompt initiation of insulin therapy. Oral agents should not be used to treat diabetes in pregnancy. Patients with a diagnosis of gestational diabetes will benefit from postpartum follow-up as they are at increased risk for developing type 2 diabetes.

THYROID DISEASE (See also Chap. 330)   In pregnancy, the estrogen-induced increase in thyroxine-binding globulin causes an increase in circulating levels of total T_3 and total T_4. The normal range of circulating levels of free T_4, free T_3, and thyroid stimulating hormone (TSH) remain unaltered by pregnancy.

The thyroid gland normally enlarges during pregnancy. Maternal hyperthyroidism occurs at a rate of approximately 2 per 1000 pregnancies and is generally well tolerated by pregnant women. Clinical signs and symptoms should alert the physician to the occurrence of this disease. Many of the physiologic adaptations to pregnancy may mimic subtle signs of hyperthyroidism. Although pregnant women are able to tolerate mild hyperthyroidism without adverse sequelae, more severe hyperthyroidism can cause spontaneous abortion or premature labor, and thyroid storm is associated with a significant risk of maternal mortality.

℞ **TREATMENT**   *Hyperthyroidism* in pregnancy should be aggressively evaluated and treated. The treatment of choice is propylthiouracil. Because it crosses the placenta, the minimum effective dose should be used to maintain free T_4 in the upper normal range. Methimazole crosses the placenta to a greater degree than propylthiouracil and has been associated with fetal aplasia cutis. Radioiodine should not be used during pregnancy, either for scanning or treatment, because of effects on the fetal thyroid. In emergent circumstances, additional treatment with beta blockers and a saturated solution of potassium iodide may be necessary. Hyperthyroidism is most difficult to control in the first trimester of pregnancy and easiest to control in the third trimester.

The goal of therapy for *hypothyroidism* is to maintain the serum TSH in the normal range, and thyroxine is the drug of choice. Children born to women with an elevated serum TSH (and a normal total thyroxine) during pregnancy have impaired performance on neuropsychologic tests. During pregnancy, the dose of thyroxine required to keep the TSH in the normal range rises. In one study, the mean replacement dose of thyroxine required to maintain the TSH in the normal range was 0.1 mg daily before pregnancy, and it increased to 0.15 mg daily during pregnancy.

DISORDERS OF CALCIUM METABOLISM (See also Chap. 340) Serum *total* calcium concentration decreases throughout gestation due to a reduction in serum albumin concentration, while serum *ionized* calcium remains unchanged during pregnancy. Circulating parathyroid hormone concentration is slightly reduced throughout the course of pregnancy. Pregnancy has been described as a state of physiologic absorptive hypercalciuria. Estrogen and increased production of 1,25-dihydroxyvitamin D by both the kidney and the placenta mediate the increased absorption of calcium during pregnancy. Due to the fetal requirements for calcium, the National Institutes of Health has recommended that pregnant women receive 1500 mg/d of elemental calcium, slightly higher than the recommended daily intake of 1200 mg/d for nonpregnant adults.

HEMATOLOGIC DISORDERS

Pregnancy has been described as a state of physiologic anemia. Part of the reduction in hemoglobin concentration is dilutional, but iron and folate deficiencies are the major causes of correctable anemia during pregnancy. Folic acid food supplementation implemented in 1998 has reduced the risk of fetal neural tube defects.

In populations at high risk for hemoglobinopathies (Chap. 106), hemoglobin electrophoresis should be performed as part of the prenatal screen. Hemoglobinopathies can be associated with increased maternal and fetal morbidity and mortality. Management is tailored to the specific hemoglobinopathy and is generally the same for both pregnant and nonpregnant women. Prenatal diagnosis of hemoglobinopathies in the fetus is readily available and should be discussed with prospective parents either prior to or early in pregnancy.

Thrombocytopenia occurs commonly during pregnancy. The majority of cases are benign gestational thrombocytopenias, but the differential diagnosis should include immune thrombocytopenia (Chap. 116) and preeclampsia. Maternal thrombocytopenia may also be caused by catastrophic obstetric events such as retention of a dead fetus, sepsis, abruptio placenta, and amniotic fluid embolism.

NEOPLASTIC DISEASES

Maternal neoplasms are rarely, if ever, transmitted to the fetus. The three most common cancers in pregnant women are cervical cancer (~1 case per 1000 pregnancies, depending on the country), breast cancer (~2 cases per 10,000 pregnancies), and lymphomas (Hodgkin's disease or non-Hodgkin's lymphomas). Cervical cancer may be missed when its early sign, vaginal bleeding, is attributed to the pregnancy. Pregnant women with vaginal bleeding should be examined, and suspicious cervical lesions biopsied. Conization is generally performed only after the first trimester because of the abortion risk.

Breast lumps may also be attributed to change associated with pregnancy. However, women with a dominant mass should undergo diagnostic evaluation (mammogram, ultrasound, biopsy). Resection of the primary lesion is safe, but radiation therapy is unsafe at any time during pregnancy. The fetus cannot be shielded from internal scattering of radiation; therapeutic doses are associated with spontaneous abortion, increased perinatal death, and defects in central nervous system and/or cognitive function. Tamoxifen is not safe for pregnant women.

Lymphoma is usually diagnosed on the basis of adenopathy or constitutional symptoms (fever, sweats, or weight loss). Staging eval-

uation is not undertaken during the first trimester; women in the first trimester should be counseled about termination of the pregnancy. Single-agent chemotherapy can be used in the second or third trimester as a temporizing measure. Vinblastine or doxorubicin have been used most commonly. Early induction of labor may permit the physician to maximize the survival chances of both the fetus and the mother. Survival rates for 28-week-old fetuses are about 75% and about 90% for 32-week-old fetuses.

Cancer survivors of reproductive age may desire children. Pregnancy may increase the risk of melanoma recurrence but does not influence breast cancer recurrence. Cancer treatment may deplete oocytes. Oocyte retrieval and storage of fertilized or nonfertilized eggs before cancer treatment may permit conception after the cancer has been treated successfully.

GASTROINTESTINAL AND LIVER DISEASE

Up to 90% of pregnant women experience nausea and vomiting during the first trimester of pregnancy. Occasionally, hyperemesis gravidarum requires hospitalization to prevent dehydration, and sometimes parenteral nutrition is required.

Crohn's disease may be associated with exacerbations in the second and third trimesters. Ulcerative colitis is associated with disease exacerbations in the first trimester and during the early postpartum period. Medical management of these diseases during pregnancy is identical to the management in the nonpregnant state (Chap. 287).

Exacerbation of gall bladder disease is commonly observed during pregnancy. In part this may be due to pregnancy-induced alteration in the metabolism of bile and fatty acids. Intrahepatic cholestasis of pregnancy is generally a third-trimester event. Profound pruritus may accompany this condition and may be associated with increased fetal mortality. It has been suggested that placental bile salt deposition may contribute to progressive uteroplacental insufficiency. Therefore, regular fetal surveillance should be undertaken once the diagnosis of intrahepatic cholestasis is made. Favorable results with ursodiol have been reported.

Acute fatty liver is a rare complication of pregnancy. Frequently confused with the HELLP syndrome (see "Preeclampsia," above) and severe preeclampsia, the diagnosis of acute fatty liver of pregnancy may be facilitated by imaging studies and laboratory evaluation. Acute fatty liver of pregnancy is generally characterized by markedly increased levels of bilirubin and ammonia and by hypoglycemia. Management of acute fatty liver of pregnancy is supportive; recurrence in subsequent pregnancies has been reported.

All pregnant women should be screened for hepatitis B. This information is important for pediatricians after delivery of the infant. All infants receive hepatitis B vaccine. Infants born to mothers who are carriers of hepatitis B surface antigen should also receive hepatitis B immune globulin as soon after birth as possible and preferably within the first 72 h.

INFECTIONS

BACTERIAL INFECTIONS Other than bacterial vaginosis, the most common bacterial infections during pregnancy involve the urinary tract (Chap. 280). Many pregnant women have asymptomatic bacteriuria, most likely due to stasis caused by progestational effects on ureteral and bladder smooth muscle and to compression effects of the enlarging uterus. In itself, this condition is not associated with an adverse outcome of pregnancy. However, if asymptomatic bacteriuria is left untreated, symptomatic pyelonephritis may occur. Indeed, approximately 75% of cases of pregnancy-associated pyelonephritis are the result of untreated asymptomatic bacteriuria. All pregnant women should be screened with a urine culture for asymptomatic bacteriuria at the first prenatal visit. Subsequent screening with nitrite/leukocyte esterase strips is indicated for high-risk women, such as those with sickle cell trait or a history of urinary tract infections. All women with positive screens should be treated.

Because of the association between bacterial vaginosis and preterm delivery, screening for bacterial vaginosis has been used in an effort to reduce risk. However, standard treatment for bacterial vaginosis does not reduce the risk of preterm delivery.

Abdominal pain and fever during pregnancy create a clinical dilemma. The diagnosis of greatest concern is intrauterine amniotic infection. While amniotic infection most commonly follows rupture of the membranes, this is not always the case. In general, antibiotic therapy is not recommended as a temporizing measure in these circumstances. If intrauterine infection is suspected, induced delivery with concomitant antibiotic therapy is generally indicated. Intrauterine amniotic infection is most often caused by pathogens such as *Escherichia coli* and group B streptococcus. In high-risk patients at term or in preterm patients, routine intrapartum prophylaxis of group B streptococcal disease is recommended. Penicillin G and ampicillin are the drugs of choice. In penicillin-allergic patients, clindamycin is recommended.

Postpartum infection is a significant cause of maternal morbidity and mortality. While rare after vaginal delivery, postpartum endomyometritis develops in 5% of patients having elective repeat cesarean section and in 25% of patients after emergency cesarean section following prolonged labor. Prophylactic antibiotics should be given to all patients undergoing cesarean section. As most cases of postpartum endomyometritis are polymicrobial, broad-spectrum antibiotic coverage with a penicillin, aminoglycoside, and metronidazole is recommended (Chap. 167). Most cases resolve within 72 h. Women who do not respond to antibiotic treatment for postpartum endomyometritis should be evaluated for septic pelvic thrombophlebitis. Imaging studies may be helpful in establishing the diagnosis, which is primarily a clinical diagnosis of exclusion. Patients with septic pelvic thrombophlebitis generally have tachycardia out of proportion to their fever and respond rapidly to intravenous administration of heparin.

All patients are screened prenatally for gonorrhea and chlamydial infections, and the detection of either should result in prompt treatment. Ceftriaxone and azithromycin are the agents of choice (Chaps. 147 and 179).

VIRAL INFECTIONS   **Cytomegalovirus Infection**   Viral infection in pregnancy presents a significant challenge. The most common cause of congenital viral infection in the United States is cytomegalovirus (CMV) (Chap. 185). As many as 50 to 90% of women of childbearing age have antibodies to CMV, but only rarely does CMV reactivation result in neonatal infection. More commonly, primary CMV infection during pregnancy creates a risk of congenital CMV. No currently accepted treatment of CMV during pregnancy has been demonstrated to protect the fetus effectively. Moreover, it is impossible to predict which fetus will sustain life-threatening CMV infection. Severe CMV disease in the newborn is characterized most often by petechiae, hepatosplenomegaly, and jaundice. Chorioretinitis, microcephaly, intracranial calcifications, hepatitis, hemolytic anemia, and purpura may also develop. Central nervous system involvement resulting in the development of psychomotor, ocular, auditory, and dental abnormalities over time have been described.

Rubella (See also Chap. 195)   Rubella virus is a known teratogen; first-trimester rubella carries a high risk of fetal anomalies, though the risk decreases significantly later in pregnancy. Congenital rubella may be diagnosed by percutaneous umbilical blood sampling with the detection of IgM antibodies in fetal blood. All pregnant women should be screened for their immune status to rubella. Indeed, all women of childbearing age, regardless of pregnancy status, should have their immune status for rubella verified and be immunized if necessary. The incidence of congenital rubella in the United States is extremely low.

Herpesvirus (See also Chap. 182)   The acquisition of genital herpes during pregnancy is associated with spontaneous abortion, pre-

maturity, and congenital and neonatal herpes. A recent cohort study of pregnant women without evidence of previous herpes infection demonstrated that approximately 2% of the women acquired a new herpes infection during the pregnancy. Approximately 60% of the newly infected women had no clinical symptoms. Infection occurred equally in all three trimesters. If herpes seroconversion occurred early in pregnancy, the risk of transmission to the newborn was very low. In women who acquired genital herpes shortly before delivery, the risk of transmission was high. The risk of active genital herpes lesions at term can be reduced by prescribing acyclovir for the last 4 weeks of pregnancy to women who have had their first episode of genital herpes during the pregnancy. However, whether or not this strategy results in less viral shedding or enhanced fetal protection at delivery remains to be determined.

Herpesvirus infection in the newborn can be devastating. Disseminated neonatal herpes carries with it high mortality and morbidity rates from central nervous system involvement. It is recommended that pregnant women with active genital herpes lesions at the time of presentation in labor be delivered by cesarean section.

Parvovirus (See also Chap. 187)   Parvovirus infection (human parvovirus B19) may occur during pregnancy. It rarely causes sequelae, but susceptible women infected during pregnancy may be at risk for fetal hydrops secondary to erythroid aplasia and profound anemia.

Toxoplasmosis (See also Chap. 217)   In the United States, approximately 70% of women of childbearing age are susceptible to *Toxoplasma*. Most primary infections of toxoplasmosis in the United States come from eating undercooked meat. The diagnosis of congenital toxoplasmosis is possible through sampling of fetal umbilical blood. If there is no evidence of placental/fetal infection, single-drug treatment with spiramycin is recommended. Triple-drug therapy with spiramycin, pyrimethamine, and sulfa is recommended if there is evidence of fetal infection and the woman does not wish to terminate the pregnancy or cannot terminate it because of advanced gestational age. Prenatal treatment has been shown to reduce the number of infants with severe infection.

Human Immunodeficiency Virus (See also Chap. 309)   The predominant cause of HIV infection in children is transmission of the virus from the mother to the newborn during the perinatal period. Exposures, which increase the risk of mother-to-child transmission, include vaginal delivery, preterm delivery, trauma to the fetal skin, and maternal bleeding. Additionally, recent infection with high maternal viral load, low maternal CD4+T cell count, prolonged labor, prolonged length of membrane rupture, and the presence of other genital tract infections, such as syphilis or herpes, increase the risk of transmission. Breast feeding may also transmit HIV to the newborn and is therefore contraindicated in most developed countries for HIV-infected mothers. There is no clear evidence to suggest that the course of HIV disease is altered by pregnancy. There is also no clear evidence to suggest that uncomplicated HIV disease adversely impacts pregnancy other than by its inherent infection risk.

℞ **TREATMENT**   The majority of cases of mother-to-child (vertical) transmission of HIV-1 occur during the intrapartum period. Mechanisms of vertical transmission include infection after rupture of the membranes and direct contact of the fetus with infected secretions or blood from the maternal genital tract. In women with HIV infection who are not receiving antiretroviral therapy, the rate of vertical transmission is approximately 25%. Cesarean section and treatment with zidovudine, administered both before and during delivery, decrease the rate of vertical transmission. In a meta-analysis, zidovudine treatment of both the mother during the prenatal and intrapartum periods and of the neonate at birth reduced the risk of vertical transmission to 7.3%. The combination of elective cesarean section plus zidovudine treatment reduced the risk of vertical transmission to 2%. The role of multiple drug therapy during pregnancy has not yet been established, pending safety data for the neonate.

SUMMARY

Maternal mortality has decreased steadily during the past 60 years. The maternal death rate has decreased from nearly 600/100,000 live births in 1935 to 8.5/100,000 live births in 1996. The most common causes of maternal death in the United States today are, in decreasing order of frequency, thromboembolic disease, hypertension, ectopic pregnancy, and hemorrhage. With improved diagnostic and therapeutic modalities as well as with advances in the treatment of infertility, more patients with medical complications will be seeking, and be in need of, complex obstetric care. Improving outcome of pregnancy in these women will be best obtained by assembling a team of internists and specialists in maternal-fetal medicine (high-risk obstetrics) to counsel these patients about the risks of pregnancy and to plan their treatment prior to conception. The importance of preconception counseling cannot be overstated. It is the responsibility of all physicians caring for women in the reproductive age group to assess their patient's reproductive plans as part of their overall health evaluation.

BIBLIOGRAPHY

Brown ZA et al: The acquisition of herpes simplex virus during pregnancy. N Engl J Med 337:509, 1997

Caritis S et al: Low dose aspirin to prevent preeclampsia in women at high risk. N Engl J Med 338:701, 1998

Gleicher N (ed): *Principles and Practice of Medical Therapy in Pregnancy*, 3d ed. Stamford, CT, Appleton/Lange, 1998

Haddow JE et al: Maternal thyroid deficiency during pregnancy and subsequent neuropsychological development of the child. N Engl J Med 41:549, 1999

Hirsch DR et al: Pulmonary embolism and deep venous thrombosis during pregnancy or oral contraceptive use: Prevalence of factor V Leiden. Am Heart J 131:1145, 1996

International Perinatal HIV Group: The mode of delivery and the risk of vertical transmission of human immunodeficiency virus type 1—a meta-analysis of 15 prospective cohort studies. N Engl J Med 325:1371, 1999

Jones DC, Hayslett JP: Outcome of pregnancy in women with moderate or severe renal insufficiency. N Engl J Med 335:226, 1996

Lipscomb KJ et al: Outcome of pregnancy in women with Marfan's syndrome. Br J Obstet Gynecol 104:201, 1997

Mandel SJ et al: Increased need for thyroxine during pregnancy in women with primary hypothyroidism. N Engl J Med 323:91, 1990

Ridker PM et al: Factor V Leiden mutation as a risk factor for recurrent pregnancy loss. Ann Intern Med 128:1000, 1998

Scott LL et al: Acyclovir suppression to prevent cesarean delivery after first episode genital herpes. Obstet Gynecol 87:69, 1996

8

Mehul T. Dattani, Charles G. D. Brook

ADOLESCENT HEALTH PROBLEMS

Adolescence marks the transition from childhood to adulthood. It is a time of dramatic physical and psychological change. Adolescents are particularly prone to risk-taking behaviors. In the United States, 73% of deaths among adolescents and young adults result from motor vehicle and other accidents, homicide, and suicide. As a result of sexual maturation, adolescents begin to experiment sexually and, consequently, are susceptible to sexually transmitted diseases (STDs) and unwanted pregnancies. For adolescents with underlying disease, the psychological consequences can be as important as the physical disabilities; denial or resentment of disease is common and can hamper treatment. Adolescence is also a time when many lifelong health-relevant behaviors are established, including dietary habits, exercise patterns, tobacco and alcohol use, and interactions with the health care system. The physician, working together with parents, can help to guide adolescents through this dynamic period of life.

PUBERTY

Puberty encompasses (1) the adolescent growth spurt, (2) development of secondary sexual characteristics, (3) attainment of fertility, and (4) establishment of individual sexual identity.

There is wide variation in the timing of puberty. Signs of puberty are first evident between 9 and 14 years of age (mean 11.5) in 95% of American boys (Fig. 8-1A). In girls, puberty begins earlier, with 95% of American girls entering puberty between 8 and 12 years of age (mean 10.5) (Fig. 8-1B). The age of menarche in girls from developed countries has decreased by approximately 2 to 3 months per decade over the past 100 to 150 years. This trend is likely the result of improvements in socioeconomic conditions, nutritional status, and general health and well-being. Currently in the United States, the average age of menarche is 12.8 years. Genetic factors also influence the course of puberty. Data from twin studies indicate that the average age of

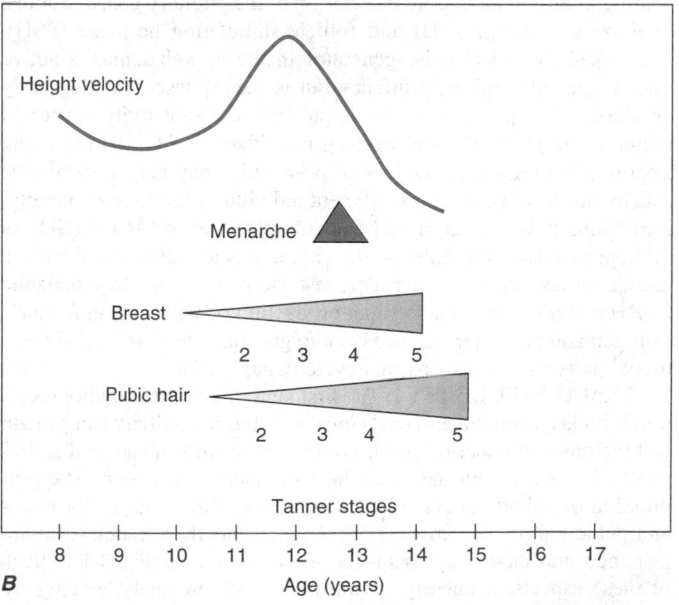

FIGURE 8-1 *A.* Pubertal events in males. Sexual maturity ratings for genitalia and pubic hair and divided into five stages *(From Marshall and Tanner, 1970).* *B.* Pubertal events in females. Sexual maturity ratings for breast development and pubic hair are divided into five stages *(From Marshall and Tanner, 1969).*

menarche is more similar in identical twin sisters than in nonidentical twins. Secondary sexual development occurs earlier in girls of Asian and African-Caribbean heritage than in girls of European heritage. Recognition of the progressively earlier onset of puberty, the ethnic variations, and wide age distribution in the timing of puberty is important for identifying precocious or delayed puberty and for counseling adolescents and parents about the natural course of physiologic changes.

HORMONAL CHANGES Puberty is accompanied by dramatic changes in multiple hormonal systems including alterations in adrenal steroid production, maturation of the reproductive axis, and increased production and action of growth hormone (GH). Serum GH levels increase early in puberty as a consequence of the rise in gonadal steroids. GH in turn increases the level of insulin-like growth factor 1 (IGF-1), which enhances linear bone growth (Chap. 328). The prolonged pubertal exposure to gonadal steroids ultimately causes epiphyseal closure and limits further bone growth. Appetite increases in association with the growth spurt, and sleep patterns change with a tendency to stay up later and a desire to sleep later into the morning.

The development of secondary sexual characteristics is initiated by *adrenarche*, which usually occurs between 6 and 8 years of age and marks the time when the adrenal gland begins to produce greater amounts of androgens. Despite the search for hormonal mediators, the mechanism that controls adrenarche is unknown. It may well result from adrenal cell differentiation, characterized by the growth of the innermost zone of the adrenal cortex, the zona reticularis, which is the principal site of dehydroepiandrosterone (DHEA) production. The increase in adrenal androgen (DHEA, androstenedione) secretion precedes activation of the reproductive axis. Nonetheless, adrenarche and gonadarche are independent events: children with Addison's disease enter puberty at the normal time, and children with premature adrenarche achieve gonadarche at the expected age.

The sexual maturation process is greatly accelerated by the activation of the hypothalamic-pituitary axis, leading to gonadal stimulation and the production of sex steroids. The hypothalamic-pituitary-gonadal axis is controlled predominantly by gonadotropin-releasing hormone (GnRH), a decapeptide produced by the arcuate nucleus of the mediobasal hypothalamus. GnRH is released in a pulsatile fashion, leading in turn to the pulsatile secretion of the pituitary gonadotropins, luteinizing hormone (LH) and follicle-stimulating hormone (FSH). The so-called GnRH pulse-generator in the hypothalamus is active during fetal life and early infancy but is then quiescent during early childhood. In the early stages of puberty, the sensitivity to steroid inhibition is gradually lost, causing reactivation of GnRH secretion. Leptin, a hormone produced by adipose cells, may play a permissive role in this process, as leptin-deficient individuals fail to enter puberty. Early puberty is characterized by nocturnal surges of LH and FSH. As the reproductive axis matures, the characteristic patterns of feedback regulation are acquired. In males, testosterone inhibits hypothalamic GnRH and pituitary gonadotropin production (Chap. 335); in females, estrogen and progesterone feed back to generate the characteristic hormonal patterns of the menstrual cycle (Chap. 336).

FEMALE PUBERTY The first sign of ovarian estradiol secretion is breast development, or *thelarche*. Pubic and axillary hair growth and the onset of apocrine sweat production result from adrenal androgen secretion, though they may be facilitated by estrogen. The progression of puberty is classified according to Tanner stages for breast and pubic hair development: stage 1 represents the preadolescent appearance, and stage 5 represents the adult appearance (Fig. 8-1*A*). Each of these aspects of puberty should be staged separately, as they are controlled by different underlying endocrine mechanisms. Concurrent with these outward signs of puberty are the changes in the size and shape of the uterus. The pubertal growth spurt is dependent on estradiol secretion, which leads to increased GH secretion. This in turn results in a doubling of the growth rate, and peak height velocity is

usually coincident with breast stage 3. After menarche, a girl usually grows only an additional 5 cm.

MALE PUBERTY In boys, growth of the testes is usually the first sign of puberty, reflecting the effects of pulsatile gonadotropin secretion on seminiferous tubule volume and, to some degree, Leydig cell mass. Testosterone is converted to dihydrotestosterone by 5-α reductase. Both hormones act via the androgen receptor to induce growth of the external genitalia and pubic hair (Fig. 8-1; Chap. 338). The growth spurt in boys occurs at a testicular volume of about 10 to 12 mL (as measured by a Prader orchidometer). Testosterone also deepens the voice and increases muscle growth. Dihydrotestosterone stimulates prostate growth and beard growth and initiates recession of the temporal hairline. Although boys enter puberty approximately 6 to 12 months later than girls, they are potentially fertile at an earlier stage of puberty. Aromatization of testosterone to estradiol increases GH secretion, which acts synergistically with testosterone to induce a greater peak height velocity in boys than in girls.

DISORDERS OF PUBERTY *Precocious puberty* is usually defined as an early onset of puberty in boys younger than 9 years or in girls younger than 8 years of age. Some authorities suggest that the lower limits of normal in girls be revised downward to age 7 for Caucasians and age 6 for African-American girls. *Premature thelarche* refers to breast development in the absence of other signs of puberty. It occurs most commonly in girls between infancy and 3 years of age and usually resolves spontaneously. Causes of precocious puberty are divided into central *gonadotropin-dependent* forms and peripheral *gonadotropin-independent* forms (Table 8-1). Central precocious puberty is much more common in girls than in boys, and the majority of these cases involve idiopathic activation of spontaneous GnRH pulses. It

Table 8-1   Causes of Precocious and Delayed Puberty

I. Causes of precocious puberty
  A. Central (gonadotropin-dependent)
    1. Idiopathic
    2. CNS tumor or inflammatory states
    3. Hypothalamic hamartoma
  B. Peripheral (gonadotropin-independent)
    1. Females
      a. McCune-Albright syndrome
      b. Congenital adrenal hyperplasia
      c. Aromatase excess syndrome
      d. Exogenous estrogen
      e. Hypothyroidism
    2. Males
      a. Congenital adrenal hyperplasia
      b. Activating LH receptor mutations
      c. hCG-secreting tumor
      d. Exogenous androgens
      e. Hypothyroidism
II. Causes of pubertal delay
  A. Constitutional delay
  B. Chronic diseases (asthma, gastrointestinal problems, renal failure)
  C. Malnutrition
  D. Excessive exercise
  E. Anorexia nervosa
  F. Hypothalamic-pituitary causes of pubertal failure (low gonadotropins)
    1. Congenital defects (Kallmann syndrome, congenital adrenal hypoplasia, pituitary hypoplasia)
    2. CNS tumors and their treatment (radiotherapy and surgery)
    3. Hemochromatosis
  G. Gonadal causes of pubertal failure (elevated gonadotropins)
    1. Females
      a. Chemotherapy or radiotherapy
      b. Turner syndrome
      c. Premature menopause
    2. Males
      a. Chemotherapy or radiotherapy
      b. Anorchia
      c. Bilateral undescended testes
      d. Orchitis

NOTE: CNS, central nervous system; hCG, human chorionic gonadotropin; LH, luteinizing hormone.

can also be caused by a variety of central nervous system tumors, structural lesions, and inflammatory conditions.

Delayed puberty is defined as the 3% of girls and boys who have not developed the first signs of puberty by 13.2 and 14.2 years, respectively. It is most commonly due to delayed activation of the hypothalamic-pituitary-gonadal axis (Table 8-1). Most individuals who meet this definition will progress through puberty normally, but at a later age. Short stature and delayed skeletal maturation are commonly seen in association with delayed puberty. Growth delay may have been evident earlier in childhood; the diagnosis of *constitutional delay of growth and puberty* can be suspected from a delayed bone age in a short child who is otherwise well. Individuals who experience delays in puberty may be emotionally as well as physically immature relative to their peers.

The main diagnostic challenge in delayed puberty is to distinguish those with constitutional delay, who will progress through puberty at a later age, from those with an underlying pathologic process. LH and FSH responses to GnRH do not differentiate constitutional delay from pathologic causes of *hypogonadotropic hypogonadism* (Chap. 335). Thus, constitutional delay is a diagnosis of exclusion and requires ongoing evaluation during development to assure that normal growth and development occur at a later time. Reassurance without hormonal treatment is appropriate for most individuals with presumed constitutional delay of puberty. Alternatively, an anabolic steroid (e.g., 50 to 100 mg per month testosterone enanthate, intramuscularly) in boys or estrogen (5 to 10 mg/d ethinyl estradiol, orally) in girls may be useful to induce growth and secondary sexual characteristics appropriate for age. Low-dose oral oxandrolone (2.5 mg/d), an anabolic steroid that is not aromatized to estrogen, is also used for boys because it does not accelerate skeletal maturation when used for short periods. After treatment for a year or more, hormonal treatments can be stopped and the function of the reproductive axis can be reassessed.

PSYCHOLOGICAL CHANGES AND SOCIAL FACTORS

The adolescent years are characterized by a multitude of psychological changes, including (1) the development of abstract thinking, (2) greater independence from family, (3) the formation of a personal and sexual identity, (4) the establishment of a system of values, and (5) an increase in socialization. For most adolescents, these transitions occur relatively smoothly. For others, however, these years can be frustrating and tumultuous; parents and clinicians must be attuned to the needs of those who show signs of struggling with emotional, sexual, and social issues.

Young people tend to share their feelings openly, one of which is ambivalence. These contradictory feelings most often involve both a desire for greater autonomy and, at the same time, a need to cling to the emotional and physical security provided by the family. Adolescents are granted increasing responsibilities but still lack some of the social and legal privileges of adults. This feature of adolescence can lead to conflict and challenges to parental authority.

Adolescents have a strong desire to establish an identity that is increasingly independent of the family. This new identity is strongly influenced by peer groups, some of which are institutionalized (e.g., team sports). Role confusion is quite common in adolescence, and some young people move from one intense allegiance to another with alarming speed. These transitional arrangements are eventually replaced by more permanent attachments to individuals.

In an attempt to alleviate some of the transitions associated with adolescence, many cultures have traditionally used "rites of passage" to acknowledge and accelerate an adolescent's evolution to adulthood. Among Native American Great Plains cultures, for example, a boy was sent away from the village at the time of puberty to fast and receive a vision from a spirit; upon returning to the community, he took his place among the adult men. Similarly, it was traditional in many societies for girls to be secluded at the time of the first menstruation before returning a "full-grown woman." These rites provide a public recognition of the end of childhood, and the ritual leaves the young person with the conviction that he or she has undergone a personal transformation. A relative lack of these coming-of-age rituals in western cultures may contribute to the sense of alienation experienced by some adolescents in this part of the world.

During adolescence, gender identity must be renegotiated. Though prepubertal children have a relatively secure view of themselves as either a boy or a girl, experimentation with gender roles is a common feature of adolescence. For example, adolescents may explore, at least in fantasy, alternative gender roles (e.g., cross-dressing), homosexuality, or relationships with older men or women.

The hormonal changes of puberty influence behavior as well as causing physical changes. Rising levels of testosterone in boys and the increase in adrenal and ovarian androgens in girls increase libido. The mean age of sexual intercourse varies widely within and among cultures, but ranges between ages 15 and 18 for most groups. Boys generally report sexual intercourse about 1 year earlier than girls.

ADOLESCENT VIOLENCE

Adolescents and young adults are subject to much greater rates of violence, both as victims and perpetrators. Males are involved in violence much more commonly than females and account for >90% of homicides involving those 10 to 17 years of age. Ethnic and racial differences in rates of adolescent violence have been noted consistently. African Americans, Hispanics, and Native Americans are much more likely to be victims and perpetrators of lethal violence than are people of Asian or European ancestry. The origins of different rates of violence are complex. Higher rates of lethal aggression are associated with low socioeconomic status, high housing density, increased population turnover in neighborhoods, single-parent households, and socially disorganized communities. In many cases, these factors interact; increased violence leads to high population turnover and social disorganization.

Gangs represent a potentially volatile environment that is characterized by power struggles, initiation and detachment rituals, battles over territory, and escalating violence associated with retaliation. The increase in lethal violence has been attributed in part to easier access to firearms and a greater willingness to use firearms. A Centers for Disease Control and Prevention study in 1995 found that about one-fourth of students had carried a weapon to school during the preceding month and 8 to 10% had carried a gun. Many adolescents lack the abstract reasoning skills required to understand social mores and the consequence of gun use. Though firearms do not cause violence, handguns in particular provide a facile means to a lethal outcome; widespread reduction in access to handguns is essential to curb the current trend in adolescent homicide and serious injury.

Aggressive behavior can often be recognized in early childhood; bullying is a precursor to later antisocial behavior. Child abuse, antisocial parents, inadequate child-rearing practices, and dysfunctional interpersonal interactions between parents or among siblings are associated with aggressive behavior. The physician, along with teachers, clergy, and others in positions of authority, should be alert to a pattern of aggressive behavior or problems in the home. Though these issues are not easily remedied, appropriate interventions to improve family functioning and parenting may interrupt a pattern of violence, which is all too often perpetuated by the adolescent.

HEALTH PROBLEMS

Adolescence is generally a healthy period and is often accompanied by a feeling of immortality, which leads to risk-taking. When diseases of childhood or the consequences of their treatment extend into adolescence, or when disease strikes during adolescence, the sense of unfairness may be overwhelming. Anger and denial can lead to poor compliance with therapeutic regimens.

Table 8-2 Medical Disorders for Which Adolescents Are at Increased Risk

Cancer and hematologic disorders	Orthopedic disorders
Hodgkin's disease, lymphomas	Osteosarcoma, Ewing's sarcoma
Acute myelogenous leukemia, acute	Fractures
lymphoblastic leukemia	Legg-Calvé-Perthes disease (slipped capital
Ovarian cysts/cancer, testicular cancer	femoral epiphysis)
Survivors of childhood cancers, secondary	Osgood-Schlatter disease (osteochondrosis of
cancers	tibial tuberosity)
Sickle cell anemia	Scoliosis
Hemophilias	Rheumatologic disorders
Infectious diseases	Juvenile rheumatoid arthritis
Sexually transmitted diseases (see text)	Connective tissue diseases (e.g., systemic
HIV	lupus erythematosus)
Chlamydia, gonorrhea, syphilis	Vasculitis (e.g., Takayasu's arteritis,
Human papilloma virus	Kawasaki's disease)
Pelvic inflammatory disease	Endocrine disorders
Toxic shock syndrome	Type 1 diabetes mellitus
Meningococcal infection	Polycystic ovarian syndrome
Tuberculosis	Delayed puberty
Infectious mononucleosis	Turner syndrome
Pertussis	Klinefelter syndrome
Rubella	Graves' disease
Parvovirus	Neurologic disorders
Cardiac disorders	Becker muscular dystrophy
Survivors of congenital heart disease	Migraine headaches
Atrial septal defect, bicuspid aortic valve,	Temporal lobe epilepsy
pulmonary stenosis	Multiple sclerosis
Hypertrophic cardiomyopathy	Friedreich's ataxia
Marfan syndrome	Germinomas
Hypertension	Meningitis
Respiratory disorders	Psychiatric and behavioral disorders
Asthma	Depression
Cystic fibrosis	Substance abuse
Tobacco abuse	Antisocial behavior
Renal disorders	Excessive risk-taking
Survivors of childhood renal failure	Eating disorders
Glomerulonephritis, interstitial nephritis	
Gastrointestinal disorders	
Celiac disease	
Crohn's disease	

Relatively few diseases are unique to adolescents. Rather, diseases of childhood, including many inherited disorders and infectious diseases, extend into the adolescent period. Similarly, many of the disorders that affect teenagers are also seen in the adult population. The presentation and management of asthma, for example, is similar in adolescents and adults. Some of the diseases with relatively increased prevalence during adolescence are summarized in Table 8-2. These diseases should be borne in mind when considering the differential diagnosis. For example, when an adolescent presents with exertional chest pain, dyspnea, and syncope, hypertrophic cardiomyopathy or congenital heart disease should be considered as likely diagnoses, whereas coronary artery disease would be more likely in an adult.

SEXUALLY TRANSMITTED DISEASES Sexually active adolescents are at greater risk of acquiring STDs than their adult counterparts (Chap. 132). Prevention of STDs in adolescence depends on adequate sexual education coupled with access to appropriate clinical services. Early age of first sexual intercourse is associated with (1) an increased number of lifetime sexual partners; (2) an increased risk of acquiring chronic STDs, such as herpes simplex, HIV, and hepatitis B; and (3) cervical cancer in women. In addition, pelvic inflammatory disease in adolescent females increases the likelihood of future ectopic pregnancy, tubal infertility, and chronic pelvic inflammation. A low rate of barrier contraceptive use, combined with ignorance about the acquisition and prevention of infectious diseases, also contributes to the increased risk of STDs among adolescents. Screening for STDs is recommended in sexually active teens (Table 8-3). Adolescents with sexually transmitted infections, particularly those who deny sexual activity, may be victims of sexual abuse.

CHILD SEXUAL ABUSE Child sexual abuse is defined as the involvement of developmentally immature children and adoles-

cents in sexual activities they do not comprehend, to which they are unable to give consent, or that violate social taboos or family roles. In a U.S. study in 1985, sexual abuse during childhood was reported by 27% of adult females and 16% of adult males. Females are more likely than males to have been sexually abused by a family member. Although there is a paucity of literature on male sexual abuse, it is probably more common than generally recognized. The psychological trauma appears to be similar for boys and girls. Sexual abuse during adolescence may merge with peer sexual assault, or "date rape." Sexual abuse in adolescent girls can be associated with a constant fear of pregnancy. Teenage pregnancy or STD may, in fact, be the first indication of ongoing abuse.

Psychological consequences of child sexual abuse often involve behavioral problems, psychiatric disturbances, or adjustment difficulties at the onset of adolescence, even though the actual abuse may have taken place at a younger age. Child sexual abuse may lead to low self-esteem and/or a degree of sexual disinhibition. The cognitive maturation that occurs with adolescence may bring about the realization and expression of these feelings. Young women who have been sexually abused have significantly higher rates of early-onset consensual sexual activity, teenage pregnancy, multiple sexual partners, unprotected intercourse, STDs, and later sexual assault. Poor psychological outcome is related to the duration of abuse, the extent to which the abuse involves violence or coercion, and the perception that the child has cooperated with the abuser, with ensuing feelings of guilt. The impact of these sequelae can be reduced by supportive peer and family relationships. Disclosure of the abuse may help to ameliorate some of the psychological traumas associated with abuse.

SUBSTANCE ABUSE Substance abuse and drug misuse among adolescents is a significant cause of morbidity and mortality (Chaps. 386 to 389). The prevalence rates vary widely by region, ethnic group, age, and gender. The age of initiation into substance abuse has gradually declined. In 1997, rates among American teenagers for substance use or abuse, at some stage during their lifetimes, were: cigarettes smoking (70%), alcohol use (79%), marijuana use (47%), cocaine use (8%), anabolic steroids (4%), injected illegal drugs (2%), and other illegal drugs (17%), e.g., lysergic acid (LSD), phencyclidine (PCP), methylenedioxymethamphetamine (ecstasy), methamphetamine (ice), or heroin.

The forms of substance abuse change continuously. Anabolic steroids, for example, are now used by 3 to 5% of male high school seniors, with a 10% prevalence rate among male adolescent athletes. In addition to their use by athletes in an effort to increase muscle strength, nonathletes use anabolic steroids with a goal of achieving a more virile appearance. In contrast to popular views, anabolic steroids do not appear to enhance performance except at very high doses, which are associated with significant side effects (Chap. 335). Other performance-enhancing agents include human growth hormone and erythropoietin (EPO), but the high cost of these hormones limits their use.

In addition to the direct effect on health, substance abuse is associated with other risk-taking behaviors. The relationship of alcohol use and motor vehicle accidents, for example, is well documented. However, drug and alcohol use are also correlated with many other problems during adolescence including violence, suicide, depression, STD,

Table 8-3 Health Maintenance during Adolescence

History/counseling
  Review physical and psychological changes associated with puberty and
    adolescence
  Assess habits including tobacco, alcohol, anabolic steroids, illegal drugs
  Inquire about sexual activity and preference
  Review strategies to prevent unwanted pregnancies and STDs
  Provide guidance regarding injury prevention, particularly related to motor
    vehicles, sports and recreation, weapons
  Encourage development of health maintenance including diet and exercise
  Inquire regarding history of emotional, sexual, or physical abuse
  Review school attendance; assess decline in performance or evidence of
    learning disabilities
Examination
  Comprehensive physical examination at least every 3 years
  Evaluate progression of growth and puberty
  Yearly screening for hypertension[a]
  Yearly body mass index (BMI),[b] consider features of eating disorders
  Review symptoms and signs of depression or risk of suicide
Laboratory testing
  Screen for hyperlipidemia in those at increased risk[c]
  Screen sexually active adolescents for STDs,[d] including chlamydia,
    gonorrhea using urinary tests or pelvic examination; consider syphilis in
    those with other STDs
  HIV in those at increased risk (Chap. 309)
Immunizations[e] (Chaps. 122, 132)
  Review previous immunizations and tuberculin testing
  Measles/mumps/rubella (MMR), tetanus toxoid at age 11 to 12,
    if indicated
  Varicella vaccine, in the absence of childhood chickenpox
  Hepatitis B
  Influenza vaccine in those with underlying respiratory or cardiac disease

---

[a] See Update on the Task Force Report (1987) on High Blood Pressure in Children and Adolescents: A Working Group Report from the High Blood Pressure Education Program. NIH Publication No. 96-3790, 1996 (www.nhibi.nih.gov/health/prof/heart/hbp/hbp_ped.pdf).

[b] See Clinical guidelines on the identification, evaluation, and treatment of overweight and obesity in adults (www.nhibi.nih.gov/guidelines/obesity/ob_gdlns.pdf).

[c] See protocol developed by the Expert Panel on Blood Cholesterol Levels in Children and Adolescents (amhrt.org/Heart_and_Stroke_A_Z_Guide/cholk.html).

[d] See Centers for Disease Control and Prevention 1998 Guidelines for Treatment of Sexually Transmitted Diseases (aepo-xdv-www.epo.cdc.gov/wonder/prevguid/p0000480/body002.htm).

[e] See Centers for Disease Control and Prevention Recommendations of the Advisory Committee on Immunization Practices (ACIP) www.cdc.gov/nip/publications/ACIP-list.htm.

NOTE: STDs, sexually tansmitted diseases.
SOURCE: Adapted from Guidelines for Adolescent Preventive Services (GAPS) (www.ama-assn.org/adolhlth/recomend/monogrf1.htm)

and unwanted pregnancies. Therefore, the presence of one form of risky behavior should prompt consideration of others.

SUICIDAL BEHAVIOR AND DEPRESSION After motor vehicle accidents and homicide, suicide is the third leading cause of death in adolescents, and the rate has risen almost fourfold over the past 50 years. In 1988, the suicide rate among 15- to 19-year olds was 11.3 in 100,000. The causes for increased rates of suicide are not well understood, but one theory holds that modern society fosters increased social isolation and alienation. Nearly one-fourth of adolescents acknowledge seriously considering suicide, and 8% have actually attempted it. Attempted suicide is three times more common in females than males, with drug overdose or wrist-cutting being the most common means of suicide attempt. Completed suicide is three to five times more common in teenage boys than girls and usually involves firearms, hanging, or jumping from heights. Suicide is rare before puberty. Risk factors for suicide among adolescents include prior attempt of suicide, a history of depression or other major psychiatric disorder, history of substance abuse, medical illness, family history of suicidal behavior, and knowing someone who has committed suicide. Unfortunately, these and other risk factors are relatively common among nonsuicidal youth as well, making suicide difficult to predict in individual cases. Stressful events can precipitate depression and increase risk of suicide; these can include the death of a relative or friend, disciplinary crisis,

rejection or humiliation, school difficulty, and anxiety about homosexuality. Apparently impulsive actions may be harbingers of more serious underlying mood disturbances, personality disorders, or substance abuse.

Major depression occurs in 4 to 6% of adolescents, and the *DSM-IV* criteria for diagnosis are the same as in adults (Chap. 385). Every depressed or suicidal adolescent should undergo psychiatric examination, whether hospitalized or not. Comprehensive evaluation requires exploration of the adolescent's history of mental health problems, symptoms of depression, level of functioning in school, interactions with friends and family, and evaluation for comorbid disorders. Indications for hospitalization include imminent risk of suicide as evidenced by an identified plan and access to lethal means, recurrent suicide attempts, the presence of severe depression or psychosis, substance abuse, and the need to remove the individual from an overwhelmingly stressful environment.

ADOLESCENT EATING DISORDERS Many adolescents have voracious appetites in response to the increased energy and caloric requirements generated by the growth spurt. The unique physical, psychological, and social transitions of adolescence provide a context for the development and perpetuation of eating patterns. Adolescents with a body mass index (BMI), measured as weight (kg)/height (m^2), greater than the 95th percentile for age and gender are overweight, and those between the 85th and 94th percentiles are at risk for becoming overweight. Based on the NHANES III survey for 1988 to 1994, there was evidence for a 6% increase in the prevalence of overweight adolescents compared to the previous decade. The increasing prevalence of obesity is multifactorial and involves patterns of eating behavior as well as alterations in activity level (Chap. 77). Physical activity among both girls and boys tends to decline steadily during adolescence. Regular involvement in enjoyable forms of exercise should be encouraged to help promote lifelong habits that involve physical activity.

Eating disorders such as anorexia nervosa or bulimia nervosa often have their onset during adolescence (Chap. 78). Control over dietary intake is perhaps one of the first mechanisms that adolescents use to establish autonomy and achieve independence from family. The majority of female adolescents and young adults in western cultures report feeling discontented with their body shape. Surveys of normal adolescent populations disclose a surprisingly high frequency of dieting and abnormal eating patterns. For instance, up to 79% binge, 70% consider themselves fat, 11% induce vomiting, 5% abuse laxatives, and about 3% meet diagnostic criteria for anorexia or bulimia nervosa. Eating disorders also occur in males, but much less frequently than in females.

PHYSICIAN–ADOLESCENT RELATIONSHIP

The transition from the pediatrician to an adult medical practice can be difficult for adolescents, their parents, and their physicians. The emergence of adolescent medicine as a specialty practice has helped to facilitate this transition and to focus on the special needs of this group. When adolescents transfer to an adult-based practice, the physician should first establish a relationship with the patient and his or her parents. Previous medical history should be reviewed and medical records obtained. The need for the teenager to be seen alone, and office policies concerning confidentiality, should be discussed and agreed to with the parent(s) and adolescent together.

Legal issues related to the medical care of minors arise frequently, and laws vary in different countries and from state to state (Chap. 2). As a general rule, anyone who has reached the age of majority (usually 18 years) may consent to treatment. Under this age, a parent or legal guardian must consent for medical intervention. However, there are several exceptions to this requirement. The delivery of medical care is generally accepted in an emergency, but it is important to document the nature of the emergency and any efforts to notify parents. Emancipated minors may also provide consent. This group includes those fulfilling adult roles (e.g., military service), married teens, and those who are financially independent and living separately from their parents. In addition, when the health of a minor is potentially endangered by disorders for which they may be reluctant to seek parental consent, such as substance abuse, pregnancy, or STD, mature minors may generally provide consent. In these circumstances, the caregiver must assess the minor's maturity, ability to understand the risks and benefits of treatment, and capacity to provide informed consent. Mature or emancipated minors do not need to reveal consent or treatment to their parents.

Obtaining a medical history from an adolescent includes many elements that are distinct from an adult history. It should include, for example, schoolwork, home environment, and relationships with parents, siblings, and peers. Adolescents often lack knowledge about medical issues and may be reluctant to discuss sensitive topics with authority figures. Most will be nervous, even when these issues do not pertain. It can be useful, therefore, to provide printed forms or questionnaires. These not only serve to gather information in a relatively nonthreatening manner but also provide an indication of the kinds of issues that might be discussed with the physician. It is difficult to predict the topics that are paramount to the adolescent. Some may be preoccupied with concerns about the onset of acne, whereas others fear HIV or pregnancy. Adolescents may harbor guilt about sexual abuse or feel overwhelmed by peer pressure to engage in certain activities. The physician is well positioned to assist with many of these issues, if there is trust and an indication of interest and understanding. Because of these types of questions, it is important to interview the adolescent in private. Some parents will resist this approach, but it is necessary if the adolescent is to volunteer information that he or she is unwilling to discuss in the presence of parents. It is useful to reinforce the fact that conversations will be kept confidential. Adolescents are sometimes willing to bring concerns to the attention of nurses or other caregivers before raising these issues with a physician. It is helpful, therefore, to have another health care provider interact with the patient, if only briefly. In addition to direct questioning, general conversation about topical issues or inquiries about school or peers may provide insight into an adolescent's interests, activities, and potential risk factors. Because of the prevalence of substance abuse, risk-taking behavior, suicide, sexual orientation crises, STDs, unwanted pregnancies, sexual abuse, depression, and eating disorders in the teenage years, these topics warrant specific inquiry as part of routine health assessment. The interview should also include adequate time for education, health care guidance, and counseling. It is also useful to provide written information about topics that are pertinent to the care of the adolescent.

The physical examination of the adolescent, while incorporating many elements of the adult examination, has several unique features. Foremost among these is the assessment of growth and sexual development. In addition to questionnaires that allow the adolescent an opportunity to self-assess stages of pubertal development, the examination can be made less stressful by using it as opportunity to explain normal physiology. The issue of when to perform a pelvic examination as part of the routine health maintenance is controversial. Some advocate pelvic examinations in all sexually active young women as a means to detect STDs and for Pap smears. With the advent of urinary screening tests for chlamydia and gonorrhea, others suggest that pelvic examinations are not routinely necessary in the absence of specific indications. When a pelvic examination is performed, the patient should be asked whether she prefers her mother or a member of the health care team as an observer. The physical examination should also focus on diseases that tend to present during adolescence (Table 8-2).

Disorders such as hypertension, hyperlipidemia, and obesity are often first detected during adolescence. Strategies for disease prevention also include immunization, avoidance of cigarette smoking or excessive alcohol use, establishing good dietary habits, and engaging in regular exercise. General guidelines for adolescent preventive services (GAPS) are summarized in Table 8-3.

SUMMARY

The term *adolescent* is derived from a Latin phrase meaning "to grow up." Adolescence is, in many ways, the culmination of development, with the achievement of identity and reproductive competence. Though these processes are triggered by internal physiologic events, they are intimately intertwined with the family and social environment. Physicians have an important role to facilitate these transitions by providing information and managing the diseases of adolescents. Moreover, it should be remembered that many adolescents view physicians as role models and will seek objective and informed advice about issues that reach beyond medicine.

BIBLIOGRAPHY

ELLIOTT DS et al: *Violence in American Schools: A New Perspective*. New York, Cambridge University Press, 1998

EMANS SJ et al: *Pediatric and Adolescent Gynecology*, 4th ed. Philadelphia, Lippincott-Raven, 1998

FINKELHOR D et al: Sexual abuse in a national survey of adult men and women: Prevalence, characteristics, and risk factors. Child Abuse Negl 14:19, 1990

GRUMBACH MM, STYNE DM: Puberty: Ontogeny, neuroendocrinology, physiology, and disorders, in *Williams Textbook of Endocrinology*, 9th ed, JD Wilson, DW Foster, HM Kronenberg, PR Larsen (eds). Philadelphia, Saunders, 1998, pp 1509–1625

Guidelines for adolescent preventive services (GAPS). Arch Pediatr Adolesc Med 51:123, 1997

JELLINEK MS, SNYDER JB: Depression and suicide in children and adolescents. Pediatr Rev 19:255, 1998

KANN L et al: Youth risk behavior surveillance—United States, 1997. MMWR CDC Surveill Summ 47:1, 1998

KAPLOWITZ PB et al: Reexamination of the age limit for defining when puberty is precocious in girls in the United States: Implications from evaluation and treatment. Pediatrics 104:936, 1999

MARSHALL WA, TANNER JM: Variations in pattern of pubertal changes in girls. Arch Dis Child 44:291, 1969

———, ———: Variations in the pattern of pubertal changes in boys. Arch Dis Child 45:13, 1970

SHAFER MB: Annual pelvic examination in the sexually active adolescent female: What are we doing and why are we doing it? J Adolesc Health 23:68, 1998

9   *Neil M. Resnick*

GERIATRIC MEDICINE

Of all the people who have ever lived to age 65, more than half are now alive. This statistic has important demographic and economic implications, and its impact on medical care is also substantial.

BIOLOGY OF AGING

Numerous molecular concomitants of aging have been described. For instance, there is an increase in chromosome structural abnormalities, DNA cross-linking, and frequency of single-strand breaks; a decline in DNA methylation; and loss of DNA telomeric sequences. The primary structure of proteins is unaltered, but posttranslational changes, such as deamidation, oxidation, cross-linking, and nonenzymatic glycation, increase. Mitochondrial structure also deteriorates, albeit not universally.

However, the biologic changes are clearer than the mechanisms that mediate them. In fact, although the senescent phenotype appears to be ubiquitous, biologists disagree about whether senescence even exists beyond zoos and civilized societies and whether it occurs at all in many species. There is little evolutionary rationale for a process that happens after reproduction is complete, particularly one associated with such a long and complex course. In nature, senescence is most notable for its absence; nearly all animals die of predation, disease, or environmental hazards rather than aging. The argument that different species have different maximum life spans can be explained without invoking a specific aging process: while growth and development are based on a genetic template, aging may reflect merely the accumulation of random damage rather than a specific mechanism.

If aging exists as a distinct process, there is consensus that the mechanisms are likely multifactorial, environmentally influenced, and species-specific, if not organ- and cell-specific, making the paucity of available human data particularly problematic. As a result, there are nearly as many theories of aging as investigators. Most theories overlap or are not mutually exclusive, and none is completely compatible with the dearth of data. As a group, the theories can be divided into two broad categories, based on whether they attribute aging to a genetic program or to progressive and random damage to homeostatic systems.

Enthusiasm for genetic theories of aging is fueled by several observations, including the dramatic species-specific differences in maximal life span, the strong correlation with survival among monozygotic compared to dizygotic twins, and the fact that single mutations can prolong life span by more than 50% in some nematodes and mice. However, all genetic theories must account for the fact that evolutionary selection pressure is minimal following completion of reproduction. Three genetic theories have recently been advanced, but few relevant data have yet been accrued. The first theory suggests that, since animals usually succumb to natural forces long before reaching their maximal life span, aging might reflect mutations that impair long-term survival. These mutations would accumulate in the genome because there is no selection pressure to delete them. A second theory, "pleiotropic antagonism," proposes that aging may be caused by the late and deleterious effects of genes that are conserved because of the survival advantages they confer prior to reproduction. The third theory applies to ecological niches where extrinsic hazards are relatively low. In such an environment, evolution might select for mutations that retard the aging process since these might allow an animal to produce and protect many more litters. In support of this theory, the rate of aging in an isolated clan of Virginia opossums was calculated to be roughly half of that seen in their less fortunate cousins.

The "random damage" theories are based on the possibility that the balance between ongoing damage and repair is disrupted. The theories differ in the emphasis placed on increased damage (e.g., by free radicals, oxidation, or glycation) versus deficient repair, as well as in the mechanisms that might mediate each. However, all share the observation that cell and organ repair capacity declines with age. Some 40 years ago, Hayflick and Moorehead observed that the number of replications among cultured cells is finite. Subsequent research revealed that this replicative senescence was due to arrest of the cell cycle at the G_1/S phase, the point at which DNA synthesis begins. Recently, cell replication has also been linked to the length of telomeric DNA. Present at the termini of chromosomes, telomeric DNA prevents chromosomal instability, fragmentation, and rearrangement; anchors chromosomes to nuclear matrix; and provides a buffer between coding regions of DNA and the ends of the chromosomes. In addition, telomeric DNA is necessary for cell division. With each cell division, however, roughly 50 of the total 2000 base pairs of the telomere are lost. Telomeric shortening might thus result in loss of gene accessibility, which is necessary to repair ongoing cell damage caused by metabolism. Together with cytoplasmic factors mediating arrest of DNA synthesis, telomeric shortening could also limit the cell's ability to divide and thereby replace cells lost to apoptosis.

Many mechanisms previously postulated to mediate aging have not been borne out, including the somatic mutation theory (in which aging would result from cumulative spontaneous mutations), the error catastrophe theory (in which aging would result from errors in the synthesis of proteins critical to the synthesis of genetic material or protein-synthesizing machinery), and the intrinsic mutagenesis theory (in which aging is the result of ongoing intrinsic DNA rearrangements).

To date, the only intervention known to delay aging is caloric restriction. The salutary effect of restricting caloric intake by 30 to 40% has been documented in multiple species, from single-cell organisms to rodents. In rodents, it not only increases average life expectancy and maximum life span but also delays the onset of some typical age-associated diseases as well as deterioration of physiologic systems (e.g., immune responsiveness, glucose metabolism, muscle atrophy). Moreover, its impact is evident in both mitotic and postmitotic cells, in gene expression, and in protein turnover and cross-linking. Although the mechanism is still not determined, it is specific to caloric restriction rather than to reduction of any dietary component (e.g., fat intake) or supplements with vitamins or antioxidants. Unfortunately, adequate data from primates are not yet available, and the effect of caloric restriction in humans is still unknown.

PRINCIPLES OF GERIATRIC MEDICINE

Despite the biologic controversy, from a physiologic standpoint human aging is characterized by progressive constriction of the homeostatic reserve of every organ system. This decline, often referred to as *homeostenosis*, is evident by the third decade and is gradual and progressive, although the rate and extent of decline vary. The decline of each organ system (Table 9-1) appears to occur independently of changes in other organ systems and is influenced by diet, environment, and personal habits as well as by genetic factors.

Several important principles follow from these facts: (1) Individuals become more dissimilar as they age, belying any stereotype of aging; (2) an *abrupt* decline in any system or function is always due to disease and not to "normal aging"; (3) "normal aging" can be attenuated by modification of risk factors (e.g., increased blood pressure, smoking, sedentary lifestyle); and (4) "healthy old age" is not an oxymoron. In fact, *in the absence of disease, the decline in homeostatic reserve causes no symptoms and imposes few restrictions on activities of daily living regardless of age.*

Appreciation of these facts may make it easier to understand the striking increases that have occurred in life expectancy. Average life expectancy is now 17 years at age 65, 11 years at age 75, 6 years at age 85, 4 years at age 90, and 2 years at age 100. Moreover, the bulk of these years is characterized by a lack of significant impairment (Table 9-2). Even beyond age 85, only 30% of people are impaired in any activity required for daily living and only 20% reside in a nursing home. Yet, as individuals age they are more likely to suffer from disease, disability, and the side effects of drugs, all of which, when combined with the decrease in physiologic reserve, make the older person more vulnerable to environmental, pathologic, and pharmacologic challenges.

The following concepts underlie the remainder of the chapter:

1. Disease presentation is often atypical in the elderly, especially in those more than 75 to 80 years old. Homeostatic strain caused by onset of a new disease often leads to symptoms associated with a different organ system, particularly one compromised by preexisting disease. For example, fewer than one-fourth of older patients with hyperthyroidism present with goiter, tremor, and exophthalmos; more likely are atrial fibrillation, confusion, depression, syncope, and weakness. Significantly, because the "weakest link" is so often the brain, the lower urinary tract, or the cardiovascular or musculoskeletal system, a limited number of presenting symptoms predominate—acute confusion, depression, incontinence, falling, and syncope—no matter what the underlying disease. Thus for the most common geriatric syndromes, regardless of the presenting symptom, the differential diagnosis is often largely similar. The corollary is equally important: The organ system usually associated with a particular symptom is less likely to be the source of that symptom in older individuals than in younger ones. Compared with middle-aged individuals, for example, acute confusion in older patients is less often due to a new brain lesion,

Table 9-1 Selected Age-Related Changes and Their Consequences

Organ/System	Age-Related Physiologic Change[a]	Consequences of Age-Related Physiologic Change	Consequences of Disease, not Age
General	↑ Body fat	↑ Volume of distribution for fat-soluble drugs	Obesity
	↓ Total body water	↓ Volume of distribution for water-soluble drugs	Anorexia
Eyes/ears	Presbyopia	↓ Accommodation	
	Lens opacification	↑ Susceptibility to glare	Blindness
		Need for increased illumination	
	↓ High-frequency acuity	Difficulty discriminating words if background noise is present	Deafness
Endocrine	Impaired glucose homeostasis	↑ Glucose level in response to acute illness	Diabetes mellitus
	↓ Thyroxine clearance (and production)	↓ T_4 dose required in hypothyroidism	Thyroid dysfunction
	↑ ADH, ↓ renin, and ↓ aldosterone		↓ Na^+, ↑ K^+
	↓ Testosterone		Impotence
	↓ Vitamin D absorption and activation	Osteopenia	Osteomalacia, fracture
Respiratory	↓ Lung elasticity and ↑ chest wall stiffness	Ventilation/perfusion mismatch and ↓ P_{O_2}	Dyspnea, hypoxia
Cardiovascular	↓ Arterial compliance and ↑ systolic BP →LVH	Hypotensive response to ↑ HR, volume depletion, or loss of atrial contraction	Syncope
	↓ β-adrenergic responsiveness	↓ Cardiac output and HR response to stress	Heart failure
	↓ Baroreceptor sensitivity and ↓ SA node automaticity	Impaired blood pressure response to standing, volume depletion	Heart block
Gastrointestinal	↓ Hepatic function	Delayed metabolism of some drugs	Cirrhosis
	↓ Gastric acidity	↓ Ca^{2+} absorption on empty stomach	Osteoporosis, B_{12} deficiency
	↓ Colonic motility	Constipation	Fecal impaction
	↓ Anorectal function		Fecal incontinence
Hematologic/immune system	↓ Bone marrow reserve(?)		Anemia
	↓ T cell function	False-negative PPD response	
	↑ Autoantibodies	False-positive rheumatoid factor, antinuclear antibody	Autoimmune disease
Renal	↓ GFR	Impaired excretion of some drugs	↑ Serum creatinine
	↓ Urine concentration/dilution (see also "Endocrine")	Delayed response to salt or fluid restriction/overload; nocturia	↓ ↑ Na^+
Genitourinary	Vaginal/urethral mucosal atrophy	Dyspareunia, bacteriuria	Symptomatic UTI
	Prostate enlargement	↑ Residual urine volume	Urinary incontinence; urinary retention
Musculoskeletal	↓ Lean body mass, muscle		Functional impairment
	↓ Bone density	Osteopenia	Hip fracture
Nervous system	Brain atrophy	Benign senescent forgetfulness	Dementia, delirium
	↓ Brain catechol synthesis		Depression
	↓ Brain dopaminergic synthesis	Stiffer gait	Parkinson's disease
	↓ Righting reflexes	↑ Body sway	Falls
	↓ Stage 4 sleep	Early wakening, insomnia	Sleep apnea

[a] Changes generally observed in healthy elderly subjects free of symptoms and detectable disease in the organ system studied. The changes are usually important only when the system is stressed or other factors are added (e.g., drugs, disease, or environmental challenge); they rarely result in symptoms otherwise. Abbreviations: T_4, thyroxine; BP, blood pressure; HR, heart rate; ADH, antidiuretic hormone; GFR, glomerular filtration rate.

depression to a psychiatric disorder, incontinence to bladder dysfunction, falling to a neuropathy, or syncope to heart disease.

2. Because of decreased physiologic reserve, older patients often develop symptoms at an earlier stage of their disease (Fig. 9-1). For example, heart failure may be precipitated by mild hyperthyroidism, cognitive dysfunction by mild hyperparathyroidism, urinary retention by mild prostatic enlargement, and nonketotic hyperosmolar coma by mild glucose intolerance. Paradoxically, therefore, treatment of the underlying disease may be easier because it is frequently less advanced at the time of presentation. A corollary is that drug side effects can occur with drugs and drug doses unlikely to produce side effects in younger people (Chap. 71). For instance, an antihistamine (e.g., diphenhydramine) may cause confusion, loop diuretics may precipitate urinary incontinence, digoxin may induce depression even with normal serum levels, and over-the-counter sympathomimetics may precipitate urinary retention in men with mild prostatic obstruction.

Table 9-2 Life Expectancy and Number of Remaining Years Free of Dependency in Activities of Daily Living

Age	Life Expectancy[a], av		Disability-Free Years Remaining	
	Men	Women	Men	Women
65–69	13	20	9	11
70–74	12	16	8	8
75–79	10	13	7	7
80–84	7	10	5	5
≥85	7	8	3	3

[a] For independent noninstitutionalized elderly men and women in Massachusetts. Longevity and disability-free longevity are surprisingly long and must be incorporated into treatment decisions. All figures rounded to nearest year. See text for more recent data on longevity alone.
SOURCE: S Katz et al: N Engl J Med 309:1218, 1983.

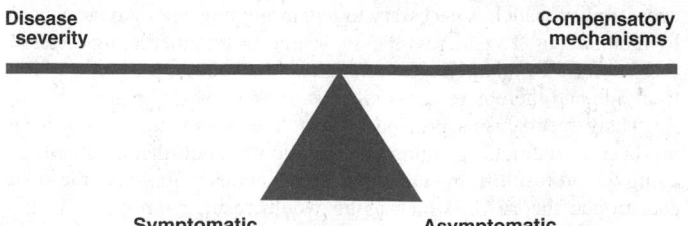

FIGURE 9-1 Even mild organ system dysfunction may cause symptoms if compensatory mechanisms are impaired. (*From NM Resnick: JAMA 276:1832, 1996.*)

Unfortunately, the predisposition to develop symptoms at an earlier stage of disease is often offset by the change in illness behavior that occurs with age. Raised at a time when symptoms and debility were accepted as normal consequences of aging, the elderly are less likely to seek attention until symptoms become disabling. Thus, any symptom, particularly those associated with a change in functional status, must be taken seriously and evaluated promptly.

3. Since many homeostatic mechanisms may be compromised concurrently, there are usually multiple abnormalities amenable to treatment, and small improvements in each may yield dramatic benefits overall. For instance, cognitive impairment in patients with Alzheimer's disease may respond much better to interventions that alleviate comorbidity than to prescription of donepezil (Fig. 9-2). Similar approaches apply to most other geriatric syndromes, including falls, incontinence, depression, delirium, syncope, and fracture. In each case, substantial functional improvement can result from treating the contributing factors even if—as in Alzheimer's disease—the disease itself is largely untreatable.

4. Many findings that are abnormal in younger patients are relatively common in older people—e.g., bacteriuria, premature ventricular contractions, low bone mineral density, impaired glucose tolerance, and uninhibited bladder contractions. However, they may not be responsible for a particular symptom but only be incidental findings that result in missed diagnoses and misdirected therapy. For instance, the finding of bacteriuria should not end the search for a source of fever in an acutely ill older patient, nor should an elevated random blood sugar—especially in an acutely ill patient—be incriminated as the cause of neuropathy. On the other hand, certain other abnormalities must not be dismissed as due to old age—e.g., there is no anemia, impotence, depression, or confusion of old age.

5. Because symptoms in older people are often due to multiple causes, the diagnostic "law of parsimony" often does not apply. For instance, fever, anemia, retinal embolus, and a heart murmur prompt almost a reflex diagnosis of infective endocarditis in a younger patient but may reflect aspirin-induced blood loss, a cholesterol embolus, insignificant aortic sclerosis, and a viral illness in an older patient. Moreover, even when the diagnosis is correct, treatment of a single disease in an older patient is unlikely to result in cure. For instance, in a younger patient, incontinence due to involuntary bladder contractions is treated effectively with a bladder relaxant medication. However, in an older patient with the same condition but who also has fecal impaction, takes medications that cloud the sensorium, and suffers from arthritis-associated impairments of mobility and manual dexterity, treatment of the bladder spasms alone is unlikely to restore continence. On the other hand, disimpaction, discontinuation of the offending medications, and treatment of the arthritis are likely to restore continence without the need for a bladder relaxant. Failure to recognize these principles often leads to prescribing "ineffective" therapy and to unjustified therapeutic nihilism towards older patients.

6. Because the older patient is more likely to suffer the adverse consequences of disease, treatment—and even prevention—may be equally or even more effective. For instance, the survival benefits of exercise, as well as thrombolysis and beta-blocker therapy after a myocardial infarction, are as impressive in older patients as in younger ones; and treatment of hypertension and transient ischemic attacks, as well as immunization against influenza and pneumococcal pneumonia, are more effective in older patients. In addition, prevention in older patients must often be seen in a broader context. For instance, although interventions to increase bone density may be limited in older patients, fracture may still be prevented by efforts to improve balance, strengthen legs, reduce peripheral edema, treat other contributing medical conditions, replete nutritional deficits, eliminate environmental hazards, and remove adverse medications—not so much those that affect bone metabolism, but rather those that induce orthostasis, confusion, and extrapyramidal stiffness.

In summary, optimal treatment of the older patient generally requires treating much more than the organ system usually associated

FIGURE 9-2 Although young and old patients may appear to suffer equally from Alzheimer's disease, its extent in older patients is often magnified by comorbidity and drug use. Identification and treatment of these contributing factors will improve the older patient's function even though the Alzheimer's disease is inadequately treatable. CHF, congestive heart failure; COPD, chronic obstructive pulmonary disease. *(From Resnick and Marcantonio.)*

with the disease or symptom, and often permits ignoring that system entirely.

EVALUATION Evaluation of the older patient can be time-consuming, even when it is tailored to the problem. Yet, such initial investment can reduce subsequent morbidity and resource utilization and enhance patient and physician satisfaction. Additionally, the assessment can often be accomplished over several visits. Moreover, much can be gleaned from questionnaires filled out by the patient or caregiver in advance as well as from observation. For instance, greeting the patient in the waiting room allows the physician to note affective and cognitive response, the strength of the handshake, the ease of rising from a chair without using the arms, the length and steadiness of the stride, and the ability to follow directions to the examining room and to sit down safely in the examining room chair. Observing the patient dress or undress can also enhance detection of impaired cognition, fine motor skills, balance, and judgment. Such observations often provide more information than standard examinations and can shorten the clinical evaluation.

HISTORY TAKING IN ELDERLY PATIENTS Most older patients are able to provide a reliable medical history; however, a multitude of complaints may make obtaining a history more difficult. If the patient is unable to comprehend or communicate, data should be sought from family, friends, and caregivers. The history should also include drug ingestion; dietary patterns; falling, incontinence, sexual dysfunction, depression and anxiety.

Advance Directives All older patients should be asked whether they have drafted advance health care directives, and, if they have, a copy should be placed in the record. Such directives may consist of a health care proxy or durable power of attorney for health care, in which patients designate a surrogate decision-maker who makes health care decisions if the patient cannot, and/or a living will or medical directive, in which patients specify their desires for treatment in specific situations if they cannot communicate at the critical time.

Whether or not the patient has formally drafted these directives, it is useful to indicate in the record who should make health care decisions if the patient is no longer able to do so. Patients should then be encouraged to discuss their thoughts with the physician as well as the designated proxy. It is not feasible to cover all possible future complications in such discussions. Ascertaining patients' perspectives on specific interventions, such as resuscitation or intubation, is also difficult because preferences will likely differ depending on prognosis.

For instance, a patient may not be interested in feeding tube placement following a massive stroke with little chance of recovery but would prefer the same intervention if it is short-term and helps ensure more rapid and complete recovery from an intercurrent illness such as pneumonia. More useful is a discussion that uses open-ended questions and empathic comments to elicit the patient's values and goals. Moreover, for any given condition, preferences may differ depending on baseline clinical status. For robust elderly individuals, recovery is a realistic goal, albeit the odds of complications are higher than for younger individuals. For the frail elderly patient with comorbidity that impairs functional status, reduction or alleviation of symptoms may be the goal. For patients with advanced dementia or terminal illness, palliation may be the most appropriate strategy. In each situation, however, early elicitation of a patient's preferences and values—when the patient can still state them—can often help both physicians and families in subsequent difficult decisions by giving surrogate decision-makers the sense that they are doing as the patient would have wanted.

PHYSICAL EXAMINATION Certain features of the examination should receive special attention, depending in part on clues from the history. Weight and postural blood pressure should be measured at most visits. Vision and hearing should be checked; if hearing is impaired, excess cerumen should be removed from the external auditory canals prior to audiologic referral. Denture fit should be assessed, and the oral cavity should be inspected with the dentures removed. Although thyroid disease becomes more common with age, the sensitivity and specificity of related findings are substantially lower than in younger individuals; consequently, the physical examination can rarely corroborate or exclude thyroid dysfunction in older patients. The breasts should not be overlooked, since older women are more likely to have breast cancer and less likely to do breast self-examination. The systolic murmur of aortic sclerosis is common and may be difficult to differentiate from aortic stenosis, especially since the presence of a fourth heart sound in an elderly person does not imply significant cardiac disease, and the carotid upstroke normally increases owing to age-related arterial stiffening.

In inactive patients and those with fecal or urinary incontinence, one should check for fecal impaction. In patients with urinary incontinence—especially men—a distended bladder must be looked for, since it may be the only finding in urinary retention; perineal sensation and the bulbocavernosus reflex should also be tested. Patients who fall should be observed standing up from a chair, bending down, reaching up, walking 10 feet, turning, returning, and sitting again; abnormalities of gait and balance should be evaluated with the patient's eyes open and closed and in response to a sternal push. It should be appreciated that "frontal release signs" (e.g., "snout," "glabellar," or palmomental reflexes) and absent ankle jerks and vibratory sense in the feet may be normal in the elderly.

MENTAL STATUS EXAMINATION In addition to evaluating mood and affect, some form of cognitive testing is essential in all elderly patients, even if it involves only checking different components of the history for consistency. People with mild degrees of dementia usually retain their social graces and may mask intellectual impairment by a cheerful and cooperative manner. Thus, the examiner should always probe for content. For patients who follow the news, one can ask what stories they are particularly interested in and why; the same applies to reading, social events—even the soap operas on television.

If there is any suspicion of a cognitive deficit after this kind of conversational probing, further questioning is indicated. An examination that tests only orientation as to person, place, and time is insufficient to detect mild or moderate intellectual impairment. As a quick screen, simply assessing orientation and asking the patient to draw a clock with the hands at a set time (e.g., 10 min before 2:00) can be very informative regarding cognitive status, visuospatial deficits, ability to comprehend and execute instructions in logical sequence, and presence or absence of perseveration. For slightly more detailed examinations, many practical mental status tests are available. The most widely used is the Mini-Mental Status Examination of Folstein (Chap. 24), which provides a numerical score that can be obtained in 5 to 10 min. Regardless of the test employed, the total score is less useful diagnostically than is knowledge of the specific domain of the deficit. As a general rule, disproportionate difficulty with immediate recall (e.g., of a list of three items) suggests depression, while predominant difficulty with recalling the items 5 min later suggests dementia. For patients with deficits of attention—recognized by inability to spell simple words backwards, repeat five digits, or recite the months of the year backwards—delirium is probably present, and the accuracy of the remainder of the test is dubious. However, the test can be interpreted accurately only in the context of a comprehensive evaluation.

EVALUATION OF FUNCTIONAL CAPACITY Medical problem lists, a standard tool for assessing and following younger patients, often prove inadequate for older patients. Heart failure, stroke, and prostate cancer can describe a bedbound institutionalized person as well as a Supreme Court justice. Thus, it is essential to ascertain the patient's degree of functional incapacity owing to both medical and psychosocial problems. The functional assessment includes determination of the patient's ability to perform basic activities of daily life (ADL), which are those needed for personal self-care, as well as the ability to perform more complex tasks required for independent living, the instrumental activities of daily living (IADL). ADLs include bathing, dressing, toileting, feeding, getting in and out of chairs and bed, and walking. IADLs include shopping, cooking, money management, housework, using a telephone, and traveling outside the home. For frail patients, an assessment in the home by a trained observer may be required, but for most patients a questionnaire dealing with these activities can be completed by the family or patient. In either case, the physician must determine the cause of any impairment and whether it can be treated. Assessment should conclude with determination of the socioeconomic circumstances and social support systems.

MANAGEMENT OF COMMON GERIATRIC CONDITIONS

Diseases more common in the elderly are covered elsewhere in the text. The medical problems discussed below do not usually present as clear-cut organ-specific diagnoses and are most common in the frail elderly, especially those over 80 years of age.

INTELLECTUAL IMPAIRMENT The predominant causes of impaired mentation in older patients are delirium, dementia, and depression. Each condition is covered elsewhere in the text in detail (Chaps. 24 and 362), but their management in the elderly is discussed here.

Differentiating the causes of impaired mentation is important, but in older patients they frequently coexist. Thus, the most important first step is to search for and correct all factors that may contribute to cognitive impairment, even in patients with dementia (Fig. 9-2). Evidence of dangerous behavior should also be sought (e.g., leaving the stove on, wandering, and getting lost), and plans should be devised to deal with it. Although there is no specific pharmacologic treatment for Alzheimer's disease and agents such as donepezil are of limited efficacy, this does not mean that the physician has no further role in treating the patient and family. In addition to discontinuing all nonessential medications and treating new intercurrent illness, the physician should help the family and patient predict and deal with the disease; indeed, the family often needs the physician's support more than the patient does.

℞ TREATMENT Community services should be suggested as needed, including a visiting nurse, a home health aide to assist with personal hygiene, a homemaker to assist with housework, meal delivery, transportation services, day health centers, and respite care to ease the burden on family members. Support groups such as the

Alzheimer's Association are often of value to the family and help them to anticipate problems. Signs of patient abuse by an overstressed caregiver should be watched for. Legal counsel should be recommended to help the patient and family devise plans for ongoing management and ultimate disposition of assets not already obtained; advance directives should be sought as soon as possible while the patient can still participate.

Finally, abrupt worsening of mentation or the onset of disruptive behavior should always prompt a search for new illness or medication. Exacerbation of cognitive dysfunction may occur with mild infections (e.g., subungual toe abscess, vaginitis, or pressure ulcer); with "therapeutic" levels of many drugs; with use of nonprescribed drugs or alcohol; with modest abnormalities of serum sodium, calcium, glucose, or thyroxine; with mild hypoxia; with borderline nutritional deficiencies; with subdural hematoma or "minor" stroke; and with the development of fecal impaction, urinary retention, pain, or change in environment, particularly in frail older patients. However, if a cause is not found and behavior does not respond to environmental manipulation (e.g., ignoring the behavior, distracting the patient, addressing situational "triggers," and providing a calm environment), low doses of an antipsychotic medication may be helpful (e.g., haloperidol 0.25 to 2 mg/d orally; see below).

DEPRESSION Depression of significant degree occurs in 5 to 10% of community-dwelling elderly but is often overlooked. At highest risk are individuals with recent medical illness (e.g., stroke or fracture), bereavement, lack of social supports, recent nursing home admission, or psychiatric history (including alcohol abuse). The diagnosis requires the presence of a depressed mood for at least two consecutive weeks plus at least four of the following eight symptoms: sleep disturbance, lack of interest, feelings of guilt, decreased energy, decreased concentration, decreased appetite, psychomotor agitation/retardation, and suicidal ideation. Also helpful diagnostically are a personal or family history of depression, anhedonia (loss of pleasure), and past response to an antidepressant. It is essential to bear in mind that depression in older patients is often caused or contributed to by drugs or a systemic illness. Although "subsyndromal" depression (fewer than four of the above symptoms) also causes substantial morbidity and health resource utilization, it appears to be less responsive than major depression to therapy.

RX **TREATMENT** For the hospitalized patient in whom acute depression delays recovery or rehabilitation—when correction of medical and pharmacologic contributing factors is ineffective and there is no prior history of mania or major depression—methylphenidate, 5 to 10 mg at 8 A.M. and noon (to avoid insomnia) is often very effective, with benefits discernible within a few days. For patients with major depression, there is no ideal antidepressant drug. All are about equally effective, but the side effects differ (see below and Chap. 385). Consequently, one should become familiar with one or two agents for patients with psychomotor retardation (e.g., sertaline, desipramine) and for those with agitation (e.g., nortriptyline or nefazodone). Because of its potent anticholinergic and orthostatic side effects, amitriptyline should be avoided whenever possible in older patients. Initial low dosages should be increased slowly to avoid serious side effects; low doses of each medication (e.g., nortriptyline, 10 to 50 mg daily; desipramine, 25 to 75 mg daily; or sertraline 50 to 150 mg daily) are often effective in the elderly. Careful follow-up is required to anticipate and minimize anticholinergic side effects, orthostatic hypotension, sedating effects, confusion, bizarre mental symptoms, cardiovascular complications, and drug overdose with suicidal intent. Adverse drug reactions should not be assumed to be due to the aging process.

Cautious use of the monoamine oxidase inhibitors is sometimes of benefit when other antidepressants are ineffective. Neither monoamine oxidase inhibitors nor selective serotonin reuptake inhibitors should be used in combination with the cyclic compounds. Electroconvulsive therapy has been successful and is usually well tolerated by elderly patients who remain severely depressed despite drug treatment, particularly if they also have delusions.

URINARY INCONTINENCE **Transient Incontinence** (Table 9-3) Because urinary continence requires adequate mobility, mentation, motivation, and manual dexterity—in addition to integrated control of the lower urinary tract—problems outside the bladder can result in incontinence.

1. *Delirium.* A clouded sensorium impedes recognition of both the need to void and the location of the nearest toilet; once delirium clears, incontinence resolves.
2. *Infection.* Symptomatic urinary tract infection commonly causes or contributes to incontinence; asymptomatic infection does not.
3. *Atrophic urethritis/vaginitis.* Atrophic urethritis/vaginitis, characterized by the presence of vaginal telangiectasia, petechiae, erythema, or friability, commonly contributes to incontinence in women and responds to a several-month course of low-dose estrogen or vaginal estrogen creams.
4. *Pharmaceutical.* The drugs most commonly causing transient incontinence are listed in Table 9-4.
5. *Psychologic.* Depression and psychosis are uncommon but treatable causes.
6. *Excess urine output.* Excess urine output may overwhelm the ability to reach a toilet in time. Causes include diuretics, alcohol, excess fluid intake, and metabolic abnormalities (e.g., hyperglycemia, hypercalcemia, diabetes insipidus); nocturnal incontinence may also result from mobilization of peripheral edema.
7. *Restricted mobility.* If mobility cannot be improved, access to a urinal or commode may restore continence. (See "Immobility," below.)
8. *Stool impaction.* This is a common cause of urinary incontinence, especially in hospitalized or immobile patients. Although the mechanism is unknown, a clue to its presence is the coexistence of both urinary and fecal incontinence. Disimpaction restores continence.

Established Incontinence (Table 9-3) The causes of established incontinence include irreversible functional deficits, such as *end-stage* Alzheimer's disease, and intrinsic lower urinary tract dysfunction. Lower urinary tract dysfunction should be sought after transient causes have been excluded.

Detrusor Overactivity This disorder (involuntary bladder contraction) accounts for two-thirds of geriatric incontinence in both sexes, regardless of whether patients are demented. Detrusor overactivity can be diagnosed presumptively in a woman when leakage occurs in the absence of stress maneuvers or urinary retention and is preceded by the abrupt onset of an intense urge to urinate that cannot

Table 9-3 Classification of Incontinence

TRANSIENT

Delirium/confusional state
Infection—urinary (symptomatic)
Atrophic urethritis/vaginitis
Pharmaceuticals
Psychological, especially depression
Excessive urine output (e.g., CHF, hyperglycemia)
Restricted mobility
Stool impaction

ESTABLISHED

Detrusor overactivity
Detrusor underactivity
Urethral obstruction
Urethral incompetence

NOTE: CHF, congestive heart failure.
SOURCE: Adapted from NM Resnick: Medical Grand Rounds 3:281, 1984.

Table 9-4 Commonly Used Medications that May Affect Continence

Type of Medication	Examples	Potential Effects on Continence
Sedatives/hypnotics	Long-acting benzodi-azepines (e.g., diazepam, flurazepam)	Sedation, delirium, immobility
Alcohol		Polyuria, frequency, urgency, sedation, delirium, immobility
Anticholinergics	Dicyclomine, diso-pyramide, sedating antihistamines	Urinary retention, overflow incontinence, delirium, impaction
Antipsychotics	Thioridazine, haloperidol	Anticholinergic actions, sedation, rigidity, immobility
Tricyclic antidepressants	Amitriptyline, desipramine	Anticholinergic actions, sedation
Antiparkinsonians	Trihexyphenidyl, benztropine mesylate (not L-dopa/selegiline)	Anticholinergic actions, sedation
Narcotic analgesics	Opiates	Urinary retention, fecal impaction, sedation, delirium
α-Adrenergic antagonists	Prazosin, terazosin, doxazosin	Urethral relaxation may precipitate stress incontinence in women
α-Adrenergic agonists	Nasal decongestants	Urinary retention in men
Calcium channel blockers	All dihydropyridines[a]	Urinary retention; nocturnal diuresis due to fluid retention
Potent diuretics	Furosemide, bumetanide	Polyuria, frequency, urgency
Angiotensin-converting enzyme inhibitors	Captopril, enalapril, lisinopril	Drug-induced cough can precipitate stress incontinence in women and in some men with prior prostatectomy
Vincristine		Urinary retention

[a] Examples include nifedipine, nicardipine, israpidine, felodipine, nimodipine.
SOURCE: Adapted from NM Resnick, in *Current Medical Diagnosis and Treatment*, LT Tierney et al (eds), Norwalk, Appleton & Lange, 1993.

be forestalled. In men, the symptoms are similar, but since detrusor overactivity often coexists with urethral obstruction, urodynamic testing should be done if prescription of a bladder relaxant is planned. Because detrusor overactivity may also be due to bladder stones or tumor, the abrupt onset of otherwise unexplained urge incontinence—especially if accompanied by perineal/suprapubic discomfort or sterile hematuria—should prompt cystoscopy and cytologic examination.

℞ **TREATMENT** The cornerstone of treatment is behavioral therapy with or without biofeedback. Patients without dementia are instructed to void every 1 to 2 h (while awake only) and to suppress urgency in between; once daytime continence is restored, the interval between voiding can be progressively increased. Demented patients are "prompted" to void at similar intervals. When drugs are necessary, they should be added to these regimens and monitored to avoid inducing urinary retention. Effective drugs include oxybutynin (2.5 to 5 mg three or four times daily, or sustained release, 5 to 20 mg once daily), dicyclomine (10 to 30 mg three times daily), tolterodine (1 to 2 mg twice daily), and imipramine or doxepin (25 to 100 mg at bedtime). If prescribed for older patients, DDAVP should be used cautiously—especially in the setting of renal insufficiency or heart failure—and it probably should not be given to patients with

hyponatremia or urine output >2500 mL/d. Alternative treatments, such as neuromodulation, are under investigation.

Indwelling catheterization is rarely indicated for detrusor overactivity. If all measures fail, an external collection device or protective pad or undergarment may be required.

Stress Incontinence This disorder, the second most common cause of established incontinence in older women (it is rare in men), is characterized by symptoms and evidence of *instantaneous* leakage of urine in response to stress. Leakage is worse or occurs only during the day unless another abnormality (e.g., detrusor overactivity) is also present. On examination, with the bladder full and the perineum relaxed, instantaneous leakage upon coughing strongly suggests stress incontinence, especially if it reproduces symptoms and if urinary retention has been excluded by a postvoiding residual determination; a several-second delay suggests that leakage is instead caused by an involuntary bladder contraction induced by coughing.

℞ **TREATMENT** Surgery is the most effective treatment. For women who can comply indefinitely, pelvic muscle exercises are an option for mild to moderate stress incontinence, but they often require specialized training using vaginal cones or biofeedback. If not contraindicated, an α-adrenergic agonist (e.g., phenylpropanolamine) is also helpful in such cases, especially if combined with estrogen. Occasionally, a pessary or even a tampon (for women with vaginal stenosis) provides some relief.

Urethral Obstruction Rarely present in women, urethral obstruction (due to prostatic enlargement, urethral stricture, bladder neck contracture, or prostate cancer) is the second most common cause of established incontinence in older men. It can present as dribbling incontinence after voiding, urge incontinence due to detrusor overactivity (which coexists in two-thirds of cases), or overflow incontinence due to urinary retention. Renal ultrasound is recommended to exclude hydronephrosis in men whose postvoiding residual volume exceeds 100 to 200 mL; in older men for whom surgery is planned, urodynamic confirmation of obstruction is strongly advised.

℞ **TREATMENT** Surgical decompression is the most effective treatment for obstruction, especially if there is urinary retention. For a nonoperative candidate, intermittent or indwelling catheterization is used; a condom catheter is contraindicated when urinary retention is present. For a man with prostatic obstruction who is not in retention, treatment with an α-adrenergic antagonist (e.g., terazosin 5 to 10 mg daily) may lessen symptoms in a few weeks. The 5α-reductase inhibitor finasteride may also ameliorate symptoms in a third or more of patients, but its impact is modest and not apparent for many months. Combined treatment with both agents has proved no better than treatment with an alpha blocker alone in most men.

Detrusor Underactivity Whether idiopathic or due to sacral lower motor nerve dysfunction, this is the least common cause of incontinence (<10% of cases). When it causes incontinence, detrusor underactivity is associated with urinary frequency, nocturia, and frequent leakage of small amounts. The elevated postvoiding residual volume (generally >450 mL) distinguishes it from detrusor overactivity and stress incontinence, but only urodynamic testing (rather than cystoscopy or intravenous urography) differentiates it from urethral obstruction in men; such testing is not usually required in women, in whom obstruction is rare.

℞ **TREATMENT** For the patient with a poorly contractile bladder, augmented voiding techniques (e.g., double voiding or applying suprapubic pressure) are often effective; pharmacologic agents (e.g., bethanechol) are rarely effective. If further emptying is needed or for the patient with an acontractile bladder, intermittent or indwelling catheterization is the only option. Antibiotics should be used for symptomatic upper tract infection, or as prophylaxis for recurrent symptomatic infections only in a patient using intermittent catheterization; they should not be used as prophylaxis with an indwelling catheter.

FALLS Falls are a major problem for elderly people, especially women. Some 30% of community-dwelling elderly individuals fall each year, and the proportion increases with age. Nonetheless, falling must *not* be viewed as accidental, inevitable, or untreatable.

Causes of Falls Balance and ambulation require a complex interplay of cognitive, neuromuscular, and cardiovascular function and the ability to adapt rapidly to an environmental challenge. With age, balance becomes impaired and sway increases. The resulting vulnerability predisposes the older person to fall when challenged by an additional insult to *any* of these systems. Thus, a seemingly minor fall may be due to a serious problem, such as pneumonia or a myocardial infarction.

Much more commonly, however, falls are due to the complex interaction between a variably impaired patient and an environmental challenge. While a warped floorboard may pose little problem for a vigorous, unmedicated, alert person, it may be sufficient to precipitate a fall and hip fracture in the patient with impaired vision, strength, balance, or cognition. Thus, falls in older people are rarely due to a single cause, and effective prevention entails a comprehensive assessment of the patient's intrinsic deficits (usually diseases and medications), the routine activities, and the environmental obstacles.

Intrinsic deficits are those that impair sensory input, judgment, blood pressure regulation, reaction time, and balance and gait (Table 9-5). Medications and alcohol use are among the most common, significant, and reversible causes of falling. Other treatable contributors include postprandial hypotension (which peaks 30 to 60 min after a meal), insomnia, urinary urgency, foot problems, and peripheral edema [which can burden impaired leg strength and gait with an additional 2 to 5 kg (5 to 10 lb)].

Environmental obstacles are listed in Table 9-6. Since most falls occur in or around the home, a visit by a visiting nurse, physical therapist, or physician often reaps substantial dividends.

Complications of Falls and Treatment One out of four people who fall suffers serious injury. About 5% of falls result in fractures, and an equal proportion cause serious soft tissue damage. Falls are the sixth leading cause of death for older people and a contributing factor in 40% of admissions to nursing homes. Resultant hip problems and fear of falls are major causes of loss of independence.

Subdural hematoma is a treatable but easily overlooked complication of falls that must be considered in any elderly patient presenting with new neurologic signs, including confusion alone, even in the absence of a headache. Dehydration, electrolyte imbalance, pressure sores, rhabdomyolysis, and hypothermia may also occur and endanger the patient's life following a fall.

The risk of falling is related to the number of contributory conditions. Because the relationship is multiplicative rather than additive, however, even minor improvement in a number of these factors will reduce the risk substantially. In addition, gait training by a physical therapist often alleviates fear of falling. Ensuring the availability of phones at floor level, a portable phone, or a lightweight radio call system is also important, as is detection and treatment of osteoporosis.

IMMOBILITY The main causes of immobility are weakness, stiffness, pain, imbalance, and psychological problems. Weakness may result from disuse of muscles, malnutrition, electrolyte disturbances, anemia, neurologic disorders, or myopathies. The most common cause of stiffness in the elderly is osteoarthritis; however, Parkinson's disease, rheumatoid arthritis, gout, pseudogout, and antipsychotic drugs such as haloperidol may also contribute. Pain, whether from bone (e.g., osteoporosis, osteomalacia, Paget's disease, metastatic bone cancer, trauma), joints (e.g., osteoarthritis, rheumatoid arthritis, gout), bursa, muscle (e.g., polymyalgia rheumatica, intermittent claudication, or "pseudoclaudication"), or foot problems may immobilize the patient.

Imbalance and fear of falling are major causes of immobilization. Imbalance may result from general debility, neurologic causes (e.g., stroke; loss of postural reflexes; peripheral neuropathy due to diabetes mellitus, alcohol, or malnutrition; and vestibulocerebellar abnormalities), orthostatic or postprandial hypotension, or drugs (e.g., diuretics, antihypertensives, neuroleptics, and antidepressants) or may occur following prolonged bed rest. Psychological conditions such as severe anxiety or depression may also contribute to immobilization.

Consequences In addition to thrombophlebitis and pulmonary embolus, there are multiple hazards of bed rest in the elderly. Decon-

Table 9-5   Intrinsic Risk Factors for Falling, and Possible Interventions

Risk Factor	Interventions	
	Medical	Rehabilitative or Environmental
Reduced visual acuity, dark adaptation, and perception	Refraction; cataract extraction	Home safety assessment
Reduced hearing	Removal of cerumen; audiologic evaluation	Hearing aid if appropriate (with training); reduction in background noise
Vestibular dysfunction	Avoidance of drugs affecting the vestibular system; neurologic or ear, nose, and throat evaluation, if indicated	Habituation exercises
Proprioceptive dysfunction, cervical degenerative disorders, and peripheral neuropathy	Screening for vitamin B_{12} deficiency and cervical spondylosis	Balance exercises; appropriate walking aid; correctly sized footwear with firm soles; home safety assessment
Dementia	Detection of reversible causes; avoidance of sedative or centrally acting drugs	Supervised exercise and ambulation; home safety assessment
Musculoskeletal disorders	Appropriate diagnostic evaluation	Balance-and-gait training; muscle-strengthening exercises; appropriate walking aid; home safety assessment
Foot disorders (calluses, bunions, deformities, edema)	Shaving of calluses; bunionectomy; treatment of edema	Trimming of nails; appropriate footwear
Postural hypotension	Assessment of medications; rehydration; possible alteration in situational factors (e.g., meals, change of position)	Dorsiflexion exercises; pressure-graded stockings; elevation of head of bed; use of tilt table if condition is severe
Use of medications (sedatives: benzodiazepines, phenothiazines, antidepressants; antihypertensives; others: antiarrhythmics, anticonvulsants, diuretics, alcohol)	Steps to be taken: 1. Attempted reduction in the total number of medications taken 2. Assessment of risks and benefits of each medication 3. Selection of medication, if needed, that is least centrally acting, least associated with postural hypotension, and has shortest action 4. Prescription of lowest effective dose 5. Frequent reassessment of risks and benefits	

SOURCE: After ME Tinetti and M Speechley, N Engl J Med 320:1055, 1989.

Table 9-6 Environmental Factors Affecting the Risk of Falling

Environmental Area or Factor	Objective and Recommendations
All areas	
Lighting	Adequacy of illumination (older people need twice as much as younger people); absence of glare and shadows; accessible switches at room entrances; night light in bedroom, hall, bathroom
Floors	Nonskid backing for throw rugs; carpet edges tacked down; carpets with shallow pile; nonskid wax on floors; cords out of walking path; small objects (e.g., clothes, shoes) off floor
Stairs	Lighting sufficient, with switches at top and bottom of stairs; securely fastened bilateral handrails that stand out from wall; top and bottom steps marked with bright, contrasting tape; stair rises of no more than 6 in; steps in good repair; no objects stored on steps
Kitchen	Items stored so that reaching up and bending over are not necessary; secure step stool available if climbing is necessary; firm, nonmovable table
Bathroom	Grab bars for tub, shower, and toilet; nonskid decals or rubber mat in tub or shower; shower chair with handheld shower; nonskid rugs; raised toilet seat; door locks removed to ensure access in an emergency
Yard and entrances	Repair of cracks in pavement, holes in lawn; removal of rocks, tools, and other tripping hazards; well-lit walkways, free of ice and wet leaves; stairs and steps as above
Institutions	All the above; bed at proper height (not too high or low); spills on floor cleaned up promptly; appropriate use of walking aids and wheelchairs
Footwear	Shoes with firm, nonskid, nonfriction soles; low heels (unless person is accustomed to high heels); avoidance of walking in stocking feet or loose slippers

SOURCE: After ME Tinetti and M Speechley, N Engl J Med 320:1055, 1989.

ditioning of the cardiovascular system occurs within days and involves fluid shifts, fluid loss, decreased cardiac output, decreased peak oxygen uptake, and increased resting heart rate. Striking changes also occur in skeletal muscle. At the cellular level, intracellular ATP and glycogen concentrations decrease, rates of protein degradation increase, and contractile velocity and strength decline, while at the whole-muscle level, atrophy, weakness, and shortening are seen. Pressure sores are another serious complication; mechanical pressure, moisture, friction, and shearing forces all predispose to their development. As a result, within days of being confined to bed, the risk of postural hypotension, falls, and skin breakdown rises. Moreover, these changes usually take weeks to months to reverse.

TREATMENT The most important step is preventive—to avoid bedrest whenever possible. When it cannot be avoided, several measures can be employed to minimize its consequences. Patients should be positioned as close to the upright position as possible several times daily. Range-of-motion exercises should begin immediately, and the skin over pressure points should be inspected frequently. Isometric and isotonic exercises should be performed while the patient is in bed, and whenever possible patients should assist their own positioning, transferring, and self-care. As mobility becomes feasible, graduated ambulation should begin. For individuals confined to a wheelchair, ring-shaped devices ("donuts") should not be used to prevent pressure ulcers since they cause venous congestion and edema and actually increase the risk.

If a pressure ulcer develops, therapy depends on its stage. Stage 1 ulcers are characterized by nonblanchable erythema of intact skin; stage 2 lesions involve an ulcer of the epidermis, dermis, or both; stage 3 ulcers extend to the subcutaneous tissue; and stage 4 lesions involve muscle, bone, and/or the supporting tissues. For stage 1 lesions, eliminating excess pressure and ensuring adequate nutrition and hygiene

are sufficient. For the remaining types, the caregiver must also ensure that the wound stays clean and moist; thus, if saline dressings are used they should be changed when they are damp rather than dry. Synthetic dressings are more expensive than saline but are more effective because they require fewer changes (with less disruption of reepithelialization) and protect against contamination. Because bacterial colonization of pressure ulcers is universal, swab cultures should not be performed and topical treatment should be considered only for patients whose ulcers have not healed after 2 weeks of therapy. By contrast, associated cellulitis, osteomyelitis, or sepsis requires systemic therapy after cultures of blood and the wound border (by needle aspiration or biopsy) have been obtained. Surgical or enzymatic debridement is required for stage 3 and 4 lesions. In addition to a daily multivitamin, prescribing vitamin C (500 mg twice daily) is also useful. For debilitated patients, special mattresses are beneficial, including those that reduce pressure (e.g., static air mattress or foam) and those that relieve it (e.g., dynamic units that sequentially inflate and deflate).

In addition to treating all identified factors that contribute to immobility, consultation with a physical therapist should be sought. Installing handrails, lowering the bed, and providing chairs of proper height with arms and rubber skid guards may allow the patient to be safely mobile in the home. A properly fitted cane or walker may be helpful.

IATROGENIC DRUG REACTIONS For several reasons, older patients are two or three times more likely to have adverse drug reactions (Chap. 71). Drug clearance is often markedly reduced. This is due to a decrease in renal plasma flow and glomerular filtration rate and a reduced hepatic clearance. The last is due to a decrease in activity of the drug-metabolizing microsomal enzymes and an overall decline in blood flow to the liver with aging. The volume of distribution of drugs is also affected, since the elderly have a decrease in total-body water and a relative increase in body fat. Thus, water-soluble drugs become more concentrated, and fat-soluble drugs have longer half-lives. In addition, serum albumin levels decline, particularly in sick patients, so that there is a decrease in protein binding of some drugs (e.g., warfarin, phenytoin), leaving more free (active) drug available.

In addition to impaired drug clearance, which alters pharmacokinetics, older patients have altered responses to similar serum drug levels, a phenomenon known as *altered pharmacodynamics*. They are more sensitive to some drugs (e.g., opiates, anticoagulants) and less sensitive to others (e.g., β-adrenergic agents). Finally, the older patient with multiple chronic conditions is likely to be taking several drugs, including nonprescribed agents. Thus, adverse drug reactions and dosage errors are more likely to occur, especially if the patient has visual, hearing, or memory deficits.

Precautions to Avoid Drug Toxicity • *Drug selection and administration* Before initiating treatment, the physician should first ensure that the symptom requiring treatment is not itself due to another drug. For example, antipsychotic agents can cause symptoms that mimic depression (flat affect, restlessness, and pacing); such symptoms should prompt lowering of the dose rather than initiation of an antidepressant. In addition, drug therapy should be employed only after nonpharmacologic means have been considered or tried and only when the benefit clearly outweighs the risk.

Once pharmacotherapy has been decided upon, it should begin at less than the usual adult dosage and the dose should be increased slowly. However, given the marked variability in pharmacokinetics and pharmacodynamics in the elderly, dose escalation should continue until either a successful endpoint is reached or an intolerable side effect is encountered. The final dosage schedule should be kept as simple as possible, and the number of pills should be kept as low as possible. Serum drug levels are often useful in older patients, especially for monitoring drugs with narrow therapeutic indices such as phenytoin, theophylline, quinidine, aminoglycosides, lithium, and psychotropic agents such as nortriptyline. However, toxicity can occur even with "normal" therapeutic levels of some drugs (e.g., digoxin, phenytoin).

Over-the-counter agents   Nearly three-quarters of the elderly regularly use nonprescribed drugs, many of which cause significant symptoms and/or interact with other medications. Frequent offenders include nonprescribed agents for insomnia (all of which are anticholinergics), and nonsteroidal anti-inflammatory drugs (NSAIDs), which can hamper control of hypertension in addition to causing renal dysfunction and gastrointestinal bleeding. Gingko biloba, increasingly used as a "memory booster," may interfere with previously stable anticoagulation regimens. Because older patients often consider such agents "nostrums" rather than drugs, the physician must ask about them directly.

Sedative-hypnotics   If nonpharmacologic treatment of insomnia is unsuccessful, low-dose and short-term or intermittent use of an intermediate-acting agent whose metabolism is not affected by age (e.g., oxazepam, 10 to 30 mg/d) may be useful. Because of the increased risk of confusion and other adverse effects, benzodiazepines with either short (e.g., triazolam) or long duration of action (e.g., flurazepam and diazepam) should be avoided. Barbiturates should be avoided for the same reasons. An antidepressant should not be prescribed for insomnia unless the patient is depressed.

Antibiotics   Serum creatinine is not a good index of renal function in old people; however, when it is elevated, special care must be taken with the administration of drugs normally excreted by the kidneys. Concentrations of relevant antibiotics should be measured directly.

Cardiac drugs   In older patients, digitalis, procainamide, and quinidine have prolonged half-lives and narrow therapeutic windows; toxicity is common at the usual dosages. For example, digoxin toxicity—especially anorexia, confusion, or depression—can occur even with therapeutic digoxin levels.

H₂ receptor antagonists   Most of these agents interfere with hepatic metabolism of other drugs, and all can produce confusion in the elderly. Because they are renally excreted, lower doses should be used to minimize the risk of toxicity in older individuals.

Antipsychotics and tricyclic antidepressants   These drugs can produce anticholinergic side effects in old people (e.g., confusion, urinary retention, constipation, dry mouth). These can be minimized by switching to a nonanticholinergic agent (e.g., sertraline or nefazodone) or one with less anticholinergic effect (e.g., olanzapine, desipramine). In general, the least potent agents for psychosis (e.g., chlorpromazine) have the most sedating and anticholinergic effects and are the most likely to induce postural hypotension. By contrast, the most potent antipsychotic agents (e.g., haloperidol) have the least sedating, anticholinergic, and hypotensive side effects but cause extrapyramidal side effects, including dystonia, akathisia, rigidity, and tardive dyskinesia. The newer potent antipsychotics (e.g., risperidone, olanzapine, quetiapine, and clozapine) are relative exceptions to this rule. More specific for serotonin than dopamine D₂ receptors, these medications may be safer for older demented patients, especially those with hallucinations associated with Lewy body dementia or in those receiving therapy for Parkinson's disease. Unfortunately, even these newer drugs lose their specificity at the higher doses that are commonly required in clinical practice. Thus all of these agents are potentially toxic. Moreover, since both depression and agitation often remit spontaneously, cautious discontinuation of these drugs should be considered periodically.

Glaucoma medications   Both topical beta blockers and carbonic anhydrase inhibitors can cause systemic side effects. The latter can cause malaise and anorexia independent of the induced metabolic acidosis.

Anticoagulants   Elderly patients benefit from anticoagulation as much as do younger individuals but are more vulnerable to serious bleeding and drug interactions. Hence, more careful monitoring and less aggressive anticoagulation are advisable.

Analgesics   Both propoxyphene and meperidine are associated with a disproportionate risk of delirium, and propoxyphene also increases the risk of hip fracture. Of the NSAIDs, indomethacin is most likely to induce confusion, fluid retention, and gastrointestinal bleeding. Each of these agents should be avoided in the elderly.

Avoidance of overtreatment   Drugs are frequently not indicated in some common clinical situations. For instance, antibiotics need not be given for asymptomatic bacteriuria unless obstructive uropathy, other anatomic abnormalities, or stones are also present. Ankle edema is often due to venous insufficiency, drugs such as NSAIDs or some calcium antagonists, or even inactivity or malnutrition in chairbound patients. Diuretics are usually not indicated unless edema is associated with heart failure. Fitted, pressure gradient stockings are often helpful. Regular exercise is much more useful for claudication than is pentoxifylline. Finally, since older patients generally tolerate aspirin and other NSAIDs less well than do younger patients, localized pain should be treated when possible with local measures such as injection, physical therapy, heat, ultrasound, or transcutaneous electrical stimulation (Chap. 12).

PREVENTION

Much can be done to prevent the progression and even the onset of disease in older people. Dietary inadequacies should be corrected. Daily calcium intake should approximate 1500 mg, and most elderly people should take 400 to 800 IU of vitamin D daily (contained in one to two multivitamin tablets). Tobacco and alcohol use should be minimized, since the benefits of discontinuing these accrue even to individuals over age 65. The importance of reviewing all of a patient's medications and discontinuing them whenever feasible cannot be overemphasized.

Hypertension, whether isolated systolic hypertension or combined systolic and diastolic hypertension, should be treated. Treatment reduces the risk of stroke and the risk of death due to cardiovascular causes substantially in this age group and may also reduce the risk of cognitive impairment. These benefits have been achieved using *low doses* of a thiazide-like diuretic (e.g., chlorthalidone, 12.5 to 25 mg/d) as the first step (alone effective in almost half of patients) and adding low-dose reserpine (0.05 to 0.1 mg/d) or atenolol (25 to 50 mg/d) only as needed. Benefits are dramatic, side effects are minimal, cost is trivial, and concerns about potential toxicity have not been borne out.

Because of the prevalence, functional impact, and ease of treatment, glaucoma should be screened for, and visual and auditory impairment should be corrected. Dentures should be assessed for their fit, and oral lesions beneath them should be detected.

Because thyroid dysfunction is more prevalent in the elderly, difficult to detect clinically, and treatable, serum levels of thyroid-stimulating hormone should be measured at least once in asymptomatic older people and probably every 3 to 5 years thereafter. Serum cholesterol is worth measuring in patients with established coronary heart disease, but in those without apparent disease, screening for hypercholesterolemia is controversial. It seems reasonable to screen those who would be willing to comply with therapy, whose quality of life is good (from the patient's viewpoint), whose life expectancy exceeds several years (long enough to potentially benefit from therapy), and whose other risk factors—for which benefit of treatment has been definitely established—have already been addressed. A Papanicolaou test should be done in women who have not had one before, since the incidence of both preventable cervical carcinoma and associated death increases with age, especially in this group; it should be repeated triennially in all older women unless two previous tests have been normal. Screening for colon cancer is warranted until a minimum age of 80 to 85, at least in the community-dwelling elderly, although the optimal method is unclear. Immunizations for influenza, pneumococcal pneumonia, and tetanus should be current. Purified protein derivative (PPD) testing should be done on residents of chronic care facilities and on others at high risk of tuberculosis; those who have recently converted probably should be treated. Since responsiveness wanes with age, the test, if negative, should be repeated in a week to increase the chances of detecting all exposed patients. Because older women with breast cancer are more likely to die *of* it than *with* it, screening mammography is indicated every 1 to 2 years at least until age 75 and thereafter if a positive finding would result in therapeutic intervention. The relative risks and benefits of low-dose aspirin and (for women) estrogen replacement therapy have not yet been elucidated sufficiently in the elderly to warrant routine use, but they should be considered on an individual basis.

Exercise should be encouraged not only because of its beneficial effects on blood pressure, cardiovascular conditioning, glucose homeostasis, bone density, insomnia, functional status, and even longevity, but also because it may improve mood and social interaction, reduce constipation, and prevent falls. Resistance training should be encouraged as much as a walking program. Spinal flexion exercises should be avoided in patients with osteopenia; consultation with a physical therapist may be helpful.

Measures should be taken to prevent falling, as outlined in Tables 9-5 and 9-6. Now that alendronate has proved effective in preventing vertebral and hip fractures in older women, bone density should be measured in women who are willing to take the drug and who do not already take estrogen. Counseling about driving is important, especially for patients with cognitive impairment.

Perhaps the most valuable preventive measure in old people is to take a careful history, focusing not only on the "chief complaint" but also on common and often hidden conditions such as falls, confusion, depression, alcohol abuse, sexual dysfunction, and incontinence. In addition, one should always identify the complications for which the specific patient is at risk and take steps to avert them. For instance, a patient with cognitive impairment who smokes is at risk not only for lung cancer but also for starting a fire, and a patient who requires narcotics is at risk for fecal impaction, delirium, urinary retention, and confusion. Community-dwelling patients who are at highest risk of rapid deterioration and institutionalization and who should be monitored more closely include those over age 80, those who live alone, those who are bereaved or depressed, and those who are intellectually impaired.

BIBLIOGRAPHY

BURGIO KL et al: Behavioral vs. drug treatment for urge urinary incontinence in older women: A randomized controlled trial. JAMA 280:1995, 1998

Clinical Practice Guideline: *Recognition and Initial Assessment of Alzheimer's Disease and Related Dementias.* AHCPR Publication No. 97-0702. U.S. Dept. Health and Human Services, Public Health Service. Rockville, MD, Agency for Health Care Policy and Research, 1997

CLOSE J et al: Prevention of Falls in the Elderly Trial (PROFET). A randomized controlled trial. Lancet 353:93, 1999

COUNCIL ON ETHICAL AND JUDICIAL AFFAIRS, AMA: Medical futility in end-of-life care. JAMA 281:937, 1999

ERSHLER WB, LONGO DL: The biology of aging. Cancer 80:1284, 1997

GILLICK M et al: A patient-centered approach to advance medical planning in the nursing home. J Am Geriatr Soc 47:227, 1999

GUI Z et al: Cognitive impairment, drug use, and the risk of hip fracture in persons over 75 years old: A community-based prospective study. Am J Epidemiol 148:887, 1998

GUEYFFIER F et al: Antihypertensive drugs in very old people: A subgroup meta-analysis of randomised controlled trials. Lancet 353:793, 1999

IKEGAMI N: Functional assessment and its place in health care. N Engl J Med 332:598, 1995

INOUYE S et al: A multicomponent intervention to prevent delirium in hospitalized older patients. N Engl J Med 340:669, 1999

LEBOWITZ BD et al: Diagnosis and treatment of depression in late life. Consensus statement update. JAMA 278:1186, 1997

MILLER KE et al: The geriatric patient: A systematic approach to maintaining health. Am Family Phys 61:1089, 2000

OUSLANDER JG, SCHNELLE JF: Incontinence in the nursing home. Ann Intern Med 122: 438, 1995

REYNOLDS CF et al: Treating insomnia in older adults. JAMA 281:1034, 1999

RESNICK NM, MARCANTONIO ER: How should clinical care of the aged differ? Lancet 350:1157, 1997

SALZMAN C: *Clinical Geriatric Psychopharmacology*, 3d ed. Baltimore, Williams & Wilkins, 1998

SINGER PA et al: Quality end-of-life care. Patients' perspectives. JAMA 281:163, 1999

VESTAL R: Aging and pharmacology. Cancer 80:1302, 1997

YANCIK R, RIES LA: Aging and cancer in America: Demographic and epidemiologic perspectives. Hem Onc Clin N Am 14:17, 2000

10   *Maureen T. Connelly, Thomas S. Inui*

PRINCIPLES OF DISEASE PREVENTION

PERSPECTIVES ON PREVENTION

The primary goals of prevention in medicine are to prolong life, to decrease morbidity, and to improve quality of life—all with the available resources. Working in partnership with patients, physicians play critical roles as educators, managers of access to screening and intervention services, and interpreters of divergent recommendations for promoting health. Despite evidence of the effectiveness of many preventive services in prolonging healthy life and decreasing medical costs, physicians frequently do not integrate appropriate preventive practices into their care. Obstacles to providing optimal preventive care include lack of appropriate training, doubt about the effectiveness of preventive interventions, skepticism about patients' commitment to change, limited reimbursement and time, and conflicting professional recommendations. Success achieved for populations may not be visible to individuals, and physicians may not appreciate the cumulative benefit of their efforts. Despite considerable success in some areas, such as the reduction of smoking by U.S. adults from 40 to 25% in the last 35 years, effective behavior change in other domains is often elusive, challenging and frustrating physicians and patients alike.

DEFINITIONS   This chapter will be devoted to a discussion of *primary* and *secondary* prevention. *Primary prevention*, including various forms of health promotion and vaccination, is care intended to minimize risk factors and the subsequent incidence of disease. *Secondary prevention* is screening for detection of early disease, for example the use of mammography to detect preclinical breast cancer. While the term secondary prevention is also sometimes used for the prevention of recurrent episodes of an existing illness, most would consider this activity to be *tertiary prevention*, care intended to ameliorate the course of established disease.

Deciding what types of primary and secondary preventive care clinicians should offer to their patients is not a trivial matter. The United States Preventive Services Task Force (USPSTF), The Canadian Task Force on the Periodic Health Examination, and the American College of Physicians, among other organizations, have critically reviewed the strength of available evidence for preventive practices and have made recommendations. Adopting an evidence-based approach to the development of preventive practices policy is an essential step to assuaging provider concerns about the validity of particular recommendations, to identifying the specific basis of controversies in prevention, and to reassuring patients that certain interventions will do more good than harm.

PRIMARY PREVENTION

RISK MODIFICATION   Of the more than 2 million deaths that occur in the United States each year, as many as half may be due to preventable causes (Table 10-1). Life-style and behavior play a central role in the primary causes of morbidity and mortality for adults—coronary heart disease, cancer, and injuries.

Tobacco   The largest potentially modifiable risk to health is the abuse of tobacco products. Responsible for more than 400,000 deaths each year and an estimated annual cost to society as high as $50 billion, tobacco abuse accounts for a substantial fraction of cardiovascular, cancer, and pulmonary morbidity and mortality. Recent evidence also suggests that passive exposure to tobacco smoke results in chronic pulmonary disease, cardiovascular disease, and lung cancer for some adults. Because of the addictive properties of nicotine, preventing the initiation of tobacco abuse is the tobacco control intervention of choice. Most adult smokers acquire their habit as teenagers, and primary efforts to discourage initial tobacco use must engage younger

Table 10-1 Actual Causes of Preventable Deaths in the United States in 1990

Cause	Deaths	
	Estimated No.*	Percentage of Total Deaths
Tobacco	400,000	19
Diet/activity patterns	300,000	14
Alcohol	100,000	5
Microbial agents	90,000	4
Toxic agents	60,000	3
Firearms	35,000	2
Sexual behavior	30,000	1
Motor vehicles	25,000	1
Illicit use of drugs	20,000	<1
TOTAL	1,060,000	50

* Composite approximation drawn from studies that use different approaches to derive estimates, ranging from actual counts (e.g., firearms) to population attributable risk calculations (e.g., tobacco). Numbers over 100,000 are rounded to the nearest 100,000; those over 50,000 are rounded to the nearest 10,000; those below 50,000 are rounded to the nearest 5000.

SOURCE: McGinnis JM, Foege WH: Actual cases of death in the United States. JAMA 270:2207, 1993.

audiences. However, smoking cessation extends life, even in individuals who quit after age 65 or those with established disease.

Counseling regarding the health risks of tobacco and methods for quitting is advised by all prevention advisory panels. Because 70% of smokers come into contact with health professionals each year, the medical encounter provides an opportunity to address the health implications of tobacco abuse. Although 70% of smokers say that they want to stop smoking, many are not ready to make an immediate change. The role of the provider is to motivate smokers to attempt cessation, reduce barriers to smoking cessation, and advise effective methods for cessation, including an expanding array of pharmacotherapeutic agents. Ninety percent of successful quitters will stop smoking without the aid of programmatic interventions. Setting a date to quit, arranging follow-up visits or phone calls during the initial quitting period, providing literature, and considering the use of nicotine replacement systems and other effective medications, such as bupropion, are all interventions that may improve the quitting success rate. Compared to placebo, nicotine replacement systems and bupropion have approximately twice the success rate at 6 months.

Diet Mounting evidence suggests that modification of caloric intake, particularly the quality of calories, can result in decreased morbidity and mortality from cardiovascular disease, cancer, and diabetes. Excess weight is an independent risk factor for coronary disease, in addition to its contribution to the incidence of diabetes, hyperlipidemia, and hypertension. Between 20 and 30% of Americans are overweight, defined as 20% above the acceptable body-mass index (kg/m²), and more than 40% of certain subpopulations, such as black, Native American, and Mexican-American women, are overweight. Despite concern about the risk of weight cycling, the health hazards of obesity appear to outweigh the potential harm of repeated weight loss and gain.

Americans derive excess calories from fats, particularly saturated fats, rather than from more beneficial sources such as complex carbohydrates, monounsaturated fats, and fiber. Since intake of saturated fat correlates with cholesterol level, and coronary heart disease is reduced by 2 to 3% for every 1% reduction in plasma cholesterol level, dietary modification will play a central role in decreasing the primary cause of mortality in America. Excess dietary fat intake has also been associated with breast, colon, prostate, and lung cancer in epidemiologic studies. The once widely accepted goals of reducing calories from all fats to 30% and from saturated fat to 10% have been challenged as the impact of types of fat (not simply fat itself) on morbidity and mortality is further elucidated. Increasing the intake of dietary fiber, such as from plant, legume, and grain sources, may contribute specifically to a decrease in colon cancer incidence.

Dietary sodium restriction may benefit those who have salt-sensitive hypertension, although the need for such restriction in the general population is unclear. Calcium and vitamin D are protective against osteoporosis, particularly in young women prior to reaching menopause, and evidence suggests that females at all ages have an inadequate intake. Menstruating women are at risk for iron-deficiency anemia. To achieve the recommended daily intake of vitamins and minerals, a varied diet including fish, lean meats, dairy products, whole grains, and five to six servings of fruits and vegetables daily is recommended, rather than the use of vitamin supplements. However, certain nutrients, such as adequate folate to prevent neural tube defects in developing fetuses, are not readily obtained from the typical American diet and may be best found in supplements. While evidence supporting the use of antioxidants such as vitamins E and C is still incomplete, the recommended quantities of these micronutrients can be obtained from a balanced diet.

Alcohol and Drugs The use of alcohol and drugs accounts for more than 100,000 deaths annually. While the ability of health care providers to prevent the initiation of such behaviors has not been proven, screening for exposure and addiction could potentially direct medical effort to the prevention of alcohol and drug-associated problems such as injury, violence, and medical complications of drug abuse. Although instruments such as the CAGE questionnaire have proven to be valuable for detection of alcohol abuse, no comparable brief screening strategy is available for the routine identification of illicit drug abuse. Health care providers screen inadequately for both disorders, despite evidence for effective early treatment of addictions and their complications. Reviewing recent data that moderate alcohol consumption may lower the risk of heart disease may open a discussion with patients about appropriate use. Legal implications of identifying illicit drug use may hinder detection of this problem. When screening for these disorders is feasible, interventions that have proven effective include brief counseling, referral to ambulatory and in-patient treatment programs, use of 12-step and other community organizations, and appropriate use of medications such as methadone for heroin abuse.

Physical Activity Not only can increased physical activity decrease obesity, but avoiding a sedentary life-style can also decrease the incidence of cardiac disease, hypertension, diabetes, and osteoporotic fracture. It is estimated that only 22% of U.S. adults engage in at least light to moderate physical activity, such as walking for 30 min three to five times per week. A full quarter of the population pursues no vigorous physical activity at all. The magnitude of benefit derived from physical activity may be as great as a 35% reduction in coronary heart disease, and even light exercise is preferable to no exercise. At present, the intensity, frequency, duration, and type of physical activity required to achieve optimal cardiac benefit remain unclear. While earlier studies suggested that vigorous exercise was needed to achieve maximal risk reduction, recent studies suggest that regular moderate-intensity activity, such as walking for exercise on most days, is associated with a reduced risk of cardiac events. A sudden onset of vigorous activity in the unfit may increase the risk for myocardial infarction and sudden death. Patients should be informed that, despite previous physical inactivity, the incremental adoption of a regular fitness program can decrease their risk of cardiovascular and other diseases to the level of those who have remained fit throughout their lives. Successful exercise programs are integrated into daily routines, self-directed, and injury-free.

Sexual Behavior Because of the substantial risks of infectious diseases and unwanted pregnancy from unprotected sexual activity, patients should be strongly advised to use barrier methods for all high-risk practices such as oral, anal, and vaginal intercourse as well as additional contraceptive methods when pregnancy would not be welcome.

Environment Physicians should adopt a broad construction of environmental risks to health, considering the physical, social, and occupational environments of their patients. Taking a complete exposure history, focusing on home, work, neighborhood, hobbies, and

Table 10-2   Recommendations for Preventive Medical Care for the General Population, Age 25 and Older

Screening
  Blood pressure
  Height and weight
  Pap smear if history of sexual activity and cervix present
  FOBT and/or sigmoidoscopy[a]
  Mammography ± breast exam[b]
  Assess for problem drinking
  Total blood cholesterol (men age 35 to 64, women age 45 to 64)
  Vision screening[c]
  Assess for hearing impairment[c]
Counseling
  Tobacco cessation
  Avoidance of alcohol and drugs when driving, swimming, boating
  Limitation of fat, cholesterol
  Maintenance of caloric balance
  Emphasis on grains, fruits, vegetables in diet
  Adequate calcium
  Physical activity
  Lap/shoulder belts
  Motorcycle and bicycle helmets
  Smoke detectors
  Storage or removal of firearms
  STD prevention
  Dental visits, fluoride, flossing
  Contraception
  Fall prevention[c]
  CPR training for household[c]
  Hot water heater at <120°[c]
Immunization
  Tetanus-diphtheria (Td)
  Pneumococcal vaccine[c]
  Influenza vaccine[c]
  Rubella serology or vaccination[d]
Chemoprophylaxis
  Discussion of hormone replacement therapy with perimenopausal women
  Multivitamin with folic acid[d]

---

[a] After age 49
[b] After age 49; evidence conflicting after age 69[d]
[c] Ages 65+
[d] Women of childbearing years
SOURCE: Adapted from the U.S. Preventive Services Task Force *Guide to Clinical Preventive Services.* Consult full report for details and recommendations for high-risk individuals.

dietary habits, can help direct interventions and recommendations. While local circumstances will dictate specific risks to which patients should be alerted, such as regional infectious diseases or particular toxic exposures produced by local industry, certain general recommendations should be adopted universally for health promotion.

Since skin cancers, the vast majority of them secondary to sun exposure, constitute the most common form of malignancy, all patients should be counseled to avoid sun overexposure and to use sunscreens. Patients should be encouraged to consider potential toxin exposures, such as those due to air pollution, household smoking, or carbon monoxide and radon gases, and be informed of the medical symptoms and consequences of such exposures. Proper food preparation and storage decrease the incidence of food-borne infectious disease.

Unintended injury constitutes a significant preventable burden of morbidity and mortality and is the leading cause of death for the general population under 40. Automobile accidents are the leading cause of unintentional injuries. The risk of being involved in a disabling traffic accident may be as high as 30% in the course of an individual's lifetime, and 50% of deaths from automobile accidents could be prevented with regular seatbelt use. Physicians should recommend seatbelt use, as well as helmet use for motorcycle and bicycle riders, since evidence supports a higher likelihood of use among patients who receive such advice. Clinicians should also recommend against operating

a motor vehicle after drinking, since alcohol (and illicit drugs) is a clear-cut risk cofactor.

Smoke detectors are underused, being found in only 80% of homes. Since most deaths due to fire occur in the residential setting, patients should be encouraged to install at least one on each floor of their home.

Attention to health hazards in the workplace can identify those at risk and prevent long-term consequences of exposure. Evaluation of the work environment should include questions about exposure to metals, dusts, fibers, chemicals, fumes, radiation, loud noises, extreme temperatures, and biologic agents.

Community and family violence, particularly through the misuse of firearms, is the second leading cause of death from unintentional injury. Firearms, especially handguns, are far more likely to injure a family member than an intruder and are associated with increased rates of suicide and harm to children. Patients should be encouraged to remove their weapons from the home and should be informed of the risks associated with improper security and storage of firearms. At a minimum, trigger locks may prevent accidental injury from firearms. While community and family violence are epidemic in the United States, interventions to curtail violent behavior are not well established. Screening for exposure to relationship violence, developing plans for safe havens, and referrals to appropriate community and government agencies can prevent continued abuse.

IMMUNIZATION As many as 70,000 deaths due to influenza, pneumococcal infections, and hepatitis B occur in the United States annually. Despite good availability and evidence for the cost-effectiveness of recommended vaccinations for adults, only 40% or fewer members of target populations are immunized. Factors explaining poor adherence to adult immunization guidelines include lack of confidence in vaccine efficacy among providers and patients, underestimation of the severity of the target diseases, incomplete reimbursement, lack of systems to identify and vaccinate high-risk populations, and the absence of an adult requirement for vaccination equivalent to our vaccination policies for school-age children. Table 10-2 lists recommended adult immunizations.

CHEMOPROPHYLAXIS There is significant supportive evidence for the use of certain medications in primary prevention. Therapy of this nature in the otherwise healthy person, however, is not risk-free. The use of aspirin for the prevention of cardiovascular disease or colorectal cancer, for example, is supported by evidence from cohort and, in the case of cardiovascular disease, randomized controlled trials. The potential for cerebral bleeds and gastrointestinal intolerance, however, must be balanced against a patient's individual risk for the target diseases. Although no randomized trials have measured the impact on mortality, postmenopausal hormone replacement therapy is another therapy given to healthy women for the prevention of future disease (coronary heart disease and osteoporosis), as well as to control menopausal symptoms. These benefits must be weighed against the risks of possible breast and endometrial cacinoma. Patient involvement in the decision-making process, perhaps even informed consent, is recommended to ensure compliance, proper use of medication, and sustained monitoring for side effects.

SECONDARY PREVENTION

SCREENING Widespread screening for the presence of existing diseases should meet the following criteria:

1. The targeted disease must be sufficiently burdensome to the population that a screening program is warranted. Minor changes in relative risk should have a substantial impact on the absolute risk within the population.
2. The target disease must have a well-understood natural history with a long preclinical latent period.
3. The screening method must have acceptable technical performance parameters, detecting the disease at an earlier stage than would be possible without screening and minimizing false-positive and false-negative results.
4. Efficacious treatment for the target illness must be available.

5. Early detection must improve disease outcome.
6. Cost, feasibility, and acceptability of screening and early treatment should be established.

While physicians under-provide certain screening services that have met these criteria (for example, regular mammograms for women over age 50 years), it is also the case that some prevalent screening practices today are not solidly rooted in evidence. Screening tests such as mammography in women under 50 and measurement of prostate-specific antigen have been adopted for use by many clinicians despite lack of complete current evidence that these services will decrease the risk of morbidity or mortality or improve the quality of life. See Table 10-2 recommendations of the USPSTF for screening of adults who are at average risk for target conditions. Recommendations for special-risk and vulnerable populations are available in the USPSTF *Guide*.

COMMUNITY HEALTH ADVOCACY

In addition to the direct clinical provision of preventive and health-promoting services, physicians can bring their knowledge, expertise, clinical experience, and influence to bear at the community level to promote health. Whether arguing for the denormalization of tobacco use or providing data about the health risks of local incinerators, physicians are important sources of information and support for improving health beyond the clinical office. Such activities are consistent with the overall objective of caring for patients and may have a substantial impact on decreasing the prevalence of the root causes of disease.

BIBLIOGRAPHY

BROWN AI, GARBER AM: A concise review of the cost effectiveness of coronary heart disease prevention. Med Clin N Am 84:279, 2000

FEDSON DS: Adult immunization: Summary of the National Vaccine Advisory Committee Report. JAMA 272:1133, 1994

GOLDSTEIN MG, NIAURA R: Methods to enhance smoking cessation after myocardial infarction. Med Clin N Am 84:63, 2000

HENSRUD DD: Clinical preventive medicine in primary care: Background and practice. Mayo Clin Proc 75:165, 2000

LEMAITRE RN et al: Leisure-time physical activity and the risk of primary cardiac arrest. Arch Intern Med 159:686, 1999

POPE AM, RALL DP (eds): *Environmental Medicine: Integrating a Missing Element into Medical Education.* Washington, DC, National Academy Press, 1995

SMOKING CESSATION CLINICAL PRACTICE GUIDELINE PANEL AND STAFF. The Agency for Health Care Policy and Research Smoking Cessation Clinical Practice Guideline. JAMA 275:1270, 1996

SOX HC: Preventive health services in adults. N Engl J Med 330:1589, 1994

U.S. PREVENTIVE SERVICES TASK FORCE: *Guide to Clinical Preventive Services*, 2d ed. Baltimore, Williams & Wilkins, 1995

WILLETT WC: Diet and health: What should we eat? Science 264:532, 1994

11 *Adriane Fugh-Berman*

ALTERNATIVE MEDICINE

Alternatives to conventional medicine will always exist. Defined by its outsider status, alternative therapies of one era may be conventional therapies in another. Radiation treatment and the use of transcutaneous electrical nerve stimulation (TENS), now widely used in medicine, were once unconventional therapies. Even leeches have made a minor comeback; hirudin, a potent anticoagulant secreted by leeches, has been approved by the U.S. Food and Drug Administration (FDA) as an antithrombotic agent. Alternative medicine is any approach to a health problem that is different from those used by conventional medical practitioners; many alternative therapies complement rather than supplant conventional medicine.

Alternative medicine ranges from systems with distinct disease theories, diagnostic methods, and multiple treatment options (including traditional Chinese medicine and Ayurvedic medicine) to single-

component panaceas, such as bee pollen (Table 11-1). While conventional western medicine is primarily based upon physiology and pathophysiology, alternative therapies may be based on alternative paradigms (e.g., eastern concepts of energy, called "qi" in Chinese medicine or "prana" in Ayurvedic medicine) or may be based on unproven biochemical hypotheses (e.g., high doses of vitamin C). Although many unconventional therapies are not supported by rigorous prospective clinical trials, "alternative" is not synonymous with "unproven." Data from well-designed and well-executed clinical studies support the use of certain alternative medicines in some settings (see below).

The use of unconventional therapies is widespread. In 1997, a telephone survey found that 42% of English-speaking adults in the United States used some sort of alternative therapy. Usage is especially high among people of color, reflecting the fact that, for many, alternative therapies *are* traditional medicine. Patients who use alternative medicine do so most often at opposite ends of the disease spectrum: either for symptom relief in mild or chronic illnesses or for life-threatening conditions (typically as adjuncts to conventional medicine).

PLACEBO OR NONSPECIFIC EFFECTS To what extent does the *placebo effect* explain the popularity of alternative medicine? Now more commonly called *nonspecific effects*, this phenomenon encompasses numerous factors including the environment, the relationship between the patient and the practitioner, beliefs and expectations (of both the patient and practitioner), natural history of the disease, and individual variability. The nature of the placebo effect is itself under investigation.

It may be assumed that nonspecific effects enhance positive outcomes of both unconventional and conventional therapies. However, scientific evaluation must be the primary determinant of the physician's attitude toward alternative therapies.

HERBAL MEDICINE *Herbalism* (also called *phytomedicine*, *phytotherapy*, or *botanical medicine*) is the medicinal use of plants or plant constituents. The use of plants as medicine predates even human evolution; great apes have been noted to consume specific medicinal plants when they are ill. Many of the drugs in clinical practice are derived from plants, as are the majority of analgesics: lidocaine and novocaine from the coca plant (*Erythroxylum coca*); opioids from the poppy (*Papaver somniferum*); aspirin from meadowsweet (*Spirea ulmaria*), whence the "spir" part of its name derives. The progestin component of oral contraceptives comes from the Mexican yam (*Diascorea villosa*); digoxin comes from foxglove (*Digitalis lanata*); cromolyn sodium is a khellin derivative from the Ayurvedic herb *Ammi visnaga*; and warfarin is a derivative of dicoumarin, from sweet clover (*Melilotus officinalis*). The ipecac that is kept in the medicine cabinet for poisonings comes from the root of a South American shrub (*Cephaelis ipecacuanha*); the benzoin that attaches bandages to skin is a gum resin from *Styrax benzoin*; and the witch hazel used to soothe hemorrhoids is an extract of *Hamamelis virginiana*. Fungi also have contributed to pharmaceuticals: penicillin was isolated from the fungus *Penicillium notatum*, cephalosporins were derived from a marine fungus (*Cephalosporium acremonium*), and lovastatin was derived from the fungus *Aspergillus terreus*.

Essentially every culture has a tradition of herbal medicine. In western herbalism, herbs are often used singly but may sometimes be combined. Chinese herbal medicine utilizes complex mixtures of many herbs, sometimes combined with animal materials. Herbs may be used to treat or prevent disease. As preventives, "tonics" support the function of specific organs, and "adaptogens" are nonspecific treatments that facilitate a return to homeostasis.

Some clinical trial data support the use of Saint John's wort (SJW) for depression, kava for anxiety, saw palmetto for benign prostatic hyperplasia (BPH), and ginkgo for increasing cerebral blood flow. Evidence also supports the use of garlic for lowering cholesterol, hawthorn to improve cardiac function, and echinacea for treating (but not preventing) upper respiratory infections.

Saint John's Wort (*Hypericum perforatum*) A meta-analysis of the use of SJW for mild to moderate depression examined 23 ran-

Table 11-1 Some Alternative Medicines

Type	Description
Ayurvedic medicine	The major East Indian traditional medicine system, utilizing pulse and tongue diagnosis; treatments include diet, exercise, herbs, oil massages, and elimination regimens (utilizing emetics, diarrheals, etc.)
Aromatherapy	The use of essential plant oils (distilled concentrates) in massage, baths, or inhalation
Alexander technique	A movement therapy that emphasizes efficient use of muscles to relieve pain, decrease skeletal strain, and improve posture
Acupuncture	A Chinese medical practice that involves the insertion of hair-thin needles into non-anatomic energy channels called meridians
Anthroposophic medicine	A spiritually based system of medicine that incorporates herbs, homeopathy, diet, and a movement therapy called eurythmy
Bach flower remedies	Dilute flower infusions used to treat emotional conditions
Biofeedback	The use of machinery that translates physiologic processes into audio or visual signals
Chiropractic	Adjustment of spinal vertebrae in an effort to affect neuromuscular function
Cranial sacral therapy	Gentle manipulation of the cranium and spine
Curanderismo	A spiritual healing tradition common in Mexican-American communities that utilizes ritual cleansing, herbs, and incantations
Espiritismo/Mesa Blanca/spiritism	A religious system, common in Puerto Rico and Cuba, that utilizes mediums; therapies include herbs and oils
Dance therapy	Therapeutic method that uses movement to facilitate emotional expression and release
Feldenkrais bodywork	Highly structured movement sequences that emphasize proper head positioning
Guided imagery	The use of imagination to invoke specific images that affect physiologic function
Hydropathy	Treatment utilizing water at various temperatures, sometimes aerated or under pressure, sometimes with added salts or other substances
Hypnosis	The induction of an altered state of mind within which a subject becomes receptive to specific suggestions
Massage	The use of specific gliding and kneading strokes and friction to achieve muscle relaxation
Meditation	A process by which one tries to achieve awareness without thought
Music therapy	Singing, playing instruments, or listening to music
Naturopathy	A mixture of modalities that may include herbs, homeopathy, acupuncture, hydropathy, diet, and exercise
Native American medicine	Diverse systems, many of which incorporate prayer, chant, music, healing ceremonies, counseling, herbs, laying on of hands, and smudging (ritual cleansing with smoke from sacred plants)
Reflexology/zone therapy	Manual stimulation of points on the hands or feet, believed to affect distant organs
Rolfing/structural integration	A manual therapy that attempts to realign the body by deep tissue manipulation of fasciae
Santeria	A Latin American spiritist system derived from the Yoruba tribe (of southern Nigeria); santeros are believed to communicate with saints
Shiatsu/acupressure	Finger pressure at points along nonanatomic meridians
Siddha medicine	An East Indian medical system (prevalent among Tamil-speaking people) utilizing breathing techniques, incantations, herbs, and muppu (a tri-salt preparation)
T'ai chi ch'uan	Chinese dance-like exercises described as a "moving meditation"
Therapeutic touch	Secular version of the laying on of hands, described as a "healing meditation"
Tibetan medicine	A medical system that utilizes diagnosis by pulse and urine examination; therapies include herbs, diet, and massage
Traditional Chinese medicine	A medical system that utilizes examination of the tongue and pulses for diagnosis and acupuncture, herbal mixtures, massage, exercise, and diet as therapeutics
Trager bodywork	Light massage combined with gentle passive movements to help patients maximize freedom of movement
Unani medicine	An East Indian medical system, derived from Persian medicine, practiced primarily in the Muslim community
Yoga	An Indian practice that includes postures (asanas), breathing exercises (pranayama), and cleansing practices (kriyas)

domized trials (20 were double-blind) with a total of 1757 outpatients. In 15 placebo-controlled trials, SJW was found to be significantly more effective than placebo. In eight treatment-controlled trials, clinical improvement in those receiving SJW did not differ significantly from those receiving tricyclic antidepressants. The trials in this meta-analysis were heterogeneous and used varying diagnostic criteria and dosages of SJW.

Most clinical trials have been done with extracts of the flowering-tops standardized to 0.3% hypericin (long thought to be the most active compound in SJW). However, hyperforin is most likely the prime active agent, and extracts standardized to 3% hyperforin have been tested in clinical trials and are available. The usual dose of both of these preparations is 300 mg tid.

In vitro, a high concentration of SJW inhibits the uptake of serotonin, norepinephrine, and dopamine. Among neurotransmitters, its strongest binding affinity is to γ-aminobutyric acid (GABA) A and B receptors. Although SJW demonstrates monoamine oxidase (MAO) inhibition in vitro, this effect has not been demonstrated in vivo, nor have there been any reported cases of MAO inhibitor–associated hypertensive crises in humans using SJW (the herb may, however, potentiate serotonin reuptake inhibitors). Side effects of SJW include gastrointestinal symptoms, fatigue, and photosensitization.

Ginkgo (*Ginkgo biloba*) Ginkgo leaf extracts have been proposed for treating Alzheimer's or multi-infarct dementia. In several randomized controlled trials, a small but statistically significant effect after 3 to 6 months of treatment with 40 to 80 mg tid of standardized *G. biloba* extract (containing 22 to 27% flavonoid glycosides and 5 to 7% terpene lactones) was noted on objective measures of cognitive function in patients with Alzheimer's disease. Ginkgo appears to have vasoregulatory and antioxidant effects as well as inhibiting platelet-activating factor (PAF). Serious intracerebral bleeding associated with ginkgo use has been reported, including two subdural hematomas, one intracerebral hemorrhage, one subarachnoid hemorrhage, and one case of spontaneous hyphema. In most cases, these patients were receiving concurrent anticoagulant drugs.

Kava (*Piper methysticum*) Used in Polynesia as a ceremonial beverage, the roots and rhizomes of kava are used medicinally for anxiety and insomnia in Europe and in North America. Several placebo-controlled trials have shown significant anxiolytic activity of kava products (standardized to 70% kavalactones), usually in a dose of 70 mg tid. *Kavalactones* (also called *kavapyrones*) are muscle relaxants; they include kawain, dihydrokawain, methysticin, and dihydromethysticin (the latter two are potent inhibitors of norepinephrine uptake).

Therapeutic doses may result in mild gastrointestinal complaints or allergic skin reactions (incidence ~1.5%). Chronic use of high-dose kava may result in *kava dermopathy*, a reversible ichthyosiform eruption that is often accompanied by eye irritation.

Ginseng (*Panax ginseng* and other *Panax* species) Ginseng is a popular herb in both western and eastern medicine. The place of ginseng root in the treatment of specific conditions remains to be shown in clinical trials. Ginseng contains ginsenosides, polyacetylenes, and sesquiterpenes. It appears to have some glucocorticoid-like actions and hypoglycemic activity and also affects neurotransmitter activity. Glucocorticoid administration blocks the effect of ginsenosides both in vitro and in vivo; ginsenosides increase adrenal cyclic AMP in intact but not hypophysectomized rats, so effects on adrenal secretion appear to be through the pituitary gland. Several cases of postmenopausal uterine bleeding have been reported from ginseng use, although ginseng does not contain known phytoestrogens.

Saw Palmetto (*Serenoa repens*) Saw palmetto fruits were used as food by Native Americans; their most common use today is to treat BPH. A systemic review of randomized controlled trials of extracts of the fruit *S. repens* (alone or in combination with other herbs) identified 18 randomized trials (16 double-blind) that included 2939 men and lasted 4 to 48 weeks. Compared with placebo, *S. repens* improved urinary symptom scores, nocturia, and peak urine flow. In two studies that compared finasteride with *S. repens*, improvements in urinary symptoms scores were similar. Adverse effects due to *S. repens* were mild and infrequent.

Saw palmetto is usually administered in liposterolic extracts standardized to 70 to 95% free fatty acids; the usual dose is 160 mg bid. Saw palmetto appears to have multiple mechanisms of action including inhibition of 5α-reductase and inhibition of dihydrotestosterone binding to cytosolic androgen receptors.

Pollen/Bee Pollen Pollen may be collected directly from plants or their pollinators; bee pollen is flower pollen collected from bees. A double-blind placebo-controlled trial of a mixed-pollen extract in 60 patients with BPH found that subjective improvement was significantly better in the treated group; there was a significant decrease in residual urine and in diameter of the prostate on ultrasound. However, flow rate and volume were unchanged. Allergic reactions, hypereosinophilia, and eosinophilic gastroenteritis have been associated with bee pollen intake.

Echinacea Species Echinacea roots are used to treat or prevent infections. The three species used commercially are *Echinacea purpurea*, *E. angustifolia*, and *E. pallida*. A systemic review of 16 trials (8 prevention and 8 treatment trials on upper respiratory tract infections) with a total of 3396 participants found a wide variation in preparations and methodologic quality of trials. Although many available studies reported positive results of echinacea compared to placebo, reviewers concluded that the evidence is not strong enough to recommend a specific dose, product, or preparation.

Immunomodulatory effects are attributed to five classes of compounds in echinacea preparations: caffeic acid derivatives, alkylamides, polyacetylenes, glycoproteins, and polysaccharides. The alkylamides are regarded as the most active chemical constituent. Echinacea stimulates both humoral and cellular immunity; theoretically, it could worsen symptoms in atopic individuals or those with autoimmune disease.

Adverse Effects of Herbs Herbs have pharmacologic effects and can be associated with adverse effects or interactions. Many medicinal herbs (and pharmaceutical drugs) are therapeutic at one dose and toxic at another. The relative dearth of reports of adverse events and interactions attributed to herbal products reflects a combination of underreporting and the relatively nontoxic nature of most herbal usage.

The most dangerous plants used medicinally are aconite and any herbs containing unsaturated pyrrolizidine alkaloids (saturated pyrrolizidine alkaloids lack toxicity). Several herbs that do not contain pyrrolizidine alkaloids have also shown hepatotoxicity.

Aconite (*Aconitum* spp.), sometimes used in Chinese herb mixtures to treat pain or heart failure, contains aconitine and other C_{19} diterpenoid alkaloids. Proper curing of aconite reduces alkaloids by 90%, but even appropriately cured aconite can result in serious, sometimes fatal, cardiac arrhythmias. The first symptoms of aconite poisoning occur within 90 min of ingestion; the majority of patients present with neurologic symptoms (most commonly oral numbness or burning), progressing to peripheral paresthesia and generalized muscle weakness. Nausea and vomiting are also common.

Cardiovascular effects include bradycardia, hypotension, and arrhythmias (including ventricular or supraventricular tachycardia, bidirectional tachycardia, sinus bradycardia with first-degree heart block, bundle branch block with junctional escape rhythm, or torsade de pointes). Other symptoms may include chest pain, abdominal pain,

diarrhea, hyperventilation, respiratory distress, dizziness, sweating, confusion, headache, and excessive lacrimation. No specific antidote for aconite is known, and treatment is mainly supportive. Atropine may be given if symptoms of cholinergic excess are apparent. Antiarrhythmics are often helpful, but characteristically, electrical cardioversion is markedly unsuccessful in aconite poisoning.

Unsaturated pyrrolizidine alkaloids are hepatotoxic; children may be especially sensitive. Unsaturated pyrrolizidine alkaloids occur in comfrey (*Symphytum*), borage (*Borago officinalis*) leaf (seed oils are safe), coltsfoot (*Tussilago farfara*), and species of *Crotalaria* and *Senecio*. Liver toxicity has also been associated with chaparral (*Larrea divaricata*), germander (*Teucrium chamaedrys*), and a Chinese medicine called *jin bu huan* (which contains 36% levo-tetrahydropalmitine, a chemical present in *Stephania* and *Corydalis* genera).

Drug Interactions One of the most serious herb-drug interactions is increased risk of bleeding when warfarin is combined with anticoagulant herbs: cases of bleeding have been reported with ginkgo (*G. biloba*), garlic (*Allium sativum*), and the Chinese herbs danshen (*Salvia miltiorrhiza*) and dong quai (*Angelica sinensis*). The soluble fibers guar gum and psyllium can slow or reduce the absorption of many drugs, and anthranoid-containing laxatives, including senna (*Cassia senna* and *C. angustifolia*) and cascara sagrada (*Rhamnus purshiana*), can also reduce the absorption of many drugs. An Ayurvedic syrup, shankhapushpi, has been associated with reduced levels of phenytoin. Licorice (*Glycyrrhiza glabra*) can potentiate both oral and topical glucocorticoids.

Several herbs can interact with psychotropic drugs; the herb yohimbe (*Pausinystalia yohimbe*) (also available as the drug yohimbine; both forms are used to treat impotence) increases the risk of hypertension when combined with tricyclic antidepressants. Extrapyramidal effects have occurred in patients ingesting neuroleptics and betel nut (*Areca catechu*); mania has been induced in depressed patients who mix antidepressants and *P. ginseng*; and SJW (*H. perforatum*) combined with a serotonin reuptake inhibitor may produce a mild "serotonin syndrome" (with symptoms of nausea, vomiting, and confusion); the full-blown syndrome may include myoclonus, agitation, fever, abdominal cramping, and hypertension (Chap. 385).

Adulterants and Contaminants Herbal products may be contaminated, mislabeled, or contain misidentified plants. Medicinal plants from India and Sri Lanka can be contaminated with toxigenic fungi, including *Aspergillus* and *Fusarium*. Heavy metals have been detected in some Asian herbal products (metals are sometimes deliberately used in the preparation of Ayurvedic herbal medicines). Without any mention on the label, pharmaceutical drugs may also be incorporated into herbal products, a particular problem in Chinese herbal preparations imported from Hong Kong and Taiwan. Nonsteroidal anti-inflammatory drugs and benzodiazepines have been found in Chinese herbal products, including Miracle Herb, Tung Shueh, and Chuifong Toukuwan (since 1974 this notorious brand has incorporated at least 10 different drugs into the preparation). The absence of standard manufacturing practices creates risks that are difficult to quantify.

ACUPUNCTURE Acupuncture was recognized in western medical texts a century ago; Sir William Osler's *Principles and Practice of Medicine*, first published in 1892, recommended acupuncture for both sciatica and lumbago; and the 1901 edition of *Gray's Anatomy* noted the use of acupuncture for sciatica.

Stimulation of acupuncture points may be done by needles, finger pressure, electrical stimulation, or heat (usually applied by a smoldering cone or rod of "moxa," made of the herb mugwort, *Artemisia vulgaris*). Acupuncture is effective in the treatment of nausea and vomiting. In 27 of 33 controlled trials, superiority of acupuncture point stimulation over placebo for nausea and vomiting of various etiologies was demonstrated. In substance abusers, the therapy may reduce withdrawal symptoms, but evidence is lacking about whether acupuncture has any long-term effect in preventing recidivism. An analysis of 16 randomized controlled trials of acupuncture for smoking cessation showed no beneficial effect of acupuncture over sham or no treatment. Limited preliminary data suggest a possible beneficial effect for acupuncture in stroke rehabilitation. Although acupuncture is known to stimulate endorphin release, and its use for pain is better accepted than for other conditions, controlled clinical trials of pain treatment have had mixed results.

Risks Inadequately sterilized acupuncture needles have been linked to infections, including HIV infection and an epidemic of hepatitis B. Two cases of fatal *Staphylococcus* sepsis have been reported. More than 100 cases of pneumothorax have been reported. Rare cases both of spinal trauma and cardiac tamponade (caused by penetration of a congenital sternal foramen) have been reported.

HOMEOPATHY Originated in the early nineteenth century by Samuel Hahnemann, a German physician, homeopathy is based on the "doctrine of similars"; animal, vegetable, or mineral substances that cause symptoms in a well person are used to treat those same symptoms in a sick person. For example, poison ivy (*Rhus toxicodendron*) is used to treat varicella (chickenpox). Because conventional treatments aim to counter rather than reproduce symptoms, practitioners of homeopathy refer to conventional medicine as "allopathy."

Usually, remedies are used in highly dilute concentrations, and homeopaths believe that the most dilute remedies are the most potent. If analyzed chemically, many homeopathic remedies contain no detectable levels of the original substance. It is difficult to conceive of a scientifically testable hypothesis that could explain the putative effects of homeopathic medicine where a preparation containing few or no molecules of an active agent are said to have pharmacologic effects. A meta-analysis of 89 placebo-controlled trials of homeopathy found that the odds ratio was 2.45 (CI, 2.05 to 2.93) in favor of homeopathy over placebo. The quality of these studies was not uniform, and the studies with the best methodologic quality yielded significantly less positive results.

Risks A case of pancreatitis associated with intake of homeopathic medication has been reported. Potentially toxic levels of arsenic and cadmium have been found in "low potency" (less dilute) homeopathic preparations.

SPINAL MANIPULATION Therapeutic manipulation of the body has ancient roots; Hippocrates, Aesculapius, and Galen all used some form of it. A physician, Andrew Taylor Still, originated osteopathy in 1892. Daniel David Palmer invented chiropractic in 1895. A meta-analysis of nine methodologically acceptable studies of spinal manipulation for low-back pain found a definite improvement at 3 weeks for patients with uncomplicated, acute back pain. For patients with chronic pain or sciatic nerve irritation, chiropractic was not helpful.

A meta-analysis of cervical manipulation for neck pain concluded that manipulation, in combination with other treatment, may produce short-term pain relief.

Risks Complications of spinal manipulation include vertebrobasilar accidents, disc herniations, vertebral fracture, spinal cord compression, and cauda equina syndrome. More than 80% of serious complications from chiropractic occur after cervical manipulation. It is impossible to determine the true rate of complications from chiropractic manipulations, but estimates vary from 1 in 400,000 to between 3 and 6 per 10 million. The incidence of cauda equina syndrome is thought to be less than 1 per 10 million manipulations.

MASSAGE Several studies support the use of massage for reducing lymphedema; the technique matches the effectiveness of uniform-pressure pneumatic devices.

Numerous studies in hospital settings describe the use of infant massage to decrease hospital stays of premature babies. A meta-analysis of randomized trials found that massage interventions improved daily weight gain by 5 g, while gentle, still touch did not show a benefit. Methodologic concerns about the blinding undermine the conclusions.

Risks Massage has been used in an effort to prevent pressure sores, but it is not clearly effective and may increase tissue trauma when done over bony prominences.

MIND/BODY THERAPIES **Biofeedback** Biofeedback uses instruments to translate information on physiologic function into audio or visual signals that patients use as cues to help them learn to affect functions not normally thought to be under voluntary control. Commonly used modalities include electromyographic (EMG) feedback of skeletal muscle contraction, thermal feedback of skin temperature (an indirect measure of peripheral blood flow), electroencephalographic (EEG) feedback, electrodermal response (EDR) (feedback of sweat gland activity on the fingers), and perineometry (feedback of contraction of pelvic floor muscles and anal sphincter).

Biofeedback treatment modalities may be combined. For example, for urinary incontinence, biofeedback may be used to measure pelvic muscle activity through urethral sphincter pressure and electromyography, circumvaginal muscle manometry and electromyography, and anorectal manometry and electromyography. Detrusor pressure feedback may be measured by cystometry, and feedback on intraabdominal pressure may be used to help patients learn to simultaneously contract pelvic muscles while relaxing abdominal muscles (to avoid putting excess pressure on the bladder). Clinical trials support the use of biofeedback in the treatment of urinary incontinence (stress, urge, or mixed), fecal incontinence, migraine, tension headaches, and in stroke rehabilitation.

Hypnosis Traditional hypnosis utilizes the induction of a deep trance state to enhance suggestibility. Several clinical trials indicate that hypnosis is effective in chemotherapy-associated nausea and may be helpful in the treatment of irritable bowel syndrome and pain syndromes. Numerous uncontrolled trials suggest a beneficial effect of hypnosis on smoking cessation, but controlled trials are less impressive. A meta-analysis of hypnosis in nine randomized controlled trials of hypnotherapy found significant heterogeneity among the results of the individual studies, with conflicting results for the effectiveness of hypnotherapy compared to no treatment or to advice. Hypnotherapy was not more effective than rapid smoking (an aversive therapy in which cigarettes are smoked in quick succession) or psychological treatment.

DIETARY SUPPLEMENTS The fundamental principles of good nutrition are to eat a balanced variety of foods and to maintain a balance of calories taken in with calories burned through activity. Dietary supplements have become a large and lucrative business that promotes the idea that our food is somehow lacking in specific nutrients and that additional intake of any number of food components will treat or prevent specific diseases, improve athletic and sexual performance, and make us live longer. These claims are largely either untested or unproven (Table 11-2). Unfortunately, the *Dietary Supplement Health and Education Act* (DSHEA) of 1994 prevents the FDA from monitoring the quality or safety of dietary supplements before marketing. Supplements do not even have to be dietary components to be sold as dietary supplements (the availability of over-the-counter hormones, including DHEA, progesterone topical creams, and organ extracts is particularly worrisome).

Even vitamin and mineral supplementation may have unexpected results. For example, high dietary consumption of carrots, sweet potatoes, greens, and other foods rich in β-carotene is associated with decreased risk of cardiovascular disease and cancer. However, two large prospective randomized controlled trials of β-carotene [the Alpha Tocopherol Beta Carotene (ATBC) Cancer Prevention Study and the Beta-Carotene and Retinal Efficacy Trial (CARET)] found that β-carotene increased rates of lung cancer in supplemented groups. The ATBC trial also failed to show a benefit in terms of cardiovascular disease, and β-carotene supplementation has been disappointing in other trials. β-carotene may well be a dietary marker for more beneficial carotenoids (including lycopene, lutein, α-carotene, and β-cryptoxanthin) that typically occur in mixtures in foods.

Similarly, while dietary intake of vitamin E is associated with a reduced risk of coronary heart disease and several observational studies (including the Health Professionals Follow-Up Study and the Nurses Health Study) found a protective effect of supplemental vitamin E, prospective placebo-controlled trials have had mixed results.

Table 11-2   Some Commonly Used Dietary Supplements

Supplement	Clinical Trial Evidence	Toxicities	Comments
Arginine	Preliminary evidence of improvement in intermittent claudication and improved endothelial function in arteries.	Very safe.	
Vitamin A	Derivatives used to treat certain epithelial cell cancers, acne, and psoriasis. Decreases childhood mortality and measles mortality (in developing countries).	Headaches, nausea, bone pain; liver toxicity at high doses (>50,000 IU qd). Teratogenic; pregnant women should avoid supplements containing >5000 IU qd.	Vitamin A deficiency is unusual in North America. Megadoses have significant toxicity.
Riboflavin (vitamin B$_2$)	High doses of riboflavin may help in migraine prophylaxis.	Very safe	
Pantothenic acid	Preliminary evidence of benefit in hyperlipidemia.	Very safe. High doses can cause diarrhea.	
Vitamin B$_6$ (pyridoxine)	Improves symptoms in carpal tunnel syndrome, premenstrual syndrome, and nausea and vomiting of pregnancy.	Although more common at doses >200 mg qd, doses as low as 50 mg qd can cause sensory neuropathy.	
Vitamin B$_{12}$ (cobalamin)	With folic acid, preliminary evidence that B$_{12}$ may decrease bronchial squamous metaplasia in smokers.	Very safe.	B$_{12}$ deficiency is common in North America, especially in the elderly and those on proton pump inhibitors. In the absence of macrocytosis or anemia, deficiency may cause psychiatric symptoms.
Thiamine (B$_1$)	Possible benefit in CHF but no large prospective trials.	Very safe.	Marginal deficiency is common (symptoms include weakness, parasthesia, and depression). Administer thiamine IV first when treating alcohol toxicity (IV glucose may cause life-threatening lactic acidosis in a thiamine-deficient patient).
Niacin (vitamin B$_3$)	Nicotinic acid lowers serum triglycerides, lowers LDL, and increases HDL.	Flushing, itching, rashes, gastrointestinal effects, and fatigue. Should not be used by those with impaired hepatic function or in those on beta blockers. Sustained-release preparations are hepatotoxic and should never be used.	Niacinamide is ineffective for hypercholesterolemia
Vitamin C	Preliminary evidence of improved endothelial function in arteries of patients with CHF. No evidence of benefit in advanced cancer or colds.	Diarrhea at high doses; increases iron absorption.	Epidemiologically, vitamin C intake or serum levels are associated with lower risk of nephrolithiasis, gall bladder disease, and some cancers. High serum levels are associated with lower serum lead levels.
Calcium	Reduces bone loss; lowers risk of recurrence of colorectal adenomas; may help premenstrual syndrome. Mixed results on treatment of hypertension; reduces risk of pregnancy-induced hypertension.	Relatively safe. Extremely high doses can cause milk alkali syndrome or hypercalcemia (symptoms may include lax muscle tone, nausea, constipation, large urine volume, later confusion, coma, death).	Although dietary intake of calcium reduces renal stone formation, supplemental calcium (especially taken between meals) may increase risk.
β-Carotene	Increases risk of lung cancer in smokers; may increase risk of cardiovascular disease; no effect on risk of type 2 diabetes; mixed results on prevention of cervical intraepithelial neoplasia; may decrease oral leukoplakia.	Hypercarotenosis (benign yellowing of the skin). In general, supplementation appears harmful; there is no risk to consuming foods high in β-carotene.	Dietary intake of foods high in carotenoids associated with decreased risk of cardiovascular disease and cancer (see text).
Vitamin D (calciferol)	Analogues are used to treat osteoporosis, renal osteodystrophy, hypocalcemia, and psoriasis and are being studied as cancer treatments.	In high doses may cause weakness, fatigue, headache, vomiting, hypercalcemia, hypercalciuria, and impaired renal function.	Marginal deficiency is common. Sunscreen use prevents vitamin D conversion in the skin. Fortification is required in milk but not other dairy products.
Vitamin E (α-tocopherol)	Ineffective in preventing lung cancer, reducing cardiovascular deaths, or reducing angina; may increase risk of pancreatic cancer; may reduce risk of myocardial infarction and risk of prostate cancer	Increases risk of hemorrhagic stroke.	Large doses of α-tocopherol displace γ-tocopherol in tissues.
Dehydroepiandrosterone (DHEA)	May be helpful in lupus and menopausal symptoms.	Acne and hirsutism (in women).	High serum levels are associated with decreased cardiovascular disease in men; increased cardiovascular disease in women; and increased risk of postmenopausal breast cancer.
Coenzyme Q10	Trials are mixed on whether it benefits CHF.	Very safe. Occasionally causes gastrointestinal upset.	
Iron	In iron-deficient individuals, supplementation reduces symptoms in restless legs syndrome; increases verbal learning and memory in adolescents, and increases growth in children.	High body stores of iron are associated with increased risk of cardiovascular disease. In iron-replete young children, supplementation may impair growth.	Supplementation should be discouraged unless deficiency exists.
Melatonin	Mixed results in jet lag or sleep disorders, not well examined in other indications	May cause depression. Safety of long-term use not established.	High-dose melatonin is under study as an adjunctive cancer treatment.
Magnesium	Mixed results in trials on hypertension and cardiovascular disease; may decrease arrhythmias; may help in migraine prophylaxis.	Toxic in high doses (causing hyporeflexia), later cardiac arrest); can cause diarrhea at relatively low doses; renal patients should avoid supplementation	

(continued)

Table 11-2 Some Commonly Used Dietary Supplements—*(continued)*

Supplement	Clinical Trial Evidence	Toxicities	Comments
Glucosamine	Effective in osteoarthritis	Very safe; may cause gastrointestinal discomfort.	
Chondroitin	Preliminary evidence of benefit in osteoarthritis	Very safe	
Fish oil	Lowers blood pressure in hypertensives; mixed results on reduction of coronary restenosis, may help psoriasis and rheumatoid arthritis, retards renal failure in IgA nephropathy, improved lung function in cystic fibrosis; improves symptoms in inflammatory bowel disease. Lowers VLDL, increases LDL, no effect on HDL or total cholesterol.	Relatively safe. May cause gastrointestinal discomfort, fishy breath, anticoagulant effects.	Dietary sources of fish oil include salmon, mackerel, sardines, and bluefish.
Selenium	Reduces prostate, lung, and colon cancer incidence; no effect on skin cancer.	Dizziness, nausea, metallic taste, garlicky breath. Very high doses (>4 mg qd) can cause loss of hair and nails, skin lesions, tooth decay, and peripheral neuropathy.	
Carnitine	Improves exercise tolerance and time to ST-segment depression in patients with angina; preliminary evidence of improvement in left ventricular dysfunction.	Relatively safe; L-carnitine occasionally causes diarrhea or agitation. D-carnitine can cause muscle pain and weakness	
Zinc	No evidence of benefit in leg ulcers. Mixed results on zinc lozenges for cold symptoms. Reduces respiratory infections and diarrhea in developing countries. Preliminary evidence of increased cell-mediated immunity in elderly.	In high doses, nausea, vomiting, diarrhea, abdominal pain; can cause copper depletion.	
Chromium	Preliminary evidence of benefit in diabetes; appears to increase HDL. No effect on body composition or strength in nondeficient individuals.	Oral chromium is safe. Occupational exposure to high doses of airborne chromium may cause dermatitis, skin and nasal septum lesions, and increased incidence of lung cancer.	

NOTE: CHF, congestive heart failure; HDL, high-density lipoprotein; LDL, low-density lipoprotein; VLDL, very low density lipoprotein.

In the Cambridge Heart Antioxidant Study (CHAOS), a placebo-controlled trial of vitamin E supplementation in patients with coronary artery disease, vitamin E supplementation reduced nonfatal myocardial infarction but did not appear to decrease cardiovascular deaths or all-cause mortality. In the ATBC study, vitamin E failed to protect male smokers with a previous myocardial infarction from major coronary events and significantly increased risk of death from hemorrhagic stroke. Although vitamin E improves endothelium-dependent vasodilation significantly and attenuates the development of nitrate tolerance, prospective trials have found no benefit of vitamin E for angina.

Vitamin E is not a single compound; the term applies to eight related compounds in two groups, the tocopherols and the tocotrienols. Most North American dietary sources of vitamin E are composed of two-thirds γ-tocopherol and one-third α-tocopherol. γ-Tocopherol neutralizes both oxygen and nitrogen free radicals, while α-tocopherol is selective for oxygen free radicals. Most vitamin E supplements, however, contain only D- or D,L-α-tocopherol, and large doses of α-tocopherol displace γ-tocopherol in plasma and tissues.

While it is possible that tomorrow's trendy carotenoid or tocopherol will be more successful than yesterday's, it is more likely that carotenoids and tocopherols are most beneficial when consumed in the naturally occurring mixtures of nutrients found in foods.

Dietary supplements that are safe under one set of conditions may be harmful under other conditions. For example, nearly all physiologic reactions that generate free radicals are oxidation-reduction reactions, capable of either generating free radicals or reducing free radicals. While low doses of vitamin C and other substances have antioxidant effects, high levels may actually have a prooxidant effect.

There is clinical trial evidence supporting the supplemental use of some vitamins, minerals, and amino acids (Table 11-2); but at high doses these supplements should be treated with the same respect given pharmaceuticals.

SUMMARY The incorporation of science into medicine began only in the middle of the nineteenth century; *evidence-based medicine* is a recent term and still not necessarily standard practice. There is no such thing as objective care of a patient. There are many ways in which we physicians communicate goals and our own beliefs in our therapies; it is likely that a substantial proportion of benefit from even rational interventions is due to nonspecific effects.

Many of our patients take alternative medicines; physicians need to adopt an open-minded, nonjudgmental attitude toward the practice. Inquire about all the medications and supplements a patient is taking. Increasingly, data are available to help guide decision-making about alternative medicines. A thorough knowledge of all therapies a patient is utilizing may help explain unexpected findings and is an important component of a holistic approach to patient care.

Conventional medicine often casts a wary eye on therapies outside its boundaries, but it is incumbent upon physicians to evaluate evidence regarding alternative therapies with the same rigor with which we evaluate conventional therapies. Scientific evidence from controlled clinical trials supports specific applications of alternative medicine, and some therapies considered alternative today may well be incorporated into conventional medicine in the future.

BIBLIOGRAPHY

DeSmet AGM et al: *Adverse Effects of Herbal Drugs*, vol. 3. Berlin, Springer-Verlag, 1997

Ernst E (ed): *Complementary Medicine: An Objective Appraisal*. Oxford, Butterworth-Heinemann, 1996

Fugh-Berman A: *5 Minute Clinical Consult to Herbs and Dietary Supplements*. Philadelphia, Lippincott, Williams & Wilkins, in press

———: *Alternative Medicine: What Works*. Baltimore, Williams & Wilkins, 1997

Jonas WB, Levin JS (eds): *Essentials of Complementary and Alternative Medicine*. Philadelphia, Lippincott Williams & Wilkins, 1999

Kaptchuk TJ, Eisenberg DM: Chiropractic: Origins, controversies, and contributions. Arch Intern Med 158:2215, 1998

Linde K et al: Are the clinical effects of homeopathy placebo effects? A meta-analysis of placebo-controlled trials. Lancet 350:834, 1997

Schulz V et al: *Rational Phytotherapy*, 3d ed. Berlin, Springer, 1998

Shils ME et al: *Modern Nutrition in Health and Disease*, 9th ed. Baltimore, Williams & Wilkins, 1999

Vandenbroucke JP: Medical journals and the shaping of medical knowledge. Lancet 352:2001, 1998

Section 1
PAIN

12   *Howard L. Fields, Joseph B. Martin*

PAIN: PATHOPHYSIOLOGY AND MANAGEMENT

The task of medicine is to preserve and restore health and to relieve suffering. Understanding pain is essential to both these goals. Because pain is universally understood as a signal of disease, it is the most common symptom that brings a patient to a physician's attention. The function of the pain sensory system is to detect, localize, and identify tissue-damaging processes. Since different diseases produce characteristic patterns of tissue damage, the quality, time course, and location of a patient's pain complaint and the location of tenderness provide important diagnostic clues and are used to evaluate the response to treatment.

THE PAIN SENSORY SYSTEM

Pain is an unpleasant sensation localized to a part of the body. It is often described in terms of a penetrating or tissue-destructive process (e.g., stabbing, burning, twisting, tearing, squeezing) and/or of a bodily or emotional reaction (e.g., terrifying, nauseating, sickening). Furthermore, any pain of moderate or higher intensity is accompanied by anxiety and the urge to escape or terminate the feeling. These properties illustrate the duality of pain: it is both sensation and emotion. When acute, pain is characteristically associated with behavioral arousal and a stress response consisting of increased blood pressure, heart rate, pupil diameter, and plasma cortisol levels. In addition, local muscle contraction (e.g., limb flexion, abdominal wall rigidity) is often present.

THE PRIMARY AFFERENT NOCICEPTOR A peripheral nerve consists of the axons of three different types of neurons: primary sensory afferents, motor neurons, and sympathetic postganglionic neurons (Fig. 12-1). The cell bodies of primary afferents are located in the dorsal root ganglia in the vertebral foramina. The primary afferent axon bifurcates to send one process into the spinal cord and the other to innervate tissues. Primary afferents are classified by their diameter, degree of myelination, and conduction velocity. The largest-diameter fibers, A-beta (Aβ), respond maximally to light touch and/or moving stimuli; they are present primarily in nerves that innervate the skin. In normal individuals, the activity of these fibers does not produce pain. There are two other classes of primary afferents: the small-diameter myelinated A-delta (Aδ) and the unmyelinated (C fiber) axons (Fig. 12-1). These fibers are present in nerves to the skin and to deep somatic and visceral structures. Some tissues, such as the cornea, are innervated only by Aδ and C afferents. Most Aδ and C afferents respond maximally only to intense (painful) stimuli and produce the subjective experience of pain when they are electrically stimulated; this defines them as *primary afferent nociceptors* (*pain receptors*). The ability to detect painful stimuli is completely abolished when Aδ and C axons are blocked.

Individual primary afferent nociceptors can respond to several different types of noxious stimuli. For example, most nociceptors respond to heating, intense mechanical stimuli such as a pinch, and application of irritating chemicals.

Sensitization When intense, repeated, or prolonged stimuli are applied in the presence of damaged tissue or inflammation, the threshold for activating primary afferent nociceptors is lowered and the frequency of firing is higher for all stimulus intensities. Inflammatory mediators such as bradykinin, some prostaglandins, and leukotrienes contribute to this process, which is called *sensitization*. In sensitized tissues normally innocuous stimuli can produce pain. Sensitization is a clinically important process that contributes to tenderness, soreness, and hyperalgesia. A striking example of sensitization is sunburned skin, in which severe pain can be produced by a gentle slap on the back or a warm shower.

Under normal conditions, viscera are relatively insensitive to noxious mechanical and thermal stimuli. Hollow viscera do generate significant discomfort when distended. Furthermore, when affected by a disease process with an inflammatory component, deep structures such as joints or hollow viscera characteristically become exquisitely sensitive to mechanical stimulation.

A large proportion of Aδ and C afferents innervating viscera are completely insensitive in normal noninjured, noninflamed tissue. That is, they cannot be activated by known mechanical or thermal stimuli and are not spontaneously active. However, in the presence of inflammatory mediators, these afferents become sensitive to mechanical stimuli. Such afferents have been termed *silent nociceptors*, and their characteristic properties may explain how under pathologic conditions the relatively insensitive deep structures can become the source of severe and debilitating pain and tenderness.

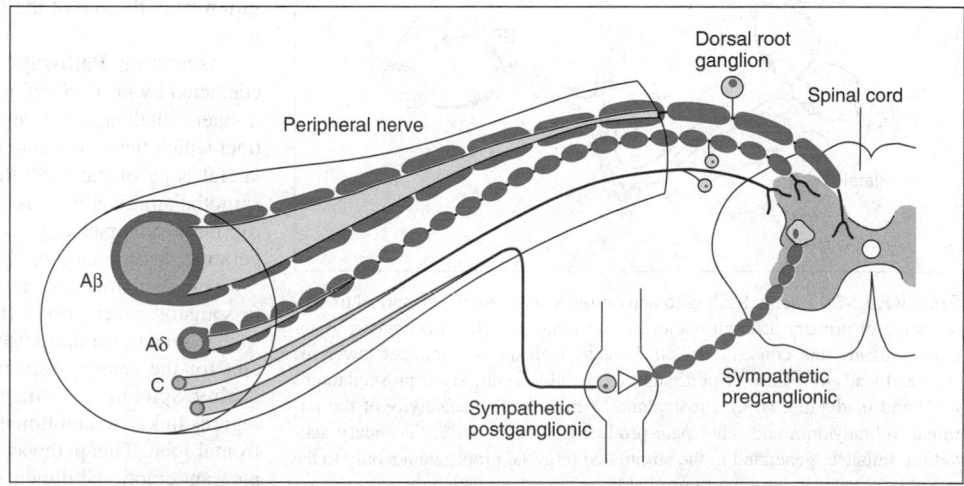

FIGURE 12-1 Components of a typical cutaneous nerve. There are two distinct functional categories of axons: primary afferents with cell bodies in the dorsal root ganglion, and sympathetic postganglionic fibers with cell bodies in the sympathetic ganglion. Primary afferents include those with large-diameter myelinated (Aβ), small-diameter myelinated (Aδ), and unmyelinated (C) axons. All sympathetic postganglionic fibers are unmyelinated.

Nociceptor-Induced Inflammation   One important concept to emerge in recent years is that afferent nociceptors also have a neuroeffector function. Most nociceptors contain polypeptide mediators that are released from their peripheral terminals when they are activated (Fig. 12-2). An example is substance P, an 11-amino-acid peptide. Substance P is released from primary afferent nociceptors and has multiple biologic activities. It is a potent vasodilator, degranulates mast cells, is a chemoattractant for leukocytes, and increases the production and release of inflammatory mediators. Interestingly, depletion of substance P from joints reduces the severity of experimental arthritis. Primary afferent nociceptors are not simply passive messengers of threats to tissue injury but also play an active role in tissue protection through these neuroeffector functions.

CENTRAL PATHWAYS FOR PAIN   The Spinal Cord and Referred Pain   The axons of primary afferent nociceptors enter the spinal cord via the dorsal root. They terminate in the dorsal horn of the spinal gray matter (Fig. 12-3). The terminals of primary afferent

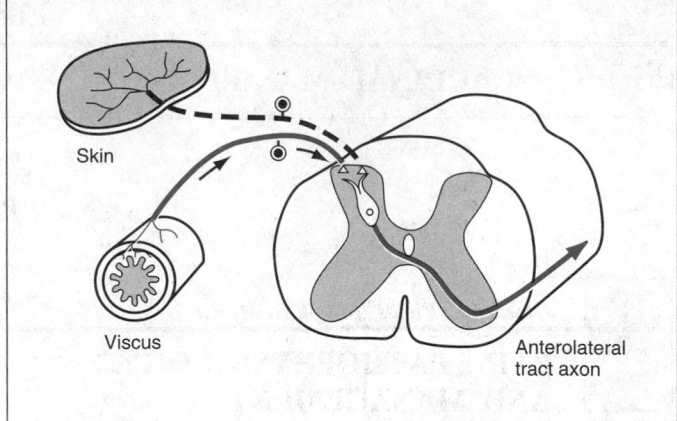

FIGURE 12-3   The convergence-projection hypothesis of referred pain. According to this hypothesis, visceral afferent nociceptors converge on the same pain-projection neurons as the afferents from the somatic structures in which the pain is perceived. The brain has no way of knowing the actual source of input and mistakenly "projects" the sensation to the somatic structure.

axons contact spinal neurons that transmit the pain signal to brain sites involved in pain perception. The axon of each primary afferent contacts many spinal neurons, and each spinal neuron receives convergent inputs from many primary afferents.

From a clinical standpoint, the convergence of many sensory inputs to a single spinal pain-transmission neuron is of great importance because it underlies the phenomenon of referred pain. All spinal neurons that receive input from the viscera and deep musculoskeletal structures also receive input from the skin. The convergence patterns are determined by the spinal segment of the dorsal root ganglion that supplies the afferent innervation of a structure. For example, the afferents that supply the central diaphragm are derived from the third and fourth cervical dorsal root ganglia. Primary afferents with cell bodies in these same ganglia supply the skin of the shoulder and lower neck. Thus sensory inputs from both the shoulder skin and the central diaphragm converge on pain-transmission neurons in the third and fourth cervical spinal segments. *Because of this convergence and the fact that the spinal neurons are most often activated by inputs from the skin, activity evoked in spinal neurons by input from deep structures is mislocalized by the patient to a place that is roughly coextensive with the region of skin innervated by the same spinal segment.* Thus inflammation near the central diaphragm is usually reported as discomfort near the shoulder. This spatial displacement of pain sensation from the site of the injury that produces it is known as *referred pain.*

Ascending Pathways for Pain   A majority of spinal neurons contacted by primary afferent nociceptors send their axons to the contralateral thalamus. These axons form the contralateral spinothalamic tract which lies in the anterolateral white matter of the spinal cord, the lateral edge of the medulla, and the lateral pons and midbrain. The spinothalamic pathway is crucial for pain sensation in humans. Interruption of this pathway produces permanent deficits in pain and temperature discrimination.

Spinothalamic tract axons connect to thalamic neurons that project to somatosensory cortex (Fig. 12-4). This pathway from spinal cord to thalamus to somatosensory cortex appears to be particularly important for the sensory aspects of pain, i.e., its location, intensity, and quality. Spinothalamic tract axons also connect to thalamic and cortical regions linked to emotional responses, such as the cingulate gyrus and frontal lobe. This pathway is thought to subserve the affective or unpleasant emotional dimension of pain.

PAIN MODULATION   The pain produced by similar injuries is remarkably variable in different situations and in different people. For example, athletes have been known to sustain serious fractures with only minor pain, and Beecher's classic World War II survey

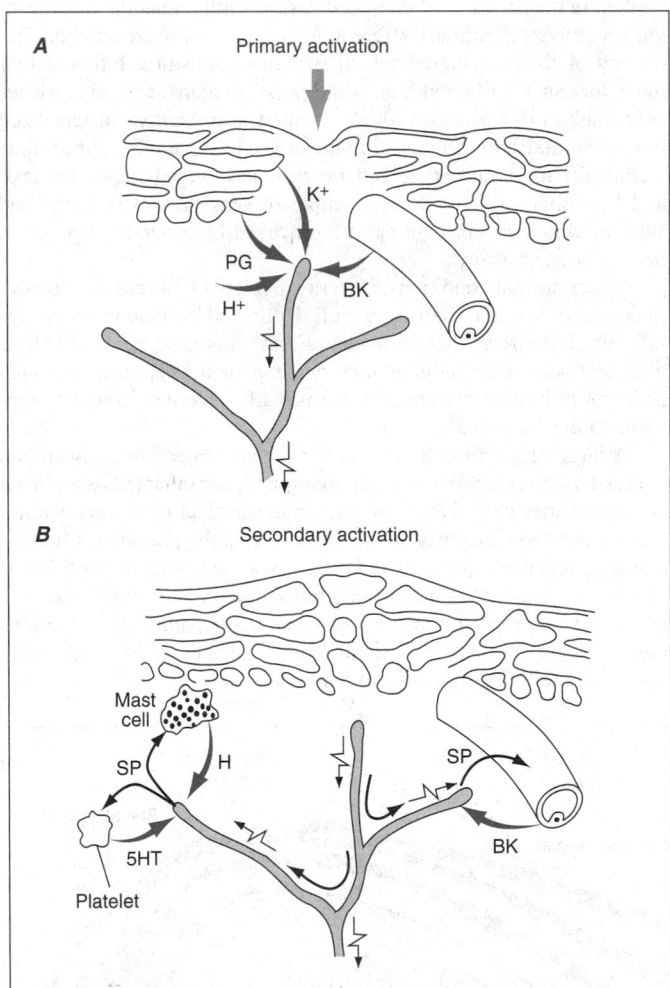

FIGURE 12-2   Events leading to activation, sensitization, and spread of sensitization of primary afferent nociceptor terminals. *A.* Direct activation by intense pressure and consequent cell damage. Cell damage induces lower pH (H⁺) and leads to release of potassium (K⁺) and to synthesis of prostaglandins (PG) and bradykinin (BK). Prostaglandins increase the sensitivity of the terminal to bradykinin and other pain-producing substances. *B.* Secondary activation. Impulses generated in the stimulated terminal propagate not only to the spinal cord but also into other terminal branches where they induce the release of peptides, including substance P (SP). Substance P causes vasodilation and neurogenic edema with further accumulation of bradykinin. Substance P also causes the release of histamine (H) from mast cells and serotonin (5HT) from platelets.

FIGURE 12-4 *A.* Transmission system for nociceptive messages. Noxious stimuli activate the sensitive peripheral ending of the primary afferent nociceptor by the process of transduction (1). The message is then transmitted over the peripheral nerve to the spinal cord, where it synapses with cells of origin of the two major ascending pain pathways, the spinothalamic and spinoreticulothalamic. The message is relayed in the thalamus to both the frontal (F Cx) and the somatosensory cortex (SS Cx). *B.* Pain-modulation network. Inputs from frontal cortex and hypothalamus (Hyp.) activate cells in the midbrain that control spinal pain-transmission cells via cells in the medulla.

revealed that many men were unbothered by battle injuries that would have produced agonizing pain in civilian patients. Furthermore, even the suggestion of relief can have a significant analgesic effect (placebo). On the other hand, many patients find even minor injuries (such as venipuncture) unbearable, and the expectation of pain has been demonstrated to induce pain *without a noxious stimulus.*

The powerful effect of expectation and other psychological variables on the perceived intensity of pain implies the existence of brain circuits that can modulate the activity of the pain-transmission pathways. Although there are probably several circuits that can modulate pain, only one has been studied extensively. This circuit has links in the hypothalamus, midbrain, and medulla, and it selectively controls spinal pain-transmission neurons through a descending pathway (Fig. 12-4).

There is good evidence that this pain-modulating circuit contributes to the pain-relieving effect of opioid analgesic medications. Each of the component structures of the pathway contains opioid receptors and is sensitive to the direct application of opioid drugs. Furthermore, lesions of the system reduce the analgesic effect of systemically administered opioids such as morphine. Along with the opioid receptor, the component nuclei of this pain-modulating circuit contain endogenous opioid peptides such as the enkephalins and β-endorphin.

The most reliable way to activate this endogenous opioid-mediated modulating system is by prolonged pain and/or fear. There is evidence that pain-relieving endogenous opioids are released following operative procedures and in patients given a placebo for pain relief.

Pain modulation is bidirectional. Pain-modulating circuits not only produce analgesia but are also capable of increasing pain. Both pain-inhibiting and pain-facilitating neurons in the medulla project to and control spinal pain-transmission neurons. Since pain-transmission neurons can be activated by modulatory neurons, it is theoretically possible to generate a pain signal with no peripheral noxious stimulus. Some such mechanism could account for the finding that pain can be induced by suggestion alone and may provide a framework for understanding how psychological factors can contribute to chronic pain.

NEUROPATHIC PAIN The normal nervous system transmits coded signals that result in pain. Thus lesions of the peripheral or central nervous system may result in a loss or impairment of pain sensation. Paradoxically, damage or dysfunction of the nervous system can produce pain. For example, damage to peripheral nerves, as occurs in diabetic neuropathy, or to primary afferents, as in herpes zoster, can result in pain that is referred to the body region innervated by the damaged nerves. Though rare, pain may also be produced by damage to the central nervous system, particularly the spinothalamic pathway or thalamus. Such neuropathic pains are often severe and are notoriously intractable to standard treatments for pain.

Neuropathic pains typically have an unusual burning, tingling, or electric shock-like quality and may be triggered by very light touch. These features are rare in other types of pain. On examination, a sensory deficit is characteristically present in the area of the patient's pain.

A variety of mechanisms contribute to neuropathic pain. As with sensitized primary afferent nociceptors, damaged primary afferents, including nociceptors, become highly sensitive to mechanical stimulation and begin to generate impulses in the absence of stimulation. There is evidence that this increased sensitivity and spontaneous activity is due to an increased concentration of sodium channels. Damaged primary afferents may also develop sensitivity to norepinephrine. Interestingly, spinal pain-transmission neurons cut off from their normal input may also become spontaneously active. Thus both central and peripheral nervous system changes may contribute to neuropathic pain.

Sympathetically Maintained Pain A certain percentage of patients with peripheral nerve injury develop a severe burning pain (causalgia) in the region innervated by the nerve. The pain typically begins after a delay of hours to days or even weeks. The pain is accompanied by swelling of the extremity, periarticular osteoporosis, and arthritic changes in the distal joints. A similar syndrome called *reflex sympathetic dystrophy* can be produced without obvious nerve damage by a variety of injuries, including fractures of bone, soft tissue trauma, myocardial infarction, and stroke (Chap. 366). Although the pathophysiology of this condition is poorly understood, the pain can be relieved within minutes by blocking the sympathetic nervous system. This implies that sympathetic activity activates nociceptors even if they are not obviously damaged. These results also suggest that the sympathetic nervous system can, under some circumstances, play an active role in inflammation.

℞ TREATMENT The ideal treatment for any pain is to remove the cause. Sometimes this is possible, but more often after diagnosis and initiation of appropriate treatments for the cause, there is a lag period before the pain subsides. Furthermore, some conditions are so painful that rapid and effective analgesia is essential (e.g., the postoperative state, burns, trauma, cancer, sickle cell crisis). Analgesic medications are a first line of treatment in these cases, and their use should be familiar to all practitioners.

Aspirin, Acetaminophen, and Nonsteroidal Anti-Inflammatory Agents (NSAIDS) These drugs are considered together because they are used for similar problems and may have a similar mechanism of action (Table 12-1). All these compounds inhibit cyclooxygenase (COX), and, except for acetaminophen, all have anti-inflammatory actions, especially at higher dosages. They are particularly effective for mild to moderate headache and for pain of musculoskeletal origin.

Since they are effective for these common types of pains and are available without prescription, COX inhibitors are by far the most commonly used analgesics. They are absorbed well from the gastrointestinal tract and, with occasional use, side effects are minimal. With chronic use, gastric irritation is a common side effect of aspirin and NSAIDs and is the problem that most frequently limits the dose that can be given. Gastric irritation is most severe with aspirin, which may cause erosion of the gastric mucosa, and because aspirin irreversibly acetylates platelets and interferes with coagulation of the blood, gas-

Table 12-1 Drugs for Relief of Pain

NONNARCOTIC ANALGESICS: USUAL DOSES AND INTERVALS

Generic Name	Dose, mg	Interval	Comments
Acetylsalicylic acid	650 PO	q 4 h	Enteric-coated preparations available
Acetaminophen	650 PO	q 4 h	Side effects uncommon
Ibuprofen	400 PO	q 4–6 h	Available without prescription
Naproxen	250–500 PO	q 12 h	Delayed effects may be due to long half-life
Fenoprofen	200 PO	q 4–6 h	Contraindicated in renal disease
Indomethacin	25–50 PO	q 8 h	Gastrointestinal side effects common
Ketorolac	15–60 IM	q 4–6 h	Available for parenteral use (IM)
Rofecoxib	12.5–25 PO	q 24 h	FDA approved for pain management
Celecoxib	100–200 PO	q 12–24 h	Useful for arthritis

NARCOTIC ANALGESICS: USUAL DOSES AND INTERVALS

Generic Name	Parenteral Dose, mg	PO Dose, mg	Comments
Codeine	30–60 q 4 h	30–60 q 4 h	Nausea common
Oxycodone	—	5–10 q 4–6 h	Usually available with acetaminophen or aspirin
Morphine	10 q 4 h	60 q 4 h	
Morphine sustained release	—	30–200 bid to tid	Oral slow-release preparation
Hydromorphone	1–2 q 4 h	2–4 q 4 h	Shorter acting than morphine sulfate
Levorphanol	2 q 6–8 h	4 q 6–8 h	Longer acting than morphine sulfate; absorbed well PO
Methadone	10 q 6–8 h	20 q 6–8 h	Delayed sedation due to long half-life
Meperidine	75–100 q 3–4 h	300 q 4 h	Poorly absorbed PO; normeperidine a toxic metabolite
Butorphanol	—	1–2 q 4 h	Intranasal spray
Fentanyl	2.5–10 q 72 h	—	Transdermal patch
Tramadol		50–100 q4–6 h	Mixed opioid/adrenergic action

ANTICONVULSANTS AND ANTIARRHYTHMICS

Generic Name	PO Dose, mg	Interval
Phenytoin	300	daily/qhs
Carbamazepine	200–300	q 6 h
Clonazepam	1	q 6 h
Mexiletine	150–300	q 6–12 h
Gabapentin	600–1200	q 8 h

ANTIDEPRESSANTS

Generic Name	Uptake Blockade 5-HT	Uptake Blockade NE	Sedative Potency	Anticholinergic Potency	Orthostatic Hypotension	Cardiac Arrhythmia	Average Dose, mg/day	Range, mg/day
Doxepin	++	+	High	Moderate	Moderate	Less	200	75–400
Amitriptyline	++++	++	High	Highest	Moderate	Yes	150	25–300
Imipramine	++++	++	Moderate	Moderate	High	Yes	200	75–400
Nortriptyline	+++	++	Moderate	Moderate	Low	Yes	100	40–150
Desipramine	+++	++++	Low	Low	Low	Yes	150	50–300
Venlafaxine	+++	++	Low	None	None	No	150	75–400

NOTE: 5-HT, serotonin; NE, norepinephrine.

trointestinal bleeding is a risk. The NSAIDs are less problematic in this regard. Although toxic to the liver when taken in a high dose, acetaminophen rarely produces gastric irritation and does not interfere with platelet function. Table 12-1 lists the dosages and durations of action of the commonly used drugs of this class.

The introduction of a parenteral form of NSAID, ketorolac, extends the usefulness of this class of compounds in the management of acute severe pain. Ketorolac is sufficiently potent and rapid in onset to supplant opioids for many patients with acute severe headache and musculoskeletal pain.

There are two major classes of COX: COX 1 is constitutively expressed, and COX 2 is induced in the inflammatory state. COX 2–selective drugs have recently been introduced for the treatment of arthritis and are associated with a significant reduction of gastric irritation. Whether COX 2-selective drugs have analgesic actions equivalent to other NSAIDs remains to be demonstrated.

Opioid Analgesics Opioids are the most potent pain-relieving drugs currently available. Furthermore, of all analgesics, they have the broadest range of efficacy, providing the most reliable method for rapidly relieving pain. Although side effects are common, they are usually not serious except for respiratory depression and can be reversed rapidly with the narcotic antagonist naloxone. The physician should not hesitate to use opioid analgesics in patients with acute severe pain. Table 12-1 lists the most commonly used opioid analgesics.

Opioids produce analgesia by actions in the central nervous system. They activate pain-inhibitory neurons and directly inhibit pain-transmission neurons. Most of the commercially available opioid analgesics act at the same opioid receptor (mu receptor), differing mainly in potency, speed of onset, duration of action, and optimal route of administration. Although the dose-related side effects (sedation, respiratory depression, pruritus, constipation) are similar among the different opioids, some side effects are due to accumulation of nonopioid metabolites that are unique to individual drugs. One striking example of this is normeperidine, a metabolite of meperidine. Normeperidine produces hyperexcitability and seizures that are not reversible with naloxone. Normeperidine accumulation is much greater in patients with renal failure.

The most rapid relief with opioids is obtained by intravenous administration; relief with oral administration is significantly slower. Common acute side effects include nausea, vomiting, and sedation. The most serious side effect is respiratory depression. Patients with any form of respiratory compromise must be kept under close observation following opioid administration; an oxygen saturation monitor may be useful. The opioid antagonist, naloxone, should be readily available. These effects are dose-related, and there is great variability among patients in the doses that relieve pain and produce side effects. Because of this, initiation of therapy requires titration to optimal dose and interval. The most important principle is to provide adequate pain relief. This requires asking the patient whether the drug has relieved the pain and, if so, when the relief wears off. *The most common error made by physicians in managing severe pain with opioids is to prescribe an inadequate dose. Since many patients are reluctant to complain, this practice leads to needless suffering.* In the absence of sedation at the expected time of peak effect, a physician should not hesitate to repeat the initial dose to achieve satisfactory pain relief.

An innovative approach to the problem of achieving adequate pain relief is the use of patient-controlled analgesia (PCA). PCA requires a device that delivers a baseline continuous dose of an opioid drug, and preprogrammed additional doses whenever the patient pushes a button. The device can be programmed to limit the total hourly dose so that overdosing is impossible. The patient can then titrate the dose to the optimal level. This approach is used most extensively for the management of postoperative pain, but there is no reason why it should not be used for any hospitalized patient with persistent severe pain. PCA is also used for short-term home care of patients with intractable pain, such as is caused by metastatic cancer.

Many physicians, nurses, and patients have a certain trepidation about using opioids that is based on an exaggerated fear of patients becoming addicted. In fact, there is a vanishingly small chance of patients becoming addicted to narcotics as a result of their appropriate medical use.

The availability of new routes of administration has extended the usefulness of opioid analgesics. Most important is the availability of spinal administration. Opioids can be infused through a spinal catheter placed either intrathecally or epidurally. By applying opioids directly to the spinal cord, regional analgesia can be obtained using a relatively low total dose. In this way, such side effects as sedation, nausea, and respiratory depression can be minimized. This approach has been used extensively in obstetric procedures and for lower-body postoperative pain. Opioids can also be given intranasally (butorphanol), rectally, and transdermally (fentanyl), thus avoiding the discomfort of frequent injections in patients who cannot be given oral medication.

Opioid and cyclooxygenase inhibitor combinations When used in combination, opioids and COX inhibitors have additive effects. Because a lower dose of each can be used to achieve the same degree of pain relief and their side effects are nonadditive, such combinations can be used to lower the severity of dose-related side effects. Fixed-ratio combinations of an opioid with acetaminophen carry a special risk. Dose escalation as a result of increased severity of pain or decreased opioid effect as a result of tolerance may lead to levels of acetaminophen that are toxic to the liver.

CHRONIC PAIN

PATIENT EVALUATION Managing patients with chronic pain is intellectually and emotionally challenging. The patient's problem is often difficult to diagnose: such patients are demanding of the physician's time and often appear emotionally distraught. The traditional medical approach of seeking an obscure organic pathology is usually unhelpful. On the other hand, psychological evaluation and behaviorally based treatment paradigms are frequently helpful, particularly in the setting of a multidisciplinary pain-management center.

There are several factors that can cause, perpetuate, or exacerbate chronic pain. First, of course, the patient may simply have a disease that is characteristically painful for which there is presently no cure. Arthritis, cancer, migraine headaches, fibromyalgia, and diabetic neuropathy are examples of this. Second, there may be secondary perpetuating factors that are initiated by disease and persist after that disease has resolved. Examples include damaged sensory nerves, sympathetic efferent activity, and painful reflex muscle contraction. Finally, a variety of psychological conditions can exacerbate or even cause pain.

There are certain areas to which special attention should be paid in the medical history. Because depression is the most common emotional disturbance in patients with chronic pain, patients should be questioned about their mood, appetite, sleep patterns, and daily activity. A simple standardized questionnaire, such as the Beck Depression Inventory, can be a useful screening device. It is important to remember that major depression is a common, treatable, and potentially fatal illness.

Other clues that a significant emotional disturbance is contributing to a patient's chronic pain complaint include: pain that occurs in multiple unrelated sites; a pattern of recurrent, but separate, pain problems beginning in childhood or adolescence; pain beginning at a time of emotional trauma, such as the loss of a parent or spouse; a history of physical or sexual abuse; and past or present substance abuse.

On examination, special attention should be paid to whether the patient guards the painful area and whether certain movements or postures are avoided because of pain. Discovering a mechanical component to the pain can be useful both diagnostically and therapeutically. Painful areas should be examined for deep tenderness, noting whether this is localized to muscle, ligamentous structures, or joints. Chronic myofascial pain is very common, and in these patients deep palpation may reveal highly localized trigger points that are firm bands or knots in muscle. If injection of local anesthetic into these trigger points relieves the pain, it supports the diagnosis. A neuropathic component to the pain is indicated by evidence of nerve damage, such as sensory impairment, exquisitely sensitive skin, weakness and muscle atrophy, or loss of deep tendon reflexes. Evidence suggesting sympathetic nervous system involvement includes the presence of diffuse swelling, changes in skin color and temperature, and hypersensitive skin and joint tenderness compared with the normal side. Relief of the pain with a sympathetic block is diagnostic.

A guiding principle in evaluating patients with chronic pain is to assess both emotional and organic factors before initiating therapy. Addressing these issues together, rather than waiting to "rule out" organic causes of the pain, improves compliance in part because it assures patients that a psychological evaluation does not mean that the physician is questioning the validity of their complaint. Even when an organic cause for a patient's pain can be found, it is still wise to look for other factors. For example, cancer patients with painful bony metastases may also have pain due to nerve damage and significant depression. Optimal therapy requires that each of these factors be looked for and treated.

TREATMENT Once the evaluation process has been completed and the likely causative and exacerbating factors identified, an explicit treatment plan should be developed. An important part of this process is to identify specific and realistic functional goals for therapy, such as getting a good night's sleep, being able to go shopping, or returning to work. A multidisciplinary approach that utilizes medications, counseling, physical therapy, nerve blocks, and even surgery may be required to improve the patient's quality of life. This may require referral to a pain clinic; however, this is not necessary for all chronic pain patients. For some, pharmacologic management alone can provide significant help.

Antidepressant Medications The tricyclic antidepressants (Table 12-1) are extremely useful for the management of patients with chronic pain. Although developed for the treatment of depression, the tricyclics have a spectrum of dose-related biologic activities that include the production of analgesia in a variety of clinical conditions. Although the mechanism is unknown, the analgesic effect of tricyclics has a more rapid onset and occurs at a lower dose than is typically required for the treatment of depression. Furthermore, patients with chronic pain who are not depressed obtain pain relief with antidepressants. There is evidence that tricyclic drugs potentiate opioid analgesia, so they are useful adjuncts for the treatment of severe persistent pain such as occurs with malignant tumors. Table 12-2 lists some of the painful conditions that respond to tricyclics. Tricyclics are of particular

Table 12-2 Painful Conditions That Respond to Tricyclic Antidepressants

Postherpetic neuralgia[a]	Rheumatoid arthritis[a,b]
Diabetic neuropathy[a]	Chronic low back pain[b]
Tension headache[a]	Cancer
Migraine headache[a]	

[a] Controlled trials demonstrate analgesia.
[b] Controlled studies indicate benefit but not analgesia.
SOURCE: From HL Fields: *Pain.* New York, McGraw-Hill, 1987.

value in the management of neuropathic pain such as occurs in diabetic neuropathy and postherpetic neuralgia, for which there are few other therapeutic options.

The tricyclics that have been shown to relieve pain have significant side effects (Table 12-1; Chap 385). Unfortunately, some of the serotonin-selective reuptake inhibitors such as fluoxetine (Prozac) that have fewer and less serious side effects have not been shown to provide pain relief. On the other hand, venlafaxine (Effexor), a nontricyclic antidepressant that blocks both serotonin and norepinephrine reuptake, appears to be useful in patients who cannot tolerate tricyclics.

Anticonvulsants and Antiarrhythmics (Table 12-1) These drugs are useful primarily for patients with neuropathic pain. Phenytoin (Dilantin) and carbamazepine (Tegretol) were first shown to relieve the pain of trigeminal neuralgia. This pain has a characteristic brief, shooting, electric shock-like quality. In fact, anticonvulsants seem to be helpful largely for pains that have such a lancinating quality. A new-generation anticonvulsant, gabapentin (Neurontin), which increases brain γ-aminobutyric acid levels, is effective for a broad range of neuropathic pains.

Antiarrhythmic drugs such as low-dose lidocaine and mexiletine (Mexitil) are also effective for neuropathic pains. These drugs block the spontaneous activity of primary afferent nociceptors that appears when they are damaged.

Chronic Opioid Medication The long-term use of opioids is accepted for patients with pain due to malignant disease. Although its use for chronic pain of nonmalignant origin is controversial, it is clear that for many such patients opioid analgesics are the only option available for obtaining effective relief. This is understandable since opioids are the most potent and have the broadest range of efficacy of any analgesic medications. Although addiction is rare in patients who first use opioids for pain relief, some degree of tolerance and physical dependence are likely to occur with long-term use. Therefore, before embarking on opioid therapy, other options should be explored, and the limitations and risks of opioids should be explained to the patient. It is also important to point out that some opioid analgesic medications have mixed agonist-antagonist properties (e.g., pentazocine and butorphanol). From a practical standpoint, this means that they may worsen pain by inducing an abstinence syndrome in patients who are physically dependent on other opioid analgesics.

With long-term outpatient use of orally administered opioids it is desirable to use long-acting compounds such as levorphanol, methadone, or sustained-release morphine (Table 12-1). The pharmacokinetic profile of these drugs enables prolonged pain relief, minimizes side effects such as sedation that are associated with high peak plasma levels, and, perhaps, reduces the likelihood of rebound pain associated with a rapid fall in plasma opioid concentration. Constipation is a virtually universal side effect of opioid use and should be treated expectantly.

It is worth emphasizing, in conclusion, that many patients, especially those with chronic pain, seek medical attention primarily because they are suffering and because only physicians can provide the medications required for their relief. A primary responsibility of all physicians is to minimize the physical and emotional discomfort of their patients. Familiarity with pain mechanisms and analgesic medications is an important step toward accomplishing this aim.

BIBLIOGRAPHY

BARON R et al: Causalgia and reflex sympathetic dystrophy: Does the sympathetic nervous system contribute to the generation of pain? Muscle Nerve 22:678, 1999

DEVOR M et al (eds): Proceedings of the Ninth World Congress on Pain. Seattle IASP Press, 1160 pp, 2000

FIELDS HL et al: Postherpetic neuralgia: Irritable nociceptors and deafferentation. Neurobiol Dis 5:209, 1998

——— et al: Peripheral neuropathic pain: An approach to management, in *Textbook of Pain*, 4th ed, PD Wall, R Melzack (eds). London, Churchill Livingston, 1999

FORT J: Celecoxib, a COX-2–specific inhibitor: The clinical data. Am J Orthop 28(3 Suppl):13, 1999

GEBHART GF (ed): *Visceral Pain*. Seattle, IASP Press, 1995

MARKOWITZ JS, PATRICK KS: Venlafaxine-tramadol similarities. Med Hypotheses 51:167, 1998

ROWBOTHAM MC et al: Gabapentin for the treatment of postherpetic neuralgia: A randomized controlled trial. JAMA 280:1837, 1998

STEIN C: The control of pain in peripheral tissue by opioids. N Engl J Med 332:1685, 1995

WALL PD, MELZACK R (eds): *Textbook of Pain*, 4th ed. London, Churchill Livingstone, 1999

WILLIS WD (ed): *Hyperalgesia and Allodynia*. New York, Raven, 1992

———, COGGESHALL RE: *Sensory Mechanism of the Spinal Cord*. New York, Plenum, 1991

---

13 *Thomas H. Lee*

CHEST DISCOMFORT AND PALPITATIONS

CHEST DISCOMFORT

Chest discomfort is one of the most common challenges for clinicians in the office or emergency department. The differential diagnosis includes conditions affecting organs throughout the thorax and abdomen, with prognostic implications that vary from benign to life-threatening (Table 13-1). Failure to recognize potentially serious conditions such as acute ischemic heart disease, aortic dissection, or pulmonary embolism can lead to serious complications, including death. Conversely, overly conservative management of low-risk patients leads to unnecessary hospital admissions, tests, and procedures.

CAUSES OF CHEST DISCOMFORT **Myocardial Ischemia and Injury** (See also Chap. 244) Myocardial ischemia occurs when the oxygen supply to the heart is not sufficient to meet metabolic needs. This mismatch can result from a decrease in oxygen supply, a rise in demand, or both. The most common underlying cause of myocardial ischemia is obstruction of coronary arteries by atherosclerosis; in the presence of such obstruction, transient ischemic episodes are usually precipitated by an increase in oxygen demand as a result of physical exertion. However, ischemia can also result from psychological stress, fever, or large meals or from compromised oxygen delivery due to anemia, hypoxia, or hypotension. Ventricular hypertrophy due to valvular heart disease, hypertrophic cardiomyopathy, or hypertension can predispose the myocardium to ischemia because of impaired penetration of blood flow from epicardial coronary arteries to the endocardium.

Angina pectoris The chest discomfort of myocardial ischemia is a visceral discomfort that is usually described as a heaviness, pressure,

Table 13-1 Differential Diagnoses of Patients Admitted to Hospital with Acute Chest Pain Ruled Not Myocardial Infarction

Diagnosis	Percent
Gastroesophageal disease	42
Gastroesophageal reflux	(30)
Esophageal motility disorders	(13)
Peptic ulcer	(10)
Gallstones	(5)
Ischemic heart disease	31
Chest wall syndromes	28
Pericarditis	4
Pleuritis/pneumonia	2
Pulmonary embolism	2
Lung cancer	1.5
Aortic aneurysm	1
Aortic stenosis	1
Herpes zoster	1

SOURCE: Fruergaard P et al: Eur Heart J 17:1028, 1996.

or squeezing (Table 13-2). Other common adjectives for anginal pain are burning and aching. Some patients deny any "pain" but may admit to dyspnea or a vague sense of anxiety. The word "sharp" is sometimes used by patients to describe intensity rather than quality.

The location of angina pectoris is usually retrosternal; most patients do not localize the pain to any small area. The discomfort may radiate to the neck, jaw, teeth, arms, or shoulders, reflecting the common origin in the posterior horn of the spinal cord of sensory neurons supplying the heart and these areas. Some patients present with aching in sites of radiated pain as their only symptoms of ischemia. Occa-

Table 13-2 Typical Clinical Features of Major Causes of Acute Chest Discomfort

Condition	Duration	Quality	Location	Associated Features
Angina	More than 2 and less than 10 min	Pressure, tightness, squeezing, heaviness, burning	Retrosternal, often with radiation to or isolated discomfort in neck, jaw, shoulders, or arms—frequently on left	Precipitated by exertion, exposure to cold, psychologic stress. S4 gallop or mitral regurgitation murmur during pain
Unstable angina	10–20 min	Similar to angina but often more severe	Similar to angina	Similar to angina, but occurs with low levels of exertion or even at rest
Acute myocardial infarction	Variable; often more than 30 min	Similar to angina but often more severe	Similar to angina	Unrelieved by nitroglycerin. May be associated with evidence of heart failure or arrhythmia
Aortic stenosis	Recurrent episodes as described for angina	As described for angina	As described for angina	Late-peaking systolic murmur radiating to carotid arteries
Pericarditis	Hours to days; may be episodic	Sharp	Retrosternal or toward cardiac apex; may radiate to left shoulder	May be relieved by sitting up and leaning forward. Pericardial friction rub
Aortic dissection	Abrupt onset of unrelenting pain	Tearing or ripping sensation; knifelike	Anterior chest, often radiating to back, between shoulder blades	Associated with hypertension and/or underlying connective tissue disorder, e.g., Marfan syndrome. Murmur of aortic insufficiency, pericardial rub, pericardial tamponade, or loss of peripheral pulses
Pulmonary embolism	Abrupt onset; several minutes to a few hours	Pleuritic	Often lateral, on the side of the embolism	Dyspnea, tachypnea, tachycardia, and hypotension
Pulmonary hypertension	Variable	Pressure	Substernal	Dyspnea, signs of increased venous pressure including edema and jugular venous distention
Pneumonia or pleuritis	Variable	Pleuritic	Unilateral, often localized	Dyspnea, cough, fever, rales, occasional rub
Spontaneous pneumothorax	Sudden onset; several hours	Pleuritic	Lateral to side of pneumothorax	Dyspnea, decreased breath sounds on side of pneumothorax
Esophageal reflux	10–60 min	Burning	Substernal, epigastric	Worsened by postprandial recumbency. Relieved by antacids
Esophageal spasm	2–30 min	Pressure, tightness, burning	Retrosternal	Can closely mimic angina
Peptic ulcer	Prolonged	Burning	Epigastric, substernal	Relieved with food or antacids
Gallbladder disease	Prolonged	Burning, pressure	Epigastric, right upper quadrant, substernal	May follow meal
Musculoskeletal disease	Variable	Aching	Variable	Aggravated by movement. May be reproduced by localized pressure on examination
Herpes zoster	Variable	Sharp or burning	Dermatomal distribution	Vesicular rash in area of discomfort
Emotional and psychiatric conditions	Variable; may be fleeting	Variable	Variable; may be retrosternal	Situational factors may precipitate symptoms. Anxiety or depression often detectable with careful history

sional patients report epigastric distress with ischemic episodes. Less common is radiation to below the umbilicus or to the back.

Stable angina pectoris usually develops gradually with exertion, emotional excitement, or after heavy meals. Rest or treatment with sublingual nitroglycerin typically leads to relief within several minutes. In contrast, pain that is fleeting (lasting only a few seconds) is rarely ischemic in origin. Similarly, pain that lasts for several hours is unlikely to represent angina, particularly if the patient's electrocardiogram does not show evidence of ischemia.

Anginal episodes can be precipitated by any physiologic or psychological stress that induces tachycardia. Most myocardial perfusion occurs during diastole, when there is minimal pressure opposing coronary artery flow from within the left ventricle. Since tachycardia decreases the percentage of the time in which the heart is in diastole, it decreases myocardial perfusion.

Unstable angina and myocardial infarction (See also Chaps. 243 and 244)   Patients with these acute ischemic syndromes usually complain of symptoms similar in quality to angina pectoris, but more prolonged and severe. The onset of these syndromes may occur with the patient at rest, and sublingual nitroglycerin may lead to transient or no relief. Accompanying symptoms may include diaphoresis, dyspnea, nausea, and light-headedness.

The physical examination may be completely normal in patients with chest discomfort due to ischemic heart disease. Careful auscultation during ischemic episodes may reveal a third or fourth heart sound, reflecting myocardial systolic or diastolic dysfunction. A transient murmur of mitral regurgitation suggests ischemic papillary muscle dysfunction. Severe episodes of ischemia can lead to pulmonary congestion and even pulmonary edema.

Other cardiac causes   Myocardial ischemia caused by hypertrophic cardiomyopathy, aortic stenosis, or other conditions leads to angina pectoris similar to that caused by coronary atherosclerosis. In such cases, a systolic murmur or other findings usually suggest abnormalities other than coronary atherosclerosis that may be contributing to the patient's symptoms.

Pericarditis (See also Chap. 239)   The pain in pericarditis is believed to be due to inflammation of the adjacent parietal pleura, since most of the pericardium is believed to be insensitive to pain. Thus, infectious pericarditis, which usually involves adjoining pleura surfaces, tends to be associated with pain, while conditions that cause only local inflammation (e.g., myocardial infarction or uremia) and cardiac tamponade tend to result in mild or no chest pain.

The adjacent parietal pleura receives its sensory supply from several sources, so the pain of pericarditis can be experienced in areas ranging from the shoulder and neck to the abdomen and back. Most typically, the pain is retrosternal and is aggravated by coughing, deep breaths, or changes in position—all of which lead to movements of pleural surfaces. The pain is often worse in the supine position and relieved by sitting upright and leaning forward. Less common is a steady aching discomfort that mimics acute myocardial infarction.

Diseases of the Aorta (See also Chap. 247)   *Aortic dissection* is a potentially catastrophic condition that is due to spread within the wall of the aorta of a subintimal hematoma. The hematoma may begin with a tear in the intima of the aorta or with rupture of the vasa vasorum within the aortic media. This syndrome can occur with trauma to the aorta, including motor vehicle accidents or medical procedures in which catheters or intraaortic balloon pumps damage the intima of the aorta. Nontraumatic aortic dissections are rare in the absence of hypertension and/or conditions associated with deterioration of the elastic or muscular components of the media within the aorta's wall. Cystic medial degeneration is a feature of several inherited connective tissue diseases, including Marfan and Ehlers-Danlos syndromes. About half of all aortic dissections in women under 40 years of age occur during pregnancy.

Almost all patients with acute dissections present with severe chest pain, although some patients with chronic dissections are identified without associated symptoms. Unlike the pain of ischemic heart disease, symptoms of aortic dissection tend to reach peak severity immediately, often causing the patient to collapse from its intensity. The adjectives used to describe the pain reflect the process occurring within the wall of the aorta—"ripping" and "tearing"—and the location usually correlates with the site and extent of the dissection. Thus, dissections that begin in the ascending aorta and extend to the descending aorta tend to cause pain in the front of the chest that extends into the back, between the shoulder blades.

Physical findings may also reflect extension of the aortic dissection that compromises flow into arteries branching off the aorta. Thus, loss of a pulse in one or both arms, cerebrovascular accident, or paraplegia can all be catastrophic consequences of aortic dissection. Hematomas that extend proximally and undermine the coronary arteries or aortic valve apparatus may lead to acute myocardial infarction or acute aortic insufficiency. Rupture of the hematoma into the pericardial space leads to pericardial tamponade.

Another abnormality of the aorta that can cause chest pain is a *thoracic aortic aneurysm*. Aortic aneurysms are frequently asymptomatic but can cause chest pain and other symptoms by compressing adjacent structures. This pain tends to be steady, deep, and sometimes severe.

Pulmonary Embolism (See also Chap. 261)   Chest pain due to pulmonary embolism is believed to be due to distention of the pulmonary artery or infarction of a segment of the lung adjacent to the pleura. Massive pulmonary emboli may lead to substernal pain that is suggestive of acute myocardial infarction. More commonly, smaller emboli lead to focal pulmonary infarctions that cause pain that is lateral and pleuritic. Associated symptoms include dyspnea and, occasionally, hemoptysis. Tachycardia is usually present.

Pneumonia or Pleuritis   Lung diseases that damage and cause inflammation of the pleura of the lung usually cause a sharp, knifelike pain that is aggravated by inspiration or coughing.

Gastrointestinal Conditions   Esophageal pain from acid reflux from the stomach, spasm, obstruction, or injury can be difficult to discern from myocardial syndromes. Acid reflux typically causes a deep burning discomfort that may be exacerbated by alcohol, aspirin, or some foods; this discomfort is often relieved by antacid or other acid-reducing therapies. Acid reflux tends to be exacerbated by lying down and may be worse in early morning when the stomach is empty of food that might otherwise absorb gastric acid.

Esophageal spasm may occur in the presence or absence of acid reflux, and leads to a squeezing pain indistinguishable from angina. Prompt relief of esophageal spasm is often provided by antianginal therapies such as sublingual nifedipine, further promoting confusion between these syndromes. Chest pain can also result from injury to the esophagus, such as a Mallory-Weiss tear caused by severe vomiting.

Chest pain can result from diseases of the gastrointestinal tract below the diaphragm, including *peptic ulcer disease*, *biliary disease*, and *pancreatitis*. These conditions usually cause abdominal pain as well as chest discomfort; symptoms are not likely to be associated with exertion. The pain of ulcer disease typically occurs 60 to 90 min after meals, when postprandial acid production is no longer neutralized by food in the stomach. Cholecystitis usually causes a pain that is described as aching, occurring an hour or more after meals.

Neuromusculoskeletal Conditions   *Cervical disk disease* can cause chest pain by compression of nerve roots. Pain in a dermatomal distribution can also be caused by *intercostal muscle cramps* or by *herpes zoster*. Chest pain symptoms due to herpes zoster may occur before skin lesions are apparent.

Costochondral and chondrosternal syndromes are the most common causes of anterior chest musculoskeletal pain. Only occasionally are physical signs of costochondritis such as swelling, redness, and warmth (Tietze's syndrome) present. The pain of such syndromes is usually fleeting and sharp, but some patients experience a dull ache that lasts for hours. Direct pressure on the chondrosternal and costochondral junctions may reproduce the pain from these and other musculoskeletal syndromes. Arthritis of the shoulder and spine and bursitis may also cause chest pain. Some patients who have these conditions and myocardial ischemia blur and confuse symptoms of these syndromes.

Emotional and Psychiatric Conditions As many as 10% of patients who present to emergency departments with acute chest pain have panic disorder or other emotional conditions. The symptoms in these populations are highly variable, but frequently the discomfort is described as visceral tightness or aching that lasts more than 30 min. Some patients offer other atypical descriptions, such as pain that is fleeting, sharp, and/or localized to a small region. The electrocardiogram in patients with emotional conditions may be difficult to interpret if hyperventilation causes ST-T-wave abnormalities. A careful history may elicit clues of depression, prior panic attacks, somatization, agoraphobia, or other phobias.

Approach to the Patient

The evaluation of the patient with chest discomfort must accommodate two goals—determining the diagnosis and assessing the safety of the immediate management plan. The latter issue is often dominant when the patient has acute chest discomfort, such as patients seen in the emergency department. In such settings, the clinician must focus on questions such as the safety of discharge to home, admission to a noncoronary care unit facility, or immediate exercise testing. Table 13-3 displays a sequence of questions that can be used in the evaluation of the patient with chest discomfort, with the diagnostic entities that are most important for consideration at each stage of the evaluation.

Acute Chest Discomfort In patients with acute chest discomfort, the clinician must first assess the patient's respiratory and hemodynamic status. If either is compromised, initial management should focus on stabilizing the patient before the diagnostic evaluation is pursued. If, however, the patient does not require emergent interventions, then a focused history, physical examination, and laboratory evaluation should be performed to assess the patient's risk of life-threatening conditions, including acute ischemic heart disease, aortic dissection, and pulmonary embolism.

The *history* should include questions about the quality and location of the chest discomfort (Table 13-2). The patient should also be asked about the nature of onset of the pain and its duration. Myocardial ischemia is usually associated with a gradual intensification of symptoms over a period of minutes. Pain that is fleeting or that lasts hours without being associated with electrocardiographic changes is not likely to be ischemic in origin.

The *physical examination* should include evaluation of blood pressure in both arms and of pulses in both legs. Poor perfusion of a limb

may be due to an aortic dissection that has compromised flow to an artery branching from the aorta. Chest auscultation may reveal diminished breath sounds; a pleural rub; or evidence of pneumothorax, pulmonary embolism, pneumonia, or pleurisy. The cardiac examination should seek pericardial rubs, systolic and diastolic murmurs, and third or fourth heart sounds.

An *electrocardiogram* is an essential test for adults with chest discomfort that is not due to an obvious traumatic cause. The presence of electrocardiographic changes consistent with ischemia or infarction (Chap. 226) is associated with high risks of acute myocardial infarction or unstable angina (Table 13-4); such patients should be admitted to a unit with electrocardiographic monitoring and the capacity to respond to a cardiac arrest. The absence of such changes does not exclude acute ischemic heart disease, but the risk of life-threatening complications is low for patients with normal electrocardiograms or only nonspecific ST-T-wave changes. If these patients are not considered appropriate for immediate discharge, they are often candidates for early or immediate exercise testing.

Markers of myocardial injury are often obtained in the emergency department evaluation of acute chest discomfort. The most commonly used markers are creatine kinase (CK), CK-MB, and the cardiac troponins (I and T). Single values of these markers do not have high sensitivity for acute myocardial infarction or for prediction of complications. Hence, decisions to discharge patients home should not be made on the basis of single negative values of these tests.

Provocative tests for coronary artery disease are not appropriate for patients with ongoing chest pain. In such patients, rest myocardial perfusion scans can be considered; a normal scan reduces the likelihood of coronary artery disease. Clinicians frequently employ therapeutic trials with sublingual nitroglycerin or antacids, and a common error is to assume that a response to either of these interventions clarifies the diagnosis. While such information is often helpful, the patient's response may be due to the placebo effect. Hence, myocardial ischemia should never be considered excluded solely because of a response to antacid therapy. Similarly, failure of nitroglycerin to relieve pain does not exclude the diagnosis of coronary disease.

If the patient's history or examination is consistent with aortic dissection, imaging studies to evaluate the aorta must be pursued promptly because of the high risk of catastrophic complications with this condition. A chest x-ray is not sufficient to exclude this diagnosis. Appropriate tests include a chest computed tomography scan with contrast or a magnetic resonance imaging scan in patients who are hemodynamically stable, or a transesophageal echocardiogram in pa-

Table 13-3 Considerations in the Assessment of the Patient with Chest Pain

1. Could the chest discomfort be due to an acute, potentially life-threatening condition that warrants immediate hospitalization and aggressive evaluation?

Acute ischemic heart disease	Pulmonary embolism
Aortic dissection	Spontaneous pneumothorax

2. If not, could the discomfort be due to a chronic condition likely to lead to serious complications?

Stable angina
Aortic stenosis
Pulmonary hypertension

3. If not, could the discomfort be due to an acute condition that warrants specific treatment?

Pericarditis
Pneumonia/pleuritis
Herpes zoster

4. If not, could the discomfort be due to another treatable chronic condition?

Esophageal reflux	Cervical disk disease
Esophageal spasm	Arthritis of the shoulder or spine
Peptic ulcer disease	Costochondritis
Gallbladder disease	Other musculoskeletal disorders
Other gastrointestinal conditions	Anxiety state

Table 13-4 Prevalence of Myocardial Infarction and Unstable Angina Among Subsets of Patients with Acute Chest Pain in the Emergency Department

Finding	Prevalence of Myocardial Infarction, %	Prevalence of Unstable Angina, %
ST elevation ($\geq$1 mm) or Q waves on ECG not known to be old	79	12
Ischemia or strain on ECG not known to be old (ST depression $\geq$1 mm or ischemic T waves)	20	41
None of the preceding ECG changes but a prior history of angina or myocardial infarction (history of heart attack or nitroglycerin use)	4	51
None of the preceding ECG changes and no prior history of angina or myocardial infarction (history of heart attack or nitroglycerin use)	2	14

NOTE: ECG, electrocardiogram.
SOURCE: Unpublished data from Brigham and Women's Hospital Chest Pain Study, 1997–1999.

tients who are less stable. Aortic angiography is no longer a first test at most institutions.

Acute pulmonary embolism should be considered in patients with respiratory symptoms, pleuritic chest pain, hemoptysis, or a history of venous thromboembolism or coagulation abnormalities. Initial tests usually include a lung scan and/or pulmonary arteriography.

If patients with acute chest discomfort show no evidence of life-threatening conditions, the clinician should then focus on serious chronic conditions with the potential to cause major complications, the most common of which is stable angina. Early use of treadmill exercise testing for such patients, whether in the office or the emergency department, is now an accepted management strategy for low-risk patients. Exercise testing is not appropriate, however, for patients who (1) report pain that is believed to be ischemic occurring at rest or (2) have electrocardiographic changes consistent with ischemia not known to be old.

Patients with sustained chest discomfort who do not have evidence for life-threatening conditions should be evaluated for evidence of conditions likely to benefit from acute treatment (Table 13-3). Pericarditis may be suggested by the history, physical examination, and electrocardiogram (Table 13-2). Clinicians should carefully assess blood pressure patterns and consider echocardiography in such patients to detect evidence of impending pericardial tamponade. Chest x-rays can be used to evaluate the possibility of pulmonary disease.

GUIDELINES AND CRITICAL PATHWAYS FOR ACUTE CHEST PAIN

Guidelines for the initial evaluation for patients with acute chest pain have been developed by the American College of Emergency Physicians (ACEP) and other organizations. The ACEP statement describes *rules* and *guidelines* about the data that should be recorded as part of the evaluation, and the actions that should follow from certain findings (Table 13-5). In the ACEP framework, *rules* are actions that are general principles of good practice, while *guidelines* are actions that should be considered but are not always followed. Hence, failure to follow a guideline is not necessarily improper care.

Other organizations, including the Agency for Health Care Policy and Research (AHCPR) and the National Heart Attack Alert Program, have also issued guidelines for management of patients with a high probability of acute ischemic heart disease. In these and other guidelines, patients with possible or probable acute myocardial infarction as suggested by the description of their pain or electrocardiographic findings are expected to be admitted to the hospital. The AHCPR guidelines for unstable angina note that not all patients with that syndrome require admission but recommend that patients with unstable angina be monitored electrocardiographically during their evaluation; that those with ongoing rest pain should be placed at bed rest during the initial phase of stabilization. The ACEP policy statement indicates that patients who are discharged should be given a referral for follow-up care and instructions regarding treatment and circumstances that require a return to the emergency department.

Many medical centers have adopted critical pathways and other forms of guidelines to increase efficiency. These guidelines emphasize two strategies:

- Triage to non-coronary care unit monitored facilities such as intermediate care units or chest pain units of patients with a low risk for complications, such as patients without new ischemic changes on their electrocardiograms and without ongoing chest pain. Such patients can usually be safely observed in non-coronary care unit settings, undergo early exercise testing, or be discharged home. Risk stratification can be assisted through use of prospectively validated multivariate algorithms that have been published for acute ischemic heart disease and its complications.
- Shortening lengths of stay in the coronary care unit and hospital. Recommendations regarding the minimum length of stay in a monitored bed for a patient who has no further symptoms have decreased in recent years to 12 h or less if exercise testing or other risk stratification technologies are available.

NONACUTE CHEST DISCOMFORT   The management of patients who do not require admission to the hospital or who no longer require inpatient observation should seek to identify the cause of the symptoms and the likelihood of major complications. Cost-effectiveness analyses support use of noninvasive testing for coronary disease, such as exercise electrocardiography and stress echocardiography. These tests serve both to diagnose coronary disease and to identify patients with high-risk forms of coronary disease who may benefit from revascularization. Gastrointestinal causes of chest pain can be evaluated via endoscopy or radiology studies. Emotional and psychiatric conditions warrant appropriate evaluation and treatment; randomized trial data indicate that cognitive therapy and group interventions lead to decreases in symptoms for such patients.

PALPITATIONS

Palpitations are characterized by an awareness of the beating of the heart. Patients commonly describe "pounding" or "fluttering" heart beats or report a sensation that the heart is stopping or skipping beats. These symptoms may be caused by a change in the heart's rhythm or rate or by an increase in the force of its contractions. In many cases, this awareness reflects lack of competing sensory stimuli, such as when a person is lying in bed, unable to sleep.

Palpitations are often manifestations of psychiatric conditions, the most common of which are depression and panic disorder. For example, in one study of outpatients referred for ambulatory electrocardiographic monitoring to evaluate palpitations, 19% were found to have a psychiatric disorder. Patients with psychiatric disorders were more likely than other patients to report that their palpitations lasted longer than 15 min or were accompanied by ancillary symptoms. In this study, physicians usually recognized the emotional basis of the patients' symptoms but frequently did not refer the patient for specific therapy.

Palpitations can also be caused by virtually any cardiac arrhythmia as well as by other cardiac and noncardiac conditions. A markedly enlarged left ventricle can cause awareness of the heart beat by contact with the chest wall. Any condition associated with increased catecholamine levels can lead to palpitations both by increasing the forcefulness of cardiac contractions and by increasing the rate of premature beats.

Palpitations can be intermittent or sustained and regular or irregular. Patients with this complaint should be asked to describe their palpitations' onset, duration, associated symptoms and the circumstances in which they occur. Abrupt onset and termination after several minutes may reflect a sustained ventricular or supraventricular tachyarrhythmia. Gradual onset and termination of a pounding heart beat is more consistent with sinus tachycardia. Patients should try to replicate the rhythm of their palpitations by tapping on a table. This maneuver can help the physician determine the nature of any cardiac arrhythmia. Patients should also be taught to take their pulse so that they can more accurately report their approximate heart rate and whether the rhythm was regular.

DIFFERENTIAL DIAGNOSIS   Patients who report "skipped" beats or a "flopping" sensation often have atrial or ventricular extrasystoles (Chap. 230). These premature beats are followed by a compensatory pause, and the first heart beat after the pause may be unusually strong due to increased left ventricular volume and enhanced contractility (a phenomenon called *postextrasystolic potentiation*). Sustained bursts of rapid heart beats may be due to ventricular or supraventricular tachyarrhythmias. A sustained irregular rhythm suggests atrial fibrillation.

Conditions that cause marked left ventricular enlargement such as aortic regurgitation can cause an awareness of the heart beat that is sometimes positional. Presumably because of associated arrhythmias, hypertrophic cardiomyopathy, mitral valve prolapse, and other cardiac structural abnormalities are also associated with palpitations.

Palpitations can also be a prominent symptom in noncardiac conditions, including thyrotoxicosis, hypoglycemia, pheochromocytoma,

Table 13-5 Evaluation of Acute Chest Pain: Excerpts from the Clinical Policy of the American College of Emergency Physicians (1995)

Variable	Finding	Action Rule[a]	Action Guideline[b]
HISTORY			
Pain	Ongoing *and* severe *and* crushing *and* substernal *or* same as previous pain diagnosed as MI	IV access Supplemental oxygen ECG Aspirin Nitrates Management of ongoing pain Admit	Serum cardiac markers CXR Anticoagulation
	Severe *or* pressure *or* substernal *or* exertional *or* radiating to jaw, neck, shoulder, or arm	ECG	IV access Supplemental oxygen Cardiac monitor Serum cardiac markers CXR Nitrates Management of ongoing pain Admit
	Tearing, severe, and radiating to back	Large-bore IV access Supplemental oxygen Cardiac monitor CXR ECG	Differential upper extremity blood pressures Aortic imaging Management of ongoing pain Admit
	Similar to that of previous pulmonary embolus	IV access Supplemental oxygen Cardiac monitor ABG and oximetry Anticoagulation/pulmonary vascular imaging ECG	CXR Admit
	Indigestion or burning epigastric	None	ECG
	Pleuritic	None	CXR ECG
ASSESSMENT			
Associated symptoms	Syncope or near-syncope	ECG	Cardiac monitor Hct
	Shortness of breath, dyspnea on exertion, paroxysmal nocturnal dyspnea, or orthopnea	ECG	ABG/oximetry CXR
Past medical history	Previous MI, coronary artery bypass surgery, angioplasty, cocaine use within last 96 h, previous positive cardiac diagnostic studies	ECG	
	Major risk factors for coronary artery disease		ECG
	Pericarditis/myocarditis	ECG	Serum cardiac markers CXR Echocardiography Consult/admit
	Unstable angina—new-onset, exertional	ECG Aspirin	IV access Supplemental oxygen Cardiac monitor Nitrates Consult/admit
	Unstable angina—ongoing or recurrent ischemia	IV access Supplemental oxygen Cardiac monitor	Serial serum cardiac markers CXR Cardiac imaging
	ECG showing new ST segment depressions or T wave inversions consistent with ischemia	Anticoagulation Aspirin Nitrates Management of ongoing pain Admit	Serial ECGs Beta blockers

(continued)

Table 13-5—*(continued)*

Variable	Finding	Rule[a]	Guideline[b]
		Action	
	High clinical suspicion of MI with nondiagnostic ECG	IV access Supplemental oxygen Cardiac monitor Anticoagulation Aspirin Nitrates Management of ongoing pain Admit	Serial serum cardiac markers CXR Cardiac imaging Serial ECGs Magnesium therapy Beta blockers
	High clinical suspicion of MI with diagnostic ECG of bundle branch block	IV access Supplemental oxygen Cardiac monitor Assessment for thrombolytic therapy or other reperfusion techniques Anticoagulation Aspirin Nitrates Management of ongoing pain Admit	Serial serum cardiac markers CXR Cardiac imaging Serial ECGs Magnesium therapy if not given thrombolytics Beta blockers
	Aortic dissection	Large-bore IV access Supplemental oxygen Cardiac monitor Blood type and cross-match ECG Management of blood pressure/cardiac contractility Management of ongoing pain Immediate surgical consultation Admit	Aortic imaging

[a] Rule: An action reflecting principles of good practice in most situations. There may be circumstances when a rule need not or cannot be followed; in these situations, it is advisable that deviation from the rule be justified in writing. Inability to comply with rules should be incorporated in institutional policies.
[b] Guideline: An action that may be considered, depending on the patient, the circum-

stances, or other factors. Thus, guidelines are not always followed, and there is no implication that failure to follow a guideline is improper.
NOTE: MI, myocardial infarction; ECG, electrocardiogram; CXR; chest x-ray; ABG, arterial blood gases; Hct, hematocrit.
SOURCE: American College of Emergency Physicians.

and fever. The physiologic basis of palpitations with these conditions is either arrhythmia or increased catecholamine levels leading to greater myocardial contractility. Drugs that can precipitate arrhythmias and palpitations include tobacco, coffee, tea, alcohol, epinephrine, ephedrine, aminophylline, and atropine.

Approach to the Patient

The first goal in the evaluation of patients with palpitations is to exclude the possibility of life-threatening arrhythmias. The risk for such arrhythmias is highest in patients with coronary artery disease, congestive heart failure, or other structural cardiac abnormalities. The history, physical examination, and electrocardiogram should therefore be focused on stratifying patients according to the risk of such conditions. Palpitations are also more likely to reflect serious arrhythmias if they are associated with symptoms that suggest hemodynamic compromise, such as syncope, light-headedness, dizziness, or shortness of breath.

The most common first test after the initial evaluation of palpitations is continuous electrocardiographic (Holter) monitoring. This test is especially useful if patients have palpitations on a daily basis. For patients with more sporadic palpitations, a variety of new technologies have become available to allow capture of electrocardiographic tracings at the time of their symptoms. These technologies include loop recorders, that can freeze the last several minutes of data when the patient presses a button, and telephonic monitors, which can be used to "call in" tracings when symptoms occur. If episodes are associated with physical stress, exercise electrocardiography can be used in an attempt to elicit an arrhythmia.

Most patients with palpitations do not have evidence of major arrhythmias or abnormal physiologic conditions associated with increased catecholamine levels. Patients with emotional or psychological causes of palpitations should be evaluated for possible cognitive and

pharmaceutical therapy. Drugs and medications that may precipitate palpitations should be eliminated or reduced. A trial of beta blockers is often successful in reducing premature beats and symptoms. Regardless of the cause and treatment, the clinician should remain aware that palpitations are extremely bothersome symptoms for patients. Reassurance that a comprehensive evaluation has been performed and that the palpitations do not adversely affect the patient's prognosis is a critical part of the patient's care.

BIBLIOGRAPHY

AMERICAN COLLEGE OF EMERGENCY PHYSICIANS: Clinical policy for the initial approach to adults presenting with a chief complaint of chest pain, with no history of trauma. Ann Emerg Med 25:274, 1995

BARSKY AJ et al: Somatized psychiatric disorder presenting as palpitations. Arch Intern Med 156:1102, 1996

BRAUNWALD E et al: *Unstable Angina: Diagnosis and Management. Clinical Practice Guideline Number 10* (amended). AHCPR Publication No. 94-0602. Rockville, MD, Agency for Health Care Policy and Research and National Heart, Lung, and Blood Institute, Public Health Service, U.S. Department of Health and Human Services, May 1994

FARKOUH ME et al: A clinical trial of a chest-pain observation unit for patients with unstable angina. N Engl J Med 339:1882, 1998

KUNTZ KM et al: Cost-effectiveness of diagnostic strategies for patients with chest pain. Ann Intern Med 130:709, 1999

NICHOL G et al: A critical pathway for management of patients with acute chest pain at low risk for myocardial ischemia. Recommendations and potential impact. Ann Intern Med 127:996, 1997

VAN PESKI-OOSTERBAAN AS et al: Cognitive-behavioral therapy for noncardiac chest pain: A randomized trial. Am J Med 106:424, 1999

WEBER BE, KAPOOR WN: Evaluation and outcomes of patients with palpitations. Am J Med 100:138, 1996

ABDOMINAL PAIN

The correct interpretation of acute abdominal pain is challenging. Since proper therapy may require urgent action, the unhurried approach suitable for the study of other conditions is sometimes denied. Few other clinical situations demand greater judgment, because the most catastrophic of events may be forecast by the subtlest of symptoms and signs. A meticulously executed, detailed history and physical examination is of great importance. The etiologic classification in Table 14-1, although not complete, forms a useful basis for the evaluation of patients with abdominal pain.

The diagnosis of "acute or surgical abdomen" is not an acceptable one because of its often misleading and erroneous connotation. The most obvious of "acute abdomens" may not require operative intervention, and the mildest of abdominal pains may herald an urgently correctable lesion. Any patient with abdominal pain of recent onset requires early and thorough evaluation and accurate diagnosis.

SOME MECHANISMS OF PAIN ORIGINATING IN THE ABDOMEN Inflammation of the Parietal Peritoneum

The pain of parietal peritoneal inflammation is steady and aching in character and is located directly over the inflamed area, its exact reference being possible because it is transmitted by somatic nerves supplying the parietal peritoneum. The intensity of the pain is dependent

Table 14-1 Some Important Causes of Abdominal Pain

PAIN ORIGINATING IN THE ABDOMEN

1. Parietal peritoneal inflammation
   a. Bacterial contamination, e.g., perforated appendix, pelvic inflammatory disease
   b. Chemical irritation, e.g., perforated ulcer, pancreatitis, mittelschmerz
2. Mechanical obstruction of hollow viscera
   a. Obstruction of the small or large intestine
   b. Obstruction of the biliary tree
   c. Obstruction of the ureter
3. Vascular disturbances
   a. Embolism or thrombosis
   b. Vascular rupture
   c. Pressure or torsional occlusion
   d. Sickle cell anemia
4. Abdominal wall
   a. Distortion or traction of mesentery
   b. Trauma or infection of muscles
5. Distention of visceral surfaces, e.g., hepatic or renal capsules

PAIN REFERRED FROM EXTRAABDOMINAL SOURCE

1. Thorax, e.g., pneumonia, referred pain from coronary occlusion
2. Spine, e.g., radiculitis from arthritis
3. Genitalia, e.g., torsion of the testicle

METABOLIC CAUSES

1. Exogenous
   a. Black widow spider bite
   b. Lead poisoning and others
2. Endogenous
   a. Uremia
   b. Diabetic ketoacidosis
   c. Porphyria
   d. Allergic factors (C′1 esterase inhibitor deficiency)

NEUROGENIC CAUSES

1. Organic
   a. Tabes dorsalis
   b. Herpes zoster
   c. Causalgia and others
2. Functional

on the type and amount of material to which the peritoneal surfaces are exposed in a given time period. For example, the sudden release into the peritoneal cavity of a small quantity of *sterile* acid gastric juice causes much more pain than the same amount of grossly contaminated neutral feces. Enzymatically active pancreatic juice incites more pain and inflammation than does the same amount of sterile bile containing no potent enzymes. Blood and urine are often so bland as to go undetected if exposure of the peritoneum has not been sudden and massive. In the case of bacterial contamination, such as in pelvic inflammatory disease, the pain is frequently of low intensity early in the illness until bacterial multiplication has caused the elaboration of irritating substances.

The rate at which the irritating material is applied to the peritoneum is important. Perforated peptic ulcer may be associated with entirely different clinical pictures dependent only on the rapidity with which the gastric juice enters the peritoneal cavity.

The pain of peritoneal inflammation is invariably accentuated by pressure or changes in tension of the peritoneum, whether produced by palpation or by movement, as in coughing or sneezing. The patient with peritonitis lies quietly in bed, preferring to avoid motion, in contrast to the patient with colic, who may writhe incessantly.

Another characteristic feature of peritoneal irritation is tonic reflex spasm of the abdominal musculature, localized to the involved body segment. The intensity of the tonic muscle spasm accompanying peritoneal inflammation is dependent on the location of the inflammatory process, the rate at which it develops, and the integrity of the nervous system. Spasm over a perforated retrocecal appendix or perforated ulcer into the lesser peritoneal sac may be minimal or absent because of the protective effect of overlying viscera. A slowly developing process often greatly attenuates the degree of muscle spasm. Catastrophic abdominal emergencies such as a perforated ulcer may be associated with minimal or no detectable pain or muscle spasm in obtunded, seriously ill, debilitated elderly patients or in psychotic patients.

Obstruction of Hollow Viscera The pain of obstruction of hollow abdominal viscera is classically described as intermittent, or colicky. Yet the lack of a truly cramping character should not be misleading, because distention of a hollow viscus may produce steady pain with only very occasional exacerbations. It is not nearly as well localized as the pain of parietal peritoneal inflammation.

The colicky pain of obstruction of the small intestine is usually periumbilical or supraumbilical and is poorly localized. As the intestine becomes progressively dilated with loss of muscular tone, the colicky nature of the pain may diminish. With superimposed strangulating obstruction, pain may spread to the lower lumbar region if there is traction on the root of the mesentery. The colicky pain of colonic obstruction is of lesser intensity than that of the small intestine and is often located in the infraumbilical area. Lumbar radiation of pain is common in colonic obstruction.

Sudden distention of the biliary tree produces a steady rather than colicky type of pain; hence the term *biliary colic* is misleading. Acute distention of the gallbladder usually causes pain in the right upper quadrant with radiation to the right posterior region of the thorax or to the tip of the right scapula, and distention of the common bile duct is often associated with pain in the epigastrium radiating to the upper part of the lumbar region. Considerable variation is common, however, so that differentiation between these may be impossible. The typical subscapular pain or lumbar radiation is frequently absent. Gradual dilatation of the biliary tree, as in carcinoma of the head of the pancreas, may cause no pain or only a mild aching sensation in the epigastrium or right upper quadrant. The pain of distention of the pancreatic ducts is similar to that described for distention of the common bile duct but, in addition, is very frequently accentuated by recumbency and relieved by the upright position.

Obstruction of the urinary bladder results in dull suprapubic pain, usually low in intensity. Restlessness without specific complaint of pain may be the only sign of a distended bladder in an obtunded patient. In contrast, acute obstruction of the intravesicular portion of the ureter is characterized by severe suprapubic and flank pain that radiates to the penis, scrotum, or inner aspect of the upper thigh. Obstruction of the ureteropelvic junction is felt as pain in the costovertebral angle, whereas obstruction of the remainder of the ureter is associated with flank pain that often extends into the same side of the abdomen.

Vascular Disturbances   A frequent misconception, despite abundant experience to the contrary, is that pain associated with intra-abdominal vascular disturbances is sudden and catastrophic in nature. The pain of embolism or thrombosis of the superior mesenteric artery or that of impending rupture of an abdominal aortic aneurysm certainly may be severe and diffuse. Yet, just as frequently, the patient with occlusion of the superior mesenteric artery has only mild continuous diffuse pain for 2 or 3 days before vascular collapse or findings of peritoneal inflammation appear. The early, seemingly insignificant discomfort is caused by hyperperistalsis rather than peritoneal inflammation. Indeed, absence of tenderness and rigidity in the presence of continuous, diffuse pain in a patient likely to have vascular disease is quite characteristic of occlusion of the superior mesenteric artery. Abdominal pain with radiation to the sacral region, flank, or genitalia should always signal the possible presence of a rupturing abdominal aortic aneurysm. This pain may persist over a period of several days before rupture and collapse occur.

Abdominal Wall   Pain arising from the abdominal wall is usually constant and aching. Movement, prolonged standing, and pressure accentuate the discomfort and muscle spasm. In the case of hematoma of the rectus sheath, now most frequently encountered in association with anticoagulant therapy, a mass may be present in the lower quadrants of the abdomen. Simultaneous involvement of muscles in other parts of the body usually serves to differentiate myositis of the abdominal wall from an intraabdominal process that might cause pain in the same region.

REFERRED PAIN IN ABDOMINAL DISEASES   Pain referred to the abdomen from the thorax, spine, or genitalia may prove a vexing diagnostic problem, because diseases of the upper part of the abdominal cavity such as acute cholecystitis or perforated ulcer are frequently associated with intrathoracic complications. A most important, yet often forgotten, dictum is that the possibility of intrathoracic disease must be considered in every patient with abdominal pain, especially if the pain is in the upper part of the abdomen. Systematic questioning and examination directed toward detecting myocardial or pulmonary infarction, pneumonia, pericarditis, or esophageal disease (the intrathoracic diseases that most often masquerade as abdominal emergencies) will often provide sufficient clues to establish the proper diagnosis. Diaphragmatic pleuritis resulting from pneumonia or pulmonary infarction may cause pain in the right upper quadrant and pain in the supraclavicular area, the latter radiation to be distinguished from the referred subscapular pain caused by acute distention of the extrahepatic biliary tree. The ultimate decision as to the origin of abdominal pain may require deliberate and planned observation over a period of several hours, during which repeated questioning and examination will provide the diagnosis.

Referred pain of thoracic origin is often accompanied by splinting of the involved hemithorax with respiratory lag and decrease in excursion more marked than that seen in the presence of intraabdominal disease. In addition, apparent abdominal muscle spasm caused by referred pain will diminish during the inspiratory phase of respiration, whereas it is persistent throughout both respiratory phases if it is of abdominal origin. Palpation over the area of referred pain in the abdomen also does not usually accentuate the pain and in many instances actually seems to relieve it. Thoracic and abdominal disease frequently coexist and may be difficult or impossible to differentiate.

For example, the patient with known biliary tract disease often has epigastric pain during myocardial infarction, or biliary colic may be referred to the precordium or left shoulder in a patient who has suffered previously from angina pectoris. →*For an explanation of the radiation of pain to a previously diseased area, see Chap. 12.*

Referred pain from the spine, which usually involves compression or irritation of nerve roots, is characteristically intensified by certain motions such as cough, sneeze, or strain and is associated with hyperesthesia over the involved dermatomes. Pain referred to the abdomen from the testicles or seminal vesicles is generally accentuated by the slightest pressure on either of these organs. The abdominal discomfort is of dull aching character and is poorly localized.

METABOLIC ABDOMINAL CRISES   Pain of metabolic origin may simulate almost any other type of intraabdominal disease. Several mechanisms may be at work. In certain instances, such as hyperlipidemia, the metabolic disease itself may be accompanied by an intraabdominal process such as pancreatitis, which can lead to unnecessary laparotomy unless recognized. C'1 esterase deficiency associated with angioneurotic edema is often associated with episodes of severe abdominal pain. Whenever the cause of abdominal pain is obscure, a metabolic origin always must be considered. Abdominal pain is also the hallmark of familial Mediterranean fever (Chap. 289).

The problem of differential diagnosis is often not readily resolved. The pain of porphyria and of lead colic is usually difficult to distinguish from that of intestinal obstruction, because severe hyperperistalsis is a prominent feature of both. The pain of uremia or diabetes is nonspecific, and the pain and tenderness frequently shift in location and intensity. Diabetic acidosis may be precipitated by acute appendicitis or intestinal obstruction, so if prompt resolution of the abdominal pain does not result from correction of the metabolic abnormalities, an underlying organic problem should be suspected. Black widow spider bites produce intense pain and rigidity of the abdominal muscles and back, an area infrequently involved in intraabdominal disease.

NEUROGENIC CAUSES   Causalgic pain may occur in diseases that injure sensory nerves. It has a burning character and is usually limited to the distribution of a given peripheral nerve. Normal stimuli such as touch or change in temperature may be transformed into this type of pain, which is frequently present in a patient at rest. The demonstration of irregularly spaced cutaneous pain spots may be the only indication of an old nerve lesion underlying causalgic pain. Even though the pain may be precipitated by gentle palpation, rigidity of the abdominal muscles is absent, and the respirations are not disturbed. Distention of the abdomen is uncommon, and the pain has no relationship to the intake of food.

Pain arising from spinal nerves or roots comes and goes suddenly and is of a lancinating type (Chap. 16). It may be caused by herpes zoster, impingement by arthritis, tumors, herniated nucleus pulposus, diabetes, or syphilis. It is not associated with food intake, abdominal distention, or changes in respiration. Severe muscle spasm, as in the gastric crises of tabes dorsalis, is common but is either relieved or is not accentuated by abdominal palpation. The pain is made worse by movement of the spine and is usually confined to a few dermatomes. Hyperesthesia is very common.

Psychogenic pain conforms to none of the aforementioned patterns. Mechanism is hard to define. The most common problem is the hysterical adolescent or young person who develops abdominal pain and who frequently loses an appendix or other organs because of it. Ovulation or some other natural event that causes brief mild abdominal discomfort may be experienced as an abdominal catastrophe.

Psychogenic pain varies enormously in type and location but usually has no relation to meals. It is often markedly accentuated during the night. Nausea and vomiting are rarely observed. Spasm is seldom induced in the abdominal musculature and, if present, does not persist, especially if the attention of the patient can be distracted. Persistent localized tenderness is rare, and if found, the muscle spasm in the area is inconsistent or absent. Shallow respiration is the most common breathing abnormality; anxiety may produce a smothering or choking sensation. It occurs in the absence of thoracic splinting or change in the respiratory rate.

Approach to the Patient

Few abdominal conditions require such urgent operative intervention that an orderly approach need be abandoned, no matter how ill the patient. Only those patients with exsanguinating hemorrhage must be rushed to the operating room immediately, but in such instances, only a few minutes are required to assess the critical nature of the problem. Under these circumstances, all obstacles must be swept aside, adequate venous access for fluid replacement obtained, and the operation begun. Many patients of this type have died in the radiology department or the emergency room while awaiting such unnecessary examinations as electrocardiograms or abdominal films. *There are no contraindications to operation when massive hemorrhage is present.* This situation fortunately is relatively rare.

Nothing will supplant an orderly, painstakingly *detailed history*, which is far more valuable than any laboratory or radiographic examination. This kind of history is laborious and time-consuming, making it not especially popular, even though a reasonably accurate diagnosis can be made on the basis of the history alone in the majority of cases. Computer-aided diagnosis of abdominal pain provides no advantage over clinical assessment alone. In cases of *acute* abdominal pain, a diagnosis is readily established in most instances, whereas success is not so frequent in patients with *chronic* pain. Irritable bowel syndrome is one of the most common causes of abdominal pain and must always be kept in mind (Chap. 288). The *chronological sequence of events* in the patient's history is often more important than emphasis on the location of pain. If the examiner is sufficiently open-minded and unhurried, asks the proper questions, and listens, the patient will usually provide the diagnosis. Careful attention should be paid to the extraabdominal regions that may be responsible for abdominal pain. An accurate menstrual history in a female patient is essential. Narcotics or analgesics should *not* be withheld until a definitive diagnosis or a definitive plan has been formulated; obfuscation of the diagnosis by adequate analgesia is unlikely.

In the examination, simple critical inspection of the patient, e.g., of facies, position in bed, and respiratory activity, may provide valuable clues. The amount of information to be gleaned is directly proportional to the *gentleness* and thoroughness of the examiner. Once a patient with peritoneal inflammation has been examined brusquely, accurate assessment by the next examiner becomes almost impossible. Eliciting rebound tenderness by sudden release of a deeply palpating hand in a patient with suspected peritonitis is cruel and unnecessary. The same information can be obtained by gentle percussion of the abdomen (rebound tenderness on a miniature scale), a maneuver that can be far more precise and localizing. Asking the patient to cough will elicit true rebound tenderness without the need for placing a hand on the abdomen. Furthermore, the forceful demonstration of rebound tenderness will startle and induce protective spasm in a nervous or worried patient in whom true rebound tenderness is not present. A palpable gallbladder will be missed if palpation is so brusque that voluntary muscle spasm becomes superimposed on involuntary muscular rigidity.

As in history taking, there is no substitute for sufficient time spent in the examination. Abdominal signs may be minimal but nevertheless, if accompanied by consistent symptoms, may be exceptionally meaningful. Abdominal signs may be virtually or totally absent in cases of pelvic peritonitis, so careful *pelvic and rectal examinations are mandatory in every patient with abdominal pain.* Tenderness on pelvic or rectal examination in the absence of other abdominal signs can be

14 Abdominal Pain
69

caused by operative indications such as perforated appendicitis, diverticulitis, twisted ovarian cyst, and many others.

Much attention has been paid to the presence or absence of peristaltic sounds, their quality, and their frequency. Auscultation of the abdomen is one of the least revealing aspects of the physical examination of a patient with abdominal pain. Catastrophes such as strangulating small intestinal obstruction or perforated appendicitis may occur in the presence of normal peristalsis. Conversely, when the proximal part of the intestine above an obstruction becomes markedly distended and edematous, peristaltic sounds may lose the characteristics of borborygmi and become weak or absent, even when peritonitis is not present. It is usually the severe chemical peritonitis of sudden onset that is associated with the truly silent abdomen. Assessment of the patient's state of hydration is important.

Laboratory examinations may be of great value in assessment of the patient with abdominal pain, yet with few exceptions they rarely establish a diagnosis. Leukocytosis should never be the single deciding factor as to whether or not operation is indicated. A white blood cell count greater than $20,000/\mu L$ may be observed with perforation of a viscus, but pancreatitis, acute cholecystitis, pelvic inflammatory disease, and intestinal infarction may be associated with marked leukocytosis. A normal white blood cell count is not rare in cases of perforation of abdominal viscera. The diagnosis of anemia may be more helpful than the white blood cell count, especially when combined with the history.

The urinalysis may reveal the state of hydration or rule out severe renal disease, diabetes, or urinary infection. Blood urea nitrogen, glucose, and serum bilirubin levels may be helpful. Serum amylase levels may be increased by many diseases other than pancreatitis, e.g., perforated ulcer, strangulating intestinal obstruction, and acute cholecystitis; thus, elevations of serum amylase do not rule out the need for an operation. The determination of the serum lipase may have greater accuracy than that of the serum amylase.

Plain and upright or lateral decubitus radiographs of the abdomen may be of value in cases of intestinal obstruction, perforated ulcer, and a variety of other conditions. They are usually unnecessary in patients with acute appendicitis or strangulated external hernias. In rare instances, barium or water-soluble contrast study of the upper part of the gastrointestinal tract may demonstrate partial intestinal obstruction that may elude diagnosis by other means. If there is any question of obstruction of the colon, oral administration of barium sulfate should be avoided. On the other hand, in cases of suspected colonic obstruction (with perforation), contrast enema may be diagnostic.

In the absence of trauma, peritoneal lavage has been replaced as a diagnostic tool by ultrasound, computed tomography (CT), and laparoscopy. Ultrasonography has proved to be useful in detecting an enlarged gallbladder or pancreas, the presence of gallstones, an enlarged ovary, or a tubal pregnancy. Laparoscopy is especially helpful in diagnosing pelvic conditions, such as ovarian cysts, tubal pregnancies, salpingitis, and acute appendicitis. Radioisotopic scans (HIDA) may help differentiate acute cholecystitis from acute pancreatitis. A CT scan may demonstrate an enlarged pancreas, ruptured spleen, or thickened colonic or appendiceal wall and streaking of the mesocolon or mesoappendix characteristic of diverticulitis or appendicitis.

Sometimes, even under the best circumstances with all available aids and with the greatest of clinical skill, a definitive diagnosis cannot be established at the time of the initial examination. Nevertheless, despite lack of a clear anatomic diagnosis, it may be abundantly clear to an experienced and thoughtful physician and surgeon that on clinical grounds alone operation is indicated. Should that decision be questionable, watchful waiting with repeated questioning and examination will often elucidate the true nature of the illness and indicate the proper course of action.

BIBLIOGRAPHY

BOHNER H et al: Simple data from history and physical examination help to exclude bowel obstruction and to avoid radiographic studies in patients with acute abdominal pain. Eur J Surg 164:777, 1998

CERVERO F, LAIRD JM: Visceral pain. Lancet 353:2145, 1999

DAVIES AH et al: Ultrasonography in the acute abdomen. Br J Surg 78:1178, 1991

MARCO CA et al: Abdominal pain in geriatric emergency patients: Variables associated with adverse outcome. Acad Emerg Med 5:1163, 1998

SCOTT HJ, ROSIN RD: The influence of diagnostic and therapeutic laparoscopy on patients presenting with an acute abdomen. J R Soc Med 86:699, 1993

TAIT IS et al: Do patients with abdominal pain wait unduly long for analgesia? J R Coll Surg Edinb 44:181, 1999

TAOUREL P et al: Acute abdomen of unknown origin: Impact of CT on diagnosis and management. Gastrointest Radiol 17:287, 1992

15   *Neil H. Raskin, Stephen J. Peroutka*

HEADACHE, INCLUDING MIGRAINE AND CLUSTER HEADACHE

CSF	cerebrospinal fluid	MELAS *m*itochondrial
CT	computed tomography	*e*ncephalomyopathy, *l*actic *a*cidosis, and
ESR	erythrocyte sedimentation rate	*s*troke-like episodes
FDA	Food and Drug Administration	MRI magnetic resonance imaging
FHM	Familial hemiplegic migraine	NSAIDs nonsteroidal anti-
5-HT	5-hydroxytryptamine	inflammatory drugs
MAOIs monoamine oxidase		PET positron emission tomography
inhibitors		SNS sympathetic nervous system

Few of us are spared the experience of head pain. As many as 90% of individuals have at least one headache per year. Severe, disabling headache is reported to occur at least annually by 40% of individuals worldwide. A useful classification of the many causes of headache is shown in Table 15-1. Headache is usually a benign symptom, but occasionally it is the manifestation of a serious illness such as brain tumor, subarachnoid hemorrhage, meningitis, or giant cell arteritis. In emergency settings, approximately 5% of patients with headache are found to have a serious underlying neurologic disorder. Therefore, it is imperative that the serious causes of headache be diagnosed rapidly and accurately.

PAIN-SENSITIVE STRUCTURES OF THE HEAD

Pain is most commonly due to tissue injury resulting in stimulation of peripheral nociceptors in an intact nervous system. Pain can also result from damage to or anomalous activation of pain-sensitive pathways of the peripheral or central nervous system. Headache may originate from either or both mechanisms. Relatively few cranial structures are pain-sensitive: the scalp, middle meningeal artery, dural sinuses, falx cerebri, and the proximal segments of the large pial arteries. The ventricular ependyma, choroid plexus, pial veins, and much of the brain parenchyma are pain-insensitive. Electrical stimulation of the midbrain in the region of the dorsal raphe has resulted in migraine-like headaches. Thus, whereas most of the brain is insensitive to electrode probing, a site in the midbrain represents a possible source of headache generation. Sensory stimuli from the head are conveyed to the central nervous system via the trigeminal nerves for structures above the tentorium in the anterior and middle fossae of the skull and via the first three cervical nerves for those in the posterior fossa and the inferior surface of the tentorium.

Headache can occur as the result of (1) distention, traction, or dilation of intracranial or extracranial arteries; (2) traction or displacement of large intracranial veins or their dural envelope; (3) compression, traction, or inflammation of cranial and spinal nerves; (4) spasm, inflammation, or trauma to cranial and cervical muscles; (5) meningeal irritation and raised intracranial pressure; or (6) other possible mechanisms such as activation of brainstem structures.

GENERAL CLINICAL CONSIDERATIONS

The quality, location, duration, and time course of the headache and the conditions that produce, exacerbate, or relieve it should be carefully reviewed. Ascertaining the *quality* of cephalic pain is occasionally helpful for diagnosis. Most tension-type headaches are described as tight "bandlike" pain or as dull, deeply located, and aching pain. Jabbing, brief, sharp cephalic pain, often occurring multifocally (ice pick–like pain), is the signature of a benign, nondescript disorder. A throbbing quality and tight muscles about the head, neck, and shoulder girdle are common nonspecific accompaniments of vascular headaches.

Pain *intensity* rarely has diagnostic value, although from the patient's perspective, it is the single aspect of pain that is most important. Although meningitis, subarachnoid hemorrhage, and cluster headache produce intense cranial pain, most patients entering emergency departments with the most severe headache of their lives usually have migraine. Contrary to common belief, the headache produced by a brain tumor is not usually distinctive or severe.

Data regarding *location* of headache may be informative. If the source is an extracranial structure, as in giant cell arteritis, the correspondence with the site of pain is fairly precise. Inflammation of an extracranial artery causes pain and exquisite tenderness localized to the site of the vessel. Lesions of paranasal sinuses, teeth, eyes, and upper cervical vertebrae induce less sharply localized pain, but pain that is still referred in a regional distribution. Intracranial lesions in the posterior fossa cause pain that is usually occipitonuchal, and supratentorial lesions most often induce frontotemporal pain.

Duration and *time-intensity* curves of headaches are diagnostically useful. A ruptured aneurysm results in head pain that peaks in an instant, thunderclap-like; much less often, unruptured aneurysms may signal their presence in the same way. Cluster headache attacks reach their peak over 3 to 5 min, remain at maximal levels for about 45 min, and then taper off. Migraine attacks build up over hours, are maintained for several hours to days, and are characteristically relieved by sleep. Sleep disruption and early morning headaches that improve during the day are characteristics of headaches produced by brain tumors.

The analysis of facial pain requires a different approach. Trigeminal and, less commonly, glossopharyngeal neuralgia are frequent causes of facial pain (Chap. 367). "Neuralgias" are painful disorders characterized by paroxysmal, fleeting, often electric shock–like episodes that are frequently caused by demyelinating lesions of nerves (the trigeminal or glossopharyngeal nerves in cranial neuralgias). Certain maneuvers characteristically trigger paroxysms of pain. However, the most common cause of facial pain by far is dental; provocation by hot, cold, or sweet foods is typical. The application of a cold stimulus will repeatedly induce dental pain, whereas in neuralgic disorders, a refractory period usually occurs after the initial response so that pain cannot be repeatedly induced.

The effect of eating on facial pain may provide insight into its cause. Is it the chewing, swallowing, or taste of the food that elicits pain? Chewing points toward trigeminal neuralgia, temporomandibular joint dysfunction, or giant cell arteritis ("jaw claudication"), whereas swallowing *and* taste provocation point toward glossopharyngeal neuralgia. Pain upon swallowing is common among patients with carotidynia (see below) because the inflamed, tender carotid artery abuts the esophagus during deglutition.

Many patients with facial pain do not experience stereotypic neuralgias; the term *atypical facial pain* has been used in this setting.

Table 15-1 International Headache Society Classification of Headache

1. **Migraine**
   Migraine without aura
   Migraine with aura
   Ophthalmoplegic migraine
   Retinal migraine
   Childhood periodic syndromes that may be precursors to or associated
     with migraine
   Migrainous disorder not fulfilling above criteria
2. **Tension-type headache**
   Episodic tension-type headache
   Chronic tension-type headache
3. **Cluster headache and chronic paroxysmal hemicrania**
   Cluster headache
   Chronic paroxysmal hemicrania
4. **Miscellaneous headaches not associated with structural lesion**
   Idiopathic stabbing headache
   External compression headache
   Cold stimulus headache
   Benign cough headache
   Benign exertional headache
   Headache associated with sexual activity
5. **Headache associated with head trauma**
   Acute posttraumatic headache
   Chronic posttraumatic headache
6. **Headache associated with vascular disorders**
   Acute ischemic cerebrovascular disorder
   Intracranial hematoma
   Subarachnoid hemorrhage
   Unruptured vascular malformation
   Arteritis
   Carotid or vertebral artery pain
   Venous thrombosis
   Arterial hypertension
   Other vascular disorder
7. **Headache associated with nonvascular intracranial disorder**
   High CSF pressure
   Low CSF pressure
   Intracranial infection

7. **Headache associated with nonvascular intracranial disorder (cont.)**
   Sarcoidosis and other noninfectious inflammatory diseases
   Related to intrathecal injections
   Intracranial neoplasm
   Associated with other intracranial disorder
8. **Headache associated with substances or their withdrawal**
   Headache induced by acute substance use or exposure
   Headache induced by chronic substance use or exposure
   Headache from substance withdrawal (acute use)
   Headache from substance withdrawal (chronic use)
9. **Headache associated with noncephalic infection**
   Viral infection
   Bacterial infection
   Other infection
10. **Headache associated with metabolic disorder**
    Hypoxia
    Hypercapnia
    Mixed hypoxia and hypercapnia
    Hypoglycemia
    Dialysis
    Other metabolic abnormality
11. **Headache or facial pain associated with disorder of facial or cranial
    structures**
    Cranial bone
    Eyes
    Ears
    Nose and sinuses
    Teeth, jaws, and related structures
    Temporomandibular joint disease
12. **Cranial neuralgias, nerve trunk pain, and deafferentation pain**
    Persistent (in contrast to ticlike) pain of cranial nerve origin
    Trigeminal neuralgia
    Glossopharyngeal neuralgia
    Nervus intermedius neuralgia
    Superior laryngeal neuralgia
    Occipital neuralgia
    Central causes of head and facial pain other than tic douloureux
13. **Headache not classifiable**

NOTE: CSF, cerebrospinal fluid.
SOURCE: After Olesen, 1988.

Vague, poorly localized, continuous facial pain is characteristic of nasopharyngeal carcinoma; a burning pain often develops as deafferentation occurs and evidence of cranial neuropathy appears. Burning facial pain may also occur with tumors of the fifth cranial nerve (meningioma or schwannoma) or with lesions of the pons that interrupt the dorsal root entry zone of the nerve (multiple sclerosis). In patients with facial pain, the finding of objective sensory loss is an important clue to a serious underlying disorder. Occasionally, the cause of a pain problem cannot be resolved promptly, necessitating periodic follow-up until further signs appear.

CLINICAL EVALUATION OF ACUTE, NEW-ONSET HEADACHE

Patients who present with their first severe headache raise entirely different diagnostic possibilities than those with recurrent headaches over many years. In new-onset and severe headaches, the probability of finding a potentially serious cause is considerably greater than in recurrent headache. When a patient complains of an acute, new-onset headache, a number of causes should be considered including meningitis, subarachnoid hemorrhage, epidural or subdural hematoma, glaucoma, and purulent sinusitis. Clinical features of acute, new-onset headache caused by serious underlying conditions are summarized in Table 15-2.

A complete neurologic examination is an essential first step in the evaluation. In most cases, an abnormal examination should be followed by a computed tomography (CT) or a magnetic resonance imaging (MRI) study. As a screening procedure for intracranial pathology in this setting, CT and MRI methods appear to be equally sensitive.

A general evaluation of acute headache might include the investigation of cardiovascular and renal status by blood pressure monitoring and urine examination; eyes by fundoscopy, intraocular pressure measurement, and refraction; cranial arteries by palpation; and cervical spine by the effect of passive movement of the head and imaging.

The psychological state of the patient should also be evaluated since a relationship exists between head pain and depression. Many patients in chronic daily pain cycles become depressed; moreover, there is a greater-than-chance coincidence of migraine with both bipolar (manic depressive) and unipolar major depressive disorders. Drugs with antidepressant actions are also effective in the prophylactic treatment of both tension-type headache and migraine.

Underlying recurrent headache disorders may be activated by pain that follows otologic or endodontic surgical procedures. Treatment of the headache problem is largely ineffective until the cause of the primary problem is addressed. Thus, pain about the head as the result of

Table 15-2 Headache Symptoms That Suggest a Serious
Underlying Disorder

"Worst" headache ever
First severe headache
Subacute worsening over days or weeks
Abnormal neurologic examination
Fever or unexplained systemic signs
Vomiting precedes headache
Induced by bending, lifting, cough
Disturbs sleep or present immediately upon awakening
Known systemic illness
Onset after age 55

diseased tissue or trauma may reawaken an otherwise quiescent migrainous syndrome.

Serious underlying conditions that are associated with headache are described below and in Table 15-3.

MENINGITIS   In general, acute, severe headache with stiff neck and fever suggests meningitis. Lumbar puncture is mandatory. Often there is striking accentuation of pain with eye movement. Meningitis is particularly easy to mistake for migraine in that the cardinal symptoms of pounding headache, photophobia, nausea, and vomiting are present. →*A detailed discussion of meningitis can be found in Chaps. 372 to 374.*

INTRACRANIAL HEMORRHAGE   In general, acute, severe headache with stiff neck but without fever suggests subarachnoid hemorrhage. A ruptured aneurysm, arteriovenous malformation, or intraparenchymal hemorrhage may also present with only headache. Rarely, if the hemorrhage is small or below the foramen magnum, the head CT scan can be normal. Therefore, a lumbar puncture may be required to make the definitive diagnosis of a subarachnoid hemorrhage. →*A detailed discussion of intracranial hemorrhage can be found in Chap. 361.*

BRAIN TUMOR   Approximately 30% of patients with brain tumors consider headache to be their chief complaint. The head pain is usually nondescript—an intermittent deep, dull aching of moderate intensity, which may worsen with exertion or change in position and may be associated with nausea and vomiting. This pattern of symptoms results from migraine far more often than from brain tumor. Headache of brain tumor disturbs sleep in about 10% of patients. Vomiting that precedes the appearance of headache by weeks is highly characteristic of posterior fossa brain tumors. A history of amenorrhea or galactorrhea should lead one to question whether a prolactin-secreting pituitary adenoma (or the polycystic ovary syndrome) is the source of headache. Headache arising de novo in a patient with known malignancy suggests either cerebral metastases and/or carcinomatous meningitis. Head pain appearing abruptly after bending, lifting, or coughing can be the clue to a posterior fossa mass (or a Chiari malformation). →*A detailed discussion of brain tumors can be found in Chap. 370.*

TEMPORAL ARTERITIS   (See also Chaps. 28 and 317) Temporal (giant cell) arteritis is an inflammatory disorder of arteries that frequently involves the extracranial carotid circulation. This is a common disorder of the elderly; its annual incidence is 77:100,000 in individuals aged 50 and older. The average age of onset is 70 years,

and women account for 65% of cases. About half of patients with untreated temporal arteritis develop blindness due to involvement of the ophthalmic artery and its branches; indeed, the ischemic optic neuropathy induced by giant cell arteritis is the major cause of rapidly developing bilateral blindness in patients over 60 years of age. Because treatment with glucocorticoids is effective in preventing this complication, prompt recognition of this disorder is important.

Typical presenting symptoms include headache, polymyalgia rheumatica (Chap. 317), jaw claudication, fever, and weight loss. Headache is the dominant symptom and often appears in association with malaise and muscle aches. Head pain may be unilateral or bilateral and is located temporally in 50% of patients but may involve any and all aspects of the cranium. Pain usually appears gradually over a few hours before peak intensity is reached; occasionally, it is explosive in onset. The quality of pain is only seldom throbbing; it is almost invariably described as dull and boring with superimposed episodic ice pick–like lancinating pains similar to the sharp pains that appear in migraine. Most patients can recognize that the origin of their head pain is superficial, external to the skull, rather than originating deep within the cranium (the pain site for migraineurs). Scalp tenderness is present, often to a marked degree; brushing the hair or resting the head on a pillow may be impossible because of pain. Headache is usually worse at night and is often aggravated by exposure to cold. Reddened, tender nodules or red streaking of the skin overlying the temporal arteries may be found in patients with headache, as is tenderness of the temporal or, less commonly, the occipital arteries.

The erythrocyte sedimentation rate (ESR) is often, though not always, elevated; a normal ESR does not exclude giant cell arteritis. A temporal artery biopsy and the initiation of prednisone at 80 mg daily for the first 4 to 6 weeks should be instituted when clinical suspicion is high. The prevalence of migraine among the elderly is substantial, considerably higher than that of giant cell arteritis. Migraineurs often report amelioration of their headaches with prednisone, so that one must be cautious about interpreting the therapeutic response.

GLAUCOMA   Glaucoma may present with a prostrating headache associated with nausea and vomiting. The history will usually reveal that the headache started with severe eye pain. On physical examination, the eye is often red with a fixed, moderately dilated pupil. →*A detailed discussion of glaucoma can be found in Chap. 28.*

OTHER CAUSES OF HEADACHE   **Systemic Illness** There is hardly any illness that is never manifested by headache; however, some illnesses are frequently associated with headache. These include infectious mononucleosis, systemic lupus erythematosus, chronic pulmonary failure with hypercapnia (early morning headaches), Hashimoto's thyroiditis, inflammatory bowel disease, many of the illnesses associated with HIV, and the acute blood pressure elevations that occur in pheochromocytoma and in malignant hypertension. The last two examples are the exceptions to the generalization that hypertension per se is a very uncommon cause of headache; diastolic pressures of at least 120 mmHg are requisite for hypertension to cause headache. Persistent headache and fever are often the manifestations of an acute systemic viral infection; if the neck is supple in such a patient, lumbar puncture may be deferred. Some drugs and drug-withdrawal states, e.g., oral contraceptives, ovulation-promoting medications, and glucocorticoid withdrawal, are also associated with headache in some individuals.

Idiopathic Intracranial Hypertension (Pseudotumor Cerebri) Headache, clinically resembling that of brain tumor, is a common presenting symptom of pseudotumor cerebri, a disorder of raised intracranial pressure probably resulting from impaired cerebrospinal fluid CSF absorption by the arachnoid villi. Transient visual obscurations and papilledema with enlarged blind spots and loss of peripheral visual fields are additional manifestations. Most patients are young, female, and obese. They often have a history of exposure to provoking agents such as vitamin A and glucocorticoids. →*Treatment of idiopathic intracranial hypertension is discussed in Chap. 28.*

Table 15-3   Symptoms of Serious Underlying Causes of Headache

Cause	Symptoms
Meningitis	Nuchal rigidity, headache, photophobia, and prostration; may not be febrile. Lumbar puncture is diagnostic.
Intracranial hemorrhage	Nuchal rigidity and headache; may not have clouded consciousness or seizures. Hemorrhage may not be seen on CT scan. Lumbar puncture shows "bloody tap" that does not clear by the last tube. A fresh hemorrhage may not be xanthochromic.
Brain tumor	May present with prostrating pounding headaches that are associated with nausea and vomiting. Should be suspected in progressively severe new "migraine" that is invariably unilateral.
Temporal arteritis	May present with a unilateral pounding headache. Onset generally in older patients (>50 years) and frequently associated with visual changes. The erythrocyte sedimentation rate is the best screening test and is usually markedly elevated (i.e., >50). Definitive diagnosis can be made by arterial biopsy.
Glaucoma	Usually consists of severe eye pain. May have nausea and vomiting. The eye is usually painful and red. The pupil may be partially dilated.

Cough A male-dominated (4:1) syndrome, cough headache is characterized by transient, severe head pain upon coughing, bending, lifting, sneezing, or stooping. Head pain persists for seconds to a few minutes. Many patients date the origins of the syndrome to a lower respiratory infection accompanied by severe coughing or to strenuous weight-lifting programs. Headache is usually diffuse but is lateralized in about one-third of patients. The incidence of serious intracranial structural anomalies causing this condition is about 25%; the Chiari malformation (Chap. 368) is a common cause. Thus, MRI is indicated for most patients with cough headache. The benign disorder may persist for a few years; it responds dramatically to indomethacin at doses ranging from 50 to 200 mg daily. Approximately half of patients will also show a response to therapeutic lumbar puncture with removal of 40 mL of CSF.

Many patients with migraine note that attacks of headache may be provoked by *sustained* physical exertion, such as during the third mile of a 5-mile run. Such headaches build up over hours, in contrast to cough headache. The term *effort migraine* has been used for this syndrome to avoid the ambiguous term *exertional headache*.

Lumbar Puncture Headache following lumbar puncture (Chap. 356) usually begins within 48 h but may be delayed for up to 12 days. Its incidence is between 10 and 30%. Head pain is dramatically positional; it begins when the patient sits or stands upright; there is relief upon reclining or with abdominal compression. The longer the patient is upright, the longer the latency before head pain subsides. It is worsened by head shaking and jugular vein compression. The pain is usually a dull ache but may be throbbing; its location is occipitofrontal. Nausea and stiff neck often accompany headache, and occasional patients report blurred vision, photophobia, tinnitus, and vertigo. The symptoms resolve over a few days but may on occasion persist for weeks to months.

Loss of CSF volume decreases the brain's supportive cushion, so that when a patient is upright there is probably dilation and tension placed on the brain's anchoring structures, the pain-sensitive dural sinuses, resulting in pain. Intracranial hypotension often occurs, but severe lumbar puncture headache may be present even in patients who have normal CSF pressure.

Treatment with intravenous caffeine sodium benzoate given over a few minutes as a 500-mg dose will promptly terminate headache in 75% of patients; a second dose given in 1 h brings the total success rate to 85%. An epidural blood patch accomplished by injection of 15 mL of autologous whole blood rarely fails for those who do not respond to caffeine. The mechanism for these treatment effects is not straightforward. The blood patch has an *immediate* effect, making it unlikely that sealing off a dural hole with blood clot is its mechanism of action.

Postconcussion Following seemingly trivial head injuries and particularly after rear-end motor vehicle collisions, many patients report varying combinations of headache, dizziness, vertigo, and impaired memory. Anxiety, irritability and difficulty with concentration are other hallmarks of this syndrome. Symptoms may remit after several weeks or persist for months and even years after the injury. Postconcussion headaches may occur whether or not a person was rendered unconscious by head trauma. Typically, the neurologic examination is normal with the exception of the behavioral abnormalities, and CT or MRI studies are unrevealing. Chronic subdural hematoma may on occasion mimic this disorder. Although the cause of postconcussive headache disorder is not known, it should not in general be viewed as a primary psychological disturbance. It often persists long after the settlement of pending lawsuits. The treatment is symptomatic support. Repeated encouragement that the syndrome eventually remits is important.

Coital Headache This is another male-dominated (4:1) syndrome. Attacks occur periorgasmically, are very abrupt in onset, and subside in a few minutes if coitus is interrupted. These are nearly always benign events and usually occur sporadically; if they persist for hours or are accompanied by vomiting, subarachnoid hemorrhage must be excluded (Chap. 361).

PRINCIPAL CLINICAL VARIETIES OF RECURRENT HEADACHE

There is usually little difficulty in diagnosing the serious types of headaches listed above because of the clues provided by the associated symptoms and signs. It is when headache is chronic, recurrent, and unattended by other important signs of disease that the physician faces a challenging and unique medical problem. The following sections describe a variety of headache types, ranging from the most common (e.g., tension-type headache) to rare causes of recurrent headache.

TENSION-TYPE HEADACHE The term *tension-type headache* is still commonly used to describe a chronic head pain syndrome characterized by bilateral tight, bandlike discomfort. Patients may report that the head feels as if it is in a vise or that the posterior neck muscles are tight. The pain typically builds slowly, fluctuates in severity, and may persist more or less continuously for many days. Exertion does not usually worsen the headache. The headache may be episodic or chronic (i.e., present more than 15 days per month). Tension-type headache is common in all age groups, and females tend to predominate. In some patients, anxiety or depression coexist with tension headache.

The pathophysiologic basis of tension-type headache remains unknown. Some investigators believe that periodic tension headache is biologically indistinguishable from migraine, whereas others believe that tension-type headache and migraine are two distinct clinical entities. Abnormalities of cervical and temporal muscle contraction are likely to exist, but the exact nature of the dysfunction has not yet been elucidated.

Relaxation almost always relieves tension-type headaches. Patients should be encouraged to find a means of relaxation, which, for a given individual, could include bed rest, massage, and/or formal biofeedback training. Pharmacologic treatment consists of either simple analgesics and/or muscle relaxants. Ibuprofen and naproxen sodium are useful treatments for most individuals. When simple over-the-counter analgesics such as acetaminophen, aspirin, ibuprofen, and/or other nonsteroidal anti-inflammatory drugs (NSAIDs) alone fail, the addition of butalbital and caffeine (in a combination compound such as Fiorinal, Fioricet) to these analgesics may be effective. A list of commonly used analgesics for tension-type headaches is presented in Table 15-4. For chronic tension-type headache, prophylactic therapy is recommended. Low doses of amitriptyline (10 to 50 mg at bedtime) can provide effective prophylaxis.

MIGRAINE Migraine, the most common cause of vascular headache, afflicts approximately 15% of women and 6% of men. A useful definition of migraine is a benign and recurring syndrome of headache, nausea, vomiting, and/or other symptoms of neurologic dysfunction in varying admixtures (Table 15-5). Migraine can often be recognized by its activators (red wine, menses, hunger, lack of sleep, glare, estrogen, worry, perfumes, let-down periods) and its deactivators (sleep, pregnancy, exhiliration, sumatriptan). A classification of the many subtypes of migraine, as defined by the International Headache Society, is shown in Table 15-1.

Severe headache attacks, regardless of cause, are more likely to be described as throbbing and associated with vomiting and scalp tenderness. Milder headaches tend to be nondescript—tight, bandlike discomfort often involving the entire head—the profile of tension-type headache.

Pathogenesis • *Genetic basis of migraine* Migraine has a definite genetic predisposition. Specific mutations leading to *rare* causes of vascular headache have been identified (Table 15-6). For example, the MELAS syndrome consists of a *m*itochondrial *e*ncephalomyopathy, *l*actic *a*cidosis, and *s*troke-like episodes and is caused by an A → G point mutation in the mitochondrial gene encoding for tRNA$^{Leu(UUR)}$ at nucleotide position 3243. Episodic migraine-like headaches are another common clinical feature of this syndrome, especially early in the

Table 15-4 Drugs Effective in the Treatment of Tension-Type Headache

Drug	Trade Name	Dosage
NONSTEROIDAL ANTI-INFLAMMATORY AGENTS		
Acetaminophen	Tylenol, generic	650 mg PO q4–6h
Aspirin	Generic	650 mg PO q4–6h
Diclofenac	Cataflam, generic	50–100 mg q4–6h (max 200 mg/d)
Ibuprofen	Advil, Motrin, Nuprin, Generic	400 mg PO q3–4h
Naprosyn sodium	Aleve, Anaprox, generic	220–550 mg bid
COMBINATION ANALGESICS		
Acetaminophen, 325 mg, *plus* butalbital, 50 mg	Phrenelin, generic	1–2 tablets; max 6 per day
Acetaminophen, 650 mg, *plus* butalbital, 50 mg	Phrenelin Forte	1 tablet; max 6 per day
Acetaminophen, 325 mg, *plus* butalbital, 50 mg, *plus* caffeine, 40 mg	Fioricet; Esgic, generic	1–2 tablets; max 6 per day
Acetaminophen, 500 mg, *plus* butalbital, 50 mg, *plus* caffeine, 40 mg	Esgicplus	1–2 tablets; max 6 per day
Aspirin, 325 mg, *plus* butalbital, 50 mg, *plus* caffeine, 40 mg	Fiorinal	1–2 tablets; max 6 per day
Aspirin, 650 mg, *plus* butalbital, 50 mg	Axotal	1 tablet q4h; max 6 per day
PROPHYLACTIC MEDICATIONS		
Amitriptyline	Elavil, generic	10–50 mg at bedtime
Doxepin	Sinequan, generic	10–75 mg at bedtime
Nortriptyline	Pamelor, generic	25–75 mg at bedtime

course of the disease. The genetic pattern of mitochondrial disorders is unique, since only mothers transmit mitochondrial DNA. Thus, all children of mothers with MELAS syndrome are affected with the disorder.

Familial hemiplegic migraine (FHM) is characterized by episodes of recurrent hemiparesis or hemiplegia during the aura phase of a migraine headache. Other associated symptoms may include hemianesthesia or paresthesia; hemianopic visual field disturbances; dysphasia; and variable degrees of drowsiness, confusion, and/or coma. In severe attacks, these symptoms can be quite prolonged and persist for days or weeks, but characteristically they last for only 30 to 60 min and are followed by a unilateral throbbing headache.

Approximately 50% of cases of FHM appear to be caused by mutations within the CACNL1A4 gene on chromosome 19, which encodes a P/Q type calcium channel subunit expressed only in the central nervous system. The gene is very large (>300 kb in length) and consists of 47 exons. Four distinct point mutations have been identified within the gene (in five different families) that cosegregate with the clinical diagnosis of FHM. Analysis of haplotypes in the two families with the same mutation suggest that each mutation arose independently

Table 15-5 Symptoms Accompanying Severe Migraine Attacks in a Group of 500 Patients

Symptom	Patients Affected, %
Nausea	87
Photophobia	82
Lightheadedness	72
Scalp tenderness	65
Vomiting	56
Visual disturbances	36
Photopsia	26
Fortification spectra	10
Paresthesias	33
Vertigo	33
Alteration of consciousness	18
Syncope	10
Seizure	4
Confusional state	4
Diarrhea	16

SOURCE: From Raskin, 1988.

rather than representing a founder effect. Thus, certain subtypes of FHM are caused by mutations in the CACNL1A4 gene. The function of the CACNL1A4 gene remains unknown, but it is likely to play a role in calcium-induced neurotransmitter release and/or contraction of smooth muscle. Different mutations within this gene are the cause of another neurogenetic disorder, episodic ataxia type 2 (Chap. 364).

In a genetic association study, a *Nco*I polymorphism in the gene encoding the D_2 dopamine receptor (DRD2) was overrepresented in a population of patients with migraine with aura compared to a control group of nonmigraineurs, suggesting that susceptibility to migraine with aura is modified by certain DRD2 alleles. In a Sardinian population, an association between different DRD2 alleles and migraine has also been demonstrated. Therefore, these initial studies suggest that variations in dopamine receptor regulation and/or function may alter susceptibility to migraine since molecular variations within the DRD2 gene have been associated with variations in dopaminergic function. However, since not all individuals with certain DRD2 genotypes suffer from migraine with aura, additional genes or factors must also be involved. Migraine is likely to be a complex disorder with polygenic inheritance and a strong environmental component.

The vascular theory of migraine It was widely held for many years that the headache phase of migrainous attacks was caused by extracranial vasodilatation and that the neurologic symptoms were produced by intracranial vasoconstriction (i.e., the "vascular" hypothesis of migraine). Regional cerebral blood flow studies have shown that in patients with classic migraine there is, during attacks, a modest cortical hypoperfusion that begins in the visual cortex and spreads forward at a rate of 2 to 3 mm/min. The decrease in blood flow averages 25 to 30% (insufficient to explain symptoms on the basis of ischemia) and progresses anteriorly in a wavelike fashion independent of the topography of cerebral arteries. The wave of hypoperfusion persists for 4 to 6 h, appears to follow the convolutions of the cortex, and does not cross the central or lateral sulcus, progressing to the frontal lobe via the insula. Perfusion of subcortical structures is normal. Contralateral neurologic symptoms appear during temporoparietal hypoperfusion; at times, hypoperfusion persists in these regions after symptoms cease. More often, frontal spread continues as the headache phase begins. A few patients with classic migraine show no flow abnormalities; an occasional patient has developed focal ischemia sufficient to cause symptoms. However, focal ischemia does not appear to be *necessary* for focal symptoms to occur.

The ability of these changes to induce the symptoms of migraine has been questioned. Specifically, the decrease in blood flow that is observed does not appear to be significant enough to cause focal neurologic symptoms. Second, the increase in blood flow per se is not painful, and vasodilatation alone cannot account for the local edema and focal tenderness often observed in migraineurs. Moreover, in migraine without aura, no flow abnormalities are usually seen. Thus, it is unlikely that simple vasoconstriction and vasodilatation are the fundamental pathophysiologic abnormalities in migraine. However, it is clear that cerebral blood flow is altered during certain migraine attacks, and these changes may explain some, but clearly not all, of the clinical syndrome of migraine.

The neuronal theory of migraine In 1941, the psychologist KS Lashley charted his own *fortification spectrum*, which is a migraine aura characterized by a slowly enlarging visual scotoma with luminous edges (see below). He was able to estimate that the evolution of his own scotoma proceeded across the occipital cortex at a rate of 3 mm/

min. He speculated that a wavefront of intense excitation followed by a wave of complete inhibition of activity were propagated across the visual cortex. In 1944, the phenomenon that has come to be known as *spreading depression* was described by the Brazilian physiologist Leão in the cerebral cortex of laboratory animals. It is a slowly moving (2 to 3 mm/min), potassium-liberating depression of cortical activity, preceded by a wavefront of increased metabolic activity that can be produced by a variety of experimental stimuli, including hy-

Table 15-6 Status of Migraine Genetics

Gene (Locus)	Function of Gene	Clinical Syndrome	Comment
tRNA$^{Leu(UUR)}$ (mitochondrial)	Unknown	MELAS syndrome	Extremely rare syndrome
CACNL1A4 (19p13)	P/Q calcium channel regulating neurotransmitter release	Familial hemiplegic migraine (FHM)	Mutations account for approximately 50% of FHM cases
DRD2 (11q23)	G protein–coupled D$_2$ receptor for dopamine	Migraine	Positive association reported in two independent laboratories

poxia, mechanical trauma, and the topical application of potassium. These observations suggest that neuronal abnormalities, most likely initiated in the brainstem, could be the cause of a migraine attack. More recently, both cortical and brainstem changes have been observed in positron emission tomography (PET) scan studies of migraine. Thus, the existence of a specific "brainstem generator" for migraine remains an intriguing possibility that might represent the pathophysiologic basis of migraine.

The trigeminovascular system in migraine Activation of cells in the trigeminal nucleus caudalis in the medulla (a pain-processing center for the head and face region) results in the release of vasoactive neuropeptides, including substance P and calcitonin gene–related peptide (CGRP), at vascular terminations of the trigeminal nerve. These peptide neurotransmitters have been proposed to induce a sterile inflammation that activates trigeminal nociceptive afferents originating on the vessel wall, further contributing to the production of pain. This mechanism also provides a potential mechanism for the soft tissue swelling and tenderness of blood vessels that attend migraine attacks. However, numerous pharmacologic agents that are effective in preventing or reducing inflammation in this animal model (e.g., selective 5-HT$_{1D}$ agonists, NK-1 antagonists, endothelin antagonists) have failed to demonstrate any clinical efficacy in recent migraine trials.

5-Hydroxytryptamine in migraine Pharmacologic and other data point to the involvement of the neurotransmitter 5-hydroxytryptamine (5-HT; also know as serotonin) in migraine. Approximately 40 years ago, methysergide was found to antagonize certain peripheral actions of 5-HT and was introduced as the first drug capable of preventing migraine attacks. Subsequently, it was found that platelet levels of 5-HT fall consistently at the onset of headache and that drugs that cause 5-HT to be released may trigger migrainous episodes. Such changes in circulating 5-HT levels proved to be pharmacologically trivial, however, and interest in the humoral role of 5-HT in migraine declined.

More recently, interest in the role of 5-HT in migraine has been renewed due to the introduction of the triptan class of antimigraine drugs. The triptans are designed to stimulate selectively a particular subpopulation of 5-HT receptors. Molecular cloning studies have demonstrated that at least 14 specific 5-HT receptors exist in humans. The triptans (e.g., naratriptan, rizatriptan, sumatriptan, and zolmitriptan) are potent agonists of 5-HT$_{1B}$, 5-HT$_{1D}$, and 5-HT$_{1F}$ receptors and are less potent at 5-HT$_{1A}$ and 5-HT$_{1E}$ receptors. A growing body of data indicates that the antimigraine efficacy of the triptans relates to their ability to stimulate 5-HT$_{1B}$ receptors, which are located both on blood vessels and nerve terminals. Selective 5-HT$_{1D}$ receptor agonists have, thus far, failed to demonstrate clinical efficacy in migraine. Triptans that are weak 5-HT$_{1F}$ agonists are also effective in migraine; however, only 5-HT$_{1B}$ efficacy is currently thought to be essential for antimigraine efficacy.

Physiologically, electrical stimulation near dorsal raphe neurons can result in migraine-like headaches. Blood flow in the pons and midbrain increases focally during migraine headache episodes; this alteration probably results from increased activity of cells in the dorsal raphe and locus caeruleus. There are projections from the dorsal raphe that terminate on cerebral arteries and alter cerebral blood flow. There are also major projections from the dorsal raphe to important visual centers, including the lateral geniculate body, superior colliculus, ret-

ina, and visual cortex. These various serotonergic projections may represent the neural substrate for the circulatory and visual characteristics of migraine. The dorsal raphe cells stop firing during deep sleep, and sleep is known to ameliorate migraine; the antimigraine prophylactic drugs also inhibit activity of the dorsal raphe cells through a direct or indirect agonist effect.

Recent PET scan studies have demonstrated that midbrain structures near the dorsal raphe are differentially activated during a migraine attack. In one study of acute migraine, an injection of sumatriptan relieved the headache, but did not alter the brainstem changes noted on the PET scan. These data suggest that a "brainstem generator" may be the cause of migraine and that certain antimigraine medications may not interfere with the underlying pathologic process in migraine.

Dopamine in migraine A growing body of biologic, pharmacologic, and genetic data support a role for dopamine in the pathophysiology of certain subtypes of migraine. Most migraine symptoms can be induced by dopaminergic stimulation. Moreover, there is dopamine receptor hypersensitivity in migraineurs, as demonstrated by the induction of yawning, nausea, vomiting, hypotension, and other symptoms of a migraine attack by dopaminergic agonists at doses that do not affect nonmigraineurs. Conversely, dopamine receptor antagonists are effective therapeutic agents in migraine, especially when given parenterally or concurrently with other antimigraine agents. As noted above, recent genetic data also suggest that molecular variations within dopamine receptor genes play a modifying role in the pathophysiology of migraine with aura. Therefore, modulation of dopaminergic neurotransmission should be considered in the therapeutic management of migraine.

The sympathetic nervous system in migraine Biochemical changes occur within the sympathetic nervous system (SNS) of migraineurs before, during, and between migraine attacks. Factors that activate the SNS are all trigger factors for migraine. Specific examples include environmental changes (e.g., stress, sleep patterns, hormonal shifts, hypoglycemia) and agents that cause release and a secondary depletion of peripheral catecholamines [e.g., tyramine, phenylethylamine, fenfluramine, m-chlorophenylpiperazine (mCPP) and reserpine]. By contrast, effective therapeutic approaches to migraine share an ability to mimic and/or enhance the effects of norepinephrine in the peripheral SNS. For example, norepinephrine itself, sympathomimetics (e.g., isometheptene), monoamine oxidase inhibitors (MAOIs) and reuptake blockers alleviate migraine. Dopamine antagonists, prostaglandin synthesis inhibitors, and adenosine antagonists are pharmacologic agents effective in the acute treatment of migraine. These drugs block the negative feedback inhibition or norepinephrine release induced by endogenous dopamine, prostaglandins, and adenosine. Therefore, migraine susceptibility may relate to genetically based variations in the ability to maintain adequate concentrations of certain neurotransmitters within postganglionic sympathetic nerve terminals. This hypothesis has been called the *empty neuron theory* of migraine.

Clinical Features • *Migraine without aura (common migraine)* In this syndrome no focal neurologic disturbance precedes the recurrent headaches. Migraine without aura is by far the more frequent type of vascular headache. The International Headache Society criteria for migraine include moderate to severe head pain, pulsating quality, unilateral location, aggravation by walking stairs or similar routine activity, attendant nausea and/or vomiting, photophobia and phonophobia, and multiple attacks, each lasting 4 to 72 h.

Migraine with aura (classic migraine) In this syndrome headache is associated with characteristic premonitory sensory, motor, or visual symptoms. Focal neurologic disturbances are more common during headache attacks than as prodromal symptoms. Focal neurologic disturbances without headache or vomiting have come to be known as *migraine equivalents* or *migraine accompaniments* and appear to occur more commonly in patients between the ages of 40 and 70 years. The term *complicated migraine* has generally been used to describe migraine with dramatic transient focal neurologic features or a migraine attack that leaves a persisting residual neurologic deficit.

The most common premonitory symptoms reported by migraineurs are visual, arising from dysfunction of occipital lobe neurons. Scotomas and/or hallucinations occur in about one-third of migraineurs and usually appear in the central portions of the visual fields. A highly characteristic syndrome occurs in about 10% of patients; it usually begins as a small paracentral scotoma, which slowly expands into a "C" shape. Luminous angles appear at the enlarging outer edge, becoming colored as the scintillating scotoma expands and moves toward the periphery of the involved half of the visual field, eventually disappearing over the horizon of peripheral vision. The entire process lasts 20 to 25 min. This phenomenon is pathognomonic for migraine, and has never been described in association with a cerebral structural anomaly. It is commonly referred to as a *fortification spectrum* because the serrated edges of the hallucinated "C" seemed to resemble a "fortified town with bastions all round it"; "spectrum" is used in the sense of an apparition or specter.

Basilar migraine Symptoms referable to a disturbance in brainstem function, such as vertigo, dysarthria, or diplopia, occur as the only neurologic symptoms of the attack in about 25% of patients. A dramatic form of basilar migraine (Bickerstaff's migraine) occurs primarily in adolescent females. Episodes begin with total blindness accompanied or followed by admixtures of vertigo, ataxia, dysarthria, tinnitus, and distal and perioral paresthesia. In about one-quarter of patients, a confusional state supervenes. The neurologic symptoms usually persist for 20 to 30 min and are generally followed by a throbbing occipital headache. This basilar migraine syndrome is now known also to occur in children and in adults over age 50. An altered sensorium may persist for as long as 5 days and may take the form of confusional states superficially resembling psychotic reactions. Full recovery after the episode is the rule.

Carotidynia The carotidynia syndrome, sometimes called *lower-half headache* or *facial migraine*, is most common among older patients, with the incidence peaking in the fourth through sixth decades. Pain is usually located at the jaw or neck, although sometimes periorbital or maxillary pain occurs; it may be continuous, deep, dull, and aching, and it becomes pounding or throbbing episodically. There are often superimposed sharp, ice pick–like jabs. Attacks occur one to several times per week, each lasting several minutes to hours. Tenderness and prominent pulsations of the cervical carotid artery and soft tissue swelling overlying the carotid are usually present ipsilateral to the pain; many patients also report throbbing ipsilateral headache concurrent with carotidynia attacks as well as between attacks. Dental trauma is a common precipitant of this syndrome. Carotid artery involvement also appears to be common in the more traditional forms of migraine; over 50% of patients with frequent migraine attacks are found to have carotid tenderness at several points on the side most often involved during hemicranial migraine attacks.

℞ TREATMENT

Nonpharmacologic Approaches for All Migraineurs Migraine can often be managed to some degree by a variety of nonpharmacologic approaches (Table 15-7). The measures that apply to a given individual should be used routinely since they provide a simple, cost-effective approach to migraine management. Patients with mi-

Table 15-7 Nonpharmacologic Approaches to Migraine

Identify and then avoid trigger factors such as:
  Alcohol (e.g., red wine)
  Foods (e.g., chocolate, certain cheeses, monosodium glutamate, nitrate-
    containing foods)
  Hunger (avoid missing meals)
  Irregular sleep patterns (both lack of sleep and excessive sleep)
  Organic odors
  Sustained exertion
  Acute changes in stress levels
  Miscellaneous (glare, flashing lights)
Attempt to manage environmental shifts
  Time zone shifts
  High altitude
  Barometric pressure changes
  Weather changes
Assess menstrual cycle relationship

graine do not encounter more stress than headache-free individuals; overresponsiveness to stress appears to be the issue. Since the stresses of everyday living cannot be eliminated, lessening one's response to stress by various techniques is helpful for many patients. These include yoga, transcendental meditation, hypnosis, and conditioning techniques such as biofeedback. For most patients, this approach is, at best, an adjunct to pharmacotherapy. Avoidance of migraine trigger factors may also provide significant prophylactic benefits (Table 15-7). Unfortunately, these measures are unlikely to prevent all migraine attacks. When these measures fail to prevent an attack, then pharmacologic approaches are needed to abort an attack.

Pharmacologic Treatment of Acute Migraine The mainstay of pharmacologic therapy is the judicious use of one or more of the many drugs that are effective in migraine. The selection of the optimal regimen for a given patient depends on a number of factors, the most important of which is the severity of the attack (Table 15-8). Mild migraine attacks can usually be managed by oral agents; the average efficacy rate is 50–70%. Severe migraine attacks may require parenteral therapy. Most drugs effective in the treatment of migraine are members of one of three major pharmacologic classes: anti-inflammatory agents, 5-HT1 agonists, and dopamine antagonists.

Table 15-9 lists specific drugs effective in migraine. In general, an adequate dose of whichever agent is chosen should be used as soon as possible after the onset of an attack. If additional medication is required within 60 min because symptoms return or have not abated, the initial dose should be increased for subsequent attacks. Migraine therapy must be individualized for each patient; a standard approach for all patients is not possible. A therapeutic regimen may need to be constantly refined and personalized until one is identified that provides

Table 15-8 A Staged Approach to Migraine Pharmacotherapy

Stage	Diagnosis	Therapies
Mild migraine	Occasional throbbing headaches	NSAIDs
		Combination analgesics
	No major impairment of functioning	Oral 5-HT$_1$ agonists
Moderate migraine	Moderate or severe headaches	Oral, nasal, or SC 5-HT$_1$ agonists
	Nausea common	Oral dopamine antagonists
	Some impairment of functioning	
Severe migraine	Severe headaches >3 times per month	SC, IM, or IV 5-HT$_1$ agonists
	Significant functional impairment	IM or IV dopamine antagonists
	Marked nausea and/or vomiting	Prophylactic medications

NOTE: NSAIDs, nonsteroidal anti-inflammatory drugs; 5-HT, 5-hydroxytryptamine.

Table 15-9 Drugs Effective in Acute Treatment of Migraine

Drug	Trade Name	Dosage
NSAIDs		
Acetaminophen, aspirin, caffeine	Excedrin Migraine	Two tablets or caplets q6h (max 8 per day)
5-HT₁ AGONISTS		
Oral		
Ergotamine	Ergomar	One 2-mg sublingual tablet at onset and q1/2h (max 3 per day, 5 per week)
Ergotamine 1 mg, caffeine 100 mg	Ercaf, Wigraine	One or two tablets at onset, then one tablet q1/2h (max 6 per day, 10 per week)
Naratriptan	Amerge	2.5-mg tablet at onset; may repeat once after 4 h
Rizatriptan	Maxalt Maxalt-MLT	5- to 10-mg tablet at onset; may repeat after 2 h (max 30 mg/d)
Sumatriptan	Imitrex	50- to 100-mg tablet at onset; may repeat after 2 h (max 200 mg/d)
Zolmitriptan	Zomig Zomig Rapimelt	2.5-mg tablet at onset; may repeat after 2 h (max 10 mg/d)
Nasal		
Dihydroergotamine	Migranal Nasal Spray	Prior to nasal spray, the pump must be primed 4 times; one spray (0.5 mg) per nostril is administered followed, in 15 min, by a second spray per nostril
Sumatriptan	Imitrex Nasal Spray	5- to 20-mg spray as 4 sprays of 5 mg per nostril or a single 20-mg spray (may repeat once after 2 h, not to exceed a dose of 40 mg/d)
Parenteral		
Dihydroergotamine	DHE-45	1 mg IV, IM, or SC at onset and q1h (max 3 mg/d, 6 mg per week)
Sumatriptan	Imitrex Injection	6 mg SC at onset (may repeat once after 1 h for max of two doses in 24 h)
DOPAMINE ANTAGONISTS		
Oral		
Metoclopramide	Reglan,[a] generic[a]	5–10 mg/d
Prochlorperazine	Compazine,[a] generic[a]	1–25 mg/d
Parenteral		
Chlorpromazine	Generic[a]	0.1 mg/kg IV at 2 mg/min; max 35 mg/d
Metoclopramide	Reglan,[a] generic	10 mg IV
Prochlorperazine	Compazine,[a] generic[a]	10 mg IV
OTHER		
Oral		
Acetaminophen, 325 mg, *plus* dichloralphenazone, 100 mg, *plus* isometheptene, 65 mg	Midrin, Duradrin, generic	Two capsules at onset followed by 1 capsule q1h (max 5 capsules)
Nasal		
Butorphanol	Stadol[a]	1 mg (1 spray in 1 nostril), may repeat if necessary in 1–2 h
Parenteral		
Narcotics	Generic[a]	Multiple preparations and dosages; see Table 12-1.

[a] Not specifically indicated by the U.S. Food and Drug Administration for migraine.
NOTE: NSAIDs, nonsteroidal anti-inflammatory drugs; 5-HT, 5-hydroxytryptamine.

the patient with rapid, complete, and consistent relief with minimal side effects.

Nonsteroidal anti-inflammatory agents Both the severity and duration of a migraine attack can be reduced significantly by anti-inflammatory agents. Indeed, many undiagnosed migraineurs are self-treated with nonprescription anti-inflammatory agents (Table 15-4). A general consensus is that NSAIDs are most effective when taken early in the migraine attack. However, the effectiveness of anti-inflammatory agents in migraine is usually less than optimal in moderate or severe migraine attacks. The combination of acetaminophen, aspirin, and caffeine (Excedrin Migraine) has been approved for use by the U.S. Food and Drug Administration (FDA) for the treatment of mild to moderate migraine. The combination of aspirin and metoclopramide has been show to be equivalent to a single dose of sumatriptan. Major side effects of NSAIDs include dyspepsia and gastrointestinal irritation.

5-HT₁ agonists • ORAL Stimulation of 5-HT₁ receptors can stop an acute migraine attack. Ergotamine and dihydroergotamine are nonselective receptor agonists, while the series of drugs known as triptans are selective 5-HT₁ receptor agonists. A variety of triptans (e.g., naratriptan, rizatriptan, sumatriptan, zolmitriptan) are now available for the treatment of migraine (Table 15-9).

Each of the triptan class of drugs has similar pharmacologic properties, but varies slightly in terms of clinical efficacy. Rizatriptan appears to be the fastest acting and most efficacious of the triptans currently available in the United States. Sumatriptan and zolmitriptan have similar rates of efficacy as well as time to onset, whereas naratriptan is the slowest acting and the least efficacious. Clinical efficacy appears to be related more to the t_{max} (time to peak plasma level) than to the potency, half-life, or bioavailability (Table 15-10). This observation is in keeping with a significant body of data indicating that faster-acting analgesics are more efficacious than slower-acting agents.

Unfortunately, monotherapy with a selective oral 5-HT₁ agonist does not result in rapid, consistent, and complete relief of migraine in all patients. Triptans are not effective in migraine with aura unless given after the aura is completed and the headache initiated. Side effects, although often mild and transient, occur in up to 89% of patients. Moreover, 5-HT₁ agonists are contraindicated in individuals with a history of cardiovascular disease. Recurrence of headache is a major limitation of triptan use, and occurs at least occasionally in 40 to 78% of patients.

Ergotamine preparations offer a nonselective means of stimulating 5-HT₁ receptors. A nonnauseating dose of ergotamine should be sought since a dose that provokes nausea is too high and may intensify head pain. Except for a sublingual formulation of ergotamine (Ergomar), oral formulations of ergotamine also contain 100 mg caffeine (theoretically to enhance ergotamine absorption and possibly to add additional vasoconstrictor activity). The average oral ergotamine dose for a migraine attack is 2 mg. Since the clinical studies demonstrating the efficacy of ergotamine in migraine predated the clinical trial methodologies used with the triptans, it is difficult to assess the clinical efficacy of ergotamine versus the triptans. In general, ergotamine appears to have a much higher incidence of nausea than triptans, but less headache recurrence.

NASAL The fastest acting nonparenteral antimigraine therapies that can be self-administered include nasal formulations of dihydroer-

Table 15-10 Comparative Pharmacology of Oral Triptans[a]

Drug and Dose	t_{max}, h	$t_{1/2}$, h	Oral Bioavailability, %	Clinical Efficacy at 2 h, %
Rizatriptan, 10 mg	1–2	2–3	45	71
Zolmitriptan, 2.5 mg	2	2.5–3	44	65
Sumatriptan, 50 mg	2–3	2	14	61
Naratriptan, 2.5 mg	2–4	5–6	68	45

[a] Data adapted from package inserts approved by the U.S. Food and Drug Administration.

gotamine (Migranal) or sumatriptan (Imitrex Nasal). The nasal sprays result in substantial blood levels within 30 to 60 min. However, the nasal formulations suffer from inconsistent dosing, poor taste, and variable efficacy. Although in theory the nasal sprays might provide faster and more effective relief of a migraine attack than oral formulations, their reported efficacy is only approximately 50 to 60%.

PARENTERAL Parenteral administration of drugs such as dihydroergotamine (DHE-45 Injectable) and sumatriptan (Imitrex SC) is approved by the FDA for the rapid relief of a migraine attack. Peak plasma levels of dihydroergotamine are achieved 3 min after intravenous dosing, 30 min after intramuscular dosing, and 45 min after subcutaneous dosing. If an attack has not already peaked, subcutaneous or intramuscular administration of 1 mg dihydroergotamine suffices for about 80 to 90% of patients. Sumatriptan, 6 mg subcutaneously is effective in approximately 70 to 80% of patients.

Dopamine antagonists • *ORAL* Oral dopamine antagonists should be considered as adjunctive therapy in migraine. Drug absorption is impaired during migrainous attacks because of reduced gastrointestinal motility. Delayed absorption occurs in the absence of nausea and is related to the severity of the attack and not its duration. Therefore, when oral NSAIDs and/or triptan agents fail, the addition of a dopamine antagonist such as metoclopramide, 10 mg, should be considered to enhance gastric absorption. In addition, dopamine antagonists decrease nausea/vomiting and restore normal gastric motility.

PARENTERAL Parenteral dopamine antagonists (e.g., chlorpromazine, prochlorperazine, metoclopramide) can also provide significant acute relief of migraine; they can be used in combination with parenteral 5-HT$_1$ agonists. A common intravenous protocol used for the treatment of severe migraine is the administration over 2 min of a mixture of 5 mg of prochlorperazine and 0.5 mg of dihydroergotamine.

Other medications for acute migraine • *ORAL* The combination of acetaminophen, dichloralphenazone, and isometheptene (i.e., Midrin, Duradrin, generic), one to two capsules, has been classified by the FDA as "possibly" effective in the treatment of migraine. Since the clinical studies demonstrating the efficacy of this combination analgesic in migraine predated the clinical trial methodologies used with the triptans, it is difficult to assess the clinical efficacy of this sympathomimetic compound in comparison to other agents.

NASAL A nasal preparation of butorphanol is available for the treatment of acute pain. As with all narcotics, the use of nasal butorphanol should be limited to a select group of migraineurs, as described below.

PARENTERAL Narcotics are effective in the acute treatment of migraine. For example, intravenous meperidene (Demerol), 50 to 100 mg, is given frequently in the emergency room. This regimen "works" in the sense that the pain of migraine is eliminated. However, this regimen is clearly suboptimal in patients with recurrent headache for two major reasons. First, narcotics do not treat the underlying headache mechanism; rather, they act at the thalamic level to alter pain sensation. Second, the recurrent use of narcotics can lead to significant problems. In patients taking oral narcotics such as oxycodone (Percodan) or hydrocodone (Vicoden), narcotic addiction can greatly confuse the treatment of migraine. The headache that results from narcotic craving and/ or withdrawal can be difficult to distinguish from chronic migraine. Therefore, it is recommended that narcotic use in migraine be limited to patients with severe, but infrequent, headaches that are unresponsive to other pharmacologic approaches.

Prophylactic Treatment of Migraine A substantial number of drugs are now available that have the capacity to stabilize migraine (Table 15-11). The decision of whether to use this approach depends on the frequency of attacks and on how well acute treatment is working. The occurrence of at least three attacks per month could be an indication for this approach. Drugs must be taken daily and there is usually a lag of at least 2 to 6 weeks before an effect is seen. The

Table 15-11 Drugs Effective in the Prophylactic Treatment of Migraine

Drug	Trade Name	Dosage
β-Adrenergic agents		
Propranolol	Inderal	80–320 mg qd
	Inderal LA	
Timolol	Blocadren	20–60 mg qd
Anticonvulsants		
Sodium valproate	Depakote	250 mg bid (max 1000 mg/d)
Tricyclic antidepressants		
Amitriptyline	Elavil,[a] generic	10–50 mg qhs
Nortriptyline	Pamelor,[a] generic	25–75 mg qhs
Monoamine oxidase inhibitors		
Phenelzine	Nardil[a]	15 mg tid
Isocarboxazid	Marplan[a]	10 mg qid
Serotonoergic drugs		
Methysergide	Sansert	4–8 mg qd
Cyproheptadine	Periactin[a]	4–16 mg qd
Other		
Verapamil	Calan[a]	40–240 mg qd
	Isoptin[a]	

[a] Not specifically indicated for migraine by the U.S. Food and Drug Administration.

drugs that have been approved by the FDA for the prophylactic treatment of migraine include propranolol, timolol, sodium valproate, and methysergide. In addition, a number of other drugs appear to display prophylactic efficacy. This group of drugs includes amitriptyline, nortriptyline, verapamil, phenelzine, isocarbazid, and cyproheptadine. Phenelzine and methysergide are usually reserved for recalcitrant cases because of their serious potential side effects. Phenelzine is an MAOI; therefore, tyramine-containing foods, decongestants, and meperidine are contraindicated. Methysergide may cause retroperitoneal or cardiac valvular fibrosis when it is used for more than 8 months, thus monitoring is required for patients using this drug; the risk of the fibrotic complication is about 1:1500 and is likely to reverse after the drug is stopped.

The probability of success with any one of the antimigraine drugs is 50 to 75%; thus, if one drug is assessed each month, there is a good chance that effective stabilization will be achieved within a few months. Many patients are managed adequately with low-dose amitriptyline, propranolol, or valproate. If these agents fail or lead to unacceptable side effects, then methysergide or phenelzine can be used. Once effective stabilization is achieved, the drug is continued for 5 to 6 months and then slowly tapered to assess the continued need. Many patients are able to discontinue medication and experience fewer and milder attacks for long periods, suggesting that these drugs may alter the natural history of migraine.

CLUSTER HEADACHE A variety of names have been used for this condition, including *Raeder's syndrome*, *histamine cephalalgia*, and *sphenopalatine neuralgia*. *Cluster headache* is a distinctive and treatable vascular headache syndrome. The episodic type is most common and is characterized by one to three short-lived attacks of periorbital pain per day over a 4- to 8-week period, followed by a pain-free interval that averages 1 year. The chronic form, which may begin de novo or several years after an episodic pattern has become established, is characterized by the absence of sustained periods of remission. Each type may transform into the other. Men are affected seven to eight times more often than women; hereditary factors are usually absent. Although the onset is generally between ages 20 and 50, it may occur as early as the first decade of life. Propranolol and amitriptyline are largely ineffective. Lithium is beneficial for cluster headache and ineffective in migraine. The cluster syndrome is thus clinically, genetically, and therapeutically different from migraine. Nevertheless, mixed features of the two disorders are occasionally present, suggesting some common elements to their pathogenesis.

Clinical Features Periorbital or, less commonly, temporal pain begins without warning and reaches a crescendo within 5 min. It is often excruciating in intensity and is deep, nonfluctuating, and explosive in quality; only rarely is it pulsatile. Pain is strictly unilateral and usually affects the same side in subsequent months. Attacks last from 30 min to 2 h; there are often associated symptoms of homolateral lacrimation, reddening of the eye, nasal stuffiness, lid ptosis, and nausea. Alcohol provokes attacks in about 70% of patients but ceases to be provocative when the bout remits; this on-off vulnerability to alcohol is pathognomonic of cluster headache. Only rarely do foods or emotional factors precipitate pain, in contrast to migraine.

There is a striking periodicity of attacks in at least 85% of patients. At least one of the daily attacks of pain recurs at about the same hour each day for the duration of a cluster bout. Onset is nocturnal in about 50% of the cases, and then the pain usually awakens the patient within 2 h of falling asleep.

Pathogenesis No consistent cerebral blood flow changes accompany attacks of pain. Perhaps the strongest evidence for a central mechanism is the periodicity of attacks; the existence of a central mechanism is also suggested by the observation that autonomic symptoms that accompany the pain are bilateral and are more severe on the painful side. The hypothalamus may be the site of activation in this disorder. The posterior hypothalamus contains cells that regulate autonomic functions, and the anterior hypothalamus contains cells (in the suprachiasmatic nuclei) that constitute the principal circadian pacemaker in mammals. Activation of both is necessary to explain the symptoms of cluster headache. The pacemaker is modulated via serotonergic dorsal raphe projections. It can be concluded tentatively that both migraine and cluster headache result from abnormal serotonergic neurotransmission, albeit at different loci.

℞ TREATMENT The most satisfactory treatment is the administration of drugs to prevent cluster attacks until the bout is over. Effective prophylactic drugs are prednisone, lithium, methysergide, ergotamine, sodium valproate, and verapamil. Lithium (600 to 900 mg daily) appears to be particularly useful for the chronic form of the disorder. A 10-day course of prednisone, beginning at 60 mg daily for 7 days followed by a rapid taper, may interrupt the pain bout for many patients. When ergotamine is used, it is most effective when given 1 to 2 h before an expected attack. Patients must be educated regarding the early symptoms of ergotism when ergotamine is used daily; a weekly limit of 14 mg should be adhered to.

For the attacks themselves, oxygen inhalation (9 L/min via a loose mask) is the most effective modality; 15 min of inhalation of 100% oxygen is often necessary. Sumatriptan, 6 mg subcutaneously, will usually shorten an attack to 10 to 15 min.

BIBLIOGRAPHY

BRESLAU N: Psychiatric comorbidity in migraine. Cephalalgia 18(Suppl 22): 56, 1998

CAO Y et al: Functional MRI-BOLD of visually triggered headache in patients with migraine. Arch Neurol 56:548, 1999

COUCH JR: Headache to worry about. Med Clin North Am 77:141, 1993

EDLOW JA, CAPLAN LR: Avoiding pitfalls in the diagnosis of subarachnoid hemorrhage. N Engl J Med 342:29, 2000

FRISHBERG BM: The utility of neuroimaging in the evaluation of headache in patients with normal examination. Neurology 44:1191, 1994

GERVIL et al: The relative role of genetic and environmental factors in migraine without aura. Neurology 53:995, 1999

GOADSBY PJ: Serotonin 5-HT 1B/1D receptor agonists in migraine. CNS Drugs 10:271, 1998

LANCE JW, GOADSBY PJ: *Mechanism and Management of Headache*, 6th ed. London, Butterworth Scientific, 1998

LIPTON RB: Pharmacologic profile and clinical efficacy of rizatriptan. Headache 39 (Suppl 1):S9, 1999

——— et al: Efficacy and safety of acetaminophen, aspirin and caffeine in alleviating migraine pain. Three double-blind, randomized, placebo-controlled trials. Arch Neurol 55:210, 1998

MAY A et al: Hypothalamic activation in cluster headache attacks. Lancet 352:275, 1998

——— et al: Correlation between structural and functional changes in brain in an idiopathic headache syndrome. Nature Med 5:836, 1999

MOSKOWITZ MA, COUTRER FM: Attacking migraine headache from beginning to end. Neurology 49:1193, 1997

OLESEN C et al: Pregnancy outcome following prescription for sumatriptan. Headache 40: 20, 2000

OLESEN J: Headache Classification Committee of the International Headache Society. Classification and diagnostic criteria for headache disorders, cranial neuralgia, and facial pain. Cephalalgia 8(Suppl 7): 1, 1988

OPHOFF RA et al: Familial hemiplegic migraine and episodic ataxia type-2 are caused by mutations in the Ca²⁺ channel gene CACNL1A4. Cell 87:543, 1996

PASCUAL J et al: Cough, exertional, and sexual headaches: An analysis of 72 benign and symptomatic cases. Neurology 46:1520, 1996

PEROUTKA SJ: Dopamine and migraine. Neurology 49:650, 1997

——— et al: Clinical susceptibility to migraine with aura is modified by dopamine D2 receptor (DRD2) *Nco*I alleles. Neurology 49:201, 1997

RASKIN NH: *Headache*, 2d ed. New York, Churchill Livingstone, 1988

SCHWARTZ BS et al: Epidemiology of tension-type headache. JAMA 279:381, 1998

SILBERSTEIN SD et al: Classification of daily and near-daily headaches: Field trial of revised IHS criteria. Neurology 47:871, 1996

TOUNIER-LASSERVE E: CACNA1A mutations: Hemiplegic migraine, episodic ataxia type 2, and the others. Neurology 53:3, 1999

---

16 *John W. Engstrom*

BACK AND NECK PAIN

AAA	abdominal aortic aneurysm	MRI	magnetic resonance imaging
ALBP	acute low back pain	NSAIDs	nonsteroidal anti-inflammatory
CLBP	chronic low back pain		drugs
CPGs	clinical practice guidelines	PT	physical therapy
CSF	cerebrospinal fluid	RA	rheumatoid arthritis
CT	computed tomography	SLR	straight leg–raising
EMG	electromyography	TOS	thoracic outlet syndrome

The importance of back and neck pain in our society is underscored by the following: (1) the annual societal cost of back pain in the United States is estimated to be between $20 and $50 billion; (2) back symptoms are the most common cause of disability in patients under 45 years of age; (3) 50% of working adults, in one survey, admitted to having a back injury each year; and (4) approximately 1% of the U.S. population is chronically disabled because of back pain.

The enormous economic pressure to provide rational and efficient care of patients with back pain has resulted in clinical practice guidelines (CPGs) for these patients. CPGs are algorithms which guide evaluation or treatment at specific steps in patient care. CPGs for *acute low back pain* (ALBP) are based upon incomplete evidence (see algorithms, Fig. 16-6) but represent an attempt to standardize common medical practice. Major revisions in CPGs for back pain can be anticipated in the future. Management of patients with *chronic low back pain* (CLBP) is complex and not amenable to a simple algorithmic approach at this time.

ANATOMY OF THE SPINE

The anterior portion of the spine consists of cylindrical vertebral bodies separated by intervertebral disks and held together by the anterior and posterior longitudinal ligaments. The intervertebral disks are composed of a central gelatinous nucleus pulposus surrounded by a tough cartilagenous ring, the annulus fibrosis; disks are responsible for 25% of spinal column length (Figs. 16-1 and 16-2). The disks are largest in the cervical and lumbar regions where movements of the spine are greatest. The disks are elastic in youth and allow the bony vertebrae to move easily upon each other. Elasticity is lost with age. The function of the anterior spine is to absorb the shock of typical body movements such as walking and running.

The posterior portion of the spine consists of the vertebral arches and seven processes. Each arch consists of paired cylindrical pedicles anteriorly and paired laminae posteriorly (Fig. 16-1). The vertebral arch gives rise to two transverse processes laterally, one spinous pro-

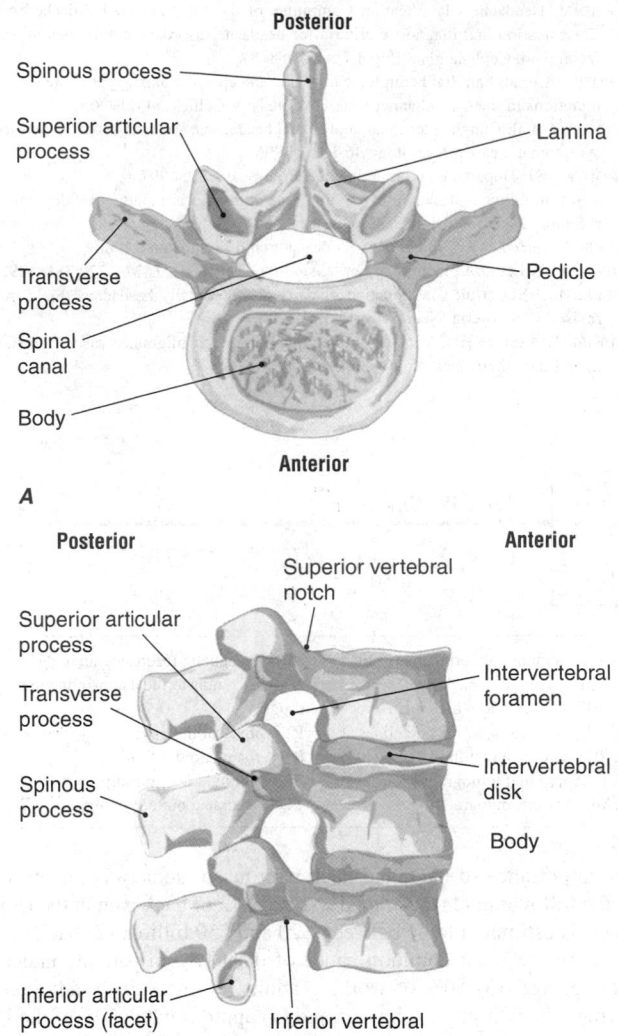

FIGURE 16-1 Vertebral anatomy. (*From Andrea Gauthier Cornuelle and Diane H. Gronefeld, Radiographic Anatomy Positioning. New York, McGraw-Hill, 1998, with permission.*)

cess posteriorly, plus two superior and two inferior articular facets. The functions of the posterior spine are to protect the spinal cord and nerves within the spinal canal and to stabilize the spine by providing sites for the attachment of muscles and ligaments. The contraction of muscles attached to the spinous and transverse processes produces a system of pulleys and levers that results in flexion, extension, and lateral bending movements of the spine. Normal upright posture in humans places the center of gravity anterior to the spine. The graded contraction of well-developed paraspinal muscles attached to the laminae, transverse processes, and spinous processes is necessary to maintain normal upright posture.

The nerve roots exit at a level above their respective vertebral bodies in the cervical region (the C7 nerve root exits at the C6-C7 level) and below their respective vertebral bodies in the thoracic and lumbar regions (the T1 nerve root exits at the T1-T2 level). The spinal cord ends at the L1 or L2 level of the bony spine. Consequently, the lumbar nerve roots follow a long intraspinal course and can be injured anywhere from the upper lumbar spine to their exit at the intervertebral foramen. For example, it is common for disk herniation at the L4-L5 level to produce compression of the S1 nerve root (Fig. 16-3). In contrast, cervical nerve roots follow a short intraspinal course and exit at the level of their respective spinal cord segments (upper cervical) or one segment below the corresponding levels (lower cervical cord).

Cervical spine pathology can result in spinal cord compression, but lumbar spine pathology cannot.

Pain-sensitive structures in the spine include the vertebral body periosteum, dura, facet joints, annulus fibrosus of the intervertebral disk, epidural veins, and the posterior longitudinal ligament. Damage to these nonneural structures may cause pain. The nucleus pulposus of the intervertebral disk is not pain-sensitive under normal circumstances. Pain sensation is conveyed by the sinuvertebral nerve that arises from the spinal nerve at each spine segment and reenters the spinal canal through the intervertebral foramen at the same level. Disease of these diverse pain-sensitive spine structures may explain many cases of back pain without nerve root compression. The lumbar and cervical spine possess the greatest potential for movement and injury.

Approach to the Patient

Types of Back Pain An understanding of the nature of the pain as described by the patient is the essential first step in evaluation. Attention is also focused on identification of risk factors for serious underlying diseases that require specific evaluation.

Local pain is caused by stretching of pain-sensitive structures that compress or irritate sensory nerve endings. The site of the pain is near the affected part of the back.

Pain referred to the back may arise from abdominal or pelvic viscera. The pain is usually described as primarily abdominal or pelvic but is accompanied by back pain and usually unaffected by posture. The patient may occasionally complain of back pain only.

Pain of spine origin may be located in the back or referred to the buttocks or legs. Diseases affecting the upper lumbar spine tend to refer pain to the lumbar region, groin, or anterior thighs. Diseases affecting the lower lumbar spine tend to produce pain referred to the buttocks, posterior thighs, or rarely the calves or feet. Provocative injections into pain-sensitive structures of the spine (diskography) may produce leg pain that does not follow a dermatomal distribution. The exact pathogenesis of this "sclerotomal" pain is unclear, but it may explain many instances in which combined back and leg pain is unaccompanied by evidence of nerve root compression.

Radicular back pain is typically sharp and radiates from the spine to the leg within the territory of a nerve root (see "Lumbar Disk Disease," below). Coughing, sneezing, or voluntary contraction of abdominal muscles (lifting heavy objects or straining at stool) may elicit the radiating pain. The pain may increase in postures that stretch the nerves and nerve roots. Sitting stretches the sciatic nerve (L5 and S1 roots) because the nerve passes posterior to the hip. The femoral nerve (L2, L3, and L4 roots) passes anterior to the hip and is not stretched by sitting. The description of the pain alone often fails to distinguish clearly between sclerotomal pain and radiculopathy.

Pain associated with muscle spasm, although of obscure origin, is commonly associated with many spine disorders. The spasms are accompanied by abnormal posture, taut paraspinal muscles, and dull pain.

Back pain at rest or unassociated with specific postures should raise the index of suspicion for an underlying serious cause (e.g., spine tumor, fracture, infection, or referred pain from visceral structures). Knowledge of the circumstances associated with the onset of back pain is important when weighing possible serious underlying causes for the pain. Some patients involved in accidents or work-related injuries may exaggerate their pain for the purpose of compensation or for psychological reasons.

Examination of the Back A physical examination that includes the abdomen and rectum is advisable. Back pain referred from visceral organs may be reproduced during palpation of the abdomen (pancreatitis, abdominal aortic aneurysm) or percussion over the costovertebral angles (pyelonephritis, adrenal disease, L1-L2 transverse process fracture).

The normal spine (Fig. 16-2) displays a thoracic kyphosis, lumbar lordosis, and cervical lordosis. Exaggeration of these normal alignments may result in hyperkyphosis (lameback) of the thoracic spine or hyperlordosis (swayback) of the lumbar spine. Spasm of lumbar paraspinal muscles results in flattening of the usual lumbar lordosis. Inspection may reveal lateral curvature of the spine (scoliosis) or an asymmetry in the appearance of the paraspinal muscles, suggesting muscle spasm. Taut paraspinal muscles limit the motion of the lumbar spine. Back pain of bony spine origin is often reproduced by palpation or percussion over the spinous process of the affected vertebrae.

Forward bending is frequently limited by paraspinal muscle spasm. Flexion of the hips is normal in patients with lumbar spine disease, but flexion of the lumbar spine is limited and sometimes painful. Lateral bending to the side opposite the injured spinal element may stretch the damaged tissues, worsen pain, and limit motion. Hyperextension of the spine (with the patient prone or standing) is limited when nerve root compression or bony spine disease is present.

Pain from hip disease may mimic the pain of lumbar spine disease. The first movement is typically internal rotation of the hip. Manual internal and external rotation at the hip with the knee and hip in flexion (Patrick sign) may reproduce the pain, as may percussion of the heel (of an outstretched leg) with the palm of the examiner's hand.

In the supine position passive flexion of the thigh on the abdomen while the knee is extended produces stretching of the L5 and S1 nerve roots and the sciatic nerve because the nerve passes posterior to the hip. Passive dorsiflexion of the foot during the maneuver adds to the stretch. While flexion to at least 80° is normally possible without causing pain, tight hamstrings commonly limit motion, may result in pain, and are readily identified by the patient. This *straight leg–raising (SLR) sign* is positive if the maneuver reproduces the patient's usual back or limb pain. Eliciting the SLR sign in the sitting position may help determine if the finding is reproducible. The patient may describe pain in the low back, buttocks, posterior thigh, or lower leg, but the key feature is reproduction of the patient's usual pain. The *crossed* SLR sign is positive when performance of the maneuver on one leg reproduces the patient's pain symptoms in the opposite leg or buttocks. The nerve or nerve root lesion is always on the side of the pain. The *reverse* SLR sign is elicited by standing the patient next to the examination table and passively extending each leg while the patient continues to stand. This maneuver stretches the L2-L4 nerve roots and the femoral nerve because the nerves pass anterior to the hip. The reverse SLR test is positive if the maneuver reproduces the patient's usual back or limb pain.

The neurologic examination includes a search for weakness, muscle atrophy, focal reflex changes, diminished sensation in the legs, and signs of spinal cord injury. Findings with specific nerve root lesions are shown in Table 16-1 and are discussed below.

Laboratory Studies Routine laboratory studies such as a complete blood count, erythrocyte sedimentation rate, chemistry panel, and urinalysis are rarely needed for the initial evaluation of acute (<3 months), nonspecific, low back pain. If risk factors for a serious underlying disease are present, then laboratory studies (guided by the history and examination) are indicated (Fig. 16-6B).

Plain films of the lumbar or cervical spine are helpful when risk factors for vertebral fracture (trauma, chronic steroid use) are present. *In the absence of risk factors, routine x-rays of the lumbar spine in the setting of acute, nonspecific, low back pain are expensive and rarely helpful.* Magnetic resonance imaging (MRI) and computed tomography (CT)-myelography have emerged as the radiologic tests of choice for evaluation of most serious diseases involving the spine. In general, the definition of soft tissue structures by MRI is superior, whereas CT-myelography provides optimal imaging of bony lesions in the region of the lateral recess and intervertebral foramen and is tolerated by claustrophobic patients. With rare exceptions, conventional myelography and bone scan are inferior to MRI and CT-myelography.

Electromyography (EMG) can be used to assess the functional

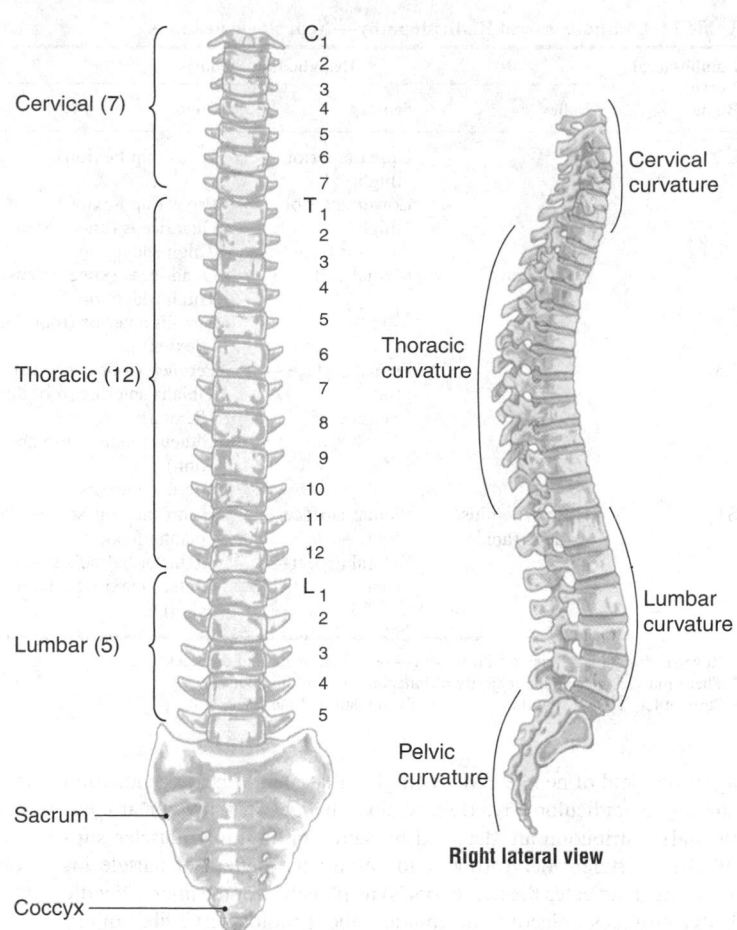

FIGURE 16-2 Spinal column. (*From Andrea Gauthier Cornuelle and Diane H. Gronefeld, Radiographic Anatomy Positioning. New York, McGraw-Hill, 1998, with permission.*)

integrity of the peripheral nervous system (Chap. 357) in the setting of back pain. Sensory nerve conduction studies are normal when focal sensory loss is due to nerve root damage because the nerve roots are proximal to the nerve cell bodies in the dorsal root ganglia. The di-

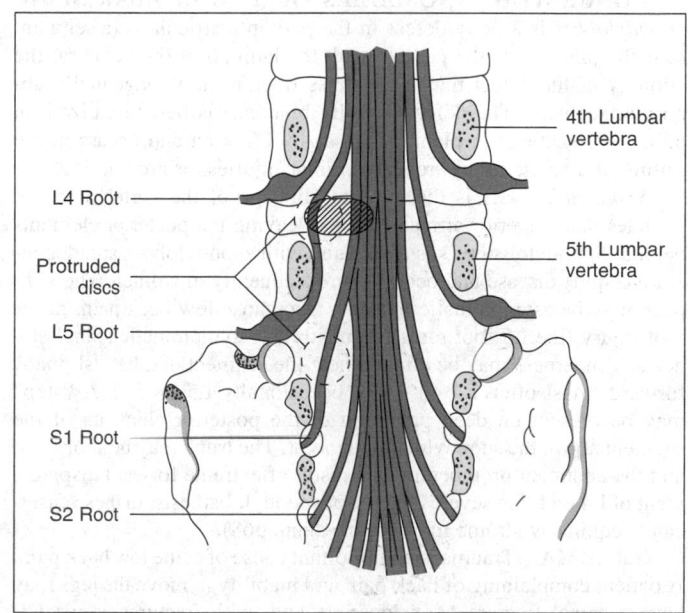

FIGURE 16-3 Locations of compression of lumbar and sacral roots by herniated disks. (*From RD Adams, M Victor, A Ropper, Principles of Neurology, 7th ed. New York, McGraw-Hill, 1997, with permission.*)

Table 16-1 Lumbosacral Radiculopathy—Neurologic Features

Lumbosacral Nerve Roots	Examination Findings			
	Reflex	Sensory	Motor	Pain Distribution
L2[a]	—	Upper anterior thigh	Psoas (hip flexion)	Anterior thigh
L3[a]	—	Lower anterior thigh Anterior knee	Psoas (hip flexion) Quadriceps (knee extension) Thigh adduction	Anterior thigh, knee
L4[a]	Quadriceps (knee)	Medial calf	Quadriceps (knee extension)[b] Thigh adduction Tibialis anterior (foot dorsiflexion)	Knee, medial calf
L5[c]	—	Dorsal surface—foot Lateral calf	Peroneii (foot eversion)[b] Tibialis anterior (foot dorsiflexion) Gluteus medius (hip abduction) Toe dorsiflexors	Lateral calf, dorsal foot, posterolateral thigh, buttocks
S1[c]	Gastrocnemius/soleus (ankle)	Plantar surface—foot Lateral aspect—foot	Gastrocnemius/soleus (foot plantar flexion)[b] Abductor hallucis (toe flexors)[b] Gluteus maximus (hip extension)	Bottom foot, posterior calf, posterior thigh, buttocks

[a] Reverse straight leg–raising sign present—see "Examination of the Back."
[b] These muscles receive the majority of innervation from this root.
[c] Straight leg–raising sign present—see "Examination of the Back."

agnostic yield of needle EMG is higher than that of nerve conduction studies for radiculopathy. Denervation changes in a myotomal (segmental) distribution are detected by sampling multiple muscles supplied by different nerve roots and nerves; the pattern of muscle involvement indicates the nerve root(s) responsible for the injury. Needle EMG provides objective information about motor nerve fiber injury when the clinical evaluation of weakness is limited by pain or poor effort. EMG and nerve conduction studies will be normal when only limb pain or sensory nerve root injury or irritation is present. Mixed nerve somatosensory evoked potentials and F-wave studies are of uncertain value in the evaluation of radiculopathy.

CAUSES OF BACK PAIN

CONGENITAL ANOMALIES OF THE LUMBAR SPINE

Spondylolysis is a bony defect in the pars interarticularis (a segment near the junction of the pedicle with the lamina) of the vertebra; the etiology of the defect may be a stress fracture in a congenitally abnormal segment. The defect (usually bilateral) is best visualized on oblique projections in plain x-rays or by CT scan and occurs in the setting of a single injury, repeated minor injuries, or growth.

Spondylolisthesis is the anterior slippage of the vertebral body, pedicles, and superior articular facets, leaving the posterior elements behind. Spondylolisthesis is associated with spondylolysis and degenerative spine disease and occurs more frequently in women. The slippage may be asymptomatic but may also cause low back pain, nerve root injury (the L5 root most frequently), or symptomatic spinal stenosis. Tenderness may be elicited near the segment that has "slipped" forward (most often L4 on L5 or occasionally L5 on S1). A "step" may be present on deep palpation of the posterior elements of the segment above the spondylolisthetic joint. The trunk may be shortened and the abdomen protuberant as a result of extreme forward displacement of L4 on L5 in severe degrees of spondylolisthesis. In these cases, cauda equina syndrome may occur (Chap. 368).

TRAUMA

Trauma is an important cause of acute low back pain. A patient complaining of back pain and inability to move the legs may have a spinal fracture or dislocation, and, with fractures above L1, spinal cord compression. In such cases care must be taken to avoid further damage to the spinal cord or nerve roots. The back should be immobilized pending results of plain x-rays.

Sprains and Strains

The terms *low back sprain*, *strain*, or *mechanically induced muscle spasm* are used for minor, self-limited injuries associated with lifting a heavy object, a fall, or a sudden deceleration such as occurs in an automobile accident. These terms are used loosely and do not clearly describe a specific anatomic lesion. The pain is usually confined to the lower back, and there is no radiation to the buttocks or legs. Patients with low back pain and paraspinal muscle spasm often assume unusual postures.

Vertebral Fractures

Most traumatic fractures of the lumbar vertebral bodies result from compression or flexion injuries producing anterior wedging or compression. With more severe trauma, the patient may sustain a fracture-dislocation or a "burst" fracture involving not only the vertebral body but posterior elements as well. Traumatic vertebral fractures are caused by falls from a height (a pars interarticularis fracture of the L5 vertebra is common), sudden deceleration in an automobile accident, or direct injury. Neurologic impairment is commonly associated with these injuries, and early surgical treatment is indicated (Chap. 369).

When fractures are atraumatic, the bone is presumed to be weakened by a pathologic process. The cause is usually postmenopausal (type 1) or senile (type 2) osteoporosis (Chap. 342). Underlying systemic disorders such as osteomalacia, hyperparathyroidism, hyperthyroidism, multiple myeloma, metastatic carcinoma, or glucocorticoid use may also weaken the vertebral body. The clinical context, neurologic signs, and x-ray appearance of the spine establish the diagnosis. Antiresorptive drugs including biphosphatonates, alendronate, transdermal estrogen, and tamoxifen have been shown to reduce the risk of osteoporotic fractures.

LUMBAR DISK DISEASE

This disorder is a common cause of chronic or recurrent low back and leg pain. Disk disease is most likely to occur at the L4-L5 and L5-S1 levels, but upper lumbar levels are involved occasionally. The cause of the disk injury is often unknown; the risk is increased in overweight individuals. Degeneration of the nucleus pulposus and the annulus fibrosus increases with age and may be asymptomatic or painful. A sneeze, cough, or trivial movement may cause the nucleus pulposus to prolapse, pushing the frayed and weakened annulus posteriorly. In severe disk disease, the nucleus may protrude through the annulus (herniation) or become extruded to lie as a free fragment in the spinal canal.

The mechanism by which intervertebral disk injury causes back pain is controversial. The inner annulus fibrosus and nucleus pulposis are normally devoid of innervation. Inflammation and production of proinflammatory cytokines within the protruding or ruptured disk may trigger or perpetuate back pain. Ingrowth of nociceptive (pain) nerve fibers into inner portions of diseased intervertebral disk may be responsible for chronic "diskogenic" pain. Nerve root injury (*radiculopathy*) from disk herniation may be due to compression, inflammation, or both; pathologically, varying degrees of demyelination and axonal loss are usually present.

The symptoms of a ruptured intervertebral disk include back pain, abnormal posture, limitation of spine motion (particularly flexion), or radicular pain. A dermatomal pattern of sensory loss or a reduction in or loss of a deep tendon reflex is more suggestive of a specific root lesion than the pattern of pain. Motor findings (focal weakness, muscle atrophy, or fasciculations) occur less frequently than sensory or reflex changes, but a myotomal pattern of involvement can suggest specific nerve root injury. Lumbar disk disease is usually unilateral (Fig. 16-4), but bilateral involvement does occur with large central disk herniations that compress several nerve roots at the same level. Clinical manifestations of specific lumbosacral nerve root lesions are summarized in Table 16-1. There is evidence to suggest that lumbar disk herniation with a nonprogressive nerve root deficit can be managed conservatively (i.e., nonsurgically) with a successful outcome. The size of the disk protrusion may naturally decrease over time.

Degeneration of the intervertebral disk without frank extrusion of disk tissue may give rise to low back pain only. There may be referred pain in the leg, buttock, or hip with little or no discomfort in the back and no signs of nerve root involvement. Lumbar disk syndromes are usually unilateral, but large central disk herniations can cause bilateral symptoms and signs and may produce a cauda equina syndrome.

Breakaway weakness describes a variable power of muscle contraction by a patient who is asked to provide maximal effort. The weakness may be due to pain or a combination of pain and underlying true weakness. Breakaway weakness without pain is due to lack of effort; patients who exhibit breakaway weakness should be asked if testing a specific muscle is painful. In uncertain cases, EMG can determine whether or not true weakness is present.

The differential diagnosis of lumbar disk disease includes a variety of serious and treatable conditions, including epidural abscess, hematoma, or tumor. Fever, constant pain uninfluenced by position, sphincter abnormalities, or signs of spinal cord disease suggest an etiology other than lumbar disk disease. Bilateral absence of ankle reflexes can be a normal finding in old age or a sign of bilateral S1 radiculopathy. An absent deep tendon reflex or focal sensory loss may reflect injury to a nerve root, but other sites of injury along the nerve must also be considered. For example, an absent knee reflex may be due to a femoral neuropathy rather than an L4 nerve root injury. A focal decrease in sensation over the foot and distal lateral calf may result from a peroneal or lateral sciatic neuropathy rather than an L5 nerve root injury. Focal muscle atrophy may reflect loss of motor axons from a nerve root or peripheral nerve injury, an anterior horn cell disease, or disuse.

An MRI scan or CT-myelogram is necessary to establish the location and type of pathology. Simple MRI yields exquisite views of intraspinal and adjacent soft tissue anatomy and is more likely to establish a specific anatomic diagnosis than plain films or myelography. Bony lesions of the lateral recess or intervertebral foramen may be seen with optimal clarity on CT-myelographic studies.

The correlation of neuroradiologic findings to symptoms, particularly pain, is often problematic. As examples, contrast-enhancing tears in the annulus fibrosus or disk protrusions are widely accepted as common sources of back pain. However, one recent study found that over half of asymptomatic adults have annular tears on lumbar spine MR imaging, nearly all of which demonstrate contrast enhancement. Furthermore, asymptomatic disk protrusions are common in adults, and many of these abnormalities enhance with contrast. These observations strongly suggest that MRI findings of disk protrusion, tears in the annulus fibrosus, or contrast enhancement are common incidental findings that by themselves should not dictate management decisions for patients with back pain. The presence or absence of persistent disk herniation 10 years after surgical or conservative treatment has no bearing on a successful clinical outcome.

There are four indications for intervertebral disk surgery: (1) progressive motor weakness from nerve root injury demonstrated on clinical examination or EMG, (2) bowel or bladder disturbance or other signs of spinal cord disease, (3) incapacitating nerve root pain despite conservative treatment for at least 4 weeks, and (4) recurrent incapacitating pain despite conservative treatment. The latter two criteria are more subjective and less well established than the others. Surgical treatment should also be considered if the pain and/or neurologic findings do not substantially improve over 4 to 12 weeks.

Surgery is preceded by MRI scan or CT-myelogram to define the

FIGURE 16-4 Lumbar herniated disk; left S1 radiculopathy. Sagittal T1-weighted image on the left with arrows outlining disk margins. Sagittal T2 image on the right reveals a protruding disk at the L5-S1 level (*arrows*), which displaces the central thecal sac.

location and type of pathology. The usual surgical procedure is a partial hemilaminectomy with excision of the involved and prolapsed intervertebral disk. Arthrodesis of the involved lumbar segments is considered only in the presence of significant spinal instability (i.e., degenerative spondylolisthesis or isthmic spondylolysis).

OTHER CAUSES OF LOW BACK PAIN *Spinal stenosis* is an anatomic diagnosis reflecting a narrowed lumbar or cervical spinal canal. Classic *neurogenic claudication* occurs in the setting of moderate to severe spinal stenosis and typically consists of back and buttock or leg pain induced by walking or standing. The pain is relieved by sitting. Symptoms in the legs are usually bilateral. Focal weakness, sensory loss, or reflex changes may occur when associated with radiculopathy. Unlike vascular claudication, the symptoms are often provoked by standing without walking. Unlike lumbar disk disease, the symptoms are usually relieved by sitting. Severe neurologic deficits, including paralysis and urinary incontinence, occur rarely. Spinal stenosis usually results from acquired (75%), congenital, or mixed acquired/congenital factors. Congenital forms (achondroplasia, idiopathic) are characterized by short, thick pedicles that produce both spinal canal and lateral recess stenosis. Acquired factors that may contribute to spinal stenosis include degenerative diseases (spondylosis, spondylolisthesis, scoliosis), trauma, spine surgery (postlaminectomy, fusion), metabolic or endocrine disorders (epidural lipomatosis, osteoporosis, acromegaly, renal osteodystrophy, hypoparathyroidism), and Paget's disease. MRI or CT-myelography provide the best definition of the abnormal anatomy (Fig. 16-5).

Conservative treatment includes nonsteroidal anti-inflammatory drugs (NSAIDs), exercise programs, and symptomatic treatment of acute pain exacerbations. Surgical therapy is considered when medical therapy does not relieve pain sufficiently to allow for activities of daily living or when significant focal neurologic signs are present. Between 65 and 80% of properly selected patients treated surgically experience >75% relief of back and leg pain. Up to 25% develop recurrent stenosis at the same spinal level or an adjacent level 5 years after the initial surgery; recurrent symptoms usually respond to a second surgical decompression.

Facet joint hypertrophy can produce unilateral radicular symptoms, due to bony compression, that are indistinguishable from disk-related radiculopathy. Patients may exhibit stretch signs, focal motor weakness, hyporeflexia, or sensory loss. Hypertrophic superior or in-

FIGURE 16-5 Spinal stenosis. Sagittal T2 fast spin echo magnetic resonance imaging of a normal (left) and stenotic (right) lumbar spine, revealing multifocal narrowing (arrows) of the cerebrospinal fluid spaces surrounding the nerve roots within the thecal sac.

ferior facets can often be visualized radiologically. Foraminotomy results in long-term relief of leg and back pain in 80 to 90% of patients.

Lumbar adhesive arachnoiditis with radiculopathy is the result of a fibrotic process following an inflammatory response to local tissue injury within the subarachnoid space. The fibrosis results in nerve root adhesions, producing back and leg pain associated with motor, sensory, and reflex changes. Myelography-induced arachnoiditis has become rare with the abandonment of oil-based contrast. Other causes of arachnoiditis include multiple lumbar operations, chronic spinal infections, spinal cord injury, intrathecal hemorrhage, intrathecal injection of steroids and anesthetics, and foreign bodies. The spine MRI appearance of arachnoiditis includes nerve roots clumping together centrally and adherent to the dura peripherally, or loculations of cerebrospinal fluid (CSF) within the thecal sac that obscure nerve root visualization. Treatment is often unsatisfactory. Microsurgical lysis of adhesions, dorsal rhizotomy, and dorsal root ganglionectomy have resulted in poor outcomes. Dorsal column stimulation for pain relief has produced varying results. Epidural steroid injections have been of limited value.

ARTHRITIS   Arthritis is a major cause of spine pain.

Spondylosis   Osteoarthritic spine disease typically occurs in later life and primarily involves the cervical and lumbosacral spine. Patients often complain of back pain that is increased by motion and associated with stiffness or limitation of motion. The relationship between clinical symptoms and radiologic findings is usually not straightforward. Pain may be prominent when x-ray findings are minimal; alternatively, large osteophytes can be seen in asymptomatic patients in middle and later life. Hypertrophied facets and osteophytes may compress nerve roots in the lateral recess or intervertebral foramen. Osteophytes arising from the vertebral body may cause or contribute to central spinal canal stenosis. Loss of intervertebral disk height reduces the vertical dimensions of the intervertebral foramen; the descending pedicle may compress the nerve root exiting at that level. Osteoarthritic changes in the lumbar spine may rarely compress the cauda equina.

Ankylosing Spondylitis (See also Chap. 315)   This distinctive arthritic spine disease typically presents with the insidious onset of low back and buttock pain. Patients are often males below age 40. Associated features include morning back stiffness, nocturnal pain, pain unrelieved by rest, an elevated sedimentation rate, and the histocompatibility antigen HLA-B27. The differential diagnosis includes tumor and infection. Onset at a young age and back pain characteristically improving with exercise suggest ankylosing spondylitis. Loss of the normal lumbar lordosis and exaggeration of thoracic kyphosis are seen as the disease progresses. Inflammation and erosion of the outer fibers of the annulus fibrosus at the point of contact with the vertebral body are followed by ossification and bone growth. Bony growth (syndesmophyte) bridges adjacent vertebral bodies and results in reduced spine mobility in all planes. The radiologic hallmarks of the disease are periarticular destructive changes, sclerosis of the sacroiliac joints, and bridging of vertebral bodies by bone to produce the fused "bamboo spine." Similar restricted movement may accompany Reiter's syndrome, psoriatic arthritis, and chronic inflammatory bowel disease. Stress fractures through the spontaneously ankylosed posterior bony elements of the rigid, osteoporotic spine may result in focal spine pain, spinal cord compression or cauda equina syndrome. Occasional atlantoaxial subluxation with spinal cord compression occurs. Bilateral ankylosis of the ribs to the spine and a decrease in the height of axial thoracic structures may cause marked impairment of respiratory function.

OTHER DESTRUCTIVE DISEASES   **Neoplasm** (See also Chap. 370)   Back pain is the most common neurologic symptom among patients with systemic cancer. One-third of patients with undiagnosed back or neck pain and known systemic cancer have epidural extension or metastasis of tumor, and one-third have pain associated with vertebral metastases alone. About 11% have back pain unrelated to metastatic disease. Metastatic carcinoma (breast, lung, prostate, thyroid, kidney, gastrointestinal tract), multiple myeloma, and non-Hodgkin's and Hodgkin's lymphomas frequently involve the spine. Back pain may be the presenting symptom because the primary tumor site may be overlooked or asymptomatic. The pain tends to be constant, dull, unrelieved by rest, and worse at night. In contrast, mechanical low back pain is usually improved with rest. Plain x-rays usually, though not always, show destructive lesions in one or several vertebral bodies without disk space involvement. MRI or CT-myelography are the studies of choice in the setting of suspected spinal metastasis, but the trend of evidence favors the use of MRI. The procedure of choice is the study most rapidly available because the patient may worsen during a diagnostic delay.

Infection   *Vertebral osteomyelitis* is usually caused by staphylococci, but other bacteria or the tubercle bacillus (Pott's disease) may be the responsible organism. A primary source of infection, most often from the urinary tract, skin, or lungs, can be identified in 40% of patients. Intravenous drug use is a well-recognized risk factor. Back pain exacerbated by motion and unrelieved by rest, spine tenderness over the involved spine segment, and an elevated erythrocyte sedimentation rate are the most common findings. Fever or elevated white blood cell count are found in a minority of patients. Plain radiographs may show a narrowed disk space with erosion of adjacent vertebrae; these diagnostic changes may take weeks or months to appear. MRI and CT are sensitive and specific for osteomyelitis; MRI definition of soft tissue detail is exquisite. CT scan may be more readily available and better tolerated by some patients with severe back pain.

Spinal epidural abscess (Chap. 368) presents with back pain (aggravated by palpation or movement) and fever. The patient may exhibit nerve root injury or spinal cord compression accompanied by a sensory level, incontinence, or paraplegia. The abscess may track over multiple spinal levels and is best delineated by spine MRI.

Osteoporosis and Osteosclerosis   Considerable loss of bone may occur with or without symptoms in association with medical disorders, including hyperparathyroidism, chronic glucocorticoid use, or immobilization. Compression fractures occur in up to half of patients with severe osteoporosis. The risk of osteoporotic vertebral fracture is 4.5 times greater over 3 years among patients with a baseline fracture compared with osteoporotic controls. The sole manifestation of a compression fracture may be focal lumbar or thoracic aching (often after a trivial injury) that is exacerbated by movement. Other patients experience thoracic or upper lumbar radicular pain. Focal spine tenderness is common. When compression fractures are found, treatable risk factors should be sought. Compression fractures above the midthoracic region suggest malignancy.

Osteosclerosis is readily identifiable on routine x-ray studies (e.g., Paget's disease) and may or may not produce back pain. Spinal cord or nerve root compression may result from bony encroachment on the spinal canal or intervertebral foramina. Single dual-beam photon absorptiometry or quantitative CT can be used to detect small changes in bone mineral density. →*For further discussion of these bone disorders, see Chaps. 341 to 343.*

REFERRED PAIN FROM VISCERAL DISEASE Diseases of the pelvis, abdomen, or thorax may produce referred pain to the posterior portion of the spinal segment that innervates the diseased organ. Occasionally, back pain may be the first and only sign. In general, pelvic diseases refer pain to the sacral region, lower abdominal diseases to the lumbar region (around the second to fourth lumbar vertebrae), and upper abdominal diseases to the lower thoracic or upper lumbar region (eighth thoracic to the first and second lumbar vertebrae). Local signs (pain with spine palpation, paraspinal muscle spasm) are absent, and minimal or no pain accompanies normal spine movements.

Low Thoracic and Upper Lumbar Pain in Abdominal Disease Peptic ulcer or tumor of the posterior stomach or duodenum typically produces epigastric pain (Chaps. 285 and 90), but midline back or paraspinal pain may occur if retroperitoneal extension is present. Back pain due to peptic ulcer may be precipitated by ingestion of an orange, alcohol, or coffee and relieved by food or antacids. Fatty foods are more likely to induce back pain associated with biliary disease. Diseases of the pancreas may produce back pain to the right of the spine (head of the pancreas involved) or to the left (body or tail involved). Pathology in retroperitoneal structures (hemorrhage, tumors, pyelonephritis) may produce paraspinal pain with radiation to the lower abdomen, groin, or anterior thighs. A mass in the iliopsoas region often produces unilateral lumbar pain with radiation toward the groin, labia, or testicle. The sudden appearance of lumbar pain in a patient receiving anticoagulants suggests retroperitoneal hemorrhage.

Isolated low back pain occurs in 15 to 20% of patients with a contained rupture of an abdominal aortic aneurysm (AAA). The classic clinical triad of abdominal pain, shock, and back pain in an elderly man occurs in fewer than 20% of patients. Two of these three features are present in two-thirds of patients, and hypotension is present in half. Ruptured AAA has a high mortality rate; the typical patient is an elderly male smoker with back pain. The diagnosis is initially missed in at least one-third of patients because the symptoms and signs can be nonspecific. Common misdiagnoses include nonspecific back pain, diverticulitis, renal colic, sepsis, and myocardial infarction. A careful abdominal examination revealing a pulsatile mass (present in 50 to 75% of patients) is an important physical finding.

Lumbar Pain with Lower Abdominal Diseases Inflammatory bowel disorders (colitis, diverticulitis) or colonic neoplasms may produce lower abdominal pain, midlumbar back pain, or both. The pain may have a beltlike distribution around the body. A lesion in the transverse or initial descending colon may refer pain to the middle or left back at the L2-L3 level. Sigmoid colon disease may refer pain to the upper sacral or midline suprapubic regions or left lower quadrant of the abdomen.

Sacral Pain in Gynecologic and Urologic Disease Pelvic organs rarely cause low back pain, except for gynecologic disorders involving the uterosacral ligaments. The pain is referred to the sacral region. Endometriosis or uterine carcinoma may invade the uterosacral ligaments; malposition of the uterus may cause uterosacral ligament traction. The pain associated with endometriosis begins during the premenstrual phase and often continues until it merges with menstrual pain. Malposition of the uterus (retroversion, descensus, and prolapse) may lead to sacral pain after standing for several hours.

Menstrual pain may be felt in the sacral region. The poorly localized, cramping pain can radiate down the legs. Other pelvic sources of low back pain include neoplastic invasion of pelvic nerves, radiation necrosis, and pregnancy. Pain due to neoplastic infiltration of nerves is typically continuous, progressive in severity, and unrelieved by rest at night. Radiation therapy of pelvic tumors may produce sacral pain from late radiation necrosis of tissue or nerves. Low back pain with radiation into one or both thighs is common in the last weeks of pregnancy.

Urologic sources of lumbosacral back pain include chronic prostatitis, prostate carcinoma with spinal metastasis, and diseases of the kidney and ureter. Lesions of the bladder and testes do not usually produce back pain. The diagnosis of metastatic prostate carcinoma is established by rectal examination, spine imaging studies (MRI or CT), and measurement of prostate-specific antigen (PSA) (Chap. 95). Infectious, inflammatory, or neoplastic renal diseases may result in ipsilateral lumbosacral pain, as can renal artery or vein thrombosis. Ureteral obstruction due to renal stones may produce paraspinal lumbar pain.

Postural Back Pain There is a group of patients with chronic, nonspecific low back pain in whom no anatomic or pathologic lesion can be found despite exhaustive investigation. These individuals complain of vague, diffuse back pain with prolonged sitting or standing that is relieved by rest. The physical examination is unrevealing except for "poor posture." Imaging studies and laboratory evaluations are normal. Exercises to strengthen the paraspinal and abdominal muscles are sometimes therapeutic.

Psychiatric Disease Chronic low back pain (CLBP) may be encountered in patients with compensation hysteria, malingering, substance abuse, chronic anxiety states, or depression. Many patients with CLBP have a history of psychiatric illness (depression, anxiety, substance abuse) or childhood trauma (physical or sexual abuse) that antedates the onset of back pain. Preoperative psychological assessment has been used to exclude patients with marked psychological impairment who are at high risk for a poor surgical outcome. It is important to be certain that the back pain in these patients does not represent serious spine or visceral pathology in addition to the impaired psychological state.

Unidentified The cause of low back pain occasionally remains unclear. Some patients have had multiple operations for disk disease but have persistent pain and disability. The original indications for surgery may have been questionable with back pain only, no definite neurologic signs, or a minor disk bulge noted on CT or MRI. Scoring systems based upon neurologic signs, psychological factors, physiologic studies, and imaging studies have been devised to minimize the likelihood of unsuccessful surgical explorations and to avoid selection of patients with psychological profiles that predict poor functional outcomes.

℞ TREATMENT   Acute Low Back Pain A practical approach to the management of low back pain is to consider acute and chronic presentations separately. ALBP is defined as pain of less than 3 months' duration. Full recovery can be expected in 85% of adults with ALBP unaccompanied by leg pain. Most of these patients exhibit "mechanical" symptoms—pain that is aggravated by motion and relieved by rest.

Observational, population-based studies have been used to justify a minimalist approach to individual patient care. These studies share a number of limitations: (1) a true placebo control group is often lacking; (2) patients who consult different provider groups (generalists, orthopedists, neurologists) are assumed to have similar etiologies for their back pain; (3) no information is provided about the details of treatment within each provider group or between provider groups; and (4) no attempt to tabulate serious causes of ALBP is made. The appropriateness of specific diagnostic procedures or therapeutic interventions for low back pain cannot be assessed from these studies.

The proposed algorithms (Fig. 16-6) for management of ALBP in adults draw considerably from published guidelines. However, it must be emphasized that current CPGs for the treatment of low back pain are based on incomplete evidence—for example, there is a paucity of well-designed studies documenting the natural history of disk lesions associated with a focal neurologic deficit. Guidelines should not substitute for sound clinical judgment.

The initial assessment excludes serious causes of spine pathology that require urgent intervention, including infection, cancer, and

FIGURE 16-6 Algorithms for management of acute low back pain, age ≥18 years. *A.* Symptoms <3 months, first 4 weeks. *B.* Possible serious etiology.

trauma. Risks factors for a possible serious underlying cause of back pain include: age > 50 years, prior diagnosis of cancer or other serious medical illness, bed rest without relief, duration of pain >1 month, urinary incontinence or recent nocturia, focal leg weakness or numbness, pain radiating into the leg(s) from the back, intravenous drug use, chronic infection (pulmonary or urinary), pain increasing with standing and relieved by sitting, history of spine trauma, and glucocorticoid use. Clinical signs associated with a possible serious etiology include unexplained fever, well-documented and unexplained weight loss, positive SLR sign or reverse SLR sign, crossed SLR sign, percussion tenderness over the spine or costovertebral angle, an abdominal mass (pulsatile or nonpulsatile), a rectal mass, focal sensory loss (saddle anesthesia or focal limb sensory loss), true leg weakness, spasticity, and asymmetric leg reflexes. Laboratory studies are unnecessary unless a serious underlying cause (Fig. 16-6, Algorithms *A* and *B*) is suspected. Plain spine films are rarely indicated in the first month of symptoms unless a spine fracture is suspected.

The roles of bed rest, early exercise, and traction in the treatment of acute uncomplicated low back pain have been the subject of recent prospective studies. Clinical trials fail to demonstrate any benefit of prolonged (>2 days) bed rest for ALBP. There is evidence that bed rest is also ineffective for patients with sciatica or for acute back pain with findings of nerve root injury. Theoretical advantages of early ambulation for ALBP include maintenance of cardiovascular conditioning, improved disk and cartilage nutrition, improved bone and muscle strength, and increased endorphin levels. A recent trial did not show benefit from an early vigorous exercise program, but the benefits of less vigorous exercise or other exercise programs remain unknown. The early resumption of normal physical activity (without heavy manual labor) is likely to be beneficial. Well-designed clinical studies of traction that include a sham traction group have failed to show a benefit of traction for ALBP. Despite this knowledge, one survey of physicians' perceptions of effective treatment identified strict bed rest for >3 days, trigger point injections (see below), and physical therapy (PT) as beneficial for more than 50% of patients with ALBP. In many instances, the behavior of treating physicians does not reflect the current medical literature.

Proof is lacking to support the treatment of acute back and neck pain with acupuncture, transcutaneous electrical nerve stimulation, massage, ultrasound, diathermy, or electrical stimulation. Cervical collars can be modestly helpful by limiting spontaneous and reflex neck movements that exacerbate pain. Evidence regarding the efficacy of ice or heat is lacking, but these interventions are optional given the

FIGURE 16-6—*(continued)* *C.* Management weeks 4–12. ①, entry point from Algorithm D postoperatively or if patient declines surgery. *D.* Surgical options. (NSAIDs, nonsteroidal anti-inflammatory drugs; CBC, complete blood count; ESR, erythrocyte sedimentation rate; UA, urinalysis; EMG, electromyography; NCV, nerve conduction velocity studies; MRI, magnetic resonance imaging; CT, computed tomography; CNS, central nervous system.)

lack of negative evidence, low cost, and low risk. Biofeedback has not been studied rigorously. Facet joint, trigger point, and ligament injections are not recommended in the treatment of ALBP.

A beneficial role for specific exercises or modification of posture has not been validated by rigorous clinical studies. As a practical matter, temporary suspension of activity known to increase mechanical stress on the spine (heavy lifting, prolonged sitting, bending or twisting, straining at stool) may be helpful.

Patient education is an important part of treatment. Studies reveal that patient satisfaction and the likelihood of follow-up increase when patients are educated about prognosis, treatment methods, activity modifications, and strategies to prevent future exacerbations. In one study, patients who felt they did not receive an adequate explanation for their symptoms wanted more diagnostic tests. Evidence for the efficacy of structured education programs ("back school") is inconclusive; in one controlled study, patients attending back school had a shorter duration of sick leave during the initial episode but not during subsequent episodes. Recent large, controlled, randomized studies of back school for primary prevention of low back injury and pain have failed to demonstrate a benefit.

Medications used in the treatment of ALBP include NSAIDs, acetaminophen, muscle relaxants, and opioids. NSAIDs are superior to placebo for back pain relief. Acetaminophen is superior to placebo in the treatment of other types of pain but has not been compared against placebo for low back pain. Muscle relaxants provide short-term (4 to 7 days) benefit compared with placebo, but drowsiness often limits their daytime use. The efficacy of muscle relaxants compared to NSAIDs or in combination with NSAIDs is unclear. Opioid analgesics have not been shown to be more effective than NSAIDs or acetaminophen for relief of ALBP or likelihood of return to work. Short-term use of opioids in selected patients unresponsive to or intolerant of acetaminophen or NSAIDs may be helpful. There is no evidence to support the use of oral glucocorticoids or tricyclic antidepressants in treatment of ALBP.

The role of diagnostic and therapeutic nerve root blocks for patients with acute back or neck pain remains controversial. Equivocal data suggests that epidural steroids may occasionally produce short-term pain relief in patients with ALBP and radiculopathy, but proof is lacking for pain relief beyond 1 month. Epidural anesthetics, steroids, or opioids are not indicated as initial treatment for ALBP without radiculopathy. Diagnostic selective nerve root blocks have been advocated to determine if pain originates from a nerve root. However, these studies may be falsely positive due to a placebo effect, in patients with a painful lesion located distally along the peripheral nerve, or from anesthesia of the sinuvertebral nerve. Therapeutic selective nerve root blocks are an option after brief conservative measures fail, particularly when temporary relief of pain may be important for patient function. Needle position is confirmed under fluoroscopic guidance with nonionic contrast before injection of glucocorticoid and local anesthetic.

A short course of spinal manipulation or PT for symptomatic relief of uncomplicated ALBP is an option. A prospective, randomized study comparing PT, chiropractic manipulation, and education interventions for patients with ALBP found modest trends toward benefit with both PT and chiropractic manipulation at 1 year. Costs per year were equivalent in the PT/chiropractic group and ~$280 less for the group treated with the education booklet alone. The extent to which this modest improvement in symptoms and outcome is worth the cost must be determined for each patient. Extended duration of treatment or treatment of patients with radiculopathy is of unknown value and carries potential risk. The appropriate frequency or duration of spinal manipulation has not been addressed adequately.

Chronic Low Back Pain CLBP is defined as pain lasting longer than 12 weeks. Patients with CLBP account for 50% of back pain costs. Overweight individuals appear to be at particular risk. Other risk factors include: female gender, older age, prior history of back pain, restricted spinal mobility, pain radiating into a leg, high levels of psychological distress, poor self-rated health, minimal physical activity, smoking, job dissatisfaction, and widespread pain. Combinations of these premorbid factors have been used to predict which individuals with ALBP are likely to develop CLBP. The initial approach to these patients is similar to that for ALBP, and the differential diagnosis of CLBP includes most of the conditions described in this chapter. Treatment of this heterogeneous group of patients is directed toward the underlying cause when possible; the ultimate goal is to restore function to the greatest extent possible.

Many conditions that produce CLBP can be identified by the combination of neuroimaging and electrophysiologic studies. Spine MRI or CT-myelography are the techniques of choice but are generally not indicated within the first month after initial evaluation in the absence of risk factors for a serious underlying cause. Imaging studies should be performed only in circumstances where the results are likely to influence surgical or medical treatment.

Diskography is of questionable value in the evaluation of back pain. No additional anatomic information is provided beyond what is available by MRI. Reproduction of the patient's typical pain with the injection is often used as evidence that a specific disk is the pain generator, but it is not known whether this information has any value in selecting candidates for surgery. There is no proven role for thermography in the assessment of radiculopathy.

The diagnosis of nerve root injury is most secure when the history, examination, results of imaging studies, and the EMG are concordant. The correlation between CT and EMG for localization of nerve root injury is between 65 and 73%. Up to one-third of asymptomatic adults have a disk protrusion detected by CT or MRI scans. Thus, surgical intervention based solely upon radiologic findings and pain increases the likelihood of an unsuccessful outcome.

CLBP can be treated with a variety of conservative measures. Acute and subacute exacerbations are managed with NSAIDs and comfort measures. There is no good evidence to suggest that one NSAID is more effective than another. Bed rest should not exceed 2 days. Activity tolerance is the primary goal, while pain relief is secondary. Exercise programs can reverse type II muscle fiber atrophy in paraspinal muscles and strengthen trunk extension. Supervised, intensive physical exercise or "work hardening" regimens (under the guidance of a physical therapist) have been effective in returning some patients to work, improving walking distances, and diminishing pain. The benefit can be sustained with home exercise regimens; compliance with the exercise regimen strongly influences outcome. The role of manipulation, back school, or epidural steroid injections in the treatment of CLBP is unclear. Up to 30% of "blind" epidural steroid injections miss the epidural space even when performed by an experienced anesthesiologist. There is no strong evidence to support the use of acupuncture or traction in this setting. A reduction in sick leave days, long-term health care utilization, and pension expenditures may offset the initial expense of multidisciplinary treatment programs. In one study comparing 3 weeks of hydrotherapy versus routine ambulatory care, hydrotherapy resulted in diminished duration and intensity of back pain, reduced analgesic drug consumption, improved spine mobility, and improved functional score. Functional score returned to baseline at the 9-month follow-up, but all other beneficial effects were sustained. Percutaneous electrical nerve stimulation (PENS) has been shown to provide significant short-term relief of CLBP, but additional studies regarding long-term efficacy and cost are necessary.

PAIN IN THE NECK AND SHOULDER

Approach to the Patient

In one recent epidemiologic survey, the 6-month prevalence of disabling neck pain was 4.6% among adults. Neck pain commonly arises from diseases of the cervical spine and soft tissues of the neck. Neck pain arising from the cervical spine is typically precipitated by neck movements and may be accompanied by focal spine tenderness and limitation of motion. Pain arising from the brachial plexus, shoulder, or peripheral nerves can be confused with cervical spine disease, but the history and examination usually identify a more distal origin for the pain. Cervical spine trauma, disk disease, or spondylosis may be asymptomatic or painful and can produce a myelopathy, radiculopathy, or both. The nerve roots most commonly affected are C7 and C6.

TRAUMA TO THE CERVICAL SPINE   Unlike injury to the low back, trauma to the cervical spine (fractures, subluxation) places the spinal cord at risk for compression. Motor vehicle accidents, violent crimes, or falls account for 87% of spinal cord injuries, which can have devastating consequences (Chap. 369). Emergency immobilization of the neck prior to complete assessment is mandatory to minimize further spinal cord injury from movement of unstable cervical spine segments.

Whiplash injury is due to trauma (usually automobile accidents) causing cervical musculoligamental sprain or strain due to hyperflexion or hyperextension. This diagnosis should not be applied to patients with fractures, disk herniation, head injury, or altered consciousness. One prospective study found that 18% of patients with whiplash injury had persistent injury-related symptoms 2 years after the car accident. Such patients were older, had a higher incidence of inclined or rotated head position at impact, greater intensity of initial neck and head pain, greater number of initial symptoms, and more osteoarthritic changes on cervical spine x-rays at baseline compared to patients who ultimately recovered. Objective data on the pathology of neck soft tissue injuries is lacking. Patients with severe initial injury are at increased risk for poor long-term outcome.

CERVICAL DISK DISEASE   Herniation of a lower cervical disk is a common cause of neck, shoulder, arm, or hand pain. Neck pain (worse with movement), stiffness, and limited range of neck motion are common. With nerve root compression, pain may radiate into a shoulder or arm. Extension and lateral rotation of the neck narrows the intervertebral foramen and may reproduce radicular symptoms (Spurling's sign). In young individuals, acute cervical nerve root compression from a ruptured disk is often due to trauma. Subacute radiculopathy is less likely to be related to a specific traumatic incident and may involve both disk disease and spondylosis. Cervical disk herniations are usually posterolateral near the lateral recess and intervertebral foramen. The usual patterns of reflex, sensory, and motor changes that accompany specific cervical nerve root lesions are listed in Table 16-2. When evaluating patients with suspected cervical radiculopathy it is important to consider the following: (1) overlap in function between adjacent nerve roots is common, (2) the anatomic pattern of pain is the most variable of the clinical features, and (3) the distribution of symptoms and signs may be evident in only part of the injured nerve root territory.

Surgical management of cervical herniated disks usually consists of an anterior approach with diskectomy followed by anterior interbody fusion. A simple posterior partial laminectomy with diskectomy is an alternative approach. The risk of subsequent radiculopathy or myelopathy at cervical segments adjacent to the fusion is 3% per year and 26% at 10 years. Although the risk is sometimes portrayed as a late complication of cervical surgery, it may also reflect the natural history of degenerative cervical spine disease in this subpopulation of patients.

CERVICAL SPONDYLOSIS   Osteoarthritis of the cervical spine may produce neck pain that radiates into the back of the head, shoulders, or arms. Arthritic or other pathologic conditions of the upper cervical spine may be the source of headaches in the posterior occipital region (supplied by the C2-C4 nerve roots). Cervical spondylosis with osteophyte formation in the lateral recess or hypertrophic facet joints may produce a monoradiculopathy (Fig. 16-7). Narrowing of the spinal canal by osteophytes, ossification of the posterior longitudinal ligament, or a large central disk may compress the cervical spinal cord. In some patients, a combination of radiculopathy and myelopathy occur. An electrical sensation elicited by neck flexion and radiating down the spine from the neck (Lhermitte's symptom) usually indicates cervical or upper thoracic (T1-T2) spinal cord involvement. When little or no neck pain accompanies the cord compression, the diagnosis may be confused with amyotrophic lateral sclerosis (Chap. 365), multiple sclerosis (Chap. 371), spinal cord tumors (Chap. 368), or syringomyelia (Chap. 368). The possibility of this treatable cervical spinal cord disease must be considered even when the patient presents with leg complaints only. Furthermore, lumbar radiculopathy or polyneuropathy may mask an associated cervical myelopathy. MRI or CT-myelography can define the anatomic abnormalities, and EMG and nerve conduction studies can quantify the severity and localize the levels of motor nerve root injury.

OTHER CAUSES OF NECK PAIN Rheumatoid arthritis (RA) (Chap. 312) of the cervical apophyseal joints results in neck pain, stiffness, and limitation of motion. In typical cases with symmetric inflammatory polyarthritis, the diagnosis of RA is straightforward. In advanced RA, synovitis of the atlantoaxial joint (C1-C2; Fig. 16-2) may damage the transverse ligament of the atlas, producing forward displacement of the atlas on the axis (atlantoaxial subluxation). Radiologic evidence of atlantoaxial subluxation occurs in 30% of patients with RA. Not surprisingly, the degree of subluxation correlates with the severity of erosive disease. When subluxation is present, careful neurologic assessment is important to identify early signs of myelopathy. Occasional patients develop high spinal cord compression leading to quadriparesis, respiratory insufficiency, and death. Although low back pain is common among RA patients, the frequency of facet disease, fracture, and spondylolisthesis is no greater than among age- and sex-matched controls with mechanical low back pain.

Ankylosing spondylitis can cause neck pain and on occasion atlantoaxial subluxation; when spinal cord compression is present or threatened, surgical intervention is indicated. Herpes zoster produces neck and posterior occipital pain in a C2-C3 distribution prior to the outbreak of vesicles. Neoplasms metastatic to the cervical spine, infections (osteomyelitis and epidural abscess), and metabolic bone diseases may also be the cause of neck pain. Neck pain may also be referred from the heart in the setting of coronary artery ischemia (cervical angina syndrome).

THORACIC OUTLET The thoracic outlet is an anatomic region containing the first rib, the subclavian artery and vein, the brachial plexus, the clavicle, and the lung apex. Injury to these structures may result in posture or task-related pain around the shoulder and supraclavicular region. There are at least three subtypes of thoracic outlet syndrome (TOS). *True neurogenic TOS* results from compression of the lower trunk of the brachial plexus by an anomalous band of tissue connecting an elongate transverse process at C7 with the first rib. Neurologic deficits include weakness of intrinsic muscles of the hand and diminished sensation on the palmar aspect of the fourth and fifth digits. EMG and nerve conduction studies confirm the diagnosis. Definitive treatment consists of surgical division of the anomalous band compressing either the lower trunk of the brachial plexus or ventral rami of the C8 or T1 nerve roots. The weakness and wasting of intrinsic hand muscles typically does not improve, but surgery halts the insidious progression of weakness. The *arterial TOS* results from compression of the subclavian artery by a cervical rib; the compression results in poststenotic dilatation of the artery and thrombus formation. Blood pressure is reduced in the affected limb, and signs of emboli may be present in the hand; neurologic signs are absent. Noninvasive ultrasound techniques confirm the diagnosis. Treatment is with thrombolysis or anticoagulation (with or without embolectomy) and surgical excision of the cervical rib compressing the subclavian artery or vein. The *disputed TOS* includes a large number of patients with chronic arm and shoulder pain of unclear cause. The lack of sensitive and specific findings on physical examination or laboratory markers for this condition frequently results in diagnostic uncertainty. The role of surgery in disputed TOS is controversial; conservative approaches often include multidisciplinary pain management. Treatment is often unsuccessful.

BRACHIAL PLEXUS AND NERVES Pain from injury to the brachial plexus or arm peripheral nerves can occasionally be confused with pain of cervical spine origin. Neoplastic infiltration of the lower trunk of the brachial plexus may produce shoulder pain radiating down the arm, numbness of the fourth and fifth fingers, and weakness of intrinsic hand muscles innervated by the ulnar and median nerves.

Table 16-2   Cervical Radiculopathy—Neurologic Features

Cervical Nerve Roots	Examination Findings			
	Reflex	Sensory	Motor	Pain Distribution
C5	Biceps	Over lateral deltoid	Supraspinatus[a] (initial arm abduction) Infraspinatus[a] (arm external rotation) Deltoid[a] (arm abduction) Biceps (arm flexion)	Lateral arm, medial scapula
C6	Biceps	Thumb, index fingers Radial hand/ forearm	Biceps (arm flexion) Pronator teres (internal forearm rotation)	Lateral forearm, thumb, index finger
C7	Triceps	Middle fingers Dorsum forearm	Triceps[a] (arm extension) Wrist extensors[a] Extensor digitorum[a] (finger extension)	Posterior arm, dorsal forearm, lateral hand
C8	Finger flexors	Little finger Medial hand and forearm	Abductor pollicis brevis (abduction D1) First dorsal interosseous (abduction D2) Abductor digiti minimi (abduction D5)	4th and 5th fingers, medial forearm
T1	Finger flexors	Axilla and medial arm	Abductor pollicis brevis (abduction D1) First dorsal interosseous (abduction D2) Abductor digiti minimi (abduction D5)	Medial arm, axilla

[a] These muscles receive the majority of innervation from this root.

FIGURE 16-7 Cervical spondylosis; left C6 radiculopathy. *A.* Sagittal T2 fast spin echo magnetic resonance imaging reveals a hypointense osteophyte that protrudes from the C5-C6 level into the thecal sac, displacing the spinal cord posteriorly (*white arrow*). *B.* Axial 2-mm section from a 3-D volume gradient echo sequence of the cervical spine. The high signal of the right C5-C6 intervertebral foramen contrasts with the narrow high signal of the left C5-C6 intervertebral foramen produced by osteophytic spurring (*arrows*).

Postradiation fibrosis (breast carcinoma is the most common setting) or a Pancoast tumor of the lung (Chap. 88) may produce similar findings. A Horner's syndrome is present in two-thirds of patients with a Pancoast tumor. Suprascapular neuropathy may produce severe shoulder pain, weakness, and wasting of the supraspinatous and infraspinatous muscles. *Acute brachial neuritis* is often confused with radiculopathy. It consists of the acute onset of severe shoulder or scapular pain followed over days to weeks by weakness of the proximal arm and shoulder girdle muscles innervated by the upper or middle trunks or cords of the brachial plexus. The onset is often preceeded by an infection or immunization. Separation of this syndrome from cervical radiculopathy is important because slow, complete recovery of brachial neuritis occurs in 75% of patients after 2 years and in 89% after 3 years. Occasional cases of carpal tunnel syndrome produce pain and paresthesia extending into the forearm, arm, and shoulder resembling a C5 or C6 root lesion. Lesions of the radial or ulnar nerve can mimic a radiculopathy at C7 or C8, respectively. EMG and nerve conduction studies can accurately localize lesions to the nerve roots, brachial plexus, or nerves. →*For further discussion of peripheral nerve disorders, see Chap. 377.*

SHOULDER   Pain in the shoulder region can be difficult to separate clearly from neck pain. If the symptoms and signs of radiculopathy are absent, then the differential diagnosis includes mechanical shoulder pain (tendonitis, bursitis, rotator cuff tear, dislocation, adhesive capsulitis, and cuff impingement under the acromion) and referred pain (subdiaphragmatic irritation, angina, Pancoast tumor). Mechanical pain is often worse at night, associated with local shoulder tenderness, and aggravated by abduction, internal rotation, or extension of the arm. The pain of shoulder disease may at times radiate into the arm or hand, but the sensory, motor, and reflex changes that indicate disease of the nerve roots, plexus, or peripheral nerves are absent.

℞ **TREATMENT**   A paucity of well-designed clinical trials exists for the treatment of neck pain. Symptomatic treatment of neck pain can include the use of analgesic medications and/or a soft cervical collar. Current indications for cervical disk surgery are similar to those for lumbar disk surgery; because of the risk of spinal cord injury with cervical spine disease, an aggressive approach is generally indicated whenever spinal cord injury is threatened. Surgical management of cervical herniated disks usually consists of an anterior approach with diskectomy followed by anterior interbody fusion. A simple posterior partial laminectomy with diskectomy is an acceptable alternative approach. The cumulative risk of subsequent radiculopathy or myelopathy at cervical segments adjacent to the fusion is approximately 3% per year and 26% per decade. Although this risk is sometimes portrayed as a late complication of surgery, it may also reflect the natural history of degenerative cervical spine disease. Nonprogressive cervical radiculopathy (associated with a focal neurologic deficit) due to a herniated cervical disk may be treated conservatively with a high rate of success. Cervical spondylosis with bony, compressive cervical radiculopathy is generally treated with surgical decompression to interrupt the progression of neurologic signs. Cervical spondylotic myelopathy is typically managed with either anterior decompression and fusion or laminectomy. Outcomes in both surgical groups vary, but late functional deterioration occurs in 20 to 30% of patients; a prospective, controlled study comparing different surgical interventions is sorely needed.

BIBLIOGRAPHY

ANDERSSON GBJ et al: A comparison of osteopathic spinal manipulation with standard care for patients with low back pain. N Engl J Med 341(19):1426, 1999

BEURSKENS AJ et al: Efficacy of traction for non-specific low back pain: A randomised clinical trial. Lancet 346:1596, 1995

BIGOS SJ: Perils, pitfalls, and accomplishments of guidelines for treatment of back problems. Neurol Clin North Am 17(1):179, 1999

CAREY TS et al: The outcomes and costs of care for acute low back pain among patients seen by primary care practitioners, chiropractors, and orthopedic surgeons. N Engl J Med 333:913, 1995

CASSIDY JD et al: Effect of eliminating compensation for pain and suffering on the outcome of insurance claims for whiplash injury. N Engl J Med 342:1179, 2000

CHERKIN DC et al: A comparison of physical therapy, chiropractic manipulation, and provision of an educational booklet for the treatment of patients with low back pain. JAMA 339(15):1021, 1998

DALTROY LH et al: A controlled trial of an educational program to prevent low back injuries. N Engl J Med 337:322, 1998

FRANKLIN GM et al: Outcome of surgery for thoracic outlet syndrome in Washington state workers' compensation. Neurology 54:1252, 2000

LAUDER TD et al: Effect of history and exam in predicting electrodiagnostic outcome among patients with suspected lumbosacral radiculopathy. Am J Phys Med Rehabil 79(1):60, 75, 2000

MALMIVAARA A et al: The treatment of acute low back pain—bed rest, exercises, or ordinary activity? N Engl J Med 332:351, 1995

STADNIK TW et al: Annular tears and disk herniation: Prevalence and contrast enhancement on MR images in the absence of low back pain or sciatica. Radiology 206(1): 49, 1998

VROOMEN PCAJ et al: Lack of effectiveness of bed rest for sciatica. N Engl J Med 40(6): 418, 1999

Section 2

ALTERATIONS IN BODY TEMPERATURE

17   *Charles A. Dinarello, Jeffrey A. Gelfand*

FEVER AND HYPERTHERMIA

Body temperature is controlled by the hypothalamus. Neurons in both the preoptic anterior hypothalamus and the posterior hypothalamus receive two kinds of signals: one from peripheral nerves that reflect warmth/cold receptors and the other from the temperature of the blood bathing the region. These two types of signals are integrated by the thermoregulatory center of the hypothalamus to maintain normal temperature. In a neutral environment, the metabolic rate of humans consistently produces more heat than is necessary to maintain the core body temperature at 37°C. Therefore, the hypothalamus controls temperature by mechanisms of heat loss.

A normal body temperature is ordinarily maintained, despite environmental variations, because the hypothalamic thermoregulatory center balances the excess heat production derived from metabolic activity in muscle and the liver with heat dissipation from the skin and lungs. According to recent studies of healthy individuals 18 to 40 years of age, the mean oral temperature is 36.8° ± 0.4°C (98.2° ± 0.7°F), with low levels at 6 A.M. and higher levels at 4 to 6 P.M. The maximum normal oral temperature is 37.2°C (98.9°F) at 6 A.M. and 37.7°C (99.9°F) at 4 P.M.; these values define the 99th percentile for healthy individuals. In light of these studies, *an A.M. temperature of >37.2°C (98.9°F) or a P.M. temperature of >37.7°C (99.9°F) would define a fever.* The normal daily temperature variation is typically 0.5°C (0.9°F). However, in some individuals recovering from a febrile illness, this daily variation can be as great as 1.0°C. During a febrile illness, diurnal variations are usually maintained but at higher levels. Daily temperature swings do not occur in patients with hyperthermia (see below). Rectal temperatures are generally 0.4°C (0.7°F) higher than oral readings. The lower oral readings are probably attributable to mouth breathing, which is a particularly important factor in patients with respiratory infections and rapid breathing. Lower esophageal temperatures closely reflect core temperature. Tympanic membrane (TM) thermometers measure radiant heat energy from the tympanic membrane and nearby ear canal and display that absolute value (unadjusted mode) or a value automatically calculated from the absolute reading on the basis of nomograms relating the radiant temperature measured to actual core temperatures obtained in clinical studies (adjusted mode). These measurements, although convenient, may be more variable than directly determined oral or rectal values. Studies in adults show that readings are lower with unadjusted-mode than with adjusted-mode TM thermometers and that unadjusted-mode TM values are 0.8°C (1.6°F) lower than rectal temperatures.

In women who menstruate, the A.M. temperature is generally lower in the 2 weeks before ovulation; it then rises by about 0.6°C (1°F) with ovulation and remains at that level until menses occur. Seasonal variation in body temperature has been described but may reflect a metabolic change and is not common. Body temperature is elevated in the postprandial state, but this elevation does not represent fever. Pregnancy and endocrinologic dysfunction also affect body temperature. The daily temperature variation appears to be fixed in early childhood; in contrast, elderly individuals can exhibit a reduced ability to develop fever, with only a modest fever even in severe infections.

FEVER VERSUS HYPERTHERMIA

FEVER Fever is an elevation of body temperature that exceeds the normal daily variation and occurs *in conjunction with an increase in the hypothalamic set point*—for example, from 37°C to 39°C. This shift of the set point from "normothermic" to febrile levels very much resembles the resetting of the home thermostat to a higher level in order to raise the ambient temperature in a room. Once the hypothalamic set point is raised, neurons in the vasomotor center are activated and vasoconstriction commences. The individual first notices vasoconstriction in the hands and feet. Shunting of blood away from the periphery to the internal organs essentially decreases heat loss from the skin, and the person feels cold. For most fevers, body temperature increases by 1 to 2°C. Shivering, which increases heat production from the muscles, may begin at this time; however, shivering is not required if heat conservation mechanisms raise blood temperature sufficiently. Heat production from the liver also increases. In humans, behavioral instincts (e.g., putting on more clothing or bedding) lead to a reduction of exposed surfaces, which helps raise body temperature.

The processes of heat conservation (vasoconstriction) and heat production (shivering and increased metabolic activity) continue until the temperature of the blood bathing the hypothalamic neurons matches the new thermostat setting. Once that point is reached, the hypothalamus maintains the temperature at the febrile level by the same mechanisms of heat balance that are operative in the afebrile state. When the hypothalamic set point is again reset downward (due to either a reduction in the concentration of pyrogens or the use of antipyretics), the processes of heat loss through vasodilation and sweating are initiated. Behavioral changes triggered at this time include the removal of insulating clothing or bedding. Loss of heat by sweating and vasodilation continues until the blood temperature at the hypothalamic level matches the lower setting.

A fever of >41.5°C (106.7°F) is called *hyperpyrexia*. This extraordinarily high fever can develop in patients with severe infections but most commonly occurs in patients with central nervous system hemorrhages. In the preantibiotic era, fever due to a variety of infectious diseases rarely exceeded 106°F, and there has been speculation that this natural "thermal ceiling" is mediated by neuropeptides functioning as central antipyretics.

In some rare cases, the hypothalamic set point is elevated as a result of local trauma, hemorrhage, tumor, or intrinsic hypothalamic malfunction. The term *hypothalamic fever* is sometimes used to describe elevated temperature caused by abnormal hypothalamic function. However, most patients with hypothalamic damage have *sub*normal, not *supra*normal, body temperatures. These patients do not respond properly to mild environmental temperature changes. For example, when exposed to only mildly cold conditions, their core temperature falls quickly rather than over the normal period of a few hours. In the very few patients in whom elevated core temperature is suspected to be due to hypothalamic damage, diagnosis depends on the demonstration of other abnormalities in hypothalamic function, such as the production of hypothalamic releasing factors, abnormal response to cold, and absence of circadian temperature and hormonal rhythms.

HYPERTHERMIA Hyperthermia is characterized by *an unchanged (normothermic) setting of the thermoregulatory center* in conjunction with an uncontrolled increase in body temperature that exceeds the body's ability to lose heat. Exogenous heat exposure and endogenous heat production are two mechanisms by which hyperthermia can result in dangerously high internal temperatures. Excessive heat production can easily cause hyperthermia despite physiologic and behavioral control of body temperature. For example, over-insulating clothing can result in an elevated core temperature, and work or exercise in hot environments can produce heat faster than peripheral mechanisms can lose it.

Although most patients with elevated body temperature have fever, there are a few circumstances in which elevated temperature represents not fever but hyperthermia (Table 17-1). *Heat stroke*, caused by thermoregulatory failure in association with a warm environment, may be categorized as exertional or nonexertional. *Exertional heat stroke* typically occurs in younger individuals exercising at ambient temperatures and/or humidities that are higher than normal. Even in normal individuals, dehydration or the use of common medications (e.g., over-the-counter antihistamines with anticholinergic side effects) may help to precipitate exertional heat stroke. *Nonexertional* or *classic heat stroke* typically occurs in elderly individuals, particularly during heat waves. For example, in Chicago in July 1995, 465 deaths were certified as heat related. The elderly, the bedridden, persons taking anticholinergic or antiparkinsonian drugs or diuretics, and individuals confined to poorly ventilated and non-air-conditioned environments are most susceptible.

Drug-induced hyperthermia has become increasingly common as a result of the increased use of prescription psychotropic drugs and illicit drugs. Drug-induced hyperthermia may be caused by monoamine oxidase inhibitors, tricyclic antidepressants, and amphetamines and by the illicit use of phencyclidine, lysergic acid diethylamide (LSD), or cocaine.

Table 17-1 Causes of Hyperthermia Syndromes

Heat stroke
  Exertional: Exercise in higher-than-normal heat and/or humidity
  Nonexertional: Anticholinergics, including antihistamines; antiparkinsonian drugs; diuretics; phenothiazines
Drug-induced hyperthermia
  Amphetamines; monoamine oxidase inhibitors; cocaine; phencyclidine; tricyclic antidepressants; LSD
Neuroleptic malignant syndrome
  Phenothiazines; butyrophenones, including haloperidol and bromperidol; fluoxetine; loxapine; tricyclic dibenzodiazepines; metoclopramide; domperidone; thiothixene; molindone
Malignant hyperthermia
  Inhalational anesthetics; succinylcholine
Endocrinopathy
  Thyrotoxicosis
  Pheochromocytoma

SOURCE: After FJ Curley, RS Irwin, JM Rippe et al (eds): *Intensive Care Medicine*, 3d ed. Boston, Little, Brown, 1996.

Malignant hyperthermia occurs in individuals with an inherited abnormality of skeletal-muscle sarcoplasmic reticulum that causes a rapid increase in intracellular calcium levels in response to halothane and other inhalational anesthetics or to succinylcholine. Elevated temperature, increased muscle metabolism, rigidity, rhabdomyolysis, acidosis, and cardiovascular instability develop rapidly. This condition is often fatal. The *neuroleptic malignant syndrome* can occur with phenothiazines and other drugs such as haloperidol and is characterized by muscle rigidity, autonomic dysregulation, and hyperthermia. This disorder appears to be caused by the inhibition of central dopamine receptors in the hypothalamus, which results in increased heat generation and decreased heat dissipation. Thyrotoxicosis and pheochromocytoma can also cause increased thermogenesis.

It is important to distinguish between fever and hyperthermia since hyperthermia can be rapidly fatal and characteristically does not respond to antipyretics. However, there is no rapid way to make this distinction. Hyperthermia is often diagnosed on the basis of the events immediately preceding the elevation of core temperature—e.g., heat exposure or treatment with drugs that interfere with thermoregulation. However, in addition to the clinical history of the patient, the physical aspects of some forms of hyperthermia may alert the clinician. For example, in patients with heat stroke syndromes and in those taking drugs that block sweating, the skin is hot but dry. Moreover, antipyretics do not reduce the elevated temperature in hyperthermia, whereas in fever—and even in hyperpyrexia—adequate doses of either aspirin or acetaminophen usually result in some decrease in body temperature.

PYROGENS   The term *pyrogen* is used to describe any substance that causes fever. *Exogenous* pyrogens are derived from outside the patient; most are microbial products, microbial toxins, or whole microorganisms. The classic example of an exogenous pyrogen is the lipopolysaccharide endotoxin produced by all gram-negative bacteria. Endotoxins are potent not only as pyrogens but also as inducers of various pathologic changes in gram-negative infections. Another group of potent bacterial pyrogens is produced by gram-positive organisms and includes the enterotoxins of *Staphylococcus aureus* and the group A and B streptococcal toxins, also called *superantigens*. One staphylococcal toxin of clinical importance is the toxic shock syndrome toxin associated with isolates of *S. aureus* from patients with toxic shock syndrome. Like the endotoxins of gram-negative bacteria, the toxins produced by staphylococci and streptococci cause fever in experimental animals when injected intravenously at concentrations of <1 μg/kg of body weight. Endotoxin is a highly pyrogenic molecule in humans: a dose of 2 to 3 ng/kg produces fever and generalized symptoms of malaise in volunteers.

PYROGENIC CYTOKINES   Cytokines are small proteins (molecular mass, 10,000 to 20,000 Da) that regulate immune, inflammatory, and hematopoietic processes. For example, stimulation of lymphocyte proliferation during an immune response to vaccination is the result of the cytokines interleukin (IL) 2, IL-4, and IL-6. Another cytokine, granulocyte colony-stimulating factor, stimulates granulocytopoiesis in the bone marrow. Some cytokines cause fever and hence are called *pyrogenic cytokines*. From a historic point of view, the field of cytokine biology began in the 1940s with laboratory investigations into fever induction by products of activated leukocytes. These fever-producing molecules were called *endogenous pyrogens*. When endogenous pyrogens were purified from activated leukocytes, they were shown to possess various biologic activities, which are now recognized as the properties of the various cytokines.

The known pyrogenic cytokines include IL-1, IL-6, tumor necrosis factor (TNF), ciliary neurotropic factor (CNTF), and interferon (IFN) α. Others probably exist. Each cytokine is encoded by a separate gene, and each pyrogenic cytokine has been shown to cause fever in laboratory animals and in humans. When injected into humans, IL-1, IL-6, and TNF produce fever at low doses (10 to 100 ng/kg).

The synthesis and release of endogenous pyrogenic cytokines are induced by a wide spectrum of exogenous pyrogens, most of which have recognizable bacterial or fungal sources. Viruses also induce pyrogenic cytokines by infecting cells. However, in the absence of microbial infection, inflammation, trauma, tissue necrosis, or antigen-antibody complexes can induce the production of IL-1, TNF, and/or IL-6, which—individually or in combination—trigger the hypothalamus to raise the set point to febrile levels. The cellular sources of pyrogenic cytokines are primarily monocytes, neutrophils, and lymphocytes, although many other types of cells can synthesize these molecules when stimulated.

ELEVATION OF THE HYPOTHALAMIC SET POINT BY CYTOKINES   During fever, levels of prostaglandin E_2 (PGE_2) are elevated in hypothalamic tissue and the third cerebral ventricle. The concentrations of PGE_2 are highest near the circumventricular vascular organs (organum vasculosum of lamina terminalis)—networks of enlarged capillaries surrounding the hypothalamic regulatory centers. Destruction of these organs reduces the ability of pyrogens to produce fever. Most studies in animals have failed to show, however, that pyrogenic cytokines pass from the circulation into the brain itself. Thus, it appears that both exogenous and endogenous pyrogens interact with the endothelium of these capillaries and that this interaction is the first step in initiating fever—i.e., in raising the set point to febrile levels.

The key events in the production of fever are illustrated in Fig. 17-1. As has been mentioned, several cell types can produce pyrogenic cytokines. Pyrogenic cytokines such as IL-1, IL-6, and TNF are released from the cells and enter the systemic circulation. Although the systemic effects of these circulating cytokines lead to fever by inducing the synthesis of PGE_2, they also induce PGE_2 in peripheral tissues. The increase in PGE_2 in the periphery accounts for the nonspecific myalgias and arthralgias that often accompany fever. However, it is the induction of PGE_2 in the brain that starts the process of raising the hypothalamic set point for core temperature.

There are four receptors for PGE_2, and each signals the cell in different ways. Of the four receptors, the third (EP-3) is essential for fever: when the gene for this receptor is deleted in mice, no fever follows the injection of IL-1 or endotoxin. Deletion of the other PGE_2 receptor genes leaves the fever mechanism intact. Although PGE_2 is essential for fever, it is not a neurotransmitter. Rather, the release of PGE_2 from the brain side of the hypothalamic endothelium triggers the PGE_2 receptor on glial cells, and this stimulation results in the rapid release of cyclic adenosine 5′-monophosphate (cyclic AMP), which is a neurotransmitter. As shown in Fig. 17-1, the release of cyclic AMP from the glial cells activates neuronal endings from the thermoregulatory center that extend into the area. The elevation of cyclic AMP is thought to account for changes in the hypothalamic set point either directly or indirectly by inducing the release of monoamine

FIGURE 17-1 Chronology of events required for the induction of fever.

neurotransmitters. Since receptors for endotoxin are in many ways similar to IL-1 receptors, the activation of endotoxin receptors on the hypothalamic endothelium also results in PGE_2 production and fever.

PRODUCTION OF CYTOKINES IN THE CENTRAL NERVOUS SYSTEM Several viral diseases produce active infection in the brain. Glial and possibly neuronal cells synthesize IL-1, TNF, and IL-6. CNTF is also synthesized by neural as well as neuronal cells. What role in the production of fever is played by these cytokines produced in the brain itself? In experimental animals, the concentrations of cytokine required to cause fever are several orders of magnitude lower with direct injection into the brain than with intravenous injection. Therefore, central nervous system production of these cytokines apparently can raise the hypothalamic set point, bypassing the circumventricular organs involved in fever caused by circulating cytokines. Central nervous system cytokines may account for the hyperpyrexia of central nervous system hemorrhage, trauma, or infection.

Approach to the Patient

History It is in the diagnosis of a febrile illness that the science and art of medicine come together. In no other clinical situation is a meticulous history more important. Painstaking attention must be paid to the chronology of symptoms in relation to the use of prescription drugs (including drugs or herbs taken without a physician's supervision) or treatments such as surgical or dental procedures. The exact nature of any prosthetic materials and/or implanted devices should be ascertained. A careful occupational history should include exposures to animals; toxic fumes; potential infectious agents; possible antigens; or other febrile or infected individuals in the home, workplace, or school. A history of the geographic areas in which the patient has lived and a travel history should include locations during military service. Information on unusual hobbies, dietary proclivities (such as raw or poorly cooked meat, raw fish, and unpasteurized milk or cheeses), and household pets should be elicited, as should that on sexual orientation and practices, including precautions taken or omitted. Attention should be directed to the use of tobacco, marijuana, intravenous drugs, or alcohol; trauma; animal bites; tick or other insect bites; and prior transfusions, immunizations, drug allergies, or hypersensitivities. A careful family history should include information on family members with tuberculosis, other febrile or infectious diseases, arthritis or collagen vascular disease, or unusual familial symptomatology such as deafness, urticaria, fevers and polyserositis, bone pain, or anemia. Ethnic origin may be critical. For example, blacks are more likely than persons in other groups to have hemoglobinopathies. Turks, Arabs, Armenians, and Sephardic Jews are especially likely to have familial Mediterranean fever.

Physical Examination A meticulous physical examination should be repeated on a regular basis. All the vital signs are relevant. The temperature may be taken orally or rectally, but the site used should be consistent. Axillary temperatures are notoriously unreliable. Particular attention should be paid to daily (or sometimes more frequent) physical examination, which should continue until the diagnosis is certain and the anticipated response has been achieved. Special attention should be paid to the skin, lymph nodes, eyes, nail beds, cardiovascular system, chest, abdomen, musculoskeletal system, and nervous system. Rectal examination is imperative. The penis, prostate, scrotum, and testes should be examined carefully and the foreskin, if present, retracted. Pelvic examination must be part of every complete physical examination of a woman, with a search for such causes of fever as pelvic inflammatory disease and tubo-ovarian abscess.

Laboratory Tests Few signs and symptoms in medicine have as many diagnostic possibilities as fever. If the history, epidemiologic situation, or physical examination suggests more than a simple viral illness or streptococcal pharyngitis, then laboratory testing is indicated. The tempo and complexity of the workup will depend on the pace of the illness, diagnostic considerations, and the immune status of the host. If findings are focal or if the history, epidemiologic setting, or physical examination suggests certain diagnoses, the laboratory examination can be focused. If fever is undifferentiated, the diagnostic nets must be cast farther, and certain guidelines are indicated, as follows.

Clinical pathology The workup should include a complete blood count; a differential count should be performed manually or with an instrument sensitive to the identification of eosinophils, juvenile or band forms, toxic granulations, and Döhle bodies, the last three of which are suggestive of bacterial infection. Neutropenia may be present with some viral infections, particularly parvovirus B19 infection; drug reactions; systemic lupus erythematosus; typhoid; brucellosis; and infiltrative diseases of the bone marrow, including lymphoma, leukemia, tuberculosis, and histoplasmosis. Lymphocytosis may occur with typhoid, brucellosis, tuberculosis, and viral disease. Atypical lymphocytes are documented in many viral diseases, including infection with Epstein-Barr virus, cytomegalovirus, or HIV; dengue; rubella; varicella; measles; and viral hepatitis. This abnormality also occurs in serum sickness and toxoplasmosis. Monocytosis is a feature of typhoid, tuberculosis, brucellosis, and lymphoma. Eosinophilia may be associated with hypersensitivity drug reactions, Hodgkin's disease, adrenal insufficiency, and certain metazoan infections. If the febrile illness appears to be severe or is prolonged, the smear should be examined carefully for malarial or babesial pathogens (where appropriate) as well as for classic morphologic features, and the erythrocyte sedimentation rate should be determined. Urinalysis, with examination of urinary sediment, is indicated. It is axiomatic that any abnormal fluid accumulation (pleural, peritoneal, joint), even if previously sampled, merits reexamination in the presence of undiagnosed fever. Joint fluids should be examined for bacteria as well as crystals. Bone marrow biopsy (not simple aspiration) for histopathologic studies (as well as culture) is indicated when marrow infiltration by pathogens or tumor cells is possible. Stool should be inspected for occult blood; an inspection for fecal leukocytes, ova, or parasites also may be indicated.

Chemistry Electrolyte, glucose, blood urea nitrogen, and creatinine levels should be measured. Liver function tests are usually indicated if efforts to identify the cause of fever do not point to the involvement of another organ. Additional assessments (e.g., measurement of creatinine phosphokinase or amylase) can be added as the workup progresses.

Microbiology Smears and cultures of specimens from the throat, urethra, anus, cervix, and vagina should be assessed when there are no localizing findings or when findings suggest the involvement of the pelvis or the gastrointestinal tract. If respiratory tract infection is suspected, sputum evaluation (Gram's staining, staining for acid-fast bacilli, culture) is indicated. Cultures of blood, abnormal fluid collections, and urine are indicated when fever is thought to reflect more than uncomplicated viral illness. Cerebrospinal fluid should be examined and cultured if meningismus, severe headache, or a change in mental status is noted.

Radiology A chest x-ray is usually part of the evaluation for any significant febrile illness.

Outcome of Diagnostic Efforts In most cases of fever, either the patient recovers spontaneously or the history, physical examination, and initial screening laboratory studies lead to a diagnosis. When fever continues for 2 to 3 weeks, during which time repeat physical examinations and laboratory tests are unrevealing, the patient is provisionally diagnosed as having fever of unknown origin (Chap. 125).

TREATMENT **The Decision to Treat Fever** Most fevers are associated with self-limited infections, most commonly of viral origin. In these cases, the general cause of the fever is easily identified. The routine use of antipyretics given automatically as "standing," "routine," or "prn" orders to treat low-grade fevers in adult patients on hospital wards is entirely unacceptable. This practice masks not only fever but also other important clinical indicators of a patient's course. The assumption underlying any decision to reduce fever with antipyretics is that there is no diagnostic benefit to be gained by allowing the fever to persist. However, there may be such a diagnostic benefit. For example, the daily highs and lows of normal temperature are exaggerated in most fevers, but the usual times of peak and trough temperatures may be reversed in typhoid fever and disseminated tuberculosis. Temperature-pulse dissociation (relative bradycardia) occurs in typhoid fever, brucellosis, leptospirosis, some drug-induced fevers, and factitious fever. In newborns, the elderly, patients with chronic renal failure, and patients taking glucocorticoids, fever may not be present despite infection, or core temperature may be hypothermic. Hypothermia is observed in patients with septic shock.

Some febrile diseases have characteristic patterns. With *relapsing* fevers, febrile episodes are separated by intervals of normal temperature; when paroxysms occur on the first and third days, the fever is called *tertian*. *Plasmodium vivax* causes tertian fevers. *Quartan* fevers are associated with paroxysms on the first and fourth days and are seen with *P. malariae*. Other relapsing fevers are related to *Borrelia* infections and rat-bite fever, which are both associated with days of fever followed by a several-day afebrile period and then a relapse of days of fever. Pel-Ebstein fever, with fevers lasting 3 to 10 days followed by afebrile periods of 3 to 10 days, is classic for Hodgkin's disease and other lymphomas. Another characteristic fever is that of cyclic neutropenia, in which fevers occur every 21 days and accompany the neutropenia. There is no periodicity of fever in patients with familial Mediterranean fever.

Mechanisms of Antipyretic Agents   The synthesis of PGE_2 depends on the constitutively expressed enzyme cyclooxygenase. The substrate for cyclooxygenase is arachidonic acid released from the cell membrane, and this release is the rate-limiting step in the synthesis of PGE_2. Inhibitors of cyclooxygenase are potent antipyretics. The antipyretic potency of various drugs is directly correlated with the inhibition of brain cyclooxygenase. Acetaminophen is a poor cyclooxygenase inhibitor in peripheral tissue and is without noteworthy anti-inflammatory activity; in the brain, however, acetaminophen is oxidized by the p450 cytochrome system, and the oxidized form inhibits cyclooxygenase activity.

Oral aspirin and acetaminophen are equally effective in reducing fever in humans. Nonsteroidal anti-inflammatory agents (NSAIDs) such as indomethacin and ibuprofen are also excellent antipyretics. Chronic high-dose therapy with antipyretics such as aspirin or the NSAIDs used in arthritis does not reduce normal core body temperature. Thus, PGE_2 appears to play no role in normal thermoregulation.

As effective antipyretics, glucocorticoids act at two levels. First, similar to the cyclooxygenase inhibitors, glucocorticoids reduce PGE_2 synthesis by inhibiting the activity of phospholipase A_2, which is needed to release arachidonic acid from the cell membrane. Second, glucocorticoids block the transcription of the mRNA for the pyrogenic cytokines.

Drugs that interfere with vasoconstriction (phenothiazines, for example) can act as antipyretics, as can drugs that block muscle contractions. However, these agents are not true antipyretics since they can also reduce core temperature independently of hypothalamic control.

Indications and Regimens for the Treatment of Fever   The objectives in treating fever are first to reduce the elevated hypothalamic set point and second to facilitate heat loss. There is no evidence that fever itself facilitates the recovery from infection or acts as an adjuvant to the immune system. In fact, peripheral PGE_2 production is a potent immunosuppressant. Hence, treating fever and its symptoms does no harm and does not slow the resolution of common viral and bacterial infections. Reducing fever with antipyretics also reduces systemic symptoms of headache, myalgias, and arthralgias.

Oral aspirin and NSAIDs effectively reduce fever but can ad-

versely affect platelets and the gastrointestinal tract. Therefore, acetaminophen is preferred to all of these agents as an antipyretic. In children, acetaminophen must be used because aspirin increases the risk of Reye's syndrome. If the patient cannot take oral antipyretics, parenteral preparations of NSAIDs and rectal suppository preparations of various antipyretics can be used.

Treatment of fever in some patient groups is recommended. Fever increases the demand for oxygen (i.e., for every increase of 1°C over 37°C, there is a 13% increase in oxygen consumption) and can aggravate preexisting cardiac, cerebrovascular, or pulmonary insufficiency. Elevated temperature can induce mental changes in patients with organic brain disease. Children with a history of febrile or nonfebrile seizure should be aggressively treated to reduce fever, although it is unclear what triggers the febrile seizure and there is no correlation between absolute temperature elevation and onset of a febrile seizure in susceptible children.

In hyperpyrexia, the use of cooling blankets facilitates the reduction of temperature; however, cooling blankets should not be used without oral antipyretics. In hyperpyretic patients with central nervous system disease or trauma, reducing core temperature mitigates the ill effects of high temperature on the brain.

Treating Hyperthermia   A high core temperature in a patient with an appropriate history (e.g., environmental heat exposure or treatment with anticholinergic or neuroleptic drugs, tricyclic antidepressants, succinylcholine, or halothane) along with appropriate clinical findings (dry skin, hallucinations, delirium, pupil dilation, muscle rigidity, and/or elevated levels of creatine phosphokinase) suggests hyperthermia. The attempt to lower the already normal hypothalamic set point is of little use. Physical cooling with sponging, fans, cooling blankets, and even ice baths should be initiated immediately in conjunction with the administration of intravenous fluids and appropriate pharmacologic agents (see below). If insufficient cooling is achieved by external means, internal cooling can be achieved by gastric or peritoneal lavage with iced saline. In extreme circumstances, hemodialysis or even cardiopulmonary bypass with cooling of blood may be performed.

Malignant hyperthermia should be treated immediately with cessation of anesthesia and intravenous administration of dantrolene sodium. The recommended dose of dantrolene is 1 to 2.5 mg/kg of body weight given intravenously every 6 h for at least 24 to 48 h—until oral dantrolene can be administered, if needed. Procainamide should also be administered to patients with malignant hyperthermia because of the likelihood of ventricular fibrillation in this syndrome. Dantrolene at similar doses is indicated in the neuroleptic malignant syndrome and in drug-induced hyperthermia and may even be useful in the hyperthermia of thyrotoxicosis. The neuroleptic malignant syndrome may also be treated with bromocriptine, levodopa, amantadine, or nifedipine or by induction of muscle paralysis with curare and pancuronium. Tricyclic antidepressant overdose may be treated with physostigmine.

BIBLIOGRAPHY

ATKINS E: Pathogenesis of fever. Physiol Rev 40:580, 1960

BREDER CD et al: Interleukin-1 immunoreactive innervation of the human hypothalamus. Science 240:321, 1988

COCEANI F et al: Prostaglandin E_2 fever: A continuing debate. Yale J Biol Med 59:169, 1986

FLOWER RJ et al: Inhibition of prostaglandin synthetase in brain explains the anti-pyretic activity of paracetamol (4-acetamidophenol). Nature 240:410, 1972

MACKOWIAK PA: Carl Reinhold August Wunderlich and the evolution of clinical thermometry. Clin Infect Dis 18:458, 1994

——: Concepts of fever. Arch Intern Med 158:1870, 1998

—— et al: A critical appraisal of 98.6°F, the upper limit of the normal body temperature, and other legacies of Carl Reinhold August Wunderlich. JAMA 268:1578, 1992

USHIKUBI F et al: Impaired febrile response in mice lacking the prostaglandin E receptor subtype EP3. Nature 395:281, 1998

WOLFF SM: Biological effects of bacterial endotoxins in man. J Infect Dis 128:733, 1973

YANG RB et al: Toll-like receptor-2 mediates lipopolysaccharide-induced cellular signalling. Nature 395:284, 1998

18

Elaine T. Kaye, Kenneth M. Kaye

FEVER AND RASH

The acutely ill patient with fever and rash often presents a diagnostic challenge for physicians. The distinctive appearance of an eruption in concert with a clinical syndrome may facilitate a prompt diagnosis and the institution of life-saving therapy or critical infection-control interventions.

Approach to the Patient

A thorough history of patients with fever and rash includes the following relevant information: immune status, medications taken within the previous month, specific travel history, immunization status, exposure to domestic pets and other animals, history of animal or arthropod bites, existence of cardiac abnormalities, presence of prosthetic material, recent exposure to ill individuals, and exposure to sexually transmitted diseases. The history should also include the site of onset of the rash and its direction and rate of spread.

A thorough physical examination entails close attention to the rash, with an assessment and precise definition of its salient features. First, it is critical to determine the *type* of lesions that make up the eruption. *Macules* are flat lesions defined by an area of changed color (i.e., a blanchable erythema). *Papules* are raised, solid lesions <5 mm in diameter; *plaques* are lesions >5 mm in diameter with a flat, plateau-like surface; and *nodules* are lesions >5 mm in diameter with a more rounded configuration. *Wheals* (urticaria, hives) are papules or plaques that are pale pink and may appear annular (ringlike) as they enlarge; classic (nonvasculitic) wheals are transient, lasting only 24 to 48 h in any defined area. *Vesicles* (<5 mm) and *bullae* (>5 mm) are circumscribed, elevated lesions containing fluid. *Pustules* are raised lesions containing purulent exudate; vesicular processes such as varicella or herpes simplex may evolve to pustules. *Nonpalpable purpura* is a flat lesion that is due to bleeding into the skin; if <3 mm in diameter, the purpuric lesions are termed *petechiae*; if >3 mm, they are termed *ecchymoses. Palpable purpura* is a raised lesion that is due to inflammation of the vessel wall (vasculitis) with subsequent hemorrhage. An *ulcer* is a defect in the skin extending at least into the upper layer of the dermis, and an *eschar* (tâche noire) is a necrotic lesion covered with a black crust.

Other pertinent features of rashes include their *configuration* (i.e., annular or target), the *arrangement* of their lesions, and their *distribution* (i.e., central or peripheral). →*For further discussion, see Chaps. 55 and 57.*

CLASSIFICATION OF RASH This chapter reviews rashes that reflect systemic disease but does not include localized skin eruptions (i.e., cellulitis, impetigo) that may also be associated with fever (Chap. 128). Rashes are classified herein on the basis of the morphology and distribution of lesions. For practical purposes, this classification system is based on the most typical disease presentations. However, morphology may vary as rashes evolve, and the presentation of diseases with rashes is subject to many variations (Chap. 57). For instance, the classic petechial rash of Rocky Mountain spotted fever (RMSF) may initially consist of blanchable erythematous macules distributed peripherally; at times, the rash associated with RMSF may not be predominantly acral, or a rash may not develop at all.

Diseases with fever and rash may be classified by type of eruption: centrally distributed maculopapular, peripheral, confluent desquamative erythematous, vesiculobullous, urticarial, nodular, purpuric, ulcerated, or eschars (Table 18-1). For a more detailed discussion of each disease associated with a rash, the reader is referred to the chapter dealing with that specific disease. (Reference chapters and color plates are cited in the text and listed in Table 18-1.)

Centrally Distributed Maculopapular Eruptions Centrally distributed rashes, in which lesions are primarily truncal, are the most common type of eruption. The rash of *measles* (rubeola) starts at the hairline 2 to 3 days into the illness and moves down the body, sparing the palms and soles (Chap. 194). It begins as discrete erythematous lesions, which become confluent as the rash spreads. Koplik's spots (1- to 2-mm white or bluish lesions with an erythematous halo on the buccal mucosa) are pathognomonic for measles and are generally seen during the first 2 days of symptoms. They should not be confused with Fordyce's spots (ectopic sebaceous glands), which have no erythematous halos and are found in the mouth of healthy individuals. Koplik's spots may briefly overlap with the measles exanthem.

German measles (rubella) also spreads from the hairline downward; unlike that of measles, however, the rash of rubella tends to clear from originally affected areas as it migrates and may be pruritic (Chap. 195). Forchheimer spots (palatal petechiae) may develop but are nonspecific since they also develop in mononucleosis (Chap. 184) and scarlet fever (Chap. 140). Postauricular and suboccipital adenopathy and arthritis are common among adults with German measles. Exposure of pregnant women to ill individuals should be avoided, as rubella causes severe congenital abnormalities. Numerous strains of enteroviruses (Chap. 193), primarily echoviruses and coxsackieviruses, cause nonspecific syndromes of fever and eruptions that may mimic rubella or measles. Patients with infectious mononucleosis caused by Epstein-Barr virus or with primary infection caused by HIV (Chap. 309) may exhibit pharyngitis, lymphadenopathy, and a nonspecific maculopapular exanthem.

The rash of *erythema infectiosum* (fifth disease), which is caused by human parvovirus B19, primarily affects children 3 to 12 years old; it develops after fever has resolved as a bright blanchable erythema on the cheeks ("slapped cheeks") with perioral pallor (Chap. 187). A more diffuse rash (often pruritic) appears the next day on the trunk and extremities and then rapidly develops into a lacy reticular eruption that may wax and wane (especially with temperature change) over 3 weeks. Adults with fifth disease often have arthritis, and fetal hydrops can develop in association with this condition in pregnant women.

Exanthem subitum (roseola) is most common among children under 3 years of age (Chap. 185). As in erythema infectiosum, the rash usually appears after fever has subsided. It consists of 2- to 3-mm rose-pink macules and papules that rarely coalesce, occur initially on the trunk and sometimes on the extremities (sparing the face), and fade within 2 days.

Though drug reactions have many manifestations, including urticaria, exanthematous *drug-induced eruptions* (Chap. 59) are most common and are often difficult to distinguish from viral exanthems. Eruptions elicited by drugs are usually more intensely erythematous and pruritic than viral exanthems, but this distinction is not reliable. A history of new medications and an absence of prostration may help to distinguish a drug-related rash from an eruption of another etiology. Rashes may persist for up to 2 weeks after administration of the offending agent is discontinued. Certain populations are more prone than others to drug rashes. Of HIV-infected patients, 50 to 60% develop a rash in response to sulfa drugs; 50 to 100% of patients with mononucleosis due to Epstein-Barr virus develop a rash when given ampicillin.

Rickettsial illnesses (Chap. 177) should be considered in the evaluation of individuals with centrally distributed maculopapular eruptions. The usual setting for *epidemic typhus* is a site of war or natural disaster in which people are exposed to body lice. A diagnosis of recrudescent typhus should be considered in European immigrants to the United States. However, an indigenous form of typhus, presumably transmitted by flying squirrels, has been reported in the southeastern United States. *Endemic typhus* or *leptospirosis* (the latter caused by a spirochete; Chap. 174) may be seen in urban environments where rodents proliferate. Outside the United States, other rickettsial diseases cause a spotted-fever syndrome and should be considered in residents

Table 18-1 Diseases Associated with Fever and Rash

Disease	Etiology	Description	Group Affected/ Epidemiologic Factors	Clinical Syndrome	Chapter/Color Atlas Reference
CENTRALLY DISTRIBUTED MACULOPAPULAR ERUPTIONS					
Measles (rubeola, first disease)	Paramyxovirus	Discrete lesions that become confluent as rash spreads from hairline downward, sparing palms and soles; lasts ≥3 days; Koplik's spots	Nonimmune individuals	Cough, conjunctivitis, coryza, severe prostration	194
German measles (rubella, third disease)	Togavirus	Spreads from hairline downward, clearing as it spreads; Forchheimer spots	Nonimmune individuals	Adenopathy, arthritis	195
Erythema infectiosum (fifth disease)	Human parvovirus B19	Bright-red "slapped-cheek" appearance followed by diffuse lacy reticular rash that waxes and wanes over 3 weeks	Most common in children aged 3–12 years; occurs in winter and spring	Mild fever; arthritis in adults	187/IID-40
Exanthem subitum (roseola, sixth disease)	Human herpesvirus 6	Diffuse maculopapular eruption (sparing face); resolves within 2 days	Usually affects children <3 years old	Rash following resolution of fever; similar to Boston exanthem (echovirus 16)	185
Primary HIV infection	HIV	Nonspecific diffuse macules and papules; may be urticarial; oral or genital ulcers in some cases	Individuals recently infected with HIV	Pharyngitis, adenopathy, arthralgias	309
Infectious mononucleosis	Epstein-Barr virus	Diffuse maculopapular eruption (10–15% of cases; 90% if ampicillin is given); urticaria in some cases; periorbital edema (50%); palatal petechiae (25%)	Adolescents, young adults	Hepatosplenomegaly, pharyngitis, cervical lymphadenopathy, atypical lymphocytosis, heterophile antibody	184
Other viral exanthems	Echoviruses 2, 4, 9, 11, 16, 19, and 25; coxsackieviruses A9, B1, and B5	Skin findings mimicking rubella or measles	Affect children more commonly than adults	Nonspecific viral syndromes	193
Exanthematous drug-induced eruption	Drugs (antibiotics, anticonvulsants, diuretics, etc.)	Intensely pruritic, bright-red macules and papules, symmetric on trunk and extremities; may become confluent	Occurs 2–3 d after exposure in those previously sensitized; otherwise, after 2–3 weeks (but can occur anytime, even after drug is discontinued)	Variable findings: fever and eosinophilia	59
Epidemic typhus	*Rickettsia prowazekii*	Maculopapular eruption appears in axillae, spreads to trunk and later to extremities; usually spares face, palms, soles; evolves from blanchable macules to confluent eruption with petechiae; rash evanescent in recrudescent typhus (Brill-Zinsser disease)	Exposure to body lice; occurrence of recrudescent typhus as relapse after 30–50 years	Headache, myalgias; 10–40% mortality if untreated; milder clinical presentation in recrudescent form	177
Endemic (murine) typhus	*Rickettsia typhi*	Maculopapular eruption, usually sparing palms, soles	Exposure to rat or cat fleas	Headache, myalgias	177
Scrub typhus	*Rickettsia tsutsugamushi*	Diffuse macular rash starting on trunk; eschar at site of mite bite	Endemic in South Pacific, Australia, Asia; transmitted by mites	Headache, myalgias, regional adenopathy; mortality up to 30% if untreated	177
Rickettsial spotted fevers	*Rickettsia conorii* (boutonneuse fever), *Rickettsia australis* (North Queensland tick typhus), *Rickettsia sibirica* (Siberian tick typhus)	Eschar at site of bite; maculopapular (rarely, vesicular and petechial) eruption on proximal extremities, spreading to trunk and face	Exposure to ticks; *R. conorii* in Mediterranean region, India, Africa; *R. australis* in Australia; *R. sibirica* in Siberia, Mongolia	Headache, myalgias, regional adenopathy	177
Ehrlichiosis	*Ehrlichia* spp.	Maculopapular eruption (40% of cases), involves trunk and extremities; may be petechial	Tick-borne; most common in U.S. Southeast and southern Midwest	Headache, myalgias, leukopenia	177
Leptospirosis	*Leptospira interrogans*	Maculopapular eruption; conjunctivitis; scleral hemorrhage in some cases	Exposure to water contaminated with animal urine	Myalgias; aseptic meningitis; *fulminant form*: icterohemorrhagic fever (Weil's disease)	174

(continued)

Table 18-1—(continued)

Disease	Etiology	Description	Group Affected/ Epidemiologic Factors	Clinical Syndrome	Chapter/Color Atlas Reference
Lyme disease	*Borrelia burgdorferi*	Papule expanding to erythematous annular lesion with central clearing (ECM; average diameter, 15 cm), sometimes with concentric rings, sometimes with indurated or vesicular center; multiple secondary ECM lesions in some cases	Bite of tick vector	Headache, myalgias, chills, photophobia occurring acutely; CNS disease, myocardial disease, arthritis weeks to months later in some cases	176/IID-46
Typhoid fever	*Salmonella typhi*	Blanchable erythematous macules and papules, 2–4 mm, usually on trunk (rose spots)	Ingestion of contaminated food or water (rare in U.S.)	Variable abdominal pain and diarrhea; headache, myalgias, hepatosplenomegaly	156
Rat-bite fever (sodoku)	*Spirillum minus*	Eschar at site of bite; then blotchy violaceous or red-brown rash involving trunk and extremities	Rate bite; primarily found in Asia; rare in U.S.	Regional adenopathy, recurrent fevers if untreated	127
Relapsing fever	*Borrelia* spp.	Central rash at end of febrile episode; petechiae in some cases	Exposure to ticks or body lice	Recurrent fever, headache, myalgias, hepatosplenomegaly	175
Erythema marginatum (rheumatic fever)	Group A *Streptococcus*	Erythematous annular papules and plaques occurring as polycyclic lesions in waves over trunk, proximal extremities; evolving and resolving within hours	Patients with rheumatic fever	Pharyngitis preceding polyarthritis, carditis, subcutaneous nodules, chorea	235
Systemic lupus erythematosus	Autoimmune disease	Macular and papular erythema, often in sun-exposed areas; discoid lupus lesions (local atrophy, scale, pigmentary changes); periungual telangiectasis; malar rash; vasculitis sometimes causing urticaria, palpable purpura; oral erosions in some cases	Most common in young to middle-aged women; flares precipitated by sun exposure	Arthritis; cardiac, pulmonary, renal, hematologic, and vasculitic disease	311/IIE-61, IIE-62
Still's disease	Autoimmune disease	Transient 2- to 5-mm erythematous papules appearing at height of fever on trunk, proximal extremities; lesions evanescent	Children and young adults	High spiking fever, polyarthritis, splenomegaly; erythrocyte sedimentation rate, >100 mm/h	326
Arcanobacterial pharyngitis	*Arcanobacterium (Corynebacterium) haemolyticum*	Diffuse, erythematous, maculopapular eruption involving trunk and proximal extremities; may desquamate	Children and young adults	Exudative pharyngitis, lymphadenopathy	141

PERIPHERAL ERUPTIONS

Disease	Etiology	Description	Group Affected/ Epidemiologic Factors	Clinical Syndrome	Chapter/Color Atlas Reference
Chronic meningococcemia, disseminated gonococcal infection[a]	—	—	—	—	146, 147
RMSF	*Rickettsia rickettsii*	Rash beginning on wrists and ankles and spreading centripetally; appears on palms and soles later in disease; lesion evolution from blanchable macules to petechiae	Tick vector; widespread but more common in southeastern and southwest-central U.S.	Headache, myalgias, abdominal pain; mortality up to 40% if untreated	177/IID-45
Secondary syphilis	*Treponema pallidum*	Coincident primary chancre in 10% of cases; copper-colored, scaly papular eruption, diffuse but prominent on palms and soles; rash never vesicular in adults; condyloma latum, mucous patches, and alopecia in some cases	Sexually transmitted	Fever, constitutional symptoms	172/IID-48, IID-50
Atypical measles	Paramyxovirus	Maculopapular eruption beginning on distal extremities and spreading centripetally; may evolve into vesicles or petechiae; edema of extremities; Koplik's spots absent	Individuals contracting measles who received killed measles vaccine between 1963 and 1967 in U.S.	Headache, nodular pneumonia	194
Hand-foot-and-mouth disease	Coxsackievirus A16	Tender vesicles, erosions in mouth; 0.25-cm papules on hands and feet with rim of erythema evolving into tender vesicles	Summer and fall; primarily children under 10 years; multiple family members	Transient fever	193/IID-39

(continued)

Table 18-1 Diseases Associated with Fever and Rash—(continued)

Disease	Etiology	Description	Group Affected/ Epidemiologic Factors	Clinical Syndrome	Chapter/Color Atlas Reference
Erythema multiforme	Drugs, infection, idiopathic causes	Target lesions (central erythema surrounded by area of clearing and another rim of erythema) up to 2 cm; symmetric on knees, elbows, palms, soles; may become diffuse; may involve mucosal surfaces	Drug intake (i.e., sulfa, phenytoin, penicillin); herpes simplex or *Mycoplasma pneumoniae* infection	Varies with predisposing factor	—,[b] IIE-67
Rat-bite fever (Haverhill fever)	*Streptobacillus moniliformis*	Maculopapular eruption over palms, soles, and extremities, tends to be more severe at joints; eruption may become generalized; may be purpuric; may desquamate	Rat bite, ingestion of contaminated food	Myalgias; arthritis (50%); fever recurrence in some cases	127
Bacterial endocarditis	*Streptococcus, Staphylococcus,* etc.	*Subacute course:* Osler's nodes (tender pink nodules on finger or toe pads); petechiae on skin and mucosa; splinter hemorrhages. *Acute course (S. aureus):* Janeway lesions (painless erythematous or hemorrhagic macules, usually on palms and soles)	Abnormal heart valve, intravenous drug use	New heart murmur	126/IID-58

CONFLUENT DESQUAMATIVE ERYTHEMAS

Disease	Etiology	Description	Group Affected/ Epidemiologic Factors	Clinical Syndrome	Chapter/Color Atlas Reference
Scarlet fever (second disease)	Group A *Streptococcus* (pyrogenic exotoxins A, B, C)	Diffuse blanchable erythema beginning on face and spreading to trunk and extremities; circumoral pallor; "sandpaper" texture to skin; accentuation of linear erythema in skin folds (Pastia's lines); enanthem of white evolving into red "strawberry" tongue; desquamation in second week	Most common in children aged 2–10 years; usually follows group A streptococcal pharyngitis	Fever, pharyngitis, headache	140
Kawasaki disease	Idiopathic causes	Rash similar to scarlet fever (scarlatiniform) or erythema multiforme; fissuring of lips, strawberry tongue; conjunctivitis; edema of hands, feet; desquamation later in disease	Children under 8 years	Cervical adenopathy, pharyngitis, coronary artery vasculitis	57, 317
Streptococcal toxic shock syndrome	Group A *Streptococcus* (associated with pyrogenic exotoxin A or certain M types)	When present, rash often scarlatiniform	May occur in setting of severe group A streptococcal infections, such as necrotizing fasciitis, bacteremia, pneumonia	Multiorgan failure, hypotension; 30% mortality rate	140
Staphylococcal toxic shock syndrome	*S. aureus* (toxic shock syndrome toxin 1, enterotoxin B or C)	Diffuse erythema involving palms; pronounced erythema of mucosal surfaces, conjunctivitis; desquamation 7–10 days into illness	Colonization with toxin-producing *S. aureus*	Fever >39°C (102°F), hypotension, multiorgan dysfunction	139
Staphylococcal scalded-skin syndrome	*S. aureus,* phage group II	Diffuse tender erythema, often with bullae and desquamation; Nikolsky's sign	Colonization with toxin-producing *S. aureus*; occurs in children under 10 (termed "Ritter's disease" in neonates) or adults with renal dysfunction	Irritability; nasal or conjunctival secretions	139
Exfoliative erythroderma syndrome	Underlying psoriasis, eczema, drug eruption, mycosis fungoides	Diffuse erythema (often scaling) interspersed with lesions of underlying condition	Usually occurs in adults over age 50; more common in men	Fever, chills (i.e., difficulty with thermoregulation); lymphadenopathy	56, 59
Toxic epidermal necrolysis	Drugs, other causes (infection, neoplasm, graft-vs.-host disease)	Diffuse erythema or target-like lesions progressing to bullae, with sloughing and necrosis of entire epidermis; Nikolsky's sign	Uncommon in children; more common in patients with HIV infection or graft-vs.-host disease	Dehydration, sepsis sometimes resulting from lack of normal skin integrity; 25% mortality	59

(continued)

Table 18-1—(continued)

Disease	Etiology	Description	Group Affected/ Epidemiologic Factors	Clinical Syndrome	Chapter/Color Atlas Reference
VESICULOBULLOUS ERUPTIONS					
Hand-foot-and-mouth syndrome[c]; staphylococcal scalded-skin syndrome, toxic epidermal necrolysis[d]	—	—	—	—	—[b]
Varicella (chicken-pox)	Varicella-zoster virus	Macules (2–3 mm) evolving into papules, then vesicles (sometimes umbilicated), on an erythematous base ("dewdrops on a rose petal"); pustules then forming and crusting; lesions appearing in crops; may involve scalp, mouth; intensely pruritic	Usually affects children; 10% of adults susceptible; most common in late winter and spring	Malaise; mild disease in healthy children; more severe disease with complications in adults and immuno-compromised children	183/IID-36
Disseminated herpes-virus infection	Varicella-zoster virus or herpes simplex virus (HSV)	Individual lesions similar for varicella-zoster and HSV; *zoster cutaneous dissemination*: >25 lesions extending outside involved dermatome; *HSV*: extensive, progressive mucocutaneous lesions in some cases; HSV lesions sometimes disseminate in eczematous skin (eczema herpeticum); HSV visceral dissemination may occur with only limited skin lesions	Immunosuppressed individuals, eczema	Visceral organ involvement (especially of liver) may occur	183, 373/IID-37
Rickettsialpox	*Rickettsia akari*	Eschar found at site of mite bite; generalized rash involving face, trunk, extremities; may involve palms and soles; <100 papules and plaques (2–10 mm); top of lesions develop vesicles that may evolve into pustules	Seen in urban settings; transmitted by mouse mites	Headache, myalgias, regional adenopathy; mild disease	177
Disseminated *Vibrio vulnificus* infection	*V. vulnificus*	Erythematous lesions evolving into hemorrhagic bullae and then into necrotic ulcers	Patients with cirrhosis, diabetes, renal failure; exposure by ingestion of contaminated saltwater seafood	Hypotension; 50% mortality	159
Ecthyma gangrenosum	*Pseudomonas aeruginosa*, other gram-negative rods, fungi	Indurated plaque evolving into hemorrhagic bulla or pustule that sloughs, resulting in eschar formation; erythematous halo; most common in axillary, groin, perianal regions	Usually affects neutropenic patients; occurs in up to 28% of individuals with *Pseudomonas* bacteremia	Clinical signs of sepsis	155/IID-57C
URTICARIAL ERUPTIONS					
Urticarial vasculitis	Serum sickness, often due to infection (including hepatitis B, enterovirus, parasitic), drugs (including penicillins, sulfonamides, salicylates, barbiturates); connective-tissue disease; idiopathic causes	Erythematous, circumscribed areas of edema; occasionally indurated; pruritic or burning; lesions sometimes purpuric; individual lesions lasting up to 5 days	In serum sickness, occurs 8–14 days after antigen exposure in nonsensitized individuals; may occur within 36 h in sensitized individuals	Malaise, lymphadenopathy, myalgias, arthralgias	317[b]/IIA-14A
NODULAR ERUPTIONS					
Disseminated infection	Fungi (e.g., candidiasis, histoplasmosis, cryptococcosis, sporotrichosis, coccidioidomycosis); mycobacteria	Subcutaneous nodules (up to 3 cm); fluctuance, draining common with mycobacteria; necrotic nodules (extremities, periorbital or nasal regions) common with *Aspergillus*, *Mucor*	Immunocompromised hosts (i.e., bone marrow transplant recipients, patients undergoing chemotherapy, HIV-infected patients, alcoholics)	Features vary with organism	—[b]

(continued)

Table 18-1 Diseases Associated with Fever and Rash—*(continued)*

Disease	Etiology	Description	Group Affected/ Epidemiologic Factors	Clinical Syndrome	Chapter/Color Atlas Reference
Erythema nodosum (septal panniculitis)	Infections (e.g., streptococcal, fungal, mycobacterial, yersinial); drugs (e.g., sulfas, penicillins, oral contraceptives); sarcoidosis; idiopathic causes	Large, violaceous, nonulcerative, subcutaneous nodules; exquisitely tender; usually on lower legs but also on upper extremities	More common in females aged 15–30	Arthralgias (50%); features vary with associated condition	—[b], IIE-70
Sweet's syndrome (acute febrile neutrophilic dermatosis)	Yersinial infection; lymphoproliferative disorders; idiopathic causes	Tender red or blue edematous nodules giving impression of vesiculation; usually on face, neck, upper extremities; when on lower extremities, may mimic erythema nodosum	More common in women and in persons aged 30–60; 20% of cases associated with malignancy (men and women equally affected in this group)	Headache, arthralgias, leukocytosis	57
Bacillary angiomatosis	*Bartonella henselae* or *Bartonella quintana*	Many forms, including erythematous, smooth vascular nodules; friable, exophytic lesions; erythematous plaques (may be dry, scaly); subcutaneous nodules (may be erythematous)	Usually in HIV infection	Peliosis of liver and spleen in some cases; lesions may involve multiple organs; bacteremia	163

PURPURIC ERUPTIONS

Disease	Etiology	Description	Group Affected/ Epidemiologic Factors	Clinical Syndrome	Chapter/Color Atlas Reference
RMSF, rat-bite fever, endocarditis[c]; epidemic typhus[e]	—	—	—	—	—[b]
Acute meningococcemia	*Neisseria meningitidis*	Petechiae rapidly becoming numerous, sometimes enlarging and becoming vesicular; trunk, extremities most commonly involved; may appear on face, hands, feet; may include purpura fulminans reflecting DIC (see below)	Most common in children, individuals with asplenia or terminal complement component deficiency (C5-C8)	Hypotension, meningitis (sometimes preceded by upper respiratory infection)	146/IID-44
Purpura fulminans	Severe DIC	Large ecchymoses with sharply irregular shapes evolving into hemorrhagic bullae and then into black necrotic lesions	Individuals with sepsis (e.g., involving *N. meningitidis*), malignancy, or massive trauma; asplenic patients at high risk for sepsis	Hypotension	124, 146
Chronic meningococcemia	*N. meningitidis*	Variety of recurrent eruptions, including pink maculopapular; nodular (usually on lower extremities); petechial (sometimes developing vesicular centers); purpuric areas with pale blue-gray centers	Individuals with complement deficiencies	Fevers, sometimes intermittent; arthritis, myalgias, headache	146
Disseminated gonococcal infection	*Neisseria gonorrhoeae*	Papules (1–5 mm) evolving over 1–2 days into hemorrhagic pustules with gray necrotic centers; hemorrhagic bullae occurring rarely; lesions (usually fewer than 40) distributed peripherally near joints (more commonly on upper extremities)	Sexually active individuals (more often females), some with complement deficiency	Low-grade fever, tenosynovitis, arthritis	147/IID-60
Enteroviral petechial rash	Usually echovirus 9 or coxsackievirus A9	Disseminated petechial lesions (may also be maculopapular, vesicular, or urticarial)	Often occurs in outbreaks	Pharyngitis, headache; aseptic meningitis with echovirus 9	193
Viral hemorrhagic fever	Arboviruses and arenaviruses	Petechial rash	Residence in or travel to endemic areas	Triad of fever, shock, hemorrhage from mucosa or gastrointestinal tract	198, 199
Thrombotic thrombocytopenic purpura	Idiopathic causes	Petechiae	Usually affects young adults; more common in women; hemolytic-uremic syndrome seen in children after gastroenteritis caused by *Escherichia coli* O157:H7	Fever, hemolytic anemia, thrombocytopenia, neurologic and renal dysfunction; coagulation studies normal	57, 108, 116

(continued)

Table 18-1—*(continued)*

Disease	Etiology	Description	Group Affected/ Epidemiologic Factors	Clinical Syndrome	Chapter/Color Atlas Reference
Cutaneous small-vessel vasculitis (leukocytoclastic vasculitis)	Infections (including group A *Streptococcus*, viral hepatitis), drugs, chemicals, food allergens, idiopathic causes	Palpable purpuric lesions appearing in crops on legs or other dependent areas; may become vesicular or ulcerative; usually resolve over 3–4 weeks	Occurs in a wide spectrum of diseases, including connective tissue disease, cryoglobulinemia, malignancy, Henoch-Schönlein purpura (HSP; more common in children)	Fever, malaise, arthralgias, myalgias; systemic vasculitis in some cases; renal, joint, and gastrointestinal involvement commonly seen in HSP	57/IIE-71
ERUPTIONS WITH ULCERS AND/OR ESCHARS					
Scrub typhus, rickettsial spotted fevers, rat-bite fever[e]; rickettsialpox, ecthyma gangrenosum[f]	—	—	—	—	—[b]
Tularemia	*Francisella tularensis*	Ulceroglandular form: erythematous, tender papule evolves into necrotic, tender ulcer with raised borders; in 35% of cases, eruptions (maculopapular, vesiculopapular, acneiform, urticarial, erythema nodosum, or erythema multiforme) may occur	Exposure to ticks, biting flies, infected animals	Fever, headache, lymphadenopathy	161
Anthrax	*Bacillus anthracis*	Pruritic papule enlarging and evolving into a 1- to 3-cm painless ulcer surrounded by vesicles and then developing a central eschar with edema; residual scar	Exposure to infected animals or animal products	Lymphadenopathy, headache	141

[a] See "Purpuric eruptions."
[b] See etiology-specific chapters.
[c] See "Peripheral eruptions."
[d] See "Confluent desquamative erythemas."

[e] See "Centrally distributed maculopapular eruptions."
[f] See "Vesiculobullous eruptions."
NOTE: DIC, disseminated intravascular coagulation; ECM, erythema chronicum migrans; RMSF, Rocky Mountain spotted fever.

of or travelers to endemic areas. Similarly, *typhoid fever*, a nonrickettsial disease caused by *Salmonella typhi* (Chap. 156), is usually acquired during travel outside the United States.

Some centrally distributed maculopapular eruptions have distinctive features. Erythema chronicum migrans (ECM), the rash of Lyme disease (Chap. 176), typically manifests as singular or multiple annular plaques. Untreated ECM lesions usually fade within a month but may persist for more than a year. *Erythema marginatum*, the rash of acute rheumatic fever (Chap. 235), has a distinctive pattern of enlarging and shifting transient annular lesions.

Collagen vascular diseases may cause fever and rash. Patients with *systemic lupus erythematosus* (Chap. 311) typically develop a sharply defined, erythematous eruption in a butterfly distribution on the cheeks (malar rash) as well as many other skin manifestations. *Still's disease* (Chap. 326) manifests as an evanescent salmon-colored rash on the trunk and proximal extremities that coincides with fever spikes.

Peripheral Eruptions These rashes are alike in that they are most prominent peripherally or begin in peripheral (acral) areas before spreading centripetally. Early diagnosis and therapy are critical in RMSF (Chap. 177) because of its grave prognosis if untreated. Lesions evolve from macular to petechial, start on the wrists and ankles, spread centripetally, and appear on the palms and soles only later in the disease. The rash of *secondary syphilis* (Chap. 172), which may be diffuse but is prominent on the palms and soles, should be considered in the differential diagnosis of pityriasis rosea, especially in sexually active patients. *Atypical measles* (Chap. 194) is seen in individuals contracting measles who received the killed measles vaccine between 1963 and 1967 in the United States and who were not subsequently protected with the live vaccine. *Hand-foot-and-mouth disease* (Chap. 193) is distinguished by tender vesicles distributed peripherally and in the mouth; outbreaks commonly occur within families. The classic target lesions of *erythema multiforme* appear symmetrically on the elbows, knees, palms, and soles. In relatively severe cases, these lesions may spread diffusely and involve mucosal surfaces. Lesions may develop on the hands and feet in *endocarditis* (Chap. 126).

Confluent Desquamative Erythemas These eruptions consist of diffuse erythema frequently followed by desquamation. The eruptions caused by group A *Streptococcus* or *Staphylococcus aureus* are toxin mediated. Certain disease features may provide diagnostic clues. *Scarlet fever* (Chap. 140) usually follows pharyngitis; patients have a facial flush, a "strawberry" tongue, and accentuated petechiae in body folds (Pastia's lines). *Kawasaki disease* (Chaps. 57 and 317) presents in the pediatric population as fissuring of the lips, a strawberry tongue, conjunctivitis, adenopathy, and sometimes cardiac abnormalities. *Streptococcal toxic shock syndrome* (Chap. 140) manifests with hypotension, multiorgan failure, and often a severe group A streptococcal infection (e.g., necrotizing fasciitis). *Staphylococcal toxic shock syndrome* (Chap. 139) also presents with hypotension and multiorgan failure, but usually only *S. aureus* colonization—not a severe *S. aureus* infection—is documented. *Staphylococcal scalded-skin syndrome* (Chap. 139) is seen primarily in children and in immunocompromised adults. Generalized erythema is often evident during the prodrome of fever and malaise; profound tenderness of the skin is distinctive. In the exfoliative stage, the skin can be induced to form bullae with light lateral pressure (Nikolsky's sign). In a mild form, a scarlatiniform eruption mimics scarlet fever, but the patient does not exhibit a strawberry tongue or circumoral pallor. In contrast to the staphylococcal scalded-skin syndrome, in which the cleavage plane is superficial in the epidermis, *toxic epidermal necrolysis* (Chap. 59) involves sloughing of the entire epidermis, resulting in severe disease. *Exfoliative erythroderma syndrome* (Chaps. 56 and 59) is a serious reaction associated with systemic toxicity that is often due to eczema, psoriasis, mycosis fungoides, or a severe drug reaction.

Vesiculobullous Eruptions *Varicella* (Chap. 183) is highly contagious, often occurring in winter or spring. At a given time within a given region of the body, varicella lesions are in different stages of

101

development. In immunocompromised hosts, varicella vesicles may lack the characteristic erythematous base or may appear hemorrhagic. *Rickettsialpox* (Chap. 177) is often documented in urban settings and is characterized by vesicles. It can be distinguished from varicella by an eschar at the site of the mouse-mite bite and the papule/plaque base of each vesicle. Disseminated *Vibrio vulnificus* infection (Chap. 159) or *ecthyma gangrenosum* due to *Pseudomonas aeruginosa* (Chap. 155) should be considered in immunosuppressed individuals with sepsis and hemorrhagic bullae.

Urticarial Eruptions Individuals with classic urticaria ("hives") usually have a hypersensitivity reaction without associated fever. In the presence of fever, urticarial eruptions are usually due to *urticarial vasculitis* (Chap. 317). Unlike individual lesions of classic urticaria, which last up to 48 h, these lesions may last up to 5 days. Etiologies include serum sickness (often induced by drugs such as penicillins, sulfas, salicylates, or barbiturates), connective-tissue disease (e.g., systemic lupus erythematosus or Sjögren's syndrome), and infection (e.g., with hepatitis B virus, coxsackievirus A9, or parasites). Malignancy may be associated with fever and chronic urticaria (Chap. 57).

Nodular Eruptions In immunocompromised hosts, nodular lesions often represent disseminated infection. Patients with disseminated *candidiasis* (often due to *Candida tropicalis*) may have a triad of fever, myalgias, and eruptive nodules (Chap. 205). Disseminated *cryptococcosis* lesions (Chap. 204) may resemble molluscum contagiosum. Necrosis of nodules should raise the suspicion of *aspergillosis* (Chap. 206) or *mucormycosis* (Chap. 207). *Erythema nodosum* presents with exquisitely tender nodules on the lower extremities. *Sweet's syndrome* (Chap. 57) should be considered in individuals with multiple nodules and plaques, often so edematous that they give the appearance of vesicles or bullae. Sweet's syndrome may affect either healthy individuals or persons with lymphoproliferative disease.

Purpuric Eruptions *Acute meningococcemia* (Chap. 146) classically presents in children as a petechial eruption, but initial lesions may appear as blanchable macules or urticaria. RMSF should be considered in the differential diagnosis of acute meningococcemia. *Echovirus 9 infection* (Chap. 193) may mimic acute meningococcemia; patients should be treated as if they have bacterial sepsis since prompt differentiation of these conditions may be impossible. Large ecchymotic areas of *purpura fulminans* (Chaps. 124 and 146) reflect severe underlying disseminated intravascular coagulation, which may be due to infectious or noninfectious causes. The lesions of *chronic meningococcemia* (Chap. 146) may have a variety of morphologies, including petechial. Purpuric nodules may develop on the legs and resemble erythema nodosum but lack its exquisite tenderness. Lesions of *disseminated gonococcemia* (Chap. 147) are distinctive, sparse, countable hemorrhagic pustules, usually located near joints. The lesions of chronic meningococcemia and those of gonococcemia may be indistinguishable in terms of appearance and distribution. *Viral hemorrhagic fever* (Chaps. 198 and 199) should be considered in patients with an appropriate travel history and a petechial rash. *Thrombotic thrombocytopenic purpura* (Chaps. 57, 108, and 116) is a noninfectious cause of fever and petechiae. *Cutaneous small-vessel vasculitis* (*leukocytoclastic vasculitis*) typically manifests as palpable purpura and has a wide variety of causes (Chap. 57).

Eruptions with Ulcers or Eschars The presence of an ulcer or eschar in the setting of a more widespread eruption can provide an important diagnostic clue. For example, the presence of an eschar may suggest the diagnosis of scrub typhus or rickettsialpox in the appropriate setting. In other illnesses (e.g., anthrax), an ulcer or eschar may be the only skin manifestation.

BIBLIOGRAPHY

CHERRY JD: Contemporary infectious exanthems. Clin Infect Dis 16:199, 1993
———: Cutaneous manifestations of systemic infections, in *Textbook of Pediatric Infectious Diseases*, vol. 1, 3d ed, RD Feigin and JD Cherry (eds). Philadelphia, Saunders, 1992, pp 755–782

FREEDBERG IM et al (eds): *Fitzpatrick's Dermatology in General Medicine*, 5th ed. New York, McGraw-Hill, 1999
HURWITZ S (ed): *Clinical Pediatric Dermatology*. Philadelphia, Saunders, 1981
LEVIN S, GOODMAN LJ: An approach to acute fever and rash (AFR) in the adult. Curr Clin Top Infect Dis 15:19, 1995
LOTTI T et al: Cutaneous small-vessel vasculitis. J Am Acad Dermatol 39:667, 1998
SCHLOSSBERG D: Fever and rash. Infect Dis Clin North Am 10:101, 1996
WEBER DJ, COHEN MS: The acutely ill patient with fever and rash, in *Principles and Practice of Infectious Diseases*, vol 1, 4th ed, GL Mandell et al (eds). New York, Churchill Livingstone, 1995, pp 549–561
WENNER HA: Virus diseases associated with cutaneous eruptions. Prog Med Virol 16: 269, 1973

---

19   *Tamar F. Barlam, Dennis L. Kasper*

APPROACH TO THE ACUTELY ILL INFECTED FEBRILE PATIENT

The physician treating the acutely ill febrile patient must be able to recognize infections that require emergent attention. If such infections are not adequately evaluated and treated at initial presentation, the opportunity to alter an adverse outcome may be lost. In this chapter, the clinical presentations of and approach to patients with relatively common infectious disease emergencies are discussed. These infectious processes are discussed in detail in other chapters. →*Noninfectious causes of fever are not covered in this chapter; information on the approach to fever of unknown origin, including that eventually shown to be of noninfectious etiology, is presented in Chap. 125.*

GENERAL CONSIDERATIONS

APPEARANCE A physician must have a consistent approach to acutely ill patients. Even before the history is elicited and a physical examination performed, an immediate assessment of the patient's general appearance yields valuable information. The perceptive physician's subjective sense that a patient is septic or toxic often proves accurate. Visible agitation or anxiety in a febrile patient can be a harbinger of critical illness.

HISTORY Presenting symptoms are frequently nonspecific. In addition to a general description of symptoms, it is important to obtain a sense of disease progression. Detailed questions should be asked about the onset and duration of symptoms and about changes in severity or rate of progression over time. Host factors and comorbid conditions may enhance the risk of infection with certain organisms or of a more fulminant course than is usually seen. Lack of splenic function, alcoholism with significant liver disease, intravenous drug use, HIV infection, diabetes, malignancy, and chemotherapy all predispose to specific infections and frequently to increased severity. The patient should be questioned about factors that might help identify a nidus for invasive infection, such as recent upper respiratory tract infections, influenza, or varicella; prior trauma; disruption of cutaneous barriers due to lacerations, burns, surgery, or decubiti; and the presence of foreign bodies, such as nasal packing after rhinoplasty, barrier contraceptives, tampons, arteriovenous fistulas, or prosthetic joints. Travel, contact with pets or other animals, or activities that might result in tick exposure can lead to diagnoses that would not otherwise be considered. Recent dietary intake, medication use, social contact with ill individuals, vaccination history, and menstrual history may be relevant. A review of systems should focus on any neurologic signs or sensorium alterations, rashes or skin lesions, and focal pain or tenderness and should also include a general review of respiratory, gastrointestinal, or genitourinary symptoms. It is especially important to determine the duration and progression of these symptoms in order to gain an appreciation of the pace and urgency of the process.

A complete physical examination should be performed, with special attention to some areas that are sometimes given short shrift in routine examinations. Assessment of the patient's general appearance and vital signs, skin and soft tissue examination, and the neurologic evaluation are of particular importance.

PHYSICAL EXAMINATION A complete physical examination should be performed, with special attention to some areas that are sometimes given short shrift in routine examinations. Assessment of the patient's general appearance and vital signs, skin and soft tissue examination, and the neurologic evaluation are of particular importance.

The patient may appear either anxious and agitated or lethargic and apathetic. Fever is usually present, although the elderly and compromised hosts, such as those who are uremic or cirrhotic and patients who are taking glucocorticoids or nonsteroidal anti-inflammatory agents, may be afebrile despite serious underlying infection. Measurement of blood pressure, heart rate, and respiratory rate helps determine the degree of hemodynamic and metabolic compromise. The patient's airway must be evaluated to rule out the risk of obstruction from an invasive oropharyngeal infection.

The etiologic diagnosis may become evident in the context of a thorough skin examination. Petechial rashes are typically seen with meningococcemia or Rocky Mountain spotted fever (RMSF); erythroderma is usual with toxic shock syndrome (TSS) and drug fever. The soft tissue and muscle examination is critical. Areas of erythema or duskiness, edema, and tenderness may indicate underlying necrotizing fasciitis, myositis, or myonecrosis. The neurologic examination must include a careful assessment of mental status for signs of early encephalopathy. Evidence of nuchal rigidity or focal neurologic findings should be sought. Focal findings, depressed mental status, or papilledema should be evaluated by brain imaging prior to lumbar puncture, which, in this setting, could initiate herniation.

SPECIFIC PRESENTATIONS

For most infections, there is time for careful evaluation, diagnostic testing, and consultation with other physicians. However, the infections considered below according to common clinical presentation can have rapidly catastrophic outcomes, and their immediate recognition can be life-saving. Recommended therapeutic regimens are presented in Table 19-1.

SEPSIS WITHOUT AN OBVIOUS FOCUS OF PRIMARY INFECTION These patients initially have a brief prodrome of nonspecific symptoms and signs that progresses quickly to hemodynamic instability with hypotension, tachycardia, tachypnea, or respiratory distress. A patient may display altered mental status. Disseminated intravascular coagulation (DIC) with clinical evidence of a hemorrhagic diathesis is a poor prognostic sign.

Septic Shock (See also Chap. 124) Patients with bacteremia leading to septic shock may have a primary site of infection (e.g., pneumonia, pyelonephritis, or cholangitis) that is not evident initially. Elderly patients with comorbid conditions, hosts compromised by malignancy and neutropenia, or patients who have recently undergone a surgical procedure or hospitalization are at increased risk for an adverse outcome. Gram-negative bacteremia with organisms such as *Pseudomonas aeruginosa*, *Aeromonas hydrophila*, or *Escherichia coli* and gram-positive infection with organisms such as *Staphylococcus aureus* or group A streptococci can present as intractable hypotension and multiorgan failure. Treatment can usually be initiated empirically on the basis of the presentation (Table 124-3).

Overwhelming Infection in Asplenic Patients (See also Chap. 124) Patients without splenic function are at risk for overwhelming bacterial sepsis. Asplenic patients succumb to sepsis at 600 times the rate of the general population; 50 to 70% of cases occur within the first 2 years after splenectomy, with a mortality rate of up to 80%. However, in the asplenic individual, an increased risk of overwhelming sepsis continues throughout life. In asplenia, encapsulated bacteria cause the majority of infections, and adults are at lower risk than children because they are more likely to have antibody to these organisms. *Streptococcus pneumoniae* infection is most common, but the risk of infection with *Haemophilus influenzae* or *Neisseria meningitidis* is also high. Severe clinical manifestations of infections due to *E. coli*, *S. aureus*, group B streptococci, *P. aeruginosa*, *Capnocytophaga*, *Babesia*, and *Plasmodium* have been described.

Babesiosis (See also Chap. 214) A history of recent travel to endemic areas should raise the possibility of infection with *Babesia*. Between 1 and 4 weeks after a tick bite, the patient experiences chills, fatigue, anorexia, myalgia, arthralgia, nausea, and headache; ecchymosis and/or petechiae are occasionally seen. The tick that most commonly transmits *Babesia*, *Ixodes scapularis*, also transmits *Borrelia burgdorferi* (the agent of Lyme disease) and *Ehrlichia*, and co-infection can occur, resulting in more severe disease. Infection with the European species *Babesia divergens* is more frequently fulminant than that due to the U.S. species *B. microti*, causing a febrile syndrome with hemolysis, jaundice, hemoglobinemia, and renal failure and a mortality rate of >50%. Severe babesiosis is especially common in asplenic hosts but does occur in hosts with normal splenic function.

Other Sepsis Syndromes Tularemia (Chap. 161) is seen throughout the United States, but primarily in Arkansas, Oklahoma, and Missouri, in association with wild rabbit, tick, and tabanid fly contact. The uncommon typhoidal form can be associated with gram-negative septic shock and a mortality rate of >30%. In the United States, plague (Chap. 162) is found primarily in New Mexico, Arizona, and Colorado after contact with ground squirrels, prairie dogs, or chipmunks. The septic form is particularly rare and is associated with shock, multiorgan failure, and a 30% mortality rate. These rare infections should be considered in the appropriate epidemiologic setting.

SEPSIS WITH SKIN MANIFESTATIONS (See also Chap. 18) Maculopapular rashes may reflect early meningococcal or rickettsial disease but are usually associated with nonemergent infections. Exanthems are usually viral.

Petechiae Petechial rashes caused by viruses are seldom associated with hypotension or a toxic appearance, although severe measles can be an exception. In other settings, petechial rashes require more urgent attention.

Meningococcemia (See also Chap. 146) Almost three-quarters of patients with bacteremic *N. meningitidis* infection have a rash. Meningococcemia most often affects young children (i.e., those 6 months to 5 years old, often in daycare). However, sporadic cases and outbreaks occur in schools (grade school through college) and army barracks. Between 10 and 20% of all cases have a fulminant course, with shock, DIC, and multiorgan failure. Of these patients, 50 to 60% die, and survivors often require extensive debridement or amputation of gangrenous extremities. Patients may exhibit fever, headache, nausea, vomiting, myalgias, change in mental status, and meningismus. However, the rapidly progressive form of disease is not usually associated with meningitis. The rash is initially pink, blanching, and maculopapular, appearing on the trunk and extremities, but then becomes hemorrhagic, forming petechiae. Petechiae are first seen at the ankles, wrists, axillae, mucosal surfaces, and palpebral and bulbar conjunctiva, with subsequent spread to the lower extremities and trunk. A cluster of petechiae may be seen at pressure points, e.g., where a blood pressure cuff has been inflated. In rapidly progressive meningococcemia, the petechial rash quickly becomes purpuric **(Plate IID-44)** and patients develop DIC. Hypotension with petechiae for <12 h is associated with significant mortality. The mortality rate can exceed 90% in patients without meningitis who have rash, hypotension, and a normal or low white blood cell count and erythrocyte sedimentation rate. A better prognosis has been reported in cases where antibiotics are given before admission by the primary care provider. This observation suggests that early initiation of treatment may be life-saving.

Rocky Mountain spotted fever (See also Chap. 177) RMSF occurs throughout the United States. A history of tick bite is common; however, if such a history is lacking, a history of travel or outdoor activity (e.g., camping in tick-infested areas) can be ascertained. RMSF is caused by *Rickettsia rickettsii*. For the first 3 days, headache, fever, malaise, myalgias, nausea, vomiting, and anorexia are present. By day 3, half of patients have skin findings. Blanching macules develop initially on the wrists and ankles and then spread over the legs and trunk. The lesions become hemorrhagic and are frequently pete-

Table 19-1 Common Infectious Disease Emergencies

Clinical Syndrome	Possible Etiologies	Treatment	Comments	Reference Chapter(s)
Sepsis without a clear focus				
Gram-negative sepsis	*Pseudomonas* spp., gram-negative enteric bacilli	Piperacillin/tazobactam (3.75 g q4h) *or* Ceftazidime (2 g q8h) *plus* Tobramycin (5 mg/kg per day)	See Table 124-3.	124, 155
Gram-positive sepsis	*Staphylococcus* spp., *Streptococcus* spp.	Vancomycin (1 g q12h) *plus* Gentamicin (5 mg/kg per day)	If a β-lactam-sensitive strain is identified, antibiotics should be altered.	124, 139, 140
Overwhelming post-splenectomy sepsis	*Streptococcus pneumoniae, Haemophilus influenzae, Neisseria meningitidis*	Ceftriaxone (2 g q12h)[a]	If the isolate is penicillin-sensitive, penicillin is the drug of choice.	124
Babesiosis	*Babesia microti* (U.S.), *B. divergens* (Europe)	Clindamycin (600 mg tid) *plus* Quinine (650 mg tid)	Treatment with doxycycline (100 mg bid) for potential coinfection with *Borrelia burgdorferi* or *Ehrlichia* spp. may be prudent.	212, 214
Sepsis with skin findings Petechiae				
Meningococcemia	*N. meningitidis*	Penicillin (4 million units q4h) *or* Ceftriaxone (2 g q12h)	If both meningococcemia and Rocky Mountain spotted fever are being considered, use chloramphenicol (50–75 mg/kg per day in four divided doses). *Do not add doxycycline to a regimen including a β-lactam agent.*	146, 177
Rocky Mountain spotted fever	*Rickettsia rickettsii*	Doxycycline (100 mg bid)		
Purpura fulminans	*S. pneumoniae, H. influenzae, N. meningitidis*	Ceftriaxone (2 g q12h)[a]	If the isolate is penicillin-sensitive, penicillin is the drug of choice.	124, 146
Erythroderma: toxic shock syndrome	Group A *Streptococcus, Staphylococcus aureus*	Penicillin (2 million units q4h) *or* Oxacillin (2 g q4h) *plus* Clindamycin (600 mg q8h)	Site of toxigenic bacteria should be debrided; if necessary, intravenous immunoglobulin can be used in severe cases.	139, 140
Sepsis with soft tissue findings Necrotizing fasciitis	Group A *Streptococcus,* mixed aerobic/anaerobic flora	Penicillin (2 million units q4h) *plus* Clindamycin (600 mg q8h) *plus* Gentamicin (5 mg/kg per day)	Urgent surgical evaluation is critical.	128, 140
Clostridial myonecrosis	*Clostridium perfringens*	Penicillin (2 million units q4h) *plus* Clindamycin (600 mg q8h)	Urgent surgical evaluation is critical.	145
Neurologic infections Bacterial meningitis	*S. pneumoniae, N. meningitidis*	Ceftriaxone (2 g q12h)[a]	If the isolate is penicillin-sensitive, penicillin is the drug of choice. If the patient is >50 years old, add ampicillin for *Listeria* coverage.	372
Suppurative intracranial infections	*Staphylococcus* spp., *Streptococcus* spp., anaerobes, gram-negative bacilli	Oxacillin (2 g q4h)[b] *plus* Metronidazole (500 mg tid) *plus* Ceftriaxone (2 g q12h)	Urgent surgical evaluation is critical.	372
Brain abscess	*Streptococcus* spp., anaerobes, *Staphylococcus* spp.	Penicillin (4 million units q4h) *or* Oxacillin (2 g q4h)[b] *plus* Metronidazole (500 mg tid)	Surgical evaluation is essential.	372
Cerebral malaria	*Plasmodium falciparum*	Quinine (650 mg tid for 3 days) *plus* Tetracycline (250 mg tid for 7 days)	Do not use glucocorticoids.	212, 214
Spinal epidural abscess	*Staphylococcus* spp.	Oxacillin (2 g q4h)[c]	Surgical evaluation is essential.	368
Focal infections Acute bacterial endocarditis	*S. aureus,* β-hemolytic streptococci, HACEK group,[d] *Neisseria* spp., *S. pneumoniae*	Ceftriaxone (2 g q12h) *plus* Vancomycin (1 g q12h)	Adjust treatment when culture data become available. Surgical evaluation is essential.	126

[a] If resistant pneumococci are prevalent, add vancomycin (1 g q12h).
[b] Vancomycin (1 g q12h) should replace oxacillin if methicillin-resistant strains are highly prevalent.
[c] In HIV-infected intravenous drug users with suspected spinal epidural abscess, empirical therapy must cover gram-negative rods and methicillin-resistant *S. aureus.*

[d] *Haemophilus aphrophilus, H. paraphrophilus, H. parainfluenzae, Actinobacillus actinomycetemcomitans, Cardiobacterium hominis, Eikenella corrodens,* and *Kingella kingae.*

chial. The rash spreads to palms and soles later in the course (**Plate IID-45**). The centripetal spread is a classic feature of RMSF. However, 10 to 15% of patients with RMSF never develop a rash. The patient can be hypotensive and develop noncardiogenic pulmonary edema, confusion, lethargy, and encephalitis progressing to coma. The cerebrospinal fluid (CSF) contains 10 to 100 cells/μL, usually with a predominance of mononuclear cells. The CSF glucose level is often normal; the protein concentration may be slightly elevated. Renal and hepatic injury and bleeding secondary to vascular damage are noted. Untreated infection has a mortality rate of 30%.

Purpura Fulminans (See also Chaps. 124 and 146) This is the cutaneous manifestation of DIC and presents as large ecchymotic areas and hemorrhagic bullae. Progression of petechiae to purpura and ecchymoses is associated with congestive heart failure, septic shock, acute renal failure, acidosis, hypoxia, hypotension, and death. Purpura fulminans has primarily been associated with *N. meningitidis* but, in the splenectomized patient, has been described in association with *S. pneumoniae* and *H. influenzae*.

Ecthyma Gangrenosum Septic shock caused by *P. aeruginosa* and *A. hydrophila* can be associated with ecthyma gangrenosum (**Plate IID-57C**): hemorrhagic vesicles surrounded by a rim of erythema with central necrosis and ulceration. These gram-negative bacteremias are most common among patients with neutropenia, extensive burns, and hypogammaglobulinemia.

Other Emergent Infections Associated with Rash *Vibrio vulnificus* and other noncholera *Vibrio* bacteremic infections (Chap. 159) can cause focal skin lesions and overwhelming sepsis in the host with liver disease. After ingestion of contaminated shellfish, there is a sudden onset of malaise, chills, fever, and hypotension. The patient develops bullous or hemorrhagic skin lesions, usually on the lower extremities, and 75% of patients have leg pain. The mortality rate can be as high as 50%. *Capnocytophaga canimorsus* (Chap. 127) can cause septic shock in asplenic patients. Infection with this fastidious gram-negative rod typically presents after a dog bite as fever, chills, myalgia, vomiting, diarrhea, dyspnea, confusion, and headache. Findings can include an exanthem or erythema multiforme (**Plate IIE-67**), cyanotic mottling or peripheral cyanosis, petechiae, and ecchymosis. About 30% of patients with this fulminant form die of overwhelming sepsis and DIC, and survivors may require amputation to treat gangrene.

Erythroderma TSS (Chaps. 139 and 140) is usually associated with erythroderma. The patient presents with fever, malaise, myalgias, nausea, vomiting, diarrhea, and confusion. There is a sunburn-type rash that may be subtle and patchy but is usually diffuse and is found on the face, trunk, and extremities. Erythroderma, which desquamates after 1 to 2 weeks, is more common in *Staphylococcus*-associated than in *Streptococcus*-associated TSS. Hypotension develops rapidly after onset of symptoms, often within hours. Multiorgan failure is seen. Often there is no indication of a primary focal infection. Colonization rather than overt infection of the vagina or a postoperative wound, for example, is typical with staphylococcal TSS, and the mucosal areas appear hyperemic but not infected. Early renal failure may distinguish this syndrome from other septic shock syndromes. Clinical evaluation constitutes the diagnosis because TSS is defined by the clinical criteria of fever, rash, hypotension, and multiorgan involvement. The mortality rate is 5% for menstruation-associated TSS, 10 to 15% for nonmenstrual TSS, and 30 to 70% for streptococcal TSS.

SEPSIS WITH A SOFT TISSUE/MUSCLE PRIMARY FOCUS (See also Chap. 128) **Necrotizing Fasciitis** This infection may arise at a site of minimal trauma or postoperative incision and may also be associated with recent varicella, childbirth, or muscle strain. The most common causes of necrotizing fasciitis are group A streptococci alone (Chap. 140) and a mixed facultative and anaerobic flora (Chap. 128). Diabetes mellitus, peripheral vascular disease, and intravenous drug use are associated risk factors. Use of nonsteroidal anti-inflammatory agents adversely affects granulocyte chemotaxis, phagocytosis, and bacterial killing, allowing progression of skin or soft tissue infections. The patient may have bacteremia and hypotension without other organ-system failure. Physical findings are minimal

compared to the severity of pain and the degree of fever. The examination is often unremarkable except for soft tissue edema and erythema. The infected area is red, hot, shiny, swollen, and exquisitely tender. In untreated infection, the overlying skin develops blue-gray patches after 36 h, and cutaneous bullae and necrosis develop after 3 to 5 days. Necrotizing fasciitis due to a mixed flora, but not that due to group A streptococci, can be associated with gas production. Without treatment, pain decreases because of thrombosis of the small blood vessels and destruction of the peripheral nerves—an ominous sign. The mortality rate is >30% overall, >70% in association with TSS, and nearly 100% without surgical intervention. Life-threatening necrotizing fasciitis may also be due to *Clostridium perfringens* (Chap. 145); in this condition, the patient is extremely toxic and the mortality rate is high. Within 48 h, rapid tissue invasion and systemic toxicity associated with hemolysis and death ensue. The distinction between this entity and clostridial myonecrosis is made by muscle biopsy.

Clostridial Myonecrosis (See also Chap. 145) Myonecrosis is often associated with trauma or surgery but can be spontaneous. The incubation period is usually 12 to 24 h long, and massive necrotizing gangrene develops within hours of onset. Systemic toxicity, shock, and death can occur within 12 h. The patient's pain and toxic appearance are out of proportion to physical findings. On examination, the patient is febrile, apathetic, tachycardic, and tachypneic and may express a feeling of impending doom. Hypotension and renal failure develop later, and hyperalertness is evident preterminally. The skin over the affected area is bronze-brown, mottled, and edematous. Bullous lesions with serosanguineous drainage and a mousy or sweet odor can be present. Crepitus can occur secondary to gas production in muscle tissue. The mortality rate is >65% with spontaneous myonecrosis, which is often associated with *C. septicum* and underlying malignancy. The mortality rates associated with trunk and limb infection are 63% and 12%, respectively, and any delay in surgical treatment increases the risk of death.

NEUROLOGIC INFECTIONS WITH OR WITHOUT SEPTIC SHOCK **Bacterial Meningitis** (See also Chap. 372) Bacterial meningitis is one of the most common infectious emergencies involving the central nervous system. Although hosts with cell-mediated immune deficiency, including transplant recipients, diabetic patients, the elderly, and cancer patients treated with certain chemotherapeutic agents, are at particular risk for *Listeria monocytogenes* meningitis, most cases in adults are due to *S. pneumoniae* (30 to 50%) and *N. meningitidis* (10 to 35%). An early presentation of headache, meningismus, and fever is classic but is seen in only half of patients. The elderly can present without fever or meningeal signs despite lethargy and confusion. Cerebral dysfunction is evidenced by confusion, delirium, and lethargy that can progress to coma. The presentation is fulminant, with sepsis and brain edema, in some cases; papilledema at presentation is unusual and suggests another diagnosis (e.g., an intracranial lesion). Focal signs, including cranial nerve palsies (IV, VI, VII), can be seen in 10 to 20% of cases; 50 to 60% of patients have bacteremia. A poor neurologic outcome is associated with coma at any time during the course or with a CSF glucose level of <0.6 mmol/L (<10 mg/dL). Mortality is associated with coma, respiratory distress, shock, a CSF protein level of >2.5 g/L, a peripheral white blood cell count of <5000/μL, and a serum sodium level of <135 mmol/L.

Suppurative Intracranial Infections (See also Chap. 372) Other rare intracranial lesions that present with sepsis and hemodynamic instability are subdural empyema, septic cavernous sinus thrombosis, and septic superior sagittal sinus thrombosis. Rapid recognition of the toxic patient with central neurologic signs is crucial to improvement of the dismal prognosis of these entities.

Subdural empyema This infection arises from the paranasal sinus in 60 to 70% of cases. Microaerophilic streptococci and staphylococci are the predominant etiologic organisms. The patient is toxic, with fever, headache, and nuchal rigidity. Of all patients, 75% have focal signs and 6 to 20% die.

Septic cavernous sinus thrombosis This condition follows a facial or sphenoid sinus infection; 70% of cases are due to staphylococci and the remainder to aerobic or anaerobic streptococci. A unilateral or retroorbital headache progresses to a toxic appearance and fever within days. Three-quarters of patients have unilateral periorbital edema that becomes bilateral and then progresses to ptosis, proptosis, ophthalmoplegia, and papilledema. The mortality rate is as high as 30%.

Septic thrombosis of the superior sagittal sinus This infection spreads from the ethmoid or maxillary sinuses. Its bacterial causes include *S. pneumoniae*, other streptococci, and staphylococci. The fulminant course is characterized by headache, nausea, vomiting, rapid progression to confusion and coma, nuchal rigidity, and brainstem signs. If the sinus is totally thrombosed, the mortality rate exceeds 80%.

Brain Abscess (See also Chap. 372) Brain abscess often occurs without systemic signs. Almost half of patients are afebrile, and presentations are more consistent with a space-occupying lesion in the brain; 70% have headache, 50% have focal neurologic signs, and 25% have papilledema. Abscesses can present as single or multiple lesions resulting from contiguous foci or hematogenous infection, such as unrecognized endocarditis. The infection progresses over several days from cerebritis to an abscess with a mature capsule. Abscesses arising hematogenously are especially apt to rupture into the ventricular space, causing a sudden and severe deterioration in clinical status and high mortality. Otherwise, mortality is low but morbidity is high (30 to 55%). Patients presenting with stroke and a parameningeal infectious focus, such as sinusitis or otitis, may have a brain abscess, and physicians must maintain a high level of suspicion. Prognosis worsens in patients with a fulminant course, delayed diagnosis, abscess rupture into the ventricles, multiple abscesses, or abnormal neurologic status at presentation.

Cerebral Malaria (See also Chap. 214) This entity should be urgently considered if patients who have recently traveled to areas endemic for malaria present with a febrile illness and lethargy or other neurologic signs. Fulminant malaria is caused by *Plasmodium falciparum* and is associated with temperatures of >40°C (>104°F), hypotension, jaundice, adult respiratory distress syndrome, and bleeding. By definition, any patient with a change in mental status or repeated seizure in the setting of fulminant malaria has cerebral malaria. In adults this nonspecific febrile illness progresses to coma over several days; occasionally, coma occurs within hours and death within 24 h. Nuchal rigidity and photophobia are rare. On physical examination, symmetric encephalopathy is typical, and upper motor neuron dysfunction with decorticate and decerebrate posturing can be seen with advanced disease. Unrecognized infection results in a 30% mortality rate.

Spinal Epidural Abscesses (See also Chap. 368) Patients with spinal epidural abscesses often present with back pain and develop neurologic deficits late in their course. At-risk patients include those with diabetes mellitus; intravenous drug use; recent spinal trauma, surgery, or epidural anesthesia; and other comorbid conditions, such as HIV infection. The thoracic or lumbar spine is the most common location, and staphylococci are the most common etiologic agents; in HIV-infected intravenous drug users, therapy must cover gram-negative rods and methicillin-resistant *S. aureus*. If a patient gives a history of antecedent back pain and has new neurologic symptoms, this diagnosis must immediately be considered. Almost 60% of patients have fever and almost 90% have back pain. Paresthesia, bowel and bladder dysfunction, radicular pain, and weakness are frequent neurologic complaints, and examination of the patient may reveal abnormal reflexes and motor and sensory deficits. Rapid recognition and treatment, including immediate drainage, can prevent or minimize permanent neurologic sequelae.

FOCAL SYNDROMES WITH A FULMINANT COURSE
Infection at virtually any primary focus (e.g., osteomyelitis, pneumonia, pyelonephritis, or cholangitis) can result in bacteremia and sepsis.

TSS has been associated with focal infections such as septic arthritis, peritonitis, sinusitis, and wound infection. Death occurs secondary to septic shock or toxin production with hemodynamic instability and multiorgan failure. Rapid clinical deterioration and death can be associated with destruction of the primary site of infection, as is seen in endocarditis and in necrotizing infections of the oropharynx (in which edema suddenly compromises the airway).

Rhinocerebral Mucormycosis (See also Chap. 207) Patients with diabetes or malignancy are at risk for invasive rhinocerebral mucormycosis. Patients present with low-grade fever, dull sinus pain, diplopia, decreased mental status, decreased ocular motion, chemosis, proptosis, dusky or necrotic nasal turbinates, and necrotic hard-palate lesions that respect the midline. Without rapid recognition and intervention, the process continues an inexorable invasive course with high mortality.

Acute Bacterial Endocarditis (See also Chap. 126) This entity presents with a much more aggressive course than subacute endocarditis. Bacteria such as *S. aureus*, *S. pneumoniae*, *L. monocytogenes*, *Haemophilus* spp., and streptococci of groups A, B, and G attack native valves. Mortality rates range from 10 to 40%. The host may have comorbid conditions such as underlying malignancy, diabetes mellitus, intravenous drug use, or alcoholism. The patient presents with fever, fatigue, and malaise <2 weeks after onset of infection. On physical examination, a changing murmur and congestive heart failure may be noted. Hemorrhagic macules on palms or soles (*Janeway lesions*) sometimes develop. Petechiae, Roth's spots, splinter hemorrhages, and splenomegaly are unusual. Rapid valvular destruction, particularly of the aortic valve, results in pulmonary edema and hypotension. Myocardial abscesses can form, eroding through the septum or into the conduction system and causing life-threatening arrhythmias or high-degree conduction block. Large friable vegetations can result in major arterial emboli, metastatic infection, or tissue infarction. Emboli can lead to stroke, change in mental status, visual disturbances, aphasia, ataxia, headache, meningismus, brain abscess, cerebritis, spinal cord infarct with paraplegia, arthralgia, osteomyelitis, splenic abscess, septic arthritis, and hematuria. Rapid intervention is crucial for a successful outcome.

DIAGNOSTIC WORKUP OF THE ACUTELY ILL PATIENT

After a quick clinical assessment, diagnostic material should be obtained rapidly and antibiotic and supportive treatment begun. In the sepsis syndromes, blood (for cultures; baseline complete blood count with differential; measurement of serum electrolytes, blood urea nitrogen, serum creatinine, and serum glucose; and liver function tests) can be obtained at the time an intravenous line is placed and before antibiotics are administered. For patients with possible acute endocarditis, three sets of blood cultures should be performed. Asplenic patients should have a blood smear examined to confirm the presence of Howell-Jolly bodies (indicating the absence of splenic function) and a buffy coat examined for bacteria; these patients can have >10^6 organisms per milliliter of blood (compared to 10^4/mL in patients with an intact spleen). Blood smears from patients with possible cerebral malaria or babesiosis must be examined for the diagnosis and quantitation of parasitemia. Blood smears may also be diagnostic in ehrlichiosis.

Patients with meningitis should have CSF obtained before the initiation of antibiotic therapy. *If focal neurologic signs, abnormal mental status, or papilledema mandates brain imaging before a lumbar puncture, antibiotics should be administered prior to imaging but after blood for cultures has been drawn.* If CSF cultures are negative, laboratory examination of CSF by latex agglutination or immunoprecipitation can be attempted to make an etiologic diagnosis. However, blood cultures will provide the diagnosis in 50 to 70% of cases.

Focal abscesses necessitate immediate computed tomography or magnetic resonance imaging as part of an evaluation for surgical intervention. Other diagnostic procedures, such as cultures of wounds or scraping of skin lesions, should not delay the initiation of treatment for more than minutes. Once emergent evaluation, diagnostic procedures, and (if appropriate) surgical consultation (see below) have been completed, other laboratory tests can be conducted. Appropriate radiography, computed axial tomography, magnetic resonance imaging, urinalysis, erythrocyte sedimentation rate determination, and transthoracic or transesophageal echocardiography may all prove important.

℞ **TREATMENT** Table 19-1 lists first-line treatments for the infections considered in this chapter. (For a more detailed discussion of treatment, see specific chapters.) In addition to the initiation of parenteral antibiotic therapy, several of these infections require urgent surgical attention. General surgery for possible necrotizing fasciitis or myonecrosis, neurosurgical evaluation for subdural empyema or spinal epidural abscess, otolaryngologic surgery for possible mucormycosis, and cardiothoracic surgery for critically ill patients with acute endocarditis are as important as the rapid commencement of antibiotic therapy. For infections such as necrotizing fasciitis and clostridial myonecrosis, rapid surgical intervention supercedes other diagnostic or therapeutic maneuvers.

Acutely ill febrile patients require close observation, aggressive supportive measures, and—in most cases—admission to intensive care units. Adjunctive treatments, such as intravenous immunoglobulin administration for TSS, can be considered after initial stabilization. The most important task of the physician is to recognize the acute infectious emergency and proceed with appropriate urgency.

BIBLIOGRAPHY

ASTIZ ME et al: Septic shock. Lancet 351:1501, 1998

BARQUET N et al: Prognostic factors in meningococcal disease—development of a bedside predictive model and scoring system. JAMA 278:491, 1997

DAVIES HD et al: Invasive group A streptococcal infections in Ontario, Canada. N Engl J Med 335:547, 1996

DRAGE LA: Life-threatening rashes: Dermatologic signs of four infectious diseases. Mayo Clin Proc 74:68, 1999

MATHISEN GE et al: Brain abscess. Clin Infect Dis 25:763, 1997

NEWTON CRJC et al: Neurological manifestations of falciparum malaria. Ann Neurol 43:695, 1998

QUAGLIARELLO VJ et al: Treatment of bacterial meningitis. N Engl J Med 336:709, 1997

| 20 | *Daniel F. Danzl* |

HYPOTHERMIA AND FROSTBITE

HYPOTHERMIA

Accidental hypothermia occurs when there is an unintentional drop in the body's core temperature below 35°C (95°F). At this temperature, many of the compensatory physiologic mechanisms to conserve heat begin to fail. *Primary accidental hypothermia* is a result of the direct exposure of a previously healthy individual to the cold. The mortality rate is much higher for those patients who develop *secondary hypothermia* as a complication of a serious systemic disorder.

CAUSES Primary accidental hypothermia is geographically and seasonally pervasive. Although most cases occur in the winter months and in colder climates, it is surprisingly common in warmer regions as well. In the United States, hypothermia accounts for more than 700 deaths each year, half of which occur in people age 65 or older.

Multiple variables make individuals at the extremes of age, the elderly and neonates, particularly vulnerable to hypothermia (Table 20-1). The elderly have diminished thermal proprioception and are more susceptible to immobility, malnutrition, and systemic illnesses that interfere with heat generation or conservation. Dementia, psychiatric illness, and socioeconomic factors often compound these problems by impeding adequate measures to prevent hypothermia. Neonates have high rates of heat loss because of their increased

Table 20-1 Risk Factors for Hypothermia

Age extremes	Endocrine-related
Elderly	Hypoglycemia
Neonates	Hypothyroidism
Outdoor exposure	Adrenal insufficiency
Occupational	Hypopituitarism
Sports-related	Neurologic-related
Inadequate clothing	Stroke
Drugs and intoxicants	Hypothalamic disorders
Ethanol	Parkinson's disease
Phenothiazines	Spinal cord injury
Barbiturates	Multisystem
Anesthetics	Malnutrition
Neuromuscular blockers	Sepsis
Others	Shock
	Hepatic or renal failure
	Burns and exfoliative dermatologic disorders
	Immobility or debilitation

surface-to-mass ratio and their lack of effective shivering and adaptive behavioral responses. In addition, malnutrition can contribute to heat loss because of diminished subcutaneous fat and because of its association with depleted energy stores used for thermogenesis.

Individuals whose occupations or hobbies entail extensive exposure to cold weather are clearly at increased risk for hypothermia. Military history is replete with hypothermic tragedies. Hunters, sailors, skiers, and climbers also are at great risk of exposure, whether it involves injury, changes in weather, or lack of preparedness.

Ethanol causes vasodilatation (which increases heat loss), reduces thermogenesis and gluconeogenesis, and may impair judgment or lead to obtundation. Hypothermia is not an uncommon feature in Wernicke's encephalopathy and may mask its other manifestations. A number of medications are associated with altered thermal regulation. Phenothiazines, barbiturates, benzodiazepines, cyclic antidepressants, and many other medications reduce centrally-mediated vasoconstriction. Up to one-quarter of patients admitted to an intensive care unit because of drug overdose are hypothermic. Anesthetics can block the shivering responses; their effects may be compounded when patients are not covered adequately in the operating or recovery rooms.

Several types of endocrine dysfunction can lead to hypothermia. Hypothyroidism—particularly when extreme, as in myxedema coma—reduces the metabolic rate and impairs thermogenesis and behavioral responses. Myxedema is more common in women than in men and may be occult. Adrenal insufficiency and hypopituitarism can also increase susceptibility to hypothermia. Hypoglycemia, most commonly caused by insulin or oral hypoglycemic drugs, is associated with hypothermia, in part the result of neuroglycopenic effects on hypothalamic function. Increased osmolality and metabolic derangements associated with uremia, diabetic ketoacidosis, and lactic acidosis can lead to altered hypothalamic thermoregulation.

Neurologic injury from trauma, cerebrovascular accident, subarachnoid hemorrhage, or hypothalamic lesions increases susceptibility to hypothermia. Agenesis of the corpus callosum, or Shapiro syndrome, is one cause of episodic hypothermia, characterized by profuse perspiration followed by a rapid fall in temperature. Acute spinal cord injury disrupts the autonomic pathways that lead to shivering and prevents cold-induced reflex vasoconstrictive responses.

Hypothermia associated with sepsis is a poor prognostic sign. Hepatic failure causes decreased glycogen stores and gluconeogenesis, as well as a diminished shivering response. In acute myocardial infarction associated with low cardiac output, hypothermia may be reversed after adequate resuscitation. With extensive burns, psoriasis, erythrodermas, and other skin diseases, increased peripheral blood flow leads to excessive heat loss.

THERMOREGULATION Heat loss occurs through five mechanisms: radiation (55 to 65% of heat loss), conduction (10 to 15% of heat loss, but much greater in cold water), convection (increase in the wind), respiration, and evaporation (which are affected by the ambient temperature and the relative humidity).

The preoptic anterior hypothalamus normally orchestrates thermoregulation (Chap. 17). The immediate defense of thermoneutrality is via the autonomic nervous system (Chap. 72), whereas delayed control is mediated by the endocrine system. Autonomic nervous system responses include the release of norepinephrine, increased muscle tone, and shivering, leading to thermogenesis and an increase in the basal metabolic rate. Cutaneous cold thermoreception causes direct reflex vasoconstriction to converse heat. Prolonged exposure to cold also stimulates hypothalamic release of thyrotropin releasing hormone; this leads to increased levels of thyroid stimulating hormone (TSH), which stimulates the thyroid gland to produce thyroxine, a hormone that increases metabolic rate.

CLINICAL PRESENTATION   In most cases of hypothermia, the history of exposure to environmental factors, such as prolonged exposure to the outdoors without adequate clothing, makes the diagnosis straightforward. In urban settings, however, the presentation is often more subtle and the clinician may focus on other disease processes, toxin exposures, or psychiatric diagnoses.

After initial stimulation by hypothermia, there is progressive depression of all organ systems. The timing of the appearance of these clinical manifestations varies widely (Table 20-2). Without knowing the core temperature, it can be difficult to interpret other vital signs. For example, a tachycardia disproportionate to the core temperature suggests secondary hypothermia resulting from hypoglycemia, hypovolemia, or a toxin overdose. Because carbon dioxide production declines progressively, the respiratory rate should be low; persistent hyperventilation suggests a central nervous system (CNS) lesion or one of the organic acidoses. A markedly depressed level of consciousness in a patient with mild hypothermia should raise suspicion of an overdose or CNS dysfunction due to infection or trauma.

Physical examination findings can also be altered by hypothermia. For instance, the assumption that areflexia is solely attributable to hypothermia can obscure and delay the diagnosis of a spinal cord injury. Patients with hypothermia may be confused or combative; these symptoms abate more rapidly with rewarming than with the use of restraints. A classic example of maladaptive behavior in patients with hypothermia is paradoxical undressing, which involves the inappropriate removal of clothing in response to a cold stress. The cold-induced ileus and abdominal rectus spasm can mimic, or mask, the presentation of an acute abdomen (Chap. 14).

When a patient in hypothermic cardiac arrest is first discovered, cardiopulmonary resuscitation is indicated, unless (1) a do-not-resuscitate status is verified, (2) obviously lethal injuries are identified, or (3) the depression of a frozen chest wall is not possible. As the resuscitation proceeds, the prognosis is grave if there is evidence of widespread cell lysis, as reflected by potassium levels exceeding 10 mEq/L. Other findings that may preclude continuing resuscitation include a core temperature <12°C, a pH <6.5, or evidence of intravascular thrombosis with a fibrinogen value <50 mg/dL. The decision to terminate resuscitation before rewarming the patient to 35°C is extremely difficult. There are no validated prognostic indicators for recovery from hypothermia. A history of asphyxia with secondary cooling is the most important negative predictor of survival.

DIAGNOSIS AND STABILIZATION   Hypothermia is confirmed by measuring the core temperature, preferably at two sites. Rectal probes should be placed to a depth of 15 cm and not adjacent to cold feces. A simultaneous esophageal measurement will be falsely high during heated inhalation therapy. The probe should be placed 24 cm below the larynx. The greatest discordance between the readings is usually during the transition phase before effective rewarming. Relying solely on infrared tympanic thermography is not advisable.

After a diagnosis of hypothermia is established, cardiac monitoring should be instituted, along with attempts to limit further heat loss. If the patient is in ventricular fibrillation, one sequence of 3 defibrillation attempts (2 J/kg) should be administered. If unsuccessful, active re-

Table 20-2   Physiologic Changes Associated with Hypothermia

Severity of Hypothermia	Body Temperature	Central Nervous System	Cardiovascular	Respiratory	Renal and Endocrine	Neuromuscular
Mild	35°C (95°F)–32.2°C (90°F)	Linear depression of cerebral metabolism; amnesia; apathy; dysarthria; impaired judgment; maladaptive behavior	Tachycardia, then progressive bradycardia; cardiac-cycle prolongation; vasoconstriction; increase in cardiac output and blood pressure	Tachypnea, then progressive decrease in respiratory minute volume; declining oxygen consumption; bronchorrhea; bronchospasm	Diuresis; increase in catecholamines, adrenal steroids, triiodothyronine and thyroxine; increase in metabolism with shivering	Increased preshivering muscle tone, then fatiguing, shivering-induced thermogenesis; ataxia
Moderate	<32.2°C (90°F)–28°C (82.4°F)	EEG abnormalities; progressive depression of level of consciousness; pupillary dilatation; paradoxical undressing; hallucinations	Progressive decrease in pulse and cardiac output; increased atrial and ventricular arrhythmias; nonspecific and suggestive (J-wave) electrocardiographic changes; prolonged systole	Hypoventilation; 50% decrease in carbon dioxide production per 8°C drop in temperature; absence of protective airway reflexes; 50% decrease in oxygen consumption	50% increase in renal blood flow; renal autoregulation intact; impaired insulin action	Hyporeflexia; diminishing shivering-induced thermogenesis; rigidity
Severe	<28°C (82.4°F)	Loss of cerebrovascular autoregulation; decline in cerebral blood flow; coma; loss of ocular reflexes; progressive decrease in EEG	Progressive decreases in blood pressure, heart rate, and cardiac output; reentrant dysrhythmias; decreased ventricular arrhythmia threshold; asystole	Pulmonic congestion and edema; 75% decrease in oxygen consumption; apnea	Decrease in renal blood flow parallels decrease in cardiac output; extreme oliguria; poikilothermia; 80% decrease in basal metabolism	No motion; decreased nerve-conduction velocity; peripheral areflexia

warming should be continued past 30° to 32°C. Supplemental oxygenation is always warranted, since tissue oxygenation is adversely affected by the leftward shift of the oxyhemoglobin dissociation curve. Pulse oximetry may be unreliable in patients with vasoconstriction. If protective airway reflexes are absent, gentle endotracheal intubation should be performed. Adequate pre-oxygenation will prevent ventricular arrhythmias.

Insertion of a gastric tube prevents dilatation secondary to decreased bowel motility. Indwelling bladder catheters facilitate monitoring of cold-induced diuresis. Dehydration is commonly encountered with chronic hypothermia, and most patients benefit from a bolus of crystalloid. Normal saline containing 5% dextrose is preferable to lactated Ringer's solution, as the liver in hypothermic patients inefficiently metabolizes lactate. The placement of a pulmonary artery catheter, although of potential value, risks perforation of the less compliant pulmonary artery. The use of a central venous catheter should be avoided because of right atrial irritability.

Arterial blood gases should not be corrected for temperature (Chap. 50). This is termed the ectothermic or alpha-stat approach, which maximizes enzymatic function and maintains the normal distribution of charged metabolic intermediates. An uncorrected pH of 7.42 and a P_{CO_2} of 40 mmHg reflects appropriate alveolar ventilation and acid-base balance at any core temperature. Acid-base imbalances should be corrected gradually, since the bicarbonate buffering system is inefficient. When the P_{CO_2} increases 10 mmHg at 28°C, it doubles the pH decline of 0.08 that is normally induced at 37°C.

The severity of anemia may be underestimated because the hematocrit increases 2% for each 1°C drop in temperature. White blood cell sequestration and bone marrow suppression are common, potentially masking an infection. Although hypokalemia is more common in chronic hypothermia, hyperkalemia also occurs; the expected electrocardiographic changes can be obscured by hypothermia. Patients with renal insufficiency, metabolic acidoses, or rhabdomyolysis are most at risk for electrolyte disturbances.

Coagulopathies are common because cold inhibits the enzymatic reactions required for activation of the intrinsic cascade. In addition, the production of thromboxane B_2 by platelets is temperature-dependent, and platelet function is impaired. The administration of platelets and fresh frozen plasma is, therefore, not effective. The prothrombin or partial thromboplastin times reported by the laboratory appear deceptively normal and contrast with the observed coagulopathy. This contradiction appears because all coagulation tests are routinely performed at 37°C, and the enzymes are thus rewarmed.

REWARMING STRATEGIES The key initial decision is whether to rewarm the patient passively or actively. *Passive external rewarming* simply involves covering and insulating the patient in a warm environment. With the head covered, the rate of rewarming is usually 0.5° to 2.0°C per hour. This technique is ideal for previously healthy patients who develop acute, mild primary accidental hypothermia. The patient must have sufficient fuel and glycogen to support endogenous thermogenesis.

There are reservations about the application of heat directly to the extremities of patients with chronic severe hypothermia. Extinguishing peripheral vasoconstriction in the dehydrated patient may precipitate core temperature "afterdrop"—the continual decline in the core temperature after removal of the patient from the cold. This phenomenon results from conductive temperature equilibration and a circulatory convective mechanism. Rewarming frostbitten extremities before stabilization of the core temperature causes a significant core temperature afterdrop. In contrast, truncal heat application may minimize the risk of afterdrop.

Active rewarming is necessary under the following circumstances: core temperature <32°C (poikilothermia), cardiovascular instability, age extremes, CNS dysfunction, endocrine insufficiency, or any suspicion of secondary hypothermia. *Active external rewarming* is best accomplished with forced-air heating blankets. Other options include radiant heat sources and hot packs. Monitoring a patient with hypothermia in a heated tub is extremely difficult. Electric blankets should be avoided because vasoconstricted skin is easily burned. Widely available *active core rewarming* options include heated inhalation, heated infusion, and lavage (gastric, colonic, mediastinal, thoracic, pleural). The therapeutic options also include hemodialysis, venovenous, and continuous arteriovenous rewarming, in addition to formal cardiopulmonary bypass.

Arteriovenous anastomoses (AVA) rewarming provides exogenous heat by immersion of the hands, forearms, feet, and calves in 44° to 45°C water. Airway rewarming with heated humidified oxygen (40° to 45°C) is a convenient option via mask or endotracheal tube. Although airway rewarming provides less heat than some other forms of active core rewarming, it eliminates respiratory heat loss and adds 1° to 2°C to the overall rewarming rate. Crystalloids should be heated to 40° to 42°C. The quantity of heat provided is significant only during massive volume resuscitations. The most efficient method for heating and delivering fluid or blood is with a countercurrent in-line heat exchanger. Heated irrigation of the gastrointestinal tract or bladder transfers minimal heat because of the limited available surface area. These methods should be reserved for patients in cardiac arrest and then used in combination with all available active rewarming techniques. Closed thoracic lavage is far more efficient in severely hypothermic patients with cardiac arrest. The hemithoraces are irrigated through two large-bore thoracostomy tubes that are inserted into the left or both of the hemithoraces. Thoracostomy tubes should not be placed in the left chest of a spontaneously perfusing patient for purposes of rewarming. Peritoneal lavage with the dialysate at 40° to 45°C efficiently transfers heat when delivered through two catheters with outflow suction. Like peritoneal dialysis, standard hemodialysis is especially useful for patients with electrolyte abnormalities, rhabdomyolysis, or toxin ingestions.

With extracorporeal venovenous rewarming, the blood is removed from a central venous catheter, heated to 40°C, and returned through a second central or peripheral venous catheter. Continuous arteriovenous rewarming involves the use of percutaneously inserted femoral arterial and contralateral femoral venous 8.5 Fr catheters. The blood pressure must be at least 60 mmHg. Heparin-bonded tubing obviates the need for systemic anticoagulation. Full circulatory support with an oxygenator can only be provided through formal cardiopulmonary bypass (CPB). Femoral flow rates of 2 to 3 L/min elevate the core temperature 1° to 2°C every 3 to 5 min. CPB should be considered in nonperfusing patients without documented contraindications to resuscitation. Circulatory support may also be the only effective option in patients with completely frozen extremities, or those with significant tissue destruction coupled with rhabdomyolysis.

There is no evidence that extremely rapid rewarming improves survival in perfusing patients. The best strategy is usually a combination of passive, truncal active, and active core rewarming techniques.

DRUG THERAPY When a patient is hypothermic, target organs and the cardiovascular system respond minimally to most medications. Moreover, cumulative doses can cause toxicity during rewarming because of increased binding of drugs to proteins, and impaired metabolism and excretion. As an example, the administration of repeated doses of digoxin or insulin would be ineffective while the patient is hypothermic, and the residual drugs are potentially toxic during rewarming.

Any pharmacologic manipulation of the depressed and vasoconstricted cardiovascular system should generally be avoided. If the hypotension does not respond to crystalloid infusion and rewarming, low-dose dopamine (2 to 5 μg/kg per min) support should be considered. Atrial arrhythmias should initially be monitored without intervention, as the ventricular response will be slow, and most will convert spontaneously during rewarming. When indicated, bretylium tosylate is the class III ventricular antiarrhythmic of choice. During ventricular fibrillation, it should initially be administered at a dose of 10 mg/kg. Bretylium uniquely increases the ventricular arrhythmia threshold at low temperatures, although the wisdom of prophylaxis is unresolved.

Initiating empirical therapy for adrenal insufficiency is usually not warranted unless there is a history suggesting steroid dependence, hypoadrenalism, or a failure to rewarm with standard therapy. However, the administration of parenteral levothyroxine to euthyroid patients with hypothermia is potentially hazardous. Because laboratory results can be delayed and confounded by the presence of the sick euthyroid syndrome (Chap. 330), historical clues or physical findings suggestive of hypothyroidism should be sought. When myxedema is the cause of hypothermia, the relaxation phase of the Achilles reflex is prolonged more than the contraction phase.

Hypothermia obscures most of the symptoms and signs of infection, notably fever and leukocytosis. Shaking rigors from infection may be mistaken for shivering. Except in mild cases, extensive cultures and repeated physical examinations are essential. Unless an infectious source is identified, empirical antibiotic prophylaxis is most warranted in the elderly, neonates, and immunocompromised patients.

Preventive measures should be discussed with high-risk individuals, such as the elderly or people whose work frequently exposes them to extreme cold. The importance of layered clothing and headgear, adequate shelter, increased caloric intake, and the avoidance of ethanol should be emphasized, along with access to rescue services.

FROSTBITE

Peripheral cold injuries include both freezing and nonfreezing injuries to tissue. Frostbite occurs when the tissue temperature drops below 0°C. Ice crystal formation subsequently distorts and destroys the cellular architecture. Once the vascular endothelium is damaged, stasis progresses rapidly to microvascular thrombosis. Tissue freezes quickly when in contact with thermal conductors such as metal or volatile solutions. Other predisposing factors include constrictive clothing or boots, immobility, or vasoconstrictive medications.

Clinically, it is most practical to classify frostbite as superficial or deep. Superficial does not entail tissue loss. Classically, frostbite is retrospectively graded like a burn once the resultant pathology is demarcated over time. First-degree frostbite causes only anesthesia and erythema. The appearance of superficial vesiculation surrounded by edema and erythema is considered second degree (**Plates IIA-18, IIA-19**). Hemorrhagic vesicles reflect a serious injury to the microvasculature, and indicate third-degree frostbite. Fourth-degree injuries damage subcuticular, muscular, and osseous tissues.

PATHOPHYSIOLOGY   Peripheral cold injury involves a cascade of events. Endothelial cells are very susceptible to cold injury. In the prefreeze phase, plasma leaks and there is the development of microvascular vasoconstriction. The radiation of heat from underlying tissues initially prevents crystallization. The freeze phase usually begins with extracellular fluid crystallization. Water exits the cell and causes intracellular dehydration, hyperosmolality, and ultimately cellular shrinkage and demise. Damaged tissue releases thromboxane A_2 and prostaglandin $F_{2\alpha}$, which produce platelet aggregation, leukocyte immobilization, and vasoconstriction.

After the tissue thaws, the second phase of the cascade causes progressive dermal ischemia. The microvasculature begins to collapse, arteriovenous shunting increases tissue pressures, and there is progressive formation of edema. Finally, thrombosis, ischemia, and superficial necrosis appear. The development of mummification and demarcation may take weeks to months.

CLINICAL PRESENTATION   The initial presentation of frostbite can be deceptively benign. The symptoms always include a sensory deficiency affecting light touch, pain, and temperature perception. The acral areas and distal extremities are the most common insensate areas. Some patients complain of a clumsy or "chunk of wood" sensation in the extremity.

Deep frostbitten tissue can appear waxy, mottled, yellow, or violaceous-white. Favorable presenting signs include some warmth or sensation with normal color. The injury is often superficial if the subcutaneous tissue is pliable or if the dermis can be rolled over boney prominences.

The two most common nonfreezing peripheral cold injuries are *chilblain (pernio)* and *immersion (trench) foot*. Chilblain results from neuronal and endothelial damage induced by repetitive exposure to dry cold. Young females, particularly those with a history of Raynaud's phenomenon, are most at risk. Persistent vasospasticity and vasculitis can cause erythema, mild edema, and pruritus. Eventually plaques, blue nodules, and ulcerations develop. These lesions typically involve the dorsa of the hands and feet. In contrast, immersion (trench) foot results from repetitive exposure to wet cold above the freezing point. The feet initially appear cyanotic, cold, and edematous. The subsequent development of bullae is often indistinguishable from frostbite. This vesiculation rapidly progresses to ulceration and liquefaction gangrene. Patients with milder cases complain of hyperhidrosis, cold sensitivity, and painful ambulation for many years.

Various ancillary tests have been used in an attempt to diagnose the severity of peripheral cold injuries. None consistently predicts the extent of injury at presentation. For example, angiography and magnetic resonance imaging can demonstrate the patency of large vessels but not the microvasculature. Ultrasonography and digital plethysmography are also insensitive. Thermography and technetium scintigraphy help evaluate perfusion several days after rewarming.

℞ **TREATMENT**   Frozen tissue should be rapidly and completely thawed by immersion in circulating water at 37° to 40°C. Rapid rewarming often produces an initial hyperemia. The early formation of clear distal large blebs is more favorable than smaller proximal dark hemorrhagic blebs. A common error is the premature termination of thawing, since the reestablishment of perfusion is intensely painful. Parenteral narcotics will be necessary with deep frostbite. If cyanosis persists after rewarming, the tissue compartment pressures should be monitored carefully.

Numerous experimental antithrombotic and vasodilatory treatment regimens have been evaluated. There is no conclusive evidence that dextran, heparin, steroids, calcium channel blockers, or hyperbaric oxygen salvage tissue. A treatment protocol for frostbite is summarized in Table 20-3.

Unless infection develops,

Table 20-3   Treatment for Frostbite

Before Thawing	During Thawing	After Thawing
Remove from environment	Consider parenteral analgesia and ketorolac	Gently dry and protect part; elevate; pledgets between toes, if macerated
Prevent partial thawing and refreezing	Administer ibuprofen, 400 mg PO	If clear vesicles are intact, the fluid will reabsorb in days; if broken, debride and dress with antibiotic or sterile aloe vera ointment
Stabilize core temperature and treat hypothermia	Immerse part in 37°–40°C (thermometer-monitored) circulating water containing an antiseptic soap until distal flush (10–45 min)	Leave hemorrhagic vesicles intact to prevent infection
Protect frozen part—no friction or massage	Encourage patient to gently move part	Continue ibuprofen 400 mg PO (12 mg/kg per day) q8–12h
Address medical or surgical conditions	If pain is refractory, reduce water temperature to 33°–37°C	Consider tetanus and streptococcal prophylaxis; elevate part Hydrotherapy at 37°C

any decision regarding debridement or amputation should be deferred until there is clear evidence of demarcation, mummification, and sloughing. The most common symptomatic sequelae reflect neuronal injury and the persistently abnormal sympathetic tone, including paresthesias, thermal misperception, and hyperhidrosis. Delayed findings include nail deformities, cutaneous carcinomas, and epiphyseal damage in children.

BIBLIOGRAPHY

DANZL DF: Accidental hypothermia, in *Emergency Medicine: Concepts and Clinical Practice*, 4th ed, P Rosen et al (eds). St. Louis, Mosby, 1998, p 963

DANZL DF, POZOS RS: Current concepts: Accidental hypothermia. N Engl J Med 331: 1756, 1994

GIESBRECHT GG, BRISTOW GK: Recent advances in hypothermia research. Ann NY Acad Sci 813:676, 1997

MCADAMS TR et al: Frostbite: An orthopedic perspective. Am J Orthop 28:21, 1999

WEINBERG AD: The role of inhalation rewarming in the early management of hypothermia. Resuscitation 36:101, 1998

Section 3
NERVOUS SYSTEM DYSFUNCTION

21

Robert B. Daroff, Mark D. Carlson

FAINTNESS, SYNCOPE, DIZZINESS, AND VERTIGO

Syncope is defined as transient loss of consciousness due to reduced cerebral blood flow. Syncope is associated with postural collapse and spontaneous recovery. It may occur suddenly, without warning, or may be preceded by symptoms of varying duration. These include faintness or lightheadedness, "dizziness" without true vertigo, a feeling of warmth, diaphoresis, nausea, and visual blurring occasionally proceeding to blindness. These presyncopal symptoms may increase in severity until loss of consciousness occurs or may resolve prior to loss of consciousness if the cerebral ischemia is corrected. The differentiation of syncope from seizure is an important, sometimes difficult, diagnostic problem.

Syncope may be benign when it occurs as a result of normal cardiovascular reflex effects on heart rate and vascular tone or malignant when due to a life-threatening arrhythmia. Syncope may occur as a single event or may be recurrent. Recurrent, unexplained syncope, particularly in an individual with structural heart disease, is associated with a high risk for death (40% mortality within 2 years).

SYNCOPE

At the beginning of a syncopal attack, the patient is nearly always in the upright position, either sitting or standing. A cardiac etiology, such as an arrhythmia, is exceptional in this respect. The patient is warned of the impending faint by a sense of "feeling bad," of giddiness, and of movement or swaying of the floor or surrounding objects. The patient becomes confused and may yawn, visual spots and dimming may occur, and the ears may ring. Nausea and vomiting sometimes accompany these symptoms. There is a striking pallor or ashen gray color of the face, and generalized perspiration ensues. In some patients, a gradual onset with presyncopal symptoms may allow time for protection against injury; in others the syncope is sudden and without warning. The onset varies from instantaneous to 10 to 30 s, rarely longer.

The depth and duration of unconsciousness vary. Sometimes the patient remains partly aware of the surroundings, or there may be profound coma. The patient may remain in this state for seconds or minutes. Usually the patient lies motionless with skeletal muscles relaxed, but a few clonic jerks of the limbs and face may occur shortly after consciousness is lost. Sphincter control is usually maintained, in contrast to a seizure. The pulse is feeble or apparently absent, the blood pressure may be low or undetectable, and breathing may be almost imperceptible. Once the patient is in a horizontal position, gravity no longer hinders the flow of blood to the brain. The strength of the pulse may then improve, color begins to return to the face, breathing becomes quicker and deeper, and consciousness is regained. There is usually an immediate recovery of consciousness. Some patients, however, may be keenly aware of physical weakness, and rising too soon may precipitate another faint. In other patients, particularly those with tachyarrhythmias, there may be no residual symptoms following the initial syncope. Headache and drowsiness, which with mental confusion are the usual sequelae of a seizure, do not follow a syncopal attack.

PATHOPHYSIOLOGY The more common types of faint are reducible to a few simple mechanisms. Syncope results from a sudden impairment of brain metabolism, usually brought about by hypotension with reduction of cerebral blood flow. Several mechanisms subserve circulatory adjustments to the upright posture. Approximately three-fourths of the systemic blood volume is contained in the venous bed, and any interference in venous return may lead to a reduction in cardiac output. Cerebral blood flow may still be maintained, as long as systemic arterial vasoconstriction occurs, but when this adjustment fails, serious hypotension with resultant cerebral underperfusion to less than half of normal results in syncope. Normally, the pooling of blood in the lower parts of the body is prevented by: (1) pressor reflexes that induce constriction of peripheral arterioles and venules, (2) reflex acceleration of the heart by means of aortic and carotid reflexes, and (3) improvement of venous return to the heart by activity of the muscles of the limbs. Placing a normal person on a tilt table to relax the muscles and tilting upright slightly diminishes cardiac output and allows the blood to accumulate in the legs to a slight degree; this may then be followed by a slight transitory fall in systolic arterial pressure and, in patients with defective vasomotor reflexes, may produce faints.

CAUSES OF SYNCOPE Transiently decreased cerebral blood flow is usually due to one of three general mechanisms: disorders of vascular tone or blood volume, cardiovascular disorders including cardiac arrhythmias, or cerebrovascular disease (Table 21-1). Not infrequently, however, the cause of syncope is multifactorial.

Disorders of Vascular Tone or Blood Volume Disorders of autonomic control of the heart and circulation account for at least half of syncopal episodes. These disorders share common pathophysiologic mechanisms: a cardioinhibitory component (e.g., bradycardia due to increased efferent vagal activity), a vasodepressor component (e.g., inappropriate vasodilatation due to sympathetic withdrawal), or both.

Vasovagal (vasodepressor, neurocardiogenic) syncope This form of syncope is the common faint that may be experienced by normal persons and accounts for approximately half of all episodes of syncope. It is frequently recurrent and commonly precipitated by a hot or crowded environment, alcohol, extreme fatigue, severe pain, hunger, prolonged standing, and emotional or stressful situations. Episodes are often preceded by a presyncopal prodrome lasting seconds

Table 21-1   Causes of Syncope

I. Disorders of vascular tone or blood volume
  A. Vasovagal (vasodepressor, neurocardiogenic)
  B. Postural (orthostatic) hypotension
    1. Drug induced (especially antihypertensive or vasodilator drugs)
    2. Peripheral neuropathy (diabetic, alcoholic, nutritional, amyloid)
    3. Idiopathic postural hypotension
    4. Multisystem atrophies
    5. Physical deconditioning
    6. Sympathectomy
    7. Acute dysautonomia (Guillain-Barré syndrome variant)
    8. Decreased blood volume (adrenal insufficiency, acute blood loss, etc.)
  C. Carotid sinus hypersensitivity
  D. Situational
    1. Cough
    2. Micturition
    3. Defecation
    4. Valsalva
    5. Deglutition
  E. Glossopharyngeal Neuralgia
II. Cardiovascular disorders
  A. Cardiac arryhthmias (Chaps. 229 and 230)
    1. Bradyarrhythmias
      a. Sinus bradycardia, sinoatrial block, sinus arrest, sick-sinus syndrome
      b. Atrioventricular block
    2. Tachyarrhythmias
      a. Supraventricular tachycardia with structural cardiac disease
      b. Atrial fibrillation associated with the Wolff-Parkinson-White syndrome
      c. Atrial flutter with 1:1 atrioventricular conduction
      d. Ventricular tachycardia
  B. Other cardiopulmonary etiologies
    1. Pulmonary embolism
    2. Pulmonary hypertension
    3. Atrial myxoma
    4. Myocardial disease (massive myocardial infarction)
    5. Left ventricular myocardial restriction or constriction
    6. Pericardial constriction or tamponade
    7. Aortic outflow tract obstruction
    8. Aortic valvular stenosis
    9. Hypertrophic obstructive cardiomyopathy
III. Cerebrovascular disease (Chap. 361)
  A. Vertebrobasilar insufficiency
  B. Basilar artery migraine
IV. Other disorders that may resemble syncope
  A. Metabolic
    1. Hypoxia
    2. Anemia
    3. Diminished carbon dioxide due to hyperventilation
    4. Hypoglycemia
  B. Psychogenic
    1. Anxiety attacks
    2. Hysterical fainting
  C. Seizures

to minutes. Vasovagal syncope rarely occurs in the supine position. The individual is usually sitting or standing and experiences weakness, nausea, diaphoresis, lightheadedness, blurred vision, and often a forceful heart beat with tachycardia followed by cardiac slowing prior to loss of consciousness. The individual appears pallid and has decreasing blood pressure prior to syncope. The duration of unconsciousness is rarely longer than a few minutes if the conditions that provoke the episode are reversed. Consciousness is usually regained shortly after assuming a recumbent posture, but unconsciousness may be prolonged if an individual remains upright. Although commonly benign, vasovagal syncope can be associated with prolonged asystole and hypotension, resulting in injury.

Vasovagal syncope occurs in the setting of increased sympathetic activity and venous pooling. Under these conditions, vigorous myocardial contraction of a relatively empty left ventricle activates ventricular mechanoreceptors and vagal afferent nerve fibers, inhibiting sympathetic efferent activity and increasing parasympathetic efferent activity. The resultant vasodilatation and bradycardia induce hypotension and syncope.

The central nervous system (CNS) mechanisms responsible for vasovagal syncope are not clear. Animal studies, not confirmed in humans, suggest that endogenous opiates (endorphins) may play a role. Serotonin (5-hydroxytryptamine) participates in blood pressure regulation and may also be involved in inhibition of sympathetic efferent activity (and arterial vasodilatation) associated with vasovagal syncope.

Although the reflex involving myocardial mechanoreceptors is the mechanism usually accepted as responsible for vasovagal syncope, other reflexes may also be operative. Patients with transplanted (denervated) hearts have experienced cardiovascular responses identical to those present during vasovagal syncope. This should not be possible if the response depends solely on the reflex mechanisms described above unless the transplanted heart has become reinnervated. Moreover, vasovagal syncope often occurs in response to stimuli (fear, emotional stress, or pain) that may not be associated with venous pooling in the lower extremities, which suggests a cognitive or cortical component to the reflex. Thus, a variety of afferent and efferent responses may cause vasovagal syncope.

Postural (orthostatic) hypotension   This occurs in patients who have a chronic defect in, or variable instability of, vasomotor reflexes. Systemic arterial blood pressure falls on assumption of upright posture due to loss of vasoconstriction reflexes in resistance and capacitance vessels of the lower extremities. Although the syncopal attack differs little from vasodepressor syncope, the effect of posture is critical. Sudden rising from a recumbent position or standing quietly are precipitating circumstances. *Orthostatic hypotension may be the cause of syncope in up to 30% of the elderly; polypharmacy with antihypertensive or antidepressant drugs is often a contributor in these patients.*

Postural syncope may occur in otherwise normal persons with defective postural reflexes. Patients with *idiopathic postural hypotension* may be identified by a characteristic response to upright tilt on a table. Initially, the blood pressure diminishes slightly before stabilizing at a lower level. Shortly thereafter, the compensatory reflexes fail and the systemic arterial pressure falls precipitously. The condition is often familial.

Orthostatic hypotension, often accompanied by disturbances in sweating, impotence, and sphincter difficulties, is also a primary feature of the autonomic nervous system disorders discussed in Chap. 366 and listed in Table 366-1. The most common causes of neurogenic orthostatic hypotension are chronic diseases of the peripheral nervous system that involve postganglionic unmyelinated fibers (e.g., diabetic, nutritional, and amyloid polyneuropathy). Much less common are the multisystem atrophies, which are CNS disorders in which orthostatic hypotension is associated with (1) parkinsonism (Shy-Drager syndrome), (2) progressive cerebellar degeneration, or (3) a more variable parkinsonian and cerebellar syndrome (striatonigral degeneration). Very rarely, an acute postganglionic dysautonomia has been reported that appears to represent a variant of Guillain-Barré syndrome (Chap. 378).

There are several additional causes of postural syncope: (1) After physical deconditioning (such as after prolonged illness with recumbency, especially in elderly individuals with reduced muscle tone) or after prolonged weightlessness, as in space flight; (2) after sympathectomy that has abolished vasopressor reflexes; and (3) in patients receiving antihypertensive or vasodilator drugs and those who are hypovolemic because of diuretics, excessive sweating, diarrhea, vomiting, hemorrhage, or adrenal insufficiency.

Carotid sinus hypersensitivity   Syncope due to carotid sinus hypersensitivity is precipitated by pressure on the carotid sinus baroreceptors, which are located just cephalad to the bifurcation of the common carotid artery. This typically occurs in the setting of shaving, a tight collar, or turning the head to one side. Carotid sinus hypersensitivity occurs predominantly in men, most of whom are 50 years of age or older. Activation of carotid sinus baroreceptors gives rise to

21   Faintness, Syncope, Dizziness, and Vertigo   **113**

Activation of carotid sinus baroreceptors gives rise to impulses carried via the nerve of Hering, a branch of the glossopharyngeal nerve, to the medulla oblongata. These afferent impulses activate efferent sympathetic nerve fibers to the heart and blood vessels, cardiac vagal efferent nerve fibers, or both. In patients with carotid sinus hypersensitivity, these responses may cause sinus arrest or atrioventricular (AV) block (a cardioinhibitory response), vasodilatation (a vasodepressor response), or both (a mixed response). Although originally described in 1933, the mechanisms responsible for the syndrome are not clear, and validated diagnostic criteria do not exist; some authorities have questioned its very existence.

Situational syncope A variety of activities, including cough, deglutition, micturition, and defecation, are associated with syncope in susceptible individuals. These syndromes are caused, at least in part, by abnormal autonomic control and may involve a cardioinhibitory response, a vasodepressor response, or both. Cough, micturition, and defecation are associated with maneuvers (such as Valsalva, straining, and coughing) that may contribute to hypotension and syncope by decreasing venous return. Increased intracranial pressure secondary to the increased intrathoracic pressure may also contribute by decreasing cerebral blood flow.

Cough syncope typically occurs in men with chronic bronchitis or chronic obstructive lung disease during or immediately after prolonged coughing fits. Micturition syncope occurs predominantly in middle-aged and older men, particularly those with prostatic hypertrophy and obstruction of the bladder neck; loss of consciousness usually occurs at night during or immediately after voiding. Deglutition and defecation syncope occur in men and women. Deglutition syncope may be associated with esophageal disorders, particularly esophageal spasm. In some individuals, particular foods and carbonated or cold beverages initiate episodes by activating esophageal sensory receptors that trigger reflex sinus bradycardia or AV block. Defecation syncope is probably secondary to a Valsalva maneuver in older individuals with constipation.

Glossopharyngeal neuralgia Syncope due to glossopharyngeal neuralgia is preceded by pain in the oropharynx, tonsillar fossa, or tongue. Loss of consciousness is usually associated with asystole rather than vasodilatation. The mechanism is thought to involve activation of afferent impulses in the glossopharyngeal nerve which terminate in the nucleus solitarius of the medulla and, via collaterals, activate the dorsal motor nucleus of the vagus nerve.

Cardiovascular Disorders Cardiac syncope results from a sudden reduction in cardiac output, caused most commonly by a cardiac arrhythmia. In normal individuals, heart rates between 30 and 180 beats per minutes (bpm) do not reduce cerebral blood flow, especially if the person is in the supine position. As the heart rate decreases, ventricular filling time and stroke volume increase to maintain normal cardiac output. At rates below 30 bpm, stroke volume can no longer increase to compensate adequately for the decreased heart rate. At rates greater than approximately 180 bpm, ventricular filling time is inadequate to maintain adequate stroke volume. In either case, cerebral hypoperfusion and syncope may occur. Upright posture, cerebrovascular disease, anemia, and coronary, myocardial, or valvular disease all reduce the tolerance to alterations in rate.

Bradyarrhythmias (Chap. 229) may occur as a result of an abnormality of impulse generation (e.g., sinoatrial arrest) or impulse conduction (e.g., AV block). Either may cause syncope if the escape pacemaker rate is insufficient to maintain cardiac output. Syncope due to bradyarrhythmias may occur abruptly, without presyncopal symptoms, and recur several times daily. Patients with *sick sinus syndrome* may have sinus pauses (>3 s), and those with syncope due to high-degree AV block (*Stokes-Adams-Morgagni syndrome*) may have evidence of conduction system disease (e.g., prolonged PR interval, bundle branch block). However, the arrhythmia is often transitory, and the surface electrocardiogram or continuous electrocardiographic monitor (Holter monitor) taken later may not reveal the abnormality. The *bradycardia-tachycardia syndrome* is a common form of sinus node dysfunction in which syncope generally occurs as a result of marked sinus pauses

following termination of paroxysmal supraventricular tachycardia. Drugs are a common cause for bradyarrhythmias, particularly in patients with underlying structural heart disease. Digoxin, β-adrenergic receptor antagonists, calcium channel blockers, and many antiarrhythmic drugs may suppress sinoatrial node impulse generation or slow AV nodal conduction.

Syncope due to a *tachyarrhythmia* (Chap. 230) is usually preceded by palpitation or lightheadedness but may occur abruptly with no warning symptoms. *Supraventricular tachyarrhythmias* are unlikely to cause syncope in individuals with structurally normal hearts but may do so if they occur in patients with: (1) heart disease that also compromises cardiac output, (2) cerebrovascular disease, (3) a disorder of vascular tone or blood volume, or (4) a rapid ventricular rate. These tachycardias result most commonly from paroxysmal atrial flutter, atrial fibrillation, or reentry involving the AV node or accessory pathways that bypass part or all of the AV conduction system. Patients with the *Wolff-Parkinson-White syndrome* may experience syncope when a very rapid ventricular rate occurs due to reentry across an accessory AV connection.

In patients with structural heart disease, ventricular tachycardia, sometimes associated with ventricular fibrillation, is a common cause of syncope, particularly in patients with a prior myocardial infarction. Patients with aortic valvular stenosis and hypertrophic obstructive cardiomyopathy are also at risk for ventricular tachycardia. Individuals with abnormalities of ventricular repolarization (prolongation of the QT interval) are at risk to develop polymorphic ventricular tachycardia (*torsade de pointes*). Those with the inherited form of this syndrome often have a family history of sudden death in young individuals. Genetic markers can identify some patients with familial long-QT syndrome but the clinical utility of these markers remains unproven. Drugs (i.e., certain antiarrhythmics and erythromycin) and electrolyte disorders (i.e., hypokalemia, hypocalcemia, hypomagnesemia) can prolong the QT interval and predispose to torsade de pointes. Antiarrhythmic medications may precipitate ventricular tachycardia, particularly in patients with structural heart disease.

In addition to arrythmias, syncope may also occur with a variety of structural cardiovascular disorders. Episodes are usually precipitated when the cardiac output cannot increase to compensate adequately for peripheral vasodilatation. Peripheral vasodilatation may be appropriate, such as following exercise, or may occur due to inappropriate activation of left ventricular mechanoreceptor reflexes, as occurs in aortic outflow tract obstruction (aortic valvular stenosis or hypertrophic obstructive cardiomyopathy). Obstruction to forward flow is the most common reason that cardiac output cannot increase. Pericardial tamponade is a rare cause of syncope. Syncope occurs in up to 10% of patients with massive pulmonary embolism and may occur with exertion in patients with severe primary pulmonary hypertension. The cause is an inability of the right ventricle to provide appropriate cardiac output in the presence of obstruction or increased pulmonary vascular resistance. Loss of consciousness is usually accompanied by other symptoms such as chest pain and dyspnea. Atrial myxoma, a prosthetic valve thrombus, and, rarely, mitral stenosis may impair left ventricular filling, decrease cardiac output, and cause syncope.

Cerebrovascular Disease Cerebrovascular disease alone rarely causes syncope but may lower the threshold for syncope in patients with other causes. The vertebrobasilar arteries, which supply brainstem centers responsible for maintaining consciousness, are usually involved when cerebrovascular disease causes or contributes to syncope. An exception is the rare patient with tight bilateral carotid stenosis and recurrent syncope, often precipitated by standing or walking. Most patients who experience lightheadedness or syncope due to cerebrovascular disease also have symptoms of focal neurologic ischemia, such as arm or leg weakness, diplopia, ataxia, dysarthria, or sensory disturbances. Basilar artery migraine is a rare disorder that causes syncope in adolescents.

DIFFERENTIAL DIAGNOSIS Anxiety Attacks and the Hyperventilation Syndrome Anxiety, such as occurs in panic attacks, is frequently interpreted as a feeling of faintness or dizziness resembling presyncope. The symptoms are not accompanied by facial pallor and are not relieved by recumbency. The diagnosis is made on the basis of the associated symptoms such as a feeling of impending doom, air hunger, palpitations, and tingling of the fingers and perioral region. Attacks can often be reproduced by hyperventilation, resulting in hypocapnia, alkalosis, increased cerebrovascular resistance, and decreased cerebral blood flow. The release of epinephrine in anxiety states also contributes to the symptoms.

Seizures A seizure may be heralded by an aura, which is caused by a focal seizure discharge and hence has localizing significance. The aura is usually followed by a rapid return to normal or by a loss of consciousness. Injury from falling is frequent in a seizure and rare in syncope, because only in seizures are protective reflexes abolished instantaneously. Tonic-convulsive movements are characteristic of seizures and usually do not occur with syncope, although, as stated above, brief tonic-clonic seizure-like activity can accompany fainting episodes. The period of unconsciousness tends to be longer in seizures than in syncope. Urinary incontinence is frequent in seizures and rare in syncope. The return of consciousness is prompt in syncope, slow after a seizure. Mental confusion, headache, and drowsiness are common sequelae of seizures; physical weakness with a clear sensorium characterizes the postsyncopal state. Repeated spells of unconsciousness in a young person at a rate of several per day or month are more suggestive of epilepsy than syncope.

Hypoglycemia Severe hypoglycemia is usually due to a serious disease such as a tumor of the islets of Langerhans; advanced adrenal, pituitary, or hepatic disease; or to excessive administration of insulin.

Acute Hemorrhage Hemorrhage, usually within the gastrointestinal tract, is an occasional cause of syncope. In the absence of pain and hematemesis, the cause of the weakness, faintness, or even unconsciousness may remain obscure until the passage of a black stool.

Hysterical Fainting The attack is usually unattended by an outward display of anxiety. Lack of change in pulse and blood pressure or color of the skin and mucous membranes distinguish it from the vasodepressor faint.

Approach to the Patient

The diagnosis of syncope is often challenging. The cause may only be apparent at the time of the event, leaving few, if any, clues when the patient is seen later by the physician. In dealing with patients who have fainted, the physician should think first of those causes of fainting that constitute a therapeutic emergency. Among them are massive internal hemorrhage or myocardial infarction, which may be painless, and cardiac arrythmias. In elderly persons, a sudden faint, without obvious cause, should arouse the suspicion of complete heart block or a tachyarrhythmia, even though all findings are negative when the patient is seen.

An algorithmic approach to syncope is presented in Fig. 21-1. A careful history is the most important diagnostic tool, both to suggest the correct cause and to exclude other important potential causes (Table 21-1). Although no single element of the history is specific for a particular etiology of syncope, the nature of the events and their time course immediately prior to, during, and after an episode often provide valuable etiologic clues. Loss of consciousness in particular situations, such as during venipuncture, micturition, or in association with volume depletion, suggests an abnormality of vascular tone. The position of the patient at the time of the syncopal episode is very important; syncope in the supine position is unlikely to be vasovagal and suggests an arrhythmia or a seizure. Syncope due to carotid sinus syndrome may occur when the individual is wearing a shirt with a tight collar, turning the head (turning to look while driving in reverse), or manipulating the neck (as in shaving). The patient's medications must be

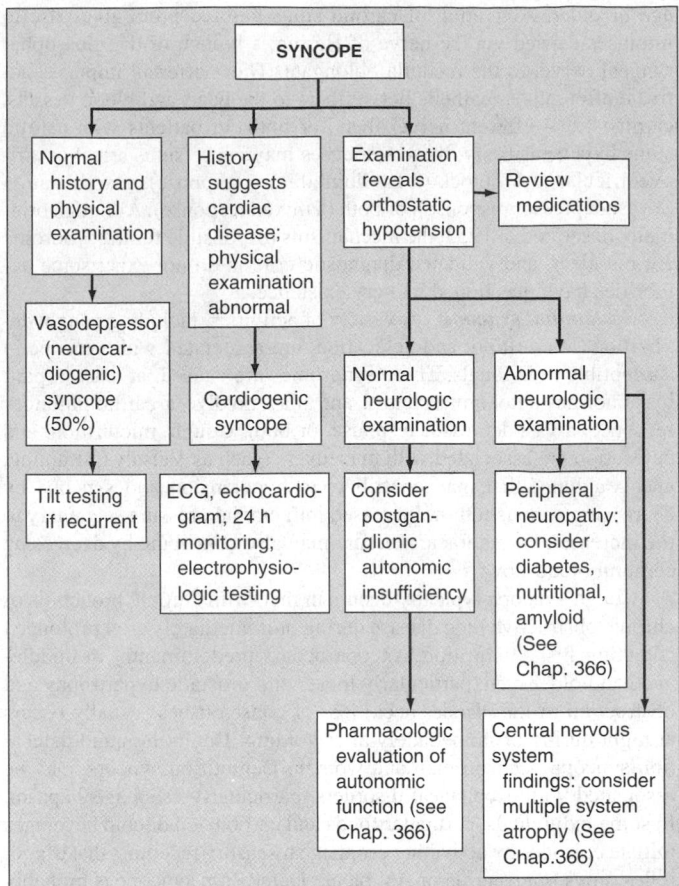

FIGURE 21-1 Approach to the patient with syncope.

noted, including nonprescription drugs or health store supplements, with particular attention to recent changes.

The physical examination should include evaluation of heart rate and blood pressure in the supine, sitting, and standing positions. In patients with unexplained recurrent syncope, an attempt to reproduce an attack may assist in diagnosis. Anxiety attacks induced by hyperventilation can be reproduced readily by having the patient breathe rapidly and deeply for 2 to 3 min. Cough syncope may be reproduced by inducing the Valsalva maneuver. Carotid sinus massage should generally be avoided, even in patients with suspected carotid sinus hypersensitivity; it is a risky procedure that can cause a transient ischemic attack (TIA) or stroke in susceptible individuals.

Diagnostic Tests The choice of diagnostic tests should be guided by the history and the physical examination. Measurements of serum electrolytes, glucose, and the hematocrit may help to establish the cause of syncope. Cardiac enzymes should be evaluated if myocardial ischemia is suspected. Blood and urine toxicology screens may reveal the presence of alcohol or other drugs. In patients with possible adrenocortical insufficiency, plasma aldosterone and mineralocorticoid levels should be obtained.

Although the surface electrocardiogram is unlikely to provide a definitive diagnosis, it may provide clues to the cause of syncope *and should be performed in almost all patients*. The presence of conduction abnormalities (PR prolongation and bundle branch block) suggests a bradyarrhythmia, whereas pathologic Q waves or prolongation of the QT interval suggests a ventricular tachyarrhythmia. Inpatients should undergo continuous electrocardiographic monitoring; outpatients should wear a Holter monitor for 24 to 48 h. Whenever possible, symptoms should be correlated with the occurrence of arrhythmias. Continuous electrocardiographic monitoring may establish the cause of syncope in as many as 15% of patients. Cardiac event monitors may be useful in patients with infrequent symptoms, particularly in patients with presyncope. The presence of a late potential on a signal-averaged electrocardiogram is associated with increased risk for ventricular tacharrhythmias in patients with a prior myocardial infarction. Low-voltage (visually inapparent) T wave alternans is also associated with development of sustained ventricular arrhythmias.

Invasive cardiac electrophysiologic testing provides diagnostic and prognostic information regarding sinus node function, AV conduction, and supraventricular and ventricular arrhythmias. Abnormal findings include prolongation of the sinus node recovery time, prolongation of the histoventricle (HV) interval, induction of a supraventricular arrhythmia associated with hypotension, or induction of a supraventricular arrhythmia. Prolongation of the sinus node recovery time (>1500 ms) is a specific finding (85 to 100%) for diagnosis of sinus node dysfunction but has a low sensitivity; continuous electrocardiographic monitoring is usually more effective for diagnosing this abnormality. Prolongation of the HV interval and conduction block below the His bundle indicate that His-Purkinje disease may be responsible for syncope. Although an HV interval >100 ms is abnormal, this finding is not common in patients with syncope, and some patients with shorter intervals are also at risk for AV block. Programmed stimulation for ventricular arrhythmias is most useful in patients who have experienced a myocardial infarction; the sensitivity and specificity of this technique is lower in patients with normal hearts or those with heart disease other than coronary artery disease.

Upright tilt table testing is indicated for recurrent syncope, a single syncopal episode that caused injury, or a single syncopal event in a "high-risk" setting (pilot, commercial vehicle driver, etc.), whether or not there is a history of preexisting heart disease or prior vasovagal episodes. In susceptible patients, upright tilt at an angle between 60 and 80° for 30 to 60 min induces a vasovagal episode. The protocol can be shortened if upright tilt is combined with intravenous administration of drugs that cause venous pooling or increase adrenergic stimulation (isoproterenol, nitroglycerin, edrophonium, or adenosine). The sensitivity and specificity of tilt table testing is difficult to ascertain because of the lack of validated criteria. Moreover, the reflexes responsible for vasovagal syncope can be elicited in most, if not all, individuals given the appropriate stimulus. The reported accuracy of the test ranges from 30 to 80%, depending on the population studied and the techniques used. Whereas the reproducibility of a negative test is 85 to 100%, the reproducibility of a positive tilt table test is only between 62 and 88%.

A variety of other tests may be useful to determine the presence of structural heart disease that may cause syncope. The echocardiogram with Doppler examination detects valvular, myocardial, and pericardial abnormalities. The echocardiogram is the "gold standard" for the diagnosis of hypertrophic cardiomyopathy and atrial myxoma. Cardiac cine magnetic resonance (MR) imaging provides an alternative noninvasive modality that may be useful for patients in whom diagnostic-quality echocardiographic images cannot be obtained. This test is also indicated for patients suspected of having arrhythmogenic right ventricular dysplasia or right ventricular outflow tract ventricular tachycardia. Both are associated with right ventricular structural abnormalities that are better visualized on MR imaging than by echocardiogram. Exercise testing may detect ischemia or exercise-induced arrhythmias. In some patients, cardiac catheterization may be necessary to diagnose the presence or severity of coronary artery disease or valvular abnormalities. Ultrafast computed tomographic scan, ventilation-perfusion scan, or pulmonary angiography are indicated in patients in whom syncope may be due to pulmonary embolus.

In possible cases of cerebrovascular syncope, a variety of neuroimaging tests may be indicated, including Doppler ultrasound studies of the carotid and vertebrobasilar systems, MR imaging, MR angiography, and x-ray angiography of the cerebral vasculature (Chaps. 358 and 361). Electroencephalography is indicated if seizures are suspected.

$\mathrm{R_X}$ **TREATMENT** The treatment of syncope is directed toward the underlying cause. This discussion will focus on the treatment

of disorders of autonomic control. →*Arrythmias are discussed in Chaps. 229 and 230, valvular heart diseases in Chap. 236, and cerebrovascular disorders in Chap. 361.*

Certain precautions should be taken regardless of the cause of syncope. At the first sign of symptoms, patients should make every effort to avoid injury should they lose consciousness. Patients with frequent episodes, or those who have experienced syncope without warning symptoms should avoid situations in which sudden loss of consciousness might result in injury (e.g., climbing ladders, swimming alone, operating heavy machinery, driving). Patients should lower their head to the extent possible, and preferably should lie down. Lowering the head by bending at the waist should be avoided because it may further compromise venous return to the heart. When appropriate, family members or other close contacts should be educated as to the problem. This will ensure appropriate therapy and may prevent delivery of inappropriate therapy (chest compressions associated with cardiopulmonary resuscitation) that may inflict trauma.

Patients who have lost consciousness should be placed in a position that maximizes cerebral blood flow, offers protection from trauma, and secures the airway. Whenever possible, the patient should be placed supine with the head turned to the side to prevent aspiration and the tongue from blocking the airway. Assessment of the pulse and direct cardiac auscultation may assist in determining if the episode is associated with a bradyarrhythmia or tachyarrhythmia. Clothing that fits tightly around the neck or waist should be loosened. Peripheral stimulation, such as by sprinkling cold water on the face, may be helpful. Patients should not be given anything by mouth or be permitted to rise until the sense of physical weakness has passed.

Patients with vasovagal syncope should be instructed to avoid situations or stimuli that have caused them to lose consciousness. Episodes associated with intravascular volume depletion may be prevented by salt and fluid loading prior to provocative events. β-Adrenoceptor antagonists, the most widely used agents, mitigate the increase in myocardial contractility that stimulates left ventricular mechanoreceptors and also block central serotonin receptors. Disopyramide, a vagolytic with negative inotropic properties, and another vagolytic, transdermal scopolamine, are used to treat vasovagal syncope. Paroxetine, a serotonin reuptake inhibitor used for depression, appears to be an effective treatment, as are theophylline and ephedrine. Midodrine, an α agonist, has been a first-line agent for some patients. Permanent cardiac pacing is effective for patients with frequent episodes of vasovagal syncope and is indicated for those with prolonged asystole associated with vasovagal episodes.

Patients with orthostatic hypotension should be instructed to rise slowly and systematically (supine to seated, seated to standing) from the bed or a chair. Movement of the legs prior to rising facilitates venous return from the lower extremities. Whenever possible, medications that aggravate the problem (vasodilators, diuretics, etc.) should be discontinued. Elevation of the head of the bed [20 to 30 cm (8 to 12 in.)] and use of elastic stockings may help.

Therapeutic modalities include devices that prevent lower limb blood pooling, such as an antigravity or g suit or elastic stockings; salt loading; and a variety of pharmacologic agents including sympathomimetic amines, monamine oxidase inhibitors, beta blockers, and levodopa. →*The treatment of orthostatic hypotension secondary to central or peripheral disorders of the autonomic nervous system is discussed in Chap. 366.*

Glossopharyngeal neuralgia is treated with carbamazepine, which is effective for the syncope as well as for the pain. Patients with carotid sinus syndrome should be instructed to avoid clothing and situations that stimulate carotid sinus baroreceptors. Patients should turn their entire body, rather than just their head, to look to one side. Those with intractable syncope due to the cardioinhibitory response to carotid sinus stimulation should undergo permanent pacemaker implantation.

Patients with syncope should be hospitalized when the episode may have resulted from a life-threatening abnormality or if recurrence with significant injury seems likely. These individuals should be admitted to a bed with continuous electrocardiographic monitoring. Patients who are known to have a normal heart and for whom the history strongly suggests vasovagal or situational syncope may be treated as outpatients if the episodes are neither frequent nor severe.

DIZZINESS AND VERTIGO

Dizziness is a common and often vexing symptom. Patients use the term to encompass a variety of sensations, including those that seem semantically appropriate (e.g., lightheadedness, faintness, spinning, giddiness, etc.) and those that are misleadingly inappropriate, such as mental confusion, blurred vision, headache, or tingling. Moreover, some individuals with gait disorders complain of dizziness despite the absence of vertigo or other abnormal cephalic sensations. The causes include peripheral neuropathy, myelopathy, spasticity, parkinsonian rigidity, and cerebellar ataxia. In this context, the term *dizziness* is being used to describe disturbed mobility. There may be mild associated lightheadedness, particularly with impaired sensation from the feet or poor vision; this is known as *multiple-sensory-defect dizziness* and occurs in elderly individuals who complain of dizziness only during ambulation. Decreased position sense (secondary to neuropathy or myelopathy) and poor vision (from cataracts or retinal degeneration) create an overreliance on the aging vestibular apparatus. A less precise but sometimes comforting designation to patients is *benign dysequilibrium of aging.* Thus, a careful history is necessary to determine exactly what a patient who states, "Doctor, I'm dizzy," is experiencing. After eliminating the misleading symptoms or gait disturbance, "dizziness" usually means either *faintness* (presyncope) or *vertigo* (an illusory or hallucinatory sense of movement of the body or environment, most often a feeling of spinning). Operationally, dizziness is classified into three categories: (1) faintness, (2) vertigo, and (3) miscellaneous head sensations.

FAINTNESS   Prior to an actual faint (syncope), there are often prodromal presyncopal symptoms (faintness) reflecting ischemia to a degree insufficient to impair consciousness (see above).

VERTIGO   Vertigo is usually due to a disturbance in the vestibular system. The end organs of this system, situated in the bony labyrinths of the inner ears, consist of the three semicircular canals and the otolithic apparatus (utricle and saccule) on each side. The canals transduce angular acceleration, while the otoliths transduce linear acceleration and static gravitational forces, the latter providing a sense of head position in space. The neural output of the end organs is conveyed to the vestibular nuclei in the brainstem via the eighth cranial nerve. The principal projections from the vestibular nuclei are to the nuclei of cranial nerves III, IV, and VI, the spinal cord, the cerebral cortex, and the cerebellum. The vestibuloocular reflex (VOR) serves to maintain visual stability during head movement and depends on direct projections from the vestibular nuclei to the sixth cranial nerve (abducens) nuclei in the pons and, via the medial longitudinal fasciculus, to the third (oculomotor) and fourth (trochlear) cranial nerve nuclei in the midbrain. These connections account for the nystagmus (to-and-fro oscillation of the eyes) that is an almost invariable accompaniment of vestibular dysfunction. The vestibular nerves and nuclei project to areas of the cerebellum (primarily the flocculus and nodulus) that modulate the VOR. The vestibulospinal pathways assist in the maintenance of postural stability. Projections to the cerebral cortex, via the thalamus, provide conscious awareness of head position and movement.

The vestibular system is one of three sensory systems subserving spatial orientation and posture; the other two are the visual system (retina to occipital cortex) and the somatosensory system that conveys peripheral information from skin, joint, and muscle receptors. The three stabilizing systems overlap sufficiently to compensate (partially or completely) for each other's deficiencies. Vertigo may represent either physiologic stimulation or pathologic dysfunction in any of the three systems.

Physiologic Vertigo   This occurs when (1) the brain is confronted with a mismatch among the three stabilizing sensory systems; (2) the vestibular system is subjected to unfamiliar head movements to which it has never adapted, such as in seasickness; or (3) unusual head/neck positions, such as the extreme extension when painting a ceiling. Intersensory mismatch explains carsickness, height vertigo, and the visual vertigo most commonly experienced during motion picture chase scenes; in the latter, the visual sensation of environmental movement is unaccompanied by concomitant vestibular and somatosensory movement cues. *Space sickness*, a frequent transient effect of active head movement in the weightless zero-gravity environment, is another example of physiologic vertigo.

Pathologic Vertigo   This results from lesions of the visual, somatosensory, or vestibular systems. Visual vertigo is caused by new or incorrect spectacles or by the sudden onset of an extraocular muscle paresis with diplopia; in either instance, CNS compensation rapidly counteracts the vertigo. Somatosensory vertigo, rare in isolation, is usually due to a peripheral neuropathy that reduces the sensory input necessary for central compensation when there is dysfunction of the vestibular or visual systems.

The most common cause of pathologic vertigo is vestibular dysfunction. The vertigo is frequently accompanied by nausea, jerk nystagmus, postural unsteadiness, and gait ataxia. Since vertigo increases with rapid head movements, patients tend to hold their heads still.

Labyrinthine dysfunction   This causes severe rotational or linear vertigo. When rotational, the hallucination of movement, whether of environment or self, is directed away from the side of the lesion. The fast phases of nystagmus beat away from the lesion side, and the tendency to fall is toward the side of the lesion.

When the head is straight and immobile, the vestibular end organs generate a tonic resting firing frequency that is equal from the two sides. With any rotational acceleration, the anatomic positions of the semicircular canals on each side necessitate an increased firing rate from one and a commensurate decrease from the other. This change in neural activity is ultimately projected to the cerebral cortex, where it is summed with inputs from the visual and somatosensory systems to produce the appropriate conscious sense of rotational movement. After cessation of movement, the firing frequencies of the two end organs reverse; the side with the initially increased rate decreases, and the other side increases. A sense of rotation in the opposite direction is experienced; since there is no actual head movement, this hallucinatory sensation is *physiologic postrotational vertigo.*

Any disease state that changes the firing frequency of an end organ, producing unequal neural input to the brainstem and ultimately the cerebral cortex, causes vertigo. The symptom can be conceptualized as the cortex inappropriately interpreting the abnormal neural input from the brainstem as indicating actual head rotation. Transient abnormalities produce short-lived symptoms. With a fixed unilateral deficit, central compensatory mechanisms ultimately diminish the vertigo. Since compensation depends on the plasticity of connections between the vestibular nuclei and the cerebellum, patients with brainstem or cerebellar disease have diminished adaptive capacity, and symptoms may persist indefinitely. Compensation is always inadequate for severe fixed bilateral lesions despite normal cerebellar connections: these patients are permanently symptomatic.

Acute unilateral labyrinthine dysfunction is caused by infection, trauma, and ischemia. Often, no specific etiology is uncovered, and the nonspecific terms *acute labyrinthitis, acute peripheral vestibulopathy,* or *vestibular neuritis* are used to describe the event. The attacks are brief and leave the patient for some days with a mild positional vertigo. Infection with herpes simplex virus type 1 has been implicated. It is impossible to predict whether a patient recovering from the first bout of vertigo will have recurrent episodes.

Acute bilateral labyrinthine dysfunction is usually the result of toxins such as drugs or alcohol. The most common offending drugs are the aminoglycoside antibiotics which damage the fine hair cells of the vestibular end organs and may cause a permanent disorder of equilibrium.

Recurrent unilateral labyrinthine dysfunction, in association with signs and symptoms of cochlear disease (progressive hearing loss and tinnitus), is usually due to Ménière's disease (Chap. 29). When auditory manifestations are absent, the term *vestibular neuronitis* denotes recurrent monosymptomatic vertigo. TIAs of the posterior cerebral circulation (vertebrobasilar insufficiency) very infrequently cause recurrent vertigo without concomitant motor, sensory, visual, cranial nerve, or cerebellar signs.

Positional vertigo is precipitated by a recumbent head position, either to the right or to the left. Benign paroxysmal positional (or positioning) vertigo (BPPV) of the posterior semicircular canal is particularly common. Although the condition may be due to head trauma, usually no precipitating factors are identified. It generally abates spontaneously after weeks or months. The vertigo and accompanying nystagmus have a distinct pattern of latency, fatigability, and habituation that differs from the less common central positional vertigo (Table 21-2) due to lesions in and around the fourth ventricle. Moreover, the pattern of nystagmus in posterior canal BPPV is distinctive. The lower eye displays a large-amplitude torsional nystagmus, and the upper eye has a lesser degree of torsion combined with upbeating nystagmus. If the eyes are directed to the upper ear, the vertical nystagmus in the upper eye increases in amplitude.

Vertigo of vestibular nerve origin may occur with diseases that involve the nerve in the petrous bone or the cerebellopontine angle. Except that it is less severe and less frequently paroxysmal, it has many of the characteristics of labyrinthine vertigo. The adjacent auditory division of the eighth cranial nerve also may be affected, which explains the frequent association of vertigo with tinnitus and deafness. The function of the eighth cranial nerve may be disturbed by tumors of the lateral recess (especially schwannomas), less frequently by meningeal inflammation in this region and, rarely, by an abnormal vessel that compresses the nerve.

Schwannomas involving the eighth cranial nerve (*acoustic neuroma*) grow slowly and produce such a gradual reduction of labyrinthine output that central compensatory mechanisms can prevent or minimize the vertigo; auditory symptoms of hearing loss and tinnitus are the most common manifestations. While lesions of the brainstem or cerebellum can cause acute vertigo, associated signs and symptoms usually permit distinction from a labyrinthine etiology (Table 21-3). However, labyrinthine ischemia, presumably due to occlusion of the labyrinthine branch of the internal auditory artery, may be the sole manifestation of vertebrobasilar insufficiency; patients with this syndrome present with the abrupt onset of severe vertigo, nausea and vomiting without tinnitus or hearing loss. Occasionally, an acute lesion of the vestibulocerebellum may present with monosymptomatic vertigo indistinguishable from a labyrinthopathy.

Vestibular epilepsy, vertigo secondary to temporal lobe epileptic activity, is rare and almost always intermixed with other epileptic manifestations.

Psychogenic vertigo, usually a concomitant of panic attacks or

Table 21-3   Differentiation of Peripheral and Central Vertigo

Sign or Symptom	Peripheral (Labyrinth)	Central (Brainstem or Cerebellum)
Direction of associated nystagmus	Unidirectional; fast phase opposite lesion[a]	Bidirectional or unidirectional
Purely horizontal nystagmus without torsional component	Uncommon	Common
Vertical or purely torsional nystagmus	Never present	May be present
Visual fixation	Inhibits nystagmus and vertigo	No inhibition
Severity of vertigo	Marked	Often mild
Direction of spin	Toward fast phase	Variable
Direction of fall	Toward slow phase	Variable
Duration of symptoms	Finite (minutes, days, weeks) but recurrent	May be chronic
Tinnitus and/or deafness	Often present	Usually absent
Associated central abnormalities	None	Extremely common
Common causes	Infection (labyrinthitis), Ménière's, neuronitis, ischemia, trauma, toxin	Vascular, demyelinating, neoplasm

[a] In Ménière's disease, the direction of the fast phase is variable.

agoraphobia (fear of large open spaces, crowds, or leaving the safety of home), should be suspected in patients so "incapacitated" by their symptoms that they adopt a prolonged housebound status. Most patients with organic vertigo attempt to function despite their discomfort. Organic vertigo is accompanied by nystagmus; a psychogenic etiology is almost certain when nystagmus is absent during a vertiginous episode.

Miscellaneous Head Sensations   This designation is used, primarily for purposes of initial classification, to describe dizziness that is neither faintness nor vertigo. Cephalic ischemia or vestibular dysfunction may be of such low intensity that the usual symptomatology is not clearly identified. For example, a small decrease in blood pressure or a slight vestibular imbalance may cause sensations different from distinct faintness or vertigo but that may be identified properly during provocative testing techniques. Other causes of dizziness in this category are hyperventilation syndrome, hypoglycemia, and the somatic symptoms of a clinical depression; these patients should have normal neurologic examinations and vestibular function tests.

Approach to the Patient

The most important diagnostic tool is a careful history focused on the meaning of "dizziness" to the patient. Is it faintness? Is there a sensation of spinning? If either of these is affirmed and the neurologic examination is normal, appropriate investigations for the multiple etiologies of cephalic ischemia or vestibular dysfunction are undertaken.

When the meaning of "dizziness" is uncertain, provocative tests may be helpful. These office procedures simulate either cephalic ischemia or vestibular dysfunction. Cephalic ischemia is obvious if the dizziness is duplicated during maneuvers that produce orthostatic hypotension. Further provocation involves the Valsalva maneuver, which decreases cerebral blood flow and should reproduce ischemic symptoms.

The simplest provocative test for vestibular dysfunction is rapid rotation and abrupt cessation of movement in a swivel chair. This always induces vertigo that the patients can compare with their symptomatic dizziness. The intense induced vertigo may be unlike the spontaneous symptoms, but shortly thereafter, when the vertigo has all but subsided, a lightheadedness supervenes that may be identified as "my

Table 21-2   Benign Paroxysmal Positional Vertigo (BPPV) and Central Positional Vertigo

Features	BPPV	Central
Latency[a]	3–40 s	None: immediate vertigo and nystagmus
Fatigability[b]	Yes	No
Habituation[c]	Yes	No
Intensity of vertigo	Severe	Mild
Reproducibility[d]	Variable	Good

[a] Time between attaining head position and onset of symptoms.
[b] Disappearance of symptoms with maintenance of offending position.
[c] Lessening of symptoms with repeated trials.
[d] Likelihood of symptom production during any examination session.

dizziness." When this occurs, the dizzy patient, originally classified as suffering from "miscellaneous head sensations," is now properly diagnosed as having mild vertigo secondary to a vestibulopathy.

Patients with symptoms of positional vertigo should be appropriately tested (Table 21-2); positional testing is more sensitive with special spectacles that preclude visual fixation (Frenzel lenses).

A final provocative test, requiring the use of Frenzel lenses, is vigorous head shaking in the horizontal plane for about 10 s. If nystagmus develops after the shaking stops, even in the absence of vertigo, vestibular dysfunction is demonstrated. The maneuver can then be repeated in the vertical plane. If the provocative tests establish the dizziness as a vestibular symptom, an evaluation of vestibular vertigo is undertaken.

Evaluation of Patients with Pathologic Vestibular Vertigo
The evaluation depends on whether a central etiology is suspected (Table 21-3). If so, MR imaging of the head is mandatory. Such an examination is rarely helpful in cases of recurrent monosymptomatic vertigo with a normal neurologic examination. Typical BPPV requires no investigation after the diagnosis is made (Table 21-2).

Vestibular function tests serve to (1) demonstrate an abnormality when the distinction between organic and psychogenic is uncertain, (2) establish the side of the abnormality, and (3) distinguish between peripheral and central etiologies. The standard test is electronystagmography (calorics), where warm and cold water (or air) are applied, in a prescribed fashion, to the tympanic membranes, and the slow-phase velocities of the resultant nystagmus from the right and left ears are compared. A velocity decrease from one side indicates hypofunction ("canal paresis"). An inability to induce nystagmus with ice water denotes a "dead labyrinth." Some institutions have the capability of quantitatively determining various aspects of the vestibuloocular reflex using computer-driven rotational chairs and precise oculographic recording of the eye movements.

Hyperventilation is the cause of dizziness in many anxious individuals; tingling of the hands and face may be absent. Forced hyperventilation for 1 min is indicated for patients with enigmatic dizziness and normal neurologic examinations. Similarly, depressive symptoms (which patients usually insist are "secondary" to the dizziness) must alert the examiner to a clinical depression as the *cause*, rather than the effect, of the dizziness.

CNS disease can produce dizzy sensations of all types. Consequently, a neurologic examination is always required even if the history or provocative tests suggest a cardiac, peripheral vestibular, or psychogenic etiology. Any abnormality on the neurologic examination should prompt appropriate neurodiagnostic studies.

℞ **TREATMENT**   Treatment of acute vertigo consists of bed rest and vestibular suppressant drugs such as antihistaminics (meclizine, dimenhydrinate, promethazine), or a tranquilizer with GABA-ergic effects (diazepam). If the vertigo persists beyond a few days, most authorities advise ambulation in an attempt to induce central compensatory mechanisms, despite the short-term discomfort to the patient. Chronic vertigo of labyrinthine origin may be treated with a systematized vestibular rehabilitation program to facilitate central compensation (see also Table 21-4).

BPPV is often self-limited but, when persistent, responds dramatically to specific repositioning exercise programs designed to empty particulate debris from the posterior semicircular canal. One of these exercises, the Epley procedure, is graphically demonstrated, in four languages, on a website for use in both physician's offices and self-treatment (www.charite.de/ch/neuro/vertigo.html).

Prophylactic measures to prevent recurrent vertigo are variably effective. Antihistamines are commonly utilized. Ménière's disease may respond to a diuretic or, more effectively, to a very low salt diet (1 g/day).

There are a variety of inner ear surgical procedures for refractory Ménière's disease, but these are only rarely necessary.

Table 21-4   Treatment of Vertigo

Agent	Dose[a]
Antihistamines	
Meclizine	25–50 mg 3 times/day
Dimenhydrinate	50 mg 1–2 times/day
Promethazine[b]	25–50 mg/d
Anticholinergic[c]	
Scopolamine transdermal patch	1.5 mg over 3 days
Sympathomimetic	
Ephedrine	25 mg/d
Benzodiazepine	
Diazepam	2.5 mg 1–3 times/day
Combination preparation	
Ephedrine and promethazine	25 mg/d of each
Exercise therapy	
Repositioning maneuvers[d]	
Vestibular rehabilitation[e]	
Other	
Diuretics or low-salt (1 g/d) diet[f]	
Inner ear surgery[g]	

[a] Usual starting dose in adults; maintenance dose can be increased by a factor of 2–3.
[b] Also has strong antiemetic effect.
[c] For motion sickness only.
[d] For benign paroxysmal positional vertigo.
[e] For vertigo other than Ménière's and positional.
[f] For Ménière's disease.
[g] For refractory cases of Ménière's disease.

BIBLIOGRAPHY

ARBUSOW V et al: Distribution of herpes simplex virus Type I in human geniculate and vestibular ganglia: Implications for vestibular neuritis. Ann Neurol 46:416, 1999

BALOH RW: Vertigo. Lancet 352:1841, 1998

BALOH RW: The dizzy patient: Presence of vertigo points to vestibular cause. Post Grad Med 105:161, 1999

BÜTTNER U et al: The direction of nystagmus is important for the diagnosis of central paroxysmal positional nystagmus (cPPV). Neuro-ophthalmology 21:97, 1999

CONNOLLY SJ et al: The North American Vasovagal Pacemaker Study (VPS). A randomized trial of permanent cardiac pacing for the prevention of vasovagal syncope. J Am Coll Cardiol 33:16, 1999

DIGIROLAMO E et al: Effects of paroxetine hydrochloride, a selective serotonin reuptake inhibitor, on refractory vasovagal syncope: A randomized double-blind, placebo controlled study. J Am Coll Cardiol 33:1227, 1999

FURMAN JM, CASS SP: Benign paroxysmal positional vertigo. N Engl J Med 3418:590, 1999

HERDMAN SJ et al: Vestibular rehabilitation of patients with vestibular hypofunction or with benign positional vertigo. Curr Opin Neurol 13:39, 2000

HOFFMAN RM et al: Evaluating dizziness. Am J Med 107:468, 1999

LINZER M et al: Diagnosing syncope—Part 1: Value of history, physical examination, and electrocardiography. Ann Intern Med 126:989, 1997

——— et al: Diagnosing syncope—Part 2: Unexplained syncope. Ann Intern Med 127:76, 1997

RADTKE A et al: A modified Epley's procedure for self-treatment of benign paroxysmal positional vertigo. Neurology 53:1358, 1999

TROOST BT: Dizziness and vertigo, in *Neurology in Clinical Practice*, 3d ed, WG Bradley et al (eds). Boston, Butterworth-Heinemann, 2000, chap 18

TUSA RJ: The dizzy patient: Disturbances of the vestibular system. In *Neuro-ophthalmology*, 3d ed, JS Glaser (ed). New York, Lippincott Williams & Wilkins, 2000, chap 18

22   *Richard K. Olney, Michael J. Aminoff*

WEAKNESS, MYALGIAS, DISORDERS OF MOVEMENT, AND IMBALANCE

Normal motor function requires integrated muscle activity with appropriate modulation by neuronal activity in the cerebral cortex, basal ganglia, cerebellum, and spinal cord. Symptoms and signs of motor system dysfunction may include weakness, fatigue, myalgias, spasms, cramps, dyskinetic movement, ataxia, imbalance, or disorders in the initiation or planning of movement.

WEAKNESS

Weakness is a reduction in normal power of one or more muscles. Patients may use the term differently; thus one or more specific examples of weakness should be elicited during the history. Increased fatigability or limitation in function due to pain is often confused with weakness by patients. *Increased fatigability* is the inability to sustain the performance of an activity that should be normal for a person of the same age, gender, and size.

Weakness is described commonly by severity and distribution. Paralysis and the suffix "-plegia" indicate weakness that is so severe that it is complete or nearly complete. "Paresis" refers to weakness that is mild or moderate. The prefix "hemi-" refers to one half of the body, "para-" to both legs, and "quadri-" to all four limbs.

Tone is the resistance of a muscle to passive stretch. Central nervous system (CNS) abnormalities that cause weakness generally produce *spasticity*, an increase in tone due to upper motor neuron disease. Spasticity is velocity-dependent, has a sudden release after reaching a maximum (the "clasp-knife" phenomenon), and predominantly affects antigravity muscles (i.e., upper limb flexors and lower limb extensors). Spasticity is distinct from rigidity and paratonia, two other types of increased tone. *Rigidity* is increased tone that is present throughout the range of motion (a "lead pipe" or "plastic" stiffness) and affects flexors and extensors equally. In some patients, rigidity has a cogwheel quality that is enhanced by voluntary movement of the contralateral limb (reinforcement). Rigidity occurs with certain extrapyramidal disorders. *Paratonia*, also referred to as *gegenhalten*, is increased tone that varies irregularly in a manner that may seem related to the degree of relaxation, is present throughout the range of motion, and affects flexors and extensors equally. Paratonia usually results from disease of the frontal lobes. Weakness with decreased tone (flaccidity) or normal tone occurs with disorders of the *motor unit*, that is, a single lower motor neuron and all of the muscle fibers it innervates.

Three basic patterns of weakness can usually be recognized based on the signs summarized in Table 22-1. One results from upper motor neuron pathology, and the other two from disorders of the motor unit (lower motor neuron and myopathic weakness). Fasciculations and early atrophy help to distinguish lower motor neuron (neurogenic) weakness from myopathic weakness. A *fasciculation* is a visible or palpable twitch within a single muscle due to the spontaneous discharge of one motor unit. Neurogenic weakness also produces more prominent hypotonia and greater depression of tendon reflexes than myopathic weakness.

PATHOGENESIS Upper Motor Neuron Weakness This pattern of weakness results from disorders that affect the upper motor neurons or their axons in the cerebral cortex, subcortical white matter, internal capsule, brainstem, or spinal cord (Fig. 22-1). Both the pyramidal and bulbospinal pathways contribute to normal strength, tone, coordination, and gait. Upper motor neuron lesions produce weakness through decreased activation of the lower motor neurons. In general, distal muscle groups are affected more severely than proximal ones, and axial movements are spared unless the lesion is severe and bilateral. With corticobulbar involvement, weakness is usually observed

FIGURE 22-1 The corticospinal and bulbospinal upper motor neuron pathways. Upper motor neurons have their cell bodies in layer V of the primary motor cortex (the precentral gyrus, or Brodmann's area 4) and in the premotor and supplemental motor cortex (area 6). The upper motor neurons in the primary motor cortex are somatotopically organized as illustrated on the right side of the figure.

Axons of the upper motor neurons descend through the subcortical white matter and the posterior limb of the internal capsule. Axons of the *pyramidal* or *corticospinal system* descend through the brainstem in the cerebral peduncle of the midbrain, the basis pontis, and the medullary pyramids. At the cervicomedullary junction, most pyramidal axons decussate into the contralateral corticospinal tract of the lateral spinal cord, but 10 to 30% remain ipsilateral in the anterior spinal cord. Pyramidal neurons make direct monosynaptic connections with lower motor neurons. They innervate most densely the lower motor neurons of hand muscles and are involved in the execution of learned, fine movements. Corticobulbar neurons are similar to corticospinal neurons but innervate brainstem motor nuclei.

Bulbospinal upper motor neurons influence strength and tone but are not part of the pyramidal system. The descending *ventromedial bulbospinal pathways* originate in the tectum of the midbrain (tectospinal pathway), the vestibular nuclei (vestibulospinal pathway), and the reticular formation (reticulospinal pathway). These pathways influence axial and proximal muscles and are involved in the maintenance of posture and integrated movements of the limbs and trunk. The descending *ventrolateral bulbospinal pathways*, which originate predominantly in the red nucleus (rubrospinal pathway), facilitate distal limb muscles. The bulbospinal system is sometimes referred to as the *extrapyramidal upper motor neuron system*. In all figures, nerve cell bodies and axon terminals are shown, respectively, as closed circles and forks.

only in the lower face and tongue; extraocular, upper facial, pharyngeal, and jaw muscles are almost always spared. With bilateral corticobulbar lesions, *pseudobulbar palsy* often develops, in which dysarthria, dysphagia, dysphonia, and emotional lability accompany bilateral facial weakness. Spasticity accompanies upper motor neuron weakness but may not be present in the acute phase.

Upper motor neuron lesions also affect the ability to perform rapid repetitive movements. Such movements are slow and coarse, but nor-

Table 22-1 Signs That Distinguish Patterns of Weakness

Sign	Upper Motor Neuron	Lower Motor Neuron	Myopathic
Atrophy	None	Severe	Mild
Fasciculations	None	Common	None
Tone	Spastic	Decreased	Normal/decreased
Distribution of weakness	Pyramidal/regional	Distal/segmental	Proximal
Tendon reflexes	Hyperactive	Hypoactive/absent	Normal/hypoactive
Babinski's sign	Present	Absent	Absent

mal rhythmicity is maintained. Finger-nose-finger and heel-knee-shin are performed slowly but adequately.

Lower Motor Neuron Weakness   This pattern results from disorders of cell bodies of lower motor neurons in the brainstem motor nuclei and the anterior horn of the spinal cord, or from dysfunction of the axons of these neurons as they pass to skeletal muscle (Fig. 22-2).

Lower motor weakness is produced by a decrease in the number of motor units that can be activated, through a loss of the α motor neurons or disruption of their connections to muscle. With a decreased number of motor units, fewer muscle fibers are activated with full effort and maximum power is reduced. Loss of γ motor neurons does not cause weakness but decreases tension on the muscle spindles. Muscle tone and tendon reflexes depend on γ motor neurons, muscle spindles, spindle afferent fibers, and the α motor neurons. A tap on a tendon stretches muscle spindles and activates the primary spindle afferent fibers. These monosynaptically stimulate the α motor neurons in the spinal cord, producing a brief muscle contraction, which is the familiar tendon reflex.

When a motor unit becomes diseased, especially in anterior horn cell diseases, it may spontaneously discharge, producing a fasciculation. These isolated small twitches may be seen or felt clinically or recorded by electromyography (EMG) (Chap. 357). When α motor neurons or their axons degenerate, the denervated muscle fibers spontaneously discharge in a manner that cannot be seen or felt but can be recorded with EMG. These small single muscle fiber discharges are called *fibrillation potentials*. If significant lower motor neuron weakness is present, recruitment of motor units is delayed or reduced, with

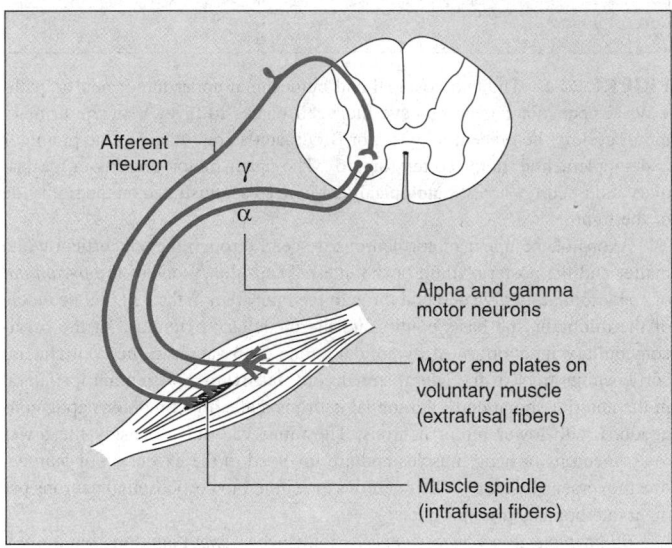

FIGURE 22-2   Lower motor neurons are divided into α and γ types. γ motor neurons are smaller than α motor neurons and innervate the intrafusal muscle fibers of the muscle spindle. Activation of the γ motor neuron increases the tension on muscle spindles and facilitates stretch reflexes and other local reflex mechanisms that activate a muscle through the α motor neurons. Each muscle is innervated by many (usually several hundred) α motor neurons.

Lower motor neuron axons exit the brainstem in certain cranial nerves and the spinal cord in the ventral roots. The ventral roots fuse with the dorsal roots at the intervertebral foramen to form spinal nerves. For innervation of limb muscles, several adjacent spinal nerves fuse to form plexuses before dividing into peripheral nerves. Most peripheral nerves branch one or more times as they innervate different muscles. Each α motor axon extensively arborizes just before reaching the many muscle fibers that it innervates.

The α motor neuron receives direct excitatory input from corticomotoneurons and primary muscle spindle afferents. The α and γ motor neurons also receive excitatory input from other descending upper motor neuron pathways, segmental sensory inputs, and interneurons. The α motor neurons receive direct inhibition from Renshaw cell interneurons, and other interneurons indirectly inhibit the α and γ motor neurons.

fewer than normal activated at a given discharge frequency. This contrasts with upper motor neuron weakness, in which a normal number of motor units are activated at a given frequency but in which the maximum discharge frequency is decreased.

Myopathic Weakness   This pattern of weakness is produced by disorders within the motor unit that affect the muscle fibers or the neuromuscular junctions.

Two types of muscle fibers exist. Type I muscle fibers are rich in mitochondria and oxidative enzymes, produce relatively low force, but have low energy demands that can be supplied by ongoing aerobic metabolism. They produce sustained postural and nonforceful movements. Type II muscle fibers are rich in glycolytic enzymes, can produce relatively high force, but have high energy demands that cannot be supplied for long by ongoing aerobic metabolism. Thus, these units can be activated maximally for only brief periods of time to produce high-force movements.

For graded voluntary movements, type I muscle fibers are activated earlier in recruitment. For each muscle fiber, if the nerve terminal releases a normal number of acetylcholine molecules presynaptically and a sufficient number of postsynaptic acetylcholine receptors are opened, the end plate reaches threshold and thereby generates an action potential that spreads across the muscle fiber membrane and into the transverse tubular system. This electrical excitation activates intracellular events that produce an energy-dependent contraction of the muscle fiber (excitation-contraction coupling).

Myopathic weakness is produced by a decrease in the number or contractile force of muscle fibers activated within the motor unit. With muscular dystrophies, inflammatory myopathies, or myopathies with muscle fiber necrosis, decreased numbers of muscle fibers survive within many motor units. As demonstrated with EMG, the size of each motor unit action potential is decreased so that motor units must be recruited more rapidly than normal to produce the power necessary for a certain movement. Neuromuscular junction diseases, such as myasthenia gravis, produce weakness in a similar manner, although the loss of muscle fibers within the motor unit is functional rather than actual. Furthermore, the number of muscle fibers activated can vary over time, depending on the state of rest of the neuromuscular junctions. Thus, fatigable weakness is suggestive of myasthenia gravis or another neuromuscular junction disease. Some myopathies produce weakness through loss of contractile force of muscle fibers or through relatively selective involvement of the type II muscle fibers. These may not affect the size of individual motor unit action potentials observed with EMG and are detected by a discrepancy between the electrical activity and force of a muscle.

Integrated Movements   Most purposeful movements require the integrated coordination of many muscle groups. Consider a simple movement, such as grasping a ball. The primary movement is a flexion of the thumb and fingers of one hand, with opposition of the thumb and little finger. This requires the contraction of several muscles, including flexor digitorum superficialis, flexor digitorum profundus, flexor pollicis longus, flexor pollicis brevis, opponens pollicis, and opponens digiti minimi. These prime movers for this action are called *agonists*. In order for the grasping to be smooth and forceful, the thumb and finger extensors need to relax at the same rate as the flexors contract. The muscles that act in a directly opposing manner to the agonists are *antagonists*. A secondary action of the thumb and finger flexors is to flex the wrist; because wrist flexion tends to weaken finger flexion if both occur, activation of wrist extensors assists the grasping movement. Muscles that produce such complementary movements are *synergists*. Finally, the arm needs to be held in a stable position as the grasp occurs, so that the ball is not knocked away before it is secured. Muscles that stabilize the arm position are *fixators*.

The coordination of activity by agonists, antagonists, synergists, and fixators is regulated by a three-level hierarchy of motor control. The lowest level of control is mediated through segmental reflexes in the spinal cord. These reflexes facilitate agonists and reciprocally inhibit the antagonists. Spinal segments also control rhythmic patterns of movement that involve more than a single pair of agonists and antagonists. For example, the lumbosacral spinal cord contains the basic programming for cyclical stepping movements that involve the synergistic activation of different muscle groups over time. The intermediate level of control is mediated through the descending bulbospinal pathways, which integrate visual, proprioceptive, and vestibular feedback into the execution of an action. For example, the locomotor center in the midbrain is required to modify the cyclical stepping movements in order that balance be maintained and forward movement occur. The highest level of control is mediated by the cerebral cortex. Superimposition of this highest level of control is necessary for activities such as walking to be goal-directed. Precise movements that are learned and improved through practice are also initiated and controlled by the motor cortex. Although only the agonists are directly activated, during the course of a complex sequence of actions such as playing the piano, the sequential activation of different groups of agonists for each note or chord is a part of the learned motor program. Further, the execution of these actions also involves input from the basal ganglia and cerebellar hemispheres to facilitate agonists, synergists, and fixators and to inhibit undesired antagonists.

Apraxia is a disorder of planning and initiating a skilled or learned movement (Chap. 25). Unilateral apraxia of the right hand may be due to a lesion of the left frontal lobe (especially anterior or inferior), the left temporoparietal region (especially the supramarginal gyrus), or their connections. Left body apraxia is produced by lesions of these regions in the right hemisphere or by lesions in the corpus callosum that disconnect the right temporoparietal or frontal regions from those on the left. Bilateral apraxia is often due to bilateral frontal lobe lesions or diffuse bilateral hemispheric disease.

Approach to the Patient

The mode of onset, distribution, and associated features of weakness should be carefully defined. When there is a discrepancy between the history and physical findings, it is usually because the patient complains of weakness, whereas symptoms are actually due to other causes, such as incoordination or pain limiting effort. Power may be examined in a variety of ways. The patient is asked to push or pull in a specified direction against resistance, and the strength in each muscle group is graded from 0 to 5 by the scale developed by the Medical Research Council (Table 22-2). A second method is indirect testing through observation of task performance such as holding the arms outstretched. This is especially useful in detecting mild, asymmetric upper motor neuron weakness through the observation of a downward drift with pronation of the forearm on one side. A third method is functional testing, which involves quantitation of activities. Common tests include counting the number of times a person can perform a deep-knee bend or step on a stool or chair, or timing the length of time the arms can be held abducted to 90 degrees. When performed serially, functional tests provide useful estimates of changes in the patient's status over time.

Other elements of the motor examination include appraisal of muscular bulk, inspection for fasciculations, and assessment of tone. Fasciculations are most easily determined by observing relaxed limbs that are illuminated from behind, but they can also be palpated as irregular low-amplitude twitches within the muscle. Tone is assessed by passive movement of each limb at its various joints and at several different speeds. In the clinical context of weakness, tone may be spastic or

Table 22-2 Medical Research Council Grading of Strength

Grade	Definition
5	Normal strength
4	Active movement against gravity and resistance
3	Active movement against gravity (no resistance from physician)
2	Active movement with gravity eliminated (no resistance from physician)
1	Flicker or trace contraction
0	No visible or palpable contraction

flaccid. The presence of cogwheel rigidity, lead-pipe rigidity, or paratonia suggests a disorder of integrated movements, rather than true weakness.

Hemiparesis Hemiparesis results from an upper motor neuron lesion above the midcervical spinal cord; most lesions that produce hemiparesis are located above the foramen magnum. The presence of language disorders, cortical sensory disturbances, cognitive abnormalities, disorders of visual-spatial integration, apraxia, or seizures indicates a cortical lesion. Homonymous visual field defects reflect either a cortical or a subcortical hemispheric lesion. A "pure motor" hemiparesis of the face, arm, and/or leg is due to a small, discrete lesion in the posterior limb of the internal capsule, cerebral peduncle, or upper pons. Some brainstem lesions produce the classic findings of ipsilateral cranial nerve signs and contralateral hemiparesis. These "crossed paralyses" are discussed further in Chap. 361. The absence of cranial nerve signs or facial weakness suggests that a hemiparesis is due to a lesion in the high cervical spinal cord, especially if associated with ipsilateral loss of proprioception and contralateral loss of pain and temperature sense (the Brown-Séquard syndrome). However, most spinal cord lesions produce quadriparesis or paraparesis.

Acute or episodic hemiparesis usually has a vascular pathogenesis, either ischemia or a primary hemorrhage (Chap. 361). Less commonly, hemorrhage may occur into brain tumors (Chap. 370) or from rupture of normal vessels due to trauma (Chap. 369); the trauma may be trivial in patients who are anticoagulated or elderly. Less likely possibilities include a focal inflammatory lesion from multiple sclerosis (Chap. 371), abscess, or sarcoidosis (Chap. 318). Evaluation begins immediately with a computed tomography (CT) scan of the brain (Fig. 22-3). If CT is normal and an ischemic stroke is unlikely, magnetic resonance imaging (MRI) of the brain or cervical spine may be indicated.

Subacute hemiparesis that evolves over days or weeks has a long differential diagnosis. A common cause is subdural hematoma; this readily treatable condition must always be considered, especially in elderly or anticoagulated patients, even in the absence of a history of trauma (Chap. 369). Infectious possibilities include cerebral bacterial abscess (Chap. 372), fungal granuloma or meningitis (Chap. 374), and parasitic infection. Weakness from malignant primary and metastatic neoplasms may evolve over days to weeks (Chap. 370). AIDS (Chap. 309) may present with subacute hemiparesis due to toxoplasmosis or primary CNS lymphoma. Noninfectious inflammatory processes, such as multiple sclerosis (Chap. 371) or, less commonly, sarcoidosis, are further considerations. If the brain MRI is normal and if cortical and hemispheric signs are not present, MRI of the cervical spine may be required.

Chronic hemiparesis that evolves over months is usually due to a neoplasm (Chap. 370), an unruptured arteriovenous malformation (Chap. 361), a chronic subdural hematoma (Chap. 369), or a degenerative disease (Chaps. 363 to 366). The initial diagnostic test is often an MRI of the brain, especially if the clinical findings suggest brainstem pathology. If MRI of the brain is normal, the possibility of a foramen magnum or high cervical spinal cord lesion should be considered.

Paraparesis An intraspinal lesion at or below the upper thoracic spinal cord level is most commonly responsible. A sensory level over the trunk identifies the approximate level of the cord lesion. Paraparesis can also result from lesions at other locations that disturb upper motor neurons (especially parasagittal lesions and hydrocephalus) and lower motor neurons (anterior horn cell disorders, cauda equina syndromes, and occasionally peripheral neuropathies).

Acute or episodic paraparesis due to spinal cord disease may be difficult to distinguish from disorders affecting lower motor neurons or cerebral hemispheres. Recurrent episodes of paraparesis are often due to multiple sclerosis or to vascular malformations of the spinal cord. With acute spinal cord disease, the upper motor neuron deficit

DISTRIBUTION OF WEAKNESS

Hemiparesis | Paraparesis | Quadriparesis | Monoparesis | Distal | Proximal | Restricted

Alert → Yes / No

UMN signs | LMN signs* | UMN signs | LMN signs*

Cortical signs → Yes / No

UMN signs | LMN signs*

EMG and NCS

UMN pattern | LMN pattern | Myopathic pattern

Brain CT or MRI† | **Spinal MRI‡** | Anterior horn, root, or peripheral nerve disease | Muscle or neuromuscular junction disease

* or signs of myopathy
† If no abnormality detected, consider spinal MRI.
‡ If no abnormality detected, consider myelogram or brain MRI.

FIGURE 22-3 An algorithm for the initial work-up of a patient with weakness. CT, computed tomography; EMG, electromyography; LMN, lower motor neuron; MRI, magnetic resonance imaging; NCS, nerve conduction studies; UMN, upper motor neuron.

is usually associated with incontinence and a sensory disturbance of the lower limbs that extends rostrally to a level on the trunk; tone is typically flaccid, and tendon reflexes absent. In such cases, the diagnostic approach starts with an imaging study of the spinal cord (Fig. 22-3). Compressive lesions (particularly epidural tumor, abscess, or hematoma), spinal cord infarction (proprioception is usually spared), an arteriovenous fistula or other vascular anomaly, and transverse myelitis, among other causes may be responsible (Chap. 368). Diseases of the cerebral hemispheres that produce acute paraparesis include anterior cerebral artery ischemia (shoulder shrug also affected), superior sagittal sinus or cortical venous thrombosis, and acute hydrocephalus. If upper motor neuron signs are associated with drowsiness, confusion, seizures, or other hemispheric signs but not a sensory level over the trunk, the diagnostic approach starts with an MRI of the brain. Paraparesis is part of the cauda equina syndrome, which may result from trauma to the low back, a midline disk herniation, or intraspinal tumor; although sphincters are affected, hip flexion is often spared, as is sensation over the anterolateral thighs. Rarely, paraparesis is caused by a rapidly evolving peripheral neuropathy such as Guillain-Barré syndrome or by a myopathy. In such cases, electrophysiologic studies are diagnostically helpful and refocus the subsequent evaluation (Chaps. 378 and 381).

Subacute or chronic paraparesis with spasticity is caused by upper motor neuron disease. When paraparesis evolves over weeks or months with lower limb sensory loss and sphincter involvement, possible spinal cord disorders include multiple sclerosis, intraparenchymal tumor, chronic spinal cord compression from degenerative disease of the spine, subacute combined degeneration due to vitamin B_{12} deficiency, viral infections (especially human T cell leukemia/lymphoma virus I), and hereditary or other degenerative diseases. Primary progressive multiple sclerosis usually presents in the fourth or fifth decade as progressive paraparesis (Chap. 371). Gliomas of the spinal cord typically produce a progressive myelopathy that is painful (Chap. 370). The clinical approach begins with an MRI of the spinal cord. If the imaging

study is normal and spasticity is present, MRI of the brain may be indicated. If hemispheric signs are present, parasagittal meningioma or chronic hydrocephalus is likely and MRI of the brain is the initial test. Progression over months to years is typical of degenerative disorders such as primary lateral sclerosis (Chap. 365) and hereditary disorders such as familial spastic paraparesis and adrenomyeloneuropathy (Chap. 368). In the rare situations when a chronic paraparesis is due to a lower motor neuron or myopathic etiology, the localization is usually suspected on clinical grounds by the absence of spasticity and confirmed by EMG and nerve conduction tests.

Quadriparesis or Generalized Weakness Generalized weakness may be due to disorders of the central nervous system or of the motor unit. Although the terms *quadriparesis* and *generalized weakness* are often used interchangeably, quadriparesis is more often chosen when an upper motor neuron cause is suspected and generalized weakness when a disease of the motor unit is likely. Weakness from CNS disorders is usually associated with changes in consciousness or cognition, with increased muscle tone and muscle stretch reflexes, and with alterations of sensation. Most neuromuscular causes of intermittent weakness are associated with normal mental function, diminished muscle tone, and hypoactive muscle stretch reflexes. Exceptions are some causes of acute quadriparesis due to upper motor neuron disorders in which transient hypotonia is present. The major causes of intermittent weakness are listed in Table 22-3. A patient with generalized fatigability without objective weakness may have the *chronic fatigue syndrome* (Chap. 384).

Acute quadriparesis Acute quadriparesis with onset over minutes may result from disorders of upper motor neurons (e.g., anoxia, hypotension, brainstem or cervical cord ischemia, trauma, and systemic metabolic abnormalities) or muscle (electrolyte disturbances, certain inborn errors of muscle energy metabolism, toxins, or periodic paralyses). Onset over hours to weeks may, in addition to the above, be due to lower motor neuron disorders. Guillain-Barré syndrome (Chap. 378) is the most common lower motor neuron weakness that progresses over days to several weeks; the finding of an elevated protein level in the cerebrospinal fluid is helpful but may be absent early in the course. If stupor or coma is present, the evaluation begins with

Table 22-3   Causes of Episodic Generalized Weakness

1. Electrolyte disturbances, e.g., a. hypokalemia, b. hyperkalemia, c. hypercalcemia, d. hypernatremia, e. hyponatremia, f. hypophosphatemia, g. hypermagnesemia
2. Muscle disorders
   a. Channelopathies (periodic paralyses)
   b. Metabolic defects of muscle (impaired carbohydrate or fatty acid utilization; abnormal mitochondrial function
3. Neuromuscular junction disorders
   a. Myasthenia gravis
   b. Lambert-Eaton myasthenic syndrome
4. Central nervous system disorders
   a. Transient ischemic attacks of the brainstem
   b. Transient global cerebral ischemia
   c. Multiple sclerosis

a CT scan of the brain. If upper motor neuron signs are present but the patient is alert, the initial test is usually an MRI of the cervical cord. If weakness is lower motor neuron, myopathic, or uncertain in origin, the clinical approach starts with blood studies for muscle enzymes and electrolytes and an EMG and nerve conduction study.

Subacute or chronic quadriparesis When quadriparesis due to upper motor neuron disease develops over weeks, months, or years, the distinction between disorders of the cerebral hemispheres, brainstem, and cervical spinal cord is usually possible by clinical criteria alone. The diagnostic approach begins with an MRI of the clinically suspected site of pathology. Lower motor neuron disease usually presents with weakness that is most profound distally, whereas myopathic weakness is typically proximal; the evaluation then begins with EMG and nerve conduction studies.

Monoparesis This is usually due to lower motor neuron disease, with or without associated sensory involvement. Upper motor neuron weakness occasionally presents with a monoparesis of distal and nonantigravity muscles. Myopathic weakness is rarely limited to one limb.

Acute monoparesis Distinguishing between upper and lower motor neuron disorders may be difficult clinically because tone and reflexes are frequently decreased in both at presentation. If the weakness is predominantly in distal and nonantigravity muscles and not associated with sensory impairment or pain, focal cortical ischemia is likely (Chap. 361); in this setting, diagnostic possibilities are similar to those for acute hemiparesis. Sensory loss and pain usually accompany acute lower motor neuron weakness. The distribution of weakness is commonly localized to a single nerve root or peripheral nerve within one limb but occasionally reflects involvement of the brachial or lumbosacral plexus. If lower motor neuron weakness is suspected, or if the pattern of weakness is uncertain, the clinical approach begins with an EMG and nerve conduction study.

Subacute or chronic monoparesis Weakness with atrophy of one limb that develops over weeks or months is almost always lower motor neuron in origin. If the weakness is associated with numbness, a peripheral nerve or spinal root origin is likely; uncommonly, the brachial or lumbosacral plexus is affected. If numbness is absent, anterior horn cell disease is likely. In either case, an electrodiagnostic study is indicated. If upper rather than lower motor neuron signs are present, a tumor, vascular malformation, or other cortical lesion affecting the precentral gyrus may be responsible. Alternatively, if the leg is affected, a small thoracic cord lesion, often a tumor or multiple sclerosis, may be present. In these situations, the approach begins with an imaging study of the suspicious area.

Distal Weakness Involvement of two or four limbs distally suggests lower motor neuron or peripheral nerve disease. Acute distal lower limb weakness occurs occasionally from an acute toxic polyneuropathy or cauda equina syndrome. Distal symmetric weakness usually develops over weeks, months, or years and is due to metabolic, toxic, hereditary, degenerative, or inflammatory diseases of peripheral nerves (Chap. 377). With peripheral nerve disease, weakness is usually less severe than numbness. Anterior horn cell disease may begin distally but is typically asymmetric and is not associated with numbness (Chap. 365). Rarely, myopathies also present with distal weakness (Chap. 381). The first step in evaluation is an electrodiagnostic study (Fig. 22-3).

Proximal Weakness Proximal weakness of two or four limbs suggests a disorder of muscle or, less commonly, neuromuscular junction or anterior horn cell. Myopathy often produces symmetric weakness of the pelvic or shoulder girdle muscles (Chap. 381). Diseases of the neuromuscular junction (such as myasthenia gravis) may present with symmetric proximal weakness (Chap. 380), often associated with ptosis, diplopia, or bulbar weakness and fluctuating in severity during the day. Extreme fatigability present in some cases of myasthenia gravis may even suggest episodic weakness, but strength rarely returns fully to normal. The proximal weakness of anterior horn cell disease is most often asymmetric, but may be symmetric if familial (Chap. 365). Numbness does not occur with any of these diseases. The evaluation usually begins with determination of the serum creatine kinase level and electrophysiologic studies.

Weakness in a Restricted Distribution In some patients, weakness does not fit any of the above patterns. Examples include weakness limited to the extraocular, hemifacial, bulbar, or respiratory muscles. If unilateral, restricted weakness is usually due to lower motor neuron or peripheral nerve disease, such as in a facial palsy (Chap. 367) or an isolated superior oblique muscle paresis (Chap. 28). Relatively symmetric weakness of extraocular or bulbar muscles is usually due to a myopathy (Chap. 381) or neuromuscular junction disorder (Chap. 380). Bilateral facial palsy with areflexia suggests Guillain-Barré syndrome (Chap. 378). Worsening of relatively symmetric weakness with fatigue is characteristic of neuromuscular junction disorders (Chap. 380). Asymmetric bulbar weakness is usually due to motor neuron disease. Weakness limited to respiratory muscles is uncommon and is usually due to motor neuron disease, myasthenia gravis, or polymyositis/dermatomyositis (Chap. 382).

MYALGIAS, SPASMS, AND CRAMPS

Spontaneous or exercise-related discomfort from muscles is usually benign and is rarely caused by a definable neuromuscular disease. However, a number of disorders of the motor system are characteristically painful. Some terms for muscular discomfort or involuntary contractions, such as myalgias, spasms, and cramps, are often used interchangeably by patients but have a more specific meaning to physicians. Other terms, such as aching, heaviness, and stiffness, are less specific. *Myalgias* are pains that are felt in muscle; the term does not imply an involuntary contraction. *Spasms* and *cramps* refer to episodes of involuntary contraction of one or more muscles. Cramps are usually painful, whereas spasms are not necessarily uncomfortable.

MYALGIAS Proximal or generalized weakness associated with myalgias is usually due to an inflammatory, metabolic, endocrine, or toxic myopathy (Chap. 381). Spontaneous myalgias not accompanied by objective weakness are often without a clear cause unless associated with a well-defined systemic illness. Myalgias are a common manifestation of fever or infection, especially influenza. Muscle pains and stiffness with elevated serum creatine kinase concentration is common in hypothyroidism, even in patients without objective weakness. *Polymyalgia rheumatica* (Chap. 317) is characterized by diffuse myalgias and joint stiffness that predominantly affect the pelvic and shoulder girdles in a patient over 50 years of age who has anorexia, mild weight loss, and low-grade fever. Limitation of activity from the myalgias and joint stiffness also leads to disuse atrophy and may give the impression of weakness. However, EMG, serum creatine kinase levels, and muscle biopsy are normal. The erythrocyte sedimentation rate is elevated in most patients, and features of giant-cell arteritis are present in 25%. Diffuse myalgias are common in many rheumatologic diseases, in which the diagnosis and treatment are based on other symptoms and signs. Myalgias are occasionally present in dermatomyositis/polymyositis, but most patients have weakness without significant pain. *Fibromyalgia* (fibrositis, fibromyositis) is associated with pain and tenderness of muscle and adjacent connective tissue (Chap. 325). Fatigue, insomnia, and depression are often present, but objective weakness, elevation of serum creatine kinase level, or elevation of the erythrocyte sedimentation rate does not occur. The diagnosis is dependent upon identifying characteristic focal "trigger points."

Focal Myalgias Focal muscle pain is often traumatic. Rupture of muscle tendons such as the biceps or gastrocnemius muscle may produce visible muscle shortening. Many such tears resolve without surgery but leave an abnormal appearance to the muscle belly. Nontraumatic focal muscle pain is often related to adjacent nonmuscular disorders (e.g., unilateral gastrocnemius pain due to deep venous thrombosis). Rarely, focal muscle pain may be caused by ischemic infarction or bacterial myositis, if acute, or by neoplasm, parasitic infection, sarcoidosis, or other inflammation or infection, if subacute or chronic.

Exertional Myalgias   Myalgias following unaccustomed, strenuous physical activity occur in normal individuals are often associated with laboratory evidence for muscle damage, such as an elevation of serum creatine kinase, edema of muscles on MRI, necrosis of muscle fibers on biopsy, and rarely myoglobinuria. Similar symptoms and laboratory abnormalities characterize certain metabolic disorders of muscle, such as carnitine palmitoyl transferase and glycolytic pathway enzyme deficiencies. The association of objective weakness during an episode of myalgias suggests a metabolic muscle disease. The development of an acute contracture (the inability to relax a muscle due to energy depletion) with the myalgias suggests a metabolic muscle disease with a glycolytic enzyme deficiency (Chap. 383). Exertional myalgias with muscle fiber necrosis also occur in muscular dystrophy with partial deficiency of dystrophin, and certain mitochondrial cytopathies (Chap. 383). Exertional myalgias with elevated creatine kinase concentration but without weakness also occur in hypothyroidism, and when confined to the legs may be due to vascular or neurogenic intermittent claudication. Most patients with exertional myalgias and no weakness do not have a definable abnormality.

SPASMS AND CRAMPS   Involuntary contraction of muscle may occur with disorders of the CNS, lower motor neuron, or muscle. Contractions that originate within the CNS and are associated with upper motor neuron signs are usually referred to as spasms and generally affect the flexors or extensors of one or more limbs. Those that originate within the CNS and are not associated with upper motor neuron signs include movement disorders discussed below, as well as the rare stiff-person syndrome and tetanus. Muscle rigidity from active muscle contraction can occur in the malignant hyperthermia syndrome, usually associated with general anesthesia. In the neuroleptic malignant syndrome, muscle rigidity arises from CNS overactivity and is present in muscle. Involuntary contractions that originate in the lower motor neurons are usually cramps, occasionally tetany, or rarely neuromyotonia. Spasms that originate in muscle or muscle membrane are usually a delayed relaxation after voluntary contraction, either myotonia or rarely a contracture. These conditions may be difficult to distinguish clinically but are often well characterized by EMG studies.

Stiff-Person Syndrome   This rare syndrome is characterized by slowly progressive muscle stiffness and superimposed spasms. The stiffness commonly begins in the low back and spreads over months up the spine and into the limbs but not into the jaw. The gait becomes stiff, and there is hyperlordosis of the lumbar spine. Spasms are often produced by startle. Emotional stress tends to worsen the stiffness as well as the frequency and severity of spasms. The spontaneous motor activity disappears during sleep. The syndrome is often associated with diabetes mellitus and can be paraneoplastic, accompanying Hodgkin's lymphoma, small cell cancer of the lung, and breast cancer. Most patients have a serum antibody against glutamic acid decarboxylase, an enzyme responsible for synthesis of the inhibitory neurotransmitter γ-aminobutyric acid (GABA). Stiffness results from loss of descending brainstem or segmental spinal inhibitory influences on the lower motor neurons. EMG studies reveal continuous motor unit activity that is similar to voluntary effort with preservation of the silent period to muscle stretch. Stiffness and spasms typically respond partially to treatment with baclofen or benzodiazepines.

Tetanus   This rare hyperexcitable state results from exposure to tetanus toxin in patients infected with *Clostridium tetani* (Chap. 143). Painful spasms typically begin with jaw closure (trismus) and soon become generalized. EMG studies reveal continuous motor unit activity that is similar to voluntary effort except for loss of the silent period to muscle stretch.

Cramps   These are the most common type of involuntary muscle contraction. Cramps are a painful contraction of a single muscle that produces a palpable knot within the muscle for seconds to minutes and is relieved by passive stretch of the muscle or spontaneously. EMG

studies reveal motor unit activity that has too high a discharge frequency to be voluntary. If cramps are associated with weakness, the weakness is almost always lower motor neuron in origin. When strength is normal, no definable condition is usually found, although dehydration, hypothyroidism, or uremia is occasionally present. If prominent, membrane stabilizing drugs, such as carbamazepine, may provide symptomatic benefit.

Tetany   Tetany is characterized by contraction of distal muscles of the hands (carpal spasm with extension of interphalangeal joints and adduction and flexion of the metacarpophalangeal joints) and feet (pedal spasm) and is associated with tingling around the mouth and distally in the limbs. Tetany with carpopedal spasms is a common manifestation of hypocalcemia or respiratory alkalosis (even from hyperventilation). EMG studies reveal single or more often grouped motor unit discharges at low discharge frequency.

Neuromyotonia (Isaac's Syndrome)   Neuromyotonia is characterized by muscle stiffness at rest that persists during sleep and by delayed relaxation after voluntary effort. Distal limb muscles are usually affected most severely, but all skeletal muscle may be involved. Gait may be stiff, and close inspection of the muscle reveals undulation of the overlying skin due to continuous muscle fiber contractions (myokymia). The continuous muscle fiber activity generates heat, and excessive sweating is common. EMG studies commonly reveal myokymic discharges, especially in familial cases. Rarely, EMGs record high-frequency neuromyotonic discharges. Autoantibodies against voltage-gated potassium channels have been demonstrated in some cases, and plasma exchange may be effective.

Myotonia   This is a nonpainful delay in the relaxation of muscle after voluntary activity. Delay in opening the hand after a forceful grip (grip myotonia) is common. These disorders are usually familial and worsen in cold weather. EMG demonstrates a waxing and waning discharge of individual muscle fibers.

Contracture   A painful inability to relax a muscle after voluntary activity due to energy depletion characterizes certain metabolic disorders with failure of energy production, such as myophosphorylase deficiency (McArdle's disease). EMG studies reveal electrical silence.

MOVEMENT DISORDERS

Movement disorders are neurologic syndromes in which abnormal movements (or *dyskinesias*) occur due to a disturbance of fluency and speed of voluntary movement or the presence of unintended extra movements. Because they are so distinct from the pyramidal disorders that cause upper motor neuron weakness, movement disorders are often referred to as *extrapyramidal diseases*. *Hyperkinetic movement disorders* are those in which an excessive amount of spontaneous motor activity is seen or in which abnormal involuntary movements occur. *Hypokinetic movement disorders* are characterized by *akinesia* or *bradykinesia*, in which purposeful motor activity is absent or reduced. This is often described as "poverty of movement."

PATHOGENESIS   Movement disorders result from disease of the basal ganglia, paired subcortical gray matter structures consisting of the caudate and the putamen (which together are called the striatum), the internal and external segments of the globus pallidus, the subthalamic nucleus, and the substantia nigra. The major interconnections and neurotransmitters involved in basal ganglia circuits are illustrated in Fig. 22-4A. An understanding of this circuitry can explain, in part, the perturbation that occurs in both the hypo- and hyperkinetic disorders. *Parkinson's disease* (Chap. 363), the prototypic hypokinetic movement disorder, results from a loss of dopaminergic neurons in the substantia nigra pars compacta. This leads to less excitation of striatal neurons that express the D_1 type of dopamine receptors and less inhibition of D_2 striatal neurons, both contributing to reduced facilitation of cortically initiated movement (Fig. 22-4B). The resting tremor of Parkinson's disease is less readily explained by this model but may result from effects on cholinergic interneurons in the striatum. *Huntington's disease* (Chap. 362), a hyperkinetic movement disorder, may be explained by selective loss of D_2 striatal neurons, resulting in

| NORMAL | PARKINSON'S DISEASE | HUNTINGTON'S CHOREA |

FIGURE 22-4 Basal ganglia circuits. *A.* Normal interaction. The striatum (caudate and putamen) receives glutamatergic afferents from the sensorimotor cortex and dopaminergic afferents from the substantia nigra pars compacta. The striatum has direct and indirect projections to the major outflow nuclei of the basal ganglia, the globus pallidus interna and the substantia nigra pars reticulata. The direct pathway from the striatum is GABA-ergic and inhibits the output nuclei. By contrast, the indirect pathway, which is more complex, facilitates the output nuclei. The output nuclei project to the ventral anterior and ventral lateral nuclei of the thalamus via inhibitory GABA neurotransmission. The thalamic nuclei in turn have glutamatergic, excitatory projections to cortical neurons. Thus, the direct pathway disinhibits (facilitates) thalamocortical projections that reinforce cortically initiated movement, whereas the indirect pathway is more complex and has the opposite effect. The direct and indirect pathways are influenced also by input from the substantia nigra pars compacta. This dopaminergic input on the striatum excites the direct pathway

neurons that predominantly express D_1 dopamine receptors and inhibits the indirect pathway neurons that predominantly express D_2 dopamine receptors. Striatal activity is further modulated by cholinergic interneurons within the striatum, which are functionally antagonistic to the dopaminergic projections.

B. Parkinson's disease results from a loss of dopaminergic projections from the substantia nigra pars compacta to the striatum. Loss of D_1 receptor stimulation results in disinhibition of the output nuclei by the direct pathway. Loss of D_2 receptor inhibition results in excitation of the output nuclei by the indirect pathway. Thus, inhibition of the thalamus is abnormally increased, and cortically initiated movements are not facilitated.

C. Huntington's chorea results from loss of striatal neurons that express D_2 receptors and normally project GABA-ergic inhibition to the globus pallidus externa. This causes disinhibition of the thalamus and excess thalamocortical excitation of movements. GABA, γ-aminobutyric acid; Glu, glutamate; ⟶ excitatory; dashed arrow, ······>, inhibitory.

disinhibition of cortically initiated movements without normal feedback control. The pathogenesis of hemiballismus is similar—a direct lesion of the glutamatergic neurons in the subthalamic nucleus (usually from a stroke) leads to disinhibition of thalamocortical projections.

Approach to the Patient

An algorithm for the interpretation of abnormal movements is illustrated in Fig. 22-5. The initial step is to determine if the movement disorder is due to an excess or a poverty of movement (i.e., a hyperkinetic or a hypokinetic movement disorder).

Hyperkinetic Movement Disorders Abnormal involuntary movements are divided into those that are rhythmical and those that are irregular. Those that are rhythmical are termed *tremors*, with the uncommon exception of *palatal and segmental myoclonus*. Tremors are divided into three types: rest, postural, and intention tremor. A *rest tremor* is maximal at rest and becomes less prominent with activity. It is characteristic of parkinsonism, a hypokinetic movement disorder, and is therefore commonly associated with bradykinesia and cogwheel rigidity. A rest tremor that develops acutely is usually due to toxins [such as exposure to 1-methyl-4-phenyl-1,2,3,6-tetrahydropyridine (MPTP)] or dopamine blocking drugs (such as phenothiazines). If insidious in onset, the diagnostic approach is the same as for Parkinson's disease (Chap. 363). A *postural tremor* is maximal while limb posture is actively maintained against gravity; it is lessened by rest and is not markedly enhanced during voluntary movement toward a target. A postural tremor that develops acutely is usually due to toxic or metabolic factors (for example, hyperthyroidism) or stress. The insidious onset of a postural tremor suggests a benign or familial essential tremor

(Chap. 363). An *intention tremor* is most prominent during voluntary movement toward a target and is not present during postural maintenance or at rest. It is a sign of cerebellar disease (Chap. 364). *Asterixis*, which may superficially resemble a tremor, is an intermittent inhibition of muscle contraction that occurs with metabolic encephalopathy (Chap. 376). This leads, for example, to a momentary and repetitive partial flexion of the wrists during attempted sustained wrist extension.

Involuntary movements that are irregular are characterized further by their speed and site of occurrence and by whether they can be suppressed voluntarily. The slowest are athetosis and dystonia. *Athetosis* is a slow, writhing, sinuous movement that occurs nearly continuously in distal muscles. *Dystonia* is a slowly varying but nearly continuous deviation of posture about one or more joints; it may occur in a proximal or distal limb or in axial structures. Dystonia is a more sustained deviation of posture than athetosis, although these two phenomena overlap considerably. The further evaluation of athetosis and dystonia are discussed in Chap. 363.

Among the rapid irregular movements, *tics* are controlled with voluntary effort, while the others are not. Tics often occur repetitively in a single location but are sometimes multifocal (Chap. 363).

Chorea, hemiballismus, and myoclonus are rapid, irregular jerks that cannot be consciously suppressed. *Hemiballismus* is the most distinctive among them. It is manifest as a sudden and often violent flinging movement of a proximal limb, usually an arm (Chap. 363). Hemiballismus usually develops acutely due to infarction of the contralateral subthalamic nucleus but occasionally develops subacutely or chronically due to other lesions of this nucleus.

Chorea is a rapid, jerky, irregular movement that tends to occur

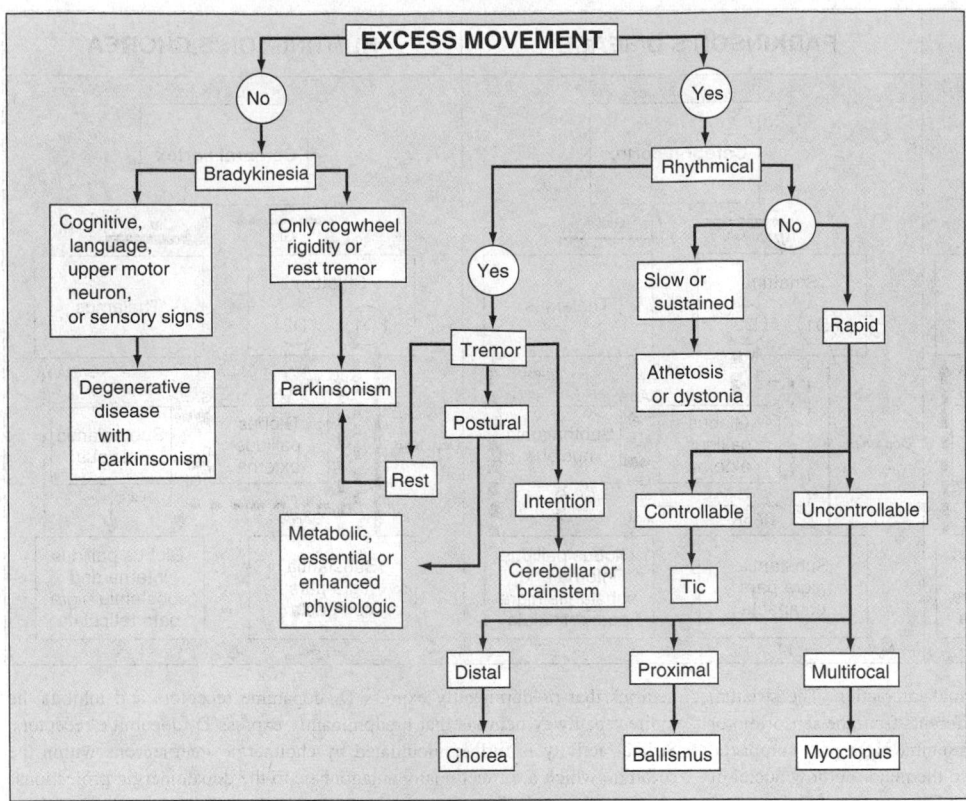

FIGURE 22-5 An algorithm for interpretation of abnormal movements.

in the distal limbs or face but may also occur in proximal limb and axial structures. Acute or subacute onset is usually toxic due to excess levodopa or dopamine-agonist therapy or, less often, neuroleptics, birth control pills, pregnancy (chorea gravidarum), hyperthyroidism, or the antiphospholipid syndrome. In children, it may be associated with rheumatic fever and, in such cases, is referred to as *Sydenham's chorea*. The gradual onset of chorea is typical of degenerative neurologic diseases, such as Huntington's chorea (Chap. 362).

Myoclonus is a rapid, brief, irregular movement that is usually multifocal. Myoclonus can occur spontaneously at rest, in response to sensory stimuli, or with voluntary movements. It is a symptom that occurs in a wide variety of metabolic and neurologic disorders. Posthypoxic intention myoclonus is a special myoclonic syndrome that occurs as a sequel to transient cerebral anoxia. Myoclonus may result from lipid storage disease, encephalitis, Creutzfeldt-Jakob disease, or metabolic encephalopathies due to respiratory failure, chronic renal failure, hepatic failure, or electrolyte imbalance. Myoclonus is also a feature of certain types of epilepsy, as discussed in Chap. 360. *Palatal and segmental myoclonus* are uncommon rhythmic forms of myoclonus that may resemble tremor; they are caused by structural disease of the brainstem or spinal cord at the level of the abnormal movement.

Hypokinetic Movement Disorders   These syndromes are manifest as bradykinesia, with a masked, expressionless facial appearance, loss of associated limb movements during walking, and rigid en bloc turning. If bradykinesia is associated only with a rest tremor, cogwheel rigidity, or impairment of postural reflexes (especially with a tendency to fall backwards), Parkinson's disease is likely (Chap. 363). If cognitive, language, upper motor neuron, sensory, or autonomic signs are also present, a *multisystem degenerative neurologic disease* is present. →*These disorders are discussed in Chaps. 363, 364, and 366.*

IMBALANCE AND DISORDERS OF GAIT

Imbalance is the impaired ability to maintain the intended orientation of the body in space. It is generally manifest as difficulty in maintaining an upright posture while standing or walking; a severe imbalance may also affect the ability to maintain posture while seated. Patients with imbalance commonly complain of a feeling of unsteadiness or dysequilibrium. Whereas imbalance and unsteadiness are synonymous, *dysequilibrium* implies the additional component of impaired spatial orientation even while lying down. Patients with dysequilibrium commonly also experience *vertigo*, defined as an hallucination of rotatory movement.

PATHOGENESIS   Imbalance and Limb Ataxia   Imbalance results from disorders of the spinal cord (spinocerebellar) or vestibular sensory input, the integration of these inputs in the brainstem or midline cerebellum, or the motor output to the spinal neurons that control axial and proximal muscles. Limb ataxia results from disorders of the spinocerebellar and corticopontocerebellar inputs, the integration of these inputs in the intermediate and lateral cerebellum, or the output to the spinal neurons (via the red nucleus and rubrospinal tract) or to the cortex. These pathways ensure adequate speed, fluency, and integration of limb movements. The lateral cerebellar hemispheres coordinate a complex feedback circuit that modulates cortically initiated limb movement.

Sensory ataxia is caused by lesions that affect the peripheral sensory fibers, dorsal root ganglia cells, posterior columns of the spinal cord, lemniscal system in the brainstem, thalamus, or parietal cortex; relevant anatomy is discussed in Chap. 23. Impairment of the proprioceptive sensory feedback to the cerebellum, basal ganglia, and cortex produces sensory ataxia. Sensory ataxia results in imbalance and disturbs the fluency and integration of movements that can be partially alleviated by visual feedback.

Disorders of Gait   Walking is one of the most complicated motor activities. Essentially all structures discussed in this chapter participate in normal walking. Cyclical stepping movements produced by the lumbosacral spinal cord centers are modified by cortical, basal ganglionic, brainstem, and cerebellar influences based on proprioceptive, vestibular, and visual feedback.

_____ *Approach to the Patient* _____

Examination of coordination, balance, and gait is typically performed at the same time. The finger-nose-finger and the heel-knee-shin maneuvers are observed for signs of incoordination in general and dysmetria in particular. *Dysmetria* consists of irregular errors in the amplitude and force of limb movements. This is accentuated near the target or point of intention and hence termed *intention tremor*. The patient is also asked to maintain the arms outstretched against a resistance that is suddenly removed; excessive *rebound* indicates cerebellar dysfunction. The ability of the patient to rapidly and repetitively tap the hands and feet is assessed for speed and rhythmicity. Errors in rhythm (irregular rate, velocity, or force) indicate *dysdiadochokinesia*. Slow, coarse, but rhythmical movements indicate upper motor neuron disorders. The patient is asked to demonstrate how to comb the hair or brush the teeth to assess the ability to initiate and execute a simple sequence of activity. Balance is examined by having the patient stand stationary with the feet together. If this position can be maintained, the eyes are closed for 5 to 10 s. Accentuation of sway or actual loss of balance is assessed. If balance is momentarily lost, several trials may be necessary to determine if the loss is consistently in the same direction. Walking along an uncrowded space, such as a hallway, is observed. Symmetry of arm swing and various phases of the gait cycle are observed. Walking is then performed for several steps on the heels, on the toes, and in tandem.

Imbalance An algorithm for interpretation of imbalance is presented in Fig. 22-6.

Cerebellar ataxia results from disorders of the cerebellum or of its afferent inputs or efferent projections. Abnormalities of the midline cerebellar vermis or the flocculonodular lobe produce truncal ataxia which is usually revealed during the process of rising from a chair, assuming the upright stance with the feet together, or performing some other activity while standing. Once a desired position is reached, imbalance may be surprisingly mild. As walking begins, the imbalance recurs. Patients usually learn to lessen the imbalance by walking with the legs widely separated. The imbalance is usually not lateralized and may be accompanied by symmetric nystagmus.

Abnormalities of the intermediate and lateral portions of the cerebellum typically produce impaired limb movements rather than truncal ataxia. If involvement is asymmetric, lateralized imbalance is common and usually associated with asymmetric nystagmus. Clinical signs of cerebellar limb ataxia include dysmetria, intention tremor,

FIGURE 22-6 An algorithm for evaluation of imbalance.

dysdiadochokinesia, and abnormal rebound. Muscle tone is often modestly reduced; this contributes to the abnormal rebound due to decreased activation of segmental spinal cord reflexes and also to pendular reflexes, i.e., a tendency for a tendon reflex to produce multiple swings to and fro after a single tap. →*For further discussion of cerebellar diseases, see Chap. 364.*

Imbalance with vestibular dysfunction is characterized by a consistent tendency to fall to one side. The patient commonly complains of vertigo rather than imbalance, especially if the onset is acute. Acute vertigo associated with lateralized imbalance but no other neurologic signs is often due to disorders of the semicircular canal (Chap. 21); the presence of other neurologic signs suggests brainstem ischemia (Chap. 361) or multiple sclerosis (Chap. 371). When the vestibular dysfunction is peripheral, positional nystagmus and vertigo tend to resolve if a provocative position is maintained (extinction) or repeated (habituation). Lateralized imbalance of gradual onset or persisting for more than 2 weeks, accompanied by nystagmus, may result from lesions of the semicircular canal or vestibular nerve, brainstem, or cerebellum.

Imbalance with sensory ataxia is characterized by marked worsening when visual feedback is removed. The patient can often assume the upright stance with feet together cautiously with eyes open. With eye closure, balance is rapidly lost (positive Romberg sign) in various directions at random. Sensory examination reveals impairment of proprioception at the toes and ankles, usually associated with an even more prominent abnormality of vibratory perception. Prompt evaluation for vitamin B$_{12}$ deficiency is important, as this disorder is reversible if recognized early (Chap. 368). Depression or absence of reflexes

points to peripheral nerve disorders (Chap. 377). Spasticity with extensor plantar responses suggests posterior column and spinal cord disorders (Chap. 368). Rarely, sensory ataxia produces lateralized imbalance. In these cases, the disorder is usually in the parietal lobe or thalamus (Chap. 23), but may also be due to an asymmetric sensory neuropathy (Chap. 377) or posterior column disease (Chap. 368).

Sensory limb ataxia is similar to cerebellar limb ataxia but is markedly worse when the eyes are closed. Examination also reveals abnormal proprioception and vibratory perception. The approach focuses on localizing the proprioceptive impairment to the peripheral nerves (Chap. 377), the posterior columns of the spinal cord (Chap. 368), or rarely the parietal lobe.

Other forms of imbalance occur, but the fundamental problem is usually a primary disorder of strength, extrapyramidal function, or cortical initiation of movement.

Abnormal Gait Each of the disorders discussed in this chapter produces a characteristic gait disturbance. If the neurologic examination is normal except for an abnormal gait, diagnosis may be difficult even for the experienced clinician.

Hemiparetic gait characterizes spastic hemiparesis. In its most severe form, an abnormal posture of the limbs is produced by spasticity. The arm is adducted and internally rotated, with flexion of the elbow, wrist, and fingers and with extension of the hip, knee, and ankle. Forward swing of the spastic leg during walking requires abduction and circumduction at the hip, often with contralateral tilt of the trunk to prevent the toes catching on the floor as the leg is advanced. In its mildest form, the affected arm is held in a normal position, but swings less than the normal arm. The affected leg is flexed less than the normal leg during its forward swing and is more externally rotated. A hemiparetic gait is a common residual sign of a stroke (Chap. 361).

Paraparetic gait is a walking pattern in which both legs are moved in a slow, stiff manner with circumduction, similar to the leg movement in a hemiparetic gait. In many patients, the legs tend to cross with each forward swing ("scissoring"). A paraparetic gait is a common sign of spinal cord disease (Chap. 368) and also occurs in cerebral palsy.

Steppage gait is produced by weakness of ankle dorsiflexion. Because of the partial or complete foot drop, the leg must be lifted higher than usual to avoid catching the toe on the floor during the forward swing of the leg. If unilateral, steppage gait is usually due to L5 radiculopathy, sciatic neuropathy, or peroneal neuropathy (Chap. 377). If bilateral, it is the common result of a distal polyneuropathy or lumbosacral polyradiculopathy (Chap. 377).

Waddling gait results from proximal lower limb weakness, most often from myopathy (Chap. 381) but occasionally from neuromuscular junction disease (Chap. 380) or a proximal symmetric spinal muscular atrophy (Chap. 365). With weakness of hip flexion, the trunk is tilted away from the leg that is being moved to lift the hip and provide extra distance between the foot and the floor, and the pelvis is rotated forward to assist with forward motion of the leg. Because pelvic girdle weakness is customarily bilateral, the pelvic lift and rotation alternates from side to side, giving the waddling appearance to the gait.

Parkinsonian gait is characterized by a forward stoop, with modest flexion at the hips and knees. The arms are flexed at the elbows and adducted at the shoulders, often with a 4- to 6-Hz resting pronation-supination tremor but little other movement, even during walking. Walking is initiated slowly by leaning forward and maintained with short rapid steps, during which the feet shuffle along the floor. The pace tends to accelerate (festination) as the upper body gradually leans further ahead of the feet, whether movement is forward (propulsion) or backward (retropulsion). The postural instability leads to falls (Chap. 363).

Apraxic gait results from bilateral frontal lobe disease with impaired ability to plan and execute sequential movements. This gait superficially resembles that of parkinsonism, in that the posture is stooped and any steps taken are short and shuffling. However, initiation and maintenance of walking are impaired in a different manner. Each movement that is required for walking can usually be performed, if tested in isolation while sitting or lying. However, when asked to step forward while standing, a long pause often occurs before any attempt is made to flex at the hip and advance, as if the patient is "glued to the ground." Once walking is initiated, it is not maintained, even in an abnormal festinating manner. Rather, after one or several steps are taken, walking is stopped for several seconds or longer. The process is then repeated. Dementia and incontinence may coexist.

Choreoathetotic gait is characterized by an intermittent, irregular movement that disrupts the smooth flow of a normal gait. Flexion or extension movements at the hip are common and unpredictable but readily observed as a pelvic lurch (Chap. 363).

Cerebellar ataxic gait is a broad-based gait disorder in which the speed and length of stride varies irregularly from step to step. With midline cerebellar disease, as in alcoholics, posture is erect but the feet are separated; lower limb ataxia is commonly present as well. Assumption of a particular stance or a change in position may cause instability, yet balance can usually be maintained well with the eyes open or closed. Walking may be rapid, but cadence is irregular. Although patients commonly lack confidence in the stability of their walking, only minimal support is often required for reassurance. With disease of the cerebellar hemispheres, limb ataxia and nystagmus are commonly present as well (Chap. 364).

Sensory ataxic gait may resemble a cerebellar gait, with its broad-based stance and difficulty with change in position. However, although balance may be maintained with the eyes open, loss of visual input through eye closure results in rapid loss of balance with a fall (positive Romberg sign), unless the physician assists the patient.

Vestibular gait is one in which the patient consistently tends to fall to one side, whether walking or standing. Cranial nerve examination demonstrates an obviously asymmetric nystagmus. The possibilities of unilateral sensory ataxia and hemiparesis are excluded by the findings of normal proprioception and strength (Chap. 21).

Astasia-abasia is a typical hysterical gait disorder. Although the patient usually has normal coordination of leg movements in bed or while sitting, the patient is unable to stand or walk without assistance. If distracted, stationary balance is sometimes maintained and several steps are taken normally, followed by a dramatic demonstration of imbalance with a lunge toward the examiner's arms or a nearby bed.

BIBLIOGRAPHY

ADAMS RD et al: *Principles of Neurology*, 6th ed. McGraw-Hill, New York, 1997

KANDEL ER et al: *Principles of Neural Science*, 4th ed, McGraw-Hill, New York, 2000

ZEHR EP, STEIN RB: What functions do reflexes serve during human locomotion? Prog Neurobiol 58:185, 1999

---

23   *Arthur K. Asbury*

NUMBNESS, TINGLING, AND SENSORY LOSS

NORMAL SENSATION   Normal somatic sensation reflects a continuous day and night monitoring process that occupies considerable moment-to-moment nervous system capacity. Little of this activity reaches consciousness under ordinary conditions. In contrast, disordered sensation, particularly if experienced as painful, is alarming and dominates the sufferer's attention. Abnormalities of sensation, especially if painful, tend to make those suffering seek medical help. The physician must be able to recognize abnormal sensations by how they are described, know their type and likely site of origin, and understand their implications. →*For a consideration of pain, see Chap. 12.*

Positive and Negative Phenomena   Abnormal sensory phenomena may be divided into two categories, positive and negative. The prototypical positive phenomenon is tingling (pins-and-needles), and the principal negative phenomenon is numbness. In addition to tingling, positive sensory phenomena include other altered sensations that are often described as pricking, bandlike, lightning-like shooting feelings (lancinations), aching, knifelike, twisting, drawing, pulling, tightening, burning, searing, electrical, or raw feelings. These descriptors are frequently the actual words used by patients. Such sensations may or may not be experienced as painful.

Positive phenomena usually result from trains of impulses generated at a site or sites of lowered threshold or heightened excitability along a sensory pathway, either peripheral or central. The nature and severity of an abnormal sensation depend on the number, rate, timing, and distribution of ectopic impulses and the type and function of nervous tissue in which they arise. Because positive phenomena represent excessive activity in sensory pathways, they are not necessarily associated with any sensory deficit (loss) upon examination.

Negative phenomena represent loss of sensory function and are characterized by diminished or absent feeling, often experienced as numbness. In contrast to positive phenomena, negative phenomena are accompanied by abnormal findings on sensory examination. In disorders affecting peripheral sensation, it is estimated that at least half the afferent axons innervating a given site are lost or functionless before sensory deficit can be demonstrated by clinical examination. This estimate probably varies according to how rapidly sensory nerve fibers have lost function. If the rate of loss is slow and chronic, lack of cutaneous feeling may be unnoticed by the patient and difficult to demonstrate on examination, even though few sensory fibers are functioning. Rapidly evolving sensory abnormality usually evokes both positive and negative phenomena and is readily recognized by patients. Subclinical degrees of sensory dysfunction not demonstrable on clinical sensory examination may be revealed by sensory nerve conduction studies or somatosensory cerebral evoked potentials (Chap. 357). Sensory symptoms may be either positive or negative, but sensory signs on examination are always a measure of negative phenomena.

Terminology Words used to characterize sensory disturbance are descriptive and have been arrived at mainly by convention. Paresthesia and dysesthesia are general terms used to denote sensory symptoms (positive phenomena) and are usually stated in the plural form. *Paresthesias* usually refer to tingling or pins-and-needles sensations but may also include a wide variety of other abnormal sensations, excepting pain. Sometimes "paresthesias" carry the implication that the abnormal sensations are perceived without an apparent stimulus. *Dysesthesia* is a more general term used to subsume all types of abnormal sensations, even painful ones, whether a stimulus is evident or not.

While dysesthesias and paresthesias refer to sensations described by patients, another set of terms refers to sensory abnormalities found on examination. These include *hypesthesia* or *hypoesthesia* (reduction of cutaneous sensation to a specific type of testing such as pressure, light touch, and warm or cold stimuli); *anesthesia* (complete absence of skin sensation to the same stimuli plus pinprick); and *hypalgesia* (referring to reduced pain perception, i.e., nociception, such as the pricking quality elicited by a pin). *Hyperesthesia* means pain in response to touch. Similarly, *allodynia* describes the situation in which a nonpainful stimulus, once perceived, is experienced as painful, even excruciating. An example is elicitation of a painful sensation by application of a vibrating tuning fork. *Hyperalgesia* denotes severe pain in response to a mildly noxious stimulus, and *hyperpathia*, a broad term, encompasses all the phenomena described by hyperesthesia, allodynia, and hyperalgesia. With hyperpathia, the threshold for a sensory stimulus is increased and the perception is delayed but once felt, is unduly painful.

Disorders of deep sensation, arising from muscle spindles, tendons, and joints, affect proprioception (position sense). Manifestations include imbalance (particularly with eyes closed or in the dark), clumsiness of precision movements, and unsteadiness of gait, which are referred to collectively as *sensory ataxia* (Chap. 22). Other findings on examination usually, but not invariably, include reduced or absent joint position and vibratory sensibility and absent deep tendon reflexes in the affected limbs. Romberg's sign is positive, which means that the patient sways or topples when asked to stand with feet close together and eyes closed. In severe states of deafferentation involving deep sensation, the patient cannot walk or stand unaided or even sit unsupported. Continuous, sometimes wormlike involuntary movements, called *pseudoathetosis*, of the outstretched hands and fingers occur, particularly with eyes closed. Such patients are severely disabled.

Anatomy of Sensation Cutaneous afferent innervation is conveyed by a rich variety of receptors, both naked nerve endings (nociceptors and thermoreceptors) and encapsulated terminals (mechanoreceptors). Each type of receptor has its own set of sensitivities to specific stimuli, size and distinctness of receptive fields, and adaptational qualities. Much of the knowledge about these receptors has come from the development of techniques to study single intact nerve fibers intraneurally in awake unanesthetized human subjects. It is possible not only to record from single nerve fibers, large or small, but also to stimulate single fibers in isolation. A single impulse, whether elicited by a natural stimulus or evoked by electrical microstimulation, in a large myelinated afferent fiber may be both perceived and localized.

Afferent fibers of all sizes in peripheral nerve trunks traverse the dorsal roots and enter the dorsal horn of the spinal cord (Fig. 23-1). From there the smaller fibers take a different route to the parietal cortex than the larger fibers. The polysynaptic projections of the smaller fibers

(unmyelinated and small myelinated), which subserve mainly nociception, temperature sensibility, and touch, cross and ascend in the opposite anterior and lateral columns of the spinal cord, through the brainstem, to the ventral posterolateral (VPL) nucleus of the thalamus, and ultimately project to the postcentral gyrus of the parietal cortex (Chap. 12). This is referred to as the *spinothalamic pathway*, or *anterolateral system*. The larger fibers, which subserve tactile and position sense and kinesthesia, project rostrally in the posterior column on the same side of the spinal cord and make their first synapse in the gracile or cuneate nuclei of the lower medulla. The second-order neuron decussates and ascends in the medial lemniscus located medially in the medulla and in the tegmentum of the pons and midbrain and synapses in the VPL. The third-order neuron projects to parietal cortex; this large fiber system is referred to as the *posterior column–medial lemniscal pathway* (lemniscal, for short). Note that although the lemniscal and the anterolateral pathways both project up the spinal cord to the thalamus, it is the (crossed) anterolateral pathway that is referred to as the *spinothalamic tract*, by convention.

Although the fiber types and functions that make up the spinothalamic and lemniscal systems are relatively well known, it has been found that many other fibers, particularly those associated with touch, pressure, and position sense, ascend in a diffusely distributed pattern both ipsilaterally and contralaterally in the anterolateral quadrants of the spinal cord. This explains why an individual with a complete lesion of the posterior columns of the spinal cord may have little sensory deficit on examination.

FIGURE 23-1 Schematic diagram of lemniscal and spinothalamic pathways. Note that the large fibers that subserve proprioception and discriminative touch ascend ipsilaterally as the lemniscal pathway in the posterior column of the spinal cord, and that the small fibers that subserve pain, thermal sensation, and crude touch ascend contralaterally as the spinothalamic pathway in the anterior and lateral columns of the spinal cord (insert). SS CTX, somatosensory cortex; Thal, thalamus; VPL, ventral posterolateral nucleus.

Table 23-1 Testing Primary Sensation

Sense	Test Device	Endings Activated	Fiber Size Mediating	Central Pathway
Pain	Pinprick	Cutaneous nociceptors	Small	SpTh, also D
Temperature, heat	Warmed metal object	Cutaneous thermoreceptors for hot	Small	SpTh
Temperature, cold	Cold metal object	Cutaneous thermoreceptors for cold	Small	SpTh
Touch	Cotton wisp, fine brush	Cutaneous mechanoreceptors, also naked endings	Large and small	Lem, also D and SpTh
Vibration	Tuning fork, 128 Hz	Mechanoreceptors, especially pacinian corpuscles	Large	Lem, also D
Joint position	Passive movement of specific joints	Joint capsule and tendon endings, muscle spindles	Large	Lem, also D

NOTE: D, diffuse ascending projections in ipsilateral and contralateral anterolateral columns; SpTh, spinothalamic projection, contralateral; Lem, posterior column and lemniscal projection, ipsilateral.

EXAMINATION OF SENSATION The main tasks of the sensory examination are tests of primary sensation. By convention these include the sense of pain, touch, vibration, joint position, and thermal sensation, both hot and cold (Table 23-1). Detailed descriptions of how to perform the various tests of the sensory examination can be found in standard texts (see "Bibliography").

Some general principles pertain. First, the examiner must depend on subjective patient response, particularly when using cutaneous stimuli (pin, touch, vibration, warm or cold). This factor may complicate the interpretation of the sensory examination. Second, with complaints of numbness, patients should be asked to outline on themselves the borders of numb areas. Third, some patients are only partially examinable. In a stuporous patient, sensory examination is reduced to observing the briskness of withdrawal in response to a pinch or other noxious stimulus. Comparison of response on one side of the body to the other is essential. In the alert but uncooperative patient, cutaneous sensation may be unexaminable. However, it is usually possible to get some idea of proprioceptive function by noting the patient's best performance of movements requiring balance and precision. Fourth, sensory examination of a patient who has no neurologic complaints should be abbreviated and may consist of pin, touch, and vibration testing in the hands and feet plus evaluation of stance and gait, including the Romberg maneuver. Evaluation of stance and gait also tests the integrity of motor and cerebellar systems.

Primary Sensation (See Table 23-1) The sense of pain is usually tested with a pin, asking the patient to focus on the pricking or unpleasant quality of the stimulus and not just the pressure or touch sensation elicited. Areas of hypalgesia should be mapped by proceeding radially from the most hypalgesic site (Figs. 23-2 and 23-3).

Temperature sensation, to both hot and cold, is probably best tested with water flasks filled with water of the desired temperature, using a thermometer to verify the temperature. This is impractical in most settings. An alternative way to test cold sensation is to touch a metal object, such as a tuning fork at room temperature, to the skin. For testing warm temperatures, the tuning fork or other metal object may be held under warm water of the desired temperature and then used. Both cold and warm should be tested because different receptors respond to each.

Touch is usually tested with a wisp of cotton or a fine camelhair brush. In general, it is better to avoid testing touch on hairy skin because of the profusion of sensory endings that surround each hair follicle.

Joint position testing is a measure of proprioception, one of the most important functions of the sensory system. With the patient keeping eyes closed, joint position is tested in the great toe and in the fingers. If errors are made in recognizing the direction of passive movements of the toe or the finger, more proximal joints should be

tested. A test of proximal joint position sense, primarily at the shoulder, is performed by asking the patient to bring the two index fingers together with the arms extended and the eyes closed. Normal individuals should be able to do this quite accurately, with errors of a centimeter or less.

The sense of vibration is tested with a tuning fork, preferably a large one that vibrates at 128 Hz. Vibration is usually tested at bony prominences, beginning distally at the malleoli of the ankles, and at the knuckles. If abnormalities are found, more proximal sites can be examined. Vibratory thesholds at the same site in the patient and the examiner can be compared for control purposes.

Quantitative Sensory Testing Effective sensory testing devices have been developed over the past two decades. Quantitative sensory testing is particularly useful for serial evaluation of cutaneous sensation in clinical trials. Threshold testing for touch and vibratory and thermal sensation is the most widely used application.

Cortical Sensation Cortical sensory testing includes two-point discrimination, touch localization, and bilateral simultaneous stimu-

FIGURE 23-2 Anterior view of dermatomes (*left*) and cutaneous areas supplied by individual peripheral nerves (*right*). (*Modified from MB Carpenter and J Sutin, in Human Neuroanatomy, 8th ed, Baltimore, Williams & Wilkins, 1983.*)

FIGURE 23-3 Posterior view of dermatomes *(left)* and cutaneous areas supplied by individual peripheral nerves *(right). (Modified from MB Carpenter and J Sutin, in Human Neuroanatomy, 8th ed, Baltimore, Williams & Wilkins, 1983.)*

lation and tests for graphesthesia and stereognosis, to name the most commonly used methods. Abnormalities of these sensory tests, in the presence of normal primary sensation in an alert cooperative patient, signify a lesion of the parietal cortex or thalamocortical projections to the parietal lobe. If primary sensation is altered, these cortical discriminative functions will usually be abnormal, too. Comparisons should always be made between analogous sites on the two sides of the body because the deficit with a specific parietal lesion is likely to be hemilateral. Side-to-side comparisons hold true for all cortical sensory testing.

Two-point discrimination is tested by special calipers, the points of which may be set from 2 mm to several centimeters apart and then applied simultaneously to the site to be tested. The pulp of the fingertips is a common site to test; a normal individual can distinguish about 3-mm separation of points there.

Touch localization is usually carried out by light pressure with the examiner's fingertip, asking the patient, whose eyes are closed, to identify the site of touch. It is usual to ask the patient to touch the same site with a fingertip.

Bilateral simultaneous stimulation at analogous sites (e.g., the dorsa of both hands) can be carried out to determine whether the perception of touch is extinguished consistently on one side or the other. The phenomenon is referred to as *extinction* on bilateral simultaneous stimulation.

Graphesthesia means the capacity to recognize with eyes closed letters or numbers drawn by the examiner's fingertip on the palm of the hand. Once again, the comparison of one side with the other is of prime importance. Inability to recognize numbers or letters is termed *agraphesthesia.*

Stereognosis refers to the ability to identify common objects by palpation, recognizing their shape, texture, and size. Common standard objects are the best test objects, such as a marble, a paper clip, or coins. Patients with normal stereognosis should be able to distinguish a dime from a penny and a nickel from a quarter without looking. Patients should only be allowed to feel the object with one hand at a time. If they are unable to identify it in one hand, it should be placed in the other for comparison. Individuals unable to identify common objects and coins in one hand who can do so in the other are said to have *astereognosis* of the abnormal hand.

LOCALIZATION OF SENSORY ABNORMALITIES

Sensory symptoms and signs can result from lesions at almost any level of the nervous system, including parietal cortex, deep white matter, thalamus, brainstem, spinal cord, spinal root, peripheral nerve, and sensory receptor. Noting the distribution and nature of sensory symptoms and signs is the most important way to localize their source. The extent, configuration, symmetry, quality, and severity are the key observations.

Dysesthesias without sensory findings by examination can be difficult to interpret. To illustrate, tingling dysesthesias in an acral distribution (hands and feet) can have more than one interpretation. Distal dysesthesias can be systemic in origin, e.g., secondary to hyperventilation, or can be induced by a medication, such as the diuretic acetazolamide. Distal dysesthesias can also be an early event in an evolving polyneuropathy or can herald a myelopathy, such as with vitamin B_{12} deficiency. Sometimes distal dysesthesias have no definable basis. In contrast, dysesthesias that correspond to a particular peripheral nerve territory denote a lesion of that nerve trunk. For instance, dysesthesias restricted to the fifth digit and the adjacent one-half of the fourth finger on one hand reliably point to disorder of the ulnar nerve, most commonly at the elbow.

Nerve and Root In focal nerve trunk lesions severe enough to cause a deficit, sensory abnormalities are readily mapped and generally have discrete boundaries (Figs. 23-2 and 23-3). Root lesions, referred to as radicular, are frequently accompanied by deep, aching pain along the course of the related nerve trunk. With compression of a fifth lumbar (L5) or first sacral (S1) root, as may occur with a ruptured intervertebral disc, sciatica is a frequent manifestation. With a lesion affecting a single root, sensory deficit in the distribution of that root is often minimal or not demonstrable at all. This is because adjacent root territories overlap extensively.

Polyneuropathies are generally graded, distal, and symmetric in distribution of deficit (Chap. 377). Dysesthesias begin in the toes and ascend symmetrically, followed by numbness. When dysesthesias reach the knees, they have usually also appeared in the fingertips. The process appears to be nerve length–dependent, and the deficit is often described as "stocking-glove" in type. Although most polyneuropathies are pansensory and affect all modalities of sensation, selective sensory dysfunction according to nerve fiber size may occur. In polyneuropathies that affect small nerve fibers selectively, the hallmark is burning, painful dysesthesias with reduced pinprick and thermal sensation but with sparing of proprioception, motor function, and even deep tendon jerks. Touch is variably involved, but when spared, the sensory pattern is referred to as *sensory dissociation.* Sensory dissociation patterns can be seen with spinal cord lesions (see below) as well as with small fiber neuropathies. In contrast to small fiber polyneuropathies, large fiber polyneuropathies are characterized by position sense deficit, imbalance, absent tendon jerks, and variable motor dysfunction but preservation of most cutaneous sensation. Dysesthesias, if present at all, tend to be tingling or bandlike.

Spinal Cord (See Chap. 368) If the spinal cord is transected, all sensation is lost below the level of transection. Bladder and bowel function are also lost, as is motor function. Hemisection of the spinal cord produces the Brown-Séquard syndrome, which involves absent pain and temperature sensation on the opposite side below the lesion, and loss of proprioceptive sensation and loss of motor power on the same side below the lesion (see Figs. 23-1 and 368-1). Dissociated sensory deficit patterns (see above) are also a sign of spinothalamic tract involvement in the spinal cord, especially if the deficit is unilateral and has an upper level on the torso. Bilateral spinothalamic tract involvement occurs with lesions affecting the center of the spinal cord, such as happens with expansion of the central canal in syringomyelia. Sensory dissociation is characteristic of syringomyelia.

Brainstem   Harlequin patterns of sensory disturbance, in which one side of the face and the opposite side of the body are affected, localize to the lateral medulla. Here a small lesion may damage both the ipsilateral descending trigeminal tract and ascending spinothalamic fibers subserving the opposite arm, leg, and hemitorso (see "Lateral medullary syndrome" in Fig. 361-7). In the tegmentum of the pons and midbrain, where the lemniscal and spinothalamic tracts merge, a lesion here causes pansensory loss on the contralateral body.

Thalamus   Hemisensory disturbance with tingling numbness from head to foot is often thalamic in origin but can also be anterior parietal. If abrupt in onset, the lesion is likely to be due to a small stroke (lacunar infarction), particularly if localized to the thalamus. Occasionally, with lesions affecting the VPL or adjacent white matter, a syndrome of thalamic pain, also called *Déjerine-Roussy syndrome*, may ensue. This persistent unrelenting hemipainful state is often described in dramatic terms such as "like the flesh is being torn from my limbs" or "as though that side is bathed in acid" (Chap. 12).

Cortex   With lesions of the parietal lobe, either of the cortex or of subjacent white matter, the most prominent symptoms are contralateral hemineglect, hemi-inattention, and a tendency not to use the affected hand and arm. Tests of primary sensation may be normal or altered. Anterior parietal infarction may present as a pseudothalamic syndrome with crossed hemilateral loss of primary sensation. Dysesthesias or a sense of numbness may also occur, and rarely a painful state.

Focal Sensory Seizures   These are generally due to lesions in or near the postcentral gyrus. Symptoms of focal sensory seizures are usually combinations of numbness and tingling, but frequently additional more complex sensations are present, such as a rushing feeling, a sense of warmth, a sense of movement without visible motion, or other unpleasant dysesthesias. Duration of seizures is variable; they may be transient, lasting only seconds, or they may persist for hours. Focal motor features (clonic jerking) may supervene, and seizures can become generalized with loss of consciousness. Likely sites of symptoms are unilaterally in the lips, face, digits, or foot, and symptoms may spread as in a Jacksonian march. On occasion, symptoms may occur in a symmetric bilateral fashion, for instance, in both hands; this results from involvement of the second sensory area (unilaterally) located in the rolandic area at and just above the Sylvian fissure.

BIBLIOGRAPHY

Adams RD et al: *Principles of Neurology*, 6th ed. New York, McGraw-Hill, 1997

Bassetti C et al: Sensory syndromes in parietal stroke. Neurology 43:1942, 1993

Mogydros I et al: Mechanisms of paresthesias arising from healthy axons. Muscle Nerve 23:310, 2000

Ochoa JL: Positive sensory symptoms in neuropathy: Mechanisms and aspects of treatment, in *Peripheral Nerve Disorders*, AK Asbury, PK Thomas (eds). Oxford, Butterworth-Heinemann, 1995, pp 44–58

Remy P et al: Somatosensory cortical activations are suppressed in patients with tactile extinction. Neurology 52:571, 1999

Ross RT: *How to Examine the Nervous System*, 3d ed. Stamford, Appleton & Lange, 1999

Rowbotham MC, Fields HL: The relationship of pain, allodynia and thermal sensation in post-herpetic neuralgia. Brain 119:347, 1996

Simon RP et al: *Clinical Neurology*, 4th ed. Stamford, Appleton & Lange, 1999

Yarnitsky D: Quantitative sensory testing. Muscle Nerve 20:198, 1997

24

Allan H. Ropper

ACUTE CONFUSIONAL STATES AND COMA

Confusional states and coma are among the most common problems in general medicine. They account for a substantial portion of admissions to emergency wards and are a frequent cause of distress on all hospital services. Because clouding of consciousness and a diminished level of consciousness frequently coexist and result from many of the same diseases, they are presented together here, but from a medical perspective they have different clinical characteristics and physiologic explanations.

The basis of consciousness has long been a topic of great interest to psychologists and philosophers and is the subject of a vast literature. Physicians have been mainly concerned with impairments in the level of consciousness (coma, stupor, drowsiness) and with alterations of consciousness, meaning an inability to think coherently, i.e., with accustomed clarity and speed. The latter, broadly termed *confusion* relates to lessened awareness, perception, apperception (the interpretation of perceptions), thinking, expression in language and action, and all forms of intellection that are dependent on the continuous integration of mental processes. Normal awareness provides a background to our inner mental life, which flows from infancy to death like a "stream of thought," to use William James's metaphor. Self-awareness requires that a person experience these thoughts and be able to reflect and operate upon them.

Almost all instances of diminished alertness can be traced to widespread abnormalities of the cerebral hemispheres or to reduced activity of a special thalamocortical alerting system termed the *reticular activating system* (RAS). The proper functioning of this system, its ascending projections to the cortex, the cortex itself, and corticothalamic connections are required to maintain alertness and coherence of thought.

THE CONFUSIONAL STATE   Confusion is a mental and behavioral state of reduced comprehension, coherence, and capacity to reason. Inattention, as defined by the inability to sustain uninterrupted thought and actions, and disorientation are its earliest outward signs. As the state of confusion worsens, there are more global mental failings, including impairments of memory, perception, comprehension, problem solving, language, praxis, visuospatial function, and various aspects of emotional behavior that are each attributable to particular regions of the brain. In other instances an apparent confusional state may arise from an isolated deficit in mental function such as an impairment of language (*aphasia*), loss of memory (*amnesia*), or lack of appreciation of spatial relations of self and the external environment (*agnosia*), but the attributes of the problem are then quite different (Chap. 25). Confusion is also a feature of dementia, in which case the chronicity of the process, as in the instance of Alzheimer's disease, distinguishes it from an acute encephalopathy (Chap. 26).

The confused patient is usually subdued, not inclined to speak, and is physically inactive. A state of confusion that is accompanied by agitation, hallucinations, tremor, and illusions (misperceptions of environmental sight, sound, or touch) is termed *delirium*, as typified by delirium tremens from alcohol or drug withdrawal. In psychiatric circles, delirium often refers, albeit imprecisely, to all acute states of confusion with clouding of consciousness and incoherence of thought.

Approach to the Patient

Confusion and delirium always signify a disorder of the nervous system. They may be the major manifestation of a head injury; a seizure; drug toxicity (or drug withdrawal); a metabolic disorder resulting from hepatic, renal, pulmonary or cardiac failure; a systemic infection; meningitis or encephalitis; or a chronic dementing disease.

The search for these manifold causes begins with a careful history emphasizing the patient's condition before the onset of confusion. The clinical examination should focus on signs of diminished attentiveness, disorientation, and drowsiness and on the presence of localizing neurologic signs. From the clinical data the clinician is directed to the appropriate laboratory tests discussed further on. Often, even after all diagnostic tests are completed, one may still not know the cause of a confusional state. The proper approach is to observe the patient in the hospital for a number of days under stable conditions. New clues may appear or an obscure confusion perhaps related to a medication, may clear up, while other causes such as renal or hepatic failure may worsen and lead to coma.

Orientation and memory are tested by asking the patient in a forthright manner the date, inclusive of month, day, year, and day of week; the precise place; and some items of generally acknowledged and universally known information (the names of the President and Vice President, a recent national catastrophe, the state capital). Further probing may be necessary to reveal a defect—why is the patient in the hospital; what is his or her address, zip code, telephone number, social security number? Problems of increasing complexity may be pursued, but they usually provide little additional information. Attention and coherence of thought can be gauged by the clarity of and speed of responses while the history is being given but are examined more explicitly by having the patient repeat strings of numbers (most adults easily retain seven digits forward and four backward), spell a word such as "world" backwards, and perform serial calculations—tests of serial subtraction of 3 from 30 or 7 from 100 are useful. It is the inability to sustain coherent mental activity in performing tasks such as these that exposes the most subtle confusional states.

Other salient neurologic findings are the level of alertness, which fluctuates if there is drowsiness; indications of focal damage of the cerebrum such as hemiparesis, hemianopia, and aphasia; or adventitious movements of myoclonus or partial convulsions. The language of the confused patient may be disorganized and rambling, even to the extent of incorporating paraphasic words. These features, along with impaired comprehension that is due mainly to inattention, may be mistaken for aphasia.

One of the most specific signs of a metabolic encephalopathy is asterixis, which is an arrhythmic flapping tremor that is typically elicited by asking the patient to hold the arms outstretched with the wrists and hands fully extended. After a few seconds, there is a large jerking lapse in the posture of the hand and then a rapid return to the original position. The same movements can be appreciated in any tonically held posture, even of the tongue, and in extreme form the movements may intrude on voluntary limb motion. Bilateral asterixis always signifies a metabolic encephalopathy, e.g., from hepatic failure, hypercapnia, or from drug ingestion, especially with anticonvulsant medications. Myoclonic jerking and tremor in an awake patient are typical of uremic encephalopathy or the use of antipsychotic drugs such as lithium, phenothiazines, or butyrophenones; myoclonus with coma may also signify anoxic cerebral damage.

Confusion in the postoperative period is common but at times so subtle as to escape attention. Cardiac and orthopedic procedures are particularly likely to produce disorientation or delirium in susceptible patients. Often a careful history will reveal that a mild but compensated dementia existed prior to the operation. Medications, particularly those with anticholinergic activity (including meperidine), inadvertent withdrawal from sleeping pills or alcohol, fever, and any of the endogenous metabolic derangements listed above may be responsible, or a stroke may have occurred.

Frequently confusion cannot be attributed to any single factor and it clears in several days. In many cases, particularly in the elderly, transient confusion and drowsiness arise with a febrile infection of the urinary tract, lungs, blood, or peritoneum. The term *septic encephalopathy* is currently used to describe this association, but the mechanism by which infection or inflammation leads to cerebral dysfunction is unknown. Fever can also alter brain function in a way that makes preexisting focal signs worse.

Distinguishing dementia from an acute confusional state is a great problem, especially in the elderly, since the two may coexist if a fever, other acute medical problem, or a poorly tolerated medication supervenes in a mildly demented patient, producing a so-called beclouded dementia. The memory loss of dementia brings about a confusional state that varies little in severity from hour to hour and day to day. Poor mental performance is derived mainly from incomplete recollection, inadequate access to names and ideas, and the inability to retain new information, thus affecting orientation and factual knowledge. In contrast to the acute confusional states, attention, alertness, and coherence are preserved until the most advanced stages. Eventually dementia produces a chronic confusion with breakdown of all types of mental performance, and the distinction from an acute encephalopathy depends mainly on the longstanding nature of the condition.

Treatment of the confusional state requires that all unnecessary medication be stopped, metabolic alterations be rectified, and infection be treated. Skilled nursing and a quiet room with a window are important. Careful explanations should be given at regular intervals to the family. In the elderly, regular reorientation and active measures to avoid risk factors (sleep deprivation, immobility, and vision and hearing impairments) reduce the number and severity of episodes of delirium in hospitalized patients.

COMA AND RELATED DISORDERS OF CONSCIOUSNESS The unnatural situation of reduced alertness and responsiveness represents a continuum that in severest form is called *coma,* a deep sleeplike state from which the patient cannot be aroused. *Stupor* defines lesser degrees of unarousability in which the patient can be awakened only by vigorous stimuli, accompanied by motor behavior that leads to avoidance of uncomfortable or aggravating stimuli. *Drowsiness,* which is familiar to all persons, simulates light sleep and is characterized by easy arousal and the persistence of alertness for brief periods. Drowsiness and stupor are usually attended by some degree of confusion. In clinical practice these terms should be supplemented by a narrative description of the level of arousal and of the type of responses evoked by various stimuli precisely as observed at the bedside. Such an account is preferable to ambiguous terms such as semicoma or obtundation, the definitions of which differ between physicians.

Several other neurologic conditions render patients apparently unresponsive and simulate coma, and certain other subsyndromes of coma must be considered separately because of their special significance. Among the latter, the *vegetative state* signifies an awake but unresponsive state. Most of these patients were earlier comatose and after a period of days or weeks emerge to an unresponsive state in which their eyelids are open, giving the appearance of wakefulness. Yawning, grunting, swallowing, as well as limb and head movements persist, but there are few, if any, meaningful responses to the external and internal environment—in essence, an "awake coma." Although respiratory and autonomic functions are retained, the term "vegetative" is nonetheless unfortunate as it is subject to misinterpretation by lay persons. Always there are accompanying signs that indicate extensive damage in both cerebral hemispheres, e.g., decerebrate or decorticate limb posturing and absent responses to visual stimuli (see below). Cardiac arrest and head injuries are the most common causes of the vegetative state (Chaps. 369 and 376). The prognosis for regaining mental faculties once the vegetative state has supervened for several months is almost nil hence the term *persistent vegetative state.* Most instances of dramatic recovery, when investigated carefully, are found to yield to the usual rules for prognosis, but it must be acknowledged that rare instances of awakening to a condition of dementia and paralysis have been documented.

Certain other clinical states are prone to be misinterpreted as stupor or coma. *Akinetic mutism* refers to a partially or fully awake patient who is able to form impressions and think but remains immobile and mute, particularly when unstimulated. The condition may result from damage in the regions of the medial thalamic nuclei, the frontal lobes (particularly situated deeply or on the orbitofrontal surfaces), or from hydrocephalus. The term *abulia* is used to describe a mental and physical slowness and lack of impulse to activity that is in essence a mild form of akinetic mutism, with the same anatomic origins. *Catatonia* is a curious hypomobile and mute syndrome associated with a major psychosis. In the typical form patients appear awake with eyes open but make no voluntary or responsive movements, although they blink spontaneously, swallow, and may not appear distressed. As often, the eyes are half-open as if the patient is in a fog or light sleep. There are signs that indicate voluntary attempts to appear less than fully responsive, though it may take some ingenuity on the part of the examiner to demonstrate these. Eyelid elevation is actively resisted, blinking occurs in response to a visual threat, and the eyes move concomitantly with head rotation, all signs belying a brain lesion. It is characteristic but not invariable for the limbs to retain the posture, no matter how bizarre, in which they have been placed by the examiner ("waxy flexibility," or catalepsy.) Upon recovery, such patients have some memory of events that occurred during their catatonic stupor. The appearance is superficially similar to akinetic mutism, but clinical evidence of brain damage is lacking.

The *locked-in state* describes a pseudocoma in which an awake patient has no means of producing speech or volitional limb, face, and pharyngeal movements in order to indicate that he or she is awake, but vertical eye movements and lid elevation remain unimpaired, thus allowing the patient to signal. Such individuals have written entire treatises using Morse code. Infarction or hemorrhage of the ventral pons, which transects all descending corticospinal and corticobulbar pathways, is the usual cause. A similar awake but deefferented state occurs as a result of total paralysis of the musculature in severe cases of Guillain-Barré syndrome (Chap. 378), critical illness neuropathy (Chap. 376), and pharmacologic neuromuscular blockade.

THE ANATOMY AND PHYSIOLOGY OF UNCONSCIOUSNESS   To the extent that all complex waking behaviors require the widespread participation of the cerebral cortex, consciousness cannot exist without the activity of these structures. A loosely grouped aggregation of neurons located in the upper brainstem and medial thalamus, the RAS, maintains the cerebral cortex in a state of wakeful consciousness. It follows that the principal causes of coma are (1) lesions that damage a substantial portion of the RAS; (2) destruction of large portions of both cerebral hemispheres; and (3) suppression of thalamocerebral function by drugs, toxins, or by internal metabolic derangements such as hypoglycemia, anoxia, azotemia, or hepatic failure.

The classic animal experiments of Moruzzi and Magoun, published in 1949, and subsequent human clinicopathologic observations have established that the regions of the reticular formation that are critical to the maintenance of wakefulness extend from the caudal midbrain to the lower thalamus. A most important practical consideration derives from the anatomic proximity of the RAS to structures that are concerned with pupillary function and eye movements. Pupillary enlargement and loss of vertical and adduction movements of the globes suggest that upper brainstem damage may be the source of coma. Although circumscribed lesions confined to one or both cerebral hemispheres do not affect the brainstem RAS, a large mass on one side of the brain may cause coma by secondarily compressing the upper brainstem and consequently producing abnormalities of the pupils and eye movements (see discussion of transtentorial herniation below). This type of indirect effect is most typical of cerebral hemorrhages and of rapidly expanding tumors within a cerebral hemisphere. In all cases the degree of diminished alertness also relates to the rapidity of evolution and the extent of compression of the RAS.

The neurons of the RAS are thought to project rostrally to the cortex primarily via thalamic relay nuclei that in turn exert a tonic influence on the activity of the entire cerebral cortex. The behavioral arousal effected by somesthetic, auditory, and visual stimuli depends upon the rich reciprocal innervation that the RAS receives from these sensory systems. The relays between the RAS and the thalamic and cortical areas utilize a variety of neurotransmittors. Of these, the effect of arousal on acetylcholine and on the biogenic amines has been studied more extensively. Cholinergic fibers connect the midbrain to other areas of the upper brainstem, thalamus, and cortex. Serotonin and norepinephrine also subserve important functions in regulation of the sleep-wake cycle (Chap. 27). Their roles in arousal and coma have not been clearly established, although the alerting effects of amphetamines are likely to be mediated by catecholamine release.

Coma Due to Cerebral Mass Lesions and Herniations   The cranial cavity is separated into compartments by infoldings of the dura—the two cerebral hemispheres are separated by the falx, and the anterior and posterior fossae by the tentorium. *Herniation* refers to displacement of brain tissue away from a mass and into a compartment that it normally does not occupy. Many of the signs associated with coma, and indeed coma itself, can be attributed to these tissue shifts. Herniation can be *transfalcial* (displacement of the cingulate gyrus under the falx and across the midline), *transtentorial* (displacement of the medial temporal lobe into the tentorial opening), and *foraminal* (downward forcing of the cerebellar tonsils into the foramen magnum; Fig. 24-1).

Uncal transtentorial herniation refers to impaction of the anterior medial temporal gyrus (the uncus) into the anterior portion of the tentorial opening. The displaced tissue compresses the third nerve as it traverses the subarachnoid space and results in enlargement of the ipsilateral pupil (putatively because the fibers subserving parasympathetic pupillary function are located peripherally in the nerve). The coma that follows may be due to lateral compression of the midbrain against the opposite tentorial edge by the displaced parahippocampal gyrus (Fig. 24-2). In some cases the lateral displacement causes compression of the opposite cerebral peduncle, producing a Babinski response and hemiparesis contralateral to the original hemiparesis (the Kernohan-Woltman sign). In addition to compressing the upper brainstem, tissue shifts, including herniations, may compress major blood vessels, particularly the anterior and posterior cerebral arteries as they pass over the tentorial reflections, thus producing brain infarctions. The distortions may also entrap portions of the ventricular system, resulting in regional hydrocephalus.

Central transtentorial herniation denotes a symmetric downward movement of the upper thalamic region through the tentorial opening. Miotic pupils and drowsiness are the heralding signs. Both temporal and central herniations are thought to cause progressive compression of the brainstem from above: first the midbrain, then the pons, and finally the medulla. The result is a sequential appearance of neurologic signs that corresponds to the affected level.

A direct relationship between the various configurations of transtentorial herniations and coma is, at best, tenuous. The orderly pro-

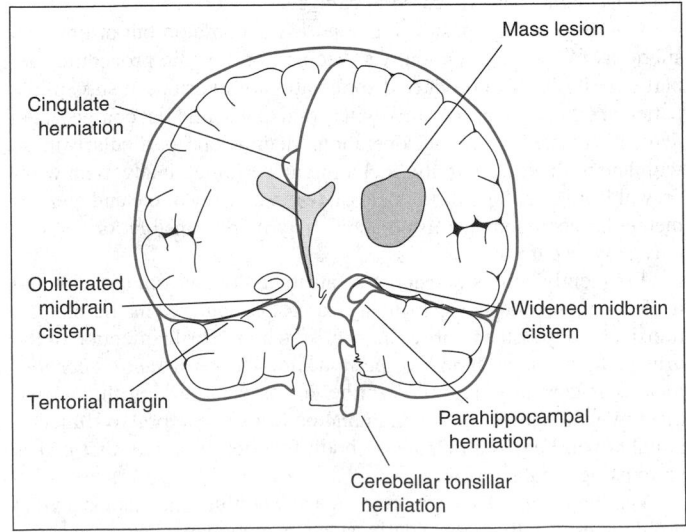

FIGURE 24-1   Herniation.

gression of signs from midbrain to medulla is often bypassed in catastrophic lesions where all brainstem functions are lost almost simultaneously. It is also clear that displacement of deep brain structures by a mass in any direction, with or without herniation, compresses the region of the RAS and results in coma. Furthermore, drowsiness and stupor typically occur with moderate lateral shifts at the level of the diencephalon (thalami) well before transtentorial or other herniations are evident. Lateral shift is easily quantified on axial images of computed tomography (CT) and magnetic resonance imaging (MRI) scans (Fig. 24-2). In cases of *acutely appearing masses*, a fairly consistent and simple relationship exists between the degree of horizontal displacement of midline structures and the level consciousness. Specifically, horizontal displacement of the pineal calcification of 3 to 5 mm is generally associated with drowsiness, 6 to 8 mm with stupor, and >9 mm with coma. At the same time, intrusion of the medial temporal lobe into the tentorial opening may be apparent as an obliteration of the cisterns that surround the upper brainstem.

FIGURE 24-2 Coronal *(A)* and axial *(B)* magnetic resonance images from a stuporous patient with a left third nerve palsy as a result of large left-sided subdural hematoma (seen as a gray-white rim). The upper midbrain and lower thalamic regions are compressed and displaced laterally to the right, and there is transtentorial herniation of the medial temporal lobe structures, including the uncus anteriorly. The lateral ventricle opposite to the hematoma has become enlarged as a result of compression of the third ventricle.

Coma and Confusional States Due to Metabolic Disorders A large variety of systemic metabolic abnormalities cause coma by interrupting the delivery of energy substrates (hypoxia, ischemia, hypoglycemia) or by altering neuronal excitability (drug and alcohol intoxication, anesthesia, and epilepsy). The same metabolic abnormalities that produce coma may in milder form induce widespread cortical dysfunction and an acute confusional state. Thus, in metabolic encephalopathies, clouded consciousness and coma are a continuum. Neuropathologic changes in the various metabolic failures are variable— very evident in hypoxia-ischemia, manifest as astrocytic changes in hepatic coma, and negligible in renal and other metabolic encephalopathies.

Cerebral neurons are fully dependent on cerebral blood flow (CBF) and the related delivery of oxygen and glucose. CBF approximates 75 mL per 100 g/min in gray matter and 30 mL per 100 g/min in white matter (mean = 55 mL per 100 g/min); oxygen consumption is 3.5 mL per 100 g/min, and glucose utilization is 5 mg per 100 g/min. Brain stores of glucose provide energy for approximately 2 min after blood flow is interrupted, and oxygen stores last 8 to 10 s after the cessation of blood flow. Simultaneous hypoxia and ischemia exhaust glucose more rapidly. The electroencephalogram (EEG) rhythm in these circumstances becomes diffusely slowed, typical of metabolic encephalopathies, and as conditions of substrate delivery worsen, eventually all recordable brain electrical activity ceases. In almost all instances of metabolic encephalopathy, the global metabolic activity of the brain is reduced in proportion to the degree of unconsciousness.

Conditions such as hyponatremia, hyperosmolarity, hypercapnia, hypercalcemia, and hepatic and renal failure are associated with a variety of alterations in neurons and astrocytes. It should be stated at the outset that the reversible effects of these conditions on the brain are not understood, but they may in different circumstances impair energy supplies, change ion fluxes across neuronal membranes, and cause neurotransmitter abnormalities. For example, the high brain ammonia concentration that is associated with hepatic coma interferes with cerebral energy metabolism and with the Na+, K+-ATPase pump, increases the number and size of astrocytes, alters nerve cell function, and causes increased concentrations of potentially toxic products of ammonia metabolism; it may also result in abnormalities of neurotransmitters, including possible "false" neurotransmitters that may be active at receptor sites. Apart from hyperammonemia, which of these mechanisms is of critical importance is not clear. The mechanism of the encephalopathy of renal failure is also not known. Unlike ammonia, urea itself does not produce central nervous system (CNS) toxicity. A multifactorial causation has been proposed, including increased permeability of the blood-brain barrier to toxic substances such as organic acids and an increase in brain calcium or cerebrospinal fluid (CSF) phosphate content. Likewise, the basis of confusion and drowsiness that commonly accompanies the septic state has not been clarified.

Coma and seizures are a common accompaniment of any large shifts in sodium and water balance. These changes in osmolarity may be the result of a number of systemic medical disorders including diabetic ketoacidosis, the nonketotic hyperosmolar state, and hyponatremia from any cause (e.g., water intoxication, excessive secretion of antidiuretic hormone or atrial natriuretic peptides). The volume of brain water correlates with the level of consciousness in these states, but other factors also play a role. Sodium levels below 125 mmol/L induce confusion, and below 115 mmol/L are associated with coma and convulsions. In hyperosmolar coma the serum osmolarity generally exceeds 350 mosmol/L. *As in most other metabolic encephalopathies, the severity of neurologic change depends to a large degree on the rapidity with which the serum changes occur.* Hypercapnia depresses the level of consciousness in proportion to the rise in CO_2 tension in the blood and depends very much on the rapidity of change. The pathophysiology of other metabolic encephalopathies such as hypercalcemia, hypothyroidism, vitamin B_{12} deficiency, and hypothermia are incompletely understood but must also reflect derangements of CNS biochemistry and membrane function.

Epileptic Coma Although all metabolic derangements in some way alter neuronal electrophysiologic function, epilepsy is the only primary excitatory disturbance of brain electrical activity that is encountered in clinical practice. Continuous, generalized electrical discharges of the cortex (*seizures*) are associated with coma even in the absence of epileptic motor activity (*convulsions*). The self-limited coma that follows seizures, termed the *postictal state*, may be due to exhaustion of energy reserves or effects of locally toxic molecules that are the byproduct of seizures. The postictal state produces a pattern of continuous, generalized slowing of the background EEG activity similar to that of other metabolic encephalopathies.

Pharmacologic Coma This class of encephalopathy is in large measure reversible and leaves no residual damage providing hypoxia does not supervene. Many drugs and toxins are capable of depressing nervous system function. Some produce coma by affecting both the brainstem nuclei, including the RAS, and the cerebral cortex. The combination of cortical and brainstem signs, which occurs in certain drug overdoses, may lead to an incorrect diagnosis of structural brainstem disease.

Approach to the Patient

The diagnosis and management of coma depend on knowledge of its main causes (see "Differential Diagnosis," below) and on interpretation of salient clinical signs, notably brainstem reflexes and motor function. Acute respiratory and cardiovascular problems should be attended to prior to neurologic assessment. A complete medical evaluation, except for the vital signs, funduscopy, and examination for nuchal rigidity, may be deferred until the neurologic evaluation has established the severity and nature of coma.

History In many cases, the cause of coma is immediately evident (e.g., trauma, cardiac arrest, or known drug ingestion). In the remainder, historic information about the onset of coma is often sparse, but certain historic points are especially useful: (1) the circumstances and rapidity with which neurologic symptoms developed; (2) the details of any immediately preceding medical and neurologic symptoms (confusion, weakness, headache, fever, seizures, dizziness, double vision, or vomiting); (3) the use of medications, illicit drugs, or alcohol; and (4) chronic liver, kidney, lung, heart, or other medical disease. Direct interrogation or telephone calls to family and observers on the scene are an important part of the initial evaluation. Ambulance technicians often provide the most useful information in an enigmatic case.

General Physical Examination The temperature, pulse, respiratory rate and pattern, and blood pressure should be measured quickly as the evaluation is getting under way. Fever suggests a systemic infection, bacterial meningitis, or encephalitis; only rarely is it attributable to a brain lesion that has disturbed temperature-regulating centers. A slight elevation in temperature may follow vigorous convulsions. High body temperature, 42 to 44°C, associated with dry skin should arouse the suspicion of heat stroke or anticholinergic drug intoxication. Hypothermia is observed with bodily exposure to lowered environmental temperature; alcoholic, barbiturate, sedative, or phenothiazine intoxication; hypoglycemia; peripheral circulatory failure; or hypothyroidism. Hypothermia itself causes coma only when the temperature is <31°C. Tachypnea may indicate acidosis or pneumonia. Aberrant respiratory patterns that may reflect brainstem disorders are discussed below. Marked hypertension, a sign of hypertensive encephalopathy or a rapid rise in intracranial pressure, may occur acutely after head injury. Hypotension is characteristic of coma from alcohol or barbiturate intoxication, internal hemorrhage, myocardial infarction, sepsis, profound hypothyroidism, or Addisonian crisis. The funduscopic examination is invaluable in detecting subarachnoid hemorrhage (subhyaloid hemorrhages), hypertensive encephalopathy (exudates, hemorrhages, vessel-crossing changes, papilledema), and increased intracranial pressure (papilledema). Generalized cutaneous petechiae suggest thrombotic thrombocytopenic purpura, meningococcemia, or a bleeding diathesis from which an intracerebral hemorrhage arises.

Neurologic Assessment The patient should be observed first without examiner intervention. Patients who toss about, reach up toward the face, cross their legs, yawn, swallow, cough, or moan are close to being awake. Lack of restless movements on one side or an outturned leg at rest suggests a hemiplegia. Intermittent twitching movements of a foot, finger, or facial muscle may be the only sign of seizures. Multifocal myoclonus almost always indicates a metabolic disorder, particularly azotemia, anoxia, or drug ingestion (lithium and haloperidol are particularly prone to cause this sign), or the rarer conditions of spongiform encephalopathy and Hashitmoto disease. In a drowsy and confused patient bilateral asterixis is a certain sign of metabolic encephalopathy or drug ingestion.

The terms *decorticate rigidity* and *decerebrate rigidity*, or "posturing," describe stereotyped arm and leg movements occurring spontaneously or elicited by sensory stimulation. Flexion of the elbows and wrists and supination of the arm (decortication) suggests severe bilateral damage rostral to the midbrain, whereas extension of the elbows and wrists with pronation (decerebration) indicates damage to motor tracts in the midbrain or caudal diencephalon. The less frequent combination of arm extension with leg flexion or flaccid legs is associated

with lesions in the pons. These concepts have been adapted from animal work and cannot be applied with the same precision to coma in humans. In fact, acute and widespread cerebral disorders of any type, regardless of location, frequently cause limb extension, and almost all such extensor posturing becomes predominantly flexor as time passes. Thus, posturing alone cannot be utilized for precise anatomic localization. Posturing may also be unilateral and may coexist with purposeful limb movements, usually reflecting incomplete damage to the motor system.

Level of Arousal and Elicited Movements If the patient is not aroused by a conversational volume of voice, a sequence of increasingly intense stimuli is used to determine the patient's threshold of arousal and the optimal motor response of each limb. It should be recognized that the results of this testing may vary from minute to minute and that serial examinations are most useful. Tickling the nostrils with a cotton wisp is a moderate stimulus to arousal—all but deeply stuporous and comatose patients will move the head away and rouse to some degree. Using the hand to remove an offending stimulus such as this one represents an even lesser degree of unresponsiveness.

Responses to noxious stimuli should be appraised critically. Stereotyped posturing indicates severe dysfunction of the corticospinal system. Abduction-avoidance movement of a limb is usually purposeful and denotes an intact corticospinal system extending from the contralateral cortex to the ipsilateral spinal cord. Pressure on the knuckles or bony prominences and pinprick are humane forms of noxious stimulus; pinching the skin causes unsightly ecchymoses and is generally not necessary but may be useful in eliciting abduction withdrawal movements of the limbs. Conversely, consistent (obligatory) adduction and flexion of stimulated limbs may be reflexive in origin and implies damage to the corticospinal system. Brief clonus or twitching may occur at the end of extensor posturing movements and should not be mistaken for convulsions.

Brainstem Reflexes Assessment of brainstem damage is essential to the localization of the lesion in coma (Fig. 24-3). The brainstem reflexes that are conveniently assessed are pupillary responses to light, spontaneous and elicited eye movements, corneal responses, and the respiratory pattern. As a rule, when these brainstem activities are preserved, particularly the pupil reactions and eye movements, coma must necessarily be ascribed to bilateral hemispheral disease. The converse, however, is not always true as a mass in the hemispheres may be the proximate cause of coma but nonetheless produce brainstem signs.

Pupils Pupillary reactions are examined with a bright, diffuse light (not an ophthalmoscope); if the response is absent, this should be confirmed by observation through a magnifying lens. Reaction to light is often difficult to appreciate in pupils <2 mm in diameter, and bright room lighting mutes pupillary reactivity. Normally reactive and round pupils of midsize (2.5 to 5 mm) essentially exclude midbrain damage, either primary or secondary to compression. One unreactive and enlarged pupil (>6 mm) or one that is poorly reactive signifies a compression or stretching of the third nerve from the effects of a mass above. Enlargement of the pupil contralateral to a mass may occur but is infrequent. It may be found in cases of subdural hematoma or brain hemorrhage, possibly as a result of compression of the midbrain or third nerve against the opposite tentorial margin. An oval and slightly eccentric pupil is a transitional sign that accompanies early midbrain–third nerve compression. The most extreme pupillary sign, bilaterally dilated and unreactive pupils, indicates severe midbrain damage, usually from compression by a mass or from ingestion of drugs with anticholinergic activity. The use of mydriatic eye drops, by a previous examiner or self-administered by the patient, and direct ocular trauma are among the causes of misleading pupillary enlargement.

Unilateral miosis in coma has been attributed to dysfunction of sympathetic efferents originating in the posterior hypothalamus and descending in the tegmentum of the brainstem to the cervical cord. Reactive and bilaterally small (1 to 2.5 mm) but not pinpoint pupils are seen in metabolic encephalopathies or in deep bilateral hemispheral lesions such as hydrocephalus or thalamic hemorrhage. Very small but reactive pupils (<1 mm) characterize narcotic or barbiturate overdoses

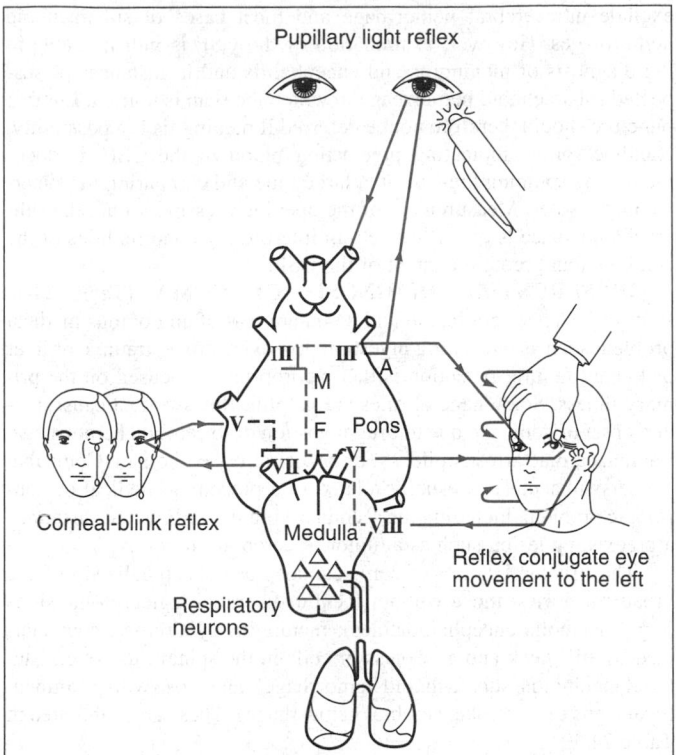

FIGURE 24-3 Brainstem reflexes in the coma examination. Midbrain and third nerve function are tested by pupillary reaction to light, pontine function by spontaneous and reflex eye movements and corneal responses, and medullary function by respiratory and pharyngeal responses.

Reflex conjugate, horizontal eye movements are dependent on the medial longitudinal fasciculus (MLF) interconnecting the sixth and contralateral third nerve nuclei. Head rotation (oculocephalic reflex) or caloric stimulation of the labyrinths (oculovestibular reflex) elicits contraversive eye movements (for details see text).

but also occur with extensive pontine hemorrhage. The response to naloxone and the presence of reflex eye movements (see below) distinguish these. The unilaterally small pupil of the Horner syndrome is detected by failure of the pupil to enlarge in the dark. It is an occasional finding with a large cerebral hemorrhage that affects the thalamus.

Ocular movements Eye movements are the second sign of importance in determining if the brainstem has been damaged. Abnormalities, implicate both midbrain and pontine functions, thus permitting the analysis of a large portion of the brainstem. The eyes are first observed by elevating the lids and noting the resting position and spontaneous movements of the globes. Lid tone, tested by lifting the eyelids and noting their resistance to opening and the speed of closure, is reduced progressively as coma deepens. Horizontal divergence of the eyes at rest is normal in drowsiness. As coma deepens, the ocular axes may become parallel again. An abducted eye indicates a medial rectus paresis due to third nerve dysfunction and has the same significance as pupillary enlargement. An adducted eye indicates lateral rectus paresis due to a sixth nerve lesion and, when bilateral, is often a sign of increased intracranial pressure. With few exceptions, vertical separation of the ocular axes (one eye lower than the other, i.e. skew deviation) results from pontine or cerebellar lesions but may also be a manifestation of a partial third nerve palsy.

Spontaneous eye movements in coma often take the form of conjugate horizontal roving. This finding alone exonerates the midbrain and pons and has the same meaning as normal reflex eye movements (see below). Cyclic vertical downward movements are seen in some circumstances. "Ocular bobbing" describes a brisk downward and slow upward movement of the eyes associated with loss of horizontal eye movements and is diagnostic of bilateral pontine damage, characteristically from thrombosis of the basilar artery. "Ocular dipping" is a

slower, arrhythmic downward movement followed by a faster upward movement in patients with normal reflex horizontal gaze; it usually indicates diffuse cortical anoxic damage. The eyes may turn down and inward as a result of thalamic and upper midbrain lesions, typically with thalamic hemorrhage or dilatation of the third ventricle from hydrocephalus. Conjugate horizontal ocular deviation to one extreme at rest indicates damage to the pons on the side of the gaze paresis or a lesion in the frontal lobe on the opposite side. This phenomenon may be summarized by the following maxim: *The eyes look toward a hemispheral lesion and away from a brainstem lesion.* On rare occasions, the eyes may turn paradoxically away from the side of a deep hemispheral lesion ("wrong-way eyes"). Many other complex and interesting eye movements are known but do not have the same salience in coma as the ones already mentioned.

Oculocephalic reflexes are automatic movements of the eyes elicited by moving the head from side to side or vertically. As the activity of the hemispheres is subdued from whatever cause, eye movements are evoked in the direction opposite to the head movement (Fig. 24-3). These movements, called somewhat inappropriately "doll's eyes" (which more accurately refers to the reflex elevation of the eyelids with flexion of the neck) are suppressed by visual fixation, which requires the patient to be awake. Induced adduction of the globes tends to be less complete than abduction, hence subtle abnormalities in the doll's-eye manuever should be interpreted with caution. Oculocephalic reflexes are generated by brainstem mechanisms originating in the labyrinths and in cervical proprioceptors and require the undiminished activity of the third nerve nucleus in the midbrain, the contralateral sixth nerve nucleus in the pons, and the medial longitudinal fasciculus (MLF) that runs virtually the length of the brainstem and links the two. Preservation of reflex eye movements (particularly adduction) therefore informs the examiner that coma is probably not due to an upper brainstem lesion and by implication that the origin of unconsciousness lies in the cerebral diencephalic structures. However, the opposite—the absence of eye movements—may signify either damage within the brainstem or profound metabolic depression of all neuronal function including the brainstem nuclei. Metabolic causes of depressed neuronal function include overdoses of phenytoin, tricyclic antidepressants, barbiturates, alcohol, phenothiazines, diazepam, and neuromuscular blocking agents. The presence of normal pupillary size and light reaction will distinguish most drug-induced comas from structural brainstem damage.

Thermal, or "caloric," stimulation of the vestibular apparatus (oculovestibular response) provides a more intense stimulus that may be used to confirm the absence of the oculocephalic reflex but gives fundamentally the same information. The test is performed by irrigating the external auditory canal with cool water in order to induce convection currents in the labyrinths. After a brief latency, the result is tonic deviation of both eyes (lasting 30 to 120 s) to the side of cool-water irrigation. The integrity of the third and sixth nerve complexes and brainstem pathways from the labyrinths to the midbrain are thereby confirmed, thus excluding a brainstem lesion as the cause of coma. If the cerebral hemispheres are functioning, as in catatonic or hysterical pseudocoma, an obligate rapid corrective nystagmus is generated away from the side of tonic deviation. (The acronym "COWS" has been used to remind generations of medical students of the direction of compensatory nystagmus—"cold water opposite, warm water same"). The absence of this nystagmus despite conjugate deviation of the globes signifies that the cerebral hemispheres are damaged or profoundly suppressed.

By touching the cornea with a wisp of cotton, a response consisting of brief bilateral lid closure is normally observed. Although the corneal reflexes are rarely useful alone, they may corroborate eye-movement abnormalities because they also depend on the integrity of pontine pathways. The response is lost if the reflex connections between the fifth (afferent) and both seventh (efferent) cranial nerves within the pons are damaged. CNS depressant drugs diminish or eliminate the corneal responses soon after reflex eye movements are paralyzed but before the pupils become unreactive to light. The corneal (and pharyngeal) response may be lost for a time on the side of an acute hemiplegia.

Respiration Respiratory patterns have received much attention in coma diagnosis but are of less localizing value in comparison to other brainstem signs. Shallow, slow, but regular breathing suggests metabolic or drug depression. Cheyne-Stokes respiration in its classic cyclic form, ending with a brief apneic period, signifies bihemispheral damage or metabolic suppression and commonly accompanies light coma. Rapid, deep (Kussmaul) breathing usually implies metabolic acidosis but may also occur with pontomesencephalic lesions and, of course, severe pneumonia. Agonal gasps reflect bilateral lower brainstem damage and are well known as the terminal respiratory pattern of severe brain damage. A number of other cyclic breathing variations are of lesser significance for localization.

LABORATORY STUDIES AND IMAGING The following studies are most useful in the diagnosis of confusional states and coma: chemical-toxicologic analysis of blood and urine, cranial CT or MRI, EEG, and CSF examination. Arterial blood-gas analysis is helpful in patients with lung disease and acid-base disorders. Chemical blood determinations are obtained routinely to disclose metabolic, toxic, or drug-induced encephalopathies. The metabolic aberrations commonly encountered in clinical practice require measurements of electrolytes, glucose, calcium, osmolarity, and renal (blood urea nitrogen) and hepatic (NH_3) function. Toxicologic analysis is necessary in any case of coma where the diagnosis is not immediately clear. However, the presence of exogenous drugs or toxins, especially alcohol, does not exclude the possibility that other factors, particularly head trauma, are also contributing to the clinical state. An ethanol level of 43 mmol/L (200 mg/dL) in nonhabituated patients generally causes confusion and impaired mental activity and of >65 mmol/L (300 mg/dL) is associated with stupor. The development of tolerance may allow the chronic alcoholic to remain awake at levels >87 mmol/L (400 mg/dL).

The increased availability of CT and MRI has focused attention on causes of coma that are radiologically detectable (e.g., hemorrhages, tumors, or hydrocephalus). Resorting primarily to this approach, although at times expedient, is imprudent because most cases of coma (and confusion) are metabolic or toxic in origin. The notion that a normal CT scan excludes anatomic lesions as the cause of coma is also erroneous. Bilateral hemisphere infarction, small brainstem lesions, encephalitis, meningitis, mechanical shearing of axons as a result of closed head trauma, absent cerebral perfusion associated with brain death, sagittal sinus thrombosis, and subdural hematomas that are isodense to adjacent brain are some of the lesions that may not be visible. Nevertheless, if the source of coma remains unknown, a scan should be obtained.

The EEG is useful in metabolic or drug-induced confusional states but is rarely diagnostic, with the important exceptions of coma due to clinically unrecognized seizures, to herpesvirus encephalitis and Creutzfeldt-Jakob disease. The amount of background slowing of the EEG is a useful reflection of the severity of any diffuse encephalopathy. Predominant high-voltage slowing (δ or triphasic waves) in the frontal regions is typical of metabolic coma, as from hepatic failure, and widespread fast (β) activity implicates sedative drugs (diazepines, barbiturates). A pattern of "α coma," defined by widespread, variable 8- to 12-Hz activity, superficially resembles the normal α rhythm of waking but is unresponsive to environmental stimuli. It results from pontine or diffuse cortical damage and has a poor prognosis. Most importantly, EEG recordings reveal coma that is due to persistent epileptic discharges that are not clinically manifested as convulsions. Normal α activity on the EEG may also alert the clinician to the locked-in syndrome or to hysteria or catatonia.

Lumbar puncture is used more judiciously than in prior decades in cases of coma or confusion because neuroimaging scans effectively exclude intracerebral hemorrhage and most cases of subarachnoid hemorrhages. However, examination of the CSF is indispensable in the diagnosis of meningitis and encephalitis and in instances of suspected subarachnoid hemorrhage in which the scan is normal. Lumbar puncture should therefore not be deferred if meningitis is a possibility. Xanthochromia, indicating preexisting blood in the CSF, is documented by spinning the CSF in a large tube and comparing the supernatant to water. Measurement of the opening pressure within the subarachnoid space is of further help in interpreting abnormalities of the cell count and protein content of the CSF.

DIFFERENTIAL DIAGNOSIS OF COMA (Table 24-1) In most instances confusion and coma are part of an obvious medical problem such as overt drug ingestion, hypoxia, stroke, trauma, or liver or kidney failure. Attention is then appropriately focused on the primary illness. Some general rules are helpful. Illnesses that cause sudden onset of coma are due to drug ingestion or to cerebral hemorrhage, trauma, cardiac arrest, epilepsy, or basilar artery embolism. Coma that appears subacutely is usually related to a preceding medical or neurologic problem, including the secondary brain swelling that surrounds a preexisting lesion such as a tumor or cerebral infarction.

The structural causes of coma can also be conceptualized in three broad categories: those without focal or lateralizing neurologic signs (e.g., metabolic encephalopathies); meningitis syndromes, characterized by stiff neck and an excess of cells in the spinal fluid (e.g., bacterial meningitis, subarachnoid hemorrhage); and those with prominent focal signs (e.g., stroke, cerebral hemorrhage). These are elaborated in Table 24-1.

Table 24-1 Approach to the Differential Diagnosis of Coma

1. Diseases that cause no focal or lateralizing neurologic signs, usually with normal brainstem functions; CT scan and cellular content of the CSF are normal
   a. Intoxications: alcohol, sedative drugs, opiates, etc.
   b. Metabolic disturbances: anoxia, hyponatremia, hypernatremia, hypercalcemia, diabetic acidosis, nonketotic hyperosmolar hyperglycemia, hypoglycemia, uremia, hepatic coma, hypercarbia, addisonian crisis, hypo- and hyperthyroid states, profound nutritional deficiency
   c. Severe systemic infections: pneumonia, septicemia, typhoid fever, malaria, Waterhouse-Friderichsen syndrome
   d. Shock from any cause
   e. Postseizure states, status epilepticus, subclinical epilepsy
   f. Hypertensive encephalopathy, eclampsia
   g. Severe hyperthermia, hypothermia
   h. Concussion
   i. Acute hydrocephalus
2. Diseases that cause meningeal irritation with or without fever, and with an excess of WBCs or RBCs in the CSF, usually without focal or lateralizing cerebral or brainstem signs; CT or MRI shows no mass lesion
   a. Subarachnoid hemorrhage from ruptured aneurysm, arteriovenous malformation, occasionally trauma
   b. Acute bacterial meningitis
   c. Some forms of viral encephalitis
   d. Miscellaneous: Fat embolism, cholesterol embolism, carcinomatous and lymphamatous meningitis, etc.
3. Diseases that cause focal brainstem or lateralizing cerebral signs, with or without changes in the CSF; CT and MRI are abnormal
   a. Hemispheral hemorrhage (basal ganglionic, thalamic) or infarction (large middle cerebral artery territory) with secondary brainstem compression
   b. Brainstem infarction due to basilar artery thrombosis or embolism
   c. Brain abscess, subdural empyema
   d. Epidural and subdural hemorrhage, brain contusion
   e. Brain tumor with surrounding edema
   f. Cerebellar and pontine hemorrhage and infarction
   g. Widespread traumatic brain injury
   h. Metabolic coma (see above) with preexisting focal damage
   i. Miscellaneous: cortical vein thrombosis, herpes simplex encephalitis, multiple cerebral emboli due to bacterial endocarditis, acute hemorrhagic leukoencephalitis, acute disseminated (postinfectious) encephalomyelitis, thrombotic thrombocytopenic purpura, cerebral vasculitis, gliomatous cerebri, pituitary apoplexy, intravascular lymphoma, etc.

NOTE: CT, computed tomography; CSF, cerebrospinal fluid; WBCs, white blood cells; RBCs, red blood cells; MRI, magnetic resonance imaging.

Cerebrovascular diseases cause the greatest difficulty in coma diagnosis. These are described in more detail in Chap. 361 but may be summarized as follows: (1) basal ganglia and thalamic hemorrhage (acute but not instantaneous onset, vomiting, headache, hemiplegia, and characteristic eye signs); (2) pontine hemorrhage (sudden onset, pinpoint pupils, loss of reflex eye movements and corneal responses, ocular bobbing, posturing, hyperventilation, and excessive sweating); (3) cerebellar hemorrhage (occipital headache, vomiting, gaze paresis, and inability to stand); (4) basilar artery thrombosis (neurologic prodrome or warning spells, diplopia, dysarthria, vomiting, eye movement and corneal response abnormalities, and asymmetric limb paresis); and (5) subarachnoid hemorrhage (precipitous coma after headache and vomiting). The most common stroke, infarction in the territory of the middle cerebral artery, does not cause coma acutely but the surrounding edema may expand and act as a mass in a limited number of patients with large infarcts. The syndrome of acute hydrocephalus may accompany many intracranial diseases, particularly subarachnoid hemorrhage. Acute symmetric enlargement of both lateral ventricles causes headache and sometimes vomiting that may progress quickly to coma, with extensor posturing of the limbs, bilateral Babinski signs, small nonreactive pupils, and impaired vertical oculocephalic movements in the vertical direction.

If the history and examination do not suggest a large cerebral lesion or meningitic syndrome or a metabolic or drug cause, then information obtained from CT or MRI may be needed as outlined in Table 24-1. As mentioned earlier, the majority of medical causes of coma can be established without a neuroimaging study.

BRAIN DEATH   This is a state in which there has been cessation of cerebral blood flow; as a result, global ischemia of the brain occurs while respiration is maintained by artificial means and the heart continues to function. It is the only type of brain damage that is unequivocally recognized as death. Many roughly equivalent criteria have been advanced for the diagnosis of brain death, and it is essential to adhere to those endorsed as standards by the local medical community. Ideal criteria are simple, can be conducted at the bedside, and allow no chance of diagnostic error. They contain three essential elements: (1) widespread cortical destruction shown by deep coma—unresponsiveness to all forms of stimulation; (2) global brainstem damage demonstrated by absent pupillary light reaction and the loss of oculovestibular and corneal reflexes; and (3) lower brainstem destruction indicated by complete apnea. The pulse rate is also invariant and unresponsive to atropine. Most patients have diabetes insipidus, but in some it develops only hours or days after the clinical signs of brain death. The pupils are often enlarged and may be mid-sized but should not be constricted. The absence of deep tendon reflexes is not required because the spinal cord may remain functional.

The proof that apnea is due to irreversible medullary damage requires that the P_{CO_2} be high enough to stimulate respiration during a test of spontaneous breathing (apnea test). This can be done safely in most patients by the use, prior to removing the ventilator, of diffusion oxygenation. This is accomplished by preoxygenation with 100% oxygen and then sustained during the test by a tracheal cannula connected to an oxygen supply. CO_2 tension increases approximately 0.3 to 0.4 kPa/min (2 to 3 mmHg/min) during apnea. At the end of the period of observation, typically several minutes in duration, arterial P_{CO_2} should be at least >6.6 to 8.0 kPa (50 to 60 mmHg) for the test to be valid.

The possibility of profound drug-induced or hypothermic depression of the nervous system should be excluded, and some period of observation, usually 6 to 24 h, is desirable during which this state is shown to be sustained. It is particularly advisable to delay clinical testing for up to 24 h if a cardiac arrest has caused brain death or if the inciting disease is not known. An isoelectric EEG may be used as a confirmatory test for total cerebral damage but is not absolutely necessary. Radionuclide brain scanning, cerebral angiography, or transcranial Doppler measurements may also be used to demonstrate the absence of cerebral blood flow, but with the exception of the latter, they are cumbersome and have not been correlated extensively with pathology.

There is no compelling reason to demonstrate brain death except when organ transplantation is involved. Although it is largely accepted in western society that the respirator can be disconnected from a brain-dead patient, problems frequently arise because of inadequate explanation and preparation of the family by the physician. Moreover, there is no proscription in reasonable medical practice to removing such support from patients who are not brain dead but whose condition is nonetheless hopeless and are likely to live for only a brief time.

℞ **TREATMENT**   The immediate goal in acute coma is the prevention of further nervous system damage. Hypotension, hypoglycemia, hypercalcemia, hypoxia, hypercapnia, and hyperthermia should be corrected rapidly and assiduously. An oropharyngeal airway is adequate to keep the pharynx open in drowsy patients who are breathing normally. Tracheal intubation is indicated if there is apnea, upper airway obstruction, hypoventilation, or emesis, or if the patient is liable to aspirate because of coma. Mechanical ventilation is required if there is hypoventilation or if there is an intracranial mass and a need to induce hypocapnia in order to lower intracranial pressure (ICP) as described below. Intravenous access is established and naloxone and dextrose are administered if narcotic overdose or hypoglycemia are even remote possibilities, and thiamine is given with glucose in order to avoid eliciting Wernicke disease in malnourished patients. In cases of suspected basilar thrombosis with brainstem ischemia, intravenous heparin or a thrombolytic agent is often utilized, keeping in mind that cerebellar and pontine hemorrhages resemble basilar artery occlusion. Physostigmine, when used by experienced physicians and with careful monitoring, may awaken patients with anticholinergic-type drug overdose, but many physicians believe that this is justified only to treat cardiac arrhythmias resulting from these overdoses. The use of benzodiazepine antagonists offers some prospect of improvement after overdoses of soporific drugs and has transient benefit in hepatic encephalopathy. Intravenous administration of hypotonic solutions should be monitored carefully in any serious acute brain illness because of the potential for exacerbating brain swelling. Cervical spine injuries must not be overlooked, particularly prior to attempting intubation or the evaluation of oculocephalic responses. Headache accompanied by fever and meningismus indicates an urgent need for examination of the CSF to diagnose meningitis, and it is worth reemphasizing that lumbar puncture should not be delayed while awaiting a CT scan. If the lumbar puncture in a case of suspected meningitis is delayed for any reason, an antibiotic such as a third-generation cephalosporin should be administered as soon as possible, preferably after obtaining blood cultures.

Enlargement of one pupil usually indicates secondary midbrain or third nerve compression by a hemispherical mass and requires that ICP be reduced (Chap. 376). Surgical evacuation of the mass may be appropriate in some cases (e.g., subdural and epidural hematoma.). Medical management to reduce ICP begins with the infusion of normal saline (safe because it is slightly hyperosmolar to serum). Therapeutic hyperventilation may be used to reduce ICP by inducing an arterial P_{CO_2} of 3.7 to 4.2 kPa (28 to 32 mmHg), but its effects are brief. Hyperosmolar therapy with mannitol or an equivalent agent is the mainstay of ICP reduction. It is used simultaneously with hyperventilation in critical cases. A ventricular puncture is necessary to decompress hydrocephalus if medical measures fail to improve alertness. The routine use of high-dose barbiturates and other neuronal-sparing agents soon after cardiac arrest or head trauma has not been shown in clinical studies to be beneficial, and glucocorticoids, although often still used, have no proven value except in cases of brain tumor with edema.

PROGNOSIS   The prediction of the outcome of coma must be considered in reference to long-term care and medical resources. One hopes to avoid the emotionally painful, hopeless outcomes associated with patients who are left severely disabled or vegetative. Several general rules pertain. The uniformly pessimistic outcome of the persistent vegetative state has already been mentioned. Children and young adults may have ominous early clinical findings such as abnormal brainstem reflexes and yet recover, so that temporization in offering a prognosis in this group of patients is wise. Metabolic comas have a far better prognosis than traumatic comas. All schemes for prognosis in adults should be taken as approximate indicators, and medical judgments must be tempered by factors such as age, underlying systemic disease, and general medical condition. In an attempt to collect prognostic information from large numbers of patients with head injury, the Glasgow Coma Scale was devised; empirically it has predictive value in cases of brain trauma (Chap. 369). For anoxic and metabolic coma, clinical signs such as the pupillary and motor responses after 1 day, 3 days, and 1 week have been shown to have predictive value (Chap. 376). The absence of the cortical waves of the somatosensory evoked potentials has also proved a strong indicator of poor outcome in coma from any cause.

BIBLIOGRAPHY

CELESIA GG et al: Persistent vegetative state—report of the American Neurological Association Committee on Ethical Affairs. Ann Neurol 33:386, 1993

FISHER CM: The neurological examination of the comatose patient. Acta Neurol Scand 45(Suppl 36):4, 1969

INOUYE SK et al: A multicomponent intervention to prevent delirium in hospitalized older patients. N Engl J Med 340:669, 1999

IVAN L, BRUCE D: *Coma*. Springfield, IL, Charles C Thomas, 1982

JENNETT B, PLUM F: Persistent vegetative state after brain damage. Lancet 1:734, 1972

PLUM F, POSNER J: *The Diagnosis of Stupor and Coma*, 3d ed. Philadelphia, Davis, 1980

ROPPER AH: Lateral displacement of the brain and level of consciousness in patients with an acute hemispheral mass. N Engl J Med 314:953, 1986

———: *Neurological and Neurosurgical Intensive Care*, 3d ed. New York, Raven, 1992

SAPOSNIK G et al: Spontaneous and reflex movements in brain death. Neurol 54:221, 2000

YOUNG BY, PIGOTT SE: Neurobiological basis of consciousness. Arch Neurol 56:153, 1999

——— et al: *Coma and Impaired Consciousness*. New York, McGraw-Hill, 1998

25	*M.-Marsel Mesulam*

APHASIAS AND OTHER FOCAL CEREBRAL DISORDERS

The cerebral cortex of the human brain contains approximately 20 billion neurons spread over an area of 2 m^2. The *primary sensory* areas provide an obligatory portal for the entry of sensory information into cortical circuitry, whereas the *primary motor* areas provide a final common pathway for coordinating complex motor acts. The primary sensory and motor areas constitute <10% of the cerebral cortex. The rest is subsumed by unimodal, heteromodal, paralimbic, and limbic areas, collectively known as the *association cortex* (Fig. 25-1). The association cortex mediates the integrative processes that subserve cognition, emotion, and comportment. A systematic testing of these mental functions is necessary for the effective clinical assessment of the association cortex and its diseases.

According to current thinking, there are no centers for "hearing words," "perceiving space," or "storing memories." Cognitive and behavioral functions (domains) are coordinated by intersecting *large-scale neural networks* that contain interconnected cortical and subcortical components. The network approach to higher cerebral function has at least four implications of clinical relevance: (1) a single domain such as language or memory can be disrupted by damage to any one of several areas, as long as these areas belong to the same network; (2) damage confined to a single area can give rise to multiple deficits, involving the functions of all networks that intersect in that region; (3) damage to a network component may give rise to minimal or tran-

FIGURE 25-1 Lateral (*top*) and medial (*bottom*) views of the cerebral hemispheres. The numbers refer to the Brodmann cytoarchitectonic designations. Area 17 corresponds to primary visual cortex, 41–42 to primary auditory cortex, 1–3 to primary somatosensory cortex, and 4 to primary motor cortex. The rest of the cerebral cortex contains association areas. AG, angular gyrus; B, Broca's area; CC, corpus callosum; CG, cingulate cortex; DLPFC, dorsolateral prefrontal cortex; FEF, frontal eye fields (premotor cortex); FG, fusiform gyrus; IPL, inferior parietal lobule; ITG, inferior temporal gyrus; LG, lingual gyrus; MPFC, medial prefrontal cortex; MTG, middle temporal gyrus; OFC, orbitofrontal cortex; PHG, parahippocampal gyrus; PPC, posterior parietal cortex; PSC, peristriate cortex; SC, striate cortex; SMG, supramarginal gyrus; SPL, superior parietal lobule; STG, superior temporal gyrus; STS, superior temporal sulcus; TP, temporopolar cortex; W, Wernicke's area.

sient deficits if other parts of the network undergo compensatory reorganization; and (4) individual anatomic sites within a network display a relative (but not absolute) specialization for different behavioral aspects of the relevant function. Five anatomically defined large-scale networks are most relevant to clinical practice: a perisylvian network for language; a parietofrontal network for spatial cognition; an occipitotemporal network for face and object recognition; a limbic network for retentive memory; and a prefrontal network for attention and comportment.

THE LEFT PERISYLVIAN NETWORK FOR LANGUAGE: APHASIAS AND RELATED CONDITIONS Language allows the communication and reshaping of thoughts and experiences by linking them to arbitrary symbols known as words. The neural substrate of language is composed of a distributed network centered in the perisylvian region of the *left* hemisphere. The posterior pole of this network is known as *Wernicke's area* and includes the posterior third of the superior temporal gyrus and a surrounding rim of the inferior parietal lobule. An essential function of Wernicke's area is to transform sensory inputs into their neural word representations so that these can establish the distributed associations that give the word its meaning. The anterior pole of the language network, known as *Broca's area*, includes the posterior part of the inferior frontal gyrus and a surrounding rim of prefrontal heteromodal cortex. An essential function of this area is to transform neural word representations into their articulatory sequences so that the words can be uttered in the form of spoken language. The sequencing function of Broca's area also appears to involve the ordering of words into sentences that contain a meaning-appropriate *syntax* (grammar). Wernicke's and Broca's areas are

Table 25-1   Clinical Features of Aphasias and Related Conditions

	Comprehension	Repetition of Spoken Language	Naming	Fluency
Wernicke's	Impaired	Impaired	Impaired	Preserved or increased
Broca's	Preserved (except grammar)	Impaired	Impaired	Decreased
Global	Impaired	Impaired	Impaired	Decreased
Conduction	Preserved	Impaired	Impaired	Preserved
Nonfluent (motor) transcortical	Preserved	Preserved	Impaired	Impaired
Fluent (sensory) transcortical	Impaired	Preserved	Impaired	Preserved
Isolation	Impaired	Echolalia	Impaired	No purposeful speech
Anomic	Preserved	Preserved	Impaired	Preserved except for word-finding pauses
Pure word deafness	Impaired only for spoken language	Impaired	Preserved	Preserved
Pure alexia	Impaired only for reading	Preserved	Preserved	Preserved

interconnected with each other and with additional perisylvian, temporal, prefrontal, and posterior parietal regions, making up a neural network subserving the various aspects of language function. Damage to any one of these components or to their interconnections can give rise to language disturbances (*aphasia*). Aphasia should be diagnosed only when there are deficits in the formal aspects of language such as naming, word choice, comprehension, spelling, and syntax. Dysarthria and mutism do not, by themselves, lead to a diagnosis of aphasia. The language network shows a left hemisphere dominance pattern in the vast majority of the population. In approximately 90% of right handers and 60% of left handers, aphasia occurs only after lesions of the left hemisphere. In some individuals no hemispheric dominance for language can be discerned, and in some others (including a small minority of right handers) there is a right hemisphere dominance for language. A language disturbance occurring after a right hemisphere lesion in a right hander is called *crossed aphasia*.

Clinical Examination   The clinical examination of language should include the assessment of naming, spontaneous speech, comprehension, repetition, reading, and writing. A deficit of naming (*anomia*) is the single most common finding in aphasic patients. When asked to name common objects (pencil or wristwatch) or their parts (eraser, lead, stem, band), the patient may fail to come up with the appropriate word, may provide a circumlocutious description of the object ("the thing for writing"), or may come up with the wrong word (*paraphasia*). If the patient offers an incorrect but legitimate word ("pen" for "pencil"), the naming error is known as a *semantic paraphasia*; if the word approximates the correct answer but is phonetically inaccurate ("plentil" for "pencil"), it is known as a *phonemic paraphasia*. Asking the patient to name body parts, geometric shapes, and component parts of objects (lapel of coat, cap of pen) can elicit mild forms of anomia in patients who can otherwise name common objects. In most anomias, the patient cannot retrieve the appropriate name when shown an object but can point to the appropriate object when the name is provided by the examiner. This is known as a one-way (or retrieval-based) naming deficit. A two-way naming deficit exists if the patient can neither provide nor recognize the correct name, indicating the presence of a language comprehension impairment. *Spontaneous speech* is described as "fluent" if it maintains appropriate output volume, phrase length, and melody or as "nonfluent" if it is sparse, halting, and average phrase length is below four words. The examiner should also note if the speech is paraphasic or circumlocutious; if it shows a relative paucity of substantive nouns and action verbs versus function words (prepositions, conjunctions); and if word order, tenses, suffixes, prefixes, plurals, and possessives are appropriate. *Comprehension* can be tested by assessing the patient's ability to follow conversation, by asking yes-no questions ("Can a dog fly?", "Does it snow

in summer?") or asking the patient to point to appropriate objects ("Where is the source of illumination in this room?"). Statements with embedded clauses or passive voice construction ("If a tiger is eaten by a lion, which animal stays alive?") help to assess the ability to comprehend complex syntactic structure. Commands to close or open the eyes, stand up, sit down, or roll over should not be used to assess overall comprehension since appropriate responses aimed at such axial movements can be preserved in patients who otherwise have profound comprehension deficits.

Repetition is assessed by asking the patient to repeat single words, short sentences, or strings of words such as "No ifs, ands, or buts." The testing of repetition with tongue-twisters such as "hippopotamus" or "Irish constabulary" provides a better assessment of dysarthria and pallilalia than aphasia. Aphasic patients may have little difficulty with tongue-twisters but have a particularly hard time repeating a string of function words. It is important to make sure that the number of words does not exceed the patient's attention span. Otherwise, the failure of repetition becomes a reflection of the narrowed attention span rather than an indication of an aphasic deficit. *Reading* should be assessed for deficits in reading aloud as well as comprehension. *Writing* is assessed for spelling errors, word order, and grammar. *Alexia* describes an inability to either read aloud or comprehend single words and simple sentences; *agraphia* (or dysgraphia) is used to describe an acquired deficit in the spelling or grammar of written language.

The correspondence between individual deficits of language function and lesion location does not display a rigid one-to-one relationship and should be conceptualized within the context of the distributed network model. Nonetheless, the classification of aphasic patients into specific clinical syndromes helps to determine the most likely anatomic distribution of the underlying neurologic disease and has implications for etiology and prognosis (Table 25-1). Aphasic syndromes can be divided into "central" syndromes, which result from damage to the two epicenters of the language network (Broca's and Wernicke's areas), and "disconnection" syndromes, which arise from lesions that interrupt the functional connectivity of these centers with each other and with the other components of the language network. The syndromes outlined below are idealizations; pure syndromes occur rarely.

Wernicke's aphasia   Comprehension is impaired for spoken and written language. Language output is fluent but is highly paraphasic and circumlocutious. The tendency for paraphasic errors may be so pronounced that it leads to strings of neologisms, which form the basis of what is known as "jargon aphasia." Speech contains large numbers of function words (e.g., prepositions, conjunctions) but few substantive nouns or verbs that refer to specific actions. The output is therefore voluminous but uninformative. For example, a patient attempts to describe how his wife accidentally threw away something important, perhaps his dentures: "We don't need it anymore, she says. And with it when that was downstairs was my teethtick . . . a . . . den . . . dentith . . . my dentist. And they happened to be in that bag . . . see? How could this have happened? How could a thing like this happen . . . So she says we won't need it anymore . . . I didn't think we'd use it. And now if I have any problems anybody coming a month from now, four months from now, or six months from now, I have a new dentist. Where my two . . . two little pieces of dentist that I use . . . that I . . . all gone. If she throws the whole thing away . . . visit some friends of hers and she can't throw them away."

Gestures and pantomime do not improve communication. The patient does not seem to realize that his or her language is incomprehensible and may appear angry and impatient when the examiner fails to decipher the meaning of a severely paraphasic statement. In some patients this type of aphasia can be associated with severe agitation and paranoid behaviors. One area of comprehension that may be preserved is the ability to follow commands aimed at axial musculature. The dissociation between the failure to understand simple questions ("What is your name") in a patient who rapidly closes his or her eyes, sits up, or rolls over when asked to do so is characteristic of Wernicke's aphasia and helps to differentiate it from deafness, psychiatric disease, or malingering. Patients with Wernicke's aphasia cannot express their thoughts in meaning-appropriate words and cannot decode the meaning of words in any modality of input. This aphasia therefore has expressive as well as receptive components. Repetition, naming, reading, and writing are also impaired.

The lesion site most commonly associated with Wernicke's aphasia is the posterior portion of the language network and tends to involve at least parts of Wernicke's area. An embolus to the inferior division of the middle cerebral artery, and to the posterior temporal or angular branches in particular, is the most common etiology (Chap. 361). Intracerebral hemorrhage, severe head trauma, or neoplasm are other causes. A coexisting right hemi- or superior quadrantanopia is common, and mild right nasolabial flattening may be found, but otherwise the examination is often unrevealing. The paraphasic, neologistic speech in an agitated patient with an otherwise unremarkable neurologic examination may lead to the suspicion of a primary psychiatric disorder such as schizophrenia or mania, but the other components characteristic of acquired aphasia and the absence of prior psychiatric disease usually settle the issue. Some patients with Wernicke's aphasia due to intracerebral hemorrhage or head trauma may improve as the hemorrhage or the injury heals. In most other patients, prognosis for recovery is guarded.

Broca's aphasia Speech is nonfluent, labored, interrupted by many word-finding pauses, and usually dysarthric. It is impoverished in function words but enriched in meaning-appropriate nouns and verbs. Abnormal word order and the inappropriate deployment of *bound morphemes* (word endings used to denote tenses, possessives, or plurals) lead to a characteristic agrammatism. Speech is telegraphic and pithy but quite informative. In the following passage, a patient with Broca's aphasia describes his medical history: "I see . . . the dotor, dotor sent me . . . Bosson. Go to hospital. Dotor . . . kept me beside. Two, tee days, doctor send me home."

Output may be reduced to a grunt or single word ("yes" or "no"), which is emitted with different intonations in an attempt to express approval or disapproval. In addition to fluency, naming and repetition are also impaired. Comprehension of spoken language is intact, except for syntactically difficult sentences with passive voice structure or embedded clauses. Reading comprehension is also preserved, with the occasional exception of a specific inability to read small grammatical words such as conjunctions and pronouns. The last two features indicate that Broca's aphasia is not just an "expressive" or "motor" disorder and that it may also involve a comprehension deficit for function words and syntax. Patients with Broca's aphasia can be tearful, easily frustrated, and profoundly depressed. Insight into their condition is

preserved, in contrast to Wernicke's aphasia. Even when spontaneous speech is severely dysarthric, the patient may be able to display a relatively normal articulation of words when singing. This dissociation has been used to develop specific therapeutic approaches (melodic intonation therapy) for Broca's aphasia. Additional neurologic deficits usually include right facial weakness, hemiparesis or hemiplegia, and a buccofacial apraxia characterized by an inability to carry out motor commands involving oropharyngeal and facial musculature (e.g., patients are unable to demonstrate how to blow out a match or suck through a straw). Visual fields are intact. The cause is most often infarction of Broca's area (the inferior frontal convolution; Fig. 25-1) and surrounding anterior perisylvian and insular cortex, due to occlusion of the superior division of the middle cerebral artery (Chap. 361). Mass lesions including tumor, intracerebral hemorrhage, or abscess may also be responsible. Small lesions confined to the posterior part of Broca's area may lead to a nonaphasic and often reversible deficit of speech articulation, usually accompanied by mild right facial weakness. When the cause of Broca's aphasia is stroke, recovery of language function generally peaks within 2 to 6 months, after which time further progress is limited.

Global aphasia Speech output is nonfluent, and comprehension of spoken language is severely impaired. Naming, repetition, reading, and writing are also impaired. This syndrome represents the combined dysfunction of Broca's and Wernicke's areas and usually results from strokes that involve the entire middle cerebral artery distribution in the left hemisphere. Most patients are initially mute or say a few words, such as "hi" or "yes." Related signs include right hemiplegia, hemisensory loss, and homonymous hemianopia. Occasionally, a patient with a lesion in Wernicke's area will present with a global aphasia that soon resolves into Wernicke's aphasia.

Conduction aphasia Speech output is fluent but paraphasic, comprehension of spoken language is intact, and repetition is severely impaired. Naming and writing are also impaired. Reading aloud is impaired, but reading comprehension is preserved. The lesion sites spare Broca's and Wernicke's areas but may induce a functional disconnection between the two so that neural word representations formed in Wernicke's area and adjacent regions cannot be conveyed to Broca's area for assembly into corresponding articulatory patterns. Occasionally, a Wernicke's area lesion gives rise to a transient Wernicke's aphasia that rapidly resolves into a conduction aphasia. The paraphasic output in conduction aphasia interferes with the ability to express meaning, but this deficit is not nearly as severe as the one displayed by patients with Wernicke's aphasia. Associated neurologic signs in conduction aphasia vary according to the primary lesion site.

Nonfluent transcortical aphasia (transcortical motor aphasia) The features are similar to Broca's aphasia, but repetition is intact and agrammatism may be less pronounced. The neurologic examination may be otherwise intact, but a right hemiparesis can also exist. The lesion site disconnects the intact language network from prefrontal areas of the brain and usually involves the anterior watershed zone between anterior and middle cerebral artery territories or the supplementary motor cortex in the territory of the anterior cerebral artery.

Fluent transcortical aphasia (transcortical sensory aphasia) Clinical features are similar to those of Wernicke's aphasia, but repetition is intact. The lesion site disconnects the intact core of the language network from other temporoparietal association areas. Associated neurologic findings may include hemianopia. Cerebrovascular lesions (e.g., infarctions in the posterior watershed zone) or neoplasms that involve the temporoparietal cortex posterior to Wernicke's area are the most common causes.

Isolation aphasia This rare syndrome represents a combination of the two transcortical aphasias. Comprehension is severely impaired, and there is no purposeful speech output. The patient may parrot fragments of heard conversations (*echolalia*), indicating that the neural mechanisms for repetition are at least partially intact. This condition represents the pathologic function of the language network when it is isolated from other regions of the brain. Broca's and Wernicke's areas tend to be spared, but there is damage in surrounding frontal, parietal, and temporal cortex. Lesions are patchy and can be associated with anoxia, carbon monoxide poisoning, or complete watershed zone infarctions.

Anomic aphasia This form of aphasia may be considered the "minimal dysfunction" syndrome of the language network. Articulation, comprehension, and repetition are intact, but confrontation naming, word finding, and spelling are impaired. Speech is enriched in function words but impoverished in substantive nouns and verbs denoting specific actions. Language output is fluent but paraphasic, circumlocutious, and uninformative. The lesion sites can be anywhere within the left hemisphere language network, including the middle and inferior temporal gyri. *Anomic aphasia is the single most common language disturbance seen in head trauma, metabolic encephalopathy, and Alzheimer's disease.* The language impairment of Alzheimer's disease almost always leads to fluent aphasias (e.g., anomic, Wernicke's, conduction, or fluent transcortical aphasia). The insidious onset and relentless progression of nonfluent language disturbances (Broca's or nonfluent transcortical aphasia) can be seen in *primary progressive aphasia*, a degenerative syndrome most commonly associated with focal nonspecific neuronal loss or Pick's disease.

Pure word deafness This is not a true aphasic syndrome because the language deficit is modality-specific. The most common lesions are either bilateral or left-sided in the superior temporal gyrus. The net effect of the underlying lesion is to interrupt the flow of information from the unimodal auditory association cortex to Wernicke's area. Patients have no difficulty understanding written language and can express themselves well in spoken or written language. They have no difficulty interpreting and reacting to environmental sounds since primary auditory cortex and subcortical auditory relays are intact. Since auditory information cannot be conveyed to the language network, however, it cannot be decoded into neural word representations and the patient reacts to speech as if it were in an alien tongue that cannot be deciphered. Patients cannot repeat spoken language but have no difficulty naming objects. In time, patients with pure word deafness teach themselves lip reading and may appear to have improved. There may be no additional neurologic findings, but agitated paranoid reactions are frequent in the acute stages. Cerebrovascular lesions are the most frequent cause.

Pure alexia without agraphia This is the visual equivalent of pure word deafness. The lesions (usually a combination of damage to the left occipital cortex and to a posterior sector of the corpus callosum—the splenium) interrupt the flow of visual input into the language network. There is usually a right hemianopia, but the core language network remains unaffected. The patient can understand and produce spoken language, name objects in the left visual hemifield, repeat, and write. However, the patient acts as if illiterate when asked to read even the simplest sentence because the visual information from the written words (presented to the intact left visual hemifield) cannot reach the language network. Objects in the left hemifield may be named accurately because they activate nonvisual associations in the right hemisphere, which, in turn, can access the language network through transcallosal pathways anterior to the splenium. Patients with this syndrome may also lose the ability to name colors, although they can match colors. This is known as a *color anomia*. The most common etiology of pure alexia is a vascular lesion in the territory of the posterior cerebral artery or an infiltrating neoplasm in the left occipital cortex that involves the optic radiations as well as the crossing fibers of the splenium. Since the posterior cerebral artery also supplies medial temporal components of the limbic system, the patient with pure alexia may also experience an amnesia, but this is usually transient because the limbic lesion is unilateral.

Aphemia There is an acute onset of severely impaired fluency (often mutism), which cannot be accounted by corticobulbar, cerebellar, or extrapyramidal dysfunction. Recovery is the rule and involves an intermediate stage of hoarse whispering. Writing, reading, and comprehension are intact, so this is not a true aphasic syndrome. Partial lesions of Broca's area or subcortical lesions that undercut its connections with other parts of the brain may be present. Occasionally, the

lesion site is on the medial aspects of the frontal lobes and may involve the supplementary motor cortex of the left hemisphere.

Apraxia This generic term designates a complex motor deficit that cannot be attributed to pyramidal, extrapyramidal, cerebellar, or sensory dysfunction and that does not arise from the patient's failure to understand the nature of the task. The form that is most frequently encountered in clinical practice is known as *ideomotor apraxia*. Commands to perform a specific motor act ("cough," "blow out a match") or to pantomime the use of a common tool (a comb, hammer, straw, or toothbrush) in the absence of the real object cannot be followed. The patient's ability to comprehend the command is ascertained by demonstrating multiple movements and establishing that the correct one can be recognized. Some patients with this type of apraxia can imitate the appropriate movement (when it is demonstrated by the examiner) and show no impairment when handed the real object, indicating that the sensorimotor mechanisms necessary for the movement are intact. Some forms of ideomotor apraxia represent a disconnection of the language network from pyramidal motor systems: commands to execute complex movements are understood but cannot be conveyed to the appropriate motor areas, even though the relevant motor mechanisms are intact. *Buccofacial apraxia* involves apraxic deficits in movements of the face and mouth. *Limb apraxia* encompasses apraxic deficits in movements of the arms and legs. Ideomotor apraxia is almost always caused by lesions in the left hemisphere and is commonly associated with aphasic syndromes, especially Broca's aphasia and conduction aphasia. Its presence cannot be ascertained in patients with language comprehension deficits. The ability to follow commands aimed at axial musculature ("close the eyes," "stand up") is subserved by different pathways and may be intact in otherwise severely aphasic and apraxic patients. Patients with lesions of the anterior corpus callosum can display a special type of ideomotor apraxia confined to the left side of the body. Since the handling of real objects is not impaired, ideomotor apraxia, by itself, causes no limitation of daily living activities.

Ideational apraxia refers to a deficit in the execution of a goal-directed sequence of movements in patients who have no difficulty executing the individual components of the sequence. For example, when asked to pick up a pen and write, the sequence of uncapping the pen, placing the cap at the opposite end, turning the point towards the writing surface, and writing may be disrupted, and the patient may be seen trying to write with the wrong end of the pen or even with the removed cap. These motor sequencing problems are usually seen in the context of confusional states and dementias rather than focal lesions associated with aphasic conditions. *Limb-kinetic apraxia* involves a clumsiness in the actual use of tools that cannot be attributed to sensory, pyramidal, extrapyramidal, or cerebellar dysfunction. This condition can emerge in the context of focal premotor cortex lesions or *corticobasal ganglionic degeneration*.

Gerstmann's syndrome The combination of *acalculia* (impairment of simple arithmetic), *dysgraphia* (impaired writing), *finger anomia* (an inability to name individual fingers such as the index or thumb), and *right-left confusion* (an inability to tell whether a hand, foot, or arm of the patient or examiner is on the right or left side of the body) is known as Gerstmann's syndrome. In making this diagnosis it is important to establish that the finger and left-right naming deficits are not part of a more generalized anomia and that the patient is not otherwise aphasic. When Gerstmann's syndrome is seen in isolation, it is commonly associated with damage to the inferior parietal lobule (especially the angular gyrus) in the left hemisphere.

Aprosodia Variations of melodic stress and intonation influence the meaning and impact of spoken language. For example, the two statements "He *is* clever." and "He is clever?" contain an identical word choice and syntax but convey vastly different messages because of differences in the intonation and stress with which the statements are uttered. This aspect of language is known as *prosody*. Damage to perisylvian areas in the right hemisphere can interfere with speech prosody and can lead to syndromes of aprosodia. Ross has pointed out that damage to right hemisphere regions corresponding to Wernicke's area yields a greater impairment in the decoding of speech prosody, whereas damage to right hemisphere regions corresponding to Broca's area yields a greater impairment in the ability to introduce meaning-appropriate prosody into spoken language. The latter deficit is the most common type of aprosodia identified in clinical practice—the patient produces grammatically correct language with accurate word choice but the statements are uttered in a monotone that interferes with the ability to convey the intended stress and affect. Patients with this type of aprosodia give the mistaken impression of being depressed or indifferent.

Subcortical aphasias   Damage to subcortical components of the language network (e.g., the striatum and thalamus of the left hemisphere) can also lead to aphasia. The resulting syndromes contain combinations of deficits in the various aspects of language but rarely fit the specific patterns described in Table 25-1. An anomic aphasia accompanied by dysarthria or a fluent aphasia with hemiparesis should raise the suspicion of a subcortical lesion site.

THE PARIETOFRONTAL NETWORK FOR SPATIAL ORIENTATION: NEGLECT AND RELATED CONDITIONS

Hemispatial Neglect   Adaptive orientation to significant events within the extrapersonal space is subserved by a large-scale network containing three major cortical components. The *cingulate cortex* provides access to a limbic-motivational mapping of the extrapersonal space, the *posterior parietal cortex* to a sensorimotor representation of salient extrapersonal events, and the *frontal eye fields* to motor strategies for attentional behaviors (Fig. 25-2). Subcortical components of this network include the striatum and the thalamus. Contralesional hemispatial neglect represents one outcome of damage to any of the cortical or subcortical components of this network. *The traditional view that hemispatial neglect always denotes a parietal lobe lesion is inaccurate.* In keeping with this anatomic organization, the clinical manifestations of neglect display three behavioral components: sensory events (or their mental representations) within the neglected hemispace have a lesser impact on overall awareness; there is a paucity of exploratory and orienting acts directed toward the neglected hemispace; and the patient behaves as if the neglected hemispace was motivationally devalued.

According to one model of spatial cognition, the right hemisphere directs attention within the *entire* extrapersonal space, whereas the left hemisphere directs attention mostly within the contralateral right hemispace. Consequently, unilateral left hemisphere lesions do not give rise to much contralesional neglect since the ipsilateral attentional mechanisms of the right hemisphere can compensate for the loss of the *contralaterally* directed attentional functions of the left hemisphere. Unilateral right hemisphere lesions, however, give rise to severe contralesional left hemispatial neglect because the unaffected left hemisphere does not contain ipsilateral attentional mechanisms. This model is consistent with clinical experience, which shows that contralesional neglect is more common, severe, and lasting after damage to the right hemisphere than after damage to the left hemisphere. Severe neglect for the right hemispace is rare, even in left handers with left hemisphere lesions.

Patients with severe neglect may fail to dress, shave, or groom the left side of the body; may fail to eat food placed on the left side of the tray; and may fail to read the left half of sentences. When the examiner draws a large circle [12 to 16 cm (5 to 6 in.) in diameter] and asks the patient to place the numbers 1 to 12 as if the circle represented the face of a clock, there is a tendency to crowd the numbers on the right side and leave the left side empty. When asked to copy a simple line drawing, the patient fails to copy detail on the left; and when asked to write, there is a tendency to leave an unusually wide margin on the left.

Two bedside tests that are useful in assessing neglect are *simultaneous bilateral stimulation* and *visual target cancellation*. In the former, the examiner provides either unilateral or simultaneous bilat-

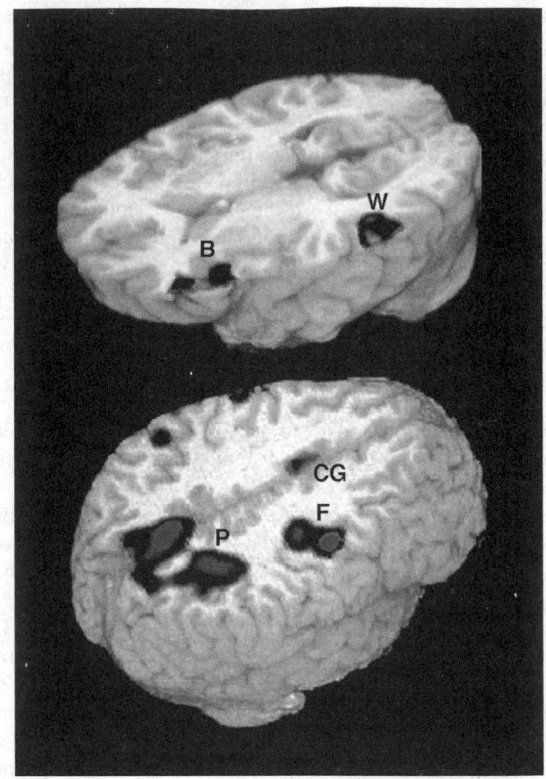

FIGURE 25-2   Functional magnetic resonance imaging of language and spatial attention in neurologically intact subjects. The dark areas show regions of task-related significant activation. (*Top*) The subjects were asked to determine if two words were synonymous. This language task led to the simultaneous activation of the two epicenters of the language network, Broca's area (B) and Wernicke's area (W). The activations are exclusively in the left hemisphere. (*Bottom*) The subjects were asked to shift spatial attention to a peripheral target. This task led to the simultaneous activation of the three epicenters of the attentional network, the posterior parietal cortex (P), the frontal eye fields (F), and the cingulate gyrus (CG). The activations are predominantly in the right hemisphere. (*Figure courtesy of Darren Gitelman, MD.*)

eral stimulation in the visual, auditory, and tactile modalities. Following right hemisphere injury, patients who have no difficulty detecting unilateral stimuli on either side experience the bilaterally presented stimulus as coming only from the right. This phenomenon is known as *extinction* and is a manifestation of the sensory-representational aspect of hemispatial neglect. In the target detection task, targets (e.g., A's) are interspersed with foils (e.g., other letters of the alphabet) on a 21.5 × 28.0 cm (8.5 × 11 in.) sheet of paper and the patient is asked to circle all the targets. A failure to detect targets on the left is a manifestation of the exploratory deficit in hemispatial neglect. Hemianopia, by itself, does not interfere with performance in this task since the patient is free to turn the head and eyes to the left. The normal tendency in target detection tasks is to start from the left upper quadrant and move systematically in horizontal or vertical sweeps. Some patients show a tendency to start the process from the right and proceed in a haphazard fashion. This represents a subtle manifestation of left neglect, even if the patient eventually manages to detect all the appropriate targets. Some patients with neglect may also deny the existence of hemiparesis and may even deny ownership of the paralyzed limb, a condition known as *anosognosia*.

Cerebrovascular lesions and neoplasms in the right hemisphere are the most common causes of hemispatial neglect. Depending on the site of the lesion, the patient with neglect may also have hemiparesis, hemihypesthesia, and hemianopia on the left, but these are not invariant findings. The majority of patients display considerable improvement of hemispatial neglect, usually within the first several weeks.

Bálint's Syndrome, Simultanagnosia, Dressing Apraxia, and Construction Apraxia   Bilateral involvement of the network for spatial attention, especially its parietal components, leads to a state of severe spatial disorientation known as *Bálint's syndrome*. Bálint's syndrome involves deficits in the orderly visuomotor scanning of the environment (*oculomotor apraxia*) and in accurate manual reaching toward visual targets (*optic ataxia*). The third and most dramatic component of Bálint's syndrome is known as *simultanagnosia* and reflects an inability to integrate visual information in the center of gaze with more peripheral information. The patient gets stuck on the detail that falls in the center of gaze without attempting to scan the visual environment for additional information. The patient with simultanagnosia "misses the forest for the trees." Complex visual scenes cannot be grasped in their entirety, leading to severe limitations in the visual identification of objects and scenes. For example, a patient who is shown a table lamp and asked to name the object may look at its circular base and call it an ash tray. Some patients with simultanagnosia report that objects they look at may suddenly vanish, probably indicating an inability to look back at the original point of gaze after brief saccadic displacements. Movement and distracting stimuli greatly exacerbate the difficulties of visual perception. Simultanagnosia can sometimes occur without the other two components of Bálint's syndrome.

A modification of the letter cancellation task described above can be used for the bedside diagnosis of simultanagnosia. In this modification, some of the targets (e.g., A's) are made to be much larger than the others [7.5 to 10 cm vs. 2.5 cm (3 to 4 in. vs. 1 in.) in height], and all targets are embedded among foils. Patients with simultanagnosia display a counterintuitive but characteristic tendency to miss the larger targets (Fig. 25-3). This occurs because the information needed for the identification of the larger targets cannot be confined to the immediate line of gaze and requires the integration of visual information across a more extensive field of view. The greater difficulty in the detection of the larger targets also indicates that poor acuity is not responsible for the impairment of visual function and that the problem is central rather than peripheral. Bálint's syndrome results from bilateral dorsal parietal lesions; common settings include watershed infarction between the middle and posterior cerebral artery territories, hypoglycemia, sagittal sinus thrombosis, or atypical forms of Alzheimer's disease. In patients with Bálint's syndrome due to stroke, bilateral visual field defects (usually inferior quadrantanopias) are common.

Another manifestation of bilateral (or right sided) dorsal parietal lobe lesions is *dressing apraxia*. The patient with this condition is unable to align the body axis with the axis of the garment and can be seen struggling as he or she holds a coat from its bottom or extends his or her arm into a fold of the garment rather than into its sleeve. Lesions that involve the posterior parietal cortex also lead to severe

difficulties in copying simple line drawings. This is known as a *construction apraxia* and is much more severe if the lesion is in the right hemisphere. In some patients with right hemisphere lesions, the drawing difficulties are confined to the left side of the figure and represent a manifestation of hemispatial neglect; in others, there is a more universal deficit in reproducing contours and three-dimensional perspective. Dressing apraxia and construction apraxia represent special instances of a more general disturbance in spatial orientation.

THE OCCIPITOTEMPORAL NETWORK FOR FACE AND OBJECT RECOGNITION: PROSOPAGNOSIA AND OBJECT AGNOSIA   Perceptual information about faces and objects is initially encoded in primary (striate) visual cortex and adjacent (upstream) peristriate visual association areas. This information is subsequently relayed first to the downstream visual association areas of occipitotemporal cortex and then to other heteromodal and paralimbic areas of the cerebral cortex. Bilateral lesions in the fusiform and lingual gyri of occipitotemporal cortex disrupt this process and interfere with the ability of otherwise-intact perceptual information to activate the distributed multimodal associations that lead to the recognition of faces and objects. The resultant face and object recognition deficits are known as *prosopagnosia* and *visual object agnosia*.

The patient with prosopagnosia cannot recognize familiar faces, including, sometimes, the reflection of his or her own face in the mirror. This is not a perceptual deficit since prosopagnosic patients can easily tell if two faces are identical or not. Furthermore, a prosopagnosic patient who cannot recognize a familiar face by visual inspection alone can use auditory cues to reach appropriate recognition if allowed to listen to the person's voice. The deficit in prosopagnosia is therefore modality-specific and reflects the existence of a lesion that prevents the activation of otherwise intact multimodal templates by relevant visual input. Damasio has pointed out that the deficit in prosopagnosia is not limited to the recognition of faces but that it can also extend to the recognition of individual members of larger generic object groups. For example, prosopagnosic patients characteristically have no difficulty with the generic identification of a face as a face or of a car as a car, but they cannot recognize the identity of an individual face or the make of an individual car. This reflects a visual recognition deficit for proprietary features that characterize individual members of an object class. When recognition problems become more generalized and extend to the generic identification of common objects, the condition is known as visual object agnosia. In contrast to prosopagnosic patients, those with object agnosia cannot recognize a face as a face or a car as a car. It is important to distinguish visual object agnosia from anomia. The patient with anomia cannot name the object but can describe its use. In contrast, the patient with visual agnosia is unable either to name a visually presented object or to describe its use. The characteristic lesions in prosopagnosia and visual object agnosia consist of bilateral infarctions in the territory of the posterior cerebral arteries. Associated deficits can include visual field defects (especially superior quadrantanopias) or a centrally based color blindness known as achromatopsia. Rarely, the responsible lesion is unilateral. In such cases, prosopagnosia is associated with lesions in the right hemisphere and object agnosia with lesions in the left.

THE LIMBIC NETWORK FOR MEMORY: AMNESIAS   Limbic and paralimbic areas (such as the hippocampus, amygdala, and entorhinal cortex), the anterior and medial nuclei of the thalamus, the medial and basal parts of the striatum, and the hypothalamus collectively constitute a distributed network known as the *limbic system*. The behavioral affiliations of this network include the coordination of emotion, motivation, autonomic tone, and endocrine function. An additional area of specialization for the limbic network, and the one which is of most relevance to clinical practice, is that of declarative (conscious) memory for recent episodes and experiences. A disturbance in this function is known as *amnestic state*. In the absence of deficits in motivation, attention, language, or visuospatial function, the clinical diagnosis of a persistent global amnestic state is always as-

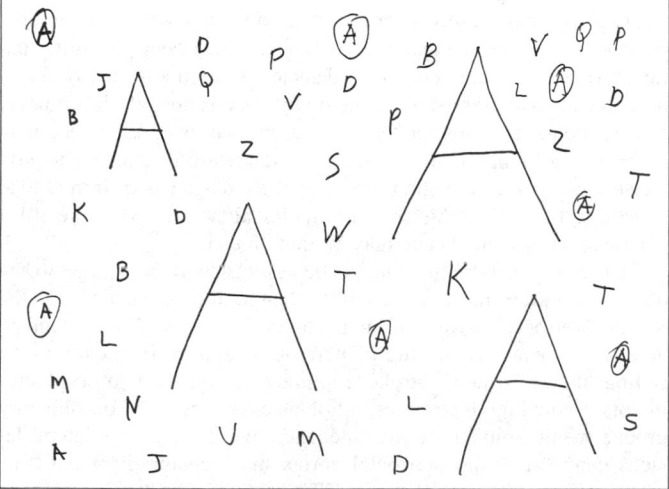

FIGURE 25-3   A 70-year-old woman with a 2-year history of degenerative dementia was asked to circle all the A's. She detects most of the small targets but ignores the larger ones. This is a manifestation of simultanagnosia.

sociated with bilateral damage to the limbic network, usually within the hippocampo-entorhinal complex or the thalamus.

The memory disturbance in the amnestic state is multimodal and includes retrograde and anterograde components. The *retrograde amnesia* involves an inability to recall experiences that occurred before the onset of the amnestic state. Relatively recent events are more vulnerable to retrograde amnesia than more remote events. A patient who comes to the emergency room complaining that he cannot remember his identity but who can remember the events of the previous day is almost certainly not suffering from a neurologic cause of memory disturbance. The second and most important component of the amnestic state is the *anterograde amnesia*, which indicates an inability to store, retain, and recall new knowledge. Patients with amnestic states cannot remember what they ate a few minutes ago or the details of an important event they may have experienced a few hours ago. In the acute stages, there may also be a tendency to fill in memory gaps with inaccurate, fabricated, and often implausible information. This is known as *confabulation*. Patients with the amnestic syndrome forget that they forget and tend to deny the existence of a memory problem when questioned.

The patient with an amnestic state is almost always disoriented, especially to time. Accurate temporal orientation and accurate knowledge of current news rule out a major amnestic state. Memory can be tested with a list of four to five words read aloud by the examiner up to five times or until the patient can immediately repeat the entire list without intervening delay. In the next phase of testing, the patient is allowed to concentrate on the words and to rehearse them internally for 1 min before being asked to recall them. Accurate performance in this phase indicates that the patient is motivated and sufficiently attentive to hold the words on-line for at least 1 min. The final phase of the testing involves a retention period of 5 to 10 min, during which the patient is engaged in other tasks. Adequate recall at the end of this interval requires off-line storage, retention, and retrieval. Amnestic patients fail this phase of the task and may even forget that they were given a list of words to remember. Accurate recognition of the words by multiple choice in a patient who cannot recall them indicates a less severe memory disturbance that affects mostly the retrieval stage of memory.

Many neurologic diseases can give rise to an amnestic state. These include tumors (of the sphenoid wing, posterior corpus callosum, thalamus, or medial temporal lobe), infarctions (in the territories of the anterior or posterior cerebral arteries), head trauma, herpes simplex encephalitis, Wernicke-Korsakoff encephalopathy, paraneoplastic limbic encephalitis, and degenerative dementias such as Alzheimer's or Pick's disease. The one common denominator of all these diseases is that they lead to the bilateral lesions within one or more components in the limbic network, most commonly the hippocampus, entorhinal cortex, the mammillary bodies of the hypothalamus, and the limbic thalamus. Occasionally, unilateral left-sided lesions can give rise to an amnestic state, but the memory disorder tends to be transient. Depending on the nature and distribution of the underlying neurologic disease, the patient may also have visual field deficits, eye movement limitations, or cerebellar findings. In many patients, such as those with *transient global amnesia* (Chap. 26), there are no associated neurologic findings; this sometimes leads incorrectly to the diagnosis of a psychiatric disorder.

Although the limbic network is the site of damage for amnestic states, it is almost certainly not the storage site for memories. Memories are stored in widely distributed form throughout the association cortex. The role attributed to the limbic network is to bind these distributed fragments into coherent events and experiences that can sustain conscious recall. Damage to the limbic network does not necessarily destroy memories but interferes with their conscious (declarative) recall in coherent form. The individual fragments of information remain preserved despite the limbic lesions and can sustain what is known as *implicit memory*. For example, patients with amnestic states can acquire new motor or perceptual skills, even though they may have no conscious knowledge of the experiences that led to the acquisition of these skills.

THE PREFRONTAL NETWORK FOR ATTENTION AND COMPORTMENT

Approximately one-third of all the cerebral cortex in the human brain is located in the frontal lobes. The frontal lobes can be subdivided into motor-premotor, dorsolateral prefrontal, medial prefrontal, and orbitofrontal components. The terms *frontal lobe syndrome* and *prefrontal cortex* refer only to the last three of these four components. These are the parts of the cerebral cortex that show the greatest phylogenetic expansion in primates and especially in humans. The dorsolateral prefrontal, medial prefrontal, and orbitofrontal areas, and the subcortical structures with which they are interconnected (i.e., the head of the caudate and the dorsomedial nucleus of the thalamus), collectively make up a large-scale network that coordinates exceedingly complex aspects of human cognition and comportment.

The prefrontal network plays an important role in behaviors that require an integration of thought with emotion and motivation. There is no simple formula for summarizing the diverse functional affiliations of the prefrontal network. Its integrity appears important for the simultaneous awareness of context, options, consequences, relevance, and emotional impact so as to allow the formulation of adaptive inferences, decisions, and actions. Damage to this part of the brain impairs mental flexibility, reasoning, hypothesis formation, abstract thinking, foresight, judgment, the on-line (attentive) holding of information, and the ability to inhibit inappropriate responses. Behaviors impaired by prefrontal cortex lesions, especially those related to the manipulation of mental content, are often referred to as "executive functions."

Even very large bilateral prefrontal lesions may leave all sensory, motor, and basic cognitive functions intact while leading to isolated but dramatic alterations of personality and comportment. The most common clinical manifestations of damage to the prefrontal network take the form of two relatively distinct syndromes. In the *frontal abulic syndrome*, the patient shows a loss of initiative, creativity, and curiosity and displays a pervasive emotional blandness and apathy. In the *frontal disinhibition syndrome*, the patient becomes socially disinhibited and shows severe impairments of judgment, insight, and foresight. The dissociation between intact intellectual function and a total lack of even rudimentary common sense is striking. Despite the preservation of all essential memory functions, the patient cannot learn from experience and continues to display inappropriate behaviors without appearing to feel emotional pain, guilt, or regret when such behaviors repeatedly lead to disastrous consequences. The impairments may emerge only in real-life situations when behavior is under minimal external control and may not be apparent within the structured environment of the medical office. Testing judgment by asking patients what they would do if they detected a fire in a theater or found a stamped and addressed envelope on the road is not very informative since patients who answer these questions wisely in the office may still act very foolishly in the more complex real-life setting. The physician must therefore be prepared to make a diagnosis of frontal lobe disease on the basis of historic information alone even when the office examination of mental state may be quite intact.

The abulic syndrome tends to be associated with damage to the dorsolateral prefrontal cortex, and the disinhibition syndrome with the medial prefrontal or orbitofrontal cortex. These syndromes tend to arise almost exclusively after bilateral lesions, most frequently in the setting of head trauma, stroke, ruptured aneurysms, hydrocephalus, tumors (including metastases, glioblastoma, and falx or olfactory groove meningiomas), or focal degenerative diseases. Unilateral lesions confined to the prefrontal cortex may remain silent until the pathology spreads to the other side. The emergence of developmentally primitive reflexes such as grasping, rooting, and sucking are seen primarily in patients with large structural lesions that extend into the premotor components of the frontal lobes or in the context of metabolic encephalopathies. The vast majority of patients with prefrontal lesions and frontal lobe behavioral syndromes do not display these reflexes.

Damage to the frontal lobe disrupts a variety of attention-related functions including working memory (the transient on-line holding of information), concentration span, verbal fluency, the scanning and retrieval of stored information, the inhibition of immediate but inappropriate responses, and mental flexibility. The capacity for focusing on a trend of thought and the ability to voluntarily shift the focus of attention from one thought or stimulus to another can become impaired. Digit span (which should be seven forward and five reverse) is decreased; the recitation of the months of the year in reverse order (which should take less than 15 s) is slowed; and the number of words starting with a, f, or s that can be generated in 1 min (normally 12 or more per letter) is diminished even in nonaphasic patients. Characteristically, there is a progressive slowing of performance as the task proceeds; e.g., the patient asked to count backwards by 3s may say "100, 97, 94 . . . 91, . . . 88," etc., and may not complete the task. In go–no go tasks (where the instruction is to raise the finger upon hearing one tap but to keep it still upon hearing two taps), the patient shows a characteristic inability to keep still in response to the "no go" stimulus; mental flexibility (tested by the ability to shift from one criterion to another in sorting or matching tasks) is impoverished; distractibility by irrelevant stimuli is increased; and there is a pronounced tendency for impersistence and perseveration.

These attentional deficits disrupt the orderly registration and retrieval of new information and lead to *secondary* memory deficits. Such memory deficits can be differentiated from the *primary* memory impairments of the amnestic state by showing that they improve when the attentional load of the task is decreased. Working memory (also known as immediate memory) is an attentional function based on the temporary on-line holding of information. It is closely associated with the integrity of the prefrontal network and the ascending reticular activating system. Retentive memory, on the other hand, depends on the stable (off-line) storage of information and is associated with the integrity of the limbic network. The distinction of the underlying neural mechanisms is illustrated by the observation that severely amnestic patients who cannot remember events that occurred a few minutes ago may have intact if not superior working memory capacity as shown in tests of digit span.

Lesions in the caudate nucleus or in the dorsomedial nucleus of the thalamus (subcortical components of the prefrontal network) can also produce a frontal lobe syndrome. This is one reason why the mental state changes associated with degenerative basal ganglia diseases, such as Parkinson's or Huntington's disease, may take the form of a frontal lobe syndrome. Because of its widespread connections with other regions of association cortex, one essential computational role of the prefrontal network is to function as an integrator, or "orchestrator," for other networks. Bilateral multifocal lesions of the cerebral hemispheres, none of which are individually large enough to cause specific cognitive deficits such as aphasia or neglect, can collectively interfere with the connectivity and integrating function of prefrontal cortex. A frontal lobe syndrome is the single most common behavioral profile associated with a variety of bilateral multifocal brain diseases including metabolic encephalopathy, multiple sclerosis, vitamin B_{12} deficiency, and others. In fact, the vast majority of patients with the clinical diagnosis of a frontal lobe syndrome tend to have lesions that do not involve prefrontal cortex but involve either the subcortical components of the prefrontal network or its connections with other parts of the brain. In order to avoid making a diagnosis of "frontal lobe syndrome" in a patient with no evidence of frontal cortex disease, it is advisable to use the diagnostic term *frontal network syndrome*, with the understanding that the responsible lesions can lie anywhere within this distributed network.

The patient with frontal lobe disease raises potential dilemmas in differential diagnosis: the abulia and blandness may be misinterpreted as depression, and the disinhibition as mania or acting-out. Appropri-ate intervention may be delayed while a treatable tumor keeps expanding. An informed approach to frontal lobe disease and its comportmental manifestations may help to avoid such errors.

CARING FOR THE PATIENT WITH DEFICITS OF HIGHER CEREBRAL FUNCTION Some of the deficits described in this chapter are so complex that they may bewilder not only the patient and family but also the physician. It is imperative to carry out a systematic clinical evaluation in order to characterize the nature of the deficits and explain them in lay terms to the patient and family. Such an explanation can allay at least some of the anxieties, address the mistaken impression that the deficit (e.g., social disinhibition or inability to recognize family members) is psychologically motivated, and lead to practical suggestions for daily living activities. The consultation of a skilled neuropsychologist may aid in the formulation of diagnosis and management. Patients with simultanagnosia, for example, may benefit from the counterintuitive instruction to stand back when they cannot find an item so that a greater search area falls within the immediate field of gaze. In some patients, the history may be more important than the bedside examination. For example, patients with frontal lobe disease can be extremely irritable and abusive to spouses and yet display all the appropriate social graces during the visit to the medical office.

Reactive depression is common in patients with higher cerebral dysfunction and should be treated. These patients may be sensitive to the usual doses of antidepressants or anxiolytics and deserve a careful titration of dosage. Brain damage may cause a dissociation between feeling states and their expression, so that a patient who may superficially appear jocular could still be suffering from an underlying depression that deserves to be treated. In many cases, agitation may be controlled with reassurance. In other cases, treatment with benzodiazepines or sedating antidepressants may become necessary. The use of neuroleptics for the control of agitation should be reserved for refractory cases since extrapyramidal side effects are frequent in patients with coexisting brain damage.

Spontaneous improvement of cognitive deficits due to acute neurologic lesions is common. It is most rapid in the first few weeks but may continue for up to 2 years, especially in young individuals with single brain lesions. The mechanisms for this recovery are incompletely understood. Some of the initial deficits appear to arise from remote dysfunction (diaschisis) in parts of the brain that are interconnected with the site of initial injury. Improvement in these patients may reflect, at least in part, a normalization of the remote dysfunction. Other mechanisms may involve functional reorganization in surviving neurons adjacent to the injury or the compensatory use of homologous structures, e.g., the right superior temporal gyrus with recovery from Wernicke's aphasia. In some patients with large lesions involving Broca's and Wernicke's areas, only Wernicke's area may show contralateral compensatory reorganization (or bilateral functionality), giving rise to a situation where a lesion that should have caused a global aphasia becomes associated with a residual Broca aphasia. Prognosis for recovery from aphasia is best when Wernicke's area is spared. Cognitive rehabilitation procedures have been used in the treatment of higher cortical deficits. There are few controlled studies, but some do show a benefit of rehabilitation in the recovery from hemispatial neglect and aphasia. Some types of deficits may be more prone to recovery than others. For example, patients with nonfluent aphasias are more likely to benefit from speech therapy than patients with fluent aphasias and comprehension deficits. In general, lesions that lead to a denial of illness (e.g., anosognosia) are associated with cognitive deficits that are more resistant to rehabilitation. The recovery of higher cortical dysfunction is rarely complete. Periodic neuropsychological assessment is necessary for quantifying the pace of the improvement and for generating specific recommendations for cognitive rehabilitation, modifications in the home environment, and the timetable for returning to school or work.

BIBLIOGRAPHY

DAMASIO AR, DAMASIO H: Aphasia and the neural basis of language, in *Principles of Behavioral and Cognitive Neurology*, 2d ed. M-M Mesulam (ed). New York, Oxford University Press, 2000, pp 294–315

GITELMAN DR et al: A large-scale distributed network for covert spatial attention. Further anatomical delineation based on stringent behavioral and cognitive controls. Brain 122:1093, 1999

HEISS W-D et al: Differential capacity of left and right hemispheric areas for compensation of poststroke aphasia. Ann Neurol 45:430, 1999

LEIGUARDA RC, MARSDEN CD: Limb apraxias. Higher-order disorders of sensorimotor integration. Brain 123:860, 2000

MESULAM M-M: Behavioral neuroanatomy: Large-scale networks, association cortex, frontal syndromes, the limbic system and hemispheric specializations, in *Principles of Behavioral and Cognitive Neurology*, 2d ed, M-M Mesulam (ed). New York, Oxford University Press, 2000, pp 1–120

————: From sensation to cognition. Brain 121:1031, 1998

26	*Thomas D. Bird*

MEMORY LOSS AND DEMENTIA

AD Alzheimer's disease	EEG electroencephalogram
CADASIL cerebral autosomal dominant arteriopathy with subcortical infarcts and leukoencephalopathy	FTD Frontotemporal dementia
	HD Huntington's disease
	LTP Long-term potentiation
CJD Creutzfeldt-Jakob disease	MMSE mini-mental status exam
CNS central nervous system	MRI magnetic resonance imaging
CREB cyclic AMP-responsive element binding protein	PD Parkinson's disease
	SPECT single photon emission computed tomography
CSF cerebrospinal fluid	
CT Computed tomography	TGA Transient global amnesia
EDTA ethylene diaminetetraacetic acid	VDRL Venereal Disease Research Laboratory

DEFINITION Dementia is a serious and common problem that affects more than 4 million Americans and costs society more than $50 billion annually. Ten percent of persons over age 70 and 20 to 40% of individuals over age 85 have clinically identifiable memory loss. Dementia is a syndrome with many causes. A simple definition of dementia is a deterioration in cognitive abilities that impairs the previously successful performance of activities of daily living. Memory is the most common and most important cognitive ability that is lost. Other mental faculties may also be affected such as attention, judgment, comprehension, orientation, learning, calculation, problem solving, mood, and behavior. Agitation or withdrawal, hallucinations, delusions, insomnia, and loss of inhibitions are also common. Individuals with mental retardation and psychosis may become demented if a decline in intellectual function occurs. Many common forms of dementia are progressive, but some dementing illnesses are static and unchanging. Dementia is a chronic condition, whereas delirium is an acute confusional state associated with a change in level of consciousness (ranging from lethargy to agitation).

Memory is a complex function of the brain that has fascinated philosophers and scientists for centuries. Memory is currently viewed as a mental process that uses several storage buffers of differing capacity and duration (Table 26-1). Sensory memory lasts for about 250 ms in the visual mode (iconic memory) and 1 to 2 s in the auditory mode (echoic memory). Immediate (short-term or primary) memory has a duration of about half a minute and a limited capacity of approximately 5 to 10 items. Immediate memory is highly vulnerable to distraction, requiring attention and vigilance to maintain the content. It is often tested at the bedside by asking the patient to recall several digits forward and backward. Recent, or secondary, memory has been called both "short-term" and "long-term." It has a duration of minutes to weeks and exhibits a larger storage capacity than immediate memory. On entering this buffer, information undergoes a process of consolidation of variable duration. Recent memory is commonly tested in the clinical setting by asking a patient to recall three words after 3 to 5 min. Remote, or long-term, memory stores information lasting weeks to a lifetime and contains most of our personal experiences and knowledge. Some information appears to be stored accurately for an indefinite time, whereas other items fade or become distorted. Memory function includes registration (encoding or acquisition), retention (storage or consolidation), stabilization, and retrieval (decoding or recall). Registration and retrieval are conscious processes. Animal experiments have shown that long-term memory requires new protein synthesis, and the stabilization process probably involves physical changes at neuronal synapses.

Several additional classifications of memory are sometimes used by psychologists, particularly in reference to the content or use of the memory stores. Reference memory refers to a filing system that contains recent and remote information gained from previous experience. Working memory refers to an active process that is being updated continually by current experience. Episodic memory contains information about events occurring in a specific place and time. Semantic memory contains unchanging facts, principles, associations, and rules (for example, state capitals and the number of days in a week). Declarative (explicit) memory refers to facts about the world and past personal events that must be consciously retrieved to be remembered. Procedural (implicit) memory, in contrast, is involved in learning and retaining a skill or procedure such as how to ride a bicycle, get dressed, or drive a car. Abilities stored in procedural memory become automatic and do not require conscious implementation.

Finally, the term *executive function* refers to mental activity involved in planning, initiating, and regulating behavior. It is considered the central organizing function of the brain that results in systematic, goal-directed activity. Executive functions are active in nonroutine situations where reflex or automatic behavior is not adequate. The anatomic and physiologic substrates of executive function are presumed to involve the frontal lobes (Chap. 25). Deficits in executive function occur frequently in patients with dementia.

FUNCTIONAL ANATOMY AND PATHOGENESIS Dementia results from disorders of cerebral neuronal circuits and is a result of the total quantity of neuronal loss combined with the specific location of such loss (Chap. 25). The anatomic basis of memory was initially clarified from study of the alcohol/thiamine deficiency syndrome of Korsakoff and the consequences of temporal lobe surgery performed for the treatment of epilepsy. In Korsakoff's syndrome lesions in the hypothalamus, mammillary bodies, and dorsomedial nuclei of the thalamus showed that these areas were important for learning, recall, and recognition. Unilateral temporal lobe surgery for epilepsy produced mild to moderate amnesia for either verbal or nonverbal material. Bilateral medial temporal lobe excision involving the hippocampal formation, the parahippocampal gyrus, and part of the amygdala produced a severe anterograde learning disorder, i.e., an inability to store new memories, often with retained ability to recall old ones. The components of the medial temporal lobe memory system include the hippocampus and adjacent cortex, including the entorhinal, perirhinal, and parahippocampal regions (Fig. 26-1). This includes a circular pathway of neurons from the entorhinal cortex to the dentate gyrus, CA3 and CA1 neurons of the hippocampus to the subiculum, and back to the entorhinal cortex; this pathway is heavily damaged in Alzheimer's disease (AD). This system is fast, has limited capacity, and performs a crucial function at the time of learning and establishing declarative memory. Its role continues after learning during a lengthy period of reorganization and consolidation whereby memory stored in neocortex eventually becomes independent of the medial temporal lobe memory system. This process, by which the burden of long-term (permanent) memory storage is gradually assumed by neocortex, assures that the medial temporal lobe system is always available for the acquisition of new information. Recent functional brain imaging studies indicate that learning and memory involve many of the same regions of the cortex that process sensory information and control motor output. The forms of perceptual and motor learning that can occur without conscious recollections are mediated in part by contractions and expansions of representations in the sensory and motor cortex. One study, for example, has shown that the cortical representation of the fingers of the left hand of musical string players is larger than that in control individuals, suggesting that the representation of different parts of the body in the primary somatosensory cortex of humans depends on use and changes to conform to the current needs and experiences of the individual. Discrete cortical regions exist in

Table 26-1 Classification of Memory

Type	Time Interval	Test/Example	Probable Cerebral Location
Sensory			
Iconic (visual)	<1 s	After image	Visual cortex
Echoic (auditory)	1–2 s	Cough/dog bark	Auditory cortex
Immediate (primary/working)	30 s	Digit span	Perisylvian cortex, frontal lobe
Recent (secondary/reference)	Minutes–weeks/months	Recall 3 words after 3–5 min	Hippocampus, mamillothalamic tract, dorsomedial thalamus
Declarative (explicit)			
Episodic		Recall trip last week	Limbic system and association cortex
Semantic		Recall names of months	
Procedural (implicit)		Ride a bike	Amygdala, cerebellum, association cortex, frontal lobe, ? other
		Get dressed	
Remote (reference)	Months–years	Recall high school graduation	Association cortex, ? other

SOURCE: Modified from K Erickson: West J Med 152:159, 1990.

which object knowledge (such as words related to color, animals, tools, or action) is organized as a distributed system in which the attributes of an object are stored close to the regions of the cortex that mediate perception of those attributes (Chap. 25). That is, brain regions active during object identification are partly dependent on the intrinsic properties of the object. Procedural (implicit) memory appears to involve centers outside the hippocampus such as amygdala, cerebellum, and sensory cortex. Different frontal regions are activated for different kinds of memory storage. Functional magnetic resonance imaging (MRI) studies show that the magnitude of focal activation in left prefrontal-temporal regions or right prefrontal-bilateral parahippocampal regions predicts how well verbal or visual stimuli, respectively, will be remembered.

Biochemically, the cholinergic system plays an important role in memory. Anticholinergic agents such as atropine and scopolamine interfere with memory. Choline acetyl transferase (the enzyme catalyzing the formation of acetylcholine) and nicotinic cholinergic receptors are known to be deficient in the cortex of patients with AD. The brains of patients with AD show severe neuronal loss in the nucleus basalis of Meynert, a major source of cholinergic input to the cerebral cortex. These findings form the basis for the use of cholinesterase inhibitors in the treatment of AD, with benefit presumably arising from increased available levels of acetylcholine. Behavior and mood are modulated by noradrenergic, serotonergic, and dopaminergic pathways; and norepinephrine has been shown to be reduced in the brainstem locus coeruleus in patients with AD. Neurotrophins are also postulated to play a role in memory in part by preserving cholinergic neurons.

Long-term potentiation (LTP), which refers to a long-lasting enhancement of synaptic transmission resulting from repetitive stimulation of excitatory synapses, is presumed to be involved in memory acquisition and storage. LTP occurs in the hippocampus and is mediated by N-methyl-D-aspartate (NMDA) receptors as well as cyclic AMP-responsive element

binding protein (CREB). Gene knockout mouse models have been useful in the definition of secondary messenger systems that play a role in hippocampal LTP. For example, disruption of either calcium/calmodulin-dependent protein kinase or cytoplasmic tyrosine kinase (fyn) results in deficient hippocampal LTP and impaired spatial learning. In contrast, mice in which a neuronal glycoprotein thy-1 has been inactivated show regionally selective impairment of LTP but intact spatial learning, suggesting that LTP in the entorhinal projection to the dentate gyrus of the hippocampus (Fig. 26-1) may not be necessary for some forms of spatial learning. Disruption of hippocampal levels of CREB impairs long-term memory in rats.

Most diseases causing dementia do not have highly restricted regions of pathology. Disorders such as AD appear to eventually rep-

FIGURE 26-1 The principal connections of the hippocampus. Afferent connections (*blue arrows*) from the cingulate gyrus (cortical association fibers) and amygdala converge on the entorhinal cortex (part of the parahippocampal gyrus) and connect with the hippocampus via a polysynaptic circuit (*black arrows*) from dentate to CA3, CA1, and subiculum neurons with output back to the entorhinal cortex. Efferent connections (*broken arrows*) are principally via the fornix to the anterior nucleus of the thalamus, septal nuclei, and mamillary body.

Table 26-2   Differential Diagnosis of Dementia

MOST COMMON CAUSES OF DEMENTIA

Alzheimer's disease	Alcoholism[a]
Vascular dementia	Parkinson's disease
Multi-infarct	Drug/medication intoxication[a]
Diffuse white matter disease (Binswanger's)	

LESS COMMON CAUSES OF DEMENTIA

Vitamin deficiencies	Toxic disorders
Thiamine (B₁): Wernicke's encephalopathy[a]	Drug, medication, and narcotic poisoning[a]
B₁₂ (pernicious anemia)[a]	Heavy metal intoxication[a]
Nicotinic acid (pellagra)[a]	Dialysis dementia (aluminum)
Endocrine and other organ failure	Organic toxins
Hypothyroidism[a]	Psychiatric
Adrenal insufficiency and Cushing's syndrome[a]	Depression (pseudodementia)[a]
Hypo- and hyperparathyroidism[a]	Schizophrenia[a]
Renal failure[a]	Conversion reaction[a]
Liver failure[a]	Degenerative disorders
Pulmonary failure[a]	Huntington's disease
Chronic infections	Pick's disease
HIV	Diffuse Lewy body disease
Neurosyphilis[a]	Progressive supranuclear palsy (Steel-Richardson
Papovavirus (progressive multifocal leukoencepha-	syndrome)
lopathy)	Multisystem degeneration (Shy-Drager syndrome)
Prion (Creutzfeldt-Jakob and Gerstmann-Sträussler-	Hereditary ataxias (some forms)
Scheinker diseases)	Motor neuron disease [amyotrophic lateral sclerosis
Tuberculosis, fungal, and protozoal[a]	(ALS); some forms]
Sarcoidosis[a]	Frontotemporal dementia
Whipple's disease[a]	Cortical basal degeneration
Head trauma and diffuse brain damage	Multiple sclerosis
Dementia pugilistica	Adult Down's syndrome with Alzheimer's
Chronic subdural hematoma[a]	ALS–Parkinson's–Dementia complex of Guam
Postanoxia	Miscellaneous
Postencephalitis	Vasculitis[a]
Normal-pressure hydrocephalus[a]	CADASIL
Neoplastic	Acute intermittent porphyria[a]
Primary brain tumor[a]	Recurrent nonconvulsive seizures[a]
Metastatic brain tumor[a]	Additional conditions in children or adolescents
Paraneoplastic limbic encephalitis	Hallervorden-Spatz disease
	Subacute sclerosing panencephalitis
	Metabolic disorders (e.g., Wilson's and Leigh's dis-
	eases, leukodystrophies, lipid storage diseases, mito-
	chondrial mutations)

[a] Potentially reversible dementia.

resent relatively diffuse neuronal deterioration throughout the cerebral cortex, whereas multi-infarct dementia associated with recurrent strokes causes more focal damage in a random patchwork of cortical regions. Diffuse white matter damage may disrupt intracerebral connections and cause dementia syndromes such as those associated with leukodystrophies, multiple sclerosis, and Binswanger's disease. Subcortical structures such as the caudate, putamen, thalamus, and substantia nigra also modulate cognition and behavior in ways that are not yet well understood. Some investigators distinguish between cortical and subcortical types of dementia. A cortical dementia such as AD primarily presents as memory loss and is often associated with aphasia or other disturbance of language. Patients with subcortical dementia such as Huntington's disease (HD) are less likely to have memory and language problems and more likely to have difficulties with attention, judgment, awareness, and behavior. Both the clinical and anatomic characteristics of the cortical and subcortical dementias show considerable overlap, and the conditions are often not distinct.

Lesions of some relatively specific cortical-subcortical pathways may have significant effects on behavior (Chap. 25). The dorsolateral prefrontal cortex has connections with the dorsolateral caudate, globus pallidus, and thalamus. Lesions of these pathways result in poor organization and planning, perseveration, and decreased cognitive flexibility with impaired judgment. The lateral orbital frontal cortex connects with the ventromedial caudate, globus pallidus, and thalamus. Lesions of these connections cause irritability, impulsiveness, and distractibility. The anterior cingulate cortex connects with the nucleus accumbens, globus pallidus, and thalamus. Interruption of these con-

nections produces apathy and poverty of speech or even akinetic mutism.

The single strongest risk factor for dementia is increasing age. The prevalence of disabling memory loss increases with each decade over age 50 and is associated most often with the microscopic changes of AD at autopsy. Slow accumulation of mutations in neuronal mitochondria is also hypothesized to contribute to the increasing prevalence of dementia with age. Yet many centenarians have intact memory function and no evidence of clinically significant dementia. Whether dementia is an inevitable consequence of normal human aging remains controversial.

DIFFERENTIAL DIAGNOSIS The many causes of dementia are listed in Table 26-2. The frequency of each condition depends on the age group under study, the country of origin, and perhaps racial or ethnic variations. AD is the most common cause of dementia in western countries, affecting more than half of demented patients. Vascular disease is the second most common cause of dementia in the United States, affecting 10 to 20%; but it is more common than AD in some Asian countries. Dementia associated with chronic alcoholism and Parkinson's disease (PD) represent the next two most common categories. Chronic intoxications including those resulting from prescription drugs are an important, potentially treatable cause of dementia. Other disorders listed in the table are uncommon but important because many are reversible. The classification of dementing illnesses into two broad groups of reversible and irreversible disorders is a useful approach to the differential diagnosis of dementia.

Subtle cumulative memory loss is a natural part of aging. This frustrating experience, often the source of jokes and humor, is referred to as *benign forgetfulness of the elderly*. Benign means that it is not so progressive or serious that it impairs reasonably successful and productive daily functioning, although the distinction between benign and more significant memory loss can be difficult to make. A proportion of persons with benign memory loss progress to frank dementia, usually caused by AD. It remains unclear why some individuals show progression and others do not. It was once assumed that a cumulative loss of hippocampal neurons with normal aging might underlie this forgetfulness, but recent quantitative neuronal counts indicate that this "natural" neuronal loss may not occur.

Alzheimer's disease is a slowly progressive dementing illness associated with diffuse cortical atrophy and specific neuropathologic hallmarks of amyloid plaques and neurofibrillary tangles. Although quite common in the elderly, it remains a diagnosis of exclusion to be confirmed definitively only at autopsy. The clinical diagnosis of AD established by experienced neurologists proves to be correct at autopsy approximately 85 to 90% of the time. →*This condition is described in greater detail in Chap. 362.*

Two major types of vascular dementia can be identified (Chap.

362). The first, often called multi-infarct dementia, results from an accumulation of discrete cerebral strokes that produce disabling deficits of memory, behavior, and other cognitive abilities. Such patients usually give a history of sudden, separate stroke episodes with stepwise deterioration. On examination, focal neurologic deficits such as hemiparesis, unilateral Babinski reflex, aphasia, or visual field defect are common. Brain imaging shows multiple areas of stroke, which may have been ischemic or hemorrhagic. A second, more subtle and insidious type of vascular dementia, Binswanger's disease, is a dementing illness associated with diffuse, subcortical white matter damage often occurring in patients with chronic hypertension and/or severe atherosclerosis. The white matter changes are dramatically visualized by MRI and have also been called leukoareosis. The pathogenesis of Binswanger's disease is unknown. Because AD and vascular dementia are common, occasional patients may have both conditions.

An inherited form of vascular dementia is CADASIL (cerebral autosomal dominant arteriopathy with subcortical infarcts and leukoencephalopathy). It is caused by a mutation in the notch 3 gene and produces characteristic dense bodies in the media of arterioles in brain and skin. Affected persons have diffuse white matter deficits on brain MRI associated with migraine and recurrent stroke without hypertension.

Frontotemporal dementia (FTD) may represent 10 to 20% of persons with presenile dementia (onset before age 65). Initial symptoms are behavioral, such as disinhibition, apathy, or agitation with relatively intact memory. Brain imaging studies show focal lobar atrophy of the frontal and/or temporal lobes. Pick's disease is a form of FTD. Some cases are familial and associated with neuronal neurofibrillary tangle formation and mutations in the tau gene.

Dementia commonly accompanies chronic alcoholism (Chap. 387). This situation may be a result of associated malnutrition, especially of B vitamins and particularly thiamine. However, other as yet poorly defined aspects of chronic alcohol ingestion may also produce cerebral damage and atrophy. A rare idiopathic syndrome of dementia and seizures with degeneration of the corpus callosum has been reported primarily in male Italian drinkers of red wine (Marchiafava-Bignami disease).

Thiamine (vitamin B_1) deficiency causes Wernicke's encephalopathy. The clinical presentation is a malnourished individual (frequently but not necessarily alcoholic) with confusion, ataxia, and diplopia from ophthalmoplegia (Charcot's triad). Thiamine deficiency damages the thalamus, mammillary bodies, midline cerebellum, periaquaductal gray matter of the midbrain, and peripheral nerves. Damage to medial thalamic regions correlates most closely with memory loss. Prompt administration of parenteral thiamine (100 mg intravenously for 3 days followed by daily oral dosage) may reverse the disease if given in the first few days of symptom onset. However, prolonged untreated thiamine deficiency can result in an irreversible dementia/amnestic syndrome (Korsakoff's psychosis) or even death.

In Korsakoff's syndrome, the patient is unable to recall new information despite normal immediate memory, attention span, and level of consciousness. Memory for new events is seriously impaired, whereas memory of knowledge prior to the illness is relatively intact. Patients are easily confused, disoriented, and incapable of recalling new information for more than a brief interval. Superficially, they may be conversant, entertaining, able to perform simple tasks, and follow immediate commands. Confabulation is common, although not always present, and may result in obviously erroneous statements and elaborations. There is no specific treatment because the previous thiamine deficiency has produced irreversible damage to the medial thalamic nuclei and mammillary bodies. Mammillary body atrophy may be visible on high-resolution MRI.

Vitamin B_{12} deficiency, as can occur in pernicious anemia, causes a macrocytic anemia and may also damage the nervous system (Chaps. 107 and 368). Neurologically it most commonly produces a spinal cord syndrome (myelopathy) affecting the posterior columns (loss of position and vibratory sense) and the lateral corticospinal tracts (hyperactive tendon reflexes and Babinski responses); it also damages peripheral nerves, resulting in sensory loss with depressed tendon reflexes. Damage to cerebral myelinated fibers may also cause dementia. The mechanism of neurologic damage is unclear but may be related to a deficiency of S-adenosylmethionine (required for methylation of myelin phospholipids) due to reduced methionine synthase activity or accumulation of methylmalonate and propionate, providing abnormal substrates for fatty acid synthesis in myelin. The neurologic signs of vitamin B_{12} deficiency are usually associated with macrocytic anemia, but on occasion may occur in its absence. Treatment with parenteral vitamin B_{12} (1000 μg intramuscularly daily for a week, weekly for a month, and monthly for life for pernicious anemia) stops progression of the disease if instituted promptly, but reversal of advanced nervous system damage will not occur.

Deficiency of nicotinic acid (pellagra) is associated with sun-exposed skin rash, glossitis, and angular stomatitis (Chap. 75). Severe dietary deficiency of nicotinic acid along with other B vitamins such as pyridoxine may result in spastic paraparesis, peripheral neuropathy, fatigue, irritability, and dementia. This syndrome has been seen in prisoner-of-war and concentration camps. Low serum folate levels appear to be a rough index of malnutrition, but isolated folate deficiency has not been proven to be a specific cause of dementia.

Approximately 20% of patients with PD (Chap. 363) eventually develop dementia. Treatment with L-dopa neither accelerates nor prevents this process. Some PD patients with dementia have cytoplasmic neuronal inclusions (Lewy bodies) or AD changes in the cerebral cortex, but others have no specific identifiable cortical pathology. Progressive supranuclear palsy is a dementing illness associated with parkinsonian features of rigidity, bradykinesia, and postural instability. Resting tremor is often absent, there is a vertical gaze palsy, and patients are resistant to treatment with L-dopa.

Infections of the central nervous system (CNS) usually cause delirium and other acute neurologic syndromes (Chap. 24). However, some chronic CNS infections such as tuberculosis or cryptococcosis may produce a dementing illness (Chap. 374). Between 20 and 30% of patients in the advanced stages of infection with HIV become demented (Chap. 309). Cardinal features include psychomotor retardation, apathy, and impaired memory. This condition may result from secondary opportunistic infections but can also be caused by direct involvement of CNS neurons with HIV, where there is a multinucleated giant cell encephalitis and diffuse pallor of white matter. The neuronal toxicity may be mediated by cytokines or the direct neurotoxic effect of the gp 120 envelope glycoprotein. In the absence of CNS opportunistic infection, elevated β_2-microglobulin in cerebrospinal fluid (CSF) is a useful marker for HIV dementia. Herpes simplex encephalitis (Chap. 373) has a predilection for the inferior temporal lobes and may present as subacute confusion and disorientation but more often as an acute syndrome rather than a chronic dementia. Computed tomography (CT), MRI, and electroencephalogram (EEG) may all demonstrate the temporal lobe location of the lesions. CSF usually shows increased protein and a lymphocytic pleocytosis. CNS syphilis (Chap. 172) was a common cause of dementia in the preantibiotic era; it is uncommon now but can still be encountered in individuals with multiple sex partners. Characteristic CSF changes consist of pleocytosis, increased protein, and a positive Venereal Disease Research Laboratory (VDRL) test.

Prion disorders such as Creutzfeldt-Jakob disease (CJD) (Chap. 375) are rare conditions (approximately 1 per million population) that commonly produce dementia. CJD is typically a rapidly progressive disease associated with dementia, rigidity, and myoclonus, causing death in less than 1 to 2 years. These clinical characteristics may also rarely be seen in AD, and the differential diagnosis usually depends on the slower progression of AD and the markedly abnormal periodic EEG discharges seen in CJD. Ataxia or cortical blindness may also accompany CJD. The transmissible agent, or prion, consists principally of an abnormal isoform of a host-encoded protein, the prion protein, which has undergone a physical conformational change and accumulates in affected brains. Bovine spongiform encephalopathy in the United Kingdom is thought to have resulted from cattle feed containing sheep tissues contaminated with infectious prions. Immunoassay for a 14-3-3 brain protein in CSF may be a useful marker for transmissible spongiform encephalopathies in patients with dementia.

Primary and metastatic neoplasms of the CNS (Chap. 370) usually produce focal neurologic findings and seizures rather than dementia. However, if tumor growth begins in the frontal or temporal lobes, the initial manifestations may be memory loss or behavioral changes. A rare paraneoplastic syndrome of dementia associated with occult carcinoma (usually small cell lung cancer) has been termed *limbic encephalitis* (Chap. 101). In this syndrome, confusion, agitation, seizures, poor memory, and frank dementia may occur in association with sensory neuropathy. The CSF often shows an increase in cells and protein. There is neuronal loss and perivascular lymphocytic infiltration in the hippocampus, amygdala, and cingulate and frontal cortex. Circulating antineuronal nuclear antibodies may be present. There is no specific treatment.

The syndrome of normal-pressure hydrocephalus (Chap. 362) is frequently discussed but difficult to diagnose. Clinically, a triad of memory loss, gait disturbance, and bladder incontinence is typical. The gait abnormality is often the initial symptom, and the dementia is usually mild. On imaging studies, the lateral ventricles are enlarged but there is minimal or no cortical atrophy. Lumbar puncture shows a normal or slightly elevated opening pressure with normal CSF. The condition may be idiopathic or the result of previous meningitis or subarachnoid blood from a ruptured aneurysm or head trauma. The pathogenetic mechanism is presumably a block of normal CSF flow over the convexity and delayed absorption into the venous system, with resulting stretch and distortion of white matter tracts within the corona radiata. Some individuals improve with ventricular shunting but many do not. The condition is difficult to distinguish from AD (Chap. 362).

A nonconvulsive seizure disorder may underlie a syndrome of confusion, clouding of consciousness, and garbled speech. Psychiatric disease is often suspected, but an EEG demonstrates the seizure discharges. If recurrent or persistent, the condition may be termed *complex partial status epilepticus*. The cognitive disturbance often responds to anticonvulsant therapy. The etiology may be previous small strokes or head trauma; some cases are idiopathic.

It is important to recognize systemic diseases that indirectly affect the brain and produce chronic confusion or dementia. Such conditions include dysthyroid states (especially hypothyroidism), vasculitis, and hepatic, renal, or pulmonary disease. Hepatic encephalopathy may begin with irritability and confusion and slowly progress to agitation, lethargy, and coma (Chap. 376).

Isolated angiitis of the CNS (CNS granulomatous angiitis) (Chaps. 317 and 361) occasionally causes a chronic encephalopathy associated with confusion, disorientation, and clouding of consciousness. Headache is common, and strokes and cranial neuropathies may occur. Brain imaging studies may be normal or nonspecifically abnormal. Studies of CSF reveal a mild pleocytosis or elevation in the protein level in half of the cases. Cerebral angiography often shows multifocal stenosis and narrowing of vessels. A few patients have only small-vessel disease that is not revealed on angiography. The angiographic appearance is not specific and may be mimicked by atherosclerosis, infection, or other causes of vascular disease. Brain or meningeal biopsy demonstrates abnormal arteries with endothelial cell proliferation and infiltrates of mononuclear cells. Autoantibodies and immune complexes are not present, and a cell-mediated process appears most likely. The prognosis is poor, but some patients respond to glucocorticoids or chemotherapy.

Chronic metal intoxications may also produce a dementing syndrome. The key to diagnosis is the elicitation of a history of exposure at work, home, or even as a consequence of a medical procedure such as dialysis. Lead poisoning has highly variable neurologic manifesta-

tions. Fatigue, depression, and confusion may be associated with episodic abdominal pain and peripheral neuropathy. Gray lead lines may appear in the gums. There is usually an associated anemia with basophilic stippling of red cells. The clinical presentation can resemble that of acute intermittent porphyria, including elevated levels of urine porphyrins as a result of the inhibition of δ-aminolevulinic acid dehydratase. Chronic lead poisoning from inadequately fired glazed pottery has been reported. The treatment is chelation therapy with agents such as ethylene diaminetetraacetic acid (EDTA). Chronic mercury poisoning may produce dementia, peripheral neuropathy, ataxia, and a fine tremulousness that may progress to a cerebellar intention tremor or choreoathetosis. The confusion and memory loss of chronic arsenic intoxication is also associated with nausea, weight loss, peripheral neuropathy, pigmentation and scaling of the skin, and transverse white lines of the fingernails (Mee's lines). Treatment is chelation therapy with dimercaprol (BAL). Aluminum poisoning has been best documented with the dialysis dementia syndrome in which water used during renal dialysis was contaminated with excessive amounts of aluminum. This resulted in a progressive encephalopathy associated with confusion, memory loss, agitation, and, later, lethargy and stupor. Speech arrest and myoclonic jerking was common and associated with severe and generalized EEG changes. The condition was often fatal. There were no specific pathologic findings, but elevated brain aluminum content was documented. The condition has been eliminated by use of deionized water for dialysis. Although aluminum injected into experimental animals may produce neurofibrillary tangles, patients with dialysis dementia had neither tangles nor amyloid plaques, and there has been no direct association of aluminum poisoning with AD.

Recurrent head trauma in professional boxers may lead to dementia, sometimes called the "punch drunk" syndrome or *dementia pugilistica*. The symptoms can be progressive and may begin late in a boxer's career or even long after retirement. The severity of the syndrome correlates with the length of the boxing career and the total number of bouts. Early in the condition there occurs a personality change associated with social instability and sometimes paranoia and delusions. Later, memory loss progresses to full dementia, often associated with parkinsonian signs and ataxia or intention tremor. At autopsy, the cerebral cortex may show changes similar to AD, although neurofibrillary tangles are usually more predominant than amyloid plaques (which are usually diffuse rather than neuritic). There may also be loss of neurons in the substantia nigra. Chronic subdural hematoma is also occasionally associated with dementia, often in the context of underlying cortical atrophy from conditions such as AD or HD. In these latter cases, evacuation of the subdural hematoma does not alter the underlying degenerative process.

Head injury (Chap. 369) may also be associated with temporary amnesia. The memory disturbance may include events that occurred both before the injury (retrograde amnesia) and during the postinjury period (posttraumatic or anterograde amnesia). Retrograde amnesia after severe head injury may extend back for hours or weeks before the injury; remote memory is usually intact. As patients recover, the extent of retrograde amnesia shrinks and may disappear. Often, retrograde amnesia causes permanent inability to recall the few minutes before the head injury, implying disruption of the immediate memory system and failure to register long-term memory. The length of posttraumatic amnesia generally corresponds to the length of the postconcussive confusional state, but posttraumatic amnesia may persist even in the presence of normal immediate memory and digit span. The duration of posttraumatic amnesia indicates the severity of head injury; the ability to learn new material is often the last cognitive deficit to recover. There are reports of recovery from retrograde amnesia occurring months or years after the initial brain insult; the recovery is sometimes stimulated by hypnosis, amobarbital interview, or electrical stimulation. One theory of such recovery envisions a resetting of distorted patterns of neuronal matrices subserving memory.

Transient global amnesia (TGA) is characterized by sudden onset of complete anterograde loss of memory and learning abilities, usually occurring in persons over age 50. Onset of memory loss may occur in the context of an emotional stimulus or physical exertion. During the attack the individual is alert and communicative, general cognition seems intact, and there are no other neurologic signs or symptoms. The patient may seem confused and repeatedly ask about present events. The ability to form new memories returns after a period of hours, and the individual returns to normal but has no recall for the period of the attack. Frequently no cause can be determined, but cerebrovascular disease, epilepsy (7% in one study), migraine, or cardiac arrhythmia sometimes may be implicated. A Mayo Clinic review of 277 patients with TGA found a past history of migraine in 14% and cerebrovascular disease in 11%, but these conditions were not temporally related to the TGA episodes. About one-fourth of the patients had recurrent attacks, but they were not at increased risk for subsequent stroke. Rare instances of permanent memory loss after sudden onset have been reported.

Psychogenic amnesia for personally important memories is common, although whether this amnesia results from deliberate avoidance of unpleasant memories or from unconscious repression may be impossible to establish. The event-specific amnesia is particularly common after violent crimes such as homicide of a close relative or friend or sexual abuse. It also may occur with severe drug or alcohol intoxication and sometimes with schizophrenia. More prolonged psychogenic amnesia occurs in fugue states that also commonly follow severe emotional stress. The patient with a fugue state suffers from a sudden loss of personal identity and may be found wandering far from home. In contrast to organic amnesia, fugue states are associated with amnesia for personal identity and events closely associated with the personal past. At the same time, memory for other recent events and the ability to learn and use new information are preserved. The episodes usually last hours or days and occasionally weeks or months while the patient takes on a new identity. On recovery, there is a residual amnesic gap for the period of the fugue.

Psychiatric diseases may mimic dementia. Severely depressed individuals may appear demented, a phenomenon called *pseudodementia*. Unlike cortical dementias, memory and language are usually intact when carefully tested in depressed persons. The patients may feel confused and are unable to accomplish routine tasks. Vegetative symptoms are common, such as insomnia, lack of energy, poor appetite, and concern with bowel function. The psychosocial milieu may suggest prominent reasons for depression. The patients respond to antidepressant treatment. Schizophrenia is usually not difficult to distinguish from dementia, but occasionally the distinction can be problematic. (Kraepelin's original term for schizophrenia was *dementia praecox*.) Schizophrenia usually has a much earlier age of onset (second and third decades) than most dementing illnesses. It is associated with intact memory, and the delusions and hallucinations of schizophrenia are usually more complex and bizarre than those of dementia. Some individuals with chronic schizophrenia develop an unexplained progressive dementia late in life that is not related to AD. Memory loss may also be part of a conversion reaction. In this situation, patients commonly complain bitterly of memory loss, but careful cognitive testing either does not confirm the deficits or demonstrates inconsistent or unusual patterns of cognitive problems. The patients' behavior and "wrong" answers to questions often indicate that they both understand the question and know the answer.

Clouding of cognition by chronic drug or medication use, often prescribed by physicians, is an important cause of dementia. Sedatives, tranquilizers, and analgesics used to treat insomnia, pain, anxiety, or agitation may cause confusion, memory loss, and lethargy, especially in the elderly. Discontinuation of such medication often improves mentation.

Approach to the Patient

The approach to the patient with dementia should always keep two major questions in the forefront: What is the most accurate diagnosis, and is there a treatable or reversible condition? A broad overview of this approach is shown in Table 26-3.

History The history should concentrate on the onset, duration, and tempo of the memory loss. Acute or subacute confusion may represent delirium and suggests intoxication, infection, or metabolic derangement. An elderly person with slowly progressive memory loss over several years is likely to have AD. Initial symptoms often are difficulty with managing money, driving, shopping, following instructions, or finding one's way around town. A change in personality with disinhibition and intact memory may suggest FTD. A history of sudden stroke with an irregular stepwise progression suggests multi-infarct dementia. Stroke is also commonly associated with a history of hypertension, atrial fibrillation, peripheral vascular disease, and diabetes. Rapid progression with rigidity and myoclonus suggests CJD. Seizures may indicate stroke or neoplasm. Trouble in walking may suggest PD or normal-pressure hydrocephalus, especially the latter when associated with bladder incontinence. A history of multiple sex partners or intravenous drug use may indicate CNS infection, especially with HIV. A history of recurrent head trauma could indicate chronic subdural hematoma, dementia pugilistica, or normal-pressure hydrocephalus. Alcoholism may suggest malnutrition and thiamine deficiency. A remote history of gastric surgery resulting in loss of intrinsic factor might indicate vitamin B$_{12}$ deficiency. Certain occupations such as working in a battery or chemical factory might indicate heavy metal intoxication. Careful review of medication intake, especially of sedatives and tranquilizers, may raise the issue of chronic drug intoxication. A positive family history of dementia would be

Table 26-3 Evaluation of the Patient with Dementia

Routine Evaluation	Optional Focused Tests	Occasionally Helpful Tests
History	HIV	EEG
Physical examination	Chest x-ray	Parathyroid function
Laboratory tests	Lumbar puncture	Adrenal function
Thyroid function (TSH)	Liver function	Urine heavy metals
Vitamin B$_{12}$	Renal function	RBC sedimentation rate
Complete blood count	Urine toxin screen	Angiogram
Electrolytes	Psychometric testing	Brain biopsy
VDRL	Apolipoprotein E	SPECT
CT/MRI		

DIAGNOSTIC CATEGORIES

Reversible Causes	Irreversible/Degenerative Dementias	Psychiatric Disorders
Examples	Examples	Depression
Hypothyroidism	Alzheimer's	Schizophrenia
Thiamine deficiency	Pick's	Conversion reaction
Vitamin B$_{12}$ deficiency	Huntington's	
Normal-pressure	Diffuse Lewy body disease	
hydrocephalus	Multi-infarct	
Chronic infection	Leukoencephalopathies	
Brain tumor	Parkinson's	
Drug intoxication		

Associated Treatable Conditions
Depression
Seizures
Insomnia
Agitation
Caregiver "burnout"
Drug side effects

elicited in HD, familial AD, and inherited FTD. The recent death of a loved one, insomnia, or poor appetite suggest depression.

Physical Examination A careful examination is essential to document the dementia, look for other signs of nervous system involvement, and search for clues suggesting other systemic disease. Cognitive function should be assessed in terms of orientation, recent and remote memory, and calculation. Many of the simple, commonly used bedside tests of cognitive function (such as serial 7s, digits forward and backward) are most useful when they are performed normally; this makes the diagnosis of dementia unlikely. Mistakes on these simple tests are more difficult to interpret and are of less diagnostic importance. Drawing a clock and the trail-making test are frequently used tests of immediate memory and visual-spatial abilities. The mini-mental status exam (MMSE) is an easily administered 30-points test of cognitive function (Table 26-4). It is used to quickly indicate a dementing process, provide a rough assessment of its severity, and follow progression of the illness. The MMSE is influenced by culture and education and is less useful in the early and late stages of dementia. Language function should be tested by the ability to read, write, comprehend, and name objects. Resting tremor, cogwheel rigidity, bradykinesia, and festinating gait indicate a parkinsonian syndrome. Gait ataxia or apraxia (inability to initiate and coordinate steps in a sequential fashion) suggests normal-pressure hydrocephalus. Confusion, sixth cranial nerve paresis, and ataxia suggests thiamine deficiency. Myoclonic jerks are present in CJD but also occur in AD. Hemiparesis or other focal neurologic deficits may occur in multi-infarct dementia or brain tumor. Bilateral hyperactive tendon reflexes, Babinski responses, and loss of vibration and position sensation suggest a myelopathy, such as occurs in vitamin B_{12} deficiency. Stocking-glove sensory loss and diminished tendon reflexes suggest a peripheral neuropathy, which could indicate underlying diabetes, vitamin deficiency, or heavy metal intoxication. Dry cool skin, hair loss, and bradycardia suggest hypothyroidism. Confusion associated with repetitive stereotyped movements may indicate ongoing seizure activity. Hearing impairment or visual loss may produce confusion and disorientation misinterpreted as dementia. Such sensory deficits are common in the elderly.

Laboratory Tests The use of multiple laboratory tests in the evaluation of dementia is controversial. The physician does not want to miss a treatable cause, yet no single treatable cause stands out as common; thus a screen must employ multiple different tests, each of which has a low yield. Therefore, cost/benefit ratios are difficult to assess, and many laboratory screening algorithms for dementia discourage multiple tests. Nevertheless, even a test with only a 1 to 2% positive rate is probably worth undertaking if the alternative is missing a reversible or treatable cause of dementia. Table 26-3 lists most screening tests for dementia. Neuroimaging studies (CT and MRI) are especially controversial because of their cost. However, they are clearly of value to identify primary and secondary neoplasms, locate areas of infarction, or suggest normal-pressure hydrocephalus or diffuse white matter disease. They also lend support to the diagnosis of AD, especially if there is hippocampal atrophy in addition to diffuse cortical atrophy, and focal lobar atrophy may suggest FTD. However, attempts to relate cognition to neuroimaging measures of atrophy and white matter changes have shown only modest correlations. A diagnosis of AD is reached primarily by exclusion of other causes of dementia. (The indications for apolipoprotein E testing for AD are discussed in Chap. 362.) Serum levels of vitamin B_{12} and TSH, complete blood count, electrolyte measurements, and a VDRL test are reasonable routine screening measures because they detect treatable conditions. Lumbar puncture need not be done routinely in the evaluation of dementia but is indicated if CNS infection is a serious consideration, for example, in patients with delirium, fever, or nuchal rigidity. CSF levels of tau protein are increased and those of Aβ amyloid are decreased in some patients with AD; however, the clinical usefulness of these changes is not yet clear. Formal psychometric testing is not necessary in every patient with dementia but can be used to document the severity of dementia, suggest psychogenic causes, and provide a semiquantitative method for following the disease course. EEG is rarely helpful except to suggest CJD (repetitive bursts of diffuse high voltage sharp waves) or an underlying nonconvulsive seizure disorder (epileptiform discharges). Brain biopsy (including meninges) is not commonly advised except to diagnose vasculitis, potentially treatable neoplasms, unusual infections (such as sarcoid), or in young persons where the diagnosis is in doubt. Angiography is not likely to be of use except when multiple strokes or cerebral vasculitis is a possible cause of the dementia.

TREATMENT The two major goals of management are, first, to treat any correctable cause of the dementia and, second, to provide comfort and support to the patient and caregivers. Treatment of underlying causes might include thyroid replacement for hypothyroidism; vitamin therapy for thiamine and B_{12} deficiency; antibiotics for opportunistic infections; ventricular shunting for normal-pressure hydrocephalus; and appropriate surgical, radiation, and/or chemotherapy for CNS neoplasms. Removal of sedating or cognition-impairing drugs and medications is often beneficial. If the patient is depressed rather than demented (pseudodementia), the depression should be vigorously treated. Patients with degenerative diseases such as AD and HD may also be depressed, and that portion of their condition may respond to antidepressant therapy. Antidepressants should be used with caution in demented patients because they may produce delirium. Antidepressants that have a low incidence of cognitive side effects, such as selective serotonin reuptake inhibitors, and tricyclic antidepressants with low anticholinergic activity such as desipramine and nortriptyline, are advisable. Anticonvulsants are used to control seizures. Agitation, hallucinations, delusions, and confusion are difficult to treat. These behavioral problems represent major causes for nursing home placement and institutionalization. Drugs such as phenothiazines, resperidone, haloperidol, and benzodiazepines may ameliorate the behavior problems but have untoward side effects such as sedation, rigidity, and dyskinesias. Medications that may calm agitation and insomnia without worsening dementia include low-dose haloperidol (0.5 to 2 mg), trazodone, buspirone, and propranolol. Olanzapine is increasingly used for patients with hallucinations. When patients do not respond, it is usually a mistake to advance to higher doses or to use anticholinergics or sedatives (such as barbiturates or benzodiazepines).

Table 26-4   The Mini-Mental Status Examination

	Points
Orientation	
Name: season/date/day/month/year	5 (1 for each name)
Name: hospital/floor/town/state/country	5 (1 for each name)
Registration	
Identify three objects by name and ask patient to repeat	3 (1 for each object)
Attention and calculation	
Serial 7s; subtract from 100 (e.g., 93–86–79–72–65)	5 (1 for each subtraction)
Recall	
Recall the three objects presented earlier	3 (1 for each object)
Language	
Name pencil and watch	2 (1 for each object)
Repeat "No ifs, ands, or buts"	1
Follow a 3-step command (e.g., "Take this paper, fold it in half, and place it on the table")	3 (1 for each command)
Write "close your eyes" and ask patient to obey written command	1
Ask patient to write a sentence	1
Ask patient to copy a design (e.g., intersecting pentagons)	1
Total	30

Cholinesterase inhibitors are being used to treat AD, and other drugs, such as estrogen, anti-inflammatory agents, and vitamin E are being investigated for the treatment or prevention of AD. These approaches are reviewed in Chap. 362.

A proactive approach has been shown to reduce the occurrence of delirium in hospitalized patients. This scheme includes frequent orientation, cognitive activities, sleep enhancement measures, vision and hearing aids, and correction of dehydration.

Nondrug behavior therapy has an important place in the management of dementia. The primary goal is to make the life of the patient with dementia comfortable, uncomplicated, and safe. Preparing lists, schedules, calendars, and labels can be helpful. It is also useful to stress familiar routines, short-term tasks, brief walks, and simple physical exercises. For many patients with dementia, the memory for facts is worse than that for routine activities, and they still may be able to take part in remembered physical activities such as walking, bowling, dancing, and golf. Patients with dementia usually object to losing control over familiar tasks such as driving, cooking, and handling finances. Attempts to help or take over may be greeted with complaints, depression, or anger. Hostile responses on the part of the caretaker are useless and sometimes harmful. Explanation, reassurance, distraction, and calm statements are more productive responses in this setting. Eventually, tasks such as finances and driving must be assumed by others, and the patient will conform and adjust. Safety is an important issue that includes not only driving but the environment of the kitchen, bathroom, and sleeping area. These areas need to be monitored, supervised, and made as safe as possible. A move to a retirement home, assisted-living center, or nursing home can initially increase confusion and agitation. Repeated reassurance, reorientation, and careful introduction to the new personnel will help to smooth the process. Provision of activities that are known to be enjoyable to the patient can be of considerable benefit. Attention should also be paid to frustration and depression in family members and caregivers. Caregiver guilt and burn-out are common. Family members often feel overwhelmed and helpless and may vent their frustrations on the patient, each other, and healthcare providers. Caregivers should be encouraged to take advantage of day-care facilities and respite breaks. Education and counseling about dementia are important. Local and national support groups can be of considerable help, such as the Alzheimer's Disease and Related Disorders Association.

BIBLIOGRAPHY

BOWEN J et al: Progression to dementia in patients with isolated memory loss. Lancet 349:763, 1998

CHUI H, ZHANG Q: Evaluation of dementia: A systematic study of the usefulness of the American Academy of Neurology's Practice Parameters. Neurology 49:925, 1997

COREY-BLOOD J et al: Diagnosis and evaluation of dementia. Neurology 45:211, 1995

DESMOND DW et al: Frequency and clinical determinants of Dementia after ischemic stroke. Neurology 54:1124, 2000

FLEMING KC, EVANS JM: Pharmacologic therapies in dementia. Mayo Clin Proc 70:1116, 1995

GALTON CJ et al: Atypical and typical presentations of Alzheimer's disease: A clinical, neuropsychological, neuroimaging and pathological study of 13 cases. Brain 123:484, 2000

INOUYE S et al: A multicomponent intervention to prevent delirium in hospitalized older patients. N Engl J Med 340:669, 1999

JIANG Y et al: Complementary neural mechanisms for tracking items in human working memory. Science 287:643, 2000

KAYE J: Diagnostic challenges in dementia. Neurology 51(Suppl 1):S45, 1998

MARTIN LM, FLEMING KC et al: Recognition and management of anxiety and depression in elderly patients. Mayo Clin Proc 70:999, 1995

MILNER B et al: Cognitive neuroscience and the study of memory. Neuron 20:445, 1998

PICCINI C et al: Treatable and reversible dementias: An update. J Neurol Sci 153:172, 1998

27

Charles A. Czeisler, John W. Winkelman, Gary S. Richardson

SLEEP DISORDERS

EEG	electroencephalogram	NREM	non-rapid-eye-movement
EMG	electromyogram	RBD	REM sleep behavior disorder
EOG	electrooculogram	REM	rapid-eye-movement
FDA	Food and Drug Administration	RLS	restless legs syndrome
GABA	γ-aminobutyric acid	SCN	suprachiasmatic nuclei
LH	luteinizing hormone	SSRIs	selective serotonin reuptake inhibitors
MSLT	multiple sleep latency test	VLPO	ventrolateral preoptic

Disturbed sleep is among the most frequent health complaints physicians encounter. More than one-half of adults in the United States experience at least intermittent sleep disturbances. For most, it is an occasional night of poor sleep and/or daytime sleepiness. However, at least 15 to 20% of adults report chronic sleep disturbance or misalignment of circadian timing, which can lead to serious impairment of daytime functioning. In addition, such problems may contribute to or exacerbate medical or psychiatric conditions. Thirty years ago, many such complaints were treated with hypnotic medications without further diagnostic evaluation. Since then, a distinct class of sleep and arousal disorders has been identified, and the field of sleep disorders medicine is now an established clinical discipline. However, most physicians still only receive, on average, 1 h of education in sleep disorders in their medical school curriculum.

PHYSIOLOGY OF SLEEP AND WAKEFULNESS

Most adults sleep 7 to 8 h per night, although the timing, duration, and internal structure of sleep vary among healthy individuals and as a function of age. At the extremes, infants and the elderly have frequent interruptions of sleep. In the United States, adults of intermediate age tend to have one consolidated sleep episode per day, although in some cultures sleep may be divided into a midafternoon nap and a shortened night sleep. Two principal neurobiologic systems govern the sleep-wake cycle: one that actively generates sleep and sleep-related processes and another that times sleep within the 24-h day. Either intrinsic abnormalities in these systems or extrinsic disturbances (environmental, drug- or illness-related) can lead to sleep or circadian rhythm disorders.

STATES AND STAGES OF SLEEP States and stages of human sleep are defined on the basis of characteristic patterns in the electroencephalogram (EEG), the electrooculogram (EOG—a measure of eye-movement activity), and the surface electromyogram (EMG) measured on the chin and neck. The continuous recording of this array of electrophysiologic parameters to define sleep and wakefulness is termed *polysomnography*.

Polysomnographic profiles define two states of sleep: (1) rapid-eye-movement (REM) sleep, and (2) non-rapid-eye-movement (NREM) sleep. NREM sleep is in turn subdivided into four stages, characterized by increasing arousal threshold and slowing of the cortical EEG. REM sleep is characterized by a low-amplitude, mixed-frequency EEG similar to that of NREM stage 1 sleep. The EOG shows bursts of REM similar to those seen during eyes-open wakefulness. Chin EMG activity is absent, reflecting the brainstem-mediated muscle atonia that is characteristic of that state.

ORGANIZATION OF HUMAN SLEEP Normal nocturnal sleep in adults displays a consistent organization from night to night (Fig. 27-1). After sleep onset, sleep usually progresses through NREM stages 1 to 4 within 45 to 60 min. Slow-wave sleep predominates in the first third of the night and comprises 15 to 25% of total nocturnal

FIGURE 27-1 Plots of the stages of REM sleep (solid bars), the four stages of NREM sleep, and wakefulness over the course of the entire night for representative young (*upper panel*, age 23) and older (*lower panel*, age 68) adult men. The recording in the older subject illustrates the reduction of slow-wave sleep, frequent spontaneous awakenings, early sleep onset, and early morning awakening that are characteristic features of sleep in older people, even in the absence of specific medical or psychiatric pathology. (*From the Circadian, Neuroendocrine, and Sleep Disorders Section, Endocrine Division, Brigham and Womens' Hospital.*)

sleep time in young adults. The percentage of slow-wave sleep is influenced by several factors, most notably age (see below). Prior sleep deprivation increases the rapidity of sleep onset and both the intensity and amount of slow-wave sleep.

The first REM sleep episode usually occurs in the second hour of sleep. More rapid onset of REM sleep in a young adult (particularly if less than 30 min) may suggest pathology such as endogenous depression, narcolepsy, circadian rhythm disorders, or drug withdrawal. NREM and REM alternate through the night with an average period of 90 to 110 min (the "ultradian" sleep cycle). Overall, REM sleep constitutes 20 to 25% of total sleep, and NREM stages 1 and 2 are 50 to 60% (increasing in elderly subjects).

Age has a profound impact on sleep state organization (Fig. 27-1). Slow-wave sleep is most intense and prominent during childhood, decreasing sharply at puberty and across the second and third decades of life. After age 30, there is a progressive, almost linear decline in the amount of slow-wave sleep, and the amplitude of delta EEG activity comprising slow-wave sleep is reduced. In the otherwise healthy older person, slow-wave sleep may be completely absent, particularly in males.

A different age profile exists for REM sleep. In infancy, REM sleep may comprise 50% of total sleep time, and the percentage is inversely proportional to developmental age. The amount of REM sleep falls off sharply over the first postnatal year as a mature REM-NREM cycle develops. During the rest of life into extreme old age, REM sleep occupies a relatively constant percentage of total sleep time.

NEUROANATOMY OF SLEEP Lesion studies in animals and neurologic diseases in humans have suggested distinct neuroanatomic sites in the generation of normal sleep and wakefulness. Experimental studies in animals have variously implicated the medullary reticular formation, the thalamus, and the basal forebrain in the generation of sleep, while the brainstem reticular formation, the midbrain, the subthalamus, the thalamus, and the basal forebrain have all been suggested to play a role in the generation of wakefulness or EEG arousal (Chap. 24).

Current hypotheses suggest that the capacity for sleep and wakefulness generation is distributed along an axial "core" of neurons extending from the brainstem rostrally to the basal forebrain. Complex commingling of neuronal groups occurs at many points along this brainstem-forebrain axis. It was recently discovered that a cluster of γ-aminobutyric acid (GABA) and galaninergic ventrolateral preoptic (VLPO) neurons, which innervate monoaminergic cell groups in the tuberomammillary nucleus that contribute to the ascending arousal system, are activated during sleep. This has led to the hypothesis that

these hypothalamic VLPO neurons may play a key role in sleep regulation.

Moreover, the neuroanatomic correlates of REM sleep appear to be discretely localized. Specific regions in the pons are associated with the neurophysiologic correlates of REM sleep. Small lesions in the dorsal pons result in the loss of the descending muscle inhibition normally associated with REM sleep; microinjections of the cholinergic agonist carbachol into the pontine reticular formation appear to produce a state with all of the features of REM sleep. These experimental manipulations are mimicked by pathologic conditions in humans and animals. In narcolepsy, for example, abrupt, complete, or partial paralysis (cataplexy) occurs in response to a variety of stimuli. In dogs with this condition, physostigmine, a central cholinesterase inhibitor, increases the frequency of cataplectic attacks, while atropine decreases their frequency. Conversely, in REM sleep behavior disorder (see below), patients suffer from incomplete motor inhibition during REM sleep, resulting in involuntary, occasionally violent movement during REM sleep.

NEUROCHEMISTRY OF SLEEP Early experimental studies that focused on the raphe nuclei of the brainstem appeared to implicate serotonin as the primary sleep-promoting neurotransmitter, while catecholamines were considered to be responsible for wakefulness. Subsequent work has demonstrated that the raphe-serotonin system may facilitate sleep but is not necessary for its expression. Extensive pharmacologic studies of sleep and wakefulness suggest roles for other neurotransmitters as well. Cholinergic neurotransmission is known to play a role in REM sleep generation. The alerting influence of caffeine implicates adenosine, whereas the hypnotic effect of benzodiazepines and barbiturates suggests a role for endogenous ligands of the GABA$_A$ receptor complex.

A variety of sleep-promoting substances have been identified, although it is not known whether or not they are involved in the endogenous sleep-wake regulatory process. These include prostaglandin D$_2$, delta sleep–inducing peptide, muramyl dipeptide, interleukin 1, fatty acid primary amides, and melatonin. The hypnotic effect of these substances is commonly limited to NREM or slow-wave sleep, although peptides that increase REM sleep have also been reported. Many putative "sleep factors," including interleukin 1 and prostaglandin D$_2$, are immunologically active as well, suggesting a link between immune function and sleep-wake states.

PHYSIOLOGY OF CIRCADIAN RHYTHMICITY The sleep-wake cycle is the most evident of the many 24-h rhythms in humans. Prominent daily variations also occur in endocrine, thermoregulatory, cardiac, pulmonary, renal, gastrointestinal, and neurobehavioral functions. However, in evaluating a daily variation, it is important to distinguish between those rhythmic components passively evoked by periodic environmental or behavioral changes (e.g., the increase in blood pressure and heart rate upon assumption of the upright posture) and those actively driven by an endogenous oscillatory process (e.g., the circadian variation in plasma cortisol that persists under a variety of environmental and behavioral conditions).

The suprachiasmatic nuclei (SCN) of the hypothalamus act as the central neural pacemaker driving endogenous circadian rhythms in mammals. Bilateral destruction of these nuclei results in a loss of endogenous circadian rhythmicity that can only be restored by transplantation of the same structure from a donor animal. The genetically determined period of this endogenous neural oscillator, which averages ~24.2 h in humans, is normally synchronized to the 24-h period of the environmental light-dark cycle. Entrainment of mammalian circadian rhythms by the light-dark cycle is mediated via the retinohypothalamic tract, a monosynaptic pathway that links the retina to the SCN. Humans are exquisitely sensitive to the resetting effects of light, even at low intensity.

The timing and internal architecture of sleep are directly coupled to the output of the endogenous pacemaker. Paradoxically, the endogenous circadian rhythms of sleep tendency, sleepiness, and REM sleep propensity all peak near the habitual wake time, just after the nadir of the endogenous circadian temperature cycle, whereas the circadian wake propensity rhythm peaks 1 to 3 h before the habitual bedtime. These rhythms are thus timed to oppose the homeostatic decline of sleep tendency during the habitual sleep episode and the rise of sleep tendency throughout the usual waking day, respectively. Misalignment of the output of the endogenous circadian pacemaker with the desired sleep-wake cycle can, therefore, induce insomnia, as well as decrements of alertness and neurobehavioral performance in night-shift workers and after jet lag.

BEHAVIORAL CORRELATES OF SLEEP STATES AND STAGES Polysomnographic staging of sleep correlates with behavioral changes during specific states and stages. During the transitional state between wakefulness and sleep (stage 1 sleep), subjects may respond to faint auditory or visual signals without "awakening." Furthermore, memory incorporation is inhibited at the onset of NREM stage 1 sleep, and individuals aroused from that transitional sleep stage frequently deny having been asleep. Such transitions occur spontaneously after chronic partial sleep deprivation (e.g., 4 to 6 h of sleep per night) and acute total sleep deprivation (e.g., 24 h of wakefulness), notwithstanding attempts to remain continuously awake (see "Shift-Work Sleep Disorder," below).

Awakenings from REM sleep are associated with recall of vivid dream imagery more than 80% of the time. The reliability of dream recall increases with REM sleep episodes occurring later in the night. Imagery may also be reported after NREM sleep interruptions, though these typically lack the detail and vividness of REM sleep dreams. The incidence of NREM sleep dream recall can be increased by selective REM sleep deprivation, suggesting that REM sleep and dreaming per se are not inexorably linked.

PHYSIOLOGIC CORRELATES OF SLEEP STATES AND STAGES All major physiologic systems are influenced by sleep. Changes in cardiovascular function include a decrease in blood pressure and heart rate during NREM, and particularly during slow-wave sleep. During REM sleep, phasic activity (bursts of eye movements) is associated with variability in both blood pressure and heart rate mediated principally by the vagus. Cardiac dysrhythmias may occur selectively during REM sleep. Respiratory function also changes (Chap. 263). In comparison to relaxed wakefulness, respiratory rate becomes more regular during NREM sleep (especially slow-wave sleep) and tonic REM sleep and becomes very irregular during phasic REM sleep. Minute ventilation decreases in NREM sleep out of proportion to the decrease in metabolic rate at sleep onset, resulting in a higher P_{CO_2}.

Endocrine function also varies with sleep. The most prominent changes are apparent in neuroendocrine parameters. Slow-wave sleep is associated with secretion of growth hormone, while sleep in general is associated with augmented secretion of prolactin. Sleep has a complex effect on the secretion of luteinizing hormone (LH): during puberty, sleep is associated with increased LH secretion, whereas sleep in the mature woman inhibits LH secretion in the early follicular phase of the menstrual cycle. Sleep onset (and probably slow-wave sleep) is associated with inhibition of thyroid-stimulating hormone and of the adrenocorticotropic hormone–cortisol axis, an effect that is superimposed on the circadian rhythms in the two systems.

The pineal hormone melatonin is secreted predominantly at night in both day- and night-active species, reflecting the direct modulation of pineal activity by the circadian pacemaker through a circuitous neural pathway from the SCN to the pineal gland. Melatonin secretion is not dependent upon the occurrence of sleep, persisting in individuals kept awake at night. In addition, exogenous melatonin increases sleepiness and may potentiate sleep when administered to good sleepers

attempting to sleep during daylight hours at a time when endogenous melatonin levels are low. However, there is little evidence to support the use of melatonin as a hypnotic in such individuals during nighttime hours, when endogenous melatonin levels are high and sleep is already consolidated. A large-scale, double-blind clinical trial is needed to evaluate the efficacy of melatonin as a sleep-promoting therapeutic for patients with insomnia.

Sleep is also associated with alterations of thermoregulatory function. NREM sleep is associated with an attenuation of thermoregulatory responses to either heat or cold stress, and animal studies of thermosensitive neurons in the hypothalamus document an NREM-sleep-dependent reduction of the thermoregulatory set-point. REM sleep is associated with complete absence of thermoregulatory responsiveness, effectively resulting in functional poikilothermy. However, the potential adverse impact of this failure of thermoregulation is blunted by inhibition of REM sleep by extreme ambient temperatures.

DISORDERS OF SLEEP AND WAKEFULNESS

Approach to the Patient

Patients may seek help from a physician because of one of several symptoms: (1) an acute or chronic inability to sleep adequately at night (insomnia); (2) chronic fatigue, sleepiness, or tiredness during the day; or (3) a behavioral manifestation associated with sleep itself. Complaints of insomnia or excessive daytime sleepiness should be viewed as symptoms (much like fever or pain) of underlying disorders. Knowledge of the differential diagnosis of these presenting complaints is essential to identify the underlying medical disorder. Only then can appropriate treatment, rather than nonspecific approaches (e.g., over-the-counter sleeping aids) be applied. Diagnoses of exclusion, such as primary insomnia, should be made only after other diagnoses have been ruled out. Table 27-1 outlines the diagnostic and therapeutic approach to the patient with a complaint of excessive daytime sleepiness.

A careful history is essential in the evaluation of the patient with a sleep complaint. In particular, the duration, severity, and consistency of the complaint are important, along with the patient's estimate—in the case of an insomnia complaint—of the consequences of reported sleep loss on subsequent waking function. Information from a friend or family member can be an invaluable aid in assessing the symptoms and the severity of the complaint for daytime functioning, as some patients may be unaware of, or will underreport, such potentially embarrassing symptoms as heavy snoring or falling asleep while driving.

Completion by the patient of a day-by-day sleep-work-drug log for at least 2 weeks can help the physician better understand the nature of the complaint. Work times and sleep times (including daytime naps and nocturnal awakenings) as well as drug and alcohol use, including caffeine and hypnotics, should be noted each day. The sleep times should be plotted to facilitate recognition of circadian rhythm sleep disorders such as delayed sleep phase syndrome (see below).

Polysomnography is necessary for the diagnosis of specific disorders such as narcolepsy and sleep apnea and may be of utility in other settings as well. In addition to the three electrophysiologic variables used to define sleep states and stages, the standard clinical polysomnogram includes measures of respiration (respiratory effort, air flow, and oxygen saturation), anterior tibialis EMG, and electrocardiogram. Evaluation of penile tumescence during nocturnal sleep can also help determine whether the cause of erectile dysfunction in a patient is psychogenic or organic (Chap. 51).

INSOMNIA Insomnia is the complaint of inadequate sleep; it can be classified according to the nature of sleep disruption and the duration of the complaint. The nature of the sleep disruption provides important information about the possible etiology of the insomnia and is also central to the selection of specific and appropriate treatment.

Table 27-1   Evaluation of the Patient with the Complaint of Excessive Daytime Somnolence

Findings on History and Physical Examination	Diagnostic Evaluation	Diagnosis	Therapy
Obesity, snoring, hypertension	Polysomnography with respiratory monitoring	Obstructive sleep apnea	Continuous positive airway pressure; ENT surgery (e.g., uvulopalatopharyngoplasty); dental appliance; pharmacologic therapy (e.g., protriptyline); weight loss; (see Chap. 264)
Cataplexy, hypnogogic hallucinations, sleep paralysis, family history	Polysomnography with multiple sleep latency test	Narcolepsy-cataplexy syndrome	Stimulants (e.g., methylphenidate, pemoline); REM-suppressant antidepressants (e.g., protriptyline); genetic counseling
Restless legs syndrome, disturbed sleep, predisposing medical condition (e.g., anemia or renal failure)	Polysomnography with bilateral anterior tibialis EMG	Periodic limb movements of sleep	Treatment of predisposing condition, if possible; dopamine agonists (e.g., levodopa-carbidopa); benzodiazepines (e.g., clonazepam)
Disturbed sleep, predisposing medical conditions (e.g., asthma) and/or predisposing medical therapies (e.g., theophylline)	Sleep-wake diary	Insomnias (see text)	Treatment of predisposing condition and/or change in therapy, if possible; behavioral therapy; short-acting benzodiazepine receptor agonist (e.g., zolpidem)

NOTE: ENT, ears, nose, throat; REM, rapid eye movement; EMG, electromyogram.

Insomnia is subdivided into difficulty falling asleep (*sleep onset insomnia*), frequent or sustained awakenings (*sleep maintenance insomnia*), early morning awakenings (*sleep offset insomnia*), or persistent sleepiness despite sleep of adequate duration (*nonrestorative sleep*). Similarly, the duration of the symptom is an important determinant of the nature of appropriate treatment. An insomnia complaint lasting one to several nights (within a single episode) is termed *transient insomnia*. Transient insomnia is typically the result of situational stress or a change in sleep schedule or environment (e.g., jet lag). *Short-term insomnia* lasts from a few days to 3 weeks. Disruption of this duration is usually associated with more protracted stress, such as recovery from surgery or short-term illness. *Long-term insomnia*, or *chronic insomnia*, lasts for months or years and, in contrast with short-term insomnia, requires a thorough evaluation of underlying causes (see below). Chronic insomnia is often a waxing and waning disorder, with spontaneous or stressor-induced exacerbations.

While an occasional night of poor sleep, typically in the setting of stress or excitement about external events, is both common and without lasting consequences, persistent insomnia can have important adverse consequences in the form of impaired daytime function and increased risk of injury due to accidents. There is also clear evidence of increased risk of the development of major depression with insomnia of at least 1 year's duration. In addition, there is emerging evidence that individuals with chronic insomnia have increased utilization of health care resources, even after controlling for comorbid medical and psychiatric disorders.

Extrinsic Insomnia   A number of sleep disorders are the result of extrinsic factors that interfere with sleep. *Transient situational insomnia* can occur after a change in the sleeping environment (e.g., in an unfamiliar hotel or hospital bed) or before or after a significant life event, such as a change of occupation, loss of a loved one, illness, or anxiety over a deadline or examination. Increased sleep latency, frequent awakenings from sleep, and early morning awakening can all occur. Recovery generally occurs rapidly, usually within a few weeks. Treatment is usually symptomatic, with intermittent use of hypnotics and resolution of the underlying stress. *Inadequate sleep hygiene* is characterized by a behavior pattern prior to sleep and/or a bedroom

environment that is not conducive to sleep. Noise and/or light in the bedroom can interfere with sleep, as can a bed partner with periodic limb movements during sleep or one who snores loudly. Clocks can heighten the anxiety about the time it has taken to fall asleep. Drugs that act on the central nervous system, large meals, vigorous exercise, or hot showers just before sleep may interfere with sleep onset. Many individuals participate in stressful work-related activities in the evening, producing a state incompatible with sleep onset. In preference to hypnotic medications, patients should be counseled to avoid stressful activities before bed, develop a soporific bedtime ritual, and to prepare and reserve the bedroom environment for sleeping. Consistent, regular rising times should be maintained daily, including weekends.

Psychophysiologic Insomnia   Persistent *psychophysiologic insomnia* is a behavioral disorder in which patients are preoccupied with a perceived inability to sleep adequately at night. The sleep disturbance is often triggered by an emotionally stressful event; however, the poor sleep habits and beliefs about sleep acquired during the stressful period persist long after the initial incident. Such patients become hyperaroused by their own persistent efforts to sleep and/or the sleep environment, and the insomnia is a conditioned or learned response. They may be able to fall asleep more easily at unscheduled times (when not trying) or outside the home environment. Polysomnographic recording in patients with psychophysiologic insomnia reveals an objective sleep disturbance, often with an abnormally long sleep latency; frequent nocturnal awakenings; and an increased amount of stage 1 transitional sleep. Rigorous attention should be paid to sleep hygiene and correction of counterproductive, arousing behaviors before bedtime. Behavioral therapies are the treatment modality of choice for psychophysiologic insomnia, with only intermittent use of medications. When patients are awake longer than 20 min, they should read or perform other relaxing activities to distract themselves from insomnia-related anxiety. In addition, bedtime and waketime should be scheduled to restrict time in bed to be equal to their perceived total sleep time. This will generally produce sleep deprivation, greater sleep drive, and, eventually, better sleep. Time in bed can then be gradually expanded.

Medication-, Drug-, or Alcohol-Dependent Insomnia   Disturbed sleep can result from ingestion of a wide variety of agents. Caffeine is perhaps the most common pharmacologic cause of insomnia. It produces increased latency to sleep onset, more frequent arousals during sleep, and a reduction in total sleep time for up to 8 to 14 h after ingestion. As few as three to five cups of coffee can significantly disturb sleep in some patients; therefore, a 1- to 2-month trial without caffeine should be attempted in patients with these symptoms. Similarly, alcohol and nicotine can interfere with sleep, despite the fact that many patients use them to relax and promote sleep. Although alcohol can increase drowsiness and shorten sleep latency, even moderate amounts of alcohol increase awakenings in the second half of the night. In addition, alcohol ingestion prior to sleep is contraindicated in patients with sleep apnea because of the inhibitory effects of alcohol on upper airway muscle tone. Acutely, amphetamines and cocaine suppress both REM sleep and total sleep time, which return to normal with chronic use. Withdrawal leads to a REM sleep rebound.

A number of prescribed medications can produce insomnia. Antidepressants, sympathomimetics, and glucocorticoids are common causes. In addition, severe rebound insomnia can result from the acute withdrawal of hypnotics, especially following the use of high doses of benzodiazepines with a short half-life. For this reason, hypnotic doses should be low to moderate, the total duration of hypnotic therapy should usually be limited to 2 to 3 weeks, and prolonged drug tapering is encouraged.

Altitude Insomnia Sleep disturbance is a common consequence of exposure to high altitude. Periodic breathing of the Cheyne-Stokes type occurs during NREM sleep about half the time at high altitude, with restoration of a regular breathing pattern during REM sleep. Both hypoxia and hypocapnia are thought to be involved in the development of periodic breathing. Frequent awakenings and poor quality sleep characterize altitude insomnia, which is generally worst on the first few nights at high altitude but may persist. Treatment with acetazolamide can decrease time spent in periodic breathing and substantially reduce hypoxia during sleep.

Restless Legs Syndrome (RLS) Patients with this sensory-motor disorder report a creeping or crawling dysesthesia deep within the calves or feet, or sometimes even in the upper extemities, that is associated with an irresistible urge to move the affected limbs. For most patients with RLS, the dysesthesias and restlessness are much worse in the evening or night compared to the daytime and frequently interfere with the ability to fall asleep. The disorder is exacerbated by inactivity and temporarily relieved by movement. In contrast, paresthesia secondary to peripheral neuropathy persists with activity. The severity of this chronic disorder may wax and wane with time and can be exacerbated by sleep deprivation, caffeine, and pregnancy. The prevalence is thought to be 5% of adults. Roughly one-third of patients will have multiple affected family members, possibly with an autosomal dominant pattern. Iron deficiency and renal failure may actually cause RLS, which is then considered secondary RLS. The symptoms of RLS are exquisitely sensitive to dopaminergic drugs (e.g., L-dopa or dopamine agonists). Narcotics, benzodiazepines, and certain anticonvulsants may also be of therapeutic value. Most patients with restless legs also experience periodic limb movement disorder during sleep, although the reverse is not the case.

Periodic Limb Movement Disorder *Periodic limb movement disorder*, previously known as *nocturnal myoclonus*, is the principal objective polysomnographic finding in 17% of patients with insomnia and 11% of those with excessive daytime somnolence (Fig. 27-2). It is often unclear whether it is an incidental finding or the cause of disturbed sleep. Stereotyped, 0.5- to 5.0-s extensions of the great toe and dorsiflexion of the foot recur every 20 to 40 s during NREM sleep, in episodes lasting from minutes to hours. Most such episodes occur during the first half of the night. The disorder occurs in a wide variety of sleep disorders (including narcolepsy, sleep apnea, REM sleep behavior disorder, and various forms of insomnia) and may be associated with frequent arousals and an increased number of sleep-stage transitions. The incidence increases with age: 44% of people over age 65 without a sleep complaint have >five periodic leg movements per hour of sleep. The pathophysiology is not well understood, though individuals with high spinal transections can exhibit periodic leg movements during sleep, suggesting the existence of a spinal generator. Polysomnography with bilateral surface EMG recording of the anterior tibialis is used to establish the diagnosis. Treatment options include dopaminergic medications or benzodiazepines.

FIGURE 27-2 Polysomnographic recordings of a patient with (*A*) obstructive sleep apnea and one with (*B*) periodic limb movement of sleep. Note the snoring and reduction in air flow in the presence of continued respiratory effort, associated with the subsequent oxygen desaturation (upper panel). Periodic limb movements occur with a relatively constant intermovement interval and are associated with changes in the EEG and heart rates acceleration (lower panel). Abbreviations: R.A.T., right anterior tibialis; L.A.T., left anterior tibialis. *(From the Circadian, Neuroendocrine, and Sleep Disorders Section, Endocrine Division, Brigham and Womens' Hospital.)*

Insomnia Associated with Mental Disorders Approximately 80% of patients with psychiatric disorders describe sleep complaints. There is considerable heterogeneity, however, in the nature of the sleep disturbance both between conditions and among patients with the same condition.

Depression can be associated with sleep onset insomnia, sleep maintenance insomnia, and/or early morning wakefulness. However, hypersomnia occurs in some depressed patients, especially adolescents and those with either bipolar or seasonal (fall/winter) depression (Chap. 385). Indeed, sleep disturbance is an important vegetative sign of depression and may commence before any mood changes are perceived by the patient. Consistent polysomnographic findings in depression include decreased REM sleep latency, lengthened first REM sleep episode, and shortened first NREM sleep episode; however, these findings are not specific for depression, and the extent of these changes varies with age and symptomatology. Depressed patients also show decreased slow-wave sleep and reduced sleep continuity.

In *mania* and *hypomania*, sleep latency is increased and total sleep time can be reduced. Patients with *anxiety disorders* tend not to show the changes in REM sleep and slow-wave sleep seen in endogenously depressed patients. Finally, *chronic alcoholics* lack slow-wave sleep, have decreased amounts of REM sleep (as an acute response to alcohol), and have frequent arousals throughout the night. This is associated with impaired daytime alertness. The sleep of chronic alcoholics may remain disturbed for years after discontinuance of alcohol usage. Sleep architecture and physiology are disturbed in *schizophrenia* (with a decreased amount of stage 4 sleep and a lack of augmentation of REM sleep following REM sleep deprivation); chronic schizophrenics often show day-night reversal, sleep fragmentation, and insomnia.

Insomnia Associated with Neurologic Disorders A variety of neurologic diseases result in sleep disruption through both indirect, nonspecific mechanisms (e.g., pain in cervical spondylosis or low back pain) or by impairment of central neural structures involved in the generation and control of sleep itself.

For example, *dementia* from any cause has long been associated with disturbances in the timing of the sleep-wake cycle, often characterized by nocturnal wandering and an exacerbation of symptomatology at night (so-called sundowning).

Epilepsy may rarely present as a sleep complaint (Chap. 360). Often the history is of abnormal behavior, at times with convulsive movements, during sleep, and the differential diagnosis includes REM sleep behavior disorder, sleep apnea syndrome, and periodic movements of sleep (see above). Diagnosis requires nocturnal EEG recording. Other neurologic diseases associated with abnormal movements, such as *Parkinson's disease, hemiballismus, Huntington's chorea*, and *Gilles de la Tourette syndrome*, are also associated with disrupted sleep, presumably through secondary mechanisms. However, the abnormal movements themselves are greatly reduced during sleep. Headache syndromes may show sleep-associated exacerbations (*migraine* or *cluster headache*) (Chap. 15) by unknown mechanisms.

Fatal familial insomnia is a rare hereditary disorder caused by bilateral degeneration of anterior and dorsomedial nuclei of the thalamus. Insomnia is a prominent early symptom. Progressively, the syndrome produces autonomic dysfunction, dysarthria, myoclonus, coma, and death. The pathogenesis is a mutation in the prion protein (Chap. 375).

Insomnia Associated with Other Medical Disorders   A number of medical conditions are associated with disruptions of sleep. The association is frequently nonspecific, e.g., that between sleep disruption and chronic pain from rheumatologic disorders. Attention to this association is important in that sleep-associated symptoms are the presenting complaint of many such patients. Treatment of the underlying medical disorder or symptom is the most useful approach to such patients. As noted above, sleep disruption can also result from the appropriate use of drugs such as glucocorticoids.

Among the most prominent associations is that between sleep disruption and *asthma*. In many asthmatics there is a prominent daily variation in airway resistance that results in marked increases in asthmatic symptoms at night, especially during sleep. In addition, treatment of asthma with theophylline-based compounds, adrenergic agonists, or glucocorticoids can independently disrupt sleep. When sleep disruption is a prominent side effect of asthma treatment, inhaled steroids (e.g., beclomethasone) that do not disrupt sleep may provide a useful alternative.

Cardiac ischemia may also be associated with sleep disruption. The ischemia itself may result from increases in sympathetic tone as a result of sleep apnea. Patients may present with complaints of nightmares or vivid, disturbing dreams, with or without awareness of the more classic symptoms of angina or of the sleep disordered breathing. Treatment of the sleep apnea may substantially improve the angina and the nocturnal sleep quality. *Paroxysmal nocturnal dyspnea* can also occur as a consequence of sleep-associated cardiac ischemia that causes pulmonary congestion exacerbated by the recumbent posture.

Chronic obstructive pulmonary disease is also associated with sleep disruption, as is *cystic fibrosis, menopause, hyperthyroidism, gastroesophageal reflux, chronic renal failure*, and *liver failure*.

EVALUATION OF DAYTIME SLEEPINESS Daytime impairment due to sleep loss may be difficult to quantify in the clinical setting for several reasons. First, sleepiness is not necessarily proportional to subjectively assessed sleep deprivation. In obstructive sleep apnea, for example, the repeated brief interruptions of sleep associated with resumption of respiration at the end of apneic episodes result in significant waking impairment, despite the fact that the patient may be unaware of the sleep fragmentation. Second, subjective descriptions of waking impairment vary from patient to patient. Patients may describe themselves as "sleepy," "fatigued," or "tired" and may have a clear sense of the meaning of those terms, while others may use the same terms to describe a completely different condition. Third, sleepiness, particularly when profound, may affect judgment in a manner analogous to ethanol, such that subjective awareness of the condition and the consequent cognitive and motor impairment is reduced. Fi-

nally, patients may be reluctant to admit that sleepiness is a problem, both because they are generally unaware of what constitutes normal alertness and because sleepiness is generally viewed pejoratively, ascribed more often to a deficit in motivation than to an inadequately addressed physiologic sleep need.

In assessing sleepiness in the clinical setting, specific questioning about the occurrence of sleep episodes during normal waking hours, both intentional and unintentional, can overcome the inconsistencies among subjective characterizations and help to interpret the adverse impact of sleepiness on daytime function. Specific areas to be addressed include the occurrence of inadvertent sleep episodes while driving or in other safety-related settings, sleepiness while at work or school (and the relationship of sleepiness to work and school performance), and the effect of sleepiness on social and family life. Evidence for significant daytime impairment [in association either with the diagnosis of a primary sleep disorder, such as narcolepsy or sleep apnea, or with imposed or self-selected sleep-wake schedules (see "Shift-Work Sleep Disorder," below)] raises the question of the physician's responsibility to notify motor vehicle licensing authorities of the increased risk of sleepiness-related vehicle accidents. As with epilepsy, legal requirements vary from state to state, and existing legal precedents do not provide a consistent interpretation of the balance between the physician's responsibility and the patient's right to privacy. At a minimum, physicians should document discussions with the patient regarding the increased risk of operating a vehicle, as well as a recommendation that driving be suspended until successful treatment or schedule modification can be instituted.

The distinction between fatigue and sleepiness can be useful in the differentiation of patients with complaints of fatigue or tiredness in the setting of disorders such as fibromyalgia, chronic fatigue syndrome (Chap. 384), or endocrine deficiencies such as hypothyroidism or Addison's disease. While patients with these disorders can typically distinguish their daytime symptoms from the sleepiness that occurs with sleep deprivation, substantial overlap can occur. This is particularly true when the primary disorder also results in chronic sleep disruption (e.g., sleep apnea in hypothyroidism) or in abnormal sleep (e.g., fibromyalgia).

While clinical evaluation of the complaint of excessive sleepiness is usually adequate, objective quantification is sometimes necessary for diagnostic purposes or for the evaluation of treatment response. Assessment of daytime functioning as an index of the adequacy of sleep can be made with the multiple sleep latency test (MSLT), which involves repeated measurement of sleep latency (time to onset of sleep) under standardized conditions during a day following quantified nocturnal sleep. The average latency across four to six tests (administered every 2 h across the waking day) is taken as an objective measure of daytime sleep tendency. Disorders of sleep that result in pathologic daytime somnolence can be reliably distinguished with the MSLT. In addition, the multiple measurements of sleep onset may identify direct transitions from wakefulness to REM sleep that are suggestive of specific pathologic conditions (e.g., narcolepsy).

NARCOLEPSY Narcolepsy is both a disorder of the ability to sustain wakefulness voluntarily and a disorder of REM sleep regulation (Table 27-2). The classic "narcolepsy tetrad" consists of excessive daytime somnolence plus three specific symptoms related to an intrusion of REM sleep characteristics (e.g., muscle atonia, vivid dream imagery) into the transition between wakefulness and sleep: (1) sudden weakness or loss of muscle tone without loss of consciousness, often elicited by emotion (cataplexy); (2) hallucinations at sleep onset (hypnogogic hallucinations) or upon awakening (hypnopompic hallucinations); and (3) muscular paralysis upon awakening (sleep paralysis). The severity of cataplexy varies, as patients may have two to three attacks per day or per decade. The extent and duration of an attack may also vary, from a transient sagging of the jaw lasting a few seconds to rare cases of flaccid paralysis of the entire voluntary musculature for up to 20 to 30 min. Symptoms of narcolepsy typically begin in the second decade, although the onset ranges from ages 5 to 50.

Symptom	Prevalence, %
Excessive daytime somnolence	100
Disturbed sleep	87
Cataplexy	76
Hypnagogic hallucinations	68
Sleep paralysis	64
Memory problems	50

SOURCE: Modified from TA Roth, L Merlotti in SA Burton et al (eds), *Narcolepsy 3rd International Symposium: Selected Symposium Proceedings,* Chicago, Matrix Communications, 1989.

Once established, the disease is chronic without remissions. Secondary forms of narcolepsy have been described (e.g., after head trauma).

Narcolepsy affects about 1 in 4000 people in the United States and appears to have a genetic basis. Recently, two independent discoveries have revealed that hypothalamic neurons containing the neuropeptide orexin (hypocretin) may play an important role in the regulation of sleep/wakefulness: (1) a mutation in the orexin (hypocretin) receptor 2 gene has been associated with canine narcolepsy; and (2) orexin "knockout" mice that are genetically unable to produce this neuropeptide exhibit a phenotype, as assessed by behavioral and electrophysiologic criteria, that is similar to human narcolepsy. In addition, modafinil, a drug recently approved by the U.S. Food and Drug Administration (FDA) for the treatment of narcolepsy, activates orexin-containing neurons. However, the inheritance pattern of narcolepsy in humans is more complex than that of the canine model. A high rate of discordance in identical twins indicates that one or more nonheritable factors contributes to its development. First-degree relatives of narcoleptic patients nonetheless have about a 1% incidence of narcolepsy, much higher than the general population but much lower than is seen in the animal models. Of note, nearly all narcoleptics with cataplexy are positive for the human leukocyte antigen DQB*0106 (ordinarily found in 20 to 30% of the general population) (Chap. 306).

Diagnosis   Definition of the essential and distinctive features of narcolepsy has continued to evolve, and the diagnostic criteria continue to be a matter of debate. Certainly, objective verification of excessive daytime somnolence, typically with MSLT mean sleep latencies <8 min, is an essential if nonspecific diagnostic feature. Other conditions that cause excessive sleepiness, such as sleep apnea or chronic sleep restriction, must be rigorously excluded. The other objective diagnostic feature of narcolepsy is the presence of REM sleep in at least two of the naps during the MSLT. This excessive REM "pressure" is also manifested by the appearance of REM sleep immediately or within minutes after sleep onset in 50% of narcoleptic patients, a rarity in unaffected individuals maintaining a conventional sleep-wake schedule. The REM-related symptoms of the classic narcolepsy tetrad are variably present. There is increasing evidence that narcoleptics with cataplexy (one-half to two-thirds of patients) may represent a more homogeneous group than those without this symptom. However, a history of cataplexy can be difficult to establish reliably. Hypnogogic and hypnopompic hallucinations and sleep paralysis are often found in nonnarcoleptic individuals and may be present in only one-half of narcoleptics. Nocturnal sleep disruption is commonly observed in narcolepsy but is also a nonspecific symptom. Similarly, history of "automatic behavior" during wakefulness (a trance-like state during which simple motor behaviors persist) is not specific for narcolepsy and serves principally to corroborate the presence of daytime somnolence.

℞ **TREATMENT**   The treatment of narcolepsy is symptomatic. Somnolence is treated with stimulants. Methylphenidate has long been considered the drug of choice by most; the usual initial dose is 10 mg bid, increasing as needed to a maximum of 20 mg qid. Pemoline, frequently used as an alternative due to its longer half-life, may be less effective and has recently been associated with fatal hepatic failure in several children. Dextroamphetamine, 10 mg bid, and methamphetamine are also frequently used alternatives. Recently, modafinil, a novel wake-promoting agent, has been approved by the FDA for treatment of the excessive daytime somnolence in narcolepsy; the dose is 200–400 mg/d given as a single dose. It is a long-acting agent that may cause fewer side effects than other medications.

Treatment of the REM-related phenomena cataplexy, hypnogogic hallucinations, and sleep paralysis requires the potent REM sleep suppression produced by antidepressant medications. The tricyclic antidepressants [e.g., protriptyline (10–40 mg/d) and clomipramine (25–50 mg/d)] and the selective serotonin reuptake inhibitors (SSRIs) [e.g., fluoxetine (10–20 mg/d)] are commonly used for this purpose in the United States. Efficacy of the antidepressants is limited largely by anticholinergic side effects (tricyclics) and by sleep disturbance and sexual dysfunction (SSRIs). Adequate nocturnal sleep time and planned daytime naps (when possible) are important preventative measures in narcolepsy.

SLEEP APNEA SYNDROMES   Respiratory dysfunction during sleep is a common, serious cause of excessive daytime somnolence as well as of disturbed nocturnal sleep. An estimated 2 to 5 million people in the United States have a reduction or cessation of breathing for 10 to 150 s, from thirty to several hundred times every night during sleep. These episodes may be due to either an occlusion of the airway (*obstructive sleep apnea*), absence of respiratory effort (*central sleep apnea*), or a combination of these factors (*mixed sleep apnea*) (Fig. 27-2). Failure to recognize and treat these conditions appropriately may lead to: significant, and often disabling, impairment of daytime alertness; increased risk of sleep-related motor vehicle accidents; hypertension and other serious cardiovascular complications; and increased mortality. Sleep apnea is particularly prevalent in overweight men and in the elderly, yet it is estimated to remain undiagnosed in 80 to 90% of affected individuals. This is unfortunate since effective treatments are available. →*Readers are referred to Chap. 263 for a comprehensive review of the diagnosis and treatment of patients with these conditions.*

PARASOMNIAS   The term *parasomnia* refers to abnormal behaviors that arise from, or occur during, sleep. A continuum of parasomnias arise from NREM sleep, from brief confusional arousals to sleepwalking and night terrors. The presenting complaint is usually related to the behavior itself, but the parasomnias can disturb sleep continuity or lead to mild impairments in daytime alertness. Only one parasomnia is known to occur in REM sleep, i.e., REM sleep behavior disorder (RBD; see below).

Sleepwalking (Somnambulism)   Patients affected by this disorder carry out automatic motor activities that range from simple to complex. Individuals may leave the bed, walk, urinate inappropriately, eat, or exit from the house while remaining only partially aware. Full arousal may be difficult, and some patients may respond to attempted awakening with agitation or even violence. Sleepwalking arises from stage 3 or 4 NREM sleep and is most common in children and adolescents, when these sleep stages are most robust. Episodes are usually isolated but may be recurrent in 1 to 6% of patients. The cause is unknown, though it has a familial basis in roughly one-third of cases.

Sleep Terrors   This disorder, also called *pavor nocturnus*, occurs primarily in young children during the first several hours after sleep onset, in stages 3 and 4 of NREM sleep. The child suddenly screams, exhibiting autonomic arousal with sweating, tachycardia, and hyperventilation. The individual may be difficult to arouse and rarely recalls the episode on awakening in the morning. Recurrent attacks are rare, and treatment is usually by way of reassurance of parents. Both sleep terrors and sleepwalking represent abnormalities of arousal. In contrast, *nightmares* (dream anxiety attacks) occur during REM sleep and cause full arousal, with intact memory for the unpleasant episode.

REM Sleep Behavior Disorder RBD is a rare condition that is distinct from other parasomnias in that it occurs during REM sleep. It primarily afflicts men of middle age or older, many of whom have a history of prior neurologic disease. In fact, over one-third of patients will go on to develop Parkinson's disease within 10 to 20 years. Presenting symptoms are of agitated or violent behavior during sleep, reported by a bed partner. In contrast to typical somnambulism, injury to patient or bed partner is not uncommon, and, upon awakening, the patient reports vivid, often unpleasant, dream imagery. The principal differential diagnosis is that of nocturnal seizures, which can be excluded with polysomnography. In RBD, seizure activity is absent on the EEG, and disinhibition of the usual motor atonia is observed in the EMG during REM sleep, at times associated with complex motor behaviors. The pathogenesis is unclear, but damage to brainstem areas mediating descending motor inhibition during REM sleep may be responsible. In support of this hypothesis are the remarkable similarities between RBD and the sleep of animals with bilateral lesions of the pontine tegmentum in areas controlling REM sleep motor inhibition. Treatment with clonazepam provides sustained improvement in almost all reported cases.

Sleep Bruxism Bruxism is an involuntary, forceful grinding of teeth during sleep that affects 10 to 20% of the population. The patient is usually unaware of the problem. The typical age of onset is 17 to 20 years, and spontaneous remission usually occurs by age 40. Sex distribution appears to be equal. Treatment is dictated by the risk of dental injury. In many cases, the diagnosis is made during dental examination, damage is minor, and no treatment is indicated. In more severe cases, treatment with a rubber tooth guard is necessary to prevent disfiguring tooth injury. Stress management or, in some cases, biofeedback can be useful when bruxism is a manifestation of psychological stress. There are anecdotal reports of benefit using benzodiazepines.

Sleep Enuresis Bedwetting, like sleepwalking and night terrors, is another parasomnia that occurs during slow-wave sleep in the young. Before age 5 or 6, nocturnal enuresis should probably be considered a normal feature of development. The condition usually improves spontaneously at puberty, has a prevalence in late adolescence of 1 to 3%, and is rare in adulthood. The age threshold for initiation of treatment depends on parental and patient concern about the problem. Persistence of enuresis into adolescence or adulthood may reflect a variety of underlying conditions. In older patients with enuresis a distinction must be made between primary and secondary enuresis, the latter being defined as bedwetting in patients who have been fully continent for 6 to 12 months. Treatment of primary enuresis is reserved for patients of appropriate age (older than 5 or 6 years) and consists of bladder training exercises and behavioral therapy. Urologic abnormalities are more common in primary enuresis and must be assessed by urologic examination. Important causes of secondary enuresis include emotional disturbances, urinary tract infections or malformations, cauda equina lesions, epilepsy, sleep apnea, and certain medications. Symptomatic pharmacotherapy is usually accomplished with intranasal desmopressin, or oral oxybutynin chloride or imipramine.

Miscellaneous Parasomnias Other clinical entities fulfill the definition of a parasomnia in that they occur selectively during sleep and are associated with some degree of sleep disruption. Examples include *jactatio capitis nocturna* (nocturnal headbanging), sleep talking, nocturnal paroxysmal dystonia, and nocturnal leg cramps.

CIRCADIAN RHYTHM SLEEP DISORDERS

A subset of patients presenting with either insomnia or hypersomnia may have a disorder of sleep *timing* rather than sleep *generation*. Disorders of sleep timing can either be organic (i.e., due to an intrinsic defect in the circadian pacemaker or its input from entraining stimuli) or environmental (i.e., due to a disruption of exposure to entraining

stimuli from the environment). Regardless of etiology, the symptoms reflect the influence of the underlying circadian pacemaker on sleep-wake function. Thus, effective therapeutic approaches should aim to entrain the oscillator at an appropriate phase.

RAPID TIME-ZONE CHANGE (JET LAG) SYNDROME
More than 60 million people experience transmeridian air travel annually, which is often associated with excessive daytime sleepiness, sleep onset insomnia, and frequent arousals from sleep, particularly in the latter half of the night. Gastrointestinal discomfort is common. The syndrome is transient, typically lasting 2 to 14 d depending on the number of time zones crossed, the direction of travel, and the traveler's age and phase-shifting capacity. Travelers who spend more time outdoors reportedly adapt more quickly than those who remain in hotel rooms, presumably due to bright (outdoor) light exposure.

SHIFT-WORK SLEEP DISORDER More than 7 million workers in the United States regularly work at night, either on a permanent or rotating schedule. In addition, each week millions of Americans elect to remain awake at night to meet deadlines, drive long distances, or participate in recreational activities, leading to both sleep loss and misalignment of their circadian rhythms with respect to their sleep-wake cycle. Chronic shift workers have higher rates of cardiac, gastrointestinal, and reproductive disorders. Studies of regular night-shift workers indicate that the circadian timing system usually fails to adapt successfully to such inverted schedules. This leads to a misalignment between the desired work-rest schedule and the output of the pacemaker and in disturbed daytime sleep. Consequent sleep deprivation, increased length of time awake prior to work, and misalignment of circadian phase produce decreased alertness and performance, increased reaction time, and increased risk of performance lapses, thereby resulting in greater safety hazards among night workers and other sleep-deprived individuals.

Sleep onset is associated with marked attenuation in perception of both auditory and visual stimuli and lapses of consciousness. The sleepy individual may thus attempt to perform routine and familiar motor tasks during the transition state between wakefulness and sleep (stage 1 sleep) in the absence of adequate sensory input from the environment. Motor vehicle operators are especially vulnerable to sleep-related accidents since the sleep-deprived driver or operator often fails to heed the warning signs of fatigue. Such attempts to override the powerful biologic drive for sleep by the sheer force of will can yield a catastrophic outcome when sleep processes intrude involuntarily upon the waking brain. Such intrusions typically last only seconds but are known on occasion to persist for longer durations. These frequent brief intrusions of stage 1 sleep into behavioral wakefulness are a major component of the impaired psychomotor performance seen with sleepiness. Such intrusions and their associated performance lapses, which are preceded by a markedly increased subjective sense of sleepiness, will inevitably occur if the need for sleep is not satiated. There is a marked increase in the risk of sleep-related, fatal-to-the-driver highway crashes in the early morning and late afternoon hours, coincident with peaks in the daily rhythm of sleep tendency.

Safety programs should promote education about sleep and increase awareness of the hazards associated with night work and should be aimed at minimizing both circadian disruption and sleep deprivation. The work schedule should minimize: (1) exposure to night work, (2) the frequency of shift rotation so that shifts do not rotate more than once every 2 to 3 weeks, (3) the number of consecutive night shifts, and (4) the duration of night shifts. In fact, shift durations of greater than 18 h should be universally recognized as increasing the risk of sleep-related errors and performance lapses. Caffeine is undoubtedly the most widely used wake-promoting drug, but it cannot forestall sleep indefinitely and does not protect users from sleep-related performance lapses. Postural changes, exercise, and strategic placement of nap opportunities can sometimes temporarily reduce the risk of fatigue-related performance lapses. Properly timed exposure to bright light can facilitate rapid adaptation to night-shift work, where feasible. An adequate number of safe highway rest areas, shoulder rumble strips, and strict enforcement and compliance monitoring of hours-of-service policies are needed to reduce the risk of sleep-related transportation crashes. Such steps can lead to improvements in performance and to reduced accident rates both at work and on the roadways.

DELAYED SLEEP PHASE SYNDROME Delayed sleep phase syndrome is characterized by: (1) reported sleep onset and wake times intractably later than desired, (2) actual sleep times at nearly the same clock hours daily, and (3) essentially normal all-night polysomnography except for delayed sleep onset. Patients exhibit an abnormally delayed endogenous circadian phase, with the temperature minimum during the constant routine occurring later than normal. This delayed phase could be due to: (1) an abnormally long intrinsic period of the endogenous circadian pacemaker; (2) an abnormally reduced phase-advancing capacity of the pacemaker; or (3) an irregular prior sleep-wake schedule, characterized by frequent nights when the patient chooses to remain awake well past midnight (for social, school, or work reasons). In most cases, it is difficult to distinguish among these factors, since patients with an abnormally long intrinsic period are more likely to "choose" such late-night activities because they are unable to sleep at that time. Patients tend to be young adults. This self-perpetuating condition can persist for years and does not usually respond to attempts to reestablish normal bedtime hours.

Treatment methods involving bright-light phototherapy during the morning hours or melatonin administration in the evening hours show promise in these patients, although the relapse rate among such patients is very high.

ADVANCED SLEEP PHASE SYNDROME Advanced sleep phase syndrome is the converse of the delayed sleep phase syndrome and tends to occur in the elderly. Patients with this condition report excessive daytime sleepiness during the evening hours, when they have great difficulty remaining awake, even in social settings. The patients awaken from 3 to 5 A.M. each day, often several hours before their desired wake times. Although such patients have not been studied extensively, familial inheritance of this condition has been reported. Some of these patients may benefit from bright-light phototherapy during the evening hours, designed to reset the circadian pacemaker to a later hour.

NON-24-H SLEEP-WAKE DISORDER This condition can occur when the maximal phase-advancing capacity of the circadian pacemaker is not adequate to accommodate the difference between the 24-h geophysical day and the intrinsic period of the pacemaker in the patient. Alternatively, patients' self-selected exposure to artificial light may drive the circadian pacemaker to a longer than 24-h schedule. Affected patients are not able to maintain a stable phase relationship between the output of the pacemaker and the 24-h day. Such patients typically present with an incremental pattern of successive delays in sleep onsets and wake times, progressing in and out of phase with local time. When the patient's endogenous rhythms are out of phase with the local environment, insomnia coexists with excessive daytime sleepiness. Conversely, when the endogenous rhythms are in phase with the local environment, symptoms remit. The intervals between symptomatic periods may last several weeks to several months. Blind individuals unable to perceive light are particularly susceptible to this disorder. Melatonin administration has been reported to improve sleep, and in some cases even to induce synchronization of the circadian pacemaker.

MEDICAL IMPLICATIONS OF CIRCADIAN RHYTHMICITY Understanding the role of circadian rhythmicity in the pathophysiology of illness may lead to improvements in diagnosis and treatment. For example, prominent circadian variations have been reported in the incidence of *acute myocardial infarction*, *sudden cardiac death*, and *stroke*, the leading causes of death in the United States. Platelet aggregability is increased after arising in the early morning hours, coincident with the peak incidence of these cardiovascular events. A better understanding of the possible role of circadian rhythmicity in the acute destabilization of a chronic condition such as atherosclerotic disease could improve the understanding of the pathophysiology.

Diagnostic and therapeutic procedures may also be affected by the time of day at which data are collected. Examples include blood pressure, body temperature, the dexamethasone suppression test, and plasma cortisol levels. The timing of chemotherapy administration has been reported to have an effect on the outcome of treatment. Few physicians realize the extent to which routine measures are affected by the time (or sleep/wake state) when the measurement is made.

In addition, both the toxicity and effectiveness of drugs can vary during the day. For example, more than a fivefold difference has been observed in mortality rates following administration of toxic agents to experimental animals at different times of day. Anesthetic agents are particularly sensitive to time-of-day effects. Finally, the physician must be increasingly aware of the public health risks associated with the ever-increasing demands made by the duty-rest-recreation schedules in our round-the-clock society.

BIBLIOGRAPHY

ALDRICH MS: Diagnostic aspects of narcolepsy. Neurology 50:S2, 1998

CAJOCHEN C et al: EEG and ocular correlates of circadian melatonin phase and human performance decrements during sleep loss. Am J Physiol 277:R640, 1999

CHEMELLI RM et al: Narcolepsy in orexin knockout mice: Molecular genetics of sleep regulation. Cell 98:437, 1999

CHESSON A JR et al: Practice parameters for the evaluation of chronic insomnia. An American Academy of Sleep Medicine report. Standards of Practice Committee of the American Academy of Sleep Medicine. Sleep 23:237, 2000

CZEISLER CA et al: Exposure to bright light and darkness to treat physiologic maladaptation to night work. N Engl J Med 322:1253, 1990

——— et al: Stability, precision, and near-24-hour period of the human circadian pacemaker. Science 284:2177, 1999

DIJK D-J et al: Ageing and the circadian and homeostatic regulation of human sleep during forced desynchrony of rest, melatonin and temperature rhythms. J Physiol (Lond) 516:611, 1999

DUNLAP JC: Molecular bases for circadian clocks. Cell 96:271, 1999

FARNEY RJ, WALKER JM: Office management of common sleep-wake disorders. Med Clin North Am 79:391, 1995

FOGEL RB, WHITE DP: Obstructive sleep apnea. Adv Int Med 45:351, 2000

FRANKLIN KA et al: Sleep apnea and nocturnal angina. Lancet 345:1085, 1995

KRYGER MH et al (eds): *Principles and Practice of Sleep Medicine*, 3d ed. Philadelphia, Saunders, 2000

LIN L et al: The sleep disorder canine narcolepsy is caused by a mutation in the hypocretin (orexin) receptor 2 gene. Cell 98:365, 1999

MORIN CM et al: Behavioral and pharmacological therapies for late-life insomnia: A randomized controlled trial. JAMA 28:991, 1999

MONTPLAISIR J et al: Restless legs syndrome improved by pramipexole: A double-blind randomized trial. Neurology 52:938, 1999

OLSON EJ et al: Rapid eye movement sleep behavior disorder: Demographic, clinical and laboratory findings in 93 cases. Brain 123:331, 2000

REDLINE S, STROHL KP: Recognition and consequences of obstructive sleep apnea hypopnea syndrome. Clin Chest Med 19:1, 1998

SCHENCK CH, MAHOWALD MW: Long-term, nightly benzodiazepine treatment of injurious parasomnias and other disorders of disrupted nocturnal sleep in 170 adults. Am J Med 100:333, 1996

28 | *Jonathan C. Horton*

DISORDERS OF THE EYE

THE HUMAN VISUAL SYSTEM

The visual system provides a supremely efficient means for the rapid assimilation of information from the environment to aid in the guidance of behavior. The act of seeing begins with the capture of images focused by the cornea and lens upon a light-sensitive membrane in the back of the eye, called the *retina*. The retina is actually part of the brain, banished to the periphery to serve as a transducer for the conversion of patterns of light energy into neuronal signals. Light is absorbed by photopigment in two types of receptors: rods and cones. In the human retina there are 100 million rods and 5 million cones. The rods operate in dim (scotopic) illumination. The cones function under daylight (photopic) conditions. The cone system is specialized for color perception and high spatial resolution. The majority of cones are located within the macula, the portion of the retina serving the central 10° of vision. In the middle of the macula a small pit termed the *fovea*, packed exclusively with cones, provides best visual acuity.

Photoreceptors hyperpolarize in response to light, activating bipolar, amacrine, and horizontal cells in the inner nuclear layer. After processing of photoreceptor responses by this complex retinal circuit, the flow of sensory information ultimately converges upon a final common pathway: the ganglion cells. These cells translate the visual image impinging upon the retina into a continuously varying barrage of action potentials that propagates along the primary optic pathway to visual centers within the brain. There are a million ganglion cells in each retina, and hence a million fibers in each optic nerve.

Ganglion cell axons sweep along the inner surface of the retina in the nerve fiber layer, exit the eye at the optic disc, and travel through the optic nerve, optic chiasm, and optic tract to reach targets in the brain. The majority of fibers synapse upon cells in the lateral geniculate body, a thalamic relay station. Cells in the lateral geniculate body project in turn to the primary visual cortex. This massive afferent retinogeniculocortical sensory pathway provides the neural substrate for visual perception. Although the lateral geniculate body is the main target of the retina, separate classes of ganglion cells project to other subcortical visual nuclei involved in different functions. The pupillary reflex is mediated by input to the pretectal olivary nuclei in the midbrain. These pretectal nuclei send their output to the ipsilateral and contralateral Edinger-Westphal nuclei of the oculomotor nuclear complex. Cells in the Edinger-Westphal nuclei provide parasympathetic innervation to the iris sphincter via an interneuron in the ciliary ganglion. Circadian rhythms are timed by a retinal projection to the suprachiasmatic nucleus. Visual orientation and eye movements are served by retinal input to the superior colliculus. Gaze stabilization and optokinetic reflexes are governed by a group of small retinal targets known collectively as the *brainstem accessory optic system*. Finally, there is a sizeable retinal projection to the pulvinar, a large thalamic visual nucleus of obscure function.

The eyes must be rotated constantly within their orbits to place and maintain targets of visual interest upon the fovea. This activity, called *foveation*, or looking, is governed by an elaborate efferent motor system. Each eye is moved by six extraocular muscles, supplied by cranial nerves from the oculomotor (III), trochlear (IV), and abducens (VI) nuclei. Activity in these ocular motor nuclei is coordinated by pontine and midbrain mechanisms for smooth pursuit, saccades, and gaze stabilization during head and body movements. Large regions of the frontal and parietooccipital cortex control these brainstem eye movement centers by providing descending supranuclear input.

Visual function can be disturbed in myriad ways. The eyes are mounted in a prominent position on the head, where they are vulnerable to trauma, exposure, and infection. Vision can be damaged by diseases intrinsic to the eye, such as glaucoma, cataract, or retinal detachment. Many neurologic diseases produce ocular symptoms, because extensive areas of the cortex, thalamus, cerebellum, and brainstem are devoted to visual perception or to the execution of eye movements. In genetic disorders, eye manifestations are common and often help the clinician to recognize a rare syndrome. Finally, the eyes are affected frequently by acquired systemic diseases.

The eye is a specialized organ, requiring unique optical instruments for proper examination. The slit lamp and ophthalmoscope proffer a beautiful, magnified view of the transparent anatomy of the eye and afford the only opportunity for direct inspection of blood vessels in a living subject. Some physicians do not acquire sufficient facility with these instruments to care for patients with eye problems. This is regrettable, for although it may be determined that a patient requires referral to an ophthalmologist, the initial evaluation of ocular symptoms lies within the purview of all physicians, and the assessment of visual acuity, pupils, eye movements, visual fields, and the fundi remain part of any general physical examination.

CLINICAL ASSESSMENT OF VISUAL FUNCTION

REFRACTIVE STATE In approaching the patient with reduced vision, the first step is to decide whether refractive error is responsible. In *emmetropia*, parallel rays from infinity are focused perfectly upon the retina. Sadly, this condition is enjoyed by only a minority of the population. In *myopia*, the globe is too long, and light rays come to a focal point in front of the retina. Near objects can be seen clearly, but distant objects require a diverging lens in front of the eye. In *hyperopia*, the globe is too short, and hence a converging lens is used to supplement the refractive power of the eye. In *astigmatism*, the corneal surface is not perfectly spherical, necessitating a cylindrical corrective lens. In recent years it has become possible to correct refractive error with the excimer laser by performing either LASIK (laser in situ keratomileusis) or PRK (photorefractive keratectomy) to alter the curvature of the cornea.

With the onset of middle age, *presbyopia* develops as the lens within the eye becomes unable to increase its refractive power to accommodate upon near objects. To compensate for presbyopia, the emmetropic patient must use reading glasses. The patient already wearing glasses for distance correction usually switches to bifocals. The only exception is the myopic patient, who may achieve clear vision at near simply by removing glasses containing the distance prescription.

Refractive errors usually develop slowly and remain stable after adolescence, except in unusual circumstances. For example, the acute onset of diabetes mellitus can produce sudden myopia because of fluid imbibition and swelling of the lens induced by hyperglycemia. Testing vision through a pinhole aperture is a useful way to screen quickly for refractive error. If the visual acuity is better through a pinhole than with the unaided eye, the patient needs a refraction to obtain best corrected visual acuity.

VISUAL ACUITY The Snellen chart is used to test acuity at a distance of 6 m (20 ft). For convenience, a scale version of the Snellen chart, called the Rosenbaum card, is held at 36 cm (14 in) from the patient (Fig. 28-1). All subjects should be able to read the 6/6 m (20/20 ft) line with each eye using their refractive correction, if any. Patients who need reading glasses because of presbyopia must wear them for accurate testing with the Rosenbaum card. If 6/6 (20/20) acuity is

ROSENBAUM POCKET VISION SCREENER

	Point	Jaeger	distance equivalent
95			20/800
874			20/400
2843	26	16	20/200
638 EШƎ XOO	14	10	20/100
8745 ƎШШ OXO	10	7	20/70
63925 ШEƎ XOX	8	5	20/50
428365 ШEШ OXO	6	3	20/40
374258 ƎШƎ XXO	5	2	20/30
937826 ШmE XOO	4	1	20/25
428739 EШm OOX	3	1+	20/20

Card is held in good light 14 inches from eye. Record vision for each eye separately with and without glasses. Presbyopic patients should read thru bifocal segment. Check myopes with glasses only.

DESIGN COURTESY J. G. ROSENBAUM, M.D.

PUPIL GAUGE (mm.)

2 3 4 5 6 7 8 9

FIGURE 28-1 The Rosenbaum card is a miniature, scale version of the Snellen chart for testing visual acuity at near. When the visual acuity is recorded, the Snellen distance equivalent should bear a notation indicating that vision was tested at near, not at 6 m (20 ft), or else the Jaeger number system should be used to report the acuity.

An eye with no light perception has no pupillary response to direct light stimulation. If the retina or optic nerve is only partially injured, the direct pupillary response will be weaker than the consensual pupillary response evoked by shining a light into the other eye. This *relative afferent pupillary defect* (Marcus Gunn pupil) can be elicited with the swinging flashlight test (Fig. 28-2). It is an extremely useful sign in retrobulbar optic neuritis and other optic nerve diseases, where it may be the sole objective evidence for disease.

Subtle inequality in pupil size, up to 0.5 mm, is a fairly common finding in normal persons. The diagnosis of essential or physiologic anisocoria is secure as long as the relative pupil asymmetry remains constant as ambient lighting varies. Anisocoria that increases in dim light indicates a sympathetic paresis of the iris dilator muscle. The triad of miosis with ipsilateral ptosis and anhidrosis constitutes Horner's syndrome, although anhidrosis is an inconstant feature. Brainstem stroke, carotid dissection, or neoplasm impinging upon the sympathetic chain are occasionally identified as the cause of Horner's syndrome, but most of cases are idiopathic.

Anisocoria that increases in bright light suggests a parasympathetic palsy. The first concern is an oculomotor nerve paresis. This possibility is excluded if the eye movements are full and the patient has no ptosis or diplopia. Acute pupillary dilation (mydriasis) can occur from damage to the ciliary ganglion in the orbit. Common mechanisms are in-

FIGURE 28-2 The swinging flashlight test shows a relative afferent pupil defect (Marcus Gunn pupil) in the left eye. *A.* With the patient fixating on a distant target and background lighting dim, the pupils are equal and relatively large. *B.* Shining a flashlight into the right eye evokes equal, strong constriction of both pupils. *C.* Swinging the flashlight over to the damaged left eye causes dilation of both pupils, although they remain smaller than in *A.* Swinging the flashlight back over to the healthy right eye would result in symmetric constriction back to the appearance shown in *B.* Note that the pupils always remain equal; the damage to the left retina/optic nerve is revealed by weaker bilateral pupil constriction to a flashlight in the left eye compared with the right eye. *(From P Levatin, Arch Ophthalmol 62:768, 1959.)*

not present in each eye, the deficiency in vision must be explained. For acuity worse than 6/240 (20/800), the ability to count fingers, see hand motions, or perceive a bright light should be recorded. Legal blindness is defined by the Internal Revenue Service as a best corrected acuity of 6/60 (20/200) or less in the better eye, or a binocular visual field subtending 20° or less. For driving the laws vary by state, but most require a corrected acuity of 6/12 (20/40) in at least one eye. Patients with a homonymous hemianopia should not drive.

PUPILS The pupils should be tested individually in dim light with the patient fixating upon a distant target. If they respond briskly to light, there is no need to check the near response, because isolated loss of constriction (miosis) to accommodation does not occur. For this reason, the ubiquitous abbreviation PERRLA (pupils equal, round, and reactive to light and accommodation) implies a wasted effort with the last step. However, it is important to test the near response if the light response is poor or absent. Light-near dissociation occurs with neurosyphilis (Argyll Robertson pupil), lesions of the dorsal midbrain (obstructive hydrocephalus, pineal region tumors), and after aberrant regeneration (oculomotor nerve palsy, Adie's tonic pupil).

fection (herpes zoster, influenza), trauma (blunt, penetrating, surgical), or ischemia (diabetes, temporal arteritis). After denervation of the iris sphincter the pupil does not respond well to light, but the response to near is often relatively intact. When the near stimulus is removed, the pupil redilates very slowly compared with the normal pupil, hence the term *tonic pupil*. In Adie's syndrome, a tonic pupil occurs in conjunction with weak or absent tendon reflexes in the lower extremities. This benign disorder, which occurs predominantly in healthy young women, is assumed to represent a mild dysautonomia. Tonic pupils are also associated with Shy-Drager syndrome, segmental hypohidrosis, diabetes, and amyloidosis. Occasionally, a tonic pupil is discovered incidentally in an otherwise completely normal, asymptomatic individual. The diagnosis is confirmed by placing a drop of dilute (0.125%) pilocarpine into each eye. Denervation hypersensitivity produces pupillary constriction in a tonic pupil, whereas the normal pupil shows no response. Pharmacologic dilation from accidental or deliberate instillation of anticholinergic agents (atropine, scopolamine drops) into the eye can also produce pupillary mydriasis. In this situation, normal strength (1%) pilocarpine causes no constriction.

Both pupils are affected equally by systemic medications. They are small with narcotic use (morphine, heroin) and large with anticholinergics (scopolamine). Parasympathetic agents (pilocarpine, demecarium bromide) used to treat glaucoma produce miosis. In any patient with an unexplained pupillary abnormality, a slit-lamp examination is helpful to exclude surgical trauma to the iris, an occult foreign body, perforating injury, intraocular inflammation, adhesions (synechia), angle-closure glaucoma, and iris sphincter rupture from blunt trauma.

EYE MOVEMENTS AND ALIGNMENT   Eye movements are tested by asking the patient with both eyes open to pursue a small target such as a penlight into the cardinal fields of gaze. Normal ocular versions are smooth, symmetric, full, and maintained in all directions without nystagmus. Saccades, or quick refixation eye movements, are assessed by having the patient look back and forth between two stationary targets. The eyes should move rapidly and accurately in a single jump to their target. Ocular alignment can be judged by holding a penlight directly in front of the patient at about 1 m. If the eyes are straight, the corneal light reflex will be centered in the middle of each pupil. To test eye alignment more precisely, the cover test is useful. The patient is instructed to gaze upon a small fixation target in the distance. One eye is covered suddenly while observing the second eye. If the second eye shifts to fixate upon the target, it was misaligned. If it does not move, the first eye is uncovered and the test is repeated on the second eye. If neither eye moves, the eyes are aligned orthotropically. If the eyes are orthotropic in primary gaze but the patient complains of diplopia, the cover test should be performed with the head tilted or turned in whatever direction elicits the patient's diplopia. With practice the examiner can detect an ocular deviation (heterotropia) as small as 1 to 2° with the cover test. Deviations can be measured by placing prisms in front of the misaligned eye to determine the power required to neutralize the fixation shift evoked by covering the other eye.

STEREOPSIS   Stereoacuity is determined by presenting targets with retinal disparity separately to each eye using polarized images. The most popular office tests measure a range of thresholds from 800 to 40 seconds of arc. Normal stereoacuity is 40 seconds of arc. If a patient achieves this level of stereoacuity, one is assured that the eyes are aligned orthotropically and that vision is intact in each eye. Random dot stereograms have no monocular depth cues and provide an excellent screening test for strabismus and amblyopia in children.

COLOR VISION   The retina contains three classes of cones, with visual pigments of differing peak spectral sensitivity: red (560 nm), green (530 nm), and blue (430 nm). The red and green cone pigments are encoded on the X chromosome; the blue cone pigment on chromosome 7. Mutations of the blue cone pigment are exceedingly rare. Mutations of the red and green pigments cause congenital X-linked color blindness in 8% of males. Affected individuals are not truly color blind; rather, they differ from normal subjects in how they perceive color and how they combine primary monochromatic lights to match a given color. Anomalous trichromats have three cone types, but a mutation in one cone pigment (usually red or green) causes a shift in peak spectral sensitivity, altering the proportion of primary colors required to achieve a color match. Dichromats have only two cone types and will therefore accept a color match based upon only two primary colors. Anomalous trichromats and dichromats have 6/6 (20/20) visual acuity, but their hue discrimination is impaired. Ishihara color plates can be used to detect red-green color blindness. The test plates contain a hidden number, visible only to subjects with color confusion from red-green color blindness. Because color blindness is almost exclusively X-linked, it is worth screening only male children.

The Ishihara plates are often used to detect acquired defects in color vision, although they are intended as a screening test for congenital color blindness. Acquired defects in color vision frequently result from disease of the macula or optic nerve. For example, patients with a history of optic neuritis often complain of color desaturation long after their visual acuity has returned to normal. Color blindness can also occur from bilateral strokes involving the ventral portion of the occipital lobe (cerebral achromatopsia). Such patients can perceive only shades of gray and may also have difficulty recognizing faces (prosopagnosia). Infarcts of the dominant occipital lobe sometimes give rise to color anomia. Affected patients can discriminate colors, but they cannot name them.

VISUAL FIELDS   Vision can be impaired by damage to the visual system anywhere from the eyes to the occipital lobes. One can localize the site of the lesion with considerable accuracy by mapping the visual field deficit by finger confrontation and then correlating it with the topographic anatomy of the visual pathway (Fig. 28-3). More quantitative data can be obtained by formal perimetric examination of the visual fields. In kinetic perimetry, the patient faces a tangent screen or a hemispheric bowl (Goldmann perimeter) while the examiner moves a small light target from the periphery towards the center. Such manual techniques have largely been supplanted by computer-driven perimeters (Humphrey, Octopus) that present a target of variable intensity at fixed positions in the visual field (Fig. 28-3A). By generating an automated printout of light thresholds, these static perimeters provide a sensitive means of detecting scotomas in the visual field. They are also useful for serial assessment of visual function in chronic diseases such as glaucoma or pseudotumor cerebri.

The crux of visual field analysis is to decide whether a lesion is before, at, or behind the optic chiasm. If a scotoma is confined to one eye, it must be due to a lesion anterior to the chiasm, involving either the optic nerve or retina. Retinal lesions produce scotomas that correspond optically to their location in the fundus. For example, a superior-nasal retinal detachment results in an inferior-temporal field cut. Damage to the macula causes a central scotoma (Fig. 28-3B).

Optic nerve disease produces characteristic patterns of visual field loss. Glaucoma selectively destroys axons that enter the superotemporal or inferotemporal poles of the optic disc, resulting in arcuate scotomas shaped like a Turkish scimitar, which emanate from the blind spot and curve around fixation to end flat against the horizontal meridian (Fig. 28-3C). This type of field defect mirrors the arrangement of the nerve fiber layer in the temporal retina. The superb acuity of humans is achieved by thrusting aside all retinal elements at the fovea except photoreceptors, to minimize absorption and scattering of light. To avoid passing over the fovea, axons from cells in the temporal retina must follow an indirect course arching around the fovea to reach the optic disc. Arcuate or nerve fiber layer scotomas also occur from optic neuritis, ischemic optic neuropathy, optic disc drusen, and branch retinal artery or vein occlusion.

Damage to the entire upper or lower pole of the optic disc causes an altitudinal field cut that follows the horizontal meridian (Fig. 28-3D). This pattern of visual field loss is typical of ischemic optic

Monocular Prechiasmal Field Defects:

A — Normal Field Right Eye (blind spot) — 30°
B — Central Scotoma — 30°
C — Nerve-Fiber Bundle (Arcuate) Scotoma — 30°
D — Altitudinal Scotoma — 30°
E — Ceco-central Scotoma — 30°
F — Enlarged Blind-Spot with Peripheral Constriction — 30°

Binocular Chiasmal or Postchiasmal Field Defects:

(Left eye) (Right eye)

G — Junctional Scotoma — 30°
H — Bitemporal Hemianopia — 30°
I — Homonymous Hemianopia — 30°
J — Superior Quadrantanopia — 30°
K — Inferior Quadrantanopia — 30°
L — Homonymous Hemianopia with Macular Sparing — 30°

Right   Left

Optic Nerve
Optic Chiasm
Optic Tract
Lateral Geniculate Body
Optic Radiations
Primary Visual Cortex

FIGURE 28-3 Ventral view of the brain, correlating patterns of visual field loss with the sites of lesions in the visual pathway. The visual fields overlap partially, creating 120° of central binocular field flanked by a 40° monocular crescent on either side. The visual field maps in this figure were done with a computer-driven perimeter (Humphrey Instruments, Carl Zeiss, Inc.). It plots the retinal sensitivity to light in the central 30° using a gray scale format. Areas of visual field loss are shown in black. The examples of common monocular, prechiasmal field defects are all shown for the right eye. By convention, the visual fields are always recorded with the left eye's field on the left, and the right eye's field on the right, just as the patient sees the world.

neuropathy but also occurs from retinal vascular occlusion, advanced glaucoma, and optic neuritis.

About half the fibers in the optic nerve originate from ganglion cells serving the macula. Damage to papillomacular fibers causes a cecocentral scotoma encompassing the blind spot and macula (Fig. 28-3E). If the damage is irreversible, pallor eventually appears in the temporal portion of the optic disc. Temporal pallor from a cecocentral scotoma may develop in optic neuritis, nutritional optic neuropathy,

A **B**

FIGURE 28-4 Pituitary adenoma: Coronal precontrast (*A*) and postcontrast (*B*) T1-weighted MRI through the sella turcica shows a large tumor (T) arising from the pituitary fossa. The optic chiasm (*black arrows*) is elevated and compressed, producing a visual field defect resembling that shown in Fig. 28-3*H*. There is peripheral enhancement around the mass due to displaced normal pituitary tissue (*white arrows*) and heterogeneous enhancement of the mass itself. The patient presented with decreased vision in both eyes of several years duration and optic pallor.

toxic optic neuropathy, Leber's hereditary optic neuropathy, and compressive optic neuropathy. It is worth mentioning that the temporal side of the optic disc is slightly more pale than the nasal side in most normal individuals. Therefore, it can sometimes be difficult to decide whether the temporal pallor visible on fundus examination represents a pathologic change. Pallor of the nasal rim of the optic disc is a less equivocal sign of optic atrophy.

At the optic chiasm, fibers from nasal ganglion cells decussate into the contralateral optic tract. Crossed fibers are damaged more by compression than uncrossed fibers. As a result, mass lesions of the sellar region cause a temporal hemianopia in each eye. Tumors anterior to the optic chiasm, such as meningiomas of the tuberculum sella, produce a junctional scotoma characterized by an optic neuropathy in one eye and a superior temporal field cut in the other eye (Fig. 28-3*G*). More symmetric compression of the optic chiasm by a pituitary adenoma (Fig. 28-4), meningioma, craniopharyngioma, glioma, or aneurysm results in a bitemporal hemianopia (Fig. 28-3*H*). The insidious development of a bitemporal hemianopia often goes unnoticed by the patient and will escape detection by the physician unless each eye is tested separately.

It is difficult to localize a postchiasmal lesion accurately, because injury anywhere in the optic tract, lateral geniculate body, optic radiations, or visual cortex can produce a homonymous hemianopia, i.e., a temporal hemifield defect in the contralateral eye and a matching nasal hemifield defect in the ipsilateral eye (Fig. 28-3*I*). A unilateral postchiasmal lesion leaves the visual acuity in each eye unaffected, although the patient may read the letters on only the left or right half of the eye chart. Lesions of the optic radiations tend to cause poorly matched or incongruous field defects in each eye. Damage to the optic radiations in the temporal lobe (Meyer's loop) produces a superior quadrantic homonymous hemianopia (Fig. 28-3*J*), whereas injury to the optic radiations in the parietal lobe results in an inferior quadrantic homonymous hemianopia (Fig. 28-3*K*). Lesions of the primary visual cortex give rise to dense, congruous hemianopic field defects. Occlusion of the posterior cerebral artery supplying the occipital lobe is a frequent cause of total homonymous hemianopia. Some patients with hemianopia after occipital stroke have macular sparing, because the macular representation at the tip of the occipital lobe is supplied by collaterals from the middle cerebral artery (Fig. 28-3*L*). Destruction of both occipital lobes produces cortical blindness. This condition can be distinguished from bilateral prechiasmal visual loss by noting that the pupil responses and optic fundi remain normal.

Corneal Abrasions These are seen best by placing a drop of fluorescein in the eye and looking with the slit lamp using a cobalt-blue light. A penlight with a blue filter will suffice if no slit lamp is available. Damage to the corneal epithelium is revealed by yellow fluorescence of the exposed basement membrane underlying the epithelium. It is important to check for foreign bodies. To search the conjunctival fornices, the lower lid should be pulled down and the upper lid everted. A foreign body can be removed with a moistened cotton-tipped applicator after placing a drop of topical anesthetic, such as proparacaine, in the eye. Alternatively, it may be possible to flush the foreign body from the eye by irrigating copiously with saline or artificial tears. If the corneal epithelium has been abraded, antibiotic ointment and a patch should be applied to the eye. A drop of an intermediate-acting cycloplegic, such as cyclopentolate hydrochloride 1%, helps to reduce pain by relaxing the ciliary body. The eye should be reexamined the next day. Minor abrasions may not require patching and cycloplegia.

Subconjunctival Hemorrhage This results from rupture of small vessels bridging the potential space between the episclera and conjunctiva. Blood dissecting into this space can produce a spectacular red eye, but vision is not affected and the hemorrhage resolves without treatment. Subconjunctival hemorrhage is usually spontaneous but can occur from blunt trauma, eye rubbing, or vigorous coughing. Occasionally it is a clue to an underlying bleeding disorder.

Pinguecula This is a small, raised conjunctival nodule at the temporal or nasal limbus. In adults such lesions are extremely common and have little significance, unless they become inflamed (pinguecu-litis). A *pterygium* resembles a pinguecula but has crossed the limbus to encroach upon the corneal surface. Removal is justified when symptoms of irritation or blurring develop, but recurrence is a common problem.

Blepharitis This refers to inflammation of the eyelids. The most common form occurs in association with acne rosacea or seborrheic dermatitis. The eyelid margins are usually colonized heavily by staphylococcus. Upon close inspection, they appear greasy, ulcerated, and crusted with scaling debris that clings to the lashes. Treatment consists of warm compresses, strict eyelid hygiene, and topical antibiotics such as erythromycin. An external *hordeolum* (sty) is caused by staphylococcal infection of the superficial accessory glands of Zeis or Moll located in the eyelid margins. An internal hordeolum occurs after suppurative infection of the oil-secreting meibomian glands within the tarsal plate of the eyelid. Systemic antibiotics, usually tetracyclines, are sometimes necessary for treatment of meibomian gland inflammation (meibomitis) or chronic, severe blepharitis. A *chalazion* is a painless, granulomatous inflammation of a meibomian gland that produces a pealike nodule within the eyelid. It can be incised and drained, or injected with glucocorticoids. Basal cell, squamous cell, or meibomian gland carcinoma should be suspected for any nonhealing, ulcerative lesion of the eyelids.

Dacrocystitis An inflammation of the lacrimal drainage system, this can produce epiphora (tearing) and ocular injection. Gentle pressure over the lacrimal sac evokes pain and reflux of mucus or pus from the tear puncta. Dacrocystitis usually occurs after obstruction of the lacrimal system. It is treated with topical and systemic antibiotics, followed by probing or surgery to reestablish patency. *Entropion* (inversion of the eyelid) or *ectropion* (sagging or eversion of the eyelid) can also lead to epiphora and ocular irritation.

Conjunctivitis This is the most common cause of a red, irritated eye. Pain is minimal, and the visual acuity is reduced only slightly. The most common viral etiology is adenovirus infection. It causes a watery discharge, mild foreign-body sensation, and photophobia. Bacterial infection tends to produce a more mucopurulent exudate. Mild cases of infectious conjunctivitis are usually treated empirically with broad-spectrum topical ocular antibiotics, such as sulfacetamide 10%, polymixin-bacitracin-neomycin, or trimethoprim-polymixin combination. Smears and cultures are usually reserved for severe, resistant, or recurrent cases of conjunctivitis. To prevent contagion, patients should be admonished to wash their hands frequently, not to touch their eyes, and to avoid direct contact with others.

Allergic Conjunctivitis This condition is extremely common and often mistaken for infectious conjunctivitis. Three forms of allergic conjunctivitis are recognized, with closely overlapping manifestations. *Hay fever conjunctivitis* has a seasonal incidence, related to the release of airborne antigens into the air by plants. IgE-mediated activation of mast cells in the conjunctiva causes itching, redness, and edema. *Vernal conjunctivitis* is also seasonal, becoming worse during warm months. It affects exclusively children or adolescents and is more common in boys. The cause is unknown, but airborne antigens are thought to trigger symptoms. Itching, photophobia, epiphora, and mucous discharge are typical. The palpebral conjunctiva may become hypertropic with giant excrescences called cobblestone papillae. Irritation from contact lenses or any chronic foreign body can also induce formation of cobblestone papillae. *Atopic conjunctivitis* occurs in subjects with atopic dermatitis or asthma. Symptoms caused by allergic conjunctivitis can be alleviated with cold compresses, topical vasoconstrictors, antihistamines, and mast-cell stabilizers such as cromolyn sodium. Topical glucocorticoid solutions provide dramatic relief of immune-mediated forms of conjunctivitis, but their long-term use is ill-advised because of the complications of glaucoma, cataract, and secondary infection. Topical nonsteroidal anti-inflammatory agents (NSAIDs) such as ketorolac tromethamine are a better alternative.

Keratoconjunctivitis Sicca Also known as dry eye, it produces a burning, foreign-body sensation, injection, and photophobia. In mild cases the eye appears surprisingly normal, but tear production measured by wetting of a filter paper (Schirmer strip) is deficient. A variety of systemic drugs, including antihistaminic, anticholinergic, and psychotropic medications, result in dry eye by reducing lacrimal secretion. Disorders that involve the lacrimal gland directly, such as sarcoidosis or Sjögren's syndrome, also cause dry eye. Patients may develop dry eye after radiation therapy if the treatment field includes the orbits. Problems with ocular drying are also common after lesions affecting cranial nerves V or VII. Corneal anesthesia is particularly dangerous, because the absence of a normal blink reflex exposes the cornea to injury without pain to warn the patient. Dry eye is managed by frequent and liberal application of artificial tears and ocular lubricants. In severe cases the tear puncta can be plugged or cauterized to reduce lacrimal outflow.

Keratitis This is a threat to vision because of the risk of corneal clouding, scarring, and perforation. Worldwide, the two leading causes of blindness from keratitis are trachoma from chlamydial infection and vitamin A deficiency related to malnutrition. In the United States, contact lenses play a major role in corneal infection and ulceration. They should not be worn by anyone with an active eye infection. In evaluating the cornea, it is important to differentiate between a superficial infection (*keratoconjunctivitis*) and a deeper, more serious ulcerative process. The latter is accompanied by greater visual loss, pain, photophobia, redness, and discharge. Slit-lamp examination shows disruption of the corneal epithelium, a cloudy infiltrate or abscess in the stroma, and an inflammatory cellular reaction in the anterior chamber. In severe cases, pus settles at the bottom of the anterior chamber, giving rise to a hypopyon. Immediate empirical antibiotic therapy should be initiated after corneal scrapings are obtained for Gram's stain, Giemsa stain, and cultures. Fortified topical antibiotics are most effective, supplemented with subconjunctival antibiotics as required. The most frequent bacterial pathogens are *Staphylococcus*, *Strepto-*

coccus (particularly *S. pneumoniae*), *Pseudomonas*, Enterobacteriaceae, *Haemophilus*, and *Neisseria*. For *Neisseria*, systemic antibiotics should be given in addition to topical antibiotics to eliminate systemic infection. A fungal etiology should always be considered in the patient with keratitis. Fungal infection is common in warm humid climates, especially after penetration of the cornea by plant or vegetable material.

Herpes Simplex The *herpes viruses* are a major cause of blindness from keratitis. Most adults in the United States have serum antibodies to herpes simplex, indicating prior viral infection (Chap. 182). Primary ocular infection is generally caused by herpes simplex type 1, rather than type 2. It manifests as a unilateral follicular blepharoconjunctivitis, easily confused with adenoviral conjunctivitis unless telltale vesicles appear on the periocular skin or conjunctiva. A dendritic pattern of corneal epithelial ulceration revealed by fluorescein staining is pathognomonic for herpes infection but is seen in only a minority of primary infections. Recurrent ocular infection arises from reactivation of the latent herpes virus. Viral eruption in the corneal epithelium may result in the characteristic herpes dendrite. Involvement of the corneal stroma produces edema, vascularization, and iridocyclitis. Herpes keratitis is treated with topical antiviral agents, cycloplegics, and oral acyclovir. Topical glucocorticoids are effective in mitigating corneal scarring but must be used with extreme caution because of the danger of corneal melting and perforation. Topical glucocorticoids also carry the risk of prolonging infection and inducing glaucoma.

Herpes Zoster Herpes zoster from reactivation of latent varicella (chickenpox) virus causes a dermatomal pattern of painful vesicular dermatitis. Ocular symptoms can occur after zoster eruption in any branch of the trigeminal nerve but are particularly common when vesicles form on the nose, reflecting nasociliary (V1) nerve involvement (Hutchinson's sign). Herpes zoster ophthalmicus produces corneal dendrites, which can be difficult to distinguish from those seen in herpes simplex. Stromal keratitis, anterior uveitis, raised intraocular pressure, ocular motor nerve palsies, acute retinal necrosis, and postherpetic scarring and neuralgia are other common sequelae. Herpes zoster ophthalmicus is treated with antiviral agents and cycloplegics. In severe cases, glucocorticoids may be added to prevent permanent visual loss from corneal scarring.

Episcleritis This is an inflammation of the episclera, a thin layer of connective tissue between the conjunctiva and sclera. Episcleritis resembles conjunctivitis but is a more localized process and discharge is absent. Most cases of episcleritis are idiopathic, but some occur in the setting of an autoimmune disease. *Scleritis* refers to a deeper, more severe inflammatory process, frequently associated with a connective tissue disease such as rheumatoid arthritis, lupus erythematosus, polyarteritis nodosa, Wegener's granulomatosis, or relapsing polychondritis. The inflammation and thickening of the sclera can be diffuse or nodular. In anterior forms of scleritis, the globe assumes a violet hue and the patient complains of severe ocular tenderness and pain. With posterior scleritis the pain and redness may be less marked, but there is often proptosis, choroidal effusion, reduced motility, and visual loss. Episcleritis and scleritis should be treated with NSAIDs. If these agents fail, topical or even systemic glucocorticoid therapy may be necessary, especially if an underlying autoimmune process is active.

Uveitis Involving the anterior structures of the eye, this is called *iritis* or *iridocyclitis*. The diagnosis requires slit-lamp examination to identify inflammatory cells floating in the aqueous humor or deposited upon the corneal endothelium (keratic precipitates). Anterior uveitis develops in sarcoidosis, ankylosing spondylitis, juvenile rheumatoid arthritis, inflammatory bowel disease, psoriasis, Reiter's syndrome, and Behçet's disease. It is also associated with herpes infections, syphilis, Lyme disease, onchocerciasis, tuberculosis, and leprosy. Although anterior uveitis can occur in conjunction with many diseases, no cause is found to explain the majority of cases. For this reason, laboratory evaluation is usually reserved for patients with recurrent or severe anterior uveitis. Treatment is aimed at reducing inflammation and scarring by judicious use of topical glucocorticoids. Dilation of the pupil reduces pain and prevents the formation of synechiae.

Posterior Uveitis This is diagnosed by observing inflammation of the vitreous, retina, or choroid on fundus examination. It is more likely than anterior uveitis to be associated with an identifiable systemic disease. Some patients have panuveitis, or inflammation of both the anterior and posterior segments of the eye. Posterior uveitis is a manifestation of autoimmune diseases such as sarcoidosis, Behçet's disease, Vogt-Koyanagi-Harada syndrome, and inflammatory bowel disease (**see Plate IV-1**). It also accompanies diseases such as toxoplasmosis, onchocerciasis, cysticercosis, coccidioidomycosis, toxocariasis, and histoplasmosis; infections caused by organisms such as *Candida*, *Pneumocystis carinii*, *Cryptococcus*, *Aspergillus*, herpes, and cytomegalovirus (**see Plate IV-2**); and other diseases such as syphilis, Lyme disease, tuberculosis, cat-scratch disease, Whipple's disease, and brucellosis. In multiple sclerosis, chronic inflammatory changes can develop in the extreme periphery of the retina (pars planitis or intermediate uveitis).

Acute Angle-Closure Glaucoma This is a rare and frequently misdiagnosed cause of a red, painful eye. Susceptible eyes have a shallow anterior chamber, either because the eye has a short axial length (hyperopia) or a lens enlarged by the gradual development of cataract. When the pupil becomes mid-dilated, the peripheral iris blocks aqueous outflow via the anterior chamber angle and the intraocular pressure rises abruptly, producing pain, injection, corneal edema, obscurations, and blurred vision. In some patients, ocular symptoms are overshadowed by nausea, vomiting, or headache, prompting a fruitless workup for abdominal or neurologic disease. The diagnosis is made by measuring the intraocular pressure during an acute attack or by performing gonioscopy to reveal the narrowed chamber angle by means of a specially mirrored contact lens. Acute angle closure is treated with oral or intravenous acetazolamide, topical beta blockers, apraclonidine, and pilocarpine to induce miosis. If these measures fail, a laser can be used to create a hole in the peripheral iris to relieve pupillary block. Many physicians are reluctant to dilate patients routinely for fundus examination because they fear precipitating an angle-closure glaucoma. The risk is actually remote and more than outweighed by the potential benefit to patients of discovering a hidden fundus lesion visible only through a fully dilated pupil. Moreover, a single attack of angle closure after pharmacologic dilation rarely causes any permanent damage to the eye and serves as an inadvertent provocative test to identify patients with narrow angles who would benefit from prophylactic laser iridectomy.

Endophthalmitis This occurs from bacterial, viral, fungal, or parasitic infection of the internal structures of the eye. It is usually acquired by hematogenous seeding from a remote site. Chronically ill, diabetic, or immunosuppressed patients, especially those with a history of indwelling intravenous catheters or positive blood cultures, are at greatest risk for endogenous endophthalmitis. Although most patients have ocular pain and injection, visual loss is sometimes the only symptom. Septic emboli, from a diseased heart valve or a dental abscess, that lodge in the retinal circulation can give rise to endophthalmitis. White-centered retinal hemorrhages (Roth's spots) are considered pathognomonic for subacute bacterial endocarditis, but they also appear in leukemia, diabetes, and many other conditions. Endophthalmitis also occurs as a complication of ocular surgery, occasionally months or even years after the operation. An occult penetrating foreign body or unrecognized trauma to the globe should be considered in any patient with unexplained intraocular infection or inflammation.

TRANSIENT OR SUDDEN VISUAL LOSS

Amaurosis Fugax This term refers to a transient ischemic attack of the retina. Because neural tissue has a high rate of metabolism, interruption of blood flow to the retina for more than a few seconds results in *transient monocular blindness*, a term used interchangeably with amaurosis fugax. Patients describe a rapid fading of vision like a curtain descending, sometimes affecting only a portion of the visual field. Amaurosis fugax usually occurs from an embolus that becomes stuck within a retinal arteriole (**see Plate IV-3**). If the embolus breaks up or passes, flow is restored and vision returns quickly to normal without permanent damage. With prolonged interruption of blood flow, the inner retina suffers infarction. Ophthalmoscopy reveals zones of whitened, edematous retina following the distribution of branch retinal arterioles. Complete occlusion of the central retinal artery produces arrest of blood flow and a milky retina with a cherry-red fovea (**see Plate IV-4**). Emboli are composed of either cholesterol (Hollenhorst plaque), calcium, or platelet-fibrin debris. The most common source is an atherosclerotic plaque in the carotid artery or aorta, although emboli can also arise from the heart, especially in patients with diseased valves, atrial fibrillation, or wall motion abnormalities.

In rare instances, amaurosis fugax occurs from low central retinal artery perfusion pressure in a patient with a critical stenosis of the ipsilateral carotid artery and poor collateral flow via the circle of Willis. In this situation, amaurosis fugax develops when there is a dip in systemic blood pressure or a slight worsening of the carotid stenosis. Sometimes there is contralateral motor or sensory loss, indicating concomitant hemispheric cerebral ischemia.

Retinal arterial occlusion also occurs rarely in association with retinal migraine, lupus erythematosus, anticardiolipin antibodies (**see Plate IV-4**), anticoagulant deficiency states (protein S, protein C, and antithrombin III deficiency), pregnancy, intravenous drug abuse, blood dyscrasias, dysproteinemias, and temporal arteritis.

Amaurosis fugax warns of a patient at high risk for stroke. The carotid arteries should be studied by ultrasound. Endarterectomy for a stenosis of ≥60%, even in asymptomatic patients, has been shown to reduce the subsequent rate of ipsilateral stroke (Chap. 361). Therapy with aspirin, warfarin, or other anticoagulants is appropriate in selected patients. If no carotid lesion is found, cardiac ultrasound should be performed. Ambulatory electrocardiographic monitoring may reveal that intermittent atrial fibrillation is giving rise to emboli.

Marked *systemic hypertension* causes sclerosis of retinal arterioles, splinter hemorrhages, focal infarcts of the nerve fiber layer (cotton-wool spots), and leakage of lipid and fluid (hard exudate) into the macula (**see Plate IV-5**). In hypertensive crisis, sudden visual loss can result from vasospasm of retinal arterioles and consequent retinal ischemia. In addition, acute hypertension may produce visual loss from ischemic swelling of the optic disc. Patients with acute hypertensive retinopathy should be treated by lowering the blood pressure. However, the blood pressure should not be reduced precipitously, because there is a danger of optic disc infarction from sudden hypoperfusion.

Impending *branch* or *central retinal vein occlusion* can produce prolonged visual obscurations that resemble those described by patients with amaurosis fugax. The veins appear engorged and phlebitic, with numerous retinal hemorrhages (**see Plate IV-6**). In some patients, venous blood flow recovers spontaneously, while others evolve a frank obstruction with extensive retinal bleeding ("blood and thunder" appearance), infarction, and visual loss. Venous occlusion of the retina is often idiopathic, but hypertension, diabetes, and glaucoma are prominent risk factors. The benefit of treatment with anticoagulants is unproven and carries the risk of hemorrhage into the vitreous. Polycythemia, thrombocythemia, or other factors leading to an underlying hypercoagulable state should be corrected.

Anterior Ischemic Optic Neuropathy (AION) This is caused by insufficient blood flow through the posterior ciliary arteries supplying the optic disc. It produces sudden, painless, monocular visual loss, although patients occasionally report premonitory obscurations. The optic disc appears swollen and surrounded by nerve fiber layer splinter hemorrhages (**see Plate IV-7**). AION is divided into two forms: arteritic and nonarteritic. The nonarteritic form of AION is most common. No specific cause can be identified, although diabetes and hypertension are frequent risk factors. No treatment is available. About

5% of patients, especially those over age 60, develop the arteritic form of AION in conjunction with giant cell (temporal) arteritis (Chap. 317). It is urgent to recognize arteritic AION so that high doses of glucocorticoids can be instituted immediately to prevent blindness in the second eye. Symptoms of polymyalgia rheumatica may be present, and the sedimentation rate is usually elevated. In a patient with visual loss from suspected arteritic AION, temporal artery biopsy is helpful to confirm the diagnosis, but glucocorticoids should be started without waiting for the biopsy to be completed. The diagnosis of arteritic AION is difficult to sustain in the face of a normal sedimentation rate and a negative temporal artery biopsy, but such cases do occur rarely.

Posterior Ischemic Optic Neuropathy This is an infrequent cause of acute visual loss. It is induced by the combination of severe anemia and hypotension, causing infarction of the retrobulbar optic nerve. Cases have been reported after major blood loss during surgery, exsanguinating trauma, gastrointestinal bleeding, and renal dialysis. The fundus usually appears normal, although optic disc swelling develops if the process extends far enough anteriorly. Vision can be salvaged in some patients by prompt blood transfusion and reversal of hypotension.

Optic Neuritis This is a common inflammatory disease of the optic nerve. In the Optic Neuritis Treatment Trial (ONTT), the mean age of patients was 32 years, 77% were female, 92% had ocular pain (especially with eye movements), and 35% had optic disc swelling. In most patients, the demyelinating event was retrobulbar and the ocular fundus appeared normal on initial examination (see Plate IV-8), although optic disc pallor slowly developed over subsequent months.

Virtually all patients experience a gradual recovery of vision after a single episode of optic neuritis, even without treatment. This rule is so reliable that failure of vision to improve considerably after a first attack of optic neuritis casts doubt upon the original diagnosis. Treatment of optic neuritis is controversial because the favorable prognosis for visual recovery has made it difficult to demonstrate any benefit from glucocorticoids. The ONTT showed that patients treated with a conventional dose of oral glucocorticoids (prednisone, 1 mg/kg per day for 14 days) did no better than patients treated with a placebo. A recent Danish trial of oral high-dose methylprednisolone (500 mg daily for 5 days, followed by a 10-day taper) reported a slight response at 1 and 3 weeks but none at 8 weeks. From these studies, it is apparent that oral glucocorticoids have little to offer in the treatment of optic neuritis. According to the ONTT, even high-dose intravenous methylprednisolone (250 mg every 6 h for 3 days) followed by oral prednisone (1 mg/kg per day for 11 days) makes no difference in final acuity (measured 6 months after the attack), although the recovery of visual function occurs more rapidly.

For some patients, optic neuritis remains an isolated event. However, the ONTT showed that the 5-year cumulative probability of developing clinically definite multiple sclerosis following optic neuritis is 30%. Remarkably, intravenous glucocorticoids were associated with a reduced rate of development of multiple sclerosis over a 2-year follow-up period, especially in the subgroup of patients with multiple foci of demyelination on their magnetic resonance (MR) scan. However, by the end of a 3-year follow-up period, patients treated with intravenous glucocorticoids versus placebo showed no difference in the rate of multiple sclerosis. Moreover, intravenous glucocorticoids did not reduce the likelihood of subsequent attacks of optic neuritis. To summarize, the organizers of the ONTT recommend an MR scan in patients with optic neuritis. If two or more foci of demyelination are found or visual loss is severe, they suggest treatment with intravenous glucocorticoids. The potential benefits of intravenous glucocorticoids are: (1) a slightly faster recovery of visual function, and (2) a potential reduction in the risk of subsequent neurologic events that would signify multiple sclerosis. Critics of the ONTT have questioned these recommendations, pointing out that: (1) visual outcome is the same in the long run, (2) evidence indicating a reduced risk of eventual multiple sclerosis with intravenous glucocorticoid treatment is based upon follow-up data in a rather small number of patients, and (3) the protection against multiple sclerosis is transient, and no longer apparent beyond 2 years of follow-up. In cases of unilateral optic neuritis, the decision whether to obtain an MR scan or to treat with intravenous glucocorticoids should be based upon clinical judgment and careful discussion with the patient. In cases of bilateral, simultaneous optic neuritis, the rationale for intravenous glucocorticoids is stronger.

Leber's Hereditary Optic Neuropathy This is a disease of young men, characterized by onset over a few weeks of painless, severe, central visual loss in one eye, followed weeks or months later by the same process in the other eye. Acutely, the optic disc appears mildly plethoric with surface capillary telangiectases, but no vascular leakage on fluorescein angiography. Eventually optic atrophy ensues. There is no treatment. Leber's optic neuropathy is caused by a point mutation at codon 11778 in the mitochondrial gene encoding nicotinamide adenine dinucleotide dehydrogenase (NADH) subunit 4. Subsequently, additional mutations responsible for the disease have been identified, most in mitochondrial genes encoding proteins involved in electron transport. Mitochrondrial mutations causing Leber's neuropathy are inherited from the mother by all her children, but usually only sons develop symptoms. This curious male predilection is a mystery.

Toxic Optic Neuropathy This can result in acute visual loss with bilateral optic disc swelling and central or cecocentral scotomas. Such cases have been reported to result from exposure to ethambutol, methyl alcohol (moonshine), ethylene glycol (antifreeze), or carbon monoxide. In toxic optic neuropathy, visual loss can also develop gradually and produce optic atrophy without a phase of acute optic disc edema (see Plate IV-9). Many agents have been implicated as a cause of toxic optic neuropathy, but the evidence supporting the association for many is weak. The following is a partial list of potential offending drugs or toxins: disulfiram, ethchlorvynol, chloramphenicol, amiodarone, monoclonal anti-CD3 antibody, ciprofloxacin, digitalis, streptomycin, lead, arsenic, thallium, D-penicillamine, isoniazid, emetine, and sulfonamides. Deficiency states, induced either by starvation, malabsorption, or alcoholism, can lead to insidious visual loss. Thiamine, vitamin B_{12}, and folate levels should be checked in any patient with unexplained, bilateral central scotomas and optic pallor.

Papilledema This connotes bilateral optic disc swelling from raised intracranial pressure (see Plate IV-10). Headache is a frequent, but not invariable, accompaniment. All other forms of optic disc swelling, e.g., from optic neuritis or ischemic optic neuropathy, should be called "optic disc edema." This convention is arbitrary but serves to avoid confusion. Often it is difficult to differentiate papilledema from other forms of optic disc edema by fundus examination alone. Transient visual obscurations are a classic symptom of papilledema. They can occur in only one eye or simultaneously in both eyes. They usually last seconds but can persist for minutes if the papilledema is fulminant. Obscurations follow abrupt shifts in posture or happen spontaneously. When obscurations are prolonged or spontaneous, the papilledema is more threatening. Visual acuity is not affected by papilledema unless the papilledema is severe, long-standing, or accompanied by macular edema and hemorrhage. Visual field testing shows enlarged blind spots and peripheral constriction (Fig. 28-3F). With unremitting papilledema, peripheral visual field loss progresses in an insidious fashion while the optic nerve develops atrophy. In this setting, reduction of optic disc swelling is an ominous sign of a dying nerve rather than an encouraging indication of resolving papilledema.

Evaluation of papilledema requires computed tomography (CT) or MR imaging to exclude an intracranial lesion. MR angiography is appropriate in selected cases to search for a dural venous sinus occlusion or an arteriovenous shunt. If neuroradiologic studies are negative, the subarachnoid opening pressure should be measured by lumbar puncture. An elevated pressure, with normal cerebrospinal fluid, points by exclusion to the diagnosis of *pseudotumor cerebri* (idiopathic intracranial hypertension). The majority of patients are young, female, and obese. Treatment with a carbonic anhydrase inhibitor such as acetazolamide lowers intracranial pressure by reducing the production of cerebrospinal fluid. Weight reduction is vital but often unsuccessful.

If acetazolamide and weight loss fail, and visual field loss is progressive, lumboperitoneal shunting or optic nerve sheath fenestration should be undertaken without delay to prevent blindness. Occasionally, emergency surgery is required for sudden blindness caused by fulminant papilledema.

Optic Disc Drusen These are refractile deposits within the substance of the optic nerve head (**see Plate IV-11**). They are unrelated to drusen of the retina, which occur in age-related macular degeneration. Optic disc drusen are most common in people of northern European descent, with an incidence of 0.3 to 0.4%. Their diagnosis is obvious when they are visible as glittering particles upon the surface of the optic disc. However, in many patients they are hidden beneath the surface, producing an elevated optic disc with blurred margins that is easily mistaken for papilledema. It is important to recognize pseudo-papilledema due to optic disc drusen to avoid an unneccessary evaluation for papilledema. Ultrasound or CT scanning are sensitive for detection of buried optic disc drusen because they contain calcium. In most patients, optic disc drusen are an incidental, innocuous finding, but they can produce visual obscurations. On perimetry they give rise to enlarged blind spots and arcuate scotomas from damage to the optic disc. With increasing age, drusen tend to become more exposed on the disc surface as optic atrophy develops. Hemorrhage, choroidal neovascular membrane, and AION are more likely to occur in patients with optic disc drusen. No treatment for drusen is available.

Vitreous Degeneration This occurs in all individuals with advancing age, leading to chronic and acute visual symptoms. Opacities develop in the vitreous, casting annoying shadows upon the retina. As the eye moves, these distracting "floaters" move synchronously, with a slight lag caused by inertia of the vitreous gel. Vitreous traction upon the retina causes mechanical stimulation, resulting in perception of flashing lights. This photopsia is brief and confined to one eye, in contrast to the bilateral, prolonged scintillations of cortical migraine. Contraction of the vitreous can result in sudden separation from the retina, heralded by an alarming shower of floaters and photopsia. This process, known as *vitreous detachment*, is a frequent involutional event in the elderly. It is not harmful unless it damages the retina. A careful examination of the dilated fundus is mandatory in any patient complaining of floaters or photopsia to search for peripheral tears or holes. If such a lesion is found, laser application or cryotherapy can forestall a retinal detachment. Occasionally a tear ruptures a retinal blood vessel, causing vitreous hemorrhage and sudden loss of vision. On attempted ophthalmoscopy the fundus is hidden by a dark red haze of blood. Ultrasound is required to examine the interior of the eye for a retinal tear or detachment. If the hemorrhage does not resolve spontaneously, the vitreous can be removed surgically. Vitreous hemorrhage also occurs from the fragile neovascular vessels that proliferate on the surface of the retina in diabetes, sickle cell anemia, and other ischemic ocular diseases.

Retinal Detachment This produces symptoms of floaters, flashing lights, and a scotoma in the peripheral visual field corresponding to the detachment (**see Plate IV-12**). If the detachment includes the fovea, there is an afferent pupil defect and the visual acuity is reduced. In most eyes, retinal detachment starts with a hole, flap, or tear in the peripheral retina (rhegmatogenous retinal detachment). Patients with peripheral retinal thinning (lattice degeneration) are particularly vulnerable to this process. Once a break has developed in the retina, liquified vitreous is free to enter the subretinal space, separating the retina from the pigment epithelium. The combination of vitreous traction upon the retinal surface and passage of fluid behind the retina leads inexorably to detachment. Patients with a history of myopia, trauma, or prior cataract extraction are at greatest risk for retinal detachment. The diagnosis is confirmed by ophthalmoscopic examination of the dilated eye.

Classic Migraine (See also Chap. 15) This usually occurs with a visual aura lasting about 20 min. In a typical attack, a small central disturbance in the field of vision marches toward the periphery, leaving a transient scotoma in its wake. The expanding border of migraine scotoma has a scintillating, dancing, or zig-zag edge, resembling the bastions of a fortified city, hence the term "fortification spectra." Patients' descriptions of fortification spectra vary widely and can be confused with amaurosis fugax. Migraine patterns usually last longer and are perceived in both eyes, whereas amaurosis fugax is briefer and occurs in only one eye. Migraine phenomena also remain visible in the dark or with the eyes closed. Generally they are confined to either the right or left visual hemifield, but sometimes both fields are involved simultaneously. Patients often have a long history of stereotypic attacks. After the visual symptoms recede, headache develops in most patients.

Transient ischemic attacks from *vertebrobasilar insufficiency* result in acute homonymous visual symptoms. Many patients mistakenly describe symptoms in their left or right eye, when in fact they are occurring in the left or right hemifield of both eyes. Interruption of blood supply to the visual cortex causes a sudden fogging or graying of vision, occasionally with flashing lights or other positive phenomena that mimic migraine. Cortical ischemic attacks are briefer in duration than migraine, occur in older patients, and are not followed by headache. There may be associated signs of brainstem ischemia, such as diplopia, vertigo, numbness, weakness, or dysarthria.

Stroke This occurs when interruption of blood supply from the posterior cerebral artery to the visual cortex is prolonged. The only finding on examination is a homonymous visual field defect that stops abruptly at the vertical meridian. Occipital lobe stroke is usually due to thrombotic occlusion of the vertebrobasilar system, embolus, or dissection. Lobar hemorrhage, tumor, abscess, and arteriovenous malformation are other common causes of hemianopic cortical visual loss.

Factitious (Functional, Nonorganic) Visual Loss This is claimed by hysterics or malingerers. The latter comprise the vast majority, seeking sympathy, special treatment, or financial gain by feigning loss of sight. The diagnosis is suspected when the history is atypical, physical findings are lacking or contradictory, inconsistencies emerge on testing, and a secondary motive can be identified. In our litigious society, the fraudulent pursuit of recompense has spawned an epidemic of factitious visual loss.

CHRONIC VISUAL LOSS

Cataract This is a clouding of the lens sufficient to reduce vision. Most cataracts develop slowly as a result of aging, leading to gradual impairment of vision. The formation of cataract occurs more rapidly in patients with a history of ocular trauma, uveitis, or diabetes mellitus. Cataracts are acquired in a variety of genetic diseases, such as myotonic dystrophy, neurofibromatosis type 2, and galactosemia. Radiation therapy and glucocorticoid treatment can induce cataract as a side effect. The cataracts associated with radiation or glucocorticoids have a typical posterior subcapsular location. Cataract can be detected by noting an impaired red reflex when viewing light reflected from the fundus with an ophthalmoscope or by examining the dilated eye using the slit lamp.

The only treatment for cataract is surgical extraction of the opacified lens. Over a million cataract operations are performed each year in the United States. The operation is generally done under local anesthesia on an outpatient basis. Remarkable technical innovations have made it possible to aspirate the cataract while leaving the lens capsule intact (extracapsular cataract extraction), rather than removing the entire lens with its capsule (intracapsular cataract extraction). A plastic or silicone intraocular lens is then placed within the empty lens capsule in the posterior chamber, substituting for the natural lens, and leading to rapid recovery of sight. More than 95% of patients who undergo cataract extraction can expect an improvement in vision. In many patients, the lens capsule remaining in the eye after cataract extraction eventually turns cloudy, causing a secondary loss of vision. A small opening is made in the lens capsule with a laser to restore clarity.

Glaucoma This is a slowly progressive, insidious optic neuropathy, usually associated with chronic elevation of intraocular pressure.

In Americans of African descent it is the leading cause of blindness. The mechanism whereby raised intraocular pressure injures the optic nerve is not understood. Axons entering the inferotemporal and superotemporal aspects of the optic disc are damaged first, producing typical nerve fiber bundle or arcuate scotomas on perimetric testing. As fibers are destroyed, the neural rim of the optic disc shrinks and the physiologic cup within the optic disc enlarges (see Plate IV-13). This process is referred to colloquially as pathologic "cupping." The cup-to-disc diameter is expressed as a ratio, e.g., 0.2/1. The cup-to-disc ratio ranges widely in normal individuals, making it difficult to diagnose glaucoma reliably simply by observing an unusually large or deep optic cup. Careful documentation of serial prospective examinations is helpful. In the patient with physiologic cupping, the large cup remains stable, whereas in the patient with glaucoma it expands relentlessly over the years. Detection of visual field loss on formal perimetry also contributes to the diagnosis of glaucoma. Finally, most patients with glaucoma have raised intraocular pressure. However, a surprising number of patients with typical glaucomatous cupping and visual field loss have intraocular pressures that apparently never exceed the normal limit of 20 mmHg (so-called low-tension glaucoma).

In acute angle-closure glaucoma, the eye is red and painful due to abrupt, severe elevation of intraocular pressure. Such cases account for only a handful of patients with glaucoma. Most patients with glaucoma have open, nonoccludable anterior chamber angles. The cause of raised intraocular pressure in these patients is uncertain. Recent studies have implicated mutations in a gene encoding a glycoprotein expressed in the trabecular meshwork. This structure serves as a filter to drain aqueous from the eye. Because the elevation of intraocular pressure develops gradually and is less marked than in angle-closure glaucoma, there is no pain or ocular injection. The central visual field and foveal acuity are spared until end-stage disease is reached. For these reasons, severe and irreversible damage can occur before either the patient or physician recognizes the diagnosis. Screening of patients for glaucoma by noting the cup-to-disc ratio on ophthalmoscopy and by measuring intraocular pressure (using a Schiotz, Tonopen, air-puff, or Goldmann tonometer) is vital. Glaucoma is treated with topical adrenergic agonists (epinephrine, dipivefrin, apraclonidine, brimonidine), cholinergic agonists (pilocarpine), beta blockers (betaxolol, carteolol, levobunolol, metipranolol, and timolol), and prostaglandin analogues (latanaprost). Occasionally, systemic absorption of beta blocker from eye drops can be sufficient to cause side effects of bradycardia, hypotension, heart block, bronchospasm, impotence, or depression. Topical or oral carbonic anhydrase inhibitors are used to lower intraocular pressure by reducing aqueous production. Laser treatment of the trabecular meshwork in the anterior chamber angle improves aqueous outflow from the eye. If medical or laser treatments fail to halt optic nerve damage from glaucoma, a filter must be constructed surgically (trabeculectomy) to release aqueous from the eye in a controlled fashion.

Macular Degeneration This is a major cause of gradual, painless, bilateral central visual loss in the elderly. The old term, "senile macular degeneration," misinterpreted by many patients as an unflattering reference, has been replaced with "age-related macular degeneration." It occurs in a nonexudative (dry) form and an exudative (wet) form. The nonexudative process begins with the accumulation of extracellular deposits, called drusen, underneath the retinal pigment epithelium. On ophthalmoscopy, they are pleomorphic but generally appear as small discrete yellow lesions clustered in the macula (see Plate IV-14). With time they become larger, more numerous, and confluent. The retinal pigment epithelium becomes focally detached and atrophic, causing visual loss by interfering with photoreceptor function. There is currently no way to prevent the development of age-related macular degeneration. Concoctions of various vitamins (A, C, and E) and minerals (zinc, copper, and selenium) have been marketed, without good evidence that they retard the process of macular degeneration.

Exudative macular degeneration, which develops in only a minority of patients, occurs when neovascular vessels from the choroid grow through defects in Bruch's membrane into the potential space beneath the retinal pigment epithelium. Leakage from these vessels produces elevation of the retina and pigment epithelium, with distortion (metamorphopsia) and blurring of vision. Although onset of these symptoms is usually gradual, bleeding from subretinal choroidal neovascular membranes sometimes causes acute visual loss. The neovascular membranes can be difficult to see on fundus examination because they are beneath the retina. Fluorescein or indocyanine green angiography is extremely useful for their detection. In some patients, prompt laser ablation of choroidal neovascular membranes seen on fluorescein angiography can halt the exudative process. However, the neovascular membranes frequently recur, requiring constant vigilance and repeated photocoagulation.

Major or repeated hemorrhage under the retina from neovascular membranes results in fibrosis, development of a round (disciform) macular scar, and permanent loss of central vision. Surgical attempts to remove subretinal membranes in age-related macular degeneration have not improved vision in most patients. However, outcomes have been more encouraging for patients with choroidal neovascular membranes from ocular histoplasmosis syndrome.

Central Serous Chorioretinopathy This primarily affects males between the ages of 20 and 50. Leakage of serous fluid from the choroid causes small, localized detachment of the retinal pigment epithelium and the neurosensory retina. These detachments produce acute or chronic symptoms of metamorphopsia and blurred vision when the macula is involved. They are difficult to visualize with a direct ophthalmoscope because the detached retina is transparent and only slightly elevated. Diagnosis of central serous chorioretinopathy is made easily by fluorescein angiography, which shows dye streaming into the subretinal space. The cause of central serous chorioretinopathy is unknown. Symptoms may resolve spontaneously if the retina reattaches, but recurrent detachment is common. Laser photocoagulation has benefited some patients with this condition.

Diabetic Retinopathy A rare disease until 1921, when the discovery of insulin resulted in a dramatic improvement in life expectancy for patients with diabetes mellitus, it is now a leading cause of blindness in the United States. The retinopathy of diabetes takes years to develop but eventually appears in nearly all cases. Regular surveillance of the dilated fundus is crucial for any patient with diabetes. In advanced diabetic retinopathy, the proliferation of neovascular vessels leads to blindness from vitreous hemorrhage, retinal detachment, and glaucoma (see Plate IV-15). These complications can be avoided in most patients by administration of panretinal laser photocoagulation at the appropriate point in the evolution of the disease. →*For further discussion of the manifestations and management of diabetic retinopathy, see Chap. 333.*

Retinitis Pigmentosa This is a general term for a disparate group of rod and cone dystrophies characterized by progressive night blindness (nyctalopia), visual field constriction with a ring scotoma, loss of acuity, and an abnormal electroretinogram (ERG). It occurs sporadically or in an autosomal recessive, dominant, or X-linked pattern. Irregular black deposits of clumped pigment in the peripheral retina, called bone spicules because of their vague resemblance to the spicules of cancellous bone, give the disease its name (see Plate IV-16). The name is actually a misnomer because retinitis pigmentosa is not an inflammatory process. Most cases are due to a mutation in the gene for rhodopsin, the rod photopigment, or in the gene for peripherin, a glycoprotein located in photoreceptor outer segments. There is no effective treatment for retinitis pigmentosa. Vitamin A (15,000 IU/day) slightly retards the deterioration of the ERG but has no beneficial effect upon visual acuity or visual fields. Some forms of retinitis pigmentosa occur in association with rare, hereditary systemic diseases (olivopontocerebellar degeneration, Bassen-Kornzweig disease, Kearns-Sayre syndrome, Refsum's disease). Chronic treatment with chloroquine, hydroxychloroquine, and phenothiazines (especially thioridazine) can produce visual loss from a toxic retinopathy that resembles retinitis pigmentosa.

Epiretinal Membrane This is a fibrocellular tissue that grows across the inner surface of the retina, causing metamorphopsia and reduced visual acuity from distortion of the macula. With the ophthalmoscope one can see a crinkled, cellophane-like membrane on the retina. Epiretinal membrane is most common in patients over 50 years of age and is usually unilateral. Most cases are idiopathic, but some occur as a result of hypertensive retinopathy, diabetes, retinal detachment, or trauma. When visual acuity is reduced to the level of about 6/24 (20/80), vitrectomy and surgical peeling of the membrane to relieve macular puckering are recommended. Contraction of an epiretinal membrane sometimes gives rise to a *macular hole*. Most macular holes, however, are caused by local vitreous traction within the fovea. Vision is usually depressed to the level of 6/30 (20/100) or worse. Vitrectomy may improve visual acuity in some patients with macular hole. Fortunately, fewer than 10% of patients with a macular hole develop a hole in their other eye.

Melanoma and Other Tumors Melanoma is the most common primary tumor of the eye (**see Plate IV-17**). It causes photopsia, an enlarging scotoma, and loss of vision. A small melanoma is often difficult to differentiate from a benign choroidal nevus. Careful serial examinations are required to document a malignant pattern of growth. Treatment of melanoma is controversial. Options include enucleation, local resection, and irradiation. *Metastatic tumors* to the eye outnumber primary tumors of uveal origin. Breast and lung carcinoma have a special propensity to spread to the choroid or iris. Leukemia and lymphoma also commonly invade ocular tissues. Sometimes their only sign on eye examination is cellular debris in the vitreous, which can masquerade as a chronic posterior uveitis. *Retrobulbar tumor* of the optic nerve (meningioma, glioma) or *chiasmal tumor* (pituitary adenoma, meningioma) produces gradual visual loss with few objective findings, except for optic disc pallor. Rarely, sudden expansion of a pituitary adenoma from infarction and bleeding (*pituitary apoplexy*) causes acute retrobulbar visual loss, with headache, nausea, and ocular motor nerve palsies. In any patient with visual field loss or optic atrophy, CT or MR scanning should be considered if the cause remains unknown after careful review of the history and thorough examination of the eye (Fig. 28-4).

PROPTOSIS

When the globes appear asymmetric, the clinician must first decide which eye is abnormal. Is one eye recessed within the orbit (*enophthalmos*) or is the other eye protuberant (*exophthalmos*, or *proptosis*)? A small globe or a Horner's syndrome can give the appearance of enophthalmos. True enophthalmos occurs commonly after trauma, from atrophy of retrobulbar fat, or fracture of the orbital floor. The position of the eyes within the orbits is measured using a Hertel exophthalmometer, a hand-held instrument that records the position of the anterior corneal surface relative to the lateral orbital rim. If this instrument is not available, relative eye position can be judged by bending the patient's head forward and looking down upon the orbits. A proptosis of only 2 mm in one eye is detectable from this perspective. The development of proptosis implies a space-occupying lesion in the orbit. A CT or MR scan should be obtained in any patient with proptosis, unless the diagnosis of Graves' ophthalmopathy is certain.

Graves' Ophthalmopathy This is the leading cause of proptosis in adults (Chap. 330). The proptosis is often asymmetric and can even appear to be unilateral. Orbital inflammation and engorgement of the extraocular muscles, particularly the medial rectus and the inferior rectus, account for the protrusion of the globe. Corneal exposure, lid retraction, conjunctival injection, restriction of gaze, diplopia, and visual loss from optic nerve compression are cardinal symptoms. Acute Graves' ophthalmopathy should be treated with oral prednisone (60 mg/day) for 1 month, followed by a taper over several months. Chronic manifestations can be managed by topical lubricants, eyelid surgery,

eye muscle surgery, or radiation treatment. Optic nerve compression should be relieved promptly with glucocorticoids and orbital decompression to prevent permanent visual loss.

Orbital Pseudotumor This is an idiopathic, inflammatory orbital syndrome, frequently confused with Graves' ophthalmopathy. Symptoms are pain, limited eye movements, proptosis, and congestion. Evaluation for sarcoidosis, Wegener's granulomatosis, and other types of orbital vasculitis or collagen-vascular disease is negative. Imaging often shows swollen eye muscles (orbital myositis) with enlarged tendons. By contrast, in Graves' ophthalmopathy the tendons of the eye muscles are usually spared. The Tolosa-Hunt syndrome may be regarded as an extension of orbital pseudotumor through the superior orbital fissure into the cavernous sinus. The diagnosis of orbital pseudotumor is difficult. Biopsy of the orbit frequently yields nonspecific evidence of fat infiltration by lymphocytes, plasma cells, and eosinophils. A dramatic response to a therapeutic trial of systemic glucocorticoids indirectly provides the best confirmation of the diagnosis.

Orbital Cellulitis This causes pain, lid erythema, proptosis, conjunctival chemosis, restricted motility, decreased acuity, afferent pupillary defect, fever, and leukocytosis. It often arises from a paranasal sinus, especially by contiguous spread of infection from the ethmoid sinus through the thin lamina papyracea of the medial orbit. A history of recent upper respiratory tract infection, chronic sinusitis, thick mucous secretions, or dental disease is significant in any patient with suspected orbital cellulitis. Blood cultures should be obtained, but they are usually negative. Most patients respond to empiric therapy with broad-spectrum intravenous antibiotics. Occasionally, orbital cellulitis follows an overwhelming course, with massive proptosis, blindness, septic cavernous sinus thrombosis, and meningitis. To avert this disaster, orbital cellulitis should be managed aggressively in the early stages, with immediate antibiotic therapy and imaging of the orbits. Prompt surgical drainage of an orbital abscess or paranasal sinusitis is indicated if optic nerve function deteriorates despite antibiotics.

Tumors Tumors of the orbit cause painless, progressive proptosis. The most common primary tumors are hemangioma, lymphangioma, neurofibroma, dermoid cyst, adenoid cystic carcinoma, optic nerve glioma, optic nerve meningioma, and benign mixed tumor of the lacrimal gland. Metastatic tumor to the orbit occurs frequently in breast carcinoma, lung carcinoma, and lymphoma. Diagnosis by fine-needle aspiration followed by urgent radiation therapy can sometimes preserve vision.

Carotid Cavernous Fistulas With anterior drainage through the orbit these produce proptosis, diplopia, glaucoma, and tortuous, red conjunctival vessels. Direct fistulas usually result from trauma. They are easily diagnosed because of the dramatic signs produced by high-flow, high-pressure shunting. Indirect fistulas, or dural arteriovenous malformations, are more likely to occur spontaneously, especially in older women. The signs are more subtle and the diagnosis is frequently missed. The combination of slight proptosis, diplopia, enlarged muscles, and an injected eye is often mistaken for thyroid ophthalmopathy. A bruit heard upon auscultation of the head, or reported by the patient, is a valuable diagnostic clue. Imaging shows an enlarged superior ophthalmic vein in the orbits. Carotid cavernous shunts can be eliminated by intravascular embolization.

PTOSIS

Blepharoptosis This is an abnormal drooping of the eyelid. Unilateral or bilateral ptosis can be congenital, from dysgenesis of the levator palpebrae superioris, or from abnormal insertion of its aponeurosis into the eyelid. Acquired ptosis can develop so gradually that the patient is unaware of the problem. Inspection of old photographs is helpful in dating the onset. A history of prior trauma, eye surgery, contact lens use, diplopia, systemic symptoms (e.g., dysphagia or peripheral muscle weakness), or a family history of ptosis should be sought. Fluctuating ptosis that worsens late in the day is typical of myasthenia gravis. Examination should focus upon evidence for proptosis, eyelid masses or deformities, inflammation, pupil inequality, or limitation of motility. The width of the palpebral fissures is measured in primary gaze to quantitate the degree of ptosis. The ptosis will be underestimated if the patient is compensating by lifting the brow with the frontalis muscle.

Mechanical Ptosis   This occurs in many elderly patients from stretching and redundancy of eyelid skin and subcutaneous fat (dermatochalasis). The extra weight of these sagging tissues causes the lid to droop. Enlargement or deformation of the eyelid from infection, tumor, trauma, or inflammation also results in ptosis on a purely mechanical basis.

Aponeurotic Ptosis   This is an acquired dehiscence or stretching of the aponeurotic tendon, which connects the levator muscle to the tarsal plate of the eyelid. It occurs commonly in older patients, presumably from loss of connective tissue elasticity. Aponeurotic ptosis is also a frequent sequela of eyelid swelling from infection or blunt trauma to the orbit, cataract surgery, or hard contact lens usage.

Myogenic Ptosis   The causes of *myogenic ptosis* include myasthenia gravis (Chap. 380) and a number of rare myopathies that manifest with ptosis. The term *chronic progressive external ophthalmoplegia* refers to a spectrum of systemic diseases caused by mutations of mitochrondrial DNA. As the name implies, the most prominent findings are symmetric, slowly progressive ptosis and limitation of eye movements. In general, diplopia is a late symptom because all eye movements are reduced equally. In the *Kearns-Sayre* variant, retinal pigmentary changes and abnormalities of cardiac conduction develop. Peripheral muscle biopsy shows characteristic "ragged-red fibers." *Oculopharyngeal dystrophy* is a distinct autosomal dominant disease with onset in middle age, characterized by ptosis, limited eye movements, and trouble swallowing. *Myotonic dystrophy*, another autosomal dominant disorder, causes ptosis, ophthalmoparesis, cataract, and pigmentary retinopathy. Patients have muscle wasting, myotonia, frontal balding, and cardiac abnormalities.

Neurogenic Ptosis   This results from a lesion affecting the innervation to either of the two muscles that open the eyelid: Müller's muscle or the levator palpebrae superioris. Examination of the pupil helps to distinguish between these two possibilities. In Horner's syndrome, the eye with ptosis has a smaller pupil and the eye movements are full. In an oculomotor nerve palsy, the eye with the ptosis has a larger, or a normal, pupil. If the pupil is normal but there is limitation of adduction, elevation, and depression, a pupil-sparing oculomotor nerve palsy is likely (see next section). Rarely, a lesion affecting the small, central subnucleus of the oculomotor complex will cause bilateral ptosis with normal eye movements and pupils.

DOUBLE VISION

The first point to clarify is whether diplopia persists in either eye after covering the fellow eye. If it does, the diagnosis is monocular diplopia. The cause is usually intrinsic to the eye and therefore has no dire implications for the patient. Corneal aberrations (e.g., keratoconus, pterygium), uncorrected refractive error, cataract, or foveal traction may give rise to monocular diplopia. Occasionally it is a symptom of malingering or psychiatric disease. Diplopia alleviated by covering one eye is binocular diplopia and is caused by disruption of ocular alignment. Inquiry should be made into the nature of the double vision (purely side-by-side versus partial vertical displacement of images), mode of onset, duration, intermittency, diurnal variation, and associated neurologic or systemic symptoms. If the patient has diplopia while being examined, motility testing should reveal a deficiency corresponding to the patient's symptoms. However, subtle limitation of ocular excursions is often difficult to detect. For example, a patient with a slight left abducens nerve paresis may appear to have full eye movements, despite a complaint of horizontal diplopia upon looking to the left. In this situation, the cover test provides a more sensitive method for demonstrating the ocular malalignment. It should be conducted in primary gaze, and then with the head turned and tilted in each direction. In the above example, a cover test with the head turned to the right will maximize the fixation shift evoked by the cover test.

Occasionally, a cover test performed in an asymptomatic patient during a routine examination will reveal an ocular deviation. If the eye movements are full and the ocular misalignment is equal in all directions of gaze (concomitant deviation), the diagnosis is strabismus. In this condition, which affects about 1% of the population, fusion is disrupted in infancy or early childhood. To avoid diplopia, vision is suppressed from the nonfixating eye. In some children, this leads to impaired vision (amblyopia, or "lazy" eye) in the deviated eye.

Binocular diplopia occurs from a wide range of processes: infectious, neoplastic, metabolic, degenerative, inflammatory, and vascular. One must decide if the diplopia is neurogenic in origin or due to restriction of globe rotation by local disease in the orbit. Orbital pseudotumor, myositis, infection, tumor, thyroid disease, and muscle entrapment (e.g., from a blowout fracture) cause restrictive diplopia. The diagnosis is confirmed by performing a forced duction test in the office. After applying topical anesthesia, the physician grasps the eye with forceps and pulls it toward the direction of deficient motion. If rotation of the globe is prevented by tethering, a restrictive process is at work. The utility of this test is limited by its unpopularity with patients; in practice, the diagnosis of restriction is made by recognizing other associated signs and symptoms of local orbital disease.

Myasthenia Gravis (See also Chap. 380)   This is a major cause of diplopia. The diplopia is often intermittent, variable, and not confined to any single ocular motor nerve distribution. The pupils are always normal. Fluctuating ptosis may be present. Many patients have a purely ocular form of the disease, with no evidence of systemic muscular weakness. The diagnosis can be confirmed by an intravenous edrophonium injection or by an assay for antiacetylcholine receptor antibodies. Negative results from these tests do not exclude the diagnosis. *Botulism* from food or wound poisoning can mimic ocular myasthenia.

After restrictive orbital disease and myasthenia gravis are excluded, a lesion of a cranial nerve supplying innervation to the extraocular muscles is the most likely cause of binocular diplopia.

Oculomotor Nerve   The third cranial nerve innervates the medial, inferior, and superior recti; inferior oblique; levator palpebrae superioris; and the iris sphincter. Total palsy of the oculomotor nerve causes ptosis, a dilated pupil, and leaves the eye "down and out" because of the unopposed action of the lateral rectus and superior oblique. This combination of findings is obvious. More challenging is the diagnosis of an early or partial oculomotor nerve palsy. In this setting, any combination of ptosis, pupil dilation, and weakness of the eye muscles supplied by the oculomotor nerve may be encountered. Frequent serial examinations during the evolving phase of the palsy and a high index of suspicion help ensure that the diagnosis is not missed. The advent of an oculomotor nerve palsy with any degree of pupil involvement in an otherwise healthy patient, especially when accompanied by pain, raises the specter of a circle of Willis aneurysm. If an MR scan shows no compressive lesion, an arteriogram must be performed to rule out an aneurysm of either the posterior communicating artery or the basilar artery. If the pupil is entirely normal, with all other components of an oculomotor palsy present, aneurysm is so rare that an angiogram is seldom indicated.

A lesion of the oculomotor nucleus in the rostral midbrain produces signs that differ from those caused by a lesion of the nerve itself. There is bilateral ptosis because the levator muscle is innervated by a single central subnucleus. There is also weakness of the contralateral superior rectus, because it is supplied by the oculomotor nucleus on the other side. Occasionally both superior recti are weak. Isolated nuclear oculomotor palsy is quite rare. Usually neurologic examination reveals additional signs to suggest brainstem damage from infarction, hemorrhage, tumor, or infection.

Injury to structures surrounding fascicles of the oculomotor nerve descending through the midbrain has given rise to a number of classic eponymic designations. In *Nothnagel's syndrome*, injury to the superior cerebellar peduncle causes ipsilateral oculomotor palsy and contralateral cerebellar ataxia. In *Benedikt's syndrome*, injury to the red nucleus results in ipsilateral oculomotor palsy and contralateral tremor, chorea, and athetosis. *Claude's syndrome* incorporates features of both the aforementioned syndromes, by injury to both the red nucleus and the superior cerebellar peduncle. Finally, in *Weber's syndrome*, injury to the cerebral peduncle causes ipsilateral oculomotor palsy with contralateral hemiparesis.

In the subarachnoid space the oculomotor nerve is vulnerable to aneurysm, meningitis, tumor, infarction, and compression. In cerebral herniation the nerve becomes trapped between the edge of the tentorium and the uncus of the temporal lobe. Oculomotor palsy can also occur from midbrain torsion and hemorrhages during herniation. In the cavernous sinus, oculomotor palsy arises from carotid aneurysm, carotid cavernous fistula, cavernous sinus thrombosis, tumor (pituitary adenoma, meningioma, metastasis), herpes zoster infection, and the Tolosa-Hunt syndrome.

The etiology of an isolated, pupil-sparing oculomotor palsy often remains obscure, even after neuroimaging and extensive laboratory testing. Most cases are thought to result from microvascular infarction of the nerve, somewhere along its course from the brainstem to the orbit. Usually the patient complains of pain. Diabetes, hypertension, and vascular disease are major risk factors. Spontaneous recovery over a period of months is the rule. If this fails to occur, or if new findings develop, the diagnosis of microvascular oculomotor nerve palsy should be reconsidered. Aberrant regeneration is common when the oculomotor nerve is injured by trauma or compression (tumor, aneurysm). Miswiring of sprouting fibers to the levator muscle and the rectus muscles results in elevation of the eyelid upon downgaze or adduction. The pupil also constricts upon attempted adduction, elevation, or depression of the globe. Aberrant regeneration is not seen after oculomotor palsy from microvascular infarct and hence vitiates that diagnosis.

Trochlear Nerve   The fourth cranial nerve originates in the midbrain, just caudal to the oculomotor nerve complex. Fibers exit the brainstem dorsally and cross to innervate the contralateral superior oblique. The principal actions of this muscle are to depress and to intort the globe. A palsy therefore results in hypertropia and excyclotorsion. The cyclotorsion is seldom noticed by patients. Instead, they complain of vertical diplopia, especially upon reading or looking down. The vertical diplopia is also exacerbated by tilting the head toward the side with the muscle palsy, and alleviated by tilting it away. This "head tilt test" is a cardinal diagnostic feature.

Isolated trochlear nerve palsy occurs from all the causes listed above for the oculomotor nerve, except aneurysm. The trochlear nerve is particularly apt to suffer injury after closed head trauma. The mechanism is unknown, but the free edge of the tentorium may impinge upon the nerve during a concussive blow. Most isolated trochlear nerve palsies are idiopathic and hence diagnosed by exclusion as "microvascular." Spontaneous improvement occurs over a period of months in most patients. A base-down prism (conveniently applied to the patient's glasses as a stick-on Fresnel lens) may serve as a temporary measure to alleviate diplopia. If the palsy does not resolve, the eyes can be realigned by surgically adjusting other eye muscles.

Abducens Nerve   The sixth cranial nerve innervates the lateral rectus muscle. A palsy produces horizontal diplopia, worse on gaze to the side of the lesion. A nuclear lesion has different consequences, because the abducens nucleus contains interneurons that project via the medial longitudinal fasciculus to the medial rectus subnucleus of the contralateral oculomotor complex. Therefore, an abducens nuclear lesion produces a complete lateral gaze palsy, from weakness of both the ipsilateral lateral rectus and the contralateral medial rectus. *Foville's syndrome* following dorsal pontine injury includes lateral gaze palsy, ipsilateral facial palsy, and contralateral hemiparesis in-

curred by damage to descending corticospinal fibers. *Millard-Gubler syndrome* from ventral pontine injury is similar, except for the eye findings. There is lateral rectus weakness only, instead of gaze palsy, because the abducens fascicle is injured rather than the nucleus. Infarct, tumor, hemorrhage, vascular malformation, and multiple sclerosis are the most common etiologies of brainstem abducens palsy.

After leaving the ventral pons, the abducens nerve runs forward along the clivus to pierce the dura at the petrous apex, where it enters the cavernous sinus. Along its subarachnoid course it is susceptible to meningitis, tumor (meningioma, chordoma, carcinomatous meningitis), subarachnoid hemorrhage, trauma, and compression by aneurysm or dolichoectatic vessels. At the petrous apex, mastoiditis can produce deafness, pain, and ipsilateral abducens palsy (*Gradenigo's syndrome*). In the cavernous sinus, the nerve can be affected by carotid aneurysm, carotid cavernous fistula, tumor (pituitary adenoma, meningioma, nasopharyngeal carcinoma), herpes infection, and Tolosa-Hunt syndrome.

Unilateral or bilateral abducens palsy is a classic sign of raised intracranial pressure. The diagnosis can be confirmed if papilledema is observed on fundus examination. The mechanism is still debated but is probably related to rostral-caudal displacement of the brainstem. The same phenomenon accounts for abducens palsy from low intracranial pressure (e.g., after lumbar puncture, spinal anesthesia, or spontaneous dural cerebrospinal fluid leak).

Treatment of abducens palsy is aimed at prompt correction of the underlying cause. However, the cause remains obscure in many instances, despite diligent evaluation. As mentioned above for isolated trochlear or oculomotor palsy, most cases are assumed to represent microvascular infarcts because they often occur in the setting of diabetes or other vascular risk factors. Some cases may develop as a postinfectious mononeuritis (e.g., following a viral flu). Patching one eye or applying a temporary prism will provide relief of diplopia until the palsy resolves. If recovery is incomplete, eye muscle surgery can nearly always realign the eyes, at least in primary position. A patient with an abducens palsy that fails to improve should be reevaluated for an occult etiology (e.g., chordoma, carcinomatous meningitis, carotid cavernous fistula, myasthenia gravis).

Multiple Ocular Motor Nerve Palsies   These should not be attributed to spontaneous microvascular events affecting more than one cranial nerve at a time. This remarkable coincidence does occur, especially in diabetic patients, but the diagnosis is made only in retrospect after exhausting all other diagnostic alternatives. Neuroimaging should focus on the cavernous sinus, superior orbital fissure, and orbital apex, where all three ocular motor nerves are in close proximity. In the diabetic or compromised host, fungal infection (*Aspergillus, Mucorales, Cryptococcus*) is a frequent cause of multiple nerve palsies. In the patient with systemic malignancy, carcinomatous meningitis is a likely diagnosis. Cytologic examination may be negative despite repeated sampling of the cerebrospinal fluid. The cancer-associated Lambert-Eaton myasthenic syndrome can also produce ophthalmoplegia. Giant cell (temporal) arteritis occasionally manifests as diplopia from ischemic palsies of extraocular muscles. Fisher syndrome, an ocular variant of Guillain-Barré, can produce ophthalmoplegia with areflexia and ataxia. Often the ataxia is mild, and the areflexia is overlooked because the physician's attention is focused upon the eyes.

Supranuclear Disorders of Gaze   These are often mistaken for multiple ocular motor nerve palsies. For example, Wernicke's encephalopathy can produce nystagmus and a partial deficit of horizontal and vertical gaze that mimics a combined abducens and oculomotor nerve palsy. The disorder occurs in malnourished or alcoholic patients and can be reversed by giving thiamine. Infarct, hemorrhage, tumor, multiple sclerosis, encephalitis, vasculitis, and Whipple's disease are other important causes of supranuclear gaze palsy.

The *frontal eye field* of the cerebral cortex is involved in generation of saccades to the contralateral side. After hemispheric stroke, the eyes usually deviate towards the lesioned side because of the unopposed action of the frontal eye field in the normal hemisphere. With time, this deficit resolves. Seizures generally have the opposite effect: the eyes deviate conjugately away from the irritative focus. *Parietal lesions* disrupt smooth pursuit of targets moving toward the side of the lesion. Bilateral parietal lesions produce *Balint's syndrome*, characterized by impaired eye-hand coordination (optic ataxia), difficulty initiating voluntary eye movements (ocular apraxia), and visuospatial disorientation (simultanagnosia).

Horizontal Gaze Descending cortical inputs mediating horizontal gaze ultimately converge at the level of the pons. Neurons in the paramedian pontine reticular formation are responsible for controlling conjugate gaze toward the same side. They project directly to the ipsilateral abducens nucleus. A lesion of either the paramedian pontine reticular formation or the abducens nucleus causes an ipsilateral conjugate gaze palsy. Lesions at either locus produce nearly identical clinical syndromes, with the following exception: vestibular stimulation (oculocephalic maneuver or caloric) will succeed in driving the eyes conjugately to the side in a patient with a lesion of the paramedian pontine reticular formation, but not in a patient with a lesion of the abducens nucleus.

Internuclear ophthalmoplegia This results from damage to the medial longitudinal fasciculus ascending from the abducens nucleus in the pons to the oculomotor nucleus in the midbrain (hence, "internuclear"). Damage to fibers carrying the conjugate signal from abducens interneurons to the contralateral medial rectus motoneurons results in a failure of adduction on attempted lateral gaze. For example, a patient with a left internuclear ophthalmoplegia will have slowed or absent adducting movements of the left eye. A patient with bilateral injury to the medial longitudinal fasciculus will have bilateral internuclear ophthalmoplegia. Multiple sclerosis is the most common cause, although tumor, stroke, trauma, or any brainstem process may be responsible. *One-and-a half syndrome* is due to a combined lesion of the medial longitudinal fasciculus and the abducens nucleus on the same side. The patient's only horizontal eye movement is abduction of the eye on the other side.

Vertical Gaze This is controlled at the level of the midbrain. The neuronal circuits affected in disorders of vertical gaze are not well elucidated, but lesions of the rostral interstitial nucleus of the medial longitudinal fasciculus and the interstitial nucleus of Cajal cause supranuclear paresis of upgaze, downgaze, or all vertical eye movements. Distal basilar artery ischemia is the most common etiology. *Skew deviation* refers to a vertical misalignment of the eyes, usually constant in all positions of gaze. The finding has poor localizing value because skew deviation has been reported after lesions in widespread regions of the brainstem and cerebellum.

Parinaud's syndrome Also known as dorsal midbrain syndrome, this is a distinct supranuclear vertical gaze disorder from damage to the posterior commissure. It is a classic sign of hydrocephalus from aqueductal stenosis. Pineal region tumors (germinoma, pineoblastoma), cysticercosis, and stroke also cause Parinaud's syndrome. Features include loss of upgaze (and sometimes downgaze), convergence-retraction nystagmus on attempted upgaze, downwards ocular deviation ("setting sun" sign), lid retraction (Collier's sign), skew deviation, pseudoabducens palsy, and light-near dissociation of the pupils. Disorders of vertical gaze, especially downwards saccades, are an early feature of progressive supranuclear palsy. Smooth pursuit is affected later in the course of the disease. Parkinson's disease, Huntington's chorea, and olivopontocerebellar degeneration can also affect vertical gaze.

Nystagmus This is a rhythmical oscillation of the eyes, occurring physiologically from vestibular and optokinetic stimulation or pathologically in a wide variety of diseases. Abnormalities of the eyes or optic nerves, present at birth or acquired in childhood, can produce a complex, searching nystagmus with irregular pendular (sinusoidal) and jerk features. This nystagmus is commonly referred to as *congenital sensory nystagmus*. It is a poor term, because even in children with congenital lesions, the nystagmus does not appear until several months

of age. *Congenital motor nystagmus*, which looks similar to congenital sensory nystagmus, develops in the absence of any abnormality of the sensory visual system. Visual acuity is also reduced in congenital motor nystagmus, probably by the nystagmus itself, but seldom below a level of 20/200.

Jerk nystagmus This is characterized by a slow drift off the target, followed by a fast corrective saccade. By convention, the nystagmus is named after the quick phase. Jerk nystagmus can be downbeat, upbeat, horizontal (left or right), and torsional. The pattern of nystagmus may vary with gaze position. Some patients will be oblivious to their nystagmus. Others will complain of blurred vision, or a subjective, to-and-fro movement of the environment (oscillopsia) corresponding to their nystagmus. Fine nystagmus may be difficult to see upon gross examination of the eyes. Observation of nystagmoid movements of the optic disc on ophthalmoscopy is a sensitive way to detect subtle nystagmus. The slit lamp is also useful.

Gaze-evoked nystagmus This is the most common form of jerk nystagmus. When the eyes are held eccentrically in the orbits, they have a natural tendency to drift back to primary position. The subject compensates by making a corrective saccade to maintain the deviated eye position. Many normal patients have mild gaze-evoked nystagmus. Exaggerated gaze-evoked nystagmus can be induced by drugs (sedatives, anticonvulsants, alcohol); muscle paresis; myasthenia gravis; demyelinating disease; and cerebellopontine angle, brainstem, and cerebellar lesions.

Vestibular nystagmus Vestibular nystagmus results from dysfunction of the labyrinth (Méniére's disease), vestibular nerve, or vestibular nucleus in the brainstem. Peripheral vestibular nystagmus often occurs in discrete attacks, with symptoms of nausea and vertigo. There may be associated tinnitus and hearing loss. Sudden shifts in head position may provoke or exacerbate symptoms.

Downbeat nystagmus Downbeat nystagmus occurs from lesions near the craniocervical junction (Chiari malformation, basilar invagination). It has also been reported in brainstem or cerebellar stroke, lithium or anticonvulsant intoxication, alcoholism, and multiple sclerosis. *Upbeat nystagmus* is associated with damage to the pontine tegmentum, from stroke, demyelination, or tumor.

Opsoclonus This rare, dramatic disorder of eye movements consists of bursts of consecutive saccades (saccadomania). When the saccades are confined to the horizontal plane, the term *ocular flutter* is preferred. It can occur from viral encephalitis, trauma, or a paraneoplastic effect of neurobastoma, breast carcinoma, and other malignancies. It has also been reported as a benign, transient phenomenon in otherwise healthy patients.

BIBLIOGRAPHY

ALBERT DM, JAKOBIEC FA (eds): *Principles and Practice of Ophthalmology*, 2d ed. Philadelphia, Saunders, 1999

AVERBUCH-HELLER L et al: A double-blind controlled study of gabapentin and baclofen as treatment of acquired nystagmus. Ann Neurol 41:818, 1997

BARTALENA L et al: Relation between therapy for hyperthyroidism and the course of Graves' ophthalmopathy. N Engl J Med 338:73, 1998

BECK RW et al: A randomized controlled trial of corticosteroids in the treatment of acute optic neuritis. N Engl J Med 326:581, 1992

BURDE RM et al: *Clinical Decisions in Neuro-ophthalmology*, 2d ed. St. Louis, Mosby, 1992

GASS JD: *Stereoscopic Atlas of Macular Diseases*, 4th ed. St. Louis, Mosby, 1996

GOLD DH, WEINGEIST TA (eds): *The Eye in Systemic Disease*. Philadelphia, Lippincott, 1990

INZITARI D et al for the North American Symptomatic Carotid Endarterectomy Trial Collaborators: The causes and risks of stroke in patients with asymptomatic internal carotid artery stenosis. N Engl J Med 342:1693, 2000

KRACHMER JH et al: *Cornea*. St. Louis, Mosby, 1997

LEIBOWITZ HM, WARING GO (eds): *Corneal Disorders. Clinical Diagnosis and Management*. Philadelphia, Saunders, 1998

LEIBOWITZ HM: The red eye. N Engl J Med 343:345, 2000

LEIGH RJ, ZEE DS: *The Neurology of Eye Movements*, 3d ed. Oxford, Oxford Univ Press, 1999

MILLER NR, NEWMAN NJ: *Walsh and Hoyt's Clinical Neuroophthalmology*, 5th ed. Baltimore, Williams & Wilkins, 1998

NATHAN J et al: Molecular genetics of inherited variation in human color vision. Science 232:203, 1986

NEITZ M, NEITZ J: Molecular genetics of color vision and color vision defects. Arch Ophthal 118:691, 2000

OPTIC NEURITIS STUDY GROUP: The 5-year risk of MS after optic neuritis. Experience of the optic neuritis treatment trial. Neurology 49:1404, 1997

————: Visual function 5 years after optic neuritis. Experience of the optic neuritis treatment trial. Arch Ophthalmol 115:1545, 1997

POLANSKY JR, NGUYEN TD: The TIGR gene, pathogenic mechanisms, and other recent advances in glaucoma genetics. Curr Opin Ophthalmol 9:15, 1998

SELLEBJERG F et al: A randomized, controlled trial of oral high-dose methylprednisolone in acute optic neuritis. Neurology 52:1479, 1999

SINGH G et al: A mitochondrial DNA mutation as a cause of Leber's hereditary optic neuropathy. N Engl J Med 320:1300, 1989

SPENCER WH (ed): Ophthalmic Pathology. An Atlas and Textbook, 4th ed. Philadelphia, Saunders, 1996

THOMKE F, HOPF HC: Isolated superior oblique palsies with electrophysiologically documented brainstem lesions. Muscle Nerve 23:267, 2000

VAUGHN D et al: *General Ophthalmology*, 15th ed. Norwalk, Appleton & Lange, 1999

WEBER J et al: Selective intra-arterial fibrinolysis of acute central retinal artery occlusion. Stroke 29:2076, 1998

29 *Anil K. Lalwani, James B. Snow, Jr.*

DISORDERS OF SMELL, TASTE, AND HEARING

SMELL

The sense of smell determines the flavor and palatability of food and drink. It serves, along with the trigeminal system, as a monitor of inhaled chemicals, including dangerous substances such as natural gas, smoke, and air pollutants. Loss of or decreased ability to smell affects approximately 1% of people under age 60 and more than half of the population beyond this age.

DEFINITIONS *Smell* is the perception of odor by the nose. *Taste* is the perception of salty, sweet, sour, or bitter by the tongue. Related sensations during eating such as somatic sensations of coolness, warmth, and irritation are mediated through the trigeminal, glossopharyngeal, and vagal afferents in the nose, oral cavity, tongue, pharynx, and larynx. *Flavor* is the complex interaction of taste, smell, and somatic sensation.

Terms relating to disorders of smell include *anosmia*, an absence of the ability to smell; *hyposmia*, a decreased ability to smell; *hyperosmia* (an increased sensitivity to an odorant); *dysosmia* (distortion in the perception of an odor); *phantosmia*, perception of an odorant where none is present; and *agnosia*, inability to classify, contrast, or identify odor sensations verbally, even though the ability to distinguish between odorants or to recognize them may be normal. An odor stimulus is referred to as an *odorant*. Each category of smell dysfunction can be further subclassified as total (applying to all odorants) or partial (dysfunction of only select odorants).

PHYSIOLOGY OF SMELL The *olfactory neuroepithelium* is located in the superior part of the nasal cavities. It contains an orderly arrangement of bipolar olfactory receptor cells, microvillar cells, sustentacular cells, and basal cells. The dendritic process of the bipolar cell has a bulb-shaped knob, or vesicle, that projects into the mucous layer and bears six to eight cilia. It is the cilia that contain the odorant receptors. The arrangement of cilia increases overall exposure to the environment and translates into each bipolar cell containing 56 cm^2 (9 in.^{2}) of surface area to receive stimulus.

The microvillar cells are located adjacent to the receptor cells on the surface of the neuroepithelium. The sustentacular cells, unlike their counterparts in the respiratory epithelium, are not specialized to secrete mucus. Although they form a tight barrier separating the neurons from the outside environment, their complete function is unknown. The basal cells are progenitors of other cell types in the olfactory neuroepithelium, including the bipolar receptor cells. There is a regular turnover of the bipolar receptor cells, which function as the primary sensory neurons. In addition, with injury to the cell body or its axon, the receptor cell is replaced by a differentiated basal cell which reestablishes a central neural connection. Hence these primary sensory neurons are unique among sensory systems in that they are regularly replaced and regenerate after injury.

The unmyelinated axons of the receptor cells form the fila of the olfactory nerve, pass through the cribriform plate, and terminate within spherical masses of neuropil, termed *glomeruli*, in the olfactory bulb. The glomeruli are the focus of a high degree of convergence of information, since many more fibers enter than leave them. The main second-order neurons are the mitral cells. The primary dendrite of each mitral cell extends into a single glomerulus. Axons of the mitral cells project along with the axons of adjacent tufted cells to the limbic system, including the anterior olfactory nucleus, the prepiriform cortex, the periamygdaloid cortex, the olfactory tubercle, the nucleus of the lateral olfactory tract, and the corticomedial nucleus of the amygdala. Cognitive awareness of smell requires stimulation of the prepiriform cortex or the amygdaloid nuclei.

A secondary potential site of olfactory chemosensation is located in the epithelium of the vomeronasal organ, a tubular structure that opens on the ventral aspect of the nasal septum. Sensory neurons located in the vomeronasal organ detect pheromones, nonvolatile chemical signals that in lower mammals trigger innate and stereotyped reproductive and social behaviors, as well as neuroendocrine changes. The neurons from the organ project to the accessory olfactory bulbs and not the main olfactory bulb, as in the olfactory neuroepithelium. Whether humans use the vomeronasal organ to detect and respond to chemical signals from others remains controversial. Recent work in delineating the molecular pathology of Kallman syndrome suggests that development of the olfactory and vomeronasal system is required for normal sexual maturation (Chap. 335).

The sensation of smell begins with introduction of an odorant to the cilia of the bipolar neuron. Most odorants are hydrophobic; as they move from the air phase of the nasal cavity to the aqueous phase of the olfactory mucous, they are transported toward the cilia by small water-soluble proteins called *odorant-binding proteins* and reversibly bind to receptors on the cilia surface. Binding causes conformational changes in the receptor protein, which induces a chain of biochemical events and results in generation of action potentials in the primary neurons. Transduction depends on the activation of G protein–coupled second messengers. Intensity appears to be coded by the amount of firing in the afferent neurons.

Basic elements of the genetic coding involved in smell are now becoming understood. Olfactory receptor proteins belong to the large family of G protein–coupled receptors that also includes rhodopsins; α- and β-adrenergic receptors; muscarinic acetylcholine receptors; and neurotransmitter receptors for dopamine, serotonin, and substance P. Members of the G protein–coupled receptors are characterized by the presence of 7 putative α-helical transmembrane domains composed of 20 to 28 hydrophobic amino acid residues. In mammals, there are probably 300 to 1000 olfactory receptor genes belonging to 20 different families located on various chromosomes in clusters. The receptor genes are present at more than 25 different human chromosomal locations. The gene clusters have likely risen as a result of repeated duplication of individual genes or clusters of genes. Each olfactory neuron seems to express only one or, at most, a few receptor genes thus providing the molecular basis of odor discrimination. While the receptors are expressed in several tissues, including the olfactory neuroepithelium and mammalian germ cells, their primary role appears to be odorant recognition and discrimination. Bipolar cells that express similar receptors appear to be scattered across discrete spatial zones.

These similar cells converge on a select few number of glomeruli in the olfactory bulb. The result is a potential spatial map of how we receive odor stimulus, much like the tonotopic organization of how we perceive sound.

DISORDERS OF THE SENSE OF SMELL Disorders of the sense of smell are caused by conditions that interfere with the access of the odorant to the olfactory neuroepithelium (transport loss), injure the receptor region (sensory loss), or damage central olfactory pathways (neural loss). At the present time, there are no clinical tests to differentiate these different types of olfactory losses. Fortunately, the history of the disease provides important clues to the cause. The leading causes of olfactory disorders are summarized in Table 29-1; the most common etiologies are head trauma and viral infections. Head trauma is a frequent cause of anosmia in children and young adults, whereas viral etiologies predominate in older adults.

Cranial trauma is followed by unilateral or bilateral impairment of smell in up to 15% of cases; anosmia is more common than hyposmia. Olfactory dysfunction is more common when trauma is associated with loss of consciousness, moderately severe head injury (grades II to V), and skull fracture. Frontal injuries and fractures disrupt the cribriform plate and olfactory axons that perforate it. Sometimes there is an associated cerebrospinal fluid (CSF) rhinorrhea resulting from a tearing of the dura overlying the cribriform plate and paranasal sinuses. Anosmia may also follow blows to the occiput. Once traumatic anosmia develops, it is usually permanent; only 10% of patients ever improve or recover. Perversion of the sense of smell may occur as a transient phase in the recovery process.

Viral infections destroy the olfactory neuroepithelium, which is replaced by respiratory epithelium. Parainfluenza virus type 3 appears to be especially detrimental to human olfaction. HIV infection is associated with subjective distortion of taste and smell, which may become more severe as the disease progresses. The loss of taste and smell may play an important role in the development and progression of HIV-associated wasting. Congenital anosmias are rare but important. Kallmann syndrome is an X-linked disorder characterized by congenital anosmia and hypogonadotropic hypogonadism resulting from a failure of migration from the olfactory placode of olfactory receptor neurons and neurons synthesizing gonadotropin-releasing hormone (Chap. 328). The responsible gene (*KAL*) has been cloned. Anosmia can also occur in albinos. The receptor cells are present but are hypoplastic, lack cilia, and do not project above the surrounding supporting cells.

Meningioma of the inferior frontal region is the most frequent neoplastic cause of anosmia; loss of smell may be the only neurologic abnormality at presentation. Rarely, anosmia can occur with glioma of the frontal lobe. Occasionally, pituitary adenomas, craniopharyn-giomas, suprasellar meningiomas, and aneurysms of the anterior part of the circle of Willis extend forward and damage olfactory structures. These tumors and hamartomas may also induce seizures with olfactory hallucinations, indicating involvement of the uncus of the temporal lobe.

Dysosmia, subjective distortions of olfactory perception, may occur with intranasal disease that partially impairs smell or may represent a phase in the recovery from a neurogenic anosmia. Most dysosmic disorders consist of disagreeable or foul odors, and they may be accompanied by distortions of taste. Dysosmia is associated with depression.

Approach to the Patient

The history of the onset and course of the disorder is often paramount in establishing an etiology. Unilateral anosmia is rarely a complaint and is only recognized by separate testing of smell in each nasal cavity. Bilateral anosmia, on the other hand, brings patients to medical attention. Anosmic patients usually complain of a loss of the sense of taste even though their taste thresholds may be within normal limits. In actuality, they are complaining of a loss of flavor detection, which is mainly an olfactory function. The physical examination should include a complete examination of the ears, upper respiratory tract, and head and neck. A neurologic examination emphasizing the cranial nerves and cerebellar and sensorimotor function is essential. The patient's general mood should be assessed, and any signs of depression should be noted.

The sensory evaluation of olfactory function is necessary to corroborate the patient's complaint, evaluate the efficacy of treatment, and assess the degree of permanent impairment. The degree to which qualitative sensations are present can be assessed by any of several methods. The Odor Stix test uses a commercially available odor-producing magic marker–like pen held approximately 8 to 15 cm (3 to 6 in.) from the patient's nose to check for gross perception of the odorant. Another gross perception of odorant test, the 30-cm alcohol test, uses a freshly opened isopropyl alcohol packet held approximately 30 cm (12 in.) from the patient's nose. There is a commercially available scratch-and-sniff card containing three odors available for testing olfaction grossly. A superior test is the University of Pennsylvania Smell Identification Test (UPSIT). This consists of a 40-item, forced choice, microencapsulated odor, scratch-and-sniff paradigm. For example, one of the items reads, "This odor smells most like (a) chocolate, (b) banana, (c) onion, or (d) fruit punch," and the patient is instructed to answer one of the alternatives. The test is highly reliable, is sensitive to age and sex differences, and provides an accurate quantitative determination of the olfactory deficit. Persons with a total loss of smell function score in the range of 7 to 19 out of 40. The average score for total anosmics is slightly higher than that expected on the basis of chance because of the inclusion of some odorants that act by trigeminal stimulation.

The second step is to establish a detection threshold for the odorant phenyl ethyl alcohol, using a graduated stimulus. Sensitivity for each side of the nose is determined with a detection threshold for phenyl ethyl methyl ethyl carbinol. Nasal resistance can also be measured with anterior rhinomanometry for each side of the nose.

Computed tomography (CT) or magnetic resonance imaging (MRI) of the head is required to rule out paranasal sinusitis, neoplasms of the anterior cranial fossa, nasal cavity, or paranasal sinuses and unsuspected fractures of the anterior cranial fossa. Bone abnormalities are best seen with CT. MRI is useful in evaluating olfactory bulbs, ventricles, and other soft tissue of the brain. Coronal CT is optimal for assessing cribriform plate, anterior cranial fossa, and sinus anatomy.

Techniques have been developed to biopsy the olfactory neuroepithelium, but in view of the widespread degeneration of the olfactory neuroepithelium and intercalation of respiratory epithelium in the ol-

Table 29-1 Causes of Olfactory Dysfunction

Transport Olfactory Losses	Neural Olfactory Losses
Allergic rhinitis	AIDS
Bacterial rhinitis and sinusitis	Alcoholism
Congenital Abnormality (encephalocele)	Alzheimer's disease
Nasal neoplasms	Chemical toxins
Nasal polyps	Cigarette smoke
Nasal septal deviation	Depression
Nasal surgery	Diabetes mellitus
Viral infections	Drugs
Sensory Olfactory Losses	Huntington's chorea
Drugs	Hypothyroidism
Neoplasms	Kallmann syndrome
Radiation therapy	Korsakoff's psychosis
Toxic chemical exposure	Malnutrition
Viral infections	Neoplasm
	Neurosurgery
	Parkinson's disease
	Trauma
	Vitamin B_{12} deficiency
	Zinc deficiency

factory area of adults with no apparent olfactory dysfunction, biopsy material must be interpreted cautiously.

R̲x̲ **TREATMENT** Therapy for patients with transport olfactory losses due to allergic rhinitis, bacterial rhinitis and sinusitis, polyps, neoplasms, and structural abnormalities of the nasal cavities can be undertaken rationally and with a high likelihood for improvement. Allergy management, antibiotic therapy, topical and systemic glucocorticoid therapy, and surgery for nasal polyps, deviation of the nasal septum, and chronic hyperplastic sinusitis are frequently effective in restoring the sense of smell.

There is no treatment with demonstrated efficacy for sensorineural olfactory losses. Fortunately, spontaneous recovery often occurs. Zinc and vitamin therapy (especially with vitamin A) are advocated by some. Profound zinc deficiency can produce loss and distortion of the sense of smell but is not a clinically important problem except in very limited geographic areas (Chap. 75). The epithelial degeneration associated with vitamin A deficiency can cause anosmia, but in western societies the prevalence of vitamin A deficiency is low. Exposure to cigarette smoke and other airborne toxic chemicals can cause metaplasia of the olfactory epithelium. Spontaneous recovery can occur if the insult is discontinued. Patient counseling is therefore helpful in these cases.

As mentioned above, more than half of people over age 60 suffer from olfactory dysfunction. No effective treatment exists for presbyosmia, but patients are often reassured to learn that this problem is common in their age group. In addition, early recognition and counseling can help patients to compensate for the loss of smell. The incidence of natural gas–related accidents is disproportionately high in the elderly, perhaps due in part to the gradual loss of smell. Mercaptan, the pungent odor in natural gas, is an olfactory stimulant and does not activate taste receptors. Many elderly with olfactory dysfunction experience a decrease in flavor sensation and find it necessary to hyperflavor food, usually by increasing the amount of salt in their diet. The physician can assist patients in developing healthy strategies to deal with the decreased sense of smell.

TASTE

Compared with disorders of smell, gustatory disorders are uncommon and their pathogenesis poorly understood. Many patients with a loss of olfactory sensitivity also complain of a loss of the sense of taste. On testing, most of these patients have normal detection thresholds for taste.

DEFINITIONS Disturbances of the sense of taste may be categorized as *total ageusia*—total absence of gustatory function or inability to detect the qualities of sweet, salt, bitter, or sour; *partial ageusia*—ability to detect some of but not all the qualitative gustatory sensations; *specific ageusia*—inability to detect the taste quality of certain substances; *total hypogeusia*—decreased sensitivity to all tastants; *partial hypogeusia*—decreased sensitivity to some tastants; and *dysgeusia* or *phantogeusia*—distortion in the perception of a tastant, i.e., the perception of the wrong quality when a tastant is presented or the perception of a taste when there has been no tastant ingested. Confusions of sour and bitter are common and, at times, may be semantic misunderstandings. Frequently, however, they have physiologic or pathophysiologic bases. Other taste quality confusions occur between sour and salty and bitter. It may be possible to differentiate between the loss of flavor recognition in patients with olfactory losses who complain of a loss of taste as well as smell by asking if they are able to taste sweetness in sodas, saltiness in potato chips, etc.

PHYSIOLOGY OF TASTE The taste receptor cells are located in the taste buds, spherical groups of cells arranged in a pattern resembling the segments of a citrus fruit. At the surface, the taste bud has a pore into which microvilli of the receptor cells project. Unlike

the olfactory system, the receptor cell is not the primary neuron. Instead, gustatory afferent nerve fibers contact individual taste receptor cells. Transduction depends on activation of G protein–coupled second messengers but differs in details for each taste quality.

The sense of taste is mediated through the facial, glossopharyngeal, and vagal nerves. The gustatory system consists of at least five receptor populations. Taste buds are located in the papillae along the lateral margin and dorsum of the tongue at the junction of the dorsum and the base of the tongue, and in the palate, epiglottis, larynx, and esophagus. The chorda tympani branch of the facial nerve subserves taste from the anterior two-thirds of the tongue. The posterior third of the tongue is supplied by the lingual branch of the glossopharyngeal nerve. Afferents from the palate travel with the greater superficial petrosal nerve to the geniculate ganglion and then via the facial nerve to the brainstem. The internal branch of the superior laryngeal nerve of the vagus nerve contains the taste afferents from the larynx, including the epiglottis and esophagus.

The central connections of the nerves terminate in the brainstem in the nucleus of the tractus solitarius. The central pathway from the nucleus of the tractus solitarius projects to the ipsilateral parabrachial nuclei of the pons. Two divergent pathways project from the parabrachial nuclei. One ascends to the gustatory relay in the dorsal thalamus, synapses, and continues to the cortex of the insula. There is also evidence for a direct pathway from the parabrachial nuclei to the cortex. (Olfaction and gustation appear to be unique among sensory systems in that at least some fibers bypass the thalamus.) The other pathway from the parabrachial nuclei goes to the ventral forebrain, including the lateral hypothalamus, substantia innominata, central nucleus of the amygdala, and the stria terminalis.

Tastants gain access to the receptor cells through the taste pore. Four classes of taste are recognized: sweet, salt, sour, and bitter. Individual gustatory afferent fibers almost always respond to a number of different chemicals. Response patterns of gustatory afferent axons can be grouped into classes based on the stimulus chemical that produces the largest response. For example, for sucrose–best response neurons, the second-best stimulus is almost always sodium chloride. The fact that individual gustatory afferent fibers respond to a large number of different chemicals led to the *across-fiber-pattern* theory of gustatory coding, while the best-stimulus analysis led to the concept of *labeled* afferents. It appears that labeled fibers are important for establishing gross quality, but the across-fiber pattern within a best-stimulus category, and perhaps among categories, is needed for discriminating chemicals within qualities. For example, sweetness may be carried by sucrose-best neurons, but the differentiation of sucrose and fructose may require a comparison of the relative activity among sucrose-best, salt-best, and quinine-best neurons. As with olfaction and other sensory systems, intensity appears to be encoded by the quantity of neural activity.

DISORDERS OF THE SENSE OF TASTE Disorders of the sense of taste are caused by conditions that interfere with the access of the tastant to the receptor cells in the taste bud (transport loss), injure receptor cells (sensory loss), or damage gustatory afferent nerves and central gustatory pathways (neural loss) (Table 29-2). *Transport gustatory losses* result from xerostomia due to many causes, including Sjögren's syndrome, radiation therapy, heavy-metal intoxication, and bacterial colonization of the taste pore. *Sensory gustatory losses* are caused by inflammatory and degenerative diseases in the oral cavity; a vast number of drugs, particularly those that interfere with cell turnover such as antithyroid and antineoplastic agents; radiation therapy to the oral cavity and pharynx; viral infections; endocrine disorders; neoplasms; and aging. *Neural gustatory losses* occur with neoplasms, trauma, and surgical procedures in which the gustatory afferents are injured. Taste buds degenerate when their gustatory afferents are transected but remain when their somatosensory afferents are severed. Patients with renal disease have increased thresholds for sweet and sour tastes, which resolves with dialysis.

A side effect of medication is the single most common cause of taste dysfunction in clinical practice. The mechanism may be a change

Table 29-2   Causes of Gustatory Dysfunction

Transport Gustatory Losses	Neural Gustatory Losses
Drugs	Diabetes mellitus
Heavy-metal intoxication	Hypothyroidism
Radiation therapy	Oral neoplasms
Sjögren's syndrome	Oral surgery
Xerostomia	Radiation therapy
Sensory Gustatory Losses	Renal disease
Aging	Trauma
Candidiasis	Upper respiratory tract infections
Drugs (antithyroid and antineoplastic)	
Endocrine disorders	
Herpes infection	
Oral neoplasm	
Pemphigus	
Radiation therapy	
Viral infections	

in the composition of saliva, an effect on receptor function or signal transduction, or disruption of the central processing of gustatory input. Unfortunately, the responsible mechanism is not well understood for most medications. Xerostomia, regardless of the etiology, can be associated with taste dysfunction. It is associated with poor oral clearance, poor dental hygeine, and can adversely affect the oral mucosa, all leading to dysgeusia. However, severe salivary gland failure does not necessarily lead to taste complaints. Xerostomia, along with the use of antibiotics or glucocorticoids, and compromised immune function can lead to overgrowth of *Candida*; overgrowth alone, without thrush or overt signs of infection can be associated with bad taste or hypogeusia. When taste dysfunction occurs in a patient at risk for fungal overgrowth, a trial of nystatin or other anti-fungal medication is warranted.

Upper respiratory infections and head trauma can lead to both smell and taste dysfunction; taste is more likely to improve than smell. The mechanism of taste disturbance in these situations is not well understood. Trauma to the chorda tympani branch of the facial nerve during middle ear surgery or third molar extractions is relatively common and can cause dysgeusia. Bilateral chorda tympani injuries are usually associated with hypogeusia, whereas unilateral lesions produce only limited symptoms, perhaps because responses from taste receptors are disinhibited by the glossopharyngeal nerve.

Finally, aging itself may be associated with reduced taste sensitivity. The taste dysfunction may be limited to a single compound and may be mild. While many older patients may acknowledge loss of taste when asked, they are unlikely to seek medical attention for taste disturbance alone.

Approach to the Patient

Patients who complain of loss of taste should be evaluated for both gustatory and olfactory function. Clinical assessment of taste is not as well developed or standardized as that of smell. The first step is to perform suprathreshold whole-mouth taste testing for quality, intensity, and pleasantness perception of four taste qualities: sweet, salty, sour, and bitter. Most commonly used reagents for taste testing are sucrose, citric acid or hydrochloric acid, caffeine or quinine (sulfate or hydrochloride), and sodium chloride. The taste stimuli should be freshly prepared. For quantification, detection thresholds are obtained by applying graduated dilutions to the tongue quandrants or by whole-mouth sips. Electric taste testing (*electrogustometry*) is used clinically to identify taste deficits in specific quandrants of the tongue, following precise applications of stimuli. Regional gustatory testing may also be performed to assess for the possibility of loss localized to one or more receptor fields as a result of a peripheral or central lesion.

Once there is objective evidence of a disorder of taste, it is important to establish an anatomic diagnosis before proceeding to an etiologic diagnosis. The history of the disease often provides important clues to the cause. For example, absence of taste on the anterior two-thirds of the tongue associated with a facial paralysis indicates that the lesion is proximal to the juncture of the chorda tympani branch with the facial nerve in the mastoid.

TREATMENT   Therapy for gustatory loss is limited. Nonetheless, some etiologies of taste dysfunction are amenable to intervention. Taste disturbance related to drugs can often be resolved by changing the prescribed medication. Xerostomia can be treated with artificial saliva, providing some benefits to patients with a disturbed salivary milieu. Oral pilocarpine may be beneficial for a variety of forms of xerostomia. Appropriate treatment of bacterial and fungal infections of the oral cavity can be of great help in improving taste function. Taste dysfunction following trauma may resolve spontaneously without intervention and is more likely to do so than posttraumatic smell dysfunction. Altered taste due to surgical stretch injury of chorda tympani nerve usually improves within 3 to 4 months, while dysfunction is usually permanent with transection of the nerve. In most patients with idiopathic cases of altered taste sensitivity, the problem either remains stable or worsens. Zinc and vitamin therapy for gustatory losses is advocated by some but lacks demonstrated efficacy. No effective therapeutic strategies exist for the sensorineural disorders of taste.

HEARING

Hearing loss is one of the most common sensory disorders in humans. Nearly 10% of the adult population has some hearing loss. For many, this impairment presents early in life. However, hearing loss can present at any age. Between 30 and 35% of individuals over the age of 65 have a hearing loss of sufficient magnitude to require a hearing aid.

PHYSIOLOGY OF HEARING (Fig. 29-1)   Hearing occurs by air conduction and bone conduction. In air conduction, sound waves reach the ear by propagation in air, enter the external auditory canal, and set the tympanic membrane in motion, which in turn moves the malleus, incus, and stapes of the middle ear. Movement of the footplate of the stapes causes pressure changes in the fluid-filled inner ear eliciting a traveling wave in the basilar membrane of the cochlea. The tympanic membrane and the ossicular chain in the middle ear serve as an impedence-matching mechanism, improving the efficiency of energy transfer from air to the fluid-filled inner ear. Hearing by bone conduction occurs when the sounding source, in contact with the head, results in vibration of the bones of the skull, including the temporal bone, producing a traveling wave in the basilar membrane.

Stereocilia of the hair cells of the organ of Corti, which rests on the basilar membrane, are in contact with the tectorial membrane and are deformed by the traveling wave. A point of maximal displacement of the basilar membrane is determined by the frequency of the stimulating tone. High-frequency tones cause maximal displacement of the basilar membrane near the base of the cochlea. As the frequency of the stimulating tone decreases, the point of maximal displacement moves toward the apex of the cochlea.

The inner and outer hair cells of the organ of Corti have different innervation patterns, but both are mechanoreceptors. The afferent innervation relates principally to the inner hair cells, and the efferent innervation relates principally to outer hair cells. The motility of the outer hair cells alters the micromechanics of the inner hair cells creating a cochlear amplifier, which explains the exquisite sensitivity and frequency selectivity of the cochlea.

The current concept of cochlear transduction is that displacement of the tips of the stereocilia allows potassium to flow into the cell, resulting in its depolarization. The potassium influx opens calcium channels near the base of the cell, stimulating transmitter release. The neurotransmitter at the hair cell and cochlear nerve dendrite interface is thought to be glutamate. The action potential in the eighth nerve occurs 0.5 ms after the onset of the cochlear microphonic potential.

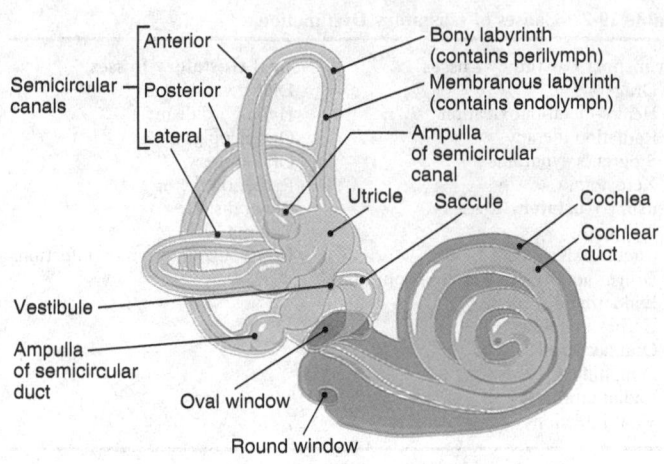

FIGURE 29-1 *A.* Drawing of modified coronal section through external ear and temporal bone, with structures of the middle and inner ear demonstrated. *B.* High-resolution view of inner ear.

Each of the cochlear nerve neurons can be activated at a frequency and intensity specific for that cell. This specificity is maintained at each point of the central auditory pathway: dorsal and ventral cochlear nuclei, trapezoid body, superior olivary complex, lateral lemniscus, inferior colliculus, medial geniculate body, and auditory cortex. At low frequencies, individual auditory nerve fibers can respond more or less synchronously with the stimulating tone. At higher frequencies, phase-locking occurs so that neurons alternate in response to particular phases of the cycle of the sound wave. Intensity is encoded by the amount of neural activity in individual neurons, the number of neurons that are active, and the specific neurons that are activated.

GENETIC CAUSES OF HEARING LOSS More than half of childhood hearing impairment is thought to be hereditary; hereditary hearing impairment (HHI) can also manifest later in life. HHI may be classified as either nonsyndromic, when hearing loss is the only clinical abnormality, or syndromic, when hearing loss is associated with anomalies in other organ systems. Nearly two-thirds of HHIs are nonsyndromic and the remaining one-third are syndromic. Between 70 and 80% of nonsyndromic HHI is inherited in an autosomal recessive manner; another 15 to 20% is autosomal dominant. Less than 5% is X-linked or maternally inherited via the mitochondria.

Over 60 loci harboring genes for nonsyndromic HHI have been mapped, with equal numbers of dominant and recessive modes of inheritance; 14 different genes have been cloned (Table 29-3). The hearing genes fall into the categories of structural proteins (MYO7A, MYO15, TECTA, DIAPH1), transcription factors (POU3F4, POU4F3), ion channels (KCNQ4, PDS), and gap junction proteins (Cx26, Cx30, Cx31). Several of these genes, including connexin 26 (Cx26), TECTA, and MYO7A, cause both autosomal dominant and recessive forms of nonsyndromic HHI. In general, the hearing loss associated with dominant genes has its onset in adolescence or adulthood and varies in severity, whereas the hearing loss associated with recessive inheritance is congenital and profound. Connexin 26 is particularly important because it is associated with nearly 20% of cases of childhood deafness; in heterozygotes the onset of hearing loss may be in adolescence or adulthood. Two frame-shift mutations, 30delG and 167delT, account for >50% of the cases, making population screening feasible. The 167delT mutation is highly prevalent in Ashkenazi Jews; it is predicted that 1 in 1765 individuals in this population will be homozygous and affected. The hearing loss can also vary among the members of the same family, suggesting that other genes or factors likely influence the auditory phenotype.

The contribution of genetics to presbycusis (see below) is also becoming better understood. In addition to connexin 26, several other nonsyndromic genes are associated with hearing loss that progresses with age. It is likely that presbycusis has both environmental and genetic components.

Over 200 syndromes are associated with hearing loss. Common syndromic forms of hearing loss include Usher syndrome (retinitis pigmentosa and hearing loss), Waardenburg syndrome (pigmentary abnormality and hearing loss), Pendred syndrome (thyroid organification defect and hearing loss), Alport syndrome (renal disease and hearing loss), Jervell and Lange-Nielsen syndrome (prolonged QT interval and hearing loss), neurofibromatosis type 2 (bilateral acoustic schwannoma), and mitochondrial disorders [mitochondrial encephalopathy, lactic acidosis, and stroke-like episodes (MELAS); myoclonic epilepsy and ragged red fibers (MERRF); progressive external ophthalmoplegia (PEO)].

Rapid progress in understanding the basis of these and related disorders has revealed a fascinating complexity, including evidence for genetic heterogeneity (different genes resulting in a similar clinical phenotype), allelic disorders (distinct phenotypes associated with different mutations in the same gene), and polygenic modifiers (Chap. 65).

DISORDERS OF THE SENSE OF HEARING Hearing loss can result from disorders of the auricle, external auditory canal, middle ear, inner ear, or central auditory pathways (Fig. 29-2). *In general, lesions in the auricle, external auditory canal, or middle ear cause conductive hearing losses, whereas lesions in the inner ear or eighth nerve cause sensorineural hearing losses.*

Conductive Hearing Loss This results from obstruction of the external auditory canal by cerumen, debris, and foreign bodies; swelling of the lining of the canal; atresia of the ear canal; neoplasms of the canal; perforations of the tympanic membrane; disruption of the ossicular chain, as occurs with necrosis of the long process of the incus in trauma or infection; otosclerosis; or fluid, scarring, or neoplasms in the middle ear.

Cholesteatoma, i.e., the presence of stratified squamous epithelium in the middle ear or mastoid, occurs frequently in adults. A cholesteatoma is a benign, slowly growing lesion that destroys bone and normal ear tissue. Major theories of pathogenesis of acquired cholesteatoma include traumatic implantation and invasion, immigration and invasion through a perforation, and metaplasia following chronic infection and irritation. On examination, there is often a perforation filled with cheesy white squamous debris. A chronically draining ear that fails to respond to appropriate antibiotic therapy should raise the suspicion of a cholesteatoma. Conductive hearing loss secondary to ossicular erosion is common. Surgery is required to remove this insidiously growing and destructive disease process.

Conductive hearing loss in the presence of a normal ear canal and intact tympanic membrane is suggestive of ossicular pathology. Fixation of the stapes from *otosclerosis* is a common cause of low-frequency conductive hearing loss. It occurs with equal frequency in men and women and has a simple autosomal dominant inheritance with incomplete penetrance. Hearing impairment usually presents between the late teens to the forties. In women, the hearing loss is often first noticeable during pregnancy, as the otosclerotic process is accelerated during pregnancy. A hearing aid or a short outpatient surgical procedure (stapedectomy) can provide adequate auditory rehabilitation. Extension of otosclerosis beyond the stapes footplate to involve the cochlea (cochlear otosclerosis) can lead to mixed or sensorineural hearing loss. Fluoride therapy to prevent hearing loss associated with cochlear otosclerosis remains controversial.

Eustachian tube dysfunction is extremely common in adults and may predispose to acute otitis media (AOM) or serous otitis media (SOM). Trauma, AOM, or chronic otitis media are the usual factors responsible for tympanic membrane perforation. While small perforations often heal spontaneously, larger defects usually require surgical intervention. Tympanoplasty is highly effective (>90%) in the repair of tympanic membrane perforations. Otoscopy is usually sufficient to diagnose AOM, SOM, chronic otitis media, cerumen impaction, tympanic membrane perforation, and eustachian tube dysfunction.

Table 29-3 Nonsyndromic Genes and Loci

Locus	Gene	Function	Inheritance
DFNB1	GBJ2 (Cx26)	Forms gap junctions, or plasma membrane channels, with connexins	AR
DFNB2	MYO7A	Moves different macromolecular structures relative to actin filaments	AR
DFNB3	MYO15	Organizes actin in hair cells	AR
DFNB4	PDS	Encodes highly hydrophobic proteins containing the sulphate transporter signature	AR
DFNB9	OTOF	Involved in trafficking of membrane vesicles	AR
DFNB21	TECTA	Includes an amino-terminal hydrophobic signal sequence for translocation across the membrane and a carboxy-terminal hydrophobic region characteristic of precursors of glycosylphosphatidyl-inositol-linked membrane-bound proteins	AR
DFNA1	DIAPH1	Involved in cytokinesis and establishment of cell polarity	AD
DFNA2	GJB3 (Cx31)	Forms gap junction protein	AD
	KCNQ4	Forms potassium channel	
DFNA3	GJB2 (Cx26)	Forms gap junctions, or plasma membrane channels, with connexins	AD
	GBJ6 (Cx30)		
DFNA5	DFNA5	Unknown; related to a gene that is upregulated in estrogen receptor–negative breast carcinomas	AD
DFNA8/12	TECTA	Includes an amino-terminal hydrophobic signal sequence for translocation across the membrane and a carboxy-terminal hydrophobic region characteristic of precursors of glycosylphosphatidyl-inositol-linked membrane-bound proteins	AD
DFNA9	COCH	Involved in hemostasis, complement system, immune system, and extracellular matrix assembly	AD
DFNA11	MYO7A	Moves different macromolecular structures relative to actin filaments	AD
DFNA15	POU4F3	Serves as a critical developmental regulator for the determination of cellular phenotypes	AD
DFN3	POU3F4	Serves as a critical developmental regulator for the determination of cellular phenotypes	X-linked

NOTE: AD, autosomal dominant; AR, autosomal recessive.

Sensorineural Hearing Loss Damage to the hair cells of the organ of Corti may be caused by intense noise, viral infections, ototoxic drugs (e.g., salicylates, quinine and its synthetic analogues, aminoglycoside antibiotics, loop diuretics such as furosemide and ethacrynic acid, and cancer chemotherapeutic agents such as cisplatin), fractures of the temporal bone, meningitis, cochlear otosclerosis (see above), Ménière's disease, and aging. Congenital malformations of the inner ear may be the cause of hearing loss in some adults. Genetic predisposition alone or in concert with environmental influences may also be responsible.

Presbycusis (age-associated hearing loss) is the most common cause of sensorineural hearing loss in adults. In the early stages, it is characterized by symmetric, gentle to sharply sloping high-frequency hearing loss. With progression, the hearing loss involves all frequencies. More importantly, the hearing impairment is associated with significant loss in clarity. There is a loss of discrimination for phonemes, recruitment (abnormal growth of loudness), and particular difficulty in understanding speech in noisy environments. Hearing aids may provide limited rehabilitation once the word recognition score deteriorates below 50%. Significant advancements and improvements in cochlear implants have made them the treatment of choice when hearing aids prove inadequate (<30% word recognition score with optimal amplification).

Ménière's disease is characterized by episodic vertigo, fluctuating sensorineural hearing loss, tinnitus, and aural fullness. Tinnitus and/or deafness may be absent during the initial attacks of vertigo, but they invariably appear as the disease progresses and are increased in severity during an acute attack. The annual incidence of Ménière's disease is 0.5 to 7.5 per 1000; onset is most frequently in the fifth decade of life but may also occur in young adults or the elderly. Histologically, there is distention of the endolymphatic system (endolymphatic hydrops) leading to degeneration of vestibular and cochlear hair cells. This may result from endolymphatic sac dysfunction secondary to infection, trauma, autoimmune disease, inflammatory causes, or tumor; an idiopathic etiology constitutes the largest category and is most accurately referred to as Ménière's disease. Although any pattern of hearing loss can be observed, typically, low-frequency, unilateral sensorineural hearing impairment is present. MRI should be obtained to exclude retrocochlear pathology such as cerebellopontine angle tumors or demyelinating disorders. Therapy is directed towards the control of vertigo. A low-salt diet is the mainstay of treatment of the control of rotatory vertigo. Diuretics, a short course of glucocorticoids, and intratympanic gentamicin may also be useful adjuncts in recalcitrant cases. Surgical therapy of vertigo is reserved for unresponsive cases and includes endolymphatic sac decompression, labyrinthectomy, and vestibular nerve section. Both labyrinthectomy and vestibular nerve section abolish rotatory vertigo in >90% of the cases. Unfortunately, there is no effective therapy for hearing loss, tinnitus, or aural fullness associated with Ménière's disease.

Sensorineural hearing loss may also result from any neoplastic, vascular, demyelinating, infectious, or degenerative disease or trauma affecting the central auditory pathways. Human immunodeficiency virus leads to both peripheral and central auditory system pathology and is associated with sensorineural hearing impairment.

An individual can have both conductive and sensory hearing loss termed *mixed hearing loss*. Mixed hearing losses are due to pathology that can affect the middle and inner ear simultaneously such as otosclerosis involving the ossicles and the cochlea, head trauma, chronic otitis media, cholesteatoma, middle ear tumors, and some inner ear malformations.

Trauma resulting in temporal bone fractures may be associated

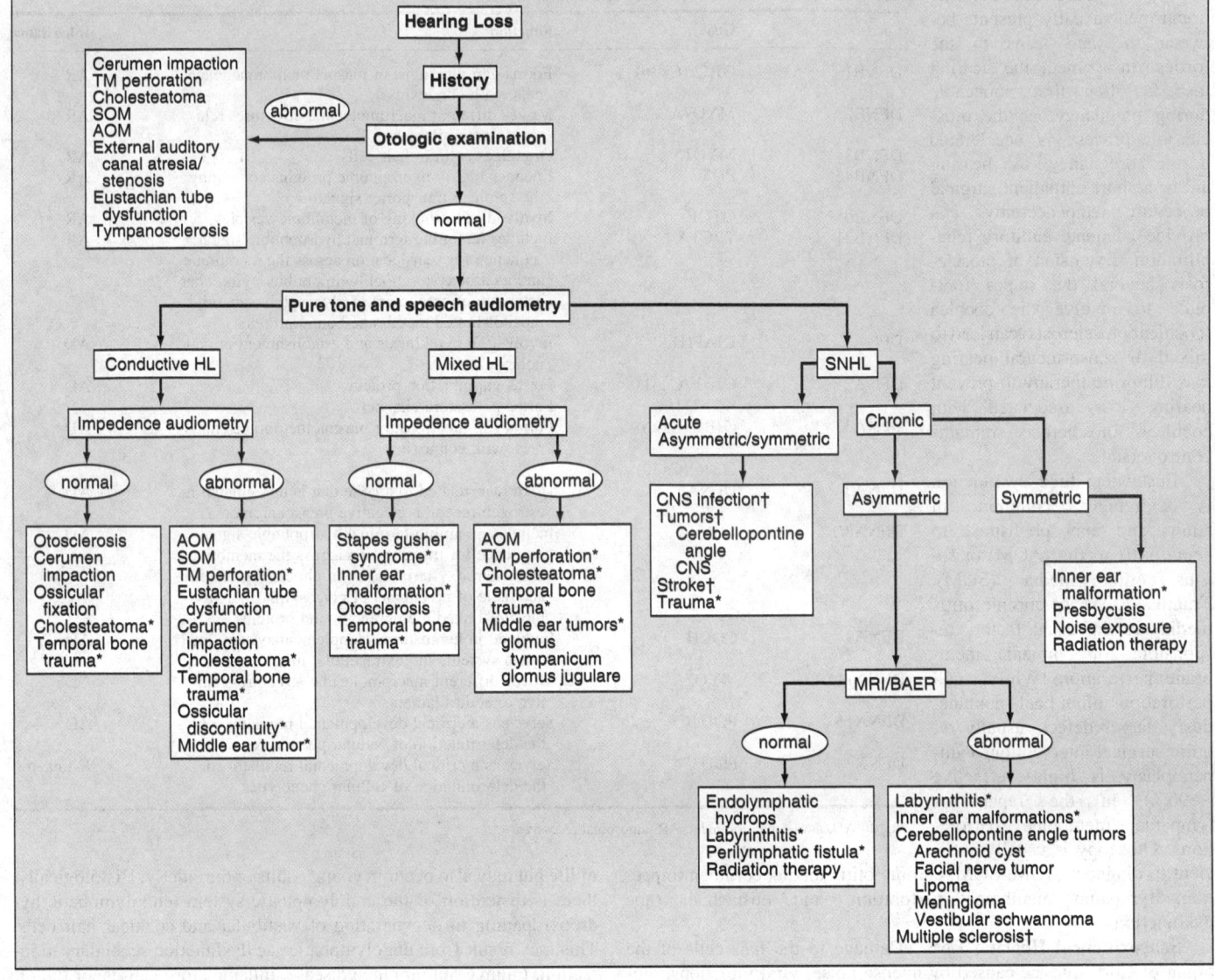

FIGURE 29-2 An algorithm for the approach to hearing loss. HL, hearing loss; SNHL, sensorineural hearing loss; TM, tympanic membrane; SOM, serous otitis media; AOM, acute otitis media; *, CT scan of temporal bone; †, MRI scan.

with conductive, sensorineural, and mixed hearing loss. If the fracture spares the inner ear, there may simply be conductive hearing loss due to rupture of the tympanic membrane or disruption of the ossicular chain. These abnormalities are amenable to surgical correction. Profound hearing loss and severe vertigo are associated with temporal bone fractures involving the inner ear. A perilymphatic fistula associated with leakage of inner-ear fluid into the middle ear can occur and may require surgical repair. An associated facial nerve injury is not uncommon. CT is best suited to assess fracture of the traumatized temporal bone, evaluate the ear canal, and determine the integrity of the ossicular chain and the involvement of the inner ear. CSF leaks that accompany temporal bone fractures are usually self-limited; the use of prophylactic antibiotics is controversial.

Tinnitus is defined as the perception of a sound when there is no sound in the environment. It may have a buzzing, roaring, or ringing quality and may be pulsatile (synchronous with the heartbeat). Tinnitus is often associated with either a conductive or sensorineural hearing loss. The pathophysiology of tinnitus is not well understood. The cause of the tinnitus can usually be determined by finding the cause of the associated hearing loss. Tinnitus may be the first symptom of a serious condition such as a vestibular schwannoma. Pulsatile tinnitus requires evaluation of the vascular system of the head to exclude vascular tumors such as glomus jugulare tumors, aneurysms, and stenotic arterial lesions; it may also occur with SOM.

Approach to the Patient

The goals in the evaluation of a patient with auditory complaints are to determine: (1) the nature of the hearing impairment (conductive vs. sensorineural), (2) the severity of the impairment (mild, moderate, severe, profound), (3) the anatomy of the impairment (external ear, middle ear, inner ear, or central auditory pathway pathology, and (4) the etiology. Initially, the history and the physical examination are critical in the identification of the underlying pathology leading to the auditory deficit. The history should elicit characteristics of the hearing loss, including the duration of deafness, nature of onset (sudden vs. insidious), rate of progression (rapid vs. slow), and involvement of the ear (unilateral vs. bilateral). The presence or absence of tinnitus, vertigo, imbalance, aural fullness, otorrhea, headache, facial nerve dysfunction, and head and neck paresthesias should be ascertained. Information regarding head trauma, exposure to ototoxins, occupational or recreational noise exposure, and family history of hearing impairment may also be important. A sudden onset of unilateral hearing loss, with or without tinnitus, may represent a viral infection of the inner ear or a vascular accident. Patients with unilateral hearing loss (sensory or conductive) usually complain of reduced hearing, poor sound localization, and difficulty hearing clearly with background noise. Gradual progression of a hearing deficit is common with otosclerosis, noise-induced hearing loss, vestibular schwannoma, or Ménière's disease.

Small vestibular schwannomas typically present with asymmetric hearing impairment, tinnitus, and imbalance (rarely vertigo); cranial neuropathy, in particular of the trigeminal or facial nerve, may accompany larger tumors. In addition to hearing loss, Ménière's disease may be associated with episodic vertigo, tinnitus, and aural fullness. Hearing loss with otorrhea is most likely due to chronic otitis media or cholesteatoma.

Family history may be crucial in delineating a genetic basis of hearing impairment. The history may also help identify environmental risk factors that lead to hearing impairment in a family. Sensitivity to aminoglycoside ototoxicity, maternally transmitted through a mitochondrial mutation, can be ascertained through a careful family history (Chap. 67). Susceptibility to noise-induced hearing loss or age-related hearing loss (presbycusis) may also be genetically determined.

The physical examination should evaluate the auricle, external ear canal, and tympanic membrane. The external ear canal of the elderly is often dry and fragile; it is preferable to clean cerumen with wall-mounted suction and cerumen loops and to avoid irrigation. In examining the eardrum, the topography of the tympanic membrane is more critical than the presence or absence of the highly touted light reflex. In addition to the pars tensa (the lower two-thirds of the eardrum), the pars flaccida above the short process of the malleus should also be examined for retraction pockets that may be evidence of chronic eustachian tube dysfunction or cholesteatoma. Insufflation of the ear canal is necessary to assess tympanic membrane mobility and compliance. Careful inspection of the nose, nasopharynx, and upper respiratory tract is indicated. Unilateral serous effusion in the adult should prompt a fiberoptic examination of the nasopharynx to exclude neoplasms. Cranial nerves should be carefully evaluated with special attention to facial and trigeminal nerves, which are commonly disturbed with tumors involving the cerebellopontine angle.

The Weber and Rinne tuning fork tests are used to differentiate conductive from sensorineural hearing losses and to confirm the findings of audiologic evaluation. Rinne's test compares the ability to hear by air conduction with the ability to hear by bone conduction. The tines of a vibrating tuning fork are held near the opening of the external auditory canal, and then the stem is placed on the mastoid process; for direct contact, it may be placed on teeth or dentures. The patient is asked to indicate whether the tone is louder by air conduction or bone conduction. Normally, and in the presence of sensorineural hearing loss, a tone is heard louder by air conduction than by bone conduction; however, with conductive hearing loss of ≥30 dB (see "Audiologic Assessment," below), the bone-conduction stimulus is perceived as louder than the air-conduction stimulus. The Rinne test is most sensitive in detecting mild conductive hearing losses if a 256-Hz tuning fork is used. The Weber test may be performed with a 256- or 512-Hz fork. The stem of a vibrating tuning fork is placed on the head in the midline and the patient asked whether the tone is heard in both ears or better in one ear than in the other. With a unilateral conductive hearing loss, the tone is perceived in the affected ear. With a unilateral sensorineural hearing loss, the tone is perceived in the unaffected ear. As a general rule, a 5-dB difference in hearing between the two ears is required for lateralization. The combined information from the Weber and Rinne tests permits a tentative conclusion as to whether a conductive or sensorineural hearing loss is present; however, these tests are associated with significant false-positive and -negative responses and therefore should be utilized only as screening tools.

LABORATORY ASSESSMENT OF HEARING Audiologic Assessment The minimum audiologic assessment for hearing loss should include the measurement of pure tone air-conduction and bone-conduction thresholds, speech reception threshold, discrimination score, tympanometry, acoustic reflexes, and acoustic-reflex decay. This test battery provides a comprehensive screening evaluation of the whole auditory system and allows one to determine whether further differentiation of a sensory (cochlear) from a neural (retrocochlear) hearing loss is indicated.

Pure tone audiometry assesses hearing acuity for pure tones. The test is administered by an audiologist and is performed in a sound-attenuated chamber. The pure tone stimulus is delivered with an audiometer, an electronic device that allows the presentation of specific frequencies (generally between 250 and 8000 Hz) at specific intensities. Air and bone conduction thresholds are established for each ear. Air conduction thresholds are established by presenting the stimulus in air with the use of headphones. Bone conduction thresholds are accomplished by placing the stem of a vibrating tuning fork or an oscillator of an audiometer in contact with the head. In the presence of a hearing loss, broad-spectrum noise is presented to the nontest ear for *masking* purposes so that responses are based on perception from the ear under test.

The responses are measured in decibels. An *audiogram* is a plot of intensity in decibels required to achieve threshold versus frequency. A decibel (dB) is equal to 20 times the logarithm of the ratio of the sound pressure required to achieve threshold in the patient to the sound pressure required to achieve threshold in a normal hearing person. Therefore, a change of 6 dB represents doubling of sound pressure, and a change of 20 dB represents a ten-fold change in sound pressure. Loudness, which depends on the frequency, intensity, and duration of a sound, doubles with approximately each 10-dB increase in sound pressure level. Pitch, on the other hand, does not directly correlate with frequency. The perception of pitch changes slowly in the low and high frequencies. In the middle tones, which are important for human speech, pitch varies more rapidly with changes in frequency.

Pure tone audiometry establishes the presence and severity of hearing impairment, unilateral vs. bilateral involvement, and the type of hearing loss. Conductive hearing losses with a large mass component, as is often seen in middle-ear effusions, produce elevation of thresholds that predominate in the higher frequencies. Conductive hearing losses with a large stiffness component, as in fixation of the footplate of the stapes in early otosclerosis, produce threshold elevations in the lower frequencies. Often, the conductive hearing loss involves all frequencies, suggesting involvement of both stiffness and mass. In general, sensorineural hearing losses such as presbycusis affect higher frequencies more than lower frequencies. An exception is Ménière's disease, which is characteristically associated with low-frequency sensorineural hearing loss. Noise-induced hearing loss has an unusual pattern of hearing impairment in which the loss at 4000 Hz is greater than at higher frequencies. Vestibular schwannomas characteristically affect the higher frequencies, but any pattern of hearing loss can be observed.

Speech recognition requires greater synchronous neural firing than is necessary for appreciation of pure tones. *Speech audiometry* tests the clarity with which one hears. The *speech reception threshold* (SRT) is defined as the intensity at which speech is recognized as a meaningful symbol and is obtained by presenting two-syllable words with an equal accent on each syllable. The intensity at which the patient can repeat 50% of the words correctly is the SRT. Once the SRT is determined, discrimination or word recognition ability is tested by presenting one-syllable words at 25 to 40 dB above the speech reception threshold. The words are phonetically balanced in that the phonemes (speech sounds) occur in the list of words at the same frequency that they occur in ordinary conversational English. An individual with normal hearing or conductive hearing loss can repeat 88 to 100% of the phonetically balanced words correctly. Patients with a sensorineural hearing loss have variable loss of discrimination depending on the severity of hearing loss and the site of lesion. Further, as a general rule, neural lesions are associated with more deterioration in discrimination ability than are lesions in the inner ear. For example, in a patient with mild asymmetric sensorineural hearing loss, a clue to the diagnosis of vestibular schwannoma is the presence of greater than expected deterioration in discrimination ability. Deterioration in discrimination ability at higher intensities above the SRT also suggests a lesion in the eighth nerve or central auditory pathways.

Tympanometry measures the impedance of the middle ear to sound and is particularly useful in the identification and diagnosis of middle-ear effusions. A sounding source and microphone are introduced into the ear canal with an airtight seal. The amount of sound that is absorbed through the middle ear or reflected from the middle ear is measured at the microphone. In conductive hearing losses, more sound is reflected than in the normal middle ear. The pressure in the ear canal can be increased or decreased from atmospheric pressure. A *tympanogram* is the graphic representation of change in impedance or compliance as the pressure in the ear canal is changed. It provides information about the status of the tympanic membrane and the ossicular chain. Normally, the middle ear is most compliant at atmospheric pressure, and the compliance decreases as the pressure is increased or decreased; this pattern is seen with normal hearing or in the presence of sensorineural hearing loss. Compliance that does not change with change in pressure suggests middle-ear effusion. With a negative pressure in the middle ear, as with eustachian tube obstruction, the point of maximal compliance occurs with negative pressure in the ear canal. A tympanogram in which no point of maximal compliance can be obtained is most commonly seen with discontinuity of the ossicular chain. A reduction in the maximal compliance peak can be seen in otosclerosis.

During tympanometry, an intense tone (80 dB above the hearing threshold) elicits contraction of the stapedius muscle. The change in compliance of the middle ear with contraction of the stapedius muscle can be detected. The presence or absence of this *acoustic reflex* is important in the anatomic localization of facial nerve paralysis as well as hearing loss. Normal or elevated acoustic reflex thresholds in an individual with significant sensorineural hearing impairment suggests a cochlear hearing loss. Assessment of *acoustic reflex decay* helps differentiate sensory from neural hearing losses. In neural hearing loss, the reflex adapts or decays with time.

Otoacoustic emissions (OAE) can be measured with sensitive microphones inserted into the external auditory canal. The emissions may be spontaneous or evoked with sound stimulation. The presence of OAEs indicates that the outer hair cells of the organ of Corti are intact and can be used to assess auditory thresholds and to distinguish sensory from neural hearing losses.

Evoked Responses   *Electrocochleography* measures the earliest evoked potentials generated in the cochlea and the auditory nerve. Receptor potentials recorded include the cochlear microphonic, generated by the outer hair cells of the organ of Corti, and the summating potential, generated by the inner hair cells in response to sound. The whole nerve action potential representing the composite firing of the first-order neurons can also be recorded during electrocochleography. Clinically, the test is useful in the diagnosis of Ménière's disease where an elevation of the ratio of summating potential to action potential is seen.

Brainstem auditory evoked responses (BAERs) are useful in differentiating the site of sensorineural hearing loss (Chap. 356). In response to sound, five distinct electrical potentials arising from different stations along the peripheral and central auditory pathway can be recorded with computer averaging from scalp surface electrodes. BAERs are valuable in situations in which patients cannot or will not give reliable voluntary thresholds. They are also used to assess the integrity of the auditory nerve and brainstem in various clinical situations, including intraoperative monitoring and in determination of brain death.

Imaging Studies   The choice of radiologic tests is largely determined by whether the goal is to evaluate the bony anatomy of the external, middle, and inner ear or to image the auditory nerve and brain. Axial and coronal CT of the temporal bone with fine 1-mm cuts is ideal for determining the caliber of the external auditory canal, integrity of the ossicular chain, and presence of middle-ear or mastoid disease; it can also detect inner-ear malformations. CT is also ideal for the detection of bone erosion often seen in the presence of chronic otitis media and cholesteatoma. MRI is superior to CT for imaging of retrocochlear pathology such as vestibular schwannoma, meningioma, other lesions of the cerebellopontine angle, demyelinating lesions of the brainstem, and brain tumors. Recent experience suggests that both CT and MRI are equally capable of identifying inner-ear malformations and assessing cochlear patency for preoperative evaluation of patients for cochlear implantation.

TREATMENT   In general, conductive hearing losses are amenable to surgical intervention and correction, while sensorineural hearing losses are permanent. The diagnosis of conductive hearing loss is usually straightforward, and the etiology of the conductive deficit is often apparent on physical examination. Atresia of the ear canal can be surgically repaired, often with significant improvement in hearing. Tympanic membrane perforations due to chronic otitis media or trauma can be repaired with an outpatient tympanoplasty. Likewise, conductive hearing loss associated with otosclerosis can be treated by stapedectomy, which is successful in 90 to 95% of cases. Tympanostomy tubes allow the prompt return of normal hearing in individuals with middle-ear effusions. Hearing aids are effective and well-tolerated in patients with conductive hearing losses.

Patients with mild, moderate, and severe sensorineural hearing losses are regularly rehabilitated with hearing aids of varying configuration and strength. Hearing aids have been improved to provide greater fidelity and have been miniaturized. The current generation of hearing aids can be placed entirely within the ear canal, thus reducing the stigma associated with their use. In general, the more severe the hearing impairment, the larger the hearing aid required for auditory rehabilitation. Digital hearing aids lend themselves to individual programming, and multiple and directional microphones at the ear level may be helpful in noisy surroundings. Since all hearing aids amplify noise as well as speech, the only absolute solution to the problem found thus far is to place the microphone closer to the speaker than the noise source. This arrangement is not possible with a self-contained, cosmetically acceptable device. It is cumbersome and requires a user-friendly environment.

In many situations, including lectures and the theater, hearing-impaired persons benefit from assistive devices that are based on the principle of having the speaker closer to the microphone than any source of noise. Assistive devices include infrared and FM transmission as well as an electromagnetic loop around the room for transmission to the individual's hearing aid. Hearing aids with telecoils can also be used with properly equipped telephones in the same way.

In the event that the hearing aid provides inadequate rehabilitation, cochlear implants are appropriate. Criteria for implantation include severe to profound hearing loss with word recognition score ≤30% under best aided conditions. Children with congenital and acquired profound hearing impairment are also appropriate candidates for cochlear implantation. Worldwide, more than 20,000 deaf individuals (including 4000 children) have received cochlear implants. Cochlear implants are neural prostheses that convert sound energy to electrical energy and can be used to stimulate the auditory division of the eighth nerve directly. In most cases of profound hearing impairment, the auditory hair cells are lost but the ganglionic cells of the auditory division of the eighth nerve are preserved. Cochlear implants consist of electrodes that are inserted into the cochlea through the round window, speech processors that extract acoustical elements of speech for conversion to electrical currents, and a means of transmitting the electrical energy through the skin. Patients with implants experience sound that helps with speech reading, allows open-set word recognition, and helps in modulating the person's own voice. Usually, within 3 months after implantation, adult patients can understand speech without visual cues. With the current generation of multichannel cochlear implants, nearly 75% of patients are able to converse on the telephone. It is anticipated that improvements in the electrode design and speech processors will permit further enhancement in understanding speech, especially in the presence of background noise.

For individuals who have had both eighth nerves destroyed by trauma or bilateral vestibular schwannomas (e.g., neurofibromatosis type 2), brainstem auditory implants placed near the cochlear nucleus may provide auditory rehabilitation. It is hoped that additional advances may provide benefits similar to those with the cochlear implant.

Tinnitus can often accompany hearing loss. The treatment of tinnitus is particularly problematic. Therapy is usually directed towards minimizing the appreciation of tinnitus. Relief of the tinnitus may be obtained by masking it with background music. Hearing aids are also helpful in tinnitus suppression, as are tinnitus maskers, devices that present a sound to the affected ear that is more pleasant to listen to than the tinnitus. The use of a tinnitus masker is often followed by several hours of inhibition of the tinnitus. Antidepressants have also shown beneficial effect in helping patients deal with tinnitus.

Tinnitus and background noise can significantly affect understanding of speech in individuals with hearing impairment. Hard-of-hearing individuals often benefit from a reduction in unnecessary noise (e.g., radio or television) to enhance the signal-to-noise ratio. Speech comprehension is aided by lip reading; therefore, the impaired listener should be seated so that the face of the speaker is well illuminated and can be seen at all times. Speaking directly into the ear is occasionally helpful, but usually more is lost in communication than gained when the speaker's face cannot be seen. Speech should be slow enough to make each word distinct, but overly slow speech is distracting and loses contextual and speech-reading benefits. Although speech should be in a loud, clear voice, one should be aware that in sensorineural hearing losses in general and in elderly hard-of-hearing persons in particular, recruitment (the ability to hear loud sounds normally loud) may be troublesome. Above all, optimal communication cannot take place without both parties giving it their full and undivided attention.

PREVENTION Conductive hearing losses may be prevented by prompt and appropriate antibiotic therapy of adequate duration for AOM and by ventilation of the middle ear with tympanostomy tubes in middle-ear effusions lasting 12 weeks or longer. Loss of vestibular function and deafness due to aminoglycoside antibiotics can largely be prevented by careful monitoring of serum peak and trough levels.

Some 10 million Americans have noise-induced hearing loss, and 20 million are exposed to hazardous noise in their employment. Noise-induced hearing loss can be prevented by avoidance of exposure to loud noise or by regular use of ear plugs or fluid-filled ear muffs to attenuate intense sound. Noise-induced hearing loss results from recreational as well as occupational activities and begins in adolescence. High-risk activities for noise-induced hearing loss include wood and metal working with electrical equipment and target practice and hunting with small firearms. All internal-combustion and electric engines, including snow and leaf blowers, snowmobiles, outboard motors, and chain saws, require protection of the user with hearing protectors. Virtually all noise-induced hearing loss is preventable through education, which should begin before the teenage years. Programs of industrial conservation of hearing are required when the exposure over an 8-h period averages 85 dB on the A scale. Workers in such noisy environments can be protected with preemployment audiologic assessment, the mandatory use of hearing protectors, and annual audiologic assessments.

ACKNOWLEDGMENT
The authors wish to acknowledge Dr. Joseph B. Martin, who was the coauthor of this chapter in the 14th edition.

BIBLIOGRAPHY

AIBA T et al: Effect of zinc sulfate on sensorineural olfactory disorder. Acta Otolaryngol Suppl (Stockh) 538:202, 1998

BALLENGER JJ, SNOW JB (eds): *Otorhinolaryngology Head and Neck Surgery*, 15th ed. Baltimore, Williams & Wilkins, 1995

DOTY RL et al: Smell identification ability: Changes with age. Science 226:1441, 1984

FIRESTEIN S, SHEPHERD GM: Interaction of anionic and cationic currents leads to a voltage dependence in the odor response of olfactory receptor neurons. J Neurophysiol 73:562, 1995

GETCHELL TV et al: *Smell and Taste in Health and Disease.* New York, Raven, 1991

KALINEC F et al: A membrane-based force generation mechanism in auditory sensory cells. Proc Natl Acad Sci USA 89:8671, 1992

LALWANI AK, CASTELEIN CM: Cracking the auditory genetic code: Nonsyndromic hereditary hearing impairment. Am J Otol 20(1):115, 1999

MORELL RJ et al: Mutations in the connexin 26 gene (GJB2) among Ashkenazi Jews with nonsyndromic recessive deafness. N Engl J Med 339:1500, 1998

OGAWA T, RUTKA J: Olfactory dysfunction in head injured workers. Acta Otolaryngol Suppl (Stockh) 540:50, 1999

RUGARLI EI et al: Kallmann syndrome and the link between olfactory and reproductive development. Am J Hum Genet 65:943, 1999

RUSSLER KJ et al: A zonal organization of odorant receptor gene expression in the olfactory epithelium. Cell 73:597, 1993

SHARON D et al: Primate evolution of an olfactory receptor cluster: Diversification by gene conversion and recent emergence of pseudogenes. Genomics 61:24, 1999

WARCHOL ME et al: Regenerative proliferation in inner ear sensory epithelia from adult guinea pigs and humans. Science 259:1619, 1993

WILLEMS PJ: Genetic causes of hearing loss. N Engl J Med 342:1101, 2000

30 *Marlene Durand, Michael Joseph*

INFECTIONS OF THE UPPER RESPIRATORY TRACT

Infections of the upper respiratory tract include some of the most common infectious diseases encountered by internists and other primary-care physicians. Pharyngitis, laryngitis, rhinitis, sinusitis, otitis externa, and otitis media account for millions of visits to physicians annually. Although these infections are usually mild enough to be treated on an outpatient basis, the primary-care physician must be able to recognize their serious complications, such as peritonsillar abscess from pharyngitis, subperiosteal abscess from frontal sinusitis, and temporal-bone osteomyelitis from invasive otitis externa. The physician must also identify potentially life-threatening infections of the head and neck, such as epiglottitis, Ludwig's angina, and rhinocerebral mucormycosis.

INFECTIONS OF THE NOSE AND FACE

Skin infections that commonly affect the nose and face include folliculitis, furunculosis, impetigo, and erysipelas. These are discussed in detail elsewhere (Chap. 128, in particular Table 128-1).

Infection of the mucosal surface of the nose is most commonly due to respiratory viruses (e.g., rhinovirus) and presents as acute rhinitis. There are several rare, chronic intranasal infections. *Ozena*, or atrophic rhinitis, is characterized by atrophied mucosa overlaid by foul-smelling dry crusts (Greek *ozein*, "stench"). *Klebsiella ozaenae* is often isolated from nasal cultures, but whether it is a cause of illness or merely a colonizer is unclear. Intranasal irrigation with aminoglycosides (e.g., tobramycin ophthalmic solution) or oral administration of ciprofloxacin has resulted in clinical improvement in some cases. *Klebsiella rhinoscleromatis* causes *rhinoscleroma*, a chronic granulomatous disease of the upper respiratory tract mucosa that is seen in inhabitants of parts of Africa, Asia, and Latin America; it has been described in two patients positive for HIV. Mikulicz cells (foamy histiocytes) are seen in the submucosa of biopsy specimens. Rhinoscleroma can be treated with streptomycin, trimethoprim-sulfamethoxazole, a quinolone, or tetracycline for 2 months. *Pseudomonas mallei* causes *glanders*, a respiratory disease of horses. Infection is rare in humans; nasal inoculation may produce a purulent nasal discharge followed by granulomatous intranasal lesions that ulcerate. Treatment is with sulfadiazine.

Neonatal congenital syphilis may present as rhinitis (snuffles), and the generalized osteochondritis that follows may result in a "saddle-nose" deformity. In *leprosy, Mycobacterium leprae* infiltrates the nasal mucosa and may cause chronic nasal congestion and nosebleeds. Involvement of the nasal cartilage may also result in a saddle nose.

Rhinosporidium seeberi is a fungus-like organism, not yet cultured, that causes *rhinosporidiosis*. Pedunculated nasal masses that grow over months or years cause obstruction and a foul odor and must be surgically excised. *Blastomyces dermatitidis*, a fungus prevalent in the Mississippi and Ohio River valleys, usually causes pulmonary disease but may cause chronic ulcerative lesions of the skin and nasal mucosa. *Mucormycosis*, a life-threatening fungal illness that occurs primarily in diabetic patients, may present as black eschars in the nasal cavity (see "Fungal Sinusitis").

THE COMMON COLD

The common cold is a mild, self-limited viral infection of the upper respiratory tract. Adults average two to four colds per year and children six to eight. The most common causes are rhinovirus (40% of cases) and coronavirus (at least 10%), but parainfluenza virus, respiratory syncytial virus, influenza virus, and adenoviruses also account for some cases. Rhinovirus alone has more than 100 different immunotypes, and this diversity has hampered efforts to identify an effective therapy or vaccine. There is no specific treatment for the common cold, although antihistamines, decongestants, and ipratropium bromide nasal spray provide some relief of symptoms. One study found that zinc gluconate lozenges, taken every 2 h, may reduce the duration of symptoms but are associated with nausea in 20% of patients. The value of vitamin C in preventing colds has not been proved.

SINUSITIS

The paranasal sinuses are aerated cavities in the bones of the face that develop as outpouches of the nasal cavity and communicate with this cavity throughout life. The maxillary and ethmoid sinuses are present at birth; the frontal and sphenoid sinuses develop after ages 2 and 7, respectively. Like the nose, the sinuses are lined with respiratory epithelium that includes mucus-producing goblet cells and ciliated cells. The mucous blanket is carried toward the sinus openings (ostia) at a speed of up to 1 cm/min by the beating of the cilia. The ostia are small; the ethmoid sinus ostia, for example, are only 1 to 2 mm in diameter. Delay in the mucociliary transport time or—more important—obstruction of the ostia may lead to retained secretions and sinusitis.

Sinusitis is a common problem. In the United States, this infection accounts for millions of office visits annually. The most common type, maxillary sinusitis, is followed in frequency by ethmoid, frontal, and sphenoid sinusitis. A viral infection of the upper respiratory tract is the most common precursor of sinusitis, although only about 0.5% of such infections are complicated by clinically evident acute bacterial sinusitis. Sinusitis develops primarily through ostial obstruction due to mucosal edema. Viral upper respiratory infections also increase the amount of mucus produced and may damage ciliated cells, thereby delaying mucus transport time. Allergic rhinitis is another common cause of ostial obstruction, either by mucosal edema or by polyps. Nasotracheal or nasogastric intubation can result in obstruction of the ostia and is a major risk factor for nosocomial sinusitis in intensive care units. Dental infections may cause 5 to 10% of all cases of maxillary sinusitis; the roots of the upper back teeth (second bicuspid, first and second molars) abut the floor of the maxillary sinus. Other causes of sinusitis include barotrauma from deep-sea diving or airplane travel, mucus abnormalities (e.g., cystic fibrosis), and chemical irritants. Foreign bodies, tumors (e.g., midline granuloma, intranasal lymphoma, or squamous cell carcinoma), and granulomatous diseases (e.g., Wegener's granulomatosis or rhinoscleroma) may all cause sinusitis secondary to obstruction.

ACUTE BACTERIAL SINUSITIS Manifestations Symptoms of acute sinusitis include purulent nasal or postnasal drainage, nasal congestion, and sinus pain or pressure whose location depends on the sinus involved. Maxillary sinus pain is often perceived as being located in the cheek or upper teeth; ethmoid sinus pain, between the eyes or retroorbital; frontal sinus pain, above the eyebrow; and sphenoid sinus pain, in the upper half of the face or retroorbital with radiation to the occiput. Sinus pain is frequently worse when the patient bends over or is supine. Fever develops in about half of patients with acute maxillary sinusitis.

Diagnosis The diagnosis of bacterial sinusitis may be difficult, as symptoms may resemble those of the inciting viral upper respiratory infection. The persistence of cold symptoms for 7 to 10 days (or longer than usual for a particular patient) is the most consistent clinical feature of bacterial sinusitis, according to some authors. Four-view sinus x-rays are helpful in the diagnosis of acute sinusitis: radiologic opacity, an air-fluid level, or ≥4 mm of sinus mucosal thickening correlates well with active bacterial infection. Computed tomography (CT) of the sinus is much more sensitive than routine radiography, particularly for ethmoid and sphenoid disease. Its use should be reserved for complicated cases and for cases in hospitalized patients, however. In light of the finding that sinus CT often shows reversible acute changes in patients with common colds, it is apparent that routine early use of CT would lead to overdiagnosis of bacterial sinusitis.

Etiology The bacteriology of acute community-acquired maxillary sinusitis has been well defined by studies using direct sinus puncture and aspiration. In children and adults, *Streptococcus pneumoniae* and *Haemophilus influenzae* (not type b), the most common pathogens, cause about one-third and one-fourth of cases, respectively. In children, *Moraxella catarrhalis* is also important, accounting for 20% of cases. Rhinoviruses, influenza viruses, and parainfluenza viruses are found alone or with bacteria in one-fifth of adult cases.

℞ **TREATMENT** Empirical therapy for acute bacterial sinusitis should be directed against the common bacterial pathogens; sinus puncture is not indicated in routine cases, and cultures of nasal drainage are not very reliable. Amoxicillin (500 mg orally, three times daily for 10 to 14 days) or trimethoprim-sulfamethoxazole may be effective in the treatment of first-time cases.[1] Other effective but more expensive antibiotics include amoxicillin/clavulanate, cefuroxime axetil, and clarithromycin. Treatment should be given for 1 to 2 weeks. Intravenous administration of antibiotics may be necessary for the treatment of patients with severe disease who appear toxic. In nosocomial sinusitis, *Staphylococcus aureus* and gram-negative bacilli are most common, and sinus cultures are indicated as an aid in tailoring therapy. Initial broad-spectrum intravenous therapy (e.g., with nafcillin and ceftriaxone) should be adjusted on the basis of culture results. Surgery to widen the ostia and drain thick secretions may be essential in severe acute sinusitis, particularly when ethmoid, frontal, or sphenoid disease fails to respond to initial intravenous therapy.

CHRONIC BACTERIAL SINUSITIS Manifestations Chronic sinusitis is characterized by symptoms of sinus inflammation lasting ≥3 months. Most experts believe that this condition is caused by dysfunction of the mucociliary blanket, usually as a result of repeated past infections, rather than by the persistence of bacterial infection. Patients report constant sinus pressure, nasal congestion, and postnasal drainage, especially in the morning. A temperature of ≥38°C (≥100.5°F) is rare and may signify a superimposed acute bacterial infection. Many patients also note a change in nasal discharge (to thick and green) with acute exacerbations.

---

[1]The dosages and durations of antimicrobial therapy given in this chapter are appropriate for adults with normal renal function and should be adjusted for children, for patients with impaired renal function, and in light of the response to treatment.

Diagnosis Sinus CT should be used in all cases of chronic sinusitis to define the extent of disease and to help exclude other diagnoses, such as an obstructing tumor. Patients should be evaluated for allergies and immunodeficiencies (e.g., hypogammaglobulinemia). Evaluation by an otolaryngologist is essential, as this specialist will be able to obtain additional information by an office nasal endoscopic examination. Surgery, now usually done endoscopically, may be necessary to correct blockage of the sinus ostia. This blockage occurs most often in the osteomeatal complex that drains the maxillary, frontal, and anterior ethmoid sinuses. Samples of sinus secretions obtained intraoperatively should be cultured for anaerobes, aerobes, and fungi. Fungal sinusitis may mimic chronic bacterial infection (see "Fungal Sinusitis").

Etiology The bacteriology of chronic sinusitis is not well defined. Nearly all patients with chronic disease, especially those who have had prior sinus surgery, have sinus cultures positive for bacteria. Such cultures may represent colonization rather than infection, however. Patients who have received multiple courses of antibiotics may be colonized by *S. aureus* or by *Pseudomonas* and other gram-negative bacilli. Anaerobes have been isolated from 100% of sinus specimens in some studies but from as few as 2% in others.

℞ **TREATMENT** The need for antibiotic therapy must be assessed on an individual basis, with antibiotics chosen in light of recent culture results.

COMPLICATIONS OF BACTERIAL SINUSITIS Orbital complications of sinusitis, such as orbital cellulitis and orbital abscess, usually arise from ethmoid sinusitis, since the ethmoid is separated from the orbit by only a very thin bone (the lamina papyracea). Patients present with fever, unilateral periorbital edema and erythema, conjunctival injection and chemosis, and proptosis. Eye movement may be decreased; with orbital abscess, the eye is often fixed in the "down and out" position. CT or magnetic resonance imaging (MRI) should be used to rule out an orbital abscess. Treatment of orbital infections should include immediate drainage of any abscess, intravenous administration of broad-spectrum antibiotics—e.g., nafcillin (1.5 to 2.0 g every 4 h) plus ceftriaxone (2 g/d)—for at least 7 days, and a consideration of sinus drainage surgery.

Another extracranial complication of sinusitis is frontal subperiosteal abscess (Pott's puffy tumor) from frontal sinusitis. Patients present with a tender doughy swelling over the forehead. Treatment consists of surgical drainage of the abscess and the frontal sinus and 6 weeks of intravenous antibiotic therapy directed at the isolated organisms.

Intracranial complications such as epidural abscess, subdural empyema, meningitis, cerebral abscess, and dural-vein thrombophlebitis may result from sinusitis, particularly from frontal or sphenoid infections. Because the sphenoid sinus sits between the two cavernous sinuses, sphenoid sinusitis is a major cause of cavernous sinus thrombophlebitis.

FUNGAL SINUSITIS Fungal sinusitis is categorized as noninvasive or invasive. *Noninvasive* disease is chronic and occurs in immunocompetent hosts. It has two forms that are analogous to the noninvasive pulmonary diseases of aspergilloma and allergic bronchopulmonary aspergillosis. A fungus ball (aspergilloma) inside a sinus may cause symptoms of obstruction without invading the mucosa. Typically, only one sinus (often maxillary) is affected, and patients have unilateral symptoms and opacification of only that sinus on CT. Treatment is surgical only, unless special fungal stains show tissue invasion on histopathology. Allergic fungal sinusitis was first described in 1983 and is seen mainly in patients with a history of nasal polyposis and asthma. It is characterized by extremely thick sinus mucus ("allergic mucin") that, on histopathologic examination, is found to contain numerous Charcot-Leyden crystals, eosinophils, and rare fungal hyphae. There is no evidence of tissue invasion. Surgical removal of the inspissated mucus is often curative. Antifungal therapy is not indicated.

Invasive fungal sinusitis presents differently in immunocompetent and immunocompromised hosts. In immunocompromised individuals, fungal disease has an acute presentation. Rhinocerebral mucormycosis is a life-threatening infection due to fungi of the order Mucorales (*Rhizopus, Rhizomucor, Mucor, Absidia, Cunninghamella*). Mucormycosis usually involves diabetic patients (70% of cases), half of whom are in ketoacidosis at presentation. Other patients at risk include those with hematologic malignancies, transplant recipients, and patients receiving chronic glucocorticoid or iron chelation (deferoxamine) therapy. Mucormycosis in patients taking deferoxamine is generally due to *Cunninghamella* and is almost always fatal. Symptoms and signs of mucormycosis may be explained by the fungal predilection for blood vessels and nerves and for invasion into the orbital apex and cavernous sinus, with consequent compromise of cranial nerves II through VI. Patients most frequently present with unilateral ocular findings of 1 to 5 days' duration that may mimic bacterial orbital cellulitis: lid swelling and erythema (sometimes bluish in appearance), ptosis, proptosis, decreased extraocular movement, and impaired vision. Retroorbital or periorbital pain is a prominent complaint. There may be either increased or decreased sensation in the first division of the fifth cranial nerve on the involved side; facial palsy with involvement of cranial nerve VII has also been described. Patients may be afebrile and appear nontoxic. Individuals in whom mucormycosis is a consideration should undergo an immediate examination by an otolaryngologist, who will look for intranasal black eschars or necrotic turbinates. If found, these sites should be biopsied and frozen tissue sections examined by a pathologist. In rare cases, the nasal passage appears normal, but biopsy of the middle turbinate reveals invasive fungi. The finding of tissue invasion by broad-based, nonseptate hyphae necessitates extensive surgical debridement and intravenous therapy with amphotericin B or liposomal amphotericin (Chaps. 200 and 207). *Aspergillus* and other filamentous fungi may also cause invasive sinus disease.

Immunocompetent hosts with invasive fungal sinusitis, in contrast, have slowly progressive disease. Fungi in ethmoid and sphenoid sinuses may invade the orbital apex, causing proptosis, ptosis, limitation of eye movement, and decreased vision. Patients may mistakenly be treated with glucocorticoids for presumed optic neuritis or orbital pseudotumor until sinus disease is recognized and biopsies are undertaken. Treatment consists of surgical debridement of the involved sinuses and prolonged intravenous therapy with amphotericin B. In all cases of invasive fungal sinusitis, follow-up CT and MRI should be conducted frequently to evaluate the progression of disease.

Mortality from invasive fungal sinusitis is high, even among immunocompetent hosts.

EAR AND MASTOID INFECTIONS

AURICULAR CELLULITIS AND PERICHONDRITIS
Auricular cellulitis usually presents as a swollen, erythematous, hot, tender ear. The lobule is especially swollen and red. There may be a history of minor trauma to the ear (e.g., involving earrings, cotton swabs, or scratching). Treatment consists of warm compresses and intravenous administration of antibiotics active against *S. aureus* and streptococci—e.g., cefazolin (1 g every 8 h) or nafcillin.

Perichondritis, an infection of the perichondrium of the ear, is often accompanied by infection of the underlying cartilage of the pinna (chondritis). Associated interruption of the blood supply to the cartilage may lead to ear deformity. Patients present with a swollen, hot, red, and exquisitely tender pinna, usually with sparing of the lobule. The most common antecedents of the infection are burns, significant trauma to the ear (e.g., as a result of boxing), or ear piercing through the pinna. *Pseudomonas aeruginosa* and *S. aureus* are the most common pathogens. Perichondritis should be treated with antibiotics, such as intravenous ticarcillin/clavulanic acid (3.1 g every 4 h) or intravenous nafcillin plus oral ciprofloxacin, for several weeks. Incision and drainage may be helpful for culture and for resolution of infection, which is often slow. This infection must be distinguished from relapsing polychondritis, a rheumatologic condition (Chap. 325).

OTITIS EXTERNA   The external auditory canal is about 2.5 cm long and is lined by skin. Beneath this skin is cartilage in the lateral half of the canal, temporal bone in the medial half. The skin in the bony portion lacks a subcutaneous layer and is attached directly to the periosteum, an important feature in the pathogenesis of invasive otitis externa (see below). Cerumen, secreted by glands, acidifies the canal and suppresses bacterial growth. However, desquamated skin and retained moisture make the canal especially susceptible to the hydrophilic organism *P. aeruginosa*.

Acute otitis externa, or swimmer's ear, occurs mostly in the summer and may be due to a decrease in canal acidity and resulting bacterial overgrowth. The ear is pruritic and painful, and the canal appears swollen and red. The most common pathogens are *P. aeruginosa*, *S. aureus*, and streptococci. Treatment consists of cleansing of the ear with alcohol–acetic acid mixtures and the administration of topical antibiotic ear drops, such as polymyxin-neomycin (4 drops four times daily for 5 days). Herpes zoster in the external canal causes severe otalgia and is often accompanied by ipsilateral facial paralysis due to the involvement of the geniculate ganglion of cranial nerve VII (Ramsay Hunt syndrome). Reports suggest that treatment with intravenous acyclovir decreases the incidence of permanent facial-nerve palsy, but the results of relevant controlled trials have not yet been published.

Chronic otitis externa causes pruritus rather than ear pain and is often due to irritation from either repeated minor trauma to the canal (e.g., scratching or use of cotton swabs) or drainage of a chronic middle-ear infection. In the latter situation, treatment of chronic otitis media with oral antibiotics will also cover this condition.

Invasive ("malignant") otitis externa is a potentially life-threatening infection, almost always due to *P. aeruginosa*, that slowly invades from the external canal into adjacent soft tissues, mastoid, and temporal bone and eventually spreads across the base of the skull. It occurs primarily in diabetic patients whose diabetes, unlike that of patients with mucormycosis, is usually under control. There is a history of weeks to months of ear pain and drainage, often misdiagnosed as chronic otitis media (an entity that is rarely painful). Examination reveals an edematous canal, with granulation tissue in the posterior wall about halfway down the canal (the region of the cartilage-bone junction). Trismus or partial facial paralysis (cranial nerve VII) is evident in some instances. Cranial nerves IX, X, and XI are occasionally affected as well. Fever is rare in invasive otitis externa and, when it does develop, is usually low-grade.

Laboratory studies generally reveal a normal white blood cell count but a high erythrocyte sedimentation rate. CT and MRI studies are essential for defining the extent of bone and soft-tissue involvement. CT shows bony destruction of the skull base in advanced cases. For culture, biopsies of granulation tissue in the canal or of deeper tissues are preferable to swab specimens of ear drainage, which may be unreliable. In nearly all cases, antibiotics should be withheld until a deep-tissue specimen is obtained for culture and pathologic examination. Once this specimen has been collected, empirical therapy with intravenous antibiotics active against *Pseudomonas*—e.g., ticarcillin (3 g every 4 h), piperacillin, or ceftazidime, plus an aminoglycoside)—may be started intraoperatively. To avoid ototoxicity, ciprofloxacin should be substituted for the aminoglycoside if cultures grow a *Pseudomonas* strain that is sensitive to this drug. In more than 95% of cases, *P. aeruginosa* is the pathogen involved; in the remaining cases, the pathogens include *Staphylococcus epidermidis*, *Aspergillus*, *Fusobacterium*, and *Actinomyces*. Systemic antibiotic treatment should be continued for 6 to 8 weeks. In early cases due to sensitive *Pseudomonas* strains, oral ciprofloxacin alone (750 mg twice daily for 6 weeks) may follow the initial 2 weeks of combination intravenous therapy.

ACUTE OTITIS MEDIA   The middle ear is connected to the nasopharynx via the eustachian tube. When this tube is blocked, fluid collects in the middle-ear and mastoid cavities, providing a culture medium for any bacteria present. Acute otitis media (AOM), or middle-ear infection, may result. Viral upper respiratory infections, which can cause edema of the eustachian tube mucosa, often precede or accompany episodes of AOM. Otitis media, like upper respiratory tract infections, is most common in fall, winter, and spring. The incidence of AOM declines with age. More than two-thirds of children under age 3 have had at least one episode of AOM; the prevalence among adults is only 0.25%.

Symptoms include ear pain, fever, and decreased hearing acuity. On examination, the tympanic membrane moves poorly with insufflation and is usually red, opaque, bulging, or retracted. Spontaneous perforations of the tympanic membrane and otorrhea are occasionally documented.

The bacteriology of AOM has been delineated for pediatric disease: *S. pneumoniae* (35%), *H. influenzae* (25%), and *M. catarrhalis* (15%) are the most common organisms. Viruses, either alone or with bacteria, are found in one-quarter of pediatric cases. Small studies of AOM in adults have also found *S. pneumoniae* (21%) and *H. influenzae* (26%) to be the most common pathogens. More than 90% of *H. influenzae* infections are due to nontypable strains: those due to type b may be accompanied by bacteremia or meningitis.

℞ **TREATMENT**   Treatment of otitis media is empirical, as diagnostic tympanocentesis is indicated only for patients who appear toxic, who are immunocompromised, or whose infection is refractory to initial therapy. Although about one-third of *H. influenzae* strains and at least three-quarters of *M. catarrhalis* strains are β-lactamase producers, most authorities still find amoxicillin therapy to be successful in routine cases. Other drugs effective against most β-lactamase-positive strains include amoxicillin/clavulanate (875 mg by mouth twice daily for 7 to 10 days), trimethoprim-sulfamethoxazole, erythromycin/sulfisoxazole, clarithromycin, and second-generation oral cephalosporins (e.g., loracarbef, cefpodoxime proxetil, and cefuroxime axetil). Penicillin resistance in pneumococci, now a major problem, is not mediated by β-lactamase (Chap. 138). Strains exhibiting intermediate resistance may respond to therapy with high-dose amoxicillin or to clindamycin, erythromycin, or trimethoprim-sulfamethoxazole. Quinolones such as levofloxacin, although not approved for use in children, may be effective in adults. Serious infections or those due to highly resistant strains require treatment with parenteral ceftriaxone or vancomycin. Adjunctive treatment of AOM with antihistamines is of no proven benefit.

Recurrent episodes of AOM in children are due to the same pathogens that cause primary AOM (*S. pneumoniae*, *H. influenzae*, and *M. catarrhalis*). Most early recurrences (75%), however, are not relapses but are due to different organisms or to different strains of the organism that caused the initial episode. The pattern of recurrent AOM in adults is presumably similar but has not been well studied. Treatment for recurrent AOM should include drugs with activity against resistant strains. Patients with frequent recurrences (e.g., three episodes within 6 months) may benefit from antibiotic prophylaxis with once-daily amoxicillin or sulfisoxazole during the winter months, although this benefit must be weighed against the risk of selecting more antibiotic-resistant strains of bacteria.

SEROUS OTITIS MEDIA   Otitis media with effusion, or serous otitis media, is characterized by the persistence of middle-ear fluid for several months without other signs of infection. This condition is associated with a 25-dB hearing loss in the affected ear. Cultures of middle-ear fluid are usually negative. Although some clinical trials have found that effusions resolve sooner in antibiotic-treated children than in controls, antibiotics are generally not recommended because the risk of increasing antibiotic resistance in the population is thought to outweigh the small benefit observed. Adenoidectomy, myringotomy, or tympanostomy tubes have been shown to decrease the duration of effusion in children.

CHRONIC SUPPURATIVE OTITIS MEDIA In chronic suppurative otitis media, patients have painless hearing loss and intermittent purulent ear drainage. On examination, there is a central perforation in the tympanic membrane and purulent drainage from the middle ear. If a cholesteatoma is present, the perforation is peripheral. Culture of draining fluid reveals *P. aeruginosa* (40%), *S. aureus* (20%), *Klebsiella* (20%), and other enteric gram-negative bacilli. Anaerobes are found in 50% of cases, usually in mixed culture with aerobes. CT should be used to help evaluate a surgically treatable nidus of infection, such as a cholesteatoma or mastoid sequestrum. For therapeutic purposes, patients are divided into two groups: those with and without cholesteatoma. Those in the former group are cured with surgical excision of the cholesteatoma. Those without cholesteatoma require repeated courses of topical antibiotic drops for relapse of "active" (draining) disease, and true cures are rare. The role of systemic antibiotics is unclear. In one study, a course of intravenous antibiotics produced long-term success in 78% of children without cholesteatoma who had persistent otorrhea despite topical and oral antibiotic therapy.

Tuberculous otitis media is rare and is frequently misdiagnosed. It mimics nontuberculous chronic suppurative otitis media, but ear drainage fails to respond to routine antibiotics. On examination, the tympanic membrane often has multiple perforations, and "pearly" or "flabby" tissue is seen in the middle ear. Only 30% of patients have evidence of active tuberculosis on chest x-ray. Treatment is the same as for other types of extrapulmonary tuberculosis.

MASTOIDITIS The mastoid is the portion of the temporal bone posterior to the ear that contains a honeycomb of air cells lined with respiratory epithelium. These air cells connect with the middle ear. Fluid in the middle ear, a prelude to otitis media, is almost always accompanied by fluid in the mastoid. True mastoiditis, however, has become rare in the antibiotic era, probably because of prompt treatment of otitis media.

Mastoiditis is characterized by erosion of the bony partitions between the mastoid air cells. Patients with acute mastoiditis present with pain, tenderness, and swelling over the mastoid. When there is an overlying subperiosteal abscess or cellulitis, the pinna is pushed out and forward. CT may show bony destruction or a drainable mastoid abscess.

The reported bacteriology of mastoiditis has varied. Some cases involve organisms similar to those implicated in AOM (*S. pneumoniae*, *H. influenzae*); others are attributable to *S. aureus* and gram-negative bacilli, including *Pseudomonas*. Ideally, therapy should be guided by the results of cultures of middle-ear fluid obtained by tympanocentesis. Initial broad-spectrum therapy, such as that with intravenous ticarcillin/clavulanate plus gentamicin or ciprofloxacin, can later be narrowed.

COMPLICATIONS OF OTITIS MEDIA AND MASTOIDITIS Extracranial complications include hearing loss, labyrinthitis and resulting vertigo, and facial-nerve palsy. Additional complications from mastoiditis develop when infection tracks under the periosteum of the temporal bone to cause a subperiosteal abscess or breaks through the mastoid tip to cause a neck abscess deep to the sternocleidomastoid muscle (Bezold's abscess). Intracranial complications include epidural abscess, dural venous thrombophlebitis (usually sigmoid sinus), meningitis, and brain abscess.

INFECTIONS OF THE ORAL CAVITY AND PHARYNX

ORAL CAVITY INFECTIONS The oral cavity extends from the lips to the circumvallate papillae of the tongue and is heavily colonized with viridans streptococci and anaerobes. These organisms can cause several infections in this area. *Gingivitis* is an infection of the gums, the earliest form of periodontal disease. Anaerobes residing in the mouth, especially anaerobic gram-negative rods such as *Prevotella*

intermedia, are the most common pathogens. Patients with *Vincent's angina*, also called *acute necrotizing ulcerative gingivitis* or *trench mouth*, have halitosis and ulcerations of the interdental papillae. Oral anaerobes are the cause, and therapy with oral penicillin plus metronidazole or with clindamycin alone is effective in both this condition and gingivitis.

Ludwig's angina is a rapidly spreading, life-threatening cellulitis of the sublingual and submandibular spaces that usually starts in an infected lower molar. Patients are febrile and may drool the secretions they cannot swallow. A brawny, boardlike edema in the sublingual area pushes the tongue up and back. Airway obstruction may result as the infection spreads to the supraglottic tissues. Treatment with intravenous antibiotics active against streptococci and oral anaerobes—e.g., ampicillin/sulbactam (3 g every 6 h) or high-dose penicillin plus metronidazole—should be followed by oral antibiotic therapy, with a total treatment duration of 14 days. Airway monitoring is also essential. Intubation or tracheostomy may be necessary.

Noma, or *cancrum oris*, is a fulminant gangrenous infection of the oral and facial tissues that occurs in severely malnourished and debilitated patients and is especially common among children. Beginning as a necrotic ulcer in the gingiva of the mandible, noma is caused by oral anaerobes, especially fusospirochetal organisms (e.g., *Fusobacterium nucleatum*). It is treated with high-dose penicillin, debridement, and correction of the underlying malnutrition.

Herpes simplex commonly causes cold sores of the lips but may also cause painful vesicles on the tongue and buccal mucosa. Primary infection may require intravenous hydration and should be treated with acyclovir. *Thrush*, or oropharyngeal candidiasis, is an infection caused by *Candida* spp. such as *C. albicans*. It occurs in neonates, patients who have received prolonged antibiotic therapy, and immunocompromised patients. More than 90% of patients with AIDS develop thrush. Patients with thrush report a "burning" tongue or "raw" throat and, on examination, have white plaques on the tongue and oral mucosa. Treatment consists of topical antifungal agents (clotrimazole, nystatin) or oral fluconazole. Therapy for fluconazole-resistant thrush in patients with AIDS may be difficult; itraconazole oral solution or amphotericin B oral suspension may be effective.

PHARYNGITIS Most cases of pharyngitis are thought to be viral. Many occur as part of common colds caused by rhinovirus, coronavirus, or parainfluenza virus. Patients have a scratchy or sore throat as well as coryza and cough. The pharynx is inflamed and edematous, but no exudate is evident. Influenza virus and adenovirus may cause a particularly severe sore throat, along with fever and myalgias. In infection with either of the latter viruses, there is pharyngeal erythema and edema; however, adenovirus infection also commonly causes an exudate, thus mimicking streptococcal pharyngitis. *Infectious mononucleosis* due to Epstein-Barr virus often causes a severe sore throat. Exudative pharyngitis or tonsillitis is documented in half of mononucleosis cases and may also mimic streptococcal infection. *Herpangina*, caused by coxsackievirus, is characterized by fever, sore throat, myalgias, and a vesicular enanthem on the soft palate between the uvula and the tonsils. There are usually only two to six lesions, which begin as small papules that vesiculate and then ulcerate. Fever and nonexudative pharyngitis are common symptoms of the acute retroviral syndrome that develops several weeks after infection with HIV.

The most important bacterial cause of pharyngitis is group A *Streptococcus* (*S. pyogenes*). This organism is responsible for about 15% of all cases of pharyngitis and can cause important complications, both suppurative (peritonsillar and retropharyngeal abscess) and nonsuppurative (scarlet fever, streptococcal toxic shock syndrome, rheumatic fever, acute poststreptococcal glomerulonephritis). Fever, severe sore throat, cervical adenopathy, and inflammation of the tonsils and pharynx (which are covered with exudate) are classic findings. However, many cases of streptococcal pharyngitis are mild, with minimal erythema and no exudate, and mimic the pharyngitis of the common cold. Although some patients may in fact have viral pharyngitis and may simply be colonized with group A streptococci, these individuals must nevertheless be treated for presumed streptococcal pharyngitis. Diagnosis is made by culture. Rapid antigen tests are now available. These tests are less sensitive than they are specific: a positive test may be considered equivalent to a positive culture, but a negative test requires culture confirmation. Either a single dose of intramuscular benzathine penicillin (1.2 million units) or a 10-day course of oral penicillin (250 mg four times daily) or erythromycin is necessary to eradicate the organism. Sensitivity to erythromycin should be verified if this agent is used, as an increase in erythromycin resistance has been noted, especially in Europe. Other antibiotics active against streptococci may be used (e.g., amoxicillin, cefuroxime), and one trial showed that 4 days of cefuroxime therapy was as effective as 10 days of penicillin treatment in eradicating the organism. However, studies of the prevention of rheumatic fever are available only for penicillin (Chap. 235).

Other bacterial causes of pharyngitis include groups C and G *Streptococcus, Neisseria gonorrhoeae* (Chap. 147), *Arcanobacterium haemolyticum, Yersinia enterocolitica,* and—very rarely—*Corynebacterium diphtheriae* (Chap. 141). In addition, *Mycoplasma pneumoniae* (Chap. 178) and *Chlamydia pneumoniae* (Chap. 179) can cause pharyngitis.

A peritonsillar abscess (*quinsy*) may follow untreated streptococcal pharyngitis. Oral anaerobes also play a role in quinsy. Patients have a severe sore throat and speak with a "hot-potato" voice. Examination reveals pronounced unilateral peritonsillar swelling and erythema causing deviation of the uvula. Immediate aspiration by an otolaryngologist is required in conjunction with antibiotic therapy—e.g., ampicillin/sulbactam (3 g intravenously every 6 h), penicillin plus metronidazole, or clindamycin.

LARYNGITIS, CROUP, AND EPIGLOTTITIS

LARYNGITIS   Laryngitis is characterized by hoarseness. Most cases of acute laryngitis are caused by viruses (rhinovirus, influenza virus, parainfluenza virus, coxsackievirus, adenovirus, or respiratory syncytial virus). Acute laryngitis may also be associated with group A *Streptococcus* and *M. catarrhalis.* Laryngitis must be differentiated from epiglottitis (see below). The goal of treatment is merely the relief of symptoms except when throat cultures are positive for group A *Streptococcus* (in which case penicillin should be used).

Chronic laryngitis due to infection is rare and must be distinguished from hoarseness of neoplastic etiology. *Tuberculous laryngitis* may be mistaken for laryngeal cancer when assessed by direct laryngoscopy. Laryngeal and supraglottic lesions include mucosal hyperemia and thickening, nodules, and ulcerations. In one study, a history of fever and night sweats was rare, and the most common chest radiographic finding was apical thickening and fibrosis. Biopsy reveals granulomas with acid-fast bacilli. Cultures should be performed to confirm the diagnosis and evaluate the sensitivities of the pathogen. Laryngeal tuberculosis is highly contagious and should be managed with the same precautions and therapy used for active pulmonary disease (Chap. 169). Fungal infections causing laryngitis include histoplasmosis (Chap. 201), blastomycosis (Chap. 203), and candidiasis (Chap. 205). *Histoplasma* and *Blastomyces* may cause nodules on the larynx, with or without ulcerations. *Candida* may cause laryngitis, along with thrush, in immunosuppressed patients or in patients with chronic mucocutaneous candidiasis.

CROUP   Croup, or acute laryngotracheobronchitis, is an infection of the upper and lower respiratory tract that causes marked subglottic edema. It mainly affects 2- and 3-year-old children and usually follows the onset of upper respiratory tract infection by 1 to 2 days. Symptoms include fever, hoarseness, a "seal's bark" cough, and inspiratory stridor. The most common etiology is parainfluenza virus, although croup may also be caused by other respiratory viruses (e.g., influenza or respiratory syncytial virus).

Croup must be differentiated from epiglottitis (see below). Epiglottitis usually progresses more rapidly and produces a more toxic appearance. Neck x-rays may be helpful but do not reliably exclude epiglottitis. In croup, the anterior-posterior neck x-ray shows subglottic edema (the "hourglass sign"); in epiglottitis, the lateral neck view shows a thick epiglottis.

Patients with severe croup should be hospitalized, monitored for hypoxemia through pulse oximetry, and watched for airway obstruction requiring intubation. Humidification is commonly prescribed, but few controlled trials have assessed its benefit. Nebulized racemic epinephrine provides temporary (2-h) improvement in patients with marked stridor, but such patients must be observed for rebound edema. Glucocorticoid therapy, either nebulized or parenteral, is clearly beneficial, and its effects are often evident within 1 h. One trial found that treatment with a single dose of either intramuscular dexamethasone or nebulized budesonide reduced the need for hospitalization of children with moderately severe croup by more than 50%.

EPIGLOTTITIS   Acute epiglottitis (supraglottis) is a life-threatening, rapidly progressive cellulitis of the epiglottis that may cause complete airway obstruction. It begins as a cellulitis between the tongue base and the epiglottis that pushes the epiglottis posteriorly. The epiglottis itself then becomes swollen, threatening the airway. Before the introduction of *H. influenzae* type b (Hib) vaccine, epiglottitis was most common among children 2 to 4 years old. The disease is now rare in children, since the vaccine has reduced the incidence of invasive disease due to Hib by more than 95%. The incidence in adults has not changed.

The typical young child with epiglottitis has a several-hour history of fever, irritability, dysphonia, and dysphagia and presents sitting forward and drooling. Adolescents and adults usually have a less fulminant presentation, with symptoms (especially sore throat) of 1 or 2 days' duration. Adults may present with dyspnea (25%), drooling (15%), and stridor (10%). Epiglottitis constitutes a medical emergency, as airway occlusion may occur suddenly. Lateral neck films showing an enlarged epiglottis (the "thumb sign") are helpful if positive but may be falsely negative. The value of obtaining these films has also been questioned because doing so may cause a critical delay in securing the airway. Direct viewing of the pharynx by use of a tongue blade should not be attempted, as immediate laryngospasm and airway obstruction may result. Instead, a child with suspected epiglottitis should be transported—while sitting up—to the operating room for visualization of the epiglottis with a fiberoptic laryngoscope, with preparations made for immediate airway control. If the epiglottis is cherry-red, an uncuffed endotracheal tube should be placed. Diagnosis in adults is also made by direct viewing of the epiglottis with a flexible fiberoptic laryngoscope, again only after preparations are made to secure the airway.

All patients must be closely monitored in an intensive care unit and should be given antibiotics active against *H. influenzae.* Before Hib vaccine became available, this organism was responsible for nearly all pediatric cases and was isolated from the blood of almost 100% of the affected children. In adults, blood cultures are positive in about 25% of cases, all of which are due to *H. influenzae.* Other pathogens isolated from the pharynx of adults with epiglottitis include *H. parainfluenzae, S. pneumoniae,* group A *Streptococcus,* and (rarely) *S. aureus*; the correlation between throat and epiglottis cultures is unclear, however. Children may be treated with intravenous cefuroxime, ceftriaxone, ampicillin/sulbactam, or trimethoprim-sulfamethoxazole. Adults may be treated for at least 7 days with cefuroxime, ampicillin/sulbactam (3 g intravenously every 6 h), or nafcillin plus ceftriaxone; those highly allergic to penicillin may be given clindamycin plus either trimethoprim-sulfamethoxazole or ciprofloxacin. If the patient with *H. influenzae* epiglottitis has household contacts that include an unvaccinated child under age 4, all members of the household and the patient

DEEP NECK INFECTIONS

Deep neck infections may be life-threatening because of airway compromise, involvement of the carotid sheath, or spread into the mediastinum.

SUBMANDIBULAR SPACE INFECTIONS See *Ludwig's angina* above (under "Oral Cavity Infections").

LATERAL PHARYNGEAL SPACE INFECTIONS The lateral pharyngeal space, also called the parapharyngeal or pharyngomaxillary space, is in the superior lateral portion of the neck and extends from the hyoid bone to the base of the skull. It lies deep to the lateral wall of the pharynx and is lateral to the tonsil and carotid sheath and medial to the parotid gland. Infection in this space may follow tonsillitis, pharyngitis with adenoid involvement, parotitis, mastoiditis, or periodontal infection.

On presentation, most patients appear toxic and have fever, sore throat, pain on swallowing, and leukocytosis. Infection confined to the posterior (retrostyloid) portion of the lateral pharyngeal space causes swelling of the lateral pharyngeal wall, which may be missed because it is behind the palatopharyngeal arch. Involvement of the anterior portion of this space causes medial displacement of the tonsil, swelling over the parotid gland, and trismus. Rigidity of the neck or torticollis toward the opposite side may develop. Diagnosis is confirmed by CT with contrast.

Treatment includes securing of the airway, surgical drainage in the operating room, and administration for at least 10 days of intravenous antibiotics active against streptococci and oral anaerobes (e.g., ampicillin/sulbactam, 3 g every 6 h). Major complications result from involvement of the carotid sheath and the vessels it contains. These complications are frequently fatal and include jugular vein thrombophlebitis, erosion into the carotid artery, and mediastinitis. Jugular vein thrombophlebitis is characterized by high fevers, chills, and neck tenderness at the angle of the mandible. When it is caused by *Fusobacterium necrophorum*, it may be accompanied by sepsis and septic pulmonary emboli (*Lemierre's syndrome*). Erosion into the carotid artery is usually heralded by repeated small bleeds into the mouth. The involvement of adjacent cranial nerves may result in ipsilateral Horner's syndrome, hoarseness, or unilateral tongue paresis. Extension of infection along the carotid sheath into the posterior mediastinum results in mediastinitis and a mortality of 50%. MRI is useful in delineating carotid and jugular involvement.

RETROPHARYNGEAL SPACE INFECTIONS The retropharyngeal space lies between the pharynx and the prevertebral fascia and extends from the base of the skull into the mediastinum. Infection in this space may result from the spread of lateral pharyngeal space infection or from the lymphatic spread of infection in more cephalad sites (posterior sinuses, adenoids, nasopharynx) to the retropharyngeal lymph nodes. Retropharyngeal abscess is most common among infants and young children, probably because the retropharyngeal nodes later involute. Retropharyngeal abscess may also follow trauma to the posterior pharynx (e.g., endoscopy in adults, lollipop-stick perforation in children) or may result from anterior extension of infection from cervical osteomyelitis.

Symptoms include fever, marked difficulty and pain with swallowing, and a "hot-potato" voice. Physical examination may document drooling, nuchal rigidity, and bulging of the posterior pharyngeal wall. Advanced cases include dyspnea and stridor. Diagnosis may be confirmed by a lateral neck soft-tissue x-ray or CT scan. Treatment requires securing of the airway and emergency surgical drainage. Intravenous antibiotics should be given; the agents chosen should be active against streptococci, oral anaerobes, *S. aureus*, and *H. influenzae* (e.g., ampicillin/sulbactam alone or clindamycin plus ceftriaxone). Potential complications include airway obstruction, intraoral rupture of the abscess causing aspiration pneumonia, and mediastinitis.

BIBLIOGRAPHY

CHOW AW: Life-threatening infections of the head and neck. Clin Infect Dis 14:991, 1992

DEL BECCARO MA et al: Bacteriology of acute otitis media: A new perspective. J Pediatr 120:81, 1992

DESHAZO RD et al: Fungal sinusitis. N Engl J Med 337:254, 1997

HARRIS JP, DARROW DH: Complications of chronic otitis media, in *Surgery of the Ear and Temporal Bone*, JB Nadol Jr, HF Schuknecht (eds). New York, Raven Press, 1993, p 171

JOHNSON DW et al: A comparison of nebulized budesonide, intramuscular dexamethasone, and placebo for moderately severe croup. N Engl J Med 339:498, 1998

KLEIN JO: Otitis externa, otitis media, mastoiditis, in *Principles and Practice of Infectious Diseases*, 4th ed, GL Mandell et al (eds). New York, Churchill Livingstone, 1995, p 579

LIM DJ (ed): Recent advances in otitis media: Report of the Sixth Research Conference. Ann Otol Rhinol Laryngol 107(Suppl 174):1, 1998

MAYO-SMITH MF et al: Acute epiglottitis. An 18-year experience in Rhode Island. Chest 108:1640, 1995

TALMOR M et al: Acute paranasal sinusitis in critically ill patients: Guidelines for prevention, diagnosis, and treatment. Clin Infect Dis 25:1441, 1997

TIERNEY MR, BAKER AS: Infections of the head and neck in diabetes mellitus. Infect Dis Clin North Am 9:195, 1995

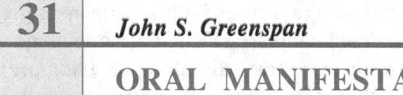

31   *John S. Greenspan*

ORAL MANIFESTATIONS OF DISEASE

A thorough oral examination, to include the oral and pharyngeal soft tissues as well as the teeth, is an important part of the physical examination. The common oral diseases are due to infection by bacteria, fungi, or viruses. The complex development of the orofacial structures leads to close interposition of diverse tissues, which are prone to developmental anomalies, growth disturbances, and neoplasia.

DISEASES OF THE TEETH

DENTAL CARIES, PULPAL AND PERIAPICAL DISEASE, AND COMPLICATIONS Dental caries is a destructive disease of the hard tissues of the teeth due to infection with *Streptococcus mutans* and other bacteria. In the United States, fewer than half of those 17 years and younger now have carious lesions, although in many segments of the population and in developing countries the disease is more common. Artificial fluoridation of water to a level of 1 part per million, fluoride-containing toothpastes, and topical fluoride administration have reduced the incidence. Conversely, retention of teeth and the aging of the population have led to an increase in root caries. Increasing numbers of individuals surviving cancer therapy and other special populations (diabetic patients and those with xerostomia due to Sjögren's syndrome or to medications) may experience severe caries unless appropriate topical fluoride prophylaxis is used. Treatment of caries involves removal of the softened and infected hard tissues, sealing of the exposed dentine, and restoration of the lost tooth structure with silver amalgam, composite plastic, gold, or porcelain.

If the carious lesion progresses, infection of the dental pulp may occur, causing *acute pulpitis*. The tooth may become sensitive to hot or cold. When severe continuous throbbing pain ensues, pulp damage is irreversible, and root canal therapy becomes necessary. The contents of the pulp chamber and root canals are removed, followed by thorough cleaning, antisepsis, and filling with an inert material. Alternatively, extraction of the tooth may be indicated.

If the pulpitis is not treated successfully, infection may spread beyond the tooth apex into the periodontal ligament. Acute inflammation causes pain on chewing or on percussion, and a *periapical abscess* may form. Chronic inflammation may be painless or produce only slight pain, and a *periapical granuloma* may form within the alveolar bone. Proliferation of epithelial cell rests may convert the granuloma into a *periapical cyst*. Periapical radiolucencies may occur with the granuloma or the cyst but not with the abscess, unless it forms as a complication of one or two lesions. The pus in the periapical abscess may track through the alveolar bone into soft tissues, causing cellulitis and bacteremia, or may discharge into the oral cavity (*parulis* or *gumboil*), into the maxillary sinus, or through the skin of the face or submandibular area. A severe form of cellulitis, *Ludwig's angina*, originates from an infected mandibular molar, involves the submandibular space, and extends throughout the floor of the mouth, with elevation of the tongue, dysphagia, and difficulty breathing. Glottal edema may occur, necessitating tracheotomy.

EFFECT OF SYSTEMIC FACTORS ON TEETH
Enamel hypoplasia of the primary and/or permanent teeth, manifested by alterations ranging from white spots to gross defects in the surface structure of the crowns, may be caused by disturbances of calcium and phosphate metabolism such as are found in vitamin D–resistant rickets, hypoparathyroidism, gastroenteritis, and celiac disease. Premature birth or high fevers may also give rise to enamel hypoplasia. Tetracycline, when given during the second half of pregnancy, in infancy, and in childhood up to 8 years of age, causes both a permanent discoloration of the teeth and enamel hypoplasia. Daily ingestion of more than 1.5 mg fluoride can result in enamel discoloration (*mottling*). Larger teeth are associated with maternal diabetes, maternal hypothyroidism, and large birth size. Tooth size is reduced in Down's syndrome. Systemic disease may give rise to pain that simulates pulpal disease. Maxillary sinusitis is frequently manifested as pain in the maxillary teeth, including sensitivity to thermal changes and percussion. Angina pectoris may result in pain referred to the lower jaw, probably through the vagus nerve.

PERIODONTAL DISEASES

In adults, chronic destructive periodontal disease (*pyorrhea*) is responsible for more loss of teeth than caries, particularly in the aged. However, the prevalence and incidence of periodontal disease also appears to be declining in the United States. The most common form of periodontal disease starts as inflammation of the marginal gingiva (*gingivitis*), which is painless, although the gingiva may bleed on brushing. The disease spreads to involve the periodontal ligament, alveolar bone is slowly resorbed, and periodontal ligament attachment between tooth and bone is lost. The soft tissue separates from the tooth surface, causing "pocket" formation with bleeding on probing and during chewing. Acute inflammation may become superimposed on this chronic process, with the production of pus and the formation of a *periodontal abscess*. Ultimately, extreme bone loss, tooth mobility, and recurrent abscess formation lead to tooth exfoliation or may mandate tooth extraction.

Gingivitis and periodontitis are infections associated with the accumulation of *bacterial plaque*, which may become mineralized (*calculus*) and can be prevented by appropriate *oral hygiene* measures, including tooth brushing, flossing, antibacterial mouth rinses, and the removal of impacted food debris. Poorly fabricated or deteriorated restorations may contribute through overextended or inadequate margins. Therapy consists of removal of plaque and calculus, debridement of the pocket lining and superficial infected cementum, and elimination of other contributing factors.

Periodontal disease appears to be a group of conditions, including *adult periodontitis*, associated with *Porphyromonas gingivalis*, *Prevotella intermedia*, and other gram-negative organisms. *Localized juvenile periodontitis* (LJP) causes rapid, severe pocketing and bone loss and is associated with *Actinobacillus actinomycetemcomitans*, *Capnocytophaga*, *Eikenella corrodens*, and other anaerobes. *Acute necrotizing ulcerative gingivitis* (ANUG) involves sudden inflammation

of the gingivae with necrosis, tissue loss, pain, bleeding, and halitosis and is associated with *P. intermedia* and spirochetes. ANUG and an aggressive and rapid form of periodontitis (*necrotizing ulcerative periodontitis*) are seen in association with HIV infection. Some of these cases progress to a destructive gangrene-like lesion of oral soft tissues and bone (*necrotizing stomatitis*) resembling the *noma* seen in severely malnourished populations. Therapy involves local antibacterial measures, debridement, and, in severe cases, systemic antibiotics effective against anaerobes.

Host factors may be involved in the pathogenesis of periodontal disease in other populations as well. Severe periodontal disease may occur in persons with *Down's syndrome* and *diabetes mellitus*. During pregnancy there may be severe gingivitis and the formation of localized *pyogenic granulomas*. Certain drugs, notably the anticonvulsant *phenytoin* and the calcium channel blocker *nifedipine*, cause *fibrous hyperplasia* of the gingiva, which may cover the teeth, interfere with eating, and be unsightly. *Idiopathic familial gingival fibromatosis* may appear similar. Surgery may correct both conditions; change in medication may reverse the drug-induced form. The oral cavity is a significant reservoir for *Helicobacter pylori*. Uncontrolled diabetes mellitus leads to an exacerbation of oral infection, notably periodontal disease. In individuals genetically predisposed to diabetes, periodontal disease may also precipitate or exacerbate the diabetes. Oral infection has been proposed to contribute to coronary atherosclerosis as well as pregnancy outcomes such as premature labor and low birthweight.

Periapical and periodontal bacterial infections can cause transient bacteremia after tooth extraction and even routine dental prophylaxis. Antibiotic coverage is appropriate in patients with heart valves susceptible to infection or those with prosthetic joints.

DISEASES OF THE ORAL MUCOSA

INFECTIONS Most oral mucosal diseases involve microorganisms (Table 31-1).

PIGMENTED LESIONS See Table 31-2

DERMATOLOGIC DISEASES See Tables 31-1, -2, and -3 and Chaps. 55 to 60

DISEASES OF THE TONGUE See Table 31-4

HALITOSIS See Table 31-5

HIV DISEASE AND AIDS (See Table 31-6 and also Chaps. 191 and 309) Immunosuppression induced by HIV infection predisposes to numerous oral infections, neoplasms, and autoimmune and idiopathic lesions. *Oral candidiasis* (**Plate IID-43**) and *hairy leukoplakia* (**Plate IID-42**) [a benign epithelial hyperplasia associated with Epstein-Barr virus (EBV)] are common features of HIV disease and often precede or accompany full-blown AIDS. Oral Kaposi's sarcoma and lymphoma are diagnostic of AIDS. Oral candidiasis is easily treated with topical or systemic antifungals: nystatin oral pastilles, clotrimazole oral troches, nystatin vaginal tablets used orally, fluconazole, and ketoconazole. While most oral lesions of HIV disease are also found in the general population. Necrotizing ulcerative periodontal disease and hairy leukoplakia are strongly associated with HIV infection and are otherwise very rare.

HEMATOLOGIC AND NUTRITIONAL DISEASE Gingival bleeding, necrotic ulcers, and enlargement due to malignant infiltrates are seen in all forms of leukemia, particularly *monocytic leukemia*. In *agranulocytosis* severe oral mucosal ulcers are seen, while in *thrombocytopenia* oral petechiae, ecchymoses, and gingival bleeding occur. In *Plummer-Vinson syndrome* (Chap. 105), atrophy of oral mucosa, particularly the tongue papillae, causes redness and soreness as well as dysphagia and is associated with increased susceptibility to oral cancer. A smooth tongue can also be seen in *pernicious anemia* (Chap. 107). Severe oral mucositis with ulcers, candidiasis, bacterial infections, and xerostomia complicate radiation therapy for head and neck cancers. Chemotherapy may also cause mucositis. Although now rarely seen in the United States, oral features of vitamin deficiency include oral mucositis and ulcers, glossitis, and burning sensations in the tongue (*B group vitamin deficiency*) and petechiae, gingival swell-

Table 31-1   Vesicular, Bullous, or Ulcerative Lesions of the Oral Mucosa

Condition	Usual Location	Clinical Features	Course
VIRAL DISEASES			
Primary acute herpetic gingivo-stomatitis (herpes simplex virus type 1, rarely type 2)	Lip and oral mucosa	Labial vesicles that rupture and crust, and intraoral vesicles that quickly ulcerate; extremely painful; acute gingivitis, fever, malaise, foul odor, and cervical lymphadenopathy; occurs primarily in infants, children, and young adults	Heals spontaneously in 10–14 days unless secondarily infected
Recurrent herpes labialis	Mucocutaneous junction of lip, perioral skin	Eruption of groups of vesicles that may coalesce then rupture and crust; painful to pressure or spicy foods	Lasts about 1 week, but condition may be prolonged if secondary infection occurs
Recurrent intraoral herpes simplex	Palate and gingiva	Small vesicles that rupture and coalesce; painful	Heal spontaneously in about 1 week
Chickenpox (varicella-zoster virus)	Gingiva and oral mucosa	Skin lesions may be accompanied by small vesicles on oral mucosa that rupture to form shallow ulcers; may coalesce to form large bullous lesions that ulcerate; mucosa may have generalized erythema	Lesions heal spontaneously within 2 weeks
Herpes zoster (reactivation of varicella-zoster virus)	Cheek, tongue, gingiva, or palate	Unilateral vesicular eruption and ulceration in linear pattern following sensory distribution of trigeminal nerve or one of its branches	Gradual healing without scarring; postherpetic neuralgia is common
Infectious mononucleosis (Epstein-Barr virus)	Oral mucosa	Fatigue, sore throat, malaise, low-grade fever, and enlarged cervical lymph nodes; numerous small ulcers usually appear several days before lymphadenopathy; gingival bleeding and multiple petechiae at junction of hard and soft palates	Oral lesions disappear during convalescence
Warts (papillomavirus)	Anywhere on skin and oral mucosa	Single or multiple papillary lesions, with thick, white keratinized surfaces containing many pointed projections; cauliflower lesions covered with normal-colored mucosa or multiple pink or pale bumps (focal epithelial hyperplasia)	Lesions grow rapidly and spread
Herpangina (coxsackievirus A; also possibly coxsackievirus B and echovirus)	Oral mucosa, pharynx, tongue	Sudden onset of fever, sore throat, and oropharyngeal vesicles, usually in children under 4 years, during summer months; diffuse pharyngeal congestion and vesicles (1–2 mm), grayish-white surrounded by red areola; vesicles enlarge and ulcerate	Incubation period 2–9 days; fever for 1–4 days; recovery uneventful
Hand, foot, and mouth disease (type A coxsackieviruses)	Oral mucosa, pharynx, palms, and soles	Fever, malaise, headache with oropharyngeal vesicles that become painful, shallow ulcers	Incubation period 2–18 days; lesions heal spontaneously in 2–4 weeks
Primary HIV infection	Gingiva, palate, and pharynx	Acute gingivitis and oropharyngeal ulceration, associated with febrile illness resembling mononucleosis and including lymphadenopathy	Followed by HIV seroconversion, asymptomatic HIV infection, and usually ultimately by HIV disease
BACTERIAL OR FUNGAL DISEASES			
Acute necrotizing ulcerative gingivitis ("trench mouth," Vincent's infection)	Gingiva	Painful, bleeding gingiva characterized by necrosis and ulceration of gingival papillae and margins plus lymphadenopathy and foul odor	Continued destruction of tissue followed by remission, but may recur
Prenatal (congenital) syphilis	Palate, jaws, tongue, and teeth	Gummatous involvement of palate, jaws, and facial bones; Hutchinson's incisors, mulberry molars, glossitis, mucous patches, and fissures of corners of mouth	Tooth deformities in permanent dentition irreversible
Primary syphilis (chancre)	Lesion appears where organism enters body; may occur on lips, tongue, or tonsillar area	Small papule developing rapidly into a large, painless ulcer with indurated border; unilateral lymphadenopathy; chancre and lymph nodes containing spirochetes; serologic tests positive by third to fourth weeks	Healing of chancre in 1–2 months, followed by secondary syphilis in 6–8 weeks
Secondary syphilis	Oral mucosa frequently involved with mucous patches, primarily on palate, also at commissures of mouth	Maculopapular lesions of oral mucosa, 5–10 mm in diameter with central ulceration covered by grayish membrane; eruptions occurring on various mucosal surfaces and skin accompanied by fever, malaise, and sore throat	Lesions may persist from several weeks to a year
Tertiary syphilis	Palate and tongue	Gummatous infiltration of palate or tongue followed by ulceration and fibrosis; atrophy of tongue papillae produces characteristic bald tongue and glossitis	Gumma may destroy palate, causing complete perforation

(continued)

Condition	Usual Location	Clinical Features	Course
Gonorrhea	Lesions may occur in mouth at site of inoculation or secondarily by hematogenous spread from a primary focus elsewhere	Earliest symptoms are burning or itching sensation, dryness, or heat in mouth followed by acute pain on eating or speaking; tonsils and oropharynx most frequently involved; oral tissues may be diffusely inflamed or ulcerated; saliva develops increased viscosity and fetid odor; submaxillary lymphadenopathy with fever in severe cases	Lesions may resolve with appropriate antibiotic therapy
Tuberculosis	Tongue, tonsillar area, soft palate	A solitary, irregular ulcer covered by a persistent exudate; ulcer has an undermined, firm border	Lesions may persist
Cervicofacial actinomycosis	Swellings in region of face, neck, and floor of mouth	Infection may be associated with an extraction, jaw fracture, or eruption of molar tooth; in acute form resembles an acute pyogenic abscess, but contains yellow "sulfur granules" (gram-positive mycelia and their hyphae)	Acute form may last a few weeks; chronic form lasts months or years; prognosis excellent; actinomycetes respond to antibiotics (tetracyclines or penicillin) but not to antifungal drugs
Histoplasmosis	Any area in mouth, particularly tongue, gingiva, or palate	Numerous small nodules that may ulcerate; hoarseness and dysphagia may occur because of lesions in larynx, usually associated with fever and malaise	May be fatal
Candidiasis	Any area of oral mucosa	Pseudomembranous form has white patches that are easily wiped off leaving red, bleeding, sore surface; erythematous form is flat and red; rarely, candidal leukoplakia appears as white patch in tongue that does not rub off; angular cheilitis due to *Candida* involves sore cracks and redness at angle of mouth; *Candida* seen on KOH preparation in all forms	Responds to antifungals

DERMATOLOGIC DISEASES

Condition	Usual Location	Clinical Features	Course
Mucous membrane pemphigoid	Primarily mucous membranes of the oral cavity, but may also involve the eyes, urethra, vagina, and rectum	Painful, grayish-white collapsed vesicles or bullae with peripheral erythematous zone; gingival lesions desquamate, leaving ulcerated area	Protracted course with remissions and exacerbations; involvement of different sites occurs slowly; glucocorticoids may temporarily reduce symptoms but do not control the disease
Erythema multiforme (Stevens-Johnson syndrome)	Primarily the oral mucosa and skin of hands and feet	Intraoral ruptured bullae surrounded by an inflammatory area; lips may show hemorrhagic crusts; the "iris," or "target," lesion on the skin is pathognomonic; patient may have severe signs of toxicity	Onset very rapid; condition may last 1–2 weeks; may be fatal; acute episodes respond to steroids
Pemphigus vulgaris	Oral mucosa and skin	Ruptured bullae and ulcerated oral areas; mostly in older adults	With repeated recurrence of bullae, toxicity may lead to cachexia, infection, and death within 2 years; often controllable with steroids
Lichen planus	Oral mucosa and skin	White striae in mouth; purplish nodules on skin at sites of friction; occasionally causes oral mucosal ulcers and erosive gingivitis	Protracted course, may respond to topical steroids

OTHER CONDITIONS

Condition	Usual Location	Clinical Features	Course
Recurrent aphthous ulcers	Anywhere on nonkeratinized oral mucosa (lips, tongue, buccal mucosa, floor of mouth, soft palate, oropharynx)	Single or clusters of painful ulcers with surrounding erythematous border; lesions may be 1–2 mm in diameter in crops (herpetiform), 1–5 mm (minor), or 5–15 mm (major)	Lesions heal in 1–2 weeks but may recur monthly or several times a year; topical steroids give symptomatic relief; systemic glucocorticoids may be needed in severe cases; a tetracycline oral suspension may decrease severity of herpetiform ulcers
Behçet's syndrome	Oral mucosa, eyes, genitalia, gut, and CNS	Multiple aphthous ulcers in mouth; inflammatory ocular changes, ulcerative lesions on genitalia; inflammatory bowel disease and CNS disease	Ulcers may persist for several weeks and heal without scarring
Traumatic ulcers	Anywhere on oral mucosa; dentures frequently responsible for ulcers in vestibule	Localized, discrete ulcerated lesion with red border; produced by accidental biting of mucosa, penetration by a foreign object, or chronic irritation by a denture	Lesions usually heal in 7–10 days when irritant is removed, unless secondarily infected

Table 31-2 Pigmented Lesions of the Oral Mucosa

Condition	Usual Location	Clinical Features	Course
Oral melanotic macule	Any area of the mouth	Discrete or diffuse localized, brown to black macule	Remains indefinitely
Diffuse melanin pigmentation	Any area of the mouth	Diffuse pale to dark-brown pigmentation; may be physiologic ("racial") or due to smoking	Remains indefinitely
Nevi	Any area of the mouth	Discrete, localized, brown to black pigmentation	Remains indefinitely
Malignant melanoma	Any area of the mouth	Can be flat and diffuse, painless, brown to black, or can be raised and nodular	Expands and invades early; metastasis leads to death
Addison's disease	Any area in mouth but mostly on buccal mucosa	Blotches or spots of bluish-black to dark-brown pigmentation occurring early in the disease, accompanied by diffuse pigmentation of skin; other symptoms of adrenal insufficiency	Condition controlled by steroid therapy
Peutz-Jeghers syndrome	Any area in mouth	Dark-brown spots on lips, buccal mucosa, with characteristic distribution of pigment around lips, nose, eyes, and on hands; concomitant intestinal polyposis	Pigmented lesions remain indefinitely; polyps may become malignant
Drug ingestion (tranquilizers, oral contraceptives, antimalarials)	Any area in mouth	Brown, black, or gray areas of pigmentation	Disappears following cessation of drug
Amalgam tattoo	Gingiva and mucobuccal fold	Small blue-black pigmented areas associated with embedded amalgam particles in soft tissues; these may show up on radiographs as radiopaque particles in some cases	Remains indefinitely
Heavy metal pigmentation (bismuth, mercury, lead)	Gingival margin	Thin blue-black pigmented line along gingival margin; due to prior treatment for syphilis with bismuth or mercury or to accidental absorption of lead	Long-lasting
Black hairy tongue	Dorsum of tongue	Elongation of filiform papillae of tongue, which take on a brown to black coloration	Long-lasting but may disappear spontaneously
Fordyce's "disease"	Buccal and labial mucosa	Aggregation of numerous small yellowish spots just beneath mucosal surface; no symptoms; due to hyperplasia of sebaceous glands	Remains without apparent change indefinitely

Table 31-3 White Lesions of Oral Mucosa

Condition	Usual Location	Clinical Features	Course
Lichen planus	Buccal mucosa, tongue, gingiva, and lips; skin	Striae, white plaques, red areas, ulcers in mouth; purplish papules on skin; may be asymptomatic, sore, or painful; lichenoid drug reactions may look similar	Protracted; responds to topical steroids
White sponge nevus	Oral mucosa, vagina, anal mucosa	Painless white thickening of epithelium; adolescent/early adult onset; familial	Benign and permanent
Smoker's leukoplakia and smokeless tobacco lesions	Any area of oral mucosa, sometimes related to location of habit	White patch that may become firm, rough, or red-fissured and ulcerated; may become sore and painful but usually painless	Occasionally premalignant; may or may not resolve on cessation of habit
Nicotinic stomatitis	Palate in pipe smokers	White nodular elevations on hard palate with central red areas	Benign; usually resolves on cessation of pipe smoking
Frictional keratosis	Any area in mouth	Elevated white lesion due to hyperkeratosis and thickening of the oral epithelium secondary to chronic irritation	Removal of irritant leads to healing in 2–3 weeks
Candidiasis ("candidosis," "moniliasis")	Any area in mouth	*Pseudomembranous type* ("thrush"): creamy white curdlike patches that reveal a raw, bleeding surface when scraped; found in sick infants, debilitated elderly patients receiving high doses of glucocorticoids or broad-spectrum antibiotics, or in patients with AIDS	Responds favorably to antifungal therapy and correction of predisposing causes where possible
		Erythematous type: flat, red, sometimes sore areas, same groups of patients	Course same as for pseudomembranous type
		Candidal leukoplakia: nonremovable white thickening of epithelium due to *Candida*	Responds to prolonged antifungals
		Angular cheilitis: sore fissures at corner of mouth	Responds to topical antifungals
Hairy leukoplakia	Usually lateral tongue, rarely elsewhere on oral mucosa	White areas ranging from small and flat to extensive and "hairy"; found in HIV carriers in all risk groups for AIDS; rarely causes discomfort	Due to EBV; many patients develop AIDS; responds to high dose acyclovir but recurs
Chemical burns	Any area in mouth	White slough due to necrosis of epithelium and underlying connective tissue caused by contact with agents (e.g., aspirin) applied locally or the use of undiluted sodium perborate or hydrogen peroxide as a mouthwash; removal of slough leaves a raw, painful surface	Lesion heals in several weeks if not secondarily infected

Table 31-4   Alterations of the Tongue

Type of Change	Clinical Features
SIZE OR MORPHOLOGY CHANGES	
Macroglossia	Enlarged tongue that may be part of a syndrome found in developmental conditions such as Down's syndrome; may be due to tumor (hemangioma or lymphangioma), metabolic disease (such as primary amyloidosis), or endocrine disturbance (such as acromegaly or cretinism)
Fissured ("scrotal") tongue	Dorsal surface and sides of tongue covered by painless shallow or deep fissures that may collect debris and become irritated
Median rhomboid glossitis	Congenital abnormality of tongue with ovoid, denuded area in median posterior portion of the tongue; may be associated with candidiasis and may respond to antifungals
COLOR CHANGES	
"Geographic" tongue (benign migratory glossitis)	Asymptomatic inflammatory condition of the tongue, with rapid loss and regrowth of filiform papillae, leading to appearance of denuded red patches "wandering" across the surface of the tongue
Hairy tongue	Elongation of filiform papillae of the medial dorsal surface area due to failure of keratin layer of the papillae to desquamate normally; brownish-black coloration may be due to staining by tobacco, food, or chromogenic organisms
"Strawberry" and "raspberry" tongue	Appearance of tongue during scarlet fever due to the hypertrophy of fungiform papillae plus changes in the filiform papilla
"Bald" tongue	Atrophy may be associated with xerostomia, pernicious anemia, iron-deficiency anemia, pellagra, or syphilis; may be accompanied by painful burning sensation; may be an expression of erythematous candidiasis and respond to antifungals

ing, bleeding, and ulceration as well as loosening of teeth (*scurvy* of vitamin C deficiency).

DISEASES OF THE SALIVARY GLANDS

The major and minor salivary glands can be involved in mumps, sarcoidosis, tuberculosis, lymphoma, and Sjögren's syndrome (Chap. 314). The latter may cause dry eyes and dry mouth (*xerostomia*) and be associated with features of connective tissue diseases, including rheumatoid arthritis or systemic lupus erythematosus. Xerostomia may also be due to medications such as diuretics, antihistamines, or tricylic antidepressants as well as radiation therapy for head and neck cancer. Without lysozyme-rich saliva, *cervical or incisal caries* and oral candidiasis may develop. Management includes fluoride mouth rinses and topical applications, saliva substitutes, salivary stimulation with sugarless candies, and the avoidance of sugar-containing drinks or food. Candidiasis is treated with nystatin or other antifungals. Salivary stones (*sialolithiasis*), usually in the duct of a major salivary gland, cause *sialoadenitis* with pain and swelling, often on eating, especially tart foods such as lemons.

The most common neoplasm of the salivary glands is the *pleomorphic adenoma*, which is benign but will recur unless fully resected; malignant tumors include *mucoepidermoid carcinoma*, *adenoid cystic carcinoma*, and *adenocarcinoma*. The pleomorphic adenoma causes a firm, slowly growing mass in the parotid, palate, or cheek, whereas malignant tumors grow faster and can cause ulceration and invade

Table 31-5   Causes of Halitosis

1. Lower respiratory tract infection
   a. Bronchiectasis
   b. Lung abscess
2. Oral infection
   a. Acute primary herpetic gingivostomatitis
   b. Acute necrotizing ulcerative gingivitis
   c. Periodontal disease
   d. Caries
3. Smoking
4. Hepatic failure (fishy odor)
5. Azotemia (ammoniacal or urinary odor)
6. Diabetic ketoacidosis (sweet, fruity odor)
7. *H. pylori* gastric infection
8. Esophageal cancer
9. Metal poisoning (garlicky)

nerves, producing numbness or facial paralysis.

NEUROLOGIC DISTURBANCES AND OROFACIAL PAIN

The mouth and face may be the site of pain from a number of vascular, neurologic, muscle/connective tissue, or joint conditions. Interdisciplinary diagnosis and management programs involving neurologists, restorative dentists, oral surgeons, otorhinolaryngologists, and other specialists, together with new imaging techniques to diagnose or exclude organic lesions, have begun to clarify this complex field. *Temporal arteritis* causes pain in the face, jaws, and tongue and may mimic temporomandibular joint disease. Glucocorticoids may provide relief. *Myofascial pain* is a dull, constant ache with local tenderness in the muscles of the jaws and difficulty in opening the mouth. Teeth clenching and grinding (*bruxism*) may play a role. *Arthralgia* of the temporomandibular joint causes local pain, which may extend to the face and head. Both myofascial pain and arthralgia can be relieved with heat, rest, and anti-inflammatory agents. Displacement of the meniscus or condyle may cause pain, clenching, or locking of the mandible in the open position. The joint may become involved in *osteoarthritis* with minimal symptoms, whereas *rheumatoid arthritis* causes pain and swelling in the joint and limitation of movement. *Ankylosis* may occur, necessitating condylectomy (Chap. 312).

Trigeminal neuralgia (tic douloureux) causes sudden, severe, unilateral lancinating pain initiated by touching a "trigger zone" or occurring spontaneously. Confusion with pulpal or periapical pain is common, leading to inappropriate endodontic or surgical therapy. Many cases respond to carbamazepine and phenytoin, but for a few,

Table 31-6   Oral Lesions of HIV Disease and AIDS

I. Fungal
   A. Candidiasis
      1. Pseudomembranous
      2. Erythematous
      3. Angular cheilitis
   B. Histoplasmosis
   C. Cryptococcosis
II. Bacterial
   A. Acute necrotizing ulcerative gingivitis
   B. Necrotizing ulcerative periodontitis
   C. Necrotizing stomatitis
   D. *Mycoabacterium avium* complex and tuberculosis
   E. Stomatitis due to enteric organisms
III. Viral
   A. Herpes simplex
   B. Herpes zoster
   C. Hairy leukoplakia
   D. Warts
IV. Neoplastic
   A. Kaposi's sarcoma
   B. Lymphoma
V. Other
   A. Recurrent aphthous ulcers
   B. Immune thrombocytopenic purpura
   C. Xerostomia
   D. Salivary gland enlargement

surgical intervention to decompress the trigeminal nerve is indicated. Similar symptoms in the distribution of the ninth cranial nerve (tongue, pharynx, soft palate) are due to *glossopharyngeal neuralgia*, which may be triggered by swallowing and may produce referred pain in the temporomandibular joint. *Postherpetic neuralgia* may follow trigeminal herpes zoster (Chap. 367) and cause burning, aching, and long-lasting pain. *Facial palsy* is usually unilateral and may be due to trauma, surgical intervention, tumor, or infection of the seventh cranial nerve. *Bell's palsy* is a form with acute onset and unknown cause, possibly viral infection such as herpes zoster. The corner of the mouth droops, and there may be difficulty in speech, eating, and in closing the eye. The symptoms usually disappear spontaneously, but residual facial immobility and lip drooping may persist. Abnormal or reduced *taste sensation* may be due to xerostomia, disturbances of the facial and glossopharyngeal nerves or their central connections, aging, or the wearing of dentures. Disease involving the hypoglossal nerve may cause atrophy of the tongue muscles with protrusion, if bilateral, or deviation toward the affected side, if unilateral. Numb chin (mental neuropathy) may be a sign of primary neural disease, but in the cancer patient it is often a harbinger of tumor relapse or progression.

BIBLIOGRAPHY

BARKER FG et al: The long-term outcome of microvascular decompression for trigeminal neuralgia. N Engl J Med 334:1077, 1996

GREENSPAN D, GREENSPAN JS: HIV-related oral disease. Lancet 348:729, 1996

REGEZI JA, SCIUBBA JJ (eds): *Oral Pathology: Clinical Pathologic Correlations*. 3d ed. Philadelphia, Saunders, 1999

STAMM JW (ed): Periodontal diseases and human health: New directions in periodontal medicine. Ann Periodontal 3:1, 1998

THYLSTRUP A, FEJERSKOV O (eds): *Textbook of Clinical Cariology*, 2d ed. Copenhagen, Munksgaard, 1994

Section 5
ALTERATIONS IN CIRCULATORY AND RESPIRATORY FUNCTIONS

32

Roland H. Ingram, Jr., Eugene Braunwald

DYSPNEA AND PULMONARY EDEMA

DYSPNEA

Breathing is controlled by central and peripheral mechanisms that adjust ventilation appropriate to increased metabolic demands during physical activity and increase ventilation in excess of metabolic demands in conditions such as anxiety and fear. A normal resting person is unaware of the act of breathing, and while he or she may become conscious of breathing during mild to moderate exertion, no discomfort is experienced. However, during and following exhausting exertion, an individual may become unpleasantly aware of breathing yet feel reasonably assured that the sensation will be transitory and is appropriate to the level of exercise. Therefore, as a cardinal symptom of diseases affecting the cardiorespiratory system, *dyspnea* is defined as an *abnormally uncomfortable awareness of breathing*.

Although dyspnea is not painful in the usual sense of the word, it is, like pain, involved with both the perception of a sensation and the reaction to that perception. Patients experience a number of uncomfortable sensations related to breathing and use an even larger number of verbal expressions to describe these sensations, such as "cannot get enough air," "air does not go all the way down," "smothering feeling or tightness or tiredness in the chest," and a "choking sensation." It may be necessary, therefore, to review the patient's history meticulously in order to ascertain whether the more abstruse descriptions do, in fact, represent dyspnea. Once it is established that a patient does have dyspnea, it is of paramount importance to define the circumstances in which it occurs and to assess associated symptoms. There are situations in which breathing appears labored but in which dyspnea does not occur. For example, the hyperventilation associated with metabolic acidemia is rarely accompanied by dyspnea. On the other hand, patients with apparently normal breathing patterns may complain of shortness of breath.

QUANTITATION OF DYSPNEA The gradation of dyspnea is based on the amount of physical exertion required to produce the sensation. In assessing the severity of dyspnea, it is important to obtain a clear understanding of the patient's general physical condition, work history, and recreational habits. For example, the development of dyspnea in a trained runner upon running 2 mi may signify a much more serious disturbance than a similar degree of breathlessness in a sedentary person upon running a fraction of this distance. Interindividual variation in perception must also be considered. Some patients with severe disease may complain of only mild dyspnea; others with mild disease may experience more severe shortness of breath. Some patients with lung or heart disease may have such reduced capabilities due to other disease (e.g., peripheral vascular insufficiency or severe osteoarthritis of the hips or knees) that exertional dyspnea is precluded despite serious impairment of pulmonary or cardiac function.

Some patterns of dyspnea are not directly related to physical exertion. Sudden and unexpected dyspneic episodes at rest can be associated with pulmonary emboli, spontaneous pneumothorax, hypercapnea secondary to breath holding, or anxiety. Nocturnal episodes of severe paroxysmal dyspnea are characteristic of left ventricular failure. Dyspnea upon assuming the supine posture, *orthopnea* (see below and Chap. 232), thought to be mainly characteristic of congestive heart failure, may also occur in some patients with asthma and chronic obstruction of the airways and is a regular finding in the rare occurrence of bilateral diaphragmatic paralysis. *Trepopnea* is used to describe the unusual circumstance in which dyspnea occurs only in a lateral decubitus position, most often in patients with heart disease, while *platypnea* is dyspnea that occurs only in the upright position. Positional alterations in ventilation-perfusion relationships (Chap. 250) have been invoked to explain these patterns.

MECHANISMS OF DYSPNEA (See Fig. 32-1) Dyspnea occurs whenever the work of breathing is excessive. Increased force generation is required of the respiratory muscles to produce a given volume change if the chest wall or lungs are less compliant or if resistance to airflow is increased. Increased work of breathing also occurs when the ventilation is excessive for the level of activity. Although an individual is more apt to become dyspneic when the work of breathing is increased, the work theory does not account for the perceptual difference between a deep breath with a normal mechanical load and a normal-sized breath with an increased mechanical load. The work might be the same with both breaths, but the normal one with the increased load will be associated with discomfort. In fact, with respiratory loading, such as adding a resistance at the mouth, there is an increase in respiratory center output that is disproportionate to the increase in the work of breathing. It has been postulated that whenever the force that muscles actually generate during breathing approaches some fraction of their maximal force-generating ability, which may vary among individuals, dyspnea ensues due to transduction of mechanical to neural stimuli.

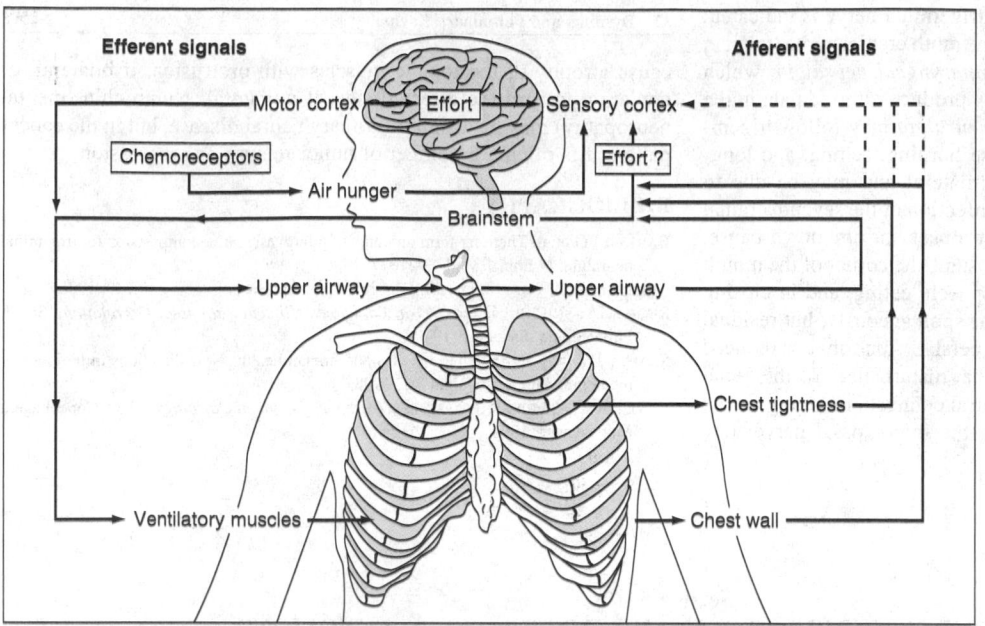

FIGURE 32-1 Efferent and afferent signals that contribute to the sensation of dyspnea. There is evidence that the sense of respiratory effort arises from a signal transmitted from the motor cortex to the sensory cortex simultaneously with the outgoing motor command to the ventilatory muscles. The motor output of the brainstem may also contribute to the sense of effort, as shown in the arrow from the brainstem to the sensory cortex. The sense of air hunger arises, in part, from increased respiratory activity within the brainstem, and the sensation of chest tightness probably results from stimulation of vagal-irritant receptors. While afferent information from airway, lung, and chest-wall receptors probably passes through the brainstem before reaching the sensory cortex, the dashed lines indicate uncertainty about whether some afferents bypass the brainstem and project directly to the sensory cortex. *(From HL Manning, RM Schwartzstein, Pathophysiology of dyspnea. N Engl J Med 333:1547, 1995, with permission.)*

In all likelihood, several different mechanisms operate to different degrees in the various clinical situations in which dyspnea occurs. In some circumstances, dyspnea is evoked by stimulation of receptors in the upper respiratory tract; in others it may originate from receptors in the lungs, airways, respiratory muscles, chest wall, or some combination of these structures. In any event, dyspnea is characterized by an excessive or abnormal activation of the respiratory centers in the brainstem. This activation comes about from stimuli transmitted from or through a variety of structures and pathways, including (1) intrathoracic receptors via the vagi; (2) afferent somatic nerves, particularly from the respiratory muscles and chest wall, but also from other skeletal muscles and joints; (3) chemoreceptors in the brain, aortic and carotid bodies, and elsewhere in the circulation; (4) higher (cortical) centers; and perhaps (5) afferent fibers in the phrenic nerves. In general, despite the interindividual variations described above, there is a reasonable correlation between the severity of dyspnea and the magnitude of disturbances of pulmonary or cardiac function that are responsible.

The mechanisms responsible for dyspnea may vary in different conditions (Table 32-1).

DIFFERENTIAL DIAGNOSIS   Obstructive Disease of Airways (See also Chaps. 252 and 258)   Obstruction to airflow can be present anywhere from the extrathoracic airways out to the small airways in the periphery of the lung. Large extrathoracic airway obstruction can occur acutely, as with aspiration of food or a foreign body or with angioedema of the glottis. An allergic history together with a few scattered hives should raise the possibility of glottic edema. Acute upper airway obstruction is a medical emergency. More chronic forms can occur with tumors or with fibrotic stenosis following tracheostomy or prolonged endotracheal intubation. Whether acute or chronic, the cardinal symptom is dyspnea, and the characteristic signs are stridor and retraction of the supraclavicular fossae with *inspiration*.

Obstruction of intrathoracic airways can occur acutely and intermittently or can be present chronically with worsening during respiratory infections. Acute intermittent obstruction with wheezing is typical of *asthma* (Chap. 252). Chronic cough with expectoration is typical of *chronic bronchitis* (Chap. 258) and *bronchiectasis* (Chap. 256). Most often there are prolongation of expiration and coarse rhonchi that are generalized in chronic bronchitis and may be localized in the case of bronchiectasis. Intercurrent infection results in worsening of the cough, increased expectoration of purulent sputum, and more severe dyspnea. During such episodes, the patient may complain of nocturnal paroxysms of dyspnea with wheezing relieved by cough and expectoration of sputum. Despite the fact that severe limitation of expiratory flow and hyperinflation of the lung are characteristic of these diseases, the sensory experience is often that of an inability to take in a sufficiently deep breath rather than difficulty in exhaling.

The patient with predominant *emphysema* is characterized by many years of exertional dyspnea progressing to dyspnea at rest (Chap. 258). Although a parenchymal disease by definition, emphysema is invariably accompanied by obstruction of airways.

Diffuse Parenchymal Lung Diseases (See also Chap. 259)   This category includes a large number of diseases ranging from acute pneumonia to chronic disorders such as sarcoidosis and the various forms of *pneumoconiosis* (Chap. 254). History, physical findings, and radiographic abnormalities often provide clues to the diagnosis. The patients are often tachypneic with arterial P_{CO_2} and P_{O_2} values below normal. Exertion often further reduces the arterial P_{O_2}. Lung volumes are decreased, and the lungs are stiffer, i.e., less compliant than normal.

Pulmonary Vascular Occlusive Diseases (See also Chap. 261)   Repeated episodes of dyspnea at rest often occur with recurrent pulmonary emboli. Evidence of a source for emboli, such as phlebitis of a lower extremity or the pelvis, is quite helpful in leading the physician to suspect the diagnosis. Arterial blood gases are most often abnormal, but lung volumes are frequently normal or only minimally abnormal.

Diseases of the Chest Wall or Respiratory Muscles (See also Chap. 263)   The physical examination establishes the presence of a

Table 32-1   Possible Mechanisms of Dyspnea in Selected Conditions

Condition	Mechanism
Asthma	Increased sense of effort
	Stimulation of irritant receptors in airways
Neuromuscular disease	Increased sense of effort
COPD	Increased sense of effort
	Hypoxia
	Hypercapnia
	Dynamic airway compression
Mechanical ventilation	Afferent mismatch
	Factors associated with the underlying condition
Pulmonary embolism	Stimulation of pressure receptors in pulmonary vasculature or right atrium (possible)

NOTE: COPD, chronic obstructive pulmonary disease.
SOURCE: From HL Manning, RM Schwartzstein, Pathophysiology of dyspnea. N Engl J Med 333:1547, 1995, with permission.

chest wall disease such as severe kyphoscoliosis, pectus excavatum, or ankylosing spondylitis. Although all three of these deformities may be associated with dyspnea, only severe kyphoscoliosis regularly interferes with ventilation sufficiently to produce chronic cor pulmonale and respiratory failure.

Both weakness and paralysis of respiratory muscles can lead to respiratory failure and dyspnea (Chap. 263), but most often the signs and symptoms of the neurologic or muscular disorder are more prominently manifested in other systems.

Heart Disease In patients with cardiac disease, exertional dyspnea occurs most commonly as a consequence of an elevated pulmonary capillary pressure, which in turn may be due to left ventricular dysfunction (Chaps. 231 and 232), reduced left ventricular compliance, and mitral stenosis. The elevation of hydrostatic pressure in the pulmonary vascular bed tends to upset the Starling equilibrium (see "Pulmonary Edema," below) with resulting transudation of liquid into the interstitial space, reducing the compliance of the lungs and stimulating J (juxtacapillary) receptors in the alveolar interstitial space. When it is prolonged, pulmonary venous hypertension results in thickening of the walls of small pulmonary vessels and an increase in perivascular cells and fibrous tissue, causing a further reduction in compliance. The competition for space among vessels, airways, and increased liquid within the interstitial space compromises the lumina of small airways, increasing the airways' resistance. Diminution in compliance and an increase in the airways' resistance increase the work of breathing. In advanced congestive heart failure, usually involving elevation of both pulmonary and systemic venous pressures, hydrothorax may develop, interfering further with pulmonary function and intensifying dyspnea.

Orthopnea, i.e., dyspnea in the supine position, is the result of the alteration of gravitational forces when this position is assumed, which elevates pulmonary venous and capillary pressures. These, in turn, increase the pulmonary closing volume (Chap. 250) and reduce the vital capacity.

Paroxysmal (nocturnal) dyspnea Also known as *cardiac asthma*, this condition is characterized by attacks of severe shortness of breath that generally occur at night and usually awaken the patient from sleep. The attack is precipitated by stimuli that aggravate previously existing pulmonary congestion; frequently, the total blood volume is augmented at night because of the reabsorption of edema from dependent portions of the body during recumbency. A sleeping patient can tolerate relatively severe pulmonary engorgement and may awaken only when actual pulmonary edema and bronchospasm have developed, with the feeling of suffocation and with wheezing respirations.

Two other forms of nocturnal dyspnea must be distinguished from that due to heart failure. Chronic bronchitis is characterized by mucus hypersecretion and, after a few hours sleep, secretions can accumulate and produce dyspnea and wheezing, both of which are relieved by cough and expectoration of sputum. Asthma patients have circadian variations in their degree of airway obstruction. The obstruction becomes most severe between 2 A.M. and 4 A.M. and can be sufficiently severe that the patient awakens with a sense of suffocation, extreme dyspnea, and wheezing. Although there is a prominent inflammatory component to nocturnal asthma, inhaled bronchodilators usually improve symptoms quickly.

Cheyne-Stokes respiration → *See Chap. 232*

Diagnosis The diagnosis of cardiac dyspnea depends on the recognition of heart disease on the basis of the clinical examination supplemented by noninvasive testing. There may be a history of antecedent myocardial infarction; third and fourth heart sounds may be audible; and/or there may be evidence of left ventricular enlargement, jugular neck vein distention, and/or peripheral edema. Often there are radiographic signs of heart failure, with evidence of interstitial edema, pulmonary vascular redistribution, and accumulation of liquid in the septal planes and pleural cavity. Transthoracic echocardiography is particularly useful in establishing the diagnosis of structural heart disease, which can be responsible for dyspnea. Specifically, left atrial and/or left ventricular dilatation, left ventricular hypertrophy, a reduced left ventricular ejection fraction, and disorders of left ventricular

wall motion may be clues to the presence of a cardiac etiology of otherwise unexplained dyspnea.

DIFFERENTIATION BETWEEN CARDIAC AND PULMONARY DYSPNEA In most patients with dyspnea there is obvious clinical evidence of disease of the heart and/or lungs. Like patients with cardiac dyspnea, patients with chronic obstructive lung disease may also waken at night with dyspnea, but, as pointed out above, this is usually associated with sputum production; the dyspnea is relieved after these patients rid themselves of secretions. The difficulty in the distinction between cardiac and pulmonary dyspnea may be compounded by the coexistence of diseases involving both organ systems.

In patients in whom the etiology of dyspnea is not clear, it is desirable to carry out pulmonary function testing, for these tests may be helpful in determining whether dyspnea is produced by heart disease, lung disease, abnormalities of the chest wall, or anxiety (Chap. 250). In addition to the usual means of assessing patients for heart disease, determination of the ejection fraction at rest and during exercise by echocardiography or radionuclide ventriculography is helpful in the differential diagnosis of dyspnea. The left ventricular ejection fraction is depressed in left ventricular failure, while the right ventricular ejection fraction may be low at rest or may decline during exercise in patients with severe lung disease. Both left and right ventricular ejection fractions are normal at rest and during exercise in dyspnea due to anxiety or malingering. Careful observation during the performance of an exercise treadmill test will often help in the identification of the patient who is malingering or whose dyspnea is secondary to anxiety. Under these circumstances, the patient usually complains of severe shortness of breath but appears to be breathing either effortlessly or totally irregularly. Cardiopulmonary testing, in which the patient's maximal functional exercise capacity is assessed while measurements of the electrocardiogram, blood pressure, oxygen consumption, arterial saturation (oximetry), and ventilation are carried out, is useful in the differentiation between cardiac and pulmonary dyspnea (Table 32-2).

ANXIETY NEUROSIS Dyspnea experienced by a patient with an anxiety neurosis is difficult to evaluate. The signs and symptoms of acute and chronic hyperventilation do not serve to distinguish between anxiety neurosis and other processes, such as recurrent pulmonary emboli. Another potentially confusing situation is seen when chest pain and electrocardiographic changes accompany the hyperventilation syndrome. When present and attributable to this condition, often referred to as *neurocirculatory asthenia* (Chap. 13), the chest pain is often sharp, fleeting, and in various loci, and the electrocardio-

Table 32-2 Patterns of Abnormality in Cardiopulmonary Exercise Testing[a]

Cardiovascular limitation
    Heart rate ≥85% of predicted maximum
    Low anaerobic threshold
    Reduced maximal oxygen consumption
    Drop in blood pressure with exercise
    Arrhythmias or ischemic changes on ECG
    Does not achieve maximal predicted ventilation
    Does not have significant desaturation
Respiratory limitation
    Achieves or exceeds maximal predicted ventilation
    Significant desaturation (<90%)
    Stable or increase dead space–to–tidal volume ratio
    Development or bronchospasm with falling FEV_1
    Does not achieve 85% of predicted maximal heart rate
    No ischemic ECG changes

[a] All features will not be present in a particular case, and there may be elements of both cardiovascular and respiratory causes of shortness of breath. One looks for the predominant pattern in assessing the etiology of the patient's exercise limitation.
NOTE: ECG, electrocardiogram; FEV_1, forced expiratory volume in 1 s.
SOURCE: From RM Schwartzstein, GE Thibault, in L Goldman, E Braunwald (eds): *Primary Cardiology.* Philadelphia, Saunders, 1998

graphic changes are most often seen during repolarization. Frequent sighing respirations and an irregular breathing pattern point to a psychogenic origin of the dyspnea. Anxiety and depression in association with heart or lung disease can serve to intensify dyspnea symptoms beyond what would be expected for a given degree of dysfunction.

PULMONARY EDEMA (See Table 32-3)

CARDIOGENIC PULMONARY EDEMA (See Table 32-3, IA) An increase in pulmonary venous pressure, which results initially in engorgement of the pulmonary vasculature, is common in most instances of dyspnea in association with congestive heart failure. The lungs become less compliant, the resistance of small airways increases, and there is an increase in lymphatic flow that apparently serves to maintain a constant pulmonary extravascular liquid volume. Mild tachypnea is present. If the increase in intravascular pressure is sufficient both in magnitude and duration, there is a net gain of liquid in the extravascular space, i.e., *interstitial* edema. At this point symptoms worsen, tachypnea increases, gas exchange deteriorates further, and radiographic changes, such as Kerley B lines and loss of distinct vascular margins, are seen. At this stage, the capillary endothelial intercellular junctions widen and allow passage of macromolecules into the interstices.

Table 32-3   Classification of Pulmonary Edema Based on Initiating Mechanism

I. Imbalance of Starling forces
  A. Increased pulmonary capillary pressure
    1. Increased pulmonary venous pressure without left ventricular failure (e.g., mitral stenosis)
    2. Increased pulmonary venous pressure secondary to left ventricular failure
    3. Increased pulmonary capillary pressure secondary to increased pulmonary arterial pressure (so-called overperfusion pulmonary edema)
  B. Decreased plasma oncotic pressure
    1. Hypoalbuminemia
  C. Increased negativity of interstitial pressure
    1. Rapid removal of pneumothorax with large applied negative pressures (unilateral)
    2. Large negative pleural pressures due to acute airway obstruction alone with increased end-expiratory volumes (asthma)
II. Altered alveolar-capillary membrane permeability (acute respiratory distress syndrome)
  A. Infectious pneumonia—bacterial, viral, parasitic
  B. Inhaled toxins (e.g., phosgene, ozone, chlorine, Teflon fumes, nitrogen dioxide, smoke)
  C. Circulating foreign substances (e.g., snake venom, bacterial endotoxins)
  D. Aspiration of acidic gastric contents
  E. Acute radiation pneumonitis
  F. Endogenous vasoactive substances (e.g., histamine, kinins)
  G. Disseminated intravascular coagulation
  H. Immunologic—hypersensitivity pneumonitis, drugs (nitrofurantoin), leukoagglutinins
  I. Shock lung in association with nonthoracic trauma
  J. Acute hemorrhagic pancreatitis
III. Lymphatic insufficiency
  A. After lung transplant
  B. Lymphangitic carcinomatosis
  C. Fibrosing lymphangitis (e.g., silicosis)
IV. Unknown or incompletely understood
  A. High-altitude pulmonary edema
  B. Neurogenic pulmonary edema
  C. Narcotic overdose
  D. Pulmonary embolism
  E. Eclampsia
  F. After cardioversion
  G. After anesthesia
  H. After cardiopulmonary bypass

SOURCE: From Braunwald et al., with permission.

Further elevations in intravascular pressure disrupt the tight junctions between alveolar lining cells, and *alveolar* edema ensues, with outpouring of liquid that contains both red blood cells and macromolecules. With yet more severe disruption of the alveolar-capillary membrane, edematous liquid floods the alveoli and airways. At this point, full-blown clinical pulmonary edema with bilateral wet rales and rhonchi occurs, and the chest radiograph may show diffuse haziness of the lung fields with greater density in the more proximal hilar regions. Typically, the patient is anxious and perspires freely, and the sputum is frothy and blood-tinged. Gas exchange is more severely compromised with worsening hypoxia. Without effective treatment (described in Chap. 232), progressive acidemia, hypercapnia, and respiratory arrest ensue.

The earlier sequence of liquid accumulation described above follows the Starling law of capillary–interstitial liquid exchange:

$$\text{Liquid accumulation} = K[(P_c - P_{IF}) - \sigma(\pi_{pl} - \pi_{IF})] - Q_{lymph}$$

where K = hydraulic conductance (directly proportional to membrane surface area and inversely proportional to membrane thickness)
  P_c = mean intracapillary pressure
  π_{IF} = oncotic pressure of interstitial liquid
  σ = reflection coefficient of macromolecules
  P_{IF} = mean interstitial liquid pressure
  π_{pl} = oncotic pressure of the plasma
  Q_{lymph} = lymphatic flow

The pressures tending to move liquid out of the vessel are P_c and π_{IF}, which are normally more than offset by pressures tending to move liquid back into the vasculature, i.e., the algebraic sum of P_{IF} and π_{pl}. Implicit in the preceding equation is that lymphatic flow can increase in the case of imbalance of forces and result in no net accumulation of interstitial liquid. Further elevations in P_c not only increase the outward movement of liquid in each capillary region but also recruit more of the capillary bed, which increases K. These two effects lead to liquid filtration that exceeds clearance capability by the lymphatics, and liquid accumulates in the loose interstitial spaces of the lung. Even greater increases in P_c open first the loose endothelial intercellular junctions and later the tight alveolar intercellular junctions with an increase in permeability to macromolecules. This secondary disruption of both the function and structure of the alveolar-capillary membrane leads to alveolar flooding.

NONCARDIOGENIC PULMONARY EDEMA (See Table 32-3, IB IC, II, III, and IV) Several clinical conditions are associated with pulmonary edema based on an imbalance of Starling forces other than through primary elevations of pulmonary capillary pressure. Although diminished plasma oncotic pressure in hypoalbuminemic states (e.g., severe liver disease, nephrotic syndrome, protein-losing enteropathy) might be expected to lead to pulmonary edema, the balance of forces normally so strongly favors resorption that even in these conditions some elevation of capillary pressure is usually necessary before interstitial edema develops. Increased negativity of interstitial pressure has been implicated in the genesis of unilateral pulmonary edema following rapid evacuation of a large pneumothorax. In this situation, the findings may be apparent only by radiography, but occasionally the patient experiences dyspnea with physical findings localized to the edematous lung. It has been proposed that large negative intrapleural pressures during acute severe asthma may be associated with the development of interstitial edema. Lymphatic blockade secondary to fibrotic and inflammatory diseases or lymphangitic carcinomatosis may lead to interstitial edema. In such instances, both clinical and radiographic manifestations are dominated by the underlying disease process.

Other conditions characterized by increases in the interstitial liquid content of the lungs appear to be associated primarily with disruption of the alveolar-capillary membranes. Any number of spontaneously occurring or environmental toxic insults, including diffuse pulmonary infections, aspiration, and shock (particularly due to sepsis and hemorrhagic pancreatitis and following cardiopulmonary bypass), are associated with diffuse pulmonary edema that clearly does not have a hemodynamic origin. →*These conditions, which may lead to the acute respiratory distress syndrome, are discussed in Chap. 265.*

Other Forms of Pulmonary Edema There are three forms of pulmonary edema whose precise mechanism remains unexplained. *Narcotic overdose* is a well-recognized antecedent to pulmonary edema. Although illicit use of parenteral heroin is the most frequent cause, parenteral and oral overdoses of legitimate preparations of morphine, methadone, and dextropropoxyphene have also been associated with pulmonary edema. The earlier idea that injected impurities lead to the disorder is untenable. Available evidence suggests that there are alterations in the permeability of alveolar and capillary membranes rather than an elevation of pulmonary capillary pressure.

Exposure to high altitude in association with severe physical exertion is a well-recognized setting for pulmonary edema in unacclimatized yet otherwise healthy persons. Acclimatized high-altitude natives also develop this syndrome upon return to high altitude after a relatively brief sojourn at low altitudes. The syndrome is far more common in persons under the age of 25 years. The mechanism for high-altitude pulmonary edema (HAPE) remains obscure, and studies have been conflicting, some suggesting pulmonary venous constriction and others indicating pulmonary arteriolar constriction as the prime mechanisms. A role for hypoxia at high altitude is suggested by the fact that patients respond to the administration of oxygen and/or return to lower altitudes. Hypoxia per se does not alter permeability of the alveolar-capillary membrane. Hence increased cardiac output and pulmonary arterial pressures with exercise combined with hypoxic pulmonary arteriolar constriction, which is more prominent in young persons, may combine to make this an example of prearteriolar, high-pressure pulmonary edema.

Neurogenic pulmonary edema has been described in patients with central nervous system disorders and without apparent preexisting left ventricular dysfunction. Although most experimental equivalents have implicated sympathetic nervous system activity, the mechanism whereby sympathetic efferent activity leads to pulmonary edema is a matter of speculation. It is known that a massive adrenergic nervous discharge leads to peripheral vasoconstriction with elevation of blood pressure and shifts of blood to the central circulation. In addition, it is probable that a reduction in left ventricular compliance also occurs, and both factors serve to increase left atrial pressures sufficiently to induce pulmonary edema on a hemodynamic basis. Some experimental evidence suggests that stimulation of adrenergic receptors increases capillary permeability directly, but this effect is relatively minor as compared with the imbalance of Starling forces.

TREATMENT OF PULMONARY EDEMA See Chap. 232

BIBLIOGRAPHY

BARTSCH P. High altitude pulmonary edema. Respiration 64:435, 1997

BRAUNWALD E et al: Clinical aspects of heart failure; High-output heart failure; Pulmonary edema, in *Heart Disease*, 6th ed, E Braunwald, D Zipes, P Libby (eds). Philadelphia, Saunders, 2001

KOSOWSKY JM et al: Continuous and bilevel positive airway pressure in the treatment of acute cardiogenic pulmonary edema. Am J Emerg Med 18:91, 2000

MANNING HL, SCHWARTZSTEIN RM: Mechanisms of dyspnea, in *Dyspnea*, DA Mahler (ed), *Lung Biology in Health and Disease*, vol III. New York, Marcel Dekker, 1998, pp 63–95

RIETVELD S: Symptom perception in asthma: A multidisciplinary review. J Asthma 35: 13, 1998

SACCHETTI AD, HARRIS RH. Acute cardiogenic pulmonary edema. What's the latest in emergency treatment? Postgrad Med 103:145–7, 153–4, 160–2, 1998

SCHWARTZSTEIN RM: Language of dyspnea, in *Dyspnea*, DA Mahler (ed), *Lung Biology in Health and Disease*, vol III. New York, Marcel Dekker, 1998, pp 35–62

STULBARG MS, ADAMS L: Dyspnea, in *Textbook of Respiratory Medicine*, 3d ed. Murray JF, Nadel JA (eds). Philadelphia, Saunders, 2000, pp 541–552

33

Steven E. Weinberger, Eugene Braunwald

COUGH AND HEMOPTYSIS

COUGH

Cough is an explosive expiration that provides a normal protective mechanism for clearing the tracheobronchial tree of secretions and foreign material. When excessive or bothersome, it is also one of the most common symptoms for which medical attention is sought. Reasons for the latter include discomfort from the cough itself, interference with normal lifestyle, and concern for the cause of the cough, especially fear of cancer or AIDS.

MECHANISM Coughing may be initiated either voluntarily or reflexively. As a defensive reflex it has both afferent and efferent pathways. The *afferent limb* includes receptors within the sensory distribution of the trigeminal, glossopharyngeal, superior laryngeal, and vagus nerves. The *efferent limb* includes the recurrent laryngeal nerve and the spinal nerves. The cough starts with a deep inspiration followed by glottic closure, relaxation of the diaphragm, and muscle contraction against a closed glottis. The resulting markedly positive intrathoracic pressure causes narrowing of the trachea. Once the glottis opens, the large pressure differential between the airways and the atmosphere coupled with tracheal narrowing produces rapid flow rates through the trachea. The shearing forces that develop aid in the elimination of mucus and foreign materials.

ETIOLOGY Cough can be initiated by a variety of airway irritants, which enter the tracheobronchial tree by inhalation (smoke, dust, fumes) or by aspiration (upper airway secretions, gastric contents, foreign bodies). When cough is due to irritation by upper airway secretions (as with postnasal drip) or gastric contents (as with gastroesophageal reflux), the initiating factor may go unrecognized and the cough can be persistent. Additionally, prolonged exposure to such irritants may initiate airway inflammation, which can itself trigger cough and sensitize the airway to other irritants. Cough associated with gastroesophageal reflux is due only in part to aspiration of gastric contents, whereas vagally mediated reflex mechanisms appear to be responsible in many patients.

Any disorder resulting in inflammation, constriction, infiltration, or compression of airways can be associated with cough. Inflammation commonly results from airway infections, ranging from viral or bacterial bronchitis to bronchiectasis. In viral bronchitis, airway inflammation sometimes persists long after resolution of the typical acute symptoms, thereby producing a prolonged cough, lasting for weeks. Pertussis infection is also a possible cause of persistent cough in adults; however, diagnosis is generally made on clinical grounds (Chap. 152). Asthma is a common cause of cough. Although the clinical setting commonly suggests when a cough is secondary to asthma, some patients present with cough in the absence of wheezing or dyspnea, thus making the diagnosis more subtle ("cough variant asthma"). A neoplasm infiltrating the airway wall, such as bronchogenic carcinoma or a carcinoid tumor, is commonly associated with cough. Airway infiltration with granulomas may also trigger a cough, as seen with endobronchial sarcoidosis or tuberculosis. Compression of airways results from extrinsic masses, including lymph nodes, mediastinal tumors, and aortic aneurysms.

Examples of parenchymal lung disease potentially producing cough include interstitial lung disease, pneumonia, and lung abscess. Congestive heart failure may be associated with cough, probably as a consequence of interstitial as well as peribronchial edema. A nonproductive cough complicates the use of angiotensin-converting enzyme (ACE) inhibitors in 5 to 20% of patients taking these agents. Onset is usually within 1 week of starting the drug but can be delayed up to 6 months. Although the mechanism is not known with certainty, it may

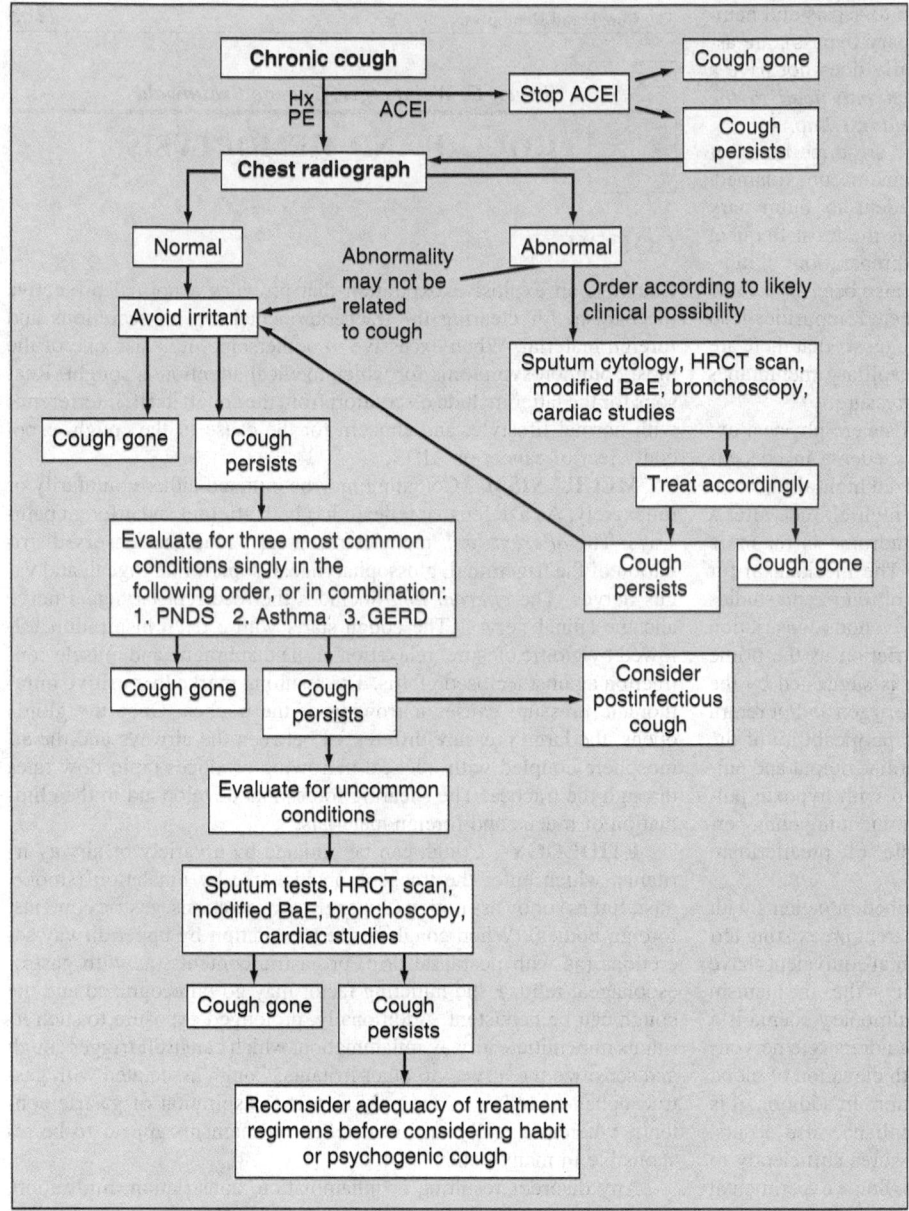

FIGURE 33-1 An algorithm for the evaluation of chronic cough. ACEI, angiotensin-converting enzyme inhibitor; BaE, barium esophagography; GERD, gastroesophageal reflux disease; HRCT, high-resolution computed tomography; Hx, history; PE, physical examination; PNDS, postnasal drip syndrome. *(Reproduced from Irwin, with permission.)*

relate to accumulation of bradykinin or substance P, both of which are degraded by ACE.

The most common causes of cough can be categorized according to the duration of the cough. Acute cough (<3 weeks) is most often due to upper respiratory infection (especially the common cold, acute bacterial sinusitis, and pertussis), but more serious disorders, such as pneumonia, pulmonary embolus, and congestive heart failure, can also present in this fashion. Chronic cough (>3 weeks) in a smoker raises the possibilities of chronic obstructive lung disease or bronchogenic carcinoma. In a nonsmoker who has a normal chest radiograph and is not taking an ACE inhibitor, the most common causes of chronic cough are postnasal drip, asthma, and gastroesophageal reflux.

_____ *Approach to the Patient* _____

A detailed *history* frequently provides the most valuable clues for etiology of the cough. Particularly important questions include:

1. Is the cough acute or chronic?
2. At its onset, were there associated symptoms suggestive of a respiratory infection?

3. Is it seasonal or associated with wheezing?
4. Is it associated with symptoms suggestive of postnasal drip (nasal discharge, frequent throat clearing, a "tickle in the throat") or gastroesophageal reflux (heartburn or sensation of regurgitation)? (The absence of such suggestive symptoms does not exclude either of these diagnoses, particularly in the case of gastroesophageal reflux.)
5. Is it associated with fever or sputum? If sputum is present, what is its character?
6. Does the patient have any associated diseases or risk factors for disease (e.g., cigarette smoking, risk factors for infection with HIV, environmental exposures)?
7. Is the patient taking an ACE inhibitor?

The general *physical examination* may point to a nonpulmonary cause of cough, such as heart failure, primary nonpulmonary neoplasm, or AIDS. Examination of the oropharynx may provide suggestive evidence for postnasal drip, including oropharyngeal mucus or erythema, or a "cobblestone" appearance to the mucosa. Auscultation of the chest may demonstrate inspiratory stridor (indicative of upper airway disease), rhonchi or expiratory wheezing (indicative of lower airway disease), or inspiratory crackles (suggestive of a process involving the pulmonary parenchyma, such as interstitial lung disease, pneumonia, or pulmonary edema).

Chest radiography may be particularly helpful in suggesting or confirming the cause of the cough. Important potential findings include the presence of an intrathoracic mass lesion, a localized pulmonary parenchymal infiltrate, or diffuse interstitial or alveolar disease. An area of honeycombing or cyst formation may suggest bronchiectasis, while symmetric bilateral hilar adenopathy may suggest sarcoidosis.

Pulmonary function testing (Chap. 250) is useful for assessing the functional abnormalities that accompany certain disorders producing cough. Measurement of forced expiratory flow rates can demonstrate reversible airflow obstruction characteristic of asthma. When asthma is considered but flow rates are normal, bronchoprovocation testing with methacholine or cold-air inhalation can demonstrate hyperreactivity of the airways to a bronchoconstrictive stimulus. Measurement of lung volumes and diffusing capacity is useful primarily for demonstration of a restrictive pattern, often seen with any of the diffuse interstitial lung diseases.

If *sputum* is produced, gross and microscopic examination may provide useful information. Purulent sputum suggests chronic bronchitis, bronchiectasis, pneumonia, or lung abscess. Blood in the sputum may be seen in the same disorders, but its presence also raises the question of an endobronchial tumor. Gram and acid-fast stains and cultures may demonstrate a particular infectious pathogen, while sputum cytology may provide a diagnosis of a pulmonary malignancy.

More specialized studies are helpful in specific circumstances. *Fiberoptic bronchoscopy* is the procedure of choice for visualizing an endobronchial tumor and collecting cytologic and histologic specimens. Inspection of the tracheobronchial mucosa can demonstrate endobronchial granulomas often seen in sarcoidosis, and endobronchial biopsy of such lesions or transbronchial biopsy of the lung interstitium can confirm the diagnosis. Inspection of the airway mucosa by bronchoscopy can also demonstrate the characteristic appearance of endobronchial Kaposi's sarcoma in patients with AIDS. *High-resolution computed tomography* (HRCT) can confirm the presence of interstitial disease and frequently suggests a diagnosis based on the pattern of disease. It is the procedure of choice for demonstrating dilated airways and confirming the diagnosis of bronchiectasis.

A diagnostic algorithm for evaluation of chronic cough is presented in Fig. 33-1.

COMPLICATIONS Common complications of coughing include chest and abdominal wall soreness, urinary incontinence, and exhaustion. On occasion, paroxysms of coughing may precipitate syncope (cough syncope; Chap. 21), consequent to markedly positive intrathoracic and alveolar pressures, diminished venous return, and decreased cardiac output. Although cough fractures of the ribs may occur in otherwise normal patients, their occurrence should at least raise the possibility of pathologic fractures, which are seen with multiple myeloma, osteoporosis, and osteolytic metastases.

℞ TREATMENT Definitive treatment of cough depends on determining the underlying cause and then initiating specific therapy. Elimination of an exogenous inciting agent (cigarette smoke, ACE inhibitors) or an endogenous trigger (postnasal drip, gastroesophageal reflux) is usually effective when such a precipitant can be identified. Other important management considerations are treatment of specific respiratory tract infections, bronchodilators for potentially reversible airflow obstruction, chest physiotherapy to enhance clearance of secretions in patients with bronchiectasis, and treatment of endobronchial tumors or interstitial lung disease when such therapy is available and appropriate.

Symptomatic or nonspecific therapy of cough should be considered when: (1) the cause of the cough is not known or specific treatment is not possible, and (2) the cough performs no useful function or causes marked discomfort. An irritative, nonproductive cough may be suppressed by an antitussive agent, which increases the latency or threshold of the cough center. Such agents include codeine (15 mg qid) or nonnarcotics such as dextromethorphan (15 mg qid). These drugs provide symptomatic relief by interrupting prolonged, self-perpetuating paroxysms. However, a cough productive of significant quantities of sputum should usually not be suppressed, since retention of sputum in the tracheobronchial tree may interfere with the distribution of ventilation, alveolar aeration, and the ability of the lung to resist infection.

Other agents working by a variety of mechanisms have also been used to control cough, but objective information assessing their benefit is meager. The inhaled anticholinergic agent, ipratropium bromide (2 to 4 puffs qid), has been used with the rationale of inhibiting the efferent limb of the cough reflex. Inhaled glucocorticoids, ideally administered with a spacer and dosed according to the particular agent, have been used for patients in whom airway inflammation is thought to be playing a role in the cough.

HEMOPTYSIS

Hemoptysis is defined as the expectoration of blood from the respiratory tract, a spectrum that varies from blood-streaking of sputum to coughing up large amounts of pure blood. *Massive hemoptysis* is variably defined as the expectoration of >100 to >600 mL over a 24-h period, although the patient's estimation of the amount of blood is notoriously unreliable. Expectoration of even relatively small amounts of blood is a frightening symptom and can be a marker for potentially serious disease, such as bronchogenic carcinoma. Massive hemoptysis, on the other hand, can represent an acutely life-threatening problem. Large amounts of blood can fill the airways and the alveolar spaces, not only seriously disturbing gas exchange but potentially causing the patient to suffocate.

ETIOLOGY Because blood originating from the nasopharynx or the gastrointestinal tract can mimic blood coming from the lower respiratory tract, it is important to determine initially that the blood is not coming from one of these alternative sites. Clues that the blood is originating from the gastrointestinal tract include a dark red appearance and an acidic pH, in contrast to the typical bright red appearance and alkaline pH of true hemoptysis.

The bronchial arteries, which are part of the high-pressure systemic circulation, originate either from the aorta or from intercostal arteries and are the source of bleeding in bronchitis or bronchiectasis or with endobronchial tumors.

An etiologic classification of hemoptysis can be based on the site of origin within the lungs (Table 33-1). The most common site of bleeding is the airways, i.e., the tracheobronchial tree, which can be affected by inflammation (acute or chronic bronchitis, bronchiectasis) or by neoplasm (bronchogenic carcinoma, endobronchial metastatic carcinoma, or bronchial carcinoid tumor). Blood originating from the pulmonary parenchyma can be either from a localized source, such as an infection (pneumonia, lung abscess, tuberculosis), or from a process diffusely affecting the parenchyma (as with a coagulopathy or with an autoimmune process such as Goodpasture's syndrome). Disorders primarily affecting the pulmonary vasculature include pulmonary embolic disease and those conditions associated with elevated pulmonary venous and capillary pressures, such as mitral stenosis or left ventricular failure.

Although the relative frequency of the different etiologies of hemoptysis varies from series to series, most recent studies indicate that bronchitis and bronchogenic carcinoma are the two most common causes. Despite the lower frequency of tuberculosis and bronchiectasis seen in recent compared to older series, these two disorders still represent the most common causes of massive hemoptysis in several series. Even after extensive evaluation, a sizable proportion of patients (up to 30% in some series) have no identifiable etiology for their hemoptysis. These patients are classified as having idiopathic or cryp-

Table 33-1 Differential Diagnosis of Hemoptysis

Source other than the lower respiratory tract
  Upper airway (nasopharyngeal) bleeding
  Gastrointestinal bleeding
Tracheobronchial source
  Neoplasm (bronchogenic carcinoma, endobronchial metastatic tumor, Kaposi's sarcoma, bronchial carcinoid)
  Bronchitis (acute or chronic)
  Bronchiectasis
  Broncholithiasis
  Airway trauma
  Foreign body
Pulmonary parenchymal source
  Lung abscess
  Pneumonia
  Tuberculosis
  Mycetoma ("fungus ball")
  Goodpasture's syndrome
  Idiopathic pulmonary hemosiderosis
  Wegener's granulomatosis
  Lupus pneumonitis
  Lung contusion
Primary vascular source
  Arteriovenous malformation
  Pulmonary embolism
  Elevated pulmonary venous pressure (esp. mitral stenosis)
  Pulmonary artery rupture secondary to balloon-tip pulmonary artery catheter manipulation
Miscellaneous/rare causes
  Pulmonary endometriosis
  Systemic coagulopathy or use of anticoagulants or thrombolytic agents

SOURCE: Adapted from SE Weinberger, *Principles of Pulmonary Medicine*, 3d ed, Philadelphia, Saunders, 1998.

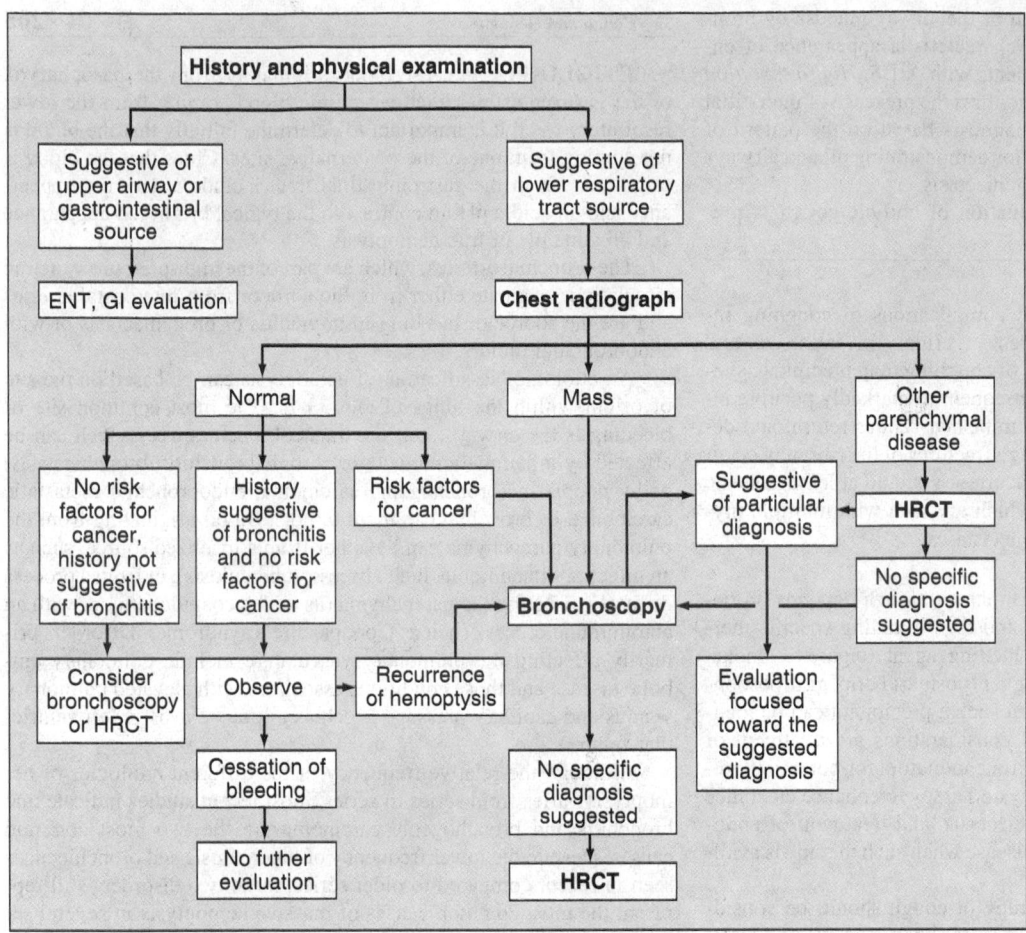

FIGURE 33-2 An algorithm for the evaluation of non-massive hemoptysis. HRCT, high-resolution computed tomography.

The figure shows boxes:
- History and physical examination
  - Suggestive of upper airway or gastrointestinal source → ENT, GI evaluation
  - Suggestive of lower respiratory tract source → Chest radiograph
    - Normal
      - No risk factors for cancer, history not suggestive of bronchitis → Consider bronchoscopy or HRCT
      - History suggestive of bronchitis and no risk factors for cancer → Observe → Cessation of bleeding → No futher evaluation; Recurrence of hemoptysis → Bronchoscopy
      - Risk factors for cancer
    - Mass → Bronchoscopy → No specific diagnosis suggested → HRCT
    - Other parenchymal disease
      - Suggestive of particular diagnosis → Evaluation focused toward the suggested diagnosis
      - HRCT → No specific diagnosis suggested → Bronchoscopy

togenic hemoptysis, and subtle airway or parenchymal disease is presumably responsible for the bleeding.

Approach to the Patient

The *history* is extremely valuable. Hemoptysis that is described as blood-streaking of mucopurulent or purulent sputum often suggests bronchitis. Chronic production of sputum with a recent change in quantity or appearance favors an acute exacerbation of chronic bronchitis. Fever or chills accompanying blood-streaked purulent sputum suggests pneumonia, whereas a putrid smell to the sputum raises the possibility of lung abscess. When sputum production has been chronic and copious, the diagnosis of bronchiectasis should be considered. Hemoptysis following the acute onset of pleuritic chest pain and dyspnea is suggestive of pulmonary embolism.

A history of previous or coexisting disorders should be sought, such as renal disease (seen with Goodpasture's syndrome or Wegener's granulomatosis), lupus erythematosus (with associated pulmonary hemorrhage from lupus pneumonitis), or a previous malignancy (either recurrent lung cancer or endobronchial metastasis from a nonpulmonary primary tumor). In a patient with AIDS, endobronchial or pulmonary parenchymal Kaposi's sarcoma should be considered. Risk factors for bronchogenic carcinoma, particularly smoking and asbestos exposure, should be sought. Patients should be questioned about previous bleeding disorders, treatment with anticoagulants, or use of drugs that can be associated with thrombocytopenia.

The *physical examination* may also provide helpful clues to the diagnosis. For example, examination of the lungs may demonstrate a pleural friction rub (pulmonary embolism), localized or diffuse crackles (parenchymal bleeding or an underlying parenchymal process associated with bleeding), evidence of airflow obstruction (chronic bron-

chitis), or prominent rhonchi, with or without wheezing or crackles (bronchiectasis). Cardiac examination may demonstrate findings of pulmonary arterial hypertension, mitral stenosis, or heart failure. Skin examination may reveal Kaposi's sarcoma, arteriovenous malformations of Osler-Rendu-Weber disease, or lesions suggestive of systemic lupus erythematosus.

Diagnostic evaluation of hemoptysis starts with a chest radiograph to look for a mass lesion, findings suggestive of bronchiectasis (Chap. 256), or focal or diffuse parenchymal disease (representing either focal or diffuse bleeding or a focal area of pneumonitis). Additional initial screening evaluation often includes a complete blood count, a coagulation profile, and assessment for renal disease with a urinalysis and measurement of blood urea nitrogen and creatinine levels. When sputum is present, examination by Gram and acid-fast stains (along with the corresponding cultures) is indicated.

Fiberoptic bronchoscopy is particularly useful for localizing the site of bleeding and for visualization of endobronchial lesions. When bleeding is massive, rigid bronchoscopy is often preferable to fiberoptic bronchoscopy because of better airway control and greater suction capability. In patients with suspected bronchiectasis, HRCT is now the diagnostic procedure of choice, having replaced bronchography.

A diagnostic algorithm for evaluation of nonmassive hemoptysis is presented in Fig. 33-2.

TREATMENT The rapidity of bleeding and its effect on gas exchange determine the urgency of management. When the bleeding is confined to either blood-streaking of sputum or production of small amounts of pure blood, gas exchange is usually preserved; establishing a diagnosis is the first priority. When hemoptysis is massive, maintaining adequate gas exchange, preventing blood from spilling into unaffected areas of lung, and avoiding asphyxiation are the highest priorities. Keeping the patient at rest and partially suppressing cough may help the bleeding to subside. If the origin of the blood is known and is limited to one lung, the bleeding lung should be placed in the dependent position, so that blood is not aspirated into the unaffected lung.

With massive bleeding, the need to control the airway and maintain adequate gas exchange may necessitate endotracheal intubation and mechanical ventilation. In patients in danger of flooding the lung contralateral to the side of hemorrhage despite proper positioning, isolation of the right and left mainstem bronchi from each other can be achieved by selectively intubating the nonbleeding lung (often with bronchoscopic guidance) or by using specially designed double-lumen endotracheal tubes. Another option involves inserting a balloon catheter through a bronchoscope by direct visualization and inflating the balloon to occlude the bronchus leading to the bleeding site. This technique not only prevents aspiration of blood into unaffected areas but also may promote tamponade of the bleeding site and cessation of bleeding.

Other available techniques for control of significant bleeding include laser phototherapy, electrocautery, embolotherapy, and surgical resection of the involved area of lung. With bleeding from an endobronchial tumor, the neodymium:yttrium-aluminum-garnet (Nd:YAG) laser can often achieve at least temporary hemostasis by coagulating the bleeding site. Electrocautery, which uses an electric current for thermal destruction of tissue, can be used similarly for management of bleeding from an endobronchial tumor. Embolotherapy involves an arteriographic procedure in which a vessel proximal to the bleeding site is cannulated, and a material such as Gelfoam is injected to occlude the bleeding vessel. Surgical resection is a therapeutic option either for the emergent therapy of life-threatening hemoptysis that fails to respond to other measures or for the elective but definitive management of localized disease subject to recurrent bleeding.

BIBLIOGRAPHY

COUGH

FAHEY T et al: Quantitative systematic review of randomized control trials comparing antibiotic with placebo for acute cough in adults. BMJ 316:906, 1998

IRWIN RS (ed): Managing cough as a defense mechanism and as a symptom: A consensus panel report of the American College of Chest Physicians. Chest 114 (Suppl): 133S, 1998

——— et al: Appropriate use of antitussives and protussives. A practical review. Drugs 46:80, 1993

IRWIN RS et al: The cough reflex and its relation to gastroesophageal reflux. Am J Med 108:735, 2000

IRWIN RS, WIDDICOMBE J: Cough, in *Textbook of Respiratory Medicine*, 3d ed., Murray JF, Nadel JA (eds). Philadelphia, Saunders, 2000, pp 553–566

ISRAILI ZH, HALL WD: Cough and angioneurotic edema associated with angiotensin-converting enzyme inhibitor therapy. Ann Intern Med 117:234, 1992

WRIGHT SW et al: Pertussis infection in adults with persistent cough. JAMA 273:1044, 1995

HEMOPTYSIS

CAHILL BC, INGBAR DH: Massive hemoptysis: Assessment and management. Clin Chest Med 15:147, 1994

FERNANDO HC et al: Role of bronchial artery embolization in the management of hemoptysis. Arch Surg 133:862, 1998

HIRSHBERG B et al: Hemoptysis: Etiology, evaluation, and outcome in a tertiary referral hospital. Chest 112:440, 1997

PRIMACH SL et al: Diffuse pulmonary hemorrhage: Clinical, pathologic and imaging features. AJR 164:295, 1995

34 *Patrick T. O'Gara, Eugene Braunwald*

APPROACH TO THE PATIENT WITH A HEART MURMUR

Auscultation of the heart constitutes the final step in the cardiovascular examination and, for many patients with established or suspected cardiac disease, represents a defining moment in the doctor-patient relationship. The examiner must bring to this exercise an integrated approach that incorporates pertinent information from several sources. The auscultatory findings must be interpreted in the context of the history and general physical examination and with the observations made regarding the venous wave forms and major arterial pulses. In this way, abnormalities of heart sounds, adventitious sounds, and murmurs can be placed in their proper perspective.

In many patients, a heart murmur is the only or the most conspicuous finding on physical examination. The recognition of a heart murmur usually leads to additional testing, such as electrocardiography, chest radiography, and echocardiography, and may result in referral to a cardiologist. The differential diagnosis of a heart murmur should begin with an unbiased and systematic evaluation of its major attributes: timing, duration, intensity, quality, frequency, configuration, location, radiation, and response to maneuvers (see Table 225-1). Laboratory testing can be pursued thereafter to clarify any remaining ambiguity and to provide additional anatomic and physiologic information that will impact on patient management.

Heart murmurs are defined in terms of their timing within the cardiac cycle. *Systolic murmurs* begin with or after the first heart sound (S_1) and terminate at or before the component $(A_2$ or $P_2)$ of the second heart sound (S_2) that corresponds to their side of origin (left or right). *Diastolic murmurs* begin with or after the associated component of S_2 and end at or before the subsequent S_1. *Continuous murmurs* are not confined to either phase of the cardiac cycle but rather begin in systole and proceed through S_2 into all or part of diastole.

The appropriate timing of heart murmurs is the first critical step in their identification. The distinction between S_1 and S_2, and, therefore, systole and diastole, is usually a straightforward process but can be difficult in the setting of a tachyarrhythmia, in which case the heart sounds can be distinguished by simultaneous palpation of the carotid arterial pulse. The upstroke should closely follow S_1. The principal causes of heart murmurs are shown in Table 34-1, and the critical importance of the timing of heart murmurs in the differential diagnosis is shown in Fig. 34-1.

SYSTOLIC HEART MURMURS

Systolic heart murmurs derive from the increased turbulence associated with (1) enhanced or accelerated flow across a normal semilunar valve, through a normal ventricular outflow tract, or into a dilated great vessel, (2) normal flow across a structurally abnormal semilunar valve or through a narrowed ventricular outflow tract, (3) flow across an incompetent atrioventricular valve, and (4) flow across the interventricular septum. One approach to their differential diagnosis further subdivides these murmurs according to their time of onset and duration within the systolic phase of the cardiac cycle.

EARLY SYSTOLIC MURMURS Early systolic murmurs begin with S_1 and extend for a variable period of time, ending well before S_2. Their causes are relatively few in number. *Acute severe mitral regurgitation* into a normal-sized, relatively noncompliant left atrium results in an early and attenuated systolic murmur that is decrescendo in configuration and usually best heard at or just medial to the apical impulse (Chap. 236). These characteristics reflect the rapid rise in left atrial pressure caused by the sudden volume load into a nondilated chamber and contrast sharply with the auscultatory features of chronic mitral regurgitation. Clinical settings in which this occurs include: (1) papillary muscle rupture complicating acute myocardial infarction, (2) infective endocarditis, (3) rupture of chordae tendineae, and (4) blunt chest wall trauma.

Acute mitral regurgitation from papillary muscle rupture usually accompanies an inferior, posterior, or lateral infarction. The murmur is associated with a precordial thrill in approximately one-half of cases and is to be distinguished from that associated with postinfarction ventricular septal rupture. The latter is more commonly (90%) accompanied by a thrill at the left sternal edge, is holosystolic, and complicates anterior infarctions as often as inferior-posterior damage. The recognition of either of these mechanical defects mandates aggressive medical stabilization and emergent surgical intervention (Chap. 243).

The other potential causes of acute severe mitral regurgitation may be distinguished on the basis of associated findings. Spontaneous chordal rupture usually occurs on a substrate of myxomatous replacement, such as that underlying most forms of mitral valve prolapse (Chap. 236). This lesion may be part of a more generalized process, as can occur with the Marfan or Ehlers-Danlos syndromes, or it may be an isolated phenomenon. Infective endocarditis is associated with fever, peripheral embolic lesions, and positive blood cultures and most

ORGANIC SYSTOLIC MURMURS

Midsystolic
  Aortic
    Obstructive
      Supravalvular—supraaortic stenosis, coarctation of the aorta
      Valvular—AS and sclerosis
      Subvalvular—discrete or HOCM
    Increased flow, hyperkinetic states, AR, complete heart block
    Dilatation of ascending aorta, atheroma, aortitis, aneurysm of aorta
  Pulmonary
    Obstructive
      Supravalvular—pulmonary arterial stenosis
      Valvular—pulmonic valve stenosis
      Subvalvular—infundibular stenosis
    Increased flow, hyperkinetic states, left-to-right shunt (e.g., ASD, VSD)
    Dilatation of pulmonary artery
Holosystolic (regurgitant)
  Atrioventricular valve regurgitation (MR, TR)
  Left-to-right shunt at ventricular level (VSD)

EARLY DIASTOLIC MURMURS

Aortic regurgitation
  Valvular; rheumatic deformity; perforation, postendocarditis, posttraumatic, postvalvulotomy
  Dilatation of valve ring: aorta dissection, annuloectasia, cystic medial necrosis, hypertension
  Widening of commissures: syphilis
  Congenital: bicuspid valve, with VSD
Pulmonic regurgitation
  Valvular: postvalvulotomy, endocarditis, rheumatic fever, carcinoid
  Dilatation of valve ring: pulmonary hypertension; Marfan syndrome
  Congenital: isolated or associated with tetralogy of Fallot, VSD, pulmonic stenosis

MIDDIASTOLIC MURMURS

Mitral stenosis
Carey-Coombs murmur (middiastolic apical murmur in acute rheumatic fever)
Increased flow across nonstenotic mitral valve (e.g., MR, VSD, PDA, high-output states, and complete heart block)
Tricuspid stenosis
Increased flow across nonstenotic tricuspid valve (e.g., TR, ASD, and anomalous pulmonary venous return)
Left and right atrial tumors

CONTINUOUS MURMURS

Patent ductus arteriosus	Proximal coronary artery stenosis
Coronary AV fistula	Mammary souffle
Ruptured aneurysm of sinus of Valsalva	Pulmonary artery branch stenosis
Aortic septal defect	Bronchial collateral circulation
Cervical venous hum	Small (restrictive) ASD with MS
Anomalous left coronary artery	Intercostal AV fistula

NOTE: AR, aortic regurgitation; AS, aortic stenosis; ASD, atrial septal defect; AV, arteriovenous; HOCM, hypertrophic obstructive cardiomyopathy; MR, mitral regurgitation; MS, mitral stenosis; PDA, patent ductus arteriosus; TR, tricuspid regurgitation; VSD, ventricular septal defect.
SOURCE: E Braunwald, in *Heart Disease*, 4th ed, E. Braunwald (ed), Philadelphia, Saunders, 1992.

commonly occurs on a previously abnormal valvular apparatus (Chap. 126). Trauma is usually self-evident but may be disarmingly trivial (Chap. 240). It can result in papillary muscle contusion and rupture, chordal interruption, or leaflet avulsion or perforation.

Echocardiography should be performed in all cases of suspected acute severe mitral regurgitation to define the responsible mechanism, estimate the severity, and provide a preliminary assessment as to the feasibility of surgical repair (versus replacement).

Other causes of early systolic murmurs include congenital, small muscular ventricular septal defects. The duration of the murmur is attenuated by the closure of the defect during systolic contraction. The murmur is localized to the left sternal edge and is commonly of grade

IV/VI or V/VI intensity. Signs of pulmonary hypertension or left ventricular volume overload are absent. Patients with anatomically large, uncorrected ventricular septal defects accompanied by pulmonary hypertension may also have murmurs confined to early systole. The elevated pulmonary vascular resistance attenuates the degree of shunting as pressures within the right and left ventricles equalize during the latter half of systole.

Tricuspid regurgitation with normal pulmonary artery pressures, such as that caused by infective endocarditis in injection drug users, may produce an early systolic murmur. The murmur is soft, best heard at the lower left sternal edge, and may accentuate with inspiration (Carvallo's sign). Regurgitant $c-v$ waves may be visible in the jugular venous pulse.

MIDSYSTOLIC MURMURS   Midsystolic murmurs begin at a short interval following S_1, end before S_2, and are usually crescendo-decrescendo in configuration (Fig. 34-1C). Semilunar valve stenosis is the classic prototype. With aortic valve stenosis, the murmur is usually loudest in the second right intercostal space (aortic area) and radiates along the carotid arteries (Chap. 236). The intensity of the murmur varies directly with the cardiac output; aortic valve stenosis with severe heart failure may produce a misleadingly soft systolic murmur. With a normal cardiac output, a systolic thrill is usually indicative of severe stenosis with a peak gradient in excess of 50 to 60 mmHg. An accompanying early systolic ejection click may be audible in younger patients with a bicuspid valve; its presence localizes the ob

FIGURE 34-1 Diagram depicting principal heart murmurs. *A.* Presystolic murmur of mitral or tricuspid stenosis. *B.* Holosystolic (pansystolic) murmur of mitral or tricuspid regurgitation or of ventricular septal defect. *C.* Aortic ejection murmur beginning with an ejection click and fading before the second heart sound. *D.* Systolic murmur in pulmonic stenosis spilling through the aortic second sound, pulmonic valve closure being delayed. *E.* Aortic or pulmonary diastolic murmur. *F.* Long diastolic murmur of mitral stenosis following the opening snap. *G.* Short middiastolic inflow murmur following a third heart sound. *H.* Continuous murmur of patent ductus arteriosus. (*Adapted from P Wood, Diseases of the Heart and Circulation, Philadelphia, Lippincott, 1968, with permission.*)

struction to the valvular (as opposed to the sub- or supravalvular) level. The midsystolic murmur of aortic stenosis may be well transmitted to the apex, especially in older patients, where it becomes less harsh and slightly higher pitched (Gallavardin effect). The murmur of aortic stenosis should increase following a postpremature beat, whereas a mitral regurgitant murmur would not be expected to change in intensity.

Sclerosis of the aortic valve produces a murmur of similar location, radiation, and configuration, albeit without the usual signs of hemodynamic significance. The carotid upstroke is well preserved, the murmur peaks in midsystole and is not accompanied by a thrill, and only a modest gradient is estimated by Doppler echocardiography. Noncritical sclerodegenerative thickening of the aortic valve leaflets is perhaps the most common cause of a midsystolic murmur in older adults. The similar midsystolic murmur of pulmonic valve stenosis, usually introduced by an ejection click, is best appreciated in the second and third left intercostal spaces (pulmonic area). The murmur lengthens and the intensity of P_2 diminishes with increasing degrees of stenosis. A midsystolic murmur in the aortic position can also be detected in hyperdynamic states (fever, thyrotoxicosis, pregnancy, anemia) and in the presence of isolated aortic regurgitation with the augmented flow into a dilated proximal aorta.

Crescendo-decrescendo midsystolic murmurs usually of grade II/VI intensity heard in the pulmonic area may be innocent if unaccompanied by any other signs of cardiac disease in children or young adults. They may also reflect enhanced flow into a normal pulmonary artery in hyperkinetic states or augmented flow into a dilated pulmonary artery. The latter may occur with an atrial septal defect, in which case splitting of S_2 is usually abnormal (fixed). Still's murmur is a vibratory, medium frequency, mid-systolic murmur heard best between the lower left sternal edge and the apex in normal children and young adults. It is generated by vibrations of the pulmonic valve leaflets at their attachments or by vibrations of a left ventricular false tendon.

The midsystolic murmur of hypertrophic cardiomyopathy (Chap. 238) is usually loudest between the left sternal edge and apex, of grade II/VI to III/VI intensity, and crescendo-decrescendo in configuration. In contrast to aortic valve stenosis, the murmur does *not* radiate into the neck and the carotid upstrokes are brisk and full and may even be bifid. The intensity of the murmur associated with hypertrophic cardiomyopathy increases following maneuvers that decrease left ventricular volume (strain phase of the Valsalva maneuver, standing, amyl nitrite) or increase myocardial contractility (inotropic therapy). Conversely, the intensity of the systolic murmur decreases with maneuvers that increase ventricular volume (squatting, passive leg raising), impair contractility (beta-adrenoreceptor blockade), or raise preload and systemic afterload (squatting). Among these several maneuvers, auscultation in the standing and squatting positions, if possible, is perhaps the most sensitive technique to elicit a dynamic change in the intensity of the murmur associated with hypertrophic obstructive cardiomyopathy.

LATE SYSTOLIC MURMURS A late systolic murmur begins well after the onset of ejection and is usually best heard at the left ventricular apex or between the apex and the left sternal edge. When introduced by a nonejection click, it is usually indicative of systolic prolapse of the mitral valve leaflet(s) into the left atrium. The click and murmur move closer to S_1 following maneuvers that decrease left ventricular volume (standing, Valsalva) and move oppositely upon increases in volume (leg raising, squatting). The intensity of the murmur augments with increases in systemic afterload (squatting, pressor agents) and decrease with vasodilation (amyl nitrite). Isometric exercise, which also delays the onset of the murmur, accentuates the intensity.

HOLOSYSTOLIC MURMURS These murmurs, also termed *pansystolic murmurs*, begin with S_1 and continue through systole to S_2 (Fig. 34-1B). They are, with rare exception, indicative of atrioventricular valve regurgitation or of a ventricular septal defect; the differential diagnosis is shown in Fig. 34-2. The murmur of mitral regurgitation is loudest at the left ventricular apex. Its radiation reflects the direction of the regurgitant jet. With a flail posterior mitral leaflet

due to ruptured chordae tendineae, for example, the jet is directed anterosuperiorly, and the murmur radiates prominently to the base of the heart, where it might be confused with aortic valve stenosis unless the carotid upstrokes are carefully examined. Conversely, a flail anterior leaflet is associated with a posteriorly directed jet, which radiates into the axilla and the back. It may even strike the spine and be transmitted to the base of the neck. Severe mitral regurgitation is usually associated with a systolic thrill, a soft S_3, and a short diastolic rumbling murmur best appreciated in the left lateral decubitus position.

The holosystolic murmur of tricuspid regurgitation is generally softer (grades I to III/VI) than that of mitral regurgitation, is loudest at the left lower sternal edge, and increases in intensity upon inspiration. Associated signs include prominent "$c-v$" waves in the jugular venous pulse, systolic hepatic pulsations, and peripheral edema. Among the several causes of tricuspid regurgitation, annular dilatation from right ventricular enlargement in the setting of pulmonary artery hypertension is the most common.

Ventricular septal defect (Chap. 234) also produces a holosystolic murmur, the intensity of which varies inversely with the anatomic size of the defect. It is usually accompanied by a palpable thrill along the mid-left sternal border. The murmur of a ventricular septal defect is louder than that due to tricuspid regurgitation and does not share the latter's inspiratory increase in intensity or associated peripheral signs.

DIASTOLIC HEART MURMURS

Like systolic murmurs, diastolic murmurs also can be subcategorized according to their time of onset.

EARLY DIASTOLIC MURMURS (Fig. 34-1E) Early diastolic murmurs result from semilunar valve incompetence and begin at the valve closure sound (A_2 or P_2), which reflects their site of origin. They are generally high pitched and decrescendo in configuration, especially in states of chronic regurgitation, in which their duration is a crude index of the severity of the lesion. The murmur of aortic regurgitation is generally, but not always, best heard in the second intercostal space at the left sternal edge. There is a tendency for the murmur associated with primary valvular pathology (e.g., rheumatic deformity, congenital bicuspid valve, endocarditis) to radiate more prominently along the *left* sternal border and to be well transmitted to the apex, while the murmur associated with primary aortic root pathology (e.g., annuloaortic ectasia, aortic dissection) radiates more often along the right sternal edge. It is occasionally necessary to examine the patient sitting forward in full expiration to appreciate the murmur, a maneuver that brings the aortic root closer to the anterior chest wall. Severe aortic regurgitation may be accompanied by a lower-pitched mid- to late-diastolic murmur at the apex (Austin Flint murmur), which is generally thought to reflect turbulence at the mitral inflow area from the mixing of the regurgitant (aortic) and forward (mitral) streams, and should be distinguished from mitral stenosis (see above). In the absence of significant heart failure, chronic severe aortic regurgitation is accompanied by several peripheral signs of significant diastolic runoff, including a wide systemic pulse pressure and water-hammer carotid upstrokes (Corrigan's pulse).

The murmur associated with *acute* aortic regurgitation is notably shorter in duration, lower pitched, and can be difficult to appreciate in the presence of tachycardia. Peripheral signs of significant diastolic runoff may be absent. These attributes reflect the abrupt rise in diastolic pressure within the noncompliant left ventricle, with a correspondingly rapid decline in the aortic diastolic–left ventricular pressure gradient.

The murmur of pulmonic valve regurgitation (Graham Steell murmur) begins with a loud (palpable) pulmonic closure sound (P_2) and is best heard in the pulmonic area with radiation along the left sternal border. Typically, it is high pitched, with a decrescendo quality, and is indicative of significant pulmonary artery hypertension with a diastolic pulmonary artery–right ventricular pressure gradient. Its in-

FIGURE 34-2 Differential diagnosis of holosystolic murmur (regurgitant). S_1, first heart sound; S_2, second heart sound; A_2, aortic component of the second heart sound; P_2, pulmonary component of the second heart sound (echo-Doppler evaluation should be considered for differential diagnosis). [*From C Chatterjee, in K Chatterjee et al (eds), Cardiology: An Illustrated Text/Reference, Philadelphia, Lippincott, 1991, with permission.*]

crease in intensity upon inspiration is one means by which to distinguish it from aortic regurgitation. Signs of right ventricular pressure and volume overload are also usually present. With significant mitral stenosis, an early decrescendo diastolic murmur along the left sternal border is not uncommon and is almost always due to aortic rather than

pulmonic regurgitation, despite the co-existence of pulmonary artery hypertension.

Pulmonic valve regurgitation in the absence of pulmonary artery hypertension can occur on a congenital basis and rarely with infective endocarditis. In these instances, the early diastolic murmur is softer and lower pitched than the classic Graham Steell murmur. It begins at or even after P_2, which should be easily separable from A_2 and thus produce appreciation of an early diastolic pause.

MIDDIASTOLIC MURMURS

Middiastolic murmurs usually result from obstruction and/or augmented flow across the antrioventricular valves. The classic example is that of mitral stenosis due to rheumatic deformity (Fig. 34-1F). In the absence of extensive calcification, the first heart sound (S_1) is loud and the murmur begins after the opening snap; the time interval between S_2 and the opening snap is inversely related to the left atrial–left ventricular pressure gradient. The murmur is low pitched and best heard with the bell of the stethoscope over the apex, particularly in the left lateral decubitus position. While its intensity does not reflect the severity of the obstruction accurately, the duration of the murmur does provide some indication as to the magnitude of the obstruction. A longer murmur denotes persistence of a left atrioventricular pressure gradient over a greater proportion of the diastolic time interval. Presystolic accentuation of the murmur (Fig. 34-1A) is frequently appreciated in the presence of sinus rhythm and reflects a further increase in transmitral flow consequent to mechanical atrial systole.

The murmur associated with tricuspid stenosis shares many of these features, but it is best heard at the lower left sternal border and, like most right-sided events, increases in intensity upon inspiration. The observant examiner may discern a prolonged y descent in the jugular venous pulse. Signs of right heart failure may predominate.

There are several other causes of mid-diastolic murmurs that are important to distinguish from mitral stenosis. *Left atrial myxomas* (Chap. 240) may masquerade as mitral stenosis, but the diastolic murmur is not accompanied by an opening snap or pre-systolic accentuation. Augmented flow across the mitral valve in diastole, such as occurs with severe mitral regurgitation or with large left to right intra-cardiac (ventricular septal defect) or great vessel (patent ductus arteriosus) shunts may produce a short, low pitched mid-diastolic apical murmur. The murmur usually follows a soft S_3 that is lower pitched and later in timing than the opening snap (Fig. 34-1G). Severe tricuspid regurgitation can also result in enhanced diastolic tricuspid flow and produce a right-sided filling complex similar to that which accompanies severe mitral regurgitation. The Austin Flint murmur of severe aortic regurgitation has been previously described and occurs in the presence of chronic severe aortic regurgitation.

FIGURE 34-3 Algorithm for the evaluation of a cardiac murmur. (*From Bonow et al.*)

Continuous murmurs begin in systole, peak near S_2, and continue into all or part of diastole (Fig. 34-1*H*). Accordingly, they reflect the persistence of flow between two chambers during both phases of the cardiac cycle. The differential diagnosis of continuous murmurs is shown in Table 34-1. Two innocent variants are the cervical venous hum and the mammary souffle. The former is audible in healthy children and young adults in the right supraclavicular fossa and can be abolished by compression over the internal jugular vein. Its diastolic component may be louder than its systolic counterpart. A mammary souffle represents augmented arterial flow through engorged breasts and becomes audible during the late third trimester of pregnancy or in the early postpartum period. Firm pressure with the diaphragm of the stethoscope can eliminate the diastolic portion of the murmur. The murmur dissipates with time after delivery.

The classic continuous murmur is that due to a patent ductus arteriosus. It is best heard at or just above and to the left of the pulmonic area and may be audible in the back. Over time, a large uncorrected shunt may lead to elevation of the pulmonary vascular resistance, with resultant pulmonary artery hypertension and diminution or elimination of the diastolic component. A continuous murmur can also signify a ruptured congenital sinus of Valsalva aneurysm, which occurs either spontaneously or as a complication of infective endocarditis. Here, a high-pressure fistula is created between the aorta and a cardiac chamber, usually the right atrium or ventricle. The murmur is loudest along the right or left sternal border and is frequently accompanied by a thrill. Notably, the diastolic component is louder than the systolic component. It can be difficult to distinguish continuous murmurs from the temporally separate systolic and diastolic murmurs of mixed aortic valve disease or isolated severe aortic regurgitation. The emphasis is on the envelopment of S_2 by continuous murmurs and a gap between the to-and-fro murmurs of aortic valve disease.

A variety of other lesions can result in continuous murmurs. A coronary arteriovenous fistula sometimes produces a faint, continuous murmur with a louder diastolic component at the left sternal border or left ventricular apex. Severe atherosclerotic disease of a major systemic artery may produce a continuous bruit, the presence of which signifies very high-grade obstruction. Patients with peripheral pulmonary (branch) stenosis or with pulmonary atresia with extensive bronchial collaterals may also have continuous murmurs best heard in the back or along the lateral thoracic cage. Similar findings are present in patients with severe aortic coarctation, a lesion that should be identifiable on the basis of weak and delayed lower extremity pulses and upper extremity hypertension. The continuous murmurs emanate from the enlarged collateral (intercostal) arteries.

Approach to the Patient

It is widely recognized that, despite the importance placed on them by medical schools and training program directors, the auscultatory skills of medical students and residents have declined considerably since the advent of Doppler echocardiography. Recent surveys indicate that trainees fail to correctly identify up to 80% of adventitious sounds and murmurs. Diagnostic errors are as frequent among third-year medical residents as they are for first-year residents. Few training programs provide a dedicated educational curriculum for cardiac auscultation. In the aggregate, these deficiencies lead to an over-reliance on the use of echocardiography and increase the costs of evaluating patients with heart murmurs.

In many patients the cause of a heart murmur can be readily elucidated from careful assessment of the murmur itself, as described in this chapter, when considered in the light of the history, general physical examination, and other features of the cardiac examination, as described in Chap. 225. When the diagnosis is in doubt, or when additional pathoanatomic and physiologic data are necessary in assessing the patient and planning treatment, transthoracic Doppler echocardiography is of great value in identifying not only the etiology of the murmur but also the severity of the responsible lesion (Fig. 34-3).

The majority of heart murmurs are midsystolic and soft (Grades I to II/VI). When such a murmur occurs in an asymptomatic child or young adult *without* other evidence of heart disease on clinical examination, it is usually benign and echocardiography is not generally required. On the other hand, echocardiographic examination is indicated in patients with loud systolic murmurs ($\geq$III/VI), especially those that are holosystolic or late systolic, in most patients with diastolic or continuous murmurs, and in patients with additional unexplained abnormal physical findings on cardiac examination.

BIBLIOGRAPHY

BRAUNWALD E, PERLOFF JK: Physical examination of the heart, in *Heart Disease*, 6th ed, E Braunwald, D Zipes, P Libby (eds). Philadelphia, Saunders, 2001

BONOW RO et al: ACC/AHA guidelines for the management of patients with valvular heart disease: a report of the American College of Cardiology/American Heart Association Task Force on Practice Guidelines (committee on Management of Patients with Valvular Heart Disease). J Am Coll Cardiol 32(5):1486, 1998

ETCHELLS E et al: Does this patient have an abnormal systolic heart murmur? JAMA 277(7):564, 1997

GREWE K et al: Differentiation of cardiac murmurs by auscultation. Curr Probl Cardiol 13:699, 1988

LEMBO NJ et al: Bedside diagnosis of systolic murmurs. N Engl J Med 318(24):1572, 1988

MANGIONE S, NIEMAN LZ: Cardiac auscultatory skills of internal medicine and family practice trainees. A comparison of diagnostic proficiency. JAMA 278(9):717, 1997

MURGO JP: Systolic ejection murmurs in the era of modern cardiology. What do we really know? J Am Coll Cardiol 32:1596, 1998

O'ROURKE RA: Approach to the patient with a heart murmur, in *Primary Cardiology*, L Goldman, E Braunwald (eds). Philadelphia, Saunders, 1998

SHAVER JA: Cardiac auscultation: A cost-effective diagnostic skill. Curr Probl Cardiol 20:441, 1995

35 *Gordon H. Williams*

APPROACH TO THE PATIENT WITH HYPERTENSION

DEFINITION Since there is no dividing line between normal and high blood pressure, arbitrary levels have been established to define persons who have an increased risk of developing a morbid cardiovascular event and/or will benefit from medical therapy. These definitions should take into account not only the level of diastolic pressure but also systolic pressure, age, sex, race, and concomitant diseases. For example, patients with a diastolic pressure >90 mmHg have a significant reduction in morbidity and mortality rate if they receive adequate therapy. These, then, are patients who have hypertension and who should be considered for treatment.

The level of *systolic* pressure is also important in assessing the influence of arterial pressure on cardiovascular morbidity. Some data suggest that it may be more important than diastolic pressure. For example, males with normal diastolic pressures (<82 mmHg) but elevated systolic pressures (>158 mmHg) have a cardiovascular mortality rate 2.5 times higher than individuals who have similar diastolic pressures but whose systolic pressures clearly are normal (<130 mmHg). A reduction in mortality and morbidity with treatment, specifically in the elderly, has been documented in these patients. This beneficial effect results mainly from a reduction in strokes and occurs in women as well. Other significant demographic factors that modify the influence of blood pressure on the frequency of morbid cardiovascular events are age, race, and sex, with young black males being most adversely affected by hypertension.

When hypertension is suspected, blood pressure should be measured at least twice during two separate examinations after the initial screening. In adults, a *diastolic* pressure below 85 mmHg is considered to be normal; one between 85 and 89 mmHg is high normal; one of 90 to 99 mmHg represents stage 1 or mild hypertension; one of 100 to 109 mmHg represents stage 2 or moderate hypertension; and one of ≥110 mmHg represents stage 3 or severe hypertension. A *systolic* pressure below 130 mmHg indicates normal blood pressure; one between 130 and 139 mmHg indicates high normal; one between 140 and 159 mmHg indicates stage 1 or mild hypertension; one between 160 and 179 mmHg indicates stage 2 or moderate hypertension; and one ≥180 mmHg indicates stage 3 or severe hypertension. Increasing use of 12- or 24-h blood pressure monitoring may provide additional useful information in patients who are difficult to classify. However, normal values for this procedure and its usefulness in relation to therapeutic outcomes are not currently known. A useful classification of hypertension derived from the Joint Committee on Detection, Evaluation, and Treatment of High Blood Pressure is shown in Table 35-1.

Arterial pressure fluctuates in most persons, whether they are normotensive or hypertensive. Patients who are classified as having *labile hypertension* are those who sometimes, but not always, have arterial pressures in the hypertensive range. These patients are often considered to have borderline hypertension.

Sustained hypertension can become accelerated or enter a malignant phase, although that is unusual in treated patients. Though a patient with *malignant hypertension* often has a blood pressure above 200/140, the condition is defined by the presence of papilledema, usually accompanied by retinal hemorrhages and exudates, rather than by the absolute pressure level. *Accelerated hypertension* is defined as a significant recent increase over previous hypertensive levels associated with evidence of vascular damage on funduscopic examination but without papilledema.

PATIENT EVALUATION In evaluating patients with hypertension, the initial history, physical examination, and laboratory tests should be directed at (1) uncovering correctable secondary forms of hypertension (Chap. 246), (2) establishing a pretreatment baseline, (3) assessing factors that may influence the type of therapy or be changed adversely by therapy, (4) determining if target organ damage is present, and (5) determining whether other risk factors for the development of arteriosclerotic cardiovascular disease are present (Chap. 241). Ideally, this evaluation would also determine the underlying mechanism(s) in essential hypertension, particularly if such information leads to a more specific therapeutic program. Unfortunately, at present this aspect of the evaluation is limited by lack of knowledge of some of the underlying mechanisms, by uncertainty as to the correct treatment for a distinct subset even if the underlying mechanisms are known, or by the prohibitive cost of defining a subset of hypertensive patients even if specific therapy were available. However, with the accumulation of additional information, this sixth component of the evaluation of patients with hypertension may become increasingly important.

Symptoms and Signs Most patients with hypertension have no specific symptoms referable to their blood pressure elevation and are identified only in the course of a physical examination. When symptoms do bring the patient to the physician, they fall into three categories. They are related to (1) the elevated pressure itself, (2) the hypertensive vascular disease, and (3) the underlying disease, in the case of secondary hypertension. Though popularly considered a symptom of elevated arterial pressure, headache is characteristic only of severe hypertension; most commonly such headaches are localized to the occipital region and are present when the patient awakens in the morning but subside spontaneously after several hours. Other complaints that may be related to elevated blood pressure include dizziness, palpitations, easy fatigability, and impotence. Complaints referable to vascular disease include epistaxis, hematuria, blurring of vision owing to retinal changes, episodes of weakness or dizziness due to transient cerebral ischemia, angina pectoris, and dyspnea due to cardiac failure. Pain due to dissection of the aorta or to a leaking aneurysm is an occasional presenting symptom.

Examples of symptoms related to the underlying disease in secondary hypertension are polyuria, polydipsia, and muscle weakness secondary to hypokalemia in patients with primary aldosteronism or weight gain, and emotional lability in patients with Cushing's syndrome. The patient with a pheochromocytoma may present with episodic headaches, palpitations, diaphoresis, and postural dizziness.

History A strong family history of hypertension, along with the reported finding of intermittent pressure elevation in the past, favors the diagnosis of essential hypertension. Secondary hypertension often develops before the age of 35 or after 55. A history of use of adrenal steroids or estrogens is of obvious significance. A history of repeated urinary tract infections suggests chronic pyelonephritis, although this condition may occur in the absence of symptoms; nocturia and polydipsia suggest renal or endocrine disease, while trauma to either flank or an episode of acute flank pain may be a clue to the presence of renal injury. A history of weight gain is compatible with Cushing's syndrome, and one of weight loss is compatible with pheochromocytoma. A number of aspects of the history aid in determining whether vascular disease has progressed to a dangerous stage. These include angina pectoris and symptoms of cerebrovascular insufficiency, congestive heart failure, and/or peripheral vascular insufficiency. Other risk factors that should be asked about include cigarette smoking, diabetes mellitus, lipid disorders, and a family history of early deaths due to cardiovascular disease. Finally, aspects of the patient's lifestyle that could contribute to the hypertension or affect its treatment should be assessed, including diet, physical activity, family status, work, and educational level.

Physical Examination The physical examination starts with the patient's general appearance. For instance, are the round face and truncal obesity of Cushing's syndrome present? Is muscular development in the upper extremities out of proportion to that in the lower extremities, suggesting coarctation of the aorta? The next step is to compare the blood pressures and pulses in the two upper extremities and in the supine and standing positions (for at least 2 min). A rise in diastolic pressure when the patient goes from the supine to the standing position is most compatible with essential hypertension; a fall, in the absence of antihypertensive medications, suggests secondary forms of hypertension. The patient's height and weight should be recorded. Detailed examination of the ocular fundi is mandatory, as funduscopic findings provide one of the best indications of the duration of hypertension and of prognosis. A useful guide is the Keith-Wagener-Barker classification of funduscopic changes (Table 35-2); the specific changes in each fundus should be recorded and a grade assigned. Palpation and auscultation of the carotid arteries for evidence of stenosis or occlusion are important; narrowing of a carotid artery may be a manifestation of hypertensive vascular disease, and it may also be a clue to the presence of a renal arterial lesion, since these two lesions may occur together. In examination of the heart and lungs, evidence of left ventricular

Table 35-1 Classification of Blood Pressure for Adults Aged 18 Years and Older

Category	Systolic Pressure, mmHg	Diastolic Pressure, mmHg
Optimal	<120	<80
Normal	<130	<85
High normal	130–139	85–89
Hypertension[a]		
Stage 1 (mild)	140–159	90–99
Stage 2 (moderate)	160–179	100–109
Stage 3 (severe)	180–209	110–119

[a] Based on the average of ≥2 readings taken at each of two or more visits after an initial screening.

NOTE: Classification of blood pressure for adults aged 18 years and older not taking antihypertensive drugs and not acutely ill. When systolic and diastolic pressures fall into different categories, the higher category should be selected to classify the individual's blood pressure status.

SOURCE: The Sixth Report of the Joint National Committee on Prevention, Detection, Evaluation, and Treatment of High Blood Pressure.

Table 35-2   Classification of Hypertensive and Arteriolosclerotic Retinopathy

| | Hypertension | | | | | Arteriolosclerosis | |
| | Arterioles | | | | | | |
Degree	General Narrowing, AV ratio[a]	Focal Spasm[b]	Hemorrhages	Exudates	Papilledema	Arteriolar Light Reflex	AV Crossing Defects[c]
Normal	3:4	1:1	0	0	0	Fine yellow line, red blood column	None
Grade I	1:2	1:1	0	0	0	Broadened yellow line, red blood column	Mild depression of vein
Grade II	1:3	2:3	0	0	0	Broad yellow line, "copper wire," blood column not visible	Depression or humping of vein
Grade III	1:4	1:3	+	+	0	Broad white line, "silver wire," blood column not visible	Right-angle deviation, tapering, and disappearance of vein under arteriole; distal dilation of vein
Grade IV	Fine, fibrous cords	Obliteration of distal flow	+	+	+	Fibrous cords, blood column not visible	Same as grade III

[a] Ratio of arteriolar to venous diameters.
[b] Ratio of diameters of region of spasm to proximal arteriole.
[c] Arteriolar length and tortuosity increase with severity.

hypertrophy and cardiac decompensation should be sought. Is there a left ventricular lift? Are third and fourth heart sounds present? Are there pulmonary rales? A third heart sound and pulmonary rales are unusual in uncomplicated hypertension. Their presence suggests ventricular dysfunction. Chest examination also includes a search for extracardiac murmurs and palpable collateral vessels that may result from coarctation of the aorta.

The most important part of the abdominal examination is auscultation for bruits originating in stenotic renal arteries. Bruits due to renal arterial narrowing nearly always have a diastolic component or may be continuous and are best heard just to the right or left of the midline above the umbilicus or in the flanks; they are present in many patients with renal artery stenosis due to fibrous dysplasia and in 40 to 50% of those with functionally significant stenosis due to arteriosclerosis. The abdomen should also be palpated for an abdominal aneurysm and for the enlarged kidneys of polycystic renal disease. The femoral pulses must be carefully felt, and, if they are decreased and/or delayed in comparison with the radial pulse, the blood pressure in the lower extremities must be measured. Even if the femoral pulse is normal to palpation, arterial pressure in the lower extremities should be recorded at least once in patients in whom hypertension is discovered before the age of 30 years. Finally, examination of the extremities for edema and a search for evidence of a previous cerebrovascular accident and/or other intracranial pathology should be performed.

Laboratory Investigation   There is controversy as to what laboratory studies should be performed in patients presenting with hypertension. In general, the disagreement centers on how extensively the patient should be evaluated for secondary forms of hypertension or subsets of essential hypertension. The *basic* laboratory studies that should be performed in all patients with sustained hypertension are described in (Table 35-3). →*The secondary studies that should be added if (1) the initial evaluation indicates a form of secondary hypertension and/or (2) arterial pressure is not controlled after initial therapy are discussed in Chap. 246.*

Renal status is evaluated by assessing the presence of protein, blood, and glucose in the urine and measuring serum creatinine and/or blood urea nitrogen. Microscopic examination of the urine is also helpful. The serum potassium level should be measured both as a screen for mineralocorticoid-induced hypertension and to provide a baseline before diuretic therapy is begun. A blood glucose determination is helpful both because diabetes mellitus may be associated with accelerated arteriosclerosis, renal vascular disease, and diabetic nephropathy in patients with hypertension and because primary aldosteronism, Cushing's syndrome, and pheochromocytoma all may be associated with hyperglycemia. Furthermore, since antihypertensive therapy with diuretics, for example, can raise the blood glucose level,

it is important to establish a baseline. The possibility of hypercalcemia may also be investigated. Serum cholesterol, high-density lipoprotein cholesterol, and triglyceride levels identify other factors that predispose to the development of arteriosclerosis.

An electrocardiogram should be obtained in all cases to permit assessment of cardiac status, particularly if left ventricular hypertrophy is present, and to provide a baseline. The echocardiogram is more sensitive than either the electrocardiogram or physical examination in determining whether cardiac hypertrophy is present. However, a complete, detailed echocardiographic study is expensive. Thus, in some circumstances, a cheaper, limited echocardiogram may be a useful addition to the *baseline* evaluation of a hypertensive patient, particularly as left ventricular hypertrophy is an independent cardiovascular risk factor and its presence suggests the need for vigorous antihypertensive therapy. Furthermore, while a substantial increase in arterial pressure usually correlates with the presence of left ventricular hypertrophy, a mild increase may not. Thus, one cannot use the blood pressure as a surrogate marker for the presence or absence of left ventricular hypertrophy. On the other hand, because of the cost of an echo-

Table 35-3   Laboratory Tests for Evaluation of Hypertension

BASIC TESTS FOR INITIAL EVALUATION

1. Always included
   a. Urine for protein, blood, and glucose
   b. Microscopic urinalysis
   c. Hematocrit
   d. Serum potassium
   e. Serum creatinine and/or blood urea nitrogen
   f. Fasting glucose
   g. Total cholesterol
   h. Electrocardiogram
2. Usually included, depending on cost and other factors
   a. Thyroid-stimulating hormone
   b. White blood cell count
   c. HDL and LDL cholesterol and triglycerides
   d. Serum calcium and phosphate
   e. Chest x-ray; limited echocardiogram

SPECIAL STUDIES TO SCREEN FOR SECONDARY HYPERTENSION

1. Renovascular disease: angiotensin-converting enzyme inhibitor radionuclide renal scan, renal duplex Doppler flow studies, and MRI angiography
2. Pheochromocytoma: 24-h urine assay for creatinine, metanephrines, and catecholamines
3. Cushing's syndrome: overnight dexamethasone suppression test or 24-h urine cortisol and creatinine
4. Primary aldosteronism: plasma aldosterone: renin activity ratio

NOTE: HDL, high-density lipoprotein; LDL, low-density lipoprotein; MRI, magnetic resonance imaging.

cardiogram and the uncertainty as to whether the resultant information would modify therapy, it is unclear that routine *follow-up* echocardiograms during therapy are justified. Furthermore, there are no data to suggest that reversal of left ventricular hypertrophy produces benefits beyond that conferred by blood pressure reduction. The chest roentgenogram may also be helpful by providing the opportunity to identify aortic dilation or elongation and the rib notching that occurs in coarctation of the aorta.

Certain clues from the history, physical examination, and basic laboratory studies may suggest an unusual cause for the hypertension and dictate the need for special studies as outlined in Chap 246.

 TREATMENT   See Chap. 246.

BIBLIOGRAPHY

BERLOWITZ DR et al: Inadequate management of blood pressure in a hypertensive population. N Engl J Med 339:1967, 1998

KAPLAN N: Systemic hypertension: Mechanisms and diagnosis, in *Heart Disease*, 6th ed, E Braunwald, D Zipes, P Libby (eds). Philadelphia, Saunders 2001

MOSTERD A et al: Trends in the prevalence of hypertension, antihypertensive therapy, and left ventricular hypertrophy from 1950 to 1989. N Engl J Med 340:1221, 1999

REEVES RA: Does this patient have hypertension? How to measure blood pressure. JAMA 273:1211, 1995

THE SIXTH REPORT OF THE JOINT NATIONAL COMMITTEE ON PREVENTION, DETECTION, EVALUATION, AND TREATMENT OF HIGH BLOOD PRESSURE. Arch Intern Med. 157:2413, 1997

WEBER MA et al: Diagnosis of mild hypertension by ambulatory blood pressure monitoring. Circulation 90:2291, 1994

1999 WORLD HEALTH ORGANIZATION—INTERNATIONAL SOCIETY OF HYPERTENSION GUIDELINES FOR THE MANAGEMENT OF HYPERTENSION. J Hypertens 17:151, 1999

36   *Eugene Braunwald*

HYPOXIA AND CYANOSIS

HYPOXIA

The fundamental purpose of the cardiorespiratory system is to deliver O_2 (and substrates) to the cells and to remove CO_2 (and other metabolic products) from them. Proper maintenance of this function depends on intact cardiovascular and respiratory systems and a supply of inspired gas containing adequate O_2. When hypoxia occurs consequent to respiratory failure, Pa_{CO_2} usually rises (Chap. 250), and the hemoglobin-oxygen (Hb-O_2) dissociation curve (see Fig. 106-2) is displaced to the right. Under these conditions, the Pa_{O_2} declines. Arterial hypoxemia, i.e., a reduction of O_2 saturation of arterial blood (Sa_{O_2}), and consequent cyanosis are likely to be more marked when such depression of Pa_{O_2} results from pulmonary disease than when the depression occurs as the result of a decline in the fraction of oxygen in inspired air (Fi_{O_2}). In this situation Pa_{CO_2} falls secondary to anoxia-induced hyperventilation and the Hb-O_2 dissociation curve is displaced to the left, limiting the decline in Sa_{O_2}.

CAUSES OF HYPOXIA   Anemic Hypoxia   Any reduction in the hemoglobin concentration of the blood is attended by a corresponding decline in the O_2-carrying capacity of the blood. In anemic hypoxia, the Pa_{O_2} is normal; but as a consequence of the reduction of the hemoglobin concentration, the absolute quantity of O_2 transported per unit volume of blood is diminished. As the anemic blood passes through the capillaries and the usual quantity of O_2 is removed from it, the P_{O_2} in the venous blood declines to a greater degree than would normally be the case.

Carbon Monoxide Intoxication (See also Chap. 396)   Hemoglobin that is combined with carbon monoxide (carboxyhemoglobin, COHb) is unavailable for O_2 transport. In addition, the presence of COHb shifts the Hb-O_2 dissociation curve to the left (see Fig. 106-2) so that O_2 is unloaded only at lower tensions. By such formation of COHb, a given degree of reduction in O_2-carrying power produces a far greater degree of tissue hypoxia than the equivalent reduction in hemoglobin due to simple anemia.

Respiratory Hypoxia   Arterial unsaturation is a common finding in advanced pulmonary disease. The most common cause of respiratory hypoxia is ventilation-perfusion mismatch, which results from perfusion of poorly ventilated alveoli. As discussed in Chap. 250, it may also be caused by hypoventilation, and it is then associated with an elevation of Pa_{CO_2}. These two forms of respiratory hypoxia may be recognized because they are usually correctable by inspiring 100% O_2 for several minutes. A third cause is shunting of blood across the lung from right to left by perfusion of nonventilated portions of the lung, as in pulmonary atelectasis or through arteriovenous connections in the lung. The low Pa_{O_2} in this situation is correctable only in part by an Fi_{O_2} of 100%.

Hypoxia Secondary to High Altitude   As one ascends rapidly to 3000 m (approximately 10,000 ft), the alveolar P_{O_2} declines to about 60 mmHg, and impaired memory and other cerebral symptoms of hypoxia may develop. At higher altitudes, arterial saturation declines rapidly and symptoms become more serious; and at 5000 m (approximately 15,000 ft) unacclimatized individuals usually cease to be able to function normally.

Hypoxia Secondary to Right-to-Left Extrapulmonary Shunting   From a physiologic viewpoint, this cause of hypoxia resembles intrapulmonary right-to-left shunting but is caused by congenital cardiac malformations such as tetralogy of Fallot, transposition of the great arteries, and Eisenmenger's syndrome (Chap. 234). As in pulmonary right-to-left shunting, the Pa_{O_2} cannot be restored to normal with inspiration of 100% O_2.

Circulatory Hypoxia   As in anemic hypoxia, the Pa_{O_2} is usually normal, but venous and tissue P_{O_2} values are reduced as a consequence of reduced tissue perfusion. Generalized circulatory hypoxia occurs in heart failure (Chap. 232) and in most forms of shock (Chap. 38).

Specific Organ Hypoxia   Decreased perfusion of any organ resulting in localized circulatory hypoxia may occur secondary to organic arterial obstruction or as a consequence of vasoconstriction (Chap. 248). The latter is seen in the upper extremities in Raynaud's phenomenon. Ischemic hypoxia with accompanying pallor occurs in organic arterial obliterative disease. Localized hypoxia also may result from venous obstruction and the resultant congestion and reduced arterial inflow. Edema, which increases the distance through which O_2 diffuses before it reaches cells, also can cause localized hypoxia. In an attempt to maintain adequate perfusion to more vital organs, constriction may reduce perfusion in all limbs in patients with heart failure or hypovolemic shock.

Increased O_2 Requirements   If the O_2 consumption of the tissues is elevated without a corresponding increase in perfusion, tissue hypoxia ensues and the P_{O_2} in venous blood becomes reduced. Ordinarily, the clinical picture of patients with hypoxia due to an elevated metabolic rate is quite different from that in other types of hypoxia; the skin is warm and flushed, owing to increased cutaneous blood flow that dissipates the excessive heat produced, and cyanosis is usually absent.

Exercise is a classic example of increased tissue O_2 requirements. These increased demands are normally met by several mechanisms operating simultaneously: (1) increasing the cardiac output and ventilation and thus O_2 delivery to the tissues; (2) preferentially directing the blood to the exercising muscles by changing vascular resistances in various circulatory beds, directly and/or reflexly; (3) increasing O_2 extraction from the delivered blood and widening the arteriovenous O_2 difference; and (4) reducing the pH of the tissues and capillary blood, thereby unloading more O_2 from hemoglobin. If the capacity of these mechanisms is exceeded, then hypoxia, especially of the exercising muscles, will result.

Improper Oxygen Utilization   Cyanide (Chap. 396) and several other similarly acting poisons cause cellular hypoxia. The tissues are unable to utilize O_2, and as a consequence, the venous blood tends to have a high O_2 tension. This condition has been termed *histotoxic hypoxia*.

EFFECTS OF HYPOXIA Changes in the central nervous system, particularly the higher centers, are especially important consequences of hypoxia. Acute hypoxia causes impaired judgment, motor incoordination, and a clinical picture closely resembling that of acute alcoholism. When hypoxia is long-standing, fatigue, drowsiness, apathy, inattentiveness, delayed reaction time, and reduced work capacity occur. As hypoxia becomes more severe, the centers of the brainstem are affected, and death usually results from respiratory failure. With the reduction of Pa_{O_2}, cerebrovascular resistance decreases and cerebral blood flow increases, increasing O_2 delivery to the brain as a compensatory mechanism. However, when the reduction of Pa_{O_2} is accompanied by hyperventilation and a reduction of Pa_{CO_2}, cerebrovascular resistance rises, cerebral blood flow falls, and hypoxia is intensified. Hypoxia also causes pulmonary arterial constriction, which shunts blood away from poorly ventilated areas toward better-ventilated portions of the lung. However, it also increases pulmonary vascular resistance and right ventricular afterload.

Glucose is normally broken down to pyruvic acid. However, the further breakdown of pyruvate and the generation of adenosine triphosphate (ATP) consequent to it require O_2; and in the presence of hypoxia increasing proportions of pyruvate are reduced to lactic acid, which cannot be broken down further, causing metabolic acidosis. Under these circumstances, the total energy obtained from the breakdown of carbohydrate is greatly reduced, and the quantity of energy available for the production of ATP becomes inadequate.

An important component of the respiratory response to hypoxia originates in special chemosensitive cells in the carotid and aortic bodies, and in the respiratory center in the brainstem. The stimulation of these cells by hypoxia increases ventilation, with a loss of CO_2, and leads to respiratory alkalosis. When combined with the metabolic acidosis resulting from the production of lactic acid, the serum bicarbonate level declines (Chap. 50).

Diminished P_{O_2} in any tissue results in local vasodilatation, and the diffuse vasodilatation that occurs in generalized hypoxia raises the cardiac output. In patients with underlying heart disease, the requirements of the peripheral tissues for an increase of cardiac output with hypoxia may precipitate congestive heart failure. In patients with ischemic heart disease, a reduced Pa_{O_2} may intensify myocardial ischemia and further impair left ventricular function.

One of the important mechanisms of compensation for chronic hypoxia is an increase in the hemoglobin concentration and in the number of red blood cells in the circulating blood, i.e., the development of polycythemia secondary to erythropoietin production (Chap. 110).

CYANOSIS

Cyanosis refers to a bluish color of the skin and mucous membranes resulting from an increased quantity of reduced hemoglobin, or of hemoglobin derivatives, in the small blood vessels of those areas. It is usually most marked in the lips, nail beds, ears, and malar eminences. Cyanosis, especially if developed recently, is more commonly detected by a family member than the patient. The florid skin characteristic of polycythemia vera (Chap. 110) must be distinguished from the true cyanosis discussed here. A cherry-colored flush, rather than cyanosis, is caused by COHb (Chap. 396). The degree of cyanosis is modified by the color of the cutaneous pigment and the thickness of the skin, as well as by the state of the cutaneous capillaries. The accurate clinical detection of the presence and degree of cyanosis is difficult, as proved by oximetric studies. In some instances, central cyanosis can be detected reliably when the Sa_{O_2} has fallen to 85%; in others, particularly in dark-skinned persons, it may not be detected until it has declined to 75%. In the latter case, examination of the mucous membranes in the oral cavity and the conjunctivae rather than examination of the skin is more helpful in the detection of cyanosis.

The increase in the quantity of reduced hemoglobin in the mucocutaneous vessels that produces cyanosis may be brought about either by an increase in the quantity of venous blood as the result of dilatation of the venules and venous ends of the capillaries or by a reduction in the Sa_{O_2} in the capillary blood. In general, cyanosis becomes apparent when the mean capillary concentration of reduced hemoglobin exceeds 40 g/L (4 g/dL). It is the *absolute* rather than the *relative* quantity of reduced hemoglobin that is important in producing cyanosis. Thus, in a patient with severe anemia, the relative amount of reduced hemoglobin in the venous blood may be very large when considered in relation to the total amount of hemoglobin in the blood. However, since the concentration of the latter is markedly reduced, the *absolute* quantity of reduced hemoglobin may still be small, and therefore patients with severe anemia and even *marked* arterial desaturation do not display cyanosis. Conversely, the higher the total hemoglobin content, the greater is the tendency toward cyanosis; thus, patients with marked polycythemia tend to be cyanotic at higher levels of Sa_{O_2} than patients with normal hematocrit values. Likewise, local passive congestion, which causes an increase in the total amount of reduced hemoglobin in the vessels in a given area, may cause cyanosis. Cyanosis also is observed when nonfunctional hemoglobin such as methemoglobin or sulfhemoglobin (Chap. 106) is present in blood.

Cyanosis may be subdivided into central and peripheral types. In the *central* type, the Sa_{O_2} is reduced or an abnormal hemoglobin derivative is present, and the mucous membranes and skin are both affected. *Peripheral* cyanosis is due to a slowing of blood flow and abnormally great extraction of O_2 from normally saturated arterial blood. It results from vasoconstriction and diminished peripheral blood flow, such as occurs in cold exposure, shock, congestive failure, and peripheral vascular disease. Often in these conditions the mucous membranes of the oral cavity or those beneath the tongue may be spared. Clinical differentiation between central and peripheral cyanosis may not always be simple, and in conditions such as cardiogenic shock with pulmonary edema there may be a mixture of both types.

DIFFERENTIAL DIAGNOSIS Central Cyanosis (Table 36-1) Decreased Sa_{O_2} results from a marked reduction in the Pa_{O_2}. This reduction may be brought about by a decline in the FI_{O_2} without sufficient compensatory alveolar hyperventilation to maintain alveolar P_{O_2}. Cyanosis does not occur to a significant degree in an ascent to an altitude of 2500 m (8000 ft) but is marked in a further ascent to 5000 m (16,000 ft). The reason for this difference becomes clear on studying

Table 36-1   Causes Of Cyanosis

CENTRAL CYANOSIS

Decreased arterial oxygen saturation
  Decreased atmospheric pressure—high altitude
  Impaired pulmonary function
    Alveolar hypoventilation
    Uneven relationships between pulmonary ventilation and perfusion
      (perfusion of hypoventilated alveoli)
    Impaired oxygen diffusion
  Anatomic shunts
    Certain types of congenital heart disease
    Pulmonary arteriovenous fistulas
    Multiple small intrapulmonary shunts
  Hemoglobin with low affinity for oxygen
Hemoglobin abnormalities
  Methemoglobinemia—hereditary, acquired
  Sulfhemoglobinema—acquired
  Carboxyhemoglobinemia (not true cyanosis)

PERIPHERAL CYANOSIS

Reduced cardiac output
Cold exposure
Redistribution of blood flow from extremities
Arterial obstruction
Venous obstruction

the S shape of the Hb-O_2 dissociation curve (see Fig. 106-1). At 2500 m (8000 ft) the FI_{O_2} is about 120 mmHg, the alveolar P_{O_2} is approximately 80 mmHg, and the Sa_{O_2} is nearly normal. However, at 5000 m (16,000 ft) the FI_{O_2} and alveolar P_{O_2} are about 85 and 50 mmHg, respectively, and the Sa_{O_2} is only about 75%. This leaves 25% of the hemoglobin in the arterial blood in the reduced form, an amount likely to be associated with cyanosis in the absence of anemia. Similarly, a mutant hemoglobin with a low affinity for O_2 (e.g., Hb Kansas) causes lowered Sa_{O_2} saturation and resultant central cyanosis (Chap. 106).

Seriously *impaired pulmonary function*, through perfusion of unventilated or poorly ventilated areas of the lung or alveolar hypoventilation, is a common cause of central cyanosis (Chap. 250). This condition may occur acutely, as in extensive pneumonia or pulmonary edema, or chronically with chronic pulmonary diseases (e.g., emphysema). In the last situation, secondary polycythemia is generally present, and clubbing of the fingers may occur. However, in many types of chronic pulmonary disease with fibrosis and obliteration of the capillary vascular bed, cyanosis does not occur because there is relatively little perfusion of underventilated areas.

Another cause of reduced Sa_{O_2} is *shunting of systemic venous blood into the arterial circuit*. Certain forms of congenital heart disease are associated with cyanosis (Chap. 234). Since blood flows from a higher-pressure to a lower-pressure region, for a cardiac defect to result in a right-to-left shunt, it must ordinarily be combined with an obstructive lesion distal to the defect or with elevated pulmonary vascular resistance. The most common congenital cardiac lesion associated with cyanosis in the adult is the combination of ventricular septal defect and pulmonary outflow tract obstruction (*tetralogy of Fallot*). The more severe the obstruction, the greater the degree of right-to-left shunting and resultant cyanosis. In patients with patent ductus arteriosus, pulmonary hypertension, and right-to-left shunt, *differential cyanosis* results; that is, cyanosis occurs in the lower but not in the upper extremities. →*The mechanisms for the elevated pulmonary vascular resistance that may produce cyanosis in the presence of intra- and extracardiac communications without pulmonic stenosis (Eisenmenger syndrome) are discussed in Chap. 234.*

Pulmonary arteriovenous fistulae (Chap. 57) may be congenital or acquired, solitary or multiple, microscopic or massive. The severity of cyanosis produced by these fistulae depends on their size and number. They occur with some frequency in hereditary hemorrhagic telangiectasia. Sa_{O_2} reduction and cyanosis may also occur in some patients with cirrhosis, presumably as a consequence of pulmonary arteriovenous fistulas or portal vein–pulmonary vein anastomoses.

In patients with cardiac or pulmonary right-to-left shunts, the presence and severity of cyanosis depend on the size of the shunt relative to the systemic flow as well as on the Hb-O_2 saturation of the venous blood. With increased extraction of O_2 from the blood by the exercising muscles, the venous blood returning to the right side of the heart is more unsaturated than at rest, and shunting of this blood or its passage through lungs incapable of normal oxygenation intensifies the cyanosis. Also, since the systemic vascular resistance falls with exercise, the right-to-left shunt is augmented by exercise in patients with congenital heart disease and communications between the two sides of the heart. Secondary polycythemia occurs frequently in patients with arterial O_2 unsaturation and contributes to the cyanosis.

Cyanosis can be caused by small amounts of circulating methemoglobin and by even smaller amounts of sulfhemoglobin (Chap. 106). Although they are uncommon causes of cyanosis, these abnormal hemoglobin pigments should be sought by spectroscopy when cyanosis is not readily explained by malfunction of the circulatory or respiratory systems. Generally, digital clubbing does not occur with them. The diagnosis of methemoglobinemia can be suspected if the patient's blood remains brown after being mixed in a test tube and exposed to air.

Peripheral Cyanosis   Probably the most common cause of peripheral cyanosis is the normal vasoconstriction resulting from exposure to cold air or water. When cardiac output is low, as in severe congestive heart failure or shock, cutaneous vasoconstriction occurs as a compensatory mechanism so that blood is diverted from the skin to more vital areas such as the central nervous system and heart (Chap. 232), and intense cyanosis associated with cool extremities may result. Even though the arterial blood is normally saturated, the reduced volume flow through the skin and the reduced P_{O_2} at the venous end of the capillary result in cyanosis.

Arterial obstruction to an extremity, as with an embolus, or arteriolar constriction, as in cold-induced vasospasm (Raynaud's phenomenon, Chap. 248), generally results in pallor and coldness, but there may be associated cyanosis. Venous obstruction, as in thrombophlebitis, dilates the subpapillary venous plexuses and thereby intensifies cyanosis.

Approach to the Patient

Certain features are important in arriving at the cause of cyanosis:

1. The history, particularly the onset (cyanosis present since birth is usually due to congenital heart disease), and possible exposure to drugs or chemicals that may produce abnormal types of hemoglobin.

2. Clinical differentiation of central as opposed to peripheral cyanosis. Objective evidence by physical or radiographic examination of disorders of the respiratory or cardiovascular systems. Massage or gentle warming of a cyanotic extremity will increase peripheral blood flow and abolish peripheral but not central cyanosis.

3. The presence or absence of clubbing of the digits (see below). Clubbing without cyanosis is frequent in patients with infective endocarditis and ulcerative colitis; it may occasionally occur in healthy persons, and in some instances it may be occupational, e.g., in jackhammer operators. The combination of cyanosis and clubbing is frequent in patients with congenital heart disease and right-to-left shunting and is seen occasionally in persons with pulmonary disease such as lung abscess or pulmonary arteriovenous fistulae. In contrast, peripheral cyanosis or acutely developing central cyanosis is *not* associated with clubbed digits.

4. Determination of Pa_{O_2} tension and Sa_{O_2} and spectroscopic and other examinations of the blood for abnormal types of hemoglobin (critical in the differential diagnosis of cyanosis).

CLUBBING

The selective bullous enlargement of the distal segments of the fingers and toes due to proliferation of connective tissue, particularly on the dorsal surface, is termed *clubbing*; there is increased sponginess of the soft tissue at the base of the nail. Clubbing may be hereditary, idiopathic, or acquired and associated with a variety of disorders, including cyanotic congenital heart disease, infective endocarditis, and a variety of pulmonary conditions (among them primary and metastatic lung cancer, bronchiectasis, lung abscess, cystic fibrosis, and mesothelioma), as well as with some gastrointestinal diseases (including regional enteritis, chronic ulcerative colitis, and hepatic cirrhosis).

Clubbing in patients with primary and metastatic lung cancer, mesothelioma, bronchiectasis, and hepatic cirrhosis may be associated with *hypertrophic osteoarthropathy*. In this condition, the subperiosteal formation of new bone in the distal diaphyses of the long bones of the extremities causes pain and symmetric arthritis-like changes in the shoulders, knees, ankles, wrists, and elbows. The diagnosis of hypertrophic osteoarthropathy may be confirmed by bone radiographs. Although the mechanism of clubbing is unclear, it appears to be secondary to a humoral substance that causes dilation of the vessels of the fingertip.

BEALL CM: Tibetan and Andean patterns of adaptation to high-altitude hypoxia. Hum Biol 72:201, 2000

BEITNER-JOHNSON D et al: Regulation of gene expression by hypoxia: A molecular approach. Respir Physiol 110:87, 1997

FISHMAN AP: Approach to the patient with respiratory symptoms: Cyanosis and clubbing, in *Fishman's Pulmonary Diseases and Disorders*, 3d ed, Fishman AP et al (eds). Philadelphia, Saunders, 1998, pp 382–3

GALLEY HF, WEBSTER NR: Acidosis and tissue hypoxia in the critically ill: How to measure it and what does it mean? Crit Rev Clin Lab Sci 36:35, 1999

GRIFFEY RT et al: Cyanosis. J Emerg Med 18:369, 2000

GRIFKA RG: Cyanotic congenital heart disease with increased pulmonary blood flow. Pediatr Clin North Am 46:405, 1999

SEVERINHAUS JW: Uses of high altitude for studies of effects of hypoxia. Adv Exp Med Biol 454:17, 1998

TISSUE HYPOXIA: How to detect, how to correct, how to prevent? Third European Consensus Conference in Intensive Care Medicine. J Crit Care 12:39, 1997

WALDMAN JD, WERNLY JA. Cyanotic congenital heart disease with decreased pulmonary blood flow in children. Pediatr Clin North Am 46:385, 1999

37   *Eugene Braunwald*

EDEMA

Edema is defined as a clinically apparent increase in the interstitial fluid volume, which may expand by several liters before the abnormality is evident. Therefore, a weight gain of several kilograms usually precedes overt manifestations of edema, and a similar weight loss from diuresis can be induced in a slightly edematous patient before "dry weight" is achieved. *Ascites* (Chap. 46) and *hydrothorax* refer to accumulation of excess fluid in the peritoneal and pleural cavities, respectively, and are considered to be special forms of edema. *Anasarca* refers to gross, generalized edema.

Depending on its cause and mechanism, edema may be localized or have a generalized distribution; it is recognized in its generalized form by puffiness of the face, which is most readily apparent in the periorbital areas, and by the persistence of an indentation of the skin following pressure; this is known as "pitting" edema. In its more subtle form, it may be detected by noting that after the stethoscope is removed from the chest wall, the rim of the bell leaves an indentation on the skin of the chest for a few minutes. When the ring on a finger fits more snugly than in the past or when a patient complains of difficulty in putting on shoes, particularly in the evening, edema may be present.

PATHOGENESIS   About one-third of the total-body water is confined to the extracellular space. Approximately 25% of the latter, in turn, is composed of the plasma volume, and the remainder is interstitial fluid.

Starling Forces   The forces that regulate the disposition of fluid between these two components of the extracellular compartment are frequently referred to as the *Starling forces* (see p. 202). The hydrostatic pressure within the vascular system and the colloid oncotic pressure in the interstitial fluid tend to promote movement of fluid from the vascular to the extravascular space. In contrast, the colloid oncotic pressure contributed by the plasma proteins and the hydrostatic pressure within the interstitial fluid, referred to as the *tissue tension*, promote the movement of fluid into the vascular compartment. Consequently there is a movement of water and diffusible solutes from the vascular space at the arteriolar end of the capillaries.

Fluid is returned from the interstitial space into the vascular system at the venous end of the capillary and by way of the lymphatics, and unless these channels are obstructed, lymph flow tends to increase with increases in net movement of fluid from the vascular compartment to the interstitium. These flows are usually balanced so that a steady state exists in the sizes of the intravascular and interstitial compartments, and yet a large exchange between them occurs. However, should any one of the hydrostatic or oncotic pressure gradients be altered significantly, a further net movement of fluid between the two components of the extracellular space will take place. The development of edema then depends on one or more alterations in the Starling forces so that there is increased flow of fluid from the vascular system into the interstitium or into a body cavity.

Edema due to increase in capillary pressure may result from an elevation of venous pressure due to obstruction in venous drainage. This increase in capillary pressure may be generalized, as occurs in congestive heart failure. The Starling forces may be imbalanced when the colloid oncotic pressure of the plasma is reduced, owing to any factor that may induce hypoalbuminemia, such as saline expansion, malnutrition, liver disease, loss of protein into the urine or into the gastrointestinal tract, or a severe catabolic state.

Capillary Damage   Edema may also result from damage to the capillary endothelium, which increases its permeability and permits the transfer of protein into the interstitial compartment. Injury to the capillary wall can result from drugs, viral or bacterial agents, and thermal or mechanical trauma. Increased capillary permeability may also be a consequence of a hypersensitivity reaction and is characteristic of immune injury. Damage to the capillary endothelium is presumably responsible for inflammatory edema, which is usually nonpitting, localized, and accompanied by other signs of inflammation—redness, heat, and tenderness.

To formulate a hypothesis about the pathophysiology of an edematous state, it is important to discriminate between the *primary* events, such as localized or generalized venous or lymphatic obstruction, reduction of cardiac output, hypoalbuminemia, trapping of fluid in spaces such as the pleural or peritoneal cavities, or an increase in capillary permeability, and the predictable *secondary* consequences, which include the renal retention of salt and water in an attempt to restore the plasma volume when the latter has been reduced, as in venous obstruction (see below). Both the primary event and the secondary consequences contribute to the formation of edema. In some cases the primary event is the renal retention of salt and water. Examples are renal failure, nephrotic syndrome, glomerulonephritis, and early hepatic failure.

Reduction of Effective Arterial Volume   In many forms of edema the *effective arterial blood volume*, an as yet poorly defined parameter of the filling of the arterial tree, is reduced, and as a consequence a series of physiologic responses designed to restore it to normal are set into motion. A key element of these responses is the retention of salt and therefore of water, principally by the renal proximal tubule (Fig. 37-1), and in many instances this repairs the deficit of the effective arterial blood volume; often this deficit is repaired without the development of overt edema. If, however, the retention of salt and water is insufficient to restore and maintain the effective arterial blood volume, the stimuli are not dissipated, the retention of salt and water continues, and edema may ultimately develop. This sequence of events is operative in dehydration and hemorrhage. Although in these conditions there is a reduction of effective arterial blood volume and activation of the entire sequence shown in the center of Fig. 37-2, including the diminished excretion of salt and water, because the net sodium and water balance is negative rather than positive, edema does *not* occur. In most conditions that lead to edema, the mechanisms responsible for maintaining a normal effective osmolality in the body fluids operate efficiently so that sodium retention promotes thirst and secretion of the antidiuretic hormone. In edematous states, isotonic expansion of the extracellular fluid space may be massive, while the intracellular fluid volume is unchanged.

Reduced Cardiac Output   A reduction of cardiac output, whatever the cause, is associated with a lowering of the effective arterial blood volume as well as of renal blood flow, constriction of the efferent renal arterioles, and an elevation of the filtration fraction, i.e., the ratio of glomerular filtration rate to renal plasma flow. In severe heart failure

FIGURE 37-1 Effect of hemodynamic changes on proximal tubule solute transport: a summary. Hemodynamic mechanisms by which a reduction of effective arterial volume causes salt and water retention and thereby contributes to the formation of edema. *(From Seldin DW et al, Semin Nephrol 11:212, 1991, with permission.)*

there is a reduction in the glomerular filtration rate. Activation of the sympathetic nervous system and of the renin-angiotensin systems are responsible for renal vasoconstriction. The finding that α-adrenergic blocking agents and/or angiotensin-converting enzyme (ACE) inhibitors augment renal blood flow and induce diuresis supports the role of these two systems in elevating renal vascular resistance and salt and water retention.

Renal Factors Reduced cardiac output lowers effective arterial blood volume. There is increased tubular reabsorption of glomerular filtrate in both the proximal and distal tubules (Fig. 37-1). Alterations in intrarenal hemodynamics appear to play a significant role. Heart failure and other conditions, such as nephrotic syndrome and cirrhosis that reduce effective arterial blood volume, cause renal efferent arteriolar constriction. This, in turn, reduces the hydrostatic pressure while the increased filtration fraction raises the colloid osmotic pressure in the peritubular capillaries, thus enhancing salt and water reabsorption in the proximal tubule as well as in the ascending limb of the loop of Henle.

In addition, the diminished renal blood flow characteristic of states in which the effective arterial blood volume is reduced is translated by the renal juxtaglomerular cells into a signal for increased renin release (Chap. 331). The mechanisms responsible for this release include a baroreceptor response: reduced renal perfusion results in incomplete filling of the renal arterioles and diminished stretch of the juxtaglomerular cells, a signal that provides for the elaboration or release, or both, of renin. A second mechanism for renin release involves the macula densa; as a result of reduced glomerular filtration, the so-

dium chloride load reaching the distal renal tubules is reduced. This is sensed by the macula densa, which signals the neighboring juxtaglomerular cells to secrete renin. A third mechanism involves the sympathetic nervous system and circulating catecholamines. Activation of the β-adrenergic receptors in the juxtaglomerular cells stimulates renin release. These three mechanisms generally act in concert.

The Renin-Angiotensin-Aldosterone (RAA) System (See Chap. 331) Renin, an enzyme with a molecular weight of about 40,000, acts on its substrate, angiotensinogen, an α_2 globulin synthesized by the liver, to release angiotensin I, a decapeptide, which is broken down to angiotensin II (AII), an octapeptide. This has generalized vasoconstrictor properties; it is especially active on the efferent arterioles and independently increases Na^+ reabsorption in the proximal tubule. The RAA system has long been recognized as a hormone system. However, it also operates locally. Both circulating and intrarenally produced AII contribute to renal vasoconstriction and to salt and water retention. These renal effects of AII are mediated by activation of AII type 1 receptors, which can be blocked by specific antagonists such as losartan. AII also enters the circulation and stimulates the production of aldosterone by the zona glomerulosa of the adrenal cortex. In patients with heart failure, not only is aldosterone secretion elevated but the biologic half-life of aldosterone is prolonged, which further increases the plasma level of the hormone. A depression of hepatic blood flow, particularly during exercise, secondary to a reduction in cardiac output, is responsible for the reduced hepatic catabolism of aldosterone. Aldosterone, in turn, enhances Na^+ reabsorption (and K^+ excretion) by the collecting tubule. The activation of the RAA system is most striking in the early phase of acute, severe heart failure and is less intense in patients with chronic, stable, compensated heart failure.

Although increased quantities of aldosterone are secreted in heart failure and in other edematous states and although blockade of the action of aldosterone by spironolactone (an aldosterone antagonist) or amiloride (a blocker of epithelial Na^+ channels) often induces a moderate diuresis in edematous states, persistent augmented levels of aldosterone (or other mineralocorticoids) alone do not always promote accumulation of edema, as witnessed by the lack of striking fluid retention in most instances of primary aldosteronism (Chap. 331). Furthermore, although normal individuals retain some salt and water with the administration of potent mineralocorticoids, such as deoxycorticosterone acetate or fludrocortisone, this accumulation is self-limiting, despite continued exposure to the steroid, a phenomenon known as *mineralocorticoid escape*. The failure of normal individuals who receive large doses of mineralocorticoids to accumulate large quantities of extracellular fluid and to develop edema is probably a consequence of an increase in glomerular filtration rate (pressure natriuresis) and through the action of natriuretic substance(s) (see below). The continued secretion of aldosterone may be more important in the accumulation of fluid in edematous states because patients with edema secondary to heart failure, nephrotic syndrome, and cirrhosis are generally unable to repair the deficit in effective arterial blood volume. As a consequence they do not develop pressure natriuresis.

Blockade of the RAA system, by blocking AII receptors or inhibiting ACE, reduces efferent arteriolar resistance and increases renal blood flow. This action (combined in patients with heart failure with a rise in cardiac output secondary to afterload reduction) as well as reduction in the secretion of aldosterone cause diuresis. However, in patients with moderate or severe impairment of renal function or with renal artery stenosis, interference with the RAA system can cause paradoxical sodium retention due to intensification of renal failure.

Arginine Vasopressin (AVP) and Endothelin (See also Chap. 329) The secretion of AVP occurs in response to increased intracellular osmolar concentration and by stimulating V_2 receptors increases the reabsorption of free water in the renal distal tubule and collecting duct, thereby increasing total-body water. Circulating AVP is elevated in many patients with heart failure secondary to a nonosmotic stimulus associated with decreased effective arterial volume. Such patients fail to show the normal reduction of AVP with a reduction of osmolality, contributing to hyponatremia and edema formation.

Endothelin This is a potent peptide vasoconstrictor released by endothelial cells; its concentration is elevated in heart failure and contributes to renal vasoconstriction, Na+ retention, and edema in heart failure.

Natriuretic Peptides Atrial distention and/or a sodium load cause release into the circulation of atrial natriuretic peptide (ANP), a polypeptide; a high-molecular-weight precursor of ANP is stored in secretory granules within atrial myocytes. Release of ANP causes (1) excretion of sodium and water by augmenting glomerular filtration rate, inhibiting sodium reabsorption in the proximal tubule, and inhibiting release of renin and aldosterone; and (2) arteriolar and venous dilatation by antagonizing the vasoconstrictor actions of AII, AVP, and sympathetic stimulation. Thus, ANP has the capacity to oppose sodium retention and arterial pressure elevation in hypervolemic states.

The closely related brain natriuretic peptide (BNP) is stored primarily in cardiac ventricular myocardium and is released when ventricular diastolic pressure rises. Its actions are similar to those of ANP. Circulating levels of ANP and BNP are elevated in congestive heart failure but obviously not sufficient to prevent edema formation. In addition, in edematous states (particularly heart failure), there is abnormal resistance to the actions of natriuretic peptides.

CLINICAL CAUSES OF EDEMA Obstruction of Venous (and Lymphatic) Drainage of a Limb In this condition the hydrostatic pressure in the capillary bed upstream to the obstruction increases so that an abnormal quantity of fluid is transferred from the vascular to the interstitial space. Since the alternative route (i.e., the lymphatic channels) may also be obstructed, an increased volume of interstitial fluid in the limb develops, i.e., there is a trapping of fluid in the extremity, causing local edema at the expense of the blood volume in the remainder of the body, thereby reducing effective arterial blood volume and leading to the consequences shown in Fig. 37-2.

When venous and lymphatic drainage are obstructed in a limb, fluid accumulates in the interstitium at the expense of plasma volume. The latter stimulates the retention of salt and water until the deficit in plasma volume has been corrected. Tissue tension rises in the affected limb until it counterbalances the primary alterations in the Starling forces, at which time no further fluid accumulates. The net effect is a local increase in the volume of interstitial fluid. This same sequence occurs in ascites and hydrothorax, in which fluid is trapped or accumulates in the cavitary space, depleting the intravascular volume and leading to secondary salt and fluid retention, as already described.

Congestive Heart Failure (See also Chap. 232) In this disorder the defective systolic emptying of the chambers of the heart and/or the impairment of ventricular relaxation promotes an accumulation of blood in the heart and venous circulation at the expense of the effective arterial volume, and the aforementioned sequence of events (Fig. 37-2) is initiated. In mild heart failure, a small increment of total blood

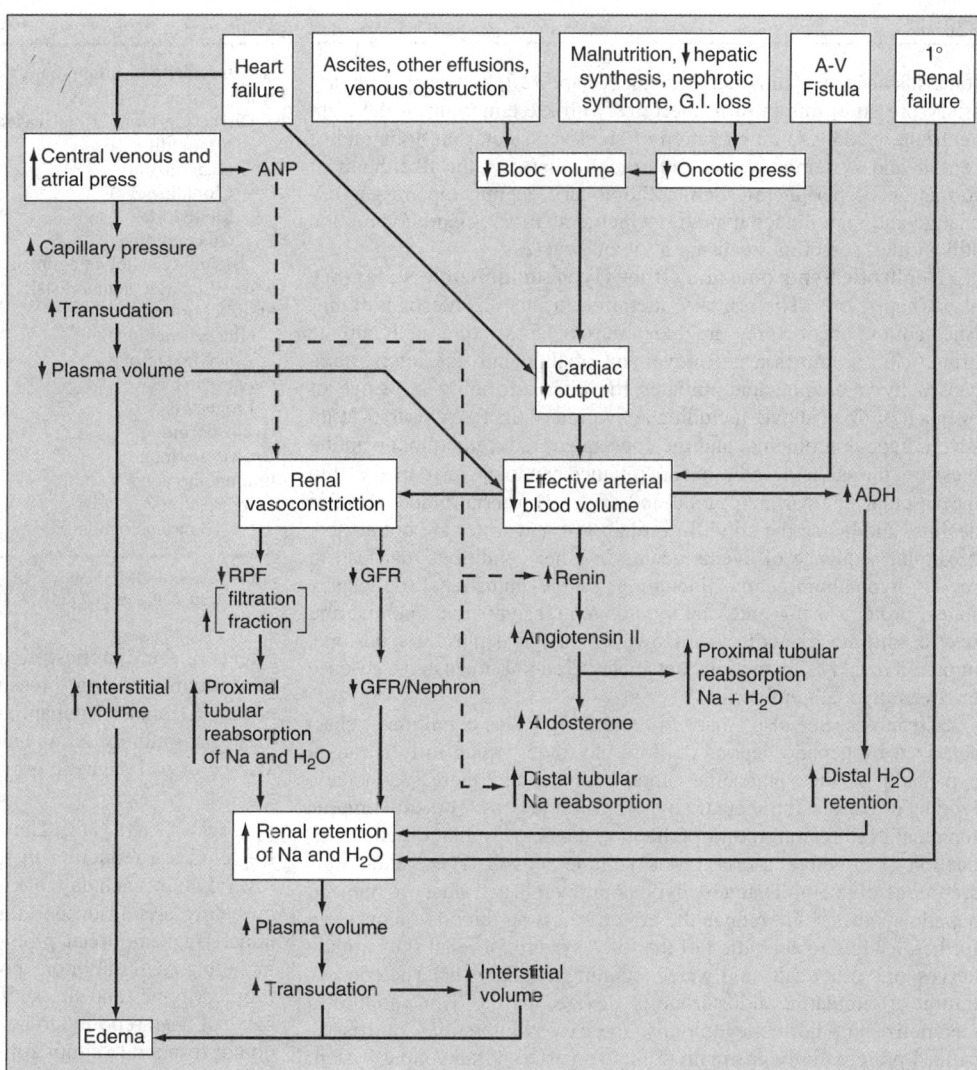

FIGURE 37-2 Sequence of events leading to the formation and retention of salt and water and the development of edema. ANP, atrial natriuretic peptide; RPF, renal plasma flow; GFR, glomerular filtration rate. Inhibitory influences are shown by broken lines. ADH, antidiuretic hormone.

volume may repair the deficit of arterial volume and establish a new steady state. Through the operation of Starling's law of the heart, an increase in the volume of blood within the chambers of the heart promotes a more forceful contraction and may thereby increase the cardiac output (See Fig. 232-1). However, if the cardiac disorder is more severe, retention of fluid cannot repair the deficit in effective arterial blood volume. The increment in blood volume accumulates in the venous circulation, and the increase in capillary and lymphatic hydrostatic pressures promotes the formation of edema. In heart failure, a reduction occurs in baroreflex-mediated inhibition of the vasomotor center, which causes activation of renal vasoconstrictor nerves and the RAA system, causing sodium and water retention.

Incomplete ventricular emptying (systolic heart failure) and/or inadequate ventricular relaxation (diastolic heart failure) both lead to an elevation of ventricular diastolic pressure. If the impairment of cardiac function involves the right ventricle, pressures in the systemic veins and capillaries may rise, thereby augmenting the transudation of fluid into the interstitial space and enhancing the likelihood of peripheral edema in the presence of the accumulation of sodium and water, as described above. The elevated systemic venous pressure is transmitted to the thoracic duct with consequent reduction of lymph drainage, further increasing the accumulation of edema.

If the impairment of cardiac function (incomplete ventricular emptying and/or inadequate relaxation) involves the left ventricle primarily, then pulmonary venous and capillary pressures rise [leading in some instances to pulmonary edema (Chap. 32)], as does pulmonary artery pressure; this in turn interferes with the emptying of the right ventricle, leading to an elevation of right ventricular diastolic and of central and systemic venous pressures, enhancing the likelihood of formation of peripheral edema. Pulmonary edema impairs gas exchange and may induce hypoxia, which embarrasses cardiac function still further, sometimes causing a vicious cycle.

Nephrotic Syndrome and Other Hypoalbuminemic States (See also Chap. 274) The primary alteration in this disorder is a diminished colloid oncotic pressure due to massive losses of protein into the urine. This promotes a net movement of fluid into the interstitium, causes hypovolemia, and initiates the edema-forming sequence of events described above, including activation of the RAA system. With severe hypoalbuminemia and the consequent reduced colloid osmotic pressure, the salt and water that are retained cannot be restrained within the vascular compartment, total and effective arterial blood volumes decline, and hence the stimuli to retain salt and water are not abated. A similar sequence of events occurs in other conditions that lead to *severe* hypoalbuminemia, including severe nutritional deficiency states, protein-losing enteropathy, congenital hypoalbuminemia, and severe, chronic liver disease. However, in the nephrotic syndrome, impaired renal Na$^+$ excretion contributes to edema, even in the absence of severe hypoalbuminemia.

Cirrhosis (See also Chaps. 46 and 299) This condition is characterized by hepatic venous outflow blockade, which in turn causes expansion of the splanchnic blood volume and increased hepatic lymph formation. Intrahepatic hypertension acts as a potent stimulus for renal Na$^+$ retention and perhaps systemic vasodilation and a reduction of effective arterial blood volume as well. These alterations are frequently complicated by hypoalbuminemia secondary to reduced hepatic synthesis and reduce the effective arterial blood volume even further, leading to activation of the RAA system, of renal sympathetic nerves, and other salt- and water-retaining mechanisms. The concentration of circulating aldosterone is elevated by the liver's failure to metabolize this hormone. Initially, the excess interstitial fluid is localized preferentially upstream to the congested portal venous system and obstructed hepatic lymphatics, i.e., in the peritoneal cavity. In later stages, particularly when there is severe hypoalbuminemia, peripheral edema may develop. The excess production of prostaglandins (PGE$_2$ and PGI$_2$) in cirrhosis attenuates renal Na$^+$ retention. When the synthesis of these substances is inhibited by nonsteroidal anti-inflammatory agents, renal function deteriorates and Na$^+$ retention increases.

Drug-Induced Edema A large number of widely used drugs can cause edema (Table 37-1). Mechanisms include renal vasoconstriction (nonsteroidal anti-inflammatory agents and cyclosporine), arteriolar dilatation (vasodilators), augmented renal sodium reabsorption (steroid hormones) and capillary damage (interleukin 2).

Idiopathic Edema This syndrome, which occurs almost exclusively in women, is characterized by periodic episodes of edema (unrelated to the menstrual cycle), frequently accompanied by abdominal distention. Diurnal alterations in weight occur with orthostatic retention of sodium and water, so that the patient may weigh several pounds more after having been in the upright posture for several hours. Such large diurnal weight changes suggest an increase in capillary permeability that appears to fluctuate in severity and to be aggravated by hot weather. There is some evidence that a reduction in plasma volume occurs in this condition with secondary activation of the RAA system and impaired suppression of AVP release. Idiopathic edema should be distinguished from cyclical or premenstrual edema, in which the sodium and water retention may be secondary to excessive estrogen stimulation. There are also some cases in which the edema appears to be "diuretic-induced." It has been postulated that in these patients, chronic diuretic administration leads to mild blood volume depletion, which causes chronic hyperreninemia and juxtaglomerular hyperplasia. Salt-retaining mechanisms appear to overcompensate for the direct

Table 37-1 Drugs Associated with Edema Formation

Nonsteroidal anti-inflammatory drugs
Antihypertensive agents
  Direct arterial/arteriolar vasodilators
    Minoxidil
    Hydralazine
    Clonidine
    Methyldopa
    Guanethidine
  Calcium channel antagonists
  α-Adrenergic antagonists
Steroid hormones
  Glucocorticoids
  Anabolic steroids
  Estrogens
  Progestins
Cyclosporine
Growth hormone
Immunotherapies
  Interleukin 2
  OKT3 monoclonal antibody

SOURCE: From GM Chertow, GE Thibault, Approach to the patient with edema, in L Goldman, E Braunwald (eds): *Primary Cardiology.* Philadelphia, Saunders, 1998.

effects of the diuretics. *Acute* withdrawal of diuretics can then leave the sodium-retaining forces unopposed, leading to fluid retention and edema. Decreased dopaminergic activity and reduced urinary kallikrein and kinin excretion have been reported in this condition and may also be of pathogenetic importance.

TREATMENT The treatment of idiopathic cyclic edema includes a reduction in salt intake, rest in the supine position for several hours each day, the wearing of elastic stockings (which are put on before arising in the morning), and an attempt to understand any underlying emotional problems. A variety of pharmacologic agents including ACE inhibitors, progesterone, the dopamine receptor agonist bromocriptine, and the sympathomimetic amine dextroamphetamine have all been reported to be useful when administered to patients who do not respond to simpler measures. Diuretics may be helpful initially but may lose their effectiveness with continuous administration; accordingly, they should be employed sparingly, if at all. Discontinuation of diuretics paradoxically leads to diuresis in "diuretic-induced" edema, described above.

DIFFERENTIAL DIAGNOSIS

The differences between the three major causes of generalized edema are shown in Table 37-2.

Localized edema can usually be readily differentiated from generalized edema. The great majority of patients with generalized edema suffer from advanced cardiac, renal, hepatic, or nutritional disorders. Consequently, the differential diagnosis of generalized edema should be directed toward identifying or excluding these several conditions.

LOCALIZED EDEMA (See also Chap. 248) Edema originating from inflammation or hypersensitivity is usually readily identified. Localized edema due to venous or lymphatic obstruction may be caused by thrombophlebitis, chronic lymphangitis, resection of regional lymph nodes, filariasis, etc. Lymphedema is particularly intractable because restriction of lymphatic flow results in increased protein concentration in the interstitial fluid, a circumstance that aggravates retention of fluid.

EDEMA OF HEART FAILURE (See also Chap. 232) The presence of heart disease, as manifested by cardiac enlargement and gallop rhythm, together with evidence of cardiac failure, such as dyspnea, basilar rales, venous distention, and hepatomegaly, usually provides an indication on clinical examination that edema results from heart failure. Noninvasive tests such as echocardiography and radionuclide angiography may be helpful in establishing the diagnosis of heart failure.

Table 37-2 Principal Causes of Generalized Edema: History, Physical Examination, and Laboratory Findings

Organ System	History	Physical Examination	Laboratory Findings
Cardiac	Dyspnea with exertion prominent—often associated with orthopnea—or paroxysmal nocturnal dyspnea	Elevated jugular venous pressure, ventricular (S_3) gallop; occasionally with displaced or dyskinetic apical pulse; peripheral cyanosis, cool extremities, small pulse pressure when severe	Elevated urea nitrogen–to–creatinine ratio common; elevated uric acid; serum sodium often diminished; liver enzymes occasionally elevated with hepatic congestion
Hepatic	Dyspnea infrequent, except if associated with significant degree of ascites; most often a history of ethanol abuse	Frequently associated with ascites; jugular venous pressure normal or low; blood pressure lower than in renal or cardiac disease; one or more additional signs of chronic liver disease (jaundice, palmar erythema, Dupuytren's contracture, spider angiomata, male gynecomastia; asterixis and other signs of encephalopathy) may be present	If severe, reductions in serum albumin, cholesterol, other hepatic proteins (transferrin, fibrinogen); liver enzymes elevated, depending on the cause and acuity of liver injury; tendency toward hypokalemia, respiratory alkalosis; macrocytosis from folate deficiency
Renal	Usually chronic: may be associated with uremic signs and symptoms, including decreased appetite, altered (metallic or fishy) taste, altered sleep pattern, difficulty concentrating, restless legs or myoclonus: dyspnea can be present, but generally less prominent than in heart failure	Blood pressure may be elevated; hypertensive or diabetic retinopathy in selected cases; nitrogenous fetor; periorbital edema may predominate; pericardial friction rub in advanced cases with uremia	Albuminuria, hypoalbuminemia; sometimes, elevation of serum creatinine and urea nitrogen; hyperkalemia, metabolic acidosis, hyperphosphatemia, hypocalcemia, anemia (usually normocytic)

NOTE: S_3, third heart sound.

SOURCE: From GM Chertow, GE Thibault, Approach to the patient with edema, in L Goldman, E Braunwald (eds): *Primary Cardiology.* Philadelphia, Saunders, 1998.

EDEMA OF THE NEPHROTIC SYNDROME (See also Chap. 274) Marked proteinuria (>3.5 g/d), hypoalbuminemia (<35 g/L), and in some instances hypercholesterolemia are present. This syndrome may occur during the course of a variety of kidney diseases, which include glomerulonephritis, diabetic glomerulosclerosis, and hypersensitivity reactions. A history of previous renal disease may or may not be elicited.

EDEMA OF ACUTE GLOMERULONEPHRITIS AND OTHER FORMS OF RENAL FAILURE The edema occurring during the acute phases of glomerulonephritis is characteristically associated with hematuria, proteinuria, and hypertension. Although some evidence supports the view that the fluid retention is due to increased capillary permeability, in most instances the edema in this disease results from primary retention of sodium and water by the kidneys owing to renal insufficiency. This state differs from congestive heart failure in that it is characterized by a normal (or sometimes even increased) cardiac output and a normal arterial–mixed venous oxygen difference. Patients with edema due to renal failure commonly have evidence of pulmonary congestion on chest roentgenograms before cardiac enlargement is significant, but they usually do not develop orthopnea. Patients with chronic impairment of renal function may also develop edema due to primary renal retention of sodium and water.

EDEMA OF CIRRHOSIS (See also Chap. 299) Ascites and biochemical and clinical evidence of hepatic disease (collateral venous channels, jaundice, and spider angiomas) characterize edema of hepatic origin. The ascites is frequently refractory to treatment because it collects as a result of a combination of obstruction of hepatic lymphatic drainage, portal hypertension, and hypoalbuminemia. Edema may also occur in other parts of the body in these patients as a result of hypoalbuminemia. Furthermore, the sizable accumulation of ascitic fluid may increase intraabdominal pressure and impede venous return from the lower extremities; hence, it tends to promote accumulation of edema in this region as well.

EDEMA OF NUTRITIONAL ORIGIN A diet grossly deficient in protein over a prolonged period may produce hypoproteinemia and edema. The latter may be intensified by the development of beriberi heart disease, also of nutritional origin, in which multiple peripheral arteriovenous fistulas result in reduced effective systemic perfusion and effective arterial blood volume, thereby enhancing edema formation (Chap. 75). Edema may actually become intensified when these famished subjects are first provided with an adequate diet. The ingestion of more food may increase the quantity of salt ingested, which is then retained along with water. So-called "refeeding edema"

may also be linked to increased release of insulin, which directly increases tubular sodium reabsorption. In addition to hypoalbuminemia, hypokalemia and caloric deficits may be involved in the edema of starvation.

OTHER CAUSES OF EDEMA These include hypothyroidism, in which the edema (myxedema) may be located typically in the pretibial region and which may also be associated with periorbital puffiness. Exogenous hyperadrenocortism, pregnancy, and administration of estrogens and vasodilators, particularly the calcium antagonist nifedipine, may also all cause edema.

DISTRIBUTION OF EDEMA The distribution of edema is an important guide to the cause. Thus, edema limited to one leg or to one or both arms is usually the result of venous and/or lymphatic obstruction. Edema resulting from hypoproteinemia characteristically is generalized, but it is especially evident in the very soft tissues of the eyelids and face and tends to be most pronounced in the morning because of the recumbent posture assumed during the night. Less common causes of facial edema include trichinosis, allergic reactions, and myxedema. Edema associated with heart failure, on the other hand, tends to be more extensive in the legs and to be accentuated in the evening, a feature also determined largely by posture. When patients with heart failure have been confined to bed, edema may be most prominent in the presacral region. Unilateral edema occasionally results from lesions in the central nervous system affecting the vasomotor fibers on one side of the body; paralysis also reduces lymphatic and venous drainage on the affected side.

ADDITIONAL FACTORS IN DIAGNOSIS The color, thickness, and sensitivity of the skin are significant. Local tenderness and increase in temperature suggest inflammation. Local cyanosis may signify a venous obstruction. In individuals who have had repeated episodes of prolonged edema, the skin over the involved areas may be thickened, indurated, and often red.

Measurement or estimation of the venous pressure is of importance in evaluating edema. Elevation in an isolated part of the body usually reflects localized venous obstruction. Generalized elevation of systemic venous pressure usually indicates the presence of congestive heart failure. Ordinarily, a significant generalized increase in venous pressure can be recognized by the level at which cervical veins collapse (Chap. 225). In patients with obstruction of the superior vena cava, edema is confined to the face, neck, and upper extremities, where the venous pressure is elevated compared with that in the lower extremities. Measurement of venous pressure in the upper extremities is also useful in patients with massive edema of the lower extremities and ascites; it is elevated in the upper extremities when the edema is on a cardiac basis (e.g., constrictive pericarditis or tricuspid stenosis) but is normal when it is secondary to cirrhosis. Severe heart failure may cause ascites that may be distinguished from the ascites caused by hepatic cirrhosis by the jugular venous pressure, which usually is elevated in heart failure and normal in cirrhosis.

Determination of the concentration of serum albumin aids importantly in identifying those patients in whom edema is due, at least in part, to diminished intravascular colloid oncotic pressure. The presence of proteinuria also affords useful clues. The absence of proteinuria excludes nephrotic syndrome but cannot exclude nonproteinuric causes of renal failure. Slight to moderate proteinuria is the rule in patients with heart failure.

Approach to the Patient

An important first question is whether the edema is localized or generalized. If it is localized, those phenomena that may be responsible should be concentrated upon. Hydrothorax and ascites are forms of localized edema. Either may be a consequence of local venous or lymphatic obstruction, as in inflammatory or neoplastic disease.

If the edema is generalized, it should be determined, first, if there is serious hypoalbuminemia, e.g., serum albumin <25 g/L. If so, the history, physical examination, urinalysis, and other laboratory data will help evaluate the question of cirrhosis, severe malnutrition, protein-losing gastroenteropathy, or the nephrotic syndrome as the underlying disorder. If hypoalbuminemia is not present, it should be determined if there is evidence of congestive heart failure of a severity to promote generalized edema. Finally, it should be determined whether the patient has an adequate urine output, or if there is significant oliguria or even anuria.→*These abnormalities are discussed in Chaps. 47, 269, and 270.*

BIBLIOGRAPHY

ANAND IS et al: Studies of body water and sodium, renal function, hemodynamic indexes, and plasma hormones in untreated congestive heart failure. Circulation 80:299, 1989

BRATER DC: Diuretic therapy. N Engl J Med 339:387, 1998

DISKIN CJ et al: Edema, oncotic pressure, and free entropy: Novel considerations for treatment of edema through attention to thermodynamics. Nephron 78:131, 1998

GOLDEN MHN: Protein deficiency, energy deficiency, and the oedema of malnutrition. Lancet 1:1261, 1982

LEIER C, BOUDOULAS H: Renal disorders and heart disease, in *Heart Disease,* 6th ed, E Braunwald, D Zipes, P Libby (eds). Philadelphia, Saunders, 2001

MILLER JA et al: Control of extracellular fluid volume and the pathophysiology of edema formation, in *The Kidney,* 6th ed, BM Brenner (ed). Philadelphia, Saunders, 2000, pp 795–865

SCHRIER RW, FASSETT RG: A critique of the overfill hypothesis of sodium and water retention in the nephrotic syndrome. Kidney Int 53:1111, 1998

STREETEN DH: Idiopathic edema. Pathogenesis, clinical features, and treatment. Endocrinol Metab Clin North Am 24:531, 1995

38   *Ronald V. Maier*

SHOCK

Shock is the clinical syndrome that results from inadequate tissue perfusion. Irrespective of cause, the hypoperfusion-induced imbalance between the delivery of and requirements for oxygen and substrate leads to cellular dysfunction. The cellular injury created by the inadequate delivery of oxygen and substrates also induces the production and release of inflammatory mediators that further compromise perfusion through functional and structural changes within the microvasculature. This leads to a vicious cycle in which impaired perfusion is responsible for cellular injury which causes maldistribution of blood flow, further

Table 38-1   Classification of Shock

Hypovolemic	Septic
Traumatic	Hyperdynamic
Cardiogenic	Hypodynamic
Intrinsic	Neurogenic
Compressive	Hypoadrenal

compromising cellular perfusion; the latter causes multiple organ failure and, if the process is not interrupted, leads to the death of the patient. The clinical manifestations of shock are the result, in part, of sympathetic neuroendocrine responses to hypoperfusion as well as the breakdown in organ function induced by severe cellular dysfunction.

When very severe and/or persistent, inadequate oxygen delivery leads to irreversible cell injury, and only rapid restoration of oxygen delivery can reverse the progression of the shock state. The fundamental approach to management, therefore, is to recognize overt and impending shock in a timely fashion and to intervene emergently to restore perfusion. Except in cases of cardiogenic shock, this requires the expansion or reexpansion of blood volume. Control of any inciting pathologic process, e.g., continued hemorrhage, impairment of cardiac function, or infection, must occur simultaneously.

Clinical shock is usually accompanied by hypotension, i.e., a mean arterial pressure <60 mmHg in previously normotensive persons. Multiple classification schemes have been developed in an attempt to synthesize the seemingly dissimilar processes leading to shock. Strict adherence to a classification scheme may be difficult from a clinical standpoint because of the frequent combination of two or more causes of shock in any individual patient, but the classification shown in Table 38-1 provides a useful reference point from which to discuss and further delineate the underlying processes. The individual classes are discussed below.

PATHOGENESIS AND ORGAN RESPONSE

MICROCIRCULATION   Normally when cardiac output falls, systemic vascular resistance rises to maintain a level of systemic pressure that is adequate to allow perfusion of the heart and brain at the expense of other tissues, especially muscle, skin, and the gastrointestinal tract. Systemic vascular resistance is determined primarily by the luminal diameter of arterioles. The metabolic rates of the heart and brain are high, and their stores of energy substrate are low. These organs are critically dependent on a continuous supply of oxygen and nutrients, and neither tolerates severe ischemia for more than brief periods. Autoregulation, i.e., the maintenance of blood flow over a wide range of perfusion pressures, is critical in sustaining cerebral and coronary perfusion despite significant hypotension. However, when mean arterial pressure drops to ≤60 mmHg, flow to these organs falls and their function deteriorates.

Arteriolar vascular smooth muscle has both α- and β-adrenergic receptors (Chap. 72). The α_1 receptors mediate vasoconstriction, while the β_2 receptors mediate vasodilation. Efferent sympathetic fibers release norepinephrine, which acts primarily on α_1 receptors in one of the most fundamental compensatory responses to reduced perfusion pressure. Other constrictor substances that are increased in most forms of shock include angiotensin II, vasopressin, endothelin-1, and thromboxane A_2. Both norepinephrine and epinephrine are released by the adrenal medulla, and the concentrations of these catecholamines in the blood stream rise. Circulating vasodilators in shock include prostacyclin (PGI_2), nitric oxide (NO), and, importantly, products of local metabolism such as adenosine that match flow to the metabolic needs of the tissue. The balance between these various vasoconstrictor and vasodilator influences acting upon the microcirculation determines local perfusion.

Transport to cells depends on microcirculatory flow; capillary permeability; the diffusion of oxygen, carbon dioxide, nutrients, and products of metabolism through the interstitium; and the exchange of these products across cell membranes. Impairment of the microcirculation, which is central to the pathophysiologic responses in the late stages of all forms of shock, results in the derangement of cellular metabolism, which is ultimately responsible for organ failure.

The normal response to mild or moderate hypovolemia is an attempt at restitution of intravascular volume through alterations in hydrostatic pressure and osmolarity. Constriction of arterioles leads to reductions in both the capillary hydrostatic pressure and the number of capillary beds perfused, thereby limiting the capillary surface area across which filtration occurs. When filtration is reduced while intravascular oncotic pressure remains constant or rises, there is net reabsorption of fluid into the vascular bed, in accord with Starling's law of capillary-interstitial liquid exchange (Chap. 32). Metabolic changes (including hyperglycemia and elevations in the products of glycolysis, lipolysis, and proteolysis) raise extracellular osmolarity, leading to an osmotic gradient between cells and interstitium that increases interstitial and intravascular volume at the expense of intracellular volume.

CELLULAR RESPONSES Interstitial transport of nutrients is impaired, leading to a decline of intracellular high-energy phosphate stores. Mitochondrial dysfunction and uncoupling of oxidative phosphorylation are the most likely causes for decreased amounts of ATP. As a consequence, there is an accumulation of anaerobic metabolites including hydrogen ions, lactate, and other products of anaerobic metabolism. As shock progresses, these vasodilator metabolites override vasomotor tone, causing further hypotension and hypoperfusion. Dysfunction of cell membranes is thought to represent a common end-stage pathophysiologic pathway in the various forms of shock. Normal cellular transmembrane potential falls, and there is an associated increase in intracellular sodium and water, leading to cell swelling, which interferes further with microvascular perfusion.

NEUROENDOCRINE RESPONSE Hypovolemia, hypotension, and hypoxia are sensed by baroreceptors and chemoreceptors, which contribute further to an autonomic response that attempts to restore blood volume, maintain central perfusion, and mobilize metabolic substrates. Hypotension disinhibits the vasomotor center, resulting in increased adrenergic output and reduced vagal activity. Release of norepinephrine induces peripheral and splanchnic vasoconstriction, a major contributor to the maintenance of central organ perfusion, while reduced vagal activity increases the heart rate and cardiac output. The effects of circulating epinephrine released by the adrenal medulla in shock are largely metabolic, causing increased glycogenolysis and gluconeogenesis and reduced pancreatic insulin release.

Severe pain and other severe stress cause the hypothalamic release of adrenocorticotropic hormone (ACTH). This stimulates cortisol secretion, which contributes to decreased peripheral uptake of glucose and amino acids, enhances lipolysis, and increases gluconeogenesis. Increased pancreatic secretion of glucagon during stress accelerates hepatic gluconeogenesis and further elevates blood glucose concentration. These hormonal actions act synergistically in the maintenance of blood volume. The importance of the cortisol response to stress is illustrated by the profound circulatory collapse that occurs in hypoadrenal patients (see below).

Renin release is increased in response to adrenergic discharge and reduced perfusion of the juxtaglomerular apparatus in the kidney. Renin induces the formation of angiotensin I, which is then converted to angiotensin II, an extremely potent vasoconstrictor and stimulator of aldosterone release by the adrenal cortex and of vasopressin by the posterior pituitary. Aldosterone contributes to the maintainance of intravascular volume by enhancing renal tubular reabsorption of sodium, resulting in the excretion of a low-volume, concentrated, sodium-free urine. Vasopressin has a direct action on vascular smooth muscle, contributing to vasoconstriction, and acts on the distal renal tubules to enhance water reabsorption.

CARDIOVASCULAR RESPONSE Three variables—ventricular filling (preload), the resistance to ventricular ejection (afterload), and myocardial contractility—are paramount in controlling stroke volume (Chap. 231). Cardiac output, the major determinant of tissue perfusion, is the product of stroke volume and heart rate. Hy-

povolemia leads to decreased ventricular preload, which in turn reduces the stroke volume. An increase in heart rate is a useful but limited compensatory mechanism to maintain cardiac output. A shock-induced reduction in myocardial compliance is frequent, reducing ventricular end-diastolic volume and hence stroke volume at any given ventricular filling pressure. Restoration of intravascular volume then returns stroke volume to normal but only at elevated filling pressures. In addition, sepsis, ischemia, myocardial infarction, severe tissue trauma, hypothermia, general anesthesia, prolonged hypotension, and acidemia may all impair myocardial contractility and also reduce the stroke volume at any given ventricular end-diastolic volume. The resistance to ventricular ejection is influenced importantly by the systemic vascular resistance, which is elevated in most forms of shock. However, resistance is depressed in the early hyperdynamic stage of septic shock (see below), thereby allowing the cardiac output to be maintained.

The venous system contains nearly two-thirds of the total circulating blood volume, most in the small veins, and serves as a dynamic reservoir for autoinfusion of blood. Active venoconstriction as a consequence of α-adrenergic activity is an important compensatory mechanism for the maintenance of venous return and therefore of ventricular filling during shock. On the other hand, venous dilatation, as occurs in neurogenic shock, reduces ventricular filling and hence stroke volume and cardiac output (see below).

PULMONARY RESPONSE The response of the pulmonary vascular bed to shock parallels that of the systemic vascular bed, and the relative increase in pulmonary vascular resistance, particularly in septic shock, may exceed that of the systemic vascular resistance. Shock-induced tachypnea reduces tidal volume and increases both dead space and minute ventilation. Relative hypoxia and the subsequent tachypnea induce a respiratory alkalosis. Recumbency and involuntary restriction of ventilation secondary to pain reduce functional residual capacity and may lead to atelectasis. Shock is recognized as a major cause of acute lung injury and subsequent acute respiratory distress syndrome (ARDS; Chap. 265). These disorders are characterized by noncardiogenic pulmonary edema secondary to diffuse pulmonary capillary endothelial and alveolar epithelial injury, hypoxemia, and bilateral diffuse pulmonary infiltrates. Hypoxemia results from perfusion of underventilated and nonventilated alveoli. Loss of surfactant and lung volume in combination with increased interstitial and alveolar edema reduce lung compliance. The work of breathing and the oxygen requirements of respiratory muscles increase.

RENAL RESPONSE Acute renal failure (Chap. 269), a serious complication of shock and hypoperfusion, occurs less frequently than heretofore because of early aggressive volume repletion. Acute tubular necrosis is now more frequently seen as a result of the interactions of shock, sepsis, the administration of nephrotoxic agents (such as aminoglycosides and angiographic contrast media), and rhabdomyolysis; the latter may be particularly severe in skeletal muscle trauma. The physiologic response of the kidney to hypoperfusion is to conserve salt and water. In addition to decreased renal blood flow, increased afferent arteriolar resistance accounts for diminished glomerular filtration rate, which together with increased ADH and aldosterone is responsible for reduced urine formation. Toxic injury causes necrosis of tubular epithelium and tubular obstruction by cellular debris with back-leak of filtrate. The depletion of renal ATP stores that occurs with prolonged renal hypoperfusion is related to subsequent impairment of renal function.

METABOLIC DERANGEMENTS During shock, there is disruption of the normal cycles of carbohydrate, lipid, and protein metabolism. Through the citric acid cycle, alanine in conjunction with lactate (which is converted from pyruvate in the periphery in the presence of oxygen deprivation) enhances the hepatic production of glucose. With reduced availability of oxygen, the breakdown of glucose to pyruvate and ultimately lactate represents an inefficient cycling of substrate with minimal net energy production. An elevated plasma

Table 38-2 Normal Hemodynamic Parameters

Parameter	Calculation	Normal Values
Cardiac output (CO)	$SV \times HR$	4–8 L/min
Cardiac index (CI)	CO/BSA	2.6–4.2 (L/min)/m²
Stroke volume (SV)	CO/HR	50–100 mL/beat
Systemic vascular resistance (SVR)	$[(MAP - RAP)/CO] \times 80$	700–1600 dynes · s/cm⁵
Pulmonary vascular resistance (PVR)	$[(PAP_m - PCWP)/CO] \times 80$	20–130 dynes · s/cm⁵
Left ventricular stroke work (LVSW)	$SV(MAP - PCWP) \times 0.0136$	60–80 g-m/beat
Right ventricular stroke work (RVSW)	$SV(PAP_m - RAP)$	10–15 g-m/beat

NOTE: HR, heart rate; BSA, body surface area; MAP, mean arterial pressure; RAP, right atrial pressure; PAP_m, pulmonary artery pressure—mean; PCWP, pulmonary capillary wedge pressure.

lactate/pyruvate ratio is consistent with anaerobic metabolism and reflects inadequate tissue perfusion. Decreased clearance of exogenous triglycerides coupled with increased hepatic lipogenesis causes a significant rise in serum triglyceride concentrations. There is increased protein catabolism, a negative nitrogen balance, and, if the process is prolonged, severe muscle wasting.

INFLAMMATORY RESPONSES Activation of an extensive network of proinflammatory mediator systems plays a significant role in the progression of shock and contributes importantly to the development of organ injury and failure.

Multiple humoral mediators are activated during shock and tissue injury. The complement cascade, activated through both the classic and alternate pathways, generates the anaphylatoxins C3a and C5a. Direct complement fixation to injured tissues can progress to the C5-C9 attack complex, causing further cell damage. Activation of the coagulation cascade causes microvascular thrombosis, with subsequent lysis leading to repeated episodes of ischemia and reperfusion. Components of the coagulation system, such as thrombin, are potent proinflammatory mediators that cause expression of adhesion molecules on endothelial cells and activation of neutrophils, leading to microvascular injury. Coagulation also activates the kallekrein-kininogen cascade, contributing to hypotension.

Eicosanoids are vasoactive and immunomodulatory products of arachidonic acid metabolism that include cyclooxygenase-derived prostaglandins and thromboxane A_2 as well as lipoxygenase-derived leukotrienes and lipoxins. Thromboxane A_2 is a potent vasoconstrictor that contributes to the pulmonary hypertension and acute tubular necrosis of shock. PGI_2 and prostaglandin E_2 are potent vasodilators that enhance capillary permeability and edema formation. The cysteinyl leukotrienes LTC_4 and LTD_4 are pivotal mediators of the vascular sequelae of anaphylaxis, as well as of shock states resulting from sepsis or tissue injury. LTB_4 is a potent neutrophil chemoattractant and secretagogue that stimulates the formation of reactive oxygen species. Lipoxins are endogenous autocoids that inhibit leukotriene-mediated responses. Platelet-activating factor, an ether-linked, arachidonyl-containing phospholipid mediator, also carries potent bioactivities that include pulmonary vasoconstriction, bronchoconstriction, systemic vasodilation, increased capillary permeability, and the priming of macrophages and neutrophils to produce enhanced levels of inflammatory mediators.

Tumor necrosis factor (TNF) α, produced by activated macrophages, reproduces many components of the shock state including hypotension, lactic acidosis, and respiratory failure. Interleukin (IL) 1 is also produced by tissue-fixed macrophages and is critical to the inflammatory response occurring in hypoperfusion and septic states. Chemokines also participate in the systemic inflammatory response. For example, IL-8 is a potent neutrophil chemoattractant and activator that upregulates adhesion molecules on the neutrophil to enhance aggregation and adherence to the vascular endothelium. The endothelium normally produces nitric oxide (NO), a potent vasodilator. The inflammatory response stimulates the inducible isoform of NO synthase (iNOS), which is thought to overexpress toxic NO and oxygen-derived free radicals and contributes to the hyperdynamic cardiovascular response that occurs in sepsis.

Multiple inflammatory cells, including neutrophils, macrophages, and platelets, are a major contributor to inflammation-induced injury. Margination of activated neutrophils in the microcirculation is a common pathologic finding in shock, causing secondary injury due to the release of potentially toxic oxygen radicals and proteases. Adhesion molecules are expressed on the surface of the endothelium and on cytokine-stimulated neutrophils. Tissue-fixed macrophages produce virtually all major components of the inflammatory response and orchestrate the progression and duration of the response.

Approach to the Patient

The underlying problem in all forms of shock is inadequate tissue perfusion and an imbalance between delivery and cellular needs of oxygen and metabolic substrate. It is important to recognize the onset of hypoperfusion at the earliest possible time in order to institute aggressive resuscitation and correction of the underlying etiology.

Monitoring Patients in shock require care in an intensive care unit. Careful and continuous assessment of the physiologic status is necessary. Arterial pressure through an indwelling line, pulse, and respiratory rate should be monitored continuously; a Foley catheter should be inserted to follow urine flow; and mental status assessed frequently.

Although there is ongoing debate as to the indications for using the flow-directed pulmonary artery catheter (PAC, Swan-Ganz catheter) in the management of patients in shock, most intensivists believe that the ability to predict the hemodynamic profiles of patients in shock accurately without a PAC is poor. The PAC is placed percutaneously via the subclavian or jugular vein through the central venous circulation and right heart into the pulmonary artery. There are ports both proximal in the right atrium and distal in the pulmonary artery to provide access for infusions and for cardiac output measurements. Right atrial and pulmonary artery pressures are measured, and the pulmonary capillary wedge pressure (PCWP) serves as an approximation of the left atrial pressure. Normal hemodynamic parameters are shown in Table 228-3 and Table 38-2.

Cardiac output is determined by the thermodilution technique, and high-resolution thermistors can also be used to determine right ventricular end-diastolic volume to monitor further the response of the right heart to fluid resuscitation. A PAC with an oximeter port offers the additional advantage of on-line monitoring of the mixed venous oxygen saturation, an important index of tissue perfusion. Systemic and pulmonary vascular resistances are calculated as the ratio of the pressure drop across these vascular beds to the cardiac output (Chap. 228). Determinations of oxygen content in arterial and venous blood, together with cardiac output and hemoglobin concentration allow calculation of oxygen delivery, oxygen consumption, and oxygen-extraction ratio (Table 38-3). The hemodynamic patterns associated with the various form of shock are shown in Table 38-4.

In resuscitation from shock, it is critical to restore tissue perfusion and optimize oxygen delivery, hemodynamics, and cardiac function rapidly. A goal of therapy is to achieve normal mixed venous oxygen saturation and arteriovenous oxygen-extraction ratio. To enhance oxygen delivery, red cell mass, arterial oxygen saturation, and cardiac output may be augmented singly or simultaneously. An increase in oxygen delivery not accompanied by an increase in oxygen consumption implies that oxygen availability is adequate and that oxygen consumption is not flow-dependent. Conversely, an elevation of oxygen consumption with increased cardiac output implies that the oxygen supply is inadequate. A reduction in systemic vascular resistance accompanying an increase in cardiac output indicates that compensatory vasoconstriction is reversing due to improved tissue perfusion. The determination of stepwise expansion of blood volume on cardiac performance allows identification of the optimum preload.

SPECIFIC FORMS OF SHOCK

HYPOVOLEMIC SHOCK This most common form of shock results either from the loss of red blood cell mass and plasma from hemorrhage or from the loss of plasma volume alone arising from extravascular fluid sequestration or gastrointestinal, urinary, and insensible losses. The signs and symptoms of nonhemorrhagic hypovolemic shock are the same as those of hemorrhagic shock, although they may have a more insidious onset. The normal physiologic response to hypovolemia is to maintain perfusion of the brain and heart while restoring an effective circulating blood volume. There is an increase in sympathetic activity, hyperventilation, collapse of venous capacitance vessels, release of stress hormones, and expansion of intravascular volume through the recruitment of interstitial and intracellular fluid and reduction of urine output.

Mild hypovolemia ($\leq$20% of the blood volume) generates mild tachycardia but relatively few external signs, especially in a supine resting young patient (Table 38-5). With moderate hypovolemia (~20 to 40% of the blood volume) the patient becomes increasingly anxious and tachycardic; although normal blood pressure may be maintained in the supine position, there may be significant postural hypotension and tachycardia. If hypovolemia is severe ($\geq$~40% of the blood volume), the classic signs of shock appear; the blood pressure declines and becomes unstable even in the supine position, and the patient develops marked tachycardia, oliguria, and agitation or confusion. Perfusion of the central nervous system is well maintained until shock becomes severe. Hence, mental obtundation is an ominous clinical sign. The transition from mild to severe hypovolemic shock can be insidious or extremely rapid. If severe shock is not reversed rapidly, especially in elderly patients and those with comorbid illnesses, death is imminent. A very narrow time frame separates the derangements found in severe shock that can be reversed with aggressive resuscitation from those of progressive decompensation and irreversible cell injury.

Diagnosis Hypovolemic shock is readily diagnosed when there are signs of hemodynamic instability and the source of volume loss is obvious. The diagnosis is more difficult when the source of blood loss is occult, as into the gastrointestinal tract, or when plasma volume alone is depleted. After acute hemorrhage, hemoglobin and hematocrit values do not change until compensatory fluid shifts have occurred or exogenous fluid is administered. Thus, an initial normal hematocrit does not disprove the presence of significant blood loss. Plasma losses cause hemoconcentration, and free water loss leads to hypernatremia. These findings should suggest the presence of hypovolemia.

It is essential to distinguish between hypovolemic and cardiogenic shock (see below) because definitive therapy differs significantly. Both forms are associated with a reduced cardiac output and a compensatory sympathetic mediated response characterized by tachycardia and elevated systemic vascular resistance. However, the findings in cardiogenic shock of jugular venous distention, rales, and an S_3 gallop distinguish it from hypovolemic shock and signify that volume expansion is undesirable.

℞ TREATMENT Initial resuscitation requires rapid reexpansion of the circulating blood volume along with interventions to control ongoing losses. In accordance with Starling's law (Chap. 231), stroke volume and cardiac output rise with the increase in preload. After resuscitation, the compliance of the ventricles may remain reduced due to increased interstitial fluid in the myocardium. Therefore, elevated filling pressures are required to maintain adequate ventricular performance.

Volume resuscitation is initiated with the rapid infusion of isotonic saline or a balanced salt solution such as Ringer's lactate through large-bore intravenous lines. No distinct benefit from the use of colloid has been demonstrated. The infusion of 2 to 3 L over 10 to 30 min should restore normal hemodynamic parameters. Continued hemodynamic instability implies that shock has not been reversed and/or that there are significant ongoing blood or volume losses. Continuing blood loss, with hemoglobin concentrations declining to $\leq$100 g/L (10 g/dL), should initiate blood transfusion, preferably as fully cross-matched blood. In extreme emergencies, type-specific or O-negative packed red cells may be transfused. In the presence of severe and/or prolonged hypovolemia, inotropic support with dopamine or dobutamine (Chap. 72) may be required to maintain adequate ventricular performance, after blood volume has been restored. Infusion of norepinephrine to increase arterial pressure by raising peripheral resistance is inappropriate, other than as a temporizing measure in severe shock while blood volume is reexpanded.

Successful resuscitation also requires support of respiratory function. Supplemental oxygen should be provided, and endotracheal intubation may be necessary to maintain arterial oxygenation. Following

Table 38-3 Oxygen Transport Calculations

Parameter	Calculation	Normal Values
Oxygen-carrying capacity of hemoglobin		1.39 mL/g
Plasma O_2 concentration		$P_{O_2} \times 0.0031$
Arterial O_2 concentration (Ca_{O_2})	$1.39\ Sa_{O_2} + 0.0031\ Pa_{O_2}$	20 vol%
Venous O_2 concentration (Cv_{O_2})	$1.39\ Sv_{O_2} + 0.0031\ Pv_{O_2}$	15.5 vol%
Arteriovenous O_2 difference ($Ca_{O_2} - Cv_{O_2}$)	$1.39\ (Sa_{O_2} - Sv_{O_2}) + 0.0031\ (Pa_{O_2} - Pv_{O_2})$	3.5 vol%
Oxygen delivery (D_{O_2})	$Ca_{O_2} \times CO\ (L/min) \times 10\ (dL/L)$ $1.39\ Sa_{O_2} \times CO \times 10$	800–1600 mL/min
Oxygen uptake (V_{O_2})	$(Ca_{O_2} - Cv_{O_2}) \times CO \times 10$ $1.39\ (Sa_{O_2} - Sv_{O_2}) \times CO \times 10$	150–400 mL/min
Oxygen delivery index ($D_{O_2}I$)	D_{O_2}/BSA	520–720 (mL/min)/m²
Oxygen uptake index ($V_{O_2}I$)	V_{O_2}/BSA	115–165 (mL/min)/m²
Oxygen extraction ratio (O_2ER)	$[1 - (\dot{V}_{O_2}/\dot{D}_{O_2})] \times 100$	22–32%

NOTE: F_{O_2}, partial pressure of oxygen; Sa_{O_2}, saturation of hemoglobin with O_2 in arterial blood; Pa_{O_2}, partial pressure of O_2 in arterial blood; Sv_{O_2}, saturation of hemoglobin with O_2 in venous blood; Pv_{O_2}, partial pressure of O_2 in venous blood; CO, Cardiac output; BSA, body surface area.

Table 38-4 Physiologic Characteristics of the Various Forms of Shock

Type of Shock	CVP and PCWP	Cardiac Output	Systemic Vascular Resistance	Venous O_2 Saturation
Hypovolemic	↓	↓	↑	↓
Cardiogenic	↑	↓	↑	↓
Septic				
Hyperdynamic	↓↑	↑	↓	↑↓
Hypodynamic	↓↑	↓	↑↓	↓
Traumatic	↓	↓	↑↓	↓
Neurogenic	↓	↓	↓	↓
Hypoadrenal	↓↑	↓	=↓	↓

NOTE: CVP, central venous pressure; PCWP, pulmonary capillary wedge pressure.

Table 38-5 Hypovolemic Shock

Mild (<20% Blood Volume)	Moderate (20–40% Blood Volume)	Severe (>40% Blood Volume)
Cool extremities	Same, plus:	Same, plus:
Increased capillary refill time	Tachycardia	Hemodynamic instability
Diaphoresis	Tachypnea	Marked tachycardia
Collapsed veins	Oliguria	Hypotension
Anxiety	Postural changes	Mental status deterioration (coma)

resuscitation from isolated hemorrhagic shock, end-organ damage is frequently less than following septic or traumatic shock. This may be due to the absence of the massive activation of inflammatory mediator response systems and the consequent nonspecific organ injury seen in the latter conditions.

TRAUMATIC SHOCK   Shock following trauma is, in large measure, due to hypovolemia. However, even when hemorrhage has been controlled, patients can continue to suffer loss of plasma volume into the interstitium of injured tissues. These fluid losses are compounded by injury-induced inflammatory responses, which contribute to the secondary microcirculatory injury. This causes secondary tissue injury and maldistribution of blood flow, intensifying tissue ischemia and leading to multiple organ system failure. Trauma to the heart, chest, or head can also contribute to the shock. For example, pericardial tamponade or tension pneumothorax impairs ventricular filling, while myocardial contusion depresses myocardial contractility.

TREATMENT   Inability to maintain a systolic blood pressure ≥90 mmHg after trauma-inudced hypovolemia is associated with a mortality rate of ~50%. To prevent decompensation of homeostatic mechanisms, therapy must be promptly administered.

The initial management of the seriously injured patient requires attention to the "ABCs" of resuscitation: assurance of an airway (A), adequate ventilation (breathing, B), and establishment of an adequate blood volume to support the circulation (C). Control of hemorrhage requires immediate attention. Early stabilization of fractures, debridement of devitalized or contaminated tissues, and evacuation of hematomata all reduce the subsequent inflammatory response to the initial insult and minimize subsequent organ injury.

INTRINSIC CARDIOGENIC SHOCK   This form of shock is caused by failure, often sudden, of the heart as an effective pump. It occurs most commonly as a complication of acute myocardial infarction (AMI; Chap. 243), but it may also be seen in patients with severe brady- or tachyarrhythmias, valvular heart disease, or in the terminal stage of chronic heart failure of any cause, including ischemic heart disease and dilated cardiomyopathy. Cardiogenic shock is characterized by a low cardiac output, diminished peripheral perfusion, pulmonary congestion, and elevation of systemic vascular resistance and pulmonary vascular pressures. Acute right heart failure can arise as the result of right ventricular infarction or may complicate the acute respiratory distress syndrome and severe pulmonary hypertension of any etiology. As a consequence of right ventricular failure, left ventricular preload falls, and this, in turn, reduces systemic perfusion. In contrast to other forms of shock, absolute or relative hypovolemia is usually not present in cardiogenic shock.

The ineffective contractile activity of either the right or left side of the heart leads to the accumulation of blood in the venous circulation upstream to the failing ventricle. Cardiogenic shock with left-sided heart failure increases fluid in the lungs that can overwhelm the capacity of the pulmonary lymphatics and causes interstitial and sometimes alveolar edema. Interstitial lung edema usually occurs at pulmonary capillary pressures >18 mmHg, and overt pulmonary alveolar edema develops at pressures >24 mmHg (Chap. 32). Pulmonary edema impacts cardiac function further by impairing diffusion of oxygen, setting up a vicious cycle. The increase in interstitial and intraalveolar fluid causes a progressive reduction in lung compliance, thereby increasing the work of ventilation while increasing perfusion of poorly ventilated alveoli.

In establishing the diagnosis of cardiogenic shock, a history of cardiac disease or of AMI is of value. Associated physical findings include those of hemodynamic instability, peripheral vasoconstriction, and pulmonary and/or systemic venous congestion, as well as findings specific to the underlying cardiac abnormalities. An electrocardiogram may provide evidence of AMI or preexisting cardiac disease. The chest

x-ray may show pulmonary edema and cardiomegaly. Transthoracic or transesophageal echocardiograms assist in the diagnosis of structural abnormalities and/or functional impairment of contractility. Serum cardiac markers will support the diagnosis of acute cardiac injury. Hemodynamic monitoring is usually necessary. Placement of a PAC is helpful and will show a reduced cardiac output and an elevated PCWP, and direct measurement of right atrial pressure allows calculation of systemic vascular resistance which is elevated.

TREATMENT   For all forms of cardiogenic shock, preload, afterload, and contractility should be modified using the information provided by the PAC. A PCWP of 15 to 20 mmHg should be the initial goal. If the PCWP is excessively elevated, inotropic agents may provide significant reduction. The goal is to increase contractility without significant increases in heart rate. Dopamine and norepinephrine exert both inotropic and vasoconstrictor actions (Chap. 72) that are useful in the presence of persistent hypotension. Dobutamine, a positive inotropic agent with vasodilator properties, may be substituted when arterial pressure has been restored. Pulmonary congestion may be responsive to intravenous furosemide. Patients with an inadequate response to these measures can be supported by using intraaortic balloon counterpulsation to permit recovery of myocardial function. Additional measures to consider in cases of refractory cardiogenic shock include urgent myocardial revascularization in patients with AMI (Chap. 243), correction of anatomic cardiac defects such as rupture of the papillary muscles of the interventricular septum, the placement of ventricular assist devices, and even urgent cardiac transplantation.

COMPRESSIVE CARDIOGENIC SHOCK   With compression, the heart and surrounding structures are less compliant and, thus, normal filling pressures generate inadequate diastolic filling. Blood or fluid within the poorly distensible pericardial sac may cause tamponade (Chap. 239). Any cause of increased intrathoracic pressure, such as tension pneumothorax, herniation of abdominal viscera through a diaphragmatic hernia, or excessive positive pressure ventilation to support pulmonary function, can also cause compressive cardiogenic shock. Acute right heart failure with a sudden decline in cardiac output can be caused by pulmonary embolism obstructing right ventricular outflow and impairing left ventricular filling. Although initially responsive to increased filling pressures produced by volume expansion, as compression increases, cardiogenic shock occurs.

The diagnosis of compressive cardiogenic shock is most frequently based on clinical findings, the chest radiograph, and an echocardiogram. The diagnosis of compressive cardiac shock may be more difficult to establish in the setting of trauma when hypovolemia and cardiac compression are present simultaneously. The classic findings of pericardial tamponade include the triad of hypotension, neck vein distention, and muffled heart sounds (Chap. 239). Pulsus paradoxus, i.e., an inspiratory reduction in systolic pressure >10 mmHg, may also be noted. The diagnosis is confirmed by echocardiography, and treatment consists of immediate pericardiocentesis. A tension pneumothorax produces ipsilateral decreased breath sounds, tracheal deviation away from the affected thorax, and jugular venous distention. Radiographic findings include increased intrathoracic volume, depression of the diaphragm of the affected hemithorax, and shifting of the mediastinum to the contralateral side. Chest decompression must be carried out immediately. Release of air and restoration of normal cardiovascular dynamics is both diagnostic and therapeutic.

SEPTIC SHOCK (See also Chap. 124)   This form of shock is caused by the systemic response to a severe infection. It occurs most frequently in elderly or immunocompromised patients and in those who have undergone an invasive procedure in which bacterial contamination has occurred. Infections of the lung, abdomen, or urinary tract are most common, and approximately half of the patients have bacteremia. Gram-positive and -negative bacteria, viruses, fungi, rickettsiae, and protozoa have all been reported to produce the clinical picture of septic shock, and the overall response is generally independent of the specific type of invading organism. The clinical findings in septic shock are a consequence of the combination of metabolic and circulatory derangements driven by the systemic infection and the release of toxic components of the infectious organisms, e.g., the endotoxin of gram-negative bacteria or the exotoxins and enterotoxins of gram-positive bacteria. Organism toxins lead to the release of cytokines, including IL-1 and TNF-α, from tissue macrophages. Tissue factor expression and fibrin deposition are increased, and disseminated intravascular coagulation may develop. The inducible form of NO synthase is stimulated, and NO, a powerful vasodilator, is released. Hemodynamic changes in septic shock occur in two characteristic patterns: early, or hyperdynamic, and late, or hypodynamic, septic shock.

Hyperdynamic Response In hyperdynamic septic shock, tachycardia is present, the cardiac output is normal, and the systemic vascular resistance is reduced while the pulmonary vascular resistance is elevated. The extremities are usually warm. However, splanchnic vasoconstriction with decreased visceral flow is present. The venous capacitance is increased, which decreases venous return. With volume expansion cardiac output becomes supranormal. Myocardial contractility is depressed in septic shock by mediators including NO, IL-1, and/or TNF-α. Inflammatory mediator–induced processes include increased capillary permeability and continued loss of intravascular volume.

In septic shock, in contrast to other types of shock, total oxygen delivery may be increased while oxygen extraction is reduced due to maldistribution of microcirculatory perfusion and impaired utilization. In this setting the presence of a normal mixed venous oxygen saturation is not indicative of adequate peripheral perfusion, and even though the cardiac output may be elevated, it is still inadequate to meet the total metabolic needs. The toxicity of the infectious agents and their byproducts and the subsequent metabolic dysfunction drive the progressive deterioration of cellular and organ function. Acute respiratory distress syndrome, thrombocytopenia, and neutropenia are common complications.

Hypodynamic Response As sepsis progresses, vasoconstriction occurs and the cardiac output declines. The patient usually becomes markedly tachypneic, febrile, diaphoretic, and obtunded, with cool, mottled, and often cyanotic extremities. Oliguria, renal failure, and hypothermia develop; there may be striking increases in serum lactate.

TREATMENT Aggressive volume expansion with a crystalloid solution to a PCWP of approximately 15 mmHg and the restoration of arterial oxygenation with inspired oxygen and frequently with mechanical ventilation are the highest priorities. In the presence of hypodynamic septic shock, augmentation of cardiac output may require inotropic support with dopamine or norepinephrine in the presence of hypotension or with dobutamine if arterial pressure is normal. Antibiotics should be administered, either appropriate for the results of cultures or empirical therapy based on the likely source of infection. Surgical debridement or drainage may also be necessary to control the infection.

NEUROGENIC SHOCK Interruption of sympathetic vasomotor input after a high cervical spinal cord injury, inadvertent cephalad migration of spinal anesthesia, or severe head injury may result in neurogenic shock. In addition to arteriolar dilatation, venodilation causes pooling in the venous system, which decreases venous return and cardiac output. The extremities are often warm, in contrast to the usual vasoconstriction-induced coolness in hypovolemic or cardiogenic shock. Treatment involves a simultaneous approach to the relative hypovolemia and to the loss of vasomotor tone. Large volumes of fluid may be required to restore normal hemodynamics. Once hemorrhage has been ruled out, norepinephrine may be necessary to augment vascular resistance.

HYPOADRENAL SHOCK (See also Chap. 331) The normal host response to the stress of illness, operation, or trauma requires that the adrenal glands hypersecrete cortisol in excess of that normally required. Hypoadrenal shock occurs in settings in which unrecognized adrenal insufficiency complicates the host response to the stress induced by acute illness or major surgery. Adrenocortical insufficiency may occur as a consequence of the chronic administration of high doses of exogenous glucocorticoids. Recent studies have shown that prolonged stays in a critical state in an intensive care setting may also induce a relative hypoadrenal state. Other, less common causes include adrenal insufficiency secondary to idiopathic atrophy, tuberculosis, metastatic disease, bilateral hemorrhage, and amyloidosis. The shock produced by adrenal insufficiency is characterized by reductions in systemic vascular resistance, hypovolemia, and reduced cardiac output. The diagnosis of adrenal insufficiency may be established by means of an ACTH stimulation test (Chap. 331).

TREATMENT In the hemodynamically unstable patient, dexamethasone sodium phosphate, 4 mg, should be given intravenously. This agent is preferred because unlike hydrocortisone it does not interfere with the ACTH stimulation test. If the diagnosis of adrenal insufficiency has been established, hydrocortisone, 100 mg every 6 to 8 h, can be given and tapered to a maintenance level as the patient achieves hemodynamic stability. Simultaneous volume resuscitation and pressor support is required.

ADJUNCTIVE THERAPIES

As described above, the sympathomimetic amines dobutamine, dopamine, and norepinephrine are widely used in the treatment of all forms of shock. The clinical pharmacology of these agents is described in Chap. 72.

POSITIONING Positioning of the patient may be a valuable adjunct in the initial treatment of hypovolemic shock. Elevating the foot of the bed (i.e., placing it on "shock blocks") and assumption of the Trendelenburg position without flexion at the knees are effective but may increase work of breathing and risk for aspiration. Simply elevating both legs may be the optimal approach.

PNEUMATIC ANTISHOCK GARMENT (PASG) The PASG and the military antishock trousers (MAST) are inflatable external compression devices that can be wrapped around the legs and abdomen and have been widely used in the prehospital setting as a means of providing temporary support of central hemodynamics in shock. They cause an increase in systemic vascular resistance and blood pressure by arterial compression, without causing a significant change in cardiac output. While the use of PASG has been recommended in noncardiogenic forms of shock, the most appropriate use appears to be as a means to tamponade bleeding and augment hemostasis. Inflation of the suit provides splinting of fractures of the pelvis and lower extremities and arrests hemorrhage from fractures.

REWARMING Hypothermia is a potential adverse consequence of massive volume resuscitation. The infusion of large volumes of refrigerated blood products and room-temperature crystalloid solutions can rapidly drop core temperatures if fluid is not run through warming devices. Hypothermia may depress cardiac contractility and thereby further impair cardiac output and oxygen delivery. Hypothermia, particularly temperatures $<35°$ C, directly impairs the coagulation pathway, sometimes causing a significant coagulopathy. Rapid rewarming significantly decreases the requirement for blood products and an improvement in cardiac function. The most effective method for rewarming is extracorporeal countercurrent warmers through femoral artery and vein cannulation. This process does not require a pump and can rewarm from $30°$ to $36°$C in <30 min.

BIBLIOGRAPHY

Astiz ME, Rackow EC: Septic shock. Lancet 351:1501, 1998

Choi PT et al: Crystalloids vs. colloids in fluid resuscitation: A systematic review. Crit Care Med 27:200, 1999

Connors AF Jr et al: The effectiveness of right heart catheterization in the initial care of critically ill patients. JAMA 276:889, 1996

Dries DJ: Hypotensive resuscitation [editorial]. Shock 6:311, 1996

Hebert PC et al: A multicenter, randomized, controlled clinical trial of transfusion requirements in critical care. Transfusion Requirements in Critical Care Investigators, Canadian Critical Care Trials Group. N Engl J Med 340:409, 1999

HECKBERT SR et al: Outcome after hemorrhagic shock in trauma patients. J Trauma 45: 545, 1998

LEVY B et al: Comparison of norepinephrine and dobutamine to epinephrine for hemodynamics, lactate metabolism, and gastric tonometric variables in septic shock: A prospective, randomized study. Intensive Care Med 23:282, 1997

MIRA JP et al: Association of TNF2, a TNF-alpha promoter polymorphism, with septic shock susceptibility and mortality: A multicenter study. JAMA 282:561, 1999

Practice parameters for hemodynamic support of sepsis in adult patients in sepsis. Task Force of the American College of Critical Care Medicine, Society of Critical Care Medicine. Crit Care Med. 27:639, 1999

WHEELER AP, BERNARD GR: Treating patients with severe sepsis. N Engl J Med 340: 207, 1999

39   Robert J. Myerburg, Agustin Castellanos

CARDIOVASCULAR COLLAPSE, CARDIAC ARREST, AND SUDDEN CARDIAC DEATH

CPR	cardiopulmonary resuscitation	PEA	pulseless electrical activity
EF	ejection fraction	PVCs	premature ventricular contractions
ICD	implantable cardioverter-defibrillator	SCD	sudden *cardiac* death
LV	left ventricular	VF	ventricular fibrillation
MIs	myocardial infarctions	VT	ventricular tachycardia

OVERVIEW AND DEFINITIONS

The vast majority of naturally occurring sudden deaths are caused by cardiac disorders. The magnitude of sudden *cardiac* death (SCD) as a public health problem is highlighted by estimates that more than 300,000 deaths occur each year in the United States by this mechanism, accounting for 50% of all cardiac deaths. SCD is a direct consequence of cardiac arrest, which is often reversible if responded to promptly. Since resuscitation techniques and emergency rescue systems are available to save patients who have out-of-hospital cardiac arrest, which was uniformly fatal in the past, understanding the SCD problem has practical importance.

SCD must be defined carefully. In the context of time, "sudden" is defined, for most clinical and epidemiologic purposes, as 1 h or less between the onset of the terminal clinical event, or an abrupt change in clinical status, and death. An exception is unwitnessed deaths in which pathologists may expand the definition of time to 24 h after the victim was last seen to be alive and stable.

Because of community-based interventions, victims may remain biologically alive for days or even weeks after a cardiac arrest that has resulted in irreversible central nervous system damage. Confusion in terms can be avoided by adhering strictly to definitions of death, cardiac arrest, and cardiovascular collapse (Table 39-1). Death is biologically, legally, and literally an absolute and irreversible event. Death may be delayed in a survivor of cardiac arrest, but "survival after sudden death" is an irrational term. Currently, the accepted definition of SCD is *natural death due to cardiac causes*, heralded by abrupt loss of consciousness within *1 h* of the onset of acute symptoms, in an individual who may have known *preexisting* heart disease but in whom the *time* and *mode* of death are *unexpected*. When biologic death of the cardiac arrest victim is delayed because of interventions, the relevant pathophysiologic event remains the sudden and unexpected cardiac arrest that leads ultimately to death, even though delayed by artificial methods. The language used should reflect the fact that the index event was a cardiac arrest and that death was due to its delayed consequences.

Table 39-1   Distinction Between Death, Cardiac Arrest, and Cardiovascular Collapse

Term	Definition	Qualifiers or Exceptions
Death	Irreversible cessation of all biologic functions	None
Cardiac arrest	Abrupt cessation of cardiac pump function which may be reversible by a prompt intervention but will lead to death in its absence	Rare spontaneous reversions; likelihood of successful interventions relates to mechanism of arrest, clinical setting, and prompt return of circulation
Cardiovascular collapse	A sudden loss of effective blood flow due to cardiac and/or peripheral vascular factors which may reverse spontaneously (e.g., neurocardiogenic syncope; vasovagal syncope) or only with interventions (e.g., cardiac arrest)	Nonspecific term which includes cardiac arrest and its consequences and also events which characteristically revert spontaneously

ETIOLOGY, INITIATING EVENTS, AND CLINICAL EPIDEMIOLOGY

Clinical and epidemiologic studies have identified populations at high risk for SCD. In addition, a large body of pathologic data provides information on the underlying *structural abnormalities* in victims of SCD, and studies of clinical physiology have begun to identify a group of *transient functional factors* that may convert a long-standing underlying structural abnormality from a stable to an unstable state (Table 39-2). This information is developing into an understanding of the causes and mechanisms of SCD.

Cardiac disorders constitute the most common causes of sudden *natural* death. After an initial peak incidence of sudden death between birth and 6 months of age (the sudden infant death syndrome), the incidence of sudden death declines sharply and remains low through childhood and adolescence. Among adolescents and young adults, the incidence of SCD is approximately 1 per 100,000 population per year. The incidence begins to increase in adults over the age of 30 years, reaching a second peak in the age range of 45 to 75 years, when the incidence approximates 1 to 2 per 1000 per year among the unselected adult population. Increasing age within this range is a powerful risk factor for sudden *cardiac* death, and the proportion of cardiac causes among all sudden natural deaths increases dramatically with advancing years. From 1 to 13 years of age, only one of five sudden *natural* deaths is due to cardiac causes. Between 14 and 21 years of age, the proportion increases to 30%, and then to 88% in the middle-aged and elderly.

Young and middle-aged men and women have very different susceptibilities to SCD, but the gender differences decrease with advancing age. In the 45- to 64-year-old age group, the male SCD excess is nearly 7:1. It falls to 2:1 or less in the 65- to 74-year-old age group. The difference in risk for SCD parallels the risks for other manifestations of coronary heart disease in men and women. As the gender gap for manifestations of coronary heart disease closes in the seventh and eighth decades of life, the excess risk of SCD in males also narrows. Despite the lower incidence among younger women, coronary risk factors such as cigarette smoking, diabetes, hyperlipidemia, and hypertension are highly influential, and SCD remains an important clinical and epidemiologic problem.

Hereditary factors contribute to the risk of SCD, but largely in a nonspecific manner; they represent expressions of the hereditary predisposition to coronary heart disease. A few specific syndromes, such as congenital long QT interval syndromes (Chap. 230), right ventricular dysplasia, and the syndrome of right bundle branch block and non-ischemic ST-segment elevations (Brugada syndrome), are char-

STRUCTURAL CAUSES

I. Coronary heart disease
   A. Coronary artery abnormalities
      1. Chronic atherosclerotic lesions
      2. Acute (active) lesions (plaque fissuring, platelet aggregation, acute thrombosis)
      3. Anomalous coronary artery anatomy
   B. Myocardial infarction
      1. Healed
      2. Acute
II. Myocardial hypertrophy
   A. Secondary
   B. Hypertrophic cardiomyopathy
      1. Obstructive
      2. Nonobstructive
III. Dilated cardiomyopathy—primary muscle disease
IV. Inflammatory and infiltrative disorders
   A. Myocarditis
   B. Noninfectious inflammatory diseases
   C. Infiltrative diseases
V. Valvular heart disease
VI. Electrophysiologic abnormalities, structural
   A. Anomalous pathways in Wolff-Parkinson-White syndrome
   B. Conducting system disease
   C. Membrane channel structure (e.g., congenital long QT syndrome)

FUNCTIONAL CONTRIBUTING FACTORS

I. Alterations of coronary blood flow
   A. Transient ischemia
   B. Reperfusion after ischemia
II. Low cardiac output states
   A. Heart failure
      1. Chronic
      2. Acute decompensation
   B. Shock
III. Systemic metabolic abnormalities
   A. Electrolyte imbalance (e.g., hypokalemia)
   B. Hypoxemia, acidosis
IV. Neurophysiologic disturbances
   A. Autonomic fluctuations: central, neural, humoral
   B. Receptor function
V. Toxic responses
   A. Proarrhythmic drug effects
   B. Cardiac toxins (e.g., cocaine, digitalis intoxication)
   C. Drug interactions

acterized by specific hereditary risk of SCD. There are also recent data suggesting a familial predispositon to SCD as a specific pattern of coronary heart disease expression.

The major categories of structural causes of, and functional factors contributing to, the SCD syndrome are listed in Table 39-2. Worldwide, and especially in western cultures, coronary atherosclerotic heart disease is the most common structural abnormality associated with SCD. Up to 80% of all SCDs in the United States are due to the consequences of coronary atherosclerosis. The cardiomyopathies (dilated and hypertrophic, collectively; Chap. 239) account for another 10 to 15% of SCDs, and all the remaining diverse etiologies cause only 5 to 10% of these events. Transient ischemia in the previously scarred or hypertrophied heart, hemodynamic and fluid and electrolyte disturbances, fluctuations in autonomic nervous system activity, and transient electrophysiologic changes caused by drugs or other chemicals (e.g., proarrhythmia) have all been implicated as mechanisms responsible for transition from electrophysiologic stability to instability. In addition, reperfusion of ischemic myocardium may cause transient electrophysiologic instability and arrhythmias.

PATHOLOGY   Data from postmortem examinations of SCD victims parallel the clinical observations on the prevalence of coronary heart disease as the major structural etiologic factor. More than 80% of SCD victims have pathologic findings of coronary heart disease. The pathologic description often includes a combination of long-standing, extensive atherosclerosis of the epicardial coronary arteries and

acute active coronary lesions, which include a combination of fissured or ruptured plaques, platelet aggregates, hemorrhage, and thrombosis. In one study, chronic coronary atherosclerosis involving two or more major vessels with ≥75% stenosis was observed in 75% of the victims. In another study, atherosclerotic plaque fissuring, platelet aggregates, and/or acute thrombosis were observed in 95 of 100 individuals who had pathologic studies after SCD.

As many as 70 to 75% of males who die suddenly have prior myocardial infarctions (MIs), but only 20 to 30% have recent acute MIs. A high incidence of left ventricular (LV) hypertrophy coexists with prior MIs.

CLINICAL DEFINITION OF FORMS OF CARDIOVASCULAR COLLAPSE (Table 39-1)   *Cardiovascular collapse* is a general term connoting loss of effective blood flow due to acute dysfunction of the heart and/or peripheral vasculature. Cardiovascular collapse may be caused by vasodepressor syncope (vasovagal syncope, postural hypotension with syncope, neurocardiogenic syncope—Chap. 21), a transient severe bradycardia, or cardiac arrest. The latter is distinguished from the transient forms of cardiovascular collapse in that it usually requires an intervention to achieve resuscitation. In contrast, vasodepressor syncope and many primary bradyarrhythmic syncopal events are transient and non-life-threatening, with spontaneous return of consciousness.

The most common electrical mechanism for true cardiac arrest is ventricular fibrillation (VF), which is responsible for 65 to 80% of cardiac arrests. Severe persistent bradyarrhythmias, asystole, and pulseless electrical activity (an organized electrical activity without mechanical response, formerly called electomechanical dissociation) cause another 20 to 30%. Sustained ventricular tachycardia (VT) with hypotension is a less common cause. Acute low cardiac output states, having precipitous onset, also may present clinically as a cardiac arrest. The causes include massive acute pulmonary emboli, internal blood loss from ruptured aortic aneurysm, intense anaphylaxis, cardiac rupture after myocardial infarction, and unexpected fatal arrhythmia due to electrolyte disturbances.

CLINICAL CHARACTERISTICS OF CARDIAC ARREST

PRODROME, ONSET, ARREST, DEATH   SCD may be presaged by days, weeks, or months of increasing angina, dyspnea, palpitations, easy fatigability, and other nonspecific complaints. However, these *prodromal complaints* are generally predictive of any major cardiac event; they are not specific for predicting SCD.

The *onset of the terminal event*, leading to cardiac arrest, is defined as an acute change in cardiovascular status preceding cardiac arrest by up to 1 h. When the onset is instantaneous or abrupt, the probability that the arrest is cardiac in origin is >95%. Continuous ECG recordings, fortuitously obtained at the onset of a cardiac arrest, commonly demonstrate changes in cardiac electrical activity in the minutes or hours before the event. There is a tendency for the heart rate to increase and for advanced grades of premature ventricular contractions (PVCs) to evolve. Most cardiac arrests that are caused by VF begin with a run of sustained or nonsustained VT, which then degenerates into VF.

Sudden unexpected loss of effective circulation may be separated into "arrhythmic events" and "circulatory failure." Arrhythmic events are characterized by a high likelihood of patients being awake and active immediately prior to the event, are dominated by VF as the electrical mechanism, and have a short duration of terminal illness (<1 h). In contrast, circulatory failure deaths occur in patients who are inactive or comatose, have a higher incidence of asystole than VF, have a tendency to a longer duration of terminal illness, and are dominated by noncardiac events preceding the terminal illness.

The onset of cardiac arrest may be characterized by typical symptoms of an acute cardiac event, such as prolonged angina or the pain of onset of MI, acute dyspnea or orthopnea, or the sudden onset of palpitations, sustained tachycardia, or light-headedness. However, in many patients, the onset is precipitous, with minimal forewarning.

Cardiac arrest is, by definition, abrupt. Mentation may be impaired in patients with sustained VT during the onset of the terminal event. However, complete loss of consciousness is a *sine qua non* in cardiac arrest. Although rare spontaneous reversions occur, it is usual that cardiac arrest progresses to death within minutes (i.e., SCD has occurred) if active interventions are not undertaken promptly.

The probability of achieving successful resuscitation from cardiac arrest is related to the interval from onset to institution of resuscitative efforts, the setting in which the event occurs, the mechanism (VF, VT, pulseless electrical activity, asystole), and the clinical status of the patient prior to the cardiac arrest. Those settings in which it is possible to institute prompt cardiopulmonary resuscitation (CPR) provide a better chance of a successful outcome. However, the outcome in intensive care units and other in-hospital environments is heavily influenced by the patient's preceding clinical status. The immediate outcome is good for cardiac arrest occurring in the intensive care unit in the presence of an acute cardiac event or transient metabolic disturbance, but the outcome for patients with far-advanced chronic cardiac disease or advanced noncardiac diseases (e.g., renal failure, pneumonia, sepsis, diabetes, cancer) is not much more successful in hospital than in the out-of-hospital setting.

The success rate for initial resuscitation and survival to hospital discharge after an out-of-hospital cardiac arrest depends in part on the mechanism of the event. When the mechanism is VT, the outcome is best; VF is the next most successful; and asystole and pulseless electrical activity generate dismal outcome statistics (Fig. 39-1). Advanced age also influences adversely the chances of successful resuscitation.

Progression to biologic death is a function of the mechanism of cardiac arrest and the length of the delay before interventions. VF or asystole without CPR within the first 4 to 6 min has a poor outcome, and there are few survivors among patients who had no life support activities for the first 8 min after onset. Outcome statistics are improved by lay bystander intervention (basic life support—see below) prior to definitive interventions (advanced life support—defibrillation) and even more by early defibrillation. In regard to the latter, the notion that deployment of automatic external defibrillators in communities

(e.g., police vehicles, large buildings, stadiums, etc.) will result in improved survival is currently being evaluated.

Death during the hospitalization after a successfully resuscitated cardiac arrest relates closely to the severity of central nervous system injury. Anoxic encephalopathy and infections subsequent to prolonged respirator dependence account for 60% of the deaths. Another 30% occur as a consequence of low cardiac output states that fail to respond to interventions. Recurrent arrhythmias are the least common cause of death, accounting for only 10% of in-hospital deaths.

In the setting of acute MI, it is important to distinguish between primary and secondary cardiac arrests. *Primary* cardiac arrests refer to those that occur in the absence of hemodynamic instability, and *secondary* cardiac arrests are those that occur in patients in whom abnormal hemodynamics dominate the clinical picture before cardiac arrest. The success rate for immediate resuscitation in primary cardiac arrest during acute MI in a monitored setting should approach 100%. In contrast, as many as 70% of patients with secondary cardiac arrest succumb immediately or during the same hospitalization.

IDENTIFICATION OF PATIENTS AT RISK FOR SUDDEN CARDIAC DEATH Primary prevention of cardiac arrest depends on the ability to identify individual patients at high risk. One must view the problem in the context of the total number of events and the population pools from which they are derived. The annual incidence of SCD among an unselected adult population is 1 to 2 per 1000 population (Fig. 39-2A), largely reflecting the prevalence of those coronary heart disease patients among whom SCD is the first clinically recognized manifestation (20 to 25% of first coronary events are SCD). The incidence (percent per year) increases progressively with the addition of identified coronary risk factors to populations free of prior coronary events. The most powerful factors are age, elevated blood pressure, LV hypertrophy, cigarette smoking, elevated serum cholesterol level, obesity, and nonspecific electrocardiographic abnormalities. These coronary risk factors are not specific for SCD but rather represent increasing risk for all coronary deaths. The proportion of coronary deaths that are sudden remains at approximately 50% in all risk categories. Despite the marked *relative* increased risk of SCD with addition of multiple risk factors (from 1 to 2 per 1000 population per year in an unselected population to as much as 50 to 60 per 1000 in subgroups having multiple risk factors for coronary artery disease), the *absolute* incidence remains relatively low when viewed as the relationship between the number of individuals who have a preventive intervention and the number of events that can be prevented. Specifically, a 50% reduction in annual SCD risk would be a huge *relative* decrease but would require an intervention in up to 200 unselected individuals to prevent one sudden death. These figures highlight the importance of primary prevention of coronary heart disease. Control of coronary risk factors may be the only practical method to prevent SCD in major segments of the population, because of the paradox that the majority of events occur in the large unselected subgroups rather than in the specific high-risk subgroups (compare "Events/Year" with "Percent/Year" in Fig. 39-2A). Under most conditions of higher level of risk, particularly those indexed to a recent major cardiovascular event (e.g., MI, recent onset of heart failure, survival after out-of-hospital cardiac arrest), the highest risk of sudden death occurs within the initial 6 to 18 months and then decreases toward baseline risk of the underlying disease (Fig. 39-2B). Accordingly, preventive interventions are most likely to be effective when initiated early.

For patients with acute or prior clinical manifestations of coronary heart disease, high-risk subgroups having a much higher ratio of SCD risk to population base can be identified. The acute, convalescent, and chronic phases of MI provide large population subsets with more highly focused risk (Chap. 243). The potential risk of cardiac arrest from the onset through the first 72 h after acute MI (the acute phase) may be as high as 15 to 20%. The highest risk of SCD in relation to MI is found in the subgroup that has experienced sustained VT or VF during the convalescent phase (3 days to 8 weeks) after MI. A greater than 50% mortality in 6 to 12 months has been observed among these patients, when managed with conservative medical therapy, and

	Ventricular fibrillation	Ventricular tachycardia	Asystole / Brady-arrhythmia	TOTAL
Out-of-hospital cardiac arrests	220	24	108	352
	↓ (40%)	↓ (88%)	↓ (9%)	↓ (33%)
Resuscitated and hospitalized	87	21	9	117
	↓ (59%)	↓ (76%)	↓ (−)	↓ (57%)
Discharged	51	16	0	67

FIGURE 39-1 Initial electrophysiologic mechanisms recorded during out-of-hospital cardiac arrest. The figures highlighted by the boxes indicate the number of patients in each of three mechanism categories (ventricular fibrillation, ventricular tachycardia, and bradyarrhythmia/asystole). In each category, the data indicate the number of prehospital cardiac arrests (*top*), the number of patients successfully resuscitated in the field and transferred to the hospital alive (*middle*), and the number of patients who survived to be discharged from hospital (*bottom*). The percentages in parentheses indicate survivals between each level of care for each category. (*Modified from RJ Myerburg et al: Clinical, electrophysiologic, and hemodynamic profile of patients resuscitated from prehospital cardiac arrest. Am J Med 68:568, 1980, with permission.*)

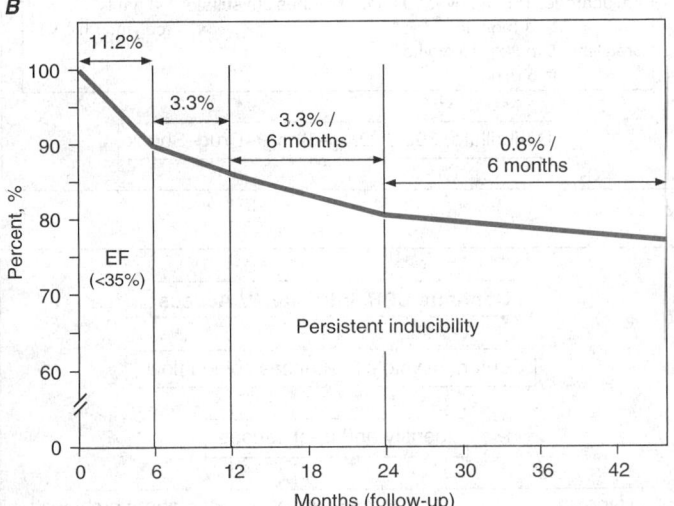

B

FIGURE 39-2 *A.* Incidence of sudden and nonsudden cardiac deaths in population subgroups, and the relation of total number of events per year to incidence figures. Approximations of subgroup incidence figures, and the related population pool from which they are derived, are presented. Approximately 50% of all cardiac deaths are sudden and unexpected. The incidence triangle on the left ("Percent/Year") indicates the approximate percentage of sudden and nonsudden deaths in each of the population subgroups indicated, ranging from the lowest percentage in unselected adult populations (0.1 to 2% per year) to the highest percentage in patients with VT or VF during convalescence after an MI (approximately 50% per year). The triangle on the right indicates the total number of events per year in each of these groups, to reflect incidence in context with the size of the population subgroups. The highest risk categories identify the smallest number of total annual events, and the lowest incidence category accounts for the largest number of events per year. (EF, ejection fraction; VT, ventricular tachycardia; VF, ventricular fibrillation; MI, myocardial infarction.) *B.* Time dependence of risk among survivors of out-of-hospital cardiac arrest. Recurrence risk is highest in the first 6 months of the index event. Survival is expressed as a percentage. High risk is best predicted initially by an ejection fraction ≤ 35% during the first 6 months, and subsequently persistent inducibility of VT during electrophysiologic testing becomes an added major risk. *n* = 101 at *t* = 0. *[After T Furukawa et al, in RJ Myerburg et al, Circulation 85(Suppl 1):2, 1992. Reproduced with permission of the American Heart Association.]*

at least 50% of the deaths are sudden. Aggressive intervention techniques may reduce this incidence.

After the acute phase of MI, long-term risk for total mortality and SCD are predicted by a number of factors. The most important for both SCD and non-SCD is the extent of myocardial damage sustained during the acute event. This is measured by the degree of reduction in the ejection fraction (EF), functional capacity, and/or the occurrence of heart failure. Increasing *frequency* of postinfarction PVCs, with a plateau above the range of 10 to 30 PVCs per hour on 24-h ambulatory

monitor recordings, also indicates increased risk, but advanced *forms* (salvos, nonsustained VT) may be more powerful predictors. PVCs interact strongly with decreased left ventricular EF. The combination of frequent PVCs, salvos or nonsustained VT, and an EF ≤ 35% identifies patients who have an annual risk of greater than 20%. The risk falls off sharply with decreasing PVC frequency and the absence of advanced forms, as well as with higher EF. Despite the risk implications of postinfarction PVCs, improved outcome as a result of PVC suppression has not been demonstrated (Chap. 230).

The extent of underlying disease due to any cause and/or prior clinical expression of risk of SCD (i.e., survival after out-of-hospital cardiac arrest not associated with acute MI) identify patients at very high risk for subsequent (recurrent) cardiac arrest. Survival after out-of-hospital cardiac arrest predicts up to a 30% 1-year recurrent cardiac arrest rate in the absence of specific interventions (see below).

A general rule is that the risk of SCD is approximately one-half the total cardiovascular mortality rate. As shown in Fig. 39-2A, the very high risk subgroups provide more focused population fractions ("Percent/Year") for predicting cardiac arrest or SCD; but the impact on the overall population, indicated by the absolute number of preventable events ("Events/Year"), is considerably smaller. The requirements for achieving a major population impact are effective prevention of the underlying diseases and/or new epidemiologic probes that will allow better resolution of subgroups within large general populations.

℞ TREATMENT The individual who collapses suddenly is managed in four stages: (1) the initial response and basic life support; (2) advanced life support; (3) postresuscitation care; and (4) long-term management. The initial response and basic life support can be carried out by physicians, nurses, paramedical personnel, and trained lay persons. There is a requirement for increasingly specialized skills as the patient moves through the stages of advanced life support, postresuscitation care, and long-term management.

Initial Response and Basic Life Support The initial response will confirm whether a sudden collapse is indeed due to a cardiac arrest. Observations for respiratory movements, skin color, and the presence or absence of pulses in the carotid or femoral arteries will promptly determine whether a life-threatening cardiac arrest has occurred. As soon as a cardiac arrest is suspected or confirmed, contacting an emergency rescue system (e.g., 911) should be the immediate priority.

Agonal respiratory movements may persist for a short time after the onset of cardiac arrest, but it is important to observe for severe stridor with a persistent pulse as a clue to aspiration of a foreign body or food. If this is suspected, a Heimlich maneuver (see below) may dislodge the obstructing body. A precordial blow, or "thump," delivered firmly by the clenched fist to the junction of the middle and lower third of the sternum may occasionally revert VT or VF, but there is concern about converting VT *to* VF. Therefore, it has been recommended to use precordial thumps as an advanced life support technique when monitoring and defibrillation are available. This conservative application of the technique remains controversial.

The third action during the initial response is to clear the airway. The head is tilted back and chin lifted so that the oropharynx can be explored to clear the airway. Dentures or foreign bodies are removed, and the Heimlich maneuver is performed if there is reason to suspect that a foreign body is lodged in the oropharynx. If respiratory arrest precipitating cardiac arrest is suspected, a second precordial thump is delivered after the airway is cleared.

Basic life support, more popularly known as CPR, is intended to maintain organ perfusion until definitive interventions can be instituted. The elements of CPR are the maintenance of ventilation of the lungs and compression of the chest. Mouth-to-mouth respiration may be used if no specific rescue equipment is immediately available (e.g., plastic oropharyngeal airways, esophageal obturators, masked Ambu bag). Conventional ventilation techniques during CPR require the lungs to be inflated 10 to 12 times per minute, i.e., once every fifth chest compression when two persons are performing the resuscitation and twice in succession every 15 chest compressions when one person is carrying out both ventilation and chest wall compression.

Chest compression is based on the assumption that cardiac compression allows the heart to maintain a pump function by sequential filling and emptying of its chambers, with competent valves maintaining forward direction of flow. The palm of one hand is placed over the lower sternum, with the heel of the other resting on the dorsum of the lower hand. The sternum is depressed, with the arms remaining straight, at a rate of approximately 80 to 100 per minute. Sufficient force is applied to depress the sternum 3 to 5 cm, and relaxation is abrupt.

Advanced Life Support Advanced life support is intended to achieve adequate ventilation, control cardiac arrhythmias, stabilize blood pressure and cardiac output, and restore organ perfusion. The activities carried out to achieve these goals include (1) intubation with an endotracheal tube, (2) defibrillation/cardioversion and/or pacing, and (3) insertion of an intravenous line. Ventilation with O_2 (room air if O_2 is not immediately available) may promptly reverse hypoxemia and acidosis. The speed with which defibrillation/cardioversion is carried out is an important element for successful resuscitation. When possible, immediate defibrillation should precede intubation and insertion of an intravenous line; CPR should be carried out while the defibrillator is being charged. As soon as a diagnosis of VT or VF is obtained, a 200-J shock should be delivered. Additional shocks at higher energies, up to a maximum of 360 J, are tried if the initial shock does not successfully abolish VT or VF. Epinephrine, 1 mg intravenously, is given after failed defibrillation, and attempts to defibrillate are repeated. The dose of epinephrine may be repeated after intervals of 3 to 5 min (see Fig. 39-3A).

If the patient is less than fully conscious upon reversion, or if two or three attempts fail, prompt intubation, ventilation, and arterial blood gas analysis should be carried out. Intravenous $NaHCO_3$, which was formerly used in large quantities, is no longer considered routinely necessary and may be dangerous in larger quantities. However, the patient who is persistently acidotic after successful defibrillation and intubation should be given 1 meq/kg $NaHCO_3$ initially and an additional 50% of the dose repeated every 10 to 15 min.

After initial unsuccessful defibrillation attempts, or with persistent electrical instability, a bolus of 1 mg/kg lidocaine is given intravenously (Chap. 243), and the dose is repeated in 2 min in those patients who have persistent ventricular arrhythmias or remain in VF. This is followed by a continuous infusion at a rate of 1 to 4 mg/min. If lidocaine fails to provide control, other antiarrhythmic therapies should be tried. For persistent, hemodynamically unstable ventricular arrhythmias, intravenous amiodarone has emerged as the treatment of choice (150 mg over 10 min, followed by 1 mg/min for up to 6 h, and 0.5 mg/min thereafter) (Fig. 39-3A). Intravenous procainamide (loading infusion of 100 mg/5 min to a total dose of 500 to 800 mg, followed by continuous infusion at 2 to 5 mg/min) may be tried for persisting, hemodynamically stable arrhythmias; or bretylium tosylate (loading dose 5 to 10 mg/kg in 5 min; maintenance dose 0.5 to 2 mg/min) may be tried as an alternative for unstable arrhythmias. Intravenous calcium gluconate is no longer considered safe or necessary for routine administration. It is used only in patients in whom acute hyperkalemia is known to be the triggering event for resistant VF, in the presence of known hypocalcemia, or in patients who have received toxic doses of calcium channel antagonists.

Cardiac arrest secondary to bradyarrhythmias or asystole is managed differently (Fig. 39-3B). The patient is promptly intubated, CPR is continued, and an attempt is made to control hypoxemia and acidosis. Epinephrine and/or atropine are given intravenously or by an intracardiac route. External pacing devices are now available to attempt to establish a regular rhythm, but the prognosis is generally very poor in this form of cardiac arrest, even with successful electrical pac-

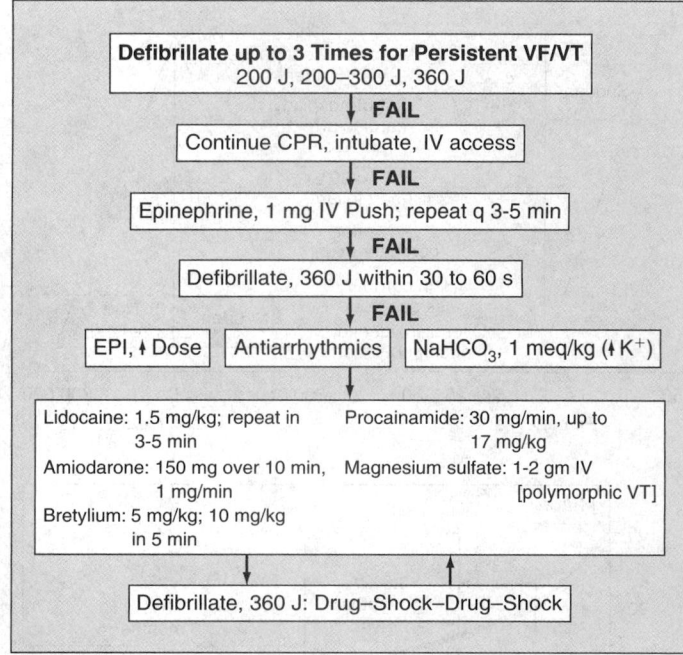

FIGURE 39-3 Management of cardiac arrest. *A.* The algorithm of ventricular fibrillation or hypotensive ventricular tachycardia begins with defibrillation attempts. If that fails, it is followed by epinephrine and then antiarrhythmic drugs. See text for details. *B.* The algorithms for bradyarrhythmia/asystole *(left)* or pulseless electrical activity *(right)* is dominated first by continued life support and a search for reversible causes. Subsequent therapy is nonspecific and accompanied by a low success rate. See text for details.

ing. Pulseless electrical activity (PEA) is treated similarly to bradyarrhythmias, but its outcome is also dismal. The one exception is bradyarrhythmic/asystolic cardiac arrest secondary to airway obstruction. This form of cardiac arrest may respond promptly to removal of foreign bodies by the Heimlich maneuver or, in hospitalized patients, by intubation and suctioning of obstructing secretions in the airway.

Postresuscitation Care This phase of management is determined by the clinical setting of the cardiac arrest. *Primary* VF in acute MI (Chap. 243) is generally very responsive to life-support techniques and easily controlled after the initial event. Patients are maintained on a lidocaine infusion at the rate of 2 to 4 mg/min for 24 to 72 h after the event. In the in-hospital setting, respirator support is usually not necessary or is needed for only a short time, and hemodynamics stabilize promptly after defibrillation or cardioversion. In *secondary* VF in acute MI (those events in which hemodynamic abnormalities predispose to the potentially fatal arrhythmia), resuscitative efforts are less often successful, and in those patients who are successfully resuscitated, the recurrence rate is high. The clinical picture and outcome are dominated by hemodynamic instability and the ability to control hemodynamic dysfunction. Bradyarrhythmias, asystole, and pulseless electrical activity are commonly secondary events in hemodynamically unstable patients.

The outcome after in-hospital cardiac arrest associated with *noncardiac* diseases is poor, and in the few successfully resuscitated patients, the postresuscitation course is dominated by the nature of the underlying disease. Patients with cancer, renal failure, acute central nervous system disease, and uncontrolled infections, as a group, have a survival rate of less than 10% after in-hospital cardiac arrest. Some major exceptions are patients with transient airway obstruction, electrolyte disturbances, proarrhythmic effects of drugs, and severe metabolic abnormalities, most of whom may have an excellent chance of survival if they can be resuscitated promptly and maintained while the transient abnormalities are being corrected.

Long-Term Management after Survival of Out-of-Hospital Cardiac Arrest   Patients who do not suffer irreversible injury of the central nervous system and who achieve hemodynamic stability should have extensive diagnostic and therapeutic testing to guide long-term management. This aggressive approach is driven by the fact that statistics from the 1970s indicated survival after out-of-hospital cardiac arrest was followed by a 30% recurrent cardiac arrest rate at 1 year, 45% at 2 years, and a total mortality rate of almost 60% at 2 years. Historical comparisons suggest that these dismal statistics may be significantly improved by newer interventions, but the magnitude of the improvement is unknown because of the lack of concurrently controlled intervention studies.

Among those patients in whom an acute transmural MI is the cause of out-of-hospital cardiac arrest, the management is the same as in any other patient who suffers cardiac arrest during the acute phase of a documented MI (Chap. 243). For almost all other categories of patients, however, extensive diagnostic studies are carried out to determine etiology, functional impairment, and electrophysiologic instability as guides to future management. In general, patients who have out-of-hospital cardiac arrest due to chronic ischemic heart disease, without an acute MI, are evaluated to determine whether transient ischemia or chronic electrophysiologic instability was the more likely cause of the event. If there is reason to suspect an ischemic mechanism, coronary revascularization by angioplasty or bypass surgery, plus drugs (most commonly beta blockers), are used to reduce ischemic burden.

Electrophysiologic instability has been identified by the use of programmed electrical stimulation to determine whether sustained VT or VF can be induced (Chap. 230). If so, this information can be used as a baseline against which to evaluate drug efficacy for prevention of inducibility. The rationale for this approach is the assumption that suppression of inducibility predicts long-term benefit by the drug that achieves such suppression. For patients for whom successful drug therapy could not be identified by this technique, insertion of an implantable cardioverter-defibrillator (ICD), antiarrhythmic surgery (e.g., coronary bypass surgery aneurysmectomy, cryoablation), or empiric amiodarone therapy have been recommended (Chap. 230). Primary surgical success, defined as surviving the procedure and reverting to a noninducible status without drug therapy, is better than 90% when patients are selected for ability to be mapped in the operating room. However, only a small fraction of patients meet the criteria. In addition, VT/VF *cannot* be induced in a number of survivors of cardiac arrest (30 to 50%), and inducible arrhythmias can be suppressed by drugs in no more than 20 to 30% of those whose arrhythmias can be induced. Because of these limitations of drug therapy and surgical approaches, ICD therapy has evolved into the most commonly used strategy for cardiac arrest survivors. ICDs have long been recognized to have very good success rates for sensing and reverting life-threatening arrhythmias, but improvement in long-term total survival outcomes remained lacking until a number of studies solidified the benefit of ICD therapy for specific subgroups. After empiric amiodarone therapy had been suggested to be as good as, or better than, conventional antiarrhythmic drug therapy for survivors of cardiac arrest, ICDs were demonstrated to be superior to amiodarone. Moreover, ICDs were also found to be superior for high risk patients with VT after myocardial infarction.

BIBLIOGRAPHY

AKHTAR M et al: Implantable cardioverter-defibrillator therapy for prevention of sudden cardiac death. Cardiol Clin 11:97, 1993

CUMMINS RO et al: Improving survival from sudden cardiac arrest: The "chain of survival" concept. Circulation 83:1832, 1991

EMERGENCY CARDIAC CARE COMMITTEE AND SUBCOMMITTEES, AMERICAN HEART ASSOCIATION: Guidelines for cardiopulmonary resuscitation and emergency cardiac care. JAMA 268:2172, 1992

EWY GA, ORNATO JP: Emergency Cardiac Care Task Force 1: Cardiac arrest. J Am Coll Cardiol 35:832, 2000

JOSLYN et al: Survival from out-of-hospital cardiac arrest: Effects of patient age and presence of 911 Emergency Medical Services phone access. Am J Emerg Med 11:200, 1993

KANNEL WB, SCHATZKIN A: Sudden death: Lessons from subsets in population studies. J Am Coll Cardiol 5(Suppl 6):141B, 1985

MYERBURG RJ, CASTELLANOS A: Cardiac arrest and sudden cardiac death, in *Heart Disease*, 6th ed, E Braunwald et al (eds). Philadelphia, Saunders, 2001

MYERBURG RJ, CASTELLANOS A et al: Epidemiology, transient risk, and intervention assessment. Ann Intern Med 119:1187, 1993

ORNATO JP: Use of adrenergic agonists during CPR in adults. Ann Emerg Med 22:411, 1993

WILBER DJ et al: Out-of-hospital cardiac arrest: Use of electrophysiologic testing in the prediction of long-term outcome. N Engl J Med 318:19, 1988

Section 6
ALTERATIONS IN GASTROINTESTINAL FUNCTION

40   *Raj K. Goyal*

DYSPHAGIA

Dysphagia is defined as a sensation of "sticking" or obstruction of the passage of food through the mouth, pharynx, or esophagus. It should be distinguished from other symptoms related to swallowing. *Aphagia* signifies complete esophageal obstruction, which is usually due to bolus impaction and represents a medical emergency. *Difficulty in initiating a swallow* occurs in disorders of the voluntary phase of swallowing. However, once initiated, swallowing is completed normally. *Odynophagia* means painful swallowing. Frequently, odynophagia and dysphagia occur together. *Globus pharyngeous* is the sensation of a lump lodged in the throat. However, no difficulty is encountered when swallowing is performed. *Misdirection of food*, resulting in nasal regurgitation and laryngeal and pulmonary aspiration of food during swallowing, is characteristic of oropharyngeal dysphagia. *Phagophobia*, meaning fear of swallowing, and *refusal to swallow* may occur in hysteria, rabies, tetanus, and pharyngeal paralysis due to fear of aspiration. Painful inflammatory lesions that cause odynophagia may also cause refusal to swallow. Some patients may feel the food as it goes down the esophagus. This esophageal sensitivity is not associated with either food sticking or obstruction, however. Similarly, the *feeling of fullness in the epigastrium* that occurs after a meal or after swallowing air should not be confused with dysphagia.

PHYSIOLOGY OF SWALLOWING   The process of swallowing begins with a voluntary (oral) phase during which a bolus of food is pushed into the pharynx by the contraction of the tongue. The bolus then activates oropharyngeal sensory receptors that initiate the involuntary (pharyngeal and esophageal) phase, or deglutition reflex. The deglutition reflex is a complex series of events and serves both to propel food through the pharynx and the esophagus and to prevent its entry into the airway. When the bolus is propelled backward by the tongue, the larynx moves forward and the upper esophageal sphincter opens. As the bolus moves into the pharynx, contraction of the superior pharyngeal constrictor against the contracted soft palate initiates a peristaltic contraction that proceeds rapidly downward to move the bolus through the pharynx and the esophagus. The lower esophageal sphincter opens as the food enters the esophagus and remains open until the peristaltic contraction has swept the bolus into the stomach. Peristaltic contraction in response to a swallow is called *primary peristalsis*. It involves inhibition followed by sequential contraction of muscles along the entire swallowing passage. The inhibition that precedes the peristaltic contraction is called *deglutitive inhibition*. Local distention of the esophagus from food activates intramural reflexes in the smooth muscle and results in *secondary peristalsis*, which is limited to the thoracic esophagus. *Tertiary contractions* are nonperistaltic because they occur simultaneously over a long segment of the esophagus. Tertiary contractions may occur in response to a swallow or esophageal distention, or they may occur spontaneously.

PATHOPHYSIOLOGY OF DYSPHAGIA   The normal transport of an ingested bolus through the swallowing passage depends on the size of the ingested bolus; the luminal diameter of the swallowing passage; the force of peristaltic contraction; and deglutitive inhibition, including normal relaxation of upper and lower esophageal sphincters during swallowing. Dysphagia caused by a large bolus or luminal narrowing is called *mechanical dysphagia*, whereas dysphagia due to weakness of peristaltic contractions or to impaired deglutitive inhibition causing nonperistaltic contractions and impaired sphincter relaxation is called *motor dysphagia*.

Mechanical Dysphagia   Mechanical dysphagia can be caused by a very large food bolus, intrinsic narrowing, or extrinsic compression of the lumen. In an adult, the esophageal lumen can distend up to 4 cm in diameter. When the esophagus cannot dilate beyond 2.5 cm in diameter, dysphagia to normal solid food can occur. Dysphagia is always present when the esophagus cannot distend beyond 1.3 cm. Circumferential lesions produce dysphagia more consistently than do lesions that involve only a portion of circumferences of the esophageal wall, as uninvolved segments retain their distensibility. The causes of mechanical dysphagia are listed in Table 40-1. Common causes include carcinoma, peptic and other benign strictures, and lower esophageal ring.

Motor Dysphagia   Motor dysphagia may result from difficulty in initiating a swallow or from abnormalities in peristalsis and deglutitive inhibition due to diseases of the esophageal striated or smooth muscle.

Diseases of the striated muscle involve the pharynx, upper esophageal sphincter, and cervical esophagus. The striated muscle is innervated by a somatic component of the vagus with cell bodies of the lower motor neurons located in the nucleus ambiguus. These neurons are cholinergic and excitatory and are the sole determinant of the muscle activity. Peristalsis in the striated muscle segment is due to sequential central activation of neurons innervating muscles at different levels along the esophagus. Motor dysphagia of the pharynx results from neuromuscular disorders causing muscle paralysis, simultaneous nonperistaltic contraction, or loss of opening of the upper esophageal sphincter. Loss of opening of the upper sphincter is caused by paralysis of geniohyoid and other suprahyoid muscles or loss of deglutitive inhibition of the cricopharyngeus muscle. Because each side of the pharynx is innervated by ipsilateral nerves, a unilateral lesion of motor neurons leads to unilateral pharyngeal paralysis. Although lesions of striated muscle also involve the cervical part of the esophagus, the clinical manifestations of pharyngeal dysfunction usually overshadow those due to esophageal involvement.

Diseases of the smooth-muscle segment involve the thoracic part of the esophagus and the lower esophageal sphincter. The smooth muscle is innervated by the parasympathetic component of the vagal preganglionic fibers and postganglionic neurons in the myenteric ganglia. The vagal pathway consists of parallel excitatory and inhibitory pathways that use acetylcholine and nitric oxide as neurotransmitters, respectively. The activation of inhibitory nerves causes inhibition that is followed by rebound contraction. These pathways are involved in the resting tone of the lower esophageal sphincter as well as swallow-induced lower esophageal sphincter opening and inhibition followed by peristaltic contractions in the esophageal body. Dysphagia results when the peristaltic contractions are weak or nonperistaltic or when the lower sphincter fails to relax normally. Loss of contractile power occurs due to muscle weakness, as in scleroderma. The nonperistaltic contractions and impaired relaxation of the lower esophageal sphincter result from a defect in inhibitory vagal innervation and account for dysphagia in achalasia.

The causes of motor dysphagia are also listed in Table 40-1. Important causes are pharyngeal paralysis, cricopharyngeal achalasia, scleroderma of the esophagus, achalasia, and diffuse esophageal spasm and related motor disorders.

Approach to the Patient

History   The history can provide a presumptive diagnosis in over 80% of patients. The type of food causing dysphagia provides useful information. Difficulty only with solids implies mechanical dysphagia with a lumen that is not severely narrowed. In advanced obstruction, dysphagia occurs with liquids as well as solids. In contrast, motor dysphagia due to achalasia and diffuse esophageal spasm is equally affected by solids and liquids from the very onset. Patients with scleroderma have dysphagia to solids that is unrelated to posture and to liquids while recumbent but not upright. When peptic stricture develops in patients with scleroderma, dysphagia becomes more persistent.

The duration and course of dysphagia are helpful in diagnosis. Transient dysphagia may be due to an inflammatory process. Progressive dysphagia lasting a few weeks to a few months is suggestive of carcinoma of the esophagus. Episodic dysphagia to solids lasting several years indicates a benign disease characteristic of a lower esophageal ring.

The site of dysphagia described by the patient helps to determine the site of esophageal obstruction; the lesion is at or below the perceived location of dysphagia.

Associated symptoms provide important diagnostic clues. Nasal regurgitation and tracheobronchial aspiration with swallowing are hallmarks of pharyngeal paralysis or a tracheoesophageal fistula. Tracheobronchial aspiration unrelated to swallowing may be secondary to achalasia, Zenker's diverticulum, or gastroesophageal reflux.

Severe weight loss that is out of proportion to the degree of dysphagia is highly suggestive of carcinoma. When hoarseness precedes dysphagia, the primary lesion is usually in the larynx. Hoarseness following dysphagia may suggest involvement of the recurrent laryngeal nerve by extension of esophageal carcinoma. Sometimes hoarseness may be due to laryngitis secondary to gastroesophageal reflux. Association of laryngeal symptoms and dysphagia also occurs in various neuromuscular disorders. Hiccups may rarely occur with a lesion in

Table 40-1 Causes of Dysphagia

MECHANICAL DYSPHAGIA	MOTOR (NEUROMUSCULAR) DYSPHAGIA

I. Luminal
 A. Large bolus
 B. Foreign body
II. Intrinsic narrowing
 A. Inflammatory condition causing edema and swelling
  1. Stomatitis
  2. Pharyngitis, epiglottitis
  3. Esophagitis
   a. Viral (herpes simplex, varicella-zoster, cytomegalovirus)
   b. Bacterial
   c. Fungal (candidal)
   d. Mucocutaneous bullous diseases
   e. Caustic, chemical, thermal injury
 B. Webs and rings
  1. Pharyngeal (Plummer-Vinson syndrome)
  2. Esophageal (congenital, inflammatory)
  3. Lower esophageal mucosal ring (Schatzki ring)
 C. Benign strictures
  1. Peptic
  2. Caustic and pill-induced
  3. Inflammatory (Crohn's disease, candidal, mucocutaneous lesions)
  4. Ischemic
  5. Postoperative, postirradiation
  6. Congenital
 D. Malignant tumors
  1. Primary carcinoma
   a. Squamous cell carcinoma
   b. Adenocarcinoma
   c. Carcinosarcoma
   d. Pseudosarcoma
   e. Lymphoma
   f. Melanoma
   g. Kaposi's sarcoma
  2. Metastatic carcinoma
 E. Benign tumors
  1. Leiomyoma
  2. Lipoma
  3. Angioma
  4. Inflammatory fibroid polyp
  5. Epithelial papilloma
III. Extrinsic compression
 A. Cervical spondylitis
 B. Vertebral osteophytes
 C. Retropharyngeal abscess and masses
 D. Enlarged thyroid gland
 E. Zenker's diverticulum
 F. Vascular compression
  1. Aberrant right subclavian artery
  2. Right-sided aorta
  3. Left atrial enlargement
  4. Aortic aneurysm
 G. Posterior mediastinal masses
 H. Pancreatic tumor, pancreatitis
 I. Postvagotomy hematoma and fibrosis
	I. Difficulty in initiating swallowing reflex
	 A. Paralysis of the tongue
	 B. Oropharyngeal anesthesia
	 C. Lack of saliva (e.g., Sjögren's syndrome)
	 D. Lesions of sensory components of vagus and glossopharyngeal nerves
	 E. Lesions of swallowing center
	II. Disorders of pharyngeal and esophageal striated muscle
	 A. Muscle weakness
	  1. Lower motor neuron lesion (bulbar paralysis)
	   a. Cerebrovascular accident
	   b. Motor neuron disease
	   c. Poliomyelitis, postpolio syndrome
	   d. Polyneuritis
	   e. Amyotrophic lateral sclerosis
	   f. Familial dysautonomia
	  2. Neuromuscular
	   a. Myasthenia gravis
	  3. Muscle disorders
	   a. Polymyositis
	   b. Dermatomyositis
	   c. Myopathies (myotonic dystrophy, oculopharyngeal myopathy)
	 B. Nonperistaltic contractions or impaired deglutitive inhibition
	  1. Pharynx and upper esophagus
	   a. Rabies
	   b. Tetanus
	   c. Extrapyramidal tract disease
	   d. Upper motor neuron lesions (pseudobulbar paralysis)
	  2. Upper esophageal sphincter (UES)
	   a. Paralysis of suprahyoid muscles (causes same as paralysis of pharyngeal musculature)
	   b. Cricopharyngeal achalasia
	III. Disorders of esophageal smooth muscle
	 A. Paralysis of esophageal body causing weak contractions
	  1. Scleroderma and related collagen-vascular diseases
	  2. Hollow visceral myopathy
	  3. Myotonic dystrophy
	  4. Metabolic neuromyopathy (amyloid, alcohol?, diabetes?)
	  5. Achalasia (classical)
	 B. Nonperistaltic contractions or impaired deglutitive inhibition
	  1. Esophageal body
	   a. Diffuse esophageal spasm
	   b. Achalasia (vigorous)
	   c. Variants of diffuse esophageal spasm
	  2. Lower esophageal sphincter
	   a. Achalasia
	    (1) Primary
	    (2) Secondary
	     (a) Chagas' disease
	     (b) Carcinoma
	     (c) Lymphoma
	     (d) Neuropathic intestinal pseudoobstruction syndrome
	     (e) Toxins and drugs
	   b. Lower esophageal muscular (contractile) ring

the distal portion of the esophagus. Unilateral wheezing with dysphagia indicates a mediastinal mass involving the esophagus and a large bronchus.

Chest pain with dysphagia occurs in diffuse esophageal spasm and related motor disorders. Chest pain resembling diffuse esophageal spasms may occur in esophageal obstruction due to a large bolus. A prolonged history of heartburn and reflux preceding dysphagia indicates peptic stricture. A history of prolonged nasogastric intubation, ingestion of caustic agents, ingestion of pills without water, previous radiation therapy, or associated mucocutaneous diseases may provide the cause of esophageal stricture. If odynophagia is present, candidal or herpes esophagitis or pill-induced esophagitis should be suspected.

In patients with AIDS or other immunodeficiency states, esophagitis due to opportunistic infections such as *Candida*, herpes simplex virus, or cytomegalovirus and tumors such as Kaposi's sarcoma and lymphoma should be suspected.

Physical Examination Physical examination is important in motor dysphagia due to skeletal muscle, neurologic, and oropharyngeal diseases. Signs of bulbar or pseudobulbar palsy, including dysarthria, dysphonia, ptosis, tongue atrophy, and hyperactive jaw jerk, in addition to evidence of generalized neuromuscular disease, should be sought. The neck should be examined for thyromegaly or a spinal abnormality. A careful inspection of the mouth and pharynx should disclose lesions that may interfere with passage of food because of pain or obstruction. Changes in the skin and extremities may suggest a diagnosis of scleroderma and other collagen-vascular diseases or mucocutaneous diseases such as pemphigoid or epidermolysis bullosa, which may involve the esophagus. Cancer spread to lymph nodes and liver may be evident. Pulmonary complications of acute aspiration pneumonia or chronic aspiration may be present.

Diagnostic Procedures Dysphagia is nearly always a symptom of organic disease rather than a functional complaint. If oropharyngeal dysphagia is suspected, videofluoroscopy of oropharyngeal swallowing should be obtained. If mechanical dysphagia is suspected on clinical history, barium swallow, esophagogastroscopy and endoscopic biopsies are the diagnostic procedures of choice. Barium swallow and esophageal motility studies are diagnostic tests for motor dysphagia. Esophagogastroscopy may be needed in patients with motor dysphagia to exclude an associated structural abnormality (Chap. 284).

BIBLIOGRAPHY

GOYAL RK, SIVARAO DV: Functional anatomy and physiology of swallowing and esophageal motility, in *The Esophagus*, 3d ed, DO Castell, JE Richter (eds). Philadelphia, Lippincott Williams &Wilkins, 1999, pp 1–31

SPECHLER SJ: American Gastroenterological Association medical position statement on treatment of patients with dysphagia caused by benign disorders of the distal esophagus. Gastroenterology 117:229, 1999

———: American Gastroenterological Association technical review on treatment of patients with dysphagia caused by benign disorders of the distal esophagus. Gastroenterology 117:233, 1999

41 *William L. Hasler*

NAUSEA, VOMITING, AND INDIGESTION

Nausea is the subjective feeling of a need to vomit. Vomiting (emesis) is the oral expulsion of upper gastrointestinal contents resulting from contractions of gut and thoracoabdominal wall musculature. *Vomiting* is contrasted with regurgitation, the effortless passage of gastric contents into the mouth. *Rumination* is the repeated regurgitation of stomach contents, which are often rechewed and then reswallowed. In contrast to vomiting, these phenomena often exhibit some volitional control. *Indigestion* is a nonspecific term that encompasses a variety of upper abdominal complaints including nausea, vomiting, heartburn, regurgitation, and dyspepsia (upper abdominal discomfort or pain). Individuals with ulcer-like dyspepsia report epigastric burning or gnawing discomfort. Dysmotility-like dyspepsia is characterized by postprandial fullness, bloating, eructation (belching), anorexia (loss of appetite), and early satiety (an inability to complete a meal due to premature fullness).

NAUSEA AND VOMITING

MECHANISMS Vomiting is coordinated by the brain stem and is effected by neuromuscular responses in the gut, pharynx, and thoracoabdominal wall. The mechanisms underlying nausea are poorly understood. Because nausea requires conscious perception, the sensation is probably mediated by the cerebral cortex. Electroencephalographic studies show activation of temporofrontal cortical regions with induction of nausea.

Coordination of Emesis Animal studies suggested that vomiting was coordinated by a single locus in the medullary reticular formation. However, further work has shown that no one "vomiting center" exists and that several brain stem nuclei initiate emesis, including the nucleus tractus solitarius; the dorsal vagal and phrenic nuclei; medullary nuclei that regulate respiration; and nuclei that control pharyngeal, facial, and tongue movements. The neurotransmitters involved in coordinating emesis are uncertain; however, neurokinin NK_1, serotonin, and vasopressin pathways are postulated.

Somatic and visceral muscles exhibit stereotypic responses during emesis. Inspiratory thoracic and abdominal wall muscles contract, producing high intrathoracic and intraabdominal pressures that facilitate expulsion of gastric contents. The gastric cardia herniates across the diaphragm, and the larynx moves upward to promote oral propulsion

of the vomitus. Under normal conditions, distally migrating upper gut contractions are regulated by an electrical phenomenon, the slow wave, which cycles at 3 cycles per minute in the stomach and 11 cycles per minute in the duodenum. With emesis, slow waves are replaced by orally propagating spike activity, which induces retrograde contractions that assist in the oral expulsion of small intestinal contents.

Activators of Emesis Emetic stimuli act at several anatomic sites. Emesis provoked by noxious thoughts or smells originates in the cerebral cortex, whereas cranial nerves mediate vomiting after gag reflex activation. Motion sickness and inner ear disorders act on the labyrinthine apparatus, while gastric irritants and emetogenic anticancer agents such as cisplatin stimulate gastroduodenal vagal afferent nerves. Nongastric visceral afferents are activated by small intestinal and colonic obstruction and mesenteric ischemia. The area postrema, a medullary nucleus, responds to bloodborne emetic stimuli and is termed the *chemoreceptor trigger zone*. Many emetic drugs act on the area postrema as do bacterial toxins and metabolic disorders such as uremia, hypoxia, and ketoacidosis.

Neurotransmitters that mediate induction of vomiting are selective for these anatomic sites. Labyrinthine disorders stimulate vestibular cholinergic muscarinic M_1 and histaminergic H_1 receptors, whereas gastroduodenal vagal afferent stimuli activate serotonin 5-HT_3 receptors. The area postrema is richly served by nerve fibers acting on diverse receptor subtypes including 5-HT_3, M_1, H_1, and dopamine D_2. Optimal pharmacologic management of the patient with vomiting requires an understanding of these pathways.

DIFFERENTIAL DIAGNOSIS Nausea and vomiting are caused by conditions within and outside the gut as well as by drugs and circulating toxins (Table 41-1).

Intraperitoneal Disorders Visceral obstruction and inflammation of hollow and solid viscera may produce vomiting as the main symptom. Gastric obstruction results from ulcer disease and malignancy, whereas small bowel and colonic obstructions occur as a consequence of adhesions, benign or malignant tumors, volvulus, intussusception, or inflammatory diseases such as Crohn's disease. The superior mesenteric artery syndrome, occurring after weight loss or prolonged bed rest, results when the duodenum is compressed by the overlying superior mesenteric artery. Abdominal irradiation evokes emesis by impairing intestinal contractile function and by inducing strictures. Biliary colic causes nausea likely by action on visceral afferent nerves. Vomiting with pancreatitis, cholecystitis, and appendicitis is due to localized visceral irritation and induction of ileus. Enteric infections with viruses or bacteria such as *Staphylococcus aureus* and *Bacillus cereus* are among the most common causes of acute vomiting, especially in children. Opportunistic infections such as cytomegalovirus or herpes simplex induce emesis in immunocompromised individuals.

Disorders of gastrointestinal motor function also commonly cause nausea and vomiting. Gastroparesis is defined as a delay in emptying of food from the stomach and occurs after vagotomy for peptic ulcer, with pancreatic adenocarcinoma, or in systemic diseases such as diabetes, scleroderma, and amyloidosis. Idiopathic gastroparesis develops in the absence of systemic illness and may follow a viral prodrome suggesting an infectious etiology. Intestinal pseudoobstruction is characterized by disruption of intestinal and colonic motor activity and leads to intestinal retention of food residue and secretions, bacterial overgrowth, nutrient malabsorption, and development of nausea, vomiting, bloating, pain, and alteration of bowel pattern. Intestinal pseudoobstruction may be idiopathic, may be inherited as a familial visceral myopathy or neuropathy, or may result from systemic disease or be a paraneoplastic consequence of malignancy (especially small cell lung carcinoma).

Extraperitoneal Disorders Myocardial infarction and congestive heart failure are cardiac causes of nausea and vomiting. Nausea and vomiting occur after 25% of surgical operations, both within and outside the peritoneum. Postoperative emesis is more common after laparotomy and orthopedic surgery than after laparoscopy and is more prevalent in women. Increased intracranial pressure from tumors, bleeding, abscess, or obstruction to cerebrospinal fluid outflow produces prominent vomiting with or without concurrent nausea. Motion sickness, labyrinthitis, and Ménière's disease evoke symptoms via labyrinthine pathways. Cyclic vomiting syndrome is a rare disorder of unknown etiology that produces episodes of intractable nausea and vomiting, usually in children. The syndrome shows a strong association with migraine headaches, suggesting that some cases may be migraine variants. Patients with psychiatric illnesses, including anorexia nervosa, bulimia nervosa, and depression, may report significant nausea. Psychogenic vomiting occurs most commonly in women with other emotional problems.

Table 41-1 Causes of Nausea and Vomiting

Intraperitoneal	Extraperitoneal	Medications/Metabolic Disorders
Obstructing disorders	Cardiopulmonary disease	Drugs
Pyloric obstruction	Cardiomyopathy	Cancer chemotherapy
Small bowel obstruction	Myocardial infarction	Antibiotics
Colonic obstruction	Labyrinthine disease	Cardiac antiarrhythmics
Superior mesenteric artery syndrome	Motion sickness	Digoxin
Enteric infections	Labyrinthitis	Oral hypoglycemics
Viral	Malignancy	Oral contraceptives
Bacterial	Intracerebral disorders	Endocrine/metabolic disease
Inflammatory diseases	Malignancy	Pregnancy
Cholecystitis	Hemorrhage	Uremia
Pancreatitis	Abscess	Ketoacidosis
Appendicitis	Hydrocephalus	Thyroid and parathyroid disease
Hepatitis	Psychiatric illness	Adrenal insufficiency
Impaired motor function	Anorexia and bulimia nervosa	Toxins
Gastroparesis	Depression	Liver failure
Intestinal pseudoobstruction	Psychogenic vomiting	Ethanol
Functional dyspepsia	Postoperative vomiting	
Gastroesophageal reflux	Cyclic vomiting syndrome	
Biliary colic		
Abdominal irradiation		

Medications and Metabolic Disorders Drugs are frequent causes of vomiting and may act on the stomach (analgesics, erythromycin) or area postrema (digoxin, opiates, anti-Parkinsonian drugs). Agents that cause emesis include antibiotics, antiarrhythmics, antihypertensives, oral hypoglycemics, and contraceptives. Cancer chemotherapy causes vomiting that is acute (within hours of administration), delayed (after 1 or more days), or anticipatory. Acute emesis resulting from highly emetogenic agents such as cisplatin is mediated by 5-HT$_3$ pathways, whereas delayed emesis is independent of 5-HT$_3$. Anticipatory nausea often responds better to anxiolytic therapy than to antiemetics.

Metabolic disorders are in the differential diagnosis in certain settings. Pregnancy is the most prevalent endocrinologic cause of nausea, occurring in 70% of women in the first trimester. Hyperemesis gravidarum is a severe form of nausea of pregnancy that can produce significant fluid loss and electrolyte disturbances. Uremia, ketoacidosis, adrenal insufficiency, as well as parathyroid and thyroid disease are other metabolic causes of emesis.

Circulating toxins evoke symptoms through effects on the area postrema. Endogenous toxins are generated in fulminant liver failure, whereas exogenous enterotoxins may be produced by enteric bacterial infection. Ethanol intoxication is a common toxic cause of nausea and vomiting.

Approach to the Patient

History and Physical Examination The history helps determine the etiology of unexplained nausea and vomiting. Drugs and toxins often cause acute symptoms, while established illnesses evoke chronic complaints. Vomiting within 1 h of eating characterizes pyloric obstruction, whereas emesis in the late postprandial period is reported with intestinal obstruction. Gastroparesis can produce nausea within minutes of food consumption but, in severe cases, leads to vomiting of meal residue ingested hours or days previously. Blood in the vomitus raises suspicion of an ulcer or malignancy; feculent emesis is noted with distal intestinal or colonic obstruction. Bilious vomiting excludes gastric obstruction, whereas emesis of undigested food is consistent with a pharyngoesophageal process such as Zenker's diverticulum or achalasia. Relief of abdominal pain by emesis characterizes small bowel obstruction, but vomiting has no effect on pancreatitis or cholecystitis pain. Pronounced weight loss raises concern about malignancy or obstruction. Fevers suggest inflammation, while an intracranial source is considered if there are headaches or visual field changes. Vertigo or tinnitus indicate labyrinthine disease.

The physical examination complements the history. Abdominal auscultation may reveal absent bowel sounds with ileus. High-pitched rushes suggest bowel obstruction, while a succession splash on abrupt lateral movement of the patient is found with gastroparesis or pyloric obstruction. Tenderness or involuntary guarding raises suspicion of inflammation, whereas fecal blood suggests mucosal injury from ulcer, ischemia, or tumor. Neurologic etiologies present with papilledema, visual field loss, or focal neural abnormalities. Neoplasm is suggested by palpable masses or adenopathy.

The history and examination can characterize complications of emesis. Reports of lightheadedness with demonstration of orthostatic hypotension and reduced skin turgor indicate intravascular fluid loss. Hematemesis, especially with repeated vomiting, suggests a Mallory-Weiss tear of the gastroesophageal junction, while pulmonary abnormalities raise concern for aspiration of vomitus.

Diagnostic Testing With intractable symptoms or an elusive diagnosis, selected diagnostic tests can direct clinical management. Electrolyte replenishment is indicated if hypokalemia or metabolic alkalosis is found. Detection of iron-deficiency anemia mandates a search for mucosal injury. Pancreaticobiliary disease is suggested by abnormal pancreatic enzymes or liver biochemistries, whereas endocrinologic or rheumatologic etiologies are diagnosed by specific hormone or serologic testing. If lumenal obstruction is considered, supine and upright abdominal radiographs may show intestinal air-fluid levels with reduced colonic air. Ileus is characterized by diffusely dilated air-filled bowel loops.

If initial testing is unrevealing, additional anatomic studies may be indicated. Upper endoscopy detects ulcer disease or gastroesophageal malignancy, and small bowel barium radiography diagnoses partial small bowel obstruction. Colonoscopy or barium enema can detect colonic obstruction. Ultrasound or computed tomography of the abdomen defines intraperitoneal inflammatory processes, while computed tomography or magnetic resonance imaging of the head can delineate intracranial sources of nausea and vomiting.

Gastrointestinal motility testing may detect a functional gastrointestinal disorder responsible for symptoms when investigation of anatomic abnormalities is negative. Gastroparesis is most commonly diagnosed with gastric scintigraphy, by which emptying of a radiolabeled meal is measured. A noninvasive means of quantitating gastric slow wave activity with cutaneous electrodes placed over the stomach, electrogastrography, has been proposed as an alternate means of diagnosing abnormal gastric emptying. With intestinal pseudoobstruction, small bowel barium radiography often suggests the diagnosis. Manometry of the small intestine may provide confirmation of the diagnosis as well as complementary information by characterizing the motor abnormality as neuropathic or myopathic based on contractile patterns. Such investigation can obviate the need for open biopsy of the intestine to evaluate for smooth muscle or neuronal degeneration.

℞ **TREATMENT　General Principles**　Therapy of vomiting is tailored to the underlying disease, with the medical or surgical correction of abnormalities if possible. Hospitalization is considered for severe dehydration, especially if oral fluid replenishment cannot be sustained. Once oral intake is tolerated, nutrients are restarted as liquids that are low in fat, as lipids delay gastric emptying. Foods high in indigestible residues are avoided because these also prolong gastric retention.

Antiemetic Medications　Drugs that act on the central nervous system serve as antiemetic agents (Table 41-2). Antihistamines such as meclizine and dimenhydrate and anticholinergic drugs such as scopolamine act on labyrinthine-activated pathways and are useful in the treatment of motion sickness and inner ear disorders. Phenothiazine and butyrophenone dopamine D_2 antagonists are used to treat emesis evoked by area postrema stimuli and are effective for many medication, toxic, and metabolic etiologies. Dopamine antagonists freely cross the blood-brain barrier and may cause anxiety, dystonic reactions, hyperprolactinemic effects (galactorrhea and sexual dysfunction), and irreversible tardive dyskinesia.

Other drug classes have antiemetic properties. Serotonin 5-HT_3 antagonists such as ondansetron and granisetron are useful in the treatment of postoperative vomiting and after radiation therapy but are mainly used to prevent cancer chemotherapy-induced emesis. The usefulness of 5-HT_3 antagonists to control other causes of refractory emesis is less well established. Antidepressant drugs are established therapeutic options for patients with functional bowel disorders such as irritable bowel syndrome. Low-dose tricyclic antidepressants provide moderate symptomatic benefit in patients with unexplained nausea of a functional nature.

Gastrointestinal Motor Stimulants　Drugs that stimulate gastric emptying are indicated for gastroparesis (Table 41-2). Cisapride, a serotonin 5-HT_4 agonist that stimulates cholinergic nerves in the stomach, has become the preferred drug for outpatient management of gas-troparesis. The drug is well tolerated but exhibits very rare drug interactions with selected antibiotics, antifungals, and other agents that predispose to fatal cardiac arrhythmias. Metoclopramide, a combined 5-HT_4 agonist and D_2 antagonist, is efficacious in the treatment of gastroparesis, but anti-dopaminergic side effects limit its use in 20% of patients. Erythromycin, a macrolide antibiotic, potently increases gastroduodenal motility by action on receptors for motilin, an endogenous stimulant of fasting motor activity. Erythromycin may be most useful when given intravenously to inpatients with refractory gastroparesis; however, oral forms of the drug also have some effect. Domperidone, a D_2 antagonist not available in the United States, has prokinetic and antiemetic effects but does not cross into most other brain regions; thus, anxiety and dystonic reactions are rare. The main side effects of domperidone are induction of hyperprolactinemia through effects on pituitary regions served by a porous blood-brain barrier.

Patients with refractory upper gut motility disorders pose significant therapeutic challenges. Liquid suspensions of prokinetic drugs may be beneficial inasmuch as liquids empty from the stomach more rapidly than pills. Metoclopramide can be administered subcutaneously in patients who do not respond to oral drugs. Intestinal pseudoobstruction may respond to the somatostatin analogue octreotide, which induces propagative small intestinal motor complexes. Placement of a feeding jejunostomy reduces hospitalizations and improves overall health in some patients with gastroparesis who do not respond to drug therapy. Surgical options are limited for refractory cases, but postvagotomy gastroparesis may improve with near-total resection of the stomach. Electrical pacing of the stomach may also be useful.

Selected Clinical Settings　Cancer chemotherapeutic agents such as cisplatin are intensely emetogenic. Given prophylactically, 5-HT_3 antagonists prevent chemotherapy-induced acute vomiting in most cases (Table 41-2). Optimal antiemetic effects often are obtained with a 5-HT_3 antagonist in combination with a glucocorticoid. In high doses, metoclopramide is effective in controlling chemotherapy-evoked emesis, whereas benzodiazepines such as lorazepam are most useful in reducing anticipatory nausea and vomiting. In contrast, delayed emesis 1 to 5 days after chemotherapy is more refractory to treatment. Agents that act as neurokinin NK_1 antagonists in the brain stem may be potent antiemetic and antinausea drugs during both the acute and the delayed periods after chemotherapy. Cannabinoids such as tetrahydrocannabinol have been advocated for cancer-associated emesis, but these drugs produce significant side effects and are no more effective than antidopaminergic agents.

The clinician should exercise caution in the management of the patient with nausea of pregnancy. Studies of the teratogenic effects of available antiemetic agents have provided conflicting results. Few controlled trials have been performed in the nausea of pregnancy, although antihistamines such as meclizine and antidopaminergics such as prochlorperazine are more efficacious than placebo. As a consequence, alternative therapies such as pyridoxine or ginger have been recommended.

INDIGESTION

MECHANISMS　Most patients with indigestion have symptoms of a functional nature that result from gastroesophageal

Table 41-2　Treatment of Nausea and Vomiting

Treatment	Mechanism	Examples	Clinical Indications
Antiemetic agents	Antihistaminergic	Dimenhydrate, meclizine	Motion sickness, inner ear disease
	Anticholinergic	Scopolamine	Motion sickness, inner ear disease
	Antidopaminergic	Prochlorperazine, droperidol	Medication-, toxin-, or metabolic-induced emesis
	5-HT_3 antagonist	Ondansetron, granisetron	Chemotherapy- and radiation-induced emesis, postoperative emesis
	Tricyclic antidepressant	Amitriptyline, nortriptyline	Functional nausea
Prokinetic agents	5-HT_4 agonist	Cisapride	Gastroparesis functional dyspepsia, gastroesophageal reflux disease, intestinal pseudoobstruction
	5-HT_4 agonist and antidopaminergic	Metoclopramide	Gastroparesis, functional dyspepsia
	Motilin agonist	Erythromycin	Gastroparesis, ? Intestinal pseudoobstruction
	Peripheral antidopaminergic	Domperidone	Gastroparesis, functional dyspepsia
	Somatostatin analogue	Octreotide	Intestinal pseudoobstruction
Special settings	Benzodiazepines	Lorazepam	Anticipatory nausea and vomiting with chemotherapy
	Glucocorticoids	Methylprednisolone, dexamethasone	Chemotherapy-induced emesis
	Cannabinoids	Tetrahydrocannabinol	?Chemotherapy-induced emesis

acid reflux or from gastric abnormalities including dysfunctional motor activity and afferent hypersensitivity; these symptoms comprise the syndrome functional dyspepsia. Some cases are a consequence of a more serious organic illness.

Gastroesophageal Acid Reflux Acid reflux results from selected physiologic defects. In scleroderma and pregnancy, lower esophageal sphincter (LES) tone is low, but most patients with acid reflux have normal LES pressures. Many individuals show frequent transient LES relaxations during which acid bathes the esophagus. The role of hiatal hernias is controversial—although most reflux patients exhibit hiatal hernias, most individuals with hiatal hernias do not have excess heartburn.

Gastric Motor Dysfunction Disturbed gastric motility is purported to cause acid reflux in some patients with indigestion. Delayed gastric emptying also is found in 25 to 50% of individuals with functional dyspepsia. The relation of these defects to symptom induction is uncertain as many studies show poor correlation between symptom severity and the degree of motor dysfunction. Abnormal gastric fundic relaxation may cause dyspeptic symptoms such as bloating, fullness, nausea, and early satiety.

Visceral Afferent Hypersensitivity Disturbed gastric sensory function also may cause functional dyspepsia. Visceral afferent hypersensitivity was first demonstrated in patients with irritable bowel syndrome who had heightened perception of rectal balloon inflation without changes in rectal compliance. Patients with dyspepsia may experience discomfort with fundic distention to lower pressures than healthy control subjects.

Other Factors *Helicobacter pylori* has a clear etiologic role in peptic ulcer disease, but ulcers cause only a minority of cases of dyspepsia. The importance of *H. pylori* in the genesis of functional dyspepsia is controversial, but most investigators believe it is of minor importance. Analgesics cause dyspepsia; nitrates, calcium channel blockers, theophylline, and progesterone promote acid reflux. Other exogenous factors that induce acid reflux include ethanol, tobacco, and caffeine via LES relaxation. Finally, functional dyspepsia is exacerbated by stress, suggesting a pathogenic role for psychological factors.

DIFFERENTIAL DIAGNOSIS **Functional Causes** Gastroesophageal reflux disease (GERD) is prevalent in Western society. Heartburn is reported once monthly by 40% of Americans and daily by 7%. Functional dyspepsia, defined as ≥3 months of dyspepsia without an organic cause, also is common. Nearly 25% of the populace has abdominal discomfort at least six times yearly, consistent with functional dyspepsia, but only 10 to 20% consult physicians. The clinician must distinguish these illnesses, which have a benign course, from conditions that have deleterious consequences.

Ulcer Disease In most cases of GERD, the esophagus is not damaged. However, 5% of patients develop esophageal ulcers, and some form esophageal strictures. Functional dyspepsia is the cause of symptoms in 60% of individuals with dyspepsia. However, 15 to 25% of cases stem from ulcers of the stomach or duodenum. The most common causes of ulcer disease are gastric infection with *H. pylori* and use of nonsteroidal anti-inflammatory drugs. Other rare causes of gastroduodenal ulcer include Crohn's disease and Zollinger-Ellison syndrome, a condition resulting from gastrin overproduction by an endocrine tumor (Chap. 285).

Malignancy Patients with dyspepsia often seek care because of fear of cancer. However, <2% of cases result from gastroesophageal malignancy. Esophageal squamous cell carcinoma occurs most often in those patients with histories of tobacco or ethanol intake. Other risk factors include prior caustic ingestion, achalasia, and the hereditary disorder tylosis. Esophageal adenocarcinoma usually complicates long-standing acid reflux. Eight to 20% of patients with GERD exhibit glandular mucosal metaplasia of the squamous epithelium in the lower esophagus, termed *Barrett's metaplasia*. This condition predisposes to esophageal adenocarcinoma. Gastric malignancies include adenocarcinoma, which is more prevalent in certain Asian societies, and lymphoma (see Chap. 90).

Other Causes Alkaline reflux esophagitis produces GERD-like symptoms in patients who have had surgery for peptic ulcer disease. Opportunistic fungal or viral esophageal infections may produce heartburn or chest discomfort but more often cause painful swallowing. Although biliary colic is in the differential diagnosis of dyspepsia, most patients with true biliary colic report discrete episodes of right upper quadrant or epigastric pain rather than chronic burning discomfort, nausea, and bloating. Lactose intolerance resulting from intestinal lactase deficiency produces gas, bloating, discomfort, and diarrhea. Lactase deficiency occurs in 15% of Caucasians of northern European descent but is more common in African Americans and Asians. Pancreatic disease (chronic pancreatitis and malignancy), hepatocellular carcinoma, celiac sprue, Ménétrier's disease, infiltrative diseases (sarcoidosis and eosinophilic gastroenteritis), mesenteric ischemia, thyroid and parathyroid disease, and abdominal wall strain cause dyspepsia. Extraperitoneal etiologies of indigestion include congestive heart failure and tuberculosis.

Approach to the Patient

History and Physical Examination GERD classically produces heartburn, a substernal warmth beginning in the epigastrium that moves toward the neck. Heartburn often is exacerbated by meals and may awaken the patient. Associated symptoms include regurgitation of acid and water brash, the reflex release of salty salivary secretions into the mouth. Atypical symptoms include pharyngitis, asthma, cough, bronchitis, hoarseness, and chest pain that mimics angina. Some patients with acid reflux on esophageal pH testing do not report heartburn and instead note abdominal pain or other symptoms.

Individuals with ulcer-like dyspepsia have epigastric gnawing or burning that is relieved by meals or acid suppression. Dysmotility-like dyspepsia is a fullness or pain that is aggravated by eating and associated with nausea, bloating, eructation, and early satiety. There is overlap among the different dyspepsia subclasses and with other functional disorders such as irritable bowel syndrome.

The physical examination of individuals with functional causes of indigestion is usually normal. In atypical GERD, pharyngeal erythema and wheezing over the lung fields may be present. Poor dentition may occur with prolonged acid regurgitation. Patients with functional dyspepsia may have epigastric tenderness or abdominal distension.

Discrimination between functional and organic causes of indigestion mandates exclusion of selected historical and examination features. Odynophagia suggests esophageal infection, while dysphagia promotes concern about a benign or malignant esophageal blockage. Other features that raise alarm include unexplained weight loss, recurrent vomiting with evidence of dehydration, occult or gross gastrointestinal bleeding, and a palpable mass or adenopathy.

Diagnostic Testing Because indigestion is prevalent in the community and because most cases result from functional illness, a general principle of diagnostic testing is to perform only limited and directed testing of selected individuals.

Once alarm factors are excluded, patients with typical GERD do not need further evaluation and are treated empirically. Upper endoscopy is indicated to exclude mucosal injury in patients with atypical symptoms, symptoms unresponsive to acid-suppressing drugs, or alarm factors. In patients with >5 years of heartburn, endoscopy is performed to screen for Barrett's metaplasia. Upper gastrointestinal barium radiography has a slightly higher sensitivity for detecting strictures and rings than endoscopy; however, benign esophageal obstructions may be dilated with an endoscopic approach. Ambulatory esophageal pH testing is considered for atypical symptoms such as unexplained chest pain and for the symptoms that are unresponsive to appropriate medications. Esophageal manometry is most commonly ordered when surgical treatment of GERD is considered. A low LES pressure may predict failure with drug therapy and identify patients who may require surgery. The demonstration of disordered esophageal body peristalsis may affect the decision to operate or modify the type of operation chosen. Manometry with provocative testing may clarify the diagnosis in patients with atypical symptoms. Blinded perfusion of saline and then acid into the esophagus, known as the Bernstein test, can delineate whether unexplained chest discomfort results from acid reflux.

The approach to unexplained dyspepsia is dependent on the patient's age, symptom profile, and findings on examination. In individuals <45 years of age without alarm factors, blood serology for *H. pylori* is obtained to exclude the organism as a cause of ulcer disease. Upper endoscopy in this patient subset is reserved for those who fail to respond to treatment of *H. pylori*-positive or -negative dyspepsia. Upper endoscopy is performed as the initial diagnostic test in any individual with alarm factors or in patients >45 years of age because of the elevated risk of gastroesophageal malignancy with advancing age.

Further testing is indicated only if other factors are present. If there is blood loss, a blood count is obtained to exclude anemia. Thyroid chemistries or calcium levels screen for metabolic disease. With suspected pancreaticobiliary causes, blood is obtained for amylase, lipase, and liver chemistry determination. If biochemical abnormalities are found, abdominal ultrasound or computed tomography may give important information. Patients with dysmotility-like dyspepsia may selectively exhibit delayed gastric emptying; thus, gastric scintigraphy can be considered when drug treatment fails. Hydrogen breath testing after lactose ingestion may be performed for suspected lactase deficiency.

R̥ **TREATMENT   General Principles**   In mild dyspepsia, reassurance that a careful evaluation revealed no serious organic disease may be the only intervention required. Drugs that cause acid reflux or dyspepsia should be stopped if possible. Patients with GERD should limit ethanol, caffeine, chocolate, and tobacco use because of their effects on the LES. Other measures with efficacy in GERD include ingestion of a low-fat diet, avoidance of snacks before bedtime, and elevation of the head of the bed.

Specific therapy for organic diseases should be offered when possible. In disorders such as biliary colic, surgery is appropriate; whereas lactase deficiency and celiac sprue respond to special diets. Some illnesses such as peptic ulcer disease require specific medical regimens to effect cure. However, as most patients present with functional causes of indigestion, medications that reduce gastric acid, stimulate upper gut motility, or blunt gastric sensitivity are indicated.

Acid Suppressing or Neutralizing Medications   Drugs that reduce or neutralize gastric acid are the most prescribed agents for GERD. Histamine H_2 receptor antagonists such as cimetidine, ranitidine, famotidine, and nizatidine are useful in the treatment of mild to moderate GERD. For uncomplicated heartburn, H_2 receptor antagonists are given for 4 weeks before endoscopy is considered. For severe symptoms or for many cases of erosive or ulcerative esophagitis, proton pump inhibitors such as omeprazole and lansoprazole are needed. These drugs, which inhibit gastric H^+, K^+-ATPase, are more potent than H_2 receptor antagonists. Liquid antacids are useful for short-term control of mild GERD but are less effective for severe disease unless given at high doses that produce side effects (diarrhea with magnesium-containing agents and constipation with aluminum-containing agents). Sucralfate is a salt of aluminum hydroxide and sucrose octasulfate and buffers acid and binds pepsin and bile salts. Its efficacy in GERD and functional dyspepsia is unproven.

Acid suppressing drugs are advocated for first-line therapy of *H. pylori* negative dyspepsia, especially with ulcer-like symptoms. Ranitidine is of benefit in the treatment of functional dyspepsia versus placebo. In young patients without alarm symptoms, a 4-week trial of an H_2 receptor antagonist or proton pump inhibitor is given. Endoscopy is performed only if symptoms do not improve.

***Helicobacter pylori* Eradication**   Regimens to eradicate *H. pylori* are recommended for young patients with dyspepsia without alarm symptoms in whom the bacterium has been detected by serology. Several drug combinations show efficacy, but most include 10 to 14 days of a proton pump inhibitor or bismuth subsalicylate in concert with two antibiotics. If symptoms resolve, no further intervention is required. Most patients who respond to this "treatment-first" approach have underlying ulcer disease. The usefulness of *Helicobacter* eradication in patients with functional dyspepsia is unproven, but evidence suggests that <15% of cases relate to *H. pylori*. No evidence demonstrates that *H. pylori* eradication is useful in the treatment of GERD.

Gastrointestinal Motor Stimulants   Cisapride is superior to placebo in treating GERD and can be prescribed as sole therapy or as an adjunct to an acid-suppressing drug. Other motor stimulants such as metoclopramide, erythromycin, and domperidone are of limited use in the treatment of GERD.

Prokinetic agents are frequently used for treatment of functional dyspepsia. Cisapride and domperidone relieve symptoms more effectively than placebo. In general, these drugs are more potent than acid-reducing agents in the treatment of functional dyspepsia and may be given instead of acid suppressants as the initial empirical treatment of young patients with dyspepsia without alarm symptoms who are not infected with *H. pylori*. Patients with dysmotility-like dyspepsia may respond preferentially to motor-stimulating drugs.

Other Options   In patients with GERD who do not respond to drug therapy, antireflux surgery may be offered. Operations include the Nissen fundoplication, in which the proximal stomach is wrapped completely around the LES to increase LES pressure, and the Belsey procedure, in which the wrap encircles 270° of the circumference of the LES. The latter is selected if esophageal peristalsis is suboptimal when a 360° wrap might cause dysphagia. Fundoplications can be performed laparoscopically, thereby reducing the morbidity and the postoperative recuperation period.

Some patients with functional dyspepsia do not respond to acid suppressants or prokinetic drugs but may respond to low-dose tricyclic antidepressant therapy. The mechanism of action of these agents in functional dyspepsia is unknown but may involve blunting of visceral pain processing in the brain. Gas and bloating may be the most troubling symptoms in some patients with indigestion and can be difficult to treat. Successes with dietary exclusion of gas-producing foods such as legumes and use of the surface-active compound simethicone or the gas-absorptive agent activated charcoal have been reported. Psychological treatments have been proposed for functional dyspepsia; however, convincing data on their efficacy are lacking.

BIBLIOGRAPHY

BLUM AL et al: Lack of effect of treating *Helicobacter pylori* infection in patients with nonulcer dyspepsia. Omeprazole plus clarithromycin and amoxicillin effect one year after treatment (OCAY) study group. N Engl J Med 339:1928, 1998

CAMILLERI M et al: Measurement of gastrointestinal motility in the GI laboratory. Gastroenterology 115:747, 1998

DEVAULT KR, CASTELL DO: Guidelines for the diagnosis and treatment of gastroesophageal reflux disease. Practice Parameters Committee of the American College of Gastroenterology. Arch Intern Med 155:2165, 1995

FINNEY JS et al: Meta-analysis of antisecretory and gastrokinetic compounds in functional dyspepsia. J Clin Gastroenterol 26:312, 1998

JANTUNEN IT et al: An overview of randomised studies comparing 5-HT$_3$ receptor antagonists to conventional anti-emetics in the prophylaxis of acute chemotherapy-induced vomiting. Eur J Cancer 33:66, 1997

LACROIX R et al: Nausea and vomiting during pregnancy. Am J Obstet Gynecol 182:931, 2000

MITCHELSON F: Pharmacological agents affecting emesis: A review (part I). Drugs 43:295, 1992

PRAKASH C et al: Tricyclic antidepressants for functional nausea and vomiting: Clinical outcome in 37 patients. Dig Dis Sci 43:1951, 1998

RICHTER JE: Typical and atypical presentations of gastroesophageal reflux disease. The role of esophageal testing in the diagnosis and management. Gastroenterol Clin North Am 25:75, 1996

TALLEY NJ et al: AGA technical review: Evaluation of dyspepsia. Gastroenterology 114:582, 1998

DIARRHEA AND CONSTIPATION

Diarrhea and constipation are exceedingly common and together exact an enormous toll in terms of morbidity, loss of work productivity, and consumption of medical resources. Worldwide, more than one billion people suffer one or more episodes of acute diarrhea each year. Among the 100 million persons affected annually by acute diarrhea in the United States, nearly half must restrict activities, 10% consult physicians, 250,000 require hospitalization, and roughly 3000 die (primarily the elderly). The economic burden to society is estimated at more than $20 billion. Because of poor sanitation and more limited access to health care, acute infectious diarrhea remains one of the most common causes of mortality in developing countries, particularly among children, accounting for 5 to 8 million deaths per year. Population statistics on chronic diarrhea and constipation are more uncertain, perhaps due to variable definitions and reporting, but the frequency of these conditions is also high. Based on United States population surveys, prevalence rates for chronic diarrhea range from 2 to 7% and for chronic constipation from 3 to 17%. Diarrhea and constipation are among the most common patient complaints faced by internists and primary care physicians, and they account for nearly 50% of referrals to gastroenterologists.

Although diarrhea and constipation may present as mere nuisance symptoms at one extreme, they can be severe or life-threatening at the other. Even mild symptoms may signal a serious underlying gastrointestinal lesion, like colorectal cancer, or systemic disorder, like thyroid disease. Given the heterogeneous causes and potential severity of these common complaints, it is imperative for clinicians to appreciate the pathophysiology, etiologic classification, diagnostic strategies, and therapeutic principles of diarrhea and constipation so that rational and cost-effective care can be delivered.

NORMAL PHYSIOLOGY

The human small intestine and colon perform important functions including the secretion and absorption of water and electrolytes, the storage and subsequent transport of intraluminal contents aborally, and the salvage of some nutrients after bacterial metabolism of carbohydrate that are not absorbed in the small intestine. The main motor functions are summarized in Table 42-1. Alterations in fluid and electrolyte handling contribute significantly to diarrhea. Alterations in motor and sensory functions of the human colon result in highly prevalent syndromes such as irritable bowel syndrome, chronic diarrhea, and chronic constipation.

NEURAL CONTROL   The small intestine and colon have intrinsic and extrinsic innervation. The *intrinsic innervation* also called the enteric nervous system, comprises myenteric, submucosal, and mucosal neuronal layers. The function of these layers is modulated by interneurons through the actions of neurotransmitter amines or peptides, including acetylcholine, opioids, norepinephrine, serotonin, ATP, and nitric oxide. The myenteric plexus regulates smooth muscle function, and the submucosal plexus affects secretion and absorption.

Table 42-1   Normal Gastrointestinal Motility: Functions at Different Anatomic Levels

Stomach and small bowel	Colon: Irregular mixing, absorption, transit
Synchronized MMCs in fasting	
Accommodation, trituration, mixing, transit	Ascending, transverse: reservoirs
Stomach, ~3 h	Descending: conduit
Small bowel, ~3 h	Sigmoid/rectum: volitional reservoir
Ileal reservoir empties boluses	

NOTE: MMC, migrating motor complex.

The *extrinsic innervations* of the small intestine and colon are part of the autonomic nervous system and also modulate both motor and secretory functions. The parasympathetic nerve supply conveys both visceral sensory as well as excitatory pathways to the motor components of the colon. Parasympathetic fibers via the vagus nerve reach the small intestine and proximal colon along the branches of the superior mesenteric artery. The distal colon is supplied by sacral parasympathetic nerves (S_{2-4}) via the pelvic plexus; these fibers course through the wall of the colon as ascending intracolonic fibers as far as, and in some instances including, the proximal colon. The chief excitatory neurotransmitters controlling motor function are acetylcholine and the tachykinins, such as substance P. The sympathetic nerve supply modulates motor functions and reaches the small intestine and colon alongside the arterial arcades of the superior and inferior mesenteric vessels. Sympathetic input to the gut is generally excitatory to sphincters and inhibitory to nonsphincteric muscle. Visceral afferents convey sensation from the gut to the central nervous system; initially, they course along sympathetic fibers, but as they approach the spinal cord they separate, have cell bodies in the dorsal root ganglion, and enter the dorsal horn of the spinal cord. Afferent signals are conveyed to the brain along the lateral spinothalamic tract and the nociceptive dorsal column pathway and are then perceived. Other afferent fibers synapse in the prevertebral ganglia and reflexly modulate intestinal motility.

INTESTINAL FLUID ABSORPTION AND SECRETION On an average day, 9 L of fluid enters the gastrointestinal tract; approximately 1 L of residual fluid reaches the colon; the stool excretion of fluid constitutes about 0.2 L/d. The colon has a large capacitance and functional reserve and may recover up to four times its usual volume of 0.8 L/d, provided the rate of flow permits reabsorption to occur. Thus, the colon can partially compensate for intestinal absorptive or secretory disorders.

In the colon, sodium absorption is predominantly electrogenic, and uptake takes place at the apical membrane; it is also compensated by the pumping out functions of the basolateral sodium pump. A variety of neural and non-neural mediators regulate colonic fluid and electrolyte balance, including cholinergic, adrenergic and serotonergic mediators. Angiotensin and aldosterone also influence colonic absorption, reflecting the common embryologic development of the distal colonic epithelium and the renal tubules.

ILEOCOLONIC STORAGE AND SALVAGE The distal ileum acts as a reservoir, emptying intermittently by bolus movements. This action allows time for salvage of fluids, electrolytes, and nutrients. Segmentation by haustra compartmentalizes the colon and facilitates mixing, retention of residue, and formation of solid stools. In health, the ascending and transverse regions of colon function as reservoirs (average transit, 15 h), and the descending colon acts as a conduit (average transit, 3 h). The colon is efficient at conserving sodium and water, a function that is particularly important in sodium-depleted patients in whom the small intestine alone is unable to maintain sodium balance. Diarrhea or constipation may result from alteration in the reservoir function of the proximal colon, or the propulsive function of the left colon. Constipation may also result from disturbances of the rectal or sigmoid reservoir, typically as a result of dysfunction of the pelvic floor or the coordination of defecation.

SMALL INTESTINAL MOTILITY During fasting, the motility of the small intestine is characterized by a cyclical event called the migrating motor complex (MMC), which serves to clear nondigestible residue from the small intestine. This organized, propagated series of contractions lasts on average 4 min, occurs every 60 to 90 min, and usually involves the entire small intestine. After food ingestion, the small intestine produces irregular, mixing contractions of relatively low amplitude, except in the distal ileum where more powerful contractions occur intermittently and empty the ileum by bolus transfers.

Resting	**Straining**
Pubis	Pubis
Puborectalis	Puborectalis
External anal sphincter	External anal sphincter
Coccyx	Coccyx

Continence requires
Contraction of puborectalis
Maintenance of anorectal angle
Normal rectal sensation
Contraction of sphincter

Defecation requires
Relaxation of puborectalis
Straightening of anorectal angle
Relaxation of sphincter

FIGURE 42-1 Mechanisms involved in continence and defecation. Note the importance of pelvic floor and anal sphincter functions.

COLONIC MOTILITY AND TONE The small intestinal MMC only rarely continues into the colon. However, short duration or phasic contractions mix colonic contents, and high amplitude propagated contractions (HAPCs) are sometimes associated with mass movements through the colon and occur approximately five times per day, usually on awakening in the morning and postprandially. Increased frequency of HAPCs may result in diarrhea. The predominant phasic contractions are irregular and nonpropagated and serve as a "mixing" function.

Colonic tone refers to the background contractility upon which phasic contractile activity (typically contractions lasting less than 15 s) is superimposed. It is an important cofactor in the colon's capacitance (volume accommodation) and sensation.

COLONIC MOTILITY AFTER MEAL INGESTION After meal ingestion, colonic phasic and tonic contractility increase for a period of approximately 2 h. The initial phase (about 10 min) is mediated by the vagus nerve in response to mechanical distention of the stomach. The subsequent response of the colon requires caloric stimulation and is at least in part mediated by hormones, e.g., gastrin and serotonin.

DEFECATION Tonic contraction of the puborectalis muscle, which forms a sling around the rectoanal junction, is important to maintain continence; during defecation, sacral parasympathetic nerves relax this muscle, facilitating the straightening of the rectoanal angle (Fig. 42-1). Distention of the rectum results in transient relaxation of the internal anal sphincter via intrinsic and reflex sympathetic innervation. As sigmoid and rectal contractions increase the pressure within the rectum, the rectosigmoid angle opens by more than 15°. Voluntary relaxation of the external anal sphincter (striated muscle innervated by the pudendal nerve) permits the evacuation of feces; this evacuation process can be augmented by an increase in intraabdominal pressure created by the Valsalva maneuver.

DIARRHEA

DEFINITION Diarrhea is loosely defined as passage of abnormally liquid or unformed stools at an increased frequency. For adults on a typical Western diet, stool weight exceeding 200 g/d can generally be considered diarrheal. Because of the fundamental importance of duration to diagnostic considerations, diarrhea may be further defined as *acute* if <2 weeks, *persistent* if 2 to 4 weeks, and *chronic* if >4 weeks in duration.

Two common conditions, usually associated with the passage of stool totaling <200 g/d, must be distinguished from diarrhea, as diagnostic and therapeutic algorithms differ. *Pseudodiarrhea*, or the frequent passage of small volumes of stool, often is associated with rectal urgency and accompanies the irritable bowel syndrome or anorectal disorders like proctitis. *Fecal incontinence* is the involuntary discharge of rectal contents and is most often caused by neuromuscular disorders or structural anorectal problems. Diarrhea and urgency, especially if severe, may aggravate or cause incontinence. Pseudodiarrhea and fecal incontinence occur at prevalence rates comparable to or higher than that of chronic diarrhea and should always be considered in patients complaining of "diarrhea." A careful history and physical examination generally allow these conditions to be discriminated from true diarrhea.

ACUTE DIARRHEA More than 90% of cases of acute diarrhea are caused by infectious agents; these cases are often accompanied by vomiting, fever, and abdominal pain. The remaining 10% or so are caused by medications, toxic ingestions, ischemia, and other conditions.

Infectious Agents Most infectious diarrheas are acquired by fecal-oral transmission via direct personal contact or, more commonly, via ingestion of food or water contaminated with pathogens from human or animal feces. In the immunologically competent person, the resident fecal microflora, containing more than 500 taxonomically distinct species, are rarely the source of diarrhea and may actually play a role in suppressing the growth of ingested pathogens. Acute infection or injury occurs when the ingested agent overwhelms the host's mucosal immune and nonimmune (gastric acid, digestive enzymes, mucus secretion, peristalsis, and suppressive resident flora) defenses. Established clinical associations with specific enteropathogens may offer diagnostic clues.

In the United States, high risk groups are recognized:

1. *Travelers.* Nearly 40% of tourists to endemic regions of Latin America, Africa, and Asia develop so-called traveler's diarrhea, most commonly due to enterotoxigenic *Escherichia coli* as well as to *Campylobacter*, *Shigella*, and *Salmonella*. Visitors to Russia (especially St. Petersburg) may have increased risk of *Giardia*-associated diarrhea; visitors to Nepal may acquire *Cyclospora*. Campers, backpackers, and swimmers in wilderness areas may become infected with *Giardia*.

2. *Consumers of certain foods.* Diarrhea closely following food consumption at a picnic, banquet, or restaurant may suggest infection with *Salmonella*, *Campylobacter*, or *Shigella* from chicken; enterohemorrhagic *E. coli* (O157:H7) from undercooked hamburger; *Bacillus aureus* from fried rice; *Staphylococcus aureus* or *Salmonella* from mayonnaise or creams; *Salmonella* from eggs; and *Vibrio* species, *Salmonella*, or acute hepatitis A or B from seafood, especially if raw.

3. *Immunodeficient persons.* Individuals at risk for diarrhea include those with either primary immunodeficiency (e.g., IgA deficiency, common variable hypogammaglobulinemia, chronic granulomatous disease) or the much more common secondary immunodeficiency states (e.g., AIDS, senescence, pharmacologic suppression). Common enteropathogens often cause a more severe and protracted diarrheal illness; and, particularly in persons with AIDS, opportunistic infections, such as by *Mycobacterium* species, certain viruses (cytomegalovirus, adenovirus, and herpes simplex), and protozoa (*Cryptosporidium*, *Isospora belli*, Microsporidia, and *Blastocystis hominis*) may also play a role (Chap. 309). In patients with AIDS, agents transmitted venereally per rectum (e.g., *Neisseria gonorrhoeae*, *Treponema pallidum*, *Chlamydia*) may contribute to proctocolitis.

4. *Daycare participants and their family members.* Infections with *Shigella*, *Giardia*, *Cryptosporidium*, rotavirus, and other agents are very common and should be considered.

5. *Institutionalized persons.* Infectious diarrhea is one of the most frequent categories of nosocomial infections in many hospitals and long-term care facilities; the causes are a variety of microorganisms but most commonly *Clostridium difficile.*

The pathophysiology underlying acute diarrhea by infectious agents produces specific clinical features that may also be helpful in diagnosis (Table 42-2). Profuse watery diarrhea secondary to small bowel hypersecretion occurs with ingestion of preformed bacterial toxins, enterotoxin-producing bacteria, and enteroadherent pathogens. Diarrhea associated with marked vomiting and minimal or no fever may occur abruptly within a few hours after ingestion of the former two types; vomiting is usually less, and abdominal cramping or bloating is greater; fever is higher with the latter. Cytotoxin-producing and invasive microorganisms all cause high fever and abdominal pain. Invasive bacteria and *Entamoeba histolytica* often cause bloody diarrhea (referred to as *dysentery*). *Yersinia* invades the terminal ileal and proximal colon mucosa and may cause especially severe abdominal pain with tenderness mimicking acute appendicitis.

Finally, infectious diarrhea may be associated with systemic manifestations. Reiter's syndrome (arthritis, urethritis, and conjunctivitis) may accompany or follow infections by *Salmonella, Campylobacter, Shigella,* and *Yersinia.* Yersiniosis may also lead to an autoimmune-type thyroiditis, pericarditis, and glomerulonephritis. Both enterohemorrhagic *E. coli* (O157:H7) and *Shigella* can lead to the *hemolytic-uremic syndrome* with an attendant high mortality rate. Acute diarrhea can also be a major symptom of several systemic infections including *viral hepatitis, listeriosis, legionellosis,* and *toxic shock syndrome.*

Other Causes Side effects from medications are probably the most common noninfectious cause of acute diarrhea, and etiology may be suggested by a temporal association between use and symptom onset. Although innumerable medications may produce diarrhea, some of the more frequently incriminated include antibiotics, cardiac antidysrhythmics, antihypertensives, nonsteroidal anti-inflammatory drugs, certain antidepressants, chemotherapeutic agents, bronchodilators, antacids, and laxatives. Occlusive or nonocclusive *ischemic colitis* typically occurs in persons older than 50 years of age, often presents as acute lower abdominal pain preceding watery, then bloody diarrhea, and generally results in acute inflammatory changes in the sigmoid or left colon while sparing the rectum. Acute diarrhea may accompany colonic *diverticulitis* and *graft-versus-host disease.* Acute diarrhea, often associated with systemic compromise, can follow ingestion of toxins including organophosphate insecticides, amanita and other mushrooms, arsenic, and preformed environmental toxins in seafoods, like ciguatera and scombroid. The conditions causing chronic diarrhea can also be confused with acute diarrhea early in their course. This confusion may occur with inflammatory bowel disease and some of the other inflammatory chronic diarrheas that may have an abrupt rather than insidious onset and exhibit features that mimic infection.

Approach to the Patient

The decision to evaluate acute diarrhea depends on its severity and duration and on various host factors (Fig. 42-2). Most episodes of acute diarrhea are mild and self-limited, and they do not justify the cost and potential morbidity of diagnostic or pharmacologic interventions. Indications for evaluation include profuse diarrhea with dehydration, grossly bloody stools, fever ≥38.5° C, duration >48 h without improvement, new community outbreaks, associated severe abdominal pain in patients older than 50 years of age, and elderly (≥70 years) or immunocompromised patients. In some patients with moderately severe febrile diarrhea with fecal leukocytes (or increased fecal levels of the leukocyte proteins lactoferrin or calprotectin) present or with dysentery, a diagnostic evaluation might be eschewed in favor of an empiric antibiotic trial (see below).

The cornerstone of diagnosis in those suspected of severe acute infectious diarrhea is microbiologic analysis of the stool. Workup includes cultures for bacterial and viral pathogens, direct inspection for ova and parasites, and immunoassays for certain bacterial toxins (*C. difficile*), viral antigens (rotavirus), and protozoal antigens (*Giardia,*

Table 42-2 Association between Pathobiology of Causative Agents and Clinical Features in Acute Infectious Diarrhea

Pathobiology/Agents	Incubation Period	Vomiting	Abdominal Pain	Fever	Diarrhea
Toxin producers					
Preformed toxin					
Bacillus cereus, Staphylococcus aureus, Clostridium perfringens	1–8 h 8–24 h	3–4+	1–2+	0–1+	3–4+, watery
Enterotoxin					
Vibrio cholerae, enterotoxigenic *Escheria coli, Klebsiella pneumoniae, Aeromonas* species	8–72 h	2–4+	1–2+	0–1+	3–4+, watery
Enteroadherent					
Enteropathogenic and enteroadherent, *E. coli, Giardia* organisms, cryptosporidiosis, helminths	1–8 d	0–1+	1–3+	1–2+	1–2+, watery
Cytotoxin-producers					
Clostridium difficile	1–3 d	0–1+	3–4+	1–2+	1–3+, usually watery, occasionally bloody
Hemorrhagic *E. coli*	12–72 h	0–1+	3–4+	1–2+	1–3+, initially watery, quickly bloody
Invasive organisms					
Minimal inflammation					
Rotavirus and Norwalk agent	1–3 d	1–2+	2–3+	3–4+	1–3+, watery
Variable inflammation					
Salmonella, Campylobacter, and *Aeromonas* species, *Vibrio parahaemolyticus, Yersinia*	12 h–11 d	0–3+	2–4+	3–4+	1–4+, watery or bloody
Severe inflammation					
Shigella species, enteroinvasive *E. coli, Entamoeba histolytica*	12 h–8 d	0–1+	3–4+	3–4+	1–2+, bloody

SOURCE: Adapted from DW Powell, in T Yamada (ed): *Textbook of Gastroenterology,* 2d ed. Philadelphia, Lippincott, 1995; and DR Syndman, in SL Gorbach (ed): *Infectious Diarrhea.* London, Blackwell, 1986.

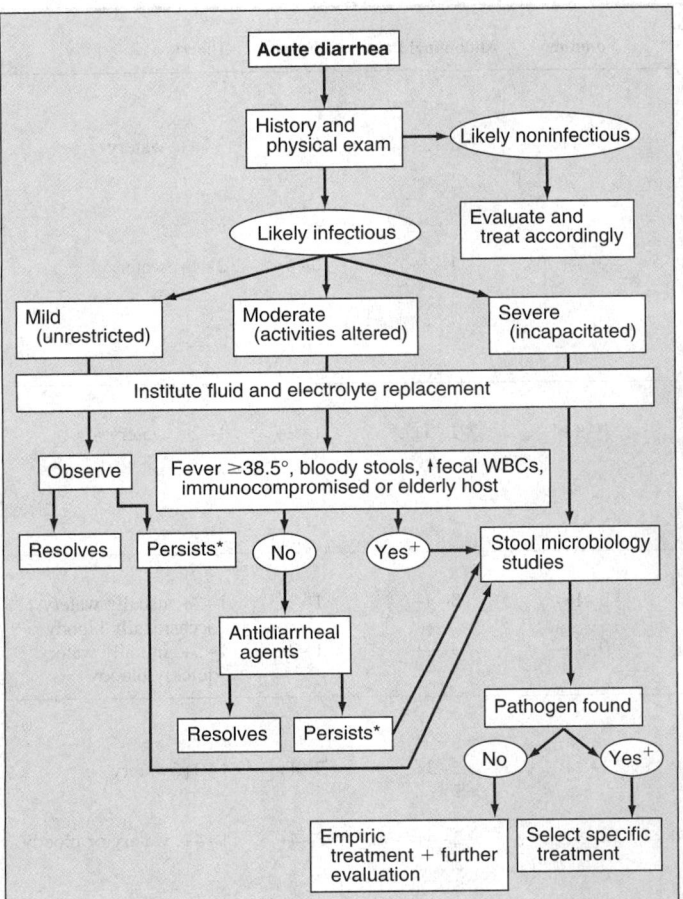

*Consider empiric Rx with metronidazole before eval;
+Consider empiric Rx with quinolone before eval.

FIGURE 42-2 Algorithm for the management of acute diarrhea. Consider empiric Rx before evaluation with (*) metronidazole and (†) with quinolone.

E. histolytica). The aforementioned clinical and epidemiologic associations may assist in focusing the evaluation. If a particular pathogen or set of possible pathogens is so implicated, then either the whole panel of routine studies may not be necessary or, in some instances, special cultures may be appropriate as for enterohemorrhagic and other types of *E. coli*, *Vibrio* species, and *Yersinia*. Molecular diagnosis of pathogens in stool can be made by identification of unique DNA sequences; and evolving microarray technologies could lead to a more rapid, sensitive, specific, and cost-effective diagnostic approach in the future.

Persistent diarrhea is commonly due to *Giardia*, but additional causative organisms that should be considered include *C. difficile* (especially if antibiotics had been administered), *E. histolytica*, *Cryptosporidium*, *Campylobacter*, and others. If stool studies are unrevealing, then flexible sigmoidoscopy with biopsies and upper endoscopy with duodenal aspirates and biopsies may be indicated.

Structural examination by sigmoidoscopy, colonoscopy, or abdominal CT scanning (or other imaging approaches) may be appropriate in patients with uncharacterized persistent diarrhea to exclude inflammatory bowel disease, or as an initial approach in patients with suspected noninfectious acute diarrhea such as might be caused by ischemic colitis, diverticulitis, or partial bowel obstruction.

TREATMENT   Fluid and electrolyte replacement are of central importance to all forms of acute diarrhea. Fluid replacement alone may suffice for mild cases. Oral sugar-electrolyte solutions (sport drinks or designed formulations) should be instituted promptly with

severe diarrhea to limit dehydration, which is the major cause of death. Profoundly dehydrated patients, especially infants and the elderly, require intravenous rehydration.

In moderately severe nonfebrile and nonbloody diarrhea, antimotility antisecretory agents like loperamide can be useful adjuncts to control symptoms. Such agents should be avoided with febrile dysentery, which may be exacerbated or prolonged by them. Bismuth subsalicylate may reduce symptoms of vomiting and diarrhea but should not be used to treat immunocompromised patients because of the risk of bismuth encephalopathy.

Judicious use of antibiotics is appropriate in selected instances of acute diarrhea and may reduce its severity and duration (Fig. 42-2). Many physicians treat moderately to severely ill patients with febrile dysentery empirically without diagnostic evaluation using a quinolone, such as ciprofloxacin (500 mg bid for 3 to 5 d). Empiric treatment can also be considered for suspected giardiasis with metronidazole (250 mg qid for 7d). Selection of antibiotics and dosage regimens is otherwise dictated by specific pathogens and conditions found (Chaps. 131, 153, 156–162). Antibiotic coverage is indicated whether or not a causative organism is discovered in patients that are immunocompromised, have mechanical heart valves or recent vascular grafts, or are elderly. Antibiotic prophylaxis is indicated for certain patients traveling to high-risk countries in whom the likelihood or seriousness of acquired diarrhea would be especially high, including those with immunocompromise, inflammatory bowel disease, or gastric achlorhydria. Use of trimethoprim/sulfamethoxazole or ciprofloxacin may reduce bacterial diarrhea in such travelers by 90%.

CHRONIC DIARRHEA   Diarrhea lasting more than 4 weeks warrants evaluation to exclude serious underlying pathology. In contrast to acute diarrhea, most of the many causes of chronic diarrhea are noninfectious. The classification of chronic diarrhea by pathophysiologic mechanism facilitates a rational approach to management (Table 42-3).

Secretory Causes   Secretory diarrheas are due to derangements in fluid and electrolyte transport across the enterocolic mucosa. They are characterized clinically by watery, large-volume fecal outputs that are typically painless and persist with fasting. Because there is no malabsorbed solute, stool osmolality is accounted for by normal endogenous electrolytes with no fecal osmotic gap.

Medications   Side effects from regular ingestion of drugs and toxins are the most common secretory causes of chronic diarrhea. Hundreds of prescription and over-the-counter medications (see "Other Causes of Acute Diarrhea," above) may produce unwanted diarrhea. Surreptitious or habitual use of stimulant laxatives [e.g., senna, cascara, bisacodyl, ricinoleic acid (castor oil)] must also be considered. Chronic ethanol consumption may cause a secretory-type diarrhea due to enterocyte injury with impaired sodium and water absorption as well as to rapid transit and other alterations. Inadvertent ingestion of certain environmental toxins (e.g., arsenic) may lead to chronic rather than acute forms of diarrhea. Certain bacterial infections may occasionally persist and be associated with a secretory-type diarrhea.

Bowel resection, mucosal disease, or enterocolic fistula   These conditions may result in a secretory-type diarrhea because of inadequate surface for resorption of secreted fluids and electrolytes. Unlike other secretory diarrheas, this subset of conditions tends to worsen with eating. With disease (e.g., Crohn's ileitis) or resection of <100 cm of terminal ileum, dihydroxy bile acids may escape absorption and stimulate colonic secretion (cholorrheic diarrhea). This mechanism may contribute to so-called *idiopathic secretory diarrhea*, in which bile acids are functionally malabsorbed from a normal-appearing terminal ileum. Partial bowel obstruction, ostomy stricture, or fecal impaction may paradoxically lead to increased fecal output due to hypersecretion.

Hormones   Although uncommon, the classic examples of secretory diarrhea are those mediated by hormones. *Metastatic gastrointestinal carcinoid tumors* or, rarely, *primary bronchial carcinoids* may

Table 42-3 Major Causes of Chronic Diarrhea According to Predominant Pathophysiologic Mechanism

Secretory causes	**Inflammatory causes**
Exogenous stimulant laxatives	Idiopathic inflammatory bowel
Chronic ethanol ingestion	disease (Crohn's chronic ulcera-
Other drugs and toxins	tive colitis)
Endogenous laxatives (dihydroxy	Microscopic and collagenous co-
bile acids)	litis
Idiopathic secretory diarrhea	Immune-related mucosal disease
Certain bacterial infections	(1° or 2° immunodeficiencies,
Bowel resection, disease, or fis-	food allergy, eosinophilic gas-
tula (↓ absorption)	troenteritis, graft-vs-host dis-
Partial bowel obstruction or fecal	ease)
impaction	Infections (invasive bacteria, vi-
Hormone-producing tumors (car-	ruses, and parasites)
cinoid, vipoma, medullary can-	Radiation injury
cer of thyroid, mastocytosis,	Gastrointestinal malignancies
gastrinoma, colorectal villous	**Dysmotile causes**
adenoma)	Visceral neuromyopathies
Addison's disease	Hyperthyroidism
Congenital electrolyte absorption	Drugs (prokinetic agents)
defects	**Factitial causes**
Osmotic causes	Munchausen
Osmotic laxatives (Mg^{2+}, PO_4^{3-},	Bulimia
SO_4^{2-})	
Lactase and other disaccharide	
deficiencies	
Nonabsorbable carbohydrates	
(sorbitol, lactulose, polyethyl-	
ene glycol)	
Steatorrheal causes	
Intraluminal maldigestion (pan-	
creatic exocrine insufficiency,	
bacterial overgrowth, liver dis-	
ease)	
Mucosal malabsorption (celiac	
sprue, Whipple's disease, infec-	
tions, abetalipoproteinemia, is-	
chemia)	
Postmucosal obstruction (1° or 2°	
lymphatic obstruction)	

produce watery diarrhea alone or as part of the carcinoid syndrome that comprises episodic flushing, wheezing, dyspnea, and right-sided valvular heart disease. Diarrhea is due to the release into the circulation of potent intestinal secretagogues including serotonin, histamine, prostaglandins, and various kinins. Pellagra-like skin lesions may rarely occur as the result of serotonin overproduction with niacin depletion. *Gastrinoma*, one of the most common neuroendocrine tumors, most typically presents with refractory peptic ulcers, but diarrhea occurs in up to one-third of cases and may be the only clinical manifestation in 10%. While various secretagogues released with gastrin may play a role, the diarrhea most often results from fat maldigestion owing to pancreatic enzyme inactivation by low intraduodenal pH. The watery diarrhea hypokalemia achlorhydria (WDHA) syndrome, also called *pancreatic cholera*, is due to a non-β cell pancreatic adenoma, referred to as a VIPoma, that secretes vasoactive intestinal peptide (VIP) and a host of other peptide hormones including pancreatic polypeptide, secretin, gastrin, gastrin-inhibitory polypeptide, neurotensin, calcitonin, and prostaglandins. The secretory diarrhea is often massive with stool volumes >3 L/d; daily volumes as high as 20 L have been reported. Life-threatening dehydration, neuromuscular dysfunction from associated hypokalemia, hypomagnesemia, or hypercalcemia, flushing, and hyperglycemia may accompany vipoma. *Medullary carcinoma of the thyroid* may present with watery diarrhea caused by calcitonin, other secretory peptides, or prostaglandins. This tumor occurs sporadically or, in 25 to 50% of cases, as a feature of multiple endocrine neoplasia type IIa with pheochromocytomas and hyperparathyroidism. Prominent diarrhea is often associated with metastatic disease and poor prognosis. *Systemic mastocytosis*, which may be associated with the skin lesion urticaria pigmentosa, may cause diarrhea that is either secretory and mediated by histamine, or inflammatory and due

to intestinal filtration by mast cells. Large *colorectal villous adenomas* may rarely be associated with a secretory diarrhea that may cause hypokalemia, can be inhibited by NSAIDs, and is apparently mediated by prostaglandins.

Congenital defects in ion absorption Rarely, these defects cause watery diarrhea from birth and include defective Cl^-/HCO_3^- exchange (*congenital chloridorrhea*) with alkalosis and defective Na^+/H^+ exchange with acidosis. Some hormone deficiencies may be associated with watery diarrhea, such as occurs with adrenocortical insufficiency (Addison's disease) that may be accompanied by hyperpigmentation.

Osmotic Causes Osmotic diarrhea occurs when ingested, poorly absorbable, osmotically active solutes draw enough fluid lumenward to exceed the resorptive capacity of the colon. Fecal water output increases in proportion to such a solute load. Osmotic diarrhea characteristically ceases with fasting or with discontinued oral intake of the offending agent.

Osmotic laxatives Ingestion of magnesium-containing antacids, health supplements, or laxatives may induce osmotic diarrhea typified by a stool osmotic gap: $2([Na] + [K]) \ll 290$ mosm/kg. Anionic laxatives containing sulfates or phosphates produce osmotic diarrhea without an osmotic gap, as sodium accompanies the anionic solutes; direct measurement of stool sulfates and phosphates may be necessary to confirm the cause of diarrhea.

Carbohydrate malabsorption Carbohydrate malabsorption due to acquired or congenital defects in brush-border disaccharidases and other enzymes leads to osmotic diarrhea with a low pH. One of the most common causes of chronic diarrhea in adults is *lactase deficiency*, which affects three-fourths of non-Caucasians worldwide and 5 to 30% of persons in the United States; most learn to avoid milk products without an intervention. Some sugars, such as sorbitol, are universally malabsorbed, and diarrhea ensues with ingestion of ample medications, gum, or candies sweetened with these nonabsorbable sugars. Lactulose, used to acidify stools in patients with hepatic failure, also causes diarrhea on this basis.

Steatorrheal Causes Fat malabsorption may lead to greasy, foul-smelling, difficult-to-flush diarrhea often associated with weight loss and nutritional deficiencies due to concomitant malabsorption of amino acids and vitamins. Increased fecal output is caused by the osmotic effects of fatty acids, especially after bacterial hydroxylation, and, to a lesser extent, by the burden of neutral fat. Quantitatively, steatorrhea is defined as stool fat exceeding the normal 7 g/d; daily fecal fat averages 15 to 25 g with small intestinal diseases and often exceeds 40 g with pancreatic exocrine insufficiency. Intraluminal maldigestion, mucosal malabsorption, or lymphatic obstruction may produce steatorrhea.

Intraluminal maldigestion This condition most commonly results from pancreatic exocrine insufficiency, which occurs when >90% of pancreatic secretory function is lost. *Chronic pancreatitis*, usually a sequela of ethanol abuse, most frequently causes pancreatic insufficiency. Other causes include *cystic fibrosis*, *pancreatic duct obstruction*, and rarely, *somatostatinoma*. Bacterial overgrowth in the small intestine may deconjugate bile acids and alter micelle formation that impair fat digestion; it occurs with stasis from a blind-loop, small bowel diverticulum, or dysmotility and is especially likely in the elderly. Finally, cirrhosis or biliary obstruction may lead to mild steatorrhea due to deficient intraluminal bile acid concentration.

Mucosal malabsorption Mucosal malabsorption occurs from a variety of enteropathies, but most prototypically and perhaps most commonly from *celiac sprue*. This gluten-sensitive enteropathy characterized by villous atrophy and crypt hyperplasia in the proximal small bowel often presents with fatty diarrhea associated with multiple nutritional deficiencies of varying severity and affects all ages. *Tropical sprue* may produce a similar histologic and clinical syndrome, but it occurs in residents of or travelers to tropical climates; its often abrupt onset and response to antibiotics suggest an infectious etiology. *Whipple's disease*, due to the actinomycete *Treponema whippleii* and histiocytic infiltration of the small bowel mucosa, is a less common cause of steatorrhea that most typically occurs in young or middle-aged men; it is frequently associated with arthralgias, fever, lymphadenopathy, and extreme fatigue and may affect the central nervous system and endocardium. A similar clinical and histologic picture results from *Mycobacterium avium intracellulare* infection in patients with AIDS. *Abetalipoproteinemia* is a rare defect of chylomicron formation and fat malabsorption in children associated with acanthocytic erythrocytes, ataxia, and retinitis pigmentosa. Several other conditions may cause mucosal malabsorption including infections, especially with protozoa like *Giardia*, numerous medications (e.g., colchicine, cholestyramine, neomycin), and chronic ischemia.

Postmucosal lymphatic obstruction   The pathophysiology of this condition, which is due to the rare *congenital intestinal lymphangiectasia* or to *acquired lymphatic obstruction* secondary to trauma, tumor, or infection, leads to the unique constellation of fat malabsorption with enteric losses of protein (often causing edema) and lymphocytes (with resultant lymphocytopenia) that enter the portal circulation directly. Carbohydrate and amino acid absorption are preserved.

Inflammatory Causes   Inflammatory diarrheas are generally accompanied by pain, fever, bleeding, or other manifestations of inflammation. The mechanism of diarrhea may not only be exudation but, depending on lesion site, may include fat malabsorption, disrupted fluid/electrolyte absorption, and hypersecretion or hypermotility from release of cytokines and other inflammatory mediators. The unifying feature on stool analysis is the presence of leukocytes or leukocyte-derived proteins such as calprotectin. With severe inflammation, exudative protein loss can lead to anasarca (generalized edema). Any middle-aged or older person with chronic inflammatory-type diarrhea, especially with blood, should be carefully evaluated to exclude a colorectal or large enteric tumor.

Idiopathic inflammatory bowel disease   The illnesses in this category, which include *Crohn's disease* and *chronic ulcerative colitis*, are among the most common organic causes of chronic diarrhea in adults and range in severity from mild to fulminant and life threatening. They may be associated with uveitis, polyarthralgias, cholestatic liver disease (primary sclerosing cholangitis), and various skin lesions (erythema nodosum, pyoderma gangrenosum). *Microscopic colitis*, including *collagenous colitis*, is an increasingly recognized cause of chronic watery diarrhea; biopsy of a normal appearing colorectum is required for histologic diagnosis.

Primary or secondary forms of immunodeficiency   Immunodeficiency may lead to prolonged infectious diarrhea. With common variable *hypogammaglobulinemia*, diarrhea is particularly prevalent and often the result of giardiasis.

Eosinophilic gastroenteritis   Eosinophil infiltration of the mucosa, muscularis, or serosa at any level of the gastrointestinal tract may cause diarrhea, pain, vomiting, or ascites. Affected patients often have an atopic history, Charcot-Leyden crystals due to extruded eosinophil contents may be seen on microscopic inspection of stool, and peripheral eosinophilia is present in 50 to 75% of patients. While hypersensitivity to certain foods occurs in adults, true food allergy causing chronic diarrhea is rare.

Other causes   Chronic inflammatory diarrhea may be caused by *radiation enterocolitis*, *chronic graft-versus-host disease*, *Behcet's syndrome*, and *Cronkite-Canada syndrome*, among others.

Dysmotile Causes   Rapid transit may accompany many diarrheas as a secondary or contributing phenomenon, but primary dysmotility is an unusual etiology of true diarrhea. Stool features often suggest a secretory diarrhea, but mild steatorrhea up to 14 g of fat per day can be produced by maldigestion from rapid transit alone. *Hyperthyroidism*, *carcinoid syndrome*, and certain drugs (e.g., prostaglandins, prokinetic agents) may produce hypermotility with resultant diarrhea. Primary visceral neuromyopathies or idiopathic acquired intestinal pseudo-obstruction may lead to stasis with secondary bacterial overgrowth causing diarrhea. *Diabetic diarrhea*, often accompanied by peripheral and generalized autonomic neuropathies, may occur in part because of intestinal dysmotility.

The exceedingly common *irritable bowel syndrome* (10% point prevalence, 1 to 2% per year incidence) is characterized by disturbed intestinal and colonic motor and sensory responses to various stimuli. Symptoms of stool frequency typically cease at night, alternate with periods of constipation, are accompanied by abdominal pain relieved with defecation, and rarely result in weight loss or true diarrhea.

Factitial Causes   Factitial diarrhea accounts for up to 15% of unexplained diarrheas referred to tertiary care centers. Either as a form of *Munchausen syndrome* (deception or self-injury for secondary gain) or *bulimia*, some patients covertly self-administer laxatives alone or in combination with other medications (e.g., diuretics) or surreptitiously add water or urine to stool sent for analysis. Such patients are typically women, often with histories of psychiatric illness and disproportionately from careers in health care. Hypotension and hypokalemia are common co-presenting features. Such patients often deny this possibility when confronted, but they do benefit from psychiatric counseling when they acknowledge their behavior.

Approach to the Patient

The laboratory tools available to evaluate the very common problem of chronic diarrhea are extensive, and many are costly and invasive. As such, the diagnostic evaluation must be rationally directed by a careful history and physical examination, and simple triage tests are often warranted before complex investigations are launched (Fig. 42-3). The history, physical examination, and routine blood studies should attempt to characterize the mechanism of diarrhea, identify diagnostically helpful associations, and assess the patient's fluid/electrolyte and nutritional status. Patients should be questioned about the onset, duration, pattern, aggravants (especially diet), relieving factors, and stool characteristics of their diarrhea. The presence or absence of fecal incontinence, fever, weight loss, pain, certain exposures (travel, medications, contacts with diarrhea), and common extraintestinal manifestations (skin changes, arthralgias, oral aphtha) should be noted. Physical findings may offer clues such as a thyroid mass, wheezing, heart murmurs, edema, hepatomegaly, abdominal masses, lymphadenopathy, mucocutaneous abnormalities, perianal fistulae, or anal sphincter laxity. Peripheral blood counts may reveal leukocytosis that suggests inflammation; anemia that reflects blood loss or nutritional deficiencies; or eosinophilia that may occur with parasitoses, neoplasia, collagen-vascular disease, allergy, or eosinophilic gastroenteritis. Blood chemistries may demonstrate electrolyte, hepatic, or other metabolic disturbances.

A therapeutic trial is often appropriate, definitive, and highly cost-effective when a specific diagnosis is suggested on the initial physician encounter. For example, chronic watery diarrhea, which ceases with fasting in an otherwise healthy young adult, may justify a trial of a lactose-restricted diet; bloating and diarrhea persisting since a mountain backpacking trip may warrant a trial of metronidazole for likely giardiasis; and postprandial diarrhea persisting since an ileal resection might be treated with cholestyramine before further evaluation. Persistent symptoms require additional investigation.

Certain diagnoses may be suggested on the initial encounter, e.g., idiopathic inflammatory bowel disease; however, additional focused evaluations may be necessary to confirm the diagnosis and characterize the severity or extent of disease so that treatment can be best guided. Patients suspected of having irritable bowel syndrome should be initially evaluated with proctosigmoidoscopy and mucosal biopsies; those with normal findings might be reassured and, as indicated, treated empirically with antispasmodics, antidiarrheals, bulk agents, anxiolytes, or antidepressants. Any patient who presents with chronic diarrhea and hematochezia should be evaluated with stool microbiologic studies and colonoscopy.

In an estimated two-thirds of cases, the cause for chronic diarrhea remains unclear after the initial encounter, and further testing is required. Quantitative stool collection and analyses can yield important objective data that may establish a diagnosis or characterize the type of diarrhea as a triage for focused additional studies (Fig. 42-3). If stool weight exceeds 200 g/d, additional stool analyses should be performed that might include electrolyte concentration, pH, occult blood testing, leukocyte inspection (or leukocyte protein assay), fat quantitation, and laxative screens.

For secretory diarrheas (watery, normal osmotic gap), possible medication-related side effects or surreptitious laxative use should be reconsidered. Microbiologic studies should be done including fecal bacterial cultures (including media for *Aeromonas* and *Pleisiomonas*), inspection for ova and parasites, and *Giardia* antigen assay (the most sensitive test for giardiasis). Small bowel bacterial overgrowth can be excluded by intestinal aspirates with quantitative cultures or with glucose or xylose breath tests involving measurement of breath hydrogen or other metabolite (e.g., $^{14}CO_2$). However, interpretation of these breath tests may be confounded by disturbances of intestinal transit. When suggested by history or other findings, screens for peptide hormones should be pursued (e.g., serum gastrin, VIP, calcitonin, and thyroid hormone/thyroid stimulating hormone, or urinary 5-hydroxyindolacetic acid and histamine). Upper endoscopy and colonoscopy with biopsies and small bowel barium x-rays are helpful to rule out structural or occult inflammatory disease.

Further evaluation of osmotic diarrhea should include tests for lactose intolerance and magnesium ingestion, the two most common causes. Low fecal pH suggests carbohydrate malabsorption; lactose malabsorption can be confirmed by lactose breath testing or by a therapeutic trial with lactose exclusion and observation of the effect of lactose challenge (e.g., a quart of milk). Lactase determination on small bowel biopsy is generally not available. If fecal Mg^{2+} or laxative levels are elevated, then inadvertent or surreptitious ingestion should be considered and psychiatric help should be sought.

For those with proven fatty diarrhea, endoscopy with small bowel biopsy (including aspiration for *Giardia* and quantitative cultures) should be performed; if this procedure is unrevealing, a small bowel radiograph is often an appropriate next step. If small bowel studies are negative or if pancreatic disease is suspected, pancreatic exocrine insufficiency should be excluded with direct tests, such as the secretin-cholecystokinin stimulation test, or by indirect tests, such as assay of fecal chymotrypsin activity or a bentiromide test.

Chronic inflammatory-type diarrheas should be suspected by the presence of blood or leukocytes in the stool. Such findings warrant stool cultures, inspection for ova and parasites, *C. difficile* toxin assay, colonoscopy with biopsies, and if indicated, small bowel oral contrast studies.

TREATMENT Treatment of chronic diarrhea depends on the specific etiology and may be curative, suppressive, or empiric. If the cause can be eradicated, treatment is curative as with resection of a colorectal cancer, antibiotic administration for Whipple's disease, or discontinuation of an offending drug. For many chronic conditions, diarrhea can be controlled by suppression of the underlying mechanism. Examples include elimination of dietary lactose for lactase deficiency or gluten for celiac sprue, use of glucocorticoids or other antiinflammatory agents for idiopathic inflammatory bowel diseases, adsorptive agents such as cholestyramine for ileal bile acid malabsorption, proton pump inhibitors such as omeprazole for the gastric hypersecretion of gastrinomas, somatostatin analogues such as octreotide for malignant carcinoid, prostaglandin inhibitors such as indomethacin for medullary carcinoma of the thyroid, and pancreatic enzyme replacement for pancreatic insufficiency. When the specific cause or mechanism of chronic diarrhea evades diagnosis, empiric therapy may be beneficial. Mild opiates such as diphenoxylate or loperamide are often helpful in mild or moderate watery diarrhea. For those with more severe diarrhea, codeine or tincture of opium may be beneficial. Such antimotility agents should be avoided with inflammatory bowel disease, as toxic megacolon may be precipitated. Clonidine, an α_2-adrenergic agonist, may allow control of diabetic diarrhea. For all patients with chronic diarrhea, fluid and electrolyte repletion is an important component of management (see "Acute Diarrhea," above). Replacement of fat-soluble vitamins may also be necessary in patients with chronic steatorrhea.

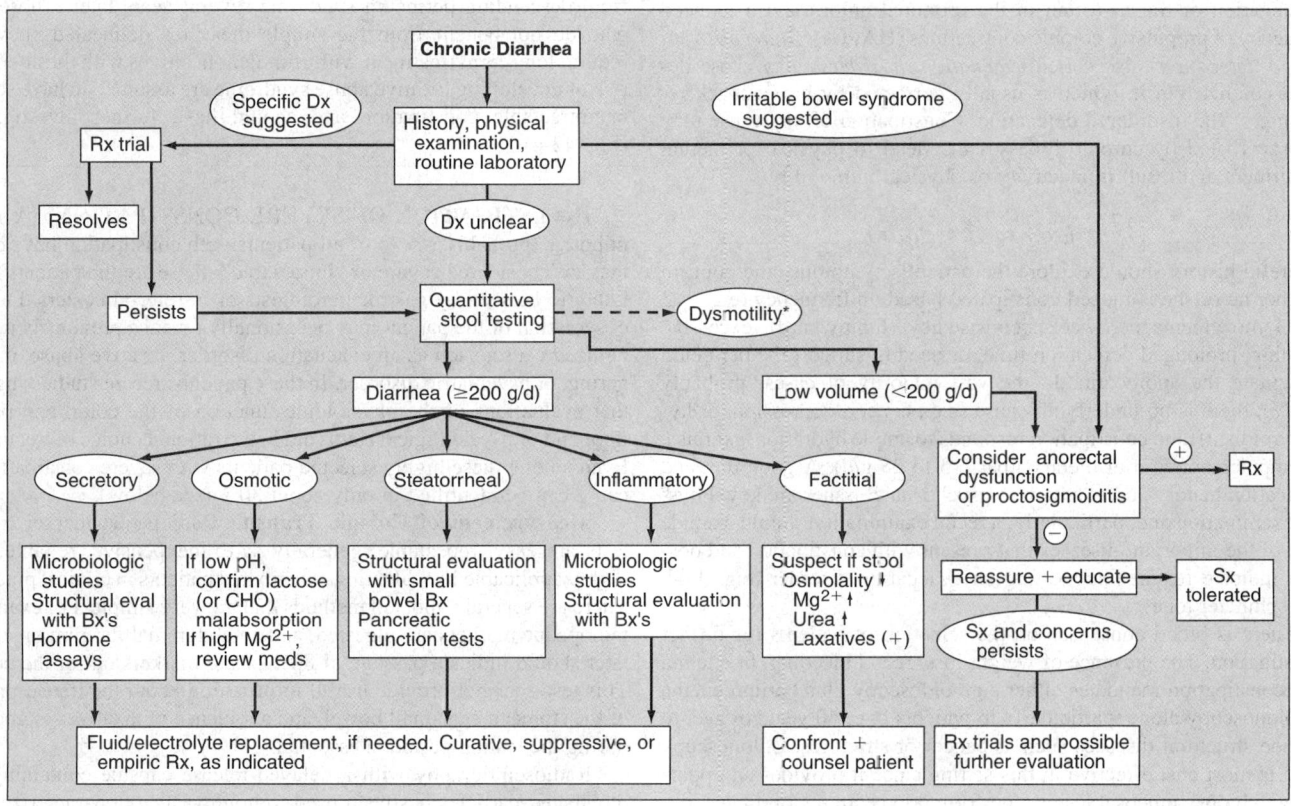

FIGURE 42-3 Algorithm for the management of chronic diarrhea.* Dysmotility presents variable stool profile.

CONSTIPATION

DEFINITION Constipation is a common complaint in clinical practice and usually refers to persistent, difficult, infrequent, or seemingly incomplete defecation. Because of the wide range of normal bowel habits, constipation is difficult to define precisely. Most persons have at least three bowel movements per week; however, stool frequency alone is not a sufficient criterion for the diagnosis of constipation because many constipated patients describe a normal frequency of defecation but subjective complaints of excessive straining, hard stools, lower abdominal fullness, and a sense of incomplete evacuation. The individual patient's symptoms must be analyzed in detail to ascertain what is meant by "constipation" or "difficulty" with defecation.

Stool form and consistency are well correlated with the time elapsed from the preceding defecation. Hard, pellety stools occur with slow transit, while loose watery stools are associated with rapid transit. Small, pellety stools are more difficult to expel than large ones.

The perception of hard stools or excessive straining is more difficult to assess objectively, and the need for enemas or digital disimpaction is a clinically useful way to corroborate the patient's perceptions of difficult defecation.

Psychosocial factors may also be important. A person whose parents attached great importance to daily defecation will become greatly concerned when he or she misses a daily bowel movement; some children withhold stool to gain attention; and some adults are simply too busy or too embarrassed to interrupt their work when the call to have a bowel movement is sensed.

CAUSES Pathophysiologically, chronic constipation generally results from inadequate fiber intake or from disordered colonic transit or anorectal function as a result of a neurogastroenterologic disturbance, certain drugs, or in association with a large number of systemic diseases that affect the gastroinestinal tract (Table 42-4). Constipation of recent onset may be a symptom of significant organic disease such as tumor or stricture. In *idiopathic constipation*, a subset of patients exhibit delayed emptying of the ascending and transverse colon with prolongation of transit (often in the proximal colon) and a reduced frequency of propulsive colonic contractions (HAPCs). *Outlet obstruction to defecation* (also called *evacuation disorders*) may cause delayed colonic transit, which is usually corrected by biofeedback retraining of the disordered defecation. Constipation of any cause may be exacerbated by chronic illnesses that lead to physical or mental impairment and result in inactivity or physical immobility.

Approach to the Patient

A careful history should explore the patient's symptoms and confirm whether he or she is indeed constipated based on frequency (e.g., <3 bowel movements per week), consistency (lumpy/hard), excessive straining, prolonged defecation time, or need to support the perineum or digitate the anorectum. In the vast majority of cases (probably >90%), there is no underlying cause (e.g., cancer, depression, or hypothyroidism), and constipation responds to ample hydration, exercise, and supplementation of dietary fiber (15 to 25 g/d). A good diet and medication history and attention to psychosocial issues are key. Physical examination and, particularly, a rectal examination should exclude most of the important diseases that present with constipation and possibly indicate features suggesting an evacuation disorder (e.g., high anal sphincter tone).

There is broad consensus on the selection of patients for further investigation. The presence of weight loss, rectal bleeding, or anemia with constipation mandates either sigmoidoscopy plus barium enema or colonoscopy alone, particularly in patients over 40 years of age, to exclude structural diseases such as cancer or strictures. Colonoscopy alone is most cost effective in this setting since it provides an opportunity to biopsy mucosal lesions, perform polypectomy, or dilate strictures. Barium enema has advantages over colonoscopy in the patient

Table 42-4 Causes of Constipation in Adults

Types of Constipation and Causes	Examples
Recent Onset	
Colonic obstruction	Neoplasm: stricture: ischemic, diverticular, inflammatory
Anal sphincter spasm	Anal fissure, painful hemorrhoids
Medications	
Chronic	
Irritable bowel syndrome	Constipation–predominant, alternating
Medications	Ca^{2+} blockers, antidepressants
Colonic pseudo-obstruction	Slow transit constipation, megacolon (rare Hirschsprung's, Chagas)
Disorders of rectal evacuation	Pelvic floor dysfunction, anismus, descending perineum syndrome, rectal mucosal prolapse, rectocele
Endocrinopathies	Hypothyroidism, hypercalcemia, pregnancy
Psychiatric disorders	Depression, eating disorders, drugs
Neurologic disease	Parkinsonism, multiple sclerosis, spinal cord injury
Generalized muscle disease	Progressive systemic sclerosis

with isolated constipation, since it is less costly and identifies colonic dilatation and all significant mucosal lesions or strictures that are likely to present with constipation. Melanosis coli, or pigmentation of the colon mucosa, indicates the use of anthraquinone laxatives such as cascara or senna; however, this is usually apparent from a careful history. An unexpected disorder such as megacolon or cathartic colon may also be detected by colonic radiographs. Measurement of serum calcium and thyroid stimulating hormone levels will identify rare patients with metabolic disorders.

Patients with more troublesome constipation may not respond to fiber alone and may be helped by a bowel training regimen: taking an osmotic laxative and evacuating with enema or glycerine suppository as needed. After breakfast, a distraction-free 15 to 20 min on the toilet without straining is encouraged. Excessive straining may lead to development of hemorrhoids, and, if there is weakness of the pelvic floor or injury to the pudendal nerve, may result in obstructed defecation from descending perineum syndrome several years later. Those few who do not benefit from the simple measures delineated above or require long-term treatment with stimulant laxatives with the attendant risk of developing laxative abuse syndrome are assumed to have severe or intractable constipation and should have further investigation (Fig. 42-4).

INVESTIGATION OF SEVERE CONSTIPATION A small minority (probably <5%) of all patients with constipation have cases that are considered severe or "intractable"; these are the patients most likely to be seen by gastroenterologists or in referral centers. Further observation of the patient may occasionally reveal a previously unrecognized cause, such as an evacuation disorder, laxative abuse, malingering, or psychiatric disorder. In these patients, recent studies suggest that evaluations of the physiologic function of the colon and pelvic floor and of psychological status aid in the rational choice of treatment. Even among these highly selected patients with severe constipation, a cause can be identified in only about 30% (see below).

Measurement of Colonic Transit Radiopaque marker transit tests are easy, repeatable, generally safe, inexpensive, reliable, and highly applicable in evaluating constipated patients in clinical practice. There are several validated methods that are very simple. For example, radiopaque markers are ingested, and an abdominal flat film taken 5 d later should indicate passage of 80% of the markers out of the colon. This test does not provide useful information about the transit profile of the stomach and small bowel, and avoidance of laxatives or enemas during the testing period is essential.

Radioscintigraphy with a delayed-release capsule containing radiolabeled particles has been used to noninvasively characterize normal, accelerated, or delayed colonic function over 24 to 48 h with low

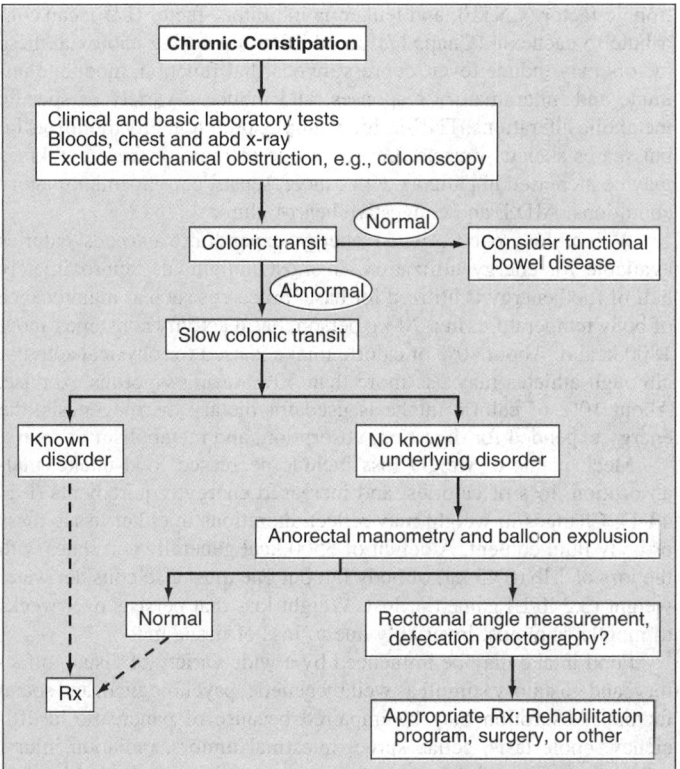

Chronic Constipation

Clinical and basic laboratory tests
Bloods, chest and abd x-ray
Exclude mechanical obstruction, e.g., colonoscopy

Colonic transit — (Normal) → Consider functional bowel disease

(Abnormal)

Slow colonic transit

Known disorder / No known underlying disorder

Anorectal manometry and balloon explusion

Normal / Rectoanal angle measurement, defecation proctography?

Rx

Appropriate Rx: Rehabilitation program, surgery, or other

FIGURE 42-4 Algorithm for the management of constipation.

radiation exposure. This approach simultaneously assesses gastric, small bowel, and colonic transit. The disadvantages are the greater cost and the need for specific materials prepared in a nuclear medicine laboratory.

Anorectal and Pelvic Floor Tests Pelvic floor dysfunction is suggested by the inability to evacuate the rectum, a feeling of persistent rectal fullness, rectal pain, the need to extract stool from the rectum digitally, application of pressure on the posterior wall of the vagina, support of the perineum during straining, and excessive straining. These significant symptoms should be contrasted with the sense of incomplete rectal evacuation, which is common in irritable bowel syndrome.

Patients with clinically suspected obstruction of defecation should also be evaluated by a psychologist to identify eating disorders or a "need to control," to provide stress management or relaxation training, and to identify depression.

A simple clinical test in the office to document a nonrelaxing puborectalis muscle is to have the patient strain to expel the index finger during a digital rectal exam. Motion of the puborectalis posteriorly during straining indicates proper coordination of the pelvic floor muscles.

Measurement of perineal descent is relatively easy to gauge clinically by placing the patient in the left decubitus position and watching the perineum to assess either paucity or lack of descent (<1.5 cm, a sign of pelvic floor dysfunction) or perineal ballooning during straining relative to bony landmarks (>4 cm, suggesting excessive perineal descent).

A useful overall test of evacuation is the balloon expulsion test. A urinary catheter is placed in the rectum, the balloon is inflated to 50 ml with water, and a determination is made about whether the patient can expel it while seated on a toilet or in the left lateral decubitus position. In the lateral position, the weight needed to facilitate expulsion of the balloon (normal, 0 to 200 g) is determined.

Anorectal manometry is not often contributory in the evaluation of patients presenting with severe constipation, except when an excessively high resting or squeeze anal sphincter tone suggests anismus (anal sphincter spasm). This test also identifies rare syndromes, such

as adult Hirschsprung's disease, by the absence of the rectoanal inhibitory reflex or the presence of occult incontinence.

Defecography (a dynamic barium enema including lateral views obtained during barium expulsion) reveals "soft abnormalities" in many patients; the most relevant findings are the measured changes in rectoanal angle, anatomic defects of the rectum, and enteroceles or rectoceles. In a very small proportion of patients, significant anatomic defects associated with intractable constipation respond best to surgical treatment. These defects include severe intussusception with complete outlet obstruction due to funnel-shaped plugging at the anal canal or an extremely large rectocele that is preferentially filled during attempts at defecation instead of expulsion of the barium through the anus. In summary, defecography requires an interested and experienced radiologist, and abnormalities are not pathognomonic for pelvic floor dysfunction. More commonly, outlet obstruction results from a nonrelaxing puborectalis muscle, which impedes rectal emptying, rather than from defects identified by defecography.

Dynamic imaging studies such as proctography during defecation or scintigraphic expulsion of artificial stool help measure perineal descent and the rectoanal angle during rest, squeezing and straining, and scintigraphic expulsion quantitates the amount of "artificial stool" emptied. Failure of the rectoanal angle to increase significantly ($\sim15°$) during straining confirms pelvic floor dysfunction.

Neurologic testing (EMG) is more helpful in the evaluation of patients with incontinence than of those with symptoms suggesting obstructed defecation. The absence of neurologic signs in the lower extremities suggests that any documented denervation of the puborectalis results from pelvic (e.g., obstetric) injury or from stretching of the pudendal nerve by chronic, long-standing straining.

Ultrasonography identifies sphincter or rectal wall defects and may help select patients for surgical correction. Spinal-evoked responses during electrical rectal stimulation or stimulation of external anal sphincter contraction by applying magnetic stimulation over the lumbosacral cord identify patients with limited sacral neuropathies with sufficient residual nerve conduction to attempt biofeedback training.

In summary, a balloon expulsion test is an important screening test for anorectal dysfunction. If positive, an anatomic evaluation of the rectum or anal sphincters and an assessment of pelvic floor relaxation are the tools for evaluating patients in whom obstructed defecation is suspected.

TREATMENT After the cause of constipation is characterized, a treatment decision can be made. Slow transit constipation requires aggressive medical or surgical treatment; anismus or pelvic floor dysfunction usually responds to biofeedback management (Fig. 42-4). However, only about 30% of patients with severe constipation are found to have such a physiologic disorder.

Patients with slow transit constipation are treated with bulk, osmotic, and stimulant laxatives, including fiber, psyllium, milk of magnesia, lactulose, polyethylene glycol (colonic lavage solution), and bisacodyl. If a 2- to 3-month trial of medical therapy fails and patients continue to have documented slow transit constipation unassociated with obstructed defecation, colectomy with ileorectostomy is indicated. The decision to resort to surgery is facilitated in the presence of megacolon and megarectum. The complications after surgery include small bowel obstruction (11%) and fecal soiling, particularly at night during the first postoperative year.

Patients who have a combined disorder should pursue pelvic floor retraining (biofeedback and muscle relaxation), psychological counseling, and dietetic advice first, followed by colectomy and ileorectostomy if colonic transit studies do not normalize with biofeedback alone. In patients with pelvic floor dysfunction alone, biofeedback training has a 70 to 80% success rate, measured by the acquisition of comfortable stool habits. Attempts to manage pelvic floor dysfunction with operations (internal anal sphincter or puborectalis muscle division) have achieved only mediocre success and have been largely abandoned.

BIBLIOGRAPHY

AMERICAN GASTROENTEROLOGICAL ASSOCIATION MEDICAL POSITION STATEMENT. Guidelines for the evaluation and management of chronic diarrhea. Gastroenterology 116:1461, 1991

CAMILLERI M et al: Clinical management of intractable constipation. Ann Intern Med 121:520, 1994

DUPONT HL and PRACTICE PARAMETERS COMMITTEE OF THE AMERICAN COLLEGE OF GASTROENTEROLOGY: Guidelines on acute infectious diarrhea in adults. Am J Gastroenterol 92:1962, 1997

FINE KD, SCHILLER LR: AGA technical review on the evaluation and management of chronic diarrhea. Gastroenterology 116:1461, 1999

LOCKE GR: The epidemiology of functional gastrointestinal disorders in North America. Gastroenterol Clin North Am 25:1, 1996

PROANO M et al: Transit of solids through the human colon: regional quantification in the unprepared bowel. Am J Physiol 1990;258:G856-62.

ROHNER P et al: Etiological agents of infectious diarrhea: Implications for requests for microbial culture. J Clin Microbiol 35:1427, 1997

SUAREZ FL et al: Bismuth subsalicylate markedly decreases hydrogen sulfide release in the human colon. Gastroenterology 114:923, 1998

SURRENTI E et al: Audit of constipation in a tertiary-referral gastroenterology practice. Am J Gastroenterol 90:1471, 1995

---

43 Carol M. Reife

WEIGHT LOSS

Significant unintentional weight loss in a previously healthy individual is often a harbinger of underlying systemic disease. During the routine medical history, therefore, inquiry should always be made about changes in weight; loss of 5% of body weight over 6 to 12 months should prompt further evaluation.

PHYSIOLOGY OF WEIGHT REGULATION   The normal individual maintains weight at a remarkably stable "set point," given the wide variation in daily caloric intake and level of activity. Because of the physiologic importance of maintaining energy stores, voluntary weight loss is difficult to achieve and sustain.

Appetite and metabolism are regulated by an intricate network of neural and hormonal factors. The hypothalamic feeding and satiety centers play a central role in these processes (Chap. 77). Neuropeptides, like corticotropin-releasing hormone (CRH), α-melanocyte stimulating hormone (α-MSH), and cocaine and amphetamine-related transcript (CART) induce anorexia by acting centrally on satiety centers. Epinephrine and norepinephrine cause a decrease in food intake and an increase in metabolic rate (Chap. 72). Amphetamines and related drugs used to suppress appetite act by releasing norepinephrine in the central nervous system. The gastrointestinal peptides glucagon, somatostatin, and particularly cholecystokinin induce a decrease in food intake by acting through a vagal mechanism to signal satiety. Hypoglycemia decreases levels of insulin which reduces glucose utilization and inhibits activity of the satiety center.

Leptin plays a central role in the long-term maintenance of weight homeostasis (Chap. 77). Leptin is produced by adipose tissue and acts on the hypothalamus to decrease food intake and increase energy expenditure. It suppresses expression of hypothalamic neuropeptide Y, a potent appetite stimulatory peptide. In parallel, leptin increases the expression of α-MSH, which decreases appetite by acting on the MC4R melanocortin receptor. Thus, leptin activates a series of downstream neural pathways that alter food-seeking behavior and metabolism. However, leptin deficiency, which occurs in conjunction with the loss adipose tissue, stimulates appetite and induces other adaptive responses including inhibition of hypothalamic thyrotropin releasing hormone (TRH) and gonadotropin releasing hormone (GnRH).

A variety of cytokines, including tumor necrosis factor α (TNF-α), interleukin (IL) (IL-6), IL-1, interferon γ (IFN-γ), ciliary neurotrophic factor (CNTF), and leukemia inhibitory factor (LIF), can contribute to cachexia (Chap. 17). In addition to causing anorexia, these factors may induce fever, depress myocardial function, modulate immune and inflammatory responses, and induce a variety of specific metabolic alterations. TNF-α, for example, preferentially mobilizes fat but spares skeletal muscle. Levels of one or more of these cytokines may be increased in patients with cancer, sepsis, chronic inflammatory conditions, AIDS, and congestive heart failure.

Weight loss occurs when energy expenditure exceeds calories available for energy utilization. In most individuals, approximately half of food energy is utilized for basal processes such as maintenance of body temperature. In a 70-kg person, basal activity consumes about 1800 kcal/d. About 40% of caloric intake is used for physical activity, although athletes may use more than 50% during vigorous exercise. About 10% of caloric intake is used for dietary thermogenesis, the energy expended for digestion, absorption, and metabolism of food.

Mechanisms of weight loss include decreased food intake, malabsorption, loss of calories, and increased energy requirements (Fig. 43-1). Changes in weight may reflect alterations in either tissue mass or body fluid content. A deficit of 3500 kcal generally correlates with the loss of 1 lb (0.45 kg) of body fat, but one must also consider water weight (2.2 lb/L) gained or lost. Weight loss that persists over weeks to months is almost invariably due to loss of tissue mass.

Food intake may be influenced by a wide variety of visual, olfactory, and gustatory stimuli as well by genetic, psychological, and social factors. Absorption may be impaired because of pancreatic insufficiency, cholestasis, celiac sprue, intestinal tumors, radiation injury, inflammatory bowel disease, infection, or medication effect. Manifestations of these disease processes may be suggested by changes in stool frequency and consistency. Calories also may be lost due to vomiting or diarrhea, glucosuria in diabetes mellitus, or fistulous drainage. Resting energy expenditure decreases with age and can be affected by thyroid status. Beginning at about age 60, body weight declines by an average of 0.5% per year. Body composition is also affected by aging; adipose tissue increases and lean muscle mass decreases with age.

SIGNIFICANCE OF WEIGHT LOSS   Unintentional weight loss, especially in the elderly, is not uncommon and is associated with increased morbidity and mortality rates, even after comorbid conditions have been taken into account. Prospective studies indicate that significant involuntary weight loss is associated with a mortality rate of 25% over the next 18 months. Retrospective studies of significant weight loss in the elderly document mortality rates of 9 to 38% over a 2- to 3-year period.

Cancer patients with weight loss have decreased performance status, response to chemotherapy, and median survival (Chap. 79).

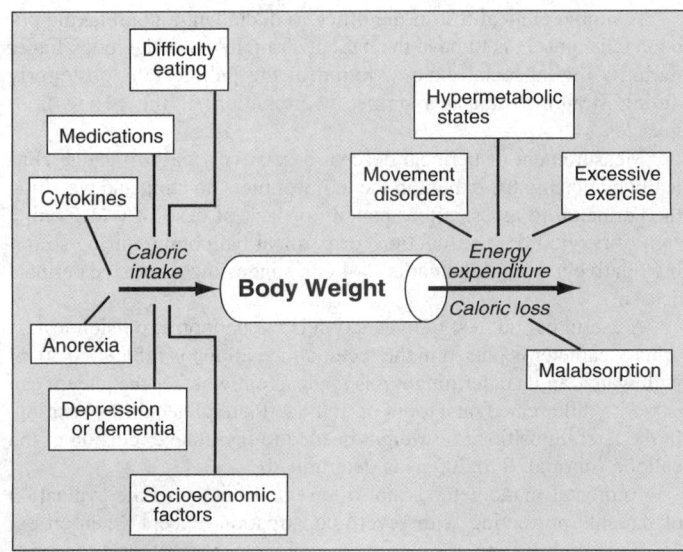

FIGURE 43-1   Energy balance and pathophysiology of weight loss.

Marked degrees of weight loss also predispose to infection. Patients undergoing elective surgery, who have lost more than 10 lb (4.5 kg) in 6 months, have higher surgical mortality rates. Vitamin and nutrient deficiencies also can accompany significant weight loss (Chap. 74).

CAUSES OF WEIGHT LOSS The list of possible causes of weight loss is extensive (Table 43-1). In the elderly, the most common causes of weight loss are depression, cancer, and benign gastrointestinal disease. Lung and gastrointestinal cancer are the most common malignancies in patients presenting with weight loss. In younger individuals, diabetes mellitus, hyperthyroidism, psychiatric disturbances including eating disorders, and infection, especially with HIV, should be considered.

The cause of involuntary weight loss is rarely occult. Careful history and physical examination, in association with directed diagnostic testing, will identify the cause of weight loss in 75% of patients. The etiology of weight loss will not be found in the remaining patients, despite extensive testing. Patients with negative evaluations tend to have lower mortality rates than those found to have organic disease.

Patients with medical causes of weight loss usually have signs or symptoms that suggest involvement of a particular organ system. Gastrointestinal tumors, including those of the pancreas and liver, may affect food intake early in the course of illness, causing weight loss before other symptoms are apparent. Lung cancer may present with post-obstructive pneumonia, dyspnea, or cough and hemoptysis; however, it may be silent and should be considered even in those without a history of cigarette smoking. Depression and isolation can cause profound weight loss, especially in the elderly. Chronic pulmonary disease and congestive heart failure can produce anorexia and may also increase resting energy expenditure. Weight loss may be the presenting sign of infectious diseases such as HIV infection, tuberculosis, endocarditis, and fungal and parasitic infections. Hyperthyroidism or pheochromocytoma increase metabolism; elderly patients with apathetic hyperthyroidism may present with weight loss alone. New onset diabetes mellitus is often accompanied by weight loss, reflecting glucosuria and loss of the anabolic actions of insulin. Adrenal insufficiency may be suggested by increased pigmentation, hyponatremia, and hyperkalemia.

Table 43-1 Causes of Weight Loss

Cancer	Medications
Endocrine and metabolic	Antibiotics
causes	Nonsteroidal anti-inflammatory drugs
Hyperthyroidism	Serotonin reuptake inhibitors
Diabetes mellitus	Metformin
Pheochromocytoma	Levodopa
Adrenal insufficiency	ACE inhibitors
Gastrointestinal disorders	Other drugs
Malabsorption	Disorders of the mouth and teeth
Obstruction	Age-related factors
Pernicious anemia	Physiologic changes
Cardiac disorders	Decreased taste and smell
Chronic ischemia	Functional disabilities
Chronic congestive heart	Neurologic causes
failure	Stroke
Respiratory disorders	Parkinson's disease
Emphysema	Neuromuscular disorders
Chronic obstructive pul-	Dementia
monary disease	Social Causes
Renal insufficiency	Isolation
Rheumatologic disease	Economic hardship
Infections	Psychiatric and behavioral causes
HIV	Depression
Tuberculosis	Anxiety
Parasitic infection	Bereavement
Subacute bacterial endo-	Alcoholism
carditis	Eating disorders
	Increased activity or exercise
	Idiopathic

Table 43-2 Screening Tests for Evaluation of Involuntary Weight Loss

Initial testing	Additional testing
CBC	HIV test
Electrolytes, calcium, glucose	Upper and/or lower gastrointesti-
Renal and liver function tests	nal endoscopy
Urinalysis	Abdominal CT scan or MRI
TSH	Chest CT scan
Chest x-ray	
Recommended cancer screening	

Approach to the Patient

Before extensive evaluation is undertaken, it is important to confirm that weight loss has occurred. Almost half of patients who claim significant weight loss have no actual change in weight when it is measured objectively. If weight loss is present, efforts should be made to determine the time interval over which it has occurred. In the absence of documentation, changes in belt notch size or the fit of clothing may help confirm loss of weight. Not infrequently, patients who have actually sustained significant weight loss are unaware that it has occurred. Routine documentation of weight during office visits is therefore important.

The review of systems should focus on signs or symptoms that are associated with disorders that commonly cause weight loss. These include fever, pain, shortness of breath or cough, palpitations, changes in pattern of urination, and evidence of neurologic disease. Gastrointestinal disturbances, including difficulty eating, dysphagia, anorexia, nausea, and change in bowel habits, should be sought. Use of cigarettes, alcohol, and all medications should be reviewed, and patients should be questioned about previous illness or surgery as well as diseases in family members. Risk factors for HIV infection should be assessed. Signs of depression, evidence of dementia, and social factors, including financial issues that might affect food intake, should be considered.

Physical examination should begin with weight determination and documentation of vital signs. The skin should be examined for pallor, jaundice, turgor, scars from prior surgery, and stigmata of systemic disease. The search for oral thrush or dental disease, thyroid gland enlargement, adenopathy, and respiratory or cardiac abnormalities and a detailed examination of the abdomen often lead to clues for further evaluation. Rectal examination, including prostate exam and testing of stool for occult blood, should be performed in men; and all women should have a pelvic examination, even if they have had a hysterectomy. Neurologic examination should include mental status assessment and screening for depression.

Laboratory testing should confirm or exclude possible diagnoses elicited from the history and physical examination (Table 43-2). An initial phase of testing should include a complete blood count with differential, serum chemistry tests including glucose, electrolytes, renal and liver tests, calcium, thyroid stimulating hormone (TSH), urinalysis, and chest x-ray. Patients at risk for HIV infection should have HIV antibody testing. In all cases, recommended cancer screening tests appropriate for the gender and age group, such as mammograms and Pap smears, should be updated (Chap. 80). If gastrointestinal signs or symptoms are present, upper and/or lower endoscopy and abdominal imaging with either computed tomography (CT) or magnetic resonance imaging (MRI) have a relatively high yield, consistent with the high prevalence of gastrointestinal disorders in patients with weight loss. If an etiology of weight loss is not found, careful clinical follow-up, rather than persistent undirected testing, is reasonable.

BIBLIOGRAPHY

FISCHER J, JOHNSON MA: Low body weight and weight loss in the aged. J Am Diet Assoc 90:1697, 1990

FLIER JS, MARATOS-FLIER E: Obesity and the hypothalamus: Novel peptides for new pathways. Cell 92:437, 1998

GAZEWOOD JD, MEHR DR: Diagnosis and management of weight loss in the elderly. J Fam Pract 47:19, 1998

MARTON KI et al: Involuntary weight loss: Diagnostic and prognostic significance. Ann Intern Med 95:568, 1981

RABINOVITZ M et al: Unintentional weight loss: A retrospective analysis of 154 cases. Arch Intern Med 146:186, 1986

REIFE CM: Involuntary weight loss. Med Clin North Am 79:299, 1995

THOMPSON MP, MORRIS LK: Unexplained weight loss in the ambulatory elderly. J Am Geriatr Soc 39:497, 1991

WALLACE JI et al: Involuntary weight loss in older outpatients: incidence and clinical significance. J Am Geriatr Soc 43:329, 1995

44　*Loren Laine*

GASTROINTESTINAL BLEEDING

Bleeding from the gastrointestinal (GI) tract may present in 5 ways. *Hematemesis* is vomitus of red blood or "coffee-grounds" material. *Melena* is black, tarry, foul-smelling stool. *Hematochezia* is the passage of bright red or maroon blood from the rectum. *Occult GI bleeding (GIB)* may be identified in the absence of overt bleeding by special examination of the stool (e.g., guaiac testing). Finally, patients may present only with *symptoms of blood loss or anemia* such as light-headedness, syncope, angina, or dyspnea.

SOURCES OF GASTROINTESTINAL BLEEDING

UPPER GASTROINTESTINAL SOURCES OF BLEEDING (Table 44-1)　The annual incidence of hospital admissions for upper GIB (UGIB) in the United States and Europe is approximately 0.1%, with a mortality rate of ~10%. Patients rarely die from exsanguination; rather, they die due to decompensation from other underlying illnesses. The mortality rate for patients under 60 years of age in the absence of malignancy or organ failure is <1%.

Peptic ulcers are the most common cause of UGIB, accounting for about 50% of cases. Mallory-Weiss tears account for 5 to 15% of cases. The proportion of patients bleeding from varices varies widely from ~5 to 30%, depending on the population. Hemorrhagic or erosive gastropathy [e.g., due to nonsteroidal anti-inflammatory drugs (NSAIDs) or alcohol] and erosive esophagitis often cause mild UGIB, but major bleeding is rare.

Peptic Ulcers　Clinical features that predict poorer outcome include hemodynamic instability, the number of units of blood transfused, red blood in the emesis and the stool, increasing age, and the presence of concurrent illness. Characteristics of the ulcer at endoscopy also provide important prognostic information. One-third of patients with active bleeding or a non-bleeding visible vessel have further bleeding that requires urgent surgery if they are treated conservatively.

Table 44-1　Sources of Bleeding in Patients Hospitalized for Acute UGIB

Sources of Bleeding	Proportion of Patients (%)
Ulcers	35–62
Varices	4–31
Mallory-Weiss tears	4–13
Gastroduodenal erosions	3–11
Erosive esophagitis	2–8
Malignancy	1–4
No source identified	7–25

SOURCE: Data from Rockall et al; GF Longstreth: Am J Gastroenterol 90:206, 1995; EM Vreeburg et al: Am J Gastroenterol 92:236, 1997; and L Laine: West J Med 155:274, 1991.

These patients clearly benefit from endoscopic therapy with bipolar electrocoagulation, heater probe, or injection therapy (e.g., absolute alcohol, 1:10,000 epinephrine), with reductions in bleeding, hospital stay, mortality rate, and costs. In contrast, patients with clean-based ulcers have rates of recurrent bleeding approaching zero. If there is no other reason for hospitalization, such patients may be discharged on the first hospital day, following stabilization. Patients without clear-based ulcers should usually remain in the hospital for 3 days, since most episodes of recurrent bleeding occur within 3 days.

Various pharmacologic agents have been assessed in the past for the treatment of ulcer bleeding without clearcut benefit. However, in recent controlled trials in Europe and Asia, high-dose intravenous omeprazole used to raise intragastric pH to 6 to 7 and enhance clot stability decreased further bleeding (but not mortality), even after the use of appropriate endoscopic therapy.

Approximately one-third of patients with a bleeding ulcer will rebleed within the next 1 to 2 years. Prevention of recurrent bleeding focuses on the three main factors in ulcer pathogenesis, *Helicobacter pylori*, NSAIDs, and acid. Eradication of *H. pylori* in patients with bleeding ulcers dramatically decreases rates of rebleeding to < 5%. If a bleeding ulcer develops in a patient taking NSAIDs, the NSAIDs should be discontinued if possible. If NSAIDs must be continued, initial treatment should be with a proton pump inhibitor, and subsequent prophylactic therapy with a proton pump inhibitor or misoprostol should be continued as long as the patient is taking NSAIDs. Changing from a standard NSAID to a COX-2-specific inhibitor should markedly lower the risk of recurrent UGIB. Patients with bleeding ulcers unrelated to *H. pylori* or NSAIDs should remain on full-dose antisecretory therapy indefinitely. →*Peptic ulcers are discussed in Chap. 285.*

Mallory-Weiss Tears　The classic history is vomiting, retching, or coughing preceding hematemesis, especially in an alcoholic patient. Bleeding from these tears, which are usually on the gastric side of the gastroesophageal junction, stops spontaneously in 80 to 90% of patients and recurs in only 0 to 5%. Endoscopic therapy is effective for actively bleeding Mallory-Weiss tears. Angiographic therapy with intra-arterial infusion of vasopressin or embolization also may be useful. Rarely, operative therapy with oversewing of the tear may be required. →*Mallory-Weiss tears are discussed in Chap. 284.*

Esophageal Varices　Patients with UGIB and clinical evidence suggesting the possibility of liver disease should undergo early endoscopy to determine if varices are the sources of bleeding, because patients with variceal hemorrhage have poorer outcomes than patients with other sources of UGIB. Endoscopic therapy at this time decreases further bleeding, and repeated sessions with endoscopic therapy to eradicate esophageal varices significantly reduces rebleeding and mortality. Endoscopic ligation therapy is the endoscopic therapy of choice for esophageal varices because it has less rebleeding, a lower mortality rate, fewer local complications, and requires fewer treatment sessions to achieve variceal eradication as compared to sclerotherapy.

Acute treatment with octreotide (50 μg bolus and 50 μg/h intravenous infusion for 2 to 5 days) or somatostatin may help in the control of acute bleeding, and these agents have replaced vasopressin as the medical therapy of choice for acute variceal bleeding. Over the long term, treatment with nonselective beta blockers (e.g., propranolol) has also been shown to decrease recurrent bleeding from esophageal varices. These agents commonly are given along with chronic endoscopic therapy.

In patients who have persistent or recurrent bleeding despite endoscopic and medical therapy, more invasive therapy is warranted. Transjugular intrahepatic portosystemic shunt (TIPS) decreases rebleeding more effectively than endoscopic therapy, although hepatic encephalopathy is more common and the mortality rates are comparable. Most patients with TIPS have shunt stenosis within 1 to 2 years and require re-instrumentation. Therefore, TIPS is most appropriate for patients with more severe liver disease and those in whom transplant is anticipated. Patients with milder, well-compensated cirrhosis probably should undergo decompressive surgery (e.g., distal spleno-renal shunt).

Portal hypertension is also responsible for bleeding from gastric varices, ectopic varices in the small and large intestine, and portal hypertensive gastropathy and enterocolopathy.

Hemorrhagic and Erosive Gastropathy ("Gastritis") Hemorrhagic and erosive gastropathy or gastritis refers to endoscopically visualized subepithelial hemorrhages and erosions. These are mucosal lesions and thus do not cause major bleeding. They develop in various clinical settings, the most important of which are ingestion of NSAIDs, alcohol, and stress. Half of patients who chronically ingest NSAIDs have erosions (15 to 30% have ulcers), while up to 20% of actively drinking alcoholic patients with symptoms of UGIB have evidence of subepithelial hemorrhages or erosions.

Stress-related gastric mucosal injury occurs only in extremely sick patients: those who have experienced serious trauma, major surgery, burns covering more than one-third of the body surface area, major intracranial disease, and severe medical illness (ventilator dependency, coagulopathy). Significant bleeding probably does not develop unless ulceration occurs. The mortality rate in these patients is quite high because of their serious underlying illnesses.

The incidence of bleeding from stress-related gastric mucosal injury or ulceration has decreased dramatically in recent years, most likely due to better care of critically ill patients. Pharmacologic prophylaxis for bleeding may be considered in the high-risk patients mentioned above. The best clinical data suggest that intravenous H$_2$-receptor antagonist therapy is the treatment of choice, although sucralfate also is effective. Prophylactic therapy decreases bleeding, but it does not lower the mortality rate.

Other Causes Other, less frequent causes of UGIB include erosive duodenitis, neoplasms, aortoenteric fistulas, vascular lesions [including hereditary hemorrhagic telengectasias (Osler-Weber-Rendu) and gastric antral vascular ectasia ("watermelon stomach")], Dieulafoy's lesion (in which an aberrant vessel in the mucosa bleeds from a pinpoint mucosal defect), prolapse gastropathy (prolapse of proximal stomach into esophagus with retching, especially in alcoholics), and hemobilia and hemosuccus pancreaticus (bleeding from the bile duct or pancreatic duct).

SMALL INTESTINAL SOURCES OF BLEEDING Small intestinal sources of bleeding (bleeding from sites beyond the reach of the standard upper endoscope) are difficult to diagnose and are responsible for the majority of cases of obscure GIB. Fortunately, small intestinal bleeding is uncommon. The most common causes are vascular ectasias and tumors (e.g., adenocarcinoma, leiomyoma, lymphoma, benign polyps, carcinoid, metastases, and lipoma). Other less common causes include Crohn's disease, infection, ischemia, vasculitis, small bowel varices, diverticula, Meckel's diverticula, duplication cysts, and intussusception. NSAIDs induce small intestinal erosions and ulcers and may be a relatively common cause of chronic, obscure GIB.

Meckel's diverticulum is the most common cause of significant lower GIB (LGIB) in children, decreasing in frequency as a cause of bleeding with age. In adults younger than 40 to 50 years, small bowel tumors often account for obscure GIB, while in patients older than 50 to 60 years, vascular ectasias are usually responsible.

Vascular ectasias should be treated with endoscopic therapy if possible. Surgical therapy can be used for vascular ectasias isolated to a segment of the small intestine when endoscopic therapy is unsuccessful; estrogen/progesterone compounds may also be tried. Isolated lesions, such as tumors, diverticula, or duplications, generally are treated with surgical resection.

COLONIC SOURCES OF BLEEDING The incidence of hospitalizations for LGIB is about one-fifth that for UGIB. Hemorrhoids are probably the most common cause of LGIB; anal fissures also cause minor bleeding and pain. If these local anal processes, which rarely require hospitalization, are excluded, the most common causes of LGIB in adults are diverticula, vascular ectasias (especially

in the proximal colon of patients > 70 years), neoplasms (adenomatous polyps and adenocarcinoma), and colitis—most commonly infectious or idiopathic inflammatory bowel disease, but occasionally ischemic or radiation-induced. Uncommon causes include post-polypectomy bleeding, solitary rectal ulcer syndrome, NSAID-induced ulcers or colitis, other neoplasms, trauma, ectopic varices (most commonly rectal), lymphoid nodular hyperplasia, vasculitis, and aortocolic fistulas. In children and adolescents, the most common colonic causes of significant GIB are inflammatory bowel disease and juvenile polyps.

Diverticular bleeding is abrupt in onset, usually painless, sometimes massive, and often from the right colon; minor and occult bleeding is not characteristic. Clinical reports suggest that bleeding colonic diverticula stop bleeding spontaneously in approximately 80% of patients, and rebleed in 20 to 25% of patients. Intraarterial vasopressin may halt the bleeding, at least temporarily. If bleeding persists or recurs, segmental surgical resection is indicated.

Bleeding from right colonic vascular ectasias in the elderly may be overt or occult; it tends to be chronic and only occasionally is hemodynamically significant. Endoscopic hemostatic therapy may be useful in the treatment of vascular ectasias, as well as discrete bleeding ulcers and post-polypectomy bleeding, while endoscopic polypectomy, if possible, is used for bleeding colonic polyps. Surgical therapy is generally required for major, persistent, or recurrent bleeding from the wide variety of colonic sources of GIB that cannot be treated medically or endoscopically.

Approach to the Patient

Measurement of the heart rate and blood pressure is the best way to assess a patient with GIB. Clinically significant bleeding leads to postural changes in heart rate or blood pressure, tachycardia, and, finally, recumbent hypotension. Patients also may have a vasovagal reaction with bradycardia during bleeding episodes.

In contrast, the hemoglobin does not fall immediately with acute GIB, due to proportionate reductions in plasma and red cell volumes (i.e., "people bleed whole blood"). Thus, hemoglobin may be normal or only minimally decreased at the initial presentation of a severe bleeding episode. As extravascular fluid enters the vascular space to restore volume, the hemoglobin falls, but this process may take up to 72 h. Patients with slow, chronic GIB may have very low hemoglobin values despite normal blood pressure and heart rate. With the development of iron deficiency anemia, the mean corpuscular volume will be low and red blood cell distribution width will be increased.

Differentiation of Upper from Lower GIB Hematemesis indicates an upper GI source of bleeding (above the ligament of Treitz). Melena indicates that blood has been present in the GI tract for at least 14 h. Thus, the more proximal the bleeding site, the more likely melena will occur. Hematochezia usually represents a lower GI source of bleeding, although an upper GI lesion may bleed so rapidly that blood does not remain in the bowel long enough for melena to develop. When hematochezia is the presenting symptom of UGIB, it is associated with hemodynamic instability and dropping hemoglobin. Bleeding lesions of the small bowel may present as melena or hematochezia.

A non-bloody nasogastric aspirate may be seen in up to 16% of patients with UGIB—usually from a duodenal source. Even a bile-stained appearance does not exclude a bleeding post-pyloric lesion since reports of bile in the aspirate are incorrect in about 50% of cases. Testing of aspirates that are not grossly bloody for occult blood is of no clinical value. Other clues to UGIB include hyperactive bowel sounds and an elevated BUN (due to volume depletion and absorbed blood proteins).

Diagnostic Evaluation of the Patient with GIB • Upper GIB (Fig. 44-1) The history and physical exam seldom are diagnostic of the source of GIB. Upper endoscopy is the test of choice in patients

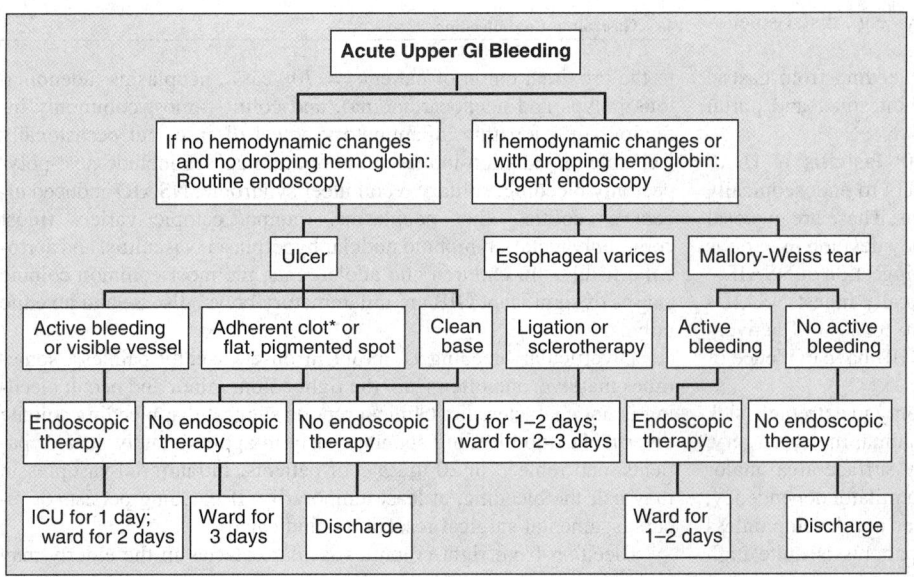

FIGURE 44-1 Suggested algorithm for patients with acute UGIB. Recommendations on level of care and time of discharge assume patient is stabilized without further bleeding or other concomitant medical problems. Upper GI endoscopy is the major diagnostic and therapeutic tool. *Some authors suggest endoscopic therapy for adherent clots.

with UGIB, and should be performed urgently in patients with hemodynamic instability (hypotension, tachycardia, or postural changes in heart rate or blood pressure). Early routine endoscopy is also beneficial in cases of milder bleeding for management decisions. Patients with major bleeding and high risk endoscopic findings (varices, ulcers with active bleeding or a visible vessel) benefit from endoscopic hemostatic therapy, while patients with low-risk lesions (e.g., clean based ulcers, non-bleeding Mallory-Weiss tears, erosive or hemorrhagic gastropathy) who have stable vital signs and hemoglobin, and no other medical problems, can be discharged home.

Lower GIB (Fig. 44-2) Patients with presumed LGIB may undergo early sigmoidoscopy for the detection of obvious, low-lying lesions. However, the procedure is difficult with brisk bleeding, and it often is impossible to identify the area of bleeding. Sigmoidoscopy

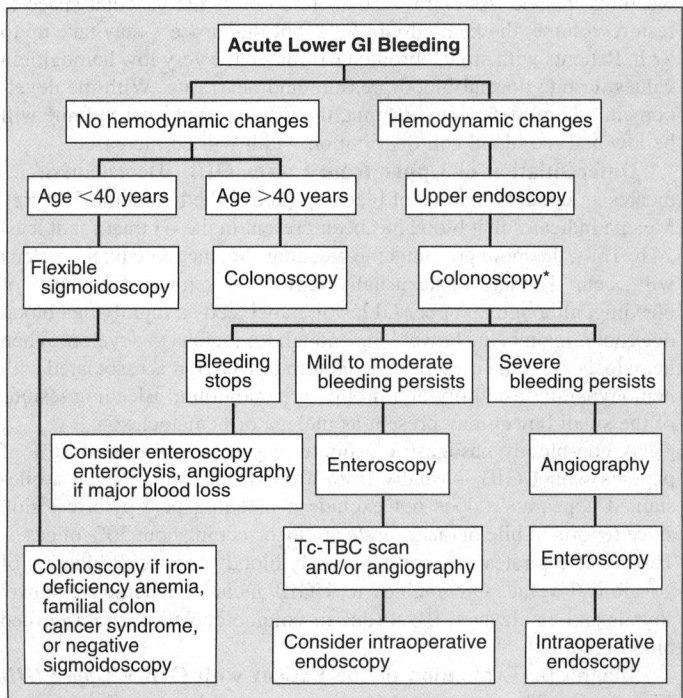

FIGURE 44-2 Suggested algorithm for patients with acute LGIB. *If massive bleeding does not allow time for colonic lavage, proceed to angiography.

is useful primarily in patients < 40 years with relatively minor bleeding. Patients with hematochezia and hemodynamic instability should have upper endoscopy to rule out an upper GI source before evaluation of the lower GI tract.

Colonoscopy after an oral lavage solution is the procedure of choice in patients with LGIB unless bleeding is too massive or unless sigmoidoscopy has disclosed an obvious actively bleeding lesion. ^{99M}Tc-labeled red cell scan allows repeated imaging for up to 24 h and may identify the general location of bleeding. However, radionuclide scans should be interpreted with caution because results are highly variable. In active LGIB, angiography can detect the site of bleeding (extravasation of contrast into the gut) and permits treatment with intraarterial infusion of vasopressin or embolization. Even after bleeding has stopped, angiography may identify lesions with abnormal vasculature such as vascular ectasias or tumors.

GIB of obscure origin Obscure GIB is defined as recurrent acute or chronic bleeding for which no source has been identified by routine endoscopic and contrast studies. Push enteroscopy, with a specially designed enteroscope or a pediatric colonoscope to inspect the entire duodenum and part of the jejunum, is generally the next step. Push enteroscopy may identify probable bleeding sites in 20 to 40% of patients with obscure GIB. If enteroscopy is negative or unavailable, a specialized radiographic examination of the small bowel (e.g., enteroclysis) should be performed.

Patients with recurrent bleeding who require transfusions or repeated hospitalizations warrant further investigations. ^{99M}Tc-labeled red blood cell scintigraphy should be employed. Angiography is useful even if bleeding has subsided, since it may disclose vascular anomalies or tumor vessels. ^{99M}Tc-pertechnetate scintigraphy for diagnosis of Meckel's diverticulum should be done, especially in the evaluation of young patients with LGIB. When all tests are unrevealing, intraoperative endoscopy is indicated in patients with severe recurrent or persistent bleeding requiring repeated transfusions.

Occult GIB Occult GIB is manifested by either a positive test for fecal occult blood or iron deficiency anemia. Unless a patient has upper GI symptoms, evaluation of occult bleeding generally should begin with colonoscopy, particularly in patients older than 40 years. If evaluation of the colon is negative, some perform upper endoscopy only if iron deficiency anemia or upper GI symptoms are present, while others recommend upper endoscopy in all patients since up to 25 to 40% of these patients have some abnormality noted on upper endoscopy. If standard endoscopic tests are unrevealing, enteroscopy and/or enteroclysis may be considered in patients with iron-deficiency anemia.

BIBLIOGRAPHY

COOK DJ et al: Endoscopic therapy for acute non-variceal upper gastrointestinal hemorrhage—a meta-analysis. Gastroenterology 102:139, 1992

—— et al: A comparison of sucralfate and ranitidine for the prevention of upper gastrointestinal bleeding in patients requiring mechanical ventilation. N Engl J Med 338: 791, 1998

LAINE L, PETERSON WL: Bleeding peptic ulcer. N Engl J Med 331:717, 1994

MOLONEY M, WILKINSON M: Early administration of somatostatin and efficacy of sclerotherapy in acute oesophageal bleeds: The European Acute Bleeding Oesophageal Variceal Episodes (ABOVE) randomised trial. Gastrointest Endosc 51:372, 2000

ROCKALL TA et al: Incidence of and mortality from acute upper gastrointestinal haemorrhage in the United Kingdom. BMJ 311:222, 1995

ROCKEY DC: Occult gastrointestinal bleeding. N Engl J Med 341:38, 1999

JAUNDICE

ALT	alanine aminotransferase	MRCP	magnetic resonance
AST	aspartate aminotransferase		cholangiopancreatography
CMV	cytomegalovirus	PSC	primary sclerosing cholangitis
CT	computed tomography	TPN	total parenteral nutrition
EBV	Epstein-Barr virus	UDP	uridine-diphosphate
ERCP	endoscopic retrograde		
	cholangiopancreatography		

Jaundice, or icterus, is a yellowish discoloration of tissue resulting from the deposition of bilirubin. Tissue deposition of bilirubin occurs only in the presence of serum hyperbilirubinemia and is a sign of either liver disease or, less often, a hemolytic disorder. The degree of serum bilirubin elevation can be estimated by physical examination. Slight increases in serum bilirubin are best detected by examining the sclerae which have a particular affinity for bilirubin due to their high elastin content. The presence of scleral icterus indicates a serum bilirubin of at least 3.0 mg/dL. The ability to detect scleral icterus is made more difficult if the examining room has fluorescent lighting. If the examiner suspects scleral icterus, a second place to examine is underneath the tongue. As serum bilirubin levels rise, the skin will eventually become yellow in light-skinned patients and even green if the process is long-standing; the green color is produced by oxidation of bilirubin to biliverdin.

The differential diagnosis for yellowing of the skin is limited. In addition to jaundice, it includes carotenoderma, the use of the drug quinacrine, and excessive exposure to phenols. Carotenoderma is the yellow color imparted to the skin by the presence of carotene; it occurs in healthy individuals who ingest excessive amounts of vegetables and fruits that contain carotene, such as carrots, leafy vegetables, squash, peaches, and oranges. Unlike jaundice, where the yellow coloration of the skin is uniformly distributed over the body, in carotenoderma the pigment is concentrated on the palms, soles, forehead, and nasolabial folds. Carotenoderma can be distinguished from jaundice by the sparing of the sclerae. Quinacrine causes a yellow discoloration of the skin in 4 to 37% of patients treated with it. Unlike carotene, quinacrine can cause discoloration of the sclerae.

Another sensitive indicator of increased serum bilirubin is darkening of the urine, which is due to the renal excretion of conjugated bilirubin. Patients often describe their urine as tea or cola colored. Bilirubinuria indicates an elevation of the direct serum bilirubin fraction and therefore the presence of liver disease.

Increased serum bilirubin levels occur when an imbalance exists between bilirubin production and clearance. A logical evaluation of the patient who is jaundiced requires an understanding of bilirubin production and metabolism.

PRODUCTION AND METABOLISM OF BILIRUBIN (See also Chap. 294) Bilirubin, a tetrapyrrole pigment, is a break-down product of heme (ferroprotoporphyrin IX). About 70 to 80% of the 250 to 300 mg of bilirubin produced each day is derived from the breakdown of hemoglobin in senescent red blood cells. The remainder comes from prematurely destroyed erythroid cells in bone marrow and from the turnover of hemoproteins such as myoglobin and crytochromes found in tissues throughout the body.

The formation of bilirubin occurs in reticuloendothelial cells, primarily in the spleen and liver. The first reaction, catalyzed by the enzyme heme oxygenase, oxidatively cleaves the α bridge of the porphyrin group and opens the heme ring. The end products of this reaction are biliverdin, carbon monoxide, and iron. The second reaction, catalyzed by the cytosolic enzyme biliverdin reductase, reduces the central methylene bridge of biliverdin and converts it to bilirubin. Bilirubin formed in the reticuloendothelial cells is virtually insoluble in water. To be transported in blood, it must be solubilized. This is ac-

complished by its reversible, noncovalent binding to albumin. Unconjugated bilirubin bound to albumin is transported to the liver, where it, but not the albumin, is taken up by hepatocytes via a process that at least partly involves carrier-mediated membrane transport.

In the cytosol of the hepatocyte, unconjugated bilirubin is coupled predominantly to the protein ligandin (formerly called the Y protein). Ligandin was initially thought to be a transport protein facilitating the movement of bilirubin from the sinusodial membrane to the endoplasmic reticulum. It is now thought to slow the cytosolic diffusion of bilirubin and to reduce its efflux back into serum. In the endoplasmic reticulum, bilirubin is solubilized by conjugation to glucuronic acid, forming bilirubin monoglucuronide and diglucuronide. The conjugation of glucuronic acid to bilirubin is catalyzed by bilirubin uridine-diphosphate (UDP) glucuronosyltransferase.

The now hydrophilic bilirubin conjugates diffuse from the endoplasmic reticulum to the canalicular membrane, where bilirubin monoglucuronide and diglucuronide are actively transported into canalicular bile by an energy-dependent mechanism involving the multiple organic ion transport protein/multiple drug resistance protein. The conjugated bilirubin excreted into bile drains into the duodenum and passes unchanged through the proximal small bowel. Conjugated bilirubin is not taken up by the intestinal mucosa. When the conjugated bilirubin reaches the distal ileum and colon, it is hydrolyzed to unconjugated bilirubin by bacterial β-glucuronidases. The unconjugated bilirubin is reduced by normal gut bacteria to form a group of colorless tetrapyrroles called urobilinogens. About 80 to 90% of these products are excreted in feces, either unchanged or oxidized to orange derivatives called urobilins. The remaining 10 to 20% of the urobilinogens are passively absorbed, enter the portal venous blood, and are re-excreted by the liver. A small fraction (usually less than 3 mg/dL) escapes hepatic uptake, filters across the renal glomerulus, and is excreted in urine.

MEASUREMENT OF SERUM BILIRUBIN The terms direct- and indirect-reacting bilirubin are based on the original van den Bergh reaction. This assay, or a variation of it, is still used in most clinical chemistry laboratories to determine the serum bilirubin level. In this assay, bilirubin is exposed to diazotized sulfanilic acid, splitting into two relatively stable dipyrrylmethene azopigments that absorb maximally at 540 nm, allowing for photometric analysis. The direct fraction is that which reacts with diazotized sulfanilic acid in the absence of an accelerator substance such as alcohol. The direct fraction provides an approximate determination of the conjugated bilirubin in serum. The total serum bilirubin is the amount that reacts after the addition of alcohol. The indirect fraction is the difference between the total and the direct bilirubin and provides an estimate of the unconjugated bilirubin in serum.

With the van den Bergh method, the normal serum bilirubin concentration usually is <1 mg/dL (17 μmol/L). Up to 30%, or 0.3 mg/dL (5.1 μmol/L), of the total may be direct-reacting (conjugated) bilirubin. Total serum bilirubin concentrations are between 0.2 and 0.9 mg/dL in 95% of a normal population.

Several new techniques, although less convenient to perform, have added considerably to our understanding of bilirubin metabolism. First, they demonstrate that in normal people or those with Gilbert's syndrome, almost 100% of the serum bilirubin is unconjugated; less than 3% is monoconjugated bilirubin. Second, in jaundiced patients with hepatobiliary disease, the total serum bilirubin concentration measured by these new, more accurate methods is lower than the values found with diazo methods. This suggests that there are diazo-positive compounds distinct from bilirubin in the serum of patients with hepatobiliary disease. Third, these studies indicate that in jaundiced patients with hepatobiliary disease, monoglucuronides of bilirubin predominate over the diglucuronides. Fourth, part of the direct-reacting bilirubin fraction includes conjugated bilirubin that is covalently linked to albumin. This albumin-linked bilirubin fraction (*delta fraction* or *biliprotein*) represents an important fraction of total

FIGURE 45-1 Evaluation of the patient with jaundice. ERCP, endoscopic retrograde cholangiopancreatography; CT, computed tomography; ALT, alanine aminotransferase; AST, aspartate aminotransferase; SMA, smooth muscle antibody; AMA, antimitochondrial antibody; LKM, liver-kidney microsomal antibody; SPEP, serum protein electrophoresis; CMV, cytomegalovirus; EBV, Epstein-Barr virus.

serum bilirubin in patients with cholestasis and hepatobiliary disorders. Albumin-bound conjugated bilirubin is formed in serum when hepatic excretion of bilirubin glucuronides is impaired and the glucuronides are present in serum in increasing amounts. By virtue of its tight binding to albumin, the clearance rate of albumin-bound bilirubin from serum approximates the half-life of albumin, 12 to 14 days, rather than the short half-life of bilirubin, about 4 h.

The prolonged half-life of albumin-bound conjugated bilirubin explains two previously unexplained enigmas in jaundiced patients with liver disease: (1) that some patients with conjugated hyperbilirubinemia do not exhibit bilirubinuria during the recovery phase of their disease because the bilirubin is bound to albumin and therefore not filtered by the renal glomeruli and (2) that the elevated serum bilirubin level declines more slowly than expected in some patients who otherwise appear to be recovering satisfactorily. Late in the recovery phase of hepatobiliary disorders, all the conjugated bilirubin may be in the albumin-linked form. Its value in serum falls slowly because of the long half-life of albumin.

MEASUREMENT OF URINE BILIRUBIN Unconjugated bilirubin is always bound to albumin in the serum, is not filtered by the kidney, and is not found in the urine. Conjugated bilirubin is filtered at the glomerulus and the majority is reabsorbed by the proximal tubules; a small fraction is excreted in the urine. Any bilirubin found in the urine is conjugated bilirubin. The presence of bilirubinuria implies the presence of liver disease. A urine dipstick test (Ictotest) gives the same information as fractionation of the serum bilirubin. This test is very accurate. A false-negative test is possible in patients with prolonged cholestasis due to the predominance of conjugated bilirubin covalently bound to albumin.

THE EVALUATION OF JAUNDICE The bilirubin present in serum represents a balance between input from production of bilirubin and hepatic/biliary removal of the pigment. Hyperbilirubinemia may result from (1) overproduction of bilirubin; (2) impaired uptake, conjugation, or excretion of bilirubin; or (3) regurgitation of unconjugated or conjugated bilirubin from damaged hepatocytes or bile ducts. An increase in unconjugated bilirubin in serum results from either overproduction, impairment of uptake, or conjugation of bilirubin. An increase in conjugated bilirubin is due to decreased excretion into the bile ductules or backward leakage of the pigment. The initial steps in evaluating the patient with jaundice are to determine (1) whether the hyperbilirubinemia is predominantly conjugated or unconjugated in nature, and (2) whether other biochemical liver tests are abnormal. The thoughtful interpretation of limited data will allow for a rational evaluation of the patient (Fig. 45-1). This discussion will focus solely on the evaluation of the adult patient with jaundice.

ISOLATED ELEVATION OF SERUM BILIRUBIN Unconjugated Hyperbilirubinemia The differential diagnosis of an isolated unconjugated hyperbilirubinemia is limited (Table 45-1). The critical determination is whether the patient is suffering from a hemolytic process resulting in an overproduction of bilirubin (hemolytic disorders and ineffective erythropoiesis) or from impaired hepatic uptake/conjugation of bilirubin (drug effect or genetic disorders).

Hemolytic disorders that cause excessive heme production may be either inherited or acquired. Inherited disorders include spherocytosis, sickle cell anemia, and deficiency of red cell enzymes such as pyruvate kinase and glucose-6-phosphate dehydrogenase. In these conditions, the serum bilirubin rarely exceeds 5 mg/dL. Higher levels may occur when there is coexistent renal or hepatocellular dysfunction, or in acute hemolysis such as a sickle cell crisis. In evaluating jaundice in patients with chronic hemolysis, it is important to remember the high incidence of pigmented (calcium bilirubinate) gallstones found in these patients, which increases the likelihood of choledocholithiasis as an alternative explanation for hyperbilirubinemia.

Acquired hemolytic disorders include microangiopathic hemolytic anemia (e.g., hemolytic-uremic syndrome), paroxysmal nocturnal hemoglobinuria, and immune hemolysis. Ineffective erythropoiesis occurs in cobalamin, folate, and iron deficiencies.

In the absence of hemolysis, the physician should consider a problem with the hepatic uptake or conjugation of bilirubin. Certain drugs, including rifampicin and probenecid, may cause unconjugated hyperbilirubinemia by diminishing hepatic uptake of bilirubin. Impaired bilirubin conjugation occurs in three genetic conditions: *Crigler-Najjar*

Table 45-1 Causes of Isolated Hyperbilirubinemia

45 Jaundice 257

I. Indirect hyperbilirubinemia
  A. Hemolytic disorders
    1. Inherited
      a. Spherocytosis, elliptocytosis
        Glucose-6-phosphate dehydrogenase and pyruvate kinase deficiencies
      b. Sickle cell anemia
    2. Acquired
      a. Microangiopathic hemolytic anemias
      b. Paroxysmal nocturnal hemoglobinuria
      c. Immune hemolysis
  B. Ineffective erythropoiesis
    1. Cobalamin, folate, and iron deficiencies
  C. Drugs
    1. Rifampicin, probenecid, ribavirin
  D. Inherited conditions
    1. Crigler-Najjar types I and II
    2. Gilbert's syndrome
II. Direct hyperbilirubinemia
  A. Inherited conditions
    1. Dubin-Johnson syndrome
    2. Rotor's syndrome

syndrome, types I and II, and *Gilbert's syndrome. Crigler-Najjar type I* is an exceptionally rare condition found in neonates and characterized by severe jaundice (bilirubin > 20 mg/dL) and neurologic impairment due to kernicterus, frequently leading to death in infancy or childhood. These patients have a complete absence of bilirubin UDP glucuronosyltransferase activity, usually due to mutations in the critical 3' domain of the UDP glucuronosyltransferase gene, and are totally unable to conjugate, hence cannot excrete bilirubin. The only effective treatment is orthotopic liver transplantation. Use of gene therapy and allogeneic hepatocyte infusion are experimental approaches of future promise for this devastating disease.

Crigler-Najjar type II is somewhat more common than type I. Patients live into adulthood with serum bilirubin levels that range from 6 to 25 mg/dL. In these patients, mutations in the bilirubin UDP glucuronosyltransferase gene cause reduced but not completely absent activity of the enzyme. Bilirubin UDP glucuronosyltransferase activity can be induced by the administration of phenobarbital, which can reduce serum bilirubin levels in these patients. Despite marked jaundice, these patients usually survive into adulthood, although they may be susceptible to kernicterus under the stress of intercurrent illness or surgery.

Gilbert's syndrome is also marked by the impaired conjugation of bilirubin due to reduced bilirubin UDP glucuronosyltransferase activity. Molecular analyses show that Gilbert's syndrome is due to reduced expression of UDP glucuronosyltransferase activity caused by lengthening of the TATAA box from A(TA)$_6$ TAA to A(TA)$_7$ TAA in the promoter element of the gene. This results in mild unconjugated hyperbilirubinemia with serum levels almost always less than 6 mg/dL. The serum levels may fluctuate and jaundice is often identified only during periods of fasting. Unlike both Crigler-Najjar syndromes, Gilbert's syndrome is very common. The reported incidence is 3 to 7% of the population with males predominating over females by a ratio of 2–7:1.

Conjugated Hyperbilirubinemia Elevated conjugated hyperbilirubinemia is found in two rare inherited conditions: *Dubin-Johnson syndrome* and *Rotor's syndrome* (Table 45-1). Patients with both conditions present with asymptomatic jaundice, typically in the second generation of life. The defect in Dubin-Johnson syndrome is a point mutation in the gene for the canalicular multispecific organic anion transporter. These patients have altered excretion of bilirubin into the bile ducts. Rotor's syndrome seems to be a problem with the hepatic storage of bilirubin. Differentiating between these syndromes is possible, but clinically unnecessary, due to their benign nature.

ELEVATION OF SERUM BILIRUBIN WITH OTHER LIVER TEST ABNORMALITIES

The remainder of this chapter will focus on the evaluation of the patient with a conjugated hyperbilirubinemia in the setting of other liver test abnormalities. This group of patients can be divided into those with a primary hepatocellular process and those with intra- or extrahepatic cholestasis. Being able to make this differentiation will guide the physician's evaluation (Fig. 45-1). This differentiation is made on the basis of the history and physical examination as well as the pattern of liver test abnormalities.

History A complete medical history is perhaps the single most important part of the evaluation of the patient with unexplained jaundice. Important considerations include the use of or exposure to any chemical or medication, either physician-prescribed or over-the-counter, such as herbal and vitamin preparations and other drugs such as anabolic steroids. The patient should be carefully questioned about possible parenteral exposures, including transfusions, intravenous and intranasal drug use, tattoos, and sexual activity. Other important questions include recent travel history, exposure to people with jaundice, exposure to possibly contaminated foods, occupational exposure to hepatotoxins, alcohol consumption, the duration of jaundice, and the presence of any accompanying symptoms such as arthralgias, myalgias, rash, anorexia, weight loss, abdominal pain, fever, pruritis, and changes in the urine and stool. While none of these latter symptoms are specific for any one condition, they can suggest a particular diagnosis. A history of arthralgias and myalgias predating jaundice suggests hepatitis, either viral or drug-related. Jaundice associated with the sudden onset of severe right upper quadrant pain and shaking chills suggests choledocholithiasis and ascending cholangitis.

Physical Examination The general assessment should include assessment of the patient's nutritional status. Temporal and proximal muscle wasting suggests longstanding diseases such as pancreatic cancer or cirrhosis. Stigmata of chronic liver disease, including spider nevi, palmar erythema, gynecomastia, caput medusae, Dupuytren's contractures, parotid gland enlargement, and testicular atrophy are commonly seen in advanced alcoholic (Laennec's) cirrhosis and occasionally in other types of cirrhosis. An enlarged left supraclavicular node (Virchow's node) or periumbilical nodule (Sister Mary Joseph's nodule) suggest an abdominal malignancy. Jugular venous distention, a sign of right-sided heart failure, suggests hepatic congestion. Right pleural effusion, in the absence of clinically apparent ascites, may be seen in advanced cirrhosis.

The abdominal examination should focus on the size and consistency of the liver, whether the spleen is palpable and hence enlarged, and whether there is ascites present. Patients with cirrhosis may have an enlarged left lobe of the liver which is felt below the xiphoid and an enlarged spleen. A grossly enlarged nodular liver or an obvious abdominal mass suggests malignancy. An enlarged tender liver could be viral or alcoholic hepatitis or, less often, an acutely congested liver secondary to right-sided heart failure. Severe right upper quadrant tenderness with respiratory arrest on inspiration (Murphy's sign) suggests cholecystitis or, occasionally, ascending cholangitis. Ascites in the presence of jaundice suggests either cirrhosis or malignancy with peritoneal spread.

Laboratory Tests When the physician encounters a patient with unexplained jaundice, there are a battery of tests that are helpful in the initial evaluation. These include total and direct serum bilirubin with fractionation, aminotransferases, alkaline phosphatase, albumin, and prothrombin time tests. Enzyme tests [alanine aminotransferase (ALT), aspartate aminotransferase (AST), and alkaline phosphatase] are helpful in differentiating between a hepatocellular process and a cholestatic process (see Table 293-1 and Fig. 45-1), a critical step in determining what additional workup is indicated. Patients with a hepatocellular process generally have a disproportionate rise in the aminotransferases compared to the alkaline phosphatase. Patients with a cholestatic process have a disproportionate rise in the alkaline phosphatase compared to the aminotransferases. The bilirubin can be prominently elevated in both hepatocellular and cholestatic conditions and therefore is not necessarily helpful in differentiating between the two.

In addition to the enzyme tests, all jaundiced patients should have additional blood tests, specifically an albumin and a prothrombin time, to assess liver function. A low albumin suggests a chronic process such as cirrhosis or cancer. A normal albumin is suggestive of a more acute process such as viral hepatitis or choledocholithiasis. An elevated prothrombin time indicates either vitamin K deficiency due to prolonged jaundice and malabsorption of vitamin K or significant hepatocellular dysfunction. The failure of the prothrombin time to correct with parenteral administration of vitamin K indicates severe hepatocellular injury.

The results of the bilirubin, enzyme, albumin, and prothrombin time tests will usually indicate whether a jaundiced patient has a hepatocellular or a cholestatic disease. The causes and evaluation of each of these is quite different.

Hepatocellular Conditions   Hepatocellular diseases that can cause jaundice include viral hepatitis, drug or environmental toxicity, alcohol, and end-stage cirrhosis from any cause (Table 45-2). Wilson's disease should be considered in young adults. Autoimmune hepatitis is typically seen in young to middle-aged women, but may affect men and women of any age. Alcoholic hepatitis can be differentiated from viral and toxin-related hepatitis by the pattern of the aminotransferases. Patients with alcoholic hepatitis typically have an AST:ALT ratio of at least 2:1. The AST rarely exceeds 300 U/L. Patients with acute viral hepatitis and toxin-related injury severe enough to produce jaundice typically have aminotransferases greater than 500 U/L, with the ALT greater than or equal to the AST. The degree of aminotransferase elevation can occasionally help in differentiating between hepatocellular and cholestatic processes. While ALT and AST values less than 8 times normal may be seen in either hepatocellular or cholestatic liver disease, values 25 times normal or higher are seen primarily in acute hepatocellular diseases. Patients with jaundice from cirrhosis can have normal or only slight elevations of the aminotransferases.

When the physician determines that the patient has a hepatocellular disease, appropriate testing for acute viral hepatitis includes a hepatitis A IgM antibody, a hepatitis B surface antigen and core IgM antibody, and a hepatitis C viral RNA test. It can take many weeks for the hepatitis C antibody to become detectable, making it an unreliable test if acute hepatitis C is suspected. Depending on circumstances, studies for hepatitis D, E, Epstein-Barr virus (EBV), and cytomegalovirus (CMV) may be indicated. Ceruloplasmin is the initial screening test for Wilson's disease. Testing for autoimmune hepatitis usually includes an antinuclear antibody and measurement of specific immunoglobulins.

Drug-induced hepatocellular injury can be classified either as predictable or unpredictable. Predictable drug reactions are dose-dependent and affect all patients who ingest a toxic dose of the drug in question. The classic example is acetaminophen hepatotoxicity. Unpredictable or idiosyncratic drug reactions are not dose-dependent and occur in a minority of patients. A great number of drugs can cause

Table 45-2   Hepatocellular Conditions That May Produce Jaundice

Viral hepatitis
  Hepatitis A, B, C, D, and E
  Epstein-Barr virus
  Cytomegalovirus
  Herpes simplex
Alcohol
Drug toxicity
  Predictable, dose-dependent, e.g., acetaminophen
  Unpredictable, idosyncratic, e.g., isoniazid
Environmental toxins
  Vinyl chloride
  Jamaica bush tea—pyrrolizidine alkaloids
  Wild mushrooms—Amanita phalloides or verna
Wilson's disease
Autoimmune hepatitis

idiosyncratic hepatic injury. Environmental toxins are also an important cause of hepatocellular injury. Examples include industrial chemicals such as vinyl chloride, herbal preparations containing pyrrolizidine alkaloids (Jamaica bush tea), and the mushrooms Amanita phalloides or verna containing highly hepatotoxic amatoxins.

Cholestatic Conditions   When the pattern of the liver tests suggests a cholestatic disorder, the next step is to determine whether it is intra- or extrahepatic cholestasis (Fig. 45-1). Distinguishing intrahepatic from extrahepatic cholestasis may be difficult. History, physical examination, and laboratory tests are often not helpful. The next appropriate test is an ultrasound. The ultrasound is inexpensive, does not expose the patient to ionizing radiation, and can detect dilation of the intra- and extrahepatic biliary tree with a high degree of sensitivity and specificity. The absence of biliary dilatation suggests intrahepatic cholestasis, while the presence of biliary dilatation indicates extrahepatic cholestasis. False-negative results occur in patients with partial obstruction of the common bile duct or in patients with cirrhosis or primary sclerosing cholangitis (PSC) where scarring prevents the intrahepatic ducts from dilating.

Although ultrasonography may indicate extrahepatic cholestasis, it rarely identifies the site or cause of obstruction. The distal common bile duct is a particularly difficult area to visualize by ultrasound because of overlying bowel gas. Appropriate next tests include computed tomography (CT) and endoscopic retrograde cholangiopancreatography (ERCP). CT scanning is better than ultrasonography for assessing the head of the pancreas and for identifying choledocholithiasis in the distal common bile duct, particularly when the ducts are not dilated. ERCP is the gold standard for identifying choledocholithiasis. It is performed by introducing a side-viewing endoscope perorally into the duodenum. The ampulla of Vater is visualized and a catheter is advanced through the ampulla. Injection of dye allows for the visualization of the common bile duct and the pancreatic duct. The success rate for cannulation of the common bile duct ranges from 80 to 95%, depending on the operator's experience. Beyond its diagnostic capabilities, ERCP allows for therapeutic interventions, including the removal of common bile duct stones and the placement of stents. In patients in whom ERCP is unsuccessful, transhepatic cholangiography can provide the same information. Magnetic resonance cholangiopancreatography (MRCP) is a rapidly developing, noninvasive technique for imaging the bile and pancreatic ducts; this may replace ERCP as the initial diagnostic test in cases where the need for intervention is felt to be small.

In patients with apparent *intrahepatic cholestasis*, the diagnosis is often made by serologic testing in combination with percutaneous liver biopsy. The list of possible causes of intrahepatic cholestasis is long and varied (Table 45-3). A number of conditions that typically cause a hepatocellular pattern of injury can also present as a cholestatic variant. Both hepatitis B and C can cause a cholestatic hepatitis (fibrosing cholestatic hepatitis) that has histologic features that mimic large duct obstruction. This disease variant has been reported in patients who have undergone solid organ transplantation. Hepatitis A, alcoholic hepatitis, EBV, and CMV may also present as cholestatic liver disease.

Drugs may cause intrahepatic cholestasis, a variant of drug-induced hepatitis. Drug-induced cholestasis is usually reversible after eliminating the offending drug, although it may take many months for cholestasis to resolve. Drugs most commonly associated with cholestasis are the anabolic and contraceptive steroids. Cholestatic hepatitis has been reported with chlorpromazine, imipramine, tolbutamide, sulindac, cimetidine, and erythromycin estolate. It also occurs in patients taking trimethoprim, sulfamethoxazole, and penicillin-based antibiotics such as ampicillin, dicloxacillin, and clavulinic acid. Rarely, cholestasis may be chronic and associated with progressive fibrosis despite early discontinuation of the drug. Chronic cholestasis has been associated with chlorpromazine and prochlorperazine.

Primary biliary cirrhosis is a disease predominantly of middle-aged women in which there is a progressive destruction of interlobular bile ducts. The diagnosis is made by the presence of the antimitochondrial antibody that is found in 95% of patients. *Primary sclerosing*

Table 45-3 Cholestatic Conditions That May Produce Jaundice

I. Intrahepatic
  A. Viral hepatitis
    1. Fibrosing cholestatic hepatitis—hepatitis B and C
    2. Hepatitis A, Epstein-Barr virus, cytomegalovirus
  B. Alcoholic hepatitis
  C. Drug toxicity
    1. Pure cholestasis—anabolic and contraceptive steroids
    2. Cholestatic hepatitis—chlorpromazine, erythromycin estolate
    3. Chronic cholestasis—chlorpromazine and prochlorperazine
  D. Primary biliary cirrhosis
  E. Primary sclerosing cholangitis
  F. Vanishing bile duct syndrome
    1. Chronic rejection of liver tranplants
    2. Sarcoidosis
    3. Drugs
  G. Inherited
    1. Benign recurrent cholestasis
  H. Cholestasis of pregnancy
  I. Total parenteral nutrition
  J. Nonhepatobiliary sepsis
  K. Benign postoperative cholestasis
  L. Paraneoplastic syndrome
  M. Venoocclusive disease
  N. Graft-versus-host disease
II. Extrahepatic
  A. Malignant
    1. Cholangiocarcinoma
    2. Pancreatic cancer
    3. Gallbladder cancer
    4. Ampullary cancer
    5. Malignant involvement of the porta hepatis lymph nodes
  B. Benign
    1. Choledocholithiasis
    2. Primary sclerosing cholangitis
    3. Chronic pancreatitis
    4. AIDS cholangiopathy

cholangitis (PSC) is characterized by the destruction and fibrosis of larger bile ducts. The disease may involve only the intrahepatic ducts and present as intrahepatic cholestasis. However, in 65% of patients with PSC, both intra- and extrahepatic ducts are involved. The diagnosis of PSC is made by ERCP. The pathognomonic findings are multiple strictures of bile ducts with dilatations proximal to the strictures. Approximately 75% of patients with PSC have inflammatory bowel disease.

The *vanishing bile duct syndrome* and *adult bile ductopenia* are rare conditions in which there are a decreased number of bile ducts seen in liver biopsy specimens. The histologic picture is similar to that found in primary biliary cirrhosis. This picture is seen in patients who develop chronic rejection after liver transplantation and in those who develop graft-versus-host disease after bone marrow transplantation. Vanishing bile duct syndrome also occurs in rare cases of sarcoidosis, in patients taking certain drugs including chlorpromazine, and idiopathically. There are also familial forms of intrahepatic cholestasis, including the *familial intrahepatic cholestatic syndromes, I–III*. Benign recurrent cholestasis is an autosomal recessive disease that appears to be due to mutations in a P type ATPase, which probably acts as a bile acid transporter. The disease is marked by recurrent episodes of jaundice and pruritis; the episodes are self-limited but can be debilitating. *Cholestasis of pregnancy* occurs in the second and third trimesters and resolves after delivery. Its cause is unknown, but the condition is probably inherited and cholestasis can be triggered by estrogen administration.

Other causes of intrahepatic cholestasis include total parenteral nutrition (TPN), nonhepatobiliary sepsis, benign postoperative chole-

stasis, and a paraneoplastic syndrome associated with a number of different malignancies, including Hodgkin's disease, medullary thyroid cancer, hypernephroma, renal sarcoma, T cell lymphoma, prostate cancer, and several GI malignancies. In patients developing cholestasis in the intensive care unit, the major considerations should be sepsis, shock liver, and TPN jaundice. Jaundice occurring after bone marrow transplantation is most likely due to venoocclusive disease or graft-versus-host disease.

Causes of *extrahepatic cholestasis* can be split into malignant and benign (Table 45-3). Malignant causes include pancreatic, gallbladder, ampullary, and cholangiocarcinoma. The latter is most commonly associated with PSC and is exceptionally difficult to diagnose because its appearance is often identical to PSC. Pancreatic and gallbladder tumors, as well as cholangiocarcinoma, are rarely resectable and have poor prognoses. Ampullary carcinoma has the highest surgical cure rate of all the tumors that present as painless jaundice. Hilar lymphadenopathy due to metastases from other cancers may cause obstruction of the extrahepatic biliary tree.

Choledocholithiasis is the most common cause of extrahepatic cholestasis. The clinical presentation can range from mild right upper quadrant discomfort with only minimal elevations of the enzyme tests to ascending cholangitis with jaundice, sepsis, and circulatory collapse. PSC may occur with clinically important strictures limited to the extrahepatic biliary tree. In cases where there is a dominant stricture, patients can be effectively managed with serial endoscopic dilatations. Chronic pancreatitis rarely causes strictures of the distal common bile duct, where it passes through the head of the pancreas. AIDS cholangiopathy is a condition, usually due to infection of the bile duct epithelium with CMV or cryptosporidium, which has a cholangiographic appearance similar to PSC. These patients usually present with greatly elevated serum alkaline phosphatase levels, mean of 800 IU/L, but the bilirubin is often near normal. These patients do not typically present with jaundice.

SUMMARY The goal of this chapter is not to provide an encyclopedic review of all of the conditions that can cause jaundice. Rather, it is intended to provide a framework that helps a physician to evaluate the patient with jaundice in a logical way (Fig. 45-1).

Simply stated, the initial step is to obtain appropriate blood tests to determine if the patient has an isolated elevation of serum bilirubin. If so, is the bilirubin elevation due to an increased unconjugated or conjugated fraction? If the hyperbilirubinemia is accompanied by other liver test abnormalities, is the disorder hepatocellular or cholestatic? If cholestatic, is it intra- or extrahepatic? All of these questions can be answered with a thoughtful history, physical examination, and interpretation of laboratory and radiologic tests and procedures.

BIBLIOGRAPHY

BERG CL et al: Bilirubin metabolism and the pathophysiology of jaundice, in *Schiff's Diseases of the Liver*, 8th ed, ER Schiff et al (eds). Philadelphia, Lippincott, 1999

BERK PD, NOYER C (eds): Bilirubin metabolism and the hereditary hyperbilirubinemias. Semin Liv Dis 14:321, 1994

BLANCKAERT N, FEVERY J: Physiology and pathophysiology of bilirubin metabolism, in *Hepatology: A Textbook of Liver Disease*, 3d ed, D Zakin, TD Boyer (eds). Philadelphia, Saunders, 1997

FOX IJ et al: Treatment of the Crigler-Najjar syndrome type I with hepatocyte transplantation. N Engl J Med 338:1422, 1998

PRATT DS, KAPLAN MM: Laboratory tests, in *Schiff's Diseases of the Liver*, 8th ed, ER Schiff et al (eds). Philadelphia, Lippincott, 1999

TRAUNER M et al: Molecular pathogenesis of cholestasis. N Engl J Med 339:1217, 1998

WEISS JS et al: The clinical importance of a protein-bound fraction of serum bilirubin in patients with hyperbilirubinemia. N Engl J Med 309:147, 1983

ZIMMERMAN HJ: *Hepatoxicity: The Adverse Effects of Drugs and Other Chemicals on the Liver*, 2d ed. Philadelphia, Lippincott Williams & Wilkins, 1999

46   *Robert M. Glickman*

ABDOMINAL SWELLING AND ASCITES

ABDOMINAL SWELLING   Abdominal swelling or distention is a common problem in clinical medicine and may be the initial manifestation of a systemic disease or of otherwise unsuspected abdominal disease. *Subjective* abdominal enlargement, often described as a sensation of fullness or bloating, is usually transient and is often related to a functional gastrointestinal disorder when it is not accompanied by objective physical findings of increased abdominal girth or local swelling. *Obesity* and lumbar lordosis, which may be associated with prominence of the abdomen, may usually be distinguished from true increases in the volume of the peritoneal cavity by history and careful physical examination.

Clinical History   Abdominal swelling may first be noticed by the patient because of a progressive increase in belt or clothing size, the appearance of abdominal or inguinal hernias, or the development of a localized swelling. Often, considerable abdominal enlargement has gone unnoticed for weeks or months, either because of coexistent obesity or because the ascites formation has been insidious, without pain or localizing symptoms. Progressive abdominal distention may be associated with a sensation of "pulling" or "stretching" of the flanks or groins and vague low back pain. Localized pain usually results from involvement of an abdominal organ (e.g., a passively congested liver, large spleen, or colonic tumor). Pain is uncommon in cirrhosis with ascites, and when it is present, pancreatitis, hepatocellular carcinoma, or peritonitis should be considered. Tense ascites or abdominal tumors may produce increased intraabdominal pressure, resulting in indigestion and heartburn due to gastroesophageal reflux or dyspnea, orthopnea, and tachypnea from elevation of the diaphragm. A coexistent pleural effusion, more commonly on the right, presumably due to leakage of ascitic fluid through lymphatic channels in the diaphragm, also may contribute to respiratory embarrassment. The patient with diffuse abdominal swelling should be questioned about increased alcohol intake, a prior episode of jaundice or hematuria, or a change in bowel habits. Such historic information may provide the clues that will lead one to suspect an occult cirrhosis, a colonic tumor with peritoneal seeding, congestive heart failure, or nephrosis.

Physical Examination   A carefully executed general physical examination can yield valuable clues concerning the etiology of abdominal swelling. Thus palmar erythema and spider angiomas suggest an underlying cirrhosis, while supraclavicular adenopathy (Virchow's node) should raise the question of an underlying gastrointestinal malignancy.

Inspection of the abdomen is important. By noting the abdominal contour, one may be able to distinguish localized from generalized swelling. The tensely distended abdomen with tightly stretched skin, bulging flanks, and everted umbilicus is characteristic of ascites. A prominent abdominal venous pattern with the direction of flow away from the umbilicus often is a reflection of portal hypertension; venous collaterals with flow from the lower part of the abdomen toward the umbilicus suggest obstruction of the inferior vena cava; flow downward toward the umbilicus suggests superior vena cava obstruction. "Doming" of the abdomen with visible ridges from underlying intestinal loops is usually due to intestinal obstruction or distention. An epigastric mass, with evident peristalsis proceeding from left to right, usually indicates underlying pyloric obstruction. A liver with metastatic deposits may be visible as a nodular right upper quadrant mass moving with respiration.

Auscultation may reveal the high-pitched, rushing sounds of early intestinal obstruction or a succussion sound due to increased fluid and gas in a dilated hollow viscus. Careful auscultation over an enlarged liver occasionally reveals the harsh bruit of a vascular tumor, especially a hepatocellular carcinoma, or the leathery friction rub of a surface nodule. A venous hum at the umbilicus may signify portal hypertension and an increased collateral blood flow around the liver. A fluid wave and flank dullness that shifts with change in position of the patient are important signs that indicate the presence of peritoneal fluid. In obese patients, small amounts of fluid may be difficult to demonstrate; on occasion, the fluid may be detected by abdominal percussion with patients on their hands and knees. Small amounts of ascites often can only be detected by ultrasound examination of the abdomen, which can detect as little as 100 mL of fluid. Careful percussion should serve to distinguish generalized abdominal enlargement from localized swelling due to an enlarged uterus, ovarian cyst, or distended bladder. Percussion also can outline an abnormally small or large liver. Loss of normal liver dullness may result from massive hepatic necrosis; it also may be a clue to free gas in the peritoneal cavity, as from perforation of a hollow viscus.

Palpation is often difficult with massive ascites, and ballottement of overlying fluid may be the only method of palpating the liver or spleen. A slightly enlarged spleen in association with ascites may be the only evidence of an occult cirrhosis. When there is evidence of portal hypertension, a soft liver suggests that obstruction to portal flow is extrahepatic; a firm liver suggests cirrhosis as the likely cause of the portal hypertension. A very hard or nodular liver is a clue that the liver is infiltrated with tumor, and when accompanied by ascites, it suggests that the latter is due to peritoneal seeding. The presence of a hard periumbilical nodule (Sister Mary Joseph's nodule) suggests metastatic disease from a pelvic or gastrointestinal primary tumor. A pulsatile liver and ascites may be found in tricuspid insufficiency.

An attempt should be made to determine whether a mass is solid or cystic, smooth or irregular, and whether it moves with respiration. The liver, spleen, and gallbladder should descend with respiration unless they are fixed by adhesions or extension of tumor beyond the organ. A fixed mass not descending with respiration may indicate that it is retroperitoneal. Tenderness, especially if localized, may indicate an inflammatory process such as an abscess; it also may be due to stretching of the visceral peritoneum or tumor necrosis. Rectal and pelvic examinations are mandatory; they may reveal otherwise undetected masses due to tumor or infection.

Radiographic and laboratory examinations are essential for confirming or extending the impressions gained on physical examination. Upright and recumbent films of the abdomen may demonstrate the dilated loops of intestine with fluid levels characteristic of intestinal obstruction or the diffuse abdominal haziness and loss of psoas margins suggestive of ascites. Ultrasonography is often of value in detecting ascites, determining the presence of a mass, or evaluating the size of the liver and spleen. Computed tomography (CT) scanning provides similar information. CT scanning is often necessary to visualize the retroperitoneum, pancreas, and lymph nodes. A plain film of the abdomen may reveal the distended colon of otherwise unsuspected ulcerative colitis and give valuable information as to the size of the liver and spleen. An irregular and elevated right side of the diaphragm may be a clue to a liver abscess or hepatocellular carcinoma. Studies of the gastrointestinal tract with barium or other contrast media are usually necessary in the search for a primary tumor.

ASCITES   The evaluation of a patient with ascites requires that the cause of the ascites be established. In most cases ascites appears as part of a well-recognized illness, that is, cirrhosis, congestive heart failure, nephrosis, or disseminated carcinomatosis. In these situations, the physician should determine that the development of ascites is indeed a consequence of the basic underlying disease and not due to the presence of a separate or related disease process. This distinction is necessary even when the cause of ascites seems obvious. For example, when the patient with compensated cirrhosis and minimal ascites develops progressive ascites that is increasingly difficult to control with sodium restriction or diuretics, the temptation is to attribute the worsening of the clinical picture to progressive liver disease. However, an occult hepatocellular carcinoma, portal vein thrombosis, spontaneous bacterial peritonitis, or even tuberculosis may be responsible for the decompensation. The disappointingly low success in diagnosing tuberculous peritonitis or hepatocullar carcinoma in the patient with cirrhosis and ascites reflects the too-low index of suspicion for the development of such superimposed conditions. Similarly, the patient with congestive heart failure may develop ascites from a disseminated carcinoma with peritoneal seeding.

Diagnostic paracentesis (50 to 100 mL) should be part of the routine evaluation of the patient with ascites. The fluid should be examined for its gross appearance; protein content, cell count, and differential cell count should be determined; and Gram's and acid-fast stains and culture should be performed. Cytologic and cell-block examination may disclose an otherwise unsuspected carcinoma. Table 46-1 presents some of the features of ascitic fluid typically found in various disease states. In some disorders, such as cirrhosis, the fluid has the characteristics of a transudate (<25 g protein per liter and a specific gravity of <1.016); in others, such as peritonitis, the features are those of an exudate. Rather than the total protein content of ascites, many authors prefer the use of a *serum-ascites albumin gradient (SAG)* to characterize ascites. The gradient correlates directly with portal pressure. A gradient >1.1 g/dL (high gradient) is characteristic of uncomplicated cirrhotic ascites and differentiates ascites due to portal hypertension from ascites not due to portal hypertension >95% of the time. A gradient <1.1 g/dL (low gradient) suggests that the ascites is not due to portal hypertension with >95% accuracy and mandates a search for other causes (Table 46-1). Although there is variability of the ascitic fluid in any given disease state, some features are sufficiently characteristic to suggest certain diagnostic possibilities. For example, blood-stained fluid with >25 g protein per liter is unusual in uncomplicated cirrhosis but is consistent with tuberculous peritonitis or neoplasm. Cloudy fluid with a predominance of polymorphonuclear cells and a positive Gram's stain are characteristic of bacterial peritonitis; if most cells are lymphocytes, tuberculosis should be suspected. The complete examination of each fluid is most important, for occasionally only one finding may be abnormal. For example, if the fluid is a typical transudate but contains >250 white blood cells per microliter, the finding should be recognized as atypical for cirrhosis and should warrant a search for tumor or infection. This is especially true in the evaluation of cirrhotic ascites where occult peritoneal infection may be present with only minor elevations in the white blood cell count of the peritoneal fluid (300 to 500 cells per microliter). Since Gram's stain of the fluid may be negative in a high proportion of such cases, careful culture of the peritoneal fluid is mandatory. Bedside innoculation of blood culture flasks with ascitic fluid results in a dramatically increased incidence of positive cultures when bacterial infection is present (90 versus 40% positivity with conventional cultures done by the laboratory). Direct visualization of the peritoneum (laparoscopy) may disclose peritoneal deposits of tumor, tuberculosis, or metastatic disease of the liver. Biopsies are taken under direct vision, often adding to the diagnostic accuracy of the procedure.

Chylous ascites refers to a turbid, milky, or creamy peritoneal fluid due to the presence of thoracic or intestinal lymph. Such a fluid shows Sudan-staining fat globules microscopically and an increased triglyceride content by chemical examination. Opaque milky fluid usually has a triglyceride concentration of >1000 mg/dL. A turbid fluid due to leukocytes or tumor cells may be confused with chylous fluid (pseudochylous), and it is often helpful to carry out alkalinization and ether extraction of the specimen. Alkali tend to dissolve cellular proteins and thereby reduce turbidity; ether extraction leads to clearing if the turbidity of the fluid is due to lipid. Chylous ascites is most often the result of lymphatic obstruction from trauma, tumor, tuberculosis, filariasis (Chap. 221), or congenital abnormalities. It also may be seen in the nephrotic syndrome.

Rarely, ascitic fluid may be *mucinous* in character, suggesting either pseudomyxoma peritonei (Chap. 289) or rarely a colloid carcinoma of the stomach or colon with peritoneal implants.

On occasion, ascites may develop as a seemingly isolated finding in the absence of a clinically evident underlying disease. Then, a care-

Table 46-1 Characteristics of Ascitic Fluid in Various Disease States

Condition	Gross Appearance	Protein, g/dL	Serum-Ascites Albumin Gradient, g/dL	Red Blood Cells, >10,000/μL	White Blood Cells, per μL	Other Tests
Cirrhosis	Straw-colored or bile-stained	<25 (95%)	>1.1	1%	<250 (90%);[a] predominantly mesothelial	
Neoplasm	Straw-colored, hemorrhagic, mucinous, or chylous	>25 (75%)	<1.1	20%	>1000 (50%); variable cell types	Cytology, cell block, peritoneal biopsy
Tuberculous peritonitis	Clear, turbid, hemorrhagic, chylous	>25 (50%)	<1.1	7%	>1000 (70%); usually >70% lymphocytes	Peritoneal biopsy, stain and culture for acid-fast bacilli
Pyogenic peritonitis	Turbid or purulent	If purulent, >25	<1.1	Unusual	Predominantly polymorphonuclear leukocytes	Positive Gram's stain, culture
Congestive heart failure	Straw-colored	Variable, 15–53	>1.1	10%	<1000 (90%); usually mesothelial, mononuclear	
Nephrosis	Straw-colored or chylous	<25 (100%)	<1.1	Unusual	<250; mesothelial, mononuclear	If chylous, ether extraction, Sudan staining
Pancreatic ascites (pancreatitis, pseudocyst)	Turbid, hemorrhagic, or chylous	Variable, often >25	<1.1	Variable, may be blood-stained	Variable	Increased amylase in ascitic fluid and serum

[a] Because the conditions of examining fluid and selecting patients were not identical in each series, the percentage figures (in parentheses) should be taken as an indication of the order of magnitude rather than as the precise incidence of any abnormal finding.

ful analysis of ascitic fluid may indicate the direction the evaluation should take. A useful framework for the workup starts with an analysis of whether the fluid is classified as a high (transudate) or low (exudate) gradient fluid. *High gradient (transudative) ascites* of unclear etiology is most often due to occult cirrhosis, right-sided venous hypertension raising hepatic sinusoidal pressure, or hypoalbuminemic states such as nephrosis or protein-losing enteropathy. Cirrhosis with well-preserved liver function (normal albumin) resulting in ascites invariably is associated with significant portal hypertension (Chap. 298). Evaluation should include liver function tests, liver-spleen scan, or other hepatic imaging procedure (i.e., CT or ultrasound) to detect nodular changes in the liver or a colloid shift of isotope to suggest portal hypertension. On occasion, a wedged hepatic venous pressure can be useful to document portal hypertension. Finally, if clinically indicated, a liver biopsy will confirm the diagnosis of cirrhosis and perhaps suggest its etiology. Other etiologies may result in hepatic venous congestion and resultant ascites. Right-sided cardiac valvular disease and particularly constrictive pericarditis should raise a high index of suspicion and may require cardiac imaging and cardiac catheterization for definitive diagnosis. Hepatic vein thrombosis is evaluated by visualizing the hepatic veins with imaging techniques (Doppler ultrasound, angiography, CT scans, magnetic resonance imaging) to demonstrate obliteration, thrombosis, or obstruction by tumor. Uncommonly, transudative ascites may be associated with benign tumors of the ovary, particularly fibroma (Meigs' syndrome) with ascites and hydrothorax.

Low gradient (exudative) ascites should initiate an evaluation for primary peritoneal processes, most importantly infection and tumor. Routine bacteriologic culture of ascitic fluid often yields a specific organism causing infectious peritonitis. Tuberculous peritonitis (Table 46-1) is best diagnosed by peritoneal biopsy, either percutaneously or via laparoscopy. Histologic examination invariably shows granulomata that may contain acid-fast bacilli. Since cultures of peritoneal fluid and biopsies for tuberculosis may require 6 weeks, characteristic histology with appropriate stains allows antituberculosis therapy to be started promptly. Similarly, the diagnosis of peritoneal seeding by tumor can usually be made by cytologic analysis of peritoneal fluid or by peritoneal biopsy if cytology is negative. Appropriate diagnostic studies can then be undertaken to determine the nature and site of the primary tumor. Pancreatic ascites (Table 46-1) is invariably associated with an extravasation of pancreatic fluid from the pancreatic ductal system, most commonly from a leaking pseudocyst. Ultrasound or CT examination of the pancreas followed by visualization of the pancreatic duct by direct cannulation [viz., endoscopic retrograde cholangiopancreatography (ERCP)] usually discloses the site of leakage and permits resective surgery to be carried out.

An analysis of the physiologic and metabolic factors involved in the production of ascites (detailed in Chap. 298), coupled with a complete evaluation of the nature of the ascitic fluid, invariably discloses the etiology of the ascites and permits appropriate therapy to be instituted.

ACKNOWLEDGMENT
Dr. Kurt J. Isselbacher was the co-author of this chapter in previous editions.

BIBLIOGRAPHY

LIPSKY MS, STERNBACH MR: Evaluation and initial management of patients with ascites. Am Fam Physician 54:1327, 1996

MCHUTCHISON JG: Differential diagnosis of ascites. Semin Liver Dis 17:191, 1997

PARSONS SL et al: Malignant ascites. Br J Surg 83:6, 1996

PINTO PC et al: Large volume paracentesis in nonedematous patients with tense ascites: Its effect on intravascular volume. Hepatology 8:207, 1988

RECTOR WG JR, REYNOLDS TB: Superiority of the serum: ascites albumin difference over the ascites total protein concentration in separation of "transudative" and "exudative" ascites. Am J Med 77:83, 1988

RUNYON BA: Management of adult patients with ascites caused by cirrhosis. Hepatology 27:264, 1998

———— et al: The serum-ascites albumin gradient in the differential diagnosis of ascites. Ann Intern Med 117:215, 1992

Section 7
ALTERATIONS IN RENAL AND URINARY TRACT FUNCTION

47

Bradley M. Denker, Barry M. Brenner

AZOTEMIA AND URINARY ABNORMALITIES

Body homeostasis is maintained predominantly through the cellular processes that together comprise normal kidney function. Disturbances to any of these functions can lead to a constellation of abnormalities that may be detrimental to survival. The clinical manifestations of these diseases will depend upon the pathophysiology of the renal injury and will often be initially identified as a complex of symptoms, abnormal physical findings, and laboratory changes that will allow the identification of specific syndromes. These renal syndromes (summarized in Table 47-1) may arise as the consequence of a systemic illness or can occur as a primary renal disease. Nephrologic syndromes usually consist of several elements that reflect the underlying pathologic processes and the duration of the disease and typically include one or more of the following features: (1) disturbances in urine volume (oliguria, anuria, polyuria); (2) abnormalities of urine sediment [red blood cells (RBC); white blood cells, casts, and crystals]; (3) abnormal excretion of serum proteins (proteinuria); (4) reduction in glomerular filtration rate (GFR) (azotemia); (5) presence of hypertension and/or expanded total body volume (edema); (6) electrolyte abnormalities, or (7) in some syndromes, fever/pain. The combination of these findings should permit identification of one of the major nephrologic syndromes (Table 47-1) and will allow the differential diagnoses to be narrowed and the appropriate diagnostic evaluation and therapeutic course to be determined. Each of these syndromes and their associated diseases are discussed in more detail in subsequent chapters. This chapter will focus on several aspects of renal abnormalities that are critically important to distinguishing these processes: (1) reduction in GFR leading to azotemia, (2) alterations of the urinary sediment and/or protein excretion, and (3) abnormalities of urinary volume.

AZOTEMIA

ASSESSMENT OF GLOMERULAR FILTRATION RATE
Monitoring the GFR is important in both the hospital and outpatient settings, and several different methodologies are available (discussed below). In most acute clinical circumstances a measured GFR is not available, and it is necessary to estimate the GFR from the serum creatinine level in order to provide appropriate doses of drugs that are excreted into the urine. Serum creatinine is the most widely used marker for GFR and is related directly to the urine creatinine excretion and inversely to the serum creatinine (U_{Cr}/P_{Cr}). Based upon this relationship and some important caveats (discussed below), the GFR will fall proportionately with the increase in P_{Cr}. Failure to account for GFR

Table 47-1 Initial Clinical and Laboratory Data Base for Defining Major Syndromes in Nephrology

Syndromes	Important Clues to Diagnosis	Findings That Are Common	Location of Discussion of Diseases Causing Syndrome
Acute or rapidly progressive renal failure	Anuria Oliguria Documented recent decline in GFR	Hypertension, hematuria Proteinuria, pyuria Casts, edema	Chaps. 269, 274, 277, 281
Acute nephritis	Hematuria, RBC casts Azotemia, oliguria Edema, hypertension	Proteinuria Pyuria Circulatory congestion	Chaps. 273, 274, 275
Chronic renal failure	Azotemia for >3 months Prolonged symptoms or signs of uremia Symptoms or signs of renal osteodystrophy Kidneys reduced in size bilaterally Broad casts in urinary sediment	Hematuria, proteinuria Casts, oliguria Polyuria, nocturia Edema, hypertension Electrolyte disorders	Chaps. 268, 270
Nephrotic syndrome	Proteinuria >3.5 g per 1.73 m² per 24 h Hypoalbuminemia Hyperlipidemia Lipiduria	Casts Edema	Chap. 274
Asymptomatic urinary abnormalities	Hematuria Proteinuria (below nephrotic range) Sterile pyuria, casts		Chap. 274
Urinary tract infection	Bacteriuria >10⁵ colonies per milliliter Other infectious agent documented in urine Pyuria, leukocyte casts Frequency, urgency Bladder tenderness, flank tenderness	Hematuria Mild azotemia Mild proteinuria Fever	Chap. 280
Renal tubule defects	Electrolyte disorders Polyuria, nocturia Symptoms or signs of renal osteodystrophy Large kidneys Renal transport defects	Hematuria "Tubular" proteinuria Enuresis	Chaps. 276, 277
Hypertension	Systolic/diastolic hypertension	Proteinuria Casts Azotemia	Chaps. 35, 246, 278
Nephrolithiasis	Previous history of stone passage or removal Previous history of stone seen by x-ray Renal colic	Hematuria Pyuria Frequency, urgency	Chap. 279
Urinary tract obstruction	Azotemia, oliguria, anuria Polyuria, nocturia, urinary retention Slowing of urinary stream Large prostate, large kidneys Flank tenderness, full bladder after voiding	Hematuria Pyuria Enuresis, dysuria	Chap. 281

reductions in drug dosing can lead to significant morbidity and mortality from drug toxicities (e.g., digoxin, aminoglycosides). In the outpatient setting, serial determinations of GFR are helpful for following the progression of chronic renal insufficiency, but again, the serum creatinine is often used as a surrogate for GFR (although much less accurate; see below). In patients with chronic progressive renal insufficiency there is an approximately linear relationship between $1/P_{Cr}$ and time. The slope of this line will remain constant for an individual patient, and when values are obtained that do not fall on this line, an investigation for a superimposed acute process (e.g., volume depletion, drug reaction) should be initiated. It should be emphasized that the signs and symptoms of uremia will develop at significantly different levels of serum creatinine depending upon the patient (size, age, and sex), the underlying renal disease, existence of concurrent diseases, and true GFR. In general, patients do not develop symptomatic uremia until renal insufficiency is usually quite severe (GFR < 15 mL/min) and in some patients it does not occur until the GFR < 5 mL/min.

A reduced GFR leads to retention of nitrogenous waste products (azotemia) such as serum urea nitrogen and creatinine. Azotemia may result from reduced renal perfusion, intrinsic renal disease, or postrenal processes (ureteral obstruction; see below and Fig. 47-1). Precise determination of GFR is problematic as both commonly used markers (urea and creatinine) have characteristics that affect their accuracy as markers of clearance. Urea clearance is generally an underestimate of GFR because of tubule urea reabsorption and may be as low as one-half of GFR measured by other techniques.

Creatinine is a small, freely filtered solute that varies little from day to day (since it is derived from muscle metabolism of creatine).

However, serum creatinine can increase acutely from dietary ingestion of cooked meat. Creatinine can be secreted by the proximal tubule through an organic cation pathway. There are many clinical settings where a creatinine clearance is not available, and decisions concerning drug dosing must be made based on the serum creatinine. A formula that allows an estimate of creatinine clearance in men that accounts for age-related decreases in GFR, body weight, and sex has been derived by Cockcroft-Gault:

$$\text{Creatinine clearance (mL/min)} = \frac{(140 - \text{age}) \times \text{lean body weight (kg)}}{\text{plasma creatinine (mg/dL)} \times 72}$$

This value should be multiplied 0.85 for women, since a lower fraction of the body weight is composed of muscle. The gradual loss of muscle from chronic illness, chronic use of glucocorticoids, or malnutrition can mask significant changes in GFR with small or imperceptible changes in serum creatinine. More accurate determinations of GFR are available using inulin clearance or radionuclide-labeled markers such as ¹²⁵I-iothalamate or EDTA. These methods are highly accurate due to precise quantitation and the absence of any renal reabsorption/secretion and should be used to follow GFR in patients in whom creatinine is not likely to be a reliable indicator (patients with decreased muscle mass secondary to age, malnutrition, concurrent illnesses).

Approach to the Patient

Once it has been established that GFR is reduced, the physician must decide if this represents acute or chronic renal failure. The clinical

FIGURE 47-1 Approach to the patient with azotemia. (WBC, white blood cell; RBC, red blood cell; GBM, glomerular basement membrane.)

be affected by reductions in cardiac output from peripheral vasodilatation (sepsis, drugs) or profound renal vasoconstriction [severe heart failure, hepatorenal syndrome, drugs (such as nonsteroidal anti-inflammatory drugs (NSAIDs)]. True, or "effective," hypovolemia leads to a fall in mean arterial pressure, which in turn triggers a series of neural and humoral responses that include activation of the sympathetic nervous and renin-angiotensin-aldosterone systems and ADH release. GFR is maintained by prostaglandin-mediated relaxation of afferent arterioles and angiotensin II–mediated constriction of efferent arterioles. Once the mean arterial pressure falls below 80 mmHg, there is a steep decline in GFR.

Blockade of prostaglandin production by NSAIDs can result in severe vasoconstriction and acute renal failure under these circumstances. Angiotensin-converting enzyme (ACE) inhibitors decrease efferent arteriolar tone and can decrease glomerular capillary perfusion pressure. Patients on NSAIDs and/or ACE inhibitors are most susceptible to hemodynamically mediated acute renal failure when blood volume is reduced for any reason. Patients with renal artery stenosis are dependent upon efferent arteriolar vasoconstriction for maintenance of glomerular filtration pressure and are particularly susceptible to precipitous decline in GFR when given ACE inhibitors.

Prolonged renal hypoperfusion can lead to acute tubular necrosis (ATN; an intrinsic renal disease discussed below). The urinalysis and urinary electrolytes can be useful in distinguishing prerenal azotemia from ATN (Table 47-2). The urine of patients with prerenal azotemia can be predicted from the stimulatory actions of norepinephrine, angiotensin II, ADH, and low tubule fluid flow on salt and water reabsorption from the urine. In prerenal conditions the tubules are intact, leading to a concentrated urine (>500 mosm), avid Na retention (urine Na concentration <20 mM/L; fractional excretion of Na <1%), and U_{Cr}/P_{Cr} > 40 (Table 47-2). The prerenal urine sediment is usually normal or has occasional hyaline and granular casts, while the sediment of ATN is usually filled with cellular debris and muddy brown granular casts.

Intrinsic Renal Disease When prerenal and postrenal azotemia have been excluded as etiologies of renal failure, an intrinsic parenchymal renal disease is present. Intrinsic renal disease can arise from processes involving large renal vessels, microvasculature and glomeruli, or tubulointerstitium. Ischemic and toxic ATN account for about 90% of acute intrinsic renal failure. As outlined in Fig. 47-1, the clinical setting and urinalysis are helpful in separating the possible etiologies of acute intrinsic renal failure. Prerenal azotemia and ATN are part of a spectrum of renal hypoperfusion; evidence of structural tubule injury is present in ATN, whereas prompt reversibility occurs with prerenal azotemia upon restoration of adequate renal perfusion. Thus, ATN can often be distinguished from prerenal azotemia by urinalysis and urine electrolyte composition (Table 47-2 and Fig. 47-1). Ischemic ATN is observed most frequently in patients who have undergone ma-

situation, history, and laboratory data often make this an easy distinction. However, the laboratory abnormalities characteristic of chronic renal failure, including anemia, hypocalcemia, and hyperphosphatemia, are often also present in patients presenting with acute renal failure. Radiographic evidence of renal osteodystrophy (Chap. 270) would be seen only in chronic renal failure but is a very late finding, and these patients are usually on dialysis. The urinalysis and renal ultrasound can occasionally facilitate distinguishing acute from chronic renal failure. An approach to the evaluation of azotemic patients is shown in Fig. 47-1. Patients with advanced chronic renal insufficiency often have some proteinuria, nonconcentrated urine (isosthenuria), and small kidneys on ultrasound characterized by increased echogenicity and cortical thinning. Treatment should be directed toward slowing the progression of renal disease and providing symptomatic relief for edema, acidosis, anemia, and hyperphosphatemia, as discussed in Chap. 270. Acute renal failure (Chap. 269) can result from processes affecting renal blood flow (prerenal azotemia), intrinsic renal diseases (affecting vessels, glomeruli, or tubules), or postrenal processes (obstruction to urine flow in ureters, bladder, or urethra) (Chap. 281).

Prerenal Failure Decreased renal perfusion accounts for 40 to 80% of acute renal failure and, if appropriately treated, is readily reversible. The etiologies of prerenal azotemia include any cause of decreased circulating blood volume including volume loss (gastrointestinal hemorrhage, burns, diarrhea, diuretics), volume sequestration (pancreatitis, peritonitis, rhabdomyolysis), or decreased effective circulating volume (cardiogenic shock, sepsis). Renal perfusion can also

Table 47-2   Laboratory Findings in Acute Renal Failure

Index	Prerenal Azotemia	Oliguric Acute Renal Failure
BUN/P_{Cr} Ratio	>20:1	10–15:1
Urine sodium (U_{Na}), meq/L	<20	>40
Urine osmolality, mosmol/L H_2O	>500	<350
Fractional excretion of sodium $$FE_{Na} = \frac{U_{Na} \times P_{Cr} \times 100}{P_{Na} \times U_{Cr}}$$	<1%	>2%
Urine/plasma creatinine (U_{Cr}/P_{Cr})	>40	<20

NOTE: BUN, Blood urea nitrogen; P_{Cr}, plasma creatinine; U_{Na}, urine sodium concentration; P_{Na}, plasma sodium concentration; U_{Cr}, urine creatinine concentration.

jor surgery, trauma, severe hypovolemia, overwhelming sepsis, or extensive burns. Nephrotoxic ATN complicates the administration of many common medications, usually by inducing a combination of intrarenal vasoconstriction, direct tubule toxicity, and/or tubular obstruction. The kidney is vulnerable to toxic injury by virtue of its rich blood supply (25% of cardiac output) and its ability to concentrate and metabolize toxins. A diligent search for hypotension and nephrotoxins will usually uncover the specific etiology of ATN. Discontinuation of nephrotoxins and stabilizing blood pressure will often suffice without the need for dialysis while the tubules recover. →*An extensive list of potential drugs and toxins implicated in ATN can be found in Chap. 269.*

Processes that involve the tubules and interstitium can lead to acute renal failure. These include drug-induced interstitial nephritis (especially antibiotics, NSAIDs, and diuretics), severe infections (both bacterial and viral), systemic diseases (e.g., systemic lupus erythematosus), or infiltrative disorders (e.g., sarcoid, lymphoma, or leukemia). A list of drugs associated with allergic interstitial nephritis can be found in Chap. 277. The urinalysis usually shows mild to moderate proteinuria, hematuria, and pyuria (approximately 75% of cases) and occasionally white blood cell casts. The finding of RBC casts in interstitial nephritis has been reported but should prompt a search for glomerular diseases. Occasionally renal biopsy will be needed to distinguish among these possibilities. The finding of eosinophils in the urine is suggestive of allergic interstitial nephritis and is optimally observed by using a Hansel stain. The absence of eosinophiluria, however, does not exclude the possibility of acute interstitial nephritis.

Occlusion of large renal vessels including arteries and veins is an uncommon cause of acute renal failure. A significant reduction in GFR by this mechanism suggests bilateral processes or a unilateral process in a patient with a single functioning kidney. Renal arteries can be occluded with atheroemboli, thromboemboli, in situ thrombosis, aortic dissection, or vasculitis. Atheroembolic renal failure can occur spontaneously but is most often associated with recent aortic instrumentation. The emboli are cholesterol-rich and lodge in medium and small renal arteries leading to an eosinophil-rich inflammatory reaction. Atheroembolic acute renal failure often has a normal urinalysis but may contain eosinophils and casts. The diagnosis can be confirmed by renal biopsy, but this is often unnecessary when other stigmata of atheroemboli are present (livedo reticularis, distal peripheral infarcts, eosinophilia). Renal artery thrombosis may lead to mild proteinuria and hematuria, whereas renal vein thrombosis typically induces heavy proteinuria and hematuria. →*These vascular catastrophes often require angiography for confirmation and are discussed in Chap. 278.*

Diseases of glomeruli (glomerulonephritis or vasculitis) and the renal microvasculature (hemolytic uremic syndromes, thrombotic thrombocytopenic purpura, or malignant hypertension) usually present with various combinations of glomerular injury: proteinuria, hematuria, reduced GFR, and alterations of Na excretion leading to hypertension, edema, and circulatory congestion (acute nephritic syndrome). These findings may occur as primary renal diseases or as renal manifestations of systemic diseases. The clinical setting and other laboratory data will help distinguish primary renal from systemic diseases. The finding of RBC casts in the urine is an indication for early renal

biopsy (Fig. 47-1) as the pathologic pattern has important implications for diagnosis, prognosis, and treatment. Hematuria without RBC casts can also be an indication of glomerular disease, and this evaluation is summarized in Fig. 47-2. →*A detailed discussion of glomerulonephritis and diseases of the microvasculature can be found in Chap. 274.*

Postrenal Azotemia   Urinary tract obstruction accounts for fewer than 5% of cases of acute renal failure, but it is usually reversible and must be ruled out early in the evaluation (Fig. 47-1). Since a single kidney is capable of adequate clearance, acute renal failure from obstruction requires obstruction at the urethra or bladder outlet, bilateral ureteral obstruction, or unilateral obstruction in a patient with a single functioning kidney. Obstruction is usually diagnosed by the presence of ureteral dilatation on renal ultrasound. However, early in the course of obstruction or if the ureters are unable to dilate (such as encasement by pelvic tumors), the ultrasound examination may be negative. →*The specific urologic conditions that cause obstruction are discussed in Chap. 281.*

Oliguria and Anuria   *Oliguria* refers to a 24-h urine output of <500 mL, and *anuria* is the complete absence of urine formation. Anuria can be caused by total urinary tract obstruction, total renal artery or vein occlusion, and shock (manifested by severe hypotension and intense renal vasoconstriction). Cortical necrosis, ATN, and rapidly progressive glomerulonephritis can occasionally cause anuria. Oliguria can accompany any cause of acute renal failure and carries a more serious prognosis for renal recovery in all conditions except prerenal azotemia. *Nonoliguria* refers to urine output in excess of

FIGURE 47-2   Approach to the patient with hematuria. (RBC, red blood cell; WBC, white blood cell; GBM, glomerular basement membrane; ANCA, antineutrophil cytoplasmic antibody; VDRL, venereal disease research laboratory; ASLO, antistreptolysin O; UA, urinalysis; IVP, intravenous pyelography; CT, computed tomography.)

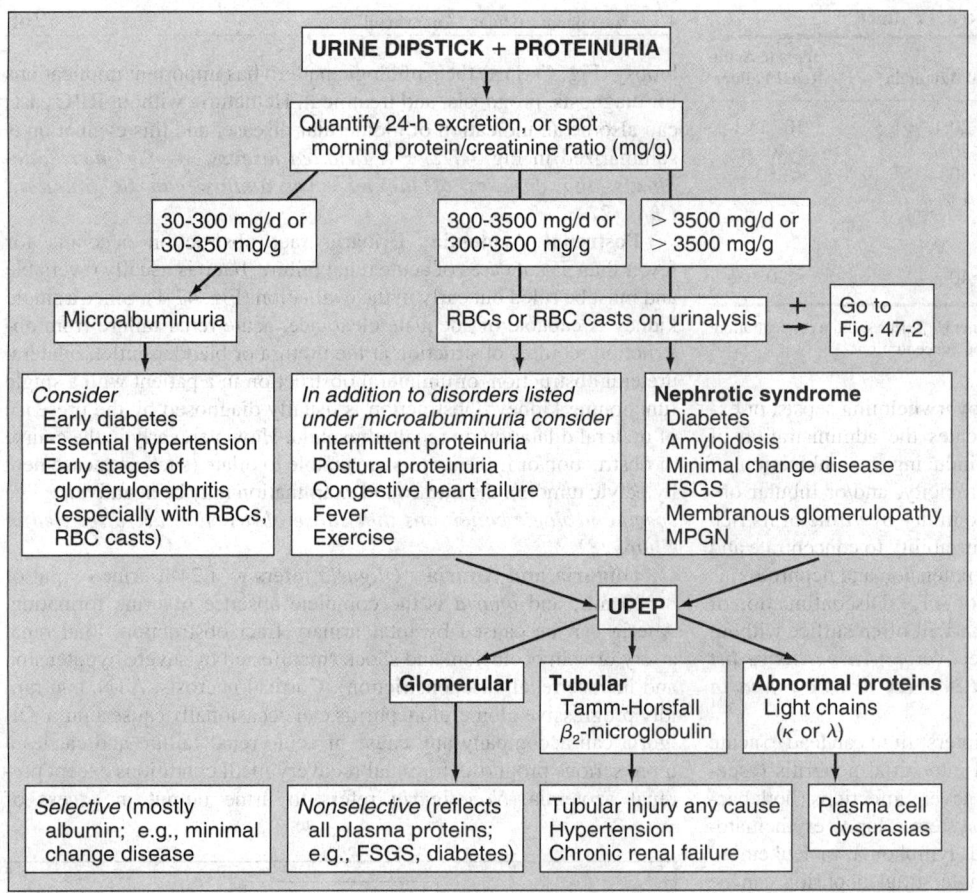

FIGURE 47-3 Approach to the patient with proteinuria. Investigation of proteinuria is often initiated by a positive dipstick on routine urinalysis. Conventional dipsticks detect predominantly albumin and cannot detect urinary albumin levels of 30 to 300 mg/d. However, more exact determination of proteinuria should employ a 24-h urine collection or a spot morning protein/creatinine ration (mg/g). The pattern of proteinuria on UPEP (urine protein electrophoresis) can be classified as "glomerular," "tubular," or "abnormal" depending upon the origin of the urine proteins. Glomerular proteinuria is due to abnormal glomerular permeability. "Tubular proteins" such as Tamm-Horsfall are normally produced by the renal tubule and shed into the urine. Abnormal circulating proteins such as kappa or lambda light chains are readily filtered because of their small size. (RBC, red blood cell; FSGS, focal segmental glomerulosclerosis; MPGN, membranoproliferative glomerulonephritis.)

---

500 mL/day in patients with acute or chronic azotemia. With nonoliguric ATN, disturbances of potassium and hydrogen balance are less severe than in oliguric patients and recovery to normal renal function is usually more rapid.

ABNORMALITIES OF THE URINE

PROTEINURIA The evaluation of proteinuria is shown schematically in Fig. 47-3 and is typically initiated after colorimetric detection of proteinuria by dipstick examination. Current methods for measuring proteinuria vary significantly. The dipstick measurement detects mostly albumin and gives false-positive results when pH > 7.0 and the urine is very concentrated or contaminated with blood. A very dilute urine may obscure significant proteinuria on dipstick examination, and proteinuria that is not predominantly albumin will be missed. This is particularly important for the detection of Bence Jones proteins in the urine of patients with multiple myeloma. Tests to measure total urine concentration accurately rely on precipitation with sulfosalicylic or trichloracetic acids. Currently, ultrasensitive dipsticks are available to measure microalbuminuria (30 to 300 mg/d), an early marker of glomerular disease that has been shown to predict glomerular injury in early diabetic nephropathy (Fig. 47-3).

The magnitude of proteinuria and the protein composition in the urine depend upon the mechanism of renal injury leading to protein losses. Large amounts of plasma proteins normally course through the glomerular capillaries but do not enter the urinary space. Both charge and size selectivity prevent virtually all of albumin, globulin, and other large-molecular-weight proteins from crossing the glomerular wall. However, if this barrier is disrupted, there can be leakage of plasma proteins into the urine (glomerular proteinuria; Fig. 47-3). Smaller proteins (<20 kDa) are freely filtered but are readily reabsorbed by the proximal tubule. Normal individuals excrete less than 150 mg/d of total protein and only about 30 mg/d of albumin. The remainder of the protein in the urine is secreted by the tubules (Tamm-Horsfall, IgA, and urokinase) or represents small amounts of filtered β_2-microglobulin, apoproteins, enzymes, and peptide hormones. Another mechanism of proteinuria occurs when there is excessive production of an abnormal protein that exceeds the capacity of the tubule for reabsorption. This most commonly occurs with plasma cell dyscrasias such as multiple myeloma and lymphomas that are associated with monoclonal production of immunoglobulin light chains.

The normal glomerular endothelial cell forms a barrier penetrated by pores of about 100 nm that holds back cells and other particles but offers little impediment to passage of most proteins. The glomerular basement membrane traps most large proteins (>100 kDa), while the foot processes of epithelial cells (podocytes) cover the urinary side of the glomerular basement membrane and produce a series of narrow channels (slit diaphragms) to allow molecular passage of small solutes and water (Fig. 47-4). The channels are coated with anionic glycoproteins that are rich in glutamate, aspartate, and sialic acid, which are negatively charged at physiologic pH. This negatively charged barrier impedes the passage of anionic molecules such as albumin. Some glomerular diseases, such as minimal change disease, cause fusion of glomerular epithelial cell foot processes, resulting in predominantly "selective" (Fig. 47-3) loss of albumin. Other glomerular diseases can present with disruption of the basement membrane and slit diaphragms (e.g., by immune complex deposition), resulting in large amounts of protein losses that include albumin and other plasma proteins. The fusion of foot processes causes increased pressure across the capillary basement membrane, resulting in areas with larger pore sizes. The combination of increased pressure and larger pores results in significant proteinuria ("nonselective"; Fig. 47-3).

When the total daily excretion of protein exceeds 3.5 g, there is often associated hypoalbuminemia, hyperlipidemia, and edema (nephrotic syndrome; Table 47-1). However, total daily urinary protein excretion greater than 3.5 g can occur without the other features of the nephrotic syndrome in a variety of other renal diseases (Fig. 47-3). Plasma cell dyscrasias (multiple myeloma) can be associated with large amounts of excreted light chains in the urine, which may not be detected by dipstick (which detects mostly albumin). The light chains produced from these disorders are filtered by the glomerulus and overwhelm the reabsorptive capacity of the proximal tubule. A sulfosalicylic acid precipitate that is out of proportion to the dipstick estimate is suggestive of light chains (Bence Jones protein), and light chains typically redissolve upon warming of the precipitate. Renal failure

Urinary Space

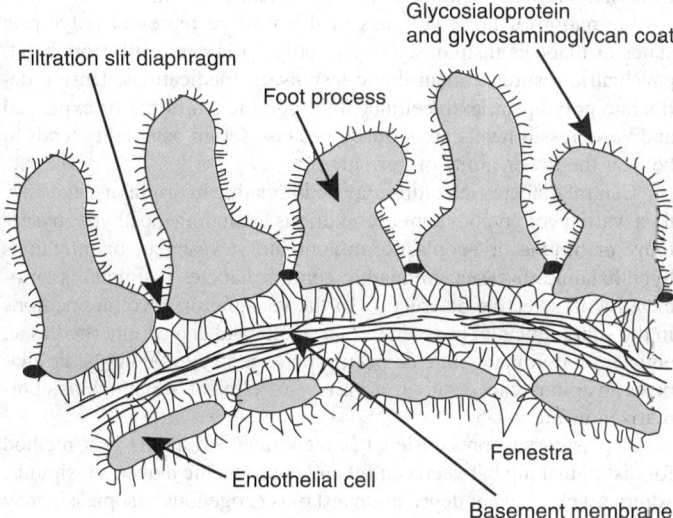

Capillary Lumen

FIGURE 47-4 Diagram showing normal structures separating the capillary lumen and urinary space in the glomerulus. In the process of glomerular filtration, an ultrafiltrate of plasma traverses the capillary wall through endothelial fenestrae, basement membrane, and filtration slit diaphragms (now known to contain the protein nephrin). Proteins are restricted from access to the urinary space by the filtration slit diaphragm and by negatively charged glycosialoproteins and glycosaminoglycans, which coat the glomerular epithelial cell foot processes as well as glomerular endothelial cells lining the capillary lumen.

from these disorders occurs through a variety of mechanisms including tubule obstruction (cast nephropathy) and light chain deposition (Chap. 275).

Hypoalbuminemia in nephrotic syndrome occurs through excessive urinary losses, increased renal catabolism, and inadequate hepatic synthesis. The resulting decrease in plasma oncotic pressure contributes to edema formation by altering the Starling forces and favoring fluid movement from capillaries to interstitium. The resulting homeostatic mechanisms designed to correct the decrease in effective intravascular volume contribute to edema formation in some patients. These mechanisms include activation of the renin-angiotensin system, antidiuretic hormone, and the sympathetic nervous system, which contribute to excessive renal salt and water reabsorption and can contribute to unrelenting edema.

The severity of edema correlates with the degree of hypoalbuminemia and is modified by other factors such as heart disease or peripheral vascular disease. The diminished plasma oncotic pressure and urinary losses of regulatory proteins appear to stimulate hepatic lipoprotein synthesis. The resulting hyperlipidemia results in lipid bodies (fatty casts, oval fat bodies) in the urine. Other proteins are lost in the urine, leading to a variety of metabolic disturbances. These include thyroxine-binding globulin, cholecalciferol-binding protein, transferrin, and metal-binding proteins. A hypercoagulable state frequently accompanies severe nephrotic syndrome due to urinary losses of antithrombin III, reduced serum levels of proteins S and C, hyperfibrinogenemia, and enhanced platelet aggregation. Some patients develop severe IgG deficiency with resulting defects in immunity. Many diseases (some listed in Fig. 47-3) and drugs can cause the nephrotic syndrome, and a complete list can be found in Chap. 274.

HEMATURIA, PYURIA, AND CASTS Isolated hematuria without proteinuria, other cells, or casts is often indicative of bleeding from the urinary tract. Normal red blood cell excretion is up to 2 million RBCs per day. Hematuria is defined as two to five RBCs per high-power field (HPF) and can be detected by dipstick. Common causes of isolated hematuria include stones, neoplasms, tuberculosis, trauma, and prostatitis. Gross hematuria with blood clots is almost never indicative of glomerular bleeding; rather, it suggests a postrenal

source in the urinary collecting system. Evaluation of patients presenting with microscopic hematuria is outlined in Fig. 47-2. A single urinalysis with hematuria is common and can result from menstruation, viral illness, allergy, exercise, or mild trauma. Annual urinalysis of servicemen over a 10-year period showed an incidence of 38%. However, persistent or significant hematuria (>three RBCs/HPF on three urinalyses, or single urinalysis with >100 RBCs, or gross hematuria) identified significant renal or urologic lesions in 9.1% of over 1000 patients. Even patients who are chronically anticoagulated should be investigated as outlined in Fig. 47-2. The suspicion for urogenital neoplasms in patients with isolated painless hematuria (nondysmorphic RBCs) increases with age. Neoplasms are rare in the pediatric population, and isolated hematuria is more likely to be "idiopathic" or associated with a congenital anomaly. Hematuria with pyuria and bacteriuria is typical of infection and should be treated with antibiotics after appropriate cultures. Acute cystitis or urethritis in women can cause gross hematuria. Hypercalciuria and hyperuricosuria are also risk factors for unexplained isolated hematuria in both children and adults. In some of these patients (50 to 60%), reducing calcium and uric acid excretion through dietary interventions can eliminate the microscopic hematuria.

Isolated microscopic hematuria can be a manifestation of glomerular diseases. The RBCs of glomerular origin are often dysmorphic when examined by phase-contrast microscopy. Irregular shapes of RBCs may also occur due to pH and osmolarity changes found in the distal tubule. There is, however, significant observer variability in detecting dysmorphic RBCs, especially if a phase-contrast microscope is not available. The most common etiologies of isolated glomerular hematuria are IgA nephropathy, hereditary nephritis, and thin basement membrane disease. IgA nephropathy and hereditary nephritis can have episodic gross hematuria. A family history of renal failure is often present in patients with hereditary nephritis, and patients with thin basement membrane disease often have other family members with microscopic hematuria. A renal biopsy is needed for the definitive diagnosis of these disorders, which are discussed in more detail in Chap. 275. Hematuria with dysmorphic RBCs, RBC casts, and protein excretion >500 mg/d is virtually diagnostic of glomerulonephritis. RBC casts form as RBCs that enter the tubular fluid become trapped in a cylindrical mold of gelled Tamm-Horsfall protein. Even in the absence of azotemia, these patients should undergo serologic evaluation and renal biopsy as outlined in Fig. 47-2.

Isolated pyuria is unusual since inflammatory reactions in the kidney or collecting system are also associated with hematuria. The presence of bacteria suggests infection, and white blood cell casts with bacteria are indicative of pyelonephritis. White blood cells and/or white blood cell casts may also be seen in tubulointerstitial processes such as interstitial nephritis, systemic lupus erythematosus, and transplant rejection. In chronic renal diseases, degenerated cellular casts called *waxy casts* can be seen in the urine. *Broad casts* are thought to arise in the dilated tubules of enlarged nephrons that have undergone compensatory hypertrophy in response to reduced renal mass (i.e., chronic renal failure). A mixture of broad casts typically seen with chronic renal failure together with cellular casts and RBCs may be seen in smoldering processes such as chronic glomerulonephritis with active glomerulitis.

ABNORMALITIES OF URINE VOLUME

The volume of urine produced varies depending upon the fluid intake, renal function, and physiologic demands of the individual. See "Azotemia," above, for discussion of decreased (oliguria) or absent urine production (anuria). →*The physiology of water formation and renal water conservation are discussed in Chap. 268.*

POLYURIA By history, it is often difficult for patients to distinguish urinary frequency (often of small volumes) from polyuria, and a 24-h urine collection is needed for evaluation (Fig. 47-5). It is

FIGURE 47-5 Approach to the patient with polyuria. (Osm, osmolality; ATN, acute tubular necrosis.)

necessary to determine if the polyuria represents a solute or water diuresis and if the diuresis is appropriate for the clinical circumstances. The average person excretes between 600 and 800 mosmol of solutes per day, primarily as urea and electrolytes. The urine osmolality can help distinguish a solute from water diuresis. If the urine output is >3 L/d (arbitrarily defined as polyuria) and the urine is dilute (<250 mosmol/L), then total mosmol excretion is normal and a water diuresis is present. This circumstance could arise from polydipsia, inadequate secretion of vasopressin (central diabetes insipidus), or failure of renal tubules to respond to vasopressin (nephrogenic diabetes insipidus). If the urine volume is >3 L/d and urine osmolality is >300 mosmol/L, then a solute diuresis is clearly present and a search for the responsible solute(s) is mandatory.

Excessive filtration of a poorly reabsorbed solute such as glucose, mannitol, or urea can depress reabsorption of NaCl and water in the proximal tubule and lead to enhanced excretion in the urine. Poorly controlled diabetes mellitus is the most common cause of a solute diuresis, leading to volume depletion and serum hypertonicity. Since the urine Na concentration is less than that of blood, more water than Na is lost, causing hypernatremia and hypertonicity. Common iatrogenic solute diuresis occurs from mannitol administration, radiocontrast media, and high-protein feedings (enterally or parenterally), leading to increased urea production and excretion. Less commonly, excessive Na loss may occur from cystic renal diseases, Bartter's syndrome, or during the course of a tubulointerstitial process (such as resolving ATN). In these so-called salt-wasting disorders, the tubule damage results in direct impairment of Na reabsorption and indirectly reduces the responsiveness of the tubule to aldosterone. Usually, the Na losses are mild, and the obligatory urine output is less than 2 L/d

(resolving ATN and postobstructive diuresis are exceptions and may be associated with significant natriuresis and polyuria.)

Formation of large volumes of dilute urine represent polydipsic states or diabetes insipidus. Primary polydipsia can result from habit, psychiatric disorders, neurologic lesions, or medications. During deliberate polydipsia, extracellular fluid volume is normal or expanded and vasopressin levels are reduced because serum osmolality tends to be near the lower limits of normal.

Central diabetes insipidus may be idiopathic in origin or secondary to a variety of hypothalamic conditions including posthypophysectomy or trauma or neoplastic, inflammatory, vascular, or infectious hypothalamic diseases. Idiopathic central diabetes insipidus is associated with selective destruction of the vasopressin-secreting neurons in the supraoptic and paraventricular nuclei and can be inherited as an autosomal dominant trait or occur spontaneously. Nephrogenic diabetes insipidus can occur in a variety of clinical situations as summarized in Fig. 47-5.

A plasma vasopressin level is recommended as the best method for distinguishing between central and nephrogenic diabetes insipidus. Alternatively, a water deprivation test plus exogenous vasopressin may also distinguish primary polydipsia from central and nephrogenic diabetes insipidus. →*For a detailed discussion, see Chap. 329.*

BIBLIOGRAPHY

ANDERSON S et al: Renal and systemic manifestations of glomerular disease, in *Brenner & Rector's The Kidney*, 6th ed, BM Brenner (ed). Philadelphia, Saunders, 2000, pp 1871–1900.

BERL T, ROBERTSON GL: Pathophysiology of water metabolism, in *Brenner & Rector's The Kidney*, 6th ed, BM Brenner (ed). Philadelphia, Saunders, 2000, pp 66–924

BICHET DG: Nephrogenic diabetes insipidus. Am J Med 105(5):431, 1998

GROSSFELD GD, CARROLL PR: Evaluation of asymptomatic microscopic hematuria. Urol Clin North Am 25(4):661, 1998

KASISKE BL, KEANE WF: Laboratory assessment of renal disease: Clearance, urinalysis and renal biopsy, in *Brenner & Rector's The Kidney*, 6th ed, BM Brenner (ed). Philadelphia, Saunders, 2000, pp 129–1170

KESTILA M et al: Positively cloned gene for a novel glomerular protein—nephrin—is mutated in congenital nephrotic syndrome. Mol Cell 1(4):575, 1998

MARIANI AJ et al: The significance of adult hematuria: 1000 hematuria evaluations including a risk-benefit and cost-effectiveness analysis. J Urol 141:350, 1989

NOLAN CR, ANDERSON RJ: Hospital-acquired acute renal failure. J Am Soc Nephrol 9: 710, 1998

48

Philippe E. Zimmern, John D. McConnell

INCONTINENCE AND LOWER URINARY TRACT SYMPTOMS

PHYSIOLOGY OF VOIDING

Normal bladder filling depends on unique elastic properties of the bladder wall that allow it to increase in volume at a pressure lower than that of the bladder neck and urethra (otherwise incontinence would occur). Despite provocative maneuvers such as coughing, voluntary bladder contractions do not occur. Emptying is dependent on the integrity of a complex neuromuscular network that causes relaxation of the urethral sphincter a few milliseconds before the onset of the detrusor (bladder muscle) contraction. With normal, sustained detrusor contraction, the bladder empties completely. A bladder that can fill and empty in this manner has a normal detrusor muscle and is described as *stable* according to conventional terminology.

Since the voluntary control of micturition depends on the neural connections between the cerebral cortex and the brainstem, disruption of these pathways (brain tumor, stroke, head trauma, Parkinson's disease) impairs the ability to suppress and control bladder contractions.

A bladder contraction without voluntary effort characterizes an unstable bladder. Bladder or detrusor instability of neurologic origin is termed *detrusor hyperreflexia*. Conversely, the detrusor muscle that cannot contract during voiding is called *noncontractile*; underactivity of the detrusor due to a lesion of the sacral cord or pelvic nerves is termed *detrusor areflexia*.

Contrary to common belief, the center that controls normal micturition is not in the spinal cord but in the brainstem. Proper coordination (*synergia*) between the detrusor and urethral sphincters requires an intact neural (autonomic and somatic nervous systems) communication between bladder and urethra. Injury to the upper spinal cord, for example, can cause dyssynergia between bladder and urethra that results in urge incontinence, residual urine retention, bladder wall changes (trabeculation and fibrosis), and possibly renal insufficiency.

A simple way to classify voiding dysfunction is to determine whether it is primarily a *storage failure* or an *emptying failure* by asking two questions:

Is the voiding dysfunction due to the bladder or outlet (bladder neck or urethra) (failure to store)?
Is there neurologic dysfunction (failure to empty)?

Bladder storage and emptying problems may coexist in the same individual and can cause similar lower urinary tract symptoms (LUTS).

LOWER URINARY TRACT SYMPTOMS IN MEN The most common cause of LUTS in men of middle age and older is prostatic hyperplasia, which causes obstruction to urine flow by encroachment on the urethral lumen (Chap. 95). Histologically, 50 to 80% of the prostatic volume is composed of stromal tissue (smooth muscle), while the remainder is glandular. The transitional zone, which is responsible for benign prostatic growth, comprises 10 to 15% of the prostate at the end of puberty but increases in volume after age 40. However, prostatic enlargement is not always accompanied by symptoms because the direction of growth can be outward, so that little change may occur in urine flow. Alternatively, men with early histologic evidence of prostatic hyperplasia can experience significant voiding symptoms. In this circumstance, increased tone of the prostatic smooth muscle and enhanced prostatic tension within a nondistensible capsule can cause obstruction.

In response to obstruction, the bladder smooth-muscle cells hypertrophy to generate the higher pressures necessary for voiding, and the increase in bladder muscle mass leads to reduced elasticity, or compliance, and decreased bladder capacity. Detrusor dysfunction from bladder outlet obstruction can cause any combination of the LUTS described above. When the obstruction progresses, infiltration of extracellular matrix between the smooth-muscle bundles of the bladder wall can result in a hypocontractile or acontractile bladder (bladder failure).

Other complications such as urinary tract infections or bladder stones secondary to the large postvoid residuals (stasis) and upper tract damage (hydronephrosis, reflux) can develop during the course of the obstructive process. Although prostatic hyperplasia is the most common cause of bladder outlet obstruction in men, other sources of obstruction include prostate cancer, urethral stricture, and lack of proper sphincteric relaxation (neurologic cause). Nonobstructive causes of LUTS include diabetic neuropathy, which can affect the parasympathetic nerves of the bladder. Decreased sensation of bladder fullness leads to incomplete emptying and overdistention of the bladder and, in turn, to increased frequency and nocturia due to bladder overflow; these symptoms are frequently made worse by the polydipsia/polyuria of diabetes mellitus. At times, storage symptoms can be caused by other neurologic causes such as stroke, multiple sclerosis, or Parkinson's disease.

The International Prostate Symptom Score (IPSS) is used to assess the severity of LUTS:

Decreased force of stream—over the past month how often have you had a weak urinary stream?

Intermittency—over the past month how often have you found you stopped and started again several times when urinating?
Incomplete emptying—over the past month how often have you had a sensation of not emptying your bladder completely after finishing urination?
Straining—over the past month how often have you had to push or strain to begin urination?

The IPSS also assesses the impact of storage symptoms:

Frequency—over the past month how often have you had to urinate again within 2 h after urinating?
Urgency—over the past month how often have you found it difficult to postpone urination?
Nocturia—over the past month how many times did you typically get up to urinate between going to bed and getting up in the morning? (Range: none to five or more times.)

Except for nocturia, the answers range from 0 (not at all) to 5 (almost always). A total score of <8 indicates minimal voiding dysfunction; a total score of ≥13 is usually required to enroll patients in drug studies for the management of benign prostatic hyperplasia (BPH); and symptom scores >23 suggest significant bladder outlet obstruction. Because similar symptoms can result from neurologic causes, the IPSS questionnaire cannot be used to make the diagnosis of prostatic hyperplasia but is useful only as an index of severity and of the response to treatment.

LOWER URINARY TRACT SYMPTOMS IN WOMEN Urethral obstruction is an uncommon cause of LUTS in women. A careful bimanual examination and passage of a urethral catheter are sufficient to exclude urethral stenosis, which is usually secondary to prior instrumentation or operative procedures, and urethral cancer. Urinary tract infection (cystitis) is more prevalent in women and must be excluded by urinalysis. Multiple sclerosis should be considered in middle-aged women presenting with frequency, urgency, or incontinence. In addition to many of the same disorders that produce voiding symptoms in men, estrogen deficiency, frequency-urgency syndrome, and interstitial cystitis (IC) with minimal pain must be considered. Cystocele and pelvic prolapse can cause urinary frequency secondary to impairment of bladder emptying.

EVALUATION Men and women with LUTS and concomitant neurologic disease should undergo a complete urodynamic evaluation. In the absence of neurologic disease, men with LUTS most commonly have prostatic hyperplasia. However, it is necessary to exclude prostate cancer, especially if there is a positive family history, an abnormal prostate examination, or an elevated level of prostate-specific antigen (PSA). In both sexes bladder cancer can also cause storage symptoms and is suggested by microscopic hematuria and/or abnormal urine cytology. Usually, a detailed genitourinary history, a symptom assessment, a careful neurologic examination including rectal examination and assessment of the bulbocavernosus reflex, measurements of urine flow and postvoid residual urine volume (by bladder ultrasound), and limited laboratory evaluation (urinalysis, urine culture, PSA levels, urine cytology, urea/creatinine levels, as indicated) should be sufficient to direct therapy. More complex investigations of the lower urinary tract (cystoscopy, voiding cystography, urodynamics) and upper urinary tract (pyelogram or ultrasonography) are sometimes indicated. →*For therapy of BPH, see Chap. 95.*

INCONTINENCE

Incontinence is a condition where involuntary loss of urine is objectively demonstrated and is a social or hygienic problem. A common variant, *stress incontinence*, denotes involuntary loss of urine with physical exercise (coughing, sneezing, sports, sexual activity). *Urge incontinence* is an involuntary loss of urine associated with a strong desire to void, and *overflow incontinence* is an involuntary loss of urine when the elevation of intravesical pressure with bladder overfilling or distention exceeds the maximal urethral pressure. Loss of urine through channels other than the urethra is rare (ectopic ureter, fistulae) but causes total or continuous incontinence.

INCONTINENCE IN WOMEN   Among noninstitutionalized women 60 years of age and older, 25 to 30% have urinary incontinence daily or weekly, and approximately half of institutionalized women are incontinent more than once a day. The annual cost of caring for incontinent persons is very high and, if not well managed, can be associated with complications such as decubitus ulcers.

Stress urinary incontinence (SUI) is secondary to urethral hypermobility or, less commonly (<10%), to intrinsic sphincteric deficiency (ISD). In the continent woman the bladder neck and proximal urethra are supported by the anterior vaginal wall and its lateral attachment to the levator muscles. Anterior vaginal wall relaxation causes urethral hypermobility, usually due to aging and/or estrogen deficiency or a prior traumatic delivery or pelvic surgery. Paradoxically, women can have clinical evidence of urethral hypermobility but no stress urinary incontinence.

Some women have an anatomically normal urethra and bladder neck but still have SUI due to damage to the internal sphincter (fixed, rigid, or "pipestem" urethra), due to prior anti-incontinence surgery, pelvic radiation or trauma, or neurologic disorders that cause denervation of the urethra. Urethral hypermobility and ISD can coexist in some patients and cause persistence (or rapid recurrence) of incontinence after a simple bladder neck suspension procedure that fixes the hypermobility but leaves the sphincter untreated.

Urge incontinence can be present alone or in association with SUI (mixed incontinence). The cause of the unsuppressible or uninhibited bladder contractions is usually idiopathic, but bacterial cystitis, bladder tumor, bladder outlet obstruction, and neurogenic bladder must be excluded. Overflow incontinence is due either to bladder outlet obstruction (rare in women), an acontractile bladder (diabetic neuropathy, multiple sclerosis), excessive smooth-muscle relaxation from drugs (anticholinergic medications), or psychogenic retention.

INCONTINENCE IN MEN   In men incontinence is less common than obstruction, but urgency and urge incontinence can occur as the result of bladder outlet obstruction (as from prostatic hyperplasia) that impairs detrusor smooth-muscle function and leads to detrusor instability. Men with neurogenic bladders (diabetic neuropathy, multiple sclerosis, Parkinson's disease, stroke) can develop urge incontinence. Other causes such as bacterial cystitis or bladder tumor must be excluded. SUI in men is usually the result of distal sphincteric damage, for example, as the result of radical prostatectomy for prostate cancer.

INCONTINENCE IN THE ELDERLY   Transient urinary incontinence is common in the elderly. A mnemonic devised by Resnick delineates its numerous causes, namely *d*elirium, *i*nfection, *a*trophic urethritis, *p*harmacologic, *p*sychological, *e*xcessive urine output (hyperglycemia, congestive heart failure), *r*estricted mobility, and *s*tool impaction (DIAPPERS). Urge incontinence is the next most common disorder in this age group and is attributed to the progressive loss of the modulating influence of the frontal lobes of the cortex on the micturition center in the brainstem.

EVALUATION   The evaluation of urinary incontinence in women should include history and quality-of-life assessment, voiding diary, physical examination including pelvic examination, urinalysis and urine culture, and measurement of postvoid residual urine volume. For patients with an unclear history or after prior pelvic or anti-incontinence procedures, evaluation may include cystoscopy, urodynamic evaluation, and imaging studies (lower and/or upper urinary tract). The history should define the onset, duration, evolution, and triggering events of leakage. Prior treatments with medications, frequent voiding schedules, and exercise regimens should be noted. Severity of incontinence is denoted by recording the type and number of pads used per day or at night and how the incontinence affects daily activities (incontinence-impact questionnaire). The amount and type of fluid consumed, sexual history (hormonal status, deliveries, venereal diseases), gastrointestinal function (fecal incontinence, constipation), and past urologic history (bed-wetting, surgeries) must also be documented. The physical examination should place special emphasis on the abdominal, genital, pelvic (associated prolapses), and neurologic systems. SUI must be demonstrated by asking the patient to cough, strain, or even stand or squat. While leakage during a cough confirms SUI, leakage after a cough is due to bladder instability (stress-induced instability). SUI in the absence of urethral hypermobility raises the suspicion of a sphincteric defect. More complex testing is needed to determine whether the urethral anatomy is normal (evaluation of urethral mobility, lateral view of the urethra on the voiding cystourethrogram, cystoscopy), whether urethral function is normal with adequate closure (leak point pressure, urethral profilometry, videourodynamics), or whether bladder function is normal (bladder volume based on home diary, filling cystometrogram).

TREATMENT   Mild stress incontinence can be treated nonoperatively with medications, estrogen replacement, or biofeedback techniques. Modalities such as urethral plugs and anterior vaginal wall prostheses are under investigation. Moderate to severe stress incontinence responds to surgical procedures aimed at supporting the anterior vaginal wall (vaginal, laparoscopic, or abdominal operations) or enhancing urethral closure when stress incontinence is secondary to internal sphincter deficiency (periurethral injection of fat or collagen, autologous or cadaveric fascial sling, synthetic sling, or insertion of an artificial urinary sphincter).

Urge incontinence responds to the management of its cause. When it is due to neurogenic or idiopathic causes, anticholinergic agents are partially effective, although side effects such as mouth dryness, blurring of vision, or constipation can limit their usefulness. Better tolerated medications are now available including slow-release oxybutinin (Ditropan XL), which is administered as 5- to 10-mg tablets once daily, and the more specific antimuscarinic agent, tolterodine (Detrol), which is usually given as 2 mg orally twice daily. Fluid restriction (which must be undertaken only with great caution) and bladder retraining with biofeedback may also be helpful. More aggressive intervention with bladder augmentation or urinary diversion are seldom necessary in the absence of neurologic disease.

BLADDER PAIN

Painful bladder disease is a general term for any bladder pathology that causes suprapubic, urethral, or pelvic pain. IC is the most common cause of bladder pain, but endometriosis, bacterial cystitis, and outlet obstruction that causes bladder instability can mimic the symptoms of IC.

INTERSTITIAL CYSTITIS   IC is a severe, chronic bladder disorder that causes frequency, nocturia, and suprapubic pain. The disorder usually affects women and is rare in blacks. Routine urine culture is uniformly negative, and the symptoms do not respond to antibiotic therapy. The etiology is probably multifactorial (Table 48-1). Current hypotheses as to etiology include autoimmune reaction against bladder antigens, deficiency in the glycosaminoglycan layer of the bladder surface allowing presumed toxins to penetrate the mucosa, mast cell infiltration and activation leading to the histamine release, and local bladder wall damage from bacteria.

The National Institutes of Health has established a series of criteria to define IC clinically (Table 48-2). The diagnosis is one of exclusion—infection, radiation cystitis, urethral diverticula, herpes simplex, and malignancy must be excluded. Cystoscopy under anesthesia may be used for the following: (1) reveal glomerulations (submucosal vascular anomalies) or the infrequent Hunner's ulcer suggestive of IC; (2) make it possible to estimate bladder capacity (an important guide to treatment); (3) allow biopsy of the bladder wall when indicated; and (4) by bladder filling, sometimes provide therapeutic benefit with a

Table 48-1 Consensus Criteria for Diagnosis of Interstitial Cystitis

Automatic Exclusions
  Less than 18 years old
  Benign or malignant bladder tumors
  Radiation cystitis
  Bacterial cystitis
  Vaginitis
  Cyclophosphamide cystitis
  Symptomatic urethral diverticulum
  Uterine, cervical, vaginal, or urethral cancers
  Active herpes
  Bladder or lower urethral calculi
  Waking frequency less than five times in 12 h
  Nocturia less than twice nightly
  Symptoms relieved by antibiotics, urinary antiseptics, urinary analgesics
    (e.g., phenazopyridine hydrochloride)
  Duration less than 12 months
  Involuntary bladder contractions (urodynamics)
  Capacity greater than 400 mL, absence of sensory urgency
Automatic Inclusions
  Hunner's ulcer
Positive Factors
  Pain on bladder filling relieved by emptying
  Pain (suprapubic, pelvic, urethral, vaginal, or perineal)
  Glomerulations after hydrodistention on cystoscopy

Table 48-2 Possible Causes of Interstitial Cystitis

Infection	Allergic/immune/autoimmune
Fastidious bacteria	causes
Latent viruses	Neurogenic disturbances
Dysfunctional bladder epithelium	Bladder mastocytosis
Defective glycosaminoglycan layer	Psychosomatic
Abnormal intercellular junctions	Others
Toxic substances in urine	Food intolerance
	Endocrine causes

reduction in pain level and urinary frequency up to 6 months or rarely longer.

EVALUATION Chronic urinary frequency and bladder pain affect the quality of life to an extreme degree, though most patients experience a waxing and waning evolution; only 10% of patients have a consistent progression in symptoms. Evaluation should include a detailed history; physical examination designed to exclude neurologic and gynecologic pathology; voiding cystogram to exclude urethral defects; and urodynamic testing to eliminate a neurogenic bladder, bladder instability, or outlet obstruction and to document sensory instability. Referral to specialists may be indicated to exclude adnexal pathology, endometriosis, or bowel dysfunction or to utilize modern pain management techniques to prevent drug addiction.

[Rx] **TREATMENT** Empirical treatments that have been used include oral medications (amitriptyline, hydroxyzine, pentosanpolysulfate) and intravesical agents (dimethyl sulfoxide, chlorpactin, heparin). These measures may improve the urinary symptoms and occasionally reduce pain but do not modify the long-term course. Surgical intervention (augmentation cystoplasty, urinary diversion) is indicated in fewer than 5% of cases because this is a non-life-threatening, chronic disease with occasional spontaneous remissions. "Last-resort" interventions such as removal of the bladder and urethra are not a guarantee of success because some patients continue to experience pelvic pain afterwards.

BIBLIOGRAPHY

BARRY MJ et al: The American Urological Association symptom index for benign prostatic hyperplasia. The measurement committee of the American Urological Association. J Urol 148:1549, 1992

CHAI TB, STEERS WD: Neurophysiology of micturition and continence. Urol Clin North Am 23:221, 1996

DUPONT MC et al: Diagnosis of stress urinary incontinence. An overview. Urol Clin North Am 23:407, 1996

HAAB F et al: Female stress urinary incontinence due to intrinsic sphincteric deficiency: Recognition and management. J Urol 156:3, 1996

HOLTGREWE HL The evaluation and management of the adult male with lower urinary tract symptoms. Urology 51(Suppl):1, 1998

LEACH GE et al: Female stress urinary incontinence: Clinical Guidelines Panel summary report on surgical management of female stress urinary incontinence. J Urol 158:875, 1997

RESNICK N: Geriatric incontinence. Urol Clin North Am 23:55, 1996

SIMON LJ et al: The Interstitial Cystitis Data Base Study: Concepts and preliminary baseline descriptive statistics. Urology 49(Suppl 5A):64, 1997

WALSH PC et al (eds): *Campbell's Urology*, 7th ed. Philadelphia, Saunders, 1998

49	*Gary G. Singer, Barry M. Brenner*

FLUID AND ELECTROLYTE DISTURBANCES

ACE	angiotensin-converting enzyme	NSAIDs	nonsteroidal anti-inflammatory drugs
AVP	arginine vasopressin		
BUN	blood urea nitrogen	ODS	osmotic demyelination syndrome
CCD	cortical collecting duct		
CDI	central diabetes insipidus	RBCs	red blood cells
ECF	extracellular fluid	RTA	renal tubular acidosis
GFR	glomerular filtration rate	SIADH	syndrome of inappropriate antidiuretic hormone secretion
11β-HSDH	11β-hydroxysteroid dehydrogenase		
		TEPD	transepithelial potential difference
ICF	intracellular fluid		
MCD	medullary collecting duct	TTKG	transtubular K$^+$ concentration gradient
NDI	nephrogenic diabetes insipidus		

SODIUM AND WATER

COMPOSITION OF BODY FLUIDS Water is the most abundant constituent in the body, comprising approximately 50% of body weight in women and 60% in men. This difference is attributable to differences in the relative proportions of adipose tissue in men and women. Total body water is distributed in two major compartments—55 to 75% is intracellular [intracellular fluid (ICF)], and 25 to 45% is extracellular [extracellular fluid (ECF)]. The ECF is further subdivided into intravascular (plasma water) and extravascular (interstitial) spaces in a ratio of 1:3.

The solute or particle concentration of a fluid is known as its *osmolality* and is expressed as milliosmoles per kilogram of water (mosmol/kg). Water crosses cell membranes to achieve osmotic equilibrium (ECF osmolality = ICF osmolality). The extracellular and intracellular solutes or osmoles are markedly different due to disparities in permeability and the presence of transporters and active pumps. The major ECF particles are Na$^+$ and its accompanying anions Cl$^-$ and HCO$_3^-$, whereas K$^+$ and organic phosphate esters (ATP, creatine phosphate, and phospholipids) are the predominant ICF osmoles. Solutes that are restricted to the ECF or the ICF determine the *effective osmolality* (or *tonicity*) of that compartment. Since Na$^+$ is largely restricted to the extracellular compartment, total body Na$^+$ content is a reflection of ECF volume. Likewise, K$^+$ and its attendant anions are predominantly limited to the ICF and are necessary for normal cell function. Therefore, the number of intracellular particles is relatively constant, and a change in ICF osmolality is usually due to a change in ICF water content. However, in certain situations, brain cells can vary the number of intracellular solutes in order to defend against large water shifts. This process of *osmotic adaptation* is important in the defense of cell volume and occurs in chronic hyponatremia and hypernatremia. This response is mediated initially by transcellular shifts of K$^+$ and Na$^+$, followed by synthesis, import, or export of organic solutes (so-called osmolytes) such as inositol, betaine, and glutamine.

During chronic hyponatremia, brain cells lose solutes, thereby defending cell volume and diminishing neurologic symptoms. The converse occurs during chronic hypernatremia. Certain solutes, such as urea, do not contribute to water shift across cell membranes and are known as *ineffective osmoles*.

Fluid movement between the intravascular and interstitial spaces occurs across the capillary wall and is determined by the Starling forces—capillary hydraulic pressure and colloid osmotic pressure. The transcapillary hydraulic pressure gradient exceeds the corresponding oncotic pressure gradient, thereby favoring the movement of plasma ultrafiltrate into the extravascular space. The return of fluid into the intravascular compartment occurs via lymphatic flow.

WATER BALANCE (See also Chap. 268)   The normal plasma osmolality is 275 to 290 mosmol/kg and is kept within a narrow range by mechanisms capable of sensing a 1 to 2% change in tonicity. To maintain a steady state, water intake must equal water excretion. Disorders of water homeostasis result in hypo- or hypernatremia. Normal individuals have an obligate water loss consisting of urine, stool, and evaporation from the skin and respiratory tract. Gastrointestinal excretion is usually a minor component of total water output, except in patients with vomiting, diarrhea, or high enterostomy output states. Evaporative or insensitive water losses are important in the regulation of core body temperature. Obligatory renal water loss is mandated by the minimum solute excretion required to maintain a steady state. Normally, about 600 mosmols must be excreted per day, and since the maximal urine osmolality is 1200 mosmol/kg a minimum urine output of 500 mL/d is required for neutral solute balance.

Water Intake   The primary stimulus for water ingestion is *thirst*, mediated either by an increase in effective osmolality or a decrease in ECF volume or blood pressure. *Osmoreceptors*, located in the anterolateral hypothalamus, are stimulated by a rise in tonicity. Ineffective osmoles, such as urea and glucose, do not play a role in stimulating thirst. The average osmotic threshold for thirst is approximately 295 mosmol/kg and varies among individuals. Under normal circumstances, daily water intake exceeds physiologic requirements.

Water Excretion   In contrast to the ingestion of water, its excretion is tightly regulated by physiologic factors. The principal determinant of renal water excretion is *arginine vasopressin* (AVP; formerly antidiuretic hormone), a polypeptide synthesized in the supraoptic and paraventricular nuclei of the hypothalamus and secreted by the posterior pituitary gland. The binding of AVP to V_2 receptors on the basolateral membrane of principal cells in the collecting duct activates adenylyl cyclase and initiates a sequence of events that leads to the insertion of water channels into the luminal membrane. These water channels that are specifically activated by AVP are encoded by the *aquaporin-2* gene (Chap. 329). The net effect is passive water reabsorption along an osmotic gradient from the lumen of the collecting duct to the hypertonic medullary interstitium. The major stimulus for AVP secretion is hypertonicity. Since the major ECF solutes are Na^+ salts, effective osmolality is primarily determined by the plasma Na^+ concentration. An increase or decrease in tonicity is sensed by hypothalamic osmoreceptors as a decrease or increase in cell volume, respectively, leading to enhancement or suppression of AVP secretion. The osmotic threshold for AVP release is 280 to 290 mosmol/kg, and the system is sufficiently sensitive that plasma osmolality varies by no more than 1 to 2%.

Nonosmotic factors that regulate AVP secretion include *effective circulating* (arterial) *volume*, nausea, pain, stress, hypoglycemia, pregnancy, and numerous drugs. The hemodynamic response is mediated by baroreceptors in the carotid sinus. The sensitivity of these receptors is significantly lower than that of the osmoreceptors. In fact, depletion of blood volume sufficient to result in a decreased mean arterial pressure is necessary to stimulate AVP release, whereas small changes in effective circulating volume have little effect. In the setting of hypovolemia, the osmotic regulation of AVP remains intact. However, the

osmotic threshold, or set point, for AVP release is decreased, and the sensitivity is increased.

To maintain homeostasis and a normal plasma Na^+ concentration, the ingestion of solute-free water must eventually lead to the loss of the same volume of electrolyte-free water. Three steps are required for the kidney to excrete a water load: (1) filtration and delivery of water (and electrolytes) to the diluting sites of the nephron; (2) active reabsorption of Na^+ and Cl^- without water in the thick ascending limb of the loop of Henle and, to a lesser extent, in the distal nephron; and (3) maintenance of a dilute urine due to impermeability of the collecting duct to water in the absence of AVP. Abnormalities of any of these steps can result in impaired free water excretion, and eventual hyponatremia.

SODIUM BALANCE   Sodium is actively pumped out of cells by the Na^+,K^+-ATPase pump. As a result, 85 to 90% of all Na^+ is extracellular, and the ECF volume is a reflection of total body Na^+ content. Normal volume regulatory mechanisms ensure that Na^+ loss balances Na^+ gain. If this does not occur, conditions of Na^+ excess or deficit ensue and are manifest as edematous or hypovolemic states, respectively. It is important to distinguish between disorders of osmoregulation and disorders of volume regulation since water and Na^+ balance are regulated independently. Changes in Na^+ concentration generally reflect disturbed water homeostasis, whereas alterations in Na^+ content are manifest as ECF volume contraction or expansion and imply abnormal Na^+ balance.

Sodium Intake   Individuals eating a typical western diet consume approximately 150 mmol of NaCl daily. This normally exceeds basal requirements. As noted above, sodium is the principal extracellular cation. Therefore, dietary intake of Na^+ results in ECF volume expansion, which in turn promotes enhanced renal Na^+ excretion to maintain steady state Na^+ balance.

Sodium Excretion (See also Chap. 268)   The regulation of Na^+ excretion is multifactorial and is the major determinant of Na^+ balance. A Na^+ deficit or excess is manifest as a decreased or increased effective circulating volume, respectively. Changes in effective circulating volume tend to lead to parallel changes in glomerular filtration rate (GFR). However, tubule Na^+ reabsorption, and not GFR, is the major regulatory mechanism controlling Na^+ excretion. Almost two-thirds of filtered Na^+ is reabsorbed in the proximal convoluted tubule—this process is electroneutral and isoosmotic. Further reabsorption (25 to 30%) occurs in the thick ascending limb of the loop of Henle via the apical Na^+-K^+-$2Cl^-$ cotransporter—this is an active process and is also electroneutral. Distal convoluted tubule reabsorption of Na^+ (5%) is mediated by the *thiazide-sensitive* Na^+-Cl^- *cotransporter*. Final Na^+ reabsorption occurs in the cortical and medullary collecting ducts, the amount excreted being reasonably equivalent to the amount ingested per day (Chap. 268).

HYPOVOLEMIA

ETIOLOGY   True volume depletion, or hypovolemia, generally refers to a state of combined salt and water loss exceeding intake, leading to ECF volume contraction. The loss of Na^+ may be renal or extrarenal (Table 49-1).

Renal   Many conditions are associated with excessive urinary NaCl and water losses, including diuretics. Pharmacologic diuretics inhibit specific pathways of Na^+ reabsorption along the nephron with a consequent increase in urinary Na^+ excretion. Enhanced filtration of non-reabsorbed solutes, such as glucose or urea, can also impair tubular reabsorption of Na^+ and water, leading to an osmotic or solute diuresis. This often occurs in poorly controlled diabetes mellitus and in patients receiving high-protein hyperalimentation. Mannitol is a diuretic that produces an osmotic diuresis because the renal tubule is impermeable to mannitol. Many tubule and interstitial renal disorders are associated with Na^+ wasting. Excessive renal losses of Na^+ and water may also occur during the diuretic phase of acute tubular necrosis (Chap. 269) and following the relief of bilateral urinary tract ob-

I. ECF volume contracted
   A. Extrarenal Na⁺ loss
      1. Gastrointestinal
         (vomiting, nasogastric suction, drainage, fistula, diarrhea)
      2. Skin/respiratory
         (insensible losses, sweat, burns)
      3. Hemorrhage
   B. Renal Na⁺ and water loss
      1. Diuretics
      2. Osmotic diuresis
      3. Hypoaldosteronism
      4. Salt-wasting nephropathies
   C. Renal water loss
      1. Diabetes insipidus (central or nephrogenic)
II. ECF volume normal or expanded
   A. Decreased cardiac output
      1. Myocardial, valvular, or pericardial disease
   B. Redistribution
      1. Hypoalbuminemia
         (hepatic cirrhosis, nephrotic syndrome)
      2. Capillary leak
         (acute pancreatitis, ischemic bowel, rhabdomyolysis)
   C. Increased venous capacitance
      1. Sepsis

NOTE: ECF, extracellular fluid.

struction. The natriuresis and water diuresis associated with these two conditions are often short-lived and an appropriate response to a state of ECF volume expansion that ensued as a result of prior oliguria. However, ongoing losses in the absence of adequate replacement fluids may eventually lead to a state of hypovolemia. Chronic renal insufficiency is associated with a diminished ability to regulate renal salt and water excretion appropriately (Chap. 270). Therefore, patients with a GFR of less than 25 mL/min have an obligatory renal Na⁺ loss that may result in progressive ECF volume depletion if Na⁺ intake is restricted. Finally, mineralocorticoid deficiency (hypoaldosteronism) causes salt wasting in the presence of normal intrinsic renal function.

Massive renal water excretion can also lead to hypovolemia. The ECF volume contraction is usually less severe since two-thirds of the volume lost is intracellular. Conditions associated with excessive urinary water loss include *central diabetes insipidus* (CDI) and *nephrogenic diabetes insipidus* (NDI). These two disorders are due to impaired secretion of and renal unresponsiveness to AVP, respectively, and are discussed below.

Extrarenal Nonrenal causes of hypovolemia include fluid loss from the gastrointestinal tract, skin, and respiratory system and third space accumulations (burns, pancreatitis, peritonitis). Approximately 9 L of fluid enters the gastrointestinal tract daily, 2 L by ingestion and 7 L by secretion. Almost 98% of this volume is reabsorbed so that fecal fluid loss is only 100 to 200 mL/d. Impaired gastrointestinal reabsorption or enhanced secretion leads to volume depletion. Since gastric secretions have a low pH (high H⁺ concentration) and biliary, pancreatic, and intestinal secretions are alkaline (high HCO_3^- concentration), vomiting and diarrhea are often accompanied by metabolic alkalosis and acidosis, respectively.

Water evaporation from the skin and respiratory tract contributes to thermoregulation. These *insensible losses* amount to 500 mL/d. During febrile illnesses, prolonged heat exposure, or exercise, increased salt and water loss from skin, in the form of sweat, can be significant and lead to volume depletion. The Na⁺ concentration of sweat is normally 20 to 50 mmol/L and decreases with profuse sweating due to the action of aldosterone. Since sweat is hypotonic, the loss of water exceeds that of Na⁺. The water deficit is minimized by enhanced thirst. Nevertheless, ongoing Na⁺ loss is manifest as hypovolemia. Enhanced evaporative water loss from the respiratory tract may be associated with hyperventilation, especially in mechanically ventilated febrile patients.

Certain conditions lead to fluid sequestration in a *third space*. This compartment is extracellular but is not in equilibrium with either the ECF or the ICF. The fluid is effectively lost from the ECF and can result in hypovolemia. Examples include the bowel lumen in gastrointestinal obstruction, subcutaneous tissues in severe burns, retroperitoneal space in acute pancreatitis, and peritoneal cavity in peritonitis. Finally, severe hemorrhage from any source can result in volume depletion.

PATHOPHYSIOLOGY ECF volume contraction is manifest as a decreased plasma volume and hypotension. Hypotension is due to decreased venous return (preload) and diminished cardiac output; it triggers baroreceptors in the carotid sinus and aortic arch and leads to activation of the sympathetic nervous system and the renin-angiotensin system. The net effect is to maintain mean arterial pressure and cerebral and coronary perfusion. In contrast to the cardiovascular response, the renal response is aimed at restoring the ECF volume by decreasing the GFR and filtered load of Na⁺ and, most importantly, by promoting tubular reabsorption of Na⁺. Increased sympathetic tone increases proximal tubular Na⁺ reabsorption and decreases GFR by causing preferential afferent arteriolar vasoconstriction. Sodium is also reabsorbed in the proximal convoluted tubule in response to increased angiotensin II and altered peritubular capillary hemodynamics (decreased hydraulic and increased oncotic pressure). Enhanced reabsorption of Na⁺ by the collecting duct is an important component of the renal adaptation to ECF volume contraction. This occurs in response to increased *aldosterone* and AVP secretion, and suppressed *atrial natriuretic peptide* secretion.

CLINICAL FEATURES A careful history is often helpful in determining the etiology of ECF volume contraction (e.g., vomiting, diarrhea, polyuria, diaphoresis). Most symptoms are nonspecific and secondary to electrolyte imbalances and tissue hypoperfusion and include fatigue, weakness, muscle cramps, thirst, and postural dizziness. More severe degrees of volume contraction can lead to end-organ ischemia manifest as oliguria, cyanosis, abdominal and chest pain, and confusion or obtundation. Diminished skin turgor and dry oral mucous membranes are poor markers of decreased interstitial fluid. Signs of intravascular volume contraction include decreased jugular venous pressure, postural hypotension, and postural tachycardia. Larger and more acute fluid losses lead to hypovolemic shock, manifest as hypotension, tachycardia, peripheral vasoconstriction, and hypoperfusion—cyanosis, cold and clammy extremities, oliguria, and altered mental status.

DIAGNOSIS A thorough history and physical examination are generally sufficient to diagnose the etiology of hypovolemia. Laboratory data usually confirm and support the clinical diagnosis. The blood urea nitrogen (BUN) and plasma creatinine concentrations tend to be elevated, reflecting a decreased GFR. Normally, the BUN:creatinine ratio is about 10:1. However, in *prerenal azotemia*, hypovolemia leads to increased urea reabsorption and a proportionately greater elevation in BUN than plasma creatinine, and a BUN:creatinine ratio of 20:1 or higher. An increased BUN (relative to creatinine) may also be due to increased urea production that occurs with hyperalimentation (high-protein), glucocorticoid therapy, and gastrointestinal bleeding.

Volume depletion may be associated with hyponatremia, hypernatremia, or a normal plasma Na⁺ concentration, depending on the tonicity of the fluid lost, the presence of thirst, and the access to water. Hypokalemia is common in settings of increased renal or gastrointestinal K⁺ loss, and hyperkalemia occurs in renal failure, adrenal insufficiency, and certain types of metabolic acidosis. Metabolic alkalosis occurs with diuretic-induced hypovolemia and in cases of vomiting or nasogastric suction. In contrast, metabolic acidosis is associated with renal failure, tubulointerstitial disorders, adrenal insufficiency, diarrhea, diabetic ketoacidosis, and lactic acidosis. Since albumin and erythrocytes are confined to the intravascular compartment, ECF volume contraction often leads to a relative elevation in hematocrit (hemoconcentration) and plasma albumin concentration.

The appropriate response to hypovolemia is enhanced renal Na^+ and water reabsorption, which is reflected in the urine composition. Therefore, the urine Na^+ concentration should usually be less than 20 mmol/L except in conditions associated with impaired Na^+ reabsorption, as in acute tubular necrosis (Chap. 269). Another exception is hypovolemia due to vomiting, since the associated metabolic alkalosis and increased filtered HCO_3^- impair proximal Na^+ reabsorption. In this case, the urine Cl^- is low (<20 mmol/L). The urine osmolality and specific gravity in hypovolemic subjects are generally greater than 450 mosmol/kg and 1.015, respectively, reflecting the presence of enhanced AVP secretion. However, in hypovolemia due to diabetes insipidus, urine osmolality and specific gravity are indicative of inappropriately dilute urine.

℞ **TREATMENT**   The therapeutic goals are to restore normovolemia with fluid similar in composition to that lost and to replace ongoing losses. Symptoms and signs, including weight loss, can help estimate the degree of volume contraction and should also be monitored to assess response to treatment. Mild volume contraction can usually be corrected via the oral route. More severe hypovolemia requires intravenous therapy. Isotonic or normal saline (0.9% NaCl or 154 mmol/L Na^+) is the solution of choice in normonatremic and mildly hyponatremic individuals and should be administered initially in patients with hypotension or shock. Severe hyponatremia may require hypertonic saline (3.0% NaCl or 513 mmol/L Na^+). Hypernatremia reflects a proportionally greater deficit of water than Na^+, and its correction will therefore require a hypotonic solution such as half-normal saline (0.45% NaCl or 77 mmol/L Na^+) or 5% dextrose in water. Patients with significant hemorrhage, anemia, or intravascular volume depletion may require blood transfusion or colloid-containing solutions (albumin, dextran). Hypokalemia may be present initially or may ensue as a result of increased urinary K^+ excretion; it should be corrected by adding appropriate amounts of KCl to replacement solutions.

HYPONATREMIA

ETIOLOGY   A plasma Na^+ concentration less than 135 mmol/L usually reflects a hypotonic state. However, plasma osmolality may be normal or increased in some cases of hyponatremia, referred to as *pseudohyponatremia*. Plasma is 93% water, the remaining 7% consisting of plasma proteins and lipids. Since Na^+ ions are dissolved in plasma water, increasing the nonaqueous phase artificially lowers the Na^+ concentration measured per liter of plasma (except when Na^+-sensitive glass electrodes are used). The plasma osmolality and the Na^+ concentration remain normal. This type of hyponatremia has little clinical significance, except to ascertain the cause of the hyperproteinemia or hyperlipidemia. Isotonic or slightly hypotonic hyponatremia may complicate transurethral resection of the prostate or bladder because large volumes of isoosmotic (mannitol) or hypoosmotic (sorbital or glycine) bladder irrigation solution can be absorbed and result in a dilutional hyponatremia. The metabolism of sorbitol and glycine to CO_2 and water may lead to hypotonicity if the accumulated fluid and solutes are not rapidly excreted. Hypertonic hyponatremia is usually due to hyperglycemia or, occasionally, intravenous administration of mannitol. Relative insulin deficiency causes myocytes to become impermeable to glucose. Therefore, during poorly controlled diabetes mellitus, glucose is an effective osmole and draws water from muscle cells, resulting in hyponatremia. Plasma Na^+ concentration falls by 1.4 mmol/L for every 100 mg/dL rise in the plasma glucose concentration.

Most causes of hyponatremia are associated with a low plasma osmolality (Table 49-2). In general, hypotonic hyponatremia is due either to a primary water gain (and secondary Na^+ loss) or a primary Na^+ loss (and secondary water gain). In the absence of water intake or

Table 49-2   Causes of Hyponatremia

I. Pseudohyponatremia
  A. Normal plasma osmolality
    1. Hyperlipidemia
    2. Hyperproteinemia
    3. Posttransurethral resection of prostate/bladder tumor
  B. Increased plasma osmolality
    1. Hyperglycemia
    2. Mannitol
II. Hypoosmolal hyponatremia
  A. Primary Na^+ loss (secondary water gain)
    1. Integumentary loss: sweating, burns
    2. Gastrointestinal loss: vomiting, tube drainage, fistula, obstruction, diarrhea
    3. Renal loss: diuretics, osmotic diuresis, hypoaldosteronism, salt-wasting nephropathy, postobstructive diuresis, nonoliguric acute tubular necrosis
  B. Primary water gain (secondary Na^+ loss)
    1. Primary polydipsia
    2. Decreased solute intake (e.g., beer potomania)
    3. AVP release due to pain, nausea, drugs
    4. Syndrome of inappropriate AVP secretion
    5. Glucocorticoid deficiency
    6. Hypothyroidism
    7. Chronic renal insufficiency
  C. Primary Na^+ gain (exceeded by secondary water gain)
    1. Heart failure
    2. Hepatic cirrhosis
    3. Nephrotic syndrome

hypotonic fluid replacement, hyponatremia is usually associated with hypovolemic shock due to a profound sodium deficit and transcellular water shift. Contraction of the ECF volume stimulates thirst and AVP secretion. The increased water ingestion and impaired renal excretion result in hyponatremia. It is important to note that *diuretic-induced hyponatremia* is almost always due to thiazide diuretics. Loop diuretics decrease the tonicity of the medullary interstitium and impair maximal urinary concentrating capacity. This limits the ability of AVP to promote water retention. In contrast, thiazide diuretics lead to Na^+ and K^+ depletion, and AVP-mediated water retention. In the presence of a large K^+ deficit, transcellular ion exchange (K^+ exits and Na^+ enters cells) may contribute to hyponatremia. Hyponatremia can also occur by a process of *desalination*. This occurs when the urine tonicity (the sum of the concentrations of Na^+ and K^+) exceeds that of administered intravenous fluids (including isotonic saline). This accounts for some cases of acute postoperative hyponatremia and cerebral salt wasting after neurosurgery.

Hyponatremia in the setting of ECF volume expansion is usually associated with edematous states, such as congestive heart failure, hepatic cirrhosis, and the nephrotic syndrome. These disorders all have in common a decreased effective circulating arterial volume, leading to increased thirst and increased AVP levels. Additional factors impairing the excretion of solute-free water include a reduced GFR, decreased delivery of ultrafiltrate to the diluting site (due to increased proximal fractional reabsorption of Na^+ and water), and diuretic therapy. The degree of hyponatremia often correlates with the severity of the underlying condition and is an important prognostic factor. Oliguric acute and chronic renal failure may be associated with hyponatremia if water intake exceeds the ability to excrete equivalent volumes.

Hyponatremia in the absence of ECF volume contraction, decreased effective circulating arterial volume, or renal insufficiency is usually due to increased AVP secretion resulting in impaired water excretion. Ingestion or administration of water is also required since high levels of AVP alone are usually insufficient to produce hyponatremia. This disorder, commonly termed the *syndrome of inappropriate antidiuretic hormone secretion* (SIADH), is the most common cause of normovolemic hyponatremia and is due to the nonphysiologic release of AVP from the posterior pituitary or an ectopic source (Chap. 329). Renal free water excretion is impaired while the regulation of

Na+ balance is unaffected. The most common causes of SIADH include neuropsychiatric and pulmonary diseases, malignant tumors, major surgery (postoperative pain), and pharmacologic agents. Severe pain and nausea are physiologic stimuli of AVP secretion; these stimuli are inappropriate in the absence of hypovolemia or hyperosmolality. A variety of central nervous system disorders may be associated with SIADH, such as meningitis, encephalitis, hemorrhage, stroke, psychosis, primary and metastatic tumors, and acute porphyria. Pneumonia, empyema, tuberculosis, and acute respiratory failure can be complicated by hyponatremia secondary to SIADH. Hypoxemia, hypercarbia, and positive-pressure ventilation are all nonosmotic stimuli for AVP release. Various tumors, notably oat cell carcinoma of the lung, have been demonstrated to secrete AVP ectopically. Many drugs either stimulate AVP release or potentiate its actions on the kidney. The pattern of AVP secretion can be used to classify SIADH into four subtypes: (1) erratic autonomous AVP secretion (ectopic production); (2) normal regulation of AVP release around a lower osmolality set point or *reset osmostat* (cachexia, malnutrition); (3) normal AVP response to hypertonicity with failure to suppress completely at low osmolality (incomplete pituitary stalk section); and (4) normal AVP secretion with increased sensitivity to its actions or secretion of some other antidiuretic factor (rare).

Hormonal excess or deficiency may cause hyponatremia. Adrenal insufficiency (Chap. 331) and hypothyroidism (Chap. 330) may present with hyponatremia and should not be confused with SIADH. Although decreased mineralocorticoids may contribute to the hyponatremia of adrenal insufficiency, it is the cortisol deficiency that leads to hypersecretion of AVP both indirectly (secondary to volume depletion) and directly (cosecreted with corticotropin-releasing factor). The mechanisms by which hypothyroidism leads to hyponatremia include decreased cardiac output and GFR and increased AVP secretion in response to hemodynamic stimuli.

Finally, hyponatremia may occur in the absence of AVP or renal failure if the kidney is unable to excrete the dietary water load. In psychogenic or primary polydipsia, compulsive water consumption may overwhelm the normally large renal excretory capacity of 12 L/d (Chap. 329). These patients often have psychiatric illnesses and may be taking medications, such as phenothiazines, that enhance the sensation of thirst by causing a dry mouth. The maximal urine output is a function of the minimum urine osmolality achievable and the mandatory solute excretion. Metabolism of a normal diet generates about 600 mosmol/d, and the minimum urine osmolality in humans is 50 mosmol/kg. Therefore, the maximum daily urine output will be about 12 L (600 ÷ 50 = 12). A solute excretion rate of greater than ~750 mosmol/d is, by definition, an *osmotic diuresis*. A low-protein diet may yield as few as 250 mosmol/d, which translates into a maximal urine output of 5 L/d at a minimum urine tonicity of 50 mosmol/kg. Beer drinkers typically have a poor dietary intake of protein and electrolytes and consume large volumes (of beer), which may exceed the renal excretory capacity and result in hyponatremia. This phenomenon is referred to as *beer potomania*.

CLINICAL FEATURES   The clinical manifestations of hyponatremia are related to osmotic water shift leading to increased ICF volume, specifically brain cell swelling or cerebral edema. Therefore, the symptoms are primarily neurologic, and their severity is dependent on the rapidity of onset and absolute decrease in plasma Na+ concentration. Patients may be asymptomatic or complain of nausea and malaise. As the plasma Na+ concentration falls, the symptoms progress to include headache, lethargy, confusion, and obtundation. Stupor, seizures, and coma do not usually occur unless the plasma Na+ concentration falls acutely below 120 mmol/L or decreases rapidly. As described above, adaptive mechanisms designed to protect cell volume occur in chronic hyponatremia. Loss of Na+ and K+, followed by organic osmolytes, from brain cells decreases brain swelling due to secondary transcellular water shifts (from ICF to ECF). The net effect is to minimize cerebral edema and its symptoms. Hospitalized patients with hyponatremia have an increased mortality rate compared to normonatremic control subjects. However, the excess mortality is usually

attributed to the underlying disorder rather than the electrolyte disturbance.

DIAGNOSIS   Hyponatremia is not a disease but a manifestation of a variety of disorders. The underlying cause can often be ascertained from an accurate history and physical examination, including an assessment of ECF volume status and effective circulating arterial volume. The differential diagnosis of hyponatremia, an expanded ECF volume, and decreased effective circulating volume includes congestive heart failure, hepatic cirrhosis, and the nephrotic syndrome. Hypothyroidism and adrenal insufficiency tend to present with a near-normal ECF volume and decreased effective circulating arterial volume. All of these diseases have characteristic signs and symptoms. Patients with SIADH are usually euvolemic.

Four laboratory findings often provide useful information and can narrow the differential diagnosis of hyponatremia: (1) the plasma osmolality, (2) the urine osmolality, (3) the urine Na+ concentration, and (4) the urine K+ concentration. Since ECF tonicity is determined primarily by the Na+ concentration, most patients with hyponatremia have a decreased plasma osmolality. If the plasma osmolality is not low, pseudohyponatremia must be ruled out. The appropriate renal response to hypoosmolality is to excrete the maximum volume of dilute urine, i.e., urine osmolality and specific gravity of less than 100 mosmol/kg and 1.003, respectively. This occurs in patients with primary polydipsia. If this is not present, it suggests impaired free water excretion due to the action of AVP on the kidney. The secretion of AVP may be a physiologic response to hemodynamic stimuli or it may be inappropriate in the presence of hyponatremia and euvolemia. Since Na+ is the major ECF cation and is largely restricted to this compartment, ECF volume contraction represents a deficit in total body Na+ content. Therefore, volume depletion in patients with normal underlying renal function results in enhanced tubule Na+ reabsorption and a urine Na+ concentration less than 20 mmol/L. The finding of a urine Na+ concentration greater than 20 mmol/L in hypovolemic hyponatremia implies a salt-wasting nephropathy, diuretic therapy, hypoaldosteronism, or occasionally vomiting. Both the urine osmolality and the urine Na+ concentration can be followed serially when assessing response to therapy.

SIADH is characterized by hypoosmotic hyponatremia in the setting of an inappropriately concentrated urine (urine osmolality greater than 100 mosmol/kg). Patients are typically normovolemic and have normal Na+ balance. They tend to be mildly volume expanded secondary to water retention and have a urine Na+ excretion rate equal to intake (urine Na+ concentration usually greater than 40 mmol/L). By definition, they have normal renal, adrenal, and thyroid function and usually have normal K+ and acid-base balance. SIADH is often associated with hypouricemia due to the uricosuric state induced by volume expansion. In contrast, hypovolemic patients tend to be hyperuricemic secondary to increased proximal urate reabsorption.

CLINICAL APPROACH   See Fig. 49-1.

Rx **TREATMENT**   The goals of therapy are twofold: (1) to raise the plasma Na+ concentration by restricting water intake and promoting water loss; and (2) to correct the underlying disorder. Mild asymptomatic hyponatremia is generally of little clinical significance and requires no treatment. The management of asymptomatic hyponatremia associated with ECF volume contaction should include Na+ repletion, generally in the form of isotonic saline. The direct effect of the administered NaCl on the plasma Na+ concentration is trivial. However, restoration of euvolemia removes the hemodynamic stimulus for AVP release, allowing the excess free water to be excreted. The hyponatremia associated with edematous states tends to reflect the severity of the underlying disease and is usually asymptomatic. These patients have increased total body water that exceeds the increase in total body Na+ content. Treatment should include restriction of Na+ and water intake, correction of hypokalemia, and promotion of water loss in excess of Na+. The latter may require the use of loop diuretics

FIGURE 49-1 Algorithm depicting clinical approach to hyponatremia. ECF, extracellular fluid; SIADH, syndrome of inappropriate antidiuretic hormone secretion.

with replacement of a proportion of the urinary Na⁺ loss to ensure net free water excretion. Dietary water restriction should be less than the urine output. Correction of the K⁺ deficit may raise the plasma Na⁺ concentration by favoring a shift of Na⁺ out of cells as K⁺ moves in. Water restriction is also a component of the therapeutic approach to hyponatremia associated with primary polydipsia, renal failure, and SIADH (Chap. 329).

The rate of correction of hyponatremia depends on the absence or presence of neurologic dysfunction. This, in turn, is related to the rapidity of onset and magnitude of the fall in plasma Na⁺ concentration. In asymptomatic patients, the plasma Na⁺ concentration should be raised by no more than 0.5 to 1.0 mmol/L per hour and by less than 10 to 12 mmol/L over the first 24 h. Acute or severe hyponatremia (plasma Na⁺ concentration <110 to 115 mmol/L) tends to present with altered mental status and/or seizures and requires more rapid correction. Severe symptomatic hyponatremia should be treated with hypertonic saline, and the plasma Na⁺ concentration should be raised by 1 to 2 mmol/L per hour for the first 3 to 4 h or until the seizures subside. Once again, the plasma Na⁺ concentration should probably be raised by no more than 12 mmol/L during the first 24 h. The quantity of Na⁺ required to increase the plasma Na⁺ concentration by a given amount can be estimated by multiplying the deficit in plasma Na⁺ concentration by the total body water. Under normal conditions, total body water is 50 or 60% of lean body weight in women or men, respectively. Therefore, to raise the plasma Na⁺ concentration from 105 to 115 mmol/L in a 70-kg man requires 420 mmol [(115 − 105) × 70 × 0.6] of Na⁺. The risk of correcting hyponatremia too rapidly is the development of the *osmotic demyelination syndrome* (ODS). This is a neurologic disorder characterized by flaccid paralysis, dysarthria, and dys-

phagia. The diagnosis is usually suspected clinically and can be confirmed by appropriate neuroimaging studies. There is no specific treatment for the disorder, which is associated with significant morbidity and mortality. Patients with chronic hyponatremia are most susceptible to the development of ODS, since their brain cell volume has returned to near normal as a result of the osmotic adaptive mechanisms described above. Therefore, administration of hypertonic saline to these individuals can cause sudden osmotic shrinkage of brain cells. In addition to rapid or overcorrection of hyponatremia, risk factors for ODS include prior cerebral anoxic injury, hypokalemia, and malnutrition, especially secondary to alcoholism. Water restriction in primary polydipsia and intravenous saline therapy in ECF volume–contracted patients may also lead to overly rapid correction of hyponatremia as a result of AVP suppression and a brisk water diuresis. This can be prevented by administration of water or use of an AVP analogue to slow down the rate of free water excretion. →*For further discussion, see Chap. 329.*

HYPERNATREMIA

ETIOLOGY   Hypernatremia is defined as a plasma Na⁺ concentration greater than 145 mmol/L. Since Na⁺ and its accompanying anions are the major effective ECF osmoles, hypernatremia is a state of hyperosmolality. As a result of the fixed number of ICF particles, maintenance of osmotic equilibrium in hypernatremia results in ICF volume contraction. Hypernatremia may be due to primary Na⁺ gain or water deficit. The two components of an appropriate response to hypernatremia are increased water intake stimulated by thirst and the excretion of the minimum volume of maximally concentrated urine reflecting AVP secretion in response to an osmotic stimulus.

In practice, the majority of cases of hypernatremia result from the loss of water. Since water is distributed between the ICF and the ECF in a 2:1 ratio, a given amount of solute-free water loss will result in a twofold greater reduction in the ICF compartment than the ECF compartment. For example, consider three scenarios: the loss of 1 L of water, isotonic NaCl, or half-isotonic NaCl. If 1 L of water is lost, the ICF volume will decrease by 667 mL, whereas the ECF volume will fall by only 333 mL. Due to the fact that Na⁺ is largely restricted to the ECF, this compartment will decrease by 1 L if the fluid lost is isoosmotic. One liter of half-isotonic NaCl is equivalent to 500 mL of water (one-third ECF, two-thirds ICF) plus 500 mL of isotonic saline (all ECF). Therefore, the loss of 1 L of half-isotonic saline decreases the ECF and ICF volumes by 667 mL and 333 mL, respectively.

The degree of hyperosmolality is typically mild unless the thirst mechanism is abnormal or access to water is limited. The latter occurs in infants, the physically handicapped, patients with impaired mental status, in the postoperative state, and in intubated patients in the intensive care unit. On rare occasions, impaired thirst may be due to *primary hypodipsia.* This usually occurs as a result of damage to the hypothalamic osmoreceptors that control thirst and tends to be associated with abnormal osmotic regulation of AVP secretion. Primary hypodipsia may be due to a variety of pathologic changes including granulomatous disease, vascular occlusion, and tumors. A subset of hypodipsic hypernatremia, referred to as *essential hypernatremia,* does not respond to forced water intake. This appears to be due to a specific osmoreceptor defect resulting in nonosmotic regulation of AVP release. Thus, the hemodynamic effects of water loading lead to AVP suppression and excretion of dilute urine.

The source of free water loss is either renal or extrarenal. Nonrenal loss of water may be due to evaporation from the skin and respiratory tract (insensible losses) or loss from the gastrointestinal tract. Insensible losses are increased with fever, exercise, heat exposure, and severe burns and in mechanically ventilated patients. Furthermore, the Na⁺ concentration of sweat decreases with profuse perspiration, thereby increasing solute-free water loss. Diarrhea is the most common gastrointestinal cause of hypernatremia. Specifically, osmotic diarrheas (induced by lactulose, sorbitol, or malabsorption of carbohydrate) and viral gastroenterites result in water loss exceeding that of

Na+ and K+. In contrast, secretory diarrheas (e.g., cholera, carcinoid, VIPoma) have a fecal osmolality (twice the sum of the concentrations of Na+ and K+) similar to that of plasma and present with ECF volume contraction and a normal plasma Na+ concentration or hyponatremia.

Renal water loss is the most common cause of hypernatremia and is due to drug-induced or osmotic diuresis or diabetes insipidus (Chap. 329). Loop diuretics interfere with the countercurrent mechanism and produce an isoosmotic solute diuresis. This results in a decreased medullary interstitial tonicity and impaired renal concentrating ability. The presence of non-reabsorbed organic solutes in the tubule lumen impairs the osmotic reabsorption of water. This leads to water loss in excess of Na+ and K+, known as an osmotic diuresis. The most frequent cause of an osmotic diuresis is hyperglycemia and glucosuria in poorly controlled diabetes mellitus. Intravenous administration of mannitol and increased endogenous production of urea (high-protein diet) can also result in an osmotic diuresis. Hypernatremia secondary to non-osmotic urinary water loss is usually due to: (1) CDI or neurogenic diabetes insipidus characterized by impaired AVP secretion, or (2) NDI resulting from end-organ (renal) resistance to the actions of AVP. The most common cause of CDI is destruction of the neurohypophysis. This may occur as a result of trauma, neurosurgery, granulomatous disease, neoplasms, vascular accidents, or infection. In many cases, CDI is idiopathic and may occasionally be hereditary. The familial form of the disease is inherited in an autosomal dominant fashion and has been attributed to mutations in the propressophysin (AVP precursor) gene. NDI may be either inherited or acquired. Congenital NDI is an X-linked recessive trait due to mutations in the V_2 receptor gene. Mutations in the autosomal aquaporin-2 gene may also result in NDI. The aquaporin-2 gene encodes the water channel protein whose membrane insertion is stimulated by AVP. The causes of sporadic NDI are numerous and include drugs (especially lithium), hypercalcemia, hypokalemia, and conditions that impair medullary hypertonicity (e.g., papillary necrosis or osmotic diuresis). Pregnant women, in the second or third trimester, may develop NDI as a result of excessive elaboration of vasopressinase by the placenta.

Finally, although infrequent, a primary Na+ gain may cause hypernatremia. For example, inadvertent administration of hypertonic NaCl or NaHCO₃ or replacing sugar with salt in infant formula can produce this complication.

CLINICAL FEATURES As a consequence of hypertonicity, water shifts out of cells, leading to a contracted ICF volume. A decreased brain cell volume is associated with an increased risk of subarachnoid or intracerebral hemorrhage. Hence, the major symptoms of hypernatremia are neurologic and include altered mental status, weakness, neuromuscular irritability, focal neurologic deficits, and occasionally coma or seizures. Patients may also complain of polyuria or thirst. For unknown reasons, patients with polydipsia from CDI tend to prefer ice-cold water. The signs and symptoms of volume depletion are often present in patients with a history of excessive sweating, diarrhea, or an osmotic diuresis. The mortality rate associated with a plasma Na+ concentration greater than 180 mmol/L is very high. As with hyponatremia, the severity of the clinical manifestations is related to the acuity and magnitude of the rise in plasma Na+ concentration. Chronic hypernatremia is generally less symptomatic as a result of adaptive mechanisms designed to defend cell volume. Brain cells initially take up Na+ and K+ salts, later followed by accumulation of organic osmolytes such as inositol. This serves to restore the brain ICF volume towards normal.

DIAGNOSIS A complete history and physical examination will often provide clues as to the underlying cause of hypernatremia. Relevant symptoms and signs include the absence or presence of thirst, diaphoresis, diarrhea, polyuria, and the features of ECF volume contraction. The history should include a list of current and recent medications, and the physical examination is incomplete without a thorough mental status and neurologic assessment. Measurement of urine volume and osmolality are essential in the evaluation of hyperosmolality. The appropriate renal response to hypernatremia is the excretion of the minimum volume (500 mL/d) of maximally concentrated urine

(urine osmolality >800 mosmol/kg). These findings suggest extrarenal or remote renal water loss or administration of hypertonic Na+ salt solutions. The presence of a primary Na+ excess can be confirmed by the presence of ECF volume expansion and natriuresis (urine Na+ concentration usually >100 mmol/L). Many causes of hypernatremia are associated with polyuria and a submaximal urine osmolality. The product of the urine volume and osmolality, i.e., the solute excretion rate, is helpful in determining the basis of the polyuria (see above). To maintain a steady state, total solute excretion must equal solute production. As stated above, individuals eating a normal diet generate ~600 mosmol/d. Therefore, daily solute excretion in excess of 750 mosmol defines an osmotic diuresis. This can be confirmed by measuring the urine glucose and urea. In general, both CDI and NDI present with polyuria and hypotonic urine (urine osmolality <250 mosmol/kg). The degree of hypernatremia is usually mild unless there is an associated thirst abnormality. The clinical history, physical examination, and pertinent laboratory data can often rule out causes of acquired NDI. CDI and NDI can generally be distinguished by administering the AVP analogue desmopressin (10 μg intranasally) after careful water restriction. The urine osmolality should increase by at least 50% in CDI and will not change in NDI. Unfortunately, the diagnosis may sometimes be difficult due to partial defects in AVP secretion and action.

CLINICAL APPROACH See Fig. 49-2.

℞ TREATMENT The therapeutic goals are to stop ongoing water loss by treating the underlying cause and to correct the water deficit. The ECF volume should be restored in hypovolemic patients. The quantity of water required to correct the deficit can be calculated from the following equation:

$$\text{Water deficit} = \frac{\text{plasma Na}^+ \text{ concentration} - 140}{140} \times \text{total body water}$$

In hypernatremia due to water loss, total body water is approxi-

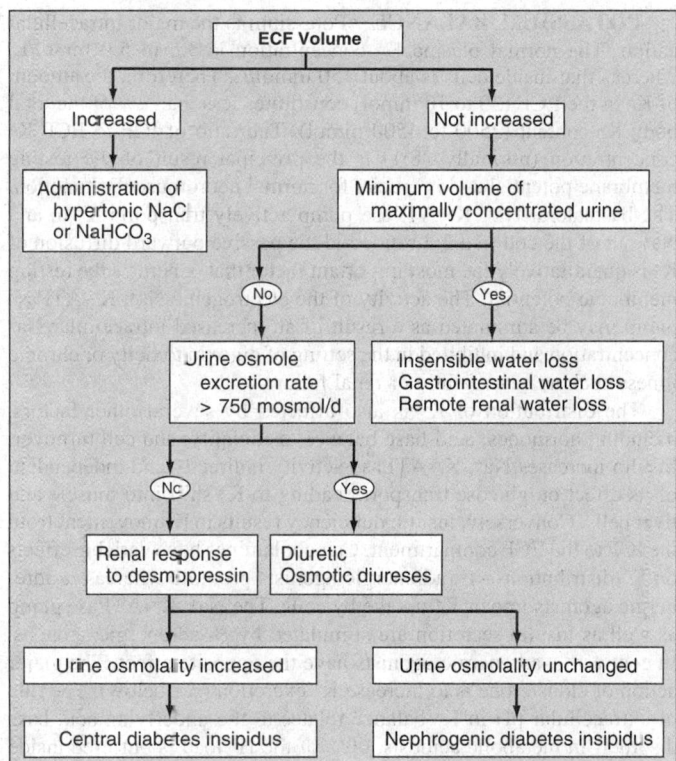

FIGURE 49-2 Algorithm depicting clinical approach to hypernatremia.

mately 50 and 40% of lean body weight in men and women, respectively. For example, a 50-kg woman with a plasma Na$^+$ concentration of 160 mmol/L has an estimated free water deficit of 2.9 L $\{[(160 - 140) \div 140] \times (0.4 \times 50)\}$. As in hyponatremia, rapid correction of hypernatremia is potentially dangerous. In this case, a sudden decrease in osmolality could potentially cause a rapid shift of water into cells that have undergone osmotic adaptation. This would result in swollen brain cells and increase the risk of seizures or permanent neurologic damage. Therefore, the water deficit should be corrected slowly over at least 48 to 72 h. When calculating the rate of water replacement, ongoing losses should be taken into account, and the plasma Na$^+$ concentration should be lowered by 0.5 mmol/L per hour and by no more than 12 mmol/L over the first 24 h. The safest route of administration of water is by mouth or via a nasogastric tube (or other feeding tube). Alternatively, 5% dextrose in water or half-isotonic saline can be given intravenously. The appropriate treatment of CDI consists of administering desmopressin intranasally (Chap. 329). Other options for decreasing urine output include a low-salt diet in combination with low-dose thiazide diuretic therapy. In some patients with partial CDI, drugs that either stimulate AVP secretion or enhance its action on the kidney have been useful. These include chlorpropamide, clofibrate, carbamazepine, andnonsteroidal anti-inflammatory drugs (NSAIDs). The concentrating defect in NDI may be reversible by treating the underlying disorder or eliminating the offending drug. Symptomatic polyuria due to NDI can be treated with a low-Na$^+$ diet and thiazide diuretics as described above. This induces mild volume depletion, which leads to enhanced proximal reabsorption of salt and water and decreased delivery to the site of action of AVP, the collecting duct. By impairing renal prostaglandin synthesis, NSAIDs potentiate AVP action and thereby increase urine osmolality and decrease urine volume. Amiloride may be useful in patients with NDI who need to be on lithium. The nephrotoxicity of lithium requires the drug to be taken up into collecting duct cells via the amiloride-sensitive Na$^+$ channel.

POTASSIUM

POTASSIUM BALANCE   Potassium is the major intracellular cation. The normal plasma K$^+$ concentration is 3.5 to 5.0 mmol/L, whereas that inside cells is about 150 mmol/L. Therefore, the amount of K$^+$ in the ECF (30 to 70 mmol) constitutes less than 2% of the total body K$^+$ content (2500 to 4500 mmol). The ratio of ICF to ECF K$^+$ concentration (normally 38:1) is the principal result of the resting membrane potential and is crucial for normal neuromuscular function. The basolateral Na$^+$, K$^+$-ATPase pump actively transports K$^+$ in and Na$^+$ out of the cell in a 2:3 ratio, and the passive outward diffusion of K$^+$ is quantitatively the most important factor that generates the resting membrane potential. The activity of the electrogenic Na$^+$, K$^+$-ATPase pump may be stimulated as a result of an increased intracellular Na$^+$ concentration and inhibited in the setting of digoxin toxicity or chronic illness such as heart failure or renal failure.

The distribution of K$^+$ is also affected by several other factors, including hormones, acid-base balance, osmolality, and cell turnover. Insulin increases Na$^+$, K$^+$-ATPase activity indirectly and independent of its effect on glucose transport, leading to K$^+$ shift into muscle and liver cells. Conversely, insulin deficiency results in K$^+$ movement from the ICF to the ECF compartment. Catecholamines have variable effects on K$^+$ distribution—β_2-adrenergic agonists promote whereas α-adrenergic agonists impair K$^+$ uptake by cells. The Na$^+$, K$^+$-ATPase pump as well as insulin secretion are stimulated by β_2-adrenergic agonists. In contrast, α-adrenergic agonists have the opposite effect. The major action of aldosterone is to increase K$^+$ excretion (see below). The role of extracellular pH in K$^+$ balance relates to the underlying acid-base disorder. In metabolic acidosis, 60% of the H$^+$ load is buffered inside cells. To maintain electroneutrality, the H$^+$ ion must either be accompanied by an anion or exchanged for intracellular K$^+$ (leading to hy-

perkalemia). Organic acidoses are not usually associated with a pH-related K$^+$ shift, since anions such as lactate and β-hydroxybutyrate can be readily taken up by the cell. The converse, movement of K$^+$ into cells, may be seen with metabolic alkalosis. However, this is less important due to diminished intracellular buffering. Primary respiratory disturbances in acid-base balance result in minimal transcellular K$^+$ shifts. In hyperosmolal states, K$^+$ diffuses out of cells along with water due to *solvent drag*. The concentration gradient favoring K$^+$ movement out of cells is also increased as a result of ICF water loss. Tissue destruction or breakdown results in the release of intracellular K$^+$, whereas the production of new cells shifts K$^+$ out of the ECF. Finally, moderate to severe exercise may be associated with K$^+$ release from muscle, leading to glycogenolysis and local vasodilatation. This is usually transient but may affect the plasma K$^+$ concentration if patients repeatedly clench and unclench their fist prior to venipuncture.

The K$^+$ intake of individuals on an average western diet is 40 to 120 mmol/d or approximately 1 mmol/kg per day, 90% of which is absorbed by the gastrointestinal tract. Maintenance of the steady state necessitates matching K$^+$ ingestion with excretion. Initially, extrarenal adaptive mechanisms, followed later by urinary excretion, prevent a doubling of the plasma K$^+$ concentration that would occur if the dietary K$^+$ load remained in the ECF compartment. Immediately following a meal, most of the absorbed K$^+$ enters cells as a result of the initial elevation in the plasma K$^+$ concentration and facilitated by insulin release and basal catecholamine levels. Eventually, however, the excess K$^+$ is excreted in the urine (see below). The regulation of gastrointestinal K$^+$ handling is not well understood. The amount of K$^+$ lost in the stool can increase from 10 to 50 or 60% (of dietary intake) in chronic renal insufficiency. In addition, colonic secretion of K$^+$ is stimulated in patients with large volumes of diarrhea, resulting in potentially severe K$^+$ depletion.

POTASSIUM EXCRETION   (See also Chap. 268)   Renal excretion is the major route of elimination of dietary and other sources of excess K$^+$. The filtered load of K$^+$ (GFR $\times$ plasma K$^+$ concentration = 180 L/d $\times$ 4 mmol/L = 720 mmol/d) is 10- to 20-fold greater than the ECF K$^+$ content. Some 90% of filtered K$^+$ is reabsorbed by the proximal convoluted tubule and loop of Henle. Proximally, K$^+$ is reabsorbed passively with Na$^+$ and water, whereas the luminal Na$^+$-K$^+$-2Cl$^-$ cotransporter mediates K$^+$ uptake in the thick ascending limb of the loop of Henle. Therefore, K$^+$ delivery to the distal nephron [distal convoluted tubule and cortical collecting duct (CCD)] approximates dietary intake. Net distal K$^+$ secretion or reabsorption occurs in the setting of K$^+$ excess or depletion, respectively. The cell responsible for K$^+$ secretion in the late distal convoluted tubule (or connecting tubule) and CCD is the principal cell. Virtually all regulation of renal K$^+$ excretion and total body K$^+$ balance occurs in the distal nephron. The driving force for K$^+$ secretion is a favorable electrochemical gradient across the luminal membrane of the principal cell. As a result of the action of the basolateral Na$^+$, K$^+$-ATPase pump, the intracellular K$^+$ concentration far exceeds that of the fluid in the lumen of the CCD. The electrical gradient is created by electrogenic Na$^+$ reabsorption leading to a lumen-negative transepithelial potential difference (TEPD), favoring K$^+$ secretion. The generation of a lumen-negative TEPD depends on the relative rates of reabsorption of Na$^+$ and its accompanying anion (primarily Cl$^-$). Equimolar reabsorption of Na$^+$ and Cl$^-$ at equivalent rates is electroneutral, whereas reabsorption of Na$^+$ in excess of Cl$^-$ is electrogenic. The cellular uptake of Na$^+$ by the principal cell occurs via an apical Na$^+$ channel and is driven by a low intracellular Na$^+$ concentration relative to that in the lumen of the CCD. The mechanism and regulation of distal nephron Cl$^-$ transport is less clear. Obviously, factors that impact on either Na$^+$ or Cl$^-$ reabsorption by the principal cell will influence the TEPD. Potassium secretion is regulated by two physiologic stimuli—aldosterone and hyperkalemia. Aldosterone is secreted by the zona glomerulosa cells of the adrenal cortex in response to high renin and angiotensin II or hyperkalemia. The actions of aldosterone on the principal cell include enhanced apical membrane Na$^+$ conductivity, stimulation of the basolateral Na$^+$, K$^+$-ATPase, and increased luminal K$^+$ channels. The plasma K$^+$ concentration, independent of aldosterone, can directly affect K$^+$ secretion. In addition to the K$^+$ concentration in the lumen of the CCD, renal K$^+$ loss depends on the urine flow rate, a function of daily solute excretion (see above). Since excretion is equal to the product of concentration and volume, increased distal flow rate can significantly enhance urinary K$^+$ output. Finally, in severe K$^+$ depletion, secretion of K$^+$ is reduced and reabsorption, via apical H$^+$, K$^+$-ATPase pumps in cortical and medullary collecting ducts, is upregulated.

HYPOKALEMIA

ETIOLOGY (See Table 49-3) Hypokalemia, defined as a plasma K$^+$ concentration < 3.5 mmol/L, may result from one (or more) of the following: decreased net intake, shift into cells, or increased net loss. Diminished intake is seldom the sole cause of K$^+$ depletion since urinary excretion can be effectively decreased to less than 15 mmol/d as a result of net K$^+$ reabsorption in the distal nephron. With the exception of the urban poor and certain cultural groups, the amount of K$^+$ in the diet almost always exceeds that excreted in the urine. However, dietary K$^+$ restriction may exacerbate the hypokalemia secondary to increased gastrointestinal or renal loss. An unusual cause of decreased K$^+$ intake is ingestion of clay (geophagia), which binds dietary K$^+$ and iron. This custom was previously common among African Americans in the American South.

Redistribution into Cells Movement of K$^+$ into cells may transiently decrease the plasma K$^+$ concentration without altering total body K$^+$ content. For any given cause, the magnitude of the change is relatively small, often less than 1 mmol/L. However, a combination of factors may lead to a significant fall in the plasma K$^+$ concentration and may amplify the hypokalemia due to K$^+$ wasting. Alkalosis, especially that due to a primary increase in plasma HCO$_3^-$ (metabolic alkalosis), is often associated with hypokalemia. This occurs as a result

Table 49-3 Causes of Hypokalemia

I. Decreased intake
   A. Starvation
   B. Clay ingestion
II. Redistribution into cells
   A. Acid-base
      1. Metabolic alkalosis
   B. Hormonal
      1. Insulin
      2. β_2-Adrenergic agonists (endogenous or exogenous)
      3. α-Adrenergic antagonists
   C. Anabolic state
      1. Vitamin B$_{12}$ or folic acid (red blood cell production)
      2. Granulocyte-macrophage colony stimulating factor (white blood cell production)
      3. Total parenteral nutrition
   D. Other
      1. Pseudohypokalemia
      2. Hypothermia
      3. Hypokalemic periodic paralysis
      4. Barium toxicity
III. Increased loss
   A. Nonrenal
      1. Gastrointestinal loss (diarrhea)
      2. Integumentary loss (sweat)
   B. Renal
      1. Increased distal flow: diuretics, osmotic diuresis, salt-wasting nephropathies
      2. Increased secretion of potassium
         a. Mineralocorticoid excess: primary hyperaldosteronism, secondary hyperaldosteronism (malignant hypertension, renin-secreting tumors, renal artery stenosis, hypovolemia), apparent mineralocorticoid excess (licorice, chewing tobacco, carbenoxolone), congenital adrenal hyperplasia, Cushing's syndrome, Bartter's syndrome
         b. Distal delivery of non-reabsorbed anions: vomiting, nasogastric suction, proximal (type 2) renal tubular acidosis, diabetic ketoacidosis, glue-sniffing (toluene abuse), penicillin derivatives
         c. Other: amphotericin B, Liddle's syndrome, hypomagnesemia

of K$^+$ redistribution as well as excessive renal K$^+$ loss. Treatment of diabetic ketoacidosis with insulin may lead to hypokalemia due to stimulation of the Na$^+$-H$^+$ antiporter and (secondarily) the Na$^+$, K$^+$-ATPase pump. Furthermore, uncontrolled hyperglycemia often leads to K$^+$ depletion from an osmotic diuresis (see below). Stress-induced catecholamine release and administration of β_2-adrenergic agonists directly induce cellular uptake of K$^+$ and promote insulin secretion by pancreatic islet β cells. *Hypokalemic periodic paralysis* is a rare condition characterized by recurrent episodic weakness or paralysis (Chap. 381). Since K$^+$ is the major ICF cation, anabolic states can potentially result in hypokalemia due to a K$^+$ shift into cells. This may occur following rapid cell growth seen in patients with pernicious anemia treated with vitamin B$_{12}$ or with neutropenia after treatment with granulocyte-macrophage colony stimulating factor. Massive transfusion with thawed washed red blood cells (RBCs) could cause hypokalemia since frozen RBCs lose up to half of their K$^+$ during storage.

Nonrenal Loss of Potassium Excessive sweating may result in K$^+$ depletion from increased integumentary and renal K$^+$ loss. Hyperaldosteronism, secondary to ECF volume contraction, enhances K$^+$ excretion in the urine (Chap. 331). Normally, K$^+$ lost in the stool amounts to 5 to 10 mmol/d in a volume of 100 to 200 mL. Hypokalemia subsequent to increased gastrointestinal loss can occur in patients with profuse diarrhea (usually secretory), villous adenomas, VIPomas, or laxative abuse. However, the loss of gastric secretions does not account for the moderate to severe K$^+$ depletion often associated with vomiting or nasogastric suction. Since the K$^+$ concentration of gastric fluid is 5 to 10 mmol/L, it would take 30 to 80 L of vomitus to achieve a K$^+$ deficit of 300 to 400 mmol typically seen in these patients. In fact, the hypokalemia is primarily due to increased renal K$^-$ excretion. Loss of gastric contents results in volume depletion and metabolic alkalosis, both of which promote kaliuresis. Hypovolemia stimulates aldosterone release, which augments K$^+$ secretion by the principal cells. In addition, the filtered load of HCO$_3^-$ exceeds the reabsorptive capacity of the proximal convoluted tubule, thereby increasing distal delivery of NaHCO$_3$, which enhances the electrochemical gradient favoring K$^+$ loss in the urine.

Renal Loss of Potassium In general, most cases of chronic hypokalemia are due to renal K$^+$ wasting. This may be due to factors that increase the K$^+$ concentration in the lumen of the CCD or augment distal flow rate. As described above, distal nephron K$^+$ secretion is driven by a lumen-negative TEPD, affected by aldosterone and the relative rates of reabsorption of Na$^+$ and its accompanying anion(s). Mineralocorticoid excess commonly results in hypokalemia (Chap. 331). *Primary hyperaldosteronism* is due to dysregulated aldosterone secretion by an adrenal adenoma (Conn's syndrome) or carcinoma or to adrenocortical hyperplasia. In a rare subset of patients, the disorder is familial (autosomal dominant) and aldosterone levels can be suppressed by administering low doses of exogenous glucocorticoid. The molecular defect responsible for *glucocorticoid-remediable hyperaldosteronism* is a rearranged gene (due to a chromosomal crossover), containing the 5'-regulatory region of the 11β-hydroxylase gene and the coding sequence of the aldosterone synthase gene. Consequently, mineralocorticoid is synthesized in the zona fasciculata and regulated by corticotropin. A number of conditions associated with hyperreninemia result in secondary hyperaldosteronism and renal K$^+$ wasting. High renin levels are commonly seen in both renovascular and malignant hypertension. Renin-secreting tumors of the juxtaglomerular apparatus are a rare cause of hypokalemia. Other tumors that have been reported to produce renin include renal cell carcinoma, ovarian carcinoma, and Wilms' tumor. Hyperreninemia may also occur secondary to decreased effective circulating arterial volume.

In the absence of elevated renin or aldosterone levels, enhanced distal nephron secretion of K$^+$ may result from increased production of non-aldosterone mineralocorticoids in *congenital adrenal hyperplasia* (Chap. 331). Glucocorticoid-stimulated kaliuresis does not normally occur due to the conversion of cortisol to cortisone by 11β-

hydroxysteroid dehydrogenase (11β-HSDH). Therefore, 11β-HSDH deficiency or suppression allows cortisol to bind to the aldosterone receptor and leads to the *syndrome of apparent mineralocorticoid excess*. Drugs that inhibit the activity of 11β-HSDH include glycyrrhetinic acid, present in licorice, chewing tobacco, and carbenoxolone. The presentation of Cushing's syndrome may include hypokalemia if the capacity of 11β-HSDH to inactivate cortisol is overwhelmed by persistently elevated glucocorticoid levels.

Liddle's syndrome is a rare familial (autosomal dominant) disease characterized by hypertension, hypokalemic metabolic alkalosis, renal K^+ wasting, and suppressed renin and aldosterone secretion (Chap. 331). Increased distal delivery of Na^+ with a non-reabsorbable anion (not Cl^-) enhances the lumen-negative TEPD and K^+ secretion. Classically, this is seen with *proximal (type 2) renal tubular acidosis* (RTA) and vomiting, associated with bicarbonaturia. Diabetic keto-acidosis and toluene abuse (glue-sniffing) can lead to increased delivery of β-hydroxybutyrate and hippurate, respectively, to the CCD and to renal K^+ loss. High doses of penicillin derivatives administered to volume-depleted patients may likewise promote renal K^+ secretion as well as an osmotic diuresis. *Classic distal (type 1) RTA* is associated with hypokalemia due to increased renal K^+ loss, the mechanism of which is uncertain. Amphotericin B causes hypokalemia due to increased distal nephron permeability to Na^+ and K^+ and to renal K^+ wasting.

Bartter's syndrome is a disorder characterized by hypokalemia, metabolic alkalosis, hyperreninemic hyperaldosteronism secondary to ECF volume contraction, and juxtaglomerular apparatus hyperplasia (Chap. 331). Finally, diuretic use and abuse are common causes of K^+ depletion. Carbonic anhydrase inhibitors, loop diuretics, and thiazides are all kaliuretic. The degree of hypokalemia tends to be greater with long-acting agents and is dose-dependent. Increased renal K^+ excretion is due primarily to increased distal solute delivery and secondary hyperaldosteronism (due to volume depletion).

CLINICAL FEATURES   The clinical manifestations of K^+ depletion vary greatly between individual patients, and their severity depends on the degree of hypokalemia. Symptoms seldom occur unless the plasma K^+ concentration is less than 3 mmol/L. Fatigue, myalgia, and muscular weakness of the lower extremities are common complaints and are due to a lower (more negative) resting membrane potential. More severe hypokalemia may lead to progressive weakness, hypoventilation (due to respiratory muscle involvement), and eventually complete paralysis. Impaired muscle metabolism and the blunted hyperemic response to exercise associated with profound K^+ depletion increase the risk of rhabdomyolysis. Smooth-muscle function may also be affected and manifest as paralytic ileus.

The electrocardiographic changes of hypokalemia (Fig. 226-19) are due to delayed ventricular repolarization and do not correlate well with the plasma K^+ concentration. Early changes include flattening or inversion of the T wave, a prominent U wave, ST-segment depression, and a prolonged QU interval. Severe K^+ depletion may result in a prolonged PR interval, decreased voltage and widening of the QRS complex, and an increased risk of ventricular arrhythmias, especially in patients with myocardial ischemia or left ventricular hypertrophy. Hypokalemia may also predispose to digitalis toxicity. Epidemiologic studies have linked a low-K^+ diet with an increased prevalence of hypertension, particularly among African Americans. Furthermore, in patients with essential hypertension, systemic blood pressure may be lowered by K^+ supplementation. The mechanism of the hypertensive effect of K^+ depletion is not certain but may relate to enhanced distal NaCl reabsorption.

Hypokalemia is often associated with acid-base disturbances related to the underlying disorder. In addition, K^+ depletion results in intracellular acidification and an increase in net acid excretion or new HCO_3^- production. This is a consequence of enhanced proximal HCO_3^- reabsorption, increased renal ammoniagenesis, and increased distal H^+ secretion. This contributes to the generation of metabolic alkalosis frequently present in hypokalemic patients. NDI (see above) is not uncommonly seen in K^+ depletion and is manifest as polydipsia and polyuria. Glucose intolerance may also occur with hypokalemia and has been attributed to either impaired insulin secretion or peripheral insulin resistance.

DIAGNOSIS   In most cases, the etiology of K^+ depletion can be determined by a careful history. Diuretic and laxative abuse as well as surreptitious vomiting may be difficult to identify but should be excluded. Rarely, patients with a marked leukocytosis (e.g., acute myeloid leukemia) and normokalemia may have a low measured plasma K^+ concentration due to white blood cell uptake of K^+ at room temperature. This *pseudohypokalemia* can be avoided by storing the blood sample on ice or rapidly separating the plasma (or serum) from the cells. After eliminating decreased intake and intracellular shift as potential causes of hypokalemia, examination of the renal response can help to clarify the source of K^+ loss. The appropriate response to K^+ depletion is to excrete less than 15 mmol/d of K^+ in the urine, due to increased reabsorption and decreased distal secretion. Hypokalemia with minimal renal K^+ excretion suggests that K^+ was lost via the skin or gastrointestinal tract or that there is a remote history of vomiting or diuretic use. As described above, renal K^+ wasting may be due to factors that either increase the K^+ concentration in the CCD or increase the distal flow rate (or both). The ECF volume status, blood pressure, and associated acid-base disorder may help to differentiate the causes of excessive renal K^+ loss. A rapid and simple test designed to evaluate the driving force for net K^+ secretion is the *transtubular K^+ concentration gradient* (TTKG). The TTKG is the ratio of the K^+ concentration in the lumen of the CCD ($[K^+]_{CCD}$) to that in peritubular capillaries or plasma ($[K^+]_P$). The validity of this measurement depends on three assumptions: (1) few solutes are reabsorbed in the medullary collecting duct (MCD), (2) K^+ is neither secreted nor reabsorbed in the MCD, and (3) the osmolality of the fluid in the terminal CCD is known. Significant reabsorption or secretion of K^+ in the MCD seldom occurs, except in profound K^+ depletion or excess, respectively. When AVP is acting ($OSM_U \geq OSM_P$), the osmolality in the terminal CCD is the same as that of plasma, and the K^+ concentration in the lumen of the distal nephron can be estimated by dividing the urine K^+ concentration ($[K^+]_U$) by the ratio of the urine to plasma osmolality (OSM_U/OSM_P):

$$[K^+]_{CCD} = [K^+]_U \div (OSM_U/OSM_P)$$

$$TTKG = \frac{[K^+]_{CCD}}{[K^+]_P} = \frac{[K^+]_U \div (OSM_U/OSM_P)}{[K^+]_P}$$

Hypokalemia with a TTKG greater than 4 suggests renal K^+ loss due to increased distal K^+ secretion. Plasma renin and aldosterone levels are often helpful in differentiating the various causes of hyperaldosteronism. Bicarbonaturia and the presence of other non-reabsorbed anions also increase the TTKG and lead to renal K^+-wasting.

CLINICAL APPROACH   See Fig. 49-3.

TREATMENT   The therapeutic goals are to correct the K^+ deficit and to minimize ongoing losses. With the exception of periodic paralysis, hypokalemia resulting from transcellular shifts rarely requires intravenous K^+ supplementation, which can lead to rebound hyperkalemia. It is generally safer to correct hypokalemia via the oral route. The degree of K^+ depletion does not correlate well with the plasma K^+ concentration. A decrement of 1 mmol/L in the plasma K^+ concentration (from 4.0 to 3.0 mmol/L) may represent a total body K^+ deficit of 200 to 400 mmol, and patients with plasma levels under 3.0 mmol/L often require in excess of 600 mmol of K^+ to correct the deficit. Furthermore, factors promoting K^+ shift out of cells (e.g., insulin deficiency in diabetic ketoacidosis) may result in underestimation of the K^+ deficit. Therefore, the plasma K^+ concentration should be monitored frequently when assessing the response to treatment. Potassium chloride is usually the preparation of choice and will promote more rapid correction of hypokalemia and metabolic alkalosis. Potas-

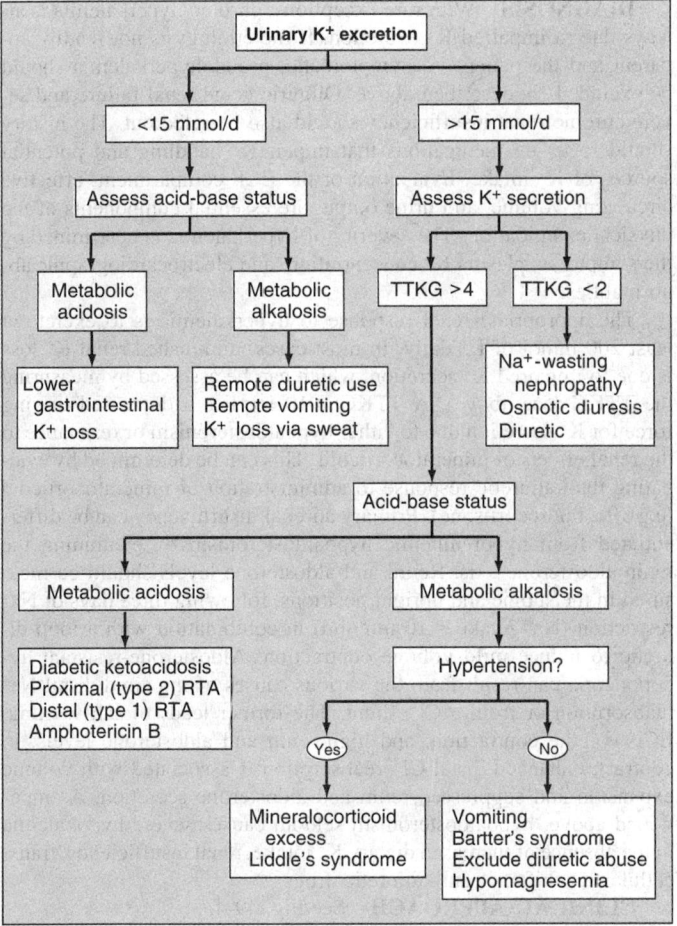

FIGURE 49-3 Algorithm depicting clinical approach to hypokalemia. TTKG, transtubular K^+ concentration gradient; RTA, renal tubular acidosis.

sium bicarbonate and citrate (metabolized to HCO_3^-) tend to alkalinize the patient and would be more appropriate for hypokalemia associated with chronic diarrhea or RTA.

Patients with severe hypokalemia or those unable to take anything by mouth require intravenous replacement therapy with KCl. The maximum concentration of administered K^+ should be no more than 40 mmol/L via a peripheral vein or 60 mmol/L via a central vein. The rate of infusion should not exceed 20 mmol/h unless paralysis or malignant ventricular arrhythmias are present. Ideally, KCl should be mixed in normal saline since dextrose solutions may initially exacerbate hypokalemia due to insulin-mediated movement of K^+ into cells. Rapid intravenous administration of K^+ should be used judiciously and requires close observation of the clinical manifestations of hypokalemia (electrocardiogram and neuromuscular examination).

HYPERKALEMIA

ETIOLOGY Hyperkalemia, defined as a plasma K^+ concentration >5.0 mmol/L, occurs as a result of either K^+ release from cells or decreased renal loss. Increased K^+ intake is rarely the sole cause of hyperkalemia since the phenomenon of *potassium adaptation* ensures rapid K^+ excretion in response to increases in dietary consumption. Iatrogenic hyperkalemia may result from overzealous parenteral K^+ replacement or in patients with renal insufficiency. *Pseudohyperkalemia* represents an artificially elevated plasma K^+ concentration due to K^+ movement out of cells immediately prior to or following venipuncture. Contributing factors include prolonged use of a tourniquet with or without repeated fist clenching, hemolysis, and marked leukocytosis or thrombocytosis. The latter two result in an elevated serum K^+ concentration due to release of intracellular K^+ following clot formation. Pseudohyperkalemia should be suspected in an otherwise

asymptomatic patient with no obvious underlying cause. If proper venipuncture technique is used and a plasma (not serum) K^+ concentration is measured, it should be normal. Intravascular hemolysis, tumor lysis syndrome, and rhabdomyolysis all lead to K^+ release from cells as a result of tissue breakdown. Metabolic acidoses, with the exception of those due to the accumulation of organic anions, can be associated with mild hyperkalemia resulting from intracellular buffering of H^+ (see above). As previously described (p. 278), insulin deficiency and hypertonicity (e.g., hyperglycemia) promote K^+ shift from the ICF to the ECF. The severity of exercise-induced hyperkalemia is related to the degree of exertion. It is due to release of K^+ from muscles and is usually rapidly reversible, often associated with rebound hypokalemia. Treatment with beta blockers rarely causes hyperkalemia but may contribute to the elevation in plasma K^+ concentration seen with other conditions. *Hyperkalemic periodic paralysis* (Chap. 381) is a rare autosomal dominant disorder characterized by episodic weakness or paralysis, precipitated by stimuli that normally lead to mild hyperkalemia (e.g., exercise). The genetic defect appears to be a single amino acid substitution due to a mutation in the gene for the skeletal muscle Na^+ channel. Hyperkalemia may occur with severe digitalis toxicity due to inhibition of the Na^+, K^+-ATPase pump. Depolarizing muscle relaxants such as succinylcholine can increase the plasma K^+ concentration, especially in patients with massive trauma, burns, or neuromuscular disease.

Chronic hyperkalemia is virtually always associated with decreased renal K^+ excretion due to either impaired secretion or diminished distal solute delivery (Table 49-4). The latter is seldom the only cause of impaired K^+ excretion but may significantly contribute to hyperkalemia in protein-malnourished (low urea excretion) and ECF volume–contracted (decreased distal NaCl delivery) patients. Decreased K^+ secretion by the principal cells results from either impaired Na^+ reabsorption or increased Cl^- reabsorption, both of which give rise to a diminished (less lumen-negative) TEPD in the CCD. *Hyporeninemic hypoaldosteronism* is a syndrome characterized by euvolemia or ECF volume expansion and suppressed renin and aldosterone levels (Chaps. 331 and 333). This disorder is commonly seen in mild renal insufficiency, diabetic nephropathy, or chronic tubulointerstitial disease. Patients frequently have an impaired kaliuretic response to exogenous mineralocorticoid administration, suggesting that enhanced distal Cl^- reabsorption (electroneutral Na^+ reabsorption) may account for many of the findings of hyporeninemic hypoaldosteronism. NSAIDs inhibit renin secretion and the synthesis of vasodilatory renal prostaglandins. The resultant decrease in GFR and K^+ secretion is often manifest as hyperkalemia. As a rule, the degree of hyperkalemia due to hypoaldosteronism is mild in the absence of increased K^+ intake or renal dysfunction. Angiotensin-converting enzyme (ACE) inhibitors block the conversion of angiotensin I to angiotensin II, resulting in

Table 49-4 Causes of Hyperkalemia

I. Renal failure
II. Decreased distal flow (i.e., decreased effective circulating arterial volume)
III. Decreased K^+ secretion
  A. Impaired Na^+ reabsorption
    1. Primary hypoaldosteronism: adrenal insufficiency, adrenal enzyme deficiency (21-hydroxylase, 3β-hydroxysteroid dehydrogenase, corticosterone methyl oxidase)
    2. Secondary hypoaldosteronism: hyporeninemia, drugs (ACE inhibitors, NSAIDs, heparin)
    3. Resistance to aldosterone: pseudohypoaldosteronism, tubulointerstitial disease, drugs (K^+-sparing diuretics, trimethoprim, pentamidine)
  B. Enhanced Cl^- reabsorption (chloride shunt)
    1 Gordon's syndrome
    2. Cyclosporine

NOTE: ACE, angiotensin-converting enzyme; NSAIDs, nonsteroidal anti-inflammatory drugs.

impaired aldosterone release. Patients at increased risk of ACE inhibitor–induced hyperkalemia include those with diabetes mellitus, renal insufficiency, decreased effective circulating arterial volume, bilateral renal artery stenosis, or concurrent use of K^+-sparing diuretics or NSAIDs.

Decreased aldosterone synthesis may be due to *primary adrenal insufficiency* (Addison's disease) or congenital adrenal enzyme deficiency (Chap. 331). Heparin (including low-molecular-weight heparin) inhibits production of aldosterone by the cells of the zona glomerulosa and can lead to severe hyperkalemia in a subset of patients with underlying renal disease; diabetes mellitus; or those receiving K^+-sparing diuretics, ACE inhibitors, or NSAIDs. *Pseudohypoaldosteronism* is a rare familial disorder characterized by hyperkalemia, metabolic acidosis, renal Na^+ wasting, hypotension, high renin and aldosterone levels, and end-organ resistance to aldosterone. The gene encoding the mineralocorticoid receptor is normal in these patients, and the electrolyte abnormalities can be reversed with suprapharmacologic doses of an exogenous mineralocorticoid (e.g., 9α-fludrocortisone) or an inhibitor of 11β-HSDH (e.g., carbenoxolone). The kaliuretic response to aldosterone is impaired by K^+-sparing diuretics. Spironolactone is a competitive mineralocorticoid antagonist, whereas amiloride and triamterene block the apical Na^+ channel of the principal cell. Two other drugs that impair K^+ secretion by blocking distal nephron Na^+ reabsorption are trimethoprim and pentamidine. These antimicrobial agents may contribute to the hyperkalemia often seen in patients infected with HIV who are being treated for *Pneumocystis carinii* pneumonia.

Hyperkalemia frequently complicates acute oliguric renal failure due to increased K^+ release from cells (acidosis, catabolism) and decreased excretion. Increased distal flow rate and K^+ secretion per nephron compensate for decreased renal mass in chronic renal insufficiency. However, these adaptive mechanisms eventually fail to maintain K^+ balance when the GFR falls below 10 to 15 mL/min or oliguria ensues. Otherwise asymptomatic urinary tract obstruction is an often overlooked cause of hyperkalemia. Other nephropathies associated with impaired K^+ excretion include drug-induced interstitial nephritis, lupus nephritis, sickle cell disease, and diabetic nephropathy.

Gordon's syndrome is a rare condition characterized by hyperkalemia, metabolic acidosis, and a normal GFR. These patients are usually volume-expanded with suppressed renin and aldosterone levels as well as refractory to the kaliuretic effect of exogenous mineralocorticoids. It has been suggested that these findings could all be accounted for by increased distal Cl^- reabsorption (electroneutral Na^+ reabsorption), also referred to as a *Cl^- shunt*. A similar mechanism may be partially responsible for the hyperkalemia associated with cyclosporine nephrotoxicity. *Hyperkalemic distal (type 4) RTA* may be due to either hypoaldosteronism or a Cl^- shunt (aldosterone-resistant).

CLINICAL FEATURES Since the resting membrane potential is related to the ratio of the ICF to ECF K^+ concentration, hyperkalemia partially depolarizes the cell membrane. Prolonged depolarization impairs membrane excitability and is manifest as weakness, which may progress to flaccid paralysis and hypoventilation if the respiratory muscles are involved. Hyperkalemia also inhibits renal ammoniagenesis and reabsorption of NH_4^+ in the thick ascending limb of the loop of Henle. Thus, net acid excretion is impaired and results in metabolic acidosis, which may further exacerbate the hyperkalemia due to K^+ movement out of cells.

The most serious effect of hyperkalemia is cardiac toxicity, which does not correlate well with the plasma K^+ concentration. The earliest electrocardiographic changes include increased T-wave amplitude, or peaked T waves. More severe degrees of hyperkalemia result in a prolonged PR interval and QRS duration, atrioventricular conduction delay, and loss of P waves. Progressive widening of the QRS complex and merging with the T wave produces a sinewave pattern. The terminal event is usually ventricular fibrillation or asystole.

DIAGNOSIS With rare exceptions, chronic hyperkalemia is always due to impaired K^+ excretion. If the etiology is not readily apparent and the patient is asymptomatic, pseudohyperkalemia should be excluded, as described above. Oliguric acute renal failure and severe chronic renal insufficiency should also be ruled out. The history should focus on medications that impair K^+ handling and potential sources of K^+ intake. Evaluation of the ECF compartment, effective circulating volume, and urine output are essential components of the physical examination. The severity of hyperkalemia is determined by the symptoms, plasma K^+ concentration, and electrocardiographic abnormalities.

The appropriate renal response to hyperkalemia is to excrete at least 200 mmol of K^+ daily. In most cases, diminished renal K^+ loss is due to impaired K^+ secretion, which can be assessed by measuring the TTKG (see above). A TTKG <10 implies a decreased driving force for K^+ secretion due to either hypoaldosteronism or resistance to the renal effects of mineralocorticoid. This can be determined by evaluating the kaliuretic response to administration of mineralocorticoid (e.g., 9α-fludrocortisone). Primary adrenal insufficiency can be differentiated from hyporeninemic hypoaldosteronism by examining the renin-aldosterone axis. Renin and aldosterone levels should be measured in the supine and upright positions, following three days of Na^+ restriction (Na^+ intake <10 mmol/d) in combination with a loop diuretic to induce mild volume contraction. Aldosterone-resistant hyperkalemia can result from the various causes of impaired distal Na^+ reabsorption or from a Cl^- shunt. The former leads to salt wasting, ECF volume contraction, and high renin and aldosterone levels. In contrast, enhanced distal Cl^- reabsorption is associated with volume expansion and suppressed renin and aldosterone secretion. As mentioned above, hypoaldosteronism seldom causes severe hypokalemia in the absence of increased dietary K^+ intake, renal insufficiency, transcellular K^+ shifts, or antikaliuretic drugs.

CLINICAL APPROACH See Fig. 49-4.

TREATMENT The approach to therapy depends on the degree of hyperkalemia as determined by the plasma K^+ concentration, associated muscular weakness, and changes on the electrocardiogram. Potentially fatal hyperkalemia rarely occurs unless the plasma K^+ concentration exceeds 7.5 mmol/L and is usually associated with profound weakness and absent P waves, QRS widening, or ventricular arrhythmias on the electrocardiogram.

Severe hyperkalemia requires emergent treatment directed at minimizing membrane depolarization, shifting K^+ into cells, and promoting K^+ loss. In addition, exogenous K^+ intake and antikaliuretic drugs should be discontinued. Administration of calcium gluconate decreases membrane excitability. The usual dose is 10 mL of a 10% solution infused over 2 to 3 min. The effect begins within minutes but is short-lived (30 to 60 min), and the dose can be repeated if no change in the electrocardiogram is seen after 5 to 10 min. Insulin causes K^+ to shift into cells by mechanisms described previously and will temporarily lower the plasma K^+ concentration. Although glucose alone will stimulate insulin release from normal pancreatic β cells, a more rapid response generally occurs when exogenous insulin is administered (with glucose to prevent hypoglycemia). A commonly recommended combination is 10 to 20 units of regular insulin and 25 to 50 g of glucose. Obviously, hyperglycemic patients should not be given glucose. If effective, the plasma K^+ concentration will fall by 0.5 to 1.5 mmol/L in 15 to 30 min and the effect will last for several hours. Alkali therapy with intravenous $NaHCO_3$ can also shift K^+ into cells. This is safest when administered as an isotonic solution of 3 ampules per liter (134 mmol/L $NaHCO_3$) and ideally should be reserved for severe hyperkalemia associated with metabolic acidosis. Patients with end-stage renal disease seldom respond to this intervention and may not tolerate the Na^+ load and resultant volume expansion. When administered parenterally or in nebulized form, β_2-adrenergic agonists promote cellular uptake of K^+ (see above). The onset of action is 30 min, lowering the plasma K^+ concentration by 0.5 to 1.5 mmol/L, and the effect lasts 2 to 4 h.

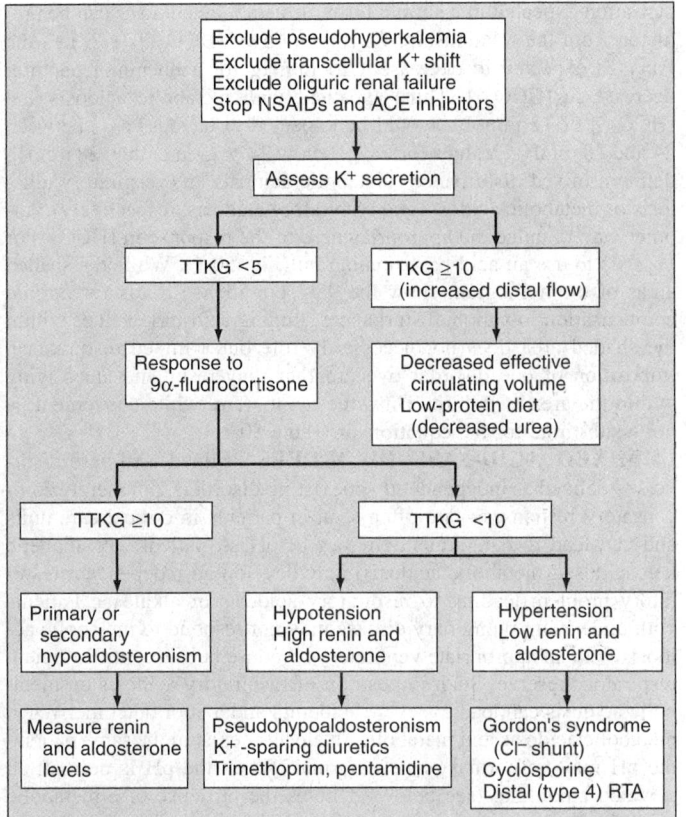

FIGURE 49-4 Algorithm depicting clinical approach to hyperkalemia. NSAID, nonsteroidal anti-inflammatory drug; ACE, angiotensin-converting enzyme; RTA, renal tubular acidosis; TTKG, transtubular K^+ concentration gradient.

Removal of K^+ can be achieved using diuretics, cation-exchange resin, or dialysis. Loop and thiazide diuretics, often in combination, may enhance K^+ excretion if renal function is adequate. Sodium polystyrene sulfonate is a cation-exchange resin that promotes the exchange of Na^+ for K^+ in the gastrointestinal tract. Each gram binds 1 mmol of K^+ and releases 2 to 3 mmol of Na^+. When given by mouth, the usual dose is 25 to 50 g mixed with 100 mL of 20% sorbitol to prevent constipation. This will generally lower the plasma K^+ concentration by 0.5 to 1.0 mmol/L within 1 to 2 h and last for 4 to 6 h. Sodium polystyrene sulfonate can also be administered as a retention enema consisting of 50 g of resin and 50 mL of 70% sorbitol mixed in 150 mL of tap water. The sorbitol should be omitted from the enema in postoperative patients due to the increased incidence of sorbitol-induced colonic necrosis, especially following renal transplantation. The most rapid and effective way of lowering the plasma K^+ concentration is hemodialysis. This should be reserved for patients with renal failure and those with severe life-threatening hyperkalemia unresponsive to more conservative measures. Peritoneal dialysis also removes K^+ but is only 15 to 20% as effective as hemodialysis. Finally, the underlying cause of the hyperkalemia should be treated. This may involve dietary modification, correction of metabolic acidosis, cautious volume expansion, and administration of exogenous mineralocorticoid.

BIBLIOGRAPHY

SODIUM AND WATER

ABRAHAM WT, SCHRIER RW: Body fluid volume regulation in health and disease. Adv Intern Med 39:23, 1994

BERL T, ROBERTSON GL: Pathophysiology of water metabolism, in *Brenner & Rector's The Kidney*, 6th ed, BM Brenner (ed). Philadelphia, Saunders, 2000, pp 866–924

FUJIWARA TM et al: Molecular biology of diabetes insipidus. Ann Rev Med 46:331, 1995

GINES P et al: Vasopressin in pathophysiological states. Semin Nephrol 14:384, 1994

GOLDSZMIDT MA, ILIESCU EA: DDAVP to prevent rapid correction in hyponatremia. Clin Nephrol 53:226, 2000

GULLANS SR, VERBALIS JG: Control of brain volume during hyperosmolar and hypoosmolar conditions. Ann Rev Med 44:289, 1993

KNEPPER MA et al: Role of aquaporins in water balance. Curr Opin Nephrol Hypertens 6:367, 1997

KUMAR S, BERL T: Sodium. Lancet 352:220, 1998

MCKENNA K, THOMPSON C: Osmoregulation in clinical disorders of thirst appreciation. Clin Endocrinol 49:139, 1998

STERNS RH et al: Neurologic sequelae after treatment of severe hyponatremia: A multicenter perspective. J Am Soc Nephrol 4:1522, 1994

VERBALIS JG: Adaptation to acute and chronic hyponatremia: Implications for symptomatology, diagnosis, and therapy. Semin Nephrol 18:3, 1998

POTASSIUM

DEFRONZO RA, SMITH JD: Clinical disorders of hyperkalemia, in *Clinical Disorders of Fluid and Electrolyte Metabolism*, 5th ed, RG Narins (ed). New York, McGraw-Hill, 1994, pp 697–754

FIELD MJ et al: Regulation of renal potassium metabolism, in *Clinical Disorders of Fluid and Electrolyte Metabolism*, 5th ed, RG Narins (ed). New York, McGraw-Hill, 1994, pp 147–174

HALPERIN ML, KAMEL KS: Potassium. Lancet 352:135, 1998

KUPIN WL, NARINS RG: The hyperkalemia of renal failure: Pathophysiology, diagnosis, and therapy. Contrib Nephrol 102:1, 1993

SCHEINMAN SJ et al: Genetic disorders of renal electrolyte transport. N Engl J Med 340:1177, 1999

WHITE PC: Disorders of aldosterone biosynthesis and action. N Engl J Med 331:250, 1994

WINGO CS, WEINER ID: Disorders of potassium balance, in *Brenner & Rector's The Kidney*, 6th ed, BM Brenner (ed). Philadelphia, Saunders, 2000, pp 998–1035

---

50   *Thomas D. DuBose, Jr.*

ACIDOSIS AND ALKALOSIS

NORMAL ACID-BASE HOMEOSTASIS

Systemic arterial pH is maintained between 7.35 and 7.45 by extracellular and intracellular chemical buffering together with respiratory and renal regulatory mechanisms. The control of arterial CO_2 tension (Pa_{CO_2}) by the central nervous system and respiratory systems and the control of the plasma bicarbonate by the kidneys stabilize the arterial pH by excretion or retention of acid or alkali. The metabolic and respiratory components that regulate systemic pH are described by the Henderson-Hasselbalch equation:

$$pH = 6.1 + \log \frac{HCO_3^-}{Pa_{CO_2} \times 0.0301}$$

Under most circumstances, CO_2 production and excretion are matched, and the usual steady-state Pa_{CO_2} is maintained at 40 mmHg. Underexcretion of CO_2 produces hypercapnia, and overexcretion causes hypocapnia. Nevertheless, production and excretion are again matched at a new steady-state Pa_{CO_2}. Therefore, the Pa_{CO_2} is regulated primarily by neural respiratory factors (Chap. 263) and is not subject to regulation by the rate of CO_2 production. Hypercapnia is usually the result of hypoventilation rather than of increased CO_2 production. Increases or decreases in Pa_{CO_2} represent derangements of neural respiratory control or are due to compensatory changes in response to a primary alteration in the plasma $[HCO_3^-]$.

Primary changes in Pa_{CO_2} can cause acidosis or alkalosis, depending on whether Pa_{CO_2} is above or below the normal value of 40 mmHg (respiratory acidosis or alkalosis, respectively). Primary alteration of Pa_{CO_2} evokes cellular buffering and renal adaptation, a slow process that becomes more efficient with time. A primary change in the plasma $[HCO_3^-]$ as a result of metabolic or renal factors results in compensatory changes in ventilation that blunt the changes in blood pH that would occur otherwise. Such respiratory alterations are referred to as *secondary*, or compensatory, changes, since they occur in response to primary metabolic changes.

The kidneys regulate plasma $[HCO_3^-]$ through three main processes: (1) "reabsorption" of filtered HCO_3^-, (2) formation of titratable acid, and (3) excretion of NH_4^+ in the urine. The kidney filters approximately 4000 mmol of HCO_3^- per day. To reabsorb the filtered load of HCO_3^-, the renal tubules must therefore secrete 4000 mmol of hydrogen ions. Between 80 and 90% of HCO_3^- is reabsorbed in the proximal tubule. The distal nephron reabsorbs the remainder and secretes protons, as generated from metabolism, to defend systemic pH. While this quantity of protons, 40 to 60 mmol/d, is small, it must be secreted to prevent chronic positive H^+ balance and metabolic acidosis. This quantity of secreted protons is represented in the urine as titratable acid and NH_4^+. Metabolic acidosis in the face of normal renal function increases NH_4^+ production and excretion. NH_4^+ production and excretion are impaired in chronic renal failure, hyperkalemia, and renal tubular acidosis.

In sum, these regulatory responses, including chemical buffering, the regulation of Pa_{CO_2} by the respiratory system, and of $[HCO_3^-]$ by the kidneys, act in concert to maintain a systemic arterial pH between 7.35 and 7.45.

DIAGNOSIS OF GENERAL TYPES OF DISTURBANCES

The most common clinical disturbances are simple acid-base disorders, i.e., metabolic acidosis or alkalosis or respiratory acidosis or alkalosis. Since compensation is not complete, the pH is abnormal in simple disturbances. More complicated clinical situations can give rise to mixed acid-base disturbances.

SIMPLE ACID-BASE DISORDERS Primary respiratory disturbances (primary changes in Pa_{CO_2}) invoke compensatory metabolic responses (secondary changes in $[HCO_3^-]$), and primary metabolic disturbances elicit predictable compensatory respiratory responses. Physiologic compensation can be predicted from the relationships displayed in Table 50-1. Primary changes in Pa_{CO_2} or $[HCO_3^-]$ alter systemic pH and cause acidosis or alkalosis. To illustrate, metabolic acidosis due to an increase in endogenous acids (e.g., ketoacidosis) lowers extracellular fluid $[HCO_3^-]$ and decreases extracellular pH. This stimulates the medullary chemoreceptors to increase ventilation and to return the ratio of $[HCO_3^-]$ to Pa_{CO_2}, and thus pH, toward normal, although not to normal. The degree of respiratory com-

Table 50-1 Prediction of Compensatory Responses on Simple Acid-Base Disturbances

Disorder	Prediction of Compensation
Metabolic acidosis	$Pa_{CO_2} = (1.5 \times HCO_3^-) + 8$
	or
	Pa_{CO_2} will $\downarrow$ 1.25 mmHg per mmol/L $\downarrow$ in $[HCO_3^-]$
	or
	$Pa_{CO_2} = [HCO_3^-] + 15$
Metabolic alkalosis	Pa_{CO_2} will $\uparrow$ 0.75 mmHg per mmol/L $\uparrow$ in $[HCO_3^-]$
	or
	Pa_{CO_2} will $\uparrow$ 6 mmHg per 10-mmol/L $\uparrow$ in $[HCO_3^-]$
	or
	$Pa_{CO_2} = [HCO_3^-] + 15$
Respiratory alkalosis	
Acute	$[HCO_3^-]$ will $\downarrow$ 2 mmol/L per 10-mmHg $\downarrow$ in Pa_{CO_2}
Chronic	$[HCO_3^-]$ will $\downarrow$ 4 mmol/L per 10-mmHg $\downarrow$ in Pa_{CO_2}
Respiratory acidosis	
Acute	$[HCO_3^-]$ will $\uparrow$ 1 mmol/L per 10-mmHg $\uparrow$ in Pa_{CO_2}
Chronic	$[HCO_3^-]$ will $\downarrow$ 4 mmol/L per 10-mmHg $\uparrow$ in Pa_{CO_2}

pensation expected in a simple form of metabolic acidosis can be predicted from the relationship: $Pa_{CO_2} = (1.5 \times [HCO_3^-]) + 8$, i.e., the Pa_{CO_2} is expected to decrease 1.25 mmHg for each mmol per liter decrease in $[HCO_3^-]$. Thus, a patient with metabolic acidosis and $[HCO_3^-]$ of 12 mmol/L would be expected to have a Pa_{CO_2} between 24 and 28 mmHg. Values for Pa_{CO_2} below 24 or greater than 28 mmHg define a mixed disturbance (metabolic acidosis and respiratory alkalosis or metabolic acidosis and respiratory acidosis, respectively). Another way to judge the appropriateness of the response in $[HCO_3^-]$ or Pa_{CO_2} is to use an acid-base nomogram (Fig. 50-1). While the shaded areas of the nomogram show the 95% confidence limits for normal compensation in simple disturbances, finding acid-base values within the shaded area does not necessarily rule out a mixed disturbance. Imposition of one disorder over another may result in values lying within the area of a third. Thus, the nomogram, while convenient, is not a substitute for the equations in Table 50-1.

MIXED ACID-BASE DISORDERS Mixed acid-base disorders—defined as independently coexisting disorders, not merely compensatory responses—are often seen in patients in critical care units and can lead to dangerous extremes of pH. A patient with diabetic ketoacidosis (metabolic acidosis) may develop an independent respiratory problem leading to respiratory acidosis or alkalosis. Patients with underlying pulmonary disease may not respond to metabolic acidosis with an appropriate ventilatory response because of insufficient respiratory reserve. Such imposition of respiratory acidosis on metabolic acidosis can lead to severe acidemia and a poor outcome. When metabolic acidosis and metabolic alkalosis coexist in the same patient, the pH may be normal or near normal. When the pH is normal, an elevated anion gap (see below) denotes the presence of a metabolic acidosis. A diabetic patient with ketoacidosis may have renal dysfunction resulting in simultaneous metabolic acidosis. Patients who have ingested an overdose of drug combinations such as sedatives and salicylates may have mixed disturbances as a result of the acid-base response to the individual drugs (metabolic acidosis mixed with respiratory acidosis or respiratory alkalosis, respectively). Even more complex are triple acid-base disturbances. For example, patients with metabolic acidosis due to alcoholic ketoacidosis may develop metabolic alkalosis due to vomiting and superimposed respiratory alkalosis due to the hyperventilation of hepatic dysfunction or alcohol withdrawal.

DIAGNOSIS OF ACID-BASE DISORDERS Care should be taken when measuring blood gases to obtain the arterial blood sample without using excessive heparin. In the determination of arterial blood gases by the clinical laboratory, both pH and Pa_{CO_2} are measured, and the $[HCO_3^-]$ is calculated from the Henderson-Hasselbalch equation. This calculated value should be compared with the measured $[HCO_3^-]$ (total CO_2) on the electrolyte panel. These two values should agree within 2 mmol/L. If they do not, the values may not have been drawn simultaneously, a laboratory error may be present, or an error could have been made in calculating the $[HCO_3^-]$. After verifying the blood acid-base values, one can then identify the precise acid-base disorder.

The most common causes of acid-base disorders should be kept in mind while probing the history for clues about the etiology. For example, established chronic renal failure is expected to cause a metabolic acidosis, and chronic vomiting frequently causes metabolic alkalosis. Patients with pneumonia, sepsis, or cardiac failure frequently have respiratory alkalosis, and patients with chronic obstructive pulmonary disease or a sedative drug overdose often display a respiratory acidosis. The drug history is important since loop or thiazide diuretics may cause metabolic alkalosis, and the carbonic anhydrase inhibitor, acetazolamide, can result in metabolic acidosis.

Blood for electrolytes and arterial blood gases should be drawn simultaneously prior to therapy, since an increase in $[HCO_3^-]$ occurs with metabolic alkalosis and respiratory acidosis. Conversely, a decrease in $[HCO_3^-]$ occurs in metabolic acidosis and respiratory alkalosis.

Metabolic acidosis leads to hyperkalemia as a result of cellular shifts in which H⁺ is exchanged for K⁺ or Na⁺. For each decrease in blood pH of 0.10, the plasma [K⁺] should rise by 0.6 mmol/L. This relationship is not invariable. Diabetic ketoacidosis, lactic acidosis, diarrhea, and renal tubular acidosis (RTA) are often associated with potassium depletion because of urinary K⁺ wasting.

Anion Gap All evaluations of acid-base disorders should include a simple calculation of the anion gap (AG); it represents those unmeasured anions in plasma (normally 10 to 12 mmol/L) and is calculated as follows: $AG = Na^+ - (Cl^- + HCO_3^-)$. The unmeasured anions include anionic proteins, phosphate, sulfate, and organic anions. When acid anions, such as acetoacetate and lactate, accumulate in extracellular fluid, the AG increases, causing a high-AG acidosis. An increase in the AG is most often due to an increase in unmeasured anions and less commonly is due to a decrease in unmeasured cations (calcium, magnesium, potassium). In addition, the AG may increase with an increase in anionic albumin, either because of increased albumin concentration or alkalosis, which alters albumin charge. A decrease in the AG can be due to: (1) an increase in unmeasured cations; (2) the addition to the blood of abnormal cations, such as lithium (lithium intoxication) or cationic immunoglobulins (plasma cell dyscrasias); (3) a reduction in the major plasma anion albumin concentration (nephrotic syndrome); (4) a decrease in the effective anionic charge on albumin by acidosis; or (5) hyperviscosity and severe hyperlipidemia, which can lead to an underestimation of sodium and chloride concentrations.

In the face of a normal serum albumin, a high AG is usually due to non-chloride-containing acids that contain inorganic (phosphate, sulfate), organic (ketoacids, lactate, uremic organic anions), exogenous (salicylate or ingested toxins with organic acid production), or unidentified anions. By definition, therefore, a high-AG acidosis has two identifying features: a low [HCO₃⁻] and an elevated AG. The latter is present even if an additional acid-base disorder is superimposed to modify the [HCO₃⁻] independently. Simultaneous metabolic acidosis of the high-AG variety plus either chronic respiratory acidosis or metabolic alkalosis represents such a situation in which [HCO₃⁻] may be normal or even high. However, the AG is elevated, and [Cl⁻] is depressed.

Similarly, normal values for [HCO₃⁻], Pa$_{CO_2}$, and pH do not ensure the absence of an acid-base disturbance. For instance, an alcoholic who has been vomiting may develop a metabolic alkalosis with a pH of 7.55, Pa$_{CO_2}$ of 48 mmHg, [HCO₃⁻] of 40 mmol/L, [Na⁺] of 135, [Cl⁻] of 80, and [K⁺] of 2.8. If such a patient were then to develop a superimposed alcoholic ketoacidosis with a β-hydroxybutyrate concentration of 15 mM, arterial pH would fall to 7.40, [HCO₃⁻] to 25 mmol/L, and the Pa$_{CO_2}$ to 40 mmHg. Although these blood gases are normal, the AG is elevated at 30 mmol/L, indicating a mixed metabolic alkalosis and metabolic acidosis.

METABOLIC ACIDOSIS

Metabolic acidosis can occur because of an increase in endogenous acid production (such as lactate and ketoacids), loss of bicarbonate (as in diarrhea), or accumulation of endogenous acids (as in renal failure). Metabolic acidosis has profound effects on the respiratory, cardiac, and nervous systems. The fall in blood pH is accompanied by a char-

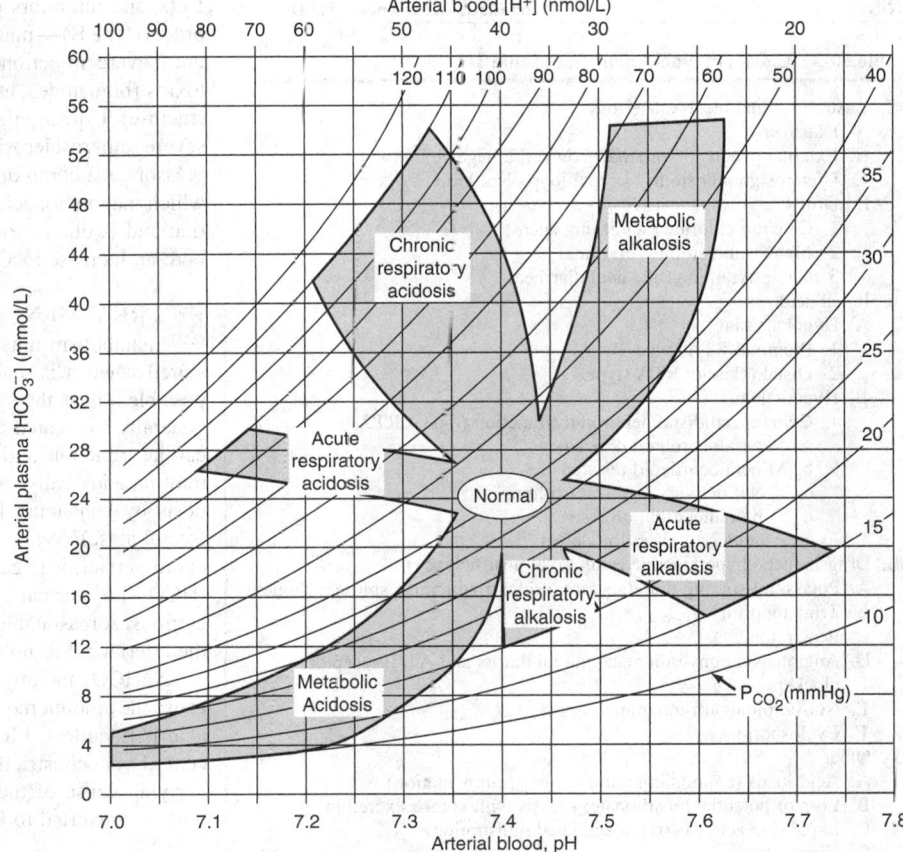

FIGURE 50-1 Acid-base nomogram. Shown are the 90% confidence limits of the normal respiratory and metabolic compensations for primary acid-base disturbances. (*From DuBose, used with permission.*)

acteristic increase in ventilation, especially the tidal volume (Kussmaul respiration). Intrinsic cardiac contractility may be depressed, but inotropic function can be normal because of catecholamine release. Both peripheral arterial vasodilation and central venoconstriction can be present; the decrease in central and pulmonary vascular compliance predisposes to pulmonary edema with even minimal volume overload. Central nervous system function is depressed, with headache, lethargy, stupor, and, in some cases, even coma. Glucose intolerance may also occur.

There are two major categories of clinical metabolic acidosis: high-AG and normal-AG, or hyperchloremic acidosis (Table 50-2 and Table 50-3).

Rx **TREATMENT** Treatment of metabolic acidosis with alkali should be reserved for severe acidemia except when the patient has no "potential HCO₃⁻" in plasma. Potential [HCO₃⁻] can be estimated from the increment (Δ) in the anion gap (ΔAG = patient's AG − 10). It must be determined if the acid anion in plasma is metabolizable (i.e. β-hydroxybutyrate, acetoacetate, and lactate) or nonmetabolizable (anions that accumulate in chronic renal failure and after toxin ingestion). The latter requires return of renal function to replenish the [HCO₃⁻] deficit, a slow and often unpredictable process. Consequently, patients with a normal AG acidosis (hyperchloremic acidosis), a slightly elevated AG (mixed hyperchloremic and AG acidosis), or an AG attributable to a nonmetabolizable anion in the

Table 50-2   Causes of High-Anion-Gap Metabolic Acidosis

Lactic acidosis	Toxins
Ketoacidosis	Ethylene glycol
Diabetic	Methanol
Alcoholic	Salicylates
Starvation	Renal failure (acute and chronic)

Table 50-3 Causes of Non-Anion-Gap Acidosis

I. Gastrointestinal bicarbonate loss
  A. Diarrhea
  B. External pancreatic or small-bowel drainage
  C. Ureterosigmoidostomy, jejunal loop, ileal loop
  D. Drugs
    1. Calcium chloride (acidifying agent)
    2. Magnesium sulfate (diarrhea)
    3. Cholestyramine (bile acid diarrhea)
II. Renal acidosis
  A. Hypokalemia
    1. Proximal RTA (type 2)
    2. Distal (classic) RTA (type 1)
  B. Hyperkalemia
    1. Generalized distal nephron dysfunction (type 4 RTA)
      a. Mineralocorticoid deficiency
      b. Mineralocorticoid resistance
      c. ↓ Na$^+$ delivery to distal nephron
      d. Tubulointerstitial disease
      e. Ammonium excretion defect
III. Drug-induced hyperkalemia (with renal insufficiency)
  A. Potassium-sparing diuretics (amiloride, triamterene, spironolactone)
  B. Trimethoprim
  C. Pentamidine
  D. Angiotensin-converting enzyme inhibitors and AT-II receptor blockers
  E. Nonsteroidal anti-inflammatory drugs
  F. Cyclosporine
IV. Other
  A. Acid loads (ammonium chloride, hyperalimentation)
  B. Loss of potential bicarbonate: ketosis with ketone excretion
  C. Expansion acidosis (rapid saline administration)
  D. Hippurate
  E. Cation exchange resins

NOTE: RTA, renal tubular acidosis; AT-II, angiotensin-II receptor blockers.

face of renal failure should receive alkali therapy, either orally (NaHCO$_3$ or Shohl's solution) or intravenously (NaHCO$_3$), in an amount necessary to slowly increase the plasma [HCO$_3^-$] into the 20 to 22 mmol/L range.

Controversy exists, however, in regard to the use of alkali in patients with a pure AG acidosis owing to accumulation of a metabolizable organic acid anion (ketoacidosis or lactic acidosis). In general, severe acidosis (pH < 7.20) warrants the intravenous administration of 50 to 100 meq of NaHCO$_3$, over 30 to 45 min, during the initial 1 to 2 h of therapy. Provision of such modest quantities of alkali in this situation seems to provide an added measure of safety, but it is essential to monitor plasma electrolytes during the course of therapy, since the [K$^+$] may decline as pH rises. The goal is to increase the [HCO$_3^-$] to 10 meq/L and the pH to 7.25, not to increase these values to normal.

HIGH-ANION-GAP ACIDOSES   There are four principal causes of a high-AG acidosis: (1) lactic acidosis, (2) ketoacidosis, (3) ingested toxins (Table 50-2), and (4) acute and chronic renal failure. Initial screening to differentiate the high-AG acidoses should include: (1) a probe of the history for evidence of drug and toxin ingestion and measurement of arterial blood gas to detect coexistent respiratory alkalosis (salicylates); (2) determination of whether diabetes mellitus is present (diabetic ketoacidosis); (3) a search for evidence of alcoholism or increased levels of β-hydroxybutyrate (alcoholic ketoacidosis); (4) observation for clinical signs of uremia and determination of the blood urea nitrogen (BUN) and creatinine (uremic acidosis); (5) inspection of the urine for oxalate crystals (ethylene glycol); and (6) recognition of the numerous clinical settings in which lactate levels may be increased (hypotension, shock, cardiac failure, leukemia, cancer, and drug or toxin ingestion).

Lactic Acidosis   An increase in plasma L-lactate may be secondary to poor tissue perfusion (type A)—circulatory insufficiency (shock, circulatory failure), severe anemia, mitochondrial enzyme de-

fects, and inhibitors (carbon monoxide, cyanide)—or to aerobic disorders (type B)—malignancies, diabetes mellitus, renal or hepatic failure, severe infections (cholera, malaria), seizures, AIDS, or drugs/toxins (biguanides, ethanol, methanol, isoniazid, AZT analogues, and fructose). Unrecognized bowel ischemia or infarction in a patient with severe atherosclerosis or cardiac decompensation receiving vasopressors is a common cause of lactic acidosis. D-Lactic acid acidosis, which may be associated with jejunoileal bypass or intestinal obstruction and is due to formation of D-lactate by gut bacteria, may cause both an increased AG and hyperchloremia.

℞ **TREATMENT**   The underlying condition that disrupts lactate metabolism must first be corrected; tissue perfusion must be restored when it is inadequate. Vasoconstrictors should be avoided, if possible, since they may worsen tissue perfusion. Alkali therapy is generally advocated for acute, severe acidemia (pH < 7.1) to improve cardiac function and lactate utilization. However, NaHCO$_3$ therapy may paradoxically depress cardiac performance and exacerbate acidosis by enhancing lactate production (HCO$_3^-$ stimulates phosphofructokinase). While the use of alkali in moderate lactic acidosis is controversial, it is generally agreed that attempts to return the pH or [HCO$_3^-$] to normal by administration of exogenous NaHCO$_3$ are deleterious. A reasonable approach is to infuse sufficient NaHCO$_3$ to raise the arterial pH to no more than 7.2 over 30 to 40 min.

NaHCO$_3$ therapy can cause fluid overload and hypertension because the amount required can be massive when accumulation of lactic acid is relentless. Fluid administration is poorly tolerated because of central venoconstriction, especially in the oliguric patient. If the underlying cause of the lactic acidosis can be remedied, blood lactate will be converted to HCO$_3^-$ and may result in an overshoot alkalosis.

Ketoacidosis • *Diabetic ketoacidosis*   This condition is caused by increased fatty acid metabolism and the accumulation of ketoacids (acetoacetate and β-hydroxybutyrate). Diabetic ketoacidosis usually occurs in insulin-dependent diabetes mellitus in association with cessation of insulin or an intercurrent illness, such as an infection, gastroenteritis, pancreatitis, or myocardial infarction, which increases insulin requirements temporarily and acutely. The accumulation of ketoacids accounts for the increment in the AG and is accompanied most often by hyperglycemia [glucose > 17 mmol/L (300 mg/dL)]. It should be noted that since insulin prevents production of ketones, bicarbonate therapy is rarely needed except with extreme acidemia (pH < 7.1), and then in only limited amounts (see "Treatment" for lactic acidosis). →*The management of this condition is described in Chap. 333.*

Alcoholic ketoacidosis   Chronic alcoholics can develop ketoacidosis when alcohol consumption is abruptly curtailed; it is usually associated with binge drinking, vomiting, abdominal pain, starvation, and volume depletion. The glucose concentration is low or normal, and acidosis may be severe because of elevated ketones, predominantly β-hydroxybutyrate. Mild lactic acidosis may coexist because of alteration in the redox state. The nitroprusside ketone reaction (Acetest) can detect acetoacetic acid but not β-hydroxybutyrate, so that the degree of ketosis and ketonuria can be underestimated. Typically, insulin levels are low, and concentrations of triglyceride, cortisol, glucagon, and growth hormone are increased.

℞ **TREATMENT**   Extracellular fluid deficits should be repleted by intravenous administration of saline and glucose (5% dextrose in 0.9% NaCl). Hypophosphatemia, hypokalemia, and hypomagnesemia may coexist and should be corrected. Hypophosphatemia usually emerges 12 to 24 h after admission, may be exacerbated by glucose infusion, and, if severe, may induce rhabdomyolysis. Upper gastrointestinal hemorrhage, pancreatitis, and pneumonia may accompany this disorder.

Drug- and Toxin-Induced Acidosis • *Salicylates*   (See also Chap. 396)   Salicylate intoxication in adults usually causes respiratory alkalosis, mixed metabolic acidosis–respiratory alkalosis, or a pure high-AG metabolic acidosis. In the latter example, which is less common, only a portion of the AG is due to the salicylates. Lactic acid production is also often increased.

TREATMENT This should begin with vigorous gastric lavage with isotonic saline (not NaHCO$_3$) followed by administration of activated charcoal. In the acidotic patient, to facilitate removal of salicylate, intravenous NaHCO$_3$ is administered in amounts adequate to alkalinize the urine and to maintain urine output (urine pH > 7.5). While this form of therapy is straightforward in acidotic patients, a coexisting respiratory alkalosis may make this approach hazardous. Acetazolamide may be administered when an alkaline diuresis cannot be achieved, but this drug can cause systemic metabolic acidosis if HCO$_3^-$ is not replaced. Hypokalemia may occur with an alkaline diuresis from NaHCO$_3$ and should be treated promptly and aggressively. Glucose-containing fluids should be administered because of the danger of hypoglycemia. Excessive insensible fluid losses may cause severe volume depletion and hypernatremia. If renal failure prevents rapid clearance of salicylate, hemodialysis can be performed against a bicarbonate dialysate.

Alcohols Under most physiologic conditions, sodium, urea, and glucose generate the osmotic pressure of blood. Plasma osmolality is calculated according to the following expression: $P_{osm} = 2Na^+ + Glu + BUN$ (all in mmol/L), or, using conventional laboratory values in which glucose and BUN are expressed in milligrams per deciliter: $P_{osm} = 2Na^+ + Glu/18 + BUN/2.8$. The calculated and determined osmolality should agree within 10 to 15 mmol/kg H$_2$O. When the measured osmolality exceeds the calculated osmolality by more than 15 to 20 mmol/kg H$_2$O, one of two circumstances prevails. Either the serum sodium is spuriously low, as with hyperlipidemia or hyperproteinemia (pseudohyponatremia), or osmolytes other than sodium salts, glucose, or urea have accumulated in plasma. Examples include mannitol, radiocontrast media, isopropyl alcohol, ethylene glycol, ethanol, methanol, and acetone. In this situation, the difference between the calculated osmolality and the measured osmolality (*osmolar gap*) is proportional to the concentration of the unmeasured solute. With an appropriate clinical history and index of suspicion, identification of an osmolar gap is helpful in identifying the presence of poison-associated AG acidosis.

Ethylene glycol (See also Chap. 396) Ingestion of ethylene glycol (commonly used in antifreeze) leads to a metabolic acidosis and severe damage to the central nervous system, heart, lungs, and kidneys. The increased AG and osmolar gap are attributable to ethylene glycol and its metabolites, oxalic acid, glycolic acid, and other organic acids. Lactic acid production increases secondary to inhibition of the tricarboxylic acid cycle and altered intracellular redox state. Diagnosis is facilitated by recognizing oxalate crystals in the urine, the presence of an osmolar gap in serum, and a high-AG acidosis. Treatment should not be delayed while awaiting measurement of ethylene glycol levels in this setting.

TREATMENT This includes the prompt institution of a saline or osmotic diuresis, thiamine and pyridoxine supplements, fomepizole or ethanol, and hemodialysis. The intravenous administration of the new alcohol dehydrogenase inhibitor, fomepizole (4-methylpyrazole; 7 mg/kg as a loading dose), or ethanol intravenously to achieve a level of 22 mmol/L (100 mg/dL) serves to lessen toxicity because they compete with ethylene glycol for metabolism by alcohol dehydrogenase. Fomepizole, although expensive, offers the advantages of a predictable decline in ethylene glycol levels without the adverse effects, such as excessive obtundation, associated with ethyl alcohol infusion.

Methanol (See also Chap. 396) The ingestion of methanol (wood alcohol) causes metabolic acidosis, and its metabolites formaldehyde and formic acid cause severe optic nerve and cental nervous system

damage. Lactic acid, ketoacids, and other unidentified organic acids may contribute to the acidosis. Due to its low molecular weight (32 Da), an osmolar gap is usually present.

TREATMENT This is similar to that for ethylene glycol intoxication, including general supportive measures, fomepizole or ethanol administration, and hemodialysis.

Renal Failure (See also Chaps. 269 and 270) The hyperchloremic acidosis of moderate renal insufficiency is eventually converted to the high-AG acidosis of advanced renal failure. Poor filtration and reabsorption of organic anions contribute to the pathogenesis. As renal disease progresses, the number of functioning nephrons eventually becomes insufficient to keep pace with net acid production. Uremic acidosis is characterized, therefore, by a reduced rate of NH$_4^+$ production and excretion, primarily due to decreased renal mass. [HCO$_3^-$] rarely falls below 15 mmol/L, and the AG rarely exceeds 20 mmol/L. The acid retained in chronic renal disease is buffered by alkaline salts from bone. Despite significant retention of acid (up to 20 mmol/d), the serum [HCO$_3^-$] does not decrease further, indicating participation of buffers outside the extracellular compartment. Chronic metabolic acidosis results in significant loss of bone mass due to reduction in bone calcium carbonate. Chronic acidosis also increases urinary calcium excretion, proportional to cumulative acid retention.

TREATMENT Both uremic acidosis and the hyperchloremic acidosis of renal failure require oral alkali replacement to maintain the [HCO$_3^-$] between 20 and 24 mmol/L. This can be accomplished with relatively modest amounts of alkali (1.0 to 1.5 mmol/kg body weight per day). It is assumed that alkali replacement prevents the harmful effects of H$^+$ balance on bone and prevents or retards muscle catabolism. Sodium citrate (Shohl's solution) or NaHCO$_3$ tablets are equally effective alkalinizing salts. Citrate enhances the absorption of aluminum from the gastrointestinal tract and should never be given together with aluminum-containing antacids because of the risk of aluminum intoxication. When hyperkalemia is present, furosemide (60 to 80 mg/d) should be added.

HYPERCHLOREMIC METABOLIC ACIDOSES Alkali can be lost from the gastrointestinal tract in diarrhea or from the kidneys (renal tubular acidosis, RTA). In these disorders (Table 50-3), reciprocal changes in [Cl$^-$] and [HCO$_3^-$] result in a normal AG. In pure hyperchloremic acidosis, therefore, the increase in [Cl$^-$] above the normal value approximates the decrease in [HCO$_3^-$]. The absence of such a relationship suggests a mixed disturbance.

In diarrhea, stools contain a higher [HCO$_3^-$] and decomposed HCO$_3^-$ than plasma so that metabolic acidosis develops along with volume depletion. Instead of an acid urine pH (as anticipated with systemic acidosis), urine pH is usually around 6 because metabolic acidosis and hypokalemia increase renal synthesis and excretion of NH$_4^+$, thus providing a urinary buffer that increases urine pH. Metabolic acidosis due to gastrointestinal losses with a high urine pH can be differentiated from RTA (Chap. 276) because urinary NH$_4^+$ excretion is typically low in RTA and high with diarrhea. Urinary NH$_4^+$ levels can be estimated by calculating the urine anion gap (UAG): UAG = [Na$^+$ + K$^+$]$_u$ − [Cl$^-$]$_u$. When [Cl$^-$]$_u$ > [Na$^+$ + K$^+$], the urine ammonium level is appropriately increased, suggesting an extrarenal cause of the acidosis.

Loss of functioning renal parenchyma by progressive renal disease leads to hyperchloremic acidosis when the glomerular filtration rate (GFR) is between 20 and 50 mL/min and to uremic acidosis with a high AG when the GFR falls to <20 mL/min. Such a progression occurs commonly with tubulointerstitial forms of renal disease, but hyperchloremic metabolic acidosis can persist with advanced glomerular disease. In advanced renal failure, ammoniagenesis is reduced in proportion to the loss of functional renal mass, and ammonium accumulation and trapping in the outer medullary collecting tubule may also be impaired. Because of adaptive increases in K^+ secretion by the collecting duct and colon, the acidosis of chronic renal insufficiency is typically normokalemic.

Proximal RTA (type 2 RTA) is most often due to generalized proximal tubular dysfunction manifested by glycosuria, generalized aminoaciduria, and phosphaturia (Fanconi syndrome). With a low plasma $[HCO_3^-]$, the urine pH is acid (pH < 5.5). The fractional excretion of $[HCO_3^-]$ may exceed 10 to 15% when the serum HCO_3^- > 20 mmol/L. Since HCO_3^- is not reabsorbed normally in the proximal tubule, therapy with $NaHCO_3$ will enhance renal potassium wasting and hypokalemia.

The typical findings in classic distal RTA (type 1 RTA) (Chap. 276) include hypokalemia, hyperchloremic acidosis, low urinary NH_4^+ excretion (positive UAG, low urine $[NH_4^+]$), and inappropriately high urine pH (pH > 5.5). Such patients are unable to acidify the urine below a pH of 5.5. Most patients have hypocitraturia and hypercalciuria, so that nephrolithiasis, nephrocalcinosis, and bone disease are common. In type 4 RTA, hyperkalemia is disproportionate to the reduction in GFR because of coexisting dysfunction of potassium and acid secretion. Urinary ammonium excretion is invariably depressed, and renal function may be compromised, for example, due to diabetic nephropathy, amyloidosis, or tubulointerstital disease. →*See Chap. 276 for the pathophysiology, diagnosis, and treatment of RTA.*

Hyporeninemic Hypoaldosteronism (See also Chap. 331) This condition typically causes hyperchloremic metabolic acidosis, most commonly in older adults with diabetes mellitus or tubulointerstitial disease and renal insufficiency. Patients usually have mild to moderate renal insufficiency and acidosis, with elevation in serum $[K^+]$ (5.2 to 6.0 mmol/L), concurrent hypertension, and congestive heart failure. Both the metabolic acidosis and the hyperkalemia are out of proportion to impairment in GFR. Nonsteroidal anti-inflammatory drugs—trimethoprim, pentamidine, and ACE-inhibitors—can also cause hyperkalemia with hyperchloremic metabolic acidosis in patients with renal insufficiency (Table 50-3).

METABOLIC ALKALOSIS

Metabolic alkalosis is manifested by an elevated arterial pH, an increase in the serum $[HCO_3^-]$, and an increase in Pa_{CO_2} as a result of compensatory alveolar hypoventilation. It is often accompanied by hypochloremia and hypokalemia. The patient with a high $[HCO_3^-]$ and a low $[Cl^-]$ has either metabolic alkalosis or chronic respiratory acidosis. As shown in Table 50-1, the Pa_{CO_2} increases 6 mmHg for each 10-mmol/L increase in the $[HCO_3^-]$ above normal. Stated differently, in the range of $[HCO_3^-]$ from 10 to 40 mmol/L, the predicted Pa_{CO_2} is approximately equal to the $[HCO_3^-]$ + 15. The arterial pH establishes the diagnosis, since it is increased in metabolic alkalosis and decreased or normal in respiratory acidosis. Metabolic alkalosis frequently occurs in association with other disorders such as respiratory acidosis or alkalosis or metabolic acidosis.

PATHOGENESIS Metabolic alkalosis occurs as a result of net gain of $[HCO_3^-]$ or loss of nonvolatile acid (usually HCl by vomiting) from the extracellular fluid. Since it is unusual for alkali to be added to the body, the disorder involves a generative stage, in which the loss of acid usually causes alkalosis, and a maintenance stage, in which the kidneys fail to compensate by excreting HCO_3^- because of volume contraction, a low GFR, or depletion of Cl^- or K^+.

Under normal circumstances, the kidneys have an impressive capacity to excrete HCO_3^-. Continuation of metabolic alkalosis represents a failure of the kidneys to eliminate HCO_3^- in the usual manner. For HCO_3^- to be added to the extracellular fluid, it must be administered exogenously or synthesized endogenously, in part or entirely by the kidneys. The kidneys will retain, rather than excrete, the excess alkali and maintain the alkalosis if (1) volume deficiency, chloride deficiency, and K^+ deficiency exist in combination with a reduced

GFR, which augments distal tubule H^+ secretion; or (2) hypokalemia exists because of autonomous hyperaldosteronism. In the first example, alkalosis is corrected by administration of NaCl and KCl, while in the latter it is necessary to repair the alkalosis by pharmacologic or surgical intervention, not with saline administration.

DIFFERENTIAL DIAGNOSIS To establish the cause of metabolic alkalosis (Table 50-4), it is necessary to assess the status of the extracellular fluid volume (ECFV), the recumbent and upright blood pressure, the serum $[K^+]$, and the renin-aldosterone system. For example, the presence of chronic hypertension and chronic hypokalemia in an alkalotic patient suggests either mineralocorticoid excess or that the hypertensive patient is receiving diuretics. Low plasma renin activity and normal urine $[Na^+]$ and $[Cl^-]$ in a patient who is not taking diuretics indicate a primary mineralocorticoid excess syndrome. The combination of hypokalemia and alkalosis in a normotensive, nonedematous patient can be due to Bartter's or Gitelman's syndrome, magnesium deficiency, vomiting, exogenous alkali, or diuretic ingestion. Determination of urine electrolytes (especially the urine $[Cl^-]$) and screening of the urine for diuretics may be helpful. If the urine is alkaline, with an elevated $[Na^+]$ and $[K^+]$ but low $[Cl^-]$, the diagnosis is usually either vomiting (overt or surreptitious) or alkali ingestion.

Table 50-4   Causes of Metabolic Alkalosis

I. Exogenous HCO_3^- loads
   A. Acute alkali administration
   B. Milk-alkali syndrome
II. Effective ECFV contraction, normotension, K^+ deficiency, and secondary hyperreninemic hyperaldosteronism
   A. Gastrointestinal origin
      1. Vomiting
      2. Gastric aspiration
      3. Congenital chloridorrhea
      4. Villous adenoma
      5. Combined administration of sodium polystyrene sulfonate (Kayexalate) and aluminum hydroxide
   B. Renal origin
      1. Diuretics
      2. Edematous states
      3. Posthypercapnic state
      4. Hypercalcemia/hypoparathyroidism
      5. Recovery from lactic acidosis or ketoacidosis
      6. Nonreabsorbable anions including penicillin, carbenicillin
      7. Mg^{2+} deficiency
      8. K^+ depletion
      9. Bartter's syndrome (loss of function mutations in TALH)
      10. Gitelman's syndrome (loss of function mutation in Na^+-Cl^- cotransporter in DCT)
III. ECFV expansion, hypertension, K^+ deficiency, and mineralocorticoid excess
   A. High renin
      1. Renal artery stenosis
      2. Accelerated hypertension
      3. Renin-secreting tumor
      4. Estrogen therapy
   B. Low renin
      1. Primary aldosteronism
         a. Adenoma
         b. Hyperplasia
         c. Carcinoma
      2. Adrenal enzyme defects
         a. 11β-Hydroxylase deficiency
         b. 17α-Hydroxylase deficiency
      3. Cushing's syndrome or disease
      4. Other
         a. Licorice
         b. Carbenoxolone
         c. Chewer's tobacco
         d. Lydia Pincham tablets
IV. Gain of function mutation of renal sodium channel with ECFV expansion, hypertension, K^+ deficiency, and hyporeninemic-hypoaldosteronism
   A. Liddle's syndrome

NOTE: ECFV, extracellular fluid volume; TALH, thick ascending limb of Henle's loop; DCT, distal convoluted tubule.

If the urine is relatively acid and has low concentrations of Na^+, K^+, and Cl^-, the most likely possibilities are prior vomiting, the posthypercapnic state, or prior diuretic ingestion. If, on the other hand, neither the urine sodium, potassium, nor chloride concentrations are depressed, magnesium deficiency, Bartter's or Gitelman's syndrome, or current diuretic ingestion should be considered. Bartter's syndrome is distinguished from Gitelman's syndrome because of hypocalciuria and hypomagnesemia in the latter disorder. The genetic and molecular basis of these two disorders has been elucidated recently (Chap. 276).

Alkali Administration Chronic administration of alkali to individuals with normal renal function rarely, if ever causes alkalosis. However, in patients with coexistent hemodynamic disturbances, alkalosis can develop because the normal capacity to excrete HCO_3^- may be exceeded or there may be enhanced reabsorption of HCO_3^-. Such patients include those who receive oral or intravenous HCO_3^-, acetate loads (parenteral hyperalimentation solutions), citrate loads (transfusions), or antacids plus cation-exchange resins (aluminum hydroxide and sodium polystyrene sulfonate).

METABOLIC ALKALOSIS ASSOCIATED WITH ECFV CONTRACTION, K⁺ DEPLETION, AND SECONDARY HYPERRENINEMIC HYPERALDOSTERONISM **Gastrointestinal Origin** Gastrointestinal loss of H^+ from vomiting or gastric aspiration results in retention of HCO_3^-. The loss of fluid and NaCl in vomitus or nasogastric suction results in contraction of the ECFV and an increase in the secretion of renin and aldosterone. Volume contraction causes a reduction in GFR and an enhanced capacity of the renal tubule to reabsorb HCO_3^-. During active vomiting, there is continued addition of HCO_3^- to plasma in exchange for Cl^-, and the plasma $[HCO_3^-]$ exceeds the reabsorptive capacity of the proximal tubule. The excess $NaHCO_3$ reaches the distal tubule, where secretion is enhanced by an aldosterone and the delivery of the poorly reabsorbed anion, HCO_3^-. Because of contraction of the ECFV and hypochloremia, Cl^- is avidly conserved by the kidney. Correction of the contracted ECFV with NaCl and repair of K^+ deficits corrects the acid-base disorder.

Renal Origin • *Diuretics* (See also Chap. 232) Drugs that induce chloruresis, such as thiazides and loop diuretics (furosemide, bumetanide, torsemide, and ethracrynic acid), acutely diminish the ECFV without altering the total body bicarbonate content. The serum $[HCO_3^-]$ increases. The chronic administration of diuretics tends to generate an alkalosis by increasing distal salt delivery, so that K^+ and H^+ secretion are stimulated. The alkalosis is maintained by persistence of the contraction of the ECFV, secondary hyperaldosteronism, K^+ deficiency, and the direct effect of the diuretic (as long as diuretic administration continues). Repair of the alkalosis is achieved by providing isotonic saline to correct the ECFV deficit.

Bartter's syndrome and Gitelman's syndrome See Chap. 276.

Nonreabsorbable anions and magnesium deficiency Administration of large quantities of nonreabsorbable anions, such as penicillin or carbenicillin, can enhance distal acidification and K^+ secretion by increasing the transepithelial potential difference (lumen negative). Mg^{2+} deficiency results in hypokalemic alkalosis by enhancing distal acidification through stimulation of renin and hence aldosterone secretion.

Potassium depletion Chronic K^+ depletion may cause metabolic alkalosis by increasing urinary acid excretion. Both NH_4^+ production and absorption are enhanced and HCO_3^- reabsorption is stimulated. Chronic K^+ deficiency upregulates the renal H^+, K^+-ATPase to increase K^+ absorption at the expense of enhanced H^+ secretion. Alkalosis associated with severe K^+ depletion is resistant to salt administration, but repair of the K^+ deficiency corrects the alkalosis.

After treatment of lactic acidosis or ketoacidosis When an underlying stimulus for the generation of lactic acid or ketoacid is removed rapidly, as with repair of circulatory insufficiency or with insulin therapy, the lactate or ketones are metabolized to yield an equivalent amount of HCO_3^-. Other sources of new HCO_3^- are additive with the original amount generated by organic anion metabolism to create a surfeit of HCO_3^-. Such sources include (1) new HCO_3^- added to the blood by the kidneys as a result of enhanced acid excretion

during the preexisting period of acidosis, and (2) alkali therapy during the treatment phase of the acidosis. Acidosis-induced contraction of the ECFV and K^+ deficiency act to sustain the alkalosis.

Posthypercapnia Prolonged CO_2 retention with chronic respiratory acidosis enhances renal HCO_3^- absorption and the generation of new HCO_3^- (increased net acid excretion). If the Pa_{CO_2} is returned to normal, metabolic alkalosis results from the persistently elevated $[HCO_3^-]$. Alkalosis develops if the elevated Pa_{CO_2} is abruptly returned toward normal by a change in mechanically controlled ventilation. Associated ECFV contraction does not allow complete repair of the alkalosis by correction of the Pa_{CO_2} alone, and alkalosis persists until Cl^- supplementation is provided.

METABOLIC ALKALOSIS ASSOCIATED WITH ECFV EXPANSION, HYPERTENSION, AND HYPERALDOSTERONISM Mineralocorticoid administration or excess production [primary aldosteronism of Cushing's syndrome and adrenal cortical enzyme defects (Chap. 331)] increases net acid excretion and may result in metabolic alkalosis, which may be worsened by associated K^+ deficiency. ECFV expansion from salt retention causes hypertension and antagonizes the reduction in GFR and/or increases tubule acidification induced by aldosterone and by K^+ deficiency. The kaliuresis persists and causes continued K^+ depletion with polydipsia, inability to concentrate the urine, and polyuria. Increased aldosterone levels may be the result of autonomous primary adrenal overproduction or of secondary aldosterone release due to renal overproduction of renin. In both situations, the normal feedback of ECFV on net aldosterone production is disrupted, and hypertension from volume retention can result.

Liddle's syndrome (Chap. 276) results from increased activity of collecting duct Na^+ channel (ENaC) and is a rare inherited disorder associated with hypertension due to volume expansion manifested as hypokalemic alkalosis and normal aldosterone levels.

Symptoms With metabolic alkalosis, changes in central and peripheral nervous system function are similar to those of hypocalcemia (Chap. 340); symptoms include mental confusion, obtundation, and a predisposition to seizures, paresthesia, muscular cramping, tetany, aggravation of arrhythmias, and hypoxemia in chronic obstructive pulmonary disease. Related electrolyte abnormalities include hypokalemia and hypophosphatemia.

℞ **TREATMENT** This is primarily directed at correcting the underlying stimulus for HCO_3^- generation. If primary aldosteronism is present, correction of the underlying cause will reverse the alkalosis. $[H^+]$ loss by the stomach or kidneys can be mitigated by the use of H_2 receptor blockers, H^+, K^+-ATPase inhibitors, or the discontinuation of diuretics. The second aspect of treatment is to remove the factors that sustain HCO_3^- reabsorption, such as ECFV contraction or K^+ deficiency. Although K^+ deficits should be repaired, NaCl therapy is usually sufficient to reverse the alkalosis if ECFV contraction is present, as indicated by a low urine $[Cl^-]$.

If associated conditions preclude infusion of saline, renal HCO_3^- loss can be accelerated by administration of acetazolamide, a carbonic anhydrase inhibitor, which is usually effective in patients with adequate renal function but can worsen K^+ losses. Dilute hydrochloric acid (0.1 N HCl) is also effective but can cause hemolysis. Alternatively, acidification can also be achieved with oral NH_4Cl, which should be avoided in the presence of liver disease. Hemodialysis against a dialysate low in $[HCO_3^-]$ and high in $[Cl^-]$ can be effective when renal function is impaired.

RESPIRATORY ACIDOSIS

Respiratory acidosis can be due to severe pulmonary disease, respiratory muscle fatigue, or abnormalities in ventilatory control and is recognized by an increase in Pa_{CO_2} and decrease in pH (Table 50-5). In acute respiratory acidosis, there is an immediate compensatory el-

Table 50-5 Respiratory Acid-Base Disorders

I. Alkalosis
  A. Central nervous system
     stimulation
     1. Pain
     2. Anxiety, psychosis
     3. Fever
     4. Cerebrovascular accident
     5. Meningitis, encephalitis
     6. Tumor
     7. Trauma
  B. Hypoxemia or Tissue hypoxia
     1. High altitude, ↓ Pa_{CO_2}
     2. Pneumonia, pulmonary
        edema
     3. Aspiration
     4. Severe anemia
  C. Drugs or hormones
     1. Pregnancy, progesterone
     2. Salicylates
     3. Nikethamide
  D. Stimulation of chest receptors
     1. Hemothorax
     2. Flail chest
     3. Cardiac failure
     4. Pulmonary embolism
  E. Miscellaneous
     1. Septicemia
     2. Hepatic failure
     3. Mechanical hyperventilation
     4. Heat exposure
     5. Recovery from metabolic
        acidosis

II. Acidosis
  A. Central
     1. Drugs (anesthetics,
        morphine, sedatives)
     2. Stroke
     3. Infection
  B. Airway
     1. Obstruction
     2. Asthma
  C. Parenchyma
     1. Emphysema
     2. Pneumoconiosis
     3. Bronchitis
     4. Adult respiratory
        distress syndrome
     5. Barotrauma
  D. Neuromuscular
     1. Poliomyelitis
     2. Kyphoscoliosis
     3. Myasthenia
     4. Muscular dystrophies
  E. Miscellaneous
     1. Obesity
     2. Hypoventilation
     3. Permissive hypercapnia

evation (due to cellular buffering mechanisms) in HCO_3^-, which increases 1 mmol/L for every 10-mmHg increase in Pa_{CO_2}. In chronic respiratory acidosis (24 h), renal adaptation increases the $[HCO_3^-]$ by 4 mmol/L for every 10-mmHg increase in Pa_{CO_2}. The serum HCO_3^- usually does not increase above 38 mmol/L.

The clinical features vary according to the severity and duration of the respiratory acidosis, the underlying disease, and whether there is accompanying hypoxemia. A rapid increase in Pa_{CO_2} may cause anxiety, dyspnea, confusion, psychosis, and hallucinations and may progress to coma. Lesser degrees of dysfunction in chronic hypercapnia include sleep disturbances, loss of memory, daytime somnolence, personality changes, impairment of coordination, and motor disturbances such as tremor, myoclonic jerks, and asterixis. Headaches and other signs that mimic raised intracranial pressure, such as papilledema, abnormal reflexes, and focal muscle weakness, are due to vasoconstriction secondary to loss of the vasodilator effects of CO_2.

Depression of the respiratory center by a variety of drugs, injury, or disease can produce respiratory acidosis. This may occur acutely with general anesthetics, sedatives, and head trauma or chronically with sedatives, alcohol, intracranial tumors, and the syndromes of sleep-disordered breathing, including the primary alveolar and obesity-hypoventilation syndromes (Chaps. 263 and 264). Abnormalities or disease in the motor neurons, neuromuscular junction, and skeletal muscle can cause hypoventilation via respiratory muscle fatigue. Mechanical ventilation, when not properly adjusted and supervised, may result in respiratory acidosis, particularly if CO_2 production suddenly rises (because of fever, agitation, sepsis, or overfeeding) or alveolar ventilation falls because of worsening pulmonary function. High levels of positive end-expiratory pressure in the presence of reduced cardiac output may cause hypercapnia as a result of large increases in alveolar dead space (Chap. 266). Permissive hypercapnia is being used with increasing frequency because of studies suggesting lower mortality rates than with conventional mechanical ventilation, especially with severe central nervous system or heart disease. Although the potential

beneficial effects of permissive hypercapnia may be mitigated by correction of the acidemia, it seems prudent, nevertheless, to keep the pH in the range of 7.2 to 7.3 by administration of $NaHCO_3$.

Acute hypercapnia follows sudden occlusion of the upper airway or generalized bronchospasm as in severe asthma, anaphylaxis, inhalational burn, or toxin injury. Chronic hypercapnia and respiratory acidosis occur in end-stage obstructive lung disease. Restrictive disorders involving both the chest wall and the lungs can cause respiratory acidosis because the high metabolic cost of respiration causes ventilatory muscle fatigue. Advanced stages of intrapulmonary and extrapulmonary restrictive defects present as chronic respiratory acidosis.

The diagnosis of respiratory acidosis requires, by definition, the measurement of Pa_{CO_2} and arterial pH. A detailed history and physical examination often indicate the cause. Pulmonary function studies (Chap. 250), including spirometry, diffusion capacity for carbon monoxide, lung volumes, and arterial Pa_{CO_2} and O_2 saturation, usually make it possible to determine if respiratory acidosis is secondary to lung disease. The workup for nonpulmonary causes should include a detailed drug history, measurement of hematocrit, and assessment of upper airway, chest wall, pleura, and neuromuscular function.

℞ **TREATMENT** The management of respiratory acidosis depends on its severity and rate of onset. Acute respiratory acidosis can be life-threatening, and measures to reverse the underlying cause should be undertaken simultaneously with restoration of adequate alveolar ventilation. This may necessitate tracheal intubation and assisted mechanical ventilation. Oxygen administration should be titrated carefully in patients with severe obstructive pulmonary disease and chronic CO_2 retention who are breathing spontaneously (Chap. 258). When oxygen is used injudiciously, these patients may experience progression of the respiratory acidosis. Aggressive and rapid correction of hypercapnia should be avoided, because the falling Pa_{CO_2} may provoke the same complications noted with acute respiratory alkalosis (i.e., cardiac arrhythmias, reduced cerebral perfusion, and seizures). The Pa_{CO_2} should be lowered gradually in chronic respiratory acidosis, aiming to restore the Pa_{CO_2} to baseline levels and to provide sufficient Cl^- and K^+ to enhance the renal excretion of HCO_3^-.

Chronic respiratory acidosis is frequently difficult to correct, but measures aimed at improving lung function (Chap. 258) can help some patients and forestall further deterioration in most.

RESPIRATORY ALKALOSIS

Alveolar hyperventilation decreases Pa_{CO_2} and increases the HCO_3^-/Pa_{CO_2} ratio, thus increasing pH (Table 50-5). Nonbicarbonate cellular buffers respond by consuming HCO_3^-. Hypocapnia develops when a sufficiently strong ventilatory stimulus causes CO_2 output in the lungs to exceed its metabolic production by tissues. Plasma pH and $[HCO_3^-]$ appear to vary proportionately with Pa_{CO_2} over a range from 40 to 15 mmHg. The relationship between arterial $[H^+]$ concentration and Pa_{CO_2} is about 0.7 mmol/L per mmHg (or 0.01 pH unit/mmHg), and that for plasma $[HCO_3^-]$ is 0.2 mmol/L per mmHg. Hypocapnia sustained longer than 2 to 6 h is further compensated by a decrease in renal ammonium and titratable acid excretion and a reduction in filtered HCO_3^- reabsorption. Full renal adaptation to respiratory alkalosis may take several days and requires normal volume status and renal function. The kidneys appear to respond directly to the lowered Pa_{CO_2} rather than to alkalosis per se. In chronic respiratory alkalosis a 1-mmHg fall in Pa_{CO_2} causes a 0.4- to 0.5-mmol/L drop in $[HCO_3^-]$ and a 0.3-mmol/L fall (or 0.003 rise in pH) in $[H^+]$.

The effects of respiratory alkalosis vary according to duration and severity but are primarily those of the underlying disease. Reduced cerebral blood flow as a consequence of a rapid decline in Pa_{CO_2} may cause dizziness, mental confusion, and seizures, even in the absence of hypoxemia. The cardiovascular effects of acute hypocapnia in the conscious human are generally minimal, but in the anesthetized or mechanically ventilated patient, cardiac output and blood pressure may fall because of the depressant effects of anesthesia and positive-pressure ventilation on heart rate, systemic resistance, and venous return. Cardiac arrhythmias may occur in patients with heart disease as a result of changes in oxygen unloading by blood from a left shift in the hemoglobin-oxygen dissociation curve (Bohr effect). Acute respiratory alkalosis causes intracellular shifts of Na^+, K^+, and PO_4^- and reduces free $[Ca^{2+}]$ by increasing the protein-bound fraction. Hypocapnia-induced hypokalemia is usually minor.

Chronic respiratory alkalosis is the most common acid-base disturbance in critically ill patients and, when severe, portends a poor prognosis. Many cardiopulmonary disorders manifest respiratory alkalosis in their early to intermediate stages, and the finding of normocapnia and hypoxemia in a patient with hyperventilation may herald the onset of rapid respiratory failure and should prompt an assessment to determine if the patient is becoming fatigued. Respiratory alkalosis is common during mechanical ventilation.

The hyperventilation syndrome may be disabling. Paresthesia, circumoral numbness, chest wall tightness or pain, dizziness, inability to take an adequate breath, and, rarely, tetany may themselves be sufficiently stressful to perpetuate the disorder. Arterial blood-gas analysis demonstrates an acute or chronic respiratory alkalosis, often with hypocapnia in the range of 15 to 30 mmHg and no hypoxemia. Central nervous system diseases or injury can produce several patterns of hyperventilation and sustained Pa_{CO_2} levels of 20 to 30 mmHg. Hyperthyroidism, high caloric loads, and exercise raise the basal metabolic rate, but ventilation usually rises in proportion so that arterial blood gases are unchanged and respiratory alkalosis does not develop. Salicylates are the most common cause of drug-induced respiratory alkalosis as a result of direct stimulation of the medullary chemoreceptor (Chap. 396). The methylxanthines, theophylline, and aminophylline stimulate ventilation and increase the ventilatory response to CO_2. Progesterone increases ventilation and lowers arterial Pa_{CO_2} by as much as 5 to 10 mmHg. Therefore, chronic respiratory alkalosis is a common feature of pregnancy. Respiratory alkalosis is also prominent in liver failure, and the severity correlates with the degree of hepatic insufficiency. Respiratory alkalosis is often an early finding in gram-negative septicemia, before fever, hypoxemia, or hypotension develop.

The diagnosis of respiratory alkalosis depends on measurement of arterial pH and Pa_{CO_2}. The plasma $[K^+]$ is often reduced and the $[Cl^-]$ increased. In the acute phase, respiratory alkalosis is not associated with increased renal HCO_3^- excretion, but within hours net acid excretion is reduced. In general, the HCO_3^- concentration falls by 2.0 mmol/L for each 10-mmHg decrease in Pa_{CO_2}. Chronic hypocapnia reduces the serum $[HCO_3^-]$ by 5.0 mmol/L for each 10-mmHg decrease in Pa_{CO_2}. It is unusual to observe a plasma $HCO_3^- < 12$ mmol/L as a result of a pure respiratory alkalosis.

When a diagnosis of respiratory alkalosis is made, its cause should be investigated. The diagnosis of hyperventilation syndrome is made by exclusion. In difficult cases, it may be important to rule out other conditions such as pulmonary embolism, coronary artery disease, and hyperthyroidism.

℞ **TREATMENT** The management of respiratory alkalosis is directed toward alleviation of the underlying disorder. If respiratory alkalosis complicates ventilator management, changes in dead space, tidal volume, and frequency can minimize the hypocapnia. Patients with the hyperventilation syndrome may benefit from reassurance, rebreathing from a paper bag during symptomatic attacks, and attention to underlying psychological stress. Antidepressants and sedatives are not recommended. β-Adrenergic blockers may ameliorate peripheral manifestations of the hyperadrenergic state.

BIBLIOGRAPHY

ALPERN RJ et al: Metabolic alkalosis, in *The Kidney: Physiology and Pathophysiology*, 2d ed, DW Seldin, G Giebisch (eds). New York, Raven, 1992, pp 2733–2758

DuBOSE TD JR: Acid-base disorders, in *Brenner and Rector's The Kidney*, 6th ed, BM Brenner (ed). Philadelphia, Saunders, 2000, pp 925–997

——, ALPERN RJ: Renal tubular acidosis, in *The Metabolic and Molecular Bases of Inherited Disease*, 8th ed, CR Scriver et al (eds). New York, McGraw-Hill, 2001

FALL PJ: A stepwise approach to acid-base disorders: Practical patient evaluation for metabolic acidosis and other conditions. Postgrad Med 107:249–50, 253–4, 257–8, 2000

GALLA JH: Metabolic alkalosis. J Am Soc Nephrol 11:369, 2000

MADIAS NE, COHEN JJ: Respiratory alkalosis and acidosis, in *The Kidney: Physiology and Pathophysiology*, 2d ed, DW Seldin, G Giebisch (eds). New York, Raven, 1992, pp 2733–2758

Section 8
ALTERATIONS IN SEXUAL FUNCTION AND REPRODUCTION

51 *Kevin T. McVary*

ERECTILE DYSFUNCTION

Erectile dysfunction (ED) affects 10 to 25% of middle-aged and elderly men. Demographic changes, the popularity of newer treatments, and greater acceptance of ED by patients and society have led to increased diagnosis and associated health care expenditures for the management of this common disorder. Impairment of erectile function has a profound impact on the well-being of affected men. Because many patients are reluctant to initiate discussion of sexual function, the physician should address this topic directly to elicit a history of ED.

PHYSIOLOGIC CONTROL OF ERECTION AND MALE SEXUAL FUNCTION

Normal male sexual function requires (1) an intact libido, (2) the ability to achieve and maintain penile erection, (3) ejaculation, and (4) detumescence. *Libido* refers to sexual desire and is influenced by a variety of visual, olfactory, tactile, auditory, imaginative and hormonal stimuli. Sex steroids, particularly testosterone, act to increase libido. Libido can be diminished by hormonal or psychiatric disorders or by medications.

The major anatomic structures of the penis that are involved in erectile function include the three corpora, which consist of the paired cavernosa and a single spongiosum that encloses the urethra. A collagenous sheath, called the *tunica albuginea*, individually surrounds each corpora. The micro-architecture of the corpora is composed of a mass of smooth muscle (trabecula) which contains a network of endothelial-lined vessels (lacunar spaces).

Penile tumescence leading to erection depends on the increased flow of blood into the lacunar network after complete relaxation of the arteries and corporal smooth muscle. Subsequent compression of the trabecular smooth muscle against the fibroelastic tunica albuginea causes a passive closure of the emissary veins and accumulation of blood in the corpora. In the presence of a full erection and a competent valve mechanism, the corpora become noncompressible cylinders from which blood does not escape.

The central nervous system exerts an important influence by either stimulating or antagonizing spinal pathways that mediate erectile function and ejaculation. The erectile response is mediated by a combination of central (psychogenic) and peripheral (reflexogenic) innervation. Sensory nerves that originate from receptors in the penile skin and glans converge to form the dorsal nerve of the penis, which travels to the S2-S4 dorsal root ganglia via the pudendal nerve. Parasympathetic nerve fibers to the penis arise from neurons in the intermediolateral columns of S2-S4 sacral spinal segments. Sympathetic innervation originates from the T-11 to the L-2 spinal segments and descends through the hypogastric plexus.

Neural input to smooth muscle tone is crucial to the initiation and maintenance of an erection. There is also an intricate interaction between the corporal smooth muscle cell and its overlying endothelial cell lining (Fig. 51-1A). Nitric oxide, which induces vascular relaxation, promotes erection and is opposed by endothelin-1 (ET-1), which mediates vascular contraction. Nitric oxide is synthesized from L-arginine by nitric oxide synthase, and is released from the nonadrenergic, noncholinergic (NANC) autonomic nerve supply to act postjunctionally on smooth muscle cells. Nitric oxide increases the production of cyclic 3′,5′-guanosine monophosphate (cyclic GMP), which interacts with protein kinase G and decreases intracellular calcium, causing relaxation of the smooth muscle (Fig. 51-1B). Cyclic GMP is gradually broken down by phosphodiesterase type 5 (PDE-5). Inhibitors of PDE-5, such as the oral medication sildenafil, maintain erections by reducing the breakdown of cyclic GMP. However, if nitric oxide is not produced at some level, the addition of PDE-5 inhibitor is not effective, as the drug facilitates but does not initiate the initial enzyme cascade. In addition to nitric oxide, vasoactive prostaglandins (PGE₁, PGF₂α) are synthesized within the cavernosal tissue and increase cyclic AMP levels, also leading to relaxation of cavernosal smooth muscle cells.

Ejaculation is stimulated by the sympathetic nervous system, which results in contraction of the epididymis, vas deferens, seminal vesicles, and prostate, causing seminal fluid to enter the urethra. Seminal fluid emission is followed by rhythmic contractions of the bulbocavernosus and ischiocavernosus muscles, leading to ejaculation. *Premature ejaculation* is usually related to anxiety or a learned behavior and is amenable to behavioral therapy or treatment with medications such as selective serotonin reuptake inhibitors (SSRIs). *Retrograde ejaculation* results when the internal urethral sphincter does not close, and it may occur in men with diabetes or after surgery involving the bladder neck.

Detumescence is mediated by released norepinephrine from the sympathetic nerves, release of endothelin from the vascular surface, and contraction of smooth muscle induced by activation of postsynaptic α-adrenergic receptors. These events increase venous outflow and restore the flaccid state. Venous leak can cause premature detumescence and is thought to be caused by insufficient relaxation of the corporal smooth muscle rather than a specific anatomic defect. *Priapism* refers to a persistent and painful erection and may be associated with sickle cell anemia, hypercoagulable states, spinal cord injury, or injection of vasodilator agents into the penis.

ERECTILE DYSFUNCTION

EPIDEMIOLOGY In the Massachusetts Male Aging Study (MMAS), a community-based survey of men between the ages of 40 and 70, 52% of responders reported some degree of ED. Complete ED occurred in 10% of respondents, moderate ED occurred in 25%, and minimal ED in 17%. The incidence of moderate or severe ED more than doubled between the ages of 40 and 70. In the National Health and Social Life Survey (NHSLS), which was a nationally representative sample of men and women age 18 to 59 years, 10% of men reported being unable to maintain an erection (corresponding to the proportion of men in the MMAS reporting severe ED). Incidence was highest among men in the 50 to 59 age group (21%) and among men who were poor (14%), divorced (14%), and less educated (13%).

The incidence of ED is also higher among men with certain medical disorders. In the MMAS, ED correlated with the presence of diabetes mellitus, heart disease, hypertension, and decreased HDL levels. Medications used to treat diabetes or cardiovascular disease are additional risk factors (see below). There is a higher incidence of ED among men who have undergone radiation or surgery for cancer of the prostate and in those with a lower spinal cord injury. Psychological causes of ED include depression and anger. The NHSLS found a higher incidence of ED among men who reported fair-to-poor health or experienced stress from unemployment or other causes. ED is not considered a normal part of the aging process. Nonetheless, it is associated with certain physiologic and psychological changes related to age.

PATHOPHYSIOLOGY ED may result from three basic mechanisms: (1) failure to initiate (psychogenic, endocrinologic, or neurogenic); (2) failure to fill (arteriogenic); or (3) failure to store (venoocclusive dysfunction) adequate blood volume within the lacunar network. The inability to initiate an erection may have psychogenic, endocrinologic, or neurogenic etiologies. These categories are not mutually exclusive, and multiple factors contribute to ED in many patients. For example, diminished filling pressure can lead secondarily to venous leak. Psychogenic factor frequently co-exist with other etiologic factors and should be considered in all cases. Diabetic, atherosclerotic, and drug-related causes account for >80% of cases of ED in older men.

Vasculogenic The most frequent organic cause of ED is a disturbance of blood flow to and from the penis. Atherosclerotic or traumatic arterial disease can decrease flow to the lacunar spaces, resulting in decreased rigidity and an increased time to full erection. Excessive

FIGURE 51-1 Pathways that control erection and detumescence. *A.* Erection is mediated by cholinergic parasympathetic pathways, and nonadrenergic, noncholinergic (NANC) pathways, which release nitric oxide (NO). Endothelial cells also release NO, which induces vascular smooth muscle cell relaxation, allowing enhanced blood flow, and leading to erection. Detumescence is mediated by sympathetic pathways that release norepinephrine and stimulate α-adrenergic pathways, leading to contraction of vascular smooth muscle cells. Endothelin, released from endothelial cells, also induces contraction. *B.* Biochemical pathways of NO synthesis and action. Sildenafil enhances erectile function by inhibiting phosphodiesterase type 5 (PDE-5), thereby maintaining high levels of cyclic 3′,5′-guanosine monophosphate (cyclic GMP). NOS, nitric oxide synthase; iCa²⁺, intracellular calcium.

outflow through the veins, despite adequate inflow, may also contribute to ED. In this case, the achieved perfusion pressures cannot compensate for the unrestricted outflow needed to ensure adequate erection. This situation may be due to insufficient relaxation of trabecular smooth muscle and may occur in anxious individuals with excessive adrenergic tone or in those with damaged parasympathetic outflow. Structural alterations to the fibroelastic components of the corpora may cause a loss of compliance and an inability to compress the tunical veins. This condition may result from aging, increased cross-leaking of collagen fibers induced by nonenzymatic glycosylation, hypoxia, or altered synthesis of collagen associated with hypercholesterolemia. Fibroelastic structures can also be damaged by surgery, radiation, or trauma to the penis.

Neurogenic Disorders that affect the sacral spinal cord or the autonomic fibers to the penis preclude nervous system relaxation of penile smooth muscle, thus leading to ED. In patients with spinal cord injury, the degree of ED depends on the completeness and level of the lesion. Patients with incomplete lesions or injuries to the upper part of the spinal cord are more likely to retain erectile capabilities than those with complete lesions or injuries to the lower part. Although 75% of patients with spinal cord injuries have some erectile capability, only 25% have erections sufficient for penetration. Other neurologic disorders commonly associated with ED include multiple sclerosis and peripheral neuropathy. The latter is often due to either diabetes or alcoholism. Pelvic surgery may cause ED through disruption of the autonomic nerve supply.

Endocrinologic Androgens increase libido, but their exact role in erectile function remains unclear. Individuals with castrate levels of testosterone can achieve erections from visual or sexual stimuli. Nonetheless, normal levels of testosterone appear to be important for erectile function, particularly in older males. Androgen replacement therapy can improve depressed erectile function when it is secondary to hypogonadism; it is not useful for ED when endogenous testosterone levels are normal. Increased prolactin may decrease libido by suppressing gonadotropin-releasing hormone (GnRH), and it also leads to decreased testosterone levels. Treatment of hyperprolactinemia with dopamine agonists can restore libido and testosterone.

Diabetic ED occurs in 35 to 75% of men with diabetes mellitus. Pathologic mechanisms are primarily related to diabetes-associated vascular and neurologic complications. Diabetic macrovascular complications are mainly related to age, whereas microvascular complications correlate with the duration of diabetes and the degree of glycemic control (Chap. 333). Individuals with diabetes also have reduced amounts of nitric oxide synthase in both endothelial and neural tissues.

Psychogenic Two mechanisms contribute to the inhibition of erections in psychogenic ED. First, psychogenic stimuli to the sacral cord may inhibit reflexogenic responses, thereby blocking activation of vasodilator outflow to the penis. Second, excess sympathetic stimulation in an anxious man may increase penile smooth muscle tone. The most common causes of psychogenic ED are performance anxiety, depression, relationship conflict, loss of attraction, sexual inhibition, conflicts over sexual preference, sexual abuse in childhood, and fear of pregnancy or sexually transmitted disease. Almost all patients with ED, even when it has a clear-cut organic basis, develop a psychogenic component as a reaction to ED.

Medication-Related Medication-induced ED (Table 51-1) is estimated to occur in 25% of men seen in general medical outpatient clinics. Among the antihypertensive agents, the thiazide diuretics and beta blockers have been implicated most frequently. Calcium channel blockers and angiotensin-converting enzyme inhibitors are less frequently cited. These drugs may act directly at the corporal level (e.g., calcium channel blockers) or indirectly by reducing pelvic blood pressure, which is important in the development of penile rigidity. Alpha adrenergic blockers are less likely to cause ED. Estrogens, GnRH agonists, H2 antagonists, and spironolactone cause ED by suppressing gonadotropin production or by blocking androgen action. Antidepressant and antipsychotic agents—particularly neuroleptics, tricyclics, and SSRIs—are associated with erectile, ejaculatory, orgasmic, and

Table 51-1 Drugs Associated with Erectile Dysfunction

Classification	Drugs
Diuretics	Thiazides
	Spironolactone
Antihypertensives	Calcium channel blockers
	Methyldopa
	Clonidine
	Reserpine
	β-Blockers
	Guanethidine
Cardiac/anti-hyperlipidemics	Digoxin
	Gemfibrozil
	Clofibrate
Antidepressants	Selective serotonin reuptake inhibitors
	Tricyclic antidepressants
	Lithium
	Monoamine oxidase inhibitors
Tranquilizers	Butyrophenones
	Phenothiazines
H2 antagonists	Ranitidine
	Cimetidine
Hormones	Progesterone
	Estrogens
	Corticosteroids
	GnRH agonists
	5α-Reductase inhibitors
	Cyproterone acetate
Cytotoxic agents	Cyclophosphamide
	Methotrexate
	Roferon-A
Anticholinergics	Disopyramide
	Anticonvulsants
Recreational	Ethanol
	Cocaine
	Marijuana

sexual desire difficulties. Digoxin induces ED via blockade of the Na^+,K^+-ATPase pump, resulting in a net increase in intracellular calcium and increased corporal smooth muscle tone.

Although many medications can cause ED, patients frequently have concomitant risk factors that confound the clinical picture. If there is a strong association between the institution of a drug and the onset of ED, alternative medications should be considered. Otherwise, it is often practical to treat the ED without attempting multiple changes in medications, as it may be difficult to establish a causal role for the drug.

CLINICAL EVALUATION A good physician-patient relationship helps to unravel the possible causes of ED, many of which require discussion of personal and sometimes embarrassing topics. For this reason, a primary care provider is often ideally suited to initiate the evaluation. A complete medical and sexual history should be taken in an effort to assess whether the cause of ED is organic, psychogenic, or multifactorial (Fig. 51-2). Initial questions should focus on the onset of symptoms, the presence and duration of partial erections, and the progression of ED. A history of nocturnal or early morning erections is useful for distinguishing physiologic from psychogenic ED. Nocturnal erections occur during rapid eye movement (REM) sleep and require intact neurologic and circulatory systems. Organic causes of ED are generally characterized by a gradual and persistent change in rigidity or the inability to sustain nocturnal, coital, or self-stimulated erections. The patient should also be questioned about the presence of penile curvature or pain with coitus. It is also important to address libido, as decreased sexual drive and ED are sometimes the earliest signs of endocrine abnormalities (e.g., increased prolactin, decreased testosterone levels). It is useful to ask whether the problem is confined to coitus with one or other partners; ED arises not uncommonly in association with new or extramarital sexual relationships. Situational ED, as opposed to consistent ED, suggests psychogenic causes. Ejac-

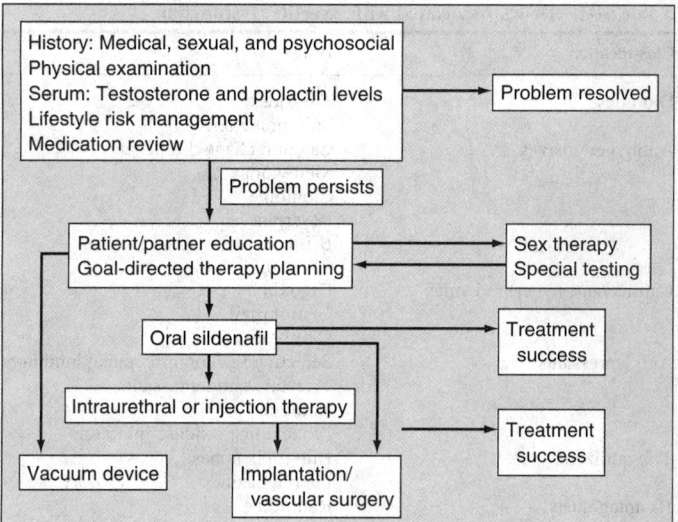

FIGURE 51-2   Algorithm for the evaluation and management of patients with ED.

ulation is much less commonly affected than erection, but questions should be asked about whether ejaculation is normal, premature, delayed, or absent. Relevant risk factors should be identified, such as diabetes mellitus, coronary artery disease, lipid disorders, hypertension, peripheral vascular disease, smoking, alcoholism, and endocrine or neurologic disorders. The patient's surgical history should be explored with an emphasis on bowel, bladder, prostate, or vascular procedures. A complete drug history is also important, as medications constitute a major source of reversible ED. Social changes that may precipitate ED are also crucial to the evaluation, including health worries, spousal death, divorce, relationship difficulties, and financial concerns.

The physical examination is an essential element in the assessment of ED. Signs of hypertension as well as evidence of thyroid, hepatic, hematologic, cardiovascular, or renal diseases should be sought. An assessment should be made of the endocrine and vascular systems, the external genitalia, and the prostate gland. The penis should be carefully palpated along the corpora to detect fibrotic plaques. Reduced testicular size and loss of secondary sexual characteristics are suggestive of hypogonadism. Neurologic examination should include assessment of anal sphincter tone, the bulbocavernosus reflex, and testing for peripheral neuropathy.

Selected laboratory testing is recommended in all cases. Although hyperprolactinemia is uncommon, a serum prolactin level should be measured, as decreased libido and/or erectile dysfunction may be the presenting symptoms of a prolactinoma or other mass lesions of the sella (Chap. 328). The serum testosterone level should be measured and, if low, gonadotropins should be measured to determine whether hypogonadism is primary (testicular) or secondary (hypothalamic-pituitary) in origin (Chap. 335). Serum chemistries, CBC, and lipid profiles may be of value, if not performed recently, as they can yield evidence of anemia, diabetes, hyperlipidemia, or other systemic diseases associated with ED. Determination of serum PSA should be conducted according to recommended clinical guidelines (Chap. 95).

Additional diagnostic testing is rarely necessary in the evaluation of ED. However, in selected patients, specialized testing may provide insight into pathologic mechanisms of ED and aid in the selection of treatment options. Optional specialized testing includes: (1) studies of nocturnal penile tumescence and rigidity; (2) vascular testing (in-office injection of vasoactive substances, penile Doppler ultrasound, penile angiography, dynamic infusion cavernosography/cavernosometry); (3) neurologic testing (biothesiometry–graded vibratory perception; somatosensory evoked potentials); and (4) psychological diagnostic

tests. The information potentially gained from these procedures must be balanced against their invasiveness and cost.

R₍ₓ₎ TREATMENT   Patient Education   Patient and partner education is essential in the treatment of ED. In goal-directed therapy, education facilitates understanding of the disease, results of the tests, and selection of treatment. Discussion of treatment options helps to clarify how treatment is best offered, and to stratify first- and second-line therapies. Patients with high-risk lifestyle issues, such as smoking, alcohol abuse, or recreational drug use, should be counseled on the role these factors play in the development of ED.

Oral Agents   Sildenafil is the only approved and effective oral agent for the treatment of ED. Sildenafil has markedly improved the management of ED because it is effective for the treatment of a broad range of causes of ED, including psychogenic, diabetic, vasculogenic, post-radical prostatectomy (nerve-sparing procedures), and spinal cord injury. Sildenafil is a selective and potent inhibitor of PDE-5, the predominant phosphodiesterase isoform found in the penis. It is administered in doses of 25, 50, or 100 mg, and enhances erections after sexual stimulation. The onset of action is approximately 60 to 90 min. Reduced initial doses should be considered for patients who are elderly, have renal insufficiency, or are taking medications that inhibit the CYP3A4 metabolic pathway in the liver (e.g., erythromycin, cimetidine, ketoconazole, and, possibly, itraconazole and mibefradil), as they may increase the serum concentration of sildenafil. The drug does not affect ejaculation, orgasm, or sexual drive. Side effects associated with sildenafil include headaches (19%), facial flushing (9%), dyspepsia (6%) and nasal congestion (4%). Approximately 7% of men may experience transient altered color vision (blue halo effect). Sildenafil is contraindicated in men receiving nitrate therapy for cardiovascular disease, including agents delivered by oral, sublingual, transnasal, or topical routes. These agents can potentiate its hypotensive effect and may result in profound shock. Likewise, amyl/butyl nitrates (poppers) may have a fatal synergistic effect on blood pressure. Sildenafil should also be avoided in patients with congestive heart failure and cardiomyopathy because of the risk of vascular collapse. Because sexual activity leads to an increase in physiologic expenditure [5 to 6 metabolic equivalents (METS)], physicians have been advised to exercise caution in prescribing any drug for sexual activity to those with active coronary disease, heart failure, borderline hypotension, hypovolemia, and to those on complex antihypertensive regimens.

Androgen Therapy   Testosterone replacement is used to treat both primary and secondary causes of hypogonadism (Chap. 335). Androgen supplementation in the setting of normal testosterone is rarely efficacious and is discouraged. Methods of androgen replacement include parenteral administration of long-acting testosterone esters (enanthate and cypionate), oral preparations (17 α-alkylated derivatives), and transdermal patches (Chap. 335). The long-acting 17 β-hydroxy esters of testosterone are the safest, most cost-effective, and practical preparations available. The administration of 200 to 300 mg intramuscularly every 2 to 3 weeks provides a practical option but is far from an ideal physiologic replacement. Oral androgen preparations have the potential for hepatotoxicity and should be avoided. Transdermal delivery of testosterone more closely mimics physiologic testosterone levels, but it is unclear whether this translates into improved sexual function. Because testosterone gradually decreases into the hypogonadal range by 24 hours, patches need to replaced daily. Testosterone therapy is contraindicated in men with androgen-sensitive cancers and may be inappropriate for men with bladder neck obstruction. It is generally advisable to measure PSA before giving androgen. Hepatic function should be tested before and during testosterone therapy.

Vacuum Constriction Devices   Vacuum constriction devices (VCD) are a well-established, noninvasive therapy. They are a reasonable treatment alternative for select patients who cannot take sildenafil or do not desire other interventions. VCD draw venous blood into the penis and use a constriction ring to restrict venous return and maintain tumescence. Adverse events with VCD include pain, numbness, bruising, and altered ejaculation. Additionally, many patients complain that the devices are cumbersome and that the induced erections have a non-physiologic appearance.

Intraurethral Alprostadil If a patient fails to respond to oral agents, a reasonable next choice is intraurethral or self-injection or vasoactive substances. Intraurethral prostaglandin E$_1$ (alprostadil), in the form of a semisolid pellet (doses of 125 to 1000 μg), is delivered with an applicator. Approximately 65% of men receiving intraurethral alprostadil respond with an erection when tested in the office, but only 50% of those achieve successful coitus at home. Intraurethral insertion is associated with a markedly reduced incidence of priapism in comparison to intracavernosal injection.

Intracavernosal Self-Injection Injection of synthetic formulations of alprostadil is effective in 70 to 80% of patients with ED, but discontinuation rates are high because of the invasive nature of administration. Doses range between 1 and 40 μg. Injection therapy is contraindicated in men with a history of hypersensitivity to the drug and in men at risk for priapism (hypercoagulable states, sickle cell disease). Side effects include local adverse events, prolonged erections, pain, and fibrosis with chronic use. Various combinations of alprostadil, phentolamine, and/or papaverine are sometimes used.

Surgery A less frequently used form of therapy for ED involves the surgical implantation of a semi-rigid or inflatable penile prosthesis. These surgical treatments are invasive, associated with potential complications, and generally reserved for treatment of refractory ED. Despite their high cost and invasiveness, penile prostheses are associated with high rates of patient satisfaction.

Sex Therapy A course of sex therapy may be useful for addressing specific interpersonal factors that may affect sexual functioning. Sex therapy generally consists of in-session discussion and at-home exercises specific to the person and the relationship. It is preferable if therapy includes both partners, provided the patient is involved in an ongoing relationship.

BIBLIOGRAPHY

ABRAMOWICZ M et al: Drugs that cause sexual dysfunction. Med Let 29:65, 1987
BURNETT AL et al: Nitric oxide: A physiologic mediator of penile erection. Science 257: 401, 1992
FELDMAN HA et al: Impotence and its medical and psychosocial correlates: Results of the Massachusetts Male Aging Study. J Urol 151:54, 1994
GOLDSTEIN I et al: Oral sildenafil in the treatment of erectile impotence. N Engl J Med 338:1397, 1998
KWAN M et al: The nature of androgen action on male sexuality: A combined laboratory–self-report study on hypogonadal men. J Clin Endocrinol Metab 57:557, 1983
LAUMANN AO et al: Sexual dysfunction in the United States. JAMA 81:553, 1999
LEVY A et al: Non-surgical management of erectile dysfunction. Clin Endocrinol (oxf) 52:253, 2000
LUE TF: Drug therapy: Erectile dysfunction. N Engl J Med 342:1802, 2000
NIH CONSENSUS CONFERENCE ON IMPOTENCE: JAMA 270:83, 1993
PADMA-NATHAN H et al: Treatment of men with erectile dysfunction with transurethral alprostadil. N Engl J Med 336:1, 1997
SAENZ DE TEJADA I et al: Impaired neurogenic and endothelium-mediated relaxation of penile smooth muscle from diabetic men with impotence. N Engl J Med 320:1025, 1989

52 *Bruce R. Carr, Karen D. Bradshaw*

DISTURBANCES OF MENSTRUATION AND OTHER COMMON GYNECOLOGIC COMPLAINTS IN WOMEN

Complaints related to the female reproductive tract can be categorized as disorders of menstruation, pelvic pain, disturbances in sexual function, or infertility. However, a single disorder, e.g., leiomyoma of the uterus, can present with symptoms referable to any one or more of these categories. Furthermore, sexual dysfunction can interdigitate with other problems in several ways. On the one hand, in women with complaints related to other reproductive tract functions, the underlying problem may actually be severe sexual dysfunction or marital conflict. Alternatively, women with severe organic disorders of the pelvis, e.g., pelvic inflammatory disease or endometriosis, may present with sexual dysfunction such as dyspareunia that in fact is only a minor manifestation of the underlying disease.

Since normal reproductive function depends on the integrated action of the central nervous system, the endocrine glands, and the reproductive organs, menstrual cycle abnormalities, sexual dysfunction, and infertility may be the result of systemic and psychological disorders as well as of primary defects in the endocrine and reproductive organs. The endocrine and physiologic control—normal and abnormal—of puberty, reproductive life, and menopause are discussed in Chap. 336. The focus of this chapter is on the initial evaluation of women with disturbances of the reproductive tract.

DISTURBANCES IN MENSTRUATION Disorders of menstruation can be divided into abnormal uterine bleeding and amenorrhea.

Abnormal Uterine Bleeding The menstrual cycle is defined as the interval between the onset of one bleeding episode and the onset of the next. In normal women the cycle averages 28 $\pm$ 3 days, the mean duration of menstrual flow is 4 $\pm$ 2 days, and the average blood loss is 35 to 80 mL. Between menarche and menopause most women experience one or more episodes of abnormal uterine bleeding, here defined as any bleeding pattern outside the normal ranges of frequency, duration, and/or amount of blood loss. The decision to evaluate a patient depends on the severity and frequency of the abnormal bleeding pattern.

When vaginal bleeding occurs, it should first be determined whether the blood is derived from the uterine endometrium. Rectal, bladder, cervical, and vaginal sources of bleeding must be excluded. Once the bleeding is established to be uterine in origin, a pregnancy-related disorder (such as threatened or incomplete abortion or ectopic pregnancy) must be ruled out by physical examination and appropriate laboratory tests. It should also be remembered that uterine bleeding may also be the initial or principal manifestation of a generalized bleeding diathesis. The remaining causes of abnormal uterine bleeding can be divided into those associated with ovulatory or anovulatory cycles.

Ovulatory cycles Menstrual bleeding with ovulatory cycles is spontaneous, regular in onset, predictable in duration and amount of flow, and frequently associated with discomfort; it is the consequence of progesterone withdrawal at the end of the luteal (postovulatory) phase and requires prior estrogen priming of the endometrium during the follicular (preovulatory) phase of the cycle. When deviations from an established pattern of menstrual flow occur but the cycles are still regular, the usual cause is disease of the outflow tract. For example, regular, prolonged, excessive bleeding episodes can result from abnormalities of the uterus such as submucous leiomyomas, adenomyosis, or endometrial polyps. On the other hand, cyclic, predictable menstruation characterized by spotting or light bleeding suggests obstruction of the outflow tract as with uterine synechiae or scarring of the cervix. Intermittent bleeding between cyclic ovulatory menses is often due to cervical or endometrial lesions.

Anovulatory cycles Uterine bleeding that is irregular in occurrence, unpredictable as to amount and duration of flow, and usually painless is called *dysfunctional or anovulatory uterine bleeding*. This type of bleeding is the result of a failure of normal follicular maturation with consequent anovulation and may be either transient or chronic. Transient disruption of ovulatory cycles occurs most often in the early menarcheal years, during the perimenopausal period, or as the consequence of a variety of stresses and intercurrent illnesses. Persistent dysfunctional uterine bleeding during the reproductive years can occur in several organic diseases that affect ovarian function and is most often due to estrogen breakthrough bleeding. Estrogen breakthrough bleeding occurs when estrogen stimulation of the endometrium is continuous and is not interrupted by cyclic progesterone withdrawal, as can occur in polycystic ovarian disease.

Amenorrhea *Amenorrhea* is defined either as failure of menarche by age 16, regardless of the presence or absence of secondary sexual characteristics, or as the absence of menstruation for 6 months in a woman with previous periodic menses. Amenorrhea in a woman who has never menstruated is termed *primary amenorrhea*; cessation of menses is termed *secondary amenorrhea*. Because some disorders can cause both primary and secondary amenorrhea, we prefer a functional classification based on the nature of the underlying defect, namely, anatomic defects of the outflow tract (uterus, cervix, or vagina), ovarian failure, and chronic anovulation.

Anatomic defects of the outflow tract include congenital defects of the vagina, imperforate hymen, transverse vaginal septa, cervical stenosis, intrauterine adhesions (synechiae), absence of the vagina or uterus, and uterine maldevelopment. The diagnosis of an anatomic defect is usually made by physical examination but may be confirmed by demonstrating failure of bleeding following administration of estrogen plus a progestogen for 21 days. Pelvic ultrasonography, magnetic resonance imaging, hysterosalpingogram, or hysteroscopy may be helpful in defining the defect.

Causes of *ovarian failure* include gonadal dysgenesis, deficiency of 17α-hydroxylase, resistant ovary syndrome, and premature ovarian failure. Ovarian failure encompasses disorders in which the ovary is deficient in germ cells and those in which the germ cells are resistant to follicle-stimulating hormone (FSH). The diagnosis of ovarian failure as the cause of amenorrhea is confirmed by an elevated plasma FSH level.

Women with *chronic anovulation* fail to ovulate spontaneously but have the capability of ovulating with appropriate therapy. In some women with chronic anovulation, total estrogen production is adequate, but it is not secreted in a cyclic fashion. In others, estrogen production is deficient.

Women who have adequate estrogen production and demonstrate withdrawal bleeding after progestogen challenge often have polycystic ovarian disease (see Fig. 336-8). Other causes include hormone-secreting ovarian and adrenal tumors. Women with deficient or absent estrogen production, and therefore with absence of withdrawal bleeding after progestogen administration, usually have hypogonadotropic hypogonadism due to organic or functional disorders of the pituitary or central nervous system such as brain tumors, pituitary tumors (especially prolactin-secreting adenomas), primary hypopituitarism, or Sheehan's syndrome.

PELVIC PAIN Pelvic pain may originate in the pelvis or be referred from another region of the body. A pelvic source is suggested by the history (e.g., dysmenorrhea and dyspareunia) and physical findings, but a high index of suspicion must be entertained for extrapelvic disorders that refer to the pelvis, such as appendicitis, diverticulitis, cholecystitis, intestinal obstruction, and urinary tract infections (Chap. 14).

"Physiologic" Pelvic Pain • *Pain associated with ovulation ("mittelschmerz")* Many women experience low abdominal discomfort with ovulation, typically a dull aching pain at midcycle in one lower quadrant lasting from minutes to hours. It is rarely severe or incapacitating. The pain may result from peritoneal irritation by follicular fluid released into the peritoneal cavity at ovulation. The onset at midcycle and short duration of pain suggest this diagnosis.

Premenstrual or menstrual pain In normal ovulatory women, somatic symptoms during the few days prior to menses may be insignificant or disabling. Such symptoms include edema, breast engorgement, and abdominal bloating or discomfort. A symptom complex of cyclic irritability, depression, and lethargy is known as the *premenstrual syndrome* (PMS). PMS appears to be caused by changes in gonadal steroid levels. Although there is no consensus about therapy, randomized, controlled trials suggest significant improvement with the daily use of serotonin-reuptake inhibitors.

Severe or incapacitating uterine cramping during ovulatory menses and in the absence of demonstrable disorders of the pelvis is termed *primary dysmenorrhea*. Primary dysmenorrhea is caused by prostaglandin-induced uterine ischemia and is treated with prostaglandin synthetase inhibitors and/or oral contraceptive agents.

Pelvic Pain due to Organic Causes Severe dysmenorrhea associated with disease of the pelvis is termed *secondary dysmenorrhea*. Organic causes of pelvic pain can be classified as (1) uterine, (2) adnexal, (3) vulvar or vaginal, and (4) pregnancy-associated.

Uterine pain Pain of uterine etiology is often chronic and continuous and increases in intensity during menstruation and intercourse. Causes include leiomyomas of the uterus (particularly submucous and degenerating leiomyomas), adenomyosis, and cervical stenosis. Infections of the uterus associated with intrauterine manipulation following dilatation and curettage or with the insertion of intrauterine devices can also cause pelvic pain (Chap. 336). Pelvic pain due to endometrial or cervical cancer is usually a late manifestation (Chap. 336).

Adnexal pain The most common cause of pain in the adnexae (fallopian tubes and ovaries) is infection (Chap. 133). Acute salpingo-oophoritis presents as low abdominal pain, fever, and chills; begins a few days after a menstrual period; and is usually due to chlamydial or gonococcal disease with or without a superimposed pyogenic infection. Chronic pelvic inflammatory disease results from either a single episode or multiple episodes of infection and may present as infertility associated with chronic pelvic pain that increases in intensity with menses and intercourse. On physical examination, cervical motion tenderness, adnexal tenderness, and adnexal thickening and/or masses may be present. Pelvic inflammatory disease may become a surgical emergency if peritonitis results from rupture of a tuboovarian abscess. Ovarian cysts or neoplasms may cause pelvic pain that becomes more severe with torsion or rupture of the mass, and ectopic pregnancy must be considered in the differential diagnosis (see below). Endometriosis involving fallopian tubes, ovaries, or peritoneum may cause both chronic low abdominal pain and infertility; the magnitude of tissue involvement does not always correlate with the severity of symptoms. Endometriosis pain typically increases with menstruation and, if the posterior ligaments of the uterus are involved, with intercourse.

Vulvar or vaginal pain Pain in these areas is most often due to infectious vaginitis caused by *Monilia*, *Trichomonas*, or bacteria and is characteristically associated with vaginal discharge and pruritus. Herpetic vulvitis, other dermatologic conditions of the vulva, condyloma acuminatum, and cysts or abscesses of Bartholin's glands may also cause vulvar pain.

Pregnancy-associated disorders Pregnancy must be considered in the differential diagnosis of pelvic pain during the reproductive years. Threatened abortion or incomplete abortion often presents with uterine cramping, bleeding, or passage of tissue following a period of amenorrhea. Ectopic pregnancy may be insidious in presentation or result in abrupt intraperitoneal hemorrhage and maternal death.

Evaluation of Pelvic Pain The evaluation of pelvic pain requires a careful history and pelvic examination. This often leads to the correct diagnosis and institution of appropriate treatment. If the pain is severe and the diagnosis is unclear, the workup should follow that outlined for the acute abdomen (Chap. 14). A culdocentesis may be indicated if a ruptured ectopic pregnancy is suspected. If there is a question of an adnexal mass or if the patient is so obese as to preclude a thorough pelvic examination, abdominal or vaginal sonography may be useful. Serial human chorionic gonadotropin (hCG) measurements may help in establishing a diagnosis of tubal pregnancy and are useful in determining if an intrauterine pregnancy is viable. Finally, diagnostic laparoscopy and laparotomy may be indicated with pain of undetermined etiology.

SEXUAL DYSFUNCTION Some women with sexual dysfunction describe minor complaints related to the reproductive tract as a means of bringing sexual problems to the attention of the physician. Alternatively, sexual dysfunction may be thought to be the cause of low abdominal discomfort or dyspareunia when the actual etiology is organic. However, more and more women seek medical advice because of sexual problems that interface in provenance between medicine, psychiatry, and sociology.

The normal sexual response begins with sexual arousal, which causes genital vasocongestion that results in vaginal lubrication in preparation for intromission. The lubrication is due to the formation of a transudate in the vagina and in conjunction with genital congestion produces the so-called orgasmic platform prior to orgasm. Sexual stimuli (visual, tactile, auditory, and olfactory) as well as healthy vaginal tissue are prerequisites for genital vasocongestion and vaginal lubrication. During the second stage of the sexual response, involuntary contractions of the muscles of the pelvis result in a pleasurable cortical sensory phenomenon known as orgasm. Direct or indirect stimulation of the clitoris is important in the production of the female orgasm. In simple terms, sexual dysfunction can be due to interference with the arousal or orgasmic phases of the sexual response. Either disorder can be due to an organic or functional cause or both.

Illnesses that impair neurologic function such as diabetes mellitus or multiple sclerosis can prevent normal sexual arousal. Local pelvic diseases such as vaginitis, endometriosis, and salpingo-oophoritis may preclude normal sexual response because of resulting dyspareunia. Debilitating systemic diseases such as cancer and cardiovascular diseases may inhibit normal sexual response indirectly.

More commonly, failure of a normal sexual response is due to psychological factors that impair sexual arousal. Such problems include misinformation, e.g., the perception of sexual satisfaction as bad, or feelings of guilt about previous psychologically traumatic events such as incest, rape, or unwanted pregnancy. In addition, women who have had previous hysterectomy or mastectomy may perceive themselves as "incomplete." Stresses such as anxiety, depression, fatigue, and marital or interpersonal conflicts may lead to failure of the vasocongestive response and prevent normal vaginal lubrication. Women with such experiences may be unable to achieve normal sexual response unless they receive professional counseling. Such problems are approached by attempting to identify and reduce the causative stresses.

Failure to achieve orgasm is a specific form of sexual dysfunction. In the absence of orgasm many women enjoy sexual encounters to variable degrees because of the pleasure derived from closeness in a cherished relationship, particularly with a loving partner. However, for other women sexual relations with rare or absent orgasms are frustrating and unsatisfying. In many instances, failure of orgasm is due to insufficient clitoral stimulation and may be rectified by appropriate counseling and patient education.

A specific entity, "vaginismus," painful, involuntary contractions of the musculature surrounding the entrance to the vagina, is a rare cause of dyspareunia. It is a conditioned response to a previous real or imagined frightening or traumatic sexual experience. Treatment is directed to elimination of the conditioned response by progressive vaginal dilation by the patient in conjunction with marital therapy.

REPRODUCTION Infertility is discussed in detail in Chap. 54. The approach to infertile couples always involves evaluation of both the man and woman. The history should address the frequency of intercourse, the sexual responses of both, the use of contraceptives or lubricants, prior pregnancies, interval to conception and outcome of pregnancy, previous or past medical illnesses, and all medications taken.

Male-associated factors account for a third of infertility problems. Therefore, one of the first procedures in the workup of infertile couples should be a semen analysis. The initial evaluation of the woman includes documentation of normal ovulatory cycles. A history of regular, cyclic, predictable, spontaneous menses usually indicates ovulatory cycles, which may be confirmed by basal body temperature graphs, properly timed endometrial biopsies, or plasma progesterone measurements during the luteal phase of the cycle. Also, the diagnosis of luteal-phase dysfunction (low progesterone secretion during the luteal phase) can be established by these methods. Transvaginal ultrasonography is useful for evaluating follicular development.

The most common cause of infertility in women is tubal disease, usually due to infection (pelvic inflammatory disease) or endometriosis. Tubal disease can be evaluated by obtaining a hysterosalpingogram or by diagnostic laparoscopy. Tubal diseases can usually be treated by laparoscopic tuboplasty and lysis of adhesions.

In many instances of infertility, it is now possible to use assisted reproductive technologies including in vitro fertilization and embryo transfer, gamete intrafallopian tube transfer, transfer of cryopreserved ova and embryos, donor oocytes or donor sperm, and ovarian hyperstimulation with clomiphene citrate or gonadotropins followed by intrauterine insemination.

The desire for contraception is also a frequent cause for women to seek medical treatment or evaluation. The most widely used methods for fertility control include (1) rhythm and withdrawal techniques, (2) barrier methods, (3) intrauterine devices, (4) oral steroid contraceptives, (5) sterilization, and (6) abortion. →*These methods and their complications are discussed in Chap. 54.*

BIBLIOGRAPHY

CARR BR, BLACKWELL RE: *Textbook of Reproductive Medicine*, 2d ed. Stamford, CT, Appleton & Lange, 1998

CUNNINGHAM FG et al: *Williams Obstetrics*, 20th ed. Stamford, CT, Appleton & Lange, 1998

FORDNEY DS: Dyspareunia and vaginismus. Clin Obstet Gynecol 21:205, 1978

HERBST AL et al: *Comprehensive Gynecology*, 2d ed. St. Louis, Mosby, 1992

HAMMOND DC: Screening for sexual dysfunction. Clin Obstet Gynecol 27:732, 1984

HATCHER RA et al: *Contraceptive Technology*, 17th ed. New York, Ardent Media, 1998

MASTERS W, JOHNSON V: *Human Sexual Response*. Boston, Little, Brown, 1966

ROSEN RJ et al: Prevention of sexual dysfunction in women. J Sex Med Ther 19:171, 1993

SCHMIDT PJ et al: Differential behavioral effects of gonadal steroids in women with and in those without premenstrual syndrome. N Engl J Med 338:209, 1998

SEIPPEL L, BÄCKSTRÖM T: Luteal-phase estradiol relates to symptom severity in patients with premenstrual syndrome. J Clin Endocrinol Metab 83:1988, 1998

SPEROFF L et al: *Clinical Gynecologic Endocrinology and Infertility*, 5th ed. Baltimore, Williams & Wilkins, 1994

53 David A. Ehrmann

HIRSUTISM AND VIRILIZATION

Hirsutism, defined as excessive male-pattern hair growth, affects approximately 10% of women of reproductive age. Hirsutism may be mild, essentially representing a variation of normal hair growth, or rarely it may be the harbinger of a serious underlying condition. It is often idiopathic but may be caused by several conditions associated with androgen excess, such as polycystic ovarian syndrome (PCOS) or congenital adrenal hyperplasia (CAH) (Table 53-1). Cutaneous manifestations commonly associated with hirsutism include acne and male-pattern balding (androgenic alopecia). *Virilization*, on the other hand, refers to the state in which androgen levels are sufficiently high to cause additional signs and symptoms such as deepening of the voice, breast atrophy, increased muscle bulk, clitoromegaly, and increased libido; virilization is an ominous sign that suggests the possibility of an ovarian or adrenal neoplasm.

HAIR FOLLICLE GROWTH AND DIFFERENTIATION

Hair can be categorized as either *vellus* (fine, soft, and not pigmented) or *terminal* (long, coarse, and pigmented). The number of hair follicles does not change over an individual's lifetime, but the follicle size and type of hair can change in response to numerous factors, particularly androgens. Androgens are necessary for terminal hair and sebaceous gland development and mediate differentiation of pilosebaceous units (PSUs) into either a terminal hair follicle or a sebaceous gland. In the former case, androgens transform the vellus hair into a terminal hair; in the latter, the sebaceous component proliferates and the hair remains vellus.

There are three phases in the cycle of hair growth: (1) *anagen*

Table 53-1 Causes of Hirsutism

Gonadal hyperandrogenism
  Ovarian hyperandrogenism
  Polycystic ovary syndrome/functional ovarian hyperandrogenism
  Ovarian steroidogenic blocks
  Syndromes of extreme insulin resistance
  Ovarian neoplasms
Adrenal hyperandrogenism
  Premature adrenarche
  Functional adrenal hyperandrogenism
  Congenital adrenal hyperplasia (nonclassic and classic)
  Abnormal cortisol action/metabolism
  Adrenal neoplasms
Other endocrine disorders
  Cushing's syndrome
  Hyperprolactinemia
  Acromegaly
Peripheral androgen overproduction
  Obesity
  Idiopathic
Pregnancy-related hyperandrogenism
  Hyperreactio luteinalis
  Thecoma of pregnancy
Drugs
  Androgens
  Oral contraceptives containing androgenic progestins
Drugs associated with hypertrichosis
  Minoxidil
  Phenytoin
  Diazoxide
  Cyclosporine
True hermaphroditism

(growth phase), (2) *catagen* (involution phase), and (3) *telogen* (rest phase). Depending on the body site, hormonal regulation may play an important role in the hair growth cycle. For example, the eyebrows, eyelashes, and vellus hairs are androgen-insensitive, whereas the axillary and pubic areas are sensitive to low doses of androgens. Hair growth on the face, chest, upper abdomen, and back requires greater levels of androgens and is therefore more characteristic of the pattern typically seen in males. Androgen excess in women leads to increased hair growth in most androgen-sensitive sites but will manifest with loss of hair in the scalp region, in part by reducing the time hairs spend in anagen phase.

Although androgen excess underlies most cases of hirsutism, there is only a modest correlation between androgen levels and the quantity of hair growth. This is due to the fact that hair growth from the follicle depends on local factors and variability in end-organ sensitivity, as well as circulating androgen concentrations. Genetic factors and ethnic background also influence hair growth. In general, dark-haired individuals tend to be more hirsute than blonde or fair individuals. Asians and Native Americans have relatively sparse hair in regions sensitive to high androgen levels, whereas people of Mediterranean descent are more hirsute. For these reasons, family history and ethnic background are important considerations when assessing the etiology and severity of hirsutism.

CLINICAL ASSESSMENT Historic elements relevant to the assessment of hirsutism include the age of onset and rate of progression of hair growth and associated symptoms or signs (e.g., acne). Depending on the cause, excess hair growth is typically first noted during the second and third decades. The growth is usually slow but progressive. Sudden development and rapid progression of hirsutism suggests the possibility of an androgen-secreting neoplasm, in which case findings of virilization may also be present.

The age of onset of menstrual cycles (menarche) and the pattern of the menstrual cycle should be ascertained; irregular cycles from the time of menarche onward are more likely to result from ovarian rather than adrenal androgen excess. Associated symptoms such as galactor-

rhea should prompt evaluation for hyperprolactinemia (Chap. 328) and possibly hypothyroidism (Chap. 330). Hypertension, striae, easy bruising, centripetal weight gain, and weakness suggest hypercortisolism (Cushing's syndrome; Chap. 331). Rarely, patients with growth hormone excess (i.e., acromegaly) will present with hirsutism. Use of medications such as phenytoin, minoxidil, or cyclosporine may be associated with androgen-independent causes of excess hair growth (i.e., hypertrichosis). A family history of infertility and/or hirsutism may indicate disorders such as nonclassic congenital adrenal hyperplasia (CAH), a disorder particularly common in Ashkenazi Jews, among others (Chap. 331).

Physical examination should include measurement of height, weight, and calculation of body mass index (BMI). A BMI >25 kg/m^2 is indicative of excess weight for height, and values >30 kg/m^2 are often seen in association with hirsutism. Notation should be made of blood pressure. Cutaneous signs sometimes associated with androgen excess and insulin resistance include acanthosis nigricans and skin tags.

An objective clinical assessment of hair distribution and quantity is central to the evaluation in any woman presenting with hirsutism. This assessment permits the distinction between hirsutism and hypertrichosis and provides a baseline reference point to gauge the response to treatment. *Hypertrichosis* refers to the excessive growth of androgen-independent hair which is vellus, prominent in nonsexual areas, and most commonly familial or caused by metabolic disorders (e.g., thyroid disturbances, anorexia nervosa) or medications (e.g., phenytoin, minoxidil or cyclosporine).

A simple and commonly used method to grade hair growth is the modified scale of Ferriman and Gallwey (Fig. 53-1), where each of nine androgen-sensitive sites is graded from 0 to 4. Approximately 95% of Caucasian women have a score below 8 on this scale; thus, it is normal for most women to have some hair growth in androgen-sensitive sites. Scores above 8 suggest an excess of androgen-mediated hair growth, a finding that should be assessed further by hormonal evaluation (see below). In racial/ethnic groups that are less likely to manifest hirsutism (e.g., Asian women), additional cutaneous evidence of androgen excess should be sought, including pustular acne or thinning hair.

HORMONAL EVALUATION Androgens are secreted by both the ovaries and adrenal glands in response to their respective tropic hormones, luteinizing hormone (LH) and adrenocorticotropic hormone (ACTH). The principal circulating steroids involved in the etiology of hirsutism are androstenedione, dehydroepiandrosterone (DHEA) and its sulfated form (DHEAS), and testosterone. The ovaries and adrenal glands normally contribute about equally to testosterone production. Further, approximately half of the total testosterone originates from direct glandular secretion, and the remainder is derived from the peripheral conversion of androstenedione and DHEA (Chap. 335).

Although it is the most important circulating androgen, testosterone is, in effect, the penultimate androgen in mediating hirsutism; it is converted to the more potent dihydrotestosterone (DHT) by the enzyme 5α-reductase, which is located in the pilosebaceous unit. DHT has a higher affinity for, and slower dissociation from, the androgen receptor. The local production of DHT allows it to serve as the primary mediator of androgen action at the level of the pilosebaceous unit. There are two isoenzymes of 5α-reductase: type 2 is found in the prostate gland and in hair follicles, whereas type 1 is primarily found in sebaceous glands.

One approach to testing for hyperandrogenemia is depicted in Fig. 53-2. This involves measuring blood levels of testosterone and DHEAS. It is also important to measure the level of free (or unbound) testosterone, because it is the fraction of testosterone that is not bound to its carrier protein, sex-hormone binding globulin (SHBG), that is biologically available. Hyperinsulinemia and/or androgen excess decrease hepatic production of SHBG, often resulting in levels of total testosterone within the high-normal range at a time when the free hormone is substantially elevated. Because adrenal androgens are readily

FIGURE 53-1 Hirsutism scoring scale of Ferriman and Gallwey. The nine body areas possessing androgen-sensitive areas are graded from 0 (no terminal hair) to 4 (frankly virile) to obtain a total score. A normal hirsutism score is less than 8. *(Reproduced from Ehrmann et al., 2000.)*

suppressed by low doses of glucocorticoids, the dexamethasone androgen-suppression test may broadly distinguish ovarian from adrenal androgen overproduction. A blood sample is obtained before and after administering dexamethasone (0.5 mg orally every 6 h for 4 days). An adrenal source is suggested by suppression of plasma free testosterone into the normal range; incomplete suppression suggests ovarian androgen excess.

A baseline plasma total testosterone level >12 nmol/L (>3.5 ng/mL) usually indicates a virilizing tumor, whereas a level >7 nmol/L (>2 ng/mL) is suggestive. A basal DHEAS level >18.5 μmol/L (>7000 μg/L) suggests an adrenal tumor. Although DHEAS has been proposed as a "marker" of predominant adrenal androgen excess, it is not unusual to find modest elevations in DHEAS among women with PCOS. Computed tomography (CT) or magnetic resonance imaging (MRI) should be used to localize an adrenal mass, and ultrasound will usually suffice to identify an ovarian mass, if clinical evaluation and hormonal levels suggest these possibilities.

PCOS is the most common cause of ovarian androgen excess (Chap. 336). However, the increased ratio of LH to follicle-stimulating hormone that is often seen in carefully studied patients with PCOS may not be exhibited in up to half of these women due to the pulsatility of gonadotropins. If performed, ultrasound shows enlarged ovaries and/or increased stroma in many women with PCOS. However, polycystic ovaries may also be found in women without clinical or laboratory features of PCOS. Therefore, polycystic ovaries are a relatively insensitive and nonspecific finding for the diagnosis of ovarian hyperandrogenism. Though it is not widely used, gonadotropin-releasing hormone agonist testing can be used to make a specific diagnosis of ovarian hyperandrogenism. A peak 17-hydroxyprogesterone level ≥7.8 nmol/L (≥2.6 μg/L), after the administration of 100 μg nafarelin (or 10 μg/kg leuprolide) subcutaneously, is virtually diagnostic of ovarian hyperandrogenism.

Nonclassic CAH is most commonly due to 21-hydroxylase deficiency but can also be caused by autosomal recessive defects in other steroidogenic enzymes necessary for adrenal corticosteroid synthesis (Chap. 331). Because of the enzyme defect, the adrenal gland cannot secrete glucocorticoids efficiently (especially cortisol). This results in diminished negative feedback inhibition of ACTH, leading to compensatory hyperplasia of the adrenal cortex and accumulation of steroid precursors proximal to the enzyme defect. These precursors are subsequently converted to androgen.

Deficiency of 21-hydroxylase can be reliably excluded by determining a morning 17-hydroxyprogesterone level <6 nmol/L (<2 μg/L) (drawn in the follicular phase). Alternatively, 21-hydroxylase deficiency can be diagnosed by measurement of 17-hydroxyprogesterone 1 h after administration of 250 μg of synthetic ACTH (cosyntropin) intravenously. Measurement after ACTH is slightly more cumbersome, though the results obtained in this manner are highly reproducible and can be compared to published nomograms.

TREATMENT Treatment of hirsutism may be accomplished pharmacologically and by mechanical means of hair removal. Nonpharmacologic treatments should be considered in all patients, either as the only treatment or as an adjunct to drug therapy.

Nonpharmacologic treatments include (1) bleaching; (2) depilatory (removal from the skin surface) such as shaving and chemical treatments; or (3) epilatory (removal of the hair including the root) such as plucking, waxing, electrolysis, and laser therapy. Despite perceptions to the contrary, shaving does not increase the rate or density of hair growth. Chemical depilatory treatments may be useful for mild hirsutism that affects only limited skin areas, though they can cause skin irritation. Wax treatment removes hair temporarily but is uncomfortable. Electrolysis is effective for more permanent hair removal, particularly in the hands of a skilled electrologist. Laser phototherapy appears to be efficacious for hair removal. It delays hair regrowth and causes permanent hair removal in some patients. The long-term effects and complications associated with laser treatment are being evaluated.

Pharmacologic therapy for androgen excess is directed at interrupting one or more of the steps in the pathway leading to its expression: (1) suppression of adrenal and/or ovarian androgen production; (2) enhancement of androgen-binding to plasma-binding proteins, particularly SHBG; (3) impairment of the peripheral conversion of androgen precursors to active androgen; and (4) inhibition of androgen action at the target tissue level. Attenuation of hair growth is typically not evident until 4 to 6 months after initiation of medical treatment and, in most cases, leads to a modest reduction in hair growth.

Combination estrogen-progestin therapy, in the form of an oral contraceptive, is usually the first-line endocrine treatment for hirsutism and acne, after cosmetic and dermatologic management. The estrogenic component of most oral contraceptives currently in use is either ethinyl estradiol or mestranol. The suppression of LH leads to reduced

Physical examination
·Body mass index/body fat distribution
·Blood pressure
·Assessment of hair growth
    Type (vellus vs terminal)
    Distribution   } Ferriman-
    Quantity   Gallwey Score
·Assessment of hair loss/alopecia
·Acne
·Features of virilization
    Clitoromegaly
    Increased muscle mass
·Features of other endocrine disorders
    Cushingoid features
    Galactorrhea
    Acanthosis nigricans, skin tags   } Evaluate
    Acromegaly

History
·Growth/sexual development
·Menstrual history
·Medication
·Family history of hirsutism

No ← Hirsutism significant   Virilization Rapid progression

(Yes)

Reassurance Nonpharmacologic approaches   Rule out ovarian or adrenal neoplasm

Laboratory Evaluation
·Total, free testosterone
·DHEAS

Normal   Increased   Marked elevation
Total testosterone >7 nmol/L (>2 ng/mL)
DHEAS >18.5 μmol/L (>7000 μg/L)

Treat empirically
or
Consider further testing
·Dexamethasone suppression → adrenal vs ovarian causes
·GnRH agonist test → assess PCOS/ovarian hyperandrogenism
·ACTH stimulation → assess nonclassic CAH

Final diagnosis

Idiopathic   ·Nonclassic CAH   ·PCOS
                  ·Functional adrenal   ·Functional ovarian
Other causes   hyperandrogenism   hyperandrogenism
see Table 53-1

FIGURE 53-2 Algorithm for the evaluation and differential diagnosis of hirsutism. ACTH, adrenocorticotropic hormone; CAH, congenital adrenal hyperplasia; DHEAS, sulfated form of dehydroepiandrosterone; GnRH, gonadotropin-releasing hormone; PCOS, polycystic ovarian syndrome.

production of ovarian androgens. The reduced androgen levels also result in a dose-related increase in SHBG, thereby lowering the fraction of unbound plasma testosterone. Combination therapy has also been demonstrated to decrease DHEAS, perhaps by reducing ACTH levels. Estrogens also have a direct, dose-dependent suppressive effect on sebaceous cell function.

The choice of a specific oral contraceptive should be predicated on the progestational component, as progestins vary in their suppressive effect on SHBG levels and in their androgenic potential. Ethynodiol diacetate has relatively low androgenic potential, whereas progestins such as norgestrel and levonorgestrel are particularly androgenic, as judged from their attenuation of the estrogen-induced increase in SHBG. Norgestimate exemplifies the newer generation of progestins that are virtually nonandrogenic. Oral contraceptives are contraindicated in women with a history of thromboembolic disease or in women with breast cancer or other estrogen-dependent cancers (Chap. 336). There is a relative contraindication to the use of oral contraceptives in smokers or in those with hypertension or a history of migraine headaches. In most trials, estrogen-progestin therapy alone improves the extent of acne by a maximum of 50 to 70%. In con-

trast, the effect on hair growth may not be evident for 6 months, and the maximum effect may require 9 to 12 months owing to the length of the hair growth cycle. Improvements in hirsutism are typically in the range of 20%, and often there is little more than arrest of further progression of hair growth.

Adrenal androgens are more sensitive than cortisol to the suppressive effects of glucocorticoids. Therefore, glucocorticoids are the mainstay of treatment in patients with CAH. Although glucocorticoids have been reported to restore ovulatory function in some women with PCOS, this effect is highly variable. Because of side effects from excessive glucocorticoids, low doses should be used. Dexamethasone (0.2 to 0.5 mg) or prednisone (5 to 10 mg) should be given at bedtime to achieve maximal suppression by inhibiting the nocturnal surge of ACTH.

Cyproterone acetate is the prototypic antiandrogen. It acts mainly by competitive inhibition of the binding of testosterone and DHT to the androgen receptor. In addition, it may act to enhance the metabolic clearance of testosterone by inducing hepatic enzymes. Although not available for use in the United States, cyproterone acetate is widely used in Canada, Mexico, and Europe. Cyproterone (50 to 100 mg) is given on days 1 to 15 and ethinyl estradiol (50 μg) is given on days 5 to 26 of the menstrual cycle. Side effects of cyproterone acetate include irregular uterine bleeding, nausea, headache, fatigue, weight gain, and decreased libido.

Spironolactone, usually used as a mineralocorticoid antagonist, is also a weak antiandrogen. It is almost as effective as cyproterone acetate when used at high enough doses (100 to 200 mg daily). Patients should be monitored intermittently for hyperkalemia or hypotension, though these side effects are uncommon. Pregnancy should be avoided because of the risk of feminization of a male fetus. Spironolactone can also cause menstrual irregularity. It is often used in combination with an oral contraceptive, which helps in prevention of pregnancy and suppression of ovarian androgen production.

Flutamide is a potent nonsteroidal antiandrogen that is effective in treating hirsutism, but concerns about the induction of hepatocellular dysfunction have limited its use. Finasteride is a competitive inhibitor of 5α-reductase type 2. Beneficial effects on hirsutism have been reported, but the prominence of 5α-reductase type 1 in the pilosebaceous unit appears to account for its limited efficacy. Finasteride would also be expected to impair sexual differentiation in a male fetus, and thus it should be used in women who may become pregnant.

A prospective, randomized trial comparing low-dose flutamide, finasteride, and combination cyproterone acetate–ethinyl estradiol demonstrated relative superiority of flutamide and cyproterone acetate–ethinyl estradiol in the treatment of hirsutism. Ultimately, the choice of any specific agent(s) must be tailored to the unique needs of the patient being treated. As noted previously, pharmacologic treatments for hirsutism should be used in conjunction with nonpharmacologic approaches. Patients should be reminded about the relatively slow and usually modest responses to pharmacologic treatment. It is also helpful to review the pattern of female hair distribution in the normal population to dispel unrealistic expectations.

DIERICKX C et al: A clinical overview of hair removal using lasers and light sources. Dermatol Clin 17:357, 1999

EHRMANN DA, ROSENFIELD RL: Clinical review: An endocrinologic approach to the patient with hirsutism. J Clin Endocrinol Metab 71:1, 1990

——— et al: Polycystic ovary syndrome as a form of functional ovarian hyperandrogenism due to dysregulation of androgen secretion. Endocr Rev 16:322, 1995

——— et al: Hyperandrogenism, hirsutism, and polycystic ovarian syndrome, in *Endocrinology*, 4th ed, LJ DeGroot et al (eds). Philadelphia, Saunders, 2000, chap 160

PAUS R, COTSARELIS G: The biology of hair follicles. N Engl J Med 341:491, 1999

RITTMASTER RS: Antiandrogen treatment of polycystic ovary syndrome. Endocrinol Metab Clin North Am 28:409, 1999

VENTUROLI S et al: A prospective randomized trial comparing low dose flutamide, finasteride, ketoconazole, and cyproterone acetate–estrogen regimens in the treatment of hirsutism. J Clin Endocrinol Metab 84:1304, 1999

54   *Janet E. Hall*

INFERTILITY AND FERTILITY CONTROL

FDA	Food and Drug Administration	IUI	intrauterine insemination
FSH	follicle-stimulating hormone	IVF	in vitro fertilization
GnRH	gonadotropin-releasing hormone	LH	luteinizing hormone
hCG	human chorionic gonadotropin	PCOS	polycystic ovarian syndrome
ICSI	intracytoplasmic sperm injection	STDs	sexually transmitted diseases
IUD	intrauterine device		

The concept of reproductive choice is now firmly entrenched in developed countries and has dramatically altered reproductive behavior. The availability of effective contraceptive methods prevents unintended pregnancies and gives women the option of pursuing educational and career opportunities without interruption. Population control also has important economic and social implications. Infertility, on the other hand, can be accompanied by substantial stress and disappointment. Fortunately, the ability to diagnose and to treat various causes of infertility now provides an array of effective new approaches to this condition.

INFERTILITY

DEFINITION AND PREVALENCE   *Infertility* is defined as the inability to conceive after 12 months of unprotected sexual intercourse. In a study of 5574 English and American women who ultimately conceived, pregnancy occurred in 50% within 3 months, 72% within 6 months, and 85% within 12 months. These findings are consistent with predictions based on *fecundability*, the probability of achieving pregnancy in one menstrual cycle (approximately 20 to 25% in healthy young couples). Assuming a fecundability of 0.25, 98% of couples should conceive within 13 months. Based on this definition, the National Survey of Family Growth reports a 14% rate of infertility in the United States in married women aged 15 to 44. The infertility rate has remained relatively stable over the past 30 years, although the proportion of couples without children has risen, reflecting a trend to delay childbearing. This trend has important implications because of an age-related decrease in fecundability, which begins at age 35, and decreases markedly after age 40.

CAUSES OF INFERTILITY   There is a spectrum of infertility, ranging from reduced conception rates or the need for medical intervention to irreversible causes of infertility (*sterility*). Infertility can be attributed primarily to male factors in 25%, female factors in 58%, and is unexplained in about 17% of couples (Fig. 54-1). Not uncommonly, both male and female factors contribute to infertility.

——— *Approach to the Patient* ———

Initial Evaluation   In all couples presenting with infertility, the initial evaluation includes discussion of the appropriate timing of in-

tercourse and a description of the range of investigations that may be required. A brief description of infertility treatment options, including adoption, should be reviewed. Initial investigations are focused on determining whether the primary cause of the infertility is male, female, or both. These investigations include a semen analysis in the male, confirmation of ovulation in the female, and, in the majority of situations, documentation of tubal patency in the female. Although frequently used in the past, recent studies have not supported the efficacy of postcoital testing of sperm interaction with cervical mucus as a routine component of initial testing. Strategies for further evaluation are described below and in Chaps. 335 and 336. In some cases, after an extensive workup excluding all male and female factors, a specific cause cannot be identified and infertility may ultimately be classified as unexplained.

Psychological Aspects of Infertility   Infertility is invariably associated with psychological stress related not only to the diagnostic and therapeutic procedures themselves but also to repeated cycles of hope and loss associated with each new procedure or cycle of treatment that does not result in the birth of a child. These feelings are often combined with a sense of isolation from friends and family. Counseling and stress-management techniques should be introduced early in the evaluation of infertility. In addition to the psychological benefits of stress management, it is possible that stress contributes to infertility in some couples (e.g., impaired ovulation). Importantly, infertility and its treatment do not appear to be associated with long-term psychological sequelae.

Female Causes   Abnormalities in menstrual function constitute the most common cause of female infertility. These disorders, which include ovulatory dysfunction and abnormalities of the uterus or outflow tract, may present as amenorrhea (absence of menses) or as irregular or short menstrual cycles. A careful history and physical examination and a limited number of laboratory tests will help to determine whether the abnormality is: (1) hypothalamic or pituitary [low follicle-stimulating hormone (FSH), luteinizing hormone (LH), and estradiol with or without an increase in prolactin]; (2) polycystic ovarian syndrome (PCOS; irregular cycles and hyperandrogenism in the absence of other causes of androgen excess); (3) ovarian (low estradiol with increased FSH); or (4) uterine or outflow tract abnormality. The frequency of these diagnoses depends on whether the amenorrhea is primary or occurs after normal puberty and menarche (Fig. 54-1). →*The approach to further evaluation of these disorders is described in detail in Chap. 52.*

Ovulatory dysfunction   In women with a history of regular menstrual cycles, *evidence of ovulation* should be sought by using urinary ovulation predictor kits (they reflect the preovulatory gonadotropin surge but do not confirm ovulation), basal body temperature charts, or a mid-luteal phase progesterone level. The mid-luteal phase progesterone increase (usually >3 ng/mL) confirms ovulation and corpus luteum function and is responsible for the rise in basal body temperature [0.3°C (>0.6°F) for 10 days]. An endometrial biopsy to exclude luteal phase insufficiency is no longer considered an essential part of the infertility workup for most patients. Even in the presence of ovulatory cycles, evaluation of *ovarian reserve* is recommended for women over 35 by measurement of FSH on day 3 of the cycle or in response to clomiphene, an estrogen antagonist (see below). An FSH level <10 IU/mL on cycle day 3 predicts adequate ovarian oocyte reserve. Inhibin B, an ovarian hormone that selectively suppresses FSH, is being investigated as an additional marker of ovarian reserve.

Tubal disease   This may result from pelvic inflammatory disease (PID), appendicitis, endometriosis, pelvic adhesions, tubal surgery, and previous use of an intrauterine device (IUD). However, a cause is not identified in up to 50% of patients with documented tubal factor infertility. Because of the high prevalence of tubal disease, testing should occur early in the majority of couples with infertility. Subclinical infections with *Chlamydia trachomatis* may be an underdiagnosed cause of tubal infertility and requires the treatment of both partners.

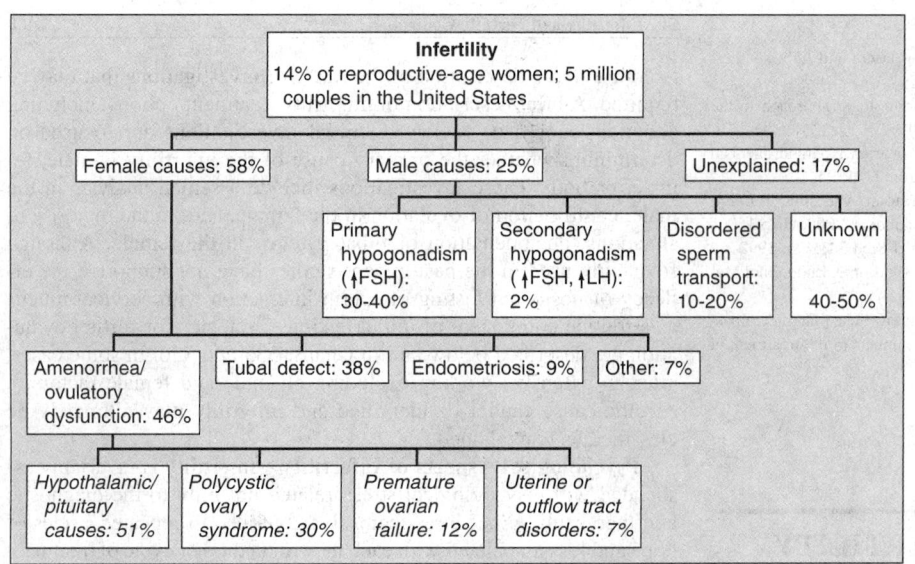

FIGURE 54-1 Causes of infertility. FSH, follicle-stimulating hormone; LH, luteinizing hormone.

A hysterosalpingogram (HSG) is the most common screening test and will determine the presence of tubal patency and identify potential abnormalities of the uterine cavity.

Endometriosis Endometriosis is defined as the presence of endometrial glands or stroma outside the endometrial cavity and uterine musculature. Its presence is suggested by a history of dyspareunia (painful intercourse), worsening dysmenorrhea that often begins before menses, or by a thickened rectovaginal septum or deviation of the cervix on pelvic examination. The pathogenesis of the infertility associated with endometriosis is unclear but may involve indirect effects on the normal endometrium as well as the direct effects of adhesions in advanced disease. Endometriosis is often clinically silent, however, and can only be excluded definitively by laparoscopy.

Male Causes Known causes of male infertility include primary testicular disease, disorders of sperm transport, and hypothalamic-pituitary disease resulting in secondary hypogonadism. However, the etiology is not ascertained in up to half of men with suspected male factor infertility (Fig. 54-1). The key initial diagnostic test is a *semen analysis*. Although 95% confidence limits can be used to define normal semen parameters, data relating sperm counts to fecundability are more useful. Such studies suggest that sperm counts of <20 million/mL, with a motility of less than 40%, are associated with an increased risk of infertility. Analysis of sperm morphology is less well validated, but >40% normal forms are usually present in fertile men. Successful in vitro fertilization (IVF) can usually be accomplished with >14% normal forms (using strict Kruger criteria), whereas low fertilization is seen with <4% normal forms. Other tests such as the hamster egg penetration test and the zona-binding assay are not of proven value.

Testosterone levels should be measured if the sperm count is low on repeated examination or if there is clinical evidence of hypogonadism. A low testosterone level may result from *primary gonadal deficiency*; in this condition, levels of LH and FSH will be elevated. Less commonly, low testosterone and decreased spermatogenesis result from hypothalamic or pituitary disease, in which case the LH and FSH levels will be low (Chap. 335).

Abnormalities of spermatogenesis may have a genetic component. Y chromosome microdeletions and substitutions are increasingly recognized as a cause of *azoospermia* (absence of sperm) or *oligospermia* (low sperm count). Microdeletions (Yq6 region) have also been identified in a subset of men with elevated FSH levels or otherwise idiopathic infertility. Several candidate genes have been identified including *DAZ* (deleted in azoospermia) and *YRRM* (Y chromosome RNA recognition motif).

Acquired disorders of the testes are often associated with impaired spermatogenesis with relatively preserved Leydig cell function; thus,

testosterone levels may be normal. Such abnormalities include viral orchitis (especially mumps) and other infectious causes such as tuberculosis or sexually transmitted diseases (STDs), chemotherapy (especially the alkylating agents cyclophosphamide and chlorambucil), ionizing radiation, and drugs that may impair fertility directly or through inhibition of testicular androgen production or action. Anabolic androgen abuse should be considered in a well-androgenized man with low gonadotropins and testosterone but a suppressed sperm count. Prolonged elevation of testicular temperature may impair spermatogenesis, e.g., after an acute febrile illness or in association with varicocele. A potential role for environmental toxins as a cause of impaired spermatogenesis has been suggested based on an apparent decrease in sperm counts over the past several decades, but a direct cause-and-effect relationship has not been established.

Secondary hypogonadism Low gonadotropin levels, associated with low testosterone, may signal the presence of a pituitary macroadenoma or hypothalamic tumor (in both cases prolactin levels may be elevated; Chap. 328) or may be the first presentation of hemochromatosis (Chap. 345) or other systemic illness. Recent studies have identified several genetic causes of gonadotropin-releasing hormone (GnRH) deficiency (*KAL* and *DAX-1*), as well as mutations that lead to isolated gonadotropin deficiency (GnRH receptor, LHβ, FSHβ mutations) (Chap. 328).

Disordered sperm transport Patients with low sperm counts and normal hormonal levels may be found to have obstructive abnormalities of the vas deferens or epididymus. The most common causes of vas deferens obstruction are previous vasectomy or accidental ligation during inguinal surgery. Patency rates with microsurgical reversal techniques are high in the first 3 years after vasectomy but decrease markedly thereafter. Congenital absence of the vas deferens can be diagnosed by a deficiency of fructose in the ejaculate and is often associated with an abnormality of the cystic fibrosis transmembrane regulator (*CFTR*) gene. Young's syndrome, characterized by inspissated secretions, can also preclude normal sperm transport.

℞ TREATMENT The treatment of infertility should be tailored to the problems unique to each couple (Table 54-1). In many situations, including unexplained infertility, mild to moderate endometriosis, and/or borderline semen parameters, a stepwise approach to infertility is optimal, beginning with low-risk interventions and moving to more invasive, higher risk interventions only if necessary. After determination of all infertility factors and their correction, if possible, this approach might include, in increasing order of complexity: (1) expectant management, (2) clomiphene citrate (see below) with or without intrauterine insemination (IUI), (3) gonadotropins with or without IUI, and (4) IVF. The time used to complete the evaluation, correction, and expectant management can be longer in women <30, but this process should be advanced rapidly in women >35. In some situations expectant management will not be appropriate.

Ovulatory Dysfunction Treatment of ovulatory dysfunction should first be directed at identification of the etiology of the disorder to allow specific management when possible. Dopamine agonists, for example, may be indicated in patients with hyperprolactinemia (Chap. 328); lifestyle modification may be successful in women with low body weight or a history of intensive exercise (Chap. 78).

Pulsatile GnRH is highly effective for restoring ovulation in patients with hypothalamic amenorrhea. When administered subcutaneously by an automated pump at a physiologic dose and frequency, pulsatile GnRH induces normal LH and FSH dynamics. Direct comparisons between pulsatile GnRH and gonadotropin treatment for ovulation induction indicate similar pregnancy rates; pulsatile GnRH is associated with lower rates of multiple gestation and virtually no risk of ovarian hyperstimulation.

Clomiphene citrate is a nonsteroidal estrogen antagonist that increases FSH and LH levels by blocking estrogen negative feedback at the hypothalamus. The efficacy of clomiphene for ovulation induction is highly dependent on patient selection. It induces ovulation in ~60% of women with PCOS and is the initial treatment of choice in these patients. The starting dose is 50 mg daily for 5 days beginning on day 5 of a spontaneous cycle or after a progestin-induced withdrawal bleed. The dose can be increased to 150 mg, if necessary, in subsequent cycles, and human chorionic gonadotropin (hCG) can be added as the ovulatory stimulus. In women with PCOS, the use of insulin-sensitizing agents, such as metformin appears to be particularly effective in combination with clomiphene.

Table 54-1 Treatment Approaches for Various Causes of Infertility

	Surgery	Clomiphene	Gonadotropins	Pulsatile GnRH	IUI	Donor Sperm	IVF	ICSI	Donor Egg
FEMALE									
Ovulatory dysfunction									
Hypothalamic-pituitary			✔	✔					
Polycystic ovary syndrome		✔	✔	✔					
Premature ovarian failure									✔
Tubal disease	✔						✔		
Endometriosis	✔	✔		✔	✔		✔		
MALE									
Primary hypogonadism					✔	✔		✔	
Secondary hypogonadism			✔	✔					
Disorders of sperm transport	✔						✔	✔	
Unexplained		✔	✔		✔		✔		

NOTE: GnRH, gonadotropin-releasing hormone; IUI, intrauterine insemination; IVF, in vitro fertilization; ICSI, intracytoplasmic sperm injection.

Gonadotropins are highly effective for ovulation induction in women with hypogonadotropic hypogonadism and PCOS. Gonadotropins are also used to induce multiple follicular recruitment in unexplained infertility and in older reproductive-aged women, particularly in conjunction with IUI. Disadvantages include a significant risk of multiple gestation and the risk of ovarian hyperstimulation, a side effect that is more common in women with PCOS. However, careful monitoring and a conservative approach to ovarian stimulation reduce these risks; gonadotropin stimulation is an effective and safe treatment when applied by experienced practitioners. Currently available gonadotropins include urinary preparations of LH and FSH, highly purified FSH, and recombinant FSH. Though FSH is the key component, there is growing data that the addition of some LH (or hCG) may improve results, particularly in hypogonadotropic patients.

None of these methods are effective in women with premature ovarian failure in whom donor oocyte or adoption are the methods of choice.

Tubal Disease If hysterosalpingography suggests a tubal or uterine cavity abnormality, or if a patient is ≥35 at the time of initial evaluation, laparoscopy with tubal lavage is recommended, often with a hysteroscopy. Although tubal reconstruction may be attempted if tubal disease is identified, it is generally being replaced by the use of IVF, as these patients are at increased risk of developing an ectopic pregnancy.

Endometriosis Though 60% of women with minimal or mild endometriosis may conceive within 1 year without treatment, laparoscopic resection or ablation appear to improve conception rates. Medical management of advanced stages of endometriosis is widely used for symptom control but has not been shown to enhance fertility (Chap. 336). In moderate to severe endometriosis, conservative surgery is associated with pregnancy rates of 50 and 39% respectively, compared with rates of 25 and 5% with expectant management alone. In some patients, IVF may be the treatment of choice.

Male Factor Infertility The treatment options for male factor infertility have expanded greatly in recent years. Secondary hypogonadism is highly amenable to treatment with pulsatile GnRH or gonadotropins (Chap. 335). In vitro techniques have provided new opportunities for patients with primary testicular failure and disorders of sperm transport. Choice of initial treatment options depends on sperm concentration and motility. Expectant management should be attempted initially in men with mild male factor infertility (sperm count of 15 to 20 × 10⁶/mL and normal motility). Moderate male factor infertility (10 to 15 × 10⁶/mL and 20 to 40% motility) should begin with IUI alone or in combination with treatment of the female partner with clomiphene or gonadotropins, but it may require IVF with or without intracytoplasmic sperm injection (ICSI). For men with a severe defect (sperm count of <10 × 10⁶/mL, 10% motility), IVF with ICSI or donor sperm should be used.

Assisted Reproductive Technologies The development of assisted reproductive technologies (ART) has dramatically altered the treatment of male and female infertility. IVF is indicated for patients with many causes of infertility that have not been successfully managed with more conservative approaches. IVF or ICSI is often the treatment of choice in couples with a significant male factor or tubal disease, whereas IVF using donor oocytes is used in patients with premature ovarian failure and in women of advanced reproductive age. Success rates depend on the age of the woman and the cause of the infertility and are generally 18 to 24% per cycle when initiated in women <40. In women >40, there is a marked decrease in both the number of oocytes retrieved and their ability to be fertilized. Though often effective, IVF is expensive and requires careful monitoring of ovulation induction and invasive techniques including the aspiration of multiple follicles. IVF is associated with a significant risk of multiple gestation (29% twins, 7% triplets, and 0.6% higher order multiples). More recently developed blastocyst transfer protocols decrease the number of transfers but increase pregnancy rates.

CONTRACEPTION

Though various forms of contraception are widely available, approximately 30% of births in the United States are the result of unintended pregnancy. Teenage pregnancies continue to represent a serious public health problem in the United States, with >1 million unintended pregnancies each year—a significantly greater incidence than in other industrialized nations (Chap. 8).

Contraceptive methods are widely used (Table 54-2). Only 15% of couples report having unprotected sexual intercourse in the past 3 months. A reversible form of contraception is used by >50% of couples. Sterilization (in either the male or female) has been employed as a permanent form of contraception by about 25% of couples. Preg-

Table 54-2 Effectiveness of Different Forms of Contraception

Method of Contraception	Theoretical Effectiveness[a]	Actual Effectiveness[a]	Percent Continuing Use at 1 year[b]	Contraceptive Methods used by U.S. women[c]
Barrier methods				
Condoms	98	88	63	19
Diaphragm	94	82	58	2
Cervical cap	94	82	50	<1
Spermacides	97	79	43	1
Sterilization				
Male	99.9	99.9	100	10
Female	99.8	99.6	100	15
Intrauterine device				1
Copper T380	99	97	78	
Progestasert	98	97	81	
Oral contraceptive pill			72	26
Combination	99.9	97		
Progestin only	99.5	97		
Long-acting progestins				
Depo-Provera	99.7	99.7	70	<1
Norplant	99.96	99.96	85	1

[a] Adapted from Trussel J et al, Obstet Gynecol 76:558, 1990.
[b] Adapted from Contraceptive Technology Update. Contraceptive Technology, Feb. 1996, vol 17, No 1, pp 13–24.
[c] Adapted from 1995 Ortho Birth Control Survey. Raritan, NJ, Ortho Pharmaceutical, 1996. 20% used no method, 5% used other.

nancy termination is relatively safe when directed by health care professionals but is rarely the option of choice.

No single contraceptive method is ideal, although all are safer than carrying a pregnancy to term. The effectiveness of a given method of contraception is dependent on the efficacy of the method itself, compliance, and appropriate use. Knowledge of the advantages and disadvantages of each contraceptive is essential for counseling an individual about the methods that are safest and most consistent with his or her lifestyle. Discrepancies between theoretical and actual effectiveness emphasize the importance of patient education and compliance when considering various forms of contraception (Table 54-2).

BARRIER METHODS Barrier contraceptives, such as condoms, diaphragms, cervical caps, and spermicides, are easily available, reversible, and have fewer side effects than hormonal methods. However, their effectiveness is highly dependent on compliance and proper use (Table 54-2). A major advantage of barrier contraceptives is the protection provided against STDs (Chap. 132). Consistent use is associated with a decreased risk of gonorrhea, nongonococcal urethritis, and genital herpes, probably due in part to the concomitant use of spermicides. Condom use also reduces the transmission of HIV infection. Natural membrane condoms may be less effective than latex condoms, and petroleum-based lubricants can degrade condoms and decrease their efficacy for preventing HIV infection. A highly effective female condom, which also provides protection against STDs, was approved in 1994 but has not achieved widespread use.

STERILIZATION Sterilization is the method of birth control most frequently chosen by fertile men and multiparous women >30 (Table 54-2). Sterilization refers to a procedure that prevents fertilization by surgical interruption of the fallopian tubes in women or the vas deferens in men. Although tubal ligation and vasectomy are potentially reversible, these procedures should be considered permanent and should not be undertaken without careful patient counseling.

Several methods of *tubal ligation* have been developed, all of which are highly effective with a 10-year cumulative pregnancy rate of 1.85 per 100 women. However, when pregnancy does occur, the risk of ectopic pregnancy may be as high as 30%. The success rate of tubal reanastomosis depends on the method used—the clip, silastic band, and modified Pomeroy procedures are easier to reverse than the Irving, Uchida, and electrocoagulation methods. Even after successful reversal, the risk of ectopic pregnancy remains great. In addition to prevention of pregnancy, tubal ligation reduces the risk of ovarian cancer, possibly by limiting the upward migration of potential carcinogens.

Vasectomy is an outpatient surgical procedure that has little risk and is highly effective. The development of azoospermia may be delayed for 2 to 6 months, and other forms of contraception must be used until two sperm-free ejaculations provide proof of sterility. Reanastomosis may restore fertility in 30 to 50% of men, but the success rate appears to decline with time after vasectomy and may be influenced by nonmechanical factors such as the development of anti-sperm antibodies.

INTRAUTERINE DEVICES IUDs inhibit pregnancy primarily through a spermicidal effect caused by a sterile inflammatory reaction produced by the presence of a foreign body in the uterine cavity. There may also be effects on cervical mucus sperm transport through the oviduct. IUDs provide a high level of efficacy in the absence of systemic metabolic effects. An additional advantage is that ongoing motivation is not required to ensure efficacy once the device has been placed. However, only 1% of women in the United States use this method compared to a utilization rate of 15 to 30% in much of Europe and Canada. This relatively low utilization rate continues despite evidence that the newer devices are not associated with increased rates of pelvic infection and infertility, as occurred with earlier devices. Screening for STD should be performed prior to insertion, and an IUD should not be used in women at high risk for development of STD or in women at high risk for bacterial endocarditis. In addition, the IUD may not be effective in women with uterine leiomyomas because they alter the size or shape of the uterine cavity. IUD use is associated with increased menstrual blood flow, although this is less pronounced with the progesterone-releasing IUD than the copper-containing device.

HORMONAL METHODS No male hormonal contraceptive methods are currently approved in the United States. However, hormonal methods of male contraception, including GnRH-mediated suppression of the hypothalamic-pituitary-gonadal axis in combination with testosterone replacement, are under investigation.

Oral Contraceptive Pills Because of their ease of use and efficacy, oral contraceptive pills are the most widely used form of hormonal contraception. They act by suppressing ovulation, changing cervical mucus, and altering the endometrium. The current formulations are made from synthetic estrogens and progestins. The estrogen component of the pill consists of ethinyl estradiol or mestranol, which is metabolized to ethinyl estradiol. Multiple synthetic progestins are used. Norethindrone and its derivatives are used in many formulations. Low-dose norgestimate and third-generation progestins (desogestrel, gestodene) have a less androgenic profile; levonorgestrel appears to be the most androgenic of the progestins and should be avoided in patients with hyperandrogenic symptoms. The three major formulations of oral contraceptives include: (1) fixed-dose estrogen-progestin combination, (2) phasic estrogen-progestin combination, and (3) progestin only. Each of these formulations is administered daily for 3 weeks followed by a week of no medication during which menstrual bleeding generally occurs.

Current doses of ethinyl estradiol range from 20 to 50 μg. However, indications for the 50-μg dose are rare, and the majority of formulations contain 35 μg of ethinyl estradiol. The reduced estrogen and progesterone content in the second- and third-generation pills has decreased both side effects and risks associated with oral contraceptive use. At the currently used doses, patients must be cautioned not to miss pills due to the potential for ovulation. Side effects, including break-through bleeding, amenorrhea, and weight gain, are often responsive to a change in formulation. There is no evidence that low-dose oral contraceptives increase the risk of cardiovascular disease in women <30 or in nonsmoking women without additional risk factors. However, the risk of myocardial infarction and stroke in women who smoke is increased by the use of oral contraceptives. The risk of developing hypertension is increased somewhat, even with the low-dose preparations. An increased risk of venous thromboembolism occurs with all oral contraceptives and may be even greater with the third-generation preparations. The factor V Leiden mutation and other thrombophilic disorders (Chap. 117) are important risk factors for venous thrombosis during oral contraceptive therapy. However, biochemical or genetic screening for these disorders before starting oral contraceptives is not cost-effective at present. In most studies, oral contraceptive use has not been shown to increase the risk of breast cancer, but there is a slight increase in the risk of cervical cancer. Risks for endometrial and ovarian cancer are decreased in oral contraceptive users.

Previous thromboembolic events or stroke are absolute contraindications for the use of oral contraceptive pills. A history of hormone-dependent tumors and liver disease are also contraindications. Oral contraceptive pills should not be given in pregnancy or in women with undiagnosed uterine bleeding or amenorrhea.

The microdose progestin-only minipill is less effective as a contraceptive, having a pregnancy rate of 2 to 7 per 100 women-years. However, it may be appropriate for women with cardiovascular disease or for women who cannot tolerate synthetic estrogens.

Injectable Contraceptives Depot medroxyprogesterone acetate (Depo-Provera) and Norplant (Table 54-2) act primarily by inhibiting ovulation and causing changes in the endometrium and cervical mucus that result in decreased implantation and sperm transport. Depo-Provera is effective for 3 months, but return of fertility after discontinuation may be delayed for up to 12 to 18 months. Norplant requires surgical insertion but is effective for up to 5 years afer insertion; fertility is possible shortly after its removal. The U.S. Food and Drug Administration (FDA) has recently approved the use of covered rods in addition to the capsules. Amenorrhea, irregular bleeding, and weight gain are the most common adverse effects associated with both injectable forms of contraception. An injectable progestin/estrogen combination con-

traceptive will be available soon. It requires monthly injection, but irregular bleeding and weight gain are less common. A major advantage of the injectable progestin-based contraceptives is the apparent lack of increased arterial and venous thromboembolic events.

POSTCOITAL CONTRACEPTION Postcoital contraceptive methods prevent implantation or cause regression of the corpus luteum and are highly efficacious if used appropriately. Although postcoital contraception is not specifically licensed for use in the United States, an FDA notice published in 1997 indicated that certain oral contraceptive pills could be used within 72 h of unprotected intercourse [Ovral (2 tablets 12 h apart) and Lo/Ovral (4 tablets 12 h apart)]. The Preven Emergency Contraceptive Kit contains four combination tablets (50 mg ethinyl estradiol and 0.25 mg levonorgestrel) and a pregnancy kit to rule out pregnancy before taking the pills. Side effects are common with these high doses of hormones and include nausea, vomiting, and breast soreness. Recent studies suggest that 600 mg mifepristone (RU486), a progesterone receptor antagonist, may be equally as effective or more effective than hormonal regimens, with fewer side effects. Mifepristone is not currently available in the United States.

BIBLIOGRAPHY

ABMA JC et al and the National Center for Health Statistics: Fertility, family planning, and women's health: New data from the 1995 Survey of Family Growth. Vital Statistics: Series 23, No. 10

BARBIERI RL: Assisted reproduction, in *Reproductive Endocrinology: Physiology, Pathophysiology and Clinical Management*, SSc Yen, RB Jaffe, RL Barbieri (eds). Philadelphia, Saunders, pp 594–621, 1999

—— et al: The safety of third-generation oral contraceptives. J Clin Endocrinol Metab 84:1822, 1999

BHASIN S et al: Y-chromosome microdeletions and male infertility. Ann Intern Med 29: 261, 1997

COLLINS JA: Unexplained infertility, in *Infertility: Evaluation and Treatment*, WR Keye et al (eds). Philadelphia, Saunders, 1995, pp 249–262

GLASIER A: Emergency postcoital contraception. N Engl J Med 337:1058, 1997

TRUSSELL J, VAUGHAN B: Contraceptive failure, method-related discontinuation and resumption of use: Results from the 1995 National Survey of Family Growth. Fam Plann Perspect 31:64, 1999

WANG C, SWERDLOFF R: Medical treatment of male infertility, in *Infertility: Evaluation and Treatment*, WR Keye et al (eds). Philadelphia, Saunders, 1995, pp 143–150

Section 9

ALTERATIONS IN THE SKIN

55

Thomas J. Lawley, Kim B. Yancey

APPROACH TO THE PATIENT WITH A SKIN DISORDER

The challenge of examining the skin lies in distinguishing normal from abnormal, significant findings from trivial ones, and in integrating pertinent signs and symptoms into an appropriate differential diagnosis. The fact that the largest organ in the body is visible is both an advantage and a disadvantage to those who examine it. It is advantageous because no special instrumentation, other than a magnifying glass, is necessary and because the skin can be biopsied with little morbidity. However, the casual observer can be overwhelmed by a variety of stimuli and overlook important, subtle signs of skin or systemic disease. For instance, the sometimes minor differences in color and shape that distinguish a malignant melanoma (**see Plate IIC-30**) from a benign pigmented nevus (**see Plate IIC-28**) can be difficult to recognize. To aid in the interpretation of skin lesions, a variety of descriptive

terms have been developed to characterize cutaneous lesions (Tables 55-1 and 55-2 and Fig. 55-1) and to formulate a differential diagnosis (Table 55-3). For instance, the finding of large numbers of scaling papules, usually indicative of a primary skin disease, places the patient in a different diagnostic category than would hemorrhagic papules, which may indicate vasculitis or sepsis (**see Plates IIE-71 and IID-44, respectively**). It is important to differentiate primary skin lesions from secondary skin changes. If the examiner focuses on linear erosions overlying an area of erythema and scaling, he or she may incorrectly assume that the erosion is the primary lesion and the redness and scale are secondary, while the correct interpretation would be that the patient has a pruritic eczematous dermatitis and the erosions have been caused by scratching.

Approach to the Patient

In examining the skin it is usually advisable to assess the patient before taking a history. This way, the entire cutaneous surface is sure to be evaluated, and objective findings can be integrated with relevant historic data. Four basic features of any cutaneous lesion must be noted

Table 55-1   Descriptions of Primary Skin Lesions

Macule: A flat, colored lesion, <2 cm in diameter, not raised above the surface of the surrounding skin. A "freckle," or ephelid, is a prototype pigmented macule.

Patch: A large (>2 cm), flat lesion with a color different from the surrounding skin. This differs from a macule only in size.

Papule: A small, solid lesion, <1 cm in diameter, raised above the surface of the surrounding skin and hence palpable (e.g., a closed comedone, or white-head, in acne).

Nodule: A larger (1–5 cm), firm lesion raised above the surface of the surrounding skin. This differs from a papule only in size (e.g., dermal nevus).

Tumor: A solid, raised growth >5 cm in diameter.

Plaque: A large (>1 cm), flat-topped, raised lesion; edges may either be distinct (e.g., in psoriasis) or gradually blend with surrounding skin (e.g., in eczematous dermatitis).

Vesicle: A small, fluid-filled lesion, <1 cm in diameter, raised above the plane of surrounding skin. Fluid is often visible, and the lesions are often translucent [e.g., vesicles in allergic contact dermatitis caused by *Toxicodendron* (poison ivy)].

Pustule: A vesicle filled with leukocytes. Note: The presence of pustules does not necessarily signify the existence of an infection.

Bulla: A fluid-filled, raised, often translucent lesion >1 cm in diameter.

Cyst: A soft, raised, encapsulated lesion filled with semisolid or liquid contents.

Wheal: A raised, erythematous papule or plaque, usually representing short-lived dermal edema.

Telangiectasia: Dilated, superficial blood vessels.

Table 55-2   Common Dermatologic Terms

Lichenification: A distinctive thickening of the skin that is characterized by accentuated skin-fold markings and that feels thick and firm on palpation.

Crust: Dried exudate of body fluids that may be either yellow (serous exudate) or red (hemorrhagic exudate).

Milia: Small, firm, white papules that are filled with keratin (and may in part resemble pustules).

Erosion: Loss of epidermis without an associated loss of dermis.

Ulcer: Loss of epidermis and at least a portion of the underlying dermis.

Excoriations: Linear, angular erosions that may be covered by crust and are caused by scratching.

Atrophy: An acquired loss of substance. In the skin, this may appear as a depression with intact epidermis (i.e., loss of dermal or subcutaneous tissue) or as sites of shiny, delicate, wrinkled lesions (i.e., epidermal atrophy).

Scar: A change in the skin secondary to trauma or inflammation. Sites may be erythematous, hypopigmented, or hypertrophic depending on their age or character. Sites on hair-bearing areas may be characterized by destruction of hair follicles.

Pruritus: A sensation that elicits the desire to scratch. Pruritus is often the predominant symptom of inflammatory skin diseases (e.g., atopic dermatitis, allergic contact dermatitis); it is also commonly associated with xerosis and aged skin. Systemic conditions that can be associated with pruritis include chronic renal disease, cholestasis, pregnancy, malignancy, polycythemia vera, and delusions of parasitosis.

---

and considered in the examination of skin: the distribution of the eruption, the type(s) of primary lesion, the shape of individual lesions, and the arrangement of the lesions. In the initial examination it is important that the patient be disrobed as completely as possible. This will minimize chances of missing important individual skin lesions and make it possible to assess the distribution of the eruption accurately. The patient should first be viewed from a distance of about 1.5 to 2 m (4 to 6 ft) so that the general character of the skin and the distribution of lesions can be evaluated. Indeed, distribution of lesions often correlates highly with diagnosis (Fig. 55-2). For example, a hospitalized patient with a generalized erythematous exanthem is more likely to have a drug eruption than is a patient with a similar rash limited to the sun-exposed portions of the face. The presence or absence of lesions on mucosal surfaces should also be determined. Once the distribution of the lesions has been established, the nature of the primary lesion must be determined. Thus, when lesions are distributed on elbows, knees, and scalp, the most likely possibility based solely on distribution is psoriasis or dermatitis herpetiformis **(see Plates IIA-3 and IIE-68, respectively).** The primary lesion in psoriasis is a scaly papule that soon forms erythematous plaques covered with a white scale, whereas that of dermatitis herpetiformis is an urticarial papule that quickly becomes a small vesicle. In this manner, identification of the primary lesion directs the examiner toward the proper diagnosis. Secondary changes in skin can also be quite helpful. For example, scale represents excessive epidermis, while crust is the result of an inadequate or discontinuous epithelial cell layer. Palpation of skin lesions can also yield insight into the character of an eruption. Thus red papules on the lower extremities that blanch with pressure can be a manifestation of many different diseases, but hemorrhagic red papules that do not blanch with pressure indicate palpable purpura characteristic of necrotizing vasculitis **(see Plate IIE-71).**

The shape of lesions is also an important feature. Flat, round, erythematous papules and plaques are common in many cutaneous diseases. However, target-shaped lesions that consist in part of erythematous plaques are specific for erythema multiforme **(see Plate IIE-67).** In the same way, the arrangement of individual lesions is important. Erythematous papules and vesicles can occur in many conditions, but their arrangement in a specific linear array suggests an external etiology such as allergic contact **(see Plate IIA-8)** or primary irritant dermatitis. In contrast, lesions with a generalized arrangement are common and suggest a systemic etiology.

As in other branches of medicine, a complete history should be obtained to emphasize the following features:

1. Evolution of lesions
   a. Site of onset
   b. Manner in which eruption progressed or spread
   c. Duration
   d. Periods of resolution or improvement in chronic eruptions
2. Symptoms associated with the eruption
   a. Itching, burning, pain, numbness
   b. What, if anything, has relieved symptoms
   c. Time of day when symptoms are most severe
3. Current or recent medications (prescribed as well as over-the-counter)
4. Associated systemic symptoms (e.g., malaise, fever, arthralgias)
5. Ongoing or previous illnesses
6. History of allergies
7. Presence of photosensitivity
8. Review of systems

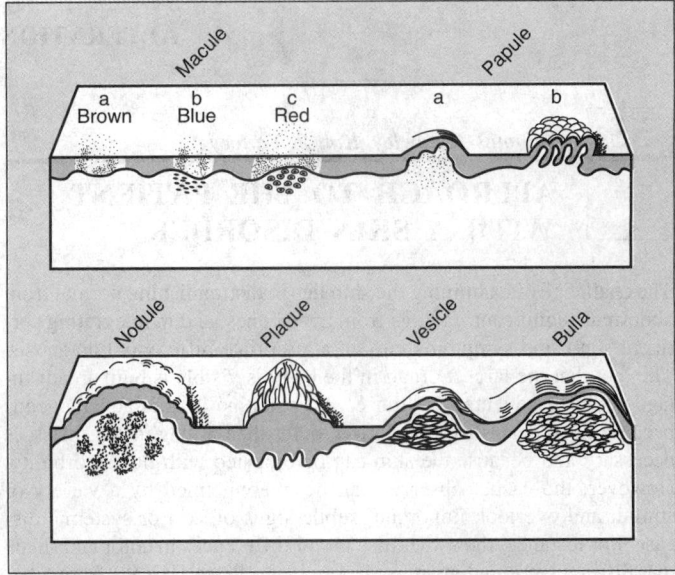

FIGURE 55-1 A schematic representation of several common primary skin lesions (see Table 55-1).

Table 55-3   Selected Common Dermatologic Conditions[a]

Diagnosis	Common Distribution	Usual Morphology	Diagnosis	Common Distribution	Usual Morphology
Acne vulgaris	Face, upper back	Open and closed comedones, erythematous papules, pustules, cysts	Seborrheic keratosis	Trunk, face	Brown plaques with adherent, greasy scale; "stuck on" appearance
Rosacea	Blush area of cheeks, nose, forehead, chin	Erythema, telangiectasias, papules, pustules	Folliculitis	Any hair-bearing area	Follicular pustules
Seborrheic dermatitis	Scalp, eyebrows, perinasal	Erythema with greasy yellow-brown scale	Impetigo	Anywhere	Papules, vesicles, pustules, often with honey-colored crusts
Atopic dermatitis	Antecubital and popliteal fossae; may be widespread	Patches and plaques of erythema, scaling, and lichenification; pruritus	Herpes simplex	Lips, genitalia	Grouped vesicles progressing to crusted erosions
Stasis dermatitis	Ankles, lower legs	Patches of erythema and scaling on background of hyperpigmentation associated with signs of venous insufficiency	Herpes zoster	Dermatomal, usually trunk but may be anywhere	Vesicles limited to a dermatome (often painful)
Dyshidrotic eczema	Palms, soles, sides of fingers and toes	Deep vesicles	Varicella	Face, trunk, relative sparing of extremities	Lesions arise in crops and quickly progress from erythematous macules to papules to vesicles to pustules to crusts
Allergic contact dermatitis	Anywhere	Localized erythema, vesicles, scale, and pruritus, e.g., fingers, earlobes—nickel; dorsal aspect of foot—shoe dermatitis; exposed surfaces—poison ivy dermatitis; etc.	Pityriasis rosea	Trunk (Christmas tree pattern) herald patch followed by multiple smaller lesions	Symmetric erythematous patches with a collarette of trailing scale
Psoriasis	Elbows, knees, scalp, lower back, fingernails (may be generalized)	Papules and plaques covered with silvery scale; nails have pits	Tinea versicolor	Chest, back, abdomen, proximal extremities	Scaly hyper- or hypopigmented macules
Lichen planus	Wrists, ankles, mouth (may be widespread)	Violaceous flat-topped papules and plaques	Candidiasis	Groin, beneath breasts, vagina, oral cavity	Erythematous macerated areas with satellite pustules; white, friable patches on mucous membranes
Keratosis pilaris	Extensor surfaces of arms and thighs, buttocks	Keratotic follicular papules with surrounding erythema	Dermatophytosis	Feet, groin, beard, or scalp	Varies with site, e.g., tinea corporis—scaly annular patch
Melasma	Forehead, cheeks, temples, upper lip	Tan to brown patches	Scabies	Groin, axillae, between fingers and toes, beneath breasts	Excoriated papules, burrows, pruritus
Vitiligo	Periorificial, trunk, extensor surfaces of extremities, flexor wrists, axillae	Chalk-white macules	Insect bites	Anywhere	Erythematous papules with central puncta
			Cherry angioma	Trunk	Red, blood-filled papules
			Keloid	Anywhere (site of previous injury)	Firm tumor, pink, purple, or brown
Actinic keratosis	Sun-exposed areas	Skin-colored or red-brown macule or papule with dry, rough, adherent scale	Dermatofibroma	Anywhere	Firm red to brown nodule that shows dimpling of overlying skin with lateral compression
Basal cell carcinoma	Face	Papule with pearly, telangiectatic border on sun-damaged skin	Acrochordons (skin tags)	Groin, axilla, neck	Fleshy papules
Squamous cell carcinoma	Face, especially lower lip, ears	Indurated and possibly hyperkaratotic lesions often showing ulceration and/or crusting	Urticaria	Anywhere	Wheals, sometimes with surrounding flare, pruritus
			Transient acantholytic dermatosis	Trunk, especially anterior chest	Erythematous papules
			Xerosis	Extensor extremities, especially legs	Dry, erythematous, scaling patches, pruritus

[a] See Color Plates for specific examples and additional information.

DIAGNOSTIC TECHNIQUES   Many skin diseases can be diagnosed on gross clinical appearance, but sometimes relatively simple diagnostic procedures can yield valuable information. In most instances, they can be performed at the bedside with a minimum of equipment.

Skin Biopsy   A skin biopsy is a straightforward minor surgical procedure; however, it is important to biopsy the anatomic site most likely to yield diagnostic findings. This decision may require expertise in skin diseases and knowledge of superficial anatomic structures in selected areas of the body. In this procedure, a small area of skin is anesthetized with 1% lidocaine with or without epinephrine. The skin lesion in question can be excised with a scalpel or removed by punch biopsy. In the latter technique, a punch is pressed against the surface of the skin and rotated with downward pressure until it penetrates to the subcutaneous tissue. The circular biopsy is then lifted with forceps, and the bottom is cut with iris scissors. Biopsy sites may or may not need suture closure, depending on size and location.

KOH Preparation   A potassium hydroxide (KOH) preparation is performed on scaling skin lesions when a fungal etiology is suspected. The edge of such a lesion is scraped gently with a scalpel blade, and the removed scale is collected on a glass microscope slide and treated with 1 to 2 drops of a solution of 10 to 20% KOH. KOH dissolves keratin and allows easier visualization of fungal elements. Brief heating of the slide accelerates dissolution of keratin. When the preparation is viewed under the microscope, the refractile hyphae will be seen more easily when the light intensity is reduced. This technique can be utilized to identify hyphae in dermatophyte infections (see Plate IID-51), pseudohyphae and budding yeast in *Candida* infections (see Plate IID-43), and fragmented hyphae and spores in tinea versicolor. The same sampling technique

FIGURE 55-2 *A–D.* The distribution of some common dermatologic diseases and lesions.

can be used to obtain scale for culture of selected pathogenic organisms.

Tzanck Smear A Tzanck smear is a cytologic technique most often used in the diagnosis of herpesvirus infections [simplex or varicella-zoster (**see Plates IID-36 and IID-37**)]. An early vesicle, not a pustule or crusted lesion, is unroofed, and the base of the lesion is scraped gently with a scalpel blade. The material is placed on a glass slide, air-dried, and stained with Giemsa or Wright's stain. Multinucleated giant cells suggest the presence of herpes, but culture or immunofluorescence testing must be performed to identify the specific virus.

Diascopy Diascopy is designed to assess whether a skin lesion will blanch with pressure as, for example, in determining whether a red lesion is hemorrhagic or simply blood-filled. For instance, a hemangioma (**see Plate IIA-17**) will blanch with pressure, whereas a purpuric lesion caused by necrotizing vasculitis (**see Plate IIE-71**) will not. Diascopy is performed by pressing a microscope slide or magnifying lens against a specified lesion and noting the amount of blanching that occurs. Granulomas often have an "apple jelly" appearance on diascopy.

Wood's Light A Wood's lamp generates 360-nm ultraviolet (or "black") light that can be used to aid the evaluation of certain skin disorders. For example, a Wood's lamp will cause erythrasma (a superficial, intertriginous infection caused by *Corynebacterium minutissimum*) to show a characteristic coral red color, and wounds colonized by *Pseudomonas* to appear pale blue. Tinea capitis caused by certain dermatophytes such as *Microsporum canis* or *M. audouini* exhibits a yellow fluorescence. Pigmented lesions of the epidermis such as freckles are accentuated, while dermal pigment such as postinflammatory hyperpigmentation fades under a Wood's light. Vitiligo (**see Plate IIA-11**) appears totally white under a Wood's lamp, and previously unsuspected areas of involvement often become apparent. A Wood's lamp may also aid in the demonstration of tinea versicolor and in recognition of ash leaf spots in patients with tuberous sclerosis.

Patch Tests Patch testing is designed to document sensitivity to a specific antigen. In this procedure, a battery of suspected allergens is applied to the patient's back under occlusive dressings and allowed to remain in contact with the skin for 48 h. The dressings are removed, and the area is examined for evidence of delayed hypersensitivity reactions (e.g., erythema, edema, or papulovesicles). This test is best performed by physicians with special expertise in patch testing and is often helpful in the evaluation of patients with chronic dermatitis.

BIBLIOGRAPHY

ARNDT KA et al (eds): *Cutaneous Medicine and Surgery, An Integrated Program in Dermatology*. Philadelphia, Saunders, 1996

CHAMPION RH et al (eds): *Textbook of Dermatology*, 6th ed. Oxford, Blackwell Scientific, 1999

FREEDBERG IM et al (eds): *Fitzpatrick's Dermatology in General Medicine*, 5th ed. New York, McGraw-Hill, 1999

56   Robert A. Swerlick, Thomas J. Lawley

ECZEMA, PSORIASIS, CUTANEOUS INFECTIONS, ACNE, AND OTHER COMMON SKIN DISORDERS

ECZEMA AND DERMATITIS

Eczema, or dermatitis, is a reaction pattern that presents with variable clinical and histologic findings and is the final common expression for a number of disorders, including atopic dermatitis, allergic contact and irritant contact dermatitis, dyshidrotic eczema, nummular eczema, lichen simplex chronicus, asteatotic eczema, and seborrheic dermatitis. Primary lesions may include papules, erythematous macules, and vesicles, which can coalesce to form patches and plaques. In severe eczema, secondary lesions from infection or excoriation, marked by weeping and crusting, may predominate. Long-standing dermatitis is often dry and is characterized by thickened, scaling skin (*lichenification*).

ATOPIC DERMATITIS   Atopic dermatitis (AD) is the cutaneous expression of the atopic state, characterized by a family history of asthma, hay fever, or dermatitis in up to 70% of patients. The criteria for the diagnosis of atopic eczema are shown in Table 56-1. The prevalence of atopic dermatitis is increasing worldwide, with a point prevalence in Norwegian school children as high as 23%.

The etiology of AD is only partially defined. There is a clear genetic predisposition. When both parents are affected by AD, over 80% of their children manifest the disease. When only one parent is affected, the prevalence drops to slightly over 50%. A number of genes have been tentatively linked to AD including genes coding for IgE, the high-affinity IgE receptor, mast cell tryptase, and interleukin (IL) 4. Patients with AD may display a variety of immunoregulatory abnormalities including increased IgE synthesis; increased specific IgE to foods, aeroallergens, bacteria, and bacterial products; increased expression of CD23 (low-affinity IgE receptor) on monocytes and B cells; impaired delayed type hypersensitivity reactions; and increased type II and decreased type I cytokine responses.

The clinical presentation often varies with age. Half of patients with AD present within the first year of life, and 80% present by 5 years of age. Some 80% ultimately coexpress allergic rhinitis or asthma later in life. The infantile pattern is characterized by weeping inflammatory patches and crusted plaques that occur on the face, neck, extensor surfaces, and groin. The childhood and adolescent pattern is

Table 56-1   Clinical Criteria for the Diagnosis of Atopic Dermatitis

1. Pruritus and scratching
2. Course marked by exacerbations and remissions
3. Lesions typical of eczematous dermatitis
4. Personal or family history of atopy (asthma, allergic rhinitis, food allergies, or eczema)
5. Clinical course lasting longer than 6 weeks

marked by dermatitis of flexural skin, particularly in the antecubital and popliteal fossae (**see Plate IIA-4**). AD may resolve spontaneously in adults, but the dermatitis will persist into adult life in over half of individuals affected as children. The distribution of lesions may be similar to those seen in childhood. However, adults affected with AD frequently have localized disease, manifesting as hand eczema or lichen simplex chronicus (see below).

Pruritus is a prominent characteristic of AD, and many of the cutaneous findings in affected patients are secondary to rubbing and scratching. Other cutaneous stigmata of AD are perioral pallor, an extra fold of skin beneath the lower eyelid (Dennie's line), increased palmar markings, and increased incidence of cutaneous infections, particularly with *Staphylococcus aureus*. Atopic individuals often have dry itchy skin, abnormalities in cutaneous vascular responses, and, in some instances, elevations in serum IgE.

Histologic examinaton of the skin affected by AD may demonstrate features of acute or chronic dermatitis. Immunopathology shows activated, memory T helper cells, which express the cutaneous lymphocyte antigen, the ligand for the inducible endothelial cell adhesion molecule E-selectin. AD skin lesions may also demonstrate IgE-bearing CD1a+ positive Langerhans cells, and these cells have been implicated in AD disease pathophysiology through mediation of hypersensitivity responses to environmental antigens.

TREATMENT   Therapy of AD should be based on avoidance of cutaneous irritants, adequate cutaneous hydration, judicious use of low- or midpotency topical glucocorticoids, and prompt treatment of secondarily infected skin lesions. Patients should be instructed to bathe using warm, but not hot, water and to limit their use of soap. Immediately after bathing while the skin is still moist, the skin should be lubricated with a low- or midpotency topical glucocorticoid in a cream or ointment base. Potent fluorinated topical glucocorticoids should not be used on the face or intertriginous areas. It takes a minimum of 30 g of glucocorticoid ointment to cover the entire body surface of an average adult.

Crusted and weeping skin lesions should be treated with systemic antibiotics with activity against *S. aureus* since secondary infection often exacerbates eczema. The frequency of macrolide-resistant organisms makes the use of penicillinase-resistant penicillins or cephalosporins preferable. Dicloxacillin or cephalexin (250 mg four times daily for 7 to 10 days) is generally adequate to decrease heavy colonization. As an adjunct, the use of triclosan-containing antibacterial washes and intermittent nasal mupirocin may be useful as prophylactic measures. The role of dietary allergens in atopic dermatitis is controversial, and there is little evidence that they play any role outside of infancy.

Control of pruritus is essential for treatment, since AD often represents "an itch that rashes." Antihistamines are useful to control the pruritus, but sedation may limit their usefulness. Unlike their effects in urticaria, nonsedating antihistamines are of little use since the effectiveness of antihistamines in the treatment of pruritus associated with AD is primarily related to their sedative effects as opposed to any specific action on histamine-mediated pathways.

Treatment with systemic glucocorticoids should be limited to severe exacerbations unresponsive to conservative topical therapy. In the patient with chronic AD, therapy with systemic glucocorticoids will generally clear the skin only briefly, but cessation of the systemic therapy will invariably be accompanied by return, if not worsening, of the dermatitis. Patients who do not respond to conventional therapies should be considered for patch testing to rule out allergic contact dermatitis. Immunotherapy with aeroallergens has not proven useful in AD, unlike its effect in allergic rhinitis and extrinsic asthma.

CONTACT DERMATITIS   Contact dermatitis is an inflammatory process in skin caused by an exogenous agent or agents that directly or indirectly injure the skin. This injury may be caused by an inherent characteristic of a compound—irritant contact dermatitis (ICD). An example of ICD would be dermatitis induced by a concentrated acid or base. Agents that cause allergic contact dermatitis (ACD) induce an antigen-specific immune response. The clinical lesions of contact dermatitis may be acute (wet and edematous) or chronic (dry, thickened, and scaly), depending on the persistence of the insult (see Plate IIA-8). The most common presentation of contact dermatitis is hand eczema, and it is frequently related to occupational exposures. Occupation-related contact dermatitis represents a significant proportion of occupation-induced injury, affecting over 60,000 persons annually.

ICD is generally strictly demarcated and often localized to areas of thin skin (eyelids, intertriginous areas) or to areas where the irritant was occluded. Lesions may range from minimal skin erythema to areas of marked edema, vesicles, and ulcers. Chronic low-grade irritant dermatitis is the most common type of ICD and the most common area of involvement is the hands (see below). The most common irritants encountered are chronic wet work, soaps, and detergents. Treatment should be directed to avoidance of irritants and use of protective gloves or clothing.

ACD is a manifestation of delayed type hypersensitivity mediated by memory T lymphocytes in the skin. The most common cause of ACD is exposure to plants, specifically to members of the family Anacardiaceae; including the genera *Toxicodendrun*, *Anacardium*, *Gluta*, *Mangifera*, and *Semecarpus*. Poison ivy, poison oak, and poison sumac are members of the genus *Toxicodendron* and cause an allergic reaction marked by erythema, vesiculation, and severe pruritus. The eruption is often linear, corresponding to areas where plants have touched the skin. However, other allergens may be more difficult to identify, especially if the exposure is chronic and the skin becomes thickened and scaly. The sensitizing antigen common to these plants is urushiol, an oleoresin containing the active ingredient pentadecyl-catechol. The oleoresin may adhere to skin, clothing, tools, and pets, and contaminated articles may cause dermatitis even after prolonged storage. Blister fluid does not contain urushiol and is not capable of inducing skin eruption in exposed subjects.

TREATMENT   If ACD is suspected and an offending agent is identified and removed, the eruption will resolve. Usually, treatment with high-potency fluorinated topical glucocorticoids is enough to relieve symptoms while the ACD runs its course. For those patients who require systemic therapy, a tapering course over 2 to 3 weeks given as single morning doses is the preferred method.

Identification of a contact allergen can be a difficult and time-consuming task. Patients with dermatitis unresponsive to conventional therapy or with an unusual and patterned distribution should be suspected of having ACD. They should be questioned carefully regarding occupational exposures, topical medicaments, and oral medications. Common sensitizers include preservatives in topical preparations, nickel sulfate, potassium dichromate, thimerosal in ocular preparations, neomycin sulfate, fragrances, formaldehyde, and rubber-curing agents. Patch testing is helpful in identifying these agents, but should not be attempted on patients with widespread active dermatitis or on those taking systemic glucocorticoids.

HAND ECZEMA   Hand eczema is a very common, chronic skin disorder. It represents a large proportion of occupation-associated skin disease. It may be associated with other cutaneous disorders such as atopic dermatitis or may occur by itself. Similar to other forms of dermatitis, both exogenous and endogenous factors play important roles in the expression of hand dermatitis. Chronic, excessive exposure to water and detergents may initiate or aggravate this disorder. It may present with dryness and cracking of the skin of the hands as well as with variable amounts of erythema and edema. Often, the dermatitis will begin under rings where water and irritants are trapped. A variant

of hand dermatitis, dyshidrotic eczema, presents with multiple, intensely pruritic, small papules and vesicles occurring on the thenar and hypothenar eminences and the sides of the fingers (see Plate IA-5). Lesions tend to occur in crops that slowly form crusts and heal.

The evaluation of a patient with hand eczema should include an assessment of potential occupation-associated exposures. Predominant involvement of the dorsal surface of the hands with sparing of the palmar surface suggests a possible contact dermatitis. The history should be directed to identifying possible irritant or allergen exposures. The use of rubber gloves to protect dermatitic skin is sometimes associated with the development of delayed type hypersensitivity reactions to agents used for cross-linking rubber. Such reactions can be detected by patch testing. Less commonly, patients may manifest hand dermatitis as a consequence of developing immediate type hypersensitivity reactions to latex. These are of particular concern since these patients are at risk for anaphylactic reactions. The most sensitive method of detection is the use of scratch testing with latex extract. However, this should be done with extreme caution only in a setting where an anaphylactic reaction can be treated. A latex radioallergo-sorbent test is available but is only about 60% sensitive.

TREATMENT   Therapy of hand dermatitis is directed toward avoidance of irritants, identification of possible contact allergens, treatment of coexistent infection, and application of topical glucocorticoids. Whenever possible, the hands should be protected by gloves, preferably vinyl. Most patients can be treated with cool moist compresses (dressings) to dry and debride acute inflammatory lesions and to decrease swelling, followed by application of a mid- to high-potency topical glucocorticoid in a cream or ointment base. As with atopic dermatitis, treatment of secondary infection by staphylococci or streptococci is essential for good control. Additionally, patients with hand dermatitis should be examined for dermatophyte infection by KOH preparation and culture (see below).

NUMMULAR ECZEMA   Nummular eczema is characterized by circular or oval "coinlike" lesions. Initially, this eruption consists of small edematous papules that become crusted and scaly. The most common locations are on the trunk or the extensor surfaces of the extremities, particularly on the pretibial areas or dorsum of the hands. It occurs more frequently in men and is most commonly seen in middle age. The etiology of nummular eczema is unknown. Whether nummular eczema represents a variant of atopic eczema is controversial. The treatment of nummular eczema is similar to that for other forms of dermatitis.

LICHEN SIMPLEX CHRONICUS   Lichen simplex chronicus may represent the end stage of a variety of pruritic and eczematous disorders. It consists of a well-circumscribed plaque or plaques with lichenified or thickened skin due to chronic scratching or rubbing. Common areas involved include the posterior nuchal region, dorsum of the feet, or ankles. Treatment of lichen simplex chronicus centers around breaking the cycle of chronic itching and scratching, which often occur during sleep. High-potency topical glucocorticoids are helpful in alleviating pruritus in most cases, but in recalcitrant cases, application of topical glucocorticoids under occlusion or intralesional injection of glucocorticoids may be required. Oral antihistamines such as hydroxyzine (10 to 50 mg every 6 h) or tricyclic antidepressants with antihistaminic activity such as doxepin (10 to 25 mg at bedtime) are useful as antipruritics primarily due to their sedating action, and are particularly useful at bedtime (see above). Patients need to be counseled regarding driving or operating heavy equipment after taking these medications due to their potentially potent sedative activity.

ASTEATOTIC ECZEMA   Asteatotic eczema, also known as xerotic eczema or "winter itch," is a mildly inflammatory variant of dermatitis that develops most commonly on the lower legs of elderly individuals during dry times of year. Fine cracks, with or without erythema, characteristically develop on the anterior surface of the lower extremities. Pruritus is variable. Asteatotic eczema responds well to avoidance of irritants, rehydration of the skin, and application of topical emollients.

STASIS DERMATITIS AND STASIS ULCERATION

Stasis dermatitis develops on the lower extremities secondary to venous incompetence and chronic edema. Early findings in stasis dermatitis consist of mild erythema and scaling associated with pruritus. The typical initial site of involvement is the medial aspect of the ankle, often over a distended vein (**see Plate IIA-7**). As the disorder progresses, the dermatitis becomes progressively pigmented, due to chronic erythrocyte extravasation leading to cutaneous hemosiderin deposition. As with other forms of dermatitis, stasis dermatitis may become acutely inflamed, with crusting and exudate. Chronic stasis dermatitis is often associated with dermal fibrosis that is recognized clinically as brawny edema of the skin. Stasis dermatitis is often complicated by secondary infection and contact dermatitis. Severe stasis dermatitis may precede the development of stasis ulcers.

Rx **TREATMENT** Avoidance of irritants and use of emollients and/or midpotency topical glucocorticoids are the cornerstones of therapy for stasis dermatitis. Control of chronic edema is important to prevent leg ulcers. Patients should be encouraged to elevate the affected extremity when sitting. A compression stocking with a gradient of at least 30 to 40 mmHg is most effective for edema control and is much more effective for preventing chronic edema than is antiembolism hose.

Stasis ulcers are difficult to treat, and resolution of these lesions is slow even under the best of circumstances. It is extremely important to elevate the affected limb as much as possible. The ulcer should be kept clear of necrotic material by gentle debridement and covered with a semipermeable dressing under pressure. Glucocorticoids should not be applied to ulcers, since they may retard healing. Secondarily infected lesions should be treated with appropriate oral antibiotics, but it should be noted that all ulcers will become colonized with bacteria, and the purpose of antibiotic therapy should not be to clear all bacterial growth. Some ulcers may take months to heal or require skin grafting.

SEBORRHEIC DERMATITIS

Seborrheic dermatitis is a common, chronic disorder, characterized by greasy scales overlying erythematous patches or plaques. The most common location is in the scalp where it may be recognized as severe dandruff. On the face, seborrheic dermatitis affects the eyebrows, eyelids, glabella, nasolabial fold, or ears (**see Plate IIA-6**). Scaling within the external ear is often mistaken for a chronic fungal infection (otomycosis), and postauricular dermatitis often becomes macerated and tender. Additionally, seborrheic dermatitis may develop in the central chest, axilla, groin, submammary folds, and gluteal cleft. Rarely, it may cause a widespread generalized dermatitis. Seborrheic dermatitis is usually symptomatic, with patients complaining of itching or burning.

Seborrheic dermatitis may be evident within the first few weeks

of life, and within this context it occurs in the scalp ("cradle cap"), face, or groin. It is rarely seen in children beyond infancy but becomes evident again during adult life. Although it is frequently seen in patients with Parkinson's disease, in those who have had cerebrovascular accidents, and in those with human immunodeficiency virus (HIV) infection, the overwhelming majority of individuals with seborrheic dermatitis have no underlying disorder.

Rx **TREATMENT** Treatment with low-potency topical glucocorticoids in conjunction with shampoos containing coal tar and/or salicylic acid is generally sufficient to control activity of this disorder. High-potency topical glucocorticoid solutions (betamethasone or fluocinonide) are effective for control of scalp involvement. Fluorinated topical glucocorticoids should not be used on the face since this is often associated with the development of rebound worsening and steroid-induced rosacea or atrophy.

PAPULOSQUAMOUS DISORDERS (Table 56-2)

PSORIASIS Psoriasis is one of the most common dermatologic diseases, affecting up to 1 to 2% of the world's population. It is a chronic inflammatory skin disorder clinically characterized by erythematous, sharply demarcated papules and rounded plaques, covered by silvery micaceous scale. The skin lesions of psoriasis are variably pruritic. Traumatized areas often develop lesions of psoriasis (Koebner or isomorphic phenomenon). Additionally, other external factors may exacerbate psoriasis including infections, stress, and medications (lithium, beta blockers, and antimalarials).

The most common variety of psoriasis is called *plaque type*. Patients with plaque-type psoriasis will have stable, slowly growing plaques, which remain basically unchanged for long periods of time. The most common areas for plaque psoriasis to occur are the elbows, knees, gluteal cleft, and the scalp. Involvement tends to be symmetric. *Inverse psoriasis* affects the intertriginous regions including the axilla, groin, submammary region, and navel, it also tends to affect the scalp, palms, and soles. The individual lesions are sharply demarcated plaques (**see Plate IIA-3**) but may be moist due to their location. Plaque psoriasis generally develops slowly and runs an indolent course. It rarely remits spontaneously.

Eruptive psoriasis (guttate psoriasis) is most common in children and young adults. It develops acutely in individuals without psoriasis or in those with chronic plaque psoriasis. Patients present with many small erythematous, scaling papules, frequently after upper respiratory tract infection with β-hemolytic streptococci. The differential diagnosis should include pityriasis rosea and secondary syphilis. Patients with psoriasis may also develop pustular lesions. These may be localized to the palms and soles or may be generalized and associated with fever, malaise, diarrhea, and arthralgias.

Table 56-2 Papulosquamous Disorders

	Clinical Features	Other Notable Features	Histologic Features
Psoriasis	Sharply demarcated, erythematous plaques with mica-like scale; predominantly elbows, knees, and scalp; atypical forms may localize to intertriginous areas; eruptive forms may be associated with infection (Reiter's syndrome)	May be aggravated by certain drugs, infection; severe forms seen associated with HIV	Acanthosis, vascular proliferation
Lichen planus	Purple polygonal papules marked by severe pruritus; lacy white markings, especially associated with mucous membrane lesions	Certain drugs may induce: thiazides, antimalarial drugs	Interface dermatitis
Pityriasis rosea	Rash often preceded by herald patch; oval to round plaques with trailing scale; most often affects the trunk, and eruption lines up in skin folds give a "fir tree"-like appearance; generally spares palms and soles	Variable pruritus; self-limited resolving in 2–8 weeks; may be imitated by secondary syphilis	Pathologic features often nonspecific
Dermatophytosis	Polymorphous appearance depending on dermatophyte, body site, and host response; sharply defined to ill-demarcated scaly plaques with or without inflammation; may be associated with hair loss	KOH preparation may show branching hyphae; culture helpful	Hyphae and neutrophils in stratum corneum

About half of all patients with psoriasis have fingernail involvement, appearing as punctate pitting, nail thickening, or subungual hyperkeratosis. About 5 to 10% of patients with psoriasis have associated joint complaints, and these are most often found in patients with fingernail involvement. Although some have the coincident occurrence of classic rheumatoid arthritis (Chap. 312), many have joint disease that falls into one of three types associated with psoriasis: (1) asymmetric inflammatory arthritis most commonly involving the distal and proximal interphalangeal joints and less commonly the knees, hips, ankles, and wrists; (2) a seronegative rheumatoid arthritis–like disease; a significant portion of these patients go on to develop a severe destructive arthritis; or (3) disease limited to the spine (psoriatic spondylitis).

The etiology of psoriasis is still poorly understood. There is clearly a genetic component to psoriasis. Over 50% of patients with psoriasis report a positive family history, and a 65 to 72% concordance among monozygotic twins has been reported in twin studies. Psoriasis has been linked to HLA-Cw6 and, to a lesser extent, to HLA-DR7. Evidence has accumulated clearly indicating a role for T cells in the pathophysiology of psoriasis. Stimulation of immune function with cytokines such as IL-2 has been associated with abrupt worsening of preexisting psoriasis, and bone marrow transplantation has resulted in clearance of disease. Psoriatic lesions are characterized by infiltration of skin with activated memory T cells, with CD8+ cells predominating in the epidermis. Agents that inhibit activated T cell function are often effective for the treatment of severe psoriasis. Presumably, cytokines from activated T cells elaborate growth factors that stimulate keratinocyte hyperproliferation.

℞ **TREATMENT**   Treatment of psoriasis depends on the type, location, and extent of disease. All patients should be instructed to avoid excess drying or irritation of their skin and to maintain adequate cutaneous hydration. Most patients with localized plaque-type psoriasis can be managed with midpotency topical glucocorticoids, although their long-term use is often accompanied by loss of effectiveness (tachyphylaxis). Crude coal tar (1 to 5% in an ointment base) is an old but useful method of treatment in conjunction with ultraviolet light therapy. A topical vitamin D analogue (calcipitriol) is also efficacious in the treatment of psoriasis.

Ultraviolet light is an effective therapy for patients with widespread psoriasis. The ultraviolet B (UV-B) spectrum is effective alone, or may be combined with coal tar (Goeckerman regimen) or anthralin (Ingram regimen). Natural sunlight or an artificial light source can be used. The combination of the ultraviolet A (UV-A) spectrum with either oral or topical psoralens (PUVA) is also extremely effective for the treatment of psoriasis, but long-term use may be associated with an increased incidence of squamous cell cancer and melanoma of the skin.

Various other agents can be used for widespread psoriatic disease.

Methotrexate is an effective agent, especially in patients with associated psoriatic arthritis. Liver toxicity from long-term use limits its use to patients with widespread disease not responsive to less aggressive modalities. The synthetic retinoid, acetretin, has been shown to be effective in some patients with severe psoriasis but is a potent teratogen, thus limiting its use in women with childbearing potential. The evidence implicating psoriasis as a T cell–mediated disorder has created a new perspective relating to the treatment of psoriasis. Based on this presumed disease mechanism, immunomodulatory therapy utilizing cyclosporine has proven to be highly effective in selected patients with severe, crippling, and potentially life-threatening disease.

LICHEN PLANUS   Lichen planus (LP) is a papulosquamous disorder in which the primary lesions are pruritic, polygonal, flat-topped, violaceous papules. Close examination of the surface of these papules often reveals a network of gray lines (Wickham's striae). The skin lesions may occur anywhere but have a predilection for the wrists, shins, lower back, and genitalia (see Plate IIA-9). Involvement of the scalp may lead to hair loss. LP commonly involves mucous membranes, particularly the buccal mucosa, where it can present as a white netlike eruption. Its etiology is unknown, but cutaneous eruptions clinically resembling LP have been observed after administration of numerous drugs, including diuretics, gold, antimalarials, penicillamine, and phenothiazines, and in patients with skin lesions of chronic graft-versus-host disease. Additionally, LP associated with abnormal liver function has been correlated with viral hepatitis, particularly hepatitis C infection. The course of LP is variable, but most patients have spontaneous remissions 6 months to 2 years after the onset of disease. Topical glucocorticoids are the mainstay of therapy.

PITYRIASIS ROSEA   Pityriasis rosea (PR) is a papulosquamous eruption of unknown etiology that occurs more commonly in the spring and fall. Its first manifestation is the development of a 2- to 6-cm annular lesion (the herald patch). This is followed in a few days to a few weeks by the appearance of many smaller annular or papular lesions with a predilection to occur on the trunk (see Plate IIA-13). The lesions are generally oval, with their long axis parallel to the skin-fold lines. Individual lesions may range in color from red to brown and have a trailing scale. PR shares many clinical features with the eruption of secondary syphilis, but palm and sole lesions are extremely rare in PR and common in secondary syphilis. The eruption tends to be moderately pruritic and lasts 3 to 8 weeks. Treatment is generally directed at alleviating pruritus and consists of oral antihistamines, midpotency topical glucocorticoids, and, in some cases, the use of UV-B phototherapy.

CUTANEOUS INFECTIONS (Table 56-3)

IMPETIGO AND ECTHYMA   Impetigo is a common superficial bacterial infection of skin caused by group A β-hemolytic streptococci (Chap. 140) or *S. aureus* (Chap. 139). The primary lesion is a

Table 56-3   Common Skin Infections

	Clinical Features	Etiologic Agent	Treatment
Impetigo	Honey-colored crusted papules, plaques, or bullae	Group A *Streptococcus* and *Staphylococcus aureus*	Systemic or topical anti-staphylococcal antibiotics
Dermatophytosis	Inflammatory or noninflammatory annular scaly plaques; may have hair loss; groin involvement spares scrotum; hyphae on KOH preparation	*Trichophyton*, *Epidermophyton*, or *Microsporum* sp.	Topical azoles, systemic griseofulvin, or azoles
Candidiasis	Inflammatory papules and plaques with satellite pustules, frequently in intertriginous areas; may involve scrotum; pseudohyphae on KOH preparation	*Candida albicans* and other *Candida* species	Topical nystatin or azoles; systemic azoles for resistant disease
Tinea versicolor	Hyperpigmented or hypopigmented scaly patches on the trunk; characteristic mixture of hyphae and spores on KOH preparation ("spaghetti and meatballs")	KOH preparation may show branching hyphae; culture helpful	Topical selenium sulfide lotion or azoles

brown honey-colored crust (see Plate IID-38). Lesions caused by staphylococci may be tense, clear bullae, and this less common form of the disease is called *bullous impetigo*. Lesions may occur on normal skin or in areas already affected by another skin disease. Ecthyma is a variant of impetigo that generally occurs on the lower extremities and causes punched-out ulcerative lesions. Treatment of both ecthyma and impetigo involves gentle debridement of adherent crusts, which is facilitated by the use of soaks and topical antibiotics, in conjunction with appropriate oral antibiotics.

ERYSIPELAS AND CELLULITIS See Chap. 128

DERMATOPHYTOSIS Dermatophytes are fungi that infect skin, hair, and nails and include members of the genera *Trichophyton*, *Microsporum*, and *Epidermophyton*. Infection of the foot (tinea pedis) is most common and is often chronic; it is characterized by variable erythema and edema, scaling, pruritus, and occasionally vesiculation. Involvement may be widespread or localized, but almost invariably the web space between the fourth and fifth toes is affected. Infection of the nails (tinea unguium) occurs in many patients with tinea pedis and is characterized by opacified, thickened nails and subungual debris. The groin is the next most commonly involved area (tinea cruris), with males affected much more often than females. It presents as a scaling erythematous eruption that spares the scrotum. Microscopic examination of either untreated tinea pedis or tinea cruris scale after digestion with KOH preparation will generally demonstrate hyphae.

Dermatophyte infection of the scalp (tinea capitis) has returned in epidemic proportions, particularly affecting inner city children. The predominant organism is *T. tonsurans*. This organism can produce an inflammatory or relatively noninflammatory infection that may present with either well-defined or irregular, diffuse areas of mild scaling and hair loss. Tinea corporis, or infection on non-hair-bearing skin, may have a variable appearance, depending on the extent of the associated inflammatory reaction (see Plate IID-51). It may have the typical annular appearance of "ringworm" or appear as deep inflammatory nodules (on the scalp known as a *kerion*) or granulomas. KOH examination of scale or hair from patients with tinea capitis or inflammatory tinea corporis often does not reveal hyphae, and diagnosis may require culture or biopsy.

℞ **TREATMENT** Both topical and systemic therapies may be used to treat dermatophyte infection. Treatment depends on the site involved and the type of infection. Topical therapy is generally effective for uncomplicated tinea corporis, tinea cruris, and limited tinea pedis. It is not effective as monotherapy for tinea capitis or tinea unguium. Topical imidazoles (miconazole, ketoconazole, econazole, clotrimazole, oxiconazole, and sulconazole), triazoles (terconazole), and allylamines (terbinafine and naftifine) may all be effective topical therapies for dermatophyte infections. Haloprogin, undecylic acid, ciclopirox-olamine, and tolnaftate are also effective, but nystatin is not active against dermatophytes. Treatment should continue until the patient is clear of infection by clinical examination and culture. Tinea pedis often requires longer treatment courses and is associated with a high relapse rate.

Griseofulvin is the drug of choice for dermatophyte infections requiring systemic therapy. A daily dose of 500 mg of microsized or 350 mg of ultramicrosized griseofulvin administered with a fatty meal is an adequate dose for most dermatophyte infections. The duration of therapy may be as short as 2 weeks for uncomplicated tinea corporis but may be as long as 6 to 12 months for nail infections. The most common side effects of griseofulvin are gastrointestinal distress and headache. Dermatophyte infection of hair-bearing areas (e.g., tinea capitis) requires systemic antifungal therapy. The usual adult dose of griseofulvin is 1 g of microsized or 0.5 g of ultramicrosized given daily, and treatment should be continued for 6 to 8 weeks. Children should be treated with 15 to 20 mg/kg as a single daily dose given with a fatty meal. The adjunctive use of topical antifungal agents in addition to systemic therapy may be useful, but topical therapy alone

is not adequate. Markedly inflammatory tinea capitis may result in scarring and hair loss, and systemic or topical glucocorticoids may be helpful in preventing this sequela. Recent studies in children have also suggested that both itraconazole (3 to 5 mg/kg for 6 to 10 weeks) and terbinafine (125 mg/d for 6 weeks) may be effective treatments for tinea capitis.

Until recently, griseofulvin was the recommended therapy for dermatophyte infection of the nails. However, despite prolonged treatment, cure rates were poor. Itraconazole given as either continuous daily therapy (200 mg/d for 3 months) or pulses (200 mg twice daily for 1 week per month for 3 consecutive months) has been shown to be a safe and effective therapy. Itraconazole has the potential for interactions with other drugs requiring the P450 enzyme system for metabolism. Similarly, terbinafine (250 mg/d for 3 months) has shown similar cure rates. Only limited data are available on the dosing and effectiveness of the newer antifungal agents in tinea corporis, tinea cruris, and uncomplicated tinea pedis.

TINEA VERSICOLOR Tinea versicolor is caused by a non-dermatophyte dimorphic fungus that is a normal inhabitant of the skin. As the yeast form *Pityrosporum orbiculare*, it generally does not cause disease (except for folliculitis in certain individuals). However, in some individuals, it converts to the hyphal form and causes characteristic lesions. The expression of infection is promoted by heat and humidity. The typical lesions consist of oval scaly macules, papules, and patches concentrated on the chest, shoulders, and back but only rarely on the face or distal extremities. On dark skin, they often appear as hypopigmented areas, while on light skin, they are slightly hyperpigmented. In some darkly pigmented individuals, they may only appear as scaling patches. A KOH preparation from scaling lesions will demonstrate a confluence of short hyphae and round spores (so-called spaghetti and meatballs). Solutions containing sulfur, salicylic acid, or selenium sulfide will clear the infection if used daily for a week and then intermittently thereafter. Treatment with a single 400-mg dose of ketoconazole is also effective.

CANDIDIASIS Candidiasis is a fungal infection caused by a related group of yeasts, whose manifestations may be localized to the skin, or rarely, may be systemic and life-threatening. The causative organism is usually *Candida albicans*, but may also be *C. tropicalis*, *C. parapsilosis*, or *C. krusei*. These organisms are normal saprophytic inhabitants of the gastrointestinal tract but may overgrow (usually due to broad-spectrum antibiotic therapy) and cause disease at a number of cutaneous sites. Other predisposing factors include diabetes mellitus, chronic intertrigo, oral contraceptive use, and cellular immune deficiency. Candidiasis is a very common infection in HIV-infected individuals (Chap. 309). The oral cavity is commonly involved. Lesions may occur on the tongue or buccal mucosa (thrush) and appear as white plaques (see Plate IID-43). Microscopic examination of scrapings demonstrate both pseudohyphae and yeast forms. Fissured, macerated lesions at the corners of the mouth (perlèche) are often seen in individuals with poorly fitting dentures and may also be associated with candidal infection. Additionally, candidal infections have an affinity for sites that are chronically wet and macerated and may occur around nails (onycholysis and paronychia) and in intertriginous areas. Intertriginous lesions are characteristically edematous, erythematous, and scaly, with scattered "satellite pustules." In males, there is often involvement of the penis and scrotum as well as the inner aspect of the thighs. In contrast to dermatophyte infections, candidal infections are frequently accompanied by a marked inflammatory response. Diagnosis of candidal infection is based upon the clinical pattern and demonstration of yeast on KOH preparation, or culture.

℞ **TREATMENT** Treatment routinely involves removing any predisposing factors such as antibiotic therapy or chronic wetness and the use of appropriate topical or systemic antifungal therapy. Effective topical agents include nystatin or topical azoles (miconazole, clotrimazole, econazole, or ketoconazole). These agents are generally effective in clearing mucous membrane or glabrous skin involvement in nonimmunosuppressed patients. The associated inflammatory response that often accompanies candidal infection on glabrous skin should be treated with a mild glucocorticoid lotion or cream (2.5% hydrocortisone). Systemic therapy is generally reserved for immunosuppressed patients or individuals with chronic or recurrent disease who fail to respond to or tolerate appropriate topical therapy. Vulvovaginal candidiasis may respond to treatment with a single dose of fluconazole (150 mg). Chronic recurrent oral or vaginal candidiasis may be treated with weekly to monthly oral fluconazole (150 to 200 mg) in conjunction with topical therapy.

WARTS   Warts are cutaneous neoplasms that are caused by papilloma viruses. Over 50 different human papilloma viruses (HPV) have been described, and this number will almost certainly continue to grow. Typical verruca vulgaris lesions are sessile, dome-shaped, usually about a centimeter in diameter, and their surface is made up of many small filamentous projections. The HPV that cause typical verruca vulgaris also cause typical plantar warts, flat warts (or verruca plana), and filiform warts in intertriginous areas. Plantar warts are endophytic and are covered by thick keratin. Paring of the wart will generally demonstrate a central core of keratinized debris and punctate bleeding points. Filiform warts are most commonly seen on the face, neck, and skin folds and present as papillomatous lesions on a narrow base. Flat warts are only slightly elevated and have a velvety, nonverrucous surface. They have a propensity for the face, arms, and legs and are often spread by shaving.

Multiple HPV types have been associated with genital tract lesions. They generally begin as small papillomas that may grow to form large fungating lesions. In women, they may involve either the labia, perineum, or perianal skin. Additionally, the mucosa of the vagina, urethra, and anus can be involved, as well as the cervical epithelium. In men, the lesions often occur initially in the coronal sulcus, but may be seen on the shaft of the penis, the scrotum, perianal skin, or in the urethra.

Within the past decade, appreciable evidence has accumulated that suggests HPV plays a role in the development of neoplasia of the uterine cervix and external genitalia (Chap. 97). HPV types 16 and 18 have been most intensely studied, while recent evidence also implicates other types. Lesions may initially appear as small, flat, velvety, hyperpigmented papules occurring on the genitalia or perianal skin. Histologic examination of biopsies from affected sites may reveal changes associated with typical warts and/or features typical of intraepidermal carcinoma (Bowen's disease). Squamous cell carcinomas associated with HPV infections have also been observed in extragenital skin (Chap. 86). This is most commonly seen in patients immunosuppressed after organ transplantation.

℞ **TREATMENT**   There are many modalities available to treat warts, but no single therapy is universally effective. Factors that influence the choice of therapy include the location of the wart, extent of disease, the age and immunologic status of the patient, and the patient's desire for therapy. Perhaps the most useful and convenient method for treating warts in almost any location is cryotherapy with liquid nitrogen. Equally effective, but requiring much more patient compliance, is the use of keratolytic agents such as salicylic acid plasters or combinations of lactic acid and salicylic acid. For genital warts, application of podophyllin solution is moderately effective but may be associated with marked local reactions in certain individuals. Dilute preparations of purified podophyllin permit physician-directed by patient-applied use, facilitating treatment of mucosal warts. Topical imiquimod, a potent inducer of local cytokine release, has also been approved for use in genital warts. Other topical agents that are used include trichloracetic acid or cantharidin. Electrodessication and curettage or CO_2 laser excision are also effective therapies but require local anesthesia. Recurrence of warts appears to be common to all

these modalities because viral genomic material is present in normal-appearing skin adjacent to the clinical lesions.

Treatment of warts should be tempered by the observation that an overwhelming majority of warts in normal individuals resolve spontaneously within 1 to 2 years. Also, only an extremely small proportion of warts is associated with neoplasia, and those are almost exclusively located on the genitalia or perianal skin.

HERPES SIMPLEX   →*See Chap. 182*
HERPES ZOSTER   →*See Chap. 183*

ACNE

ACNE VULGARIS   Acne vulgaris is a self-limited disorder primarily of teenagers and young adults, although perhaps 10 to 20% of adults may continue to experience some form of the disorder. The permissive factor for the expression of the disease in adolescence is the increase in sebum release by sebaceous glands after puberty. Small cysts, called *comedones*, form in hair follicles due to blockage of the follicular orifice by retention of sebum and keratinous material. The activity of lipophilic yeast (*Pityrosporum orbiculare*) and bacteria (*Proprionobacterium acnes*) within the comedones releases free fatty acids from sebum, causes inflammation within the cyst, and results in rupture of the cyst wall. An inflammatory foreign-body reaction develops as a result of extrusion of oily and keratinous debris from the cyst.

The clinical hallmark of acne vulgaris is the comedone, which may be closed (whitehead) or open (blackhead). Closed comedones appear as 1- to 2-mm pebbly white papules, which are accentuated when the skin is stretched. They are the precursors of inflammatory lesions of acne vulgaris. The contents of closed comedones are not easily expressed. Open comedones, which rarely result in inflammatory acne lesions, have a large dilated follicular orifice and are filled with easily expressible oxidized, darkened, oily debris. Comedones are usually accompanied by inflammatory lesions: papules, pustules, or nodules.

The earliest lesions seen in early adolescence are generally mildly inflamed or noninflammatory comedones on the forehead. Subsequently, more typical inflammatory lesions develop on the cheeks, nose, and chin **(see Plate IIA-1)**. The most common location for acne is the face, but involvement of the chest and back is not uncommon. Most disease remains mild and does not lead to scarring. However, a small number of patients develop large inflammatory cysts and nodules, which may drain and result in significant scarring.

Exogenous and endogenous factors can alter the expression of acne vulgaris. Friction and trauma may rupture preexisting microcomedones and elicit inflammatory acne lesions. This is commonly seen with headbands or chin straps of athletic helmets. Application of comedogenic topical agents in cosmetics or hair preparations or chronic topical exposure to certain industrial compounds that are comedogenic may elicit or aggravate acne. Glucocorticoids, applied topically or administered systemically in high doses, may also elicit acne. Other systemic medications such as lithium, isoniazid, halogens, phenytoin, and phenobarbital may produce acneiform eruptions, or aggravate preexisting acne.

℞ **TREATMENT**   Treatment of acne vulgaris is directed toward elimination of comedones by normalization of follicular keratinization, decreasing sebaceous gland activity, decreasing the population of lipophilic bacteria and yeast, and decreasing inflammation. Acne vulgaris may be treated with either local or systemic medications. Minimal to moderate, pauci-inflammatory disease may respond adequately to local therapy alone. Although areas affected with acne should be kept clean, there is little evidence to suggest that removal of surface oils plays an important role in therapy. Overly vigorous scrubbing may aggravate acne due to mechanical rupture of comedones. Topical agents such as retinoic acid, benzoyl peroxide, or salicylic acid may alter the pattern of epidermal desquamation, preventing the formation of comedones and aiding in the resolution of preexisting cysts. Topical antibacterial agents such as benzoyl peroxide, azelaic acid, topical erythromycin (with or without zinc), clindamycin, or tetracycline are also useful adjuncts to therapy.

Patients with moderate to severe acne with a prominent inflammatory component will benefit from the addition of systemic therapy. Oral tetracyclines or erythromycin in doses of 250 to 1000 mg/d will decrease follicular colonization with some of the lipophilic organisms. They also appear to have an anti-inflammatory effect independent of their antibacterial effect. Female patients who do not respond to oral antibiotics may benefit from hormonal therapy. Women placed on oral contraceptives containing ethinyl estradiol and norgestimate have demonstrated improvement in their acne when compared to a placebo control.

Severe nodulocystic acne not responsive to oral antibiotics, hormonal therapy, or topical therapy may be treated with the synthetic retinoid isotretinoin. It is used at doses of 0.5 to 2.0 mg/kg as a single daily dose for 15 to 20 weeks. The use of this drug is limited by its teratogenicity, and female patients must be screened for pregnancy prior to initiating therapy, maintain a method of birth control during therapy, and be screened for pregnancy during treatment. Patients receiving this medication develop extremely dry skin and cheilitis and must be followed for development of hypertriglyceridemia.

ACNE ROSACEA Acne rosacea is an inflammatory disorder predominantly affecting the central face. It is seen almost exclusively in adults, only rarely affecting patients under 30 years of age. Rosacea is seen more often in women, but those most severely affected are men. It is characterized by the presence of erythema, telangiectases, and superficial pustules (**see Plate IIA-2**), but is not associated with the presence of comedones. Rosacea only rarely involves the chest or back.

There is a relationship between the tendency for pronounced facial flushing and the subsequent development of acne rosacea. Often, individuals with rosacea initially demonstrate a pronounced flushing reaction. This may be in response to heat, emotional stimuli, alcohol, hot drinks, or spicy foods. As the disease progresses, the flush persists longer and longer and may eventually become permanent. Papules, pustules, and telangiectases can become superimposed on the persistent flush. Rosacea of very long standing may lead to connective tissue overgrowth, particularly of the nose (rhinophyma). Rosacea may also be complicated by various inflammatory disorders of the eye, including keratitis, blepharitis, iritis, and recurrent chalazion. These ocular problems are potentially sight-threatening and warrant ophthalmologic evaluation.

TREATMENT Acne rosacea can generally be treated effectively with oral tetracycline in doses ranging from 250 to 1000 mg/d. Topical metronidazole or sodium sulfacetamide has also been shown to be effective. In addition, the use of low-potency, nonfluorinated topical glucocorticoids, particularly after cool soaks, is helpful in alleviating facial erythema. Fluorinated topical glucocorticoids should be avoided since chronic use of these preparations may actually elicit rosacea. Topical therapy is not effective treatment for ocular disease.

BIBLIOGRAPHY

ARNDT KA et al (eds): *Cutaneous Medicine and Surgery: An Integrated Program in Dermatology*. Philadelphia, Saunders, 1996

BATA-CSORGO Z et al: Intralesional T-lymphocyte activation as a mediator of psoriatic epidermal hyperplasia. J Invest Dermatol 105:89S, 1995

BOS JD, DERIE MA: The pathogenesis of psoriasis: Immunological facts and speculations. Immunol Today 20:40, 1999

COHEN DE: Occupational dermatoses, in *Handbook of Occupational Safety and Health*, 2d ed, LJ DiBerardinis (ed). New York, Wiley, 1999, p 697

FREEDBURG IM et al (eds): *Fitzpatrick's Dermatology in General Medicine*, 5th ed. New York, McGraw-Hill, 1999

GOTTLIEB SL et al: Response of psoriasis to a lymphocyte-selective toxin (DAB389 IL-2) suggests a primary immune, but not keratinocyte, pathogenic basis. Nat Med 1:442, 1995

HANAFIN JM et al: Recombinant interferon gamma therapy for atopic dermatitis. J Am Acad Dermatol 28:189, 1993

PETO R, ZUR HAUSEN H: *Viral Etiology of Cervical Cancer. Banbury Report*. Cold Spring Harbor, NY, Cold Spring Harbor Laboratory, 1986

57 *Jean L. Bolognia, Irwin M. Braverman*

SKIN MANIFESTATIONS OF INTERNAL DISEASE

ACE angiotensin-converting enzyme	MEN multiple endocrine neoplasia
AV arteriovenous	MSH melanocyte-stimulating
BCEs basal cell epitheliomas	hormone
CALM café au lait macules	NAME *n*evus, *a*trial myxoma,
CNS central nervous system	*m*yxoid neurofibroma, and *e*phelides
CREST *c*alcinosis cutis, *R*aynaud's	(freckles) syndrome
phenomenon, *e*sophageal dysmotility,	NF neurofibromatosis
*s*clerodactyly, and *t*elangiectasia	NSAIDs nonsteroidal anti-
CTCL cutaneous T cell lymphoma	inflammatory drugs
DIC disseminated intravascular	OCA oculocutaneous albinism
coagulation	PAN polyarteritis nodosa
DM dermatomyositis	PCR polymerase chain reaction
EED erythema elevatum diutinum	PCT porphyria cutanea tarda
EM erythema multiforme	PMLE polymorphous light eruption
JRA juvenile rheumatoid arthritis	POEMS *p*olyneuropathy;
LAMB *l*entigines, *a*trial myxomas,	*o*rganomegaly (liver, spleen, lymph
*m*ucocutaneous myxomas, and *b*lue	nodes); *e*ndocrinopathies (impotence,
nevi	gynecomastia); *M*-protein; and *s*kin
LCV leukocytoclastic vasculitis	changes
LEOPARD *l*entigines; *E*CG	PVA poikiloderma vasculare
abnormalities, primarily conduction	atrophicans
defects, *o*cular hypertelorism;	PXE pseudoxanthoma elasticum
*p*ulmonary stenosis and subaortic	SSSS staphylococcal scalded-skin
valvular stenosis; *a*bnormal genitalia	syndrome
(cryptorchidism, hypospadias);	TEN toxic epidermal necrolysis
*r*etardation of growth; and *d*eafness	TSS toxic shock syndrome
(sensorineural)	

It is now a generally accepted concept in medicine that the skin can show signs of internal disease. Therefore, in textbooks of medicine one finds a chapter describing in detail the major systemic disorders that can be identified by cutaneous signs. The underlying assumption of such a chapter is that the clinician has been able to identify the disorder in the patient and needs only to read about it in the textbook. In reality, concise differential diagnoses and the identification of these disorders are actually difficult for the nondermatologist because he or she is not well versed in the recognition of cutaneous lesions or their spectrum of presentations. Therefore, the authors of this chapter have decided to cover this particular topic of cutaneous medicine not by discussing individual disorders but by describing and discussing the various presenting clinical signs and symptoms that indicate the presence of these disorders. Concise differential diagnoses will be generated in which the significant diseases will be briefly discussed and distinguished from the more common disorders that have no significance for internal diseases. The latter disorders are reviewed in table form and always need to be excluded when considering the former. For a detailed description of individual diseases, the reader should consult a dermatologic text.

PAPULOSQUAMOUS SKIN LESIONS (Table 57-1)   When an eruption is characterized by elevated lesions, papules (<1 cm) or plaques (>1 cm), in association with scale, it is referred to as *papulosquamous*. The most common papulosquamous diseases—*psoriasis, tinea, pityriasis rosea*, and *lichen planus*—are primary cutaneous disorders (Chap. 56). When psoriatic lesions are accompanied by arthritis, the possibility of psoriatic arthritis or *Reiter's disease* should be considered. A history of oral ulcers, conjunctivitis, uveitis, and/or urethritis points to the latter diagnosis. In *guttate psoriasis* there is an acute onset of small, widely scattered, uniform lesions, often in association with a streptococcal infection. Lithium, beta blockers, HIV infection, and a rapid taper of systemic glucocorticoids are also known to exacerbate psoriasis.

Whenever the diagnosis of pityriasis rosea or lichen planus is made, it is important to review the patient's medications because the

Table 57-1   Selected Causes of Papulosquamous Skin Lesions

1. Primary cutaneous disorders
   a. Psoriasis[a]
   b. Tinea[a]
   c. Pityriasis rosea[a]
   d. Lichen planus[a]
   e. Parapsoriasis
   f. Bowen's disease (squamous cell carcinoma in situ)[b]
2. Drugs
3. Systemic diseases
   a. Lupus erythematosus[c]
   b. Cutaneous T cell lymphoma
   c. Secondary syphilis
   d. Reiter's disease
   e. Sarcoidosis[d]

[a] Discussed in detail in Chap. 56.
[b] Associated with chronic sun exposure and exposure to arsenic.
[c] See also "Red Lesions" in "Papulonodular Skin Lesions."
[d] See also "Red-Brown Lesions" in "Papulonodular Skin Lesions."

eruption can be treated by simply discontinuing the offending agent. Pityriasis rosea–like drug eruptions are seen most commonly with beta blockers, angiotensin-converting enzyme (ACE) inhibitors, gold, and metronidazole, while the drugs that can produce a lichenoid eruption include gold, antimalarials, thiazides, quinidine, phenothiazines, sulfonylureas, and ACE inhibitors. Lichen planus–like lesions are also observed in chronic graft-versus-host disease.

Parapsoriasis is an intermediate disease, for it can remain solely as a primary cutaneous disease or it can progress to cutaneous T cell lymphoma (CTCL) after a latency period of as long as 40 years. There are several forms of parapsoriasis, including small plaque (0.5 to 5 cm), large plaque (>6 cm), and retiform. The lesions of both small plaque and large plaque parapsoriasis are thin and salmon-pink in color with fine white scale. In small plaque forms, the lesions are commonly on the trunk but can be widely scattered. In large plaque forms, the most common location is the "girdle" area, and fine wrinkling secondary to epidermal atrophy is often seen. Retiform parapsoriasis forms a netlike pattern, and the individual papules are red-brown and flat-topped. The latter two forms of parapsoriasis, large plaque and retiform, can progress to CTCL.

A clue to the development of *CTCL* within lesions of large plaque or retiform parapsoriasis is an increase in the palpable component of the plaque (increased infiltration). In its early stages, CTCL may be confused with ezcema or psoriasis, but it often fails to respond to the appropriate therapy for those inflammatory diseases. The diagnosis of CTCL is established by skin biopsy in which collections of atypical T lymphocytes are found in the epidermis and dermis. As the disease progresses, cutaneous tumors and lymph node involvement may appear.

In *secondary syphilis* there are scattered red-brown papules with thin scale. The eruption often involves the palms and soles and can resemble pityriasis rosea. Associated findings are helpful in making the diagnosis and include annular plaques on the face, nonscarring alopecia, condyloma lata (broad-based and moist), and mucous patches as well as lymphadenopathy, malaise, fever, headache, and myalgias. The interval between the primary chancre and the secondary stage is usually 4 to 8 weeks, and spontaneous resolution without appropriate therapy is seen.

ERYTHRODERMA (Table 57-2) *Erythroderma* is the term used when the majority of the skin surface is erythematous (red in color). There may be associated scale, erosions, or pustules as well as shedding of the hair and nails. Potential systemic manifestations include fever, chills, hypothermia, reactive lymphadenopathy, peripheral edema, hypoalbuminemia, and high-output cardiac failure. The major etiologies of erythroderma are (1) *cutaneous diseases* such as psoriasis and dermatitis (Table 57-3); (2) *drugs*; (3) *systemic diseases*, most commonly CTCL; and (4) *idiopathic*. In the first three groups, the

Table 57-2   Causes of Erythroderma

1. Primary cutaneous disorders
   a. Psoriasis[a]
   b. Dermatitis (atopic, stasis, contact, seborrheic)[a]
   c. Pityriasis rubra pilaris
2. Drugs
3. Systemic diseases
   a. Cutaneous T cell lymphoma
   b. Lymphoma
4. Idiopathic

[a] Discussed in detail in Chap. 56.

location and description of the initial lesions, prior to the development of the erythroderma, aid in the diagnosis. For example, a history of red scaly plaques on the elbows and knees would point to psoriasis. It is also important to examine the skin carefully for a migration of the erythema and associated secondary changes such as pustules or erosions. Migratory waves of erythema studded with superficial pustules are seen in *pustular psoriasis*.

Drug-induced erythroderma (exfoliative dermatitis) may begin as a morbilliform eruption (Chap. 59) or may arise as diffuse erythema. Fever and peripheral eosinophilia often accompany the eruption, and occasionally there is an associated allergic interstitial nephritis. A number of drugs can produce an erythroderma, including penicillins, sulfonamides, carbamazepine, phenytoin, gold, allopurinol, and captopril. While reactions to anticonvulsants can lead to a pseudolymphoma syndrome, reactions to allopurinol may be accompanied by hepatitis, gastrointestinal bleeding, and nephropathy.

The most common malignancy that is associated with erythroderma is CTCL; in some series, up to 25% of the cases of erythroderma were due to CTCL. The patient may progress from isolated plaques and tumors, but more commonly the erythroderma is present throughout the course of the disease (Sézary syndrome). In the Sézary syndrome, there are circulating atypical T lymphocytes, pruritus, and lymphadenopathy. In cases of erythroderma where there is no apparent cause (idiopathic), longitudinal follow-up is mandatory to monitor for the possible development of CTCL. There have been isolated case reports of erythroderma secondary to some solid tumors—lung, liver, prostate, thyroid, and colon—but it is usually in a late stage of the disease.

ALOPECIA (Table 57-4) The two major forms of alopecia are scarring and nonscarring. In *scarring alopecia* there is associated fibrosis, inflammation, and loss of hair follicles. A smooth scalp with a decreased number of follicular openings is usually observed clinically, but in some cases the changes are seen only in biopsy specimens from the affected areas. In *nonscarring alopecia* the hair shafts are gone, but the hair follicles are preserved, explaining the reversible nature of nonscarring alopecia.

Primary cutaneous disorders are the most common causes of nonscarring alopecia and they include *telogen effluvium, androgenetic alopecia, alopecia areata, tinea capitis*, and *traumatic alopecia* (Table 57-5). In women with androgenetic alopecia, an elevation in circulating levels of androgens may be seen as a result of ovarian or adrenal gland dysfunction. When there are signs of virilization, such as a deepened voice and enlarged clitoris, the possibility of an ovarian or adrenal gland tumor should be considered.

Exposure to various *drugs* can also cause diffuse hair loss, usually by inducing a telogen effluvium. An exception is the anagen effluvium observed with antimitotic agents such as daunorubicin. Alopecia is a side effect of the following drugs: warfarin, heparin, propylthiouracil, carbimazole, vitamin A, isotretinoin, acetretin, lithium, beta blockers, colchicine, and amphetamines. Fortunately, spontaneous regrowth usually follows discontinuation of the offending agent.

Less commonly, nonscarring alopecia is associated with *lupus erythematosus* and *secondary syphilis*. In systemic lupus there are two forms of alopecia—one is scarring secondary to discoid lesions (see below) and the other is nonscarring. The latter form may be diffuse

Table 57-3 Erythroderma (Primary Cutaneous Disorders)

	Initial Lesions	Location of Initial Lesions	Other Findings	Diagnostic Aids	Treatment
Psoriasis[a]	Pink-red, silvery scale, sharply demarcated	Elbows, knees, scalp, presacral area	Nail dystrophy, arthritis, pustules	Skin biopsy	Oral retinoid ± PUVA; UV-B; methotrexate; cyclosporine
Dermatitis[a]					
Atopic	Acute: Erythema, fine scale, crust, indistinct borders Chronic: Lichenification (increased skin markings)	Antecubital and popliteal fossae, neck, hands	Pruritus Family history of atopy, including asthma, allergic rhinitis or conjunctivitis, and atopic dermatitis Rule out secondary infection with *S. aureus* Rule out superimposed irritant contact dermatitis	Skin biopsy	Topical glucocorticoids, tar, and antipruritics; oral antihistamines; open wet dressings; UV-B + UV-A; PUVA; oral/IM glucocorticoids Topical or oral antibiotics
Stasis	Erythema, crusting, excoriations	Lower extremities	Pruritus, lower extremity edema History of venous ulcers, thrombophlebitis, and/or cellulitis Rule out cellulitis Rule out superimposed contact dermatitis, e.g., topical neomycin	Skin biopsy	Topical glucocorticoids; open wet dressings; leg elevation; pressure stockings
Contact	Local: Erythema, crusting, vesicles, and bullae	Depends on offending agent	Irritant—onset often within hours Allergic—delayed-type hypersensitivity; lag time of 48 h	Patch testing	Remove irritant or allergen; topical glucocorticoids; oral antihistamines; oral/IM glucocorticoids
	Systemic: Erythema, fine scale, crust	Generalized	Patient has history of allergic contact dermatitis to topical agent and then receives systemic medication that is structurally related, e.g., ethylenediamine (topical) aminophylline (IV)	Patch testing	Same as local
Seborrheic	Pink-red, greasy scale	Scalp, nasolabial folds, eyebrows, intertriginous zones	Flares with stress, HIV infection Associated with Parkinson's disease	Skin biopsy	Topical glucocorticoids and imidazoles
Pityriasis rubra pilaris	Orange-red, perifollicular papules	Generalized, but characteristic "skip" areas of normal skin	Wax-like keratoderma Rule out cutaneous T cell lymphoma	Skin biopsy	Isotretinoin or acetretin; methotrexate

[a] Discussed in detail in Chap. 56.

NOTE: PUVA, *p*soralens + *u*ltraviolet *A* irradiation; UV-B, *u*ltraviolet *B*; UV-A, *u*ltraviolet *A*; IM, intramuscular; IV, intravenous.

Table 57-4 Causes of Alopecia

I. Nonscarring alopecia	II. Scarring alopecia
A. Primary cutaneous disorders	A. Primary cutaneous disorders
1. Telogen effluvium	1. Cutaneous lupus
2. Androgenetic alopecia	2. Lichen planus
3. Alopecia areata	3. Folliculitis decalvans
4. Tinea capitis	4. Linear scleroderma (morphea)
5. Traumatic alopecia	5. Traumatic alopecia[a]
B. Drugs	B. Systemic diseases
C. Systemic diseases	1. Lupus erythematosus
1. Lupus erythematosus	2. Sarcoidosis
2. Secondary syphilis	3. Cutaneous metastases
3. Hypothyroidism	
4. Hyperthyroidism	
5. Hypopituitarism	
6. Deficiencies of protein, iron, biotin, and zinc	
7. HIV infection	

[a] Also referred to as follicular degeneration.

and involve the entire scalp, or it may localized to the frontal scalp and result in multiple short hairs ("lupus hairs"). Scattered, poorly circumscribed patches of alopecia with a "moth-eaten" appearance are a manifestation of the secondary stage of syphilis. Diffuse thinning of the hair is also associated with hypothyroidism, hyperthyroidism, and HIV infection (Table 57-4).

Scarring alopecia is more frequently the result of a primary cutaneous disorder such as *lichen planus*, *folliculitis decalvans*, *cutaneous lupus*, or *linear scleroderma* (*morphea*) than it is a sign of systemic disease. Although the scarring lesions of *discoid lupus* can be seen in patients with systemic lupus, in the majority of cases the disease process is limited to the skin. Less common causes of scarring alopecia include *sarcoidosis* (see "Papulonodular Skin Lesions") and cutaneous *metastases*.

In the early phases of discoid lupus, lichen planus, and folliculitis decalvans, there are circumscribed areas of alopecia. Fibrosis and subsequent loss of follicles are observed primarily in the center of the individual lesions, while the inflammatory process is most prominent at the periphery. The areas of active inflammation in discoid lupus are

Table 57-5 Nonscarring Alopecia (Primary Cutaneous Disorders)

	Clinical Characteristics	Pathogenesis	Treatment
Telogen effluvium	Diffuse shedding of normal hairs Follows either major stress (high fever, severe infection) or change in hormones (post partum) Reversible without treatment	Stress causes the normally asynchronous growth cycles of individual hairs to become synchronous; therefore, large numbers of growing (anagen) hairs simultaneously enter the dying (telogen) phase	Observation; discontinue any drugs that have alopecia as a side effect; must exclude underlying metabolic causes, e.g., hypothyroidism, hyperthyroidism
Androgenetic alopecia	Miniaturization of hairs along the midline of the scalp Recession of the anterior scalp line in men and some women	Increased sensitivity of affected hairs to the effects of testosterone Increased levels of circulating androgens (ovarian or adrenal source in women)	If no evidence of hyperandrogen state, then topical minoxidil ± tretinoin; finasteride[a]; hair transplant
Alopecia areata	Well-circumscribed, circular areas of hair loss, 2–5 cm in diameter In extensive cases, coalescence of lesions and/or involvement of other hair-bearing surfaces of the body Pitting of the nails	The germinative zones of the hair follicles are surrounded by T lymphocytes Occasional associated diseases: hyperthyroidism, hypothyroidism, vitiligo, Down's syndrome	Topical anthralin; intralesional glucocorticoids; topical contact sensitizers
Tinea	Varies from scaling with minimal hair loss to discrete patches with "black dots" (broken hairs) to boggy plaque with pustules (kerion)	Invasion of hairs by dermatophytes, most commonly *Trichophyton tonsurans*	Oral griseofulvin plus 2.5% selenium sulfide or ketoconazole shampoo; examine family members
Traumatic alopecia	Broken hairs Irregular outline	Traction with curlers, rubber bands, braiding Exposure to heat or chemicals Mechanical pulling (trichotillomania)	Discontinuation of offending hair style or chemical treatments; trichotillomania may require hair clipping and observation of shaved hairs or biopsy for diagnosis, followed by psychotherapy

[a] To date, FDA-approved for men.

Table 57-6 Causes of Figurate Skin Lesions

I. Primary cutaneous disorders
  A. Tinea
  B. Urticaria
  C. Erythema annulare centrifugum
  D. Granuloma annulare
  E. Psoriasis
II. Systemic diseases
  A. Migratory
    1. Erythema migrans
    2. Erythema gyratum repens
    3. Erythema marginatum
    4. Pustular psoriasis
    5. Necrolytic migratory erythema (glucagonoma syndrome)[a]
  B. Nonmigratory
    1. Sarcoidosis
    2. Subacute lupus erythematosus
    3. Secondary syphilis
    4. Cutaneous T cell lymphoma (e.g., mycosis fungoides)

[a] Migratory erythema with erosions; favors lower extremities and girdle area.

erythematous with scale, whereas the areas of previous inflammation are often hypopigmented with a rim of hyperpigmentation. In lichen planus the peripheral perifollicular macules are usually violet-colored. Complete examination of the skin and oral mucosa combined with a biopsy and direct immunofluorescence microscopy will aid in distinguishing these two entities. The peripheral active lesions in folliculitis decalvans are perifollicular pustules; these patients can develop a reactive arthritis.

FIGURATE SKIN LESIONS (Table 57-6) In *figurate* eruptions, the lesions form rings and arcs that are usually erythematous but can be flesh-colored to brown. Most commonly, they are due to primary cutaneous diseases such as *tinea*, *urticaria*, *erythema annulare centrifugum*, and *granuloma annulare* (Chaps. 56 and 58). An underlying systemic illness is found in a second, less common group of migratory annular erythemas. It includes *erythema gyratum repens*, *erythema migrans*, *erythema marginatum*, and *necrolytic migratory erythema*.

In erythema gyratum repens, one sees hundreds of mobile concentric arcs and wavefronts that resemble the grain in wood. A search for an underlying malignancy is mandatory in a patient with this eruption. Erythema migrans is the cutaneous manifestation of Lyme disease, which is caused by the spirochete *Borrelia burgdorferi*. In the initial stage (3 to 30 days after tick bite), a single annular lesion is usually seen, which can expand to ≥10 cm in diameter. Within several days, approximately half the patients develop multiple smaller erythematous lesions at sites distant from the bite. Associated symptoms include fever, headache, photophobia, myalgias, arthralgias, and malar rash. Erythema marginatum is seen in patients with rheumatic fever, primarily on the trunk. Lesions are pink-red in color, flat to mildly elevated, and transient.

There are additional cutaneous diseases that present as annular eruptions but lack an obvious migratory component. Examples include *CTCL*, *annular cutaneous lupus*, also referred to as *subacute lupus*, *secondary syphilis*, and *sarcoidosis* (see "Papulonodular Skin Lesions").

ACNE (Table 57-7) *Acne vulgaris* and *acne rosacea* are the two major forms of acne (Chap. 56). Estrogens decrease sebaceous gland activity, whereas androgens enhance sebum production. Therefore,

Table 57-7 Causes of Acneiform Eruptions

I. Primary cutaneous disorders
  A. Acne vulgaris
  B. Acne rosacea
II. Drugs
III. Systemic diseases
  A. Increased androgen production
    1. Adrenal origin, e.g., Cushing's disease, 21-hydroxylase deficiency
    2. Ovarian origin, e.g., polycystic ovary disease
  B. Cryptococcosis, disseminated
  C. Dimorphic fungi
  D. Behçet's disease

acne vulgaris in an adult, especially if it is of recent onset, may be a reflection of increased levels of circulating *androgens*. Dysfunction of the ovary or adrenal gland, e.g., polycystic ovary disease or Cushing's syndrome, can lead to the hormonal imbalance. Examination of the patient for signs such as hirsutism, androgenetic alopecia, hypertension, and redistribution of subcutaneous fat will aid in the diagnosis.

Exacerbations of acne vulgaris follow the ingestion of several *drugs*, such as anabolic steroids, glucocorticoids, lithium, and iodides as well as the application of oil-containing compounds. Acne-like lesions can be seen in patients with Behçet's disease (see "Ulcers"), and in immunocompromised hosts, disseminated fungal infections (e.g., cryptococcosis) may present as an acneiform eruption.

Patients with the carcinoid syndrome have episodes of flushing of the head, neck, and sometimes the trunk. Resultant skin changes of the face, in particular telangiectasias, may mimic the clinical appearance of acne rosacea.

PUSTULAR LESIONS *Acneiform eruptions* (see "Acne") and *folliculitis* represent the most common pustular dermatoses. An important consideration in the evaluation of perifollicular pustules is a determination of the associated pathogen, e.g., normal flora, *Staphylococcus aureus, Pityrosporum*. Noninfectious forms of folliculitis include HIV-associated eosinophilic folliculitis and folliculitis secondary to drugs such as glucocorticoids and lithium. Administration of high-dose oral glucocorticoids can result in a widespread eruption of perifollicular pustules on the trunk, characterized by lesions in the same stage of development. With regard to underlying systemic diseases, pustules are a characteristic component of pustular psoriasis and can be seen in septic emboli of bacterial or fungal origin (see "Purpura").

TELANGIECTASIAS (Table 57-8) In order to distinguish the various types of telangiectasias, it is important to examine the shape and configuration of the dilated blood vessels. *Linear telangiectasias* are seen on the face of patients with *actinically damaged skin* and *acne rosacea* and they are found on the legs of patients with *venous hypertension* and *essential telangiectasia*. Patients with an unusual form of *mastocytosis* (telangiectasia macularis eruptiva perstans), the *carcinoid* syndrome (see "Acne"), and *ataxia-telangiectasia* also have linear telangiectasias. In ataxia-telangiectasia, linear telangiectasias appear on the bulbar conjunctiva during childhood. Eventually, there is involvement of the ears, eyelids, cheeks, and/or flexural areas such as the antecubital and popliteal fossae. Lastly, linear telangiectasias are found in areas of cutaneous inflammation. For example, lesions of discoid lupus frequently have telangiectasias within them.

Poikiloderma is a term used to describe a patch of skin with (1) reticulated hypo- and hyperpigmentation, (2) wrinkling secondary to epidermal atrophy, and (3) telangiectasias. Poikiloderma does not imply a single disease entity—it is seen in skin damaged by *ionizing radiation*, in the disorders *poikiloderma vasculare atrophicans* (PVA) and *xeroderma pigmentosum*, as well as in patients with connective-tissue diseases, primarily *dermatomyositis* (DM). PVA is a precursor lesion of CTCL, and the areas of poikiloderma usually begin in the flexural areas of the axillae and groin.

In *scleroderma*, the dilated blood vessels have a unique configuration and are known as *mat telangiectasias*. The lesions are broad macules that usually measure 2 to 7 mm in diameter but occasionally are larger. Mats have a polygonal or oval shape, and their erythematous color may be uniform or the result of delicate telangiectasias. The most common locations for mat telangiectasias are the face, oral mucosa, and hands—peripheral sites that are prone to intermittent ischemia. The CREST (*c*alcinosis cutis, *R*aynaud's phenomenon, *e*sophageal dysmotility, *s*clerodactyly, and *t*elangiectasia) variant of scleroderma (Chap. 313) is associated with a chronic course and anticentromere antibodies. Mat telangiectasias are an important clue to the diagnosis of the CREST syndrome as well as systemic scleroderma, for they may be the only cutaneous finding.

Periungual telangiectasias are pathognomonic signs of the three major connective tissue diseases—*lupus erythematosus, scleroderma*, and *DM*. They are easily visualized by the naked eye and occur in at least two-thirds of these patients. In both DM and lupus there is associated nailfold erythema, and in DM the erythema is often accompanied by "ragged" cuticles and fingertip tenderness. Under 10× magnification, the blood vessels in the nailfolds of lupus patients are tortuous and resemble "glomeruli," whereas in scleroderma and DM there is a loss of capillary loops and those that remain are markedly dilated.

In *hereditary hemorrhagic telangiectasia* (Osler-Rendu-Weber disease), the lesions usually appear during adulthood and are most commonly seen on the mucous membranes, face, and distal extremities, including under the nails. They represent arteriovenous (AV) malformations of the dermal microvasculature, are dark red in color, and are usually slightly elevated. When the skin is stretched over an individual lesion, an eccentric punctum with radiating legs is seen. Although the degree of systemic involvement varies in this autosomal dominant disease (due to mutations in either the endoglin or activin receptor–like kinase gene), the major symptoms are recurrent epistaxis and gastrointestinal bleeding. The fact that these mucosal telangiectasias are actually AV communications helps to explain their tendency to bleed.

HYPOPIGMENTATION (Table 57-9) Disorders of hypopigmentation are classified as either diffuse or localized. The classic ex-

---

Table 57-8 Causes of Telangiectasias

I. Primary cutaneous disorders	II. Systemic diseases
A. Linear	A. Linear
1. Acne rosacea	1. Carcinoid
2. Actinically damaged skin	2. Ataxia-telangiectasia
3. Venous hypertension	3. Mastocytosis
4. Essential telangiectasia	B. Poikiloderma
B. Poikiloderma	1. Dermatomyositis
1. Ionizing radiation	2. Xeroderma pigmentosum
2. Poikiloderma vasculare atrophicans	3. Cutaneous T cell lymphoma
C. Spider angioma	C. Mat
1. Idiopathic	1. Scleroderma
2. Pregnancy	D. Periungual
	1. Lupus erythematosus
	2. Scleroderma
	3. Dermatomyositis
	E. Papular
	1. Hereditary hemorrhagic telangiectasia
	F. Spider angioma
	1. Cirrhosis

Table 57-9 Causes of Hypopigmentation

I. Primary cutaneous disorders	II. Systemic diseases
A. Diffuse	A. Diffuse
1. Generalized vitiligo	1. Oculocutaneous albinism
B. Localized	a. Hermansky-Pudlak syndrome[a]
1. Idiopathic guttate hypomelanosis	b. Chédiak–Higashi syndrome[b]
2. Postinflammatory[b]	B. Localized
3. Tinea (pityriasis) versicolor	1. Vogt-Koyanagi-Harada
4. Vitiligo	2. Scleroderma
5. Chemical leukoderma	3. Melanoma-associated leukoderma
6. Nevus depigmentosus	4. Tuberous sclerosis
7. Piebaldism	5. Hypomelanosis of Ito/mosaicism
	6. Sarcoidosis
	7. Tuberculoid and indeterminate leprosy
	8. Cutaneous T cell lymphoma

[a] Platelet storage defect and restrictive lung disease secondary to deposits of ceroid-like material.
[b] Giant lysosomal granules and recurrent infections.

ample of *diffuse hypopigmentation* is *oculocutaneous albinism* (OCA). The most common forms are due to mutations in the tyrosinase gene (type I) or the *P* gene (type II); patients with type IA OCA have a total lack of enzyme activity. At birth, different forms of OCA can appear similar—white hair, gray-blue eyes, and pink-white skin. However, the patients with no tyrosinase activity maintain this phenotype, whereas those with decreased activity or *P* gene mutations will acquire some pigmentation of the eyes, hair, and skin as they age. The degree of pigment formation is also a function of racial background, and the pigmentary dilution is readily apparent when patients are compared to their first-degree relatives.

The ocular findings in OCA correlate with the degree of hypopigmentation and include decreased visual acuity, nystagmus, photophobia, and monocular vision. Generalized vitiligo, phenylketonuria, and homocystinuria are other unusual causes of diffuse pigmentary dilution. In generalized vitiligo, melanocytes are not found in affected skin, whereas in OCA they are present but have decreased activity. Appropriate laboratory tests exclude the other disorders of metabolism.

The differential diagnosis of *localized hypomelanosis* includes the following primary cutaneous disorders: *idiopathic guttate hypomelanosis, postinflammatory hypopigmentation, tinea (pityriasis) versicolor, vitiligo, chemical leukoderma, nevus depigmentosus* (see below), and *piebaldism* (Table 57-9). In this group of diseases, the areas of involvement are macules or patches with a decrease or absence of pigmentation. Patients with vitiligo also have an increased incidence of several autoimmune disorders, including hypothyroidism, Graves' disease, pernicious anemia, Addison's disease, uveitis, alopecia areata, chronic mucocutaneous candidiasis, and the polyglandular autoimmune syndromes (types I and II). Diseases of the thyroid gland are the most frequently associated disorders, occurring in up to 30% of patients with vitiligo. Circulating autoantibodies are often found, and the most common ones are antithyroglobulin, antimicrosomal, and antiparietal cell antibodies.

There are three systemic diseases that should be considered in a patient with skin findings suggestive of vitiligo—*Vogt-Koyanagi-Harada syndrome, scleroderma,* and *melanoma-associated leukoderma.* A history of aseptic meningitis, nontraumatic uveitis, tinnitus, hearing loss, and/or dysacousis points to the diagnosis of the Vogt-Koyanagi-Harada syndrome. In these patients, the face and scalp are the most common locations of pigment loss. The vitiligo-like leukoderma seen in patients with scleroderma has a clinical resemblance to idiopathic vitiligo that has begun to repigment as a result of treatment; that is, perifollicular macules of normal pigmentation are seen within areas of depigmentation. The basis of this leukoderma is unknown; there is no evidence of inflammation in areas of involvement, but it can resolve if the underlying connective tissue disease becomes inactive. In contrast to idiopathic vitiligo, melanoma-associated leukoderma often begins on the trunk, and its appearance should prompt a search for metastatic disease. The possibility exists that the destruction of normal melanocytes is the result of an immune response against malignant melanocytes.

There are two systemic disorders that may have the cutaneous findings of piebaldism (Table 57-10). They are *Hirschsprung's disease* and *Waardenburg's syndrome.* A possible explanation for both disorders is an abnormal embryonic migration or survival of two neural crest–derived elements, one of them being melanocytes and the other myenteric ganglion cells (Hirschsprung's disease) or auditory nerve cells (Waardenburg's syndrome). The latter syndrome is characterized by congenital sensorineural hearing loss, dystopia canthorum (lateral displacement of the inner canthi but normal interpupillary distance), heterochromic irises, and a broad nasal root, in addition to the piebaldism. Patients with Waardenburg's syndrome have been shown to have mutations in two genes that encode DNA-binding proteins, *PAX-3* and *MITF,* while patients with Hirschsprung's disease and white spotting have mutations in one of three genes—endothelin 3, endothelin B receptor, and *SOX-10.*

In *tuberous sclerosis,* the earliest cutaneous sign is an ash leaf spot. These lesions are often present at birth and are usually multiple; however, detection may require Wood's lamp examination, especially in fair-skinned individuals. The pigment within them is reduced but not absent. The average size is 1 to 3 cm, and the common shapes are polygonal and lance-ovate. Examination of the patient for additional cutaneous signs such as adenoma sebaceum (multiple angiofibromas of the face), ungual and gingival fibromas, fibrous plaques of the forehead, and connective tissue nevi (shagreen patches) is recommended. It is important to remember that an ash leaf spot on the scalp will result in *poliosis,* which is a circumscribed patch of gray-white hair. Internal manifestations include seizures, mental retardation, central nervous system (CNS) and retinal hamartomas, renal angiomyolipomas, and cardiac rhabdomyomas. The latter can be detected in up to 60% of children (<18 years) with tuberous sclerosis by echocardiography.

Nevus depigmentosus is a stable, well-circumscribed hypomelanosis that is present at birth. There is usually a single circular or rectangular lesion, but occasionally the nevus has a dermatomal or whorled pattern. It is important to distinguish this more common entity from ash leaf spots especially when there are multiple lesions. In *hypomelanosis of Ito,* swirls and streaks of hypopigmentation run parallel to one another in a pattern that resembles a marble cake. Lesions may progress or regress with time, and in up to a third of patients, associated abnormalities are found including in the musculoskeletal system (asymmetry), the CNS (seizures and mental retardation), and the eyes (strabismus and hypertelorism). Chromosomal mosaicism has been detected in these patients; this lends support to the hypothesis that the pattern is the result of the migration of two clones of primordial melanocytes, each with a different pigment potential.

Localized areas of decreased pigmentation are commonly seen as a result of cutaneous inflammation (Table 57-10) and have been observed in the skin overlying active lesions of sarcoidosis (see "Papulonodular Skin Lesions") as well as in CTCL. Cutaneous infections also present as disorders of hypopigmentation, and in *tuberculoid leprosy* there are a few asymmetric patches of hypomelanosis that have associated anesthesia, anhidrosis, and alopecia. Biopsy specimens of the palpable border show dermal granulomas that lack *Mycobacterium leprae* organisms.

HYPERPIGMENTATION (Table 57-11) Disorders of hyperpigmentation are also divided into two groups—localized and diffuse. The *localized* forms are due to an epidermal alteration, a proliferation of melanocytes, or an increase in pigment production. Both seborrheic keratoses and acanthosis nigricans belong to the first group. *Seborrheic keratoses* are common lesions, but in one clinical setting they are a sign of systemic disease, and that setting is the sudden appearance of multiple lesions, often with an inflammatory base and in association with acrochordons (skin tags) and acanthosis nigricans. This is termed the *sign of Leser-Trélat* and signifies an internal malignancy. *Acanthosis nigricans* can also be a reflection of an internal malignancy, most commonly of the gastrointestinal tract, and it appears as velvety hyperpigmentation, primarily in flexural areas. In the majority of patients, acanthosis nigricans is associated with obesity, but it may be a reflection of an endocrinopathy such as acromegaly, Cushing's syndrome, the Stein-Leventhal syndrome, or insulin-resistant diabetes mellitus (type A, type B, and lipoatrophic forms).

A proliferation of melanocytes results in the following pigmented lesions: *lentigo, melanocytic nevus,* and *melanoma* (Chap. 86). In an adult, the majority of lentigines are related to sun exposure, which explains their distribution. However, in the Peutz-Jeghers and LEOPARD [*l*entigines; *E*CG abnormalities, primarily conduction defects; *o*cular hypertelorism; *p*ulmonary stenosis and subaortic valvular stenosis; *a*bnormal genitalia (cryptorchidism, hypospadias); *r*etardation of growth; and *d*eafness (sensorineural)] syndromes, lentigines do serve as a clue to systemic disease. In the multiple lentigines or *LEOPARD syndrome,* hundreds of lentigines develop during childhood and are scattered over the entire surface of the body. The lentigines in patients with *Peutz-Jeghers syndrome* are located primarily around the nose and mouth, on the hands and feet, and within the oral cavity.

Table 57-10 Hypopigmentation (Primary Cutaneous Disorders, Localized)

	Clinical Characteristics	Wood's Lamp Examination (UV-A; Peak = 365 nm)	Skin Biopsy Specimen	Pathogenesis	Treatment
Idiopathic guttate hypomelanosis	Common; acquired; 1 to 4 mm in diameter Shins and extensor forearms	Less enhancement than vitiligo	Abrupt decrease in epidermal melanin content	Possible somatic mutations as a reflection of aging; UV exposure	None
Postinflammatory hypopigmentation	Can develop within active lesions, as in subacute lupus, or after the lesion fades, as in dermatitis	Depends on particular disease Usually less enhancement than in vitiligo	Type of inflammatory infiltrate depends on specific disease	Block in transfer of melanin from melanocytes to keratinocytes could be secondary to edema or decrease in contact time Destruction of melanocytes if inflammatory cells attack basal layer	Treat underlying inflammatory disease
Tinea (pityriasis) versicolor	Common disorder Upper trunk and neck Shawl-like distribution Young adults Macules have fine white scale when scratched	Golden fluorescence	Hyphae and budding yeast in stratum corneum	Invasion of stratum corneum by the yeast *Pityrosporum* Yeast is lipophilic and produces C_9 and C_{11} dicarboxylic acids which in vitro inhibit tyrosinase	Selenium sulfide 2.5%; topical imidazoles; oral imidazoles or triazoles
Vitiligo	Acquired; progressive Symmetric areas of complete pigment loss Periorificial—around mouth, nose, eyes, nipples, umbilicus, anus Other areas—flexor wrists, extensor distal extremities Segmental form is less common—unilateral, dermatomal-like	More apparent Chalk-white	Absence of melanocytes Mild inflammation	Possible autoimmune phenomenon that results in destruction of melanocytes—humoral and/or cellular Alternative hypothesis is self-destruction of melanocytes and circulating antibodies or cytotoxic T cells as a secondary phenomenon	Topical glucocorticoids; PUVA; UV-B; transplants; depigmentation if widespread
Chemical leukoderma	Similar appearance to vitiligo Often begins on hands Satellite lesions in areas not exposed to chemicals	More apparent Chalk-white	Decreased number or absence of melanocytes	Exposure to chemicals that selectively destroy melanocytes, in particular, phenols and catechols (germicides; adhesives) Release of cellular antigens and activation of circulating lymphocytes may explain satellite phenomenon	Avoid exposure to offending agent, then treat as vitiligo
Piebaldism	Autosomal dominant Congenital, stable White forelock Areas of hypomelanosis contain normally pigmented and hyperpigmented macules of various sizes Symmetric involvement of central forehead, ventral trunk, and mid regions of upper and lower extremities	Enhancement of leukoderma and hyperpigmented macules	Hypomelanotic areas—few to no melanocytes	Defect in migration of melanoblasts from neural crest to ventral skin or failure of melanoblasts to survive or differentiate in these areas Mutations within the c-*kit* proto-oncogene that encodes the tyrosine kinase receptor for mast/stem cell growth factor	None; occasionally transplants

NOTE: PUVA, *p*soralens + *u*ltraviolet *A* irradiation; UV-B, *u*ltraviolet B.

While the pigmented macules on the face may fade with age, the oral lesions persist. However, similar intraoral lesions are also seen in Addison's disease and as a normal finding in darkly pigmented individuals. Patients with this autosomal dominant syndrome (due to mutations in a novel serine threonine kinase gene) have multiple benign polyps of the gastrointestinal tract, testicular tumors, and an increased risk of developing gastrointestinal (primarily colon), breast, and gynecologic cancers.

Lentigines are also seen in association with cardiac myxomas and have been described in two syndromes whose findings overlap: *LAMB* (*l*entigines, *a*trial myxomas, *m*ucocutaneous myxomas, and *b*lue nevi) *syndrome* and *NAME* [*n*evus, *a*trial myxoma, *m*yxoid neurofibroma, and *e*phelides (freckles)] *syndrome*. These patients can also have ev-

idence of endocrine overactivity in the form of Cushing's syndrome, acromegaly, or sexual precocity.

The third type of localized hyperpigmentation is due to a local increase in pigment production, and it includes *ephelides* and café au lait macules (CALM). The latter are most commonly associated with two disorders—neurofibromatosis (NF) and McCune-Albright syndrome. *CALM* are flat, uniformly light brown in color, and can vary in size from 0.5 to 12 cm. Approximately 80% of adult patients with *type I NF* will have six or more CALM measuring 1.5 cm or greater in diameter. Additional findings are discussed in the section on neurofibromas (see "Papulonodular Skin Lesions"). In comparison with NF, the CALM in patients with *McCune-Albright syndrome* [polyostotic fibrous dysplasia with precocious puberty in females due to

Table 57-11 Causes of Hyperpigmentation

I. Primary cutaneous disorders
  A. Localized
    1. Epidermal alteration
      a. Seborrheic keratosis
      b. Acanthosis nigricans (obesity)
      c. Pigmented actinic keratosis
    2. Proliferation of melanocytes
      a. Lentigo
      b. Nevus
      c. Melanoma
    3. Increased pigment production
      a. Ephelides (freckles)
      b. Café au lait macule
  B. Localized and diffuse
    1. Drugs
II. Systemic diseases
  A. Localized
    1. Epidermal alteration
      a. Seborrheic keratoses (sign of Leser-Trélat)
      b. Acanthosis nigricans (endocrine disorders, paraneoplastic)
    2. Proliferation of melanocytes
      a. Lentigines (Peutz-Jeghers and LEOPARD syndromes; xeroderma pigmentosum)
      b. Nevi [Carney complex (LAMB and NAME syndromes)][a]
    3. Increased pigment production
      a. Café au lait macules (neurofibromatosis, McCune-Albright syndrome[b])
      b. Urticaria pigmentosa[c]
    4. Dermal pigmentation
      a. Incontinentia pigmenti
      b. Dyskeratosis congenita
  B. Diffuse
    1. Endocrinopathies
      a. Addison's disease
      b. Nelson syndrome
      c. Ectopic ACTH syndrome
    2. Metabolic
      a. Porphyria cutanea tarda
      b. Hemochromatosis
      c. Vitamin B_{12}, folate deficiency
      d. Pellagra
      e. Malabsorption, Whipple's disease
    3. Melanosis secondary to metastatic melanoma
    4. Autoimmune
      a. Biliary cirrhosis
      b. Scleroderma
      c. POEMS syndrome
      d. Eosinophilia-myalgia syndrome
    5. Drugs and metals

[a] Also lentigines.
[b] Polyostotic fibrous dysplasia.
[c] See also "Papulonodular Skin Lesions."

mosaicism for an activating mutation in a G protein ($G_s\alpha$) gene] are usually larger, more irregular in outline, and tend to respect the midline. CALM have also been associated with pulmonary stenosis (Watson syndrome), tuberous sclerosis, the LEOPARD syndrome, and ataxia telangiectasia, but a few such lesions can be found in normal individuals.

In incontinentia pigmenti, dyskeratosis congenita, and bleomycin pigmentation, the areas of localized hyperpigmentation form a pattern—swirled in the first, reticulated in the second, and flagellate in the third. Patients with the X-linked dominant disorder *incontinentia pigmenti* can have linear blisters and verrucous papules during infancy. During childhood, parallel swirls and streaks of hyperpigmentation appear on the trunk, and occasionally streaks of hypopigmentation appear on the extremities. Associated findings include seizures, mental retardation, retinal vascular abnormalities, and delayed or impaired dentition. Biopsy specimens of the streaks will show pigment within dermal macrophages ("incontinent pigment"). In *dyskeratosis congenita*, atrophic reticulated hyperpigmentation is seen on the neck, thighs,

and trunk and is accompanied by nail dystrophy, pancytopenia, and leukoplakia of the oral and anal mucosa. The latter often develops into squamous cell carcinoma. In addition to the flagellate pigmentation (linear streaks) on the trunk, patients receiving bleomycin often have hyperpigmentation on the elbows, knees, and small joints of the hand.

Localized hyperpigmentation is seen as a side effect of several other *systemic medications*, including those that produce fixed drug reactions [phenolphthalein, nonsteroidal anti-inflammatory drugs (NSAIDs), sulfonamides, and barbiturates] and those that can complex with melanin (antimalarials). Fixed drug eruptions recur in the same location as circular areas of erythema that can become bullous and then resolve as brown macules. The eruption usually appears within hours of administration of the offending agent, and common locations include the genitalia, extremities, and perioral region. Chloroquine and hydroxychloroquine produce gray-brown to blue-black discoloration of the shins, hard palate, and face, while blue macules can be seen on the lower extremities and in sites of inflammation with prolonged minocycline administration. Estrogen in oral contraceptives can induce melasma—symmetric brown patches on the face, especially the cheeks, upper lip, and forehead. Similar changes are seen in pregnancy, in patients receiving hydantoin, and in the adult form of Gaucher's disease. In the latter group there is also hyperpigmentation of the distal lower extremities.

In the *diffuse* forms of hyperpigmentation, the darkening of the skin may be of equal intensity over the entire body or may be accentuated in sun-exposed areas. The causes of diffuse hyperpigmentation can be divided into four groups—endocrine, metabolic, autoimmune, and drugs. The endocrinopathies that frequently have associated hyperpigmentation include *Addison's disease*, *Nelson syndrome*, and *ectopic ACTH syndrome*. In these diseases, the increased pigmentation is diffuse but is accentuated in the palmar creases, sites of friction, scars, and the oral mucosa. An overproduction of the pituitary hormones α-MSH (melanocyte-stimulating hormone) and ACTH can lead to an increase in melanocyte activity. These peptides are products of the proopiomelanocortin gene and exhibit homology; e.g., α-MSH and ACTH share 13 amino acids. A minority of the patients with Cushing's disease or hyperthyroidism have generalized hyperpigmentation.

The metabolic causes of hyperpigmentation include *porphyria cutanea tarda* (PCT), *hemochromatosis*, *vitamin B_{12} deficiency*, *folic acid deficiency*, *pellagra*, *malabsorption*, and *Whipple's disease*. In patients with PCT (see "Vesicles/Bullae"), the skin darkening is seen in sun-exposed areas and is a reflection of the photoreactive properties of porphyrins. The increased level of iron in the skin of patients with hemochromatosis stimulates melanin pigment production and leads to the classic bronze color. Patients with pellagra have a brown discoloration of the skin, especially in sun-exposed areas, as a result of nicotinic acid (niacin) deficiency. In the areas of increased pigmentation, there is a thin varnish-like scale. These changes are also seen in patients who are vitamin B_6 deficient, have functioning carcinoid tumors (increased consumption of niacin), or take isoniazid. Approximately 50% of the patients with Whipple's disease have an associated generalized hyperpigmentation in association with diarrhea, weight loss, arthritis, and lymphadenopathy. A diffuse slate-blue color is seen in patients with melanosis secondary to metastatic melanoma. Although there is a debate as to whether the color is due to single-cell metastases in the dermis or to a widespread deposition of melanin resulting from the high concentration of circulating melanin precursors, there is more evidence to support the latter.

Of the autoimmune diseases associated with diffuse hyperpigmentation, *biliary cirrhosis* and *scleroderma* are the most common, and occasionally, both disorders are seen in the same patient. The skin is dark brown in color, especially in sun-exposed areas. In biliary cirrhosis the hyperpigmentation is accompanied by pruritus, jaundice, and xanthomas, whereas in scleroderma it is accompanied by sclerosis of the extremities, face, and, less commonly, the trunk. Additional clues to the diagnosis of scleroderma are telangiectasias, calcinosis cutis, Raynaud's phenomenon, and distal ulcerations (see "Telangiectasias"). The differential diagnosis of cutaneous sclerosis with hyperpigmentation includes the POEMS [*p*olyneuropathy; *o*rganomegaly (liver, spleen, lymph nodes); *e*ndocrinopathies (impotence, gynecomastia); *M*-protein; and *s*kin changes] syndrome. The skin changes include hyperpigmentation, skin thickening, hypertrichosis, and angiomas.

In the late 1980s, an epidemic of the eosinophilia-myalgia syndrome was described that was presumably due to contaminated L-tryptophan preparations. In addition to maculopapular eruptions and alopecia, large areas of scleroderma-like induration were observed with overlying hyperpigmentation.

Diffuse hyperpigmentation that is due to *drugs* or *metals* can result from one of several mechanisms—induction of melanin pigment formation, complexing of the drug or its metabolites to melanin, and deposits of the drug in the dermis. Busulfan, cyclophosphamide, long-term, high-dose ACTH, and inorganic arsenic induce pigment production. Complexes containing melanin or hemosiderin plus the drug or its metabolites are seen in patients receiving chlorpromazine and minocycline. The sun-exposed skin as well as the conjunctivae of patients on long-term, high-dose chlorpromazine can become blue-gray in color. Patients taking minocycline may develop a diffuse blue-gray, muddy appearance in sun-exposed areas in addition to pigmentation of the mucous membranes, teeth, nails, bones, and thyroid. Administration of amiodarone can result in both a phototoxic eruption (exaggerated sunburn) and/or a brown or blue-gray discoloration of sun-exposed skin. Biopsy specimens of the latter show yellow-brown granules in dermal macrophages, which represent intralysosomal accumulations of lipids, amiodarone, and its metabolites. Actual deposits of a particular drug or metal in the skin are seen with silver (argyria), where the skin appears blue-gray in color; gold (chrysiasis), where the skin has a brown to blue-gray color; and clofazimine, where the skin appears reddish brown. The associated hyperpigmentation is accentuated in sun-exposed areas, and discoloration of the eye is seen with gold (sclerae) and clofazimine (conjunctivae).

VESICLES/BULLAE (Table 57-12) Depending on their size, cutaneous blisters are referred to as *vesicles* (<0.5 cm) or *bullae* (>0.5 cm). The primary blistering disorders include *pemphigus vulgaris, pemphigus foliaceus, pemphigus erythematosus, paraneoplastic pemphigus, bullous pemphigoid, herpes gestationis, cicatricial pemphigoid, epidermolysis bullosa acquisita, linear IgA disease*, and *dermatitis herpetiformis* (Chap. 58).

Vesicles and bullae are also seen in *contact dermatitis*, both allergic and irritant forms (Chap. 56). When there is a linear arrangement of vesicular lesions, an exogenous cause should be suspected. Bullous disease secondary to the ingestion of drugs can take one of several forms, including phototoxic eruptions, isolated bullae, toxic epidermal necrolysis, and erythema multiforme (Chap. 59). Clinically, phototoxic eruptions resemble an exaggerated sunburn with diffuse erythema and bullae in sun-exposed areas. The most commonly associated drugs are thiazides, doxycycline, sulfonamides, NSAIDs, and psoralens. The development of a phototoxic eruption is dependent on the doses of both the drug and UV-A irradiation.

Toxic epidermal necrolysis (TEN) is characterized by bullae that arise on widespread areas of erythema and then slough. This results in large areas of denuded skin. The associated morbidity, such as sepsis, and mortality are relatively high and are a function of the extent of epidermal necrosis. In addition, these patients may also have involvement of the mucous membranes and intestinal tract. Drugs are the primary cause of TEN, and the most common offenders are phenytoin, barbiturates, sulfonamides, penicillins, and NSAIDs. Severe acute graft-versus-host disease (grade 4) also can resemble TEN.

In *erythema multiforme* (EM), the primary lesions are pink-red macules and edematous papules, the centers of which may become vesicular. The clue to the diagnosis of EM, as opposed to a drug-induced morbilliform exanthem, is the development of a "dusky" violet color or petechiae in the center of the lesions. Target or iris lesions are also characteristic of EM and arise as a result of active centers and borders in combination with centrifugal spread. However, iris lesions need not be present to make the diagnosis of EM. Preferred sites of involvement include the distal extremities and mucous membranes (oral, nasal, ocular, and genital). Hemorrhagic crusts of the lips are characteristic of EM as well as herpes simplex, pemphigus vulgaris, and paraneoplastic pemphigus. Fever, malaise, myalgias, sore throat, and cough may precede or accompany the eruption. The lesions of EM usually resolve over 3 to 6 weeks but may be recurrent.

Drugs can induce EM, in particular sulfonamides, phenytoin, barbiturates, penicillins, and carbamazepine, but they do not cause the majority of cases, especially in young adults. Infections with herpes simplex are the most common cause of EM in this age group, and the lesions appear 7 to 12 days after the viral eruption. Other infectious agents associated with EM include *Mycoplasma pneumoniae*, dimorphic fungi, and several viruses (echovirus, coxsackievirus, Epstein-Barr, and influenza). EM can also follow vaccinations with BCG, poliomyelitis, or vaccinia viruses; radiation therapy; and exposure to environmental toxins.

In addition to primary blistering disorders and hypersensitivity reactions, bacterial and viral infections can lead to vesicles and bullae. The most common infectious agents are herpes simplex (Chap. 182), herpes varicella-zoster (Chap. 183), and staphylococci (Chap. 139).

Staphylococcal scalded-skin syndrome (SSSS) and *bullous impetigo* are two blistering disorders associated with staphylococcal (phage group II) infection. In SSSS, the initial findings are redness and tenderness of the central face, neck, trunk, and intertriginous zones. This is followed by short-lived flaccid bullae and a slough or exfoliation of the superficial epidermis. Crusted areas then develop, characteristically around the mouth. SSSS is distinguished from TEN by the following features: younger age group, more superficial site of blister formation, no oral lesions, shorter course, less morbidity and mortality, and an association with staphylococcal exfoliative toxin ("exfoliatin"), not drugs. A rapid diagnosis of SSSS versus TEN can be made by a frozen section of the blister roof or exfoliative cytology of the blister contents. In SSSS the site of staphylococcal infection is usually extracutaneous (conjunctivitis, rhinorrhea, otitis media, pharyngitis, tonsillitis), and the cutaneous lesions are sterile, whereas in bullous impetigo the skin lesions are the site of infection. Impetigo is more localized than SSSS

Table 57-12 Causes of Vesicles/Bullae

I. Primary cutaneous diseases	II. Systemic diseases
A. Primary blistering diseases (autoimmune)	A. Autoimmune
1. Pemphigus[a]	1. Paraneoplastic pemphigus[a]
2. Bullous pemphigoid[b]	B. Infections
3. Herpes gestationis[b]	1. Cutaneous emboli[b]
4. Cicatricial pemphigoid[b]	C. Metabolic
5. Dermatitis herpetiformis[b,c]	1. Diabetic bullae[a,b]
6. Linear IgA disease[b]	2. Porphyria cutanea tarda[b]
7. Epidermolysis bullosa acquisita[b,d]	3. Porphyria variegata[b]
B. Secondary blistering diseases	4. Pseudoporphyria[b]
1. Contact[a]	5. Bullous dermatosis of hemodialysis[b]
2. Erythema multiforme[a,b]	D. Ischemia
3. Toxic epidermal necrolysis[b]	1. Coma bullae
C. Infections	
1. Varicella/zoster[a,e]	
2. Herpes simplex[a,e]	
3. Enteroviruses, e.g., hand-foot-and-mouth disease	
4. Staphylococcal scalded-skin syndrome[a,f]	
5. Bullous impetigo[a]	

[a] Intraepidermal.
[b] Subepidermal.
[c] Associated with gluten enteropathy.
[d] Associated with inflammatory bowel disease.
[e] Also systemic.
[f] In adults, associated with renal failure and immunocompromised state.

and usually presents with honey-colored crusts. Occasionally, superficial purulent blisters also form. *Cutaneous emboli* from gram-negative infections may present as isolated bullae, but the base of the lesion is purpuric or necrotic, and it may develop into an ulcer (see "Purpura").

Several metabolic disorders are associated with blister formation, including diabetes mellitus, renal failure, and porphyria. Local hypoxia secondary to decreased cutaneous blood flow can also produce blisters, which explains the presence of bullae over pressure points in comatose patients (coma bullae). In *diabetes mellitus*, tense bullae with clear viscous fluid arise on normal skin. The lesions can be as large as 6 cm in diameter and are located on the distal extremities. There are several types of porphyria, but the most common form with cutaneous findings is *PCT*. In sun-exposed areas (primarily the face and hands), the skin is very fragile, and trauma leads to erosions and tense vesicles. These lesions then heal with scarring and formation of milia; the latter are firm, 2- to 3-mm white or yellow papules that represent epidermoid inclusion cysts. Associated findings can include hypertrichosis of the lateral malar region (males) or face (females) and, in sun-exposed areas, hyperpigmentation and firm sclerotic plaques. An elevated level of urinary uroporphyrins confirms the diagnosis and is due to a decrease in uroporphyrinogen decarboxylase activity. Precipitating agents include alcohol, iron, chlorinated hydrocarbons, and hepatitis C infection.

The differential diagnosis of PCT includes (1) *porphyria variegata*—the skin signs of PCT plus the systemic findings of acute intermittent porphyria; it has a diagnostic plasma porphyrin fluorescence emission at 626 nm; (2) *drug-induced bullous photosensitivity* (pseudoporphyria)—the clinical and histologic findings are similar to PCT, but porphyrins are normal; etiologic agents include naproxen, furosemide, tetracycline, and nalidixic acid; (3) *bullous dermatosis of hemodialysis*—the same appearance as PCT, but porphyrins are usually normal or occasionally borderline elevated; patients have chronic renal failure and are on hemodialysis; (4) PCT associated with hepatomas, hepatic carcinomas, and hemodialysis; and (5) *epidermolysis bullosa acquisita* (Chap. 58).

EXANTHEMS (Table 57-13) Exanthems are characterized by an acute generalized eruption. The two most common presentations are erythematous macules and papules (morbilliform) and confluent blanching erythema (scarlatiniform). *Morbilliform* eruptions are usually due to either *drugs* or *viral infections*. For example, up to 5% of the patients receiving penicillins, sulfonamides, phenytoin, or gold will develop a maculopapular eruption. Accompanying signs may include pruritus, fever, eosinophilia, and transient lymphadenopathy. Similar maculopapular eruptions are seen in the classic childhood viral exanthems, including (1) *rubeola* (measles)—a prodrome of coryza, cough, and conjunctivitis followed by Koplik's spots on the buccal mucosa;

the eruption begins behind the ears, at the hairline, and on the forehead and then spreads down the body, often becoming confluent; (2) *rubella*—it begins on the forehead and face and then spreads down the body; it resolves in the same order and is associated with retroauricular and suboccipital lymphadenopathy; and (3) *erythema infectiosum* (fifth disease)—erythema of the cheeks is followed by a reticulated pattern on extremities; it is secondary to a parvovirus B19 infection, and an associated arthritis is seen in adults.

Both measles and rubella are seen in unvaccinated young adults, and an atypical form of measles is seen in adults immunized with either killed measles vaccine or killed vaccine followed in time by live vaccine. In contrast to classic measles, the eruption of atypical measles begins on the palms, soles, wrists, and knuckles, and the lesions may become purpuric. The patient with atypical measles can have pulmonary involvement and be quite ill. Rubelliform and roseoliform eruptions are also associated with *Epstein-Barr virus* (5 to 15% of patients), *echovirus*, *coxsackievirus*, and *adenovirus* infections. Detection of specific IgM antibodies or fourfold elevations in IgG antibodies allows the proper diagnosis. Occasionally, a maculopapular eruption is the result of a drug-viral interaction. For example, about 95% of the patients with infectious mononucleosis who are given ampicillin will develop a rash.

Of note, early in the course of infections with *Rickettsia* and *meningococcus*, prior to the development of purpura, the lesions may be erythematous macules and papules. This is also the case in chickenpox prior to the development of vesicles. Maculopapular eruptions are associated with early *HIV infection*, early secondary *syphilis*, *typhoid fever*, and *acute graft-versus-host disease*. In the last, lesions frequently begin on the palms and soles; the macular rose spots of typhoid fever involve primarily the anterior trunk.

The prototypic *scarlatiniform* eruption is seen in *scarlet fever* and is due to an erythrotoxin produced by group A β-hemolytic streptococcal infections, most commonly pharyngitis. This eruption is characterized by diffuse erythema, which begins on the neck and upper trunk, and red perifollicular puncta. Additional findings include a white strawberry tongue (white coating with red papillae) followed by a red strawberry tongue (red tongue with red papillae); petechiae of the palate; a facial flush with circumoral pallor; linear petechiae in the antecubital fossae; and desquamation of the involved skin, palms, and soles 5 to 20 days after onset of the eruption. A similar desquamation of the palms and soles is seen in toxic shock syndrome, Kawasaki's disease, and after severe febrile illnesses. Certain strains of staphylococci also produce an erythrotoxin that leads to the same clinical findings as in streptococcal scarlet fever, except that the antistreptolysin O titers are not elevated.

In *toxic shock syndrome* (TSS), staphylococcal (phage group I) infections produce an exotoxin (TSST-1) that causes the fever and rash, as well as enterotoxins. Initially, the majority of cases were reported in menstruating women who were using tampons. However, other sites of infection, including wounds and vaginitis, may produce TSS. The diagnosis of TSS is based on clinical criteria (Chap. 139), and three of these involve mucocutaneous sites. The clinical criteria are (1) fever; (2) diffuse erythema of the skin; (3) desquamation of the palms and soles 1 to 2 weeks after onset of illness; (4) hypotension; and (5) involvement of three or more organ systems, including the gastrointestinal tract, muscles, kidney, liver, CNS, hematologic (thrombocytopenia), and mucous membranes. The latter is characterized as hyperemia of the vagina, oropharynx, or conjunctivae. Similar systemic findings have been described in *streptococcal toxic shock–like syndrome* (Chap. 140), and although an exanthem is seen less often than in TSS due to a staphylococcal infection, the underlying infection is often in the soft tissue.

The cutaneous eruption in *Kawasaki's disease* (mucocutaneous lymph node syndrome) (Chap. 317) is polymorphous, but the two most common forms are morbilliform and scarlatiniform. The majority of cases are seen in children less than 5 years of age, but adult cases have been reported. The diagnosis is based on a fever lasting more than 5 days plus four of the five following criteria: (1) bilateral conjunctival

Table 57-13 Causes of Exanthems

I. Morbilliform
  A. Drugs
  B. Viral
    1. Rubeola (measles)
    2. Rubella
    3. Erythema infectiosum
    4. Epstein-Barr, echovirus, coxsackievirus, and adenovirus
    5. Early HIV
  C. Bacterial
    1. Typhoid fever
    2. Early secondary syphilis
    3. Early *Rickettsia*
    4. Early meningococcus
  D. Acute graft-versus-host disease
  E. Kawasaki's disease
II. Scarlatiniform
  A. Scarlet fever
  B. Toxic shock syndrome
  C. Kawasaki's disease

Table 57-14 Causes of Urticaria

I. Primary cutaneous disorders
  A. Acute and chronic urticaria
  B. Physical urticaria
    1. Dermatographism
    2. Solar urticaria[a]
    3. Cold urticaria[a]
    4. Cholinergic urticaria[a]
  C. Angioedema (hereditary and acquired)[a]
II. Systemic diseases
  A. Urticarial vasculitis
  B. Hepatitis B or C infection
  C. Serum sickness
  D. Angioedema (hereditary and acquired)

[a] Also systemic.

---

injection; (2) exanthem; (3) cervical lymphadenopathy, usually unilateral; (4) erythema and edema of the hands and feet followed by desquamation; and (5) diffuse erythema of the oropharynx, red strawberry tongue, and erosions with crusting on the lips. This clinical picture can resemble TSS and scarlet fever, but clues to the diagnosis of Kawasaki's disease are the cervical lymphadenopathy, lip erosions, and increased platelets. The most serious associated systemic finding in this disease is coronary aneurysm secondary to arteritis. Aneurysms may lead to sudden death, primarily within the first 30 days of the illness. Scarlatiniform eruptions are also seen in the early phase of SSSS (see "Vesicles/Bullae") and as reactions to drugs.

URTICARIA (Table 57-14) *Urticaria* (hives) are transient lesions that are composed of a central wheal surrounded by an erythematous halo. Individual lesions are round, oval, or figurate and are often pruritic. *Acute* and *chronic* urticaria have a wide variety of allergic etiologies. Less common systemic causes of urticaria are mastocytosis (urticaria pigmentosa), hyperthyroidism, malignancy, and juvenile rheumatoid arthritis (JRA). In JRA, the lesions coincide with the fever spike and are transient but not migratory as in erythema marginatum.

The common *physical urticarias* include dermographism, solar urticaria, cold urticaria, and cholinergic urticaria. Patients with *dermographism* exhibit linear wheals following minor pressure or scratching of the skin. It is a common disorder, affecting approximately 5% of the population. *Solar urticaria* characteristically occur within minutes of sun exposure and are a skin sign of one systemic disease—erythropoietic protoporphyria. In addition to the urticaria, these patients have subtle pitted scarring of the nose and hands. *Cold urticaria* are precipitated by exposure to the cold, and therefore exposed areas are usually affected. In some cases, the disease is associated with abnormal circulating proteins—more commonly cryoglobulins and less commonly cryofibrinogens and cold agglutinins. Additional systemic symptoms include wheezing and syncope, thus explaining the need for these patients to avoid swimming in cold water. *Cholinergic urticaria* are precipitated by heat, exercise, or emotion and are characterized by small wheals with relatively large flares. They are occasionally associated with wheezing.

Whereas urticaria are the result of dermal edema, subcutaneous edema leads to the clinical picture of *angioedema*. Sites of involvement include the eyelids, lips, tongue, larynx, and gastrointestinal tract as well as the subcutaneous tissue. Angioedema occurs alone or in combination with urticaria, including urticarial vasculitis and the physical urticarias. Both acquired and hereditary (autosomal dominant) forms of angioedema occur (Chap. 310), and in the latter, urticaria is rarely seen.

Urticarial vasculitis is an immune complex disease that may be confused with simple urticaria. In contrast to simple urticaria, individual lesions tend to last longer than 24 h and usually develop central petechiae that can be observed even after the urticarial phase has resolved. The patient may also complain of burning rather than pruritus. On biopsy, there is a leukocytoclastic vasculitis of the small blood vessels. Although many cases of urticarial vasculitis are idiopathic in origin, it can be a reflection of an underlying systemic illness such as lupus erythematosus, Sjögren's syndrome, or hereditary complement deficiency. There is a spectrum of urticarial vasculitis that ranges from purely cutaneous to multisystem involvement. The most common systemic signs and symptoms are arthralgias and/or arthritis, nephritis, and crampy abdominal pain, with asthma and chronic obstructive lung disease seen less often. Hypocomplementemia occurs in one- to two-thirds of patients, even in the idiopathic cases. Urticarial vasculitis can also be seen in patients with *hepatitis B* and *hepatitis C* infections, *serum sickness*, and *serum sickness–like illnesses*.

PAPULONODULAR SKIN LESIONS (Table 57-15) In the *papulonodular diseases*, the lesions are elevated above the surface of the skin and may coalesce to form plaques. The location, consistency, and color of the lesions are the keys to their diagnosis; this section is organized on the basis of color.

White Lesions In *calcinosis cutis* there are firm white to white-yellow papules with an irregular surface. When the contents are dis-

Table 57-15 Papulonodular Skin Lesions According to Color Groups

I. White
  A. Calcinosis cutis
II. Skin-colored
  A. Rheumatoid nodules
  B. Neurofibromas (von Recklinghausen's disease)
  C. Angiofibromas (tuberous sclerosis, MEN syndrome, type 1)
  D. Neuromas (MEN syndrome, type 2b)
  E. Adnexal tumors
    1. Basal cell epitheliomas (basal cell nevus syndrome)
    2. Tricholemmomas (Cowden disease)
  F. Osteomas (Gardner syndrome)
  G. Primary cutaneous disorders
    1. Epidermal inclusion cysts
    2. Lipomas
III. Pink/translucent[a]
  A. Amyloidosis
  B. Papular mucinosis
IV. Yellow
  A. Xanthomas
  B. Tophi
  C. Necrobiosis lipoidica
  D. Pseudoxanthoma elasticum
  E. Sebaceous adenomas (Torre syndrome)
V. Red[a]
  A. Papules
    1. Angiokeratomas (Fabry's disease)
    2. Bacillary angiomatosis (primarily in AIDS)
  B. Papules/plaques
    1. Cutaneous lupus
    2. Lymphoma cutis
    3. Leukemia cutis
  C. Nodules
    1. Panniculitis
    2. Cutaneous polyarteritis nodosa
    3. Systemic vasculitis
  D. Primary cutaneous disorders
    1. Arthropod bites
    2. Cherry hemangiomas
    3. Infections, e.g., erysipelas, sporotrichosis
    4. Polymorphous light eruption
    5. Lymphocytoma cutis (pseudolymphoma)
VI. Red-brown[a]
  A. Sarcoidosis
  B. Sweet's syndrome
  C. Urticaria pigmentosa
  D. Erythema elevatum diutinum (chronic leukocytoclastic vasculitis)
  E. Lupus vulgaris
VII. Blue
  A. Venous malformations (blue rubber bleb syndrome)
  B. Primary cutaneous disorders
    1. Venous lake
    2. Blue nevus
VIII. Violaceous
  A. Lupus pernio (sarcoidosis)
  B. Lymphoma cutis
  C. Cutaneous lupus
IX. Purple
  A. Kaposi's sarcoma
  B. Angiosarcoma
  C. Palpable purpura
X. Brown-black[b]
XI. Any color
  A. Metastases

[a] May have darker hue in more darkly pigmented individuals.
[b] See also "Hyperpigmentation."
NOTE: MEN, multiple endocrine neoplasia.

charged, a chalky white material is seen. *Dystrophic* calcification is seen at sites of previous inflammation or damage to the skin. It develops in acne scars as well as on the distal extremities of patients with scleroderma and in the subcutaneous tissue and intermuscular fascial planes in DM. The latter is more extensive and is more commonly seen in children. An elevated calcium phosphate product, as in secondary hyperparathyroidism, can lead to nodules of *metastatic* calcinosis cutis, which tend to be subcutaneous and periarticular. This form is often accompanied by calcification of muscular arteries and subsequent ischemic necrosis (calciphylaxis).

Skin-Colored Lesions   There are several types of skin-colored lesions, including epidermoid inclusion cysts, lipomas, rheumatoid nodules, neurofibromas, angiofibromas, neuromas, and adnexal tumors such as tricholemmomas. Both *epidermoid inclusion cysts* and *lipomas* are very common mobile subcutaneous nodules—the former are rubbery and compressible and drain cheeselike material (sebum and keratin) if incised. Lipomas are firm and somewhat lobulated on palpation. When extensive facial epidermoid inclusion cysts develop in childhood or there is a family history of such lesions, the patient should be examined for other signs of Gardner syndrome, including osteomas and desmoid tumors. *Rheumatoid nodules* are firm, 0.5- to 4-cm nodules that tend to localize around pressure points, especially the elbows. They are seen in approximately 20% of patients with rheumatoid arthritis and 6% of patients with Still's disease. Biopsies of the nodules show palisading granulomas. Similar lesions that are smaller and shorter-lived are seen in rheumatic fever.

Neurofibromas (benign Schwann cell tumors) are soft papules or nodules that exhibit the "button-hole" sign, that is, they invaginate into the skin with pressure in a manner similar to a hernia. Single lesions are seen in normal individuals, but multiple neurofibromas, usually in combination with six or more CALM measuring >1.5 cm (see "Hyperpigmentation") and multiple Lisch nodules, are seen in von Recklinghausen's disease (NF type I). Lisch nodules are 1-mm yellow-brown spots within the iris that are best observed with slit-lamp examination. Additional manifestations include axillary freckling and peripheral and CNS tumors (Chap. 370). In some patients the neurofibromas are localized and unilateral, whereas in others they are limited to the CNS.

Angiofibromas are firm, pink to skin-colored papules that measure from 3 mm to several centimeters in diameter. When they are located on the central cheeks (adenoma sebaceum) or multiple fibromas are seen around the nails, the patient has tuberous sclerosis. It is an autosomal disorder due to mutations in two different genes, and the associated findings are discussed in the section on ash leaf spots as well as in Chap. 370. Multiple facial angiofibromas have also been observed in patients with multiple endocrine neoplasia (MEN) syndrome, type 1.

Neuromas (benign proliferations of nerve fibers) are also firm, skin-colored papules. They are more commonly found at sites of amputation and as rudimentary supernumerary digits. However, when there are multiple neuromas on the eyelids, lips, distal tongue, and/or oral mucosa, the patient should be investigated for other signs of the MEN syndrome, type 2b. Associated findings include marfanoid habitus, protuberant lips, intestinal ganglioneuromas, and medullary thyroid carcinoma (>75% of patients; Chap. 339).

Adnexal tumors are derived from pluripotential cells of the epidermis that can differentiate toward hair, sebaceous, apocrine, or eccrine glands or remain undifferentiated. *Basal cell epitheliomas* (BCEs) are examples of adnexal tumors that have little or no evidence of differentiation. Clinically, they are translucent papules with rolled borders, telangiectasias, and central erosion. BCEs commonly arise in sun-damaged skin of the head and neck. When a patient has multiple BCEs, especially prior to age 30, the possibility of the basal cell nevus syndrome should be raised. It is inherited as an autosomal dominant trait and is associated with jaw cysts, palmar and plantar pits, frontal bossing, medulloblastomas and calcification of the falx cerebri and

diaphragma sellae. *Tricholemmomas* are also skin-colored adnexal tumors but differentiate toward hair follicles and can have a wartlike appearance. The presence of multiple tricholemmomas on the face and cobblestoning of the oral mucosa points to the diagnosis of Cowden's disease (multiple hamartoma syndrome) due to mutations in the *PTEN* gene. Internal organ involvement (in decreasing order of frequency) includes fibrocystic disease and carcinoma of the breast, adenomas and carcinomas of the thyroid, and gastrointestinal polyposis. Keratoses of the palms, soles, and dorsa of the hands are also seen.

Pink Lesions   The cutaneous lesions associated with primary systemic *amyloidosis* are pink in color and translucent. Common locations are the face, especially the periorbital and perioral regions, and flexural areas. On biopsy, homogeneous deposits of amyloid are seen in the dermis and in the walls of blood vessels; the latter lead to an increase in vessel wall fragility. As a result, petechiae and purpura develop in clinically normal skin as well as in lesional skin following minor trauma, hence the term "pinch purpura." Amyloid deposits are also seen in the striated muscle of the tongue and result in macroglossia.

Even though specific mucocutaneous lesions are rarely seen in secondary amyloidosis and are present in only about 30% of the patients with primary amyloidosis, a rapid diagnosis of systemic amyloidosis can be made by an examination of abdominal subcutaneous fat. By special staining, deposits are seen around blood vessels or individual fat cells in 40 to 50% of patients. There are also three forms of amyloidosis that are limited to the skin and that should not be construed as cutaneous lesions of systemic amyloidosis. They are macular amyloidosis (upper back), lichenoid amyloidosis (usually lower extremities), and nodular amyloidosis. In macular and lichenoid amyloidosis, the deposits are composed of altered epidermal keratin. Recently, macular and lichenoid amyloidosis have been associated with MEN syndrome, type 2a.

Patients with *multicentric reticulohistiocytosis* also have pink-colored papules and nodules on the face and mucous membranes as well as on the extensor surface of the hands and forearms. They have a polyarthritis that can mimic rheumatoid arthritis clinically. On histologic examination, the papules have characteristic giant cells that are not seen in biopsies of rheumatoid nodules. Pink to skin-colored papules that are firm, 2 to 5 mm in diameter, and often in a linear arrangement are seen in patients with *papular mucinosis*. This disease is also referred to as *lichen myxedematosus* or *scleromyxedema*. The latter name comes from the brawny induration of the face and extremities that may accompany the papular eruption. Biopsy specimens of the papules show localized mucin deposition, and serum protein electrophoresis demonstrates a monoclonal spike of IgG, usually with a λ light chain.

Yellow Lesions   Several systemic disorders are characterized by yellow-colored cutaneous papules or plaques—hyperlipidemia (xanthomas), gout (tophi), diabetes (necrobiosis lipoidica), pseudoxanthoma elasticum, and Torre syndrome (sebaceous tumors). Eruptive xanthomas are the most common form of *xanthomas*, and are associated with hypertriglyceridemia (types I, III, IV, and V). Crops of yellow papules with erythematous halos occur primarily on the extensor surfaces of the extremities and the buttocks, and they spontaneously involute with a fall in serum triglycerides. Increased β-lipoproteins (primarily types II and III) result in one or more of the following types of xanthoma: xanthelasma, tendon xanthomas, and plane xanthomas. Xanthelasma are found on the eyelids, whereas tendon xanthomas are frequently associated with the Achilles and extensor finger tendons; plane xanthomas are flat and favor the palmar creases, face, upper trunk, and scars. Tuberous xanthomas are frequently associated with hypertriglyceridemia, but they are also seen in patients with hypercholesterolemia (type II) and are found most frequently over the large joints or hand. Biopsy specimens of xanthomas show collections of lipid-containing macrophages (foam cells).

Patients with several disorders, including biliary cirrhosis, can have a secondary form of hyperlipidemia with associated tuberous and planar xanthomas. However, patients with myeloma have *normoli-*

pemic flat xanthomas. This latter form of xanthoma may be ≥12 cm in diameter and is most frequently seen on the upper trunk or side of the neck. It is also important to note that the most common setting for eruptive xanthomas is uncontrolled diabetes mellitus. The least specific sign for hyperlipidemia is xanthelasma, because at least 50% of the patients with this finding have normal lipid profiles.

In *tophaceous gout* there are deposits of monosodium urate in the skin around the joints, particularly those of the hands and feet. Additional sites of *tophi* formation include the helix of the ear and the olecranon and prepatellar bursae. The lesions are firm, yellow in color, and occasionally discharge a chalky material. Their size varies from 1 mm to 7 cm, and the diagnosis can be established by polarization of the aspirated contents of a lesion. Lesions of *necrobiosis lipoidica* are found primarily on the shins (90%), and patients can have diabetes mellitus or develop it subsequently. Characteristic findings include a central yellow color, atrophy (transparency), telangiectasias, and an erythematous border. Ulcerations can also develop within the plaques. Biopsy specimens show necrobiosis of collagen, granulomatous inflammation, and obliterative endarteritis.

In *pseudoxanthoma elasticum* (PXE) there is an abnormal deposition of calcium on the elastic fibers of the skin, eye, and blood vessels. In the skin, the flexural areas such as the neck, axillae, antecubital fossae, and inguinal area are the primary sites of involvement. Yellow papules coalesce to form reticulated plaques that have an appearance similar to that of plucked chicken skin. In severely affected skin, hanging, redundant folds develop. Some patients have a more subtle macular form of the disease, and careful inspection is required. Biopsy specimens of involved skin show swollen and irregularly clumped elastic fibers with deposits of calcium. In the eye, the calcium deposits in Bruch's membrane lead to angioid streaks and choroiditis; in the arteries of the heart, kidney, gastrointestinal tract, and extremities, the deposits lead to angina, hypertension, gastrointestinal bleeding, and claudication, respectively. Long-term administration of D-penicillamine can lead to PXE-like skin changes as well as elastic fiber alterations in internal organs.

Adnexal tumors that have differentiated toward sebaceous glands include sebaceous adenoma, sebaceous epithelioma, sebaceous carcinoma, and sebaceous hyperplasia. Except for sebaceous hyperplasia, which is commonly seen on the face, these tumors are fairly rare. Patients with Torre syndrome have *sebaceous adenomas*, and in the majority of cases there are multiple such tumors. These patients can also have sebaceous carcinomas and sebaceous hyperplasia as well as keratoacanthomas. The internal manifestations of Torre syndrome include *multiple* carcinomas of the gastrointestinal tract (primarily colon) as well as cancers of the larynx, genitourinary tract, and endometrium. Some patients also have a strong family history of cancer.

Red Lesions Cutaneous lesions that are red in color have a wide variety of etiologies; in an attempt to simplify their identification, they will be subdivided into papules, papules/plaques, and subcutaneous nodules. Common red papules include *arthropod bites* and *cherry hemangiomas*; the latter are small, bright-red, dome-shaped papules that represent benign proliferation of capillaries. In patients with AIDS, the development of multiple red hemangioma-like lesions points to bacillary angiomatosis, and biopsy specimens show clusters of bacilli that stain positive with the Warthin-Starry stain; the pathogens have been identified as *Bartonella henselae* and *B. quintana*. Disseminated visceral disease is seen primarily in immunocompromised hosts but can occur in immunocompetent individuals.

Multiple *angiokeratomas* are seen in Fabry's disease, an X-linked recessive lysosomal storage disease that is due to a deficiency of α-galactosidase A. The lesions are red to red-blue in color and can be quite small in size (1 to 3 mm), with the most common location being the lower trunk. Associated findings include chronic renal failure, peripheral neuropathy, and corneal opacities (cornea verticillata). Electron photomicrographs of angiokeratomas and clinically normal skin demonstrate lamellar lipid deposits in fibroblasts, pericytes, and endothelial cells that are diagnostic of this disease. Widespread acute eruptions of erythematous papules are discussed in the section on exanthems.

There are several infectious diseases that present as erythematous papules or nodules in a sporotrichoid pattern, that is, in a linear arrangement along the lymphatic channels. The two most common etiologies are *Sporothrix schenckii* (sporotrichosis) and *M. marinum* (atypical mycobacteria). The organisms are introduced as a result of trauma, and a primary inoculation site is often seen in addition to the lymphatic nodules. Additional causes include *Nocardia*, *Leishmania*, and other dimorphic fungi; culture of lesional tissue will aid in the diagnosis.

The diseases that are characterized by erythematous plaques with scale are reviewed in the papulosquamous section, and the various forms of dermatitis are discussed in the section on erythroderma. Additional disorders in the differential diagnosis of red papules/plaques include *erysipelas*, *polymorphous light eruption* (PMLE), *lymphocytoma cutis*, *cutaneous lupus*, *lymphoma cutis*, and *leukemia cutis*. The first three diseases represent primary cutaneous disorders. PMLE is characterized by erythematous papules and plaques in a primarily sun-exposed distribution—dorsum of the hand, extensor forearm, and face. Lesions follow exposure to UV-B and/or UV-A, and in northern latitudes PMLE is most severe in the late spring and early summer. A process referred to as "hardening" occurs with continued UV exposure, and the eruption fades, but in temperate climates it will recur in the spring. PMLE must be differentiated from cutaneous lupus, and this is accomplished by histologic examination and direct immunofluorescence of the lesions. Lymphocytoma cutis (pseudolymphoma) is a *benign* polyclonal proliferation of lymphocytes in the skin that presents as infiltrated pink-red to red-purple papules and plaques; it must be distinguished from lymphoma cutis.

Several types of red plaques are seen in patients with systemic *lupus*, including (1) erythematous urticarial plaques across the cheeks and nose in the classic butterfly rash; (2) erythematous discoid lesions with fine or "carpet-tack" scale, telangiectasias, central hypopigmentation, peripheral hyperpigmentation, follicular plugging, and atrophy located on the face, scalp, external ears, arms, and upper trunk; and (3) psoriasiform or annular lesions of subacute lupus with hypopigmented centers located on the face, extensor arms, and upper trunk. Additional cutaneous findings include (1) a violaceous flush on the face and V of the neck; (2) urticarial vasculitis (see "Urticaria"); (3) lupus panniculitis (see below); (4) diffuse alopecia; (5) alopecia secondary to discoid lesions; (6) periungual telangiectasias and erythema; (7) erythema multiforme–like lesions that may become bullous; and (8) distal ulcerations secondary to Raynaud's phenomenon, vasculitis, or livedoid vasculitis. Patients with only discoid lesions usually have the form of lupus that is limited to the skin. However, 2 to 10% of these patients eventually develop systemic lupus. Direct immunofluorescence of involved skin shows deposits of IgG or IgM and C3 in a granular distribution along the dermal-epidermal junction.

In *lymphoma cutis* there is a proliferation of malignant lymphocytes or histiocytes in the skin, and the clinical appearance resembles that of lymphocytoma cutis—infiltrated pink-red to red-purple papules and plaques. Lymphoma cutis can occur anywhere on the surface of the skin, whereas the sites of predilection for lymphocytomas include the malar ridge, tip of the nose, and earlobes. Patients with non-Hodgkin's lymphomas have specific cutaneous lesions more often than those with Hodgkin's disease, and occasionally, the skin nodules precede the development of extracutaneous non-Hodgkin's lymphoma or represent the only site of involvement. Arcuate lesions are sometimes seen in lymphoma and lymphocytoma cutis as well as in CTCL. *Leukemia cutis* has the same appearance as lymphoma cutis, and specific lesions are seen more commonly in monocytic leukemias than in lymphocytic or granulocytic leukemias. Cutaneous chloromas (granulocytic sarcomas) may precede the appearance of circulating blasts in acute nonlymphocytic leukemia and, as such, represent a form of aleukemic leukemia cutis.

Common causes of erythematous subcutaneous nodules include inflamed epidermoid inclusion cysts, acne cysts, and furuncles. *Panniculitis*, an inflammation of the fat, also presents as subcutaneous nodules and is frequently a sign of systemic disease. There are several forms of panniculitis, including erythema nodosum, erythema induratum, lupus profundus, lipomembranous lipodermatosclerosis, α_1-antitrypsin deficiency, facticial, and fat necrosis secondary to pancreatic disease. Except for erythema nodosum, these lesions may break down and ulcerate or heal with a scar. The shin is the most common location for the nodules of erythema nodosum, whereas the calf is the most common location for lesions of erythema induratum. In erythema nodosum the nodules are initially red but then develop a blue color as they resolve. Patients with erythema nodosum but no underlying systemic illness can still have fever, malaise, leukocytosis, arthralgias, and/or arthritis. However, the possibility of an underlying illness should be excluded, and the most common associations are streptococcal infections, upper respiratory infections, sarcoidosis, and inflammatory bowel disease. The less common associations include tuberculosis, histoplasmosis, coccidioidomycosis, psittacosis, drugs (oral contraceptives, sulfonamides, aspartame, bromides, iodides), cat-scratch fever, and infections with *Yersinia*, *Salmonella*, and *Chlamydia*.

In some patients, erythema induratum/nodular vasculitis is an idiopathic disease; however, in approximately 25 to 70% of patients, polymerase chain reaction (PCR) analysis will demonstrate *M. tuberculosis* complex DNA. The lesions of lupus profundus are found primarily on the upper arms and buttocks (sites of abundant fat) and are seen in both the cutaneous and systemic forms of lupus. The overlying skin may be normal, erythematous, or have the changes of discoid lupus. The subcutaneous fat necrosis that is associated with pancreatic disease is presumably secondary to circulating lipases and is seen in patients with pancreatic carcinoma as well as in patients with acute and chronic pancreatitis. In this disorder there may be an associated arthritis, fever, and inflammation of visceral fat. Histologic examination of deep incisional biopsy specimens will aid in the diagnosis of the particular type of panniculitis.

Subcutaneous erythematous nodules are also seen in *cutaneous polyarteritis nodosa* (PAN) and as a manifestation of *systemic vasculitis*, e.g., systemic PAN, allergic granulomatosis, or Wegener's granulomatosis (Chap. 317). Cutaneous PAN presents with painful subcutaneous nodules and ulcers within a red-purple, netlike pattern of livedo reticularis. The latter is due to slowed blood flow through the superficial horizontal venous plexus. The majority of lesions are found on the lower extremity, and while arthralgias and myalgias may accompany cutaneous PAN, there is no evidence of systemic involvement. In both the cutaneous and systemic forms of vasculitis, skin biopsy specimens of the associated nodules will show the changes characteristic of a vasculitis; the size of the vessel involved will depend on the particular disease.

Red-Brown Lesions   The cutaneous lesions in *sarcoidosis* (Chap. 318) are classically red to red-brown in color, and with diascopy (pressure with a glass slide) a yellow-brown residual color is observed that is secondary to the granulomatous infiltrate. The waxy papules and plaques may be found anywhere on the skin, but the face is the most common location. Usually there are no surface changes, but occasionally the lesions will have scale. Biopsy specimens of the papules show "naked" granulomas in the dermis, i.e., granulomas surrounded by a minimal number of lymphocytes. Other cutaneous findings in sarcoidosis include annular lesions with an atrophic or scaly center, papules within scars, hypopigmented macules and papules, alopecia, acquired ichthyosis, erythema nodosum, and lupus pernio (see below). Additional physical findings are peripheral lymphadenopathy and parotid and lacrimal gland enlargement. When there is cutaneous involvement of the hands, radiographs will often show lytic lesions in the underlying bone.

The differential diagnosis of sarcoidosis includes foreign-body

granulomas produced by chemicals such as beryllium and zirconium, late secondary syphilis, and *lupus vulgaris*. Lupus vulgaris is a form of cutaneous tuberculosis that is seen in previously infected and sensitized individuals. There is often underlying active tuberculosis elsewhere, usually in the lungs or lymph nodes. At least 90% of the lesions occur in the head and neck area and are red-brown plaques with a yellow-brown color on diascopy. Secondary scarring and squamous cell carcinomas can develop within the plaques. Cultures or PCR analysis of the lesions should be done because it is rare for the acid-fast stain to show bacilli within the dermal granulomas.

Sweet's syndrome is characterized by red to red-brown plaques and nodules that are frequently painful and occur primarily on the head, neck, and upper extremities. The patients also have fever, neutrophilia, and a dense dermal infiltrate of neutrophils in the lesions. In approximately 10% of the patients there is an associated malignancy, most commonly acute nonlymphocytic leukemia. Sweet's syndrome has also been reported with lymphoma, chronic leukemia, myeloma, myelodysplastic syndromes, and solid tumors (primarily of the genitourinary tract). The differential diagnosis includes neutrophilic eccrine hidradenitis and atypical forms of pyoderma gangrenosum. Extracutaneous sites of involvement include joints, muscles, eye, kidney (proteinuria, occasionally glomerulonephritis), and lung (neutrophilic infiltrates). The idiopathic form of Sweet's syndrome is seen more often in women, following a respiratory tract infection.

A generalized distribution of red-brown macules and papules is seen in the form of mastocytosis known as *urticaria pigmentosa* (Chap. 310). Each lesion represents a collection of mast cells in the dermis, with hyperpigmentation of the overlying epidermis. Stimuli such as rubbing cause these mast cells to degranulate, and this leads to the formation of localized urticaria (Darier's sign). Additional symptoms can result from mast cell degranulation and include headache, flushing, diarrhea, and pruritus. Mast cells also infiltrate various organs such as the liver, spleen, and gastrointestinal tract in up to 30 to 50% of patients with urticaria pigmentosa, and accumulations of mast cells in the bones may produce either osteosclerotic or osteolytic shadows on radiographs. In the majority of these patients, however, the internal involvement remains fairly static. A subtype of chronic leukocytoclastic vasculitis, *erythema elevatum diutinum* (EED), also presents with papules that are red-brown in color. The papules coalesce into plaques on the extensor surfaces of knees, elbows, and the small joints of the hand. Flares of EED have been associated with streptococcal infections.

Blue Lesions   Lesions that are blue in color are the result of either vascular ectasias and tumors or melanin pigment in the dermis. *Venous lakes* (ectasias) are compressible dark-blue lesions that are found commonly in the head and neck region. *Venous malformations* are also compressible blue papules and nodules that can occur anywhere on the body, including the oral mucosa. When they are multiple rather than single congenital lesions, the patient may have the blue rubber bleb syndrome or Mafucci's syndrome. Patients with the blue rubber bleb syndrome also have vascular anomalies of the gastrointestinal tract that may bleed, whereas patients with Mafucci's syndrome have associated dyschondroplasia and osteochondromas. *Blue nevi* (moles) are seen when there are collections of pigment-producing nevus cells in the dermis. These benign papular lesions are dome-shaped and occur most commonly on the dorsum of the hand or foot.

Violaceous Lesions   Violaceous papules and plaques are seen in *lupus pernio*, *lymphoma cutis*, and *cutaneous lupus*. Lupus pernio is a particular type of sarcoidosis that involves the tip of the nose and the earlobes, with lesions that are violaceous in color rather than red-brown. This form of sarcoidosis is associated with involvement of the upper respiratory tract. The plaques of lymphoma cutis and cutaneous lupus may be red or violaceous in color and were discussed above.

Purple Lesions   Purple-colored papules and plaques are seen in vascular tumors, such as *Kaposi's sarcoma* (Chap. 309) and *angiosarcoma*, and when there is extravasation of red blood cells into the skin in association with inflammation, as in *palpable purpura* (see "Purpura"). Patients with congenital or acquired AV fistulas and venous hypertension can develop purple papules on the lower extremities that can resemble Kaposi's sarcoma clinically and histologically; this condition is referred to as pseudo-Kaposi sarcoma (acral angiodermatitis). Angiosarcoma is found most commonly on the scalp and face of elderly patients or within areas of chronic lymphedema and presents as purple papules and plaques. In the head and neck region the tumor often extends beyond the clinically defined borders and may be accompanied by facial edema.

Brown and Black Lesions Brown- and black-colored papules are reviewed in "Hyperpigmentation."

Cutaneous Metastases These are discussed last because they can have a wide range of colors. Most commonly they present as either firm, skin-colored subcutaneous nodules or firm, red to red-brown papulonodules. The lesions of lymphoma cutis range from pink-red to plum in color, whereas metastatic melanoma can be pink, blue, or black in color. Cutaneous metastases develop from hematogenous or lymphatic spread and are most often due to the following primary carcinomas: in men, lung, colon, melanoma, and oral cavity; and in women, breast, colon, and lung. These metastatic lesions may be the initial presentation of the carcinoma, especially when the primary site is the lung, kidney, or ovary.

PURPURA (Table 57-16) *Purpura* are seen when there is an extravasation of red blood cells into the dermis, and as a result, the lesions do not blanch with pressure. This is in contrast to those erythematous or violet-colored lesions that are due to localized vasodilatation—they do blanch with pressure. Purpura (≥ 3 mm) and petechiae (≤ 2 mm) are divided into two major groups, palpable and nonpalpable. The most frequent causes of *nonpalpable* petechiae and purpura are primary cutaneous disorders such as *trauma*, *solar purpura*, and *capillaritis*. Less common causes are *steroid purpura* and *livedoid vasculitis* (see "Ulcers"). Solar purpura are seen primarily on the extensor forearms, while glucocorticoid purpura secondary to potent topical steroids or endogenous or exogenous Cushing's syndrome can be more widespread. In both cases there is alteration of the supporting connective tissue that surrounds the dermal blood vessels. In contrast, the petechiae that result from capillaritis are found primarily on the lower extremities. In capillaritis there is an extravasation of erythrocytes as a result of perivascular lymphocytic inflammation. The petechiae are bright red, 1 to 2 mm in size, and scattered within annular or coin-shaped yellow-brown macules. The yellow-brown color is caused by hemosiderin deposits within the dermis.

Table 57-16 Causes of Purpura

I. Primary cutaneous disorders	c. Thrombotic thrombocytopenic purpura
A. Nonpalpable	d. Warfarin reaction
1. Trauma	4. Emboli
2. Solar purpura	a. Cholesterol
3. Steroid purpura	b. Fat
4. Capillaritis	5. Possible immune complex
5. Livedoid vasculitis[a]	a. Gardner-Diamond syndrome (autoerythrocyte sensitivity)
II. Systemic diseases	
A. Nonpalpable	b. Waldenström's hypergammaglobulinemic purpura
1. Clotting disturbances	B. Palpable
a. Thrombocytopenia (including ITP)	1. Vasculitis
b. Abnormal platelet function	a. Leukocytoclastic vasculitis
c. Clotting factor defects	b. Polyarteritis nodosa
2. Vascular fragility	2. Emboli[b]
a. Amyloidosis	a. Acute meningococcemia
b. Ehlers-Danlos syndrome	b. Disseminated gonococcal infection
c. Scurvy	c. Rocky Mountain spotted fever
3. Thrombi	d. Ecthyma gangrenosum
a. Disseminated intravascular coagulation	
b. Monoclonal cryoglobulinemia	

[a] Also associated with systemic diseases.
[b] Bacterial, fungal, or parasitic.
NOTE: ITP, idiopathic thrombocytopenic purpura.

Systemic causes of nonpalpable purpura fall into several categories, and those secondary to clotting disturbances and vascular fragility will be discussed first. The former group includes *thrombocytopenia* (Chap. 116), *abnormal platelet function* as is seen in uremia, and *clotting factor defects*. The initial site of presentation for thrombocytopenia-induced petechiae is the distal lower extremity. Capillary fragility leads to nonpalpable purpura in patients with systemic *amyloidosis* (see "Papulonodular Skin Lesions"), disorders of collagen production such as *Ehlers-Danlos syndrome*, and *scurvy*. In scurvy there are flattened corkscrew hairs with surrounding hemorrhage on the lower extremities, in addition to gingivitis. Vitamin C is a cofactor for lysyl hydroxylase, an enzyme involved in the posttranslational modification of procollagen that is necessary for cross-link formation.

In contrast to the previous group of disorders, the purpura seen in the following group of diseases are associated with thrombi formation within vessels. It is important to note that these thrombi are demonstrable in skin biopsy specimens. This group of disorders includes disseminated intravascular coagulation (DIC), monoclonal cryoglobulinemia, thrombotic thrombocytopenic purpura, and reactions to warfarin. DIC is triggered by several types of infection (gram-negative, gram-positive, viral, and rickettsial) as well as by tissue injury and neoplasms. Widespread purpura and hemorrhagic infarcts of the distal extremities are seen. Similar lesions are found in purpura fulminans, which is a form of DIC associated with fever and hypotension that occurs more commonly in children following an infectious illness such as varicella, scarlet fever, or an upper respiratory tract infection. In both disorders, hemorrhagic bullae can develop in involved skin.

Monoclonal cryoglobulinemia is associated with multiple myeloma, Waldenström's macroglobulinemia, lymphocytic leukemia, and lymphoma. Purpura, primarily of the lower extremities, and hemorrhagic infarcts of the fingers and toes are seen in these patients. Exacerbations of disease activity can follow cold exposure or an increase in serum viscosity. Biopsy specimens show precipitates of the cryoglobulin within dermal vessels. Similar deposits have been found in the lung, brain, and renal glomeruli. Patients with *thrombotic thrombocytopenic purpura* can also have hemorrhagic infarcts as a result of intravascular thromboses. Additional signs include thrombocytopenic purpura, fever, and microangiopathic hemolytic anemia (Chap. 108).

Administration of *warfarin* can result in painful areas of erythema that become purpuric and then necrotic with an adherent black eschar. This reaction is seen more often in women and in areas with abundant subcutaneous fat—breasts, abdomen, buttocks, thighs, and calves. The erythema and purpura develop between the third and tenth day of therapy, most likely as a result of a transient imbalance in the levels of anticoagulant and procoagulant vitamin K–dependent factors. Continued therapy does not exacerbate preexisting lesions, and patients with an inherited or acquired deficiency of protein C are at increased risk for this particular reaction as well as for purpura fulminans.

Purpura secondary to *cholesterol emboli* are usually seen on the lower extremities of patients with atherosclerotic vascular disease. They often follow anticoagulant therapy or an invasive vascular procedure such as an arteriogram but also occur spontaneously from disintegration of atheromatous plaques. Associated findings include livedo reticularis, gangrene, cyanosis, subcutaneous nodules, and ischemic ulcerations. Multiple step sections of the biopsy specimen may be necessary to demonstrate the cholesterol clefts with the vessels. Petechiae are also an important sign of *fat embolism* and occur primarily on the upper body 2 to 3 days after a major injury. By using special fixatives, the emboli can be demonstrated in biopsy specimens of the petechiae. Emboli of tumor or thrombus are seen in patients with atrial myxomas and marantic endocarditis.

In the *Gardner-Diamond syndrome* (autoerythrocyte sensitivity), female patients develop large ecchymoses within areas of painful, warm erythema. An episode of significant trauma frequently precedes the onset of this syndrome. Intradermal injections of autologous erythrocytes or phosphatidyl serine derived from the red cell membrane can reproduce the lesions in some patients; however, there are instances where a reaction is seen at an injection site of the forearm but not in the midback region. The latter has led some observers to view Gardner-Diamond syndrome as a cutaneous manifestation of severe emotional stress. *Waldenström's hypergammaglobulinemic purpura* is a chronic disorder characterized by petechiae on the lower extremities. There are circulating complexes of IgG–anti-IgG molecules, and exacerbations are associated with prolonged standing or walking.

Palpable purpura are further subdivided into vasculitic and embolic. In the group of vasculitic disorders, *leukocytoclastic vasculitis* (LCV), also known as *allergic vasculitis*, is the one most commonly associated with palpable purpura (Chap. 317). *Henoch-Schönlein purpura* is a subtype of acute LCV that is seen primarily in children and adolescents following an upper respiratory infection. The majority of lesions are found on the lower extremities and buttocks. Systemic manifestations include fever, arthralgias (primarily of the knees and ankles), abdominal pain, gastrointestinal bleeding, and nephritis. Direct immunofluorescence examination shows deposits of IgA within dermal blood vessel walls. In *polyarteritis nodosa*, specific cutaneous lesions result from a vasculitis of arterial vessels rather than postcapillary venules as in LCV. The arteritis leads to ischemia of the skin, and this explains the irregular outline of the purpura (see below).

Several types of infectious emboli can give rise to palpable purpura. These embolic lesions are usually *irregular* in outline as opposed to the lesions of leukocytoclastic vasculitis, which are *circular* in outline. The irregular outline is indicative of a cutaneous infarct, and the size corresponds to the area of skin that received its blood supply from that particular arteriole or artery. The palpable purpura in LCV are circular because the erythrocytes simply diffuse out evenly from the postcapillary venules as a result of inflammation. Infectious emboli are most commonly due to gram-negative cocci (meningococcus, gonococcus), gram-negative rods (Enterobacteriaceae), and gram-positive cocci (staphylococcus). Additional causes include *Rickettsia* and, in immunocompromised patients, *Candida* and opportunistic fungi.

The embolic lesions in *acute meningococcemia* are found primarily on the trunk, lower extremities, and sites of pressure, and a gun-metal-gray color often develops within them. Their size varies from 1 mm to several centimeters, and the organisms can be cultured from the lesions. Associated findings include a preceding upper respiratory tract infection, fever, meningitis, DIC, and, in some patients, a deficiency of the terminal components of complement. In *disseminated gonococcal infection* (arthritis-dermatitis syndrome), a small number of papules and vesicopustules with central purpura or hemorrhagic necrosis are found over the joints of the distal extremities. Additional symptoms include arthralgias, tenosynovitis, and fever. To establish the diagnosis, a Gram stain of these lesions should be performed. *Rocky mountain spotted fever* is a tick-borne disease that is caused by *R. rickettsii*. A several-day history of fever, chills, severe headache, and photophobia precedes the onset of the cutaneous eruption. The initial lesions are erythematous macules and papules on the wrists, ankles, palms, and soles. With time, the lesions spread centripetally and become purpuric.

Lesions of *ecthyma gangrenosum* begin as edematous, erythematous papules or plaques and then develop central purpura and necrosis. Bullae formation also occurs in these lesions, and they are frequently found in the girdle region. The organism that is classically associated with ecthyma gangrenosum is *Pseudomonas aeruginosa*, but other gram-negative rods such as *Klebsiella*, *Escherichia coli*, and *Serratia* can produce similar lesions. In immunocompromised hosts, the list of potential pathogens is expanded to include *Candida* and opportunistic fungi.

ULCERS The approach to the patient with a cutaneous ulcer, is outlined in Table 57-17. →*Peripheral vascular diseases of the extremities are reviewed in Chap. 248, as is Raynaud's phenomenon.*

Livedoid vasculitis (atrophie blanche) represents a combination of a vasculopathy with intravascular thrombosis. Purpuric lesions and

Table 57-17 Causes of Cutaneous Ulcers

I. Primary cutaneous disorders
  A. Peripheral vascular disease (Chap. 248)
    1. Venous
    2. Arterial
  B. Livedoid vasculitis[a]
  C. Squamous cell carcinoma, e.g., within scars
  D. Infections, e.g., ecthyma caused by *Streptococcus* (Chap. 140)
II. Systemic diseases
  A. Lower legs
    1. Leukocytoclastic vasculitis[b]
    2. Hemoglobinopathies (Chap. 106)
    3. Cryoglobulinemia,[b] cryofibrinogenemia
    4. Cholesterol emboli[b]
    5. Necrobiosis lipoidica[c]
    6. Antiphospholipid syndrome (Chap. 117)
    7. Neuropathic[d] (Chap. 333)
  B. Hands and feet
    1. Raynaud's phenomenon (Chap. 248)
  C. Generalized
    1. Pyoderma gangrenosum
    2. Calciphylaxis (Chap. 341)
    3. Infections, e.g., dimorphic fungi, chronic herpes varicella–zoster
    4. Lymphoma
  D. Mucosal
    1. Behçet's syndrome (Chap. 316)
    2. Erythema multiforme
    3. Primary blistering disorders (Chap. 58)
    4. Lupus erythematosus
    5. Inflammatory bowel disease

[a] Also associated with systemic diseases.
[b] Reviewed in section on "Purpura."
[c] Reviewed in section on "Papulonodular Skin Lesions."
[d] Favors plantar surface of the foot.

livedo reticularis are found in association with painful ulcerations of the lower extremities. These ulcers are often slow to heal, but when they do, irregularly shaped white scars are formed. The majority of cases are secondary to venous hypertension, but possible underlying illnesses include cryofibrinogenemia and disorders of hypercoagulability, e.g., the antiphospholipid syndrome (Chap. 117).

In *pyoderma gangrenosum*, the border of the ulcers has a characteristic appearance of an undermined necrotic bluish edge and a peripheral erythematous halo. The ulcers often begin as pustules that then expand rather rapidly to a size as large as 20 cm. Although these lesions are most commonly found on the lower extremities, they can arise anywhere on the surface of the body, including sites of trauma (pathergy). An estimated 30 to 50% of cases are idiopathic, and the most common associated disorders are ulcerative colitis and Crohn's disease. Less commonly, it is associated with chronic active hepatitis, seropositive rheumatoid arthritis, acute and chronic granulocytic leukemia, polycythemia vera, and myeloma. Additional findings in these patients, even those with idiopathic disease, are cutaneous anergy and a benign monoclonal gammopathy. Because the histology of pyoderma gangrenosum is nonspecific, the diagnosis is made clinically by excluding less common causes of similar-appearing ulcers such as necrotizing vasculitis, Meleney's ulcer (synergistic infection at a site of trauma or surgery), dimorphic fungi, cutaneous amebiasis, spider bites, and facticial. In the myeloproliferative disorders, the ulcers may be more superficial with a pustulobullous border, and these lesions provide a connection between classic pyoderma gangrenosum and acute febrile neutrophilic dermatosis (Sweet's syndrome).

FEVER AND RASH The major considerations in a patient with a fever and a rash are inflammatory diseases versus infectious diseases. In the hospital setting, the most common scenario is a patient who has a drug rash plus a fever secondary to an underlying infection. However, it should be emphasized that a drug reaction can lead to both a cutaneous eruption and a fever ("drug fever"). Additional inflammatory diseases that are often associated with a fever include pustular psoriasis, erythroderma, and Sweet's syndrome. Lyme disease, secondary syphilis, and viral and bacterial exanthems (see "Exanthems") are examples of infectious diseases that produce a rash and a fever. Lastly, it is important to determine whether or not the cutaneous lesions represent septic emboli (see "Purpura"). Such lesions usually have evidence of ischemia in the form of purpura, necrosis, or impending necrosis (gunmetal-gray color). In the patient with thrombocytopenia, however, purpura can be seen in inflammatory reactions such as morbilliform drug eruptions and infectious lesions.

BIBLIOGRAPHY

ARNDT KA et al: *Cutaneous Medicine and Surgery*. Philadelphia, Saunders, 1996

BRAVERMAN IM: *Skin Signs of Systemic Disease*, 3d ed. Philadelphia, Saunders, 1998

CALLEN JP: *Dermatology Clinics*, vol 8, no 2: *Skin Signs of Internal Disease II*. Philadelphia, Saunders, 1990

————, JORIZZO JL: *Dermatology Clinics*, vol 7, no 3: *Skin Signs of Internal Disease*. Philadelphia, Saunders, 1989

CHAMPION RH et al (eds): *Textbook of Dermatology*, 6th ed. Oxford, Blackwell Scientific, 1998

ELDER D et al: *Lever's Histopathology of the Skin*, 8th ed. Philadelphia, Lippincott, 1997

LITT JZ, PAWLAK WA JR: *Drug Eruption Reference Manual 1999*. New York, Parthenon, 1999

SYBERT VP: *Genetic Skin Disorders*. New York, Oxford University Press, 1997

ZURCHER K, KREBS A: *Cutaneous Drug Reactions*, 2d ed. Basel, Karger, 1992

58 *Kim B. Yancey, Thomas J. Lawley*

IMMUNOLOGICALLY MEDIATED SKIN DISEASES

BP	bullous pemphigoid	PF	pemphigus foliaceus
BPAG	bullous pemphigoid antigen	PG	pemphigoid gestationis
CP	cicatricial pemphigoid	PNP	paraneoplastic pemphigus
DH	dermatitis herpetiformis	PV	pemphigus vulgaris
DLE	discoid lupus erythematosus	SCLE	subacute cutaneous lupus
EBA	epidermolysis bullosa		erythematosus
	acquisita	SLE	systemic lupus erythematosus
LE	lupus erythematosus		

A number of immunologically mediated skin diseases and cutaneous manifestations of immunologically mediated systemic disorders are now recognized as distinct entities with relatively consistent clinical, histologic, and immunopathologic findings. Many of these disorders are due to autoimmune mechanisms. Clinically, they are characterized by morbidity (pain, pruritus, disfigurement) and in some instances by mortality (largely due to loss of epidermal barrier function and/or secondary infection). The major features of the more common immunologically mediated skin diseases are summarized in this chapter (Table 58-1).

PEMPHIGUS VULGARIS Pemphigus vulgaris (PV) is a blistering skin disease seen predominantly in elderly patients. Patients with PV have an increased incidence of the HLA-DR4 and -DRw6 serologically defined haplotypes. This disorder is characterized by the loss of cohesion between epidermal cells (a process termed *acantholysis*) with the resultant formation of intraepidermal blisters. Clinical lesions of PV typically consist of flaccid blisters on either normal-appearing or erythematous skin. These blisters rupture easily, leaving denuded areas that may crust and enlarge peripherally **(Plate IIE-69).** Substantial portions of the body surface may be denuded in severe cases. Manual pressure to the skin of these patients may elicit the separation of the epidermis (Nikolsky's sign). This finding, while characteristic of PV, is not specific to this disorder and is also seen in toxic epidermal necrolysis, Stevens-Johnson syndrome, and a few other skin diseases. Lesions in PV typically present on the oral mucosa, scalp, face, neck, axilla, and trunk. In half or more of patients, lesions begin in the mouth; approximately 90% of patients have oromucosal involvement at some time during the course of their disease. Involvement of other mucosal surfaces (e.g., pharyngeal, laryngeal, esophageal, con-

junctival, vulval, or rectal) can occur in severe disease. Pruritus may be a feature of early pemphigus lesions; extensive denudation may be associated with severe pain. Lesions usually heal without scarring, except at sites complicated by secondary infection or mechanically induced dermal wounds. Nonetheless, postinflammatory hyperpigmentation is usually present at sites of healed lesions for some time.

Biopsies of early lesions demonstrate intraepidermal vesicle formation secondary to loss of cohesion between epidermal cells (i.e., acantholytic blisters). Blister cavities contain acantholytic epidermal cells, which appear as round homogeneous cells containing hyperchromatic nuclei. Basal keratinocytes remain attached to the epidermal basement membrane, hence blister formation is within the suprabasal portion of the epidermis. Lesional skin may contain focal collections of intraepidermal eosinophils within blister cavities; dermal alterations are slight, often limited to an eosinophil-predominant leukocytic infiltrate. Direct immunofluorescence microscopy of lesional or intact patient skin shows deposits of IgG on the surface of keratinocytes; in contrast, deposits of complement components are typically found in lesional but not uninvolved skin. Deposits of IgG on keratinocytes are derived from circulating autoantibodies directed against cell-surface antigens. Circulating autoantibodies can be demonstrated in 80 to 90% of PV patients by indirect immunofluorescence microscopy; monkey esophagus is the optimal substrate for demonstration of these autoantibodies. Patients with PV have IgG autoantibodies directed against desmogleins (Dsgs), transmembrane desmosomal glycoproteins that belong to the cadherin supergene family of calcium-dependent adhesion molecules. While Dsg3 is specifically recognized by PV autoantibodies, approximately 50% of PV sera also contain IgG against Dsg1. Most patients with early PV and only mucosal involvement have only anti-Dsg3 autoantibodies, whereas most patients with advanced disease (i.e., involvement of skin and mucosa) have both anti-Dsg3 and anti-Dsg1 autoantibodies. Recent studies have shown that the anti-Dsg autoantibody profile in these patients' sera as well as the tissue distribution of Dsg3 and Dsg1 determine the site of blister formation in patients with pemphigus. Experimental studies have also shown that these autoantibodies are pathogenic (i.e., responsible for blister formation) and that their titer correlates with disease activity.

PV can be life-threatening. Prior to the availability of glucocorticoids, the mortality ranged from 60 to 90%; the current mortality is approximately 5%. Common causes of morbidity and mortality are infection and complications of treatment with glucocorticoids. Bad prognostic factors include advanced age, widespread involvement, and the requirement for high doses of glucocorticoids (with or without other immunosuppressive agents) for control of disease. The course of PV in individual patients is variable and difficult to predict. Some patients achieve remission (40% of patients in some series), but others may require long-term treatment or succumb to complications of their disease or its treatment. The mainstay of treatment is systemic glucocorticoids. Patients with moderate to severe disease are usually started on prednisone, 60 to 80 mg/d. If new lesions continue to appear after 1 to 2 weeks of treatment, the dose should be increased. Many regimens combine an immunosuppressive agent with systemic glucocorticoids for control of PV. The two most frequently used are either azathioprine (1 mg/kg per day) or cyclophosphamide (1 mg/kg per day). It is important to bring severe or progressive disease under control quickly to lessen the severity and/or duration of this disorder.

PEMPHIGUS FOLIACEUS Pemphigus foliaceus (PF) is distinguished from PV by several features. In PF, acantholytic blisters are located high within the epidermis, usually just beneath the stratum corneum. Hence PF is a more superficial blistering disease than PV. The distribution of lesions in the two disorders is much the same, except that in PF mucous membrane lesions are very rare. Patients with PF rarely demonstrate intact blisters but rather exhibit shallow erosions associated with erythema, scale, and crust formation. Mild cases of PF resemble severe seborrheic dermatitis; severe PF may cause extensive exfoliation. Sun exposure (ultraviolet irradiation) may

Table 58-1 Immunologically Mediated Blistering Diseases

Disease	Clinical	Histology	Immunopathology	Autoantigens[a]
Pemphigus foliaceus	Crusts and shallow erosions on scalp, central face, upper chest, and back	Acantholytic blister formed in superficial layer of epidermis	Cell surface deposits of IgG on keratinocytes	Dsg1
Pemphigus vulgaris	Flaccid blisters, denuded skin, oromucosal lesions	Acantholytic blister formed in suprabasal layer of epidermis	Cell surface deposits of IgG on keratinocytes	Dsg3 (plus Dsg1 in some patients)
Bullous pemphigoid	Large tense blisters on flexor surfaces, oral mucosal blisters and erosions	Blister formed in subepidermal region, usually eosinophil rich	Linear band of IgG and/or C3 in epidermal BMZ[a]	BPAG1, BPAG2
Pemphigoid gestationis	Pruritic, urticarial plaques, rimmed by vesicles and bullae on the trunk and extremities	Teardrop-shaped, subepidermal blisters in dermal papillae; eosinophil-rich infiltrate	Linear band of C3 in epidermal BMZ	BPAG2 (plus BPAG1 in some patients)
Linear IgA disease	Pruritic small papules on extensor surfaces; occasionally larger, arciform blisters	Subepidermal blister with neutrophils in dermal papillae	Linear band of IgA in epidermal BMZ	BPAG2 (see text for specific details)
Cicatricial pemphigoid	Erosive and/or blistering lesions of mucous membranes and possibly the skin; scarring of some sites	Subepidermal blister that may or may not include an inflammatory infiltrate	Linear band of IgG, IgA, and/or C3 in epidermal BMZ	BPAG2, laminin 5, or others
Epidermolysis bullosa acquisita	Blisters, erosions, scars, and milia on sites exposed to trauma; widespread, inflammatory, tense blisters may be seen initially	Subepidermal blister that may or may not include an inflammatory infiltrate	Linear band of IgG and/or C3 in epidermal BMZ	Type VII collagen
Dermatitis herpetiformis	Extremely pruritic small papules and vesicles on elbows, knees, buttocks, and posterior neck	Subepidermal blister with neutrophils in dermal papillae	Granular deposits of IgA in dermal papillae	

[a] Autoantigens bound by these patients' autoantibodies are defined as follows: Dsg1, desmoglein 1; Dsg3, desmoglein 3; BPAG1, bullous pemphigoid antigen 1; BPAG2, bullous pemphigoid antigen 2; BMZ, basement membrane zone.

be an aggravating factor. A blistering skin disease endemic to south central Brazil known as *fogo selvagem*, or *Brazilian pemphigus*, is clinically, histologically, and immunopathologically indistinguishable from PF.

Patients with PF have immunopathologic features in common with PV. Specifically, direct immunofluorescence microscopy of perilesional skin demonstrates IgG on the surface of keratinocytes. As in PV, patients with PF frequently have circulating IgG autoantibodies against keratinocyte cell surface antigens. Guinea pig esophagus is the optimal substrate for indirect immunofluorescence microscopy studies of sera from patients with PF. In PF, autoantibodies are directed against Dsg1, a 160-kDa desmosomal cadherin. As noted for PV, the autoantibody profile in patients with PF (i.e., anti-Dsg1) and the normal tissue distribution of this autoantigen (i.e., low expression in oral mucosa) is thought to account for the distribution of lesions in this disease.

Although pemphigus has been associated with several autoimmune diseases, its association with thymoma and/or myasthenia gravis is particularly notable. To date, more than 30 cases of thymoma and/or myasthenia gravis have been reported in association with pemphigus, usually with PF. Patients may also develop pemphigus as a consequence of drug exposure. The most frequently implicated agent is penicillamine; other offenders include captopril, rifampin, piroxicam, penicillin, and phenobarbital. Drug-induced pemphigus usually resembles PF rather than PV; autoantibodies in these patients have the same antigenic specificity as they do in other pemphigus patients. In most patients, lesions resolve following discontinuation of the drug; however, some patients require treatment with systemic glucocorticoids and/or immunosuppressive agents.

PF is generally a far less severe disease than PV and carries a better prognosis. Localized disease can be treated conservatively with topical or intralesional glucocorticoids; more active cases can usually be controlled with systemic glucocorticoids.

PARANEOPLASTIC PEMPHIGUS Paraneoplastic pemphigus (PNP) is an autoimmune acantholytic mucocutaneous disease associated with an occult or confirmed neoplasm. Patients with PNP typically show painful mucosal erosive lesions in association with pruritic papulosquamous eruptions that often progress to blisters. Palm and sole involvement is common in these patients and raises the possibility that prior reports of neoplasia-associated erythema multiforme actually may have represented unrecognized cases of PNP. Biopsies of lesional skin from these patients show varying combinations of acantholysis, keratinocyte necrosis, and vacuolar-interface dermatitis. Direct immunofluorescence microscopy of patient skin shows deposits of IgG and complement on the surface of keratinocytes and (variably) similar immunoreactants in the epidermal basement membrane zone. Patients with PNP have IgG autoantibodies against cytoplasmic proteins that are members of the plakin family (e.g., desmoplakins I and II, bullous pemphigoid antigen 1, envoplakin, periplakin, and plectin) and cell-surface proteins that are members of the cadherin family (e.g., Dsg3 and Dsg1). Because immunoadsorption of anti-Dsg3 IgG is sufficient to eliminate the ability of PNP sera to induce blisters in an experimental passive transfer animal model, these particular autoantibodies are thought to play a key pathogenic role in blister formation in these patients.

Although PNP is generally resistant to conventional therapies (i.e., those used to treat PV), patients may improve (or even remit) following resection of underlying neoplasms. The predominant neoplasms associated with this disorder are non-Hodgkin's lymphoma, chronic lymphocytic leukemia, Castleman's disease, thymoma, and spindle cell tumors.

BULLOUS PEMPHIGOID Bullous pemphigoid (BP) is an autoimmune subepidermal blistering disease usually seen in the elderly. Lesions typically consist of tense blisters on either normal-appearing or erythematous skin (**Plate IIE-72**). The lesions are usually distributed over the lower abdomen, groin, and flexor surface of the extremities; oral mucosal lesions are found in 10 to 40% of patients. Pruritus may be nonexistent or severe. As lesions evolve, tense blisters tend to rupture and be replaced by flaccid lesions or erosions with or without surmounting crust. Nontraumatized blisters heal without scarring. The major histocompatibility complex class II allele HLA-DQβ1*0301 is prevalent in patients with BP. Despite isolated reports, several studies have shown that patients with BP do not have an increased incidence of malignancy in comparison with appropriately age- and sex-matched controls.

While biopsies of early lesional skin demonstrate subepidermal blisters, the histologic features depend on the character of the particular lesion. Lesions on normal-appearing skin generally show a sparse perivascular leukocytic infiltrate with some eosinophils; conversely, biopsies of inflammatory lesions typically show an eosinophil-rich infiltrate within the papillary dermis at sites of vesicle formation and in perivascular areas. In addition to eosinophils, cell-rich lesions also contain mononuclear cells and neutrophils. It is not always possible to distinguish BP from other subepidermal blistering diseases by routine histologic techniques.

Immunopathologic studies have broadened our understanding of this disease and aided its diagnosis. Direct immunofluorescence microscopy of normal-appearing perilesional skin shows linear deposits of IgG and/or C3 in the epidermal basement membrane. The sera of approximately 70% of these patients contain circulating IgG autoantibodies that bind the epidermal basement membrane of normal human skin in indirect immunofluorescence microscopy. An even higher percentage of patients shows reactivity to the epidermal side of 1 M NaCl split skin [an alternative immunofluorescence microscopy test substrate that is commonly used to distinguish circulating IgG anti-basement membrane autoantibodies in patients with BP from those in patients with similar, yet different, subepidermal blistering diseases (e.g., epidermolysis bullosa acquisita, see below)]. No correlation exists between the titer of these autoantibodies and disease activity. In BP, circulating autoantibodies recognize 230- and (in approximately 70% of BP patients) 180-kDa hemidesmosome-associated proteins in basal keratinocytes [i.e., bullous pemphigoid antigen (BPAG)1 and BPAG2, respectively]. Autoantibodies are thought to develop against these antigens (more specifically, initially against BPAG2), deposit in situ, and activate complement that subsequently produces dermal mast cell degranulation and granulocyte-rich infiltrates that cause tissue damage and blister formation.

BP may persist for months to years, with exacerbations or remissions. Although extensive involvement may result in widespread erosions and compromise cutaneous integrity, the mortality rate is low even in the absence of treatment. Nonetheless, deaths may occur in elderly and/or debilitated patients. The mainstay of treatment is systemic glucocorticoids. Patients with local or minimal disease can sometimes be controlled with topical glucocorticoids alone; patients with more extensive lesions generally respond to systemic glucocorticoids either alone or in combination with immunosuppressive agents. Patients will usually respond to prednisone, 40 to 60 mg/d. In some instances, azathioprine (1 mg/kg per day) or cyclophosphamide (1 mg/kg per day) are necessary adjuncts.

PEMPHIGOID GESTATIONIS Pemphigoid gestationis (PG), also known as herpes gestationis, is a rare, nonviral, subepidermal blistering disease of pregnancy and the puerperium. PG may begin during any trimester of pregnancy or present shortly after delivery. Lesions are usually distributed over the abdomen, trunk, and extremities; mucous membrane lesions are rare. Skin lesions in these patients may be quite polymorphic and consist of erythematous urticarial papules and plaques, vesiculopapules, and/or frank bullae. Lesions are almost always very pruritic. Severe exacerbations of PG frequently occur after delivery, typically within 24 to 48 h. PG tends to recur in subsequent pregnancies, often beginning earlier during such gestations. Brief flare-ups of disease may occur with resumption of menses and may develop in patients later exposed to oral contraceptives. Occasionally, infants of affected mothers demonstrate transient skin lesions.

Biopsies of early lesional skin show teardrop-shaped subepidermal vesicles forming in dermal papillae in association with an eosinophil-rich leukocytic infiltrate. Differentiation of PG from other subepidermal bullous diseases by light microscopy is often difficult. However, direct immunofluorescence microscopy of perilesional skin from PG patients reveals the immunopathologic hallmark of this disorder—linear deposits of C3 in the epidermal basement membrane zone. These deposits develop as a consequence of complement activation produced by low titer IgG anti-basement membrane zone autoantibodies. Recent studies have shown that the majority of PG sera contain autoantibodies that recognize BPAG2, the same 180-kDa hemidesmosome-associated protein that is targeted by autoantibodies in roughly 70% of patients with BP—a subepidermal bullous disease that resembles PG morphologically, histologically, and immunopathologically.

The goals of therapy in patients with PG are to prevent the development of new lesions, relieve intense pruritus, and care for erosions at sites of blister formation. Most patients require treatment with moderate doses of daily glucocorticoids (i.e., 20 to 40 mg of prednisone) at some point in their course. Mild cases (or brief flare-ups) may be controlled by vigorous use of potent topical glucocorticoids. Although PG was once thought to be associated with an increased risk of fetal morbidity and mortality, the best evidence now suggests that these infants may only be at increased risk of being slightly premature or "small for dates." Current evidence suggests that there is no difference in the incidence of uncomplicated live births in PG patients treated with systemic glucocorticoids and in those managed more conservatively. If systemic glucocorticoids are administered, newborns are at risk for development of reversible adrenal insufficiency.

DERMATITIS HERPETIFORMIS Dermatitis herpetiformis (DH) is an intensely pruritic, papulovesicular skin disease characterized by lesions symmetrically distributed over extensor surfaces (i.e., elbows, knees, buttocks, back, scalp, and posterior neck) **(Plate IIE-68)**. The primary lesion in this disorder is a papule, papulovesicle, or urticarial plaque. Because pruritus is prominent, patients may present with excoriations and crusted papules but no observable primary lesions. Patients sometimes report that their pruritus has a distinctive burning or stinging component; the onset of such local symptoms reliably heralds the development of distinct clinical lesions 12 to 24 h later. Almost all DH patients have an associated, usually subclinical, gluten-sensitive enteropathy (Chap. 286), and more than 90% express the HLA-B8/DRw3 and HLA-DQw2 haplotypes. DH may present at any age, including childhood; onset in the second to fourth decades is most common. The disease is typically chronic.

Biopsy of early lesional skin reveals neutrophil-rich infiltrates within dermal papillae. Neutrophils, fibrin, edema, and microvesicle formation at these sites are characteristic of early disease. Older lesions may demonstrate nonspecific features of a subepidermal bulla or an excoriated papule. Because the clinical and histologic features of this disease can be variable and resemble other subepidermal blistering disorders, the diagnosis is confirmed by direct immunofluorescence microscopy of normal-appearing perilesional skin. Such studies demonstrate granular deposits of IgA (with or without complement components) in the papillary dermis and along the epidermal basement membrane zone. IgA deposits in the skin are unaffected by control of disease with medication; however, these immunoreactants may diminish in intensity or disappear in patients maintained for long periods on a strict gluten-free diet (see below). Patients with granular deposits of IgA in their epidermal basement membrane zone typically do not have circulating IgA anti-basement membrane autoantibodies and should be distinguished from individuals with linear IgA deposits at this site (see below).

Although most DH patients do not report overt gastrointestinal symptoms or laboratory evidence of malabsorption, biopsies of small bowel usually reveal blunting of intestinal villi and a lymphocytic infiltrate in the lamina propria. As is true for patients with celiac disease, this gastrointestinal abnormality can be reversed by a gluten-free diet. Moreover, if maintained, this diet alone may control the skin disease and eventuate in clearance of IgA deposits from these patients' epidermal basement membrane zone. Subsequent gluten exposure in such patients alters the morphology of their small bowel, elicits a flare-up of their skin disease, and is associated with the reappearance of IgA in their epidermal basement membrane zone. Additional evidence that DH develops as a consequence of dietary gluten exposure is the demonstration of IgA anti-endomysial antibodies in these patients' sera (as found in the sera of patients with ordinary gluten-sensitive enteropathy). Recent studies have shown that such autoantibodies are directed against tissue transglutaminase. Patients with DH also have an increased incidence of thyroid abnormalities, achlorhydria, atrophic gastritis, and antigastric parietal cell antibodies. These associations likely relate to the high frequency of the HLA-B8/DRw3 haplotype in these patients, since this marker is commonly linked to autoimmune disorders. The mainstay of treatment of DH is dapsone, a sulfone. Patients respond rapidly (24 to 48 h) to dapsone but require careful pretreatment evaluation and close follow-up to ensure that complications are avoided or controlled. All patients on more than 100 mg/d dapsone will have some hemolysis and methemoglobinemia. These are expected pharmacologic side effects of this agent. Gluten restriction can control DH and lessen dapsone requirements; this diet must rigidly exclude gluten to be of maximal benefit. Many months of dietary restriction may be necessary before a beneficial result is achieved. Good dietary counselling by a trained dietitian is essential.

LINEAR IgA DISEASE Linear IgA disease, once considered a variant form of dermatitis herpetiformis, is actually a separate and distinct entity. Clinically, these patients may resemble patients with typical cases of DH, BP, or other subepidermal blistering diseases. Lesions typically consist of papulovesicles, bullae, and/or urticarial plaques, predominantly on extensor (as seen in "classic" DH), central, or flexural sites. Oral mucosal involvement occurs in some patients. Severe pruritus resembles that in patients with DH. Patients with linear IgA disease do not have an increased frequency of the HLA-B8/DRw3 haplotype or an associated enteropathy and hence are not candidates for a gluten-free diet.

The histologic alterations in early lesions may be virtually indistinguishable from those in DH. However, direct immunofluorescence microscopy of normal-appearing perilesional skin reveals linear deposits of IgA (and often C3) in the epidermal basement membrane zone. Most patients with linear IgA disease demonstrate circulating IgA anti-basement membrane autoantibodies against epitopes in the extracellular domain of BPAG2, a transmembrane protein found in hemidesmosomes of basal keratinocytes. These patients generally respond to treatment with dapsone, 50 to 150 mg/d.

EPIDERMOLYSIS BULLOSA ACQUISITA EBA is a rare, noninherited, polymorphic, subepidermal blistering disease. (The inherited form is discussed in Chap. 351.) Patients with classic or noninflammatory EBA have blisters on noninflamed skin, atrophic scars, milia, nail dystrophy, and oral lesions. Because lesions generally occur at sites exposed to minor trauma, classic EBA is considered to be a mechanobullous disease. Other patients with EBA have widespread inflammatory, scarring, bullous lesions and oromucosal involvement that resembles severe BP. Some patients present with an inflammatory bullous disease that evolves into the classic noninflammatory form of this disorder. In general, EBA is chronic; associations with multiple myeloma, amyloidosis, inflammatory bowel disease, and diabetes mellitus have been reported. The HLA-DR2 haplotype is found with increased frequency in these patients.

The histology of lesional skin varies depending on the character of the lesion being studied. Noninflammatory bullae show subepidermal blisters with a sparse leukocytic infiltrate and resemble those in patients with porphyria cutanea tarda. Inflammatory lesions consist of a subepidermal blister and neutrophil-rich leukocytic infiltrates in the superficial dermis. EBA patients have continuous deposits of IgG (and frequently C3 as well as other complement components) in a linear pattern within the epidermal basement membrane zone. Ultrastructurally, these immunoreactants are found in the sublamina densa region in association with anchoring fibrils, wheat stack–like structures that extend from the lamina densa into the underlying papillary dermis. Approximately 25 to 50% of EBA patients have circulating IgG anti-basement membrane autoantibodies directed against type VII collagen—the collagen species that comprises anchoring fibrils. Such IgG autoantibodies bind the dermal side of 1 M NaCl split skin (in contrast to IgG autoantibodies in patients with BP that bind either epidermal or both sides of this indirect immunofluorescence microscopy test substrate).

Treatment of EBA is generally unsatisfactory. Some patients with inflammatory EBA may respond to systemic glucocorticoids, either alone or in combination with immunosuppressive agents. Other patients (especially those with neutrophil-rich inflammatory lesions) may respond to dapsone. The chronic, noninflammatory form of this disease is largely resistant to treatment, although some patients may respond to cyclosporine.

CICATRICIAL PEMPHIGOID Cicatricial pemphigoid (CP) is a rare, acquired, subepithelial blistering disease characterized by erosive lesions of mucous membranes and skin that result in scarring of at least some sites of involvement. Immunopathologically, perilesional mucosa and skin of patients with CP demonstrate in situ deposits of immunoreactants in epithelial basement membranes. Common sites of involvement include the oral mucosa (especially the gingiva) and conjunctiva; other sites that may be affected include the nasopharyngeal, laryngeal, esophageal, urogenital, and rectal mucosa. Skin lesions (present in about one-third of patients) tend to predominate on the scalp, face, and upper trunk and generally consist of a few scattered erosions or tense blisters on an erythematous or urticarial base. CP is typically a chronic and progressive disorder. Serious complications may arise as a consequence of ocular, laryngeal, esophageal, or urogenital lesions. Erosive conjunctivitis may result in shortened fornices, symblephara, ankyloblepharon, entropion, corneal opacities, and (in severe cases) blindness. Similarly, erosive lesions of the larynx may cause hoarseness, pain, and tissue loss that if unrecognized and untreated may eventuate in complete destruction of the airway. Esophageal lesions may result in stenosis and/or strictures that may place patients at risk for aspiration. Strictures may also complicate urogenital involvement.

Biopsies of lesional tissue generally demonstrate subepithelial vesiculobullae and a mononuclear leukocytic infiltrate. Neutrophils and eosinophils may be seen in biopsies of early lesions; older lesions may demonstrate a scant leukocytic infiltrate and fibrosis. Direct immunofluorescence microscopy of perilesional tissue typically demonstrates deposits of IgG, IgA, and/or C3 in these patients' epithelial basement membranes. Because many of these patients show no evidence of circulating anti-basement membrane autoantibodies, testing of perilesional skin is important diagnostically. Although CP was once thought to be a single nosologic entity, it is now largely regarded as a disease phenotype that may develop as a consequence of an autoimmune reaction against a variety of different molecules in epithelial basement membranes (e.g., BPAG2, laminin 5, type VII collagen, and other antigens yet to be completely defined). Treatment of CP is largely dependent upon sites of involvement. Due to potentially severe complications, ocular, laryngeal, esophageal, and/or urogenital involvement require aggressive systemic treatment with dapsone, prednisone, or the latter in combination with another immunosuppressive agent (e.g., azathioprine or cyclophosphamide). Less threatening forms of the disease may be managed with topical or intralesional glucocorticoids.

AUTOIMMUNE SYSTEMIC DISEASES WITH PROMINENT CUTANEOUS FEATURES

DERMATOMYOSITIS The cutaneous manifestations of dermatomyositis (Chap. 382) are often distinctive but at times may resemble those of systemic lupus erythematosus (SLE) (Chap. 311), scleroderma (Chap. 313), or other overlapping connective tissue diseases (Chap. 313). The extent and severity of cutaneous disease may or may not correlate with the extent and severity of the myositis. Patients with severe muscle involvement may have relatively minor skin changes, whereas patients with marked skin involvement may have mild muscle disease. The cutaneous manifestations of dermatomyositis are similar whether the disease appears in childhood or old age, except that calcification of subcutaneous tissue is a common late sequela in childhood dermatomyositis.

The cutaneous signs of dermatomyositis may precede or follow the development of myositis by weeks to years. Cases lacking muscle involvement (i.e., dermatomyositis sine myositis) have also been reported. The most common manifestation is a purple-red discoloration of the upper eyelids, sometimes associated with scaling ("heliotrope" erythema; **Plate IIE-63**) and periorbital edema. Erythema on the cheeks and nose in a "butterfly" distribution may resemble the eruption in SLE. Erythematous or violaceous scaling patches are common on the upper anterior chest, posterior neck, scalp, and the extensor surfaces of the arms, legs, and hands. Erythema and scaling may be particularly prominent over the elbows, knees, and the dorsal interphalangeal joints. Approximately one-third of patients have violaceous, flat-topped papules over the dorsal interphalangeal joints that are pathognomonic of dermatomyositis (Gottron's sign or Gottron's papules; **Plate IIE-65**). These lesions can be contrasted with the erythema and scaling on the dorsum of the fingers in some patients with SLE, which spares the skin over the interphalangeal joints. Periungual telangiectasia may be prominent, and a lacy or reticulated erythema may be associated with fine scaling on the extensor surfaces of the thighs and upper arms. Other patients, particularly those with long-standing disease, develop areas of hypopigmentation, hyperpigmentation, mild atrophy, and telangiectasia known as *poikiloderma vasculare atrophicans*. Poikiloderma is rare in both SLE and scleroderma and thus can serve as a clinical sign that distinguishes dermatomyositis from these two diseases. Cutaneous changes may be similar in scleroderma and dermatomyositis and may include thickening and binding down of the skin of the hands (sclerodactyly) as well as Raynaud's phenomenon. However, the presence of severe muscle disease, Gottron's papules, heliotrope erythema, and poikiloderma serve to distinguish patients with dermatomyositis. Skin biopsy of erythematous, scaling lesions of dermatomyositis may reveal only mild nonspecific inflammation but sometimes may show changes indistinguishable from those found in SLE, including epidermal atrophy, hydropic degeneration of basal keratinocytes, edema of the upper dermis, and a mild mononuclear cell infiltrate. Direct immunofluorescence microscopy of lesional skin is usually negative, although granular deposits of immunoglobulin(s) and complement in the epidermal basement membrane zone have been described in some patients. Treatment should be directed at the systemic disease. In the few instances where adjunctive cutaneous therapy is desirable, topical glucocorticoids are sometimes useful. These patients should avoid exposure to ultraviolet irradiation and use photoprotective measures such as sunscreens.

LUPUS ERYTHEMATOSUS The cutaneous manifestations of lupus erythematosus (LE) (Chap. 311) can be divided into acute, subacute, and chronic (i.e., discoid LE) types. *Acute cutaneous LE* is characterized by erythema of the nose and malar eminences in a "butterfly" distribution (**Plate IIE-61**). The erythema is often sudden in onset, accompanied by edema and fine scale, and correlated with systemic involvement. Patients may have widespread involvement of the face as well as erythema and scaling of the extensor surfaces of the extremities and upper chest. These acute lesions, while sometimes evanescent, usually last for days and are often associated with exacerbations of systemic disease. Skin biopsy of acute lesions may show only a sparse dermal infiltrate of mononuclear cells and dermal edema. In some instances, cellular infiltrates around blood vessels and hair follicles are notable, as is hydropic degeneration of basal cells of the epidermis. Direct immunofluorescence microscopy of lesional skin frequently reveals deposits of immunoglobulin(s) and complement in the epidermal basement membrane zone. Treatment is aimed at control

of systemic disease; photoprotection in this, as well as in other forms of LE, is very important.

Subacute cutaneous lupus erythematosus (SCLE) is characterized by a widespread photosensitive, nonscarring eruption. About half of these patients have SLE in which severe renal and central nervous system involvement is uncommon. SCLE may present as a papulosquamous eruption that resembles psoriasis or annular lesions that resemble those seen in erythema multiforme. In the papulosquamous form, discrete erythematous papules arise on the back, chest, shoulders, extensor surfaces of the arms, and the dorsum of the hands; lesions are uncommon on the face, flexor surfaces of the arms, and below the waist. The slightly scaling papules tend to merge into large plaques, some with a reticulate appearance. The annular form involves the same areas and presents with erythematous papules that evolve into oval, circular, or polycyclic lesions. The lesions of SCLE are more widespread but have less tendency for scarring than do lesions of discoid LE. Skin biopsy reveals a dense mononuclear cell infiltrate around hair follicles and blood vessels in the superficial dermis, combined with hydropic degeneration of basal cells in the epidermis. Direct immunofluorescence microscopy of lesional skin reveals deposits of immunoglobulin(s) in the epidermal basement membrane zone in about half these cases. A particulate pattern of IgG deposition around basal keratinocytes has recently been associated with SCLE. Most SCLE patients have anti-Ro antibodies. Local therapy is usually unsuccessful, and most patients require treatment with aminoquinoline antimalarials. Low-dose therapy with oral glucocorticoids is sometimes necessary; photoprotective measures against both ultraviolet B and A wavelengths are very important.

Discoid lupus erythematosus (DLE) is characterized by discrete lesions, most often on the face, scalp, or external ears. The lesions are erythematous papules or plaques with a thick, adherent scale that occludes hair follicles (follicular plugging). When the scale is removed, its underside will show small excrescences that correlate with the openings of hair follicles and is termed a "carpet tack" appearance. This finding is relatively specific for DLE. Long-standing lesions develop central atrophy, scarring, and hypopigmentation but frequently have erythematous, sometimes raised borders at the periphery (**Plate IIE-62**). These lesions persist for years and tend to expand slowly. Only 5 to 10% of patients with DLE meet the American Rheumatism Association criteria for SLE. However, typical discoid lesions are frequently seen in patients with SLE. Biopsy of DLE lesions shows hyperkeratosis, follicular plugging, and atrophy of the epidermis. The dermal-epidermal junction reveals hydropic degeneration of basal keratinocytes, and a mononuclear cell infiltrate surrounding hair follicles and blood vessels. Direct immunofluorescence microscopy demonstrates immunoglobulin(s) and complement deposits at the basement membrane zone in about 90% of cases. Treatment is focused on control of local cutaneous disease and consists mainly of photoprotection and topical or intralesional glucocorticoids. If local therapy is ineffective, use of aminoquinoline antimalarials may be indicated.

SCLERODERMA AND MORPHEA The skin changes of scleroderma (Chap. 313) usually begin on the hands, feet, and face, with episodes of recurrent nonpitting edema. Sclerosis of the skin begins distally on the fingers (sclerodactyly) and spreads proximally, usually accompanied by resorption of bone of the fingertips, which may have punched out ulcers, stellate scars, or areas of hemorrhage (**Plate IIE-66**). The fingers may actually shrink in size and become sausage-shaped, and since the fingernails are usually unaffected, the nails may curve over the end of the fingertips. Periungual telangiectasias are usually present, but periungual erythema is rare. In advanced cases, the extremities show contractures and calcinosis cutis. Face involvement includes a smooth, unwrinkled brow, taut skin over the nose, shrinkage of tissue around the mouth, and perioral radial furrowing (**Plate IIE-64**). Matlike telangiectasias are often present, particularly on the face and hands. Involved skin feels indurated, smooth, and bound to underlying structures; hyperpigmentation and hypopigmentation are also often present. Raynaud's phenomenon, i.e., cold-induced blanching, cyanosis, and reactive hyperemia, is present in almost all patients and can precede development of scleroderma by many years. The combination of calcinosis cutis, Raynaud's phenomenon, esophageal dysmotility, sclerodactyly, and telangiectasia has been termed the *CREST syndrome*. Anticentromere antibodies have been reported in a very high percentage of patients with the CREST syndrome but in only a small minority of patients with scleroderma. Skin biopsy reveals thickening of the dermis and homogenization of collagen bundles. Direct immunofluorescence microscopy of lesional skin is usually negative.

Morphea, which has been called *localized scleroderma*, is characterized by localized thickening and sclerosis of skin, usually affecting young adults or children. Morphea begins as erythematous or flesh-colored plaques that become sclerotic, develop central hypopigmentation, and demonstrate an erythematous border. In most cases, patients have one or a few lesions, and the disease is termed *localized morphea*. In some patients, widespread cutaneous lesions may occur, without systemic involvement. This form is called *generalized morphea*. Most patients with morphea do not have autoantibodies. Skin biopsy of morphea is indistinguishable from that of scleroderma. Linear scleroderma is a limited form of disease that presents in a linear, bandlike distribution and tends to involve deep as well as superficial layers of skin. Scleroderma and morphea are usually quite resistant to therapy. For this reason, physical therapy to prevent joint contractures and to maintain function is employed and is often helpful.

Diffuse fasciitis with eosinophilia is a clinical entity that can sometimes be confused with scleroderma. There is usually the sudden onset of swelling, induration, and erythema of the extremities frequently following significant physical exertion. The proximal portions of extremities (arms, forearms, thighs, legs) are more often involved than are the hands and feet. While the skin is indurated, it is usually not bound down as in scleroderma; contractures may occur early secondary to fascial involvement. The latter may also cause muscle groups to be separated (i.e., the "groove sign") and veins to appear depressed (i.e., sunken veins). These skin findings are accompanied by peripheral blood eosinophilia, increased erythrocyte sedimentation rate, and sometimes hypergammaglobulinemia. Deep biopsy of affected areas of skin reveals inflammation and thickening of the deep fascia overlying muscle. An inflammatory infiltrate composed of eosinophils and mononuclear cells is usually found. Patients with eosinophilic fasciitis appear to be at increased risk to develop bone marrow failure or other hematologic abnormalities. While the ultimate course of eosinophilic fasciitis is uncertain, many patients respond favorably to treatment with prednisone in doses ranging from 40 to 60 mg/d.

The *eosinophilia-myalgia syndrome*, a disorder reported in epidemic numbers in 1989 and linked to ingestion of L-tryptophan manufactured by a single company in Japan, is a multisystem disorder characterized by debilitating myalgias and absolute eosinophilia in association with varying combinations of arthralgias, pulmonary symptoms, and peripheral edema. In a later phase (i.e., 3 to 6 months after initial symptoms), these patients often develop localized sclerodermatous skin changes, weight loss, and/or neuropathy (Chap. 313). The precise cause of this syndrome, which may resemble other sclerotic skin conditions, is unknown. However, the implicated lots of L-tryptophan contained the contaminant 1,1-ethylidene bis[tryptophan]. This contaminant may be pathogenic or a marker for another substance that provokes the disorder.

BIBLIOGRAPHY

AMAGAI M: Pemphigus: Autoimmunity to epidermal cell adhesion molecules. Adv Dermatol 11:319, 1996

———— et al: Antibodies against desmoglein 3 (pemphigus vulgaris antigen) are present in sera from patients with paraneoplastic pemphigus and cause acantholysis in vivo in neonatal mice. J Clin Invest 102:775, 1998

ANHALT GJ et al: Paraneoplastic pemphigus: An autoimmune mucocutaneous disease associated with neoplasia. N Engl J Med 323:1729, 1990

BRAVERMAN IM: Connective tissue diseases, in *Skin Signs of Systemic Disease*, 3d ed. Philadelphia, Saunders, 1998

FINE JD: Management of acquired bullous skin disease. N Engl J Med 333:1475, 1995

HALL RP: Dermatitis herpetiformis. J Invest Dermatol 99:873, 1992

LIU Z et al: A passive transfer model of the organ-specific autoimmune disease, bullous pemphigoid, using antibodies generated against the hemidesmosomal antigen, BP180. J Clin Invest 92:2480, 1993

MAHONEY MG et al: Explanations for the clinical and microscopic localization of lesions in pemphigus foliaceus and vulgaris. J Clin Invest 103:461, 1999

STANLEY JR: Cell adhesion molecules as targets of autoantibodies in pemphigus and pemphigoid, bullous diseases due to defective epidermal cell adhesion. Adv Immunol 53:291, 1992

YANCEY KB: Adhesion molecules. II: Interactions of keratinocytes with epidermal basement membrane. J Invest Dermatol 104:1008, 1995

| 59 | *Robert S. Stern, Olivier M. Chosidow, Bruce U. Wintroub* |

CUTANEOUS DRUG REACTIONS

Cutaneous reactions are among the most frequent adverse reactions to drugs. Prompt recognition of these reactions, drug withdrawal, and appropriate therapeutic interventions can minimize toxicity. This chapter focuses on adverse cutaneous reactions to drugs other than topical agents and reviews the incidence, patterns, and pathogenesis of cutaneous reactions to drugs and other therapeutic agents.

USE OF PRESCRIPTION DRUGS IN THE UNITED STATES More than 1.5 billion prescriptions for 60,000 drug products, which include over 2000 different active agents, are dispensed each year in the United States. Hospital inpatients alone annually receive about 120 million courses of drug therapy, and half of adult Americans receive prescription drugs on a regular outpatient basis. Many additional patients use over-the-counter medicines that may cause adverse cutaneous reactions.

INCIDENCE OF CUTANEOUS REACTIONS Although adverse drug reactions are common, it is difficult to ascertain their incidence, seriousness, and ultimate health effects. Available information comes from evaluations of hospitalized patients, epidemiologic surveys, premarketing studies, and voluntary reporting, most notably to the U.S. Food and Drug Administration's Medwatch System. None of these efforts provides comprehensive comparable data on the risk of cutaneous reactions associated with most medicines.

In one study about 2% of medical inpatients had skin reactions consisting of rash, urticaria, or pruritus during hospitalization. The overall reaction rate per course of drug therapy was about 3:1000. Among inpatients, penicillins, sulfonamides, and blood products accounted for two-thirds of cutaneous reactions. Among outpatients, reaction rates for many antibiotics were comparable to those observed in inpatients. Fluoroquinolones are notable causes of cutaneous reactions not observed in earlier studies. Reaction rates for selected commonly used antibiotics are summarized in Table 59-1. Most cutaneous reactions occur within 2 weeks of exposure to a drug. The risk of

Table 59-1 Rates (per 1000 Recipients) of Skin Reactions to Selected Medications

Drug	Reaction Rate
Trimethoprim-sulfamethoxazole	21
Fluoroquinolones	5
Amoxicillin (Augmentin)	12
Other penicillins	11
Tetracyclines	5
Macrolides	6

SOURCE: Adapted from van der Linden et al.

allergic reactions does not vary greatly with age or sex. Among outpatients, the risk of a reaction to an antibiotic was comparable for first and subsequent courses of a given drug.

The distribution of morphologic patterns of drug eruptions cared for within a Finnish hospital dermatology department with a special interest in fixed drug eruptions included exanthematous reactions (32%), urticaria and/or angioedema (20%), fixed drug eruptions (34%), erythema multiforme (2%), Stevens-Johnson syndrome (SJS; 1%), exfoliative dermatitis (1%), and photosensitivity reactions (3%). Other studies suggest that about 80% of all cutaneous reactions are morbilliform or erythematous, 10 to 15% are urticaria or angioedema, and all other types of reactions are relatively rare.

The relative risk of SJS and toxic epidermal necrolysis (TEN), perhaps the most important severe cutaneous reactions, has been quantified in an international case control study and case series. Sulfonamide antibiotics, allopurinol, amine antiepileptic drugs (phenytoin and carbamazepine), and lamotrigine (a new antiepileptic) are associated with the highest risk of these reactions.

PATHOGENESIS OF DRUG REACTIONS

Untoward cutaneous responses to drugs can arise as a result of immunologic or nonimmunologic mechanisms. Immunologic reactions require activation of host immunologic pathways and are designated *drug allergy*. Drug reactions occurring through nonimmunologic mechanisms may be due to activation of effector pathways, overdosage, cumulative toxicity, side effects, ecologic disturbance, interactions between drugs, metabolic alterations, exacerbation of preexisting dermatologic conditions, or inherited protein or enzyme deficiencies. It is often not possible to specify the responsible drug or pathogenic mechanism because the skin responds to a variety of stimuli through a limited number of reaction patterns. The mechanism of many drug reactions is unknown.

IMMUNOLOGIC DRUG REACTIONS Drugs frequently elicit an immune response, but only a small number of individuals experience clinical hypersensitivity reactions. For example, most patients exposed to penicillin develop demonstrable antibodies to penicillin but do not manifest drug reactions when exposed to penicillin. Multiple factors determine the capacity of a drug to elicit an immune response, including the molecular characteristics of the drug and host effects.

Increases in *molecular* size and complexity are associated with increased immunogenicity, and macromolecular drugs such as protein or peptide hormones are highly antigenic. Most drugs are small organic molecules <1000 Da in size, and the capacity of such small molecules to elicit an immune response depends on their ability to act as haptens, i.e., to form stable, usually covalent, bonds with tissue macromolecules, an extremely rare event.

Route of administration of a drug or simple chemical can influence the nature of the *host* immune response. For example, topical application of antigens tends to induce delayed hypersensitivity, and exposure to antigens via oral or nasal cavities stimulates production of secretory immunoglobins, IgA and IgE, and occasionally IgM. Frequency of sensitization through intravenous administration of drugs varies, but anaphylaxis is a more likely consequence with this route of exposure than following oral administration.

The degree of drug exposure and individual variability in absorption and metabolism of a given agent may alter immunogenic load. The variable degree of in vivo acetylation of hydralazine provides a clinical example of this phenomenon. Hydralazine produces a lupuslike syndrome associated with antinuclear antibody formation more frequently in patients who acetylate the drug slowly. Frequent highdose and interrupted courses of therapy are also important risk factors for development of drug allergy.

Pathogenesis of Allergic Drug Reactions • *IgE-Dependent Reactions* IgE-dependent drug reactions are usually manifest in the skin and gastrointestinal, respiratory, and cardiovascular systems

(Chap. 310). Primary symptoms and signs include pruritus, urticaria, nausea, vomiting, cramps, bronchospasm, and laryngeal edema and, on occasion, anaphylactic shock with hypotension and death. Immediate reactions may occur within minutes of drug exposure, and accelerated reactions occur hours or days after drug administration. Accelerated reactions are usually urticarial and may include laryngeal edema. Penicillin and related drugs are the most frequent causes of IgE-dependent reactions. Release of chemical mediators such as histamine, adenosine, leukotrienes, prostaglandins, platelet-activating factor, enzymes, and proteoglycans from sensitized tissue, mast cells, or circulating basophilic leukocytes results in vasodilation and edema. Release is triggered when polyvalent drug protein conjugates crosslink IgE molecules fixed to sensitized cells. The clinical manifestations are determined by interaction of the released chemical mediator with its target organ, i.e., skin, respiratory, gastrointestinal, and/or cardiovascular systems. Certain routes of administration favor different clinical patterns (i.e., oral route: gastrointestinal effects; intravenous route: circulatory effects).

Immune-complex–dependent reactions Serum sickness is produced by circulating immune complexes and is characterized by fever, arthritis, nephritis, neuritis, edema, and an urticarial, papular, or purpuric rash (Chap. 317). The syndrome requires an antigen that remains in the circulation for prolonged periods so that when antibody is synthesized, circulating antigen-antibody complexes are formed. Serum sickness was first described following administration of foreign sera, but drugs are now the usual cause. Drugs that produce serum sickness include the penicillins, sulfonamides, thiouracils, cholecystographic dyes, phenytoin, aminosalicylic acid, heparin, and antilymphocyte globulin. Cephalosporin administration in febrile children is associated with a high risk of a clinically similar reaction, but the mechanism of this reaction is unknown. In classic serum sickness, symptoms develop 6 days or more after exposure to a drug, the latent period representing the time needed to synthesize antibody. The antibodies responsible for immune-complex–dependent drug reactions are largely of the IgG or IgM class. Vasculitis, a relatively rare cutaneous complication of drugs, may also be a result of immune complex deposition (Chap. 317).

Cytotoxicity and delayed hypersensitivity Cytotoxicity and delayed hypersensitivity mechanisms may be important in the etiology of morbilliform exanthema, hypersensitivity syndrome, SJS, or TEN, but this is not proven. Systemic manifestations occur frequently. The nature of the antigen leading to cytotoxic reactions is unknown, but it is likely that different T lymphocyte populations are activated. T_H1 type cells will lead to the production of interleukin (IL)-2 and interferon (IFN)-γ and subsequent activation of cytotoxic T cells. In early lesions of morbilliform exanthema or TEN, histopathologic studies have shown expression of HLA-DR and intercellular adhesion molecule (ICAM-1) by keratinocytes, CD4 cells (in the dermis), and CD8 T cells (in the epidermis) and apoptosis of keratinocytes (facilitated by tumor necrosis factor α secretion and *fas*-ligand expression). T_H2 type cells produce cytokines such as IL-5, which may be involved in hypersensitivity syndrome (see below).

NONIMMUNOLOGIC DRUG REACTIONS Nonimmunologic mechanisms are responsible for the majority of drug reactions; however, only the most important mechanisms will be discussed.

Nonimmunologic Activation of Effector Pathways Drug reactions may result from nonimmunologic activation of effector pathways by three mechanisms: First, drugs may release mediators directly from mast cells and basophils and present as anaphylaxis, urticaria, and/or angioedema. Urticarial anaphylactic reactions induced by opiates, polymyxin B, tubocurarine, radiocontrast media, and dextrans may occur by this mechanism. Second, drugs may activate complement in the absence of antibody. This is an additional mechanism through which radiocontrast media may act. Third, drugs such as aspirin and other nonsteroidal anti-inflammatory agents (NSAIDs) may alter pathways of arachidonic acid metabolism and induce urticaria.

Phototoxicity Phototoxic reactions may be drug-induced or may occur in metabolic disorders in which a photosensitizing chemical is overproduced. A phototoxic reaction occurs when enough chromophore (drug or metabolic product) absorbs sufficient radiation to cause a reaction or interaction with target tissue. Drug-induced phototoxic reactions can occur on first exposure. The incidence of phototoxicity is a direct function of the concentration of sensitizer and the amount of light of the appropriate wavelengths. At least three distinct photochemical mechanisms have been described: (1) the reaction between the excited state of a phototoxic molecule and a biologic target may cause formation of a covalent photoaddition product, (2) the phototoxic molecule may form stable photoproducts that are toxic to biologic substrates, and (3) radiation of a phototoxic molecule may result in transfer of energy to oxygen molecules and cause formation of toxic oxygen species, such as singlet oxygen superoxide anion, or hydroxyl radicals. Interaction of these reactive species with biologic targets produces photooxidized molecules. Phototoxic injury is usually manifest as a sunburn-like reaction.

Exacerbation of Preexisting Diseases A variety of agents can exacerbate preexisting diseases. For example, lithium can exacerbate acne and psoriasis in a dose-dependent manner. Beta-blocking agents and IFN-α may induce psoriasis. Withdrawal of glucocorticoids can exacerbate psoriasis or atopic dermatitis.

Inherited Enzyme or Protein Deficiencies Specific genetically determined defects in the ability of an individual to detoxify toxic reactive drug metabolites may predispose such individuals to the development of severe drug reactions, especially hypersensitivity syndrome, and perhaps TEN associated with use of sulfonamides and anticonvulsants.

Alterations of Immunologic Status Alterations in patients' immunologic status may also modify the risk of cutaneous reactions. Bone marrow transplant patients, HIV-infected persons, and persons with Epstein-Barr virus infection are at higher risk of developing cutaneous reactions to drugs. Skin reactions to trimethoprim-sulfamethoxazole are seen in about a third of HIV-infected users of this drug, but desensitization can be accomplished. Dapsone, trimethoprim alone, and amoxicillin-clavulanate are also frequent causes of drug eruptions in HIV-infected patients. The advent of highly active antiretroviral therapy (HAART) may have decreased the risk of cutaneous reactions in HIV patients (Chap. 309).

A CLINICAL CLASSIFICATION OF CUTANEOUS DRUG REACTIONS

URTICARIA/ANGIOEDEMA *Urticaria* is a skin reaction characterized by pruritic, red wheals. Lesions may vary from a small point to a large area. Individual lesions rarely last more than 24 h. When deep dermal and subcutaneous tissues are also swollen, this reaction is known as *angioedema*. Angioedema may involve mucous membranes and may be part of a life-threatening anaphylactic reaction. Urticarial lesions, along with pruritus and morbilliform (or maculopapular) eruptions, are among the most frequent types of cutaneous reactions to drugs.

Drug-induced urticaria may be caused by three mechanisms: an IgE-dependent mechanism, circulating immune complexes (serum sickness), and nonimmunologic activation of effector pathways. IgE-dependent urticarial reactions usually occur within 36 h but can occur within minutes. Reactions occurring within minutes to hours of drug exposure are termed *immediate reactions*, whereas those that occur 12 to 36 h after drug exposure are designated *accelerated reactions*. Immune-complex–induced urticaria associated with serum sickness usually occurs from 6 to 12 days after first exposure. In this syndrome, the urticarial eruption may be accompanied by fever, hematuria, arthralgias, hepatic dysfunction, and neurologic symptoms.

Certain drugs, such as NSAIDs, angiotensin-converting enzyme (ACE) inhibitors, and radiographic dyes, may induce urticarial reactions, angioedema, and anaphylaxis in the absence of drug-specific antibody. Although ACE inhibitors, aspirin, penicillin, and blood products are the most frequent causes of urticarial eruptions, urticaria has been observed in association with nearly all drugs. Drugs also may cause chronic urticaria, which lasts more than 6 weeks. Aspirin frequently exacerbates this problem.

The treatment of urticaria or angioedema depends on the severity of the reaction and the rate at which it is evolving. In severe cases, especially with respiratory or cardiovascular compromise, epinephrine is the mainstay of therapy, but its effect is reduced in patients using beta blockers. For more seriously affected patients, treatment with systemic glucocorticoids, sometimes intravenously administered, are helpful. In addition to drug withdrawal, for patients with only cutaneous symptoms and without symptoms of angioedema or anaphylaxis, oral antihistamines are usually sufficient.

PHOTOSENSITIVITY ERUPTIONS Photosensitivity eruptions are usually most marked in sun-exposed areas but may extend to sun-protected areas. Phototoxic reactions are more common with some drugs. Photoallergic reactions to systemically administered drugs are very rare. Phototoxic reactions usually resemble sunburn and can occur with the first exposure to a drug. Their severity depends on the tissue level of the drug, the extent of exposure to light, and the efficiency of the photosensitizer (Chap. 60).

Orally administered phototoxic drugs include many fluoroquinolones, chlorpromazine, tetracycline, thiazides, and at least two NSAIDs (benoxaprofen and piroxicam). The majority of the common phototoxic drugs have action spectrums in the long-wave ultraviolet A (UV-A) range. Phototoxic reactions abate with removal of either the drug or ultraviolet radiation. Because UV-A and visible light, which trigger these reactions, are not easily absorbed by nonopaque sunscreens and are transmitted through window glass, these reactions may be difficult to block.

Photosensitivity reactions are treated by avoiding exposure to ultraviolet light (sunlight) and treating the reaction as one would a sunburn. Rarely, individuals develop persistent reactivity to light, necessitating long-term avoidance of sun exposure.

PIGMENTATION CHANGES Drugs may cause a variety of pigmentary changes in the skin. Some drugs stimulate melanocytic activity and increase pigmentation. Drug deposition can also lead to pigmentation; this phenomenon occurs with heavy metals. Phenothiazines may be deposited in the skin and cause a slate-gray color. Antimalarial drugs may cause a slate-gray or yellow pigmentation. Long term minocycline use may cause slate-gray hyperpigmentation, especially in areas of chronic inflammation. Inorganic arsenic, once used to treat psoriasis, is associated with diffuse macular pigmentation. Other heavy metals that cause pigmentary changes include silver, gold, bismuth, and mercury. Long-term use of phenytoin can produce a chloasma-like pigmentation in women. Certain cytostatic agents can also cause pigmentary changes. Histologic examination is often diagnostic for drug deposition diseases.

Zidovudine (AZT) is a frequent cause of pigmentation, especially of the nails (Chap. 309). Nicotinic acid in large doses may cause brown pigmentation, and oral contraceptives may produce chloasma. In addition, amiodarone may cause violaceous hyperpigmentation that is increased in sun-exposed skin. Drugs such as heavy metals, copper antimalarial and arsenical agents, and ACTH also may discolor oral mucosa.

VASCULITIS Cutaneous necrotizing vasculitis often presents as palpable purpuric lesions that may be generalized or limited to the lower extremities or other dependent areas (Chap. 317). Urticarial lesions, ulcers, and hemorrhagic blisters also occur. Vasculitis may involve other organs, including the liver, kidney, brain, and joints. Drugs are only one cause of vasculitis, with infection and collagen vascular disease responsible for the majority of cases.

Propylthiouracil induces a cutaneous vasculitis that is accompanied by leukopenia and splenomegaly. Direct immunofluorescent changes in these lesions suggest immune-complex deposition. Drugs implicated in vasculitic eruptions include allopurinol, thiazides, sulfonamides, penicillin, and some NSAIDs.

HYPERSENSITIVITY SYNDROME Initially described with phenytoin, hypersensitivity syndrome presents as an erythematous eruption that may become purpuric and is accompanied by many of the following features: fever, facial and periorbital edema, tender generalized lymphadenopathy, leukocytosis (often with atypical lymphocytes and eosinophils), hepatitis, and sometimes nephritis or pneumonitis. The cutaneous reaction usually begins 1 to 6 weeks after phenytoin is begun and usually resolves with drug cessation, but symptoms, especially hepatitis, may persist. The eruption recurs with rechallenge, and cross-reactions among aromatic anticonvulsants, including phenytoin, carbamazepine, and barbiturates, are frequent. With phenytoin, an increased risk of this syndrome is associated with an inherited deficiency of epoxide hydrolase, an enzyme required for metabolism of a toxic intermediate arene oxide that is formed during metabolism of phenytoin by the cytochrome P450 system. Other drugs causing this syndrome include lamotrigine, dapsone, allopurinol, sulfonamides, minocycline, and sulfones. Systemic glucocorticoids (prednisone, 0.5 to 1.0 mg/kg) seem to reduce symptoms. Mortality as high as 10% has been reported.

WARFARIN NECROSIS OF THE SKIN This rare reaction occurs usually between the third and tenth days of therapy with warfarin derivatives, usually in women. Lesions are sharply demarcated, erythematous, indurated, and purpuric and may resolve or progress to form large, irregular, hemorrhagic bullae with eventual necrosis and slow-healing eschar formation.

Development of the syndrome is unrelated to drug dose or underlying condition. Favored sites are breasts, thighs, and buttocks. The course is not altered by discontinuation of the drug after onset of the eruption. Similar reactions have been associated with heparin. Warfarin reactions are associated with protein C deficiency. Protein C is a vitamin K–dependent protein with a shorter half-life than other clotting proteins and is in part responsible for control of fibrinolysis. Since warfarin inhibits synthesis of vitamin K–dependent coagulation factors, warfarin anticoagulation in heterozygotes for protein C deficiency causes a precipitous fall in circulating levels of protein C, permitting hypercoagulability and thrombosis in the cutaneous microvasculature, with consequent areas of necrosis. Heparin-induced necrosis may have clinically similar features but is probably due to heparin-induced platelet aggregation with subsequent occlusion of blood vessels.

Warfarin-induced cutaneous necrosis is treated with vitamin K and heparin. Vitamin K reverses the effects of warfarin, and heparin acts as an anticoagulant. Treatment with protein C concentrates may also be helpful in individuals with deficiencies of protein C, the predisposing factor for development of these reactions.

MORBILLIFORM REACTIONS Morbilliform or maculopapular eruptions are the most common of all drug-induced reactions, often start on the trunk or areas of pressure or trauma, and consist of erythematous macules and papules that are frequently symmetric and may become confluent. Involvement of mucous membranes, palms, and soles is variable; the eruption may be associated with moderate to severe pruritus and fever.

The pathogenesis is unclear. A hypersensitivity mechanism has been suggested, although these reactions do not always recur following drug rechallenge. Diagnosis is rarely assisted by laboratory or patch testing; differentiation from viral exanthem is the principal differential diagnostic consideration. Unless the suspect drug is essential it should be discontinued. Occasionally these eruptions may decrease or fade with continued use of the responsible drug.

Morbilliform reactions usually develop within 1 week of initiation of therapy and last 1 to 2 weeks; however, reactions to some drugs, especially penicillin and drugs with long half-lives, may begin more than 2 weeks after therapy has begun and last as long as 2 weeks after therapy has ceased.

Morbilliform eruptions are usually treated by discontinuing the

suspect medications symptomatically. Oral antihistamines, emollients, and soothing baths are useful for treatment of pruritus. Short courses of potent topical glucocorticoids can reduce inflammation and symptoms and are probably helpful. The beneficial effect of systemic glucocorticoids relative to risk is less clear.

FIXED DRUG REACTIONS These reactions are characterized by one or more sharply demarcated, erythematous lesions in which hyperpigmentation results after resolution of the acute inflammation; with rechallenge, the lesion recurs in the same (i.e., "fixed") location. Lesions often involve the lips, hands, legs, face, genitalia, and oral mucosa and cause burning. Most patients have multiple lesions. Patch testing is useful to establish the etiology. Fixed drug eruptions have been associated with phenolphthalein, sulfonamides, tetracyclines, phenylbutazone, NSAIDs, and barbiturates. Although cross-sensitivity appears to occur between different tetracycline compounds, cross-sensitivity was not elicited when different sulfonamide compounds were administered to patients as part of provocation testing.

LICHENOID DRUG ERUPTIONS A lichenoid cutaneous reaction, clinically and morphologically indistinguishable from lichen planus, is associated with a variety of drugs and chemicals. Eosinophils are more common when the reaction is drug-induced. Gold and antimalarials are most often associated with this eruption. Antihypertensive agents, including beta blockers and captopril, have also been reported to cause lichenoid reactions.

BULLOUS ERUPTIONS Blisters accompany a wide variety of cutaneous reactions, including fixed drug eruptions, severe morbilliform eruptions in dependent areas of the body, and phototoxic reactions. SJS and TEN are the most serious and important bullous reactions to drugs. Nalidixic acid and furosemide cause blistering eruptions indistinguishable from the primary bullous diseases. A pemphigus foliaceus–like eruption is seen with penicillamine.

PUSTULAR ERUPTIONS Acute generalized exanthematous pustulosis is often associated with exposure to drugs, most notably antibiotics. Usually beginning on the face or intertriginous areas, small nonfollicular pustules overlying erythematous and edematous skin may coalesce and lead to superficial ulceration. Fever is present and differentiating this eruption from TEN in its initial stages may be difficult. Acute generalized exanthematous pustulosis often begins within a few days of initiating drug treatment.

ERYTHEMA MULTIFORME Erythema multiforme is an acute, self-limited inflammatory disorder of skin and mucous membranes characterized by distinctive iris or target lesions, usually acrally distributed and often associated with sore throat, mucosal lesions, and malaise. Classic erythema multiforme usually has nondrug causes, most commonly herpes simplex infection, and must be differentiated from true SJS, which is usually drug related.

STEVENS-JOHNSON SYNDROME SJS is a blistering disorder that is usually more severe than erythema multiforme. Initial presentation is often a sore throat, malaise, and fever. Within a few days, in addition to erosions of multiple mucous membranes, small blisters developing on dusky or purpuric macules or atypical target lesions characterize this eruption. Total percent of body surface area blistering and eventual detachment is less than 10%. Overlap SJS/TEN shares characteristics of both SJS and TEN, with 10 to 30% of body surface area exhibiting epidermal detachment.

TOXIC EPIDERMAL NECROLYSIS TEN is the most serious cutaneous drug reaction and may be fatal. Drugs are usually the cause of TEN. Onset is generally acute and is characterized by fever >39°C (102.2°F), blisters or ulcers of multiple mucous membranes, malaise, and epidermal necrosis involving >30% of body surface area. Intestinal and pulmonary involvement is associated with a poor prognosis, as is a greater extent of epidermal detachment and older age. About 30% of affected persons die. Many treatments affecting immune response or cytokines (thalidomide) or apoptosis (intravenous immunoglobulin) have been advocated, but none have been shown to be efficacious in well-controlled trials. In spite of its theoretical potential benefits, thalidomide therapy increases TEN-associated mortality. Supportive treatment in burn units is helpful in reducing morbidity and mortality.

DRUGS OF SPECIAL INTEREST

PENICILLIN   The incidence of cutaneous reactions to penicillin is about 1%. About 85% of cutaneous reactions to penicillin are morbilliform, and about 10% are urticaria or angioedema.

IgG, IgM, and IgE antibodies can be produced; IgG and IgM anti-penicillin antibodies play a role in the development of hemolytic anemia, whereas anaphylaxis and serum sickness appear to be due to IgE antibodies in serum.

In patients with suspected IgE-mediated reactions to penicillin for whom future treatment is anticipated, accurate tests for sensitization are available. Current practice is to perform skin testing with a commercially available penicilloyl determinant preparation (Pre-pen, Kremers-Urban) and with fresh penicillin and, if possible, with another source of minor (nonpenicilloyl) determinants such as aged or base-treated penicillin. Antibodies to minor determinants are common in patients experiencing anaphylaxis, but testing with major determinants alone detects most patients at risk for anaphylaxis.

About one-fourth of patients with positive history of penicillin allergy have a positive skin test, while 6% (3 to 10%) with no history of penicillin sensitivity demonstrate a positive skin response to penicillin. Administering penicillin to those patients with a positive skin test produces reactions in a high proportion (50 to 100%); conversely, only a few patients (0.5%) with a negative skin test react to the drug, and reactions tend to be mild and to occur late. Since a false-negative skin test may occur during or just after an acute reaction, testing should be performed either prospectively or several months after a suspected reaction. As many as 80% of patients lose anaphylactic sensitivity and IgE antibody after several years. Radioallergosorbent tests and other in vitro tests offer no advantage over properly performed skin testing. Some cross-reactivity between penicillin and nonpenicillin β-lactam antibiotics (e.g., cephalosporins) occurs, but the majority of penicillin-allergic patients will tolerate cephalosporins. Persons who have negative skin tests to penicillin rarely develop reactions to cephalosporins.

In the face of a positive clinical history of penicillin reaction, another drug should be chosen. If this is not feasible or prudent (e.g., in a pregnant patient with syphilis or with enterococcal endocarditis), skin testing with penicillin is warranted. If skin tests are negative, cautious administration of penicillin is acceptable, although some recommend desensitization of such patients if the reaction was likely to be IgE-mediated. In those with positive skin tests, desensitization is mandatory if therapeutic use of β-lactam antibiotics is to be undertaken. Various protocols are available, including oral and parenteral approaches. Oral desensitization appears to have lower risk of serious anaphylactic reactions during desensitization. However, desensitization carries the risk of anaphylaxis regardless of how it is performed. After desensitization, many patients experience non-life-threatening IgE-mediated untoward reactions to penicillin during their course of therapy. Desensitization is not effective in those with exfoliative dermatitis or morbilliform reactions due to penicillin.

NONSTEROIDAL ANTI-INFLAMMATORY DRUGS   NSAIDs, including aspirin and indomethacin (indometacin), cause two broad categories of allergic-like symptoms in susceptible individuals: (1) approximately 1% of persons experience urticaria or angioedema, and (2) about half as many (0.5%) experience rhinosinusitis and asthma; however, about 10% of adults with asthma and one-third of individuals with nasal polyposis and sinusitis may respond adversely to aspirin.

Urticaria/angioedema may be delayed up to 24 h and may occur at any age. The rhinosinusitis-asthma syndrome generally develops within 1 h of drug administration. In young patients, the reaction pattern often begins as watery rhinorrhea, which can be complicated by nasal and sinus infection, and polyposis, bloody discharge, and nasal eosinophilia. In many individuals with this syndrome, asthma that can be life-threatening eventually ensues whenever NSAIDs are subsequently ingested, and symptoms may persist despite avoidance of these drugs. Proof of the association of symptoms and NSAID use requires either clear-cut history of symptoms following drug ingestion or an oral challenge. For the latter to be performed with relative safety, (1) asthma must be under good control, (2) the procedure must be conducted in a hospital setting by experienced personnel capable of recognizing and treating acute respiratory responses, and (3) the challenge should begin with very low doses (i.e., not >30 mg) of aspirin and increase every 1 to 2 h in doubling doses as tolerated to 650 mg.

While cross-reactivity between NSAIDs is common, it is not immunologic, and patients who are sensitive to NSAIDs cannot be identified by assessment of IgE antibody to aspirin, lymphocyte sensitization, or in vitro immunologic testing.

RADIOCONTRAST MEDIA   Large numbers of patients are exposed to radiocontrast agents. High-osmolality radiocontrast media are about five times more likely to induce urticaria (1%) or anaphylaxis than newer low-osmolality media. Severe reactions are rare with either type of contrast media. About one-third of those with mild reactions to previous exposure rereact on reexposure. In most cases, these reactions are probably not immunologic. Pretreatment with prednisone and diphenhydramine reduces reaction rates. Persons with a reaction to a high-osmolality contrast media should be given low-osmolality media if later contrast studies are required.

ANTICONVULSANTS   Of the anticonvulsants, the single orally administered agent with the highest risk of severe adverse cutaneous reactions is the antiseizure medicine lamotrigine. Older anticonvulsants, including phenytoin and carbamazepine, are also associated with many types of severe reactions and a high incidence of less severe reactions, particularly in children. In addition to SJS, TEN, and the hypersensitivity syndrome discussed above, the aromatic anticonvulsants can induce a pseudolymphoma syndrome and induce gingival hyperplasia.

SULFONAMIDES   Sulfonamides have perhaps the highest risk of causing cutaneous eruptions and are the drugs most frequently implicated in SJS and TEN. The combination of sulfamethoxazole and trimethoprim frequently induces adverse cutaneous reactions in patients with AIDS (Chap. 309). Desensitization is often successful in AIDS patients with morbilliform eruptions but is a high-risk procedure in AIDS patients who manifest erythroderma, fever, or a bullous reaction in response to their earlier sulfonamide exposure.

AGENTS USED IN CANCER CHEMOTHERAPY   Since many agents used in cancer chemotherapy inhibit cell division, rapidly proliferating elements of the skin, including hair, mucous membranes, and appendages, are sensitive to their effects; as a result, stomatitis and alopecia are among the most frequent dose-dependent side effects of chemotherapy. Onychodystrophy (dystrophic changes in nails) is also seen with bleomycin, hydroxyurea (hydroxycarbamide), and 5-fluorouracil. Sterile cellulitis and phlebitis and ulceration of pressure areas occur with many of these agents. Urticaria, angioedema, exfoliative dermatitis, and erythema of the palms and soles have also been seen, as has local and diffuse hyperpigmentation.

GLUCOCORTICOIDS   Both systemic and topical glucocorticoids cause a variety of skin changes, including acneiform eruptions, atrophy, striae, and other stigmata of Cushing's syndrome, and in sufficiently high doses can retard wound healing. Patients using glucocorticoids are at higher risk for bacterial, yeast, and fungal skin infections that may be misinterpreted as drug eruptions but are instead drug side effects.

CYTOKINE THERAPY   Alopecia is a common complication of IFN-α. Induction or exacerbation of various immune-mediated disorders (psoriasis, lichen planus, lupus erythematosus) has been also reported with this agent. IFN-β injection has been associated with local necrosis of the skin. Granulocyte colony stimulating factor may induce various neutrophilic dermatosis, including Sweet's syndrome, pyo-

Table 59-2 Clinical and Laboratory Findings Associated with More Serious Drug-Induced Cutaneous Clinical Findings

Cutaneous
Confluent erythema
Facial edema or central facial involvement
Skin pain
Palpable purpura
Skin necrosis
Blisters or epidermal detachment
Positive Nikolsky's sign
Mucous membrane erosions
Urticaria
Swelling of tongue

General
High fever [temperature >40°C (>104°F)]
Enlarged lymph nodes
Arthralgias or arthritis
Shortness of breath, wheezing, hypotension

Laboratory results
Eosinophil count >1000/μL
Lymphocytosis with atypical lymphocytes
Abnormal liver function tests

SOURCE: Adapted from Roujeau and Stern.

derma gangrenosum, neutrophilic eccrine hidradenitis, and vasculitis, and can exacerbate psoriasis.

IL-2 is associated with frequent cutaneous reactions including exanthema, facial edema, xerosis, and pruritus. Cases of pemphigus vulgaris, linear IgA disease, psoriasis, and vitiligo have also been described in association with this drug.

ANTIMALARIAL AGENTS Antimalarial agents are used as therapy for several skin diseases, including the skin manifestations of lupus and polymorphous light eruption, but they can also induce cutaneous reactions. Although also used to treat porphyria cutanea tarda at low doses, in patients with asymptomatic porphyria cutanea tarda, higher doses of chloroquine increase porphyrin levels to such an extent that they may exacerbate the disease.

Pigmentation disturbances, including black pigmentation of the face, mucous membranes, and pretibial and subungual areas, occur with antimalarials. Quinacrine (mepacrine) causes generalized, cutaneous yellow discoloration.

GOLD Chrysotherapy has been associated with a variety of dose-related dermatologic reactions (including maculopapular eruptions), which can develop as long as 2 years after initiation of therapy and require months to resolve. Erythema nodosum, psoriasiform dermatitis, vaginal pruritus, eruptions similar to those of pityriasis rosea, hyperpigmentation, and lichenoid eruptions resembling those seen with antimalarial agents have been reported. After a cutaneous reaction, it is sometimes possible to reinstitute gold therapy at lower doses without recurrence of the dermatitis.

DIAGNOSIS OF DRUG REACTIONS

Possible causes of an adverse reaction can be assessed as definite, probable, possible, or unlikely based on six variables: (1) previous experience with the drug in the general population, (2) alternative etiologic candidates, (3) timing of events, (4) drug levels or evidence of

Table 59-3 Clinical Features of Selected Severe Cutaneous Reactions Often Induced by Drugs

Diagnosis	Mucosal Lesions	Typical Skin Lesions	Frequent Signs and Symptoms	Alternative Causes not Related to Drugs
Stevens-Johnson syndrome	Erosions usually at ≥two sites	Small blisters on dusky purpuric macules or atypical targets; rare areas of confluence; detachment ≤10% of body surface area	10–30% of cases involve fever	Postinfectious erythema multiforme major (especially in the case of infection with herpes simplex or mycoplasma)
Toxic epidermal necrolysis[a]	Erosions usually at ≥two sites	Individual lesions like those seen in Stevens-Johnson syndrome; confluent erythema; outer layer of epidermis separates readily from basal layer with lateral pressure; large sheet of necrotic epidermis; total detachment of >30% of body surface area	Nearly all cases involve fever, "acute skin failure," leukopenia	
Hypersensitivity syndrome	Infrequent	Severe exanthematous rash (may become purpuric), exfoliative dermatitis	30–50% of cases involve fever, lymphadenopathy, hepatitis, nephritis, carditis, eosinophilia, atypical lymphocytes	Cutaneous lymphoma
Acute generalized exanthematous pustulosis	About 50% erosions mouth, tongue	Initially nonfollicular small pustules overlying edematous erythema, sometimes leading to superficial ulcers	Fever, burning, pruritus, facial swelling, leukocytosis, hypocalcemia	Infection
Serum sickness or reactions resembling serum sickness	Absent	Morbilliform lesions, sometimes with urticaria	Fever, arthralgias	Infection
Anticoagulant-induced necrosis	Infrequent	Erythema then purpura and necrosis, especially of fatty areas	Pain in affected areas	Disseminated intravascular coagulopathy, septicemia
Angioedema	Often involved	Urticaria or swelling of central part of face	Respiratory distress, cardiovascular collapse	Insect stings, foods

[a] Overlap of Stevens-Johnson syndrome and toxic epidermal necrolysis with features of both and attachment of 10 to 30% of body surface area may occur.

SOURCE: Adapted from Roujeau and Stern.

overdose, (5) patient reaction to drug discontinuation, and (6) patient reaction to rechallenge.

PREVIOUS EXPERIENCE Tables of relative reaction rates are available and are useful to assess the likelihood that a given drug is responsible for a given cutaneous reaction. The specific morphologic pattern of a drug reaction, however, may modify these reaction rates by increasing or decreasing the likelihood that a given drug is responsible for a given reaction. For example, since fixed eruptions due to drugs are more often seen with barbiturates than with penicillin, a fixed drug reaction in a patient taking both types of agents is more likely to be due to the barbiturate, even though penicillins have a higher overall drug reaction rate.

ALTERNATIVE ETIOLOGIC CANDIDATES A cutaneous eruption may be due to exacerbation of preexisting disease or to development of new disease unrelated to drugs. For example, a patient with psoriasis may have a flare-up of disease coincidental with administration of penicillin for streptococcal infection; in this case, infection is a more likely cause for the flare-up than drug reaction.

TIMING OF EVENTS Most drug reactions of the skin occur within 1 to 2 weeks of initiation of therapy. Hypersensitivity syndrome may occur later (up to 8 weeks) after initiating drug therapy. Fixed drug reactions and generalized exanthematous pustulosis often occur earlier (within 48 h), as do reactions of all types in persons with prior sensitization to that drug or a cross-sensitizing agent.

DRUG LEVELS Some cutaneous reactions are dependent on dosage or cumulative toxicity. For example, lichenoid dermatoses due to gold administration appear more often in patients taking high doses.

DISCONTINUATION Most adverse cutaneous reactions to drugs remit with discontinuation of the suspected agent. A reaction is considered unlikely to be drug-related if improvement occurs while the drug is continued or if a patient fails to improve after stopping the drug and appropriate therapy.

RECHALLENGE Rechallenge provides the most definitive information concerning adverse cutaneous reactions to drugs, since a reaction failing to recur on rechallenge with a drug is unlikely to be due to that agent. Rechallenge is usually impractical, however, because the need to ensure patient safety and comfort outweighs the value of the possible information derived from rechallenge.

Of special importance is the rapid recognition of reactions that may become serious or life-threatening. Table 59-2 lists clinical and laboratory features that, if present, suggest the reaction may be serious. Table 59-3 provides key features of the most serious adverse cutaneous reactions.

DIAGNOSIS OF DRUG ALLERGY

Tests for IgE responses include in vivo and in vitro methods, but such tests are available for only a limited number of drugs, including penicillins and cephalosporins, some peptide and protein drugs (insulin, xenogeneic sera), and some agents used for general anesthesia. In vivo testing is accomplished by prick puncture and/or by intradermal skin testing. A wheal-and-flare response 2×2 mm greater than that seen with a saline control within 20 min is considered indicative of IgE-mediated mast cell degranulation, provided (1) the patient is not dermographic, (2) the drug does not nonspecifically degranulate mast cells, (3) the drug concentration is not high enough to be irritating, and (4) the buffer itself does not cause wheal-and-flare responses.

Skin testing with major and minor determinants of penicillins or cephalosporins has proved useful for identifying patients at risk of anaphylactic reactions to these agents. However, skin tests themselves carry a small risk of anaphylaxis. Negative skin tests do not rule out IgE-mediated reactivity, and the risk of anaphylaxis in response to penicillin administration in patients with negative skin tests is about 1%; about two-thirds of patients with a positive skin test and history of a previous adverse reaction to penicillin experience an allergic response on rechallenge. Skin tests may be negative in allergic patients

receiving antihistamines or in those whose allergy is to determinants not present in the test reagent. Although less well studied, similar techniques can identify patients who are sensitive to protein drugs and to agents such as gallamine and succinylcholine. Most other drugs are small molecules, and skin testing with them is unreliable.

There are no generally available and reliable tests for assessing causality of non-IgE-mediated reactions, except possibly patch tests for assessment of fixed drug reactions. Therefore, diagnosis usually relies on clinical factors rather than test results.

BIBLIOGRAPHY

BASTUJI-GARIN S et al: Clinical classification of cases of toxic epidermal necrolysis, Stevens-Johnson syndrome, and erythema multiforme. Arch Dermatol 129:92, 1993

BIGBY M et al: Drug-induced cutaneous reactions. A report from the Boston Collaborative Drug Surveillance Program on 15,438 consecutive inpatients, 1975–1982. JAMA 256:3358, 1986

COOPMAN SA et al: Cutaneous disease and drug reactions in HIV infection. N Engl J Med 328:1670, 1993

ROUJEAU JC, STERN RS: Severe adverse cutaneous reactions to drugs. N Engl J Med 331: 1272, 1994

——— et al: Medication use and the risk of Stevens-Johnson syndrome or toxic epidermal necrolysis. N Engl J Med 333:1600, 1995

SCHLIENGER RG et al: Lamotrigine-associated anticonvulsant hypersensitivity syndrome. Neurology 51:1172, 1998

VAN DER LINDEN PD et al: Skin reactions to antibacterial agents in general practice. J Clin Epidemiol 51:703, 1998

VIARD I et al: Inhibition of toxic epidermal necrolysis by blockade of CD95 with human intravenous immunoglobulin. Science 282:490, 1998

60 *David R. Bickers*

PHOTOSENSITIVITY AND OTHER REACTIONS TO LIGHT

SOLAR RADIATION Sunlight is the most visible and obvious source of comfort in the environment. This natural proclivity for the sun has the beneficial results of warmth and vitamin D synthesis but also can produce pathologic consequences. Few effects of sun exposure beyond those affecting the skin have been identified, but cutaneous exposure to sunlight can evoke immunosuppressive responses and genetic changes that may be relevant to the pathogenesis of nonmelanoma skin cancer and perhaps infections such as herpes simplex.

The sun's energy encompasses a broad range from ultrashort highly energetic ionizing radiation (10^{-2} μm) to ultralong radiowaves of very low photon energy (10^7 μm). Thus, the emission spectrum ranges over nine orders of magnitude, but that reaching the earth's surface is narrow and is limited to components of the ultraviolet (UV), visible light, and portions of the infrared. The cutoff at the short end of the UV is at approximately 290 nm, because stratospheric ozone is formed by ionizing radiation of wavelengths less than 100 nm and absorbs solar energy between 120 and 310 nm, thereby preventing penetration to the earth's surface of the shorter, more energetic, potentially more harmful wavelengths of solar radiation. Indeed, concern about destruction of the ozone layer by chlorofluorocarbons released into the atmosphere has led to international agreements to reduce production of these chemicals.

Measurements of solar flux indicate that there is a twentyfold regional variation in the amount of energy at 300 nm that reaches the earth's surface. This variability relates to seasonal effects, the path of sunlight transmission through ozone and air, the altitude (4% increase for each 300 m of elevation), the latitude (increasing intensity with decreasing latitude), and the amount of cloud cover, fog, and pollution.

The major components of the photobiologic action spectrum include the UV and visible wavelengths between 290 and 700 nm. In addition, the wavelengths beyond 700 nm in the infrared primarily evoke heat, but warming of the skin may enhance biologic responses to wavelengths in the UV and visible spectrum.

The UV spectrum is arbitrarily divided into three major segments: C, B, and A. This includes the wavelengths between 10 and 400 nm. Ultraviolet C (UV-C) consists of wavelengths between 10 and 290 nm and does not reach the earth because of its absorption by stratospheric ozone. These wavelengths are not a cause of photosensitivity except in occupational settings where artificial sources of this energy are employed—e.g., for germicidal effects. Ultraviolet B (UV-B) consists of wavelengths between 290 and 320 nm. This portion of the photobiologic action spectrum is the most efficient in producing redness or erythema in human skin and hence is sometimes known as the "sunburn spectrum." Ultraviolet A (UV-A) represents those wavelengths between 320 and 400 nm and is approximately 1000-fold less efficient in producing skin hyperemia than is UV-B. The UV-A has also been divided into two parts known as UV-A 1 (340 to 400 nm) and UV-A 2 (320 to 340 nm).

The visible wavelengths between 400 and 700 nm include the familiar white light which when directed through a prism can be shown to consist of various colors including violet, indigo, blue, green, yellow, orange, and red. The energy possessed by photons in the visible spectrum is not capable of damaging human skin in the absence of a photosensitizing chemical. The absorption of energy is critical to the development of photosensitivity. Thus the *absorption spectrum* of a molecule is defined as the range of wavelengths absorbed by it, whereas the *action spectrum* for an effect of incident radiation is defined as the range of wavelengths that evoke the response.

Photosensitivity occurs when a photon-absorbing chemical (chromophore) present in the skin absorbs incident energy, becomes excited, and transfers the absorbed energy to various structures or to oxygen. The absorbed energy must be dissipated by processes including heat, fluorescence, and phosphorescence. It is important to emphasize that absorption spectra and action spectra need not be superimposable, but there must be overlap at some point to produce photosensitization.

STRUCTURE AND FUNCTION OF SKIN The skin's exposure to sunlight permits the absorption of some wavelengths and the transmission of others. Essentially, human skin is a sandwich of two distinctive compartments, the epidermis and dermis, separated by a basement membrane. The outer epidermis is a stratified squamous epithelium comprising the surface stratum corneum (a protein- and lipid-rich compact membrane), the stratum granulosum, stratum spinosum, and the basal cell layer. The basal cell layer contains a heterogeneous population of cells, a subset of which migrate upward in the process of terminal differentiation that results in the expression of specific keratin genes and the formation of the stratum corneum. Epidermal cells include resident keratinocytes and melanocytes and immigrant cells, including the immunologically active Langerhans cells, lymphocytes, polymorphonuclear leukocytes, monocytes, and macrophages, making the epidermis a major component of the immune system. Branches of sensory nerve endings also reach into this compartment.

The second major component of skin is the dermis, which is relatively large and less densely populated with cells that include fibroblasts, endothelial cells within dermal vessels, and mast cells. Tissue macrophages and sparsely distributed inflammatory cells are also present. All these cells exist within an extracellular matrix of collagen, elastin, and glycosaminoglycans. In contrast to the epidermis, rich vascularization of the dermis allows it to play an important role in temperature regulation and in inflammatory responses to skin injury.

UV RADIATION (UVR) AND SKIN The epidermis and the dermis contain several chromophores capable of interacting with incident solar energy. These interactions include reflection, refraction, absorption, and transmission. The stratum corneum is a major impediment to the transmission of UV-B, and less than 10% of incident wavelengths in this region penetrate the basement membrane. Approximately 3% of radiation below 300 nm, 20% of radiation below 360 nm, and 33% of short visible radiation reaches the basal cell layer in untanned human skin. Proteins and nucleic acids absorb intensely in the short UV-B. In contrast, UV-A 1 and 2 penetrate the epidermis efficiently to reach the dermis, where they likely produce changes in

structural and matrix proteins that contribute to the aged appearance of chronically sun-exposed skin, particularly in individuals of light complexion.

One of the consequences of UV-B absorption by DNA is the production of pyrimidine dimers. These structural changes can be repaired by mechanisms that result in their recognition and excision, and the reestablishment of normal base sequences. The efficient repair of these structural aberrations is crucial, since individuals with defective DNA repair are at high risk for the development of cutaneous cancer. For example, patients with xeroderma pigmentosum, an autosomal recessive disorder, are characterized by variably decreased repair of UV-induced photoproducts, and their skin may develop the xerotic appearance of photoaging as well as basal cell and squamous cell carcinomas and melanoma in the first two decades of life. Studies in mice using knockout gene technology have verified the importance of genes regulating these repair pathways in preventing the development of UV-induced cancer.

Cutaneous Optics and Chromophores Chromophores are endogenous or exogenous chemical components that can absorb physical energy. Endogenous chromophores of skin are of two types: (1) chemicals that are normally present, including nucleic acids, proteins, lipids, and 7-dehydrocholesterol, the precursor of vitamin D; and (2) chemicals, such as porphyrins, synthesized elsewhere in the body that circulate in the bloodstream and diffuse into the skin. Normally, only trace amounts of porphyrins are present in the skin, but in the diseases known as the porphyrias, increased amounts are released into the circulation and are transported to the skin, where they absorb incident energy both in the Soret band around 400 nm (short visible) and to a lesser extent in the red portion of the visible spectrum (580 to 660 nm). This results in structural damage to the skin that may be manifest as erythema, edema, urticaria, or blister formation (Chap. 346).

Acute Effects of Sun Exposure The immediate cutaneous consequences of sun exposure include sunburn and vitamin D synthesis.

Sunburn This very common affliction of human skin is caused by exposure to UVR. Generally speaking, the individual's ability to tolerate sunlight is inversely proportional to his or her melanin pigmentation. Melanin is a complex polymer of tyrosine that functions as an efficient neutral-density filter with broad absorbance within the UV portion of the solar spectrum. Melanin is synthesized in specialized epidermal dendritic cells termed *melanocytes* and is packaged into *melanosomes* that are transferred via dendritic processes into *keratinocytes*, where they provide photoprotection. Sun-induced melanogenesis is a consequence of increased tyrosinase activity in melanocytes that in turn may be due to a combination of eicosanoid and endothelin-1 release. Tolerance of sun exposure is a function of the efficiency of the epidermal-melanin unit and can usually be ascertained by asking an individual two questions: (1) Do you burn after sun exposure? and (2) Do you tan after sun exposure? By the answers to these questions, it is usually possible to divide the population into six skin types varying from type I (always burn, never tan) to type VI (never burn, always tan) (Table 60-1).

There are two general theories about the pathogenesis of the sunburn response. First, the lag phase in time between skin exposure and the development of visible redness (usually 4 to 12 h) suggests an epidermal chromophore that causes delayed production and/or release

Table 60-1 Skin Type and Sunburn Sensitivity

Type	Description
I	Always burn, never tan
II	Always burn, sometimes tan
III	Sometimes burn, sometimes tan
IV	Sometimes burn, always tan
V	Never burn, sometimes tan
VI	Never burn, always tan

of vasoactive mediator(s), or cytokines, that diffuse to the dermal vasculature to evoke vasodilatation. Indeed, UVR stimulates the release of numerous proinflammatory cytokines and nitric oxide by keratinocytes. Second, it is possible that the small amount of incident UV-B radiation (10% or less) that penetrates to the dermis can be absorbed directly by endothelial cells in the vasculature, thereby resulting in vasodilatation. The issue remains unresolved.

The action spectrum for sunburn erythema includes the UV-B and UV-A regions. Photons in the shorter UV-B are at least 1000-fold more efficient than photons in the longer UV-B and the UV-A in evoking the response. However, UV-A may contribute to sunburn erythema at midday when much more UV-A than UV-B is present.

The mechanism of injury remains poorly defined, but the action spectrum for UV-B erythema closely resembles the absorption spectrum for DNA after adjusting for the absorbance of incident energy by the stratum corneum. Apoptotic keratinocytes (so-called sunburn cells) are visible histologically within an hour of exposure and are maximal within 24 h. UV-A is less effective than UV-B in producing sunburn cells. Mast cells may release inflammatory mediators after exposure to UV-B and UV-A. For example, erythema doses of both UV-B and UV-A increase histamine levels in experimentally induced suction blisters of human skin that return to normal after 24 h (before visible erythema has subsided). Prostaglandin E_2 increases to approximately 150% of control levels after 24 h and then diminishes. Since prostaglandins evoke both pain and redness when injected intradermally, their presence in suction blisters after UV-B exposure suggests a role in UV-B erythema. Age-related declines occur in the amount of inflammatory mediators detectable in human skin after UV-B irradiation. UV-A erythema results in few epidermal sunburn cells, but vascular endothelial injury is greater than with UV-B. In addition, there are increased levels of arachidonic acid and of prostaglandins D_2, E_2, and I_2 that peak within 5 to 9 h and then subside before peak redness occurs. Despite evidence for the role of prostaglandins in both UV-B- and UV-A-irradiated skin, administration of nonsteroidal anti-inflammatory drugs is more effective in reducing erythema evoked by UV-B than by UV-A. UV-B also induces cutaneous matrix-degrading metalloproteinases within hours of exposure.

Vitamin D photochemistry Cutaneous exposure to UV-B causes photolysis of epidermal previtamin D_3 (7-dehydrocholesterol) to previtamin D_3, which then undergoes a temperature-dependent isomerization to form the stable hormone vitamin D_3. This compound then diffuses to the dermal vasculature and circulates systemically where it is converted to the functional hormone 1,25-dihydroxy vitamin D_3 [$1,25(OH)_2D_3$]. Vitamin D metabolites from the circulation or those produced in the skin itself can augment epidermal differentiation signaling. Aging substantially decreases the ability of human skin to produce vitamin D_3. This, coupled with the widespread use of sunscreens that filter out UV-B, has led to concern that vitamin D deficiency may become a significant clinical problem in the elderly. Indeed, studies have shown that the use of sunscreens can diminish the production of vitamin D_3 in human skin.

Chronic Effects of Sun Exposure: Nonmalignant The clinical features of photodamaged sun-exposed skin consist of wrinkling, blotchiness, telangiectasia, and a roughened, irregular, "weather-beaten" appearance. Whether these changes, which some refer to as *photoaging* or *dermatoheliosis*, represent accelerated chronologic aging or a separate and distinct process is not clear.

Within chronically sun-exposed epidermis, there is thickening (acanthosis) and morphologic heterogeneity within the basal cell layer. Higher but irregular melanosome content may be present in some keratinocytes, indicating prolonged residence of the cells in the basal cell layer. These structural changes may help to explain the leathery texture and the blotchy discoloration of sun-damaged skin.

The dermis is the major site for sun-associated chronic damage, manifest as a massive increase in thickened irregular masses of tangled elastic fibers resulting from enhanced expression of elastin genes. Collagen fibers are also abnormally clumped in the deeper dermis. Fibroblasts are increased in number and show morphologic signs suggesting activation. Degraded mast cells may be present in the dermis, the relevance of which remains unclear.

These morphologic changes, both gross and microscopic, are features of chronically sun-exposed skin. The chromophore(s), the action spectra, and the specific biochemical events orchestrating these changes are unknown.

Chronic Effects of Sun Exposure: Malignant One of the major known consequences of chronic skin exposure to sunlight is nonmelanoma skin cancer. The two types of nonmelanoma skin cancer are basal cell and squamous cell carcinoma (Chap. 86). There are three major steps for cancer induction: initiation, promotion, and progression. Chronic exposure of animal skin to artificial light sources that mimic solar UVR results in *initiation*, a step whereby structural (mutagenic) changes in DNA evoke an irreversible alteration in the target cell (keratinocyte) that begins the tumorigenic process. Exposure to a tumor initiator is believed to be a necessary but not sufficient step in the malignant process, since initiated skin cells not exposed to tumor promoters do not generally develop tumors. The second stage in tumor development is *promotion*, a multistep process whereby initiated cells are exposed to chemical and physical agents that evoke epigenetic changes that culminate in the clonal expansion of initiated cells and cause the development, over a period of weeks to months, of benign growths known as *papillomas*. Again, using transgenic animals, the importance of UV effects on the expression of additional oncogenes such as *fos* and *jun* in developing papillomas has been demonstrated. UV-B is a *complete carcinogen*, meaning that it can function as both an initiator and a promoter, leading to tumor induction. *Incomplete carcinogens* can initiate tumorigenesis but require additional skin exposure to tumor promoters to elicit tumors. The prototype tumor promoter is the phorbol ester 12-*O*-tetradecanoyl phorbol-13-acetate. Tumor promotion usually requires multiple exposures over time to evoke a neoplasm.

The final step in the malignant process is the conversion of benign precursors into malignant lesions, a process thought to require additional genetic alterations in already transformed cells. Indeed, *ras* gene mutations have been detected in a minority of human nonmelanoma skin cancers. Mutations of the tumor suppressor gene p53 also occur in sun-damaged human skin.

Sun exposure causes nonmelanoma and melanoma cancers of the skin, although the evidence is far more direct for its role in nonmelanoma (basal cell and squamous cell carcinoma) than in melanoma. Approximately 80% of nonmelanoma skin cancers develop on exposed body area, including the face, the neck, and the hands. Men of fair complexion who work outdoors are twice as likely as women to develop these types of cancers. Whites of darker complexions (e.g., Hispanics) have one-tenth the risk of developing such cancers as do light-skinned individuals. Blacks are at lowest risk for all forms of skin cancer. Between 600,000 and 800,000 individuals in the United States develop nonmelanoma skin cancer annually, and the lifetime risk for a white individual to develop such a neoplasm is estimated at approximately 15%. A consensus exists that the incidence of nonmelanoma skin cancer in the population is rising, for reasons that are unclear.

The relationship of sun exposure to melanoma is less clear-cut, but suggestive evidence supports an association. Melanomas occasionally develop by the teenage years, indicating that the latent period for tumor growth is less than that of nonmelanoma skin cancer. Melanomas are among the most rapidly increasing of all human malignancies (Chap. 86). Epidemiologic studies of immigrants of similar ethnic stock indicate that individuals born in one area or who migrated to the same locale before age 10 have higher age-specific melanoma rates than individuals arriving later. It is thus reasonable to conclude that life in a sunny climate from birth or early childhood increases the risk of melanoma. In general, risk does not correlate with cumulative sun exposure but may relate to sequelae of sun exposure in childhood. Thus, a blistering sunburn is associated with a doubling of melanoma risk at the site of the reaction.

Immunologic Effects Exposure to solar radiation influences both local and systemic immune responses. UV-B appears to be most efficient in altering immune responses, likely related to the capacity of such energy to affect antigen presentation in skin by interacting with epidermal Langerhans cells. These bone marrow–derived dendritic cells possess surface markers characteristic of monocytes and macrophages. Following skin exposure to erythema doses of UV-B, Langerhans cells undergo both morphologic and functional changes that result in decreased contact allergic responses when haptens are applied to the irradiated site. This diminished capacity for sensitization is due to the induction of antigen-specific suppressor T lymphocytes. Indeed, while the immunosuppressive effect of irradiation is limited to haptens applied to the irradiated site, the net result is systemic immune suppression to that antigen because of the induction of suppressor T cells.

Higher doses of radiation evoke diminished immunologic responses to antigens introduced either epicutaneously or intracutaneously at sites distant from the irradiated site. These suppressed responses are also associated with the induction of antigen-specific suppressor T lymphocytes and may be mediated by as yet undefined factors that are released from epidermal cells at the irradiated site. The implications of this generalized immune suppression in terms of altered susceptibility to cutaneous cancer or to infection remain to be defined.

It is known that UV-induced tumors in murine skin are antigenic and are rapidly rejected when transplanted into normal syngeneic animals. If the tumors are transplanted into animals previously exposed to subcarcinogenic doses of UV-B, they are not rejected and instead grow progressively in the recipients. This failure of irradiated animals to reject the transplanted tumors is due to the development of T suppressor cells that prevent the rejection response. While the mechanism of suppression of tumor rejection is unknown, such a response might be a critical determinant of cancer risk in human skin.

PHOTOSENSITIVITY DISEASES The diagnosis of photosensitivity requires a careful history to define the duration of the signs and symptoms, the length of time between exposure to sunlight and the development of subjective complaints, and visible changes in the skin. The age of onset also can be a helpful clue; for example, the acute photosensitivity of erythropoietic protoporphyria almost always begins in childhood, whereas the chronic photosensitivity of porphyria cutanea tarda typically begins in the fourth and fifth decades. A history of exposure to topical and systemic drugs and chemicals may provide important information. Many classes of drugs can cause photosensitivity on the basis of either phototoxicity or photoallergy. Fragrances such as musk ambrette that were previously present in numerous cosmetic products are also potent photosensitizers.

Examination of the skin may also offer important clues. Anatomic areas that are naturally protected from direct sunlight such as the hairy scalp, the upper eyelids, the retroauricular areas, and the infranasal and submental regions may be spared, whereas exposed areas show characteristic features of the pathologic process. These anatomic localization patterns are often helpful but not infallible in making the diagnosis. For example, airborne contact sensitizers that are blown onto the skin may produce dermatitis that can be difficult to distinguish from photosensitivity, despite the fact that such material may trigger skin reactivity in areas shielded from direct sunlight.

Many dermatologic conditions may be caused or aggravated by light (Table 60-2). The role of light in evoking these responses may be dependent on genetic abnormalities ranging from well-described defects in DNA repair that occur in xeroderma pigmentosum to the inherited abnormalities in heme synthesis that characterize the porphyrias. In certain photosensitivity diseases, the chromophore has been identified, whereas in the majority, the energy-absorbing agent is unknown.

Polymorphous Light Eruption After sunburn, the most common type of photosensitivity disease is *polymorphous light eruption*, the mechanism of which is unknown. Many affected individuals never seek medical attention because the condition is often transient, becoming manifest each spring with initial sun exposure but then subsiding spontaneously with continuing exposure, a phenomenon known as "hardening." The major manifestations of polymorphous light eruption include pruritic (often intensely so) erythematous papules that may coalesce into plaques on exposed areas of the face and arms or other areas as well, making the distribution spotty and uneven.

The diagnosis can be confirmed by skin biopsy and by performing phototest procedures in which skin is exposed to multiple erythema doses of UV-A and UV-B. The action spectrum for polymorphous light eruption is usually within these portions of the solar spectrum.

Treatment of this disease includes the induction of hardening by the cautious administration of UV light, either alone or in combination with photosensitizers such as the psoralens (see below).

Phototoxicity and Photoallergy These photosensitivity disorders are related to the topical or systemic administration of drugs and other chemicals. Both reactions require the absorption of energy by a drug or chemical resulting in the production of an excited-state photosensitizer that can transfer its absorbed energy to a bystander molecule or to molecular oxygen, thereby generating tissue-destructive chemical species

Phototoxicity is a nonimmunologic reaction caused by drugs and chemicals, a few of which are listed in Table 60-3. The usual clinical manifestations include erythema resembling a sunburn that quickly desquamates or "peels" within several days. In addition, edema, vesicles, and bullae may occur.

Photoallergy is distinct in that the immune system participates in the pathologic process. The excited-state photosensitizer may create

Table 60-2 Classification of Photosensitivity Diseases

Type	Disease
Genetic	Erythropoietic porphyria
	Erythropoietic protoporphyria
	Porphyria cutanea tarda—familial
	Variegate porphyria
	Hepatoerythropoietic porphyria
	Albinism
	Xeroderma pigmentosum
	Rothmund-Thompson disease
	Bloom syndrome
	Cockayne's disease
	Phenylketonuria
Metabolic	Porphyria cutanea tarda—sporadic
	Hartnup disease
	Kwashiorkor
	Pellagra
	Carcinoid syndrome
	Pseudoporphyria
Phototoxic	
Internal	Drugs
External	Drugs, plants, food
Photoallergic	
Immediate	Solar urticaria
Delayed	Drug photoallergy
	Persistent light reaction/chronic actinic dermatitis
Neoplastic and	Photoaging
degenerative	Actinic keratosis
	Melanoma and nonmelanoma skin cancer
Idiopathic	Polymorphous light eruption
	Hydroa aestivale
	Actinic reticuloid
Photoaggravated	Lupus erythematosus
	Systemic
	Subacute cutaneous
	Dermatomyositis
	Pemphigus foliaceus
	Herpes simplex
	Lichen planus actinicus
	Acne vulgaris (aestivale)
	Transient acantholytic dermatosis

Table 60-3   Phototoxic Drugs and Chemicals

	Topical	Systemic
Coal Tar Derivatives		
Acridine	+	
Anthracene	+	
Phenanthrene	+	
Drugs		
Amiodarone		+
Dacarbazine		+
Fluoroquinolones		+
5-Fluorouracil	+	+
Furosemide		+
Nalidixic acid		+
Phenothiazines		+
Psoralens	+	+
Retinoids	+/−	+
Sulfonamides		+
Sulfonylureas		+
Tetracyclines		+
Thiazides		+
Vinblastine		+
Dyes		
Anthraquinone		+
Eosin		+
Methylene blue		+
Rose bengal		+

highly unstable haptenic free radicals that bind covalently to macromolecules to form a functional antigen capable of evoking a delayed hypersensitivity response. Some of the drugs and chemicals that produce photoallergy are listed in Table 60-4. The clinical manifestations typically differ from those of phototoxicity in that an intensely pruritic eczematous dermatitis tends to predominate and evolves into lichenified, thickened, "leathery" changes in sun-exposed areas. A small subset (perhaps 5 to 10%) of patients with photoallergy may develop a persistent exquisite hypersensitivity to light even when the offending drug or chemical is identified and eliminated. Known as *persistent light reaction*, this may be incapacitating for years. Some have used the term *chronic actinic dermatitis* to encompass these chronic hyperresponsive states.

Table 60-4   Photoallergic Drugs and Chemicals

	Topical	Systemic
Antibiotics		
Sulfonamides		+
Antifungals		
Fenticlor	+	
Jadit	+	
Multifungin	+	
Diuretics		
Thiazides		+
Fragrances		
Musk ambrette	+	
6-Methylcoumarin	+	
Plant oleoresins	+	
Halogenated salicylanilides		
Bithionol	+	
Tetrachlorosalicylanilide	+	
Tribromosalicylanilide	+	
Nonsteroidal antiinflammatory agents		
Piroxicam	+	
Phenothiazines		
Chlorpromazine	+	
Promethazine	+	
Sulfonylureas		+
Sunscreens		
p-Aminobenzoic acid and esters	+	
Whitening Agents		
Stilbenes	+	

Diagnostic confirmation of phototoxicity and photoallergy often can be obtained using phototest procedures. In patients with suspected phototoxicity, determination of the minimal erythema dose (MED) while the patient is exposed to a suspected agent and then repeating the MED after discontinuation of the agent may provide a clue to the causative drug or chemical. Photopatch testing can be performed to confirm the diagnosis of photoallergy. This is a simple variant of ordinary patch testing in which a series of known photoallergens is applied to the skin in duplicate and one set is irradiated with a suberythema dose of UV-A. Development of eczematous changes at sites exposed to sensitizer and light is a positive result. The characteristic abnormality in patients with persistent light reaction is a diminished threshold to erythema evoked by UV-B. Patients with chronic actinic dermatitis may have a broad spectrum of UV hyperresponsiveness.

The management of drug photosensitivity is first and foremost to eliminate exposure to the chemical agents responsible for the reaction and to minimize sun exposure. The acute symptoms of phototoxicity may be ameliorated by cool, moist compresses, topical glucocorticoids, and systemically administered nonsteroidal antiinflammatory agents. In severely affected individuals, a rapidly tapered course of systemic glucocorticoids may be useful. Judicious use of analgesics may be necessary.

Photoallergic reactions require a similar management approach. Furthermore, individuals suffering from persistent light reactivity must be meticulously protected against light exposure. In selected patients in whom chronic systemic high-dose glucocorticoids pose unacceptable risks, it may be necessary to employ cytotoxic agents such as azathioprine or cyclophosphamide.

Porphyria   The porphyrias (Chap. 346) are a group of diseases that have in common various derangements in the synthesis of heme. Heme is an iron-chelated tetrapyrrole or porphyrin, and the nonmetal chelated porphyrins are potent photosensitizers that absorb light intensely in both the short (400 to 410 nm) and the long (580 to 650 nm) portions of the visible spectrum.

Heme cannot be reutilized and must be continuously synthesized, and the two body compartments with the largest capacity for its production are the bone marrow and the liver. Accordingly, the porphyrias originate in one or the other of these organs, with the end result of excessive endogenous production of potent photosensitizing porphyrins. The porphyrins circulate in the bloodstream and diffuse into the skin, where they absorb solar energy, become photoexcited, and evoke cutaneous photosensitivity. The mechanism of porphyrin photosensitization is known to be photodynamic or oxygen-dependent and is mediated by reactive oxygen species such as superoxide anions.

Porphyria cutanea tarda is the most common type of human porphyria and is associated with decreased activity of the enzyme uroporphyrinogen decarboxylase associated with a number of gene mutations. There are two basic types of porphyria cutanea tarda: the sporadic or acquired type, generally seen in individuals ingesting ethanol or receiving estrogens; and the inherited type, in which there is autosomal dominant transmission of deficient enzyme activity. Both forms are associated with increased hepatic iron stores.

In both types of porphyria cutanea tarda, the predominant feature is a chronic photosensitivity characterized by increased fragility of sun-exposed skin, particularly areas subject to repeated trauma such as the dorsa of the hands, the forearms, the face, and the ears. The predominant skin lesions are vesicles and bullae that rupture, producing moist erosions, often with a hemorrhagic base, that heal slowly with crusting and purplish discoloration of the affected skin. Hypertrichosis, mottled pigmentary change, and scleroderma-like induration are associated features. Biochemical confirmation of the diagnosis can be obtained by measurement of urinary porphyrin excretion, plasma porphyrin assay, and by assay of erythrocyte and/or hepatic uroporphyrinogen decarboxylase. Multiple mutations of the uroporphyrinogen decarboxylase gene have been identified in human populations, including exon skipping and base substitutions.

Treatment consists of repeated phlebotomies to diminish the excessive hepatic iron stores and/or intermittent low doses of the antimalarial drugs chloroquine and hydroxychloroquine. Long-term remission of the disease can be achieved if the patient eliminates exposure to porphyrinogenic agents.

Erythropoietic protoporphyria originates in the bone marrow and is due to a decrease in the mitochondrial enzyme ferrochelatase secondary to numerous gene mutations. The major clinical features include an acute photosensitivity characterized by subjective burning and stinging of exposed skin that often develops during or just after exposure. There may be associated skin swelling and, after repeated episodes, a waxlike scarring.

The diagnosis is confirmed by demonstration of measurement of free elevated erythrocyte protoporphyrin. Detection of increased plasma protoporphyrin helps to differentiate lead poisoning and iron-deficiency anemia, in both of which elevated erythrocyte protoporphyrin occurs in the absence of cutaneous photosensitivity and of elevated plasma protoporphyrin.

Treatment consists of reducing sun exposure and the oral administration of the carotenoid β-carotene, which is an effective scavenger of free radicals. This drug increases tolerance to sun exposure in many affected individuals, although it has no effect on deficient ferrochelatase.

An algorithm for the approach to a patient with photosensitivity is illustrated in Fig. 60-1.

PHOTOPROTECTION Since photosensitivity of the skin results from exposure to sunlight, it follows that avoidance of the sun would eliminate these disorders. Unfortunately, social pressures make this an impractical alternative for most individuals, and this has led to a search for better approaches to photoprotection.

Natural photoprotection is provided by structural proteins in the epidermis, particularly keratins and melanin. The amount of melanin and its distribution in cells is genetically regulated, and individuals of darker complexion (skin types IV to VI) are at decreased risk for the development of cutaneous malignancy.

Other forms of photoprotection include clothing and sunscreens. Clothing constructed of tightly woven sun-protective fabrics, irrespective of color, affords substantial protection. Wide-brimmed hats, long sleeves, and trousers all reduce direct exposure. Sunscreens are of two major types—chemical and physical. Chemical sunscreens are chromophores that absorb energy in the UV-B and/or UV-A regions, thereby diminishing photon absorption by the skin (Table 60-5). Sunscreens are rated for their photoprotective effect by their *sun protective factor* (SPF). The SPF is simply a ratio of the time required to produce sunburn erythema with and without sunscreen application. SPF ratings of 15 or higher provide effective protection against UV-B and, to a lesser extent, UV-A. The major categories of chemical sunscreens include *p*-aminobenzoic acid and its esters, benzophenones, anthranilates, cinnamates, and salicylates. Physical sunscreens are light-opaque mixtures containing metal particles such as titanium oxide and zinc oxide that scatter light, thereby reducing photon absorption by the skin.

In addition to light absorption, a critical determinant of the photoprotective effect of sunscreens is their ability to remain on the skin, a property known as *substantivity*. In general, the *p*-aminobenzoic acid esters formulated in moisturizing vehicles provide the greatest substantivity.

Photoprotection can also be achieved by limiting the time of exposure during the day. Since the majority of an individual's total lifetime sun exposure may occur by the age of 18, it is important to educate parents and young children about the hazards of sunlight. Simply eliminating exposure at midday will substantially reduce lifetime UV-B exposure.

PHOTOTHERAPY AND PHOTOCHEMOTHERAPY UVR can also be used therapeutically. The administration of UV-B alone or in combination with topically applied agents can induce remissions of psoriasis and atopic dermatitis.

Photochemotherapy in which topically applied or systemically administered *psoralens* are combined with UV-A (PUVA) is also effective in treating psoriasis and in the early stages of cutaneous T cell

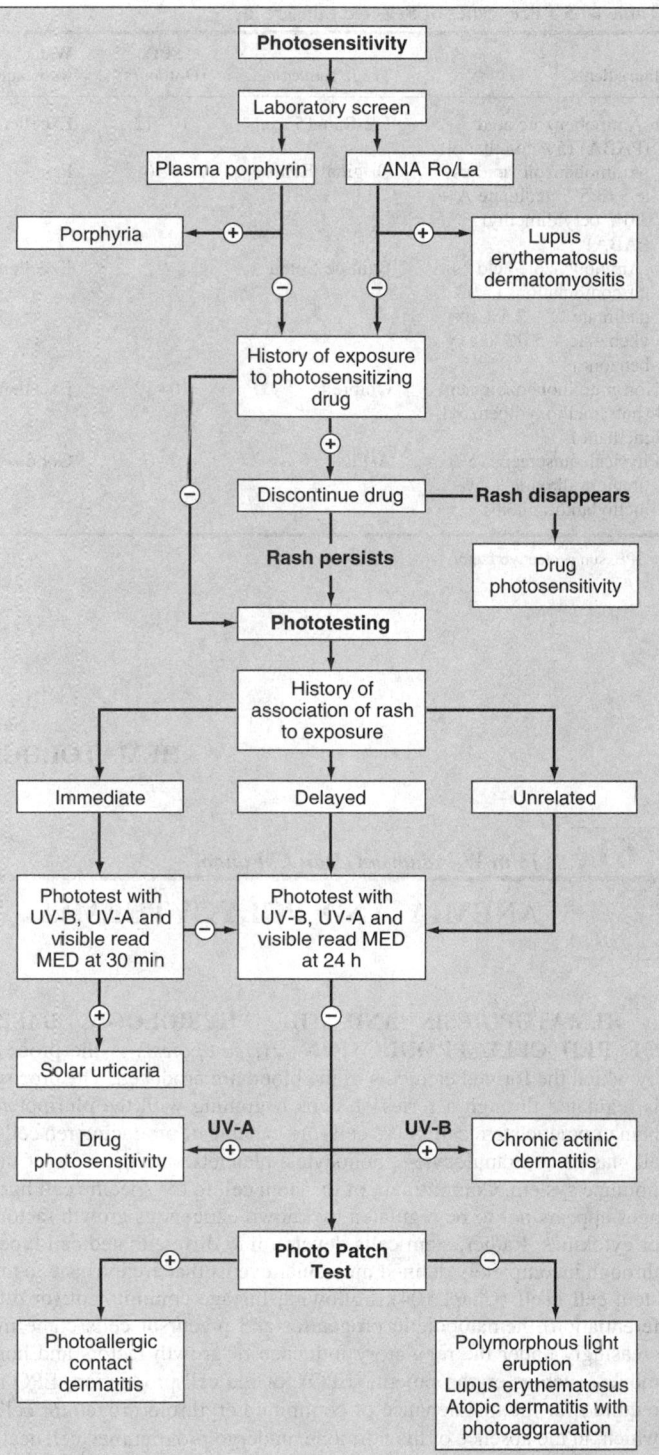

FIGURE 60-1 An algorithm for the diagnosis of a patient with photosensitivity.

lymphoma and vitiligo. Psoralens are tricyclic furocoumarins that, when intercalated into DNA and exposed to UV-A, form adducts with pyrimidine bases and eventually form DNA cross-links. These structural changes are thought to decrease DNA synthesis and relate to improvement that occurs in psoriasis. The reason that PUVA photochemotherapy is effective in cutaneous T cell lymphoma is not clear.

In addition to its effects on DNA, PUVA photochemotherapy also stimulates melanin synthesis, and this provides the rationale for its use in the depigmenting disease vitiligo. Oral 8-methoxypsoralen and UV-A appear to be most effective in this regard, but as many as 100 treat-

Ingredients	Trade Names	SPF[a] (Outdoors)	Water Resistance
p-Aminobenzoic acid (PABA) (5% in ethanol)	Pre-Sun-15	10–12	Excellent
p-Aminobenzoic acid esters (3.5% padimate A + 3.0% octyldimethyl PABA)	Original Eclipse	4–6	Fair
p-Aminobenzoic acid ester combinations (7.0% padimate O + 2.5% oxybenzone + 5.0% dioxybenzone)	Bain de Soleil	9	Excellent
Non-p-aminobenzoic acid (butylmethoxydibenzoyl methane)	Ombrelle	10–12	Excellent
Physical sunscreens (5% titanium dioxide + 5% methylanthranilate)	A-Fil	4–6	Good

[a] SPF, sun protective factor.

ments extending over 12 to 18 months may be required to promote satisfactory repigmentation.

The major side effects of UV-B phototherapy and PUVA photochemotherapy are due to the cumulative effects of photon absorption and include skin dryness, actinic keratoses, and an increased risk of nonmelanoma skin cancer. Despite these risks, the therapeutic index of these modalities is quite acceptable.

BIBLIOGRAPHY

FISHER GJ et al: Molecular basis of sun-induced premature skin aging and retinoid antagonism. Nature 379:335, 1996

GILCHREST BA et al: Mechanisms of ultraviolet light-induced pigmentation. Photochem Photobiol 63:1, 1996

GOULD JW et al: Cutaneous photosensitivity diseases induced by exogenous agents. J Am Acad Dermatol 33:551, 1995

HARBER LC, BICKERS DR: *Photosensitivity Diseases*, 2d ed. Toronto, Decker, 1989

HONIGSMANN H, STINGL G: *Therapeutic Photomedicine*. Basel, Karger, 1986

MAGNUS IA: *Dermatological Photobiology*. Oxford, Blackwell, 1976

PATHAK MA et al: Sun-protective agents: Formulations, effects, and side effects in *Dermatology in General Medicine*, 5th ed, IM Freedberg et al (eds). New York, McGraw-Hill, 1999, Chap. 248

ZIEGLER A et al: Sunburn and p53 in the onset of skin cancer. Nature 372:773, 1994

Section 10
HEMATOLOGIC ALTERATIONS

61

John W. Adamson, Dan L. Longo

ANEMIA AND POLYCYTHEMIA

HEMATOPOIESIS AND THE PHYSIOLOGIC BASIS OF RED CELL PRODUCTION *Hematopoiesis* is the process by which the formed elements of the blood are produced. The process is regulated through a series of steps beginning with the pluripotent hematopoietic stem cell. Stem cells are capable of producing red cells, all classes of granulocytes, monocytes, platelets, and the cells of the immune system. Commitment of the stem cell to the specific cell lineages appears not to be regulated by known exogenous growth factors or cytokines. Rather, stem cells develop into differentiated cell types through incompletely defined molecular events that are intrinsic to the stem cell itself (Chap. 104). Following lineage commitment (or differentiation), hematopoietic progenitor and precursor cells come increasingly under the regulatory influence of growth factors and hormones, such as erythropoietin (EPO) for red cell production. EPO is required for the maintenance of committed erythroid progenitor cells which, in the absence of the hormone, undergo programmed cell death (*apoptosis*). The regulated process of red cell production is *erythropoiesis*, and its key elements are illustrated in Fig. 61-1.

In the bone marrow, the first morphologically recognizable erythroid precursor is the pronormoblast. This cell can undergo 4 to 5 cell divisions that result in the production of 16 to 32 mature red cells. With increased EPO production, or the administration of EPO as a drug, early progenitor cell numbers are amplified and, in turn, give rise to increased numbers of erythrocytes. The regulation of EPO production itself is linked to O_2 transport.

In mammals, O_2 is transported to tissues bound to the hemoglobin contained within circulating red cells. The mature red cell is $8\mu m$ in diameter, anucleate, discoid in shape, and extremely pliable in order for it to traverse the microcirculation successfully; its membrane integrity is maintained by the intracellular generation of ATP. Normal

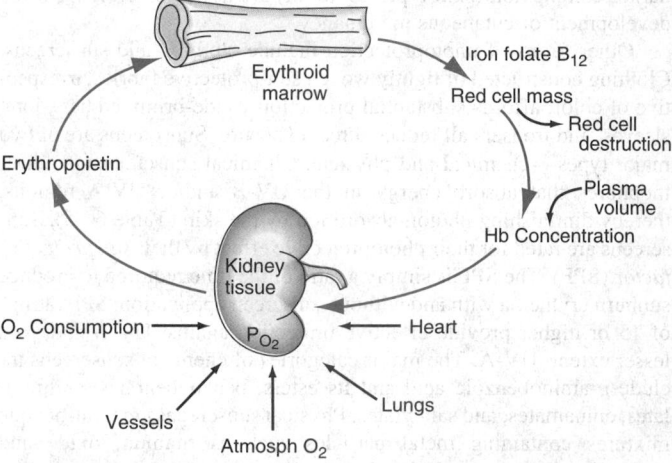

FIGURE 61-1 The physiologic regulation of red cell production by tissue oxygen tension. Hb, hemoglobin.

red cell production results in the daily replacement of 0.8 to 1% of all circulating red cells in the body. The average red cell lives 100 to 120 days. The machinery responsible for red cell production is called the *erythron*. The erythron is a dynamic organ made up of a rapidly proliferating pool of marrow erythroid precursor cells and a large mass of mature circulating red blood cells. The size of the red cell mass reflects the balance of red cell production and destruction. The physiologic basis of red cell production and destruction provides an understanding of the mechanisms that can lead to anemia.

The physiologic regulator of red cell production, the glycoprotein hormone EPO, is produced and released by peritubular capillary lining cells within the kidney. These cells are highly specialized epithelial-like cells. A small amount of EPO is produced by hepatocytes. The fundamental stimulus for EPO production is the availability of O_2 for tissue metabolic needs. Impaired O_2 delivery to the kidney can result from a decreased red cell mass (*anemia*), impaired O_2 loading of the

FIGURE 61-2 The probability that a particular hemoglobin or hematocrit value is abnormal is different in men and women.

hemoglobin molecule (*hypoxemia*), or, rarely, impaired blood flow to the kidney (renal artery stenosis). EPO governs the day-to-day production of red cells, and ambient levels of the hormone can be measured in the plasma by sensitive immunoassays—the normal level being 10 to 25 U/L. When the hemoglobin concentration falls below 100 to 120 g/L (10 to 12 g/dL), plasma EPO levels increase logarithmically in inverse proportion to the severity of the anemia. In circulation, EPO has a half-clearance time of 6 to 9 h. EPO acts by binding to specific receptors on the surface of marrow erythroid precursors, inducing them to proliferate and to mature. Under the stimulus of EPO, red blood cell production can increase four- to fivefold within a 1- to 2-week period but only in the presence of adequate nutrients, especially iron. The functional capacity of the erythron, therefore, requires normal renal production of EPO, a functioning erythroid marrow, and an adequate supply of substrates for hemoglobin synthesis. A defect in any of these key components can lead to anemia. Generally, anemia is recognized in the laboratory when a patient's hemoglobin level or hematocrit is reduced below an expected value (the normal range). The likelihood and severity of anemia are defined based on the deviation of the patient's hemoglobin/hematocrit from values expected for age- and sex-matched normal subjects. The lower ranges of distribution of hemoglobin/hematocrit values for adult males and females are shown in Fig. 61-2. The hemoglobin concentration in adults has a Gaussian distribution. The mean hematocrit value for adult males is 47% ($\pm$ SD 7) and that for adult females is 42% ($\pm$ 5). Any individual hematocrit or hemoglobin value carries with it a likelihood of associated anemia. Thus, a hematocrit of $\leq$39% in an adult male or <35% in an adult female has only about a 25% chance of being normal. Suspected low hemoglobin or hematocrit values are more easily interpreted if there are historic values for the same patient for comparison.

The critical elements of erythropoiesis—EPO production, iron availability, the proliferative capacity of the bone marrow, and effective maturation of red cell precursors—are used for the initial classification of anemia (see "Definition and Classification, below).

ANEMIA

CLINICAL PRESENTATION OF ANEMIA **Signs and Symptoms** Anemia is most often recognized by abnormal screening laboratory tests. Patients only occasionally present with advanced anemia and its attendant signs and symptoms. Acute anemia is nearly always due to blood loss or hemolysis. In fact, with acute blood loss, hypovolemia dominates the clinical picture and the hematocrit and hemoglobin levels do not reflect the volume of blood lost. Signs of vascular instability dominate with acute losses of 10 to 15% of the total blood volume. In such patients, the issue is not anemia but hy-

potension and decreased organ perfusion. When >30% of the blood volume is lost suddenly, patients are unable to compensate with the usual mechanisms of vascular contraction and changes in regional blood flow. The patient prefers to remain supine and will show postural hypotension and tachycardia if upright. If the volume of blood lost is >40% (i.e., >2 L in the average-sized adult), signs of hypovolemic shock including confusion, air hunger, diaphoresis, hypotension, and tachycardia appear (Chap. 108). Such patients have significant deficits in vital organ perfusion and require immediate volume replacement. With mild blood loss, enhanced O_2 delivery is achieved through changes in the O_2-hemoglobin dissociation curve mediated by a decreased pH or increased CO_2 (*Bohr effect*).

With acute hemolytic disease, the signs and symptoms depend on the mechanism that leads to red cell destruction. Intravascular hemolysis with release of free hemoglobin may be associated with acute back pain, free hemoglobin in the plasma and urine, and renal failure. Symptoms associated with more chronic or progressive anemia depend on the age of the patient and the adequacy of blood supply to critical organs. Symptoms associated with moderate anemia include fatigue, loss of stamina, breathlessness, and tachycardia (particularly with physical exertion). However, because of the intrinsic compensatory mechanisms that govern the O_2-hemoglobin dissociation curve, the gradual onset of anemia—particularly in young patients—may not be associated with signs or symptoms until the anemia is severe [hemoglobin <70 to 80 g/L (7 to 8 g/dL)]. When anemia develops over a period of days or weeks, the total blood volume is normal to slightly increased and changes in cardiac output and regional blood flow help compensate for the overall loss in O_2-carrying capacity. Changes in the position of the O_2-hemoglobin dissociation curve account for some of the compensatory response to anemia. With chronic anemia, intracellular levels of 2,3-bisphosphoglycerate (BPG) rise, shifting the dissociation curve to the right and facilitating O_2 unloading. This compensatory mechanism can only maintain normal tissue O_2 delivery in the face of a 20 to 30 g/L (2 to 3 g/dL) deficit in hemoglobin concentration. Finally, further protection of O_2 delivery to vital organs is achieved by the shunting of blood away from organs that are relatively rich in blood supply, particularly the kidney, gut, and skin.

Certain disorders are commonly associated with anemia. Chronic inflammatory states (e.g., infection, rheumatoid arthritis) are associated with mild to moderate anemia, whereas lymphoproliferative disorders, such as chronic lymphocytic leukemia and certain other B cell neoplasms, may be associated with autoimmune hemolysis.

Approach to the Patient

The evaluation of the patient with anemia requires a careful history and physical examination. Historic information that may be useful includes exposure to certain toxic agents or drugs and symptoms related to other disorders commonly associated with anemia. These include symptoms and signs such as bleeding, fatigue, malaise, fever, weight loss, night sweats, and other systemic symptoms. Clues to the mechanisms of anemia may be provided on physical examination by findings of infection, blood in the stool, lymphadenopathy, splenomegaly, or petechiae. Splenomegaly and lymphadenopathy suggest an underlying lymphoproliferative disease, while petechiae suggest platelet dysfunction. If it is uncertain whether a mild anemia represents an extreme normal value or an abnormal finding, past laboratory measurements may be helpful. Nutritional history related to drugs or alcohol intake and family history of anemia should always be assessed. Certain geographic backgrounds and ethnic origins are associated with an increased likelihood of an inherited disorder of the hemoglobin molecule or intermediary metabolism. Glucose-6-phosphate dehydrogenase deficiency and certain hemoglobinopathies are seen more commonly in those of middle-Eastern or African origin.

In the anemic patient, physical examination may demonstrate a forceful heartbeat, strong peripheral pulses, and a systolic "flow" murmur. The skin and mucous membranes may be pale if the hemoglobin is <80 to 100 g/L (8 to 10 g/dL). This part of the physical examination should focus on areas where vessels are close to the surface such as the mucous membranes, nail beds, and palmar creases. If the palmar creases are lighter in color than the surrounding skin when the hand is hyperextended, the hemoglobin level is usually <80 g/L (8 g/dL).

Laboratory Evaluation Table 61-1 lists the tests used in the initial workup of anemia. A routine complete blood count (CBC) is required as part of the evaluation and includes the hemoglobin, hematocrit, and red cell indices: the mean cell volume (MCV) in femtoliters, mean cell hemoglobin (MCH) in picograms per cell, and mean concentration of hemoglobin per volume of red cells (MCHC) in grams per liter (non-SI: grams per deciliter). The red cell indices are calculated as shown in Table 61-2, and the normal variations in the CBC with age are shown in Table A-7. A number of physiologic factors affect the normal CBC values including age, gender, pregnancy, smoking, and altitude. High-normal hemoglobin values may be seen in men and women who live at altitude or smoke heavily. The elevations in smokers reflect normal compensation due to the displacement of O_2 by CO in hemoglobin binding. Other important information is provided by the reticulocyte count and measurements of iron supply including the *serum iron*, the *total iron-binding capacity* (TIBC; an indirect measure of the transferrin level), and *serum ferritin*. Marked alterations in the red cell indices usually reflect disorders of maturation or iron deficiency. Clinical laboratories also provide a description of both the red and white cells, a white cell differential count, and the platelet count. In patients with severe anemia and abnormalities in red blood cell morphology, a bone marrow aspirate or biopsy may be important to assist in the diagnosis. Other tests of value in the diagnosis of specific anemias are discussed in chapters on specific disease states.

The components of the CBC also help in the classification of anemia. *Microcytosis* is reflected by a lower than normal MCV (<80), whereas high values (>100) reflect *macrocytosis*. The MCH and MCHC reflect defects in hemoglobin synthesis (*hypochromia*). Automated cell counters describe the red cell volume distribution width (RDW). The MCV (representing the peak of the distribution curve) is insensitive to the appearance of small populations of macrocytes or microcytes. An experienced laboratory technician will be able to identify minor populations of large or small cells or hypochromic cells before the red cell indices change.

Table 61-1 Laboratory Tests in Anemia Diagnosis

I. Complete blood count (CBC)	II. Reticulocyte count
A. Red blood cell count	III. Iron supply studies
1. Hemoglobin	A. Serum iron
2. Hematocrit	B. Total iron-binding
B. Red blood cell indices	capacity
1. Mean cell volume (MCV)	C. Serum ferritin, marrow
2. Mean cell hemoglobin (MCH)	iron stain
3. Mean cell hemoglobin concentration (MCHC)	IV. Marrow examination
	A. Aspirate
4. Red cell distribution width (RDW)	1. E/G ratio[a]
	2. Cell morphology
C. White blood cell count	3. Iron stain
1. Cell differential	B. Biopsy
2. Nuclear segmentation of neutrophils	1. Cellularity
	2. Morphology
D. Platelet count	
E. Cell morphology	
1. Cell size	
2. Hemoglobin content	
3. Anisocytosis	
4. Poikilocytosis	
5. Polychromasia	

[a] E/G ratio, ratio of erythroid to granulocytic precursors.

Table 61-2 Red Blood Cell Indices

Index	Normal Value
Mean cell volume (MCV) = (hematocrit $\times$ 10)/(red cell count $\times$ 10^6)	90 $\pm$ 8 fL
Mean cell hemoglobin (MCH) = (hemoglobin $\times$ 10)/(red cell count $\times$ 10^6)	30 $\pm$ 3 pg
Mean cell hemoglobin concentration = (hemoglobin $\times$ 10)/hematocrit, or MCH/MCV	33 $\pm$ 2%

Peripheral blood smear The peripheral blood smear provides important information about defects in red cell production. As a complement to the red cell indices, the blood smear also reveals variations in cell size (*anisocytosis*) and shape (*poikilocytosis*). The degree of anisocytosis usually correlates with increases in the RDW or the range of cell sizes. Poikilocytosis suggests a defect in the maturation of red cell precursors in the bone marrow or fragmentation of circulating red cells. The blood smear may also reveal *polychromasia*—red cells that are slightly larger than normal and grayish blue in color on the Wright-Giemsa stain. These cells are reticulocytes that have been prematurely released from the bone marrow, and their color represents residual amounts of ribosomal RNA. These cells appear in circulation in response to EPO stimulation or to architectural damage of the bone marrow (fibrosis, infiltration of the marrow by malignant cells, etc.) that results in their disordered release from the marrow. The appearance of nucleated red cells, Howell-Jolly bodies, target cells, sickle cells, and others may provide clues to specific disorders (**see Plates V-2, 3, 8, 9, 16, 21, 24, 26–28, 39**).

Reticulocyte count An accurate reticulocyte count is key to the initial classification of anemia. Normally, reticulocytes are red cells that have been recently released from the bone marrow. They are identified by staining with a supravital dye that precipitates the residual ribosomal RNA. These precipitates appear as blue or black punctate spots. This residual RNA is metabolized over the first 24 to 36 h of the reticulocyte's lifespan in circulation. Normally, the reticulocyte count ranges from 1 to 2% and reflects the daily replacement of 0.8 to 1.0% of the circulating red cell population. A correctly interpreted reticulocyte count provides a reliable measure of red cell production.

In the initial classification of anemia, the patient's reticulocyte count is compared with the expected reticulocyte response. In general, if the EPO and erythroid marrow responses to moderate anemia [hemoglobin <100 g/L (10 g/dL)] are intact, the red cell production rate increases to two to three times normal within 10 days following the onset of anemia. In the face of established anemia, a reticulocyte response less than two to three times normal indicates an inadequate marrow response.

In order to use the reticulocyte count to estimate marrow response, two corrections are necessary. The first correction adjusts the reticulocyte count based on the reduced number of circulating red cells. With anemia, the percentage of reticulocytes may be increased while the absolute number is unchanged. To correct for this effect, the reticulocyte percentage is multiplied by the ratio of the patient's hemoglobin or hematocrit to the expected hemoglobin/hematocrit for the age and gender of the patient (Table 61-3). This provides an estimate of the

Table 61-3 Calculation of Reticulocyte Production Index

Correction #1 for anemia:

  This correction produces the absolute reticulocyte count

  In a person whose reticulocyte count is 9%, hemoglobin 7.5 g/dL, hematocrit 23%, absolute reticulocyte count = 9 $\times$ (7.5/15)[or $\times$(23/45)] = 4.5%

Correction #2 for longer life of prematurely released reticulocytes in the blood:

  This correction produces the reticulocyte production index

  In a person whose reticulocyte count is 9%, hemoglobin 7.5 gm/dL, hematocrit 23%, reticulocyte production index

$$= 9 \times \frac{(7.5/15)(\text{hemoglobin correction})}{2 \ (\text{maturation time correction})} = 2.25$$

absolute reticulocyte count. In order to convert the corrected reticulocyte count to an index of marrow production, a further correction is required, depending on whether some of the reticulocytes in circulation have been released from the marrow prematurely. For this second correction, the peripheral blood smear is examined to see if there are polychromatophilic macrocytes present. These cells, representing prematurely released reticulocytes, are referred to as "shift" cells, and the relationship between the degree of shift (and the necessary shift correction factor) is shown in Fig. 61-3. The correction is necessary because these prematurely released cells survive as reticulocytes in circulation for >1 day, thereby providing a falsely high estimate of daily red cell production. If polychromasia is increased, the reticulocyte count, already corrected for anemia, should be divided again by a factor of 2 to account for the prolonged reticulocyte maturation time. The second correction factor varies from 1 to 3 depending upon the severity of anemia. In general, a correction of 2 is commonly used. An appropriate correction is shown in Table 61-3. If polychromatophilic cells are not seen on the blood smear, the second correction is not required. The now doubly corrected reticulocyte count is the *reticulocyte production index*, and it provides an estimate of marrow production relative to normal.

Premature release of reticulocytes is normally due to increased EPO stimulation. However, if the integrity of the bone marrow release process is lost through tumor infiltration, fibrosis, or other disorders, the appearance of nucleated red cells or polychromatophilic macrocytes should still invoke the second reticulocyte correction. The shift correction should always be applied to a patient with anemia and a very high reticulocyte count to provide a true index of effective red cell production. Patients with severe chronic hemolytic anemia may increase red cell production as much as six- to sevenfold. This measure alone, therefore, confirms the fact that the patient has an appropriate EPO response, a normally functioning bone marrow, and sufficient iron available to meet the demands for new red cell formation. If the reticulocyte production index is <2 in the face of established anemia, a defect in erythroid marrow proliferation or maturation must be present.

Tests of iron supply and storage The laboratory measurements that reflect the availability of iron for hemoglobin synthesis include the serum iron, the TIBC, and the percent transferrin saturation. The percent transferrin saturation is derived by dividing the serum iron level ($\times$ 100) by the TIBC. The normal serum iron ranges from 9 to 27 μmol/L (50 to 150 μg/dL), while the normal TIBC is 54 to 64 μmol/L (300 to 360 μg/dL); the transferrin saturation ranges from 25 to 50%. A diurnal variation in the serum iron leads to a variation in the percent transferrin saturation. The serum ferritin is used to evaluate

total-body iron stores. Adult males have serum ferritin levels that average about 100 μg/L, corresponding to iron stores of about 1 g. Adult females have lower serum ferritin levels averaging 30 μg/L, reflecting lower iron stores. A serum ferritin level of 10 to 15 μg/L represents depletion of body iron stores. However, ferritin is also an acute-phase reactant and, in the presence of acute or chronic inflammation, may rise severalfold above baseline levels. As a rule, a serum ferritin >200 μg/L means there is at least some iron in tissue stores.

Bone marrow examination A bone marrow aspirate and smear or a needle biopsy may be useful in the diagnosis of a marrow disorder such as myelofibrosis, a red cell maturation defect, or an infiltrative disease (**Plates V-5, 13–15, 19, 29, 33**). The increase or decrease of one cell lineage (myeloid vs. erythroid) compared to another is obtained by a differential count of nucleated cells in a bone marrow smear [the erythroid/granulocytic (E/G) ratio]. A patient with a hypoproliferative anemia (see below) and a reticulocyte production index <2 will demonstrate an E/G ratio of 1:2 or 1:3. In contrast, patients with hemolytic disease and a production index >3 will have an E/G ratio of at least 1:1. Maturation disorders are identified from the discrepancy between a high E/G ratio and a low reticulocyte production index (see below). Either the marrow smear or biopsy can be stained for the presence of iron stores or iron in developing red cells. The storage iron is in the form of *ferritin* or *hemosiderin*. On carefully prepared bone marrow smears, small ferritin granules can normally be seen in 10 to 20% of developing erythroblasts. Such cells are called *sideroblasts*.

Other laboratory measurements Additional laboratory tests may be of value in confirming specific diagnoses. →*For details of these tests and how they are applied in individual disorders, see Chaps. 105 to 109.*

DEFINITION AND CLASSIFICATION OF ANEMIA

Initial Classification of Anemia Classifying an anemia according to the functional defect in red cell production helps organize the subsequent use of laboratory studies. The three major classes of anemia are: (1) marrow production defects (*hypoproliferation*), (2) red cell maturation defects (*ineffective erythropoiesis*), and (3) decreased red cell survival (*blood loss/hemolysis*). This functional classification of anemia then guides the selection of specific clinical and laboratory studies designed to complete the differential diagnosis and to plan appropriate therapy. The classification is shown in Fig. 61-4. A hypoproliferative anemia is typically seen with a low reticulocyte production index together with little or no change in red cell morphology (a normocytic, normochromic anemia) (Chap. 105). Maturation disorders typically have a slight to moderately elevated reticulocyte production index that is accompanied by either macrocytic (Chap. 107) or microcytic (Chaps. 105, 106) red cell indices. Increased red blood cell destruction secondary to hemolysis results in an increase in the reticulocyte production index to at least three times normal (Chap. 108), provided sufficient iron is available for hemoglobin synthesis. Hemorrhagic anemia does not typically result in production indices of more than 2.5 times normal because of the limitations placed on expansion of the erythroid marrow by iron availability.

In the first branch point of the classification of anemia, a reticulocyte production index >2.5 indicates that hemolysis is most likely. A reticulocyte production index of <2 indicates either a hypoproliferative anemia or maturation disorder. The latter two possibilities can often be distinguished by the red cell indices, by examination of the peripheral blood smear, or by a marrow examination. If the red cell indices are normal, the anemia is almost certainly hypoproliferative in nature. Maturation disorders are characterized by ineffective red cell production and a low reticulocyte production index with bizarre red cell shapes—macrocytes or hypochromic microcytes on the peripheral blood smear. With a hypoproliferative anemia, no erythroid hyperpla-

Hematocrit (%)	Marrow normoblasts and reticulocytes (days)	Peripheral blood reticulocytes (days)
45	3.5	1.0
35	3.0	1.5
25	2.5	2.0
15	1.5	2.5

"SHIFT" correction factor

FIGURE 61-3 Correction of reticulocyte count based upon level of anemia and the circulatory life span of prematurely released reticulocytes. Erythroid cells take about 4.5 days to mature. At normal hematocrit levels, they are released to the circulation with about 1 day left as reticulocytes. However, with different levels of anemia, erythroid cells are released from the marrow prematurely. Most patients come to clinical attention with hematocrits in the mid-20s and thus, a correction factor of 2 is commonly used because the observed reticulocytes will live for 2 days in the circulation before losing their RNA.

FIGURE 61-4 The physiologic classification of anemia. CBC, complete blood count.

sia is noted in the marrow, whereas patients with ineffective red cell production have erythroid hyperplasia and an E/G ratio $\geq$1:1.

Hypoproliferative Anemias   At least 75% of all cases of anemia are hypoproliferative in nature. A hypoproliferative anemia reflects absolute or relative marrow failure in which the erythroid marrow has not proliferated appropriately for the degree of anemia. The majority of hypoproliferative anemias are due to mild to moderate iron deficiency or inflammation. A hypoproliferative anemia can result from marrow damage, iron deficiency, or inadequate EPO stimulation. The last may reflect impaired renal function, suppression of EPO production by inflammatory cytokines such as interleukin 1, or reduced tissue needs for O_2 from metabolic disease such as hypothyroidism. Only occasionally is the marrow unable to produce red cells at a normal rate, and this is most prevalent in patients with renal failure. In general, hypoproliferative anemias are characterized by normocytic, normochromic red cells, although microcytic, hypochromic cells may be observed with mild iron deficiency or long-standing chronic inflammatory disease. The key laboratory tests in distinguishing between the various forms of hypoproliferative anemia include the serum iron and iron-binding capacity, evaluation of renal and thyroid function, a marrow biopsy or aspirate to detect marrow damage or infiltrative disease, and serum ferritin to assess iron stores. Occasionally, an iron stain of the marrow will be needed to determine the pattern of iron distribution. Patients with the anemia of acute or chronic inflammation show a distinctive pattern of serum iron (low), TIBC (normal or low), percent transferrin saturation (low), and serum ferritin (normal or high). A distinct pattern of results is noted in mild to moderate iron deficiency (low serum iron, high TIBC, low percent transferrin saturation, low serum ferritin) (Chap. 105). Marrow damage by a drug, infiltrative disease such as leukemia or lymphoma, or marrow aplasia can usually be diagnosed from the peripheral blood and bone marrow morphology. With infiltrative disease or fibrosis, a marrow biopsy will likely be required.

Maturation Disorders   The presence of anemia with an inappropriately low reticulocyte production index, macro- or microcytosis on smear, and abnormal red cell indices suggests a maturation disorder. Maturation disorders are divided into two categories: nuclear maturation defects, associated with macrocytosis and abnormal marrow development, and cytoplasmic maturation defects, associated with microcytosis and hypochromia usually from defects in hemoglobin production. The low reticulocyte production index is a reflection of the ineffective erythropoiesis that results from the destruction within the marrow of developing erythroblasts. Marrow morphology shows an E/G ratio of $\geq$ 1:1, diagnostic of erythroid hyperplasia.

Nuclear maturation defects result from vitamin B_{12} or folic acid deficiency, drug damage, or myelodysplasia. Drugs that interfere with cellular DNA metabolism, such as methotrexate or alkylating agents, can produce a nuclear maturation defect. Alcohol, alone, is also capable of producing macrocytosis and a variable degree of anemia, but this is usually associated with coincident folic acid deficiency. Measurements of folic acid and vitamin B_{12} are key not only in identifying the specific vitamin deficiency but also because they reflect different pathogenetic mechanisms.

Cytoplasmic maturation defects result from severe iron deficiency or abnormalities in globin or heme synthesis. Iron deficiency occupies an unusual position in the classification of anemia. If the iron-deficiency anemia is mild to moderate, erythroid marrow proliferation is decreased and the anemia is classified as hypoproliferative. However, if the anemia is severe and prolonged, the erythroid marrow will become hyperplastic despite the inadequate iron supply, and the anemia will be classified as ineffective erythropoiesis with a cytoplasmic maturation defect. In either case, a reduced reticulocyte production index, microcytosis, and a classic pattern of iron values make the diagnosis clear and easily distinguish iron deficiency from other cytoplasmic maturation defects such as the thalassemias. Defects in heme synthesis, in contrast to globin synthesis, are less common and may be acquired or inherited (Chap. 346). Acquired abnormalities are usually associated with myelodysplasia, may lead to either a macro- or microcytic anemia, and are frequently associated with mitochondrial iron loading. In these cases, iron is taken up by the mitochondria of the developing erythroid cell but not incorporated into heme. The iron-encrusted mitochondria surround the nucleus of the erythroid cell, forming a ring. Based on the distinctive finding of so-called ringed sideroblasts on the marrow iron stain (**see Plate V-37**), patients are diagnosed as having a sideroblastic anemia—almost always reflecting myelodysplasia. Again, studies of iron parameters are helpful in the differential diagnosis and management of these patients.

Blood Loss/Hemolytic Anemia   In contrast to anemias associated with an inappropriately low reticulocyte production index, blood loss or hemolysis is associated with red cell production indices of $\geq$2.5 times normal. The stimulated erythropoiesis is reflected in the blood smear by the appearance of increased numbers of polychromatophilic macrocytes. A marrow examination is rarely indicated if the reticulocyte production index is increased appropriately. The red cell indices are typically normocytic or slightly macrocytic, reflecting the increased number of reticulocytes. Acute blood loss is not associated with an increased reticulocyte production index because of the time required to increase EPO production and, subsequently, marrow proliferation. Subacute blood loss may be associated with modest reticulocytosis because iron is lost along with the red cells. Anemia from chronic blood loss more often presents as iron deficiency than with the picture of increased red cell production.

The evaluation of blood loss anemia is usually not difficult. Most problems arise when a patient presents with an increased red cell production index from an episode of acute blood loss that went unrecognized. The cause of the anemia and increased red cell production may not be obvious. The confirmation of a recovering state may require observations over a period of 2 to 3 weeks, during which the hemoglobin concentration will be seen to rise and the reticulocyte production index fall.

Hemolytic disease, while dramatic, is among the least common forms of anemia. The ability to sustain a high reticulocyte production index reflects the ability of the erythroid marrow to compensate for hemolysis and the efficient recycling of iron from the destroyed red cells to support new hemoglobin synthesis. The level of response will depend on the severity of the anemia and the nature of the underlying disease process.

Hemolytic anemias present in different ways. Some appear suddenly as an acute, self-limited episode of intravascular or extravascular hemolysis, a presentation pattern often seen in patients with autoimmune hemolysis or with inherited defects of the Embden-Myerhof pathway or the glutathione reductase pathway. Patients with inherited disorders of the hemoglobin molecule or red cell membrane generally have a lifelong clinical history typical of the disease process. Those with chronic hemolytic disease, such as hereditary spherocytosis, may actually present not with anemia but with a complication stemming from the prolonged increase in red cell destruction such as aplastic crisis, symptomatic bilirubin gallstones, or splenomegaly.

The differential diagnosis of an acute or chronic hemolytic event requires the careful integration of family history, pattern of clinical presentation, and a number of highly specific laboratory studies (Chap. 108). Some of the more common congenital hemolytic anemias may be identified from the red cell morphology, a routine laboratory test such as hemoglobin electrophoresis, or a screen for red cell enzymes. Acquired defects in red cell survival are often immunologically mediated and require the immunoglobulin test or a cold agglutinin titer to detect the presence of hemolytic antibodies or complement-mediated red cell destruction.

TREATMENT An overriding principle is to not initiate treatment of mild to moderate anemia without a specific diagnosis. Rarely, in the acute setting, anemia may be so severe that red cell transfusions are required before a specific diagnosis is made. Whether the anemia is of acute or gradual onset, the selection of the appropriate treatment is determined by the documented cause(s) of the anemia. Often, the cause of the anemia may be multifactorial. For example, a patient with severe rheumatoid arthritis who has been taking anti-inflammatory drugs may have a hypoproliferative anemia associated with chronic inflammation as well as chronic blood loss associated with intermittent gastrointestinal bleeding. In every circumstance, it is important to evaluate the patient's iron status fully before and during the treatment of any anemia.→*Transfusion is discussed in Chap. 114; iron therapy is discussed in Chap. 105; treatment of megaloblastic anemia is discussed in Chap. 107; treatment of other entities is discussed in their respective chapters (sickle cell anemia, Chap. 106; hemolytic anemias, Chap. 108; aplastic anemia and myelodysplasia, Chap. 109).*

Therapeutic options for the treatment of anemias have expanded dramatically during the past 25 years. Blood component therapy is available and safe. Recombinant EPO as an adjunct to anemia management has transformed the lives of patients with chronic renal failure on dialysis. Improvements in the management of sickle cell crises and sickle cell anemia have also occurred. Eventually, patients with inherited disorders of globin synthesis or mutations in the globin gene, such as sickle cell disease, may benefit from the successful introduction of targeted genetic therapy (Chap. 69).

POLYCYTHEMIA

Polycythemia is defined as an increase in circulating red blood cells above normal. This increase may be real or only apparent (spurious or relative) because of a decrease in plasma volume. The term *erythrocytosis* may be used interchangeably with polycythemia, but some draw a distinction between them; erythrocytosis implies documentation of increased red cell mass, whereas polycythemia refers to any increase in red cells. Often patients with polycythemia are detected through an incidental finding of elevated hemoglobin or hematocrit levels. Concern that the hemoglobin level may be abnormally high is usually triggered at 170 g/L (17 g/dL) for men and 150 g/L (15 g/dL)

for women. Hematocrit levels >50% in men or >45% in women may be abnormal. Hematocrits >60% in men and >55% in women are almost invariably associated with increased red cell mass.

Historic features useful in the differential diagnosis include smoking history; living at high altitude; or a history of congenital heart disease, peptic ulcer disease, sleep-apnea, chronic lung disease, or renal disease.

Patients with polycythemia may be asymptomatic or experience symptoms related to the increased red cell mass or an underlying disease process that leads to increased red cell production. The dominant symptoms from increased red cell mass are thrombotic (both venous and arterial), because the blood viscosity increases logarithmically at hematocrits >55%. Manifestations range from digital ischemia to Budd-Chiari syndrome with hepatic vein thrombosis. Abdominal thromboses are particularly common. Neurologic symptoms such as vertigo, tinnitus, headache, and visual disturbances may occur. Hypertension is often present. Patients with *polycythemia vera* may have aquagenic pruritus and symptoms related to hepatosplenomegaly. Patients may have easy bruising, epistaxis, or bleeding from the gastrointestinal tract. Patients with hypoxemia may develop cyanosis on minimal exertion or have headache, impaired mental acuity, and fatigue.

The physical examination usually reveals a ruddy complexion. Splenomegaly favors polycythemia vera as the diagnosis (Chap. 110). The presence of cyanosis or evidence of a right-to-left shunt suggests congenital heart disease presenting in the adult, particularly tetralogy of Fallot or Eisenmerger syndrome (Chap. 234). Increased blood viscosity raises pulmonary artery pressure; hypoxemia can lead to increased pulmonary vascular resistance. Together these factors can produce cor pulmonale.

Polycythemia can be spurious (related to a decrease in plasma volume; Gaisbock's syndrome), primary, or secondary in origin. The secondary causes are all associated with increases in EPO levels: either a physiologically adapted appropriate elevation based upon tissue hypoxia (lung disease, high altitude, CO poisoning, high-affinity hemoglobinopathy) or an abnormal overproduction (renal disease, tumors with ectopic EPO production). A rare familial form of polycythemia is associated with normal EPO levels but mutations producing hyperresponsive EPO receptors.

Approach to the Patient

As shown in Fig. 61-5, the first step is to document the presence of an increased red cell mass using the principle of isotope dilution by administering ^{51}Cr-labeled autologous red blood cells to the patient and sampling blood radioactivity over a 2-h period. If the red cell mass is normal (<36 mL/kg in men, <32 mL/kg in women), the patient has spurious polycythemia. If the red cell mass is increased (>36 mL/kg in men, >32 mL/kg in women), serum EPO levels should be measured. If EPO levels are low or absent, the patient most likely has polycythemia vera. Ancillary tests that support this diagnosis include elevated white blood cell count, increased absolute basophil count, thrombocytosis, elevated leukocyte alkaline phosphatase levels, and elevated serum vitamin B_{12} and vitamin B_{12}-binding protein levels.

If serum EPO levels are elevated, one attempts to distinguish whether the elevation is a physiologic response to hypoxia or is related to autonomous production. Patients with low arterial O_2 saturation (<92%) should be further evaluated for the presence of heart or lung disease, if they are not living at high altitude. Patients with normal O_2 saturation who are smokers may have elevated EPO levels because of CO displacement of O_2. If carboxyhemoglobin (COHb) levels are high, the diagnosis is smoker's polycythemia. Such patients should be urged to stop smoking. Those who cannot stop smoking require phlebotomy to control their polycythemia. Patients with normal O_2 saturation who do not smoke either have an abnormal hemoglobin that does not deliver O_2 to the tissues (evaluated by finding elevated O_2-hemoglobin

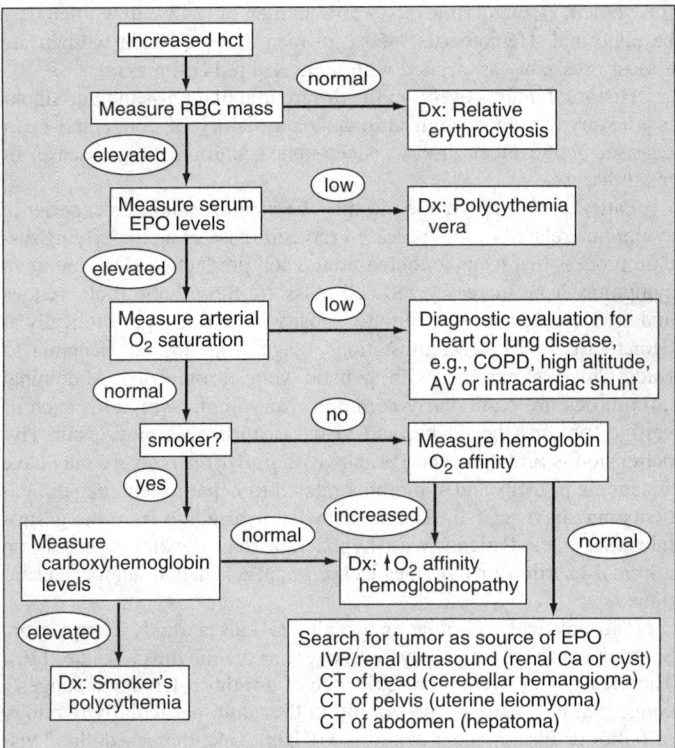

FIGURE 61-5 An approach to diagnosing patients with polycythemia. RBC, red blood cell; EPO, erythropoietin; COPD, chronic obstructive pulmonary disease; AV, atrioventricular; IVP, intravenous pyelogram; CT, computed tomography.

affinity) or have a source of EPO production that is not responding to the normal feedback inhibition. Further workup is dictated by the differential diagnosis of EPO-producing neoplasms. Hepatoma, uterine leiomyoma, and renal disease or cysts are all detectable with abdominopelvic computed tomography scans. Cerebellar hemangiomas may produce EPO, but they nearly always present with localizing neurologic signs and symptoms rather than polycythemia-related symptoms.

ACKNOWLEDGMENT
Dr. Robert S. Hillman wrote this chapter in the 14th edition, and elements of his chapter were retained here.

BIBLIOGRAPHY

HILLMAN RS, AULT KA: *Hematology in Clinical Practice.* New York, McGraw-Hill, 1998

62   *Robert I. Handin*

BLEEDING AND THROMBOSIS

Hemorrhage, intravascular thrombosis, and embolism are common clinical manifestations of many diseases. The normal hemostatic system limits blood loss by precisely regulated interactions between components of the vessel wall, blood platelets, and plasma proteins. However, when disease or trauma damages large arteries and veins, excessive bleeding may occur, despite a normal hemostatic system. Less frequently, hemorrhage is caused by an inherited or acquired disorder of the hemostatic machinery itself. A large number of such bleeding disorders have been identified.

In addition, unregulated activation of the hemostatic system may cause thrombosis and embolism, which can reduce blood flow to critical organs such as the brain and myocardium. Although we understand less about the pathophysiology of thrombosis than of hemostatic failure, certain patient groups have been identified that are particularly prone to thrombosis and embolism. These include patients who (1) are immobilized after surgery, (2) have chronic congestive heart failure, (3) have atherosclerotic vascular disease, (4) have a malignancy, or (5) are pregnant. Most of these "thrombosis-prone" patients have inherited or acquired "hypercoagulable" or "prethrombotic" disorders.

Certain information in the patient's history, such as the mode of onset and sites of bleeding, a family bleeding tendency, and a record of drug ingestion, helps establish the correct diagnosis. Physical examination can identify bleeding in the skin or joint deformities due to previous hemarthroses. Ultimately, however, bleeding disorders are diagnosed by laboratory tests. General screening tests are used first, to document a systemic disorder, and are then supplemented by specific tests of coagulation protein or platelet function to arrive at an accurate diagnosis.

The hypercoagulable or prethrombotic patient can also be identified by a careful history. Three important clues to this diagnosis are: (1) repeated episodes of thromboembolism without an obvious predisposing condition, (2) a family history of thrombosis, and (3) well-documented thromboembolism in adolescents and young adults. All of the known inherited prethrombotic disorders can be diagnosed with specific immunologic, functional, and, in some cases, genetic tests.

NORMAL HEMOSTASIS

Accurate diagnosis and treatment of patients with either bleeding or thrombosis require knowledge of the pathophysiology of hemostasis. The process can be divided into primary and secondary components and is initiated when trauma, surgery, or disease disrupts the vascular endothelial lining and blood is exposed to subendothelial connective tissue. *Primary hemostasis* is the name given to the process of platelet plug formation at sites of injury. It occurs within seconds of injury and is of prime importance in stopping blood loss from capillaries, small arterioles, and venules (Fig. 62-1). *Secondary hemostasis* consists of the reactions of the plasma coagulation system that result in fibrin formation. It requires several minutes for completion. The fibrin strands that are produced strengthen the primary hemostatic plug. This

FIGURE 62-1 Schematic presentation of the major events in primary hemostasis. The first event is platelet adhesion, the interaction of platelets with a nonplatelet surface such as vascular subendothelium. This is followed by platelet activation and secretion. Some of the products secreted by platelets are depicted. Abbreviations: ADP, adenosine diphosphate; PDGF, platelet-derived growth factor; vWF, von Willebrand factor. The final event is the binding of activated platelets to the adherent monolayer in the process of platelet aggregation.

reaction is particularly important in larger vessels and prevents bleeding from recurring hours or days after the injury. Although presented here as separate events, primary and secondary hemostasis are closely linked. For example, activated platelets accelerate plasma coagulation, and products of the plasma coagulation reaction, such as thrombin, induce platelet activation.

Effective primary hemostasis requires three critical events—platelet adhesion, granule release, and platelet aggregation. Within a few seconds of injury, platelets adhere to collagen fibrils in vascular subendothelium via a specific platelet collagen receptor, glycoprotein Ia/IIa, which is a member of the integrin family. As shown in Fig. 62-2, this interaction is stabilized by the von Willebrand factor, an adhesive glycoprotein that allows platelets to remain attached to the vessel wall despite the high shear forces generated within the vascular lumen. The von Willebrand factor accomplishes this task by forming a link between a platelet receptor site on glycoprotein Ib/IX and subendothelial collagen fibrils. The adherent platelets then release preformed granule constituents and generate de novo mediators like those depicted in Fig. 62-1.

As in other cells, platelet activation and secretion are regulated by changes in the level of cyclic nucleotides, the influx of calcium, hydrolysis of membrane phospholipids, and phosphorylation of critical intracellular proteins. The relevant pathways are depicted in Figs. 62-3 and 62-4. The binding of agonists such as epinephrine, collagen, or thrombin to platelet surface receptors activates two membrane enzymes—phospholipase C and phospholipase A_2. These enzymes catalyze the release of arachidonic acid from two of the major membrane phospholipids, phosphatidylinositol and phosphatidylcholine. Initially, a small quantity of the released arachidonic acid is converted to thromboxane A_2 (TXA_2), which, in turn, can activate phospholipase C. The formation of TXA_2 from arachidonic acid is mediated by the enzyme cyclooxygenase (Fig. 62-3). This enzyme is inhibited by aspirin and nonsteroidal anti-inflammatory drugs. Inhibition of TXA_2 synthesis is a cause of mild bleeding in some patients and is the same way some antithrombotic drugs work.

Hydrolysis of the membrane phospholipid phosphatidylinositol 4,5-bisphosphate produces diacylglycerol (DAG) and inositol triphosphate (IP_3), both of which play critical roles in platelet metabolism. IP_3 mediates the movement of calcium into the platelet cytosol and stimulates the phosphorylation of myosin light chains. The latter interact with actin to facilitate granule movement and platelet shape change. DAG activates protein kinase C, which, in turn, phosphorylates several substrates, including myosin light chain kinase and a 47-

FIGURE 62-3 Generation of thromboxane A_2 in platelets and prostacyclin (PGI_2) in endothelial cells.

kDa protein (plekstrin). Phosphorylation of these or other proteins may regulate platelet granule secretion.

A finely balanced mechanism controls the rate and extent of platelet activation (Fig. 62-3). TXA_2, a platelet product of arachidonic acid, stimulates platelet activation and secretion. In contrast, prostacyclin, an endothelial cell product of arachidonic acid metabolism, inhibits platelet activation by raising intraplatelet levels of cyclic adenosine monophosphate.

Following activation, platelets secrete their granule contents into

FIGURE 62-2 The molecular basis of platelet adhesion and aggregation. Adhesion of platelets to vascular subendothelium is facilitated by von Willebrand factor, which forms a bridge between collagen fibrils in the vessel wall and receptors on platelet glycoprotein Ib/IX (GpIb–IX). In a similar manner, platelet aggregation is mediated by fibrinogen, which links adjacent platelets via receptors on the platelet glycoprotein IIb and IIIa complex (GpIIb–IIIa).

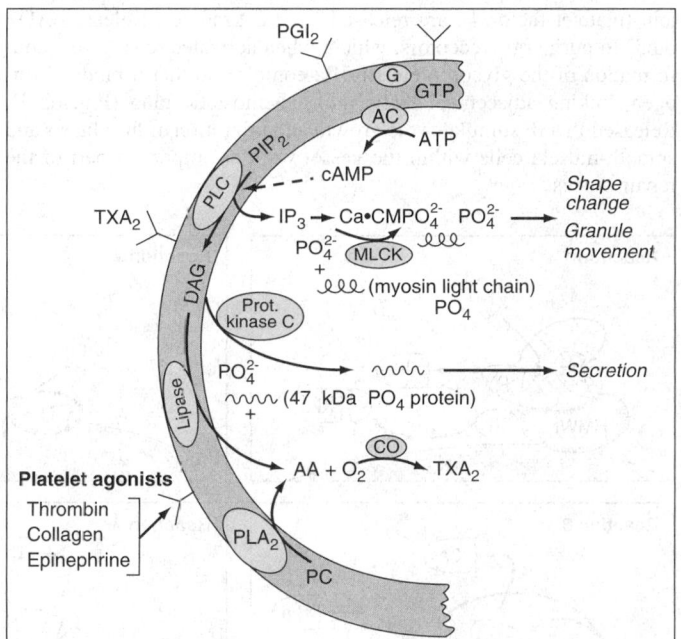

FIGURE 62-4 The biochemical basis of platelet activation and secretion. Binding of agonists such as thrombin, epinephrine, or collagen sets in motion a chain of events that hydrolyzes membrane phospholipids, inhibits adenylate cyclase, mobilizes intracellular calcium, and phosphorylates critical intracellular proteins. The net result is shape change, movement of granules to the canalicular system, generation of mediators such as thromboxane A_2, and granule secretion. Abbreviations: AC, adenylate cyclase; G, guanine nucleotide–binding protein; PIP_2, phosphatidylinositol 4,5-bisphosphate; PLC, phospholipase C; DAG, diacylglycerol; PLA_2, phospholipase A_2; PC, phosphatidylcholine; AA, arachidonic acid; CO, cyclooxygenase; O_2, oxygen; IP_3, inositol triphosphate; cAMP, cyclic AMP; Ca-CM, calcium calmodulin complex; MLCK, myosin light chain kinase.

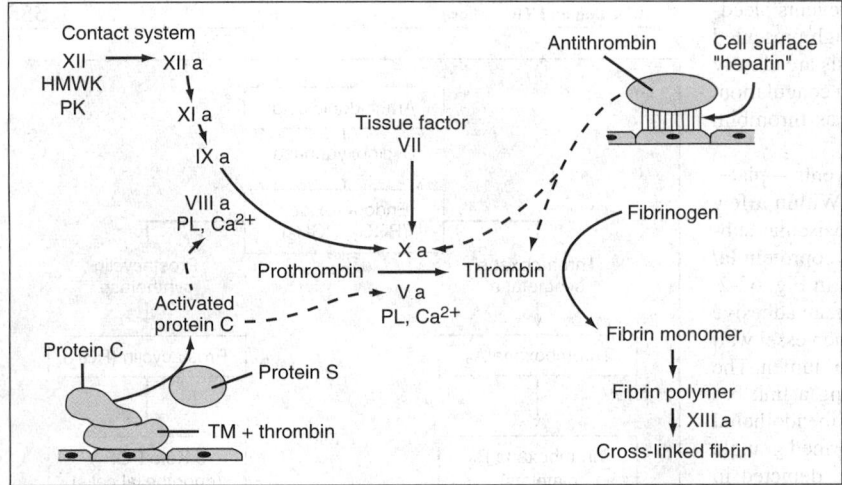

FIGURE 62-5 A schematic diagram of some of the clinically important coagulation reactions. The unactivated or precursor proteins are indicated by roman numerals, and the active form by the addition of a lowercase "a"—a standard convention. Other abbreviations: HMWK, high-molecular-weight kininogen; PK, prekallikrein; PL, phospholipid; TM, thrombomodulin; Ca^{2+}, calcium. There are two independent activation pathways, the contact system and the tissue factor–mediated or extrinsic system. They merge at the point of factor X activation and lead to the generation of thrombin, which converts fibrinogen into fibrin. These reactions are regulated by antithrombin, which forms complexes with all of the coagulation protein serine proteases except factor VII, and by the protein C–protein S system, which inactivates factors V and VIII.

plasma. Endoglycosidases and a heparin-cleaving enzyme are released from lysosomes; calcium, serotonin, and adenosine diphosphate (ADP) are released from the dense granules; and several proteins, including the von Willebrand factor, fibronectin, thrombospondin, the platelet-derived growth factor (PDGF), and a heparin-neutralizing protein (platelet factor 4), are released from α granules. Released ADP binds to purinergic receptors, which, when activated, change the conformation of the glycoprotein IIb/IIIa complex so that it binds fibrinogen, linking adjacent platelets into a hemostatic plug (Fig. 62-2). Released PDGF stimulates the growth and migration of fibroblasts and smooth-muscle cells within the vessel wall, an important part of the repair process.

As the primary hemostatic plug is being formed, plasma coagulation proteins are activated to initiate secondary hemostasis. An overall picture of the coagulation scheme, including the role of various inhibitors, is shown in Fig. 62-5. The coagulation pathway can be broken down into a series of reactions (Fig. 62-6) that culminate in the production of enough thrombin to convert a small amount of plasma fibrinogen to fibrin. Each of the reactions requires the formation of a surface-bound complex and the conversion of inactive precursor proteins into active proteases by limited proteolysis, and each is regulated by both plasma and cellular cofactors and calcium.

In *reaction 1*, the intrinsic or contact phase of coagulation, three plasma proteins, Hageman factor (factor XII), high-molecular-weight kininogen (HMWK), and prekallikrein (PK), form a complex on vascular subendothelial collagen. After binding to HMWK, factor XII is slowly converted to an active protease (XIIa), which then activates PK to kallikrein and factor XI to XIa. Kallikrein accelerates the conversion of XII to XIIa, while XIa participates in subsequent coagulation reactions. An alternative mechanism for the activation of factor XI may exist, as patients who are deficient in either factor XII, HMWK, or PK have apparently normal hemostasis and no clinical bleeding.

Reaction 2 provides a second pathway to initiate coagulation by activating factor VII to a protease. In this extrinsic or tissue-factor-dependent pathway, a complex is formed between factor VII, calcium, and tissue factor, a ubiquitous lipoprotein present in cellular membranes and exposed by cellular injury. The tissue factor–VII pathway is continuously active and makes a major contribution to basal coagulation. Factor VII and three other coagulation proteins—factors II (prothrombin), IX, and X—require calcium and vitamin K for biologic activity. These proteins are synthesized in the liver, where a vitamin K–dependent carboxylase catalyzes a unique posttranslational modification that adds a second carboxyl group to certain glutamic acid residues. Pairs of these di-γ-carboxyglutamic acid (Gla) residues bind calcium, which alters protein comformation for binding to phospholipid surfaces and confers biologic activity. Inhibition of this modification by vitamin K antagonists (e.g., warfarin) is the basis of one of the most common forms of anticoagulant therapy.

In *reaction 3*, factor X is activated by the proteases generated in the two previous reactions. In one reaction, a calcium- and lipid-dependent complex is formed between factors VIII, IX, and X. Within this complex, factor IX is first converted to IXa by factor XIa that was generated within the intrinsic pathway (reaction 1). Factor X is then activated by factor IXa in concert with factor VIII. Alternatively, both factors IX and X can be activated more directly by factor VIIa, generated via the extrinsic pathway (reaction 2). Activation of factors IX and X provides a link between the intrinsic and extrinsic coagulation pathways (Fig. 62-5).

Reaction 4, the final step, converts prothrombin to thrombin in the presence of factor V, calcium, and phospholipid. Although prothrombin conversion can take place on various natural and artificial phospholipid-rich surfaces, it proceeds several thousand times faster on the surface of activated platelets or endothelial cells. Thrombin has multiple functions in hemostasis. Although its principal role in hemostasis is the conversion

FIGURE 62-6 The major coagulation reactions are subdivided and depicted in schematic form to emphasize their similarity. They all rely on the formation of surface-bound enzyme-cofactor complexes. Abbreviations: PK, prekallikrein; K, kallikrein; HMWK, high-molecular-weight kininogen; TF, tissue factor; Ca^{2+}, calcium; PT, prothrombin; Thr, thrombin. By convention, other coagulation factors are indicated by roman numerals, with a lowercase "a" appended to indicate their active form. The ∧∧∧ is used to indicate the Gla (di-γ-carboxyglutamic acid)–containing domains of factors VII, IX, X, Xa, and PT, which bind calcium and phospholipid. Hatching is used to indicate proteins that adhere to surfaces by hydrophobic interaction.

of fibrinogen to fibrin, it also activates factors V, VIII, and XIII and stimulates platelet aggregation and secretion. Following the release of fibrinopeptides A and B from the α and β chains of fibrinogen, the modified molecule, now called *fibrin monomer*, polymerizes into an insoluble gel. The fibrin polymer is then stabilized by the cross-linking of individual chains by factor XIIIa, a plasma transglutaminase (Fig. 62-5).

Although the classic view of coagulation had clinical utility, it left several important questions unanswered: (1) Why does factor XII deficiency dramatically prolong partial thromboplastin time (PTT) but not cause bleeding? (2) Why is there heterogeneity in the bleeding symptoms of patients with factor XI deficiency? (3) Why do deficiencies in factors VIII or IX produce such dramatic bleeding even though the "extrinsic" pathway remains intact? Activation of factors IX and X by the tissue factor–VIIa complex is thought to play a major role in the initiation of hemostasis. Once coagulation is initiated by this interaction, the tissue factor pathway inhibitor (TFPI) blocks the pathway, and elements of the intrinsic pathway, particularly factors VIII and IX, become the dominant regulators of thrombin generation. This step in the pathway explains why factor XII–deficient patients are asymptomatic and why factor XI–deficient patients have only a mild to moderate bleeding diathesis (Fig. 62-7).

Clot lysis and vessel repair begin immediately after the formation of the definitive hemostatic plug. Three potential activators of the fibrinolytic system are: Hageman factor fragments, urinary plasminogen activator (uPA) or urokinase, and tissue plasminogen activator (tPA). The principal physiologic activators, tPA and uPA, diffuse from endothelial cells and convert plasminogen, adsorbed to the fibrin clot, into plasmin (Fig. 62-8). Plasmin then degrades fibrin polymer into small fragments, which are cleared by the monocyte-macrophage scavenger system. Although plasmin can also degrade fibrinogen, the reaction remains localized because (1) tPA and some forms of uPA activate plasminogen more effectively when it is adsorbed to fibrin clots; (2) any plasmin that enters the circulation is rapidly bound and neutralized by the α_2 plasmin inhibitor (patients who lack this factor have unchecked fibrinolysis and bleed); and (3) endothelial cells release a plasminogen activator inhibitor (PAI-1), which blocks the action of tPA.

Only a small quantity of each coagulation enzyme is converted to its active form. As a consequence, the hemostatic plug does not propagate beyond the site of injury. Precise regulation is important, since each milliliter of blood contains enough clotting potential to clot all the fibrinogen in the body in 10 to 15 s. Blood fluidity is maintained

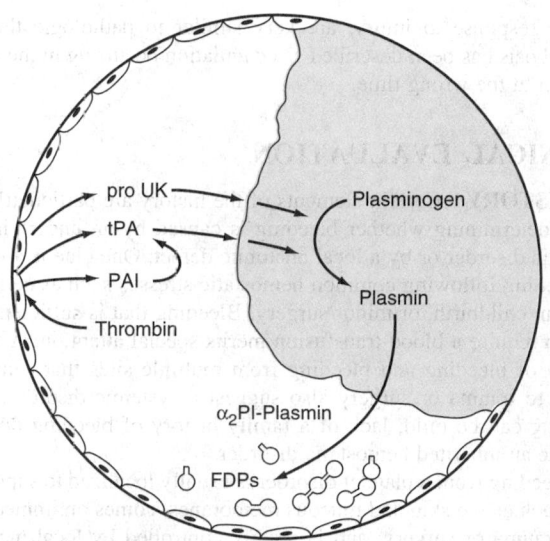

FIGURE 62-8 A schematic diagram of the fibrinolytic pathway. Tissue plasminogen activator (tPA) is released from endothelial cells, enters the fibrin clot, and activates plasminogen to plasmin. Any free plasmin is complexed with α_2 plasmin inhibitor (α_2PI). Fibrin is degraded to low-molecular-weight fragments, fibrin degradation products (FDPs).

by the flow of blood, the adsorption of coagulation factors to surfaces and their trapping in the emerging clot, and by multiple inhibitors in plasma. Antithrombin, proteins C and S, and TFPI are important inhibitors that maintain blood fluidity.

These inhibitors have distinct modes of action. Antithrombin forms complexes with all serine protease coagulation factors except factor VII (Fig. 62-5). Rates of complex formation are accelerated by heparin and heparin-like molecules on the surface of the endothelial cells. Heparin's ability to accelerate antithrombin activity is the basis for its anticoagulant action. Protein C is converted to an active protease by thrombin after it is bound to an endothelial cell protein called *thrombomodulin*. Activated protein C then inactivates the two plasma cofactors V and VIII by limited proteolysis, which slows down two critical coagulation reactions. Protein C may also stimulate the release of tPA from endothelial cells. The inhibitory function of protein C is enhanced by protein S. Reduced levels of antithrombin or proteins C and S, or dysfunctional forms of these molecules, result in a hypercoagulable or prethrombotic state. In addition, a particularly common heritable defect associated with a hypercoagulable state is the presence of a form of factor V (factor V Leiden) that is resistant to protein C inhibition. Between 20 and 50% of patients with unexplained venous thromboembolism have this defect.

Blood coagulation is not uniform throughout the body. The composition of the blood clot varies with the site of injury. Hemostatic plugs or thrombi that form in veins where blood flow is slow are rich in fibrin and trapped red blood cells and contain relatively few platelets. They are often called *red thrombi* because of their appearance in surgical and pathologic specimens. The friable ends of these red thrombi, which most often form in leg veins, can break off and embolize to the pulmonary circulation. Conversely, clots that form in arteries under conditions of high flow are predominantly composed of platelets and have little fibrin. These *white thrombi* may readily dislodge from the arterial wall and embolize to distant sites, causing temporary or permanent ischemia. These clots are a particularly common cause of embolism in the cerebral and retinal circulation, where they may lead to transient neurologic dysfunction (transient ischemic attacks), including temporary monocular blindness (amaurosis fugax), or to strokes. In addition, most episodes of myocardial infarction are due to thrombi that form after the rupture of atherosclerotic plaques within diseased coronary arteries. Hemostatic plugs, which are a phys-

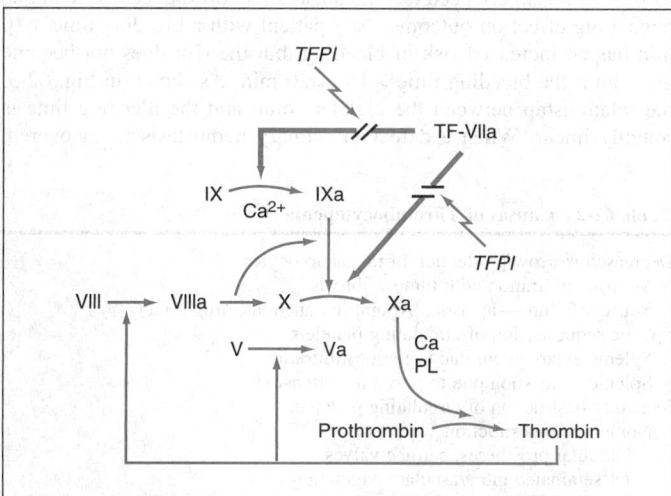

FIGURE 62-7 The contribution of the tissue factor–VIIa complex (TF-VIIa) and tissue factor pathway inhibitor (TFPI) to coagulation. Initial activation of factor IX by TF-VIIa compensates for deficiencies in the early factors, e.g., factors XII and XI. The subsequent inhibition of TF-VIIa by TFPI makes sustained activation of factor X by IXa and VIIIa critical for normal hemostasis. PL, phospholipid.

iologic response to injury, are very similar to pathologic thrombi. Thrombosis has been described as coagulation occurring in the wrong place or at the wrong time.

CLINICAL EVALUATION

HISTORY   Certain elements of the history are particularly useful in determining whether bleeding is caused by an underlying hemostatic disorder or by a local anatomic defect. One clue is a history of bleeding following common hemostatic stresses such as dental extraction, childbirth, or minor surgery. Bleeding that is sufficiently severe to require a blood transfusion merits special attention. A family history of bleeding and bleeding from multiple sites that cannot be linked to trauma or surgery also suggest a systemic disorder. Since bleeding can be mild, lack of a family history of bleeding does not exclude an inherited hemostatic disorder.

Bleeding from a platelet disorder is usually localized to superficial sites such as the skin and mucous membranes, comes on immediately after trauma or surgery, and is readily controlled by local measures (Table 62-1). In contrast, bleeding from secondary hemostatic or plasma coagulation defects occurs hours or days after injury and is unaffected by local therapy. Such bleeding most often occurs in deep subcutaneous tissues, muscles, joints, or body cavities. A careful and thorough history may establish the presence of a hemostatic disorder and guide initial laboratory testing.

PHYSICAL EXAMINATION   The most common site to observe bleeding is in the skin and mucous membranes. Collections of blood in the skin are called *purpura* and may be subdivided on the basis of the site of bleeding in the skin. Small pinpoint hemorrhages into the dermis due to the leakage of red cells through capillaries are called *petechiae* and are characteristic of platelet disorders—in particular, severe thrombocytopenia. Larger subcutaneous collections of blood due to leakage of blood from small arterioles and venules are called *ecchymoses* (common bruises) or, if somewhat deeper and palpable, *hematomas*. They are also common in patients with platelet defects and result from minor trauma. Dilated capillaries, or *telangiectasia*, may cause bleeding without any hemostatic defect. In addition, the loss of connective tissue support for capillaries and small veins that accompanies aging increases the fragility of superficial vessels, such as those on the dorsum of the hand, leading to extravasation of blood into subcutaneous tissue—*senile purpura*. Menorrhagia is sometimes a serious problem in women with severe thrombocytopenia or platelet dysfunction. Some patients with primary hemostatic defects, especially von Willebrand's disease, may have recurrent gastrointestinal hemorrhage, often associated with angiodysplasia, a common vascular malformation in the gastrointestinal tract.

Bleeding into body cavities, the retroperitoneum, or joints is a common manifestation of plasma coagulation defects. Repeated joint bleeding may cause synovial thickening, chronic inflammation, and fluid collections and may erode articular cartilage and lead to chronic joint deformity and limited mobility. Such deformities are particularly common in deficiencies of factors VIII and IX, the two sex-linked coagulation disorders referred to as the *hemophilias*. For unclear reasons, hemarthroses are much less common in patients with other plasma coagulation defects. Blood collections in various body cavities or soft tissues can cause secondary necrosis of tissues or nerve compression. Retroperitoneal hematomas can cause femoral nerve compression, and large collections of poorly coagulated blood in soft tissues occasionally mimic malignant growths—the pseudotumor syndrome. Two of the most life-threatening sites of bleeding are in the oropharynx, where bleeding can compromise the airway, and in the central nervous system. Intracerebral hemorrhage is one of the leading causes of death in patients with severe coagulation disorders. Because of their need for plasma and factor concentrates derived from multiple donors, many patients with hemophilia were infected with HIV before effective testing of donors was in place.

LABORATORY TESTS   The most important screening tests of the primary hemostatic system are (1) a *bleeding time* (a sensitive measure of platelet function), and (2) a *platelet count*. The latter correlates well with the propensity to bleed. The normal platelet count is 150,000 to 450,000/μL of blood. As long as the count is >100,000/μL, patients are usually not symptomatic and the bleeding time remains normal. Platelet counts of 50,000 to 100,000/μL cause mild prolongation of the bleeding time; bleeding occurs only from severe trauma or other stress. Patients with platelet counts <50,000/μL have easy bruising, manifested by skin purpura after minor trauma and bleeding after mucous membrane surgery. Patients with a platelet count <20,000/μL have an appreciable incidence of spontaneous bleeding, usually have petechiae, and may have intracranial or other spontaneous internal bleeding. The major causes of thrombocytopenia are outlined in Table 62-2.

Patients with qualitative platelet abnormalities have a normal platelet count and a prolonged bleeding time (Table 62-3). The bleeding time is ascertained by making a small, superficial skin incision and timing the duration of blood flow from the wounded area. By careful standardization, bleeding time is a reliable and sensitive test of platelet function. A template or an automated scalpel controls the length and depth of the incision (usually 1 mm deep by 9 mm long), and a sphygmomanometer inflated to 40 mmHg distends the capillary bed of the forearm uniformly. The bleeding time test must be performed by an experienced technician, as small differences in technique have a big effect on outcome. Any patient with a bleeding time >10 min has an increased risk of bleeding, but the risk does not become great until the bleeding time >15 or 20 min. As shown in Fig. 62-9, the relationship between the platelet count and the bleeding time is roughly linear. When a defect in primary hemostasis is uncovered,

Table 62-1   Differences in the Clinical Manifestations of Disorders of Primary and Secondary Hemostasis

Manifestations	Defects of Primary Hemostasis (Platelet Defects)	Defects of Secondary Hemostasis (Plasma Protein Defects)
Onset of bleeding after trauma	Immediate	Delayed—hours or days
Sites of bleeding	Superficial—skin, mucous membranes, nose, gastrointestinal and genitourinary tracts	Deep—joints, muscle, retroperitoneum
Physical findings	Petechiae, ecchymoses	Hematomas, hemarthroses
Family history	Autosomal dominant	Autosomal or X-linked recessive
Response to therapy	Immediate; local measures effective	Requires sustained systemic therapy

Table 62-2   Causes of Thrombocytopenia

Decreased marrow production of megakaryocytes
  Marrow infiltration with tumor, fibrosis
  Marrow failure—aplastic, hypoplastic anemias, drug effects
Splenic sequestration of circulating platelets
  Splenic enlargement due to tumor infiltration
  Splenic congestion due to portal hypertension
Increased destruction of circulating platelets
  Nonimmune destruction
    Vascular prostheses, cardiac valves
    Disseminated intravascular coagulation
    Sepsis
    Vasculitis
  Immune destruction
    Autoantibodies to platelet antigens
    Drug-associated antibodies
    Circulating immune complexes (systemic lupus erythematosus, viral agents, bacterial sepsis)

Table 62-3   Primary Hemostatic (Platelet) Disorders

Defects of platelet adhesion
    von Willebrand's disease
    Bernard-Soulier syndrome (absence or dysfunction of GpIb/IX)
Defects of platelet aggregation
    Glanzmann's thrombasthenia (absence or dysfunction of GpIIb/IIIa)
Defects of platelet release
    Decreased cyclooxygenase activity
        Drug-induced—aspirin, nonsteroidal anti-inflammatory agents
        Congenital
    Granule storage pool defects
        Congenital
        Acquired
    Uremia
    Platelet coating (e.g., penicillin or paraproteins)
Defect of platelet coagulant activity
    Scott's syndrome

ABBREVIATION: Gp, glycoprotein.

specialized testing is needed to determine the cause of the platelet dysfunction (Table 62-3). A precise diagnosis is important in determining the proper treatment. Occasional patients with a strong history of bleeding, particularly those with mild von Willebrand's disease, may have a normal bleeding time when initially tested, owing to cyclical variations in the level of the von Willebrand factor. Repeated testing may be necessary to establish an accurate diagnosis. Bleeding time is not an effective screening test for preoperative patients.

Plasma coagulation function is readily assessed with the PTT, prothrombin time (PT), thrombin time (TT), and quantitative fibrinogen determination (Fig. 62-5, Table 62-4). The PTT screens the intrinsic limb of the coagulation system and tests for the adequacy of factors XII, HMWK, PK, XI, IX, and VIII. The PT screens the extrinsic or tissue factor–dependent pathway. Both tests also evaluate the common coagulation pathway involving all the reactions that occur after the activation of factor X. Prolongation of the PT and PTT that does not resolve after the addition of normal plasma suggests a coagulation inhibitor. A specific test for the conversion of fibrinogen to fibrin is needed when both the PTT and PT are prolonged—either a TT or a clottable fibrinogen level can be employed. When abnormalities are noted in any of the screening tests, more specific coagulation factor assays can be ordered to determine the nature of the defect.

Several rare coagulation abnormalities that may be missed as they do not affect these screening tests: factor XIII deficiency, α_2 plasmin inhibitor deficiency, PAI-1 deficiency (PAI-1 is the major inhibitor of plasminogen activators), and Scott's syndrome, a platelet coagulant defect. A test for factor XIII–dependent fibrin cross-linking, such as clot solubility in 5 M urea, should be ordered when the PT and PTT

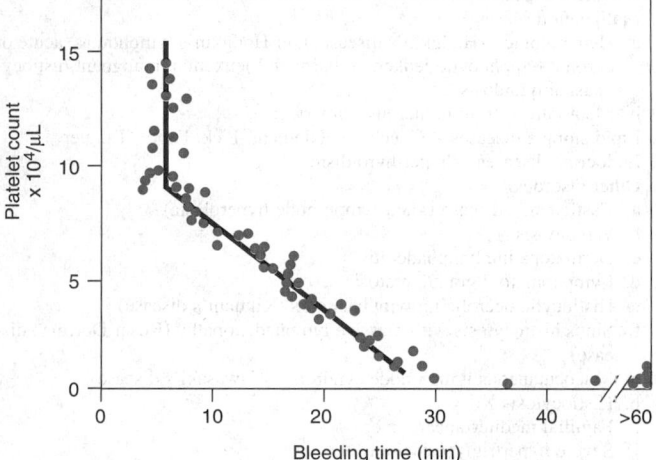

FIGURE 62-9   The relationship between the platelet count and the bleeding time. (*From LA Harker, Hemostasis Manual, 2d ed. Philadelphia, FA Davis Company, 1974.*)

Table 62-4   Relationship between Secondary Hemostatic Disorders and Coagulation Test Abnormalities

Prolonged partial thromboplastin time (PTT)
    No clinical bleeding—factors XII, HMWK, PK
    Mild or rare bleeding—factor XI
    Frequent, severe bleeding—factors VIII and IX
Prolonged prothrombin time (PT)
    Factor VII deficiency
    Vitamin K deficiency—early
    Warfarin anticoagulant ingestion
Prolonged PTT and PT
    Factor II, V, or X deficiency
    Vitamin K deficiency—late
    Warfarin anticoagulant ingestion
Prolonged thrombin time (TT)
    Mild or rare bleeding—afibrinogenemia
    Frequent, severe bleeding—dysfibrinogenemia
    Heparin-like inhibitors or heparin administration
Prolonged PT and/or PTT not corrected with normal plasma
    Specific or nonspecific inhibitor syndromes
Clot solubility in 5 M urea
    Factor XIII deficiency
    Inhibitors or defective cross-linking
Rapid clot lysis
    α_2 plasmin inhibitor

ABBREVIATIONS: HMWK, high-molecular-weight kininogen; PK, prekallikrein.

are both normal but the history of bleeding is strong. The fibrinolytic system can be assessed by measuring the rate of clot lysis with the euglobulin lysis or whole blood clot lysis tests and by measuring the levels of α_2 plasmin inhibitor and PAI-1. Scott's syndrome can be detected by measuring the serum PT, which assesses the amount of residual prothrombin.

Conditions associated with thrombosis are listed in Table 62-5. Patients suspected of having a hypercoagulable or prethrombotic disorder on the basis of clinical information should be tested with specific

Table 62-5   Thrombotic Disorders

Inherited
    Defective inhibition of coagulation factors
        Factor V Leiden (resistant to inhibition by activated protein C)
        Antithrombin III deficiency
        Protein C deficiency
        Protein S deficiency
        Prothrombin gene mutation (G40210A)
    Impaired clot lysis
        Dysfibrinogenemia
        Plasminogen deficiency
        tPA deficiency
        PAI-1 excess
    Uncertain mechanism
        Homocystinuria - ? endothelial damage
Acquired
    Diseases or syndromes
        Lupus anticoagulant/anticardiolipin antibody syndrome
        Malignancy
        Myeloproliferative disorder
        Thrombotic thrombocytopenic purpura
        Estrogen treatment
        Hyperlipidemia
        Diabetes mellitus
        Hyperviscosity
        Nephrotic syndrome
        Congestive heart failure
        Paroxysmal nocturnal hemoglobinuria
    Physiologic states
        Pregnancy (especially postpartum)
        Obesity
        Postoperative state
        Immobilization
        Old age

assays to screen for the known defects. Currently available tests can identify 50 to 60% of the cases of familial or recurrent venous thrombosis.

Inhibitor syndromes or circulating anticoagulants are usually due to antibodies that impair coagulation factor activity. They are an infrequent cause of bleeding and require specialized diagnostic testing. Inhibitors are likely when screening test abnormalities cannot be reversed by adding normal plasma to patient plasma. Antibodies against specific coagulation factors may develop in (1) postpartum women, (2) patients with autoimmune disorders such as systemic lupus erythematosus, (3) patients taking drugs such as penicillin and streptomycin, and (4) otherwise healthy elderly individuals. In addition, between 10 to 20% of patients with severe hemophilia who have received multiple plasma infusions develop inhibitory antibodies. Some patients, especially those with systemic lupus erythematosus, may also have a nonspecific form of anticoagulant antibody that interferes with phospholipid binding of coagulation factors and prolongs the PT and PTT but does not cause clinical bleeding. The presence of the lupus anticoagulant may increase the risk of thromboembolism and may cause placental infarction, recurrent midtrimester abortion, and venous and arterial thrombosis. The lupus-like anticoagulant is one manifestation of the anticardiolipin antibody syndrome. Patients may have anticardiolipin antibodies that do not prolong the PTT, but patients are still at risk from thrombosis. Occasionally, patients develop inhibitors that are not antibodies. For example, several patients with clinical bleeding have been found to have circulating mucopolysaccharides that have heparin-like activity.

BIBLIOGRAPHY

BERTINA RM: Introduction: Hypercoagulable states. Sem Hematol 34:167, 1997

COLMAN RW et al (eds): *Hemostasis and Thrombosis: Basic Principles and Clinical Practice*, 4th ed. Philadelphia, Lippincott, 1996

HANDIN RI: Diseases of the platelet and vessel wall, in *Hematology of Infancy and Childhood*, 5th ed., DG Nathan et al (eds). Philadelphia, Saunders, 1997, pp 1511–1530

———— et al (eds): *Blood: Principles and Practice of Hematology and Hematologic Oncology*, 4th ed. Philadelphia, Lippincott, 1994

MANN KC: Biochemistry and physiology of blood coagulation. Thromb Haemost 82:165, 1999

63   *Patrick H. Henry, Dan L. Longo*

ENLARGEMENT OF LYMPH NODES AND SPLEEN

This chapter is intended to serve as a guide to the evaluation of patients who present with enlargement of the lymph nodes (*lymphadenopathy*) or the spleen (*splenomegaly*). Lymphadenopathy is a rather common clinical finding in primary care settings, whereas palpable splenomegaly is less so.

LYMPHADENOPATHY

Lymphadenopathy may be an incidental finding in patients being examined for various reasons or it may be a presenting sign or symptom of the patient's illness. The physician must eventually decide whether the lymphadenopathy is a normal finding or one that requires further study, up to and including biopsy. Soft, flat, submandibular nodes (<1 cm) are often palpable in healthy children and young adults, and healthy adults may have palpable inguinal nodes of up to 2 cm, which are considered normal. Further evaluation of these normal nodes is not warranted. In contrast, if the physician believes the node(s) to be abnormal, then pursuit of a more precise diagnosis is needed.

Lymphadenopathy may be a primary or secondary manifestation of numerous disorders, as shown in Table 63-1. Many of these disorders are infrequent causes of lymphadenopathy. Analysis of lymphadenopathy in primary care practice has shown that more than two-thirds of patients have nonspecific causes or upper respiratory illnesses (viral or bacterial), and fewer than 1% have a malignancy. In one study, researchers reported that 186 of 220 patients (84%) referred for evaluation of lymphadenopathy had a "benign" diagnosis. The remaining 34 patients (16%) had a malignancy (lymphoma or metastatic adenocarcinoma). Sixty-three percent (112) of the 186 patients with benign lymphadenopathy had a nonspecific or reactive etiology (no causative agent found), and the remainder had a specific cause demonstrated, most commonly infectious mononucleosis, toxoplasmosis, or tuberculosis. Thus, the vast majority of patients with lymphadenopathy will have a nonspecific etiology requiring few diagnostic tests.

Clinical Assessment   The physician will be aided in the pursuit of an explanation for the lymphadenopathy by a careful medical history, physical examination, selected laboratory tests, and perhaps an excisional lymph node biopsy.

The *medical history* should reveal the setting in which lymphadenopathy is occurring. Symptoms such as sore throat, cough, fever,

Table 63-1   Diseases Associated with Lymphadenopathy

1. Infectious diseases
   a. Viral—infectious mononucleosis syndromes (EBV, CMV), infectious hepatitis, herpes simplex, herpesvirus-6, varicella-zoster virus, rubella, measles, adenovirus, HIV, epidemic keratoconjunctivitis, vaccinia, herpesvirus-8
   b. Bacterial—streptococci, staphylococci, cat-scratch disease, brucellosis, tularemia, plague, chancroid, melioidosis, glanders, tuberculosis, atypical mycobacterial infection, primary and secondary syphilis, diphtheria, leprosy
   c. Fungal—histoplasmosis, coccidioidomycosis, paracoccidioidomycosis
   d. Chlamydial—lymphogranuloma venereum, trachoma
   e. Parasitic—toxoplasmosis, leishmaniasis, trypanosomiasis, filariasis
   f. Rickettsial—scrub typhus, rickettsialpox
2. Immunologic diseases
   a. Rheumatoid arthritis
   b. Juvenile rheumatoid arthritis
   c. Mixed connective tissue disease
   d. Systemic lupus erythematosus
   e. Dermatomyositis
   f. Sjögren's syndrome
   g. Serum sickness
   h. Drug hypersensitivity—diphenylhydantoin, hydralazine, allopurinol, primidone, gold, carbamazepine, etc.
   i. Angioimmunoblastic lymphadenopathy
   j. Primary biliary cirrhosis
   k. Graft-vs.-host disease
   l. Silicone-associated
3. Malignant diseases
   a. Hematologic—Hodgkin's disease, non-Hodgkin's lymphomas, acute or chronic lymphocytic leukemia, hairy cell leukemia, malignant histiocytosis, amyloidosis
   b. Metastatic—from numerous primary sites
4. Lipid storage diseases—Gaucher's, Niemann-Pick, Fabry, Tangier
5. Endocrine diseases—hyperthyroidism
6. Other disorders
   a. Castleman's disease (giant lymph node hyperplasia)
   b. Sarcoidosis
   c. Dermatopathic lymphadenitis
   d. Lymphomatoid granulomatosis
   e. Histiocytic necrotizing lymphadenitis (Kikuchi's disease)
   f. Sinus histiocytosis with massive lymphadenopathy (Rosai-Dorfman disease)
   g. Mucocutaneous lymph node syndrome (Kawasaki's disease)
   h. Histiocytosis X
   i. Familial mediterranean fever
   j. Severe hypertriglyceridemia
   k. Vascular transformation of sinuses
   l. Inflammatory pseudotumor of lymph node

NOTE: EBV, Epstein-Barr virus; CMV, cytomegalovirus.

night sweats, fatigue, weight loss, or pain in the nodes should be sought. The patient's age, sex, occupation, exposure to pets, sexual behavior, and use of drugs such as diphenylhydantoin are other important historic points. For example, children and young adults usually have benign (i.e., nonmalignant) disorders, such as viral or bacterial upper respiratory infections, infectious mononucleosis, toxoplasmosis, and, in some countries, tuberculosis, which account for the observed lymphadenopathy. In contrast, after age 50 the incidence of malignant disorders increases and that of benign disorders decreases.

The *physical examination* can provide useful clues such as the extent of lymphadenopathy (localized or generalized), size of nodes, texture, presence or absence of nodal tenderness, signs of inflammation over the node, skin lesions, and splenomegaly. A thorough ear, nose, and throat (ENT) examination is indicated in adult patients with cervical adenopathy and a history of tobacco use. Localized or regional adenopathy implies involvement of a single anatomic area. Generalized adenopathy has been defined as involvement of three or more noncontiguous lymph node areas. Many of the causes of lymphadenopathy (Table 63-1) can produce localized *or* generalized adenopathy, so this distinction is of limited utility in the differential diagnosis. Nevertheless, generalized lymphadenopathy is frequently associated with nonmalignant disorders such as infectious mononucleosis [Epstein-Barr virus (EBV) or cytomegalovirus (CMV)], toxoplasmosis, AIDS, other viral infections, systemic lupus erythematosus (SLE), and mixed connective tissue disease. Acute and chronic lymphocytic leukemias and malignant lymphomas also produce generalized adenopathy in adults.

The site of localized or regional adenopathy may provide a useful clue about the cause. Occipital adenopathy often reflects an infection of the scalp, and preauricular adenopathy accompanies conjunctival infections and cat-scratch disease. The most frequent site of regional adenopathy is the neck, and most of the causes are benign—upper respiratory infections, oral and dental lesions, infectious mononucleosis, other viral illnesses. The chief malignant causes include metastatic cancer from head and neck, breast, lung, and thyroid primaries. Enlargement of supraclavicular and scalene nodes is always abnormal. Because these nodes drain regions of the lung and retroperitoneal space, they can reflect either lymphomas, other cancers, or infectious processes arising in these areas. Virchow's node is an enlarged left supraclavicular node infiltrated with metastatic cancer from a gastrointestinal primary. Metastases to supraclavicular nodes also occur from lung, breast, testis, or ovarian cancers. Tuberculosis, sarcoidosis, and toxoplasmosis are nonneoplastic causes of supraclavicular adenopathy. Axillary adenopathy is usually due to injuries or localized infections of the ipsilateral upper extremity. Malignant causes include melanoma or lymphoma and, in women, breast cancer. Inguinal lymphadenopathy is usually secondary to infections or trauma of the lower extremities and may accompany sexually transmitted diseases such as lymphogranuloma venereum, primary syphilis, genital herpes, or chancroid. These nodes may also be involved by lymphomas and metastatic cancer from primary lesions of the rectum, genitalia, or lower extremities (melanoma).

The size and texture of the lymph node(s) and the presence of pain are useful parameters in evaluating a patient with lymphadenopathy. Nodes <1.0 cm² in area (1.0 × 1.0 cm or less) are almost always secondary to benign, nonspecific reactive causes. In one retrospective analysis of younger patients (9 to 25 years) who had a lymph node biopsy, a maximum diameter of >2 cm served as one discriminant for predicting that the biopsy would reveal malignant or granulomatous disease. Another study showed that a lymph node size of 2.25 cm² (1.5 cm × 1.5 cm) was the best discriminating limit for distinguishing malignant or granulomatous lymphadenopathy from other causes of lymphadenopathy. Patients with node(s) ≤1.0 cm² should be observed after excluding infectious mononucleosis and/or toxoplasmosis unless there are symptoms and signs of an underlying systemic illness.

The texture of lymph nodes may be described as soft, firm, rubbery, hard, discrete, matted, tender, movable, or fixed. Tenderness is found when the capsule is stretched during rapid enlargement, usually secondary to an inflammatory process. Some malignant diseases such as acute leukemia may produce rapid enlargement and pain in the nodes. Nodes involved by lymphoma tend to be large, discrete, symmetric, rubbery, firm, mobile, and nontender. Nodes containing metastatic cancer are often hard, nontender, and nonmovable because of fixation to surrounding tissues. The coexistence of splenomegaly in the patient with lymphadenopathy implies a systemic illness such as infectious mononucleosis, lymphoma, acute or chronic leukemia, SLE, sarcoidosis, toxoplasmosis, cat-scratch disease, or other less common hematologic disorders. The patient's story should provide helpful clues about the underlying systemic illness.

Nonsuperficial presentations (thoracic or abdominal) of adenopathy are usually detected as the result of a symptom-directed diagnostic workup. Thoracic adenopathy may be detected by routine chest roentgenography or during the workup for superficial adenopathy. It may also be found because the patient complains of a cough or wheezing from airway compression; hoarseness from recurrent laryngeal nerve involvement; dysphagia from esophageal compression; or swelling of the neck, face, or arms secondary to compression of the superior vena cava or subclavian vein. The differential diagnosis of mediastinal and hilar adenopathy includes primary lung disorders and systemic illnesses that characteristically involve mediastinal or hilar nodes. In the young, mediastinal adenopathy is associated with infectious mononucleosis and sarcoidosis. In endemic regions, histoplasmosis can cause unilateral paratracheal lymph node involvement that mimics lymphoma. Tuberculosis can also cause unilateral adenopathy. In older patients, the differential diagnosis includes primary lung cancer (especially among smokers), lymphomas, metastatic carcinoma (usually lung), tuberculosis, fungal infection, and sarcoidosis.

Enlarged intraabdominal or retroperitoneal nodes are usually malignant. Although tuberculosis may present as mesenteric lymphadenitis, these masses usually contain lymphomas or, in young men, germ cell tumors.

Laboratory Investigation The laboratory investigation of patients with lymphadenopathy must be tailored to elucidate the etiology suspected from the patient's history and physical findings. One study from a family practice clinic evaluated 249 younger patients with "enlarged lymph nodes, not infected" or "lymphadenitis." No laboratory studies were obtained in 51%. When studies were performed, the most common were a complete blood count (33%), throat culture (16%), chest x-ray (12%), or monospot test (10%). Only eight patients (3%) had a node biopsy, and half of those were normal or reactive. The complete blood count can provide useful data for the diagnosis of acute or chronic leukemias, EBV or CMV mononucleosis, lymphoma with a leukemic component, pyogenic infections, or immune cytopenias in illnesses such as SLE. Serologic studies may demonstrate antibodies specific to components of EBV, CMV, HIV, and other viruses; *Toxoplasma gondii*; *Brucella*; etc. If SLE is suspected, then antinuclear and anti-DNA antibody studies are warranted.

The chest x-ray is usually negative, but the presence of a pulmonary infiltrate or mediastinal lymphadenopathy would suggest tuberculosis, histoplasmosis, sarcoidosis, lymphoma, primary lung cancer, or metastatic cancer and demands further investigation.

A variety of imaging techniques [computed tomography (CT), magnetic resonance imaging (MRI), ultrasound, color Doppler ultrasonography] have been employed to differentiate benign from malignant lymph nodes, especially in patients with head and neck cancer. CT and MRI are comparably accurate (65 to 90%) in the diagnosis of metastases to cervical lymph nodes. Ultrasonography has been used to determine the long (L) axis, short (S) axis, and a ratio of long to short axis in cervical nodes. An L/S ratio of <2.0 has a sensitivity and a specificity of 95% for distinguishing benign and malignant nodes in patients with head and neck cancer. This ratio has greater specificity and sensitivity than palpation or measurement of either the long or the short axis alone.

The indications for lymph node biopsy are imprecise, yet it is a valuable diagnostic tool. The decision to biopsy may be made early in a patient's evaluation or delayed for up to 2 weeks. Prompt biopsy should occur if the patient's history and physical findings suggest a malignancy; examples include a solitary, hard, nontender cervical node in an older patient who is a chronic user of tobacco; supraclavicular adenopathy; and solitary or generalized adenopathy that is firm, movable, and suggestive of lymphoma. If a primary head and neck cancer is suspected as the basis of a solitary, hard cervical node, then a careful ENT examination should be performed. Any mucosal lesion that is suspicious for a primary neoplastic process should be biopsied first. If no mucosal lesion is detected, an excisional biopsy of the largest node should be performed. Fine-needle aspiration should not be performed as the first diagnostic procedure. Most diagnoses require more tissue than such aspiration can provide and it often delays a definitive diagnosis. Fine-needle aspiration should be reserved for thyroid nodules and for confirmation of relapse in patients whose primary diagnosis is known. If the primary physician is uncertain about whether to proceed to biopsy, consultation with a hematologist or medical oncologist should be helpful. In primary care practices, fewer than 5% of lymphadenopathy patients will require a biopsy. That percentage will be considerably larger in referral practices, i.e., hematology, oncology, or otolaryngology (ENT).

Two groups have reported algorithms that they claim will identify more precisely those lymphadenopathy patients who should have a biopsy. Both reports were retrospective analyses in referral practices. The first study involved patients 9 to 25 years of age who had a node biopsy performed. Three variables were identified that predicted those young patients with peripheral lymphadenopathy who should undergo biopsy; lymph node size >2 cm in diameter and abnormal chest x-ray had positive predictive value, whereas recent ENT symptoms had negative predictive values. The second study evaluated 220 lymphadenopathy patients in a hematology unit and identified five variables [lymph node size, location (supraclavicular or non-supraclavicular), age (>40 years or <40 years), texture (nonhard or hard), and tenderness] that were utilized in a mathematical model to identify those patients requiring a biopsy. Positive predictive value was found for age >40 years, supraclavicular location, node size >2.25 cm^2, hard texture, and lack of pain or tenderness. Negative predictive value was evident for age <40 years, node size <1.0 cm^2, nonhard texture, and tender or painful nodes. Ninety-one percent of those who required biopsy were correctly classified by this model. Since both of these studies were retrospective analyses and one was limited to young patients, it is not known how useful these models would be if applied prospectively in a primary care setting.

Most lymphadenopathy patients do not require a biopsy, and at least half require no laboratory studies. If the patient's history and physical findings point to a benign cause for lymphadenopathy, then careful follow-up at a 2- to 4-week interval can be employed. The patient should be instructed to return for reevaluation if the node(s) increase in size. Antibiotics are not indicated for lymphadenopathy unless there is strong evidence of a bacterial infection. Glucocorticoids should not be used to treat lymphadenopathy because their lympholytic effect obscures some diagnoses (lymphoma, leukemia, Castleman's disease) and they contribute to delayed healing or activation of underlying infections. An exception to this statement is the life-threatening pharyngeal obstruction by enlarged lymphoid tissue in Waldeyer's ring that is occasionally seen in infectious mononucleosis.

SPLENOMEGALY

STRUCTURE AND FUNCTION OF THE SPLEEN The spleen is a reticuloendothelial organ that has its embryologic origin in the dorsal mesogastrium at about 5 weeks' gestation. It arises in a series of hillocks, migrates to its normal adult location in the left upper quadrant (LUQ), and is attached to the stomach via the gastrolienal

ligament and to the kidney via the lienorenal ligament. When the hillocks fail to unify into a single tissue mass, accessory spleens may develop in around 20% of persons. The function of the spleen has been elusive. Galen believed it was the source of "black bile" or melancholia, and the word *hypochondria* (literally, beneath the ribs) and the idiom "to vent one's spleen" attest to the beliefs that the spleen had an important influence on the psyche and emotions. In humans, its normal physiologic roles seem to be the following:

1. Maintenance of quality control over erythrocytes in the red pulp by removal of senescent and defective red blood cells. The spleen accomplishes this function through a unique organization of its parenchyma and vasculature (Fig. 63-1).
2. Synthesis of antibodies in the white pulp.
3. The removal of antibody-coated bacteria and antibody-coated blood cells from the circulation.

An increase in these normal functions may result in splenomegaly.

The spleen is composed of red pulp and white pulp, which are Malpighi's terms for the red blood–filled sinuses and reticuloendothelial cell–lined cords and the white lymphoid follicles arrayed within the red pulp matrix. The spleen is in the portal circulation. The reason for this is unknown but may relate to the fact that lower blood pressure

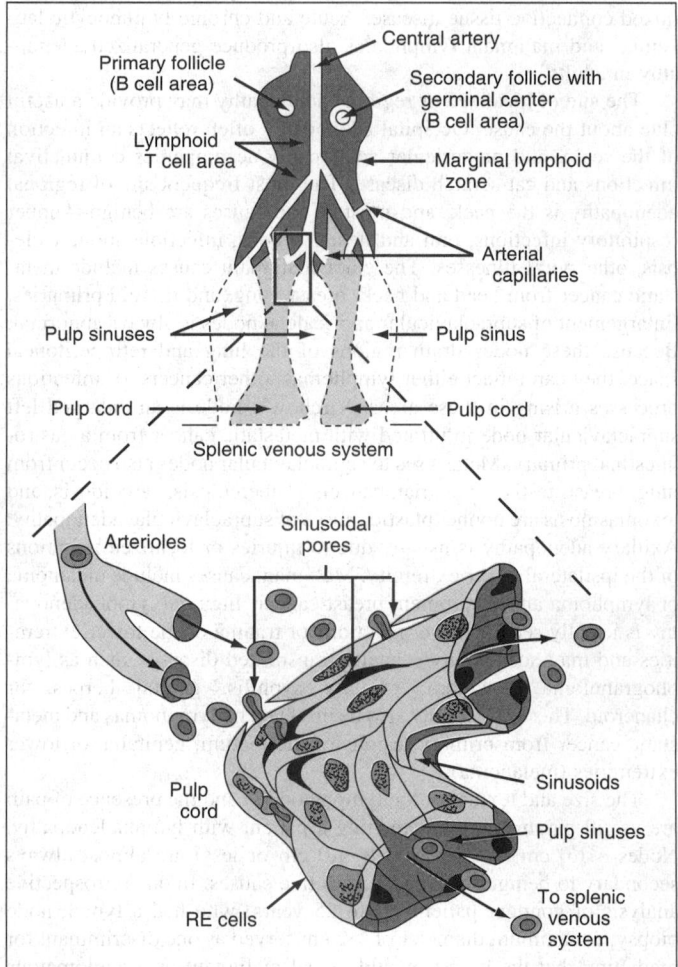

FIGURE 63-1 Schematic spleen structure. The spleen comprises many units of red and white pulp centered around small branches of the splenic artery, called central arteries. White pulp is lymphoid in nature and contains B cell follicles, a marginal zone around the follicles, and T cell–rich areas sheathing arterioles. The red pulp areas include pulp sinuses and pulp cords. The cords are dead ends. In order to regain access to the circulation, red blood cells must traverse tiny openings in the sinusoidal lining. Stiff, damaged, or old red cells cannot enter the sinuses. (*Bottom portion of figure from RS Hillman, KA Ault: Hematology in Clinical Practice. New York, McGraw-Hill, 1995.*)

allows less rapid flow and minimizes damage to normal erythrocytes. Blood flows into the spleen at a rate of about 150 mL/min through the splenic artery, which ultimately ramifies into central arterioles. Some blood goes from the arterioles to capillaries and then to splenic veins and out of the spleen, but the majority of blood from central arterioles flows into the macrophage-lined sinuses and cords. The blood entering the sinuses reenters the circulation through the splenic venules, but the blood entering the cords is subjected to an inspection of sorts. In order to return to the circulation, the blood cells in the cords must squeeze through slits in the cord lining to enter the sinuses that lead to the venules. Old and damaged erythrocytes are less deformable and are retained in the cords, where they are destroyed and their components recycled. Red cell inclusion bodies such as parasites, nuclear residua (Howell-Jolly bodies), or denatured hemoglobin (Heinz bodies) are pinched off in the process of passing through the slits, a process called *pitting*. The culling of dead and damaged cells and the pitting of cells with inclusions appear to occur without significant delay since the blood transit time through the spleen is only slightly slower than in other organs.

The spleen is also capable of assisting the host in adapting to its hostile environment. It has at least three adaptational functions: (1) clearance of bacteria and particulates from the blood, (2) the generation of immune responses to certain invading pathogens, and (3) the generation of cellular components of the blood under circumstances in which the marrow is unable to meet the needs (i.e., extramedullary hematopoiesis). The latter adaptation is a recapitulation of the blood-forming function the spleen plays during gestation. In some animals, the spleen also serves a role in the vascular adaptation to stress because it stores red blood cells (often hemoconcentrated to higher hematocrits than normal) under normal circumstances and contracts under the influence of β-adrenergic stimulation to provide the animal with an autotransfusion and improved oxygen-carrying capacity. However, the normal human spleen does not sequester or store red blood cells and does not contract in response to sympathetic stimuli. The normal human spleen contains approximately one-third of the total body platelets and a significant number of marginated neutrophils. These sequestered cells are available when needed to respond to bleeding or infection.

Approach to the Patient

Clinical Assessment The most common *symptoms* produced by diseases involving the spleen are pain and a heavy sensation in the LUQ. Massive splenomegaly may cause early satiety. Pain may result from acute swelling of the spleen with stretching of the capsule, infarction, or inflammation of the capsule. For many years, it was believed that splenic infarction was clinically silent, which at times is true. However, Soma Weiss, in his classic 1942 report of the self-observations by a Harvard medical student on the clinical course of subacute bacterial endocarditis, documented that severe LUQ and pleuritic chest pain may accompany thromboembolic occlusion of splenic blood flow. Vascular occlusion, with infarction and pain, is commonly seen in children with sickle cell crises. Rupture of the spleen, either from trauma or infiltrative disease that breaks the capsule, may result in intraperitoneal bleeding, shock, and death. The rupture itself may be painless.

A palpable spleen is the major *physical sign* produced by diseases affecting the spleen and suggests enlargement of the organ. The normal spleen is said to weigh less than 250 g, decreases in size with age, normally lies entirely within the rib cage, has a maximum cephalocaudad diameter of 13 cm by ultrasonography or maximum length of 12 cm and/or width of 7 cm by radionuclide scan, and is usually not palpable. However, a palpable spleen was found in 3% of 2200 asymptomatic, male, freshman college students. Follow-up at 3 years revealed that 30% of those students still had a palpable spleen without any increase in disease prevalence. Ten-year follow-up found no evidence for lymphoid malignancies. Furthermore, in some tropical countries (e.g., New Guinea) the incidence of splenomegaly may reach 60%. Thus, the presence of a palpable spleen does not always equate

with presence of disease. Even when disease is present, splenomegaly may not reflect the primary disease, but rather a reaction to it. For example, in patients with Hodgkin's disease, only two-thirds of the palpable spleens show involvement by the cancer.

Physical examination of the spleen utilizes primarily the techniques of palpation and percussion. Inspection may reveal a fullness in the LUQ that descends on inspiration, a finding associated with a massively enlarged spleen. Auscultation may reveal a venous hum or a friction rub.

Palpation can be accomplished by bimanual palpation, ballotment, and palpation from above (Middleton maneuver). For bimanual palpation, which is at least as reliable as the other techniques, the patient is supine with flexed knees. The examiner's left hand is placed on the lower rib cage and pulls the skin toward the costal margin, allowing the fingertips of the right hand to feel the tip of the spleen as it descends while the patient inspires slowly, smoothly, and deeply. Palpation is begun with the right hand in the left lower quadrant with gradual movement toward the left costal margin, thereby identifying the lower edge of a massively enlarged spleen. When the spleen tip is felt, the finding is recorded as centimeters below the left costal margin at some arbitrary point, i.e., 10 to 15 cm, from the midpoint of the umbilicus or the xiphisternal junction. This allows other examiners to compare findings or the initial examiner to determine changes in size over time. Bimanual palpation in the right lateral decubitus position adds nothing to the supine examination.

Percussion for splenic dullness is accomplished with any of three techniques described by Nixon, Castell, or Barkun:

1. *Nixon's method*: The patient is placed on the right side so that the spleen lies above the colon and stomach. Percussion begins at the lower level of pulmonary resonance in the posterior axillary line and proceeds diagonally along a perpendicular line toward the lower mid-anterior costal margin. The upper border of dullness is normally 6 to 8 cm above the costal margin. Dullness greater than 8 cm in an adult is presumed to indicate splenic enlargement.

2. *Castell's method*: With the patient supine, percussion in the lowest intercostal space in the anterior axillary line (8th or 9th) produces a resonant note if the spleen is normal in size. This is true during expiration or full inspiration. A dull percussion note on full inspiration suggests splenomegaly.

3. *Percussion of Traube's semilunar space*: The borders of Traube's space are the sixth rib superiorly, the left midaxillary line laterally, and the left costal margin inferiorly. The patient is supine with the left arm slightly abducted. During normal breathing, this space is percussed from medial to lateral margins, yielding a normal resonant sound. A dull percussion note suggests splenomegaly.

Studies comparing methods of percussion and palpation with a standard of ultrasonography or scintigraphy have revealed sensitivity of 56 to 71% for palpation and 59 to 82% for percussion. Reproducibility among examiners is better for palpation than percussion. Both techniques are less reliable in obese patients or patients who have just eaten. Thus, the physical examination techniques of palpation and percussion are imprecise at best. It has been suggested that the examiner perform percussion first and, if positive, proceed to palpation; if the spleen is palpable, then one can be reasonably confident that splenomegaly exists. However, not all LUQ masses are enlarged spleens; gastric or colon tumors and pancreatic or renal cysts or tumors can mimic splenomegaly.

The presence of an enlarged spleen can be more precisely determined, if necessary, by liver-spleen radionuclide scan, CT, MRI, or ultrasonography. The latter technique is the current procedure of choice for routine assessment of spleen size (normal = a maximum cephalocaudad diameter of 13 cm) because it has high sensitivity and specificity and is safe, noninvasive, quick, mobile, and less costly. Nuclear medicine scans are accurate, sensitive, and reliable but are costly, require greater time to generate data, and utilize immobile equipment. They have the advantage of demonstrating accessory

Table 63-2 Diseases Associated with Splenomegaly Grouped by Pathogenic Mechanism

ENLARGEMENT DUE TO INCREASED DEMAND FOR SPLENIC FUNCTION

Reticuloendothelial system hyperplasia (for removal of defective erythrocytes)
  Spherocytosis
  Early sickle cell anemia
  Ovalocytosis
  Thalassemia major
  Hemoglobinopathies
  Paroxysmal nocturnal hemoglobinuria
  Nutritional anemias
Immune hyperplasia
  Response to infection (viral, bacterial, fungal, parasitic)
    Infectious mononucleosis
    AIDS
    Viral hepatitis
    Cytomegalovirus
    Subacute bacterial endocarditis
    Bacterial septicemia
    Congenital syphilis
    Splenic abscess
    Tuberculosis
    Histoplasmosis
    Malaria
    Leishmaniasis
    Trypanosomiasis
    Ehrlichiosis
  Disordered immunoregulation
    Rheumatoid arthritis (Felty's syndrome)
    Systemic lupus erythematosus
    Collagen vascular diseases
    Serum sickness
    Immune hemolytic anemias
    Immune thrombocytopenias
    Immune neutropenias
    Drug reactions
    Angioimmunoblastic lymphadenopathy
    Sarcoidosis
    Thyrotoxicosis (benign lymphoid hypertrophy)
    Interleukin-2 therapy
Extramedullary hematopoiesis
  Myelofibrosis
  Marrow damage by toxins, radiation, strontium
  Marrow infiltration by tumors, leukemias, Gaucher's disease

ENLARGEMENT DUE TO ABNORMAL SPLENIC OR PORTAL BLOOD FLOW

Cirrhosis
Hepatic vein obstruction
Portal vein obstruction, intrahepatic or extrahepatic
Cavernous transformation of the portal vein
Splenic vein obstruction
Splenic artery aneurysm
Hepatic schistosomiasis
Congestive heart failure
Hepatic echinococcosis
Portal hypertension (any cause including the above): "Banti's disease"

INFILTRATION OF THE SPLEEN

Intracellular or extracellular depositions
  Amyloidosis
  Gaucher's disease
  Niemann-Pick disease
  Tangier disease
  Hurler's syndrome and other mucopolysaccharidoses
  Hyperlipidemias
Benign and malignant cellular infiltrations
  Leukemias (acute, chronic, lymphoid, myeloid, monocytic)
  Lymphomas
  Hodgkin's disease
  Myeloproliferative syndromes (e.g., polycythemia vera)
  Angiosarcomas
  Metastatic tumors (melanoma is most common)
  Eosinophilic granuloma
  Histiocytosis X
  Hamartomas
  Hemangiomas, fibromas, lymphangiomas
  Splenic cysts

UNKNOWN ETIOLOGY

Idiopathic splenomegaly
Berylliosis
Iron-deficiency anemia

---

splenic tissue. CT and MRI provide accurate determination of spleen size, but the equipment is immobile and the procedures are expensive. MRI appears to offer no advantage over CT. Changes in spleen structure such as mass lesions, infarcts, inhomogeneous infiltrates, and cysts are more readily assessed by CT, MRI, or ultrasonography. None of these techniques is very reliable in the detection of patchy infiltration (e.g., Hodgkin's disease).

Differential Diagnosis Many of the diseases associated with splenomegaly are listed in Table 63-2. They are grouped according to the presumed basic mechanisms responsible for organ enlargement:

1. Hyperplasia or hypertrophy related to a particular splenic function such as reticuloendothelial hyperplasia (work hypertrophy) in diseases such as hereditary spherocytosis or thalassemia syndromes that require removal of large numbers of defective red blood cells; immune hyperplasia in response to systemic infection (infectious mononucleosis, subacute bacterial endocarditis) or to immunologic diseases (immune thrombocytopenia, SLE, Felty's syndrome).

2. Passive congestion due to decreased blood flow from the spleen in conditions that produce portal hypertension (cirrhosis, Budd-Chiari syndrome, congestive heart failure).

3. Infiltrative diseases of the spleen (lymphomas, metastatic cancer, amyloidosis, Gaucher's disease, myeloproliferative disorders with extramedullary hematopoiesis).

The differential diagnostic possibilities are much fewer when the spleen is "massively enlarged," that is, it is palpable more than 8 cm below the left costal margin or its drained weight is ≥ 1000 g (Table 63-3). The vast majority of such patients will have non-Hodgkin's lymphoma, chronic lymphocytic leukemia, hairy cell leukemia, chronic myelogenous leukemia, myelofibrosis with myeloid metaplasia, or polycythemia vera.

Laboratory Assessment The major laboratory abnormalities accompanying splenomegaly are determined by the underlying systemic illness. Erythrocyte counts may be normal, decreased (thalassemia major syndromes, SLE, cirrhosis with portal hypertension), or increased (polycythemia vera). Granulocyte counts may be normal, decreased (Felty's syndrome, congestive splenomegaly, leukemias), or increased (infections or inflammatory disease, myeloproliferative disorders). Similarly, the platelet count may be normal, decreased when there is enhanced sequestration or destruction of platelets in an enlarged spleen (congestive splenomegaly, Gaucher's disease, immune thrombocytopenia), or increased in the myeloproliferative disorders such as polycythemia vera.

The complete blood count may reveal cytopenia of one or more blood cell types, which should suggest *hypersplenism*. This condition is characterized by splenomegaly, cytopenia(s), normal or hyperplastic bone marrow, and a response to splenectomy. The latter characteristic is less precise because reversal of cytopenia, particularly granulocytopenia, is sometimes not sustained after splenectomy. The cytopenias result from increased destruction of the cellular elements secondary to reduced flow of blood through enlarged and congested cords (congestive splenomegaly) or to immune-mediated mechanisms. In hypersplenism, various cell types usually have normal morphology on the peripheral blood smear, although the red cells may be spherocytic due to loss of surface area during their longer transit through the enlarged spleen. The increased marrow production of red cells should be reflected as an increased reticulocyte production index, although the value may be less than expected due to increased sequestration of reticulocytes in the spleen.

The need for additional laboratory studies is dictated by the differential diagnosis of the underlying illness of which splenomegaly is a manifestation.

Table 63-3 Diseases Associated with Massive Splenomegaly[a]

Chronic myelogenous leukemia	Gaucher's disease
Lymphomas	Chronic lymphocytic leukemia
Hairy cell leukemia	Sarcoidosis
Myelofibrosis with myeloid metaplasia	Autoimmune hemolytic anemia
Polycythemia vera	Diffuse splenic hemangiomatosis

[a] The spleen extends greater than 8 cm below left costal margin and/or weighs more than 1000 g.

SPLENECTOMY Splenectomy is infrequently performed for diagnostic purposes, especially in the absence of clinical illness or other diagnostic tests that suggest underlying disease. More often splenectomy is performed for staging the extent of disease in patients with Hodgkin's disease, for symptom control in patients with massive splenomegaly, for disease control in patients with traumatic splenic rupture, or for correction of cytopenias in patients with hypersplenism or immune-mediated destruction of one or more cellular blood elements. Splenectomy is necessary for routine staging of patients with Hodgkin's disease only in those with clinical stage I or II disease in whom radiation therapy alone is contemplated as the treatment. Noninvasive staging of the spleen in Hodgkin's disease is not a sufficiently reliable basis for treatment decisions because one-third of normal-sized spleens will be involved with Hodgkin's disease and one-third of enlarged spleens will be tumor-free. Although splenectomy in chronic myelogenous leukemia does not affect the natural history of disease, removal of the massive spleen usually makes patients significantly more comfortable and simplifies their management by significantly reducing transfusion requirements. Splenectomy is an effective secondary or tertiary treatment for two chronic B cell leukemias, hairy cell leukemia and prolymphocytic leukemia, and for the very rare splenic mantle cell or marginal zone lymphoma. Splenectomy in these diseases may be associated with significant tumor regression in bone marrow and other sites of disease. Similar regressions of systemic disease have been noted after splenic irradiation in some types of lymphoproliferative disease, especially chronic lymphocytic leukemia and prolymphocytic leukemia. This has been termed the *abscopal effect*. Such systemic tumor responses to local therapy directed at the spleen suggest that there may be some hormone or growth factor produced by the spleen that affects tumor cell proliferation, but this conjecture is not yet substantiated. The most common indication for splenectomy is traumatic or iatrogenic splenic rupture. In a fraction of patients with splenic rupture, peritoneal seeding of splenic fragments can lead to splenosis—the presence of multiple rests of spleen tissue not connected to the portal circulation. This ectopic spleen tissue may cause pain or gastrointestinal obstruction, as in endometriosis. A large number of hematologic, immunologic, and congestive causes of splenomegaly can lead to destruction of one or more cellular blood elements. In the majority of such cases, splenectomy can correct the cytopenias, particularly anemia and thrombocytopenia. Perhaps the only contraindication to splenectomy is the presence of marrow failure, in which the enlarged spleen is the only source of hematopoietic tissue.

The absence of the spleen has minimal long-term effects on the hematologic profile. In the immediate postsplenectomy period, there may be some leukocytosis (up to 25,000/μL) and thrombocytosis (up to $1 \times 10^6/\mu$L), but within 2 to 3 weeks, blood cell counts and survival of each cell lineage are usually normal. The chronic manifestations of splenectomy are marked variation in size and shape of erythrocytes (anisocytosis, poikilocytosis) and the presence of Howell-Jolly bodies (nuclear remnants), Heinz bodies (denatured hemoglobin), basophilic stippling, and an occasional nucleated erythrocyte in the peripheral blood. When such erythrocyte abnormalities appear in a patient whose spleen has not been removed, one should suspect splenic infiltration by tumor that has interfered with its normal culling and pitting function.

The most serious consequence of splenectomy is increased susceptibility to bacterial infections, particularly those with capsules such as *Streptococcus pneumoniae*, *Haemophilus influenzae*, and some gram-negative enteric organisms. Patients under age 20 years are particularly susceptible to overwhelming sepsis with *S. pneumoniae*, and the overall actuarial risk of sepsis in patients who have had their spleens removed is about 7% in 10 years. The case-fatality rate for pneumococcal sepsis in splenectomized patients is 50 to 80%. About 25% of patients without spleens will develop a serious infection at some time in their life. The frequency is highest within the first 3 years after splenectomy. About 15% of the infections are polymicrobial, and lung, skin, and blood are the most common sites. No increased risk of viral infection has been noted in patients who have no spleen. The susceptibility to bacterial infections relates to the inability to remove opsonized bacteria from the bloodstream and a defect in making antibodies to T cell–independent antigens such as the polysaccharide components of bacterial capsules. Pneumococcal vaccine (23-valent polysaccharide vaccine) should be administered to all patients 2 weeks before elective splenectomy. The Advisory Committee on Immunization Practices recommends that even splenectomized patients receive pneumococcal vaccine with a repeat vaccination 5 years later. Efficacy has not been proven in this setting, and the recommendation discounts the possibility that administration of the vaccine may actually lower the titer of specific pneumococcal antibodies. A more effective pneumococcal vaccine that involves T cells in the response is in development. The vaccine to *H. influenzae* should also be given to patients in whom elective splenectomy is planned. No other vaccines are routinely recommended in this setting.

Splenectomized patients should be educated to consider any unexplained fever as a medical emergency. Prompt medical attention with evaluation and treatment of suspected bacteremia may be life-saving. Routine chemoprophylaxis with oral penicillin can result in the emergence of drug-resistant strains and is not recommended.

In addition to an increased susceptibility to bacterial infections, splenectomized patients are also more susceptible to the parasitic disease babesiosis. The splenectomized patient should avoid areas where the parasite *Babesia* is endemic (e.g., Cape Cod, MA).

Surgical removal of the spleen is an obvious cause of *hyposplenism*. Patients with sickle cell disease often suffer from autosplenectomy as a result of splenic destruction by the numerous infarcts associated with sickle cell crises during childhood. Indeed, the presence of a palpable spleen in a patient with sickle cell disease after age 5 suggests a coexisting hemoglobinopathy, e.g., thalassemia or hemoglobin C. In addition, patients who receive splenic irradiation for a neoplastic or autoimmune disease are also functionally hyposplenic. The term *hyposplenism* is preferred to *asplenism* in referring to the physiologic consequences of splenectomy because asplenia is a rare, specific, and fatal congenital abnormality in which there is a failure of the left side of the coelomic cavity (which includes the splenic anlagen) to develop normally. Infants with asplenia have no spleens, but that is the least of their problems. The right side of the developing embryo is duplicated on the left so there is liver where the spleen should be, there are two right lungs, and the heart comprises two right atria and two right ventricles.

BIBLIOGRAPHY

BARKUN AN et al: The bedside assessment of splenic enlargement. Am J Med 91:512, 1991

GRAVES SA et al: Does this patient have splenomegaly? JAMA 270:2218, 1993

KAJI A et al: Imaging of cervical adenopathy. Semin Ultrasound CT MRI 18:220, 1997

MCINTYRE OR, EBAUGH FG JR: Palpable spleens: Ten year follow-up. Ann Intern Med 90:130, 1979

PANGALIS GA et al: Clinical approach to lymphadenopathy. Semin Oncol 20:570, 1993

PREVENTION OF PNEUMOCOCCAL DISEASE: Recommendations of the Advisory Committee on Immunization Practices. MMWR 46(RR-8):1, 1997

SLAP GB et al: Validation of a model to identify young patients for lymph node biopsy. JAMA 255:2768, 1986

STEINKAMP HJ et al: Cervical lymphadenopathy: Ratio of long- to short-axis diameter as a predictor of malignancy. Br J Radiol 68:266, 1995

WILLIAMSON HA JR: Lymphadenopathy in a family practice: A descriptive study of 240 cases. J Fam Pract 20:449, 1985

64   *Steven M. Holland, John I. Gallin*

DISORDERS OF GRANULOCYTES AND MONOCYTES

Leukocytes are the major cells comprising inflammatory and immune responses and include neutrophils, T and B lymphocytes, natural killer (NK) cells, monocytes, eosinophils, and basophils. These cells have specific functions, such as antibody production by B lymphocytes or destruction of bacteria by neutrophils, but in no single infectious disease is the exact role of the cell types completely established. Thus, whereas neutrophils are classically thought to be critical to host defense against bacteria, they may also play important roles in defense against viral infections.

The blood delivers leukocytes to the various tissues from the bone marrow, where they are produced. Normal blood leukocyte counts are given in the Appendix (Tables A-7 and A-8). The various leukocytes are derived from a common stem cell in the bone marrow. Three-fourths of the nucleated cells of bone marrow are committed to the production of leukocytes. Leukocyte maturation in the marrow is under the regulatory control of a number of different factors, known as colony stimulating factors and interleukins (Chap. 104). Because an alteration in the number and type of leukocytes is often associated with disease processes, total white blood count (WBC) (cells per microliter) and differential counts are informative. The lymphocytes and basophils are discussed in Chaps. 305 and 310, respectively. This chapter focuses on the neutrophils, monocytes, and eosinophils.

NEUTROPHILS

MATURATION   Important events in neutrophil life are summarized in Fig. 64-1. In normal humans, neutrophils are produced only in the bone marrow. The minimum number of stem cells necessary to support hematopoiesis is estimated to be 400 to 500. Human blood monocytes, tissue macrophages, and stromal cells produce colony stimulating factors, hormones required for the growth of monocytes and neutrophils in the bone marrow. The hematopoietic system not only produces enough neutrophils ($\sim 1.3 \times 10^{11}$ cells per 80-kg person

per day) to carry out physiologic functions but also has a large reserve stored in the marrow which can be mobilized in response to inflammation or infection. An increase in the number of blood neutrophils is called neutrophilia, and the presence of immature cells is termed a shift to the left. A decrease in the number of blood neutrophils is called neutropenia.

Neutrophils and monocytes evolve from pluripotent stem cells under the influence of cytokines and colony stimulating factors (Fig. 64-2). The proliferation phase through the metamyelocyte takes about 1 week, while the maturation phase from metamyelocyte to mature neutrophil takes another week. The myeloblast is the first recognizable precursor cell and is followed by the *promyelocyte* (**Plate V-23**). The promyelocyte evolves when the classic lysosomal granules, called the *primary* or *azurophil granules*, are produced. The primary granules contain hydrolases, elastase, myeloperoxidase, cationic proteins, and bactericidal/permeability-increasing protein, which is important for killing gram-negative bacteria. Azurophil granules also contain *defensins*, a family of cysteine-rich polypeptides with broad antimicrobial activity against bacteria, fungi, and certain enveloped viruses. The promyelocyte divides to produce the *myelocyte*, a cell responsible for the synthesis of the *specific* or *secondary granules* which contain unique (specific) constituents such as lactoferrin, vitamin B_{12}–binding proteins, membrane components of the nicotinamide-adenine dinucleotide phosphate (NADPH) oxidase required for hydrogen peroxide production, histaminase, and receptors for certain chemoattractants and adherence-promoting factors (CR3) as well as receptors for the basement membrane component, laminin. The secondary granules do not contain acid hydrolases and therefore are not classic lysosomes. Packaging of secondary granule contents during myelopoiesis is controlled by CCAAT/enhancer binding protein-ε. Secondary granule contents are readily released extracellularly, and their mobilization is important in modulating inflammation. During the final stages of maturation no cell division occurs, and the cell passes through the *metamyelocyte* stage and then to the *band* neutrophil with a sausage-shaped nucleus (**Plate V-35**). As the band cell matures, the nucleus assumes a lobulated configuration. The nucleus of neutrophils normally contains up to four segments. Excessive segmentation (more than five nuclear lobes) may be a manifestation of folate or vitamin B_{12} deficiency (**Plate V-38**). The Pelger-Hüet anomaly (**Plate V-34B**), an infrequent dominant benign inherited trait, results in neutrophils with distinctive bilobed nuclei that must be distinguished from band forms.

The physiologic role of the multilobed nucleus of neutrophils is unknown, but it may allow great deformation of neutrophils during migration into tissues at sites of inflammation.

In severe acute bacterial infection, prominent neutrophil cytoplasmic granules called *toxic granulations* are occasionally seen (**Plate V-11**). Toxic granulations are immature or abnormally staining azurophil granules. Cytoplasmic inclusions, also called *Döhle bodies* (**Plate V-35**), can be seen during infection and are fragments of ribosome-rich endoplasmic reticulum. Large neutrophil vacuoles are often present in acute bacterial infection and probably represent pinocytosed (internalized) membrane.

Neutrophils are heterogeneous in function. Monoclonal antibodies have been developed that recognize only a subset of mature neutrophils. The meaning of neutrophil heterogeneity is not known.

MARROW RELEASE AND CIRCULATING COMPARTMENTS   Specific signals, including interleukin (IL) 1, tumor necrosis factor-α (TNF-α), the colony stimulating factors, complement fragment C3e, and perhaps other cytokines mobilize leukocytes

FIGURE 64-1   Schematic events in neutrophil production, recruitment, and inflammation. The four cardinal signs of inflammation (rubor, tumor, calor, dolor) are indicated as are the interactions of neutrophils with other cells and cytokines. PMN, polymorphonuclear leukocytes; G-CSF, granulocyte colony stimulating factor; IL, interleukin; TNF-α, tumor necrosis factor.

from the bone marrow and deliver them to the blood in an unstimulated state. Under normal conditions, about 90% of the neutrophil pool is in the bone marrow, 2 to 3% in the circulation, and the remainder in the tissues (Fig. 64-3).

The circulating pool exists in two dynamic compartments: one freely flowing and one marginated. The freely flowing pool is about one-half the neutrophils in the basal state and is composed of those cells that are in the blood and not in contact with the endothelium. Marginated leukocytes are those that are in close physical contact with the endothelium (Fig. 64-4). In the pulmonary circulation, where an extensive capillary bed (~1000 capillaries per alveolus) exists, margination occurs because the capillaries are about the same size as a mature neutrophil. Therefore, neutrophil fluidity and deformability are necessary to make the transit through the pulmonary bed. Increased neutrophil rigidity and decreased deformability lead to augmented neutrophil trapping and margination in the lung. In contrast, in the systemic postcapillary venules, margination is mediated by the interaction of specific cell-surface molecules. *Selectins* are glycoproteins expressed on neutrophils and endothelial cells, among others, that cause a low-affinity interaction, resulting in "rolling" of the neutrophil along the endothelial surface. On neutrophils, the molecule L-selectin [cluster determinant (CD) 62L] binds to glycosylated proteins on endothelial cells [e.g., glycosylation-dependent cell adhesion molecule (GlyCAM1) and CD34]. Glycoproteins on neutrophils, most importantly sialyl-Lewis^x (SLe^x, CD15s), are targets for binding of selectins expressed on endothelial cells [E-selectin (CD62E) and P-selectin (CD62P)] and other leukocytes. In response to chemotactic stimuli from injured tissues (e.g., complement product C5a, leukotriene B$_4$, IL-8) or bacterial products [e.g., N-formylmethionyl-leucylphenylalanine (f-metleuphe)], neutrophil adhesiveness increases, and the cells "stick" to the endothelium through *integrins*. The integrins are leukocyte glycoproteins that exist as complexes of a common CD18 β-chain with CD11a (LFA-1), CD11b (also called either Mac-1, CR3, or the C3bi receptor), and CD11c (p150,95). CD11a/CD18 and CD11b/CD18 bind to specific endothelial receptors [intercellular adhesion molecules (ICAM) 1 and 2].

On cell stimulation, L-selectin is shed; receptors for chemoattractants and opsonins are mobilized; the phagocytes orient toward the chemoattractant source in the extravascular space, increase their motile activity (chemokinesis), and migrate directionally (chemotaxis) into tissues. The process of migration into tissues is called *diapedesis* and involves the crawling of neutrophils between postcapillary endothelial cells that open junctions between adjacent cells to permit leukocyte passage. Diapedesis involves platelet/endothelial cell adhesion molecule (PECAM) 1 (CD31), which is expressed on both the emigrating leukocyte and the endothelial cells. The endothelial responses (increased blood flow from increased vasodilation and permeability) are mediated by anaphylatoxins (e.g., C3a and C5a) as well as vasodilators such as histamine, bradykinin, serotonin, nitric oxide, vascular endothelial growth factor (VEGF), and prostaglandins E and I. Cytokines regulate some of these processes [e.g., TNF-α induction of VEGF, interferon (IFN) γ inhibition of prostaglandin E].

In the healthy adult, most neutrophils leave the body by migration through the mucous membrane of the gastrointestinal tract. Normally, neutrophils spend a short time in the circulation (half-life, 6 to 7 h).

Cell	Stage	Surface Markers^a	Characteristics
	MYELOBLAST	CD33, CD13, CD15	Prominent nucleoli
	PROMYELOCYTE	CD33, CD13, CD15	Large cell Primary granules appear
	MYELOCYTE	CD33, CD13, CD15, CD14, CD11b	Secondary granules appear
	METAMYELOCYTE	CD33, CD13, CD15, CD14, CD11b	Kidney bean–shaped nucleus
	BAND FORM	CD33, CD13, CD15, CD14, CD11b CD10, CD16	Condensed, band–shaped nucleus
	NEUTROPHIL	CD33, CD13, CD15, CD14, CD11b, CD10, CD16	Condensed, multilobed nucleus

^{a}CD= Cluster Determinant; ● Nucleolus; ● Primary granule; ○ Secondary granule.

FIGURE 64-2 Stages of neutrophil development are schematically shown. G-CSF and GM-CSF are critical to this process. Identifying cellular characteristics and specific cell-surface markers are listed for each maturational stage.

Senescent neutrophils are cleared from the circulation by macrophages in the lung and spleen. Once in the tissues, neutrophils release enzymes, such as collagenase and elastase, that help establish abscess cavities. Neutrophils ingest pathogenic materials that have been opsonized by IgG and C3b. Fibronectin and the tetrapeptide tuftsin facilitate phagocytosis.

With phagocytosis comes a burst of oxygen consumption and activation of the hexose-monophosphate shunt. A membrane-associated NADPH oxidase, consisting of membrane and cytosolic components, is assembled and catalyzes the reduction of oxygen to superoxide anion, which is then converted to hydrogen peroxide and other toxic oxygen products (e.g., hydroxyl radical). Hydrogen peroxide + chloride + neutrophil myeloperoxidase generates hypochlorous acid (bleach), hypochlorite, and chlorine. These products oxidize and halogenate microorganisms and tumor cells and, when uncontrolled, can damage host tissue. Strongly cationic proteins, defensins, and probably nitric oxide also participate in microbial killing. Other enzymes, such as lysozyme and acid proteases, help digest microbial debris. After 1 to 4 days in tissues neutrophils die. The apoptosis of neutrophils is also cytokine regulated; granulocyte colony stimulating factor (G-CSF) and IFN-γ prevent their death. Under certain conditions, such as in delayed-type hypersensitivity, monocyte accumulation occurs within 6 to 12 h of initiation of inflammation. Neutrophils, monocytes, microorganisms in various states of digestion, and altered local tissue cells make up the inflammatory exudate, pus. Myeloperoxidase confers the characteristic green color to pus and may participate in turning off

FIGURE 64-3 Schematic neutrophil distribution and kinetics between the different anatomic and functional pools.

the inflammatory process by inactivating chemoattractants and immobilizing phagocytic cells.

Neutrophils respond to certain cytokines [IFN-γ, granulocyte-macrophage colony stimulating factor (GM-CSF), IL-8] and produce cytokines and chemotactic signals [TNF-α, IL-8, macrophage inflammatory protein (MIP) 1] that modulate the inflammatory response. In the presence of fibrinogen, f-metleuphe or leukotriene B$_4$ induces IL-8 production by neutrophils, providing autocrine amplification of inflammation. *Chemokines* (*chemo*attractant cyto*kines*) are small proteins produced by many different cell types, including endothelial cells, fibroblasts, epithelial cells, neutrophils, and monocytes, that regulate neutrophil and monocyte recruitment and activation. The chemokines transduce their signals through heterotrimeric G protein–linked receptors that have seven cell membrane–spanning domains, the same type of cell-surface receptor that mediates the response to the classical chemoattractants *N*-f-metleuphe and C5a. Four major groups of chemokines are recognized based on the cysteine structure near the N terminus: C, CC, CXC, and CXXXC. The CXC cytokines like IL-8 mainly attract neutrophils; CC chemokines like MIP-1α attract lymphocytes, monocytes, eosinophils, and basophils; the C chemokine lymphotactin is T cell tropic; the CXXXC chemokine fractalkine attracts neutrophils, monocytes, and T cells. These molecules and their receptors not only regulate the trafficking and activation of inflammatory cells, but chemokine receptors serve as co-receptors for HIV infection (Chap. 309).

NEUTROPHIL ABNORMALITIES A defect in the neutrophil life cycle can lead to dysfunction and compromised host defenses. Inflammation is often depressed, and the clinical result is often recurrent and severe bacterial and fungal infections. Aphthous ulcers of mucous membranes (gray ulcers without pus) and gingivitis and periodontal disease suggest a phagocytic cell disorder. Patients with congenital phagocyte defects can have infections within the first few days of life. Skin, ear, upper and lower respiratory tract, and bone infections are common. Sepsis and meningitis are rare. In some disorders the frequency of infection is variable, and patients can go for months or even years without major infection. Aggressive management of these congenital diseases has extended the life span of patients beyond 30 years.

Neutropenia The consequences of absent neutrophils are dramatic. Susceptibility to infectious diseases increases sharply when neutrophil counts fall below 1000 cells/μL. When the absolute neutrophil count (ANC; band forms and mature neutrophils combined) falls below 500 cells/μL, control of endogenous microbial flora (e.g., mouth, gut) is impaired; when the ANC is < 200/μL, the inflammatory process is absent. Neutropenia can be due to depressed production, increased peripheral destruction, or excessive peripheral pooling. A falling neutrophil count or a significant decrease in the number of neutrophils below steady state levels, together with a failure to increase neutrophil counts in the setting of infection or other challenge, requires investigation. Acute neutropenia, such as that caused by cancer chemotherapy, is more likely to be associated with increased risk of infection than neutropenia of long duration (months to years) that reverses in response to

FIGURE 64-4 Neutrophil travel through the pulmonary capillaries is dependent on neutrophil deformability. Neutrophil rigidity (e.g., caused by C5a) enhances pulmonary trapping and response to pulmonary pathogens in a way that is not so dependent upon cell-surface receptors. Intraalveolar chemotactic factors, such as those caused by certain bacteria (e.g., *Streptococcus pneumoniae*) lead to diapedesis of neutrophils from the pulmonary capillaries into the alveolar space. Neutrophil interaction with the endothelium of the systemic postcapillary venules is dependent on molecules of attachment. The neutrophil "rolls" along the endothelium using selectins: neutrophil CD15s (sialyl-Lewis^x) binds to CD62E (E-selectin) and CD62P (P-selectin) on endothelial cells; CD62L (L-selectin) on neutrophils binds to CD34 and other molecules (e.g., GlyCAM-1) expressed on endothelium. Chemokines or other activation factors stimulate integrin-mediated "tight adhesion": CD11a/CD18 (LFA-1) and CD11b/CD18 (Mac-1, CR3) bind to CD54 (ICAM-1) and CD102(ICAM-2) on the endothelium. Diapedesis occurs between endothelial cells: CD31 (PECAM-1) expressed by the emigrating neutrophil interacts with CD31 expressed at the endothelial cell-cell junction.

infection or carefully controlled administration of endotoxin (see "Laboratory Diagnosis," below).

64 Disorders of Granulocytes and Monocytes **369**

Some causes of inherited and acquired neutropenia are listed in Table 64-1. The most common neutropenias are iatrogenic, resulting from the use of cytotoxic or immunosuppressive therapies for malignancy or control of autoimmune disorders. These drugs cause neutropenia because they result in decreased production of rapidly growing progenitor (stem) cells of the marrow. Certain antibiotics such as chloramphenicol, trimethoprim-sulfamethoxazole, flucytosine, vidarabine, and the antiretroviral drug zidovudine may cause neutropenia by inhibiting proliferation of myeloid precursors. The marrow suppression is generally dose-related and dependent on continued administration of the drug. Recombinant human G-CSF reverses this form of neutropenia.

Another important mechanism for iatrogenic neutropenia is the effect of drugs that serve as immune haptens and sensitize neutrophils or neutrophil precursors to immune-mediated peripheral destruction. This form of drug-induced neutropenia can be seen within 7 days of exposure to the drug; with previous drug exposure, resulting in preexisting antibodies, neutropenia may occur a few hours after administration of the drug. Although any drug can cause this form of neutropenia, the most frequent causes are commonly used antibiotics, such as sulfa-containing compounds, penicillins, and cephalosporins. Fever and eosinophilia also may be associated drug reactions, but often these signs are not present. Drug-induced neutropenia can be severe, but discontinuation of the sensitizing drug is sufficient for recovery, which is usually seen within 5 to 7 days and is complete by 10 days. Readministration of the sensitizing drug should be avoided, since abrupt neutropenia often will result. For this reason, diagnostic challenge should be avoided.

Autoimmune neutropenias caused by circulating antineutrophil antibodies are another form of acquired neutropenia that results in increased destruction of neutrophils. Acquired neutropenia also may be seen with viral infections, including infection with HIV. Acquired neutropenia may be cyclic in nature, occurring at intervals of several weeks. Acquired cyclic or stable neutropenia may be associated with an expansion of large granular lymphocytes (LGL), which may be T cells, NK cells, or NK-like cells. Patients with LGL lymphocytosis may have moderate blood and bone marrow lymphocytosis, neutropenia, polyclonal hypergammaglobulinemia, splenomegaly, rheumatoid arthritis, and absence of lymphadenopathy. Such patients may have a chronic and relatively stable course. Recurrent bacterial infections are frequent. Benign and malignant forms of this syndrome oc-

cur. In some patients, a spontaneous regression has occurred even after 11 years, suggesting an immunoregulatory defect as the basis for at least one form of the disorder. Glucocorticoids, cyclosporine, IFN-α, and nucleosides such as 2-chlorodeoxyadenosine each have induced remission.

Hereditary Neutropenias Hereditary neutropenias are rare and may manifest in early childhood as a profound constant neutropenia or agranulocytosis. Congenital forms of neutropenia include Kostmann's syndrome (neutrophil count <100/μL), which is often fatal; more benign chronic idiopathic neutropenia (neutrophil count of 300 to 1500/μL); the cartilage-hair hypoplasia syndrome; Shwachman's syndrome associated with pancreatic insufficiency; myelokathexis, a congenital disorder characterized by neutrophil degeneration, hypersegmentation, and myeloid hyperplasia in the marrow associated with decreased expression of bcl-X$_L$ in myeloid precursors and accelerated apoptosis; and neutropenias associated with other immune defects (X-linked agammaglobulinemia, ataxia telangiectasia, IgA deficiency). Mutations in the G-CSF receptor on chromosome 1 associated with poor response to G-CSF can occur with severe congenital neutropenia and predispose to myeloid malignancy. Hereditary cyclic neutropenia, an autosomal dominant trait, may occur in infancy and is characterized by a remarkably regular 3-week cycle. Hereditary cyclic neutropenia actually is cyclic hematopoiesis, due to mutations in the neutrophil elastase gene. Glucocorticoids and G-CSF blunt the cycling in some patients.

Maternal factors can be associated with neutropenia in the newborn. Transplacental transfer of IgG directed against antigens on fetal neutrophils can result in peripheral destruction. Drugs (e.g., thiazides) ingested during pregnancy can cause neutropenia in the newborn by either depressed production or peripheral destruction.

The presence of immunoglobulin directed toward neutrophils is seen in Felty's syndrome—a triad of rheumatoid arthritis, splenomegaly, and neutropenia (Chap. 312). Patients with Felty's syndrome who respond to splenectomy with an increase in their neutrophil count also have lower postoperative serum neutrophil-binding IgG. Some of these patients have neutropenia associated with an increased number of LGL. Splenomegaly with peripheral trapping and destruction of neutrophils is also seen in lysosomal storage diseases and in portal hypertension.

Neutrophilia Neutrophilia results from increased neutrophil production, increased marrow release, or defective margination (Table 64-2). The most important acute cause of neutrophilia is infection.

Table 64-1 Causes of Neutropenia

Decreased Production
Drug-induced—alkylating agents (nitrogen mustard, busulfan, chlorambucil, cyclophosphamide); antimetabolites (methotrexate, 6-mercaptopurine, 5-flucytosine); noncytotoxic agents [antibiotics (chloramphenicol, penicillins, sulfonamides), phenothiazines, tranquilizers (meprobamate), anticonvulsants (carbamazepine), antipsychotics (clozapine), certain diuretics, anti-inflammatory agents, antithyroid drugs, many others]
Hematologic diseases—idiopathic, cyclic neutropenia, Chédiak-Higashi syndrome, aplastic anemia, infantile genetic disorders (see text)
Tumor invasion, myelofibrosis
Nutritional deficiency—vitamin B$_{12}$, folate (especially alcoholics)
Infection—tuberculosis, typhoid fever, brucellosis, tularemia, measles, infectious mononucleosis, malaria, viral hepatitis, leishmaniasis, AIDS

Peripheral Destruction
Antineutrophil antibodies and/or splenic or lung (alveolar macrophage) trapping
Autoimmune disorders—Felty's syndrome, rheumatoid arthritis, lupus erythematosus
Drugs as haptens—aminopyrine, α-methyl dopa, phenylbutazone, mercurial diuretics, some phenothiazines
Wegener's granulomatosis

Peripheral Pooling (Transient Neutropenia)
Overwhelming bacterial infection (acute endotoxemia)
Hemodialysis
Cardiopulmonary bypass

Table 64-2 Causes of Neutrophilia

Increased Production
Idiopathic
Drug-induced—glucocorticoids
Infection—bacterial, fungal, rarely viral
Inflammation—thermal injury, tissue necrosis, myocardial and pulmonary infarction, hypersensitivity states, collagen vascular diseases
Myeloproliferative diseases—myelocytic leukemia, myeloid metaplasia, polycythemia vera
Increased Marrow Release
Glucocorticoids
Acute infection (endotoxin)
Inflammation—thermal injury
Defective Margination
Drugs—epinephrine, glucocorticoids, nonsteroidal anti-inflammatory agents
Stress, excitement, vigorous exercise
Leukocyte adhesion deficiency type 1 (integrin β chain, CD18); leukocyte adhesion deficiency type 2 (selectin ligand, CD15s, sialyl-Lewis^x)
Miscellaneous
Metabolic disorders—ketoacidosis, acute renal failure, eclampsia, acute poisoning
Drugs—lithium
Other—metastatic carcinoma, acute hemorrhage or hemolysis

Table 64-3 Types of Granulocyte and Monocyte Disorders

Function	Cause of Indicated Dysfunction		
	Drug-Induced	**Acquired**	**Inherited**
Adherence-aggregation	Aspirin, colchicine, alcohol, glucocorticoids, ibuprofen, piroxicam	Neonatal state, hemodialysis	Leukoctye adhesion deficiency types 1 and 2
Deformability		Leukemia, neonatal state, diabetes mellitus, immature neutrophils	
Chemokinesis-chemotaxis	Glucocorticoids (high dose), auranofin, colchicine (weak effect), phenylbutazone, naproxen, indomethacin, interleukin 2	Thermal injury, malignancy, malnutrition, periodontal disease, neonatal state, systemic lupus erythematosus, rheumatoid arthritis, diabetes mellitus, sepsis, influenza virus infection, herpes simplex virus infection, acrodermatitis enteropathica, AIDS	Chédiak-Higashi syndrome, neutrophil-specific granule deficiency, hyper IgE—recurrent infection (Job's) syndrome (in some patients), Down syndrome, α-mannosidase deficiency, severe combined immunodeficiency, Wiskott-Aldrich syndrome
Microbicidal activity	Colchicine, cyclophosphamide, glucocorticoids (high dose)	Leukemia, aplastic anemia, certain neutropenias, tuftsin deficiency, thermal injury, sepsis, neonatal state, diabetes mellitus, malnutrition, AIDS	Chédiak-Higashi syndrome, neutrophil-specific granule deficiency, chronic granulomatous disease, interferon γ receptor deficiency, IL-12 receptor deficiency, IL-12 deficiency

Neutrophilia from acute infection represents both increased production and increased marrow release. Increased production is also associated with chronic inflammation and certain myeloproliferative diseases. Increased marrow release and mobilization of the marginated leukocyte pool are induced by glucocorticoids. Release of epinephrine, as with vigorous exercise, excitement, or stress, will demarginate neutrophils in the spleen and lungs and double the neutrophil count in minutes. Leukocytosis with cell counts of 10,000 to 25,000/μL occurs in response to infection and other forms of acute inflammation and results from both release of the marginated pool and mobilization of marrow reserves. Persistent neutrophilia with cell counts of 30,000 to 50,000/μL or higher is called a *leukemoid reaction*, a term often used to distinguish this degree of neutrophilia from leukemia. In a leukemoid reaction, the circulating neutrophils are usually mature and not clonally derived.

Abnormal Neutrophil Function Inherited and acquired abnormalities of phagocyte function are listed in Table 64-3. The resulting diseases are best considered in terms of the functional defects of adherence, chemotaxis, and microbicidal activity. The distinguishing features of the important inherited disorders of phagocyte function are shown in Table 64-4.

Disorders of adhesion Two types of leukocyte adhesion deficiency (LAD) have been described. Both are autosomal recessive traits and result in the inability of neutrophils to exit the circulation to sites of infection, leading to leukocytosis and increased susceptibility to infection (Fig. 64-4). Patients with LAD 1 have mutations in CD18, the common component of the integrins LFA-1, Mac-1, and p150,95, leading to a defect in tight adhesion between neutrophils and the endothelium. The heterodimer formed by CD18/CD11b (Mac-1) is also the receptor for the complement-derived opsonin C3bi (CR3). The CD18 gene is located on distal chromosome 21q. Variable expression of the defect determines the severity of clinical disease. Complete lack of expression of the leukocyte adhesion proteins results in the severe phenotype in which inflammatory cytokines do not increase the expression of leukocyte adhesion proteins on neutrophils or activated T and B cells. Neutrophils (and monocytes) from patients with LAD 1 adhere poorly to endothelial cells and protein-coated surfaces and exhibit defective spreading, aggregation, and chemotaxis. Patients with LAD 1 have recurrent bacterial and fungal infections involving skin, oral and genital mucosa, and respiratory and intestinal tracts; persistent leukocytosis (neutrophil counts of 15,000 to 20,000/μL) because cells do not marginate; and, in severe cases, a history of delayed separation of the umbilical stump. Infections, especially of the skin, may become necrotic with progressively enlarging borders, slow healing, and development of dysplastic scars. The most common bacteria are *Staphylococcus aureus* and enteric gram-negative bacteria. LAD 2 is caused by an abnormality of SLe^x(CD15s), the ligand on neutrophils that interacts with selectins on endothelial cells.

Disorders of neutrophil granules The most common neutrophil defect is *myeloperoxidase deficiency*, a primary granule defect inherited as an autosomal recessive trait; the incidence is ~1 in 2000 persons. Isolated myeloperoxidase deficiency is not associated with clinically compromised defenses, because other defense systems such as hydrogen peroxide generation are amplified. Microbicidal activity of neutrophils is delayed but not absent. Myeloperoxidase deficiency may make other acquired host defense defects more serious. An acquired form of myeloperoxidase deficiency occurs in myelomonocytic leukemia and acute myeloid leukemia.

Chédiak-Higashi syndrome (CHS) is a rare disease with autosomal recessive inheritance due to defects in the lysosomal transport protein LYST, encoded by the gene *CHS1* at 1q42. This protein is required for normal packaging and disbursement of granules. Neutrophils (and all cells containing lysosomes) from patients with CHS characteristically have large granules (**Plate V-34A**). Patients with CHS have an increased number of infections resulting from many agents. CHS neutrophils and monocytes have impaired chemotaxis and abnormal rates of microbial killing due to slow rates of fusion of the lysosomal granules with phagosomes. NK cell function is also impaired.

Specific granule deficiency is a rare autosomal recessive disease in which the production of secondary granules and their contents, as well as primary granule component defensins, is defective. The defect in bacterial killing leads to severe bacterial infections. One type of specific granule deficiency is due to a mutation in the CCAAT/enhancer binding protein-ε, a regulator of expression of granule components.

Chronic granulomatous disease Chronic granulomatous disease (CGD) is a group of disorders of granulocyte and monocyte oxidative metabolism. Although CGD is rare, with an incidence of 1 in 200,000 individuals, it is an important model of defective neutrophil oxidative metabolism. Most often CGD is inherited as an X-linked recessive trait; 30% of patients inherit the disease in an autosomal recessive pattern. Mutations in the genes for the four proteins that assemble at the plasma membrane account for all patients with CGD. Two proteins (a 91-kDa protein, abnormal in X-linked CGD, and a 22-kDa protein, absent in one form of autosomal recessive CGD) form the heterodimer cytochrome b-558 in the plasma membrane. Two other proteins (47 and 67 kDa, abnormal in the other autosomal recessive forms of CGD) are cytoplasmic in origin and interact with the cytochrome after cell activation to form NADPH oxidase, required for hydrogen peroxide production. Leukocytes from patients with CGD have severely diminished hydrogen peroxide production. The genes involved in each of the defects have been cloned and sequenced and the chromosome locations identified. Patients with CGD characteristically have increased numbers of infections due to catalase-positive microorganisms (organisms that destroy their own hydrogen peroxide). When patients with CGD become infected, they often have extensive inflammatory reactions, and lymph node suppuration is common despite the administration of appropriate antibiotics. Aphthous ulcers and chronic inflammation of the nares are often present. Granulomas are frequent and can obstruct the gastrointestinal or genitourinary tracts. The excessive inflammation probably reflects failure to degrade chemoattractants and antigens, leading to persistent neutrophil accumulation. Impaired killing of intracellular microorganisms by macrophages may lead to persistent cell-mediated immunity and granuloma formation.

MONONUCLEAR PHAGOCYTES

The mononuclear phagocyte system is composed of monoblasts, promonocytes, and monocytes in addition to the structurally diverse tissue macrophages that make up what was previously referred to as the reticuloendothelial system. Macrophages are long-lived phagocytic cells capable of many of the functions of neutrophils. They are also secretory cells that participate in many immunologic and inflammatory processes distinct from neutrophils. Monocytes leave the circulation by diapedesis more slowly than neutrophils and have a half-life in the blood of 12 to 24 h.

After blood monocytes arrive in the tissues, they differentiate into macrophages ("big eaters") with specialized functions suited for specific anatomic locations. Macrophages are particularly abundant in capillary walls of the lung, spleen, liver, and bone marrow, where they function to remove microorganisms and other noxious elements from the blood. Alveolar macrophages, liver Kupffer cells, splenic macrophages, peritoneal macrophages, bone marrow macrophages, lymphatic macrophages, brain microglial cells, and dendritic macrophages all have specialized functions. Macrophage-secreted products include lysozyme, neutral proteases, acid hydrolases, arginase, complement components, enzyme inhibitors (plasmin, α_2-macroglobulin), binding proteins (transferrin, fibronectin, transcobalamin II), nucleosides, and cyto-

Table 64-4   Inherited Disorders of Phagocyte Function: Differential Features

Clinical Manifestations	Cellular or Molecular Defects	Diagnosis
CHRONIC GRANULOMATOUS DISEASES OF CHILDHOOD (70% X-LINKED, 30% AUTOSOMAL RECESSIVE)		
Severe infections of skin, ears, lungs, liver, and bone with catalase-positive microorganisms such as *S. aureus, Burkholderia cepacia, Aspergillus* spp., *Chromobacterium violaceum*; often hard to culture organism; excessive inflammation with granulomas, frequent lymph node suppuration; granulomas can obstruct GI or GU tracts; gingivitis, aphthous ulcers, seborrheic dermatitis	No respiratory burst due to the lack of one of four NADPH oxidase subunits in neutrophils, monocytes, and eosinophils	NBT test; no superoxide and H_2O_2 production by neutrophils; no chemiluminescence; immunoblot for NADPH oxidase components
CHÉDIAK-HIGASHI SYNDROME (AUTOSOMAL RECESSIVE)		
Recurrent pyogenic infections, especially with *S. aureus*; many patients get lymphoma-like illness during adolescence; periodontal disease; partial oculocutaneous albinism, nystagmus, progressive peripheral neuropathy, mental retardation in some patients	Reduced chemotaxis and phagolysosome fusion, increased respiratory burst activity, defective egress from marrow, abnormal skin window	Giant primary granules in neutrophils and other granule-bearing cells (Wright's stain)
SPECIFIC GRANULE DEFICIENCY (AUTOSOMAL RECESSIVE?)		
Recurrent infections of skin, ears, and sinopulmonary tract; delayed wound healing; decreased inflammation; bleeding diathesis	Abnormal chemotaxis, impaired respiratory burst and bacterial killing, failure to upregulate chemotactic and adhesion receptors with stimulation, defect in transcription of granule proteins	Lack of secondary (specific) granules in neutrophils (Wright's stain), no neutrophil-specific granule contents (i.e., lactoferrin), no defensins, platelet α granule abnormality
MYELOPEROXIDASE DEFICIENCY (AUTOSOMAL RECESSIVE)		
Clinically normal except in patients with underlying disease such as diabetes mellitus; then candidiasis or other fungal infections	No myeloperoxidase due to pre- and post-translational defects	No peroxidase in neutrophils
LEUKOCYTE ADHESION DEFICIENCY (AUTOSOMAL RECESSIVE)		
Type 1: Delayed separation of umbilical cord, sustained neutrophilia, recurrent infections of skin and mucosa, gingivitis, periodontal disease	Impaired phagocyte adherence, aggregation, spreading, chemotaxis, phagocytosis of C3bi-coated particles; defective production of CD18 subunit common to leukocyte integrins	Reduced phagocyte surface expression of the CD18-containing integrins with monoclonal antibodies against LFA-1 (CD18/CD11a), Mac-1 or CR3 (CD18/CD11b), p150,95 (CD18/CD11c)
Type 2: Severe mental retardation, short stature, Bombay (hh) blood phenotype, recurrent infections, neutrophilia	Impaired phagocyte rolling along endothelium	Reduced phagocyte surface expression of Sialyl-Lewis^x, with monoclonal antibodies against CD15s
HYPER IGE–RECURRENT INFECTION SYNDROME (AUTOSOMAL DOMINANT) (JOB'S SYNDROME)		
Eczematoid or pruritic dermatitis, "cold" skin abscesses, recurrent pneumonias with *S. aureus* with bronchopleural fistulas and cyst formation, mild eosinophilia, mucocutaneous candidiasis, atopy, characteristic facies, restrictive lung disease, scoliosis delayed primary dental decidiation	Reduced chemotaxis in some patients, reduced suppressor T cell activity	Clinical features, serum IgE > 2000 IU/mL, high serum anti-*S. aureus* IgE, low or no serum and salivary anti-*S. aureus* IgA
MYCOBACTERIA SUSCEPTIBILITY (AUTOSOMAL DOMINANT AND RECESSIVE FORMS)		
Severe local or disseminated infections with bacilli Calmette-Gutrin, nontuberculous mycobacteria, salmonella, historiasmosis, poor granuloma formation	Inability to kill intracellular organisms due to low IFN-γ production; mutations in IFN-γ receptors, IL-12 receptor, IL-12 p40	Low or very high levels of IFN-γ receptor 1; functional assays of cytokine production and response

kines (TNF-α; IL-1, -8, -12, and -18). IL-1 (Chaps. 17 and 305) has many functions, including initiating fever in the hypothalamus, mobilizing leukocytes from the bone marrow, activating lymphocytes and neutrophils. TNF-α is a pyrogen that duplicates many of the actions of IL-1 and plays an important role in the pathogenesis of gram-negative shock (Chap. 124). TNF-α stimulates production of hydrogen peroxide and related toxic oxygen species by macrophages and neutrophils. In addition, TNF-α induces catabolic changes that contribute to the profound wasting (cachexia) associated with many chronic diseases.

Other macrophage-secreted products include reactive oxygen and nitrogen metabolites, bioactive lipids (arachidonic acid metabolites and platelet-activating factors), chemokines, colony stimulating factors, and factors stimulating fibroblast and vessel proliferation. Macrophages help regulate the replication of lymphocytes and participate in the killing of tumors, viruses, and certain bacteria (*Mycobacterium tuberculosis* and *Listeria monocytogenes*). Macrophages are key effector cells in the elimination of intracellular microorganisms. Their ability to fuse to form giant cells that coalesce into granulomas in response to some inflammatory stimuli is important in the elimination of intracellular microbes and is under the control of IFN-γ. Nitric oxide induced by IFN-γ is an important effector against intracellular parasites including tuberculosis and *Leishmania*.

Macrophages play an important role in the immune response (Chap. 305). They process and present antigen to lymphocytes and secrete cytokines that modulate and direct lymphocyte development and function. Macrophages participate in autoimmune phenomena by removing immune complexes and other substances from the circulation. Polymorphisms in macrophage receptors for immunoglobulin (FcγRII) determine suceptibility to some infections and autoimmune diseases. In wound healing, they dispose of senescent cells, and they contribute to atheroma development. Macrophage elastase mediates development of emphysema from cigarette smoking.

DISORDERS OF THE MONONUCLEAR PHAGOCYTE SYSTEM   Many disorders of neutrophils extend to mononuclear phagocytes. Thus, drugs that suppress neutrophil production in the bone marrow can cause monocytopenia. Transient monocytopenia occurs after stress or glucocorticoid administration. Monocytosis is associated with tuberculosis, brucellosis, subacute bacterial endocarditis, Rocky Mountain spotted fever, malaria, and visceral leishmaniasis (kala azar). Monocytosis also occurs with malignancies, leukemias, myeloproliferative syndromes, hemolytic anemias, chronic idiopathic neutropenias, and granulomatous diseases such as sarcoidosis, regional enteritis, and some collagen vascular diseases. Patients with LAD, hyperimmunoglobulin E−recurrent infection (Job's) syndrome, CHS, and CGD all have defects in the mononuclear phagocyte system.

Monocyte cytokine production is impaired in some patients with disseminated nontuberculous mycobacterial infection who are not infected with HIV. Genetic defects in IFN-γ receptors 1 and 2 impair monocyte killing of intracellular parasites, as do lesions in the potent IFN-γ inducer, IL-12 and its receptor (Fig. 64-5).

Certain viral infections impair mononuclear phagocyte function. For example, influenza virus infection causes abnormal monocyte chemotaxis. Mononuclear phagocytes can be infected by HIV using CCR5, the chemokine receptor that acts as a coreceptor with CD4 for HIV. T lymphocytes produce IFN-γ, which induces FcR expression and phagocytosis and stimulates hydrogen peroxide production by mononuclear phagocytes and neutrophils. In certain diseases, such as AIDS, IFN-γ production may be deficient, while in other diseases, such as T cell lymphomas, excessive release of IFN-γ may be associated with erythrophagocytosis by splenic macrophages.

Monocytopenia occurs with acute infections, with stress, and after treatment with glucocorticoids. Monocytopenia also occurs in aplastic anemia, hairy cell leukemia, acute myeloid leukemia, and as a direct result of myelotoxic drugs.

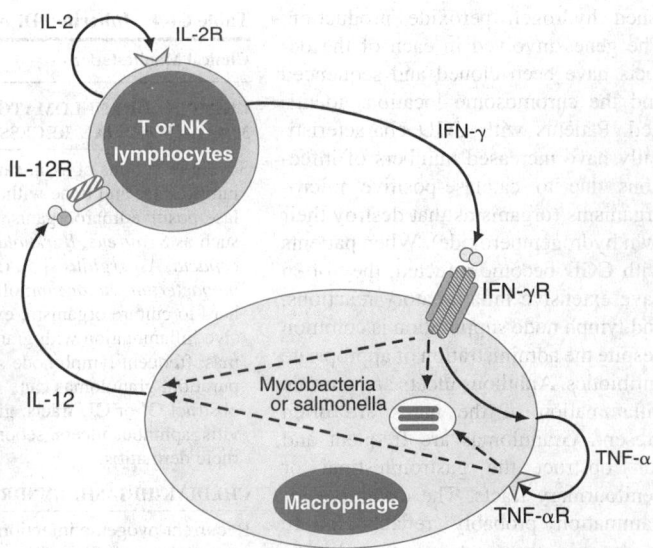

FIGURE 64-5   Lymphocyte-macrophage interactions underlying resistance to mycobacteria and other intracellular parasites such as Salmonella. Mycobacteria infect macrophages, leading to the production of IL-12, which activates T or NK cells through its receptor, leading to production of IL-1 and IFN-γ. IFN-γ acts through its receptor on macrophages to upregulate TNF-α and IL-12 and kill intracellular parasites. Mutant forms of the cytokines and receptors shown in large type have been found in severe cases of nontuberculous mycobacterial infection and salmonellosis.

EOSINOPHILS

Eosinophils and neutrophils share similar morphology, many lysosomal constituents, phagocytic capacity, and oxidative metabolism. Eosinophils express a specific chemoattractant receptor and respond to a specific chemokine, eotaxin. Little is known about the role of eosinophils. Eosinophils are much longer lived than neutrophils, and unlike neutrophils, tissue eosinophils can recirculate. During most infections, eosinophils are not important. However, in invasive helminthic infections, such as hookworm, schistosomiasis, strongyloidiasis, toxocariasis, trichinosis, filariasis, echinococcosis, and cysticercosis, the eosinophil plays a central role in host defense. Eosinophils are associated with bronchial asthma, cutaneous allergic reactions, and other hypersensitivity states.

The distinctive feature of the red-staining (Wright's stain) eosinophil granules is its crystalline core consisting of an arginine-rich protein (major basic protein) with histaminase activity, important in host defense against parasites. Eosinophil granules also contain a unique eosinophil peroxidase that catalyzes the oxidation of many substances by hydrogen peroxide and may facilitate killing of microorganisms.

Eosinophil peroxidase, in the presence of hydrogen peroxide and halide, initiates mast cell secretion in vitro and thereby promotes inflammation. Eosinophils contain cationic proteins, some of which bind to heparin and reduce its anticoagulant activity. Eosinophil-derived neurotoxin and eosinophil cationic protein are ribonucleases that can kill respiratory syncytial virus. Eosinophil cytoplasm contains Charcot-Leyden crystal protein, a hexagonal bipyramidal crystal first observed in a patient with leukemia and then in sputum of patients with asthma; this protein is lysophospholipase and may function to detoxify certain lysophospholipids.

Several factors enhance the eosinophil's function in host defense. T cell−derived factors enhance the ability of eosinophils to kill parasites. Mast cell−derived eosinophil chemotactic factor of anaphylaxis (ECFa) increases the number of eosinophil complement receptors and enhances eosinophil killing of parasites. Eosinophil colony stimulating factors (e.g., IL-5) produced by macrophages increase eosinophil production in the bone marrow and activate eosinophils to kill parasites.

EOSINOPHILIA   Eosinophilia is the presence of >500 eosinophils per microliter of blood and is common in many settings besides parasite infection. Significant tissue eosinophilia can occur without an elevated blood count. The most common cause of eosinophilia is allergic reactions to drugs (iodides, aspirin, sulfonamides, nitrofurantoin, penicillins, and cephalosporins). Allergies such as hay fever, asthma, eczema, serum sickness, allergic vasculitis, and pemphigus are associated with eosinophilia. Eosinophilia also occurs in collagen vascular diseases (e.g., rheumatoid arthritis, eosinophilic fasciitis, allergic angiitis, and periarteritis nodosa) and malignancies (e.g., Hodgkin's disease; mycosis fungoides; chronic myelogenous leukemia; and cancer of the lung, stomach, pancreas, ovary, or uterus), as well as in Job's syndrome and CGD. Eosinophilia commonly is present in the helminthic infections. IL-5 is the dominant eosinophil growth factor. Therapeutic administration of the cytokines IL-2 and GM-CSF frequently leads to transient eosinophilia. The most dramatic hypereosinophilic syndromes are Loeffler's syndrome, tropical pulmonary eosinophilia, Loeffler's endocarditis, eosinophilic leukemia, and idiopathic hypereosinophilic syndrome (50,000 to 100,000/μL).

The idiopathic hypereosinophilic syndrome represents a heterogeneous group of disorders with the common feature of prolonged eosinophilia of unknown cause and organ system dysfunction, including the heart, central nervous system, kidneys, lungs, gastrointestinal tract, and skin. The bone marrow is involved in all affected individuals, but the most severe complications involve the heart and central nervous system. Clinical manifestations and organ dysfunction are highly variable. Eosinophils are found in the involved tissues and likely cause tissue damage by local deposition of toxic eosinophil proteins such as eosinophil cationic protein and major basic protein. In the heart, the pathologic changes lead to thrombosis, endocardial fibrosis, and restrictive endomyocardiopathy. The damage to tissues in other organ systems is similar. The mechanism for the hypereosinophilia is not known. Glucocorticoids usually induce remission. In patients who do not respond to glucocorticoids, a cytotoxic agent such as hydroxyurea has been used successfully to lower the peripheral blood eosinophil counts and to improve markedly the prognosis. IFN-α also is effective in some patients, including those unresponsive to hydroxyurea. Aggressive medical and surgical approaches are used to manage patients with cardiovascular complications.

The *eosinophilia-myalgia syndrome* is a multisystem disease with prominent cutaneous, hematologic, and visceral manifestations that frequently evolves into a chronic course and can occasionally be fatal. The syndrome is characterized by eosinophilia (eosinophil count >1000/μL) and generalized disabling myalgias without other recognized causes. Eosinophil fasciitis, pneumonitis, and myocarditis; neuropathy culminating in respiratory failure; and encephalopathy may occur. The disease is caused by ingesting contaminants in L-tryptophan–containing products. Eosinophils, lymphocytes, macrophages, and fibroblasts accumulate in the affected tissues, but their role in pathogenesis is unclear. Activation of eosinophils and fibroblasts and the deposition of eosinophil-derived toxic proteins in affected tissues may contribute. IL-5 and transforming growth factor β have been implicated as potential mediators. Treatment is withdrawal of L-tryptophan–containing products and the administration of glucocorticoids. Most patients recover fully, remain stable, or show slow recovery; but the disease can be fatal in up to 5% of patients.

EOSINOPENIA   Eosinopenia occurs with stress, such as acute bacterial infection, and after treatment with glucocorticoids. The mechanism of eosinopenia of acute bacterial infection is unknown but is independent of endogenous glucocorticoids, since it occurs in animals after total adrenalectomy. There is no known adverse effect of eosinopenia.

HYPERIMMUNOGLOBULIN E-RECURRENT INFECTION SYNDROME

The hyperimmunoglobulin E–recurrent infection (HIE) syndrome or *Job's syndrome* is a rare multisystem disease in which the immune system, bone, teeth, lung and skin are affected. Abnormal chemotaxis

is a variable feature. The molecular basis for this syndrome is not known, but some cases show autosomal dominant transmission with linkage to 4q. Patients with this syndrome have characteristic facies with broad nose, kyphoscoliosis and osteoporosis, and eczema. The primary teeth erupt normally but do not deciduate, often requiring extraction. Patients develop recurrent sinopulmonary and cutaneous infections that tend to be much less inflamed than appropriate for the degree of infection and have been referred to as "cold abscesses." A high degree of suspicion is required to diagnose infections in these patients, who may appear well despite extensive disease. The cold abscesses have been considered a reflection of impaired chemotaxis with too few phagocytes arriving too late, perhaps due to a lymphocyte factor inhibiting chemotaxis. However, the chemotactic defect in these patients is variable, and the fundamental basis for the impaired defenses is complex and poorly defined.

LABORATORY DIAGNOSIS AND MANAGEMENT

Initial studies of WBC and differential and often a bone marrow examination are followed by assessment of bone marrow reserves (steroid challenge test), marginated circulating pool of cells (epinephrine challenge test), and marginating ability (endotoxin challenge test) (Fig. 64-3). In vivo assessment of inflammation is possible with a Rebuck skin window test or an in vivo blister assay, which measures the ability of leukocytes and inflammatory mediators to accumulate locally in the skin. In vitro tests of phagocyte aggregation, adherence, chemotaxis, phagocytosis, degranulation, and microbicidal activity (for *S. aureus*) may help pinpoint cellular or humoral lesions. Deficiencies of oxidative metabolism are detected with the nitroblue tetrazolium (NBT) dye test, which is based on the ability of products of oxidative metabolism to reduce yellow, soluble NBT to blue-black formazan, an insoluble material that can be seen microscopically. Studies of superoxide and hydrogen peroxide production may further define neutrophil oxidative function.

Patients with leukopenias or leukocyte dysfunction often have delayed inflammatory responses. Therefore, clinical manifestations may be minimal despite overwhelming infection, and unusual infections must always be suspected. Early signs of infection demand prompt, aggressive culturing for microorganisms, use of antibiotics, and surgical drainage of abscesses. Prolonged antibiotics are often required. In patients with CGD, prophylactic antibiotics (trimethoprim-sulfamethoxazole) diminish the frequency of life-threatening infections. Short courses of glucocorticoids may relieve gastrointestinal or genitourinary tract obstruction by granulomas in patients with CGD. Recombinant human IFN-γ, which nonspecifically stimulates phagocytic cell function, reduces the frequency of infections in patients with CGD by 70% and reduces the severity of infection. This effect of IFN-γ in CGD is additive to the effect of prophylactic antibiotics. The recommended dose is 50 μg/m^2 subcutaneously three times weekly. IFN-γ also has been used successfully in the treatment of leprosy, nontuberculous mycobacteria, and visceral leishmaniasis.

Rigorous oral hygiene reduces but does not eliminate the discomfort of gingivitis, periodontal disease, and aphthous ulcers; chlorhexidine mouthwash and tooth brushing with a hydrogen peroxide–sodium bicarbonate paste helps many patients. Oral antifungal agents (fluconazole) have reduced mucocutaneous candidiasis in patients with Job's syndrome. Androgens, glucocorticoids, lithium, and immunosuppressive therapy have been used to restore myelopoiesis in patients with neutropenia due to impaired production. Recombinant G-CSF is useful in the management of certain forms of neutropenia due to depressed neutrophil production, especially that related to cancer chemotherapy. Patients with chronic neutropenia with evidence of a good bone marrow reserve need not receive prophylactic antibiotics.

Patients with constant or cyclic neutrophil counts <500/μL may benefit from prophylactic antibiotics and G-CSF during periods of neutropenia. Oral trimethoprim-sulfamethoxazole (160/800 mg) twice daily can prevent infection. Increased numbers of fungal infections are not seen in patients with CGD on this regimen. Oral quinolones such as norfloxacin and ciprofloxacin are alternatives.

In the setting of cytotoxic chemotherapy with severe, persistent neutropenia, trimethoprim-sulfamethoxazole prevents *Pneumocystis carinii* pneumonia. These patients, and patients with phagocytic cell dysfunction, should avoid heavy exposure to airborne soil, dust, or decaying matter (mulch, manure), which are often rich in spores of *Aspergillus* or other fungi. Restriction of activities or social contact has no proven role in reducing risk of infection.

Cure of some congenital phagocyte defects is possible by bone marrow transplantation (Chap. 115). However, complications of bone marrow transplantation are still serious, and with rigorous medical care many patients with phagocytic disorders can go for years without a life-threatening infection. The identification of specific gene defects in patients with LAD 1 and CGD has led to gene therapy trials in a number of genetic white cell disorders.

BIBLIOGRAPHY

GRIMBACHER B et al: Hyper-IgE syndrome with recurrent infections—an autosomal dominant multisystem disorder. N Engl J Med 340:692, 1999

HOLLAND SM et al: Abnormal regulation of interferon-γ, interleukin-12, and tumor necrosis factor-α in human interferon-γ receptor 1 deficiency. J Infect Dis 178:1095, 1998

HOLLAND SM, GALLIN JI: Disorders of phagocytic cells, in *Inflammation: Basic Principles and Clinical Correlates*, 3d ed. JI Gallin, R Snyderman (eds). Philadelphia, Lippincott-Williams & Wilkins, 1999

HUNTER MG, AVALOS BR: Deletion of a critical internalization domain in the G-CSF receptor in acute myelogenous leukemia preceded by severe congenital neutropenia. Blood 93:440, 1999

LEKSTROM-HIMES JA et al: Neutrophil-specific granule deficiency results from a novel mutation with loss of function of the transcription factor CCAAT/enhancer binding protein-ε. J Exp Med 189:1847, 1999

LOCATI M, MURPHY PM: Chemokines and chemokine receptors: Biology and clinical relevance in inflammation and AIDS. Annu Rev Med 50:425, 1999

NEUFELD G et al: Vascular endothelial growth factor (VEGF) and its receptors. FASEB J 13:9, 1999

ROSENBERG HF: The eosinophil ribonucleases. Cell Mol Life Sci 54:795, 1998

SEMENZATO G et al: The lymphoproliferative disease of granular lymphocytes: Updated criteria for diagnosis. Blood 89:256, 1997

WINKELSTEIN JA et al: Chronic granulomatous disease: Report on a national registry of 368 patients. Medicine (Baltimore) 79:155, 2000

NOBEL PRIZE IN PHYSIOLOGY OR MEDICINE, 1990

Joseph Edward Murray was born April 1, 1919, in Milford, Massachusetts, the third child of William and Mary Murray. After high school he attended the College of Holy Cross, then entered Harvard Medical School. He received his medical degree in 1943. After an internship in surgery at the Peter Bent Brigham Hospital, Murray entered the military and was assigned to Valley Forge General Hospital where there were many badly burned World War II patients. He was there from 1944 to 1947 and during that time developed substantial expertise in both grafting and plastic surgery. After discharge he completed his residency in surgery at the Peter Bent Brigham and New York Hospitals. He then became director of the laboratory for surgical research at Harvard Medical School. In 1951 at Harvard, David Hume began a series of nine renal transplants into the thighs of recipients, but they were all ultimately rejected. During his surgical residency, Murray had carried out numerous renal autografts in dogs and concluded that transplants could function normally if the immunologic barrier could be overcome. The opportunity to test this theory in patients occurred with an end-stage renal patient who had a twin brother. The kidney transplant from the twin brother was a resounding success. The patient married his recovery room nurse, fathered two children, and lived more than seven years with the transplanted kidney.

In 1961 the Brigham team began using immunosuppressive drugs to perform kidney transplants in non-twins. The results by 1965 were 80% allograft survival at 1 year and 65% unrelated cadaveric graft survival at 1 year. Murray subsequently returned to plastic surgery with a specialty in the repair of facial defects in children. His contribution of successfully transplanting the first organ in a human was a seminal event that launched the era of organ transplantation. For this contribution he shared the Nobel Prize in Physiology or Medicine in 1990 with Donnall Thomas.

Edward Donnall Thomas was born March 15, 1920, in Mart, Texas. Thomas received his B.A. degree at the University of Texas, where he met and married his wife, Dorothy. He then attended Harvard Medical School and on graduation had his internship at the Peter Bent Brigham Hospital. This was the same time at the Brigham when Murray had been successful in transplanting kidneys. This led Thomas to believe that bone marrow tissue could also be transplanted to treat patients with aplastic anemia. Thomas then joined the staff at Mary Bassett Hospital in Cooperstown, New York, where, in collaboration with Dr. Joseph Ferrabee, Thomas showed that dogs could survive otherwise fatal radiation if their own marrow had been previously harvested and then returned to the animals following radiation. The ability to store bone marrow without loss of vitality was a major breakthrough. However, bone marrow from other animals, that is, an allogeneic graft, was not successful. Thomas and Ferrabee then treated a twin suffering from leukemia with supralethal radiation, followed by marrow infusion from the twin sibling. The use of the antimetabolite methotrexate and the availability of histocompatibility typing then allowed for non-twin allogeneic bone marrow transplantation. In March 1967 Thomas moved to the University of Washington, and in March 1969 the Thomas team performed the first bone marrow infusion from a matched brother donor to his sister who was dying of leukemia; 20 years later the woman was still in good health. In 1974 Thomas became director of medical oncology at the Fred Hutchinson Cancer Research Center, which, with his leadership, became the largest bone marrow transplant center in the world and the training site for the majority of individuals who started bone marrow transplant units worldwide. The "biological force," which was supposed to prevent tissue and organ transplant, had thus been overcome. In 1990 Murray and Thomas were rewarded as pioneers in the area of transplantation with the Nobel Prize.

REFERENCES

1. Magill FN (ed): *Nobel Prize Winners: Physiology or Medicine*, vol 3. Pasadena, Salem Press, 1993

2. Schrier RW: *A Salute to Nobel Laureates in Physiology and Medicine*, Proceedings of the Association of American Physicians. 108(1): Jan 1996

Robert W. Schrier, MD

65

J. Larry Jameson, Peter Kopp

PRINCIPLES OF HUMAN GENETICS

ACTH adrenocorticotropic hormone	RFLPs restriction fragment length
BACs bacterial artificial	polymorphisms
chromosomes	RT reverse transcriptase
CREB cyclic AMP response element	SNPs single nucleotide
binding	polymorphisms
HGP Human Genome Project	STRs short tandem repeats
HNPCC hereditary nonpolyposis	VNTRs variable number of tandem
colon cancer	repeats
MEN multiple endocrine neoplasia	YACs yeast artificial chromosomes
PCR polymerase chain reaction	

IMPACT OF GENETICS ON MEDICAL PRACTICE

New insights into the genetic basis of disease are being generated at an ever-increasing rate. This explosion of information was ignited by technological advances, such as the polymerase chain reaction (PCR) and automated DNA sequencing, and is fueled by rapid progress in the Human Genome Project (HGP). Although its promise is great, the integration of genetics into the everyday practice of medicine remains challenging. To date, the most significant impact of genetics has been to enhance our understanding of disease etiology and pathogenesis. In the near term, we can expect an even greater role for genetics in the diagnosis, prevention, and treatment of disease (Chaps. 68 and 69).

Genetic disorders are more common than generally appreciated. It is estimated, for example, that 3% of pregnancies result in a child with a genetic disease or birth defect. About 10% of all pediatric and adult hospitalization admissions involve genetic diseases. This number would increase substantially if one included complex, multifactorial genetic diseases, such as diabetes or cardiovascular disease. The prevalence of genetic diseases, combined with their severity and chronic nature, imposes a great financial, social, and emotional burden on society.

Genetics has historically focused on chromosomal and metabolic disorders, reflecting the long-standing availability of techniques to diagnose these conditions. For example, conditions such as trisomy 21 (Down syndrome) or monosomy X (Turner syndrome) can be diagnosed using cytogenetics (Chap. 66). Likewise, many metabolic disorders (e.g., phenylketonuria, familial hypercholesterolemia) have been diagnosed using biochemical analyses. Recent advances in DNA diagnostics have extended the field of genetics to include virtually all medical specialties. In cardiology, for example, the molecular basis of inherited cardiomyopathies and ion channel defects that predispose to arrhythmias is being defined (Chaps. 230 and 238). In neurology, genetics has unmasked the pathophysiology of a startling number of neurodegenerative disorders (Chap. 359). Hematology has evolved dramatically, from its incipient genetic descriptions of hemoglobinopathies to the current understanding of the molecular basis of red cell membrane defects, clotting disorders, and thrombotic disorders (Chaps. 106 and 117). It is now abundantly clear that neoplasia and the acquisition of metastatic potential can be described in genetic terms (Chaps. 81, 82, and 83).

New concepts derived from genetic studies can sometimes clarify topics that were previously opaque. For example, although many different genetic defects can cause peripheral neuropathies, disruption of the normal folding of the myelin sheaths is frequently a common final

pathway (Chap. 379). Several genetic causes of obesity appear to converge on a physiologic pathway that involves products of the proopiomelanocortin polypeptide and the MC4R receptor, thus identifying a key mechanism for appetite control (Chap. 77). A similar situation is emerging for genetically distinct forms of Alzheimer disease, several of which lead to the formation of neurofibrillary tangles (Chap. 362). Increasingly, the identification of defective genes can pinpoint cellular pathways involved in key physiologic processes. Examples include identification of the cystic fibrosis conductance regulator (*CFTR*) gene, the Duchenne's muscular dystrophy (*DMD*) gene, which encodes dystrophin, and the fibroblast growth factor receptor-3 (*FGFR3*) gene, which is responsible for achondroplastic dwarfism. Similarly, transgenic and gene "knockout" models can help to unravel the physiologic function of genes. Genetic approaches have proven invaluable for the detection of infectious pathogens and are used clinically to identify agents that are difficult to culture such as mycobacteria, viruses, and parasites (Chap. 121). In many cases, molecular genetics has improved the feasibility and accuracy of diagnostic testing, enhanced our understanding of pathophysiology, and is beginning to open new avenues for therapy, including gene therapy (Chap. 69).

It is increasingly apparent that genetic background plays some role in virtually every medical condition. This is particularly true when one considers disease susceptibility, the interaction of genetic background with the environment, host responses to illness and to pharmaceutical agents, or the metabolism of drugs. Although genetics has traditionally been viewed through the window of relatively rare single-gene diseases, many disorders such as hypertension, asthma, diabetes, susceptibility to cardiovascular disease, and mental illness are also affected by genetic background, as often evident from a patient's family history. These complex genetic traits involve the contributions of many different genes, as well as environmental factors that can modify disease risk (Chap. 68).

The astounding rate at which new genetic information is being generated creates a major challenge for physicians and other health care providers. The terminology and techniques used for discovery evolve continuously. Much genetic information presently resides in computer databases or is being published in basic science journals. The ongoing development of bioinformatics promises to simplify this seemingly daunting onslaught of new information. It is now possible, for example, to search for genetic testing centers through a web site (www.genlink.wustl.edu) that can be accessed conveniently by organ system, disease state, or gene. Monogenic disorders are summarized in a large, continuously evolving compendium, referred to as the *Online Mendelian Inheritance in Man* (OMIM; www.ncbi.nlm.nih.gov/omim/). These and other databases (www.genebank.com) will expand rapidly in conjunction with advances in the HGP.

CHROMOSOMES AND DNA REPLICATION

ORGANIZATION OF DNA INTO CHROMOSOMES

Size of the Human Genome The human genome is divided into 23 different chromosomes, including 22 autosomes (numbered 1 to 22) and the X and Y sex chromosomes. Adult cells are diploid, meaning they contain two homologous sets of 22 autosomes and a pair of sex chromosomes. Females have two X chromosomes (XX), whereas males have one X and one Y chromosome (XY). As a consequence of meiosis, germ cells (sperm or oocytes) are haploid and contain one set of 22 autosomes and one of the sex chromosomes. At the time of fertilization, the diploid genome is reconstituted by pairing of the homologous chromosomes from the mother and father. With each cell division (mitosis), chromosomes are replicated, paired, segregated, and divided into two daughter cells (Chap. 66).

FIGURE 65-1 Structure of chromatin and chromosomes. Chromatin is composed of double-stranded DNA that is wrapped around histone and nonhistone proteins forming nucleosomes. The nucleosomes are further organized into solenoid structures. Chromosomes assume their characteristic structure, with short (p) and long (q) arms at the metaphase stage of the cell cycle.

genes are about this size, the range is quite broad. For example, some genes are only a few hundred bp, whereas others, like the *DMD* gene, are extraordinarily large (2 million bp).

Structure of DNA Each gene is composed of a linear polymer of DNA. DNA is a double-stranded helix composed of four different bases: adenine (A), thymidine (T), guanine (G), and cytosine (C). Adenine is paired to thymidine, and guanine is paired to cytosine, by hydrogen bond interactions that span the double helix. DNA has several remarkable features that make it ideal for the transmission of genetic information. It is relatively stable, at least in comparison to RNA or proteins. The double-stranded nature of DNA and its feature of strict base-pair complementarity permit faithful replication during cell division. As described below, complementarity also allows the transmission of genetic information from DNA → RNA → protein (Fig. 65-2). Messenger RNA (mRNA) is encoded by the so-called sense strand of the DNA double helix and is translated into proteins by ribosomes.

The presence of four different bases provides surprising genetic diversity. In the protein-coding regions of genes, the DNA bases are arranged into codons, a triplet of bases that specifies a particular amino acid. It is possible to arrange the four bases into 64 different triplet codons (4^3). Each codon specifies 1 of the 20 different amino acids, or a regulatory signal, such as stop translation. Because there are more codons than amino acids, the genetic code is degenerate; that is, most amino acids can be specified by several different codons. By arranging the codons in different combinations and in various lengths, it is possible to generate the tremendous diversity of primary protein structure.

REPLICATION OF DNA AND MITOSIS

Genetic information in DNA is transmitted to daughter cells under two different circumstances: (1) somatic cells divide by mitosis, allowing the diploid (2*n*) genome to replicate itself completely in conjunction with cell division; and (2) germ cells (sperm and ova) undergo meiosis, a process that enables the reduction of the diploid (2*n*) set of chromosomes to the haploid state (1*n*) (Chap. 66).

Prior to mitosis, cells exit the resting, or G_0 state, and enter the cell cycle (Chap. 82). After traversing a critical checkpoint in G_1, cells undergo DNA synthesis (S phase), during which the DNA in each chromosome is replicated, yielding two pairs of sister chromatids (2*n* → 4*n*). The process of DNA synthesis requires stringent fidelity in order to avoid transmitting errors to subsequent generations of cells. Genetic abnormalities of DNA mismatch/repair include xeroderma pigmentosum, Bloom syndrome, ataxia telangiectasia, and hereditary nonpolyposis colon cancer (HNPCC), among others. Many of these disorders strongly redispose to neoplasia because of the rapid acquisition of additional mutations (Chap. 81). After completion of DNA synthesis, cells enter G_2 and progress through a second checkpoint before entering mitosis. At this stage, the chromosomes condense and are aligned along the equatorial plate at metaphase. The two identical sister chromatids, held together at the centromere, divide and migrate to opposite poles of the cell (Fig. 66-3). After formation of a nuclear membrane around the two separated sets of chromatids, the cell divides and two daughter cells are formed, thus restoring the diploid (2*n*) state.

ASSORTMENT AND SEGREGATION OF GENES DURING MEIOSIS

Meiosis occurs only in germ cells of the gonads. It shares certain features with mitosis but involves two distinct steps of

The genome is estimated to contain about 100,000 genes that are divided among the 23 chromosomes. A *gene* is a functional unit that is regulated by transcription (see below) and encodes a product, either RNA or protein, that exerts activity within the cell. Historically, genes were identified because they conferred specific traits that are transmitted from one generation to the next.

Human DNA is estimated to consist of about 3 billion base pairs (bp) of DNA per haploid genome. DNA length is normally measured in units of 1000 bp (kilobases, kb) or 1,000,000 bp (megabases, Mb). Not all DNA encodes genes. In fact, genes account for only about 10 to 15% of DNA. Much of the remaining DNA consists of highly repetitive sequences, the function of which is poorly understood. These repetitive DNA regions, along with nonrepetitive sequences that do not encode genes, may serve a structural role in the packaging of DNA into chromatin (DNA bound to histone proteins) and chromosomes (Fig. 65-1). If only 10% of DNA is expressed and there are 100,000 genes, the average gene would be about 3 kb in length. Although many cell division that reduce the chromosome number to the haploid state. In addition, there is active recombination that generates genetic diversity. During the first cell division, two sister chromatids ($2n \rightarrow 4n$) are formed for each chromosome pair and there is an exchange of DNA between homologous paternal and maternal chromosomes. This process involves the formation of *chiasmata*, structures that correspond to the DNA segments that cross over between the maternal and paternal homologues (Fig. 65-3). Usually there is at least one crossover on each chromosomal arm; recombination occurs more frequently in female meiosis than in male meiosis. Subsequently, the chromosomes segregate randomly. Because there are 23 chromosomes, there exist 2^{23} (>8 million) possible combinations of chromosomes. Together with the genetic exchanges that occur during recombination, chromosomal segregation generates tremendous diversity, and each gamete is genetically unique. The process of recombination, and the independent segregation of chromosomes, provide the foundation for performing linkage analyses, whereby one attempts to correlate the inheritance of certain chromosomal regions (or linked genes) with the presence of a disease or genetic trait (see below).

After the first meiotic division, which results in two daughter cells ($2n$), the two chromatids of each chromosome separate during a second meiotic division to yield four gametes with a haploid state ($1n$). When the egg is fertilized by sperm, the two haploid sets are combined, thereby restoring the diploid state ($2n$) in the zygote.

FIGURE 65-2 Flow of genetic information. Multiple extracellular signals activate intracellular signal cascades that result in altered regulation of gene expression through the interaction of transcription factors with regulatory regions of genes. RNA polymerase transcribes DNA into RNA that is processed to mRNA by excision of intronic sequences. The mRNA is translated into a polypeptide chain to form the mature protein after undergoing posttranslational processing. HAT, histone acetyl transferase; CBP, CREB-binding protein; CREB, cyclic AMP response element binding protein; CRE, cyclic AMP responsive element; CoA, Co activator; TAF, TBP-associated factors; GTF, general transcription factors; TBP, TATA-binding protein; TATA, TATA box; RE, response element; NH_2, aminoterminus; COOH, carboxyterminus.

REGULATION OF GENE EXPRESSION

Mechanisms that regulate gene expression play a critical role in the function of genes. The new field of *functional genomics* is based on the concept that understanding gene regulation and function will provide a better understanding of physiology and offer novel therapeutic opportunities. The transcription of genes is controlled primarily by *transcription factors* that bind to DNA sequences in the regulatory regions of genes. As described below, mutations in transcription factors cause an unexpectedly large number of genetic disorders. Gene expression is also influenced by *epigenetic events*, such as X-inactivation and imprinting, processes in which DNA methylation is associated with the silencing (i.e., suppression) of expression. Several genetic disorders, such as Prader-Willi syndrome (neonatal hypotonia, developmental delay, obesity, short stature, and hypogonadism) and Albright hereditary osteodystrophy (resistance to parathyroid hormone, short stature, brachydactyly, resistance to other hormones in certain subtypes), exhibit the consequences of genomic imprinting. Most studies of gene expression have focused on the regulatory DNA elements of genes that control transcription. However, it should be emphasized that gene expression requires a series of steps including mRNA processing, protein translation, and posttranslational modifications, all of which are actively regulated (Fig. 65-2).

STRUCTURE OF GENES A gene product is usually a protein but can occasionally consist of RNA that is not translated. *Exons* refer to the portion of genes that are eventually spliced together to form mRNA. *Introns* refer to the spacing regions between the exons that are spliced out of precursor RNAs during RNA processing (Fig. 65-2).

The gene locus also includes regions that are necessary to control its expression. The regulatory regions most commonly involve sequences upstream ($5'$) of the transcription start site, although there are also examples of control elements within introns or downstream of the coding regions of a gene. The upstream regulatory regions are also referred to as the *promoter*. The minimal promoter usually consists of a TATA box (which binds TATA-binding protein, TBP) and initiator sequences that enhance the formation of an active transcription complex. Transcriptional termination signals reside downstream, or $3'$, of a gene. Specific sequences, such as the AAUAAA sequence at the $3'$ end of the mRNA, designate the site for polyadenylation (poly-A tail), a process that influences mRNA transport to the cytoplasm, stability, and translation efficiency. A rigorous test of the regulatory region boundaries involves expressing a gene in a transgenic animal to determine whether the isolated DNA flanking sequences are sufficient to recapitulate the normal developmental, tissue-specific, and signal-responsive features of the endogenous gene. This has been accomplished for only a few genes; there are many examples in which large genomic fragments only partially reconstitute normal gene regulation in vivo, implying the presence of distant regulatory sequences. This approach is critical to our understanding of mechanisms that regulate genes and is also relevant for gene therapy strategies that require normal gene regulation (Chap. 69).

As genes are dissected with greater resolution, the number of DNA sequences and transcription factors that regulate transcription is much greater than originally anticipated. Most genes contain at least 15 to 20 discrete regulatory elements within 300 bp of the transcription start site. This densely packed promoter region often contains binding sites for ubiquitous transcription factors such as CAAT box/enhancer binding protein (C/EBP), cyclic AMP response element binding (CREB) protein, selective promoter factor 1 (Sp-1), or activator protein 1 (AP-1). However, factors involved in cell-specific expression may also bind to these sequences. For example, basic helix-loop-helix (bHLH) proteins bind to E-boxes in the promoters of myogenic genes, and ste-

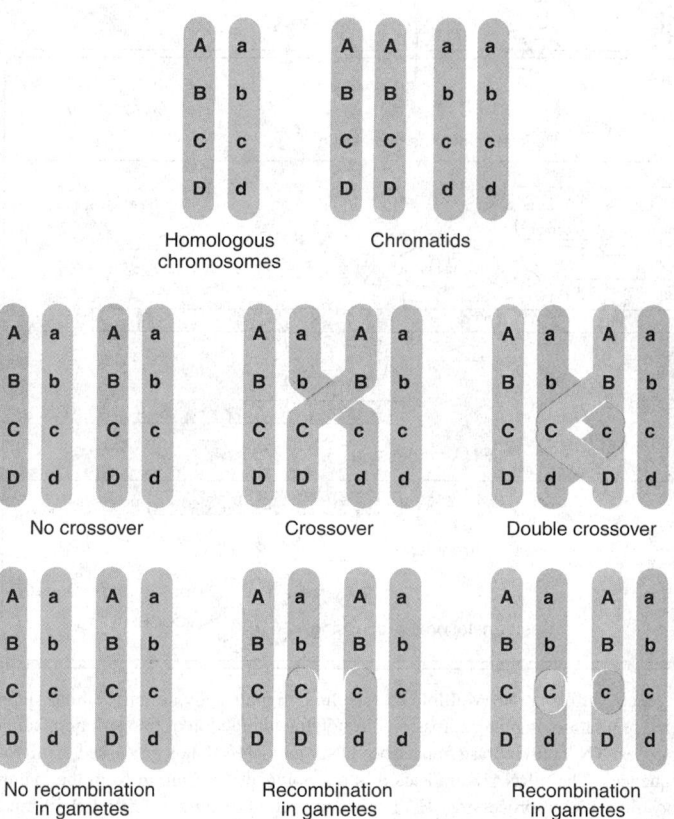

FIGURE 65-3 Crossing-over and genetic recombination. During chiasma formation, either of the two sister chromatids on one chromosome pairs with one of the chromatids of the homologous chromosome. Genetic recombination occurs through crossing-over and results in recombinant and nonrecombinant chromosome segments in the gametes. Together with the random segregation of the maternal and paternal chromosomes, recombination contributes to genetic diversity and forms the basis of the concept of linkage.

roidogenic factor 1 (SF-1) binds to a specific recognition site in the regulatory region of multiple steroidogenic enzyme genes. Key regulatory elements may also reside at some distance from the proximal promoter. The globin and the immunoglobulin genes, for example, contain *locus control regions* that are several kilobases away from the structural sequences of the gene. Specific groups of transcription factors that bind to these promoter and enhancer sequences provide a combinatorial code for regulating transcription. In this manner, relatively ubiquitous factors interact with more restricted factors to allow each gene to be expressed and regulated in a unique manner. As described below, the transcription factors that bind to DNA actually represent only the first level of regulatory control. Other proteins—*coactivators* and *corepressors*—interact with the DNA-binding transcription factors to generate large regulatory complexes. These complexes are subject to control by numerous cell-signaling pathways, including phosphorylation and acetylation. Ultimately, the recruited transcription factors interact with, and stabilize, components of the basal transcription complex that assembles at the site of the TATA box and initiator region. This basal transcription factor complex consists of >30 different proteins. Gene transcription occurs when RNA polymerase begins to synthesize RNA from the DNA template.

TRANSCRIPTIONAL ACTIVATION AND REPRESSION
Every gene is controlled uniquely, whether in its spatial or temporal pattern of expression or in its response to extracellular signals. It is estimated that transcription factors account for about 30% of expressed genes. A growing number of identified genetic diseases involve transcription factors (Table 65-1). The MODY (maturity-onset diabetes of the young) disorders are representative of this group of diseases; mu-

tations in several different islet cell–specific transcription factors cause various forms of MODY (Chap. 333).

Transcriptional activation can be divided into three main mechanisms:

1. Events that alter chromatin structure can enhance the access of transcription factors to DNA. For example, histone acetylation opens chromatin structure and is correlated with transcriptional activation.
2. Posttranslational modifications of transcription factors, such as phosphorylation, can induce the assembly of active transcription complexes. As an example, phosphorylation of CREB protein on serine 133 induces a conformational change that allows the recruitment of CREB-binding protein (CBP), a factor that integrates the actions of many transcription factors, including proteins, with histone acetyltransferase activity.
3. Transcriptional activators can displace a repressor protein. This mechanism is particularly common during development when the pattern of transcription factor expression changes dynamically.

Of course, these mechanisms are not mutually exclusive, and most genes are activated by some combination of these events.

In general, mechanisms of transcriptional repression have not been studied to the same extent as mechanisms of transcriptional activation. Nonetheless, suppression of gene expression is as important as gene activation. Some mechanisms of repression are the corollary of activation. For example, repression is often associated with histone deacetylation or protein dephosphorylation. For nuclear hormone receptors, transcriptional silencing involves the recruitment of repression complexes that contain histone deacetylase activity. Aberrant expression of repressor proteins is sometimes associated with neoplasia. The t(15;17) chromosomal translocation that occurs in promyelocytic leukemia fuses the *PML* gene to a portion of the retinoic acid receptor α (*RAR α*) gene (Table 65-1). This event causes unregulated transcriptional repression in a manner that precludes normal cellular differentiation. The addition of the RAR ligand, retinoic acid, activates the receptor, thereby relieving repression and allowing cells to differentiate and ultimately undergo apoptosis. This mechanism has therapeutic importance as the addition of retinoic acid to treatment regimens induces a higher remission rate in patients with promyelocytic leukemia (Chap. 111).

CLONING AND SEQUENCING DNA

Since the mid-1970s, eight Nobel prizes have been awarded for research that led, directly or indirectly, to major methodological advances as well as to profound insights into genetics. Examples include the discoveries of reverse transcriptase, restriction enzymes, plasmid cloning vectors, DNA sequencing, and PCR. A description of recombinant DNA techniques, the methodology used for the manipulation, analysis, and characterization of DNA segments, is beyond the scope of this chapter. As these methods are widely used in genetics and molecular diagnostics, however, it is useful to review briefly some of the fundamental principles of cloning and DNA sequencing.

CLONING OF GENES *Cloning* refers to the creation of a recombinant DNA molecule that can be propagated indefinitely. The ability to clone genes and cDNAs therefore provides a permanent and renewable source of these reagents. Cloning is essential for DNA sequencing, nucleic acid hybridization studies, expression of recombinant proteins, and other recombinant DNA procedures.

The cloning of DNA involves the insertion of a DNA fragment into a cloning vector, followed by the propagation of the recombinant DNA in a host cell. The most straightforward cloning strategy involves inserting a DNA fragment into bacterial plasmids. Plasmids are small, autonomously replicating, circular DNA molecules that propagate separately from the chromosome in bacterial cells. The process of DNA insertion relies heavily on the use of restriction enzymes, which cleave DNA at highly specific sequences (usually 4 to 6 bp in length). Restriction enzymes generate complementary, cohesive sequences at the ends of the DNA fragment, which allow them to be efficiently ligated to the plasmid vector. Because plasmids contain genes that confer resistance to antibiotics, their presence in the host cell can be used for selection and DNA amplification.

A variety of vectors and appropriate hosts are now used for cloning (Table 65-2). Many of these are used for creating *libraries*, a term that refers to a collection of DNA clones. A genomic library represents an array of clones derived from genomic DNA. These overlapping DNA fragments represent the entire genome and can ultimately be arranged according to their linear order. Genomic libraries are propagated using a variety of vectors, such as lambda (λ) phage, cosmids, bacterial artificial chromosomes (BACs), and yeast artificial chromosomes (YACs). Phage libraries have been used extensively to isolate specific genes. Cosmids, BACs, and YACs are particularly useful for studying large genes and for defining the order of genes along the chromosomes (Fig. 65-4). cDNA libraries reflect clones derived from mRNA, typically from a particular tissue source. Thus, a cDNA library from the heart contains copies of mRNA expressed specifically in cardiac myocytes, in addition to those that are expressed ubiquitously. For this reason, a heart cDNA library will be enriched with cardiac-specific gene products and will differ from cDNA libraries generated from liver or pituitary mRNAs. As an example of the complexity of a genomic library, consider that the human genome contains 3×10^9 bp and the average genomic insert in a λ phage library is about 10^4 bp. Therefore, it requires at least 3×10^5 clones to represent all of the genomic DNA. Specific clones are isolated from the several hundred thousand clones by using DNA hybridization.

With completion of the HGP, all human genes have been cloned and sequenced. As a result, many of these cloning procedures will be unnecessary or greatly facilitated by the extensive information concerning DNA markers and the sequence of DNA (see below).

NUCLEIC ACID HYBRIDIZATION
Nucleic acid *hybridization* is a fundamental principle in molecular biology that takes advantage of the fact that the two complementary strands of nucleic acids bind, or *hybridize*, to one another with very high specificity. The goal of hybridization is to detect specific nucleic acid (DNA or RNA) sequences in a complex background of other sequences. This technique is used for Southern blotting, northern blotting, and for screening libraries (see above). Further adaptation of hybridization techniques has led to the development of microarray DNA chips.

Southern Blot Southern blotting is used to analyze whether genes have been deleted or rearranged. It is also used to detect restriction fragment length polymorphisms (RFLPs). Genomic DNA is digested with restriction endonucleases and separated by gel electrophoresis. Individual fragments can then be transferred to

Table 65-1   Examples of Diseases Caused by Transcription Factor Mutations and Rearrangements

Transcription Factor Class	Disorder
Nuclear receptors	
Androgen receptor	Complete or partial androgen insensitivity
	Spinobulbar muscular atrophy
Estrogen receptor	Unfused epiphyses, osteopenia, impaired fertility
	Amplified coactivators in breast cancer
Glucocorticoid receptor	Elevated cortisol without signs of hypercortisolism; increased mineralocorticoids and androgens
Thyroid hormone receptor β	Thyroid hormone resistance
Vitamin D receptor	Vitamin D–resistant rickets type II
AHC (DAX1)	Adrenal hypoplasia congenita
DAX1	Dosage-sensitive sex reversal
SF-1	Adrenal and gonadal deficiency
Zinc finger proteins	
WT1	WAGR syndrome: Wilm's tumor, aniridia, genitourinary malformations, mental retardation
	Denys-Drash syndrome: Wilm's tumor, renal dysgenesis and failure gonadoblastomas
GLI-3	Greig cephalopolysyndactyly; polydactyly
Paired homeodomain (PAX) proteins	
PAX-2	Colobomas, renal hypoplasia
PAX-3	Waardenburg syndrome types 1 and 3
PAX-6	Aniridia, anophthalmia; autosomal dominant keratitis; Peter's anomaly: malformations of anterior chamber
Basic helix-loop-helix (bHLH) proteins	
MITF	Waardenburg syndrome type 2A
TWIST	Saethre-Chotzen syndrome: craniosynostosis, cleft palate, conductive deafness
Homeodomain proteins	
MSX1 (HOX7.1)	Tooth agenesis
MSX2 (HOX8.1)	Craniosynostosis
HOXD13	Synpolydactyly
RIEG	Rieger syndrome: craniofacial malformations, microcornea, pupillary distortion, dental abnormalities
IPF-1	Maturity-onset of diabetes mellitus type 4; pancreatic agenesis, diabetes mellitus type 2
High-mobility group (HMG) proteins	
SRY	Sex reversal
SOX-9	Campomelic dysplasia, sex reversal
Forkhead transcription factors	
HNF-4α	Maturity-onset of diabetes mellitus type 1
HNF-1α	Maturity-onset of diabetes mellitus type 3
HNF-1β	Maturity-onset of diabetes mellitus type 5
TITF2/FKHL15	Congenital hypothyroidism, cleft palate, spiky hair
POU homeodomain proteins	
POUF1 (PIT1)	Combined pituitary hormone deficiency (GH, PRL, TSH)
POU3F4/BRN4	X-linked deafness DFN3, stapes fusion
Coactivators	
CREB binding protein (CBP)	Rubenstein-Taybi syndrome
General transcription factors	
TFIIH subunits	Xeroderma pigmentosum; Cochayne syndrome; trichothiodystrophy
Cell cycle control proteins	
Rb	Retinoblastoma, other cancers
p53	Li-Fraumeni syndrome, other cancers
Transcription elongation factor	
VHL	von-Hippel–Lindau syndrome, pheochromocytoma
Chimeric proteins	
FUS—CHOP (transcription factor—b-Zip)	Mixed liposarcomas
PAX3 or 7—FKHR (paired box homeodomain—forkhead)	Alveolar rhabdomyosarcomas
EWS—ATF-1 (b-Zip)	Ewing's sarcoma
E2A—PBX1 (bHLH—homeodomain)	Acute lymphoblastic leukemia
MLL—ELL (transcription elongation)	Acute myeloid leukemia
PML—RAR (retinoid action)	Acute promyelocytic leukemia
PDGFR—ETS	Chronic myelogenous leukemia
TCR—TAL-1,2 (twist)	T cell leukemia
Ig-MYC (bHLH)	Lymphomas, leukemia

NOTE: Selected abbreviations include: AHC, adrenal hypoplasia congenita; DAX-1, dosage-sensitive sex-reversal adrenal hypoplasia congenita (critical region on the X chromosome); GLI, amplified in glioblastoma; SRY, sex-determining region Y; SOX, SRY box; HNF, hepatocyte nuclear factor; CREB, cAMP responsive element binding protein; VHL, Von Hippel–Lindau; FUS, fusion; EWS, Ewing's sarcoma; CHOP, C/EBP homologous protein; PBX, pre-B cell leukemia; MLL, mixed lineage leukemia; ELL, elongation factor homologous to MLL; PML, promyelocytic leukemia; RAR, retinoic acid receptor; PDGFR, platelet-derived growth factor receptor; TCR, T cell receptor; TAL, T cell acute leukemia.

Table 65-2   **Commonly Used Vectors for Cloning of DNA**

Vector	DNA Insert in kb	Host
Yeast artificial chromosome (YAC)	1000	*Saccharomyces cerevisiae*
Bacterial artificial chromosome (BAC)	250	*Escherichia coli*
P1 artificial chromosomes (PAC)	150	*E. coli*
Cosmid	35	*E. coli*
λ phage	15	*E. coli*
Plasmid	10	*E. coli*

NOTE: kb, kilobases.

a membrane and detected after hybridization with specific radioactive DNA probes. Because single base-pair mismatches can disrupt the hybridization of short DNA probes (oligonucleotides), a variation of the Southern blot, termed *oligonucleotide-specific hybridization* (OSH), uses short oligonucleotides to distinguish normal from mutant genes.

Northern Blot   Northern blots are used to analyze patterns and levels of gene expression in different tissues. In a northern blot, mRNA is separated on a gel and transferred to a membrane, and specific transcripts are detected using radiolabeled DNA as a probe. This technique is rapidly being supplanted by more sensitive and comprehensive methods such as reverse transcriptase (RT)–PCR and gene expression arrays on DNA chips (see below).

Microarray Technology   A rapidly evolving approach to genome-scale studies consists of *microarrays*, or *DNA chips*. These approaches consist of thousands of synthetic nucleic acid sequences aligned on thin glass or silicon surfaces. Fluorescently labeled test sample DNA or RNA is hybridized to the chip, and a computerized scanner detects sequence matches. Microarrays allow the detection of

variations in DNA sequence and are used for mutational analysis and genotyping. Alternatively, the expression pattern of large numbers of mRNA transcripts can be determined by hybridization of RNA samples to cDNA or genomic microarrays. This method has tremendous potential in the era of functional genomics. As one example, microarrays can be used to develop genetic fingerprints of different types of lymphomas, providing information useful for classification, pathophysiology, prognosis, and treatment.

THE POLYMERASE CHAIN REACTION   The PCR, introduced in 1985, has revolutionized the way DNA analyses are performed and has become a cornerstone of molecular biology and genetic analysis. In essence, PCR provides a rapid way of cloning (amplifying) specific DNA fragments in vitro (Fig. 65-5). Exquisite specificity is conferred by the use of PCR primers, which are designed for a given DNA sequence. The geometric amplification of the DNA after multiple cycles yields remarkable sensitivity. As a result, PCR can be used to amplify DNA from very small samples, including single cells. These properties also allow DNA amplification from a variety of tissue sources including blood samples, biopsies, surgical or autopsy specimens, or cells from hair or saliva. PCR can also be used to study mRNA. In this case, the enzyme RT is first used to convert the RNA to DNA, which can then be amplified by PCR. This procedure, commonly known as *RT-PCR*, is useful as a quantitative measure of gene expression.

PCR provides a key component of molecular diagnostics. It provides a strategy for the rapid amplification of DNA (or mRNA) to search for mutations by a wide array of techniques, including DNA sequencing. PCR is also used for the amplification of highly polymorphic di- or trinucleotide repeat sequences, which allow various polymorphic alleles to be traced in genetic linkage or association studies. PCR is increasingly used to diagnose various microbial pathogens (Chap. 121).

DNA SEQUENCING   DNA sequencing is now an automated procedure. Although many protocols exist, the most commonly used strategy is based on the Sanger method in which dideoxynucleotides are used to randomly terminate DNA polymerization at each of the four bases (A,G,T,C). After separating the array of terminated DNA fragments using high-resolution gel or capillary electrophoresis, it is

STS markers   1 2 3 4 5 6 7 8 9 10 11 12 13 14 15 16

YAC clones

BAC clones

Contig

Genetic locus

STS 11   Gene A   Gene B   STS 12

Gene structure

FIGURE 65-4   Overlapping genomic clones. A chromosomal region can be mapped after the cloning of DNA fragments into vectors, such as yeast artificial chromosomes (YAC) or bacterial artificial chromosomes (BAC). Sequenced-tag sites (STS) allow each clone to be characterized, and the order of clones can be determined based on overlapping sequences. A series of overlapping clones is called a contig.

Denature

Anneal primer

Primer

Repeat for 25 - 30 cycles

Primer

DNA synthesis with *Taq* polymerase

FIGURE 65-5   Polymerase chain reaction. The polymerase chain reaction (PCR) generates multiple copies of a DNA segment. After denaturing the double-stranded (ds) DNA, complementary synthetic oligonucleotide primers of about 20 bp are annealed on each side of the fragment of interest. A heat-stable polymerase then extends the oligonucleotides and synthesizes the complementary strand. This cycle is repeated 25 to 30 times. The number of DNA amplified DNA segments is thus doubled after every PCR cycle.

possible to deduce the DNA sequence by examining the progression of fragment lengths generated in each of the four nucleotide reactions. The use of fluorescently labeled dideoxynucleotides allows automated detection of the different bases and direct computer analysis of the DNA sequence. Efforts are underway to develop faster, more cost-effective DNA sequencing technologies. These include the use of mass spectrometry; detection of fluorescently labeled bases in flow cytometry; direct reading of the DNA sequence by scanning, tunneling, or atomic force microscopy; and sequence analysis using DNA chips.

TRANSGENIC MICE AS MODELS OF GENETIC DISEASE

Several organisms have been studied extensively as genetic models, including *Mus musculus* (mouse), *Drosophila melanogaster* (fruit fly), *Caenorhabditis elegans* (nematode), *Saccharomyces cerevisiae* (baker's yeast), and *Eschericia coli* (colonic bacterium). The ability to use these evolutionarily distant organisms as genetic models that are relevant to human physiology reflects a surprising conservation of genetic pathways and gene function. Transgenic mouse models have been particularly valuable, because many human and mouse genes exhibit similar structure and function and because manipulation of the mouse genome is relatively straightforward compared to those of other mammalian species.

Transgenic strategies in mice can be divided into two main approaches: (1) overexpression of a gene by random insertion into the genome, and (2) deletion or targeted mutagenesis of a gene by homologous recombination with the native endogenous gene (Fig. 65-6). Many variations of these basic approaches now exist that allow genes to be expressed in specific cell types, at different times during development, or at varying levels. Consequently, transgenic technology has emerged as a powerful strategy for defining the physiologic effects of deleting or overexpressing a gene, as well as providing unique genetic models for dissecting pathophysiology or testing therapies.

Examples of transgenic models relevant to human genetic disorders are listed in Table 65-3. Transgenic overexpression of genes is useful for studying disorders that are sensitive to gene dosage. Overexpression of *PMP22*, for example, mimics a common duplication of this gene in type IA Charcot-Marie-Tooth disease (Chap. 379). Duplication of the *PMP22* gene results in high levels of expression of peripheral myelin protein 22, and this dosage effect is responsible for the demyelinating neuropathy. Expression of the Y chromosome–specific gene, *SRY*, in XX females demonstrates that *SRY* is sufficient to induce the formation of testes. This finding confirms the pathogenic role of *SRY* translocations to the X chromosome in sex-reversed XX females. Huntington disease is an autosomal dominant disorder caused by expansion of a CAG trinucleotide repeat that encodes a polyglutamine tract. Targeted deletion of the Huntington disease (*HD*) gene does not induce the neurologic disorder. On the other hand, transgenic expression of the entire gene or of the first exon containing the expanded polyGlu repeat is sufficient to cause many features of the neurologic disorder, indicating a gain-of-function property for the ex-

Prepare DNA transgene

Inject transgene into male pronucleus of fertilized ovum

Implant ovum into pseudopregnant female

Test tail DNA of F1 generation for transgene

Breed to homozygosity

Prepare targeting construct

Select for homologous recombination in embryonic stem (ES) cells

Introduce selected ES cells into blastocyst and implant

Mixed coat color in chimeric mice

Breed to homozygosity

FIGURE 65-6 Transgenic mouse models. *Left.* Transgenic mice are generated by pronuclear injection of foreign DNA into fertilized mouse oocytes and subsequent transfer into the oviduct of pseudopregnant foster mothers. *Right.* For targeted mutagenesis (gene knockout/knockin), embryonic stem (ES) cells are transfected with the targeted (mutagenized) transgene. The transgene undergoes homologous recombination with the wild-type gene. After selection, positive ES cells are introduced into blastocysts and implanted into foster mothers. Chimeric mice can be identified based on the mixed coat color of the offspring. Heterozygous mice are bred to obtain mice homozygous for the mutant allele.

panded polyGlu-containing protein. Transgenic strategies can also be used as a precursor to gene therapy. Expression of dystrophin, the protein that is deleted in Duchenne muscular dystrophy, partially corrects the disorder in a mouse model of Duchenne's. Targeted expression of oncogenes has been valuable to study mechanisms of neoplasia and to generate immortalized cell lines. For example, expression of the simian virus 40 (SV40) large T antigen under the direction of the insulin promoter induces the formation of islet cell tumors.

Targeted deletion mutagenesis, commonly known as *gene knockout*, is performed using a targeting vector that carries a mutant version of the gene. After homologous recombination in embryonic stem (ES) cells, chimeric animals are produced by injection of ES cells into blastocysts. Subsequently, animals are bred to be heterozygous or homozygous for the mutation. In addition to their use in examining gene function, gene knockouts provide valuable animal models for many loss-of-function mutations. A variation of this strategy is to use cre recombinase to induce genetic recombination in vivo. Cre recombinase will delete genes that have been flanked by its recognition sequences, called *loxP* sites. One advantage to this approach is that transgenic expression of cre in specific tissues can be used to delete a gene in a tissue-specific or developmentally staged manner. This is particularly useful for genes that would be lethal if deleted universally or during early development.

The list of genes that have been knocked out in mice is already very large. Many of these knockouts do not have an apparent phenotype, either because of redundant functions of the other genes or because the phenotype is subtle. For example, deletion of the hypoxanthine phosphoribosyltransferase (HPRT) gene (*Hprt*) does not cause characteristic features of Lesch-Nyhan syndrome in mice because of their reliance on adenine phosphoribosyltransferase (APRT) in the purine salvage pathway. The administration of an APRT inhibitor to HPRT-deficient mice, however, results in the typical self-injurious be-

Table 65-3 Examples of Transgenic Models of Human Genetic Disorders[a]

Disease	Gene	Encoded Protein	Phenotype
TRANSGENIC MODELS			
Duchenne muscular dystrophy	DMD	Dystrophin	Rescues muscular dystrophy in the mdx mouse, a natural mutant with a DMD-like phenotype
Amyotrophic lateral sclerosis	SOD1	Mutant superoxide dismutase 1	Similar to amyotrophic lateral sclerosis: motor neuron degeneration with accumulation of mutant SOD in perikarya and neurons
Sickle cell anemia	HBB	Hemoglobin S	Sickle cell anemia when in the genetic background of deleted normal hemoglobin α and β genes
Charcot-Marie-Tooth type 1A	PMP22	Peripheral myelin protein 22	Sensorineural polyneuropathy with demyelination in the peripheral nervous system and progressive weakness of the hind legs; confirmation of dosage effect of PMP22 duplication
Huntington disease	HDH	Huntingtin with expanded polyglutamine repeat	Huntington phenotype; demonstration that expansion of the polyglutamine repeat is sufficient to induce neurologic abnormalities
Spinocerebellar ataxia	SCA1	Ataxin 1 with expanded polyglutamine repeat under control of Purkinje cell–specific Pcp2 promoter	Ataxia, loss of Purkinje cells, glial proliferation
Acromegaly	GH	Growth hormone	Giantism
Sex-reversal	SRY	Sex-reversal Y chromosome	Testis formation in XX females, confirming role of SRY in testis formation
Diabetes mellitus MODY type 2	GCK	Glucokinase	Diabetes mellitus
Insulinoma	INS-SV40 LT antigen	Targeted expression of large T antigen under control of insulin promoter	β-cell tumors; targeted oncogenesis with viral antigen
Papillary thyroid cancer	RET/PTC	RET/PTC rearrangement; tissue-specific overexpression with thyroid-specific thyroglobulin promoter	Papillary thyroid carcinoma; targeted oncogenesis using a naturally occurring rearrangement
Li-Fraumeni syndrome	p53	p53 protein (53 kDa) involved in cell cycle and apoptosis	Tumors developing at very early age with 100% penetrance
Cystic fibrosis	CFTR	Cystic fibrosis transmembrane conductance regulator	Similar to cystic fibrosis: defect in chloride transport; alterations in lung, intestinal system, pancreas; and premature death
Hemochromatosis	HFE	HFE hemochromatosis protein	Elevated plasma iron and transferrin saturation, increased hepatic iron concentration
Hemophilia A	Factor VIII	Factor VIII	Absent factor VIII; prolonged bleeding
Familial polyposis coli	APC	APC tumor suppressor protein	Intestinal polyps
Xeroderma pigmentosa	XPC XPA	Xeroderma pigmentosum C Xeroderma pigmentosum A	High susceptibility for chemical and UV light–induced skin cancer
Ataxia telangiectasia	ATM	ATM kinase (cell cycle regulator)	Growth retardation, neurologic dysfunction, infertility, defective T cell maturation, sensitivity to γ-irradiation, lymphomas
Apparent mineralocorticoid excess	HSD11B2	11β-Hydroxysteroid dehydrogenase 2	Hypertension, hypokalemia, low plasma renin activity, low aldosterone, decreased conversion of cortisol to cortisone
Glycogen storage disease type II (Pompe's disease)	GAA	Acid α-glucosidase	Accumulation of glycogen in cardiac and skeletal muscle lysosomes, muscle weakness
Obesity	MC4R	Melanocortin 4 receptor	Maturity onset of obesity, hyperphagia, hyperinsulinemia
Neurofibromatosis type 1	NF1/p53	Neurofibromin (tumor suppressor)	No tumors in +/– mice; neurofibromas in Nf1 –/– mice and soft tissue sarcomas in Nf1/p53 –/– mice
Lipoid congenital adrenal hyperplasia	StAR	Steroidogenic acute regulatory protein	Female external genitalia in males and females, death due to adrenocortical insufficiency, defects in adrenal steroids, lipid deposits in adrenal cortex
Atherosclerosis	APOE	Apolipoprotein E	Atherosclerosis, increase of VLDL and LDL, decreased efflux of LDL from macrophages
Familial hypercholesteronemia	LDLR	LDL receptor	Increased LDL and VLDL cholesterol levels, atherosclerosis, xanthomas
Prader-Willi syndrome	NDN	Necdin	Neonatal respiratory distress and lethality in mice carrying paternally inherited Ndn deletion
Polycystic kidney disease	Pkd1	PKD1 protein (protein-protein adhesion in extracellular compartment)	Pancreatic ductal cysts, massive renal cysts, perinatal lethality
TARGETED MUTAGENESIS: GENE KNOCK-IN			
Osteogenesis imperfecta	Col1a1	Collagen 1	Osteogenesis imperfecta type 4 with variability in phenotype
Gaucher disease	GD1	Glucocerebrosidase	Glucosylceramide accumulation in brain and liver; premature death
Acute lymphoblastic leukemia	BCL-ABL	Reciprocal translocation of BCL and ABL	Transgenic model using a tetracycline-responsive promoter for BCL-ABL expression

[a] A comprehensive list of transgenic mouse models and spontaneous mouse mutants can be found at the Jackson laboratory (www.jax.org/tbase). This site contains numerous links to other databases with murine and other mammalian transgenic models.

NOTE: LDL, low-density lipoprotein; VLDL, very low density lipoprotein.

havior seen in patients with Lesch-Nyhan syndrome. The phenotypes of some knockouts are quite different from their human disease counterparts. For example, deletion of the retinoblastoma (Rb) gene does not lead to retinoblastoma or other tumors that characterize the human syndrome. These examples underscore the fact that the functions of genes, and their interactions with genetic background and the environment, cannot be assumed to be identical in mice and humans. On the other hand, the deletion of many genes provides a remarkably faithful model of human disorders (Table 65-3). In addition to clarifying pathophysiology, these models facilitate the development of therapies, both genetic and pharmaceutical.

In addition to transgenic animal models, naturally occurring mutations in mice and other species continue to provide fundamental insights into human disease. A compendium of natural and transgenic animal models is provided in continuously evolving databases (Online Mendelian Inheritance in Animals OMIA: www.angis.su.oz.au/Databases/BIRX/omia/; The Jackson Library: www.jax.org/).

Human pluripotential *stem cells* have recently been developed, and, consistent with their potential for self-renewal, these cell lines express high levels of telomerase, an enzyme that is essential for allowing repeated replication of the ends of eukaryotic chromosomes. Although much remains to be learned about the properties of pluripotential stem cells, they may prove useful for transplantation, drug testing, or for other purposes.

THE HUMAN GENOME PROJECT

The HGP was initiated in the mid-1980s as an ambitious effort to characterize the human genome, culminating in a complete DNA sequence. In the United States, the National Institutes of Health (NIH) and the Department of Energy (DOE) officially launched the genome project in 1990; the project has evolved as an international effort and has also included important contributions from the private sector. The main goals include: (1) creation of genetic maps, (2) development of physical maps, and (3) determination of the complete human DNA sequence.

Some analogies help in appreciating the scope of the HGP. The 23 pairs of human chromosomes are thought to encode approximately 100,000 genes. The total length of DNA is about 3 billion bp, which is nearly 1000-fold greater than the *E. coli* genome. If the human DNA sequence were printed out, it would correspond to about 120 volumes of *Harrison's Principles of Internal Medicine*.

THE GENETIC MAP Given the size and complexity of the human genome, genetic maps have been developed to provide orientation and to delimit where a gene of interest may be located. A *genetic map* describes the order of genes and defines the position of a gene relative to other loci on the same chromosome. It is constructed by assessing how frequently two markers are inherited together by linkage studies. Distances of the genetic map are expressed in recombination units, or centimorgans (cM). One cM corresponds to a recombination frequency of 1% between two polymorphic markers; 1 cM corresponds to approximately 1 Mb of DNA (Fig. 65-3). Any polymorphic sequence variation can be useful for mapping purposes. Examples of polymorphic markers include variable number of tandem repeats (VNTRs), RFLPs, microsatellite repeats, and single nucleotide polymorphisms (SNPs); the latter two methods are now used predominantly because of the high density of markers and because they are amenable to automated procedures.

The current genetic map exists at about 1 cM resolution. A goal for the near term is to add about 100,000 SNPs to these maps. This would provide 1 SNP approximately every 100,000 bp. The addition of SNPs will facilitate automation using DNA chips and will enhance the ability to perform linkage studies of complex genetic diseases.

THE PHYSICAL MAP Cytogenetics and chromosomal banding techniques provide a relatively low-resolution microscopic view of genetic loci. Physical maps indicate the position of a locus or gene in absolute values. Sequence-tagged sites (STSs) are used as a standard unit for physical mapping and serve as sequence-specific landmarks for arranging overlapping cloned fragments in the same order as they occur in the genome. These overlapping clones, usually in YACs or BACs, allow the characterization of contiguous DNA sequences, commonly referred to as *contigs* (Fig. 65-4). The STSs consist of 200 to 500 bp, which can be retrieved from computer databases; >50,000 STSs have been mapped. The goal of achieving a high-resolution physical map of the human genome has essentially been achieved as all of the genome has been cloned into overlapping

fragments. The highest resolution physical map will provide the complete DNA sequence of each chromosome in the human genome.

STATUS OF DNA SEQUENCING The primary focus of the genome project is to obtain DNA sequence for the entire human genome as well as model organisms. The sequences of *E. coli* and many other bacteria, *S. cerevisiae*, *C. elegans*, and *D. melanogaster* have already been completed. Sequencing of the laboratory mouse genome is in progress. Although the prospect of determining the complete sequence of the human genome was a daunting prospect several years ago, technical advances in DNA sequencing and bioinformatics have led to the completion of a draft human sequence in June 2000, well in advance of the original goal of the year 2003. The current standard is to achieve 99.99% (1 error in 10,000 bp) accuracy. This level of accuracy is important for many reasons, including efforts to determine the degree of DNA sequence variation in the population. Comparisons of the DNA sequence from multiple individuals or populations will allow assessments of genetic variance in the human population. Another goal is to develop a complete set of full-length human cDNAs and to define their locations on the physical map.

ETHICAL ISSUES Implicit in the HGP is the idea and hope that identifying disease-causing genes can lead to improvements in diagnosis, prognosis, and treatment. It is estimated that most individuals harbor several serious recessive genes. However, completion of the human genome sequence, determination of the association of genetic defects with disease, and studies of genetic variation raise many new issues with implications for the individual and mankind. The controversies concerning the cloning of mammals and the establishment of human embryonic stem cells underscore the relevance of these questions. Moreover, the information gleaned from genotypic results can have quite different impacts, depending on the availability of strategies to modify the course of disease. For example, the identification of mutations that cause multiple endocrine neoplasia (MEN) type 2 or hemochromatosis allows specific interventions for affected family members. On the other hand, at present the identification of an Alzheimer or Huntington disease gene does not alter therapy. Genetic test results can generate anxiety in affected individuals and family members, and there is the possibility of discrimination on the basis of the test results. Most genetic disorders are likely to fall into an intermediate category where the opportunity for prevention or treatment is significant but limited (Chap. 68). For these reasons, the scientific components of the HGP have been paralleled by efforts to examine ethical and legal implications as new issues arise.

Many issues raised by the genome project are familiar, in principle, to medical practitioners. For example, an asymptomatic patient with increased low-density lipoprotein (LDL) cholesterol, high blood pressure, or a strong family history of early myocardial infarction, is known to be at increased risk of coronary heart disease. In such cases, it is clear that the identification of risk factors and an appropriate intervention are beneficial. Likewise, patients with phenylketonuria, cystic fibrosis, or sickle cell anemia are often identified as having a genetic disease early in life. These precedents can be helpful for adapting policies that relate to genetic information. We can anticipate similar efforts, whether based on genotypes or other markers of genetic predisposition, to be applied to many disorders. One confounding aspect of the rapid expansion of information is that our ability to make clinical predictions often lags behind genetic advances. For example, when genes that predispose to breast cancer, such as *BRCA1*, are described, they generate tremendous public interest in the potential to predict disease, but many years of clinical research are still required to rigorously establish genotype and phenotype correlations.

Whether related to informed consent, participation in research, or the management of a genetic disorder that affects an individual or their families, there is a great need for more information about fundamental principles of genetics. The pervasive nature of the role of genetics in medicine makes it imperative for physicians and other health care professionals to become more informed about genetics and to provide advice and counseling in conjunction with trained genetic counselors (Chap. 68). The application of screening and prevention strategies will therefore require intensive patient and physician education, changes in health care financing, and legislation to protect patient's rights.

TRANSMISSION OF GENETIC DISEASE

ORIGINS AND TYPES OF MUTATIONS   A *mutation* can be defined as any change in the primary nucleotide sequence of DNA regardless of its functional consequences. Some mutations may be lethal, others are less deleterious, and some may confer an evolutionary advantage. Mutations can occur in the germline (sperm or oocytes); these can be transmitted to progeny. Alternatively, mutations can occur during embryogenesis or in somatic tissues. Mutations that occur during development lead to *mosaicism*, a situation in which tissues are composed of cells with different genetic constitutions. If the germline is mosaic, a mutation can be transmitted to some progeny but not others, which sometimes leads to confusion in assessing the pattern of inheritance. Somatic mutations that do not affect cell survival can sometimes be detected because of variable phenotypic effects in tissues (e.g., pigmented lesions in McCune-Albright syndrome). Other somatic mutations are associated with neoplasia because they confer a growth advantage to cells. Epigenetic events such as altered DNA methylation may also influence gene expression. With the exception of triplet nucleotide repeats, which can expand (see below), mutations are usually stable.

Mutations are structurally diverse—they can involve the entire genome, as in triploidy (one extra set of chromosomes), or gross numerical or structural alterations in chromosomes or individual genes (Chap. 66). Large deletions may affect a portion of a gene or an entire gene, or, if several genes are involved, they may lead to a *contiguous gene syndrome*. Unequal crossing-over between homologous genes can result in fusion gene mutations, as illustrated by color blindness (Chap. 28). Mutations involving single nucleotides are referred to as *point mutations*. Substitutions are called *transitions* if a purine is replaced by another purine base (A ↔ G) or if a pyrimidine is replaced by another pyrimidine (C ↔ T). Changes from a purine to a pyrimidine, or vice versa, are referred to as *transversions*. If the DNA sequence change occurs in a coding region and alters an amino acid, it is called a *missense mutation*. Depending on the functional consequences of such a missense mutation, amino acid substitutions in different regions of the protein can lead to distinct phenotypes. *Polymorphisms* are sequence variations that have a frequency of at least 1%. Usually, they do not result in a perceptible phenotype. Often they consist of single base-pair substitutions that do not alter the protein coding sequence because of the degenerate nature of the genetic code, although it is possible that some might alter mRNA stability, translation, or the amino acid sequence. These types of silent base substitutions and SNPs are encountered frequently during genetic testing and must be distinguished from true mutations that alter protein expression or function. Small nucleotide deletions or insertions cause a shift of the codon reading frame. Most commonly, reading frame alterations result in an abnormal protein segment of variable length before termination of translation occurs at a stop codon (*nonsense mutation*). Mutations in intronic sequences or in exon junctions may destroy or create splice donor or splice acceptor sites. Mutations may also be found in the regulatory sequences of genes, resulting in reduced gene transcription.

Mutation Rates   As noted before, mutations represent an important cause of genetic diversity as well as disease. Mutation rates are difficult to determine in humans because many mutations are silent and because testing is often not adequate to detect the phenotypic consequences. Mutation rates vary in different genes but are estimated to occur at a rate of about 10^{-10}/bp per cell division. Germline mutation rates (as opposed to somatic mutations) are relevant in the transmission of genetic disease. Because the population of oocytes is established very early in development, only about 20 cell divisions are required for completed oogenesis, whereas spermatogenesis involves about 30 divisions by the time of puberty and 20 cell divisions each year thereafter. Consequently, the probability of acquiring new point mutations is much greater in the male germline than the female germline, in which rates of aneuploidy are increased (Chap. 66). Thus, the incidence of new point mutations in spermatogonia increases with paternal age (e.g., achondrodysplasia, Marfan syndrome, neurofibromatosis). It is estimated that about 1 in 10 sperm carries a new deleterious mutation. The rates for new mutations are calculated most readily for autosomal dominant and X-linked disorders and are ~10^{-5} to 10^{-6}/ locus per generation. Because most monogenic diseases are relatively rare, new mutations account for a significant fraction of cases. This is important in the context of genetic counseling, as a new mutation can be transmitted to the affected individual but does not necessarily imply that the parents are at risk to transmit the disease to other children. An exception to this is when the new mutation occurs early in germline development, leading to *gonadal mosaicism*.

Unequal Crossing-Over   Normally, DNA recombination in germ cells occurs with remarkable fidelity to maintain the precise junction sites for the exchanged DNA sequences (Fig. 65-2). However, mispairing of homologous sequences leads to unequal crossover, with gene duplication on one of the chromosomes and gene deletion on the other chromosome. A significant fraction of growth hormone (*GH*) gene deletions, for example, involve unequal crossing-over (Chap. 328). The *GH* gene is a member of a large gene cluster that includes a growth hormone variant gene as well as several structurally related chorionic somatomammotropin genes and pseudogenes (highly homologous but functionally inactive relatives of a normal gene). Because such gene clusters contain multiple homologous DNA sequences arranged in tandem, they are particularly prone to undergo recombination and, consequently, gene duplication or deletion. On the other hand, duplication of the *PMP22* gene as a result of unequal crossing-over results in increased gene dosage and type IA Charcot-Marie-Tooth disease (Chap. 379). Unequal crossing-over resulting in deletion of *PMP22* results in a distinct neuropathy called *hereditary liability to pressure palsy* (Chap. 379).

Glucocorticoid-remediable aldosteronism (GRA) is caused by a rearrangement involving the genes that encode aldosterone synthase (*CYP11B2*) and steroid 11β-hydroxylase (*CYP11B1*), normally arranged in tandem on chromosome 8q. These two genes are 95% identical, predisposing to gene duplication and deletion by unequal crossing-over. The rearranged gene product contains the regulatory regions of 11β-hydroxylase fused to the coding sequence of aldosterone synthetase. Consequently, the latter enzyme is expressed in the adrenocorticotropic hormone (ACTH)-dependent zone of the adrenal gland, resulting in overproduction of mineralocorticoids and hypertension (Chap. 331).

Gene conversion refers to a nonreciprocal exchange of homologous genetic information; it is probably more common than generally recognized. In human genetics, gene conversion has been used to explain how an internal portion of a gene is replaced by a homologous segment copied from another allele or locus; these genetic alterations may range from a few nucleotides to a few thousand nucleotides. As a result of gene conversion, it is possible for short DNA segments of two chromosomes to be identical, even though these sequences are distinct in the parents. A practical consequence of this phenomenon is that nucleotide substitutions can occur during gene conversion between related genes, often altering the function of the gene. In disease states, gene conversion often involves intergenic exchange of DNA between a gene and a related pseudogene. For example, the 21-hydroxylase gene (*CYP21A*) is adjacent to a nonfunctional pseudogene. Many of the nucleotide substitutions that are found in the *CYP21A* gene in patients with congenital adrenal hyperplasia correspond to sequences that are present in the pseudogene, suggesting gene conversion as a mechanism of mutagenesis. In addition, mitotic gene conversion has been suggested as a mechanism to explain revertant mosaicism in which an inherited mutation is "corrected" in certain cells. For example, patients with autosomal recessive generalized atrophic benign epidermolysis bullosa have acquired reverse mutations in one of the two mutated *COL17A1* alleles, leading to clinically unaffected patches of skin.

Insertions and Deletions Though many instances of insertions and deletions occur as a consequence of unequal crossing-over, there is also evidence for internal duplication, inversion, or deletion of DNA sequences. The fact that certain deletions or insertions appear to occur repeatedly as independent events suggests that specific regions within the DNA sequence predispose to these errors. For example, certain regions of the *DMD* gene appear to be hot spots for deletions.

Errors in DNA Repair Because mutations caused by defects in DNA repair accumulate as somatic cells divide, these types of mutations are particularly important in the context of neoplastic disorders (Chap. 82). Several genetic disorders involving DNA repair enzymes underscore their importance. Patients with xeroderma pigmentosum have defects in DNA damage recognition or in the nucleotide excision and repair pathway (Chap. 86). Exposed skin is dry and pigmented and is extraordinarily sensitive to the mutagenic effects of ultraviolet irradiation. More than 10 different genes have been shown to cause the different forms of xeroderma pigmentosum. This finding is consistent with the earlier classification of this disease into different complementation groups (Table 65-4) in which normal function is rescued by the fusion of cells derived from two different forms of xeroderma pigmentosum.

Ataxia telangiectasia causes large telangiectatic lesions of the face, cerebellar ataxia, immunologic defects, and hypersensitivity to ionizing radiation (Chap. 364). The discovery of the ataxia telangiectasia mutated (*ATM*) gene reveals that it is homologous to genes involved in DNA repair and control of cell cycle checkpoints. Mutations in the *ATM* gene give rise to defects in meiosis as well as increasing susceptibility to damage from ionizing radiation. Fanconi's anemia is also associated with an increased risk of multiple acquired genetic abnormalities. It is characterized by diverse congenital anomalies and a strong predisposition to develop aplastic anemia and acute myelogenous leukemia (Chap. 111). Cells from these patients are susceptible to chromosomal breaks caused by a defect in genetic recombination. At least eight different complementation groups have been identified, and several loci and genes associated with Fanconi's anemia have been mapped or cloned (Table 65-4).

HNPCC is caused by mutations in one of several different mismatch repair (MMR) genes including MutS homologue 2 (*MSH2*) and MutL homologue 1 (*MLH1*) (Chap. 90). These enzymes are involved in the detection of nucleotide mismatches and in the recognition of slipped-strand trinucleotide repeats. Germline mutations in these genes lead to microsatellite instability and a high mutation rate in colon cancer. This syndrome is characterized by autosomal dominant transmission of colon cancer, young age (<50 years) of presentation, predisposition to lesions in the proximal large bowel, and associated malignancies such as uterine cancer and ovarian cancer. Genetic screening tests for this disorder are now being used for families considered to be at risk (Chap. 68). Recognition of HNPCC allows early screening with colonoscopy and the implementation of prevention strategies using nonsteroidal anti-inflammatory drugs.

CpG and Dipyrimidine Sequences Certain DNA sequences are particularly susceptible to mutagenesis. Successive pyrimidine residues (e.g., T-T or C-C) are subject to the formation of ultraviolet light–induced photoadducts. If these pyrimidine dimers are not repaired by the nucleotide excision repair pathway, mutations will be introduced after DNA synthesis. The dinucleotide C-G, or CpG, is also a hot spot for a specific type of mutation. In this case, methylation of the cytosine is associated with an enhanced rate of deamination to uracil, which is then replaced with thymine. This C → T transition (or G → A on the opposite strand) accounts for at least one-third of point mutations associated with polymorphisms and mutations. Many of the *MSH2* mutations in HNPCC, for example, involve CpG sequences.

Table 65-4   Selected Examples of Locus Heterogeneity

Phenotype	Gene/Locus	Chromosomal Location	Protein
Hypertrophic cardiomyopathy			
CMH1	*MYH7*	14q12	Myosin heavy chain β
CMH2	*TNNT2*	1q2	Troponin-T2
CMH3	*TPM1*	15q22.1	Tropomyosin α
CMH4	*MYBPC3*	11p11q	Myosin binding protein C
Osteogenesis imperfecta			
Type 1	*COL1A1*	17q21.31-q22.05	Collagen α_1
Type 2	*COL1A2*	7q22.1	Collagen α_2
Retinitis pigmentosa			
RP1	*ORP1*	8q11-13	Oxygen-regulated photoreceptor ORP1
RP2	*RP2*	Xp11.3	RP2
RP3	*RP3*	Xp21.1	Retinitis pigmentosa GTPase regulator
Numerous other syndromic and nonsyndromic forms of RP			
Tuberous sclerosis			
TSC1	*TSC1*	9q34	Hamartin
TSC2	*TSC2*	16p13.3	Tuberin
Familial Alzheimer disease			
AD1	*APP*	21q21.3-22.05	Amyloid precursor protein
AD2 (modifying gene)	*APOE*	19q13.2	Apolipoprotein E
AD3	*PSEN1*	14q24.3	Presenilin 1
AD4	*PSEN2*	1q31-42	Presenilin 2
Familial breast cancer			
BRCA1	*BRCA1*	17q21	BRCA1 (RNA polymerase II component)
BRCA2	*BRCA2*	13q12.3	BRCA2
Xeroderma pigmentosum			
XP1	*XPA*	9q22.3	XPA
XP	*XPCC*	3p25	XPCC nucleotide excision repair protein
XP4	*ERCC2*	19q13.2-13.3	ERCC2 DNA repair protein
Fanconi anemia			
FANCA	*FAA*	16q24.3	FAA protein
FANCA	*FAB* locus	?	?
FANCC	*FAC*	9q22.3	FAC protein
FANCD	*FAD* locus	3p26-22	?
FANCE	*FAE* locus	6p22-21	?
FANCF	*FAF*	11p15	FAF/ROM
FANCG	*FAG*	9p13	FAG/XRCC9
FANCH	*FAH* locus	?	?
Polycystic kidney disease			
PKD1	*PKD1*	16p13 3-13.12	Polycystin 1
PKD2	*PKD2*	4q21-23	Polycystin 2

Certain types of mutations ($C \rightarrow T$ or $G \rightarrow A$) are relatively common. Moreover, the redundant nature of the genetic code results in overrepresentation of certain amino acid substitutions. For example, arginine codons are most likely to be converted to cysteine, tryptophan, or a stop codon when a $C \rightarrow T$ transition occurs, and to histidine or glutamine when a $G \rightarrow A$ transition occurs.

Unstable DNA Sequences *Trinucleotide repeats* may be unstable and expand beyond a critical number. Mechanistically, the expansion is thought to be caused by unequal recombination and slipped mispairing. A premutation represents a small increase in trinucleotide copy number. In subsequent generations, the expanded repeat may increase further in length and result in an increasingly severe phenotype, a process called *dynamic mutation* (see below for discussion of anticipation). Trinucleotide expansion was first recognized as a cause of the fragile X syndrome, one of the most common causes of mental retardation (Chap. 359). Other disorders arising from a similar mechanism include Huntington disease (Chap. 362), X-linked spinobulbar muscular atrophy (Chap. 365), and myotonic dystrophy (Chap. 383) (Tables 65-5 and 65-6). Malignant cells are also characterized by genetic instability, indicating a breakdown in mechanisms that regulate DNA repair and the cell cycle.

FUNCTIONAL CONSEQUENCES OF MUTATIONS Functionally, mutations can be broadly classified as gain-of-function and loss-of-function mutations. Gain-of-function mutations are typically dominant; that is, they result in phenotypic alterations when a single allele is affected. Inactivating mutations are usually recessive, and an affected individual is homozygous or compound heterozygous (i.e., carrying two different mutant alleles) for the disease-causing mutations. Alternatively, mutation in a single allele can result in *haploinsufficiency*, a situation in which one normal allele is not sufficient for a normal phenotype. This phenomenon applies, for example, to expression of rate-limiting en-

386

Table 65-5 Selected Monogenic Disorders for Which Genetic Testing Is Available

Disorder	Inheritance[a]	Gene[b]	Chapters
Oncology			
Hereditary nonpolyposis colon cancer	AD	MSH2, MLH1	81, 90
Familial adenomatous polyposis	AD	APC	81, 90
Familial breast cancer	AD	BRCA1, BRCA2	81, 89, 97
Basal cell nevus	AD	PTCH	57, 81, 89
Li-Fraumeni syndrome	AD	P53	81, 88, 89, 98
Von Hippel–Lindau syndrome	AD	VHL	81, 94, 332, 370
Retinoblastoma	AD	RB	81, 359
Familial malignant melanoma	AD	CDKN2A	81, 86
Multiple endocrine neoplasia type 1	AD	MEN1	81, 93, 339, 341
Multiple endocrine neoplasia type 2	AD	RET	81, 93, 339, 341
Ataxia telangiectasia	AR	ATM	57, 81, 308, 364
Hematology			
Spherocytosis	AD	SPTB, SLC4A1, ANK1, EPB42	108
von Willebrand's disease	AD	VWF	62, 116
Antithrombin III	AD	AT	62, 117
Factor V Leiden	AD	F5	62, 117, 261, 361
Sickle cell disease	AR	HBB	106
α Thalassemia	AR	HBA2 and others	106
β Thalassemia	AR	HBB and others	106
Familial Mediterranean fever	AR	MEFV	289
Hemophilia A	XL	F8C	117
Hemophilia B	XL	F9	117
Glucose-6-phosphate dehydrogenase deficiency	XL	G6PD	71, 108
Cardiovascular			
Hypertrophic obstructive cardiomyopathy	AD	MYH7, MYBPC3, TNNT2, TPM1	238
Long QT syndrome	AD	KCNQ1, KCNH2, SCN5A	230
Pulmonary			
Cystic fibrosis	AR	CFTR	257, 304
α_1 Antitrypsin deficiency	AR	PI	258, 300
Nephrology			
Polycystic kidney disease	AD	PKD1, PKD2	276
Nephrogenic diabetes insipidus	XL/AR	AVPR2, AQP2	49, 329
Gastrointestinal			
Hereditary hemorrhagic telangiectasia	AD	ENG	44
Peutz-Jegher syndrome	AD	STK11	90
Wilson's disease	AR	ATP7B	300, 348
Hemochromatosis	AR	HFE	345
Bone/Connective tissue			
Achondroplasia	AD	FGFR3	343
Crouzon syndrome	AD	FGFR2	343
Marfan syndrome	AD	FBN1	234, 351
Osteogenesis imperfecta	AD	COL1A1, COL1A2	351
Ehlers-Danlos syndrome	AD	Multiple genes	351
Amyloidosis	AD	TTR	238, 319
Menkes syndrome	XL	ATP7A	351, 359
Endocrinology			
Maturity-onset diabetes of the young	AD	Multiple genes	333
Neurohypophyseal diabetes insipidus	AD	AVP	49, 329
Thyroid hormone resistance	AD	THRB	330
Male-limited precocious puberty	AD	LHCGR	338
Congenital adrenal hyperplasia	AR	CYP21	53, 331, 338
Obesity	AR	MC4R, LEPR, LEP, POMC	77
Androgen insensitivity	XL	AR	338
Male-to-female sex reversal	YL	SRY	338
Metabolism			
Familial hypercholesterolemia	AD	LDLR	241, 344
Glycogen storage disease type I–VIII	AR	Multiple genes	350
Tay-Sachs disease	AR	HEXA	349, 359
Gaucher disease	AR	GBA	349
Mucopolysaccharidosis type I–VII	AR	Multiple genes	349
Phenylketonuria	AR	PAH	352
Pseudocholinesterase deficiency	AR	BCHE	71, 72
Niemann-Pick disease	AR	SMPD1, NPC1	349

(continued)

Disorder	Inheritance[a]	Gene[b]	Chapters
Neurologic			
Huntington disease	AD	*HD*	359, 362
Neurofibromatosis type I and II	AD	*NF1, NF2*	81, 359, 370
Familial Parkinson disease	AD	*SNCA, PARK2*	359, 364
Spinocerebellar ataxia type 1–12	AD	Multiple genes	359, 364
Amyotrophic lateral sclerosis	AD	*SOD1*	359, 365
Tuberous sclerosis type 1 and 2	AD	*TSC1, TSC2*	359, 370
Familial Alzheimer disease	AD	*PSEN1, PSEN2, APP, APOE*	359, 362
Malignant hyperthermia	AD	*RYR1*	17, 381, 359
Familial fatal insomnia	AD	*PRNP*	27, 359, 373
Charcot-Marie-Tooth disease	AD	Multiple genes	359, 377
Hyperkalemic periodic paralysis	AD	*SCN4A*	49, 359, 381
Hypokalemic periodic paralysis	AD	*CACNA1S*	49, 359, 381
Friedreich ataxia	AR	*FRDA1*	359, 364
Duchenne and Becker muscular dystrophy	XL	*DMD*	238, 359, 381
Fragile X syndrome	XL	*FMR1, FRAXE*	359
Adrenoleukodystrophy	XL	*ALD*	331, 359
Spinobulbar muscular atrophy	XL	*AR*	359, 364

[a] For many disorders, several different types of inheritance have been described. The most common form of transmission is listed. Additional information on these disorders, including specific mutations, can be found on-line at the Human Genome Mutation Database (HGMD) www.uwcm.ac.uk, or in the On-line Mendelian Inheritance in Man (OMIM) catalogue www.ncbi.nlm.nih.gov/Omim. An overview of available genetic tests and laboratories can be found at www.genetests.org.

[b] Only some of the genes associated with these disorders have been listed. In some instances, there is genetic heterogeneity.

NOTE: AD, autosomal dominant; AR, autosomal recessive; XL, X-linked; YL, Y-linked.

zymes in heme synthesis that cause porphyrias (Chap. 346). An increase in dosage of a gene product may also result in disease, as illustrated by the duplication of the *DAX1* gene in dosage-sensitive sex-reversal (Chap. 338). Mutation in a single allele can also result in loss of function due to a dominant-negative effect. In this case, the mutated allele interferes with the function of the normal gene product by one of several different mechanisms: (1) a mutant protein may interfere with the function of a multimeric protein complex, as illustrated by mutations in type 1 collagen (*COL1A1*, *COL1A2*) genes in osteogenesis imperfecta (Chap. 351); (2) a mutant protein may occupy binding sites on proteins or promoter response elements, as illustrated by thyroid hormone resistance, a disorder in which inactivated thyroid hormone receptor binds to target genes and functions as an antagonist of normal receptors (Chap. 330); or (3) a mutant protein can be cytotoxic as in α_1 antitrypsin deficiency (Chap. 258) or autosomal dominant neurohypophyseal diabetes insipidus (Chap. 329), in which the abnormally folded proteins are trapped within the endoplasmic reticulum and ultimately cause cellular damage.

GENOTYPE AND PHENOTYPE   Alleles, Genotypes, and Haplotypes   An observed trait is referred to as a *phenotype*; the genetic information defining the phenotype is called the *genotype*. Alternative forms of a gene or a genetic marker are referred to as alleles. Alleles may be polymorphic variants of nucleic acids that have no apparent effect on gene expression or function. In other instances, these variants may have subtle effects on gene expression, thereby conferring the adaptive advantages associated with genetic diversity. On the other hand, allelic variants may reflect mutations in a gene that clearly alter its function. The common Glu → Val sickle cell mutation (E6V) in the β-*globin* gene and the ΔF508 deletion of phenylalanine (F) in the *CFTR* gene are examples of allelic variants of these genes. Because each individual has two copies of each chromosome (one inherited from the mother and one inherited from the father), he or she can only have two alleles at a given locus. However, there can be many different alleles in the population. The normal or common allele is usually referred to as *wild type*. When alleles at a given locus are identical, the individual is *homozygous*. Inheriting such identical copies of a mutant allele occurs in many autosomal recessive disorders, particularly in circumstances of consanguinity. If the alleles are different, the individual is *heterozygous* at this locus. If two different mutant alleles are inherited at a given locus, the individual is said to be a *compound heterozygote*. *Hemizygous* is used to describe males with a mutation in an X chromosomal gene, or a female with a loss of one X chromosomal locus.

Genotypes describe the specific alleles at a particular locus. For example, there are three common alleles (E2, E3, E4) of the apolipoprotein E (*APOE*) gene. The genotype of an individual can therefore be described as *APOE3/4* or *APOE4/4* or any other variant. These designations indicate which alleles are present on the two chromosomes in the *APOE* gene at locus 19q13.2. In other cases, the genotype might be assigned arbitrary numbers (e.g., 1/2) or letters (e.g., B/b) to distinguish different alleles.

A *haplotype* refers to a group of alleles that are closely linked

Table 65-6   Selected Trinucleotide Repeat Disorders

Disease	Locus	Repeat	Triplet Length Normal	Triplet Length Disease	Inheritance	Gene Product
X-chromosomal spinobulbar muscular atrophy (SBMA)	Xq11-q12	CAG	11–34	40–62	XR	Androgen receptor
Fragile X-syndrome (FRAXA)	Xq27.3	CGG	6–50	200–300	XR	FMR-1 protein
Fragile X-syndrome (FRAXE)	Xq28	GCC	6–25	>200	XR	FMR-2 protein
Dystrophia myotonica (DM)	19q13.2-q13.3	CTG	5–30	200–1000	AD, variable penetrance	Myotonin protein kinase
Huntington disease (HD)	4p16.3	CAG	11–34	37–121	AD	Huntingtin
Spinocerebellar ataxia type 1 (SCA1)	6p21.3-21.2	CAG	19–36	39–83	AD	Ataxin 1
Spinocerebellar ataxia type 2 (SCA2)	12q24.1	CAG	15–31	34–400	AD	Ataxin 2
Spinocerebellar ataxia type 3 (SCA3); Machado Joseph disease (MD)	14q21	CAG	13–36	55–86	AD	SC3/MJD1
Spinocerebellar ataxia type 6 (SCA6, CACNAIA)	19p13.1-13.2	CAG	4–16	20–33	AD	Alpha 1A voltage-dependent calcium channel
Spinocerebellar ataxia type 7 (SCA7)	3p21.1-p12	CAG	4–19	37–>300	AD	Ataxin 7
Spinocerebellar ataxia type 8 (SCA8)	13q21	CTG	16–34	100–250	AD	?
Spinocerebellar ataxia type 12 (SCA12)	5q31	CAG	6–26	66–78	AD	Protein phosphatase 2A
Dentorubral pallidoluysiane atrophy (DRPLA)	12p	CAG	7–23	49–75	AD	Atrophin
Friedereich ataxia (FRDA1)	9q13-21	GAA	7–22	200–900	AR	Frataxin

NOTE: AD, autosomal dominant; AR, autosomal recessive; XR, X-linked recessive.

FIGURE 65-7 Point mutations causing β-thalassemia as example of allelic heterogeneity. The β-globin gene is located in the globin gene cluster. Point mutations can be located in the promoter, the CAP site, the 5′-untranslated region, the initiation codon, each of the three exons, the introns, or the polyadenylation signal. Many mutations introduce missense or nonsense mutations, whereas others cause defective RNA splicing. Not shown here are deletion mutations of the β-globin gene or larger deletions of the globin locus that can also result in thalassemia. ▼, Promoter mutations; *, CAP site; •, 5′UTR; ☐1, Initiation codon; ◆, Defective RNA processing; ✦, Missense and nonsense mutations; ☐A, Poly A signal.

together at a genomic locus. Haplotypes are useful for tracking the transmission of genomic segments within families and for detecting evidence of genetic recombination, if the crossover event occurs between the alleles (Fig. 65-3). As an example, various alleles at the histocompatibility locus antigen (HLA) on chromosome 6p are used to establish haplotypes associated with certain disease states. For example, 21-hydroxylase deficiency, complement deficiency, and hemochromatosis are each associated with specific HLA haplotypes. It is now recognized that these genes lie in close vicinity to the HLA locus, which explains why HLA associations were identified even before the disease genes were cloned and localized. In other cases, specific HLA associations with diseases such as ankylosing spondylitis (HLA-B27) or type 1 diabetes mellitus (HLA-DR4) reflect the role of specific HLA allelic variants in susceptibility to these autoimmune diseases.

Allelic Heterogeneity *Allelic heterogeneity* refers to the fact that different mutations in the same genetic locus can cause an identical or similar phenotype. For example, many different mutations of the β-globin locus can cause β-thalassemia (Fig. 65-7). In essence, allelic heterogeneity reflects the fact that many different mutations are capable of altering protein structure and function. For this reason, maps of inactivating mutations in genes usually show a near-random distribution. Exceptions include: (1) a founder effect, in which a particular mutation that does not affect reproductive capacity can be traced to a single individual; (2) "hot spots" for mutations, in which the nature of the DNA sequence predisposes to a recurring mutation; and (3) localization of mutations to certain domains that are particularly critical for protein function. Allelic heterogeneity creates a practical problem for genetic testing because one must often examine the entire genetic locus for mutations, as these can differ in each patient.

Phenotypic Heterogeneity *Phenotypic heterogeneity* occurs when more than one phenotype is caused by allelic mutations (e.g., different mutations in the same gene). For example, mutations in the *myosin VIIIA* gene can result in four distinct clinical disorders: (1) autosomal recessive deafness DFNB2, (2) autosomal dominant nonsyndromic deafness DFNA11, (3) Usher 1B syndrome [congenital deafness, retinitis pigmentosa (**Plate IV-14**)], and (4) an atypical variant of Usher's syndrome. Similarly, identical mutations in the *FGFR2* gene can result in very distinct phenotypes: Crouzon syndrome (craniofacial synostosis), or Pfeiffer syndrome (acrocephalopolysyndactyly).

Locus or Nonallelic Heterogeneity and Phenocopies *Nonallelic or locus heterogeneity* refers to the situation in which a similar disease phenotype results from mutations at different genetic loci (Ta-

ble 65-4). This often occurs when more than one gene product produces different subunits of an interacting complex or when different genes are involved in the same genetic cascade or physiologic pathway. For example, osteogenesis imperfecta can arise from mutations in two different procollagen genes (*COL1A1* or *COL1A2*) that are located on different chromosomes (Chap. 351). The effects of inactivating mutations in these two genes are similar because the protein products comprise different subunits of the helical collagen fiber. Similarly, muscular dystrophy syndromes can be caused by mutations in various genes, consistent with the fact that it can be transmitted in an X-linked (Duchenne or Becker), autosomal dominant (limb-girdle muscular dystrophy type 1), or autosomal recessive (limb-girdle muscular dystrophy type 2) manner (Chap. 383). Mutations in the X-linked *DMD* gene, which encodes dystrophin, are the most common cause of muscular dystrophy. This feature reflects the large size of the gene as well as the fact that the phenotype is expressed in hemizygous males because they only have a single copy of the X chromosome. Dystrophin is associated with a large group of additional proteins that form the membrane-associated cytoskeleton in muscle. Mutations in several components of this protein complex can also cause muscular dystrophy syndromes. Although the phenotypic features of some of these disorders are distinct, the phenotypic spectrum caused by mutations in different genes overlaps, thereby leading to nonallelic heterogeneity. It should be noted that mutations in dystrophin also cause allelic heterogeneity. For example, mutations in the *DMD* gene can cause either Duchenne or the less severe Becker muscular dystrophy, depending on the severity of the protein defect.

Recognition of nonallelic heterogeneity is important for several reasons: (1) the ability to identify disease loci in linkage studies is reduced by including patients with similar phenotypes but different genetic disorders; (2) genetic testing is more complex because several different genes need to be considered along with the possibility of different mutations in each of the candidate genes; and (3) novel information is gained about how genes or proteins interact, providing unique insights into molecular physiology.

Phenocopies refer to circumstances in which nongenetic conditions mimic a genetic disorder. For example, features of toxin- or drug-induced neurologic syndromes can resemble those seen in Huntington disease, and vascular causes of dementia share phenotypic features with familial forms of Alzheimer dementia (Chap. 362). Children born with activating mutations of the thyroid-stimulating hormone receptor (TSH-R) exhibit goiter and thyrotoxicosis similar to that seen in neonatal Graves' disease, which is caused by the transfer of maternal autoantibodies to the fetus (Chap. 330). As in nonallelic heterogeneity, the presence of phenocopies has the potential to confound linkage studies and genetic testing. Patient history and subtle differences in phenotype can often provide clues that distinguish these disorders from related genetic conditions.

Variable Expressivity and Incomplete Penetrance It is not uncommon for the same genetic mutation to cause a phenotypic spectrum illustrating the phenomenon of *variable expressivity*. This may include different manifestations of a complex disorder (e.g., MEN), the severity of the disorder (e.g., sickle cell anemia), or the age of disease onset (e.g., Alzheimer dementia). MEN-1 illustrates several of these features. Families with this autosomal dominant disorder develop tumors of the parathyroid gland, endocrine pancreas, and the pituitary gland (Chap. 339). However, the pattern of tumors in the different glands, the age at which tumors develop, and the types of hormones produced vary among affected individuals, even within a given family.

In this example, the phenotypic variability arises, in part, because of the requirement for a second mutation in the normal copy of the *MEN1* gene, as well as the large array of different cell types that are susceptible to the effects of *MEN1* gene mutations. In part, variable expression reflects the influence of other genes, or genetic background, on the effects of a particular mutation. Even in identical twins, in whom the genetic constitution is the same, one can occasionally see variable expression of a genetic disease.

Interactions with the environment can also influence the course of a disease. For example, the manifestations and severity of hemochromatosis can be influenced by iron intake (Chap. 345), and the course of phenylketonuria is affected by exposure to phenylalanine in the diet (Chap. 352). Other metabolic disorders, such as hyperlipidemias and porphyria, also fall into this category. Many mechanisms, including genetic effects and environmental influences, can therefore lead to variable expressivity. In genetic counseling, it is particularly important to recognize this variability, as one cannot always predict the course of disease, even when the mutation is known.

Penetrance is the probability of expressing the phenotype given a defined genotype; it can be complete or incomplete. For example, hypertrophic obstructive cardiomyopathy (HOCM) caused by mutations in the *myosin heavy chain β* gene is a dominant disorder with clinical features in only a subset of patients who carry the mutation (Chap. 238). Patients who have the mutation but no evidence of the disease can still transmit the disorder to subsequent generations. In this situation, the disorder is said to be *nonpenetrant* or *incompletely penetrant*. This classification depends to some degree on the criteria and techniques used for diagnosis. For disorders such as Huntington disease or familial amyotrophic lateral sclerosis, which present late in life, the rate of penetrance is influenced by the age at which the clinical assessment is performed. *Imprinting* can also modify the penetrance of a disease (see below). For example, in patients with Albright hereditary osteodystrophy, mutations in the Gsα subunit (*GNAS1* gene) are expressed clinically only in individuals who inherit the mutation from their mother (Chap. 343).

Sex-Influenced Phenotypes Certain mutations affect males and females quite differently. In some instances, this is because the gene resides on the X or Y sex chromosomes (X-linked disorders and Y-linked disorders). As a result, the phenotype of mutated X-linked genes will be expressed fully in males but variably in heterozygous females, depending on the degree of X-inactivation and the function of the gene. For example, most heterozygous female carriers of factor VIII deficiency (hemophilia A) are asymptomatic because sufficient factor VIII is produced to prevent a defect in coagulation (Chap. 117). On the other hand, some females heterozygous for the X-linked lipid storage defect caused by α-galactosidase A deficiency (Fabry disease) experience mild manifestations of painful neuropathy, as well as other features of the disease (Chap. 349). Because only males have a Y chromosome, mutations in genes such as *SRY* (which causes male-to-female sex-reversal) or *DAZ* (which causes abnormalities of spermatogenesis) are unique to males (Chap. 338).

Other diseases are expressed in a sex-limited manner because of the differential function of the gene product in males and females. Activating mutations in the luteinizing hormone receptor cause dominant male-limited precocious puberty in boys (Chap. 335). The phenotype is unique to males because activation of the receptor induces testosterone production in the testis, whereas it is functionally silent in the immature ovary. Homozygous inactivating mutations of the follicle-stimulating hormone (FSH) receptor cause primary ovarian failure in females because the follicles do not develop in the absence of FSH action. In contrast, affected males have a more subtle phenotype, because testosterone production is preserved (allowing sexual maturation) and spermatogenesis is only partially impaired (Chap. 335). In congenital adrenal hyperplasia, most commonly caused by 21-hydroxylase deficiency, cortisol production is impaired and ACTH stimulation of the adrenal gland leads to increased production of androgenic precursors (Chap. 331). In females, the increased androgen level causes ambiguous genitalia, which can be recognized at the time of birth. In males, the diagnosis may be made on the basis of adrenal insufficiency at birth, because the increased adrenal androgen level does not alter sexual differentiation, or later in childhood, because of the development of precocious puberty. Hemochromatosis is more common in males than in females, presumably because of differences in dietary iron intake and losses associated with menstruation and pregnancy in females (Chap. 345).

GENETIC LINKAGE *Genetic linkage* refers to the fact that genes are physically connected, or linked, to one another along the chromosomes. Two fundamental principles are essential for understanding the concept of a genetic linkage: (1) When two genes are close together on a chromosome, they are usually transmitted together, unless a recombination event separates them (Fig. 65-3); and (2) the odds of a crossover, or recombination event, between two linked genes is proportional to the distance that separates them. Thus, genes that are further apart are more likely to undergo a recombination event than genes that are very close together. Linkage is used in genetic counseling to predict the odds of disease gene transmission.

Polymorphisms are essential for linkage studies because they provide a means to distinguish the maternal and paternal chromosomes in an individual. On average, 1 out of every 1000 bp varies from one person to the next. Although this degree of variation seems low (99.9% identical), it means that >3 million sequence differences exist between any two unrelated individuals. This sequence variation usually has no significant functional consequence and provides much of the basis for variation in genetic traits. Although many of these sequence variations are SNPs, other variants include VNTRs or short tandem repeats (STRs). In VNTRs and STRs, the number of times a sequence is repeated is highly variable in the population. Consequently, the probability that sequences will differ on the two homologous chromosomes is high (often >70 to 90%). Most STRs, also called *polymorphic microsatellite markers*, consist of di-, tri-, or tetranucleotide repeats that can be measured readily using PCR and primers that reside on either side of the repeat sequences (Fig. 65-8). Many other methods for analyzing polymorphic variation are also available. Historically, RFLPs were used to detect sequence variations that caused changes in the recognition sites for restriction enzymes. This procedure has been largely replaced by the use of STRs. Analyses of SNPs, using DNA chips, provide a promising means for rapid analysis of genetic variation and linkage.

In order to identify a chromosomal locus that segregates with a disease, it is necessary to determine the genotype or haplotype of DNA samples from one or several pedigrees. One can then assess whether certain marker alleles cosegregate with the disease. Markers that are closest to the disease gene are less likely to undergo recombination events and therefore receive a higher linkage score. Linkage is expressed as a lod (logarithm of odds) score—the ratio of the probability that the disease and marker loci are linked rather than unlinked. Lod scores of +3 (1000:1) are generally accepted as supporting linkage, whereas a score of −2 is consistent with the absence of linkage.

An example of the use of linkage analysis is shown in Fig. 65-8. In this case, the gene for the autosomal dominant disorder, MEN-1, is known to be located on chromosome 11q13. Using positional cloning, the *MEN1* gene was identified and shown to encode menin, the function of which is poorly understood. However, the transmission of the disorder suggests that menin acts like a tumor-suppressor gene. Affected individuals inherit a mutant form of the *MEN1* gene, predisposing them to certain types of tumors (parathyroid, pituitary, pancreatic islet) (Chap. 339). In the tissues that develop a tumor, a "second hit" occurs in the normal copy of the *MEN1* gene. This somatic mutation may be a point mutation, a microdeletion, or loss of a chromosomal fragment (detected as loss of heterozygosity, LOH). Within a given family, linkage to the *MEN1* gene locus can be assessed without necessarily knowing the specific mutation in the *MEN1* gene. Using polymorphic STRs that are close to the *MEN1* gene, one can assess transmission of the different *MEN1* alleles and compare this pattern

FIGURE 65-8 CAG repeat length and linkage analysis in multiple endocrine neoplasia type 1. *Upper panel.* Detection of different alleles using polymorphic microsatellite markers. The example depicts a CAG trinucleotide repeat. PCR with primers flanking the polymorphic region results in products of variable length, depending on the number of CAG repeats. After characterization of the alleles in the parents, transmission of the paternal and maternal alleles can be determined. *Lower panel.* Genotype analysis using microsatellite markers in a family with multiple endocrine neoplasia type 1. Two microsatellite markers, A and B, are located in close proximity to the *MEN1* gene on chromosome 11q13. For each individual, the A and B alleles have been determined. Based on this analysis, the genotype A3,B4 is linked to the disease because it occurs in the two affected individuals I-1 and II-1 but not in unaffected siblings. Because the disease allele is linked to A3,B4 within the affected family, it is likely that the individual III-1 is a carrier of the mutated *MEN1* gene. Although III-5 also has the A3,B4 genotype, she has inherited the allele from her unaffected father (III-4), who is not related to the original family. The A3,B4 genotype is only associated with MEN-1 in the original family, but not in the general population. Therefore, individual III-5 is not at risk for developing the disease.

to development of the disorder to determine which allele is associated with risk of MEN-1. In the pedigree shown, the affected grandfather in generation I carries alleles 3 and 4 on the chromosome with the mutated *MEN1* gene and alleles 2 and 2 on his other chromosome 11. Consistent with linkage of the 3/4 genotype to the *MEN1* locus, his son in generation II is affected, whereas his daughter (who inherits the 2/2 genotype from her father) is unaffected. In the third generation, transmission of the 3/4 genotype indicates risk of developing MEN-1, assuming that no genetic recombination between the 3/4 alleles and the *MEN1* gene has occurred. After a specific mutation in the *MEN1* gene is identified within a family, it is possible to track transmission of the mutation itself, thereby eliminating uncertainty caused by recombination.

CHROMOSOMAL DISORDERS Chromosomal or cytogenetic disorders are caused by numerical or structural aberrations in

chromosomes. Deviations in chromosome number are common causes of abortions, developmental disorders, and malformations. →*For discussion of disorders of chromosome number and structure, see Chap. 66.*

Contiguous Gene Syndromes Large deletions or duplications may affect a portion of a gene, an entire gene, or, if several genes are involved, cause a *contiguous gene syndrome.* Syndromes associated with chromosomal deletions or duplications have a wide phenotypic spectrum that is dependent on the number of involved gene loci. For example, the cri-du-chat syndrome, one of the most common deletion disorders, is associated with deletions on the short arm of chromosome 5 that vary in size from extremely small deletions within 5p15.2 to the loss of the entire short arm. Because of the variable size of the involved deletions, the phenotype encompasses a spectrum that ranges from severe mental retardation and microcephaly to an isolated catlike cry without morphologic or mental abnormalities.

Contiguous gene syndromes have been useful for identifying the location of new disease-causing genes. Because of the variable size of gene deletions in different patients, a systemic comparison of phenotypes and locations of deletion breakpoints allows positions of particular genes to be mapped within the critical genomic region.

MONOGENIC MENDELIAN DISORDERS Monogenic human diseases are frequently referred to as *Mendelian disorders* because they obey the principles of genetic transmission originally set forth in Gregor Mendel's classic work. The mode of inheritance for a given phenotypic trait or disease is determined by pedigree analysis. All affected and unaffected individuals in the family are recorded in a pedigree using standard symbols (Fig. 65-9). The principles of allelic segregation, and the transmission of alleles from parents to children, are illustrated in Fig. 65-10. One dominant (A) allele and one recessive (a) allele can display three Mendelian modes of inheritance: autosomal dominant, autosomal recessive, and X-chromosomal. About 65% of human monogenic disorders are autosomal dominant, 25% are autosomal recessive, and 5% are X-linked (Table 65-5). Genetic testing is now available for many of these disorders and plays an increasingly important role in clinical medicine.

Autosomal Dominant Disorders Autosomal dominant disorders assume particular relevance because mutations in a single allele are sufficient to cause the disease. In contrast to recessive disorders, in which disease pathogenesis is relatively straightforward because there is loss of gene function, in dominant disorders there are various disease mechanisms, many of which are unique to the function of the genetic pathway involved.

In autosomal dominant disorders, individuals are affected in successive generations; the disease does not occur in the offspring of unaffected individuals. Males and females are affected with equal frequency because the defective gene resides on one of the 22 autosomes (Fig. 65-11A). Autosomal dominant mutations alter one of the two alleles at a given locus. Because the alleles segregate randomly at meiosis, the probability that an offspring will be affected is 50%. Un-

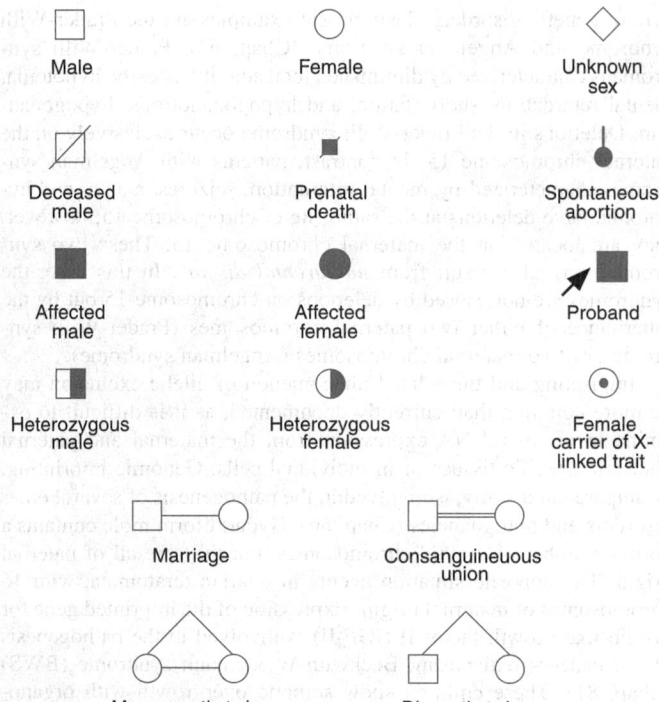

Male — Female — Unknown sex

Deceased male — Prenatal death — Spontaneous abortion

Affected male — Affected female — Proband

Heterozygous male — Heterozygous female — Female carrier of X-linked trait

Marriage — Consanguineuous union

Monozygotic twins — Dizygotic twins

FIGURE 65-9 Symbols used in pedigree analysis.

less there is a new germline mutation, an affected individual has an affected parent. Children with a normal genotype do not transmit the disorder. Due to differences in penetrance or expressivity (see above), the clinical manifestations of autosomal dominant disorders may be variable. Because of these variations, it is sometimes challenging to determine the pattern of inheritance.

It should be recognized, however, that some individuals acquire a mutated gene from an unaffected parent. De novo germline mutations occur more frequently during later cell divisions in gametogenesis, explaining why siblings are rarely affected. As noted before, new germline mutations occur more frequently in fathers of advanced age. For example, the average age of fathers with new germline mutations that cause Marfan's syndrome is approximately 37 years, whereas fathers who transmit the disease by inheritance have an average age of about 30 years.

Autosomal Recessive Disorders The clinical expression of autosomal recessive disorders is more uniform than in autosomal dominant disorders. Most mutated alleles lead to a complete or partial loss of function. They frequently involve enzymes in metabolic pathways, receptors, or proteins in signaling cascades. Though most recessive disorders are rare, the relatively high frequency of certain recessive disorders, such as sickle cell anemia, cystic fibrosis, and thalassemia, is partially explained by a selective biologic advantage for the heterozygous state (see below).

In an autosomal recessive disease, the affected individual, who can be of either sex, is a homozygote or compound heterozygote for a

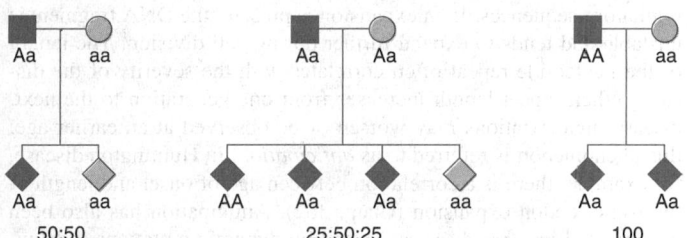

FIGURE 65-10 Segregation of alleles. Segregation of genotypes in the offspring of parents with one dominant (A) and one recessive (a) allele. The distribution of the parental alleles to their offspring depends on the combination present in the parents.

single-gene defect. With a few important exceptions, autosomal recessive diseases are rare and often occur in the context of parental consanguinity. Though heterozygous carriers of a defective allele are usually clinically normal, they may display subtle differences in phenotype that only become apparent with more precise testing or in the context of certain environmental influences. In sickle cell anemia, for example, heterozygotes are normally asymptomatic. However, in situations of dehydration or diminished oxygen pressure, sickle cell crises can also occur in heterozygotes (Chap. 106).

In most instances, an affected individual is the offspring of heterozygous parents. In this situation, there is a 25% chance that the offspring will have a normal genotype, a 50% probability of a heterozygous state, and a 25% risk of homozygosity for the recessive alleles (Fig. 65-11B). In the case of one unaffected heterozygous and one affected homozygous parent, the probability of disease increases to 50% for each child. In this instance, the pedigree analysis mimics an autosomal dominant mode of inheritance (*pseudodominance*). In contrast to autosomal dominant disorders, new mutations in recessive alleles are rarely manifest because they usually result in an asymptomatic carrier state.

X-Linked Disorders Males have only one X chromosome; consequently, a daughter always inherits her father's X chromosome in addition to one of her mother's two X chromosomes. A son inherits the Y chromosome from his father and one maternal X chromosome. Thus, the characteristic features of X-linked inheritance are (1) the absence of father-to-son transmission, and (2) the fact that all daughters of an affected male are obligate carriers of the mutant allele (Fig. 65-11C). The risk of developing disease due to a mutant X-chromosomal gene differs in the two sexes. Because males have only one X chromosome, they are hemizygous for the mutant allele; thus, they are more likely to develop the mutant phenotype, regardless of whether

A   Autosomal dominant

B   Autosomal recessive   Autosomal recessive with pseudodominance

C   X-linked

FIGURE 65-11 Dominant, recessive, and X-linked inheritance.

the mutation is dominant or recessive. A female may be either heterozygous or homozygous for the mutant allele, which may be dominant or recessive. The terms *X-linked dominant* or *X-linked recessive* are therefore only applicable to expression of the mutant phenotype in women. In addition, the expression of X-chromosomal genes is influenced by X chromosome inactivation (see below).

Y-Linked Disorders   Only a few genes are known on the Y chromosome. One such gene, the sex-region determining Y factor (*SRY*), or testis-determining factor (*TDF*), is crucial for normal male development. Normally there is infrequent exchange of sequences on the Y chromosome with the X chromosome. Because the *SRY* region is closely adjacent to the pseudoautosomal region, a chromosomal segment on the X and Y chromosomes with a high degree of homology, a crossing-over occasionally involves the *SRY* region. Translocations can result in XY females with the Y chromosome lacking the *SRY* gene or XX males harboring the *SRY* gene on one of the X chromosomes (Chap. 338). Point mutations in the *SRY* gene may also result in individuals with an XY genotype and an incomplete female phenotype. Most of these mutations occur de novo. Men with oligospermia/azoospermia frequently have microdeletions on the long arm of the Y chromosome that involve one or more of the azoospermia factor (*AZF*) genes.

EXCEPTIONS TO SIMPLE MENDELIAN INHERITANCE PATTERNS   Mitochondrial Disorders   Each mitochondrion contains several copies of a circular chromosome. Mitochondrial DNA predominantly encodes transfer RNAs and proteins that are components of the respiratory chain involved in oxidative phosphorylation and ATP generation. The mitochondrial genome is inherited through the maternal line because sperm does not contribute significant cytoplasmic components to the zygote. All children from an affected mother will inherit the disease, but it will not be transmitted from an affected father to his children. During cell replication, the proportion of wild-type and mutant mitochondria can drift; differences in the fraction of defective mitochondria are referred to as *heteroplasmia* and explain, in part, the phenotypic variability that is common in mitochondrial diseases. →*For detailed discussion of mitochondrial disorders, see Chap. 67.*

Mosaicism   Mosaicism refers to the presence of two or more genetically distinct cell lines in the tissues of an individual. It results from a mutation that occurs during embryonic, fetal, or extrauterine development. The developmental stage at which the mutation arises will determine whether germ cells and/or somatic cells are involved. Chromosomal mosaicism results from non-disjunction at an early embryonic mitotic division, leading to the persistence of more than one cell line, as exemplified by some patients with Turner syndrome (Chap. 338). Somatic mosaicism is characterized by a patchy distribution of genetically altered somatic cells. The McCune-Albright syndrome, for example, is caused by activating mutations in the stimulatory G protein α (G$_s\alpha$) that occur early in development (Chap. 343). The clinical phenotype varies depending on the tissue distribution of the mutation; manifestations include ovarian cysts that secrete sex steroids and cause precocious puberty, polyostotic fibrous dysplasia, café-au-lait skin pigmentation, growth hormone–secreting pituitary adenomas, and hypersecreting autonomous thyroid nodules (Chap. 336).

X-Inactivation, Imprinting, and Uniparental Disomy   According to traditional Mendelian principles, the parental origin of a mutant gene is irrelevant for the expression of the phenotype. Nonetheless, there are important exceptions to this rule. X-inactivation prevents the expression of most genes on one of the two X-chromosomes in every cell of a female. Gene inactivation also occurs on selected chromosomal regions of autosomes. This phenomenon, referred to as *genomic imprinting*, leads to preferential expression of an allele depending on its parental origin. It is of pathophysiologic importance in disorders where the transmission of disease is dependent on the sex of the transmitting parent and, thus, plays an important role in the expression of

certain genetic disorders. Two classic examples are the Prader-Willi syndrome and Angelman syndrome (Chap. 66). Prader-Willi syndrome is characterized by diminished fetal activity, obesity, hypotonia, mental retardation, short stature, and hypogonadotropic hypogonadism. Deletions in the Prader-Willi syndrome occur exclusively on the paternal chromosome 15. In contrast, patients with Angelman syndrome, characterized by mental retardation, seizures, ataxia, and hypotonia, have deletions at the same site of chromosome 15; however, they are located on the maternal chromosome 15. These two syndromes may also result from *uniparental disomy*. In this case, the syndromes are not caused by deletions on chromosome 15 but by the inheritance of either two paternal chromosomes (Prader-Willi syndrome), or two maternal chromosomes (Angelman syndrome).

Imprinting and the related phenomenon of allelic exclusion may be more common than currently documented, as it is difficult to examine levels of mRNA expression from the maternal and paternal alleles in specific tissues or in individual cells. Genomic imprinting, or uniparental disomy, is involved in the pathogenesis of several other disorders and malignancies (Chap. 66). Hydatidiform mole contains a normal number of diploid chromosomes, but they are all of paternal origin. The opposite situation occurs in ovarian teratomata, with 46 chromosomes of maternal origin. Expression of the imprinted gene for insulin-like growth factor II (IGF-II) is involved in the pathogenesis of the cancer-predisposing Beckwith-Wiedemann syndrome (BWS) (Chap. 81). These children show somatic overgrowth with organomegalies and hemihypertrophy, and they have an increased risk of embryonal malignancies such as Wilm's tumor. Normally only the paternally derived copy of the *IGF-II* gene is active and the maternal copy is inactive. Imprinting of the *IGF-II* gene is regulated by *H19*, which encodes an RNA transcript that is not translated into protein. Disruption or lack of *H19* methylation leads to a relaxation of *IGF-II* imprinting and expression of both alleles. Heritable changes in gene expression not associated with DNA sequence alterations are referred to as *epigenetic effects*; these changes are increasingly recognized to play a role in human diseases and possibly in aging as well (Chap. 9).

Somatic Mutations   In many cancer syndromes, there is an inherited predisposition to tumor formation. However, the neoplastic process requires the acquisition of additional somatic mutations (Chap. 81). In retinoblastoma, the tumor develops when both copies of the retinoblastoma (*RB*) gene are inactivated through two somatic events (sporadic retinoblastoma) or through a somatic loss of the normal allele in an individual with a hereditary defect in the other allele (hereditary retinoblastoma). This "two-hit" model applies to other inherited cancer syndromes such as MEN-1 (Chap. 339) and neurofibromatosis type 2 (Chap. 370). The defective allele is transmitted in a dominant pattern, though tumorigenesis results from a recessive loss of the tumor suppressor gene in an affected tissue. In other instances, the development of cancer typically requires somatic defects in multiple genes, a process termed *multistep carcinogenesis* (Chap. 82).

Nucleotide Repeat Expansion Disorders   Several diseases are associated with an increase in the number of nucleotide repeats above a certain threshold (Table 65-6). The repeats are sometimes located within the coding region of the genes, as in Huntington disease or the X-linked form of spinal and bulbar muscular atrophy (SBMA, Kennedy syndrome). In other instances, the repeats probably alter gene regulatory sequences. If an expansion is present, the DNA fragment is unstable and tends to expand further during cell division. The length of the nucleotide repeat often correlates with the severity of the disease. When repeat length increases from one generation to the next, disease manifestations may worsen or be observed at an earlier age; this phenomenon is referred to as *anticipation*. In Huntington disease, for example, there is a correlation between age of onset and length of the triplet codon expansion (Chap. 362). Anticipation has also been documented in other diseases caused by dynamic mutations in trinucleotide repeats (Table 65-6). The repeat number may also vary in a tissue-specific manner. In myotonic dystrophy, the CTG repeat may be tenfold greater in muscle tissue than in lymphocytes (Chap. 383).

POPULATION GENETICS AND AS-SOCIATION STUDIES Overview of Population Genetics In population genetics, the focus changes from alterations in an individual's genome to the distribution pattern of different genotypes of alleles in the population. In a case where there are only two alleles, A and a, the frequency of the genotypes will be $p^2 + 2pq + q^2 = 1$, with p^2 corresponding to the frequency of AA, $2pq$ to the frequency of Aa, and q^2 to aa. When the frequency of an allele is known, the frequency of the genotype can be calculated. Alternatively, one can determine an allele frequency, if the genotype frequency has been determined.

Allele frequencies vary among ethnic groups and geographical regions. For example, heterozygous mutations in the *CFTR* gene are relatively common in populations of European origin but are rare in the African population. Allele frequencies may vary because certain allelic variants confer a selective advantage. For example, heterozygotes for the sickle cell mutation, which is particularly common in West Africa, are more resistant to malarial infection because the erythrocytes of heterozygotes provide a less favorable environment for *Plasmodium* parasites. Though homozygosity for the sickle cell gene is associated with severe anemia and sickle crises (Chap. 106), heterozygotes have a higher probability of survival because of the reduced morbidity and mortality from malaria; this phenomenon has led to an increased frequency of the mutant allele. Recessive conditions are more prevalent in geographically isolated populations because of the more restricted gene pool.

Allelic Association and Linkage Disequilibrium There are two primary strategies for mapping genes that cause or increase susceptibility to human disease: (1) classic linkage can be performed based on a known genetic model (see above) or, when the model is unknown, by studying pairs of affected relatives; or (2) disease genes can be mapped using allelic association studies (Table 65-7). *Allelic association* refers to a situation in which the frequency of an allele is significantly increased or decreased in a particular disease. Linkage and association differ in several aspects. Genetic linkage is demonstrable in families or sibships. Association studies, on the other hand, compare a population of affected individuals with a control population. Association studies can be performed as case-control studies that include unrelated affected individuals and matched controls, or as family-based studies that compare the frequencies of alleles transmitted or not transmitted to affected children.

Allelic association studies are particularly useful for identifying susceptibility genes in complex diseases. When alleles at two loci occur more frequently in combination than would be predicted (based on known allele frequencies and recombination fractions), they are said to be in *linkage disequilibrium*. In Fig. 65-12, a mutation, Z, has occurred at a susceptibility locus where the normal allele is Y. The mutation is in close proximity to a genetic polymorphism with allele A or B. With time, the chromosomes carrying the A and Z alleles accumulate and represent 10% of the chromosomes in the population. The fact that the disease susceptibility gene, Z, is found preferentially, or exclusively, in association with the A allele illustrates linkage disequilibrium. Though not all chromosomes carrying the A allele carry the disease gene, the A allele is associated with an increased risk because of its possible association with the Z allele. This model implies that it may be possible in the future to identify Z directly to provide a more accurate prediction of disease susceptibility. Evidence for linkage disequilibrium can be helpful in mapping disease genes because it suggests that the two loci, in this case A and Z, are tightly linked.

Table 65-7 Genetic Approaches for Identifying Disease Genes

Method	Indications and Advantages	Limitations
Linkage analysis	Analysis of monogenic traits Suitable for genome scan Control population not required Useful for multifactorial disorders in isolated populations	Difficult to collect large informative pedigrees Difficult to obtain sufficient statistical power for complex traits
Allele-sharing methods Affected sib and relative pair analyses Sib pair analysis	Suitable for identification of susceptibility genes in polygenic and multifactorial disorders Suitable for genome scan Control population not required if allele frequencies are known Statistical power can be increased by including parents and relatives	Difficult to collect sufficient number of subjects Difficult to obtain sufficient statistical power for complex traits
Association studies Case-control studies Linkage disequilibrium Transmission distortion test	Suitable for identification of susceptibility genes in polygenic and multifactorial disorders Suitable for testing specific allelic variants of known candidate loci Does not necessarily need relatives	Requires large sample size and matched control population False-positive results in the absence of suitable control population

POLYGENIC DISEASE AND COMPLEX GENETIC TRAITS Approach to Polygenic and Multifactorial Disease The expression of many common diseases such as cardiovascular disease, hypertension, diabetes, asthma, psychiatric disorders, and certain cancers is determined by genetic background, environmental factors, and lifestyle (Table 65-8). A trait is called *polygenic* if multiple genes are thought to contribute to the phenotype or *multifactorial* if multiple genes are assumed to interact with environmental factors. Genetic models for complex traits need to account for genetic heterogeneity and interactions with other genes and the environment. Complex genetic traits may be influenced by modifying genes that are not linked to the main gene involved in the pathogenesis of the trait. This type of gene-gene interaction, or *epistasis*, plays an important role in polygenic traits that require the simultaneous presence of variations in multiple genes in order to result in a pathologic phenotype. Gene-environment interactions are relevant for many monogenic and polygenic disorders. In phenylketonuria, the phenotypic expression of the disease depends not only on the presence of the mutation in the phenylalanine hydroxylase gene but also on the exposure to the amino acid phenylalanine (Chap. 352). Another example is type 2 diabetes

Wild type: Polymorphic alleles
A = 40%; B = 60%
Wild type allele Y = 100%

Linkage disequilibrium: Allele A is associated with the mutation Z in 10%. B is never associated with the mutation Z, unless a recombination has occurred between the two loci.

Mutation Y → Z

Passage of many generations

30%   10%   60%

FIGURE 65-12 Linkage disequilibrium.

Table 65-8   Selected Multifactorial and Polygenic Disorders

Disorder	Genes or Susceptibility Loci[a]	Chromosomal Location	Other Factors
Diabetes mellitus type 1	HLA-DQB1,-DRB1 (IDDM1)	6p21	Viral infections
	Insulin VNTR (IDDM2)	11p15	Autoimmunity
	Cytotoxic T lymphocyte–associated 4 (CTLA-4, IDDM12)	2q33	
	IGF binding protein 2, -5 (IDDM13)	2q34	
	Glucokinase	7p15.1-15.3	
Diabetes mellitus type 2	Insulin promoter factor 1 (IPF1)	13q12.1	Diet
	Insulin receptor substrate (IRS-1)	2q36	Energy expenditure
	Peroxisome proliferator receptor γ	3p25	Obesity
	Sulfonylurea receptor	11p15.1	
	Amylin	12p12.3-p12.1	
	Phosphoenolpyruvate carboxykinase 1 (PEPCK1)	20q13.31	
	Hepatocyte nuclear factor 1α (HNF1A)	12q24.2	
	Cholecystokinin receptor B	11p15.5-p15.4	
	Growth hormone	17q22-q24	
	Ras-related associated with diabetes (RRAD)	16q22	
	Apolipoprotein A2	1q21-q23	
Hypertension	Angiotensinogen	1q42-43	Salt intake
	Angiotensin-converting enzyme	17q23	
	Angiotensin receptor 1	3q21-25	
	G-protein subunit 3	12p13	
	Hypertension susceptibility locus 1 (HYT1)	17q	
	Hypertension susceptibility locus 2 (HYT2)	15q	
Coronary artery disease— atherosclerosis	Low-density lipoprotein receptor	19p13.2-p13.1	Diet
	Apolipoprotein E4	19q13.2	Exercise
	Apolipoprotein (a)	6q27	Smoking
	Homocysteine	Unknown	Diabetes
	Plasminogen-activator inhibitor	7q21.3-q22	Hypertension
			Hormones
			Infection of endothelial cells
Asthma—bronchial hyperreactivity	IgE receptor	11q13	Allergens
	5q31 locus	5q32-33	Pollution
	MHC locus	6p21	
	Interleukin receptor	Xq28	
Manic-depressive psychosis	Xq26 locus	Xq26	Familial and social environment
	18p locus	18p	
	4p locus	4p	
	21q locus	21q	
	18q locus	18q	
Psoriasis	HLA-Cw6,-DR7,-B13,-Bw57, and others	6p21	Environmental stimuli
	17q locus	17q	
	16q locus	16q	
	20p locus	20p	
Systemic lupus erythematosus	HLA-DR2,-DR3	6p21	Hormones
	C4 deficiency	6p21.3	Unspecified environmental stimuli
	1q locus	1q41-q42	

[a] The relative importance of the listed susceptibility genes and loci is in part controversial among different studies, and positive associations may vary among different populations. Additional genes and loci have been associated with most of the disorders included in this table.
NOTE: IGF, insulin-like growth factor; MHC, major histocompatibility complex; VNTR, variable number of tandem repeats.

mellitus, in which genetic, nutritional, and lifestyle factors are intimately interrelated in disease pathogenesis (Chap. 333). The identification of genetic variations and environmental factors that either predispose or protect against disease is essential for predicting disease risk, designing preventive strategies, and developing novel therapeutic approaches (Chap. 68). The study of rare monogenic diseases may provide insights into genetic and molecular mechanisms that are subsequently of importance for the understanding of complex diseases. For example, the identification of the insulin promoter factor 1 in maturity-onset of diabetes type 4 was followed by the observation that it also plays a role in the pathogenesis of diabetes mellitus type 2 (Tables 65-1 and -8).

Approach to the Patient

Identifying the Disease-Causing Gene   *Genomic medicine* aims to enhance the quality of medical care through the use genotypic analysis (DNA testing) to identify genetic predisposition to disease, to select more specific pharmacotherapy, and to design individualized medical care based on genotype. Genotype can be deduced by analysis of protein (e.g., hemoglobin, apoprotein E), mRNA, or DNA. However, technological advances have made DNA analysis particularly useful because it can be readily applied to all but the largest genes (Fig. 65-13).

DNA testing is performed by mutational analysis or linkage studies in individuals at risk for a genetic disorder known to be present in a family. Mass screening programs require tests of high sensitivity and specificity to be cost-effective. Prerequisites for the success of genetic screening programs include the following: that the disorder is potentially serious; that it can be influenced at a presymptomatic stage by changes in behavior, diet, and/or pharmaceutical manipulations; and that the screening does not result in any harm or discrimination. Screening in Jewish populations for the autosomal recessive neurodegenerative storage disease Tay-Sachs has reduced the number of affected individuals. In contrast, screening for sickle cell trait/disease in African Americans has led to unanticipated problems of discrimination by health insurers and employers. Mass screening programs harbor additional potential problems. For example, screening for the most common genetic alteration in cystic fibrosis, the ΔF508 mutation with a frequency of ~70% in northern Europe, is feasible and seems to be effective. One has to keep in mind, however, that there is pronounced allelic heterogeneity and that the disease can be caused by >600 other mutations. The search for these less common mutations would substantially increase costs but not the effectiveness of the screening program as a whole. Occupational screening programs aim to detect individuals with increased risk for certain professional activities (e.g., α_1 antitrypsin deficiency and smoke or dust exposure).

Mutational analyses DNA sequence analysis is increasingly used as a diagnostic tool and significantly enhanced diagnostic accuracy. It is used for determining carrier status and for prenatal testing in monogenic disorders (Table 65-5). Certain cancer susceptibility genes, such as *BRCA1* and *BRCA2*, may identify individuals with an increased risk for the development of malignancies. The detection of mutations is an important diagnostic and prognostic tool in leukemias and lymphomas. The demonstration of the presence or absence of mutations is also relevant for the rapidly evolving field of pharmacogenetics, including the identification of differences in drug treatment response or metabolism as a function of genetic background.

A general algorithm for the approach to mutational analysis is outlined in Fig. 65-13. The importance of a detailed clinical phenotype

FIGURE 65-13 Approach to genetic disease.

Table 65-9 Methods Used for the Detection of Mutations

Method	Principle	Type of Mutation Detected
Cytogenic analysis	Unique visual appearance of various chromosomes	Numerical or structural abnormalities in chromosomes
Fluorescent in situ hybridization (FISH)	Hybridization to chromosomes with fluorescently labeled probes	Numerical or structural abnormalities in chromosomes
Southern blot	Hybridization with genomic probe or cDNA probe after digestion of high molecular DNA	Large deletion, insertion, rearrangement, expansions of triplet repeat, amplification
Polymerase chain reaction (PCR)	Amplification of DNA segment	Expansion of triplet repeats, variable number of tandem repeats (VNTR), gene rearrangements, translocations; prepare DNA for other mutation methods
Reverse transcriptase PCR (RT-PCR)	Reverse transcription, amplification of DNA segment → absence or reduction of mRNA transcription	Analyzed expressed mRNA (cDNA) sequence; detect loss of expression
DNA sequencing	Direct sequencing of PCR products / Sequencing of DNA segments cloned into plasmid vectors	Point mutations, small deletions and insertions
Single-strand conformational polymorphism (SSCP)	PCR of DNA segment: Mutations result in conformational change and altered mobility	Point mutations, small deletions and insertions
Denaturing gradient gel electrophoresis (DGGE)	PCR of DNA segment: Mutations result in conformational change and altered mobility	Point mutations, small deletions and insertions
RNAse cleavage	Cleavage of mismatch between mutated and wild-type sequence	Point mutations, small deletions and insertions
Restriction fragment length polymorphism (RFLP)	Detection of altered restriction pattern of genomic DNA (Southern blot) or PCR products	Point mutations, small deletions and insertions
Oligonucleotide specific hybridization (OSH)	Hybridization of PCR products to wild-type or mutated oligonucleotides immobilized on chips or slides	Point mutations, small deletions and insertions
Microarrays	Hybridization of PCR products to wild-type or mutated oligonucleotides	Point mutations, small deletions and insertions
Protein truncation test (PTT)	Transcription/translation of cDNA isolated from tissue sample	Mutations leading to premature truncations

cannot be overemphasized. This is the step where one should also consider the possibility of genetic heterogeneity and phenocopies. If obvious candidate genes are suggested by the phenotype, they can be analyzed directly. After identification of a mutation, it is essential to demonstrate that it segregates with the phenotype. The functional characterization of novel mutations is labor-intensive and may require analyses in vitro or in transgenic models in order to document the relevance of the genetic alteration.

Numerous techniques are available for the detection of mutations (Table 65-9). In a very broad sense, one can distinguish between techniques that allow for screening the absence or presence of known mutations (screening mode) or techniques that definitively characterize mutations. Analyses of large alterations in the genome are possible using cytogenetics, fluorescent in situ hybridization (FISH), and Southern blotting (Chap. 66).

More discrete sequence alterations rely heavily on the use of the PCR, which allows rapid gene amplification and analysis. Moreover, PCR makes it possible to perform genetic testing and mutational analysis with small amounts of DNA extracted from leukocytes or even from single cells, buccal cells, or hair roots. Screening for point mutations can be performed by numerous methods (Table 65-9); most are based on the recognition of mismatches between nucleic acid duplexes, electrophoretic separation of single- or double-stranded DNA, or sequencing of DNA fragments amplified by PCR. DNA sequencing can be performed directly on PCR products or on fragments cloned into plasmid vectors amplified in bacterial host cells.

RT-PCR may be useful to detect absent or reduced levels of mRNA expression due to a mutated allele. Protein truncation tests (PTT) can be used to detect the broad array of mutations that result in premature termination of a polypeptide during its synthesis. The isolated cDNA is transcribed and translated in vitro, and the proteins are analyzed by gel electrophoresis. Comparison of electrophoretic mobility with the wild-type protein allows detection of truncated mutants.

The majority of traditional diagnostic methods are gel-based. Novel technologies for the analysis of mutations, genetic mapping, and mRNA expression profiles are in rapid development. DNA chip technologies allow hybridization of DNA or RNA to hundreds of thousands of probes simultaneously. Microarrays are being used clinically for mutational analysis of several human disease genes, as well as for the identification of viral sequence variations. Together with the knowledge gained from the HGP, these technologies provide the foundation to expand from a focus on single genes to analyses at the scale of the genome.

ACKNOWLEDGMENTS
This chapter reflects the cumulative contributions of many past contributors to Harrison's Principles of Internal Medicine. *Most recently, this includes Dr. Joseph L. Goldstein, Dr. Michael S. Brown, Dr. Andrea Ballabio, and Dr. Arthur L. Beaudet.*

BIBLIOGRAPHY

ALBERTS B et al (eds): *Molecular Biology of the Cell*, 3d ed. New York, Garland, 1995

BRENT R: Genomic biology. Cell 100(1):169, 2000

BROWN PO, BOTSTEIN D: Exploring the new world of the genome with DNA microarrays. Nat Genet Suppl 21:33, 1999

BURLEY SK et al: Structural genomics: Beyond the Human Genome Project. Nat Genet 23:151, 1999

COLLINS FS et al: New goals for the U.S. human genome project: 1998–2003. Science 282:682, 1998

CONNOR JM, FERGUSON-SMITH M (eds): *Essential Medical Genetics*. Oxford, Blackwell Scientific, 1993

COTTON RGH, KAZAZIAN HH JR: The HUGO mutation database initiative: Issues, databases, and perspectives for the new millenium. Hum Mutat 15(1):1, 2000

DARNELL J et al (eds): *Molecular Cell Biology*, 3d ed. New York, Scientific American, 1995

Ethical, Legal, and Social Implications of Biotechnology. www.ncgr.org/gpi/

GELEHERTER TD et al (eds): *Principles of Medical Genetics*, 2d ed. Philadelphia, Lippincott, 1998

HAINES JL, PERICAK-VANCE MA (eds): Approaches to gene mapping in complex human diseases. New York, Wiley-Liss, 1998

HALUSKA MK et al: Patterns of single-nucleotide polymorphisms in candidate genes for blood-pressure homeostasis. Nat Genet 22:239, 1999

HANAKAN D, WEINBERG RA: The hallmarks of cancer. Cell 100(1):57, 2000

HARPER PS: *Practical Genetic Counseling*, 5th ed. Stoneham, MA, Butterworth-Heinemann, 1998

JAMESON JL (ed): *Principles of Molecular Medicine*. Totowa, NJ, Humana, 1998

LEWIN B: *Genes VI*. New York, Oxford, 1997

National Center for Biotechnology Information (GenBank, Medline, OMIM). www.ncbi.nlm.nih.gov

OTT J: *Analysis of Human Genetic Linkage*. Baltimore, John Hopkins, 1991

READ AP, STRACHAN T: *Human Molecular Genetics*. New York, Wiley, 1997

RIMOIN DL et al (eds): *Emery and Rimoin's Principles and Practice of Medical Genetics*, 3d ed. New York, Churchill Livingstone, 1996

SCRIVER CR et al (eds): *The Metabolic and Molecular Bases of Inherited Disease*, 8th ed. New York, McGraw-Hill, 2000

SOUTHERN EM: DNA chips: Analyzing sequence by hybridization to oligonucleotides on a large scale. Trends Genet 12:110, 1996

THOMPSON MW et al: *Genetics in Medicine*. Philadelphia, Saunders, 1993

VOGEL F, MOTULSKY AG (eds): *Human Genetics: Problems and Approaches*, 3d ed. Berlin, Springer, 1996

WRIGHT AF et al: Population choice in mapping genes for complex diseases. Nat Genet 23:397, 1999

66   *Terry Hassold, Stuart Schwartz*

CHROMOSOME DISORDERS

AS Angelman syndrome	MDS Miller-Dieker syndrome
BACs bacterial artificial chromosomes	PUBS percutaneous umbilical blood sampling
CML chronic myelogenous leukemia	PWS Prader-Willi syndrome
CMT1A Charcot-Marie-Tooth type 1A	UPD uniparental disomy
	VCF velocardiofacial syndrome
CVS chorionic villus sampling	WAGR Wilms' tumor–aniridia
FISH fluorescence in situ hybridization	complex
	YACs yeast artificial chromosomes

In humans, the normal diploid number of chromosomes is 46, consisting of 22 pairs of autosomal chromosomes (numbered 1 to 22 in decreasing size) and one pair of sex chromosomes (XX in females and XY in males). The genome is estimated to contain between 80,000 and 100,000 genes, with the smallest autosome housing between 500 and 1000 genes. Not surprisingly, duplications or deletions of even small chromosome segments have profound consequences on normal gene expression.

Deviations in the number or structure of the 46 human chromosomes are astonishingly common, despite severe deleterious consequences. Chromosomal disorders occur in an estimated 10 to 25% of all pregnancies. They are the leading cause of fetal loss and, among pregnancies surviving to term, the leading known cause of birth defects and mental retardation.

In recent years, the practice of cytogenetics has shifted from conventional cytogenetic methodology to a union of cytogenetic and molecular techniques. Formerly the province of research laboratories, *fluorescence in situ hybridization* (FISH) and related molecular cytogenetic technologies have been incorporated into everyday practice in clinical laboratories. As a result, there is an increased appreciation of the importance of "subtle" constitutional cytogenetic abnormalities, such as microdeletions and imprinting disorders, as well as previously recognized translocations and disorders of chromosome number.

VISUALIZING CHROMOSOMES

CONVENTIONAL CYTOGENETIC ANALYSIS In theory, chromosome preparations can be obtained from any actively dividing tissue by causing the cells to arrest in metaphase, the stage of the cell cycle at which chromosomes are maximally condensed. In practice, only a small number of tissues are used for routine chromosome analysis: amniocytes or chorionic villi for prenatal testing; and blood, bone marrow, or skin fibroblasts for postnatal studies. Samples of blood, bone marrow, and chorionic villi can be processed using short-term culture techniques that yield results in 1 to 3 days. Analysis of other tissue types typically involves long-term tissue culture, requiring 1 to 3 weeks of processing before cytogenetic analysis is possible.

Regardless of the culturing technique, cells are processed to recover chromosomes at metaphase or prometaphase and treated chemically or enzymatically to reveal chromosome "bands" (Fig. 66-1). Analysis of the number of chromosomes in the cell, and the distribution of bands on individual chromosomes, allows the identification of numerical or structural abnormalities. This strategy is useful for characterizing the normal chromosome complement and determining the incidence and types of major chromosome abnormalities.

Chromosomes are complex structures, consisting of the DNA double helix and chromosome-associated proteins. As for virtually all organisms, each human chromosome contains two specialized structures: a centromere and two telomeres. The *centromere*, or primary constriction, divides the chromosome into short (p) and long (q) arms and is responsible for the segregation of chromosomes during cell division. The *telomeres*, or chromosome ends, "cap" the p and q arms and are important for allowing DNA replication at the ends of the chromosomes. Prior to DNA replication, each chromosome consists of a single chromatid copy of the DNA double helix. After DNA replication and continuing until the time of cell division (including metaphase, when chromosomes are typically visualized), each chromosome consists of two identical sister chromatids (Fig. 66-1).

MOLECULAR CYTOGENETICS
The introduction of FISH methodologies in the late 1980s revolutionized the field of cytogenetics. In principle, FISH is similar to other DNA-DNA hybridization methodologies. The labeled probe DNA and the target DNA (usually metaphase chromosomes) are denatured to become single-stranded and are hybridized together. The probe is labeled with a hapten, such as biotin or digoxigenin, to allow detection with a fluorophore (e.g., FITC or rhodamine). Alternatively, many probes are already labeled with fluorophores and thus can be detected directly. After the hybridization step, the specimen is counter-stained and the preparations are visualized with a fluorescence microscope.

Types of FISH Probes   A variety of probes are available for use with FISH, including chromosome-specific paints (chromosome libraries), repetitive probes, and single-copy probes. Chromosome libraries were developed initially from flow-sorted individual chromosomes and more recently from monochromosomal human-rodent hybrids. These probes hybridize to sequences that span the entirety of the chromosome from which they are derived and, as a result, they can be used to "paint" individual chromosomes (Fig. 66-2).

Repetitive probes recognize amplified DNA sequences present in chromosomes. The most common are α-satellite DNA probes that are complementary to DNA sequences found at the centromeric regions of all human chromosomes. There are also α-satellite probes that hybridize to the centromeric regions of specific chromosomes (Fig. 66-2).

A vast number of *single-copy probes* are now available, both commercially and as a result of the human genome project. These probes can be as small as 1 kb, though normally they are packaged in cosmids (40 kb), bacterial artificial chromosomes (BACs) or P1 clones (100 to 200 kb), or yeast artificial chromosomes (YACs) (1 to 2 Mb). With the advent of the National Cancer Institute BAC initiative, these large DNA fragments will be placed at 1-Mb intervals on every chromosome, each of which can be used for FISH hybridization. Probes for a variety of microdeletion syndromes and for subtelomeric regions of individual chromosomes are commercially available (Fig. 66-2).

Applications of FISH   The majority of FISH applications involve hybridization of one or two probes of interest as an adjunctive procedure to conventional chromosomal banding techniques. In this

FIGURE 66-1   *A.* An idealized human chromosome, showing the centromere (cen), long (q) and short (p) arms, and telomeres (tel). *B.* A G-banded human karyotype from a normal (46,XX) female.

FIGURE 66-2 Examples of different applications of fluorescence in situ hybridization (FISH) to metaphase or interphase preparations. *A.* A chromosome 1–specific "paint" probe hybridizes to both normal chromosomes 1 as well as to a marker chromosome derived from chromosome 1. *B.* A repetitive DNA probe specific for centromeric α-satellite sequences on chromosome 1 hybridizes to the centromeric region of both normal chromosomes 1 as well as to a marker chromosome derived from chromosome 1. *C.* Two-color FISH used to detect a microdeletion of chromosome 15 associated with Prader-Willi syndrome. A repetitive classic satellite probe hybridizes to the short arm of chromosome 15 (large blue dots) and a probe for PML (a locus on the distal portion of chromosome 15, visualized as small black dots) are observed on both chromosomes. However, a probe for SNRPN (a locus within the PWS region of chromosome 15, small black dots) hybridizes only to the normal chromosome. The arrow points to the deleted chromosome. *D.* Interphase FISH using chromosome 13 (large blue dots) and chromosome 21 (small black dots) unique sequence probes on interphase cells from direct amniotic fluid preparations. Three chromosome 21-specific signals are observed, indicating the presence of trisomy 21 in the fetus.

regard, FISH can be utilized to identify specific chromosomes, characterize de novo duplications or deletions, and identify and clarify subtle chromosomal rearrangements. Its greatest utilization, however, is in the detection of microdeletions (see below), including those associated with Prader-Willi syndrome (PWS), Angelman syndrome (AS), William syndrome, velocardiofacial (VCF) and DiGeorge syndromes, Smith-Magenis syndrome, and Miller-Dieker syndrome (MDS) (see below). Though conventional cytogenetic studies can detect some of these microdeletions, initial detection and/or confirmation with FISH is essential. In fact, since appropriate FISH probes have become available, detection of the aforementioned syndromes has increased significantly.

In addition to metaphase FISH, cells can be analyzed at a variety of stages. *Interphase analysis*, for example, can be used to make a rapid diagnosis in instances where metaphase chromosome preparations are not yet available (e.g., amniotic fluid interphase analysis). Interphase analysis also increases the number of cells available for examination, allows for investigation of nuclear organization, and provides results when cells do not progress to metaphase. One specialized type of interphase analysis involves the application of FISH to paraffin-embedded sections, thereby preserving the architecture of the tissue.

The use of interphase FISH has increased recently, especially for analyses of amniocentesis samples. These studies are performed on uncultured amniotic fluid, typically using DNA probes specific for the chromosomes most commonly identified in trisomies (chromosomes 13, 18, 21, and the X and Y). These studies can be performed rapidly (24 to 72 h) and will ascertain about 60% of the abnormalities detected prenatally. Nevertheless, guidelines from the American College of Medical Genetics suggest that standard cytogenetic analysis be conducted on all specimens following FISH analysis.

Another area in which interphase analysis is routinely utilized is cancer cytogenetics (Chap. 81). Many site-specific translocations are associated with specific types of malignancies. For example, there are probes available for both the Abelson (Abl) oncogene and breakpoint cluster region (bcr) involved in chronic myelogenous leukemia (CML). These probes are labeled with rhodamine and FITC, respectively; the fusion of these genes in CML combines the fluorescent colors and appears as a yellow hybridization signal.

In addition to standard metaphase and interphase FISH analyses, a number of enhanced techniques have been developed for specific types of analysis, including multicolor FISH techniques, reverse painting, comparative genomic hybridization, and fiber FISH. *Spectral karyotyping* (SKY) and *multicolor FISH* (m-FISH) techniques use combinatorially labeled probes that create a unique color for individual chromosomes. In this manner, all of the chromosomes are studied simultaneously, and computer software is used to generate "pseudocolors" for the individual chromosomes. This technology is useful in the identification of unknown chromosome material (such as markers of duplications) but is most commonly used with the complex rearrangements seen in cancer specimens.

Reverse painting is accomplished by either flow-sorting a chromosome of interest or scraping the chromosome off a slide. The DNA from this chromosome (or portion of a chromosome) is extracted, amplified, labeled, and used as a FISH probe. This probe is then hybridized to a normal metaphase chromosome to identify the origin of the DNA of interest. It is also utilized to identify marker chromosomes or chromosome duplications of unknown origin.

Comparative genomic hybridization (CGH) is a method that can be used when only DNA is available from a specimen of interest. The entire DNA specimen from the sample of interest is labeled in one color (e.g., green), and the normal control DNA specimen in another color (e.g., red). These are mixed in equal amounts and hybridized to normal metaphase chromosomes. The red-to-green ratio is analyzed by a computer program, which determines where the DNA of interest may have gains or loss of material. This technique is useful in the analysis of tumors, particularly in those cases where cytogenetic analysis is not possible.

Fiber FISH is a technique in which chromosomes are mechanically stretched, using one of a variety of different methods. Fiber FISH provides a higher resolution of analysis than conventional FISH and more precise information on the chromosomal localization of a specific probe.

CYTOGENETIC TESTING IN PRENATAL DIAGNOSIS
(See also Chap. 68) The vast majority of prenatal diagnostic studies are performed to rule out a chromosomal abnormality, but cells may also be propagated for biochemical studies or molecular analyses of DNA. Three procedures are used to obtain samples for prenatal diagnosis: amniocentesis, chorionic villus sampling (CVS), and fetal blood sampling. *Amniocentesis* is the most commonly used procedure and is routinely performed at 15 to 17 weeks of gestation. On some occasions, early amniocentesis at 12 to 14 weeks is done to expedite results, though less fluid is obtained at this time. Early amniocentesis carries a greater risk of spontaneous abortion or fetal injury but provides results at an earlier stage of pregnancy.

The vast majority of amniocentesis are performed in the context of advanced maternal age, the best-known correlate of trisomy (see below). Additional reasons for referral for amniocentesis include an abnormal "triple-marker assay" and/or detection of ultrasound abnormalities. In the triple-marker assay, levels of human chorionic gonadotropin, α fetoprotein, and unconjugated estriol in the maternal serum are quantified and used to adjust the maternal age-predicted risk of a trisomy 21 or trisomy 18 fetus. Specific ultrasound abnormalities, when detected at mid-trimester, can also be associated with chromosomal defects. When a nonspecific ultrasound abnormality is present, the estimated risk of a chromosomal defect is approximately 16%. Associations of chromosomal abnormalities and specific types of abnormal ultrasound findings are listed in Table 66-1.

Chorionic villus sampling is the second most common procedure for genetic prenatal diagnosis. Because this procedure is routinely performed at about 8 to 10 weeks of gestation, it allows for an earlier detection of abnormalities and a safer pregnancy termination, if desired. CVS is a relatively safe procedure (spontaneous abortions < 0.5

Table 66-1 Frequency of Chromosome Abnormalities, Identified on the Basis of Abnormal Ultrasound Findings

	Chromosomal Abnormalities (Frequency)	
Ultrasound Finding	Average, %	Range in Different Studies, %
Abnormal ultrasound (nonspecific)	16	13–35
Omphalocele	39	26–54
Cystic hygroma	68	46–78
Congenital heart disease	30	8–40
Choroid plexus cyst	5	4–10

to 1%). Because there is an increased association of limb defects when the procedure is performed later (≥11 weeks of gestation), CVS is applicable during a very narrow window of time of gestation. CVS involves the use of a catheter inserted transvaginally; approximately 25 mg of villi are aspirated from the chorion frondosum (the fetal portion of the placenta). Care must be taken not to obtain villi from the maternal portion from the placenta to avoid compromising the analysis. The majority of the sample (the mesenchymal cells from the CVS sample) is enzymatically digested and cultured in a fashion similar to amniotic fluid cells. However, cells in the outer layer of the villi—the cytotrophoblasts—are actively dividing and can be analyzed directly. Therefore, by adding colchicine directly to these cells, a result can be obtained within 24 to 48 h. Findings from these procedures should be confirmed by analyses of cultured mesenchymal cells, as they are more reliably derived from the fetus.

Percutaneous umbilical blood sampling (PUBS) is a method for obtaining fetal blood during the second and third trimesters of pregnancy. It allows for acquisition of a blood sample, which can be used for cytogenetic studies; results can be obtained within 48 h of sampling. PUBS is carried out under ultrasound guidance. It is usually performed when ultrasound abnormalities are detected late in the second trimester. PUBS is also used when cytogenetic results from amniocentesis need clarification, such as the detection of mosaicism.

CHROMOSOME ABNORMALITIES

CHROMOSOMES IN CELL DIVISION
To understand the etiology of chromosome abnormalities, it is important to review the movement of chromosomes during cell division. In somatic tissues, chromosomes are replicated during the S-phase of the cell cycle, so that each replicated chromosome consists of two identical sister chromatids (Fig. 66-1). When the cell enters mitosis, each of the 46 chromosomes align on the metaphase plate, with the centromeres cooriented toward opposite spindle poles (Fig. 66-3). At anaphase the sister chromatids separate, with each of the daughter cells receiving one sister chromatid from each of the 46 chromosomes.

Chromosome segregation is more complicated in germ cell division, since the number of chromosomes must be reduced from 46 to 23 in the mature sperm and eggs. This is accomplished by two rounds of division—meiosis I and meiosis II (Fig. 66-3). In meiosis I, homologous chromosomes become paired and exchange genetic material, then align on the metaphase plate, and finally separate from one another. Thus, by the end of meiosis I, only 23 of the original 46 chromosomes are represented in each of the two daughter cells. Meiosis II quickly follows meiosis I and is essentially a "haploid mitosis," involving separation of the sister chromatids in each of the 23 chromosomes.

Although the fundamentals of meiosis are the same in males and females, there are important distinctions, particularly in the timing of the meiotic divisions. In males, meiosis begins with puberty and continues throughout the individual's lifetime. In females, meiosis begins prenatally, with oocytes proceeding through the first stages of meiosis I but arresting at mid-prophase. At the time of birth, the first meiotic division is suspended in oocytes. Only after ovulation many years later do oocytes complete meiosis I and proceed to the metaphase stage of meiosis II; if fertilized, the oocyte then completes the second meiotic division. Thus, in females, the first meiotic division takes at least 10 to 15 years, and possibly as many as 40 to 45 years, to complete. Maternal age-related increases in the incidence of trisomy are likely the consequence of this protracted process of cell division.

INCIDENCE AND TYPES OF CHROMOSOME ABNORMALITIES
Errors in meiosis, or in early cleavage divisions, occur with extraordinary frequency. At least 10 to 25% of all pregnancies, for example, involve chromosomally abnormal conceptions. A large proportion of these terminate in the earliest stages of pregnancy. Nevertheless, even among clinically recognized pregnancies, nearly 10%

FIGURE 66-3 Chromosome segregation in meiosis. *A.* In meiosis I (MI), each of the 23 pairs of chromosomes finds its "partner," or homologue, and exchanges genetic material (recombines) with it. At metaphase, each homologous pair aligns on the equatorial plate; at anaphase, each member of the homologous pair segregates from its partner. Thus, at the end of MI, each daughter cell contains 23 chromosomes, with each chromosome consisting of two sister chromatids. *B.* In meiosis II (MII), each chromosome aligns on the metaphase plate, and at anaphase, each of the two sister chromatids divide from one another. Thus, at the end of MII, each daughter cell (e.g., the oocyte or spermatocyte) contains 23 chromosomes, with each chromosome consisting of one sister chromatid.

In mitosis, the chromosomes behave exactly as they do in MII, except that somatically dividing cells contain 46 chromosomes, not the 23 that are present in the MII cell.

of fetuses are chromosomally unbalanced. The occurrence of different classes of chromosome abnormalities are summarized in Table 66-2 for the three types of clinically recognized pregnancies: spontaneous abortions, stillbirths, and livebirths. The commonest abnormalities are numerical, involving fetuses with additional (*trisomy*) or missing (*monosomy*) chromosomes or those with one (*triploidy*) or two (*tetraploidy*) additional sets of chromosomes. Structural chromosome abnormalities are much less common, although several of the most important clinical chromosomal disorders involve structural rearrangements (see below).

By far the most common abnormality is trisomy, which is identified in approximately 25% of spontaneous abortions and 0.3% of newborns. Trisomies for all chromosomes have now been identified in embryos or fetuses, but there is considerable variation in frequency for various chromosomes. For example, trisomy 16 is extraordinarily common, accounting for about one-third of all trisomies in spontaneous abortions, whereas trisomies 1, 5, 11, and 19 have been identified less often. Available evidence suggests two reasons for this variation: (1) some chromosomes (e.g., chromosome 16) are more likely to segregate abnormally or undergo nondisjunction during meiosis than are others; and (2) the potential for development varies widely among different trisomic conditions, with some being eliminated very early in gestation, others surviving to the time of clinical pregnancy recognition, and some (e.g., trisomies 13, 18, and 21 and sex chromosome trisomies) being compatible with survival to term.

CHROMOSOMAL SYNDROMES   While most chromosomally abnormal conceptions perish in utero (Table 66-2), several conditions are compatible with survival to term. The best-characterized of these are numerical abnormalities involving loss or gain of individual chromosomes and abnormalities resulting from unbalanced translocations. FISH and other molecular studies have led to the identification of two "new" types of chromosome abnormalities, commonly referred to as *microdeletion syndromes* and *imprinting syndromes*.

Numerical Abnormalities   Virtually all types of numerical abnormalities are eliminated prenatally, so that only those involving small, gene-poor autosomes or the sex chromosomes are identified with any frequency among live-borns. Clinically, the most important of these is *trisomy 21*, the most frequent cause of Down syndrome. Depending on the maternal age structure of the population and the utilization of prenatal testing, the incidence of trisomy 21 ranges from 1/600 to 1/1000 live births, making it the most common chromosome abnormality in live-born individuals. Like most trisomies, the incidence of trisomy 21 is highly correlated with maternal age, increasing from about 1/1500 live births for women 20 years of age to 1/30 for women 45 years of age and older.

In addition to trisomy 21, only two other autosomal trisomies, 13 and 18, occur with any frequency in livebirths. Incidence rates for trisomies 13 and 18 in live births are 1/20,000 and 1/10,000 respectively. Unlike trisomy 21, which is associated with near-normal life expectancy, both trisomies 13 and 18 are associated with death in infancy, typically occurring during the first year of life.

Three sex chromosome trisomies—the 47,XXX, 47,XXY (*Klinefelter syndrome*), and 47,XYY conditions—are quite common, with each occurring in about 1/2000 newborns. Of all the trisomic conditions, these three have the fewest phenotypic complications. In fact, with the exception of infertility in Klinefelter syndrome (Chap. 335), it is likely that most individuals with such trisomic conditions would go undetected. The additional chromosome in the 47,XYY condition is small and contains only a few genes. Most Y-linked genes are involved in testicular development or spermatogenesis. Thus, dosage imbalance of Y-linked genes has relatively little effect on other developmental processes. The 47,XYY genotype is associated with increased height. Its role in antisocial behavior, postulated initially because of an increased prevalence among some penalized populations, is unclear.

For the 47,XXX and 47,XXY conditions, the situation is different—the X chromosome contains over 1000 genes, many of them essential for normal development. How, then, are 47,XXX and 47,XXY individuals spared from the catastrophic consequences of dosage imbalance? The answer lies in the biology of X chromosome gene expression. In normal females, one of the X chromosomes is inactivated in somatic cells. The inactivation of the paternal or maternal X chromosome occurs randomly in each somatic cell and thereby serves as a mechanism of dosage compensation, ensuring that males and females have equal expression of most X-linked genes. The inactivation process occurs at the blastocyst stage of development; prior to this time both X chromosomes are active. In addition, the rules for inactivation are different for germ cells than for somatic cells: in female germ cells both X chromosomes remain active, whereas in male germ cells the X chromosome is inactivated. In addition, not all X-linked genes are inactivated. Some genes on the X chromosome "escape" the inactivating mechanism and are expressed from both X chromosomes. In disorders such as Klinefelter syndrome, some genes may be expressed from both X chromosomes, resulting in phenotypic abnormalities. Individuals with Klinefelter syndrome have small testes, hyalinized seminiferous tubules, and azoospermia or severe oligospermia (Chap. 335). Testosterone levels are variably reduced, and often there is gynecomastia and eunuchoidal body proportions. Antisocial behavior and mild mental deficiency are seen in some individuals. Females with the 47,XXX genotype are more likely to have mild mental deficiency and may be subfertile. Despite these features, sex chromosome trisomies impart relatively minor phenotypic complications in comparison to aneuploidies that involve autosomal chromosomes.

As a rule, monosomic conditions are incompatible with fetal development and, consequently, autosomal monosomies are only rarely identified in spontaneous abortions and are not found among live-born individuals. In fact, the only monosomy compatible with live birth is the 45,X condition, which causes *Turner syndrome*. The 45,X chromosome constitution occurs with surprisingly high frequency, being present in at least 1 to 2% of all pregnancies. More than 99% of all 45,X conceptions are spontaneously aborted. Thus, live-born individuals with a 45,X chromosome constitution represent a rare group of survivors. The 45,X phenotype is mild, presumably because the second copy of many X chromosomal genes is normally inactivated. Nonetheless, Turner syndrome causes gonadal dysgenesis, resulting in infertility and failure to undergo secondary sexual development. Other prominent features are more variable and include short stature, webbing of the neck, and shield-shaped chest; lymphedema; increased carrying angle at the elbow; cardiovascular and renal abnormalities; and a propensity to hypertension, glucose intolerance, and autoimmune thyroid disease (Chap. 336). Several other structural abnormalities of the X chromosome such as partial deletions, isochromosome X, or ring chromosomes can cause Turner syndrome. Mosaicism, including 45,X/45,XX, 45X/45,XXX, 45,X/45,XY, and others, also occurs (see below) and contributes to the phenotypic spectrum seen in Turner syndrome.

Because numerical abnormalities originate in meiosis (Table 66-3), affected individuals have missing or extra chromosomes in all cells. In a small proportion of cases, though, a mitotic nondisjunctional event occurs at an early stage in an individual with an initially normal chromosome constitution. Alternatively, a "normalizing" mitotic nondisjunctional event may result in a normal chromosome complement in some cells of an embryo. In either case, the embryo is a *mosaic*, with some cells bearing a normal chromosome constitution and others an aneuploid number of chromosomes. The phenotypic consequences are difficult to predict because they depend on the timing of nondisjunction and the distribution of normal and abnormal cells in different tissues. Nevertheless, mosaicism may lead to clinical abnormalities indistinguishable from those of nonmosaic individuals; for example, nearly 5% of all cases of Down syndrome involve individuals with mosaic trisomy 21, and about 15% of individuals with Turner syndrome are mosaic for various sex chromosomal constitutions as described above.

The Origin and Etiology of Numerical Abnormalities Over the past decade, a number of studies have used DNA polymorphisms to investigate the origin of different types of chromosome abnormalities (Fig. 66-4). The most thoroughly investigated types have been numerical abnormalities (Table 66-3). Sex chromosome monosomy usually results from loss of the paternal sex chromosome. This is the case regardless of whether the conception is live-born or spontaneously aborted, indicating that the parental origin of the abnormality does not affect its likelihood of surviving to term.

Trisomies show remarkable variation in parental origin. For example, paternal nondisjunction is responsible for nearly 50% of 47,XXY but only 5 to 10% of cases of trisomies 13, 14, 15, 21, and 22; it is rarely, if ever, the source of the additional chromosome in trisomy 16. Similarly, there is considerable variability in the meiotic stage of origin. For example, among maternally derived trisomies, all cases of trisomy 16 may be due to meiosis I errors, whereas for trisomy 21, one-third of cases are associated with meiosis II errors, and for trisomy 18, the majority of cases are apparently due to meiosis II nondisjunction. In spite of this variation in parental and meiotic origin, nondisjunction at maternal meiosis I appears to be the most common source of trisomy.

Molecular studies have also begun to shed light on the molecular mechanisms underlying nondisjunction, the source of trisomy and monosomy. Most, if not all, trisomies are associated with alterations in genetic recombination. This is the process by which chromosomes exchange genetic material during the first of the two meiotic divisions. In other organisms, the physical connections, or chiasmata, associated with recombination are known to hold chromosomes together at meiosis I. This mechanism is now known to be true for humans as well. Nondisjunction at meiosis I is linked to a reduced extent of crossing-over, with some cases involving outright failure of recombination between the homologous chromosomes, and others associated with distally placed exchanges. Unexpectedly—since recombination occurs at meiosis I—maternal meiosis II errors involving chromosome 21 may also be linked to altered recombination. In this instance, though, the effect involves increased—not decreased—recombination, especially in proximal 21q. Presumably, this indicates that errors scored as arising at meiosis II are, in fact, precipitated by events occurring at meiosis I.

Maternal Age and Trisomy The association between increasing maternal age and trisomy is arguably the most important etiologic factor in congenital chromosomal disorders. Among women under the age of 25, approximately 2% of all clinically recognized pregnancies are trisomic; by the age of 36, however, this figure increases to 10% and by the age of 42, to >33% (Fig. 66-5). This association between maternal age and trisomy is exerted without respect to race, geography, or socioeconomic factors and likely affects segregation of all chromosomes.

Despite the importance of increasing age, almost nothing is known about the mechanism by which aging leads to abnormal chromosomal segregation. As noted above, it is thought to originate in maternal meiosis I owing to the protracted time to completion (often ≥40 years) in females. As noted above, alterations in genetic recombination may

Table 66-2 Frequency and Distribution of Chromosome Abnormalities in Different Types of Clinically Recognizable Pregnancies

Chromosome Abnormality	Frequency of Abnormality			Probability of Surviving to Term, %
	Spontaneous Abortion	Stillbirth	Livebirth	
Trisomy, all	25.1	4.0	0.3	5
+13, 18, 21	4.5	2.7	0.14	15
+16	7.5	—	—	0
Sex chromosome monosomy (45,X)	8.7	0.1	0.01	1
Triploidy	6.4	0.2	—	0
Tetraploidy	2.4	—	—	0
Structural abnormality	2.0	0.8	0.3	45
Total abnormalities	50.0	5.1	0.6	5

Table 66-3 Studies of the Parent and Meiotic/Mitotic Stage of Origin of Human Trisomies and Sex Chromosome Monosomy

	Origin, %				
	Paternal		Maternal		
	I	II	I	II	Mitotic
TRISOMY					
2	28	—	54	13	6
7	—	—	17	26	57
15	—	15	76	9	—
16	—	1	96	3	—
18	—	—	33	56	11
21	3	5	67	22	2
22	3	—	94	3	—
XXY	46	—	38	14	3
XXX	—	6	60	16	18
MONOSOMY					
X[a]	80		20		

[a] Results pertain to nonmosaic 45,X individuals.

A. Parental origin of
trisomy 21

B. Parental origin of PWS

FIGURE 66-4 Use of DNA technology to determine the origin of chromosome abnormalities. *A.* Analysis of a chromosome 21–specific DNA polymorphism demonstrates that the trisomic individual received two chromosomes 21 from his mother and one from his father; thus, the extra chromosome 21 resulted from an error in oogenesis. *B.* Inheritance of a chromosome 15–specific DNA polymorphism in an individual with Prader-Willi syndrome (PWS). The affected individual has received two maternal, but no paternal, chromosomes 15; thus, the individual is said to have maternal uniparental disomy 15, a common cause of PWS.

explain age-related trisomy. In trisomy 21, for example, recombination patterns appear to be similarly altered in younger and older mothers of trisomic conceptions. With this in mind, it has been suggested that two distinct steps, or "hits," may be involved in maternal age-related nondisjunction. The first hit, which is age-independent, involves the establishment of a "vulnerable" recombination configuration in the fetal oocyte; the second hit, which is age-dependent, involves abnormal processing of the vulnerable bivalent structure at metaphase I. If this model is correct, it means that the nondisjunctional process is the same in younger and older women, but it occurs more frequently with aging, possibly because of age-dependent degradation of cell cycle proteins or meiotic proteins responsible for maintaining sister chromatid cohesion.

Structural Chromosome Abnormalities   Structural rearrangements involve breakage and reunion of chromosomes. Although less common than numerical abnormalities, they present additional challenges from a genetic counseling standpoint. This is because structural abnormalities, unlike numerical abnormalities, can be present in "balanced" form in clinically normal individuals but transmitted in "unbalanced" form to progeny, thereby resulting in a hereditary form of chromosome abnormality.

Rearrangements may involve exchanges of material between different chromosomes (*translocations*) or loss, gain, or rearrangements of individual chromosomes (e.g., *deletions, duplications, inversions,*

FIGURE 66-5   Estimated maternal age–adjusted rates of trisomy among all clinically recognized pregnancies (e.g., spontaneous abortions, stillbirths, and livebirths). Among women in their forties, over 25% of all pregnancies are estimated to involve a trisomic conception; the vast majority of these spontaneously abort, with only trisomies 13, 18, and 21 and sex chromosome trisomies surviving to term with any appreciable frequency.

rings or *isochromosomes*). Of particular clinical importance are translocations, which involve two basic types: Robertsonian and reciprocal. *Robertsonian rearrangements* are a special class of translocation, in which the long arms of two acrocentric chromosomes (chromosomes 13, 14, 15, 21, and 22) join together, generating a fusion chromosome that contains virtually all of the genetic material of the original two chromosomes. If the Robertsonian translocation is present in unbalanced form, a monosomic or trisomic conception ensues. For example, approximately 3% of cases of Down syndrome are attributable to unbalanced Robertsonian translocations, most often involving chromosomes 14 and 21. In this instance, the affected individual has 46 chromosomes, including one structurally normal chromosome 14, two structurally normal chromosomes 21, and one fusion 14/21 chromosome. This effect leads to a normal diploid dosage for chromosome 14 and to a triplication of chromosome 21, thus resulting in Down syndrome. Similarly, a small proportion of individuals with trisomy 13 syndrome are clinically affected because of an unbalanced Robertsonian translocation.

Reciprocal translocations involve exchanges between any two chromosomes. In this circumstance, the phenotypic consequences associated with unbalanced translocations depend on the location of the breakpoints, which dictate the amount of material that has been "exchanged" between the two chromosomes. Because most reciprocal translocations involve unique sets of breakpoints, it is difficult to predict the phenotypic consequences in any one situation. In general, severity is determined by the amount of excess or missing chromosome material in individuals with unbalanced translocations.

In addition to rearrangements between chromosomes, there are several examples of intrachromosome structural abnormalities. The most common and deleterious of these involve loss of chromosome material due to deletions. The two best-characterized deletion syndromes, *Wolf-Hirschhorn syndrome* and *cri-du-chat syndrome*, result from loss of relatively small chromosomal segments on chromosomes 4p and 5p, respectively. Nonetheless, each is associated with multiple congenital anomalies, developmental delays, profound retardation, and reduced lifespan.

Microdeletion Syndromes The term *contiguous gene syndromes* refers to genetic disorders that mimic a combination of single gene disorders. They result from the deletion of a small number of tightly clustered genes. Because they are usually too small to be detected cytogenetically, they are termed *microdeletions*. The application of molecular techniques has led to the identification of at least 18 of these microdeletion syndromes (Table 66-4). Some of the more common ones include the Wilms' tumor–aniridia complex (WAGR), MDS, and VCF syndrome. *WAGR* is characterized by mental retardation and involvement of multiple organs, including kidney (Wilm's tumor), eye (aniridia), and the genitourinary system. The cytogenetic abnormality involves a deletion of part of the short arm of chromosome 11 (11p13), which typically is detectable on well-banded chromosome preparations. In *MDS*, a disorder characterized by mental retardation, dysmorphic faces, and lissencephaly, the deletion involves chromosome 17 (17p13). Using FISH, 17p deletions have been detected in >90% of MDS patients as well as in 20% of cases of isolated lissencephaly.

Deletions involving the long arm of chromosome 22 (22q11) are the most common microdeletions identified to date, present in approximately 1/3000 newborns. VCF syndrome, the most commonly associated syndrome, consists of learning disabilities or mild mental retardation, palatal defects, a hypoplastic aloe nasi and long nose, and congenital heart defects (conotruncal defect). Some individuals with 22q11 deletion are more severely affected and present with *DiGeorge syndrome*, which involves abnormalities in the development of the third and fourth branchial arches leading to thymic hypoplasia, parathyroid hypoplasia, and conotruncal heart defects. In approximately 30% of these cases, a deletion at 22q11 can be detected with high-resolution banding; by combing conventional cytogenetics, FISH, and molecular detection techniques (i.e., Southern blotting or polymerase chain reaction analyses), these rates improve to >90%. Additional studies have demonstrated a surprisingly high frequency of 22q11 deletions in individuals with nonsyndromic conotruncal defects. Approximately 10% of individuals with a 22q11 deletion inherited it from a parent with a similar deletion.

Smith-Magenis syndrome involves a microdeletion localized to the short arm of chromosome 17 (17p11.2). Affected individuals have mental retardation, dysmorphic facial features, delayed speech, peripheral neuropathy, and behavior abnormalities. Most of these deletions can be detected with cytogenetic analysis, although FISH is available to confirm these findings. In contrast, *William syndrome*, a chromosome 7 (7q11.23) microdeletion, cannot be diagnosed with standard or high-resolution analysis; it is only detectable utilizing FISH or other molecular methods. William syndrome involves a deletion of the elastin gene and is characterized by mental retardation, dysmorphic features, a gregarious personality, premature aging, and congenital heart disease (usually supravalvular aortic stenosis).

In addition to microdeletion syndromes, there is now at least one well-described microduplication syndrome, Charcot-Marie-Tooth type 1A (CMT1A). This is a nerve conduction disease previously though to be transmitted as a simple autosomal dominant disorder. Recent molecular studies have demonstrated that affected individuals are heterozygous for duplication of a small region of chromosome 17 (17p11.2-12). Although it is not yet clear why increased gene dosage

Table 66-4 Some Commonly Identified Microdeletion and Microduplication Syndromes

Syndrome	Cytogenetic Location	Principal Features	Imprinting Effects
Langer-Giedion syndrome	8q24.1 (del)	Sparse hair, bulbous nose, variable mental retardation	No
WAGR complex	11p13 (del)	Wilms' tumor, aniridia, genitourinary disorders, mental retardation	No
Beckwith-Wiedemann syndrome	11p15 (dup)	Macrosomia, macroglossia, omphalocoele	Yes, occasionally associated with "paternal uniparental disomy" (see text)
Retinoblastoma	13q14.11 (del)	Retinoblastoma due to homozygous loss of functional RB allele	No obvious effect, although abnormal RB allele more likely to be paternal
Prader-Willi syndrome	15q11-13 (del)	Obesity, hypogonadism, mental retardation	Yes; prototypic imprinting disorder (see text)
Angelman syndrome	15q11-13 (del)	Ataxic gait	With Prader-Willi syndrome, prototypic imprinting disorder (see text)
α-Thalassemia and mental retardation	16p13.3 (del)	α-thalassemia and mental retardation, due to deletion of distal 16p, including α-globin locus	No
Smith-Magenis syndrome	17p11.2 (del)	Brachycephaly, midface hypoplasia, mental retardation	No
Miller-Dieker syndrome	17p13 (del)	Dysmorphic facies, lissencephaly	No
Charcot-Marie-Tooth syndrome type 1A	17p11.2 (dup)	Progressive neuropathy due to microduplication	No
DiGeorge syndrome/velocardiofacial syndrome	22q11 (del)	Abnormalities of third and fourth branchial arches	No

would result in CMT1A, the inheritance pattern is explained by the fact that one-half of the offspring of affected individuals inherit the duplication-carrying chromosome.

Imprinting Disorders Two other microdeletion syndromes, PWS and AS, exhibit parent-of-origin, or "imprinting," effects. For many years, it has been known that cytogenetically detectable deletions of chromosome 15 occur in a proportion of patients with PWS, as well as in those with AS. This seemed curious, as the clinical manifestations of the two syndromes are very dissimilar. PWS is characterized by obesity, hypogonadism, and mild to moderate mental retardation, whereas AS is associated with microcephaly, ataxic gait, seizures, inappropriate laughter, and severe mental retardation. New insight into the pathogenesis of these disorders has been provided by the recognition that parental origin of the deletion determines which phenotype ensues: if the deletion is paternal, the result is PWS, whereas if the deletion is maternal, the result is AS (Fig. 66-2).

This scenario is complicated further by the recognition that not all individuals with PWS or AS carry the chromosome 15 deletion. For such individuals, it turns out that the parental origin of the chromosome 15 region is again the important determinant. In PWS, for example, nondeletion patients invariably have two maternal and no paternal chromosomes 15 [*maternal uniparental disomy* (UPD)], whereas for some nondeletion AS patients the reverse is true (*paternal UPD*). This indicates that at least some genes on chromosome 15 are differently expressed, depending on which parent contributed the chromosome. Additionally, this means that normal fetal development requires the presence of one maternal and one paternal copy of chromosome 15.

Approximately 70% of PWS cases are due to paternal deletions of

15q11-q13, whereas 25% are due to maternal uniparental disomy, and about 5% are caused by mutations in a chromosome 15 imprinting center. Though 75% of the AS cases are due to maternal deletions, only 2% are due to paternal uniparental disomy. The rest of the cases are presumed to be caused by imprinting mutations (5%) or mutations in the UBE3A gene, which is one of the genes associated with AS. The UPD cases are mostly caused by meiotic nondisjunction resulting in trisomy 15, subsequently followed by a normalizing mitotic nondisjunction event ("trisomy rescue") resulting in two normal chromosomes 15, both from the same parent. *UBE3A* is the only maternally imprinted gene known in the critical region of chromosome 15. However, several paternally imprinted genes, or expressed-sequence tags (ESTs), have been identified, including *ZNF127*, *IPW*, *SNRPN*, *SNURF*, *PAR1*, and *PAR5*.

Chromosomal regions that behave in the manner observed in PWS and AS are said to be *imprinted*. This phenomenon is involved in differential expression of certain genes on different chromosomes. Chromosome 11 must be one of these with an imprinted region, since it is known that a small proportion of individuals with the *Beckwith-Wiedemann overgrowth syndrome* have two paternal but no maternal copies of this chromosome.

ACQUIRED CHROMOSOME ABNORMALITIES IN CANCER

In addition to the constitutional cytogenetic chromosomal abnormalities that are present at birth, somatic chromosomal changes can be acquired later in life and are often associated with malignant conditions. As with constitutional abnormalities, somatic changes can include the net loss of chromosomal material (due to a deletion or loss of a chromosome), net gain of material (duplication or gain of a chromosome), and relocation of DNA sequences (translocation). These chromosomal changes are intertwined with the three major categories of cancer genes: (1) *tumor-suppressor genes* that inhibit cell proliferation may be deleted; (2) *oncogenes* that activate cell proliferation may be activated by duplication, amplification, or translocation; and (3) *DNA repair genes* may also be deleted from somatic cells, thereby predisposing to the accumulation of additional DNA damage. Cytogenetic changes have been particularly well studied in (1) leukemias, e.g., Philadelphia chromosome translocation in CML[t(9;22)(q34.1; q11.2)]); and (2) lymphomas, e.g., translocations of MYC in Burkitt's [t(8;14)(q24;q32)]. These and other translocations are useful for diagnosis, classification, and prognosis. Analyses of cytogenetic changes are also proving useful in certain solid tumors. For example, a complex karyotype with Wilms' tumor, diploidy in medulloblastoma, and Her-2/neu amplification in breast cancer are poor prognostic signs. The genetic basis of malignancy, including the role of germline and somatic chromosomal alterations, is discussed further in Chap. 81.

BIBLIOGRAPHY

GELEHRTER TD et al (eds): *Principles of Medical Genetics*, 2d ed. Baltimore, Williams & Wilkins, 1998

GERSEN SL, KEAGLE MB (eds): *The Principles of Clinical Cytogenetics*. Totowa, NJ, Humana, 1999

JAMESON JL (ed): *Principles of Molecular Medicine*. Totowa, NJ, Humana, 1998

MITELMAN F: *Catalog of Chromosome Aberrations in Cancer*, 6th ed. New York, Wiley, 1998

NICHOLLS RD et al: Imprinting in Prader-Willi and Angelman syndromes. Trends Genet 14:194, 1998

RIMOIN DL et al (eds): *Emery and Rimoin's Principles and Practice of Medical Genetics*, 3d ed. New York, Churchill Livingstone, 1996

SCRIVER CR et al (eds): *The Metabolic and Molecular Bases of Inherited Disease*, 8th ed. New York, McGraw-Hill, 2001

STUMM M et al: Molecular cytogenetic techniques for the diagnosis of chromosomal abnormalities in childhood disease. Eur J Pediatr 158:531, 1999

67   *Donald R. Johns*

DISEASES CAUSED BY GENETIC DEFECTS OF MITOCHONDRIA

Mitochondrial defects play a role in several metabolic and neurodegenerative diseases as well as aging. Mitochondrial disorders have protean clinical manifestations, reflecting the fact that nearly all organ systems utilize oxidative metabolism. Clinical features often involve tissues with high energy requirements such as the central and peripheral nervous systems, the eye, muscle, kidney, and endocrine organs. The age and mode of onset and clinical course of mitochondrial diseases range widely as a result of the unusual mechanisms of mitochondrial DNA (mtDNA) replication, which is distinct from that of the nuclear genome. A maternal mode of inheritance is characteristic of many mitochondrial diseases because mtDNA is transmitted by the oocyte. Hundreds of different mtDNA mutations have been described since the first mutation was described in 1988.

STRUCTURE AND FUNCTION OF MITOCHONDRIAL DNA   Most cells contain several hundred mitochondria, though the number varies depending on the energy requirements and function of a tissue. Mitochondria are the only cellular organelles that contain their own extrachromosomal DNA. Human mtDNA is a small (16,569 bp) double-stranded, circular molecule that encodes 13 protein subunits of 4 different oxidative phosphorylation biochemical complexes. mtDNA also encodes the 24 structural RNAs (2 ribosomal RNAs and 22 transfer RNAs) required for the intramitochondrial translation of these proteins. The noncoding D (displacement)-loop is a regulatory region that controls transcription and replication. mtDNA mutations are found in each type of mitochondrial gene (Fig. 67-1).

Mitochondria probably evolved from independent organisms that became endosymbiotically incorporated into the cell. As a result, mitochondria replicate, transcribe, and translate their DNA independently of nuclear DNA. However, cellular and mitochondrial function are interdependent. Nuclear DNA-encoded proteins are also involved in oxidative phosphorylation, and the myriad macromolecular compounds required for mitochondrial structure and function (e.g., mtDNA replication, transcription, and translation) are imported from the cytoplasm into the mitochondria.

Oxidative phosphorylation and the generation of adenosine triphosphate (ATP) for energy-requiring cellular processes are the central functions of mitochondria. Alterations in mitochondrial function lead to disease pathogenesis by three main mechanisms: (1) reduction of ATP supply when mutations impair oxidative phosphorylation; (2) generation of reactive oxygen species such as H_2O_2 and $OH\cdot$ free radicals that can damage DNA, proteins, or lipids; and (3) execution of the apoptosis pathway when mitochondria release cell death–promoting factors including caspases, cytochrome c, and apoptosis-inducing factor.

Several unique features of mtDNA render it vulnerable to mutations and contribute to its role in disease. For example, mtDNA has no introns (a random mutation will therefore usually strike a coding DNA sequence) or protective histones, and it has an imperfect DNA repair system and is exposed to oxygen free radicals generated by oxidative phosphorylation. mtDNA is estimated to mutate 10 times more rapidly than nuclear DNA. Importantly, mtDNA is strictly *maternally inherited* and does not recombine, and mtDNA mutations sequentially accumulate along maternal lineages. These properties have made mtDNA sequence variation an invaluable tool for evolutionary biologists and forensic scientists.

Each mitochondrion contains 2 to 10 mtDNA molecules, and each cell contains multiple mitochondria (*polyplasmy*). Population genetic principles, as opposed to Mendelian genetics, govern mitochondrial genetics. When a new mtDNA mutation arises, cells initially harbor copies of both normal and mutant DNA sequences—a condition

▨ Ribosomal RNA genes	▨ Complex-V genes (ATP synthase)
▨ Transfer RNA genes	▨ Complex-IV genes (cytochrome-coxidase)
▨ Complex-I genes (NADH dehydrogenase)	▨ Complex-III genes (ubiquinol: cytochrome-c oxidoreductase)

FIGURE 67-1 Schematic diagram of human mitochondrial DNA and the most prominent pathogenetic mutations. Point mutations in structural and protein-coding genes are indicated inside the circle, with the clinical phenotype and the nucleotide position of the mutation. The thick arc indicates the position of the most common single deletion, which is 5 kb in length, and the thin arcs outside the circle indicate the multiple deletions. MERRF, myoclonic epilepsy with ragged red fibers; MELAS, the syndrome of mitochondrial encephalomyopathy, lactic acidosis, and strokelike episodes; LHON, Leber's hereditary optic neuropathy; NARP, neuropathy, ataxia, and retinitis pigmentosa; Leigh, maternally inherited Leigh's disease. *(Adapted from Johns, with permission.)*

known as *heteroplasmy*—which allows an otherwise lethal mutation to persist and cause disease. The presence of either completely normal or completely mutant mtDNA is known as *homoplasmy*. During cell division, mitchondria are unevenly partitioned to the daughter cells through the process of *replicative segregation*; consequently, the proportion of mutant and normal mtDNA molecules can drift. Selection pressures apply at the molecular, cellular, and organismal levels. The critical proportion of mutant mtDNA required for deleterious phenotypic expression is known as the *threshold effect*. It varies among individuals, among organ systems, and within a given tissue, depending on the delicate balance of oxidative supply and demand. These features of mtDNA segregation, combined with the uneven transmission of mitochondria to daughter cells during cell division, form much of the basis for the phenotypic diversity seen in mitochondrial diseases.

MITOCHONDRIAL DNA MUTATIONS mtDNA mutations that cause a severe, lethal impairment of oxidative phosphorylation—such as gross structural defects or point mutations in structural RNAs—are only viable if heteroplasmic. In contrast, the majority of the milder, missense mtDNA mutations in protein-coding genes are homoplasmic. mtDNA point mutations have been found in each type of mtDNA gene, but tRNA mutations predominate in severe, multisystemic mitochondrial encephalomyopathy phenotypes; protein-cod-

ing gene mutations predominate in Leber's hereditary optic neuropathy (LHON). A point mutation in the 12S ribosomal RNA gene is associated with both spontaneous and aminoglycoside-associated sensorineural deafness (Fig. 67-1).

A definitive cause-and-effect relationship between a mtDNA mutation and a clinical phenotype can be difficult to establish for several reasons: (1) mtDNA is highly polymorphic, (2) different mutations can be associated with the same phenotype or the same mutation can be associated with different phenotypes, and (3) epigenetic factors can affect clinical manifestations.

CLASSIC MITOCHONDRIAL ENCEPHALOMYOPATHY PHENOTYPES Many diseases were provisionally classified as mitochondrial disorders on the basis of abnormal mitochondrial morphology, biochemistry, or a pattern of maternal inheritance. Disease-associated mtDNA mutations are now an important diagnostic criterion. Though each classic mitochondrial encephalomyopathy phenotype has distinctive clinical features (Table 67-1), each also shares many clinical and laboratory features (Tables 67-2 and 67-3).

Mitochondrial Myopathy Mitochondrial myopathy is characterized by fixed proximal weakness with marked exercise intolerance. Fatigability and poor stamina are prominent clinical features, but a mitochondrial etiology is often considered in the context of other neurologic, somatic, or laboratory features. Frank rhabdomyolysis is rare. Electromyography documents a nonirritative myopathy, and serum creatine kinase is usually normal or slightly elevated. Skeletal muscle biopsy shows abnormal proliferating mitochondria and "ragged red fibers," a histologic hallmark of the severe biochemical defects in oxidative phosphorylation. Large mtDNA deletions and a variety of mtDNA point mutations occur in mitochondrial myopathy.

Chronic Progressive External Ophthalmoplegia (CPEO) Ptosis, ophthalmoplegia, and limb myopathy characterize CPEO. Additional clinical features (Table 67-2) may also occur along with the laboratory abnormalities characteristic of mitochondrial disorders (Table 67-3). Patients with CPEO have abnormal skeletal muscle biopsies, with ragged red fibers and ultrastructural changes. Additional somatic and central nervous system findings in conjunction with CPEO are known as the "CPEO-plus" syndromes. Kearns-Sayre syndrome is a subset of CPEO-plus that begins before age 20 and is characterized by CPEO and atypical pigmentary retinopathy; ancillary features include elevated cerebrospinal fluid protein, ataxia, or heart block.

Most patients with CPEO have large, single deletions in mtDNA that can be reliably detected by molecular genetic methods. However, skeletal muscle is required as the source of DNA because almost all single mtDNA deletions occur sporadically. The presence of pigmentary retinopathy is strongly predictive of a deletion. The mechanism of DNA deletion is unknown, though recombination or slippage during replication is plausible. The junctions of most deletions contain directly repeated sequences, including a 13-nucleotide direct repeat "hot spot" that accounts for about 25% of all deletions. Approximately half of all deletions are bound by other direct repeats; one-quarter have no apparent direct repeat. A few patients have partially duplicated

Table 67-1 Cardinal Neurologic Manifestations of Mitochondrial Diseases

Disease	Neurologic Manifestation
Chronic progressive external ophthalmoplegia	Ophthalmoplegia
Mitochondrial myopathy	Myopathy
Mitochondrial encephalomyopathy, lactic acidosis, and strokelike episodes	Strokelike episodes
Myoclonic epilepsy with ragged red fibers	Myoclonus, epilepsy
Neuropathy, ataxia, and retinitis pigmentosa	Neuropathy, ataxia, retinitis pigmentosa
Leber's hereditary optic neuropathy	Optic neuropathy

Table 67-2   Clinical Features of Mitochondrial Diseases

Neurologic manifestations	Systemic manifestations
Sensorineural hearing loss	Cardiac conduction defects
Myopathy with fatigability	Cardiomyopathy
Peripheral neuropathy	Diabetes mellitus
Myoclonus	Pseudohypoparathyroidism
Myelopathy	Short stature
Ataxia	Pigmentary retinopathy
Seizures	Lactic acidosis
Dementia	Fanconi's proximal nephron dysfunction
Vascular headache	Glomerulopathy
	Hepatic dysfunction
	Intestinal pseudo-obstruction
	Lipomas
	Pancytopenia, sideroblastic anemia
	Psychiatric disease (depression)

mtDNA molecules. A point mutation at nucleotide position 3243 has been found in many patients who lack a mtDNA deletion or duplication.

Autosomally Transmitted Multiple Mitochondrial DNA Deletions   Several families with clinical variants of CPEO have been found to harbor multiple mtDNA deletions in skeletal muscle. The autosomal inheritance of multiple mtDNA deletions implies a primary defect in a nuclear DNA gene that has secondary qualitative effects on mtDNA. Multiple mtDNA deletions can be transmitted in either an autosomal dominant or autosomal recessive mode or can occur as somatic mutations.

Thymidine phosphorylase was the first nuclear-encoded gene shown to influence the regulation and function of normal mtDNA in a trans-acting manner. Mutations in thymidine phosphorylase cause an autosomal recessive disease known as *myoneurogastrointestinal encephalomyopathy* (MNGIE). Several different nuclear loci have been linked to the autosomal dominant forms of CPEO. Tissue-specific, autosomally transmitted depletion of mtDNA represents a quantitative mtDNA defect caused by an intergenomic communication error.

Mitochondrial Encephalomyopathy, Lactic Acidosis, and Strokelike Episodes (MELAS)   This syndrome is characterized by strokelike events that cause subacute brain dysfunction, cerebral structural changes, seizures, and several other common clinical and laboratory features (Tables 67-2, 67-3). Maternal inheritance of the MELAS syndrome may be obscured because of mild clinical features in relatives. A point mutation at nucleotide 3243 in the tRNA$^{Leu(UUR)}$ gene accounts for 80% of MELAS cases. However, the clinical features of the 3243 mtDNA mutation are pleiomorphic; it is also associated with nondeletion CPEO, myopathy, deafness, diabetes, and dystonia.

Myoclonic Epilepsy with Ragged Red Fibers (MERRF) Syndrome   The MERRF syndrome consists of myoclonus, seizures, cerebellar ataxia, and mitochondrial myopathy. Pathogenetic mutations have been demonstrated at nucleotide positions 8344 and 8356 in the tRNA^{Lys} gene. Neurologic and laboratory features common to

Table 67-3   Laboratory Findings in Mitochondrial Diseases

Ragged red fibers and COX-negative fibers on skeletal muscle biopsy
Elevated serum and cerebrospinal fluid lactate concentration
Myopathic potentials on electromyography
Axonal or demyelinating peripheral neuropathy on nerve conduction studies
Sensorineural hearing loss on audiogram
Abnormal glucose tolerance test or elevated hemoglobin A_{1c}
Cardiac conduction defects
Basal ganglia calcification or focal abnormalities on MRI
Altered phosphorus magnetic resonance spectroscopy
Defects in oxidative phosphorylation on biochemical studies
Molecular genetic demonstration of mtDNA mutations

NOTE: COX, cytochrome c oxidase; MRI, magnetic resonance imaging.

other mitochondrial encephalomyopathies are seen. Maternal relatives may be asymptomatic or may have partial clinical syndromes, including lipomas in a characteristic "horse-collar" distribution, and hypertension.

Neuropathy, Ataxia, and Retinitis Pigmentosa (NARP)/Maternally Inherited Leigh's Disease   NARP is characterized by proximal weakness, sensory neuropathy, developmental delay, ataxia, seizures, dementia, and retinal pigmentary degeneration. This maternally inherited disorder is associated with two different heteroplasmic missense mutations at nucleotide position 8993 in the ATPase 6 gene. High proportions of the same mutations are also seen in maternally inherited Leigh's disease. Autosomal recessive Leigh's disease is associated with cytochrome c oxidase deficiency and is caused by a deficiency of the nuclear-encoded protein, SURF1, which is required for biogenesis of the cytochrome c oxidase complex (complex IV). The mtDNA point mutations associated with NARP, MELAS, MERRF, and other mitochondrial disorders are readily detected by molecular genetic analysis of mtDNA extracted from muscle or blood.

Leber's Hereditary Optic Neuropathy   LHON typically presents with painless, subacute, bilateral visual loss with central scotomas and dyschromatopsia. The mean age of onset is 23 years, and males are affected three to four times more commonly than females. LHON bears little clinical resemblance to the other mitochondrial disease phenotypes. It was first classified in this group on the basis of the maternal inheritance pattern. The pathophysiology of visual loss appears to involve both genetic and epigenetic (tobacco and alcohol) factors. The mtDNA mutations exhibit a high degree of genetic heterogeneity. Primary LHON-associated mtDNA mutations predominantly affect complex I genes [at nucleotide positions 11778 (ND-4 gene), 3460 (ND-1 gene), and 14484 (ND-6 gene)] (Fig. 67-1). Several other mtDNA mutations may have secondary pathogenetic roles in LHON, including a mutation at nucleotide position 13708 (ND-5 gene) of Caucasian haplogroup J mtDNA.

Genotype-phenotype correlations are beginning to emerge for the primary LHON-associated mtDNA mutations. The prognosis for visual recovery, for example, varies nearly ten-fold depending on the mutation. mtDNA mutations that cause LHON plus dystonia have also been described.

ORGAN SYSTEM MANIFESTATIONS OF MITOCHONDRIAL DISEASE   Because virtually all tissues of the body depend, to some extent, on oxidative metabolism, patients with mitochondrial disease can present to many specialists in medicine. The somatic manifestations listed in Table 67-2, first noted in association with the classic mitochondrial diseases, may be the dominant or initial clinical symptom or may be important comorbid features.

The ophthalmologic manifestations of mtDNA mutations are prominent, with involvement of virtually the entire visual axis from the lids, cornea, and extraocular muscles to the occipital cortex. The cardinal eye findings include ophthalmoplegia, optic neuropathy, and pigmentary retinopathy. Cardiovascular manifestations include dilated and hypertrophic cardiomyopathy, conduction disease and heart block, Wolff-Parkinson-White syndrome, and hypertension. The prevalence of diabetes mellitus is higher than expected in patients with mitochondrial encephalomyopathies, and it occurs in association with a variety of mtDNA mutations. Diabetes mellitus has been linked with the 3243 mtDNA point mutation, usually, but not exclusively, in association with sensorineural hearing loss.

ROLE OF MITOCHONDRIAL DNA MUTATIONS IN PREVALENT DISEASES   The role of mtDNA mutations in common, socioeconomically significant diseases is under active investigation. The genetic basis of many prevalent diseases is complex and does not follow simple, single-gene Mendelian inheritance (Chap. 65). Mitochondrial diseases, such as LHON and aminoglycoside-induced deafness, illustrate the potential for complex pathophysiologic interactions between genetic and epigenetic factors. As a result of these interactions, mtDNA mutations may be involved in subsets of common diseases, such as diabetes mellitus, in which the maternal inheritance pattern is not obvious.

The tissue-specific accumulation of somatic (noninherited) mtDNA mutations is likely relevant to some late-onset degenerative disorders, such as Alzheimer's disease and Parkinson's disease. It has been shown, for example, that as people age, mtDNA mutations accumulate in tissues, including some postmitotic tissues such as the basal ganglia and cerebral cortex. The high mutations rate and poor repair capacity of mtDNA contribute to the buildup of mtDNA mutations in postmitotic tissues or those with a slower turnover rate. Oxidative damage, as occurs with repeated episodes of ischemia and reperfusion, markedly increases the accumulation of mtDNA mutations. Environmental factors may also affect mtDNA. The anti-retroviral drug azidothymidine depletes muscle mtDNA and causes an acquired mitochondrial myopathy. Cumulative, age-dependent mitochondrial dysfunction, mediated to a significant degree by oxidative damage to mtDNA and other mitochondrial macromolecules, may be a major contributor to aging.

The unequivocal establishment of the diagnosis of a mitochondrial disease by molecular genetic methods is a prerequisite for proper genetic counseling and ultimately treatment.

BIBLIOGRAPHY

BEAL MF et al: Do defects in mitochondrial energy metabolism underlie the pathology of neurodegenerative disease? Trends Neurosci 16:125, 1993

JOHNS DR: Mitochondrial DNA and disease. N Engl J Med 333:638, 1995

SHIGENAGA MK et al: Oxidative damage and mitochondrial decay in aging. Proc Natl Acad Sci USA 91:10771, 1994

SIMON DK, JOHNS DR: Mitochondrial disorders: Clinical and genetic features. Annu Rev Med 50:111, 1999

WALLACE DC: Mitochondrial diseases in man and mouse. Science 283:1482, 1999

ZEVIANI M et al: Mitochondrial disorders. Medicine (Baltimore) 77:59, 1998

68 Susan Miesfeldt, J. Larry Jameson

SCREENING, COUNSELING, AND PREVENTION OF GENETIC DISORDERS

IMPLICATIONS OF MOLECULAR GENETICS FOR INTERNAL MEDICINE

Approximately 1 in 50 children is born with a serious congenital abnormality or mental handicap. It is known that each of us harbors mutations in several genes that can potentially lead to serious diseases. The field of medical genetics has traditionally focused on chromosomal abnormalities (Chap. 66) and Mendelian disorders (Chap. 65). However, there is genetic susceptibility to many common adult-onset diseases including atherosclerosis, hypertension, autoimmune diseases, diabetes mellitus, Alzheimer disease, psychiatric disorders, and many forms of cancer. Genetic contributions to these common disorders involve more than the ultimate expression of a disease; these genes can also influence the severity of infirmity, response to treatment, and progression of disease.

The primary care clinician is now faced with the role of recognizing and counseling patients at risk for a large number of genetically influenced illnesses. This role reflects the advances in genetic medicine that are changing the way diseases are classified, enhancing our understanding of pathophysiology, providing practical information concerning drug metabolism and therapeutic responses, and promising to allow individualized screening and health care management programs. In view of these changes, the physician must integrate personal medical history, family history, and diagnostic molecular testing into the overall care of individual patients and their families. In addition, the internist has an important role in educating patients about the indications, benefits, risks, and limitations of genetic testing in the management of diverse diseases. This is a formidable task as scientific ad-

vances in genetic medicine, and media attention to these advances, have outpaced the translation into standards of clinical care.

PRENATAL AND NEWBORN GENETIC SCREENING AND TESTING

During pregnancy and in the newborn period, genetic screening and testing are both used to detect genetic disorders (Table 68-1). *Genetic screening* refers to the search for a genetic disorder in the entire population or in a high-risk population. Screening techniques must be cost-effective, have a high positive predictive value, and should yield information that leads to disease prevention or a useful therapeutic intervention. Examples of screening tests include maternal serum markers used to detect increased risk of Down syndrome, postnatal tests for phenylketonuria, and cholesterol levels in children used to identify individuals at risk for familial hyperlipidemias. Thus, genetic screening tests do not necessarily imply DNA- or chromosome-based tests. Instead, many such tests use a surrogate biochemical marker or phenotypic feature of the underlying genetic disorder. Determination of which genetic disorders should be screened routinely depends on disease frequency, the severity of the disorder, cost of screening, and whether treatment interventions can alter the course of the disease.

Genetic testing, on the other hand, is used in an individual suspected to have a disease based on physical features, family history, or biochemical findings. Genetic testing can include the following: (1) diagnostic testing as for hemochromatosis, (2) predictive testing as for breast cancer predisposition, (3) carrier testing as for muscular dystrophy, and (4) prenatal testing as for β-thalassemia when both parents are carriers.

Depending on the disorder(s) under consideration, several different techniques are currently used for genetic screening during pregnancy. For instance, first-trimester screening for Down syndrome is performed using measurements of maternal serum pregnancy-associated plasma protein A and the free β subunit of human chorionic gonadotropin in combination with ultrasonographic measurement of nuchal translucency (at 10 to 14 weeks of gestation). Second-trimester maternal serum screening includes measurements of human chorionic gonadotropin, unconjugated estriol, α-fetoprotein, and inhibin that, in combination, increase the sensitivity of Down syndrome detection (Chap. 66). Increased α-fetoprotein levels are also associated with open neural tube defects.

Amniocentesis or *chorionic villus sampling* (CVS) is used to isolate fetal cells for chromosomal analysis or to test for specific genetic abnormalities. Amniocentesis is typically performed during the early second trimester (14 to 16 weeks' gestational age). CVS can be performed earlier (8 to 10 weeks' gestational age) and involves transcervical or transabdominal biopsy of fetal trophoblastic tissue. CVS is associated with a somewhat greater risk of spontaneous abortion (<0.5 to 1%) than amniocentesis (<0.5%) but allows for elective abortion

Table 68-1 Examples of Screening Tests for Genetic Disorders in the Newborn[a]

Disorder	Inheritance	Incidence[b]
Phenylketonuria	AR	1/10,000
Hypothyroidism	Sporadic or AR	1/4000
Galactosemia	AR	1/40,000
Maple syrup urine disease	AR	1/200,000
Homocystinuria	AR	1/200,000
Biotinidase deficiency	AR	1/100,000
Cystic fibrosis	AR	1/2000
Adrenal hyperplasia	AR	1/10,000
Hemoglobinopathy	AR	1/2500

[a] The panel of prenatal screening tests varies in different states and in different countries; additional information on screening tests is available online at: www.aap.org/policy.

[b] AR, autosomal recessive.

earlier during pregnancy. Ultrasonography is used to analyze the fetus directly at different stages of development. Preimplantation molecular diagnostic testing is now possible by isolating single cells from the 8- to 10-cell embryo. The polymerase chain reaction (PCR) is then used to test for selected single-gene disorders such as Tay-Sachs disease, cystic fibrosis, or sickle cell anemia. This testing strategy requires in vitro fertilization but has the advantage that affected embryos are not implanted.

It should be remembered that prenatal genetic testing focuses on chromosomal abnormalities (Chap. 66), along with specific genetic disorders for which there is increased risk of parental transmission. There is no guarantee that a child will be free of birth defects or other genetic disorders not included among the diagnostic tests.

The genetic counseling process should begin before prenatal testing and should include: (1) a description of the test, (2) the types of disorders that will be screened, (3) the limitations of the screening, (4) an exploration of what the parents will do with the information, and (5) an indication of when the results will be available. If a genetic disorder is identified, the full repertoire of genetic counseling skills is required (see below). The nature of the genetic disease needs to be reviewed with the parents, often on separate occasions. The counselor should also discuss the kinds of physical and emotional challenges that a genetic disease might pose for the affected individual and the family. Written information should be provided, if available. Ultimately, the parents must reach a decision to continue or terminate the pregnancy. If pregnancy is terminated, counseling should continue after the procedure. If pregnancy is continued, counseling should continue to address the medical needs of the affected fetus or child, as well as to help the family meet any challenges presented by the genetic disorder.

At the time of birth, all newborns undergo a complete physical examination to detect gross developmental abnormalities. Within 24 to 72 h of birth, blood samples from newborns are sent to a state-designated laboratory to screen for selected diseases, such as congenital hypothyroidism and a variety of inherited metabolic disorders (Table 68-1). This program represents a clear example of the benefits of selected genetic screening. The early diagnosis of phenylketonuria, for example, permits parents to introduce a phenylalanine-free diet before the development of severe neurologic sequelae (Chap. 352).

COMMON ADULT-ONSET GENETIC DISORDERS

MULTIFACTORIAL INHERITANCE The risk for many adult-onset disorders reflects the additive effects of genetic factors at multiple loci that may function independently—or in combination—with other genes or environmental factors. Our understanding of the genetic basis of these disorders is incomplete, despite the clear recognition of genetic susceptibility. In type 2 diabetes mellitus, for example, the concordance rate in monozygotic twins ranges between 50 to 90%. Diabetes or impaired glucose tolerance occurs in 40% of siblings and in 30% of the offspring of an affected individual. Despite the fact that diabetes affects 5% of the population and exhibits a high degree of heritability, there are only a few examples of genetic mutations that might account for the familial nature of the disease (most of which are rare). They include certain mitochondrial DNA disorders (Chap. 67), mutations in a cascade of genes that control pancreatic islet cell development and function (*HNF4α, HNF1α, IPF1*), insulin receptor mutations, and others (Chap. 333). Obesity and other factors that contribute to insulin resistance also represent important risk factors for type 2 diabetes. Current models for the genetic basis of type 2 diabetes propose the involvement of more than a dozen genes: some genes influence pancreatic islet development or function; others likely modulate glucose-sensing; and an important group determine insulin sensitivity, either directly by affecting insulin signaling or indirectly by regulating body weight or composition. Superimposed on this genetic background are environmental influences such as diet, exercise, pregnancy, and medications.

Identifying these susceptibility genes is a formidable task. Nonetheless, a reasonable goal for this type of disease is to identify genes that increase (or decrease) disease risk by a factor of two or more. For common diseases such as diabetes or heart disease, this level of risk has important implications for health. Much the same way that cholesterol is currently used as a biochemical marker of cardiovascular risk, we can anticipate the development of genetic panels with similar predictive power. Genetic tests for a large number of genetic disorders are now available; a web site (www.genetests.org) lists various laboratories that perform specific tests. The advent of DNA-sequencing chips represents an important technical advance that promises to make large-scale testing more feasible (Chap. 65). The decision whether or not to perform a genetic test for a particular inherited adult-onset disorder, such as hemochromatosis, multiple endocrine neoplasia (MEN) type 1, prolonged QT syndrome, or Huntington disease, is complex; it depends on the clinical features of the disorder, the desires of the patient and family, and whether the results of genetic testing will alter medical decision-making or treatment (see below).

THE FAMILY HISTORY Pending additional advances in genetic testing, the key to determining the inherited risk for common adult-onset diseases still rests in the collection and interpretation of a detailed personal and family medical history in conjunction with a directed physical examination. For example, a history of multiple family members with early-onset coronary artery diseases, glucose intolerance, and hypertension should suggest increased risk for genetic, and perhaps environmental, predisposition to insulin resistance (Chap. 333). Individual patients with this family history should be monitored for the possible development of hypertension, diabetes, and hyperlipidemia. They should be counseled about the importance of avoiding additional risk factors such as obesity and cigarette smoking.

Family history, recorded in the form of a pedigree, greatly assists the assessment of risk in the individual patient. At a minimum, pedigrees should convey health-related data on all first-degree relatives and selected second-degree relatives, including grandparents. When pedigrees appear to suggest an inherited disease, they should be extended to include additional family members. The determination of risk for an asymptomatic individual will vary depending on the size of the pedigree, the number of unaffected relatives, and the types of diagnoses within the family. For example, a woman with two first-degree relatives with breast cancer is more at risk if she has a total of three female first-degree relatives than if she has a total of eight female first-degree relatives. Additional variables that factor into the assessment of risk—and should be documented in the pedigree—include the age at diagnosis of each affected family member, present age of all family members, and the presence or absence of nonhereditary risk factors among those affected with diseases.

When assessing the personal and family history, the physician should be alert to a younger age of disease onset than is usually seen in the general population. A 30-year-old with acute myocardial infarction should be considered at risk for a hereditary trait, even if there is no family history of premature coronary artery disease (Chap. 241). The absence of the nonhereditary risk factors typically associated with a disease also raises the prospect of genetic risk factors. A personal or family history of deep vein thrombosis, in the absence of known nongenetic risk factors, might suggest a hereditary thrombotic disorder (Chap. 117). The physical examination may also provide important clues concerning the risk for a specific inherited disorder. A patient with xanthomas at a young age should prompt consideration of familial hypercholesterolemia. Some adult-onset disease-causing mutations are more prevalent in certain ethnic groups. For instance, >2% of the Ashkenazi population carry one of three specific mutations in the *BRCA1* or *BRCA2* genes. The prevalence of the factor V Leiden allele ranges from 3 to 7% in Caucasians but is much less common in Africans or Asians.

Recall of family history is often inaccurate. This is especially so when the history is remote and as families become more dispersed. It can be helpful to ask patients to fill out family history forms before or after their visits, as this provides them with an opportunity to contact relatives. Attempts should be made to confirm the illnesses reported in the family history before making management decisions. This process is often labor-intensive and ideally involves interviews of additional family members or reviewing medical records, autopsy reports, and death certificates.

Nongenetic factors associated with disease risk should also be reviewed in full, including occupation, diet, living conditions, and social habits. For example, patients at hereditary risk for heart disease should be questioned about tobacco use, diet, exercise, and lipid levels. Patients should also be asked about their health screening and prevention behaviors. These nonhereditary factors contribute to the assessment of overall risk and represent an important focus for disease prevention.

Although many inherited disorders will be suggested by the clustering of relatives with the same or related conditions, it is important to note that *disease penetrance* is incomplete for most multifactorial genetic disorders. As a result, the pedigree obtained in such families may not exhibit a clear Mendelian pattern of inheritance, as not all family members carrying the disease-associated alleles will manifest disease. Furthermore, genes associated with some of these disorders often exhibit *variable expression* of disease. For example, the breast cancer–associated gene, *BRCA1*, can predispose to several different malignancies in the same family, including cancers of the breast, ovary, and prostate (Chap. 81). For common diseases such as breast cancer, some family members without the disease-causing mutation may also develop breast cancer, representing another confounding variable in the pedigree analysis.

Some of the aforementioned features of the family history are illustrated in Fig. 68-1. The proband, a 36-year-old woman, has a strong history of breast and ovarian cancer on the paternal side of her family. The early age of onset, as well as the co-occurrence of breast and ovarian cancer in this family, suggests the possibility of an inherited mutation in *BRCA1* or *BRCA2*. It is unclear though—without genetic testing—whether her father inherited such a mutation and transmitted it to her. After appropriate genetic counseling of the proband and her family, one approach to DNA analysis in this family is to test the potentially affected 42-year-old living cousin (IV-4) for the presence of a *BRCA1* or *BRCA2* mutation. If a mutation is found, then it is possible to test for this particular alteration in the proband and other family members, if they so desire. In the example shown, if the pro-

FIGURE 68-1 A 36-year-old woman (*arrow*) seeks consultation because of her family history of cancer. The patient expresses concern that the multiple cancers in her relatives imply an inherited predisposition to develop cancer. The family history is recorded and records of the patient's relatives confirm the reported diagnoses.

band's father has inherited the *BRCA1* mutation, there is a 50:50 probability that the mutation has been transmitted to her. Genetic testing can be used to establish the absence or presence of this particular risk factor.

GENETIC TESTING FOR ADULT-ONSET DISORDERS

A critical first step before initiating genetic testing is to assure that the correct clinical diagnosis has been made, whether based on family history, characteristic physical findings, or biochemical testing. Careful clinical assessment will prevent unnecessary testing and will direct testing towards the most probable candidate genes. Many disorders exhibit the feature of *locus heterogeneity*, which refers to the fact that mutations in different genes can cause phenotypically similar disorders. For example, osteogenesis imperfecta (Chap. 351), muscular dystrophy (Chap. 383), homocystinuria (Chap. 352), and hereditary predisposition to colon cancer (Chap. 90) or breast cancer (Chap. 89) can each be caused by mutations in distinct genes. The pattern of disease transmission, clinical course, and treatment may differ significantly, depending on which gene is affected. In these cases, the choice of which genes to test is often determined by unique clinical features, the relative prevalence of mutations in various genes, or test availability.

Like all laboratory tests, there are limitations to the accuracy and interpretation of genetic tests. In addition to technical errors, genetic tests are often designed to detect only the most common mutations. In this case, a negative result must be qualified by the possibility that the individual may have a mutation that is not included in the test.

In addition to molecular testing for established disease, presymptomatic testing for susceptibility to chronic disease is being increasingly integrated into the practice of medicine. In most cases, however, the discovery of disease-associated genes has greatly outpaced studies that assess clinical outcomes and the impact of interventions. Until such outcomes-based studies are available, predictive molecular testing must be approached with caution and should be offered only to patients who have been adequately counseled and have provided informed consent (Fig. 68-2). In the majority of cases, presymptomatic testing should be offered only to individuals with a suggestive personal or family medical history or in the context of a clinical trial.

Molecular analysis is generally more informative if testing is initiated in a symptomatic family member, since the identification of a mutation can direct the testing of other at-risk family members (whether they are symptomatic or not). In the absence of additional familial or environmental risk factors, individuals who test negative for the mutation found in the affected family member can be informed that they are at general population risk for that particular disease. Furthermore, they can be reassured that they are not at risk for passing on the mutation to their children. On the other hand, asymptomatic family members who test positive for the known mutation must be informed that they are at increased risk for disease development and for transmitting the mutation to their children. Nevertheless, for most multifactorial genetic disorders, the test results cannot predict with confidence whether, or when, the disease will develop. For example, not everyone with the apolipoprotein E allele (ε4) will develop Alzheimer disease, and many individuals without this susceptibility gene can still develop the disorder (Chap. 362).

A negative test result is interpreted differently when no genetic mutation is found in a symptomatic family member. In this difficult circumstance, the test performed on a given gene may not detect all mutations in that gene (false negative) or the individual may have a mutation in a different disease-associated gene that was not tested.

Clinicians providing pretest counseling and education should assess the patient's emotional ability to cope with test results. Individuals who demonstrate signs and symptoms of psychiatric illness should have their emotional needs addressed before proceeding with molecular testing. Generally, genetic testing should not be offered at a time

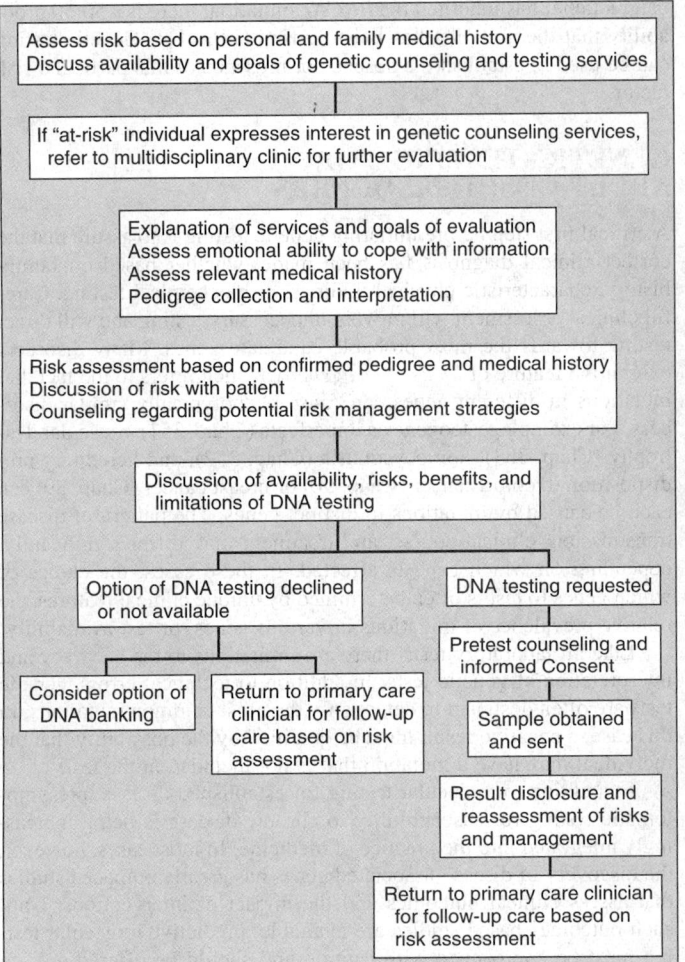

FIGURE 68-2 Algorithm for genetic counseling and testing.

of personal crisis or acute illness within the family. Patients will derive more benefit from test results if they are emotionally able to comprehend and absorb the information. It is important to assess patients' preconceived notions of their personal likelihood of disease in preparing pretest educational strategies. Often, patients harbor unwarranted fear or denial of their likelihood of genetic risk.

Genetic testing has the potential of affecting the way individual family members relate to one another, both negatively and positively. As a result, patients addressing the option of molecular testing must consider how test results might impact their relationships with relatives, spouses, and friends. In families with a known genetic mutation, those who test positive must address the impact of the disease on their present and future lifestyles; those who test negative may manifest survivor guilt. Family members are likely to differ in their emotional and social responses to the same information. Counseling should also address the potential consequences of test results on relationships with a spouse or child. Parents who are found to have a disease-associated mutation often express considerable anxiety and despair as they address the issue of risk to their children.

When a condition does not manifest until adulthood, clinicians will be faced with the question of whether at-risk children should be offered molecular testing and, if so, at what age. Several professional organizations have cautioned that genetic testing for adult-onset disorders should not be offered to children. Many of these conditions are not preventable and, consequently, such information can pose significant psychosocial risk. In addition, there is concern that testing during childhood violates a child's right to make an informed decision regarding testing upon reaching adulthood. On the other hand, testing

should be offered in childhood for disorders that may be manifest early in life, especially when management options are available. For example, children at risk for familial adenomatous polyposis (FAP) may develop polyps as early as their teens, and progression to an invasive cancer can occur by their twenties. Likewise, children at risk for MEN type 2, which is caused by mutations in the *RET* proto-oncogene, may develop medullary thyroid cancer as early as 6 years of age, and the issue of prophylactic thyroidectomy should be addressed with the parents of children with documented mutations (Chap. 339).

INFORMED CONSENT   When the issue of testing is addressed, patients should be strongly encouraged to involve other relatives in the decision-making process, as molecular diagnostics will likely have an impact on the entire family. Informed consent for molecular testing begins with detailed education and counseling. The patient must fully understand the risks, benefits, and limitations of undergoing the analysis. Informed consent should be in the form of a written document, drafted clearly and concisely in a language and format that is comprehensible to the patient, who should be made aware of the disposition of test results. Informed consent should also include a discussion of the mechanics of testing. Most molecular testing for hereditary disease involves DNA-based analysis of peripheral blood. In the majority of circumstances, test results should be given only to the individual, in person, and with a support person in the room.

Because molecular testing of an asymptomatic individual often allows prediction of future risk, the patient should understand any potential long-term medical, psychological, and social implications of this decision. In the United States, legislation affecting this area is still evolving, and it is important to explore with the patient the potential impact that test results may have on employment, future health, and life insurance coverage.

Patients should understand that alternatives to molecular analysis remain available if they decide not to proceed with this option. They should also be notified that testing is available in the future if they are not prepared to undergo analysis immediately. The option of DNA banking should be presented so that samples are readily available for future use by family members, if needed.

FOLLOW-UP CARE AFTER TESTING   Depending on the nature of the genetic disorder, posttest interventions may include (1) cautious surveillance and appropriate health care screening, (2) specific medical interventions, (3) chemoprevention, (4) risk avoidance, and (5) referral to support services. For example, patients with known pathologic mutations in *BRCA1* or *BRCA2* are offered intensive screening as well as the option of prophylactic mastectomy and/or oophorectomy. In addition, such women may be eligible for preventive treatment with agents such as tamoxifen, raloxifene, or retinoids. In contrast, those at known risk for Huntington disease are offered continued follow-up and supportive services, including physical and occupational therapy, and social services and support groups as indicated. Specific interventions will change as translational research enhances our understanding of these genetic diseases and as more is learned about the functions of the genes involved.

Individuals who test negative for a mutation in a disease-associated gene identified in an affected family member must be reminded that they may still be at risk for the disease. This is of particular importance for common diseases such as diabetes mellitus, cancer, and coronary artery disease. For example, a woman who finds that she does not carry the disease-associated mutation in *BRCA2* previously discovered in her family must be reminded that she still requires the same breast cancer screening used in the general population.

GENETIC COUNSELING AND EDUCATION

Genetic counseling should be distinguished from genetic testing and screening, even though genetic counselors are often involved in issues related to testing. Genetic counseling refers to *a communication process that deals with human problems associated with the occurrence or risk of a genetic disorder in a family.* Genetic risk assessment can be complex and often involves elements of uncertainty. Counseling therefore includes genetic education as well as psychosocial counseling. Genetic counselors may be called upon by other health care professionals (or by individual patients and families) to address a broad range of issues directly and indirectly involved with genetic disease (Table 68-2). The genetic counselor will do the following:

- Gather and document a detailed family history
- Educate the patient about general genetic principles related to disease risk, both for themselves and others in the family
- Assess and enhance the patient's ability to cope with the genetic information offered
- Discuss how nongenetic factors may relate to the ultimate expression of disease
- Address medical management issues
- Assist in determining the role of genetic testing for the individual and family
- Ensure that the patient is aware of the risks, benefits, and limitations of the various genetic testing options
- Refer the patient and other at-risk family members for additional medical and support services, if necessary

The complexity of genetic counseling and the broad scope of genetic diseases are leading to the development of specialized, multidisciplinary clinics designed to provide broad-based support and medical care for those at risk and their family members. Such multidisciplinary teams are often composed of medical geneticists, specialist physicians, genetic counselors, nurses, psychologists, social workers, and biomedical ethicists who work together to consider difficult diagnostic, treatment, and testing decisions. Such a format also provides primary care physicians with invaluable support and assistance as they follow and treat at-risk patients.

The approach to genetic counseling has important ethical, social, and financial implications. Philosophies related to genetic counseling vary widely by country and center. In North American centers, for example, counseling is generally offered in a nondirective manner, wherein patients learn to understand how their values factor into a particular medical decision. Nondirective counseling is particularly appropriate when there are no data demonstrating a clear benefit associated with a particular intervention or when an intervention is considered experimental. For example, nondirective genetic counseling is employed when a person is deciding whether or not to undergo genetic testing for Huntington disease (Chap. 362). At this time, there is no clear benefit (in terms of medical outcome) to an at-risk individual undergoing genetic testing for this disease, as its course cannot be altered by therapeutic interventions. However, testing can have an important impact on such a person's perception of the future and his or her interpersonal relationships and plans for reproduction. Therefore, the decision to pursue testing rests on the individual's belief system and values. On the other hand, a more directive approach is appropriate when a condition can be treated. In a family with FAP (associated with mutations in the *APC* gene), colon cancer screening and prophylactic colectomy should be recommended for known *APC* mutation carriers. The counselor and clinician following this family must ensure that the at-risk individuals have access to the resources necessary to adhere to these recommendations.

Genetic education is central to an individual's ability to make an informed decision regarding testing options and treatment. Although genetic counselors represent one source of genetic education, other health care providers also need to contribute to patient education. Pa-

tients at risk for genetic disease should understand fundamental medical genetic principles and terminology relevant to their situation. This includes the concept of genes, how they are transmitted, and how they confer hereditary disease risk. An adequate knowledge of patterns of inheritance will allow patients to understand the probability of disease risk for themselves and other family members. It is also important to impart the concepts of disease penetrance and expression. For complex genetic disorders, asymptomatic patients should be advised that a positive test result does not always translate into future disease development. In addition, the role of nongenetic factors, such as environmental exposures, must be discussed in the context of multifactorial disease risk and disease prevention. Finally, patients should understand the natural history of the disease as well as the potential options for intervention, including screening, prevention, and—in certain circumstances—pharmacologic treatment or prophylactic surgery.

THERAPEUTIC INTERVENTIONS BASED ON GENETIC SUSCEPTIBILITY TO DISEASE

Specific treatments are now available for an increasing number of genetic disorders, whether identified through population-based screening or directed testing (Table 68-3). A number of metabolic disorders fall into this group. For example, the complications of phenylketonuria can be mitigated by recognizing the disease early and avoiding foods that contain phenylalanine (Chap. 352). Similar principles apply to maple syrup urine disease (Chap. 352) and galactosemia (Chap. 350). Children with 21-hydroxylase deficiency present with adrenal insufficiency, usually within the first few weeks of life (Chap. 331). Because of the block in cortisol synthesis, the adrenal steroid precursors are shunted into the androgen pathway, causing ambiguous genitalia in females and premature virilization in males. In this disorder, treatment with glucocorticoid and mineralocorticoid not only corrects the hormone deficits but is also required to suppress ACTH overproduction, which otherwise worsens virilization.

Although the strategies for therapeutic interventions are best developed for childhood genetic diseases, these principles are gradually making their way into the diagnosis and management of adult-onset disorders. Hereditary hemochromatosis illustrates many of the issues raised by the potential availability of genetic screening in the adult population. For instance, it is relatively common (approximately 1 in 200 individuals of northern European descent are homozygous), and its complications are potentially preventable through phlebotomy (Chap. 345). The recent identification of the *HFE* gene, mutations of which are associated with this syndrome, has sparked interest in the use of DNA-based testing for presymptomatic diagnosis of the disorder. However, up to one-third of individuals who are homozygous for the *HFE* mutation do not have evidence of iron overload. Consequently, in the absence of a positive family history, current recommendations are phenotypic screening for evidence of iron overload followed by genetic testing. Whether genetic screening for hemochromatosis will someday be coupled to assessment of phenotypic expression awaits further studies. In contrast to the issue of population screening, it is important to test and counsel other family members when the diagnosis of hemochromatosis has been made in a proband. Testing allows the physician to exclude family members who are not at risk. It also permits presymptomatic detection of iron overload and the institution of treatment (phlebotomy) before the development of organ damage.

Preventive measures and therapeutic interventions are not restricted to metabolic disorders. Identification of familial forms of long QT syndrome, associated with ventricular arrythmias, allows early electrocardiographic testing and the use of prophylactic antiarrythmic therapy (Chap. 230). Individuals with familial hypertrophic cardiomyopathy can be screened by ultrasound, treated with beta blockers or other drugs, and counseled about the importance of avoiding strenuous exercise and dehydration (Chap. 238). Likewise, individuals with Marfan syndrome can be treated with beta blockers and monitored for

Table 68-2   Indications for Genetic Counseling

Advanced maternal (>35) or paternal (>50) age
Consanguinity
Previous history of a child with birth defects or a genetic disorder
Personal or family history suggestive of a genetic disorder
High-risk ethnic groups; known carriers of genetic mutations
Ultrasound or prenatal testing suggesting a genetic disorder

Table 68-3   Examples of Interventions Based on Genetic Testing[a]

Genetic Disorders	Interventions	Chapter
Phenylketonuria	Avoid dietary phenylalanine	352
Homocystinuria	Treatment with folic acid, pyridoxine, and vitamin B_{12}	352
Hemochromatosis	Phlebotomy	345
Wilson's disease	D-Penicillamine treatment	348
Galactosemia	Avoid dietary galactose	350
Porphyrias	Avoid precipitants	346
Glucose-6-phosphate dehydrogenase deficiency	Avoid oxidant drugs	108
21-Hydroxylase deficiency	Glucocorticoid and mineralocorticoid treatment	331
Familial Mediterranean fever	Colchicine treatment	289
Malignant hyperthermia	Avoid precipitating anesthetics	17
α_1 Antitrypsin deficiency	Avoid smoking; avoid occupational and environmental toxins	258
Hypertrophic cardiomyopathy	Echocardiographic screening; early pharmacologic intervention	238
Long QT syndrome	Electrocardiographic screening and electrophysiologic testing; early pharmacologic intervention	230
Marfan syndrome	Echocardiographic screening; prophylactic beta blockers	247, 351
Factor V Leiden	Avoid thrombogenic risk factors and oral contraceptives	117
Hemophilia A	Factor VIII replacement	117
Hemophilia B	Factor IX replacement; possible gene therapy	117
Familial hypocalciuric hypercalcemia	Avoid parathyroidectomy	341
Kallmann syndrome	Induce puberty with hormone replacement	328
Neurohypophyseal diabetes insipidus	Replace vasopressin	329
Maturity onset diabetes of the young	Screen and treat for diabetes	333
Hereditary nonpolyposis colon cancer	Early colonoscopy screening	90
Familial adenomatous polyposis	Nonsteroidal anti-inflammatory drugs; early colonoscopy screening; colectomy	90
Familial breast cancer	Consider estrogen receptor antagonists; early screening by exams and mammography; consider prophylactic mastectomy; consider risk for additional types of cancers	89
Basal cell nevus syndrome	Avoid UV light; screening and biopsies	86
Familial melanoma	Avoid UV light; screening and biopsies	86
Multiple endocrine neoplasia type 2	Prophylactic thyroidectomy; screen for pheochromocytoma and hyperparathyroidism	339

[a] See the Web site www.genetests.org for a compendium of available genetic tests.

the development of aortic aneurysms (Chap. 247). Individuals with α_1 antitrypsin deficiency can be strongly counseled to avoid cigarette smoking and exposure to environmental pulmonary and hepatotoxins. Various host genes influence the pathogenesis of certain infectious diseases in humans, including HIV (Chap. 309). The factor V Leiden allele increases risk of thrombosis (Chap. 62). Approximately 3% of the worldwide population is heterozygous for this mutation. Moreover, it is found in up to 25% of patients with recurrent deep venous thrombosis or pulmonary embolism. Women who are heterozygous or ho-

mozygous for this allele should therefore avoid the use of oral contraceptives and receive heparin prophylaxis after surgery or trauma.

The field of pharmacogenetics seeks to identify genes that alter drug metabolism or confer susceptibility to toxic drug reactions (Chap. 71). Examples include succinylcholine sensitivity, malignant hyperthermia, the porphyrias, and glucose-6-phosphase dehydrogenase (G6PD) deficiency.

As noted above, the identification of genes that increase the risk of specific types of neoplasia is rapidly changing the management of many cancers. Identifying family members with mutations that predispose to FAP or hereditary nonpolyposis colon cancer (HNPCC) can lead to recommendations of early screening by colonoscopy or prophylactic surgery (Chap. 90). Similar principles apply to familial forms of melanoma, basal cell carcinoma, and breast cancer. It should be recognized, however, that most cancers harbor several distinct genetic abnormalities by the time they acquire invasive or metastatic potential (Chaps. 81 and 82). Consequently, the major impact of genetic testing in these cases is to allow more intensive clinical screening, as it remains very challenging to predict disease penetrance or the clinical course of these diseases.

Although genetic diagnosis of these and other disorders is only beginning to be used in the clinical setting, susceptibility testing holds the promise of allowing earlier and more targeted interventions that can reduce the morbidity and mortality associated with these disorders. We can expect the availability of genetic tests to expand rapidly. A critical challenge for physicians and other health care providers is to keep pace with these advances in genetic medicine and to implement testing judiciously. Meeting this goal will enhance patient care through adequate counseling, directed testing, and appropriate interventions, with the ultimate objective being the reduction of morbidity and mortality from genetic diseases.

BIBLIOGRAPHY

BIESECKER BB, MARTEAU TM: Future of genetic counselling: An international perspective. Nat Genet 22:133, 1999

COUGHLIN SS: The intersection of genetics, public health, and preventative medicine. Am J Prev Med 16:89, 1999

FRASER FC: Genetic counseling. Am J Hum Genet 26:636, 1974

GELEHRTER TD et al: Principles of Medical Genetics, 2d ed. Baltimore, Williams & Wilkins, 1998

HARPER PS: Practical Genetic Counselling, 5th ed. Oxford, Butterworth Heinmann, 1998

McKINNON WC et al: Predisposition genetic testing for late-onset disorders in adults: Position paper of the National Society of Genetic Counselors. JAMA 278:1217, 1997

MEHLMAN MJ, KODISH ED et al: The need for anonymous genetic counseling and testing. Am J Hum Genetic 58:393, 1996

ROSENDAAL FR: Risk factors for venous thrombosis: Prevalence, risk and interaction. Semin Hematol 34:171, 1997

STEPHENSON J: "Talking" genetics glossary (www.nhgri.nih.gov/DIR/VIP/Glossary/). JAMA 281: 600, 1999

THE AMERICAN SOCIETY OF HUMAN GENETICS: Report from the ASHG Information and Education Committee: Medical school core curriculum in genetics. Am J Hum Genet 56:535, 1995

———, THE AMERICAN COLLEGE OF MEDICAL GENETICS: Points to consider: Ethical, legal and psychosocial implications of genetic testing in children and adolescents. Am J Hum Genet 57:1233, 1995

69	Mark A. Kay, David W. Russell

GENE THERAPY

AAV	adeno-associated viruses	LTRs	long terminal repeats
ADA	adenosine deaminase	MLVs	murine leukemia viruses
CNS	central nervous system	RP	retinitis pigmentosa
CSF	colony stimulating factor	TK	thymidine kinase
IFNs	interferons	VEGF	vascular endothelial growth factor
ILs	interleukins		
LDL	low-density lipoprotein		

Gene therapy is generally defined as *the delivery of nucleic acids to alter or prevent a pathologic process*. Although initially considered primarily in the context of inherited monogenic disorders, gene therapy is now recognized as a potential treatment strategy for a wide range of acquired disorders, such as cancer, neurodegenerative diseases, and infections. Gene therapy has been used in several hundred protocols. Despite early hopes that gene therapy might be quickly incorporated into medical practice, it has yielded limited success to date and remains an investigational treatment. The technical challenges associated with gene therapy are formidable, but with steady progress in vector development, definitive therapeutic milestones may soon be realized for selected disorders.

GENERAL APPROACHES TO GENE THERAPY

FORMS OF GENE THERAPY Gene therapy can be used, in principle, to modify all cells in the body, including the germ line. *Germ-line gene therapy* would allow transmission of the modified genetic information to the next generation and is not currently accepted as an appropriate therapeutic approach. For ethical reasons, opposition to germ-line gene therapy is likely to continue in the foreseeable future. *Somatic gene therapy* refers to modification of the somatic, differentiated cells of the body. It is used in an effort to correct inherited diseases such as cystic fibrosis and acquired disorders such as rheumatoid arthritis or malignancies.

Whole-organ transplantation (e.g., bone marrow, liver, and kidney) has been used for years as a strategy to replace the function of defective genes. The idea of using nonautologous cell transplantation has been revisited in the past few years, and with the advent of human embryonic stem cells, similar transplantation strategies are being considered for a variety of disorders once considered prime targets for gene therapy. Thus, the interface between gene therapy and *cell transplantation* is complementary.

The production of *genetically engineered proteins* is another area closely aligned with gene therapy. The cloning of human genes allows proteins to be produced in unlimited quantities and free of the potential contaminants associated with their purification from natural sources such as plasma. Moreover, recombinant DNA technology allows these proteins to be modified in ways that can enhance their therapeutic benefit. Examples of recombinant proteins are listed in Table 69-1. These include: (1) hormones such as insulin, growth hormone, and gonadotropins; (2) factors used to enhance blood cell production including erythropoietin, granulocyte colony stimulating factor (CSF), granulocyte-macrophage CSF, and thrombopoietin; (3) interferons (IFNs) and interleukins (ILs) used to treat a variety of autoimmune, infectious, and neoplastic diseases; (4) clotting factors VIII and IX; (5) thrombolytic agents such as tissue plasminogen activator or the antithrombotic agent hirudin; (6) recombinant antigens used for hepatitis B vaccines; and (7) humanized monoclonal antibodies used for immunosuppression or to treat specific types of malignancy. Although these recombinant proteins are an indirect form of gene therapy, they represent an important outgrowth of genetic medicine.

Long-Term versus Transient Gene Delivery Strategies for Gene Therapy The goals of gene therapy vary depending on the nature of the disease being treated. For an inherited, monogenic disorder such as hemophilia, the goal is lifelong replacement of the missing gene product. Expression of the missing secreted clotting factor, even at modest levels, might ameliorate the disease or reduce the need for exogenous treatment. For other inherited disorders, such as sickle cell anemia, strategies for gene replacement are more demanding. In this case, there is a requirement for cell-specific and exquisitely regulated expression of the transferred gene, and one is still faced with endogenous expression of the mutant form of β-globin. Long-term gene delivery strategies typically involve direct modification of host chromosomal sequences, which allows normal inheritance and stability of the delivered gene.

A growing use of gene therapy involves transient gene expression

Table 69-1 Examples of Genetically Engineered Recombinant Proteins

Recombinant Proteins	Clinical Applications[a]
Hormones/growth factors	
Growth hormone	Growth hormone deficiency
Insulin-like growth factor 1	Growth disorders resistant to growth hormone
Insulin	Diabetes mellitus
Follicle-stimulating hormone	Ovulation induction
Luteinizing hormone	Ovulation induction
Thyroid-stimulating hormone	^{131}I scanning in thyroid cancer
Leptin	Obesity
Platelet-derived growth factor	Wound healing in diabetic ulcers
Blood cell stimulatory factors	
Erythropoietin	Anemia
Granulocyte CSF	Neutropenia
Granulocyte-macrophage CSF	Neutropenia
Thrombopoietin	Thrombocytopenia
Interleukin (IL) 11	Thrombocytopenia
Cytokines	
Interferon α-2a	Hepatitis C
Interferon β-1a	Multiple sclerosis
Interferon α-2b	Follicular lymphoma
IL-2	Renal cell carcinoma
IL-2 α receptor	Immunosuppression in renal transplantation
Soluble tumor necrosis factor α receptor	Rheumatoid arthritis
Clotting factors/anticoagulants	
Factor VIII	Hemophilia A
Factor IX	Hemophilia B
Tissue-plasminogen activator	Myocardial infarction, stroke, pulmonary embolus
Hirudin	Deep vein thrombosis
Enzymes	
Adenosine deaminase	Severe combined immune deficiency (SCID)
Glucocerebrosidase	Gaucher disease
Monoclonal antibodies	
Epidermal growth factor receptor	Breast cancer
IL-2α	Immunosuppression in renal transplantation
Tumor necrosis factor	Crohn's disease
GPIIb/IIIa receptor	Prevent platelet aggregation after angioplasty
CD20	Follicular lymphoma
Vaccines	
Hepatitis B antigen vaccine	Hepatitis B

[a] The efficacy and approval of some of these agents remain under investigation.
NOTE: CSF, colony stimulating factor.

to treat a variety of diseases (Table 69-2). Gene therapy is now being considered or used for (1) killing cancer cells; (2) providing chemoprotection to normal cells; (3) preventing coronary restenosis or enhancing vascularization; (4) providing DNA-based immunization (e.g., viral DNA), in which the injection of DNA results in antigen expression and generation of an immune response; and (5) impairing viral replication. In cancer therapy, for example, the requirements for long-term gene expression and the level of gene expression are not as stringent as for gene replacement. Rather, the challenge of many cancer-based gene therapies is to achieve highly efficient gene transfer into cancer cells without expression in surrounding normal cells.

EX VIVO VERSUS IN VIVO ADMINISTRATION OF GENE THERAPY Gene therapy has been administered ex vivo for conditions in which cells can be readily harvested, manipulated in tissue culture, and then reintroduced into the patient. The ex vivo approach is potentially applicable to a variety of hematologic or immune deficiency disorders. For example, in adenosine deaminase (ADA) deficiency, the missing ADA gene has been integrated into the patient's T lymphocytes, which are then reintroduced after genetic manipulation. In familial hypercholesterolemia, an analogous approach has been

Table 69-2 Examples of Disorders Potentially Amenable to Gene Therapy

Disease	Gene Therapy Strategy
Inherited disorders	Gene addition
Cystic fibrosis	Express CFTR in pulmonary system and/or GI tract
Familial hypercholesterolemia	Express low-density lipoprotein receptor in liver
Hemophilias A and B	Express factor VIII or IX and secrete in circulation
Thalassemia	Express normal globin in red blood cells
Immunodeficiencies	Express mutant genes, such as adenosine deaminase
Metabolic disorders	Express missing enzymes or transporters
Duchenne's muscular dystrophy	Express mutant dystrophin protein in muscle cells
Retinitis pigmentosa (recessive)	Express normal protein in retina
	Gene correction
Lesch-Nyhan	Modify hypoxanthine phosphoribosyl transferase locus
Retinitis pigmentosa (dominant)	Correct missense mutation
Sickle cell disease	Correct β-globin mutation
Cystic fibrosis	Correct ΔF508 mutation in pulmonary system
Cardiovascular diseases	Modify vascular biology
Coronary artery restenosis	Block cell proliferation in vessel wall
Peripheral vascular disease	Induce angiogenesis
Hypertension	Express genes (e.g., tissue kallikrein) to induce vasodilation
Cancer	Multiples approaches
Many types	Express immunostimulants in or near malignant cells
	Express toxic genes in tumor cells (e.g., herpes simplex virus–TK)
	Express genes in normal cells to protect from chemotherapy
Infectious diseases	
Viral diseases	Express genes that block viral replication or function, including ribozymes, decoys, dominant negative proteins
Many	Express antigens as recombinant vaccines
Miscellaneous	
Rheumatoid arthritis	Express anti-inflammatory cytokines in joints
Parkinson's disease	Express genes required for L-dopa synthesis in striatum
Neurodegenerative disease	Express neurotrophic factors

NOTE: CFTR, cystic fibrous transmembrane regulator.

used for ex vivo treatment of hepatocytes. After surgical resection of liver tissue, the low-density lipoprotein (LDL) receptor gene is inserted into hepatocytes in cell culture, and the modified cells are infused back through the portal vein. Another form of ex vivo gene therapy involves the treatment of saphenous veins with oligonucleotides designed to block vascular smooth-muscle cell proliferation before using the tissue for coronary artery bypass graft.

In vivo approaches to gene therapy vary depending on the nature of the disease. In cystic fibrosis, an aerosol has been used to administer viral vectors to the lung. Factor IX expression has been achieved by introduction of the gene into muscle. Tumors have been injected directly with viral vectors expressing cytotoxic genes or immunotherapies. A major advantage of in vivo approaches is the potential to target cells that cannot easily be removed from the patient.

GENE TRANSFER VECTORS

A vector, or vehicle, is required to transfer a gene to an appropriate cell. When the goal is to add a gene (often called a *transgene*) to supply a function not present in the recipient cell, the vector typically contains DNA sequences encoding a therapeutic protein under the control of transcriptional regulatory elements necessary for gene expression (Fig. 69-1). The gene is expressed from an ectopic location as opposed to its normal chromosomal position. An alternative strategy is to correct mutant genes at their normal chromosomal location through *gene targeting*. Although this represents an ideal approach for many genetic diseases, it is far more technically demanding, and therapeutic gene-targeting efficiencies are difficult to achieve currently.

Two major classes of vectors are used for transferring nucleic acids into cells for the purposes of gene therapy: viral and nonviral vectors. *Viral vectors* have been genetically engineered so that the viruses transfer exogenous (therapeutic) nucleic acids into cells through a process called transduction. *Nonviral vectors* consist of nucleic acids that

are typically complexed with other chemicals to facilitate gene transfer. Although nonviral vectors offer improved safety by avoiding viral components, their gene transfer efficiencies are generally much lower than those of viral vectors. The major vector systems currently used in clinical trials or under development are summarized in Table 69-3.

Vectors that integrate into host chromosomes are considered ideal for lifelong gene expression, whereas episomal (unintegrated) vectors are preferred for transient gene delivery. The host range of a particular vector, in combination with the mode of delivery, will determine which cell types can be genetically modified. Also, it may be possible to alter the natural tropism of viral capsids or envelopes, as well as of nonviral vector complexes, to limit transduction to particular cell types. Transcriptional control elements, such as promoters and enhancers, can be used to regulate expression of the transgene. In some cases, the inclusion of special regulatory elements may allow gene expression to be controlled by the administration of pharmacologic agents that specifically switch the regulatory elements on or off. Many types of vectors, each exhibiting a unique set of properties, will ultimately be needed for safe and effective gene therapy of different diseases.

RETROVIRAL VECTORS Retroviral vectors based on murine leukemia viruses (MLVs) were the first vectors used in clinical gene transfer protocols and illustrate many of the principles of viral-mediated gene therapy. Typically, the vector genome consists of a transgene cassette placed between the two *cis*-acting long terminal repeats (LTRs) of the viral genome. Viral coding regions are removed from the vector genome to allow the insertion of the therapeutic gene and to prevent viral replication and toxicity to the host. The packaging capacity of MLV vectors is approximately 8 kb (including the LTRs), enough to accommodate most therapeutic cDNAs. The viral gene products needed for vector production and packaging are supplied by helper virus expression constructs.

The envelope protein of the virus interacts with specific cellular receptors to allow cellular entry of the core proteins and vector genome. After transduction, the vector gene integrates at random locations in host chromosomes and replicates with the host chromosome during cell proliferation, offering the potential for lifelong transgene expression. *Chromosomal integration* may also cause insertional mutagenesis, but no clinically relevant consequences of such events have been observed to date with replication-incompetent retroviral vectors.

Although MLV vectors are widely used, primarily because of their ability to integrate and simple production requirements, they still have significant disadvantages. Complement-mediated vector particle inactivation has largely limited their use to ex vivo applications. MLV vectors also require cell division for transduction because the vector genome can only enter the cell nucleus during mitosis, when the nuclear membrane breaks down. Since the majority of cells present in the human body are nondividing, this severely limits the potential uses of MLV-based vectors.

Promising new retroviral vectors are based on complex retroviruses (rather than the relatively simple oncoviruses such as MLV). Both lentiviral vectors and spumaviral vectors have broad host ranges, improved transduction of nondividing cells, and may function well in vivo. Although lentiviral vector production systems can be designed to eliminate the potential for replication-competent retrovirus contamination, and these vectors appear safe from a virologic standpoint, the

| Regulated promoter | Therapeutic Gene | Transgene |

| Viral DNA | | Viral DNA | Recombinant viral DNA |

Virus packaging and production in cell lines

Viral vectors

Ex vivo or in vivo transduction

Cell entry — *Expression of therapeutic gene product*

DNA integration or episomal maintenance — *Nucleus* — *Patient's transduced target cell*

FIGURE 69-1 General design of viral vectors used for gene therapy.

stigma associated with vectors based on human pathogens such as HIV may limit their acceptance.

ADENOVIRAL VECTORS Adenoviral-mediated gene expression is not lifelong, making it well suited for applications that require transient gene expression. In contrast to retroviruses, which integrate into the host genome, the adenoviral vector genome remains *episomal*, or extrachromosomal. Adenoviral vectors typically are derived from serotypes 2 or 5 and contain double-stranded DNA genomes. Wild-type adenovirus encodes over 50 peptides on overlapping gene fragments from both DNA strands. Nonessential viral genes have been removed to make room for up to 8 kb of exogenous DNA. The vector containing the therapeutic transgene is amplified in a cell line that supplies viral proteins needed for replication and packaging. Recombinant adenoviruses can be generated at high titers in the range of 10^{13} to 10^{14} particles per milliliter, a feature that is important for efficient in vivo gene therapy.

In clinical practice, adenoviral vectors are limited by relatively short durations of expression (usually several weeks) and by the synthesis of remaining cytotoxic or antigenic viral proteins that can cause an acute inflammatory response and/or a robust cellular immune response. These features of the virus ap-

pear to have contributed to hepatic failure and death in an individual receiving adenoviral-based gene therapy for ornithine transcarbamylase deficiency. On the other hand, the inflammatory properties of adenoviruses may enhance their efficacy in cancer trials, as discussed below. Several methods that eliminate the remaining viral genes have been devised recently, and these "gutted" vectors appear to exhibit much reduced toxicity and inflammatory properties in comparison to previous generations of adenoviral vectors.

ADENO-ASSOCIATED VIRUS VECTORS Adeno-associated viruses (AAV) are parvoviruses that normally require a helper virus, such as adenovirus, to mediate a productive infection. A major limitation of the AAV vector is its relatively small packaging capacity, which restricts the size of exogenous DNA to about 4.5 kb. AAV vectors have been shown to transduce cells both through episomal transgene expression and by chromosomal integration. They can also be used to modify homologous chromosomal sequences through gene targeting, which is an important strategy for the correction of genetic mutations.

Since the AAV vector genome lacks viral coding sequences, the vector itself causes little immune or inflammatory response (except for the generation of neutralizing antibodies that may limit readministration). The vector particle can be delivered to many different organs [e.g., the central nervous system (CNS), liver, lung, and muscle] by in vivo administration, and AAV vectors have been found to transduce nondividing cells efficiently. Clinical trials using AAV for the treatment of cystic fibrosis and hemophilia are underway.

OTHER VIRAL VECTORS Many other viruses are under development as vector systems, such as herpesviruses, double-stranded RNA viruses, autonomous parvoviruses, and papovaviruses. Hybrid viral vectors that use components from more than one virus are also under development, offering the potential to combine the most desirable properties of different vectors. Ultimately, vectors will be developed that utilize both viral components and synthetic functions, allowing vectors to be custom designed.

NONVIRAL VECTORS Nonviral vectors usually consist of DNA complexes with lipids, carbohydrates, proteins, and/or other synthetic chemicals to facilitate delivery or increase vector stability. Gene delivery with naked DNA is also possible but is relatively inefficient.

Table 69-3 Properties of Vectors Used for Gene Therapy

Vector	Production	Cell Cycle Effects	Expression	Gene Status	Toxicity
Retrovirus (MLV-based)	Simple but low titers ~10^6 particles/mL	Mitosis required	Persistent	Integrated	Safe
Lentivirus	Can be concentrated to ~10^9 particles/mL	Cell division not always required	Persistent	Integrated	Untested
Adenovirus	Easily produced at titers up to 10^{13}–10^{14} particles/mL	Quiescent or dividing cells	Transient	Episomal	Initial vectors toxic; gutted vectors much improved
AAV	Difficult process, but high titers possible, ~10^{12} particles/mL	Quiescent or dividing cells, DNA synthesis sometimes beneficial	Persistent or transient	Integrated or episomal, often in concatamers	Safe
Nonviral	Highly concentrated	Quiescent or dividing cells	Transient	Episomal	Variable, based on type and dose

NOTE: MLV, murine leukemia virus; AAV, adeno-associated virus.

Nonviral vectors are desirable because they eliminate the risk of viral contamination and can be produced under more controlled conditions. Their major disadvantage is low gene transfer rates, at least in relation to most viral vector systems. Because the vectors do not integrate and the majority of DNA molecules that enter the cell are rapidly degraded, only transient gene expression is possible. Examples of applications that may be well suited to gene delivery with nonviral vectors include vaccination with specific antigen genes, ex vivo treatment of vessels used for coronary artery bypass graft, and perhaps transient immune modulation for the treatment of cancer.

Nonviral vectors composed of RNA or modified nucleotides may also prove useful, if problems associated with effective delivery can be addressed. For example, antisense oligonucleotides can be used to inhibit gene expression by pairing with complementary mRNA molecules. Antisense oligonucleotides might be used, for example, to block the expression of cell cycle proteins or cytokines. Oligonucleotides with binding sites for specific DNA- or RNA-binding proteins may be designed to function as decoys that inhibit protein function. Chimeric RNA/DNA oligonucleotides have been used to introduce specific genetic modifications through gene targeting. In animal studies, this novel approach has been shown to work efficiently in the liver, and it may be used soon for clinical trials of uridine diphosphate–glucuronosyltransferase deficiency.

GENE THERAPY FOR SELECTED DISEASE CATEGORIES

LIVER AND GASTROINTESTINAL TRACT   The liver has been studied intensively as a target organ for gene therapy, in part because of the many genetic diseases amenable to gene replacement in hepatocytes. In addition, because of the regenerative capacity of the hepatocyte, integration of a vector offers the possibility of lifelong gene expression. The first hepatic gene therapy attempted in humans involved the ex vivo transplant of autologous hepatocytes transduced in culture by retroviral vectors encoding the LDL receptor as a treatment for familial hypercholesterolemia. Due to the low levels (nontherapeutic) of gene expression observed and the labor-intensive nature of the ex vivo transduction process, current strategies are geared towards in vivo gene transfer. MLV-based retroviral vectors require cell division for transduction of host cells. The use of growth factors (rather than partial hepatectomy) to stimulate hepatocellular replication can enhance the efficacy of MLV vectors. Alternative retroviral vectors based on lentiviruses may overcome these obstacles.

Adenovirus vectors are very effective at gene transfer into the liver, thus allowing for the transduction of a majority of hepatocytes. However, the early generations of these vectors exhibited dose-dependent toxicity, inflammation, and immunogenicity that limited the persistence of transgene expression. Adenoviral vectors devoid of all viral genes have been shown to transduce hepatocytes efficiently with reduced toxicity or immunogenicity. In rodents, transgene expression appears to be lifelong, but in nonhuman primates, expression declines by 90% over a 2-year period.

AAV vectors stably integrate their proviral DNA into hepatocytes in vivo with no apparent toxicity. This vector has been used in preclinical liver gene therapy studies to cure mice with hemophilia B and to partially correct the defect in dogs with hemophilia B. Hepatocyte gene transfer by AAV vectors is likely to be useful for treating a variety of metabolic diseases, such as urea cycle disorders, aminoacidopathies, disorders of carbohydrate metabolism, and lysosomal storage diseases. This strategy is particularly applicable when expression of the transgene in a relatively small percentage of hepatocytes is of therapeutic benefit.

The intestinal tract offers a large cell mass for gene therapy and is accessible by oral administration of vectors. Although a number of vectors have been tested in the gastrointestinal tract, major limitations still exist, such as the rapid turnover of the intestinal epithelial cells, the inability to target the stem or early progenitor cells, and the effects of digestive secretions on vector delivery. If these obstacles can be overcome, many diseases may be amenable to treatment by intestinal gene transfer.

THE HEMATOPOIETIC SYSTEM   Clinical trials targeting hematopoietic cells have almost exclusively taken an ex vivo approach, with gene transfer occurring outside the body, followed by reinfusion of transduced cells. The most common cellular targets are lymphocytes and hematopoietic stem cells. Because stem cells can reconstitute the entire hematopoietic system, ex vivo genetic manipulation and autologous transplantation of bone marrow or peripheral blood stem cells represents a powerful therapeutic paradigm. Long-term gene transfer to hematopoietic stem cells requires the use of integrating viral vectors to ensure that the transgene replicates with the chromosomes during the extensive cellular proliferation that occurs during hematopoiesis. Thus, most stem cell gene therapy trials have used retroviral vectors. In part, because stem cells are not actively dividing, transduction rates have been too low to be therapeutic. Despite this, recent success in treating X-linked severe combined immunodeficiency with MLV vectors encoding the cytokine receptor gamma common chain demonstrates the feasibility of this approach. The use of different envelope proteins and vectors based on lentiviruses or spumaviruses may yield greater success in stem cell transduction.

Gene transfer to hematopoietic stem cells could be used to treat diseases of erythroid, myeloid, and lymphoid cells as well as platelet disorders (since the stem cell ultimately differentiates into all these cell types). An important aspect of this approach is the level of myeloablation required to allow engraftment of ex vivo–modified stem cells. An optimal therapy would minimize myeloablation and its associated toxicity, perhaps by delivering a gene that confers a selective advantage to transduced stem cells along with the therapeutic transgene. Many of the clinical trials to date have involved genes that confer increased resistance to chemotherapeutic agents used in treating cancer. An alternative strategy is to apply gene therapy to disorders in which expression is not required in all cells to prevent clinical disease. In chronic granulomatous disease, in which there is failure of granulocytes and monocytes to generate the hydrogen peroxide needed for bacterial killing, it may be feasible to achieve a threshold level of normal cells to respond to infections. Another major area of stem cell gene therapy research is the treatment of hemoglobinopathies with vectors expressing globin genes. Although clinical trials have not begun, these efforts have helped define the problems that must be solved for successful stem cell gene therapy, especially with regard to regulating transgene expression levels. Globin gene replacement is a daunting task, since the gene must be expressed at high levels in a select subset of erythroid cells, thus requiring the inclusion of a variety of transcriptional control elements in the vector (many of which have resulted in vector instability and low viral titers).

Lymphocyte gene transfer has the potential to treat genetic immunodeficiencies and to modulate immune functions. ADA deficiency was one of the first diseases to be treated with gene therapy and employed ex vivo transduction of lymphocytes. Although this early clinical trial represented an important milestone in gene therapy, the assessment of a therapeutic effect has been complicated by concomitant treatment with the ADA protein. Replacement of the ADA gene also confers a selective advantage to ADA-deficient lymphocytes, a property that would not be generally applicable to lymphocyte gene transfer. Still, as lymphocyte transduction protocols improve, many treatments may be developed with this cellular target, especially for acquired diseases. Genetic manipulations with antibody or cytokine genes offer a multitude of possible treatments for infectious and autoimmune diseases, as well as for cancer.

PULMONARY SYSTEM   Gene therapy of the lung has concentrated primarily on treatments for cystic fibrosis. The gene for cystic fibrosis, *CFTR*, was cloned in 1989; by 1993 the first trials using adenovirus vectors were attempted in the nasal epithelium and airway. Though no clinical efficacy was demonstrated, these studies underscored the need to develop defined clinical endpoints for future trials. In addition to the adenovirus trials, clinical trials with nonviral liposome and AAV vectors also failed to demonstrate therapeutic effects. Difficulties encountered in pulmonary gene therapy include poor vector delivery due to respiratory secretions, lack of accessible vector receptors on the exposed cellular surface, transient transgene expression due to turnover of the respiratory epithelium, and vector-induced inflammation and pneumonitis. It also remains unclear which type of lung cells should be targeted with the *CFTR* gene to result in clinical benefit. As efficient and safe vectors for lung gene transfer are developed, treatments for acquired disorders such as chronic obstructive pulmonary disease may also be possible.

NERVOUS SYSTEM AND RETINA Gene transfer to the nervous system will be important for the treatment of many inherited and acquired neurologic diseases. Depending on the disorder, both glial cells and neurons may be appropriate cellular targets. Several vectors have been shown to transduce cells (including neurons) in animals after in vivo injection into the brain. Gene transfer is typically localized near the site of injection, a feature that is desirable for disorders such as Parkinson's disease, where transduction in the striatum could allow selective expression of genes involved in dopamine synthesis. Vector delivery throughout the nervous system will be more difficult to achieve, making gene therapy of global neurologic disorders problematic. The possibility of delivering neurotrophic factors to the CNS is a potential strategy for the treatment of neurodegenerative diseases, such as amyotrophic lateral sclerosis, and for facilitating recovery after spinal cord injury. Genetically modified stem cells have also been suggested as a strategy for the treatment of neurodegenerative disorders, but studies of these cells are at very early stages.

Retinitis pigmentosa (RP), a common cause of blindness from retinal degeneration, represents one class of disorders that stands to benefit from gene therapy. Though many different gene defects may cause RP, treatment of a form caused by mutation in the rod photoreceptor cGMP phosphodiesterase β-subunit gene has been studied in animal models by intraocular gene addition with adenovirus, lentivirus, and AAV vectors. In a different type of RP, progression of an autosomal dominant form of the disease was significantly slowed in a transgenic rat model using AAV vectors that express *ribozymes* (RNA enzymes) against the mutant mRNA. Ribozymes are catalytically active RNA molecules that specifically anneal to, and cleave, other RNA sequences, resulting in their selective degradation. This strategy may be useful for the treatment of other genetic diseases caused by dominant mutations. Viral vectors that express cytotoxic genes have been used to treat CNS tumors (see below).

MUSCULOSKELETAL SYSTEM Efficient gene transfer to myotubes through intramuscular injection has been demonstrated with adenoviral vectors, AAV vectors, and lentiviral vectors. In the case of AAV vectors, long-term transgene expression in muscles has been observed in several animal species. The treatment of the muscular dystrophies will require efficient delivery to multiple muscle groups throughout the body, and vector delivery to all the necessary locations remains a formidable task. In the case of Duchenne muscular dystrophy, the large size of the dystrophin cDNA also poses technical challenges in vector design. In contrast to primary diseases of muscle, success is more likely in muscle gene therapy trials aimed at the synthesis of secreted proteins, such as clotting factors. The large tissue mass and accessibility of muscle make it particularly attractive for these applications.

CARDIOVASCULAR SYSTEM The cardiovascular system (including the peripheral vasculature) has become an important target for gene therapy. Vascular wall gene delivery is being studied as a way to inhibit smooth-muscle cell proliferation and prevent restenosis. The transgenes used in this application are designed to interfere with the cell cycle or induce apoptosis in smooth-muscle cells. This approach is especially attractive if the vector can be delivered during angioplasty.

Other gene therapy strategies are used to promote the vascularization of tissues. There is some evidence for a therapeutic response in patients with critical limb ischemia due to poor peripheral vascularization who received intramuscular injection of naked DNA vectors encoding the vascular endothelial growth factor (VEGF) gene. Small amounts of the protein are secreted from the muscle, resulting in collateral vessel development that can reverse the ischemia. Patients who were expected to require limb amputation were spared this procedure after gene therapy. Similar clinical trials with the VEGF gene using nonviral and viral vectors are being studied in the context of myocardial ischemia.

CANCER Most of the gene therapy clinical trials to date have been aimed at the treatment of cancer. One approach uses gene therapy with cytokine or neoantigen genes to increase tumor immunogenicity. The vector is usually injected directly into the tumor, and there is some evidence that once the immune system is stimulated, nontransduced tumor cells may also be eliminated by the immune system. In melanoma, for example, cells have been genetically altered to express mismatched histocompatibility antigens or cytokines such as tumor necrosis factor, IFN-γ, or IL-2 in an effort to stimulate an immune response. Another approach involves the delivery of genes to tumor cells that convert a prodrug into a cytotoxic compound. Although several strategies are being developed, the most common involves the transfer of the herpes thymidine kinase (TK) gene. The TK enzyme converts gancyclovir into a thymidine analogue that interferes with DNA synthesis and causes cell death. The toxic effects also occur in adjacent nontransduced cells due to the uptake of the toxic analogue; this process is referred to as the *bystander effect*. Vectors designed to replace defective tumor-suppressor proteins with normal versions are being considered for cancer gene therapy, but it is difficult to envision success with this approach unless virtually all the tumor cells are genetically modified. Genes that control tumor growth when expressed in nontumor cells may also be effective in cancer gene therapy. The delivery of gene products that interfere with tumor angiogenesis best exemplifies this approach. Finally, lytic viral vectors that selectively replicate and kill malignant cells are being developed. One example is an adenovirus designed to replicate in cells deficient in p53, a tumor-suppressor protein that is mutated in many different cancers.

These and other related strategies have shown efficacy in animal models when tumor cells are transplanted into various anatomic locations. These models do not always emulate the natural processes that result in bonafide cancers, in part due to the tumor cells not being truly autologous in origin. Although there have been encouraging results in some of the clinical trials performed to date, efficacy has not been demonstrated definitively. In many cases the patient populations studied had advanced malignancies, and more informative results might be obtained at earlier disease stages. Still, cancer gene therapy has a promising future, and ongoing research involving tumor-specific antigens, angiogenesis, cell cycle control, and apoptosis are all likely to lead to new gene therapy approaches. Improvements in vector targeting of tumor cells and in the development of tumor-specific gene expression will also enhance future therapeutic approaches.

COAGULOPATHIES Inherited coagulopathies, especially hemophilia A and B, are promising areas of gene therapy research because even a low level of coagulation factor reconstitution can potentially benefit a patient with a severe phenotype. Although the liver is the major site of synthesis for factors VIII and IX, several other tissues may support factor synthesis and secretion into the bloodstream. AAV vectors, in particular, have shown prolonged therapeutic effects in animal models of hemophilia B when delivered to muscle or liver. Hemophilia A has been more difficult to treat, due to the larger cDNA (which approaches the packaging capacity of AAV vectors) and the requirement that expressing cells deliver the protein directly into the intravascular space. Other coagulopathies, such as factor X deficiency, are also good candidates for gene therapy. Various approaches to the treatment of hemophilia are currently in the early stages of clinical trials.

INFECTIOUS DISEASES Most infectious pathogens studied as targets for gene therapy are viral (particularly HIV), in part because they replicate inside human cells. One approach involves introducing inhibitory versions of essential viral proteins that disrupt the viral life cycle even in the presence of their normal counterparts (e.g., by disrupting the packaging of virions). Another strategy involves the expression of proteins, peptides, or even RNA transcripts that function as decoys by binding to other proteins required for viral replication and preventing them from acting on their normal viral target sites. The cellular proteins required for a pathogen's life cycle, such as receptor molecules used for viral entry, or specific proteins used for adherence of the pathogen, can also be manipulated through gene therapy; this tactic could also be applied to nonviral pathogens. Ribozymes can be engineered to cleave specific viral transcripts, thereby blocking expression of viral gene products or destroying viral genomes (in the case of RNA viruses). Because ribozymes can, in principle, be engineered to attack any RNA transcript, they are being considered as treatments for many different viral diseases. Clinical trials have begun using ribozymes to block HIV infection. Antisense oligonucleotides can also be used to interfere with viral or cellular nucleic acid sequences. Other gene therapy approaches that may be applied to infectious diseases include vaccination with specific antigens and manipulation of the immune system to enhance the clearance of pathogens.

SUMMARY

The gene can be thought of as a new pharmaceutical agent in the armamentarium used to treat disease. The availability of cloned genes has already yielded a large array of recombinant proteins for clinical use. The limited success of gene therapy to date is due primarily to difficulties inherent in the efficient and safe delivery of genes to their appropriate target cells. The field is still in its infancy, and many of the technical problems are likely to be solved by advances in vector design.

BIBLIOGRAPHY

AMADO RG, CHEN ISY: Lentiviral vectors—the promise of gene therapy within reach? Science 285:674, 1999

BLAESE M et al: T lymphocyte–directed gene therapy for ADA-SCID: Initial trial results after 4 years. Science 270:475, 1995

CAVAZZANA-CALVO M et al: Gene therapy of human severe combined immunodeficiency (SCID)-X1 disease. Science 288:669, 2000

FERRY N, HEARD JM: Liver-directed gene transfer vectors. Hum Gene Ther 9:1975, 1998

HALL SJ et al: The promise and reality of cancer gene therapy. Am J Hum Genet 61:785, 1997

HITT MM et al: Human adenovirus vectors for gene transfer into mammalian cells. Adv Pharmacol 40:137, 1997

KAY MA et al: Evidence for gene transfer and expression of blood coagulation factor IX in patients with severe hemophilia B treated with an AA vector. Nat Genet 24:257, 2000

MILLER AD: Development and applications of retroviral vectors, in *Retroviruses*, JM Coffin, SH Hughes, HE Varmus (eds). Cold Spring Harbor, NY, Cold Spring Harbor Laboratory, 1997, p 437

MORSY MA, CASKEY CT: Expanded-capacity adenoviral vectors—the helper dependent vectors. Mol Med Today 5:18, 1999

NABEL GJ: Immune recognition of malignancies: Relevance to immunotherapy. Cancer J Sci Am Suppl 1:S106, 1998

ORKIN SH, MOTULSKY AG: Report and recommendations of the panel to assess the NIH investment in research on gene therapy. www.nih.gov/news/panelrep.html

ROTH JA, CHRISTIANO RJ: Gene therapy for cancer: What have we done and where are we going? J Natl Cancer Inst 89:21, 1997

RUSSELL DW, KAY MA: Adeno-associated virus vectors and hematology. Blood 94:864, 1999

SVENSSON EC, SCHWARTZ LB: Gene therapy for vascular disease. Curr Opin Cardiol 13:369, 1998

NOBEL PRIZE IN PHYSIOLOGY OR MEDICINE, 1905

Robert Koch was born in Prussia on December 11, 1843. He was the third of thirteen children. He was a brilliant student, entering *Gymnasium* (German high school) at 8 years of age. He then matriculated into the University of Göttingen, where he studied medicine. In 1866 he graduated from medical school and started a general practice in Hamburg. His practice was interrupted by the Franco-German War. After discharge from the army, he became a public health physician in Wollstein, Germany. It was there that Koch launched his scientific career. He studied anthrax and developed techniques for the microscopy of bacteria. Earlier, Louis Pasteur had proposed the germ theory of disease, but leading pathologists, including Rudolph Virchow and Theodore Billroth, had rejected this possibility. It was Robert Koch's work on anthrax that convinced skeptics that microorganisms could cause infectious diseases. In 1880 Robert Koch moved to Berlin to become a member of the Imperial Health Office where he developed his culture plating technique, which is used basically unchanged today.

His real fame came in 1882 when he identified the tubercle bacillus as the cause of tuberculosis. Koch's postulates to incriminate microorganisms in causing an infectious disease are still the standard in microbiology. The organisms must be isolated and grown in pure culture from the infected tissue. The pure culture must then be shown to induce the disease experimentally and be recovered from the experimental animal. Koch accomplished all facets of this experimental design with tuberculosis by using a guinea pig model. He went on to study cholera in Egypt and India. In Calcutta, Koch was able to isolate a pure culture of the cholera bacterium from autopsy specimens, which was morphologically the same comma bacillus as seen in Egyptian samples. In epidemiologic studies he demonstrated that cholera could be spread by contaminated water, a finding that led to control of the dreaded disease by water filtration. Koch then returned to the study of tuberculosis. He proposed that a glycerin extract of the tubercle bacilli, tuberculin, would lead to immunization against tuberculosis. Although patients with tuberculosis, but not healthy subjects, had a generalized and local reaction to tuberculin, immunity to tuberculosis was not achieved.

Koch's early warnings about the transmission of tuberculosis from human to human went largely unheeded. Eventually, however, measures were instituted around the world to prevent the spread of tuberculosis from infected individuals' sputum to other individuals. Koch was in Africa studying tropical diseases when he heard he had been awarded the 1905 Nobel Prize in Physiology or Medicine. He received the Nobel Prize for his contributions in tuberculosis, including identifying the causative agent and advocating public health measures to decrease the spread of the disease. Robert Koch, however, made many other important contributions and clearly deserves to be regarded as one of the founding fathers of the science of bacteriology.

REFERENCES

1. Magill FN (ed): *Nobel Prize Winners: Physiology or Medicine*, vol 1. Pasadena, Salem Press, 1993
2. Schrier RW: *A Salute to Nobel Laureates in Physiology and Medicine*, Proceedings of the Association of American Physicians 108(1): Jan 1996
3. Sourkes TL: *Nobel Prize Winners in Medicine and Physiology 1901–1965*. London, Abelard-Schuman, 1967

Robert W. Schrier, MD

70

John A. Oates, Dan M. Roden, Grant R. Wilkinson

PRINCIPLES OF DRUG THERAPY

Safe and effective drug therapy requires that drugs be delivered to their molecular targets in tissues at concentrations within the range that yields efficacy without toxicity. Variability in drug effects between individual patients can thus be attributed, in part, to differences in the processes that determine these concentrations, i.e., drug disposition involving absorption, distribution, and elimination. *Pharmacokinetics* provides a quantitative description of these processes, i.e., what the body does to the drug. In addition, variability in response may also reflect differences in the drug-target interaction that affect the concentration-related effects of the drug on the body, termed *pharmacodynamics*. This chapter reviews the principles of pharmacokinetics and pharmacodynamics and their application to optimizing therapeutic regimens.

CLINICAL PHARMACOKINETICS

PLASMA LEVELS AFTER A SINGLE DOSE The levels of lidocaine in plasma following intravenous administration decline in two phases, as illustrated in Fig. 70-1; such a biphasic decline is typical for many drugs. Immediately after rapid injection, essentially all of the drug is in the plasma or central compartment, and the high initial plasma level reflects the confinement of the drug to this small volume. The drug is then transferred into an extravascular or peripheral compartment during a period called the *distribution phase*. For lidocaine, the distribution phase is virtually complete within 30 min. A phase of slower decline, the *equilibrium phase*, then occurs. During this phase, the drug levels in the plasma and in tissues change in parallel. Although this disposition profile is common to many drugs given intravenously, the characteristic parameters vary among drugs.

Distribution Phase The pharmacologic effects during the distribution phase depend on whether the concentration of drug at the receptor site is similar to that in the plasma. If that is the case, the pharmacologic effects may be intense during this period because of the high initial levels in the plasma. For example, after a small bolus

FIGURE 70-1 Concentrations of lidocaine in plasma following the administration of 50 mg intravenously. The half-life ($t_{1/2}$) of 108 min is computed as the time required for levels to fall from any given value during the equilibrium phase ($C_{initial}$) to one-half that level. C_0 is the hypothetical concentration of lidocaine in plasma at time zero if equilibrium had been achieved instantly.

dose (50 mg) of lidocaine, antiarrhythmic effects may be evident during the early distribution phase but will disappear as levels fall below those that are minimally effective, even before equilibrium between plasma and tissue is reached. Thus, a larger single dose or multiple small doses must be administered to achieve an effect that is sustained into the equilibrium phase. Toxicity resulting from high levels of some drugs during the distribution phase precludes administration of a single intravenous loading dose that will yield therapeutic levels during the equilibrium phase. For example, the administration of the entire loading dose of phenytoin as a single intravenous bolus can cause cardiovascular collapse due to the high levels during the distribution phase. If a loading dose of phenytoin is administered intravenously, it must be given slowly, e.g., at infusion rates of 25 to 50 mg/min. For similar reasons, the intravenous loading dose of many potent drugs that equilibrate rapidly with their receptors is either divided into fractional doses given at intervals or administered by infusion over a similar period.

A dose given orally results in lower plasma levels during the initial period than an intravenous bolus dose that delivers the same amount of drug to the systemic circulation. Because the drug is not absorbed instantly after oral administration and is delivered into the systemic circulation more slowly, much of it has been distributed by the time absorption is complete. Thus, procainamide, which is almost totally absorbed after oral administration, can be given orally as a single 750-mg loading dose with little risk of hypotension; in contrast, loading of this drug by the intravenous route is more safely accomplished by giving the dose in fractions of about 100 mg at 5-min intervals or by slow infusion to avoid hypotension during the distribution phase.

Some drugs are so predictably lethal when infused too rapidly that special precautions should be taken to prevent even the inadvertent occurrence. For example, solutions of potassium for intravenous administration in excess of 20 meq/L should be avoided in all but the most exceptional and carefully monitored circumstances. This minimizes the possibility of cardiac arrests, which can occur as a result of accidental increases in infusion rates of more concentrated solutions.

As these examples illustrate, excessively rapid administration of many drugs can lead to catastrophic consequences that result from high concentrations in the blood during the distribution phase.

In contrast, for some centrally active drugs, the higher concentration of drug during the distribution phase after intravenous administration is used to advantage. The use of midazolam for "IV sedation," for example, depends upon its rapid uptake by the brain during the distribution phase to produce sedation quickly, with subsequent egress from the brain during the redistribution of the drug as equilibrium is achieved.

Some drugs are distributed slowly to their sites of action during the distribution phase, i.e., concentration at the relevant receptor does not parallel that in plasma early after drug administration. For example, the level of digoxin at the receptor site (and the drug's pharmacologic effect) do not reflect plasma levels during the distribution phase. Digoxin is transported (or bound) to its cardiac receptors slowly by a process that proceeds throughout distribution. Thus, over the distribution phase of several hours, plasma levels fall while the level at the site of action and the pharmacologic effect increase. Only at the end of the distribution phase, when the drug has reached equilibrium with the receptor, does the concentration of digoxin in plasma reflect pharmacologic effect. For this reason, there should be a 6- to 8-h wait after administration before plasma levels of digoxin are measured as a guide to therapy.

Equilibrium Phase After the concentration of drug in plasma has reached a dynamic equilibrium with that in the tissues, the levels in plasma and tissues fall in parallel as the drug is eliminated from the

Table 70-1   Amount of a Drug Dose Remaining in Body over Successive Half-Lives

No. of Elapsed Half-Lives	Amount of Dose Remaining in Body, %	Amount of Dose Eliminated, %
1	50.00	50.00
2	25.00	75.00
3	12.50	87.50
4	6.25	93.75
5	3.125	96.875

FIGURE 70-2   Time course of digoxin accumulation following repeated 0.25 mg/d oral maintenance dose administration (solid line), assuming bioavailability is about 85%. The smooth (dashed line) curve depicts the pattern of accumulation following administration of an equivalent dosing rate (150 ng/min) by continuous intravenous infusion. Note that accumulation and elimination are >90% complete after four half-lives and this is independent of the dosing regimen. Also, that steady state is proportional to the dosing rate (dose/dosing interval) and the ratio of bioavailability to clearance. The temporal relationships shown apply equally well to other drugs with linear pharmacokinetics and one-compartment distribution. For comparison, the plasma concentration-time curve if only the first dose were given is also shown (dotted line). $C_{max,ss}$, maximum plasma concentration at steady state; C_{avg}, average plasma concentration; C_{min}, minimal plasma concentration.

body. Thus, the equilibrium phase is also called the *elimination phase.* During this phase, drug concentrations measured in plasma can provide a useful index of drug levels in tissues.

Most drugs are eliminated as a first-order process. This means that the time required for the plasma level of the drug to fall to one-half the original value (the half-life, $t_{1/2}$) is the same regardless of the point on the plasma level curve at which measurement begins. Another characteristic of the first-order process is that a plot of the logarithm of the plasma concentration versus time is linear. From such a plot (Fig. 70-1), it can be seen that the half-life of lidocaine is 108 min. If the half-life is known, the amount of a dose remaining in the body at any time following administration of a single dose can be calculated. Table 70-1 shows how this amount changes over five successive half-lives.

From a clinical standpoint, elimination is essentially complete when it has reached about 90%. Therefore, for practical purposes, *a first-order elimination process reaches completion after three to four half-lives.*

DRUG ACCUMULATION—LOADING AND MAINTENANCE DOSES   If a drug is given repeatedly at intervals shorter than the time required to eliminate a dose, both the amount of drug in the body and its pharmacologic effect increase with successive doses until they reach a plateau. Figure 70-2 shows the accumulation of digoxin administered in repeated maintenance doses (without a loading dose). Since the half-life of digoxin is about 1.6 days in a patient with normal renal function, 65% of a digoxin dose remains in the body at the end of 1 day. Thus, the second dose will raise the amount of digoxin in the body (and the average plasma level) to 165% of the level produced by the first dose. Each subsequent dose causes a further increase until a *steady state* is achieved. At that point, the drug dosing rate (bioavailable dose/dosage interval) is equal to the rate of elimination, with the fluctuation between peak and trough plasma levels remaining constant. If the rate of drug delivery is then altered, a new steady state will be attained. Continuous infusion of a drug at constant rate also results in progressive accumulation to a predictable steady state (Fig. 70-2). In this case, the steady-state plasma level (C_{ss}) is equivalent to the average between the peak and trough levels ($C_{avg,ss}$) produced by intermittent administration of the same amount of drug over the same period. For *all* drugs with first-order kinetics, the time required to achieve steady-state levels can be predicted from the half-life, because accumulation is a first-order process with a half-life identical to that for elimination. Thus, accumulation reaches 90% of steady-state levels at the end of three to four half-lives. This is true for either intermittent or continuous dosing (Fig. 70-2).

When a therapeutic effect is required urgently, simply administering the maintenance dose of a drug with a long half-life results in an unacceptable delay in reaching steady-state levels of the drug and its intended effect. The time required to achieve the desired pharmacologic effect may be shortened by the administration of a *loading dose*—the amount of drug that will bring the plasma concentration rapidly to the steady-state level. Therefore, if treatment with lidocaine ($t_{1/2} \sim 108$ min) were initiated by infusion at only the maintenance dose level, it would take about 4 to 8 h before the drug's maximal effect was achieved. Because ventricular arrhythmias may be life-threatening, it is not reasonable to wait that long to achieve an effective steady-state drug level. Accordingly, it would be appropriate to administer one or more loading doses at the onset of therapy, together with infusion at the rate of the maintenance dose.

Loading may be accomplished by the administration of a single loading dose or, if that would create a risk of toxicity, by the administration of the loading dose in a series of fractions of that dose over time. The latter approach is particularly appropriate for most drugs that have a low therapeutic index. A divided loading dose strategy or the administration of the loading dose in a slow intravenous infusion are particularly advisable when the drug is given intravenously. Thus, in the case of lidocaine, a common regimen is to administer an initial intravenous bolus of 1 mg/kg followed by up to three additional bolus injections of 0.5 mg/kg every 8 to 10 min as necessary, and a maintenance infusion of 2 mg/min.

Regardless of the size of the loading dose, *after maintenance therapy has been given for three to four half-lives, the amount of drug in the body is determined by the maintenance dose.* The independence of the steady state plasma levels from the loading dose is illustrated in Fig. 70-2, which shows that the elimination of the loading dose would be practically complete after three to four half-lives.

DETERMINANTS OF DRUG DISPOSITION   A number of physiologic and pathophysiologic factors determine the disposition of a drug and hence its pharmacokinetics in an individual patient. The three most important are *clearance*, a measure of the body's ability to eliminate drug; *volume of distribution*, an indication of the extent to which the drug is distributed outside of the blood compartment; and *bioavailability*, the fraction of the administered dose that reaches the systemic circulation. The elimination half-life ($t_{1/2}$), which measures the rate of drug removal from the body, is determined by the relationship between the physiologically determined clearance and volume of distribution.

Clearance   The majority of drugs are given over a prolonged period of time according to a multiple dosage regimen, e.g., x mg every y h. The clinical goal is to maintain the drug's steady-state concentration within the therapeutic range for the individual patient; if the level is too low, reduced efficacy results, whereas if it is too high, the likelihood of adverse effects increases.

Steady state is achieved when the rate of drug elimination equals the rate of drug delivery into the systemic circulation, which, if bioavailability is complete, corresponds to the rate at which the drug dose is administered:

$$\text{Dosing rate} = Cl \times C_{ss}$$
$$\text{(amt/unit time)} \quad \text{(vol/unit time)} \quad \text{(amt/vol)}$$

where Cl is clearance and C_{ss} is the steady-state concentration in plasma. Therefore, *at a given dosing rate the concentration of drug in plasma is completely dependent on its clearance.* If the drug is infused, the concentration remains constant so long as drug delivery continues; however, when the drug is given intermittently, the above relationship is expressed as:

$$\text{Dosing/dosage interval} = Cl \times C_{avg,ss}$$

where $C_{avg,ss}$ is the *average* value during the dosage interval and is equal to C_{ss} although the *actual* concentrations will be higher or lower at various points during this period. Thus, clearance determines the rate at which a drug should be administered in order to obtain a desired steady-state concentration; stated in a different fashion, steady-state drug levels can be modified either up or down by changing the dosage rate. *The clearance of the vast majority of drugs is constant over the therapeutic range of concentrations.*

Clearance is a measure of the rate at which the organs that eliminate drug from the body remove drug from the blood.

$$Cl = \text{Rate of elimination}/C$$

Accordingly, clearance reflects the volume of blood (or plasma) from which the drug would have to be removed per unit time to account for the elimination; it can be related to either total or unbound drug.

Drug elimination generally occurs as a result of metabolism and/or excretion in the liver, kidney, and possibly other organs. Clearance of drug from the body, therefore, reflects the overall contribution of each of these organs, as indicated by their individual rates of elimination normalized to the concentration of drug, and is additive.

$$Cl = Cl_{hepatic} + Cl_{renal} + Cl_{other}$$

Clearance of a drug is usually estimated following administration

of an intravenous dose ($dose_{iv}$) and measurement of the resulting total area under the curve (AUC) for the blood or plasma concentration-time curve (AUC_{iv}) from zero to infinite time.

$$Cl = dose_{iv}/AUC_{iv}$$

Table 70-2 indicates the marked differences in plasma clearance for some commonly used drugs. Some drugs such as phenobarbital and valproic acid have relatively low values (<10 mL/min), whereas others such as procainamide and lidocaine have much larger clearances (>500 mL/min). Such differences mainly reflect different rate-limiting determinants such as blood flow through the organ(s) of clearance, the extent of binding of the drug to plasma proteins, and the efficiency of the clearance process to remove drug from tissue water by metabolism and/or excretion. The data in Table 70-2 also demonstrate that the relative contributions of the two major routes of elimination, i.e., renal and nonrenal, also vary according to the individual drug. In some cases, such as amikacin, digoxin, gentamicin, lithium, and tobramycin, excretion by the kidneys is predominant. However, with many other drugs (e.g., carbamazepine, lidocaine), nonrenal elimination, which usually reflects metabolism in the liver, is more important.

Volume of Distribution The relationship between the amount of drug in the body and the concentration of drug in the plasma provides a measure of the apparent volume of distribution:

$$V = \text{amount of drug in the body}/C$$
$$\text{(vol)} \quad \text{(amt)/(amt/vol)}$$

This volume does not, except in a limited number of special cases, reflect an identifiable physiologic volume but corresponds to the virtual volume of fluid that would be required to contain all of the drug in the body at the same concentration as in the plasma. In a typical 70-kg human, plasma volume is about 3 L, blood volume around 5.5 L, and extracellular water outside the vasculature is approximately 42 L. The volume of distribution of drugs that are extensively bound to plasma proteins but are not bound to tissue components approaches plasma volume. However, for most drugs, the volume of distribution is far greater than any physiologic space. For example, the volume of distribution of digoxin is about 700 L, which obviously exceeds total body volume. This simply indicates that digoxin is largely distributed outside the vascular system and hence the proportion of the drug present in the plasma compartment is low.

The volume of distribution may be estimated by back-extrapolation of the plasma concentration-time curve to zero time (C_0) (Fig.

Table 70-2 Pharmacokinetic Parameters (Mean ± Standard Deviation) and Plasma Therapeutic Ranges of Some Commonly Used Drugs

	Cl, mL/min	V, L	$t_{1/2}$, h	Oral F, %	Urinary Excretion, %	Plasma Binding, %	Effective Plasma Level, μg/mL	Toxic Plasma Level, μg/mL
Carbamazepine	90 ± 35	98 ± 28	15 ± 5	>70	<1	74 ± 3	4	10
Digoxin	133 ± 69[a]	658 ± 196	39 ± 13	70 ± 13	60 ± 11	25 ± 5	>0.8 ng/mL	2.0 ng/mL
Ethosuximide	13 ± 3	50 ± 11	45 ± 8	—	25 ± 15	0	40	100
Gentamicin	110 ± 35[a]	22 ± 7	53 ± 25	—	>90	<10	5	peak 10 trough 2
Lidocaine	644 ± 168	77 ± 18	1.8 ± 0.4	35 ± 11	2	70 ± 5	1.5	6
Lithium	24 ± 7	46 ± 11	22 ± 8	100	95 ± 15	0	0.5 meq/L	1.5meq/L
Midazolam	462 ± 126	77 ± 42	1.9 ± 0.6	44 ± 17	56 ± 26	95 ± 2	50	200
Phenobarbital	4.3 ± 0.9	38 ± 2	99 ± 18	100	24 ± 5	51 ± 3	10	30
Phenytoin	Dose-dependent	45 ± 3	6–24	90 ± 3	2 ± 8	89 ± 23	10	20
Primidone	38 ± 8	48 ± 13	15 ± 4	92 ± 18	48 ± 16	19	8	12
Procainamide	600 ± 200[b]	133 ± 21	3.0 ± 0.6	83 ± 16	67 ± 8	16 ± 5	3	14
Quinidine	329 ± 126	189 ± 84	6.2 ± 1.8	70–80	18 ± 3	87 ± 3	2	6
Tacrolimus	49 ± 19	62 ± 22	15 ± 7	16 ± 7	<1	75–99	15	25
Theophylline	45 ± 14	35 ± 11	9.0 ± 2.1	96 ± 8	18 ± 3	56 ± 4	5	20
Valproic acid	7.7 ± 14	15 ± 5	14 ± 3	100	1.8 ± 2.4	93 ± 1	30	100

[a] Dependent on renal function.
[b] Dependent on *N*-acetylator phenotype.

NOTE: Cl, clearance; V, volume of distribution; F, bioavailability.

70-1) and dividing this into the dose of drug administered intravenously.

$$V = dose_{iv}/C_0$$

When distribution of the drug is not instantaneous, a more useful volume estimate is based on the area under the plasma-concentration time curve (AUC) and the terminal elimination half-life of the drug ($t_{1/2}$).

$$V_{area} = \frac{dose_{iv} \times t_{1/2}}{0.693 \times AUC}$$

Extent and Rate of Bioavailability   After intravenous administration, all of the administered dose reaches the systemic circulation. In contrast, with all other routes of administration, such as oral, intramuscular, and subcutaneous, there is the potential for only a part of the dose to be absorbed; this fraction (F) is termed the drug's *bioavailability*. Lack of complete bioavailability may reflect the inability of the drug to be completely released from the dosage form or vehicle, chemical destruction at the site of administration, incomplete absorption into the vascular system, and metabolism and/or excretion during translocation of the drug from its site of administration to the systemic circulation. In the case of oral dosing, this would include the intestinal epithelium and the liver and lungs. Metabolism and/or excretion by the gastrointestinal tract (F_{GI}) and liver (F_L) are collectively referred to as the *first-pass effect*, since the resulting drug elimination only occurs during drug delivery to the systemic circulation. Loss of drug because of a first-pass effect thus requires that the dosing rate appropriately take into account bioavailability. For example, after oral drug administration:

$$F_{oral} \times \text{dosing rate} = Cl \times C_{avg,ss}$$

Bioavailability and the first-pass effect are important with respect to possible differences in drug responsiveness dependent on the route of administration. For example, glyceryl trinitrate has such a large oral first-pass effect ($>99\%$) that systemic concentrations after an oral dose are negligible and no antianginal effect is present. Giving the drug by the sublingual or transdermal routes bypasses the splanchnic organs and allows essentially all of the drug to reach the systemic circulation. For drugs that are efficiently metabolized by the intestinal epithelium and/or liver, i.e., drugs with high extraction ratios in either of these organs, differences in the extent of the first-pass effect between individuals frequently explain variability in drug response. With propranolol, for example, the 15-fold variability in plasma concentrations after the same oral dose results from differences in the individual hepatic extraction ratios reflective of different levels of drug metabolizing activity.

Drug administration by nonintravenous routes involves an absorption process characterized by the plasma level increasing to a maximum value at some time after administration and then declining as the rate of drug elimination exceeds the rate of absorption. Thus, the peak concentration is lower and occurs later than after the same dose given by rapid intravenous injection. The rate of absorption can be an important consideration during the initial period after drug administration, especially for drugs with a narrow *therapeutic index*—the ratio of the toxic dose to the therapeutic dose. If absorption is too rapid, then the resulting high concentration may cause adverse effects not observed with a more slowly available formulation. At the other extreme, slow absorption is deliberately designed into "slow-release" or "sustained-release" drug formulations in order to maintain plasma concentrations essentially constant during the dosage interval, because the drug's rate of elimination is offset by an equivalent rate of absorption controlled by formulation factors.

Half-Life   The organs of elimination can only clear drug from the blood. Thus, the rate at which drug is eliminated from the body is a function of both clearance and the extent to which drug is distributed outside of the vascular compartment. The fraction of total drug in the body that is eliminated in a given time is designated the *fractional elimination constant* (k).

$$k = Cl/V$$

For example, if the volume of distribution is 10 L and clearance is 1 L/min, then one-tenth of the drug is eliminated per minute. If k is multiplied by the total amount of drug in the body, the actual rate of elimination at any given time can be determined:

Rate of elimination = $k \times$ amount in body = $k \times C \times V = Cl \times C$

This relationship, indicating that the rate of drug elimination is proportional to the drug concentration, describes a first-order, or monoexponential, process. With a few notable exceptions, the elimination of drugs used clinically is first-order.

Half-life ($t_{1/2}$) is the time that it takes for the plasma concentration or amount of drug in the body to decline by 50%. This parameter is related to k as follows:

$$t_{1/2} = 0.693/k$$

where 0.693 is the natural logarithm of $2(C_o/0.5\,C_o)$.

Because

$$k = Cl/V$$

then

$$t_{1/2} = 0.693\,(V/Cl)$$

This is an important relationship since it indicates that the rate of drug elimination, reflected by $t_{1/2}$, is dependent on both the efficiency of drug removal (Cl) and the drug's volume of distribution (V). When V remains constant, $t_{1/2}$ is a reflection of clearance. Thus, $t_{1/2}$ is shortened when rifampin induces the enzymes responsible for a drug's hepatic clearance and is lengthened when a drug's renal clearance is impaired in renal failure. However, when there are concomitant alterations in V, as occurs for some drugs in cardiac failure, $t_{1/2}$ is not an accurate measure of Cl or drug dose.

DESIGNING DOSAGE REGIMENS   Most drugs are administered as part of long-term therapy involving multiple dosing, and it is critical that the dosage regimen be optimized to the individual patient. With some drugs, the desired response, e.g., coagulation or blood pressure, is readily measurable and an individualized dosage regimen can be developed with dosage titration. However, dosage changes should be conservative ($<50\%$ for drugs with a low therapeutic index) and not more frequent than every three to four half-lives. Other drugs have little dose-related toxicity so the therapeutic window is large, e.g., penicillins and β-adrenoceptor antagonists. In these situations, effective and prolonged drug effects may be obtained by a "maximal dose" strategy. It is also possible to use this strategy to extend the duration of action of a drug, especially one that is eliminated rapidly from the body. Thus, 75 mg of captopril will result in reduced blood pressure for up to 12 h, even though the elimination half-life of this angiotensin-converting enzyme (ACE) inhibitor is about 2 h; this is because the dose raises the concentration of drug in plasma many times higher than the threshold for its pharmacologic effect.

Determination of the Maintenance Dose   The relationship between the maintenance dose and the final steady-state concentration is

Maintenance dosing rate = $F \times$ dose/dosage interval = $Cl \times C_{avg,ss}$

Thus, steady-state concentrations can be predictably increased or decreased by appropriate modification of the maintenance dosing rate to achieve a desired target value:

$$C_{target} = C_{avg,ss} = \frac{F \times dose}{Cl \times dosing\ interval}$$

In most cases, this is best achieved by changing the drug dose but not the dosing interval, e.g., by giving 250 mg every 8 h instead of 200 mg every 8 h. However, this approach is acceptable only if the resulting maximum concentration is not toxic and the trough value does not fall below the minimum effective concentration for an undesirable period of time. Alternatively, the steady state may be changed by altering the frequency of intermittent dosing but not the size of each dose. In this case, the magnitude of the fluctuations around the average steady-state level will change—the shorter the dosing interval, the smaller the difference between peak and trough levels (Fig. 70-3).

The extent of fluctuation is determined by the relationship between the dosing interval and the drug's half-life. For example, if the dosing interval is equal to the drug's half-life, then the fluctuation would be twofold, which is usually a tolerable variation. If a longer dosing interval is used, then the difference between the maximum and minimum plasma levels will be greater (Fig. 70-3). Marked fluctuations increase the likelihood of increased concentration-dependent drug effects early during the dosing interval and possible ineffectiveness at the end of the period, even though the average steady-state drug concentration is the same as that following administration at the same dosing rate but at shorter intervals.

Determination of the Loading Dose The loading dose can be estimated if both the desired plasma level (C) and the apparent volume of distribution (V) are known:

$$Loading\ dose = C_{avg,ss} \times V$$

The loading amount required to achieve steady-state plasma levels can also be determined from the fraction of drug eliminated during the dosing interval and the maintenance dose. For example, if the fraction of digoxin eliminated daily is 35% and the planned maintenance dose is 0.25 mg daily, then the loading dose to achieve steady-state levels would be (100/35) times the maintenance dose, or approximately 0.75 mg. Thus,

$$Loading\ dose = \frac{100}{\%\ of\ drug\ eliminated\ per\ dosage\ interval} \times maintenance\ dose$$

NONLINEAR DRUG ELIMINATION The elimination of some drugs (e.g., phenytoin, salicylate, propafenone, and theophylline) does not follow first-order kinetics because the clearance of these drugs changes as levels in the body fall during elimination or change after alterations in dose. Such elimination is called *concentration-dependent* or *dose-dependent*. Accordingly, the time for the concentration to fall to one-half becomes less as plasma levels fall. (This halving time is not truly a half-life, because the term *half-life* applies to first-order kinetics and is a constant.) When a drug is eliminated by first-order kinetics, the plasma level at steady state is directly related to the amount of the maintenance dose, and a doubling of the dose should lead to doubling of the steady-state plasma level. However, for drugs with dose-dependent kinetics, an increase in the dose may be accompanied by a disproportionate increase in the plasma level. For example, a threefold increase in the dose of propafenone (from 300 mg to 900 mg daily) leads to a tenfold increase in the concentration of propafenone in plasma. Changes in dosage regimens for drugs with dose-dependent kinetics should always be accompanied by surveillance for adverse effects and by measurement of the concentration of the drug in plasma during the time of transition to the new steady-state, if this is feasible.

FIGURE 70-3 Plasma concentrations of a drug with an elimination half-life of 12 h during chronic therapy using different dosage regimens for a period sufficient to reach steady state. Proportionally reducing or increasing both the size of the maintenance dose and the interval between dosage changes the magnitude of the fluctuations in plasma levels but has no effect on the average steady-state (C_{av}) value, since this depends on the dosing rate (dose/dosing interval).

INDIVIDUALIZATION OF DRUG THERAPY

EFFECTS OF RENAL DISEASE Whether a drug's dosing rate needs to be modified in patients with renal dysfunction depends on whether the drug is primarily excreted through the kidneys and whether increased drug levels, secondary to impaired renal clearance, will be associated with adverse effects. If both of these factors are present, it is likely that with decreased renal clearance the drug will accumulate to a greater extent than in patients with normal renal function and toxicity will result. This is especially true for drugs with long half-lives and narrow therapeutic indexes (e.g., digoxin). In general, over 60 to 70% of the drug must be renally excreted for dosage modification to be necessary and then only when renal function is less than about 30 to 50% of normal.

The goal of any dosing rate adjustment is to modify the dosing schedule so that the drug's plasma concentration-time profile is as similar to the desired one as possible and that the steady state is reached in about the same time as in a patient with normal renal function. To obtain the desired profile, a modification may be made by decreasing the dose while maintaining the dosage interval, keeping the dose the same but increasing the dosing interval, or a combination of these two approaches.

A drug's renal clearance is proportional to creatinine's clearance (Cl_{CR}), which may be measured directly or estimated from the serum creatinine level (C_{CR}). In men:

$$Cl_{CR} = \frac{(140 - age) \times weight\ (kg)}{72 \times C_{CR}(mg/d\ L)}\ (mL/min)$$

For women, the estimate by the above equation should be multiplied by 0.85 to reflect their smaller muscle mass. It should also be noted that this equation is not valid for patients with severe renal insufficiency ($C_{CR} < 5$ mg/dL) or when renal function is changing rapidly. For simplicity, normal creatinine clearance is conveniently considered to be 100 mL/min. Thus, if the relative contributions of renal and nonrenal elimination to systemic clearance are known, an appropriate modification of the dose in a patient with a given level of insufficiency can be estimated. For example, if the fraction of drug excreted unchanged is 0.9 and creatinine clearance is reduced to 10% of normal, the dosing rate should be reduced to 19% of normal. This modification,

Table 70-3 Drug Dosing Rate Adjustment in Renal Failure

Drug	Method	Adjustment in Renal Failure GFR, mL/min >50	10–50	<10	Dosage Increase Needed in Dialysis[b]
Allopurinol	D	Unchanged	50%	30%	Yes
	I	24 h	24–36 h	48–72 h	
Carbenicillin	I	8–12 h	12–24 h	24–48 h	Yes
Ciprofloxacin	D	Unchanged	50–75%	50%	No
Cimetidine	D	Unchanged	75%	50%	No
Digoxin	D	Unchanged	25–75%	10–25%	No
Fluconazole	I	24 h	24–48 h	48–72 h	Yes
Gentamycin	D	60–90%	30–70%	20–30%	Yes
	I	8–12 h	12 h	24 h	
Lithium	D	Unchanged	50–75%	25–50%	Yes
Penicillin G	D	Unchanged	75%	25–50%	Yes
	I	6–8 h	8–12 h	12–66 h	
Primidone	I	8	8–12 h	12–24 h	Yes
Procainamide	I	4–6 h	6–12 h	8–24 h	Yes
Tobramycin	D	60–90%	30–70%	20–30%	Yes
	I	8–12 h	12 h	24 h	
Vancomycin	I	24–72 h	72–240 h	240 h	No

[a] D is a dosage method based on administering the indicated percentage of the usual maintenance dose at the usual dosage interval. I indicates a dosage interval extension method of adjusting the dosing rate where the values given are the dosage interval in hours at which the usual maintenance dose is administered.

[b] "Yes" indicates removal of enough drug by dialysis to require a dosage supplement to ensure adequate therapeutic drug concentrations. GFR, glomerular filtration rate

which in practice would be rounded to 20%, is based on the fact that nonrenal clearance is unchanged (10% of normal clearance); renal clearance is reduced from 90% to 9% of normal Cl; thus systemic clearance is reduced to $10 + 9 = 19\%$ of normal Cl.

In clinical practice today, most decisions involving dosing adjustment in patients with renal failure use published tables of recommended dosage reduction or dosing interval lengthening based on the level of renal function indicated by Cl_{CR}, or similar information provided in the drug "label" (Table 70-3). Such modifications are, however, rigorously based on pharmacokinetic principles and are best used when resulting plasma concentration data and clinical observation are used, as necessary, to further optimize therapy for the individual patient.

Often metabolites of the drug are pharmacologically active or cause toxicity, and renal insufficiency may result in their unanticipated accumulation. Meperidine, for example, is extensively metabolized, and renal failure has little effect on its plasma concentration; however, its metabolite, normeperidine, accumulates above its usual level when renal function is impaired. Because normeperidine has greater convulsant activity than meperidine, this accumulation probably accounts for the signs of central nervous system (CNS) excitation, such as irritability, twitching, and seizures, that appear when multiple doses of meperidine are administered to patients with renal disease.

EFFECTS OF LIVER DISEASE   In contrast to the predictable decline in renal clearance of drugs in renal insufficiency, it is not possible to make a general prediction of the effect of liver disease on hepatic biotransformation of drugs (Chap. 292). Rather, the possible effects of hepatitis or cirrhosis range from impaired to increased drug clearance. Even in advanced hepatocellular disease, drug clearance is usually impaired only about two- to fivefold. The extent of such changes, however, cannot be predicted by the common tests of liver function. Consequently, even when it is suspected that drug elimination is altered in liver disease, there is no quantitative basis on which to adjust the dosage regimen other than assessment of clinical response and the concentration of the drug in plasma.

A drug's oral bioavailability may markedly increase in patients with liver disease. This is particularly the case for those drugs that normally are very well extracted by the liver and thus have a high first-pass effect. In addition, the presence of portacaval shunts may further reduce first-pass elimination and lead to higher drug concentrations reaching the systemic circulation, with the increased risk of adverse effects. For example, the oral availability for high first-pass drugs such as morphine, meperidine, midazolam, and nifedipine is almost doubled in patients with cirrhosis, compared to those with normal liver function. The size of the oral dose of such drugs should, therefore, be reduced in such patients.

EFFECTS OF CIRCULATORY INSUFFICIENCY — CARDIAC FAILURE AND SHOCK   Under conditions of decreased tissue perfusion, the cardiac output is redistributed to preserve blood flow to the heart and brain at the expense of other tissues (Chap. 38). As a result, the drug may be distributed into a smaller volume of distribution, higher drug concentrations will be present in the plasma, and the tissues that are best perfused will be exposed to these higher concentrations. If either the brain or heart is sensitive to the drug, an alteration in response will occur.

Furthermore, the decreased perfusion of the kidney and liver may impair drug clearance by these organs, directly or indirectly. Thus, in severe congestive heart failure, in hemorrhagic shock, and in cardiogenic shock, the response to the usual dose of drug may be excessive, and dosage modification may be necessary. For example, the clearance of lidocaine is reduced by about 50% in cardiac failure, and therapeutic plasma levels are achieved at infusion rates only about half those usually required. The volume of distribution of lidocaine is also reduced, meaning that the correct loading dose will be smaller than usual. Similar situations are thought to exist for procainamide, theophylline, and possibly quinidine. Unfortunately, predictors of these types of pharmacokinetic alterations are unavailable. Therefore, loading doses should be conservative, and continued therapy should be monitored closely, following clinical indicators of toxicity and plasma levels.

DISEASE-INDUCED CHANGES IN PLASMA BINDING Many drugs circulate in the plasma partly bound to plasma proteins. Since only the unbound (free) drug can distribute to the site of pharmacologic action, the therapeutic response should be related to the free rather than the total circulating plasma drug concentration. In most cases, the degree of binding is fairly constant across the therapeutic concentration range, so that the total drug levels in plasma can be used as a basis for adjusting dosage without resulting in significant error. However, conditions such as hypoalbuminemia, liver disease, and renal disease can decrease the extent of drug binding, particularly of acidic and neutral drugs so that at any total plasma level there is a greater concentration of free drug than usual and thus a risk of increased response and toxicity. By contrast, conditions that lead to an increased plasma concentration of the acute-phase reactant α_1-acid glycoprotein—such as myocardial infarction, surgery, neoplastic disease, rheumatoid arthritis, and burns—cause an increase in drug binding for the basic drugs, e.g., lidocaine and quinidine, that bind to this macromolecule, resulting in an opposite set of effects. The drugs for which changes in binding are important are those that are normally highly bound to plasma proteins (>90%), because a small alteration in the extent of binding produces a large change in the amount of unbound drug.

For many drugs, elimination and distribution are restricted largely to the unbound fraction, and so a decrease in binding leads to an increase in the clearance and distribution of the drug. The relative magnitudes of these changes are such that the net effect is a shortened half-life.

GENETIC DETERMINANTS OF THE RESPONSE TO DRUGS

Knowledge of the enzyme that catalyzes the predominant pathway of metabolism of a drug provides a basis for understanding the therapeutic consequences of variations in the genotype of that enzyme. For a number of the enzymes that metabolize drugs, there are differences (polymorphisms) in catalytic function that are genetically determined (Chap. 65). *A phenotypic trait or its corresponding gene is said to be polymorphic if there is more than one form of the trait or gene in the population.* Polymorphisms in the function of an enzyme are determined by allelic variants in its gene. Increasingly it is possible to individualize treatment based on analysis of the phenotype and/or genotype of the relevant drug-metabolizing enzyme.

Similarly, polymorphism in the receptor for a drug can determine variability in its pharmacologic effect. Genotyping those drug receptors for which polymorphisms influence response may also assist in individualizing drug therapy.

THIOPURINE S-METHYLTRANSFERASE (TPMT) The metabolism of azathioprine provides an example of the importance of genetic polymorphisms of enzymes. Azathioprine exerts its immunosuppressive action via an active metabolite, 6-mercaptopurine. Within target cells, the major pathway of inactivation of 6-mercaptopurine is by TPMT. Genetic polymorphisms in this enzyme lead to differences in inactivation of 6-mercaptopurine, with corresponding vast differences in the sensitivity of patients to the toxic and therapeutic effects of azathioprine. Homozygotes for alleles encoding inactive TPMT (0.3 to 1% of the population) predictably exhibit severe pancytopenia on standard doses of azathioprine. Heterozygotes for alleles encoding enzymes with deficient TPMT activity also experience more bone marrow suppression on "usual" doses. From a therapeutic standpoint it is likely that the bone marrow suppression in the heterozygotes has influenced the empiric determination of the "usual" dose range of azathioprine and that this results in undertreatment of some of the patients homozygous for the allele encoding a TPMT with full catalytic activity. To detect the TPMT deficient phenotype in patients anticipating therapy with azathioprine, the catalytic function of TPMT may be measured in red blood cells (if no blood or red cell transfusions have been given within 2 months). A high concordance of genotype with phenotype (~95%) suggests that analysis of genotype may be used to individualize dosing and therefore improve treatment with azathioprine (and 6-mercaptopurine) in the future.

ACETYLATION Isoniazid, hydralazine, sulfonamides, procainamide, and a number of other drugs are metabolized by acetylation of a hydrazino or amino group. This reaction is catalyzed by N-acetyl transferase-2 (NAT-2), an enzyme in the liver cytosol that transfers an acetyl group from acetyl coenzyme A to the drug. Individuals differ markedly in the rate at which drugs are acetylated, because of polymorphisms in the NAT-2 gene, resulting in a bimodal distribution of the population into "rapid acetylators" and "slow acetylators."

Acetylation phenotype can be determined by measuring the ratio of acetylated to nonacetylated forms of the probe drugs, dapsone, caffeine, or sulfamethazine, in plasma or urine following administration of a test dose of these acetylation substrates. Slow, intermediate, and rapid acetylators may be identified by these methods for phenotyping. It is also possible to identify slow acetylators by genotyping, using genomic DNA obtained from blood leukocytes.

METABOLISM BY CYTOCHROME P450 MONOOXYGENASES In healthy individuals taking no other medications, the major determinant of the rate of metabolism of drugs by the cytochrome P450 monooxygenases is genetic. Hepatic endoplasmic reticulum contains a family of cytochrome P450 (CYP) isoforms with different substrate specificities. Many drugs undergo oxidative metabolism by more than one isoform, and the steady-state concentrations of such drugs in the plasma is a function of the sum of the activities of these and other metabolizing enzymes. When a drug is metabolized by multiple pathways, the catalytic activities of the participating enzymes are regulated by a number of genes, so that the clearance rates and steady-state concentrations of the drug tend to distribute unimodally within the population. The range of activity may differ markedly ($\geq$tenfold) between different individuals, as is the case for chlorpromazine, and there is no way to predict the rate before beginning therapy.

Certain metabolic pathways show a bimodal or trimodal distribu-

tion of activity, suggesting control by a single gene, and polymorphisms in these genes have been identified. Most individuals are extensive metabolizers (EM phenotype); a smaller group have a lower ability to metabolize the drug (or no ability at all) and are called poor metabolizers (PM phenotype). Heterozygotes for genes encoding the enzymes lacking catalytic activity may be intermediate metabolizers (IM phenotype). And patients with duplicate or multiple copies of the gene may exhibit ultrarapid metabolism. These polymorphisms are of greatest clinical relevance during administration of substrate drugs for which there are no major alternative routes of elimination. The clinical consequences of the PM phenotype will then depend on the resultant accumulation of the drug or occasionally on the absence of generation of active metabolites.

The cytochrome P450 isoform CYP2D6 is polymorphically distributed in the population, and about 8 to 10% of Caucasians are deficient in this enzyme. CYP2D6 represents the main metabolic pathway for a number of drugs, including antiarrhythmic agents (propafenone, flecainide), β-adrenoceptor blockers (timolol, metoprolol, and alprenolol), tricyclic antidepressants (nortriptyline, desipramine, imipramine, clomipramine), neuroleptic drugs (perphenazine, thioridazine, and possibly haloperidol), selective serotonin reuptake inhibitors (fluoxetine and paroxetine), and certain opiates, such as codeine and dextromethorphan. Thus, codeine has a much lower analgesic effect in PM patients because of impaired production of the active metabolite, morphine. Conversely, a patient with duplicate or multiple copies of CYP2D6 will exhibit an exaggerated response to codeine. Patients with the PM phenotype experience more pronounced systemic β-adrenoceptor blockade after the administration of timolol ophthalmic solution. The catalytic activity of CYP2D6 in humans may be assessed by using a test drug, debrisoquin, which is eliminated almost entirely via hydroxylation by CYP2D6. Individuals with the PM phenotype can be identified by genotyping for the alleles that encode proteins with loss of catalytic function. There are ethnic variations in the frequency of the PM phenotype, which occurs in 5 to 10% of Caucasians but with a lesser frequency in Asians (1 to 2%).

The isoform CYP2C19 also exhibits polymorphism; it was initially detected with the hydroxylation of mephenytoin, which is used as a probe drug for the function of this P450 isoform. This enzyme catalyzes the major metabolic pathway of omeprazole, proguanil, diazepam, and citalopram. The impact of the polymorphism in CYP2C19 on treatment outcome is clearly illustrated by omeprazole. The efficacy of omeprazole (20 mg in combination with amoxicillin) in eradicating *Helicobacter pylori* is markedly reduced in persons with the homozygous EM genotype (29% cured) as compared with 100% cure in those with homozygous PM genotype. This reflects the relative lack of effect of the recommended dose of omeprazole (20 mg) on gastric acid secretion and ulcer healing in patients with the CYP2C19 EM genotype. Certainly knowledge of a patient's CYP2C19 genotype would improve therapy with this proton pump inhibitor. Impaired hydroxylation of mephenytoin is present in only 3 to 5 percent of Caucasians, but the incidence is about 20 percent in individuals of Japanese and Chinese descent.

CYP2C9 catalyzes the major pathways of metabolism of warfarin and phenytoin. There are allelic variants of the gene for this enzyme that encode proteins with loss of catalytic function. These variant alleles are associated with requirement for a very low dose of warfarin, difficulties in initiating warfarin therapy, and an increased risk of bleeding complications. Similarly, high concentrations of phenytoin in plasma and resulting adverse effects of phenytoin occur in patients with loss of function alleles for CYP2C9.

Polymorphisms in drug-metabolizing ability may be associated with large differences in the disposition of a drug among individuals, especially when the involved pathway makes a major contribution to the elimination of the drug. For example, the clearance of mephenytoin given orally differs 100- to 200-fold between individuals of the EM and PM phenotypes. As a result, the peak plasma concentrations and bioavailability after oral administration are much higher, and the rate of drug elimination much lower, in PM than in EM individuals. In PM individuals, the result is excessive drug accumulation and exaggerated pharmacologic responses, including toxicity, when usual drug dosages are administered. Individualization of drug therapy is especially critical for drugs that exhibit polymorphic drug metabolism. The increasing availability of laboratory methods to identify the PM phenotype for NAT-2, CYP2D6, and CYP2C19 by genotyping should be useful for this purpose.

INTERINDIVIDUAL VARIABILITY IN THE MOLECULAR TARGETS WITH WHICH DRUGS INTERACT The increasing emphasis on identifying molecular mechanisms of disease (Chap. 65) has important consequences for further understanding a genetic basis for individual variability in drug actions. As molecular approaches identify the role of specific gene products in human physiology, polymorphisms that alter expression or function of those gene products are being recognized; it is estimated that such polymorphisms occur in 1 in 1000 bp in the human genome. These genes in turn, are now being recognized as the molecular targets with which available and new drugs interact to produce beneficial and adverse effects.

Genome-wide searches in families with premature Alzheimer's disease identified the *APOE* locus as linked to the disease (Chap. 362). Specifically, the *E4* allele of the *APOE* gene appears associated with a worse prognosis, and this is thought to relate to reduced expression of choline acetyl transferase. Further, a therapeutic response to the choline acetyl transferase inhibitor, tacrine, appears to be more common with the prognostically more benign *APOE2* or *APOE3* alleles. Multiple polymorphisms identified in the β_2-adrenergic receptor appear to be linked to specific phenotypes in asthma and congestive heart failure, diseases in which β_2-receptor function might be expected to determine prognosis. It has been suggested that polymorphisms in the β_2 receptor may be a determinant of response to inhaled β_2-receptor agonists.

The development of marked QT prolongation and the polymorphic ventricular tachycardia, *torsade de pointes* (Chap. 230), in response to certain action potential–prolonging drugs such as quinidine used to be characterized as an "idiosyncratic" response. Advances in understanding the molecular basis of normal cardiac repolarization have resulted in identification of genes encoding ion channel proteins, the molecules whose normal function results in physiologic cardiac repolarization. Mutations in these genes cause congenital arrhythmia syndromes, such as the long QT syndrome, and block of ion channels is a common mechanism whereby drugs prolong QT intervals. Patients with mutations in these genes that remain subclinical until challenge with drugs are now recognized. In summary, continuing efforts to unravel the molecular basis of disease are likely also to provide insights into determinants of the response to drug therapy.

DRUG USE IN THE ELDERLY (See also Chap. 9) Aging results in changes in organ function, especially of the organs involved in drug disposition, as well as alterations in body size and composition. Not surprisingly, therefore, pharmacokinetics are often different in elderly individuals than in younger adults. Also, elderly patients often have multiple diseases and may therefore be taking a large number of drugs. Consequently, drug interactions, as well as an increased vulnerability to morbidity and mortality, contribute to the higher incidence of adverse drug reactions in elderly patients. Increased sensitivity of target organs and impairment of physiologic control systems, such as those involved in the regulation of the circulation, may also be a factor. Accordingly, optimization of drug therapy in the elderly, particularly in frail patients, is often difficult, as a variety of factors (often poorly defined) accentuate the usual interindividual variability in drug response.

Although many individuals preserve good renal function into old age, elderly patients as a group have an increased likelihood of impaired renal excretion of drugs. Even in the absence of kidney disease, renal clearance is generally reduced by about 35 to 50% in elderly

patients. Dosage adjustments analogous to those in patients with renal dysfunction (see above) are therefore necessary for drugs that are eliminated mainly by the kidneys, such as digoxin, aminoglycosides, lithium, and other drugs listed in Table 70-3. In this regard, it is important to recognize that the reduced muscle mass of older individuals results in a reduced rate of creatinine production; thus, a normal serum creatinine concentration can be present even though creatinine clearance is impaired.

Aging also results in a decrease in the size of and blood flow to the liver and possibly in the activity of hepatic drug-metabolizing enzymes; accordingly, the hepatic clearance of some drugs is impaired in the elderly. Unfortunately, no consistent pattern of clinical application appears to be present. Moreover, the changes are often modest relative to other causes for interindividual variability in these patients. However, even a small reduction in hepatic extraction may significantly increase the oral bioavailability of drugs with a high first-pass effect, such as propranolol and labetalol.

Impaired clearance and/or increased distribution may cause the elimination half-life of a drug to increase with aging. Thus, if a dosage modification in an elderly patient is required, it is often possible to accomplish it by decreasing the frequency of drug administration, possibly along with a reduction in dose.

Even if the pharmacokinetics of a drug are not altered, an elderly patient may require a smaller dosage because of an increase in pharmacodynamic sensitivity. Examples include increased analgesic effects of opioids, increased sedation from benzodiazepines and other CNS depressants, and increased risk of bleeding while receiving anticoagulant therapy, even when clotting parameters are well controlled. Exaggerated responses to cardiovascular drugs are also common because of the impaired responsiveness of normal homeostatic mechanisms. Such age-related changes require close monitoring of the patient's clinical response and appropriate dosage titration. Accordingly, in the elderly, initial doses should be less than the usual adult dosage and should be increased slowly. The final therapeutic regimen should be as simple as possible, and the number of different drugs used should be kept as low as possible. Also, because interindividual variability in drug responsiveness is greater in geriatric patients than in younger adults, individualization of therapy is even more critical.

INTERACTIONS BETWEEN DRUGS

The effect of some drugs can be altered markedly by the administration of other agents. Such interactions can complicate therapy by adversely increasing or decreasing the action of a drug. Drug interactions must be considered in the differential diagnosis of unexpected responses to drugs, and it should be recognized that patients often come to the physician with a legacy of drugs acquired during previous medical experiences. A meticulous drug history will minimize such unknown elements. It should include examination of the patient's medications and, if necessary, calls to the pharmacist to identify prescriptions. It should also address the use agents not often volunteered on initial questioning, such as over-the-counter drugs, health food supplements, and topical agents such as eye drops.

There are two principal types of interactions between drugs. In *pharmacokinetic interactions*, the delivery of a drug to its site of action is altered, whereas in *pharmacodynamic interactions*, the responsiveness of the target organ or system is modified.

An index of the drug interactions discussed in this chapter is provided in Table 70-4. The table includes interactions that have verified significance in patients, plus a few that are so potentially dangerous that cognizance should be taken of the experimental data or case reports suggesting they occur.

I. PHARMACOKINETIC INTERACTIONS CAUSING DIMINISHED DRUG DELIVERY A. Impaired Gastrointestinal Absorption Examples include aluminum ions, present in antacids, which form insoluble chelates with the tetracyclines, preventing absorption of these drugs. Ferrous ions similarly block tetracycline absorption. Kaolin-pectin suspensions bind digoxin, and when these substances are administered together, digoxin absorption is reduced by about one-half. However, when kaolin-pectin is administered 2 h after digoxin, digoxin absorption is unaffected.

Ketoconazole is a weak base that dissolves well only at acidic pH. Histamine H_2 receptor antagonists, such as ranitidine and cimetidine, reduce gastric acidity and thus impair the dissolution and absorption of ketoconazole. By contrast, the absorption of fluconazole is not impaired by an increase in gastric pH.

B. Induction of Hepatic Drug-Metabolizing Enzymes When a drug is eliminated largely by metabolism, an increase in the rate of its metabolism reduces its availability to sites of action. Most drugs are metabolized largely in the liver because of this organ's large mass, high blood flow, and high concentration of drug-metabolizing enzymes. The first step in the metabolism of many drugs is catalyzed by a group of cytochrome P450 mixed-function oxidases located in the endoplasmic reticulum (see "Metabolism by Cytochrome P450 Monooxygenases," above). These enzyme systems oxidize drug molecules by a variety of reactions, including aromatic hydroxylations, N-demethylations, O-demethylations, and sulfoxidations. The products of these reactions are usually more polar than the parent compound (and more readily excreted by the kidney).

The expression of some of the mixed-function oxidase (CYP) isoforms is regulated, and their content in the liver can be increased, by a number of drugs. Phenobarbital is the prototype of these inducers, and all the barbiturates in clinical use increase CYP enzyme activity. Induction with phenobarbital can occur with doses of as little as 60 mg daily. Mixed-function oxidases are also induced by rifampin, carbamazepine, phenytoin, and glutethimide and by smoking, exposure to chlorinated insecticides such as DDT, and chronic alcohol ingestion.

Table 70-4 Drug Interaction Index

Drug	Section of Chapter Describing Interaction	Drug	Section of Chapter Describing Interaction
Allopurinol	IIA	6-Mercaptopurine	IIA
Amiloride	III	Methadone	IB
Amiodarone	IIA, IIB	Methotrexate	IIB
Amphetamine	IC	Methylprednisolone	IB, IIA
Antidepressants, tricyclic (desipramine, nortriptyline, imipramine, doxepin, protriptyline, amitriptyline)	IC	Metronidazole	IB, IIA
		Metyrapone	IB
		Mexiletine	IB
		Nicardipine	IIA
Aspirin	IIB, III	Nifedipine	IIA
Atorvastatin	IIA	Nitrates	III
Azathioprine	IIA	Nonsteroidal anti-inflammatory drugs	III
Barbiturates (class)	IB		
Carbamazepine	IB, IIA		
Chlorpromazine	IC, IIA	Oral contraceptive steroids	IB
Cholestyramine	IA		
Cimetidine	IA, IIA, IIB	Phenobarbital	IB
Cisapride	IIA	Phenylbutazone	IIA, IIB
Clofibrate	IIA	Phenytoin (diphenylhydantoin)	IB, IIA
Clonidine	IC		
Codeine	IIA	Piroxicam	III
Cotrimoxazole	IIA	Potassium	III
Cyclosporine	IB, IIA, IIB	Prednisone	IB
Dexamethasone	IB	Probenecid	IIB
Digoxin	IA, IIB	Procainamide	IIB
Diltiazem	IIA	Propranolol	III
Diuretics	III	Quinidine	IB, IIA, IIB, III
Ephedrine	IC	Ranitidine	IA, IIA
Erythromycin	IIA	Rifampin	IA, IB
Ethanol	IIA	Salicylate	IIB
Fluconazole	IIA	Sildenafil	III
Fluoxetine	IIA	Simvastatin	IIA
Guanadrel	IC	Spironolactone	III
Guanethidine	IC	Tetracycline	IA
Haloperidol	IIA	Theophylline	IIA
Indomethacin	III	Thiazide diuretics	III
Isoniazid	IIA	Tolbutamide	IIA
Itraconazole	IB, IIA, IIB	Triamterene	III
Kaolin-pectin	IA	Triazolam	IIA
Ketoconazole	IA, IB, IIA	Verapamil	IB, IIA, IIB
Lidocaine	IIA	Warfarin	IB, IIA, III
Lovastatin	IIA		

Phenobarbital, rifampin, and other inducers lower plasma levels of many drugs, including warfarin, quinidine, mexiletine, verapamil, ketoconazole, itraconazole, cyclosporine, dexamethasone, methylprednisolone, prednisolone (the active metabolite of prednisone), oral contraceptive steroids, methadone, metronidazole, and metyrapone. These interactions all have obvious clinical significance. In the case of the coumarin anticoagulants, the patient is placed at major risk if the appropriate level of anticoagulation is achieved when an inducer is also being administered and the inducer is later discontinued (for example, at discharge from the hospital). The plasma levels of the coumarin anticoagulant will rise as the induction effect wears off, leading to excessive anticoagulation. There is considerable variation among individuals in the extent to which drug metabolism can be induced.

C. Inhibition of Cellular Uptake or Binding The guanidinium antihypertensive agents guanethidine and guanadrel are transported to their site of action in adrenergic neurons by an energy-requiring membrane transport system for biogenic monoamines; the physiologic function of this system is reuptake of the adrenergic neurotransmitter. Inhibitors of norepinephrine uptake prevent the uptake of the guanidinium antihypertensive agents into adrenergic neurons and thereby block their pharmacologic effects. The tricyclic antidepressants are potent inhibitors of norepinephrine uptake. Consequently, concomitant administration of clinical doses of tricyclic antidepressants, including desipramine, protriptyline, nortriptyline, and amitriptyline, almost totally abolishes the antihypertensive effects of

guanethidine and guanadrel. Although they are less potent inhibitors of norepinephrine uptake, doxepin and chlorpromazine produce dose-related antagonism of the action of the guanidinium antihypertensives.

The antihypertensive effect of clonidine is partially antagonized by tricyclic antidepressants. Clonidine lowers arterial pressure by reducing sympathetic outflow from the blood pressure–regulating centers in the hindbrain (Chap. 246). This central hypotensive action is antagonized by the tricyclic antidepressants.

II. PHARMACOKINETIC INTERACTIONS CAUSING INCREASED DRUG DELIVERY A. Inhibition of Drug Metabolism If the active form of a drug is eliminated largely by biotransformation, inhibition of its metabolism leads to reduced clearance, prolonged half-life, and accumulation of the drug during maintenance therapy. Excessive accumulation due to inhibited metabolism can lead to adverse effects.

Cimetidine is a potent inhibitor of the oxidative metabolism of many drugs, including warfarin, quinidine, nifedipine, lidocaine, theophylline, and phenytoin. Adverse reactions, many of them severe, have resulted from the administration of these drugs in conjunction with cimetidine. Cimetidine is a more potent inhibitor of mixed-function oxidases than ranitidine, whereas ranitidine is more potent as a histamine H_2 receptor antagonist. Famotidine and nizatidine are not known to produce clinically appreciable inhibition of drug metabolism.

Knowledge of the CYP isoforms that catalyze the main pathway of metabolism of a drug provides a basis for predicting and understanding drug interactions. For example, the CYP3A subfamily of isoforms catalyzes the metabolism of many drugs for which blockage of metabolism results in toxicity. Drugs that depend on CYP3A as a major route of metabolism include cyclosporine, quinidine, lovastatin, simvastatin, atorvastatin, nifedipine, lidocaine, cisapride, erythromycin, methylprednisolone, carbamazepine, midazolam, and triazolam.

The antifungal agents ketoconazole and itraconazole are potent inhibitors of enzymes in the CYP3A family. When fluconazole levels are elevated as a result of higher doses and/or renal insufficiency, this drug can also inhibit CYP3A. The macrolide antibiotics erythromycin and clarithromycin inhibit CYP3A4 to a clinically significant extent, but azithromycin does not inhibit this enzyme. Some of the calcium antagonists, diltiazem, nicardipine, and verapamil can also inhibit CYP3A, as can some of its other substrates, such as cyclosporine.

Cyclosporine can cause serious toxicity when its metabolism is inhibited by erythromycin, ketoconazole, diltiazem, nicardipine, or verapamil. A serious complication of HMG-CoA reductase inhibitors is myopathy. Fortunately, this is infrequent except in the context of interactions of a subset of the HMG-CoA reductase inhbitors with other drugs, particularly those that inhibit CYP3A4. The disposition of lovastatin is reduced markedly by drugs that inhibit CYP3A4, causing increases in plasma levels by more than tenfold. As a consequence, lovastatin has produced severe myopathy with rhabdomyolysis when administered together with erythromycin or cyclosporine. Not all of the HMG-CoA reductase inhibitors are as dependent on CYP3A4 for disposition as is lovastatin. Blocking CYP3A4 causes moderate elevations of plasma levels of simvastatin and atorvastatin (increases of severalfold), whereas elevations of the levels of fluvastatin and cerivastatin are only slight. Pravastatin disposition and plasma levels are not altered by inhibitors of CYP3A4. Cisapride can cause polymorphic ventricular tachycardia (torsade de pointes) when its metabolism is blocked by inhibitors of CYP3A, such as ketoconazole, itraconazole, clarithromycin, and erythromycin.

Whenever an inhibitor of CYP3A4 is administered to a patient, the physician should be alert to the possibility of serious interactions with drugs that are metabolized by CYP3A.

The CYP2D6 isoform that catalyzes the polymorphic metabolism of debrisoquin is markedly inhibited by quinidine and is also blocked by a number of neuroleptic drugs, such as chlorpromazine and haloperidol, and by fluoxetine. The analgesic effect of codeine depends on its metabolism to morphine via CYP2D6 in individuals with the EM phenotype. Thus, quinidine reduces the analgesic efficacy of codeine in EMs. Since desipramine is cleared largely by metabolism via CYP2D6 in EMs, its levels are increased substantially by concurrent administration of quinidine, fluoxetine, or the neuroleptic drugs that inhibit CYP2D6.

Some drugs are inactivated by mechanisms other than the hepatic drug-metabolizing enzymes. Azathioprine is converted in the body to an active metabolite, 6-mercaptopurine, which in turn is oxidized by xanthine oxidase to 6-thiouric acid. When allopurinol, a potent inhibitor of xanthine oxidase, is administered concurrently with standard doses of azathioprine or 6-mercaptopurine, life-threatening toxicity (bone marrow suppression) can result.

Other drugs that inhibit biotransformation of pharmacologic compounds (with examples of drugs whose metabolism is blocked by the inhibitor listed in parenthesis) include:

- Amiodarone (warfarin, quinidine)
- Clofibrate (phenytoin, tolbutamide)
- Excessive ingestion of ethanol (warfarin)
- Isoniazid (phenytoin)
- Metronidazole, cotrimoxazole (warfarin)
- Phenylbutazone (warfarin, phenytoin, tolbutamide)

B. Inhibition of Drug Transport Specific molecules that transport drugs into and out of cells are increasingly recognized, and

inhibition of their function can be a major cause of clinically important drug interactions. The best studied to date is P-glycoprotein, originally isolated from tumor cells displaying resistance to multiple, structurally unrelated anticancer agents. The mechanism underlying this "multidrug resistance" phenomenon is P-glycoprotein-mediated pumping of anticancer agents out of cells, thereby inhibiting their anticancer effects. P-glycoprotein is also expressed in normal tissues (the luminal aspect of intestinal and renal tubular cells, the canalicular aspect of hepatocytes, the capillary endothelium of the blood-brain barrier), where it is responsible for efflux of not only antineoplastics but also digoxin and HIV protease inhibitors. Quinidine inhibits P-glycoprotein function in vitro, and it now seems apparent that the widely recognized doubling of plasma digoxin when quinidine is coadministered reflects this action in vivo, particularly since the effects of quinidine (increased digoxin bioavailability and reduced renal and hepatic secretion) occur at the sites of P-glycoprotein expression. Many other drugs also elevate digoxin concentrations (e.g., amiodarone, verapamil, cyclosporine, itraconazole, and erythromcyin), and a similar mechanism seems likely. Reduced CNS penetration of multiple HIV protease inhibitors (with the attendant risk of facilitating a sanctuary site for the virus) appears attributable to P-glycoprotein-mediated exclusion of the drug from the CNS.

A number of drugs are secreted by the renal tubular transport systems for organic anions. Inhibition of this tubular transport system can cause excessive accumulation of a drug. Phenylbutazone, probenecid, and salicylates competitively inhibit this transport system. Salicylate, for example, reduces the renal clearance of methotrexate, an interaction that may lead to methotrexate toxicity. Renal tubular secretion contributes substantially to the elimination of penicillin, which can be inhibited by probenecid.

Inhibition of the tubular cation transport system by cimetidine impedes the renal clearance of procainamide and its active metabolite N-acetylprocainamide.

III. PHARMACODYNAMIC AND OTHER INTERACTIONS BETWEEN DRUGS Therapeutically useful interactions occur in which the effect of two drugs in combination is greater than the sum of their effects when used individually. Favorable drug combinations are described in specific therapeutic sections in this text, and this section focuses on interactions that create unwanted effects. Two drugs may act on separate components of a common process to yield effects greater than either has alone. For example, although small doses of aspirin (<1 g daily) do not alter the prothrombin time appreciably in patients who are receiving warfarin therapy, aspirin nevertheless increases the risk of bleeding in these patients because it inhibits platelet aggregation. Thus the combination of impaired functions of platelets and the clotting system, while useful for some therapeutic purposes, also increases the potential for hemorrhagic complications in patients receiving warfarin therapy.

Nonsteroidal antiinflammatory drugs (NSAIDs) cause gastric and duodenal ulcers, and, in patients treated with warfarin, the risk of bleeding from a peptic ulcer is increased almost threefold by concomitant use of a NSAID. This clearly is a serious drug interaction.

Indomethacin, piroxicam, and probably other NSAIDs antagonize the antihypertensive effects of β-adrenergic receptor blockers, diuretics, ACE inhibitors, and other drugs. The resulting elevation in blood pressure ranges from trivial to severe. Aspirin and sulindac, however, do not elevate the blood pressure in treated hypertensive patients.

Polymorphic ventricular tachycardia (torsade de pointes) during quinidine administration occurs much more frequently in patients receiving diuretics, probably owing to potassium and/or magnesium depletion.

The administration of supplemental potassium leads to more frequent and more severe hyperkalemia when potassium elimination is reduced by concurrent treatment with ACE inhibitors, spironolactone, amiloride, or triamterene.

The pharmacologic effects of sildenafil result from inhibition of the phosphodiesterase type 5 isoform that inactivates cyclic GMP in the vasculature. Nitroglycerin and related nitrates produce vasodilation by elevating cyclic GMP. Thus, coadministration of these nitrates with sildenafil will cause profound and potentially catastrophic hypotension.

CONCENTRATION OF DRUGS IN PLASMA AS A GUIDE TO THERAPY

In many cases, the plasma concentration of a drug is measured as a guide in the individualization of therapy. Genetic variation in elimination rates, interactions with other drugs, disease-induced alterations in elimination and distribution, and other factors combine to yield a wide range of plasma levels in patients given the same dose. Furthermore, the problem of noncompliance with prescribed regimens during continuing therapy is an endemic and elusive cause of therapeutic failure (see below). Clinical indicators assist in the titration of some drugs into the desired range, but no chemical determination is a substitute for careful observations of the response to treatment. However, the therapeutic and adverse effects are not precisely quantifiable for all drugs, and, in complex clinical situations, estimates of the action of a drug may be misleading. For example, previously existing neurologic disease may obscure the neurologic consequences of intoxication with phenytoin. Because clearance, half-life, accumulation, and steady-state plasma levels are difficult to predict, the measurement of plasma levels is often useful as a guide to the optimal dose. This is particularly true when there is a narrow range between the plasma levels yielding therapeutic and adverse effects. For drugs having such characteristics—e.g., digoxin, theophylline, lidocaine, aminoglycosides, cyclosporine, and anticonvulsants—dose optimization should involve modification of the standard dose on the basis of the pharmacokinetic principles described above. In certain instances, predictive nomograms and algorithms have been developed to facilitate the necessary modifications. However, the most flexible and accurate method for individualizing drug dosage appears to be a feedback approach using a small number of previously obtained plasma levels and Bayesian forecasting. In controlled studies, this type of computer-assisted dosing has been shown to improve patient care. However, the overall cost/benefit ratio of such methods in routine management still remains to be conclusively demonstrated.

For drugs with a narrow therapeutic window that exhibit first-order elimination, then, dosage adjustments may be made on the assumption that the average, maximum, and minimum steady-state concentrations are related linearly to the dosing rate. Accordingly, the dose may be adjusted on the basis of the ratio between the desired and measured concentrations:

$$\frac{C_{ss} \text{ (desired)}}{C_{ss} \text{ (measured)}} = \frac{\text{dose (new)}}{\text{dose (previous)}}$$

For drugs that have dose-dependent kinetics (e.g., phenytoin and theophylline), plasma concentrations change disproportionately more than the alteration in the dosing rate. Not only should changes in dose be small to minimize the degree of unpredictability, but plasma concentration monitoring is also critical to ensure appropriate modification.

The variability among individual responses to given plasma levels must be recognized. This is illustrated by a hypothetical population concentration-response curve (Fig. 70-4) and its relationship to the therapeutic range or therapeutic window of desired plasma levels. The defined therapeutic window should include the levels at which the intended pharmacologic effect is achieved in most patients. However, a few persons, who are sensitive to the therapeutic effects, respond to lower levels, whereas others are refractory enough to require levels that may cause adverse effects. For example, a few patients with strong seizure foci require plasma levels of phenytoin exceeding 20 μg/mL to control seizures. Dosages to achieve this effect may be appropriate if tolerated.

As also illustrated in Fig. 70-4, some patients are prone to adverse

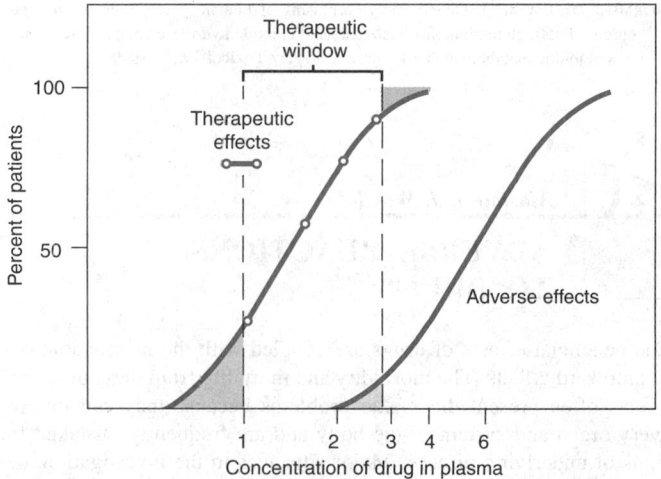

FIGURE 70-4   The cumulative percentage of patients responding to increasing levels of drug in plasma with both therapeutic and adverse effects. The therapeutic window defines the range of concentrations of drug that will achieve therapeutic effects in most patients with adverse effects in only a small percentage.

effects at levels that are tolerated by most of the population. Therefore, raising the plasma concentration of a drug to a level that has a high probability of being therapeutically effective may bring on unwanted actions in an occasional patient. Table 70-2 presents for a number of drugs the plasma concentrations that are associated with adverse and therapeutic effects in most patients. Use of this information according to the guidelines discussed should permit more effective and safer therapy for those patients who are not "average."

EFFECTIVE PARTICIPATION OF THE PATIENT IN THERAPY   Measurement of the concentration of a drug in plasma is the most effective way to detect failure to take a drug. Such "noncompliance" is a frequent problem in the long-term treatment of diseases such as hypertension and epilepsy, occurring in 25% or more of patients in therapeutic environments in which no special effort is made to involve patients in the responsibility for their own health. Occasionally, noncompliance can be uncovered by sympathetic, nonincriminating questioning, but more often it is recognized only after determining that the concentration of drug in plasma is nil or is recurrently low. Because other factors can cause plasma levels to be lower than expected, comparison with levels obtained during inpatient treatment may be required to confirm that noncompliance has occurred. Once the physician is certain of noncompliance, a nonaccusatory discussion of the problem with the patient may clarify the reason for the noncompliance and serve as a basis for more effective cooperation on the part of the patient. Many approaches have been tried to help patients exercise more responsibility for their own treatment, most based on better communication regarding the nature of the disease and the chances of success or failure of the treatment. The patient is given a chance to discuss problems associated with treatment. The process may be improved by the involvement of nurses and other paramedical personnel. Minimizing the complexity of the regimen is helpful in terms of both the number of drugs and the frequency of administration. Educating patients to assume the principal role in their own health care requires a blend of the art and science of medicine.

BIBLIOGRAPHY

BENET LZ et al: Design and optimization of dosage regimens: Pharmacokinetic data, in *Goodman and Gilman's The Pharmacological Basis of Therapeutics*, 9th ed, JG Hardman et al (eds). New York, McGraw-Hill, 1995, Appendix II, p 1707

HOLFORD N (ed): *Clinical Pharmacokinetics—Drug Data Handbook*, 3d ed. Adis International, Auckland, New Zealand, 1998

REYNOLDS DJ, ARONSON JK: ABCs of monitoring drug therapy. Making the most of plasma drug concentration measurements. BMJ 306:48, 1993

WORMHOUDT LW et al: Genetic polymorphisms of human *N*-acetyltransferase, cytochrome P450, glutathione-*S*-transferase, and epoxide hydrolase enzymes: Relevance
to xenobiotic metabolism and toxicity. Clin Rev Toxicol 29:59, 1999

71   *Alastair J. J. Wood*

ADVERSE REACTIONS TO DRUGS

The beneficial effects of drugs are coupled with the inescapable risk of untoward effects. The morbidity and mortality from these untoward effects often present diagnostic problems because they can involve every organ and system of the body and are frequently mistaken for signs of underlying disease. Major advances in the investigation, development, and regulation of drugs ensure in most instances that they are uniform, effective, and relatively safe and that their recognized hazards are publicized. However, prior to regulatory approval and marketing, new drugs are tested in relatively few patients who tend to be less sick and to have fewer concomitant diseases than those patients who subsequently receive the drug therapeutically. Because of the relatively small number of patients studied in clinical trials, and the selected nature of these patients, rare adverse effects may not be detected prior to a drug's approval, and physicians therefore need to be cautious in the prescription of new drugs and alert for the appearance of previously unrecognized adverse events.

The large number and variety of drugs available over the counter (OTC), herbal preparations, and by prescription, make it impossible for patient or physician to obtain or retain the knowledge necessary to use all drugs well. It is understandable, therefore, that many OTC drugs are used unwisely by the public and that restricted drugs may be prescribed incorrectly by physicians.

Most physicians use no more than 50 drug products in their practice, gaining familiarity with their effectiveness and safety. Most patients probably use only a limited number of OTC drugs. Nevertheless, many patients receive care and drug prescriptions from more than one physician, and in any 30-day period, many patients consume more than three different OTC drug products containing nine or more different chemical agents.

Some 25 to 50% of patients make errors in self-administration of prescribed medicines, and these errors can be responsible for adverse drug effects. Elderly patients are the group most likely to commit such errors, perhaps in part because they consume more medicines. One-third or more of patients also may not take their prescribed medications. Similarly, patients commit errors in taking OTC drugs by not reading or following the directions on the containers. Physicians must recognize that providing directions with prescriptions does not always guarantee compliance.

Every drug can produce untoward consequences, even when used according to standard or recommended methods of administration. When used incorrectly, the effectiveness may be reduced, and adverse reactions can be expected to occur more frequently. Also, the administration of several drugs concurrently may result in adverse drug interactions (Chap. 70). In the hospital, all drugs a patient is given should be under the control of a physician, and patient compliance is, in general, ensured. Errors may occur nevertheless—the wrong drug or dose may be given, or the drug may be given to the wrong patient—although improved drug distribution and administration systems have reduced this problem. On the other hand, there are no easy means for controlling how ambulatory patients take prescription or OTC drugs.

EPIDEMIOLOGY   Epidemiologic studies of adverse drug reactions have been helpful in evaluating the magnitude of the overall problem, in calculating the rate of reactions to individual drugs, and in characterizing some of the determinants of adverse drug effects.

Patients receive, on average, 10 different drugs during each hospitalization. The sicker the patient, the more drugs are given, and there is a corresponding increase in the likelihood of adverse drug reactions. When fewer than 6 different drugs are given to hospitalized patients, the probability of an adverse reaction is about 5%, but if more than 15 drugs are given, the probability is over 40%. Retrospective analyses of ambulatory patients have revealed adverse drug effects in 20%.

Thus, the magnitude of drug-induced disease is large. Of patients admitted to the medical and pediatric services of general hospitals, 2 to 5% are admitted because of illnesses attributed to drugs. The case/fatality ratio from drug-induced disease in hospitalized patients varies from 2 to 12%. Furthermore, some fetal or neonatal abnormalities are due to medicines taken by the mother during pregnancy or parturition.

A small group of widely used drugs accounts for a disproportionate number of reactions. Aspirin and other nonsteroidal anti-inflammatory drugs, analgesics, digoxin, anticoagulants, diuretics, antimicrobials, glucocorticoids, antineoplastics, and hypoglycemic agents account for 90% of reactions, although the drugs involved differ between ambulatory and hospitalized patients. Estimates of the cost of drug-related morbidity and mortality in the ambulatory setting range from $30 billion to $130 billion.

ADVERSE DRUG REACTIONS IN THE ELDERLY (See also Chap. 9)   The elderly as a group have a greater burden of disease and receive a greater number of medications than other persons. Thus, it is not surprising that adverse drug reactions occur frequently in elderly patients. The issue of whether an elderly individual is more likely to develop an adverse drug reaction than a young person with a similar number of concurrent diseases and taking the same number of drugs has not been answered unequivocally. However, in population surveys of the noninstitutionalized elderly, as many as 10% report having had at least one adverse drug reaction in the last year. The incidence appears to be even greater in hospitalized elderly patients. Although it is widely believed that the elderly are more sensitive to drugs than the young, that is not true for all drugs. For example, a consistent decrease in sensitivity to drugs acting at the β-adrenergic receptor has been demonstrated in the elderly. The consequences of adverse drug effects may differ in the elderly because of their greater likelihood of other disease. For example, use of long–half-life benzodiazepines is linked to the occurrence of hip fractures in elderly patients, perhaps reflecting both a risk of falls from these drugs and the increased incidence of osteoporosis in elderly patients. Even when a drug impairs function similarly in patients of different age groups, the poorer baseline function in elderly persons may put them at greater risk for an adverse drug reaction. When prescribing for an elderly patient, the possibility that hepatic or renal mechanisms of drug excretion may be impaired should be taken into account. Adverse drug effects in the elderly may be subtle and, as in all populations, the physician must be alert to the possibility that a patient's signs and symptoms reflect an adverse effect of medication.

ETIOLOGY   Most adverse drug reactions are preventable, and recent studies using a systems analysis approach suggest that the most common system failure associated with an adverse drug reaction is the failure to disseminate knowledge about drugs to individuals involved in prescribing and administering them. Most adverse reactions can be classified into two groups. The most frequent ones result from an exaggeration of a predicted pharmacologic action of the drug. Other adverse reactions ensue from toxic effects unrelated to the intended pharmacologic actions. The latter effects are often unpredictable, are frequently severe, and result from recognized as well as undiscovered mechanisms. Some mechanisms unrelated to the drug's primary pharmacologic activity may include direct cytotoxicity, initiation of abnormal immune responses, and perturbation of metabolic processes in individuals with genetic enzymatic defects. Further understanding of interindividual differences in the expression of the enzymes responsible for drug metabolism has contributed to the understanding of adverse drug reactions that previously were thought to be idiosyncratic (see below). Prior consideration of the factors known to modify drug action often make it possible to prevent adverse reactions of this type.

Genetic Variations in Drug Oxidation by Cytochromes There is considerable interindividual variability in drug metabolism, resulting in variability in drug concentrations (Chap. 70). The majority of drugs are oxidized by cytochrome P450s (CYP) in the liver and gut. Some of these enzymes exhibit genetic polymorphisms resulting in enzymes with absent or reduced drug metabolizing activity, which may result in concentration-dependent toxicity. Conversely, where toxicity or pharmacologic effect is produced by a metabolite, individuals with low enzyme activity may have reduced drug effect whereas those with genetically determined increased enzyme activity will have increased drug effect. Examples of such polymorphically distributed oxidation enzymes include CYP2D6, CYP2C9, and CYP2C19.

The clinical consequences of the poor metabolizer phenotype are now becoming clearer and depend on the specific consequences of excessive drug concentrations. For example, the more potent (S) isomer of warfarin is metabolized by the polymorphically distributed enzyme CYP2C9, resulting in lower (S) warfarin clearance and higher concentrations in both heterozygotes and homozygotes for the allelic variants associated with reduced enzyme activity. Recently, the clinical consequences of this polymorphism have been demonstrated in patients followed in an anticoagulant clinic. Patients who were stabilized on warfarin doses of 1.5 mg/d or less had an increased frequency of the genotypes associated with low warfarin metabolism compared to either community controls or patients requiring higher doses of warfarin (Table 71-1). In addition, the group stabilized on low-dose warfarin had a greater incidence of initial over-anticoagulation and hemorrhage than the group on the higher dose. This serves as an example of how genetic variations of a cytochrome P450 enzyme alter the response to a drug.

The oral hypoglycemic glipizide is also metabolized by CYP2C9, and excessively low blood glucose concentrations occur after usual doses in genetic CYP2C9 poor metabolizers. Another oral hypoglycemic, phenformin, produced lactic acidosis in some patients. It is now recognized that phenformin is metabolized by another polymorphically distributed oxidative enzyme, CYP2D6. Patients who have genetically determined low activity of CYP2D6 may be at particular risk from phenformin-induced lactic acidosis.

Genotypically determined variability in drug toxicity may also occur with drugs metabolized by enzymes other than cytochrome P450s. Such toxicity can be severe with the clinical use of the antimetabolites azathioprine and 6-mercaptopurine (to which it is converted in vivo). The cytotoxic thioguanine nucleotides produced in vivo are detoxified by further metabolism by xanthine oxidase and thiopurine methyltransferase (TPMT). The latter enzyme shows a trimodal distribution (Fig. 71-1). In children receiving mercaptopurine for treatment of leukemia, low activity of this enzyme is associated with excessive myelosuppression, whereas children with high TPMT levels have a poor antileukemic response. Azathioprine is currently used as a disease-modifying agent in the treatment of rheumatoid arthritis. Individuals with mutant TPMT alleles that result in impaired metabolism devel-

FIGURE 71-1 Thiopurine methyltransferase (TPMT) polymorphism: Frequency distribution of TPMT activity showing presumed genotype. *(From L Leonard: Lancet 336:225, 1990, with permission.)*

oped toxicity rapidly after beginning azathioprine and were uniformly unable to take the drug chronically. Thus the genotypic basis for drug toxicity is beginning to emerge.

Pharmacokinetic Bases for Adverse Reactions *An abnormally high drug concentration at the receptor site* (site of action) owing to pharmacokinetic variability is the usual cause of these reactions (Chap. 70). For example, a reduction in the volume of distribution, in the rate of metabolism, or in the rate of excretion all result in higher than expected concentration of drug at the receptor site, with a consequent increase in the pharmacologic effect.

Alteration in the dose-response curve due to increased receptor sensitivity results in an increase in drug effect at a given drug concentration. An example is the excessive response of elderly persons to the anticoagulant warfarin at normal or lower than normal blood levels. Such alterations in the dose-response curve may reflect altered drug sensitivity due to receptor polymorphisms, which are now being recognized. One such example is the prolonged QT syndrome, which has both a genetic basis, in individuals with abnormal potassium channels involved in cardiac repolarization, and a pharmacologic basis in individuals who receive drugs known to prolong the QT interval. Such individuals may develop torsade de pointes (Chap. 230). A large number of drugs have now been identified that can produce this potentially lethal effect (Table 71-2; also www.dml.georgetown.edu/depts/ pharmacology/torsades.html).

The shape of the dose-response curve also determines the likelihood of adverse drug reactions. Drugs with a steep dose-response curve or a narrow therapeutic index (Chap. 70) are more likely to cause dose-related toxicity because a small increase in dose produces a large change in pharmacologic effect. An increase in the dose of drugs that exhibit nonlinear kinetics, such as phenytoin (Chap. 70), may produce a proportionately greater increase in the blood level, resulting in toxicity.

Concurrent administration of other drugs may affect pharmacokinetics or pharmacodynamics. Pharmacokinetics may be affected by alterations in bioavailability, protein binding, or the rate of metabolism or excretion. Pharmacodynamics may be altered by another drug that competes for the same receptor sites, that prevents the drug from reaching its site of action, or that antagonizes or enhances the drug's pharmacologic effect. Inhibition of the metabolism of one drug by another may occur when both drugs bind to the same CYP. Therefore, as the specific CYPs responsible for the metabolism of individual drugs become known, prediction of drug interactions is put on a more rational scientific basis. An important example of such a mechanism is the inhibition of terfenadine's metabolism by inhibitors of CYP3A, such as erythromycin and systemic antimycotics. Such inhibition has resulted in torsade de pointes and lethal cardiac arrhythmia (Chap. 70).

Table 71-1 Warfarin Dose and Genotype

| Genotype, % | Distribution in Patients, % | | Community, % |
	<1.5 mg/d	>1.5 mg/d	
CYP2C9 *1/*1	19	62	60
*1/*2	33	17	20
*1/*3	28	19	17
*2/*3	14	0	2
*2/*2	6	2	0
*3/*3	0	0	1

NOTE: Warfarin dose and genotype. Distribution of CYP2D6 genotype in patients stabilized on warfarin doses of less than 1.5 mg/d and more than 1.5 mg/d compared to similar patients in the community. *1, *2, and *3 are the three genotypes. The genotype distribution in patients stabilized on > 1.5 mg/d is similar to that in the community population. However, patients stabilized on < 1.5 mg/d more frequently had genotypes other than *1/*1.

SOURCE: *Data from Aithal et al.*

Table 71-2   Clinical Manifestations of Adverse Reactions To Drugs

I. MULTISYSTEM MANIFESTATIONS

Anaphylaxis
  ACE[a] inhibitors and dialysis
  Cephalosporins
  Demeclocycline
  Dextran
  Insulin
  Intravenous immune globulin
  Iodinated drugs or contrast media
  Iron dextran
  Lidocaine
  Penicillins
  Procaine
  Streptomycin
  Sulfobromophthalein
Angioedema
  ACE[a] inhibitors
  Penicillin
  Rituximab
Drug-induced lupus erythematosus
  Acebutolol
  Asparaginase

Drug-induced lupus erythematosus (cont.)
  Barbiturates
  Bleomycin
  Cephalosporins
  Hydralazine
  Iodides
  Isoniazid
  Methyldopa
  Minocycline
  Phenolphthalein
  Phenytoin
  Procainamide
  Quinidine
  Sulfonamides
  Thiouracil
Fever
  Aminosalicylic acid
  Amphotericin B
  Antihistamines

Fever (cont.)
  Infliximab
  Interferon α
  Intravenous immune globulin
  Novobiocin
  Pamidronate
  Penicillins
  Streptokinase
Hyperpyrexia
  Antipsychotics
Increased susceptibility to infections
  Interferon α
Influenza-like reaction
  Interferon α
Neuroleptic malignant syndrome
  Antipsychotics
  Antidopaminergenics
Serum sickness
  Aspirin
  β-lactams
  Penicillins

Serum sickness (cont.)
  Propylthiouracil
  Streptokinase
  Streptomycin
  Sulfonamides
Vasculitis
  Allopurinol
  Aminopenicillins
  Hydantoins
  Penicillin
  Propylthiouracil
  Sulfonamides
  Thiazides

II. ENDOCRINE MANIFESTATIONS

Addisonian-like syndrome
  Busulfan
  Etomidate
  Ketoconazole
Galactorrhea (may also cause
    amenorrhea)
  Domperidone
  Methyldopa
  Metoclopramide
  Phenothiazines
  Reserpine
  Tricyclic antidepressants
Gynecomastia
  Calcium channel antagonists
  Clomiphene
  Digitalis
  Estrogens
  Ethionamide
  Griseofulvin

Gynecomastia (cont.)
  Isoniazid
  Methyldopa
  Phenytoin
  Reserpine
  Spironolactone
  Testosterone
Sexual dysfunction
  Impaired ejaculation
    Bethanidine
    Debrisoquin
    Guanethidine
    Thioridazine
  Decreased libido and impotence
    Beta blockers
    Clonidine
    Diuretics
    HIV-protease inhibitors
    Lithium

Sexual dysfunction (cont.)
  Decreased libido and
    impotence (cont.)
    Major tranquilizers
    Methyldopa
    Oral contraceptives
    Sedatives
  Impairment of spermatogenesis or
    oogenesis
    Cytotoxic agents
  Priapism
    Trazodone
Thyroid dysfunction (disorders caus-
  ing abnormal results on thyroid
  function tests)
  Acetazolamide
  Amiodarone
  Bromsulfophthalein
  Chlorpropamide

Thyroid dysfunction (cont.)
  Clofibrate
  Colestipol and nicotinic acid
  Dimercaprol
  Gold salts
  Iodides
  Lithium
  Oral contraceptives
  Phenindione
  Phenothiazines (long-term)
  Phenylbutazone
  Phenytoin
  Sulfonamides
  Tolbutamide
Vaginal carcinoma
  Diethylstilbestrol (given to
    mother)

III. METABOLIC MANIFESTATIONS

Hyperbilirubinemia
  Novobiocin
  Rifampin
Hypercalcemia
  Antacids with absorbable alkali
  Calcitonin
  Thiazides
  Vitamin D
Hyperglycemia
  Asparaginase
  Chlorthalidone
  Diazoxide
  Encainide
  Ethacrynic acid
  Furosemide
  Glucocorticoids
  Growth hormone
  HIV-protease inhibitors
  Niacin
  Oral contraceptives
  Phenytoin
  Pentamidine
  Thiazides
Hypoglycemia
  ACE[a] inhibitors
  Insulin
  Octreotide
  Oral hypoglycemics
  Pentamidine
  Quinine

Hyperkalemia
  ACE[a] inhibitors
  Amiloride
  Cyclosporine
  Cytotoxics
  Digitalis overdose
  Heparin
  Lithium
  NSAIDs[b]
  Pentamidine
  Potassium preparations including
    salt substitute
  Potassium salts of drugs
  Spironolactone
  Succinylcholine
  Triamterene
  Trimethoprin
Hypokalemia
  Alkali-induced alkalosis
  Amphotericin B
  Carbenoxolone
  Corticosteroids
  Diuretics
  Gentamicin
  Insulin
  Laxatives (abused)
  Mineralocorticoids, some gluco-
    corticoids
  Osmotic diuretics
  Sympathomimetic agents

Hypokalemia (cont.)
  Tetracycline (degraded)
  Theophylline
  Vitamin B$_{12}$
Hyperuricemia
  Aspirin (low dose)
  Chlorthalidone
  Cyclosporine
  Cytotoxics
  Ethacrynic acid
  Fructose (IV)
  Furosemide
  Hyperalimentation
  Pyrazinamide
  Thiazides
Hyponatremia
  Dilutional:
    Antipsychotics
    Carbamazepine
    Chlorpropamide
    Cyclophosphamide
    Desmopressin
    Diuretics
    Intravenous immune globulin
    Octreotide
    Selective serotonin reuptake in-
      hibitors
    Vincristine

Hyponatremia (cont.)
  Salt-wasting:
    Diuretics
    Enemas
    Mannitol
  Metabolic acidosis
    Acetazolamide
    Metformin
    Paraldehyde (degraded)
    Phenformin
    Salicylates
    Spironolactone
  Porphyria exacerbation
    Barbiturates
    Chlordiazepoxide
    Chlorpropamide
    Estrogens
    Glutethimide
    Griseofulvin
    Meprobamate
    Oral contraceptives
    Phenytoin
    Rifampin
    Sulfonamides

(continued)

432

IV. DERMATOLOGIC MANIFESTATIONS

Acne
- Anabolic and androgenic steroids
- Bromides
- Glucocorticoids
- Iodides
- Isoniazid
- Oral contraceptives
- Troxidone

Alopecia
- Beta blockers
- Colchicine
- Cytotoxics
- Ethionamide
- Fluconazole
- Heparin
- Interferon
- Lithium
- Oral contraceptives (withdrawal)
- Retinoids

Eczema
- Captopril
- Cream and lotion preservatives
- Lanolin
- Topical antihistamines
- Topical antimicrobials
- Topical local anesthetics

Erythema multiforme or Stevens-Johnson syndrome/toxic epidermal necrolysis
- Allopurinol
- Aminopenicillins
- Barbiturates
- Carbamazepine
- Cephalosporins
- Chlorpropamide
- Codeine
- Ethosuximide
- Imidazoles

Erythema multiforme (*cont.*)
- Iodides
- Lamotrigine
- Nalidixic acid
- Penicillins
- Phenolphthalein
- Phenylbutazone
- Phenytoin
- Piroxicam
- Quinolones
- Salicylates
- Sulfonamides
- Sulfones
- Tetracyclines
- Thiazides
- Tocainide
- Valproic acid

Erythema nodosum
- Oral contraceptives
- Penicillins
- Sulfonamides

Exfoliative dermatitis
- Barbiturates
- Gold salts
- Penicillins
- Phenylbutazone
- Phenytoin
- Quinidine
- Sulfonamides

Fixed drug eruptions
- Barbiturates
- Captopril
- Foscarnet (penile ulceration)
- Phenolphthalein
- Phenylbutazone
- Quinine
- Salicylates
- Sulfonamides

Flushing
- Nicotinic acid
- Sildenafil

Hyperpigmentation
- Amiodarone
- Bleomycin
- Busulfan
- Chloroquine and other anti-malarials
- Corticotropin
- Cyclophosphamide
- Gold salts
- Minocycline
- Oral contraceptives
- Phenothiazines
- Vitamin A (hypervitaminosis A)

Hypertrichosis
- Cyclosporine
- Minoxidil
- Phenytoin

Leg ulcers
- Hydroxyurea

Lichenoid eruptions
- Aminosalicylic acid
- Antimalarials
- Chlorpropamide
- Gold salts
- Methyldopa
- Phenothiazines

Nail changes
- Penicillamine
- Retinoids
- Tetracyclines

Photodermatitis
- Captopril
- Chlordiazepoxide
- Furosemide

Photodermatitis (*cont.*)
- Griseofulvin
- NSAIDs[b]
- Oral contraceptives
- Phenothiazines
- Sulfonamides
- Sulfonylureas
- Tetracyclines, particularly deme-clocycline
- Thiazides

Purpura (see also thrombocytopenia)
- Aspirin
- Glucocorticoids

Rashes (nonspecific)
- Allopurinol
- Ampicillin
- Barbiturates
- Indapamide
- Methyldopa
- Phenytoin

Rash
- Infliximab

Raynaud's disease or digital necrosis
- Beta blockers
- Bleomycin
- Ergot alkaloids

Skin necrosis
- Warfarin

Urticaria
- Aspirin
- Barbiturates
- Captopril
- Enalapril
- Intravenous immune globulin
- Penicillins
- Sulfonamides

V. HEMATOLOGIC MANIFESTATIONS

Agranulocytosis (see also pancytopenia)
- Aprindine
- Captopril
- Carbimazole
- Cefotaxime
- Chloramphenicol
- Clozapine
- Co-trimoxazole
- Cytotoxics
- Gold salts
- Indomethacin
- Methimazole
- Oxyphenbutazone
- Phenothiazines
- Phenylbutazone
- Propylthiouracil
- Sulfonamides
- Ticlopidine
- Tolbutamide
- Tricyclic antidepressants

Churg-Strauss syndrome
- Fluticasone propionate
- Montelukast
- Zafirlukast

Clotting and bleeding abnormalities/ hypothrombinemia
- Cefamandole
- Cefoperazone
- Ketorolac
- Mezlocillin
- Moxalactam
- Piperacillin
- Valproic acid

Eosinophilia
- Aminosalicylic acid
- Chlorpropamide
- Erythromycin estolate

Eosinophilia (*cont.*)
- Imipramine
- L-Tryptophan
- Methotrexate
- Montelukast
- Nitrofurantoin
- Procarbazine
- Sulfonamides
- Zafirlukast

Hemolytic anemia
- Aminosalicylic acid
- Cephalosporins
- Chlorpromazine
- Dapsone
- Insulin
- Isoniazid
- Levodopa
- Mefenamic acid
- Melphalan
- Methyldopa
- Penicillins
- Phenacetin
- Procainamide
- Quinidine
- Rifampin
- Sulfonamides

Hemolytic anemia (in G6PD deficiency)
- Aminosalicylic acid
- Antimalarials, e.g., primaquine
- Aspirin
- Chloramphenicol
- Co-trimoxazole
- Dapsone
- Nalidixic acid
- Nitrofurantoin
- Phenacetin
- Probenecid

Hemolytic anemia (*cont.*)
- Procainamide
- Quinidine
- Sulfonamides
- Vitamin C
- Vitamin K

Leukocytosis
- Glucocorticoids
- Lithium

Lymphadenopathy
- Phenytoin
- Primidone

Megaloblastic anemia
- Co-trimoxazole
- Folate antagonists
- Nitrous oxide (repeated or prolonged exposure)
- Oral contraceptives
- Phenobarbital
- Phenytoin
- Primidone
- Triamterene
- Trimethoprim

Pancytopenia (aplastic anemia)
- Carbamazepine
- Carbimazole
- Chloramphenicol
- Cytotoxics
- Felbamate
- Gold salts
- Mepacrine
- Mephenytoin
- Oxyphenbutazone
- Phenylbutazone
- Phenytoin
- Potassium perchlorate
- Quinacrine
- Sulfonamides

Pancytopenia (*cont.*)
- Thiouracils
- Ticlopidine
- Trimethadione
- Zidovudine (AZT)

Pure red cell aplasia
- Azathioprine
- Chlorpropamide
- Isoniazid
- Phenytoin

Thrombocytopenia (see also pancytopenia)
- Acetazolamine
- Aspirin
- Carbamazepine
- Carbenicillin
- Chlorpropamide
- Chlorthalidone
- Co-trimoxazole
- Digitoxin
- Furosemide
- Gold salts
- Heparin
- Indomethacin
- Isoniazid
- Methyldopa
- Moxalactam
- Novobiocin
- Oxyphenbutazone
- Phenylbutazone
- Phenytoin and other hydantoins
- Quinidine
- Quinine
- Thiazides
- Ticarcillin

TTP[c]
- Ticlopidine

(continued)

VI. CARDIOVASCULAR MANIFESTATIONS

Acute chest pain (nonischemic)
  Bleomycin
Angina exacerbation
  Alpha blockers
  Beta-blocker withdrawal
  Ergotamine
  Excessive thyroxine
  Hydralazine
  Methysergide
  Minoxidil
  Nifedipine
  Oxytocin
  Sumatriptan
  Vasopressin
Arrhythmias (see also prolonged QT
  torsade de pointes)
  Adenosine
  Adriamycin
  Antiarrhythmic drugs
  Astemizole
  Atropine
  Anticholinesterases
  Beta blockers
  Cisapride
  Daunorubicin
  Digitalis
  Emetine
  Erythromycin
  Guanethidine
  Ketanserin
  Lithium
  Papaverine
  Pentamidine
  Phenothiazines, particularly thiori-
    dazine

Arrhythmias *(cont.)*
  Probucol
  Sympathomimetics
  Terfenadine
  Theophylline
  Thyroid hormone
  Tricyclic antidepressants
  Verapamil
AV block
  Clonidine
  Methyldopa
  Verapamil
Cardiomyopathy
  Adriamycin
  Daunorubicin
  Emetine
  Hydroxychloroquine
  Lithium
  Phenothiazines
  Sulfonamides
  Sympathomimetics
Fluid retention/congestive heart fail-
  ure/edema
  Beta blockers
  Calcium blockers
  Carbenoxolone
  Diazoxide
  Estrogens
  Growth hormone
  NSAIDs[b]
  Mannitol
  Minoxidil
  Phenylbutazone
  Steroids
  Verapamil

Hypotension (see also arrhythmias)
  Amiodarone (perioperative)
  Calcium channel blockers, e.g.,
    nifedipine
  Citrated blood
  Diuretics
  Interleukin 2
  Levodopa
  Morphine
  Nitroglycerin
  Phenothiazines
  Protamine
  Quinidine
  Sildenafil
Hypertension
  Clonidine withdrawal
  Corticotropin
  Cyclosporine
  Erythropoietin
  Glucocorticoids
  Monoamine oxidase inhibitors
    with sympathomimetics
  NSAIDs[b] (some)
  Oral contraceptives
  Sympathomimetics
  Tricyclic antidepressants with
    sympathomimetics
Pericarditis
  Emetine
  Hydralazine
  Methysergide
  Procainamide
Pericardial effusion
  Minoxidil

Prolonged QT interval/torsade de
  pointes
  Amiodarone
  Amitriptyline
  Astemizole
  Bepridil
  Chlorpromazine
  Cisapride
  Clomipramine
  Desipramine
  Diphenylhydramine
  Disopyramide
  Doxepin
  Erythromycin
  Haloperidol
  Ibutilide
  Imipramine
  Maprotiline
  Pentamidine
  Probucol
  Procainamide
  Quinidine
  Risperidone
  Sotalol
  Terfenadine
  Trimethoprim-sulfamethoxazole
  Thioridazine
  Thiothixene
  Trifluoperazine
Thromboembolism
  Estrogen
  Oral contraceptives
Valvular heart disease
  Fenfluramine

VII. RESPIRATORY MANIFESTATIONS

Airway obstruction (bronchospasm,
  asthma; see also anaphylaxis)
  Adenosine
  Beta blockers
  Cephalosporins
  Cholinergic drugs
  NSAIDs,[b] e.g., aspirin, indo-
    methacin
  Penicillins
  Pentazocine
  Streptomycin
  Tartrazine (drugs with yellow
    dye)
Cough
  ACE[a] inhibitors

Nasal congestion
  Decongestant abuse
  Guanethidine
  Isoproterenol
  Oral contraceptives
  Reserpine
Pulmonary edema
  Contrast media
  Heroin
  Hydrochlorthiazide
  Interleukin 2
  Methadone
  Propoxyphene
Pulmonary hypertension
  Fenfluramine

Pulmonary infiltrates
  Acyclovir
  Amiodarone
  Azothioprine
  Bleomycin
  Busulfan
  Carmustine (BCNU)
  Chlorambucil
  Cyclophosphamide
  Gold
  Melphalan
  Methotrexate
  Methysergide
  Mitomycin C
  Nitrofurantoin

Pulmonary infiltrates *(cont.)*
  Procarbazine
  Sulfonamides
Respiratory depression
  Aminoglycosides
  Hypnotics
  Opiates
  Polymyxins
  Sedatives
  Trimethaphan

VIII. GASTROINTESTINAL MANIFESTATIONS

Cholestatic hepatitis
  Acetohexamide
  Anabolic steroids
  Androgens
  Chlorpropamide
  Clavulanic acid/amoxicillin
  Cyclosporine
  Erythromycin estolate
  Flucloxacillin
  Gold salts
  Methimazole
  Nitrofurantoin
  Oral contraceptives
  Phenothiazines
Constipation or ileus
  Aluminum hydroxide
  Barium sulfate
  Calcium carbonate

Constipation or ileus *(cont.)*
  Ferrous sulfate
  Ganglionic blockers
  Ion exchange resins
  Opiates
  Phenothiazines
  Tricyclic antidepressants
  Verapamil
Diarrhea or colitis
  Antibiotics (broad-spectrum)
  Clindamycin
  Cocaine
  Colchicine
  Digitalis
  Donepezil
  Guanethidine
  Lactose excipients
  Lincomycin

Diarrhea or colitis *(cont.)*
  Magnesium in antacids
  Methyldopa
  Misoprostol
  Oral contraceptives
  Purgatives
  Reserpine
  Ticlopidine
Diffuse hepatocellular damage
  Acetaminophen (paracetamol)
  Acebutolol
  Allopurinol
  Aminosalicylic acid
  Amiodarone
  Aprindine
  Bromfenae
  Carbenicillin
  Cyclophosphamide

Diffuse hepatocellular
  damage *(cont.)*
  Dapsone
  Diclofenac
  Erythromycin estolate
  Ethionamide
  Felbamate
  Glyburide
  Halothane
  HMG-CoA reductase inhibitors
  Isoniazid
  Ketoconazole
  Labetalol
  Lovastatin
  Methimazole
  Methotrexate
  Methoxyflurane
  Methyldopa

(continued)

Minocycline
Monamine oxidase inhibitors
Nefazodone
Niacin
Nifedipine
Nitrofurantoin
Oxyphenisatin
Pemoline
Phenytoin and other hydantoins
Propoxyphene
Propylthiouracil
Pyridium
Quinidine
Quinolone antibiotics
Rifampin
Salicylates
Sodium valproate
Sulfonamides
Tacrine
Tetracyclines
Tolcapone
Trazodone
Troglitazone
Verapamil
Zidovudine (AZT)
Esophagitis
  Alendronate
Fibrosing colonopathy and colonic
  stricture
  Pancreatin

Gallstones/biliary pseudolithiasis
  Ceftriaxone
  Estrogens
Malabsorption
  Aminosalicylic acid
  Antibiotics (broad-spectrum)
  Cholestyramine
  Colchicine
  Colestipol
  Cytotoxic agents
  Neomycin
  Phenobarbital
  Phenytoin
  Primidone
Nausea or vomiting
  Cytotoxic agents
  Digitalis
  Donepezil
  Estrogens
  Ferrous sulfate
  Levodopa
  Opiates
  Potassium chloride
  Tetracyclines
  Theophylline
Oral conditions
  Dental discoloration:
    Tetracycline
  Dry mouth:
    Anticholinergics

Dry mouth: (cont.)
  Brimonidine
  Clonidine
  Levodopa
  Methyldopa
  Tricyclic antidepressants
Gingival hyperplasia:
  Calcium antagonists
  Cyclosporine
  Phenytoin
Salivary gland swelling:
  Bethanidine
  Bretylium
  Clonidine
  Guanethidine
  Iodides
  Phenylbutazone
Taste disturbances
  Acetazolamide
  Biguanides
  Captopril
  Griseofulvin
  Lithium
  Metronidazole
  Penicillamine
  Rifampin
Ulceration
  Aspirin
  Cytotoxic agents
  Gentian violet

Ulceration (cont.)
  Isoproterenol (sublingual)
Pancreatitis
  Asparaginase
  Azathioprine
  Didanosine
  Estrogens
  Ethacrynic acid
  Furosemide
  Glucocorticoids
  Mercaptopurine
  Opiates
  Oral contraceptives
  Pentamidine
  Sulfonamides
  Thiazides
  Valproic acid
Peptic ulceration or hemorrhage
  Aspirin
  Ethacrynic acid
  Glucocorticoids
  NSAIDs[b]
  Reserpine (large doses)
Ulceration
  Esophageal:
    Alendronate
  Intestinal:
    Solid KCl preparations

IX. RENAL MANIFESTATIONS

Bladder dysfunction/incontinence
  Anticholinergics
  Disopyramide
  Monoamine oxidase inhibitors
  Prazosin
  Terazosin
  Tricyclic antidepressants
Calculi/crystaluria
  Acetazolamide
  Indinavir
  Vitamin D
Concentrating defect with polyuria
  (or nephrogenic diabetes insipidus)
  Demeclocycline
  Lithium
  Methoxyflurane
  Vitamin D
Hemorrhage cystitis
  Busulfan
  Carmustine
  Chlorambucil

Hemorrhage cystitis (cont.)
  Cyclophosphamide
  Extended-spectrum penicillins
  Nitrogen mustard
  Vincristine
Interstitial nephritis
  Cephalosporins
  Ciprofloxacin
  Allopurinol
  Furosemide
  NSAIDs[b]
  Penicillins, esp. methicillin
  Phenindione
  Rifampin
  Sulfonamides
  Thiazides
Nephropathies
  Analgesics (e.g., phenacetin)
Nephrotic syndrome
  Captopril
  Gold salts

Nephrotic syndrome (cont.)
  Ketoprofen
  Penicillamine
  Phenindione
  Probenecid
Obstructive uropathy
  Extrarenal:
    Methysergide
  Intrarenal:
    Acyclovir
    Cytotoxic agents
    Methotrexate
    Metyrosine
Renal dysfunction
  ACE inhibitors[a]
  Cidofovir
  Cyclosporine
  NSAIDs[b]
  Pentamidine
  Tacrolimus
  Triamterene

Renal tubular acidosis
  Acetazolamide
  Amphotericin B
  Degraded tetracycline
Tubular necrosis
  Aminoglycosides
  Amphotericin B
  Cephaloridine
  Colistin
  Cyclosporine
  Intravenous immune globulin
  Methoxyflurane
  Polymyxins
  Radioiodinated contrast medium
  Sulfonamides
  Tetracyclines

X. NEUROLOGIC MANIFESTATIONS

Aseptic meningitis
  Intravenous immune globulin
  NSAIDs
  OKT3 antibodies
  Antibiotics
CNS/vasculitis/cerebral hemorrhage
  Cocaine
  Phenylpropanolamine
Exacerbation of myasthenia
  Aminoglycosides
  D-Penicillamine
  Polymyxins
Extrapyramidal effects
  Butyrophenones, e.g., haloperidol
  Levodopa
  Methyldopa
  Metoclopramide
  Oral contraceptives
  Phenothiazines
  Reserpine
  Tricyclic antidepressants

Headache
  Bromides
  Ergotamine (withdrawal)
  Glyceryl trinitrate
  Hydralazine
  Indomethacin
  Interferon α
  Intravenous immune globulin
  Sibutramine
  Sildenafil
Peripheral neuropathy
  Amiodarone
  Chloramphenicol
  Chloroquine
  Chlorpropamide
  Cisplatin
  Clioquinol
  Clofibrate
  Demeclocycline
  Disopyramide
  Ethambutol

Peripheral neuropathy (cont.)
  Ethionamide
  Glutethimide
  Hydralazine
  Isoniazid
  Methysergide
  Metronidazole
  Mustine
  Nalidixic acid
  Nitrofurantoin
  Perhexiline
  Phenelzine
  Phenytoin
  Polymyxin, colistin
  Procarbazine
  Streptomycin
  Tolbutamide
  Tricyclic antidepressants
  Vincristine

Pseudotumor cerebri (or intracranial
  hypertension)
  Amiodarone
  Glucocorticoids, mineralocorti-
    coids
  Vitamin A (hypervitaminosis A)
  Oral contraceptives
  Tetracyclines
Seizures
  Amphetamines
  Analeptics
  Imipenem
  Interferon α
  Isoniazid
  Lidocaine
  Lithium
  Nalidixic acid
  Meperidine
  Penicillins
  Phenothiazines
  Physostigmine

(continued)

X. NEUROLOGIC MANIFESTATIONS (*cont.*)

Seizures (*cont.*)	Sleep disorders	Stroke	Tremor
Theophylline	HMG-CoA reductase inhibitors	Cocaine	β-Adrenergic agonists
Tramadol	Lovastatin	Oral contraceptives	Cyclosporine
Tricyclic antidepressants			
Vincristine			

XI. OCULAR MANIFESTATIONS

Cataracts	Color vision alteration (*cont.*)	Glaucoma	Optic neuritis (*cont.*)
Busulfan	Thiazides	Ipratropium bromide	Phenothiazines
Chlorambucil	Troxidone	Mydriatics	Phenylbutazone
Glucocorticoids	Corneal edema	Sympathomimetics	Quinine
Phenothiazines	Oral contraceptives	Optic neuritis	Streptomycin
Color vision alteration	Corneal opacities	Aminosalicylic acid	Retinopathy
Barbiturates	Chloroquine	Amiodarone	Chloroquine
Digitalis	Indomethacin	Chloramphenicol	Phenothiazines
Methaqualone	Mepacrine	Clioquinol	Uveitis/iritis
Sildenafil	Vitamin D	Ethambutol	Cidofovir
Streptomycin	Eye pain	Isoniazid	
Sulfonamides	Nifedipine	Penicillamine	

XII. EAR MANIFESTATIONS

Deafness	Deafness (*cont.*)	Deafness (*cont.*)
Aminoglycosides	Deferoxamine	Nortriptyline
Aspirin	Erythromycin	Quinine
Bleomycin	Ethacrynic acid	Vestibular disorders
Chloroquine	Furosemide	Aminoglycosides
Cidofovir	Interferon	Mustine
Cisplatin	Mustine	Quinine

XIII. MUSCULOSKELETAL MANIFESTATIONS

Arthralgias	Bone disorders (*cont.*)	Myopathy or myalgia (*cont.*)	Rhabdomyolysis
Growth hormone	Gout: see Hyperuricemia	Clofibrate	Gemfibrozil
Infiximab	Osteomalacia:	Glucocorticoids	HMG-CoA reductase inhibitors
Interferon α	Aluminum hydroxide	Growth hormone	Lovastatin
Avascular necrosis	Anticonvulsants	HMG-CoA reductase inhibitors	Tendon rupture
Glucocorticoids	Glutethimide	Infliximab	Quinolones
Bone disorders	Myopathy or myalgia	Interferon α	
Osteoporosis:	Amphotericin B	Oral contraceptives	
Glucocorticoids	Carbenoxolone	Zidovudine	
Heparin	Chloroquine		
Thyroxine	Cimetidine		

XIV. PSYCHIATRIC MANIFESTATIONS

Delirious or confusional states	Depression (*cont.*)	Hallucinatory states (*cont.*)	Schizophrenic-like or paranoid reactions (*cont.*)
Amantadine	Centrally acting antihypertensives	Meperidine	Glucocorticoids
Aminophylline	(reserpine, methyldopa,	Narcotics	Levodopa
Anticholinergics	clonidine)	Pentazocine	Lysergic acid
Antidepressants	Glucocorticoids	Tricyclic antidepressants	Monoamine oxidase inhibitors
Bromides	Isotretinoin	Hypomania, mania, or excited reactions	Tricyclic antidepressants
Cimetidine	Levodopa	Glucocorticoids	Sleep disturbances
Digitalis	Drowsiness	Levodopa	Anorexiants
Glucocorticoids	Antihistamines	Monoamine oxidase inhibitors	Levodopa
Isoniazid	Anxiolytic drugs	Sympathomimetics	Monoamine oxidase inhibitors
Levodopa	Brimonidine	Tricyclic antidepressants	Sympathomimetics
Methyldopa	Clonidine	Hypersexuality	
Penicillins	Major tranquilizers	Antiparkinsonian agents	
Phenothiazines	Methyldopa	Memory loss	
Ranitidine	Reserpine	Triazolam	
Sedatives and hypnotics	Tricyclic antidepressants	Schizophrenic-like or paranoid reactions	
Vigabatrin	Hallucinatory states	Amphetamines	
Depression	Amantadine	Bromides	
Amphetamine withdrawal	Beta blockers		
Beta blockers	Levodopa		

^a ACE, angiotensin-converting enzyme.
^b NSAID, nonsteroidal anti-inflammatory drug.

^c TTP, thrombotic thrombocytopenic purpura.

[a] ACE, angiotensin-converting enzyme.
[b] NSAID, nonsteroidal anti-inflammatory drug.
[c] TTP, thrombotic thrombocytopenic purpura.

TOXICITY UNRELATED TO A DRUG'S PRIMARY PHARMACOLOGIC ACTIVITY Cytotoxic Reactions The understanding of so-called idiosyncratic reactions has greatly improved with the recognition that many of them are due to irreversible binding of a drug or its metabolites to tissue macromolecules by co-valent bonds. Some chemical carcinogens, such as the alkylating agents, combine directly with DNA. Usually, it is only after metabolic activation of a drug to reactive metabolites that covalent binding occurs. This activation usually occurs in the microsomal mixed-function oxidase system, the hepatic enzyme system responsible for the metabolism of many drugs (Chap. 70). During the course of drug metabolism, reactive metabolites may covalently bind to tissue macromolecules, causing tissue damage. Because of the reactive nature of these metabolites, covalent binding often occurs close to the site of production. Typically that is the liver, but the mixed-function oxidase system is found in other tissues as well.

An example of this type of adverse drug reaction is the hepatotoxicity associated with isoniazid. This drug is metabolized principally by acetylation to acetylisoniazid, which is then hydrolyzed to acetylhydrazine. The further metabolism of acetylhydrazine by the mixed-function oxidase system liberates reactive metabolites that covalently bind to hepatic macromolecules, causing hepatic necrosis. The administration of drugs known to increase the activity of the mixed-function oxidase system, such as phenobarbital or rifampin, together with isoniazid results in the production of increased amounts of reactive metabolites, increased covalent binding, and a greater risk of hepatic damage.

The hepatic necrosis produced by overdosage of acetaminophen is also caused by reactive metabolites. Normally these metabolites are detoxified by combining with hepatic glutathione. When glutathione becomes exhausted, the metabolites bind instead to hepatic protein, with resultant hepatocyte damage. The hepatic necrosis produced by the ingestion of acetaminophen can be prevented, or at least attenuated, by the administration of substances such as N-acetylcysteine that reduce the binding of electrophilic metabolites to hepatic proteins. The risk of hepatic necrosis is increased in patients receiving drugs such as phenobarbital that increase the rate of drug metabolism and the rate of production of toxic metabolite(s).

It is likely, though as yet not proved, that other idiosyncratic reactions are caused by the covalent binding of reactive metabolites to tissue macromolecules, resulting either in direct cytotoxicity or in the initiation of an immune response.

Immunologic Mechanisms Most pharmacologic agents are poor immunogens because they are small molecules with molecular weights of less than 2000. Stimulation of antibody synthesis or sensitization of lymphocytes by a drug or one of its metabolites usually requires in vivo activation and covalent linkage to protein, carbohydrate, or nucleic acid.

Drug stimulation of antibody production may mediate tissue injury by one of several mechanisms. The antibody may attack the drug when the drug is covalently attached to a cell, and thereby destroy the cell. This mechanism occurs in penicillin-induced hemolytic anemia. Antibody-drug-antigen complexes may be passively adsorbed by a bystander cell, which is then destroyed by activation of complement; this occurs in quinine- and quinidine-induced thrombocytopenia. Drugs or their reactive metabolites may alter a host tissue, rendering it antigenic and eliciting autoantibodies. For example, hydralazine and procainamide can chemically alter nuclear material, stimulating the formation of anti-nuclear antibodies and occasionally causing lupus erythematosus. Autoantibodies can be elicited by drugs that neither interact with the host antigen nor have any chemical similarity to the host tissue; for example, α-methyldopa frequently stimulates the formation of antibodies to host erythrocytes, yet the drug neither attaches to the erythrocyte nor shares any chemical similarities with the antigenic determinants on the erythrocyte.

Drug-induced pure red cell aplasia (Chap. 109) is due to an immune-based drug reaction. Red cell formation in bone marrow cultures can be inhibited by phenytoin and purified IgG obtained from a patient with pure red cell aplasia associated with phenytoin.

Serum sickness (Chap. 310) results from the deposition of circulating drug-antibody complexes on endothelial surfaces. Complement activation occurs, chemotactic factors are generated locally, and an inflammatory response develops at the site of complex entrapment. Arthralgias, urticaria, lymphadenopathy, glomerulonephritis, or cerebritis may result. Penicillin is the most common cause of serum sickness today. Many drugs, particularly antimicrobial agents, induce production of IgE, which binds to mast cell membranes. Contact with a drug antigen initiates a series of biochemical events in the mast cell and results in the release of mediators that can produce the urticaria, wheezing, flushing, rhinorrhea, and (occasionally) hypotension characteristic of anaphylaxis.

Drugs may also excite cell-mediated immune responses. Topically administered substances may interact with sulfhydryl or amino groups in the skin and react with sensitized lymphocytes to produce the rash characteristic of contact dermatitis. Other types of rashes may also result from the interaction of serum factors, drugs, and sensitized lymphocytes. The role of drug-activated lymphocytes in the immune mechanisms governing destruction of visceral tissue is unknown.

Toxicity Associated with Genetically Determined Enzymatic Defects In the porphyrias, drugs that increase the activity of enzymes proximal to the deficient enzyme in the biosynthetic pathway of porphyrins can increase the quantity of porphyrin precursors that accumulate proximal to the deficient enzyme (Chap. 346). These drugs are listed in Table 71-1.

Patients with a deficiency of glucose-6-phosphate dehydrogenase (G6PD) develop hemolytic anemia in response to primaquine and a number of other drugs (Table 71-1) that do not cause hemolysis in patients with adequate quantities of this enzyme (Chap. 108).

DIAGNOSIS The manifestations of drug-induced diseases frequently resemble those of other diseases, and a given set of manifestations may be produced by different and dissimilar drugs. Recognition of the role of a drug or drugs in an illness depends on appreciation of the possible adverse reactions to drugs in any disease, on identification of the temporal relationship between drug administration and development of the illness, and on familiarity with the common manifestations of the drugs. Many associations between particular drugs and specific reactions have been described, but there is always a "first time" for a novel association, and any drug should be suspected of causing an adverse effect if the clinical setting is appropriate.

Illness related to a drug's pharmacologic action is often more easily recognized than illness attributable to immune or other mechanisms. For example, side effects such as cardiac arrhythmias in patients receiving digitalis, hypoglycemia in patients given insulin, and bleeding in patients receiving anticoagulants are more readily related to a specific drug than are symptoms such as fever or rash, which may be caused by many drugs or by other factors.

Once an adverse reaction is suspected, discontinuance of the suspected drug followed by disappearance of the reaction is presumptive evidence of a drug-induced illness. Confirming evidence may be sought by cautiously reintroducing the drug and seeing if the reaction reappears. However, that should be done only if confirmation would be useful in the future management of the patient and if the attempt would not entail undue risk. With concentration-dependent adverse reactions, lowering the dosage may cause the reaction to disappear, and raising it may cause the reaction to reappear. When the reaction is thought to be allergic, however, readministration of the drug may be hazardous, since anaphylaxis may develop. Readministration is unwise under these conditions unless no alternative drugs are available and treatment is necessary.

If the patient is receiving many drugs when an adverse reaction is suspected, the drugs likeliest to be responsible can usually be identified. All drugs may be discontinued at once, or, if that is not practical, they should be discontinued one at a time, starting with the one that is most suspect, and the patient observed for signs of improvement. The time needed for a concentration-dependent adverse effect to disappear depends on the time required for the concentration to fall below the range associated with the adverse effect, and that, in turn, depends on the initial blood level and on the rate of elimination or metabolism of the drug. Adverse effects of drugs with long half-lives, such as phenobarbital, take a considerable time to disappear.

Drugs recognized as producing a number of reactions are listed in Table 71-1. This table includes both well-documented and some less well-documented reactions, focusing on those that are sufficiently important to require consideration. This information should be used to suggest the drug likely to be causing a reaction; the absence of a drug from the table does not mean that it cannot be responsible for the reaction, however.

Serum antibody has been demonstrated in some persons with drug allergies involving cellular blood elements, as in agranulocytosis, hemolytic anemia, and thrombocytopenia. For example, both quinine and quinidine can produce platelet agglutination in vitro in the presence of complement and the serum from a patient who has developed thrombocytopenia following use of this drug.

Eliciting a drug history from patients is important for diagnosis. Attention must be directed to OTC drugs and herbal preparations as well as to prescription drugs. Each type can be responsible for adverse drug effects, and adverse interactions may occur between OTC drugs and prescribed drugs. In addition, it is common for patients to be cared for by several physicians, and duplicative, additive, counteractive, or synergistic drug combinations may therefore be administered if the physicians are not aware of the patients' drug histories. Every physician should determine what drugs a patient has been taking, at least during the preceding 30 days, before prescribing any medications. A frequently overlooked source of additional drug exposure is topical therapy; for example, a patient complaining of bronchospasm may not mention that an ophthalmic beta blocker is being used unless specifically asked. A history of previous adverse drug effects in patients is common. Since these patients have shown a predisposition to drug-induced illnesses, such a history should dictate added caution in prescribing drugs.

Patients with biochemical abnormalities such as erythrocyte G6PD deficiency can be identified. Most patients with the G6PD defect are of African or Mediterranean descent. Drug-induced hemolytic crisis can be avoided by testing for the enzyme defect before administering drugs that could cause the reaction. Similarly, persons with an abnormal serum pseudocholinesterase level may have abnormally prolonged apnea when given succinylcholine.

GENERAL COMMENTS   No drug is completely without side effects, and a side effect in one patient may be the desired pharmacologic effect in another. Current drug regulations allow physicians to have considerable confidence in the purity, bioavailability, and effectiveness of the drugs they prescribe. However, physicians have to weigh potential toxicity against possible benefits. Toxicity that would be acceptable for an effective antineoplastic agent would not be permitted in an oral contraceptive, for example. Because of the necessarily small number of patients treated in premarketing studies, rare adverse reactions may not be identified, so the first responsibility for identifying and reporting these effects must rest with the practicing clinician through the use of the various national adverse reaction reporting systems, such as those operated by the Food and Drug Administration in the United States and the Committee on Safety of Medicines in Great Britain. The publication of a newly recognized adverse reaction can in a short time stimulate many similar such reports of reactions that previously had gone unrecognized.

The prevention of adverse drug reactions first involves a high index of suspicion that the development of a new symptom or sign may be drug-related. Reduction of the dose or discontinuation of the suspected agent usually clarifies the issue in concentration-dependent toxic reactions. Physicians should be familiar with the common adverse effects of the drugs they use and, when in doubt, should consult the literature.

BIBLIOGRAPHY

AITHAL GP et al: Association of polymorphisms in the cytochrome P450 CYP2C9 with warfarin dose requirement and risk of bleeding complications. Lancet 353:717, 1999

BLACK AJ et al: Thiopurine methyltransferase genotype predicts therapy-limiting severe toxicity from azathioprine. Ann Intern Med 129:716, 1998

DAVIES DM et al: *Textbook of Adverse Drug Reactions*, 5th ed. New York, Oxford University Press, 1998

FELDMANN U: Design and analysis of drug safety studies, with special reference to sporadic drug use and acute adverse reactions. J Clin Epidemiol 46:237, 1993

LAZAROU J et al: Incidence of adverse drug reactions in hospitalized patients: A meta-analysis of prospective studies. 279:1200, 1998

LENNARD I et al: Thiopurine drugs in the treatment of childhood leukemia: The activity influence of inherited thiopurine methyltransferase activity on drug metabolism and cytotoxicity. Br J Clin Pharmacol 44:445, 1997

ROUJEAU J-C, STERN RS: Severe adverse cutaneous reactions to drugs. N Engl J Med 331:1272, 1994

WOOD AJJ: The safety of new medicines: The importance of asking the right questions. JAMA 281:1753, 1999

——— et al: Making medicines safer: The need for an independent drug safety board. N Engl J Med 25:1851, 1998

72   *Lewis Landsberg, James B. Young*

PHYSIOLOGY AND PHARMACOLOGY OF THE AUTONOMIC NERVOUS SYSTEM

ACh	acetylcholine	IP$_3$	inositol-1,4,5-trisphosphate
AMP	adenosine monophosphate	MAO	monoamine oxidase
CNS	central nervous system	NE	norepinephrine
COMT	catechol-*O*-methyltransferase	NTS	nucleus of the solitary tract
DAG	1,2-diacylglycerol	PIP$_2$	phosphatidylinositol-4,5-bisphosphate
HDL	high-density lipoprotein		

FUNCTIONAL ORGANIZATION OF THE AUTONOMIC NERVOUS SYSTEM

The autonomic nervous system innervates vascular and visceral smooth muscle, exocrine and endocrine glands, and parenchymal cells throughout the various organ systems. Functioning below the conscious level, the autonomic nervous system responds rapidly and continuously to perturbations that threaten the constancy of the internal environment. The many functions governed by this system include the distribution of blood flow and the maintenance of tissue perfusion, the regulation of blood pressure, the regulation of the volume and composition of the extracellular fluid, the expenditure of metabolic energy and supply of substrate, and the control of visceral smooth muscle and glands.

ANATOMIC ORGANIZATION   The autonomic neurons, located in ganglia outside the central nervous system (CNS), give rise to the postganglionic autonomic nerves that innervate organs and tissues throughout the body (Fig. 72-1). The activity of autonomic nerves is regulated by central neurons responsive to diverse afferent inputs. After central integration of afferent information, autonomic outflow is adjusted to permit the functioning of the major organ systems in accordance with the needs of the organism as a whole. Connections between the cerebral cortex and the autonomic centers in the brainstem coordinate autonomic outflow with higher mental functions.

The Sympathetic and Parasympathetic Divisions   The preganglionic neurons of the parasympathetic nervous system leave the CNS in the third, seventh, ninth, and tenth cranial nerves and in the second and third sacral nerves, while the preganglionic neurons of the sympathetic nervous system exit the spinal cord between the first thoracic and the second lumbar segments (Fig. 72-1). Responses to sympathetic and parasympathetic stimulation are frequently antagonistic, as exemplified by their opposing effects on heart rate and gut motility. This antagonism reflects highly coordinated interactions within the CNS; the resultant changes in parasympathetic and sympathetic activity, often reciprocal, provide more precise control of autonomic responses

FIGURE 72-1 Schematic representation of the autonomic nervous system. *(From M. Moskowitz: Clin Endocrinol Metab 6:77, 1977.)*

Parasympathetic system
from cranial nerves III, VII, IX, X
and from sacral nerves 2 and 3

Sympathetic system
from T1 L2
Preganglionic fibers — — — — —
Postganglionic fibers —————

A	Ciliary ganglion	H	Superior cervical ganglion
B	Sphenopalatine	J	Middle cervical ganglion and
	(pterygopalatine) ganglion		inferior cervical (stellate)
C	Submandibular ganglion		ganglion including T1
D	Otic ganglion		ganglion
E	Vagal ganglion cells	K	Coeliac and other
	in heart wall		abdominal ganglia
F	Vagal ganglion cells	L	Lower abdominal
	in bowel wall		sympathetic ganglia
G	Pelvic ganglia		

than could be achieved by the modulation of a single system. Moreover, both sympathetic and parasympathetic portions of the autonomic nervous system are composed of multiple function-specific subdivisions. Neurons with the various subdivisions differ neurochemically and neurophysiologically and are controlled by distinct regions within the CNS. This specialization within sympathetic and parasympathetic divisions contributes to the precision and specificity of autonomic regulation.

Neurotransmitters *Acetylcholine* (ACh) is the preganglionic neurotransmitter for both divisions of the autonomic nervous system as well as the postganglionic neurotransmitter of the parasympathetic neurons. Nerves that release ACh are said to be cholinergic. *Norepinephrine* (NE) is the neurotransmitter of the postganglionic sympathetic neurons; these nerves are said to be adrenergic. Within the sympathetic outflow, postganglionic neurons innervating the eccrine sweat glands (and perhaps some blood vessels supplying skeletal muscle) are of the cholinergic type.

THE SYMPATHETIC NERVOUS SYSTEM AND ADRENAL MEDULLA

CATECHOLAMINES All three of the naturally occurring catecholamines, NE, *epinephrine* (E), and *dopamine*, function as neurotransmitters within the CNS. NE, the neurotransmitter of postgangli-

onic sympathetic nerve endings, exerts its effects locally, in the immediate vicinity of its release. Epinephrine, the circulating hormone of the adrenal medulla, influences processes throughout the body. A peripheral dopaminergic system also exists but has not been characterized in detail.

Biosynthesis (Fig. 72-2) Catecholamines are synthesized from the amino acid tyrosine, which is sequentially hydroxylated to form dihydroxyphenylalanine (dopa), decarboxylated to form dopamine, and hydroxylated on the β position of the side chain to form NE. The initial step, the hydroxylation of tyrosine, is rate-limiting and is regulated so that synthesis of dopa is coupled to NE release. This regulation is achieved by alterations in both the activity and the amount of tyrosine hydroxylase. In the adrenal medulla and in those central neurons utilizing epinephrine as neurotransmitter, NE is *N*-methylated to epinephrine by the enzyme phenylethanolamine-*N*-methyltransferase (PNMT).

Catecholamine Metabolism The major metabolic transformations of catecholamines involve *O*-methylation at the meta-hydroxyl group and oxidative deamination. *O*-Methylation is catalyzed by the enzyme catechol-*O*-methyltransferase (COMT), and oxidative deamination is promoted by monoamine oxidase (MAO). COMT in liver and kidney is important in the metabolism of circulating catecholamines. MAO, a mitochondrial enzyme present in most tissues, including nerve endings, has a lesser role in the metabolism of circulating catecholamines but is important in regulating the catecholamine stores within the peripheral sympathetic nerve endings. The metane-

FIGURE 72-2 Catecholamine biosynthesis, release, and metabolism. Schematic representation of a peripheral sympathetic nerve ending is shown at the top; the bulbous areas on the terminal fiber represent varicosities identified by histochemical fluorescence techniques as areas of high neurotransmitter concentration. The processes of biosynthesis, release, modulation, and reuptake are shown sequentially for demonstration purposes only; in vivo they proceed concurrently. Adrenal medullary chromaffin cells are shown at the bottom of the diagram. (TH, tyrosine hydroxylase; AAD, aromatic-l-amino acid decarboxylase; DA, dopamine; DBH, dopamine-β-hydroxylase; NE, norepinephrine; PNMT, phenylethanolamine-*N*-methyltransferase; E, epinephrine; COMT, catechol-*O*-methyltransferase; NMN, normetanephrine; MAO, monoamine oxidase; DHMA, 3,4-dihydroxymandelic acid; VMA, 3-methoxy-4-hydroxymandelic acid.)

phrines and 3-methoxy-4-hydroxymandelic acid (vanilmandelic acid, VMA) are the major end products of E and NE metabolism. Homovanillic acid (HVA) is the end product of dopamine metabolism.

STORAGE AND RELEASE OF CATECHOLAMINES
In both the adrenal medulla and sympathetic nerve endings catecholamines are stored in subcellular vesicles and released by exocytosis. The large stores of catecholamines in these tissues provide an important physiologic reserve that maintains an adequate supply of catecholamines in the face of intense stimulation. A variety of substances may be stored along with catecholamines in sympathetic nerve endings and adrenal medulla and released with catecholamines during exocytosis. These substances, which may function as cotransmitters or neuromodulators, include peptides such as neuropeptide Y, substance P, and enkephalins; purines such as ATP and adenosine; and other amines such as serotonin. At the neuroeffector junction, coreleased neuromodulators modify the response to NE, while cotransmitters exert physiologic effects independent of those induced by NE.

Adrenal Medulla The adrenal medullary chromaffin tissue in a pair of normal human adrenal glands weighs about 1 g and contains approximately 6 mg catecholamines, 85% of which is epinephrine.

Catecholamine secretion, stimulated by ACh from the preganglionic sympathetic nerves, occurs after calcium influx triggers fusion of the chromaffin granule membrane and cell membrane; obliteration of the cell membrane at the point of fusion and extrusion of the entire soluble contents of the granule into the extracellular space complete the process of exocytosis (Fig. 72-2). Although the molecular mechanisms involved in the exocytotic process are only partially understood, evidence has accumulated that specific calcium-binding proteins are involved. Once bound, calcium induces a conformational change in these proteins that induces fusion of granules and docking of granules at the cell membrane.

Peripheral Sympathetic Nerve Endings The peripheral sympathetic nerve endings form a reticulum or ground plexus that brings the terminal fibers into close contact with effector cells. All the NE in peripheral tissues is in the sympathetic nerve endings, and heavily innervated tissues contain as much as 1 to 2 μg/g of tissue. NE stored in the nerve endings is in discrete subcellular particles analogous to the adrenal medullary chromaffin granules. MAO in the mitochondria of the nerve endings plays an important role in regulating the local concentration of NE (Fig. 72-2). Amines in storage vesicles are protected from oxidative deamination; amines within the cytoplasm, however, are deaminated to inactive metabolites. Release from the nerve ending occurs in response to action potentials propagated in terminal sympathetic fibers.

THE PERIPHERAL ADRENERGIC NEUROEFFECTOR JUNCTION
The peripheral sympathetic nerve endings possess an amine transport system that actively takes up amines from the extracellular fluid. Neuronal uptake or recapture of locally released NE terminates the action of the transmitter and contributes to the constancy of the NE stores.

A variety of factors alter the relationship between neuronal impulse traffic and NE release. Diminished temperature and acidosis, for example, both decrease the amount of NE released in response to sympathetic impulses. Several chemical mediators operate at the peripheral sympathetic nerve ending (referred to as *prejunctional* or *presynaptic sites*) to modify sympathetic neurotransmission by influencing the amount of NE released in response to nerve impulses. Prejunctional modulation may be either inhibitory or facilitatory. Certain modulators, such as catecholamines and ACh, may either inhibit or facilitate NE release, antagonistic effects that are mediated by different adrenergic or cholinergic receptors, respectively. Those compounds exerting an *inhibitory* effect on NE release at the prejunctional nerve ending include the following: catecholamines (α_2 receptor), ACh (muscarinic receptor), dopamine (D_2 receptor), histamine (H_2 receptor), serotonin, adenosine, enkephalins, and prostaglandins.

Catecholamines reduce NE release via prejunctional α receptors

in a classic negative-feedback system. Feedback regulation is complicated by the fact that β-receptor activation facilitates NE release.

Though both inhibitory and facilitatory effects of ACh on NE release have been described, the inhibitory effect of ACh, mediated by the muscarinic cholinergic receptor, occurs at lower ACh concentrations and is probably of greater physiologic significance.

CENTRAL REGULATION OF SYMPATHOADRENAL OUTFLOW
Brainstem Sympathetic Centers Sympathetic outflow is initiated from the reticular formation of the medulla oblongata and pons and from centers in the hypothalamus. The rostral ventral portion of the medulla, particularly the area designated the rostral ventrolateral medulla (RVLM), appears to contain especially important sympathoexcitatory areas. Descending fibers originating from all these centers synapse in the intermediolateral cell column of the spinal cord with the preganglionic sympathetic neurons. Changes in the physical and chemical properties of the extracellular fluid, including the circulating levels of hormones and substrates, also affect sympathetic nervous system outflow. The area postrema, in the floor of the fourth ventricle, along with other circumventricular organs lie outside the blood-brain barrier and may play an important role in this regard. Although the hallmark of intense sympathoadrenal stimulation is a global response (the fight-or-flight reaction of Cannon), discrete changes in sympathetic outflow to different organ systems continuously regulate many autonomic functions.

Relationship between the sympathetic nervous system and the adrenal medulla Sympathetic nervous system activity and adrenal medullary secretion are coordinated but not always congruent. During periods of intense sympathetic stimulation, such as cold exposure and exhaustive exercise, the adrenal medulla is progressively recruited, and circulating epinephrine reinforces the physiologic effects of sympathetic stimulation. In other situations, the sympathetic nervous system and the adrenal medulla are stimulated independently. The response to upright posture, for example, involves predominantly the sympathetic nervous system, while hypoglycemia stimulates only the adrenal medulla.

Sympathetic Regulation of the Cardiovascular System Stretch receptors in the systemic and pulmonary arteries and veins continuously monitor intravascular pressures; the resulting afferent impulses, after relay and integration in the brainstem, alter sympathetic activity in defense of blood pressure and blood flow to critical areas (Fig. 72-3).

Arterial baroreceptors An increase in blood pressure stimulates receptors in the carotid sinus and aortic arch. The ensuing afferent impulses, after relay within the nucleus of the solitary tract (NTS) in the brainstem, suppress the brainstem sympathetic centers (Fig. 72-3). This baroreceptor reflex arc forms a negative-feedback loop in which a rise in arterial pressure results in the inhibition of central sympathetic outflow. A brainstem noradrenergic pathway interacts with the NTS to participate in suppression of sympathetic outflow. This noradrenergic inhibitory pathway is stimulated by centrally acting α-adrenergic agonists and may be involved in the action of certain antihypertensive drugs, such as clonidine, that potentiate the baroreceptor-mediated vasodepressor response (Chap. 246). In the opposite manner, when the blood pressure falls, decreased afferent impulses diminish central inhibition, resulting in an increase in sympathetic outflow and a rise in arterial pressure.

Central venous pressure Receptors in the walls of the great veins and within the atria are also involved in the regulation of sympathetic outflow. Stimulation of these receptors by high venous pressure suppresses the brainstem sympathetic centers; when central venous pressure is low, sympathetic outflow increases. The central connections are poorly understood, but the afferent impulses are carried in the vagus (Fig. 72-3).

ASSESSMENT OF SYMPATHOADRENAL ACTIVITY
The clinical assessment of sympathoadrenal activity involves the measurement of catecholamines in plasma and of catecholamines and catecholamine metabolites in urine, and the assessment of sympathetic nerve impulse traffic by microneurography. Microneurography, util-

FIGURE 72-3 Sympathetic regulation of the circulation. Receptors in the venous and arterial circulations are stimulated by stretch, caused by an increase in pressure; afferent impulses from these receptors are carried to the central nervous system by the ninth (*IX*) and tenth (*X*) cranial nerves. The net result of these afferent impulses, after relay in the brainstem, is to inhibit central sympathetic outflow. The arterial baroreceptor reflex involves a relay in the nucleus of the tractus solitarius. (+, stimulation; −, inhibition.)

izing microelectrodes implanted in nerves supplying skeletal muscle (such as the peroneal nerve), is primarily a research tool. Quantitation of urinary catecholamines and metabolites is useful in the diagnosis of pheochromocytoma (Chap. 332).

Plasma Catecholamines Catecholamines in human plasma may be measured by radioenzymatic isotope derivative techniques or by high-performance liquid chromatography in conjunction with electrochemical detection. Plasma catecholamine measurements provide an index of sympathetic nervous system and adrenal medullary activity and have been widely used to assess sympathoadrenal activity in clinical investigation in human subjects. The usefulness of plasma catecholamine measurements, however, is compromised by factors that alter the relationship between the plasma concentration of catecholamines and the functional state of the sympathoadrenal system, and also by important regional differences in sympathetic outflow. Techniques utilizing tracer infusions of tritiated NE, which correct for changes in NE clearance when applied across a particular anatomic region, estimate regional sympathetic outflow with some precision and have helped to define differentiated sympathetic nervous system activity in the investigational setting. The clinical usefulness of plasma catecholamine levels remains limited to the evaluation of patients with autonomic insufficiency and, on occasion, patients with suspected pheochromocytoma (Chap. 332).

Basal plasma NE concentrations are in the range of 0.09 to 1.8 nmol/L (150 to 350 pg/mL); basal E levels are about 135 to 270 pmol/L (25 to 50 pg/mL). The half-time of disappearance of NE from the circulation is approximately 2 min. The plasma NE level is markedly affected by a variety of factors, including posture; accordingly, the conditions under which blood is obtained for assay must be controlled. By convention, basal plasma NE levels are those obtained through an indwelling intravenous line after the patient has rested supine in a relaxed environment for 30 min.

Plasma NE response to upright posture The predictable increase in circulating NE concentration during upright posture provides a convenient test of sympathetic nervous system function. Five minutes of quiet standing results in a two- to threefold increase in plasma NE level. A normal response requires an intact afferent system, appropriate CNS relays, and an intact peripheral sympathetic nervous system; a defect of any of these components reduces the increment in circulating NE.

Plasma E levels are also dependent on the physical and mental state of the subject. Change in plasma E with upright posture is usually small. Hypoglycemia, strenuous exercise, and various types of mental stress, however, can cause large increases in the plasma E level.

PERIPHERAL DOPAMINERGIC SYSTEM

In addition to its role as neurotransmitter in the CNS, dopamine functions as an inhibitory transmitter in the carotid body and the sympathetic ganglia. A distinct peripheral dopaminergic system is also believed to exist. Dopamine elicits a variety of responses not attributable to stimulation of classic adrenergic receptors; it relaxes the lower esophageal sphincter, delays gastric emptying, causes vasodilation in the renal and mesenteric arterial circulation, suppresses aldosterone secretion, directly stimulates renal sodium excretion, and suppresses NE release at sympathetic nerve terminals by a presynaptic inhibitory mechanism. The mediation of these dopaminergic effects in vivo is poorly understood. Dopamine does not appear to be a circulating hormone.

ADRENERGIC RECEPTORS

Catecholamines influence effector cells by interacting with specific surface *receptors* coupled to G proteins. Two major categories of response to catecholamines reflect the activation of two populations of adrenergic receptors, designated α and β. Both α and β receptors have been further divided into subtypes that serve different functions and are susceptible to differential stimulation and blockade.

α-**ADRENERGIC RECEPTORS** α-Adrenergic receptors mediate vasoconstriction, intestinal relaxation, and pupillary dilatation. Epinephrine and NE are approximately equipotent as α-receptor agonists. Distinct α_1- and α_2-receptor subtypes are also recognized. Originally the postsynaptic or postjunctional α-adrenergic receptors on effector cells were designated α_1, while the prejunctional α-adrenergic receptors on the sympathetic nerve endings were designated α_2. It is now recognized that nonneuronal (postsynaptic) processes are mediated by the α_2 receptor as well. The α_1 receptor mediates the classic α effects, including vasoconstriction; phenylephrine and methoxamine are selective α_1 agonists, and prazosin is a selective α_1 antagonist. The α_2 receptor mediates presynaptic inhibition of NE release from adrenergic nerves and other responses, including inhibition of ACh release from cholinergic nerves, inhibition of lipolysis in adipocytes, inhibition of insulin secretion, stimulation of platelet aggregation, and vasoconstriction in some vascular beds. Specific α_2 agonists include clonidine and α-methylnorepinephrine; these agents, the latter derived from α-methyldopa in vivo, exert an antihypertensive effect by interacting with α_2 receptors within the brainstem sympathetic centers that regulate blood pressure. Yohimbine is a specific α_2 antagonist.

β-**ADRENERGIC RECEPTORS** Physiologic events associated with β-adrenergic receptor responses include stimulation of heart rate and contractility, vasodilation, bronchodilation, and lipolysis. β-Receptor responses can also be divided into two types. The β_1 receptor responds equally to E and NE and mediates cardiac stimulation and lipolysis. The β_2 receptor is more responsive to E than to NE and mediates responses such as vasodilation and bronchodilation. Isoproterenol stimulates and propranolol blocks both β_1 and β_2 receptors. Other agonists and antagonists that have partial selectivity for the β_1 or β_2 receptors have been used therapeutically where the desired response involves predominantly one of the two subtypes.

Both pharmacologic and molecular genetic studies have demonstrated an additional distinct β_3-adrenergic receptor that subserves lipolysis in white and brown adipose tissue as well as the stimulation of heat production in brown adipose tissue. The human β_3-adrenergic receptor has been cloned, and a distinct polymorphism noted that may, in some populations, be associated with weight gain, insulin resistance, and type 2 diabetes mellitus. The β_3-adrenergic receptor has a much greater affinity for NE than E and, unlike the β_1 and β_2 receptors, does not undergo desensitization. Synthetic agonists for the β_3 receptor, currently under development, have a potential role in the treatment of obesity by increasing metabolic rate.

DOPAMINERGIC RECEPTORS Specific dopaminergic receptors, distinct from the classic α- and β-adrenergic receptors, are present in the CNS and peripheral nervous system and in several nonneural tissues. Two types of dopaminergic receptors serve different functions and have different second messengers. Dopamine is a potent agonist of both types of receptors; the action of dopamine is antagonized by phenothiazines and thioxanthenes. The D_1 receptor mediates vasodilation in the renal, mesenteric, coronary, and cerebral vascular beds. Fenoldopam is an agonist selective for the D_1 receptor. The D_2 receptor inhibits transmission in the sympathetic ganglia, inhibits NE release from sympathetic nerve endings by an effect on the presynaptic membrane (Fig. 72-2), inhibits prolactin release from the pituitary, and causes vomiting. Selective agonists of the D_2 receptor include bromocriptine, cabergoline, and apomorphine, while butyrophenones such as haloperidol (active within the CNS), domperidone (does not cross blood-brain barrier readily), and the benzamide sulpiride are relatively selective D_2 antagonists.

STRUCTURE AND FUNCTION OF ADRENERGIC RECEPTORS Adrenergic receptors belong to a superfamily of related membrane proteins, including the visual protein rhodopsin and the muscarinic acetylcholine receptors, that interacts with G proteins. These proteins share significant sequence homologies and, as deduced from the properties of the constituent amino acids, a similar topographic structure in the cell membrane. The postulated structure of this family of receptor proteins is shown schematically in Fig. 72-4. The characteristic features include seven membrane-spanning hydrophobic domains containing 20 to 28 amino acids each. The membrane-span-

FIGURE 72-4 Proposed structure of adrenergic receptors as deduced from primary amino acid sequences. The single protein chain contains a hydrophilic N terminus (extracellular) and C terminus (intracellular) connected by seven lipophilic membrane-spanning regions (M-1 to M-7) which are interconnected by three extracellular loops (E-I to E-III) and three cytoplasmic loops (C-I to C-III). The β_1-, β_2-, α_1-, and α_2-adrenergic receptors have appreciable sequence homologies and are believed to fit the general structural model represented. Specificity of agonist binding may be conferred by the tertiary structure of several of the membrane-spanning domains while specificity of intracellular response may be related to the length and tertiary structure of the cytoplasmic loops and C terminus. The top portion of the figure is a longitudinal representation of the receptor protein in the cell membrane; shown below is a hypothetical, more compact arrangement seen from the membrane surface. (ECF, extracellular fluid; ICF, intracellular fluid.) *(From Landsberg and Young, 1998, with permission.)*

ning domains, particularly M-7 (Fig. 72-4), appear to be important in determining the characteristic agonist binding.

Coupling of Receptor Occupancy with Cellular Response The major mediators of adrenergic (as well as many other) cellular responses are a family of regulatory proteins termed *G proteins* that, when activated, bind the nucleotide guanosine triphosphate (GTP). The best-characterized G proteins are those that stimulate or inhibit adenylyl cyclase, designated G_s or G_i, respectively (Fig. 72-5). The β_1, β_2, and D_1 receptors are coupled to G_s; receptor occupancy is therefore associated with stimulation of adenylyl cyclase and results in an increase in intracellular cyclic adenosine monophosphate (AMP), which in turn results in activation of protein kinase A and other cyclic AMP–dependent protein kinases. The resultant protein phosphorylation alters the activity of enzymes and the function of other proteins, culminating in a cellular response that is characteristic of the tissue being stimulated. The α_2, M_2 subtype of the muscarinic acetylcholine receptor and the D_2 receptor are coupled to G_i, resulting in diminished adenylyl cyclase activity and a fall in cyclic AMP. The subsequent alterations in enzyme activity and function of other proteins produce an alternate, frequently opposite, series of cellular responses. Although many α_2 responses can be explained by inhibition of adenylyl cyclase, other mechanisms may be involved as well.

The α_1-adrenergic receptor (as well as the M_1 subtype of the acetylcholine receptor) is coupled to a different G protein that activates phospholipase C; this G protein has not been as well characterized but is sometimes designated G_q. Receptor occupancy in this system stimulates phospholipase C, which catalyzes the breakdown of membrane-bound phospholipids, particularly phosphatidylinositol-4,5-bisphosphate (PIP_2) with the production of inositol-1,4,5-trisphosphate (IP_3) and 1,2-diacylglycerol (DAG), both of which act as second messengers (Fig. 72-5). IP_3 rapidly mobilizes calcium from intracellular stores within the endoplasmic reticulum, producing an increase in free cytoplasmic calcium which by itself and via calcium-calmodulin–dependent protein kinases influences cellular processes appropriate to the stimulated cell. The transient rise in calcium induced by IP_3 from the intracellular stores is reinforced in the presence of continued agonist stimulation by alterations in membrane calcium flux that result eventually in net calcium uptake from the extracellular fluid by mechanisms that have been incompletely defined.

DAG, the other second messenger produced by the action of phospholipase C on PIP_2 (as well as other membrane phospholipids), remains associated with the cell membrane and activates protein kinase C, which has different substrates than the calcium-calmodulin kinases stimulated by IP_3. Protein phosphorylation stimulated by protein kinase C contributes to the tissue-specific response in ways that remain poorly understood. Increases in intracellular calcium also potentiate the activation of protein kinase C (Fig. 72-5).

REGULATION OF ADRENERGIC RECEPTORS Prolonged exposure to α- or β-adrenergic agonists decreases the number of corresponding adrenergic receptors on effector cells. Although the biochemical mechanisms involved are obscure, internalization of the β-adrenergic receptor within the cell occurs during agonist exposure in some systems, suggesting that internal translocation contributes to the decrease in receptor number under these circumstances.

Alteration in agonist concentration may also affect the affinity of the receptor for the agonist. Adrenergic receptors that utilize adenylyl cyclase for the second messenger (β receptors, α_2 receptors) exist in high- and low-affinity states; exposure to agonist diminishes the proportion of receptors in the high-affinity state. Such alterations in adrenergic receptors induced by adrenergic agonists are termed *homologous regulation*. Agonist-induced alterations in adrenergic-receptor density and affinity are believed to contribute to the diminished physiologic response that occurs after prolonged exposure of an effector tissue to adrenergic agonist, a phenomenon known as *tachyphylaxis* or *desensitization*.

Adrenergic receptors are also influenced by factors other than adrenergic agonists, so-called *heterologous regulation*. Enhanced α-adrenergic-receptor affinity, for example, may underlie the potentiation of α-adrenergic responses that occur in response to lowered environmental temperatures. Thyroid hormones potentiate β-receptor responses by alterations in β-receptor number and in the efficiency of coupling receptor occupancy with physiologic response. Estrogen and progesterone alter the sensitivity of the myometrium to catecholamines by effects on α-adrenergic receptors. Glucocorticoids may influence adrenergic function by antagonizing agonist-induced decreases in adrenergic receptors, thereby counteracting tachyphylaxis in response to intense adrenergic stimulation.

Alterations in sensitivity to catecholamines also occur as a consequence of postreceptor changes, although the latter remain poorly characterized.

FIGURE 72-5 Interaction of autonomic agonists with membrane-bound regulatory proteins and cellular effector systems. The designations α and β refer to adrenergic receptors, DA refers to dopaminergic receptors, and M, to muscarinic receptors. G designates the GTP-associated regulatory protein which may have a stimulatory (s) or inhibitory (i) effect on adenylyl cyclase or may stimulate phospholipase C (q). [(+) designates stimulation; (−) designates inhibition; PIP_2, phosphatidylinositol-4,5-bisphosphate; DAG, 1,2-diacylglycerol; IP_3, inositol-1,4,5-trisphosphate. See text for details.]

PHYSIOLOGY OF THE SYMPATHOADRENAL SYSTEM

Catecholamines influence all of the major organ systems. The effects take place in seconds and may occur in anticipation of physiologic requirement. An increase in sympathoadrenal activity prior to strenuous exercise, for example, lessens the impact of exercise on the internal environment.

DIRECT EFFECTS OF CATECHOLAMINES Cardiovascular System Catecholamines stimulate vasoconstriction in the subcutaneous, mucosal, splanchnic, and renal vascular beds by α-receptor–mediated mechanisms. Although vasoconstriction was originally considered an α_1-receptor response, vascular tone appears to be more complexly regulated and, in many areas, involves α_2-mediated responses as well. The venous portion of the circulation, in particular, is endowed with α_2 receptors. Differential regulation of the two types of α receptors, under certain circumstances, contributes to an integrated physiologic response. Since vasoconstriction in the coronary and cerebral circulations is minimal, flow to these areas is maintained during sympathetic stimulation. Skeletal muscle vasculature contains β receptors sensitive to low circulating levels of epinephrine so that skeletal muscle blood flow is augmented during adrenal medullary activation.

The effects of catecholamines on the heart are mediated by β_1 receptors and include increase in heart rate, enhancement of cardiac contractility, and increase in conduction velocity. The increase in myocardial contractility is illustrated by a leftward and upward shift of the ventricular function curve (see Fig. 231-6) that relates cardiac work to ventricular diastolic fiber length; at any initial fiber length, catecholamines increase cardiac work. Catecholamines also enhance cardiac output by stimulating venoconstriction, enhancing venous return, and increasing the force of atrial contraction, thereby augmenting diastolic volume and hence fiber length. The acceleration of conduction in the junctional tissues results in a more synchronous, and hence more effective, ventricular contraction. Cardiac stimulation increases myocardial oxygen consumption, a major factor in the pathogenesis and treatment of myocardial ischemia.

Metabolism Catecholamines increase metabolic rate. In small mammals, mitochondrial respiration in brown adipose tissue is functionally uncoupled by NE. In a reaction unique to brown adipose tissue, NE stimulates the β_3-adrenergic receptor that activates a specific mitochondrial uncoupling protein that dissipates the proton gradient between the inner mitochondrial matrix and the cytoplasm, thereby uncoupling substrate utilization and ATP synthesis. In humans, a functional role for brown adipose tissue has not been established with certainty.

Substrate mobilization In a variety of tissues, catecholamines stimulate the breakdown of stored fuel with the production of substrate for local consumption; glycogenolysis in the heart, for example, provides substrate for immediate metabolism by the myocardium. Catecholamines also accelerate fuel mobilization in liver, adipose tissue, and skeletal muscle, liberating substrates (glucose, free fatty acids, lactate) into the circulation for use throughout the body.

Fluids and Electrolytes By a direct action on the renal tubule, NE stimulates sodium reabsorption, thereby defending extracellular fluid volume. Dopamine, in contrast, promotes sodium excretion. NE and E also promote cellular uptake of potassium.

Viscera Catecholamines affect visceral function by actions on smooth muscle and glandular epithelium. Urinary bladder and intestinal smooth muscle are relaxed while the corresponding sphincters are stimulated. Gallbladder emptying also involves sympathetic mechanisms. Catecholamine-mediated smooth-muscle contraction in the female aids ovulation and ovum transport along the fallopian tubes, and in the male provides propulsive force for the seminal fluid during ejaculation. Inhibitory α_2 receptors on cholinergic neurons within the gut contribute to intestinal relaxation. Catecholamines induce bronchodilation by a β_2-receptor mechanism.

INDIRECT EFFECTS OF CATECHOLAMINES The ultimate physiologic response induced by catecholamines involves changes in hormone secretion and in blood flow distribution, both of which support and amplify the direct effects of catecholamines.

Endocrine System Catecholamines influence the secretion of renin, insulin, glucagon, calcitonin, parathormone, thyroxine, gastrin, erythropoietin, progesterone, and, possibly, testosterone. Secretion of each of these hormones is governed by complex feedback loops. With the exception of thyroxine and the gonadal steroids, each is a polypeptide not under the direct control of the pituitary gland. Sympathoadrenal input into the secretion of these hormones provides a mechanism for regulation by the CNS and ensures a coordinated hormonal response in accord with the homeostatic needs of the organism.

Renin (See also Chap. 246) Sympathetic stimulation increases renin release by a direct β-receptor effect independent of vascular changes within the kidney. The renin response to volume depletion is sympathetically mediated and is initiated by a fall in central venous pressure. Since renin secretion activates the angiotensin-aldosterone system, angiotensin-induced vasoconstriction supports the direct effects of catecholamines on blood vessels, while aldosterone-mediated sodium reabsorption complements the direct increase in sodium reabsorption induced by sympathetic stimulation. β-receptor blocking agents suppress renin secretion.

Insulin and glucagon Stimulation of pancreatic sympathetic nerves or an elevation in circulating catecholamines suppresses insulin and increases glucagon release. Inhibition of insulin secretion is mediated by the α_2 receptor, and stimulation of glucagon is mediated by the β receptor. This combination of effects supports substrate mobilization, reinforcing the direct effects of catecholamines on hepatic glucose output and lipolysis. Although α-receptor–mediated suppression of insulin release usually predominates, a β-receptor mechanism may augment insulin secretion under some circumstances.

SYMPATHOADRENAL FUNCTION IN SELECTED PHYSIOLOGIC AND PATHOPHYSIOLOGIC STATES

Support of the Circulation   The sympathetic nervous system functions to maintain an adequate circulation. During upright posture and volume depletion, reduction of afferent venous and arterial baroreceptor impulse traffic diminishes an inhibitory input to the vasomotor center, thereby increasing sympathetic activity (Fig. 72-3) and reducing efferent vagal tone. As a result, heart rate is increased, and cardiac output is diverted from the skin, subcutaneous tissues, mucosa, and viscera. Sympathetic stimulation of the kidney increases sodium reabsorption, and sympathetically mediated venoconstriction enhances venous return (Fig. 72-6). With pronounced hypotension, the adrenal medulla is recruited and epinephrine reinforces the effects of the sympathetic nervous system.

The intense sympathoadrenal stimulation that accompanies severe volume depletion may contribute to the development of ketoacidosis in alcoholics as well as to the ketoacidosis sometimes seen in association with hyperemesis gravidarum. Catecholamine-mediated suppression of insulin and stimulation of glucagon markedly potentiate ketogenesis in these disease states. Volume resuscitation and provision of adequate glucose promptly reverse the ketoacidosis in most cases.

Congestive heart failure   The sympathetic nervous system also provides circulatory support during congestive heart failure (Chap. 232). Venoconstriction and sympathetic stimulation of the heart increase cardiac output while peripheral vasoconstriction directs blood flow to the heart and brain. The afferent signals are less clear than in simple volume depletion because the venous pressure is usually elevated. In severe heart failure, depletion of cardiac NE may impair the effectiveness of sympathetic circulatory support. On the other hand, the possibility has been raised that intense sympathetic stimulation may further impair cardiac function, suggesting possible benefit from β-adrenergic blockade. The use of beta blockers in the treatment of congestive heart failure, in fact, has increased in recent years.

Trauma and shock   In acute traumatic injury or shock, adrenal catecholamines support the circulation and mobilize substrates. In the chronic, reparative phase following injury, catecholamines also contribute to substrate mobilization and to the elevation in metabolic rate.

Exercise   Sympathetic activation during exercise increases cardiac output and ensures sufficient substrate to meet the increased metabolic needs. Central neural factors, such as anticipation, and circulatory factors, such as fall in venous pressure, trigger the sympathetic response. Mild degrees of exercise stimulate the sympathetic nervous system alone; during more severe exertion the adrenal medulla is activated as well. Cardiovascular conditioning is associated with a decrease in sympathetic nervous system activity both at rest and during exercise, in comparison with the untrained state.

Hypoglycemia (See also Chap. 334)   Hypoglycemia causes a marked increase in adrenal medullary epinephrine secretion. When glucose concentrations fall below overnight fasting levels, regulatory glucose-sensitive neurons in the CNS initiate a prompt increase in adrenal medullary secretion. The increase is especially intense at plasma glucose levels below 2.8 mmol/L (50 mg/dL), when plasma E levels increase 25 to 50 times above baseline, thereby increasing hepatic glucose output, providing alternative substrate in the form of free fatty acids, suppressing endogenous insulin release, and inhibiting insulin-mediated glucose utilization in muscle. Many clinical manifestations of hypoglycemia, such as tachycardia, palpitations, nervousness, tremor, and widened pulse pressure, are secondary to increased E secretion, and these manifestations constitute an "early warning" system in insulin-requiring diabetics. In patients with long-standing diabetes mellitus, however, the E response to hypoglycemia may be diminished or absent, leaving affected patients at greater risk to develop severe hypoglycemia.

Cold Exposure   The sympathetic nervous system plays a critical role in the maintenance of normal body temperature during exposure to a cold environment. Receptors in the skin and CNS respond to a fall in temperature by activating hypothalamic and brainstem centers that increase sympathetic activity. Sympathetic stimulation leads to vasoconstriction in the superficial vascular beds, thereby diminishing heat loss. The sympathetic response involves a complex interaction between lowered environmental temperatures and α_2-adrenergic receptors. Acclimatization during chronic cold exposure increases the capacity for metabolic heat production in response to sympathetic stimulation.

Dietary Intake   Fasting suppresses and overfeeding stimulates the sympathetic nervous system. The reduction in sympathetic activity during fasting or starvation contributes to the decrease in metabolic rate, bradycardia, and hypotension in these states. Enhanced sympathetic activity during periods of increased caloric intake contributes to the elevation in metabolic rate associated with a chronic increase in dietary intake.

Hypoxia   Chronic hypoxia is associated with stimulation of the sympathoadrenal system, and some of the cardiovascular changes attendant to hypoxia are dependent on catecholamines.

Orthostatic Hypotension   The maintenance of arterial pressure during upright posture depends on an adequate blood volume, an unimpaired venous return, and an intact sympathetic nervous system. Significant postural hypotension, therefore, often reflects extracellular fluid volume depletion or dysfunction of the circulatory reflexes. Diseases of the nervous system, such as tabes dorsalis, syringomyelia, or diabetes mellitus, may disrupt these sympathetic reflexes with resultant orthostatic hypotension. Although any antiadrenergic agent may impair the postural sympathetic response, orthostatic hypotension is most prominent with drugs that block neurotransmission within the ganglia or adrenergic neurons.

The term *idiopathic orthostatic hypotension* refers to a group of degenerative diseases involving either the pre- or postganglionic sympathetic neurons (Chaps. 21 and 365).

Treatment of orthostatic hypotension is usually unsatisfactory except in the mildest cases. There is no way of reestablishing the normal relationship between fall in venous return and sympathetic neuronal

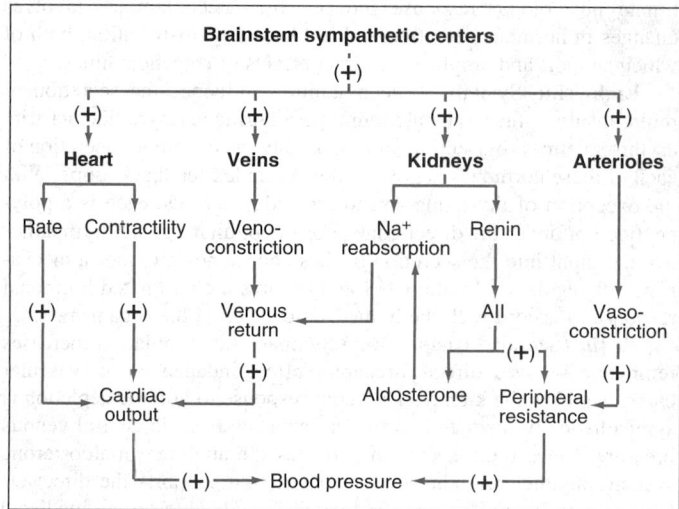

FIGURE 72-6   Sympathetic nervous system effects on blood pressure. Sympathetic stimulation (+) increases blood pressure by effects on the heart, the veins, the kidneys, and the arterioles. The net result of sympathetic stimulation is an increase in both cardiac output and peripheral resistance. AII, angiotensin II. [*From JB Young, L Landsberg, in P Sleight et al (eds), Scientific Foundations of Cardiology, London, Heinemann, 1981.*]

activation. Volume expansion with fludrocortisone and a liberal salt diet in conjunction with fitted stockings to the waist, as well as elevation of the head of the bed to avoid recumbency, will maintain plasma volume and venous return and frequently provide symptomatic improvement.

PHARMACOLOGY OF THE SYMPATHOADRENAL SYSTEM

A variety of therapeutic agents affect sympathetic nervous system function or interact with adrenergic receptors, making it possible to stimulate or suppress effects mediated by catecholamines with some degree of specificity (Table 72-1).

SYMPATHOMIMETIC AMINES Sympathomimetic amines may directly activate adrenergic receptors (direct acting) or release NE from the sympathetic nerve endings (indirect acting). Many agents have both direct and indirect effects.

Epinephrine and Norepinephrine The naturally occurring catecholamines act predominantly by the direct stimulation of adrenergic receptors. NE is employed to support the circulation and elevate the blood pressure in hypotensive states (Chap. 38). Peripheral vasoconstriction is the major effect, although cardiac stimulation occurs as well. Epinephrine, also employed as a pressor, has special usefulness in the treatment of allergic reactions, especially those associated with anaphylaxis. Epinephrine antagonizes the effects of histamine and other mediators on vascular and visceral smooth muscle and is useful in the treatment of bronchospasm.

Dopamine *Dopamine* is used in treating hypotension, shock (Chap. 38), and certain forms of heart failure (Chap. 232). At low infusion rates it exerts a positive inotropic effect both by a direct action on the cardiac β_1 receptors and by the indirect release of NE from sympathetic nerve endings in the heart. At low doses direct stimulation of dopaminergic receptors in the renal and mesenteric vasculature also results in vasodilation in the gut and kidney and facilitates sodium excretion. At

Table 72-1 Some Commonly Used Autonomic Drugs[a]

Agent	Indication	Dose and Route	Comment
ADRENERGIC AGONISTS[b]			
Epinephrine	Anaphylaxis	300–500 µg SC or IM (0.3–0.5 mL of 1/1000 solution of hydrochloride salt); 25–50 µg IV (slowly) every 5–15 min; titrate as needed	Nonselective α and β agonist; increases BP, heart rate Bronchodilation
Norepinephrine	Shock Hypotension	2–4 µg of NE base/min IV; titrate as needed	α and β_1 agonist Vasoconstriction predominates Extravasation causes tissue necrosis; infuse through IV cannula
Isoproterenol	Cardiogenic shock Bradyarrhythmias AV block	0.5–5.0 µg/min IV; titrate as needed	Nonselective β agonist Increases cardiac rate and contractility (β_1) Tachycardia limits usefulness
	Asthma	Inhalation	Dilates bronchi (β_2); cardiac stimulation also occurs
Dobutamine	Refractory CHF Cardiogenic shock	2.5–25 (µg/kg)/min IV	Selective β_1 agonist with greater effect on contractility than heart rate; a congener of dopamine but not a dopaminergic agonist
Phenylephrine	Hypotension	2–5 mg SC or IM 0.1–0.5 mg IV	Selective α_1 agonist; useful in antagonizing hypotension of spinal anesthesia
	Supraventricular tachycardia	150–800 µg slow IV push	Pressor effect induces vagotonic response; do not exceed 160 mmHg systolic BP
Terbutaline	Asthma	2.5–5.0 mg PO tid; 0.25–0.5 mg SC; inhalation every 4–5 h	Selective β_2 agonist; β_1 (cardiac) effects at higher doses (inhalation preferred route)
Bitolterol	Asthma	Inhalation every 4–6 h	Selective β_2 agonist
Salmeterol	Asthma	Inhalation bid	Selective β_2 agonist; long-acting agent for maintenance therapy
Albuterol	Asthma	2.0–4.0 mg PO tid or qid; 0.2 mg inhalation every 4–6 h	Selective β_2 agonist; β_1 effects (cardiac) at higher doses (inhalation preferred route)
Isoetharine	Asthma	Inhalation every 2–4 h	Selective β_2 agonist; some β_1 effects
Metaproterenol	Asthma	10–20 mg PO tid or qid; inhalation every 3–4 h	Selective β_2 agonist; some β_1 effects (inhalation preferred route)
Pirbuterol	Asthma	Inhalation every 4–6 h	Selective β_2 agonist; some β_1 effects
Ritodrine	Premature labor	50–350 µg/min IV	Selective β_2 agonist; hypokalemia, hyperglycemia, hypotension, cardiac stimulation may occur Neonatal hypoglycemia, hypocalcemia reported
DOPAMINERGIC AGONISTS			
Dopamine	Shock	2–5 (µg/kg)/min IV (dopaminergic range) 5–10 (µg/kg)/min IV (dopaminergic and beta range) 10–20 (µg/kg)/min IV (beta range) 20–50 (µg/kg)/min IV (alpha range)	Pharmacologic effects are dose dependent: renal and mesenteric vasodilation predominate at lower doses; cardiac stimulation and vasoconstriction develop as the dose is increased

(continued)

445

Table 72-1 Some Commonly Used Autonomic Drugs[a]—(continued)

Agent	Indication	Dose and Route	Comment
DOPAMINERGIC AGONISTS (cont.)			
Bromocriptine	Amenorrhea-galactorrhea	2.5 mg PO bid or tid	Selective agonist of D_2 receptor; inhibits prolactin secretion
	Acromegaly	5–15 mg PO tid or qid	Lowers growth hormone in a minority of patients with acromegaly
Cabergoline	Hyperprolactinemia	0.25–1.0 mg PO twice a week	Agonist at D_2 receptor; inhibits prolactin secretion
Fenoldopam	Hypertension, acute treatment	0.01–0.3 (μg/kg)/min infusion	Agonist at D_1 receptors
INHIBITORS OF CENTRAL SYMPATHETIC OUTFLOW			
Clonidine	Hypertension	0.1–0.6 mg PO bid	Selective α_2 agonist; potentiates central baroreceptor depressor reflex Abrupt discontinuation may result in withdrawal syndrome with rebound hypertension
Methyldopa	Hypertension	250–500 mg PO every 6–8 h	Metabolized by decarboxylation and β hydroxylation to α-methylnorepinephrine, a centrally active selective α_2 agonist
ADRENERGIC NEURON BLOCKING AGENTS			
Guanethidine	Hypertension	10–100 mg PO qd	Concentrated in sympathetic nerve endings; blocks release of NE in response to nerve impulses and depletes NE stores; prominent orthostatic hypotension
Bretylium	Ventricular fibrillation and tachycardia	150–300 mg IV 1–4 mg/min IV	In addition to blocking NE release, has direct effect on electrical properties of cardiac muscle
BETA-BLOCKING AGENTS			
Propranolol	Hypertension	40–160 mg PO bid (or higher)	Lipophilic, nonselective Dosage highly variable
	Angina	10–40 mg PO tid or qid	
	Myocardial infarction	60–80 mg PO tid	Prolongs survival post MI
	Arrhythmias	10–30 mg PO tid or qid; 1–3 mg IV	
	Hypertrophic cardiomyopathy	20–40 mg PO tid or qid	
	Pheochromocytoma	10–20 mg PO tid or qid; 0.5–2.0 mg IV	After alpha blockade initiated
	Essential tremor	20–80 mg PO tid	
	Migraine	20–80 mg PO bid or tid	
	Hyperthyroidism	10–60 mg PO tid or qid	
Metoprolol	Hypertension	50–200 mg PO bid	Selective β_1 (cardiac), lipophilic
	Myocardial infarction	100 mg PO bid	Prolongs survival post MI
Nadolol	Hypertension	80–320 mg PO qd	Hydrophilic, nonselective; lengthen dosage interval with renal failure
	Angina	80–240 mg PO qd	
Timolol	Hypertension	10–30 mg PO bid	Lipophilic, nonselective
	Myocardial infarction	10 mg PO bid	Prolongs survival post MI
Atenolol	Hypertension	50–100 mg PO qd	Selective β_1, hydrophilic; lengthen dosage interval with renal failure
Pindolol	Hypertension	5–30 mg PO bid	Nonselective, lipophilic with partial agonist activity
	Angina	10 mg PO qid	
Acebutolol	Hypertension	200–800 mg qid	Selective β_1, hydrophilic, partial agonist activity
	Arrhythmias	200–600 mg bid	
Penbutolol	Hypertension	20–40 mg PO qd	Nonselective

(continued)

higher infusion rates interaction with α-adrenergic receptors results in vasoconstriction, an increase in peripheral resistance, and an elevation of blood pressure.

β-Receptor Agonists *Isoproterenol*, a direct-acting β-receptor agonist, stimulates the heart, decreases peripheral resistance, and relaxes bronchial smooth muscle. It raises the cardiac output and accelerates atrioventricular conduction while increasing the automaticity of ventricular pacemakers. Isoproterenol was formerly used in the treatment of heart block and bronchoconstriction. *Dobutamine*, a congener of dopamine with relative selectivity for the β_1 receptor and with a greater effect on myocardial contractility than on heart rate, is also used in the treatment of congestive heart failure, often in combination with vasodilators (Chap. 232). In conjunction with radionuclide imaging or echocardiographic assessment of wall motion, dobutamine, as well as other investigational congeners that have a relatively greater effect on heart rate, is used in the diagnosis of demand-induced myocardial ischemia.

Selective β_2-receptor agonists The cardiac stimulation caused by nonselective β agonists, such as isoproterenol or epinephrine, is occasionally dangerous when these agents are used in the treatment of bronchoconstriction (Chap. 252). Selective β_2 agonists, administered by inhalation for bronchoconstriction, include agents with an intermediate duration of action (*metaproterenol*, *albuterol*, *terbutaline*, *pirbuterol*, *isoetharine*, and *bitolterol*) and the newer long-acting agents (*salmeterol* and *formoterol*); these drugs improve the therapeutic ratio by achieving bronchial dilatation with less activation of the cardiovascular system (Chaps. 252 and 258). Although selectivity is relative and cardiac stimulation may occur with these agents at higher dose levels, inhaled agonists at the usual doses result in relatively little cardiac stimulation. Oral administration, which is no longer preferred, is associated with more systemic β-agonist effects. *Ritodrine*, another selective β_2 agonist, is used as a tocolytic agent (as is *terbutaline*) to relax the uterus and antagonize premature labor.

α-Adrenergic Agonists *Phenylephrine* and *methoxamine* are direct-acting α agonists that elevate blood pressure by increasing peripheral vasoconstriction. They are used primarily in the treatment of hypotension and paroxysmal supraventricular tachycardia (Chap. 230), in the latter case by increasing cardiac vagal tone through reflex baroreceptor stimulation. Phenylephrine and a related proprietary compound, *phenylpropanolamine*, are common constituents of decongestant medications (often combined with antihistamines) for the treatment of allergic rhinitis and upper respiratory infections.

Miscellaneous Sympathomimetic Amines with Mixed Actions *Ephedrine* has both direct β-receptor agonist properties and an indirect effect on sympathetic nerve endings, from which it releases NE, and is used primarily as a bronchodilator. *Su-dephedrine*, a congener of ephedrine, is less potent at dilating bronchi and serves as a nasal decongestant. *Metaraminol* has both direct and indirect effects on sympathetic nerve endings and is employed in the treatment of hypotensive states.

Dopaminergic Agonists The D$_2$-receptor agonists, *bromocriptine* and *cabergoline*, are used to suppress prolactin secretion (Chap. 328). *Apomorphine*, another D$_2$-receptor agonist, is used to induce emesis. The D$_1$ receptor agonist, *fenoldapam*, has recently been approved for the short-term in-hospital treatment of severe hypertension.

ANTIADRENERGIC OR SYMPATHOLYTIC AGENTS (See also Chap. 246) **Agents Inhibiting Central Sympathetic Outflow** The antihypertensive agents *methyldopa*, *clonidine*, *guanabenz*, and *guanfacine* diminish central sympathetic outflow by stimulating a central α-adrenergic pathway (α$_2$ receptor) that diminishes vasomotor outflow. CNS side effects such as sedation are common. When administration of clonidine is stopped abruptly, a withdrawal syndrome characterized by rebound hyperactivity of the sympathetic nervous system can produce a state resembling the crises

Table 72-1   Some Commonly Used Autonomic Drugs[e]**—(continued)**

Agent	Indication	Dose and Route	Comment
BETA-BLOCKING AGENTS[c] *(cont.)*			
Betaxolol	Hypertension	15–20 mg PO qd	Selective β$_1$, hydrophilic
Carteolol	Hypertension	2.5–10 mg PO qd	Nonselective, partial agonist activity, hydrophilic; lengthen dosage interval with renal failure
Esmolol	Supraventricular tachycardia	50–200 (μg/kg)/min IV after loading dose of 500 μg/kg/min for 1 min	Selective β$_1$, very short duration of action
Sotalol	Arrythmias	80–320 mg bid	Nonselective, hydrophilic
Bisoprolol	Hypertension	5–20 mg qd	Selective β$_1$, lipophilic
Carvedilol	CHF	3.125–50 mg PO bid	Nonselective, α$_1$-blocking activity
	Hypertension	6.25–25 mg PO bid	
ALPHA-BLOCKING AGENTS			
Phenoxybenzamine	Pheochromocytoma	10–60 mg PO bid; titrate as needed	Noncompetitive, nonselective alpha blockade
Phentolamine	Pheochromocytoma	5 mg IV (after test dose of 0.5 mg)	Competitive, nonselective alpha blockade
Prazosin	Hypertension	1–5 mg PO bid or tid	Competitive, selective alpha$_1$ blockade
	CHF	2–7 mg PO qid	
Doxazosin	Hypertension Prostatism	1–16 mg PO qd	Competitive selective alpha$_1$ blockade, long duration of action
Terazosin	Hypertension Prostatism	1–5 mg PO qd	Competitive, selective alpha$_1$ blockade, long duration of action
Tamsulosin	Benign prostatic hypertrophy	0.4–0.8 PO qd	Selective α$_1$-blocking activity in prostate, predominantly α$_{1A}$
COMBINED ALPHA-BETA BLOCKING AGENT			
Labetalol	Hypertension	100–1200 mg PO bid; titrate slowly as needed; 20–80 mg IV (by increments up to 300 mg); 2 mg/min by IV infusion	Competitive α and β antagonist with relatively more activity against β receptors
DOPAMINERGIC ANTAGONIST[d]			
Metoclopramide	Diabetic gastroparesis	10–15 mg PO qid	Competitive dopaminergic antagonist with prominent cholinergic agonist activity
	Gastroesophageal reflux	10–15 mg PO qid	
	Antiemetic (cancer chemotherapy)	10 mg IV	
GANGLIONIC BLOCKING AGENT			
Trimethaphan	Hypertensive crisis (aortic dissection)	0.5–5 mg/min IV	Competitive ganglionic blocker; some direct vasodilating effects; inhibits parasympathetic as well as sympathetic nervous system
CHOLINERGIC AGENT			
Bethanechol	Urinary retention (nonobstructive)	10–20 mg PO tid or qid; 2.5 mg SC	M$_2$ receptor agonist
ANTICHOLINESTERASE AGENTS[c]			
Physostigmine	Central cholinergic blockade	1–2 mg IV (slow)	Tertiary amine; penetrates CNS well; may cause seizures; used to reverse central anticholinergic effects produced by overdose of atropine or tricyclic antidepressants
Edrophonium	Paroxysmal supraventricular tachycardia	5 mg IV (after 1.0-mg test dose)	Induces vagotonic response; rapid onset, short duration of action; effects reversed by atropine

(continued)

Table 72-1 Some Commonly Used Autonomic Drugs[a]—(continued)

Agent	Indication	Dose and Route	Comment
CHOLINERGIC BLOCKING AGENTS[f]			
Atropine	Bradycardia and hypotension	0.4–1.0 mg IV every 1–2 h	Competitive inhibition of M_1 and M_2 receptor; blocks hemodynamic changes associated with increased vagal tone
Ipratropium	Asthma Chronic obstructive pulmonary disease	500 mg by inhalation (nebulizer) tid or qid	Anticholinergic bronchodilator
Oxybutynin	Overactive bladder	5 mg PO bid or qid	Muscarinic receptor antagonist
Tolterodine	Overactive bladder	1–2 mg PO bid	Competitive muscarinic receptor antagonist

[a] Consult complete prescribing information; doses for children are not given; only the more common indications and routes of administration are listed.

[b] Dopaminergic agonists are listed separately although dopamine, at high doses, is an adrenergic agonist as well.

[c] Clinical efficacy of most beta blockers appears similar for major indications. Not all beta blockers are FDA approved for all indications listed in the table. When beta-blocking agents are discontinued, gradual dosage reduction is recommended. Both beta$_1$ selective and nonselective agents have cardioprotective effects after myocardial infarction.

[d] Neuroleptic and antipsychotic agents are also dopaminergic antagonists; these are not included in the table.

[e] A major use of cholinesterase inhibitors is in myasthenia gravis (Chap. 380). These agents, quaternary amines that do not penetrate the CNS, are not included here.

[f] A wide variety of synthetic atropine derivatives are available for the purpose of (1) diminishing GI tract motility and secretion and (2) increasing urinary bladder capacity. Their usefulness is limited by anticholinergic side effects. Some may be useful as adjuncts in the treatment of peptic ulcer disease.

NOTE: BP, blood pressure; NE; norepinephrine; AV, atrioventricular; CHF, congestive heart failure; MI, myocardial infarction; CNS, central nervous system; FDA, U.S. Food & Drug Administration; GI, gastrointestinal.

of patients with pheochromocytoma. *Opiates* also may exert a central sympatholytic effect; the sympathetic excitation of morphine withdrawal responds to clonidine and vice versa. *Propranolol* and *reserpine* may exert some sympatholytic effects at the level of the CNS.

Ganglionic Blocking Agents Ganglionic transmission may be antagonized by drugs that block the (nicotinic) cholinergic synapse between the pre- and postganglionic autonomic nerves. These agents inhibit the parasympathetic as well as the sympathetic nervous system. Only *trimethaphan* is in general clinical use; its major application is in the treatment of hypertensive crises, particularly aortic dissection, when controlled hypotension and decreased myocardial contractility are desirable (Chap. 246).

Agents Acting at the Peripheral Sympathetic Nerve Endings Adrenergic neuron-blocking agents depress the function of the peripheral sympathetic nerves by decreasing the amount of neurotransmitter released. *Guanethidine*, the prototype of this class of drugs, is concentrated in the sympathetic nerve endings by the amine-uptake mechanism. Within the terminal it blocks the release of NE in response to nerve impulses and eventually depletes the nerve of NE by displacing it from the intraneuronal storage granules. The drug was formerly useful in the management of severe hypertension, although orthostatic hypotension was a limiting side effect. *Bretylium*, an agent whose effects are similar to those of guanethidine, is employed in the treatment of ventricular fibrillation (Chap. 230). Both guanethidine and bretylium are antagonized by agents that affect the amine-uptake transport process such as sympathomimetic amines, tricyclic antidepressants, phenoxybenzamine, and phenothiazines. The antihypertensive action of guanethidine may be rapidly reversed by these drugs.

Reserpine depletes catecholamines from the peripheral sympathetic nerve endings, the brain, and the adrenal medulla. Its antihypertensive effect in humans is usually attributed to depletion of peripheral NE stores within sympathetic nerve endings. The sedation and occasionally morbid depression attending its use result from NE depletion within the CNS.

Adrenergic-Receptor Blocking Agents Adrenergic blocking agents antagonize the effects of catecholamines at the level of the peripheral tissue.

α-Adrenergic-receptor blocking agents *Phenoxybenzamine* and *phentolamine* are utilized principally in treating pheochromocytoma (Chap. 332). Phenoxybenzamine produces prolonged, noncompetitive

alpha blockade, while phentolamine leads to reversible, competitive blockade. Because of its rapid action and short duration, phentolamine is commonly used in the treatment of acute hypertensive paroxysms secondary to catecholamine excess, such as occur with pheochromocytoma. Both phentolamine and phenoxybenzamine antagonize α_1 and α_2 receptors, although phenoxybenzamine is more potent at the α_1-receptor site. *Prazosin*, an α-adrenergic blocking agent with selectivity for the α_1 receptor, possesses properties that resemble those of primary vasodilators and has been used in the treatment of essential hypertension, as an afterload-reducing agent in congestive heart failure, and as an adjunct in the treatment of pheochromocytoma (Chap. 332). *Doxazosin* and *terazosin*, long-acting selective α_1 blockers, are more useful in the treatment of essential hypertension because of better dosing schedule and less orthostatic hypotension. These agents also lower triglyceride levels and raise high-density lipoprotein (HDL) cholesterol levels. These selective α_1 blockers, along with *tamsulosin* are useful in the symptomatic treatment of urinary outflow track obstruction and prostatism because they antagonize contraction of the sphincter at the bladder trigone and the prostate smooth muscle.

β-Adrenergic-receptor blocking agents These drugs antagonize the effects of catecholamines on the heart and are useful in the treatment of angina pectoris, hypertension, and cardiac arrhythmias. The benefit of beta blockade in angina derives from the decrease in myocardial oxygen consumption following reduction in heart rate and myocardial contractility (Chap. 244). The hypotensive effect of beta blockade is not clearly understood (Chap. 246). Diminished cardiac output, decreased NE release at postganglionic sympathetic nerve endings, reduced renin secretion, and suppressed central sympathetic outflow are possible mechanisms. The efficacy of β-blocking agents in the treatment of arrhythmias depends on reduction of the rate of spontaneous depolarization of pacemaker cells in the sinus node and junctional pacemakers and on slowing conduction within the atria and atrioventricular node. Beta blockade is also effective in the symptomatic management of hyperthyroidism and the control of tachycardia and arrhythmias in patients with pheochromocytoma. β-adrenergic blocking agents are also useful in the treatment of migraine, essential tremor, idiopathic hypertrophic subaortic stenosis, and aortic dissection. Several trials have demonstrated that β-receptor blocking agents, administered long-term, diminish mortality following acute myocardial infarction. The mechanism of this cardioprotective effect may involve antiarrhythmic action, prevention of reinfarction, and reduction in infarct size (Chap. 243).

Pharmacologic properties of β-receptor blocking agents Fourteen beta-blocking agents (atenolol, acebutolol, betaxolol, bisoprolol, carvedilol, carteolol, esmolol, metoprolol, nadolol, pindolol, penbutolol, propranolol, sotalol, and timolol) are available for use in the United States. Other agents (alprenolol, bevantolol, dilevalol, oxprenolol, etc.) are in use in other countries and investigational within the United States. The utility of these agents is derived predominantly from blockade of β-adrenergic receptors.

Although much has been written about other pharmacologic properties, including cardioselectivity, membrane-stabilizing (local anesthetic) effects, intrinsic sympathomimetic (partial-agonist) activity, and lipid solubility, the clinical significance of these additional properties is small. Local anesthetic properties are most prominent with propranolol; however, membrane stabilization probably does not contribute substantially to the clinical utility. The various beta blockers do differ in their water and lipid solubility. The lipophilic agents (propranolol, metoprolol, oxprenolol, bisoprolol, carvedilol) are readily absorbed from the gastrointestinal tract, metabolized by the liver, have large volumes of distribution, and penetrate the CNS well; the hydrophilic agents (acebutolol, atenolol, betaxolol, carteolol, nadolol, sotalol) are less readily absorbed, not extensively metabolized, and have relatively long plasma half-lives. As a consequence, the hydrophilic agents may be administered once per day. Hepatic failure may prolong the plasma half-life of the lipophilic agents, whereas renal failure may prolong the action of the hydrophilic group. The degree of lipid solubility, therefore, provides a basis for choice of a particular agent in patients with hepatic or renal insufficiency. Although the hydrophilic agents penetrate the CNS less well, CNS side effects (sedation, depression, hallucinations) are well described with the hydrophilic as well as with the lipophilic agents.

Some β-adrenergic blocking agents possess β-agonist activity. This has been referred to as "intrinsic sympathomimetic activity" (ISA). Agents with partial agonist activity (pindolol, alprenolol, acebutolol, carteolol, dilevalol, oxprenolol) cause little or no depression of resting heart rate (partial agonist effect) while blocking the increase in heart rate that occurs in response to exercise or the administration of a beta agonist such as isoproterenol. The presence of partial agonist activity may be useful when bradycardia limits treatment in patients with slow resting heart rates. Pindolol also produces mild vasodilation, perhaps in part related to peripheral β_2 stimulation. Agents with partial agonist activity cause less change in blood lipid levels than agents without agonist properties. On theoretical grounds, intrinsic sympathomimetic activity would be undesirable in the treatment of thyrotoxicosis, idiopathic hypertrophic subaortic stenosis, aortic dissection, and tachyarrhythmias.

Cardioselective (β_1) adrenergic-receptor blocking agents Propranolol, the prototype of the nonselective β-adrenergic blocking agent, induces a competitive blockade of both β_1 and β_2 receptors. Other nonselective beta-blocking agents include alprenolol, carteolol, dilevalol, nadolol, oxprenolol, penbutolol, pindolol, sotalol, timolol, and carvedilol. Metoprolol, esmolol, acebutolol, atenolol, and betaxolol possess relative selectivity for the β_1 receptor. Although β_1-(cardio-) selective agents have the theoretical advantage of producing less bronchoconstriction and less peripheral vasoconstriction, a clear-cut clinical advantage of the cardioselective agents has not been decisively demonstrated, since the β_1 selectivity is only relative. Bronchoconstriction may occur when β_1-selective agents are administered in full therapeutic doses.

Adverse effects of β-receptor blocking agents Aside from the effects on the CNS, most adverse reactions to beta-blocking agents are consequences of β-adrenergic blockade. These include the precipitation of heart failure in patients in whom cardiac compensation depends on enhanced sympathetic drive; the aggravation of bronchospasm in patients with asthma; predisposition to the development of hypoglycemia in insulin-requiring diabetics (blockade of catecholamine-mediated counterregulation and antagonism of the adrenergic warning signs of hypoglycemia); the development of hyperkalemia in diabetic or uremic patients with impaired potassium tolerance; the enhancement of coronary or peripheral arterial vasospasm; and elevation in triglycerides and depression of HDL levels. The lipid (and perhaps the peripheral vascular) effects are less (or absent) in agents with partial (β_2) agonist activity or alpha-blocking properties (carvedilol).

Miscellaneous adrenergic blocking agents Labetalol, approved for use in the United States as an antihypertensive agent, is a competitive antagonist of both α- and β-adrenergic receptors. Although labetalol induces relatively more β- than α-receptor blockade, fall in peripheral resistance may be marked following acute administration of the drug. Vasodilation may be mediated in part by a partial agonist

effect on the β_2-adrenergic receptor; labetalol does not possess partial agonist activity for the β_1 (cardiac) receptor.

Metoclopramide is a dopaminergic antagonist with cholinergic agonist properties. It enhances gastric emptying, increases the tone of the lower esophageal sphincter, increases prolactin and aldosterone secretion, and antagonizes emesis induced by apomorphine. It is useful clinically in enhancing gastric emptying (in the absence of organic obstruction such as in diabetic gastroparesis), in antagonizing gastroesophageal reflux, and as an antiemetic during cancer chemotherapy.

THE PARASYMPATHETIC NERVOUS SYSTEM

ACETYLCHOLINE ACh serves as the neurotransmitter at all autonomic ganglia, at the postganglionic parasympathetic nerve endings, at the postganglionic sympathetic nerve endings innervating the eccrine sweat glands, and at the skeletal muscle end plate (neuromuscular junction). The enzyme choline acetyltransferase catalyzes the synthesis of ACh from acetyl coenzyme A (CoA) produced within the nerve ending and from choline, actively taken up from the extracellular fluid. Within the cholinergic nerve endings, ACh is stored in discrete synaptic vesicles and released in response to nerve impulses that depolarize the nerve terminals and increase calcium influx.

Cholinergic Receptors Different receptors for ACh exist on the postganglionic neurons within the autonomic ganglia and at the postjunctional autonomic effector sites. Those within the autonomic ganglia and adrenal medulla are stimulated predominantly by nicotine (*nicotinic receptors*) and those on autonomic effector cells by the alkaloid muscarine (*muscarinic receptors*). Ganglionic blocking agents antagonize the nicotinic receptors, while atropine blocks the muscarinic receptors. The muscarinic (M) receptor, furthermore, has been recently subdivided into additional types. The M_1 receptor is localized to the CNS and perhaps parasympathetic ganglia; the M_2 receptor is the nonneuronal muscarinic receptor on smooth muscle, cardiac muscle, and glandular epithelium. Bethanechol is a selective agonist of the M_2 receptor; pirenzepine, an investigational agent, is a selective antagonist of the M_1 receptor that markedly reduces gastric acid secretion. The M_2 receptor inhibits adenylyl cyclase and utilizes the regulatory G_i protein; the M_1 receptor interacts with G_q and stimulates phospholipase C (Fig. 72-5). The M_3 receptor, present on smooth muscle and secretory glands, is antagonized by atropine and utilizes phospholipase C, IP_3, and DAG as second messengers. Other subtypes have been identified by molecular biologic techniques but have not yet been fully characterized.

Acetylcholinesterase Hydrolysis of ACh by acetylcholinesterase inactivates the neurotransmitter at cholinergic synapses. This enzyme (also known as specific or true cholinesterase) is present within neurons and is distinct from butyrocholinesterase (serum cholinesterase or pseudocholinesterase). The latter enzyme is present in plasma and nonneuronal tissues and is not primarily involved in the termination of the effects of ACh at autonomic effector sites. The pharmacologic effects of anticholinesterase agents are due to inhibition of neuronal (true) acetylcholinesterase.

PHYSIOLOGY OF THE PARASYMPATHETIC NERVOUS SYSTEM The parasympathetic nervous system participates in the regulation of the cardiovascular system, the gastrointestinal tract, and the genitourinary system. Tissues such as liver, kidney, pancreas, and thyroid also receive parasympathetic innervation, suggesting a role for the parasympathetic nervous system in metabolic regulation as well, although cholinergic effects on metabolism are not well characterized.

Cardiovascular System Parasympathetic effects on the heart are mediated by the vagus nerve. ACh reduces the rate of spontaneous depolarization of the sinoatrial node and decreases heart rate. ACh also delays impulse conduction within the atrial musculature while shortening the effective refractory period, a combination of factors that may initiate or perpetuate atrial arrhythmias. At the atrioventricular node, ACh reduces conduction velocity, increases the effective refractory period, and thus diminishes the ventricular response during atrial flutter or fibrillation (Chap. 230). The decrease in inotropy induced by ACh is related to a prejunctional inhibitory effect on sympathetic nerve endings as well as to a direct inhibitory effect on the atrial myocardium. The ventricular myocardium is not much affected since innervation by cholinergic fibers is minimal. A direct cholinergic contribution to the regulation of peripheral resistance appears unlikely since parasympathetic innervation of the vasculature is not extensive. The parasympathetic nervous system, however, may influence peripheral resistance indirectly by inhibiting NE release from sympathetic nerves.

Gastrointestinal Tract   Parasympathetic innervation of the gut is via the vagus nerve and the pelvic sacral nerves. The parasympathetic nervous system increases the tone of gastrointestinal smooth muscle, enhances peristaltic activity, and relaxes the gastrointestinal sphincters. ACh stimulates exocrine secretion from the glandular epithelium and enhances the secretion of gastrin, secretin, and insulin.

Genitourinary and Respiratory Systems   Sacral parasympathetic nerves supply the urinary bladder and genitalia. ACh increases ureteral peristalsis, contracts the urinary detrusor muscle, and relaxes the trigone and sphincter, thereby playing a critical role in the coordination of urination. The respiratory tract is innervated with parasympathetic fibers derived from the vagus nerve. ACh increases tracheobronchial secretions and stimulates bronchial constriction.

PHARMACOLOGY OF THE PARASYMPATHETIC NERVOUS SYSTEM
Cholinergic Agonists   ACh itself has no therapeutic role because of its widespread effects and short duration of action. Congeners of ACh are less susceptible to hydrolysis by cholinesterase and have a narrower range of physiologic effects. Bethanechol, the only systemic cholinergic agonist in general use, stimulates gastrointestinal and genitourinary smooth muscle with minimal effect on the cardiovascular system. It is used in the treatment of urinary retention in the absence of outflow tract obstruction and, less commonly, in gastrointestinal disorders such as postvagotomy gastric atony. Pilocarpine and carbachol are topical cholinergic agonists used in the treatment of glaucoma.

Acetylcholinesterase Inhibitors   Cholinesterase inhibitors enhance the effects of parasympathetic stimulation by diminishing the inactivation of ACh. The therapeutic application of reversible cholinesterase inhibitors depends on the role of ACh as neurotransmitter at the skeletal muscle neuroeffector junction and within the CNS and includes the treatment of myasthenia gravis (Chap. 380), the termination of neuromuscular blockade following general anesthesia, and the reversal of intoxication by agents with a central anticholinergic action. Physostigmine, a tertiary amine, penetrates the CNS well, while related quaternary amines (neostigmine, pyridostigmine, ambenonium, and edrophonium) do not. Organophosphorous cholinesterase inhibitors produce irreversible cholinesterase blockade; these agents are used principally as insecticides and are primarily of toxicologic interest. With regard to the autonomic nervous system, cholinesterase inhibitors are of limited use in the treatment of intestinal and bladder smooth-muscle dysfunction such as occurs in paralytic ileus and atonic urinary bladder. Cholinesterase inhibitors induce a vagotonic response in the heart and may be useful in terminating attacks of paroxysmal supraventricular tachycardia (Chap. 230).

Cholinergic-Receptor Blocking Agents   *Atropine* blocks muscarinic cholinergic receptors, with little effect on cholinergic transmission at the autonomic ganglia and the neuromuscular junctions. Many of the CNS actions of atropine and atropine-like drugs are attributable to blockade of central muscarinic synapses. The related alkaloid, *scopolamine*, is similar to atropine but causes drowsiness, euphoria, and amnesia, effects that make it suitable as a preanesthetic medication.

Atropine increases heart rate and enhances atrioventricular conduction, actions that may be useful in combating the bradycardia or heart block associated with heightened vagal tone. In addition, atropine reverses cholinergically mediated bronchoconstriction and diminishes respiratory tract secretions. These effects contribute to its utility as a preanesthetic medication.

Atropine also decreases gastrointestinal tract motility and secretion. Although various derivatives and congeners of atropine (such as *propantheline, isopropamide,* and *glycopyrrolate*) have been advocated in patients with peptic ulcer or with diarrheal syndromes, the chronic use of such agents is limited by other manifestations of parasympathetic inhibition such as dry mouth and urinary retention. The investigational selective M_1 inhibitor pirenzepine inhibits gastric secretion at doses that have minimal anticholinergic effects at other sites; this agent may be useful in the treatment of peptic ulcer. Atropine and its congener *ipratropium,* when given by inhalation, cause bronchodilation and have been used experimentally in the treatment of asthma.

BIBLIOGRAPHY

ARNER P, HOFFSTEDT J: Adrenoceptor genes in human obesity. J Intern Med 245:667, 1999

CARON MG, LEFKOWITZ RJ: Catecholamine receptors: Structure, function and regulation. Recent Prog Horm Res 48:277, 1993

CHALMERS J, PILOWSKY P: Brainstem and bulbospinal neurotransmitter systems in the control of blood pressure. J Hypertens 9:675, 1991

ESLER M et al: Overflow of catecholamine neurotransmitters to the circulation: Source, fate, and functions. Physiol Rev 70:963, 1990

GRASSI G, ESLER M: How to assess sympathetic activity in humans. J Hypertens 17:719, 1999

JÄNIG W, MCLACHLAN EM: Specialized functional pathways are the building blocks of the autonomic nervous system. J Auton Nerv Syst 41:3, 1992

LAM YW: Clinical pharmacology of dopamine agonists. Pharmacotherapy 20:175, 2000

LOW PA: Autonomic nervous system function. J Clin Neurophysiol 10:14, 1993

NELSON H: β-Adrenergic bronchodilators. N Engl J Med 333:499, 1995

PITCHER JA et al: G protein–coupled receptor kinases. Annu Rev Biochem 67:653, 1998

RUFFOLO RR JR, HIEBLE JP: α-Adrenoceptors. Pharmacol Ther 61:1, 1994

STROSBERG AD: Structure and function of the β_3-adrenergic-receptor. Annu Rev Pharmacol Toxicol 37:421, 1997

YOUNG JB, LANDSBERG L: Catecholamines and the adrenal medulla, in *Williams' Textbook of Endocrinology,* 9th ed, JD Wilson et al (eds). Philadelphia, Saunders, 1998, p 665

73   *Johanna Dwyer*

NUTRITIONAL REQUIREMENTS AND DIETARY ASSESSMENT

Nutrients are substances that are not synthesized in the body in sufficient amounts and therefore must be supplied by the diet. Nutrient requirements for groups of healthy persons have been thoroughly defined on the basis of experimental evidence. For good health we require energy-providing nutrients (protein, fat, and carbohydrate), vitamins, minerals, and water. Specific nutrient requirements include 9 essential amino acids, several fatty acids, 4 fat-soluble vitamins, 10 water-soluble vitamins, and choline. Several inorganic substances, including four minerals, seven trace minerals, three electrolytes, and the ultratrace elements, must also be supplied in the diet (Chap. 75).

The required amounts of the essential nutrients differ by age and physiologic state. Conditionally essential nutrients are not required in the diet but must be supplied to individuals who do not synthesize them in adequate amounts, such as those with genetic defects, those having pathologic states with nutritional implications, and developmentally immature infants (Chap. 74). Many organic phytochemicals and zoochemicals present in foods have various health effects. For example, dietary fiber has been shown to have beneficial effects on gastrointestinal function.

ESSENTIAL NUTRIENT REQUIREMENTS   **Energy** For weight to remain stable, energy intake must match energy output (Chap. 77). The major categories of energy output are resting energy expenditure (REE) and physical activity; minor sources include the energy cost of metabolizing food (thermic effect of food or specific dynamic action) and shivering thermogenesis (e.g., cold-induced thermogenesis). The average energy intake is about 2800 kcal/d for American men and about 1800 kcal/d for American women, though these estimates vary with body size and activity level. Formulas for estimating REE are useful for assessing the energy needs of an individual whose weight is stable. Thus, for males, REE $= 900 + 10w$, and for females, REE $= 700 + 7w$, where w is weight in kg. The calculated REE is then adjusted for physical activity level by multiplying by 1.2 for sedentary, 1.4 for moderately active, or 1.8 for very active individuals. The final figure provides an estimate of total caloric needs in a state of energy balance.

Illness often alters energy needs. Unstressed hospitalized patients at bed rest usually require 1.2 times their REE, whereas those who are stressed, febrile, and catabolic require 1.5 to 2 times their REE (Chap. 74). Intestinal malabsorption may decrease net utilizable energy to as little as 25% of ingested energy and may necessitate feeding by parenteral routes (Chap. 76). Fever increases energy expenditure by 10 to 13% per degree Celsius above normal. Other diseases increase energy needs by varying amounts, such as burns (40 to 100%), trauma (40 to 100%), and hyperthyroidism (10 to 100%). Hypothyroidism and adrenal insufficiency decrease resting energy needs, but these alterations are corrected after adequate hormone replacement. In obese patients, weight reduction can be accomplished by reducing energy intakes by approximately 500 kcal/d to achieve a loss of 0.5 kg of fat per week, or 1000 kcal/d to lose 1 kg per week (Chap. 77).

Protein   Dietary protein consists of both essential and nonessential amino acids that are required for protein synthesis, whereas certain amino acids can also be used for energy and gluconeogenesis (Chap. 334). The nine essential amino acids are histidine, isoleucine, leucine, lysine, methionine/cystine, phenylalanine/tyrosine, threonine, tryptophan, and valine. When energy intake is inadequate, protein intake must be increased, since ingested amino acids are diverted into pathways of glucose synthesis and oxidation. In extreme energy deprivation, protein-calorie malnutrition may ensue (Chaps. 74 and 76).

For adults, the recommended dietary allowance (RDA) for protein is about 0.6 g/kg desirable body weight per day, assuming that energy needs are met and that the protein is of relatively high biologic value. Current recommendations for a healthy diet call for at least 10 to 14% of calories from protein. Biologic value tends to be highest for animal proteins, followed by proteins from legumes (beans), cereals (rice, wheat, corn), and roots. Combinations of plant proteins that complement one another in biologic value or combinations of animal and plant proteins can increase biologic value and lower total protein requirements.

Protein needs increase during growth, pregnancy, lactation, and rehabilitation during treatment of malnutrition. The tolerance of dietary protein is decreased in renal insufficiency and liver failure. Normal protein intake can precipitate encephalopathy in patients with cirrhosis of the liver (Chap. 299) or worsen uremia in those with renal failure (Chap. 270).

Fat and Carbohydrate   Fats are a concentrated source of energy and constitute on average 34% of calories in U.S. diets. However, for optimal health, fat intake should total no more than 30% of calories. Saturated fat and trans-fat should be limited to $<10\%$ of calories, and polyunsaturated fats to $<10\%$ of calories, with monounsaturated fats comprising the remainder of fat intake. At least 55% of total calories should be derived from carbohydrates. The brain requires about 100 g/d of glucose for fuel; other tissues use about 50 g/d. Over time, adaptations in carbohydrate needs are possible in hypocaloric states. For example, reduced insulin levels lead to adipose tissue breakdown and cause the body to burn more fatty acids. However, some tissues (e.g., brain and red blood cells) rely on glucose supplied either exogenously or from muscle proteolysis (Chap. 334).

Water   For adults, 1 to 1.5 mL water per kcal of energy expenditure is sufficient under usual conditions to allow for normal variations in physical activity levels, sweating, and solute load of the diet. Water losses include 50 to 100 mL/d in the feces, 500 to 1000 mL/d by evaporation or exhalation, and, depending on the renal solute load, ≥ 1000 mL/d in the urine. If external losses increase, intakes must increase accordingly to avoid underhydration. Fever increases water losses by approximately 200 mL/d per °C; diarrheal losses vary but may be as great as 5 L/d in severe diarrhea. Heavy sweating and vomiting also increase water losses. When renal function is normal and solute intakes are adequate, the kidneys can adjust to increased water intake by excreting up to 18 L/d of excess water (Chap. 329). However, obligatory urine outputs can compromise hydration status when there is inadequate intake or when losses increase in disease or kidney damage.

Infants have high requirements for water because of their large ratio of surface area to volume, the limited capacity of the immature kidney to handle high renal solute loads, and their inability to communicate their thirst. Increased water needs during pregnancy are low, perhaps an additional 30 mL/d; but during lactation, milk production increases water requirements so that approximately 1000 mL/d of additional water is needed, or 1 mL for each mL of milk produced. Special attention must be paid to the water needs of the elderly, who have reduced total body water and blunted thirst sensation and may be taking diuretics.

Other Nutrients   The vitamins and minerals required for health and the clinical disorders caused by vitamin deficiency or excess are discussed in Chap. 75.

DIETARY REFERENCE INTAKES, RECOMMENDED ALLOWANCES, AND TOLERANCES

Fortunately, human life and well-being can be maintained within a fairly wide range for most nutrients. However, the capacity for adaptation is not infinite—too much, as well as too little, intake of a nutrient may have adverse effects or alter the health benefits conferred by another nutrient (Chap. 75). Therefore, benchmark recommendations on nutrient intakes have been developed to guide clinical practice. These quantitative estimates of nutrient intakes are collectively referred to as the *dietary reference intakes* (DRIs). The DRIs supplant the RDAs, the single reference values used in the United States since 1989. DRIs include the estimated average requirement (EAR) for nutrients, as well as three other reference values used for dietary planning for individuals: the RDAs, the adequate intake (AI), and the safe upper level (UL). The current RDAs and AIs are provided in Tables 73-1 and 73-2, respectively.

Estimated Average Requirement When florid dietary deficiency diseases such as rickets, scurvy, xerophthalmia, and protein-calorie malnutrition were common, nutrient adequacy was assumed by the absence of clinical signs of a dietary deficiency disease. Later, it was determined that biochemical and other changes were evident long before the clinical deficiency became apparent. Consequently, criteria of adequacy are chosen using such biologic markers when they are available. Current efforts focus on the amount of a nutrient that reduces the risk of chronic degenerative diseases. Priority is given to sensitive biochemical, physiologic, or behavioral tests that reflect early changes in regulatory processes or maintenance of body stores of nutrients.

The EAR is the amount of a nutrient estimated to be adequate for half of the healthy individuals of a specific age and sex. The types of evidence and criteria used to establish nutrient requirements vary by nutrient, age, and physiologic group. The EAR is not an effective estimate of nutrient adequacy in individuals because it is a median requirement for a group, and the variation around this number is considerable. As the EAR specifies, 50% of individuals in a group fall below the requirement and 50% fall above it. Thus, a person with a usual intake at the EAR has a 50% risk of an inadequate intake during the reporting period. For these reasons, other standards, described below, are more useful for clinical purposes.

Recommended Dietary Allowances The RDA is the average daily dietary intake level that meets the nutrient requirements of nearly all healthy persons of a specific sex, age, life stage, or physiologic condition (such as pregnancy or lactation). The RDA is commonly used as a nutrient-intake goal for planning diets of individuals.

The RDA is defined statistically as 2 standard deviations (SD) above the EAR to ensure that the needs of any given individual are met. The RDAs are used to formulate food guides such as the U.S. Department of Agriculture (USDA) Food Guide Pyramid for individuals, food exchange lists for therapeutic diet planning, and as a standard for describing the nutritional content of processed foods and nutrient supplements. The nutrient content in a food is stated by weight or as a percent of the daily value (DV), a varient of the RDA which, for an adult, represents the highest RDA for an adult consuming 2000 kcal/d.

The risk of dietary inadequacy increases as intakes fall further below the RDA. However, the RDA is an overly generous criterion for evaluating nutrient adequacy. For example, by definition the RDA exceeds the actual requirements of all but about 2 to 3% of the population. Therefore, many people whose intakes fall below the RDA may still be getting enough of the nutrient.

Adequate Intake It is not possible to set an RDA for some nutrients that do not have an established EAR. In this circumstance, the AI is based on observed, or experimentally determined, approximations of nutrient intakes in healthy people. In the DRIs established to date, AIs rather than RDAs are proposed for infants up to age 1, as well as for calcium, vitamin D, fluoride, pantothenic acid, biotin, and choline for persons of all ages.

Tolerable Upper Levels of Nutrient Intake Excessive nutrient intake can disturb body functions and cause acute, progressive, or permanent disabilities (Chap. 75). Some diseases of nutritional excess include fluorosis, hypervitaminosis A, hypervitaminosis D, and obesity. The tolerable UL is the highest level of chronic nutrient intake (usually daily) that is unlikely to pose a risk of adverse health effects for most of the population. An uncertainty factor is applied to ensure that even very sensitive persons would not experience adverse effects at the UL dose chosen. For many nutrients, data on the adverse effects of large amounts of the nutrient are unavailable or too limited establish a UL. Therefore, the lack of a UL does *not* mean that the risk of adverse

Table 73-1 Recommended Dietary Allowances[a]

Category	Age, Years, or Condition	Weight[b] kg	Weight[b] lb	Height[b] cm	Height[b] in	Protein, g	Vitamin A, μg RE[c]	Vitamin E, mg α-TE[d]	Vitamin K, μg	Vitamin C, mg	Iron, mg	Zinc, mg	Iodine, μg	Selenium, μg
Infants	0.0–0.5	6	13	60	24	13	375	3	5	30	6	5	40	10
	0.5–1.0	9	20	71	28	14	375	4	10	35	10	5	50	15
Children	1–3	13	29	90	35	16	400	6	15	40	10	10	70	20
	4–6	20	44	112	44	24	500	7	20	45	10	10	90	20
	7–10	28	62	132	52	28	700	7	30	45	10	10	120	30
Males	11–14	45	99	157	62	45	1000	10	45	50	12	15	150	40
	15–18	66	145	176	69	59	1000	10	65	60	12	15	150	50
	19–24	72	160	177	70	58	1000	10	70	60	10	15	150	70
	25–50	79	174	176	70	63	1000	10	80	60	10	15	150	70
	51+	77	170	173	68	63	1000	10	80	60	10	15	150	70
Females	11–14	46	101	157	62	46	800	8	45	50	15	12	150	45
	15–18	55	120	163	64	44	800	8	55	60	15	12	150	50
	19–24	58	128	164	65	46	800	8	60	60	15	12	150	55
	25–50	63	138	163	64	50	800	8	65	60	15	12	150	55
	51+	65	143	160	63	50	800	8	65	60	10	12	150	55
Pregnant						60	800	10	65	70	30	15	175	65
Lactating	1st 6 months					65	1300	12	65	95	15	19	200	75
	2nd 6 months					62	1200	11	65	90	15	16	200	75

[a] This table does not include nutrients for which dietary reference intakes have recently been established. (See *Dietary Reference Intakes for Calcium, Phosphorus, Magnesium, Vitamin D, and Fluoride* and *Dietary Reference Intakes for Thiamin, Riboflavin, Niacin, Vitamin B₆, Folate, Vitamin B₁₂, Pantothenic Acid, Biotin, and Choline.* Washington DC, National Academy Press, 1997 and 1998, respectively.) The allowances, expressed as average daily intakes over time, are intended to provide for individual variations among most normal persons as they live in the United States under usual environmental stresses. Diets should be based on a variety of common foods in order to provide other nutrients for which human requirements have been less well defined.

[b] Weights and heights of Reference Adults are actual medians for the U.S. population of the designated age. The use of these figures does not imply that the height-to-weight ratios are ideal.

[c] Retinol equivalents. 1 retinol equivalent = 1 μg retinol or 6 μg β-carotene.

[d] α-Tocopherol equivalents. 1 mg d-α tocopherol = 1 α-TE.

SOURCE: Food and Nutrition Board, National Academy of Sciences–National Research Council Recommended Dietary Allowances, Revised 1989 (Abridged), reprinted with permission. Courtesy of the National Academy Press, Washington, DC.

effects from high intakes is nonexistent; caution is warranted in those who consume large amounts of such nutrients. Healthy individuals derive no established benefit from consuming nutrient levels above the RDA or AI. Individual nutrients in foods that most people eat rarely reach levels that exceed the UL. However, nutritional supplements provide more concentrated amounts of nutrients per dose and, as a result, pose a potential risk of toxicity. Nutrient supplements are labeled with "supplement facts" that express the amount of nutrient in absolute units or as the percent of the DV provided per recommended serving size. Those who use supplements should be advised that total nutrient consumption, including both food and supplements, should not exceed RDA levels.

FACTORS ALTERING NUTRIENT NEEDS The DRIs are affected by age, sex, rate of growth, pregnancy, lactation, physical activity, composition of diet, concomitant diseases, and drugs. When only slight differences exist between the requirements for nutrient sufficiency and excess, dietary planning becomes more difficult. Renal insufficiency provides one example in which protein intakes must be sufficient to maintain protein nutritional status, while avoiding exacerbation of uremic symptoms because of protein excess.

Physiologic Factors Growth, strenuous physical activity, pregnancy, and lactation increase needs for energy and several essential nutrients. Energy needs rise during pregnancy, due to the demands of fetal growth, and during lactation, because of the increased energy required for milk production. Energy needs decrease with loss of lean

body mass, the major determinant of REE. Because both health and physical activity tend to decline with age, energy needs in older persons, especially those over 70, tend to be less than those of younger persons.

Dietary Composition Dietary composition affects the biologic availability and utilization of nutrients. For example, the absorption of iron may be impaired by high amounts of calcium or lead; non-heme iron uptake may be impaired by the lack of ascorbic acid and amino acids in the meal. The absorption of calcium and magnesium is decreased by large amounts of phytates in the diet. Protein utilization by the body may be decreased when essential amino acids are not present in sufficient amounts. Animal foods, such as milk, eggs, and meat, have high biologic values with most of the needed amino acids present in adequate amounts. Plant proteins in corn (maize), soy, and wheat have lower biologic values and must be combined with other plant or animal proteins to achieve optimal utilization by the body.

Route of Administration The RDAs apply only to oral intakes. When nutrients are administered parenterally, similar values can sometimes be used for amino acids, carbohydrates, fats, sodium, chloride, potassium, and most of the vitamins, since their intestinal absorption is nearly 100% (Chap. 75). However, the oral bioavailability of most mineral elements may be only half that obtained by parenteral administration. For some nutrients that are not readily stored in the body, or

Table 73-2 Recommended Intakes for Individuals[a]

Life-Stage Group	Calcium, mg/d	Phosphorus, mg/d	Magnesium, mg/d	Vitamin D, μg/d[b,c]	Fluoride, mg/d	Thiamine, mg/d	Riboflavin, mg/d	Niacin, mg/d[d]	Vitamin B$_6$, mg/d	Folate, μg/d[e]	Vitamin B$_{12}$, μg/d	Pantothenic Acid, mg/d	Biotin, μg/d	Choline, mg/d[f]
Infants														
0–6 mo	210	100	30	5	0.01	0.2	0.3	2	0.1	65	0.4	1.7	5	125
7–12 mo	270	275	75	5	0.5	0.3	0.4	4	0.3	80	0.5	1.8	6	150
Children														
1–3 yr	500	**460**	80	5	0.7	**0.5**	**0.5**	6	**0.5**	**150**	0.9	2	8	200
4–8 yr	800	**500**	130	5	1	**0.6**	**0.6**	8	**0.6**	**200**	1.2	3	12	250
Males														
9–13 yr	1300	**1250**	240	5	2	**0.9**	**0.9**	12	**1.0**	**300**	1.8	4	20	375
14–18 yr	1300	**1250**	410	5	3	**1.2**	**1.3**	16	**1.3**	**400**	2.4	5	25	550
19–30 yr	1000	**700**	400	5	4	**1.2**	**1.3**	16	**1.3**	**400**	2.4	5	30	550
31–50 yr	1000	**700**	420	5	4	**1.2**	**1.3**	16	**1.3**	**400**	2.4	5	30	550
51–70 yr	1200	**700**	420	10	4	**1.2**	**1.3**	16	**1.7**	**400**	2.4[g]	5	30	550
>70 yr	1200	**700**	420	15	4	**1.2**	**1.3**	16	**1.7**	**400**	2.4[g]	5	30	550
Females														
9–13 yr	1300	**1250**	240	5	2	**0.9**	**0.9**	12	**1.0**	**300**	1.8	4	20	375
14–18 yr	1300	**1250**	360	5	3	**1.0**	**1.0**	14	**1.2**	**400**[h]	2.4	5	25	400
19–30 yr	1000	**700**	310	5	3	**1.1**	**1.1**	14	**1.3**	**400**[h]	2.4	5	30	425
31–50 yr	1000	**700**	320	5	3	**1.1**	**1.1**	14	**1.3**	**400**[h]	2.4	5	30	425
51–70 yr	1200	**700**	320	10	3	**1.1**	**1.1**	14	**1.5**	**400**	2.4[g]	5	30	425
>70 yr	1200	**700**	320	15	3	**1.1**	**1.1**	14	**1.5**	**400**	2.4[g]	5	30	425
Pregnancy														
≤18 yr	1300	**1250**	**400**	5	3	**1.4**	**1.4**	18	**1.6**	**600**[i]	2.6	6	30	450
19–30 yr	1000	**700**	**350**	5	3	**1.4**	**1.4**	18	**1.9**	**600**[i]	2.6	6	30	450
31–50 yr	1000	**700**	**360**	5	3	**1.4**	**1.4**	18	**1.9**	**600**[i]	2.6	6	30	450
Lactation														
≤18 yr	1300	**1250**	**360**	5	3	**1.5**	1.6	17	2.0	**500**	2.8	7	35	550
19–30 yr	1000	**700**	**310**	5	3	**1.5**	1.6	17	2.0	**500**	2.8	7	35	550
31–50 yr	1000	**700**	**320**	5	3	**1.5**	1.6	17	2.0	**500**	2.8	7	35	550

[a] This table presents recommended dietary allowances (RDAs) in bold type and adequate intakes (AIs) in ordinary type. RDAs and AIs may both be used as goals for individual intake. RDAs are set to meet the needs of almost all (97 to 98%) individuals in a group. For healthy breastfed infants, the AI is the mean intake. The AI for other life-stage and gender groups is believed to cover needs of all individuals in the group, but lack of data or uncertainty in the data prevent being able to specify with confidence the percentage of individuals covered by this intake.

[b] As cholecalciferol. 1 μg cholecalciferol = 40 IU vitamin D.

[c] In the absence of adequate exposure to sunlight.

[d] As niacin equivalents (NE). 1 mg of niacin = 60 mg of tryptophan; 0–6 months = preformed niacin (not NE).

[e] As dietary folate equivalents (DFE). 1 DFE = 1 μg food folate = 0.6 μg of folic acid from fortified food or as a supplement consumed with food = 0.5 μg of a supplement taken on an empty stomach.

[f] Although AIs have been set for choline, there are few data to assess whether a dietary

supply of choline is needed at all stages of the life cycle, and it may be that the choline requirement can be met by endogenous synthesis at some of these stages.

[g] Because 10 to 30% of older people may malabsorb food-bound B$_{12}$, it is advisable for those > 50 years to meet their RDA mainly by consuming foods fortified with B$_{12}$ or a supplement containing B$_{12}$.

[h] In view of evidence linking inadequate folate intake with neural tube defects in the fetus, it is recommended that all women capable of becoming pregnant consume 400 μg from supplements or fortified foods in addition to intake of food folate from a varied diet.

[i] It is assumed that women will continue consuming 400 μg from supplements or fortified food until their pregnancy is confirmed and they enter prenatal care, which ordinarily occurs after the end of the periconceptional period—the critical time for formation of the neural tube.

SOURCE: Food and Nutrition Board, Institute of Medicine—National Academy of Sciences Dietary Reference Intakes, 1999, reprinted with permission. Courtesy of the National Academy Press, Washington, DC.

Table 73-3 The USDA Food Guide Pyramid for Healthy Persons

Servings and Examples of Standard Portion Sizes	Lower: 1600 kcal	Moderate: about 2200 kcal	Higher: about 2800 kcal
Bread group			
1 slice bread; 1 oz. ready-to-eat cereal; ½ cup cooked cereal, rice, or pasta	6	9	22
Vegetable group			
1 cup raw leafy vegetables; ½ cup other vegetables, cooked or chopped raw; ¾ cup vegetable juice	3	4	5
Fruit group			
1 medium banana, apple, or orange; ½ cup chopped, cooked, or canned fruit; ¾ cup fruit juice	2	3	4
Milk group			
1 cup milk or yogurt, 1.5 oz natural cheese, 1 oz processed cheese	2–3[a]	2–3[a]	1–3[a]
Meat group			
2–3 oz cooked lean meat, poultry or fish; ½ cup cooked dry beans; 1 egg or 2 Tbsp. peanut butter count as 1 oz lean meat)	5	5	7
Total fat, g	53	73	93
Total added sugars, tsp	6	12	18

[a] Women who are pregnant or breastfeeding, teenagers, and young adults to age 24 need 3 servings.
SOURCE: US Department of Agriculture, Human Nutrition Information Service. *The Food Guide Pyramid*, Home and Garden Bulletin Number 252, US Department of Agriculture, Washington DC, August 1992.

cannot be stored in large amounts, timing of administration may also be important. For example, amino acids cannot be used for protein synthesis if they are not supplied together; instead they will be used for energy production.

Disease Specific dietary deficiency diseases include protein-calorie malnutrition; iron, iodine, and vitamin A deficiency; megaloblastic anemia due to vitamin B_{12} or folic acid deficiency; vitamin D deficiency rickets; and scurvy, beriberi, and pellagra (Chaps. 74 and 75). Each deficiency disease is characterized by imbalances at the cellular level between the supply of nutrients or energy and the body's nutritional needs for growth, maintenance, and other functions. Imbalances in nutrient intakes are recognized as risk factors for certain chronic degenerative diseases, such as saturated fat and cholesterol in coronary artery disease; sodium in hypertension; obesity in hormone-dependent endometrial, breast, and prostate cancers; and ethanol in alcoholism. Since the etiology and pathogenesis of these disorders are multifactorial, diet is only one of many risk factors. Osteoporosis, for example, is associated with calcium deficiency, as well as risk factors related to environment (e.g., smoking, sedentary lifestyle), physiology (e.g., estrogen deficiency), genetic determinants (e.g., defects in collagen metabolism), and drug use (chronic steroids) (Chap. 342).

DIETARY ASSESSMENT In clinical situations, nutritional assessment is an iterative process that involves: (1) screening for malnutrition, (2) assessing the diet and other data to establish either the absence or presence of malnutrition and its possible causes, and (3) planning for the most appropriate nutritional therapy. Some disease states affect the bioavailability, requirements, utilization, or excretion of specific nutrients. In these circumstances, specific measurements of various nutrients may be required to assure adequate replacement (Chap. 75).

Most health care facilities have a nutrition screening process in place for identifying possible malnutrition after hospital admission. Nutritional screening is required by the Joint Commission on Accreditation of Healthcare Organizations (JCAHO), but there are no universally recognized or validated standards, so techniques vary. The factors that are usually assessed include: abnormal weight for height or body mass index (e.g., BMI <19 or >25); reported weight change (involuntary loss or gain of >5 kg in past 6 months) (Chap. 43); diagnoses with known nutritional implications (metabolic disease, any disease affecting the gastrointestinal tract, alcoholism, and others); present therapeutic dietary prescription; chronic poor appetite; presence of chewing and swallowing problems or major food intolerances; need for assistance with preparing or shopping for food, eating, or other aspects of self care; and social isolation. Reassessment of nutrition status should occur periodically in hospitalized patients—at least once every week.

A more complete dietary assessment is indicated for patients who exhibit a high risk of malnutrition on nutrition screening. The type of assessment varies based on the clinical setting, severity of the patient's illness, and stability of his or her condition.

Acute Care Settings In acute care settings, anorexia, various diseases, test procedures, and medications can compromise dietary intake. Under such circumstances, the goal is to identify and avoid inadequate intake and assure appropriate alimentation. Dietary assessment in acute care situations focuses on what patients are currently eating, whether they are able and willing to eat, and whether they experience any problems with eating. Dietary intake assessment is based on information from observed intakes; medical record; history; clinical examination; and anthropometric, biochemical, and functional status. The objective is to gather enough information to establish the likelihood of malnutrition due to poor dietary intake or other causes in order to determine whether nutritional therapy is indicated.

Simple observations may suffice to suggest inadequate oral intake. These include dietitians' and nurses' notes, the amount of food eaten on trays, frequent tests and procedures that are likely to cause meals to be skipped, nutritionally inadequate diet orders such as clear liquids or full liquids for more than a few days, fever, gastrointestinal distress, vomiting, diarrhea, or a comatose state. Patients with diseases or treatments that involve any part of the alimentary tract are at high nutritional risk. Acutely ill patients with diet-related diseases such as diabetes need assessment because an inappropriate diet may exacerbate these conditions and adversely affect other therapies. Abnormal biochemical values [serum albumin levels <35 g/L (<3.5 mg/dL); serum cholesterol levels <3.9 mmol/L (<150 mg/dL)] are nonspecific but may also indicate a need for further nutritional assessment.

Most therapeutic diets offered in hospitals are calculated to meet individual nutrient requirements and the RDA. Exceptions include clear liquids, some full liquid diets, and test diets, which are inadequate for several nutrients and should not be used, if possible, for more than 24 h. As much as half of the food served to hospitalized patients is not eaten, and so it cannot be assumed that the intakes of hospitalized patients are adequate. The dietary assessment should therefore compare how much and what food the patient has consumed with the diet that has been provided in the hospital. Major deviations in intakes of energy, protein, fluids, or other nutrients of special concern for the patient's illness should be noted and corrected.

Nutritional monitoring is especially important for patients who are very ill and who have extended lengths of stay. Patients who are fed by special enteral and parenteral routes also require special nutritional assessment and monitoring by physicians with training in nutrition support and/or dietitians with certification in nutrition support (Chap. 76).

Ambulatory Settings The aim of dietary assessment in the outpatient setting is to determine whether the patient's usual diet is a health risk in itself or if it contributes to existing chronic disease-related problems. It also provides the basis for planning a diet that fulfills therapeutic goals while ensuring patient compliance. The outpatient dietary assessment should review the adequacy of present and usual food intakes, including vitamin and mineral supplements, medications, and alcohol, as all of these may affect the patient's nutritional status. The dietary assessment should focus on the dietary constituents that are most likely to be involved or compromised by a specific diagnosis, as well as any comorbidities that are present. More than one day's intake should be reviewed to provide a better representation of the usual diet.

There are many ways to assess the adequacy of the patient's habitual diet. These include a food guide, a food exchange list, a diet history, or a food frequency questionnaire. A commonly used food guide for healthy persons is the USDA's food pyramid, which is useful as a basis for identifying inadequate intakes of essential nutrients, as well as likely excesses in fat, saturated fat, sodium, sugar, and alcohol (Table 73-3). The guide is calculated to provide approximately 1600 kcal for sedentary women and some older adults; 2200 kcal for most children, teenage girls, active women, and many sedentary men (women who are pregnant or breastfeeding may need somewhat more); and 2800 kcal for teenage boys, most active men, and some very active women. Results provide a rough guide to food groups that may be eaten either in excess of recommendations or in insufficient quantities. Respondents who follow ethnic or unusual dietary patterns may need extra instruction on how foods should be categorized, as well as the appropriate portion sizes that constitute a serving. The process of reviewing the guide with patients helps them transition to healthier dietary patterns. For those on therapeutic diets, assessment against food exchange lists may be useful. These include, for example, the American Diabetes Association food exchange lists for diabetes, or the American Dietetic Association food exchange lists for renal disease.

Nutritional Status Assessment Full nutritional status assessment is a complex, time-consuming, and expensive process that requires considerable expertise. Candidates include seriously ill patients and those at very high nutritional risk when the cause of malnutrition is still uncertain after initial clinical evaluation and dietary assessment. Full nutritional status assessment involves multiple dimensions, including documentation of dietary intake, anthropometric measurements, biochemical measurements of blood and urine, clinical examination, health history, and functional. →*For further discussion of Nutritional Assessment, see Chap. 74.*

BIBLIOGRAPHY

COMMITTEE ON MICRONUTRIENT DEFICIENCIES, BOARD ON INTERNATIONAL HEALTH, FOOD AND NUTRITION BOARD, INSTITUTE OF MEDICINE: *Prevention of Micronutrient Deficiencies: Tools for Policymakers and Public Health Workers*, CP Howson et al (eds). Washington, National Academy Press, 1998

FOOD AND NUTRITION BOARD, COMMISSION ON LIFE SCIENCES, NATIONAL RESEARCH COUNCIL: *Recommended Dietary Allowances*, 10th ed. Washington, National Academy Press, 1989

OWEN OE et al: A reappraisal of caloric requirements in healthy women. Am J Clin Nutr 44:1, 1986

————: A reappraisal of the caloric requirements of men. Am J Clin Nutr 46:875, 1987

SADLER MJ et al (eds): *Encyclopedia of Human Nutrition*. San Diego, Academic Press, 1998

SHILS ME et al (eds): *Modern Nutrition in Health and Disease*, 9th ed. Baltimore, Williams & Wilkins, 1999

STANDING COMMITTEE ON THE SCIENTIFIC EVALUATION OF DIETARY REFERENCE INTAKES, FOOD AND NUTRITION BOARD, INSTITUTE OF MEDICINE: *Dietary Reference Intakes for Calcium, Phosphorus, Magnesium, Vitamin D, and Fluoride.* Washington, National Academy Press, 1997

74 *Charles H. Halsted*

MALNUTRITION AND NUTRITIONAL ASSESSMENT

Malnutrition is a frequent and integral component of acute and chronic illness. When recognized by appropriate clinical assessment, malnutrition is found in >50% of all hospitalized adults. It contributes to increased in-hospital morbidity and mortality in both medical and surgical patients, and leads to more frequent hospital admissions among the elderly. Malnutrition results from various combinations of starvation, including inadequate intake or abnormal gastrointestinal assim-

ilation of the diet, the stress response to acute injury or chronic inflammation, and abnormal nutrient metabolism. Nutritional assessment should be considered an integral part of the clinical evaluation and be used as a basis for nutritional support in the overall therapeutic plan.

DEFINITIONS OF MALNUTRITION In the strict sense, the term *malnutrition* includes extremes of underweight and overweight. The current chapter, however, focuses on the evaluation of the undernourished patient who presents with diminished body protein and energy stores and micronutrient deficiencies.

To the practicing physician, both outpatients and inpatients should be considered at risk for malnutrition if they meet one or more of the following criteria: (1) unintentional loss of >10% of usual body weight in the preceding 3 months, (2) body weight <90% of ideal for height, or (3) body mass index (BMI; the weight in kilograms divided by the height in square meters) <18.5. With regard to varying levels of severity, body weight <90% of ideal for height represents risk of malnutrition, body weight <85% of ideal constitutes *malnutrition,* <70% of ideal represents *severe malnutrition,* and <60% of ideal is usually incompatible with survival.

Malnutrition may be endemic in regions of famine, and two forms of severe malnutrition are recognized under conditions of inadequate food supply or distribution: *marasmus* refers to generalized starvation with loss of body fat and protein, whereas *kwashiorkor* refers to selective protein malnutrition with edema and fatty liver. The latter form occurs following restriction of dietary protein among children in settings of recurrent diarrheal illness. These distinctions, however, seldom apply to malnourished patients in more developed societies. In this setting, features of combined protein-calorie malnutrition (PCM) are more commonly seen in the context of a wide variety of acute and chronic illnesses that lead to depletion of body fat, muscle wasting, multiple signs of micronutrient deficiencies, decubitus ulcers, and life-threatening infections. An overview of the evaluation of malnutrition in the sick adult is depicted in Fig. 74-1.

PATHOPHYSIOLOGY AND ETIOLOGIES OF MALNUTRITION In simple terms, patients lose weight when: (1) the intake or gastrointestinal assimilation of dietary calories is insufficient to meet normal energy expenditure; (2) the expenditure of body energy stores is greater than energy normally consumed and assimilated by the body; or (3) the metabolism of energy supplies, protein, and other nutrients is significantly impaired by the intrinsic disease process.

Body Composition As depicted in Fig. 74-2, the human body stores between 15 and 25% of its energy as fat (greater in women than men), which is available for the metabolism of endogenous fatty acids during starvation. The remaining fat-free mass (FFM) is composed of extracellular and intracellular water, the bony skeleton, glycogen, and skeletal and visceral protein. Aside from body fat, energy reserves are also provided by intracellular glycogen and protein, which, together with intracellular water, constitute the body cell mass (BCM). Thus, in addition to the enzymes that support the normal metabolic machinery of the body, the BCM provides reserve protein for energy production by gluconeogenesis during the stress response.

The Metabolic Response to Starvation and Stress The expenditure of body stores of energy (as fat, glycogen, and protein) is different during *starvation* (due to decreased intake and/or assimilation of the diet) and *stress* (due to excessive expenditure of energy and body protein). Consequently, these events affect body compartments differently. Starvation decreases the size of all body compartments, whereas stress reduces BCM, increases extracellular water, and has variable effects on body fat.

A normal 70-kg man stores fuel at about 15 kg as fat, 6 kg as protein, and 0.4 kg as glycogen. During a 24-h fast, energy needs are met by the consumption of liver glycogen stores and the conversion of up to 75 g of body protein to glucose (by gluconeogenesis). During prolonged starvation, metabolism is supported by stores of body fat (about 150 g/d), which provides fatty acid–derived ketones, and muscle protein (about 20 g/d), which is used for gluconeogenesis. Under

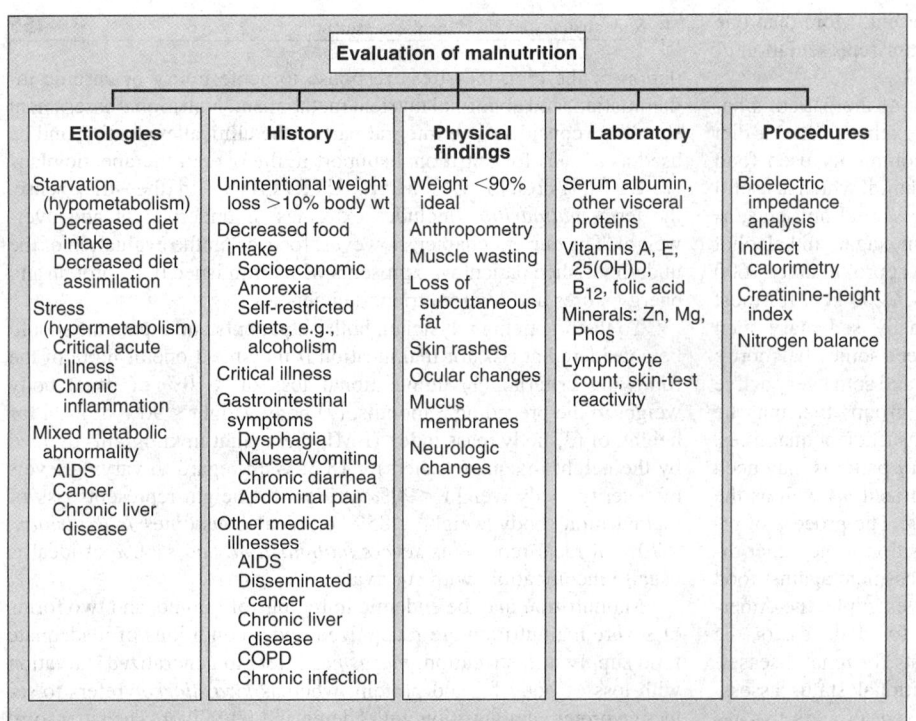

FIGURE 74-1 Conceptual framework for the nutritional assessment of sick patients. COPD, chronic obstructive pulmonary disease.

these conditions, total energy expenditure is decreased in order to conserve energy. While normal-weight individuals can sustain total fasting for about 2 months, obese individuals can fast for periods >12 months, depending on their fat stores.

The metabolic responses to the stress of acute critical illness (e.g., following accidental or surgical trauma or sepsis) significantly modify this sequence of events. In contrast to the hypometabolism, protein conservation, and reliance on body fat stores for energy needs during starvation, the acute stress response is characterized by hypermetabolism, in which the demands of accelerated energy expenditure are met by skeletal and visceral proteolysis to provide amino acid substrate for gluconeogenesis. Muscle proteolysis and gluconeogenesis are promoted by high levels of circulating catecholamines, glucagon, cortisol, and cytokines, including tumor necrosis factor (TNF) α and interleukins 1 and 6, in the setting of insulin resistance. When untreated, body protein catabolism is accelerated to 240 g/d, which is sufficient to deplete 50% of body protein stores within 3 weeks.

A more common clinical situation is the malnourished patient with

chronic illness in whom acute trauma or sepsis superimposes cytokine-mediated proteolysis with increased metabolic demands. If unchecked by appropriate therapy, the process of progressive PCM in such patients is associated with decreased cardiac and renal function, fluid retention, intestinal mucosal atrophy, loss of intracellular minerals (zinc, magnesium, and phosphorus), diminished cell-mediated immune functions, increased risk of infection, and eventual death (Fig. 74-3).

Etiologies of Malnutrition The causes of decreased dietary intake are diverse and include social and economic conditions, psychiatric diseases, neurodegenerative dementias, cytokine-mediated appetite suppression in chronic infections such as AIDS or in disseminated cancer, and self-limited food intake in abdominal pain syndromes (Table 74-1; Chap. 43). Given the central role of the gastrointestinal tract in the assimilation of nutrients, PCM is a predictable component of many chronic gastrointestinal diseases. These diseases promote starvation through decreased assimilation of the diet by: (1) blocking the transit of dietary constituents to the intestinal absorbing surface, (2) impairing normal processes of pancreatic or biliary digestion, or (3) preventing the intestinal mucosal transport of dietary constituents. Diseases that are characterized by increased catabolism of stored energy and protein include acute surgical or medical critical illness and acute or chronic inflammatory or infectious disorders affecting diverse organ systems. Other chronic diseases promote malnutrition through mixed mechanisms that contribute to abnormal nutrient metabolism. Both AIDS and disseminated malignancy, for example, cause progressive malnutrition through combinations of anorexia and futile cycles of fatty acid and glucose metabolism. Chronic obstructive pulmonary disease increases risk of malnutrition through the increased energy expenditure of labored respiration, chronic indolent bronchial infection, and the anorexic side effects of many bronchodilating drugs. Chronic liver disease is often

FIGURE 74-2 Schematic of body composition of a healthy subject. Body cell mass (BCM) is shown by shading as a composite of intracellular water, glycogen, and protein. FFM, fat-free mass. *(Adapted with permission from Heymsfield et al.)*

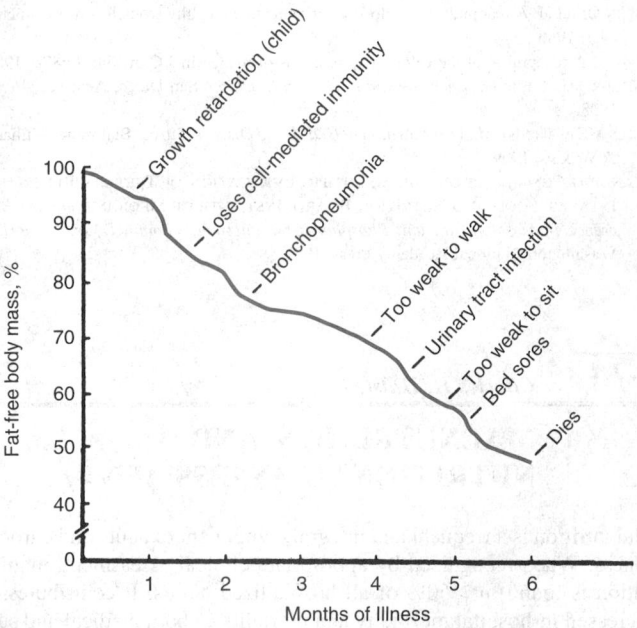

FIGURE 74-3 Hypothetical history of progressive protein-calorie malnutrition in a patient with wasting illness. *(Reproduced with permission from Heymsfield et al.)*

456

Table 74-1   Etiologies of Protein-Calorie Malnutrition

I. Starvation (hypometabolism with reliance on body fat stores)
   A. Decreased diet intake
      1. Social and economic: poverty, chronic alcoholism
      2. Psychiatric: anorexia nervosa, severe depression
      3. Neurodegenerative dementias of aging
      4. Anorexia associated with AIDS, disseminated cancer, renal failure
      5. Abdominal pain triggered by food intake: pancreatitis, intestinal ischemia
   B. Decreased assimilation of the diet
      1. Impaired transit of diet, e.g., benign or malignant esophageal, gastric, or intestinal obstruction
      2. Impaired digestion of diet, e.g., pancreatic insufficiency, short bowel syndrome
      3. Intestinal malabsorption of dietary constituents, e.g., celiac disease
II. Stress (hypermetabolism with reliance on protein stores for gluconeogenesis)
   A. Acute trauma, e.g., accident, burns, major surgery
   B. Acute sepsis
   C. Acute or chronic inflammation: pancreatitis, collagen diseases, chronic infectious disease, e.g., tuberculosis, AIDS opportunistic infections
III. Mixed mechanisms
   A. Futile metabolic cycles and anorexia, e.g., AIDS, disseminated cancer
   B. Increased energy demands, e.g., chronic obstructive pulmonary disease
   C. Abnormal metabolism and decreased biliary digestion, e.g., chronic liver disease
   D. Protein-losing enteropathy and chronic inflammation, e.g., Crohn's disease, ulcerative colitis

Table 74-2   The Patient History of Weight Loss and Malnutrition

Finding	Example/Interpretation
Involuntary diet restriction	Poverty due to inadequate income
Anorexia	Anorexia nervosa, severe depression, dementia, AIDS, cancer, chronic renal disease
Inadequate diet selection	Chronic alcoholism, fad diets, strict vegetarianism
Critical illness	Untreated stress response to trauma, burn, major surgery, sepsis
Gastrointestinal symptoms	
Dysphagia	Esophageal obstruction impairs diet transit
Nausea, vomiting	Gastric or intestinal obstruction impairs diet transit
Chronic diarrhea	Pancreatic, biliary, or intestinal mucosal disease impairs digestion and absorption Protein-losing enteropathy in inflammatory bowel disease
Chronic abdominal pain	Self-limited food intake reduces pain: e.g., pancreatitis, intestinal ischemia, inflammatory bowel disease
Other chronic medical diseases	Combinations of anorexia, increased energy demands, and abnormal nutrient metabolism: e.g., recurrent pancreatitis, AIDS, disseminated cancer, chronic liver disease, chronic obstructive pulmonary disease, chronic infectious illness

associated with PCM caused by the cumulative effects of anorexia; decreased biliary circulation; and abnormal lipid, carbohydrate, and protein metabolism. The chronic intestinal inflammation of Crohn's disease or ulcerative colitis accelerates fecal losses of protein, electrolytes, and zinc.

CLINICAL EVALUATION OF THE MALNOURISHED PATIENT

THE PATIENT HISTORY   The clinical nutritional history should include diet and weight change, socioeconomic conditions, and symptoms unique to each clinical setting (Table 74-2). Social and economic conditions that may lead to poverty include inadequate income, homelessness, and activities that restrict real income and promote involuntary diet restriction, such as drug abuse or chronic alcoholism. Anorexia, or loss of appetite, is a feature of psychiatric disorders, such as anorexia nervosa and neurodegenerative dementia in the elderly. Many self-selected, inadequate diets may promote malnutrition. During binge drinking, chronic alcoholics typically substitute more than half their daily food calories with excessive amounts of ethanol, the metabolism of which consumes energy and promotes unbalanced metabolism of fat and carbohydrates. Other inadequate diets include unbalanced and commercially promoted formulas for rapid weight loss and strict vegetarianism, which may lead to selective deficiencies of specific nutrients such as vitamin B_{12} and iron.

Digestive diseases are major causes of malnutrition, both in the inpatient and outpatient settings. The malnourished patient with digestive disease may present with symptoms of: (1) dysphagia or recurrent vomiting due to benign or malignant esophageal or gastrointestinal obstruction; (2) chronic diarrhea due to abnormal pancreatic or biliary digestion, intestinal mucosal malabsorption, or protein-losing enteropathy; or (3) recurrent abdominal pain exacerbated by eating, as occurs in patients with chronic pancreatitis, inflammatory bowel disease, or intestinal ischemia.

On the general medical service, PCM is prevalent in patients with multiple chronic illnesses that are associated with anorexia, recurrent stress, and abnormal nutrient metabolism. In addition, PCM is comorbid with chronic recurrent pancreatitis, renal failure, chronic liver disease, chronic obstructive pulmonary disease, disseminated cancer, and chronic infections such as AIDS and tuberculosis. Depending on the severity of injury or illness, critically ill surgical and medical patients predictably develop stress-related PCM if increased nutritional needs are not met after 5 to 10 days.

THE PHYSICAL EXAMINATION   A careful physical examination can both characterize and define the extent of malnutrition. Measurements of unclothed weight and height are essential for establishing the severity of malnutrition in all patients but may be confounded by the effects of fluid overload as a result of edema and ascites. The normal values for weight (in kg) and height (in cm) in men and women are provided in Table 74-3. These values can be adjusted by ±10% to account for variability in body frame.

Anthropometry   Measurements of subcutaneous fat and skeletal muscle are important to determine the severity of PCM. Using specialized calipers and a tape measure, anthropometry estimates body fat from the thickness of the skin-fold of the posterior mid-upper arm. Anthropometric measurements in healthy and malnourished adults are shown in Table 74-4. Mid-arm muscle circumference is estimated from the equation:

$$\text{Mid-arm muscle circumference} = \text{mid-upper arm circumference} - (\pi \times \text{triceps skin-fold thickness})$$
$$\text{(in cm)} \qquad\qquad\qquad\qquad \text{(in cm)}$$

The use of anthropometry is limited by the requirement for specialized calipers, the experience of the observer, and potential confounding effects of edema or dehydration.

Specific Physical Findings of Malnutrition   During the conventional physical examination, the observant and experienced clinician can identify multiple and specific findings of PCM and its associated micronutrient deficiencies (Chap. 75). A variety of nutritional deficiencies can be identified by examination of the patient's general appearance, including skin, hair, nails, mucus membranes, and neurologic system (Table 74-5). Initially, a pinch of the posterior upper arm may reveal loss of subcutaneous fat in the malnourished patient. Hollowing of the temporal muscles, wasting of upper arms and thigh muscles, easily plucked hair, and peripheral edema are all consistent with protein deficiency. Examination of the skin may reveal the papular keratitis ("goose bump rash") of vitamin A deficiency, perifollicular

Table 74-3 Ideal Weight for Height

Men				Women			
Height[a]	Weight[a]	Height	Weight	Height	Weight	Height	Weight
145	51.9	166	64.0	140	44.9	161	56.9
146	52.4	167	64.6	141	45.4	162	57.6
147	52.9	168	65.2	142	45.9	163	58.3
148	53.5	169	65.9	143	46.4	164	58.9
149	54.0	170	66.6	144	47.0	165	59.5
150	54.5	171	67.3	145	47.5	166	60.1
151	55.0	172	68.0	146	48.0	167	60.7
152	55.6	173	68.7	147	48.6	168	61.4
153	56.1	174	69.4	148	49.2	169	62.1
154	56.6	175	70.1	149	49.8		
155	57.2	176	70.8	150	50.4		
156	57.9	177	71.6	151	51.0		
157	58.6	178	72.4	152	51.5		
158	59.3	179	73.3	153	52.0		
159	59.9	180	74.2	154	52.5		
160	60.5	181	75.0	155	53.1		
161	61.1	182	75.8	156	53.7		
162	61.7	183	76.5	157	54.3		
163	62.3	184	77.3	158	54.9		
164	62.9	185	78.1	159	55.5		
165	63.5	186	78.9	160	56.2		

[a] Values are expressed in cm for height and kg for weight. To obtain height in inches, divide by 2.54. To obtain weight in pounds, multiply by 2.2.
SOURCE: Adapted from Blackburn et al.

hemorrhages of vitamin C deficiency, ecchymoses of vitamin K deficiency, the "flaky paint" lower extremity rash of zinc deficiency, hyperpigmentation of skin-exposed areas from niacin deficiency, seborrhea of essential fatty acid deficiency, spooning of nails in iron deficiency, and transverse nail pigmentation in protein deficiency. The eye examination yields conjunctival pallor of anemia, pericorneal and corneal opacities of severe vitamin A deficiency ("Bitot spots"), and nystagmus and isolated ocular muscle paresis of thiamine deficiency. The oral examination may reveal angular stomatitis and cheilosis of either riboflavin or niacin deficiency; glossitis with smooth and red tongue of riboflavin, niacin, vitamin B_{12}, or pyridoxine deficiency; and hypertrophied bleeding gums of vitamin C deficiency. Examination of the neurologic system, particularly in the setting of chronic alcohol abuse, may detect memory loss with confabulation, a wide-based gait, and past pointing, which, together with ophthalmoplegia and peripheral neuropathy, constitute the Wernicke-Korsakoff syndrome of thiamine deficiency. Other neurologic causes of dementia include pellagra due to niacin and/or tryptophan deficiency. Additional causes of peripheral neuropathy include deficiencies of pyridoxine or vitamin E; loss of distal vibratory and position sense is characteristic of the subacute combined degeneration of vitamin B_{12} deficiency.

LABORATORY ASSESSMENT Selected use of laboratory tests, most of which are widely available, is essential for characterizing and quantifying malnutrition. Laboratory findings that are often attributed to chronic disease may, in actuality, reflect the response to PCM or selected micronutrient deficiencies in the setting of chronic illness.

Table 74-4 Anthropometric Measurements in Adults

% Standard	Men	Women	Interpretation
TRICEPS SKIN-FOLD, MM			
100	12.5	16.5	Adequate
50	6.0	8.0	Borderline
20	2.5	3.0	Severe depletion
MID-ARM MUSCLE CIRCUMFERENCE, CM			
100	25.5	23.0	Adequate
80	20.0	18.5	Borderline
60	15.0	14.0	Depletion
40	10.0	9.0	Severe depletion

SOURCE: Adapted from Morgan and Weinsier.

Serum Visceral Proteins Serum albumin, which has a 2- to 3-week half-life, is a highly sensitive but nonspecific measure of PCM. A normal serum albumin level in a well-hydrated patient is inconsistent with PCM. On the other hand, a low serum albumin level must be interpreted in its clinical context, since the concentration of albumin is decreased in the setting of increased plasma volume (as seen in acute trauma or sepsis and in chronic liver, renal, or cardiopulmonary failure). The acute stress of surgery, sepsis, or other acute inflammatory illness lowers the serum albumin level because of a combination of increased circulating extracellular volume and TNF-α-mediated inhibition of albumin synthesis. Hepatic albumin synthesis is inhibited in the setting of liver cirrhosis, AIDS, and disseminated cancer, whereas albumin loss from the body is accelerated in inflammatory bowel diseases, including ulcerative colitis, Crohn's disease, and radiation enteritis. Several shorter-lived visceral proteins can also be measured for estimation of the severity of PCM. These include transferrin (1-week half-life), prealbumin or retinol-binding protein complex (2-day half-life), and fibronectin (1-day half-life). However, like the serum albumin level, the circulating level of each of these proteins is affected by the changes in extracellular volume that occur in acute and chronic illnesses.

Vitamin and Mineral Assays Specific micronutrient deficiencies can be measured by a variety of serum and red blood cell assays, often utilizing high-performance liquid chromatography or enzyme or

Table 74-5 Physical Findings of Malnutrition

Finding	Deficiency/Interpretation
General appearance	
Weight loss	Malnutrition <90% of ideal body weight
	Severe <70% of ideal body weight
Decreased temporal and proximal extremity muscle mass	Decreased skeletal protein
Decreased skin-fold thickness by "pinch test"	Decreased body fat stores
Skin, nails, and hair	
Easily plucked hair	Protein
Easy bruising, perifollicular hemorrhages	Vitamin C
"Flaky paint" rash of lower extremities	Zinc
Coarse skin, "goose bumps"	Vitamin A
Hyperpigmentation of sun-exposed areas	Niacin, tryptophan
Spooning of nails	Iron
Eyes	
Conjunctival pallor	Anemia (nonspecific)
Bitot spot	Vitamin A
Ophthalmoplegia	Thiamine
Mouth and mucus membranes	
Nasolabial seborrhea	Essential fatty acids
Glossitis (smooth, red tongue) and/or cheilosis	Riboflavin, niacin, vitamin B_{12}, pyridoxine, folate
Diminished taste	Zinc
Neurologic system	
Disorientation	Niacin, phosphorus
Confabulation	Thiamine
Cerebellar gait, past pointing	Thiamine
Peripheral neuropathy	Thiamine, pyridoxine, vitamin E
Lost vibratory, position sense	Vitamin B_{12}

microbiologic assays (Chap. 75). Commonly available assays and their interpretations are listed in Table 74-6. PCM is typically associated with low serum levels of vitamin A, zinc, and magnesium. Abnormal digestion and absorption of dietary fat are associated with deficiencies of fat-soluble vitamins A, D, and E, whereas intestinal mucosal malabsorption (as in celiac disease) is commonly associated with additional deficiencies of iron and folic acid. Chronic alcoholism is frequently associated with thiamine, folate, vitamin A, and zinc deficiencies. Vitamin B_{12} deficiency due to achlorhydria occurs in up to 15% of elderly individuals as well as in those with pernicious anemia or with diseases involving the terminal ileum. As described in Chap. 105, both folate and vitamin B_{12} deficiencies are associated with elevations in plasma homocysteine; vitamin B_{12} deficiency can also elevate the plasma level of methylmalonic acid.

Assessment of Immune Function PCM is associated with atrophy of thymic-dependent lymphoid structures and reduced T cell–mediated immunity. Conversely, B cell–mediated production of immunoglobulins is usually unaffected. Total lymphocyte count (total white cell count × fraction as lymphocytes) is often $<1000/\mu$L in PCM and may be accompanied by anergy to common skin test antigens. While sensitive for PCM, these measures of cell-mediated immunity are nonspecific and can be affected by other disorders such as acute or chronic infections, uremia, or immunosuppressive therapy.

SPECIALIZED PROCEDURES FOR NUTRITIONAL ASSESSMENT Several specialized procedures are used to assess energy and protein stores and energy expenditure in malnourished patients. These procedures may be employed during the initial nutritional assessment or may serve as an index of the efficacy of nutritional support during the treatment of malnourished patients.

Bioelectric Impedance Analysis Bioelectric impedance analysis (BIA) is a simplified and portable method for measurement of body fat, FFM, and total-body water. BIA is based on differences in the electric conductivity of a weak current between electrodes placed on the dorsal surfaces of the hands and feet. The measurement reflects differences in the impedance to electric current, which is greatest through fat and least through water. Lean body mass can be calculated as the difference between fat mass and body weight or as total-body water divided by 0.73.

Overall, BIA is most useful in assessing body fat and FFM in stable patients and in those who suffer from conditions leading to relative starvation. However, BIA can also be used to assess critically ill patients with decreased intracellular water space and BCM and expanded extracellular compartment size. Reduced BCM correlates inversely with increased metabolic rate. BIA may be confounded in AIDS patients receiving protease-inhibitor therapy, if they exhibit lipodystrophy with associated redistribution of interscapular, abdominal, and breast fat (Chap. 309).

Energy Expenditure Body weight and energy balance are sustained in health by the consumption of dietary calories in an amount equal to the daily expenditure of energy. Therefore, caloric needs can be determined from the estimated daily total energy expenditure (TEE), which is composed of basal or resting energy expenditure (REE, about 75% of total), the thermic expenditures of digestion (about 10% of total), and modest physical activity (about 15% of total). The REE is directly proportional to both the FFM and BCM and can be estimated in healthy people using the Harris and Benedict formula

Table 74-6 Commonly Available Vitamin and Mineral Assays		
Vitamin/Mineral	**Normal Range**	**Interpretation of Abnormal Result**
Vitamin A	1.30–3.15 μmol/L (37–90 μg/dL)	Low value consistent with PCM, abnormal fat digestion or malaborption, chronic liver disease. High value consistent with vitamin abuse; toxicity expressed as liver failure.
25(OH)D$_3$	25–150 nmol/L (10–60 ng/mL)	Low value consistent with abnormal fat digestion or absorption, primary rickets, chronic liver disease, osteomalacia. High value suggestive of vitamin toxicity expressed as calcinosis.
Vitamin E	12–35 μmol/L (0.5–1.5 mg/dL)	Low value consistent with abnormal fat digestion, chronic liver disease; expressed as peripheral neuropathy, tunnel vision.
Thiamine	6–60 pmol/L (0.2–2.0 μg/dL)	Low value seen in starvation, chronic alcoholism, malabsorption syndromes; expressed as Wernicke-Korsakoff syndrome, peripheral neuropathy, high-output cardiac failure.
Folate Serum	12–53 nmol/L (5–21 ng/mL)	Low levels in starvation, chronic alcoholism, intestinal malabsorption; expressed as macrocytic anemia, diarrhea, elevated homocysteine.
Red cell	>400 nmol/L (>160 ng/mL)	Same as above, but more stable and reflects tissue stores of folates.
Vitamin B$_{12}$	>104 pmol/L (>140 pg/mL)	Low level associated with gastric atrophy of aging, pernicious anemia; expressed as macrocytic anemia, neuropathy; elevated homocysteine and methylmalonic acid.
Zinc	10–21 mmol/L (65–140 μg/dL)	Low level in chronic diarrhea, PCM, alcoholic liver disease, inflammatory bowel disease, intestinal malabsorption; expressed as rash, delayed wound healing, decreased taste sensation.
Magnesium	0.72–0.99 mmol/L (1.8–2.4 mg/dL)	Low in chronic alcoholism, diabetes, intestinal malabsorption, PCM; expressed as hyperactive reflexes, hypocalcemia.
Phosphorus	0.81–1.43 mmol/L (2.5–4.4 mg/dL)	Low in starvation, chronic alcoholism, chronic diarrhea; expressed as confusion, disorientation.

NOTE: PCM, protein-calorie malnutrition.

on the basis of weight in kg (W), height in cm (H), and age in years (A):

$$\text{REE (men)} = 66.473 + 13.751 \ (W) + 5.0033 \ (H) - 6.7550 \ (A) \ \text{kcal/d}$$

$$\text{REE (women)} = 655.0955 + 9.4634 \ (W) + 1.8496 \ (H) - 4.6756 \ (A) \ \text{kcal/d}$$

A simplified bedside estimation for TEE in sick patients is 25 kcal/kg of body weight, to which is added 10% for digestion or metabolism of intravenous or enteral nutrition. In the acutely ill patient, one should include an additional 12.5% for each degree of fever over 37°C, as well as an additional multiplier commensurate with the severity of illness (e.g., 25% for general surgery, 50% for sepsis, and 100% for extensive third-degree burns).

While REE can be predicted by the Harris-Benedict equations in healthy persons, it is decreased in starvation because of hypometabolism. In contrast, REE is increased in the hypermetabolic stress that accompanies critical illness. REE and caloric requirements cannot be predicted in certain clinical conditions. These include the relatively starved, chronically ill patient admitted with a critical illness, the obese patient who develops a critical illness on the background of both increased body fat and FFM, or the patient with chronic liver disease accompanied by combinations of anorexia and ongoing hepatic inflammation. In these situations, REE can be measured accurately by the gas-exchange method of indirect calorimetry. In practice, indirect calorimetry is performed at the bedside using a mobile metabolic cart. This procedure is applicable to ventilator-independent and -dependent patients whose fractional intake of oxygen is less than 0.45. Because the goal is to reach an accurate approximation of the 24-h energy requirement, measurements must be taken at intervals during the day and must account for several variables, including food intake and activity. To calculate the energy cost of metabolism by indirect calorimetry, the volumes (V) of oxygen consumed and carbon dioxide produced are measured over a given period of time, according to the modified Weir equation where

$$REE = 3.9\, V_{O_2} + 1.1\, V_{CO_2}$$

Indirect calorimetry also provides the respiratory quotient (RQ), which is the ratio of carbon dioxide produced to oxygen consumed during the process of gas collection. The RQ decreases when fat is the predominant substrate for metabolism (as in starvation) and increases when the contribution of carbohydrate increases (as during stress with gluconeogenesis). In healthy individuals, the RQ usually falls between 0.80 and 0.90. A RQ <0.7 is consistent with active ketogenesis from endogenous fatty acid metabolism with limited generation of carbon dioxide. An RQ >1.0 indicates net lipogenesis, or the conversion of substrate carbohydrate to fat, a situation that occurs with overfeeding. Values that fall outside the range of 0.65 to 1.25 suggest an error in measurement technique.

Creatinine Excretion in the 24-h Urine Creatinine, the metabolic product of skeletal muscle creatine, is produced at a constant rate and in an amount directly proportional to skeletal muscle mass. With steady-state day-to-day renal function, each gram of creatinine in the 24-h urine collection represents 18.5 g of fat-free skeletal muscle. Since skeletal muscle is the major component of FFM and BCM, measurement of creatinine in the 24-h urine collection can be used as a relative measure of these body compartments during the initial assessment and/or during the course of nutritional support. The *creatinine coefficient* represents the amount of creatinine excreted per kilogram of body weight; it is equal to 23 mg/kg of ideal body weight in men and 18 mg/kg of ideal body weight in women. The *creatinine-height index* represents the ratio of the measured 24-h urine creatinine excretion to the value predicted by the creatinine coefficient for the patient's ideal body weight. These values can be calculated from estimation of the patient's ideal body weight (Table 74-3) or from tables that relate creatinine excretion to height in men and women (Table 74-7). In practice, the accuracy of the 24-h urine creatinine depends primarily on completeness of the urine collection. Together with variations due to fever and fluctuations in dietary intake, inaccuracies of urine collections may result in as much as 10% error in the quantitative 24-h urine creatinine measurement. The constancy of creatinine excretion depends on steady-state renal function, and unpredictable creatinine excretion may occur through feces or skin in patients with

Table 74-7 Ideal 24-h Urine Creatinine Values

Men[a]		Women[b]	
Height, cm[c]	24-h Creatinine, mg	Height, cm	24-h Creatinine, mg
157.5	1288	147.3	830
160.0	1325	149.9	851
162.6	1359	152.4	875
165.1	1386	154.9	900
167.6	1426	157.5	925
170.2	1467	160.0	949
172.7	1513	162.6	977
175.3	1555	165.1	1006
177.8	1596	167.6	1044
180.3	1642	170.2	1076
182.9	1691	172.7	1109
185.4	1739	175.3	1141
188.0	1785	177.8	1174
190.5	1831	180.3	1206
193.0	1891	182.9	1240

[a] Creatinine coefficient for men is 23 mg/kg of ideal body weight.
[b] Creatinine coefficient for women is 18 mg/kg of ideal body weight.
[c] To obtain height in inches, divide by 2.54.
SOURCE: From Blackburn et al.

serum creatinine levels >530 μmol/L (>6 mg/dL). The presence of ascites, however, apparently does not compromise the accuracy of the 24-h urine creatinine as a reflection of FFM or BCM in patients with chronic liver disease.

Urine Nitrogen Excretion and Nitrogen Balance Nitrogen balance provides an index of protein gain or loss: 1 g nitrogen is equivalent to 6.25 g protein. Nitrogen balance can be assessed by measuring the difference between nitrogen consumed through the mouth, enteral tube, or intravenous sources and nitrogen excreted in the urine, feces, and other intestinal sources. Protein requirements to achieve zero or positive balance are less in starvation states, where daily protein losses are minimized because of hypometabolism, than in clinical states of stress, where the catabolism of skeletal muscle is accelerated for gluconeogenesis. Accurate measurement of nitrogen balance requires complete measurement of nitrogen losses from all possible excretory routes. In most cases, total urine nitrogen can be calculated by dividing 24-h urinary urea nitrogen by 0.85 and assuming approximately 2 g/d for nitrogen losses in feces and sweat. On the other hand, when the clinical condition includes extensive diarrhea and/or protein losses from pancreatic or enterocutaneous fistulas, the accuracy of nitrogen balance requires measurement of total nitrogen by the modified Kjeldahl technique in both urine and enteric sources. Total nitrogen measurements are also advisable in patients with liver failure, where urinary ammonia becomes a major and alternative source of nitrogen.

INTEGRATED BEDSIDE NUTRITIONAL ASSESSMENT
Several different approaches have been developed in order to simplify the process of nutritional assessment by using selective measurements that relate malnutrition to the specific medical condition and the severity of the underlying disease process.

Subjective Global Assessment This approach incorporates historic and physical findings as a basis for nutrition assessment by the trained physician. Major components in the history include evaluation of the extent of recent weight loss, changes in dietary intake, presence of significant gastrointestinal symptoms persisting more than 2 weeks, alterations in functional status, and the metabolic demand of the patient's underlying disease. Emphasis in the physical examination is placed on findings of depletion of subcutaneous body fat; skeletal muscle wasting; typical changes in skin, mucus membranes, and neurologic examination; as well as the presence of edema. Integration of the historic and physical data permits ranking of patients according to the following categories: adequate nutrition, moderate malnutrition, or severe malnutrition. Though the developers of the subjective global assessment have reported good sensitivity and specificity, the approach is still quite dependent on the training and experience of the clinician.

Prognostic Nutritional Assessment Several paradigms have been developed to link different parameters of nutritional assessment with clinical prognosis. Each approach links specific features of malnutrition with certain measurements of cell-mediated immunity, since abnormal immune function is a common pathway for increased risk in the malnourished patient (Fig. 74-3). A surgical prognostic nutritional index predicts morbidity based on preoperative measurements of serum albumin, transferrin, triceps skin-fold thickness, and delayed hypersensitivity to skin-test antigens. Another PCM score was developed to link survival in alcoholic liver disease to both skin-fold and mid-arm muscle measurements; the creatinine-height index; values for serum albumin, transferrin, prealbumin, and retinol-binding protein; the total lymphocyte count; and the skin-test response to a series of antigens. The Maastricht index predicts survival in patients with serious gastrointestinal diseases on the basis of factors related to serum albumin, retinol-binding protein, lymphotyce count, and deviation from the patient's ideal body weight.

BIBLIOGRAPHY

BAKER JP et al: Nutritional assessment: A comparison of clinical judgment and objective measurements. N Engl J Med 306:969, 1982
BLACKBURN GL et al: Nutritional and metabolic assessment of the hospitalized patient. J Parenter Enteral Nutr 1:11, 1977
CAHILL GF: Starvation in man. N Engl J Med 282:668, 1970

HALSTED CH: Clinical nutrition education—relevance and role models. Am J Clin Nutr 67:192, 1998

HEYMSFIELD SB et al: Nutritional assessment of malnutrition by anthropomorphic methods, in *Modern Nutrition in Health and Disease*, 9th ed, ME Shils et al (eds). Philadelphia, Lea & Febiger, 1999, p 903

MENDENHALL C et al: Relationship of protein calorie malnutrition to alcoholic liver disease: A reexamination of data from two Veterans Administration Cooperative Studies. Alcohol Clin Exp Res 19:635, 1995

MORGAN SL, WEINSIER RL: *Fundamentals of Clinical Nutrition*. St. Louis, Mosby, 1998, p 167

MULLEN JL et al: Reduction of operative morbidity and mortality by combined preoperative and postoperative nutritional support. Ann Surg 192:604, 1980

NABER THJ et al: Prevalence of malnutrition in nonsurgical hospitalized patients and its association with disease complications. Am J Clin Nutr 66:1232, 1997

YANOVSKI SZ et al: Bioelectrical impedance analysis in body composition measurement: National Institutes of Health technology assessment conference statement. Am J Clin Nutr 64:524S, 1996

75   *Robert M. Russell*

VITAMIN AND TRACE MINERAL DEFICIENCY AND EXCESS

FAD flavin adenine dinucleotide	NADP NAD phosphate
FMN flavin-mononucleotide	PLP pyridoxal phosphate
HPLC high-performance liquid chromatography	RDA Recommended Dietary Allowance
LDL low-density lipoprotein	RE retinol equivalent
NAD nicotinamide adenine dinucleotide	TPN total parenteral nutrition
	VLDL very low density lipoprotein

Vitamins and trace minerals are required constituents of the human diet since they are either inadequately synthesized or not synthesized in the human body. Only small amounts of these substances are needed for carrying out essential biochemical reactions (e.g., acting as coenzymes or prosthetic groups). Overt vitamin or trace mineral deficiencies are rare in western countries due to a plentiful, varied, and inexpensive food supply; however, multiple nutrient deficiencies may appear together in persons who are ill or alcoholic. Moreover, subclinical vitamin and trace mineral deficiencies, as diagnosed by laboratory testing, are quite common in the normal population—especially the geriatric population.

Body stores of vitamins and minerals vary tremendously. For example, vitamin B_{12} and vitamin A stores are large, and an adult may not become deficient for 1 or more years after being on a depleted diet. However, folate and thiamine may become depleted within weeks when eating a deficient diet. Therapeutic modalities can deplete essential nutrients from the body; for example, hemodialysis removes water-soluble vitamins, which must be replaced by supplementation.

There are several roles for vitamins and trace minerals in diseases: (1) deficiencies of vitamins and minerals may be caused by disease states such as malabsorption; (2) both deficiency and excess of vitamins and minerals can cause disease in and of themselves (e.g., vitamin A intoxication and liver disease); and (3) vitamins and minerals in high doses may be used as drugs (e.g., niacin for hypercholesterolemia). The hematologic-related vitamins and minerals (Chaps. 105, 107) are not considered in this chapter, nor are the bone-related vitamins and minerals (vitamin D, calcium, phosphorus; Chap. 340), as they are covered elsewhere.

VITAMINS

THIAMINE (VITAMIN B_1)   Thiamine was the first B vitamin to be identified and is therefore also referred to as vitamin B_1. Thiamine pyrophosphate, the coenzyme form of thiamine, is required for branched-chain amino acid metabolism and carbohydrate metabolism (Fig. 75-1). Thiamine functions in the decarboxylation of α-ketoacids, such as pyruvate α-ketoglutarate, and branched-chain amino acids and thus is a source of energy generation. In addition, thiamine pyrophosphate acts as a coenzyme for a transketolase reaction that mediates the conversion of hexose and pentose phosphates. It has also been postulated that thiamine plays a role in peripheral nerve conduction, although the exact chemical reactions underlying this function are unknown.

Absorption and Requirements   At high doses, thiamine is absorbed by a passive mechanism; at low doses, it is absorbed by a carrier-mediated, active transport system and becomes phosphorylated in the process. Once absorbed, thiamine circulates bound to plasma proteins (mainly albumin) and erythrocytes. Storage sites for thiamine include muscle, heart, liver, kidney, and brain, although muscle is the principal storage site. The total body store of thiamine, mainly in the form of thiamine pyrophosphate, is approximately 30 mg, and its biologic half-life ranges between 9 and 18 days.

Given the fact that thiamine is involved in carbohydrate metabolism and energy generation, the Recommended Dietary Allowance (RDA) for males has been adjusted upward to account for increased energy utilization. Experiments have shown that heavy athletic training also increases thiamine utilization slightly. The RDA for thiamine is 1.2 mg/d for males and 1.1 mg/d for females. The median intake of thiamine in the United States from food alone is 2 mg/d. There is a 10% increase in the need for thiamine in pregnancy, and a small further increase in lactating females.

Primary food sources for thiamine include yeast, pork, legumes, beef, whole grains, and nuts. Milled and polished rice contain little, if any, thiamine. Thiamine deficiency is therefore more common in cultures that rely heavily on a rice-based diet. The molecule is heat-sensitive and is destroyed at pH > 8. Tea, coffee (caffeinated and decaffeinated), raw fish, and shellfish contain thiamineases, which can destroy the vitamin. Thus, drinking large amounts of tea or coffee can theoretically lower thiamine body stores.

Deficiency   Most dietary deficiency of thiamine worldwide is the result of poor dietary intake. In western countries, the primary causes of thiamine deficiency are alcoholism and chronic illness, such as cancer. Alcohol is known to interfere directly with the absorption of thiamine and with the synthesis of thiamine pyrophosphate. Malnourished individuals with alcoholic liver disease are also at increased risk of thiamine deficiency because of diminished storage sites in liver and muscle. Thiamine should always be replenished when refeeding a patient with alcoholism, as carbohydrate repletion without adequate thiamine can precipitate acute thiamine deficiency.

Thiamine deficiency in its early stage induces anorexia, irritability, apathy, and generalized weakness. Prolonged thiamine deficiency causes beriberi, which is classically categorized as wet or dry, although there is considerable overlap. In either form of beriberi, patients may complain of pain and parathesia. *Wet beriberi* presents primarily with cardiovascular symptoms, due to impaired myocardial energy metabolism and dysautonomia, and can occur after 3 months of a thiamine-deficient diet. Patients present with an enlarged heart, tachycardia, high-output congestive heart failure, peripheral edema, and peripheral neuritis. Patients with *dry beriberi* present with a symmetric peripheral neuropathy of the motor and sensory systems with diminished reflexes. The neuropathy affects the legs most markedly, and patients have difficulty rising from a squatting position.

Alcoholic patients with chronic thiamine deficiency may also have central nervous system manifestations known as *Wernicke's encephalopathy*, consisting of horizontal nystagmus, ophthalmoplegia (due to weakness of one or more extraocular muscles), cerebellar ataxia, and mental impairment (Chap. 387). When there is an additional loss of memory and a confabulatory psychosis, the syndrome is known as *Wernicke-Korsakoff syndrome*. Although this syndrome is generally described in alcoholic patients, there may be a genetic predisposition to Wernicke-Korsakoff that involves a variant transketolase isozyme.

In severely malnourished infants 2 to 3 months old, thiamine de-

Vitamin	Active derivative or cofactor form	Principal function
Thiamine	Thiamine pyrophosphatate	Coenzyme for cleavage of carbon-carbon bonds; amino acid and carbohydrate metabolism
Riboflavin	Flavin mononucleotide (FMN) and flavin adenine dinucleotide (FAD)	Cofactor for oxidation reduction reactions and covalently attached prosthetic groups for some enzymes
Niacin	Nicotanimide adenine dinucleotide phosphate (NADP) and nicotine adenine dinucleotide (NAD)	Coenzymes for oxidation and reduction reactions
Pyridoxine	Pyridoxal phosphate	Cofactor for enzymes of amino acid metabolism
Ascorbic	Ascorbic acid and dehydroascorbic acid	Participation as a redox ion in many biological oxidation and hydrogen transfer reactions
Vitamin A	Retinol, retinaldehyde, and retinoic acid	Formation of rhodopsin (vision) and glycoproteins (epithelial cell function); also regulates gene transcription
Vitamin E	Tocopherol and tocotrionols	Antioxidants
Vitamin K	Napthoquinone	Cofactor for post-translation carboxylation of many proteins including essential clotting factors

FIGURE 75-1 The structures and principal functions of some of the vitamins associated with human disorders.

ficiency may occur precipitously with sudden cardiovascular failure and collapse, resulting in death within hours. In addition, infants with thiamine deficiency may present with features suggesting meningitis, including vomiting, nystagmus, and convulsions. An aphonic presentation has also been described in which there is extreme irritability and either a very hoarse cry or total inability to emit any noise whatsoever (a silent scream).

The laboratory diagnosis of thiamine deficiency is usually made by a functional enzymatic assay of transketolase activity measured before and after the addition of thiamine pyrophosphate. A >25% stimulation by the addition of thiamine pyrophosphate (an activity coefficient of 1.25) is taken as abnormal. Thiamine or the phosphorylated esters of thiamine in serum or blood can also be measured by high-performance liquid chromatography (HPLC) to detect deficiency. Moreover, a urinary level of thiamine $<27\ \mu g$ per gram of creatinine per day is abnormal. In measuring urinary excretion of thiamine, one should make sure the patient is not taking diuretics, which increase thiamine excretion.

℞ **TREATMENT** In acute thiamine deficiency with either cardiovascular or neurologic signs, 100 mg/d of thiamine should be given parenterally for 7 days, followed by 10 mg/d orally until there is complete recovery. Cardiovascular improvement occurs in ≤ 12 h, and ophthalmoplegic improvement occurs within 24 h. Other manifestations gradually clear, although psychosis in the Wernicke-Korsakoff syndrome may be permanent or persist for several months. Consistent with this, pathologic changes occur in the cortex, cerebellum, and mammillary bodies of the thalamus. Parenteral thiamine should be given prophylactically to all chronic alcoholic patients in the emergency room, or as soon as they are admitted, to prevent precipitation of thiamine deficiency after the provision of glucose-containing solutions.

Thiamine-responsive conditions requiring pharmacologic doses of thiamine include branched-chain ketoaciduria (maple sugar urine disease), subacute necrotizing encephalopathy due to thiamine dihydrophosphate deficiency in the brain (Leigh syndrome), thiamine-responsive lactic acidosis, and thiamine-responsive megaloblastic anemia associated with diabetes mellitus and deafness (Chap. 353). The gene for this recessive disorder, *SLC19A2*, encodes a thiamine transporter.

Toxicity Although anaphylaxis has been reported after high doses of thiamine, no adverse effects have been recorded from either food or supplements at high doses. Thiamine supplements may be bought over the counter in doses of up to 50 mg/d.

RIBOFLAVIN (VITAMIN B$_2$) Riboflavin is important for the metabolism of fat, carbohydrate, and protein, reflecting its role as a respiratory coenzyme and an electron donor. Riboflavin is esterified with phosphoric acid in the body to form two coenzymes, flavin-mononucleotide (FMN) and flavin adenine dinucleotide (FAD) which are involved in a variety of cellular oxidation-reduction processes. Enzymes that contain FAD or FMN as prosthetic groups are known as *flavoenzymes* (e.g., succinic acid dehydrogenase, monoamine oxidase, glutathione reductase). Riboflavin plays an important role in niacin metabolism, since flavoenzymes act as intermediaries in the oxidation of the reduced forms of nicotinamide adenine dinucleotide (NAD) and NAD phosphate (NADP).

Riboflavin is normally absorbed by active and carrier-mediated saturable mechanisms, whereas diffusion is the principal mechanism of absorption at high concentrations. Riboflavin phosphorylation takes place mainly in the wall of the small intestine. Both FMN and FAD are bound to immunoglobulins and albumin in the circulation, and both forms are stored to some degree in liver and muscle.

Although much is known about the chemical and enzymatic reactions of riboflavin, the clinical manifestations of riboflavin deficiency are nonspecific and similar to those of other B vitamin deficiencies. Further, riboflavin deficiency usually occurs in combination with other water-soluble vitamin deficiencies (Chap. 74). Riboflavin deficiency is manifested principally by lesions of the mucocutaneous surfaces of the mouth (angular stomatitis, cheilosis, atrophic glossitis, magenta tongue, pharyngitis) and skin (seborrhea, genital dermatitis). In addition to the mucocutaneous lesions, corneal vascularization, anemia, and personality changes have been described with riboflavin deficiency.

Deficiency and Excess Riboflavin deficiency is almost always due to dietary deficiency. The requirement for riboflavin is increased during pregnancy and lactation and possibly by heavy exercise. The use of phenothiazines and antibiotics also appears to increase the need for riboflavin. Milk, other dairy products, and enriched breads and cereals are the most important dietary sources of riboflavin in the United States, although lean meat, fish, eggs, broccoli, and legumes are also good sources. Riboflavin is extremely sensitive to light, and milk should be stored in containers that protect against photodegradation. In non-milk-drinking societies (e.g., Central America), the laboratory diagnosis of riboflavin deficiency is common. Laboratory diagnosis of riboflavin deficiency can be made by measurement of red blood cell or urinary riboflavin concentrations or by measurement of erythrocyte glutathione reductase activity, with and without added FAD. A stimulation (activity coefficient) of >1.4 is diagnostic of a deficient state. The RDA for riboflavin is 1.1 to 1.3 mg/d in adults, with slightly higher recommendations for lactating and pregnant women. Rare genetic defects of flavoprotein synthesis may require pharmacologic doses of riboflavin for treatment. Because the capacity of the gastrointestinal tract to absorb riboflavin is limited ($\sim$20 mg if given in one oral dose), riboflavin toxicity has not been described. Thus, the most recent revision of the RDAs did not set an upper limit for this nutrient.

NIACIN (VITAMIN B$_3$) The term *niacin* refers to nicotinic acid and nicotinamide and their biologically active derivatives. Nicotinic acid and nicotinamide serve as precursors of two coenzymes, NAD and NADP. These coenzymes are important in numerous oxidation and reduction reactions in the body. NAD and NADP serve as cofactors for dehydrogenases and are involved in the transfer of the hydride ion in many redox reactions. Thus, niacin is important in pentose, steroid, and fatty acid biosynthesis; glycolysis; protein metabolism; and the oxidation of fuels such as lactate, pyruvate, and alcohol. In addition, NAD and NADP are active in adenine diphosphate–ribose transfer reactions involved in DNA repair and calcium mobilization.

Absorption, Metabolism, and Requirements Nicotinic acid and nicotinamide are absorbed well from the stomach and small intestine. Both forms of niacin are absorbed by a sodium-dependent, facilitated diffusion mechanism at low doses, whereas passive diffusion occurs at high doses. Some storage of NAD takes place in the liver. The amino acid tryptophan can be converted to niacin with an efficiency of 60:1 by weight. Thus, the RDA for niacin is expressed in niacin equivalents. Greater conversion of tryptophan to niacin occurs in niacin-deficient states, pregnancy, and in women using oral contraceptives. However, a lower conversion efficiency occurs if a patient is vitamin B$_6$- or riboflavin-deficient. The drug isoniazid inhibits the conversion of tryptophan to niacin. The urinary excretion products of niacin include nicotinic acid and niacin oxide; however, the major urinary metabolites are 2-pyridone and 2-methyl nicotinamide, measurements of which are used in diagnosis of niacin deficiency.

The RDA for niacin is 16 niacin equivalents per day for men and 14 niacin equivalents for women. Median intakes of niacin in the United States considerably exceed these values. Diets that are corn-based can predispose to niacin deficiency due to the low tryptophan and niacin content. Niacin bioavailability is high from beans, milk, meat, and eggs; bioavailability from cereal grains is lower. Since flour is enriched with the "free" niacin (i.e., non-coenzyme form), bioavailability is excellent.

Deficiency Niacin deficiency causes *pellagra*, which is mostly found among people eating corn-based diets in parts of China, Africa, and India. Pellagra in North America is found mainly among alcoholics; in patients with congenital defects of intestinal and kidney absorption of tryptophan (Hartnup's disease; Chap. 352); and in patients with carcinoid syndrome (Chap. 93), in which there is increased conversion of tryptophan to serotonin. The early symptoms of pellagra include loss of appetite, generalized weakness and irritability, abdominal pain, and vomiting. Epithelial cell changes then ensue with stomatitis and bright-red glossitis, followed by a characteristic skin rash that is pigmented and scaling, particularly in skin areas exposed to sunlight. This rash is known as "Casal's necklace," when it rings the

neck, and is seen in advanced cases. Vaginitis and esophagitis may also occur. Diarrhea (in part due to proctitis and in part due to malabsorption), depression, seizures, and dementia are also part of the pellagra syndrome—the four D's: *d*ermatitis, *d*iarrhea, and *d*ementia leading to *d*eath.

The diagnosis of niacin deficiency is based on low levels of the urinary metabolites 2-methyl nicotinamide and 2-pyridone. Treatment of pellagra consists of oral supplementation of 100 to 200 mg of nicotinamide or nicotinic acid three times daily for 5 days. High doses of nicotinic acid ($\geq$3 g nicotinic acid per day) are used for the treatment of elevated cholesterol levels and in the treatment of types 2, 4, and 5 hyperlipidemias (Chap. 344).

Toxicity Prostaglandin-mediated flushing has been observed at daily doses as low as 50 mg of niacin when taken as a supplement or as therapy for hypertriglyceridemia. No toxicity has been seen from niacin derived from food sources. Flushing may be accompanied by skin dryness, itching, and headache. Premedication with aspirin may alleviate these symptoms. Nausea, vomiting, and abdominal pain also occur at similar doses of niacin. Hepatic toxicity is the most serious toxic reaction due to niacin and may present as jaundice with elevated AST and ALT levels. A few cases of fulminant hepatitis requiring liver transplantation have been reported at doses of 3 to 9 g/d. Other toxic reactions include glucose intolerance, macular edema, and macular cysts. It is not clear whether sustained-release forms of nicotinic acid are more toxic than regular forms. The upper limit for daily niacin intake has been set at 35 mg. However, this upper limit does not pertain to the therapeutic use of niacin.

PYRIDOXINE (VITAMIN B$_6$) Vitamin B$_6$ refers to a family of compounds including pyridoxine, pyridoxal, pyridoxamine, and their 5'-phosphate derivatives. 5'-Pyridoxal phosphate (PLP) is a cofactor for more than 100 enzymes involved in amino acid metabolism (e.g., 5'-PLP is a cofactor for the transulfuration enzymes involved in the conversion of homocysteine to cystathionine; Chap. 352). Vitamin B$_6$ is also involved in heme and neurotransmitter synthesis and in the metabolism of glycogen, lipids, steroids, sphingoid bases, and several vitamins, including the conversion of tryptophan to niacin.

Absorption and Metabolism Approximately 75% of vitamin B$_6$ is absorbed from a mixed diet by a nonsaturable, passive process. Much of dietary vitamin B$_6$ is in the phosphorylated form, and the phosphate must be removed by intestinal alkaline phosphatase before absorption takes place. Once absorbed, the vitamin becomes rephosphorylated in the liver, where the various forms can be interconverted. In the liver, PLP binds avidly to cellular proteins and albumin. Since these binding proteins protect it from phosphatase activity, tissue levels of PLP can become quite high with continuous supplementation. Sixty mg of vitamin B$_6$ is stored in the body, and much is in the form of PLP bound to phosphorylase A in muscle. The biologic half-life of vitamin B$_6$ is 25 days.

Dietary Sources Plants contain vitamin B$_6$ in the form of pyridoxine, whereas animal tissues contain PLP and pyridoxamine phosphate. The vitamin B$_6$ contained in plants is less bioavailable than that from animal tissues. All forms of vitamin B$_6$ are labile in alkaline conditions. Rich food sources of vitamin B$_6$ include legumes, nuts, wheat bran, and meat, although the vitamin is present in all food groups. The RDA for young adults (both males and females) has been set at 1.3 mg/d. For older adults, the RDA is slightly higher (1.5 mg/d for women, 1.7 mg/d for men).

Deficiency Symptoms of vitamin B$_6$ deficiency include seborrheic dermatitis, glossitis, stomatitis, and cheilosis, as frequently seen with other B vitamin deficiencies (Chap. 74). In addition, severe vitamin B$_6$ deficiency can lead to generalized weakness, irritability, peripheral neuropathy, abnormal electroencephalograms, and personality changes including depression and confusion. In infants, diarrhea, seizures, and anemia have been reported. Microcytic, hypochromic anemia is due to diminished hemoglobin synthesis, since the first enzyme involved in heme biosynthesis (amino-levulinate synthase) requires

PLP as a cofactor (Chap. 104). In some case reports, platelet dysfunction has also been reported. Since vitamin B_6 is necessary for the conversion of homocysteine to cystathionine, it is possible that chronic low-grade vitamin B_6 deficiency may result in hyperhomocystinemia and increased risk of cardiovascular disease (Chaps. 242 and 352).

Certain medications such as isoniazid, L-dopa, penicillamine, and cycloserine interact with PLP due to a reaction with carbonyl groups. Oral contraceptives have been reported to decrease vitamin B_6 status indicators, although the mechanism for this is uncertain. Alcoholism also decreases vitamin B_6 status due to poor diet, liver disease, and the fact that acetaldehyde can compete with PLP for protein binding, leading to increased degradation and excretion. The increased ratio of aspartate aminotransferase (AST or SGOT) to alanine aminotransferase (ALT or SGPT) seen in alcoholic liver disease reflects the relative vitamin B_6 dependence of ALT. Vitamin B_6 requirements are higher in preeclampsia, eclampsia, and hemodialysis. Vitamin B_6 dependency syndromes that require pharmacologic doses of vitamin B_6 are rare, but include cystathionine β-synthase deficiency, pyridoxine-responsive (primarily sideroblastic) anemias, and gyrate atrophy with chorioretinal degeneration due to decreased activity of the mitochondrial enzyme ornithine aminotransferase. In these situations, 100 to 200 mg/d of oral vitamin B_6 are required for treatment.

High doses of vitamin B_6 have been used to treat carpal tunnel syndrome, premenstrual tension, schizophrenia, autism, and diabetic neuropathy but have not been found to be effective.

The laboratory diagnosis of vitamin B_6 deficiency is generally made on the basis of low plasma PLP values (<20 nmol/L). Other measures of vitamin B_6 deficiency include low erythrocyte levels of PLP, low plasma pyridoxal, and low urinary levels of 4-pyridoxic acid. Treatment of vitamin B_6 deficiency is 50 mg/d; higher doses of 100 to 200 mg/d are given if vitamin B_6 deficiency is related to medication use. Vitamin B_6 should not be given with L-dopa, since the vitamin interferes with the action of this drug.

Toxicity The safe upper limit for vitamin B_6 has been set at 100 mg/d, although the lowest dose at which toxicity (sensory neuropathy) has been seen is 500 mg/d. No adverse effects have been associated with high intakes of vitamin B_6 from food sources only. When toxicity occurs, it causes a severe sensory neuropathy, leaving patients unable to walk. Some cases of photosensitivity and dermatitis have also been reported.

VITAMIN C Both ascorbic acid and its oxidized product dehydroascorbic acid are biologically active. Vitamin C participates in oxidation-reduction reactions and hydrogen ion transfer reactions. As an antioxidant, vitamin C donates electrons to quench reactive free radical and oxygen species. It also acts to regenerate other antioxidants such as vitamin E, flavonoids, and glutathione. Other actions of vitamin C include promotion of nonheme iron absorption, carnitine biosynthesis, and the conversion of dopamine to norepinephrine. Vitamin C is also important for connective tissue metabolism and cross-linking and is a component of many drug-metabolizing enzyme systems, particularly the mixed-function oxidase systems. As such, the vitamin participates in the synthesis of corticosteroids, aldosterone, and the metabolism of cholesterol. Vitamin C also participates in enzymatic reactions requiring a reduced metal, although the exact molecular basis for this role has not been delineated.

Absorption and Physiology Vitamin C is absorbed by an energy-dependent, saturable transport system, and a progressively smaller proportion of the vitamin is absorbed with increasing dose. Almost complete absorption of the vitamin occurs if <100 mg is administered in a single dose; however, only 50% or less is absorbed at doses >1 g. Enhanced degradation and fecal and urinary excretion of vitamin C occur at higher intake levels. High levels of the reduced form of vitamin C are contained in white blood cells, lens tissue, and brain. The maximum body pool in adult males is approximately 1500 mg, and 3% of this body pool is turned over each day, resulting in a half-life of approximately 18 days.

Dietary Sources and Requirements Good dietary sources of vitamin C include citrus fruits, green vegetables (especially broccoli), tomatoes, and potatoes. Appreciable amounts of vitamin C may be consumed as an antioxidant food additive, and the consumption of five servings of fruits and vegetables a day provides vitamin C in excess of the RDA of 60 mg/d for males and females. Moreover, approximately 40% of the U.S. population takes vitamin C as a dietary supplement. Vitamin C requirements are increased slightly to 70 mg in pregnancy and are increased further to 90 to 95 mg/d during lactation. Smoking, hemodialysis, and stress (e.g., infection, trauma) appear to increase vitamin C requirements. "Natural forms" of vitamin C are no more bioavailable than synthetic forms.

Deficiency Vitamin C deficiency causes scurvy; in the United States, this is seen primarily among poor and elderly people and alcoholics who consume <10 mg/d of vitamin C. Vitamin C deficiency has also been described among individuals consuming macrobiotic diets. Scurvy occurs when the body pool for vitamin C drops to <300 mg/d and plasma levels drop to <11 μmol/L. Symptoms of scurvy primarily reflect impaired formation of mature connective tissue and include bleeding into skin (petechiae, ecchymoses, perifollicular hemorrhages); inflamed and bleeding gums; and manifestations of bleeding into joints, the peritoneal cavity, pericardium, and the adrenal glands. Other generalized symptoms include weakness, fatigue, and depression. In children, vitamin C deficiency may cause impaired bone growth. Laboratory diagnosis of vitamin C deficiency is made on the basis of low plasma or leukocyte levels.

Administration of vitamin C (200 mg/d) results in marked improvement in the symptoms of scurvy in a matter of several days. High-dose vitamin C supplementation (e.g., 1 to 2 g/d) has been shown to slightly decrease the symptoms and duration of upper respiratory tract infections and to improve glycemic control. Vitamin C supplementation has also been reported to be useful in Chédiak-Higashi syndrome (Chap. 64) and osteogenesis imperfecta (Chap. 351). It has been claimed that foods high in vitamin C may lower the incidence of certain cancers, particularly esophageal and gastric cancers. If proven, this effect may be due to the fact that vitamin C can prevent the conversion of nitrites and secondary amines to carcinogenic nitrosomines. However, one intervention study from China did not show vitamin C to be protective. Other chronic diseases for which diets high in vitamin C have been reported to be protective include cardiovascular disease, stroke, and cataracts. However, these studies are correlational, and no large-scale intervention studies have been reported.

Toxicity Taking >2 g of vitamin C in a single dose may result in abdominal pain, diarrhea, and nausea; doses >3 g have been reported to elevate blood levels of alanine aminotransferase, lactic acid dehydrogenase, and uric acid. Since vitamin C may be metabolized to oxalate, it has been feared that chronic, high-dose vitamin C supplementation could result in an increased prevalence of kidney stones. However, this has not been borne out in several trials, except in individual patients with preexisting renal disease. Thus, it is reasonable to advise patients with a past history of kidney stones not to take large doses of vitamin C. There is also an unproven, but possible risk that chronic high doses of vitamin C could promote iron overload in patients taking supplemental iron. High doses of vitamin C can induce hemolysis in patients with glucose-6-phosphate dehydrogenase deficiency, and doses >1 g/d can cause false-negative guaiac reactions as well as interfering with tests for urinary glucose.

BIOTIN Biotin is a water-soluble vitamin with a bicyclic structure. The vitamin plays an important role in gluconeogenesis and fatty acid synthesis and serves as a CO_2 carrier on the surface of both cytosolic and mitochondrial carboxylase enzymes. The vitamin also functions in the catabolism of specific amino acids (e.g., leucine).

Biotin in food sources is bound to protein from which it must be cleaved in order to be absorbed. The enzyme biotinidase dissociates the vitamin and facilitates its subsequent transport. Excellent food sources of biotin include liver, soy, beans, yeast, and egg yolks, although egg white contains the protein avidin that strongly binds the vitamin and reduces its bioavailability. Biotin is contained in moderate amounts in legumes, nuts, mushrooms, cauliflower, and certain cereals. Although biotin is synthesized by intestinal bacteria, the relative importance of this source in humans is uncertain. The recommended intake of biotin for adults is 30 μg/d and 35 μg/d in lactating women.

Biotin deficiency has been induced by experimental feeding of egg white diets and in patients with short bowels who received biotin-free parenteral nutrition. In the adult, biotin deficiency results in mental changes (depression, hallucinations), paresthesia, anorexia, and nausea. A scaling, seborrheic, and erythematous rash may occur around the eyes, nose, and mouth as well as on the extremities. In infants, biotin deficiency presents as hypotonia, lethargy, and apathy. In addition, the infant may develop alopecia and a characteristic rash that includes the ears. Two types of inherited infantile biotin deficiency states have been described. Multiple carboxylase deficiency syndrome is an autosomal recessive disorder that is expressed during the first week of life and is characterized by severe metabolic ketoacidosis and dermatitis. Treatment requires pharmacologic doses of biotin, using up to 10 mg/d. Late-onset infantile biotin deficiency due to absorptive and transport defects occurs between 3 and 6 months with dermatitis, seizures, ataxia, hypotonia, and variable metabolic acidosis. The laboratory diagnosis of biotin deficiency can be established based on a decreased urinary concentration.

PANTOTHENIC ACID Pantothenic acid is a component of coenzyme A and phosphopantetheine, which are involved in fatty acid metabolism and the synthesis of cholesterol, steroid hormones, and all compounds formed from isoprenoid units. In addition, pantothenic acid is involved in the acetylation of proteins. Pantothenic acid is actively transported when given at low doses, but it is passively absorbed when given at high doses. The vitamin is excreted in the urine, and the laboratory diagnosis of deficiency is made on the basis of low urinary vitamin levels.

The vitamin is ubiquitous in the food supply. Liver, yeast, egg yolks, and vegetables are particularly good sources. The recommended adequate intake for adults is 5 mg/d. Human pantothenic acid deficiency has only been demonstrated in experimental feeding of diets low in pantothenic acid or by giving a specific pantothenic acid antagonist. The symptoms of pantothenic acid deficiency are nonspecific and include gastrointestinal disturbance, depression, muscle cramps, paresthesia, ataxia, and hypoglycemia. Pantothenic acid deficiency was thought to cause the burning feet syndrome seen in prisoners of war during World War II. No toxicity of this vitamin has been reported.

CHOLINE Choline is a precursor for acetylcholine, phospholipids, and betaine. Choline is necessary for the structural integrity of cell membranes, cholinergic neurotransmission, lipid and cholesterol metabolism, and transmembrane signaling. Recently, a recommended adequate intake was set at 550 mg/d for adult males and 425 mg/d for adult females. Choline is thought to be a "conditionally essential" nutrient, in that de novo synthesis occurs in the liver and is less than the vitamin's utilization only under certain stress conditions. Choline deficiency has occurred in patients receiving parenteral nutrition devoid of choline. Deficiency results in fatty liver and elevated transaminase levels. The diagnosis of choline deficiency is made on the basis of low plasma levels.

Toxicity from choline results in hypotension, cholinergic sweating, diarrhea, salivation, and a fishy body odor. The upper limit for choline has been set at 3.5 g/d. Therapeutically, choline has been suggested for patients with dementia and for patients at high risk of cardiovascular disease, due to its ability to lower cholesterol and homocysteine levels. However, such benefits have yet to be documented.

VITAMIN A *Vitamin A*, in the strictest sense, refers to retinol. However, the oxidized metabolites, retinaldehyde and retinoic acid, are also biologically active compounds. The term *retinoids* includes synthetic molecules that are chemically related to retinol. Retinaldehyde is the essential form of vitamin A that is required for normal vision, whereas retinoic acid is necessary for normal morphogenesis, growth, and cell differentiation. Retinoic acid does not function in vision and, in contrast to retinol, is not involved in reproduction. Vitamin A also plays a role in iron utilization, humoral immunity, T

cell–mediated immunity, natural killer cell activity, and phagocytosis. Vitamin A is commercially available in esterified forms (e.g., acetate, palmitate) since it is more stable as an ester.

There are over 600 carotenoids in nature, and approximately 50 of these can be metabolized to vitamin A. β-Carotene is the most prevalent carotenoid in the food supply that has provitamin A activity. Although the breakdown of β-carotene should theoretically yield two molecules of vitamin A, the conversion of carotenoids to vitamin A, in fact, is much less efficient. It is estimated that 6 μg or greater of dietary β-carotene is equivalent to 1 μg of retinol, whereas 12 μg or greater of other dietary provitamin A carotenoids (e.g., cryptoxanthin, α-carotene) is equivalent to 1 μg of retinol.

Absorption and Metabolism Approximately 80% of preformed vitamin A is absorbed from food, and absorption is via a carrier-mediated mechanism at low concentrations and passive diffusion at high concentrations. Approximately 15 to 30% of provitamin A carotenoids are absorbed passively from the diet, and the absorption becomes much less efficient at high dosage. The absorption of both vitamin A and carotenoids are partially dependent on an adequate bile concentration within the intestinal lumen for the formation of micelles. Once a provitamin A carotene is absorbed into the epithelial cell, a small proportion of it is split to form vitamin A. At higher doses of β-carotene, the conversion to vitamin A is less efficient, thereby preventing vitamin A toxicity. The absorption of both vitamin A and intact β-carotene is via the lymphatics after chylomicron formation.

Hepatic clearance of vitamin A in chylomicrons is efficient, and the liver contains approximately 90% of the vitamin A reserves. Approximately 10 to 40% of a vitamin A dose is oxidized or conjugated in the liver and excreted in urine or bile. Of a given dose of vitamin A, approximately 50% enters the liver storage pool. Storage of vitamin A takes place in the lipid storage (Ito) cell of the liver, which is also a collagen-producing cell. The liver secretes vitamin A in the form of retinol, which is bound to retinol-binding protein. Once this has occurred, the retinol-binding protein complex interacts with a second protein, transthryetin. This trimolecular complex functions to prevent vitamin A from being filtered by the kidney glomerulus, to protect the body against the toxicity of retinol and to allow retinol to be taken up by specific cell-surface receptors that recognize retinol-binding protein. A certain amount of vitamin A enters peripheral cells even if it is not bound to retinol-binding protein. After retinol is internalized by the cell, it becomes bound to a series of cellular retinol-binding proteins, which function as sequestering and transporting agents as well as coligands for enzymatic reactions. Certain cells also contain retinoic acid–binding proteins, which have the same sequestering functions as well as enabling retinoic acid metabolism.

11-*cis*-Retinaldehyde functions as a visual pigment chromophore to capture light. Rhodopsin is composed of the protein opsin and retinaldehyde and is contained in the rod cells, whereas iodopsin is contained in cones. When the dark-adapted retina is exposed to light, the 11-*cis*-retinaldehyde contained in rhodopsin isomerizes to an all-*trans* form. This conformational change causes dissociation from the opsin, resulting in a nerve impulse and a visual response. Once the retina returns to dim light conditions, rhodopsin is regenerated.

Retinoic acid is a ligand for certain nuclear receptors that act as transcription factors. Two families of receptors (RAR and RXR receptors) are active in retinoid-mediated gene transcription. Retinoid receptors regulate transcription by binding as dimeric complexes to specific DNA sites, the retinoic acid response elements, in target genes (Chap. 327). The receptors can either stimulate or repress gene expression in response to their ligands. RAR binds all-*trans* retinoic acid and 9-*cis* retinoic acid, whereas RXR binds only 9-*cis* retinoic acid.

The retinoid receptors play an important role in controlling cell proliferation and differentiation. Retinoic acid is useful in the treatment of promyelocytic leukemia (Chap. 111). In this case, a gene rearrangement fuses the RAR to one of several other genes [e.g., t(15; 17)], causing an apparent block in cell differentiation. Treatment with retinoic acid activates the RAR, dissociating repressor complexes and leading to cell differentiation and more normal cell turnover. Retinoic acid is also used in the treatment of cystic acne because it inhibits keratinization, decreases sebum secretion, and possibly alters the inflammatory reaction (Chap. 56). RXRs dimerize with other nuclear receptors to function as coregulators of genes responsive to retinoids, thyroid hormone, and calcitriol. RXR agonists induce insulin sensitivity experimentally, perhaps because RXR is a cofactor for the peroxisome-proliferator-activated receptors (PPARs), which are targets for the thiazolidinedione drugs such as rosiglitazone and troglitazone (Chap. 333).

Dietary Sources The retinol equivalent (RE) is used to express the vitamin A value of food. One RE is defined as 1 μg of retinol (0.003491 mmol). In the past, 1 RE was considered to be equal to 6 μg of β-carotene, but additional studies indicate that 1 RE may, in fact, be equal to 12 to 20 μg of β-carotene from a dietary source. In older literature, vitamin A was often expressed in international units (IU), with 1 RE being equal to 3.33 IU of retinol and 12 IU of β-carotene, but these units are no longer in current medical or scientific use. The RDA for vitamin A is set at 1000 RE for adult males and 800 RE for adult females.

Liver and fish are excellent food sources for preformed vitamin A; vegetable sources of provitamin A carotenoids include dark-green and -colored fruits and vegetables. Diets consisting mainly of rice, wheat, maize, and tubers can produce vitamin A deficiency, as few carotenoids are contained in these foods. In areas where these foods are staples, children are particularly susceptible to vitamin A deficiency because neither breast nor cow's milk supplies enough vitamin A to prevent deficiency. Areas of the world where vitamin A deficiency is particularly prevalent include parts of Africa, South America, and Southeast Asia. Vitamin A deficiency occurs in more than 250,000 children each year, resulting in blindness and a 50% mortality rate within the year. In western countries, vitamin A deficiency is seen primarily among patients with diseases associated with fat malabsorption (e.g., celiac sprue, short-bowel syndrome). Concurrent zinc deficiency can interfere with the mobilization of vitamin A from liver stores as well as the synthesis of rhodopsin in the eye; thus vitamin A deficiency is exacerbated by concurrent zinc deficiency. Alcohol also interferes with the conversion of retinol to retinaldehyde in the eye by competing for alcohol (retinol) dehydrogenase. Drugs that interfere with the absorption of vitamin A include mineral oil, neomycin, and cholestyramine.

Deficiency Symptoms of vitamin A deficiency include hyperkeratotic skin lesions, night blindness (inability to see in dim light), dryness of the eyes, xerosis, and Bitôt spots, which are white patches of keratinized epithelium appearing on the sclera. Aggressive xerophthalmia can result in corneal ulceration. If untreated, proteolytic destruction and rupture of the cornea ensues with permanent blindness, although vitamin A treatment of patients with corneal ulcers can also result in blindness due to permanent corneal scarring. Children with vitamin A deficiency have increased mortality, primarily from infectious diseases, measles, respiratory diseases, and diarrhea. Extremely low birth weight infants (<1000 g) should be treated parenterally with 5000 IU (1500 μg or RE) of vitamin A three times a week for 4 weeks.

There are no specific deficiency signs or symptoms that result from carotenoid deficiency. However, dietary carotenoids have been suggested to protect against cataract formation, low-density lipoprotein (LDL) oxidation, and certain cancers. It was hoped that β-carotene would be an effective chemopreventive for cancer because numerous epidemiologic studies had shown that diets high in β-carotene were associated with lower incidences of cancers of the respiratory and digestive system. However, intervention studies using high doses of β-carotene actually resulted in more lung cancers than in placebo-treated groups. Non-provitamin A carotenoids, such as lutein and zeaxanthin, have been suggested to protect against macular degeneration. The non-

provitamin A carotenoid lycopene has been suggested to protect against prostate cancer. However, the effectiveness of these agents has not been proven by intervention studies, and the mechanisms underlying these purported biologic actions are unknown.

The diagnosis of vitamin A deficiency is made by measurement of serum retinol (normal range, 30 to 65 μg/dL), tests of dark adaptation, impression cytology of the conjunctiva (decreased numbers of mucous-secreting cells), or measurement of body storage pools, either directly by liver biopsy or by isotopic dilution after administering a stable isotope of vitamin A.

Vitamin A deficiency with ocular changes should be treated by administering 100,000 IU (30 mg) of vitamin A intramuscularly, or 200,000 IU (60 mg) orally. In areas of endemic vitamin A deficiency, this is followed by vitamin A capsules of 200,000 IU at 6-month intervals. Vitamin A deficiency in patients with malabsorptive diseases, who have abnormal dark adaptation or symptoms of night blindness without ocular changes, should be treated for 1 month with 50,000 IU/d (15 mg/d) orally of a water micelle preparation of vitamin A. This is followed by lower maintenance doses with the exact amount determined by monitoring serum retinol.

Toxicity Acute toxicity of vitamin A was first noted in Arctic explorers after eating polar bear liver and has been seen after administration of 150 mg in adults or 100 mg in children. Acute toxicity is manifest by increased intracranial pressure, vertigo, diplopia, bulging fontanels in children, seizures, and exfoliative dermatitis; it may result in death. Chronic vitamin A intoxication has been seen in normal adults who ingest 50,000 IU/d (15 mg/d) of vitamin A for a period of several months and in children who ingest 20,000 IU/d (6 mg/d). Manifestations include dry skin, cheilosis, glossitis, vomiting, alopecia, bone pain, hypercalcemia, lymph node enlargement, hyperlipidemia, amenorrhea, and features of pseudotumor cerebri with increased intracranial pressure and papilledema. Liver fibrosis with portal hypertension and bone demineralization may also result from chronic vitamin A intoxication. When vitamin A is provided in excess of pregnant women, congenital malformations have included spontaneous abortions, craniofacial abnormalities, and valvular heart disease. In pregnancy, the daily dose of vitamin A should not exceed 10,000 IU (3 mg). Elderly individuals appear to be more prone to vitamin A intoxication, as are alcoholics and patients with liver disease. In fact acute hepatitis may precipitate vitamin A intoxication in patients who have extremely high vitamin A stores in the liver. It should be noted that the commercially available retinoid derivatives are also toxic, including 13-*cis*-retinoic acid, which has been associated with birth defects. As a result, contraception should be continued for at least 1 year, and possibly longer, in women who have taken 13-*cis* retinoic acid.

High doses of carotenoids do not result in toxic symptoms. However, carotenemia, which is characterized by a yellowing of the skin (creases of the palms and soles) but not the sclerae, may be seen after ingestion of >30 mg of β-carotene on a daily basis. Hypothyroid patients are particularly susceptible to the development of carotenemia due to impaired breakdown of carotene to vitamin A. Reduction of carotenes from the diet results in the disappearance of skin yellowing and carotenemia over a period of 30 to 60 days.

VITAMIN D (See Chap. 340).

VITAMIN E Vitamin E is a collective name for a group of tocopherols and tocotrionols, the latter having an unsaturated side-chain. There are eight naturally occurring plant compounds with vitamin E activity. RRR-α tocopherol is the most active, while synthetic stereoisomers of vitamin E are less biologically active. Vitamin E acts as a chain-breaking antioxidant and is an efficient pyroxyl radical scavenger, which protects LDLs and polyunsaturated fats in membranes from oxidation. A network of other antioxidants (e.g., vitamin C, glutathione) and enzymes maintains vitamin E in a reduced state. Vitamin E also inhibits prostaglandin synthesis and the activities of protein kinase C and phospholipase A_2.

Absorption and Metabolism Vitamin E is a fat-soluble vitamin and requires all the processes needed for micelle formation to be absorbed. About 15 to 40% is absorbed passively from a single physiologic dose, and there is less efficient absorption at high doses. Polyunsaturated fat may inhibit absorption. Vitamin E is taken up from chylomicrons by the liver, and an hepatic α tocopherol transport protein is involved in intracellular vitamin E transport and incorporation into very low density lipoprotein (VLDL). The transport protein has particular affinity for the RRR isomeric form of α tocopherol; thus this natural isomer has the most biologic activity. In the circulation, vitamin E is bound to all lipoprotein classes and becomes widely distributed in tissues, with fat and muscle being the most important storage depots. Vitamin E metabolites are mainly excreted in feces, although some are also excreted in urine.

Requirement The RDA for vitamin E is currently 10 mg for adults. Additional vitamin E is recommended during pregnancy (12 mg/d) and lactation (14 mg/d). Vitamin E is widely distributed in the food supply. The RRR-α isomers are particularly high in sunflower oil, safflower oil, and wheat germ oil; γ tocotrionols are notably present in soybean and corn oils. Vitamin E is also found in meats, nuts, and cereal grains, and small amounts are present in fruits and vegetables. Vitamin E pills containing doses of 50 to 1000 mg are ingested by a large fraction of the U.S. population. In the older literature, 1 IU of vitamin E is equal to 1 mg all-racemic α tocopherol acetate. Diets high in polyunsaturated fats may necessitate a slightly higher requirement for vitamin E.

Dietary deficiency of vitamin E does not exist. Vitamin E deficiency is seen only in severe and prolonged malabsorptive diseases, such as celiac disease, or after small-intestinal resection, leading to short-bowel syndrome. Children with cystic fibrosis or prolonged cholestasis may develop vitamin E deficiency characterized by areflexia and hemolytic anemia. Children with abetalipoproteinemia cannot absorb or transport vitamin E and become deficient quite rapidly. A familial form of isolated vitamin E deficiency also exists, which is due to a defect in the α tocopherol transport protein. Vitamin E deficiency causes axonal degeneration of the large myelinated axons and results in posterior column and spinocerebellar symptoms. Peripheral neuropathy is initially characterized by areflexia, with progression to an ataxic gait, and by decreased vibration and position sensations. Ophthalmoplegia, skeletal myopathy, and pigmented retinopathy may also be features of vitamin E deficiency. The laboratory diagnosis of vitamin E deficiency is made on the basis of low blood levels of α tocopherol (<5 μg/mL, or <0.8 mg of α tocopherol per gram of total lipids).

TREATMENT Symptomatic vitamin E deficiency should be treated with 800 to 1200 mg of α tocopherol per day. Patients with abetalipoproteinemia may need as much as 5000 to 7000 mg/d. Children with symptomatic vitamin E deficiency should be treated with 400 mg/d orally of water-soluble esters; alternatively, 2 mg/kg per day may be administered intramuscularly. Vitamin E in high doses may protect against oxygen-induced retrolental fibroplasia and bronchopulmonary dysplasia in prematurity, as well as intraventricular hemorrhage of prematurity. Vitamin E has been suggested to increase sexual performance, to treat intermittent claudication, and to slow the aging process, but evidence for these properties is lacking. High doses (60 to 800 mg/d) of vitamin E have been shown in controlled trials to improve parameters of immune function, and there are two intervention studies showing that vitamin E at 400 to 800 mg/d may be protective against cardiovascular disease, possibly by inhibiting LDL oxidation. Also, supplemental intake of vitamin E (100 to 200 mg/d) has been associated with a decreased risk of cataracts.

Toxicity High doses of vitamin E (>800 mg/d) may reduce platelet aggregation and interfere with vitamin K metabolism and are therefore contraindicated in patients taking coumadin. Nausea, flatulence, and diarrhea have been reported at doses >1 g/d.

VITAMIN K There are two natural forms of vitamin K: vitamin K I, also known as *phylloquinone*, from vegetable and animal sources, and vitamin K II, or *menaquinone*, which is synthesized by bacterial

flora and found in hepatic tissue. *Menadione*, or vitamin K III, is a chemically synthesized pro-vitamin that can be converted to menaquinone by the liver. Phylloquinone and menaquinones differ only in their lipophilic sidechains, and both are destroyed in an alkaline pH and by ultraviolet light.

Absorption and Physiology As with other fat-soluble vitamins, vitamin K absorption is dependent on normal pancreatic function and the presence of bile salts. Phylloquinones are absorbed by a saturable energy-dependent mechanism in the proximal small intestine, whereas menaquinones are absorbed by passive diffusion in the small intestine and colon. Approximately 100 μg of vitamin K is stored in the liver as well as in lung, bone marrow, kidneys, and adrenal glands. Most vitamin K circulates bound to VLDL, although it is also carried by LDL and high-density lipoprotein (HDL). The half-life of vitamin K is only 1½ days, despite the presence of a vitamin K regeneration cycle.

Vitamin K is necessary for the posttranslational carboxylation of glutamic acid, which is necessary for calcium binding to γ-carboxylated proteins such as prothrombin (factor II); factors VII, IX, and X; protein C; protein S; and proteins found in bone (bone gla, matrix gla protein, and osteocalcin). The importance of vitamin K for bone mineralization is not known. Warfarin-type drugs inhibit γ carboxylation by preventing the conversion of vitamin K to its active hydroquinone form. Vitamin E, at high doses, may act as a vitamin K antagonist.

Dietary Sources Vitamin K is found in green leafy vegetables such as kale and spinach, but appreciable amounts are also present in butter, margarine, liver, milk, ground beef, coffee, and pears. Vitamin K is present in vegetable oils and is particularly rich in olive oil and soybean oil. The recommended intake of vitamin K is 70 μg/d in adults. The average daily intake by Americans is estimated to be approximately 100 μg/d.

Deficiency The symptoms of vitamin K deficiency are due to hemorrhage, and newborns are particularly susceptible because of low fat stores, low breast milk levels of vitamin K, sterility of the infantile intestinal tract, liver immaturity, and poor placental transport. Intracranial bleeding, as well as gastrointestinal and skin bleeding, can be seen in vitamin K–deficient infants 1 to 7 days after birth. Thus, vitamin K (1 mg intramuscularly) is given prophylactically at the time of delivery.

Vitamin K deficiency in adults may be seen in patients with chronic small-intestinal disease (e.g., celiac disease, Crohn's disease), obstructed biliary tracts, or after small-bowel resection. Broad-spectrum antibiotic treatment can precipitate vitamin K deficiency by reducing gut bacteria, which synthesize menaquinones, as well as by inhibiting the metabolism of vitamin K. The diagnosis of vitamin K deficiency is usually made on the basis of an elevated prothrombin time or reduced clotting factors. Vitamin K may also be measured directly by HPLC. In addition, undercarboxylated prothrombin and low gla levels in urine are indicative of vitamin K deficiency. Vitamin K deficiency is treated using a parenteral dose of 10 mg. For patients with chronic malabsorption, 1 to 2 mg/d of vitamin K may be given orally, or 1 to 2 mg/week can be taken parenterally. Patients with liver disease may have an elevated prothrombin time because of liver cell destruction as well as vitamin K deficiency. If an elevated prothrombin time does not improve on vitamin K therapy, it can be assumed that it is not the result of vitamin K deficiency.

Toxicity Parenteral doses of the water-soluble vitamin K derivative (menadione) have been reported to cause hemolytic anemia and hypobilirubinemia in infants. Toxicity from dietary phylloquinones and menaquinones has not been described. High doses of vitamin K can impair the actions of oral anticoagulants.

TRACE MINERALS (See Table 75-1)

ZINC Zinc is an integral component of many metalloenzymes in the body; it is involved in the synthesis and stabilization of proteins,

Table 75-1 Deficiencies and Toxicities of Metals

Element	Deficiency	Toxicity
Zinc	Growth retardation, ↓ taste and smell, alopecia, dermatitis, diarrhea, immunologic dysfunction, failure to thrive, gonadal atrophy, impaired spermatogenesis, congenital malformations	General Gastritis, sweating, fever, nausea, vomiting Occupational Respiratory distress, pulmonary fibrosis
Copper	Anemia, growth retardation, defective keratinization and pigmentation of hair, hypothermia, degenerative changes in aortic elastin, osteopenia, mental deterioration, scurvy-like changes in skeleton	General Nausea, vomiting, diarrhea, hepatic failure, tremor, mental deterioration, hemolytic anemia, renal dysfunction
Selenium	Cardiomyopathy, congestive heart failure, striated muscle degeneration	General Alopecia, nausea, vomiting, abnormal nails, emotional lability, peripheral neuropathy, lassitude, garlic odor to breath, dermatitis Occupational Lung and nasal carcinomas, liver necrosis, pulmonary inflammation
Chromium	Impaired glucose tolerance	Occupational Renal failure, dermatitis, pulmonary cancer
Manganese	Bone demineralization, ataxia, convulsions, anemia	Occupational Encephalitis-like syndrome, Parkinson-like syndrome, psychosis, pneumoconiosis

DNA, and RNA and plays a structural role in ribosomes and membranes. Zinc is necessary for the binding of steroid hormone receptors and several other transcription factors to DNA and thereby plays an important role in the regulation of gene transcription. Zinc is absolutely required for normal spermatogenesis, fetal growth, and embryonic development.

Absorption and Physiology Zinc is absorbed in the small intestine by a carrier-mediated mechanism. The absorption of zinc from the diet is inhibited by dietary phytate, fiber, oxalate, iron, and copper, as well as by certain drugs including penicillamine, sodium valproate, and ethambutol. The RDA for zinc is 15 mg in males and 12 mg in females, with an additional 3 mg in pregnancy and 4 to 7 mg during lactation. Supplemental zinc is recommended for women taking ≥60 mg/d of iron during pregnancy.

Meat, shellfish, nuts, and legumes are good sources of bioavailable zinc, whereas zinc in grains is less available for absorption. Zinc is excreted mainly in the feces but also in urine and sweat. The body contains approximately 2 g of zinc, and high concentrations are found in liver, prostate, pancreas, bone, and brain (hippocampus and cerebral cortex), where the metal may function in neural transmission.

Deficiency Mild zinc deficiency has been described in many diseases including diabetes mellitus, AIDS, cirrhosis, alcoholism, inflammatory bowel disease, malabsorption syndromes, and sickle cell anemia. In these diseases, mild chronic zinc deficiency can cause stunted growth in children, decreased taste sensation (hypogusia), impaired immune function, and night blindness due to impaired conversion of retinol to retinaldehyde. Severe chronic zinc deficiency has been described as a cause of hypogonadism and dwarfism in several Middle Eastern countries. In these children, hypopigmented hair is also part of the syndrome. Acrodermatitis enteropathica is a rare autosomal recessive disorder characterized by abnormalities in zinc absorption. Clinical manifestations include diarrhea, alopecia, muscle wasting, depression, irritability, and a rash involving the extremities, face, and perineum. The rash is characterized by vesicular and pustular crusting with scaling and erythema. In addition, hypopigmentation and corneal edema have been described in these patients. Occasional patients with Wilson's disease have developed zinc deficiency as a consequence of penicillamine therapy. Patients on long-term parenteral nutrition have developed deficiency when zinc has been omitted from the total parenteral nutrition (TPN) solution.

The diagnosis of zinc deficiency is usually made by a serum zinc level of <12 μmol/L (<70 μg/dL). Pregnancy and birth control pills may cause a slight depression in serum zinc levels, and hypoalbuminemia from any cause can result in hypozincemia. In acute stress situations, zinc may be redistributed from serum into tissues. Zinc deficiency may be treated with 60 mg elemental zinc, given orally twice a day. Zinc gluconate lozenges (13 mg elemental Zn every 2 h while awake) have been reported to reduce the duration and symptoms of the common cold in adults, but these studies are conflicting.

Toxicity Acute zinc toxicity after oral ingestion causes nausea and vomiting, fever, and respiratory distress. Zinc fumes from welding may also be toxic and cause fever, chills, excessive salivation, sweating, and headache. Chronic large doses of zinc may depress immune function and cause hypochromic anemia as a result of copper deficiency.

COPPER Copper is an integral part of numerous enzyme systems including amine oxidases, ferrooxidase (ceruloplasmin), cytochrome-c oxidase, superoxide dismutase, and dopamine hydroxylase. As such, copper plays a role in iron metabolism, melanin synthesis, and central nervous system function; the synthesis and cross-linking of elastin and collagen; and the scavenging of superoxide radicals.

Copper is absorbed in the proximal small intestine, and 90% of circulating copper is bound to ceruloplasmin. The body contains 50 to 120 mg of copper, and high concentrations are found in liver, brain, heart, spleen, kidney, and blood. The U.S. RDA is 1.5 to 3 mg of copper intake per day, although World Health Organization recommendations are somewhat lower. Dietary sources of copper include shellfish, liver, nuts, legumes, bran, and organ meats, whereas milk is a very poor source. Copper is primarily excreted in the feces, and small amounts are also excreted in urine.

Deficiency Dietary copper deficiency is relatively rare, although it has been described in premature infants fed milk diets and in infants with malabsorption. Signs and symptoms of copper deficiency include a hypochromic-normocytic anemia, osteopenia, depigmentation, mental retardation, and psychomotor abnormalities. Copper deficiency anemia has been reported in patients with malabsorptive diseases and nephrotic syndrome and in patients treated for Wilson's disease with chronic high doses of oral zinc, which can interfere with copper absorption. Menkes kinky hair syndrome is an X-linked metabolic disturbance of copper metabolism characterized by mental retardation, hypocupremia, and decreased circulating ceruloplasmin (Chap. 351). It is caused by mutations in a copper-transporting *ATP7A* gene. Children with this disease often die within 5 years due to dissecting aneurysms or cardiac rupture.

The diagnosis of copper deficiency is usually made on the basis of low serum levels of copper (<65 μg/dL) and low ceruloplasmin levels (<18 mg/dL). Serum levels of copper may be elevated in pregnancy or stress conditions since ceruloplasmin is an acute-phase reactant.

Toxicity Toxicity due to copper is usually accidental and may include nausea, vomiting, diarrhea, and hemolytic anemia. In severe cases, kidney failure, liver failure, and coma may ensue. In Wilson's disease, mutations in the copper-transporting *ATP7B* gene lead to accumulation of copper in the liver and brain, with low blood levels due to decreased ceruloplasmin (Chap. 348). Indian childhood cirrhosis is another hereditary disease characterized by extremely high copper levels in the liver. The World Health Organization recommends that adult females should not ingest >10 mg/d and males should not take in >12 mg/d of copper.

SELENIUM Selenium, in the form of selenocysteine, is a component of the enzyme glutathione peroxidase, which serves to protect proteins, cell membranes, lipids, and nucleic acids from oxidant molecules. Selenocysteine is also found in the deiodinase enzymes, which mediate the deiodination of thyroxine to the more active triiodothyronine (Chap. 330). Rich sources of selenium include seafood, muscle meat, and cereals, although the selenium content of cereal is determined by the soil concentration. Countries with low soil concentrations include parts of Scandinavia, China, and New Zealand. *Keshan disease* is an endemic cardiomyopathy found in children and young women residing in regions of China where dietary intake of selenium is low (<20 μg/d). Concomitant deficiencies of iodine and selenium may worsen the clinical manifestations of cretinism. The adult RDAs for selenium in the United States are 55 and 70 μg/d for females and males, respectively. Low blood levels of selenium in various populations have been correlated with an increase in coronary artery disease and certain cancers, although the data are not consistent. Selenosis occurs at intakes of ≥400 μg/d and can result in nausea, vomiting, loss of hair, nail changes, peripheral neuropathy, and fatigue.

CHROMIUM Chromium potentiates the action of insulin in patients with impaired glucose tolerance, presumably by increasing insulin receptor–mediated signaling. In addition, in some patients, improvement in blood lipid profiles has been reported. The usefulness of chromium supplements in muscle building are not substantiated. Rich food sources of chromium include yeast, meat, and grain products. Chromium deficiency has been reported to cause glucose intolerance, peripheral neuropathy, and confusion. The suggested intake of chromium for adults is 50 to 200 μg/d. Chromium in the trivalent state is found in supplements and is largely nontoxic; however, chromium-6 is a product of stainless steel welding and is a known pulmonary carcinogen, as well as causing liver, kidney, and central nervous system.

MAGNESIUM See Chap. 340

FLUORIDE, MANGANESE, AND ULTRATRACE ELEMENTS An essential function for *fluoride* in humans has not been described, although it is useful for the maintenance of structure in teeth and bone. An adequate intake for fluoride (on the basis of protection against dental caries) has been set at 3.1 and 3.8 mg/d in adult females and males, respectively. Adult fluorosis can occur at an intake of 10 mg/d for prolonged periods and results in mottled and pitted defects in tooth enamel as well as brittle bone (skeletal fluorosis). Much lower doses of fluoride (0.7 to 2 mg) can cause dental fluorosis or mottled enamel in infants and children.

Manganese and molybdenum deficiencies have been reported in patients with rare genetic abnormalities as well as in a few patients receiving prolonged TPN. Several manganese-specific enzymes have been identified (e.g., manganese superoxide dismutase). The estimated adequate daily dietary *manganese* intake for adults is 2 to 3 mg/d. Deficiencies of manganese have been reported to result in bone demineralization, poor growth, ataxia, and convulsions.

Ultratrace elements are those for which the need is <1 mg/d. Essentiality has not been established for most ultratrace elements, although *iodine* is clearly essential (Chap. 330). *Molybenum* is necessary for the activity of sulfite and xanthine oxidase, and molybdenum deficiency may result in skeletal and brain lesions. The minimum required daily molybdenum intake is estimated to be ~25 μg/d. There is circumstantial evidence to suggest that *arsenic* (impaired growth, infertility), *boron* (impaired energy metabolism, impaired brain function), *nickel* (impaired-growth and reproduction), *silicon* (impaired growth) and *vanadium* (impaired skeletal formation) might also be essential.

BIBLIOGRAPHY

THIAMINE

FLEMING JC et al: The gene mutated in thiamine-responsive anaemia with diabetes and deafness (TRMA) encodes a functional thiamine transporter. Nat Genet 22:305, 1999

SHIMON I et al: Improved left ventricular function after thiamine supplementation in patients with congestive heart failure receiving long-term furosemide therapy. Am J Med 98:485, 1995

WILKINSON TJ et al: The response to treatment of subclinical thiamine deficiency in the elderly. Am J Clin Nutr 66:925, 1997

RIBOFLAVIN

SOARES MJ et al: The effect of exercise on the riboflavin status of older men. Br J Nutr 69:541, 1993

ZEMPLENI J, GALLOWAY JR: Pharmacokinetics of orally and intravenously administered riboflavin in healthy humans. Am J Clin Nutr 63:54, 1996

NIACIN

GIBBONS LW et al: The prevalence of side effects with regular and sustained-release nicotinic acid. Am J Med 99:378, 1995

STERN RH et al: Pharmacodynamics and drug action: Tolerance to nicotinic acid flushing. Clin Pharmacol Ther 50:66, 1991

VITAMIN B₆

RIBAYA-MERCADO JD et al: Vitamin B-6 requirements of elderly men and women. J Nutr 121:1062, 1991

RIMM EB et al: Folate and vitamin B₆ from diet and supplements in relation to risk of coronary heart disease among women. JAMA 279:359, 1998

ROBINSON K et al: Hyperhomocysteinemia and low pyridoxal phosphate. Common and independent reversible risk factors for coronary artery disease. Circulation 92:2825, 1995

VITAMIN C

CARR AC, FREI B: Toward a new recommended dietary allowance for vitamin C based on antioxidant and health effect in humans. Am J Clin Nutr 69:1086, 1999

HEMILA H: Vitamin C intake and susceptibility to the common cold. Br J Nutr 77:59, 1997

WEBB PM et al: Gastric cancer, gastritis and plasma vitamin C: Results from an international correlation and cross-sectional study. Int J Cancer 73:684, 1997

VITAMIN A

OMENN GS et al: Effects of a combination of beta-carotene and vitamin A on lung cancer and cardiovascular disease. N Engl J Med 334:1150, 1996

RUSSELL RM et al: Hepatic injury from chronic hypervitaminosis A resulting in portal hypertension and ascites. N Engl J Med 291:435, 1974

TYSON JE et al: Vitamin A supplementation for extremely low birth weight infants. N Engl J Med 340:1962, 1999

VITAMIN E

HARDING AE et al: Spinocerebellar degeneration associated with a selective defect of vitamin E absorption. N Engl J Med 313:32, 1985

HEART OUTCOMES PREVENTION EVALUATION STUDY INVESTIGATORS: Vitamin E supplementation and cardiovascular events in high-risk patients. N Engl J Med 342:154, 2000

SANO M et al: A controlled trial of selegiline, alpha-tocopherol, or both as treatment for Alzheimer's disease. N Engl J Med 336:1216, 1997

VITAMIN K

DOWD P et al: The mechanism of action of vitamin K. Annu Rev Nutr 15:419, 1995

FESKANICH D et al: Vitamin K intake and hip fractures in women: A prospective study. Am J Clin Nutr 69:74, 1999

METALS

ANDERSON RA et al: Elevated intakes of supplemental chromium improve glucose and insulin variables in individuals with type 2 diabetes. Diabetes 46:1786, 1997

CLARK LC et al: Effects of selenium supplementation for cancer prevention in patients with carcinoma of the skin. A randomized controlled trial. JAMA 276:1957, 1996

MOSSAD SB, MACKNIN ML: Zinc gluconate lozenges for treating the common cold. A randomized, double-blind, placebo-controlled study. Ann Intern Med 125:81, 1996

ZINC INVESTIGATORS' COLLABORATIVE GROUP: BHJUTTA ZA et al: Prevention of diarrhea and pneumonia by zinc supplementation in children in developing countries: Pooled analysis of randomized controlled trials. J Pediatr 135:689, 1999

76 *Lyn Howard*

ENTERAL AND PARENTERAL NUTRITION THERAPY

Parenteral and enteral nutrition provide life-sustaining therapy for patients who cannot take adequate food by mouth and who consequently are at risk for malnutrition and its effects, including susceptibility to infection, weakness and immobility; these features predispose the patient to aspiration pneumonia, pulmonary embolism, and pressure sores, all of which delay recovery from illness and increase mortality.

The term *enteral* refers to feeding via the gut and hence includes normal eating, but in the present context implies the infusion of formulas via a tube into the upper gastrointestinal tract. *Parenteral* refers to the infusion of nutrient solutions into the bloodstream. While these are different approaches to nutritional support, their goals are the same. Where feasible, enteral nutrition is the preferred route because it sustains the digestive, absorptive, and immunologic barrier functions of the gastrointestinal tract. The cost of enteral tube feeding is about one-tenth the cost of parenteral feeding.

Several developments have made tube feeding easier and more acceptable to patients. Small-bore pliable tubes have largely replaced large-bore rubber tubes, and double-lumen tubes are now available for simultaneous gastric suction and jejunal feeding when there is concern about gastric retention and aspiration. Enteral tubes can be inserted into the stomach or jejunum through the nose or, for long-term use, directly through the abdominal wall, using endoscopic, radiologic, or surgical techniques. Once the enterocutaneous tract is established, the protruding tube can be replaced by a "button" entry port, flush with the abdominal wall.

Complete nutrition by vein with sufficient calories, amino acids, minerals, and vitamins to permit wound healing, restoration of normal body composition of a cachectic patient, or growth in children became feasible in the 1960s with the development of high-flow central vein catheters. Parental nutrition is now available in all large hospitals and for some patients at home. Adequate calories and other nutrients can be delivered in the form of high-energy, isotonic intravenous fat solutions via a peripheral vein. However, peripheral veins usually cannot sustain such infusions indefinitely, and long-term support requires central venous access.

THE DECISION PROCESS FOR USING PARENTERAL OR ENTERAL NUTRITION The decision to use specialized nutrition support should be based on the likelihood that averting or redressing malnutrition will improve the quality of life or the ability to recover from a serious illness.

Approximately 15 to 20% of hospitalized patients have evidence of malnutrition. Some malnourished patients benefit from specialized nutrition support; for others, wasting is an inevitable component of a terminal disease. Selecting the appropriate form of nutritional support for the patient requires knowledge of the potential benefits and risks of nutritional support, and the physician must inform the patient and family of these issues. A flow diagram of the steps involved in deciding whether specialized nutrition support should be undertaken and, if so, how, is depicted in Fig. 76-1. Like all life-support measures, these therapies are difficult to withdraw once started.

The first step requires consideration of the nutritional implications of the disease process. Is the condition or its treatment likely to impair appetite or food ingestion and absorption for a prolonged period of time? Because prevention of malnutrition is easier than repleting a cachectic patient, this issue must be considered in the initial evaluation (Chap. 74). The second step is to determine whether the patient is already sufficiently malnourished that lean body mass is decreased and critical functions such as healing and ventilation are impaired. The presence or absence of metabolic stress should be noted, since injury or infection can evoke the secretion of hormonal and cytokine factors that reduce the efficiency of nutrition repletion.

Weight loss without physiologic impairment is probably of no consequence. Physiologic impairment usually develops when more than 20% of body protein is lost and is more likely if key organ systems, such as the gut or liver, are directly affected by disease. Once it is recognized that the patient is malnourished or at major risk, the next question is whether specialized nutritional support will impact positively on the patient's response to the disease, improving the quality of life. While the provision of food and water is part of basic medical care, nutrition support by enteral or parenteral means is associated with risk and discomfort and should be recommended only when potential benefit exceeds risk and undertaken only with the consent of the patient.

If it is decided that preventing or treating malnutrition with specialized nutrition support would improve the prognosis and quality of life, the nutritional requirements must be determined and the route of nutrient delivery must be selected.

RISKS AND BENEFITS OF NUTRITION SUPPORT The risks are determined primarily by the route required to deliver nutrition support. Providing nutritional requirements by special attention to oral intake of food, or by adding oral liquid supplements and monitoring food intake with frequent calorie counts, is the safest and least costly approach. It is also the most metabolically efficient since normal eating initiates the cephalic phase of digestion. Tube-fed infants grow better if the cephalic phase is stimulated by having the infant suck on a pacifier.

Anorexia, impairment of swallowing, or bowel disease may limit oral intake or the absorption of oral nutrients, in which case tube enteral nutrition is the next consideration. The bowel and its associated digestive organs derive 70% of their required nutrients directly from food in the lumen. In addition, glutamine, short-chain fatty acids, and nucleotides may have particular importance in maintaining gut integrity. Enteral feeding also supports gut function by stimulating splanchnic blood flow, neuronal activity, IgA antibody release, and secretion of gastrointestinal hormones such as epidermal growth factor that stimulate gut trophic activity. All these factors support the gut as an immunologic barrier against enteric pathogens, reducing the likelihood of bacterial overgrowth. For these reasons, some enteral nutrition should always be provided if possible, even when parenteral nutrition is required to provide most of the support. In the past, bowel rest through parenteral nutrition was thought to be the cornerstone of treatment of many severe gastrointestinal disorders, but the value of some enteral nutrition is now widely accepted, and strict bowel rest is rarely appropriate. Parenteral nutrition alone is necessary in severe hemorrhagic pancreatitis, necrotizing enterocolitis, prolonged ileus, and distal bowel obstruction.

Specialized nutrition support is expensive, accounting for >1% of all health care dollars. Consequently, hard clinical endpoints such as mortality rate, incidence of major complications, and duration of hospital stay are required of risk-benefit studies. Better nitrogen balance, increased levels of serum albumin, and improved delayed hypersensitivity are softer endpoints. Table 76-1 summarizes clinical trials that evaluate the use of specialized nutrition support in different disease states.

Perioperative Nutrition There is a clear-cut association between preoperative malnutrition and poor surgical outcome, but it has been difficult to demonstrate the benefit of preoperative parenteral nutrition on the outcome of surgery in malnourished patients. However, a meta-analysis of several small studies and a large cooperative Veterans Administration study indicates that preoperative parenteral nutrition does improve the outcome of severely malnourished surgical patients. In treated patients, noninfectious complications (e.g., pulmonary emboli and delayed wound healing) are reduced in the postoperative period. Effective preoperative restoration of nutrition by the parenteral route requires at least 7 to 14 days. If feasible, a safer and less costly approach is preoperative enteral nutrition, especially if provided at home.

Immediate postoperative nutritional support is appropriate for patients who received preoperative support and for patients unlikely to resume oral feeding within 10 days. The parenteral route is commonly used because of postoperative ileus or concern about disrupting a new bowel anastomosis. However, cautious jejunal feeding is often tolerated. Specialized enteral formulas supplemented with conditionally essential nutrients may be particularly beneficial in debilitated and immunosuppressed postoperative patients (Table 76-2).

Critical Illness Very early nutrition support (within the first 48 h) improves survival and reduces infections and length of hospital stay in patients with severe head injuries, burns, and major abdominal trauma. Enteral therapy, where feasible, is superior to parenteral therapy in several randomized trials. Enteral nutrition equally benefits malnourished and well-nourished injured patients. Animal studies show that enteral feeding reduces translocation of gut bacteria and the systemic catabolic response; however, these phenomena have not been substantiated in humans. Early enteral feeding may prevent bacterial overgrowth and decrease aspiration pneumonia.

The practical issue is obtaining jejunal access in a critically ill patient, who is not easily transferred out of the intensive care unit for endoscopic or radiologic tube placement. Sometimes a nasal or percutaneous combined gastric suction and jejunal feeding tube can be inserted at the bedside. If a surgical laparotomy is indicated, a feeding tube can be placed simultaneously.

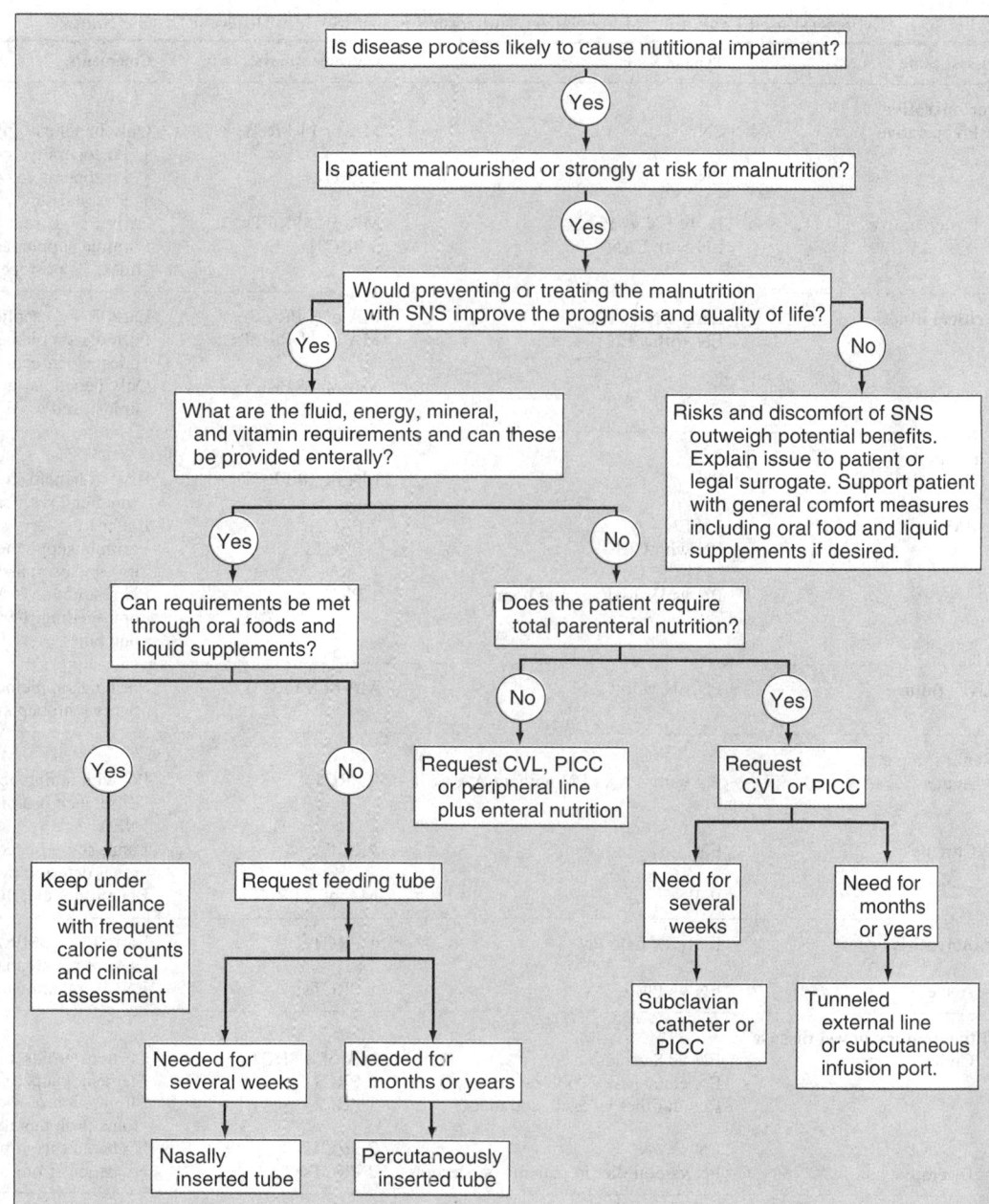

FIGURE 76-1 Should specialized nutrition support (SNS) be undertaken and if so, how? An algorithm. (PICC, peripherally inserted, central catheter; CVL, central venous line.)

Most studies of enteral feeding in critically ill patients used either a general polymeric formula or one with hydrolyzed protein. Formulas supplemented with conditionally essential nutrients reduce infections and length of hospital stay. Parenteral formulas enriched with large amounts of branched-chain amino acids (BCAA) improve nitrogen balance but do not appear to affect clinical outcome.

Cancer Cachexia Early nonrandomized studies suggested that patients with cancer cachexia benefitted from parenteral nutrition, but randomized trials demonstrated more risk than benefit for patients receiving chemotherapy or radiation. Severely malnourished cancer patients undergoing surgery benefit from preoperative parenteral nutrition, as do other malnourished patients.

In two randomized, prospective trials, patients undergoing bone marrow transplantation had better long-term survival after parenteral or enteral nutrition in the cytoreduction phase; nutrition support did not influence the initial infection rate or the frequency of graft rejection or graft-versus-host disease. Immediate morbidity is reduced if glutamine supplements are added to the parenteral nutrition solution. Par-

enteral nutrition continued at home delays return to oral feeding. For cancer patients with unresectable upper gastrointestinal cancer, enteral feeding is usually justified if it is desired by the patient and family. Parenteral feeding should be provided only if clinical improvement can be expected and when quality survival at home for several months is predicted.

Liver Failure Malnutrition is common in advanced liver disease. Patients with acute or chronic liver failure have decreased levels of BCAA and elevated levels of aromatic amino acids (AAA) in plasma and cerebrospinal fluid. Randomized, prospective trials with parenteral and enteral formulas high in BCAA and low in AAA have demonstrated better nitrogen balance and less risk of encephalopathy. One large multicenter study also reported improved survival. The BCAA-enriched formulas are expensive and should be used only in patients who have encephalopathy or who develop encephalopathy when fed a standard protein formula providing 0.8 g protein/kg per day.

Renal Failure Since renal failure is associated with impaired nitrogen excretion, it is rational to assume that protein restriction might

Table 76-1 Evidence-Based Evaluation of Specialized Nutrition Support (SNS) in Different Disease States[a]

Disease State	Type of SNS	Outcome Analysis	Comments
Perioperative			
Preoperative	PN	MA of 14 PRCTs	Only beneficial in severe PCM ↓ Postoperative complications by 10%
	EN	2 PRCTs	↓ Postoperative complications by 25%; ↓ Hospital stay
Postoperative	Early EN vs PN	MA of 8 PRCTs	Early EN ↓ septic complications
	EN with CEN	3 PRCTs	Formula supplemented with arginine, W3 FA nucleotides; ↓ postoperative complications, ↓ hospital stay
Critical illness	Early EN vs PN	MA of 8 PRCTs	Early EN ↓ septic complications
	EN with CEN	MA of 11 PRCTs	Formula supplemented with arginine, W3 FA nucleotides: ↓ infections, ↓ hospital stay
	PN	MA of 26 PRCTs	Only beneficial in severe PCM; ↓ Complications if no lipids used
Cancer			
Cachexia	PN	MA of 18 PRCTs	Risk > benefit in patients undergoing CXT or RXT, but beneficial with cancer surgery in severe PCM
BMT	PN/EN	2 PRCTs	Better long-term survival
	PN with CEN	2 PRCTs	Formula supplemented with glutamine: ↓ early mortality, ↓ hospital stay
	PN vs IV hydration at home	1 PRCT	PN resulted in less weight loss but delayed return to oral feeding. IV hydration did not result in adverse outcome
Liver failure	PN/EN with CEN	MA of 8 PRCTs	Formula supplemented with BCAA beneficial in patients with hepatic encephalopathy
Renal failure			
Acute	PN with AA vs PN without AA	2 PRCTs	PN with amino acids ↓ infectious complications. No difference if amino acids just EAA or both EAA and NEAA
Chronic	EN	PRCT	Large study of reduced protein diet did not slow rate of renal deterioration
	IDPN	MA of 2 PRCTs	Benefit not clearly established
Pancreatitis	Early vs Late PN	1 PRCT	Early PN ↓ MR and infectious complications if used in severe pancreatitis
Acute	EN vs PN	2 PRCTs	EN ↓ inflammatory response, ↓ sepsis
Inflammatory bowel disease			
Crohn's	EN vs Steroids	MA of 8 PRCTs	Corticosteroids superior to EN
	EN elemental vs polymeric	2 PRCTs	Elemental superior to polymeric
	Regular diet vs exclusion diets	1 PRCT	Elimination of foods that induce gastrointestinal symptoms prolongs remission
	EN vs PN	2 PRCTs	No benefit from bowel rest
Ulcerative colitis	PN vs oral diet in patients on steroids	2 PRCTs	No benefit from bowel rest
Short bowel syndrome	EN and CEN	PRCT, crossover design	IV HGH and oral glutamine supplements did not improve bowel function in long-term HPN patients
Pulmonary disease			
Acute, ventilated	PN and EN	2 PRCTs	↓ Glucose and ↑ fat-aided weaning process
	EN: continuous vs intermittent	1 PRCT	No difference in gastric bacterial colonization
Chronic	EN: gastric vs jejunal delivery	1 PRCT	Jejunal feeding resulted in better intake and lower incidence of pneumonia
	EN: gastric vs postpyloric delivery	1 PRCT	Equal incidence of aspiration pneumonia unless tube at Ligament of Treitz or beyond
HIV disease	PN vs EN	PRCT	PN induced greater gain of weight, fat, and H$_2$O, but gain in body cell mass was similar, EN led to better physical functioning
	PN vs dietary counseling	PRCT	Two months of home PN improved body composition and Karnofsky index but did not change survival. Patients who then continued PN had longer survival: median survival on PN 199 days, with dietary counseling 57 days

[a] Only those disease states where SNS treatment has been evaluated by meta-analysis and/or prospective randomized controlled trials.

NOTE: SNS, specialized nutrition support; PN, parenteral nutrition; MA, meta-analysis; PRCT, prospective randomized control trial; PCM, protein calorie malnutrition; Early EN, tube feeding started within 48 h of onset of acute condition; EN, tube feeding; CEN, conditionally essential nutrients; W3FA, omega 3 fatty acids; CXT, chemotherapy; RXT, radiation therapy; BMT, bone marrow transplant; BCAA, branch chain amino acids; EAA, essential amino acids; NEAA, nonessential amino acids; IDPN, intradialytic parenteral nutrition; hGH, human growth hormone; HPN, home parenteral nutrition.

Nutrient	Metabolic Function
Glutamine	Fuel for enterocyte and immunocytes; preserves hepatic glutathione
Nucleotides	Derivatives (cyclicAMP, cyclicGMP) serve as mediators for many metabolic processes
Arginine	Enhances lymphocyte cytotoxicity via nitric oxide; substrate for polyamine synthesis; promotes protein synthesis via release of human growth hormone
Branched-chain amino acids	Level in muscle regulates muscle-protein breakdown; decreased in catabolic patients, especially those with liver disease
Sulfur-containing amino acids methionine ↓ S-adenosyl methionine (SAM) ↓ Homocysteine ↓ cysteine→glutathione taurine carnitine	Glutathione, chief cytoplasmic free radical scavenger; taurine, conjugates bile salts; carnitine, transports fatty acids into mitochondria for β-oxidation; SAM donates methyl group to choline and creatine, normalizes cell wall fluidity
Short-chain fatty acids	Derived by bacterial breakdown, from soluble fibers such as pectin; fuel for enterocytes, particularly colonocytes
Omega-3 fatty acids	Promote production of prostaglandins (PG) and leukotrienes (LT) of N-3 series (PGE$_3$, LTB$_5$, etc.) and reduce production from N-6 series (PGE$_2$, LTB$_4$, etc.), which are proinflammatory

benefit patients with both acute and chronic renal failure. Patients with acute renal failure given parenteral calories and amino acids have fewer infectious complications and a better chance of leaving the hospital than similar patients given only calories. An early randomized study showed benefit when essential amino acids were the sole source of nitrogen, but in other studies, standard solutions supplying both essential and nonessential amino acids provide similar advantage. Thus, the benefit of using expensive formulas containing only essential amino acids or their keto analogues is not established. A large national study failed to show any benefit of a low-protein diet on slowing progression of renal impairment in patients on chronic dialysis. Some 15 to 20% of patients on chronic dialysis have significant nutritional impairment, usually due to profound anorexia. The anorexia may improve with stepped-up dialysis or treatment of gastritis but usually persists. The resulting growth impairment in younger patients has been treated with supplemental tube enteral nutrition. This approach has not been widely used in adult patients. Limited parenteral calories and amino acids can be provided in the last 90 min of hemodialysis treatment (intradialytic parenteral nutrition). This may improve appetite, serum protein levels, and body weight. No randomized studies have documented better survival, so the appropriateness of this regimen is not established. Standard dialysis uses glucose to provide an osmotic load, and some glucose calories are absorbed. During continuous ambulatory peritoneal dialysis, amino acids can be substituted for glucose and are also partly absorbed, offsetting the loss of endogenous amino acids into the dialysate. This approach to nutrition repletion is expensive and also awaits a randomized study.

Pancreatitis Parenteral nutrition does not improve the outcome of patients with mild or moderate pancreatitis. However, in severe pancreatitis, survival decreases as malnutrition becomes more severe. When parenteral nutrition support was delayed beyond 72 h, patients with severe pancreatitis had a threefold higher complication and mortality rate, compared to similar patients treated earlier. In the absence of severe hyperlipidemia or thrombocytopenia, intravenous lipids appear safe and are especially useful if glucose intolerance is present.

Several studies report successful enteral jejunal feeding in acute pancreatitis and, compared to parenteral nutrition, the inflammatory response and infectious complications are less.

Inflammatory Bowel Disease Evidence of nutritional deficiencies such as weight loss, growth failure, anemia, and hypoalbuminemia are common in inflammatory bowel disease (IBD), more so in Crohn's disease than in ulcerative colitis (Chap. 287). Nutrition support plays a role in correcting these nutritional deficiencies, particularly prior to elective surgery. Since IBD often improves with diversion of the fecal stream, the question is whether bowel rest and parenteral nutrition have a role as primary treatment. However, randomized, prospective studies have shown no special benefit from bowel rest. Elemental diets are not quite as effective as glucocorticoids for inducing remission in acute Crohn's disease but may be preferable in children to avoid growth impairment. Relapse is common when a regular diet is resumed. In controlled studies, remissions are prolonged if the Crohn's patient does not return to a regular diet but instead eliminates from the diet those foods that induce gastrointestinal symptoms. For the majority of Crohn's patients this leads to avoidance of cereals, yeast, green vegetables, and, early on, dairy products. Because of the possibility that diets high in omega-3 fatty acids have a beneficial effect in immune disorders by altering prostaglandin synthesis, their value in IBD is under investigation. Some studies suggest that high-fiber diets benefit IBD patients, but fiber can also cause obstruction in patients with bowel strictures.

Short Bowel Syndrome Before the advent of parenteral nutrition, patients with acute short bowel syndrome from mesenteric vascular infarction or massive small bowel surgical resection seldom survived. Parenteral nutrition has allowed many patients to survive indefinitely with only a foot or two of small intestine. In some, the remaining bowel eventually adapts and allows the absorption of adequate calories and protein. This is especially true of patients who retain their iliocecal valve and colon. However, fluid and electrolyte imbalance may persist, necessitating some parenteral fluid and electrolyte support. A gradual switch to overnight tube enteral hydration or constant sipping of an electrolyte solution may allow discontinuation of all parenteral support.

Pulmonary Disease Weight loss in patients with advanced pulmonary disease is due to increased work of breathing and poor food intake. Patients with chronic pulmonary disease who are <90% of their ideal weight have a higher 5-year mortality, independent of pulmonary status. The recommended energy intake for these patients is 1.7 times their resting energy expenditure. The use of a low-carbohydrate formula is beneficial in the weaning of patients from ventilators, but the superiority of such formulas in ambulatory patients with chronic lung disease is not established. In cystic fibrosis, malnutrition may hasten pulmonary deterioration, and enteral tube feeding enhances growth and stabilizes or improves pulmonary function, particularly in young children. Tube feeding is safest when delivered into the jejunum. Postpyloric feeding is no safer than gastric feeding.

HIV Disease Specialized nutrition support can replete body cell mass if the weight loss is due to inadequate oral intake caused by oral or esophageal disease or to inadequate intestinal absorption, which is common in HIV patients with cryptosporidosis or microsporidiosis infections (Chap. 309). The route of nutrition support has usually been parenteral, but patients respond equally well with an isocaloric semielemental oral diet. Patients using the oral supplement experience a better quality of life, and their medical costs are significantly lower. Wasting due to systemic infection and increased cytokine secretion is not redressed by specialized nutrition support. Survival, CD4+ counts, and intestinal function also are not improved by specialized nutrition support.

Pregnancy Severe hyperemesis gravidarum can make any oral or tube enteral nutrition impossible, and profound weight loss and ketosis may harm the developing fetus. The underlying mechanism of the disorder is not understood, but it is cured by abortion or delivery.

Table 76-3 Summary of Outcomes for Patients on Home Parenteral and Enteral Nutrition (HPEN)

Diagnosis	Number in Group	Age in Years	% Survival[a] on Therapy	Therapy Status, % at 1 year[b,c] Full Oral Nutrition	Continued on HPEN Rx	Died	Rehabilitation[c,d] Status, % in 1st year C	P	M	Complications[e] per Patient-Year HPEN[c]	NonHPEN[c]
HOME PARENTERAL NUTRITION											
Crohn's disease	562	36	96	70	25	2	60	38	2	0.9	1.1
Ischemic bowel disease	331	49	87	27	48	19	53	41	6	1.4	1.1
Motility disorder	299	45	87	31	44	21	49	39	12	1.3	1.1
Congenital bowel defect	172	5	94	42	47	9	63	27	11	2.1	1.0
Hyperemesis gravidarum	112	28	100	100	0	0	83	16	1	1.5	3.5
Chronic pancreatitis	156	42	90	82	10	5	60	38	2	1.2	2.5
Radiation enteritis	145	58	87	28	49	22	42	49	9	0.8	1.1
Chronic adhesive obstructions	120	53	83	47	34	13	23	68	10	1.7	1.4
Cystic fibrosis	51	17	50	38	13	36	24	66	16	0.8	3.7
Cancer	2122	44	20	26	8	63	29	57	14	1.1	3.3
AIDS	280	33	10	13	6	73	8	63	29	1.6	3.3
HOME ENTERAL NUTRITION											
Neurologic disorders of swallowing	1134	65	55	19	25	48	5	24	71	0.3	0.9
Cancer	1644	61	30	30	6	59	21	59	21	0.4	2.7

[a] Survival rates on therapy are values at 1 year, calculated by the life table method. This will differ from the percentage listed as died under Therapy Status, since all patients with known endpoints are considered in this latter measure. The ratio of observed versus expected deaths is equivalent to a Standard Mortality Ratio.

[b] Not shown are those patients who were back in hospital or who had changed therapy type by 12 months.

[c] Chi-square test, $p < .05$

[d] Rehabilitation is designated complete (C), partial (P), or minimal (M), relative to the patient's ability to sustain normal age-related activity.

[e] Complications refer only to those complications that resulted in rehospitalization.

SOURCE: Derived from North American HPEN Registry.

Temporary parenteral nutrition usually results in a successful outcome, but nausea and vomiting tend to persist, despite bowel rest.

Home Parenteral and Enteral Nutrition Some patients require long-term nutrition support, and for many this can be administered at home. Clinical outcomes of patients with severe intestinal disorders that used either parenteral or enteral nutrition are summarized in Table 76-3. Nutrition support is not usually appropriate in terminally ill patients but is an option if the patient is expected to survive for several months. Such therapy must make sense to the patient, and sufficient help must be available so the treatment can be given at home without undue hazard. Both home therapies are relatively safe, with <5% therapy-related mortality.

THE DESIGN OF INDIVIDUAL REGIMENS Fluid Requirements These can be estimated by adding the normal daily requirement (120 mL/kg of body weight for infants, 35 mL/kg of body weight for adults) to any abnormal loss. If the patient is on parenteral therapy, any enteral intake should be subtracted from the estimate (Table 76-4). Since abnormal loss of enteric fluid implies significant mineral losses, extra amounts of these nutrients, as well as fluid (Table 76-5), must be added to the parenteral formula.

Energy Requirements These can be determined as outlined in Chaps. 73 and 74. In the long run, energy expenditure dictates energy requirements, but in the early phase of nutrition repletion, requirements may not reflect expenditure. For example, malnourished patients are hypometabolic and may expend only 85 kJ/kg (20 kcal/kg) per day, but more calories are needed both for tissue repletion and because the metabolic rate increases with refeeding. Conversely, a highly stressed patient (sepsis, trauma) may expend 165 kJ/kg (40 kcal/kg) per day with a significant proportion of the calories coming from protein breakdown and gluconeogenesis and from catecholamine-induced lipolysis. Oxidation of exogenous glucose plateaus at 100 kJ/kg (25 kcal/kg) per day, and administering additional glucose induces hepatic steatosis. Providing such patients with additional calories as exogenous fat does not suppress endogenous lipolysis. Furthermore, lipid solutions are made from vegetable oil and egg phospholipid and lack apoproteins, which they acquire from endogenous lipoproteins. Initially, the artificial chylomicron may be taken up by the reticuloendothelial system enhancing its blockade. For all these reasons, modest hypocaloric glucose feeding with minimal parenteral fat is safer in the acutely stressed subject.

Parenteral lipid solutions are available as 10 or 20% isotonic solutions and are infused separately from amino acids and glucose or as a combined "three-in-one solution," obviating the need for an extra pump. Three-in-one solutions are less stable than the glucose and amino acid mix, and destabilized fat particles have the potential to coalesce into larger droplets, becoming fat emboli. For this reason, three-in-one solutions have a shorter storage life and must be mixed by a phar-

---

Table 76-4 Estimation of Daily Fluid Requirements

NORMAL 70-KG MAN

Intake
Normal requirement: 35 × 70 = ~2500 ml/d (derived from oral liquids of 1200 mL, or 5 glasses/cups per day and solid food providing 1300 mL, 1000 mL from water in food, 300 mL from water generated by metabolism of foods)

Output
Urine: 1600 mL/d
Insensible loss: 800 mL/d
Stool: 100 mL/d
[sweat loss can be up to 2 L/d; each degree of fever (C) = 200 mL/d]

TUBE ENTERAL PATIENT

58-kg woman recovering from total gastrectomy for gastric cancer and supported by jejunostomy feedings, taking nothing by mouth or intravenously but experiencing 600 mL of diarrheal losses/day:
Normal requirement 35 × 58 = ~2000 mL/d
Abnormal gastrointestinal loss 600 − 100 = 500 mL/d
Total per tube requirement = 2500 mL/d

PARENTERAL PATIENT

66-kg man with a high jejunostomy following massive bowel resection for Crohn's disease with oral intake of 2000 mL/day and jejunostomy loss of 4000 mL/day:
Normal requirement 35 × 66 = 2300 mL/d
Abnormal gastrointestinal loss (4000 − 100) minus oral intake (2000) = 1900 mL/d
Total parenteral requirement = 4200 mL/d

	L/d[b]	Na, mmol/L	K,[c] mmol/L	Cl, mmol/L	HCO$_3$,[d] mmol/L
Oral intake	2–3				
Enteric secretions					
Saliva	1–2	10	30	10	30
Gastric juice	2	60	9	90	0
Bile	2–3	150	10	90	70
Small bowel	1	100	5	100	20
Colon	Variable	40	100	15	60

[a] Enteric secretions are also rich in divalent cations (Ca, Mg, Zn, Cu), and their loss is increased by steatorrhea, a high bowel fistula, or prolonged suction.

[b] Of the 9 L/d of oral and enteric fluid presented to the upper small bowel, normally 50% is absorbed in the jejunum, 40% in the ileum, and 10% in the colon. In short bowel patients, the colon may absorb greater amounts, up to 3 L/d.

[c] Potassium losses are small except in secretions distal to the ileocecal valve. The colon ion exchange is partly controlled by aldosterone, and therefore, Na$^+$ depletion increases K$^+$ loss in the stool.

[d] Bicarbonate losses must be replaced in parenteral solutions as acetane or lactate because of potential precipitation of bicarbonate with ingredients such as calcium.

macist knowledgeable about the correct mixing sequence and safe levels of electrolytes and trace elements. Iron, for example, cannot be added to this solution.

Polyunsaturated vegetable oils are used in most enteral formulas because they are absorbed better than animal fat by a diseased gastrointestinal tract. Fat must supply the essential fatty acid requirement (1 to 4% of energy from linoleic and linolenic acid) (Table 76-6). Larger amounts (30% of energy) are safe in relatively stable patients and avoid the problems of providing large amounts of glucose (e.g., hyperglycemia and hepatic steatosis). Substituting omega-3 polyunsaturated fish oils for polyunsaturated vegetable fats may reduce the catabolic response to burn injury, trauma, and radiation by reducing the synthesis of prostaglandins that enhance the inflammatory response

Table 76-6 Daily Enteral and Parenteral Requirements of Essential Fatty Acids, Minerals, and Vitamins

Nutrient	Daily Requirement, Adult Range	
	Enteral	Parenteral
Essential fatty acids, % kcal	1–2	2–4
Calcium, g	0.8–1.2	0.2–0.4
Phosphorus, g	0.8–1.2	0.4–0.8
Potassium, g	2–5	3–4
Sodium, g	1–3	1–3
Chloride, g	25–5	3–4[a]
Magnesium, g	0.3	0.3
Iron, mg	10	1–2
Zinc, mg	15	3–12
Copper, mg	2–3	0.3–0.5
Iodine, mg	0.15	0.15
Manganese, mg	2–5	2–5
Chromium, μg	50–200	15–30
Molybdenum, μg	150–300	20–120
Selenium, μg	50–200	50–100
Ascorbic acid, mg	60	100
Thiamine, mg	1.4	3.0
Riboflavin, mg	1.6	3.6
Niacin, mg	18	40
Biotin, μg	60	60
Pantothenic acid, mg	5	15
Pyridoxine, mg	2.0	4.0
Folic acid, μg	400	400
Cobalamin, μg	3.0	5
Vitamin A, μg	1000	1000
Vitamin D, μg	10	5–10
Vitamin E, mg	8–10	10–15
Vitamin K, μg	70–140	200

[a] In addition to chloride anions there is a parenteral requirement for bicarbonate equivalents to protect normal acid-base balance. These are provided as 90 mmoL or more per day of acetate or lactate because of potential precipitation of bicarbonate with ingredients such as calcium.

(Table 76-2). Such fats are available in enteral formulas and are currently being tested in parenteral formulas.

Protein or Amino Acid Requirements The recommended dietary protein allowance of 0.8 g/kg per day is adequate for nonstressed patients, such as a starved patient with a high-grade esophageal stricture. Catabolic patients, in contrast, may require up to 1.5 g/kg per day of protein to induce positive nitrogen balance and reconstitute normal body mass. Early studies showed that recombinant human growth hormone (rHGH) increases lean body mass. However, subsequent trials have shown that it is associated with increased mortality in critically ill patients, and it should not be used in this setting.

In a stable patient the adequacy of protein support can be assessed by analyzing protein balance:

$$\text{Protein balance} = \text{protein intake} - \text{protein loss}$$

where protein loss = [(24-h urine urea nitrogen (g) + 4) × 6.25]. Over a long period, protein balance is assessed by documenting wound healing, restoration of normal body composition, or resumption of longitudinal growth. In states of disturbed protein utilization (e.g., renal and hepatic failure), azotemia and abnormal plasma amino acid patterns develop. The benefit of special enteral and parenteral solutions that correct these aberrations is only established in hepatic encephalopathy (see "Risks and Benefits of Nutrition Support").

Certain nutrients that can normally be synthesized endogenously become essential in severely ill patients when endogenous production or salvage pathways are impaired. This is true of glutamine, nucleotides, and the products of methionine metabolism (Table 76-2). Glutamine, an important fuel for the enterocyte and lymphocyte, is fairly insoluble and is absent from standard parenteral formulas and present in low concentrations in most enteral formulas. Soluble glutamine-containing dipeptides are under investigation.

Nucleotides and their related metabolic products have beneficial effects on the immune system, growth of the small intestine, lipid metabolism, and hepatic function. Nucleotides can be synthesized de novo in all cells only in small amounts, and the body therefore depends on dietary nucleotides or on salvage pathways that recycle nucleotides from purine and pyrimidine turnover. Nutritionally depleted patients benefit from formulas enriched in nucleotides.

When amino acids are infused systemically, rather than via the more physiologic portal vein, methionine, the only sulfur-containing amino acid in most parenteral solutions, is transaminated in peripheral tissues rather than transulfurated in the liver. As a result, downstream sulfur products such as carnitine, taurine, and glutathione become relatively deficient (Chap. 352). Preliminary studies suggest that the addition of an intermediate compound, *S*-adenosyl methionine, to parenteral solutions results in less cholestasis.

Mineral and Vitamin Requirements Parenteral and enteral mineral and vitamin requirements are summarized in Table 76-6. Electrolyte modifications are necessary if the patient has significant gastrointestinal losses (Table 76-5) or renal failure. Requirements of some minerals and vitamins are higher when administered parenterally for several reasons: (1) many micronutrients delivered into the systemic rather than the portal circulation are not captured by the liver and instead pass directly into the urine; (2) patients with bowel disease may have enteric loss of sodium, potassium, chloride, and bicarbonate and malabsorption of divalent cations, fat-soluble vitamins, and vitamin B$_{12}$; and (3) nutrients may adhere to the tubing and delivery bags, and exposure to oxygen and light may destroy vitamins (particularly vitamin A).

PARENTERAL NUTRITION **Infusion Technique and Patient Monitoring** Partial and short-term total parenteral nutrition can be provided via a peripheral vein if the majority of the energy is supplied by isotonic fat solutions; long-term total parenteral nutrition using glucose as the chief energy source requires administration via a central vein catheter so the hypertonic solution can be rapidly diluted

Table 76-7 Central Venous Access for Parenteral Nutrition

Type of Catheters	Advantages	Disadvantages

Peripherally inserted central catheter
  Single lumen
  Double lumen
	Insertion cost low; can be done at bedside or by vascular radiology using Doppler guidance; especially advantageous for patients with neck wounds such as tracheostomies	High incidence of skin site irritation; tendency to break at hub; patient requires assistance with weekly dressing change

Centrally inserted externalized catheter (subclavian, jugular, femoral)
  Single lumen
  Triple lumen
	Can be inserted at bedside; relatively low cost; can be changed over a guidewire if clinically indicated; catheter sepsis rate within subclavian < jugular < femoral vein	10% incidence of mechanical complication with insertion, higher if physician inexperienced; need dedicated nutrition line; multiple-lumen catheters have increased sepsis rate

Centrally inserted, tunneled catheter or subcutaneous port	More stable for long-term use; when needle out, patients with ports have less disturbance of body image and can shower and swim without risk	More expensive device requiring operating room insertion; ports require needle stick.

in a high-flow system. The preferred site for central vein infusion is the superior vena cava. Access sites and catheter choices are summarized in Table 76-7. Peripherally inserted central catheters are the most economical option for short-term parenteral nutrition. In one randomized study, the number of catheter-related infections was the same with peripherally and centrally inserted catheters. Tunneled catheters and implanted subcutaneous ports require operating room insertion and are more stable for long-term use. Central catheters should be changed when clinically indicated; routine changes are costly and hazardous. Chlorhexidine solution is a more effective local antiseptic than iodophor or alcohol. Although transparent dressings are helpful in stabilizing catheters and allow easy observation of the skin site, the incidence of catheter-related sepsis is higher than with traditional dry gauze dressings; newer transparent dressings that trap less moisture are under investigation. Catheters made from Silastic material or polyurethane are associated with lower complications than polyvinylchloride catheters. Several types of needleless systems use hub valves, and contamination rates are higher with these devices when used for long-term parenteral nutrition. Appropriate clinical and laboratory monitoring for patients on parenteral nutrition are summarized in Table 76-8.

Complications (See Table 76-9) • *Mechanical* The insertion of a central venous catheter should be done only by trained personnel under aseptic techniques. Major mechanical complications include pneumothorax; hemothorax from laceration of the subclavian artery or vein; brachial plexus injury; and malpositioning of the catheter in a cerebral vein, the azygos vein, or the right ventricle. The correct catheter position must be confirmed by x-ray before hypertonic nutrient solution is infused. Catheters can subsequently dislocate, develop leaks, or become detached from the hub and embolize into the heart or pulmonary artery. Catheter thrombosis may occur, especially if the catheter is used for withdrawing blood samples, and extension of the thrombosis to the central vein is frequently coincident with infection. Thrombosed catheters can sometimes be unblocked by urokinase treatment. The addition of low-dose heparin (1000 U/L) to limit thrombosis in parenteral catheters is controversial; no randomized, controlled studies demonstrate benefit, and heparin can contribute to loss of bone mineral, which is already a problem with long-term parenteral nutrition.

Metabolic Fluid overload can cause congestive heart failure, particularly in elderly and debilitated patients. Glucose overload can cause an osmotic diuresis or stimulate insulin secretion, which in turn promotes extracellular to intracellular shifts of potassium and phosphorous. Such shifts are most dangerous in cachectic patients with depletion of potassium and phosphorus stores and can cause arrhythmias, cardiopulmonary dysfunction, and neurologic symptoms. To avoid these problems, parenteral nutrition should be started slowly and mon-

itored carefully. Glucose content is increased gradually as the patient demonstrates tolerance of the high glucose load. Late metabolic complications include cholestatic liver disease with bile sludging and gallstone formation. The exact cause of the liver disease is not understood, but lack of enteral stimulation to bile flow and defective sulfur amino acid metabolism and cholesterol solubilization appear to play a role. Cholestasis is less likely to occur if some enteral feeding is maintained. Parenteral nutrition induces hypercalciuria, which can result in negative calcium balance and osteopenia. Hypercalciuria may have several causes, including the high fixed-acid load of infused amino acids and the bisulfite preservative in parenteral solutions. Earlier, protein hydrolysates were used as an amino acid source and were contaminated with aluminum, which blocked bone mineralization. Aluminum is still a contaminant of some additives such as calcium gluconate. Once patients on long-term parenteral nutrition change from catabolic breakdown to sustained anabolism, deficiencies of micronutrients such as essential fatty acids, trace minerals, and vitamins may develop unless they are supplied in adequate amounts (Table 76-6).

Infectious Infection of the access line rarely occurs in the first 72 h, and fever during this period is usually due to infection elsewhere or some other cause. Infection of the access line is likely if the fever defervesces when the infusion of the parenteral formula is tapered.

Positive central line cultures suggest catheter sepsis, especially if no other infectious source is identified and if the organism is *Staphylococcus* or *Candida*. Although removal of the central catheter may allow fungemia to clear spontaneously, antibiotic therapy is recommended for bacterial infections and the more invasive fungi. Catheter sepsis rates are similar in single lumen central lines dedicated to parenteral nutrition whether inserted peripherally via the subclavian vein

Table 76-8 Monitoring the Patient on Total Parenteral Nutrition

CLINICAL DATA MONITORED DAILY

Sense of well-being: symptoms suggesting fluid overload, high or low blood glucose, electrolyte imbalance, etc.

Strength as judged by graded activity: getting out of bed, walking, stair climbing

Vital signs: temperature, blood pressure, pulse rate, and respiratory rate

Fluid balance: weight; fluid input (intravenous +/− enteral) versus fluid output (urine, stool, gastric suction, etc.).

Delivery equipment for parenteral nutrition: composition of nutrient solution, tubing, pump, filter, catheter, dressing (skin checked for local infection at time of dressing change)

LABORATORY DATA

Fingerstick glucose	Three times daily until patient stable
Blood glucose Na⁺, K⁺, CL⁻, HCO₃⁻ Blood urea nitrogen	Daily until glucose infusion load and patient stable, then twice weekly
Liver function studies Serum creatinine, albumin PO₄³⁻, Ca²⁺, Mg²⁺ Hb/Hct, WBC	Baseline, then twice weekly
Clotting, INR	Baseline, then weekly
Micronutrient tests as indicated	

NOTE: Hb, hemoglobin; Hct, hematocrit; WBC, white blood cell (count); INR, international normalized ratio.

or tunneled; multiple-lumen catheters are associated with a greater incidence of sepsis. While there is no evidence to support the use of prophylactic antibiotics, recurrent catheter sepsis may be avoided if cuffs are used around the catheter exit site or small amounts of an antibiotic solution are left in the line along with a heparin lock.

ENTERAL NUTRITION Tube Placement and Patient Monitoring The types of enteral feeding tubes, methods of insertion, their clinical uses, and potential complications are outlined in Table 76-10. The different types of enteral formulas are listed in Table 76-11. Patients on enteral feeding are at risk for many of the same metabolic complications as those receiving parenteral nutrition and should be monitored in the same way (Table 76-8). Since small-bore tubes are easily displaced, tube position should be checked at intervals by aspirating and measuring the pH of the gut fluid (<4 in stomach, >6 in jejunum).

Complications • *Aspiration* The debilitated patient with poor gastric emptying and impairment of swallowing and cough mechanisms is at risk for aspiration; this is particularly so for those on respirators. Tracheal suctioning induces coughing and gastric regurgitation, and cuffs on endotracheal or tracheostomy tubes seldom provide protection against aspiration. Under these circumstances, it may be safer to use a large-bore feeding tube to allow for temporary removal of gastric contents during tracheal suction or to use jejunal feeding. Constant gastric infusion of an enteral formula is better tolerated in sick patients than intermittent bolus feeding. A continuous infusion is best achieved with a pump, especially when using fine-bore tubes that

have a greater potential to clog. If long-term feeding is anticipated, endoscopic, radiologic, or surgical placement of a gastric tube is preferred by most patients. For long-term ambulatory patients, a gastrostomy tube can be converted to a gastric "button," an access device that is flush with the skin. A nasojejunal tube reduces the risk of aspiration. However, fluoroscopically guided placement of fine-bore tubes through the pylorus is time-consuming, and such tubes frequently pull back into the stomach. A percutaneous combined gastric-suction and jejunal-feeding tube is more reliable. This can be placed radiologically, endoscopically, or surgically.

Diarrhea Enteral feeding often causes diarrhea, especially if bowel function is compromised by bowel disease or drugs. The diarrhea may be controlled by the use of continuous feeding of fiber-containing formulas or by adding an antichdinergic medication to the

Table 76-9   Complications of Total Parenteral Nutrition (TPN)

First 48 h	First 2 Weeks	3 Months Onward
MECHANICAL		

Complications from catheter insertion:
  Cephalad displacement
  Pneumothorax
  Hemothorax
Detachment of line at catheter hub
  with blood loss or air embolism
	Catheter coming out of vein, more common if Silastic
	Detachment of line at catheter hub with blood loss or air embolism
	Thrombosis
		Detachment of line at catheter hub with blood loss or air embolism
		Fractures or tears in catheter
		Catheter embedded in vein wall

METABOLIC		
Fluid overload Hyperglycemia Hypophosphatemia Hypokalemia	Cardiopulmonary failure Refeeding edema Hyperosmolar nonketotic hyperglycemic coma Acid-base imbalance Electrolyte imbalance	Essentially fatty acid deficiency Iron deficiency Vitamin deficiencies TPN metabolic bone disease TPN liver disease Zinc, copper, chromium, selenium, molybdenum, deficiency
INFECTIOUS		
	Catheter-induced sepsis Exit site infection	Catheter-induced sepsis Tunnel infections Exit site infection

Table 76-10   Enteral Feeding Tubes

Type/Insertion Technique	Clinical Uses	Potential Complications
NASOGASTRIC TUBE		
External measurement, nostril, ear, xiphisternum; tube stiffened by ice water or stylet; position verified by injecting air and auscultating, aspirating gastric acid, or by x-ray	Short-term clinical situation (weeks) or longer periods with intermittent insertion; bolus feeding simpler, but continuous drip with pump better tolerated	Aspiration; ulceration of nasal and esophageal tissues, leading to stricture
NASOJEJUNAL TUBE		
External measurement: nostril, ear, anterior superior iliac spine (medical malleolus in infants); tube stiffened by stylet and passed through pylorus under fluoroscopy or with endoscopic loop	Short-term clinical situations where gastric emptying impaired or proximal leak suspected; requires continuous drip with pump	Spontaneous pulling back into stomach (position reverified by aspirating content pH > 6); diarrhea common, fiber-containing formula may help
GASTROSTOMY TUBE		
Percutaneous placement endoscopically, radiologically, or surgically: after tract established, can be converted to a gastric "button"	Long-term clinical situations, swallowing disorders, or impaired small-bowel absorption requiring continuous drip	Aspiration; irritation around tube exit site; peritoneal leak; balloon migration and obstruction of pylorus
JEJUNOSTOMY TUBE		
Percutaneous placement endoscopically or radiologically via pylorus or surgically into jejunum sutured to abdominal wall using fine-bore tube or larger tube	Long-term clinical situations where gastric emptying impaired; requires continuous drip with pump	Clogging or displacement of tube; jejunal fistula if large-bore tube used; diarrhea
COMBINED GASTROJEJUNOSTOMY TUBE		
Percutaneous placement endoscopically, radiologically, or surgically; intragastric arm for continuous or intermittent gastric suction; jejunal arm for enteral feeding	Used for patients with impaired gastric emptying and at high risk for aspiration or patients with acute pancreatitis or proximal leaks	Clogging; irritation around tube exit site

Table 76-11 Enteral Formulas

Composition Characteristics	Clinical Indication
STANDARD ENTERAL FORMULA	

1. Complete dietary products (+)[a]
   a. Caloric density 1 kcal/mL
   b. Protein ~14% cals, caseinates, soy, lactalbumin
   c. Fat ~30% cals, corn, soy, safflower oils
   d. CHO ~60% cals, hydrolysed corn starch, maltodextrin, sucrose
   e. Recommended daily intake of all minerals and vitamins in ≥1500 kcal/d
   f. Osmolality (mosm/kg) ~300
	Suitable for most patients requiring tube feeding; flavors available for oral use

MODIFIED ENTERAL FORMULAS	
1. Caloric density 1.5–2 kcal/mL (+)	Fluid-restricted patients

2. a. High protein ~20% cals (+)
   b. Hydrolysed protein to small peptides (++)
   c. ↑ Glutamine, arginine, S-containing amino acids, nucleotides (+++)
 	
   d. ↑ Branch-chain amino acids, ↓ aromatic amino acids (+++)
   e. ↓ Protein, ↓ K, Mg, and P diets (++)
   f. ↓ Protein, ↑ essential amino acids, ↓ minerals and vitamins (+++)
	Protein malnutrition and ↓ wound healing
	 ↓ Protein digestion/absorption or allergy
	 Severely immunocompromised patients
	 Liver failure patients intolerant of 0.8 g/kg per day of regular protein
	
	 Renal failure patients
	 Renal failure patients not on dialysis

3. a. Low fat, partial MCT substitution (+)
   b. ↑ Fat >40% cals (++)
   c. ↑ Fat from MUFA (++)
   d. Fat ↑ in ω3 (fish oil) and ↓ ω6 (+++)
 4. a. Fiber provided as soy poly saccharide (+)
   b. Fiber provided as blenderized fruits and vegetables (++)
 5. ↑ Minerals (Zn) and vitamins (A and C) (++)
	Fat malabsorption
	 Pulmonary failure with ↑ P_{CO_2} on standard formulas
	 Poorly controlled diabetes mellitus
	 Immunocompromised and autoimmune disorder
	 Diarrhea/constipation
	 ↓ Binding of dilantin
	 Decubitus ulcers

[a] Cost: + inexpensive; + + moderately expensive; + + + very expensive.
NOTE: CHO, carbohydrate; MCT, medium-chain triglyceride; MUFA, monounsaturated fatty acid, ω3 or ω6 polyunsatuated fat with first double bond at carbon 3 (fish oils) or carbon 6 (vegetable oils).

formula. Diarrhea associated with enteral feeding does not necessarily imply inadequate absorption of nutrients, other than water and electrolytes. Furthermore, since luminal nutrients exert trophic effects on the gut mucosa and enhance the enteric immunologic barrier, it is often appropriate to persist with tube feeding, despite the diarrhea, even when this necessitates supplemental parenteral fluid support.

THE SCOPE AND COST OF NUTRITION SUPPORT

As many as 25% of patients entering tertiary care hospitals have central catheters placed, and 20 to 30% of these catheters are used for parenteral nutrition. The incidence of catheter-related infection reflects the severity of the underlying medical condition and varies from 2 to 30 per thousand catheter days, depending on the type of patients involved. In critically ill patients, catheter sepsis is associated with a 35% mortality rate and a high cost per survivor. Most catheter-related complications derive from faulty insertion and management of the catheter rather than defects in the device. In large tertiary care hospitals, the insertion and management of these lines by specially trained teams can reduce complications by 80%, impacting significantly on outcome and costs. A growing shift from parenteral to enteral nutrition also promises significant cost savings. Home parenteral nutrition costs approximately half as much as similar treatment in the hospital, and home enteral nutrition costs much less.

BIBLIOGRAPHY

AMERICAN COLLEGE OF PHYSICIANS: Position paper: Parenteral nutrition in patients receiving cancer chemotherapy: A meta-analysis. Ann Intern Med 110:734, 1989

ANDERSON JD et al: Enteral feeding in the critically injured patient. Nutr Clin Pract 7:117, 1992

CHARUHAS PN et al: A double-blind randomized trial comparing outpatient parenteral nutrition with intravenous hydration: Effect on resumption of oral intake after marrow transplantation. JPEN 21:157, 1997

FLYNN MB, LEIGHTTY FF: Preoperative outpatient nutritional support of patients with squamous cancer of the upper aerodigestive tract. Am J Surg 154:359, 1987

FOULKS CJ et al: An evidence-based evaluation of intradialytic parenteral nutrition. Am J Kidney Dis 33:186, 1999

GRIFFITHS AM et al: Meta-analysis of enteral nutrition as a primary treatment of active Crohn's disease. Gastroenterology 108:1056, 1995

HEYLAND DK et al: Total parenteral nutrition in the critically ill patient: A meta-analysis. JAMA 280:2013, 1998

HEYS SD et al: Enteral nutritional supplementation with key nutrients in patients with critical illness and cancer: A meta-analysis of randomized controlled clinical trials. Ann Surg 228:467, 1999

HILL GL: Body composition research: Implications for the practice of clinical nutrition. J Parenter Enter Nutr 16:197, 1992

HOWARD L et al: Current use and clinical outcome of home parenteral and enteral nutrition therapies in the United States. Gastroenterology 109:335, 1995

KALFARENTZOS F et al: Enteral nutrition is superior to parenteral nutrition in severe acute pancreatitis: Results of a randomized prospective trial. Br J Surg 84:1665, 1997

KLEIN S et al: Nutritional support in clinical practice: Review of published data and recommendations for future research directions. Am J Clin Nutr 66:683, 1997

KOTLER DP et al: Comparison of total parenteral nutrition and an oral, semielemental diet on body composition, physical function, and nutrition-related costs in patients with malabsorption due to acquired immunodeficiency syndrome. JPEN 22:120, 1998

LIPMAN TO: Clinical trials of nutrition support in cancer. Hematol Oncol Clin North Am 5:91, 1991

MELCHIOR JC et al: Improved survival by home total parenteral nutrition in AIDS patients: Follow-up of a controlled randomized prospective trial. AIDS 12:336, 1998

MOORE FA et al: Early enteral feeding, compared with parenteral, reduces postoperative septic complications. The results of a meta-analysis. Ann Surg 216:172, 1992

NAYLOR CD et al: Parenteral nutrition with branched-chain amino acids in hepatic encephalopathy: A meta-analysis. Gastroenterology 97:1033, 1989

RAAD II et al: Infectious complications of indwelling vascular catheters. Clin Infect Dis 15:197, 1992

RIORDAN AM et al: Treatment of active Crohn's disease by exclusion diet: East Anglian Multicenter Controlled Trial. Lancet 342:1131, 1993

SCOLAPIO JS et al: Effect of growth hormone, glutamine, and diet on adaption in short bowel syndrome. A randomized controlled study. Gastroenterology 113:1074, 1997

TRALLORI MA et al: Defined formula diets versus steroids in the treatment of active Crohn's disease. Scan J Gastroenterol 31:267, 1996

VETERANS ADMINISTRATION TOTAL PARENTERAL NUTRITION COOPERATIVE STUDY. Perioperative total parenteral nutrition in surgical patients. N Engl J Med 325:525, 1991

WEINSIER RL et al: Cost containment: A contribution of aggressive nutrition support in burn patients. J Burn Care Rehabil 6:436, 1985

WEISDORF S et al: Influence of prophylactic total parenteral nutrition on long-term outcome of bone marrow transplantation. Transplantation 43:833, 1987

ZIEGLER TR et al: Clinical and metabolic efficacy of glutamine-supplemented parenteral nutrition after bone marrow transplantation. Ann Intern Med 116:821, 1992

77

OBESITY

ACTH	adrenocorticotropic hormone
AgRP	Agouti-related peptide
BAT	brown adipose tissue
BMI	body mass index
CHF	congestive heart failure
LDL	low-density lipoprotein
MSH	melanocyte-stimulating hormone
NIDDM	non-insulin-dependent diabetes mellitus
NPY	neuropeptide Y
PPARγ	peroxisome proliferator-activated receptor γ
SHBG	sex hormone–binding globulin
TNF	tumor necrosis factor
UCP	uncoupling protein

In a world where food supplies are intermittent, the ability to store energy in excess of what is required for immediate use is essential for survival. Fat cells, residing within widely distributed adipose tissue depots, are adapted to store excess energy efficiently as triglyceride and, when needed, to release stored energy as free fatty acids for use at other sites. This physiologic system, orchestrated through endocrine and neural pathways, permits humans to survive starvation for as long as several months. However, in the presence of nutritional abundance and a sedentary lifestyle, and influenced importantly by genetic endowment, this system increases adipose energy stores and produces adverse health consequences.

DEFINITION AND MEASUREMENT   *Obesity* is a state of excess adipose tissue mass. Although often viewed as equivalent to increased body weight, this need not be the case—lean but very muscular individuals may be overweight by arbitrary standards without having increased adiposity. Body weights are distributed continuously in populations, so that a medically meaningful distinction between lean and obese is somewhat arbitrary. Obesity is therefore more effectively defined by assessing its linkage to morbidity or mortality.

Although not a direct measure of adiposity, the most widely used method to gauge obesity is the *body mass index* (BMI), which is equal to weight/height^2 (in kg/m^2) (Fig. 77-1). Other approaches to quantifying obesity include anthropometry (skin-fold thickness), densitometry (underwater weighing), computed tomography (CT) or magnetic resonance imaging (MRI), and electrical impedance. Using data from the Metropolitan Life Tables, BMIs for the midpoint of all heights and frames among both men and women range from 19 to 26 kg/m^2; at a similar BMI, women have more body fat than men. Based on unequivocal data of substantial morbidity, a BMI of 30 is most commonly used as a threshold for obesity in both men and women. Large-scale epidemiologic studies suggest that all-cause, metabolic, and cardiovascular morbidity begin to rise (albeit at a slow rate) when BMIs are ≥ 25, suggesting that the cut-off for obesity should be lowered. Some authorities use the term *overweight* (rather than obese) to describe individuals with BMIs between 25 or 27 and 30. A BMI between 25 and 30 should be viewed as medically significant and worthy of therapeutic intervention, especially in the presence of risk factors that are influenced by adiposity, such as hypertension and glucose intolerance.

The distribution of adipose tissue in different anatomic depots also has substantial implications for morbidity. Specifically, intraabdominal and abdominal subcutaneous fat have more significance than subcutaneous fat present in the buttocks and lower extremities. This distinction is most easily made by determining the waist-to-hip ratio, with a ratio >0.9 in women and >1.0 in men being abnormal. Many of the most important complications of obesity, such as insulin resistance, diabetes, hypertension, and hyperlipidemia, and hyperandrogenism in women, are linked more strongly to intraabdominal and/or upper body fat than to overall adiposity. The mechanism underlying this association is unknown but may relate to the fact that intraabdominal adipocytes are more lipolytically active than those from other depots. Release of free fatty acids into the portal circulation has adverse metabolic actions, especially on the liver.

PREVALENCE   Recent data from the National Health and Nutrition Examination Surveys (NHANES) show that the percent of the American adult population with obesity (BMI > 30) has increased from 14.5% (between 1976 and 1980) to 22.5% (between 1998 and 1994). As many as 50% of U.S. adults ≥20 years of age were overweight (defined as BMI > 25) between the years of 1998 and 1991. Because substantial health risks exist in many individuals with BMI between 25 and 30, the increasing prevalence of medically significant obesity raises great concern. Obesity is more common among women and in the poor; the prevalence in children is also rising at a worrisome rate.

PHYSIOLOGIC REGULATION OF ENERGY BALANCE   Substantial evidence suggests that body weight is regulated by both endocrine and neural components that ultimately influence the effector arms of energy intake and expenditure. This complex regulatory system is necessary because even small imbalances between energy intake and expenditure will ultimately have large effects on body weight. For example, a 0.3% positive imbalance over 30 years would result in a 9-kg (20-lb) weight gain. Alterations in stable weight by forced overfeeding or food deprivation induce physiologic changes that resist these perturbations: with weight loss, appetite increases and energy expenditure falls; with overfeeding, appetite falls and energy expenditure increases. This latter compensatory mechanism frequently fails, however, permitting obesity to develop when food is abundant and physical activity is limited. A major regulator of these adaptative responses is the adipocyte-derived hormone leptin, which acts through brain circuits (predominantly in the hypothalamus) to influence appetite, energy expenditure, and neuroendocrine function (see below).

Appetite is influenced by many factors that are integrated by the brain, most importantly within the hypothalamus (Fig. 77-2). Signals that impinge on the hypothalamic center include neural afferents, hormones, and metabolites. Vagal inputs are particularly important, bringing information from viscera, such as gut distention. Hormonal signals include leptin, insulin, cortisol, and gut peptides such as cholecystokinin, which signals to the brain through the vagus nerve. Metabolites, including glucose, can influence appetite, as seen by the effect of hypoglycemia to induce hunger; however, glucose is not normally a major regulator of appetite. These diverse hormonal, metabolic, and neural signals act by influencing the expression and release of various hypothalamic peptides [e.g., neuropeptide Y (NPY), Agouti-related peptide (AgRP), α melanocyte-stimulating hormone (MSH), and melanin concentrating hormone (MCH)] that are integrated with serotonergic, catecholaminergic, and opioid signaling pathways (see below). Psychological and cultural factors also appear to play a role in the final expression of appetite. Apart from rare syndromes involving leptin, its receptor, and the melanocortin system (see below), the defects in this complex appetite control network that account for common causes of obesity are not well understood.

Energy expenditure includes the following components: (1) resting or basal metabolic rate; (2) the energy cost of metabolizing and storing food; (3) the thermic effect of exercise; and (4) adaptive thermogenesis, which varies in response to chronic caloric intake (rising with increased intake). Basal metabolic rate accounts for about 70% of daily energy expenditure, whereas active physical activity contributes 5 to 10%. Thus, a significant component of daily energy consumption is fixed.

Adaptive thermogenesis occurs in *brown adipose tissue* (BAT), which plays an important role in energy metabolism in many mammals. In contrast to white adipose tissue, which is used to store energy in the form of lipids, BAT expends stored energy as heat. A mitochondrial *uncoupling protein* (UCP-1) in BAT dissipates the hydrogen ion gradient in the oxidative respiration chain and releases energy as heat. The metabolic activity of BAT is increased by a central action of leptin, acting through the sympathetic nervous system, which heavily innervates this tissue. In rodents, BAT deficiency causes obesity and diabetes; stimulation of BAT with a specific adrenergic agonist

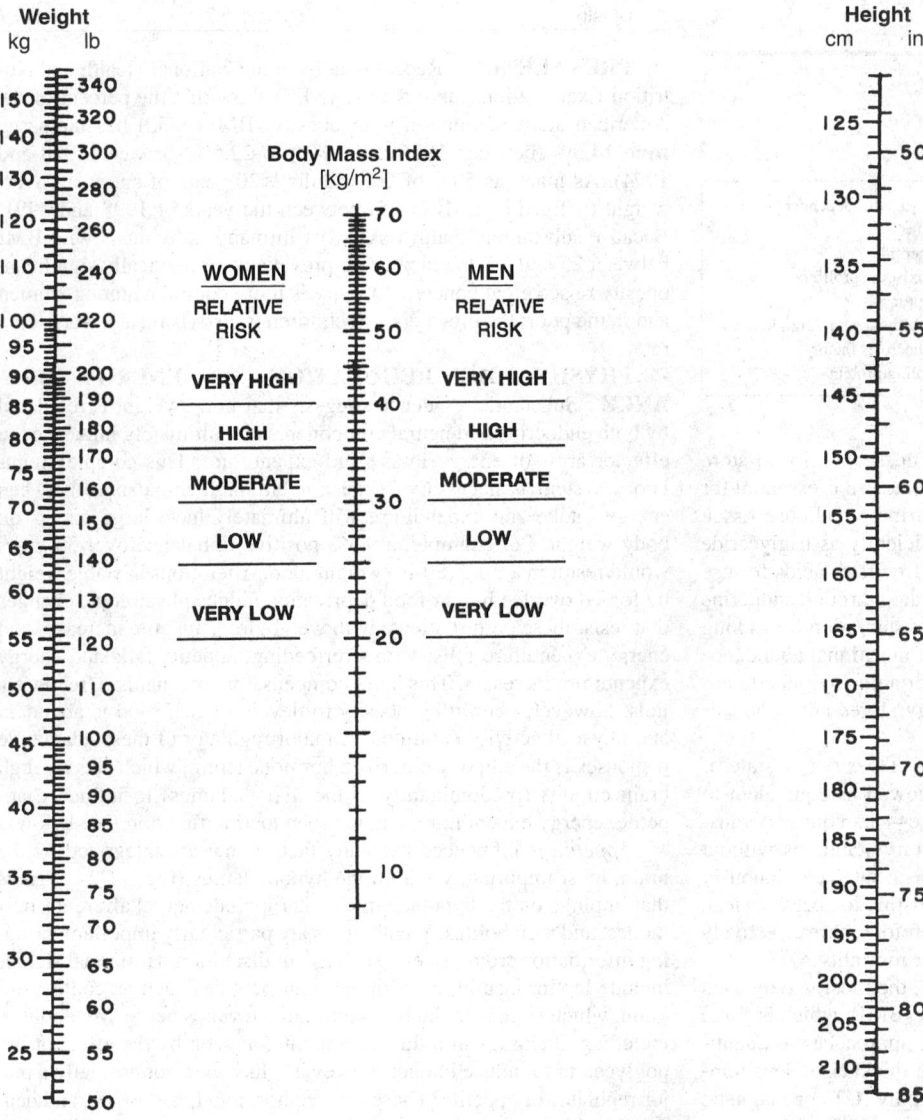

FIGURE 77-1 Nomogram for determining body mass index. To use this nomogram, place a ruler or other straight edge between the body weight (without clothes) in kilograms or pounds located on the left-hand line and the height (without shoes) in centimeters or in inches located on the right-hand line. The body mass index is read from the middle of the scale and is in metric units. (*Copyright 1978, George A. Bray, MD. Used with permission.*)

(β_3 agonist) protects against diabetes and obesity. Although BAT exists in humans (especially neonates), its physiologic role is not yet established. Homologues of UCP-1 may mediate uncoupled mitochondrial respiration in other tissues.

THE ADIPOCYTE AND ADIPOSE TISSUE Adipose tissue is composed of the lipid-storing adipose cell and a stromal/vascular compartment in which preadipocytes reside. Adipose mass increases by enlargement of adipose cells through lipid deposition, as well as by an increase in the number of adipocytes. The process by which adipose cells are derived from a mesenchymal preadipocyte involves an orchestrated series of differentiation steps mediated by a cascade of specific transcription factors. One of the key transcription factors is *peroxisome proliferator-activated receptor* γ (PPARγ), a nuclear receptor that binds the thiazoladinedione class of insulin-sensitizing drugs used in the treatment of type 2 diabetes (Chap. 333).

Although the adipocyte has generally been regarded as a storage depot for fat, it is also an endocrine cell that releases numerous molecules in a regulated fashion (Fig. 77-3). These include the energy balance-regulating hormone leptin, cytokines such as tumor necrosis factor (TNF) α, complement factors such as factor D (also known as adipsin), prothrombotic agents such as plasminogen activator inhibitor I, and a component of the blood pressure regulating system, angioten-

sinogen. These factors, and others not yet identified, play a role in the physiology of lipid homeostasis, insulin sensitivity, blood pressure control, and coagulation and are likely to contribute to obesity-related pathologies.

ETIOLOGY OF OBESITY

Though the molecular pathways regulating energy balance are beginning to be illuminated, the causes of obesity remain elusive. In part, this reflects the fact that obesity is a heterogeneous group of disorders. At one level, the pathophysiology of obesity seems simple: a chronic excess of nutrient intake relative to the level of energy expenditure. However, due to the complexity of the neuroendocrine and metabolic systems that regulate energy intake, storage, and expenditure, it has been difficult to quantitate all the relevant parameters (e.g., food intake and energy expenditure) over time in human subjects.

Role of Genes vs. Environment Obesity is commonly seen in families. Inheritance is usually not Mendelian, however, and it is difficult to distinguish the role of genes and environmental factors. Adoptees usually resemble their biologic rather than adoptive parents with respect to obesity, providing strong support for genetic influences. Likewise, identical twins have very similar BMIs whether reared together or apart, and their BMIs are much more strongly correlated than those of dizygotic twins. These genetic effects appear to relate to both energy intake and expenditure.

Whatever the role of genes, it is clear that the environment plays a key role in obesity, as evidenced by the fact that famine prevents obesity in even the most obesity-prone individual. In addition, the recent increase in the prevalence of obesity in the United States is too rapid to be due to changes in the gene pool. Cultural factors are also important—these relate to both availability and composition of the diet and to changes in the level of physical activity.

FIGURE 77-2 The factors that regulate appetite through effects on central neural circuits. Some factors that increase or decrease appetite are listed. NPY, neuropeptide Y; MCH, melanin concentrating hormone; AgRP, Agouti-related peptide; MSH, melanocyte stimulating hormone; CART, cocaine- and amphetamine-related transcript; GLP-1, glucagon-related peptide-1; CCk, cholecystokinin.

FIGURE 77-3 Factors released by the adipocyte that can affect peripheral tissues. PAI, plasminogen activator inhibitor; TNF, tumor necrosis factor.

In industrial societies, obesity is more common among poor women, whereas in underdeveloped countries, wealthier women are more often obese. In children, obesity correlates to some degree with time spent watching television. High-fat diets may promote obesity, as may diets rich in simple (as opposed to complex) carbohydrates.

Specific Genetic Syndromes Obesity in rodents has been known for many years to be caused by a number of distinct mutations distributed through the genome. Most of these single-gene mutations cause both hyperphagia and diminished energy expenditure, suggesting a link between these two parameters of energy homeostasis. Identification of the *ob* gene mutation in genetically obese (ob/ob) mice represents a major breakthrough in the field. The ob/ob mouse develops severe obesity, insulin resistance, and hyperphagia, as well as efficient metabolism (e.g., it gets fat even when given the same number of calories as lean littermates). The product of the *ob* gene is the peptide leptin, a name derived from the Greek root *leptos*, meaning thin. Leptin is secreted by adipose cells and acts through the hypothalamus. Its level of production provides an index of adipose energy stores (Fig. 77-4). High leptin levels decrease food intake and increase energy expenditure. Another mouse mutant, db/db, which is resistant to leptin, has a mutation in the leptin receptor and develops a similar syndrome. The *ob* gene is present in humans and expressed in fat. Several families with morbid, early-onset obesity due to inactivating mutations in either leptin or the leptin receptor have been described, thus demonstrating the biologic relevance of leptin in humans. The obesity in these individuals begins shortly after birth, is severe, and is accompanied by neuroendocrine abnormalities. The most prominent of these is hypogonadotropic hypogonadism, which is reversed by leptin replacement. Central hypothyroidism and growth retardation are seen in the mouse model, but their occurrence in leptin-deficient humans is less clear. To date, there is no evidence to suggest that mutations or polymorphisms in the leptin or leptin receptor genes play a prominent role in common forms of obesity.

FIGURE 77-4 The physiologic system regulated by leptin. Rising or falling leptin levels act through the hypothalamus to influence appetite, energy expenditure, and neuroendocrine function and through peripheral sites to influence systems such as the immune system.

Mutations in several other genes cause severe obesity in humans (Table 77-1), each of these syndromes is rare. Mutations in the gene encoding proopiomelanocortin (POMC) cause severe obesity through failure to synthesize α-MSH, a key neuropeptide that inhibits appetite in the hypothalamus. The absence of POMC also causes secondary adrenal insufficiency due to absence of adrenocorticotropic hormone (ACTH), as well as pale skin and red hair due to absence of MSH. Proenzyme convertase 1 (PC-1) mutations are thought to cause obesity by preventing synthesis of α-MSH from its precursor peptide, POMC. α-MSH binds to the type 4 melanocortin receptor (MC4R), a key hypothalamic receptor that inhibits eating; mutations of this receptor also cause obesity. These three genetic defects, although rare, define a pathway through which leptin (by stimulating POMC and increasing MSH) restricts food intake and limits weight (Fig. 77-5).

In addition to these human obesity genes, studies in rodents reveal several other molecular candidates for hypothalamic mediators of human obesity or leanness. The *tub* gene encodes a hypothalamic peptide of unknown function; mutation of this gene causes late-onset obesity. The *fat* gene encodes carboxypeptidase E, a peptide-processing enzyme; mutation of this gene is thought to cause obesity by disrupting production of one or more neuropeptides. AgRP is coexpressed with NPY in arcuate nucleus neurons. AgRP antagonizes α-MSH action at MC4 receptors, and its overexpression induces obesity. A putative activating mutation in the gene encoding PPARγ, the adipocyte transcription factor required for adipogenesis, has been linked to obesity in a group of German subjects.

A number of complex human syndromes with defined inheritance are associated with obesity (Table 77-2). Although specific genes are undefined at present, their identification will likely enhance our understanding of more common forms of human obesity. In the Prader-Willi syndrome, obesity coexists with short stature, mental retardation, hypogonadotropic hypogonadism, hypotonia, small hands and feet, fish-shaped mouth, and hyperphagia. Most patients have a chromosome 15 deletion (Chap. 66). Laurence-Moon-Biedl syndrome involves obesity, mental retardation, retinitis pigmentosa, polydactyly, and hypogonadotropic hypogonadism.

Other Specific Syndromes Associated with Obesity • *Cushing's syndrome* Although obese patients commonly have central obesity, hypertension, and glucose intolerance, they lack other specific stigmata of Cushing's syndrome (Chap. 331). Nonetheless, a potential diagnosis of Cushing's syndrome is often entertained. Cortisol production and urinary metabolites (17OH steroids) may be increased in simple obesity. Unlike in Cushing's syndrome, however, cortisol levels in blood and urine in the basal state and in response to CRH or ACTH are normal; the overnight 1-mg dexamethasone suppression test is normal in 90%, with the remainder being normal on a standard 2-day low-dose dexamethasone suppression test.

Hypothyroidism The possibility of hypothyroidism should be considered when evaluating obesity, but it is an uncommon cause of obesity; hypothyroidism is easily ruled out by measuring thyroid stimulating hormone (TSH). Much of the weight gain that occurs in hypothyroidism is due to myxedema (Chap. 330).

Insulinoma Patients with insulinoma often gain weight as a result of overeating to avoid hypoglycemia symptoms (Chap. 334). The increased substrate plus high insulin levels promotes energy storage in fat. This can be marked in some individuals but is modest in most.

Craniopharyngioma and other disorders involving the hypothalamus Whether through tumors, trauma, or inflammation, hypothalamic dysfunction of systems controlling satiety, hunger, and energy expenditure can cause varying degrees of obesity (Chap. 328). It is uncommon to identify a discrete anatomic basis for these disorders. Subtle hypothalamic dysfunction is probably a more common cause of obesity than can be documented using currently available techniques. Growth hormone (GH), which exerts lipolytic activity, is diminished in obesity and increases with weight loss. Despite low growth hormone levels, insulin-like growth factor (IGF) I (somato-

Table 77-1 Some Obesity Genes in Humans and Mice

Gene	Gene Product	Mechanism of Obesity	In Human	In Rodent
Lep (ob)	Leptin, a fat-derived hormone	Mutation prevents leptin from delivering satiety signal; brain perceives starvation	Yes	Yes
LepR (db)	Leptin receptor	Same as above	Yes	Yes
POMC	Proopiomelanocortin, a precursor of several hormones and neuropeptides	Mutation prevents synthesis of melanocyte-stimulating hormone (MSH), a satiety signal	Yes	Yes
MC4R	Type 4 receptor for MSH	Mutation prevents reception of satiety signal from MSH	Yes	Yes
AgRP	Agouti-related peptide, a neuropeptide expressed in the hypothalamus	Overexpression inhibits signal through MC4R	No	Yes
PC-1	Prohormone convertase 1, a processing enzyme	Mutation prevents synthesis of neuropeptide, probably MSH	Yes	No
Fat	Carboxypeptidase E, a processing enzyme	Same as above	No	Yes
Tub	Tub, a hypothalamic protein of unknown function	Hypothalamic dysfunction	No	Yes
PPARγ	Peroxisome proliferator activated receptor, a transcription factor that promotes adipogenesis and modulates insulin action	Unknown	Yes	No

medin) production is normal, suggesting that GH suppression is a compensatory response to increased nutritional supply.

Pathogenesis of Common Obesity Obesity can result from increased energy intake, decreased energy expenditure, or a combination of the two. Thus, identifying the etiology of obesity should involve measurements of both parameters. However, it is nearly impossible to perform direct and accurate measurements of energy intake in free-living individuals. Obese people, in particular, appear to underreport intake. Measurements of chronic energy expenditure have only recently become available using doubly-labeled water or metabolic chamber/rooms. In subjects at stable weight and body composition, energy intake equals expenditure. Consequently, these techniques allow determination of energy intake in free-living individuals. The level of energy expenditure differs in established obesity, during periods of weight gain or loss, and in the pre- or postobese state. Studies that fail to take note of this phenomenon are not easily interpreted.

There is increased interest in the concept of a body weight "set point." This idea is supported by physiologic mechanisms centered around a sensing system in adipose tissue that reflects fat stores, and a receptor, or "adipostat," that is in the hypothalamic centers. When fat stores are depleted, the adipostat signal is low, and the hypothalamus responds by stimulating hunger and decreasing energy expenditure to conserve energy. Conversely, when fat stores are abundant, the signal is increased, and the hypothalamus responds by decreasing hunger and increasing energy expenditure. The recent discovery of the *ob* gene, and its product leptin, provides a molecular basis for this physiologic concept (see above).

What Is the Status of Food Intake in Obesity (Do the Obese Eat More Than the Lean?) This question has stimulated much debate, due in part to the methodologic difficulties inherent in determining food intake. Many obese individuals believe that they eat small quantities of food, and this claim has often been supported by the results of food intake questionnaires. However, it is now established that average energy expenditure increases as people get more obese, due primarily to the fact that metabolically active lean tissue mass increases with obesity. Given the laws of thermodynamics, the obese person must therefore eat more than the average lean person to maintain their increased weight. It may be the case, however, that a subset of individuals who are predisposed to obesity have the capacity to become obese initially without an absolute increase in caloric consumption.

What Is the State of Energy Expenditure in Obesity? The average total daily energy expenditure is higher in obese than lean individuals when measured at stable weight. However, energy expenditure falls as weight is lost, due in part to loss of lean body mass and to decreased sympathetic nerve activity. When reduced to near-normal weight and maintained there for a while, (some) obese individuals have lower energy expenditure than (some) lean individuals. There is also a tendency for those who develop obesity as infants or children to have lower resting energy expenditure rates than those who remain lean.

The physiologic basis for variable rates of energy expenditure (at a given body weight and level of energy intake) is essentially unknown. A mutation in the human β_3 adrenergic receptor may be associated with increased risk of obesity and/or insulin resistance in certain (but not all) populations. Homologues of the BAT uncoupling protein, named UCP-2 and UCP-3, have been identified in both rodents and humans. UCP-2 is expressed widely, whereas UCP-3 is primarily expressed in skeletal muscle. These proteins may play a role in disordered energy balance.

One newly described component of thermogenesis, called *nonexercise activity thermogenesis* (NEAT), has been linked to obesity. It is the thermogenesis that accompanies physical activities other than volitional exercise, such as the activities of daily living, fidgeting, spontaneous muscle contraction, and maintaining posture. NEAT accounts for about two-thirds of the increased daily energy expenditure induced by overfeeding. The wide variation in fat storage seen in overfed individuals is predicted by the degree to which NEAT is induced. The molecular basis for NEAT and its regulation are unknown.

Leptin in Typical Obesity The vast majority of obese people have increased leptin levels but do not have mutations of either leptin or its receptor. They appear, therefore, to have a form of functional "leptin resistance." Data suggesting that some individuals produce less leptin per unit fat mass than others or have a form of relative leptin deficiency that predisposes to obesity are at present contradictory and unsettled. The mechanism for leptin resistance, and whether it can be overcome by raising leptin levels, is not yet established. Some data

FIGURE 77-5 A central pathway through which leptin acts to regulate appetite and body weight. Leptin signals through proopiomelanocortin (POMC) neurons in the hypothalamus to induce increased production of α melanocyte stimulating hormone (α-MSH), requiring the processing enzyme PC-1 (proenzyme convertase 1). α-MSH acts as an agonist on melanocortin-4 receptors to inhibit appetite, and the neuropeptide AgRp (Agouti-related peptide) acts as an antagonist of this receptor. Mutations that cause obesity in humans are indicated by the solid blue arrows.

suggest that leptin may not effectively cross the blood-brain barrier as levels rise. It is also possible that leptin signaling inhibitors are involved in the leptin-resistant state.

PATHOLOGIC CONSEQUENCES OF OBESITY

Obesity has major adverse effects on health. Morbidly obese individuals (>200% ideal body weight) have as much as a twelvefold increase in mortality. Morality rates rise as obesity increases, particularly when obesity is associated with increased intra-abdominal fat (see above). It is also apparent that the degree to which obesity affects particular organ systems is influenced by susceptibility genes that vary in the population.

Insulin Resistance and Type 2 Diabetes Mellitus Hyperinsulinemia and insulin resistance are pervasive features of obesity, increasing with weight gain and diminishing with weight loss. Insulin resistance is more strongly linked to intraabdominal fat than to fat in other depots. The molecular link between obesity and insulin resistance has been sought for many years, with the major factors under investigation being: (1) insulin itself, by inducing receptor downregulation; (2) free fatty acids, known to be increased and capable of impairing insulin action; and (3) the cytokine TNF-α, which is produced by adipocytes, overexpressed in obese adipocytes, and capable of inhibiting insulin action. Despite insulin resistance, most obese individuals do not develop diabetes, suggesting that the onset of diabetes requires an interaction between obesity-induced insulin resistance and other factors that predispose to diabetes, such as impaired insulin secretion (Chap. 333). Obesity, however, is a major risk factor for diabetes, and as many as 80% of patients with type 2 diabetes mellitus are obese. Weight loss, even of modest degree, is associated with increased insulin sensitivity and often improves glucose control in diabetes.

Reproductive Disorders Disorders that affect the reproductive axis are associated with obesity in both men and women. Male hypogonadism is associated with increased adipose tissue, often distributed in a pattern more typical of females. In men >160% ideal body weight, plasma testosterone and sex hormone–binding globulin (SHBG) are often reduced, and estrogen levels (derived from conversion of adrenal androgens in adipose tissue) are increased (Chap. 335). Gynecomastia may be seen. However, masculinization, libido, potency, and spermatogenesis are preserved in most of these individuals. Free testosterone may be decreased in morbidly obese men whose weight exceeds 200% ideal body weight.

Obesity has long been associated with menstrual abnormalities in women, particularly in women with upper body obesity (Chaps. 52 and 336). Common findings are increased androgen production, decreased SHBG, and increased peripheral conversion of androgen to estrogen. Most obese women with oligomenorrhea have the polycystic ovarian syndrome (PCOS), with its associated anovulation and ovarian hyperandrogenism; 40% of women with PCOS are obese. Interestingly, most nonobese women with PCOS are also insulin-resistant, suggesting that insulin resistance, hyperinsulinemia, or the combina-

tion of the two are causative or contribute to the ovarian pathophysiology in PCOS in both obese and lean individuals. In obese women with PCOS, weight loss or treatment with insulin-sensitizing drugs often restores normal menses, along with a fall in estrone levels and normalized gonadotropin secretion. The increased conversion of androstenedione to estrogen, which occurs to a greater degree in women with lower body obesity, may contribute to the increased incidence of uterine cancer in postmenopausal women with obesity.

Cardiovascular Disease The Framingham Study revealed that obesity was an independent risk factor for the 26-year incidence of cardiovascular disease in men and women [including coronary disease, stroke, and congestive heart failure (CHF)]. The waist/hip ratio may be the best predictor of these risks. When the additional effects of hypertension and glucose intolerance associated with obesity are included, the adverse impact of obesity is even more evident. The effect of obesity on cardiovascular mortality in women may be seen at BMIs as low as 25. Obesity, especially abdominal obesity, is associated with an atherogenic lipid profile, with increased low-density lipoprotein (LDL) cholesterol, very low density lipoprotein and triglyceride, and decreased high-density lipoprotein cholesterol (Chap. 344). Obesity is also associated with hypertension. Measurement of blood pressure in the obese requires use of a larger cuff size to avoid artifactual increases. Obesity-induced hypertension is associated with increased peripheral resistance and cardiac output, increased sympathetic nervous system tone, increased salt sensitivity, and insulin-mediated salt retention; it is often responsive to modest weight loss.

Pulmonary Disease Obesity may be associated with a number of pulmonary abnormalities. These include reduced chest wall compliance, increased work of breathing, increased minute ventilation due to increased metabolic rate, and decreased total lung capacity and functional residual capacity (Chap. 250). Severe obesity may be associated with obstructive sleep apnea and the "obesity hypoventilation syndrome" (Chap. 263). Sleep apnea can be obstructive (most common),

Table 77-2 A Comparison of Syndromes of Obesity—Hypogonadism and Mental Retardation

Feature	Prader-Willi	Laurence-Moon-Biedl	Ahlstrom	Cohen	Carpenter
Inheritance	Sporadic; two-thirds have defect	Autosomal recessive	Autosomal recessive	Probably autosomal recessive	Autosomal recessive
Stature	Short	Normal; infrequently short	Normal; infrequently short	Short or tall	Normal
Obesity	Generalized Moderate to severe Onset 1–3 yrs	Generalized Early onset, 1–2 yrs	Truncal Early onset, 2–5 yrs	Truncal Mid-childhood, age 5	Truncal, gluteal
Craniofacies	Narrow bifrontal diameter Almond-shaped eyes Strabismus V-shaped mouth High-arched palate	Not distinctive	Not distinctive	High nasal bridge Arched palate Open mouth Short philtrum	Acrocephaly Flat nasal bridge High-arched palate
Limbs	Small hands and feet Hypotonia	Polydactyly	No abnormalities	Hypotonia Narrow hands and feet	Polydactyly Syndactyly Genu valgum
Reproductive status	1° Hypogonadism	1° Hypogonadism	Hypogonadism in males but not in females	Normal gonadal function or hypogonadotrophic hypogonadism	2° Hypogonadism
Other features	Enamel hypoplasia Hyperphagia Temper tantrums Nasal speech			Dysplastic ears Delayed puberty	
Mental retardation	Mild to moderate		Normal intelligence	Mild	Slight

483

central, or mixed. Weight loss (10 to 20 kg) can bring substantial improvement, as can major weight loss following gastric bypass or restrictive surgery. Continuous positive airway pressure has been used with some success.

Gallstones Obesity is associated with enhanced biliary secretion of cholesterol, supersaturation of bile, and a higher incidence of gallstones, particularly cholesterol gallstones (Chap. 302). A person 50% above ideal body weight has about a sixfold increased incidence of symptomatic gallstones. Paradoxically, fasting increases supersaturation of bile by decreasing the phospholipid component. Fasting-induced cholecystitis is a complication of extreme diets.

Cancer Obesity in males is associated with higher mortality from cancer of the colon, rectum, and prostate; obesity in females is associated with higher mortality from cancer of the gallbladder, bile ducts, breasts, endometrium, cervix, and ovaries. Some of the latter may be due to increased rates of conversion of androstenedione to estrone in adipose tissue of obese individuals.

Bone, Joint, and Cutaneous Disease Obesity is associated with an increased risk of osteoarthritis, no doubt partly due to the trauma of added weight bearing. The prevalence of gout may also be increased (Chap. 322). Among the skin problems associated with obesity is acanthosis nigricans, manifested by darkening and thickening of the skin folds on the neck, elbows, and dorsal interphalangeal spaces. Acanthosis reflects the severity of underlying insulin resistance and diminishes with weight loss. Friability of skin may be increased, especially in skin folds, enhancing the risk of fungal and yeast infections. Finally, venous stasis is increased in the obese.

℞ **TREATMENT** Obesity is a chronic medical condition. Successful treatment, defined as the sustained attainment of normal body weight without producing unacceptable treatment-induced morbidity, is rarely achieved in clinical practice. Many approaches produce short-term weight loss, and this has clear benefits for associated morbidities such as hypertension and diabetes. Despite the fact that sustained weight loss is uncommon, enormous resources are expended in pursuit of this goal.

Treatment goals should be guided by the health risks of obesity in any given individual (Fig. 77-6). The clinician should always consider the possibility that an individual has an identified cause of obesity, such as hypothyroidism, hypercortisolism, male hypogonadism, insulinoma, or central nervous system disease that affects hypothalamic function. Although they are infrequent causes of obesity, specific therapy may be available.

Behavior Modification The principles of behavior modification provide the underpinnings for many current programs of weight reduction. Typically, the patient is requested to monitor and record the circumstances related to eating, and rewards are designed to modify maladaptive behaviors. Patients may benefit from counseling offered in a stable group setting for extended periods of time, including after weight loss.

Diet Reduced caloric intake is the cornerstone of obesity treatment. The fundamental goal is the sustained reduction of energy intake below that of energy expenditure. The difficulty in achieving this goal has led to a wide array of suggested diets that vary in recommended calorie content (from total fasting to mild reductions), as well as specific food content and form (e.g., liquid vs. solid). There is no scientific evidence to validate the utility of specific "fad diets." The main diet regimens in use follow several general facts relevant to food intake and weight loss. First, a deficit of 7500 kcal will produce a weight loss of approximately 1 kg. Therefore, eating 100 kcal/d less for a year should cause a 5-kg weight loss, and a deficit of 1000 kcal/d should cause a loss of approximately 1 kg per week. The rate of weight loss on a given caloric intake is related to the rate of energy expenditure. Because obese individuals have a higher metabolic rate than lean individuals, and because men have a higher metabolic rate than women

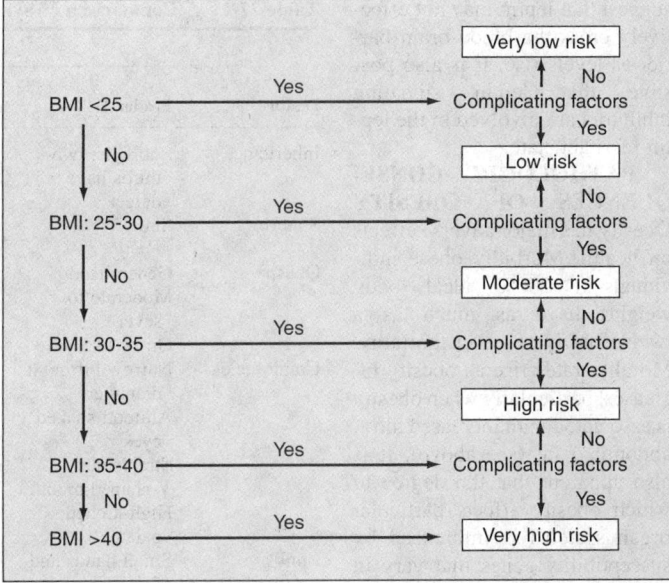

FIGURE 77-6 Risk classification algorithm. The patient is first placed into a category based on body mass index. The presence or absence of complicating factors determines the degree of health risk. Complicating factors include elevated abdominal-gluteal ratio (male: 0.95, female: 0.85), diabetes mellitus, hypertension, hyperlipidemia, male sex, and age <40. (*Copyright 1987, George A. Bray, MD. Used with permission.*)

(due to their greater lean body mass), the rate of weight loss is greater among the more obese and among men (relative to women). With chronic caloric restriction, metabolic rate diminishes, but because of reduced lean body mass (along with much greater loss in fat mass) and possibly because of other adaptations. This fall in metabolic rate with food restriction slows the rate of weight loss on a constant diet. With total starvation or diets restricted to <600 kcal/d, initial weight loss over the first week results predominantly from natriuresis and the loss of fluids.

Very low energy diets (e.g., 400 to 600 kcal/d) are widely used. The liquid protein diets popularized in the 1970s were proved to be unsafe, causing >60 deaths. Life-threatening arrhythmias were documented in the clinical research setting, a consequence of both low-quality protein and deficiencies of vitamins, minerals, and trace elements. These types of diets have now been substantially modified. A very low energy diet consisting of 45 to 70 g high-quality protein, 30 to 50 g carbohydrate, and approximately 2 g fat per day, as well as supplements of vitamins, minerals, and trace elements, appears to be safe in selected patients under medical supervision. Patients should not be started on such diets unless they are >130% of their ideal body weight. Contraindications include pregnancy, cancer, recent myocardial infarction, cerebrovascular disease, hepatic disease, or untreated psychiatric disease. When used in patients with diabetes who are receiving insulin or oral agent therapy, close supervision is required and diabetic treatment may need to be adjusted. Whenever possible, exercise regimens and behavioral modification approaches should be used in conjunction with the diet.

Advantages of very low calorie diets are the greater rate of weight loss compared to less restrictive diets, as well as the possible beneficial effect of hunger suppression brought about by the production of ketones. In patients on such diets, blood pressure, blood glucose, cholesterol, and triglyceride levels fall, and pulmonary function and exercise tolerance improve. Sleep apnea may improve within a few weeks. Complications of these very low energy diets are usually minor and include fatigue, constipation or diarrhea, dry skin, hair loss, menstrual irregularities, orthostatic dizziness, and difficulty concentrating. Cholelithiasis and pancreatitis may occur when such diets are interrupted by binge eating; gallstones have been shown to develop in as many as 25% of patients while on the diet.

Low-calorie diets, >800 kcal/d, are applicable to most patients and have fewer restrictions than the very low calorie diets. Considerable controversy has attended the question of which diet composition is most appropriate for promoting weight loss. Though commonly recommended, benefits resulting from very low fat diets are modest at best. Nonetheless, the health effects of low-fat diets—apart from curbing obesity—may be important. A diet rich in fruits, vegetables, and whole grains may promote weight loss and is preferable to low-fat diets in which large amounts of simple carbohydrates are substituted for fats. The latter may actually promote obesity. Some have advocated diets with protein replacement of simple carbohydrates in an effort to minimize insulin production. The efficacy of this strategy, aside from overall calorie reduction, is unknown.

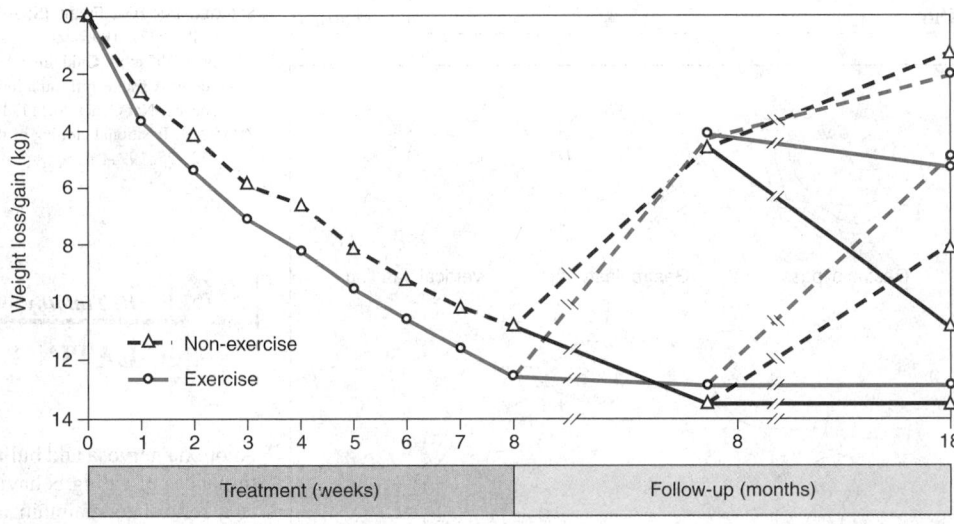

FIGURE 77-7   Weight loss and exercise. During the first 8 weeks, subjects were divided into two groups, one treated with diet and the other with diet plus exercise, with no difference in weight loss. Thereafter the subjects who exercised maintained better weight loss than those that did not. (*After KN Pavlou et al: Am J Clin Nutr 49:1115, 1989.*)

Exercise   Exercise is an important component of the overall approach to treating obesity. Increased energy expenditure is the most obvious mechanism for an effect of exercise. The impact of an exercise regimen as a sole therapy of obesity has been difficult to document. On the other hand, exercise appears to be a valuable means to sustain diet therapy (Fig. 77-7). Even if exercise had no such salutary effect, it would be valuable in the obese individual for its effects on cardiovascular tone and blood pressure. Because many obese individuals have not engaged in exercise on a regular basis and may have cardiovascular risk factors, it should be introduced gradually and under medical supervision, especially in the most obese individuals.

Drugs   Unfortunately, drug treatment of obesity is rarely efficacious. Despite short-term benefits, medication-induced weight loss is often associated with rebound weight gain after the cessation of drug use, side effects from the medications, and the potential for drug abuse. Given the need for effective therapies, many possible compounds have been evaluated. On the basis of placebo-controlled trials, the U.S. Food and Drug Administration (FDA) approved several amphetamine-like agents for short-term use. Phentermine is an amphetamine-like drug with low addictive potential that has shown modest efficacy (10 vs. 4.4 kg of weight loss over a 24-week period in well-controlled study). This class of drugs is thought to act centrally by reducing appetite. Effects on energy expenditure are less clear. Over-the-counter drugs, such as phenylpropanolamine HCl, have similar efficacy to prescription appetite suppressants in short-term studies. Drugs that promote serotonin release or inhibit serotonin reuptake, such as fenfluramine, also have modest efficacy. When fenfluramine was administered together with phentermine, as "fen-phen," the combination was widely used based on controlled trials that demonstrated modest but definite efficacy. However, the risk of primary pulmonary hypertension was increased up to 20-fold in association with this treatment. The FDA withdrew approval of the fen-phen combination in 1997 when reports suggested an association with right- and left-sided valvular heart disease. The histopathologic features of the valvular disease are similar to those seen in carcinoid syndrome and are thought to result from fenfluramine. Though the true incidence and long-term effects of these valvular lesions are currently unknown, the occurrence of this complication has been verified in multiple studies.

Sibutramine is a novel central reuptake inhibitor of both norepinephrine and serotonin. Using a once-daily dose over 24 weeks, it produced a 7% weight loss in a double-blind, placebo-controlled trial. It lowered cholesterol and triglyceride levels and exhibited similar clinical efficacy to fenfluramine. Sibutramine increases pulse and blood pressure in some patients, and long-term safety is not established. Orlistat is an inhibitor of intestinal lipase that causes modest weight loss due to drug-induced fat malabsorption. A randomized, double-blind trial over 2 years revealed modest weight loss (8.7 kg for 120 mg orlistat versus 5.8 kg from diet alone) during the first year and better maintenance of weight loss in a second year compared to the placebo-treated group (3.2 kg regained versus 5.6 kg regained for placebo). LDL cholesterol and insulin levels were also reduced. In patients with obesity and type 2 diabetes mellitus, the antidiabetic medication metformin tends to decrease body weight. The mechanism appears to involve inhibition of appetite. Thyroid hormone has little place in the treatment of obesity, as the vast majority of obese individuals are euthyroid. It promotes loss of lean body mass and raises the risk of complications from the hyperthyroid state.

β_3-Adrenergic receptor agonists may provide a new treatment approach for obesity. Drugs of this class are in clinical trials. In animals, β_3 agonists promote leanness by stimulating thermogenesis in BAT; they also stimulate lipolysis in white adipose tissue. These drugs also reduce insulin resistance and lower blood glucose in animal models by a mechanism that is not yet defined. Recombinant human leptin is also in clinical trials. In the rare cases of leptin deficiency caused by mutations of the leptin gene, the administration of recombinant leptin is highly effective. Preliminary reports suggest that the response to leptin is limited or absent in common causes of obesity (which are associated with hyperleptinemia and leptin resistance). New drugs are also being developed based on insights into central pathways that regulate body weight. These include antagonists for NPY receptors (subtypes Y1, Y5) and agonists for melanocortin 4 receptors.

Surgery   Morbid obesity, commonly defined as either 45 kg (100 lb) or 100% above ideal body weight, is estimated to increase mortality by as much as twelvefold in men between 25 and 34 years of age and sixfold between 35 and 45 years of age. Deaths from cardiovascular disease, diabetes, and accidents have been documented. In response to ineffective treatment using diet, exercise, and available drugs, surgical approaches have been tried. The potential benefits of surgery include major weight loss and improvement in hypertension, diabetes, sleep apnea, CHF, angina, hyperlipidemia, and venous disease. Many different approaches have been used, often without adequate assessment of efficacy and complications. Jejunoileal bypass surgery has largely been abandoned because of complications, which have included electrolyte disturbances, nephrolithiasis, gallstones, gastric ulcers, arthritis, and hepatic dysfunction, with cirrhosis occurring in as many as 7% of patients. Two procedures in common use today

SPIEGELMAN BM, FLIER JS: Adipogenesis and obesity: Rounding out the big picture. Cell 87:377, 1996

WILLETT WC et al: Guidelines for healthy weight. N Engl J Med 341:427, 1999

YEO et al: A frameshift mutation in MC4R associated with dominantly inherited human obesity. Nat Genet 20:111, 1998

ZHANG Y: Positional cloning of the mouse obese gene and its human homologue. Nature 372:425, 1994

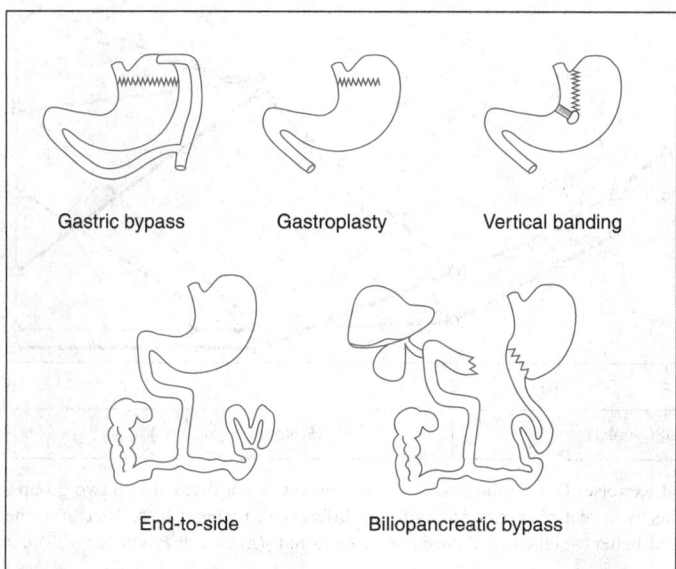

FIGURE 77-8 Examples of operative interventions used for surgical manipulation of the gastrointestinal tract.

are the vertical-banded gastroplasty and the Roux-en-Y gastric bypass (Fig. 77-8).

Following the National Institutes of Health Consensus Conference on Gastrointestinal Surgery for Severe Obesity in 1991, it was recommended that suitable patients be selected using the following criteria: (1) the presence of 45 kg (100 lb) or 100% above ideal body weight, or one or more severe medical conditions related to refractory obesity; (2) repeated failures of other therapeutic approaches; (3) at eligible weight for 3 to 5 years; (4) capability of tolerating surgery; (5) absence of alcoholism, other addictions, or major psychopathology; and (6) prior clearance by a psychiatrist. It is recommended that an appropriately experienced surgeon work together with nutritionists and other support personnel; evaluation and follow-up programs should be monitored closely.

ACKNOWLEDGMENT

The author acknowledges the contributions of Dr. George A. Bray, who wrote this chapter in the 14th edition.

BIBLIOGRAPHY

BRAY GA, GREENWAY FL: Current and potential drugs for treatment of obesity. Endocr Rev 20:805, 1999

BURTON BT et al: Report of Consensus Proceedings. Health implications of obesity: An NIH Consensus Development Conference. Int J Obesity 9:155, 1985

CONNOLLY HM et al: Valvular heart disease associated with fenfluramine-phentermine. N Engl J Med 337:581, 1997

FLIER JS: What's in a name? In search of leptin's physiologic role. J Clin Endocrinol Metab 83:1407, 1998

Gastrointestinal surgery for severe obesity: Proceedings of an NIH Consensus Development Conference, March 25–27, 1991. Am J Clin Nutr 55 (Suppl 2):615S, 1992

HEYMSFIELD SB et al: Recombinant leptin for weight loss in obese and lean adults: A randomized, controlled, dose-escalation trial. JAMA 282:1568, 1999

HOTAMISLIGIL GS et al: Tumor necrosis factor α: A key component of the obesity-diabetes link. Diabetes 43:1271, 1994

KRUDE et al: Severe early onset obesity, adrenal insufficiency and red hair pigmentation caused by POMC mutations in humans. Nat Genet 19(2):155, 1998

KUCZMARSKI RJ et al: Increasing prevalence of overweight among US adults: JAMA 272:205, 1994

LEVINE JA: Role of nonexercise activity thermogenesis in resistance to fat gain in humans. Science 283:212, 1999

MONTAGUE CT: Congenital leptin deficiency is associated with severe early onset obesity in humans. Nature 387:903, 1998

PI-SUNYER FX: Short-term medical benefits and adverse effects of weight loss. Ann Intern Med 119:722, 1993

ROSENBAUM M et al: Obesity. N Engl J Med 337:396, 1997

78   *B. Timothy Walsh*

EATING DISORDERS

Anorexia nervosa and bulimia nervosa are characterized by severe disturbances of eating behavior. The salient feature of *anorexia nervosa* is a refusal to maintain a minimally normal body weight. *Bulimia nervosa* is characterized by recurrent episodes of binge eating followed by abnormal compensatory behaviors, such as self-induced vomiting. Anorexia nervosa and bulimia nervosa are closely related. Both occur primarily among previously healthy young women who become overly concerned with body shape and weight. Many patients with bulimia nervosa have past histories of anorexia nervosa, and many patients with anorexia nervosa engage in binge eating and purging behavior. In the current diagnostic system, the critical distinction between anorexia nervosa and bulimia nervosa depends on body weight: patients with anorexia nervosa are, by definition, significantly underweight, whereas the weights of patients with bulimia nervosa are in the normal range or above.

Another syndrome of disturbed eating behavior has been described recently: *Binge eating disorder* is characterized by repeated episodes of binge eating, similar to those of bulimia nervosa, in the absence of inappropriate compensatory behavior. Patients with binge eating disorder are typically middle-aged men or women with significant obesity. They have an increased frequency of anxiety and depression compared to similarly obese patients without binge eating disorder. It is not known whether patients with binge eating disorder are at increased risk for medical complications or what treatments are most useful.

EPIDEMIOLOGY

In women, the full syndrome of anorexia nervosa occurs with a lifetime prevalence of approximately 0.5%; bulimia nervosa occurs with a lifetime prevalence of 1 to 3%. Variants of these eating disorders with only some features of anorexia nervosa or bulimia nervosa are much more common and occur in 5 to 10% of young women. Both anorexia nervosa and bulimia nervosa also occur in males but at frequencies approximately one-tenth of those in females.

Anorexia nervosa and bulimia nervosa are more prevalent in cultures where food is plentiful and in which being thin is associated with attractiveness. These disorders are more frequent among young women who place a premium on thinness, such as ballet dancers and models. The incidence of anorexia nervosa appears to have increased in recent decades. The frequency of bulimia nervosa increased dramatically in the early 1970s and 1980s but may have declined somewhat in recent years.

DIAGNOSIS

The diagnosis of eating disorders is based on the presence of characteristic behavioral, psychological, and physical attributes (Tables 78-1 and 78-2). Widely accepted diagnostic criteria are provided by the American Psychiatric Association's *Diagnostic and Statistical Manual of Mental Disorders* (DSM-IV).

ANOREXIA NERVOSA For anorexia nervosa, these criteria include weight <85% of the expected weight for age and height, which

Table 78-1 Diagnostic Criteria for Anorexia Nervosa

1. Refusal to maintain body weight at or above a minimally normal weight for age and height (e.g., weight loss leading to maintenance of body weight <85% of that expected; or failure to make expected weight gain during period of growth, leading to body weight <85% of that expected).
2. Intense fear of gaining weight or becoming fat, even though underweight.
3. Disturbance in the way in which one's body weight or shape is experienced, undue influence of body weight or shape on self-evaluation, or denial of the seriousness of the current low body weight.
4. In postmenarchal females, amenorrhea, i.e., the absence of at least three consecutive menstrual cycles. (A woman is considered to have amenorrhea if her periods occur only following hormone, e.g., estrogen, administration.)

Specify type:
  Restricting type: During the episode of anorexia nervosa, the person has not regularly engaged in binge-eating or purging behavior (i.e., self-induced vomiting or the misuse of laxatives, diuretics or enemas).
  Binge eating/purging type: During the episode of anorexia nervosa, the person has regularly engaged in binge-eating or purging behavior (i.e., self-induced vomiting or the misuse of laxatives, diuretics, or enemas).

SOURCE: From the *Diagnostic and Statistical Manual of Mental Disorders*, 4th ed, Washington, DC, American Psychiatric Association, 1994.

is roughly equivalent to a body mass index (BMI) of 18.5 kg/m² for adult women. This weight criterion is somewhat arbitrary, so that a patient who meets all other diagnostic criteria but weighs between 85 and 90% of expected would still merit the diagnosis of anorexia nervosa. Despite being underweight, patients with anorexia nervosa are irrationally afraid of gaining weight, often out of a concern that weight gain will get "out of control." They also exhibit a distortion of body image (criterion 3, Table 78-1), which may express itself in several ways. For example, despite being emaciated, patients with anorexia nervosa may believe that their body as a whole, or some part of their body, is too fat and experience additional weight loss as a highly rewarding achievement. The current diagnostic criteria require that women with anorexia nervosa not have spontaneous menses, but occasional patients with the characteristics and complications of anorexia nervosa describe regular menses. Two mutually exclusive subtypes of anorexia nervosa are specified in DSM-IV. Patients whose weight loss is maintained primarily by caloric restriction, perhaps augmented by excessive exercise, are considered to have the "restricting" subtype of anorexia nervosa. The "binge eating/purging" subtype is characterized

Table 78-2 Diagnostic Criteria for Bulimia Nervosa

1. Recurrent episodes of binge eating. An episode of binge eating is characterized by both of the following:
   a. Eating, in a discrete period of time (e.g., within any 2-h period), an amount of food that is definitely larger than most people would eat during a similar period of time and under similar circumstances.
   b. A sense of lack of control over eating during the episode (e.g., a feeling that one cannot stop eating or control what or how much one is eating).
2. Recurrent inappropriate compensatory behavior in order to prevent weight gain, such as self-induced vomiting, misuse of laxatives or diuretics, enemas, or other medications; fasting; or excessive exercise.
3. The binge eating and inappropriate compensatory behaviors both occur, on average, at least twice a week for 3 months.
4. Self-evaluation is unduly influenced by body shape and weight.
5. The disturbance does not occur exclusively during episodes of anorexia nervosa.

Specify type:
  Purging type: during the current episode of bulimia nervosa, the person has regularly engaged in self-induced vomiting or the misuse of laxatives, diuretics, or enemas.
  Nonpurging type: during the current episode of bulimia nervosa, the person has used other inappropriate compensatory behaviors such as fasting or excessive exercise but has not regularly engaged in self-induced vomiting or the misuse of laxatives, diuretics, or enemas.

SOURCE: From the *Diagnostic and Statistical Manual of Mental Disorders*, 4th ed, Washington, DC, American Psychiatric Association, 1994.

by self-induced vomiting or laxative abuse. Patients with the binge/purge subtype are more prone to develop electrolyte imbalances, are more emotionally labile, and are more likely to have other problems with impulse control, such as drug abuse.

The diagnosis of anorexia nervosa can usually be made confidently on the basis of history when significant weight loss is accomplished by restrictive dieting and excessive exercise and is accompanied by a marked reluctance to gain weight. Patients with anorexia nervosa often deny that they have a serious problem and may be brought to medical attention by concerned family or friends. In atypical presentations, other causes of significant weight loss in previously healthy young people should be considered, including inflammatory bowel disease, gastric outlet obstruction, central nervous system (CNS) tumors, and neoplasm (Chap. 43).

BULIMIA NERVOSA The critical diagnostic features of bulimia nervosa are repeated episodes of binge eating followed by inappropriate and abnormal behaviors aimed at avoiding weight gain. During binges, patients with this disorder tend to consume large amounts of sweet foods with a high fat content, such as dessert items. The most frequent compensatory behaviors are self-induced vomiting and laxative abuse, but a wide variety of techniques have been described, including the omission of insulin injections by diabetics. Typically, patients with bulimia nervosa are ashamed of their behavior and endeavor to keep their disorder hidden from family and friends. Like patients with anorexia nervosa, those with bulimia nervosa place an unusual emphasis on weight and shape as a basis for their self-esteem.

As in anorexia nervosa, there are two mutually exclusive subtypes of bulimia nervosa. Patients with the "purging" subtype utilize compensatory behaviors that directly rid the body of calories or fluids (e.g., self-induced vomiting, laxative or diuretic abuse), whereas those with the "nonpurging" subtype attempt to compensate for binges by fasting or by excessive exercise. Patients with the nonpurging subtype tend to be heavier and are less prone to fluid and electrolyte disturbances.

The diagnosis of bulimia nervosa requires a candid history from the patient detailing recurrent, large eating binges followed by the purposeful use of inappropriate mechanisms to avoid weight gain. Most patients with bulimia nervosa who present for treatment are distressed by their inability to control their eating behavior but are able to provide such details if queried in a supportive and nonjudgmental fashion.

ETIOLOGY

The fundamental etiology of the eating disorders is unknown but is believed to involve a combination of psychological, biologic, and cultural risk factors. Many of these risk factors, such as sexual or physical abuse and a family history of mood disturbance or substance abuse, are best viewed as nonspecific risk factors that increase vulnerability to a range of psychiatric disorders. Other factors appear to be more specific to the development of an eating disorder.

Patients who develop anorexia nervosa are inclined to be more obsessional and perfectionist than their peers. The disorder often begins as a diet not distinguishable at the outset from those undertaken by many adolescents and young women. As weight loss progresses, the fear of gaining weight grows; dieting becomes stricter; and psychological, behavioral, and medical aberrations increase. The fact that most cases are reported from countries where food is plentiful and where thinness, especially among women, is highly valued suggests that cultural factors play a significant role in the development of anorexia nervosa. However, it is notable that the clinical syndrome was well described over a century ago, when the cultural pressures were quite different.

Numerous physiologic disturbances, including abnormalities in a variety of neurotransmitter systems, have been described in anorexia nervosa (see below). It is difficult to distinguish neurochemical, metabolic, and hormonal changes that may have a role in the initiation or

Table 78-3 Common Characteristics of Anorexia Nervosa and Bulimia Nervosa

	Anorexia Nervosa	Bulimia Nervosa
CLINICAL CHARACTERISTICS		
Onset	Mid-adolescence	Late adolescence/early adulthood
Female:male	10:1	10:1
Prevalence in women	0.5%	1–3%
Weight	Markedly decreased	Usually normal
Menstruation	Absent	Usually normal
Binge eating	25–50%	Required for diagnosis
Mortality	~5% per decade	Low
PHYSICAL AND LABORATORY FINDINGS[a]		
Skin/extremities	Lanugo	
	Acrocyanosis	
	Edema	
Cardiovascular	Bradycardia	
	Hypotension	
Gastrointestinal	Salivary gland enlargement	Salivary gland enlargement
	Slow gastric emptying	Dental erosion
	Constipation	
	Elevated liver enzymes	
Hematopoietic	Normochromic, normocyctic anemia	
	Leukopenia	
Fluid/electrolyte	Increased BUN, creatinine	Hypokalemia
	Hyponatremia	Hypochloremia
		Alkalosis
Endocrine	Hypoglycemia	
	Low estrogen or testosterone	
	Low LH and FSH	
	Low-normal thyroxine	
	Normal TSH	
	Increased cortisol	
Bone	Osteopenia	

[a] Patients with the binge-eating/purging subtype of anorexia nervosa may also exhibit the physical and laboratory findings associated with bulimia nervosa.

NOTE: BUN, blood urea nitrogen; LH, luteinizing hormone; FSH, follicle stimulating hormone; TSH, thyroid stimulating hormone.

perpetuation of the syndrome from those that are secondary to the disorder. The resolution of most of these abnormalities with weight restoration argues against their having a critical etiologic role.

Bulimia nervosa typically begins during or following an episode of dieting, often in association with depressed mood. Patients who develop bulimia nervosa describe a higher-than-expected prevalence of childhood and parental obesity, suggesting that a predisposition towards obesity may increase vulnerability to this eating disorder. The marked increase in the number of cases of bulimia nervosa during the past 25 years and the rarity of bulimia nervosa in underdeveloped countries suggest that cultural factors are important. Several biologic abnormalities in patients with bulimia nervosa may perpetuate this disorder once it has begun. These include abnormalities of CNS serotonergic function, which is involved in the regulation of eating behavior, and disruption of peripheral satiety mechanisms, including the release of cholecystokinin (CCK) from the small intestine.

Genetic factors probably contribute to the risk of development of eating disorders, as the incidence of these disorders is greater in families with one affected member and the concordance in monozygotic twins is greater than in dizygotic twins. However, specific genes have not been identified, and the range of the estimates of heritability is large.

CLINICAL FEATURES (Table 78-3)

ANOREXIA NERVOSA Anorexia nervosa typically begins in mid to late adolescence, sometimes in association with a stressful life event such as leaving home for school. The disorder occasionally develops in early puberty, before menarche, but seldom begins after age 40. Despite being underweight, patients with anorexia nervosa rarely complain of hunger or fatigue and often exercise extensively. Further weight loss is viewed by the patient as a fulfilling accomplishment,

while weight gain is seen as a personal failure. Patients tend to become socially withdrawn and increasingly committed to work or study, dieting, and exercise. As weight loss progresses, thoughts of food dominate mental life and idiosyncratic rules develop around eating. Patients with anorexia nervosa may obsessively collect cookbooks and recipes and be drawn to food-related occupations. Despite the denial of hunger, one-quarter to one-half of patients with anorexia nervosa engage in eating binges.

Physical Features Patients with anorexia nervosa typically have few physical complaints but may note cold intolerance and constipation. Some women who develop anorexia nervosa after menarche report that their menses ceased before significant weight loss occurred. Weight and height should be measured to allow calculation of BMI (kg/m^2). Vital signs may reveal bradycardia, hypotension, and hypothermia. Soft, downy hair growth (lanugo) sometimes occurs, especially on the back, and alopecia may be seen. Salivary gland enlargement, which is associated with starvation as well as with binge eating and vomiting, may make the face appear surprisingly full in contrast to the marked general wasting. Acrocyanosis of the digits is common, and peripheral edema can be seen in the absence of hypoalbuminemia, particularly when the patient begins to regain weight. Some patients who consume large amounts of vegetables containing vitamin A develop a yellow tint to the skin (hypercarotenemia), which is especially notable on the palms.

Laboratory Abnormalities Mild normochromic, normocytic anemia is frequent, as is mild to moderate leukopenia, with a disproportionate reduction of polymorphonuclear leukocytes. Dehydration may result in slightly increased levels of blood urea nitrogen and creatinine. Serum liver enzyme levels may increase, especially during the early phases of refeeding. The level of serum proteins is usually normal. Blood sugar is often low and serum cholesterol may be moderately elevated. Gastrointestinal motility is diminished, leading to reduced gastric emptying and constipation. A range of electrolyte disturbances may develop, reflecting the degree to which the patient restricts or overconsumes fluids and whether the patient engages in purging behavior. Hypokalemic alkalosis suggests self-induced vomiting or the use of diuretics. Hyponatremia is common and may result from excess fluid intake and disturbances in the secretion of antidiuretic hormone.

Endocrine Abnormalities The regulation of virtually every endocrine system is altered in anorexia nervosa, but the most striking changes occur in the reproductive system. Amenorrhea is hypothalamic in origin and reflects diminished production of gonadotropin-releasing hormone (GnRH). When exogenous GnRH is administered in a physiologic pulsatile manner, pituitary responses of luteinizing hormone (LH) and follicle stimulating hormone (FSH) are normalized, indicating the absence of a primary pituitary abnormality. The resulting gonadotropin deficiency causes low plasma estrogen in women and reduced testosterone in men. The hypothalamic GnRH pulse generator is exquisitely sensitive, particularly in women, to body weight, stress, and exercise, each of which may contribute to hypothalamic amenorrhea in anorexia nervosa (Chap. 336). Although the mechanisms underlying these effects are unknown, the decreased adipose tissue associated with weight loss leads to a marked reduction in leptin, a hormone that plays a permissive role in GnRH production (Chap. 77). In many patients, weight gain to a specific threshold triggers restoration of the GnRH pulse generator, initially recapitulating the pubertal pattern of nocturnal gonadotropin secretion before returning to the normal adult pattern.

Serum cortisol and 24-h urine free cortisol levels are generally elevated but without characteristic clinical signs of cortisol excess. Thyroid function tests resemble the pattern seen in euthyroid sick syndrome (Chap. 330). Thyroxine (T_4) and free T_4 levels are usually in the low-normal range, triiodothyronine (T_3) levels are reduced, and reverse T_3 (rT_3) is elevated. The level of thyroid stimulating hormone (TSH) is normally or partially suppressed. Growth hormone is increased, but insulin-like growth factor 1 (IGF-1), which is produced mainly by the liver, is reduced, as it is in other conditions of starvation. Diminished bone density is routinely observed in anorexia nervosa and reflects the effects of multiple nutritional deficiencies, reduced gonadal steroids, and increased cortisol. The degree of bone density reduction is proportional to the length of the illness, and patients are at risk for the development of symptomatic fractures. The occurrence of anorexia nervosa during adolescence may lead to the premature cessation of linear bone growth and a failure to achieve expected adult height.

Cardiac Abnormalities   Cardiac output is reduced, and congestive heart failure occasionally occurs during rapid refeeding. The electrocardiogram usually shows sinus bradycardia, reduced QRS voltage, and nonspecific ST-T-wave abnormalities. Some patients develop a prolonged QT_c interval, which may predispose to serious arrhythmias.

BULIMIA NERVOSA   The typical patient presenting for treatment of bulimia nervosa is a woman of normal weight in her mid-twenties who reports binge eating and purging 5 to 10 times a week for 5 to 10 years. The disorder usually begins in late adolescence or early adulthood during or following a diet. The self-imposed caloric restriction leads to increased hunger and to overeating. In an attempt to avoid weight gain, the patient induces vomiting, takes laxatives or diuretics, or engages in some other form of compensatory behavior. Initially, patients may experience a sense of satisfaction that appealing food can be eaten without weight gain. However, as the disorder progresses, patients perceive diminished control over eating. Binges increase in size and frequency and are provoked by a variety of stimuli, such as transient depression, anxiety, or a sense that too much food has been consumed in a normal meal. Between binges, patients attempt to restrict caloric intake, which increases hunger and sets the stage for the next binge.

Although vomiting may be triggered initially by manual stimulation of the gag reflex, most patients with bulimia nervosa develop the ability to induce vomiting at will. Rarely, patients resort to the regular use of syrup of ipecac. Laxatives and diuretics are frequently taken in impressive quantities, such as 30 or 60 laxative pills on a single occasion. The resulting fluid loss produces dehydration and a feeling of emptiness but has little impact on caloric balance.

The physical abnormalities associated with bulimia nervosa primarily result from the purging behavior. Painless bilateral salivary gland hypertrophy (sialadenosis) may be noted. A scar or callus on the dorsum of the hand may develop due to repeated trauma from the teeth among patients who manually stimulate the gag reflex. Recurrent vomiting and the exposure of the lingual surfaces of the teeth to stomach acid leads to loss of dental enamel and eventually to chipping and erosion of the front teeth. Laboratory abnormalities are surprisingly infrequent, but hypokalemia, hypochloremia, and hyponatremia are observed occasionally. Repeated vomiting may lead to alkalosis, whereas repeated laxative abuse may produce a mild metabolic acidosis. Serum amylase may be mildly elevated due to an increase in the salivary isoenzyme.

Serious physical complications resulting from bulimia nervosa are rare. Oligomenorrhea and amenorrhea are more frequent than in women without eating disorders. Arrhythmias occasionally occur secondary to electrolyte disturbances. Tearing of the esophagus and rupture of the stomach, which constitute life-threatening events, have been reported. Some patients who have chronically abused laxatives or diuretics develop transient peripheral edema when this behavior ceases, presumably due to high levels of aldosterone resulting from persistent fluid and electrolyte depletion.

PROGNOSIS

The course and outcome of anorexia nervosa are highly variable. One-quarter to one-half of patients eventually recover fully, with few psychological or physical sequelae. However, many patients have persistent difficulties with weight maintenance, depression, and eating disturbances, including bulimia nervosa. The development of obesity following anorexia nervosa is rare. The long-term mortality of anorexia nervosa is among the highest associated with any psychiatric disorder. Approximately 5% of patients die per decade of follow-up, primarily due to the physical effects of chronic starvation or by suicide.

Virtually all of the physiologic abnormalities associated with anorexia nervosa are observed in other forms of starvation and markedly improve or disappear with weight gain. A worrisome exception is the reduction in bone mass, which may not recover fully, particularly when anorexia nervosa occurs during adolescence when peak bone mass is normally achieved.

The prognosis of bulimia nervosa is much more favorable. Mortality is low, and full recovery occurs in approximately 50% of patients within 10 years. Approximately 25% of patients have persistent symptoms of bulimia nervosa over many years. Few patients progress from bulimia nervosa to anorexia nervosa.

℞ TREATMENT   Anorexia Nervosa   Because of the profound physiological and psychological effects of starvation, there is a broad consensus that weight restoration to 90% of predicted weight is the primary goal in the treatment of anorexia nervosa. Unfortunately, because most patients resist this goal, its accomplishment is often accompanied by frustration for the patient, the family, and the physician. In attempting to engage the patient in treatment, it may be useful for the physician to elicit the patient's physical concerns (e.g., about osteoporosis, weakness, or fertility) and, if possible, educate the patient regarding the importance of normalizing nutritional status in order to address those concerns. The physician should attempt to reassure the patient that weight gain will not be permitted to get "out of control" but simultaneously emphasize that weight restoration is medically and psychologically imperative.

The intensity of the initial treatment, including the need for hospitalization, is determined by the patient's current weight, the rapidity of recent weight loss, and the severity of medical and psychological complications (Fig. 78-1). Hospitalization should be strongly considered for patients weighing <75% of expected, even if the results of routine blood studies are within normal limits. Acute medical problems, such as severe electrolyte imbalances, should be identified and addressed. Nutritional restoration can almost always be successfully accomplished by oral feeding, and parenteral methods are rarely required. For severely underweight patients, sufficient calories (approximately 1500 to 1800 kcal/d) should be provided initially in divided meals as food or liquid supplements to maintain weight and to permit stabilization of fluid and electrolyte balance. Calories can then be gradually increased to achieve a weight gain of 1 to 2 kg (2 to 4 lb) per week, typically requiring an intake of 3000 to 4000 kcal/d. Meals must be supervised, ideally by personnel who are firm regarding the necessity of food consumption, empathic regarding the challenges entailed, and reassuring regarding the patient's eventual recovery. Patients have great psychological difficulty complying with the need for increased caloric consumption, and the assistance of psychiatrists or psychologists experienced in the treatment of anorexia nervosa is usually necessary.

Psychiatric treatment focuses primarily on two issues. First, patients require much emotional support during the period of weight gain. Second, patients must learn to base their self-esteem, not on the achievement of an inappropriately low weight, but on the development of satisfying personal relationships and the attainment of reasonable academic and occupational goals. For younger patients, the active involvement of the family in treatment is crucial.

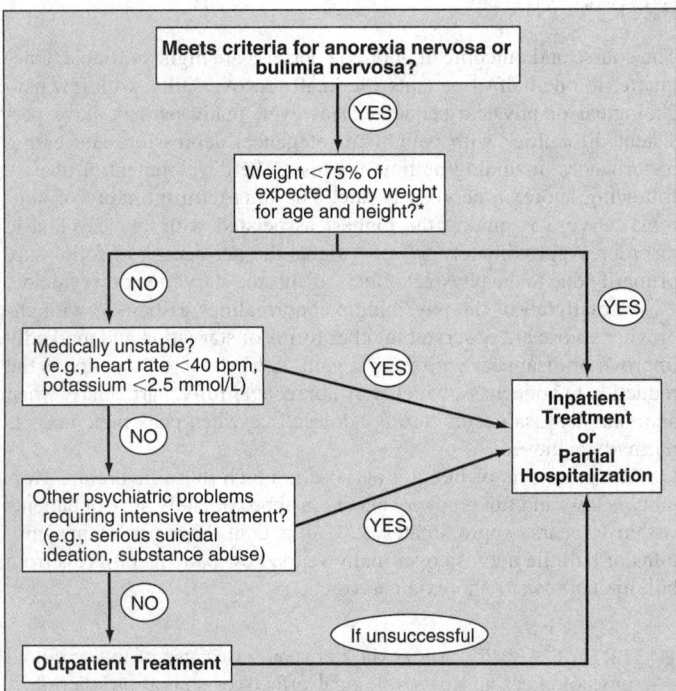

```
┌─────────────────────────────────────┐
│  Meets criteria for anorexia nervosa │
│         or bulimia nervosa?          │
└─────────────────────────────────────┘
                  │ (YES)
        ┌─────────────────────┐
        │   Weight <75% of     │
        │ expected body weight │
        │  for age and height?*│
        └─────────────────────┘
    (NO)                        (YES)
   ┌──────────────────────────┐
   │ Medically unstable?       │     ┌──────────────┐
   │ (e.g., heart rate <40 bpm,│ YES │  Inpatient   │
   │ potassium <2.5 mmol/L)    │     │  Treatment   │
   └──────────────────────────┘     │     or       │
        (NO)                         │  Partial     │
   ┌──────────────────────────┐     │Hospitalization│
   │ Other psychiatric problems│ YES └──────────────┘
   │ requiring intensive       │
   │ treatment? (e.g., serious │
   │ suicidal ideation,        │
   │ substance abuse)          │
   └──────────────────────────┘
        (NO)          If unsuccessful
   ┌──────────────────────┐
   │ Outpatient Treatment  │
   └──────────────────────┘
```

FIGURE 78-1 An algorithm for basic treatment decisions regarding patients with anorexia nervosa or bulimia nervosa. Based on the American Psychiatric Association's practice guidelines for the treatment of patients with eating disorders.* Although outpatient management may be considered for patients with anorexia nervosa weighing more than 75% of expected, there should be a low threshold for using more intensive interventions if the weight loss has been rapid or if current weight is <80% of expected.

Less severely affected patients may be treated in a partial hospitalization program where medical and psychiatric supervision is available and several meals can be monitored each day. Outpatient treatment may suffice for mildly ill patients. Weight must be monitored at frequent intervals, and explicit goals agreed on for weight gain, with the understanding that more intensive treatment will be required if the level of care initially employed is not successful.

Medical complications occasionally occur during refeeding. Most patients transiently retain excess fluid, occasionally resulting in peripheral edema. Fluid retention occurs during recovery from other forms of malnutrition and generally does not require specific treatment in the absence of cardiac, renal, or hepatic dysfunction. Congestive heart failure and acute gastric dilatation have been described when refeeding has been rapid. Transient modest elevations in serum levels of liver enzymes occasionally occur. Low levels of magnesium and phosphate should be repleted. Multivitamins should be given, and it is important to ensure adequate intake of vitamin D (400 IU/d) and calcium (1500 mg/d) to minimize bone loss.

No psychotropic medications are of established value in the treatment of anorexia nervosa; tricyclic antidepressants are contraindicated when there is prolongation of the QT_c interval. The alterations of cortisol and thyroid hormone metabolism do not require specific treatment and are corrected by weight gain. Estrogen treatment appears to have minimal impact on bone density in underweight patients but may be helpful to relieve symptoms of estrogen deficiency.

Bulimia Nervosa Bulimia nervosa can usually be treated on an outpatient basis. Cognitive behavioral therapy (CBT) is a short-term (4 to 6 months) psychological treatment that focuses on the intense concern with shape and weight, the persistent dieting, and the binge eating and purging that characterize this disorder. Patients are directed to monitor the circumstances, thoughts, and emotions associated with binge/purge episodes, to eat regularly, and to challenge their assumptions linking weight to self-esteem. CBT produces symptomatic remission in 25 to 50% of patients.

Numerous double-bind, placebo-controlled trials have documented that antidepressant medications are useful in the treatment of bulimia nervosa but are probably somewhat less effective than CBT. Although efficacy has been established for virtually all chemical classes of antidepressants, only the selective serotonin reuptake inhibitor fluoxetine (Prozac) has been approved for use in bulimia nervosa by the U.S. Food and Drug Administration. Antidepressant medications are helpful even for patients with bulimia nervosa who are not depressed, and the dose of fluoxetine recommended for bulimia nervosa (60 mg/d) is higher than that typically used to treat depression. These observations suggest that different mechanisms may underlie the utility of these medications in bulimia nervosa and in depression.

A substantial minority of patients with bulimia nervosa do not respond adequately to CBT, antidepressant medication, or their combination. More intensive forms of treatment, including hospitalization, may be required for such patients.

BIBLIOGRAPHY

AMERICAN PSYCHIATRIC ASSOCIATION: Practice guideline for the treatment of patients with eating disorders (revision). Am J Psychiatry 157(Suppl 1):1, 2000.

BECKER AE et al: Eating disorders. N Engl J Med 340:1092, 1999

DEVLIN MJ: Assessment and treatment of binge-eating disorder. Psychiatr Clin North Am 19:761, 1996

FAIRBURN CG et al: Risk factors for bulimia nervosa. A community-based case-control study. Arch Gen Psychiatry 54:509, 1997

KEEL PK et al: Long-term outcome of bulimia nervosa. Arch Gen Psychiatry 56:63, 1999

SULLIVAN PF: Mortality in anorexia nervosa. Am J Psychiatry 152:1073, 1995

WALSH BT, DEVLIN MJ: Eating disorders: Progress and problems. Science 280:1387, 1998

PART SIX

ONCOLOGY AND HEMATOLOGY

Section 1
NEOPLASTIC DISORDERS

79 *Dan L. Longo*

APPROACH TO THE PATIENT WITH CANCER

The application of current treatment techniques (surgery, radiation therapy, chemotherapy, and biological therapy) results in the cure of >50% of patients diagnosed with cancer. Nevertheless, patients experience the diagnosis of cancer as one of the most traumatic and revolutionary events that has ever happened to them. Independent of prognosis, the diagnosis brings with it a change in a person's self-image and in his or her role in the home and workplace. The prognosis of a person who has just been found to have pancreatic cancer is the same as the prognosis of the person with aortic stenosis who develops the first symptoms of congestive heart failure (median survival, about 8 months). However, the patient with heart disease may remain functional and maintain a view of him- or herself as a fully intact person with just a malfunctioning part, a diseased organ ("a bum ticker"). By contrast, the patient with pancreatic cancer has a completely altered self-image and is viewed differently by family and anyone who knows the diagnosis. He or she is being attacked and invaded by a disease that could be anywhere in the body. Every ache or pain takes on desperate significance. Cancer is an exception to the coordinated interaction among cells and organs. In general, the cells of a multicellular organism are programmed for collaboration. Many diseases occur because the specialized cells fail to perform their assigned task. Cancer takes this malfunction one step further. Not only is there a failure of the cancer cell to maintain its specialized function, but it also strikes out on its own; the cancer cell competes to survive using natural mutability and natural selection to seek advantage over normal cells in a recapitulation of evolution. One consequence of the traitorous behavior of cancer cells is that the patient feels betrayed by his or her body. The cancer patient feels that he or she, and not just a body part, is diseased.

THE MAGNITUDE OF THE PROBLEM

There is no nationwide cancer registry; therefore, the incidence of cancer is estimated on the basis of the National Cancer Institute's Surveillance, Epidemiology, and End Results (SEER) database, which tabulates cancer incidence and death figures from nine sites, accounting for about 10% of the U.S. population, and from population data from the Bureau of the Census. In 2000, 1.22 million new cases of invasive cancer (619,700 men, 600,400 women) were diagnosed and 552,200 people (284,100 men, 268,100 women) died from cancer. The percent distribution of new cancer cases and cancer deaths by site for men and women are shown in Table 79-1. Cancer incidence has been declining by about 2% each year since 1992.

The most significant risk factor for cancer overall is age; two-thirds of all cases were in people over age 65. Cancer incidence increases as the third, fourth, or fifth power of age in different sites. For the interval between birth and age 39, 1 in 62 men and 1 in 52 women will develop cancer; for the interval between ages 40 and 59, 1 in 12 men and 1 in 11 women will develop cancer; and for the interval between ages 60 and 79, 1 in 3 men and 1 in 4 women will develop cancer.

Cancer is the second leading cause of death behind heart disease.

Table 79-1 Distribution of Cancer Incidence and Deaths for 2000[a]

Male			Female		
Sites	%	Number	Sites	%	Number
CANCER INCIDENCE					
Prostate	29	180,400	Breast	30	182,800
Lung and bronchus	14	89,500	Lung and bronchus	12	74,600
Colon and rectum	10	63,600	Colon and rectum	11	66,600
Bladder	6	38,300	Endometrium	6	36,100
Lymphoma	5	31,700	Ovary	4	23,100
Melanoma	4	27,300	Lymphoma	4	23,100
Oral Cavity	3	20,200	Melanoma	3	20,400
Kidney	3	18,800	Bladder	2	14,900
Leukemia	3	16,900	Pancreas	2	14,600
Pancreas	2	13,700	Thyroid	2	13,700
All other	19	119,300	All other	22	130,500
CANCER DEATHS					
Lung and bronchus	31	89,300	Lung and bronchus	25	67,600
Prostate	11	31,900	Breast	15	40,800
Colon and rectum	10	27,800	Colon and rectum	11	28,500
Pancreas	5	13,700	Pancreas	5	14,500
Lymphoma	5	13,700	Ovary	5	14,000
Leukemia	4	12,100	Lymphoma	5	12,400
Esophagus	3	9,200	Leukemia	4	9,600
Liver and bile duct	3	8,500	Endometrium	2	6,500
			Brain	2	5,900
Bladder	3	8,100	Stomach	2	5,400
Stomach	3	7,600	Myeloma	2	5,400
All other	22	62,200	All other	21	57,500

[a] Data exclude basal and squamous cell skin cancers and carcinoma in situ except the bladder.
SOURCE: RT Greenlee et al, with permission.

Deaths from heart disease have declined 45% in the United States since 1950 and continue to decline. After a 70-year period of increases, cancer deaths began to decline in 1997 (Fig. 79-1). The five leading causes of cancer deaths are shown for various populations in Table 79-2. Along with the decrease in incidence has come an increase in survival for cancer patients. The 5-year survival for white patients was 39% in 1960–1963 and 61% in 1989–1995. Cancers are more often deadly in blacks; the 5-year survival was 48% for the 1989–1995 interval. Incidence and mortality vary among racial and ethnic groups (Table 79-3). The basis for these differences is unclear.

PATIENT MANAGEMENT

Important information is obtained from every portion of the routine history and physical examination. The duration of symptoms may reveal the chronicity of disease. The past medical history may alert the physician to the presence of underlying diseases that may affect the choice of therapy or the side effects of treatment. The social history may reveal occupational exposure to carcinogens or habits, such as smoking or alcohol consumption, that may influence the course of disease and its treatment. The family history may suggest an underlying familial cancer predisposition and point out the need to begin

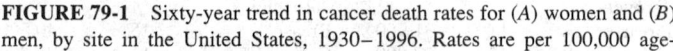

FIGURE 79-1 Sixty-year trend in cancer death rates for (*A*) women and (*B*) men, by site in the United States, 1930–1996. Rates are per 100,000 age- adjusted to the 1970 U.S. standard population. *(From Greenlee.)*

surveillance or other preventive therapy for unaffected siblings of the patient. The review of systems may suggest early symptoms of metastatic disease or a paraneoplastic syndrome.

DIAGNOSIS The diagnosis of cancer relies most heavily on invasive tissue biopsy and should never be made without obtaining tissue; no noninvasive diagnostic test is sufficient to define a disease process as cancer. Although in rare clinical settings (e.g., thyroid nodules) fine-needle aspiration is an acceptable diagnostic procedure, the diagnosis generally depends on obtaining adequate tissue to permit careful evaluation of the histology of the tumor, its grade, and its invasiveness and to yield further molecular diagnostic information, such as the expression of cell-surface markers or intracellular proteins that typify a particular cancer, or the presence of a molecular marker, such as the t(8;14) translocation of Burkitt's lymphoma. Increasing evidence links the expression of certain genes with the prognosis and response to therapy (Chaps. 81 and 82).

Occasionally a patient will present with a metastatic disease process that is defined as cancer on biopsy but has no apparent primary site of disease. Efforts should be made to define the primary site based on age, sex, sites of involvement, histology and tumor markers, and personal and family history. Particular attention should be focused on ruling out the most treatable causes (Chap. 99).

Once the diagnosis of cancer is made, the management of the patient is best undertaken as a multidisciplinary collaboration among the primary care physician, medical oncologists, surgical oncologists, radiation oncologists, oncology nurse specialists, pharmacists, social workers, rehabilitation medicine specialists, and a number of other consulting professionals working closely with each other and with the patient and family.

DEFINING THE EXTENT OF DISEASE AND THE PROGNOSIS The first priority in patient management after the diagnosis of cancer is established and shared with the patient is to determine the extent of disease. The curability of a tumor usually is inversely proportional to the tumor burden. Ideally, the tumor will be diagnosed before symptoms develop or as a consequence of screening efforts (Chap. 80). A very high proportion of such patients can be cured. However, most patients with cancer present with symptoms related to the cancer, caused either by mass effects of the tumor or by alterations associated with the production of cytokines or hormones by the tumor.

For most cancers, the extent of disease is evaluated by a variety of noninvasive and invasive diagnostic tests and procedures. This process is called *staging*. There are two types. *Clinical staging* is based on physical examination, radiographs, isotopic scans, computed tomography, and other imaging procedures;

Table 79-2 The Five Leading Primary Tumor Sites for Patients Dying of Cancer Based on Age and Sex in 1997

Rank	All Ages	Under 20	20–39	40–59	60–79	>80
			Age			
1	M,F: lung	M,F: leukemia	M: lymphoma F: breast	M: lung F: breast	M,F: lung	M,F: lung
2	M: prostate F: breast	M,F: brain	M: leukemia F: cervix	M: colorectal F: lung	M: prostate F: breast	M: prostate F: colorectal
3	M,F: colorectal	M: endocrine F: soft tissue sarcoma	M: brain F: lung	M: pancreas F: colorectal	M: colorectal	M: colorectal F: breast
4	M,F: pancreas	M: bone sarcoma F: endocrine	M: lung F: leukemia	M: lymphoma F: ovary	M,F: pancreas	M: bladder F: pancreas
5	M: lymphoma F: ovary	M: lymphoma F: bone sarcoma	M: colorectal F: brain	M: esophagus F: cervix	M: lymphoma F: ovary	M: pancreas F: lymphoma

NOTE: M, male; F, female.

492

pathologic staging takes into account information obtained during a surgical procedure, which might include intraoperative palpation, resection of regional lymph nodes and/or tissue adjacent to the tumor, and inspection and biopsy of organs commonly involved in disease spread. Pathologic staging includes histologic examination of all tissues removed during the surgical procedure. Surgical procedures performed may include a simple lymph node biopsy or more extensive procedures such as thoracotomy, mediastinoscopy, or laparotomy. Surgical staging may occur in a separate procedure or may be done at the time of definitive surgical resection of the primary tumor.

Table 79-3 Cancer Incidence and Mortality in Racial and Ethnic Groups 1990–1996

Site	White	Black	Asian/Pacific Islander	American Indian	Hispanic
INCIDENCE PER 100,000 POPULATION					
All	M: 480	M: 598	M: 326	M: 178	M: 327
	F: 352	F: 336	F: 245	F: 137	F: 243
Breast (F)	113	66	73	34	69
Colon	M: 53	M: 58	M: 47	M: 22	M: 36
	F: 37	F: 45	F: 23	F: 12	F: 20
Lung	M: 73	M: 112	M: 52	M: 25	M: 39
	F: 43	F: 46	F: 23	F: 14	F: 20
Prostate (M)	147	223	82	47	103
MORTALITY PER 100,000 POPULATION					
All	M: 209	M: 309	M: 129	M: 123	M: 132
	F: 140	F: 168	F: 84	F: 90	F: 86
Breast (F)	26	31	11	12	15
Colon	M: 22	M: 28	M: 13	M: 11	M: 13
	F: 15	F: 20	F: 9	F: 9	F: 8
Lung	M: 70	M: 101	M: 35	M: 41	M: 32
	F: 34	F: 33	F: 15	F: 20	F: 11
Prostate (M)	24	55	11	14	17

NOTE: M, male; F, female.

Knowledge of the predilection of particular tumors for spread to adjacent or distant organs helps direct the staging evaluation.

Information obtained from staging is used to define the extent of disease either as localized, as exhibiting spread outside of the organ of origin to regional but not distant sites, or as metastatic to distant sites. The most widely used system of staging is the TNM (tumor, node, metastasis) system codified by the International Union Against Cancer and the American Joint Committee on Cancer (AJCC).[1] The TNM classification is an anatomically based system that categorizes the tumor on the basis of the size of the primary tumor lesion (T1–4, where a higher number indicates a tumor of larger size), the presence of nodal involvement (usually N0 and N1 for the absence and presence, respectively, of involved nodes, although some tumors have more elaborate systems of nodal grading), and the presence of metastatic disease (M0 and M1 for the absence and presence, respectively, of metastases). The various permutations of T, N, and M scores are then broken into stages, usually designated by the roman numerals I through IV. Tumor burden increases and curability decreases with increasing stage. Other anatomic staging systems are used for some tumors, e.g., the Dukes classification for colorectal cancers, the International Federation of Gynecologists and Obstetricians (FIGO) classification for gynecologic cancers, and the Ann Arbor classification for Hodgkin's disease.

Certain tumors cannot be grouped appropriately on the basis of anatomic considerations. For example, hematopoietic tumors such as leukemia, myeloma, and lymphoma are often disseminated at presentation and do not spread in the fashion typical of solid tumors. For these tumors, other prognostic factors have been identified (Chaps. 111, 112, and 113).

In addition to tumor burden, a second major determinant of treatment outcome is the physiologic reserve of the patient. Patients who are bedridden before developing cancer are likely to fare worse, stage for stage, than fully active patients. Physiologic reserve is a determinant of how a patient is likely to cope with the physiologic stresses imposed by the cancer and its treatment. This factor is difficult to assess directly. Instead, surrogate markers for physiologic reserve are used, such as the patient's age or Karnofsky performance status (Table 79-4). Older patients and those with a Karnofsky performance status <70 have a poor prognosis unless the poor performance is a reversible consequence of the tumor.

Increasingly, biologic features of the tumor are being related to

prognosis. The expression of particular oncogenes, drug-resistance genes, apoptosis-related genes, and genes involved in metastasis are being found to influence response to therapy and prognosis. The presence of selected cytogenetic abnormalities may influence survival. Tumors with higher growth fractions, as assessed by expression of proliferation-related markers such as proliferating cell nuclear antigen (PCNA), behave more aggressively than tumors with lower growth fractions. Information obtained from studying the tumor itself will increasingly be used to influence treatment decisions.

MAKING A TREATMENT PLAN From information on the extent of disease and the prognosis and in conjunction with the patient's wishes, it is determined whether the treatment approach should be curative or palliative in intent. Cooperation among the various professionals involved in cancer treatment is of the utmost importance in treatment planning. For some cancers, chemotherapy or chemotherapy plus radiation therapy delivered before the use of definitive surgical treatment (so-called neoadjuvant therapy) may improve the outcome, as seems to be the case for locally advanced breast cancer and head and neck cancers. In certain settings in which combined modality therapy is intended, coordination among the medical oncologist, radiation oncologist, and surgeon is crucial to achieving optimal results. Sometimes the chemotherapy and radiation therapy need to be delivered sequentially, and other times concurrently. Surgical procedures may precede or follow other treatment approaches. It is best for the treat-

Table 79-4 Karnofsky Performance Index

Performance Status	Functional Capability of the Patient
100	Normal; no complaints; no evidence of disease
90	Able to carry on normal activity; minor signs or symptoms of disease
80	Normal activity with effort; some signs or symptoms of disease
70	Cares for self; unable to carry on normal activity or do active work
60	Requires occasional assistance but is able to care for most needs
50	Requires considerable assistance and frequent medical care
40	Disabled; requires special care and assistance
30	Severely disabled; hospitalization is indicated although death is not imminent
20	Very sick; hospitalization necessary; active supportive treatment is necessary
10	Moribund, fatal processes progressing rapidly
0	Dead

[1]The AJCC *Manual for Staging Cancer*, 5th edition, can be obtained from the AJCC at 55 East Erie Street, Chicago, Il, 60611.

Table 79-5 Tumor Markers

Tumor Markers	Cancer	Non-Neoplastic Conditions
HORMONES		
Human chorionic gonadotropin	Gestational trophoblastic disease, gonadal germ cell tumor	Pregnancy
Calcitonin	Medullary cancer of the thyroid	
Catecholamines	Pheochromocytoma	
ONCOFETAL ANTIGENS		
Alphafetoprotein	Hepatocellular carcinoma, gonadal germ cell tumor	Cirrhosis, hepatitis
Carcinoembryonic antigen	Adenocarcinomas of the colon, pancreas, lung, breast, ovary	Pancreatitis, hepatitis, inflammatory bowel disease, smoking
ENZYMES		
Prostatic acid phosphatase	Prostate cancer	Prostatitis, prostatic hypertrophy
Neuron-specific enolase	Small cell cancer of the lung, neuroblastoma	
Lactate dehydrogenase	Lymphoma, Ewing's sarcoma	Hepatitis, hemolytic anemia, many others
TUMOR-ASSOCIATED PROTEINS		
Prostate-specific antigen	Prostate cancer	Prostatitis, prostatic hypertrophy
Monoclonal immunoglobulin	Myeloma	Infection, MGUS[a]
CA-125	Ovarian cancer, some lymphomas	Menstruation, peritonitis, pregnancy
CA 19-9	Colon, pancreatic, breast cancer	Pancreatitis, ulcerative colitis
CD30	Hodgkin's disease, anaplastic large cell lymphoma	—
CD25	Hairy cell leukemia, adult T cell leukemia/lymphoma	—

[a] MGUS, monoclonal gammopathy of uncertain significance.

ment plan either to follow a standard protocol precisely or else to be part of an ongoing clinical research protocol evaluating new treatments. Ad hoc modifications of standard protocols are likely to compromise treatment results.

The choice of treatment approaches was formerly dominated by the local culture in both the university and the practice settings. However, it is now possible to gain access electronically to standard treatment protocols and to every approved clinical research study in North America through a personal computer interface with the Internet.[2]

The skilled physician also has much to offer the patient for whom curative therapy is no longer an option. Often a combination of guilt and frustration over the inability to cure the patient and the pressure of a busy schedule greatly limit the time a physician spends with a patient who is receiving only palliative care. Resist these forces. In addition to the medicines administered to alleviate symptoms (see below), it is important to remember the comfort that is provided by holding the patient's hand, continuing regular examinations, and taking time to talk.

MANAGEMENT OF DISEASE AND TREATMENT COMPLICATIONS   Because cancer therapies are toxic (Chap. 84), patient management involves addressing complications of both the disease and its treatment as well as the complex psychosocial problems

associated with cancer. In the short term during a course of curative therapy, the patient's functional status may decline. Treatment-induced toxicity is less acceptable if the goal of therapy is palliation. The most common side effects of treatment are nausea and vomiting (see below), febrile neutropenia (Chap. 85), and myelosuppression (Chap. 104). Therapeutic tools are now available to minimize the acute toxicity of cancer treatment.

New symptoms developing in the course of cancer treatment should always be assumed to be reversible until proven otherwise. The fatalistic attribution of anorexia, weight loss, and jaundice to recurrent or progressive tumor could result in a patient dying from a reversible intercurrent cholecystitis. Intestinal obstruction may be due to reversible adhesions rather than progressive tumor. Systemic infections, sometimes with unusual pathogens, may be a consequence of the immunosuppression associated with cancer therapy. Some drugs used to treat cancer or its complications (e.g., nausea) may produce central nervous system symptoms that look like metastatic disease or may mimic paraneoplastic syndromes such as the syndrome of inappropriate antidiuretic hormone. A definitive diagnosis should be pursued and may even require a repeat biopsy.

A critical component of cancer management is assessing the response to treatment. In addition to a careful physical examination in which all sites of disease are physically measured and recorded in a flow chart by date, response assessment usually requires periodic repeating of imaging tests that were abnormal at the time of staging. If imaging tests have become normal, repeat biopsy of previously involved tissue is performed to document complete response by pathologic criteria. Biopsies are not usually required if there is macroscopic residual disease. A *complete response* is defined as disappearance of all evidence of disease, and a *partial response* as >50% reduction in the sum of the products of the perpendicular diameters of all measureable lesions. *Progressive disease* is defined as the appearance of any new lesion or an increase of >25% in the sum of the products of the perpendicular diameters of all measurable lesions. Tumor shrinkage or growth that does not meet any of these criteria is considered *stable disease*. Some sites of involvement (e.g., bone) or patterns of involvement (e.g., lymphangitic lung or diffuse pulmonary infiltrates) are considered unmeasurable. No response is complete without biopsy documentation of their resolution but partial responses may exclude their assessment unless clear objective (though unmeasurable) progression has occurred.

Tumor markers may be useful in patient management in certain tumors. Response to therapy may be difficult to gauge with certainty. However, some tumors produce or elicit the production of markers that can be measured in the serum or urine and, in a particular patient, rising and falling levels of the marker are usually associated with increasing or decreasing tumor burden, respectively. Some clinically useful tumor markers are shown in Table 79-5. Tumor markers are not in themselves specific enough to permit a diagnosis of malignancy to be made, but once a malignancy has been diagnosed and shown to be associated with elevated levels of a tumor marker, the marker can be used to assess response to treatment.

The recognition and treatment of depression are important components of management. The incidence of depression in cancer patients is ~25% overall and may be greater in patients with greater debility. This diagnosis is likely in a patient with a depressed mood (dysphoria) and/or a loss of interest in pleasure (anhedonia) for at least 2 weeks.

---

[2]The National Cancer Institute maintains a database called PDQ (Physician Data Query) that is accessible on the Internet under the name CancerNet at wwwicic.nci.nih.gov/health.htm. Information can be obtained through a facsimile machine using CancerFax by dialing 301-402-5874. Patient information is also provided by the National Cancer Institute in at least three formats: on the Internet via CancerNet at wwwicic.nci.nih.gov/patient.htm, through the CancerFax number listed above, or by calling 1-800-4-CANCER. The quality control for the information provided through these services is rigorous.

In addition, three or more of the following symptoms are usually present: appetite change, sleep problems, psychomotor retardation or agitation, fatigue, feelings of guilt or worthlessness, inability to concentrate, and suicidal ideation. Patients with these symptoms should receive therapy. Medical therapy with a serotonin reuptake inhibitor such as fluoxetine (10 to 20 mg/d), sertraline (50 to 150 mg/d), or paroxetine (10 to 20 mg/d) or a tricyclic antidepressant such as amitriptyline (50 to 100 mg/d) or desipramine (75 to 150 mg/d) should be tried, allowing 4 to 6 weeks for response. Effective therapy should be continued at least 6 months after resolution of symptoms. If therapy is unsuccessful, other classes of antidepressants may be used. In addition to medication, psychosocial interventions such as support groups, psychotherapy, and guided imagery may be of benefit.

Many patients opt for unproven or unsound approaches to treatment when it appears that conventional medicine is unlikely to be curative. Those seeking such alternatives are often well educated and may be early in the course of their disease. Unsound approaches are usually hawked on the basis of unsubstantiated anecdotes and not only cannot help the patient but may be harmful. Physicians should strive to keep communications open and nonjudgmental, so that patients are more likely to discuss with the physician what they are actually doing. The appearance of unexpected toxicity may be an indication that a supplemental therapy is being taken.[3]

LONG-TERM FOLLOW-UP/LATE COMPLICATIONS
At the completion of treatment, sites originally involved with tumor are reassessed, usually by radiography or imaging techniques, and any persistent abnormality is biopsied. If disease persists, the multidisciplinary team discusses a new salvage treatment plan. If the patient has been rendered disease-free by the original treatment, the patient is followed regularly for disease recurrence. The optimal guidelines for follow-up care are not known. For many years, a routine practice has been to follow the patient monthly for 6 to 12 months, then every other month for a year, every 3 months for a year, every 4 months for a year, every 6 months for a year, and then annually. At each visit, a battery of laboratory and radiographic and imaging tests were obtained on the assumption that it is best to detect recurrent disease before it becomes symptomatic. However, where follow-up procedures have been examined, this assumption has been found to be untrue. Studies of breast cancer, melanoma, lung cancer, colon cancer, and lymphoma have all failed to support the notion that asymptomatic relapses are more readily cured by salvage therapy than symptomatic relapses. In view of the enormous cost of a full battery of diagnostic tests and their manifest lack of impact on survival, new guidelines are emerging for less frequent follow-up visits during which the history and physical examination are the major investigations performed.

As time passes, the likelihood of recurrence of the primary cancer diminishes. For many types of cancer, survival for 5 years without recurrence is tantamount to cure. However, important medical problems can occur in patients treated for cancer and must be examined (Chap 103). Some problems emerge as a consequence of the disease and some as a consequence of the treatment. An understanding of these disease- and treatment-related problems may help in their detection and management.

Despite these concerns, most patients who are cured of cancer return to normal lives.

SUPPORTIVE CARE
In many ways, the success of cancer therapy depends on the success of the supportive care. Failure to control the symptoms of cancer and its treatment may lead patients to abandon curative therapy. Of equal importance, supportive care is a major determinant of quality of life. Even when life cannot be prolonged, the physician must strive to preserve its quality. Quality-of-life measurements have become common end-points of clinical research studies.

Furthermore, palliative care has been shown to be cost-effective when approached in an organized fashion. A credo for oncology could be to cure sometimes, to extend life often, and to comfort always.

Pain Pain occurs with variable frequency in the cancer patient: 25 to 50% of patients present with pain at diagnosis, 33% have pain associated with treatment, and 75% have pain with progressive disease. The pain may have several causes. In about 70% of cases, pain is caused by the tumor itself—by invasion of bone, nerves, blood vessels, or mucous membranes or obstruction of a hollow viscus or duct. In about 20% of cases, pain is related to a surgical or invasive medical procedure, to radiation injury (mucositis, enteritis, or plexus or spinal cord injury), or to chemotherapy injury (mucositis, peripheral neuropathy, phlebitis, steroid-induced aseptic necrosis of the femoral head). In 10% of cases, pain is unrelated to cancer or its treatment.

Assessment of pain requires the methodical investigation of the history of the pain, its location, character, temporal features, provocative and palliative factors, and intensity (Chap. 12); a review of the oncologic history and past medical history as well as personal and social history; and a thorough physical examination. The patient should be given a 10-division visual analogue scale on which to indicate the severity of the pain. The clinical condition is often dynamic, making it necessary to reassess the patient frequently. Pain therapy should not be withheld while the cause of pain is being sought.

A variety of tools are available with which to address cancer pain. About 85% of patients will have pain relief from pharmacologic intervention. However, other modalities, including antitumor therapy (such as surgical relief of obstruction, radiation therapy, and strontium-89 or samarium-153 treatment for bone pain), neurostimulatory techniques, regional analgesia, or neuroablative procedures are effective in an additional 12% or so. Thus, very few patients will have inadequate pain relief if appropriate measures are taken.

The World Health Organization (WHO) has devised a simple and effective method for the rational titration of oral analgesia, called the *WHO ladder*. The ladder has the following three steps. (1) For mild to moderate pain, one begins with acetaminophen (650 mg every 4 h or 975 mg every 6 h), aspirin (650 mg every 4 h or 975 mg every 6 h), or a nonsteroidal anti-inflammatory agent (NSAID; e.g., ketoprofen, 25 to 60 mg every 6 h) with or without an adjuvant such as a glucocorticoid (dexamethasone) or an antidepressant (amitriptyline). (2) When pain persists or increases, an opioid such as codeine or hydrocodone (30 mg every 3 to 4 h is roughly equivalent to 10 mg of intravenous morphine) should be added (not substituted); fixed combinations such as oxycodone/acetaminophen (Percocet) or oxycodone/aspirin (Percodan) are worth testing. (3) Pain that is persistent or that is moderate to severe at the outset should be treated by increasing the potency of the opioid or using higher dosages (e.g., morphine, 15 to 30 mg every 3 to 4 h, or controlled-release morphine, 90 to 120 mg bid), and fixed opioid/NSAID combinations should be abandoned. Adjuvants may be used at all steps. The critical features of this approach are that the treatment is oral, should be given around the clock with supplemental doses as needed to control pain, and is tailored to the individual patient. Transmucosal fentanyl (in lollipop form) may aid in control of breakthrough pain. Records of pain control should be a prominent component of the medical record. When opioids are used, the patient should be placed on a prophylactic regimen to prevent constipation.

Nausea Emesis in the cancer patient is usually caused by chemotherapy (Chap. 84). Its severity can be predicted from the drugs used to treat the cancer. Three forms of emesis are recognized on the basis of their timing with regard to the noxious insult. *Acute emesis*, the most common variety, occurs within 24 h of treatment. *Delayed emesis* occurs 1 to 7 days after treatment; it is rare, but, when present, usually follows cisplatin administration. *Anticipatory emesis* occurs before administration of chemotherapy and represents a conditioned response to visual and olfactory stimuli previously associated with chemotherapy delivery.

[3]Information about unsound methods may be obtained from the National Council Against Health Fraud, Box 1276, Loma Linda, CA 92354, or from the Center for Medical Consumers and Health Care Information, 237 Thompson Street, New York, NY 10012.

Acute emesis is the best understood form. Stimuli that activate signals in the chemoreceptor trigger zone in the medulla, the cerebral cortex, and peripherally in the intestinal tract lead to stimulation of the vomiting center in the medulla, the motor center responsible for coordinating the secretory and muscle contraction activity that leads to emesis. Diverse receptor types participate in the process, including dopamine, serotonin, histamine, opioid, and acetylcholine receptors. The serotonin receptor antagonists ondansetron and granisetron are the most effective drugs against highly emetogenic agents, but they are expensive.

As with the analgesia ladder, emesis therapy should be tailored to the situation. For mildly and moderately emetogenic agents, prochlorperazine, 5 to 10 mg orally or 25 mg rectally, is effective. Its efficacy may be enhanced by administering the drug before the chemotherapy is delivered. Dexamethasone, 10 to 20 mg intravenously, is also effective and may enhance the efficacy of prochlorperazine. For highly emetogenic agents such as cisplatin, mechlorethamine, dacarbazine, and streptozocin, combinations of agents work best and administration should begin 6 to 24 h before treatment. Ondansetron, 8 mg orally every 6 h the day before therapy and intravenously on the day of therapy, plus dexamethasone, 20 mg intravenously before treatment, is an effective regimen. Like pain, emesis is easier to prevent than to alleviate.

Delayed emesis may be related to bowel inflammation from the therapy and can be controlled with oral dexamethasone and oral metoclopramide, a dopamine receptor antagonist that also blocks serotonin receptors at high dosages. The best strategy for preventing anticipatory emesis is to control emesis in the early cycles of therapy to prevent the conditioning from taking place. If this is unsuccessful, prophylactic antiemetics the day before treatment may help. Experimental studies are evaluating behavior modification.

Effusions   Fluid may accumulate abnormally in the pleural cavity, pericardium, or peritoneum. Asymptomatic malignant effusions may not require treatment. Symptomatic effusions occurring in tumors responsive to systemic therapy usually do not require local treatment but respond to the treatment for the underlying tumor. Symptomatic effusions occurring in tumors unresponsive to systemic therapy may require local treatment in patients with a life expectancy of at least 6 months.

Pleural effusions due to tumors may or may not contain malignant cells. Lung cancer, breast cancer, and lymphomas account for about 75% of malignant pleural effusions. Their exudative nature is usually gauged by an effusion/serum protein ratio of 0.5 or an effusion/serum lactate dehydrogenase ratio of 0.6. When the condition is symptomatic, thoracentesis is usually performed first. In most cases, symptomatic improvement occurs for <1 month. Chest tube drainage is required if symptoms recur within 2 weeks. Fluid is aspirated until the flow rate is <100 mL in 24 h. Then either 60 units of bleomycin or 1 g of doxycycline is infused into the chest tube in 50 mL of 5% dextrose in water; the tube is clamped; the patient is rotated on four sides, spending 15 min in each position; and, after 1 to 2 h, the tube is again attached to suction for another 24 h. The tube is then disconnected from suction and allowed to drain by gravity. If <100 mL drains over the next 24 h, the chest tube is pulled, and a radiograph taken 24 h later. If the chest tube continues to drain fluid at an unacceptably high rate, sclerosis can be repeated. Bleomycin may be somewhat more effective than doxycycline but is very expensive. Doxycycline is usually the drug of first choice. If neither doxycycline nor bleomycin is effective, talc can be used.

Symptomatic pericardial effusions are usually treated by creating a pericardial window or by stripping the pericardium. If the patient's condition does not permit a surgical procedure, sclerosis can be attempted with doxycycline and/or bleomycin.

Malignant ascites is usually treated with repeated paracentesis of small volumes of fluid. If the underlying malignancy is unresponsive to systemic therapy, peritoneovenous shunts may be inserted. Despite the fear of disseminating tumor cells into the circulation, widespread metastases are an unusual complication. The major complications are occlusion, leakage, and fluid overload. Patients with severe liver disease may develop disseminated intravascular coagulation.

Nutrition   Cancer and its treatment may lead to a decrease in nutrient intake of sufficient magnitude to cause weight loss and alteration of intermediary metabolism. The prevalence of this problem is difficult to estimate because of variations in the definition of cancer cachexia, but most patients with advanced cancer experience weight loss and decreased appetite. A variety of both tumor-derived factors (e.g., bombesin, adrenocorticotropic hormone) and host-derived factors (e.g., tumor necrosis factor, interleukins 1 and 6, growth hormone) contribute to the altered metabolism, and a vicious cycle is established in which protein catabolism, glucose intolerance, and lipolysis cannot be reversed by the provision of calories.

It remains controversial how to assess nutritional status and when and how to intervene. Efforts to make the assessment objective have included the use of a prognostic nutritional index based on albumin levels, triceps skin fold thickness, transferrin levels, and delayed-type hypersensitivity skin testing. However, a simpler approach has been to define the threshold for nutritional intervention as >10% unexplained body weight loss, serum transferrin level <1500 mg/L (150 mg/dL), and serum albumin <34 g/L (3.4 g/dL).

The decision is important, because it appears that cancer therapy is substantially more toxic and less effective in the face of malnutrition. Nevertheless, it remains unclear whether nutritional intervention can alter the natural history. Unless some pathology is affecting the absorptive function of the gastrointestinal tract, enteral nutrition provided orally or by tube feeding is preferred over parenteral supplementation. However, the risks associated with the tube may outweigh the benefits. Megestrol acetate, a progestational agent, has been advocated as a pharmacologic intervention to improve nutritional status. Research in this area may provide more tools in the future as cytokine-mediated mechanisms are further elucidated.

Psychosocial Support   The psychosocial needs of patients vary with their situation. Patients undergoing treatment experience fear, anxiety, and depression. Self-image is often seriously compromised by deforming surgery and loss of hair. Women who receive cosmetic advice that enables them to look better also feel better. Loss of control over how one spends time can contribute to the sense of vulnerability. Juggling the demands of work and family with the demands of treatment may create enormous stresses. Sexual dysfunction is highly prevalent and needs to be discussed openly with the patient. An empathetic health care team is sensitive to the individual patient's needs and permits negotiation where such flexibility will not adversely affect the course of treatment.

Cancer survivors have other sets of difficulties. Patients may have fears associated with the termination of a treatment they associate with their continued survival. Adjustments are required to physical losses and handicaps, real and perceived. Patients may be preoccupied with minor physical problems. They perceive a decline in their job mobility and view themselves as less desirable workers. They may be victims of job and/or insurance discrimination. Patients may experience difficulty reentering their normal past life. They may feel guilty for having survived and may carry a sense of vulnerability to colds and other illnesses. Perhaps the most pervasive and threatening concern is the ever-present fear of relapse (the Damocles syndrome).

Patients in whom therapy has been unsuccessful have other problems related to the end of life.

Death and Dying   The most common causes of death in patients with cancer are infection (leading to circulatory failure), respiratory failure, hepatic failure, and renal failure. Intestinal blockage may lead to inanition and starvation. Central nervous system disease may lead to seizures, coma, and central hypoventilation. About 70% of patients develop dyspnea preterminally. However, many months usually pass between the diagnosis of cancer and the occurrence of these complications, and during this period the patient is severely affected by the possibility of death. The path of unsuccessful cancer treatment usually occurs in three phases. First, there is optimism at the hope of cure; when the tumor recurs, there is the acknowledgment of an incurable disease, and the goal of palliative therapy is embraced in the hope of being able to live with disease; finally, at the disclosure of imminent death, another adjustment in outlook takes place. The patient imagines the worst in preparation for the end of life and may go through stages of adjustment to the diagnosis. These stages include denial, isolation, anger, bargaining, depression, acceptance, and hope. Of course, patients do not all progress through all the stages or proceed through them in the same order or at the same rate. Nevertheless, developing an understanding of how the patient has been affected by the diagnosis and is coping with it is an important goal of patient management.

It is best to speak frankly with the patient and the family regarding the likely course of disease. These discussions can be difficult for the physician as well as for the patient and family. The critical features of the interaction are to reassure the patient and family that everything that can be done to provide comfort will be done. They will not be abandoned. Many patients prefer to be cared for in their homes or in a hospice setting rather than a hospital. The American College of Physicians has published a book called *Home Care Guide for Cancer: How to Care for Family and Friends at Home* that teaches an approach to successful problem-solving in home care. With appropriate planning, it should be possible to provide the patient with the necessary medical care as well as the psychological and spiritual support that will prevent the isolation and depersonalization that can attend in-hospital death.

The care of dying patients may take a toll on the physician. A "burnout" syndrome has been described that is characterized by fatigue, disengagement from patients and colleagues, and a loss of self-fulfillment. Efforts at stress reduction, maintenance of a balanced life, and setting realistic goals may combat this disorder.

End-of-Life Decisions Unfortunately, a smooth transition in treatment goals from curative to palliative may not be possible in all cases because of the occurrence of serious treatment-related complications or rapid disease progression. Vigorous and invasive medical support for a reversible disease or treatment complication is assumed to be justified. However, if the reversibility of the condition is in doubt, the patient's wishes determine the level of medical care. These wishes should be elicited before the terminal phase of illness and reviewed periodically. This information can guide the physician should the patient be unable to speak for him- or herself. The family cannot be expected to make such decisions without guidance from the patient and support from the physician when surrogate decisions are required. Advance directives such as a living will or a durable power of attorney for health care provide guidance for the health care team and the family regarding the patient's wishes and may protect the patient's assets from depletion on expensive but unwanted care.

Only about 15% of the population has implemented an advance directive. Physicians should take the initiative to speak with patients and family members about advance directives.[4]

BIBLIOGRAPHY

Clinical Practice Guideline Number 9, Management of Cancer Pain. U.S. Department of Health and Human Services, Agency for Health Care Policy and Research publication no. 94-0592, 1994

GREENLEE RT et al: Cancer statistics, 2000. CA Cancer J Clin 50:7, 2000

GRUNBERG SM, HESKETH PJ: Control of chemotherapy-induced emesis. N Engl J Med 329:1790, 1993

LEVY MH: Pharmacologic treatment of cancer pain. N Engl J Med 335:1124, 1996

THERASSE P et al: New guidelines to evaluate response to treatment in solid tumors. J Natl Cancer Inst 92:205, 2000

WALSH D et al: The symptoms of advanced cancer: Relationship to age, gender, and performance status in 1000 patients. Support Care Cancer 8:175, 2000

---

[4]Information about advance directives can be obtained from the American Association of Retired Persons, 601 E Street, NW, Washington, DC 20049, 202-434-2277 or Choice in Dying, 250 West 57th Street, New York, NY 10107, 212-366-5540.

80 *Otis W. Brawley, Barnett S. Kramer*

PREVENTION AND EARLY DETECTION OF CANCER

The prevention and control of cancer is a burgeoning field because of advances in understanding the biology of carcinogenesis. The field has expanded beyond the identification and avoidance of carcinogens to include studies of specific interventions to lower cancer risk, as well as screening for early detection of cancer.

Central to the prevention and control of cancer is the concept that carcinogenesis is not an event but a process, a series of discrete cellular changes that result in progressively more autonomous cellular processes. *Primary prevention* concerns the identification and manipulation of the genetic, biologic, and environmental factors in the causal pathway. Smoking cessation, diet modification, and chemoprevention are primary prevention activities. *Secondary prevention* concerns the identification of asymptomatic neoplastic lesions combined with effective therapy. Screening is a form of secondary prevention. Screening may also be a form of primary prevention of invasive cancer; screening Pap smears are used to identify and treat preinvasive lesions of the cervix.

EDUCATION AND HEALTHFUL HABITS Public education on the avoidance of identified risk factors for cancer and encouraging healthy habits were among early efforts in cancer prevention and control. Many educational messages have come to the public through commercials in the print and electronic media and through school health courses. The physician is a potentially powerful messenger in this education campaign about the hazards of smoking, the benefits of a healthful diet, and sun avoidance.

Smoking Cessation Tobacco use through cigarettes and other means is the most avoidable risk factor for cardiovascular disease and cancer. Lung cancer mortality rates correlate with the number of cigarettes smoked per day as well as the degree of inhalation of cigarette smoke. Those who stop smoking have a lower lung cancer mortality rate than those who continue smoking, despite the persistence for years of some carcinogen-induced genetic mutations. In addition to lung cancer, cigarette smoking is a causative agent in cancers of the larynx, oropharynx, esophagus, bladder, and pancreas. Smoking cessation and avoidance have the potential to save and extend more lives than any other public health activity. About 400,000 Americans die prematurely every year because of cigarette smoking. A smoker has a one in three lifetime risk of dying prematurely of a cancer or cardiovascular or pulmonary disease caused by cigarette smoking. Indeed, more human lives are lost due to cardiovascular disease caused by smoking than from smoking-related cancer. The risk of tobacco smoke is not necessarily limited to the smoker. Epidemiologic studies suggest that environmental tobacco smoke may cause lung cancer and other pulmonary diseases in nonsmokers.

Nonsmoking persons should be encouraged not to start smoking, and persons who smoke should be encouraged to stop. Tobacco prevention is a pediatric issue. Over 80% of American smokers begin smoking before the age of 18. Nearly 20% of Americans aged 12 to 18 have smoked a cigarette in the past month. Counseling of adolescents and young adults is critical to prevent smoking. A physician's simple advice to not start smoking or to quit smoking can be of benefit. The U.S. Agency for Health Care Research and Quality recommends that physicians query patients on tobacco use on every office visit, record the answer with the vital signs, and ask smokers if they would like assistance in quitting.

Current approaches to smoking cessation recognize that smoking is an addiction (Chap. 390). The smoker who is quitting goes through a process with identifiable stages that include contemplation of quitting, an action phase in which the smoker quits, and a maintenance phase. Smokers who quit completely are more likely to be successful than those who gradually reduce the number of cigarettes smoked or change to cigarettes lower in tar or nicotine. More than 90% of the Americans who have successfully quit smoking did so on their own without participation in an organized cessation program, but cessation programs are helpful for some smokers. The Community Intervention Trial for Smoking Cessation (COMMIT) was a community-based 4-year program. One community of each of 11 matched community pairs was randomly assigned to intervention. The intervention included public education through the media and community-wide events, health care providers, worksites and other organizations, and cessation resources. COMMIT demonstrated that light smokers can benefit from simple cessation messages and cessation programs. The quit rate (fraction of the subjects followed who achieved and maintained cessation at the end of the trial) was 30.6% in the intervention communities and 27.5% in the control communities. This finding is statistically significant, but modest. The control communities enjoyed a substantial decrease in smoking through study participation. The COMMIT interventions were not successful for heavy smokers (>25 cigarettes per day). Heavy smokers need an intensive, broad-based cessation program that includes counseling, behavioral strategies, and pharmacologic adjuncts such as nicotine gum and nicotine patches.

Cigar and pipe smoking carry the same risks as tobacco smoke including lung cancer. Smokeless tobacco is the fastest growing part of the tobacco industry and represents a significant health risk. Chewing tobacco is a carcinogen linked to dental caries, gingivitis, oral leukoplakia, and oral cancer. The systemic effects of smokeless tobacco may increase risks for other cancers. Nitrosamines found in smokeless tobacco cause lung cancer in laboratory animals.

Diet Modification Dietary modification may have significant potential for lowering cancer risk in western culture. Studies of international dietary patterns and animal studies suggest that diets high in fat increase the risk for cancers of the breast, colon, prostate, and endometrium. These cancers have their highest incidence and mortalities in western countries, where fat comprises an average of 40 to 45% of the total calories consumed. In populations at low risk for these cancers, fat accounts for <20% of dietary calories.

Nonetheless, dietary fat has not been accepted by all as important in the etiology of cancers. Case-control and cohort epidemiologic studies give conflicting results. In addition, diet is a highly complex exposure to many nutrients and chemicals. Low-fat diets may render some protection through anticarcinogens found in vegetables, fruits, legumes, nuts, and grains. Substances found in these foods that may be protective include phenols, sulfur-containing compounds, flavones, and fiber.

In observational studies, dietary fiber appears protective against colonic polyps and invasive cancer of the colon. The mechanisms involved are complex and speculative. They involve binding of oxidized bile acids, a decrease in bowel transit time, and generation of soluble fiber products, such as butyrate, that may have differentiating properties. High-fiber diets may also protect against breast and prostate cancer by absorbing and inactivating dietary estrogenic and androgenic cancer promoters. Protective effects of fiber have not been proved in a prospective clinical trial.

The U.S. National Institutes of Health (NIH) Women's Health Initiative, launched in 1994, is a long-term clinical trial enrolling more than 100,000 women aged 45 to 69. It studies the potential cancer-preventing effects of a low-fat diet and vitamin supplementation. It must be stressed that the scientific evidence does not currently establish the anticarcinogenic value of vitamin, mineral, or nutritional supplements in amounts greater than that provided by a good diet.

The Polyp Prevention Trial studied 2000 elderly persons randomly assigned to a low-fat, high-fiber diet or a routine diet followed for 4 years. No significant differences in polyp formation were noted.

A simple way to decrease dietary fat and increase fiber is to consume at least 5 to 9 servings of fruits and vegetables a day. Such a diet may lower the risk of cardiac disease as well as cancer.

Sun Avoidance Nonmelanoma skin cancers (basal cell and squamous cell) are induced by cumulative exposure to ultraviolet radiation. Intermittent acute sun exposure and sun damage have been linked to melanoma. Sunburns, especially in childhood and adolescence, are associated with an increased risk of melanoma in adulthood. Reduction of sun exposure through use of protective clothing and changes in the pattern of outdoor activities can reduce skin cancer risk. Sunscreens decrease the risk of actinic keratoses, the precursor to squamous cell skin cancer, but melanoma risk may be increased. Sunscreens prevent burning and may encourage more prolonged exposure to the sun; yet they may not filter out wavelengths of energy that cause melanoma.

Educational interventions to help people assess their risk of developing skin cancer accurately have some impact. Self-examination for skin pigment characteristics associated with melanoma, such as freckling, may be useful in identifying people at high risk. People who recognize themselves as being at risk tend to be more compliant with sun-avoidance recommendations. Possible risk factors for melanoma include a propensity to sunburn, a large number of benign melanocytic nevi, and atypical nevi.

CANCER CHEMOPREVENTION Chemoprevention of cancer is a relatively new concept. It involves the use of specific natural or synthetic chemical agents to reverse, suppress, or prevent carcinogenesis before the development of invasive malignancy. While the concept that pharmacologic agents can prevent a cancer is relatively new, the idea that a compound can prevent chronic disease is not. Clinicians routinely prevent heart disease, kidney disease, and stroke by treating hypertension with pharmacologic agents. Lipid-lowering drugs are used to prevent coronary artery disease.

Improved understanding of the biology of cancer makes chemoprevention a real possibility. Cancer develops through an accumulation of genetic changes that are potential points of intervention to prevent cancer. The initial genetic changes are termed *initiation*. The alteration can be inherited or acquired through the action of physical, infectious, or chemical carcinogens. Like most human diseases, cancer arises through an interaction between genetics and environmental exposures (Table 80-1). Influences that cause the initiated cell to progress through the carcinogenic process and to change phenotypically are termed *promoters*. Promoters include hormones such as androgens, linked to prostate cancer, and estrogen, linked to breast and endometrial cancer. The distinction between an initiator and a promoter is sometimes arbitrary; some components of cigarette smoke are "complete carcinogens," acting as both initiators and promoters. Cancer can be prevented or controlled through interference with the factors that cause initiation, promotion, or progression. Compounds of interest in chemoprevention often have antimutagenic, antioxidant, or antiproliferative activity.

Before a chemoprevention strategy can become standard practice, evidence of benefit must be gathered from clinical trials. These trials are usually large, long-term, randomized, placebo-controlled, and double-blinded. They often allow for the study of drugs for prevention of multiple cancers and the study of end-points beyond cancer, such as other chronic diseases. Several large clinical trials have been completed, and a number are continuing in the twenty-first century. Only tamoxifen has been approved by the U.S. Food and Drug Administration for prevention; it lowers risk of breast cancer in high-risk women.

Multiple Cancer Site Prevention Trials The Physicians' Health Trial involves 22,071 American male physicians. Participants were randomly assigned to receive β-carotene, aspirin, and/or placebo in a 2×2 factorial design. All major medical events were recorded. In 1988, the aspirin arm was unblinded after the trial demonstrated that aspirin therapy causes a significant reduction in cardiovascular mortality. The β-carotene arm of the study stopped in 1998, and data analysis is proceeding.

The Women's Health Study, launched in 1992, is a 10-year trial involving 44,000 female nurses. Subjects are randomly assigned to β-carotene, α-tocopherol, aspirin, and/or placebo in a factorial design

Table 80-1 Carcinogens and Associated Cancers or Neoplasms

Carcinogens[a]	Associated Cancer or Neoplasm
Alkylating agents	Acute myelocytic leukemia, bladder cancer
Androgens	Prostate cancer
Aromatic amines (dyes)	Bladder cancer
Arsenic	Cancer of the lung, skin
Asbestos	Cancer of the lung, pleura, peritoneum
Benzene	Acute myelocytic leukemia
Chromium	Lung cancer
Diethylstilbestrol (prenatal)	Vaginal cancer (clear cell)
Epstein-Barr virus	Burkitt's lymphoma, nasal T cell lymphoma
Estrogens	Cancer of the endometrium, liver
Ethyl alcohol	Cancer of the liver, esophagus, head and neck
Helicobacter pylori	Gastric cancer
Hepatitis B or C virus	Liver cancer
Human immunodeficiency virus	Non-Hodgkin's lymphoma, Kaposi's sarcoma, squamous cell carcinomas (especially of the urogenital tract)
Human papilloma virus	
Human T cell lymphotropic virus type I (HTLV-I)	Adult T cell leukemia/lymphoma
Immunosuppressive agents (azathioprine, cyclosporine, glucocorticoids)	Non-Hodgkin's lymphoma
Nitrogen mustard gas	Cancer of the lung, head and neck, nasal sinuses
Nickel dust	Cancer of the lung, nasal sinuses
Phenacetin	Cancer of the renal pelvis and bladder
Polycyclic hydrocarbons	Cancer of the lung, skin (especially squamous cell carcinoma of scrotal skin)
Schistosomiasis	Bladder cancer (squamous cell)
Sunlight (ultraviolet)	Skin cancer (squamous cell and melanoma)
Tobacco (including smokeless)	Cancer of the upper aerodigestive tract, bladder
Vinyl chloride	Liver cancer (angiosarcoma)

[a] Agents that are thought to act as cancer initiators and/or promoters.

yielding eight different treatment groups. The end-points are total epithelial cancers, breast cancer, lung cancer, colon cancer, and vascular disease.

The Women's Health Initiative uses a partial factorial design that places women in 22 intervention groups. Participants can receive calcium and vitamin D supplementation, hormone replacement therapy, and counseling to increase exercise and cease smoking. Prevention of a number of cancers, cardiovascular disease, osteoporosis, and other diseases will be assessed.

Prevention of Hormonally Driven Cancers Hormonal manipulation is being tested in the primary prevention of breast and prostate cancer. Tamoxifen is an antiestrogen with partial estrogen agonistic activity in some tissues, such as endometrium and bone. One of its actions is to upregulate transforming growth factor β, which decreases breast cell proliferation. In randomized placebo-controlled trials to assess tamoxifen as an adjuvant in breast cancer treatment, this drug reduced the number of new breast cancers in the uninvolved breast by more than a third. In a randomized placebo-controlled trial involving >13,000 women at high risk, tamoxifen decreased the risk of developing cancer by 49% compared to placebo. Tamoxifen also reduced the risk of bone fractures; a small increase in risk of endometrial cancer, stroke, pulmonary emboli, and deep vein thrombosis was noted. A trial to compare tamoxifen with another selective estrogen receptor modulator, raloxifene, is ongoing.

Finasteride is a 5α-reductase inhibitor. It inhibits the conversion of testosterone to dihydrotestosterone, a more potent stimulator of prostate cell proliferation than testosterone. In an F344 rat model of carcinogen-induced prostate cancer, finasteride decreased the inci-

dence of cancers. Finasteride is being tested as a preventive agent for prostate cancer in a 10-year study involving 18,000 men age 55 and older.

Chemoprevention of Cancers of the Upper Aerodigestive Tract
Smoking causes diffuse epithelial injury in the head, neck, esophagus, and lung. Patients cured of squamous cell cancers of the lung, esophagus, head, and neck are at risk (as high as 5% per year) of developing a second cancer of the upper aerodigestive tract. Cessation of cigarette smoking does not markedly decrease the cured cancer patient's risk of second malignancy, even though it does lower the cancer risk in those who have never developed a malignancy. Smoking cessation may halt the early stages of the carcinogenic process (such as metaplasia), but it may have no effect on late stages of carcinogenesis. This "field carcinogenesis" hypothesis for cancer of the upper aerodigestive tract has made "cured" patients an important population for chemoprevention of second malignancies. A randomized, placebo-controlled clinical trial has demonstrated that adjuvant isoretinoin (13-*cis*-retinoic acid) can reduce the incidence of second primary tumors in patients treated with local therapy for head and neck cancer. However, overall survival was not improved due to mortality from recurrences of the primary tumor.

Oral leukoplakia, a premalignant lesion commonly found in smokers, has been used as an intermediate marker allowing the demonstration of chemopreventive activity in smaller, shorter-duration, randomized, placebo-controlled trials. Response was associated with upregulation of retinoic acid receptor β. Therapy with isoretinoin causes regression of oral leukoplakia. However, the lesions recur when the agent is withdrawn, suggesting the need for chronic administration of retinoids. Premalignant lesions in the oropharyngeal area have also responded to β-carotene, retinol, α-tocopherol (vitamin E), and selenium. Further study to improve the definition of the activity of these drugs is ongoing. The ability of isoretinoin to prevent second malignancies in patients cured of early-stage non-small cell lung cancer is also being assessed.

Several large-scale trials have assessed agents in the chemoprevention of lung cancer in patients at high risk. In the Alpha-Tocopherol/Beta-Carotene (ATBC) Lung Cancer Prevention Trial, participants were male smokers, aged 50 to 69 at entry. At entry, participants had smoked an average of one pack of cigarettes per day for 35.9 years. Participants received α-tocopherol, β-carotene, and/or placebo in a randomized, 2×2 factorial design. After a median follow-up of 6.1 years, lung cancer incidence and mortality were statistically significantly *increased* in those receiving β-carotene. α-Tocopherol had no significant impact on lung cancer mortality, and no evidence suggested interaction between the two drugs. Patients receiving α-tocopherol had a higher incidence of hemorrhagic stroke.

The Beta-Carotene and Retinol Efficacy Trial (CARET) involved 17,000 American smokers and workers with asbestos exposure. Entrants were randomly assigned to one of four arms and received β-carotene, retinol, and/or placebo in a 2×2 factorial design. This trial demonstrated harm from β-carotene: a lung cancer rate of 5 per 1000 subjects per year for those taking placebo and of 6 per 1000 subjects per year for those taking β-carotene. The difference was statistically significant.

These ATBC and CARET results demonstrate the importance of testing chemoprevention hypotheses before implementing them widely, because the results stand in contrast to a number of observational epidemiologic studies. In the ATBC trial, participants taking α-tocopherol had a one-third reduction in the incidence of prostate cancer, compared to those not taking α-tocopherol. Assessment of these findings continues. The Physicians' Health Trial showed neither an increased nor a decreased risk of lung cancer in those using β-carotene; fewer of its participants were smokers than those in the ATBC and CARET studies.

Chemoprevention of Colon Cancer Many of the current colon cancer prevention trials are based on the premise that most colorectal cancers develop from adenomatous polyps. These trials use adenoma recurrence or disappearance as a surrogate end-point to assess colon cancer prevention. Early clinical trial results suggest that nonsteroidal anti-inflammatory drugs (NSAIDs), such as piroxicam, sulindac, and aspirin, may prevent adenoma formation or cause regression of adenomatous polyps. The mechanism of action of NSAIDs is unknown, but they are presumed to work through the cyclooxygenase pathway. In the Physicians' Health Trial, aspirin had no effect on colon cancer incidence, although the 6-year assessment period may not have been long enough to evaluate definitively this end-point.

Epidemiologic studies suggest that diets high in calcium lower colon cancer risk. Calcium binds bile and fatty acids, which cause hyperproliferation of colonic epithelium. It is hypothesized that this effect reduces intraluminal exposure to these compounds. Early data from randomized studies suggest that calcium supplementation decreases the risk of adenomatous polyp recurrence by about 20%, even though it does not decrease the proliferative rate of the colonic epithelium. Epithelial proliferative rate may not be an adequate surrogate marker in colon cancer prevention trials.

Cyclooxygenase II inhibitors may be even more effective at colon cancer prevention.

Vaccines and Cancer Prevention A number of infectious agents have been linked to the development of cancer, leading to interest in developing vaccines to protect against these agents. The hepatitis B vaccine is quite effective in preventing hepatitis and hepatomas due to chronic hepatitis B infection. Public health officials are encouraging widespread administration of this vaccine, especially in Asia, where the disease is epidemic. In the future, human papilloma virus (HPV) vaccines could be developed to prevent cervical cancer, and *Helicobacter pylori* vaccines may be developed to prevent gastric cancer.

CANCER SCREENING Screening is a means of detecting disease early in asymptomatic individuals with the goal of decreasing morbidity and mortality. Screening for cancer is intuitively appealing and has attracted great public interest as technology has generated a number of diagnostic tests and procedures that are safe, quick, and inexpensive. While screening can potentially save lives, and has been shown clearly to do so in the case of breast, cervical, and colon cancer, it is also subject to a number of biases, which can suggest a benefit when actually there is none. Bias can even mask net harm. Early detection does not in itself confer benefit. To be of value, screening must detect disease earlier, and treatment of earlier disease must yield a better outcome than treatment at the onset of symptoms. Cause-specific mortality, rather than survival after diagnosis, is the preferred end point (see below).

Because screening is done on asymptomatic, healthy persons, it should offer substantial likelihood of benefit. A critical approach to screening is necessary to ensure that benefit results. Screening tests and their appropriate use should be carefully evaluated before their use is widely encouraged in screening programs as a matter of public policy.

Screening examinations, tests, or procedures are usually not diagnostic of cancer but instead indicate that a cancer may be present. The diagnosis is then made following a workup that includes a biopsy and pathologic confirmation.

A number of genes have been identified that predispose for a disease, and many more will be identified in the near future. Testing for these genes can define a high-risk population. The ability to predict the development of a particular cancer may some day present therapeutic options as well as ethical dilemmas. It may eventually allow for early intervention to prevent a cancer or limit its severity. People at high risk will be ideal candidates for chemoprevention and screening; however, the efficacy of these interventions in the high-risk population should be investigated. Currently, persons at high risk for a particular cancer can engage in intensive screening. While this course is clinically prudent, it is not known if it saves lives in these populations.

The Accuracy of Screening A screening test's accuracy or ability to discriminate disease is described by four indices: sensitivity, specificity, positive predictive value, and negative predictive value (Table 80-2). *Sensitivity* is the proportion of persons with the disease who test positive in the screen (i.e., the ability of the test to detect disease when it is present). *Specificity* is the proportion of persons who do not have the disease and test negative in the screening test (i.e., the ability of a test to tell that the disease is not present). The *positive predictive value* is the proportion of persons who test positive who actually have the disease. Similarly, *negative predictive value* is the proportion of who test negative and do not have the disease. The sensitivity and specificity of a test are relatively independent of the underlying prevalence (or risk) of the disease in the population screened, but the predictive values depend strongly on the prevalence of the disease (Table 80-3).

Screening is most beneficial, efficient, and economical when the target disease is common in the population being screened. To be valuable, the screening test should have a high specificity; sensitivity need not be very high, as demonstrated in Table 80-3.

Potential Biases of Screening Tests The common biases of screening are lead time, length, and selection. These biases can make a screening test seem beneficial when actually it is not (or even causes net harm). Whether beneficial or not, screening can create the false impression of an epidemic by increasing the number of cancers diagnosed. It can also give the appearance of a shift in stage, thus improving survival statistics without reducing mortality (i.e., the number of deaths from a given cancer relative to the number of people at risk for

Table 80-2   Definition of Terms

Term	Definition
Sensitivity	The proportion of persons with the condition who test positive: $a/(a + c)$
Specificity	The proportion of persons without the condition who test negative: $d/(b + d)$
Positive predictive value	The proportion of persons with a positive test who have the condition: $a/(a + b)$
Negative predictive value	The proportion of persons with a negative test who do not have the condition: $d/(c + d)$

		Condition present	Condition absent
a = true positive	Positive test	a	b
b = false positive			
c = false negative			
d = true negative	Negative test	c	d

Table 80-3   Predictive Value Relationships[a]

Positive predictive value (PPV) is a function of sensitivity, specificity, and prevalence:

$$PPV = \frac{prevalence \times sensitivity}{(prevalence \times sensitivity) + (1 - prevalence)(1 - sensitivity)}$$

PPV for a prevalence of 5 per 1000:

	PPV for a Sensitivity of, %	
Specificity	0.8	0.95
0.95	7	9
0.999	80	83

PPV for a prevalence of 1 per 10,000:

	PPV for a Sensitivity of, %	
Specificity	0.8	0.95
0.95	0.2	0.2
0.999	7	9

[a] The positive predictive value is expressed as a percentage. It is influenced by the sensitivity and specificity of the screening test and the prevalence of the disease being screened for. As shown here, for relatively uncommon diseases, such as cancer, the positive predictive value is influenced particularly strongly by the specificity of the screening test at a given prevalence.

the cancer). In such a case, the *apparent* duration of survival increases without lives being saved or life expectancy changed.

Lead-time bias occurs when a test does not influence the natural history of the disease; the patient is merely diagnosed at an earlier date. When lead-time bias occurs, survival *appears* increased, but life is not really prolonged. The screening test only prolongs the time the subject is aware of the disease and spends as a patient.

Length bias occurs when slow-growing, less aggressive cancers are detected during screening. Cancers diagnosed owing to the onset of symptoms between scheduled screenings are on average more aggressive, and treatment outcomes are not as favorable. An extreme form of length bias is termed *overdiagnosis*, the detection of "pseudo-disease." The reservoir of some undetected slow-growing tumors is large. Many of these tumors fulfill the histologic criteria of cancer but will never become clinically significant or cause death. This problem is compounded by the fact that the most common cancers appear most frequently at ages when competing causes of death are more frequent.

Selection bias must be considered in assessing the results of any screening effort. The population most likely to seek screening may differ from the general population to which the screening test might be applied. The individuals screened may have volunteered because of a particular risk factor not found in the general population, such as a strong family history. In general, volunteers for studies may be more health conscious and thus likely to have a better prognosis or lower mortality rate, irrespective of the screening result. This is termed the *healthy volunteer effect*.

Potential Drawbacks of Screening Risks associated with screening include harm caused by the screening intervention itself, harm due to the further investigation of persons with positive test results (both true and false positives), and harm from the treatment of persons with a true-positive result, even if life is extended by treatment. The diagnosis and treatment of cancers that would never have caused medical problems can lead to the harm of unnecessary treatment and give patients the anxiety of a cancer diagnosis. The psychosocial impact of cancer screening, whether the result is positive or negative, can also be substantial when applied to the entire population.

Assessment of Screening Tests Good clinical trial design can offset some biases of screening and demonstrate the relative risks and benefits of a screening test. A randomized, controlled screening trial with cause-specific mortality as the end-point provides the strongest support for a screening intervention. In a randomized trial, two like populations are randomly established. One is given the medical standard of care (which may be no screening at all), and the other receives the screening intervention being assessed. The two populations are compared over time. Efficacy for the population studied is established when the group receiving the screening test has a better cause-specific mortality rate than the control group. Studies showing a reduction in the incidence of advanced-stage disease, an improved survival, or a stage shift are weaker evidence of benefit. These latter criteria are necessary but not sufficient to establish the value of a screening test.

Although a randomized, controlled screening trial provides the strongest evidence to support the usefulness of a screening test, it is not perfect. Unless the trial is population-based, it does not remove

Table 80-4 Screening Recommendations for Asymptomatic Normal-Risk Subjects[a]

Test or Procedure	USPSTF	ACS	CTFPHC
Sigmoidoscopy	>50, periodically <50, not recommended	≥50, every 3–5 years	Insufficient evidence
Fecal occult blood testing	≥50, every year	≥50, every year	Insufficient evidence
Digital rectal examination	No recommendation	≥40, every year	Poor evidence to include or exclude
Prostate-specific antigen	Recommendation against	M: ≥50, every year	Recommendation against
Pap test	F: 18–65, every 1–3 years	F: beginning at age 18, yearly ×3 and then at physician discretion	Fair evidence to include in examination of sexually active women
Pelvic examination	Do not recommend, advise adnexal palpation during exam for other reasons	F: 18–40, every 1–3 years with Pap test; >40, every year	Not considered
Endometrial tissue sampling	Not considered	At menopause if obese or a history of unopposed estrogen use	Not considered
Breast self-examination	No recommendation	≥20, monthly	Insufficient evidence to make a recommendation
Breast clinical examination	F: >50, every year	F: 20–40, every 3 years; >40, yearly	F: >50, every year
Mammography	F: 50–75, every 1–2 years	F: ≥40, every year	F: 50–69, every year
Complete skin examination	Not recommended	20–39, every 3 years	Poor evidence to include or exclude

[a] Summary of the screening procedures recommended for the general population by U.S. Preventive Services Task Force (USPSTF), the American Cancer Society (ACS), and the Canadian Task Force on Prevention Health Care (CTFPHC). These recommendations refer to asymptomatic persons who have no risk factors, other than age or gender, for the targeted condition.
NOTE: F, female; M, male.

the issue of generalizability to the target population. Screening trials generally involve thousands of persons and last for years. Less definitive study designs are therefore often used to estimate the effectiveness of screening practices. After a randomized controlled clinical trial, in descending order of strength, evidence may be derived from:

- The findings of internally controlled trials using intervention allocation methods other than randomization (e.g., allocation determined by birth date, date of clinic visit);
- The findings of cohort or case-control analytic observational studies;
- The results of multiple time series studies with or without the intervention;
- The opinions of respected authorities based on clinical experience, descriptive studies, or consensus reports of experts (the weakest evidence because even experts can be misled by the biases described above).

Screening for Specific Cancers Widespread screening for breast, cervical, and colon cancer is beneficial for certain age groups. Special surveillance of those at high risk for a specific cancer because of a family history or a genetic risk factor may be prudent, but few studies have been carried out to assess the impact of this practice on mortality in specific high-risk populations. A number of organizations have considered whether or not to endorse routine use of certain screening tests. Because these groups have not used the same criteria to judge whether a screening test should be endorsed, they have arrived at different recommendations. The screening guidelines of the U.S. Preventive Services Task Force, the Canadian Task Force on Preventive Health Care, and the American Cancer Society are often quoted and show a range of recommendations (Table 80-4).

Breast cancer Breast self-examination, clinical breast examination by a care giver, and mammography have been advocated as useful screening tools. Only screening mammography alone and screening mammography with clinical examination have been evaluated in randomized controlled trials. A number of well-designed trials have demonstrated that annual or biennial screening with mammography or mammography plus clinical breast examination in women over the age of 50 saves lives. In these trials, the breast cancer mortality rate is decreased by about a third. Experts disagree on whether average-risk women aged 40 to 49 should receive regular screening (Table 80-4). The statistical significance of the screening effect in women aged 40 to 49 depends on the statistical test used. An analysis of eight large randomized trials showed no benefit from mammographic screening for women aged 40 to 49 when assessed 5 to 7 years after trial entry. However, a small benefit emerged 10 to 12 years after study entry. What proportion of this possible benefit is due to screening after these women turned 50 is not known. In randomized screening studies of women aged 50 to 69, the decline in mortality begins about 5 years after initiation of screening. Nearly half of women aged 40 to 49 years screened annually will have false-positive mammograms necessitating further evaluation, often including biopsy. The risk of false-positive testing should be discussed with the patient.

While no study has shown breast self-examination to decrease mortality, it is recommended as prudent by many organizations. A substantial fraction of breast cancers are first detected by the patient, even with widespread mammographic screening.

Cervical cancer Screening with Papanicolaou smears decreases cervical cancer mortality. The cervical cancer mortality rate has fallen significantly since the widespread use of the Pap smear, although this trend actually began earlier. Most screening guidelines recommend regular Pap testing for all women who are or have been sexually active or have reached the age of 18. With the onset of sexual activity comes the risk of sexual transmission of HPV, the most common etiologic factor for cervical cancer. The recommended interval for Pap screening varies from 1 to 3 years. An upper age limit at which screening ceases to be effective is not known.

Colorectal cancer Fecal occult blood testing, digital rectal examination, rigid and flexible sigmoidoscopy, radiographic barium contrast studies, and colonoscopy have been considered for colorectal cancer screening. Annual fecal occult blood testing using hydrated specimens could reduce colorectal cancer mortality by a third. The sensitivity for fecal occult blood is increased if specimens are rehydrated before testing, but at the cost of lower specificity. The false-positive rate for rehydrated fecal occult blood testing is high; 1 to 5% of persons tested have a positive result. About 2 to 10% of those with occult blood in the stool have cancer, and 20 to 30% have adenomas. The high false-positive rate of fecal occult blood testing dramatically increases the number of colonoscopies performed.

Two case-control studies suggest that regular screening of people over 50 with sigmoidoscopy decreases mortality. These types of studies are prone to selection biases. A quarter to a third of polyps can be discovered with the rigid sigmoidoscope; half are found with a 35-cm flexible scope, and two-thirds to three-quarters are found with a 60-cm scope. Diagnosis of polyposis by sigmoidoscopy should lead to evaluation of the entire colon with colonoscopy and/or barium enema. The most efficient interval for screening sigmoidoscopy is unknown. Case-control studies suggest that testing at intervals of up to 9 years may confer benefit. Most authorities feel that full colonoscopy is too cumbersome and invasive for widespread use as a screening tool in standard-risk populations. It may be suitable for subjects at extremely high risk, such as members of families with a genetic predisposition to colorectal cancer. Colonoscopy is accepted in screening persons with inflammatory bowel disease. Data are not available on digital rectal examination or barium enema as colon cancer screening tools, but both are insensitive.

Lung cancer Screening chest radiographs and sputum cytology have been evaluated as methods for lung cancer screening. No reduction in lung cancer mortality has been found in these studies, although all the controlled trials performed have had low statistical power. Even screening of high-risk subjects (smokers) has not been proved to be beneficial. Spiral computed tomography (CT) can diagnose lung cancers at early stages; however, false-positive rates are high. Ongoing studies are evaluating spiral CT screening.

Ovarian cancer Adnexal palpation, transvaginal ultrasound, and serum CA-125 determination have been considered for ovarian cancer screening. Adnexal palpation is too insensitive to detect ovarian cancer at an early enough stage to affect mortality substantially. Neither transvaginal ultrasound nor CA-125 screening has been tested in a completed randomized prospective trial. Ovarian cancer screening can lead to an invasive diagnostic workup, which may include laparotomy. In a clinical study, 0.6% of 900 adult women had a serum CA-125 level >35 U/mL. Thus, if 100,000 adult women were screened, 600 would be identified as having a high CA-125. The prevalence of ovarian cancer in the female adult population is approximately 20 per 100,000. Thus, the screening test would identify 600 women who would undergo further evaluation to identify 20 cases of ovarian cancer. Some of these 600 would only be inconvenienced by an ultrasound examination. Others would undergo an exploratory laparotomy. A large proportion of the 20 women identified as having ovarian cancer would have advanced, incurable disease and thus not benefit from screening. An NIH consensus conference in 1994 concluded that routine screening for ovarian cancer was not indicated for standard-risk women or those with a single affected family member, but that it might be worthwhile in families with genetic ovarian cancer syndromes.

Prostate cancer The most common prostate cancer screening modalities are digital rectal examination and assays for serum prostate-specific antigen (PSA). Newer serum tests, such as measurement of the ratio of bound to free serum PSA, have yet to be fully evaluated. An emphasis on PSA screening has caused prostate cancer to become the most common non-skin cancer diagnosed in American males. Screening for this disease is very prone to lead-time bias, length bias, and overdiagnosis, and substantial debate rages among experts on whether it is effective. Some experts are concerned that prostate cancer screening, more than screening for other cancers, may cause net harm. Prostate cancer screening clearly detects many asymptomatic cancers, but the ability to distinguish tumors that are lethal but still curable from those that pose little or no threat to health is limited. Men over age 50 have a very high prevalence of indolent, clinically insignificant prostate cancers. No well-designed trial has demonstrated the true benefit of prostate cancer screening and treatment, but trials are in progress.

The effectiveness of radical prostatectomy, radiation therapy, and other treatments for low-stage prostate cancer is also under study in randomized trials. Definitive treatment of cancers detected by screening may cause morbidity for some men, such as impotence and urinary incontinence, and carries a low but finite risk of death. Pending the completion of ongoing randomized trials comparing usual care to prostate screening and comparing definitive therapy to "watchful waiting," organizations have provided conflicting recommendations on prostate cancer screening (Table 80-4). After a thorough review of the literature, the American Cancer Society and the American Urologic Association changed their guidelines from a recommendation for screening to a recommendation that men be offered screening after being informed of the potential risks and benefits. A man should have a life expectancy of at least 10 years to be eligible for screening.

Endometrial cancer Transvaginal ultrasound and endometrial sampling have been advocated as screening tests for endometrial cancer. Benefit from routine screening has not been shown. Transvaginal ultrasound and endometrial sampling are indicated for workup of vaginal bleeding in postmenopausal women but are not considered as screening tests in symptomatic women.

Skin cancer Visual examination of all skin surfaces by the patient or by a health care provider is used in screening for basal and squamous cell cancers and melanoma. No prospective randomized study has been performed to look for a mortality decrease. Observational epidemiologic evidence from Scotland and Australia suggests that screening programs have caused a stage shift in melanomas diagnosed. Screening may reinforce sun avoidance and other skin cancer prevention behaviors.

BLOCK G et al: Fruit, vegetables, and cancer prevention: A review of the epidemiological evidence. Nutr Cancer 18:1, 1992

BRAWLEY OW: Prostate carcinoma incidence and patient mortality: The effects of screening and early detection. Cancer 80:1857, 1997

FISHER B et al: Tamoxifen for prevention of breast cancer: Report of the National Surgical Adjuvant Breast and Bowel Project P-1 study. J Natl Cancer Inst 90:1371, 1998

GREENWALD P et al: Chemoprevention. CA Cancer J Clin 45:31, 1995

HENSCHKE CI et al: Early Lung Cancer Action Project: Overall design and findings from baseline screening. Lancet 354:99, 1999

LIPPMAN SM et al: Cancer chemoprevention. J Clin Oncol 12:851, 1994

NATIONAL INSTITUTES OF HEALTH CONSENSUS DEVELOPMENT PANEL: Breast cancer screening for women ages 40–49. J Natl Cancer Inst 89:1015, 1997

SOX HC: Preventive health services in adults. N Engl J Med 330:1589, 1995

THE ALPHA-TOCOPHEROL, BETA CAROTENE CANCER PREVENTION STUDY GROUP: The effect of vitamin E and beta carotene on the incidence of lung cancer and other cancers in male smokers. N Engl J Med 330:1029, 1994

U.S. PREVENTIVE SERVICES TASK FORCE: Guide to Clinical Preventive Services, 2d ed. Washington, DC, Government Printing Office, 1996

81

Francis S. Collins, Jeffrey M. Trent

CANCER GENETICS

THE CLONAL NATURE OF CANCER Nearly all cancers originate from a single cell. While multiple cumulative events are invariably required to move a cell from normal to the transformed phenotype (see below and Chap. 82), the origin of tumors from a single clone of cells is a critical discriminating feature between neoplasia and hyperplasia.

CANCER IS A GENETIC DISEASE Cancer arises because of alterations in DNA that result in unrestrained cellular proliferation. Most of these alterations involve actual sequence changes in the DNA (i.e., mutation). They may arise as a consequence of random replication errors, exposure to carcinogens (e.g., radiation), or faulty DNA repair processes.

While virtually all cancer is genetic, most cancer is not inherited. Certain individuals with cancer have inherited a germline mutation that predisposes them to the cancer, but even in that situation additional somatic mutations are required for a tumor to develop. In a truly sporadic cancer, *all* of the mutations responsible for the malignant phenotype arise somatically. Such a cancer is caused by genetic alterations but has no hereditary implications.

RNA AND RNA TUMOR VIRUSES Many malignancies in animals are transmissible, and the etiologic agent is frequently a retrovirus, which possesses a single-stranded RNA genome. During the life cycle of the virus, the single-stranded RNA is converted to double-stranded DNA and is inserted at random into the host chromosome. On rare occasions the virus can be remobilized, carrying along with it an adjacent segment of host DNA. Should this host DNA contain a growth-promoting gene, then the retrovirus is potentially transforming. Although efforts to identify retroviruses in human malignancies have mostly been fruitless, retroviruses are implicated in at least one human malignancy. Human T cell lymphotropic virus (HTLV) type I causes adult T cell lymphoma/leukemia, particularly in Japan and the Caribbean (Chap. 191). Unlike animal retroviruses that induce neoplasia, HTLV-I does not contain a growth-promoting transforming oncogene. The tax protein, a 40-kDa molecule encoded in the pX region of the viral genome, induces the activation of a number of genes (including some promoting growth) through interactions with *rel* family and CREB (cyclic AMP response element binding protein) family transcription factors.

DNA tumor viruses are more commonly involved in human malignancy. Human papilloma viruses (especially types 16 and 18) cause cervical cancer (Chap. 188), and both hepatitis B and hepatitis C viruses have been implicated in hepatocellular carcinoma (Chap. 297).

In addition, the Epstein-Barr virus, a herpesvirus that causes a mild illness in children but infectious mononucleosis in nonimmune adolescents and adults, causes Burkitt's lymphoma in Africa, nasopharyngeal carcinoma in Asia, and lymphomas in the setting of immune deficiency (Chap. 184).

GENERAL CLASSES OF CANCER GENES In 1914 Boveri hypothesized that cells become malignant either because of overactivation of a gene that promotes cell division or because of loss of function of a gene that normally restrains growth. This hypothesis is largely correct, although defects in DNA repair genes are also involved. Genes that promote normal cell growth are referred to as *protooncogenes*, and activation of such genes by point mutation, amplification, or dysregulation converts them to *oncogenes*.

Genes that normally restrain growth are called *tumor suppressors* (use of the alternative designation of anti-oncogenes is to be discouraged), and unregulated cell growth arises if their function is lost. The diploid nature of mammalian cells allows certain predictions about the consequences of somatic mutations of tumor suppressor genes. Loss of one allele is unlikely to have significant consequences in most instances, as the remaining normal allele is usually sufficient for normal function. Thus, most cells of an individual with an inherited loss of function of one tumor suppressor allele are functionally normal. Only the rare cell that loses or develops a mutation in the remaining normal copy will exhibit uncontrolled growth. This model correctly predicts that the inheritance pattern of cancer in a family with a tumor suppressor gene mutation will be expressed as an autosomal dominant trait, though the cellular mechanism is recessive.

The third category of genes that contribute to malignancy is the DNA repair genes. Every cell division involves the copying of 6 billion base pairs (bp) of DNA. DNA polymerase has a finite error rate, and many environmental influences can damage DNA. As a consequence, repair systems are essential to protect the integrity of the genome. When the repair systems themselves are faulty, either on the basis of inherited or acquired mutation, the rate of accumulation of mutations throughout the genome rises as cell divisions occur. To the extent that these mutations involve oncogenes and tumor suppressor genes, the likelihood of developing malignancy increases.

MENDELIAN CANCER SYNDROMES Roughly 100 syndromes of familial cancer have been reported, though many are rare. The majority are inherited as autosomal dominant traits, although some of those associated with DNA repair abnormalities (xeroderma pigmentosum, Fanconi anemia, ataxia telangiectasia) are autosomal recessives. Most of the genes responsible for the dominantly inherited cancer syndromes are tumor suppressor genes (Table 81-1). The hallmarks of a tumor suppressor gene are as follows: (1) the germline mutation that affects one allele generally causes a loss of function; (2) tumors also show loss of the second normal allele as a result of a somatic mutation; and (3) often the *normal* function of the gene is to suppress unrestrained cellular growth or to promote differentiation.

The retinoblastoma gene (*RB*) is a paradigm of such a tumor suppressor gene. In a pedigree showing dominant inheritance of susceptibility to retinoblastoma, a loss-of-function germline mutation occurs in one allele of the *RB* gene on chromosome 13. Analysis of the DNA from the tumors invariably shows that the wild-type allele has also been lost by one of several possible mechanisms (Fig. 81-1). However, not all retinoblastoma tumors arise in the context of a strong family history. Sporadic retinoblastoma, which is usually unilateral and on average occurs at a slightly older age than familial retinoblastoma, is usually a consequence of somatic mutation in both alleles of the *RB* gene without any germline predisposition.

Another tumor suppressor gene is the p53 gene on chromosome 17p, which is frequently altered in solid tumors. p53 is somewhat unusual for a tumor suppressor gene in that missense mutations that produce a dominant negative protein product may also be growth-promoting, so that not all alterations obliterate function. Mutations in p53 are found in nearly half of human tumors. Germline mutations in

Table 81-1 Selected Tumor Suppressor Genes Responsible for Familial Cancer Syndromes

Syndrome	Gene	Chromosome Location	Tumors
Basal cell nevus	PTC	9q22.3	Basal cell cancer, jaw cysts, medulloblastoma
Familial breast/ovarian cancer	BRCA1	17q21	Breast, ovarian, colon, prostate cancer
Familial breast cancer	BRCA2	13q12-13	Breast cancer, male breast cancer
Familial melanoma	p16	9p21	Melanoma, pancreatic cancer
Familial polyposis coli	APC	5q21	Intestinal polyposis, colorectal cancer
Familial retinoblastoma	RB	13q24	Retinoblastoma, osteosarcoma
Familial Wilms' tumor	WT1	11p13	Wilms' tumor, WAGR[a]
Hereditary multiple exostoses	EXT1	11p11-13	Exostoses, chondrosarcoma
Li-Fraumeni	p53	17q13	Sarcomas, breast cancer
Neurofibromatosis type 1	NF1	17q11.2	Neurofibroma, neurofibrosarcoma, brain tumor
Neurofibromatosis type 2	NF2	22q12	Acoustic neuroma, meningioma
Tuberous sclerosis	TSC2	16p13.3	Angiofibroma, renal angiomyolipoma
Von Hippel–Lindau	VHL	3p25-26	Renal cell cancer, pheochromocytoma, retinal angioma, hemangioblastoma

[a] WAGR, Wilms' tumor, aniridia, genitourinary abnormalities, and mental retardation.

p53 have dramatic consequences, resulting in a phenotype known as the *Li-Fraumeni syndrome*, where affected individuals may develop a variety of sarcomas, brain tumors, and leukemia. Figure 81-2 illustrates a typical pedigree of this devastating disorder.

In many instances the discovery of genes responsible for familial cancer syndromes has provided insight into the normal control of cell growth. For instance, in type I neurofibromatosis—one of the more common dominant disorders of humans—positional cloning efforts uncovered a previously unknown gene on chromosome 17q that, when mutated, produces a clinical phenotype of café au lait spots, neurofibromas, Lisch nodules of the iris, and a predisposition to neurofibrosarcoma and glioma. The responsible gene, which (like many of the genes in Table 81-1) has a close homologue in yeast, is neurofibromin (*NF1*), a critical participant in the regulation of the protooncogene *ras*. As shown in Fig. 81-3, the NF1 protein is a GTPase-activating protein (GAP) that normally acts to convert *ras* from its active, growth-promoting, GTP-bound form to its inactive, GDP-bound form. Loss of both copies of *NF1* (one copy by inheritance, one by somatic mutation)

thus renders a cell vulnerable to overgrowth, since *ras* is left in the "on" position.

While most autosomal dominant inherited cancer syndromes are due to mutations in tumor suppressor genes, there are a few interesting exceptions. Multiple endocrine neoplasia type II—a dominant disorder characterized by pituitary adenomas, medullary carcinoma of the thyroid, and (in some pedigrees) pheochromocytoma—is due to gain-of-function mutations in the protooncogene *ret* on chromosome 10.

FIGURE 81-2 Pedigree of a family with the Li-Fraumeni syndrome. The affected individuals have developed sarcomas, brain tumors, leukemia, and breast cancer at an early age. All of the affected individuals were found to have a germline mutation in codon 252 of the p53 gene. (*After D Malkin et al, Science 250:1233, 1990, with permission.*)

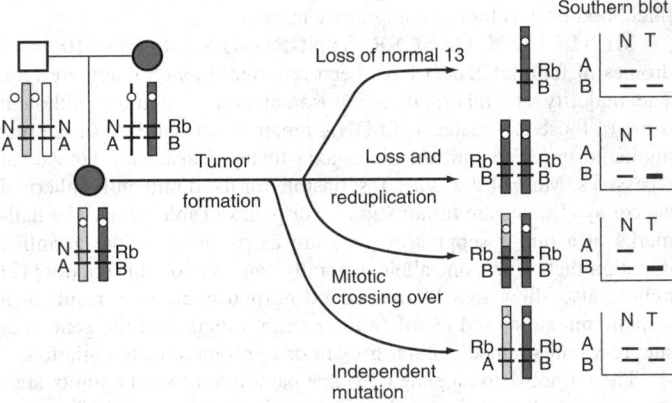

FIGURE 81-1 Diagram of possible mechanisms for tumor formation in an individual with familial retinoblastoma. On the left is shown the pedigree of an affected individual who has inherited the abnormal (Rb) allele from her affected mother. The four chromosomes of her two parents are drawn to indicate their origin. Just below the retinoblastoma locus a polymorphic marker is also analyzed in this family. The patient is AB at this locus, like her mother, whereas her father is AA. Thus the B allele must be on the chromosome carrying the retinoblastoma disease gene. Tumor formation results when the normal allele (N), which this patient inherited from her father, is inactivated. On the right are shown four possible ways in which this could occur. In each case, the resulting chromosome 13 arrangement is shown, as well as the results of a Southern blot comparing normal tissue with tumor tissue. Note that in the first three situations the normal allele (A) has been lost in the tumor tissue, which is referred to as loss of heterozygosity. (*From TD Gelehrter and FS Collins, in Principles of Medical Genetics, Baltimore, Williams & Wilkins, 1990, with permission.*)

FIGURE 81-3 The *ras* pathway. The active form of the *ras* protein binds GTP and promotes cell division. The conversion to the inactive form, which binds GDP, is catalyzed by a number of proteins including the protein product of the neurofibromatosis type I (*NF1*) gene. Thus, loss of function of NF1 has the effect of leaving *ras* in the "on" position. Alternatively, mutations in the *ras* protein that block its inactivation also predispose to cancer.

Interestingly, loss-of-function mutations in *ret* cause a totally different phenotype, Hirschsprung's disease (aganglionic megacolon) (Chaps. 339 and 289).

Dominantly inherited colon cancer is sometimes associated with familial polyposis, which is usually due to mutations in the adenomatous polyposis coli (*APC*) tumor suppressor gene on chromosome 5 (Table 81-1). However, in most colon cancer families affected individuals do not have familial polyposis, but instead the cancer arises from normal-appearing epithelium. Hereditary nonpolyposis colon cancer (HNPCC, or Lynch's syndrome) is commonly defined as the occurrence of colon cancer in at least three individuals over at least two generations and with at least one individual diagnosed under the age of 50. As many as 1 in 200 individuals in the general population may have HNPCC, although this number is somewhat controversial. Most HNPCC is due to mutations in one of four DNA mismatch repair genes (Table 81-2). All four of these genes are components of a repair system that is normally responsible for correcting errors in freshly copied DNA. Tumors in patients with HNPCC are characterized by profound genomic instability, especially for short repeated sequences called *microsatellites*. Figure 81-4 shows an example of the instability in allele sizes for dinucleotide repeats in the cancers in HNPCC. The unstable phenotype [sometimes referred to as the "mutator" phenotype, or the "RER⁺" (replication error) phenotype] probably requires loss of both copies of the particular mismatch repair gene (one inherited, one somatic), so that the mechanism is similar to that typical of a tumor suppressor gene.

MORE COMPLEX INHERITED FORMS OF CANCER

While the Mendelian forms of cancer described above have taught us much about mechanisms of cellular growth control, most forms of cancer do not follow such simple patterns of inheritance. In many instances (e.g., lung cancer), a strong environmental contribution is at work, but even in such circumstances some individuals may be genetically more susceptible to developing cancer given the appropriate exposure.

In the case of breast and ovarian cancer, circumstantial evidence indicates that a subset of affected individuals (5 to 10%) might be accounted for by dominantly inherited high-penetrance susceptibility genes; two of these genes have been identified by positional cloning. *BRCA1*, located on chromosome 17, is capable when mutated of producing a high risk (up to 85% lifelong) of breast cancer and also of ovarian cancer (50% lifelong risk). Roughly 1 in 500 women carries a germline *BRCA1* mutation, often giving rise to a strong family history. Men with *BRCA1* mutations may have a modestly increased risk of prostate cancer. An array of mutational heterogeneity has been described for *BRCA1* (Fig. 81-5), as is often the case for genetic disorders. An exception is the Ashkenazi Jewish population, where 1 in 100 individuals carries a particular 2-bp deletion (denoted 185delAG)

FIGURE 81-4 Demonstration of microsatellite instability in normal and tumor tissue from HNPCC (hereditary nonpolyposis colon cancer) patients. In each case the lane marked T contains DNA from a tumor, and the lane marked N contains DNA from normal tissue of the same patient. The marker (*D2S123*, located on chromosome 2) is a microsatellite composed of a tandem repeat of the dinucleotide CA, which varies in length from chromosome to chromosome. Normally, however, the length of the repeat is stable in somatic tissues. In this example, a polymerase chain reaction analysis has been applied to genomic DNA, and new alleles for the marker are apparent in tumors 1, 2, 5, and 7. Because the tumor tissue is defective in DNA mismatch repair, clonal abnormalities in copying of the CA repeat have arisen. Errors are also occurring in functional genes, eventually resulting in the malignant phenotype. (*From LA Aaltonen et al, Clues to the pathogenesis of familial colorectal cancer. Science 260:812, 1993, with permission.*)

of *BRCA1*, apparently as a consequence of descent from a common ancestor.

Mutations in another gene on chromosome 13, *BRCA2*, also confer a high risk of breast cancer (and a somewhat lower risk of ovarian cancer); men with *BRCA2* mutations are prone to develop breast cancer. The frequency of *BRCA2* mutations is estimated to be about half that of *BRCA1*. About 1% of Ashkenazi Jews again have a common mutation: 6174delT.

What then of the 90 to 95% of breast cancers that arise in individuals without germline alterations in *BRCA1* or *BRCA2*? Hereditary factors may still contribute to a significant fraction of these, but those factors must be weaker and therefore more difficult to discern.

GENETIC TESTING AND COUNSELING FOR CANCER SUSCEPTIBILITY

The discovery of genes like *RB*, p53, *NF1*, *ret*, the HNPCC mismatch repair genes, *BRCA1*, and *BRCA2* raises the possibility of DNA analysis to predict risk of cancer. There are many complexities associated with such testing. First, one must know the sensitivity and specificity of the test; the mutational heterogeneity for each of these genes constitutes a considerable technical challenge, as it is often necessary to sample every nucleotide of the coding region, the splice junctions, and the promoter to identify most mutations. False-positive results—i.e., sequence alterations that turn out to be benign polymorphic variants (allelic variations) rather than disease-causing mutations—can present a thorny problem. Unless proven interventions are available and the test is sensitive, specific, and relatively inexpensive, it will be inappropriate to offer such tests to the general population; the number of false-positive tests will exceed the number of true positives and a great deal of anxiety and expense will be incurred evaluating persons who are not at an increased risk. Generally, therefore, such testing is not considered except for individuals of higher-than-normal risk, usually on the basis of their family history. In deciding whether to offer such testing, it is critical to determine whether evidence exists for effective interventions to reduce the risk of cancer in those found to be at high risk. If such interventions do not exist (as is the case for Li-Fraumeni syndrome), then the value of the information is limited, and the major negative psychological consequences of this information must be seriously considered.

For conditions such as colon and breast cancer, prophylactic measures exist (total colectomy and bilateral mastectomy, respectively), but these prophylactic measures are more radical and potentially disfiguring than the surgical procedures that would be used to treat the patient if the malignancies actually occurred (segmental bowel resection and lumpectomy, respectively). Other potential negative conse-

Table 81-2 Genetic Alterations in Kindreds with Hereditary Nonpolyposis Colon Cancer (HNPCC)

Gene	Percent of Cases
MSH2	31
MLH1	33
PMS1	2
PMS2	4

SOURCE: Liu et al, *Nature Med* 2:169, 1996, with permission.

FIGURE 81-5 Germline mutations that have been reported in the *BRCA1* gene, primarily found in families with a high incidence of breast cancer, ovarian cancer, or both. The numbers refer to the exons of the gene; there is no exon 4. *(Information is provided courtesy of the Breast Cancer Information Core data base, which is accessible on the World Wide Web at www.nchgr.nih.gov/dir/lab_transfer/bic/.)*

quences of a positive genetic test include insurance and employment discrimination. One can still argue, of course, that a close relative of an individual known to carry a mutation in a cancer-causing gene is already sensitized to his or her personal risk of cancer, and that a test establishing that an individual at risk does *not* harbor the mutation can be quite useful. Testing should never be undertaken, however, without a full consideration of how the individual will handle a positive as well as a negative result.

Despite these caveats, genetic testing for some cancer syndromes already appears to have greater benefits than risks, and in those situations it is reasonable to offer testing to individuals at high risk. This would include conditions such as multiple endocrine neoplasia type 2 (Chap. 339) and von Hippel-Lindau disease (Chap. 370). More in the gray zone, although potentially applicable to much larger numbers of individuals, are tests for *BRCA1*, *BRCA2*, and the HNPCC genes. More research is urgently needed in those situations to determine the effectiveness of various interventions (life-style, diet, surveillance, or surgery). Until those answers are available, such testing should be offered only as part of a research protocol. As more susceptibility genes are identified, better answers become available about the effectiveness of interventions, and health insurance discrimination is legislatively prohibited, genetic testing will move into the mainstream of medicine. Every physician of the future will need to have the skills of a genetic counselor.

ACQUIRED MUTATIONS IN CANCER The identification of mutations in the germline of patients with heritable cancers means that the alteration is present in every cell of the body. However, in most cancers a normal cell becomes a malignant cell by a series of mutations that arise not in the germline but in somatic cells. Usually mutations must occur in several genes to give rise to neoplasia. The underlying questions are "how many mutations cause a cancer?" and "what specific genes are affected?" rather than whether or not mutational events cause cancer.

While answers to these questions are not available for every human malignancy, advances in molecular and cellular biology and epidemiologic analyses of human and experimental cancers are providing insights in cancer causation. Table 81-3 summarizes evidence from several lines of investigation pointing to a mutational basis for cancer causation. One particularly striking feature is the fact that the overall incidence of cancer increases as the fourth to sixth power of age for most malignancies (Fig. 81-6*A*). For some tumors, the shape of the age-incidence curve suggests heterogeneity in molecular mechanisms. For example, Hodgkin's disease has a bimodal age distribution, suggesting that two etiologically (and therefore mutationally) distinct forms of this disease may exist (Fig. 81-6*B*).

MULTISTEP BASIS OF CANCER From 5 to 10 accumulated mutations are thought to be necessary for a cell to move from the normal to the fully malignant phenotype. At each step the mutated cell may gain a slight growth advantage, so that it is increased in its representation relative to its neighbors. Figure 81-7, a representation of a lineage diagram hypothesized by Peter Nowell, illustrates how a single cell, afflicted with progressive alterations in tumor suppressor genes and protooncogenes, can develop into a clonal malignancy.

We are beginning to understand the precise nature of the genetic alterations responsible for some malignancies and to get a sense of the order in which they occur. Perhaps the best studied example is colon cancer, where an analysis of DNA from tissues extending from normal epithelium through adenoma to carcinoma have identified some of the genes mutated along the way (Fig. 81-8). However, the order of mutational events is far from uniform, and the diagram in Fig. 81-8 should be considered a generalization and not a defined pathway. Similar data are being accumulated for other malignancies.

MECHANISMS OF SOMATIC MUTATION OF ONCOGENES IN MALIGNANCY Cellular protooncogenes, their necessity and importance in normal cell growth, and their responsibility for transformation-associated change after removal of normal growth controls are discussed in Chap. 82. Mechanisms that upregulate (or activate) cellular protooncogenes can be grouped into three broad areas: point mutations, DNA amplification, and chromosome rearrangements.

Point Mutation One protooncogene that is commonly activated in solid tumors by point mutation is a member of the *ras* family of oncogenes; these were initially cloned from human bladder carcinoma cells and are critical regulators of normal and aberrant cell growth (Fig. 81-3). Mutations in one of the *ras* genes (H-*ras*, K-*ras*, or N-*ras*) are present in up to 85% of pancreatic cancers and 15% of all human cancers. In studies of K-*ras* (particularly in lung and colon cancer), the mutational spectrum of this gene has been identified. Remarkably, and in contrast to the diversity of mutations observed in the *BRCA1* gene (Fig. 81-5), most of these activated genes contain point mutations in codons 12 or 61 (which convey resistance to the inactivating action of GAP). The specificity of this pattern of mutation means that it has

Table 81-3 Evidence That Mutations Cause Cancer

Malignant tumors are clonal in nature
Some cancers show a Mendelian pattern of inheritance
DNA from malignant cells can in some instances transform normal cells to a malignant phenotype
Most tumors contain somatic mutations in oncogenes and/or tumor suppressor genes
Recurring sites of chromosome change are observed in cancers at the sites of genes involved in cellular growth control
Most carcinogens are mutagens
Defects in DNA repair systems increase the probability of cancer

A

B

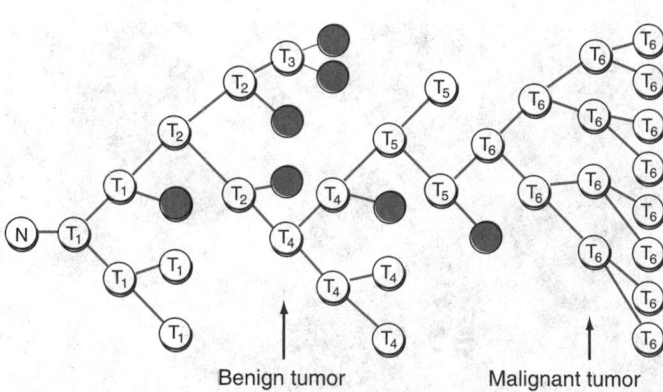

FIGURE 81-7 Multistep clonal development of malignancy. In this diagram a series of five cumulative mutations (T1, T2, T4, T5, T6), each with a modest growth advantage acting alone, eventually results in a malignant tumor. Note that not all such alterations result in progression; for example, the T3 clone is a dead end. The actual number of cumulative mutations necessary to transform from the normal to the malignant state is unknown in most tumors. *(After P Nowell, Science 194:23, 1976, with permission.)*

FIGURE 81-6 Relationship between age and cancer incidence. *A.* Age-specific incidence of skin, colon, and pancreas cancers in Canadian males. The curves appear as straight lines when plotted using logarithmic axes, fitting the multihit model of cancer (see text). *B.* For some tumor types (e.g., Hodgkin's disease), a bimodal age distribution is seen, perhaps indicative of a differing mutational basis (see text). *(From I Tannock and R Hall, The Basic Science of Oncology, 2d ed, New York, McGraw Hill, 1992, with permission.)*

The recognition of DNA amplification was greatly facilitated by the development of a procedure based on dual-color fluorescence in situ hybridization (FISH) called *comparative genomic hybridization* (CGH). DNA from tumor and normal cells is labeled with different fluorescent reporter molecules and then hybridized to normal metaphase chromosomes. Regions of duplications and deletions within tumor DNA are then demonstrated as quantifiable alterations in signal intensity at particular sites. With this technique the entire genome can be surveyed for gains and losses of DNA sequences, thus pinpointing chromosomal regions likely to contain genes important in the development or progression of cancer.

Numerous genes are known to be amplified in human malignancies. Several genes, including N-*myc* were identified because they were present within the amplified DNA sequences of a tumor and had homology to known oncogenes. Because the region amplified often extends to hundreds of thousands of base pairs, more than one oncogene may be amplified in some cancers (particularly sarcomas). Genes simultaneously amplified in many cases include *MDM2*, *GLI*, *CDK4*, *SAS*, and others implicated in cellular growth control. The clinical implications of gene amplification have been explored for some cancers [most notably *ERBB2 (HER-2/neu)* in breast cancer and N-*myc* in neuroblastoma]; demonstration of amplification of a cellular gene

potential value in diagnostic or prognostic studies of cancer. For K-*ras*, mutations may be a useful prognostic marker in lung cancer, but for most other cancers (including pancreas and colon cancer) no prognostic utility has been demonstrated. This is in part because *ras* mutations occur early in colon cancer (Fig. 81-8), being common in precancerous lesions of the bowel.

DNA Amplification The second mechanism for activation of oncogene overexpression is DNA sequence amplification. This increase in DNA sequence copy number may cause cytologically recognizable chromosome alterations referred to as *homogeneous staining regions* (HSRs), if integrated within chromosomes, or *double minutes* (dmins), if extrachromosomal in nature (Fig. 81-9).

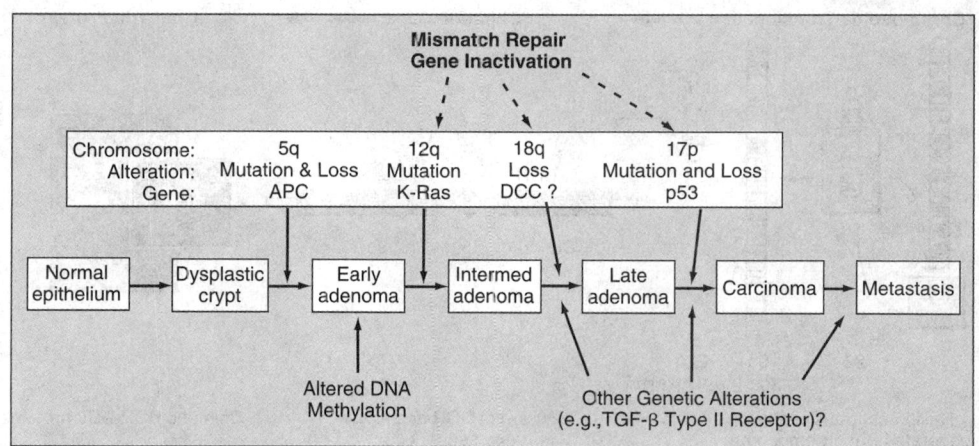

FIGURE 81-8 Progressive somatic mutational steps in the development of colon carcinoma. The accumulation of alterations in a number of different genes results in the progression from normal epithelium through early adenoma to full blown carcinoma. While the steps shown here do not always occur in this order, it is clear that an accumulation of somatic mutations is required before cancer develops. Patients with familial polyposis are already one step into this pathway, since they inherit a germline alteration of the *APC* gene.

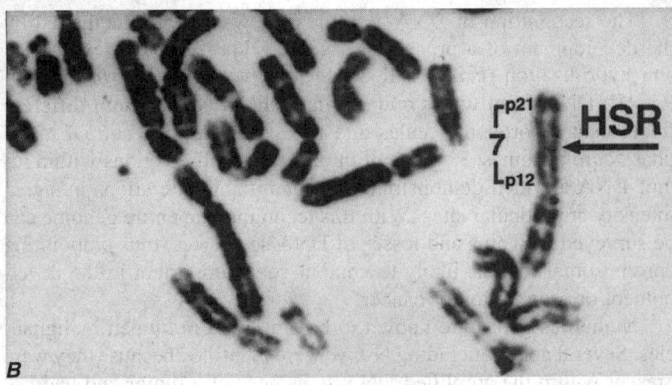

FIGURE 81-9 Representative examples of tumor cells containing cytogenetic evidence of gene amplification. *A.* Example of multiple copies of double minute (dmin) chromosomes from a patient with ovarian carcinoma. *B.* Example of a homogeneous staining region (HSR) on chromosome 7 from a patient with malignant melanoma.

is usually a predictor of poor prognosis. Once a patient has been exposed to the selective effects of chemotherapy, gene amplification may lead to drug resistance. Amplification of the dihydrofolate reductase gene may follow clinical exposure to methotrexate, a drug that inhibits the activity of the enzyme.

Chromosomal Alterations in Human Cancer Chromosomal alterations provide important clues to the genetic changes in cancers. To date, most chromosome analyses have been performed on hematopoietic cancers, although solid tumors may also have translocations. The breakpoints of several recurring chromosome abnormalities often occur at the sites of cellular protooncogenes. Translocations are particularly common in lymphoid tumors, probably because these cell types normally rearrange DNA to generate antigen receptors. Indeed, antigen receptor genes are commonly involved in the translocations, implying that an imperfect regulation of receptor gene rearrangement may be involved in the pathogenesis. An example is Burkitt's lymphoma, a B-cell tumor characterized by a reciprocal translocation between chromosomes 8 and 14. Molecular analysis of Burkitt's lymphomas demonstrated that the breakpoints occurred within or near the *myc* locus on chromosome 8 and within the immunoglobulin heavy chain locus on chromosome 14, resulting in the transcriptional activation of *myc*. Enhancer activation by translocation, although not universal, appears to play an important role in malignant progression.

Chromosome rearrangements can lead to the abnormal overexpression of a transcription factor that performs its normal function and turns on growth-related genes. The translocation may create a chimeric transcription factor that has altered function. For example, the t(15;17) of acute promyelocytic leukemia produces a retinoic acid receptor with an abnormal cell distribution that inhibits differentiation. Gene rearrangements most commonly involve transcription factors, but other components of signaling pathways may also be involved.

The first reproducible chromosome abnormality detected in human malignancy was the Philadelphia chromosome in chronic myelogenous leukemia (CML). This cytogenetic abnormality is generated by reciprocal translocation involving the *ABL* oncogene, a tyrosine kinase on chromosome 9 being placed in proximity to the *BCR* (breakpoint cluster region) on chromosome 22. Figure 81-10 illustrates the generation of the translocation and its protein product. The consequence of expression of the *BCR-ABL* gene product is the activation of signal transduction pathways, leading to cell growth independent of normal external growth factor signals.

In addition to transcription factors and signal transduction molecules, translocations may involve the overexpression of cell cycle regulatory proteins, such as cyclins, and of proteins that regulate cell death, such as bcl2. Altering control of expression of cell cycle regulatory proteins can lead to aberrant cell cycle control. The overexpression of bcl-2 can prevent the death of a cell that has endured enough genetic damage to cause its death. If such a cell survives to receive additional genetic damage, a tumor can develop. Table 81-4 lists representative examples of recurring chromosome alterations in malignancy and the associated gene(s) rearranged or dysregulated by the chromosomal change.

Technical obstacles have slowed the identification of recurring chromosome abnormalities in human solid tumors (particularly carcinomas) because of the complexity of chromosome alterations in such tumors, in contrast to the solitary, often reciprocal, nature of chromosome rearrangements in hematopoietic malignancies.

Chromosome Translocation ⟶ **Chimeric Gene** ⟶ **Chimeric Protein**

Ph¹

BCR   ABL

Chr. 22q   Chr. 9q

BCR   ABL

9   22   9q+   22q-
t(9;22)(q34;q11)

Reciprocal translocation
generates Ph¹ chromosome

Fusion of BCR and ABL
gene sequences

Chimeric BCR-ABL protein

FIGURE 81-10 Specific translocation seen in chronic myelogenous leukemia (CML). The Philadelphia chromosome (Ph) is derived from a reciprocal translocation between chromosomes 9 and 22 with the breakpoint joining the sequences of the *ABL* oncogene with the *BCR* gene. The fusion of these DNA sequences allows the generation of an entirely novel fusion protein with modified function (see text). *(Courtesy of ER Fearon and KR Cho.)*

EPIGENETIC REGULATION OF GENE EXPRESSION AND CANCER The term *epigenetic* refers

Table 81-4 Representative Oncogenes at Chromosomal Translocations

Gene (Chromosome)	Translocation	Malignancy
ABL (9q34.1)	(9;22)(q34;q11)	Chronic myelogenous leukemia
BCR (22q11)		
AML1 (21q22)	(3;21)(q26;q22)	Acute myelogenous leukemia, myelodysplasia
EAP (3q26)		
EVI1 (3q26)		
ATF1 (12q13)	(12;22)(q13;q12)	Malignant melanoma of soft parts (MMSP)
EWS (22q12)		
BCL1 (11q13.3)	(11;14)(q13;q32)	Mantle cell lymphoma
IgH (14q32)		
BCL2 (18q21.3)	(14;18)(q32;q21)	Follicular lymphoma
IgH (14q32)		
BCL3 (19q13.1)	(14;19)(q32;q13)	B cell chronic lymphocytic leukemia
IgH (14q32)		
ERG (21q22.3)	(22;21)(q12;q22)	Ewing's sarcoma
EWS (22q12)		
FLI1 (11q24)	(11;22)(q24;q12)	Ewing's sarcoma
EWS (22q12)		
LCK (1p34)	(1;7)(p34;q35)	T cell acute lymphocytic leukemia (ALL)
TCRB (7q35)		
MLL/ALL1/HRX (11q23)	(4;11)(q21;q23)	ALL
myc (8q24)	(8;14)(q24;q32)	Burkitt's lymphoma, B cell ALL
TAN1 (9q34) deletion	(7;9)(q34;q34)	T cell ALL
WT1 (11p13)	(11;22)(p13;q12)	Desmoplastic small round cell tumor (DSRCT)
EWS (22q12)		
TLS/FUS (16p11)	(12;16)(q13;p11)	Myxoid liposarcoma
CHOP (12q13)		
PAX3 (2q35)	(2;13)(q35;q14)	Alveolar rhabdomyosarcoma
FKHR/ALV(13q14)		
PAX7 (1p36)	(1;13)(p36;q14)	Alveolar rhabdomyosarcoma
KHR/ALV(13q14)		
ret (10q11.2)	(10;17)(q11.2;q23)	Papillary thyroid carcinomas

SOURCE: After Hesketh.

to mechanisms of gene regulation independent of DNA sequence. The inactivation of the second X chromosome in female cells is an example of an epigenetic mechanism that prevents gene expression from the inactivated chromosome. During embryologic development, entire regions of chromosomes from one parent are silenced and gene expression proceeds from the chromosome of the other parent. For most genes, expression occurs from both parental alleles or randomly from one parent or the other. The preferential expression of a particular gene exclusively from the allele contributed by one parent is called *parental imprinting* and is thought to be regulated by the methylation of the silenced allele.

The role of epigenetic control mechanisms in the development of human cancer is unclear. However, a general decrease in the level of DNA methylation has been noted as a common change in cancers. In addition, the loss of imprinting of the normally silent maternal allele of the insulin-like growth factor II gene at chromosome 11p15.5 has been implicated in some cases of the rare pediatric malignancy Wilms' tumor. The loss of imprinting may result in the overexpression of the growth factor and a predisposition to malignant transformation.

THE FUTURE The real challenge in oncology is to convert the growing molecular understanding of cancer into clinical advances, particularly the development of new therapies. One can anticipate that in the coming years the molecular analysis of mutations in tumors will allow stratification of malignancies into more precise subgroups than is currently possible by histologic classification, including subgroups with particularly good or bad prognoses or that have a lower or higher likelihood of responding to a particular therapy. Some of this information is already accumulating, but usually only one or two genes are assessed; the promise of the future is to obtain a detailed molecular "fingerprint" of every tumor in order to provide the maximum information about its biology and response to therapy. The application of techniques for assessing global gene expression (cDNA microarrays,

serial analysis of gene expression, or SAGE, and others) is leading to novel ways of looking at cancer that are considerably more discriminating than light microscopy, the gold standard of medical practice. The National Cancer Institute in conjunction with the National Center for Biotechnology Information have undertaken the Cancer Genome Anatomy Project (CGAP) (www.ncbi.nlm.nih.gov/ncicgap/) to collect data on the differences in gene expression between normal and malignant tissues and make it available on the Internet.

Genetics will also influence cancer prevention and early detection. The ability to identify cancer susceptibility genes presages a new era of cancer prevention, if the potential risks of such testing can be surmounted. Currently, most cancer early detection strategies (such as mammography, stool occult blood testing, or digital rectal examination) are applied to population groups. The ability to identify the individuals at highest risk and to focus preventive medicine efforts accordingly may be both better received by patients and more cost effective. Early detection strategies will be even more effective if we can develop the ability to identify very small numbers of malignant or premalignant cells at a time when the risk of metastasis is still very low.

More importantly, detailed molecular information about the regulation of the cell cycle and the interplay of tumor suppressor genes and proto-oncogenes that control it may lead to new effective therapies, based on pathophysiology rather than empiricism. Whether such strategies will rely on drugs of the traditional types or will be based on more novel strategies such as gene therapy or immunotherapy is hard to predict.

BIBLIOGRAPHY

BUNZ F et al: Disruption of p53 in human cancer cells alters the responses to therapeutic agents. J Clin Invest 104:263, 1999

BUTEL JS: Viral carcinogenesis: revelation of molecular mechanisms and etiology of human disease. Carcinogenesis 21:405, 2000

CUI H et al: Loss of imprinting in normal tissue of colorectal cancer patients with microsatellite instability. Nat Med 4:1276, 1998

EMMERT-BUCK MR et al: Molecular profiling of clinical tissue specimens: Feasibility and applications. Am J Pathol 156:1109, 2000

FEINBERG AP: DNA methylation, genomic imprinting and cancer. Curr Top Microbiol Immunol 249:87, 2000

GOLUB TR et al: Molecular classification of cancer: Class discovery and class prediction by gene expression monitoring. Science 286:531, 1999

HABER DA, FEARON ER: The promise of cancer genetics. Lancet 351(Suppl 2):S1, 1998

KORSMEYER SJ: Bcl-2 gene family and the regulation of programmed cell death. Cancer Res 59(suppl 7):1693s, 1999

LAL A et al: A public database for gene expression in human cancers. Cancer Res 59: 5403, 1999

TONIN P: Genes implicated in hereditary breast cancer syndromes. Semin Surg Oncol 18: 281, 2000

VOGELSTEIN B, KINZLER KW: The multistep nature of cancer. Trends Genet 9:138, 1993

82 Robert G. Fenton, Dan L. Longo

CELL BIOLOGY OF CANCER

Two characteristic features define a cancer: cell growth not regulated by external signals (i.e., autonomous) and the capacity to invade tissues and metastasize to and colonize distant sites (Chap. 83). The first of these features, the uncontrolled growth of abnormal cells, is a property of all neoplasms, or new growths. A neoplasm may be benign or malignant. If invasion, the second cardinal feature of cancer, is present, the neoplasm is malignant. Cancer is a synonym for *malignant neoplasm*. Cancers of epithelial tissues are called *carcinomas*; cancers of nonepithelial (mesenchymal) tissues are called *sarcomas*.

Cancer is a genetic disease, but the level of its expression is the single cell. Although some forms of cancer are heritable, most mutations occur in somatic cells and are caused by intrinsic errors in DNA replication or are induced by carcinogen exposure. A single genetic lesion is usually not sufficient to induce neoplastic transformation of a cell. The malignant phenotype is acquired only after several (5 to 10) mutations lead to derangements in a variety of gene products. Each genetic alteration may cause phenotypic changes typified by the progression in epithelial tissues from hyperplasia to adenoma to dysplasia to carcinoma in situ to invasive carcinoma. Cells have evolved mechanisms to resist neoplastic transformation (see below).

The >200 discrete cell types in the body are not equally susceptible to developing cancer. Some cells, such as cardiac myocytes, sensory receptor cells for light and sound, and lens fibers, persist throughout life without dividing or being replaced. Neoplasia in such tissues is exceedingly rare. Most differentiated tissues undergo constant renewal characterized by cell death and replacement.

In tissues with rapid turnover, such as skin, bone marrow, and gut, an individual cell is on one of two largely mutually exclusive paths: division or differentiation. Cells capable of dividing are undifferentiated (stem cells), whereas terminally differentiated cells are unable to divide. Stem cells produce daughter cells that can either become new stem cells (thus replenishing the stem cell compartment) or undergo terminal differentiation, depending on the circumstances and the environmental signals. Stem cells are distinguished from differentiating cells by different patterns of gene expression. Gene expression is the product of the tissue-specific programming interacting with environmental factors such as cell-to-cell contact; interactions with extracellular matrix; endocrine hormones; paracrine growth and differentiation factors; and stresses such as heat, oxidation, irradiation, and physical distortion or traction.

Cancer is most common in tissues with rapid turnover, especially those exposed to environmental carcinogens and whose proliferation is regulated by hormones. The most common genetic changes involve the activation of proto-oncogenes or the inactivation of tumor suppressor genes (Chap. 81). Although genetic damage is nearly universal in human cancer, cells with neoplastic features can be generated in vitro without genetic damage. Removal and in vitro culture of cells from the epiblast of a murine embryo lead to the uncontrolled proliferation of the cells and the generation of a teratocarcinoma cell line capable of producing tumors when inoculated into animals. The removal of these normal embryonic cells from their normal environment leads to uncontrolled growth. However, if the teratocarcinoma cells are reinjected into an early embryo, under the inductive influence of their normal neighbors they can differentiate into normal organs and tissues appropriate for the location where they are injected.

Thus, environmental factors exert potent effects on the gene expression of target cells. The panoply of signals received by a particular cell leads to the activation of particular sets of transcription factors. The pattern of gene expression determines whether a cell will divide, differentiate, or die.

PRINCIPLES OF CELL CYCLE REGULATION

The mechanism of cell division is substantially the same in all dividing cells and has been conserved throughout evolution. The process assures that the cell accurately duplicates its contents, especially its chromosomes. The cell cycle is divided into four phases. During M phase, the replicated chromosomes are separated and packaged into two new nuclei by mitosis and the cytoplasm is divided between the two daughter cells by cytokinesis. The other three phases of the cell cycle are called *interphase*: G1 (gap 1), a period of growth during which the cell determines its readiness to commit to DNA synthesis; S (DNA synthesis), during which the genetic material is replicated and no re-replication is permitted; and G2 (gap 2), during which the fidelity of DNA replication is determined and errors are corrected.

During S phase, DNA synthesis begins with the unfolding of chromatin and nucleosome complexes rendering DNA accessible for the addition of DNA helicase and single-strand binding proteins that help open the double helix. Replication origins are spaced roughly 100,000 nucleotide pairs apart throughout the genome. DNA polymerase and DNA primase attach to these sites and catalyze the polymerization of the DNA at a rate of about 50 nucleotides per second. DNA polymerase δ catalyzes leading-strand synthesis, while DNA polymerase α uses DNA primase–generated Okazaki fragments for lagging-strand synthesis. Topoisomerase I nicks DNA, relieving torsional tension of the replicating helix; topoisomerase II introduces double strand breaks to avoid DNA tangles. Topoisomerases are targets of many chemotherapeutic drugs. Once a DNA segment is replicated, chromatin is reassembled, and replication origins are relicensed by binding of specific proteins that prevent re-replication until the next S phase. Although this system for replication is efficient and accurate, occasional mistakes are made, and these are repaired by a variety of mechanisms. In some cancers, the mismatch repair mechanisms are defective and errors increase by 3 to 4 logs, greatly increasing the likelihood of mutations in growth regulatory genes in daughter cells.

DNA polymerase is unable to replicate the end of a DNA chain completely, resulting in loss of DNA with each replication. This problem has been solved by a mechanism that replicates tandem repeats of a six-nucleotide sequence (GGGTTA) to the ends of each chromosome. These repeated sequences are called *telomeres* and are replicated through an RNA-dependent DNA polymerase called *telomerase*. Normal somatic cells do not express telomerase, and the replicative lifetime of such cells is limited to approximately 30 cell divisions due to the progressive loss of telomere repeats; the limit imposed on somatic cell division is called the *Hayflick limit*, at which time replicative senescence occurs. Germ cells do express telomerase and have a long (possibly unlimited) replicative lifetime. The aberrant expression of telomerase in cancer cells is thought to be a component of the neoplastic process, assuring that the cell will be able to undergo many divisions without inducing senescence or genetic catastophe. Inhibition of telomerase activity in cancer cells could have antitumor effects.

The cell cycle transitions between G1 and S and between G2 and M are tightly regulated to ensure that cells are prepared to divide and to minimize errors in the replication process. Checkpoints in G1 and G2 determine whether a cell will enter S or M phase, respectively; these checkpoints are regulated by serine/threonine protein kinases (cyclin-dependent kinases, or cdk) and kinase-associated proteins called *cyclins*. The enzymatic activity of each cdk is determined by its association with a cyclin and its phosphorylation state. There are at least seven cdk family members, and a like number of cyclins, which generate a group of cdk/cyclin complexes with differing substrate specificities and times of action during the cell cycle. Cyclin expression varies with the cell cycle, and the synthesis of these proteins is transcriptionally regulated and their degradation is mediated by ubiquitin conjugation and destruction in proteasomes.

The cyclin B/cdc2 complex (also called *mitosis promoting factor*, or MPF) is the primary regulator of transition from G2 to M phase. It is activated by a cdk-activating kinase (CAK) and a phosphatase (cdc25c) that removes inhibitory phosphates. The cdc25C is the target of a DNA damage–induced kinase that inhibits its activity. DNA damage leads to phosphorylation of cdc25C and its transport out of the nucleus, away from cyclin B/cdc2. This prevents entry into M phase until DNA damage is repaired. The regulated movement of molecules into and out of the nucleus is a common control mechanism in signal transduction. Some of the substrates of cyclin B/cdc2 are defined; its phosphorylation of histone H1, nuclear lamins, and microtubule-associated proteins facilitates chromosome condensation, nuclear membrane breakdown, and spindle formation, respectively.

The checkpoint regulating transition from G1 to S is frequently disrupted in cancer. The product of the retinoblastoma tumor suppressor gene, the nuclear phosphoprotein Rb, governs the key transition referred to as the *reaction point*. A second pathway regulated by the p53 tumor suppressor interacts with the Rb pathway to ensure that cell proliferation can safely take place. Rb and p53 are inactivated by products encoded by DNA tumor viruses, including SV40 large T antigen, adenovirus E1A and E1B, and human papillomavirus E6 and E7. The Rb and p53 pathways each include other oncogenes and tumor suppressors that are frequently disrupted in cancer (Table 82-1).

Regulation of passage through the restriction point is complex. In early G1, Rb is hypophosphorylated and in a complex with the E2F transcription factor. This nuclear complex binds to the promoters of genes required for cell cycle progression and inhibits their expression. However, in mid and late G1, Rb becomes phosphorylated (at ~10 sites) by the sequential activity of the cyclin D/cdk4 and cyclin E/cdk2 complexes. Hyperphosphorylated Rb releases E2F, thus relieving transcriptional repression, and heterodimers of E2F and DP1 transcription factor family members activate several genes required for S phase progression, including dihydrofolate reluctase, thymidine kinase, DNA polymerase, and cdc2 (Fig. 82-1). In addition to its role in growth regulation, Rb is required for the in vitro differentiation of muscle cells and adipocytes. Cell cycle control and induction of differentiation are functions of Rb that contribute to tumor suppression.

The activity of cdk is also regulated by cdk inhibitors (cdki). These low-molecular-weight proteins are divided into two families: the Cip/Kip family encoding $p21^{Cip1/Waf1}$, $p27^{Kip1}$, $p57^{Kip2}$, which inhibit cdk activity broadly, and the Ink4 family encoding $p16^{INK4a}$, $p15^{INK4b}$, $p18^{INK4c}$, and $p19^{INK4d}$, which block cyclin D/cdk4 activity and inhibit Rb phosphorylation and G1/S transition. p21 is induced by p53 in response to DNA damage, causing G1 arrest to permit DNA repair. If DNA damage is too great, a cell suicide pathway is induced to eliminate cells that may be dysfunctional (see below).

The cdki can be induced by growth inhibitors such as transforming growth factor (TGF) β and can be inhibited by growth factors such as interleukin (IL) 2. Genetic alterations in cdki, especially p16 and p15, occur with high frequency in certain tumors. Alterations at the p16 locus on chromosome 9p21 have been detected in 75% of pancreatic cancers; 40 to 70% of glioblastomas; 50% of esophageal cancers; and about 20% of non-small cell lung cancers, soft tissue sarcomas, and bladder cancers. Mutations in p16 account for half of familial melanomas. Some tumors fail to express cdki because the genes are meth-

FIGURE 82-1 The retinoblastoma gene product, pRb, regulates cell cycle progression at the restriction point by sequestering the E2F transcription factor. Hypophosphorylated pRb forms an inactive complex with the E2F/DP-1 heterodimer that is bound to regulatory E2F sites of promoters of genes required for S phase. Rb recruits histone deacetylases to the promoter, rendering chromatin inaccessible to the basal transcriptional machinery. The kinase activities of cdk4/cyclin D and cdk2/cyclin E convert pRb to the hyperphosphorylated state with loss of binding pocket activity. G1 cdk activity is positively regulated by growth factors and inhibited by a variety of physiologic signals from the cell microenvironment. Hyperphosphorylated Rb dissociates from E2F/DP-1, which then associates with coactivators containing histone acetylase activity to form transcriptionally active complexes. S phase genes are expressed and cell cycle progresses.

ylated, an epigenetic mechanism for blocking transcription. Rb pathway regulation is also circumvented by overexpression of cyclin D1 [breast cancer and the t(11;14) in mantle cell lymphoma] and by mutations in cdk4 that abrogate p16 binding.

Whereas Rb, cyclin D, cdk4, and p16 are commonly altered in cancer, E2F overexpression or p21 mutations have not yet been seen. Additional study may reveal why some components of the system are susceptible to alterations and other components are not.

p53, the "guardian of the genome," is a transcription factor that is not usually called upon to act in the course of normal replication. Levels of p53 are normally kept low by its association with mdm2, which binds p53 and shuttles it out of the nucleus for degradation. However, with DNA damage, p53 is phosphorylated by the ataxia telangiectasia gene product ATM, it dissociates from mouse double minute 2 (mdm2), and its destruction is slowed, leading to increased levels. Also, p53 influences transcription to either halt cell cycle progression (e.g., through induction of p21 expression to inhibit cdk activity) to permit repair of the DNA or, if the damage is too great, to initiate cell suicide (apoptosis). p53-induced genes involved in apoptosis include death receptors (DR5) and death-inducing members of the Bcl-2 family. p53 also induces expression of mdm2, thus downregulating its own activity.

Inducers of p53 include hypoxia, DNA damage, ribonucleotide depletion, and telomere shortening. Dysregulated activity of oncogenes such as myc, which promote aberrant G1/S transition, induces p53-mediated apoptosis. A second product of the Ink4a locus is $p14^{ARF}$, encoded by an alternative reading frame (ARF) from p16. Levels of ARF are upregulated by myc and E2F. ARF binds to mdm2/p53 complexes and rescues p53 from the inhibitory effects of mdm2 with subsequent activation of p53-induced genes. This oncogene checkpoint leads to the death of renegade cells that attempt to traverse the restriction point without the right signals.

Mutation in p53 is the most common genetic alteration found in human cancer (>50%) and is the causative lesion in Li-Fraumeni familial cancer sydrome. In tumors, usually one p53 allele on chromo-

Table 82-1   Cell Cycle Regulators in Human Cancer

Gene	Genetic Change	Functional Consequences
RETINOBLASTOMA PATHWAY		
Retinoblastoma	Deletion Point mutation	Loss of growth control at restriction point; loss of G1 checkpoint; TGF-β resistance
Cyclin D	Chromosome translocation Gene amplification	Aberrant increase in cyclin D/cdk4 activity with inhibition of Rb function
Cdk4	Point mutation	Loss of $p16^{INK4a}$ binding site; deregulated cyclin D/cdk4 activity
$p16^{INK4a}$	Deletion Point mutations Methylation	Failure to regulate cyclin D/cdk4 activity; leads to Rb hyperphosphorylation and aberrant entry in S phase
P53 PATHWAY		
p53	Deletion Point mutation	Loss of $p21^{Cip1/Waf1}$-mediated checkpoint control; genomic instability; resistance to apoptosis
Mdm2	Amplification	Increased p53 degradation; failure to induce p53 stess responses
$p14^{ARF}$	Homozygous deletion	Unregulated mdm2 inhibition of p53 levels and activity; loss of oncogene checkpoint
ATM	Deletion Point mutation	Decreased activation of p53 by ionizing radiation; loss of multiple checkpoints; genomic instability

NOTE: TGF, transforming growth factor.

some 17p is deleted and the other is mutated. The mutations often involve the region between codons 120 and 290, the portion of the gene specifying the site of p53 involved in transcription. Some environmental agents cause mutations at specific sites. In 81% of hepatomas in persons from developing countries, codon 249 is mutated due to exposure to the carcinogen, aflatoxin. Codon 249 mutations occur in only 11% of hepatomas in persons from industrialized countries where aflatoxin exposure is low. Inactivation of the p53 pathway compromises cell cycle arrest, inhibits apoptosis induced by DNA damage or oncogene activation, and predisposes cells to chromosome instability.

Regardless of the pathogenesis of the tumor, most have some mechanism(s) to bypass the G1 checkpoint, avoid activation of cell suicide pathways, and propagate cells with damaged DNA. Table 82-1 summarizes some of the changes in cell cycle regulators detected in human cancers.

SIGNALING FROM OUTSIDE THE CELL TO THE NUCLEUS

The behavior of cells in the body is tightly regulated by environmental signals. The ability of a cell to respond to a specific set of signals determines whether the cell will live or die, differentiate, proliferate, or remain quiescent. In normal cells and tissues, coordinated action such as wound healing or the inflammatory response is regulated by signaling pathways that convert extracellular signals into the performance of specialized action in the responding cells. In cancer cells, the process of invading and metastasizing is influenced by signal transduction pathways activated by paracrine and autocrine factors.

The coupling of extracellular signals to cell response varies for different receptor and signaling systems. The binding of a growth factor [e.g., epidermal growth factor (EGF)] to its receptor on the cell surface produces measurable changes in the cell within seconds and elicits a sequence of events that may last for days. Rapid responses are elicited by changes in ion flux, phosphorylation events, lipid metabolism, and production of second messengers. Long-term responses are mediated by the transfer of signaling information from the receptor to the nucleus, where alterations in the pattern of gene expression result in phenotypic change. Signal transduction comprises the mechanisms by which information received at the plasma membrane is imparted to the nuclear transcriptional machinery and other cell functions. Many signal transduction pathways are perturbed in cancer cells. There are three families of cell surface receptors: ion channel–linked receptors, G protein–linked receptors, and enzyme-linked receptors. Although ion channel–linked receptors are a component of growth-related activation in many cell types, they are primarily involved in neurotransmitter signal transduction and are somewhat less important in the pathogenesis of neoplasia than the other two types and will not be discussed further.

G PROTEIN–LINKED RECEPTORS   The G protein–linked receptors traverse the plasma membrane seven times (serpentine receptors). They do not induce covalent modification of their substrates, as do enzyme-linked receptors, but generate second messenger molecules such as cyclic AMP, cyclic GMP, and calcium to activate downstream processes. Upon ligand binding, these receptors activate trimeric G proteins inducing the release of $G\alpha$ and $G\beta\gamma$ subunits, each of which elicits downstream signals. The process is terminated by GTP hydrolysis by $G\alpha$ subunits. The roles of G protein signaling pathways in human cancer include certain endocrine tumors whose cells of origin depend on cyclic AMP for growth. About half of growth hormone–secreting pituitary tumors encode mutant $G\alpha$ subunits that are defective in GTPase activity and are constitutively activated even in the absence of ligand. These $G\alpha$ subunits bind to and stimulate the activity of adenyl cyclase, leading to unregulated synthesis of cyclic AMP. Cyclic AMP binds to the repressor subunit of protein kinase A thus activating the kinase, which enters the nucleus and phosphorylates

CREB (cyclic AMP response element binding protein), a transcription factor that activates genes required for proliferation of the cancer cells. Growth stimulatory $G\alpha$ mutations have also been described in adrenal cortical tumors and endocrine tumors of the ovary. Factors involved in normal cell and tumor cell migration also stimulate cells through G protein–coupled receptors.

ENZYME-LINKED RECEPTORS   There are at least five classes of enzyme-linked receptors: receptor guanylyl cyclases, receptor tyrosine kinases, tyrosine kinase–associated receptors, receptor tyrosine phosphatases, and receptor serine/threonine kinases. The atrial natriuretic peptide receptor is a receptor guanylyl cyclase. Some disease manifestations in cancer may be related to atrial natriuretic peptide activity (such as hyponatremia), but little is known about this receptor class. Receptor phosphatases are not known to be involved in cancer. The other classes of enzyme-linked receptors are better defined and play a more important role in cancer.

Receptor Tyrosine Kinases   The receptors for most growth factors are transmembrane tyrosine kinase receptors, including platelet-derived growth factor (PDGF), fibroblast growth factors (FGFs), EGF, heregulin, insulin, insulin-like growth factors (IGF) I and II, nerve growth factor (NGF), stem cell factor, vascular endothelial growth factor, macrophage colony stimulating factors (CSF), and others. Much of what we know about receptor tyrosine kinases and the events that follow their ligation emerged from the study of the proliferation-inducing altered forms of the normal cellular genes (proto-oncogenes) that are the cancer-causing genes (oncogenes) in animal retroviruses. Although downstream events vary with the receptor/ligand combinations, the activation of the receptor follows a typical pattern. Ligand binding induces dimerization or oligomerization of receptor subunits, which activates tyrosine kinase activity and causes autophosphorylation of specific tyrosine residues in the cytoplasmic domain of the receptor. Phosphorylated tyrosine residues on the receptors or on associated adaptor proteins form docking sights for other signal transduction molecules that contain one or more *src-homology region 2*, or SH2, domains, named because the sequence was first identified in the *src* nonreceptor tyrosine kinase. Phosphorylation of tyrosine residues provides a unique amplification signal because of the rapid and specific binding of SH2 domains to p-Tyr, although p-Tyr comprises only 0.05% of total cell phosphoamino acid. These associations via SH2 domains trigger subsequent events (Fig. 82-2). Signaling is terminated by the action of p-Tyr-specific phosphatases.

Protein domain interactions between evolutionarily conserved motifs play critical roles in all forms of signal transduction, ranging from tyrosine kinase pathways, death-inducing molecules, and the association of transcription complexes on gene regulatory regions. The most common docking mechanisms are based on recognition of particular protein sequences; the SH2 domains recognize p-Tyr-containing sequences with specificity conferred by surrounding amino acid residues, the SH3 domains dock with proline-rich sequences, and the pleckstrin homology domains [pleckstrin is a major protein kinase C (PKC) substrate in platelets] lead to associations with phosphatidylinositol lipids phosphorylated in the 3 position by phosphatidylinositol 3-kinase (PI3K; see below). Some molecules that do not have docking domains are brought into association with the receptors through the activity of adaptor proteins that are composed of docking domains only. Thus, the nucleotide exchange factor son of sevenless (SOS; named for its role in *Drosophila* eye development) is brought close to the membrane to activate Ras through its association with the adaptor protein grb2 (identified because it "grabbed" p-Tyr-containing proteins).

Receptor tyrosine kinases activate many signaling pathways including phospholipase C-γ, which hydrolyzes phosphoinoside 4,5-bisphosphate (PIP2) into diacylglycerol (DAG) and inositol triphosphate (IP3). DAG together with calcium ion activates PKC, a family of serine/threonine kinases with different activation requirements, subcellular locations, and substrates in different cell types. PKC is the target of tumor-promoting phorbol esters, and its activation can influence cell proliferation, differentiation, and tumorigenesis. IP3 induces the release of intracellular calcium, which binds to calmodulin, a protein

FIGURE 82-2 *A.* Structures of receptor tyrosine kinases activated by ligand-induced dimerization. Conserved extracellular domains, a single transmembrane spanning region, and a cytoplasmic domain encoding the tyrosine kinase characterize these receptors. The insulin and insulin-like growth factor (IGF) I receptors are disulfide-linked heterotetramers of α and β chains that undergo allosteric changes upon ligand binding. In the other cases shown, ligand binding induces homo- or heterodimerization within the subfamily followed by receptor autophosphorylation on tyrosine residues. Some kinase domains contain a kinase insert (KI). Flt-1 and Flk-1 are endothelial cell–specific receptors for vascular endothelial growth factor (VEGF) and are required for embryonic blood vessel differentiation and angiogenesis in the adult. Other members of the receptor tyrosine kinase family not shown share structural similarities. *B.* Multiple tyrosine autophosphorylation sites on activated platelet-derived growth factor (PDGF) receptor β chains serve as docking sites for signal transduction molecules. These include enzymes that activate downstream substrates and docking proteins to provide SH2 or p-Tyr binding sites for other proteins. These interactions lead to the formation of a signal transduction complex whose structure determines the nature of the signal transduction pathways activated by a particular ligand. SH2, SH3, pleckstrin homology (PH), proline-rich (Pro), phospholipase C (PLC), phosphoinositol 3-kinase (PI3K), GTPase activating protein (GAP), and protein tyrosine phosphatase (PTPase) domains are shown.

that regulates the activity of many enzymes, including phosphatases. Calcium fluxes within cells can be short or prolonged, and the duration has profound physiologic effects. PI3K is a lipid kinase that generates PI(3,4)P2 and PI(3,4,5)P3, membrane lipids that act as binding sites for proteins containing PH motifs. Such proteins include Akt serine/threonine kinase, which is implicated in activating survival pathways in many cells. Src family tyrosine kinases bind to p-Tyr on activated receptors and amplify signaling information by phosphorylation of distinct protein substrates within the cell. Src activity is required for G1 progression in some cells through its induction of the transcription factor c-myc. Another consequence of receptor tyrosine kinase activation is stimulation of the Ras/MAP (mitogen-activated protein) kinase pathway that leads to activation of a number of transcription factors that regulate proliferation, differentiation, and cell survival. This pathway is frequently abnormal in cancer cells.

Ras is a 21-kDa member of a large family of proteins, including rho, rac, rab, and others, that regulate cytoskeletal changes, vesicular and nuclear transport, and proliferation and that share sequence homology with the Gα subunit of G protein–linked receptors. Ras is attached to the inner cell membrane through an isoprenyl lipid group added after translation by the enzyme farnesyl transferase. If the lipid group is not added, Ras does not localize to the membrane and cannot function normally. In unstimulated cells, Ras is bound to GDP and is inactive. Following receptor tyrosine kinase activation, the guanine nucleotide exchange factor SOS is brought to the membrane by its association with grb2. SOS removes GDP from Ras and adds GTP. GTP-bound Ras then activates a cascade ending with MAP kinase, which migrates to the nucleus and phosphorylates (activates) a number of transcription factors (Fig. 82-3). The kinetics of MAP kinase activity are critical: in PC12 rat pheochromocytoma cells, stimulation with EGF results in transient stimulation of MAP kinase activity, retention of MAP kinase in the cytoplasm, and cell proliferation; stimulation of PC12 cells with NGF induces sustained activation of MAP kinase, nuclear translocation of MAP kinase, and neuronal differentiation.

Genetic defects leading to increased signaling from receptor tyrosine kinase–linked pathways are important in the etiology and progression of human cancer. About 30% of human cancers (especially pancreatic, lung, and colon adenocarcinomas) have mutated *Ras.* The mutations usually involve codons 12, 13, or 61 and result in a Ras protein that fails to hydrolyze its bound GTP and is thus constitutively active. In the hereditary disorder, neurofibromatosis, a mutation in the gene that encodes neurofibromin, a GTPase activating protein (GAP), inhibits its ability to inactivate Ras by converting the GTP to GDP. Constitutively activated Ras results in the unregulated activity of the signaling pathways downstream of Ras, including the MAP kinase pathway and activation of PI3K. Some epithelial cancers overexpress one or more members of the receptor tyrosine kinase family. EGF receptors, IGF-I receptors, and HER-2/*neu* are overexpressed in lung, bladder, breast, head and neck, and ovarian cancers. Mutations within the Ret tyrosine kinase receptor lead to constitutive receptor dimerization and kinase activation and are responsible for the dominant inherited cancer syndromes multiple endocrine neoplasia (MEN) type 2A and type 2B and familial medullary thyroid carcinoma. Autocrine and paracrine sources of the relevant growth factors have been noted in some cases.

Tyrosine Kinase–Associated Receptors The receptors for growth hormone, prolactin, erythropoietin, thrombopoietin, most interleukins, granulocyte CSF, granulocyte-macrophage CSF, interferon-α, interferon-γ, and many other cytokines are members of the tyrosine kinase–associated receptor family. These single-transmembrane receptors contain ligand-specific subunits and shared signaling subunits. Ligand binding induces the activation of receptor-associated tyrosine kinases. Three families of kinases are known to be associated with this class of receptors: *src* family (*src, yes, fgr, fyn, lck, lyn, hck, blk,* and counting), *syk* family (*syk,* ZAP-70), and Janus family (JAK1, JAK2, JAK3, Tyk2). The Janus family kinases have receptor sites that

FIGURE 82-3 The mitogen-activated protein (MAP) kinase cascades. MAP kinase signal transduction cascades link *Ras* activation with the nucleus. The overall framework of the MAP kinase cascades is shown in the box at the left. A series of sequential protein kinase–mediated phosphorylations result in the activation of MAP kinase, which has cytoplasmic and nuclear targets. The nuclear targets of MAP kinase are transcription factors bound to their DNA recognition sites that require phosphorylation to induce transactivating functions. ERKs (extracellular signal response kinases) target the ternary complex factor (TCF), while JNK/SAPK targets c-*jun* and ATF-2. Transcription factors associated with other promoters also serve as targets for MAP kinases. Other MAP kinase cascades exist in the cell. Each pathway is activated by different stimuli, and the pattern of gene expression induced by each pathway is characteristic of that pathway. Interactions between pathways permit an integrated response to diverse signals.

act as docking sites for SH2-containing transcription factors called STATs (signal transducers and activators of transcription). Tyrosine phosphorylation of STATs induces their dimerization by SH2–p-Tyr association followed by translocation to target genes in the nucleus. A unique feature of JAK/STAT signaling is that the pathway from cell membrane to nucleus is traversed by a single dimeric molecule, as opposed to the cascade of kinase and adaptor molecules associated with membrane tyrosine kinases. The *src* family kinases can associate with receptor tyrosine kinases as well as tyrosine kinase–associated receptors, and, not surprisingly, signal transduction through either receptor class leads to the activation of similar signaling cascades. As a consequence of *src* family activation, *myc* is one of the transcription factors activated. The *syk* family usually activates the *src* family member in the receptor complex.

These receptors are often overexpressed on tumors of hematopoietic origin, and, similar to receptor tyrosine kinases, autocrine or paracrine stimulation may contribute to the neoplastic state of the tumor cell.

Serine/Threonine Kinase Receptors These receptors recognize TGF-β, bone morphogenetic factors, and other activins as ligands. Ligand binding leads to activation of the receptor kinase activity, but downstream events are not well defined. Bone morphogenetic factors are important in bone formation and in determining ventral vs. dorsal orientation in the developing embryo. TGF-β induces transformation of mesenchymal cells but inhibits the proliferation of most cell types through the induction of cdki, which block G1 progression in an Rb-dependent manner. Activation of TGF-β receptors leads to the phosphorylation of transcription factors Smad2 and Smad3, which then associate with their obligate partner Smad4. This complex, probably a heterotrimer, translocates into the nucleus where specific genes are activated. The direct path to the nucleus is analogous to the JAK/STAT signaling pathway. Smads bind to specific DNA sequences adjacent to other transcription factor sites in the promoters of target genes, leading to cooperative interaction for gene induction. TGF-β induced genes include plasminogen activator inhibitor-1 (PAI-1), collagenase I, and p15^{INK4b}.

Many cancers are resistant to growth inhibition by TGF-β, including leukemias, lymphomas, melanomas, and breast and colon cancers. Colon cancers harboring defects in DNA mismatch repair develop inactivating mutations in the extracellular domain of the TGF-β receptor. In pancreatic and colon cancers, missense mutations and loss of heterozygosity at the DPC4 locus on chromosome 18q21 are frequent. This locus has been found to encode Smad4, and its inactivation blocks TGF-β signaling. Loss of expression or loss of function of TGF-β receptors occurs in several tumor types including colon cancer and lymphomas.

Nuclear Hormone Receptors Steroids, retinoids, thyroid hormone, vitamin D, and other lipid-soluble hormones diffuse through the plasma membrane and bind to members of the nuclear hormone receptor family. Receptors for these ligands are transcription factors that reside in the nucleus. The hydrophobic nature of the ligands obviates the need for machinery to transduce signals from the cell surface to the cell interior. Steroid hormone receptors are bound as heterodimers to promoter/enhancer elements of genes; in the absence of ligand, these complexes act as transcriptional repressors. Upon ligand binding, conformational changes are induced and the active transcription factor binds to coactivating factors and transcription is induced. Coactivators tend to open chromatin structure by adding acetyl groups to histones. Histone acetylation in nucleosomal complexes permits access of promoter regions to RNA polymerase II. Transcriptional repressor complexes associate with histone deacetylases (HDAC; co-repressor complexes), and chromatin remains condensed. Nuclear hormone–induced pathways affect virtually all biologic processes. Retinoic acid receptors (RAR) provide a clear link to cancer. Retinoids bind receptors composed of an RAR subunit (α, β, γ) dimerized with a retinoid-X receptor (RXR) and activate genes that influence differentiation in many cell types.

Acute promyelocytic leukemia (APL) is associated with the t(15; 17) translocation, which fuses sequences from a novel gene PML (promyelocytic leukemia) to the RARα gene, resulting in expression of a PML-RARα fusion protein. PML-RARα binds to and represses RARα-inducible genes required for myeloid differentiation. Repression is mediated by HDAC binding to PML-RARα. The developmental arrest at the promyelocyte stage of differentiation is associated with unregulated proliferation in these cells. Patients with APL can achieve complete remission with pharmacologic doses of all-trans retinoic acid (tretinoin), the ligand for RARα. Tretinoin induces the release of HDAC, permitting coactivator binding. Drugs that inhibit HDAC activity may provide a therapeutic benefit by activating genes required for the differentiation of cancer cells.

Cell-Cell and Cell–Extracellular Matrix (ECM) Communication In addition to information conveyed by soluble mediators, cell surface receptors relay important signals between cells, such as contact inhibition, and cell-ECM signals, such as anchorage-dependent growth. In cancer, these highly organized mechanisms of intercellular interaction often become disrupted or are subsumed for the purpose of metastasizing (Chap. 83). Individual cells no longer respond to signals from their neighbors, actin filaments are highly disorganized, and adherens junctions are lost. Normal patterns of growth and differentiation are disrupted, and the potential for metastasis increases.

E-cadherins are integral membrane glycoproteins that mediate calcium-dependent homophilic adhesion as the major component of adherens junctions between epithelial cells. E-cadherin cytoplasmic domains bind complexes containing α- and β-catenins, which are structurally linked to the cytoskeleton (actin cables and intermediate filaments). β-Catenin that is not sequestered in E-cadherin complexes is rapidly phosphorylated by glycogen synthesis kinase (GSK) 3β in a complex with the APC (adenomatous polyposis coli) gene product (maps to chromosome 5, mutated in familial polyposis) and is degraded by the ubiquitin/proteosome pathway. Degradation of β-catenin can be blocked by several mechanisms, including mutations that inactivate APC and mutations in serine phosphorylation sites within β-catenin that target it for degradation. Such mutations result in increased free β-catenin, which translocates into the nucleus and binds to members of the T cell factor (TCF) family of transcription factors, influencing the expression of genes such as c-*myc* and cyclin D1 that promote progression through G1. Excess free β-catenin has been implicated in hereditary and sporadic forms of colon cancer and melanoma. Decreased expression of E-cadherin has been noted in breast, colon, prostate, gastric, and other cancers and is a marker of poor prognosis.

Epithelial cell growth and survival require attachment of cells to components of the ECM that compose basement membranes, including collagen, fibronectin, vitronectin, and laminin. The integrin family of transmembrane receptors is composed of α and β subunits that adhere to the ECM and convey information to cytoplasmic membrane-associated structures called *focal adhesions*. The complexes, whose assembly is mediated by the Rho and Rac GTPases, are sites of attachment of actin cables but are also active in cell signaling through their association with focal adhesion kinase (FAK) and Src tyrosine kinases. Integrin-ECM interactions lead to activation of the Ras/MAP kinase, PI3K, and phospholipase C-γ pathways. Detachment of epithelial and endothelial cells from ECM induces their death by a form of programmed cell death called *anoikis* (Greek, "homeless"). This molecular safeguard prevents abnormal spread of cells. Invasive cancers often avoid anoikis by activating Ras or Src, which allow anchorage-independent growth of cells by activation of Akt kinase.

REGULATION OF GENE TRANSCRIPTION

One consequence of signal transduction is the activation of sequence-specific transcription factors that regulate gene expression. Whether a cell proliferates, differentiates, or undergoes apoptosis is regulated by gene products made in response to physiologic stimuli. For some transcription factors, the ligand goes directly to the nucleus where they reside (nuclear hormone receptors). For others, activated kinases enter the nucleus and phosphorylate factors already bound to DNA (MAP kinase and AP-1 transcription factor). Some transcription factors are activated in the cytoplasm and translocate to the nucleus (STATs). NF-κB is held in the cytoplasm by the negative regulator IκB, which is phosphorylated and degraded as a consequence of signal transduction. NF-κB is then released from IκB, and NF-κB translocates to the nucleus.

Transcription factors recognize short stretches of DNA of a defined nucleotide sequence 6 to 12 base pairs in length. These recognition sites may be upstream or downstream of the transcription start site [the TATA box where the first subunit of the transcription machinery, transcription factor IID (TFIID), binds]. Transcription factors may affect transcription at sites remote from the start site by looping out large intervening DNA sequences.

Transcription factors contain specific amino acid sequences capable of recognizing the DNA sequence and usually form one of several structural motifs: helix-turn-helix, homeodomain, zinc finger, leucine zipper, and helix-loop-helix are all used as DNA-binding motifs or mediate dimerization of factors required for DNA binding. Transcription factors function in one or more of several ways. They can physically bend the DNA to permit the ordered addition of the components of the transcription machinery. Activated transcription factors bind to coactivator proteins in complexes that encode enzymatic activity leading to the acetylation of histones. This alters nucleosomal conformation and increases accessibility of DNA to transcription proteins. Transcription factors can inhibit transcription by blocking binding of a positive transcription factor or preventing the assembly of a transcription complex. They can form complexes with co-repressors and deacetylate histones. Promoters can also be made inaccessible by methylation of cytosine- and guanosine-rich sequences near promoters. The complex interaction between positive and negative transcription factors dictates the level of gene transcription. Individual genes may have ≥ 20 sites for transcription factor binding. The pattern of gene expression is determined by which factors are expressed in a given cell type.

Most genes are regulated at multiple levels, though transcription initiation is the dominant control point. The von Hippel–Lindau gene on chromosome 3p (a tumor suppressor gene involved in the pathogenesis of renal cell cancer) appears to act by inhibiting the elongation of an RNA chain after transcription initiation. A message may be spliced alternatively and encode different proteins in different cells. Transport of the message from the nucleus to the cytoplasm may be altered. Messenger RNA turnover may be accelerated. Some proteins, such as apoferritin and thymidylate synthase, regulate the translation of their own messages (and perhaps other messages) by binding to mRNA and preventing initiation of protein synthesis. Thus, there are many levels at which gene expression may be influenced.

Some transcription factors were identified because of their transforming effects when their genes, usually in mutated form, were incorporated into animal retroviral genomes; *myc, rel, fos, jun,* and others are examples of proto-oncogene transcription factors that are overexpressed in certain cancers and that contribute to the malignant phenotype of tumor cells. The mutated oncogenes are often more resistant to protein degradation and have a longer half-life than the normal cellular counterpart. Transcription factors with unusual properties may be generated by chromosome translocation that produces a chimeric protein. Novel genes may be activated that promote proliferation and inhibit apoptosis. Usually the genetic changes lead to inhibition of normal lineage-specific differentiation, resistance to apoptosis, and proliferation.

REGULATION OF CELL DEATH

The homeostasis of adult organisms requires a balance between the generation of new cells and the death of old cells. Some cells die when their telomeres no longer protect the integrity of DNA replication. Some cells die when they have sustained sufficient hypoxic, heat, oxidative, or ultraviolet irradiation damage that cannot be repaired. A cell can be killed if it becomes infected with a virus or other intracellular pathogen that destroys the cell or is recognized by the host's lymphocytes, which kill the infected cell. Multicellular organisms are models of cellular cooperation; some cells die to preserve the rest of the organism.

Genetic damage to growth-regulating genes of stem cells could be catastrophic; however, single genetic events such as activation of *myc* expression or loss of the Rb checkpoint often lead to the death of the cell by apoptosis. Apoptosis is a form of cell death initiated by extracellular or intracellular signals in which enzymes are activated to degrade nuclear DNA by making intranucleosomal cuts, causing the cell to shrink and finally break up. The core apoptosis machinery consists of a family of specialized proteases called *caspases* (they contain a cysteine at their active site and cleave substrates after *aspartic* acid residues). Like coagulation and complement systems, caspases exist as proenzymes with minimal enzymatic activity that can be rapidly induced by activators, and each enzyme acts to activate the next enzyme in the cascade. Key targets include DNA (chromatin degraded into nucleosomal multimers), nuclear lamins (nucleus shrinks and fragments), cytoskeletal regulatory proteins, DNA repair enzymes, and others. The cell shrinks, its chromatin fragments, and the cell breaks apart forming apoptotic bodies.

The latent activity of caspases is tightly regulated to prevent the death of normal cells. Assembly of initiator caspases into active complexes occurs by two main mechanisms. Members of the tumor necrosis factor (TNF) receptor superfamily, including Fas (CD95), and DR4 and DR5 death receptors encode transmembrane proteins whose cytoplasmic domains encode protein association or docking domains, called *death domains* and *death effector domains* (DED). Ligand binding induces dimerization of death domains with recruitment to the membrane of an adaptor signaling protein called *Fas-associated death domain* (FADD). FADD forms a complex with procaspase 8 mediated by DED interactions; caspase 8 is activated by self-cleavage. Caspase 8 then cleaves effector caspase 3 into active heterodimeric subunits, and death ensues (Fig. 82-4). Regulation of this pathway occurs at the level of expression of Fas receptor and ligand and the secretion of death-inducing cytokines, TNF and *t*umor necrosis factor-*r*elated *a*poptosis-*i*nducing *l*igand (TRAIL) (ligand for DR4 and -5).

The second pathway of caspase activation encompasses responses to a greater variety of noxious signals including DNA damage, growth factor deprivation, reactive oxygen damage, and heat stress. The mitochondrion plays a key role in this pathway as the storehouse of protein cofactors required for the activation of caspases. Damage within the cell is detected by the mitochondria by unknown mechanisms. The mitochondria then lose membrane potential and release cytochrome c, which forms a complex with apoptosis-activating factor (Apaf) 1. This complex binds to procaspase 9 via a caspase recruitment domain (CARD), and caspase 9 is activated. Caspase 9 then cleaves effector caspases and induces cell death. The release of cytochrome c from the mitochondria appears to be regulated by bc12.

The *bcl2* gene was discovered as the chromosome 18q contribution to the t(14;18) translocation in follicular lymphoma. The gene did not transform cells but prolonged the life of cells destined to die, greatly increasing a pool of cells available for subsequent genetic mutations. Members of the *bcl2* family fall into two groups: *bcl2* and *bcl*-X_L prevent cell death, whereas *bax*, *bad*, *bak*, and others promote cell death. The *bcl2* family members associate as homodimers or heterodimers; the combinatorial effects of the various dimers allow a fine level of control over cell survival. When any of the death promoters exist as homo- or heterodimers, the cell dies by apoptosis. When a death promoter heterodimerizes with either *bcl2* or *bcl*-X_L, cell death is prevented. Thus, the relative amounts of different *bcl2* family members determine whether a cell will survive potentially damaging insults. Furthermore, phosphorylation of *bcl2* family members by cellular kinases can alter the biologic activity of individual members, altering the balance in favor of death or survival.

In addition to its presumed role in the etiology of follicular lymphoma, *bcl2* is expressed in a number of cancers. It prevents the normal p53-mediated destruction of cells with damaged DNA and also appears to prevent the death of cells severely damaged by cancer chemotherapy. In addition, *bcl2* mediates drug resistance and contributes to neoplasia in a novel way, preventing the death that would normally eliminate the damaged cell, rather than promoting aberrant cell growth. Strategies to overcome *bcl2* function might well make available therapies more effective.

The apoptotic machinery is subject to regulation by multiple signal transduction pathways, and many of these are subverted in cancer cells to shift the balance toward survival of the malignant clone. In addition to *bcl2*, two other important links have been established between growth factor signaling and survival pathways. Activation of P13K by tyrosine kinases leads to activation of the serine/threonine kinase Akt. Akt directly promotes cell survival by phosphorylation of Bad and procaspase 9, inhibiting their apoptotic functions. Cancer cells can usurp the activity of Akt; in some cases, cells expressing a mutated Ras oncogene or increased levels of tyrosine kinase receptors (e.g., HER-2/*neu*) have upregulated the Akt pathway. An alternative genetic lesion leading to increased Akt kinase activity results in the loss of the PTEN tumor suppressor, a lipid phosphatase that normally downregulates the P13K pathway by dephosphorylating lipid second messengers. Another important pathway usurped by cancer cells involves NF-κB activation. NF-κB induces expression of the inhibitor of apoptosis (IAP) family of genes whose products inhibit caspase activity; one such, survivin, is expressed in lymphomas and other tumors.

Thus, cancer becomes more adaptive to its host from genetic events that alter apoptosis. Stimulation of proliferation or prevention of death can be complementary targets for cell transformation. Apoptosis pathways are important targets for treatment. Paclitaxel and other microtubule inhibitors induce the phosphorylation and inactivation of *bcl2*. One could make bone marrow cells highly resistant to chemotherapy-induced death by expressing a form of *bcl2* that lacks the loop domain in the BH1 region, as this is the site that is phosphorylated to inhibit *bcl2* function. Tumor cells and normal cells express DR4 and -5 receptors; however, tumor cells fail to express decoy receptors that protect normal cells from the DR4 and -5 ligand, TRAIL. Thus, therapies directed at DR4 or -5 may be tumor selective.

CELL BIOLOGY AND CANCER

For a cancer to arise, mutations must occur that affect a variety of pathways. Often the G1 cell cycle checkpoint is affected. Apoptosis

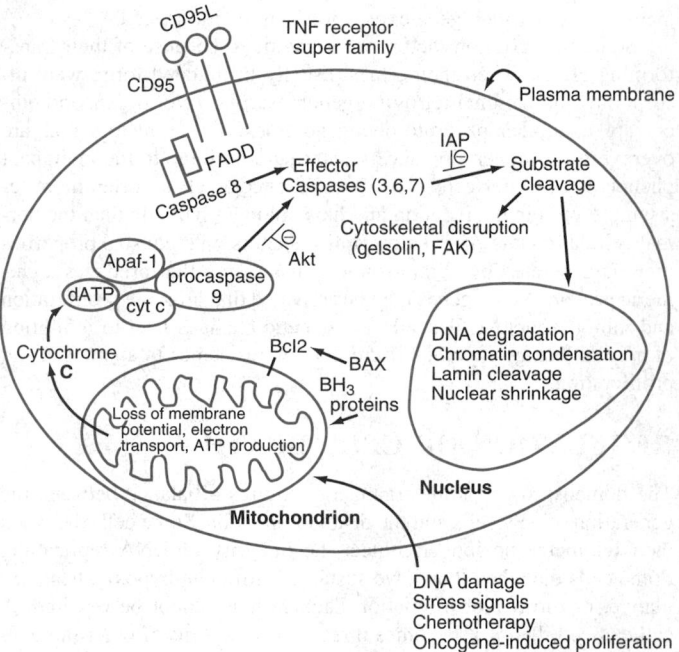

FIGURE 82-4 Mechanisms of apoptosis in eukaryotic cells. Programmed cell death is induced by two main pathways. Crosslinking of members of the tumor necrosis factor (TNF) receptor superfamily, such as CD95 (Fas) by its ligand (CD95L) lead to the binding of Fas-associated desk domain (FADD) and procaspase 8 to death domain motifs of CD95. Caspase 8 is activated by autocatalysis and subsequently cleaves and activates effector caspases such as caspase 3. Alternatively, effector caspase activation can occur when cytochrome c is released from the mitochondria in response to a variety of noxious environmental or intracellular events. The release of cytochrome c is regulated by members of the Bcl2 family, some of which form pores that traverse the mitochondrial membranes and regulate transmembrane potential. Cytochrome c, along with deoxyadenosine triphosphate (dATP), binds to Apaf-1, inducing a conformational change that permits association with procaspase 9 to form the apoptosome with subsequent activation of caspase 9. Caspase 9 activates effector caspases and the cell dies. Inhibitors of apoptosis (IAP) can inhibit caspases. One IAP member, survivin, is overexpressed in some cancer cells.

is averted by mutations in the p53 pathway or by other mechanisms. The expression of telomerase is a common feature in cancers. Over-expression of growth factors and their receptors is frequently detected. Activation of the *Ras* proto-oncogene or other changes leading to a constitutively active MAP kinase cascade are common. Changes in cytoskeleton and responsiveness to contact-mediated growth inhibition are frequent in cancer cells. Usually when a mutation occurs in one component of a signaling pathway, other mutations are seen in other pathways rather than in another component of the same pathway. The high level of mutability of cancer cells facilitates adaptation to the environment, including the development of resistance to anticancer drugs. As tumors progress, they acquire the ability to secrete proteases that aid in the escape from local barriers so that they may metastasize (Chap. 83). Discrete steps in tumor progression lead to the production of factors by the tumor cells that permit neovascularization to supply nutrients to the growing tumor. Other mutations allow the tumor to escape immune surveillance mechanisms; for example, some tumors downregulate expression of class I major histocompatibility complex antigens so that they become invisible to T cells. The wide range of changes that must occur in a single cell to permit the behavior associated with a malignant neoplasm makes it clear why carcinogenesis is a multistep process and why human cancers may have 10 or more genetic lesions that account for the biology.

The characteristic of cancer cells that has dominated clinical thinking is their uncontrolled proliferation. However, the growth fraction of most human cancers is usually not higher than the growth fraction of normal gut epithelia or normal bone marrow, and most human tumor explants are difficult to propagate for long periods of time in culture. Cancer cell lines immortal in vitro may have additional genetic lesions that permit their growth in vitro. Naturally occurring tumors growing in vivo show a Gompertzian or exponential decline in their growth fraction because the daughter cells of a division are not uniformly capable of further division. The accumulation of genetic damage, poor oxygen or nutrient supply, and other unknown factors contribute to the senescence of some tumor cells, so that by the time a tumor becomes clinically apparent at a tumor burden of 10^8 to 10^9 cells, most of the proliferative capability of the tumor is finished. Often by this time, more malignant and highly selected clonal derivatives of the tumor have metastasized to other sites where new tumor deposits with more aggressive characteristics are formed. Thus, cancer cells can be viewed as having lost the altruism that usually characterizes cell behavior in multicellular organisms. Cancer cells operate under natural selection imposed by a hostile environment. Ironically, the more successful they are at achieving independence from environmental influences, the more assured is the destruction of their host and ultimately themselves.

Many potential therapeutic agents are in clinical development based on our concepts of tumor cell biology. They include the development of growth factor and growth factor receptor antagonists; inhibitors of phosphoryl transfer to block key kinases; selective inhibitors of PKC, P13K, phospholipase C, and other targets; farnesyl transferase inhibitors that block the insertion of *Ras* into the membrane; mutant versions of proteins such as *Ras* and p53 that may make the cell vulnerable to immunologic attack if employed as a vaccine; and inhibitors of angiogenesis or the steps in metastasis that may limit tumor growth and prevent its spread. However, it seems unlikely that a single target will be the highly sought-after point of vulnerability. More likely, combinations of inhibitors will be required to improve antitumor effects. For example, the combination of chemotherapy and antibody to EGF receptors appears to produce greater antitumor effects than the sum of the effects produced individually.

BIBLIOGRAPHY

ADAMS PD, KAELIN WG: Negative control elements of the cell cycle in human cancers. Curr Opin Cell Biol 10:791, 1998

BUNZ F et al: Disruption of p53 in human cancer cells alters the responses to therapeutic agents. J Clin Invest 104:263, 1999

DOWNWARD J: Ras signaling and apoptosis. Curr Opin Genet Dev 8:49, 1998

GIACCIA AJ, KASTAN MB: The complexity of p53 modulation: Emerging patterns from divergent signals. Genes Dev 12:2973, 1998

HUNTER T: Signaling-2000 and beyond. Cell 100:113, 2000

NUNEZ G et al: Caspases: The proteases of the apoptotic pathway. Oncogene 17:3237, 1998

PORTER AC, VAILLANCOURT RR: Tyrosine kinase receptor-activated signal transduction pathways which lead to oncogenesis. Oncogene 16:1343, 1998

SGAMBATO A et al: Multiple functions of p27 (Kip1) and its alterations in tumor cells: a review. J Cell Physiol 183:18, 2000

STRUHL K: Histone acetylation and transcriptional regulatory mechanisms. Genes Dev 12:599, 1998

TAN PB, KIM SK: Signaling specificity: The RTK/RAS/MAP kinase pathway in metazoans. Trends Genet 15:145, 1999

83   *Judah Folkman*

ANGIOGENESIS

aFGF	acidic FGF	PDGF	platelet-derived growth factor
bFGF	basic FGF	TIMPs	tissue inhibitors of
COX 2	cyclooxygenase 2		metalloproteinases
HIF	hypoxia-inducible factor	uPA	urokinase plasminogen activator
IFN	interferon	VEGF	vascular endothelial growth
IL	interleukin		factor
MTD	maximum tolerated dose		

Virtually every cell in the body lives adjacent to a capillary blood vessel, or at least no further than the mean oxygen diffusion distance of 100 to 200 μm. Some cell types, such as beta cells in the pancreatic islets, fat cells, and skeletal muscle cells, are surrounded by at least two capillaries (Fig. 83-1). Capillaries of 8 to 20 μm diameter are lined by a single layer of endothelial cells. These cells cover ~1000 m², an area the size of a tennis court. The length of capillary tubing in 1 mm³ of human heart muscle is ~2500 mm, and 1 kg of fat contains ~3500 m of capillaries. During normal conditions vascular endothelial cell proliferation is barely detectable—<0.01% of endothelial cells are in cycle. Endothelial cell turnover is >1000 days and in retinal vasculature may be >5000 days. In contrast, in the normal adult bone marrow, ~6 billion cell divisions occur per hour and the turnover time is ~5 days, (i.e., the time during which bone marrow is completely replaced). Endothelial cells can emerge from their resting state and proliferate as rapidly as bone marrow cells during formation of new capillaries. This process is called *angiogenesis* and leads to *neovascularization*.

Physiologic angiogenesis is tightly regulated and of limited duration. It is essential to reproduction and embryonic development. During postnatal and adult life, angiogenesis in wound repair and in exercised muscle is restricted to days or weeks.

Pathologic angiogenesis, in contrast, is usually persistent and unabated. Angiogenesis that continues for months or years supports the growth and progression of solid tumors and leukemias, provides a conduit for the entry of inflammatory cells into sites of chronic inflammation (e.g., Crohn's disease and chronic cystitis), is the most common cause of blindness, destroys cartilage in rheumatoid arthritis, contributes to growth and hemorrhage of atherosclerotic plaques, leads to intraperitoneal bleeding in endometriosis, is the basis of life-threatening hemangiomas of infancy, and permits prostate growth in benign prostatic hypertrophy. These are just a few of the "angiogenic disease processes," which are found in almost all specialties of medicine. Angiogenesis inhibitors are a new *class* of drugs that suppress or reverse the pathologic neovascularization upon which these diseases are dependent.

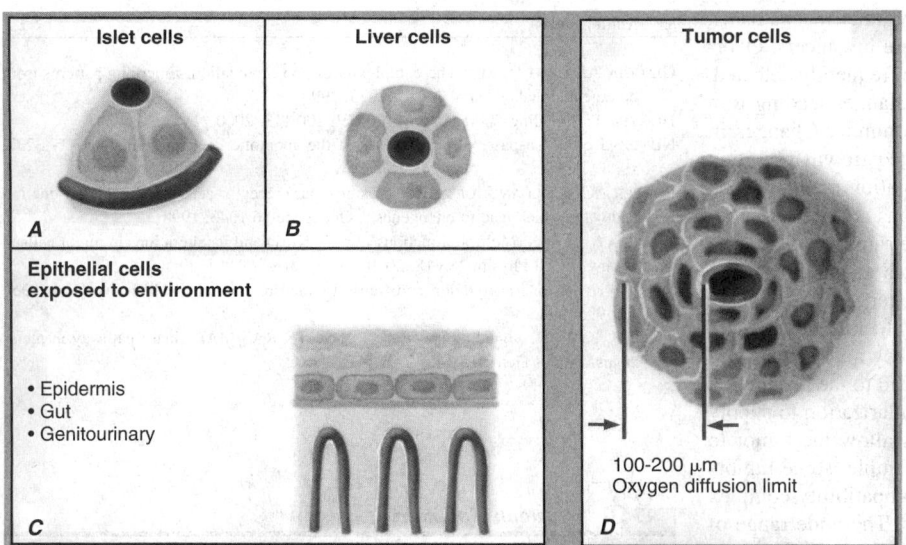

FIGURE 83-1 Diagram of three common configurations of how cells are apposed to capillary blood vessels. *A.* Islet cells are sandwiched between two capillary vessels, apical and basal. All fat cells and most skeletal cells are similar. *B.* Hepatic cells live adjacent to one capillary, and the next layer of hepatocytes are in another capillary neighborhood. Kidney, lung, and other organs are similar. *C.* Epithelial cells in the epidermis, gastrointestinal tract, and genitourinary tract are separated from vessels beneath them in dermis or submucosa but are still within the 100- to 200-μm oxygen diffusion limit. *D.* In contrast, tumor cells pile up as microcylinders around a capillary out to six or more layers. The cells at the greatest distance from the open capillary are severely hypoxic or anoxic.

NEOPLASTIC DISEASE

HISTORIC BACKGROUND Tumor hyperemia, observed during surgery since the 1870s, was for the next 100 years attributed to simple dilation of existing host vessels. Two reports, in 1939 and 1945, suggested that tumor vascularity was due to the induction of new blood vessels. This idea was dismissed by most investigators. The few who accepted it believed that new vessels were an inflammatory side effect of tumor growth.

In 1971, based on experiments carried out in the 1960s, a hypothesis was proposed that tumor growth could be angiogenesis-dependent, i.e., tumors could recruit their own private blood supply by releasing a diffusible chemical signal that stimulated angiogenesis. Tumor angiogenesis could then be a novel second target for anticancer therapy. These concepts were not accepted at the time. The conventional wisdom was that tumor neovascularization was (1) an inflammatory host response to necrotic tumor cells, (2) a host response detrimental to the tumor, or (3) "established" vasculature that could not regress. From these assumptions most scientists concluded that it was fruitless to attempt to discover an angiogenesis stimulator, to say nothing of discovering angiogenesis inhibitors. Eventual acceptance of the 1971 hypothesis was slow because it would be 2 more years before the first vascular endothelial cells were successfully cultured in vitro, 8 more years before *capillary* endothelial cells could be cultured in vitro, 11 years before the discovery of the first angiogenesis inhibitor, and 13 years before the purification of the first angiogenic protein. By the mid-1980s, after a series of reports from several laboratories demonstrating that tumor growth was angiogenesis-dependent, this hypothesis had been confirmed by genetic methods.

THE ANGIOGENIC SWITCH **The Prevascular Phase** Most human tumors arise without angiogenic activity and exist in situ as microscopic-sized lesions of 0.2 to 2 mm diameter for months to years, after which a small percentage may switch to the angiogenic phenotype. Autopsy studies of people who died of trauma but who never had cancer during their lifetime reveal that in women from 40 to 50 years of age, 39% had in situ carcinomas in their breast, but breast cancer is diagnosed in only 1% of women in this age range. In men from age 50 to 70, 46% had in situ prostate cancers at the time of death, but only 1% are diagnosed in this age range during life. In

people from age 50 to 70, >98% had small carcinomas of the thyroid (Fig. 83-2), but thyroid cancer is diagnosed in only 0.1% in this age range. In the majority of human tumors, the angiogenic phenotype appears after the malignant phenotype is recognized histologically. However, for certain human tumors (e.g., carcinoma of the cervix), the preneoplastic stage of dysplasia becomes angiogenic before the malignant phenotype is recognized histologically. When a nonangiogenic in situ carcinoma emerges in avascular epidermis or mucosa (e.g., melanoma or breast cancer), it is separated from host vessels by a basement membrane (Fig. 83-3). If a nonangiogenic tumor emerges in the midst of a vascularized tissue (e.g., an islet cell carcinoma), it may form an in situ microcylinder of tumor cells around capillary vessels (called *cooption*).

At the clinical level the angiogenic switch is recognized by expansion of tumor mass to a detectable size, local bleeding, and metastasis. For example, a positive mammogram usually represents a neovascularized tumor—a non-neovascularized in situ carcinoma is below the detectable limits of mammography. Hematuria in bladder cancer, melena in colorectal cancer, and hemoptysis in lung cancer all result from neovascularized tumors. Tumor cells are not usually shed into the circulation until after neovascularization has occurred. Furthermore, distant metastases themselves cannot be detected until they have "turned on" the angiogenic switch.

At the cellular level at least four mechanisms of the angiogenic switch have been identified in human and mouse tumors: (1) avascular in situ carcinomas can recruit their own blood supply by stimulating neovascularization in an adjacent host vascular bed—the most common process in human tumors; (2) circulating precursor endothelial cells from bone marrow may incorporate into an angiogenic focus; (3) tumors may induce host fibroblasts and/or macrophages in the tumor bed to overexpress an angiogenic factor [e.g., vascular endothelial growth factor (VEGF)]; and (4) preexisting vessels can be coopted by tumor cells. The angiogenic switch may also include combinations of these mechanisms. Once tumors have switched on angiogenesis, they rarely revert to the nonangiogenic phenotype. Neuroblastoma and retinoblastoma may be exceptions, but spontaneous loss of angiogenic activity (and tumor regression) is rare even in these two tumors. After the angiogenic switch, new microvessels converge on the tiny in situ tumor. Tumor cells grow as microcylinders, or "perivascular cuffs," around each new vessel. One endothelial cell can support from 5 to 100 tumor cells.

At the molecular level, the angiogenic switch operates as a shift in the balance of production by tumor cells of molecules that positively or negatively regulate angiogenesis. The overexpression of positive regulators of angiogenesis and the downregulation of inhibitors of angiogenesis during early tumor development are generally triggered by genetic mutations that control angiogenesis. For example, overexpression of the *ras* oncogene increases production of the angiogenic protein VEGF, while a mutation in the p53 tumor-suppressor gene or its deletion decreases production of the angiogenesis inhibitor protein, thrombospondin-1. In the normal cell wild-type p53 upregulates thrombospondin-1 and downregulates VEGF.

The angiogenic switch can be further modified by environmental conditions such as hypoxia, endogenous angiogenesis inhibitors, and genetic background of the host.

1. *Hypoxia*: After a tumor has become neovascularized, its continued expansion may lead to increased tissue pressure. This increased interstitial pressure is caused mainly by plasma that leaks from new vessels but is slow to efflux from the tumor because of a dearth of

FIGURE 83-2 *A.* Papillary carcinoma of the thyroid gland at autopsy of a patient who died of trauma and who had no cancer during lifetime. The tumor is only 0.24 mm diameter and is not angiogenic. *B.* The same magnification of a similar tumor in a different patient who also died of trauma but had no cancer diagnosed during life. This lesion is 0.5 mm and is not angiogenic. *(From Harach et al.)*

intratumoral lymphatics. Microvessels in the center of the tumor are the first to be compressed, which leads to central necrosis. Hypoxia activates an hypoxia-inducible factor (HIF-1) binding sequence in the VEGF promoter. This leads to transcription of VEGF mRNA, increased stability of VEGF message, and increased production of VEGF protein beyond what may have been triggered genetically. Tumors, therefore, do not "outgrow their blood supply" but compress it. A counterintuitive lesson is that in situ tumors arising in an avascular compartment (e.g., epidermis) are *not* hypoxic, but larger neovascularized tumors become hypoxic after compressing their blood supply. Low pH and low glucose in a tumor may also upregulate production of angiogenic factors, especially VEGF.

2. *Endogenous angiogenesis inhibitors*: At the molecular level, the angiogenic switch can also be modified by endothelial inhibitors that either circulate [e.g., interferon (IFN) β, platelet factor 4, angiostatin] or are releasable from extracellular matrix [e.g., endostatin, thrombospondin-1, and tissue inhibitors of metalloproteinases (TIMPs)]. Therapeutic administration of an endogenous angiogenesis inhibitor, such as angiostatin or endostatin, can tip the balance of the angiogenic switch so that angiogenic output of a tumor is opposed or abrogated.

3. *Genetic control of host response*: Just as the angiogenic output of a given tumor is governed by oncogenes and tumor-suppressor genes, the angiogenic response of the host is genetically regulated. It is known that hemangiomas predominate in white infants and that ocular neovascularization in macular degeneration is almost never found in black patients. The genes that regulate these effects are not yet known.

Endogenous Angiogenesis Promoters The known endogenous angiogenic promoters are listed in Table 83-1. Virtually all of these proteins are produced by different types of tumors. However, acidic FGF (aFGF), basic FGF (bFGF), VEGF, and angiopoietin-1 and -2 are the most well studied and have been found in a wide variety of human tumors.

Fibroblast growth factors aFGF and bFGF stimulate endothelial cell mitosis and migration in vitro and are among the most potent angiogenic proteins in vivo. They have high affinity for heparin and heparan sulfate. They lack a signal sequence for secretion but are stored in extracellular matrix. An unsolved problem is how bFGF is exported from tumor cells in the absence of a signal sequence. Many different cells synthesize bFGF, including tumor cells of the central nervous system, sarcomas, genitourinary tumors, and even endothelial cells in the tumor vasculature. Proteinases and heparanases are thought to mobilize bFGF from the extracellular matrix. Furthermore, some tumors recruit macrophages and activate them to secrete bFGF, while others attract mast cells, which, because of their high heparin content, sequester bFGF. bFGF is not a specific endothelial mitogen but has several cell targets including fibroblasts, smooth-muscle cells, and neurons. However, experimental tumors transfected with bFGF containing an engineered signal sequence stimulate endothelial proliferation almost to the exclusion of smooth-muscle and fibroblast proliferation. This is similar to the process in human tumors. This selective attraction of vascular endothelial cells by bFGF released from a tumor may be explained by the smooth-muscle repellant activity of angiopoietin-2 elaborated from proliferating endothelial cells in a tumor bed (see below). bFGF interferes with adhesion of leukocytes to endothelium; thus, tumors that elaborate bFGF may produce a form of local immunologic tolerance.

Abnormally elevated levels of bFGF are found in the serum and urine of cancer patients and in the cerebrospinal fluid of patients with different types of brain tumors. High bFGF levels in renal carcinoma correlate with poor outcome. Also, bFGF levels in the urine of children with Wilms' tumor correlate with stage of disease and tumor grade.

Vascular endothelial growth factor/vascular permeability factor The first proposal that tumor angiogenesis is associated with increased microvascular permeability led to the identification of vascular permeability factor (VPF). VPF was subsequently sequenced and shown to be a specific inducer of angiogenesis; it was called *vascular endothelial growth factor*. VEGF is an endothelial cell mitogen and motogen that is angiogenic in vivo. Its permeability effect on capillaries is more potent than histamine and contributes to ascites in ovarian cancer and to edema in brain tumors. Its expression correlates with blood vessel growth during embryogenesis and with angiogenesis in the female reproductive tract and in tumors. VEGF is a 40- to 45-kDa homodimeric protein with a signal sequence secreted by a wide variety of cells and by the majority of human tumor cells. For example, >60% of breast cancers overexpress VEGF. VEGF exists as five different isoforms of 121, 145, 165, 189, and 206 amino acids, of which VEGF_{165} is the predominant molecular species produced by a variety of normal and neoplastic cells. Two receptors for VEGF are found mainly on vascular endothelial cells, the 180-kDa fms-like tyrosine kinase (Flt-1) and the 200-kDa human kinase insert domain–containing receptor (KDR) and its mouse homologue, Flk-1. VEGF binds to both receptors, but KDR/Flk-1 transduces the signals for endothelial proliferation and chemotaxis. Other structural homologues of the VEGF family have recently been identified, including VEGF-B, -C,

FIGURE 83-3 *A*. Human breast cancer. Large breast duct partially lined by duct carcinoma in situ (arrow) and intense angiogenesis in the immediately adjacent periductal breast stroma. Brown-staining microvessels (antibody to von Willebrand factor) are indicated by arrowhead. Note the absence of angiogenesis in the areas of breast stroma adjacent to portions of duct lined with benign duct epithelium *(From Weidner N et al, with permission of the publisher)*. *B*. Large breast duct filled with carcinoma in situ and surrounded by new microvessels in the periductal breast stroma. Arrowhead shows invasion of microvessels through basement membrane of the duct, accompanied by invasion of tumor cells into the periductal stroma. *C*. Invasive duct carcinoma, area of highest density of microvessels. *D*. Higher power of invasive human breast carcinoma 4-μm thick section. Microvessels (brown stained with antibody to CD31) are indicated by arrowheads. *E*. 50-μm thick confocal micros- copy section showing microvessels in three dimensions (arrowheads) surrounded by tumors cells, which fill the intercapillary space. *F*. Cross-section of breast cancer in mice showing the microcylinders of tumor cells that surround each microvessel. The 100 μm thickness of these tumor microcylinders is within the range of the oxygen diffusion limit. Scanning electron microscope view of 100-μm Vibratome section of a subcutaneous MCa-IV mouse breast tumor with the skin at the top. Blood vessels appear as black holes emptied of blood and preserved in an open state by vascular perfusion of fixative. Pale necrotic regions surround perivascular rings of tumor tissue, which are ~100 μm thick. Magnification, 25×. A 10-mm scale bar would = 400 μm. *(Courtesy of Donald M. McDonald, University of California, San Francisco. Reprinted from Folkman, with permission of the publisher.)*

-D, and -E. VEGF-C stimulates lymphatic growth and binds to Flt4, which is preferentially expressed on lymphatic endothelium. Neuropilin-1, a neuronal guidance molecule, is a recently discovered receptor for $VEGF_{165}$. Neuropilin is not a tyrosine kinase receptor and is expressed on nonendothelial cells including tumor cells. This allows VEGF that is synthesized by tumor cells to bind to their surface. Surface-bound VEGF could make endothelial cells chemotactic to tumor cells or it could act in a paracrine manner to mediate cooption of tumor cells around microvessels (Fig. 83-3).

VEGF expression is upregulated by the *ras* oncogene. The farnesyl transferase inhibitors inhibit *ras* expression. One mechanism of their antitumor effect is to inhibit angiogenesis by inhibiting VEGF expression.

VEGF expression is inhibited by the von Hippel–Lindau (VHL) protein. The VHL-tumor suppressor gene is inactivated in patients with VHL disease and in most sporadic clear-cell renal carcinomas, which leads to VEGF-mediated angiogenesis. The VHL gene normally suppresses hypoxia-inducible genes including erythropoietin. When VHL is mutated or deleted, these genes are overexpressed even under normoxic conditions. This explains why renal cell carcinomas driven by mutant VHL are associated with a high hematocrit.

Experimental evidence indicates that bFGF function may be in part dependent upon VEGF. bFGF induces the expression of VEGF. The two endothelial mitogens act synergistically to stimulate capillary tube formation in vitro. Systemic administration of a soluble receptor for VEGF (flk-1) completely blocks cornea angiogenesis induced by implanted bFGF. An important implication of these studies is that angiogenesis inhibitors that block VEGF (currently in clinical trial) may also inhibit bFGF.

Angiopoietins Tie2 is a receptor found only on vascular endothelial cells. It is a specific tyrosine kinase whose ligand is angiopoietin-1. Angiopoietin-1 induces endothelial cells to recruit pericytes and smooth-muscle cells [mainly by producing platelet-derived growth factor (PDGF) BB] to become incorporated in the vessel wall. Vessels stimulated by angiopoietin-1 are not leaky and are analogous to new vessels in a healing wound. Angiopoietin-2 blocks the Tie-2 receptor and acts to repel pericytes and smooth muscle. It is produced by vascular endothelium in a tumor bed, but it is unclear how tumor cells mediate this. Nevertheless, tumor vessels remain thin "endothelial-lined tubes" even though some of these microvessels reach the diameter of venules (Fig. 83-3). A key point is that angiopoietin-2 and VEGF together increase angiogenesis. However, if VEGF is neutral-

Table 83-1 Endogenous Stimulators of Angiogenesis

Protein	Molecular Weight, kDa	Year Reported
Basic fibroblast growth factor (FGF-2)	18	1984
Acidic fibroblast growth factor (FGF-1)	16.4	1984
Angiogenin	14.1	1985
Transforming growth factor α	5.5	1986
Transforming growth factor β	25	1986
Tumor necrosis factor α	17	1987
Vascular endothelial growth factor		
VPF	40–45	1983
VEGF		1989
Platelet-derived endothelial growth factor	45	1989
Granulocyte colony-stimulating factor	17	1989
Placental growth factor	25	1991
Interleukin 8	40	1992
Hepatocyte growth factor	92	1993
Proliferin	35	1994
Angiopoietin-1	70	1996
Leptin	16	1998

NOTE: VPF, vascular permeability factor.

Table 83-2 Endogenous Inhibitors of Angiogenesis

Name	Molecular Weight, kDa	Year	Reference
Platelet factor 4		1982	Nature 297:307
Interferon alpha		1980	Science 208:516
Prolactin fragment	16	1993	Endocrinol 133:1292
Angiostatin	38	1994	Cell 88:277
Endostatin	20	1997	Cell 79:315
Antithrombin III	53	1999	Science 285:1926
Interleukin 12		1995	J Natl Cancer Inst 87:581
Inducible protein 10		1995	J Exp Med 182:155
Vasostatin	21	1998	J Exp Med 188:2349
Canstatin	24	2000	J Biol Chem 275:1209
Restin	22	1999	Biochem Biophys Res Commun 255:735
Troponin I	22	1999	Proc Natl Acad Sci 96:2645
Pigment epithelium growth factor (PEGF)	50	1999	Science 285:1926
2-methoxyestradiol		1994	Proc Natl Acad Sci 91:3964
PEX	26	1998	Cell 92:391
Id1 and Id3		1999	Nature 401:670
VEG1		1999	FASEB J 13:181
Proliferin-related protein (PRP)		1994	Science 266:1581
Meth-1, Meth-2	110, 98	1999	J Biol Chem 274:13349
Osteopontin cleaved product		1999	Trends Bio Sci 7:182
Maspin		2000	Nat Med 6:196

SOURCE: Folkman and in part from Carmeliet and Jain.

ized or withdrawn, endothelial cells in the absence of perivascular smooth muscle and pericytes undergo apoptosis and new microvessels regress. These differences indicate that angiogenesis in tumors may be more vulnerable to certain angiogenesis inhibitors than angiogenesis in healing wounds. Endostatin inhibits tumor growth in mice without delaying wound healing.

Endogenous Angiogenesis Inhibitors Certain endogenous inhibitors of angiogenesis are known to play a role in the angiogenic switch, including: IFN-α and platelet factor 4, and the class of angiostatic steroids typified by tetrahydrocortisol (Table 83-2).

thrombospondin-1 The production of thrombospondin-1 has been shown to be inversely related to the ability of a cell line to produce a tumor and vessels in vivo; loss of thrombospondin-1 production allowed non-tumorigenic cells to become tumorigenic. Thrombospondin-1 is regulated by wild-type p53. Loss of p53 function in tumor cells dramatically decreased the level of angiogenesis inhibitor. Restoration of p53 increased the inhibitor and suppressed the angiogenic activity of the tumor cells. The angiogenic switch was controlled by a negative regulator of angiogenesis generated by the tumor. The switch itself was viewed as a result of a shift in the "net balance" of angiogenesis stimulators and inhibitors. This led to the discovery of angiostatin, a second inhibitor found to be involved in the angiogenic switch.

Angiostatin, endostatin, and antiangiogenic antithrombin III Several clinical and experimental observations suggested that certain tumors may produce angiogenesis inhibitors. The removal of certain tumors (e.g., breast carcinomas, colon carcinomas, and osteogenic sarcomas) can be followed by rapid growth of distant metastases. A primary tumor can suppress metastases from a different type of tumor, e.g., a breast cancer can inhibit melanoma metastases. In melanoma, partial spontaneous regression of the primary tumor may be followed by rapid growth of metastases. Regression of small cell lung cancer by ionizing radiation may be followed by rapid growth of distant metastases. If one portion of a primary tumor is removed (e.g., cytoreductive surgery for testicular cancer), the residual tumor increases its rate of expansion. A similar phenomenon is observed in animal tumors, i.e., certain primary tumors inhibit the growth, but not the number, of their own metastases. Surgical removal of a primary tumor increases growth rate of the residual tumors. Many primary tumors can suppress the growth of a second tumor inoculation. This "resistance" to a second tumor challenge is inversely proportional to the size of the tumor inoculum and directly proportional to the size of the first tumor. A threshold size is necessary for the inhibitory effect to occur.

At least three hypotheses have been advanced to explain these diverse observations and experiments: (1) "concomitant immunity"— a primary tumor induces an immunologic response against a secondary tumor or a metastasis in the same host; (2) depletion of nutrients by the primary tumor; or (3) production of antimitotic factors from the primary tumor that directly inhibit the proliferation of the secondary tumor. However, none of these ideas offers a molecular mechanism to explain all of the experiments cited above, and overall they have not been confirmed. Concomitant immunity has been ruled out as a mechanism because tumors can suppress metastasis in mice with severe combined immunodeficiency (SCID).

Once it was realized that a tumor could generate both positive and negative regulators of angiogenesis, then it also became clear that a primary tumor, while stimulating angiogenesis in its own vascular bed, could possibly inhibit angiogenesis in the vascular bed of a distant metastasis. However, at least two conditions would be necessary: (1) the primary tumor (i.e., the first tumor to grow) would need to generate an angiogenic promoter in excess of an inhibitor in its own local vascular bed, and (2) the putative inhibitor would need to have a longer half-life in the circulation than the angiogenic promoter. Research done over the past decade has identified angiostatin, endostatin, and antiangiogenic antithrombin as negative regulators of angiogenesis.

Lewis lung carcinoma generated angiostatin, a 38-kDa cleavage product of plasminogen. Systemic administration of purified angiostatin completely inhibited growth of metastases, producing dormant tumors of microscopic size (<200 μm in diameter) in the lung, and inhibited the growth of primary tumors. Angiostatin is not secreted by tumor cells but is generated through proteolytic cleavage of circulating plasminogen by a series of enzymes released from the tumor cells. At least one of these tumor-derived enzymes, urokinase plasminogen activator (uPA), converts plasminogen to plasmin, while a phosphoglycerate kinase from hypoxic tumor cells then reduces the plasmin so that it can be converted to angiostatin by one of several different metalloproteinases. Other types of tumors have since been reported to generate angiostatin, e.g., human prostate cancer. Prostate-specific antigen generates angiostatin-like fragments from plasminogen.

Furthermore, when murine fibrosarcoma cells were transfected with angiostatin, primary subcutaneous tumors formed. Their growth was slowed in proportion to increased levels of angiostatin production by the tumor cells. In these tumors the *total angiogenic output* of the primary tumor was decreased by transfected angiostatin, which opposed the activity of the tumor's secreted angiogenic promoter in a dose-dependent manner, but never completely counteracted it. The rate of tumor growth (expansion of tumor mass) was directly proportional to the total angiogenic output of the tumor, inversely proportional to angiostatin production and to tumor cell apoptosis, and virtually independent of tumor cell proliferation.

Murine hemangioendothelioma generated endostatin, a 20-kDa cleavage product of collagen XVIII. Human non-small cell lung carcinoma generated a 53-kDa cleavage product of antithrombin III (antiangiogenic ATIII). (This tumor does not metastasize, but the circulating angiogenesis inhibitor was detected because a subcutaneous tumor suppressed the growth of a second tumor at a remote site). All three of these proteins specifically inhibit endothelial cell proliferation and not other cell types. They have no effect on tumor cells per se. Endostatin inhibits tumor angiogenesis but not wound angiogenesis. It has no effect on pregnant mice nor on normal neonatal mice. Endostatin is present in *C. elegans* as a product of collagen XVIII and so may be at least 600 million years old on an evolutionary time scale. Other endogenous angiogenesis inhibitors are presented in Table 83-2.

Angiogenesis Inhibitors in Clinical Trial Angiogenesis inhibitors are in clinical trials in the United States for patients with cancer (Table 83-3). While a few endogenous antiangiogenic proteins have entered clinical trial [e.g., angiostatin, endostatin, and interleukin (IL) 12], these are more difficult to manufacture, and it will take some time before large quantities of these inhibitors become available for large numbers of patients. The majority of angiogenesis inhibitors currently in clinical trial for cancer are antibodies or small-molecular-weight synthetic molecules that inhibit specific targets along the angiogenic pathway.

BYSTANDER MOLECULES IN THE ANGIOGENIC PATHWAY A variety of molecules in the angiogenic pathway are not strictly endothelial cell mitogens or suppressors but operate as modifiers, markers, or receptors of the angiogenic process. They include: (1) integrins $\alpha_v\beta_3$ and $\alpha_v\beta_5$, which are upregulated on proliferating endothelial cells and act as receptors for fragments of fibronectin and other matrix components; (2) ephrins, which specify arterial or venous development of capillary vessels; (3) cyclooxygenase 2 (COX 2), the production of which is stimulated by bFGF and which converts lipid precursors to prostaglandin E_2 (PGE_2), an angiogenic stimulator; (4) plasminogen activator inhibitor 1 (PAI-1), which counteracts the upregulation of uPA that is produced by growing capillaries, thus restricting proteolysis to a local event at the tip of angiogenic vessels; (5) AC133, a specific marker for circulating endothelial precursor cells, which arise from bone marrow; and (6) nitric oxide synthase, which generates nitric oxide, that induces vasodilation in the vascular bed, a possible prerequisite for sprout formation.

METASTASES ARE ANGIOGENESIS-DEPENDENT Before tumors have become neovascularized in experimental animals, tumor cells rarely, if ever, shed into the circulation and metastases are essentially nonexistent. After the primary tumor becomes neovascularized, the number of tumor cells shed into the circulation increases in proportion to the increased neovascularization. Metastases that survive at a distant site must become angiogenic to be detected. Nonangiogenic metastases remain dormant at a microscopic size (<0.2 mm) indefinitely. Therefore, angiogenesis is required at both ends of the metastatic cascade.

Table 83-3   Angiogenesis Inhibitors in Clinical Trials

Drug	Sponsor	Mechanism
PHASE I		
COL-3	Collagenex, NCI	Synthetic MMP inhibitor; tetracycline derivative
BMS-275291	Bristol-Myers Squibb	Synthetic MMP inhibitor
SU6668	Sugen	Blocks VEGF, FGF, and EGF receptor signaling
Endostatin	EntreMed	Inhibits endothelial proliferation
EMD 121974	Merck KCgaA	Blocks an endothelial integrin
Angiostatin	EntreMed	Inhibits endothelial proliferation
2-methoxy-estradiol	EntreMed	Inhibits microtubule function
PHASE II		
Squalamine	Magainin	Inhibits Na/H exchanger
TNP-470	TAP Pharm.	Fumagillin analogue; inhibits endothelial proliferation
Combretastatin	Oxigene	Apoptosis in proliferating endothelium
Interleukin-12	Genetics Inst.	Induces IFN-γ and IP-10
CAI	NCI	Inhibits calcium influx
Anti-VEGF Ab	Genentech	Monoclonal antibody to VEGF
PHASE III		
Marimastat	British Biotech	Synthetic MMP inhibitor
AG3340	Agouron	Synthetic MMP inhibitor
Neovastat	Aetema	Natural MMP inhibitor
Interferon-α	Commercially available	Inhibition of bFGF production
IM862	Cytran	Endothelial inhibitor
Thalidomide	Celgene	Unknown
SU5416	Sugen	Blocks VEGF receptor signaling

NOTE: bFGF, basic fibroblast growth factor; EGF, epidermal growth factor; IFN, interferon; IP-10, inducible protein 10; MMP, a metalloproteinase inhibitor; NCI, National Cancer Institute; VEGF, vascular endothelial growth factor.
SOURCE: From National Cancer Institute Database (updated April 14, 2000).

Clinical patterns in which metastases first present may also be explained by angiogenic mechanisms. Cancer metastases are known to present in at least four different common clinical patterns and in one rare pattern. These clinical observations have previously been unrelated to each other but may be unified by angiogenic principles from tumor-bearing animals.

1. The patient whose metastases appear, sometimes explosively, a few months after surgical removal of a primary tumor (e.g., osteogenic sarcoma) may have lost a circulating angiogenesis inhibitor generated by the primary tumor. A model for this clinical presentation is the murine Lewis lung carcinoma that generates angiostatin.

2. Metastases that are not being suppressed by the primary tumor may already be present when the primary tumor is first diagnosed. The experimental model is a Lewis lung carcinoma subline that does not generate angiostatin.

3. The "unknown," or "occult," primary describes a pattern of metastases that present in the absence of a primary tumor or before it is located. In the relevant animal model lung metastases grow so rapidly that they suppress the primary tumor. However, it has not yet been

determined whether a circulating angiogenic inhibitor is generated by the metastases.

4. If metastases do not appear until years after surgical removal of the primary tumor, the patient may harbor dormant microscopic metastases that are not angiogenic. Those that eventually switch to the angiogenic phenotype can grow to detectable metastases. An example is the node-negative breast cancer patient who develops lung metastases 10 to 15 years after resection of the primary tumor. An animal model that mimics this pattern has been developed. Surgical removal of a B-16 melanoma from a syngeneic mouse leaves numerous viable lung metastases that are not angiogenic and do not expand beyond 0.1 to 0.2 mm diameter; they remain dormant for the life of the animal. They also remain viable, as evidenced by the fact that trauma to the lung or transplantation of a small piece of lung to the subcutaneous tissue of another mouse quickly generates a lethal tumor in both cases.

5. After surgical removal of a renal cell carcinoma, metastases will sometimes regress completely or partly. While this is an uncommon clinical pattern, V2 carcinoma in the rabbit most closely resembles it. Removal of a primary tumor in the leg is followed by regression of metastases. This does not appear to be an immune reaction because fresh tumor grows successfully in the same rabbit. One explanation is that the metastases were dependent upon high production of a circulating angiogenic stimulator, such as bFGF from the primary tumor. High plasma levels of bFGF have been found to correlate with high mortality in human renal cancer.

These clinical patterns are summarized in Fig. 83-4 as a unifying guide for clinicians. The hypothesis that these clinical patterns are linked by angiogenic mechanisms requires additional confirmation in the laboratory, but it provides a direction for further research.

LEUKEMIA IS ANGIOGENESIS-DEPENDENT Leukemia was assumed not to be angiogenic because it had been thought of as "liquid tumor." However, when bone marrow biopsies from children with newly diagnosed acute lymphoblastic leukemia were stained with an antibody to von Willebrand factor to highlight vascular endothelium, microvessel density was increased six- to sevenfold when compared to children with "control" bone marrow biopsies taken at the time of diagnosis of a solid tumor. Confocal microscopy further revealed that new microvessels in leukemic bone marrow were surrounded by a perivascular cuff of tumor cells like solid tumors. bFGF in the urine of the leukemic children was approximately sevenfold higher than in controls. Acute myeloid leukemia and chronic myeloid leukemia in adults are also associated with intense bone marrow neovascularization. Cellular levels of the angiogenic factor VEGF are significantly increased in acute myeloid leukemia and provide a prognostic indicator of outcome. The close physical configuration of microvessels and bone marrow cells may facilitate a two-way para-crine pathway between vascular endothelial cells that produce mitogens for bone marrow cells [such as granulocyte colony stimulating factor (G-CSF)] and bone marrow cells that produce bFGF, a mitogen for endothelial cells.

Further work suggests that leukemia growth is dependent on angiogenesis. Murine leukemias can be suppressed or eradicated and survival of leukemia-bearing mice prolonged when they are treated with antiangiogenic therapy. The mice were treated either by systemic administration of endostatin or by chemotherapy administered on an "antiangiogenic" schedule. A conventional schedule of chemotherapy at a maximum tolerated dose was ineffective (see below).

Certain patients with multiple myeloma refractory to all conventional therapy have undergone successful remission when treated with thalidomide. This has initiated a debate about whether the beneficial effect of thalidomide is due to its antiangiogenic activity or to some other property such as its weak capacity to inhibit tumor necrosis factor (TNF-α) activity. This question arose because microvessel density did not decrease significantly in parallel with improvement of the disease. However, this result is not unexpected. In animal tumors that undergo steady regression in tumor volume as a result of antiangiogenic therapy, microvessel density (microvessels per square millimeter) may in some cases remain constant even as tumor volume is reduced by one-half, because capillary dropout and tumor cell dropout are going on at a near constant ratio. Furthermore, other effects of antiangiogenic therapy, such as the reduction of plasma leakage from tumor vessels, would not be revealed by microvessel density. Further, thalidomide is among the weakest inhibitors of TNF-α. Four other compounds that inhibit TNF-α more potently than thalidomide have no antiangiogenic effect. Pentoxifylline inhibits TNF-α at a similar potency as thalidomide, yet thalidomide inhibits cornea angiogenesis and pentoxifylline does not. Ibuprofen *increases* TNF-α in the serum of mice by twofold, yet it inhibits angiogenesis. Finally dexamethasone is a more potent inhibitor of TNF-α than thalidomide, but dexamethasone does not inhibit angiogenesis or does so only weakly.

ANTIANGIOGENIC THERAPY CIRCUMVENTS ACQUIRED DRUG RESISTANCE The emergence of drug-resistant tumor cells is a major problem accompanying almost all chemotherapy. Conventional cytotoxic chemotherapy targets the cancer cell, and it is the genetic instability and high mutation rate of these cells that are responsible in part for acquired drug resistance. However, vascular endothelial cells are genetically stable and have a low mutation rate, like bone marrow cells. Bone marrow cells do not appear to develop drug resistance against conventional chemotherapy. Thus, it is possible that tumor vessels will also maintain sensitivity to antiangiogenic therapy.

MICROVESSEL DENSITY IS A USEFUL PROGNOSTIC INDICATOR Neovascularization in human brain tumors correlates directly with tumor grade. Tumor vascularity in cutaneous melanoma also influences prognosis. Microvessel density is an independent prognostic indicator for human breast cancer. In fact, the majority of reports (52 different studies) confirm that microvessel density is a powerful and often an independent prognostic indicator for a variety of different human cancers. However, at least seven other reports fail to show the prognostic value of microvessel density. Some of these negative reports may be methodologic problems. Others may represent the co-existence of angiogenesis inhibitors and stimulators that cannot easily be measured in a tumor. Summaries of all published reports are given in (Tables 83-4 through 83-9). The best prognostic information from a histologic microsection of a tumor is obtained when the highest area of microvessel density ("hot spot") is quantified. These areas may contain the most angiogenic tumor cells, which have the highest chance of becoming an angiogenic metastasis.

Despite its usefulness as a *prognostic* marker, quantification of microvessel density is not necessarily a useful *surrogate* marker for

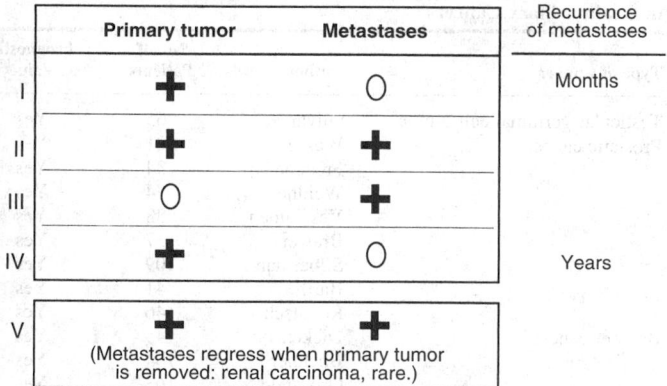

At first diagnosis:

	Primary tumor	Metastases	Recurrence of metastases
I	+	O	Months
II	+	+	
III	O	+	
IV	+	O	Years
V	+	+	

(Metastases regress when primary tumor is removed: renal carcinoma, rare.)

FIGURE 83-4 Metastatic patterns in cancer patients at the time of first diagnosis.

Table 83-4　Breast Cancer—Intratumoral Vascularization and Prognosis

Author	No. of Patients	Median Follow-up, Years	Relapse-Free Survival
Weidner	165	4.0	<.001
Bosari	180	9.0	<.03
Visscher	58	5.1	NS
Obermair	64	4.1	<.01
Ogawa	155	7.0	<.002
Fox	211	3.5	ND
Toi	125	5.1	<.01
Toi	328	4.6	<.0001
Simpson	178	6.0	0.002
Gasparini	531	6.3	<.001
Bevilacqua	211	6.6	<.0001
Obermair	230	4.6	ND
Fox	109	2.0	.04
Heimann	167	20.0	.04
Barbareschi	91	5.5	.006
Gasparini	191	5.5	<.01
Gasparini	178	5.2	<.01
Hall	87	9.5; 1.5	NS
Axelsson	220	11.5	NS
Van Hoef	93	13.0	NS

NOTE: Published positive studies. ND, not done; NS, not significant.
SOURCE: From Gasparini and Harris.

efficacy of antiangiogenic therapy. Although it is currently employed in a few early clinical trials of antiangiogenic therapy, experimental studies suggest that it will be of little value to predict efficacy of an angiogenesis inhibitor. Microvessel density is determined mainly by intercapillary distance, itself governed by the cuff thickness of tumor cells surrounding a microvessel. In experimental animals, microvessel density may remain constant as a tumor is shrinking under antiangiogenic therapy. Residual tumor cells can form cuffs around remaining vessels, so that the vessel density may not change significantly. Microvessel density also may not distinguish between benign and malignant tumors. The microvessel density in normal pituitary tissue is higher than in a pituitary adenoma, which is higher than in a pituitary carcinoma. In the normal pituitary gland, the perivascular cuff is one to two cell layers. However, in the adenoma the perivascular cuff is increased as tumor cells adapt to lower oxygen tensions. Cuff thickness is even greater in the carcinoma, thus giving the lowest microvessel density. However, for other tumors, such as breast carcinoma, microvessel density is significantly higher than in normal breast tissue. In certain animal tumors, angiogenic output exceeds the growth capacity of the tumor cells. Initial antiangiogenic therapy will lead to a reduction in microvessel density, which may then remain constant as vascular density comes into balance with tumor cell population, whether the tumor remains stable or regresses. Finally, if the first microvessel density is obtained from an open biopsy and a subsequent follow-up microvessel density is from a needle biopsy, the second density will

Table 83-5　Prognostic Value of Microvessel Density in Breast Cancer Patients Treated with Adjuvant Therapy

Author	No. of Patients	Median Follow-up, Years	Adjuvant Treatment	Relapse-Free Survival
Weidner	82	4.0	Heterogeneous	<.001
Toi	198	4.6	Heterogeneous	<.001
Gasparini	191	5.5	CD31	<.001
Macaulay	88	2.5	Tamoxifen	ND
Gasparini	178	5.2	CD31	<.001

NOTE: ND, not done.
SOURCE: From Gasparini and Harris.

Table 83-6　Prognostic Value of Microvessel Density in Non-Small Cell Lung Cancers

Author	No. of Patients	Median Follow-up, Months	Prognostic Value
Macchiarini	87	60	Yes
Yamazaki	42	71	Yes
Fontanini	253	24	Yes
Giatromanolaki	107	36	Yes
Angeletti	96	24	Yes
Apolinario	116	60	Yes
		(stage II only)	
Fontanini	470	29	Yes
Fontanini	73	47	Yes

SOURCE: From Gasparini and Harris.

be higher. This artifact is due to tissue compression by the needle biopsy.

CYTOTOXIC CHEMOTHERAPY MAY BE ANGIOGENESIS-DEPENDENT Certain cytotoxic chemotherapeutic agents may depend in part for their anticancer activity on their ability to inhibit proliferating endothelial cells. Proliferating and migrating microvascular endothelial cells are exposed to chemotherapeutic drugs before tumor cells. However, the endothelial cells have a chance to recover during the traditional 2-3 week off-therapy period designed to allow recovery of bone marrow. Recovering endothelium can resupply residual tumor cells with new vessels and with paracrine factors necessary for tumor cell survival. Tumor recurrence requires resumption of chemotherapy, which itself can lead to emergence of drug-resistant clones of tumor cells (but not of endothelial cells). The convention of *maximum tolerated dose* (MTD) virtually forces the prolonged off-therapy schedule.

If the schedule of the chemotherapeutic agent is altered (increased number of lower drug doses) to apply maximum cytotoxic pressure to the endothelial cells in the tumor bed (i.e., an "antiangiogenic schedule" instead of a "conventional schedule"), even large tumors in mice may be permanently cured. In contrast, all mice on the conventional schedule of MTD therapy died with drug-resistant tumors. The antiangiogenic schedule of the chemotherapeutic drug was more frequent but was administered at a threefold lower total lower dose per day so that bone marrow was not depressed. Thus, efficacy of cytotoxic chemotherapy can be improved (in mice) by applying new logic to an old drug. The new logic is that antiangiogenic properties of certain conventional cytotoxic agents are not revealed unless the drugs are administered frequently. Frequent administration requires lower doses.

These results in mice may help to explain why some patients who

Table 83-7　Prognostic Value of Microvessel Density in Genitourinary Cancers

Type of Cancer	Author	No. of Patients	Prognostic Value
Testicular germinal cell tumor	Olivarez	65	Yes
Prostatic cancer	Wakui	101	Yes
	Fregene	34	Yes
	Weidner	74	Yes
	Vesalainen	88	Yes
	Brawer	37	Yes
	Silberman	109	Yes
	Barth	41	Yes
	Rogatsch	46	Yes
Bladder cancer	Dickenson	45	Yes
	Bochner	164	Yes
	Grossfeld	163	Yes

NOTE: ND, not done.
SOURCE: From Gasparini and Harris.

Type of Cancer	Author	No. of Patients	Median Follow-up, Months	Prognostic Value
Esophageal	Tanigawa	43	3.1	Yes
Gastric	Maeda	124	>5	Yes
	Tanigawa	181	4.1	Yes
Colorectal	Saclarides	48	4.4	Yes
	Tomisaki	175	5.0	Yes
	Takebayashi	166	6.3	Yes
	Bossi	178	5.0	No
	Lindmark	212	4.5	Yes[a]

[a] High vascularity associated with good prognosis.
SOURCE: From Gasparini and Harris.

are receiving long-term maintenance or even palliative chemotherapy continue to have stable disease beyond the time that tumor cells would have been expected to develop drug resistance. For example, long-term stable disease has been observed in a few patients with metastatic breast cancer who have been on weekly paclitaxel for several years. Paclitaxel has been reported to have antiangiogenic activity in addition to its anticancer activity. In the future, formal clinical trials with antiangiogenic schedules of chemotherapy should be tested.

Although "fractionated" radiotherapy (i.e., increased frequency of exposures at lower doses) was found empirically to be more effective and to cause fewer side effects than higher radiation doses more widely spaced, the biologic basis of this approach may be due, in part, to the effect of ionizing radiation on endothelial cells. Conventional radiotherapy of tumor-bearing animals is greatly enhanced and with fewer side effects when the radiotherapy is administered in combination with subtherapeutic doses of angiostatin.

GUIDELINES FOR CLINICAL TRIALS OF ANGIOGENESIS INHIBITORS New guidelines are required to examine the clinical effects of angiogenesis inhibitors because this class of drugs differs so markedly from cytotoxic chemotherapy. First, end-points for efficacy require different definitions. For cytotoxic therapy, lack of tumor regression is considered a failure, and an end-point of stable disease is little valued because it has never been shown to improve patient survival. In contrast, stable disease brought about by antiangiogenic therapy may be a favorable end-point of antiangiogenic therapy if it can be shown to improve the quality or duration of life. Experience with endostatin in early phase I clinical trials shows that patients with advanced metastatic disease refractory to all conventional therapy and who have had stable disease on endostatin for up to 6 months so far have pain relief, increased appetite, normal bone marrow function, and no side effects. A similar experience has been gained from IFN-α administered daily at low dose (3 million units) for malignancies dependent upon overexpression of bFGF as their sole or main angiogenic protein (i.e., giant cell tumors of bone, angioblastoma). In fact, five of six of these patients who had failed all conven-

Table 83-9 Prognostic Value of Microvessel Density in Malignant Melanoma

Author	No. of Patients	Median Follow-up, Months	Thickness, mm	Prognostic Value
Srivastava	20	>5	0.76–4.00	Yes
Fallowfield	64	ND	0.48–18.5	Yes
Carnochan	107	>5	0.85–1.25	No
Busam	120	8.9	Invasive	No
Graham	37	>10	0.76	Yes
Vlaykova	31	>3	0.76	Yes

NOTE: ND, not done.
SOURCE: From Gasparini and Harris.

tional therapy had complete regressions of their tumors by 1 to 3 years and are now off therapy and remain tumor free. This illustrates a second difference from cytotoxic therapy: antiangiogenic therapy takes longer to achieve stable disease and tumor regression is slower. It is analogous to the use of tamoxifen or to the treatment of other chronic diseases such as tuberculosis. Nevertheless, patients enjoy a high quality of life during antiangiogenic therapy.

Third, tumor progression during a clinical trial of cytotoxic chemotherapy is considered as a failure, and patients are often discontinued from the trial. With antiangiogenic therapy, some patients with rapidly advancing metastatic disease may show some tumor progression before stable disease is achieved. In the first clinical trials of tamoxifen, some patients were discontinued early in the trials because of tumor progression. After the term *tamoxifen flare* was invented, patients stayed on long-term tamoxifen therapy for several years. Of course, very rapid tumor progression during antiangiogenic therapy requires that the inhibitor be discontinued and the patient offered a different therapy.

Fourth, unlike cytotoxic chemotherapy, antiangiogenic therapy is more effective if it is administered frequently, without gaps, for a long period of time (e.g., like tamoxifen) and at a dose that has little or no toxicity. The term *MTD* is less useful for angiogenesis inhibitors.

Fifth, angiogenesis inhibitors can be used in combination with conventional chemotherapy, radiotherapy, immunotherapy, gene therapy, or other modalities, usually without increasing side effects. Clinical trials of angiogenesis inhibitors in combination with chemotherapy or radiotherapy are already under way.

CLINICAL SIGNS IN CANCER PATIENTS BASED ON ANGIOGENESIS Certain clinical signs and symptoms from tumor neovascularization are associated with specific tumor types. For example, retinoblastomas in the posterior eye induce iris neovascularization in the anterior chamber. Some brain tumors induce angiogenesis in remote areas of the brain. Bone pain in metastatic prostate cancer may be related in part to neovascularization. A problem in the diagnosis of a primary bone tumor is that if the biopsy specimen contains only the neovascular response at the periphery of the tumor, it may be mistaken for granulation tissue or inflammation. Several cancer syndromes, such as inappropriate hormonal activity, hypercoagulation, and cachexia, are secondary to the presence of biologically active peptides released into the circulation from vascularized tumors. Therefore, an early therapeutic effect of antiangiogenic therapy could be increased appetite, weight gain, and disappearance of a cancer syndrome. The angiogenesis induced by cervical cancer may be observed by colposcopy; the appearance of telangiectasia, or "vascular spiders," in a mastectomy scar may herald local recurrence of tumor; color Doppler imaging can demonstrate neovascularization in breast cancer and other tumors; bladder carcinoma is detected by cystoscopy based, in part, on its neovascularization; and mammography may reveal the vascularized rim of a breast tumor. A wide range of radiologic signs of cancer are based on "enhancement" of lesions by radiopaque dyes sequestered transiently in the neovasculature of a tumor. Moreover, in some tumors large central areas cannot be penetrated by radiopaque dyes because of vascular compression, a situation that is unusual in prevascular tumors.

CLINICAL MISPERCEPTIONS ABOUT TUMOR ANGIOGENESIS Because angiogenesis research is such a broad and rapidly moving field (at least 30 reports each week), certain misperceptions have emerged.

One misperception is that angiogenesis is synonymous with malignancy. The presence of angiogenesis does not distinguish between a benign and a malignant tumor. Benign adrenal adenomas are highly neovascularized but appear to lack the growth potential to take advantage of the new blood vessels they have induced. Angiogenesis may not be necessary for certain tumor cells that can grow as a flat sheet between membranes, e.g., gliomatosis in the meninges. Large tumors

Table 83-10 Angiogenesis Inhibitors in U.S. Clinical Trials for Eye Disease[a]

Drug	Sponsor	Mechanism	Phase: Disease	Location
Anecortave acetate	Alcon	Angiostatic steroid	I: Macular degeneration	New York, Palo Alto, Baltimore, Cleveland
LY33531 (oral)	Lilly	Protein kinase C β inhibitor (anti-VEGF)	III: Diabetic retinopathy	U.S.
rhuFab	Genetech	Anti-VEGF	I: Macular degeneration	Boston
AG3340 (oral)	Agouron	Inhibitor of MMP-2 and -9	III: Macular degeneration	U.S.
Anti-VEGF aptamer	Gilead/ EyeTECH	Anti-VEGF	I: Macular degeneration	New York, Boston, Palo Alto

[a] Updated March, 2000.
NOTE: MMP, metalloproteinase inhibitor; VEGF, vascular endothelial growth factor.

are thought to have "established" vessels that would be refractory to antiangiogenic therapy. A few feeder vessels, usually arteries, may be observed in the midst of a histologic cross-section of a tumor and could be considered as established. However, tumor cells depend on *thin-walled microvessels* for diffusion of nutrients, growth factors, and oxygen, and it is these vessels that continue to undergo high turnover rates even in a large, slowly growing or indolent tumors. These microvessels require the continuous presence of endothelial growth factors such as VEGF. Withdrawal or blockade of VEGF leads to endothelial cell apoptosis and regression of microvessels. In both animals and humans, very large tumors have regressed in response to antiangiogenic therapy, but a longer time of therapy is required. For example, a high-grade giant cell tumor (refractory to all conventional therapy) of >1 kg in the pelvis of a 17-year-old girl underwent 90% regression after 1 year of daily systemic therapy with IFN-α (3 million units). It is commonly stated that tumors "outgrow their blood supply." This is inaccurate; growing tumors can gradually *compress* their blood supply because of increasing interstitial pressure (discussed above). These areas of vascular compression become ischemic but are not avascular. Necrosis may follow. Vessel compression also interferes with the optimal delivery of therapeutic agents. Paradoxically, antiangiogenic therapy can decrease ischemia, apparently because it decreases interstitial pressure.

Another misperception is that antiangiogenic therapy will be less effective against slowly growing tumors, because this is true for cytotoxic chemotherapeutic agents. In fact the opposite has been found in experimental animals. Slowly growing mouse tumors respond more effectively to angiogenesis inhibitors (TNP-470 or angiostatin) than do rapidly growing tumors. Rapidly growing tumors require higher doses of angiogenesis inhibitors to suppress their growth to the same extent as slowly growing tumors. While cytotoxic therapy is dependent on tumor cell cycle, antiangiogenic therapy is not. It is widely assumed that only "highly vascularized" tumors are susceptible to antiangiogenic therapy. This misperception comes from attempts to estimate the angiogenic output of a tumor from an angiogram or a gross tumor specimen. A large, dark, unstained area in an angiogram is usually due to nonfilling of compressed vessels. This is often misinterpreted as "avascular" tumor. However, at the microscopic level, histologic sections reveal high microvessel density. A large tumor observed at the operating table, such as a neurofibrosarcoma, may be a hard white mass and assumed to be "poorly vascularized," when in fact the histologic microsections show intense neovascularization.

SUMMARY: TWO CELLULAR TARGETS IN A TUMOR An important lesson from angiogenesis research is to think about a tumor as containing two cell compartments that stimulate each other: the endothelial cell compartment and the tumor cell compartment. Anticancer therapy may be more efficacious if each compartment is treated by drugs that selectively target each cell type. The mutational rate is high in the tumor cell compartment and low in the endothelial cell compartment. This is the reason why it may be possible to employ antiangiogenic therapy for the long term, together with conventional chemotherapy or other therapies and subsequently in the postchemotherapy period.

DISEASES OF OCULAR NEOVASCULARIZATION

Pathologic angiogenesis is the most common cause of blindness worldwide. Pathologic neovascularization can occur in each compartment of the eye. For example, of >21 diseases that cause pathologic neovascularization in the cornea, contact lens wear, trauma, prior surgery, herpes simplex, and herpes zoster are the most frequently associated with pathologic neovascularization. Of ~37 diseases associated with iris neovascularization, central retinal vein occlusion, neovascular glaucoma, diabetes mellitus, and retinoblastoma are the most frequent. Of 14 diseases associated with retinal neovascularization, age-related macular degeneration, diabetes mellitus, retinopathy of prematurity, central retinal vein occlusion, branch retinal vein occlusion, and sickle cell disease are the most frequent. In western countries, age-related macular degeneration and diabetic retinopathy are the diseases of ocular neovascularization that affect the most patients. The large number of diseases listed above that are associated with ocular neovascularization and that directly or indirectly cause blindness illustrates how few effective therapies are currently available. This outline also reveals how few of these therapies can be administered systemically and how great is the opportunity to employ antiangiogenic therapy in clinical trials to reduce the incidence of blindness from pathologic neovascularization.

AGE-RELATED MACULAR DEGENERATION In age-related macular degeneration, angiogenesis occurs in the choroid. In the severe form of the disease, microhemorrhages from these new vessels lead to blindness. Approximately 1.7 million individuals in the United States suffer from the severe form, which is the leading cause of blindness in those ≥64 years. Laser therapy is less effective than in diabetic retinopathy. The angiogenic protein VEGF is markedly elevated in macular degeneration and may be a major mediator of this disease. Of the five angiogenesis inhibitors currently in clinical trials for ocular neovascularization (Table 83-10), four are employed in the treatment of macular degeneration. One inhibitor is an antibody that neutralizes VEGF, and the other is a synthetic low-molecular-weight compound that targets a VEGF receptor.

DIABETIC RETINOPATHY Diabetic retinopathy affects ~1.2 million of the estimated 14 million U.S. diabetic patients. It is the leading cause of blindness in persons between ages 25 and 64. Pathologic angiogenesis occurs in the retina, and new microvessels grow into the vitreous where they bleed and cause vitreous retraction. Laser therapy is more successful than in macular degeneration, but it is painful and causes gradual obliteration of the peripheral retina and loss of accompanying visual fields. Overexpression of VEGF may also mediate diabetic retinopathy but appears to be induced by upregulation of HIF-1 secondary to hypoxia in the retina. An orally available protein kinase Cβ inhibitor of VEGF is in phase III clinical trial for diabetic retinopathy. An early primary cause of the hypoxia may be adhesion of leukocytes to endothelium in retinal vessels (by upregulation of intercellular adhesion molecule 1 on retinal microvascular endothelium), leading to slow flow or periods of no flow.

RETINOPATHY OF PREMATURITY At the time of birth, both the retina and its vascular supply are still growing. Blood vessels that supply the retina in the premature baby and in the newborn are exquisitely sensitive to changes in oxygen, a mechanism that guarantees an adequate blood supply to the growing retina. In newborn cats exposed to oxygen, VEGF levels are downregulated and vascular growth in the retina is slowed or inhibited. However, the retina continues to grow. Subsequently, when the animal is returned to room air, the mismatch between the delayed vascularization and the steadily growing retina leads to relative hypoxia, which triggers a surge of VEGF and retinal neovascularization. This may cause retinal detachment and microhemorrhage. In the United States there are currently ~180,000 cases of retinopathy of prematurity, also called *retrolental fibroplasia*.

The increased understanding of the angiogenic mechanism of retinopathy of prematurity has led to clinical trials in which infants are weaned from oxygen to room air very slowly in order to prevent the rapid rise of VEGF. A recent report showed that in newborn animals returned to room air after exposure to oxygen, pathologic neovascularization was completely prevented while normal vascular development continued if the animals were treated with angiostatin for 5 days, beginning with the first day of exposure to room air. It is not yet clear whether systemic therapy of retinopathy of prematurity will be feasible in infants.

ENDOGENOUS ANGIOGENESIS INHIBITORS IN THE EYE Normally the components of the eye that transmit light (cornea, aqueous, lens, and vitreous) are avascular. The maintenance of this avascular state is accomplished, in part, by the presence of potent inhibitors of angiogenesis. Pigment epithelium-derived factor (PEDF) is a 50-kDa serpin and is a potent angiogenesis inhibitor that is produced by retinal cells. The amount of inhibitory PEDF produced by retinal cells is directly correlated with oxygen concentrations, suggesting that its loss plays a permissive role in ischemia-driven retinal neovascularization. In other words, when oxygen is decreased PEDF is decreased and VEGF is increased. Both changes facilitate neovascularization. PEDF has the unique characteristic of inhibiting endothelial migration toward a wide variety of angiogenic inducers tested. It may be the predominant angiogenesis inhibitor in the eye. When neutralizing antibody to PEDF (but not preimmune sera) is injected into the cornea, it becomes neovascularized. PEDF has also been found in tumors.

Thrombospondin-1 has also been found in ocular tissues such as cornea and in the retina. During hypoxia-driven retinal angiogenesis in newborn mice (returned to room air after oxygen exposure), a threefold increase in expression of thrombospondin-1 was seen corresponding to peak neovascularization and peak VEGF expression. The increased thrombospondin-1 expression during ischemia-induced angiogenesis appears to be mediated by VEGF. This suggests that thrombospondin functions in a negative-feedback system to protect the eye against surges of VEGF. It is interesting that the same balance of positive and negative regulators of angiogenesis originally found in tumors operates in normal tissues and that a shift in the net balance of these regulators mediates pathologic angiogenesis as well as its return to the normal nonangiogenic state.

ANGIOGENESIS IN SKIN DISEASE

Many dermatologic diseases are associated with angiogenesis. A caveat is that, unlike neoplastic diseases, which are virtually all angiogenesis-dependent, not all nonneoplastic diseases that are angiogenic are also angiogenesis-dependent.

ANGIOGENESIS-ASSOCIATED VS. ANGIOGENESIS-DEPENDENT SKIN DISEASE In certain diseases of the skin, angiogenesis may be an important side effect that facilitates healing or otherwise protects the host. Examples include ulcerations, delayed healing of wounds, and chronic infections, in which antiangiogenic therapy could be contraindicated. A few of the dermatologic diseases known to be angiogenesis-dependent are described.

Infantile Hemangiomas Hemangiomas consist of tumor-like clusters of proliferating capillaries. They occur in 1 out of 100 new-

borns and in 1 out of 4 premature infants, and by age 1 year are present in up to 10% of infants. In the first, or proliferating, stage, the lesions grow rapidly, reaching peak growth by ~4 months. By about 1 year they may enter the involuting stage, where they stop growing, following which they regress over the next 3 to 5 years (the involuted stage) and then usually disappear. During the proliferating stage the endothelial cells overexpress bFGF, VEGF, and metalloproteinases, all of which appear in the urine at abnormally high levels. In normal skin, keratinocytes express IFN-β, an angiogenesis inhibitor of similar strength as IFN-α. IFN-α or -β inhibit overexpression of aFGF and bFGF. Glucocorticoids (prednisone, 5 mg/kg) are used as first-line therapy for hemangiomas that are destroying tissue, interfering with sight, or threatening life. A dramatic slowing and subsequent regression occur in ~30% of patients, but glucocorticoids fail in the remaining 70% (i.e., either no regression, but some slowing of the disease, or continued rapid growth of the lesions). The mechanism by which glucocorticoids act as antiangiogenic agents is not clear, but they do inhibit synthesis of metalloproteinases. When glucorticoids fail and the hemangioma is life-threatening, IFN-α is used at low dose, 3 million units/m^2 daily subcutaneously for 8 to 12 months. While ~95% of hemangiomas regress spontaneously, 5% are sight- or life-threatening. Hemangiomas in the liver, heart, airway, or brain may be associated with a 50% mortality if untreated. IFN-α is antiangiogenic on the basis of its ability to inhibit overproduction of bFGF. Urinary levels of bFGF fall toward normal as hemangiomas regress, and bFGF levels can be used as a guide to dosing of IFN-α. While IFN-α accelerates regression of hemangiomas in 85% of patients, it fails in the other 15% for unknown reasons. Many of the failures are Kaposi hemangioendotheliomas (KHE), a very aggressive form of hemangioma, often accompanied by platelet trapping and thrombocytopenia. IFN-α works well in only 50% of KHE. Regressions of hemangioma are slower with IFN-α than with glucocorticoids. In infants <1 year old, a side effect of IFN-α can be delayed walking. This occurs in ~4% of infants and can be detected early by spasticity of the lower limbs (*spastic diplegia*). It is reversible if IFN-α is discontinued; for this reason, all children on IFN-α are followed carefully by a neurologist.

A "cavernous hemangioma" is not a hemangioma but a venous malformation in which there is a dearth of smooth muscle in the wall of a large thin venous structure lined by endothelium. These never regress spontaneously, and neither glucorticoids nor IFN-α are effective. Thus an adult with a cavernous hemangioma should not be treated with IFN-α.

Verruca Vulgaris Warts are caused by infection of keratinocytes in the skin by one of many subtypes of human papillomavirus (HPV). HPV contains two genes (E6/E7) that may increase angiogenesis. The E6 gene destabilizes the p53 tumor-suppressor gene, which upregulates VEGF and downregulates thrombospondin-1, an angiogenesis inhibitor. The HPV E7 gene inactivates the tumor suppressor gene Rb. Antiangiogenic therapy may be beneficial in these lesions, which are usually highly neovascularized.

Psoriasis Psoriasis is a proliferative disorder of epidermis accompanied by increased vascularity in the dermis in the form of elongated and widened dermal capillaries. The disease is T lymphocyte mediated. Psoriatic lesions are angiogenic. The major angiogenic mediator in psoriasis appears to be VEGF, which is upregulated, as are its receptors. In patients with psoriasis, the increased vascularity induced by VEGF may act as a conduit for delivery of T lymphocytes to the epidermal target. VEGF itself may facilitate T lymphocyte targeting. When VEGF is overexpressed in a tumor vascular bed, leukocyte rolling and adhesion are enhanced.

Up to 5 million Americans have psoriasis, but ~500,000 have a severe form that requires long-term therapy, such as with methotrexate for several years. Both glucocorticoids and retinoids are weak angiogenesis inhibitors, and they may be suppressing the angiogenic component as well as the infiltration of immune cells. More potent angiogenesis inhibitors may be useful.

Basal Cell and Squamous Cell Carcinomas   Both of these skin malignancies are highly angiogenic and follow the rules for other angiogenic-dependent tumors. Inactivation of the p53 tumor-suppressor gene (in part by ultraviolet light–induced mutations) is thought to be an early event in tumorigenesis, and its inactivation downregulates the angiogenesis inhibitor thrombospondin-1 and upregulates VEGF expression. Furthermore, the normal expression of IFN-β in keratinocytes is markedly decreased, permitting upregulation of the angiogenic stimulator bFGF. These lesions comprise >90% of the ~700,000 skin cancers that are treated each year in the United States.

Cutaneous Melanoma   Melanoma in the skin begins in a radial or horizontal growth phase, which usually does not exceed a thickness of 0.75 mm. This stage is not neovascularized or is poorly neovascularized. It is analogous to the avascular phase of early in situ carcinoma. In the vertical growth phase, there are increased neovascularization, increased proliferation, and increased thickness of tumor beyond 0.75 mm, and intensity of vascularization correlates directly with increased metastatic risk and mortality. Progression of melanoma often begins with inactivation of the tumor-suppressor gene p16 and is followed later by expression of $\alpha_v\beta_3$ integrin and by expression of VEGF receptors on the melanoma cells. *Ras* mutations that upregulate VEGF expression emerge later and may be followed by expression of the angiogenic proteins, IL-8, and bFGF. This sequential onset of expression of angiogenic proteins by a tumor cell is similar to progression of breast cancer. It is not clear if or how expression of $\alpha_v\beta_3$ integrin as well as VEGF receptors on the melanoma cells themselves facilitates tumor growth, unless the VEGF is acting as an autocrine growth factor for the tumor cells, while at the same time acting as a paracrine stimulator of endothelial cells. A precedent for this mechanism has been reported for human pancreatic cancer. The angiogenesis inhibitor 2-methoxyestradiol currently in a phase I trial for breast cancer also showed efficacy against melanoma in animals.

Kaposi's Sarcoma (KS)   This lesion, which acts like a malignancy in patients with AIDS, may instead be a chronic inflammatory reactive process that is highly angiogenic. The angiogenesis is driven mainly by VEGF and hepatocyte growth factor. The tat protein of the HIV virus also plays a role in the angiogenic pathway for KS, but this is still being elucidated. The origin of KS cells is also not clear, but they appear to arise from the vascular system, possibly from smooth-muscle cells or pericytes. Two different angiogenesis inhibitors in phase II trials, thalidomide and TNP-470, a synthetic analogue of fumagillin, have shown efficacy against KS. However, there are currently too few cases to make any general conclusions.

Neurofibromatosis   These slow-growing benign skin tumors of Schwann cell origin can grow in other organs and become very large. Neurofibromas are very neovascularized and express VEGF. This may be driven by overexpression of the *ras* oncogene. The gene for neurofibromin (NF1) is a negative regulator of *ras*, and mutation of this gene increases *ras* expression. Because of their very slow growth rate and high angiogenic activity, neurofibromas illustrate a type of tumor for which long-term antiangiogenic therapy may be more effective than cytotoxic chemotherapy. They are rich in mast cells, which may enhance tumor angiogenesis by mobilization of bFGF. If a patient with a neurofibroma had abnormally high plasma or urine levels of bFGF, daily IFN-α could be used at a low dose of 3 million units/m^2 for a prolonged period of 2 to 3 years, with slow regression as a goal.

Recessive Dystrophic Epidermolysis Bullosa   This autosomal recessive disorder is characterized by subepidermal blistering, scarring, fusion of digits, and severe pruritus. Epidermis separates from dermis, in part due to a loss of collagen VII, which participates in the anchoring of these two cellular layers. Aggressive cutaneous squamous cell carcinoma, which emerges from this lesion, is the most common cause of death. Very high levels of bFGF have been found in the urine of these patients but not in patients with other blistering disorders. The source of bFGF could be its mobilization from heparan sulfate proteoglycans in the defective epidermal-dermal junction. bFGF not only stimulates angiogenesis directly but also stimulates the production of COX 2, which converts lipid precursors to prostaglandin E$_2$, another angiogenic stimulator. Keratinocyte growth is also stimulated by bFGF. Continuous keratinocyte proliferation may be a precursor to the development of squamous cell carcinoma. COX 2 inhibitors have antiangiogenic and antitumor activity in mice and may be useful in angiogenic diseases in man. Another antiangiogenic approach could be low-dose IFN-α, based on the same rationale for reducing high bFGF expression in life-threatening hemangiomas.

ANGIOGENESIS IN ARTHRITIS

The role of angiogenesis in rheumatoid arthritis and in other forms of arthritis can be most simply conceptualized as two phases: prevascular and vascular. The prevascular phase is analogous to an acute inflammatory state in which the synovium is invaded by inflammatory and immune cells, with macrophages, mast cells, and T cells predominating, among others. These cells may be the source of the angiogenic stimulators found in synovial fluid, which include VEGF, bFGF, IL-8, and hepatocyte growth factor. Activated endothelial cells can also release hepatocyte growth factor. The growth of a neovascular pannus from the synovium begins the vascular phase of arthritis. The vascular pannus can invade and destroy cartilage, a process that is enhanced by the generation of enzymatic activity, mainly metalloproteinases, at the advancing front of new proliferating endothelium. This neovascular pannus overcomes endogenous angiogenesis inhibitors in the cartilage that normally protect it from vascular invasion and maintain its avascularity. These inhibitors include, among others, TIMPs 1, 2, 3 and 4 (ranging from 21 to 29 kDa); thrombospondin-1; and troponin I. Experimental evidence that arthritis is angiogenesis-dependent is based on suppression of rat adjuvant arthritis by an angiogenesis inhibitor, TNP-470 (a synthetic analogue of fumagillin).

This somewhat simplistic model does not do justice to the complexity of the angiogenic response in arthritis, which is beyond the scope of this chapter. Nevertheless, it provides a platform to think about antiangiogenic therapy of arthritis. In principle, inhibition of neovascularization in the joint should interrupt a conduit for continuous traffic of inflammatory cells into the joint and prevent destruction of cartilage. The COX 2 inhibitors currently in wide use for arthritis have been found to be potent angiogenesis inhibitors capable of inhibiting tumor growth in mice. Other angiogenesis inhibitors currently in clinical trial for cancer may eventually also find use in antiarthritis therapy. An interesting potential candidate would be 2-methoxyestradiol.

ANGIOGENESIS IN GYNECOLOGIC DISEASE

Angiogenesis in the female reproductive tract is being actively studied because it is the principal example of physiologic angiogenesis. Angiogenesis in the ovarian follicle is driven mainly by bFGF and VEGF although other angiogenic regulatory molecules are being studied. However, while VEGF is known to be upregulated by estrogen, it is not clear whether endogenous angiogenesis inhibitors operate in combination with declining estrogen to turn off angiogenesis in the ovarian follicle. When angiogenesis is increased in any one follicle, it is suppressed in all other follicles. This is analogous to the suppression of angiogenesis in distant metastases by a primary tumor, but it is not known if the ovarian system utilizes similar endogenous inhibitors as have been discovered in various tumor systems.

A variety of diseases of the female reproductive tract are based on angiogenic processes. A few of these are mentioned here briefly to illustrate that similar molecules mediate angiogenesis in tumors and in gynecologic disease, although they may be regulated differently.

Endometriosis   In this disease, endometrial glands or stroma are present outside the uterine cavity, e.g., in the ovaries, uterine ligaments, rectovaginal septum, and pelvic peritoneum. The foci of endometrium are usually under the control of the ovarian hormones and undergo cyclic menstrual changes with periodic bleeding, which is painful and may lead to fibrosis. At least one angiogenic protein, VEGF, is known to mediate the neovascularization in these lesions. VEGF is upregulated by increased estrogen and downregulated by withdrawal of estrogen. It has been suggested that endometriotic tissue may produce its own estrogen because it contains aromatase cytochrome P450, not found in normal endometrium. Approximately 780,000 women in the United States suffer from endometriosis. No clinical trials of angiogenesis inhibitors for endometriosis are currently under way, but this class of drugs holds promise as an additional treatment of endometriosis, perhaps on a monthly basis. At least three angiogenesis inhibitors are produced in the female reproductive system: 2-methoxyestradiol, proliferin-related protein, and a 16-kDa fragment of prolactin. It would be of interest to know if any of these would be therapeutic for endometriosis.

Other Pathology   Angiogenesis may be increased in dysfunctional uterine bleeding such as breakthrough bleeding from contraceptives. The edema and ascites of the ovarian hyperstimulation syndrome is thought to be mediated by the ability of VEGF to increase vascular permeability. Preeclampsia during pregnancy may be related to abnormal vascular remodeling, although it is not clear how the hypertension and cerebral edema associated with this disease are mediated by an endothelial cell product.

Carcinoma of the Ovary, Endometrium, and Cervix   These common gynecologic tumors are all angiogenesis-dependent. As a result, they share certain characteristics discussed under "Neoplastic Disease," above. Microvessel density in histologic sections provides independent prognostic indicators of metastatic risk and/or mortality. VEGF is a major angiogenic mediator in these tumors. The ascites in ovarian carcinoma contains concentrations of VEGF of up to 100 times higher than those in serum in the same patient. Endometrial carcinoma, which can be induced by long-term tamoxifen therapy, may operate through upregulation of IL-8 in the endometrium. The potential value of angiogenesis inhibitors in the treatment of gynecologic tumors refractory to conventional therapy is suggested by two reports: (1) experimental ovarian cancer was inhibited by administration of angiostatin and endostatin, which acted synergistically; and (2) malignant ascites and growth of human ovarian cancer were inhibited in experimental animals by inhibiting a receptor for VEGF.

ANGIOGENESIS IN CARDIOVASCULAR DISEASE

Angiogenesis in the cardiovascular system occurs under three different conditions: (1) neovascularization in atherosclerotic plaques, (2) formation of collateral vessels to an area of ischemic myocardium or ischemic muscle in a limb, and (3) neovascularization at the edges of a myocardial infarction during its repair.

Angiogenesis in Atherosclerotic Plaques   Angiogenesis occurs in atherosclerotic plaques, and hypoxia is thought to be a major stimulus. The mediators of angiogenesis found in most plaques are bFGF, VEGF, transforming growth factor β (TGF-β), and PDGF-BB. Smooth-muscle cells in plaques are a source of VEGF and PDGF-BB. Macrophages, mast cells, and T cells, which are also found to infiltrate plaques, can produce bFGF and TGF-β. However, the angiogenic factor(s) directly responsible for plaque angiogenesis and the sequential order in which these factors act during the evolution of a plaque have not been worked out. The new microvessels in a plaque can be the source of intraplaque microhemorrhage. Furthermore, the production of metalloproteinases at the advancing tips of new microvessels may contribute to plaque rupture.

The evidence that atherosclerotic plaques are angiogenesis-dependent. However, some supporting experimental evidence has been obtained in transgenic mice deficient in the gene for apoliprotein E (ApoE-/-). When these mice are fed a western diet containing 0.15% cholesterol, they develop atherosclerotic plaques in the aorta over 6 months. Early plaques <250 μm thick are not neovascularized. Cells in the center of such a plaque would lie within the oxygen diffusion limit of oxygen arriving from the normal vasa vasorum or from the arterial lumen. However, intense neovascularization occurred as plaques enlarged to >250 μm. When mice were treated during the development of a plaque with either of the angiogenesis inhibitors TNP-470 (a synthetic fumagillin analogue in phase II clinical trial) or endostatin (in phase I clinical trial), total plaque area was reduced by 70% and 85%, respectively. This finding has important clinical implications.

If long-term antiangiogenic therapy inhibits plaque growth or reduces plaque microhemorrhage or rupture, then it will be important to document this in cancer patients who are receiving angiogenesis inhibitors over a period of ≥ 1 to 2 years. Furthermore, if antiangiogenic therapy blocks plaque angiogenesis, plaque growth, bleeding, or rupture, would this obviate the need for coronary collateral vessels? If so, then this would remove the theoretical concern that long-term antiangiogenic therapy for cancer might decrease collateral development. Another extenuating circumstance is that collateral vessels in general are thick-walled and coated with smooth muscle. They are less likely to undergo regression during exposure to an angiogenesis inhibitor than the thin-walled endothelial tubes, which are not covered or stabilized by smooth muscle in a tumor bed.

Therapeutic Angiogenesis in Ischemic Vascular Disease   Experimental and clinical attempts to increase angiogenesis in ischemic tissues are very recent and have generally followed two strategies: injection into the ischemic tissue of angiogenic proteins (either VEGF or FGFs) or injection of genetic material that codes for these angiogenic stimulators. The animal data show that it is possible to increase the density of new blood vessels and flow to an ischemic area beyond what can be accomplished by hypoxia defense mechanisms in the body. It is not yet clear how durable the new vessels will be once they are induced in an ischemic tissue. We understand much more about stopping angiogenesis than starting it. However, once the techniques for therapeutic angiogenesis are further developed, the clinical need could be enormous.

FUTURE DIRECTIONS

Many other diseases are dominated by the angiogenic process. These include Crohn's disease, thyroiditis, benign prostatic hypertrophy, glomerulonephritis, ectopic bone formation, keloids, and others. However, they were not included in this chapter because the evidence that they are angiogenesis-dependent is not yet sufficiently compelling.

The diseases that were included *are* more clearly angiogenesis-dependent and serve to illustrate an important direction for the future. Oncologists, dermatologists, ophthalmologists, rheumatologists, gynecologists, and cardiologists are dealing with diseases that appear on the surface to be completely different from each other. Advances in therapy of these diseases are reported at different meetings and in different journals, and the specialists who treat them rarely go to each other's meetings or talk to each other. Nevertheless, all of these diseases are dominated by pathologic angiogenesis. The angiogenesis is driven by a small but similar set of molecules, which are regulated differently in each disease. Furthermore, a new class of drugs, the angiogenesis inhibitors, is becoming available and may permit improvements in therapy for many of these diseases. Thus, angiogenesis is a unifying process that has heuristic value across many medical specialties. The "angiogenesis-dependency" of many diseases, neoplastic and nonneoplastic, is of course not sufficiently quantitative to be called a theory, but it is similar to Stephen Wolfram's definition of a theory as "a compressed package of information, applicable to many cases."

BIBLIOGRAPHY

BROWDER T et al: Antiangiogenic scheduling of chemotherapy improves efficacy against experimental drug-resistant cancer. Cancer Res 60:1878, 2000

CARMELIET P, JAIN RK: Angiogenesis in cancer and other diseases: From genes to function to therapy. Nature, in press, 2000

FOLKMAN J: Tumor angiogenesis, in *Cancer Medicine 5*, JR Holland et al (eds). Hamilton, Ontario, BC Decker, 2000, pp 132–152

GASPARINI G, HARRIS AL: Prognostic significance of tumor vascularity, in *Antiangiogenic Agents in Cancer Therapy*, BA Teicher (ed). Totowa, NJ, Humana Press, 1999, pp 317–319

HANAHAN D, FOLKMAN J: Patterns and emerging mechanisms of the angiogenic switch during tumorigenesis. Cell 86:353, 1996.

———, WEINBERG RA: The hallmarks of cancer. Cell 100:57, 2000

HARACH HR et al: Occult papillary carcinoma of the thyroid. A normal finding in Finland. A systematic autopsy study. Cancer 56:531, 1985

MASFERRER JL et al: Antiangiogenic and antitumor activities of cyclooxygenase-2 inhibitors. Cancer Res 60:1306, 2000

ROHAN RM et al: Genetic heterogeneity of angiogenesis in mice. FASEB J 14:871, 2000

SINGHAL S et al: Antitumor activity of thalidomide in refractory multiple myeloma. N Engl J Med 341:1565, 1999

WEIDNER N et al: Tumor angiogenesis and metastasis—correlation in invasive breast carcinoma. N Engl J Med 324:1, 1991

XU L et al: Inhibition of malignant ascites and growth of human ovarian carcinoma by oral administration of a potent inhibitor of the vascular endothelial growth factor receptor tyrosine kinases. Int J Oncol 16:445, 2000

YOKOYAMA Y et al: Synergy between angiostatin and endostatin: Inhibition of ovarian cancer growth. Cancer Res 60:2190, 2000

84   *Edward A. Sausville, Dan L. Longo*

PRINCIPLES OF CANCER TREATMENT

The goal of cancer treatment is first to eradicate the cancer. If this primary goal cannot be accomplished, the goal of cancer treatment shifts to palliation, the amelioration of symptoms, and preservation of quality of life while striving to extend life. The dictum *primum non nocere* is *not* the guiding principle of cancer therapy. Every cancer treatment has the potential to cause harm, and treatment may be given that produces toxicity with no benefit. The therapeutic index of many interventions is quite narrow, and most treatments are given to the point of toxicity. The guiding principle of cancer treatment is *primum succerrere*, first hasten to help. Radical surgical procedures, large-field hyperfractionated radiation therapy, high-dose chemotherapy, and maximum tolerable doses of cytokines such as interleukin (IL) 2 are all used in certain settings where 100% of the patients will experience toxicity and side effects from the intervention, and only a fraction of the patients will experience benefit. One of the challenges of cancer treatment is to use the various treatment modalities alone and together in a fashion that maximizes the chances for patient benefit.

Cancer treatments are divided into four main groups: surgery, radiation therapy (including photodynamic therapy), chemotherapy (including hormonal therapy), and biologic therapy (including immunotherapy, differentiating agents, and agents targeting cancer cell biology). The modalities are often used in combination, and agents in one category can act by several mechanisms. For example, cancer chemotherapy agents can induce differentiation, and antibodies (a form of immunotherapy) can be used to deliver radiation therapy. Surgery and radiation therapy are considered local treatments, though their effects can influence the behavior of tumor at remote sites. Chemotherapy and biologic therapy are usually systemic treatments.

Cancer behaves in many ways as an organ that regulates its own growth. However, cancers have not set an appropriate limit on how much growth should be permitted. Normal organs and cancers share the property of having a population of cells in cycle and actively renewing and a population of cells not in cycle. In cancers, cells that are not dividing are heterogeneous; some have sustained too much genetic damage to replicate but have defects in their death pathways that permit their survival; some are starving for nutrients and oxygen; and some are reversibly out of cycle poised to be recruited back into cycle and expand if needed. Severely damaged and starving cells are unlikely to kill the patient. The problem is that the cells that are reversibly not in cycle are capable of replenishing tumor cells physically removed or damaged by radiation and chemotherapy.

Tumors follow a Gompertzian growth curve (Fig. 84-1); the growth fraction of a neoplasm starts at 100% with the first transformed cell and declines exponentially over time until by the time of diagnosis at a tumor burden of 1 to 5×10^9 tumor cells, the growth fraction is usually 1 to 4%. Cancers are actually trying to limit their own growth but are not completely successful at doing so. The peak growth rate occurs before the tumor is detectable. Folkman has suggested that tumors restrict their growth by elaborating angiogenesis inhibitors (Chap. 83). Other cellular mechanisms to withdraw cells from the cell cycle probably exist as well. Several observations support the idea of autoregulation of tumor growth. Metastases can be observed to grow more rapidly than the primary tumor, consistent with the idea that an inhibitory factor slows the growth of larger tumor masses. When a tumor recurs after surgery or chemotherapy, frequently its growth is accelerated and the growth fraction of the tumor is increased. This pattern is similar to that seen in regenerating organs. Partial resection of the liver results in the recruitment of cells into the cell cycle, and the resected liver volume is replaced. Similarly, chemotherapy-damaged bone marrow increases its growth to replace cells killed by chemotherapy. However, cancers do not recognize a limit on their expansion. Monoclonal gammopathy of uncertain significance may be an example of a clonal neoplasm with intrinsic features that stop its

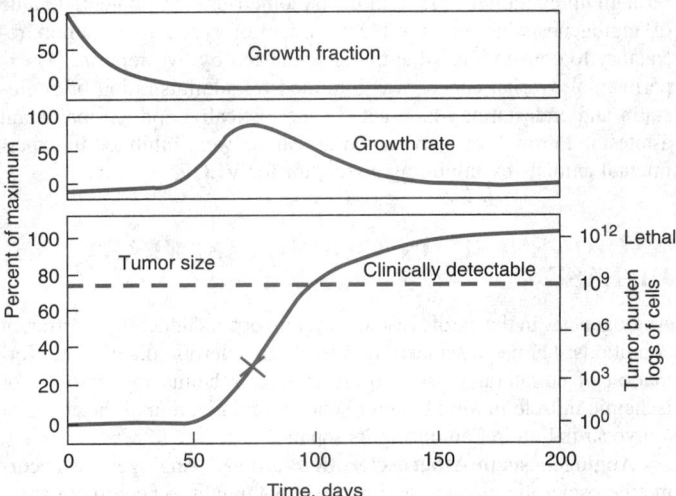

FIGURE 84-1 Gompertzian tumor growth. The growth fraction of a tumor declines exponentially over time (*top*). The growth rate of a tumor peaks before it is clinically detectable (*middle*). Tumor size increases slowly, goes through an exponential phase, and slows again as the tumor reaches the size at which it is attempting to level off. The maximum growth rate occurs at 1/e, the point at which the tumor is about 37% of its maximum size (marked with an X). Tumor becomes detectable at a burden of about 10^9 (1 cm³) and kills the patient at a tumor burden of about 10^{12} (1 kg). Efforts to treat the tumor and reduce its size can result in an increase in the growth fraction and an increase in growth rate.

growth before a lethal tumor burden is reached. A fraction of patients with this disorder go on to develop fatal multiple myeloma, but probably this occurs because of the accumulation of additional genetic lesions. Elucidation of the mechanisms that regulate this organ-like behavior may provide additional clues to cancer control and treatment.

PRINCIPLES OF CANCER SURGERY

Surgery is used in cancer prevention, diagnosis, staging, treatment (for both localized and metastatic disease), palliation, and rehabilitation.

PREVENTION Cancer can be prevented by surgery in people who have premalignant lesions resected (e.g., premalignant lesions of skin, colon, cervix) and in those who are at higher-than-normal risk of cancer from either an underlying disease (colectomy in those with pancolonic involvement with ulcerative colitis), the presence of genetic lesions (familial polyposis—colectomy; multiple endocrine neoplasia type II—thyroidectomy; familial breast or ovarian cancer—mastectomy, oophorectomy), or a developmental anomaly (orchiectomy in those with an undescended testis). In some cases, prophylactic surgery is more radical than the surgical procedures used to treat the cancer after it develops. The assessment of risk involves many factors and should be undertaken with care before advising a patient to undergo a major procedure. For breast cancer prevention, many experts use a 20% risk of developing breast cancer over the next 5 years as a threshold. However, patient fears play a major role in defining candidates for cancer prevention surgery. Counseling and education may not be enough to allay the fears of someone who has lost close family members to a malignancy.

DIAGNOSIS The ideal diagnostic procedure varies with the type of cancer, its anatomic location, and the medical condition of the patient. However, the underlying principle is to obtain as much tissue as safely possible. Tumors may be heterogeneous in appearance. Pathologists are better able to make the diagnosis when they have more tissue to examine. In addition to light-microscopic inspection of a tumor for pattern of growth, degree of cellular atypia, invasiveness, and morphologic features that aid in the differential diagnosis, sufficient tissue is of value in searching for genetic abnormalities and protein expression patterns that may aid in differential diagnosis or provide information about prognosis or likely response to treatment. Such testing requires that the tissue be handled properly (e.g., immunologic detection of proteins is more effective in fresh-frozen tissue rather than in formalin-fixed tissue); thus, coordination among the surgeon, pathologist, and primary care physician is essential to ensure that the amount of information learned from the biopsy material is maximized.

These goals are best met by an *excisional biopsy* in which the entire tumor mass is removed with a small margin of normal tissue surrounding it. If an excisional biopsy cannot be performed, *incisional biopsy* is the procedure of second choice. A wedge of tissue is removed, and an effort is made to include the majority of the cross-sectional diameter of the tumor in the biopsy to minimize sampling error. When the diagnosis is being made through an endoscope or via fluoroscopy, it may be necessary to obtain a *core-needle biopsy* of the mass; considerably less tissue is obtained and the diagnosis may be less certain. However, this procedure often provides enough information to plan a definitive surgical procedure. Least reliable in diagnosis of primary cancer is *fine-needle aspiration*. This technique generally obtains only a suspension of cells from within a mass. This approach (with stereotactic guidance of the needle) is the procedure of choice in the diagnosis of brain tumors and may be useful in diagnosing thyroid nodules and in confirming persistent or recurrent disease in a patient with known cancer, but the procedure is overutilized in primary diagnosis. It would be preferable to perform a larger open operation to obtain more tissue in most sites. The biopsy techniques that involve cutting into tumor carry with them a risk of facilitating the spread of the tumor.

STAGING As noted in Chap. 79, an important component of patient management is defining the extent of disease. Radiographic and other imaging tests can be helpful in defining the clinical stage; however, pathologic staging requires defining the extent of involvement by documenting the histologic presence of tumor in tissue biopsies obtained through a surgical procedure. Axillary lymph node sampling in breast cancer and lymph node sampling at laparotomy for lymphomas and testicular, colon, and other intraabdominal cancers provide crucial information for treatment planning and may determine the extent and nature of primary cancer treatment.

TREATMENT Surgery is perhaps the most effective means of treating cancer. About 40% of cancer patients are cured today by surgery. Unfortunately, a large fraction of patients with solid tumors (perhaps 60%) have metastatic disease that is not accessible for removal. However, even when the disease is not curable by surgery alone, the removal of tumor can obtain important benefits, including local control of tumor, preservation of organ function, debulking that permits subsequent therapy to work better, and staging information on extent of involvement. Cancer surgery aiming for cure is usually planned to excise the tumor completely with an adequate margin of normal tissue (the margin varies with the tumor and the anatomy), touching the tumor as little as possible to prevent vascular and lymphatic spread, and minimizing operative risk. Extending the procedure to resect draining lymph nodes obtains prognostic information, but such resections alone generally do not improve survival.

Increasingly, laparoscopic approaches are being taken to the primary tumor. Lymph node spread may be assessed using the *sentinel node approach*, in which the first draining lymph node a tumor would encounter is defined by injecting a dye at operation and resecting the first node to turn blue. The sentinel node evaluation is continuing to undergo clinical testing but appears to provide reliable information without the risks (lymphedema, lymphangiosarcoma) associated with resection of all the regional nodes. Advances in adjuvant chemotherapy and radiation therapy following surgery have permitted a substantial decrease in the extent of primary surgery necessary to obtain the best outcomes. Thus, lumpectomy with radiation therapy is as effective as modified radical mastectomy for breast cancer, and limb-sparing surgery followed by adjuvant radiation therapy and chemotherapy has replaced radical primary surgical procedures involving amputation and disarticulation for childhood rhabdomyosarcomas. More limited surgery is also being employed to spare organ function, as in larynx and bladder cancer. The magnitude of operations necessary to optimally control and cure cancer has also been diminished by technical advances; for example, the circular anastomotic stapler has allowed narrower (<2 cm) margins in colon cancer without compromise of local control rates, and many patients who would have had colostomies are able to maintain normal anatomy.

In some settings, e.g., bulky testicular cancer or stage III breast cancer, surgery is not the first treatment modality employed. After an initial diagnostic biopsy, chemotherapy and/or radiation therapy are delivered to reduce the size of the tumor and control clinically undetected metastatic disease, and such therapy is followed by a surgical procedure to remove residual masses. This is called *neoadjuvant therapy*. Because the sequence of treatment is critical to success and is different from the standard surgery-first approach, coordination among the surgical oncologist, radiation oncologist, and medical oncologist is crucial.

Surgery may be curative in a subset of patients with metastatic disease. Patients with lung metastases from osteosarcoma may be cured by resection of the lung lesions. In patients with colon cancer who have fewer than five liver metastases restricted to one lobe and no extrahepatic metastases, hepatic lobectomy may produce long-term disease-free survival in 25% of selected patients. Surgery can also be associated with systemic antitumor effects. In the setting of hormonally responsive tumors, oophorectomy and/or adrenalectomy may control estrogen production and orchiectomy may reduce androgen production, both with effects on metastatic tumor growth. If resection of the primary lesion takes place in the presence of metastases, any noted change in tumor behavior is most often acceleration of growth, perhaps based on the removal of a source of angiogenesis inhibitors and mass-related growth regulators in the tumor. However, on rare occasions (certain renal cancers), primary tumor resection is accompanied by regression of metastatic lesions. Similarly, splenectomy in some cases of lymphoma may be associated with regression of disease at remote sites. This phenomenon is attributed to the removal of a source of growth or angiogenic factors upon which the remote sites depend for growth.

PALLIATION　Surgery is employed in a number of ways for supportive care: insertion of central venous catheters, diagnostic evaluation of pulmonary infiltrates, control of pleural and pericardial effusions and ascites, caval interruption for recurrent pulmonary emboli, stabilization of cancer-weakened weight-bearing bones, and control of hemorrhage, among others. Surgical bypass of gastrointestinal, urinary tract, or biliary tree obstruction can alleviate symptoms and prolong survival. Surgical procedures may provide relief of otherwise intractable pain or reverse neurologic dysfunction (cord decompression). Splenectomy may relieve symptoms and reverse hypersplenism. Intrathecal or intrahepatic therapy relies on surgical placement of appropriate infusion portals. Surgery may correct other treatment-related toxicities such as adhesions or strictures.

REHABILITATION　Surgical procedures are also valuable in restoring a cancer patient to full health. Orthopedic procedures may be necessary to assure proper ambulation. Breast reconstruction can make an enormous impact on the patient's perception of successful therapy. Plastic and reconstructive surgery can correct the effects of disfiguring primary treatment.

PRINCIPLES OF RADIATION THERAPY

PHYSICAL PROPERTIES AND BIOLOGIC EFFECTS
Radiation therapy is a physical form of treatment that damages any tissue in its path. Tumor cells seem somewhat more sensitive to the lethal effects of radiation than normal tissues primarily because of differences in ability to repair sublethal DNA and other damage. In the target tissue, radiation damages DNA (usually single strand breaks) and generates free radicals from cell water that are capable of damaging cell membranes, proteins, and organelles. Radiation damage is dependent on oxygen; hypoxic cells are more resistant. Augmentation of oxygen is the basis for radiation sensitization. Sulfhydryl compounds interfere with free radical generation and may act as radiation protectors. The challenge for radiation treatment planning is to deliver the radiation to the tumor volume with as little normal tissue in the field as possible. →*Principles of radiation injury are discussed in Chap. 394.*

Therapeutic radiation is delivered in three ways: teletherapy with beams of radiation generated at a distance and aimed at the tumor within the patient, brachytherapy with encapsulated sources of radiation implanted directly into or adjacent to tumor tissues, and systemic therapy with radionuclides targeted in some fashion to a site of tumor. Teletherapy is the most commonly used form of radiation therapy.

Radiation from any source decreases in intensity as a function of the square of the distance from the source (inverse square law). Thus, if the radiation source is 5 cm above the skin surface and the tumor is 5 cm below the skin surface, the intensity of radiation in the tumor will be $5^2/10^2$, or 25% of the intensity at the skin. By contrast, if the radiation source is moved to 100 cm from the patient, the intensity of radiation in the tumor will be $100^2/105^2$, or 91% of the intensity at the skin. Teletherapy maintains intensity over a larger volume of target tissue by increasing the source-to-surface distance. In brachytherapy, the source-to-surface distance is small; thus, the effective treatment volume is small.

X-rays and *gamma rays* are the forms of radiation most commonly used to treat cancer. They are both electromagnetic, nonparticulate waves that cause the ejection of an orbital electron when absorbed. This orbital electron ejection is called *ionization*. X-rays are generated by linear accelerators; gamma rays are generated from decay of atomic nuclei in radioisotopes such as cobalt and radium. These waves behave biologically as packets of energy, called *photons*. Particulate forms of radiation are also used in certain circumstances. Electron beams have a very low tissue penetrance and are used to treat skin conditions such as mycosis fungoides. Neutron beams may be somewhat more effective than x-rays in treating salivary gland tumors. However, aside from these specialized uses, particulate forms of radiation such as neutrons, protons, and negative π mesons, which should do more tissue damage because of their higher linear energy transfer (LET) and be less dependent on oxygen, have not yet found wide applicability to cancer treatment.

A number of parameters influence the damage done to tissue by radiation. Hypoxic cells are relatively resistant. Nondividing cells are more resistant than dividing cells. In addition to these biologic parameters, physical parameters of the radiation are also crucial. The *energy* of the radiation determines its ability to penetrate tissue. Low-energy orthovoltage beams (150 to 400 kV) scatter when they strike the body, much like light diffuses when it strikes particles in the air. Such beams result in more damage to adjacent normal tissues and less radiation delivered to the tumor. Megavoltage radiation (≥ 1 MeV) has very low lateral scatter; this produces a skin-sparing effect, more homogeneous distribution of the radiation energy, and greater deposit of the energy in the tumor, or *target volume*. The tissues that the beam passes through to get to the tumor is called the *transit volume*. The maximum dose in the target volume is often the cause of complications to tissues in the transit volume, and the minimum dose in the target volume influences the likelihood of tumor recurrence. Dose homogeneity in the target volume is the goal.

Radiation is quantitated on the basis of the amount of radiation absorbed in the patient, not based upon the amount of radiation generated by the machine. A rad (radiation absorbed dose) is 100 ergs of energy per gram of tissue; a gray (Gy) is 100 rad. Radiation dose is measured by placing detectors at the body surface or calculating the dose based on radiating phantoms that resemble human form and substance. Radiation dose has three determinants: total absorbed dose, number of fractions, and time. A frequent error is to omit the number of fractions and the duration of treatment. This is analogous to saying that a runner completed a race in 20 s; without knowing how far he or she ran, the result is difficult to interpret. The time could be very good for a 200-m race or very poor for a 100-m race. Thus, a typical course of radiation therapy should be described as 4500 cGy delivered to a particular target (e.g., mediastinum) over 5 weeks in 180-cGy fractions. Most radiation treatment programs are delivered once a day, 5 days a week in 150- to 200-cGy fractions.

The killing of tumor cells in vivo by radiation is described in detail in Chap. 394. Although radiation can interfere with many cellular processes, many experts feel that a cell must undergo a double-stranded DNA break from radiation in order to be killed. The factors that influence tumor cell killing include the D_0 of the tumor (the dose required to deliver an average of one lethal hit to all the cells in a population), the D_q of the tumor (the threshold dose—a measure of the cell's ability to repair sublethal damage), hypoxia, tumor mass, growth fraction, and cell cycle time and phase (cells in late G_1 and S are more resistant). Rate of clinical response is not predictive; some cells do not die after radiation exposure until they attempt to replicate.

Compounds that incorporate into DNA and alter its stereochemistry (e.g., halogenated pyrimidines, cisplatin) augment radiation effects. Hydroxyurea, another DNA synthesis inhibitor, also potentiates radiation effects. Compounds that deplete thiols (e.g., buthionine sulfoximine) can also augment radiation effects. Hypoxia is the main factor that interferes with radiation effects.

APPLICATION TO PATIENTS　Radiation therapy can be used alone or together with chemotherapy to produce cure of localized tumors and control of the primary site of disease in tumors that have disseminated. Therapy is planned based on the use of a simulator with the treatment field or fields designed to accommodate an individual patient's anatomic features. Individualized treatment planning employs lead shielding tailored to shape the field and limit the radiation exposure of normal tissue. Often the radiation is delivered from two or three different positions. Conformal three-dimensional treatment planning is permitting the delivery of higher doses of radiation to the target volume without increasing complications in the transit volume.

Radiation therapy is a component of curative therapy for a number of diseases including breast cancer, Hodgkin's disease, head and neck cancer, prostate cancer, and gynecologic cancers. Radiation therapy can also palliate disease symptoms in a variety of settings: relief of bone pain from metastatic disease, control of brain metastases, reversal of cord compression and superior vena caval obstruction, shrinkage of painful masses, and opening threatened airways. In high-risk settings, radiation therapy can prevent the development of leptomeningeal disease and brain metastases in acute leukemia and lung cancer.

Brachytherapy involves placing a sealed source of radiation into or adjacent to the tumor and withdrawing the radiation source after a period of time precisely calculated to deliver a chosen dose of radiation to the tumor. This approach is often used to treat brain tumors and cervical cancer. The difficulty with brachytherapy is the short range of radiation effects (the inverse square law) and the inability to shape the radiation to fit the target volume. Normal tissue may receive substantial exposure to the radiation, with attendant radiation enteritis or cystitis in cervix cancer or brain injury in brain tumors.

TOXICITY Though radiation therapy is most often administered to a local region, systemic effects, including fatigue, anorexia, nausea, and vomiting, may develop related in part to the volume of tissue irradiated, dose fractionation, radiation fields, and individual susceptibility. Bone is among the most radioresistant organs, radiation effects being manifested mainly in children through premature fusion of the epiphyseal growth plate. By contrast, the male testis, female ovary, and bone marrow are the most sensitive organs. Any bone marrow in a radiation field will be eradicated by therapeutic irradiation. Organs with less need for cell renewal, such as heart, skeletal muscle, and nerves, are more resistant to radiation effects. In radiation-resistant organs, the vascular endothelium is the most sensitive component. Organs with more self-renewal as a part of normal homeostasis, such as the hematopoietic system and mucosal lining of the intestinal tract, are more sensitive. Acute toxicities include mucositis, skin erythema (ulceration in severe cases), and bone marrow toxicity. Often these can be alleviated by interruption of treatment.

Chronic toxicities are more serious. Radiation of the head and neck region usually produces thyroid failure. Cataracts and retinal damage can lead to blindness. Salivary glands stop making saliva, which leads to dental carries and poor dentition. Taste and smell can be affected. Mediastinal irradiation leads to a threefold increased risk of *fatal* myocardial infarction. Other late vascular effects include chronic constrictive pericarditis, lung fibrosis, viscus stricture, spinal cord transection, and radiation enteritis. The most serious late toxicity is the development of second solid tumors in or adjacent to the radiation fields. Such tumors can develop in any organ or tissue and occur at a rate of about 1% per year beginning in the second decade after treatment. Some organs vary in susceptibility to radiation carcinogenesis. Women under age 30 experience a 100-fold or greater increase in the incidence of breast cancer after chest or mantle field radiation; women treated after age 30 have little or no increased risk of breast cancer. No data suggest that a threshold dose of therapeutic radiation exists below which the incidence of second cancers is decreased. High rates of second tumors have been documented in people who received as little as 1000 cGy.

RADIONUCLIDES AND RADIOIMMUNOTHERAPY Nuclear medicine physicians or radiation oncologists may administer radionuclides with therapeutic effects. Iodine-131 is used to treat thyroid cancer as iodine is naturally taken up preferentially by the thyroid. It emits gamma rays that destroy the normal thyroid as well as the tumor. Strontium-89 and samarium-153 are two radionuclides that are preferentially taken up in bone, particularly sites of new bone formation. Both are capable of controlling bone metastases and the pain associated with them, but the dose-limiting toxicity is myelosuppression.

Monoclonal antibodies and other ligands can be attached to radioisotopes by conjugation (for nonmetal isotopes) or by chelation (for metal isotopes), and the targeting moiety can result in the accumulation of the radionuclide preferentially in tumor. Iodine-131-labeled anti-CD20 and yttrium-90-labeled anti-CD20 are active in B cell lymphoma, and other labeled antibodies are being evaluated. Thyroid uptake of labeled iodine is blocked by cold iodine. Dose-limiting toxicity is myelosuppression.

PHOTODYNAMIC THERAPY Some chemical structures (porphyrins, phthalocyanines) are selectively taken up by cancer cells by mechanisms not fully defined. When light, usually delivered by laser, is shone on cells containing these compounds, free radicals are generated and the cells die. Hematoporphyrins and light are being used with increasing frequency to treat skin cancer; ovarian cancer; and cancers of the lung, colon, rectum, and esophagus. Palliation of recurrent locally advanced disease can sometimes be dramatic and last many months.

PRINCIPLES OF CHEMOTHERAPY

HISTORIC BACKGROUND The treatment of patients with cancer using chemicals in the hope of causing regressions of established tumors or to slow the rate of tumor growth arose by analogy to the proposition of Ehrlich that bacteria could be killed selectively by compounds acting as "magic bullets." Candidate compounds that might have selectivity for cancer cells were suggested by the marrow-toxic effects of sulfur and nitrogen mustards and led, in the 1940s, to the first notable regressions of hematopoietic tumors following use of these compounds by Gilman and colleagues. As these compounds caused covalent modification of DNA, the structure of DNA was thereby identified as a potential target for drug design efforts. Biochemical studies demonstrating the requirement of growing tumor cells for precursors of nucleic acids led to nearly contemporaneous studies by Farber of folate analogues. The cure of patients with advanced choriocarcinoma by methotrexate in the 1950s provided further impetus to define the value of chemotherapeutic agents in many different tumor types. This resulted in efforts to understand unique metabolic requirements for biosynthesis of nucelic acids and led to the design, rational for the time, of compounds that might selectively interdict DNA synthesis in proliferating cancer cells. The capacity of hormonal manipulations including oophorectomy and orchiectomy to cause regressions of breast and prostate cancers, respectively, provided a rationale for efforts to interdict various aspects of hormone function in hormone-dependent tumors. The serendipitous finding that certain poisons derived from bacteria or plants could affect normal DNA or mitotic spindle function allowed completion of the classic armamentatrium of "cancer chemotherapy agents" with proven safety and efficacy in the treatment of certain cancers.

END-POINTS OF DRUG ACTION Chemotherapy agents may be used for the treatment of active, clinically apparent cancer. Table 84-1A lists those tumors considered curable by conventionally available chemotherapeutic agents. Most commonly, chemotherapeutic agents are used to address metastatic cancers. If a tumor is localized to a single site, serious consideration of surgery or primary radiation therapy should be given, as these treatment modalities may be curative as local treatments. Chemotherapy may be employed after the failure of these modalities to eradicate a local tumor, or as part of multimodality approaches to offer primary treatment to a clinically localized tumor. In this event, it can allow *organ preservation* when given with radiation, as in larynx or other upper airway sites; or sensitize tumors to radiation when given, for example, to patients concurrently receiving radiation for lung or cervix cancer (Table 84-1B). Chemotherapy can be administered as an *adjuvant* to surgery (Table 84-1C) or radiation, a use that may have curative potential in breast, colon, or anorectal neoplasms. In this use, chemotherapy attempts to eliminate clinically unapparent tumor that may have already disseminated.

Table 84-1 Curability of Cancers with Chemotherapy

A. Advanced cancers with possible cure
Acute lymphoid and acute myeloid leukemia (pediatric/adult)
Hodgkin's disease (pediatric/adult)
Lymphomas—certain types (pediatric/adult)
Germ cell neoplasms
  Embryonal carcinoma
  Teratocarcinoma
  Seminoma or dysgerminoma
  Choriocarcinoma
Gestational trophoblastic neoplasia
Pediatric neoplasms
  Wilm's tumor
  Embryonal rhabdomyocarcinoma
  Ewing's sarcoma
  Peripheral neuroepithelioma
  Neuroblastoma
Small cell lung carcinoma
Ovarian carcinoma

B. Advanced cancers possibly cured by chemotherapy and radiation
Squamous carcinoma (head and neck)
Squamous carcinoma (anus)
Breast carcinoma
Carcinoma of the uterine cervix
Non-small cell lung carcinoma (stage III)
Small cell lung carcinoma

C. Cancers possibly cured with chemotherapy as adjuvant to surgery
Breast carcinoma
Colorectal carcinoma[a]
Osteogenic sarcoma
Soft tissue sarcoma

D. Cancers possibly cured with "high-dose" chemotherapy with stem cell support
Relapsed leukemias, lymphoid and myeloid
Relapsed lymphomas, Hodgkin's and non-Hodgkin's
Chronic myeloid leukemia
Multiple myeloma

E. Cancers responsive with useful palliation, but not cure, by chemotherapy
Bladder carcinoma
Chronic myeloid leukemia
Hairy cell leukemia
Chronic lymphocytic leukemia
Lymphoma—certain types
Multiple myeloma
Gastric carcinoma
Cervix carcinoma
Endometrial carcinoma
Soft tissue sarcoma
Head and neck cancer
Adrenocortical carcinoma
Islet-cell neoplasms
Breast carcinoma

F. Tumor poorly responsive in advanced stages to chemotherapy
Pancreatic carcinoma
Biliary-tract neoplasms
Renal carcinoma
Thyroid carcinoma
Carcinoma of the vulva
Colorectal carcinoma
Non-small cell lung carcinoma
Prostate carcinoma
Melanoma
Hepatocellular carcinoma

[a] Rectum also receives radiation therapy.

Chemotherapy can be used in *conventional dose* regimens. In general, these doses produce reversible acute side effects primarily consisting of transient myelosuppression with or without gastrointestinal toxicity (nausea), which are readily managed. *High-dose* chemotherapy regimens are predicated on the observation that the concentration-effect curve for many anticancer agents is rather steep, and increased dose can produce markedly increased therapeutic effect, although at the cost of potentially life-threatening complications that require intensive support, usually in the form of bone marrow or stem cell support from the patient (*autologous*) or from donors matched for histocompatibility loci (*allogeneic*). High-dose regimens nonetheless have definite curative potential in defined clinical settings (Table 84-1D).

Karnofsky was among the first to champion the evaluation of a chemotherapeutic agent's benefit by carefully quantitating its effect on tumor size and using these measurements to decide objectively the basis for further treatment of a particular patient or further clinical evaluation of a drug's potential. A partial response (PR) is defined conventionally as a decrease by at least 50% in a tumor's bi-dimensional area; a complete response (CR) connotes disappearance of all tumor; progression of disease signifies increase by >25% from baseline or best response; and "stable" disease fits into none of the above categories.

If cure is not possible, chemotherapy may be undertaken with the goal of palliating some aspect of the tumor's effect on the host. Common tumors that may be meaningfully addressed with palliative intent

are listed in Table 84-1E. Usually tumor-related symptoms may manifest as pain, weight loss, or some local symptom related to the tumor's effect on normal structures. Patients treated with palliative intent should be aware of their diagnosis and the limitations of the proposed treatment, have access to suitable palliative strategies in the event that no treatment is elected, and have a suitable "performance status" [according to assessment algorithms such as the one developed by Karnofsky or by the Eastern Cooperative Oncology Group (ECOG)]. ECOG performance status 0 (PS0) patients are without symptoms; PS1 patients have mild symptoms not requiring treatment; PS2, symptoms requiring some treatment; PS3, disabling symptoms, but allowing ambulation for >50% of the day; PS4, ambulation <50% of the day. Only PS0 to PS2 patients are generally considered suitable for palliative (noncurative) treatment. If there is curative potential, even poor performance status patients may be treated, but their prognosis is usually inferior to those of good performance patients treated with similar regimens.

PATH FOR NEW DRUG DISCOVERY AND DEVELOPMENT The usefulness of any drug is governed by the extent to which a given dose causes a useful result (therapeutic effect; in the case of anticancer agents, toxicity to tumor cells) as opposed to a toxic effect. The therapeutic index is the degree of separation between toxic and therapeutic doses. Really useful drugs have large therapeutic indices, and this usually occurs when the drug target is expressed in the disease-causing compartment as opposed to the normal compartment. Classically, selective toxicity of an agent for an organ is governed by the expression of an agent's target; or differential accumulation into or elimination from compartments where toxicity is experienced or ameliorated, respectively. Current antineoplastic agents have the unfortunate property that their targets are present in both normal and tumor tissues. In the main they therefore have relatively narrow therapeutic indices.

Agents with promise for the treatment of cancer have in the past been detected empirically through screening for antiproliferative effects in animal or human tumors in rodent hosts or through inhibition of tumor cells growing in tissue culture. An optimal schedule for demonstrating antitumor activity in animals is defined in further preclinical studies, as is the optimal drug formulation for a given route and schedule. Safety testing in two species on an analogous schedule of administration defines the starting dose for a phase I trial in humans, where escalating doses of the drug are given until reversible toxicity is observed. *Dose-limiting toxicity* (DLT) defines a dose that conveys greater toxicity than would be acceptable in routine practice, allowing definition of a *maximal tolerated dose* (MTD). The occurrence of toxicity is correlated if possible with plasma drug concentrations. The MTD or a dose just lower than the MTD is usually the dose suitable for phase II trials, where a fixed dose is administered to a relatively homogeneous set of patients in an effort to define whether the drug causes regression of tumors. An "active" agent conventionally has partial response rates of at least 20 to 25% with reversible non-life-threatening side effects, and it may then be suitable for study in phase III trials to assess efficacy in comparison to standard or no therapy. Response is but the most immediate indicator of drug effect. To be clinically valuable, responses must translate into effects on *overall survival* or at least *time to progression* as important indicators of an ultimately useful drug. More recently, active efforts to quantitate effects of anticancer agents on *quality of life* as an important outcome are being developed. Cancer drug clinical trials conventionally use a toxicity grading scale where grade I toxicities do not require treatment; grade II often require symptomatic treatment but are not life-threatening; grade III toxicities are potentially life-threatening if untreated; grade IV toxicities are actually life-threatening; and grade V toxicities ultimately lead to patient death.

The process of cancer drug development is likely to evolve in significant ways in the near future as (1) the molecular analysis of human tumors defines more precisely the molecular targets that can be the focus of drug discovery efforts, and (2) clinical trials are undertaken only after means of assessing the behavior of the drug in relation to its target have been developed. The basis for optimism and anticipated change in clinical trials methodology extends from emerging understanding of the basis for cancer incidence and progression. Cancer arises from genetic lesions that cause an excess of cell growth or division, with inadequate cell death (Chap. 82). In addition, failure of cellular differentiation results in altered cellular position and capacity to proliferate while cut off from normal cell regulatory signals. An overall schema for understanding cancer progression can be seen in Fig. 84-2. Normally, cells in a differentiated state are stimulated to enter the cell cycle from a quiescent state, or "G0," or continue after completion of a prior cell division cycle in response to environmental cues including growth factor and hormonal signals. Cells progress through G1 and enter S phase after passing through "checkpoints," which are biochemically regulated transition points, to assure that the genome is ready for replication. One important checkpoint is mediated by the p53 tumor-suppressor gene product, acting through its upregulation of the p21^{WAF1} inhibitor of cyclin-dependent kinase (CDK) function, acting on CDKs 4 or 6. These molecules can also be inhibited by the p16^{INK4A} and p27^{KIP1} CDK inhibitors and, in turn, are activated by cyclins of the D family (which appear during G1) and the proper sequence of regulatory phosphorylations. Activated CDKs 4 or 6 phosphorylate and thus inactivate the product of the retinoblastoma susceptibility gene, pRb, which in its nonphosphorylated state complexes with transcription factors of the E2F family. Phosphorylated pRb re-

leases E2Fs, which activate genes important in completing DNA replication during S phase, progression through which is promoted by CDK2 acting in concert with cylins A and E. During G2, another checkpoint occurs, in which the cell assures the completion of correct DNA synthesis. Cells then progress into M phase under the influence of CDK1 and cyclin B. Cells may then go on to a subsequent division cycle or enter into a quiescent, differentiated state.

Also shown in Fig. 84-2 are the sites of action of protooncogenes, regulators of cellular proliferation that, in an active state, promote cell growth, and whose deregulation produces oncogenes, originally discovered as the genes encoded by tumor-forming viruses in animals. Oncogenes can be divided into two families: (1) those that act in the cytoplasm to disrupt normal growth factor–related signaling, including *ras, raf,* and the tyrosine kinases of the *src* and *erb*B or *sis* families; and (2) nuclear oncogenes, including *jun, fos, myc,* and *myb,* that act to alter transcriptional control of cassettes of genes. In contrast, tumor-suppressor genes, including p53 and pRb, act as cellular "brakes" whose normal function is to inhibit or prevent unregulated cellular growth. The capacity to divide indefinitely is provided by activation of *telomerase,* which allows continued replication of chromosomes by addressing the unique need of chromosome ends to be continually renewed to a proper length to allow normal mitosis. The capacity to invade and metastasize is conveyed by elaboration of *matrix metalloproteases* and *plasminogen activators* and the capacity to recruit host stromal cells at the site of invasion through tumor-induced *angiogenesis.*

As will become apparent below, currently used drugs for the treatment of cancer focus principally on the proximate biochemistry of nucleic acid and mitotic spindle structure or function. Drugs of the future may seek to replace lost function of tumor-suppressor genes; counter the action of activated oncogenes; influence the capacity of cells to die; prevent normal chromosomal end replication; actually infect cells with viruses designed to replicate in the milieu of the cancer but not the normal cell; cause differentiation of cells with exit from the cell cycle by activating the appropriate genes; and utilize immunologic strategies, including antibodies and engineered cells to be directed at novel proteins expressed on the surface of cancer cells.

BIOLOGIC BASIS FOR CANCER CHEMOTHERAPY

The classic view of how cancer chemotherapeutic agents cause regressions of tumors focused on models such as the L1210 murine leukemia system, where cancer cells grow exponentially after inoculation into the peritoneal cavity of an isogenic mouse. The interaction of drug with its biochemical target in the cancer cell was proposed to result in "unbalanced growth" that was not sustainable and therefore resulted in cell death, directly as a result of interacting with the drug's proximal target. Agents could be categorized (Fig. 84-3) as cell cycle–active, phase-specific (e.g., antimetabolites, purines, and pyrimidines in S phase; vinca alkaloids in M), and phase-nonspecific agents (e.g., alkylators, and antitumor antibiotics including the anthracyclines, actinomycin, and mitomycin), which can injure DNA at any phase of the cell cycle but appear to then block in G2 before cell division at a checkpoint in the cell cycle. Cells arrested at a checkpoint may repair DNA lesions. Checkpoints have been defined at the G1 to S transition, mediated by the tumor-suppressor gene p53 (giving rise to the characterization of p53 as a "guardian of the genome"); at the G2 to M transition, mediated by the *chk1* kinase influencing the function of CDK1; and during M phase, to ensure the integrity of the mitotic spindle. The importance of the concept of checkpoints extends from the hypothesis that repair of chemotherapy-mediated damage can occur while cells are stopped at a checkpoint; therefore, manipulation of checkpoint function emerges as an important basis of affecting resistance to chemotherapeutic agents.

Resistance to drugs was postulated to arise either from cells not being in the appropriate phase of the cell cycle or from decreased uptake, increased efflux, metabolism of the drug, or alteration of the target, e.g., by mutation or overexpression. Indeed, the *p170PGP*

FIGURE 84-2 Basis for neoplastic growth and progression. Normally cells are stimulated to enter a proliferating state through the action of growth factors, positional signals, or cytokines. Cells enter G1 under the influence of normal signaling pathways including tyrosine kinase receptors coupled to ras protooncogenes or seven-transmembrane receptors coupled through heterotrimeric guanine nucleotide binding (G) proteins, especially G$_q$ linked to calcium- and lipid-mediated signaling pathways through protein kinase C (PKC). Cells activate transcription and translation of key regulatory molecules such as the cyclins, which activate cyclin-dependent kinases (CDKs) 4 or 6. Phosphorylation of the retinoblastoma susceptibility protein (pRb) causes release of E2F transcription factors to an active state, promoting the transcription of multiple genes allowing progression through S phase, where DNA is replicated. Tumor cells possess activated oncogenes such as *erb*B1, *erb*B2, and *sis* or mutated *ras* gene products that are tonically activated, thus driving proliferation autonomously. *Raf* and the mitogen-activated kinases, MAPKK and MAPK, amplify the growth signal in a kinase cascade. "Brakes" to cell cycle progression include the p53-mediated G1 to S phase checkpoint, mediated by the CDK inhibitors p16INK4a and p21WAF1. Progression through S phase is also promoted by CDK2 acting in concert with cyclins E and A, and initiation of cell division is governed by the action of CDK1 acting in concert with cyclin B.

FIGURE 84-3 Location of drug action in the cell cycle. Cancer chemotherapy agents can be broadly described as phase-specific agents acting in S (antimetabolites) and M (spindle poisons) phase, respectively, and phase-nonspecific agents that injure their targets throughout the cycle but cause arrest of cell cycle progression at "checkpoints." The G1 checkpoint is mediated through p53 acting on CDKs 4,6, and 2, and the G2 checkpoint is mediated in part by the *chk1* kinase acting on CDK1.

(p170 P-glycoprotein; *mdr* gene product) was recognized from experiments with cells growing in tissue culture as mediating the efflux of chemotherapeutic agents in resistant cells. Certain neoplasms, particularly hematopoietic tumors, have an adverse prognosis if they express high levels of p170PGP, and modulation of this protein's function has been attempted by a variety of strategies.

Combinations of agents were proposed to afford the opportunity to affect many different targets or portions of the cell cycle at once, particularly if the toxic effects for the host of the different components of the combination were distinct. Combinations of agents were actually more effective in animal model systems than single agents, particularly if the tumor cell inoculum was high. This thinking led to the design of "combination chemotherapy" regimens, where drugs acting by different mechanisms (e.g., an alkylating agent plus an antimetabolite plus a mitotic spindle blocker) were combined. Particular combinations were chosen to emphasize drugs whose individual toxicities to the host were, if possible, distinct.

This view of cancer drug action is grossly oversimplified. Most tumors do not grow in an exponential pattern but rather follow Gompertzian kinetics, where the rate of tumor growth decreases as tumor mass increases (Fig. 84-1). Thus, a tumor has quiescent, differentiated compartments; proliferating compartments; and both well-vascularized and necrotic regions. Also, cell death is itself now understood to be a closely regulated process. *Necrosis* refers to cell death induced, for example, by physical damage with the hallmarks of cell swelling and membrane disruption. *Apoptosis*, or programmed cell death, refers to a highly ordered process whereby cells respond to defined stimuli by dying, and it recapitulates the necessary cell death observed during the ontogeny of the organism. *Anoikis* refers to death of epithelial cells after removal from the normal milieu of substrate, particularly from cell-to-cell contact. Cancer chemotherapeutic agents can cause both necrosis and apoptosis. Apoptosis is characterized by chromatin condensation (giving rise to "apoptotic bodies"); cell shrinkage; and, in

living animals, phagocytosis by surrounding stromal cells without evidence of inflammation. This process is regulated either by signal transduction systems that promote a cell's demise after a certain level of insult is achieved or in response to specific cell-surface receptors that mediate cell death signals. Modulation of apoptosis by manipulation of signal transduction pathways has emerged as a basis for understanding the actions of currently used drugs and designing new strategies to improve their use.

The current view envisions that the interaction of a chemotherapeutic drug with its target causes or is itself a signal that initiates a "cascade" of signaling steps to trigger an "execution phase" where proteases, nucleases, and endogenous regulators of the cell death pathway are activated. Effective cancer chemotherapeutic agents are efficient activators of apoptosis through signal transduction pathways (Fig. 84-4). For example, in the cytokine-mediated pathway, exogenous ligands such as the Fas ligand (FasL) bind to cell-surface receptors (CD95; Fas), or tumor necrosis factor (TNF) or its homologue Apo2L binds to its cognate receptors and directly recruits accessory molecules to activate a protease cascade (utilizing members of the caspase family of *cysteine asp*artyl prote*ases*), resulting in apoptosis. In a second pathway, growth factor deprivation elicits poorly defined signals that result in protease activation. Chemotherapeutic agents create molecular lesions (in DNA or cellular membranes) as a consequence of combining with their respective molecular targets. These lesions are sensed by a cellular "damage sensor," whose molecular nature is unclear, which leads to mitochondrial damage. Release of mitochondrial factors (e.g., APAF1, cytochrome c) promotes the activation of another set of caspases. Damage to the plasma membrane, e.g., from free radicals generated by certain chemotherapeutic agents, leads to activation of acid sphingomyelinase to release lipid components including ceramides, which then promote apoptosis through a variety of pathways including direct mitochondrial damage.

While apoptotic mechanisms are important in regulating cellular proliferation and the behavior of tumor cells in vitro, in vivo it is unclear whether all of the actions of chemotherapeutic agents to cause cell death can be attributed to apoptotic mechanisms. Loss of clonogenic survival (conventionally detecting the capacity of a few cells to survive) may predict clinical value more reliably than detection of apoptotic changes in the majority of tumor cells. However, changes in molecules that regulate apoptosis are clearly correlated with clinical outcomes (e.g., *bcl2* overexpression in certain lymphomas conveys poor prognosis; proapototic *bax* expression is associated with a better outcome in ovarian carcinoma). Further efforts to understand the relationship of cell death and cell survival mechanisms will be necessary.

CHEMOTHERAPEUTIC AGENTS USED FOR CANCER TREATMENT   Table 84-2 lists commonly used cancer chemotherapy agents and pertinent clinical aspects of their use. The drugs may be usefully grouped into three general categories: those affecting DNA, those affecting microtubules, and those acting at hormone-like receptors.

Direct DNA-Interactive Agents • *Formation of covalent DNA adducts*   Alkylating agents as a class break down, either spontaneously or after normal organ or tumor cell metabolism, to reactive intermediates that covalently modify bases in DNA. This leads to cross-linkage of DNA strands or the appearance of breaks in DNA as a result of repair efforts. "Broken" or cross-linked DNA is intrinsically unable to complete normal replication or cell division; in addition, it is a potent activator of cell cycle checkpoints and signaling pathways that can activate apoptosis. As a class, alkylating agents share similar toxicities, including myelosuppression, alopecia, gonadal dysfunction, mucositis, and pulmonary fibrosis. They differ greatly in a spectrum of normal organ toxicities.

Nitrogen mustard (mechlorethamine) is the prototypic agent of this class, decomposing rapidly in aqueous solution to yield potentially a bifunctional carbonium ion. It must be administered shortly after preparation into a rapidly flowing intravenous line. It is powerful vesicant, and infiltration may be symptomatically ameliorated by infiltration of the affected site with 1/6 *M* thiosulfate. Even without infiltration, aseptic thrombophlebitis is frequent. It can be used topically as a dilute solution in cutaneous lymphomas, with a notable incidence of hypersensitivity reactions. It causes moderate nausea after intravenous administration.

Cyclophosphamide is inactive unless metabolized by the liver to 4-hydroxyl-cyclophosphamide, which decomposes into alkylating species, as well as to chloroacetaldehyde and acrolein. The latter causes chemical cystitis, and therefore excellent hydration must be maintained while using cyclophosphamide. If severe, the cystitis may be effectively treated by mercaptoethanesulfonate (MESNA). Liver disease impairs drug activation. Sporadic interstitial pneumonitis leading to pulmonary fibrosis can accompany the use of cyclophosphamide, and high doses used in conditioning regimens for bone marrow transplant can cause cardiac dysfunction. Ifosfamide is a cyclophosphamide analogue also activated in the liver, but more slowly, and it requires mandatory coadministration of MESNA to prevent bladder injury. Central nervous system (CNS) effects, including somnolence, confusion, and psychosis, can follow ifosfamide use, and the incidence appears related to low body surface area or the presence of nephrectomy.

There are several less commonly used alkylating agents. Chlorambucil causes predictable myelosuppression, azospermia, nausea, and pulmonary side effects. Busulfan can cause profound myelosuppression, alopecia, and pulmonary toxicity but is relatively "lymphocyte sparing." Its routine use in treatment of chronic myeloid leukemia has been curtailed in favor of hydroxyurea or interferon (IFN), but it still is employed in marrow transplant preparation regimens. Melphalan shows variable oral bioavailability and undergoes extensive binding to albumin and α_1-acidic glycoprotein. Mucositis appears more prominently.

Nitrosoureas break down to carbamoylating species that not only cause a distinct pattern of DNA base pair–directed toxicity but also can covalently modify proteins. They share the feature of causing relatively delayed bone marrow toxicity, which can be cumulative and long-lasting. Streptozotocin is unique in that its glucose-like structure conveys specific toxicity to the islet cells of the pancreas (for whose derivative tumor types it is prominently indicated) as well as causing renal toxicity in the form of Fanconi's syndrome, including amino aciduria, glycosuria, and renal tubular acidosis. Methyl CCNU (lomustine) causes direct glomerular as well as tubular damage, cumulatively related to dose and time of exposure.

Procarbazine is metabolized in the liver and possibly in tumor cells to yield a variety of free radical and alkylating species. In addition to myelosuppression, it causes hypnotic and other CNS effects, including vivid nightmares. It can cause a disulfiram-like syndrome on ingestion of ethanol. Hexamethylmelamine and thiotepa can chemically give rise to alkylating species, although the nature of the DNA damage has not been well characterized in either case. Thiotepa can be used for intrathecal treatment of neoplastic meningitis. Dacarbazine (DTIC) is activated in the liver to yield the highly reactive methyl diazonium cation. It causes only modest myelosuppression from 21 to 25 days after a dose but causes prominent nausea on day 1.

Cisplatin was discovered fortuitously by observing that bacteria present in electrolysis solutions could not divide. Only the cis diamine configuration is active as an antitumor agent. It is hypothesized that in the intracellular environment, a chloride is lost from each position, being replaced by a water molecule. The resulting positively charged species is an efficient bifunctional interactor with DNA, forming Pt-base cross-links. Cisplatin requires administration with adequate hydration, including forced diuresis with mannitol to prevent kidney damage; even with the use of hydration, gradual decrease in kidney function is common. Hypomagnesemia frequently attends cisplatin use and can lead to hypocalcemia and symptomatic tetany. Other common toxicities include neurotoxicity with "stocking and glove" sensorimotor neuropathy. Hearing loss occurs in 50% of patients treated with

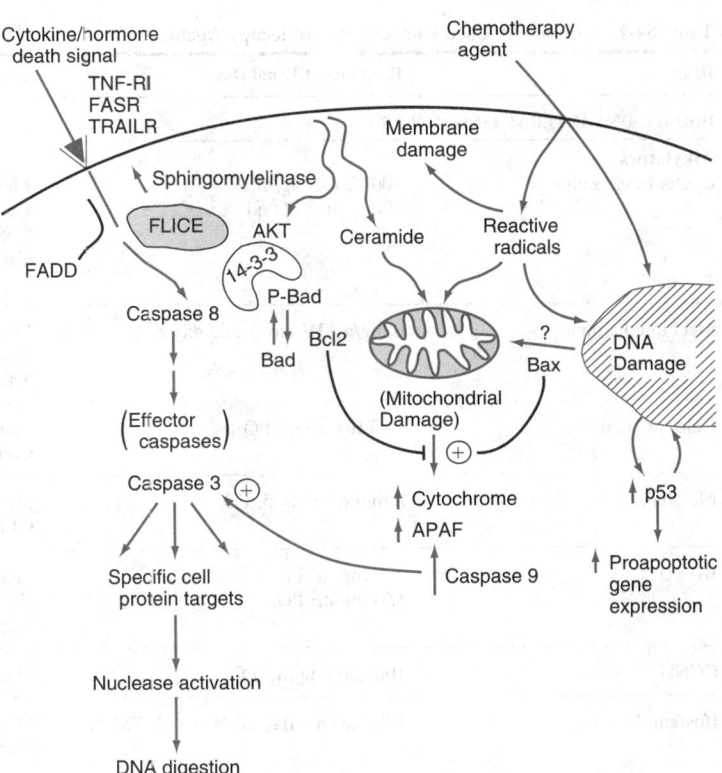

FIGURE 84-4 Integration of cell death responses. Cell death through an *apoptotic* mechanism requires active participation of the cell. In response to hormonal or cytokine death signals, receptors activate "upstream" cysteine aspartyl proteases (caspases), which then directly digest cytoplasmic and nuclear proteins, resulting in activation of "downstream" caspases; these cause activation of nucleases resulting in the characteristic DNA fragmentation that is a hallmark of apoptosis. Chemotherapy agents that create lesions in DNA seem to activate aspects of this process through a pathway that appears to result in damage to mitochondria, perhaps by activating the transcription of genes whose products can produce or modulate the toxicity of free radicals. In addition, membrane damage with activation of sphingomyelinases results in the production of ceramides that can have a direct action at mitochondria. The antiapoptotic protein *bcl2* attenuates mitochondrial toxicity, while proapoptotic gene products such as *bax* antagonize the action of *bcl2*. Damaged mitochondria release cytochrome C and "apoptosis activating factor," which can directly activate caspase 9, resulting in propagation of a direct signal to other downstream caspases through protease activation. An additional proapoptotic stimulus is the *bad* protein, which can heterodimerize with *bcl2* gene family members to antagonize apoptosis. Importantly, though, *bad* protein function can be retarded by its sequestration as phospho-*bad* through the 14-3-3 adapter proteins. The phosphorylation of *bad* is mediated by the action of the AKT kinase in a way that defines how growth factors that activate this kinase can retard apoptosis and promote cell survival.

conventional doses. Cisplatin is intensely emetogenic, requiring prophylactic antinausea agents. Myelosuppression is less evident than with other alkylating agents. Chronic vascular toxicity is a more unusual toxic phenomena, including Raynaud's syndrome and coronary artery disease. In an effort to obviate these toxicities, carboplatin was developed and clearly displays less nephro-, oto- and neurotoxicity. However, myelosuppression is more frequent, and as the drug is exclusively cleared through the kidney, adjustment of dose for creatinine clearance must be accomplished through use of various dosing nomograms.

Antitumor antibiotics and topoisomerase poisons Antitumor *antibiotics* are substances produced by bacteria that in nature appear to provide chemical defense against other hostile microorganisms. As a class they bind to DNA directly and can frequently undergo electron transfer reactions to generate free radicals in close proximity to DNA, leading to DNA damage in the form of single strand breaks or crosslinks. *Topoisomerase poisons* include natural products or semi-synthetic species derived ultimately from plants, and they modify enzymes

Table 84-2 Commonly Used Cancer Chemotherapy Agents

Drug	Examples of Usual Doses	Toxicity	Interactions, Issues
DIRECT DNA-INTERACTING AGENTS			
Alkylators			
Cyclophosphamide	400–2000 mg/m²IV 100 mg/m² PO qd	Marrow (relative platelet sparing) Cystitis Common alkylator[a] Cardiac (high dose)	Liver metabolism required to activate to phosphoramide mustard + acrolein MESNA protects against "high-dose" bladder damage
Mechlorethamine	6 mg/m² IV day 1 and day 8	Marrow Vesicant Nausea	Topical use in cutaneous lymphoma
Chlorambucil	1–3 mg/m² qd PO	Marrow Common alkylator[a]	
Melphalan	8 mg/m² qd × 5, PO	Marrow (delayed nadir) GI (high dose)	Decreased renal function delays clearance
BCNU	200 mg/m² IV 150 mg/m² PO	Marrow (delayed nadir) GI, liver (high dose) Renal	
CCNU	100–300 mg/m² PO	Marrow (delayed nadir)	
Ifosfamide	1.2 g/m² per day qd × 5 + MESNA	Myelosuppressive Bladder Neurologic Metabolic acidosis Neuropathy	Isomeric analogue of cyclophosphamide More lipid soluble Greater activity vs testicular neoplasms and sarcomas Must use MESNA
Procarbazine	100 mg/m² per day qd ×14	Marrow Nausea Neurologic Common alkylator[a]	Liver and tissue metabolism required Disulfiran-like effect with ethanol Acts as MAOI HBP after tyrosinase-rich foods
DTIC	375 mg/m² IV day 1 & day 15	Marrow Nausea Flulike	Metabolic activation
Hexamethylmelamine	260 mg/m² per day qd ×14–21 as 4 divided oral doses	Nausea Neurologic (mood swing) Neuropathy Marrow (less)	Liver activation Barbiturates enchance/cimetidine diminishes
Cisplatin	20 mg/m² qd ×5 IV 1 q3–4 weeks or 100–200 mg/m²/dose IV q3–4 weeks	Nausea Neuropathy Auditory Marrow platelets > WBCs Renal Mg²⁺, Ca²⁺	Maintain high urine flow; osmotic diuresis, monitor intake/output K⁺, Mg²⁺ Emetogenic—prophylaxis needed Full dose if CrCl > 60 mL/min and tolerate fluid push
Carboplatin	365 mg/m² IV q3–4 weeks as adjusted for CrCl	Marrow platelets > WBCs Nausea Renal (high dose)	Reduce dose according to CrCl: AUC = dose/(CrCl + 25) to AUC of 5–7 mg/mL per min
Antitumor antibiotics			
Bleomycin	15–25 mg/d qd ×5 IV bolus or continuous IV	Pulmonary Skin effects Raynaud's Hypersensitivity	Inactivate by bleomycin hydrolase (decreased in lung/skin) O₂ enhances pulmonary toxicity Cisplatin-induced decrease in CrCl may increase skin/lung toxicity Reduce dose if CrCl < 60 mL/min
Actinomycin D	10–15 μg/kg per day qd ×5 IV bolus	Marrow Nausea Mucositis Vesicant Alopecia	Radiation recall

(continued)

Table 84-2—*(continued)*

Drug	Examples of Usual Doses	Toxicity	Interactions, Issues
Mithramycin	15–20 μg/kg qd ×4–7 (hypercal-cemia) *or* 50 μg/kg qod ×3–8 (antineo-plastic)	Marrow Liver Renal Mucositis Hypocalcemia Nausea Vesicant	Acute hemorrhagic syndrome
Mitomycin C	6–10 mg/m^2 q6 weeks	Marrow Vesicant Hemolytic-uremic syndrome Lung CV—heart failure	Treat superficial bladder cancers by intravesical infusion Delayed marrow toxicity Cumulative marrow toxicity
Etoposide (VP16-213)	100–150 mg/m^2 IV qd ×3–5d *or* 50 mg/m^2 PO qd ×21d *or* up to 1500 mg/m^2/of dose (high dose with stem cell support)	Marrow (WBCs > platelet) Alopecia Hypotension Hypersensitivity (rapid IV) Nausea Mucositis (high dose)	Hepatic metabolism—renal 30% Reduce doses with renal failure Schedule-dependant (5 day better than 1 day) Late leukemogenic Accentuate antimetabolite action
Teniposide (VM-26)	150–200 mg/m^2 twice per week for 4 weeks	Marrow Alopecia	
Amsacrine	100–150 mg/m^2 IV qd ×5	Marrow Mucositis Nausea CV—arrhythmia (avoid hypokale-mia)	Decrease dose by 30% if liver or re-nal failure
Topotecan	20 mg/m^2 IV q3–4 weeks over 30 min *or* 1.5–3 mg/m^2 q3–4 weeks over 24 h *or* 0.5 mg/m^2 per day over 21 days	Marrow Mucositis Nausea Mild alopecia	Reduce dose with renal failure No liver toxicity
Irinotecan (CPT II)	100–150 mg/m^2 IV over 90 min q3–4 weeks *or* 30 mg/m^2 per day over 120 h	Diarrhea: "early onset" with cramp-ing, flushing, vomiting; "late onset" after several doses Marrow Alopecia Nausea Vomiting Pulmonary	Prodrug requires enzymatic clear-ance to active drug "SN 38" "Early diarrhea" likely due to biliary excretion Late diarrhea, use "high-dose" loper-amide (2 mg q2–4 h)
Doxorubicin and daunorubicin	45–60 mg/m^2 dose q3–4 weeks *or* 10–30 mg/m^2 dose q week *or* continuous-infusion regimen	Marrow Mucositis Alopecia Cardiovascular acute/chronic Vesicant	Heparin aggregate; coadministration increases clearance Tylenol, BCNU increase liver tox-icity Radiation recall
Idarubicin	10–15 mg/m^2 IV q 3 weeks *or* 10 mg/m^2 IV qd ×3	Marrow Cardiac (less than doxorubicin)	None established
Epirubicin	150 mg/m^2 IV q3 weeks	Marrow Cardiac	None established
Mitoxantrone	12 mg/m^2 qd ×3 *or* 12–14 mg/m^2 q3 weeks	Marrow Cardiac (less than doxorubicin) Vesicant (mild) Blue urine, sclerae, nails	Interacts with heparin Less alopecia, nausea than doxoru-bicin Radiation recall
INDIRECT DNA-INTERACTING AGENTS			
Antimetabolites Deoxycoformycin	4 mg/m^2 IV every other week	Nausea Immunosuppression Neurologic Renal	Excretes in urine Reduce dose for renal failure Inhibits adenosine deaminase

(continued)

Table 84-2   Commonly Used Cancer Chemotherapy Agents—(continued)

Drug	Examples of Usual Doses	Toxicity	Interactions, Issues
6-Mercaptopurine	75 mg/m² PO or up 500 mg/m² PO (high dose)	Marrow Liver Nausea	Variable bioavailability Metabolize by xanthine oxidase Decrease dose with allopurinol Increased toxicity with thiopurine methyltransferase deficiency
6-Thioguanine	2–3 mg/kg per day for up to 3–4 weeks	Marrow Liver Nausea	Variable bioavailability Increased toxicity with thiopurine methyltransferase deficiency
Azathioprine	1–5 mg/kg per day	Marrow Nausea Liver	Metabolizes to 6-MP, therefore reduce dose with allopurinol Increased toxicity with thiopurine methyltransferase deficiency
2-Chlorodeoxyadenosine	0.09 mg/kg per day qd ×7 as continuous infusion	Marrow Renal Fever	Notable use in hairy cell leukemia
Hydroxyurea	20–50 mg/kg (lean body weight) PO qd or 1–3 g/d	Marrow Nausea Mucositis Skin changes Rare renal, liver, lung, CNS	Decrease dose with renal failure Augments antimetabolite effect
Methotrexate	15–30 mg PO or IM qd ×3–5 or 30 mg IV days 1 and 8 or 1.5–12 g/m² per day (with leucovorin)	Marrow Liver/lung Renal tubular Mucositis	Rescue with leucovorin Excreted in urine Decrease dose in renal failure NSAIDs increase renal toxicity
5-Fluorouracil	375 mg/m² IV qd ×5 or 600 mg/m² IV days 1 and 8	Marrow Mucositis Neurologic Skin changes	Toxicity enhanced by leucovorin Dihydropyrimidine dehydrogenase deficiency increases toxicity Metabolizes in tissues
Cytosine arabinoside	100 mg/m² per day qd ×7 by continuous infusion or 1–3 g/m² dose IV bolus	Marrow Mucositis Neurologic (high dose) Conjunctivitis (high dose) Noncardiogenic pulmonary edema	Enhances activity of alkylating agents Metabolizes in tissues by deamination
Azacytidine	750 mg/m² per week or 150–200 mg/m² per day ×5–10 (bolus) or (continuous IV)	Marrow Nausea Liver Neurologic Myalgia	Use limited to leukemia Altered methylation of DNA alters gene expression
Gemcitabine	1000 mg/m² IV weekly ×7	Marrow Nausea Hepatic Fever/"flu syndrome"	
Fludarabine phosphate	25 mg/m² IV qd ×5	Marrow Neurologic Lung	Dose reduction with renal failure Metabolized to F-ara converted to F-ara ATP in cells by deoxycytidine kinase
Asparaginase	25,000 IU/m² q3–4 weeks or 6000 IU/m² per day qod for 3–4 weeks or 1000–2000 IU/m² for 10–20 days	Protein synthesis Clotting factors Glucose Albumin Hypersensitivity CNS Pancreatitis Hepatic	Blocks methotrexate action

(continued)

Table 84-2—(continued)

Drug	Examples of Usual Doses	Toxicity	Interactions, Issues
Antimitotic agents			
Vincristine	1–1.4 mg/m² per week	Vesicant Marrow Neurologic GI: ileus/constipation; bladder hypo- toxicity; SIADH Cardiovascular	Hepatic clearance Dose reduction for bilirubin >1.5 mg/dL Prophylactic bowel regimen
Vinblastine	6–8 mg/m² per week	Vesicant Marrow Neurologic (less common but similar spectrum to other vincas) Hypertension Raynaud's	Hepatic clearance Dose reduction as with vincristine
Vinorelbine	15–30 mg/m² per week	Vesicant Marrow Allergic/broncospasm (immediate) Dyspnea/cough (subacute) Neurologic (less prominent but simi- lar spectrum to other vincas)	Hepatic clearance
Paclitaxel	135–175 mg/m² per 24-h infusion or 175 mg/m² per 3-h infusion or 140 mg/m² per 96-h infusion or 250 mg/m² per 24-h infusion plus G-CSF	Hypersensitivity Marrow Mucositis Alopecia Sensory neuropathy CV conduction disturbance Nausea—infrequent	Premedicate with steroids, H_1 and H_2 blockers Hepatic clearance Dose reduction as with vincas
Docetaxel	100 mg/m² per 1-h infusion q3 weeks	Hypersensitivity Fluid retention syndrome Marrow Dermatologic Sensory neuropathy Nausea infrequent Some stomatitis	Premedicate with steroids, H_1 and H_2 blockers
Estramustine phosphate	14 mg/kg per day in 3–4 divided doses with water >2 h after meals Avoid Ca^{2+}-rich foods	Nausea Vomiting Diarrhea CHF Thrombosis Gynecomastia	

[a] Common alkylator: alopecia, pulmonary, infertility, plus teratogenesis.
NOTE: AUC, area under the curve; CHF, congestive heart failure; CNS, central nervous system; CrCl, creatinine clearance; CV, cardiovascular; G-CSF, granulocyte colony stimulating factor; GI, gastrointestinal; HBP, high blood pressure; MAOI, monoamine oxidase inhibitors; MESNA, mercaptoethanesulfonate; 6-MP, 6-mercaptopurine; NSAIDs, nonsteroidal anti-inflammatory drugs; SIADH, syndrome of inappropriate antidiuretic hormone; WBCs, white blood cells.

that regulate the capacity of DNA to unwind to allow normal replication or transcription.

Doxorubicin is the most widely active and frequently used antineoplastic agent. It can intercalate into DNA, thereby altering DNA structure, replication, and topoisomerase function. It can also undergo redox cycling by accepting electrons into its quinone ring system. It causes predictable myelosuppression, alopecia, nausea, and mucositis. In addition, it causes acute cardiotoxicity in the form of atrial and ventricular dysrhythmias, but these are rarely of clinical significance. In contrast, cumulative doses >550 mg/m² are associated with a 10% incidence of chronic cardiomyopathy. The incidence of cardiomyopathy appears to be related to schedule (peak serum concentration), with low dose, frequent treatment, or continuous infusions better tolerated than intermittent higher dose exposures. Radiation recall or interaction with radiation to cause local site complications is frequent. The drug is a powerful vesicant, with necrosis of tissue apparent 4 to 7 days after an extravasation; therefore it should be administered into a rapidly flowing intravenous line. The drug is metabolized by the liver, so doses must be reduced by 50 to 75% in the presence of liver dysfunction. Daunorubicin is closely related to doxorubicin and was actually introduced first into leukemia treament, where it remains part of curative regimens and has been shown preferable to doxorubicin owing to less mucositis and colonic damage. Idarubicin is an orally acting doxorubicin analogue, whose ultimate place in therapy is uncertain.

Bleomycin refers to a mixture of glycopeptides that have the unique feature of forming complexes with Fe^{2+} while bound to DNA. Oxidation gives rise to superoxide and hydroxyl radicals. The drug is of interest clinically as it causes little, if any, myelosuppression. The drug is cleared rapidly, but augmented skin and pulmonary toxicity in the presence of renal failure has led to the recommendation that doses be reduced by 50 to 75% in the face of a creatinine clearance <25 mL/min. Bleomycin is not a vesicant, and can be administered intravenously, intramuscularly, or subcutaneously. Common side effects include fever and chills, facial flush, and Raynaud's syndrome. Hypertension can follow rapid intravenous administration, and the incidence of anaphylaxis with early preparations of the drug has led to the practice of administering a test dose of 0.5 to 1 unit before the rest of the dose. The most feared complication of bleomycin treatment is pulmonary fibrosis, which increases in incidence at >300 cumulative units administered and is at best minimally responsive to treatment (e.g., glucocorticoids). The earliest indicator of an adverse effect is a decline in the DL_{CO}, although cessation of drug immediately upon documentation of a decrease in DL_{CO} may not prevent further decline in pulmonary function. Bleomycin is inactivated by a bleomycin hydrolase, whose concentration is diminished in skin and lung. Because bleomycin-dependent electron transport is dependent on O_2, bleomycin toxicity may become apparent after exposure to transient very high inspired P_{O_2}. Thus, during surgical procedures, patients with prior exposure to bleomycin should be maintained on the lowest inspired P_{O_2} consistent with maintaining adequate tissue oxygenation.

D-Actinomycin intercalates into DNA and appears to have less, but not absent, capacity to undergo electron transfer reactions. It causes severe myelosuppression, nausea, alopecia, and mucositis. It is a notable vesicant. Mithramycin historically was used against testicular and other neoplasms; however, in addition to causing nausea, myelosuppression, and vesicant properties, it causes an "acute hemorrhagic syndrome" consisting of platelet function defects in association with indicators of disseminated intravascular coagulation. It is used in current practice to control hypercalcemia. In addition, renal and hepatic dysfunction may complicate its use.

Mitomycin C undergoes reduction of its quinone function to generate a bifunctional DNA alkylating agent. It is a broadly active antineoplastic agent with a number of unpredictable toxicities, including delayed bronchospasm 12 to 14 h after dosing and a chronic pulmonary fibrosis syndrome more frequent at doses of 50 to 60 mg/m². Cardiomyopathy has been described, particularly in the setting of prior radiation therapy. A hemolytic-uremic syndrome carries an ultimate mortality rate of 25 to 50% and is poorly treated by conventional component support and exchange transfusion. Mitomycin is a notable vesicant and causes substantial nausea and vomiting. It can be used for intravesical instillation for curative treatment of superficial transitional bladder carcinomas and, with radiation therapy, for curative treatment of anal carcinoma.

Mitoxantrone is a synthetic compound that was designed to recapitulate features of doxorubicin but with less cardiotoxicity. It is quantitatively less cardiotoxic (comparing the ratio of cardiotoxic to therapeutically effective doses), but its status in therapy is unclear as doses of 150 mg/m² have produced evidence of 10% incidence of cardiotoxicity; it also causes alopecia.

Etoposide was synthetically derived from the plant product podophyllotoxin, and it binds directly to topoisomerase II and DNA in a reversible ternary complex. In that capacity, it stabilizes the covalent intermediate in the enzyme's action where the enzyme is covalently linked to DNA. This "alkali-labile" DNA bond was historically a first hint that an activity such as topoisomerase exists. The drug therefore causes a prominent G2 arrest, reflecting the action of a DNA damage checkpoint. Prominent clinical effects include myelosuppression, nausea, and transient hypotension related to the speed of administration of the agent. Etoposide is a mild vesicant but is relatively free from other "large organ" toxicities. Teniposide is a structural relative with unique activity in childhood lymphoblastic leukemia. When given at high doses or very frequently, topoisomerase inhibitors may cause acute leukemia associated with chromosome 11q23 abnormalities in up to 1% of exposed patients.

Camptothecin was isolated from extracts of a Chinese tree and had notable antileukemia activity. Early clinical studies with the sodium salt of the hydrolyzed camptothecin lactone showed evidence of notable toxicity with little activity. Identification of topoisomerase I as the target of camptothecins and the need to preserve lactone structure allowed additional efforts to identify active members of this series. Topoisomerase I is responsible for unwinding the DNA strand by introducing single strand breaks and allowing rotation of one strand about the other. In S phase, topoisomerase I–induced breaks that are not promptly resealed lead to progress of the replication fork off the end of a DNA strand. The DNA damage is a potent signal for induction of apoptosis. Camptothecins promote the stabilization of the DNA linked to the enzyme in a so-called cleavable complex, analogous to the action of etoposide with topoisomerase II. Topotecan is a camptothecin derivative approved for use in ovarian tumors. Toxicity is limited to myelosuppression and mucositis. CPT-11, or irinotecan, is a

camptothecin with evidence of activity in colon carcinoma. In addition to myelosuppression, it causes a secretory diarrhea, which can be treated effectively with loperamide or octreotide.

Indirect Effectors of DNA Function: Antimetabolites A broad definition of antimetabolites would include compounds with structural similarity to precursors of purines or pyrimidines or that interfere with purine or pyrimidine synthesis. Antimetabolites can cause DNA damage indirectly, through misincorporation into DNA, abnormal timing or progression through DNA synthesis, or altered function of pyrimidine and purine biosynthetic enzymes. They tend to convey greatest toxicity to cells in S phase, and the degree of toxicity increases with duration of exposure. Common toxic manifestations include stomatitis, diarrhea, and myelosuppression. Second malignancies are not associated with their use.

Methotrexate inhibits dihydrofolate reductase, which regenerates reduced folates from the oxidized folates produced when thymidine monophosphate is formed from deoxyuridine monophosphate. Without reduced folates, cells die a "thymineless" death. N^5tetrahydrofolate or N^5formyltetrahydrofolate (leucovorin) can bypass this block and rescue cells from methotrexate, which is maintained in cells by polyglutamylation. The drug and other reduced folates are transported into cells by the folate carrier, and high concentrations of drug can bypass this carrier and allow diffusion of drug directly into cells. These properties have suggested the design of "high-dose" methotrexate regimens with leucovorin rescue of normal marrow and mucosa, part of curative approaches to osteosarcoma in the adjuvant setting, and hematopoietic neoplasms of children and adults. Methotrexate is cleared by the kidney by both glomerular filtration and tubular secretion, and toxicity is augmented by renal dysfunction and drugs such as salicylates, probenecid, and nonsteroidal anti-inflammatory agents that undergo tubular secretion. With normal renal function, 15 mg/m² leucovorin will rescue 10^{-8} to 10^{-6} M methotrexate in three to four doses. However, with decreased creatinine clearance, doses of 50 to 100 mg/m² are continued until methotrexate levels are $<5 \times 10^{-8}$ M. In addition to bone marrow suppression and mucosal irritation, methotrexate can cause renal failure itself at high doses owing to crystallization in renal tubules; therefore high-dose regimens require alkalinization of urine with increased flow by hydration. Methotrexate can be sequestered in third space collections and leech back into the general circulation, causing prolonged myelosuppression. Less frequent adverse effects include reversible increases in transaminases and a hypersensitivity-like pulmonary syndrome. Chronic low-dose methotrexate can cause hepatic fibrosis. When administered to the intrathecal space, methotrexate can cause chemical arachnoiditis and CNS dysfunction. Trimetrexate is a methotrexate derivative that is not polyglutamylated and does not use the reduced folate carrier.

5-Fluorouracil (5FU) represents an early example of "rational" drug design in that it originated from the observation that tumor cells incorporate uracil more efficiently into DNA than normal cells, especially gut. 5FU is metabolized in cells to 5′FdUMP, which inhibits thymidylate synthetase (TS). In addition, misincorporation can lead to single strand breaks, and RNA can aberrantly incorporate FUMP. 5FU is metabolized by dihydropyrimidine dehydrogenase, and deficiency of this enzyme can lead to excessive toxicity from 5FU. Oral bioavailability varies unreliably. Intravenous administration leads to bone marrow suppression after short infusions but to more evidence of stomatitis after prolonged infusions. Leucovorin augments the toxicity and activity of 5FU by promoting formation of the ternary covalent complex of 5FU, the reduced folate, and TS. Less frequent toxicities include CNS dysfunction, with prominent cerebellar signs, and endothelial toxicity manifested by thrombosis, including pulmonary embolus and myocardial infarction.

Cytosine arabinoside (ara-C) is incorporated into DNA after formation of ara-CTP, resulting in S phase–related toxicity. Continuous infusion schedules allow maximal efficiency of effect, with uptake maximal at 5 to 7 μM. Ara-C can be administered intrathecally. Adverse effects include nausea, diarrhea, stomatitis, chemical conjunctivitis, and cerebellar ataxia. Gemcitabine is a cytosine derivative that is similar to ara-C in that it is incorporated into DNA after anabolism to the triphosphate, rendering DNA susceptible to breakage and repair synthesis, which differs from that in ara-C in that lesions including the analogue are very inefficiently removed. In contrast to ara-C, gemcitabine appears to have useful activity in a variety of solid tumors, with limited nonmyelosuppressive toxicities. 6-Thioguanine and 6-mercaptopurine (6MP) are used in the treatment of acute lymphoid leukemia. Although administered orally, they display very variable bioavailability. 6MP is metabolized by xanthine oxidase and therefore requires dose reduction when used with allopurinol.

Fludarabine phosphate is a prodrug of F-ara-A, which in turn was designed to diminish the susceptibility of ara-A to adenosine deaminase. Ara-A is incorporated into DNA and can cause delayed cytotoxicity even in cells with low growth fraction, including chronic lymphocytic leukemia and follicular B cell lymphoma. CNS dysfunction and T cell depletion leading to opportunistic infections can occur in addition to myelosuppression. 2-Chlorodeoxyadenosine is a similar compound with activity in hairy cell leukemia. 2-Deoxycoformycin inhibits adenosine deaminase, with resulting increase in dATP levels. This causes inhibition of ribonucleotide reductase as well as augmented susceptibility to apoptosis, particularly in T cells. Renal failure and CNS dysfunction are notable toxicities in addition to immunosuppression.

Hydroxyurea inhibits ribonucleotide reductase, resulting in S phase block. It is orally bioavailable and the drug of choice for the acute management of myeloproliferative states. Asparaginase is not classically considered an antimetabolite as it causes breakdown of extracellular asparagine required for protein synthesis in certain leukemic cells. However, it effectively stops DNA synthesis by preventing the requisite concurrent protein synthesis, and therefore it has a similar functional outcome as the classic antimetabolites. As asparaginase is a foreign protein, hypersensitivity reactions are common, as are effects on organs such as pancreas and liver that require continuing protein synthesis. This results in decreased insulin secretion with hyperglycemia, with or without hyperamylasemia and clotting function abnormalities. The latter may be associated with CNS and dural vein thrombosis.

Mitotic Spindle Inhibitors Microtubules are cellular structures that form the mitotic spindle and in interphase cells are responsible for the cellular "scaffolding" along which various motile and secretory processes occur. Microtubules are composed of repeating noncovalent multimers of a hetrodimer of α and β subunits of the protein tubulin. Vincristine binds to the tubulin dimer with the result that microtubules are disaggregated. This results in the block of growing cells in M phase; however, toxic effects in G1 and S phase are also evident. The drug is bound to blood-formed elements, leading to its occasional use as vinca-loaded platelets to treat autoimmune thrombocytopenia. The drug is metabolized by the liver, and dose adjustment in the presence of hepatic dysfunction is required. It is a powerful vesicant, and infiltration can be treated by local heat and infiltration with hyaluronidase. The drug is lethal if inadvertantly administered by the intrathecal route. At clinically used intravenous doses, neurotoxicity in the form of glove-and-stocking neuropathy is frequent. Children tolerate 2 mg/m², but adult doses may be capped at 2 mg total to lower the incidence of disabling chronic neuropathy; whether this compromises needed dose intensity in curative regimens is uncertain. Acute neuropathic effects include jaw pain, paralytic ileus, urinary retention, and the syndrome of inappropriate antidiuretic hormone secretion. Myelosuppression is not seen. Vinblastine is similar to vincristine, except that it tends to be more myelotoxic, with more frequent thrombocytopenia and also mucositis and stomatitis. Vinorelbine is a recently introduced vinca alkaloid that appears to have differences in resistance patterns in comparison to vincristine and vinblastine; it may be administered orally.

The taxanes include paclitaxel and docetaxel. These agents differ from the vinca alkaloids in that the taxanes stabilize microtubules against depolymerization. The "stabilized" microtubules function abnormally and are not able to undergo the normal dynamic changes of microtubule function necessary for cell cycle completion. Taxanes are among the most broadly active antineoplastic agents for use in solid tumors, with evidence of activity in ovarian cancer, breast cancer, Kaposi's sarcoma, and lung tumors. They are administered intravenously, and paclitaxel requires use of a cremophore-containing vehicle that can cause hypersensitiviy reactions. Premedication with regimens including dexamethasone (20 mg orally or intravenously 12 and 6 h before treatment), diphenhydramine (50 mg), and cimetidine (300 mg) both 30 min before treatment decreases but does not eliminate the risk of hypersensitivity reactions to the paclitaxel vehicle. Docetaxel uses a polysorbate 80 formulation, which can cause fluid retention in addition to hypersensitivity reactions, and dexamethasone premedication with or without antihistamines is frequently used. Paclitaxel causes hypersensitivity reactions, myelosuppression, neurotoxicity in the form of glove-and-stocking numbness, and paresthesia. Cardiac rhythm disturbances were observed in phase I and II trials, most commonly asymptomatic bradycardia but, much more rarely, varying degrees of heart block. These have not emerged as clinically significant in the majority of patients. Infrequently occurring evidence of myocardial ischemia during paclitaxel administration cannot yet be clearly related to the drug. Docetaxel causes comparable degrees of myelosuppression and neuropathy. Hypersensitivity reactions, including bronchospasm, dyspnea, and hypotension, are less frequent but occur to some degree in up to 25% of patients. Fluid retention appears to result from a vascular leak syndrome that can aggravate preexisting effusions. Rash can complicate docetaxel administration, appearing prominently as a pruritic maculopapular rash affecting the forearms, but it has also been associated with fingernail ridging, breakdown, and skin discoloration. Stomatitis appears to be somewhat more frequent than with paclitaxel.

Estramustine was originally synthesized as a mustard derivative that might be useful in neoplasms that possessed estrogen receptor sites. However, no evidence of interaction with DNA was observed. Surprisingly, the drug caused metaphase arrest, and subsequent study revealed that it binds to microtubule-associated proteins, resulting in abnormal microtubule function. Estramustine binds to estramustine-binding proteins (EMBP), which have particular presence in prostate tumor tissue. The drug is approved for treatment of metastatic prostate cancer as an oral formulation. Gastrointestinal and cardiovascular adverse effects related to the estrogen moiety occur in up to 10% of patients, including worsened heart failure and thromboembolic phenomena. Gynecomastia and nipple tenderness can also occur.

Hormonal Agents The family of steroid hormone receptor–related molecules have emerged as prominent targets for "small molecules" useful in cancer treatment. When bound to their cognate ligands, these receptors can alter gene transcription and, in certain tissues, induce apoptosis. The pharmacologic effect is a mirror or parody of the normal effects of the agent acting in nontransformed tissue, although the effects on tumors are mediated by indirect effects in some cases.

Glucocorticoids are generally given in "pulsed" high-dose exposure in leukemias and lymphomas, where they induce apoptosis in tumor cells. Cushing's syndrome or inadvertent adrenal suppression on withdrawal from high-dose glucocorticoids can be significant complications, along with infections common in immunosuppressed patients, in particular *Pneumocystis* pneumonia, which classically appears a few days after completing a course of high-dose steroids. Tamoxifen is a partial estrogen receptor antagonist; it has a tenfold greater degree of antitumor activity in breast cancer patients whose tumors express estrogen receptors than in those who have low or no levels of expression. Side effects include a somewhat increased risk of estrogen-related cardiovascular complications, such as thromboembolic phenomena, and a small increased incidence of endometrial carcinoma, which appears after chronic use. Progestational agents including medroxyprogesterone acetate, androgens including halotestin, and, paradoxically, estrogens have approximately the same degeree of activity in primary hormonal treatment of breast cancers that have elevated levels of estrogen receptors. Estrogen is not used often owing to prominent cardiovascular and uterotropic activity.

Prostate cancer is classically treated by diethylstilbesterol (DES) acting as an estrogen at the level of the hypothalamus to downregulate hypothalamic luteinizing hormone (LH) production, resulting in decreased elaboration of testosterone by the testicle. For this reason, orchiectomy is equally as effective as moderate-dose DES, inducing responses in ~80% of previously untreated patients with prostate cancer but without the prominent cardiovascular side effects of DES, including thrombosis and exacerbation of coronary artery disease. In the event that orchiectomy is not accepted by the patient, testicular androgen suppression can also be effected by luteinizing hormone–releasing hormone (LHRH) agonists such as leuprolide and goserelin. These agents cause tonic stimulation of the LHRH receptor, with the loss of its normal pulsatile activation resulting in its desensitization and decreased output of LH by the anterior pituitary. Therefore, as primary hormonal manipulation in prostate cancer one can choose orchiectomy or leuprolide, not both. The addition of actual antagonists of androgens acting at the androgen receptor, including flutamide or bicalutamide, is of uncertain additional benefit in extending overall response duration, but it clearly prevents the activation of androgen receptors by adrenal androgens, and the combined use of orchiectomy or leuprolide plus flutamide is referred to as "total androgen blockade."

Interestingly, tumors that respond to a primary hormonal manipulation may frequently respond to second and third hormonal manipulations. Thus, breast tumors that had previously responded to tamoxifen have, on relapse, notable response rates to withdrawal of tamoxifen itself or to subsequent addition of a progestin. Likewise, initial treatment of prostate cancers with leuprolide plus flutamide may be followed after disease progression by response to withrawal of flutamide. These responses may result from the removal of antagonists from mutant steroid hormone receptors that have come to depend on the presence of the antagonist as a growth-promoting influence.

Additional strategies to treat refractory breast and prostate cancers that possess steroid hormone receptors may also address adrenal capacity to produce androgens and estrogens, even after orchiectomy or oophorectomy, respectively. Thus, aminoglutethimide or ketoconazole can be used to block adrenal synthesis by interfering with the enzymes of steroid hormone metabolism. Administration of these agents requires concomitant hydrocortisone replacement and additional glucocorticoid doses administered in the event of physiologic stress. Steroid hormone–inducing "aromatase" activity may be present in tumor tissue, and second- or third-line approaches to inhibition of aromatase activity may also be effected by such agents as anastrazole and letrozole.

Humoral mechanisms can also result in complications of an underlying malignancy. Adrenocortical carcinomas can cause Cushing's syndrome as well as syndromes of androgen or estrogen excess. Mitotane can counteract these by decreasing synthesis of steroid hormones. Islet cell neoplasms can cause debilitating diarrhea, treated with the somatostatin analogue octreotide. Prolactin-secreting tumors can be effectively managed by the dopaminergic agonist bromocriptine.

An additional strategy related conceptually to the use of steroid hormones is the use of retinoids, including tretinoin, the all-*trans*-isomer of retinoic acid, or isotretinoin, the 13-*cis* isomer of retinoic acid, to cause "differentiation" by acting on the retinoid receptor, which is in the steroid hormone receptor family. In particular, tretinoin is part of curative regimens for acute promyelocytic leukemia (PML) and appears to act by causing accelerated degradation of the fusion protein created by the t(15;17) translocation fusing the retinoic acid receptor α and the PML transcription factor. Acute side effects related to differentiation of promyelocytes to mature granulocytes may result in pulmonary symptoms related to granulocyte sequestration in the pulmonary vasculature; these are treated by respiratory support and glucocorticoids. Squamous neoplasms, including those of the skin and cervix, also appear to be uniquely responsive in certain cases to retinoids.

ACUTE COMPLICATIONS OF CANCER CHEMOTHERAPY Myelosuppression The common cytotoxic chemotherapeutic agents almost invariably affect bone marrow function. Titration of this effect determines in many cases the MTD of the agent on a given schedule. The normal kinetics of blood cell turnover influence the sequence and sensitivity of each of the formed elements. Polymorphonuclear leukocytes (PMNs; $T_{1/2}$ = 6 to 8 h), platelets ($T_{1/2}$ = 5 to 7 days), and red blood cells (RBC; $T_{1/2} \sim$ 120 days) have most, less, and least susceptibility to usually administered cytotoxic agents, respectively. The *nadir count* of each cell type in response to classes of agents is characteristic. Maximal neutropenia occurs 6 to 14 days after conventional doses of anthracyclines, antifolates, and antimetabolites. Alkylating agents differ in timing of cytopenias. Nitrosoureas, DTIC, and procarbazine can display delayed marrow toxicity, first appearing 6 weeks after dosing.

Complications of myelosuppression result from the predictable sequelae of the missing cells' function. *Febrile neutropenia* refers to the clinical presentation of fever (one temperature $\geq 38.5°C$ or three readings $\geq 38°C$ but $\leq 38.5°C$ per 24 h) in a cytopenic patient with an uncontrolled neoplasm involving the bone marrow or, more usually, in a patient undergoing treatment with cytotoxic agents. Mortality from uncontrolled infection varies inversely with the PMN count. If the nadir PMN count is $>1000/\mu L$, there is little risk; if $<500/\mu L$, risk of death is markedly increased. Management of febrile neutropenia has conventionally included empirical coverage with antibiotics for the duration of neutropenia (Chap. 85). Selection of antibiotics is governed by the expected association of infections with certain underlying neoplasms; careful physical examination (with scrutiny of catheter sites, dentition, mucosal surfaces, and perirectal and genital orifices by gentle palpation); chest x-ray; and Gram stain and culture of blood, urine and sputum (if any) to define a putative site of infection. In the absence of any originating site, a broadly acting β-lactam with anti-*Pseudomonas* activity, such as ceftazidime, is begun empirically. The addition of vancomycin to cover potential cutaneous sites of origin (until these are ruled out or shown to originate from methicillin-sensitive organisms) or metronidazole or imipenem for abdominal or other sites favoring anaerobes reflects modifications tailored to individual patient presentations. The coexistence of pulmonary compromise raises a distinct set of potential pathogens, including *Legionella*, *Pneumocystis*, and fungal agents, that may require further diagnostic evaluations such as bronchoscopy with bronchoalveolar lavage. Febrile neutropenic patients can be stratified broadly into two prognostic groups. The first, with expected short duration of neutropenia and no evidence of hypotension or abdominal or other localizing symptoms, may be expected to do well even with less complex, oral regimens, e.g., ciprofloxacin plus amoxicillin/clavulinic acid. Detailed evaluation of such simple oral programs and intravenous regimens is ongoing. A less favorable prognostic group are patients with expected prolonged neutropenia, evidence of sepsis, and end-organ compromise, particularly pneumonia. These patients clearly require tailoring of their antibiotic regimen to their underlying presentation, with frequent empirical addition of antifungal agents if fever persists for 7 days without identification of an adequately treated organism or site.

Transfusion of granulocytes has no role in the management of febrile neutropenia, owing to their exceedingly short half-life, mechanical fragility, and clinical syndromes of pulmonary compromise with leukostasis after their use. Instead, *colony stimulating factors* (CSFs) are used to augment bone marrow production of PMNs. These include "early-acting" factors such as IL-1, IL-3, and stem cell factor, which act on multiple lineages, and "late-acting" lineage-specific factors such as G-CSF (granulocyte colony stimulating factor) or GM-CSF (granulocyte-macrophage colony stimulating factor), erythropoietin, thrombopoietin, IL-6, and IL-11. CSFs are overused in oncology practice. The settings in which their use has been proven effective are limited. G-CSF, GM-CSF, erythropoietin, and IL-11 are currently approved for use. The American Society of Clinical Oncology has developed practice guidelines for the use of G-CSF and GM-CSF (Table 84-3). Primary administration (i.e., shortly after completing chemo-

Preventive Uses
With the first cycle of chemotherapy (so-called primary CSF administration)
 Not needed on a routine basis
 Use if the probability of febrile neutropenia is ≤40%
 Use if patient has preexisting neutropenia or active infection
With subsequent cycles if febrile neutropenia has previously occurred (so-called secondary CSF administration)
 Not needed after short duration neutropenia without fever
 Use if patient had febrile neutropenia in previous cycle
 Use if prolonged neutropenia (even without fever) delays therapy
Therapeutic Uses
Afebrile neutropenic patients
 No evidence of benefit
Febrile neutropenic patients
 No evidence of benefit
 May feel compelled to use in the face of clinical deterioration from sepsis, pneumonia, or fungal infection, but benefit unclear
To augment dose-intensity of chemotherapy in patients with curable malignancies
 No evidence of benefit
In bone marrow or peripheral blood stem cell transplantation
 Use to mobilize stem cells from marrow
 Use to hasten myeloid recovery
In acute myeloid leukemia
 G-CSF of minor or no benefit
 GM-CSF of no benefit and may be harmful
In myelodysplastic syndromes
 Not routinely beneficial
 Use intermittently in subset with neutropenia and recurrent infection
What Dose And Schedule Should Be Used?
G-CSF: 5 μg/kg per day subcutaneously
GM-CSF: 250 μg/m² per day subcutaneously
When Should Therapy Begin And End?
When indicated, start 24–72 h after chemotherapy
Continue until absolute neutrophil count is 10,000/μL
Do not use concurrently with chemotherapy or radiation therapy

NOTE: G-CSF, granulocyte colony stimulating factor; GM-CSF, granulocyte-macrophage colony stimulating factor.
SOURCE: From the American Society of Clinical Oncology.

therapy to reduce the nadir) of G-CSF to patients receiving cytotoxic regimens associated with a 40% incidence of febrile neutropenia has reduced the incidence of febrile neutropenia in several studies by about 50%. Most patients, however, receive regimens that do not have such a high risk of expected febrile neutropenia, and therefore most patients initially should not receive G-CSF or GM-CSF. Special circumstances such as a documented history of febrile neutropenia with the regimen in a particular patient; extensive compromise of marrow by prior radiation or chemotherapy; or active, open wounds or deep-seated infection may support primary treatment with G-CSF or GM-CSF. Administration of G-CSF or GM-CSF to afebrile neutropenic patients or to patients with "low-risk" febrile neutropenia (secondary administration, use after neutropenia has developed) as defined above is not recommended, although administration to "high-risk" patients with febrile neutropenia and evidence of organ compromise is reasonable. G-CSF or GM-CSF is conventionally started 24 to 72 h after completion of chemotherapy and continued until a PMN count of 10,000/μL is achieved. Also, patients with myeloid leukemias undergoing induction therapy may have a slight reduction in the duration of neutropenia if G-CSF (not GM-CSF) is commenced after completion of therapy and may be of particular value in elderly patients, but the influence on long-term outcome has not been defined. GM-CSF probably has a more restricted utility than G-CSF, with its use currently limited to patients after autologous bone marrow transplants, although proper "head-to-head" comparisons with G-CSF have not been conducted in most instances. GM-CSF may be associated with more systemic side effects.

Dangerous degrees of thrombocytopenia do not frequently complicate the management of patients with solid tumors receiving cytotoxic chemotherapy (carboplatin-containing regimens are frequently involved), but they are frequent in patients with certain hematologic neoplasms where marrow is infiltrated with tumor. Severe bleeding related to thrombocytopenia occurs with increased frequency at platelet counts <20,000/μL and is very prevalent at counts <5000/μL. Prophylactic transfusions to keep platelets >20,000/μL are warranted in patients with leukemia (the threshold for transfusion is 10,000/μL in patients with solid tumors and no other bleeding diathesis). Careful review of medication lists to prevent exposure to nonsteroidal anti-inflammatory agents and maintenance of clotting factor levels adequate to support near-normal prothrombin and partial thromboplastin time tests are of import in minimizing the risk of bleeding in the thrombocytopenic patient. Certain cytokines in clinical investigation have shown ability to increase platelets (e.g., IL-6, IL-1, thrombopoietin), but clinical benefit and safety are not yet proven. IL-11 (oprelvekin) is approved for use in the setting of expected thrombocytopenia, but its effects on platelet counts are small and it is associated with side effects such as headache, fever, malaise, syncope, cardiac arrhythmias, and fluid retention.

Anemia associated with chemotherapy can be managed by transfusion of packed RBCs. Transfusion is not undertaken until the hemoglobin falls to <80 g/L (8 g/dL), or if compromise of end-organ function occurs or an underlying condition (e.g., coronary artery disease) calls for maintenance of hemoglobin >90 g/L (9 g/dL). Patients who are to receive therapy for >2 months on a "stable" regimen and who are likely to require continuing transfusions are also candidates for erythropoietin to maintain hemoglobin of 90 to 100 g/L (9 to 10 g/dL). In the setting of adequate iron stores and serum erythropoietin levels <100 ng/mL, erythropoietin, 150 U three times a week, can produce a slow increase in hemoglobin over about 2 months of administration. Quality of life is better at higher hemoglobin concentrations, but expense is a concern with erythropoietin use.

Nausea and Vomiting The most common side effect of chemotherapy administration is nausea, with or without vomiting. Antineoplastic agents vary in their capacity to cause nausea and vomiting. Nitrogen mustard, nitrosoureas, streptozotocin, DTIC, cisplatin, and actinomycin are highly emetogenic and produce vomiting in virtually all patients. Doxorubicin, daunorubicin, and conventional-dose cyclophosphamide are moderately emetogenic. Antimetabolites are dose- and schedule-dependent, with single doses of methotrexate and fluorouracil producing at worst anorexia; while 5-day regimens of 5-fluorouracil and high-dose methotrexate produce nausea in ~50% of patients. Other agents such as chlorambucil, melphalan, and busulfan in conventional doses produce little tendency to emesis.

Emesis is a reflex caused by stimulation of the vomiting center in the medulla. Input to the vomiting center comes from the chemoreceptor trigger zone (CTZ) and afferents from the peripheral gastrointestinal tract, cerebral cortex, and heart. In addition, a conditioned reflex may contribute to anticipatory nausea arising after repeated cycles of chemotherapy. Accordingly, antiemesis agents differ in their locus of action. Combining agents from different classes or the sequential use of different classes of agent is the cornerstone of successful management of chemotherapy-induced nausea and vomiting. Of great importance are the prophylactic administration of agents and the use of psychological techniques including the maintenance of a supportive milieu, counseling, and relaxation to augment the action of antiemetic agents.

Antidopaminergic phenothiazines act directly at the CTZ, and include prochlorperazine (Compazine), 10 mg intramuscularly or intravenously, 10 to 25 mg orally, or 25 mg per rectum every 4 to 6 h for up to four doses; and thiethylperazine (Torecan), 10 mg by all the above routes every 6 h. Haloperidol (Haldol) is a butyrophenone dopamine antagonist given at 0.5 to 1.0 mg intramuscularly or orally every 8 h. Antihistamines such as diphenhydramine (Benadryl) have little intrinsic antiemetic capacity but are frequently given to prevent or treat dystonic reactions that can complicate use of the antidopaminergic agents. Lorazepam (Ativan) is a short-acting benzodiazepine that provides an anxiolytic effect to augment the effectiveness of a variety of agents when used at 1 to 2 mg intramuscularly, intravenously, or orally every 4 to 6 h. Dexamethasone (Decadron) likewise augments the action of a variety of agents when used at 4 to 40 mg intravenously or orally, given before treatment and repeated up to 10 mg orally every 6 h four times. Metoclopramide (Reglan) acts on peripheral dopamine receptors to augment gastric emptying and is used in high doses for highly emetogenic regimens (1 to 2 mg/kg intravenously 30 min before chemotherapy and every 2 h for up to three additional doses as needed); intravenous doses of 10 to 20 mg every 4 to 6 h as needed or 50 mg orally 4 h before and 8 and 12 h after chemotherapy are used for moderately emetogenic regimens. Serotonin antagonists are useful in moderately to severely emetogenic regimens; ondansetron (Zofran) is given as 0.15 mg/kg intravenously for three doses just before and at 4 and 8 h after chemotherapy, and granisetron (Kytril) is given as a single dose of 0.01 mg/kg just before chemotherapy. δ-9-Tetrahydrocannabinol (Marinol) is a rather weak antiemetic compared to other available agents, but it may be useful for persisting nausea and is used orally at 10 mg every 3 to 4 h as needed.

Alopecia　Chemotherapeutic agents vary widely in causing alopecia, with anthracyclines, alkylating agents, and topoisomerase inhibitors reliably causing near total alopecia when given at therapeutic doses. Antimetabolites are more variably associated with alopecia. Psychologic support and the use of cosmetic resources are to be encouraged, and "chemo caps" that reduce scalp temperature to decrease the degree of alopecia should be discouraged.

Gonadal Dysfunction and Pregnancy　Cessation of ovulation and azoospermia reliably result from alkylating agent– and topoisomerase poison–containing regimens. The duration of these effects varies with age and sex. Males treated for Hodgkin's disease with mechlorethamine- and procarbazine-containing regimens are effectively sterile, while fertility usually returns after regimens including cisplatin, vinblastine or etoposide, and bleomycin for testicular cancer. Sperm banking before treatment may be considered to support patients likely to be sterilized by treatment. Females experience amenorrhea with anovulation after alkylating agent therapy but are likely to recover normal menses if treatment is completed before age 30 and unlikely to recover menses after age 35. Even those who regain menses usually experience premature menopause. As the magnitude and extent of decreased fertility can be difficult to predict, patients should be counseled to maintain effective contraception, preferably by barrier means, during and after therapy. Resumption of efforts to conceive should be considered in the context of the likely prognosis of the patient. Hormone-replacement therapy should be undertaken in women who do not have a hormonally responsive tumor.

Chemotherapy agents have variable effects on the success of pregnancy (Chap. 7). All agents tend to have increased risk of adverse outcomes when administered during the first trimester, and strategies to delay chemotherapy if possible until after this milestone should be considered if the pregnancy is to continue to term. Patients in their second or third trimester can be treated with most regimens for the common neoplasms afflicting women in their child-bearing years with the exception of antimetabolites, particularly antifolates, which have notable teratogenic or fetotoxic effects throughout pregnancy. The need for anticancer chemotherapy per se is infrequently a clear basis to recommend termination of a concurrent pregnancy, although each treatment strategy in this circumstance must be tailored to the individual needs of the patient. →*Chronic effects of cancer treatment are reviewed in Chap. 103.*

BIOLOGIC THERAPY

No postulates resembling principles have emerged from efforts to develop biologic approaches to cancer treatment. The goal of biologic therapy is to manipulate the host-tumor interaction in favor of the host. Theoretically, biologic approaches should reflect a bell-shaped dose-response curve where the maximum biologic effect is less than the MTD. Empirical trial and error has led to the discovery that a number of biologic treatment approaches may produce antitumor effects, but nearly all of them are most active at their MTD.

IMMUNE MEDIATORS OF ANTITUMOR EFFECTS　The very existence of a cancer in a person is testimony to the failure of the immune system to deal effectively with the cancer. Tumors have a variety of means of avoiding the immune system: (1) they are often only subtly different from their normal counterparts; (2) they are capable of downregulating their major histocompatibility complex antigens, effectively masking them from recognition by T cells; (3) they are inefficient at presenting antigens to the immune system; (4) they can cloak themselves in a protective shell of fibrin to minimize contact with surveillance mechanisms; and (5) they can produce a range of soluble molecules, including potential immune targets, that can distract the immune system from recognizing the tumor cell. Some of the cell products initially polarize the immune response away from cellular immunity (shifting from Th1 to Th2 responses, Chap. 305) and ultimately lead to defects in T cells that prevent their activation and cytotoxic activity. Cancer treatment further suppresses host immunity. A variety of strategies are being tested to overcome these barriers.

Cell-Mediated Immunity　The strongest evidence that the immune system can exert clinically meaningful antitumor effects comes from allogeneic bone marrow transplantation. Adoptively transferred T cells from the donor expand in the tumor-bearing host, recognize the tumor as being foreign, and mediate impressive antitumor effects (graft-versus-tumor effects). Three types of experimental interventions are being developed to take advantage of the ability of T cells to kill tumor cells.

1.　Allogeneic T cells are being transferred to cancer-bearing hosts in three major settings: in the form of allogeneic bone marrow transplantation, as pure lymphocyte transfusions following bone marrow recovery after allogeneic bone marrow transplantation, and as pure lymphocyte transfusions following immunosuppressive (but not myeloablative) therapy (so-called minitransplants). In each of these settings, the effector cells are donor T cells that recognize the tumor as being foreign, probably through minor histocompatibility differences. The main risk of such therapy is the development of graft-versus-host disease because of the minimal difference between the cancer and the normal host cells. This approach has been highly effective in hematologic cancers.

2.　Autologous T cells are being removed from the tumor-bearing host, manipulated in several ways in vitro, and given back to the patient. The two major classes of autologous T cell manipulation are: (1) to develop tumor antigen–specific T cells and expand them to large numbers over many weeks ex vivo before administration, and (2) to activate the cells with polyclonal stimulators such as anti-CD3 and anti-CD28 after a short period ex vivo and try to expand them in the host after adoptive transfer with stimulation by IL-2, for example. Short periods removed from the patient permit the cells to overcome the tumor-induced T cell defects, and such cells traffic and home to sites of disease better than cells that have been in culture for many weeks. Individual centers have successful experiences with one or the other approach but not both, and whether one is superior to the other is not known.

3.　Tumor vaccines are aimed at boosting T cell immunity. The finding that mutant oncogenes that are expressed only intracellularly can be recognized as targets of T cell killing greatly expanded the possibilities for tumor vaccine development. No longer is it difficult to find something different about tumor cells from normal cells. However, major difficulties remain in getting the tumor-specific peptides presented in a fashion to prime the T cells. Tumors themselves are very poor at presenting their own antigens to T cells at the first antigen exposure (*priming*). Priming is best accomplished by professional antigen-presenting cells (dendritic cells). Thus, a number of experimental strategies are aimed at priming host T cells against tumor-associated peptides. Vaccine adjuvants such as GM-CSF appear capable of attracting antigen-presenting cells to a skin site containing a tumor antigen. Such an approach has been documented to eradicate microscopic residual disease in follicular lymphoma and give rise to tumor-specific T cells. Purified antigen-presenting cells can be pulsed with tumor, its membranes, or particular tumor antigens and delivered as a vaccine. Tumor cells can be transfected with genes that attract antigen-presenting cells. Other ideas are also being tested. In a variation on the theme of adoptive transfer, the tumor vaccine may be given to the normal bone marrow and lymphoid cell donor of an allogeneic transplant so that the donor immune system has more cells capable of recognizing the tumor specifically. Vaccines against viral cancers (papillomavirus in cervical cancer), lymphomas, and melanomas have had modest clinical success.

Antibodies In general, antibodies are not very effective at killing cancer cells. Because the tumor seems to influence the host toward making antibodies rather than generating cellular immunity, it is inferred that antibodies are easier to defend against. Many patients can be shown to have serum antibodies directed at their tumors, but these do not appear to influence disease progression. However, the ability to grow very large quantities of high-affinity antibody directed at a tumor by the hybridoma technique has led to the application of antibodies to the treatment of cancer. The first study of a monoclonal antibody in cancer was published in 1980 and demonstrated many hurdles that needed to be overcome to make the approach successful. It seemed best to attack a determinant that was not shed or modulated by the tumor. A target that was involved in an important function for the tumor cells might be superior to a physiologically irrelevant target. Murine antibodies were not very effective because they did not mediate human effector mechanisms well and the host nearly always made antibodies against the therapeutic antibody that prevented it from finding the target.

The lessons were learned; humanized antibodies against the CD20 molecule expressed on B cell lymphomas (rituximab) and against the HER-2/neu receptor overexpressed on epithelial cancers, especially breast cancer (herceptin), have become reliable tools in the oncologists armamentarium. Each used alone can cause tumor regression (rituximab > herceptin), and both appear to potentiate the effects of combination chemotherapy given just after antibody administration. It is likely that other antibodies against other important tumor targets will be available soon. Conjugation to drugs, toxins, isotopes, photodynamic agents, and other killing moieties may also be effective. Radioconjugates are the closest to approval. Other conjugates are associated with problems that have not yet been solved (e.g., antigenicity, instability, poor tumor penetration).

Cytokines There are >70 separate proteins and glycoproteins with biologic effects in humans: IFN-α, -β, -γ; IL-1 through -18 (so far); the tumor necrosis factor (TFN) family [including lymphotoxin, TFN-related apoptosis-inducing ligand (TRAIL), CD40 ligand, and others]; and the chemokine family. Only a fraction of these has been tested against cancer; only IFN-α and IL-2 are in routine clinical use.

About 20 different genes encode IFN-α, and their biologic effects are indistinguishable. Interferon induces the expression of many genes, inhibits protein synthesis, and exerts a number of different effects on diverse cellular processes. Its antitumor effects appear to be antagonized in vitro by thymidine, suggesting that de novo thymidylate synthesis is also affected. The two recombinant forms that are commercially available are IFN-α2a and -α2b. In general, interferon antitumor effects are dose-related, and IFN is most effective at its MTD. Interferon is not curative for any tumor but can induce partial responses in follicular lymphoma, hairy cell leukemia, chronic myeloid leukemia, melanoma, and Kaposi's sarcoma. It has been used in the adjuvant setting in stage II melanoma, multiple myeloma, and follicular lymphoma. Its effects on survival are controversial. It produces fever, fatigue, a flulike syndrome, malaise, myelosuppression, and depression and can induce clinically significant autoimmune disease.

IL-2 must exert its antitumor effects indirectly through augmentation of immune function. Its biologic activity is to promote the growth and activity of T cells and natural killer (NK) cells. High doses of IL-2 can produce tumor regressions in ~20% of patients with meta-

static melanoma and renal cell cancer. About 5% of patients may experience complete remissions that are durable, unlike any other treatment for these tumors. IL-2 is associated with myriad clinical side effects: intravascular volume depletion, capillary leak syndrome, adult respiratory distress syndrome, hypotension, fever, chills, skin rash, and impaired renal and liver function. Patients may require blood pressure support and intensive care to manage the toxicity. However, once the agent is stopped, most of the toxicities reverse completely within 3 to 6 days.

BIBLIOGRAPHY

ABELOFF MD et al (eds): *Clinical Oncology*, 2d ed. Philadelphia, Churchill Livingstone, 2000

AMERICAN SOCIETY OF CLINICAL ONCOLOGY: Update of recommendations for use of hematopoietic colony-stimulating factors: Evidence-based clinical practice guidelines. J Clin Oncol 14:1957, 1996

CHABNER BA, LONGO DL (eds): *Cancer Chemotherapy and Biotherapy: Principles and Practice*, 3d ed. Philadelphia, Lippincott Williams & Wilkins, 2001

| **85** | *Robert Finberg* |

INFECTIONS IN PATIENTS WITH CANCER

ALL	acute lymphocytic leukemia	CT	computed tomography
AML	acute myelocytic leukemia	HSV	herpes simplex virus
CLL	chronic lymphocytic leukemia	MRI	magnetic resonance imaging
CMV	cytomegalovirus	PMNs	polymorphonuclear leukocytes
CNS	central nervous system	VZV	varicella-zoster virus

Infections are a common cause of death and an even more common cause of morbidity in patients with a wide variety of neoplasms. Autopsy studies show that most deaths from acute leukemia and half of deaths from lymphoma are caused directly by infection. With more intensive chemotherapy, patients with solid tumors have become more likely to die of infection rather than their underlying disease.

A physical predisposition to infection (Table 85-1) can be a result of the neoplasm's production of a break in the skin; for example, a squamous cell carcinoma may cause local invasion of the epidermis, which allows bacteria to gain access to the subcutaneous tissue and permits the development of cellulitis. The artificial closing of a normally patent orifice can also predispose to infection: Obstruction of a ureter by a tumor can cause urinary tract infection, and obstruction of the bile duct can cause cholangitis. Part of the host's normal defense against infection depends on the continuous emptying of a viscus; without emptying, a few bacteria present as a result of bacteremia or local transit can multiply and cause disease.

A similar problem can affect patients whose lymph node integrity has been disrupted by radical surgery, particularly patients who have had radical node dissections. A common clinical problem following radical mastectomy is the development of cellulitis (usually caused by streptococci or staphylococci) because of lymphedema and/or inadequate lymph drainage. In most cases, this problem can be addressed by local measures designed to prevent fluid accumulation and breaks in the skin, but antibiotic prophylaxis has been necessary in refractory cases.

A life-threatening problem common to many cancer patients is the loss of the reticuloendothelial capacity to clear microorganisms after splenectomy. Splenectomy is common in patients with Hodgkin's disease and in the management of hairy cell leukemia, chronic lymphocytic leukemia (CLL), and refractory idiopathic thrombocytopenic purpura. Even after curative therapy for the underlying disease, the lack of a spleen predisposes such patients to rapidly fatal infections.

Table 85-1 Normal Barriers to Infections

Type of Defense	Specific Lesion	Cells Involved	Organisms	Cancer Association	Disease
Physical barrier	Breaks in skin	Skin epithelial cells	Staphylococci, streptococci	Head and neck, squamous cell carcinoma	Cellulitis, extensive skin infection
Emptying of fluid collections	Occlusion of orifices: ureters, bile duct, colon	Luminal epithelial cells	Gram-negative bacilli	Renal, ovarian, biliary tree, metastatic diseases of many cancers	Rapid, overwhelming bacteremia, urinary tract infection
Lymphatic disease	Node dissection	Lymph nodes	Staphylococci, streptococci	Breast cancer surgery	Cellulitis
Splenic clearance of microorganisms	Splenectomy	Splenic reticuloendothelial cells	*Streptococcus pneumoniae, Haemophilus influenzae, Neisseria meningitidis, Babesia, Capnocytophaga canimorsus*	Hodgkin's disease, leukemia, idiopathic thrombocytopenic purpura	Rapid, overwhelming sepsis
Phagocytosis	Lack of granulocytes	Granulocytes (neutrophils)	Staphylococci, streptococci, enteric organisms	Hairy cell, acute myelocytic, and acute lymphocytic leukemias	Bacteremia
Humoral immunity	Lack of antibody	B cells	*S. pneumoniae, H. influenzae, N. meningitidis*	Chronic lymphocytic leukemia	Infections with encapsulated organisms, sinusitis, pneumonia
Cellular immunity	Lack of T cells	T cells and macrophages	*Mycobacterium tuberculosis, Listeria,* herpesviruses, fungi, other intracellular parasites	Hodgkin's disease, leukemia, T cell lymphoma	Infections with intracellular bacteria, fungi, parasites

The loss of the spleen through trauma similarly predisposes the normal host to overwhelming infection as long as 25 years after splenectomy. The splenectomized patient should be counseled about the risks of infection with certain organisms, such as the protozoan *Babesia* (Chap. 214) and *Capnocytophaga canimorsus* (formerly dysgonic fermenter 2 or DF-2), a bacterium carried in the mouths of animals (Chap. 127). Since encapsulated bacteria (*Streptococcus pneumoniae, Haemophilus influenzae,* and *Neisseria meningitidis*) are the organisms most commonly associated with postsplenectomy sepsis, splenectomized persons should be vaccinated (and revaccinated; Table 85-2) against the capsular polysaccharides of these organisms. Many clinicians recommend giving splenectomized patients a small supply of antibiotics effective against *S. pneumoniae, N. meningitidis,* and *H. influenzae* to avert rapid, overwhelming sepsis in the event that they cannot present for medical attention immediately after the onset of fever or other symptoms of bacterial infection.

The level of suspicion of infections with certain organisms should depend on the type of cancer diagnosed (Table 85-3). Diagnosis of multiple myeloma or CLL should prompt the measurement of immunoglobulin levels and the consideration of either antibody replacement or antibiotic prophylaxis. (In the case of CLL, antibiotic prophylaxis for likely pathogens has proven a cost-effective preventive measure.) Similarly, patients with acute lymphocytic leukemia (ALL), patients with non-Hodgkin's lymphoma, and all cancer patients treated with high-dose glucocorticoids (or glucocorticoid-containing chemotherapy regimens) should receive antibiotic prophylaxis for *Pneumocystis carinii* infection (Table 85-3).

In addition to exhibiting susceptibility to certain infectious organisms, patients with cancer are likely to manifest their infections in characteristic ways.

SYSTEM-SPECIFIC SYNDROMES

SKIN-SPECIFIC SYNDROMES (See Plate IID-57) Skin lesions are common in cancer patients, and their appearance may permit the diagnosis of systemic bacterial or fungal infection. While cellulitis caused by skin organisms such as *Streptococcus* or *Staphylococcus* is common, neutropenic patients and those with impaired blood or lym-

Table 85-2 Vaccination of Cancer Patients Receiving Chemotherapy

Vaccine	Use in Indicated Patients		
	Intensive Chemotherapy	Hodgkin's Disease	Bone Marrow Transplantation
Diphtheria-tetanus (diphtheria, pertussis, tetanus; DPT) for children <7 years old	Primary series and boosters as necessary	No special recommendation	12 and 24 months after transplantation
Poliomyelitis[a]	Complete primary series and boosters	No special recommendation	12 and 24 months after transplantation
Haemophilus influenzae type b	Primary series and booster for children	Immunization before treatment and booster 3 months afterward	12 and 24 months after transplantation
23-Valent pneumococcal	Every 5 years	Immunization before treatment and booster 3 months afterward	12 and 24 months after transplantation
4-Valent meningococcal	Every 5 years	Immunization before treatment and booster 3 months afterward	12 and 24 months after transplantation
Influenza	Seasonal immunization	Seasonal immunization	Seasonal immunization
Measles/mumps/rubella	Contraindicated	Contraindicated	After 24 months in patients without graft-versus-host disease
Varicella-zoster virus	Contraindicated[b]	Contraindicated	Contraindicated

[a] Live-virus vaccine is contraindicated; inactivated vaccine should be used.

[b] Contact the manufacturer for more information on use in children with acute lymphocytic leukemia.

Table 85-3 Infections and Cancer

Cancer	Underlying Immune Abnormality	Organisms Causing Infection
Multiple myeloma	Hypogammaglobulinemia	*Streptococcus pneumoniae, Haemophilus influenzae, Neisseria meningitidis*
Chronic lymphocytic leukemia	Hypogammaglobulinemia	*S. pneumoniae, H. influenzae, N. meningitidis*
Acute myelocytic or lymphocytic leukemia	Granulocytopenia, skin and mucous-membrane lesions	Extracellular gram-positive and gram-negative bacteria, fungi
Hodgkin's disease	Abnormal T cell function	Intracellular pathogens (*Mycobacterium tuberculosis, Listeria, Salmonella, Cryptococcus, Mycobacterium avium*)
Non-Hodgkin's lymphoma and acute lymphocytic leukemia	Glucocorticoid chemotherapy, T and B cell dysfunction	*Pneumocystis carinii*
Colon and rectal tumors	Local abnormalities[a]	*Streptococcus bovis* (bacteremia)
Hairy cell leukemia	Abnormal T cell function	Intracellular pathogens (*M. tuberculosis, Listeria, Cryptococcus, M. avium*)

[a] The reason for this association is not well defined.

phatic drainage may develop infections with unusual organisms. Innocent-looking macules or papules may be the first sign of bacterial or fungal sepsis in immunocompromised patients. In the neutropenic host, a macule progresses rapidly to ecthyma gangrenosum, a usually painless, round, necrotic lesion consisting of a central black or gray-black eschar with surrounding erythema. Ecthyma gangrenosum is located in nonpressure areas (as distinguished from necrotic lesions associated with lack of circulation) and is often associated with *Pseudomonas aeruginosa* bacteremia (Chap. 155) but may be caused by other bacteria.

Candidemia (Chap. 205) is also associated with a variety of skin conditions and commonly presents as a maculopapular rash. Punch biopsy of the skin may be the best method for diagnosis.

Cellulitis, an acute spreading inflammation of the skin, is most often caused by infection with group A *Streptococcus* or *Staphylococcus aureus*, virulent organisms normally found on the skin (Chap. 128). Although cellulitis tends to be circumscribed in normal hosts, it may spread rapidly in neutropenic patients [those with fewer than 500 functional polymorphonuclear leukocytes (PMNs) per microliter]. A tiny break in the skin may lead to spreading cellulitis, which is characterized by pain and erythema; in such patients, signs of infection (e.g., purulence) are often lacking. What might be a furuncle in a normal host may require amputation because of uncontrolled infection in a patient presenting with leukemia. A dramatic response to an infection that might be trivial in a normal host can mark the first sign of leukemia. Fortunately, granulocytopenic patients are likely to be infected with certain types of organisms (Table 85-4); thus the selection of an antibiotic regimen is somewhat easier than it might otherwise be. (See discussion below on the selection of antibiotics for use in neutropenic patients.) It is essential to recognize cellulitis early and to treat it aggressively. Patients who are neutropenic or have previously received antibiotics for other reasons may develop cellulitis with unusual organisms (e.g., *Escherichia coli, Pseudomonas*, or fungi). Early treatment, even of innocent-looking lesions, is essential to prevent necrosis and loss of tissue. Debridement to prevent spread may

Table 85-4 Organisms Likely to Cause Infections in Granulocytopenic Patients

Gram-positive cocci	*Enterobacter* spp.
Staphylococcus epidermidis	*Serratia* spp.
Staphylococcus aureus	*Acinetobacter* spp.[a]
Viridans *Streptococcus*	*Citrobacter* spp.
Enterococcus faecalis	Gram-positive bacilli
Streptococcus pneumoniae	Diphtheroids
Gram-negative bacilli	JK bacillus[a]
Escherichia coli	Fungi
Klebsiella spp.	*Candida* spp.
Pseudomonas aeruginosa	*Aspergillus* spp.
Non-*aeruginosa Pseudomonas* spp.[a]	

[a] Often associated with intravenous catheters.

sometimes be necessary early in the course of disease, but it can often be performed after chemotherapy, when the PMN count increases.

Sweet's syndrome, or *febrile neutrophilic dermatosis*, was originally described in women with elevated white blood cell counts. The disease is characterized by the presence of leukocytes in the lower dermis, with edema of the papillary body. Ironically, this disease now is usually seen in neutropenic patients with cancer, most often in association with acute leukemia but also in association with a variety of other malignancies. Sweet's syndrome usually presents as red or bluish-red papules or nodules that may coalesce and form sharply bordered plaques. The edema may suggest vesicles, but on palpation the lesions are solid, and vesicles probably never arise in this disease. The lesions are most common on the face, neck, and arms. On the legs, they may be confused with erythema nodosum. The development of lesions is often accompanied by high fevers and an elevated erythrocyte sedimentation rate. Both the lesions and the temperature elevation respond dramatically to glucocorticoids. Treatment begins with high doses of glucocorticoids (60 mg of prednisone per day) followed by tapered doses over the next 2 to 3 weeks.

Data indicate that *erythema multiforme* with mucous membrane involvement is often associated with herpes simplex virus (HSV) infection and is distinct from Stevens-Johnson syndrome, which is associated with drugs and tends to have a more widespread distribution. Since cancer patients are both immunosuppressed (and therefore susceptible to herpes infections) and heavily treated with drugs (and therefore subject to Stevens-Johnson syndrome), both of these conditions are common in this population.

Cytokines, which are used as adjuvants or primary treatments for cancer, can themselves cause characteristic rashes, further complicating the differential diagnosis. This phenomenon is a particular problem in bone marrow transplant recipients (Chap. 136), who, in addition to having the usual chemotherapy-, antibiotic-, and cytokine-induced rashes, are plagued by graft-versus-host disease.

CATHETER-RELATED INFECTIONS Because intravenous catheters are commonly used in cancer chemotherapy and are prone to infection (Chap. 135), they pose a major problem in the care of patients with cancer. Reviews have emphasized that some infected catheters can be treated with antibiotics while others must be removed. If the patient has a "tunneled" catheter (which consists of an entrance site, a subcutaneous tunnel, and an exit site), a red streak over the subcutaneous part of the line (the tunnel) is grounds for immediate removal of the catheter. Failure to remove catheters under these circumstances may result in extensive cellulitis and tissue necrosis.

More common than tunnel infections are exit-site infections, often with erythema around the area where the line penetrates the skin. Most authorities (Chap. 139) recommend treatment (usually with vancomycin) for an exit-site infection caused by a coagulase-negative *Staphylococcus*. Treatment of coagulase-positive staphylococcal infection is associated with a poorer outcome, and it is advisable to remove the catheter. Similarly, many clinicians remove catheters associated with infections due to *P. aeruginosa* and *Candida* species, since such infections are difficult to treat and bloodstream infections with these organisms are likely to be deadly.

GASTROINTESTINAL TRACT–SPECIFIC SYNDROMES
Upper Gastrointestinal Tract Disease • *Infections of the mouth*
The oral cavity is rich in aerobic and anaerobic bacteria (Chap. 167) that normally live in a commensal relationship with the host. The antimetabolic effects of chemotherapy cause a breakdown of host defenses, leading to ulceration of the mouth and the potential for invasion by resident bacteria. Mouth ulcerations afflict most patients receiving chemotherapy and have been associated with viridans streptococcal bacteremia. A variety of topical rinses and elixirs have been proposed to treat these ulcerations. Although some may have a local anesthetic effect, the efficacy of any of these therapies in the prevention of disease is unproven. Similarly, the efficacy of mouthwashes in the prevention of esophagitis or invasive candidiasis is doubtful. Fluconazole, on the other hand, is clearly effective in the treatment of both local infections (thrush) and systemic infections (esophagitis) due to *C. albicans*.

Noma (or *cancrum oris*), commonly seen in malnourished children, is a penetrating disease of the soft and hard tissues of the mouth and adjacent sites, with resulting necrosis and gangrene. It has a counterpart in immunocompromised patients and is thought to be due to invasion of the tissues by *Bacteroides*, *Fusobacterium*, and other normal inhabitants of the mouth. It is associated with debility, poor oral hygiene, and immunosuppression.

Viruses, particularly HSV, are a prominent cause of morbidity in immunocompromised patients, in whom they are associated with severe mucositis. The use of acyclovir, either prophylactically or therapeutically, is of value.

Esophageal infections The differential diagnosis of esophagitis (usually presenting as substernal chest pain upon swallowing) includes herpes simplex and candidiasis, both of which are readily treatable.

Lower Gastrointestinal Tract Disease Hepatic candidiasis (Chap. 205) results from seeding of the liver (usually from a gastrointestinal source) in neutropenic patients. It is most common in patients being treated for acute leukemia and usually develops around the time the neutropenia resolves. The characteristic picture is that of persistent fever unresponsive to antibiotics; abdominal pain and tenderness or nausea; and elevated serum levels of alkaline phosphatase in a patient with hematologic malignancy who has recently recovered from neutropenia. The diagnosis of this disease (which may present in an indolent manner and persist for several months) is based on the finding of yeasts or pseudohyphae in granulomatous lesions. Hepatic ultrasound or computed tomography (CT) may reveal bull's-eye lesions. In some cases, magnetic resonance imaging (MRI) reveals small lesions not visible by other imaging modalities. The pathology (a granulomatous response) and the timing (with resolution of neutropenia and an elevation in granulocyte count) suggest that the host response to *Candida* is an important component of the manifestations of disease. In many cases, although organisms are visible, cultures of biopsied material may be negative. The designation *hepatosplenic candidiasis* or *hepatic candidiasis* is a misnomer because the disease often involves the kidneys and other tissues; the term *chronic disseminated candidiasis* may be more appropriate. Because of the risk of bleeding with liver biopsy, diagnosis is often based on radiographic abnormalities. Amphotericin B is traditionally used for therapy (often for several months, until all manifestations of disease have disappeared), but fluconazole may be useful for outpatient therapy.

Typhlitis *Typhlitis*, sometimes referred to as necrotizing colitis, neutropenic colitis, necrotizing enteropathy, ileocecal syndrome, or cecitis, is a clinical syndrome of fever and right-lower-quadrant tenderness in an immunosuppressed host. This syndrome is almost always seen in neutropenic patients after chemotherapy with cytotoxic drugs. It may be more common among children than among adults and appears to be much more common among patients with acute myelocytic leukemia (AML) or ALL than among those with other types of cancer.

Physical examination reveals right-lower-quadrant tenderness, with or without rebound tenderness. Associated diarrhea (often bloody) is common, and the diagnosis can be confirmed by the finding of a thickened cecal wall on CT or ultrasonography. Plain films may reveal a right-lower-quadrant mass, but CT with contrast or MRI is a much more sensitive means of making the diagnosis. Although surgery is sometimes attempted to avoid perforation from ischemia, most cases resolve with medical therapy alone. The disease is sometimes associated with positive blood cultures (usually for aerobic gram-negative bacilli), and therapy is recommended for a broad spectrum of bacteria (particularly gram-negative bacilli, likely bowel flora). Recurrence is rare, and most patients recover uneventfully.

***Clostridium difficile*–Induced Diarrhea** Cancer patients seem to be predisposed to the development of *C. difficile* diarrhea (Chap. 145) as a consequence of chemotherapy alone. Thus, they may have positive toxin tests before receiving antibiotics. Obviously, such patients are also subject to *C. difficile*–induced diarrhea as a result of antibiotic pressure. It is worth noting that toxins other than *C. difficile* may be associated with diarrhea; therefore, the detection of nonspecific toxins in the stool—without a specific neutralization test—does not prove that *C. difficile* infection is present.

CENTRAL NERVOUS SYSTEM–SPECIFIC SYNDROMES
Meningitis While meningitis in immunocompetent adults is likely to be caused by *S. pneumoniae*, the same is not true in immunocompromised patients. As noted previously, splenectomized patients are susceptible to rapid overwhelming infection with encapsulated bacteria (including *S. pneumoniae*, *H. influenzae*, and *N. meningitidis*). Similarly, patients who are antibody-deficient (such as patients with CLL, those who have received intensive chemotherapy, or those who have undergone bone marrow transplantation) are likely to have infections with these bacteria. Other cancer patients, however, because of their defective cellular immunity, are likely to be infected with other pathogens (Table 85-3). The presentation of meningitis in patients with lymphoma, patients receiving chemotherapy (particularly with glucocorticoids) for solid tumors, and patients who have received bone marrow transplants suggests a diagnosis of cryptococcal or listerial infection.

Encephalitis The spectrum of disease resulting from viral encephalitis is expanded in immunocompromised patients. Infection with varicella-zoster virus (VZV) has been associated with encephalitis that may be caused by VZV-related vasculitis. The slow viruses (e.g., Creutzfeldt-Jakob agent) may also be associated with dementia and encephalitic presentations, and a diagnosis of progressive multifocal leukoencephalopathy should be considered when a patient who has received chemotherapy presents with dementia. Other abnormalities of the central nervous system (CNS) that may be confused with infection include normal-pressure hydrocephalus and vasculitis resulting from CNS irradiation. It may be possible to differentiate these conditions by MRI.

Brain Abscess Brain abscesses in immunocompromised patients are likely to be due to *Cryptococcus* (particularly in patients with lymphoma or those receiving glucocorticoids), *Nocardia*, or *Aspergillus*. *Aspergillus* may enter via the lungs or—like *Mucor*—may invade the hard and soft palates to cause pneumonia (see below) with or without brain abscesses.

PULMONARY INFECTIONS
Pneumonia (Chap. 255) in immunocompromised patients may be difficult to diagnose because conventional methods of diagnosis depend on the presence of neutrophils. Bacterial pneumonia in neutropenic patients may present without purulent sputum—or, in fact, without any sputum at all—and may not produce physical findings suggestive of chest consolidation (rales or egophony).

In granulocytopenic patients with persistent or recurrent fever, the chest x-ray pattern may help to localize an infection and thus to determine which investigative tests and procedures should be undertaken and which therapeutic options should be considered (Table 85-5). The difficulties encountered in the management of pulmonary infiltrates relate in part to the difficulties of performing diagnostic procedures on

| Infiltrate | Cause of Pneumonia | |
	Infectious	Noninfectious
Localized	Common bacterial pulmonary pathogens, *Legionella*, mycobacteria	Local hemorrhage or embolism, tumor
Nodular	Fungi (e.g., *Aspergillus* or *Mucor*), *Nocardia*	Recurrent tumor
Diffuse	Viruses (especially CMV), *Chlamydia*, *Pneumocystis carinii*, *Toxoplasma gondii*, mycobacteria	Congestive heart failure, radiation pneumonitis, drug-induced lung injury, diffuse alveolar hemorrhage (described after BMT)

ABBREVIATIONS: CMV, cytomegalovirus; BMT, bone marrow transplantation.

the patients involved. When platelet counts can be increased to adequate levels by transfusion, microscopic and microbiologic evaluation of the fluid obtained by endoscopic bronchial lavage is often diagnostic. Lavage fluid should be cultured for *Mycoplasma*, *Chlamydia*, *Legionella*, *Nocardia*, fungi, and more common bacterial pathogens. In addition, the possibility of *P. carinii* pneumonia should be considered, especially in patients with ALL or lymphoma who have not received prophylactic trimethoprim-sulfamethoxazole. The characteristics of the infiltrate may be helpful in decisions about further diagnostic and therapeutic maneuvers. Nodular infiltrates suggest fungal pneumonia (e.g., that caused by *Aspergillus* or *Mucor*). Such lesions may best be approached by visualized biopsy procedures.

Aspergillus species (Chap. 206) can colonize the skin and respiratory tract or cause fatal systemic illness. Although *Aspergillus* may cause aspergillomas in a previously existing cavity or may produce allergic bronchopulmonary aspergillosis, the major problem posed by this genus in neutropenic patients is invasive disease due to *A. fumigatus* or *A. flavus*. The organisms enter the host through colonization of the respiratory tract, with subsequent invasion of the blood vessels. The disease is likely to present as a thrombotic or embolic event because of the ability of the organisms to invade blood vessels. The risk of infection with *Aspergillus* correlates directly with the duration of neutropenia. In prolonged neutropenia, positive surveillance cultures for colonization of the nasopharynx with *Aspergillus* may predict the development of disease.

Patients with *Aspergillus* infection often present with pleuritic chest pain and fever, which are sometimes accompanied by cough. Hemoptysis may be an ominous sign. Chest x-rays may reveal new focal infiltrates or nodules. Chest CT may reveal a characteristic halo consisting of a mass-like infiltrate surrounded by an area of low attenuation. The presence of a "crescent sign" on a chest x-ray or a chest CT scan, in which the mass progresses to central cavitation, is characteristic of invasive *Aspergillus* infection but may develop only with the resolution of the lesions.

In addition to causing pulmonary presentations, *Aspergillus* may invade through the nose or palate, with deep sinus penetration. The appearance of a discolored area in the nasal passages or on the hard palate should prompt a search for invasive *Aspergillus*. This situation is likely to require surgical debridement. Treatment (Chap. 205) with high doses of amphotericin B has been successful in curing granulocytopenic patients of invasive *Aspergillus* infection after the return of granulocytes. Catheter infections with *Aspergillus* usually require both removal of the catheter and antifungal therapy.

Diffuse interstitial infiltrates suggest viral, parasitic, or *P. carinii* pneumonia. If the patient has a diffuse interstitial pattern on chest x-ray, it may be reasonable to institute empirical treatment with trimethoprim-sulfamethoxazole (for *Pneumocystis*) and an erythromycin derivative or a quinolone (for *Chlamydia*, *Mycoplasma*, and *Legionella*) while considering invasive diagnostic procedures. Noninvasive procedures, such as staining of sputum smears for *Pneumocystis* and serum cryptococcal antigen tests, may be helpful on occasion. In trans-

plant recipients who are seropositive for cytomegalovirus (CMV), culture of a nonpulmonary site for CMV may be worthwhile. Infections with viruses that cause only upper respiratory symptoms in immunocompetent hosts, such as respiratory syncytial, influenza, and parainfluenza viruses, may be associated with fatal pneumonitis in immunocompromised hosts. An attempt at early diagnosis by nasopharyngeal aspiration should be considered so that appropriate treatment can be instituted.

While bleomycin is the most common cause of chemotherapy-induced lung disease, other causes include alkylating agents (such as cyclophosphamide, chlorambucil, and melphalan), nitrosoureas [carmustine (BCNU), lomustine (CCNU), and methyl-CCNU], busulfan, procarbazine, methotrexate, and hydroxyurea. Both infectious and noninfectious (drug- and/or radiation-induced) pneumonitis can cause fever and abnormalities on chest x-ray; thus, the differential diagnosis of an infiltrate in a patient receiving chemotherapy encompasses a broad range of conditions (Table 85-5). Since the treatment of radiation pneumonitis (which may respond dramatically to glucocorticoids) or drug-induced pneumonitis is different from that of infectious pneumonia, a biopsy may be important in the diagnosis. Unfortunately, no definitive diagnosis can be made in approximately 30% of cases, even after bronchoscopy.

Open-lung biopsy is the "gold standard" of diagnostic techniques. Biopsy via a visualized thoracostomy can replace an open procedure in many cases. When a biopsy cannot be performed, empirical treatment can be undertaken with erythromycin (or an erythromycin derivative such as azithromycin) and trimethoprim-sulfamethoxazole (in the case of diffuse infiltrates) or with amphotericin B (in the case of nodular infiltrates). The risks should be weighed carefully in these cases. If inappropriate drugs are administered, empirical treatment may prove toxic or ineffective; either of these outcomes may be riskier than biopsy.

CARDIOVASCULAR INFECTIONS Patients with Hodgkin's disease are prone to persistent infections by *Salmonella*, sometimes (and particularly often in elderly patients) affecting a vascular site. The use of intravenous catheters deliberately lodged in the right atrium is associated with a high incidence of bacterial endocarditis (presumably related to valve damage followed by bacteremia). Nonbacterial thrombotic endocarditis has been described in association with a variety of malignancies (most often solid tumors) and may follow bone marrow transplantation as well. The presentation of an embolic event with a new cardiac murmur suggests this diagnosis. Blood cultures are negative in this disease of unknown pathogenesis.

ENDOCRINE SYNDROMES In addition to infections of the skin, gastrointestinal tract, and pulmonary system, infections of the endocrine system have been described in immunocompromised patients. *Candida* infection of the thyroid during neutropenia can be defined by indium-labeled white-cell scans or gallium scans after neutrophil counts increase. CMV infection can cause adrenalitis with or without resulting adrenal insufficiency. The presentation of a sudden endocrine anomaly in an immunocompromised patient may be a sign of infection in the involved end organ.

MUSCULOSKELETAL INFECTIONS Infection that is a result of vascular compromise (resulting in gangrene) can occur when a tumor compromises the blood supply to muscles, bones, or joints. The process of diagnosis and treatment of such infection is similar to that in normal hosts, with the following caveats: (1) In terms of diagnosis, a lack of physical findings resulting from a lack of granulocytes in the granulocytopenic patient should make the clinician more aggressive in obtaining tissue rather than relying on physical signs. (2) In terms of therapy, aggressive debridement of infected tissues may be required, but it is usually difficult to operate on patients who have recently received chemotherapy, both because of a lack of platelets (which results in bleeding complications) and because of a lack of white blood cells (which may lead to secondary infection). A blood culture positive for *Clostridium perfringens* (an organism commonly associated with gas gangrene) can have a number of meanings (Chap. 145). Bloodstream infections with intestinal organisms like *Streptococcus bovis* and *C. perfringens* may arise spontaneously from lower gastrointestinal lesions (tumor or polyps); alternatively, these lesions may be harbingers of invasive disease. The clinical setting must be considered in order to define the appropriate treatment for each case.

RENAL AND URETERAL INFECTIONS   Infections of the urinary tract are common among patients whose ureteral excretion is compromised (Table 85-1). *Candida*, which has a predilection for the kidney, can invade either from the bloodstream or in a retrograde manner (via the ureters or bladder) in immunocompromised patients. The presence of "fungus balls" or persistent candiduria suggests invasive disease. Persistent funguria (with *Aspergillus* as well as *Candida*) should prompt a search for a nidus of infection in the kidney.

Certain viruses are typically seen only in immunosuppression. BK virus (polyomavirus hominis 1) has been documented in the urine of bone marrow transplant recipients and, like adenovirus, may be associated with hemorrhagic cystitis. BK-induced cystitis usually remits with decreasing immunosuppression. Anecdotal reports have described the treatment of adenovirus with ribavirin in cases of severe hemorrhagic cystitis in immunocompromised patients.

ABNORMALITIES THAT PREDISPOSE TO INFECTION

THE LYMPHOID SYSTEM   It is beyond the scope of this chapter to detail how all the immunologic abnormalities that result from cancer or from chemotherapy for cancer lead to infections. Disorders of the immune system are discussed in other sections of this book. As has been noted, patients with antibody deficiency are predisposed to overwhelming infection with encapsulated bacteria (including *S. pneumoniae*, *H. influenzae*, and *N. meningitidis*). Infections that result from the lack of a functional cellular immune system are described in Chap. 309. It is worth mentioning, however, that patients undergoing intensive chemotherapy for any form of cancer will have not only defects due to granulocytopenia but also lymphocyte dysfunction, which may be profound. Thus, these patients—especially those receiving glucocorticoid-containing regimens—should be given prophylaxis for *P. carinii* pneumonia.

THE HEMATOPOIETIC SYSTEM   Initial studies in the 1960s revealed a dramatic increase in the incidence of infections (fatal and nonfatal) among cancer patients with a granulocyte count of <500/μL. Recent studies have cited a figure of 48.3 infections per 100 neutropenic patients (<1000 granulocytes per microliter) with hematologic malignancies and solid tumors, or 46.3 infections per 1000 days at risk.

Neutropenic patients are unusually susceptible to infection with a wide variety of bacteria; thus, antibiotic therapy should be initiated promptly to cover likely pathogens if infection is suspected. Indeed, early initiation of antibacterial agents is mandatory to prevent deaths. These patients are susceptible to gram-positive and gram-negative organisms found commonly on the skin and in the bowel (Table 85-4). Because treatment with narrow-spectrum agents leads to infection with organisms not covered by the antibiotics used, the initial regimen should target pathogens likely to be initial causes of bacterial infection in neutropenic hosts (Fig. 85-1).

℞ **TREATMENT   Antibacterial Therapy**   Hundreds of antibacterial regimens have been tested for use in neutropenic patients with cancer. Many of the relevant studies involved small populations in which the outcomes were generally good, and most lacked the statistical power to detect differences among the regimens studied. Each febrile neutropenic patient should be approached as a unique problem, with particular attention given to previous infections and recent exposures to antibiotics. Several general guidelines are useful in the initial treatment of neutropenic patients with fever (Fig. 85-1):

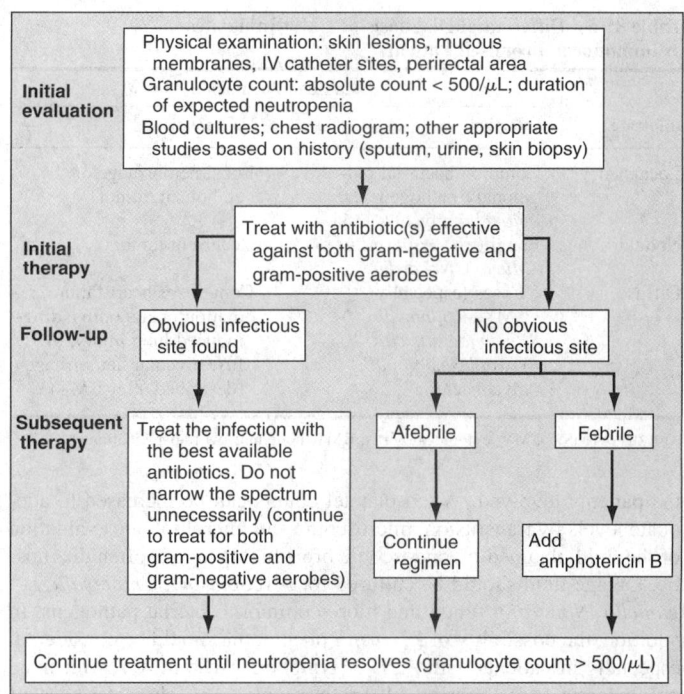

FIGURE 85-1   Diagnosis and treatment of febrile neutropenic patients: an algorithm.

1. It is necessary to use antibiotics active against both gram-negative and gram-positive bacteria (Table 85-4) in the initial regimen.
2. An aminoglycoside or an antibiotic without good activity against gram-positive organisms (e.g., ciprofloxacin) alone is not adequate in this setting.
3. The agents used should reflect both the epidemiology and the antibiotic resistance pattern of the hospital. For example, in hospitals where there is gentamicin resistance, amikacin-containing regimens should be considered; in hospitals with frequent *P. aeruginosa* infections, a regimen with the highest level of activity against this pathogen (such as tobramycin plus a semisynthetic penicillin) would be reasonable for initial therapy.
4. A single third-generation cephalosporin constitutes an appropriate initial regimen in many hospitals (if the pattern of resistance justifies its use).
5. Most standard regimens are designed for patients who have not previously received prophylactic antibiotics. The development of fever in a patient receiving antibiotics affects the choice of subsequent therapy (which should target resistant organisms and organisms known to cause infections in patients being treated with the antibiotics already administered).
6. Randomized trials have indicated that it is safe to use oral antibiotic regimens to treat "low-risk" patients with fever and neutropenia. Outpatients who are expected to remain neutropenic for <10 days and who have no concurrent medical problems (such as hypotension, pulmonary compromise, or abdominal pain) can be classified as low risk and treated with a broad-spectrum oral regimen. On the basis of large studies, it can be concluded that this therapy is safe and effective, at least when delivered in the inpatient setting. Outpatient treatment has been assessed in small studies, but data from large randomized trials demonstrating the safety of outpatient treatment of fever and neutropenia are not yet available.

The initial antibacterial regimen should be refined on the basis of culture results (Fig. 85-1). Blood cultures are the most relevant on which to base therapy; surface cultures of skin and mucous membranes may be misleading. In the case of gram-positive bacteremia or another gram-positive infection, it is important that the antibiotic be optimal for the organism isolated. If the infection is caused by certain gram-negative pathogens (such as *P. aeruginosa*), a synergistic combination of antibiotics (usually a semisynthetic penicillin, such as piperacillin, plus an aminoglycoside) may be appropriate. Although it is not desirable to leave the patient unprotected, the addition of more and more antibacterial agents to the regimen is not appropriate unless there is a clinical or microbiologic reason to do so. *Planned progressive therapy* (the serial, empirical addition of one drug after another without culture data) is not efficacious in most settings and may have unfortunate consequences. Simply adding another antibiotic for fear that a gram-negative infection is present is a dubious practice. The synergy exhibited by β-lactams and aminoglycosides against certain gram-negative organisms (especially *P. aeruginosa*) provides the rationale for using two antibiotics in this setting. Mere addition of a quinolone or another antibiotic not likely to exhibit synergy for "double coverage" has not been shown to be of benefit and may cause additional toxicities and side effects. Cephalosporins can cause bone marrow suppression, and vancomycin is associated with neutropenia in some healthy people (Chap. 137). Furthermore, the addition of multiple cephalosporins may induce β-lactamase production by some organisms; cephalosporins and double β-lactam combinations should probably be avoided altogether in *Enterobacter* infections.

Antifungal Therapy Fungal infections in cancer patients are most often associated with neutropenia. Neutropenic patients are predisposed to the development of invasive fungal infections, most commonly those due to *Candida* and *Aspergillus* species and occasionally those caused by *Fusarium*, *Trichosporon*, and *Bipolaris*. Cryptococcal infection, which is common among patients taking immunosuppressive agents, is uncommon among neutropenic patients receiving chemotherapy for AML. Invasive candidal disease is usually caused by *C. albicans* or *C. tropicalis* but can be caused by *C. krusei*, *C. parapsilosis*, and *C. glabrata*.

Most clinicians add amphotericin B to antibacterial regimens if a neutropenic patient remains febrile despite 4 to 7 days of treatment with antibacterial agents. The rationale for the empirical addition of amphotericin B is that it is difficult to culture fungi before they cause disseminated disease and that mortality from disseminated fungal infections in granulocytopenic patients is high. The imidazoles (especially fluconazole) may have prophylactic efficacy in this regard, but the spectrum of activity of the currently available azoles is narrower than that of amphotericin B. Amphotericin B is the mainstay of therapy for disseminated *Candida* or *Aspergillus* infection in the neutropenic patient. The combined use of an imidazole and amphotericin B is controversial because of the theoretical antagonistic effects of these agents. The insolubility of amphotericin B has resulted in the marketing of several amphotericin B–lipid formulations. Lipid preparations have been shown to be less toxic than the amphotericin B deoxycholate complex. However, because of the high cost of the lipid preparations, at many centers their use is reserved for patients who fail to respond to standard amphotericin B. Since the side effects of the formulations differ, unnecessary switching from one to another is not recommended.

Other Therapeutic Modalities Another way to address the problems of the febrile neutropenic patient is to replenish the neutrophil population. Although granulocyte transfusions are efficacious in the treatment of refractory gram-negative bacteremia, they do not have a documented role in prophylaxis. Because of the expense, the risk of leukoagglutinin reactions (although this risk has probably been decreased by improved cell-separation procedures), and the risk of transmission of CMV from unscreened donors, granulocyte transfusion is reserved for patients unresponsive to antibiotics. This modality is efficacious for documented gram-negative bacteremia refractory to antibiotics, particularly in situations where granulocyte numbers will be depressed for only a short period.

A variety of cytokines, including granulocyte colony-stimulating factor and granulocyte-macrophage colony-stimulating factor, enhance granulocyte recovery after chemotherapy and consequently shorten the period of maximal vulnerability to fatal infections. The role of these cytokines in routine practice is still a matter of some debate. Most authorities recommend their use only when neutropenia is both severe

and prolonged. The cytokines themselves may have adverse effects, including fever, hypoxemia, and pleural effusions or serositis in other areas. Since there is little evidence that their routine administration lessens the risk of death and since they are still expensive, the cytokines have not become the standard of care in all centers. The role of other cytokines (such as macrophage colony-stimulating factor for monocytes or interferon-γ) in preventing or treating infections in granulocytopenic patients is under investigation.

Once neutropenia has resolved, patients are not at high risk of infection. However, depending on what drugs they receive, patients who continue on chemotherapeutic protocols remain at high risk for certain diseases. Any patient receiving more than a maintenance dose of glucocorticoids (including many treatment regimens for diffuse lymphoma) should also receive prophylactic trimethoprim-sulfamethoxazole because of the risk of *P. carinii* infection; those with ALL should receive such prophylaxis for the duration of chemotherapy.

PREVENTION OF INFECTION IN CANCER PATIENTS

EFFECT OF THE ENVIRONMENT Outbreaks of fatal *Aspergillus* infection have been associated with construction projects and materials in several hospitals. The association between spore counts and risk of infection suggests the need for a high-efficiency air-handling system in hospitals that care for large numbers of neutropenic patients. The use of laminar-flow rooms and prophylactic antibiotics has decreased the number of infectious episodes in severely neutropenic patients. However, because of the expense of such a program and the failure to show that it dramatically affects mortality, most centers do not routinely use laminar flow to care for neutropenic patients. Some centers use "reverse isolation," in which health care providers and visitors to a patient who is neutropenic wear gowns and gloves. Since most of the infections these patients develop are due to organisms that colonize the patients' own skin and bowel, the validity of such schemes is dubious, and limited clinical data do not support their use. Hand washing by all staff caring for neutropenic patients should be required to prevent the spread of resistant organisms.

The presence of large numbers of bacteria (particularly *P. aeruginosa*) in certain foods, especially fresh vegetables, has led some authorities to recommend a special "low-bacteria" diet. A diet consisting of cooked and canned food is satisfactory to most neutropenic patients and does not involve elaborate disinfection or sterilization protocols. However, there are no studies to support even this type of dietary restriction. Counseling of patients to avoid leftovers, deli foods, and unpasteurized dairy products is recommended.

PHYSICAL MEASURES Although few studies address this issue, patients with cancer are predisposed to infections resulting from anatomic compromise (e.g., lymphedema resulting from node dissections after radical mastectomy). Surgeons who specialize in cancer surgery can provide specific guidelines for the care of such patients, and patients benefit from common-sense advice about how to prevent infections in vulnerable areas.

ANTIBIOTIC PROPHYLAXIS There is no consensus on the use of prophylactic antibiotics in neutropenic patients. The incidence of infection is lower among patients who receive broad-spectrum antibiotic prophylaxis than among those who do not. Because of the prolongation of neutropenia associated with the use of trimethoprim-sulfamethoxazole, some clinicians use broad-spectrum agents such as quinolones (e.g., ciprofloxacin). Either regimen can be given orally, and both have the advantage of inactivity against anaerobic organisms; thus, neither is likely to disrupt the bowel flora and permit colonization with new aerobes or *Candida*. However, both regimens have adverse effects and can lead to the selection of resistant organisms in a hospital. For these reasons, many clinicians reserve their use for patients with the longest periods of neutropenia (e.g., bone marrow transplant recipients). The same issues apply to the use of antifungal agents. While agents such as fluconazole may prevent infections with susceptible organisms (e.g., *C. albicans*), they can cause a concomitant increase in infections due to resistant fungi (e.g., *C. krusei*). Thus, the decision to use antifungal prophylaxis may vary with the fungi endemic in a given hospital. Prophylaxis for *P. carinii* is mandatory for patients with ALL and for all cancer patients receiving glucocorticoid-containing chemotherapy regimens.

VACCINATION OF CANCER PATIENTS   In general, patients undergoing chemotherapy respond less well to vaccines than normal hosts. Their greater need for vaccines thus leads to a dilemma in their management. Purified proteins and inactivated vaccines are almost never contraindicated and should be given to patients even during chemotherapy. For example, all adults should receive diphtheria-tetanus toxoid boosters at the indicated times as well as seasonal influenza vaccine. However, if possible, vaccination should not be undertaken concurrent with cytotoxic chemotherapy. If patients are expected to be receiving chemotherapy for several months and vaccination is indicated (for example, influenza vaccination in the fall), the vaccine should be given midcycle—as far as possible from the antimetabolic agents that will prevent an immune response. The meningococcal and pneumococcal polysaccharide vaccines should be given to patients before splenectomy, if possible. The Advisory Committee on Immunization Practices recommends reimmunization every 5 years for the pneumococcal vaccine; although no official stand has been taken, this recommendation seems reasonable for the meningococcal vaccine as well. The *H. influenzae* type b conjugate vaccine should be administered to all splenectomized patients; there is no current recommendation for reimmunization, but immunity appears to be much longer-lasting than that induced by polysaccharide vaccines.

In general, live virus (or live bacterial) vaccines should not be given to patients during intensive chemotherapy because of the risk of disseminated infection. Recommendations on vaccination are summarized in Table 85-2.

BIBLIOGRAPHY

DE PAUW BE, DOMPELING EC: Antibiotic strategy after the empiric phase in patients treated for a hematological malignancy. Ann Hematol 72:273, 1996

FREIFELD A et al: A double-blind trial of oral versus intravenous antibiotics for empirical therapy in low risk patients with fever and neutropenia from cancer chemotherapy. N Engl J Med 341:305, 1999

HUGHES WT et al: 1997 guidelines for the use of antimicrobial agents in neutropenic patients with unexplained fever. Clin Infect Dis 25:551, 1997

INTERNATIONAL ANTIMICROBIAL THERAPY COOPERATIVE GROUP OF THE EORTC: Oral versus intravenous antimicrobials as empirical therapy in cancer patients with fever and granulocytopenia. N Engl J Med 341:312, 1999

MALIK IA et al: Feasibility of outpatient management of fever in cancer patients with low-risk neutropenia: Results of a prospective randomized trial. Am J Med 98:224, 1995

RODRIGUEZ-ADRIAN LJ et al: The potential role of cytokine therapy for fungal infections in patients with cancer: Is recovery from neutropenia all that is needed? Clin Infect Dis 26:1270, 1998

WONG-BERINGER A et al: Lipid formulations of amphotericin B: Clinical efficacy and toxicities. Clin Infect Dis 27:603, 1998

86

Arthur J. Sober, Howard K. Koh, Gregory P. Wittenberg, Carl V. Washington, Jr.

MELANOMA AND OTHER SKIN CANCERS

Pigmented skin lesions are among the most common findings on physical examination. The challenge is to distinguish cutaneous melanomas, which may be lethal, from the remainder, which with rare exceptions are benign. Cutaneous neoplasms are depicted in Section IIB **(Plates IIB-20 to -27)** of the Color Atlas; benign and malignant pigmented lesions are in Section IIC **(Plates IIC-28 to -33)**.

MELANOMA

Melanomas originate from melanocytes, pigment cells normally present in the epidermis and sometimes in the dermis. This tumor affects approximately 44,200 individuals per year in the United States, resulting in 7300 deaths. The tumor can affect adults of all ages, even teenagers; it has distinct clinical features that make it detectable at a time when cure by surgical excision is possible; and it is located on the skin surface, where it is visible. The incidence has increased dramatically; if the incidence continues to increase at the present rate, within a decade, lifetime risk of melanoma will exceed 1%.

The reason for the increase in melanoma incidence is thought to be increased recreational sun exposure, especially early in life. Individuals of similar ethnic background who immigrate after childhood to areas of high sun exposure (e.g., Israel and Australia) have lower melanoma rates than individuals of similar age who were either born in those countries or immigrated before age 10. The individuals most susceptible to development of melanoma are those with fair complexions, red or blond hair, blue eyes, and freckles and who tan poorly and sunburn easily. Most studies link increased melanoma risk to history of sunburn. Other factors associated with increased risk include a family history of melanoma (1 in 10 melanoma patients have an affected family member); the presence of a clinically atypical mole (dysplastic nevus), a giant congenital melanocytic nevus, or a small to medium-sized congenital melanocytic nevus (see below); the presence of a higher than average number of ordinary melanocytic nevi; and immunosuppression (Table 86-1). Individuals with 50 or more moles ≥2 mm in size have a 64-fold increased risk. About 30% of melanomas arise in a nevus. Melanoma is relatively rare in heavily pigmented peoples. Dark-skinned populations (such as those of India and Puerto Rico), blacks, and East Asians have rates 10 to 20 times lower than lighter-skinned whites. In keeping with the role of sun exposure, the incidence is inversely correlated with the latitude of residence; at any latitude, however, darker-skinned persons have a lower incidence.

CLINICAL CHARACTERISTICS   There are four types of cutaneous melanoma (Table 86-2). In three of these—superficial spreading melanoma, lentigo maligna melanoma, and acral lentiginous melanoma—the lesion has a period of superficial (so-called radial) growth during which it increases in size but does not penetrate deeply. During this period, the melanoma is most capable of being cured by surgical excision. The fourth type—nodular melanoma—does not have a recognizable radial growth phase and usually presents as a deeply invasive lesion, capable of early metastasis. When tumors begin to penetrate deeply into the skin, they are in the so-called vertical growth phase. Melanomas with a radial growth phase are characterized by irregular and sometimes notched borders, variation in pigment pattern, and variation in color. An increase in size or change in color is noted by the patient in 70% of early lesions. Bleeding, ulceration, and pain are late signs and are of little help in early recognition. Nodular melanomas are dark brown-black to blue-black nodules. Melanomas are occasionally amelanotic, in which case the diagnosis is established

Table 86-1   Risk Factors for Cutaneous Melanoma

High risk (>50-fold increase in risk)
  Persistently changing mole
  Clinically atypical moles in patient with two family members with melanoma
  Adulthood (vs. childhood)
  >50 nevi ≥2 mm in diameter
Intermediate risk (~10-fold increase in risk)
  Family history of melanoma
  Sporadic clinically atypical moles
  Congenital nevi (?)
  White ethnicity (vs black or East Asian ethnicity)
  Personal history of prior melanoma
Low risk (2- to 4-fold increase in risk)
  Immunosuppression
  Sun sensitivity or excess exposure to sun

SOURCE: Adapted from AR Rhodes et al: JAMA 258:3146, 1987.

histologically after biopsy of a new or changing skin growth. Lentigo maligna melanoma is usually confined to chronically sun-damaged sites (face, neck, back of hands) in older individuals. Acral lentiginous melanoma occurs on the palms, soles, nail beds, and mucous membranes. While this type occurs in whites, it is most frequent (along with nodular melanoma) in blacks and East Asians. Superficial spreading melanoma is most frequent in whites. Melanomas arising in dysplastic nevi (see below) are usually of this type. The back is the most common site for melanoma in men. In women, the back and the lower leg (knee to ankle) are frequent sites.

PROGNOSTIC FACTORS The most important prognostic factor is the stage at the time of presentation [see the discussion of revised American Joint Cancer Commission (AJCC) stages, below]. Five-year survival for clinical stages I and II (primary tumor; no clinical evidence of disease elsewhere) is about 85%. For clinical stage III

Table 86-2 Clinical Features of Malignant Melanoma

Type	Site	Average Age at Diagnosis, Years	Duration of Known Existence, Years	Color
Lentigo maligna melanoma	Sun-exposed surfaces, particularly malar region of cheek and temple	70	5–20[a] or longer	In flat portions, shades of brown and tan predominant, but whitish gray occasionally present; in nodules, shades of reddish brown, bluish gray, bluish black
Superficial spreading melanoma	Any site (more common on upper back and, in women, on lower legs)	40–50	1–7	Shades of brown mixed with bluish red (violaceous), bluish black, reddish brown, and often whitish pink, and the border of lesion is at least in part visibly and/or palpably elevated
Nodular melanoma	Any site	40–50	Months to less than 5 years	Reddish blue (purple) or bluish black; either uniform in color or mixed with brown or black
Acral lentiginous melanoma	Palm, sole, nail bed, mucous membrane	60	1–10	In flat portions, dark brown predominantly; in raised lesions (plaques) brown-black or blue-black predominantly

[a] During much of this time, the precursor stage, lentigo maligna, is confined to the epidermis.
SOURCE: Adapted from AJ Sober, in *Pathophysiology of Dermatologic Diseases*, NA Soter, HP Baden (eds). New York, McGraw-Hill, 1984.

(clinically palpable regional nodes that contain tumor), the 5-year survival is about 50% when only one node is involved and about 15 to 20% when four or more nodes are involved. The 5-year survival for clinical stage IV (disseminated disease) is <5%. Fortunately, most melanomas are diagnosed in clinical stages I and II. Within these stages, the prognosis depends on the thickness of the primary tumor (Table 86-3). This system is based on the rationale that the likelihood of metastasis should correlate with tumor volume, with thickness being the best single index of tumor volume. Melanomas <0.76 mm thick are usually cured by surgical removal (with 5-year survival rates of 96 to 99%). Approximately 40% of primary melanomas now fall in a low-risk category (thickness <1 mm). In low-risk patients who develop metastases, the primary tumors often exhibit either microscopic features of anaplasia or a vertical growth phase. More than 50% of individuals with melanomas ≥4 mm thick will develop metastatic disease and die of their melanoma (Table 86-3). These thick tumors are almost always raised above the plane of the skin. Certain anatomic sites affect the prognosis. The favorable sites appear to be the forearm and leg (excluding feet), while unfavorable sites include scalp, hands, feet, and mucous membranes. In general, women with stage I or II disease have a better survival than men, perhaps in part because of earlier diagnosis; women frequently have melanomas on the lower leg, where self-recognition is more likely and prognosis is better. Older individuals have poorer prognoses. This finding has been explained in part by a tendency toward later diagnosis (and thus thicker tumors) in men and by a higher proportion in men of acral melanomas (palmar-plantar), which have a poorer prognosis. Melanoma may recur after many years. About 10 to 15% of first-time recurrences develop more than 5 years after treatment of the original lesion. The time to recurrence varies inversely with tumor thickness. Other prognostic factors for stages I and II melanoma include the presence of an ulcer in the primary tumor, high mitotic rate, and the presence of microscopic tumor satellites (foci of tumor ≥0.05 mm in diameter in the reticular dermis or subcutaneous fat, distinct from the main body of the tumor). The presence of microscopic satellites is also predictive of microscopic metastases to the regional lymph nodes. An

alternative prognostic scheme for clinical stages I and II melanoma, proposed by Clark, is based on the anatomic level of invasion in the skin. Level I is intraepidermal (in situ); level II penetrates the papillary dermis; level III spans the papillary dermis; level IV penetrates the reticular dermis; and level V penetrates into the subcutaneous fat. The 5-year survival for these stages averages 100, 95, 82, 71, and 49%, respectively.

NATURAL HISTORY Melanomas may spread by the lymphatic channels or the bloodstream. The earliest metastases are often to regional lymph nodes. Surgical lymphadenectomy usually controls regional disease. Liver, lung, bone, and brain are common sites of hematogenous spread, but unusual sites, such as the anterior chamber of the eye, may also be involved. Once metastatic disease is established, the likelihood of cure is low.

MANAGEMENT The entire cutaneous surface, including the scalp and mucous membranes, should be examined in each patient. Bright room illumination is important, and a 7× to 10× hand lens is helpful for evaluating variation in pigment pattern. A history of relevant risk factors should be elicited. Any suspicious lesions should be biopsied, evaluated by a specialist, or recorded by chart and/or photography for follow-up. Examination of the lymph nodes and palpation

Table 86-3 Prognosis of Melanoma by Thickness (Breslow) and AJCC Stages: 5-Year Survival Rates

AJCC Stage	Thickness Range, mm	% Overall Survival
IA (localized)	≤0.75	96
IB (localized)	0.76–1.49	87
IIA (localized)	1.5–2.49	75
	2.50–3.99	66
IIB (localized)	≥4.00	47
III (metastatic to regional nodes)		45 (one node)
		<20 (two nodes)
IV (metastatic to distant sites)		8–10[a]

[a] One-year survival.

of the abdominal viscera are part of the staging examination for suspected melanoma. The patient should be advised to have other family members screened if either melanoma or clinically atypical moles (dysplastic nevi) are present. Melanoma prevention is based on protection from the sun. Routine use of a sunblock of SPF $\geq$15, use of protective clothing, and avoiding intense midday ultraviolet exposure should be recommended. The patient should be educated in the clinical features of melanoma and advised to report any growth or other change in a pigmented lesion. Patient education brochures are available from the American Cancer Society, the American Academy of Dermatology, the National Cancer Institute, and the Skin Cancer Foundation. Self-examination at 6- to 8-week intervals may enhance the likelihood of detecting change between follow-up visits. Routine follow-up visits for melanoma patients and patients with clinically atypical moles (dysplastic nevi) may facilitate early detection of new tumors.

Precursor Lesions   Clinically atypical moles, also termed *dysplastic nevi*, occur in certain families affected by melanoma. In some families, melanomas occur nearly exclusively in the individuals with dysplastic nevi. These nevi appear to be transmitted as an autosomal dominant trait that involves chromosome 9p16. In other families, the nevi may not be present in all individuals with an increased risk of melanoma. The melanomas may arise in clinically atypical moles or in normal skin. Individuals with clinically atypical moles and two family members with melanoma have been reported to have a >50% lifetime risk for developing melanoma. Table 86-4 lists the features that are characteristic of clinically atypical moles and that differentiate them from benign acquired nevi. The number of clinically atypical moles may vary from one to several hundred. Clinically atypical moles usually differ from each other in appearance. The borders are often hazy and indistinct, and the pigment pattern is more highly varied than that in benign acquired nevi. Of the 90% of melanoma patients whose disease is regarded as sporadic (i.e., who lack a family history of melanoma), about 40% have clinically atypical moles, as compared with an estimated 5 to 10% of the population at large. The observation that at least 20% of sporadic melanomas arise in association with a clini-

cally atypical mole makes this nevus the most important precursor for melanoma.

Less frequent precursors include the giant congenital melanocytic nevus and the small congenital melanocytic nevus (although the latter relationship is disputed by some). Congenital melanocytic nevi are present at birth or appear in the neonatal period (tardive form). The giant melanocytic nevus, also called the bathing trunk, cape, or garment nevus, is a rare malformation that affects perhaps 1 in 30,000 to 1 in 100,000 individuals. These nevi are usually >20 cm in diameter and may cover more than half the body surface. Giant nevi often occur in association with multiple small congenital nevi. The borders are sharp, and hair may be present. The lesions are usually dark brown and may have darker and lighter areas. Pigment is haphazardly displayed. The surface is smooth to rugose or cerebriform and may vary from one portion of the lesion to another. A lifetime risk of melanoma development of 6% has been estimated. The risk is greatest before age 5 and next greatest between ages 5 and 10. Early detection of melanoma is difficult in these lesions because of the deep dermal or subcutaneous origin of melanoma in these lesions and because of the large and varied surface of the nevus. Prophylactic excision early in life can be accomplished by staged removal with coverage by split-thickness skin grafts. No uniform management guidelines for giant congenital nevi have been developed.

The small- to medium-sized congenital melanocytic nevus, which affects approximately 1% of persons, usually presents as a raised dark- to medium-brown lesion with a smooth or papillomatous surface. The border is sharp, and lesions may be oriented along lines of skin cleavage. Follicular hyper- and hypopigmentation may coexist in a salt-and-pepper configuration. The lesion may have an excess of coarse hairs. Melanoma may develop in these lesions but the risk is not quantitated. Considerations of body surface area suggest that the incidence of melanomas arising in small congenital melanocytic nevi is probably higher than would be expected by chance. The remnants of a nevus with histopathologic features of a congenital nevus have been observed in 2 to 6% of melanomas. The management of small- to medium-sized congenital melanocytic nevi remains controversial; prophylactic removal under local anesthesia in the early teen years is appropriate as melanomas arise later in these lesions.

Differential Diagnosis   The aim of differential diagnosis is to distinguish benign pigmented lesions from melanoma and its precursors. If melanoma is a consideration, then biopsy is appropriate. Some benign look-alikes may be removed in the process of trying to detect authentic melanoma. Table 86-5 summarizes the distinguishing features of benign lesions that may be confused with melanoma. Early detection of melanoma may be facilitated by applying the "ABCD rules": A—asymmetry, benign lesions are usually symmetric; B—border irregularity, most nevi have clear-cut borders; C—color variegation, benign lesions usually have uniform light or dark pigment; D—diameter >6 mm (the size of a pencil eraser).

Biopsy   Any pigmented cutaneous lesion that has changed in size or shape or has other features suggestive of malignant melanoma should be biopsied. The recommended technique is an excisional biopsy, as that facilitates pathologic assessment of the lesion, permits accurate measurement of thickness if the lesion is melanoma, and constitutes treatment if the lesion is benign. Shave biopsy or curettage of a suspected melanoma is contraindicated. For large lesions or lesions on anatomic sites where excisional biopsy may not be feasible (such as the face, hands, or feet), an incisional biopsy through the most nodular or darkest area of the lesion is acceptable; this should include the vertical growth phase of the primary tumor, if present. Data from prospective studies do not indicate that an incisional biopsy facilitates the spread of melanoma.

Staging   Once the diagnosis of malignant melanoma has been confirmed, the tumor must be staged to determine prognosis and treatment. The history should probe for evidence of metastatic disease, such as malaise, weight loss, headaches, visual difficulty, or bone pain. The physical examination should be directed especially to the skin, re-

Table 86-4   Clinical Features Distinguishing Atypical Moles from Benign Acquired Nevi

Clinical Feature	Clinically Atypical Moles	Benign Acquired Nevi
Color	Variable mixtures of tan, brown, black, or red/pink within a single nevus; nevi may look very different from each other	Uniformly tan or brown
Shape	Irregular borders; pigment may fade off into surrounding skin; macular portion at the edge of the nevus	Round; sharp, clear-cut borders between the nevus and the surrounding skin; may be flat or elevated
Size	Usually more than 6 mm in diameter; may be more than 10 mm; occasionally smaller than 6 mm	Usually less than 6 mm in diameter
Number	Often very many (more than 100), but occasionally may be only one	In a typical adult, 10 to 40 are scattered over the body; perhaps 15% of patients have no nevi
Location	Sun-exposed areas; the back is the most common site, but dysplastic nevi may also be seen on the scalp, breasts, and buttocks	Generally on the sun-exposed surfaces of the skin above the waist; the scalp, breasts, and buttocks are rarely involved

SOURCE: Modified from RJ Friedman et al (eds): *Cancer of the Skin.* Philadelphia, Saunders, 1991.

Table 86-5 Pigmented Lesions That Must Be Distinguished from Cutaneous Melanoma and Its Precursors

Lesion	Description
Blue nevus	Gunmetal or cerulean blue, blue-gray. Stable over time. One-half occur on dorsa of hands and feet. Lesions are usually single, small, 3 mm to <1 cm. Must be distinguished from nodular melanoma.
Compound nevus	Round or oval shape, well-demarcated, smooth-bordered. May be dome-shaped or papillomatous; colors range from flesh colored to very dark brown, with individual nevi being relatively homogeneous in color.
Hemangioma	Dome-shaped reddish, purple, blue nodule. Compression with a glass microscope slide may result in blanching. Must be distinguished from nodular melanoma.
Junctional nevus	Flat to barely raised brown lesion. Sharp border. Fine pigmentary stippling visible, especially upon magnification.
Lentigo Juvenile Solar	Flat, uniformly medium or dark brown lesion with sharp border. Solar lentigines are acquired lesions on sites of chronic solar exposure (face and backs of hands). Lesions are 2 mm to ≥1 cm. Solar lentigines have reticulate pigmentation upon magnification.
Pigmented basal cell carcinoma	Papular border. May have central ulceration. Usually on a sun-exposed surface in an older patient. Patient usually has dark brown eyes and dark brown or black hair.
Pigmented dermatofibroma	Lesion is not well demarcated visually, is firm, and dimples downward when compressed laterally. Usually on extremities. Usually <6 mm.
Seborrheic keratosis	Rough, sharp-bordered lesions that feel waxy and "stuck on"; range in color from flesh to tan, to dark brown. Presence of keratin plugs in surface is helpful for discriminating especially dark lesions from melanoma.
Subungual hematoma	Maroon (red-brown) coloration. As lesion grows out from nail fold, a curving clear area is seen.
Tattoo (medical or traumatic)	In medical tattoo, lesions are small pigmentary dots, often blue or green, which make a regular pattern (rectangle). Traumatic tattoos are irregular, and pigmentation may appear black.

gional draining lymph nodes, central nervous system, liver, and spleen. In the absence of signs or symptoms of metastasis, few laboratory or radiologic tests are indicated for staging purposes. Aside from a chest radiograph, and possibly liver function tests, no other tests or scans are routinely indicated unless the history or physical examination suggests metastasis to a specific organ. Specifically, liver-spleen scans and computed tomography have a low yield and are not cost-effective. However, once signs of metastasis exist, favored sites of spread, such as the liver, lungs, bone, and brain, should be scanned. Appropriate evaluations place patients into four clinical stages (Table 86-3).

℞ **TREATMENT Surgical Management** For a newly diagnosed cutaneous melanoma, wide surgical excision of the lesion with a margin of normal skin is necessary to remove all malignant cells and minimize local recurrence. The appropriate width of the margin is a source of controversy. Based upon clinical studies, the following margins can be recommended for primary melanoma: in situ: 0.5 cm; invasive up to 1 mm thick: 1.0 cm; 1 to 4 mm thick: 2.0 cm; >4 mm thick: at least 2 cm. For lesions on the face, hands, and feet, strict adherence to these margins must give way to individual considerations about the constraints of surgery and minimization of morbidity. In all instances, however, inclusion of subcutaneous fat in the surgical specimen facilitates adequate thickness measurement and assessment of surgical margins by the pathologist.

Elective Regional Node Dissection Elective regional node dissection in AJCC stage II disease (without palpable adenopathy) has been advocated, based on the hypothesis that melanoma metastasizes in an orderly fashion from the skin to regional lymph nodes and finally to distant sites. If that is the case, surgical excision of nodal micrometastases could theoretically provide definitive treatment at a time of relatively low tumor burden and perhaps improve survival. The efficacy of this procedure remains controversial; while some retrospective series suggest a survival benefit, randomized studies examining this question showed no survival advantage for wide local excision followed by immediate elective regional node dissection compared with wide local excision followed by delayed dissection (only if nodes became palpable). Furthermore, the procedure has associated morbidity, and some lesions, especially those on the trunk, have ambiguous nodal draining sites, making it difficult to decide which area to dissect. Results of biopsy of the first drainage node—the so-called sentinel node—predicts the likelihood of metastases in higher nodes. Sentinel nodes can be identified by injecting a blue dye or radioactive isotope around the primary tumor site. A negative biopsy result appears to obviate the need for elective regional nodal dissection. Patients with lesions <1 mm thick have an excellent prognosis and need no node dissection; at the other extreme, patients with lesions >4 mm thick have such a high risk for distant metastases that elective node dissection may not alter the ultimate clinical outcome. A subset of patients with AJCC stage II lesions of intermediate thickness may benefit from elective regional node dissection, but there is no consensus about which patients should undergo this procedure.

Adjuvant Therapy For patients who are free of disease but at high risk for metastases, adjuvant therapy that complements surgery is needed to destroy occult micrometastases, prolong disease-free survival, and improve the cure rate. Many strategies have been tried unsuccessfully. However, adjuvant interferon-α may improve disease-free and overall survival, particularly in patients with nodal metastases (stage III disease). High-dose interferon, 20 million units per square meter intravenously 5 days a week for 4 weeks followed by 10 million units per square meter subcutaneously three times a week for 11 months, has been effective in some, but not all, studies. In nearly half of patients, these doses of interferon are associated with severe toxicity, including flulike illness and decline in performance status. The toxicity reverses with lower doses and when therapy is stopped. If interferon is beneficial at all, it benefits only a small fraction of treated patients.

Treatment of Metastatic Disease Melanoma can metastasize to any organ, the brain being a particularly common site. Metastatic melanoma generally is incurable, with survival in patients with visceral metastases generally <1 year. Thus, the goal of treatment is usually palliation. Patients with soft-tissue and node metastases fare better than those with liver and brain metastases. Metastases limited to regional nodes (AJCC stage III disease) warrant a therapeutic lymph node dissection. Surgical excision of a single metastasis to the lung or to a surgically accessible brain site can prolong survival. Trials of stereotactic radiosurgery will determine its future role in the treatment of brain metastases. More often, however, patients have multiple brain metastases that require radiation therapy and glucocorticoids. Radiation therapy can provide local palliation for recurrent tumors or metastases. Patients who have advanced regional disease limited to a limb may benefit from hyperthermic limb perfusion with melphalan and tumor necrosis factor. Complete response rates >90% have been reported; responses are associated with significant palliation of symptoms.

A number of drugs and biologicals have minimal antitumor activity (15 to 20% partial response rates) in metastatic melanoma, including dacarbazine (DTIC); the nitrosoureas carmustine (BCNU), lomustine (CCNU), and semustine (methyl-CCNU); platinum analogues such as cisplatin and carboplatin; vinca alkyloids such as vincristine, vinblastine, and vindesine; the taxanes paclitaxel and docetaxel; interferon; and interleukin 2 (IL-2). Single-agent dacarbazine is considered the standard treatment. This agent has been given at a number of different doses and schedules; 250 mg/m^2 intravenously every day for 5 days every 3 weeks is a standard schedule. Dacarbazine-based combination regimens are probably more effective. Interferon and IL-2 produce response rates similar to those seen with cytotoxic agents; however, at active doses, they usually cause greater toxicity than chemotherapy.

Melanomas often express cell-surface antigens that may be recognized by host immune cells. A number of melanoma-associated antigens have been discovered. Melanoma antigens (MAGEs)-1, -2, and -3 (endogenous proteins controlled by genes on the X chromosome; there are up to 12 of these genes) and tyrosinase, an enzyme involved in melanin synthesis, are antigens that are processed into peptides and presented to T cells via HLA-A antigens on the tumor, particularly the HLA-A1 and -A2 alleles, which are expressed in about 85% of patients with melanoma. In addition, a melanoma antigen called MART is recognized in the context of class II MHC antigens. These melanoma-associated antigens alone or in combination may make it possible to develop vaccination strategies against melanoma. Such strategies include the use of purified proteins as immunogens and the use of genetically altered tumor cells to elicit a T cell response. Alternative experimental approaches include efforts to expand tumor-specific T cells (obtained either from the tumor as tumor-infiltrating lymphocytes or harvested from the peripheral blood after vaccination) in vitro and transfer them into patients in large numbers. In addition, monoclonal antibodies to tumor antigens are being tested, with some early indication of efficacy in around 15% of patients. All of these experimental approaches will need considerable further development before being applicable on a wide scale. However, once an approach is found that is active in metastatic disease, it may prove most useful as adjuvant therapy.

The absence of curative therapy for patients with metastatic melanoma underscores the importance of early detection and prevention as strategies to decrease melanoma mortality.

NONMELANOMA SKIN CANCER

Nonmelanoma skin cancer is the most common cancer in the United States, with an estimated annual incidence of more than 1,000,000 cases. Basal cell carcinomas (BCCs) account for 70 to 80% of nonmelanoma skin cancers. Squamous cell carcinomas (SCCs), while representing only about 20% of nonmelanoma skin cancers, are more significant because of their ability to metastasize; they account for most of the 2300 deaths annually. Incidence rates have risen dramatically over the past decade.

ETIOLOGY   The cause of BCC and SCC is multifactorial. Cumulative exposure to sunlight, principally the ultraviolet B (UV-B) spectrum, is the most significant factor. Other factors associated with a higher incidence of skin cancer are male sex, older age, Celtic descent, a fair complexion, a tendency to sunburn easily, and an outdoor occupation. The incidence of these tumors increases with decreasing latitude. Most tumors develop on sun-exposed areas of the head and neck. Tumors are more common on the left side of the body in the United States but on the right side in England, presumably owing to asymmetric exposure during driving. As the earth's protective ozone shield continues to thin, further increases in the incidence of skin cancer can be anticipated. In certain geographic areas, exposure to arsenic in well water or from industrial sources may significantly increase the risk of BCC and SCC. Skin cancer in affected individuals may be seen with or without other cutaneous markers of chronic arsenism (e.g., arsenical keratoses). Less common is exposure to the cyclic aromatic hydrocarbons in tar, soot, or shale. The risk of lip or oral SCC is increased with cigarette smoking. Human papillomaviruses and ultraviolet radiation may act as cocarcinogens.

Host factors associated with a high risk of skin cancer include immunosuppression induced by disease or drugs. Transplant recipients receiving chronic immunosuppressive therapy are particularly prone to SCC. The frequency of skin cancer is proportional to the duration of immunosuppression and the extent of sun exposure. Skin cancer is a not uncommon finding in patients infected with HIV, and it may be more aggressive in this setting. Other factors include ionizing radiation, thermal burns, certain scars, and chronic ulcerations. Several heritable conditions have been associated with skin cancer (e.g., albinism, xeroderma pigmentosum, and BCC nevus syndrome). Mutations in the tumor suppressor gene, *patched*, may lead to BCC.

CLINICAL PRESENTATION   Nonmelanoma skin cancers are often asymptomatic, but nonhealing ulceration, bleeding, or pain can occur.

Basal Cell Carcinoma   BCC is a malignancy arising from epidermal basal cells. The most common type is *noduloulcerative BCC*, which begins as a small, pearly nodule, often with small telangiectatic vessels on its surface. The nodule grows slowly and may undergo central ulceration. Various amounts of melanin may be present in the tumor; tumors with a heavier accumulation are referred to as *pigmented BCC*. While clinically no more aggressive than the noduloulcerative variant, the latter may be mistaken for malignant melanoma. *Superficial BCC* consists of one or several erythematous, scaling plaques that slowly enlarge. Although they are more commonly found on the trunk and extremities, the head and neck can also be affected. The lesions may be confused with benign inflammatory dermatoses, especially nummular eczema and psoriasis. *Morpheaform (fibrosing) BCC* manifests itself as a solitary, flat or slightly depressed, indurated, whitish or yellowish plaque. Borders are typically indistinct, a feature associated with a greater potential for extensive subclinical spread.

Squamous Cell Carcinoma   Primary cutaneous SCC is a malignant neoplasm of keratinizing epidermal cells. Unlike BCC, which has a very low metastatic potential, SCC can metastasize and grow rapidly. The clinical features of SCC vary widely. Commonly, SCC appears as an ulcerated nodule or a superficial erosion on the skin or lower lip, but it may present as a verrucous papule or plaque. Unlike BCC, overlying telangiectasias are uncommon. The margins of this tumor may be ill-defined, and fixation to underlying structures may occur. Cutaneous SCC may develop anywhere on the body, but it usually arises on sun-damaged skin. A related neoplasm, keratoacanthoma, typically appears as a dome-shaped papule with a central keratotic crater, expands rapidly, and commonly regresses without therapy. This lesion can be difficult to differentiate from SCC.

SCC has several premalignant forms (actinic keratosis, actinic cheilitis, and some cutaneous horns) and in situ forms (e.g., Bowen's disease) that are confined to the epidermis. Actinic keratoses and cheilitis are hyperkeratotic papules and plaques that occur on sun-exposed areas. While the potential for malignant degeneration is low in any individual lesion, the risk of SCC increases with larger numbers of lesions. Bowen's disease presents as a scaling, erythematous plaque, which may develop into invasive SCC in up to 20% of cases. Controversy exists regarding the association of Bowen's disease with internal malignancy; however, no significant relationship is noted when other predisposing factors (e.g., arsenic) are absent. Treatment of premalignant and in situ lesions reduces the subsequent risk of invasive disease.

NATURAL HISTORY   **Basal Cell Carcinoma**   The natural history of BCC is that of a slowly enlarging, locally invasive neoplasm. The degree of local destruction and risk of recurrence vary with the size, duration, and location of the tumor; the histologic subtype; the presence of recurrent disease; and various patient characteristics. Location on the central face (e.g., the nose, the nasolabial fold, or the periorbital or perioral area), the ears, or the scalp may portend a higher risk. Small nodular, pigmented, cystic, or superficial BCCs respond well to most treatments. Large nodular, noduloulcerative, and especially morpheaform BCCs may be more aggressive. The metastatic potential of BCC is about 0.0028 to 0.1%. Persons with either BCC or SCC have an increased risk of developing subsequent skin cancers.

Squamous Cell Carcinoma   The natural history of SCC depends on both tumor and host characteristics. Tumors arising on actinically damaged skin have a lower metastatic potential than those on protected surfaces. The metastatic frequency of cutaneous SCC, 0.3 to 3.7%, is lower than that of mucosal SCC. Tumors occurring on the lower lip and ear have metastatic potential approaching 13 and 11%, respectively. The metastatic potential of SCC arising in burn scars, chronic ulcerations, or the genitalia is higher. The overall metastatic rate for recurrent tumors approaches 30%. Poorly differentiated, deep tumors with perineural or lymphatic invasion often behave aggressively. Multiple tumors with rapid growth and aggressive behavior can be a therapeutic challenge in immunosuppressed patients. Regional lymph nodes are the most common site of metastasis. In patients with metastatic disease, the 5-year survival rate may be low.

℞ **TREATMENT Basal Cell Carcinoma** The treatment modalities used for BCC include electrodesiccation and curettage (ED&C), excision, cryosurgery, radiation therapy, Mohs micrographic surgery (MMS), and others. The mode of therapy chosen depends on tumor characteristics, age, medical status, preferences of the patient, and other factors. ED&C remains the method most commonly employed by dermatologists. This method is selected for low-risk tumors (e.g., a small primary tumor of a less aggressive subtype in a favorable location). Excision, which offers the advantage of histologic control, is usually selected for more aggressive tumors or those in high-risk locations, or, in many instances, for esthetic reasons. Cryosurgery using liquid nitrogen may be used in certain low-risk tumors, but it requires specialized equipment (cryoprobes) to be effective for advanced neoplasms. Radiation therapy, while not employed as often as surgical modalities, offers an excellent chance for cure in many cases of BCC. It is useful in patients not considered surgical candidates and as a surgical adjunct in high-risk tumors. Younger patients may not be good candidates for radiation therapy because of the risks of long-term carcinogenesis and radiodermatitis. MMS is a specialized type of surgical excision that permits the ultimate in histologic control and preservation of uninvolved tissue. It is preferred for lesions that are recurrent, in a high-risk location, or large and ill-defined, and where maximal tissue conservation is critical (e.g., the eyelids). Topical chemotherapy with 5-fluorouracil (5FU) cream has limited usefulness in the management of BCC and should be used only for treating superficial BCC. Intralesional 5FU is being investigated for BCC. Intralesional interferon is effective in certain primary tumors. Photodynamic therapy, which employs selective activation of a photoactive drug by visible light, may be useful in patients with numerous tumors. Lasers also have been used for the treatment of skin cancer.

Squamous Cell Carcinoma The therapy of cutaneous SCC should be based on an analysis of risk factors influencing the biologic behavior of the tumor. These include the size, location, and degree of histologic differentiation of the tumor and the age and physical condition of the patient. Surgical excision, MMS, and radiation are standard methods of treatment. Cryosurgery and ED&C have been used successfully for small primary tumors. Metastases are treated with lymph node dissection, irradiation, or both. 13-*Cis*-retinoic acid (1 mg orally every day) plus interferon (3 million units subcutaneously or intramuscularly every day) may produce a partial response in most patients. Systemic chemotherapy combinations that include cisplatin may also be palliative in some patients.

PREVENTION Since the vast majority of skin cancers are related to chronic UV-B exposure, they are largely preventable by blocking sun exposure. Emphasis should be placed on preventive measures beginning early in life. Patients must understand that damage from UV-B begins early, despite the fact that cancers develop years later. Regular use of sunscreens and protective clothing should be encouraged. Avoidance of tanning salons and sun exposure during midday (10 A.M. to 2 P.M.) is recommended. Precancerous and in situ lesions should be treated early. Early detection of small tumors affords simpler treatment modalities with higher cure rates and lower morbidity. In patients with a history of skin cancer, long-term follow-up for the detection of recurrence, metastasis, and new skin cancers should be emphasized. Chemoprophylaxis using synthetic retinoids is useful in controlling new lesions in some patients with multiple tumors.

OTHER TYPES OF CUTANEOUS CANCER

Neoplasms of cutaneous adnexa, and sarcomas of fibrous, mesenchymal, fatty, and vascular tissues make up 1 to 2% of nonmelanoma skin cancers. The recent rapid rise in the incidence of Kaposi's sarcoma is attributed to HIV infection and immunosuppressive therapy. Human herpesvirus 8 appears to be the cause of sporadic and HIV-associated Kaposi's sarcoma. Current therapy is palliative and depends on the symptoms and sites of involvement. Treatment modalities include cryosurgery, vinblastine, excision, radiation, interferon, and systemic combination chemotherapy (Chap. 309).

ACKNOWLEDGMENT
The authors wish to acknowledge Dr. Nhu-linh T. Tran, who was a co-author of this chapter in the 14th edition.

BIBLIOGRAPHY

AUTIER P et al: Sunscreen use and duration of sun exposure: A double-blind randomized trial. J Natl Cancer Inst 91:1304, 1999

BALCH CM et al: Efficacy of an elective regional lymph node dissection of 1 to 4 mm thick melanomas for persons 60 years of age and younger. Ann Surg 224:255, 1996

DRAKE LA et al: Guidelines of care of basal cell carcinoma. J Am Acad Dermatol 26: 117, 1992

——— et al: Guidelines of care for cutaneous squamous cell carcinoma. J Am Acad Dermatol 28:628, 1993

GAILANI MR et al: Developmental genes and cancer: Role of *patched* in basal cell carcinoma of the skin. J Natl Cancer Inst 89:1103, 1997

KIRKWOOD JM et al: Interferon-alpha-2b adjuvant therapy of high-risk resected cutaneous melanoma. The Eastern Cooperative Oncology Group trial EST1684. J Clin Oncol 14:7, 1996

RHODES AR: Benign neoplasias and hyperplasias of melanocytes, in *Fitzpatrick's Dermatology in General Medicine*, 5th ed, IM Freedberg et al (eds). New York, McGraw-Hill, 1999, pp 1018–1097

TOULOUKIAN CE, ROSENBERG SA: A survey of treatments used in patients with metastatic melanoma: Analysis of 189 patients referred to the National Cancer Institute. Cancer J Sci Am 5:269, 1999

87 *Everett E. Vokes*

HEAD AND NECK CANCER

Epithelial carcinomas of the head and neck arise from the mucosal surfaces in the head and neck area and typically are squamous cell in origin. This category includes tumors of the paranasal sinuses, the oral cavity, and the nasopharynx, oropharynx, hypopharynx, and larynx. Tumors of the salivary glands differ from the more common carcinomas of the head and neck in etiology, histopathology, clinical presentation, and therapy. →*Thyroid malignancies are described in Chap. 330.*

INCIDENCE AND EPIDEMIOLOGY The annual number of new cases of head and neck cancers in the United States is approximately 40,000, accounting for about 5% of adult malignancies. Head and neck cancers are more common in certain other countries, and the worldwide incidence exceeds half a million cases annually. In North America and Europe, the tumors usually arise from the oral cavity, oropharynx, or larynx, whereas nasopharyngeal cancer is more common in the Mediterranean countries and in the Far East.

ETIOLOGY AND GENETICS Alcohol and tobacco use are the most common risk factors for head and neck cancer in the United States. Smokeless tobacco is an etiologic agent for oral cancers. Other potential carcinogens include marijuana and occupational exposures such as nickel refining, exposure to textile fibers, and woodworking.

Dietary factors may contribute. The incidence of head and neck cancer is highest in people with the lowest consumption of fruits and vegetables. Certain vitamins, including dietary carotenoids, may be protective; retinoids are being tested for prevention.

Some head and neck cancers may have a viral etiology. The DNA of human papilloma virus has been detected in the tissue of oral and tonsil cancers, and Epstein-Barr virus (EBV) infection is associated with nasopharyngeal cancer. Nasopharyngeal cancer occurs endemically in some countries of the Mediterranean and Far East, where EBV antibody titers can be measured to screen high-risk populations. Nasopharyngeal cancer has also been associated with other environmental factors, such as consumption of salted fish.

No specific risk factors or environmental carcinogens have been identified for salivary gland tumors.

HISTOPATHOLOGY, CARCINOGENESIS, AND MOLECULAR BIOLOGY   Squamous cell head and neck carcinomas can be divided into well-differentiated, moderately well-differentiated, and poorly differentiated categories. Patients with poorly differentiated tumors have a worse prognosis than those with well-differentiated tumors. For nasopharyngeal cancers, the less common differentiated squamous cell carcinoma is distinguished from nonkeratinizing and undifferentiated carcinoma (lymphoepithelioma) that contains infiltrating (bystander) lymphocytes.

Salivary gland tumors can arise from the major (parotid, submandibular, sublingual) or minor salivary glands (located in the submucosa of the upper aerodigestive tract). Most parotid tumors are benign, but half of submandibular and sublingual gland tumors and most minor salivary gland tumors are malignant. Malignant tumors include mucoepidermoid and adenoidcystic carcinomas and adenocarcinomas.

The mucosal surface of the entire pharynx is exposed to alcohol and tobacco-related carcinogens and is at risk for the development of a premalignant or malignant lesion, such as erythroplakia or leukoplakia (hyperplasia, dysplasia), that can progress to invasive carcinoma. Alternatively, multiple synchronous or metachronous cancers can develop. In fact, patients with early-stage head and neck cancer are at greater risk of dying of a second malignancy than of dying from a recurrence of the primary disease.

Second head and neck malignancies are not therapy-induced but, instead, reflect the exposure of the upper aerodigestive mucosa to the same carcinogens that caused the first cancer. These second primaries develop in the head and neck area, the lung, or the esophagus.

Chromosomal deletions and other alterations, most frequently involving chromosomes 3p, 9p, 17p, and 13q, have been identified in both premalignant and malignant head and neck lesions, as have mutations in tumor suppressor genes, commonly the *p53* gene. Amplification of oncogenes is less common, but overexpression of PRAD-1/bcl-1 (cyclin D1), bcl-2, transforming growth factor β, and the epidermal growth factor receptor have been described. The latter finding correlates positively with tumor size and poor outcome and is a target for experimental treatments.

Resected tumor specimens with histopathologically negative margins ("complete resection") can have histopathologically undetectable residual tumor cells with persistent *p53* mutations at the margins. Thus, a tumor-specific *p53* mutation can be detected in some phenotypically "normal" surgical margins, indicating residual disease. Patients with such submicroscopic marginal involvement may have a worse prognosis than patients with negative margins.

CLINICAL PRESENTATION AND DIFFERENTIAL DIAGNOSIS   Most head and neck cancers occur after age 50, although these cancers can appear in younger patients, including those without known risk factors. The manifestations vary according to the stage and primary site of the tumor. Patients with nonspecific signs and symptoms in the head and neck area should be evaluated with a thorough otolaryngologic exam, particularly if symptoms persist longer than 2 to 4 weeks.

Cancer of the nasopharynx typically does not cause early symptoms. However, on occasion it may cause unilateral serous otitis media due to obstruction of the eustachian tube, unilateral or bilateral nasal obstruction, or epistaxis. Advanced nasopharyngeal carcinoma causes neuropathies of the cranial nerves.

Carcinomas of the oral cavity present as nonhealing ulcers, changes in the fit of dentures, or painful lesions. Tumors of the tongue base or oropharynx can cause decreased tongue mobility and alterations in speech. Cancers of the oropharynx or hypopharynx rarely cause early symptoms, but they may cause sore throat and/or otalgia.

Hoarseness may be an early symptom of laryngeal cancer, and persistent hoarseness requires referral to an otorhinolaryngologist for indirect laryngoscopy and/or radiographic studies. If a head and neck lesion treated initially with antibiotics does not resolve in a short period, further workup is indicated; to simply continue the antibiotic treatment may be to lose the chance of early diagnosis of a malignancy.

Advanced head and neck cancers in any location can cause severe pain, otalgia, airway obstruction, cranial neuropathies, trismus, odynophagia, dysphagia, decreased tongue mobility, fistulas, skin involvement, and massive cervical lymphadenopathy, which may be unilateral or bilateral. Some patients have enlarged lymph nodes even though no primary lesion can be detected by endoscopy or biopsy; these patients are considered to have carcinoma of unknown primary. If the enlarged nodes are located in the upper neck and the tumor cells are of squamous cell histology, the malignancy probably arose from a mucosal surface in the head or neck. Tumor cells in supraclavicular lymph nodes may also arise from a primary site in the chest or abdomen.

The physical examination should include scrutiny of all visible mucosal surfaces and palpation of the floor of mouth and tongue and of the neck. In addition to tumors themselves, leukoplakia—a white mucosal patch—or erythroplakia—a red mucosal patch—may be observed; these "premalignant" lesions can represent hyperplasia, dysplasia, or carcinoma in situ. All visible lesions should be biopsied. Further examination should be performed by the otorhinolaryngologist. Additional staging procedures include computed tomography of the head and neck to identify the extent of the disease. Patients with lymph node involvement should have chest radiography and a bone scan to screen for distant metastases. The definitive staging procedure is an endoscopic examination under anesthesia, which may include laryngoscopy, esophagoscopy, and bronchoscopy; during this procedure, multiple biopsy samples are obtained to establish a primary diagnosis, define the extent of primary disease, and identify any additional premalignant lesions or second primaries.

Head and neck tumors are classified according to the TNM system of the American Joint Committee on Cancer. This classification varies according to the specific anatomic subsite (Tables 87-1 and 87-2). Distant metastases are found in <10% of patients at initial diagnosis, but in autopsy series, microscopic involvement of the lungs, bones, or liver is more common, particularly in patients with advanced neck lymph node disease.

In patients with lymph node involvement and no visible primary, the diagnosis should be made by lymph node excision. If the results indicate squamous cell carcinoma, a panendoscopy should be performed, with biopsy of all suspicious-appearing areas and directed biopsies of common primary sites, such as the nasopharynx, tonsil, tongue base, and pyriform sinus.

℞ **TREATMENT**   Generally, patients with head and neck cancer can be categorized into three clinical groups: those with localized disease, those with locally or regionally advanced disease, and those with recurrent and/or metastatic disease. Comorbidities associated with tobacco and alcohol abuse can affect treatment outcome.

Localized Disease   Approximately one-third of patients have localized disease; that is, T1 or T2 (stage I or stage II) lesions without detectable lymph node involvement or distant metastases. These lesions are treated with curative intent by surgery or radiation. The choice of modality differs according to institutional expertise. Generally, radiation therapy is preferred for laryngeal cancer to preserve voice function, and surgery is preferred for small lesions in the oral cavity to avoid the long-term complications of radiation, such as xerostomia and dental decay. Overall 5-year survival is 60 to 90%.

Table 87-1 TNM Classification for Head and Neck Cancer (except Nasopharyngeal)

T Grade	Lip	Oral Cavity	Oropharynx	Hypopharynx	Larynx
			Primary Tumor Site		
TX			Primary tumor cannot be assessed		
T0			No evidence of primary tumor		
Tis			Carcinoma in situ		
T1	0–2 cm	0–2 cm	0–2 cm	1 site	1 site or limited to vocal cords
T2	2.1–4 cm	2.1–4 cm	2.1–4 cm	>1 site, no vocal cord fixation	>1 site or impaired cord mobility
T3	>4 cm	>4 cm	>4 cm	vocal cord paralysis	Vocal cord paralysis
T4	>4 cm with massive invasion		Massive soft tissue, bone, or cartilage invasion		

REGIONAL LYMPH NODES (N)

NX	Regional lymph nodes cannot be assessed
N0	No regional lymph node metastasis
N1	Metastasis in a single ipsilateral lymph node, 3 cm or less in greatest dimension
N2	Metastasis in a single ipsilateral lymph node, more than 3 cm but not more than 6 cm in greatest dimension; or in multiple ipsilateral lymph nodes, none more than 6 cm in greatest dimension; or in bilateral or contralateral lymph nodes, none more than 6 cm in greatest dimension
N2a	Metastasis in single ipsilateral lymph node more than 3 cm but more than 6 cm in greatest dimension
N2b	Metastasis in multiple ipsilateral lymph nodes, none more than 6 cm in greatest dimension
N2c	Metastasis in bilateral or contralateral lymph nodes, none more than 6 cm in greatest dimension
N3	Metastasis in a lymph node more than 6 cm in greatest dimension

DISTANT METASTASIS (M)

MX	Presence of distant metastasis cannot be assessed
M0	No distant metastasis
M1	Distant metastasis

STAGE GROUPING

Stage 0	Tis	N0	M0	Stage IV	T4	N0	M0
Stage I	T1	N0	M0		T4	N1	M0
Stage II	T2	N0	M0		Any T	N2	M0
Stage III	T3	N0	M0		Any T	N3	M0
	T1	N1	M0		Any T	Any N	M1
	T2	N1	M0				
	T3	N1	M0				

Locally or Regionally Advanced Disease Locally or regionally advanced disease—that is, disease with a large primary tumor and/or lymph node metastases—can also be treated with curative intent, but not with surgery or radiation therapy alone. Combined modality therapy including surgery, radiation therapy and chemotherapy is most successful. Concomitant chemotherapy and radiation therapy appears to be the most effective sequencing of treatment.

Induction chemotherapy In this strategy, patients receive chemotherapy [usually cisplatin and fluorouracil (5FU)] before surgery and radiotherapy. Most patients who receive three cycles of this combination show tumor reduction, and the response is clinically "complete" in up to half of these patients. This "sequential" multimodality therapy does not cure more patients than surgery plus radiation therapy alone. Time to recurrence may be improved but survival is similar. However, induction chemotherapy allows for organ preservation in patients with laryngeal and hypopharyngeal cancer.

Concomitant chemoradiotherapy With the concomitant strategy, chemotherapy and radiation therapy are given simultaneously rather than sequentially. Because most patients with head and neck cancer develop recurrent disease in the head and neck area, this approach is aimed at killing radiation-resistant cancer cells with chemotherapy. In addi-

tion, chemotherapy can enhance cell killing by radiation therapy. Toxicity (mucositis) is increased with concomitant chemoradiotherapy; however, meta-analysis of randomized trials documents an improvement in 5-year survival of 8% with concomitant 5FU and radiation therapy. Results seem even better with 5FU and cisplatin plus radiation

Table 87-2 Definition of TNM—Nasopharynx

PRIMARY TUMOR (T)

TX	Primary tumor cannot be assessed
T0	No evidence of primary tumor
Tis	carcinoma in situ
T1	Tumor confined to the nasopharynx
T2	Tumor extends to soft tissues of oropharynx and/or nasal fossa
T2a	without parapharyngeal extension
T2b	with parapharyngeal extension
T3	Tumor invades bony structures and/or paranasal sinuses
T4	Tumor with intracranial extension and/or involvement of cranial nerves, infratemporal fossa, hypopharynx, or orbit

REGIONAL LYMPH NODES (N)

The distribution and the prognostic impact of regional lymph node spread from nasopharynx cancer, particularly of the undifferentiated type, is different than that of other head and neck mucosal cancers and justifies use of a different N classification scheme.

NX	Regional lymph nodes cannot be assessed
N0	No regional lymph node metastasis
N1	Unilateral metastasis in lymph nodes(s), 6 cm or less in greatest dimension, above the supraclavicular fossa
N2	Bilateral metastasis in lymph node(s), 6 cm or less in greatest dimension, above the supraclavicular fossa
N3	Metastasis in a lymph node(s)
N3a	greater than 6 cm in dimension
N3b	extension to the supraclavicular fossa

STAGE GROUPING

Stage 0	Tis	N0	M0
Stage I	T1	N0	M0
Stage IIA	T2a	N0	M0
Stage IIB	T1	N1	M0
	T2	N1	M0
	T2a	N1	M0
	T2b	N0	M0
	T2b	N1	M0
Stage III	T1	N2	M0
	T2a	N2	M0
	T2b	N2	M0
	T3	N0	M0
	T3	N1	M0
	T3	N2	M0
Stage IVA	T4	N0	M0
	T4	N1	M0
	T4	N2	M0
Stage IVB	Any T	N3	M0
Stage IVC	Any T	Any N	M1

therapy. Five-year survival is 34 to 50%. The use of radiation therapy together with cisplatin has produced markedly improved survival in patients with advanced nasopharyngeal cancer. The success of concomitant chemoradiotherapy in patients with unresectable disease has led to the testing of a similar approach in patients with resectable disease in an effort to increase organ preservation.

Recurrent and/or Metastatic Disease Patients with recurrent and/or metastatic disease are, with few exceptions, treated with palliative intent. Some patients may require local or regional radiation therapy for pain control, but most are given chemotherapy. Response rates to chemotherapy average only 30 to 50%; the duration of response averages only 3 months, and the median survival time is 6 months. Therefore, chemotherapy provides transient symptomatic benefit. Drugs with single-agent activity in this setting include methotrexate, 5FU, cisplatin, paclitaxel, and docetaxel. Combinations of cisplatin and 5FU, carboplatin and 5FU, and cisplatin and paclitaxel are also used.

CHEMOPREVENTION β-carotene and *cis*-retinoic acid can lead to the regression of leukoplakia. In addition, the use of *cis*-retinoic acid may reduce the incidence of second primaries.

TREATMENT COMPLICATIONS Complications involved in the treatment of head and neck cancer are usually related to the extent of surgery. Several attempts have been made to limit the extent of surgery or to replace it with chemotherapy and radiation therapy. Acute complications of radiation include mucositis and dysphagia. Long-term complications include xerostomia, loss of taste, decreased tongue mobility, second malignancies, and dysphagia and neck fibrosis. The complications of chemotherapy vary with the regimen used but usually include myelosuppression, mucositis, nausea and vomiting, and nephrotoxicity (with cisplatin).

SALIVARY GLAND TUMORS Most benign salivary gland tumors are treated with surgical excision, and patients with invasive salivary gland tumors are treated with surgery and radiation therapy. Neutron radiation may be particularly effective. These tumors may recur regionally; adenoidcystic carcinoma has a tendency to recur along the nerve tracks. Distant metastases may occur as late as 10 to 20 years after the initial diagnosis. For metastatic disease, therapy is given with palliative intent, usually chemotherapy with doxorubicin and/or cisplatin.

BIBLIOGRAPHY

AL-SARRAF M et al: Chemoradiotherapy versus radiotherapy in patients with advanced nasopharyngeal cancer: Phase III randomized Intergroup study 0099. J Clin Oncol 16:1310, 1998

BRIZEL DM et al: Hyperfractionated irradiation with or without concurrent chemotherapy for locally advanced head and neck cancer. N Engl J Med 338:1798, 1998

CALIFANO J et al: Genetic progression model for head and neck cancer: implications for field cancerization. Cancer Res 56:2488, 1996

RICE DH: Salivary gland disorders. Neoplastic and nonneoplastic. Med Clin North Am 83:197, 1999

SHIN DM, LIPPMAN SM: Paclitaxel-based chemotherapy for recurrent and/or metastatic head and neck squamous cell carcinoma: Current and future directions. Semin Oncol 26 (Suppl 2):100, 1999

VOKES EE, ATHANASIADIS I: Chemotherapy for squamous cell carcinoma of head and neck: The future is now. Ann Oncol 7:15, 1996

VOKES EE et al: Head and neck cancer. N Engl J Med 328:184, 1993

88   *John D. Minna*

NEOPLASMS OF THE LUNG

Each year, primary carcinoma of the lung affects 94,000 males and 78,000 females in the United States, 86% of whom die within 5 years of diagnosis, making it the leading cause of cancer death in both men and women and in all races. The incidence of lung cancer peaks between ages 55 and 65 years. Lung cancer accounts for 31% of all cancer deaths in men and 25% in women. The effects of smoking cessation efforts begun 25 years ago have been seen in a slowing of the rate of age-adjusted cancer death from lung cancer in males (~70 per 100,000 male population); but, unfortunately, the rate in females is still increasing (~35 per 100,000 female population). Only 15% of patients have local disease at diagnosis; 25% have disease spread to regional lymph nodes, and >55% have distant metastases. The 5-year survival rate of patients with local disease is 50%; it is 20% for patients with regional disease and 14% overall. The 5-year overall lung cancer survival rate has nearly doubled in the last 30 years. The improvement is due to advances in combined-modality treatment with surgery, radiotherapy, and chemotherapy. Thus, primary carcinoma of the lung is a major health problem with a generally grim prognosis. However, an orderly approach to diagnosis, staging, and treatment based on knowledge of the clinical behavior of lung cancer and involving multidisciplinary input allows choice and delivery of the best therapy for potential cure or optimal palliation of individual patients.

PATHOLOGY

The term *lung cancer* is used for tumors arising from the respiratory epithelium (bronchi, bronchioles, and alveoli). Mesotheliomas, lymphomas, and stromal tumors (sarcomas) are distinct from epithelial lung cancer. Four major cell types make up 88% of all primary lung neoplasms according to the World Health Organization classification (Table 88-1). These are *squamous* or *epidermoid carcinoma*, *small cell* (also called *oat cell*) *carcinoma*, *adenocarcinoma* (including bronchioloalveolar), and *large cell* (also called *large cell anaplastic*) *carcinoma*. The remainder include undifferentiated carcinomas, carcinoids, bronchial gland tumors (including adenoid cystic carcinomas and mucoepidermoid tumors), and rarer tumor types. The various cell types have different natural histories and responses to therapy, and thus a correct histologic diagnosis by an experienced pathologist is the first step to correct treatment. In the past 25 years, for unknown reasons, adenocarcinoma has replaced squamous cell carcinoma as the most frequent histologic subtype for all sexes and races combined (Table 88-1).

Major treatment decisions are made on the basis of whether a tumor is classified histologically as a small cell carcinoma or as one of the non-small cell varieties (epidermoid, adenocarcinoma, large cell carcinoma, bronchioloalveolar carcinoma, and mixed versions of these). Some of the distinctions are summarized in Tables 88-1 and 88-2. At presentation, small cell carcinomas usually have already spread such that surgery is unlikely to be curative, and they are managed primarily by chemotherapy with or without radiotherapy. In contrast, non-small cell cancers that are found to be localized at the time of presentation may be cured with either surgery or radiotherapy. Non-small cell cancers do not respond as well to chemotherapy as small cell cancers.

Ninety percent of patients with lung cancer of all histologic types are current or former cigarette smokers. Of the annual 171,600 new cases of lung cancer, ~50% develop in former smokers. With increased success in smoking cessation efforts, the number of former smokers will grow, and these individuals will be important candidates for early detection and chemoprevention efforts. By far the most common form of lung cancer arising in lifetime nonsmokers, in women, and in young patients (<45 years) is adenocarcinoma. However, in nonsmokers with adenocarcinoma involving the lung, the possibility of other primary sites should be considered. Epidermoid and small cell cancers usually present as central masses with endobronchial growth, while adenocarcinomas and large cell cancers tend to present as peripheral nodules or masses, frequently with pleural involvement. Epidermoid and large cell cancers cavitate in ~10 to 20% of cases. Bronchioloalveolar carcinoma, a form of adenocarcinoma arising from peripheral airways, can present as a single mass; as a diffuse, multinodular lesion; or as a fluffy infiltrate.

ETIOLOGY

Most lung cancers are caused by carcinogens and tumor promoters ingested via cigarette smoking. The prevalence of smoking in the United States is 28% for males and 25% for females, age 18 years or older; 38% of high school seniors smoke. The relative risk of developing lung cancer is increased about 13-fold by active smoking and about 1.5-fold by long-term passive exposure to cigarette smoke. Chronic obstructive pulmonary disease, which is also smoking-related, further increases the risk of developing lung cancer. The lung cancer death rate is related to the total amount (often expressed in "cigarette pack-years") of cigarettes smoked, such that the risk is increased 60- to 70-fold for a man smoking two packs a day for 20 years as compared with a nonsmoker. Conversely, the chance of developing lung cancer decreases with cessation of smoking but may never return to the nonsmoker level. The increase in lung cancer rate in women is also associated with a rise in cigarette smoking. Women have a higher relative risk per given exposure than men (~1.5 fold higher), and women with lung cancer are more likely to have never smoked than men. This gender difference is likely due to a higher susceptibility to tobacco carcinogens in women.

Efforts to get people to stop smoking are mandatory. However, smoking cessation is extremely difficult, because the smoking habit represents a powerful addiction to nicotine (Chap. 390). Preventing people from starting to smoke may be more effective, an effort that needs to be targeted to children.

Although human lung cancer is not thought of as a genetic disease, various molecular genetic studies have shown the acquisition by lung cancer cells of a number of genetic lesions, including activation of dominant oncogenes and inactivation of tumor suppressor or recessive oncogenes (Chaps. 81 and 82). In fact, lung cancer cells may have to accumulate a large number (perhaps ≥10) of such lesions. For the dominant oncogenes, these include point mutations in the coding regions of the ras family of oncogenes (particularly in the K-ras gene in adenocarcinoma of the lung); amplification, rearrangement, and/or loss of transcriptional control of myc family oncogenes (c-, N-, and L-myc; changes in c-myc are found in non-small cell cancers, while changes in all myc family members are found in small cell lung cancer); and overexpression of bcl-2, Her-2/neu, and the telomerase gene (Table 88-2). Tumor mutations in ras genes are associated with a poor prognosis in non-small cell lung cancer, while tumor amplification of c-myc is associated with a poor prognosis in small cell lung cancer.

For the recessive oncogenes (tumor suppressor genes), cytogenetic and allelotyping analyses have shown allele loss involving chromosome regions 1p, 1q, 3p12-13, 3p14 (FHIT gene region), 3p21, 3p24-25, 4p, 4q, 5q, 8p, 9p (p16/CDKN2, p15,p19ARF gene cluster), 11p13, 11p15, 13q14 (retinoblastoma, rb, gene), 16q, and 17p13 (p53 gene), as well as other sites. Several candidate recessive oncogenes on chromosome 3p appear to be involved in nearly all lung cancers and may be affected early in preneoplastic lesions. The p53 and rb genes are both mutated in >90% of small cell lung cancers, while p53 is mutated in >50% and rb in 20% of non-small cell lung cancers. p16/CDKN2 is abnormal in 10% of small cell and >50% of non-small cell lung cancers. Rb and p16/CDKN2 are part of the same G1-to-S cell cycle regulatory pathway. Either one or the other of these elements appears to be mutated or to have its expression turned off (e.g., by hypermethylation of the promoter) in the large majority of lung cancers. Histologically identifiable preneoplastic lesions found in the respiratory epithelium of lung cancer patients and smokers include hyperplasia, dysplasia (progressively severe), and carcinoma in situ. 3p allele loss (hyperplasia) followed by 9p (p16/CDKN2) allele loss (hyperplasia) are the earliest events; 17p (p53) abnormalities and then ras mutations usually are found only in carcinoma in situ and invasive cancer. Thus, molecular changes involving allele loss and microsatellite alteration can be found in the earliest preneoplastic lesions and potentially even before any histologic changes are noted. Clinical trials of early diagnosis are needed to prove the usefulness of these molecular markers in the identification of very early lung cancer and in the monitoring of treatment and chemoprevention.

The large number of lesions shows that lung cancer, like other common epithelial malignancies, is a multistep process that is likely to involve both carcinogens and tumor promoters. Prevention can be directed at both processes. Lung cancer cells produce many peptide hormones and express receptors for these hormones, which can act to stimulate tumor cell growth in an "autocrine" fashion. Highly carcinogenic derivatives of nicotine are formed in cigarette smoke. Lung cancer cells of all histologic types express receptors for nicotine. Nicotine can prevent apoptosis in lung cancer cell lines. Thus, nicotine itself could be directly involved in lung cancer pathogenesis.

While lung cancer does not have a clear pattern of Mendelian inheritance, several features suggest a potential for familial association. Inherited mutations in rb (patients with retinoblastomas living to adulthood) and p53 (Li-Fraumeni syndrome) genes may develop lung cancer. First-degree relatives of lung cancer probands have a two- to threefold excess risk of lung cancer or other cancers, many of which are not smoking-related. Genetic epidemiologic studies have proposed an association between the P450 enzyme or chromosome fragility (mutagen sensitivity) genotypes and the development of lung cancer. The identification of persons at very high risk of developing lung cancer would be useful in early detection and prevention efforts.

CLINICAL MANIFESTATIONS

Lung cancer gives rise to signs and symptoms caused by local tumor growth, invasion or obstruction of adjacent structures, growth in regional nodes through lymphatic spread, growth in distant metastatic sites after hematogenous dissemination, and remote effects of tumor products (paraneoplastic syndrome). Peptide hormone secretion by the tumor or immunologic cross-reaction between tumor and normal tissue antigens can produce a variety of signs and symptoms (Chap. 100).

Although 5 to 15% of patients with lung cancer are identified while they are asymptomatic, usually as a result of a routine chest radiograph, most patients present with some sign or symptom. Central or endobronchial growth of the primary tumor may cause cough, hemoptysis, wheeze and stridor, dyspnea, and postobstructive pneumonitis (fever and productive cough). Peripheral growth of the primary tumor may cause pain from pleural or chest wall involvement, cough, dyspnea on a restrictive basis, and symptoms of lung abscess resulting from

Table 88-1 Frequency, Age-Adjusted Incidence, and Survival Rates for Different Histologic Types of Lung Cancer (All Races, Both Sexes, and All Stages)[a]

Histologic Type of Thoracic Malignancy	Frequency, %	Age-Adjusted Rate	5-year Survival Rate (All Stages)
Adenocarcinoma (and all subtypes)	32	17	17
Bronchioloalveolar carcinoma	3	1.4	42
Squamous cell (epidermoid) carcinoma	29	15	15
Small cell carcinoma	18	9	5
Large cell carcinoma	9	5	11
Carcinoid	1.0	0.5	83
Mucoepidermoid carcinoma	0.1	<0.1	39
Adenoid cystic carcinoma	<0.1	<0.1	48
Sarcoma and other soft tissue tumors	0.1	0.1	30
All others and unspecified carcinomas	11.0	6	NA
Total	100	52	14

[a] Data on histology frequency and age-adjusted incidence rates per 100,000 U.S. population are from 60,514 cases of invasive lung cancer involving all races and both sexes obtained from the data for 1983–1987 of the Surveillance, Epidemiology, and End Results (SEER) Program of the National Cancer Institute; 5-year relative survival rates for all stages, all races, and both sexes are from the SEER data on 87,128 carcinomas, 1978–1986. NA, not available.
SOURCE: Summarized from Travis et al: Cancer 75:191, 1995.

Table 88-2 Comparison of Small Cell and Non-Small Cell Lung Cancers

Feature	Small Cell	Non-Small Cell
Histology	Scant cytoplasm; small, hyperchromatic nuclei with fine chromatin pattern; nucleoli indistinct; diffuse sheets of cells	Abundant cytoplasm; pleomorphic nuclei with coarse chromatin pattern; nucleoli often prominent; glandular or squamous architecture
General neuroendocrine properties		
Dense-core granules	Present	Absent[a]
L-Dopa decarboxylase activity	High	Absent
Chromogranin	Present	Absent
Synaptophysin	Present	Absent
Neuron-specific enolase	High	Low
Creatine kinase BB isozyme	High	Low
CD56 and CD57 antigens	Present	Absent
Peptide hormone production		
Gastrin-releasing peptide gene products	Present	Absent
Other neuropeptides	ACTH, AVP, calcitonin, ANF	PTH
Autocrine loops	GRP/GRP receptor	HGF/MET
	SCF/KIT	NDF/ERBB2
Other markers		
HLA, β_2-microglobulin	Absent/low	Present
Intermediate filament pattern	"SCLC"	"Non-SCLC"
Neurofilaments	Present	Absent
Opioid receptors	Present	Present
Nicotine receptors	Present	Present
EGF receptors	Low or absent	Present
Mucin	Absent	Present in adenocarcinomas
Surfactant-associated proteins	Absent	Often present
Carcinoembryonic antigen	Present	Present
Recessive oncogene (tumor suppressor gene) and allelotype abnormalities		
3p allele loss	100%	>90%
rb mutations	~90%	~20%
p16/CDKN2 mutations/absent expression	~10%	~50%
p53 mutations/abnormal expression	>90%	>50%
4p, 4q, 5q, 8p, 11p and other allele losses	Present	Present
Microsatellite alterations	Present	Present
Dominant oncogene abnormalities		
ras mutations	<1%	~30%
myc family overexpression	>50%	10–35%
bcl-2 overexpression	>75%	>50%
Her-2/neu overexpression	<10%	~30%
Telomerase overexpression	>90%	>90%
Microsatellite alterations	35%	22%
Promoter hypermethylation (*p16*, DAP Kinase, GSTP1, MGMT, *FHIT*, *RARβ*)	10–40%	10–40%
Response to radiotherapy	Objective shrinkage in 80–90%; often complete response	Objective shrinkage in 30–50%; response uncommonly complete
Response to combination chemotherapy		
Overall regression rate	90%	40–60%
Rate of complete regression	30%	5%

[a] Ten percent of non-small cell lung cancers have populations of cells expressing neuroendocrine markers, and these are best demonstrated by immunohistochemical stains.

ABBREVIATIONS: ACTH, adrenocorticotropic hormone; ANF, atrial natriuretic factor; AVP, arginine vasopressin; CD56, neural cell adhesion molecule (NCAM)-1; CD57, Leu-7 or HNK-1; HLA, human leukocyte antigen; PTH, parathormone; SCLC, small cell lung cancer; GRP, gastrin-releasing peptide; SCF, stem cell factor; KIT, SCF receptor; HGF, hepatocyte growth factor; MET, met protooncogene, HGF receptor; NDF, neu differentiation factor or heregulin; ERBB2, her2/neu protooncogene receptor.

tumor cavitation. Regional spread of tumor in the thorax (by contiguous growth or by metastasis to regional lymph nodes) may cause tracheal obstruction, esophageal compression with dysphagia, recurrent laryngeal nerve paralysis with hoarseness, phrenic nerve paralysis with elevation of the hemidiaphragm and dyspnea, and sympathetic nerve paralysis with Horner's syndrome (enophthalmos, ptosis, miosis, and ipsilateral loss of sweating). *Pancoast's* (or *superior sulcus tumor*) *syndrome* results from local extension of a tumor (usually epidermoid) growing in the apex of the lung with involvement of the eighth cervical and first and second thoracic nerves, with shoulder pain that characteristically radiates in the ulnar distribution of the arm, often with radiologic destruction of the first and second ribs. Often Horner's syndrome and Pancoast's syndrome coexist. Other problems of regional spread include *superior vena cava syndrome* from vascular obstruction; pericardial and cardiac extension with resultant tamponade, arrhythmia, or cardiac failure; lymphatic obstruction with resultant pleural effusion; and lymphangitic spread through the lungs with hypoxemia and dyspnea. In addition, bronchioloalveolar carcinoma can spread transbronchially, producing tumor growing along multiple alveolar surfaces with impairment of gas exchange, respiratory insufficiency, dyspnea, hypoxemia, and sputum production.

Extrathoracic metastatic disease is found at autopsy in >50% of patients with epidermoid carcinoma, 80% of patients with adenocarcinoma and large cell carcinoma, and >95% of patients with small cell cancer. Lung cancer metastases may occur in virtually every organ system. Common clinical problems related to metastatic lung cancer include brain metastases with neurologic deficits; bone metastases with pain and pathologic fractures; bone marrow invasion with cytopenias or leukoerythroblastosis; liver metastases causing biochemical liver dysfunction, biliary obstruction, and pain; lymph node metastases in the supraclavicular region and occasionally in the axilla and groin; and spinal cord compression syndromes from epidural or bone metastases. Adrenal metastases are common but rarely cause adrenal insufficiency.

Paraneoplastic syndromes are common in patients with lung cancer and may be the presenting finding or first sign of recurrence. In addition, paraneoplastic syndromes may mimic metastatic disease and, unless detected, lead to inappropriate palliative rather than curative treatment. Often the paraneoplastic syndrome may be relieved with successful treatment of the tumor. In some cases, the pathophysiology of the paraneoplastic syndrome is known, particularly when a hormone with biologic activity is secreted by a tumor (Chap. 100). However, in many cases the pathophysiology is unknown. Systemic symptoms of anorexia, cachexia, weight loss (seen in 30% of patients), fever, and suppressed immunity are paraneoplastic syndromes of unknown etiology. *Endocrine syndromes* are seen in 12% of patients; hypercalcemia and hypophosphatemia resulting from the ectopic production by epidermoid tumors of parathyroid hormone (PTH) or PTH-related peptide production, hyponatremia with the syndrome of inappropriate secretion of antidiuretic hormone or possibly atrial natriuretic factor by small cell cancer, and ectopic secretion by small cell cancer of adrenocorticotropic hormone (ACTH). ACTH secretion usually results in additional electrolyte disturbances, especially hypokalemia, rather than the changes in body habitus that occur in Cushing's syndrome from a pituitary adenoma.

Skeletal–connective tissue syndromes include clubbing in 30% of cases (usually non-small cell carcinomas) and hypertrophic pulmonary osteoarthropathy in 1 to 10% of cases (usually adenocarcinomas) with periostitis and clubbing giving pain, tenderness, and swelling over the affected bones and a positive bone scan. *Neurologic-myopathic syndromes* are seen in only 1% of patients but are dramatic and include the myasthenic *Eaton-Lambert syndrome* and retinal blindness with small cell cancer, while peripheral neuropathies, subacute cerebellar degeneration, cortical degeneration, and polymyositis are seen with all lung cancer types. Many of these are caused by autoimmune responses such as the development of anti-voltage-gated calcium channel antibodies in the Eaton-Lambert syndrome (Chap. 101). Coagulation, thrombotic, or other hematologic manifestations occur in 1 to 8% of patients and include migratory venous thrombophlebitis (*Trousseau's syndrome*), nonbacterial thrombotic (marantic) endocarditis with arterial emboli, disseminated intravascular coagulation with hemorrhage, and anemia, granulocytosis, and leukoerythroblastosis. Cutaneous manifestations such as dermatomyositis and acanthosis nigricans are uncommon (≤1%), as are the renal manifestations of nephrotic syndrome or glomerulonephritis (≤1%).

DIAGNOSIS AND STAGING

EARLY DIAGNOSIS The screening of asymptomatic persons at high risk (men older than 45 years who smoke ≥40 cigarettes per day) by means of sputum cytology and chest radiographs has not improved the survival rate. Although 90% of patients whose lung cancer is detected by screening are asymptomatic, no difference was found in the survival rates of the screened and nonscreened groups. Women have not been studied. The use of low dose spiral computed tomography (CT) lung scanning may be more sensitive, particularly for peripheral lesions. However, false positive rates are high (25% have abnormal tests, only 10% of which are cancers), and survival benefit for screening has not yet been shown (Chap. 80).

ESTABLISHING A TISSUE DIAGNOSIS OF LUNG CANCER Once signs, symptoms, or screening studies suggest lung cancer, a tissue diagnosis must be established. Tumor tissue can be obtained by a bronchial or transbronchial biopsy during fiberoptic bronchoscopy; by node biopsy during mediastinoscopy; from the operative specimen at the time of definitive surgical resection; by percutaneous biopsy of an enlarged lymph node, soft tissue mass, lytic bone lesion, bone marrow, or pleural lesion; by fine-needle aspiration of thoracic or extrathoracic tumor masses using CT guidance; or from an adequate cell block obtained from a malignant pleural effusion. In most cases, the pathologist should be able to make a definite diagnosis of epithelial malignancy and make the crucial differentiation of small cell from non-small cell lung cancer.

STAGING PATIENTS WITH LUNG CANCER Lung cancer staging consists of two parts: first, a determination of the location of tumor (anatomic staging) and, second, an assessment of a patient's ability to withstand various antitumor treatments (physiologic staging). In a patient with non-small cell lung cancer, *resectability* (whether the tumor can be entirely removed by a standard surgical procedure such as a lobectomy or pneumonectomy), which depends on the anatomic stage of the tumor, and *operability* (whether the patient can tolerate such a surgical procedure), which depends on the cardiopulmonary function of the patient, are determined.

Non-Small Cell Lung Cancer The TNM International Staging System should be used for cases of non-small cell lung cancer, particularly in preparing patients for curative attempts with surgery or radiotherapy (Table 88-3). The various T (tumor size), N (regional node involvement), and M (presence or absence of distant metastasis) factors are combined to form different stage groups. At presentation, approximately one-third of patients have disease localized enough for a curative attempt with surgery or radiotherapy (patients with stage I or II disease and some with stage IIIA disease), one-third have distant

Table 88-3   TNM (Tumor, Node, Metastasis) International Staging System for Lung Cancer

Stage	TNM Descriptors	5-Year Survival Rate, %	
		Clinical Stage	Surgical-Pathologic Stage
IA	T1 N0 M0	61	67
IB	T2 N0 M0	38	57
IIA	T1 N1 M0	34	55
IIB	T2 N1 M0	24	39
IIB	T3 N0 M0	22	38
IIIA	T3 N1 M0	9	25
	T1–2–3 N2 M0	13	23
IIIB	T4 N0–1–2 M0	7	<5
	T1–2–3–4 N3 M0	3	<3
IV	Any T any N M1	1	<1

TUMOR (T) STATUS DESCRIPTOR

T0	No evidence of a primary tumor
TX	Primary tumor cannot be assessed, or tumor proven by the presence of malignant cells in sputum or bronchial washings but not visualized by imaging or bronchoscopy
TIS	Carcinoma in situ
T1	Tumor >3 cm in greatest dimension, surrounded by lung or visceral pleura, without bronchoscopic evidence of invasion more proximal than lobar bronchus (i.e., not in main bronchus)
T2	Tumor with any of following: >3 cm in greatest dimension; involves main bronchus, ≥2 cm distal to the carcina; invades visceral pleura; associated with atelectasis or obstructive pneumonitis extending to hilum but does not involve entire lung
T3	Tumor of any size that directly invades any of the following: chest wall (including superior sulcus tumors), diaphragm, mediastinal pleura, parietal pericardium; or tumor in main bronchus <2 cm distal to carina but without involvement of carina; or associated atelectasis or obstructive pneumonitis of entire lung
T4	Tumor of any size that invades any of the following: mediastinum, heart, great vessels, trachea, esophagus, vertebral body, carina; or tumor with a malignant pleural or pericardial effusion[a], or with satellite tumor nodule(s) within the ipsilateral primary-tumor lobe of the lung.

LYMPH NODE (N) INVOLVEMENT DESCRIPTOR

NX	Regional lymph nodes cannot be assessed
N0	No regional lymph node metastasis
N1	Metastasis to ipsilateral peribronchial and/or ipsilateral hilar lymph nodes, and intrapulmonary nodes involved by direct extension of the primary tumor
N2	Metastasis to ipsilateral mediastinal and/or subcarinal lymph nodes(s)
N3	Metastasis to contralateral mediastinal, contralateral hilar, ipsilateral or contralateral scalene, or supraclavicular lymph node(s)

DISTANT METASTASIS (M) DESCRIPTOR

MX	Presence of distant metastasis cannot be assessed
M0	No distant metastasis
M1	Distant metastasis present[b]

[a] Most pleural effusions associated with lung cancer are due to tumor. However, in a few patients with multiple negative cytopathologic exams of a non-bloody, non-exudative pleural or pericardial effusion that clinical judgment dictates is not related to the tumor, the effusion should be excluded as a staging element and the patient's disease staged as T1, T2, or T3.

[b] Separate metastatic pulmonary tumor nodule(s) in the ipsilateral nonprimary tumor lobe(s) of the lung are classified as M1.

SOURCE: Adapted from CF Mountain. Regional lymph node classification for lung cancer staging taken from CF Mountain and C Dresler: Chest 111:1718, 1997.

metastatic disease (stage IV disease), and one-third have local or regional disease that may or may not be amenable to a curative attempt (some patients with stage IIIA disease and others with stage IIIB disease) (see below). This staging system provides useful prognostic information.

Small Cell Lung Cancer   A simple two-stage system is used. In this system, limited-stage disease (seen in about 30% of all patients with small cell lung cancer) is defined as disease confined to one hemithorax and regional lymph nodes (including mediastinal, contralateral hilar, and usually ipsilateral supraclavicular nodes), while extensive-stage disease (seen in about 70% of patients) is defined as disease exceeding those boundaries. Clinical studies such as physical examination, x-rays, CT and bone scans, and bone marrow examination are used in staging. In part, the definition of limited-stage disease relates to whether the known tumor can be encompassed within a tolerable radiation therapy port. Thus, contralateral supraclavicular nodes, recurrent laryngeal nerve involvement, and superior vena caval obstruction can all be part of limited-stage disease. However, cardiac tamponade, malignant pleural effusion, and bilateral pulmonary parenchymal involvement generally qualify disease as extensive-stage because the organs within a curative radiation therapy port cannot safely tolerate curative radiation doses.

GENERAL STAGING PROCEDURES (See Table 88-4) All patients with lung cancer should have a complete history and physical examination, with evaluation of all other medical problems, determination of performance status and history of weight loss, and a CT scan of the chest and abdomen with contrast. Positron emission tomography (PET) scans are sensitive in detecting metastatic disease. While not done in every patient, fiberoptic bronchoscopy provides material for pathologic examination, information on tumor size, location, degree of bronchial obstruction (i.e., assesses resectability), and recurrence.

Chest radiographs and CT scans are needed to evaluate tumor size and nodal involvement; old radiographs are useful for comparison. CT scans are of use in the preoperative staging of non-small cell lung cancer to detect mediastinal nodes and pleural extension and occult abdominal disease (e.g., of the liver and adrenal glands), as well as in the planning of curative radiation therapy to allow the design of fields to encompass all the known tumor while avoiding as much normal tissue as possible. However, mediastinal nodal involvement should be documented histologically if the findings will influence therapeutic decisions. Thus, sampling of lymph nodes via mediastinoscopy or thoracotomy to establish the presence or absence of N2 or N3 nodal involvement is crucial in considering a curative surgical approach for patients with non-small cell lung cancer with clinical stage I, II, or III disease. Likewise, unless the CT-detected abnormalities are unequivocal, histology of suspicious abdominal lesions should be confirmed by procedures such as fine-needle aspiration if the patient would otherwise be considered for curative treatment. In small cell lung cancer, CT scans are used in the planning of chest radiation treatment and in the assessment of the response to chemotherapy and radiation therapy. Surgery or radiotherapy can make interpretation of conventional chest x-rays difficult; after treatment, CT scans can provide good evidence of tumor recurrence.

If signs or symptoms suggest involvement by tumor, brain CT or bone scans are performed, as well as radiography of any suspicious bony lesions. Any accessible lesions suspicious for cancer should be biopsied if a histologic diagnosis would influence treatment.

In patients presenting with a mass lesion on chest x-ray or CT scan and no obvious contraindications to a curative approach after the initial evaluation, the mediastinum must be investigated. Approaches vary among centers and include performing chest CT scan and mediastinoscopy (for right-sided tumors) or lateral mediastinotomy (for left-sided lesions) on all patients and proceeding directly to thoracotomy for staging of the mediastinum. In patients presenting with disease that is confined to the chest but not resectable, and who thus are candidates

Table 88-4   Pretreatment Staging Procedures for Patients with Lung Cancer

All Patients
Complete history and physical examination
   Determination of performance status and weight loss
Complete blood count with platelet determination
Measurement of serum electrolytes, glucose, calcium, and phosphorus; renal and liver function tests
Electrocardiogram
Skin test for tuberculosis
Chest x-ray
CT scan of chest and abdomen
CT scan of brain and radionuclide scan of bone if any finding suggests the presence of tumor metastasis in these organs
X-rays of suspicious bony lesions detected by scan or symptom
Barium-swallow radiographic examination if esophageal symptoms exist
Pulmonary function studies and arterial blood gas measurements if signs or symptoms of respiratory insufficiency are present
Biopsy of accessible lesions suspicious for cancer if a histologic diagnosis is not yet made or if treatment or staging decisions would be based on whether or not a lesion contained cancer

Patients with non-small cell lung cancer who have no contraindication to curative surgery or radiotherapy with or without chemotherapy[a]
All the above procedures, plus the following:
   Fiberoptic bronchoscopy with washings, brushings, and biopsy of suspicious areas
   Pulmonary function tests and arterial blood gas measurements
   Coagulation tests
   CT scan of brain
   If surgical resection is planned: surgical evaluation of the mediastinum at mediastinoscopy or at thoracotomy
   If the patient is a poor surgical risk or a candidate for curative radiotherapy: transthoracic fine-needle aspiration biopsy or transbronchial forceps biopsy of peripheral lesions if material from routine fiberoptic bronchoscopy is negative

Patients presenting with small cell or advanced non-small cell lung cancer
For proven small cell lung cancer, all the procedures under "All Patients," plus the following:
   Fiberoptic bronchoscopy with washings and biopsy
   CT scan of brain
   Bone marrow aspiration and biopsy (if peripheral blood counts abnormal)
For non-small cell lung cancer or cancer of unknown histology, all the procedures under "All Patients," plus the following:
   Fiberoptic bronchoscopy if indicated by hemoptysis, obstruction, pneumonitis, or no histologic diagnosis of cancer
   Biopsy of accessible lesions suspicious for tumor to obtain a histologic diagnosis or if therapy would be altered by finding of tumor
   Transthoracic fine-needle aspiration biopsy or transbronchial forceps biopsy of peripheral lesions if fiberoptic bronchoscopy is negative and no other material exists for a histologic diagnosis
   Diagnostic and therapeutic thoracentesis if a pleural effusion is present

[a] Patients with non-small cell lung cancer and extrathoracic metastatic disease, malignant pleural effusion, or intrathoracic disease beyond the bounds of a tolerable radiotherapy port.

for neoadjuvant chemotherapy plus surgery or for curative radiotherapy with or without chemotherapy, other tests are done as indicated to evaluate specific symptoms. In patients presenting with non-small cell cancer that is not curable, all the general staging procedures are done, plus fiberoptic bronchoscopy as indicated to evaluate hemoptysis, obstruction, or pneumonitis, as well as thoracentesis with cytologic examination (and chest tube drainage as indicated) if fluid is present. As a rule, a radiographic finding of an isolated lesion (such as an enlarged adrenal gland) should be confirmed as cancer by fine-needle aspiration before a curative attempt is rejected.

STAGING OF SMALL CELL LUNG CANCER   Pretreatment staging for patients with small cell lung cancer includes the initial general lung cancer evaluation with chest and abdominal CT scans (because of the high frequency of hepatic and adrenal involvement) as well as fiberoptic bronchoscopy with washings and biopsies to determine the tumor extent before therapy; brain CT scan (10% of patients have metastases); bone marrow biopsy and aspiration (20 to 30% of patients have tumor in the bone marrow); and radionuclide scans (bone) if symptoms or other findings suggest disease involvement in these areas. Chest and abdominal CT scans are very useful to evaluate and follow tumor response to therapy, and chest CT scans are helpful in planning chest radiotherapy ports.

If signs or symptoms of spinal cord compression or leptomeningitis develop at any time in lung cancer patients with disease of any histologic type, a spinal CT scan or magnetic resonance imaging (MRI) scan and examination of the cerebrospinal fluid cytology are performed. If malignant cells are detected, radiation therapy to the site of compression and intrathecal chemotherapy (usually with methotrexate) are given. In addition, a brain CT or MRI scan is performed to search for brain metastases, which often are associated with spinal cord or leptomeningeal metastases.

DETERMINATION OF RESECTABILITY AND OPERABILITY In patients with non-small cell lung cancer, the following are major contraindications to curative surgery or radiotherapy alone: extrathoracic metastases; superior vena cava syndrome; vocal cord and, in most cases, phrenic nerve paralysis; malignant pleural effusion; cardiac tamponade; tumor within 2 cm of the carina (not curable by surgery but potentially curable by radiotherapy); metastasis to the contralateral lung; bilateral endobronchial tumor (potentially curable by radiotherapy); metastasis to the supraclavicular lymph nodes; contralateral mediastinal node metastases (potentially curable by radiotherapy); and involvement of the main pulmonary artery. Most patients with small cell lung cancer have unresectable disease; however, if clinical findings suggest the potential for resection (most common with peripheral lesions), that option should be considered.

PHYSIOLOGIC STAGING Patients with lung cancer often have cardiopulmonary and other problems related to chronic obstructive pulmonary disease as well as other medical problems. To improve their preoperative condition, correctable problems (e.g., anemia, electrolyte and fluid disorders, infections, and arrhythmias) should be addressed, smoking stopped, and appropriate chest therapy instituted. Since it is not always possible to predict whether a lobectomy or pneumonectomy will be required until the time of operation, a conservative approach is to restrict resectional surgery to patients who could potentially tolerate a pneumonectomy. In addition to nonambulatory performance status, a myocardial infarction within the past 3 months is a contraindication to thoracic surgery because 20% of patients will die of reinfarction, while an infarction in the past 6 months is a relative contraindication. Other major contraindications include uncontrolled major arrhythmias, a maximum breathing capacity <40% of the predicted value, an FEV_1 (forced expiratory volume in 1 s) <1 L, CO_2 retention (which is more serious than hypoxemia), and severe pulmonary hypertension. Recommending surgery when the FEV_1 is 1.1 to 2.4 L requires careful judgment, while an FEV_1 >2.5 L usually permits a pneumonectomy. In patients with borderline pulmonary status or a question of pulmonary hypertension, split pulmonary function testing by ventilation-perfusion lung scans can define physiologic operability. The activity from quantitative scans is summed for each lung in the anterior and posterior views, and the ratio of the normal to total lung activity is multiplied by the FEV_1. Pneumonectomy usually is physiologically tolerable if this predicted value is >1 L.

℞ **TREATMENT** The overall treatment approach to patients with lung cancer is shown in Table 88-5. Patients should be encouraged to stop smoking. Those who do fare better than those who continue to smoke.

Non-Small Cell Lung Cancer: Localized Disease • Surgery In patients with non-small cell lung cancer of stages IA, IB, IIA and IIB (Table 88-3) who can tolerate operation, the treatment of choice is pulmonary resection. In stage IIIA cases where the patient's age, cardiopulmonary function, and anatomy are favorable, resection also should be considered. If a complete resection is possible, the 5-year survival rate for N1 disease is about 50%, while it is about 20% for N2 disease. However, only 20% of cases of N2 disease are technically

Table 88-5 Summary of Treatment Approach to Patients with Lung Cancer

Non-small cell lung cancer
Stages IA, IB, IIA, IIB, and some IIIA:
  Surgical resection for stages IA, IB, IIA, and IIB
  Surgical resection with complete-mediastinal lymph node dissection and consideration of neoadjuvant CRx for stage IIIA disease with "minimal N2 involvement" (discovered at thoracotomy or mediastinoscopy)
  Postoperative RT for patients found to have N2 disease if no neoadjuvant CRx given
  Discussion of risks/benefits of adjuvant CRx with individual patients
  Curative potential RT for "nonoperable" patients
Stage IIIA with selected types of stage T3 tumors:
  Tumors with chest wall invasion (T3): en bloc resection of tumor with involved chest wall and consideration of postoperative RT
  Superior sulcus (Pancoast's) (T3) tumors: preoperative RT (30–45 Gy) followed by en bloc resection of involved lung and chest wall with consideration of postoperative RT or intraoperative brachytherapy
  Proximal airway involvement (<2 cm from carina) without mediastinal nodes: sleeve resection if possible preserving distal normal lung or pneumonectomy
Stages IIIA "advanced, bulky, clinically evident N2 disease" (discovered preoperatively) and IIIB disease that can be included in a tolerable RT port:
  Curative potential RT + CRx if performance status and general medical condition are reasonable; otherwise, RT alone
  Consider neoadjuvant CRx and surgical resection for IIIA disease with advanced N2 involvement
Stage IIIB disease with carinal invasion (T4) but without N2 involvement:
  Consider pneumonectomy with tracheal sleeve resection with direct reanastomosis to contralateral mainstem bronchus
Stage IV and more advanced IIIB disease:
  RT to symptomatic local sites
  CRx for ambulatory patients
  Chest tube drainage of large malignant pleural effusions
  Consider resection of primary tumor and metastasis for isolated brain or adrenal metastases

Small cell lung cancer
  Limited stage (good performance status): combination CRx + chest RT
  Extensive stage (good performance status): combination CRx
  Complete tumor responders (all stages): prophylactic cranial RT
  Poor-performance-status patients (all stages):
    Modified-dose combination CRx
    Palliative RT

All patients
  RT for brain metastases, spinal cord compression, weight-bearing lytic bony lesions, symptomatic local lesions (nerve paralyses, obstructed airway, hemoptysis in non-small cell lung cancer and in small cell cancer not responding to CRx)
  Appropriate diagnosis and treatment of other medical problems and supportive care during CRx
  Encouragement to stop smoking
  Entrance into clinical trial, if eligible

ABBREVIATIONS: CRx, chemotherapy; RT, radiotherapy.

resectable, and most of these are discovered to be N2 only at thoracotomy. Surgery for N2 disease is the most controversial area in the surgical management of lung cancer. Patients with N2 disease can be divided into "minimal" disease (involvement of only one node with microscopic foci, usually discovered at thoracotomy or mediastinoscopy) and the more common "advanced," bulky disease, clinically obvious on CT scans and discovered preoperatively. Patients with contralateral or bilateral positive mediastinal (N3) nodes, extracapsular nodal involvement, or fixed nodes are not considered candidates for resection. Approaches that may make resection possible include chest wall resection for direct extension of tumor, tracheal sleeve pneumonectomy, and sleeve lobectomy for lesions near the carina. Neoadjuvant (preoperative) chemotherapy has response rates of 50 to 60% and causes unresectable disease to become resectable in many patients who respond (see below). Video-assisted thoracic surgery (VATS) via thoracoscopy is not usually used for curative lung cancer resection but may be useful for peripheral lesions in patients with poor lung function.

The extent of resection is a matter of surgical judgment based on findings at exploration. Conservative resection that encompasses all known tumor gives survival equal to that obtained with more extensive procedures. However, lobectomy is superior to wedge resection in reducing the rate of local recurrence. Thus, lobectomy is preferred to pneumonectomy and wedge resection. Wedge resection and segmentectomy (potentially by VATS) are reserved for patients with poor pulmonary reserve and small peripheral lesions. About 43% of all patients with lung cancer undergo thoracotomy. Of these, 76% have a definitive resection, 12% are explored only for disease extent, and 12% have a palliative procedure with known disease left behind. About 30% of patients treated with resection for cure survive for 5 years, and 15% survive for 10 years (Table 88-3). The 30-day hospital mortality rate after pulmonary resection is 3% for lobectomy and 6% for pneumonectomy. Thus, most patients thought to have a "curative" resection ultimately die of metastatic disease (usually within 5 years of surgery).

Management of occult and stage 0 carcinomas   In the uncommon situation where malignant cells are identified in a sputum or bronchial washing specimen but the chest radiograph appears normal (TX tumor stage), the lesion must be localized. More than 90% can be localized by meticulous examination of the bronchial tree with a fiberoptic bronchoscope under general anesthesia and collection of a series of differential brushings and biopsies. Often, carcinoma in situ or multicentric lesions are found in these patients. Current recommendations are for the most conservative surgical resection, allowing removal of the cancer and conservation of lung parenchyma, even if the bronchial margins are positive for carcinoma in situ. The 5-year overall survival rate for these occult cancers is ~60%. Close follow-up of these patients is indicated because of the high incidence of second primary lung cancers (5% per patient per year). One approach to in situ or multicentric lesions uses systemically administered hematoporphyrin (which localizes to tumors and sensitizes them to light) followed by bronchoscopic phototherapy.

Solitary pulmonary nodule   When a patient presents with an asymptomatic, solitary pulmonary nodule (defined as an x-ray density completely surrounded by normal aerated lung, with circumscribed margins, of any shape, usually 1 to 6 cm in greatest diameter), a decision to resect or follow the nodule must be made. Approximately 35% of all such lesions in adults are malignant, most being primary lung cancer, while <1% are malignant in nonsmokers under 35 years of age. A complete history, including a smoking history, physical examination, routine laboratory tests, chest CT scan, fiberoptic bronchoscopy, and old chest x-rays are obtained. PET scans are useful in detecting lung cancers >1.5 cm in diameter. If no diagnosis is immediately apparent, the following risk factors would all argue strongly in favor of proceeding with resection to establish a histologic diagnosis: a history of cigarette smoking; age 35 years or older; a relatively large lesion; lack of calcification; chest symptoms; associated atelectasis, pneumonitis, or adenopathy; and growth of the lesion revealed by comparison with old x-rays. At present, only two radiographic criteria are reliable predictors of the benign nature of a solitary pulmonary nodule: lack of growth over a period >2 years and certain characteristic patterns of calcification. Calcification alone does not exclude malignancy. However, a dense central nidus, multiple punctate foci, and "bull's eye" (granuloma) and "popcorn ball" (hamartoma) calcifications are all highly suggestive of a benign lesion.

When old x-rays are not available and the characteristic calcification patterns are absent, the following approach is reasonable: Nonsmoking patients younger than 35 years can be followed with serial CT every 3 months for 1 year and then yearly. If any significant growth is found, a histologic diagnosis is needed. For patients older than 35 years and all patients with a smoking history, a histologic diagnosis must be made. The sample for histologic diagnosis can be obtained either at the time of nodule resection or, if the patient is a poor oper-

ative risk, via VATS or transthoracic fine-needle biopsy. Some institutions use preoperative fine-needle aspiration on all such lesions; however, all positive lesions have to be resected, and negative cytologic findings in most cases have to be confirmed by histology on a resected specimen. While much has been made of sparing patients an operation, the high probability of finding a malignancy (particularly in smokers older than 35 years) and the excellent chance for surgical cure when the tumor is small both suggest an aggressive approach to these lesions.

The application of low-dose spiral CT scanning to high-risk populations is under investigation. The test identifies a large number of asymptomatic pulmonary nodules that require evaluation. Approximately 23% of screened high-risk patients have an abnormality, and ~12% of the detected abnormalities are lung cancer. Criteria for distinguishing cancers from nonmalignant lesions short of a lobectomy are being developed. Lesions >1 cm are usually resected; those ≤1 cm are followed for change at 3-month intervals. Although a number of early lung cancers are detected in this way, it is not yet clear that survival is improved.

Radiotherapy with curative intent   Patients with stage III disease, as well as patients with stage I or II disease who refuse surgery or are not candidates for pulmonary resection, should be considered for radiation therapy with curative intent. The decision to administer high-dose radiotherapy is based on the extent of disease and the volume of the chest that requires irradiation. Patients with distant metastases, malignant pleural effusion, or cardiac involvement are generally not considered for curative radiation treatment. The median survival period for patients with unresectable non-small cell lung cancer localized to the chest who undergo primary radiotherapy with curative intent is <1 year. However, 6% of these patients are alive at 5 years and are cured by radiotherapy alone. In addition to being potentially curative, radiotherapy, by controlling the primary tumor, may increase the quality and length of life of noncured patients. Treatment usually involves midplane doses of 55 to 60 Gy, and the major concern is the amount of lung parenchyma and other organs in the thorax included in the treatment plan, including the spinal cord, heart, and esophagus. In patients with a major degree of underlying pulmonary disease, the treatment plan may have to be compromised because of the deleterious effect of radiation on pulmonary function. The risk of radiation pneumonitis is proportional to the radiation dose and the volume of lung in the field. The full clinical syndrome (dyspnea, fever, and radiographic infiltrate corresponding to the treatment port) occurs in 5% of cases. Acute radiation esophagitis occurs during treatment but usually is self-limited, while spinal cord injury should be avoided by careful treatment planning. Continuous hyperfractionated accelerated radiation therapy (CHART) involves delivery of 36 treatments of 1.5 Gy given 3 times a day for 12 consecutive days to a total dose of 54 Gy. The 2-year survival rate increased from 20 to 29% with CHART, although more esophagitis occurred. Brachytherapy (local radiotherapy delivered by placing radioactive "seeds" in a catheter in the tumor bed) provides a way to give a high local dose while sparing surrounding normal tissue.

Combined-modality therapy with curative intent   After apparently complete resection, adjuvant radiation therapy has not been shown to improve survival. Meta-analysis of studies with post-operative radiation therapy found it to be deleterious to survival in patients with stage I and II disease.

Carcinomas of the superior pulmonary sulcus producing *Pancoast's syndrome* are usually treated with combined radiotherapy and surgery. Patients with these carcinomas should have the usual preoperative staging procedures, including mediastinoscopy and CT scans to determine tumor extent and a neurologic examination (and sometimes nerve conduction studies) to document neurologic findings. Sometimes a histologic diagnosis is not made, but the combination of tumor location and pain distribution permit a diagnostic accuracy for cancer of >90%. If mediastinoscopy is negative, two curative approaches may be used in treating a Pancoast's syndrome tumor. Preoperative irradiation [30 Gy in 10 treatments] is given to the area, followed by an en bloc resection of the tumor and involved chest wall 3 to 6 weeks later. The 3 year survival rate is 42% for epidermoid and 21% for adeno- and large cell carcinomas. The second approach involves radiotherapy alone in curative doses and standard fractionation, which leads to survival rates similar to those from combined-modality therapy.

A meta-analysis of chemotherapy in non-small cell lung cancer used updated data on 9387 individual patients from 52 randomized trials, both published and unpublished, with the main outcome measure being survival. Regimens containing cisplatin were significantly more effective than no treatment. Trials in early-stage disease comparing surgery with surgery plus chemotherapy gave a hazard ratio of 0.87 (13% reduction in risk of death at 5 years) in favor of chemotherapy. Confidence intervals of these data are wide. However, adjuvant chemotherapy is, in general, not considered standard treatment.

The most impressive benefits were obtained when chemotherapy was added to radiotherapy for locally advanced disease (stage IIIB and some stage IIIA disease) and when chemotherapy was given preoperatively in a neoadjuvant fashion in stage IIIA disease. Preoperative neoadjuvant chemotherapy is widely used for stage IIIA disease. Preoperative combined modality therapy followed by surgical resection has given promising early results. Whether the surgery adds benefit after chemoradiotherapy has not been defined. Provided the risk/benefit ratio of using chemotherapy is discussed appropriately with patients, such therapy can be given in a noninvestigational setting. For stage IIIA disease, resection followed by postoperative radiation plus chemotherapy for N2 disease, neoadjuvant chemotherapy followed by surgical resection, or neoadjuvant chemoradiotherapy followed by resection are options. For stage IIIB and bulky IIIA disease, neoadjuvant chemotherapy (2 or 3 cycles of a cisplatin-based combination) followed by chest radiation therapy (60 Gy) has improved median survival time from 10 to 14 months and the 5-year survival rate from 7 to 17% compared to results with radiation therapy alone. Administration of radiation and chemotherapy concurrently is being tested; myelotoxicity and esophagitis are increased, but survival improvement is not yet proven. Randomized clinical trials also are needed to evaluate the usefulness of the new agents with activity against non-small cell lung cancer, including the taxanes (paclitaxel and docetaxel), vinorelbine, gemcitabine, and camptothecins (topotecan and CPT-11) in both adjuvant and neoadjuvant settings.

Disseminated Non-Small Cell Lung Cancer The 70% of patients who have unresectable non-small cell cancer have a poor prognosis. Patients with performance status scores of 0 (asymptomatic), 1 (symptomatic, fully ambulatory), 2 (in bed <50% of the time), 3 (in bed >50% of the time), and 4 (bedridden) have median survival times of 34, 25, 17, 8, and 4 weeks, respectively. Standard medical management, the judicious use of pain medications, the appropriate use of radiotherapy, and outpatient chemotherapy form the cornerstone of management. Patients whose primary tumor is causing symptoms such as bronchial obstruction with pneumonitis, hemoptysis, or upper airway or superior vena cava obstruction should have radiotherapy to the primary tumor. The case for prophylactic treatment of the asymptomatic patient is to prevent major symptoms from occurring in the thorax. However, if the patient can be followed closely, it may be appropriate to defer treatment until symptoms develop. Usually a course of 30 to 40 Gy over 2 to 4 weeks is given to the tumor. Radiation therapy provides relief of intrathoracic symptoms with the following frequencies: hemoptysis, 84%; superior vena cava syndrome, 80%; dyspnea, 60%; cough, 60%; atelectasis, 23%; and vocal cord paralysis, 6%. Cardiac tamponade (treated with pericardiocentesis and radiation therapy to the heart), painful bony metastases (with relief in 66%), brain or spinal cord compression, and brachial plexus involvement may also be palliated with radiotherapy. Usually, with brain metastases and cord compression, dexamethasone (25 to 100 mg/d in four divided doses) is also given and then rapidly tapered to the lowest dosage that relieves symptoms.

Brain metastases often are isolated instances of relapse in patients with adenocarcinoma of the lung otherwise controlled by surgery or

radiotherapy. However, there is no proven value for prophylactic cranial irradiation or for CT scans of the head in asymptomatic patients.

Pleural effusions are common and are usually treated with thoracentesis. If they recur and are symptomatic, chest tube drainage with a sclerosing agent such as intrapleural talc is used. First, the chest cavity is completely drained. Xylocaine 1% is instilled (15 mL), followed by 50 mL normal saline. Then, 10 g sterile talc is dissolved in 100 mL normal saline, and this solution is injected through the chest tube. The chest tube is clamped for 4 h if tolerated, and the patient is rotated onto different sides to distribute the sclerosing agent. The chest tube is removed 24 to 48 h later, after drainage has become slight (usually <100 mL/24 h). VATS has been used to drain and treat large malignant effusions. Symptomatic endobronchial lesions that recur after surgery or radiotherapy or that develop in patients with severely compromised pulmonary function are difficult to treat with conventional therapy. Neodynium-YAG (yttrium-aluminum-garnet) laser therapy administered through a flexible fiberoptic bronchoscope (usually under general anesthesia) can provide palliation in 80 to 90% of patients even when the tumor has relapsed after radiotherapy. Local radiotherapy delivered by brachytherapy, photodynamic therapy using a photosensitizing agent, and endobronchial stents are other measures that can relieve airway obstruction from tumor.

Chemotherapy The use of chemotherapy for non-small cell lung cancer requires careful judgment to balance potential benefits and toxicity. Modest survival benefits (of 1 to 2 months), symptom palliation, and improved quality of life may accrue from combination chemotherapy. Randomized trials in advanced disease comparing supportive care with supportive care plus chemotherapy gave a hazard ratio of 0.73 (27% reduction in risk of death at 1 year) in favor of including chemotherapy. Economic analysis has found chemotherapy to be cost-effective palliation. Combination chemotherapy produces an objective tumor response in ~30 to 40% of patients; the response is complete in <5%. Median survival for chemotherapy-treated patients is 9 to 10 months, and the 1-year survival rate is 40%. Thus, in patients with non-small cell lung cancer who desire chemotherapy, it is reasonable to give chemotherapy if the patient is ambulatory, has not received prior chemotherapy, and is able to understand and accept the risk/benefit ratio from such therapy. The chemotherapy should be one of the published standard regimens, such as paclitaxel plus carboplatin, paclitaxel plus cisplatin, or vinorelbine plus cisplatin. Improved antiemetics have made treatment tolerable on an outpatient basis. New drugs with proven activity in non-small cell lung cancer include docetaxel, irinotecan, and gemcitabine. All eligible patients should be encouraged to enter clinical studies that are designed to determine the benefits and toxicities of these new treatments.

Small Cell Lung Cancer Untreated patients with small cell lung cancer have a median survival period of 6 to 17 weeks, while patients treated with combination chemotherapy have a median survival period of 40 to 70 weeks. Thus, chemotherapy with or without radiotherapy or surgery can prolong survival in patients with small cell lung cancer. The goal of treatment is to achieve a complete clinical regression of tumor documented by repeating the initial positive staging procedures, particularly fiberoptic bronchoscopy with washings and biopsy. The initial response, determined 6 to 12 weeks after the start of therapy, predicts both the median and long-term survivals and the potential for cure. Patients who achieve a complete clinical regression survive longer than patients with only partial regression, who in turn survive longer than patients with no response. Complete response is required for long-term (>3-year) survival.

After initial staging, patients are classified as having limited or extensive disease and as being physiologically able or not able to tolerate combination chemotherapy or chemoradiotherapy. The overall mortality rate from initial combination chemotherapy even in these selected patients is 1 to 5%, comparable with the operative mortality rate for pulmonary resection. Such therapy should be reserved for ambulatory patients with no prior chemotherapy or radiotherapy; no other major medical problems; and adequate heart, liver, renal, and bone marrow function. The arterial P_{O_2} on room air should be >6.6 kPa (50 mmHg), and there should be no CO_2 retention. For patients with limitations in any of these areas, the initial combined-modality therapy or chemotherapy must be modified to prevent undue toxicity. In all patients, these treatments must be coupled with supportive care for infectious, hemorrhagic, and other medical complications.

Chemotherapy The combination most widely used is etoposide plus cisplatin or carboplatin, given every 3 weeks on an outpatient basis for 4 to 6 cycles. Another active regimen is etopside, cisplatin, and paclitaxel. Increased dose intensity of chemotherapy adds toxicity without clear survival benefit. Appropriate supportive care (antiemetic therapy, administration of fluid and saline boluses with cisplatin, monitoring of blood counts and blood chemistries, monitoring for signs of bleeding or infection, and, as required, administration of erythropoietin and granulocyte colony-stimulating factor) and adjustment of chemotherapy doses on the basis of nadir granulocyte counts are essential. The initial combination chemotherapy may result in moderate to severe granulocytopenia (e.g., granulocyte counts <500 to 1500/μL) and thrombocytopenia (platelet counts <50,000 to 100,000/μL). After the initial 4 to 6 cycles of therapy, patients should be restaged to determine if they have entered a complete clinical remission, indicated by complete disappearance of all clinically evident lesions and paraneoplastic syndromes, or a partial remission, or have no response or tumor progression (seen in 10 to 20% of patients). Chemotherapy is then stopped in responding patients. More prolonged chemotherapy has not been shown to be of value. Patients whose tumors are progressing or not responding should be switched to a new, experimental chemotherapy regimen. Oral etoposide, as a single agent, has been shown to be of clinical benefit in the initial treatment of patients who are elderly or have a very poor performance status.

Radiotherapy High-dose (40 Gy) radiotherapy to the whole brain should be given to patients with documented brain metastases. Prophylactic cranial irradiation (PCI) may be given to patients with complete responses, since it significantly decreases the development of brain metastases (which occur in 60 to 80% of patients living ≥2 years who do not receive PCI), but survival benefit is small (5%). Because some studies indicate possible deficits in cognitive ability that could be related to PCI, the long-term quality of life after PCI needs to be further studied. The patient needs to be informed of the risks and benefits. In the case of symptomatic, progressive lesions in the chest or at other critical sites, if radiotherapy has not yet been given to these areas, it may be administered in full doses (e.g., 40 Gy to the chest tumor mass).

Combined-modality therapy Most patients with limited-stage small cell lung cancer should receive combined-modality therapy with etoposide plus cisplatin (or other platinum-containing regimen) and concurrent chest radiotherapy. Acute and chronic toxicities are expected with chemoradiotherapy, particularly when the chemotherapy and radiotherapy are given concurrently. However, the addition of chest radiation therapy to chemotherapy reduces the local failure rate and improves survival. Patients should be selected (limited-stage disease, a performance status of 0 to 1, and initial good pulmonary function) such that radiotherapy can be given in full doses and in a manner that does not sacrifice too much lung function. Some studies show twice-daily radiation fractions produce less toxicity and improve survival compared to once-daily treatments, but large randomized trials are still needed.

For extensive-stage disease, initial chest radiotherapy usually is not advocated. However, for favorable patients (e.g., those with a performance status of 0 to 1, good pulmonary function, and only one site of extensive disease), the addition of chest radiotherapy to chemotherapy can be considered. For all patients, if chemotherapy is inadequate to relieve local tumor symptoms, a course of radiotherapy can be added.

About 20 to 30% of patients with limited-stage disease and 1 to 5% of patients with extensive-stage disease are cured. About 50% of patients with limited-stage and 30% of patients with extensive-stage disease enter complete remission, and 90 to 95% of all patients have complete or partial responses. These responses increase the median survival period to 10 to 12 months for patients with extensive-stage disease and to 14 to 18 months for patients with limited-stage disease, as compared with 2 to 4 months for untreated patients. In addition, most patients have relief of their tumor-related symptoms and improvement of performance status. However, the maintenance of good performance status in a patient receiving outpatient chemotherapy requires judgment and skill to avoid undue therapeutic toxicity. New treatments, such as new drug combinations, very intensive initial or "reinduction" therapy with autologous bone marrow infusion, and novel ways of combining chemotherapy, radiotherapy, and surgery, should be given only in the context of an approved clinical protocol.

Although surgical resection is not routinely recommended for small cell lung cancer, occasional patients meet the usual requirements for resectability (stage I or II disease with negative mediastinal nodes). Moreover, this histologic diagnosis is made in some patients only on review of the resected surgical specimen. Such patients have been reported to have high cure rates (>25%) if adjuvant chemotherapy is used.

LUNG CANCER PREVENTION

Deterring children from taking up smoking is likely to be the most effective lung cancer prevention. Smoking cessation programs are successful in 5 to 20% of volunteers; the poor efficacy is because of the nature of nicotine addiction. Early diagnosis strategies have the problem of high false-positive rates, which add to the expense and the failure of such strategies to result in improved survival.

Chemoprevention may be an approach to reduce lung cancer risk. Patients with head and neck cancer, who are at increased risk of developing lung cancer, experienced a decrease in second cancers when given 13-cis retinoic acid. However, the drug causes significant toxicity, and its activity is not yet confirmed. Vitamin E and β-carotene supplements actually increase the risk of lung cancer. Thus, currently no strategy for chemoprevention of lung cancer has been proven effective.

BENIGN LUNG NEOPLASMS

The benign neoplasms of the lung, representing <5% of all primary tumors, include bronchial adenomas and hamartomas (90% of such lesions) and a group of very uncommon neoplasms (chondromas, fibromas, lipomas, hemangiomas, leiomyomas, teratomas, pseudolymphomas, and endometriosis). The diagnostic and primary-treatment approach is basically the same for all these neoplasms. They can present as central masses causing airway obstruction, cough, hemoptysis, and pneumonitis. The masses may or may not be visible on radiographs but usually are accessible to fiberoptic bronchoscopy. Alternatively, they can present without symptoms as solitary pulmonary nodules and thus will be evaluated as part of a solitary pulmonary nodule workup. In all cases, the extent of surgery must be determined at operation, and a conservative procedure with appropriate reconstructions is usually performed.

BRONCHIAL ADENOMAS Bronchial adenomas (80% are central) are slow-growing, endobronchial lesions; they represent 50% of all benign pulmonary neoplasms. About 80 to 90% are carcinoids, 10 to 15% are adenocystic tumors (or cylindromas), and 2 to 3% are mucoepidermoid tumors. Adenomas present in patients 15 to 60 years old (average age, 45) as endobronchial lesions and are often symptomatic for several years. Patients may have a chronic cough, recurrent hemoptysis, or obstruction with atelectasis, lobar collapse, or pneumonitis and abscess formation. Bronchial carcinoids, which usually follow a benign course, and small cell lung cancers, which are highly malignant, both express a neuroendocrine phenotype similar to the Kulchitsky cell. This cell is part of the amine precursor uptake and decarboxylation (APUD) system. Carcinoids, like small cell lung cancers, may secrete other hormones, such as ACTH or arginine vasopressin, and can cause paraneoplastic syndromes that resolve on resection. In addition, bronchial carcinoid metastases (usually to the liver) may produce the carcinoid syndrome, with cutaneous flush, bronchoconstriction, diarrhea, and cardiac valvular lesions (Chap. 93), which small cell lung cancer does not. Occasionally, pathologists may have difficulty distinguishing carcinoids from small cell lung cancers. Carcinoid tumors that have an unusually aggressive histologic appearance (referred to as *atypical carcinoids*) metastasize in 70% of cases to regional nodes, liver, or bone, compared with only a 5% rate of metastasis for carcinoids with typical histology.

Bronchial adenomas of all types, because of their endobronchial and often central location, are usually visible by fiberoptic bronchoscopy; and tissue for histologic diagnosis is obtained in this manner. Because they are hypervascular, they can bleed profusely after bronchoscopic biopsy, and this problem should be anticipated. Bronchial adenomas must be dealt with as potentially malignant and thus require removal not only for symptom relief but also because they can be locally invasive or recurrent, potentially can metastasize, and may produce paraneoplastic syndromes. Surgical excision is the primary treatment for all types of bronchial adenomas. The extent of surgery is determined at operation and should be as conservative as possible. Often bronchotomy with local excision, sleeve resection, segmental resection, or lobectomy is sufficient. Five-year survival rates after surgical resection are 95%, decreasing to 70% if regional nodes are involved. The treatment of metastatic pulmonary carcinoids is unclear because they can either be indolent or behave more like small cell lung carcinoma. Assessment of the tempo and histology of the disease in the individual patient is necessary to determine if and when chemotherapy or radiotherapy is indicated.

HAMARTOMAS Pulmonary hamartomas have a peak incidence at age 60 and are more frequent in men than in women. Histologically, they contain normal pulmonary tissue components (smooth muscle and collagen) in a disorganized fashion. They are usually peripheral, clinically silent, and benign in their behavior. Unless the radiographic findings are pathognomonic for hamartoma, with "popcorn" calcification, the lesions usually have to be resected for diagnosis, particularly if the patient is a smoker. VATS may minimize the surgical complications.

METASTATIC PULMONARY TUMORS

The lung is a frequent site of metastases from primary cancers outside the lung. Usually such metastatic disease is considered incurable. However, two special situations should be borne in mind. The first is the development of a solitary pulmonary shadow on a chest x-ray in a patient known to have an extrathoracic neoplasm. This shadow may represent a metastasis or a new primary lung cancer. Because the natural history of lung cancer is often worse than that of other primary tumors, a single pulmonary nodule in a patient with a known extrathoracic tumor is approached as though the nodule is a primary lung cancer, particularly if the patient is older than 35 years and a smoker. If a vigorous search for other sites of active cancer proves negative, the nodule is surgically resected. Second, in some cases, multiple pulmonary nodules can be resected with curative intent. This tactic is usually recommended if, after careful staging, it is found that (1) the patient can tolerate the contemplated pulmonary resection, (2) the primary tumor has been definitively and successfully treated, and (3) all known metastatic disease can be encompassed by the projected pulmonary resection. The key is selection and screening of patients to exclude those with uncontrolled primary tumors and extrapulmonary metastases. Primary tumors whose pulmonary metastases have been successfully resected for cure include osteogenic and soft tissue sarcomas; colon, rectal, uterine, cervix, and corpus tumors; head and neck, breast, testis, and salivary gland cancer; melanoma; and bladder and kidney tumors. Five-year survival rates of 20 to 30% have been found in carefully selected patients, and dramatic results have been

achieved in patients with osteogenic sarcomas, where resection of pulmonary metastases (sometimes requiring several thoracotomies) is becoming a standard curative treatment approach.

BIBLIOGRAPHY

AUPERIN A et al: Prophylactic cranial irradiation for patients with small-cell lung cancer in complete remission. N Engl J Med 341:476, 1999

CHUTE J et al: Twenty years of phase III trials for patients with extensive-stage small-cell lung cancer: Perceptible progress. J Clin Oncol 17:1794, 1999

Clinical practice guidelines for the treatment of unresectable non-small-cell lung cancer. J Clin Oncol 15:2996, 1997

HECHT SS: Tobacco smoke carcinogens and lung cancer. J Natl Cancer Inst 91:1194, 1999

HENSCHKE CI et al: Early Lung Cancer Action Project: Overall design and findings from baseline screening. Lancet 354:99, 1999

MOUNTAIN CF: Revisions in the international system for staging lung cancer. Chest 111: 1710, 1997

TURRISI AT III et al: Twice-daily compared with once-daily thoracic radiotherapy in limited small-cell lung cancer treated concurrently with cisplatin and etoposide. N Engl J Med 340:265, 1999

WAGNER H JR: Postoperative adjuvant therapy for patients with resected non-small cell lung cancer: Still controversial after all these years. Chest 117(Suppl 1):110S, 2000

WINGO PA et al: Annual report to the nation on the status of cancer, 1973–1996, with a special section on lung cancer and tobacco smoking. J Natl Cancer Inst 91:675, 1999

89 *Marc E. Lippman*

BREAST CANCER

Breast cancer is a malignant proliferation of epithelial cells lining the ducts or lobules of the breast. In the year 2000, about 185,000 cases of invasive breast cancer and 42,000 deaths occurred in the United States. Mortality from breast cancer has begun to decrease. Epithelial malignancies of the breast are the most common cause of cancer in women (excluding skin cancer), accounting for about one-third of all cancer in women. This chapter will not consider rare malignancies of the breast, including sarcomas and lymphomas. Human breast cancer is a clonal disease; a single transformed cell—the end result of a series of somatic (acquired) or germline mutations—is able to express full malignant potential. Thus, breast cancer may exist for a long period as either a noninvasive disease or an invasive but nonmetastatic disease.

GENETIC CONSIDERATIONS Not more than 10% of human breast cancers can be linked directly to germline mutations. Several genes have been implicated in familial cases. The Li-Fraumeni syndrome is characterized by inherited mutations in the p53 tumor suppressor gene, which lead to an increased incidence of breast cancer, osteogenic sarcomas, and other malignancies.

Another putative tumor suppressor gene, *BRCA-1*, has been identified at the chromosomal locus 17q21; this gene encodes a zinc finger protein, and the product therefore may function as a transcriptional factor. The gene appears to be involved in gene repair. Women who inherit a mutated allele of this gene from either parent have an approximately 60 to 80% lifetime chance of developing breast cancer and about a 33% chance of developing ovarian cancer. Men who carry a mutant allele of the gene have an increased incidence of prostate cancer but usually not of breast cancer. A third gene, termed *BRCA-2*, which has been localized to chromosome 11, is associated with an increased incidence of breast cancer in men and women.

BRCA-1 and *BRCA-2* can now be sequenced readily and germline mutations detected; patients with these mutations can be counseled appropriately. All women with strong family histories for breast cancer should be referred to genetic screening programs whenever possible, particularly women of Ashkenazi Jewish descent who have a high likelihood of a specific *BRCA-1* mutation (deletion of adenine and guanine at position 185).

Even more important than the role these genes play in inherited forms of breast cancer may be their role in sporadic breast cancer. The p53 mutation is present in approximately 40% of human breast cancers as an acquired defect. Evidence for *BRCA-1* mutation in primary breast cancer has not been reported. However, decreased expression of *BRCA-1* mRNA and abnormal cellular location of the *BRCA-1* protein have been found in some breast cancers. Loss of heterozygosity of some genes suggests that tumor-suppressor activity may be inactivated in sporadic cases of human breast cancer. Finally, one dominant oncogene plays a role in about a quarter of human breast cancer cases. The product of this gene, a member of the epidermal growth factor receptor superfamily, is called *erbB2* (HER-2, neu) and is overexpressed in these breast cancers due to gene amplification; this overexpression can transform human breast epithelium. ■

EPIDEMIOLOGY Breast cancer is a hormone-dependent disease. Women without functioning ovaries who never receive estrogen replacement do not develop breast cancer. The female to male ratio is about 150 to 1. For most epithelial malignancies, a log-log plot of incidence versus age shows a straight-line increase with every year of life. A similar plot for breast cancer shows the same straight-line increase but with a decrease in slope beginning at the age of menopause. The three dates in a woman's life that have a major impact on breast cancer incidence are age at menarche, age at first full-term pregnancy, and age at menopause. Women who experience menarche at age 16 have only 50 to 60% of the breast cancer risk of a woman having menarche at age 12; the lower risk persists throughout life. Similarly, menopause occurring 10 years before the median age of menopause (52 years), whether natural or surgically induced, reduces lifetime breast cancer risk by about 35%. Women who have a first full-term pregnancy by age 18 have a reduced (30 to 40%) risk of breast cancer compared with nulliparous women. Thus, length of menstrual life—particularly the fraction occurring before first full-term pregnancy—is a substantial component of the total risk of breast cancer. This factor can account for 70 to 80% of the variation in breast cancer frequency in different countries.

International variation in incidence has provided some of the most important clues on hormonal carcinogenesis. A woman living to age 80 in North America has one chance in nine of developing invasive breast cancer. Asian women have one-fifth to one-tenth the risk of breast cancer of women in North America or Western Europe. Asian women have substantially lower concentrations of estrogens and progesterone. These differences cannot be explained on a genetic basis, because Asian women living in a western environment have sex steroid hormone concentrations and risk identical to that of their western counterparts. These women also differ markedly in height and weight from Asian women in Asia; height and weight are critical regulators of age of menarche and have substantial effects on plasma concentrations of estrogens.

The role of diet in breast cancer etiology is controversial. While there are associative links between total caloric and fat intake and breast cancer risk, the exact role of fat in the diet is unproven. However, there is a risk associated with moderate alcohol intake; the mechanism is unknown. Recommendations favoring abstinence from alcohol must be weighed against other social pressures and the possible cardioprotective effect of moderate alcohol intake.

The potential role of exogenous hormones in breast cancer is of extraordinary importance, because millions of American women regularly use oral contraceptives and postmenopausal hormone replacement therapy (HRT). The most credible meta-analyses of oral contraceptive use suggest that these agents cause little if any increased risk of breast cancer. By contrast, oral contraceptives offer a substantial protective effect against ovarian epithelial tumors and endometrial cancers. Far more controversial are the data surrounding HRT in hy-

pogonadal and/or menopausal women. First, HRT with estrogens alone, usually in the form of equine conjugated estrogens, provides less than the physiologic equivalent of premenopausal estrogens but is associated with an increased risk of endometrial cancer, a reduction in the symptoms of estrogen deprivation, a reduction in osteoporosis and resultant hip fractures, and a one-third reduction in deaths due to cardiovascular disease. Meta-analyses suggest a small increase in breast cancer incidence, particularly with high dosages and a long duration of treatment. For the average woman, the negative effect on the breast is probably outweighed by protective effects on bone and heart. Preliminary data suggest that there is a reduction in the risk of colon cancer as well.

The addition of progestogens to HRT regimens drastically reduces the risk of endometrial cancer. It is not clear whether the protective effects against cardiovascular and osteoporotic bone diseases are altered. However, progestogens are copromoters of breast cancer in model systems, and an increased risk of breast cancer is possible.

Whether a history of previous biopsy findings of atypical hyperplasia or in situ carcinoma or strong family histories of breast cancer alter the risk-to-benefit ratios for HRT is unknown. It is likely that the average woman benefits from HRT. The risks of HRT in patients with a positive family history and patients with a remote personal history of breast cancer are unknown.

In addition to the other factors, radiation may be a risk factor in younger women. Women who have been exposed before age 30 to radiation in the form of multiple fluoroscopies (200 to 300 cGy) or treatment for Hodgkin's disease (>3600 cGy) have a substantial increase in risk of breast cancer, whereas radiation exposure after age 30 appears to have a minimal carcinogenic effect on the breast.

EVALUATION OF BREAST MASSES IN MEN AND WOMEN Because the breasts are a common site of potentially fatal malignancy in women and because they frequently provide clues to underlying systemic diseases in both men and women, examination of the breast is an essential part of the physical examination. Unfortunately, internists frequently do not examine the breast in men, and, in women, they are apt to refer this evaluation to gynecologists. Because of the association between early detection and improved outcome, it is the duty of every physician to distinguish breast abnormalities at the earliest possible stage and to institute a definite diagnostic workup. It is for this reason that all women should be trained in self-examination of the breasts. Although breast cancer in men is unusual, unilateral lesions should be evaluated in the same manner as in women, with the recognition that gynecomastia in men can sometimes begin unilaterally and is often asymmetric. Nevertheless, about as many suspicious breast lesions are now detected by screening mammography as by physical examination.

Virtually all breast cancer is diagnosed by biopsy of a nodule detected either on a mammogram or by palpation. Algorithms have been developed to enhance the likelihood of diagnosing breast cancer and reduce the frequency of unnecessary biopsy.

The Palpable Breast Mass Women should be strongly encouraged to examine their breasts monthly. The minimum benefit of this practice is the greater likelihood of detecting a mass at a smaller size, when it can be treated with more limited surgery. Breast examination by the physician should be performed in good light so as to see retractions and other skin changes. The nipple and areolae should be inspected, and an attempt should be made to elicit nipple discharge. All regional lymph node groups should be examined, and any lesions should be measured. While lesions with certain features are more likely to be cancerous (hard, irregular, tethered or fixed, or painless lesions), physical examination alone cannot exclude malignancy. Furthermore, a negative mammogram in the presence of a persistent lump in the breast does not exclude malignancy.

In premenopausal women, lesions that are either equivocal or nonsuspicious on physical examination should be reexamined in 2 to 4 weeks, during the follicular phase of the menstrual cycle. Days 5 to 7 of the cycle are the best time for breast examination. A dominant mass in a postmenopausal woman or a dominant mass that persists through a menstrual cycle in a premenopausal woman should be aspirated by fine-needle biopsy or referred to a surgeon. If nonbloody fluid is aspirated and the lesion is thereby cured, the diagnosis (cyst) and therapy have been accomplished together. Solid lesions that are persistent, recurrent, complex or bloody cysts require mammography and biopsy, although in selected patients the so-called triple diagnostic techniques (palpation, mammography, aspiration) can be used to avoid biopsy (Figs. 89-1 to 89-3). Ultrasound can be used in place of fine-needle aspiration to distinguish cysts from solid lesions. Not all solid masses are detected by ultrasound; thus, a palpable mass that is not visualized on ultrasound must be presumed to be solid.

Several points are essential in pursuing these management decision trees. First, risk factor analysis is not part of the decision structure. Second, fine-needle aspiration should be used only in centers that have proven skill in obtaining such specimens and analyzing them. Although the likelihood of cancer is low in the setting of a "triple negative" (benign-feeling lump, negative mammogram, and negative fine-needle aspiration), it is not zero, and the patient and physician must be aware of about a 1% risk of false negativity. Third, additional technologies such as magnetic resonance imaging, ultrasound, and sestamibi imaging cannot be used to exclude the need for biopsy, although in unusual circumstances they may provoke a biopsy.

The Abnormal Mammogram Screening mammography has reduced the lethality of breast cancer by promoting detection at an earlier stage. The procedure is justified on an annual basis for women over age 40.

Screening mammography should not be confused with diagnostic mammography, which is performed after a palpable abnormality has been detected. Diagnostic mammography is aimed at evaluating the rest of the breast before biopsy is performed, or occasionally is part of the triple test strategy to exclude immediate biopsy.

Subtle abnormalities that are first detected by screening mammography should be evaluated carefully by compression or magnified views. These abnormalities include clustered microcalcifications, densities (especially if spiculated), and new or enlarging architectural distortion. For some nonpalpable lesions ultrasound may be helpful either to identify cysts or to guide biopsy. If there is no palpable lesion and detailed mammographic studies are unequivocally benign, the patient should have routine follow-up appropriate to the patient's age.

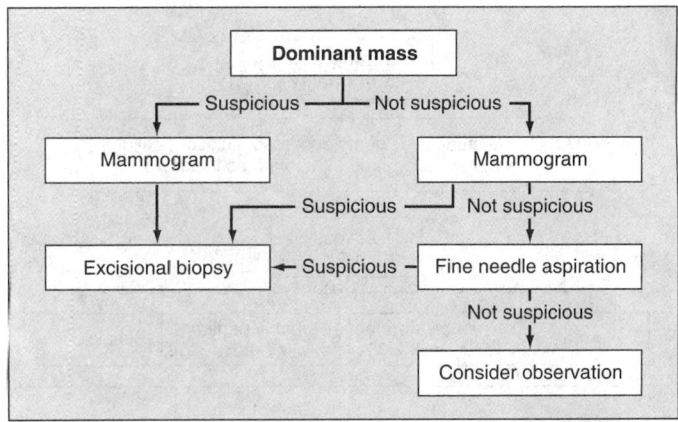

FIGURE 89-2 The "triple diagnosis" technique.

If a nonpalpable mammographic lesion has a low index of suspicion, mammographic follow-up in 3 to 6 months is reasonable. Workup of indeterminate and suspicious lesions has been rendered more complex by the advent of stereotactic biopsies. Morrow and colleagues have suggested that these procedures are indicated for lesions that require biopsy but are likely to be benign—that is, for cases in which the procedure probably will eliminate additional surgery. When a lesion is more probably malignant, open excisional biopsy should be performed with a needle localization technique. Others have proposed more widespread use of stereotactic core biopsies for nonpalpable lesions, on economic grounds and because diagnosis leads to earlier treatment planning. However, stereotactic diagnosis of a malignant lesion does not eliminate the need for definitive surgical procedures, particularly if breast conservation is attempted. For example after a breast biopsy with needle localization (i.e., local excision) of a stereotactically diagnosed malignancy, reexcision may still be necessary to achieve negative margins. To some extent, these issues are decided on the basis of referral pattern and the availability of the resources for stereotactic core biopsies. A reasonable approach is shown in Fig. 89-4.

Breast Masses in the Pregnant or Lactating Woman During pregnancy, the breast grows under the influence of estrogen, progesterone, prolactin, and human placental lactogen. Lactation is suppressed by progesterone, which blocks the effects of prolactin. After

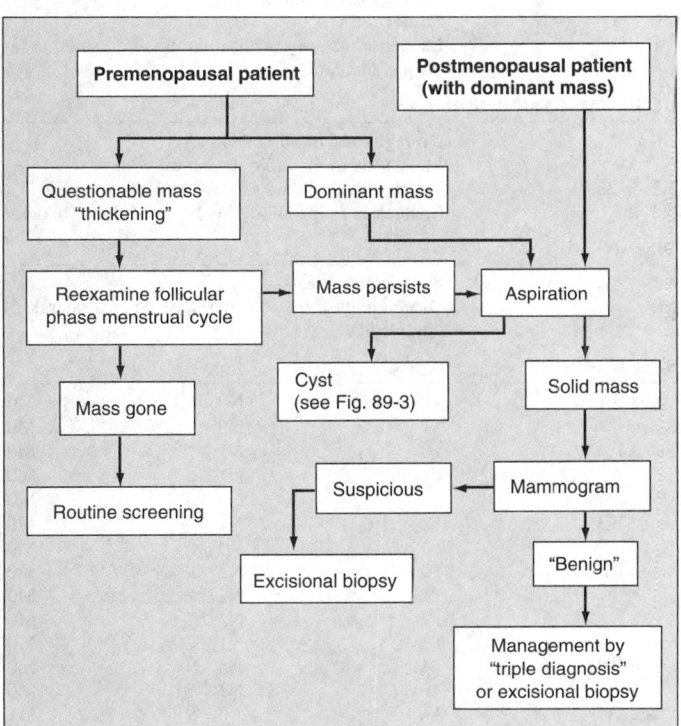

FIGURE 89-1 Approach to a palpable breast mass.

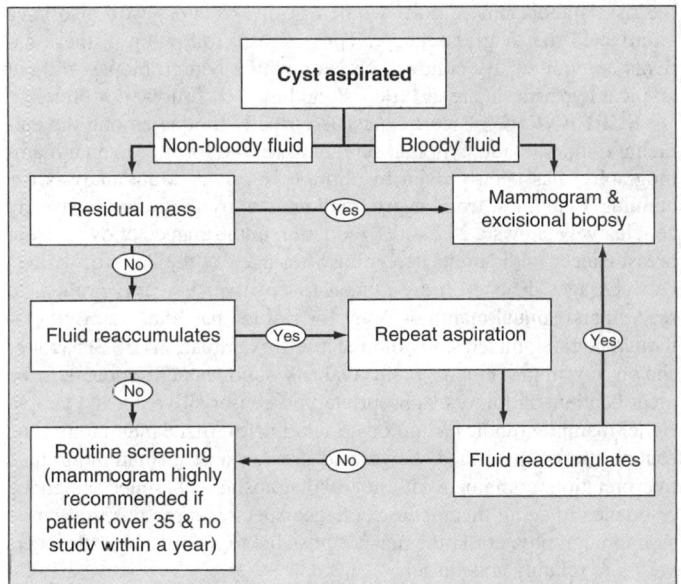

FIGURE 89-3 Management of a breast cyst.

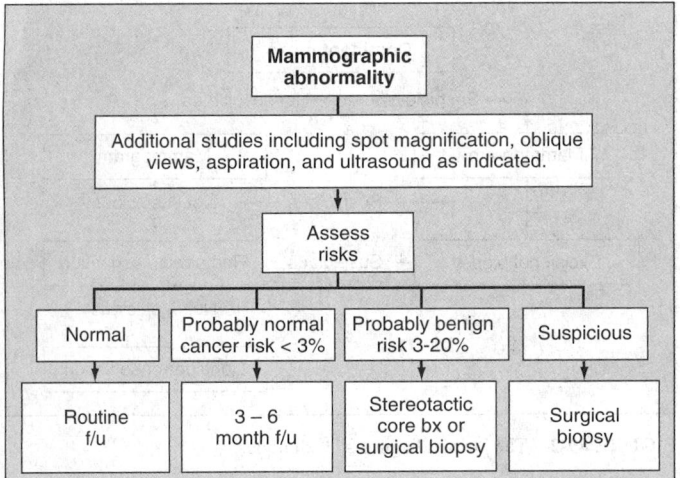

FIGURE 89-4 Approaches to abnormalities detected by mammogram. Note: f/u, follow-up.

delivery, lactation is promoted by the fall in progesterone levels, which leaves the effects of prolactin unopposed. The development of a dominant mass during pregnancy or lactation should never be attributed to hormonal changes, and biopsy should never be performed under local anesthesia. Breast cancer develops in 1 in every 3000 to 4000 pregnancies. Stage for stage, breast cancer in pregnant patients is no different from premenopausal breast cancer in nonpregnant patients. However, pregnant women often have more advanced disease because a breast mass was ignored.

Benign Breast Masses   Only about 1 in every 5 to 10 breast biopsies leads to a diagnosis of cancer, although the rate of positive biopsies varies in different countries. (These differences may be related to interpretation and availability of mammograms.) The vast majority of benign breast masses are due to "fibrocystic" disease, a descriptive term for small fluid-filled cysts and modest epithelial cell and fibrous tissues hyperplasia. However, fibrocystic disease is a histologic, not a clinical, diagnosis, and women who have had a biopsy with benign findings are at greater risk of developing breast cancer than those who have not had a biopsy. The subset of women with ductal or lobular cell proliferation (about 30% of patients), particularly the small fraction (3%) with atypical hyperplasia, have a fourfold greater risk of developing breast cancer than unbiopsied women, and the increase in the risk is about ninefold for women in this category who also have an affected first-degree relative. Thus, careful follow-up of these patients is required. By contrast, patients with a benign biopsy without atypical hyperplasia are at little risk and may be followed routinely.

SCREENING   Breast cancer is virtually unique among the epithelial tumors in adults in that screening (in the form of annual mammography) has been proven to improve survival. Meta-analysis examining outcomes from every randomized trial of mammography conclusively shows a 25 to 30% reduction in the chance of dying from breast cancer with annual screening after age 50; the data for women between ages 40 and 50 are almost as positive. It seems prudent to recommend annual mammography for women past the age of 40. Although no randomized study of breast self-examination (BSE) has ever shown any improvement in survival, its major benefit appears to be identification of tumors appropriate for conservative local therapy. Better mammographic technology, including digitized mammography, routine use of magnified views, and greater skill in mammographic interpretation, combined with newer diagnostic techniques (magnetic resonance imaging, magnetic resonance spectroscopy, positron emission tomography, etc.) may make it possible to identify breast cancers yet more reliably and earlier.

STAGING   Correct staging of breast cancer patients is of extraordinary importance. Not only does it permit an accurate prognosis,

but in many cases therapeutic decision-making is based largely on the TNM classification (Table 89-1). Comparison with historic series should be undertaken with caution, as the staging has changed in the past 10 years.

℞ TREATMENT   **Primary Breast Cancer**   A series of randomized clinical trials both in the United States and abroad have shown that breast-conserving treatments, consisting of the removal of the primary tumor by some form of lumpectomy with or without irradiating the breast, results in a survival that is as good as that after extensive procedures, such as mastectomy or modified radical mastectomy, with or without further irradiation. While breast conservation is associated with a possibility of recurrence in the breast, 10-year survival is at least as good as that after more radical surgery. Postoperative radiation to regional nodes following mastectomy is also associated with an improvement in survival. Since radiation therapy can also reduce the rate of local or regional recurrence, it should be strongly considered following mastectomy for women with high-risk primary tumors (i.e., T2 in size, positive margins, positive nodes). At present, approximately one-third of women in the United States are managed by lumpectomy. Breast-conserving surgery is not suitable for all patients; it is not generally suitable for tumors >5 cm (or for smaller tumors if the breast is small), for tumors involving the nipple areola complex, for tumors with extensive intraductal disease involving multiple quadrants of the breast, for women with a history of collagen-vascular disease, and for women who either do not have the motivation for breast conservation or do not have convenient access to radiation therapy. However, these groups probably do not account for more than one-third of patients. Thus, a great many women who undergo mastectomy could safely avoid this procedure.

An extensive intraductal component is a predictor of recurrence in the breast, and so are several clinical variables. Both axillary lymph node involvement and involvement of vascular or lymphatic channels

Table 89-1   Staging of Breast Cancer

PRIMARY TUMOR (T)

T0	No evidence of primary tumor
TIS	Carcinoma in situ
T1	Tumor ≤2 cm
T2	Tumor >2 cm but ≤5 cm
T3	Tumor >5 cm
T4	Extension to chest wall, inflammation, satellite lesions, ulcerations

REGIONAL LYMPH NODES (N)

N0	No regional lymph nodes
N1	Metastasis to movable ipsilateral nodes
N2	Metastasis to matted or fixed ipsilateral nodes
N3	Metastasis to ipsilateral internal mammary nodes

DISTANT METASTASIS (M)

M0	No distant metastasis
M1	Distant metastasis (includes spread to ipsilateral supraclavicular nodes)

STAGE GROUPING

Stage 0	TIS	N0	M0
Stage I	T1	N0	M0
Stage IIA	T0	N1	M0
	T1	N1	M0
	T2	N0	M0
Stage IIB	T2	N1	M0
	T3	N0	M0
Stage IIIA	T0	N2	M0
	T1	N2	M0
	T2	N2	M0
	T3	N1, N2	M0
Stage IIIB	T4	Any N	M0
	Any T	N3	M0
Stage IV	Any T	Any N	M1

SOURCE: Modified from the American Joint Committee on Cancer, 1992.

by metastatic tumor in the breast are associated with a higher risk of relapse in the breast but are not contraindications to breast-conserving treatment. When these patients are excluded, and when lumpectomy with negative tumor margins is achieved, breast conservation is associated with a recurrence rate in the breast of less than 10%. The survival of patients who have recurrence in the breast is somewhat worse than that of women who do not. Thus, recurrence in the breast is a negative prognostic variable for long-term survival. However, recurrence in the breast is not the *cause* of distant metastasis. If recurrence in the breast caused metastatic disease, then women treated with lumpectomy, who have a higher rate of recurrence in the breast, should have poorer survival. Most patients should consult with a radiation oncologist before making a final decision concerning local therapy. However, a multimodality clinic approach in which the surgeon, radiation oncologist, medical oncologist, and other caregivers cooperate to evaluate the patient and develop a treatment is usually considered a major advantage by patients.

Adjuvant therapy One of the significant advances in the treatment of solid tumors of adults has been the improved survival resulting from the use of systemic therapy after local management of breast cancer. More than one-third of the women who would otherwise die of metastatic breast cancer remain disease-free when treated with the appropriate systemic regimen.

PROGNOSTIC VARIABLES The most important prognostic variables are provided by *tumor staging*. The size of the tumor and the status of the axillary lymph nodes provide reasonably accurate information on the likelihood of tumor relapse. The relation of pathologic stage to 5-year survival is shown in Table 89-2. For most women, the need for adjuvant therapy can be readily defined on this basis alone. In the absence of lymph node involvement, involvement of microvessels (either capillaries or lymphatic channels) in tumors is nearly equivalent to lymph node involvement. The greatest controversy concerns women with intermediate prognoses. *There is no justification for adjuvant chemotherapy in women with tumors <1 cm in size whose axillary lymph nodes are negative.*

Other prognostic variables have been sought and some appear to influence disease-free and overall survival. What is less clear is whether they add to the information from pathologic staging.

Estrogen and progesterone receptor status are of prognostic significance. Tumors that lack either or both of these receptors are more likely to recur than tumors that have them.

Several *measures of tumor growth rate* correlate with early relapse. S-phase analysis using flow cytometry is the most accurate measure, and the indirect S-phase assessments using antigens associated with the cell cycle, such as PCNA (Ki67), are also valuable. Several studies suggest that tumors with a high proportion (more than the median) of cells in the S phase pose a greater risk of relapse and that chemotherapy offers the greatest survival benefit for these tumors. For this reason, some clinicians use S-phase assessment as a deciding factor for instituting adjuvant therapy when other pathologic features are unclear. Assessment of DNA content in the form of ploidy is of modest value, with nondiploid tumors having a somewhat worse prognosis.

Histologic classification of the tumor has also been used as a prognostic factor. Tumors with a poor nuclear grade have a higher risk of recurrence than tumors with a good nuclear grade. Semiquantitative measures such as the Elston score improve the reproducibility of this measurement.

Molecular changes in the tumor are also useful. Tumors that overexpress erbB2 (HER-2/neu) or have a mutated p53 gene have a worse prognosis. Particular interest has centered on erbB2 overexpression as measured by histochemistry. Tumors that overexpress erbB2 are more likely to respond to higher doses of doxorubicin-containing regimens. For this reason, erbB2 expression is usually worth measuring as a means of deciding on therapy.

To grow, a tumor must generate a neovasculature (Chap. 83). The presence of more microvessels in a tumor is associated with a worse prognosis.

Other variables that have also been used to evaluate prognosis include proteins associated with invasiveness, such as type IV collagenase, cathepsin D, plasminogen activator, plasminogen activator receptor, and the metastasis suppressor gene, nm23. None of these has been widely accepted as a prognostic variable for therapeutic decision-making. One problem in interpreting these prognostic variables is that most of them have not been examined in a study using a large cohort of patients.

ADJUVANT REGIMENS Selection of appropriate adjuvant chemotherapy or hormone therapy regimens is a highly controversial issue in some situations. Meta-analyses have helped to define broad limits for therapy but do not help in choosing optimal regimens or in choosing a regimen for certain subgroups of patients. A summary of recommendations is shown in Table 89-3. In general, premenopausal women for whom any form of adjuvant systemic therapy is indicated should receive chemotherapy for 6 months. The antiestrogen (tamoxifen) improves survival in premenopausal patients with positive estrogen receptor values and should be added following completion of chemotherapy. Prophylactic castration may also be associated with a substantial survival benefit (primarily in estrogen receptor–positive patients) but is not widely used in this country.

Data on postmenopausal women are also controversial. The impact of adjuvant chemotherapy is less clear-cut than in premenopausal patients, although some survival advantage has been shown. The first decision is whether chemotherapy or tamoxifen should be used. While adjuvant tamoxifen improves survival regardless of axillary lymph node status, the improvement in survival is modest for patients in whom multiple lymph nodes are involved. For this reason, it has been usual to give chemotherapy to postmenopausal patients who have no medical contraindications and who have more than one positive lymph node; tamoxifen is commonly given simultaneously or subsequently. For postmenopausal women for whom systemic therapy is warranted but who have a more favorable prognosis, tamoxifen may be used as a single agent.

Most comparisons of adjuvant chemotherapy regimens show little difference among them, although slight advantages for doxorubicin-containing regimens are usually seen.

One approach—so-called neoadjuvant chemotherapy—involves the administration of adjuvant therapy before definitive surgery and radiation therapy. Because the objective response rates of patients with breast cancer to systemic therapy in this setting exceed 75%, many patients will be "downstaged" and may become candidates for breast-conserving therapy. At least one large randomized study has failed to show any difference in survival using this approach.

Other adjuvant treatments under investigation include the use of new drugs, such as paclitaxel, and therapy based on alternative kinetic and biologic models. In such approaches, high doses of single agents are used separately in relatively dose-intensive cycling regimens. One large randomized trial for node-positive patients suggests that patients treated with doxorubicin-cyclophosphamide for four cycles followed by four cycles of paclitaxel have a substantial additional gain in survival as compared with women receiving doxorubicin-cyclophosphamide alone. Very high dose therapy with stem cell transplantation in the adjuvant setting has not proved superior.

Table 89-2 5-Year Survival Rate for Breast Cancer by Stage

Stage	5-Year Survival, %
0	99
I	92
IIA	82
IIB	65
IIIA	47
IIIB	44
IV	14

SOURCE: Modified from data of the National Cancer Institute—Surveillance, Epidemiology, and End Results (SEER).

Table 89-3 Suggested Approaches to Adjuvant Therapy

Age Group	Lymph Node Status[a]	Endocrine Receptor (ER) Status	Tumor	Recommendation
Premenopausal	Positive	Any	Any	Multidrug chemotherapy + tamoxifen if ER-positive
Premenopausal	Negative	Any	>2 cm, or 1–2 cm with other poor prognostic variables	Multidrug chemotherapy + tamoxifen if ER-positive
Postmenopausal	Positive	Negative	Any	Multidrug chemotherapy
Postmenopausal	Positive	Positive	Any	Tamoxifen with or without chemotherapy
Postmenopausal	Negative	Positive	>2 cm, or 1–2 cm with other poor prognostic variables	Tamoxifen
Postmenopausal	Negative	Negative	>2 cm, or 1–2 cm with other poor prognostic variables	Consider multidrug chemotherapy

[a] As determined by pathologic examination.

Systemic therapy of metastatic disease Nearly half of patients treated for apparently localized breast cancer develop metastatic disease. Although some of these patients can be salvaged by combinations of systemic and local therapy, most eventually succumb. Soft tissue, bony, and visceral (lung and liver) metastases each account for approximately one-third of sites of initial relapses. However, by the time of death, most patients will have bony involvement. Recurrences can appear at any time after primary therapy. Half of all initial cancer recurrences occur more than 5 years following initial therapy.

Because this diagnosis of metastatic disease alters the outlook for the patient so drastically, it should not be made without biopsy. Every oncologist has seen patients with tuberculosis, gallstones, primary hyperparathyroidism, or other nonmalignant diseases misdiagnosed and treated as though they had metastatic breast cancer. This is a catastrophic mistake and justifies biopsy for every patient at the time of initial suspicion of metastatic disease.

The choice of therapy requires consideration of local therapy needs, the overall medical condition of the patient, and the hormone receptor status of the tumor, as well as the exercise of clinical judgment. Because therapy of systemic disease is palliative, the potential toxicities of therapies should be balanced against the response rates. Several variables influence the response to systemic therapy. For example, the presence of estrogen and progesterone receptors is a strong indication for endocrine therapy, since the response rates for tumors that express both receptors may approach 70%. On the other hand, patients with short disease-free intervals, rapidly progressive visceral disease, lymphangitic pulmonary disease, or intracranial disease are unlikely to respond to endocrine therapy.

In many cases, systemic therapy can be withheld while the patient is managed with appropriate local therapy. Radiation therapy and occasionally surgery are effective at relieving the symptoms of metastatic disease, particularly when bony sites are involved. Many patients with bone-only or bone-dominant disease have a relatively indolent course. Under such circumstances, systemic chemotherapy has a modest effect, whereas radiation therapy may be effective for long periods. Other systemic treatments, such as strontium 89 and/or bisphosphonates, may provide a palliative benefit without inducing objective responses. Since the goal of therapy is to maintain well-being for as long as possible, emphasis should be placed on avoiding the most hazardous complications of metastatic disease, including pathologic fracture of the axial skeleton and spinal cord compression. New back pain in patients with cancer should be explored aggressively on an emergent basis; to wait for neurologic symptoms is a potentially catastrophic error. Metastatic involvement of endocrine organs can cause profound dysfunction, including adrenal insufficiency and hypopituitarism. Similarly, obstruction of the biliary tree or other impaired organ function

may be better managed with a local therapy than with a systemic approach.

Endocrine therapy Normal breast tissue is estrogen-dependent. Both primary and metastatic breast cancer may retain this phenotype. The best means of ascertaining whether a breast cancer is hormone-dependent is through analysis of estrogen and progesterone receptor levels on the tumor. Tumors that are positive for the estrogen receptor and negative for the progesterone receptor have a response rate of approximately 30%. Tumors that have both receptors have a response rate approaching 70%. If neither receptor is present, the objective response rates are less than 10%. Receptor analyses provide information as to the correct ordering of endocrine therapies. Because of their lack of toxicity and because some patients whose receptor analyses are reported as negative respond to endocrine therapy, an endocrine treatment should be attempted in every patient with metastatic breast cancer. Potential endocrine therapies are summarized in Table 89-4. The choice of endocrine therapy is usually determined by toxicity profile and availability. In most patients, the initial endocrine therapy is the antiestrogen tamoxifen. Newer antiestrogens that are free of agonistic effects are in clinical trial. Cases in which tumors shrink in response to tamoxifen withdrawal (as well as withdrawal of pharmacologic doses of estrogens) have been reported. Endogenous estrogen formation may be blocked by aromatase inhibitors or analogues of luteinizing hormone–releasing hormone (LHRH). Additive endocrine therapies, including treatment with progestogens, estrogens, and androgens, may also be tried in patients who respond to initial endocrine therapy; the mechanism of action of these latter therapies is unknown. However, patients who respond to one endocrine therapy have at least a 50% chance of responding to a second endocrine therapy. It is not uncommon for patients to respond to two or three sequential endocrine therapies; however, combination endocrine therapies do not appear to be superior to individual agents, and combinations of chemotherapy with endocrine therapy are not useful. The median survival of patients with metastatic disease is approximately 2 years, and many patients, particularly older persons and those with hormone-dependent disease, may respond to endocrine therapy for 3 to 5 years or longer.

Chemotherapy Unlike many other epithelial malignancies, breast cancer responds to several chemotherapeutic agents, including anthracyclines, alkylating agents, taxanes, and antimetabolites. Multiple combinations of these agents have been found to improve re-

Table 89-4 Endocrine Therapies for Breast Cancer

Therapy	Comments
Castration	For premenopausal women
Surgical	
LHRH agonists	
Antiestrogens	
Tamoxifen	Useful in pre- and postmenopausal women
"Pure" antiestrogens	Promising early clinical data
Surgical adrenalectomy	Rarely employed second-line choice
Aromatase inhibitors	Low toxicity and superiority to additive hormone therapy
High-dose progestogens	Common third line choice
Hypophysectomy	Rarely used
Additive androgens or estrogens	Plausible third-line therapies; potentially toxic

NOTE: LHRH, luteinizing hormone–releasing hormone.

sponse rates somewhat, but they have had little impact on duration of response or survival. As previously mentioned, median survival from diagnosis of metastatic disease is approximately 2 years. The choice among multidrug combinations frequently depends on whether adjuvant chemotherapy was administered and, if so, what type. While patients treated with adjuvant regimens such as cyclophosphamide, methotrexate, and fluorouracil (CMF regimens) may subsequently respond to the same combination in the metastatic disease setting, most oncologists use drugs to which the patients have not been previously exposed. Once patients have progressed after combination drug therapy, it is most common to treat them with single agents. Given the significant toxicity of most drugs, the use of a single effective agent will minimize toxicity by sparing the patient exposure to drugs that would be of little value. Unfortunately, no form of in vitro drug sensitivity testing to select the drugs most efficacious for a given patient has been demonstrated to be useful.

Most oncologists use either an anthracycline or paclitaxel following failure with the initial regimen. However, the choice has to be balanced with individual needs.

The use of a humanized antibody to *erbB2* (herceptin) combined with paclitaxel can improve response rate and survival for women whose metastatic tumors overexpress *erbB2*. The magnitude of the survival extension is modest in patients with metastatic disease. Application to adjuvant therapy may prove even more beneficial.

High-dose chemotherapy including autologous bone marrow transplantation   Autologous bone marrow transplantation combined with high doses of single agents can produce improvement even in heavily pretreated patients. However, such responses are rarely, if ever, durable and are unlikely to substantially alter the clinical course for most patients with advanced metastatic disease. Randomized trials have not been encouraging, and these approaches cannot be recommended as part of clinical care outside of research settings.

Stage III Breast Cancer   Between 10 and 25% of patients have so-called locally advanced or stage III breast cancer at diagnosis. Many of these cancers are technically operable, whereas others, particularly cancers with chest wall involvement, inflammatory breast cancers, or cancers with large matted axillary lymph nodes, cannot be managed with surgery initially. Although no randomized trials have proved the efficacy of induction chemotherapy, this approach has gained widespread use. More than 90% of patients with locally advanced breast cancer show a partial or better response to multidrug chemotherapy regimens that include an anthracycline. Early administration of this treatment reduces the bulk of the disease and frequently makes the patient a suitable candidate for salvage surgery and/or radiation therapy. These patients should be managed in multimodality clinics, if possible, to coordinate surgery, radiation therapy, and systemic chemotherapy. Such approaches produce long-term disease-free survival in about 30 to 50% of patients.

Breast Cancer Prevention   Women who have one breast cancer are at risk of developing a contralateral breast cancer at a rate of approximately 0.5% per year. When adjuvant tamoxifen is administered to these patients, the rate of development of contralateral breast cancers is reduced. In other tissues of the body, tamoxifen has estrogen-like effects that are beneficial: preservation of bone mineral density and long-term lowering of cholesterol. However, tamoxifen has estrogen-like effects on the uterus, leading to an increased risk of uterine cancer (0.75% incidence after 5 years on tamoxifen). The Breast Cancer Prevention Trial (BCPT) revealed a >40% reduction in breast cancer amongst women with a risk of at least 1.66% taking the drug for 5 years. Raloxifene has shown similar breast cancer prevention potency but may have different effects on bone and heart. The two are being compared in a prospective randomized prevention trial (the STAR trial).

Noninvasive Breast Cancer   Breast cancer develops as a series of molecular changes in the epithelial cells that lead to ever more malignant behavior. Increased use of mammography and better mammographic diagnosis have led to more frequent diagnosis of nonin-

vasive breast cancer. These lesions fall into two groups: ductal carcinoma in situ (DCIS) and lobular carcinoma in situ (lobular neoplasia). The management of both entities is controversial.

Ductal carcinoma in situ   Proliferation of cytologically malignant breast epithelial cells within the ducts is termed DCIS. Significant disagreement can occur in differentiating atypical hyperplasia from DCIS. At least one-third of the cases of untreated DCIS progress within 5 years to invasive breast cancer. For many years, the standard treatment for this disease was mastectomy. However, since treatment of this condition by lumpectomy and radiation therapy gives survival that is as good as the survival for invasive breast cancer by mastectomy, it appears paradoxical to recommend more aggressive therapy for a "less" malignant disease. In one randomized trial, the combination of wide excision plus irradiation for DCIS caused a substantial reduction in the local recurrence rate as compared with wide excision alone with negative margins, though survival is identical in the two arms. No studies have compared either of these regimens to mastectomy. Addition of tamoxifen to any DCIS surgical/radiation therapy regimen will further improve outcome.

Several prognostic features may help to identify patients at high risk for local recurrence after either lumpectomy alone or lumpectomy with radiation therapy. These include extensive disease; age less than 40; and cytologic features such as necrosis, poor nuclear grade, and comedo subtype with overexpression of erbB2. Some data suggest that adequate excision with careful determination of pathologically clear margins is associated with a low recurrence rates. When such surgery is combined with radiation therapy, recurrence (which is usually in the same quadrant) occurs with a frequency of ≤10%. Given the fact that half of these recurrences will be invasive, about 5% of the initial cohort will eventually develop invasive breast cancer. A reasonable expectation of mortality for these patients is about 1%, a figure that approximates the mortality rate for DCIS managed by mastectomy. Although this train of reasoning has not formally been proved valid, it is reasonable at present to recommend that patients who desire breast preservation, and in whom DCIS appears to be reasonably localized, be managed by adequate surgery with meticulous pathologic evaluation, followed by breast irradiation and tamoxifen. For patients with localized DCIS, there is no need for axillary lymph node dissection. More controversial is the question of what management is optimal when there is any degree of invasion. Because of a significant likelihood (10 to 15%) of axillary lymph node involvement even when the primary lesion shows only microscopic invasion, it is prudent to do at least a level 1 and 2 axillary lymph node dissection for all patients with any degree of invasion, although in centers familiar with the technique, sentinel node biopsy may be substituted. Further management is dictated by the presence of nodal spread.

Lobular neoplasia   Proliferation of cytologically malignant cells within the lobules is termed *lobular neoplasia*. Approximately 30% of patients who have had adequate local excision of the lesion develop breast cancer (usually infiltrating ductal cell carcinoma) over the next 15 to 20 years. Ipsilateral and contralateral disease are equally common. Therefore, lobular neoplasia may be a premalignant lesion that suggests an elevated risk of subsequent breast cancer, rather than a form of malignancy itself, and aggressive local management seems unreasonable. Most patients should be treated with tamoxifen for 5 years and followed with careful annual mammography and semiannual physical examinations. Additional molecular analysis of these lesions may make it possible to discriminate between patients who are at risk of further progression and who require additional therapy and those in whom simple follow-up is adequate.

Male Breast Cancer   Breast cancer is about 1/150th as frequent in men as in women. It usually presents as a unilateral lump in the breast and is frequently not diagnosed promptly. Given the small amount of soft tissue and the unexpected nature of the problem, locally advanced presentations are somewhat more common. When male

Table 89-5   Breast Cancer Surveillance Guidelines

Test	Frequency
RECOMMENDED	
History; eliciting symptoms; physical examination	q3–6 months × 3 years; q6–12 months × 2 years; then annually
Breast self-examination	Monthly
Mammography	Annually
Pelvic examination	Annually
Patient education about symptoms of recurrence	Ongoing
Coordination of care	Ongoing
NOT RECOMMENDED	
Complete blood count	
Serum chemistry studies	
Chest radiographs	
Bone scans	
Ultrasound examination of the liver	
Computed tomography of chest, abdomen, or pelvis	
Tumor marker CA 15-3	
Tumor marker CEA	

SOURCE: *Recommended Breast Cancer Surveillance Guidelines*, ASCO Education Book, Fall, 1997.

breast cancer is matched to female breast cancer by age and stage, its overall prognosis is identical. Although gynecomastia may initially be unilateral or asymmetric, any unilateral mass in a man over the age of 40 should receive a careful workup all the way through biopsy. On the other hand, bilateral symmetric breast development rarely represents breast cancer and is almost invariably due to endocrine disease or a drug effect. It should be kept in mind, nevertheless, that the risk of cancer is much greater in men with gynecomastia; in such men, gross asymmetry of the breasts should arouse suspicion of cancer. Male breast cancer is best managed by mastectomy and axillary lymph node dissection (modified radical mastectomy). Patients with locally advanced disease or positive nodes should also be treated with irradiation. Approximately 90% of male breast cancers contain estrogen receptors, and approximately 60% of cases with metastatic disease respond to endocrine therapy. There are no randomized studies exploring adjuvant therapy for male breast cancer. Two historic experiences suggest that the disease responds well to adjuvant systemic therapy, and, if not medically contraindicated, the same criteria for the use of adjuvant therapy in women should be applied to men.

The sites of relapse and spectrum of response to chemotherapeutic drugs are virtually identical for breast cancers in the two sexes.

FOLLOW-UP OF BREAST CANCER PATIENTS   Despite the availability of sophisticated and expensive imaging techniques and a wide range of serum tumor marker tests, no studies document that survival is influenced by early diagnosis of relapse. Surveillance guidelines are given in Table 89-5.

BIBLIOGRAPHY

BENICHOU J et al: Graphs to estimate an individualized risk of breast cancer. J Clin Oncol 14:103, 1996

BERRY DA: Benefits and risks of screening mammography for women in their forties: A statistical appraisal. J Natl Cancer Inst 90:1431, 1998

BRODIE AMH, NJAR VCO: Aromatase inhibitors in advanced breast cancer: Mechanism of clinical implications. J Steroid Biochem Mol Biol 66:1, 1998

EARLY BREAST CANCER TRIALISTS' COLLABORATIVE GROUP: Polychemotherapy for early breast cancer: An overview of the randomized trials. Lancet 352:930, 1998

FISHER B et al: Effect of preoperative chemotherapy on the outcome of women with operable breast cancer. J Clin Oncol 16:2672, 1998

——— et al: Lumpectomy and radiation therapy for the treatment of intraductal breast cancer: Findings from National Surgical Adjuvant Breast and Bowel Project B-17. J Clin Oncol 16:441, 1998

HARRIS J et al (eds): *Diseases of the Breast*. 2d ed. Philadelphia, Lippincott-Raven, 1999

MORROW M et al: Local control following breast-conserving surgery for invasive cancer: Results of clinical trials. J Natl Cancer Inst 87(22):1669, 1995

RAVANDI-KASHANI F, HAYES TG: Male breast cancer: A review of the literature. Eur J Cancer 34(9):1341, 1998

STOCKLER M et al: Systematic reviews of chemotherapy and endocrine therapy for metastatic breast cancer. Cancer Treat Rev 26:151, 2000

90   Robert J. Mayer

GASTROINTESTINAL TRACT CANCER

The gastrointestinal tract is the second most common noncutaneous site for cancer and the second major cause of cancer-related mortality in the United States.

ESOPHAGEAL CANCER

INCIDENCE AND ETIOLOGY   Cancer of the esophagus is a relatively uncommon but extremely lethal malignancy. The diagnosis was made in 12,300 Americans in 2000 and led to 12,100 deaths. Worldwide, the incidence of esophageal cancer varies strikingly. It occurs frequently within a geographic region extending from the southern shore of the Caspian Sea on the west to northern China on the east and encompassing parts of Iran, Central Asia, Afghanistan, Siberia, and Mongolia. High-incidence "pockets" of the disease are also present in such disparate locations as Finland, Iceland, Curaçao, southeastern Africa, and northwestern France. In North America and western Europe, the disease is far more common in blacks than whites, is more common in males than females, appears most often after age 50, and seems to be associated with a lower socioeconomic status.

A variety of causative factors have been implicated in the development of the disease (Table 90-1). In the United States, esophageal cancer cases are either squamous cell carcinomas or adenocarcinomas. The etiology of squamous cell esophageal cancer is related to excess alcohol consumption and/or cigarette smoking. The relative risk increases with the amount of tobacco smoked or alcohol consumed, with these factors acting synergistically. The consumption of whiskey is linked to a higher incidence than the consumption of wine or beer. Squamous cell esophageal carcinoma has also been associated with the ingestion of nitrites, smoked opiates, and fungal toxins in pickled vegetables, as well as mucosal damage caused by such physical insults as long-term exposure to extremely hot tea, the ingestion of lye, radiation-induced strictures, and chronic achalasia. The presence of an esophageal web in association with glossitis and iron deficiency (i.e.,

Table 90-1   Some Etiologic Factors Believed to Be Associated with Esophageal Cancer

Excess alcohol consumption
Cigarette smoking
Other ingested carcinogens
    Nitrates (converted to nitrites)
    Smoked opiates
    Fungal toxins in pickled vegetables
Mucosal damage from physical agents
    Hot tea
    Lye ingestion
    Radiation-induced strictures
    Chronic achalasia
Host susceptibility
    Esophageal web with glossitis and iron deficiency (i.e., Plummer-Vinson or Paterson-Kelly syndrome)
    Congenital hyperkeratosis and pitting of the palms and soles (i.e., tylosis palmaris et plantaris)
? Dietary deficiencies molybdenum, zinc, vitamin A
? Celiac sprue
Chronic gastric reflux (i.e., Barrett's esophagus) for adenocarcinoma

Plummer-Vinson or Paterson-Kelly syndrome) and congenital hyperkeratosis and pitting of the palms and soles (i.e., tylosis palmaris et plantaris) have each been linked with squamous cell esophageal cancer, as have dietary deficiencies of molybdenum, zinc, and vitamin A.

For unclear reasons, the incidence of squamous cell esophageal cancer has decreased in both the black and white population in the United States over the past 20 years, while the rate of adenocarcinoma has risen dramatically, particularly in white males. Adenocarcinomas arise in the distal esophagus in the presence of chronic gastric reflux and gastric metaplasia of the epithelium (Barrett's esophagus), which is more common in obese persons. Adenocarcinomas arise within dysplastic columnar epithelium in the distal esophagus. Even before frank neoplasia is detectable, aneuploidy and p53 mutations are found in the dysplastic epithelium. These adenocarcinomas behave clinically like gastric adenocarcinoma and now account for >50% of esophageal cancers.

CLINICAL FEATURES About 15% of esophageal cancers occur in the upper third of the esophagus (cervical esophagus), 40% in the middle third, and 45% in the lower third. Squamous cell carcinomas and adenocarcinomas of the esophagus cannot be distinguished radiographically or endoscopically.

Progressive dysphagia and weight loss of short duration are the initial symptoms in the vast majority of patients. Dysphagia initially occurs with solid foods and gradually progresses to include semisolids and liquids. By the time these symptoms develop, the disease is usually incurable, since difficulty in swallowing does not occur until ≥60% of the esophageal circumference is infiltrated with cancer. Dysphagia may be associated with pain on swallowing (odynophagia), pain radiating to the chest and/or back, regurgitation or vomiting, and aspiration pneumonia. The disease most commonly spreads to adjacent and supraclavicular lymph nodes, liver, lungs, and pleura. Tracheoesophageal fistulas may develop as the disease advances, leading to severe suffering. As with other squamous cell carcinomas, hypercalcemia may occur in the absence of osseous metastases, probably from parathormone-related peptide secreted by tumor cells (Chap. 100).

DIAGNOSIS Attempts at endoscopic and cytologic screening for carcinoma in patients with Barrett's esophagus, while effective as a means of detecting high-grade dysplasia, have not yet been shown to improve the prognosis in individuals found to have a carcinoma. Routine contrast radiographs effectively identify esophageal lesions large enough to cause symptoms. In contrast to benign esophageal leiomyomas, which result in esophageal narrowing with preservation of a normal mucosal pattern, esophageal carcinomas characteristically cause ragged, ulcerating changes in the mucosa in association with deeper infiltration, producing a picture resembling achalasia. Smaller, potentially resectable tumors are often poorly visualized despite technically adequate esophagograms. Because of this, esophagoscopy should be performed in all patients suspected of having an esophageal abnormality, to visualize the tumor and to obtain histopathologic confirmation of the diagnosis. Because the population of persons at risk for squamous cell carcinoma of the esophagus (i.e., smokers and drinkers) also has a high rate of cancers of the lung and the head and neck region, endoscopic inspection of the larynx, trachea, and bronchi should also be done. A thorough examination of the fundus of the stomach (by retroflexing the endoscope) is imperative as well. Endoscopic biopsies of esophageal tumors fail to recover malignant tissue in one-third of cases because the biopsy forceps cannot penetrate deeply enough through normal mucosa pushed in front of the carcinoma. Cytologic examination of tumor brushings frequently complements standard biopsies and should be performed routinely. The extent of tumor spread to the mediastinum and paraaortic lymph nodes should also be assessed by computed tomography (CT) scans of the chest and abdomen and by endoscopic ultrasound.

℞ **TREATMENT** The prognosis for patients with esophageal carcinoma is poor. Fewer than 5% of patients are alive 5 years after the diagnosis; thus, management focuses on symptom control. Surgical resection of all gross tumor (i.e., total resection) is feasible in only 40% of cases, with residual tumor cells frequently present at the resection margins. Such esophagectomies have been associated with a postoperative mortality rate of ~10% due to anastomotic fistulas, subphrenic abscesses, and respiratory complications. About 20% of patients who survive a total resection live 5 years. The outcome of primary radiation therapy (5500 to 6000 cGy) for squamous cell carcinomas is similar to that of radical surgery, sparing patients perioperative morbidity but often resulting in less satisfactory palliation of obstructive symptoms. The evaluation of chemotherapeutic agents in patients with esophageal carcinoma has been hampered by ambiguity in the definition of "response" (i.e., benefit) and the debilitated physical condition of many treated individuals. Nonetheless, significant reductions in the size of measurable tumor masses have been reported in 15 to 25% of patients given single-agent treatment and in 30 to 60% of patients treated with drug combinations that include cisplatin. Combination chemotherapy and radiation therapy as the initial therapeutic approach, either alone or followed by an attempt at operative resection, may be of benefit. When administered along with radiation therapy, chemotherapy produces a better survival outcome than radiation therapy alone. The use of preoperative chemotherapy and radiation therapy followed by esophageal resection appears to prolong survival as compared with historic controls, but randomized trials have produced inconsistent results.

For the incurable, surgically unresectable patient with esophageal cancer, dysphagia, malnutrition, and the management of tracheoesophageal fistulas loom as major issues. Approaches to palliation include repeated endoscopic dilatation, the surgical placement of a gastrostomy or jejunostomy for hydration and feeding, and endoscopic placement of an expansive metal stent to bypass the tumor. Endoscopic fulguration of the obstructing tumor with lasers appears to be the most promising of these techniques.

TUMORS OF THE STOMACH

GASTRIC ADENOCARCINOMA Incidence and Epidemiology For unclear reasons, the incidence and mortality rates for gastric cancer have decreased markedly during the past 60 years. The mortality rate from gastric cancer in the United States has dropped in men from 28 to 5.0 per 100,000 population, while in women, the rate has decreased from 27 to 2.3 per 100,000. Nonetheless, 21,500 new cases of stomach cancer were diagnosed in the United States and 13,000 Americans died of the disease in 2000. Gastric cancer incidence has decreased worldwide but remains high in Japan, China, Chile, and Ireland.

The risk of gastric cancer is greater among lower socioeconomic classes. Migrants from high- to low-incidence nations maintain their susceptibility to gastric cancer, while the risk for their offspring approximates that of the new homeland. These findings suggest that an environmental exposure, probably beginning early in life, is related to the development of gastric cancer, with dietary carcinogens considered the most likely factor(s).

Pathology About 85% of stomach cancers are adenocarcinomas, with 15% due to lymphomas and leiomyosarcomas. Gastric adenocarcinomas may be subdivided into two categories: a *diffuse type* in which cell cohesion is absent, so that individual cells infiltrate and thicken the stomach wall without forming a discrete mass; and an *intestinal type* characterized by cohesive neoplastic cells that form glandlike tubular structures. The diffuse carcinomas occur more often in younger patients, develop throughout the stomach (including the cardia), result in a loss of distensibility of the gastric wall (so-called linitis plastica or "leather bottle" appearance), and carry a poorer prognosis. Intestinal-type lesions are frequently ulcerative, more commonly appear in the antrum and lesser curvature of the stomach, and are often preceded by a prolonged precancerous process. While the incidence of diffuse carcinomas is similar in most populations, the intestinal type tends to predominate in the high-risk geographic regions and is less likely to be found in areas where the frequency of gastric cancer is declining. Thus, different etiologic factor(s) may be involved in these two subtypes. In the United States, the distal stomach is the site of origin of ~30% of gastric cancers, ~20% arise in the midportion of the stomach, and ~37% originate in the proximal third of the stomach. The remaining 13% involve the entire stomach.

Etiology   The long-term ingestion of high concentrations of nitrates in dried, smoked, and salted foods appears to be associated with a higher risk. The nitrates are thought to be converted to carcinogenic nitrites by bacteria (Table 90-2). Such bacteria may be introduced exogenously through the ingestion of partially decayed foods, which are consumed in abundance worldwide by the lower socioeconomic classes. Bacteria such as *Helicobacter pylori* may also contribute to this effect by causing chronic gastritis, loss of gastric acidity, and bacterial growth in the stomach. Loss of acidity may occur when acid-producing cells of the gastric antrum have been removed surgically to control benign peptic ulcer disease or when achlorhydria, atrophic gastritis, and even pernicious anemia develop in the elderly. Serial endoscopic examinations of the stomach in patients with atrophic gastritis have documented replacement of the usual gastric mucosa by intestinal-type cells. This process of intestinal metaplasia may lead to cellular atypia and eventual neoplasia. Since the declining incidence of gastric cancer in the United States primarily reflects a decline in distal, ulcerating, intestinal-type lesions, it is conceivable that better food preservation and the availability of refrigeration to all socioeconomic classes have decreased the dietary ingestion of exogenous bacteria.

Several additional etiologic factors have been associated with gastric carcinoma. Gastric ulcers and adenomatous polyps have occasionally been so linked, but data regarding a cause-and-effect relationship are unconvincing. The inadequate clinical distinction between benign gastric ulcers and small ulcerating carcinomas may, in part, account for this presumed association. The presence of extreme hypertrophy of gastric rugal folds (i.e., Ménétrier's disease), giving the impression of polypoid lesions, has been associated with a striking frequency of malignant transformation; such hypertrophy, however, does not represent the presence of true adenomatous polyps. Individuals with blood group A have a higher incidence of gastric cancer than persons with blood group O; this observation may be related to differences in the mucous secretion leading to altered mucosal protection from carcinogens. Duodenal ulcers are not associated with gastric cancer.

Clinical Features   Gastric cancers, when superficial and surgically curable, usually produce no symptoms. As the tumor becomes more extensive, patients may complain of an insidious upper abdominal discomfort varying in intensity from a vague, postprandial fullness to a severe, steady pain. Anorexia, often with slight nausea, is very common but is not the usual presenting complaint. Weight loss may eventually be observed, and nausea and vomiting are particularly prominent with tumors of the pylorus; dysphagia may be the major symptom caused by lesions of the cardia. There are no early physical

Table 90-2   Nitrate-Converting Bacteria as a Factor in the Causation of Gastric Carcinoma[a]

Exogenous sources of nitrate-converting bacteria:
  Bacterially contaminated food (common in lower socioeconomic classes, who have a higher incidence of the disease; diminished by improved food preservation and refrigeration)
  ? *Helicobacter pylori* infection
Endogenous factors favoring growth of nitrate-converting bacteria in the stomach:
  Decreased gastric acidity
  Prior gastric surgery (antrectomy) (15 to 20 year latency period)
  Atrophic gastritis and/or pernicious anemia
  ? Prolonged exposure to histamine H_2-receptor antagonists

---

[a] Hypothesis: Dietary nitrates are converted to carcinogenic nitrites by bacteria.

signs. A palpable abdominal mass indicates long-standing growth and predicts regional extension.

Gastric carcinomas spread by direct extension through the gastric wall to the perigastric tissues, occasionally adhering to adjacent organs such as the pancreas, colon, or liver. The disease also spreads via lymphatics or by seeding of peritoneal surfaces. Metastases to intra-abdominal and supraclavicular lymph nodes occur frequently, as do metastatic nodules to the ovary (Krukenberg's tumor), periumbilical region ("Sister Mary Joseph node") or peritoneal cul-de-sac (Blumer's shelf palpable on rectal or vaginal examination); malignant ascites may also develop. The liver is the most common site for hematogenous spread of tumor.

The presence of iron-deficiency anemia in men and of occult blood in the stool in both sexes mandate a search for an occult gastrointestinal tract lesion. A careful assessment is of particular importance in patients with atrophic gastritis or pernicious anemia. Unusual clinical features associated with gastric adenocarcinomas include migratory thrombophlebitis, microangiopathic hemolytic anemia, and acanthosis nigricans.

Diagnosis   A double-contrast radiographic examination is the simplest diagnostic procedure for the evaluation of a patient with epigastric complaints. The use of double-contrast techniques helps to detect small lesions by improving mucosal detail. The stomach should be distended at some time during every radiographic examination, since decreased distensibility may be the only indication of a diffuse infiltrative carcinoma. Although gastric ulcers can be detected fairly early, distinguishing benign from malignant lesions is difficult. The anatomic location of an ulcer is not in itself an indication of the presence or absence of a cancer.

Gastric ulcers that appear benign by radiography present special problems. Some physicians believe that gastroscopy is not mandatory if the radiographic features are typically benign, if complete healing can be visualized by x-ray within 6 weeks, and if a follow-up contrast radiograph obtained several months later shows a normal appearance. However, we recommend gastroscopic biopsy and brush cytology for all patients with a gastric ulcer in order to exclude a malignancy. Malignant gastric ulcers must be recognized before they penetrate into surrounding tissues, because the rate of cure of early lesions limited to the mucosa or submucosa is >80%. Since gastric carcinomas are difficult to distinguish clinically or radiographically from gastric lymphomas, endoscopic biopsies should be made as deep as possible, due to the submucosal location of lymphoid tumors.

The staging system for gastric carcinoma is shown in Table 90-3.

℞   TREATMENT   Complete surgical removal of the tumor with resection of adjacent lymph nodes offers the only chance for cure. However, this is possible in fewer than a third of patients. A subtotal gastrectomy is the treatment of choice for patients with distal carcinomas, while total or near-total gastrectomies are required for more proximal tumors. The inclusion of extended lymph node dissection to these procedures appears to confer an added risk for complications without enhancing survival. The prognosis following complete surgical resection depends on the degree of tumor penetration into the stomach wall and is adversely influenced by regional lymph node involvement, vascular invasion, and abnormal DNA content (i.e., aneuploidy), characteristics found in the vast majority of American patients. As a result, the probability of survival after 5 years for the 25 to 30% of patients able to undergo complete resection is ~20% for distal tumors and <10% for proximal tumors, with recurrences continuing to occur for at least 8 years after surgery. In the absence of ascites or extensive hepatic or peritoneal metastases, however, even patients whose disease is believed to be incurable by surgery should be offered an attempt at resection of the primary lesion, since reduction of tumor bulk is the best form of palliation and may enhance the probability of benefit from chemotherapy and/or radiation therapy.

Gastric adenocarcinoma is a relatively radioresistant tumor, and adequate control of the primary tumor requires doses of external beam irradiation that exceed the tolerance of surrounding structures, such as bowel mucosa and spinal cord. As a result, the major role of radiation therapy in patients has been palliation of pain. Radiation therapy alone after a complete resection does not prolong survival. In the setting of surgically unresectable disease limited to the epigastrium, patients treated with 3500 to 4000 cGy did not live longer than similar patients not receiving radiotherapy; however, survival was prolonged slightly when 5-fluorouracil (5-FU) was given in combination with radiation therapy. In this clinical setting, the 5-FU may well be functioning as a radiosensitizer.

The administration of combinations of cytotoxic drugs to patients with advanced gastric carcinoma has been associated with partial responses in 30 to 50% of cases, providing significant benefit to individuals who respond to treatment. Such drug combinations have generally included 5-FU and doxorubicin together with mitomycin-C, cisplatin, or high doses of methotrexate. Despite this encouraging response rate, complete remissions are uncommon, the partial responses are transient, and the overall influence of multidrug therapy on survival has been a source of debate. The use of prophylactic (i.e., adjuvant) chemotherapy following the complete resection of a gastric cancer has not improved survival. However, postoperative chemotherapy combined with radiation therapy has been shown to reduce the recurrence rate and prolong survival.

PRIMARY GASTRIC LYMPHOMA Primary lymphoma of the stomach is relatively uncommon, accounting for <15% of gastric malignancies and about 2% of all lymphomas. The stomach is, however, the most frequent extranodal site for lymphoma, and gastric lymphoma has increased in frequency during the past 25 years. The disease is difficult to distinguish clinically from gastric adenocarcinoma; both tumors are most often detected during the sixth decade of life; present with epigastric pain, early satiety, and generalized fatigue; and are usually characterized by ulcerations with a ragged, thickened mucosal pattern demonstrated by contrast radiographs. The diagnosis of lymphoma of the stomach may occasionally be made through cytologic brushings of the gastric mucosa but usually it requires a biopsy at gastroscopy or laparotomy. Failure of gastroscopic biopsies to detect lymphoma in a given case should not be interpreted as being conclusive, since superficial biopsies may miss the deeper lymphoid infiltrate. The macroscopic pathology of gastric lymphoma may also mimic adenocarcinoma, consisting of either a bulky ulcerated lesion localized in the corpus or antrum or a diffuse process spreading throughout the entire gastric submucosa and even extending into the duodenum. Microscopically, the vast majority of gastric lymphoid tumors are non-Hodgkin's lymphomas of B cell origin; Hodgkin's disease involving the stomach is extremely uncommon. Histologically, these tumors may range from well-differentiated, superficial processes [mucosa-associated lymphoid tissue (MALT)] to high-grade, large cell lymphomas. Infection with *H. pylori*, the same bacterium associated with the development of gastric adenocarcinoma, appears to increase the risk for gastric lymphoma in general and MALT lymphomas in particular. Gastric lymphomas spread initially to regional lymph nodes (often to Waldeyer's ring) and may then disseminate. Gastric lymphomas are staged like other lymphomas (Chap. 112).

TREATMENT Primary gastric lymphoma is a far more treatable disease than adenocarcinoma of the stomach, a fact that underscores the need for making the correct diagnosis. Antibiotic treatment to eradicate *H. pylori* infection has led to regression of about 75% of gastric MALT lymphomas and should be considered before surgery, radiation therapy, or chemotherapy are undertaken in patients having such tumors. Responding patients should undergo periodic endoscopic surveillance because it remains unclear whether the neoplastic clone is eliminated or merely suppressed. Subtotal gastrectomy, usually followed by combination chemotherapy, has led to 5-year survival rates of 40 to 60% in patients with localized high-grade lymphomas. The need for a major surgical procedure is not clear, particularly in patients with preoperative radiographic evidence of nodal involvement, for whom chemotherapy alone is effective therapy. A role for radiation therapy is not defined because most recurrences develop at sites distant from the epigastrium. If widespread disease is discovered at the time of laparotomy, combination chemotherapy should be used.

GASTRIC (NONLYMPHOID) SARCOMA Leiomyosarcomas are the most common of this group of gastric malignancies and make up 1 to 3% of gastric neoplasms. They most frequently involve the anterior and posterior walls of the gastric fundus and often ulcerate and bleed. Even those lesions that appear benign on histologic examination may behave in a malignant fashion. Leiomyosarcomas rarely invade adjacent viscera and characteristically do not metastasize to lymph nodes, but they may spread to the liver and lungs. The treatment of choice is surgical resection. Combination chemotherapy should be reserved for patients with metastatic disease.

COLORECTAL CANCER

INCIDENCE Cancer of the large bowel is second only to lung cancer as a cause of cancer death in the United States. Approximately 130,200 new cases occurred in 2000, and 56,300 deaths were due to colorectal cancer. The incidence rate has declined slightly during the past 15 years and the mortality rate has decreased in recent years, particularly in females. Colorectal cancer generally occurs in individuals ≥50 years.

POLYPS AND MOLECULAR PATHOGENESIS Most colorectal cancers, regardless of etiology, arise from adenomatous polyps. A polyp is a grossly visible protrusion from the mucosal surface and may be classified pathologically as a nonneoplastic hamartoma (*juvenile polyp*), a hyperplastic mucosal proliferation (*hyperplastic polyp*), or an adenomatous polyp. Only adenomas are clearly premalignant, and only a minority of such lesions ever develop into cancer. Population-screening studies and autopsy surveys have revealed that adenomatous polyps may be found in the colons of >30% of middle-aged or elderly people; however <1% of polyps ever become malignant. Most polyps produce no symptoms and remain clinically undetected. Occult blood in the stool may be found in <5% of patients with such lesions.

A number of molecular changes have been described in DNA ob-

Table 90-3 Staging System for Gastric Carcinoma

Stage	TNM	Features	Data from American College of Surgeons — Number of Cases, %	Data from American College of Surgeons — 5-Year Survival, %
0	TisN0M0	Node negative; limited to mucosa	1	90
IA	T1N0M0	Node negative; invasion of lamina propria or submucosa	7	59
IB	T2N0M0	Node negative; invasion of muscularis propria	10	44
II	T1N2M0 T2N1M0	Node positive; invasion beyond mucosa but within wall		
		or	17	29
	T3N0M0	Node negative; extension through wall		
IIIA	T2N2M0 T3N1-2M0	Node positive; invasion of muscularis propria or through wall	21	15
IIIB	T4N0-1M0	Node negative; adherence to surrounding tissue	14	9
IV	T4N2M0	Node positive; adherence to surrounding tissue		
		or	30	3
	T1-4N0-2M1	Distant metastases		

tained from adenomatous polyps, dysplastic lesions, and polyps containing microscopic foci of tumor cells (carcinoma in situ), which are thought to represent a multistep process in the evolution of normal colonic mucosa to life-threatening invasive carcinoma. These developmental steps towards carcinogenesis include point mutations in the K-*ras* protooncogene; hypomethylation of DNA, leading to gene activation; loss of DNA ("allelic loss") at the site of a tumor suppressor gene [the adenomatous polyposis coli (*APC*) gene] located on the long arm of chromosome 5 (5q21); allelic loss at the site of a tumor suppressor gene located on chromosome 18q [the deleted in colorectal cancer (*DCC*) gene]; and allelic loss at chromosome 17p, associated with mutations in the *p53* tumor suppressor gene (Chap. 81). Thus, the altered proliferative pattern of the colonic mucosa, which results in progression to a polyp and then to carcinoma, may involve the mutational activation of an oncogene followed by and coupled with the loss of genes that normally suppress tumorigenesis. While the present model includes five such molecular alterations, others are likely involved in the carcinogenic process. It remains uncertain whether the genetic aberrations always occur in a defined order. Based on this model, however, it is believed that neoplasia develops only in those polyps in which all of these mutational events take place.

Clinically, the probability of an adenomatous polyp becoming a cancer depends on the gross appearance of the lesion, its histologic features, and its size. Adenomatous polyps may be pedunculated (stalked) or sessile (flat-based). Cancers develop more frequently in sessile polyps. Histologically, adenomatous polyps may be tubular, villous (i.e., papillary), or tubulovillous. Villous adenomas, most of which are sessile, become malignant more than three times as often as tubular adenomas. The likelihood that any polypoid lesion in the large bowel contains invasive cancer is related to the size of the polyp, being negligible (<2%) in lesions <1.5 cm, intermediate (2 to 10%) in lesions 1.5 to 2.5 cm in size, and substantial (10%) in lesions >2.5 cm.

Following the detection of an adenomatous polyp, the entire large bowel should be visualized endoscopically or radiographically, since synchronous lesions are present in about one-third of cases. Colonoscopy should then be repeated periodically, even in the absence of a previously documented malignancy, since such patients have a 30 to 50% probability of developing another adenoma and are at a higher-than-average risk for developing a colorectal carcinoma. Adenomatous polyps are thought to require >5 years of growth before becoming clinically significant; colonoscopy need not be carried out more frequently than every 3 years.

ETIOLOGY AND RISK FACTORS Risk factors for the development of colorectal cancer are listed in Table 90-4.

Diet The etiology for most cases of large-bowel cancer appears to be related to environmental factors. The disease occurs more often in upper socioeconomic populations who live in urban areas. Mortality from colorectal cancer is directly correlated with per capita consumption of calories, meat protein, and dietary fat and oil as well as elevations in the serum cholesterol concentration and mortality from coronary artery disease. Geographic variations in incidence are unrelated to genetic differences, since migrant groups tend to assume the large-bowel cancer incidence rates of their adopted countries. Furthermore, population groups such as Mormons and Seventh Day Adventists,

Table 90-4 **Risk Factors for the Development of Colorectal Cancer**

Diet
  Animal fat
Hereditary syndromes (autosomal dominant inheritance)
  Polyposis coli
  Nonpolyposis syndrome (Lynch syndrome)
Inflammatory bowel disease
Streptococcus bovis bacteremia
Ureterosigmoidostomy
? Tobacco use

whose lifestyle and dietary habits differ somewhat from those of their neighbors, have significantly lower than expected incidence and mortality rates for colorectal cancer. Colorectal cancer has increased in Japan since that nation has adopted a more "western" diet. At least two hypotheses have been proposed to explain the relationship to diet, neither of which is fully satisfactory.

Animal fats One hypothesis is that the ingestion of animal fats leads to an increased proportion of anaerobes in the gut microflora, resulting in the conversion of normal bile acids into carcinogens. This provocative hypothesis is supported by several reports of increased amounts of fecal anaerobes in the stools of patients with colorectal cancer. Diets high in animal (but not vegetable) fats are also associated with high serum cholesterol, which is also associated with enhanced risk for the development of colorectal adenomas and carcinomas.

Fiber The observation that South African Bantus ingest a diet far higher in roughage, produce more frequent, bulkier stools, and have a lower incidence of large-bowel cancer than Americans and Europeans led to the proposal that the higher rate of colorectal cancer in western society results from low intake of dietary fiber. This theory suggests that dietary fiber accelerates intestinal transit time, thereby reducing the exposure of colonic mucosa to potential carcinogens and diluting these carcinogens because of enhanced fecal bulk. This theory has been largely discredited. Although an enhanced fiber intake increases fecal bulk, higher fiber intake has not been documented to consistently shorten stool transit time. In addition, despite the generally higher fiber intake in low-incidence countries, the environmental differences between developing and industrialized nations are myriad and include such other important dietary variables as meat and fat consumption. Furthermore, a diet low in fiber may lead to chronic constipation and diverticulosis. If a low-fiber diet were a significant risk factor in colorectal cancer, individuals with diverticulosis should be at higher risk for developing colorectal tumors; this is not the case. Finally, addition of fiber to the diet does not protect against the development of adenomatous polyps or colorectal cancer.

Thus, the weight of epidemiologic evidence implicates diet as being the major etiologic factor for colorectal cancer, particularly diets high in calories and animal fat.

HEREDITARY FACTORS AND SYNDROMES As many as 25% of patients with colorectal cancer have a family history of the disease, suggesting a hereditary predisposition. Inherited large-bowel cancers can be divided into two main groups: the well-studied but uncommon polyposis syndromes and the more common nonpolyposis syndromes (Table 90-5).

Polyposis Coli Polyposis coli (familial polyposis of the colon) is a rare condition characterized by the appearance of thousands of adenomatous polyps throughout the large bowel. It is transmitted as an autosomal dominant trait; the occasional patients with no family history probably developed the condition due to a spontaneous mutation. Polyposis coli is associated with a deletion in the long arm of chromosome 5 (including the *APC* gene) in both neoplastic (somatic mutation) and normal (germline mutation) cells. The loss of this genetic material (i.e., allelic loss) results in the absence of tumor suppressor genes whose protein products would normally inhibit neoplastic growth. The presence of soft tissue and bony tumors, congenital hypertrophy of the retinal pigment epithelium, mesenteric desmoid tumors, and of ampullary cancers in addition to the colonic polyps characterizes a subset of polyposis coli known as *Gardner's syndrome*. The appearance of malignant tumors of the central nervous system accompanying polyposis coli defines *Turcot's syndrome*. The colonic polyps in all these conditions are rarely present before puberty but are generally evident in affected individuals by age 25. If the polyposis is not treated surgically, colorectal cancer will develop in almost all patients before age 40. Polyposis coli results from a defect in the colonic mucosa leading to an abnormal proliferative pattern and an impaired DNA repair following exposure to radiation or ultraviolet light. Once the multiple polyps that constitute polyposis coli are detected, patients should undergo a total colectomy. The ileoanal anastomotic technique allows removal of the entire bowel while retaining the anal sphincter;

this appears to be the best treatment. Medical therapy with nonsteroidal anti-inflammatory drugs such as sulindac and cyclooxygenase-2 inhibitors such as celecoxib decreases the number and size of polyps in patients with polyposis coli; however, this effect on polyps is only temporary. Colectomy remains the primary therapy. The offspring of patients with polyposis coli, who often are prepubertal when the diagnosis is made in the parent, have a 50% risk for the development of this premalignant disorder and should be carefully screened by annual flexible sigmoidoscopy until age 35. Proctosigmoidoscopy is a sufficient screening procedure because polyps tend to be evenly distributed from cecum to anus, making more invasive and expensive techniques such as colonoscopy or barium enema unnecessary. Testing for occult blood in the stool is an inadequate screening maneuver. An

Table 90-5 Hereditable (Autosomal Dominant) Gastrointestinal Polyposis Syndromes

Syndrome	Distribution of Polyps	Histologic Type	Malignant Potential	Associated Lesions
Familial adenomatous polyposis	Large intestine	Adenoma	Common	None
Gardner's syndrome	Large and small intestine	Adenoma	Common	Osteomas, fibromas, lipomas, epidermoid cysts, ampullary cancers, congenital hypertrophy of retinal pigment epithelium
Turcot's syndrome	Large intestine	Adenoma	Common	Brain tumors
Nonpolyposis syndrome (Lynch syndrome)	Large intestine (often proximal)	Adenoma	Common	Endometrial and ovarian tumors
Peutz-Jeghers syndrome	Small and large intestines, stomach	Hamartoma	Rare	Mucocutaneous pigmentation; tumors of the ovary, breast, pancreas, endometrium
Juvenile polyposis	Large and small intestines, stomach	Hamartoma, rarely progressing to adenoma	Rare	Various congenital abnormalities

alternative method for identifying carriers is testing DNA from peripheral blood mononuclear cells for the presence of a mutated *APC* gene. The detection of such a germline mutation can lead to a definitive diagnosis before the development of polyps.

Hereditary Nonpolyposis Colon Cancer Hereditary nonpolyposis colon cancer (HNPCC), also known as Lynch syndrome, is another autosomal dominant trait. It is characterized by the presence of three or more relatives with histologically documented colorectal cancer, one of whom is a first-degree relative of the other two; one or more cases of colorectal cancer diagnosed before age 50 in the family; and colorectal cancer involving at least two generations. In contrast to polyposis coli, HNPCC is associated with an unusually high frequency of cancer arising in the proximal large bowel. The median age for the appearance of an adenocarcinoma is <50 years, 10 to 15 years younger than the median age for the general population. Despite having a poorly differentiated histologic appearance, the proximal colon tumors in HNPCC have a better prognosis than sporadic tumors from patients of similar age. Families with HNPCC often include individuals with multiple primary cancers; the association of colorectal cancer with either ovarian or endometrial carcinomas is especially strong in women. It has been recommended that members of such families undergo biennial colonoscopy beginning at age 25 years, with intermittent pelvic ultrasonography and endometrial biopsy offered for potentially afflicted women; such a screening strategy has not yet been validated. HNPCC is associated with germline mutations of several genes, particularly *hMSH2* on chromosome 2 and *hMLH1* on chromosome 3. These mutations lead to errors in DNA replication and are thought to result in DNA instability because of defective repair of DNA mismatches, resulting in abnormal cell growth and tumor development. Testing tumor cells for "microsatellite instability" (sequence changes reflecting defective mismatch repair) in patients under age 50 with colorectal cancer and a positive family history for colorectal or endometrial cancer may identify probands with HNPCC.

INFLAMMATORY BOWEL DISEASE (See also Chap. 287) Large-bowel cancer is increased in incidence in patients with long-standing inflammatory bowel disease. Cancers develop more commonly in patients with ulcerative colitis than in those with granulomatous colitis, but this impression may result in part from the occasional difficulty of differentiating these two conditions. The risk of colorectal cancer in a patient with inflammatory bowel disease is relatively small during the initial 10 years of the disease, but then it appears to increase at a rate of ~0.5 to 1% per year. Cancer may develop in 8 to 30% of patients after 25 years. The risk is higher in younger patients with pancolitis.

Cancer surveillance in patients with inflammatory bowel disease is unsatisfactory. Symptoms such as bloody diarrhea, abdominal cramping, and obstruction, which may signal the appearance of a tumor, are similar to the complaints caused by a flare-up of the underlying disease. In patients with a history of inflammatory bowel disease lasting 15 years or more who continue to experience exacerbations, the surgical removal of the colon can significantly reduce the risk for cancer and also eliminate the target organ for the underlying chronic gastrointestinal disorder. The value of such surveillance techniques as colonoscopy with mucosal biopsies and brushings for less symptomatic individuals with chronic inflammatory bowel disease is uncertain. The lack of uniformity regarding the pathologic criteria that characterize dysplasia and the absence of data that such surveillance reduces the development of lethal cancers have made this costly practice an area of controversy.

OTHER HIGH-RISK CONDITIONS *Streptococcus bovis* **Bacteremia** For unknown reasons, individuals who develop endocarditis or septicemia from this fecal bacteria have a high incidence of occult colorectal tumors and, possibly, upper gastrointestinal cancers as well. Endoscopic or radiographic screening appears advisable.

Ureterosigmoidostomy There is a 5 to 10% incidence of colon cancer 15 to 30 years after ureterosigmoidostomy to correct congenital extrophy of the bladder. Neoplasms characteristically are found at a site distal to the ureteral implant where colonic mucosa is chronically exposed to both urine and feces.

Tobacco Use Cigarette smoking is linked to the development of colorectal adenomas, particularly after more than 35 years of tobacco use. No biologic explanation for this association has yet been proposed.

PRIMARY PREVENTION Several orally administered compounds have been assessed as possible inhibitors of colon cancer. The most effective class of these chemopreventive agents is aspirin and other nonsteroidal anti-inflammatory drugs, which are thought to suppress cell proliferation by inhibiting prostaglandin synthesis. Regular aspirin use reduces the risk for colonic adenomas and carcinomas as well as for death from large-bowel cancer; this inhibiting effect on colonic carcinogenesis appears to increase with the duration of drug use. Oral folic acid supplements and oral calcium supplements have been found to reduce the risk of adenomatous polyps and colorectal cancers in case-control studies. While antioxidant vitamins such as ascorbic acid, tocopherols, and β-carotene are present in diets rich in fruits and vegetables, which have been associated with lower rates of colorectal cancer, they have been found to be ineffective at reducing the incidence of subsequent adenomas in patients who had undergone the removal of a colonic adenoma. Estrogen replacement therapy has been associated with a reduction in the risk of colorectal cancer in women, conceivably by an effect on bile acid synthesis and composition. The otherwise unexplained reduction in colorectal cancer mortality in women may be a result of the widespread use of estrogen replacement in postmenopausal individuals.

SCREENING The rationale for colorectal cancer screening programs is that the earlier detection of localized, superficial cancers in asymptomatic individuals will increase the surgical cure rate. Such screening programs are important for individuals having a family history of the disease in first-degree relatives. The relative risk for developing colorectal cancer increases to 1.75 in such people and may be even higher if the relative was afflicted before age 60. The use of proctosigmoidoscopy as a screening tool was based on the observation that 60% of early lesions are located in the rectosigmoid. For unexplained reasons, however, the proportion of large-bowel cancers arising in the rectum has been decreasing during the past several decades, with a corresponding increase in the proportion of cancers in the more proximal descending colon. As such, the potential for rigid proctosigmoidoscopy to detect a sufficient number of occult neoplasms to make the procedure cost-effective has been questioned. Flexible, fiberoptic sigmoidoscopes permit trained operators to visualize the colon for up to 60 cm, which enhances the capability for cancer detection. However, this technique still leaves the proximal half of the large bowel unscreened.

Most programs directed at the early detection of colorectal cancers have focused on digital rectal examinations and fecal occult blood testing. The digital examination should be part of any routine physical evaluation in adults older than age 40, serving as a screening test for prostate cancer in men, a component of the pelvic examination in women, and an inexpensive maneuver for the detection of masses in the rectum. The development of the Hemoccult test has greatly facilitated the detection of occult fecal blood. Unfortunately, even when performed optimally, the Hemoccult test has major limitations as a screening technique. About 50% of patients with documented colorectal cancers have a negative fecal Hemoccult test, consistent with the intermittent bleeding pattern of these tumors. When random cohorts of asymptomatic persons have been tested, 2 to 4% have Hemoccult-positive stools. Colorectal cancers have been found in <10% of these "test-positive" cases, with benign polyps being detected in an additional 20 to 30%. Thus, a colorectal neoplasm will not be found in most asymptomatic individuals with occult blood in their stool. Nonetheless, persons found to have Hemoccult-positive stool routinely undergo further medical evaluation, including sigmoidoscopy, barium enema, and/or colonoscopy—procedures that are not only uncomfortable and expensive but also associated with a small risk for significant complications. The added cost of these studies would appear justifiable if the small number of patients found to have occult neoplasms because of Hemoccult screening could be shown to have an improved prognosis and prolonged survival. Prospectively controlled trials addressing this issue have been performed. One of these studies, conducted at the University of Minnesota and involving >46,000 participants, reported a statistically significant reduction in mortality from colorectal cancer for individuals undergoing annual screening. However, this benefit only emerged after >13 years of follow-up and was extremely expensive to achieve, since all positive tests (most of which were false-positive) were followed by colonoscopy. Moreover, these colonoscopic examinations may have represented "chance selection" for more effective endoscopic screening and may also have provided the opportunity for cancer prevention through the removal of potentially premalignant adenomatous polyps.

Screening techniques for large-bowel cancer in asymptomatic persons remain unsatisfactory. Recommendations from governmental and private agencies are conflicting. Compliance with any screening strategy within the general population is poor. At present, the American Cancer Society suggests annual digital rectal examinations beginning at age 40, annual fecal Hemoccult screening beginning at age 50, and sigmoidoscopy (preferably flexible) every 3 to 5 years beginning at age 50 for asymptomatic individuals having no colorectal cancer risk factors. The use of colonscopy or double-contrast barium enemas for screening have not yet been systematically examined. Nonetheless, the American Cancer Society has proposed such a "total colon examination" every 10 years as an alternative to Hemoccult testing with periodic flexible sigmoidoscopy. More effective techniques for screening are needed, perhaps taking advantage of the molecular changes that have been described in these tumors. Analysis of stool for specific *ras* protooncogene mutations is being tested.

CLINICAL FEATURES **Presenting Symptoms** Symptoms vary with the anatomic location of the tumor. Since stool is relatively liquid as it passes through the ileocecal valve into the right colon, cancers arising in the cecum and ascending colon may become quite large, without resulting in any obstructive symptoms or noticeable alterations in bowel habits. Lesions of the right colon commonly ulcerate, leading to chronic, insidious blood loss without a change in the appearance of the stool. Consequently, patients with tumors of the ascending colon often present with symptoms such as fatigue, palpitations, and even angina pectoris and are found to have a hypochromic, microcytic anemia indicative of iron deficiency. Since the cancer may bleed intermittently, a random fecal occult blood test may be negative. As a result, the unexplained presence of iron-deficiency anemia in any adult (with the possible exception of a premenopausal, multiparous woman) mandates a thorough endoscopic and/or radiographic visualization of the entire large bowel (Fig. 90-1).

Since stool becomes more concentrated as it passes into the transverse and descending colon, tumors arising there tend to impede the passage of stool, resulting in the development of abdominal cramping, occasional obstruction, and even perforation. Radiographs of the abdomen often reveal characteristic annular, constricting lesions ("apple-core" or "napkin-ring") (Fig. 90-2).

Cancers arising in the rectosigmoid are often associated with hematochezia, tenesmus, and narrowing of the caliber of stool; anemia is an infrequent finding. While these symptoms may lead patients and their physicians to suspect the presence of hemorrhoids, the development of rectal bleeding and/or altered bowel habits demands a prompt digital rectal examination and proctosigmoidoscopy.

Staging, Prognostic Factors, and Patterns of Spread The prognosis for individuals having colorectal cancer is related to the depth of tumor penetration into the bowel wall and the presence of both regional lymph node involvement and distant metastases. These variables are incorporated into the staging system introduced by Dukes

FIGURE 90-1 Double-contrast air-barium enema revealing a sessile tumor of the cecum in a patient with iron-deficiency anemia and guaiac-positive stool. The lesion at surgery was a stage B adenocarcinoma.

FIGURE 90-2 Annular, constricting adenocarcinoma of the descending colon. This radiographic appearance is referred to as an "apple-core" lesion and is always highly suggestive of malignancy.

and applied to a TNM classification method, in which T represents the depth of tumor penetration, N the presence of lymph node involvement, and M the presence or absence of distant metastases (Table 90-6). Superficial lesions that do not penetrate into the muscularis or involve regional lymph nodes are designated as *stage A* (T1N0M0) disease; tumors that penetrate more deeply but have not spread to lymph nodes are *stage B* disease [subclassified as *stage B₁* (T2N0M0) if lesions are restricted to the muscularis and as *stage B₂* (T3N0M0) if lesions involve or penetrate the serosa]; regional lymph node involvement defines *stage C* (TxN1M0) disease; and metastatic spread to sites such as liver, lung, or bone indicates *stage D* (TxNxM1) disease. Unless gross evidence of metastatic disease is present, disease stage cannot be determined accurately before surgical resection and pathologic analysis of the operative specimens. It is not clear whether the detection of nodal metastases by special immunohistochemical molecular techniques has the same prognostic implications as disease detected by routine light microscopy.

Most recurrences after a surgical resection of a large-bowel cancer occur within the first 4 years, making 5-year survival a fairly reliable indicator of cure. The likelihood for 5-year survival in patients with colorectal cancer is stage-related (Table 90-6). That likelihood has improved during the past several decades when similar surgical stages have been compared. The most plausible explanation for this improvement appears to be more thorough intraoperative and pathologic staging. In particular, more exacting attention to pathologic detail has revealed that the prognosis following the resection of a colorectal cancer is not related merely to the presence or absence of regional lymph node involvement but may be more precisely assessed by the number of involved lymph nodes (one to four lymph nodes versus five or more lymph nodes). Other predictors of a poor prognosis after a total surgical resection include tumor penetration through the bowel wall into pericolic fat, poorly differentiated histology, perforation and/or tumor adherence to adjacent organs (increasing the risk for an anatomically adjacent recurrence), and venous invasion by tumor (Table 90-7). Regardless of the clinicopathologic stage, a preoperative elevation of the plasma carcinoembryonic antigen (CEA) level predicts eventual tumor recurrence. The presence of aneuploidy and specific chromosomal deletions, such as allelic loss in chromosome 18q (involving the *DCC* gene) in tumor cells, appears to predict a higher risk for metastatic spread, particularly in patients with stage B₂ (T3N0M0) disease. Conversely, the detection of microsatellite instability in tumor tissue has been associated with a more favorable outcome. In contrast to most other cancers, the prognosis in colorectal cancer is not influenced by the size of the primary lesion when adjusted for nodal involvement and histologic differentiation.

Cancers of the large bowel generally spread to regional lymph nodes or to the liver via the portal venous circulation. The liver represents the most frequent visceral site of metastatic dissemination; it is the initial site of distant spread in one-third of recurring colorectal cancers and is involved in more than two-thirds of such patients at the time of death. In general, colorectal cancer rarely metastasizes to the lungs, supraclavicular lymph nodes, bone, or brain without prior spread to the liver. A major exception to this rule occurs in patients having primary tumors in the distal rectum, from which tumor cells may spread through the paravertebral venous plexus, escaping the portal venous system and thereby reaching the lungs or supraclavicular lymph nodes without hepatic involvement. The median survival after the detection of distant metastases is 6 to 9 months (hepatomegaly, abnormal liver chemistries) to 24 to 30 months (small liver nodule initially identified by elevated CEA level and subsequent CT scan).

TREATMENT Total resection of tumor is the optimal treatment when a malignant lesion is detected endoscopically or radiographically in the large bowel. An evaluation for the presence of metastatic disease, including a thorough physical examination, chest radiograph, biochemical assessment of liver function, and measurement of the plasma CEA level, should be performed before surgery. When possible, a colonoscopy of the entire large bowel should be

Table 90-6 Staging of and Prognosis for Colorectal Cancer

Dukes	TNM	Numerical	Pathologic Description	Approximate 5-Year Survival, %
A	T1N0M0	I	Cancer limited to mucosa and submucosa	>90
B₁	T2N0M0	I	Cancer extends into muscularis	85
B₂	T3N0M0	II	Cancer extends into or through serosa	70–80
C	TxN1M0	III	Cancer involves regional lymph nodes	35–65
D	TxNxM1	IV	Distant metastases (i.e., liver, lung, etc.)	5

Table 90-7 Predictors of Poor Outcome Following Total Surgical Resection of Colorectal Cancer

Tumor spread to regional lymph nodes
Number of regional lymph nodes involved
Tumor penetration through the bowel wall
Poorly differentiated histology
Perforation
Tumor adherence to adjacent organs
Venous invasion
Preoperative elevation of CEA titer (>5.0 ng/mL)
Aneuploidy
Specific chromosomal deletion (e.g., allelic loss on chromosome 18q)

NOTE: CEA, carcinoembryonic antigen.

performed to identify synchronous neoplasms and/or polyps. The detection of metastases should not preclude surgery in patients with tumor-related symptoms such as gastrointestinal bleeding or obstruction, but it often prompts the use of a less radical operative procedure. At the time of laparotomy, the entire peritoneal cavity should be examined, with thorough inspection of the liver, pelvis, and hemidiaphragm and careful palpation of the full length of the large bowel. Following recovery from a complete resection, patients should be observed carefully for 5 years by semiannual physical examinations and yearly blood chemistry measurements. If a complete colonoscopy was not performed preoperatively, it should be carried out within the first several postoperative months. Some authorities favor measuring plasma CEA levels at 3-month intervals because of the sensitivity of this test as a marker for otherwise undetectable tumor recurrence. Subsequent endoscopic or radiographic surveillance of the large bowel, probably at triennial intervals, is indicated, since patients who have been cured of one colorectal cancer have a 3 to 5% probability of developing an additional bowel cancer during their lifetime and a >15% risk for the development of adenomatous polyps. Anastomotic ("suture-line") recurrences are infrequent in colorectal cancer patients provided the surgical resection margins were adequate and free of tumor. Periodic CT screening, chest radiographs, or more frequent colonoscopic examinations do not affect prognosis and add unnecessary costs to postoperative surveillance.

Radiation therapy to the pelvis is recommended for patients with rectal cancer because it reduces the 30 to 40% probability of regional recurrences following complete surgical resection of stage B or C tumors, especially if they have penetrated through the serosa. This alarmingly high rate of local disease recurrence is believed to be due to the fact that the contained anatomic space within the pelvis limits the extent of the resection and because the rich lymphatic network of the pelvic side wall immediately adjacent to the rectum facilitates the early spread of malignant cells into surgically inaccessible tissue. Radiation therapy, either pre- or postoperatively, reduces the likelihood of pelvic recurrences but does not appear to prolong survival. Preoperative radiotherapy is indicated for patients with large, potentially unresectable rectal cancers; such lesions may shrink enough to permit subsequent surgical removal. Radiation therapy is not effective in the primary treatment of colon cancer.

Chemotherapy in patients with advanced colorectal cancer has proven to be of only marginal benefit. 5-FU is the most effective single agent for this disease. Partial responses are obtained in 15 to 20% of patients. The probability of tumor response appears to be somewhat greater for patients with liver metastases when chemotherapy is infused directly into the hepatic artery, but intraarterial treatment is costly and toxic and does not appear to prolong survival. The concomitant administration of folinic acid (leucovorin) improves the efficacy of 5-FU in patients with advanced colorectal cancer, presumably by enhancing the binding of 5-FU to its target enzyme, thymidylate synthase. A threefold improvement in the partial response rate is noted when folinic acid is combined with 5-FU; however, the effect on survival is marginal, and the optimal dose schedule remains to be defined.

Irinotecan (CPT-11), a topoisomerase 1 inhibitor, prolongs survival when compared to supportive care in patients whose disease has progressed on 5-FU. Furthermore, the addition of irinotecan to 5-FU and leucovorin improves response rates and survival of patients with metastatic disease. Oxaliplatin, a platinum analogue, also improves the response rate when added to 5-FU and leucovorin as initial treatment of patients with metastatic disease.

Patients with solitary hepatic metastases without clinical or radiographic evidence of additional tumor involvement should be considered for partial liver resection, because such procedures are associated with 5-year survival rates of 25 to 30% when performed on selected individuals by experienced surgeons.

The administration of 5-FU and leucovorin for 6 months after re-section of tumor in patients with stage C disease leads to a 40% decrease in recurrence rates and 30% improvement in survival. Patients with stage B₂ tumors do not benefit from adjuvant therapy. In rectal cancer, the delivery of postoperative (and probably preoperative) combined modality therapy (5-FU plus radiation therapy) reduces the risk of recurrence and increases the chance of cure for patients with stages B₂ and C tumors. The 5-FU acts as a radiosensitizer when delivered together with radiation therapy.

TUMORS OF THE SMALL INTESTINE

Small-bowel tumors comprise <5% of gastrointestinal neoplasms. Because of their rarity, a correct diagnosis is often delayed. Abdominal symptoms are usually vague and poorly defined, and conventional radiographic studies of the upper and lower intestinal tract often appear normal. Small-bowel tumors should be considered in the differential diagnosis in the following situations: (1) recurrent, unexplained episodes of crampy abdominal pain; (2) intermittent bouts of intestinal obstruction, especially in the absence of inflammatory bowel disease or prior abdominal surgery; (3) intussusception in the adult; and (4) evidence of chronic intestinal bleeding in the presence of negative conventional contrast radiographs. A careful small-bowel barium study is the diagnostic procedure of choice; the diagnostic accuracy may be improved by infusing barium through a nasogastric tube placed into the duodenum (enteroclysis).

BENIGN TUMORS The histology of benign small-bowel tumors is difficult to predict on clinical and radiologic grounds alone. The symptomatology of benign tumors is not distinctive, with pain, obstruction, and hemorrhage being the most frequent symptoms. These tumors are usually discovered during the fifth and sixth decades of life, more often in the distal rather than the proximal small intestine. The most common benign tumors are adenomas, leiomyomas, lipomas, and angiomas.

Adenomas These tumors include those of the islet cells and Brunner's glands as well as polypoid adenomas. *Islet cell adenomas* are occasionally located outside the pancreas; the associated syndromes are discussed in Chap. 93. *Brunner's gland adenomas* are not truly neoplastic but represent a hypertrophy or hyperplasia of submucosal duodenal glands. These appear as small nodules in the duodenal mucosa that secrete a highly viscous alkaline mucus. Most often, this is an incidental radiographic finding not associated with any specific clinical disorder.

Polypoid Adenomas About 25% of benign small-bowel tumors are polypoid adenomas (Table 90-5). They may present as single polypoid lesions or, less commonly, as papillary villous adenomas. As in the colon, the sessile or papillary form of the tumor is sometimes associated with a coexisting carcinoma. Occasionally, patients with Gardner's syndrome develop premalignant adenomas in the small bowel; such lesions are generally in the duodenum. Multiple polypoid tumors may occur throughout the small bowel (and occasionally the stomach and colorectum) in the Peutz-Jeghers syndrome. The polyps are usually hamartomas (juvenile polyps) having a low potential for malignant degeneration. Mucocutaneous melanin deposits as well as tumors of the ovary, breast, pancreas, and endometrium are also associated with this autosomal dominant condition.

Leiomyomas These neoplasms arise from smooth-muscle components of the intestine and are usually intramural, affecting the overlying mucosa. Ulceration of the mucosa may cause gastrointestinal hemorrhage of varying severity. Cramping, intermittent abdominal pain is frequently encountered.

Lipomas These tumors occur with greatest frequency in the distal ileum and at the ileocecal valve. They have a characteristic radiolucent appearance, are usually intramural and asymptomatic, but on occasion cause bleeding.

Angiomas While not true neoplasms, these lesions are important because they frequently cause intestinal bleeding. They may take the form of telangiectasia or hemangiomas. Multiple intestinal telangiectasias occur in a nonhereditary form confined to the gastrointestinal tract or as part of the hereditary Osler-Rendu-Weber syndrome. Vascular tumors may also take the form of isolated hemangiomas, most commonly in the jejunum. Angiography, especially during bleeding, is the best procedure for evaluating these lesions.

MALIGNANT TUMORS While rare, small-bowel malignancies occur in patients with long-standing regional enteritis and celiac sprue as well as in individuals with AIDS. Malignant tumors of the small bowel are frequently associated with fever, weight loss, anorexia, bleeding, and a palpable abdominal mass. After ampullary carcinomas (many of which arise from biliary or pancreatic ducts), the most frequently occurring small-bowel malignancies are adenocarcinomas, lymphomas, carcinoid tumors, and leiomyosarcomas.

Adenocarcinomas The most common primary cancers of the small bowel are adenocarcinomas, accounting for ~50% of malignant tumors. These cancers occur most often in the distal duodenum and proximal jejunum, where they tend to ulcerate and cause hemorrhage or obstruction. Radiologically, they may be confused with chronic duodenal ulcer disease or with Crohn's disease if the patient has long-standing regional enteritis. The diagnosis is best made by endoscopy and biopsy under direct vision. Surgical resection is the treatment of choice.

Lymphomas Lymphoma in the small bowel may be primary or secondary. A diagnosis of a primary intestinal lymphoma requires histologic confirmation in a clinical setting in which palpable adenopathy and hepatosplenomegaly are absent and no evidence of lymphoma is seen on chest radiograph, CT scan, or peripheral blood smear or on bone marrow aspiration and biopsy. Symptoms referable to the small bowel are present, usually accompanied by an anatomically discernible lesion. Secondary lymphoma of the small bowel consists of involvement of the intestine by a lymphoid malignancy extending from involved retroperitoneal or mesenteric lymph nodes (Chap. 112).

Primary intestinal lymphoma accounts for ~20% of malignancies of the small bowel. These neoplasms are non-Hodgkin's lymphomas; they usually have a diffuse, large cell histology and are of T cell origin. Intestinal lymphoma involves the ileum, jejunum, and duodenum, in decreasing frequency, a pattern that mirrors the relative amount of normal lymphoid cells in these anatomic areas. The risk of small-bowel lymphoma is increased in patients with a prior history of malabsorptive conditions (e.g., celiac sprue), regional enteritis, and depressed immune function due to congenital immunodeficiency syndromes, prior organ transplantation, autoimmune disorders, or AIDS.

The development of localized or nodular masses that narrow the lumen results in periumbilical pain (made worse by eating) as well as weight loss, vomiting, and occasional intestinal obstruction. The diagnosis of small-bowel lymphoma may be suspected from the appearance on contrast radiographs of patterns such as infiltration and thickening of mucosal folds, mucosal nodules, areas of irregular ulceration, or stasis of contrast material. The diagnosis can be confirmed by surgical exploration and resection of involved segments. Intestinal lymphoma can occasionally be diagnosed by peroral intestinal mucosal biopsy, but since the disease mainly involves the lamina propria, full-thickness surgical biopsies are usually required.

Resection of the tumor constitutes the initial treatment modality. While postoperative radiation therapy has been given to some patients following a total resection, most authorities favor short-term (three cycles) systemic treatment with combination chemotherapy. The frequent presence of widespread intraabdominal disease at the time of diagnosis and the occasional multicentricity of the tumor often make a total resection impossible. The probability of sustained remission or cure is ~75% in patients with localized disease but is ~25% in individuals with unresectable lymphoma. In patients whose tumors are not resected, chemotherapy may lead to bowel perforation.

A unique form of small-bowel lymphoma, diffusely involving the entire intestine, was first described in oriental Jews and Arabs and is referred to as *immunoproliferative small intestinal disease* (IPSID), *Mediterranean lymphoma,* or *α-heavy chain disease.* This is a B cell tumor. The typical presentation includes chronic diarrhea and steator-

rhea associated with vomiting and abdominal cramps; clubbing of the digits may be observed. A curious feature in many patients with IPSID is the presence in the blood and intestinal secretions of an abnormal IgA that contains a shortened α-heavy chain and is devoid of light chains. It is suspected that the abnormal α chains are produced by plasma cells infiltrating the small bowel. The clinical course of patients with IPSID is generally one of exacerbations and remissions, with death frequently resulting from either progressive malnutrition and wasting or the development of an aggressive lymphoma. The use of oral antibiotics such as tetracycline appears to be beneficial in the early phases of the disorder, suggesting a possible infectious etiology. Combination chemotherapy has been administered during later stages of the disease, with variable results. Results are better when antibiotics and chemotherapy are combined.

Carcinoid Tumors Carcinoid tumors arise from argentaffin cells of the crypts of Lieberkühn and are found from the distal duodenum to the ascending colon, areas embryologically derived from the midgut. More than 50% of intestinal carcinoids are found in the distal ileum, with most congregating close to the ileocecal valve. Most intestinal carcinoids are asymptomatic and of low malignant potential, but invasion and metastases may occur, leading to the carcinoid syndrome (Chap. 93).

Leiomyosarcomas Leiomyosarcomas often are >5 cm in diameter and may be palpable on abdominal examination. Bleeding, obstruction, and perforation are common.

CANCERS OF THE ANUS

Cancers of the anus account for 1 to 2% of the malignant tumors of the large bowel. Most such lesions arise in the anal canal, the anatomic area extending from the anorectal ring to a zone approximately halfway between the pectinate (or dentate) line and the anal verge. Carcinomas arising proximal to the pectinate line (i.e., in the transitional zone between the glandular mucosa of the rectum and the squamous epithelium of the distal anus) are known as basaloid, cuboidal, or cloacogenic tumors; about one-third of anal cancers have this histologic pattern. Malignancies arising distal to the pectinate line have a squamous cell histology, ulcerate more frequently, and constitute ~55% of anal cancers. The prognosis for patients with basaloid and squamous cell cancers of the anus is identical when corrected for tumor size and the presence or absence of nodal spread.

The development of anal cancer is associated with infection by human papillomavirus, the same organism etiologically linked to cervical cancer. The virus is sexually transmitted. The infection may lead to anal warts (condyloma accuminata) which may progress to anal intraepithelial neoplasia and on to squamous cell carcinoma. The risk for anal cancer is increased among homosexual males, presumably related to anal intercourse. Anal cancer risk is increased in both men and women with AIDS, possibly because their immunosuppressed state permits more severe papillomavirus infection. Anal cancers occur most commonly in middle-aged persons and are more frequent in women than men. At diagnosis, patients may experience bleeding, pain, sensation of a perianal mass, and pruritus.

Radical surgery (abdominal-perineal resection with lymph node sampling and a permanent colostomy) used to be the treatment of choice for this tumor type. The 5-year survival rate after such a procedure was 55 to 70% in the absence of spread to regional lymph nodes; <20% if nodal involvement was present. An alternative therapeutic approach combining external beam radiation therapy with concomitant chemotherapy has resulted in biopsy-proven disappearance of all tumor in >80% of patients whose initial lesion was <3 cm in size. Tumor has recurred in <10% of these patients, and ~70% of patients with anal cancers can be cured with nonoperative treatment. Surgery should be reserved for the minority of individuals who are found to have residual tumor after being managed initially with radiation therapy combined with chemotherapy.

BIBLIOGRAPHY

CRUMP W et al: Lymphoma of the gastrointestinal tract. Semin Oncol 26:324, 1999

DESCH CE et al: Recommended colorectal cancer surveillance guidelines by the American Society of Clinical Oncology. J Clin Oncol 17:1312, 1999

DEVESA SS et al: Changing patterns in the incidence of esophageal and gastric carcinomas in the United States. Cancer 83:2049, 1998

FUCHS CS, MAYER RJ: Gastric carcinoma. N Engl J Med 333:32, 1995

ISAACSON PG: Gastric MALT lymphoma: From concept to cure. Ann Oncol 10:637, 1999

JÄNNE PA, MAYER RJ: Chemoprevention of colorectal cancer. N Engl J Med 342:1960, 2000

KELSEN DP et al: Chemotherapy followed by surgery compared with surgery alone for localized esophageal cancer. N Engl J Med 339:1979, 1998

LYNCH HT et al: Hereditary colorectal cancer. Semin Oncol 26:478, 1999

RYAN DP et al: Carcinoma of the anal canal. N Engl J Med 342:792, 2000

SALTZ LB et al: Irinotecan plus fluorouracil and leucovorin for metastatic colorectal cancer. N Engl J Med 343:905, 2000

91   Jules L. Dienstag, Kurt J. Isselbacher

TUMORS OF THE LIVER AND BILIARY TRACT

BENIGN LIVER TUMORS

HEPATOCELLULAR ADENOMAS Hepatocellular adenomas are benign tumors of the liver found predominantly in women in their third and fourth decades. Their preponderance in women suggests a hormonal influence in their pathogenesis, and oral contraceptives are thought to play an etiologic role. The risk of liver adenomas is increased among those who take anabolic steroids and exogenous androgens. Multiple hepatic adenomas have been associated with glycogen storage disease type I.

Hepatic adenomas occur predominantly in the right lobe of the liver, may be multiple, and are often quite large (>10 cm). Microscopically, they consist of normal or slightly atypical hepatocytes. These cells contain increased glycogen, making them appear paler and larger than normal. Clinical features include pain and the presence of a palpable mass or features of intratumor hemorrhage (pain and circulatory collapse). The diagnosis is usually made by a combination of techniques: sonography, computed tomography (CT), magnetic resonance imaging (MRI), selective hepatic arteriography, and radionuclide scans. The angiographic appearance is typically hypervascular but often also includes hypovascular regions. Technetium 99m scans usually show a defect, because phagocytosing Kupffer cells are absent. Like hepatocellular carcinomas, adenomas have a T_1-intense MRI appearance. The risk of malignant change is small; the risk is higher for large (>10 cm) and multiple adenomas.

Management involves imaging surveillance for small tumors. If the lesion is large (8 to 10 cm), near the surface, and resectable, surgical removal is appropriate. A patient with liver adenoma should stop taking oral contraceptives. Surgical resection may be required for tumors that do not shrink after oral contraceptives are stopped. Pregnancy increases the risk of hemorrhage and should be avoided in women with large adenomas. Patients with multiple large adenomas (e.g., those with glycogen-storage disease) may benefit from liver transplantation.

FOCAL NODULAR HYPERPLASIA Focal nodular hyperplasia is a benign tumor often identified incidentally on imaging studies or at laparoscopy done for other reasons. Like hepatic adenomas, it occurs predominantly in women; however, oral contraceptives are not implicated, and hemorrhage and necrosis are rare. The risk of hemorrhage, however, appears to be higher in women taking oral contra-

ceptives. Typically, the lesion is a solid tumor, often in the right lobe, with a fibrous core and stellate projections. The fibrous projections contain atypical hepatocytes, biliary epithelium, Kupffer cells, and inflammatory cells. A technetium scan will usually show a hot spot because of the presence of Kupffer cells. The lesion appears vascular on angiography, and septations may be detectable by angiography, helical CT scan, and, most reliably, by MRI, but only rarely by ultrasound. Surgery is indicated only for symptomatic lesions.

HEMANGIOMA AND OTHER BENIGN TUMORS *Hemangiomas* are the most common benign liver tumors, occurring predominantly in women and usually detected incidentally. The prevalence in the general population is in the range of 0.5 to 7.0%. These asymptomatic vascular lesions can be identified by MRI, contrast-enhanced CT, labeled red blood cell nuclide scans, or hepatic angiography. They do not need to be removed unless they are large and are producing a mass effect. Hemorrhage is rare, and malignant change does not occur.

Nodular regenerative hyperplasia consists of multiple hepatic nodules resulting from periportal hepatocyte regeneration with surrounding atrophy. It may be associated with an underlying condition such as malignancy or connective tissue disease. Portal hypertension (in the absence of cirrhosis) is the most common clinical manifestation. Other less common benign hepatic lesions include *bile duct adenomas* and *cystadenomas*.

CARCINOMAS OF THE LIVER

HEPATOCELLULAR CARCINOMA   Epidemiology and Etiology Primary hepatocellular carcinoma is one of the most common tumors in the world. It is especially prevalent in regions of Asia and sub-Saharan Africa, where the annual incidence is up to 500 cases per 100,000 population. In the United States and western Europe, it is much less common; however, the annual incidence in the United States has increased from 1.4/100,000 in the period 1976 to 1980 to 2.4/100,000 in 1991 to 1995. Hepatocellular carcinoma is up to four times more common in men than in women and usually arises in a cirrhotic liver. The incidence peaks in the fifth to sixth decades of life in western countries but one to two decades earlier in regions of Asia and Africa with a high prevalence of liver carcinoma.

The principal reason for the high incidence of hepatocellular carcinoma in parts of Asia and Africa is the frequency of chronic infection with *hepatitis B virus* (HBV) and *hepatitis C virus* (HCV). These chronic infections frequently lead to cirrhosis, which itself is an important risk factor for hepatocellular carcinoma (the risk of liver cancer in a cirrhotic liver is ~3% per year); 60 to 90% of these tumors occur in patients with macronodular cirrhosis. Studies in regions of Asia where hepatocellular carcinoma and HBV infection are prevalent have shown that the incidence of this cancer is about 100-fold higher in individuals with evidence of HBV infection than in noninfected controls. In China, the lifetime risk of developing hepatocellular carcinoma in patients with chronic hepatitis B approaches 40%. In patients with HBV infection and hepatocellular carcinoma, HBV DNA may be integrated into host genomic DNA, both in the tumor cells and in adjacent, uninvolved hepatocytes. In addition, modifications of cellular gene expression occur by insertional mutagenesis, chromosomal rearrangements, or the transcriptional transactivating activity of the X and the pre-S2 regions of the HBV genome.

HCV also leads to hepatocellular carcinoma. HCV genetic material does not become integrated into host genomic DNA. Therefore, the mechanism of HCV carcinogenesis is unclear. In Europe and Japan, HCV appears to be substantially more prevalent than HBV in cases of hepatocellular carcinoma. Both HBV and HCV can be demonstrated in some patients, but the clinical course of liver malignancy in these patients does not appear to differ from that when only one virus is implicated. One distinction in high-prevalence areas between hepatocellular carcinoma associated with HBV infection and with HCV infection is in the timing of onset. In Asia, HBV is acquired at birth via perinatal transmission, whereas HCV infection is acquired primarily during adulthood from transfused blood and injections. Correspondingly, the onset of liver carcinoma occurs one to two decades earlier in those with lifelong hepatitis B than in persons with adult-acquired hepatitis C. Retrospective analysis indicates that hepatocellular carcinoma occurs on average approximately 30 years after HCV infection and almost exclusively in patients with cirrhosis. The annual incidence of hepatocellular carcinoma in cirrhotic patients with chronic hepatitis C is 1.5 to 4%.

Any agent or factor that contributes to chronic, low-grade liver cell damage and mitosis makes hepatocyte DNA more susceptible to genetic alterations. Thus, as indicated above, *chronic liver disease* of any type is a risk factor and predisposes to the development of liver cell carcinoma. These conditions include alcoholic liver disease, α_1-antitrypsin deficiency, hemochromatosis, and tyrosinemia. In Africa and southern China, *aflatoxin B_1* is an important public health hazard. This mycotoxin appears to induce a very specific mutation at codon 249 in the tumor suppressor gene p53.

The loss, inactivation, or mutation of the p53 gene has been implicated in tumorigenesis and is the most common genetic derangement present in human cancers. Thus HBV and aflatoxin B_1 have been implicated in the pathogenesis of hepatocellular carcinoma in regions of Africa and southern China where both agents are prevalent.

In view of the male predominance of liver cancer, hormonal factors may also play a role. Hepatocellular tumors may occur with long-term androgenic steroid administration, with exposure to thorium dioxide or vinyl chloride (see below), and possibly with exposure to estrogens in the form of oral contraceptives.

Clinical and Laboratory Features Cancers of the liver initially may escape clinical recognition because they occur in patients with underlying cirrhosis, and the symptoms and signs may suggest progression of the underlying disease. The most common presenting features are abdominal *pain* with detection of an abdominal mass in the right upper quadrant. There may be a *friction rub* or *bruit* over the liver. Blood-tinged ascites occurs in about 20% of cases. Jaundice is rare, unless there is significant deterioration of liver function or mechanical obstruction of the bile ducts. Serum elevations of alkaline phosphatase and α fetoprotein (AFP) are common (see below). An abnormal type of prothrombin, des-γ-carboxy prothrombin, is made and correlates with AFP elevations.

A small percentage of patients with hepatocellular carcinoma have a *paraneoplastic syndrome*; erythrocytosis may result from erythropoietin-like activity produced by the tumor; hypercalcemia may result from secretion of a parathyroid-like hormone. Other manifestations may include hypercholesterolemia, hypoglycemia, acquired porphyria, dysfibrinogenemia, and cryofibrinogenemia.

Imaging procedures to detect liver tumors include ultrasound, CT, MRI, hepatic artery angiography (Chap. 282), and technetium scans. Ultrasound is frequently used to screen high-risk populations and should be the first test if hepatocellular carcinoma is suspected; it is less costly than scans, is relatively sensitive, and can detect most tumors >3 cm. Helical CT and MRI scans are being used with increasing frequency and have higher sensitivities.

AFP levels >500 μg/L are found in about 70 to 80% of patients with hepatocellular carcinoma. Lower levels may be found in patients with large metastases from gastric or colonic tumors and in some patients with acute or chronic hepatitis. High levels of serum AFP (>500 to 1000 μg/L) in an adult with liver disease and without an obvious gastrointestinal tumor strongly suggest hepatocellular carcinoma. A rising level suggests progression of the tumor or recurrence after hepatic resection or therapeutic approaches such as chemotherapy or chemoembolization (see below).

Percutaneous *liver biopsy* can be diagnostic if the sample is taken from an area localized by ultrasound or CT. Because these tumors tend to be vascular, percutaneous biopsies should be done with caution. Cytologic examination of ascitic fluid is invariably negative for tumor cells. Occasionally, *laparoscopy* or *minilaparotomy*, to permit liver biopsy under direct vision, may be used. This approach has the additional advantage of sometimes identifying patients who have a localized resectable tumor suitable for partial hepatectomy.

[Rx] **TREATMENT** Staging of hepatocellular carcinoma is based on tumor size (< or > 50% of the liver), ascites (absent or present), bilirubin (< or > 3), and albumin (< or >3) to establish Okuda stages I, II, and III. The Okuda system predicts clinical course better than the American Joint Cancer Commission TNM system. The natural history of each stage without treatment is: stage I, 8 months; stage II, 2 months; stage III, less than 1 month.

The course of *clinically apparent* disease is rapid; if untreated, most patients die within 3 to 6 months of diagnosis. When hepatocellular carcinoma is detected very early by serial screening of AFP and ultrasound, survival is 1 to 2 years after resection. In selected cases, therapy may prolong life. *Surgical resection* offers the only chance for cure; however, few patients have a resectable tumor at the time of presentation, because of underlying cirrhosis, involvement of both hepatic lobes, or distant metastases (common sites are lung, brain, bone, and adrenal), and the 5-year survival is low. In patients at high risk for the development of hepatocellular carcinoma, screening programs have been initiated to identify small tumors when they are still resectable. Because 20 to 30% of patients with early hepatocellular carcinoma do not have elevated levels of circulating AFP, ultrasonographic screening is recommended as well as AFP determination. In a study in the Far East, persons positive for hepatitis B surface antigen, with or without liver disease, were screened serially; a number of patients with small, subclinical tumors were identified, and surgical resection undertaken. Follow-up observation revealed a 5-year survival rate in this group of 70% and a 10-year survival rate of 50%. These Asian patients, however, were unusual in that they had minimal or no liver disease and their tumors tended to be unifocal or encapsulated. The findings are in contrast to a study in a large population of Italian patients with cirrhosis, associated in most cases with chronic HBV and/or HCV infections; screening every 3 to 12 months permitted the detection of a 3% annual incidence of cancer in this cohort but in most cases failed to achieve the goal of early detection of surgically treatable disease. No randomized study has yet shown survival benefit for screening patients at high risk of developing hepatocellular carcinoma.

Liver transplantation may be considered as a therapeutic option; tumor recurrence or metastases are the major problems. Patients who have a single lesion ≤5 cm or three or fewer lesions ≤3 cm have survival after liver transplantation that is the same as survival after transplantation for nonmalignant liver disease (Chap. 301). Other approaches include (1) hepatic artery embolization and chemotherapy (chemoembolization), (2) alcohol or radio-frequency ablation via ultrasound-guided percutaneous injection, and (3) ultrasound-guided cryoablation.

Treatment options for unresectable disease are limited. Randomized trials have not shown a survival advantage after chemoembolization. The liver cannot tolerate high doses of radiation. The disease is not responsive to chemotherapy, including newer agents such as gemcytabine. Investigative immunotherapy and gene therapy techniques have not yet been successful. Based on the presence of hormone receptors on the tumor, tamoxifen has been tested, but without success, and octreotide has had some modest activity. In patients with resectable tumors, polyprenoic acid (a retinoic acid formulation) and intra-arterial ^{131}I-labeled lipiodol have been reported to reduce the rate of recurrence.

Prevention is the preferred strategy. Hepatitis B vaccine can prevent infection and its sequelae, and a reduction in hepatocellular carcinoma has been seen in Taiwan with the introduction of universal vaccination of children. Interferon treatment reduces the incidence of hepatic failure, death, and liver cancer in patients infected with HBV.

Treatment with interferon may lower the risk of development of liver cancer in patients with hepatitis C–related cirrhosis (Chap. 297), but additional studies are needed.

OTHER MALIGNANT LIVER TUMORS

Fibrolamellar carcinoma differs from the typical hepatocellular carcinoma in that it tends to occur in young adults without underlying cirrhosis. This tumor is nonencapsulated but well circumscribed and contains fibrous lamellae; it grows slowly and is associated with a longer survival if treated. Surgical resection has resulted in 5-year survivals >50%; if the lesion is nonresectable, liver transplantation is an option, and the outcome far exceeds that observed in the nonfibrolamellar variety of liver cancer. *Hepatoblastoma* is a tumor of infancy that typically is associated with very high serum AFP levels. The lesions are usually solitary, may be resectable, and have a better 5-year survival than that of hepatocellular carcinoma. *Angiosarcoma* consists of vascular spaces lined by malignant endothelial cells. Etiologic factors include prior exposure to thorium dioxide (Thorotrast), polyvinyl chloride, arsenic, and androgenic anabolic steroids. *Epithelioid hemangioendothelioma* is of borderline malignancy; most cases are benign, but bone and lung metastases occur. This tumor occurs in early adulthood, presents with right upper quadrant pain, is heterogeneous on sonography, hypodense on CT, and without neovascularity on angiography. Immunohistochemical staining reveals expression of factor VIII antigen. In the absence of extrahepatic metastases, these lesions can be treated by surgical resection or liver transplantation.

METASTATIC TUMORS   Metastatic tumors of the liver are common, ranking second only to cirrhosis as a cause of fatal liver disease. In the United States, the incidence of metastatic carcinoma is at least 20 times greater than that of primary carcinoma. At autopsy, hepatic metastases occur in 30 to 50% of patients dying from malignant disease.

Pathogenesis   The liver is uniquely vulnerable to invasion by tumor cells. Its size, high rate of blood flow, double perfusion by the hepatic artery and portal vein, and its Kupffer cell filtration function combine to make it the next most common site of metastases after the lymph nodes. In addition, local tissue factors or endothelial membrane characteristics appear to enhance metastatic implants. Virtually all types of neoplasms except those primary in the brain may metastasize to the liver. The most common primary tumors are those of the gastrointestinal tract, lung, and breast, as well as melanomas. Less common are metastases from tumors of the thyroid, prostate, and skin.

Clinical Features   Most patients with metastases to the liver present with symptoms referable only to the primary tumor, and the asymptomatic hepatic involvement is discovered in the course of clinical evaluation. Sometimes hepatic involvement is reflected by nonspecific symptoms of weakness, weight loss, fever, sweating, and loss of appetite. Rarely, features indicating active hepatic disease, especially abdominal pain, hepatomegaly, or ascites, are present. Patients with widespread metastatic liver involvement usually have suggestive clinical signs of cancer and hepatic enlargement. Some have localized induration or tenderness, and, occasionally, a friction rub may be found over tender areas of the liver.

Results of liver biochemical tests are often abnormal, but the elevations in marker levels are often only mild and nonspecific. These signs reflect the effects of fever and wasting as well as those of the infiltrating neoplastic process itself. An increase in serum alkaline phosphatase is the most common and frequently the only abnormality. Hypoalbuminemia, anemia, and occasionally a mild elevation of aminotransferase levels may also be found with more widespread disease. Substantially elevated serum levels of carcinoembryonic antigen are usually found when the metastases are from primary malignancies in the gastrointestinal tract, breast, or lung.

Diagnosis   Evidence of metastatic invasion of the liver should be sought actively in any patient with a primary malignancy, especially of the lung, gastrointestinal tract, or breast, before resection of the primary lesion. An elevated level of alkaline phosphatase or a mass apparent on ultrasound, CT, or MRI examination of the liver may provide a presumptive diagnosis. Blind percutaneous needle biopsy of the liver will result in a positive diagnosis of metastatic disease in only 60 to 80% of cases with hepatomegaly and elevated alkaline phosphatase levels. Serial sectioning of specimens, two or three repeated biopsies, or cytologic examination of biopsy smears may increase the diagnostic yield by 10 to 15%. The yield is increased when biopsies are directed by ultrasound or CT or obtained during laparoscopy.

℞ **TREATMENT**   Most metastatic carcinomas respond poorly to all forms of treatment, which is usually only palliative. Rarely a single, large metastasis can be removed surgically. Systemic chemotherapy may slow tumor growth and reduce symptoms, but it does not alter the prognosis. Chemoembolization, intrahepatic chemotherapy, and alcohol or radio-frequency ablation may provide palliation.

CHOLANGIOCARCINOMA   Benign tumors of the extrahepatic bile ducts are extremely rare causes of mechanical biliary obstruction. Most of these are papillomas, adenomas, or cystadenomas and present with obstructive jaundice or hemobilia. Adenocarcinoma of the extrahepatic ducts is more common. There is a slight male preponderance (60%), and the incidence peaks in the fifth to seventh decades. Apparent predisposing factors include (1) some chronic hepatobiliary parasitic infestations, (2) congenital anomalies with ectactic ducts, (3) sclerosing cholangitis and chronic ulcerative colitis, and (4) occupational exposure to possible biliary tract carcinogens (employment in rubber or automotive plants). Cholelithiasis is not clearly a predisposing factor for cholangiocarcinoma. The lesions of cholangiocarcinoma may be diffuse or nodular. Nodular lesions often arise at the bifurcation of the common bile duct (Klatskin tumors) and are usually associated with a *collapsed gallbladder*, a finding that mandates cholangiography to view proximal hepatic ducts.

Patients with cholangiocarcinoma usually present with biliary obstruction, painless jaundice, pruritus, weight loss, and acholic stools. A deep-seated, vaguely localized right upper quadrant pain may be noted. Hepatomegaly and a palpable, distended gallbladder (unless the lesion is high in the duct) are frequent accompanying signs. Fever is unusual unless associated with ascending cholangitis. Because the obstructing process is gradual, the cholangiocarcinoma is often far advanced by the time it presents clinically. The diagnosis is most frequently made by cholangiography following ultrasound demonstration of dilated intrahepatic bile ducts. Any focal strictures of the bile ducts should be considered malignant until proved otherwise. Endoscopic cholangiography permits obtaining specimens for cytology (sensitivity ~60%) and insertion of stents for biliary drainage. Survival of 1 to 2 years is possible in some cases. Perhaps 20% of patients have surgically resectable tumors, but 5-year survival is only 10 to 30%. The high recurrence rate limits the value of liver transplantation. Photodynamic therapy (intravenous hematoporphyrin with cholangioscopically delivered light) has been used with promising early results.

CARCINOMA OF THE PAPILLA OF VATER   The ampulla of Vater may be involved by extension of tumor arising elsewhere in the duodenum or may itself be the site of origin of a sarcoma, carcinoid tumor, or adenocarcinoma. Papillary adenocarcinomas are associated with slow growth and a more favorable clinical prognosis than diffuse, infiltrative cancers of the ampulla, which are more frequently widely invasive. The presenting clinical manifestation is usually obstructive jaundice. Endoscopic retrograde cannulation of the pancreatic duct is the preferred diagnostic technique when ampullary carcinoma is suspected, because it allows for direct endoscopic inspection and biopsy of the ampulla and for pancreatography to exclude a pancreatic malignancy. Cancer of the papilla is usually treated by wide surgical excision. Lymph node or other metastases are present at the time of surgery in approximately 20% of cases, and the 5-year survival rate following surgical therapy in this group is only 5 to 10%. In the absence of metastases, radical pancreaticoduodenectomy (the

Whipple procedure) is associated with 5-year survival rates as high as 40%.

CANCER OF THE GALLBLADDER Most cancers of the gallbladder develop in conjunction with stones rather than polyps. In patients with gallstones, the risk for developing gallbladder cancer, while increased, is still quite low. In one study, gallbladder cancer developed in only 5 of 2583 patients with gallstones followed for a median of 13 years. In the United States, adenocarcinomas make up the vast majority of the estimated 6500 new cases of gallbladder cancer diagnosed each year. The female/male ratio is 4:1, and the mean age at diagnosis is approximately 70 years. The clinical presentation is most often one of unremitting right upper quadrant pain associated with weight loss, jaundice, and a palpable right upper quadrant mass. Cholangitis may supervene. The preoperative diagnosis of the condition has been facilitated by ultrasound and CT. CT is also useful in guiding fine-needle aspiration and biopsy.

Once symptoms have appeared, spread of the tumor outside the gallbladder by direct extension or by lymphatic or hematogenous routes is almost invariable. Over 75% of gallbladder carcinomas are unresectable at the time of surgery, the exceptions being tumors discovered incidentally at laparotomy. If the tumor is found by the pathologist, no additional therapy is required. If the tumor is noted by the surgeon on routine cholecystectomy, a second operation is generally performed to resect the adjacent liver, bile duct, and local lymph nodes. Incidental resectable gallbladder tumors have a 50% 5-year survival. The 1-year mortality rate for unresectable disease is about 95%, and <5% of patients survive 5 years. Radical operative resection does not appear to improve survival. Trials of radiation and chemotherapy in patients with gallbladder cancer have been disappointing.

BIBLIOGRAPHY

BRUIX J et al: Transarterial embolization versus symptomatic treatment in patients with advanced hepatocellular carcinoma: Results of a randomized, controlled trial in a single institution. Hepatology 27:1578, 1998

CHANG M-H et al: Universal hepatitis B vaccination in Taiwan and the incidence of hepatocellular carcinoma in children. N Engl J Med 336:1855, 1997

DE GROEN PC et al: Biliary tract cancers. N Engl J Med 341:1368, 1999

EL-SERAG HB et al: Rising incidence of hepatocellular carcinoma in the United States. N Engl J Med 340:745, 1999

LIN S-M et al: Long-term beneficial effect of interferon therapy in patients with chronic hepatitis B virus infection. Hepatology 29:971, 1999

MOR E et al: Treatment of hepatocellular carcinoma associated with cirrhosis in the era of liver transplantation. Ann Intern Med 129:643, 1998

ORTNER MA et al: Photodynamic therapy of nonresectable cholangiocarcinoma. Gastroenterology 114:536, 1998

SCHAFER DF, SORRELL MF: Hepatocellular carcinoma. Lancet 353:1253, 1999

YOSHIDA H et al: Interferon therapy reduces the risk for hepatocellular carcinoma: National surveillance program of cirrhotic and noncirrhotic patients with chronic hepatitis C in Japan. Ann Intern Med 131:174, 1999

92 *Robert J. Mayer*

PANCREATIC CANCER

INCIDENCE AND ETIOLOGY The incidence of pancreatic carcinoma in the United States has increased significantly as the median life expectancy of the American population has lengthened. The tumor results in the death of >98% of afflicted patients. 28,200 individuals died of pancreatic cancer in 2000, making it the fifth most common cause of cancer-related mortality. The disease is more common in males than in females and in blacks than in whites. It rarely develops before the age of 50.

Little is known about the causes of pancreatic cancer. Cigarette smoking is the most consistent risk factor, with the disease being two to three times more common in heavy smokers than in nonsmokers. Whether this association is due to a direct carcinogenic effect of to-

bacco metabolites on the pancreas or an as yet undefined exposure that occurs more frequently in cigarette smokers is uncertain. Patients with chronic pancreatitis are at increased risk of pancreatic cancer, as are persons with long-standing diabetes mellitus. Obesity is a risk factor for pancreatic cancer; risk is directly related to increased calorie intake. Alcohol abuse or cholelithiasis are not risk factors for pancreatic cancer. Nor is pancreatic cancer associated with coffee consumption. Mutations in K-*ras* genes have been found in >85% of specimens of human pancreatic cancer. Pancreatic cancer has been associated with mutation of the *p16*^{INK4} gene located on chromosome 9p21, a gene also implicated in the pathogenesis of malignant melanoma.

CLINICAL FEATURES More than 90% of pancreatic cancers are ductal adenocarcinomas, with islet cell tumors constituting the remaining 5 to 10%. Pancreatic cancers occur twice as frequently in the pancreatic head (70% of cases) as in the body (20%) or tail (10%) of the gland.

With the exception of jaundice, the initial symptoms associated with pancreatic cancer are often insidious and are usually present for >2 months before the cancer is diagnosed (Table 92-1). Pain and weight loss are present in >75% of patients. The pain typically has a gnawing, visceral quality, occasionally radiating from the epigastrium to the back. Pain is often a more severe problem in lesions arising in the body or tail of the gland, as such tumors may become quite large before being detected. Characteristically, the pain improves somewhat when the patient bends forward. The development of significant pain suggests retroperitoneal invasion and infiltration of the splanchnic nerves, indicating that the primary lesion is advanced and is not surgically resectable. Rarely, such pain may be transient and associated with hyperamylasemia, indicative of acute pancreatitis caused by ductal obstruction by tumor. The weight loss observed in most patients is primarily the result of anorexia, although in the initial period of the disease, subclinical malabsorption may also be a contributing factor.

Jaundice due to biliary obstruction is found in >80% of patients having tumors in the pancreatic head and is typically accompanied by dark urine, a claylike appearance of stool, and pruritus. In contrast to the "painless jaundice" sometimes observed in patients having carcinomas of the bile ducts, duodenum, or periampullary regions, most icteric individuals with ductal carcinomas of the pancreatic head will complain of significant abdominal discomfort. Although the gallbladder is usually enlarged in patients with carcinoma of the head of the pancreas, it is palpable in <50% (Courvoisier's sign). However, the presence of an enlarged gallbladder in a jaundiced patient without biliary colic should suggest malignant obstruction of the extrahepatic biliary tree.

Glucose intolerance, presumably a direct consequence of the tumor, often develops within 2 years of the clinical diagnosis. Other initial manifestations include venous thrombosis and migratory thrombophlebitis (Trousseau's syndrome), gastrointestinal hemorrhage from varices due to compression of the portal venous system by tumor, and splenomegaly caused by cancerous encasement of the splenic vein.

DIAGNOSTIC PROCEDURES (Fig. 92-1) Despite the availability of serologic tests for tumor-associated antigens, such as

Table 92-1 Presenting Signs and Symptoms of Pancreatic Carcinoma

Frequent
  Abdominal pain
  Weight loss
  Jaundice (lesions of pancreatic head only)
Infrequent
  Glucose intolerance
  Palpable gallbladder
  Migratory thrombophlebitis
  Gastrointestinal hemorrhage
  Splenomegaly

FIGURE 92-1 Carcinoma of the pancreas. *A.* Sonogram showing pancreatic carcinoma (P), dilated intrahepatic bile ducts (d), dilated portal vein (pv), and inferior vena cava (IVC). *B.* CT scan showing pancreatic carcinoma (*arrow*). *C.* Endoscopic retrograde showing abrupt cutoff of the duct of Wirsung (*arrow*). *D.* Arteriogram showing sheathing of splenic artery by tumor encasement (*arrow*).

the carcinoembryonic antigen (CEA) and CA 19-9, and noninvasive imaging techniques, such as computed tomography (CT) and ultrasonography, the early diagnosis of a potentially resectable pancreatic carcinoma remains extremely difficult. The nonspecificity of the initial symptoms and the poor sensitivity of both serologic assays and noninvasive techniques have frustrated the development of effective screening procedures. When the disease is clinically suspected in a patient having vague, persistent abdominal complaints, ultrasound should be performed to visualize the gallbladder and the pancreas, as well as upper gastrointestinal contrast radiographs to rule out a hiatal hernia or a peptic ulcer. If these studies fail to provide an explanation for the symptoms, a CT scan should be considered. It should encompass not only the pancreas but also the liver, retroperitoneal lymph nodes, and pelvis, as pancreatic cancer frequently spreads within the abdomen. While more costly than ultrasonography, CT is technically simpler, more reproducible, provides better definition of the body and tail of the pancreas, and requires less interpretive skill. CT generally detects a malignant pancreatic lesion in >80% of cases; in 5 to 15% of patients with proven pancreatic carcinoma, the CT scan shows only generalized pancreatic enlargement suggesting pancreatitis rather than malignancy. False-positive results occur in about 5 to 10% of cases where no tumor was found on laparotomy. Magnetic resonance imaging (MRI) has not been shown to be better than CT in the evaluation of pancreatic lesions. The value of positron emission tomography (PET) has not been defined. When clinical circumstances dictate additional diagnostic evaluation, endoscopic retrograde cholangiopancreatography (ERCP) with endoscopic ultrasonography (EUS) may clarify the cause of ambiguous CT or ultrasound findings. The characteristic findings are stenosis or obstruction of either the pancreatic or the common bile duct; both duct systems are abnormal in over half the cases. Carcinoma and chronic pancreatitis can be difficult to dis-

tinguish by ERCP, particularly if both diseases are present. False-negative results with ERCP are infrequent (<5%) and usually occur in the setting of islet cell, rather than ductal, carcinomas.

Selective and superselective angiography may be of value in some patients. Angiography is an effective means of detecting carcinomas in the body and tail of the pancreas by the demonstration of vascular narrowing, displacement, or occlusion by tumor. Angiography is being replaced as a diagnostic and staging procedure by spiral CT scanning with contrast imaging. This high-resolution technology predicts the resectability of the tumor if no disease is found outside the pancreas, obstruction of the superior mesenteric-portal vein confluence is absent, or tumor extension to the celiac axis and superior mesenteric arteries is not found. Radiographic staging criteria are shown in Table 92-2.

Regardless of the results of the above diagnostic studies, a histologic confirmation of pancreatic cancer is mandatory; similar findings can result from other neoplasms such as islet cell tumor or lymphoma, for which the therapeutic approach and prognosis differ from those for ductal carcinoma. In patients with unresectable disease or medical contraindications to surgical resection, tissue may be obtained through a percutaneous needle aspiration biopsy of the pancreas with CT or ultrasonographic guidance.

Unfortunately, however, even laparotomy may not provide a definitive diagnosis, because chronic pancreatitis may also produce a hard mass in the head of the pancreas indistinguishable from carcinoma by palpation. Furthermore, a superficial biopsy of such a mass may not show neoplastic tissue, revealing only evidence of pancreatitis, as the cancer is often surrounded by edematous, inflamed, and fibrotic tissue (i.e., chronic pancreatitis).

℞ **TREATMENT** Complete surgical resection of pancreatic tumors offers the only effective treatment for this disease. Unfortunately, such "curative" operations are only possible in 10 to 15% of

Table 92-2 Clinical (Radiographic) Staging of Pancreatic Cancer

Stage	Clinical/Radiographic Criteria
I	Resectable (T1–T2, selected T3,[a] NX, M0)
	No encasement of celiac axis or SMA
	Patent SMPV confluence
	No extrapancreatic disease
II	Locally advanced (T3, NX–1, M0)
	Arterial encasement (celiac axis or SMA) or venous occlusion (SMV or portal vein)
	No extrapancreatic disease
III	Metastatic (T1–3, NX–1, M1)
	Metastases typically to liver, peritoneum, and occasionally lung

[a] Resectable T3 lesions include those with isolated involvement of the SMV, portal vein, or hepatic artery without encasement of the celiac axis or SMA.

NOTE: T1, restricted to pancreas; T2, extension to duodenum, bile duct, or peripancreatic tissues; T3, extension to stomach, spleen, colon, or adjacent large vessels; NX, nodal status unknown; N0, regional nodes uninvolved; N1, regional nodes involved; M0, metastases absent; M1, metastases present; SMA, superior mesenteric artery; SMPV, superior mesenteric vein confluence with portal vein; SMV, superior mesenteric vein patients with pancreatic cancer, usually those individuals with a tumor in the pancreatic head in whom jaundice was the initial symptom. Patients considered for such a procedure should have no evidence of metastatic spread on a chest radiograph and abdominal-pelvic CT scan and should be operated on by an experienced surgeon, as mortality rates of >15% have been associated with this procedure. Curative resection is usually preceded by laparoscopic inspection of the abdomen to confirm absence of occult disease spread to the omentum, peritoneum, or liver, which would preclude curative resection. Although the potential for cure in patients with pancreatic cancer is restricted to the few who are able to undergo a complete surgical resection, the 5-year survival rate following such operations is only 10%. Nonetheless, the procedure is worth attempting, particularly for lesions in the pancreatic head, since ductal carcinomas often cannot be distinguished preoperatively from ampullary, duodenal, and distal bile duct tumors or pancreatic cyst adenocarcinomas, all of which have far higher rates of resectability and cure. Furthermore, patients who undergo resection and eventually experience disease recurrence survive three to four times longer than those whose tumor is not excised, indicating that such operations have a palliative effect. The risk for tumor recurrence is not affected by the type of operative procedure—i.e., total pancreatectomy versus pancreaticoduodenectomy ("Whipple resection")—but it is increased by the presence of lymph node metastases or tumor invasion into adjacent viscera. As a rule, pancreaticoduodenectomy or distal pancreatectomy seems preferable to total pancreatectomy because of the retention of exocrine function and avoidance of brittle diabetes.

The median survival for patients whose pancreatic cancers are surgically unresectable is 6 months. Management is directed at palliation of symptoms. Ambulatory patients having tumors in the pancreatic head should be considered for surgical diversion of the biliary system. If jaundice has already developed, therapeutic options include either nonoperative biliary decompression by endoscopic or percutaneous, transhepatic biliary drainage or surgical biliary bypass. External beam radiation in patients with unresectable tumors that have not spread beyond the pancreas does not appear to prolong survival, although a sufficient reduction in tumor size may lead to palliation of pain. However, the addition of chemotherapy with fluorouracil (5-FU) to external beam irradiation has increased the survival time for these patients, perhaps because 5-FU acts as a radiosensitizing agent. In a small patient population, a similar combination of radiation therapy and 5-FU appears to have prolonged the survival and increased the cure rate as compared to a prospectively randomized nontreatment control group of patients who had a complete surgical resection of their pancreatic cancer. This observation needs to be confirmed before it can be accepted. The possibility of administering such chemoradiation therapy at diagnosis and before surgery ("neoadjuvant" treatment), to increase the potential for resectability, is under investigation. Intraoperative radiation therapy has the potential to deliver higher doses of radiation to the tumor while sparing neighboring tissues but does not give better results than external beam treatment.

Chemotherapy in the management of patients with widely metastatic pancreatic cancer has been disappointing. Gemcitabine, a deoxycytidine analogue, produces improvement in the quality of life for patients with advanced pancreatic cancer. However, duration of survival is only moderately improved. Newer forms of treatment, including combining gemcitabine with other cytotoxic agents or therapies directed at specific molecular targets, such as K-*ras*, or p53 are being evaluated. Experimental therapy should constitute the initial treatment for consenting, ambulatory patients. →*Pancreatic endocrine tumors are discussed in Chap. 93.*

BIBLIOGRAPHY

Burris HA et al: Improvements in survival and clinical benefit with gemcitabine as first-line therapy for patients with advanced pancreatic cancer. A randomized trial. J Clin Oncol 15:2403, 1997

Conlon KC et al: Long-term survival after curative resection for pancreatic ductal adenocarcinoma. Clinicopathologic analysis of 5-year survivors. Ann Surg 223:273, 1996

Jimenez RE et al: Impact of laparoscopic staging in the treatment of pancreatic cancer. Arch Surg 135:409, 2000

Schnall S, Macdonald JS: Chemotherapy of adenocarcinoma of the pancreas. Semin Oncol 23:220, 1996

Silverman DT et al: Dietary and nutritional factors and pancreatic cancer: A case-control study based on direct interviews. J Natl Cancer Inst 86:1510, 1994

Spitz FR et al: Preoperative and postoperative chemoradiation strategies in patients treated with pancreaticoduodenectomy for adenocarcinoma of the pancreas. J Clin Oncol 15:928, 1997

Yeo CJ et al: Six-hundred-fifty consecutive pancreaticoduodenectomies in the 1990's. Ann Surg 226:248, 1997

93   *Robert T. Jensen*

ENDOCRINE TUMORS OF THE GASTROINTESTINAL TRACT AND PANCREAS

Gastrointestinal neuroendocrine tumors (NETs) are derived from the diffuse neuroendocrine system of the gastrointestinal (GI) tract, which is composed of amine- and acid-producing cells with different hormonal profiles, depending on the site of origin. The tumors they produce can be divided into carcinoid tumors and pancreatic endocrine tumors (PETs). These tumors were originally classified as APUDomas (for *a*mine *p*recursor *u*ptake and *d*ecarboxylation), as were pheochromocytomas, melanomas, and medullary thyroid carcinomas because they share certain cytochemical, pathologic, and biologic features (Table 93-1). APUDomas were thought to have a similar embryonic origin from neural crest cells, but the peptide-secreting cells are not of neuroectodermal origin.

CLASSIFICATION, PATHOLOGY, AND TUMOR BIOLOGY OF NETS

NETs are generally composed of monotonous sheets of small round cells with uniform nuclei; mitoses are uncommon. They can be tentatively identified on routine histology; however, these tumors are principally recognized by their histologic staining patterns due to shared cellular proteins. Historically, silver staining was used, and tumors were classified as showing an argentaffin reaction if they took

Table 93-1   General Characteristics of GI Neuroendocrine Tumors [Carcinoids, Pancreatic Endocrine Tumors (PETs)]

1. Share general neuroendocrine cell markers
   a. Chromogranins (A, B, C) are acidic monomeric soluble proteins found in the large secretory granules; chromogranin A is most widely used
   b. Neuron-specific enolase (NSE) is the γ-γ dimer of the enzyme enolase and is a cytosolic marker of neuroendocrine differentiation
   c. Synaptophysin is an integral membrane glycoprotein of molecular weight 38,000 found in small vesicles of neurons and neuroendocrine tumors
2. Pathologic similarities
   a. All PETs show amine precursor uptake and decarboxylation
   b. Ultrastructurally they have dense-core secretory granules (>80 nm)
   c. Histologically appear similar with few mitoses and uniform nuclei
   d. Frequently synthesize multiple peptides/amines, which can be detected immunocytochemically but may not be secreted
   e. Presence or absence of clinical syndrome or type can not be predicted by immunocytochemical studies
   f. Histologic classifications do not predict biologic behavior; only invasion or metastases establishes malignancy
3. Similarities of biologic behavior
   a. Generally slow growing, but a proportion are aggressive
   b. Secrete biologically active peptides/amines, which can cause clinical symptoms
   c. Generally have high densities of somatostatin receptors, which are used for both localization and treatment

up and reduced silver or as being argyrophilic if they did not reduce it. Immunocytochemical localization of chromogranins (A,B,C), neuron-specific enolase, or synaptophysin, which are all neuroendocrine cell markers, are now used (Table 93-1). Chromogranin A is the most widely used.

Ultrastructurally, these tumors possess electron-dense neurosecretory granules and frequently contain small clear vesicles that correspond to synaptic vesicles of neurons. NETs synthesize numerous peptides, growth factors, and bioactive amines that may be ectopically secreted, giving rise to a specific clinical syndrome (Table 93-2). The diagnosis of the specific syndrome, such as a VIPoma [vasoactive intestinal peptide (VIP)-secreting tumor], requires the clinical features of the disease and cannot be made from the immunocytochemistry results only (Table 93-1). Furthermore, pathologists cannot distinguish between benign and malignant NETs unless metastases or invasion are present.

Carcinoid tumors are frequently classified according to their anatomic area of origin (i.e., foregut, midgut, hindgut) because tumors with similar areas of origin share functional manifestations, histochemistry, and secretory products (Table 93-3). Foregut tumors generally have a low serotonin [5-hydroxytryptamine (5-HT)] content, are argentaffin-negative but argyrophilic, occasionally secrete adrenocorticotropic hormone (ACTH) or 5-hydroxytryptophan (5-HTP) causing an atypical carcinoid syndrome (Fig. 93-1), make several hormones, and may metastasize to bone. They uncommonly produce a clinical syndrome due to the secreted products. Midgut carcinoids are argentaffin-positive, have a high serotonin content, most frequently cause the typical carcinoid syndrome when they metastasize (Table 93-3, Fig. 93-1), release serotonin and tachykinins (substance P, neuropeptide K, substance K), rarely secrete 5-HTP or ACTH, and uncommonly metastasize to bone. Hindgut carcinoids (rectum and transverse and descending colon) are argentaffin-negative, often argyrophilic, rarely contain serotonin or cause the carcinoid syndrome, rarely secrete 5-HTP or ACTH, contain numerous peptides, and may metastasize to bone.

PETs can be classified into specific functional or nonfunctional syndromes (Table 93-2). Each of the functional syndromes is associated with symptoms due to the specific hormone released. In contrast,

Table 93-2   GI Neuroendocrine Tumor Syndromes

Name	Biologically Active Peptide(s) Secreted	Incidence (New Cases/ 10^6 Population Per Year)	Tumor Location	Malignant, %	Associated with MEN-1, %	Main Symptoms/Signs
I. ESTABLISHED SPECIFIC FUNCTIONAL SYNDROME						
Carcinoid Tumor						
Carcinoid syndrome	Serotonin, possibly tachykinins, motilin, prostaglandins	0.5–2	Midgut (75–87%) Foregut (2–33%) Hindgut (1–8%) Unknown (2–15%)	95–100	Rare	Diarrhea (32–84%) Flushing (63–75%) Pain (10–34%) Asthma (4–18%) Heart disease (11–41%)
Pancreatic endocrine tumor						
Zollinger-Ellison syndrome	Gastrin	0.5–1.5	Duodenum (70%) Pancreas (25%) Other sites (5%)	60–90	20–25	Pain (79–100%) Diarrhea (30–75%) Esophageal symptoms (31–56%)
Insulinoma	Insulin	1–2	Pancreas (>99%)	<10	4–5	Hypoglycemic symptoms (100%)
VIPoma (Verner-Morrison syndrome, pancreatic cholera, WDHA)	Vasoactive intestinal peptide	0.05–0.2	Pancreas (90%, adult) Other (10%, neural, adrenal, periganglionic)	40–70	6	Diarrhea (90–100%) Hypokalemia (80–100%) Dehydration (83%)
Glucagonoma	Glucagon	0.01–0.1	Pancreas (100%)	50–80	1–20	Rash (67–90%) Glucose intolerance (38–87%) Weight loss (66–96%)
Somatostatinoma	Somatostatin	Rare	Pancreas (55%) Duodenum-jejunum (44%)	>70	45	Diabetes mellitus (63–90%) Cholelithiases (65–90%) Diarrhea (35–90%)
GRFoma	Growth hormone–releasing hormone	Unknown	Pancreas (30%) Lung (54%) Jejunum (7%) Other (13%)	>60	16	Acromegaly (100%)
ACTHoma	ACTH	Rare	Pancreas (4–16%, all ectopic Cushing's)	>95	Rare	Cushing's syndrome (100%)
PET causing carcinoid syndrome	Serotonin, ? tachykinins	Rare (43 cases)	Pancreas (≤% all carcinoids)	60–88	Rare	Same as carcinoid syndrome above
PET causing hypercalcemia	PTHrP, others unknown	Rare	Pancreas (rare cause of hypercalcemia)	84	Rare	Abdominal pain due to hepatic metastases
II. POSSIBLE SPECIFIC FUNCTIONAL SYNDROME						
PET secreting calcitonin	Calcitonin	Rare	Pancreas (rare cause of hypercalcitonemia)	>80	16	Diarrhea (50%)
III. NO FUNCTIONAL SYNDROME						
PPoma/nonfunctional	None	1–2	Pancreas (100%)	>60	18–44	Weight loss (30–90%) Abdominal mass (10–30%) Pain (30–95%)

NOTE: MEN, multiple endocrine neoplasia; VIPoma, tumor-secreting vasoactive intestinal peptide; WDHA, watery diarrhea, hypokalemia, and achlorhydria syndrome; GRFoma, tumor-secreting growth hormone–releasing factor; ACTH, adrenocorticotrophic hormone; PET, pancreatic endocrine tumor; PTHrP, parathyroid hormone–related protein; PPoma, tumor secreting pancreatic polypeptide.

Table 93-3 Carcinoid Tumor Location, Frequency of Metastases, and Association with the Carcinoid Syndrome

	Location (% of Total)	Incidence of Metastases	Incidence of Carcinoid Syndrome
Foregut			
Esophagus	<1	67	—
Stomach	3.8	31	9.5
Duodenum	2.1	—	3.4
Pancreas	<1	76	20
Gallbladder	<1	56	5
Ampulla	<1	—	—
Larynx	<1	0	—
Bronchus, lung	32.5	27	13
Midgut			
Jejunum	2.3	}70	9
Ileum	17.6		9
Meckel's diverticulum	0.4	—	13
Appendix	7.6	35	<1
Colon	6.3	71	5
Liver	<1	29	—
Ovary	<1	32	50
Testis	<1	—	50
Cervix	<1	67	3
Hindgut			
Rectum	10	14	—

SOURCE: Location and incidence of metastases are from 5468 cases studied from 1973–1991, reported by Modlin and Sandor. Incidence of carcinoid syndrome is from 4349 cases studied from 1950–1971, reported by JD Godwin, Cancer 36:560, 1975.

nonfunctional PETs release no products that cause a specific clinical syndrome. "Nonfunctional" is a misnomer in the strict sense because these tumors frequently ectopically secrete a number of peptides [pancreatic polypeptide (PP) chromogranin A, neurotensin]; however, they cause no specific clinical syndrome. The symptoms caused by nonfunctional PETs are entirely due to the tumor per se.

Carcinoid tumors can occur in almost any GI tissue (Table 93-3);

however, most (70%) originate from one of four sites; bronchus, jejunum/ileum, rectum, or appendix. In the past, carcinoid tumors most frequently occurred in the appendix (i.e., 40%); however, the bronchus/lung is now the most common site (32%). Overall, the GI tract is the most common site for these tumors, comprising 74%, with the respiratory tract a distant second at 25%.

The term *pancreatic endocrine tumor*, although widely used, is also a misnomer, because these tumors can occur either almost exclusively in the pancreas (insulinomas, glucagonomas, nonfunctional PETs, PETs causing hypercalcemia) or at both pancreatic and extrapancreatic sites [gastrinomas, VIPomas, somatostatinomas, GRFomas (GRF, growth hormone–releasing factor)]. PETs are also called *islet cell tumors*; however, this term is discouraged because it is not established that many originate from the islets and many can occur at extrapancreatic sites.

The exact incidence of carcinoid tumors or PETs varies according to whether only symptomatic or all tumors are considered. The incidence of clinically significant carcinoids is 7 to 13 cases per million population per year, whereas malignant carcinoids are reported at autopsy in 21 to 84 cases per million population per year. Clinically significant PETs have a prevalence of 10 cases per million population, with insulinomas, gastrinomas, and nonfunctional PETs having an incidence of 0.5 to 2 cases per million population per year (Table 93-2); VIPomas are 2- to 8-fold less common, glucagonomas are 17- to 30-fold less common, and somatostatinomas the least common. In autopsy studies 0.5 to 1.5% of all cases have a PET; however, in fewer than 1 in 1000 cases was a functional tumor present.

Both carcinoid tumors and PETs commonly show malignant behavior (Tables 93-2, 93-3). With PETs, except for insulinomas in which <10% are malignant, 50 to 100% are malignant. With carcinoid tumors the percentage showing malignant behavior varies in different locations. For the four most common sites of occurrence the incidence of metastases varies greatly: jejunum/ileum (70%) > appendix (35%) > lung/bronchus (27%) > rectum (14%). A number of factors are important in determining survival and the aggressiveness of the tumor (Table 93-4). The presence of liver metastases is the single most im-

Table 93-4 Prognostic Factors in Neuroendocrine Tumors

Both carcinoid tumors and PETs
  Presence of liver metastases ($p < .001$)
  Extent of liver metastases ($p < .001$)
  Presence of lymph node metastases ($p < .001$)
  Depth of invasion ($p < .001$)
  Primary tumor site ($p < .001$)
  Primary tumor size ($p < .005$)
  Various histologic features
    Tumor differentiation ($p < .001$)
    High growth indices (high Ki-67 index, PCNA expression)
    High mitotic counts ($p < .001$)
    Vascular or perineural invasion
    Flow cytometric features (i.e., aneuploidy)
Carcinoid tumors
  Presence of carcinoid syndrome
  Laboratory results [urinary 5-HIAA level ($p < .01$), plasma neuropeptide K ($p < .05$), serum chromogranin A ($p < .01$)]
  Presence of a secondary malignancy
  Male gender ($p < .001$)
  Older age ($p < .01$)
  Mode of discovery (incidental > symptomatic)
PETs
  Ha-Ras oncogene or p53 overexpression
  Female gender
  MEN-1 syndrome absent
  Laboratory findings (increased chromogranin A in some studies; increased gastrin level in gastrinomas)

NOTE: PET, pancreatic endocrine tumor; MEN, multiple endocrine neoplasia; PCNA, proliferating cell nuclear antigen; Ki-67, proliferation-associated nuclear antigen recognized by Ki-67 monoclonal antibody.

FIGURE 93-1 Synthesis, secretion, and metabolism of serotonin (5-HT) in patients with typical and atypical carcinoid syndromes.

Table 93-5 Genetic Syndromes Associated with an Increased Incidence of Neuroendocrine Tumors [NETs: Carcinoids or Pancreatic Endocrine Tumors (PETs)]

Syndrome	Location of Gene Mutation and Gene Product	NETs Seen/Frequency
Multiple endocrine neoplasia type 1 (MEN-1)	11q13 (encodes 610-amino-acid protein, menin)	80–100% develop PETs, (nonfunctional > gastrinoma > insulinoma) Carcinoids: gastric (13–30%), bronchial/thymic (8%)
von Hippel-Lindau disease	3q25 (encodes 213-amino-acid protein)	12–17% develop PETs (almost always nonfunctional)
von Recklinghausen's disease [neurofibromatosis1 (NF-1)]	17q11.2 (encodes 2485-amino-acid protein, neurofibromin)	Duodenal somatostatinomas (usually nonfunctional) Rarely insulinoma, gastrinoma
Tuberous sclerosis	9q34 (TSCI) (encodes 1164-amino-acid protein, hamartin) 16p13 (TSC2) (encodes 1807-amino-acid protein, tuberin)	Uncommonly develop PETs [nonfunctional and functional (insulinoma, gastrinoma)]

portant prognostic factor for both carcinoid tumors and PETs. The size of the primary tumor is particularly important in the development of liver metastases. For example, with small-intestinal carcinoids, which are the most frequent cause of the carcinoid syndrome due to metastatic disease in the liver (Table 93-2), metastases occur in 15 to 25% if the tumor diameter is <1 cm, in 58 to 80% if it is 1 to 2 cm and in >75% if it is >2 cm. The size of the primary tumor has also been shown to be an independent predictor of the development of liver metastases for gastrinomas and other PETs. The presence of lymph node metastases, the depth of invasion, various histologic features (differentiation, mitotic rates, growth indices), and flow cytometric results such as the presence of aneuploidy are all important prognostic factors for the development of metastatic disease. The development of the carcinoid syndrome, older age, male gender, the presence of a symptomatic tumor, or greater increases in a number of tumor markers [5-hydroxyindolacetic acid (5-HIAA), neuropeptide K, chromogranin A] also adversely affect prognosis in patients with carcinoid tumors (Table 93-4). With PETs or gastrinomas, a worse prognosis is associated with female gender, overexpression of the *Ha-Ras* oncogene or p53, the absence of multiple endocrine neoplasia (MEN) type 1, and higher levels of various tumor markers (e.g., chromogranin A, gastrin).

A number of genetic disorders are associated with an increased incidence of neuroendocrine tumors (Table 93-5). Each one is caused by a loss of a possible tumor suppressor gene. The most important is MEN-1, an autosomal dominant disorder due to a defect in a 10-exon gene on 11q13, which encodes for a 610-amino-acid nuclear protein, menin (Chap. 339). In patients with MEN-1, 95 to 100% develop hyperparathyroidism due to parathyroid hyperplasia, 80 to 100% develop nonfunctional PETs, 54 to 80% develop pituitary adenomas, and bronchial carcinoids develop in 8%, thymic carcinoids in 8%, and gastric carcinoids in 13 to 30% of patients with Zollinger-Ellison syndrome. Functional PETs occur in 80% of patients with MEN-1, with 54% developing Zollinger-Ellison syndrome, 21% insulinomas, 3% glucagonomas, and 1% VIPomas. MEN-1 is present in 20 to 25% of all patients with Zollinger-Ellison syndrome, in 4% of those with insulinomas, and in <5% of those with other PETs.

Three phakomatoses associated with NETs are von Hippel–Lindau disease, von Recklinghausen's disease, or neurofibromatosis type 1 (NF-1), and tuberous sclerosis (Bourneville's disease). Von Hippel–Lindau disease is an autosomal dominant disorder due to defects in a gene on chromosome 3p25, which encodes a 213-amino-acid protein that interacts with the elongin family of proteins as a transcriptional regulator and in abnormal protein destruction (Chap. 370). In addition to cerebellar hemangioblastomas, renal cancer, and pheochromocytomas, 10 to 17% of these patients develop a PET. Most are nonfunctional, although insulinomas and VIPomas are reported. Patients with NF-1 have defects in a gene on chromosome 17q11.2 encoding for a 2845-amino-acid protein, neurofibromin, which functions in normal

cells as a suppressor of the Ras signaling cascade (Chap. 370). Up to 12% of these patients develop an upper GI carcinoid tumor, characteristically in the periampullary region (54%). Many of such tumors are classified as somatostatinomas because they contain somatostatin immunocytochemically; however, they seldom produce a clinical somatostatinoma syndrome. NF-1 has rarely been associated with insulinomas and Zollinger-Ellison syndrome. Tuberous sclerosis is caused by mutations that alter either the 1164-amino-acid protein, hamartin (TSC1), or the 1807-amino-acid protein, tuberin (TSC2) (Chap. 370). Both hamartin and tuberin interact in a pathway related to cytosolic G protein regulation. A few cases including nonfunctional and functional PETs (insulinomas and gastrinomas) have been reported (Table 93-5).

Changes in the MEN-1 gene, p16/MTS1 tumor suppressor gene, and DPC 4/Smad 4 gene; amplification of the HER-2/neu protooncogene; and deletions of unknown tumor suppressor genes on chromosomes 1 and 3p may be important in the pathogenesis of PETs. Loss of heterozygosity at the MEN-1 locus on chromosome 11q13 has been found in 93% of sporadic PETs (patients without MEN-1) and in 26 to 75% of sporadic carcinoid tumors. Mutations in the MEN-1 gene were found in 31 to 34% of sporadic gastrinomas.

CARCINOID TUMORS AND CARCINOID SYNDROME

GENERAL TUMOR CHARACTERISTICS OF THE MOST COMMON GI CARCINOID TUMORS   Appendiceal Carcinoids These occur in 1 in every 200 to 300 appendectomies, usually in the appendiceal tip. More than 90% are <1 cm in diameter; 35% have metastases. In one study of 1570 appendiceal carcinoids, 62% were localized and 27% had regional and 8% distant metastases. Half of the carcinoids between 1 and 2 cm in diameter had metastasized to lymph nodes.

Small-Intestinal Carcinoids These are frequently multiple. Between 70 and 80% are present in the ileum and 70% within 60 cm (24 in.) of the ileocecal valve; 40% are <1 cm in diameter, 32% are 1 to 2 cm, and 29% are >2 cm; and 35 to 70% are associated with metastases. They characteristically cause a marked fibrotic reaction, which can lead to intestinal obstruction. Distant metastases occur to liver in 36 to 60% of patients, to bone in 3%, and to lung in 4%. Between 15 and 25% of small (<1 cm) carcinoid tumors of the small intestine have metastases; 58 to 100% of tumors 1 to 2 cm in diameter have metastases. Carcinoids also occur in the duodenum, with 21% having metastases. In one study, no duodenal tumor <1 cm metastasized, whereas 33% of those >2 cm had metastases. Small-intestinal carcinoids are the most common cause (60 to 87%) of the carcinoid syndrome (Table 93-6).

Rectal Carcinoids Rectal carcinoids are found in 1 of every 2500 proctoscopies. Nearly all occur 4 to 13 cm above the dentate line. Most are small, with 66 to 80% being <1 cm in diameter; 5% metastasize. Tumors 1 to 2 cm in diameter metastasize in 5 to 30% of patients, and tumors >2 cm, which are uncommon, in >70%.

Bronchial Carcinoids Bronchial carcinoids are not related to smoking. A number of different classifications of bronchial carcinoid tumors are proposed. In some studies lung NETs are classified into four categories: typical carcinoid (also called bronchial carcinoid tumor, Kulchitsky cell carcinoma-I, KCC-I); atypical carcinoid (also called well-differentiated neuroendocrine carcinoma, KC-II); intermediate small cell neuroendocrine carcinoma; and small cell neuroendocarcinoma (KC-III). Another proposed classification includes three categories of lung NETs: benign or low-grade malignant (typical car-

	At Presentation	During Course of Disease
Symptoms/signs		
Diarrhea	32–73%	68–84%
Flushing	23–65%	63–74%
Pain	10%	34%
Asthma/wheezing	4–8%	3–18%
Pellagra	2%	5%
None	12%	22%
Carcinoid heart disease present	11%	14–41%
Demographics		
Male	46–59%	46–61%
Age		
Mean	57 yrs	52–54 yrs
Range	25–79 yrs	9–91 yrs
Tumor location		
Foregut	5–9%	2–33%
Midgut	78–87%	60–87%
Hindgut	1–5%	1–8%
Unknown	2–11%	2–15%

cinoid); low-grade malignant (atypical carcinoid), and high-grade malignant (poorly differentiated carcinoma of the large cell or small cell type). These different categories of lung NETs have different prognoses, varying from excellent for typical carcinoid to poor for small cell neuroendocrine carcinomas.

Gastric Carcinoids   These account for 3 of every 1000 gastric neoplasms. Three different subtypes of gastric carcinoids are noted. Each originates from gastric enterochromaffin-like (ECL) cells in the gastric mucosa. Two subtypes are associated with hypergastrinemic states: (1) chronic atrophic gastritis (type I) (80% of all gastric carcinoids); and (2) Zollinger-Ellison syndrome, almost always as part of the MEN-1 syndrome (type II) (6% of all cases). These tumors generally pursue a benign course, with 9 to 30% associated with metastases. They are usually multiple and small and infiltrate only to the submucosa. The third subtype of gastric carcinoid (type III) (sporadic) occurs without hypergastrinemia (14% of all carcinoids) and pursues an aggressive course, with 54 to 66% developing metastases. Sporadic carcinoids are usually single, large tumors; 50% have atypical histology and can be a cause of the carcinoid syndrome.

CARCINOID TUMORS WITHOUT THE CARCINOID SYNDROME   The age of patients at diagnosis ranges from 10 to 93 years, with a mean age of 63 years for carcinoid tumors of the small intestine and 66 years for those of the rectum. The presentation is diverse and related to the site of origin and extent of malignant spread. In the appendix, carcinoid tumors are usually found incidentally during surgery for suspected appendicitis. Small-intestinal carcinoids in the jejunum/ileum present with periodic abdominal pain (51%), intestinal obstruction with ileus/invagination (31%), an abdominal tumor (17%), or GI bleeding (11%). Because of the vagueness of the symptoms the diagnosis is usually delayed approximately 2 years from onset of the symptoms, with a range up to 20 years. Duodenal, gastric, and rectal carcinoids are most frequently found by chance at endoscopy. The most common symptoms of rectal carcinoids are melena/bleeding (39%), constipation (17%), and diarrhea (12%). Bronchial carcinoids are frequently discovered as a lesion on a chest radiograph, and 31% of the patients are asymptomatic. Thymic carcinoids present as anterior mediastinal masses, usually on chest radiograph of computed tomography (CT) scan. Ovarian and testicular carcinoids usually present as masses discovered on physical examination or by ultrasound. Metastatic carcinoid tumor in the liver presents frequently as hepatomegaly in a patient who may have minimal symptoms and near-normal liver function test results.

CARCINOID TUMORS WITH SYSTEMIC SYMPTOMS DUE TO SECRETED PRODUCTS   Carcinoid tumors can contain numerous GI peptides: gastrin, insulin, somatostatin, motilin, neurotensin, tachykinins (substance K, substance P, neuropeptide K), glucagon, gastrin-releasing peptide, VIP, PP, other biologically active peptides (ACTH, calcitonin, growth hormone–releasing hormone), prostaglandins, and bioactive amines (serotonin). These substances may or may not be released in sufficient amounts to cause symptoms. In patients with carcinoid tumors, elevated serum levels of PP were found in 43%, motilin in 14%, gastrin in 15%, and VIP in 6%. Foregut carcinoids are more likely to produce various GI peptides than midgut carcinoids. Ectopic ACTH production causing Cushing's syndrome is increasingly seen with foregut carcinoids (respiratory tract primarily), and in some series foregut carcinoid was the most common cause of the ectopic ACTH syndrome, accounting for 64% of all cases. Acromegaly due to GRF release occurs with foregut carcinoids, as does the somatostatinoma syndrome with duodenal carcinoids. The most common systemic syndrome is the carcinoid syndrome.

CARCINOID SYNDROME   **Clinical Features**   The cardinal features at presentation as well as during the disease course are shown in Table 93-6. Flushing and diarrhea are the two most common symptoms, occurring in up to 73% initially and in up to 89% during the course of the disease. The characteristic flush is of sudden onset: it is a deep red or violaceous erythema of the upper body (especially the neck and face), often associated with a feeling of warmth, and occasionally associated with pruritus, lacrimation, diarrhea, or facial edema. Flushes may be precipitated by stress, alcohol, exercise, or certain foods such as cheese or by certain agents such as catecholamines, pentagastrin, and serotonin reuptake inhibitors. Flushing episodes may be brief, lasting 2 to 5 min, especially initially, or they may last for hours, especially later in the disease course. Flushing is usually seen with midgut carcinoids but can also occur with foregut carcinoids. With bronchial carcinoids the flushes are frequently prolonged for hours to days, reddish in color, and associated with salivation, lacrimation, diaphoresis, diarrhea, and hypotension. The flush associated with gastric carcinoids is also reddish in color but patchy in distribution over the face and neck. It may be provoked by food and have accompanying pruritus.

Diarrhea is present in 32 to 73% of patients initially and in 68 to 84% at some time in the disease course. Diarrhea usually occurs with flushing (85% of cases). The diarrhea is usually watery, with 60% having <1 L per day or diarrhea. Steatorrhea is present in 67%, and in 46% it is >15 g/day (normal <7 g). Abdominal pain may be present with the diarrhea or independently in 10 to 34% of cases.

Cardiac manifestations occur in 11% of patients initially and in 14 to 41% at some time in the disease course. The cardiac disease is due to fibrosis involving the endocardium, primarily on the right side, although left side lesions can occur also. The dense fibrous deposits are most common on the ventricular aspect of the tricuspid valve and less common on the pulmonary valve cusps. They can result in constriction of the valves and pulmonic stenosis is usually predominant, whereas the tricuspid valve is often fixed open, resulting in regurgitation. Up to 80% of patients with cardiac lesions develop heart failure. Lesions on the left side are much less extensive, are found in 30% at autopsy, and most frequently affect the mitral valve.

Other clinical manifestations include wheezing or asthma-like symptoms (8 to 18%) and pellagra-like skin lesions (2 to 25%). A variety of noncardiac problems due to increased fibrous tissue have been reported, including retroperitoneal fibrosis causing urethral obstruction, Peyronie's disease of the penis, intrabdominal fibrosis, and occlusion of the mesenteric arteries or veins.

Pathobiology   In different studies covering 8876 patients with carcinoid tumors, carcinoid syndrome occurred in 8%, with a range of 1.4 to 18.4%. It occurs only when sufficient concentrations of tumor-secreted products reach the systemic circulation. In 91% of cases this occurs after metastasis to the liver. Rarely, the carcinoid syndrome can occur without hepatic metastases, caused by primary gut carcinoids with nodal metastases with extensive retroperitoneal invasion, pancreatic carcinoids with retroperitoneal lymph nodes, or carcinoids of the lung or ovary with direct access to the systemic circulation. All carcinoid tumors do not have the same propensity to metastasize and cause the carcinoid syndrome (Table 93-3). Midgut carcinoids account for 60 to 67% of cases of carcinoid syndrome, foregut tumors for 2 to 33%, hindgut for 1 to 8%, and unknown primary sites for 2 to 15%.

One of the main secretory products of carcinoid tumors involved in the carcinoid syndrome is serotonin [5-hydroxytryptamine (5-HT)] (Fig. 93-1), which is synthesized from tryptophan. Up to 50% of dietary tryptophan can be used in this synthetic pathway by tumor cells, which can result in inadequate supplies for conversion to niacin; hence 2 to 5% of patients can develop pellagra-like lesions. Serotonin has numerous biologic effects including stimulating intestinal secretion, inhibiting absorption, stimulating increases in intestinal motility, and stimulating fibrogenesis. While 56 to 88% of carcinoid tumors are associated with serotonin overproduction, 12 to 26% of patients do not have the carcinoid syndrome. Serotonin overproduction is noted in 90 to 100% of patients with the carcinoid syndrome. Serotonin is thought to be predominantly responsible for the diarrhea by its effects on gut motility and intestinal secretion. Serotonin receptor antagonists (especially 5-HT$_3$ antagonists) relieve the diarrhea in most patients. Prostaglandin E$_2$ and tachykinins may be important mediators of the diarrhea in some patients. Flushing is not relieved by serotonin receptor antagonists. In patients with gastric carcinoids the red, patchy pruritic flush is likely due to histamine release because it can be prevented by H$_1$ and H$_2$ receptor antagonists. Numerous studies show tachykinins are stored in carcinoid tumors and released during flushing. Octreotide can relieve the flushing induced by pentagastrin in these patients without altering stimulated increase in plasma substance P, suggesting other mediators must be involved in the flushing. Both histamine and serotonin may be responsible for the wheezing as well as the fibrotic reactions involving the heart, causing Peyronie's disease and intraabdominal fibrosis. The exact mechanism of the heart disease is unclear. The valvular heart disease caused by the appetite-suppressant drug, dexfenfluramine, is histologically indistinguishable from that observed in carcinoid disease or after long exposure to 5-HT$_2$-selective ergot drugs. Metabolites of fenfluramine have high affinity for 5-HT$_2$ receptors, whose activation is known to cause fibroblast mitogenesis. Lastly, high levels of 5-HT$_{2B}$ and 5-HT$_{2C}$ receptor transcripts are known to occur in heart valves. These observations support the conclusion that serotonin overproduction is important for the valvular changes, possibly by activating 5-HT$_2$ receptors in the endocardium.

Patients may develop either a typical or atypical carcinoid syndrome (Fig. 93-1). In patients with the typical form, characteristically caused by a midgut carcinoid tumor, the conversion of tryptophan to 5-HTP is the rate-limiting step. 5-HTP is rapidly converted to 5-HT and stored in secretory granules of the tumor or in platelets. A small amount remains in plasma and is converted to 5-HIAA, which appears in large amounts in the urine. These patients have an expanded serotonin pool size, increased blood and platelet serotonin levels, and increased urinary 5-HIAA. Some carcinoid tumors cause an atypical carcinoid syndrome thought to be due to a deficiency in the enzyme dopa decarboxylase; thus, 5-HTP cannot be converted to 5-HT (serotonin) and is secreted into the bloodstream. In these patients, plasma serotonin levels are normal but urinary levels may be increased because some 5-HTP is converted to 5-HT in the kidney. Characteristically, urinary 5-HTP and 5-HT are increased, but urinary 5-HIAA levels are only slightly elevated. Foregut carcinoids are the most likely to cause an atypical carcinoid syndrome.

One of the most life-threatening complications of the carcinoid syndrome is the development of a carcinoid crisis. This is more frequent in patients who have intense symptoms from foregut tumors or have greatly increased urinary 5-HIAA levels (i.e., >200 mg/d). The crisis may occur spontaneously or be provoked by stress, anesthesia, chemotherapy, or a biopsy. Patients develop intense flushing, diarrhea, abdominal pain, and cardiac abnormalities including tachycardia, hypertension, or hypotension. If not adequately treated, it can be fatal.

Diagnosis The diagnosis of carcinoid syndrome relies on measurement of urinary or plasma serotonin or its metabolites in the urine. The measurement of 5-HIAA is most frequently used. False-positive elevations may occur if the patient is eating serotonin-rich foods (e.g., bananas, pineapple, walnuts, pecans, avocados, or hickory nuts) or taking certain medications (e.g., cough syrup containing guaifanesin, acetaminophen, salicylates, or L-dopa). The normal range in daily urinary 5-HIAA excretion is between 2 and 8 mg. The 5-HIAA level has a 73% sensitivity and 100% specificity for carcinoid syndrome.

Most physicians use only the urinary 5-HIAA excretion rate; however, plasma and platelet serotonin levels, if available, may give additional information. Platelet serotonin levels are more sensitive than urinary 5-HIAA but are not generally available. If an atypical carcinoid syndrome is suspected and the urinary 5-HIAA is minimally elevated or normal, other urinary metabolites of tryptophan such as 5-HTP or 5-HT should be measured.

Flushing occurs in a number of other conditions or diseases including systemic mastocytosis; chronic myelogenous leukemia with increased histamine release; menopause; reactions to alcohol or glutamate; and side effects of chlorpropamide, calcium channel blockers, and nicotinic acid. None of these conditions cause an increase in urinary 5-HIAA.

The diagnosis of carcinoid tumor can be suggested by the carcinoid syndrome, by recurrent abdominal symptoms in a healthy-appearing individual, or by discovering hepatomegaly or hepatic metastases associated with minimal symptoms. Ileal carcinoids, which make up 25% of all clinically detected carcinoids, should be suspected in patients with bowel obstruction, abdominal pain, flushing, or diarrhea.

Serum chromogranin A levels are elevated in 50 to 100% of patients with carcinoid tumors, and the level correlates with tumor bulk. Serum chromogranin A levels are not specific for carcinoid tumors because they are also elevated in patients with PETs and other NETs. Plasma neuron-specific enolase levels are also used as a marker of carcinoid tumors but are less sensitive than chromogranin A, being increased in only 17 to 47% of patients.

TREATMENT Carcinoid Syndrome Treatment includes avoiding conditions that precipitate flushing, dietary supplementation with nicotinamide, treatment of heart failure with diuretics, treatment of wheezing with oral bronchodilators, and controlling the diarrhea with antidiarrheal agents such as loperamide or diphenoxylate. If patients still have symptoms, serotonin receptor antagonists or somatostatin analogues are the drugs of choice.

There are 14 subclasses of serotonin (5-HT) receptors, and antagonists for most are not available. The 5-HT$_1$ and 5-HT$_2$ receptor antagonists methysergide, cyproheptadine, and ketanserin have all been used to control the diarrhea but usually do not decrease flushing. The use of methysergide is limited because it can cause or enhance retroperitoneal fibrosis. Ketanserin diminishes diarrhea in 30 to 100% of patients. 5-HT$_3$ receptor antagonists (ondansetron, tropisetron, alosetron) can control diarrhea and nausea in up to 100% of patients and occasionally ameliorate the flushing. A combination of histamine H$_1$ and H$_2$ receptor antagonists (i.e., diphenhydramine and cimetidine or ranitidine) may control flushing in patients with foregut carcinoids.

Synthetic analogues of somatostatin (octreotide, lanreotide) are now the most widely used agents to control the symptoms of patients with carcinoid syndrome (Fig. 93-2). These drugs are effective at relieving symptoms and decreasing urinary 5-HIAA levels when self-administered every 6 to 12 h. Octreotide controls symptoms in >80% of patients, including the diarrhea and flushing, and 70% of patients show a >50% decrease in urinary 5-HIAA excretion. Patients with mild to moderate symptoms should initially be treated with 100 μg subcutaneously every 8 h. Individual responses vary, and patients have received doses as high as 3000 μg/d. About 40% of patients escape control after a median of 4 months, and the dose may need to be increased. Similar results are reported with lanreotide.

In patients with carcinoid crises, somatostatin analogues are effective at both treating the condition as well as preventing its development

FIGURE 93-2 Structure of somatostatin and synthetic analogues used for diagnostic or therapeutic indications. DOTA, 1,4,7,10-tetra-azacylododecane-N, N', N'', N'''-tetracetic acid.

during known precipitating events such as surgery, anesthesia, chemotherapy, or stress. It is recommended that octreotide (150 to 250 μg subcutaneously every 6 to 8 h) be used 24 to 48 h before anesthesia and then continued throughout the procedure.

Sustained-release preparations of both octreotide [octreotide-LAR (long-acting release)] and lanreotide [lanreotide-PR (prolonged release)] are useful. Octreotide-LAR (30 mg/month) gives a plasma level $\geq$1 ng/mL for 25 days, whereas this level would require three to six injections per day of the non-sustained-release form. Lanreotide-PR is given intramuscularly every 10 to 14 days. Both sustained-release forms are highly effective.

Short-term side effects occur in 40 to 60% of patients receiving subcutaneous somatostatin analogues. Pain at the injection site and GI side effects (59% discomfort, 15% nausea, diarrhea) are the most common. They are usually short-lived and do not interrupt treatment. Important long-term side effects include gallstone formation, steatorrhea, and poor glucose tolerance. The overall incidence of gallstones/biliary sludge is 52%, with 7% of patients having symptomatic disease requiring surgical treatment.

Interferon α is effective in controlling symptoms of the carcinoid syndrome, either alone or combined with hepatic artery embolization. The response rate is 42% for interferon α alone; when given with hepatic artery embolization, diarrhea was controlled for 1 year in 43% and flushing in 86% of patients.

Hepatic artery embolization alone or with chemotherapy (chemoembolization) has been used to control the symptoms of carcinoid syndrome. Embolization alone controls symptoms in up to 76% of patients, and chemoembolization (5-fluorouracil, doxorubicin, cisplatin, mitomycin) in 60 to 75% of patients. Hepatic artery embolization can have major side effects including nausea, vomiting, pain, and fe-

ver. In two studies, between 5 and 7% of patients died from complications of hepatic artery occlusion.

Other drugs have been used successfully in small numbers of patients to control the symptoms of carcinoid syndrome. Parachlorophenylalanine can inhibit tryptophan hydroxylase and the conversion of tryptophan to 5-HTP (Fig. 93-1). However, its severe side effects, including psychiatric disturbances, make it intolerable for long-term use. α-Methyldopa inhibits the conversion of 5-HTP to 5-HT; however, its effects are only partial.

Carcinoid Tumors (Nonmetastatic) Surgery is the only potentially curative therapy. Because the probability of metastases increases with increasing primary tumor size, the extent of surgical resection is determined accordingly. With appendiceal carcinoids, simple appendectomy is curative. With rectal carcinoids <1 cm, local resection is curative. With small-intestinal carcinoids <1 cm there is no consensus. Because 15 to 69% of small-intestinal carcinoids this size have metastases, some recommend a wide resection with *en bloc* resection of the adjacent lymph-bearing mesentery. If the carcinoid tumor is >2 cm for rectal, appendiceal, or small intestine, a full cancer operation should be done, including a right hemicolectomy for appendiceal carcinoid, an abdominoperineal or low anterior resection for rectal carcinoids, and an *en bloc* resection of adjacent lymph nodes for small-intestinal carcinoids. For carcinoids 1 to 2 cm in diameter in the appendix, a simple appendectomy is proposed by some, whereas others favor a right hemicolectomy. For 1- to 2-cm rectal carcinoids, a wide local full-thickness excision is recommended.

With type I or II gastric carcinoids, which are usually <1 cm, endoscopic removal is recommended. In type I or II gastric carcinoids if the tumor is >2 cm or if there is local invasion, some recommend total gastrectomy, others recommend antrectomy in type 1. For types I and II gastric carcinoids 1 to 2 cm, some recommend endoscopic treatment, others surgical treatment. With type III gastric carcinoids, if >2 cm, excision and regional lymph node clearance is recommended. Most tumors <1 cm are treated endoscopically.

PANCREATIC ENDOCRINE TUMORS

Functional PETs usually present with symptoms due to hormone excess. Only late in the course of the disease does the tumor itself cause prominent symptoms such as abdominal pain. In contrast, all of the symptoms due to *nonfunctional* PETs are due to the tumor. Thus, some functional PETs may present with severe symptoms with a small or undetectable primary tumor, whereas nonfunctional tumors almost always present late in their course when they are large and often metastatic. The mean delay between onset of continuous symptoms and diagnosis of a functional PET syndrome is 4 to 7 years. Therefore, the diagnoses are frequently missed for extended periods of time.

Treatment of PETs requires two different strategies. Treatment must be directed at the hormone excess state, such as the gastric acid hypersecretion in gastrinomas or hypoglycemia in insulinomas. Ectopic hormone secretion usually causes the presenting symptoms and can cause life-threatening complications. Except for insulinomas, 50% are malignant (Table 93-2); therefore treatment must also be directed against the tumor per se. These tumors are frequently not curable by surgery due to the extent of disease. Individual PETs are discussed below.

GASTRINOMA (ZOLLINGER-ELLISON SYNDROME) (See also Chap. 285) A gastrinoma is a NET secreting gastrin, a hormone that causes gastric acid hypersecretion (Zollinger-Ellison syndrome). The chronic hypergastrinemia results in marked gastric acid hypersecretion and growth of the gastric mucosa, with increased numbers of parietal cells and proliferation of gastric ECL cells. The gastric acid hypersecretion characteristically causes peptic ulcer disease, often refractory and severe, as well as diarrhea. The most common presenting symptoms are abdominal pain (70 to 100%), diarrhea (37 to 73%), and gastroesophageal reflux disease (GERD) (30 to 35%) and 10 to 20% have diarrhea only. Although peptic ulcers may occur in unusual locations, most patients have a typical duodenal ulcer. The diagnosis of gastrinoma should be considered in patients with peptic ulcer disease with diarrhea; with peptic ulcers in an unusual or in multiple locations; and with peptic ulcer disease that is refractory to treatment or persistent, associated with prominent gastric folds, associated with findings suggestive of MEN-1 (hyperparathyroidism, family history of ulcer or endocrinopathy, pituitary tumors), or without *Helicobacter pylori* present. *H. pylori* is present in >90% of patients with idiopathic peptic ulcers but is present in <50% of patients with gastrinomas. Chronic unexplained diarrhea should also suggest gastrinoma.

About 20 to 25% of patients have MEN-1, and in most cases the hyperparathyroidism is present before the gastrinoma. These patients are treated differently from those without MEN-1; therefore, MEN-1 should be sought in all patients by family history and by measuring plasma calcium and plasma hormones (parathormone, growth hormone, prolactin).

Most gastrinomas (50 to 70%) are present in the duodenum, followed by the pancreas (20 to 40%) and other intraabdominal sites (mesentery, lymph nodes, biliary tract, liver, stomach, ovary). Gastrinomas may also occur in the left ventricular septum. In MEN-1 the gastrinomas are also usually in the duodenum (70 to 90%), followed by the pancreas (10 to 30%), and they are almost always multiple. Between 60 and 90% of gastrinomas are malignant (Table 93-2) with metastatic spread to lymph nodes and liver. Distant metastases to bone occur in 12 to 30% of patients with liver metastases.

Diagnosis   The diagnosis of gastrinoma requires the demonstration of fasting hypergastrinemia and an increased basal gastric acid output (BAO; hyperchlorhydria). More than 98% of patients with gastrinomas have fasting hypergastrinemia, although in 40 to 60% the level may be less than 10 times normal. Therefore, when the diagnosis is suspected, a fasting gastrin level should be determined first. Gastric acid–suppressant drugs such as proton pump inhibitors (omeprazole, pantoprazole, lansoprazole) can suppress acid secretion sufficiently to cause hypergastrinemia and need to be discontinued for a week before the gastrin determination. If the gastrin level is elevated, document that the gastric pH <2.5; hypergastrinemia secondary to achlorydria (atrophic gastritis, pernicious anemia) is one of the most common causes of hypergastrinemia. If the fasting gastrin is >1000 ng/L; 10 times normal) and the pH <2.5, which occurs in 40 to 60% of patients with gastrinoma, the diagnosis is established after ruling out the possibility of retained antrum syndrome by history. In patients with hypergastrinemia with fasting gastrins <1000 ng/L and gastric pH <2.5, other conditions such as *H. pylori* infections, antral G cell hyperplasia/hyperfunction, gastric outlet obstruction, or, rarely, renal failure can masquerade as a gastrinoma. To establish the diagnosis in this group, a determination of BAO and a secretin provocative test should be done. In >80% of patients with gastrinomas, BAO is elevated, i.e., 15 meq/h, and the secretin provocative test is positive, i.e., >200 ng/L increase in serum gastrin level.

℞ **TREATMENT**   The gastric acid hypersecretion in patients with gastrinomas can be controlled in almost every case by oral gastric antisecretory drugs. Because of their long duration of action and potency, the proton pump inhibitors (H^+,K^+-ATPase inhibitors) are the drugs of choice. Histamine H_2-receptor antagonists are also effective, although more frequent dosing (every 4 to 8 h) and high doses are frequently required. In patients with MEN-1 with hyperparathyroidism, correction of the hyperparathyroidism increases the sensitivity to gastric antisecretory drugs and decreases the basal acid output.

With the increased ability to control acid hypersecretion, >50% of the patients who are not cured (>60% of patients) will die from tumor-related causes. At presentation, careful imaging studies are essential to localize the extent of the tumor (see below). About one-third of patients present with hepatic metastases; in <15% of those with hepatic metastases, the disease is limited so that surgical resection may be possible. Surgical cure is possible in 30% of all patients without MEN-1 or liver metastases (40% of all patients). In patients with MEN-1, long-term surgical cure is rare because the tumors are multiple, frequently with lymph node metastases. Therefore, all patients with gastrinomas without MEN-1 or a medical condition limiting life expectancy should undergo surgery.

INSULINOMAS   Insulinomas are endocrine tumors of the pancreas thought to be derived from β cells that autonomously secrete insulin, which results in hypoglycemia. The average age of occurrence is in persons 40 to 50 years old. The most common clinical symptoms are due to the effect of the hypoglycemia on the central nervous system (neuroglycemic symptoms) and include confusion, headache, disorientation, visual difficulties, irrational behavior, or even coma (Chap. 334). Also, most patients have symptoms due to excess catecholamine release secondary to the hypoglycemia, including sweating, tremor, and palpitations. Characteristically these attacks are associated with fasting.

Insulinomas are generally small (>90% are <2 cm in diameter), usually solitary (90%), and only 5 to 15% are malignant. They almost invariably occur only in the pancreas, distributed equally in the pancreatic head, body and tail. Insulinomas should be suspected in all patients with hypoglycemia, especially with a history suggesting attacks provoked by fasting or with a family history of MEN-1. Insulin is synthesized as proinsulin, which consists of a 21-amino-acid α chain and a 30-amino-acid β chain connected by a 33-amino-acid connecting peptide (C peptide). In insulinomas, in addition to elevated plasma insulin levels, elevated plasma proinsulin levels are found and C-peptide levels can be elevated.

Diagnosis   The diagnosis of insulinoma requires the demonstration of an elevated plasma insulin level at the time of hypoglycemia. Other causes of fasting hypoglycemia include inadvertent or surreptitious use of insulin or oral hypoglycemic agents, severe liver disease, alcoholism, poor nutrition, or other extrapancreatic tumors. The most reliable test for diagnosing insulinoma is a fast up to 72 h with serum glucose, C-peptide, and insulin measurements every 4 to 8 h. If at any point the patient becomes symptomatic or glucose levels are persistently <2.2 mmol/L (40 mg/dL), the test should be terminated and repeat samples for the above studies obtained before glucose is given. Some 70 to 80% of patients will develop hypoglycemia during the first 24 h and 98% by 48 h. In nonobese normal subjects, serum insulin levels should decrease to >43 pmol/L (6 μU/mL) when blood glucose decreases to ≤2.2 mmol/L (40 mg/dL) and the ratio of insulin to glucose is <0.3 (in mg/dL). In addition to having an insulin level >6 μU/ml when blood glucose is ≤40 mg/dL, some investigators also require elevated C-peptide and serum proinsulin levels and/or insulin: glucose ratio >0.3 for the diagnosis of insulinoma. The effects of surreptitious use of insulin or hypoglycemic agents may be difficult to distinguish from the symptoms of insulinomas. The combination of proinsulin levels (normal in exogenous insulin/hypoglycemic agent users), C-peptide levels (low in exogenous insulin users), antibodies to insulin (positive in exogenous insulin users), and sulfonylurea levels in serum or plasma will allow the correct diagnosis to be made.

℞ **TREATMENT**   Only 5 to 15% of insulinomas are malignant; therefore, after appropriate imaging, surgery should be performed. Between 75 and 95% of patients are cured by surgery. Before surgery the hypoglycemia can be controlled by frequent small meals and the use of diazoxide (150 to 800 mg/d). Diazoxide is a benozthiadiazide whose hyperglycemic effect is attributed to inhibition of insulin release; 50 to 60% of patients respond to diazoxide. Its side effects are sodium retention and GI symptoms such as nausea. Other agents effective in some patients to control the hypoglycemia include verapamil and diphenylhydantoin. Long-acting somatostatin analogues such as octreotide are acutely effective in 40% of patients. However, octreotide needs to be used with care because it inhibits growth hormone secretion and can lower plasma glucagon levels and so worsen the hypoglycemia.

For the 5 to 15% of patients with malignant insulinomas, the above drugs or somatostatin analogues are used initially. If they are not effective, hepatic arterial embolization, chemoembolization, or chemotherapy have been used. These will be discussed below.

GLUCAGONOMAS Glucagonomas are endocrine tumors of the pancreas that secrete excessive amounts of glucagon that causes a distinct syndrome characterized by dermatitis, glucose intolerance or diabetes, and weight loss. Glucagonomas mainly occur in persons between 45 and 70 years old. They are heralded clinically by a characteristic dermatitis (migratory necrolytic erythema; in 67 to 90%), accompanied by glucose intolerance (40 to 90%), weight loss (66 to 96%), anemia (33 to 85%), diarrhea (15 to 29%), and thromboembolism (11 to 24%). The characteristic rash usually starts as an annular erythema at intertriginous and periorificial sites, especially in the groin or buttock. It subsequently becomes raised and bullae form; when the bullae rupture, eroded areas form. The lesions can wax and wane. A characteristic laboratory finding is hypoaminoacidemia, which occurs in 26 to 100% of patients.

Glucagonomas are generally large tumors at diagnosis, with an average size of 5 to 10 cm. Between 50 and 80% occur in the pancreatic tail and 50 to 82% have evidence of metastatic spread at presentation, usually to the liver. Glucagonomas are rarely extrapancreatic and usually occur singly.

Diagnosis The diagnosis is confirmed by demonstrating an increased plasma glucagon level [normal is <150 ng/L]. In one study plasma glucagon levels were >1000 ng/L in 90%, between 500 and 1000 ng/L in 7%, and <500 ng/L in 3%. A plasma glucagon level >1000 ng/L is considered diagnostic. Other diseases causing increased plasma glucagon levels include renal failure, acute pancreatitis, hypercortisolism, hepatic failure, prolonged fasting, or familial hyperglucagonemia. Except for cirrhosis, these disorders do not usually increase plasma glucagon to >500 ng/L.

TREATMENT Metastases are present at presentation in 50 to 80% of patients, so curative surgical resection is not possible. Surgical debulking in patients with advanced disease or other antitumor treatments may be beneficial (see below). Long-acting somatostatin analogues (octreotide, lanreotide) improve the skin rash in 75% of patients and may improve the weight loss, pain, and diarrhea but not the glucose intolerance.

SOMATOSTATINOMA SYNDROME Somatostatinomas are endocrine tumors that secrete excessive amounts of somatostatin, which causes a syndrome characterized by diabetes melitus, gallbladder disease, diarrhea, and steatorrhea. The mean age of onset is 51 years. Somatostatinomas occur primarily in the pancreas and small intestine, and the frequency of the symptoms differs in each. The usual symptoms are more frequent in pancreatic than intestinal somatostatinomas: diabetes mellitus (95% vs. 21%), gallbladder disease (94% vs. 43%), diarrhea (92% vs. 38%), steatorrhea (83% vs. 12%), hypochlorhydria (86% vs. 12%), and weight loss (90% vs. 69%). Somatostatinomas occur in the pancreas in 56 to 74% of cases, with the primary location being in the pancreatic head. The tumors are usually solitary (90%) and large (mean diameter, 4.5 cm). Liver metastases are present in 69 to 84% of patients.

Somatostatin is a tetradecapeptide (Fig. 93-2), widely distributed in the central nervous system and gastrointestinal tract where it functions as a neurotransmitter or has paracrine and autocrine actions. It is a potent inhibitor of many processes, including release of almost all hormones, acid secretion, intestinal and pancreatic secretion, and intestinal absorption. Most of the clinical manifestations are directly related to these inhibitory actions.

Diagnosis In most cases somatostatinomas have been found incidentally either at the time of cholecystectomy or during endoscopy. The presence of psammoma bodies in a duodenal tumor should particularly raise suspicion. Duodenal somatostatin-containing tumors are increasingly associated with von Recklinghausen's disease. Most of these do not cause the somatostatinoma syndrome as patients are usually asymptomatic and have normal plasma somatostatin levels. The diagnosis of somatostatinoma requires elevated plasma somatostatin levels.

TREATMENT Pancreatic tumors are frequently metastatic at presentation (70 to 92%), whereas 30 to 69% of small-intestinal somatostatinomas have metastases. Symptoms are improved by octreotide treatment (Fig. 93-2).

VIPOMAS VIPomas are endocrine tumors that secrete excessive amounts of VIP, which causes a distinct syndrome characterized by large-volume diarrhea, hypokalemia, and dehydration. This syndrome is also called Verner-Morrison syndrome, pancreatic cholera, or WDHA syndrome (*w*atery *d*iarrhea, *h*ypokalemia, and *a*chlorhydria), which some patients develop. The mean age of patients is 49 years; however, the syndrome can occur in children; when it does, it is usually caused by a ganglioneuroma or ganglioneuroblastoma.

The principal symptoms are large-volume diarrhea (in 100%) severe enough to cause hypokalemia (80 to 100%), dehydration (83%), hypochlorhydria (54 to 76%), and flushing (20%). The diarrhea is secretory in nature, persists during fasting, and is almost always >1 L per day and >3 L per day in 70%. Most patients do not have accompanying steatorrhea (16%), and the increased stool volume is due to increased excretion of sodium and potassium, which, with the anions, accounts for the osmolality of the stool. Patients frequently have hyperglycemia (25 to 50%) and hypercalcemia (25 to 50%).

VIP is a 28-amino-acid peptide neurotransmitter, ubiquitously present in the central nervous system and GI tract. Its known actions include stimulation of small-intestinal chloride secretion as well as effects on smooth-muscle contractility, inhibition of acid secretion, and vasodilatory effects which explain most features of the clinical syndrome.

In adults 80 to 90% of VIPomas are pancreatic; VIP-secreting pheochromocytomas, intestinal carcinoids, and occasional ganglioneuromas account for the rest. These tumors are usually single; 50 to 75% are in the pancreatic tail and 37 to 68% have hepatic metastases at diagnosis.

Diagnosis The diagnosis requires the demonstration of an elevated plasma VIP level and the presence of large-volume diarrhea. A stool volume of <700 mL/day excludes the diagnosis of VIPoma. A number of causes of diarrhea can be excluded by fasting the patient. Other diseases that can cause secretory large-volume diarrhea include gastrinomas, chronic laxative abuse, carcinoid syndrome, systemic mastocytosis, diabetic diarrhea, AIDS, and rarely medullary thyroid cancer. Of these conditions, only VIPomas causes a marked increase in plasma VIP.

TREATMENT The most important initial treatment in these patients is to correct their dehydration, hypokalemia, and electrolyte losses with fluid and electrolyte replacement. Patients may require 5 L/day of fluid and >350 mmol/day (350 meq/day) of potassium. Because 37 to 68% of adults with VIPomas have metastatic disease in the liver at presentation, a significant number of patients cannot be cured surgically. In these patients, long-acting somatostatin analogues such as octreotide or lanreotide (Fig. 93-2) are the drugs of choice.

Octreotide will control the diarrhea in 87% of patients. In nonresponsive patients, the combination of glucocorticoids and octreotide has proved helpful in a few. Other drugs that may be helpful include prednisone (60 to 100 mg/d), clonidine, indomethacin, phenothiazines, loperamide, lidamidine, lithium, proparanolol, and metoclopramide. Treatment of advanced disease with embolization, chemoembolization, and chemotherapy may also be helpful (see below).

NONFUNCTIONAL PANCREATIC ENDOCRINE TUMORS Nonfunctional PETs are endocrine tumors that originate in the pancreas and either secrete no products or their secreted products do not cause a specific clinical syndrome. The symptoms are due entirely to the tumor per se. Nonfunctional PETs almost always secrete chromogranin A (90 to 100%), chromogranin B (90 to 100%), PP (58%), α-human chorionic gonadotropin (hCG) (40%), and β-HCG (20%), but none cause a specific syndrome. Patients with nonfunctional PETs usually present late in their disease course with invasive tumors and hepatic metastases (in 64 to 92%), and the tumors are usually large (72% >5 cm). These tumors are usually solitary except in patients with MEN-1, where they are multiple; they occur primarily in the pancreatic head; and though they do not cause a functional syndrome, they synthesize numerous peptides and cannot be distinguished from functional tumors by immunocytomchemistry.

The most common symptoms are abdominal pain (30 to 80%), jaundice (20 to 35%), and weight loss, fatigue, or bleeding; 10 to 15% are found incidentally. The average time from the beginning of symptoms to diagnosis is 5 years.

Diagnosis The diagnosis is established by histology in a patient with a PET without either clinical symptoms or elevated plasma hormone levels of one of the established syndromes (Table 93-2). Even though chromogranin A levels are elevated in almost every patient, this can be found in functional PETs, carcinoids, and other neuroendocrine disorders. Plasma PP is increased in 22 to 71% of patients and should suggest the diagnosis in a patient with a pancreatic mass because it is usually normal in patients with pancreatic adenocarcinomas. However, elevated plasma PP is not diagnostic of this tumor because it is elevated in a number of other conditions such as chronic renal failure, old age, inflammatory conditions, and diabetes.

℞ **TREATMENT** Unfortunately, surgical curative resection can be considered in only a minority of patients because 64 to 92% present with metastatic disease. Treatment needs to be directed against the tumor itself using chemotherapy, embolization, chemoembolization, or hormonal therapy (see below).

GRFOMAS GRFomas are endocrine tumors that secrete excessive amounts of GRF that causes acromegaly. The frequency is not known. GRF (also called growth hormone–releasing hormone, GHRH) is a 44-amino-acid peptide, and 25 to 44% of PETs have GRF immunoreactivity, although excess secretion is uncommon. GRFomas are lung tumors in 47 to 54% of cases, PETs in 29 to 30%, and small-intestinal carcinoids in 8 to 10% and up to 12% occur at other sites. Patients have a mean age of 38 years, and the symptoms are usually due to either acromegaly or the tumor per se. The acromegaly caused by GRFomas is indistinguishable from classic acromegaly. The pituitary abnormality is growth hormone–secreting somatotrope cell hyperplasia rather than a pituitary adenoma. The pancreatic tumors are usually large (>6 cm), and liver metastases are present in 39%. They should be suspected in any patient with acromegaly and an abdominal tumor, in a patient with MEN-1 with acromegaly, or in a patient without a pituitary adenoma with acromegaly or associated with hyperprolactinemia, which occurs in 70% of GRFomas. GRFomas are an uncommon cause of acromegaly. The diagnosis is established by performing plasma assays for GRF and growth hormone. The normal level for GRF is <5 ng/L (5 pg/mL) in men and <10 ng/L (10 pg/mL) in women. Most GRFomas have a plasma GRF level ≥300 ng/L (300 pg/mL). Patients with GRFomas also have increased plasma insulin-like growth factor 1 levels similar to those in classic acromegaly. Surgery is the treatment of choice if diffuse metastases are not present. Long-acting somatostatin analogues such as octreotide or lanreotide (Fig. 93-2) induce responses in 75 to 100% of patients.

OTHER RARE PET SYNDROMES Cushing's syndrome (ACTHoma) due to a PET occurs in 4 to 16% of all patients with ectopic Cushing's syndrome. It occurs in 5% of cases of sporadic gastrinomas, almost invariably in patients with hepatic metastases, and is an independent, poor prognostic factor. Paraneoplastic hypercal-

cemia due to PETs releasing parathyroid hormone–related peptide is rare. The tumors are usually large, and liver metastases are usually present. PETs secreting calcitonin may cause a specific clinical syndrome. In one study, half the patients had diarrhea, which disappeared with resection of the tumor. In Table 93-2, this is a possible specific disorder because so few cases have been described.

TUMOR LOCALIZATION

Localization of the primary tumor and defining the extent of the disease are essential to the proper management of all carcinoids and PETs. Numerous tumor localization methods are used in both types of NETs, including conventional imaging studies [CT scanning, magnetic resonance imaging (MRI), transabdominal ultrasound, selective angiography] and somatostatin receptor scintigraphy (SRS). In PETs, endoscopic ultrasound (EUS) and functional localization by measuring venous hormonal gradients are also reported useful. Bronchial carcinoids are usually detected by a standard chest radiography and assessed by CT. Rectal, duodenal, colonic, and gastric carcinoids are usually detected by GI endoscopy.

PETs as well as carcinoid tumors possess high-affinity somatostatin receptors in both their primary tumors and their metastases. Of the five types of somatostatin receptors (sst_{1-5}), radiolabeled octreotide binds with high affinity to sst_2, lower for sst_3 and sst_5, and has very low affinity for sst_1 and sst_4. Between 90 and 100% of carcinoid tumors and PETs express sst_2, and many also have the other four sst subtypes. Interaction with these receptors can be used to localize NETs using [^{111}In-DTPA-D-Phe^1] octreotide (Fig. 93-2) and radionuclide scanning (SRS) as well as for treatment of the hormone excess state with octreotide or lanreotide. Because of its greater sensitivity than conventional imaging and its ability to localize tumor throughout the body at one time, SRS is now the imaging modality of choice for localizing both primary and metastatic NET tumors. SRS localizes tumors in 73 to 89% of patients with carcinoids and in 56 to 100% of patients with PETs, except for insulinomas. Insulinomas are usually small and have low densities of sst receptors, which results in SRS being positive in only 12 to 50% of patients with insulinomas. Figure 93-3 shows an example of the increased sensitivity of SRS in a patient with a gastrinoma. The CT scan (Fig. 93-3, *top*) did not show any disease after primary tumor resection; however, hypergastrinemia remained, and the SRS demonstrated a metastasis in the liver (Fig. 93-3, *bottom*). Occasional false-positive responses with SRS can occur (12% in one study) because numerous other normal and abnormal cells can have high densities of sst receptors including granulomas (sarcoid, tuberculosis, etc.), thyroid diseases (goiter, thyroiditis), and activated lymphocytes (lymphomas, wound infections). For PETs located in the pancreas, EUS is highly sensitive, localizing 77 to 93% of insulinomas, which occur almost exclusively within the pancreas. EUS is less sensitive for extrapancreatic tumors. If liver metastases are identified by SRS, a CT scan or MRI is then recommended to assess the size and exact location of the metastases, because SRS does not provide reliable information on tumor size. Functional localization measuring hormone gradients after intraarterial calcium injections in insulinomas (insulin) or gastrin gradients after secretin injections in gastrinoma will be positive in 80 to 100% of patients. However, this method gives only regional localization and therefore is reserved for cases where other imaging tests are negative.

℞ **TREATMENT** **Advanced Disease (Diffuse Metastatic Disease)** The single most important prognostic factor for survival is the presence of liver metastases (Fig. 93-4). For patients with carcinoids without hepatic metastases, the 5-year survival is 80%; with limited liver metastases, it is also 80%; but with diffuse metastases, it is 50% (Fig. 93-4, *bottom*). With gastrinomas, the 5-year survival without liver metastases is 98%; with limited metastases in one hepatic lobe it is 78%; and with diffuse metastases, 16% (Fig. 93-4, *top*). A number of different modalities are effective, including cytoreductive surgery (removal of all visible tumor), treatment with chemotherapy,

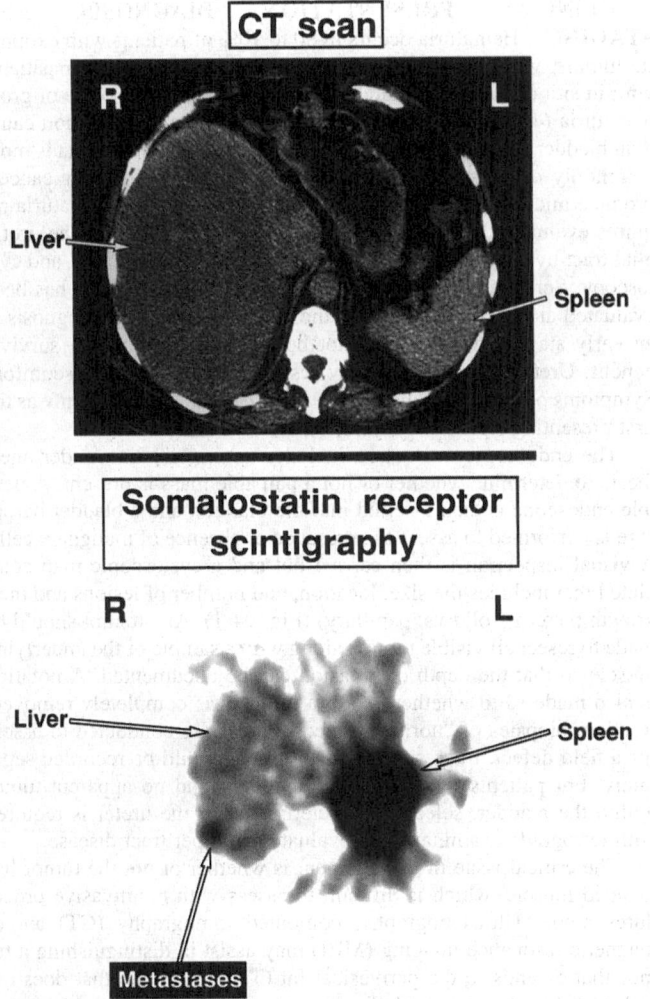

FIGURE 93-3 Ability of computed tomography (CT) (*top*) or somatostatin receptor scintigraphy (*bottom*) to localize metastatic gastrinoma in the liver in a patient with Zollinger-Ellison syndrome.

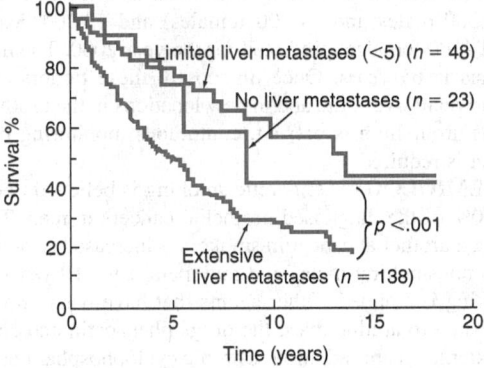

FIGURE 93-4 Effect of the presence and extent of liver metastases on survival in patients with gastrinomas (*top*) or carcinoid tumors (*bottom*). (*Top panel is drawn from data from 199 patients with gastrinomas, modified from F Yu et al: J Clin Oncol 17:615, 1999. Bottom panel is drawn from data from 209 patients with carcinoid tumors from ET Janson et al: Ann Oncol 8:685, 1997.*)

somatostatin analogues, interferon α, hepatic embolization alone or with chemotherapy (chemoembolization), radiotherapy, and liver transplantation.

Specific Antitumor Treatments Cytoreductive surgery is only possible in the 9 to 22% of patients who have limited hepatic metastases. No randomized studies have proven it extends life, but it appears to increase survival and therefore is recommended if possible.

Chemotherapy for metastatic carcinoid tumors has been disappointing, with response rates of 0 to 40% with various two- or three-drug combinations. Chemotherapy for PETs has been more successful, with tumor shrinkage reported in 30 to 70% of patients. The current regimen of choice is streptozotocin and doxorubicin.

Long-acting somatostatin analogues (octreotide, lanreotide) and interferon α rarely decrease tumor size (i.e., 0 to 17%); however, these drugs have tumoristatic effects, stopping additional growth in 50 to 95% of patients with NETs. How long tumor stabilization lasts or whether it prolongs survival has not been established.

Hepatic embolization and chemoembolization (with dacarbazine, cisplatin, doxorubicin, 5-fluorouracil, or streptozotocin) decrease tumor bulk and help control the symptoms of hormone excess. These modalities are generally reserved for patients in whom treatment with somatostatin analogues, interferon (carcinoids), or chemotherapy (PETs) fails.

Radiotherapy is being used with two different somatostatin radionuclides coupled by a DOTA-chelating group to octreotide (Fig. 93-2): [^{111}In-DTPA-D-Phe^1] octreotide (emits γ rays, internal conversion, and Auger electrons) and yttrium-90 (emits high energy β particles). The ^{111}In compound showed disease stabilization in 40% and a decrease in tumor size in 30% of patients with advanced metastatic disease.

The use of liver transplantation has been abandoned for treatment of most metastatic tumors to the liver. However, for metastatic NETs it is still a consideration. Liver transplantation in 103 cases of malignant NETs (48 were PETs, 43 were carcinoids) achieved 2- and 5-year survival rates of 60% and 47%, respectively. However, recurrence-free survival was low (<24%). Liver transplantation may be justified for younger patients with metastatic NETs limited to the liver.

BIBLIOGRAPHY

CARCINOID TUMORS AND SYNDROME

CAPLIN ME et al: Carcinoid tumour. Lancet 352:799, 1998

JENSEN RT, NORTON JA: Carcinoid tumors and the carcinoid syndrome, *Cancer: Principles and Practice of Oncology*, VT DeVita Jr, S Hellman, SA Rosenberg (eds). Philadelphia, Lippincott-Raven, 1997, pp 1704–1723

KULKE MH, MAYER RJ: Carcinoid tumors. N Engl J Med 340:858, 1999

MODLIN IM, SANDOR A: An analysis of 8305 cases of carcinoid tumors. Cancer 79:813, 1997

PANCREATIC ENDOCRINE TUMORS

FRAKER DL, JENSEN RT: Pancreatic endocrine tumors, in *Cancer: Principles and Practice of Oncology*, VT DeVita Jr, S Hellman, SA Rosenberg (eds). Philadelphia, Lippincott-Raven, 1997, pp 1678–1704

JENSEN RT, NORTON JA: Endocrine neoplasma of the pancreas, in *Textbook of Gastroenterology*, 3d ed, T Yamada et al (eds). Philadelphia, Lippincott Williams & Wilkins, 1999, pp 2193–2228

MIGNON M, JENSEN RT (eds): *Endocrine Tumors of the Pancreas: Recent Advances in Research and Management.* Basel, Karger, 1995

O'SHEA D, BLOOM SR (Guest Eds): Gastrointestinal Endocrine Tumours. Bailliere's Clin Gastroenterol 10:555, 1996

94   *Howard I. Scher, Robert J. Motzer*

BLADDER AND RENAL CELL CARCINOMAS

BLADDER CANCER

A transitional cell epithelium lines the urinary tract from the renal pelvis to the ureter, urinary bladder, and the proximal two-thirds of the urethra. Carcinomas may occur at any point, but generally 90% develop in the bladder, 8% in the renal pelvis, and 2% in the ureter or urethra. Overall, urinary bladder cancer is the fourth most common cancer in men and the ninth in women, with an estimated 53,200 new cases (38,300 males and 14,900 females) and 12,200 deaths (8100 males and 4100 females) predicted for the year 2000. The median age at diagnosis is 65 years. Once diagnosed, these tumors exhibit the tendency to recur over time and in new locations in the urothelial tract. As long as urothelium is present, continuous monitoring of the urothelial tract is required.

EPIDEMIOLOGY   Cigarette smoking is believed to contribute to up to 50% of the diagnosed urothelial cancers in men. The risk of developing a urothelial cancer in smokers is increased two- to fourfold relative to nonsmoking males and may persist for 10 years or longer after smoking is stopped. Other agents that have been implicated include exposure to aniline dyes, the drugs phenacetin and chlornaphazin, and external beam radiation. Chronic cyclophosphamide exposure increases risk nine-fold. Diets rich in meat and fat predispose to bladder cancer; ingestion of vitamin A supplements appears to be protective. Exposure to *Schistosoma haematobium*, a parasite found in many developing countries, is associated with an increase in both squamous (70%) and transitional cell (30%) carcinomas of the bladder.

PATHOLOGY   In the United States, 90 to 95% of bladder tumors diagnosed are transitional cell tumors. Pure squamous tumors with keratinization comprise 3%, adenocarcinomas 2%, and small cell tumors (with paraneoplastic syndromes) <1%. Adenocarcinomas develop primarily in the urachal remnant in the dome of the bladder or in the periurethral tissues. Some assume a signet cell histology. Lymphomas or melanomas are rare. Overall, 75% of tumors present as superficial lesions, 20% with muscle invasion, and 5% with metastatic disease. Of the transitional cell tumors, low-grade papillary lesions that grow on a central stalk are most common. They are very friable, have a tendency to bleed, and are at a high risk for recurrence, yet they rarely progress to the more lethal invasive variety. In contrast, carcinoma in situ (CIS) is a high-grade tumor that is considered a precursor of the more lethal muscle-infiltrating cancers. Tumors are rated by histologic type and grade. Grade I lesions (highly differentiated tumors) rarely progress to a higher stage, while grade III tumors usually do.

PATHOGENESIS   The multicentric nature of the disease and high rate of recurrence has led to the hypothesis that a field defect develops in the urothelium. Molecular genetic analyses of bladder tumors representing defined stages and different grades have shown a series of *primary chromosomal aberrations* associated with cancer *development*, and *secondary changes* associated with *progression* to a more advanced stage. Using paired bladder tumor and normal tissues from the same patient, 9q deletions are an early event in cancer development, while 3p and 5q deletions were more prevalent in invasive vs. superficial tumors. Deletions of 17p (*TP53* locus), 18q (the *DCC* gene locus), and the *RB* gene locus on chromosome 13q24 were seen only in invasive disease, while deletions of 3p and 11p occur in both superficial and invasive tumors. p53 overexpression correlates with a higher probability of progression to a more advanced stage and bladder cancer mortality for patients with Ta, Tis, T1 and muscle-infiltrating lesions. These factors have not been routinely used for clinical decision-making.

CLINICAL PRESENTATION, DIAGNOSIS, AND STAGING   Hematuria occurs in 80 to 90% of patients with exophytic tumors, while irritative symptoms are more common for patients with in situ disease. The bladder is the most common source of gross hematuria (40%), but benign cystitis (22%) is a more common cause than bladder cancer (15%) (Chap. 48). Microscopic hematuria is more commonly of prostatic origin (25%), while 2% of bladder cancers produce microscopic hematuria. The documentation of hematuria requires evaluation with a urinary cytology, visualization of the urothelial tract by sonography or an intravenous pyelogram (IVP), and cystoscopy. Screening of asymptomatic subjects for hematuria has been evaluated and shown to increase the frequency of tumor diagnosis at an early stage. Screening has not been shown to confer a survival benefit. Ureteral obstruction may result in flank pain or discomfort. Symptoms of metastatic disease are documented less commonly as the first presenting sign of a urothelial cancer.

The endoscopic evaluation includes an examination under anesthesia to determine whether or not a palpable mass is present. A flexible endoscope is then inserted into the bladder, and a bladder barbotage is performed to assess the presence or absence of malignant cells. A visual inspection is then carried out and a cystoscopic map completed that includes the size, location, and number of lesions and their growth pattern (solid vs. papillary) (Fig. 94-1). An attempt should be made to resect all visible tumors along with a sample of the underlying muscle so that the depth of invasion can be documented. A notation is also made as to whether or not a tumor was completely removed. Random biopsies of "normal" mucosal areas are conducted to assess for a field defect. Each site that is biopsied should be recorded separately. For patients with a positive cytology and no apparent tumor within the bladder, selective catheterization of the ureter is required with retrograde examination to evaluate for upper tract disease.

The critical issue in management is whether or not the tumor has invaded muscle, which is difficult to assess with noninvasive procedures alone. Ultrasonography, computed tomography (CT) and/or magnetic resonance imaging (MRI) may assist in distinguishing a tumor that extends to the perivesical fat (T3b) from one that does not (T3a), and to document whether or not regional lymph nodes are involved (N+). They are also important in the assessment of the upper tracts. Distal metastases are assessed by CT of the abdomen, pulmonary x-rays, or radionuclide imaging of the skeleton. The need for these studies is based in part on the local extent of the lesion.

The revised 1997 TNM (tumor, nodes, metastasis) staging system is illustrated in Fig. 94-2. Ta lesions grow as exophytic lesions, while CIS starts on the surface and tends to invade muscle. As the degree of muscle infiltration increases, the probability of nodal and subsequent distal spread also increases.

TREATMENT   Treatments are based on the extent and depth of invasion of the tumor within the primary site and the presence or probability of metastatic spread. At a minimum, the management of a tumor that has not invaded the bladder wall is a complete endoscopic resection with or without intravesical therapy. Recurrences are seen in 50% or more of cases, of which 5 to 20% will progress to a more advanced stage. The decision to recommend additional therapy is based on the histologic subtype, the number of lesions, the depth of invasion, and whether or not CIS is present. Solitary papillary lesions are generally treated by surgery alone. Intravesical therapy is usually recommended for recurrent disease.

CIS frequently follows a more aggressive course. As such, intravesical therapy is generally recommended earlier in the clinical course. The standard treatment for a tumor that has invaded muscle, either at the time of diagnosis or following treatment for superficial disease, is radical cystectomy. Depending on the findings at surgery, systemic chemotherapy may or may not be advised.

Superficial Disease   Intravesical therapies are applied in two contexts: as an adjuvant to a complete endoscopic resection to prevent recurrence, or, less commonly, to eliminate disease that cannot be controlled by endoscopic resection alone. Intravesical treatments are advised for patients with four or more recurrences in a given year,

>40% involvement of the bladder surface by tumor, the presence of diffuse CIS, or documented T1 disease. A number of agents are available, but based on randomized comparisons, Bacillus Calmette-Guerin (BCG) is considered standard. Thiotepa, doxorubicin, mitomycin-C, and interferon have also been used. Side effects include dysuria, frequency, and, depending on the drug, myelosuppression or a contact dermatitis (from mitomycin C). Rarely, intravesical BCG may produce a systemic illness associated with granulomatous infections in multiple sites that requires anti-tuberculin therapy for control. Significant BCG toxicities occur in <6% of patients.

Following endoscopic resection, patients are reevaluated at 3-month intervals to ensure that no recurrences have developed. Those with persistent disease or new tumors are generally

FIGURE 94-1 Bladder cancer map.

considered for a second course of BCG or intravesical chemotherapy. Those with persistent disease may be considered for cystectomy, although the specific indications vary. Obvious candidates are those with new invasive tumors or persistent CIS, and those with bladder function that has been compromised to the point where persistent pain, blood loss, frequency, or a severely limited bladder capacity is present. Recurrences may develop anywhere along the urothelial tract, including the renal pelvis, ureter, or urethra. In fact, one consequence of the "successful" treatment of tumors in the bladder is an increase in the frequency of extravesical recurrences.

Muscle-Infiltrating Disease The treatment of a tumor that has invaded muscle can be separated into control of the primary tumor and control of systemic disease. Radical cystectomy is considered the standard treatment, although in selected cases bladder-sparing approaches using an aggressive endoscopic resection, partial cystectomy, or a combined modality approach with resection, systemic chemotherapy, and external beam radiation therapy are used. The latter should not be considered outside of a research setting.

Radical cystectomy involves an evaluation of the pelvic lymph nodes, removal of the primary tumor, and creation of a conduit or reservoir for urinary flow. At the time of surgery, grossly abnormal lymph nodes are evaluated by frozen section. If metastases are confirmed, the procedure is often aborted unless a diversion is required for palliation of local symptoms. The results of treatment of node-positive disease are shown in Table 94-1. In males radical cystectomy involves the removal of the bladder, prostate, seminal vesicles, proximal vas deferens, and proximal urethra, with a margin of adipose tissue and peritoneum. Impotence is universal unless the *nervi erigentes*, responsible for erectile capacity, can be preserved. In females the procedure includes removal of the bladder, urethra, uterus, fallopian tubes, ovaries, anterior vaginal wall, and surrounding fascia.

Urine flow is directed through either an internal reservoir that drains to the urethra or the abdominal wall, or via a Bricker procedure in which urine flows through an ileal conduit from the ureters to the abdominal wall, where it is collected in an external appliance without an internal reservoir. A segment of colon, jejunum, or ileum can be used to bridge the gap between the ureters and the skin. Use of absorbable sutures may prevent formation of calculi at the sutures. A uretero-ileal conduit probably is the most widely used. A syndrome characterized by hypochloremic acidosis, hyperkalemia, hyponatremia, and uremia has been described when a segment of jejunum is utilized. Concurrent diseases in the bowel, such as ulcerative colitis or Crohn's disease, may hinder the use of resected bowel.

Alternatives to an external appliance include internal reservoirs that are created from detubularized bowel segments and are periodically self-catheterized by the patient. A number of procedures have been described that use either ileocecal or ileal reservoirs, which are anastamosed to either the abdominal wall or the urethra. When an anastomosis to the urethra is created, primarily in men with no urethral disease, the patient can then void in a manner that is similar to natural voiding. Several indications for urethrectomy (including CIS or exophytic tumor in the urethra and diffuse CIS in the urinary bladder) preclude the creation of a urethral anastomosis. Continent reservoirs are being applied with increasing frequency, but are still not constructed for the majority of patients, for technical or disease-related reasons. Intercurrent diseases, impaired renal function, hesitancy to prolong the surgical trauma, dilated ureters, and bowel diseases all decrease the use of continent reservoirs. Patients with ureterosigmoid diversion require periodic colonoscopy because of the risk of cancer.

Cystectomy is major surgery, and appropriate medical clearance is essential. This includes optimizing cardiac medications and nutritional status. In approximately 5 to 10% of cases, depending on the location of the tumor, a partial cystectomy is possible. This procedure can be considered when a lesion develops on the dome of the bladder where a 2-cm margin can be achieved, CIS is absent in other sites of the bladder, and bladder capacity is adequate after the tumor is removed. Carcinomas in the ureter or in the renal pelvis are treated by nephroureterectomy with a bladder cuff.

Indications for cystectomy include: (1) muscle-invading tumors not suitable for segmental resection; (2) low-stage tumors unsuitable for conservative management due to, for example, multicentric and frequent recurrences resistant to intravesical instillations; (3) high grade tumors (T1G3) associated with CIS or bladder symptoms such as frequency or hemorrhage rendering the patient a "bladder cripple." Outcomes are reported on the basis of 5-year survivals. As shown in Table 94-2, survival varies inversely with depth of invasion and lymph node status. For the majority of cases, however, extension to a single lymph node predicts a poor outcome with a median time to recurrence of 22 months. In some countries external beam radiation therapy is considered standard. This is not the case in the United States, where its role is limited to those patients deemed unfit for cystectomy or those with unresectable local disease, and as part of an experimental approach that seeks to spare the bladder.

Metastatic Disease Patients with metastatic disease include those whose tumor has recurred after definitive local treatment and those who present with metastases. A number of chemotherapeutic agents have shown activity as single agents, of which cisplatin, paclitaxel, and gemcitabine are considered most active (Table 94-3). Responses to single agents are generally incomplete and not durable. Using multidrug regimens, response rates in excess of 50% have been reported with combinations such as M-VAC (methotrexate, vinblastine, doxorubicin, and cisplatin), PT (cisplatin and paclitaxel), and gemcitabine variants. Based on randomized comparisons, M-VAC is considered standard but can be associated with significant toxicities, including neutropenia and fever; mucositis in 10 to 20%; a decrease in renal and auditory function; and a peripheral neuropathy. Alopecia is universal; fatigue can be dose-limiting in some cases. More recently 2- and 3-drug combinations based on cisplatin/carboplatin, paclitaxel, and gemcitabine have been explored. In a direct comparison to M-VAC, gemcitabine/cisplatin showed similar response proportions and

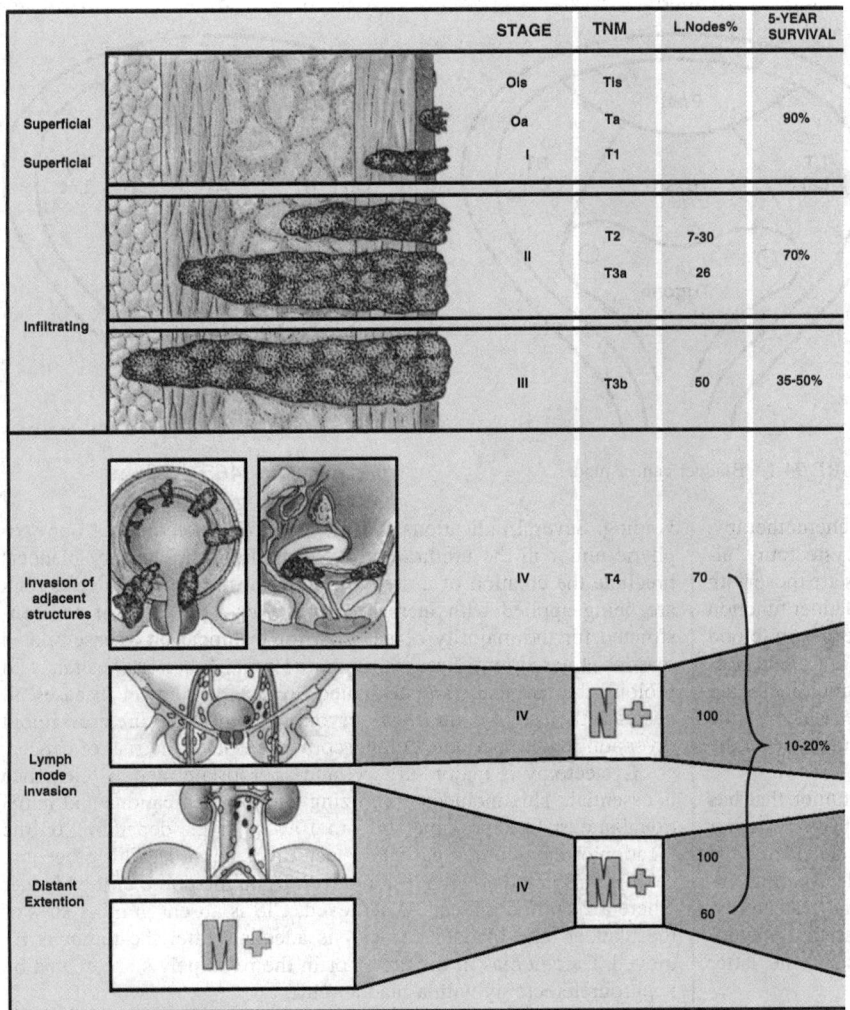

STAGE		TNM	L.Nodes%	5-YEAR SURVIVAL
Superficial	Ois	Tis		90%
	Oa	Ta		
Superficial	I	T1		
Infiltrating	II	T2	7-30	70%
		T3a	26	
	III	T3b	50	35-50%
Invasion of adjacent structures	IV	T4	70	
Lymph node invasion	IV	N+	100	10-20%
Distant Extention	IV	M+	100	
			60	

FIGURE 94-2 Bladder staging.

survival with fewer side effects. Long-term survival may be obtained in 10 to 15% of patients with metastatic disease and 20 to 25% of patients with unresectable nodal disease at presentation. In general, the proportion of patients rendered tumor-free is higher in patients with disease limited to nodal sites as opposed to visceral or bone sites. Patients with adverse features, such as a compromised performance status, visceral disease, or bone metastases, are rarely cured with chemotherapy alone. In these cases, median survivals rarely exceed 6 months.

Chemotherapy for Invasive Disease Chemotherapy can be given before (neoadjuvant) or after (adjuvant) definitive local therapy. Cumulative results of nonrandomized phase II trials have shown that the proportion of bladders rendered free of tumor varies inversely with T stage; but only 20 to 25% of bladders are tumor-free after chemotherapy alone. To date, neoadjuvant chemotherapy has not been shown to prolong life. Several groups are investigating bladder-sparing strategies but these approaches are not considered routine practice. The need for adjuvant therapy is based on a pathologic determination of risk. In general, the finding of nodal disease at surgery, extravesical tumor extension, or vascular invasion in the resected specimen are considered indications for postoperative adjuvant therapy. When administered, a minimum of four cycles at full dose is recommended.

Overview Superficial TaG1 lesions rarely progress to an invasive lesion and can be handled with an endoscopic resection. Muscle-invasive disease may require both aggressive local therapy and systemic therapy of micrometastases for cure, while metastatic urinary bladder cancer is the most lethal for the majority of patients. Only a small proportion of patients with metastatic disease can be cured with chemotherapy. Current refinements in therapy include identifying subgroups of patients with superficial disease where the intensity of follow-up can be reduced or where intravesical therapy is needed. For muscle-invasive disease, efforts are being made to identify patients for whom organ preservation is possible without compromising overall survival, as well as those with subclinical micrometastases for whom systemic therapy is needed for cure. Efforts to improve therapy include better surgical techniques and the incorporation of newly identified chemotherapeutic agents into combination regimens. For the majority of patients, combined modality approaches are essential to optimal management.

RENAL CELL CARCINOMA

Renal cell carcinoma accounts for 90 to 95% of malignant neoplasms arising from the kidney. Notable features include refractoriness to cytotoxic agents, infrequent but reproducible responses to biologic response modifiers such as interferon α and interleukin (IL) 2, and a variable clinical course for patients with metastatic disease, including anecdotal reports of spontaneous regression.

EPIDEMIOLOGY AND ETIOLOGY In the year 2000, 31,200 new cases of renal cancer were diagnosed, and 11,900 people died of the disease. The male:female ratio is 2:1. Incidence peaks between the ages of 50 and 70, although this malignancy may be diagnosed at any age. Many environmental factors have been investigated as possible contributing causes. The strongest association is with cigarette smoking (accounting for 20 to 30% of cases) and obesity. The risk is increased for patients who have acquired cystic disease of the kidney associated with end-stage renal disease.

Most cases are sporadic, although familial forms have been reported. One is associated with von Hippel-Lindau (VHL) syndrome. Nearly 35% of patients with VHL disease develop renal cell cancer. An increased incidence has also been reported for patients with tuberous sclerosis and polycystic kidney disease.

Most of the cancers arise from the epithelial cells of the proximal tubules. A number of genetic alterations have been described, of which abnormalities on chromosome 3 are most frequent. A t(3;8) translocation was first described in a pedigree of patients with the familial form of the disease, while deletions of 3p21–26 (where *VHL* maps) have been identified in familial as well as sporadic tumors. *VHL* mutations are identified in a high proportion of sporadic, nonpapillary renal cell cancers and associated cell lines.

Table 94-1 Survival of Patients with Node Positive Bladder Cancer

Series	Year	No. of Patients	5-Year Survival, %
Whitmore	1981	134	7
Smith	1983	230	4
Skinner	1984	36	35
Bosl	1991	229	19
Pagano	1991	26	4

Table 94-2 5-Year Survival in Bladder Cancer Based on Pathologic Stage

Series	No. of Patients	Year	P2, %	P3a, %	P3b, %	Operative Mortality, %
Whitmore	137	1983	60	26	11	14
Montie	99	1983	62	74	57	9
Skinner	197	1984	83	69	29	1.0
Pagano	261	1991	63	50	15	1.8

Table 94-3 Selected Single Agents with Activity in Urothelial Tract Malignancies

Agent	No. Responding/ No. Treated	Percent	95% Confidence Interval
Cisplatin	200/706	28	26–32
Methrotrexate	8/236	45	37–50
Doxorubicin	47/274	17	13–22
Vinblastine	6/38	16	4–28
Ifosfamide	28/101	28	19–37
Gallium nitrate	9/29	29	13–45
Paclitaxel	11/26	42	23–61

PATHOLOGY Renal cell neoplasia represents a heterogeneous group of tumors with distinct histopathologic, genetic, and clinical features ranging from benign to high-grade malignant. Categories include clear cell carcinoma (60% of cases), papillary (5 to 15%), chromophobic tumors (5 to 10%), oncocytomas (5 to 10%), and collecting or Bellini duct tumors (<1%). Clear cell tumors are characterized by tumor cells with clear cytoplasm and consistently show a deletion of 3p. Papillary tumors tend to be bilateral and multifocal. Trisomy 7 and/or 17 are the most frequent genetic markers. Chromophobic tumors are characterized by multiple chromosomal losses but do not exhibit 3p deletions; they also have a more indolent clinical course. Oncocytomas have a characteristic morphology including a deeply eosinophilic cytoplasm, do not exhibit 3p deletions or trisomy 7 or 17, and are considered benign neoplasms. In contrast, Bellini duct carcinomas are very rare and are thought to arise from the collecting ducts within the renal medulla. They tend to afflict younger patients and are very aggressive tumors.

CLINICAL PRESENTATION The presenting signs and symptoms include hematuria, abdominal pain, and a flank or abdominal mass. This classic triad occurs in 10 to 20% of patients. Other symptoms are fever, weight loss, anemia, and a varicocele (Table 94-4); the tumor can be found incidentally on a radiograph.

The presentation has changed over the past two decades, due to the advent and widespread use of radiologic cross-sectional imaging procedures (CT, ultrasound, MRI). The more frequent use of sensitive abdominal imaging modalities in recent years contributes to earlier detection, including incidental low-stage renal masses detected during evaluation for other medical conditions. The increasing number of incidentally discovered low-stage tumors contributes to an improved 5-year survival for patients with renal cell carcinoma and increased use of nephron-sparing surgery (partial nephrectomy).

A spectrum of paraneoplastic syndromes has been associated with these malignancies, including erythrocytosis, hypercalcemia, nonmetastatic hepatic dysfunction (Stauffers' syndrome) and acquired dysfibrinogenemia. Erythrocytosis is present at presentation in only about 3% of patients. More frequently anemia, a sign of advanced disease, is reported.

The standard evaluation of patients with suspected renal cell tu-

Table 94-4 Signs and Symptoms in Patients with Renal Cell Cancer

Presenting Sign or Symptom	Incidence, %
Classic triad: hematuria, flank pain, flank mass	10–20
Hematuria	40
Flank pain	40
Palpable mass	25
Weight loss	33
Anemia	33
Fever	20
Hypertension	20
Abnormal liver function	15
Hypercalcemia	5
Erythrocytosis	3
Neuromyopathy	3
Amyloidosis	2
Increased erythrocyte sedimentation rate	55

mors includes a CT scan of the abdomen and pelvis, a chest radiograph, urine analysis, and urine cytology. A CT of the chest is warranted if metastatic disease is suspected from the chest radiograph, as it will detect significantly smaller lesions, and their presence may influence the approach to the primary tumor. MRI is useful in evaluating the inferior vena cava in cases of suspected tumor involvement or invasion by thrombus, as well as for patients in whom iodinated contrast cannot be administered owing to either allergy or renal dysfunction. In clinical practice any solid renal masses should be considered malignant until proved otherwise and require a definitive diagnosis. If no metastases are demonstrated, surgery is indicated, even if there is invasion of the renal vein. The differential diagnosis of a renal mass includes cysts, benign neoplasms (adenoma, angiomyolipoma, oncocytoma), inflammatory lesions (pyelonephritis or abscesses), and other primary or metastatic malignant neoplasms. Other malignancies that may involve the kidney include transitional cell carcinomas of the renal pelvis, sarcoma, lymphoma, Wilms' tumor, and metastatic disease, especially from melanoma primaries. All of these are less common than renal cell carcinoma as kidney masses.

STAGING AND PROGNOSIS Two staging systems used commonly are the Robson classification and the American Joint Committee on Cancer (AJCC) staging system. According to the former, stage I tumors are confined to the kidney; stage II tumors extend through the renal capsule but are confined to Gerota's fascia; stage III tumors involve the renal vein or vena cava (stage III A) or the hilar lymph nodes (stage III B); and stage IV disease includes tumors that are locally invasive to adjacent organs (excluding the adrenal gland) or distant metastases. Five-year survival rate varies by stage: 66% for stage I, 64% for stage II, 42% for stage III, and 11% for stage IV. The prognosis for patients with stage IIIA lesions is similar to that of stage II disease, whereas the 5-year survival rate for patients with stage IIIB lesions is only 20%, closer to that of stage IV.

TREATMENT Localized Tumors The standard management for stage I or II tumors and selected cases of stage III disease is radical nephrectomy. This procedure involves en bloc removal of Gerota's fascia; its contents including the kidney, the ipsilateral adrenal gland, and adjacent hilar lymph nodes. The role of a regional lymphadenectomy is controversial. For patients with stage IIIA disease, the tumor should be resected from the renal vein or vena cava.

In selected patients who have only one kidney, a partial nephrectomy may be performed, depending on the size and location of the lesion. Partial nephrectomy may also be performed for patients with bilateral tumors, accompanied by a radical nephrectomy on the opposite side. Partial nephrectomy techniques are being applied electively to resect small masses for patients with a normal contralateral kidney. There is no proven role for adjuvant chemotherapy, immunotherapy, or radiation therapy following successful surgical removal of the tumor, even in cases with a poor prognosis.

Advanced Disease Metastatic renal cell carcinoma, for which there is no effective therapy, is associated with dismal survival. A number of options have been explored, including hormonal therapy, chemotherapy (cytotoxic agents), and immunotherapy. Responses to hormonal therapy (progestins) are rare (1 to 2%) and of short duration. No chemotherapy agent has been shown to consistently produce tumor regressions in >20% of patients.

Two biologic therapies, interferon α and IL-2, have been studied extensively for the treatment of advanced disease. Both reproducibly produce responses in 10 to 20% of patients; the response is durable in fewer than 5% of patients. It was the observation of occasional durable complete remissions that resulted in the Food and Drug Administration's approval of IL-2 as a treatment for this disease. IL-2 is usually administered by infusion of 720,000 IU/k every 8 h per day for 5 to 7 days. Toxicities from IL-2 include a capillary leakage syndrome, fever, chills, fatigue, and hypotension.

Surgery in the Setting of Metastases Nephrectomy may be indicated in highly selected cases for the alleviation of symptoms, including pain or recurrent urinary hemorrhage, and particularly if the latter is severe or associated with obstruction. Some physicians advocate the performance of a nephrectomy in the presence of metastases in the hope either that a spontaneous regression will occur or that the sensitivity to a cytokine will be increased. The observed frequency of spontaneous regression, 0.8%, coupled with the morbidity and mortality of the procedure itself, does not justify the approach. Nephrectomy in the presence of metastatic disease followed by IFN-α is associated with a modest survival benfit over IFN-α alone.

There are reports of long-term survival at rates of 15 to 50% for patients who relapse following nephrectomy at a solitary site and undergo surgical resection of the metastasis. Because renal cell tumors are radioresistant, surgical resection is also advised for palliation of solitary central nervous system metastases, repair of actual or impending fractures in weight-bearing bones, or relief of spinal cord compression.

Observation Alone Renal cell carcinoma is one of several malignancies in which spontaneous regressions have been reported anecdotally. A more frequent occurrence is prolonged periods of stable disease: up to 10% of patients with metastatic disease show no progression for >12 months. Because responses to systemic therapy are uncommon, and all systemic therapies are associated with treatment-related toxicity, an option for management in asymptomatic patients with metastases is close observation until evidence of disease progression or symptoms occur, at which time appropriate therapy is initiated. It is important to document the presence of progressive disease before initiating an experimental treatment; this will avoid attributing stable disease to the drug when it may be a feature of the tumor.

CARCINOMA OF THE RENAL PELVIS AND URETER

About 500 cases of renal pelvis and ureter cancer occur each year; nearly all are transitional cell carcinomas similar to bladder cancer in biology and appearance. This tumor also is associated with chronic phenacetin abuse and with Balkan nephropathy, a chronic interstitial nephritis endemic in Bulgaria, Greece, Bosnia-Herzegovina, and Romania.

The most common symptom is painless gross hematuria, and the disease usually is detected on IVP during the workup for hematuria. Patterns of spread are like those in bladder cancer. For disease localized to the renal pelvis and ureter, nephroureterectomy (including excision of the distal ureter with a portion of the bladder) is associated with a 5-year survival of 80 to 90% for low-grade lesions. More invasive or histologically poorly differentiated tumors are more likely to recur locally and metastasize. Metastatic disease is treated with M-VAC or CMV (cisplatin, methotrexate, vinblastine) chemotherapy, as used in bladder cancer, and the outcome is similar to that for metastatic transitional cell cancer of bladder origin.

BIBLIOGRAPHY

BASSELLI EC, GREENBERG RE: Intravesical therapy for superficial bladder cancer. Oncology 14:719, 2000

FIGLIN RA: Renal cell carcinoma: Management of advanced disease. J Urol 161:381, 1999

LINEHAN WM et al: Cancer of the kidney and ureter, in *Cancer: Principles and Practice of Oncology*, 5th ed, VT DeVita et al (eds). Philadelphia New York: Lippincott-Raven, 1997, pp 1271–1300

MOTZER RJ et al: Renal-cell carcinoma. N Engl J Med 335:865,1996

———: Systemic therapy for renal cell carcinoma. J Urol 163:408,2000

OZEN H, HALL MC: Bladder cancer. Curr Opin Oncol 12:255, 2000

REUTER VE et al. Contemporary approach to the classification of renal epithelial tumors. Sem Oncol 27:124, 2000

HYPERPLASTIC AND MALIGNANT DISEASES OF THE PROSTATE

CT computed tomography	PSAD prostate-specific antigen density
DRE digital rectal examination	PIN prostatic intraepithelial neoplasia
GnRH gonadotropin-releasing hormone	3D-CRT three-dimensional conformal radiation therapy
LH luteinizing hormone	TRUS transrectal ultrasonography
MRI magnetic resonance imaging	TURP transurethral resection of the prostate
PSA prostate-specific antigen	

The process of aging is associated with an increasing frequency of both benign and malignant alterations of the prostate gland. These conditions reflect the uncontrolled growth of both the stromal and epithelial components of the gland. Autopsies of men in the eighth decade of life show hyperplastic changes in >90% and malignant changes in >70%. Most men with benign or malignant conditions of the prostate are not diagnosed during their lifetimes. The high prevalence of these diseases, coupled with comorbid conditions and competing causes of death that are frequent in this age group, mandates a careful consideration of the risk/benefit ratio of any proposed intervention. Management is centered on the continual reassessment of the disease as it unfolds in the individual. For the benign proliferative disorders, the symptoms of urinary frequency, infection, and potential for obstruction are counterbalanced by the side effects and complications of medical or surgical therapy. For malignant disease, the risk of developing symptoms or death from cancer is balanced against treatment efficacy and treatment-related morbidity for interventions proposed at different points in the natural history.

The incidence and mortality of prostate cancer have declined over the past few years. The decline is not clearly related to any meaningful decrease in the disease or its severity. Instead, the number of cases diagnosed increased dramatically in the early 1990s based on the widespread use of serum prostate-specific antigen (PSA) levels. The test led to the diagnosis of more asymptomatic cancers, some of which may never have produced symptoms—so-called lead-time bias (Chap. 80). Screening for prostate cancer has not been proven effective in prospective randomized trials. Prostate cancer is the most common cancer diagnosis and the second leading cause of cancer death in men. In 2000, 180,400 cases were diagnosed and 31,900 men died of prostate cancer, down from the peak of 352,000 new cases in 1996. The projected lifetime risk of developing prostate cancer for a 50-year-old man is 42%, of being diagnosed is 9.5%, and of dying from prostate cancer is 2.9%.

ANATOMY

The prostate is located in the pelvis and is surrounded by the rectum, bladder, dorsal and periprostatic venous complexes, musculature of the pelvic sidewall, the urethral sphincter (responsible for passive urinary control), the pelvic plexus, and cavernous nerves (which innervate the pelvic organs and corpora cavernosa). It is divided into a peripheral zone, a central zone, and a transition zone. The anterior surface is covered by the fibromuscular stroma. Most cancers develop in the peripheral zone, while nonmalignant proliferation occurs predominantly in the transition zone. The functional unit is the glandular acinus, which consists of an epithelial compartment including epithelial, basal, and neuroendocrine cells, and a stromal compartment including fibroblasts and smooth-muscle cells. These compartments are separated by a basement membrane. PSA and prostate-specific acid phosphatase are produced in the epithelial cells. Both stromal and epithelial cells express androgen receptors and depend on androgens for growth. Additional growth regulatory signals occur via paracrine signaling between the two compartments. In cancer, the relationship between stromal and epithelial elements contributes to growth both in the primary and in metastatic sites. The major circulating androgen in the blood is testosterone, which is converted to dihydrotestosterone, the active form, by 5α-reductase. Changes in prostate size occur during two distinct periods: diffuse enlargement during puberty and in focal regions in the periurethral area after the age of 55.

DIAGNOSIS AND SCREENING

Symptoms Most cancers are asymptomatic in their early stages. By contrast, benign proliferative disorders may encroach on the urethra early in the clinical course, giving rise to symptoms of outlet obstruction such as hesitancy, intermittent voiding, diminished stream, incomplete emptying, and postvoid leakage. For the patient with symptoms, the history is focused on the urinary tract to identify other causes of voiding dysfunction. For quantification of symptoms, the preferred questionnaire is the self-administered American Urological Association (AUA) *Symptom Index* in which the symptoms can be classified as mild, moderate, or severe on the basis of seven questions (Table 95-1). This index is useful in planning and in follow-up. Over time, the resistance to the flow of urine reduces the compliance of the detrusor muscle, resulting in nocturia, urgency, and bladder instability and ultimately in urinary retention. The relationship between the signs and symptoms of obstruction and prostate size is not straightforward, and a small gland does not exclude significant blockage. In severe cases the bladder may be palpable on physical examination. Infection, tranquilizing drugs, antihistamines, or alcohol can precipitate urinary retention.

Obstructive symptoms are distinct from irritative symptoms such as frequency, dysuria, or urgency, which may occur from infectious, inflammatory, or neoplastic diseases. Conditions that can mimic cancer include acute prostatitis, granulomatous prostatitis, and prostate calculus. Prostatitis usually produces induration and/or pain and is treated with antibiotics. Prostate cancer may manifest in the same manner, and the distinction can only be established histologically, but a biopsy should not be performed before a trial of antibiotics if prostatitis is a possible diagnosis. In cases where the tumor has extended beyond the confines of the gland, symptoms of hematospermia or erectile dysfunction may occur. Prostate cancer may also present with pain secondary to bone metastases, although many patients are asymptomatic despite extensive spread. Less common presentations include myelophthisic disorders, disseminated intravascular coagulation, or spinal cord compression. The proportion of men diagnosed at these late stages has also decreased significantly as a result of PSA-based detection strategies.

Physical Examination The standard evaluation for prostatic diseases includes the digital rectal examination (DRE). It should be performed with careful attention to the size and consistency of the gland, the presence of lesions within the gland, or evidence of extension beyond its confines. Its importance can not be overemphasized. The posterior surfaces of the lateral lobes, where carcinoma begins most often, are easily palpable on DRE. Carcinoma characteristically is hard, nodular, and irregular, but induration may also be due to fibrous areas in a benign hyperplastic background or to calculi. Extraprostatic extension to the seminal vesicles can often be detected by rectal examination, while scrotal and/or lower extremity lymphedema secondary to infiltration of pelvic lymph nodes indicates extensive disease. The need for establishing a histologic diagnosis is based on the finding of an abnormal DRE or an elevated serum PSA level.

Prostate-Specific Antigen PSA is a serine protease that is produced by both nonmalignant and malignant epithelial cells. In serum, it circulates as an inactive complex with two protease inhibitors—α_1-antichymotrypsin and β_2-macroglobulin. PSA is prostate specific but not prostate cancer specific and is measured most commonly by radioimmunoassay. The normal range is 0 to 4 ng/mL; ~30% of men with a PSA in the range of 4 to 10 ng/mL and 50% of those with a PSA >10 ng/mL will have cancer. Between 20 and 25% of men with an abnormal DRE have cancer at biopsy, and 20% of men have cancer detected when the PSA is in the normal range. African American men normally have higher PSA levels, even if they do not have prostate cancer. They also have a 50% higher risk of prostate cancer. The reason for the racial differences is not known.

Several refinements have been proposed to increase the sensitivity of the test for younger men more likely to die of the disease, while reducing the frequency of diagnosing cancers of low biologic potential in elderly men more likely to die of other causes. These modifications include age-specific reference ranges, using a lower "upper" limit of normal for younger males and higher "upper" limit for older individuals. Prostate-specific antigen density (PSAD) is calculated by dividing the serum PSA level by the estimated prostate weight calculated from transrectal ultrasonography (TRUS). It was proposed to correct for the influence of benign prostatic hyperplasia (BPH) on the measured level of PSA. Values <0.10 are consistent with BPH, while values >0.15 suggest the presence of cancer. PSAD levels also increase with age.

PSA velocity is derived from calculations of the rate of change in PSA before the diagnosis of cancer was established. Increases of >0.75 ng/mL per year are suggestive of cancer. For a 50-year-old male, an increase from 2.5 to 3.9 ng/mL in a 1-year period would warrant further testing, even though the level is still in the "normal" range. Free and complexed PSA measurements are used to determine which men require a biopsy when the PSA level is in the range of 4 to 10 ng/mL. In cancer, the level of free PSA is lower. Using a 25%

Table 95-1 AUA System Index

Questions to be Answered	Not at All	Less than 1 Time in 5	Less than Half the Time	About Half the Time	More than Half the time	Almost Always
Over the past month, how often you have had a sensation of not emptying your bladder completely after you finished urinating?	0	1	2	3	4	5
Over the past month, how often have you had to urinate again less than 2 h after you finished urinating?	0	1	2	3	4	5
Over the past month, how often have you found you stopped and started again several times when you urinated?	0	1	2	3	4	5
Over the past month, how often have you found it difficult to postpone urination?	0	1	2	3	4	5
Over the past month, how often have you had a weak urinary stream?	0	1	2	3	4	5
Over the past month, how often have you had to push or strain to begin urination?	0	1	2	3	4	5
Over the past month, how many times did you most typically get up to urinate from the time you went to bed at night until the time you got up in the morning?	(None)	(1 time)	(2 times)	(3 times)	(4 times)	(5 times)
Sum of 7 circled numbers (AUA Symptom Score): ——						

The heading spans: AUA Symptom Score (Circle 1 Number on Each Line)

NOTE: AUA, American Urological Association.

SOURCE: Barry MJ et al: J Urol 148:1549, 1992. Used with permission.

FIGURE 95-1 Men who desire early detection after discussion of pros and cons with their health care providers and who have a > 10 year life expectancy.

(Modified from NCCN Prostate Practice Guidelines)

threshold of free PSA for patients with levels in the range of 4 to 10 ng/mL, specificity was improved by 20% while maintaining a sensitivity of 95%. Further refinements to increase the specificity of distinguishing benign and malignant conditions involve the determination of the ratios of free to total, complexed to total, and free to complexed PSA. Using normal ranges for free/total PSA of >0.15, for complexed/total PSA of <0.70, and for free/complexed PSA of >0.25 improved specificity in one study by 20%. These modifications are designed to reduce the frequency of biopsies in men without cancer. Figure 95-1 illustrates a diagnostic algorithm based on the DRE and PSA findings.

Transrectal Ultrasonography Most cancers are hypoechoic by ultrasonography. Unfortunately, no single finding on ultrasound permits univeral distinction between cancer and benign conditions and identification of extracapsular disease. Cancers <5 to 7 mm, those that are well differentiated, and those located in the transition zone are difficult to distinguish from the normal prostate. The primary role of ultrasound is to ensure accurate sampling of any index lesions and of the gland during biopsy. Routine sampling includes a minimum of six cores from the peripheral zone of the gland, each of which is identified and labeled separately for histologic examination. A biopsy session, defined as one that procures four or more cores from widely separated areas of the prostate, has a sensitivity of ~80% for the detection of a cancer. TRUS has also been used in the assessment of local disease extent; accuracy is limited and is generally restricted to determining whether the tumor invades the seminal vesicles. It is also used to determine the size of the gland for the calculation of PSAD and to guide the placement of radioactive seeds during implantation.

Pathology The noninvasive proliferation of epithelial cells within ducts is termed *prostatic intraepithelial neoplasia* (PIN). It is considered the precursor of cancer, but not all PIN lesions develop into invasive cancers. Nevertheless, on a genetic level, these regions are highly unstable and typically multifocal. Of the cancers identified, >95% are adenocarcinomas; the remainder include squamous cell tumors, transitional cell tumors, and, rarely, carcinosarcomas. Metastases to the prostate are rare, but in some cases, transitional cell tumors originating in the bladder or colonic lesions may invade the gland directly. In the evaluation for adenocarcinoma, each core is examined for the presence or absence of cancer. When cancer is identified, the extent and grade are assessed and the presence or absence of perineural invasion or extracapsular extension reported. Histologic grade is based most commonly on the *Gleason system*, in which the dominant and secondary glandular histologic patterns are independently assigned numbers from 1 to 5 (best to least differentiated) and summed to give a total score of 2 to 10 for each tumor. The grading is reproducible and correlates with clinical outcomes. The most poorly differentiated area of tumor (i.e., the area with the highest histologic grade) often determines biologic behavior.

STAGING

The TNM staging system (Table 95-2) includes categories for cancers identified solely on the basis of an abnormal PSA with no palpable abnormalities on DRE (T1c), those that are palpable but clinically confined to the gland (T2), and those that have extended outside of

Table 95-2   Comparison of Clinical Stage by the TNM Classification System and the Whitmore-Jewett Staging System

TNM Stage	Description	Whitmore-Jewett Stage	Description
T1a	Nonpalpable, with 5% or less of resected tissue with cancer	A1	Well differentiated tumor on few chips from 1 lobe
T1b	Nonpalpable, with >5% of resected tissue with cancer	A2	Involvement more diffuse
T1c	Nonpalpable, detected due to elevated serum PSA		
T2a	Palpable, half of one lobe or less	BIN	Palpable, < one lobe, surrounded by normal tissue
T2b	Palpable, > half of one lobe but not both lobes	B1	Palpable, < one lobe
T2c	Palpable, involves both lobes	B2	Palpable, one entire lobe or both lobes
T3a	Palpable, unilateral extra-capsular extension	C1	Palpable, outside capsule, not into seminal vesicles
T3b	Palpable, bilateral extra-capsular extension		
T3c	Tumor invades seminal vesicle(s)	C2	Palpable, seminal vesicle involved
MI	Distant metastases	D	Metastatic disease

SOURCE: Adapted from FF Schroder et al: TNM classification of prostate cancer. Prostate (Suppl) 4:129, 1992; and American Joint Committee on Cancer, 1992.

the gland (T3 and T4). The presence or absence of nodal (N) and distant metastases (M) are also recorded. Clinical staging alone is inaccurate in assessing capsular invasion and the probability of spread to nodal or more distant sites. To refine this assessment, the TNM system has been modified to incorporate the results of imaging studies such as ultrasound or magnetic resonance imaging (MRI) in the assignment of T stage.

Computed tomography (CT) scans lack sensitivity and specificity to detect extraprostatic extension and in visualization of lymph nodes. MRI is an improvement, particularly with an endorectal coil and is superior to CT. T1-weighted images demonstrate the periprostatic fat, periprostatic venous plexus, perivesicular tissues, lymph nodes, and bone marrow. T2-weighted images demonstrate the internal architecture of the prostate and seminal vesicles. Most cancers have a low signal, while the normal peripheral zone has a high signal. Nevertheless, MRI lacks sensitivity and specificity. No single test accurately predicts pathologic stage at surgery.

Another limitation of the TNM system is that the majority of men are now being diagnosed with T1c or T2 disease. Thus, to refine the prediction of local disease extent, most groups are now using multiplex staging models based on a combination of the findings of the DRE, biopsy, Gleason score, and baseline PSA (Table 95-3). Others are developing models based on the number of cores and the percentage of each core involved by tumor. This information can be used to assist patients in selecting treatments, although it remains controversial how recommendations should be affected by a particular level of probability of node-positive disease.

These same parameters are also being used to assess the probability of cure (Fig. 95-2). Some tumors that have extended beyond the confines of the gland may still be curable, while others that are still organ-confined may not. Because successful surgery removes all prostatic tissues, both benign and malignant, and radiation therapy eliminates only the malignant component, different definitions of cure are needed depending on the modality used. Thus, following surgery, the PSA level should become undetectable; following radiation therapy, it should generally fall to <1.0 ng/mL. What the models do not address is what probability of cure a patient would accept to proceed with a given approach. For example, would one categorically deny a surgical procedure to a 40-year-old male if the probability of cure was only 15%? These same models can also be used to stratify patients into risk

groups to assess outcomes of specific therapies. While this form of analysis does not replace prospective trials, it does eliminate the bias associated with the tendency to refer older and more infirm patients for radiation therapy and younger, healthier individuals for surgery.

To complete the staging evaluation, patients may undergo radionuclide bone scanning. This test is highly sensitive but relatively nonspecific, because areas of increased uptake are not always secondary to osteoblastic activity from metastases. Healing fractures, arthritis, Paget's disease, and numerous other conditions will also show abnormal uptake. True-positive bone scan results are rare if the PSA is <8 and uncommon when the PSA is <10 ng/mL. More common is a false-positive scan, which, in turn, leads to additional low-yield testing. CT scans yield little useful clinical information unless the probability of lymph node metastases is >30% using nomogram predictions; an MRI is more likely to detect pathologically significant nodal disease. Molecular diagnostics are being performed that seek to identify the presence of circulating prostate cancer cells using an assay for PSA based on reverse transcriptase polymerase chain reaction (RT-PCR) in the leukocyte fraction of the peripheral blood or bone marrow. A large proportion of men with tumors seemingly confined to the organ test positive; the significance is unclear. These procedures are in their infancy, and application is not advised on a routine basis.

TREATMENT SELECTION: THE MODEL OF CLINICAL STATES

The framework for evaluating the risks from an enlarging but nonmalignant gland, the probability that a clinically significant cancer is present in an individual with or without urinary symptoms, and the probability that a patient with cancer will develop symptoms or die of prostate cancer are provided by the clinical states model illustrated in Fig. 95-3. It includes clinically significant milestones where interventions might be considered and allows for the assessment of the prognosis of the treated patient. In the first state are patients with no cancer diagnosis. It includes patients with benign proliferative disorders or those who warrant screening on the basis of family history or a level of PSA or symptoms. In the second state are those with a cancer that is clinically confined to the gland. For these patients the issue is to determine which tumors require treatment based on their biologic potential, which can be eradicated by local means alone, and which require a combined-modality approach that includes systemic therapy to effect cure. The third state includes those who have a rising PSA level after surgery or radiation for localized disease but who have no clinically detectable lesions on scans. Next are patients with detectable metastases who have not undergone castration, and the last level is those who have detectable disease on scan despite castration. The risk of death from cancer relative to the risk of death from comorbid conditions increases over time, being greatest for the patient who has progressed after hormonal therapy.

At any point, a patient resides in only one state and remains there until the disease progresses. Thus, a patient who presents with a localized prostate cancer who has had all cancer removed surgically remains in the state of localized disease as long as his PSA remains undetectable. In this way, both time factors and that the fact that a patient has been treated are accounted for. Overall treatment effects are assessed by measuring time within a particular state. The scheme also allows a distinction between cure, elimination of all cancer cells, with an undetectable PSA and cancer control, i.e., modulating the rate of growth so that the patient dies of other causes. In this paradigm, a patient with a detectable PSA who dies of other causes having suffered no morbidity from the disease or its treatment, PSA level, is considered a therapeutic success.

MANAGEMENT BY STATES

NO CANCER DIAGNOSIS   **Screening**   The American Cancer Society (ACS) and the AUA recommend an annual DRE and a

Table 95-3 Predicted Probability of Each Pathologic Stage Based on Preoperative PSA, Clinical Stage, and Gleason Grade in the Biopsy Specimen*†

	PSA, 0.0–4.0 NG/ML			PSA, 4.1–10.0 NG/ML			PSA, 10.1–20.0 NG/ML		
	Clinical Stage			Clinical Stage			Clinical Stage		
Gleason Score	T1c	T2a	T2b	T1c	T2a	T2b	T1c	T2a	T2b
ORGAN-CONFINED DISEASE									
5	81 (76–84)	68 (63–72)	57 (50–62)	71 (67–75)	55 (51–60)	43 (38–49)	60 (54–65)	43 (38–49)	32 (26–37)
6	78 (74–81)	64 (59–68)	52 (46–57)	67 (64–70)	51 (47–54)	38 (34–43)	55 (51–59)	38 (34–43)	26 (23–31)
7	63 (58–68)	47 (41–52)	34 (29–39)	49 (45–54)	33 (29–38)	22 (18–26)	35 (31–40)	22 (18–26)	13 (11–16)
8 to 10	52 (41–62)	36 (27–45)	24 (17–32)	37 (28–46)	23 (16–31)	14 (9–19)	23 (16–32)	14 (9–19)	7 (5–11)
ESTABLISHED CAPSULAR PENETRATION									
5	18 (15–22)	30 (26–35)	40 (34–46)	27 (23–30)	41 (36–46)	50 (45–55)	35 (30–40)	50 (45–56)	57 (51–63)
6	21 (18–25)	34 (30–38)	43 (38–48)	30 (27–33)	44 (41–48)	52 (48–56)	38 (34–42)	52 (48–57)	57 (51–62)
7	31 (26–36)	45 (40–50)	51 (46–57)	40 (35–44)	52 (48–57)	54 (49–59)	45 (40–50)	55 (50–60)	51 (45–57)
8 to 10	34 (27–44)	47 (38–56)	48 (40–57)	40 (33–49)	49 (42–57)	46 (39–53)	40 (33–49)	46 (38–55)	38 (30–47)
SEMINAL VESICLE INVOLVEMENT									
5	1 (1–2)	2 (1–3)	3 (2–4)	2 (1–3)	3 (2–5)	5 (3–8)	3 (2–5)	5 (3–8)	8 (5–11)
6	1 (1–2)	2 (1–3)	3 (2–4)	2 (2–3)	3 (2–4)	5 (4–7)	4 (3–5)	5 (3–7)	7 (5–10)
7	4 (2–7)	6 (4–9)	10 (6–14)	8 (5–11)	10 (8–13)	15 (11–19)	12 (8–16)	14 (10–19)	18 (13–24)
8 to 10	9 (5–16)	12 (7–19)	17 (11–25)	15 (10–22)	19 (13–26)	24 (17–31)	20 (13–28)	22 (15–31)	25 (18–34)
LYMPH NODE INVOLVEMENT									
5	0 (0–0)	0 (0–1)	1 (0–2)	0 (0–1)	1 (0–1)	2 (1–3)	1 (0–2)	2 (1–3)	4 (1–7)
6	0 (0–1)	1 (0–1)	2 (1–3)	1 (1–2)	2 (1–3)	4 (3–6)	3 (2–5)	4 (3–6)	10 (7–13)
7	1 (1–3)	2 (1–4)	5 (2–8)	3 (2–5)	4 (3–6)	9 (6–12)	8 (5–11)	9 (6–13)	17 (12–23)
8 to 10	4 (2–7)	5 (2–9)	10 (5–17)	8 (4–12)	9 (5–13)	16 (11–24)	16 (10–24)	17 (11–25)	29 (21–38)

* Modified from Partin AW, Kattan MW, Subong ENP, et al: Combination of prostate-specific antigen, clinical stage, and Gleason score to predict pathological stage of localized prostate cancer a multi-institutional update. JAMA 277:1445, 1997. Copyright 1997 American Medical Association, with permission.
† Numbers represent percent predictive probability (95% CI).
ABBREVIATION: PSA, prostate-specific antigen.

determination of PSA level for all men aged 50 to 79. Individuals with a first-degree relative with prostate cancer and African Americans, who have a higher risk of dying of the disease, are advised to begin testing at age 45. Routine screening for prostate cancer has been advised despite a lack of prospective, randomized, controlled trials proving the benefit of the approach because the disease rarely causes symptoms until it is advanced. The more widespread use of routine DREs and PSA testing has resulted in a significant increase in the proportion of men with clinically localized tumors, a reduced frequency of nodal spread, and a decreased frequency of nodal and osseous disease at presentation. Risks of screening are unnecessary morbidity or mortality from overdetection and overtreatment. Formal clinical trials are underway, but until the studies are complete and the results available, men must make an informed decision to be screened or not.

Hyperplasia A patient with an enlarged prostate who has no symptoms and normal PSA levels generally does not require treatment. Those with symptoms such as an inability to urinate, renal insufficiency, urinary tract infection, gross hematuria, or bladder stones are candidates for prostate surgery. As the natural history is not well defined, it is not always clear whether to intervene and, if so, how. The majority of men do not develop significant obstruction, and in many, minor irritative and/or obstructive symptoms change slowly or not at all. In these cases urine flow studies can identify those whose maximum flows are normal and who are unlikely to benefit from treatment. Measuring postvoid residual volume identifies patients likely to fail a "watch and wait" approach, while pressure-flow studies may identify those with primary bladder dysfunction. A cystoscopic examination is advised for all patients with hematuria and to assess the urinary outflow tract before a surgical intervention. Imaging of the upper urinary tract by ultrasonography or intravenous pyelography should be reserved for patients with indications such as hematuria, a history of stones, or prior urinary tract problems.

Most patients are monitored and/or treated medically, after a discussion with their physicians about the degree of incapacity and/or discomfort present and the likely outcome of each potential treatment strategy. A variety of decision diagrams have been proposed. Patients who opt for deferred therapy should be evaluated on an annual basis by the reassessment of symptoms and clinical manifestations. Medical therapies include finasteride, which blocks the conversion of testosterone to dihydrotestosterone, the principal androgen in the prostate, by competitively inhibiting the 5α-reductase enzyme. A dose of 5 mg/d causes an average decrease in prostate size of ~24%, an increase in urine flow rates, and, in some, improvement in symptoms. Long-term efficacy has not been documented, but symptomatic improvement

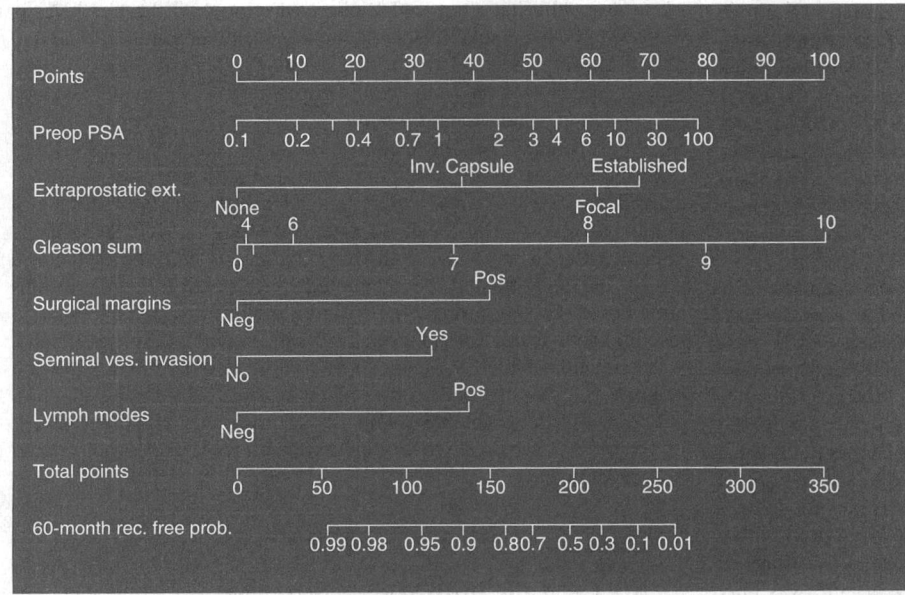

FIGURE 95-2 Kattan recurrence nomogram. (*From Kattan et al.*)

FIGURE 95-3 Clinical states. *(From Scher and Heller).*

has been documented for ≥3 years provided therapy is continued. α-Adrenergic blockers such as terazosin act by relaxing the smooth muscle of the bladder neck, increasing peak urinary flow rates and reducing symptoms. No data prove that these agents influence the progression of the disease.

Patients who do not improve or who progress on medical therapy require surgical intervention. Surgical approaches include a transurethral resection of the prostate (TURP); transurethral incision; or removal of the gland by a retropubic, suprapubic, or perineal route. Other approaches include ultrasound, coils, stents, lasers, or hyperthermia. Overall, surgery offers the best chance for improving symptoms, at the cost of the highest rate of complications. TURP is the most common surgical procedure. Transurethral incision of the prostate is of similar efficacy in men with relatively small prostates and can be performed in ambulatory settings. Open prostatectomy is usually reserved for men with massive prostates; it has the longest recovery time and the highest morbidity, particularly impotence. Transurethral incision has the least morbidity overall and is least disruptive to ejaculatory function.

Elevated PSA and No Cancer Diagnosis on Biopsy Patients who have undergone a biopsy procedure and do not have a cancer diagnosis should continue to be monitored. In some cases, a repeat biopsy session with particular attention to the transition zone is advised. The frequency of PIN is similar in men of different ethnic backgrounds around the world, while the incidence of the clinical disease varies in different ethnic groups. Prevention of progression from PIN to cancer is an area of active research. Proving the benefit of a prevention strategy is difficult because of the long-term follow-up that is necessary, the large sample sizes required to demonstrate a difference in outcome, and the absence of surrogate measures that predict for efficacy. Agents under study include the retinoids, vitamin D, selenium, soy, and modifications of dietary fat. Most are based on epidemiologic data suggesting a decreased prostate cancer risk. A large-scale, double-blind, randomized, multicenter trial of finasteride in men over age 55 has accrued 18,000 men, and follow-up is awaited.

CLINICALLY LOCALIZED DISEASE Localized prostate cancer (stages T1-2, NX or 0, M0) may require no therapy, may be curable with localized therapy, or may require combined-modality systemic and local therapy. The key is to distinguish these distinct prognostic groups. Treatment planning includes an assessment of the probability of local control, local failure, and systemic failure. The more advanced the disease, the lower the probability of local control and the higher the probability of systemic relapse. In general, these tumors are managed by watchful waiting, radical surgery, or radiation therapy. Comparisons between these approaches are limited by the lack of prospective comparative trials, referral biases, and differences in the endpoints evaluated.

Conservative Management (Watchful Waiting) The concept of watchful waiting, or deferred therapy, evolved from the recognition of the high prevalence of the disease in the population, the low probability that some cancers would affect an individual's quality-adjusted life expectancy, and the fact that morbidities associated with the local treatment options were unacceptable to many patients. Watchful waiting acknowledges the facts that the natural history of an untreated prostate cancer is to progress and that it may be difficult to monitor progression within the gland so that the "window of curability" is not

lost. That the disease is often multifocal leads to the possibility that the biopsy on which the decision to defer therapy is made may not represent accurately the malignant potential of a second unidentified cancer. Within 10 years of diagnosis, most tumors produce local symptoms such as urinary retention, incontinence, hematuria, ureteral and bowel obstruction, and pelvic pain, but these complications rarely lead to the death of the patient. Some tumors may metastasize, but few patients succumb to the disease. Case selection criteria are evolving, but in general, watchful waiting is not advised for patients with high-grade disease or for those with a >10-year life expectancy. Some physicians consider observation only for patients with low-grade tumors (Gleason score ≤6) that do not involve more than a small percentage of a single core.

Radical Prostatectomy The objective of a radical prostatectomy is the removal of all prostate tissue with a clear margin of resection, preservation of the external sphincter to maintain continence, and sparing of the autonomic nerves in the neurovascular bundle so that potency is retained. The procedure is performed through a retropubic or perineal approach. In contemporary series, hospital stays are short; mortality <0.4%; and complications such as rectal injury, deep vein thrombosis, and embolic events are rare. The procedure is recommended primarily for patients with clinically localized disease (T1c–T3a, N0 or NX, M0 or MX) who have a life expectancy of >10 years. The operation is not justified in men with a life expectancy <5 years. Properly performed, the procedure requires appropriate case selection and meticulous technique that permits the delineation of the anatomy of the gland and surrounding tissues. In one review, the overall rate of positive margins was 25%. Careful planning can reduce this rate. For example, by considering the laterality and extent of disease, it may be apparent that nerve-sparing cannot be achieved without compromising cancer control. A positive margin increases the risk of progression significantly. Through PSA-based detection, the proportion of men with positive nodes and positive margins continues to decline.

Complication rates, specifically the probability of developing a bladder neck contracture, incontinence, or impotence, vary depending on the experience of the surgeon and whether the patient or the physician is describing the outcome. Rates of incontinence based on physician reporting are 5 to 10%, compared to 19 to 31% based on independent questioning by a third party. Time is also a consideration, as full recovery of function may not occur for weeks or months following the procedure. Factors associated with incontinence include older age, functional length of the urethra, surgical technique, preservation of neurovascular bundles, and development of an anastomotic stricture. If the nerves are preserved, ~70% of men recover the ability to achieve an erection sufficient for penetration. Most men are impotent immediately after the procedure and gradually recover function over 6 to 12 months. Often the quality of the erection is decreased from preoperative levels. Nevertheless, with orally active drugs such as sildenafil, intraurethral inserts of alprostadil, and intracavernosal injections of vasodilators, many patients can achieve nearly natural erections and recover satisfactory sexual activity. Factors associated with recovery include younger age, quality of erections before the operation, and the absence of damage to the neurovascular bundles. Loss of one bundle is associated with a 75% reduction in the recovery of function.

After a successful radical prostatectomy in which all prostate tissue has been removed, serum PSA levels should become undetectable within 4 weeks, based on the half-life of 3 days. If the PSA level remains detectable or becomes detectable after having been undetectable, the patient is considered to have persistent disease or to have a recurrence. In the absence of adjuvant treatment, most patients destined to recur do so within the first 5 years after surgery. Thus, one early benchmark of "success" is the probability of freedom from PSA (or "biochemical") progression. This varies as a function of initial clinical stage, Gleason grade, and serum PSA level before surgery. In one series of 1359 men with clinical stages T1/T2 cancer followed for a mean of 44 months (range 1 to 170), the PSA relapse–free survival rates were 78% at 5 years and 73% at 10 years. In a separate series of T1c patients, 89% were free of progression at 5 years. Considered by baseline PSA levels, 95% of those with a normal level (<4 ng/mL) and 68% of those with a PSA >10 ng/mL were free of progression at 5 years. Considered by grade or Gleason sum in the biopsy specimen, 5- and 10-year PSA relapse-free survivals were 56% and 46%, respectively, for those with tumors of Gleason score of 7, and 46 to 53% at 5 years for those with tumors of Gleason score ≥8. These outcomes appear superior to those reported with watchful waiting, recognizing the limitations in comparing the results of nonrandomized selected series.

The most significant predictor of recurrence is pathologic stage. When the disease is confined to the organ and has not extended into the periprostatic soft tissue, 91 to 97% of patients remain free of progression at 5 years and 85 to 92% at 10 years. Extension to the periprostatic soft tissues (pT3a and N0) decreases PSA relapse–free probabilities to 74% and 68% at 5 and 10 years, respectively, which is decreased further to 40 to 47% and 25% if there is seminal vesicle invasion (pT3c and N0). The high frequency of extracapsular extension and positive surgical margins in patients with clinically localized prostate cancers that were presumed to be confined to the gland led to the investigation of neoadjuvant hormonal therapy. The results of several large contemporary series evaluating 3 months of hormone therapy before surgery showed that, on average, positive margins are reduced from 41% to 17%, serum PSA levels by 96%, and prostate volume by 34% with neoadjuvant hormone therapy. The surrogate of a reduction in positive margin rates was not predictive of a reduction in failure rates, as the time to PSA relapse was no different between groups receiving and not receiving hormones. As such, neoadjuvant hormonal therapy is not recommended. Several recurrence models are available that incorporate all of these factors.

Radiation Therapy   Radiation therapy can be delivered externally, by implantation of radioactive sources into the gland, or a combination of both. As is the case with surgery, outcomes vary as a function of the method, the dose, the endpoints, and whether outcomes were based on clinical or pathologic staging of the lymph nodes. Some groups report local control, and others PSA relapse–free survival, time to metastases, or overall survival. Cause-specific survivals are rarely reported. Local control can be reported on the basis of a DRE alone or the more stringent criterion of a negative biopsy at 18 to 24 months following treatment. Length of follow-up can also influence the results. To standardize reporting, the American Society of Therapeutic Radiation Oncology has developed a consensus definition of PSA relapse as three consecutive rising PSA values from the nadir value.

External beam therapy   Overall, outcomes with external beam therapy are similar for patients with T1 and T2a disease to those obtained with radical surgery. Outcomes for patients with locally advanced disease (T2bc and T3/T4) are less favorable, the result of both inadequate control of the primary tumor and the high rate of systemic failure associated with more advanced disease. For the latter group, 30 to 40% of patients relapse locally using standard doses.

Conventional techniques use simulators and CT scans of the pelvis to determine the location and shape of the target volume and the surrounding normal organs. Typical treatment plans use a four-field pelvic box designed to include the prostate, seminal vesicles, and the locally draining lymph nodes. Normal structures are protected by shaping the beams with cerrobend trim blocks. Therapy is delivered on a daily basis, excepting weekends, in 1.8- to 2.0-Gy fractions. Outcomes are dose-dependent; in one series of stage C patients, actuarial 7-year local recurrence rates were 36% for those receiving 60 to 64.9 Gy, 32% for those receiving 65 to 69.9 Gy, and 24% for those treated at ≥70 Gy. Complication rates also increase with increasing dose. Using standard doses, grade 2 or greater rectal and/or urinary symptoms requiring medication occur in 60% of cases, while late sequelae such as cystitis, hematuria, stricture, or bladder contracture occur in 7% of cases. The frequency of adverse events is significantly higher in patients who have undergone a TURP, while the frequency of rectal complications is directly related to the volume of the anterior rectal wall receiving full-

dose treatment. The frequency of erectile dysfunction is related to the quality of erections before treatment, the dose administered, and the time of assessment. Impotence is related to a disruption of the vascular supply and not the nerve fibers.

More contemporary approaches use three-dimensional conformal radiation therapy (3D-CRT) techniques with sophisticated computer-generated treatment plans to deliver the prescribed radiation dose to the entire target volume, while conforming to the anatomic boundaries of the tumor in its entire three-dimensional configuration. This treatment method has increased the ability to control the cancer through the administration of higher radiation doses, with less morbidity to the surrounding normal organs. In a series of 743 patients treated with 3D-CRT, 90% of patients receiving 75.6 or 81.0 Gy achieved a PSA nadir of ≤1 ng/mL compared with 76% and 56% of those treated with 70.2 Gy and 64.8 Gy, respectively ($p < .001$).

As is the case with surgically treated patients, pre-therapy nomograms can be used to stratify patient groups. In one series, the 5-year actuarial PSA relapse–free survival for patients with favorable prognostic indicators (stage T1/T2, pretreatment PSA of 10.0 ng/mL, and Gleason score of 6) was 85%; it was 65% for those with an intermediate prognosis (one of the prognostic indicators with a higher value) and 35% for those with unfavorable features (two or more indicators with higher values) ($p < .001$).

Tolerance of 3D-CRT has been excellent despite the use of higher radiation doses; grade 3 to 4 rectal or urinary toxicities were seen in 2.1% of patients. In contrast, among patients treated with conventional external-beam radiotherapy, the incidence of grade 3 to 4 toxicities for patients who received radiation doses of >70 Gy was 6.9%.

To improve outcomes for patients with unfavorable features, several groups have explored hormone therapy before radiation therapy. Prospective randomized trials showed improved local control and a delay in time to PSA relapse in patients receiving 2 to 3 years of treatment. The impact on survival has been less clear.

Interstitial therapy   Interstitial brachytherapy is based on the principle that the deposition of radiation energy in tissues decreases exponentially as a function of distance from the radiation source. By infiltrating tumor tissue with radioactive sources, intensive irradiation is delivered to the prostate with minimal irradiation of the surrounding tissues. In a series of 197 patients followed for a median of three years, 5-year actuarial PSA relapse–free survival for patients with pre-therapy PSA levels of 0 to 4, 4 to 10, and >10 were 98%, 90%, and 89%, respectively. Nevertheless, many physicians feel that implantation is best reserved for patients with good or intermediate prognostic features.

Overall, the procedure is well tolerated, although most patients experience urinary frequency and urgency, which can persist for several months. Incontinence has been seen in 2 to 4% of cases. Higher complication rates are observed in patients who have undergone a prior TURP or who have obstructive symptoms at baseline. Proctitis has been reported in <2% of patients. Longer follow-up will be necessary to see whether the overall frequency of impotence is lower, higher, or the same as that observed using external radiation delivery techniques.

RISING PSA   Included in the group of patients with a rising PSA and no evidence of metasatic disease on scans are those who have progressed after watchful waiting, radical prostatectomy, radiation therapy, or both surgery and radiation, with or without prior hormone exposure. For these individuals, the issue is to determine whether the rising PSA is due to local persistence or recurrence (additional therapy to the primary site might be curative) or the result of micrometastatic disease. Imaging studies such as CT, MRI, or bone scan are typically uninformative. The objective is to assess the probability of disease progressing to the point where metastases will occur or cause symptoms. This is the point in the disease where the probability of death from disease exceeds the probability of death from other causes. Difficulty in making these predictions comes from the fact that most patients with a rising PSA receive some form of therapy before the development of metastatic disease, making it virtually impossible to assess the natural history.

To estimate the probability of having a local or systemic recurrence, many investigators use the time to PSA failure or the rate of rise of PSA as predictive factors. In general, recurrences documented >1 year after primary treatment tend to be localized, while those recurring in <1 year tend to be systemic. These predictions are not hard and fast. In one series of patients with PSA recurrence after surgery who did not receive systemic therapy until metastatic disease was documented, the median time to metastatic progression was 8 years, and 63% of the patients with rising PSA values remained free of metastases at 5 years. Patients with tumors of Gleason score 8 to 10 had a probability of metastatic progression of 37%, 51%, and 71% at 3, 5, and 7 years, respectively. Combining a high-grade histology and rapid PSA doubling time, the proportion with metastases was 23%, 32%, and 53% during the same time intervals if the time to recurrence was <2 years and the PSA doubling time was >10 months and 47%, 69%, and 79% for the same recurrence interval with <10 months doubling time. For those with tumors of Gleason score 5 to 7, a PSA recurrence in the first 2 years and a doubling time of <10 months identified a group of patients with a frequency of metastases of 19%, 65%, and 85% at 3, 5, and 7 years, respectively.

FIGURE 95-4 Sites of action of different hormone therapies.

Prostascint scanning uses a radioactive antibody to prostate-specific membrane antigen (PSMA), which is highly expressed on prostate epithelial cells. For a patient who has undergone a radical prostatectomy, antibody localization to the prostatic fossa is suggestive of local recurrence, in which case external beam radiation therapy might be recommended. Others recommend that a biopsy of the urethrovesical anastamosis be obtained before considering radiation. Most, however, rely on clinical criteria with the additional caveat that the probability of durable PSA control varies inversely with the level of PSA at the start of radiation therapy. Radiation therapy is usually not recommended if the PSA level exceeds 1 to 2 ng/mL or if the PSA was persistently elevated after surgery (indicating that disease-free status was not achieved). For patients with a rising PSA after radiation therapy, a salvage prostatectomy can be considered if (1) residual disease is detected in the gland based on a repeat biopsy, (2) the tumor was amenable to surgical extirpation before radiation therapy, and (3) metastatic disease is absent on imaging studies. Unfortunately, case selection is poorly defined in most series, and morbidities have been significant. As currently performed, virtually all patients are impotent, and ~45% have either incontinence or stress incontinence. Bleeding, bladder neck contractures, and rectal injury are not uncommon.

METASTATIC DISEASE **Noncastrate** The removal or blockade of androgens by medical or surgical means is the mainstay of treatment for patients with advanced disease. Surgical orchiectomy is the "gold standard" but is the least preferred by patients. Medical therapies can be subdivided into those that result in a lowering of serum testosterone levels, e.g., gonadotropin-releasing hormone (GnRH) agonists and antagonists and estrogens, and the antiandrogens (Fig. 95-4). Inhibitors of adrenal enzyme synthesis such as ketoconazole and aminoglutethimide are typically used as second-line treatment. The antitumor effects of agents that lower serum testosterone levels are similar, but toxicities differ. Castration is associated with gynecomastia, impotence, weakness, fatigue, hot flushes, loss of muscle mass, changes in personality, anemia, depression, and loss of skeletal mass. Loss of bone mass can be reduced by coadministration of bisphosphonates.

GnRH analogues (leuprolide acetate and goserelin acetate) initially produce a rise in luteinizing hormone (LH) and follicle-stimulating hormone (FSH), followed by a downregulation of receptors in the pituitary gland, which effects a chemical castration. The initial rise in testosterone may result in a clinical flare of the disease. As such, these agents are contraindicated in men with significant obstructive symptoms, cancer-related pain, or spinal cord compromise. The flare can be prevented by pretreatment with antiandrogens. Pure GnRH antagonists that do not produce the initial rise in testosterone will shortly be available.

Diethylstilbestrol (3 mg/d) produces castrate levels of testosterone in 1 to 2 weeks and is inexpensive. Its significant cardiovascular toxicities include edema, congestive heart failure, myocardial infarction, cerebrovascular accidents, phlebitis, and pulmonary embolism. Gynecomastia, a common adverse event, can be reduced by prophylactic irradiation of the breasts. Progestational agents such as medroxyprogesterone acetate (Provera) and megestrol acetate (Megace), are inferior to conventional castration and are not used as first-line treatment. The antifungal agent ketoconazole administered at a dose of 1200 mg/d (six times the antifungal dose) produces a chemical castration in 24 h. It is absorbed in an acid environment and typically prescribed with citrus juices to improve absorption; antacids or H_2 blocking agents reduce absorption and should be avoided when the pills are administered. The effects on testosterone synthesis, however, are not sustained, and long-term use is limited by hepatotoxicity. It can be useful for the unusual patient who presents with a coagulopathy or spinal neurologic compromise and who requires a rapid response. Aminoglutethimide, a second adrenal synthesis inhibitor, was originally developed as an antiseizure medication. It is administered with hydrocortisone. Side effects include somnolence, fatigue, rash, and, after prolonged periods, hypothyroidism; its use is limited.

Nonsteroidal antiandrogens such as flutamide (Eulexin), bicalutamide (Casodex), or nilutamide (Anandron) block the binding of androgens to the receptor. They do not block the production of LH centrally, and as a result, serum testosterone levels increase. These drugs have been used clinically in several situations: (1) to block the flare from the initial rise in testosterone from GnRH use, (2) as monotherapy to preserve potency, and (3) as part of a combined androgen-blockade approach designed to simultaneously inhibit testicular and adrenal androgens. Toxicities differ among the agents but generally include gynecomastia (which can be significant), fatigue, elevations in serum transaminases, and diarrhea. The latter is the most common reason the drug is discontinued. Nilutamide is also associated with impaired adaptation to darkness, alcohol intolerance, and, rarely, pneumonitis.

Hormonal therapy is the treatment of choice, but the timing of treatment is not as clear. Early administration of hormones delays progression, but the survival benefit is less clear. It is controversial whether hormonal therapy should be initiated with a rising PSA level or whether treatment should be held until metastatic disease is detectable on scans. Most physicians recommend use of hormonal therapy with PSA elevation, based on evidence from clinical trials suggesting a survival advantage to such an approach.

A second controversy is whether a combined androgen-blockade that includes an antiandrogen is superior to castration without an antiandrogen. In randomized comparisons, both positive and negative trials have been reported but the majority have shown no difference. Some feel that the method of primary castration (GnRH analogue vs.

orchiectomy) and the class of antiandrogen (steroidal vs. nonsteroidal) may influence outcome, but this is controversial. A meta-analysis of 22 randomized trials that included 5710 patients showed an absolute 2.1% difference in mortality at 5 years. This translated into a 6.4% reduction in the annual odds of death. A similar analysis by the Blue Cross/Blue Shield Association Evidence-Based Practice Center concluded that no benefit was seen with combined androgen blockade.

Castrate The management of patients who progress on hormone therapy requires documentation of a castrate status and an evaluation for residual hormone sensitivity. For patients on hormonal therapy, this involves discontinuing all hormonal therapy to evaluate for a withdrawal response. Responses are noted within a few weeks of stopping the medication, with the exception of nilutamide and bicalutamide, both of which have a long terminal half-life. For these agents, the response may be delayed. Signs of benefit include declines in PSA level, regression of measurable disease, palliation of pain, and improvements in cancer-related anemia.

Patients who are documented to be castrated, and/or who progress after a trial of withdrawal, are often given one additional hormonal manipulation. Depending on prior hormone exposure, options include inhibitors of adrenal steroid hormone synthesis such as ketoconazole and aminoglutethimide, glucocorticoids, antiandrogens, estrogens, or progestational agents. The responses are often short-lived and do not occur in the majority of patients. Nevertheless, the response can be durable in some patients and provide significant palliation in the absence of curative therapies. Glucocorticoids have been associated with clinical benefit and declines in PSA levels in 30 to 40% of cases.

Estramustine (Emcyt) is a synthetic combination of estrogen with a nitrogen mustard moiety at C17 that affects microtubule assembly and disassembly. It has no alkylating effects in vivo. About 20% of the drug is metabolized to pure estrogenic moieties, which exert an antigonadotropin effect and which account for the side effect profile. It is often used in patients who have failed hormone therapy and has additive/synergistic effects with other drugs including the vinca alkaloids (vinblastine and navelbine), taxanes (paclitaxel, docetaxel), and the podophyllotoxins (etoposide).

Patients who progress on primary hormone therapy and after hormone withdrawal and receive one additional (second-line) intervention are considered to have "hormone-independent" or "hormone-refractory" disease. At this point, chemotherapy is often considered, although some feel it has no role in the management of prostate cancer because no single agent or combination of drugs has been shown to improve survival in a prospective randomized trial. In the absence of a proven benefit in survival, it is important to consider the specific goals of therapy before it is recommended. These goals might include palliation of symptoms, delaying progression, or inducing decreases in the PSA level. Interpreting reported outcomes with individual agents is limited in part by differences in case selection and the wide range of endpoints used.

Mitoxantrone has modest activity as a single agent and is more effective at relieving pain and improving quality of life when given together with prednisone. No effect on survival has been shown. However, mitoxantrone plus prednisone and estramustine plus vinblastine are often used to palliate symptoms of disease. The most frequently utilized contemporary regimens are weekly combinations of estramustine and a taxane (paclitaxel or docetaxel). Weekly doxorubin also provides palliation.

PALLIATION OF PAIN Pain is one of the most feared debilitating manifestations of advanced disease. Palliation of pain can be achieved with external beam radiation therapy, bone-seeking radioisotopes, cold bisphosphonates, and chemotherapy. The goals are to relieve symptoms, prevent complications, and improve quality-adjusted life expectancy. To optimize treatment selection, it is important to consider the sites and distribution of the pain and the presence or absence of neurologic compromise. Spinal cord compression is one of the most devastating complications. Once a loss of function is documented, the probability of recovery is small. Particular areas where a high index of suspicion is required are the base of the skull, which

can produce a variety of symptoms including diplopia, deafness, difficulty swallowing, dysarthria, and facial weakness; and mental nerve compression in the jaw, resulting in a numb lip and chin, which can interfere with eating. In these situations, external beam radiation together with glucocorticoids are required.

For a solitary lesion that is symptomatic and can be treated through a single port, external beam radiation therapy is the treatment of choice. Depending on the clinical situation, a single high-dose fraction (6 to 9 Gy) may be all that is necessary. The overall utility is limited by the facts that metastases are rarely solitary and that additional untreated areas often become symptomatic in a relatively short time. In other cases, wide-field portals are needed. For those with more diffuse disease, bone-seeking radioisotopes are available. ^{153}Sm-EDTMP (quadramet) emits β particles and a photon; its half-life is about 22 h. When given at 37 MBq/kg (1 mCi/kg), half the administered dose goes to bone, and 70 to 95% of patients experience decreased bone pain within 2 weeks that lasts 8 to 15 weeks. ^{89}Sr (metastron) is a pure β-emitter with a half-life of 50 days that emits a 1.46-MeV electron with a 2- to 3-mm range in bone. Used alone it has modest effects on the level of PSA but does provide a degree of palliation that is similar to external beam approaches. The results of randomized comparisons suggest a systemic effect, as fewer patients treated with the isotope developed new areas of pain or required additional radiation therapy compared to patients receiving radiation therapy alone. Cold bisphosphonates have been shown to be superior to placebo in the prevention of skeletal events for patients with breast cancer, lung cancer, and multiple myeloma. They may be active in prostate cancer as well.

ACKNOWLEDGMENT

Dr. Jean Wilson and Dr. Arthur Sagalowski were the authors of this chapter in the 14th edition and parts of their chapter have been retained here.

BIBLIOGRAPHY

BENIGN PROSTATIC HYPERPLASIA

CORDON-CARDO C et al: Distinct altered patterns of p27kip1 expression in benign prostatic hyperplasia and prostatic carcinoma. J Natl Cancer Inst 90:1284, 1998

GROSSFELD GD, COAKLEY FV: Benign prostatic hyperplasia: Clinical overview and value of diagnostic imaging. Radiol Clin North Am 38:31, 2000

McCONNELL JD et al: The effect of finasteride on the risk of acute urinary retention and the need for surgical treatment among men with benign prostatic hyperplasia. N Engl J Med 338:557, 1998

PROSTATE CANCER

ALBERTSEN PC et al: Competing risk analysis of men aged 55 to 74 years at diagnosis managed conservatively for clinically localized prostate cancer. JAMA 280:975, 1998

CARTER H et al: Prostate-specific antigen testing of older men. J Natl Cancer Inst 91: 1733, 1999

KATTAN MW et al: Postoperative nomogram for disease recurrence after radical prostatectomy for prostate cancer. J Clin Oncol 17:1499, 1999

OSOBA D et al: Health-related quality of life in men with metastatic prostate cancer treated with prednisone alone or mitxantrone and prednisone. J Clin Oncol 17:1654, 1999

POUND CR et al: Natural history of progression to metastases and death from prostate cancer in men with PSA recurrence following radical prostatectomy. JAMA 281:1591, 1999

SCHER HI, HELLER G: Clinical states in prostate cancer: Towards a dynamic model of disease progression. Urology 55:323, 2000

SELTZER MA et al: Comparison of helical computerized tomography, positron emission tomography and monoclonal antibody scans for evaluation of lymph node metastases in patients with prostate specific antigen relapse after treatment for localized prostate cancer. J Urol 162:1322, 1999

## 96	*Robert J. Motzer, George J. Bosl*

TESTICULAR CANCER

Primary germ cell tumors (GCTs) of the testis, arising by the malignant transformation of primordial germ cells, constitute 95% of all testicular neoplasms. Infrequently, GCTs arise from an extragonadal site, including the mediastinum, retroperitoneum and, very rarely, the pineal gland. This disease is notable for the young age of the afflicted patients, the totipotent capacity for differentiation of the tumor cells, and its curability; >90% of all newly diagnosed patients will be cured. Experience in the management of GCTs leads to improved outcome.

INCIDENCE AND EPIDEMIOLOGY   Nearly 6900 new cases of testicular GCT were diagnosed in the United States in 2000; the incidence of this malignancy has increased slowly over the past 40 years. The tumor occurs most frequently in men between the ages of 20 and 40. A testicular mass in a man 50 years or older should be regarded as a lymphoma until proved otherwise. GCT is at least 4 to 5 times more common in white than in African-American males, and a higher incidence has been observed in Scandinavia and New Zealand than in the United States.

ETIOLOGY AND GENETICS   Cryptorchidism is associated with a severalfold higher risk of GCT. Abdominal cryptorchid testes are at a higher risk than inguinal cryptorchid testes. Orchiopexy should be performed before puberty, if possible. Early orchiopexy reduces the risk of GCT and improves the ability to save the testis. An abdominal cryptorchid testis that cannot be brought into the scrotum should be removed. About 2% of men with GCTs of one testis will develop a primary tumor in the other testis. Testicular feminization syndromes increase the risk of testicular GCT, and Klinefelter's syndrome is associated with mediastinal GCT.

An isochromosome of the short arm of chromosome 12 [i(12p)] is pathognomonic for GCT of all histologic types. Excess 12p copy number either in the form of i(12p) or as increased 12p on aberrantly banded marker chromosomes occurs in nearly all GCT, but the gene(s) on 12p involved in the pathogenesis are not yet defined.

CLINICAL PRESENTATION   A painless testicular mass is pathognomonic for a testicular malignancy. More commonly, patients present with testicular discomfort or swelling suggestive of epididymitis and/or orchitis. In this circumstance, a trial of antibiotics is reasonable. However, if symptoms persist or a residual abnormality remains, then testicular ultrasound examination is indicated.

Ultrasound of the testis is indicated whenever a testicular malignancy is considered and for persistent or painful testicular swelling. If a testicular mass is detected, a radical inguinal orchiectomy should be performed. Because the testis develops from the gonadal ridge, its blood supply and lymphatic drainage originate in the abdomen and descend with the testis into the scrotum. An inguinal approach is taken to avoid breaching anatomic barriers and permitting additional pathways of spread.

Back pain from retroperitoneal metastases is common and must be distinguished from musculoskeletal pain. Dyspnea from pulmonary metastases occurs infrequently. Patients with increased serum levels of human chorionic gonadotropin (hCG) may present with gynecomastia. A delay in diagnosis is associated with a more advanced stage and possibly worse survival.

The staging evaluation for GCT includes a determination of serum levels of α fetoprotein (AFP) and hCG. After orchiectomy, a chest radiograph and a computed tomography (CT) scan of the abdomen and pelvis should be performed. A chest CT scan is required if pulmonary nodules, mediastinal or hilar disease is suspected. *Stage I disease* is limited to the testis, epididymis, or spermatic cord. *Stage II disease* is limited to retroperitoneal (regional) lymph nodes. *Stage III disease* is disease outside the retroperitoneum, involving supradiaphragmatic nodal sites or viscera. The staging may be "clinical"—defined solely by physical examination, blood marker evaluation, and radiographs— or "pathologic"—defined by an operative procedure.

The regional draining lymph nodes for the testis are in the retroperitoneum, and the vascular supply originates from the great vessels (for the right testis) or the renal vessels (for the left testis). As a result, the lymph nodes that are involved first by a right testicular tumor are the interaortocaval lymph nodes just below the renal vessels. For a left testicular tumor, the first involved lymph nodes are lateral to the aorta (para-aortic) and below the left renal vessels. In both cases, further nodal spread is inferior and contralateral and, less commonly, above the renal hilum. Lymphatic involvement can extend cephalad to the retrocrural, posterior mediastinal, and supraclavicular lymph nodes.

Treatment is determined by tumor histology (seminoma versus nonseminoma) and clinical stage (Table 96-1).

PATHOLOGY   GCTs are divided into nonseminoma and seminoma subtypes. Nonseminomatous GCTs are most frequent in the third decade of life and can display the full spectrum of embryonic and adult cellular differentiation. This entity comprises four histologies: embryonal carcinoma, teratoma, choriocarcinoma, and endodermal sinus (yolk sac) tumor. Choriocarcinoma, consisting of both cytotrophoblasts and syncytiophoblasts, represents malignant trophoblastic differentiation and is invariably associated with secretion of hCG. Endodermal sinus tumor is the malignant counterpart of the fetal yolk sac and is associated with secretion of AFP. Pure embryonal carcinoma may secrete AFP or hCG, or both; this pattern is biochemical evidence of differentiation. Teratoma is composed of somatic cell types derived from two or more germ layers (ectoderm, mesoderm, or endoderm). Each of these histologies may be present alone or in combination with others. Nonseminomatous GCTs tend to metastasize early to sites such as the retroperitoneal lymph nodes and lung parenchyma. One-third of patients present with disease limited to the testis (stage I), one-third with retroperitoneal metastases (stage II), and one-third with more extensive supradiaphragmatic nodal or visceral metastases (stage III).

Seminoma represents about 50% of all GCTs, has a median age in the fourth decade, and generally follows a more indolent clinical course. Most patients (70%) present with stage I disease, about 20% with stage II disease, and 10% with stage III disease; lung or other visceral metastases are rare. Radiation therapy is the treatment of choice in patients with stage I disease and stage II disease where the nodes are <5 cm in maximum diameter. When a tumor contains both seminoma and nonseminoma components, patient management is directed by the more aggressive nonseminoma component.

TUMOR MARKERS   Careful monitoring of the serum tumor markers AFP and hCG is essential in the management of patients with GCT, as these markers are important for diagnosis, as prognostic indicators, in monitoring treatment response, and in the detection of early relapse. Approximately 70% of patients presenting with disseminated nonseminomatous GCT have increased serum concentrations of AFP and/or hCG. While hCG concentrations may be increased in patients with either nonseminoma or seminoma histology, the AFP concentration is increased only in patients with nonseminoma. The presence of an increased AFP level in a patient whose tumor showed only seminoma indicates that an occult nonseminomatous component exists and that the patient should be treated accordingly for nonseminomatous GCT. The serum lactate dehydrogenase (LDH) level serves as an additional marker of all GCTs, but it is not as specific as either AFP or

Table 96-1   Germ Cell Tumor Staging and Treatment

Stage	Extent of Disease	Treatment	
		Seminoma	Nonseminoma
I	Testis only, T1, no vascular/lymphatic invasion	Radiation therapy	RPLND or observation
II	T2–4 or vascular/lymphatic invasion present	Radiation therapy	RPLND
IIA	Nodes <2 cm	Radiation therapy	RPLND or chemotherapy often followed by RPLND
IIB	Nodes 2–5 cm	Radiation therapy	RPLND +/− adjuvant chemotherapy or chemotherapy followed by RPLND
IIC	Nodes >5 cm	Chemotherapy	Chemotherapy
III	Distant metastases	Chemotherapy	Chemotherapy, often followed by surgery (biopsy or resection)

hCG. LDH levels are increased in 50 to 60% patients with metastatic nonseminoma and in up to 80% of patients with advanced seminoma.

AFP, hCG, and LDH levels should be determined before and after orchiectomy. Increased serum AFP and hCG concentrations decay according to first-order kinetics; the half-life is 24 to 36 h for hCG and 5 to 7 days for AFP. AFP and hCG should be assayed serially during and after treatment. The reappearance of hCG and/or AFP or the failure of these markers to decline according to the predicted half-life is an indicator of persistent or recurrent tumor.

℞ **TREATMENT**   **Stage I Nonseminoma**   If, after an orchiectomy (for clinical stage I disease), radiographs and physical examination show no evidence of disease, and serum AFP and hCG concentrations either are normal or are declining to normal according to the known half-life, patients may be managed by either a nerve-sparing retroperitoneal lymph node dissection (RPLND) or surveillance. The retroperitoneal lymph nodes are pathologically involved by GCT (pathologic stage II) in 20 to 50% of these patients. The choice of surveillance or RPLND is based on the pathology of the primary tumor. If the primary tumor shows no pathologic evidence for lymphatic or vascular invasion *and* is limited to the testis (T1), then either option is reasonable. If lymphatic or vascular invasion is present *or* the tumor extends into the tunica, spermatic cord, or scrotum (T2 through T4), then surveillance should not be offered. Either approach should cure >95% of patients.

A RPLND is the standard operation for removal of the regional lymph nodes of the testis (retroperitoneal nodes). The operation removes the lymph nodes ipsilateral to the primary site and the nodal groups adjacent to the primary landing zone. The standard (modified bilateral) RPLND removes all node-bearing tissue down to the bifurcation of the great vessels, including the ipsilateral iliac nodes. The major long-term effect of this operation is retrograde ejaculation and infertility. A nerve-sparing RPLND, usually accomplished by identification and dissection of individual nerve fibers, may avoid injury to the sympathetic nerves responsible for ejaculation. Normal ejaculation is preserved in approximately 90% of patients. Patients with pathologic stage I disease are observed, and only the 10% who relapse require additional therapy. If retroperitoneal nodes are found to be involved at RPLND, then a decision regarding adjuvant chemotherapy is made on the basis of the extent of retroperitoneal disease (see below).

Surveillance is an option in the management of clinical stage I disease when no vascular/lymphatic invasion is found and the primary tumor is classified as T1. Only 20 to 30% of patients have pathologic stage II disease, implying that most RPLNDs in this situation are not therapeutic. Although surveillance has not been compared to RPLND in a randomized trial, all large studies show that surveillance and RPLND lead to equivalent long-term survival rates. Patient compliance is essential if surveillance is to be successful. Patients must be carefully followed with periodic chest radiography, physical examination, CT scan of the abdomen, and serum tumor marker determinations. The median time to relapse is about 7 months, and late relapses (later than 2 years) are rare. The 70 to 80% of patients who do not relapse require no intervention after orchiectomy; treatment is reserved for those who do relapse. When the primary tumor is classified as T2 through T4 *or* lymphatic/vascular invasion is identified, nerve-sparing RPLND is preferred. About 50% of these patients have pathologic stage II disease and are destined to relapse.

Stage II Nonseminoma   Patients with limited, ipsilateral retroperitoneal adenopathy (nodes usually ≤3 cm in largest diameter) generally undergo a modified bilateral RPLND as primary management. Nearly all patients with pathologic stage II disease whose disease is completely resected by RPLND are cured. The local recurrence rate after a properly performed RPLND is very low. Depending on the extent of disease, the postoperative management options include either surveillance or two cycles of adjuvant chemotherapy. Surveillance is the preferred approach for patients with resected "low-volume" metastases (tumor nodes ≤2 cm in diameter, *and* <6 nodes are involved) because the probability of relapse is one-third or less. Because relapse occurs in ≥50% of patients with "high-volume" metastasis (>6 nodes involved, *or* any involved node >2 cm in largest diameter, *or* extranodal tumor extension), two cycles of adjuvant chemotherapy should be considered, as it results in cure in ≥98% of patients. Regimens consisting of etoposide (100 mg/m² daily on days 1 through 5) plus cisplatin (20 mg/m² daily on days 1 through 5) with or without bleomycin (30 units per day on days 2, 9, and 16) given at 3-week intervals are effective and well tolerated.

Stages I and II Seminoma   Inguinal orchiectomy followed by retroperitoneal radiation therapy cures about 98% of patients with stage I seminoma. The dose of radiation (2500 to 3000 cGy) is low and well tolerated, and the in-field recurrence rate is negligible. About 2% of patients relapse with supradiaphragmatic or systemic disease. Surveillance has been proposed as an option, and studies have shown that about 15% of patients relapse. The median time to relapse is 12 to 15 months, and late relapses during surveillance (>5 years) may be more frequent than with nonseminoma. The relapse is usually treated with chemotherapy. Surveillance for clinical stage I seminoma is generally not recommended.

Nonbulky retroperitoneal disease (stage IIA and IIB) is also treated with radiation therapy. Prophylactic supradiaphragmatic fields are not used. Relapses in the anterior mediastinum are unusual. Approximately 90% of patients achieve relapse-free survival with retroperitoneal masses <5 cm in diameter. Because at least one-third of patients with bulkier disease relapse, initial chemotherapy is preferred for stage IIC disease.

Chemotherapy for Advanced GCT   Regardless of histology, patients with stage IIC and stage III GCT are treated with chemotherapy. Combination chemotherapy programs based on cisplatin at doses of 100 to 120 mg/m² per cycle plus etoposide cure 70 to 80% of such patients, with or without bleomycin, depending on risk stratification (see below). A complete response (the complete disappearance of all clinical evidence of tumor on physical examination and radiography plus normal serum levels of AFP and hCG for 1 month or more) occurs after chemotherapy alone in about 60% of patients, and another 10 to 20% become disease-free with surgical resection of all sites of residual disease. Lower doses of cisplatin result in inferior survival rates.

The toxicity of the cisplatin/bleomycin/etoposide (BEP) regimen may be substantial. Nausea, vomiting, and hair loss occur in most patients, although nausea and vomiting have been markedly ameliorated by modern antiemetic regimens. Myelosuppression is frequent, and symptomatic bleomycin pulmonary toxicity occurs in about 5% of patients. Treatment-induced mortality due to neutropenia with septicemia or bleomycin-induced pulmonary failure occurs in 1 to 3% of patients. Dose reductions for myelosuppression are rarely indicated. Long-term permanent toxicities include nephrotoxicity (reduced glomerular filtration and persistent magnesium wasting), ototoxicity, and peripheral neuropathy. When bleomycin is administered by weekly bolus injection, Raynaud's phenomenon appears in 5 to 10% of patients. Less often, other evidence of small blood vessel damage has been reported, including transient ischemic attacks and myocardial infarction.

Risk-Directed Chemotherapy   Because not all patients are cured and treatment may cause significant toxicities, patients are stratified into "good-risk" and "poor-risk" groups according to pretreatment clinical features. For good-risk patients, the goal is to achieve maximum efficacy with minimal toxicity. For poor-risk patients, the goal is to identify more effective therapy with tolerable toxicity.

The International Germ Cell Cancer Consensus Group (IGCCCG) developed criteria to assign patients to three risk groups (good, intermediate, poor) (Table 96-2). Seminoma is either good or intermediate risk based on the absence or presence of nonpulmonary visceral metastases. Marker levels play no role in defining risk. No poor-risk category exists for seminoma. Nonseminomas have good-, intermediate-, and poor-risk categories based on the site of the primary tumor,

Risk Group	Nonseminoma	Seminoma
Good	Gonadal or retroperitoneal primary site, no nonpulmonary visceral metastases, AFP <1000 ng/mL, beta-hCG < mIU/mL, LDH <1.5 × upper limit of normal (ULN)	Any primary site, no nonpulmonary visceral metastases, any LDH are hCG levels
Intermediate	Gonadal or retroperitoneal primary site, no nonpulmonary visceral metastases, AFP 1000–10000 ng/mL, beta-hCG 5000–50000 mIU/mL, LDH 1.5–10 × ULN	Any primary site, nonpulmonary visceral metastases present, any LDH and hCG levels
Poor	Mediastinal primary site, nonpulmonary visceral metastases present, AFP ≥10000 ng/ML, beta-hCG >50,000 mIU/mL, LDH >10 × ULN	No patients classified as poor risk

the presence or absence of nonpulmonary visceral metastases, and marker levels.

For ~90% of patients with good-risk GCTs, four cycles of etoposide plus cisplatin (EP) or three cycles of BEP produce durable, complete responses, with minimal acute and chronic toxicity. Pulmonary toxicity is absent when bleomycin is not used and is rare when therapy is limited to 9 weeks; myelosuppression with neutropenic fever is less frequent; and the treatment mortality rate is negligible. About 75% of intermediate-risk patients and 45% of poor-risk patients achieve durable complete remission with four cycles of BEP, and no regimen has proved superior. More effective therapy is needed.

Postchemotherapy Surgery Resection of residual metastases after the completion of chemotherapy is an integral part of therapy. If the initial histology is nonseminoma and the marker values have normalized, all sites of residual disease should be resected. In general, residual retroperitoneal disease requires a modified bilateral RPLND, which is associated with retrograde ejaculation. Thoracotomy (unilateral or bilateral) and neck dissection are less frequently required to remove residual mediastinal, pulmonary parenchymal, or cervical nodal disease. Viable tumor (seminoma, embryonal carcinoma, yolk sac tumor, or choriocarcinoma) will be present in 15%, mature teratoma in 40%, and necrotic debris and fibrosis in 45% of resected specimens. The frequency of teratoma or viable disease is highest in residual mediastinal tumors. If necrotic debris or mature teratoma is present, no further chemotherapy is necessary. If viable tumor is present but is completely excised, two additional cycles of chemotherapy are given.

If the initial histology is seminoma, mature teratoma is rarely present, and the most frequent finding is necrotic debris. For residual retroperitoneal disease, a complete RPLND is technically difficult owing to extensive postchemotherapy fibrosis. Observation is recommended when no radiographic abnormality exists or a residual mass <3 cm is present. Controversy exists over what to do when the residual mass exceeds 3 cm in diameter. About 25% of such masses contain viable GCT. Some investigators prefer excision or biopsy, but radiation therapy and surveillance are alternatives.

Salvage Chemotherapy Of patients with advanced GCT, 20 to 30% fail to achieve a durable complete response to first-line chemotherapy. A combination of cisplatin, ifosfamide and vinblastine (VeIP) will cure about 25% of patients as a second-line therapy. Patients are more likely to achieve a durable complete response to VeIP if they had a testicular primary tumor and relapsed from a prior complete remission to first-line cisplatin-containing chemotherapy. In contrast, if the patient failed to achieve a complete response or has a primary mediastinal nonseminoma, then VeIP is rarely beneficial. Those patients are candidates for dose-intensive treatment.

Chemotherapy consisting of dose-intensive, high-dose carboplatin (≥1500 mg/m^2) plus etoposide (≥1200 mg/m^2), with or without cyclophosphamide or ifosfamide, with peripheral blood stem cell support induces a complete response in 25 to 40% of patients who have progressed after ifosfamide-containing salvage chemotherapy. About one-half of the complete responses will be durable. High-dose therapy is the treatment of choice and standard of care for this patient population. Paclitaxel is active in previously treated patients and is being studied as a new component in conventional-dose and dose-intensive salvage therapy. Cure is still possible in some relapsed patients.

EXTRAGONADAL GCT AND MIDLINE CARCINOMA OF UNCERTAIN HISTOGENESIS The prognosis and management of patients with extragonadal GCTs depends on the tumor histology and site of origin. All patients with a diagnosis of extragonadal GCT should have a testicular ultrasound examination. Nearly all patients with retroperitoneal or mediastinal seminoma achieve a durable complete response to BEP or EP. The clinical features of patients with primary retroperitoneal nonseminoma GCT are similar to those of patients with a primary of testis origin, and careful evaluation will find evidence of a primary testicular GCT in about two-thirds of cases. In contrast, a primary mediastinal nonseminomatous GCT is associated with a poor prognosis; one-third of patients are cured with standard therapy (four cycles of BEP). Patients with newly diagnosed mediastinal nonseminoma are considered to have poor-risk disease and should be considered for clinical trials testing regimens of possibly greater efficacy. In addition, mediastinal nonseminoma is associated with hematologic disorders, including acute myelogenous leukemia, myelodysplastic syndrome, and essential thrombocytosis unrelated to previous chemotherapy. These hematologic disorders are very refractory to treatment. Nonseminoma of any primary site may change into other malignant histologies such as embryonal rhabdomyosarcoma or adenocarcinoma. This is called malignant transformation. i(12p) has been identified in the transformed cell type, indicating GCT clonal origin.

A group of patients (most commonly men) with poorly differentiated tumors of unknown histogenesis, midline in distribution, and not associated with secretion of AFP or hCG has been described; a few (10 to 20%) are cured by standard cisplatin-containing chemotherapy. i(12p) is present in about 25% of such tumors (the fraction that are cisplatin-responsive), confirming their origin from primitive germ cells. This finding is also predictive of the response to cisplatin-based chemotherapy and resulting long-term survival. These tumors are heterogeneous; neuroepithelial tumors and lymphoma may also present in this fashion.

FERTILITY Infertility is an important consequence of the treatment of GCTs. Preexisting infertility or impaired fertility is often present. Azoospermia and/or oligospermia are present at diagnosis in at least 50% of patients with testicular GCTs. Ejaculatory dysfunction is associated with RPLND, and germ cell damage may result from cisplatin-containing chemotherapy. Nerve-sparing techniques to preserve the retroperitoneal sympathetic nerves have made retrograde ejaculation less likely in the subgroups of patients who are candidates for this operation. Spermatogenesis does recur in some patients after chemotherapy. However, because of the significant risk of impaired reproductive capacity, semen analysis and cryopreservation of sperm in a sperm bank should be recommended to all patients before radiation therapy, chemotherapy, or RPLND.

BIBLIOGRAPHY

Bosl GJ et al: Testicular germ-cell cancer. N Engl J Med 337:242, 1997

Chaganti RSK et al: Molecular biology of adult male germ cell tumors, in *Comprehensive Tetbook of Genitourinary Oncology*, NJ Vogelzang, PT Scardino, WO Shipley, DS Coffey (eds). Baltimore, Williams and Wilkins, 1999

Einhorn LH et al: Evaluation of optimal duration of chemitherapy in favorable-prognosis disseminated germ cell tumors: A Southeastern Cancer Study Group protocol. J Clin Oncol 7:387, 1989

INTERNATIONAL GERM CELL CANCER CONSENSUS GROUP: International Germ Cell Consensus Classification: A prognostic factor-based staging system for metastatic germ cell cancers. J Clin Oncol 15:594, 1997

LOEHRER PJ et al: Vinblastine plus ifosfamide plus cisplatin as initial salvage therapy in recurrent germ cell tumor. J Clin Oncol 16:2500, 1998

SIEGERT W et al: Germ cell tumors: dose-intensive therapy. Semin Oncol 25:215, 1998

| 97 | *Robert C. Young* |

GYNECOLOGIC MALIGNANCIES

OVARIAN CANCER

Incidence and Epidemiology Epithelial ovarian cancer is the leading cause of death from gynecologic cancer in the United States. In 2000, 23,100 new cases were diagnosed and 14,000 women died from ovarian cancer. The disease accounts for 5% of all cancer deaths in women in the United States; more women die of this disease than from cervical and endometrial cancer combined.

The age-specific incidence of the common epithelial type of ovarian cancer increases progressively and peaks in the eighth decade. Epithelial tumors, unlike germ cell and stromal tumors, are uncommon before the age of 40. Epidemiologic studies suggest higher incidences in industrialized nations and an association with disordered ovarian function, including infertility, nulliparity, frequent miscarriages, and use of ovulation-inducing drugs such as clomiphene. Each pregnancy reduces the ovarian cancer risk by about 10%, and breast feeding and tubal ligation also appear to reduce the risk. Oral contraceptives reduce the risk of ovarian cancer in patients with a familial history of cancer and in the general population. Many of these risk-reduction factors support the "incessant ovulation" hypothesis for ovarian cancer etiology, which implies that an aberrant repair process of the surface epithelium is central to ovarian cancer development. Estrogen replacement after menopause does not appear to increase the risk of ovarian cancer, although one study showed a modest increase in risk with >11 years of use.

Familial cases account for about 5% of all ovarian cancer, and a family history of ovarian cancer is a major risk factor. Compared to a lifetime risk of 1.6% in the general population, women with one affected first-degree relative have a 5% risk. In families with two or more affected first-degree relatives, the risk may exceed 50%. Three types of autosomal dominant familial cancer are recognized: (1) site-specific in which only ovarian cancer is seen, (2) families with cancer of the ovary and breast, and (3) the Lynch type II cancer family syndrome with nonpolyposis colorectal cancer, endometrial cancer, and ovarian cancer.

Etiology and Genetics In women with hereditary breast-ovarian cancer, two susceptibility loci have been identified: BRCA-1, located on chromosome 17q12-21, and BRCA-2, on 13q12-13. Both are tumor suppressor genes, and their protein products act as inhibitors of tumor growth. Both genes are large, and numerous mutations have been described; most are frameshift or nonsense mutations, and 86% produce truncated protein products. The implications of the many other mutations including many missense mutations are not known. The cumulative risk of ovarian cancer with critical mutations of BRCA-1 or -2 is 25%, compared to the lifetime risk of 50% for breast cancer for similar mutations. Men in such families have an increased risk of prostate cancer.

Cytogenetic analysis of sporadic epithelial ovarian cancers generally reveals complex karyotypic rearrangements. Structural abnormalities frequently appear on chromosomes 1 and 11, and loss of heterozygosity (LOH) is common on 3q, 6q, 11q, 13q, and 17.

Abnormalities of oncogenes are frequently found in ovarian cancer and include c-*myc*, H-*ras*, K-*ras*, and *neu*.

Ovarian tumors (usually not epithelial) are sometimes components of complex genetic syndromes. Peutz-Jeghers syndrome (mucocutaneous pigmentation and intestinal polyps) is associated with ovarian sex cord stromal tumors and Sertoli cell tumors in men. Patients with gonadal dysgenesis (46XY genotype or mosaic for Y-containing cell lines) develop gonadoblastomas, and women with nevoid basal cell carcinomas have an increased risk of ovarian fibromas.

Clinical Presentation and Differential Diagnosis Most patients with ovarian cancer are first diagnosed when the disease has already spread beyond the true pelvis. The occurrence of abdominal pain, bloating, and urinary symptoms usually indicates advanced disease. Localized ovarian cancer is generally asymptomatic. However, progressive enlargement of a localized ovarian tumor can produce urinary frequency or constipation, and rarely torsion of an ovarian mass causes acute abdominal pain or a surgical abdomen. In contrast to cervical or endometrial cancer, vaginal bleeding or discharge is rarely seen with early ovarian cancer. The diagnosis of early disease usually occurs with palpation of an asymptomatic adnexal mass during routine pelvic examination. However, most ovarian enlargements discovered this way, especially in premenopausal women, are benign functional cysts that characteristically resolve over one to three menstrual cycles. Adnexal masses in premenarchal or postmenopausal women are more likely to be pathologic. A solid, irregular, fixed pelvic mass is usually ovarian cancer. Other causes of adnexal masses include pedunculated uterine fibroids, endometriosis, benign ovarian neoplasms, and inflammatory lesions of the bowel.

Evaluation of patients with suspected ovarian cancer should include measurement of serum levels of the tumor marker CA-125. CA-125 determinants are glycoproteins with molecular masses from 220 to 1000 kDa, and a radioimmunoassay is used to determine circulating CA-125 antigen levels. Between 80 and 85% of patients with epithelial ovarian cancer have levels of CA-125 ≥35 U/mL. Other malignant tumors can also elevate CA-125 levels, including cancers of the endometrium, cervix, fallopian tubes, pancreas, breast, lung, and colon. Certain nonmalignant conditions that can elevate CA-125 levels include pregnancy, endometriosis, pelvic inflammatory disease, and uterine fibroids. About 1% of normal females have serum CA-125 levels >35 U/mL. However, in postmenopausal women with an asymptomatic pelvic mass and CA-125 levels ≥65 U/mL, the test has a sensitivity of 97% and a specificity of 78%.

Screening In contrast to patients who present with advanced disease, patients with early ovarian cancers (stages I and II) are commonly curable with conventional therapy. Thus, effective screening procedures would improve the cure rate in this disease. Although pelvic examination can occasionally detect early disease, it is a relatively insensitive screening procedure. Transvaginal sonography has replaced the slower and less sensitive abdominal sonography, but significant false-positive results are noted, particularly in premenopausal women. In one study, 67 laparotomies were required to diagnose 1 primary ovarian cancer. Doppler flow imaging coupled with transvaginal ultrasound may improve accuracy and reduce the high rate of false positives.

CA-125 has been studied as a screening tool. Unfortunately, half of women with stages I and II ovarian cancer have CA-125 levels <65 U/mL. Other nonmalignant disorders can elevate the CA-125 level, and both false-negative and -positive results have been high in most screening studies.

Attempts have been made to improve the sensitivity and specificity by combinations of procedures, commonly transvaginal ultrasound and CA-125 levels. In a screening study of 22,000 women, 42 had a positive screen and 11 had ovarian cancer (7 with advanced disease). In addition, eight women with a negative screen developed ovarian cancer. Thus, the false-positive rate would lead to a large number of unnecessary (i.e., negative) laparotomies if each positive screen resulted in a surgical exploration. The National Institutes of Health Consensus Conference recommended against screening for ovarian cancer among the general population without known risk factors for the disease. Although no evidence shows that screening saves lives, many physicians use annual pelvic examinations, transvaginal ultrasound, and CA-125 levels to screen women with a family history of ovarian cancer or breast/ovarian cancer syndromes.

Pathology Common epithelial tumors comprise most (85%) of the ovarian neoplasms. These may be benign (50%), frankly malignant (33%), or tumors of low malignant potential (16%) (tumors of borderline malignancy). Epithelial tumors of low malignant potential have the cytologic features of malignancy but do not invade the ovarian stroma. More than 75% of borderline malignancies present in early stage and generally occur in younger women. They have a much better natural history than their malignant counterpart.

There are five major subtypes of common epithelial tumors: serous (50%), mucinous (25%), endometroid (15%), clear cell (5%), and Brenner tumors (1%), the latter derived from the urothelium. Benign common epithelial tumors are almost always serous or mucinous and develop in women ages 20 to 60. They are frequently large (20 to 30 cm), bilateral, and cystic.

Malignant epithelial tumors are usually seen in women over 40. They present as solid masses, with areas of necrosis and hemorrhage. Masses >10 to 15 cm have usually already spread into the intraabdominal space. Spread eventually results in intraabdominal carcinomatosis, which leads to bowel and renal obstruction and cachexia.

Although most ovarian tumors are epithelial, two other important ovarian tumor types exist—stromal and germ cell tumors. These tumors are distinct in their cell of origin but also have different clinical presentations and natural histories and are often managed differently (see below).

Metastasis to the ovary can occur from breast, colon, gastric, and pancreatic cancers, and the Krukenberg tumor was classically described as bilateral ovarian masses from metastatic mucin-secreting gastrointestinal cancers.

Staging and Prognostic Factors Laparotomy is often the primary procedure used to establish the diagnosis. Less invasive studies useful in defining the extent of spread include chest x-rays, abdominal computed tomography scans, and abdominal and pelvic sonography. If the woman has specific gastrointestinal symptoms, a barium enema or gastrointestinal series can be performed. Symptoms of bladder or renal dysfunction can be evaluated by cystoscopy or intravenous pyelography.

A careful staging laparotomy will establish the stage and extent of disease and allow for the cytoreduction of tumor masses in patients with advanced disease. Proper laparotomy requires a vertical incision of sufficient length to ensure adequate examination of the abdominal contents. The presence, amount, and cytology of any ascites fluid should be noted. The primary tumor should be evaluated for rupture, excrescences, or dense adherence. Careful visual and manual inspection of the diaphragm and peritoneal surfaces is required. In addition to total abdominal hysterectomy and bilateral salpingo-oophorectomy, a partial omentectomy should be performed and the paracolic gutters inspected. Pelvic lymph nodes as well as para-aortic nodes in the region of the renal hilus should be biopsied. Since this surgical procedure defines stage, establishes prognosis, and determines the necessity for subsequent therapy, it should be performed by a surgeon with special expertise in ovarian cancer staging. Studies have shown that patients operated upon by gynecologic oncologists were properly staged 97% of the time, compared to 52 and 35% of cases staged by obstetricians/gynecologists and general surgeons, respectively. At the end of staging, 23% of women have stage I disease (cancer confined to the ovary or ovaries); 13% have stage II (disease confined to the true pelvis);

Stage	Ovarian	5-Year Survival, %	Endometrial	5-Year Survival, %	Cervix	5-Year Survival, %
0	—		—		Carcinoma in situ	100
I	Confined to ovary	90	Confined to corpus	89	Confined to uterus	85
II	Confined to pelvis	70	Involves corpus and cervix	80	Invades beyond uterus but not to pelvic wall	60
III	Intraabdominal spread	15–20	Extends outside the uterus but not outside the true pelvis	30	Extends to pelvic wall and/or lower third of vagina, or hydronephrosis	33
IV	Spread outside abdomen	1–5	Extends outside the true pelvis or involves the bladder or rectum	9	Invades mucosa of bladder or rectum or extends beyond the true pelvis	7

Table 97-1 Staging and Survival in Gynecologic Malignancies

47% have stage III (disease spread into but confined to the abdomen); and 16% have stage IV disease (spread outside the pelvis and abdomen). The 5-year survival correlates with stage of disease: stage I—90%, stage II—70%, stage III—15 to 20%, and stage IV—1 to 5% (Table 97-1).

Prognosis in ovarian cancer is dependent not only upon stage but on the extent of residual disease and histologic grade. Patients presenting with advanced disease but left without significant residual disease after surgery have a median survival of 39 months, compared to 17 months for those with suboptimal tumor resection.

Prognosis of epithelial tumors is also highly influenced by histologic grade but less so by histologic type. In early-stage disease, survival is better in mucinous adenocarcinoma than endometrial and serous types, and clear cell carcinomas have the worst prognosis. Although grading systems differ among pathologists, all grading systems show a better prognosis for well- or moderately differentiated tumors and a poorer prognosis for poorly differentiated histologies. Typical 5-year survivals for patients with all stages of disease are: well differentiated—88%, moderately differentiated—58%, poorly differentiated—27%.

The prognostic significance of pre- and postoperative CA-125 levels is uncertain. Serum levels generally reflect volume of disease, and high levels usually indicate unresectability and a poorer survival. Postoperative levels, if elevated, usually indicate residual disease. Nevertheless, on multivariate analysis, CA-125 is not an independent prognostic factor because of the association with volume of disease. The rate of decline of CA-125 levels during initial therapy or the absolute level after one to three cycles of chemotherapy correlates with prognosis but is not sufficiently accurate to guide individual treatment decisions. Even when the CA-125 level falls to normal after surgery or chemotherapy, "second-look" laparotomy identifies residual disease in 60% of women. Other more quantitative approaches to define prognosis include ploidy analysis and image cytometry (automated analysis of cell morphology); they remain investigational.

Genetic and biologic factors may influence prognosis. Increased tumor levels of p53 are associated with a worse prognosis in advanced disease. Epidermal growth factor receptors in ovarian cancer are associated with a high risk of progression, but the increased expression of HER-2/neu has given conflicting prognostic results, and expression of Mdr-1 has not been of prognostic value. HER-2/neu is being evaluated as a target for antibody therapy.

℞ **TREATMENT** The selection of therapy for patients with epithelial ovarian cancer depends upon the stage, extent of residual tumor, and histologic grade. In general, patients are considered in three separate treatment groups: (1) those with early (stages I and II) ovarian cancer and microscopic or no residual disease; (2) patients with advanced (stage III) disease but minimal residual tumor (<1 cm) after initial surgery; and (3) patients with bulky residual tumor and advanced (stage III or IV) disease.

Patients with stage I disease, no residual tumor, and well or moderately differentiated tumors need no adjuvant therapy after definitive surgery and 5-year survival exceeds 95%. For all other patients with early disease and those stage I patients with poor prognosis histologic grade, adjuvant therapy is probably warranted, and single-agent cisplatin or platinum-containing drug combinations used in advanced disease are appropriate. Five-year survival for this group exceeds 80%.

For the patients with advanced (stage III) disease but with limited or no residual disease after definitive cytoreductive surgery (about half of all stage III patients), the primary therapy is platinum-based combination chemotherapy. Approximately 70% of women respond to initial combination chemotherapy, and 40 to 50% have a complete regression of disease. Only about half of these patients are free of disease if surgically restaged. Although a variety of combinations are active, a randomized prospective trial of paclitaxel and cisplatin compared to cyclophosphamide and cisplatin in patients with more advanced disease demonstrated better results for the paclitaxel-cisplatin combination (response rate: 77 versus 64%; complete remission rate: 54 versus 33%, median survival: 37.5 versus 24.4 months). A subsequent trial of paclitaxel, 175 mg/m^2 by 3-h infusion, and carboplatin, dosed to an AUC (area under the curve) of 7.5, showed equal antitumor activity to paclitaxel plus cisplatin but substantially less toxicity.

Patients with advanced disease (stages III and IV) and bulky residual tumor are generally treated with a paclitaxel-platinum combination regimen as well and, while the overall prognosis is poorer, 5-year survival may reach 10 to 15%. In some instances, cytoreductive surgery can be performed after initial response to chemotherapy, and a multicenter European trial demonstrated that this strategy led to a significant improvement in progression-free interval and survival.

Historically, patients who had an excellent initial response to chemotherapy and have no clinical evidence of disease have had a second-look laparotomy. For patients with stage I ovarian cancer or for germ cell tumors, the operation rarely detects residual tumor and has been largely abandoned. Even for those with stages II and III epithelial tumors, the second-look surgical procedure itself does not prolong overall survival. Its routine use cannot be recommended. Maintenance therapy does not prevent recurrences in patients in complete remission.

Patients with advanced disease whose disease recurs after initial treatment are usually not curable but may benefit significantly from limited surgery to relieve intestinal obstruction, localized radiation therapy to relieve pressure or pain from mass lesions or metastasis, or palliative chemotherapy. The selection of chemotherapy for palliation depends upon the initial regimen and evidence of drug resistance. Patients who have a complete regression of disease that lasts ≥6 months respond to reinduction with the same agents. Patients relapsing within the first 6 months of initial therapy rarely do. Chemotherapeutic agents with >15% response rates in patients relapsing after initial combination chemotherapy include gemcitabine, topotecan, ifosfamide, etoposide, and hexamethylmelamine. Intraperitoneal chemotherapy (usually cisplatin) may be used if a small residual volume (<1 cm^3) of tumor exists. Progestational agents and antiestrogens produce responses in 5 to 15% of patients and have minimal side effects.

Borderline malignancy has a 95% 5-year survival even in stage III disease when managed with surgery. Radiation and chemotherapy are not useful.

OVARIAN GERM CELL TUMORS   Fewer than 5% of all ovarian tumors are germ cell in origin. They include teratoma, dysgerminoma, endodermal sinus tumor, and embryonal carcinoma. Germ cell tumors of the ovary generally occur in younger women (75% of ovarian malignancies in women <30), display an unusually aggressive

natural history, and are commonly cured with less extensive nonsterilizing surgery and chemotherapy. Women cured of these malignancies are able to conceive and have normal children.

These neoplasms can be divided into three major groups: (1) benign tumors (usually dermoid cysts); (2) malignant tumors that arise from dermoid cysts; and (3) primitive malignant germ cell tumors including dysgerminoma, yolk sac tumors, immature teratomas, embryonal carcinomas, and choriocarcinoma.

Dermoid cysts are teratomatous cysts usually lined by epidermis and skin appendages. They often contain hair, and calcified bone or teeth can sometimes be seen on conventional pelvic x-ray. They are almost always curable by surgical resection. Approximately 1% of these tumors have malignant elements, usually squamous cell carcinoma.

Malignant germ cell tumors are usually large (median—16 cm). Bilateral disease is rare except in dysgerminoma (10 to 15% bilaterality). Abdominal or pelvic pain in young women is the usual presenting symptom. Serum human chorionic gonadoptropin (β-hCG) and α fetoprotein levels are useful in the diagnosis and management of these patients. Before the advent of chemotherapy, extensive surgery was routine but has now been replaced by careful evaluation of extent of spread followed by resection of bulky disease and preservation of one ovary, uterus, and cervix, if feasible. This allows many affected women to preserve fertility. After surgical staging, 60 to 75% of women have stage I disease and 25 to 30% have stage III disease. Stages II and IV are infrequent.

Most of the malignant germ cell tumors are managed with chemotherapy after surgery. Regimens used in testicular cancer such as PVB (cisplatin, vinblastine, bleomycin) and BEP (bleomycin 30 units IV weekly, etoposide 100 mg/m^2 days 1 to 5, and cisplatin 20 mg/m^2 days 1 to 5), with three or four courses given at 21-day intervals, have produced 95% long-term survival in patients with stages I to III disease. This regimen is the treatment of choice for all malignant germ cell tumors except grade I, stage I immature teratoma, where surgery alone is adequate, and perhaps early-stage dysgerminoma, where surgery and radiation therapy are used.

Dysgerminoma is the ovarian counterpart of testicular seminoma. The tumor is very sensitive to radiation therapy. The 5-year disease-free survival is 100% in early-stage patients and 61% in stage III disease. Unfortunately, the use of radiation therapy makes many patients infertile. BEP chemotherapy is equally or more effective and does not cause infertility. In incompletely resected patients with dysgerminoma, the 2-year disease-free survival was 95% and infertility was not observed. Combination chemotherapy (BEP) has replaced postoperative radiation therapy as the treatment of choice in women with ovarian dysgerminoma.

OVARIAN STROMAL TUMORS   Stromal tumors make up <10% of ovarian tumors. They are named for the stromal tissue involved: granulosa, theca, Sertoli, Leydig, and collagen-producing stromal cells. The granulosa and theca cell stromal cell tumors occur most frequently in the first three decades of life. Granulosa cell tumors frequently produce estrogen and cause menstrual abnormalities, bleeding, and precocious puberty. Endometrial carcinoma can be seen in 5% of these women, perhaps related to the persistent hyperestrogenism. Sertoli and Leydig cell tumors, when functional, produce androgens with resultant virilization or hirsutism. Some 75% of these stromal cell tumors present in stage I and can be cured with total abdominal hysterectomy and bilateral salpingo-oophorectomy. Stromal tumors generally grow slowly, and recurrences can occur 5 to 10 years after initial surgery. Neither radiation therapy nor chemotherapy have been documented to be consistently effective, and surgical management remains the primary treatment.

CARCINOMA OF THE FALLOPIAN TUBE

The fallopian tube is the least common site of cancer in the female genital tract although its epithelial surface far exceeds that of the ovary, where epithelial cancer is 20 times more common. Approximately 300 new cases occur yearly; 90% are papillary serous adenocarcinomas, with the remainder being mixed mesodermal, endometroid, and transitional cell tumors. BRCA-1 and -2 mutations are found in 7% of cases. The gross and microscopic characteristics and the spread of the tumor are similar to those of ovarian cancer but can be distinguished if the tumor arises from the endosalpinx, the tubal epithelium shows a transition between benign and malignant, and the ovaries and endometrium are normal or minimally involved. The differential diagnosis includes primary or metastatic ovarian cancer, chronic salpingitis, tuberculous salpingitis, salpingitis isthmica nodosa, and cautery artifact.

Unlike patients with ovarian cancer, patients frequently present with early symptoms, usually postmenopausal vaginal bleeding, pain, and leukorrhea. Surgical staging is similar to that used for ovarian cancer, and prognosis is related to stage and extent of residual disease. Patients with stages I and II disease are generally treated with surgery alone or with surgery and pelvic radiation therapy, although radiation therapy does not clearly improve 5-year survival (5-year survival stage I: 74 versus 75%, stage II: 43 versus 48%). Patients with stages III and IV disease are treated with the same chemotherapy regimens used in advanced ovarian carcinoma, and 5-year survival is similar (stage III—20%, stage IV—5%).

UTERINE CANCER

Carcinoma of the endometrium is the most common female pelvic malignancy. Approximately 36,100 new cases are diagnosed yearly, although in most (75%) tumor is confined to the uterine corpus at diagnosis and therefore most can be cured. The 6500 deaths yearly make uterine cancer only the seventh leading cause of cancer death in females. It is primarily a disease of postmenopausal women, although 25% of cases occur in women <age 50 and 5% <age 40. The disease is common in Eastern Europe and the United States and uncommon in Asia.

Phenotypic characteristics and risk factors common in patients with endometrial cancer include obesity, altered menstruation, low fertility index, late menopause, anovulation, and postmenopausal bleeding. Exposure to unopposed estrogen from either endogenous or exogenous sources may play a central etiologic role. Women taking tamoxifen for breast cancer treatment or prevention have a twofold increased risk.

Endometrial carcinoma occurs most often in the sixth and seventh decades of life. Symptoms often include abnormal vaginal discharge (90%); abnormal bleeding (80%), which is usually postmenopausal; and leukorrhea (10%). Evaluation of such patients should include a history and physical and pelvic examinations followed by an endometrial biopsy or a fractional dilation and curettage. Outpatient procedures such as endometrial biopsy or aspiration curettage can be used but are definitive only when positive.

Between 75 and 80% of all endometrial carcinomas are adenocarcinomas, and the prognosis depends upon stage, histologic grade, and extent of myometrial invasion. Grade I tumors are highly differentiated adenocarcinomas, grade II contain some solid areas, and grade III tumors are largely solid or undifferentiated. Adenocarcinoma with squamous differentiation is seen in 10% of patients; the most differentiated form is known as *adenoacanthoma*, and the poorly differentiated form is called *adenosquamous carcinoma*. Other less common pathologies include mucinous carcinoma (5%) and papillary serous carcinoma (<10%). This latter type has a natural history similar to ovarian carcinoma and should be managed as an ovarian cancer. Rarer histologies include secretory (2%), ciliated, clear cell, and undifferentiated carcinomas.

The staging of endometrial cancer requires surgery to establish the extent of disease and the depth of myometrial invasion. Peritoneal fluid should be sampled; the abdomen and pelvis explored; and pelvic and para-aortic lymphadenectomy performed depending upon the histology, grade, and depth of invasion in the uterine specimen on frozen section. After evaluation and staging, 74% of patients are stage I, 13%

are stage II, 9% are stage III, and 3% are stage IV. Five-year survival by stage is as follows: stage I—89%, stage II—80%, stage III—30%, and stage IV—9% (Table 97-1).

Patients with uncomplicated endometrial carcinoma are effectively managed with total abdominal hysterectomy and bilateral salpingo-oophorectomy. Pre- or postoperative irradiation has been used, and although vaginal cuff recurrence is reduced, survival is not altered. In women with poor histologic grade, deep myometrial invasion, or extensive involvement of the lower uterine segment or cervix, intracavitary or external beam irradiation is warranted.

About 15% of women have endometrial carcinoma with extension to the cervix only (stage II), and management depends upon the extent of cervical invasion. Superficial cervical invasion can be managed like stage I disease, but extensive cervical invasion requires radical hysterectomy or preoperative radiotherapy followed by extrafascial hysterectomy. Once disease is outside the uterus but still confined to the true pelvis (stage III), management generally includes surgery and irradiation. Patients who have involvement only of the ovary or fallopian tubes generally do well with such therapy (5-year survivals of 80%). Other stage III patients with disease extending beyond the adnexa or those with serous carcinomas of the endometrium have a significantly poorer prognosis (5-year survival of 15%).

Patients with stage IV disease (outside the abdomen or invading the bladder or rectum) are treated palliatively with irradiation, surgery, and/or progestational agents. Progestational agents produce responses in about 25% of patients. Well-differentiated tumors respond most frequently, and response can be correlated with the level of progesterone receptor expression in the tumor. The commonly used progestational agents hydroxyprogesterone (Dilalutin), megastrol (Megace), and deoxyprogesterone (Provera) all produce similar response rates, and the antiestrogen tamoxifen (Nolvadex) produces responses in 10 to 25% of patients in a salvage setting.

Chemotherapy is not very successful in advanced endometrial carcinoma. The most active single agents with consistent response rates of ≥20% include cisplatin, carboplatin, doxorubicin, epirubicin, and paclitaxel. Combinations of drugs with or without progestational agents have generally produced response rates similar to single agents.

CERVIX CANCER

Carcinoma of the cervix was once the most common cause of cancer death in women, but over the past 30 years, the mortality rate has decreased by 50% due to widespread screening with the Pap smear. Cervix cancer trails breast, lung, colorectal, endometrium, and ovarian cancers in incidence. In 2000, ~12,800 new cases of invasive cervix cancer occurred, and >50,000 cases of carcinoma in situ were detected. There were 4600 deaths from the disease, and of those patients, ~85% had never had a Pap smear. It remains the major gynecologic cancer in underdeveloped countries. It is more common in lower socioeconomic groups, in women with early initial sexual activity and/or multiple sexual partners, and in smokers. Venereal transmission of human papilloma virus (HPV) has an important etiologic role. Over 66 types of HPVs have been isolated, and many are associated with genital warts. Those types associated with cervical carcinoma are 16, 18, 31, 45, and 51 to 53. These, along with many other types, are also associated with cervical intraepithelial neoplasia (CIN). The protein product of HPV-16, the E7 protein, binds and inactivates the tumor suppressor gene Rb, and the E6 protein of HPV-18 has sequence homology to the SV40 large T antigen and has the capacity to bind and inactivate the tumor suppressor gene p53. E6 and E7 are both necessary and sufficient to cause cell transformation in vitro. These binding and inactivation events may explain the carcinogenic effects of the viruses (Chap. 188).

Uncomplicated HPV lower genital tract infection and condylomatous atypia of the cervix can progress to CIN. This lesion precedes invasive cervical carcinoma and is classified as low-grade squamous intraepithelial lesion (SIL), high-grade SIL, and carcinoma in situ. Carcinoma in situ demonstrates cytologic evidence of neoplasia without invasion through the basement membrane, can persist unchanged for 10 to 20 years, but eventually progresses to invasive carcinoma.

The Pap smear is 90 to 95% accurate in detecting early lesions such as CIN but is less sensitive in detecting cancer when frankly invasive cancer or fungating masses are present. Inflammation, necrosis, and hemorrhage may produce false-positive smears, and colposcopic-directed biopsy is required when any lesion is visible on the cervix, regardless of Pap smear findings. The American Cancer Society recommends that women after onset of sexual activity, or >age 20, have two consecutive yearly smears. If negative, smears should be repeated every 3 years. The American College of Obstetrics and Gynecology recommends yearly Pap smears with routine annual pelvic and breast examinations. The Pap smear can be reported as normal (includes benign, reactive or reparative changes); atypical squamous cells of undetermined significance (ASCUS); low- or high-grade CIN; or frankly malignant. Women with ASCUS or low-grade CIN should have repeat smears in 3 to 6 months and be tested for HPV. Women with high-grade CIN or frankly malignant Pap smears should have colposcopic-directed cervical biopsy. Colposcopy is a technique using a binocular microscope and 3% acetic acid applied to the cervix in which abnormal areas appear white and can be biopsied directly. Cone biopsy is still required when endocervical tumor is suspected, colposcopy is inadequate, the biopsy shows microinvasive carcinoma, or when a discrepancy is noted between the Pap smear and the colposcopic findings. Cone biopsy alone is therapeutic for CIN in many patients, although a less radical electrocautery excision may be sufficient.

Approximately 80% of invasive cervix carcinomas are squamous cell tumors, 10 to 15% are adenocarcinomas, 2 to 5% are adenosquamous with epithelial and glandular structures, and 1 to 2% are clear cell mesonephric tumors.

Patients with cervix cancer generally present with abnormal bleeding or postcoital spotting that may increase to intermenstrual or prominent menstrual bleeding. Yellowish vaginal discharge, lumbosacral back pain, and urinary symptoms can also be seen.

The staging of cervical carcinoma is clinical and generally completed with a pelvic examination under anesthesia with cystoscopy and proctoscopy. Chest x-rays, intravenous pyelograms, and computed tomography are generally required, and magnetic resonance imaging (MRI) may be used to assess extracervical extension. Stage 0 is carcinoma in situ, stage I is disease confined to the cervix, stage II disease invades beyond the cervix but not to the pelvic wall or lower third of the vagina, stage III disease extends to the pelvic wall or lower third of the vagina or causes hydronephrosis, stage IV is present when the tumor invades the mucosa of bladder or rectum or extends beyond the true pelvis. Five-year survivals are as follows: stage I—85%, stage II—60%, stage III—33%, and stage IV—7% (Table 97-1).

Carcinoma in situ (stage 0) can be managed successfully by cone biopsy or by abdominal hysterectomy. For stage I disease, results appear equivalent for either radical hysterectomy or radiation therapy. Patients with stages II to IV disease are primarily managed with radical radiation therapy or combined modality therapy. Retroperitoneal lymphadenectomy has no proven therapeutic role. Pelvic exenterations, although uncommon, are performed for centrally recurrent or persistent disease. Advances have been made in the reconstruction of the vagina, bladder, and rectum following this operation.

In women with locally advanced disease (stages IIB to IVA), platinum-based chemotherapy given concomitantly with radiation therapy improves survival compared to radiation therapy alone. Cisplatin, 75 mg/m^2 over 4 h, followed by 5-fluorouracil (5-FU) 4 g given by 96-h infusion on days 1 to 5 of radiation therapy, is a common regimen. Two additional cycles of chemotherapy are given at 3-week intervals. Concurrent chemoradiotherapy reduced the risk of recurrence by 30 to 50% across wide spectrum of stages and presentations and is the treatment of choice in stages IIB to IV cervix cancer.

Chemotherapy has been used in patients with unresectable advanced disease or recurrent disease. Active agents with ≥20% response rates include cisplatin, 5-FU, ifosfamide, and irinotecan. No combination of agents has proved better than single agents. Intraarterial chemotherapy has been studied, either pre-or postoperatively, but is associated with substantial local toxicity and response rates of 20%.

GESTATIONAL TROPHOBLASTIC NEOPLASIA

Gestational choriocarcinoma accounts for <1% of female gynecologic malignancies and can be cured with appropriate chemotherapy. Deaths from this disease have become rare in the United States. The spectrum of disease ranges from benign hydatidiform mole to trophoblastic malignancy (placental-site trophoblastic tumor and choriocarcinoma).

Epidemiology   In the United States, the incidence is about 1 per 1000 pregnancies; in Asia, 2 per 1000 pregnancies. Maternal age >45 years is a risk factor for hydatidiform mole. A prior history of molar pregnancy is also a risk factor. Choriocarcinoma occurs approximately once in 25,000 pregnancies or once in 20,000 live births. Prior history of hydatidiform mole is a risk factor for choriocarcinoma. A woman with a molar pregnancy is 1000 times more likely to develop choriocarcinoma than a woman with a prior normal-term pregnancy.

Pathology and Etiology   The trophoblastic neoplasms have been divided by morphology into complete or partial hydatidiform mole, invasive mole, placental-site trophoblastomas, and choriocarcinomas. Hydatidiform moles contain clusters of villi with hydropic changes, hyperplasia of the trophoblast, and the absence of fetal vessels. Invasive moles differ only by invasion into the uterine myometrium. Placental-site trophoblastic tumors are predominately made up of cytotrophoblast cells arising from the placental implantation site. Choriocarcinomas consist of anaplastic trophoblastic tissue with both cytotrophoblastic and syncytiotrophoblastic elements and no identifiable villi.

Complete moles result from uniparental disomy in which loss of the maternal genes (23 autosomes plus X) occurs by unknown mechanisms and is followed by duplication of the paternal haploid genome (23 autosomes plus X). Uncommonly (5%), moles result from dispermic fertilization of an empty egg, resulting in either 46XY or 46XX genotype. Partial moles result from dispermic fertilization of an egg with retention of the maternal haploid set of chromosomes, resulting in diandric triploidy (Chap. 65).

Clinical Presentation   Molar pregnancies are generally associated with first-trimester bleeding, ectopic pregnancies, or threatened abortions. The uterus is inappropriately large for the length of gestation, and β-hCG levels are higher than expected. Fetal parts and heart sounds are not present. The diagnosis is generally made by the passage of grapelike clusters from the uterus, but ultrasound demonstration of the hydropic mole can be diagnostic. Patients suspected of a molar pregnancy require a chest film, careful pelvic examinations, and weekly serial monitoring of β-hCG levels.

℞   **TREATMENT**   Patients with hydatidiform moles require surgical evacuation coupled with postevacuation monitoring of β-hCG levels. In most women (80%), the β-hCG titer progressively declines within 8 to 10 days of evacuation (serum half-life is 24 to 36 h). Patients should be monitored on a monthly basis and should not become pregnant for at least a year. Patients found to have invasive mole at curettage are generally treated with hysterectomy and chemotherapy. Approximately half of patients with choriocarcinoma develop the malignancy after a molar pregnancy, and the other half develop the malignancy after abortion, ectopic pregnancy, or occasionally after a normal full-term pregnancy.

Chemotherapy is generally used for gestational trophoblastic neoplasia and is often used in hydatidiform mole if β-hCG levels rise or plateau or if metastases develop. Patients with invasive mole or choriocarcinoma require chemotherapy. Several regimens are effective, including methotrexate at 30 mg/m² intramuscularly on a weekly basis until β-hCG titers are normal. However, methotrexate (1 mg/kg) every other day for 4 days followed by leukovorin (0.1 mg/kg) intravenously 24 h after methotrexate is associated with a cure rate of ≥90% and low toxicity. Intermittent courses are continued until the β-hCG titer becomes undetectable for 3 consecutive weeks, and then patients are monitored monthly for a year.

Patients with high-risk tumors (high β-hCG levels, disease presenting ≥4 months after antecedent pregnancy, brain or liver metastasis, or failure of single-agent methotrexate) are initially treated with combination chemotherapy. MAC chemotherapy with methotrexate, actinomycin-D, and cyclophosphamide has been the most commonly used regimen, with cycles of therapy given every 3 weeks until complete remission. Other effective regimens include EMA-CO (a cyclic non-cross-resistant combination of etoposide, methotrexate, and dactinomycin alternating with cyclophosphamide and vincristine); cisplatin, bleomycin, and vinblastine; and cisplatin, etoposide, and bleomycin. EMA-CO is now the regimen of choice for patients with high-risk disease because of excellent survival rates (>80%) and less toxicity than MAC. The use of etoposide carries a 1.5% lifetime risk of acute myeloid leukemia (16-fold relative risk). Because of this problem, etoposide-containing regimens should be reserved for patients with high risk features. Patients with brain or liver metastasis are usually treated with local irradiation to metastatic sites in conjunction with chemotherapy. Long-term studies of patients cured of trophoblastic disease have not demonstrated an increased risk of maternal complications or fetal abnormalities with subsequent pregnancies.

BIBLIOGRAPHY

Barakat RR et al: Corpus epithelial tumors, in *Principles and Practice of Gynecologic Oncology*, 3d ed, WJ Hoskins et al (eds). Philadelphia, Lippincott Williams & Wilkins, 2000, pp 919–959

Hacker NF: Uterine cancer, in *Practical Gynecologic Oncology*, 2d ed, JS Berek, NF Hacker (eds). Baltimore, Williams & Wilkins, 1994, pp 285–326.

Morris M et al: Pelvic radiation with concurrent chemotherapy compared with pelvic and para-aortic radiation for high-risk cervical cancer. N Engl J Med 340:1137, 1999

Ozols RF et al: Epithelial ovarian cancer, in *Principles and Practice of Gynecologic Oncology*, 3d ed, WJ Hoskins et al (eds). Philadelphia, Lippincott, Williams & Wilkins, 2000, pp 981–1057

——— et al: Randomized phase III study of cisplatin/paclitaxel versus carboplatin/paclitaxel in optimal stage III epithelial ovarian cancer. Proc Am Soc Clin Oncol 18:356a, 1999

Soper VT: Identification and management of high-risk gestational trophoblastic disease. Semin Oncol 22:172, 1995

Stehman FB et al: Uterine cervix, in *Principles and Practice of Gynecologic Oncology*, 3d ed, WJ Hoskins et al (eds). Philadelphia, Lippincott, Williams & Wilkins, 2000, pp 841–918

VanderBurg ME et al: Intervention debulking surgery does improve survival in advanced epithelial ovarian cancer. N Engl J Med 332:629, 1995

Williams S et al: Adjuvant therapy of ovarian germ cell tumors with cisplatin, etoposide and bleomycin: A trial of the Gynecologic Oncology Group. J Clin Oncol 12:701, 1994

Young RC et al: Adjuvant therapy in stage I and stage II epithelial ovarian cancer. Results of two prospective trials. N Engl J Med 327:1021, 1990

98 *Shreyaskumar R. Patel, Robert S. Benjamin*

SOFT TISSUE AND BONE SARCOMAS AND BONE METASTASES

Sarcomas are rare (less than 1% of all malignancies) mesenchymal neoplasms that arise in bone and soft tissues. These tumors are usually of mesodermal origin, although a few are derived from neuroectoderm, and they are biologically distinct from the more common epithelial malignancies. Sarcomas affect all age groups; 15% are found in children younger than age 15, and 40% occur after age 55. Sarcomas are

one of the most common solid tumors of childhood and are the fifth most common cause of cancer deaths in children. Sarcomas may be divided into two groups, those derived from bone and those derived from soft tissues.

SOFT TISSUE SARCOMAS

Soft tissues include muscles, tendons, fat, fibrous tissue, synovial tissue, vessels, and nerves. Approximately 60% of soft tissue sarcomas arise in the extremities, with the lower extremities involved three times as often as the upper extremities. Thirty percent arise in the trunk, the retroperitoneum accounting for 40% of all trunk lesions. The remaining 10% arise in the head and neck.

INCIDENCE Approximately 7800 new cases of soft tissue sarcomas occurred in the United States in 1999. The annual age-adjusted incidence is approximately 2 per 100,000 population, but the incidence varies with age. Soft tissue sarcomas constitute 0.7% of all cancers in the general population and 6.5% of all cancers in children.

EPIDEMIOLOGY Malignant transformation of a benign soft tissue tumor is extremely rare, with the exception that malignant peripheral nerve sheath tumors (neurofibrosarcoma, malignant schwannoma) can arise from neurofibromas in patients with neurofibromatosis. Several etiologic factors have been implicated in soft tissue sarcomas.

Environmental Factors Trauma or previous injury is rarely involved, but sarcomas can arise in scar tissue resulting from a prior operation, burn, fracture, or foreign body implantation. Chemical carcinogens such as polycyclic hydrocarbons, asbestos, and dioxin may be involved in the pathogenesis.

Iatrogenic Factors Sarcomas in bone or soft tissues occur in patients who are treated with radiation therapy. The tumor nearly always arises in the irradiated field. The risk increases with time.

Viruses Kaposi's sarcoma (KS) in patients with HIV type 1, classic KS, and KS in HIV-negative homosexual men is caused by human herpes virus (HHV8) (Chap. 185). No other sarcomas are associated with viruses.

Immunologic Factors Congenital or acquired immunodeficiency, including therapeutic immunosuppression, increases risk of sarcoma.

Genetic Factors Li-Fraumeni syndrome is a familial cancer syndrome in which affected individuals have germ-line abnormalities of the tumor suppressor gene *p53* and an increased incidence of soft tissue sarcomas and other malignancies, including breast cancer, osteosarcoma, brain tumor, leukemia, and adrenal carcinoma (Chap. 81). Neurofibromatosis 1 (NF-1, peripheral form, von Recklinghausen's disease) is characterized by multiple neurofibromas and café au lait spots. Neurofibromas occasionally undergo malignant degeneration to become malignant peripheral nerve sheath tumors. The gene for NF-1 is located in the pericentromeric region of chromosome 17 and encodes neurofibromin, a tumor suppressor protein with GTPase-activating activity that inhibits Ras function (Chap. 370). Germ-line mutation of the *Rb-1* locus (chromosome 13q14) in patients with inherited retinoblastoma is associated with the development of osteosarcoma in those who survive the retinoblastoma and of soft tissue sarcomas unrelated to radiation therapy. Other soft tissue tumors, including desmoid tumors, lipomas, leiomyomas, neuroblastomas, and paragangliomas, occasionally show a familial predisposition.

Ninety percent of synovial sarcomas contain a characteristic chromosomal translocation t(X;18) (p11;q11) involving a nuclear transcription factor on chromosome 18 called *SYT* and two breakpoints on X. Patients with translocations to the second X breakpoint (*SSX2*) may have longer survival than those with translocations involving *SSX1*.

Insulin-like growth factor (IGF) type 2 is produced by some sarcomas and may act as an autocrine growth factor and as a motility factor that promotes metastatic spread. IGF-2 stimulates growth through IGF-1 receptors but its effects on motility are through different

Table 98-1 AJCC Staging System for Sarcomas

Histologic Grade (G)	Tumor Size (T)	Node Status (N)	Metastases (M)
Well differentiated (G1)	≤5 cm (T1)	Not involved (N0)	Absent (M0)
Moderately differentiated (G2)	>5 cm (T2)	Involved (N1)	Present (M1)
Poorly differentiated (G3)	Superficial fascial involvement (Ta)		
Undifferentiated (G4)	Deep fascial involvement (Tb)		

Disease Stage	5-year survival, %
Stage I	98.8
A: G1,2; T1a,b; N0; M0	
B: G1,2; T2a; N0; M0	
Stage II	81.8
A: G1,2; T2b; N0; M0	
B: G3,4; T1; N0; M0	
C: G3,4; T2a; N0; M0	
Stage III G3,4; T2b; N0; M0	51.7
Stage IV	<20
A: any G; any T; N1; M0	
B: any G; any T; any N; M1	

receptors. If secreted in large amounts, IGF-2 may produce hypoglycemia (Chaps. 100 and 334).

CLASSIFICATION Approximately 20 different groups of sarcomas are recognized on the basis of the pattern of differentiation toward normal tissue. For example, rhabdomyosarcoma shows evidence of skeletal muscle fibers with cross-striations; leiomyosarcomas contain interlacing fascicles of spindle cells resembling smooth muscle; and liposarcomas contain adipocytes. When precise characterization of the group is not possible, the tumors are called *unclassified sarcomas*. All of the primary bone sarcomas also can arise from soft tissues (e.g., extraskeletal osteosarcoma). The entity *malignant fibrous histiocytoma* includes many tumors previously classified as fibrosarcomas or as pleomorphic variants of other sarcomas and is characterized by a mixture of spindle (fibrous) cells and round (histiocytic) cells arranged in a storiform pattern with frequent giant cells and areas of pleomorphism.

For purposes of treatment, most soft tissue sarcomas can be considered together. However, some specific tumors have distinct features. For example, *liposarcoma* can have a spectrum of behaviors. Pleomorphic liposarcomas and dedifferentiated liposarcomas behave like other high-grade sarcomas; in contrast, well-differentiated liposarcomas (better termed *atypical lipomatous tumors*) lack metastatic potential, and myxoid liposarcomas metastasize infrequently but, when they do, have a predilection for unusual metastatic sites containing fat, such as the retroperitoneum, mediastinum, and subcutaneous tissue. Rhabdomyosarcomas, Ewing's sarcoma, and other small cell sarcomas tend to be more aggressive, and are more responsive to chemotherapy than other soft tissue sarcomas.

DIAGNOSIS The most common presentation is an asymptomatic mass. Mechanical symptoms referable to pressure, traction, or entrapment of nerves or muscles may be present. All new and persistent or growing masses should be biopsied, either by a cutting needle (core-needle biopsy) or by a small incision, placed so that it can be encompassed in the subsequent excision without compromising a definitive resection. Sarcomas tend to metastasize through the blood rather than the lymphatic system; lymph node metastases occur in 5%, except in synovial and epithelioid sarcomas, clear-cell sarcoma (melanoma of the soft parts), angiosarcoma, and rhabdomyosarcoma where nodal spread may be seen in 17%. The pulmonary parenchyma is the most common site of metastases. Exceptions are leiomyosarcomas arising in the gastrointestinal tract, which metastasize to the liver; myxoid liposarcomas, which seek fatty tissue; and clear-cell sarcomas, which may metastasize to bones. Central nervous system metastases are rare, except in alveolar soft part sarcoma.

Radiographic Evaluation Imaging of the primary tumor is best with plain radiographs and magnetic resonance imaging (MRI) for tumors of the extremities or head and neck and by computed tomography (CT) for tumors of the chest, abdomen, or retroperitoneal cavity. A radiograph and CT scan of the chest are important for the detection of lung metastases. Other imaging studies may be indicated, depending on the symptoms, signs, or histology.

STAGING AND PROGNOSIS The histologic grade, relationship to fascial planes, and size of the primary tumor are the most important prognostic factors. The newly revised American Joint Commission on Cancer (AJCC) staging system is shown in Table 98-1. Prognosis is related to the stage. Cure is common in the absence of metastatic disease, but a small number of patients with metastases can also be cured. Most patients with stage IV disease die within 6 to 12 months, but some patients may live with slowly progressive disease for many years.

TREATMENT AJCC stage I patients are adequately treated with surgery alone. Stage II patients require adjuvant radiation therapy. Stage III patients require adjuvant chemotherapy. Stage IV patients are managed primarily with chemotherapy with or without other modalities.

Surgery Soft tissue sarcomas tend to grow along fascial planes, with the surrounding soft tissues compressed to form a pseudocapsule that gives the sarcoma the appearance of a well-encapsulated lesion. This is invariably deceptive, because "shelling out" or marginal excision of such lesions results in a 50 to 90% probability of local recurrence. Wide excision with a negative margin, incorporating the biopsy site, is the standard surgical procedure for local disease. The adjuvant use of radiation therapy and/or chemotherapy improves the local control rate and permits the use of limb-sparing surgery with a local control rate (85 to 90%) comparable to that achieved by radical excisions and amputations. Limb-sparing approaches are indicated except when negative margins are not obtainable, when the risks of radiation are prohibitive, or when neurovascular structures are involved so that resection will result in serious functional consequences to the limb.

Radiation Therapy External beam radiation therapy is an adjuvant to limb-sparing surgery for improved local control. Preoperative radiation therapy allows the use of smaller fields and smaller doses but results in a higher rate of wound complications. Postoperative radiation therapy must be given to larger fields, as the entire surgical bed must be encompassed, and in higher doses to compensate for hypoxia in the operated field. Brachytherapy or interstitial therapy, in which the radiation source is inserted into the tumor bed, is comparable in efficacy (except in low grade lesions), less time consuming, and less expensive.

Adjuvant Chemotherapy Chemotherapy is the mainstay of treatment for Ewing's/peripheral neuroepithelial tumors (PNET) and rhabdomyosarcomas. Meta-analysis of 14 randomized trials revealed a highly significant improvement in local control and disease-free survival in favor of doxorubicin-based chemotherapy. Overall survival is improved only for extremity sarcomas, however. An alternative approach is to treat such patients preoperatively with chemotherapy (neoadjuvant therapy); the subset of patients who respond continue adjuvant therapy postoperatively, and the nonresponders can be spared the toxicity of systemic therapy to which they are unlikely to respond. Neither strategy has been proved superior.

Advanced Disease Metastatic soft tissue sarcomas are largely incurable, but up to 20% of patients who achieve a complete response become long-term survivors. The therapeutic intent, therefore, is to produce a complete remission with chemotherapy and/or surgery. Surgical resection of metastases, whenever possible, is an integral part of the management. Some patients benefit from repeated surgical excision of metastases. Despite their histologic heterogeneity, the sensitivity to chemotherapy of most soft tissue sarcomas is poor. The two most active chemotherapeutic agents are doxorubicin and ifosfamide. There is a steep dose-response relationship for these drugs in sarcomas. Dacarbazine (DTIC) in combination with doxorubicin may be more active than the single agents. Vincristine, etoposide, and dactinomycin are effective in Ewing's sarcoma and rhabdomyosarcoma, especially in children. Chondrosarcomas and leiomyosarcomas arising from the gastrointestinal tract are unresponsive to standard chemotherapeutic drugs.

BONE SARCOMAS

INCIDENCE AND EPIDEMIOLOGY Bone sarcomas are rarer than soft tissue sarcomas; they accounted for only 0.2% of all new malignancies and approximately 2500 new cases in the United States in 1999. Several benign bone lesions have the potential for malignant transformation. Enchondromas and osteochondromas can transform into chondrosarcoma; fibrous dysplasia, bone infarcts, and Paget's disease of bone can transform into either malignant fibrous histiocytoma or osteosarcoma.

CLASSIFICATION **Benign Tumors** The common benign bone tumors include enchondroma, osteochondroma, chondroblastoma, and chondromyxoid fibroma, of cartilage origin; osteoid osteoma and osteoblastoma, of bone origin; fibroma and desmoplastic fibroma, of fibrous tissue origin; hemangioma, of vascular origin; and giant cell tumor, of unknown origin.

Malignant Tumors The most common malignant tumors of bone are plasma cell tumors (Chap. 113). The four most common malignant nonhematopoietic bone tumors are osteosarcoma, chondrosarcoma, Ewing's sarcoma, and malignant fibrous histiocytoma. Rare malignant tumors include chordoma (of notochordal origin), malignant giant cell tumor and adamantinoma (of unknown origin), and hemangioendothelioma (of vascular origin).

Musculoskeletal Tumor Society Staging System Sarcomas of bone are staged according to the Musculoskeletal Tumor Society staging system based on grade and compartmental localization. A Roman numeral reflects the tumor grade: stage I is low-grade, stage II is high-grade, and stage III includes tumors of any grade that have lymph node or distant metastases. In addition, the tumor is given a letter reflecting its compartmental localization. Tumors designated A are intracompartmental (i.e., confined to the same soft tissue compartment as the initial tumor), and tumors designated B are extracompartmental (i.e., extending into the adjacent soft tissue compartment or into bone).

OSTEOSARCOMA Osteosarcoma, accounting for almost 45% of all bone sarcomas, is a spindle cell neoplasm that produces osteoid (unmineralized bone) or bone. About 60% of all osteosarcomas occur in children and adolescents in the second decade of life, and about 10% occur in the third decade of life. Osteosarcomas in the fifth and sixth decades of life are frequently secondary to either radiation therapy or transformation in a preexisting benign condition, such as Paget's disease. Males are affected 1.5 to 2 times as often as females. Osteosarcoma has a predilection for metaphyses of long bones; the most common sites of involvement are the distal femur, proximal tibia, and proximal humerus. The classification of osteosarcoma is complex, but 75% of osteosarcomas fall in the "classic" category, which include osteoblastic, chondroblastic, and fibroblastic osteosarcomas. The remaining 25% are classified as "variants" on the basis of (1) clinical characteristics, as in the case of osteosarcoma of the jaw, postradiation osteosarcoma, or Paget's osteosarcoma; (2) morphologic characteristics, as in the case of telangiectatic osteosarcoma, small cell osteosarcoma, or epithelioid osteosarcoma; or (3) location, as in parosteal or periosteal osteosarcoma. Diagnosis usually requires a synthesis of clinical, radiologic, and pathologic features. Patients typically present with

pain and swelling of the affected area. A plain radiograph reveals a destructive lesion with a moth-eaten appearance, a spiculated periosteal reaction (sunburst appearance), and a cuff of periosteal new bone formation at the margin of the soft tissue mass (Codman's triangle). A CT scan of the primary tumor is best for defining bone destruction and the pattern of calcification, whereas MRI is better for defining intramedullary and soft tissue extension. A chest radiograph and CT scan are used to detect lung metastases. Metastases to the bony skeleton should be imaged by a bone scan. Almost all osteosarcomas are hypervascular. Angiography is not helpful for diagnosis, but it is the most sensitive test for assessing the response to preoperative chemotherapy. Pathologic diagnosis is established either with a core-needle biopsy, where feasible, or with an open biopsy with an appropriately placed incision that does not compromise future limb-sparing resection. Most osteosarcomas are high-grade. The most important prognostic factor for long-term survival is response to chemotherapy. Preoperative chemotherapy followed by limb-sparing surgery (which can be accomplished in >80% of patients) followed by postoperative chemotherapy is standard management. The effective drugs are doxorubicin, ifosfamide, cisplatin, and high-dose methotrexate with leucovorin rescue. The various combinations of these agents that have been used have all been about equally successful. Long-term survival rates in extremity osteosarcoma range from 60 to 80%. Osteosarcoma is radioresistant; radiation therapy has no role in the routine management. Malignant fibrous histiocytoma is considered a part of the spectrum of osteosarcoma and is managed similarly.

CHONDROSARCOMA Chondrosarcoma, which constitutes approximately 20 to 25% of all bone sarcomas, is a tumor of adulthood and old age with a peak incidence in the fourth to sixth decades of life. It has a predilection for the flat bones, especially the shoulder and pelvic girdles, but can also affect the diaphyseal portions of long bones. Chondrosarcomas can arise de novo or as a malignant transformation of an enchondroma or, rarely, of the cartilaginous cap of an osteochondroma. Chondrosarcomas have an indolent natural history and typically present as pain and swelling. Radiographically, the lesion may have a lobular appearance with mottled or punctate or annular calcification of the cartilaginous matrix. It is difficult to distinguish low-grade chondrosarcoma from benign lesions by x-ray or histologic examination. The diagnosis is therefore influenced by clinical history and physical examination. A new onset of pain, signs of inflammation, and progressive increase in the size of the mass suggest malignancy. The histologic classification is complex, but most tumors fall within the classic category. Like other bone sarcomas, high-grade chondrosarcomas spread to the lungs. Most chondrosarcomas are resistant to chemotherapy, and surgical resection of primary or recurrent tumors, including pulmonary metastases, is the mainstay of therapy. There are two histologic variants for which this rule does not hold, however. Dedifferentiated chondrosarcoma is a low-grade tumor that dedifferentiates into a high-grade osteosarcoma or a malignant fibrous histiocytoma, a tumor that responds to chemotherapy. Mesenchymal chondrosarcoma, a rare variant composed of a small cell element, also is responsive to systemic chemotherapy and is treated like Ewing's sarcoma.

EWING'S SARCOMA Ewing's sarcoma, which constitutes approximately 10 to 15% of all bone sarcomas, is common in adolescence and has a peak incidence in the second decade of life. It typically involves the diaphyseal region of long bones and also has an affinity for flat bones. The plain radiograph may show a characteristic "onion peel" periosteal reaction with a generous soft tissue mass, which is better demonstrated by CT or MRI. This mass is composed of sheets of monotonous, small, round, blue cells and can be confused with lymphoma, embryonal rhabdomyosarcoma, and small cell carcinoma. The presence of p30/32, the product of the *mic-2* gene (which maps to the pseudoautosomal region of the X and Y chromosomes) is a cell-surface marker for Ewing's sarcoma [and other members of a family of tumors called *peripheral primitive neuroectodermal tumors*

(*PNETs*)]. Most PNETs arise in soft tissues; they include peripheral neuroepithelioma, Askin's tumor (chest wall), and esthesioneuroblastoma. Glycogen-filled cytoplasm detected by staining with periodic acid–Schiff is also characteristic of Ewing's sarcoma cells. The classic cytogenetic abnormality associated with this disease (and other PNETs) is a reciprocal translocation of the long arms of chromosomes 11 and 22, t(11;22), which creates a chimeric gene product of unknown function with components from the *fli-1* gene on chromosome 11 and *ews* on 22. This disease is very aggressive, and it is therefore considered a systemic disease. Common sites of metastases are lung, bones, and bone marrow. Systemic chemotherapy is the mainstay of therapy, often being used before surgery. Doxorubicin, cyclophosphamide or ifosfamide, etoposide, vincristine, and dactinomycin are active drugs. Local treatment for the primary tumor includes surgical resection, usually with limb salvage or radiation therapy. Patients with lesions below the elbow and below the mid-calf have a 5-year survival rate of 80% with effective treatment. Ewing's sarcoma is a curable tumor, even in the presence of obvious metastatic disease, especially in children less than 11 years old.

TUMORS METASTATIC TO BONE

Bone is a common site of metastasis for carcinomas of the prostate, breast, lung, kidney, bladder, and thyroid and for lymphomas and sarcomas. Prostate, breast, and lung primaries account for 80% of all bone metastases. Metastatic tumors of bone are more common than primary bone tumors. Tumors usually spread to bone hematogenously, but local invasion from soft tissue masses also occurs. In descending order of frequency, the sites most often involved are the vertebrae, proximal femur, pelvis, ribs, sternum, proximal humerus, and skull. Bone metastases may be asymptomatic or may produce pain, swelling, nerve root or spinal cord compression, pathologic fracture, or myelophthisis (replacement of the marrow). Symptoms of hypercalcemia may be noted in cases of bony destruction.

Pain is the most frequent symptom. It usually develops gradually over weeks, is usually localized, and often is more severe at night. When patients with back pain develop neurologic signs or symptoms, emergency evaluation for spinal cord compression is indicated (Chap. 102). Bone metastases exert a major adverse effect on quality of life in cancer patients.

Cancer in the bone may produce osteolysis, osteogenesis, or both. Osteolytic lesions result when the tumor produces substances that can directly elicit bone resorption (vitamin D–like steroids, prostaglandins, or parathyroid hormone–related peptide) or cytokines that can induce the formation of osteoclasts (interleukin 1 and tumor necrosis factor). Osteoblastic lesions result when the tumor produces cytokines that activate osteoblasts. In general, purely osteolytic lesions are best detected by plain radiography, but they may not be apparent until they are larger than 1 cm. These lesions are more commonly associated with hypercalcemia and with the excretion of hydroxyproline-containing peptides indicative of matrix destruction. When osteoblastic activity is prominent, the lesions may be readily detected using radionuclide bone scanning (which is sensitive to new bone formation), and the radiographic appearance may show increased bone density or sclerosis. Osteoblastic lesions are associated with higher serum levels of alkaline phosphatase, and, if extensive, may produce hypocalcemia. Although some tumors may produce mainly osteolytic lesions (e.g., kidney cancer) and others mainly osteoblastic lesions (e.g., prostate cancer), most metastatic lesions produce both types of lesion and may go through stages where one or the other predominates.

In older patients, particularly women, it may be necessary to distinguish metastatic disease of the spine from osteoporosis. In osteoporosis, the cortical bone may be preserved, whereas cortical bone destruction is usually noted with metastatic cancer.

Treatment of metastatic bone disease depends on the underlying malignancy and the symptoms. Some metastatic bone tumors are cur-

able (lymphoma, Hodgkin's disease), and others are treated with palliative intent. Pain may be relieved by local radiation therapy. Hormonally responsive tumors are responsive to hormone inhibition (antiandrogens for prostate cancer, antiestrogens for breast cancer). Strontium 89 and samarium 153 are bone-seeking radionuclides that can exert antitumor effects and relieve symptoms. Bisphosphonates such as pamidronate may relieve pain and inhibit bone resorption. Monthly administration prevents bone-related clinical events and may reduce the incidence of bone metastases in women with breast cancer. When the integrity of a weight-bearing bone is threatened by an expanding metastatic lesion that is refractory to radiation therapy, prophylactic internal fixation is indicated. Overall survival is related to the prognosis of the underlying tumor. Bone pain at the end of life is particularly common; an adequate pain relief regimen including sufficient amounts of narcotic analgesics is required. →*The management of hypercalcemia is discussed in Chap. 341.*

BIBLIOGRAPHY

EVANS RG et al: Multimodal therapy for the management of localized Ewing's sarcoma of pelvic and sacral bones: A report from the second intergroup study. J Clin Oncol 9:1173, 1991

PATEL SR, BENJAMIN RS: New chemotherapeutic strategies for soft tissue sarcomas. Sem Surg Oncol 17:47, 1999

———— (eds): Sarcomas. Part I. Hematol Oncol Clin North Am 9:513, 1995

———— (eds): Sarcomas. Part II. Hematol Oncol Clin North Am 9:707, 1995

WEST DC: Ewing sarcoma family of tumors. Curr Opin Oncol 12:323, 2000

99   *Richard M. Stone*

METASTATIC CANCER OF UNKNOWN PRIMARY SITE

INCIDENCE AND EPIDEMIOLOGY   The presenting findings in a patient with a newly discovered malignancy may not reveal its site of origin. Patients with cancer of unknown primary site (CUPS) present difficult diagnostic and therapeutic dilemmas. First, as additional studies may be many, costly, and/or uncomfortable for the patient, the strategy used in searching for the primary must assess what, if any, result the identification of the site of origin would have on the patient's treatment and survival. Second, while individuals with CUPS fare poorly overall (median survival is 4 to 11 months), certain subgroups of patients are more likely to benefit from treatment and, in some cases, to enjoy long disease-free survival. The literature is a poor guide for the care of such patients, owing to the heterogeneity of the tumors, the selection bias in small retrospective studies, and the variability in the definition of the syndrome and the thoroughness of the evaluation performed to identify a primary site.

No universally accepted definition of the CUPS syndrome exists. An occult neoplasm should fulfill all of the following criteria: (1) biopsy-proven malignancy; (2) unrevealing history, physical examination, chest film, abdominal and pelvic computed tomography (CT) scans, complete blood counts, chemistry survey, mammography (women), β human chorionic gonadotropin (βhCG) levels (men), α fetoprotein (AFP) levels (men), and prostate-specific antigen (PSA) levels (men); (3) histologic evaluation not consistent with a primary tumor at the biopsy site; and (4) failure of additional diagnostic studies (based only on findings from the laboratory and pathologic review) to identify the primary site. Such additional diagnostic tests could include, for example, colonoscopy in a patient whose rectal examination discloses guaiac-positive stool or a meticulous otolaryngologic examination in a patient who presents with squamous cell carcinoma in a cervical node. Many cases that fulfill the definition of CUPS offer clues that a given organ is the probable site of origin. Epidemiologic data suggest that the incidence of cancers for which the primary site is unknown is decreasing. CUPS accounts for about 2% of all cancer diagnoses—about 24,400 cases in the year 2000. Most patients with CUPS are over age 60.

BIOLOGIC CONSIDERATIONS The biologic behavior of CUPS is unique. In ~25% of patients, the primary site becomes apparent during the course of the illness; in about 57% of patients, the primary site can be diagnosed at autopsy; but in almost 20%, the primary site remains obscure even at autopsy. Cancers presenting as CUPS often display unusual patterns of metastatic spread (e.g., pancreatic cancer presenting with bony metastases). The fact that more tumor bulk is present at distant sites than in the tissue of origin suggests that the genetic lesions underlying cases of CUPS produce a distinctly aggressive phenotype. Microsattelite DNA analysis has shown that the same pattern of genetic alterations that appear in a cervical lymph node metastasis can be found in seemingly morphologically normal aerodigestive tissue. Such data imply that clinically evident metastases may be able to arise from microscopic primary lesions. Although physiologic and genetic data that might account for the distinctive natural history of CUPS neoplasms are scant, cell lines derived from such tumors may have abnormalities of chromosome 1, a finding generally associated with advanced malignancy. In some patients, the primary tumor spontaneously regresses (perhaps under immunologic attack) or necroses. In some, a primary lesion was resected years before presentation (e.g., melanoma).

CLINICAL PRESENTATION, DIAGNOSTIC EVALUATION, AND PATHOLOGY **History and Physical Examination** Patients present with a variety of symptoms and signs, including fatigue, weight loss, other systemic symptoms, pain, abnormal bleeding, abdominal swelling, subcutaneous masses, and lymphadenopathy. Once CUPS is considered, the physician's approach must involve reasonable efforts to identify the primary site or to determine the histology or subcategory of the metastatic tumor to decide on the optimal therapy. Though usually unrevealing, a thorough history and physical examination should be carried out to elicit easily obtainable clues regarding the primary site. The patient should be questioned concerning epigastric pain, which, if present, would mandate careful exclusion of pancreatic carcinoma as well as other gastrointestinal malignancies. Symptoms referable to a given location (e.g., new cough, hematochezia, hemoptysis, change in bowel habits, unusual vaginal bleeding, nipple discharge) should prompt an aggressive specific diagnostic approach. Occupational exposure to asbestos, for example, would raise the suspicion of mesothelioma. The absence of prior smoking reduces the likelihood of lung cancer but does not exclude it. A history of fulguration of a skin lesion, colonic polypectomy, dilatation and curettage, or prostate biopsy should prompt a review of the original histology.

Pathology Review The most important aspect of the workup of a patient with CUPS is the thorough evaluation of the tissue obtained at biopsy by light-microscopy, immunohistochemistry, ultrastructural studies, immunophenotyping, and karyotypic and molecular biologic analysis. First, if the original biopsy sample is inadequate for either confirmation of malignancy or the performance of additional specialized studies, rebiopsy is mandatory. The clinician must have a close working relationship with a pathologist skilled in the evaluation of tumor specimens, especially when the organ of origin is uncertain. Plans may be made to process the tissue for (1) routine light-microscopy, histochemical, and immunohistochemical analysis; (2) freezing for DNA and RNA isolation or for in situ genetic and immunologic evaluation; and (3) special fixation for ultrastructural analysis. Single-cell tumor suspensions in short-term culture permit cytogenetic analysis.

If routine histologic analysis fails to suggest the tissue of origin (e.g., gland formation in adenocarcinoma, psammoma bodies in ovarian or thyroid cancer, or spindle architecture in sarcomas), special histochemical studies may be helpful. For example, mucin positivity is helpful in recognizing a poorly differentiated adenocarcinoma. Light-microscopic analysis will show approximately 60% of CUPS tumors to be well or moderately differentiated adenocarcinomas, 30%

poorly differentiated carcinomas/adenocarcinomas, and 5% poorly differentiated malignant neoplasms not further classifiable. In the poorly differentiated neoplasms, immunohistochemical, cytogenetic, and molecular biologic studies can be extremely useful in identifying sarcomas, germ cell carcinomas, lymphomas, neuroendocrine neoplasms (including melanoma), and other tumors whose diagnosis would suggest a more specific therapeutic approach.

Immunohistochemical Analysis Antibodies to specific cell components make it possible to characterize tumors that are not identified by standard techniques. Table 99-1 provides a list of antigens

Table 99-1 Possible Pathologic Evaluation of Biopsy Specimens from Patients with Metastatic Cancer of Unknown Primary Site

Evaluation/Findings	Suggested Primary Site or Neoplasm
HISTOLOGY (HEMATOXYLIN AND EOSIN STAINING)	
Psammoma bodies, papillary configuration	Ovary, thyroid
Signet ring cells	Stomach
IMMUNOHISTOLOGY	
Leukocyte common antigen (LCA, CD45)	Lymphoid neoplasm
Leu-M1	Hodgkin's disease
Epithelial membrane antigen	Carcinoma
Cytokeratin	Carcinoma[a]
CEA	Carcinoma
HMB45	Melanoma
Desmin	Sarcoma
Thyroglobulin	Thyroid carcinoma
Calcitonin	Medullary carcinoma of the thyroid
Myoglobin	Rhabdomyosarcoma
PSA/prostatic acid phosphatase	Prostate
AFP	Liver, stomach, germ cell
Placental alkaline phosphatase	Germ cell
B, T cell markers	Lymphoid neoplasm
S-100 protein	Neuroendocrine tumor, melanoma
Gross cystic fluid protein	Breast, sweat gland
Factor VIII	Kaposi's sarcoma, angiosarcoma
FLOW CYTOMETRY	
B, T cell markers	Lymphoid neoplasm
ULTRASTRUCTURE	
Actin-myosin filaments	Rhabdomyosarcoma
Secretory granules	Neuroendocrine tumors
Desmosomes	Carcinoma
Premelanosomes	Melanoma
CYTOGENETICS	
Isochromosome 12p; 12q(−)	Germ cell
t(11;22)	Ewing's sarcoma, primitive neuroectodermal tumor
t(8;14)[b]	Lymphoid neoplasm
3p(−)	Small cell lung carcinoma; renal cell carcinoma, mesothelioma
t(X;18)	Synovial sarcoma
t(12;16)	Myxoid liposarcoma
t(12;22)	Clear cell sarcoma (melanoma of soft parts)
t(2;13)	Alveolar rhabdomyosarcoma
1p(−)	Neuroblastoma
RECEPTOR ANALYSIS	
Estrogen/progesterone receptor	Breast
MOLECULAR BIOLOGIC STUDIES	
Immunoglobulin, *bcl*-2, T-cell receptor gene rearrangement	Lymphoid neoplasm

[a] See text for discussion of cytokeratins.
[b] Or any other rearrangement involving an antigen-receptor gene.
NOTE: CEA, carcinoembryonic antigen; PSA, prostate-specific antigen; AFP, α fetoprotein.

that may be assessed in undifferentiated or poorly differentiated specimens. A diagnosis of lymphoma should be excluded by employing antibodies reactive to the leukocyte common antigen (LCA, CD45). LCA-positive tumors are lymphomas and have the same chances of responding to therapy as if the diagnosis were unambiguous. About half of patients with aggressive-histology lymphoma can be cured with combination chemotherapy (Chap. 112). The immunohistochemical detection of specific types of filament proteins is helpful in the identification of carcinomas and sarcomas. The presence of keratin suggests carcinoma; all epithelial tumors contain this protein. Specific types of cytokeratins (CK) permit a firm diagnosis. For example, ovarian cancers are CK20−/CK7+, colorectal cancers are CK20+/CK7−, and pancreaticobiliary tumors are CK20+/CK7+. However, certain sarcomas, mesotheliomas, and germ cell tumors are also keratin-positive. Sarcomas may react with antibodies to desmin. Sarcoma subgroups may be identified by expression of myoglobin (rhabdomyosarcoma) or factor VIII (angiosarcoma or Kaposi's sarcoma). Prostate, breast, and thyroid carcinomas express, respectively, PSA, gross cystic fluid protein, or thyroglobulin. The finding of AFP, βhCG, or placental alkaline phosphatase staining is very helpful in assigning a germ cell origin. The S-100 protein is present in virtually all primary and metastatic melanomas, including the amelanotic variety. However, S-100 positivity is also found in other tumors of neuroendocrine origin (e.g., small cell lung cancer, carcinoid, neuroepithelioma); a more specific marker for melanomas is the HMB45 (human melanoma black) antigen.

Other Diagnostic Approaches Electron microscopy can identify cell junctions (i.e., desmosomes, typical of epithelial cancers), neuroendocrine granules, melanosomes, and muscle filaments. Cytogenetic analysis may identify tumors with specific chromosomal translocations or other genetic abnormalities (Table 99-1). Cytogenetic abnormalities can also be determined by fluorescence in situ hybridization with chromosome-specific probes, a technique that does not require cells to divide, as is the case with traditional karyotype analysis. Fresh tissue may be required for detection of estrogen or progesterone receptors (to assess breast cancer) or antigens that are sensitive to fixation. Lineage can be assigned by analysis of DNA for signature gene rearrangements, such as those of immunoglobulin (B cell) or T cell receptor (T cell). Technological advances promise to influence the diagnosis of cancer. Isolation of mRNA from tumor specimens may permit the molecular profiling of tumors by microarray analysis of gene expression. This could lead to novel classifications of tumors based on molecular characteristics that may predict clinical behavior and/or response to specific therapies.

Additional Studies If the pathologist does not identify the likely tissue of origin, it is unlikely that additional expensive diagnostic tests will benefit the patient. In females with metastatic adenocarcinoma or poorly differentiated carcinoma, mammography should be performed, although the diagnostic yield will be quite low except in patients with axillary metastases. Magnetic resonance imaging, positron-emission tomography, or indium-111-pentreotide scanning can identify occult primary breast lesions but are expensive. The use of abdominal/pelvic CT scans leads to the identification of the primary site (often the pancreas) in up to 35% of patients but has little effect on natural history. Whether to measure serum tumor markers such as AFP, βhCG, carcinoembryonic antigen (CEA), CA-125 (associated with ovarian cancer), and PSA is controversial; value has not been proven. Numerous studies have shown a lack of benefit of contrast studies (upper gastrointestinal series, barium enema, or intravenous pyelogram) in patients with CUPS who have no specific symptoms and no findings referable to the gastrointestinal or urinary tract. Moreover, autopsy series reveal that the most likely primary site of origin includes epithelial tissues such as lung, stomach, colon, and kidney, which give rise to tumors that respond poorly to chemotherapy, minimizing the therapeutic impact of such a diagnosis.

Additional invasive diagnostic studies are indicated if the presentation strongly suggests a particular primary site. For example, radiographic evidence of lung or mediastinal involvement would mandate fiberoptic bronchoscopy to exclude lung cancer. In the relatively unusual case of metastatic squamous cell cancer presenting in an inguinal lymph node, anoscopy and colposcopy should be performed to detect carcinoma of the vulva, cervix, vagina, penis, or anus, all of which may be cured even with lymph node spread. A summary of a reasonable diagnostic approach is found in Table 99-2.

℞ **TREATMENT Prognostic Subgroups** The exclusion of treatable and potentially curable neoplasms is important. Patients with squamous cell carcinoma have a somewhat longer median survival (9 months) than do those with adenocarcinoma or unclassifiable neoplasms (4 to 6 months). If laboratory studies indicate a significant likelihood that the neoplasm is a lymphoma, germ cell tumor, sarcoma, neuroendocrine tumor, or breast or prostate cancer, then disease-appropriate therapy should be administered. Patients with lymphoma or a germ cell neoplasm may be cured with combination chemotherapy. In other malignancies, effective palliative chemotherapy (for sarcoma or a breast or neuroendocrine tumor) or hormonal therapy (for breast or prostate cancer) should be strongly considered. Although often requiring electron microscopy for diagnosis, neuroendocrine tumors (especially if anaplastic) often respond to cisplatin-based chemotherapy.

Patients in whom the primary site can be identified fare somewhat better than those in whom it remains undefined. Classification and regression tree (CART) analysis has led to a prognostic index ranging from a median survival of 40 months (those with one or two organ sites involved; not adenocarcinoma in histology; and without adrenal, bone, liver, or pleural involvement) to a median survival of 5 months (liver metastases, nonneuroendocrine histology, age ≥62). Patients may often be categorized as having one of several clinical features or syndromes suggesting a specific form of potentially beneficial therapy (Table 99-3).

Syndrome of unrecognized extragonadal germ cell cancer A subset of patients with poorly differentiated CUPS are responsive to chemotherapy. These patients display one or more of the following features: age <50; tumor involving midline structures, lung parenchyma, or lymph nodes; an elevated serum AFP or βhCG level; evidence of rapid tumor growth; or tumor responsiveness to previously administered radiotherapy or chemotherapy. Platinum-based chemotherapy has led to long-term survival in a fraction of patients with these features, especially those who have a favorable performance status at diagnosis, suggesting that their tumors behaved like germ cell neoplasms. If all patients with poorly differentiated carcinoma (including poorly differentiated adenocarcinoma) are treated with a chemotherapy regimen designed for germ cell cancer (e.g., cisplatin plus etoposide or vinblastine, often also with bleomycin) (Chap. 96), about 25% will respond completely and 33% will have a partial response. Patients whose disease does not respond to two cycles of therapy should not continue therapy. One in six patients survives >5 years without evidence of disease. Patients with poorly differentiated carcinoma or adenocarcinoma whose tumors have abnormalities of chromosome 12 similar to those described in patients with proven germ cell cancer are more likely to respond to platinum-based chemotherapy

Table 99-2 Suggested Clinical Evaluation of Patients with Metastatic Cancer of Unknown Primary Site

History: smoking history, asbestos exposure, abdominal pain
Physical examination: lymph nodes, thyroid, skin;
  Men: prostate
  Women: breasts, pelvic examination
Laboratory evaluation: stool evaluation for occult blood; urinalysis; complete blood count; liver function tests; calcium, electrolytes, creatine; measurement of serum levels of βhCG, AFP, CEA, and CA-125 (women); chest x-ray; abdominal and pelvic CT; mammography
Pathologic evaluation: see Table 99-1

NOTE: PSA, prostate-specific antigen; βhCG, β-human chorionic gonadotropin; AFP, α fetoprotein; CEA, carcinoembryonic antigen; CT, computed tomography.

Clinicopathologic Features	Suspected Primary Site	Suggested Therapy
Squamous cell carcinoma, cervical node	Head and neck cancer	Radical neck dissection; radiotherapy ± chemotherapy
Carcinoma, axillary nodes (female)	Breast cancer	Breast radiotherapy or mastectomy, systemic adjuvant therapy
Peritoneal carcinomatosis (female)	Ovarian cancer	Debulking surgery, cisplatin-based chemotherapy
Pleural effusion, adenocarcinoma cells estrogen and/or progesterone receptor positive	Breast cancer	Systemic therapy for metastatic breast cancer
Poorly differentiated cancer, age <50, lung or retroperitoneal or mediastinal mass or lymph nodes, elevated serum βhCG or AFP levels	Germ cell tumor (extragonadal)	Cisplatin/VP-16-based chemotherapy (controversial)
Bony metastases (male)	Prostate cancer	Androgen blockade (leuprolide plus flutamide)
Adenocarcinoma, liver metastases, elevated CEA level	Gastrointestinal malignancy	Surgical resection of liver lesion feasible; colonoscopy with resection (if appropriate) of tumors; 5-fluoro-uracil/leucovorin

NOTE: βhCG, β-human chorionic gonadotropin; AFP, α fetoprotein; CEA, carcinoembryonic antigen.

than are patients with a similar presentation whose tumors lack this cytogenetic abnormality.

Peritoneal carcinomatosis in women Women who present with increased abdominal girth and a pelvic mass or pain and who are found to have adenocarcinoma throughout the peritoneal cavity without a clear site of origin also may benefit from platinum-based chemotherapy. This syndrome has been termed *primary peritoneal papillary serous carcinoma* or *multifocal extraovarian serous carcinoma*. While breast cancer or a gastrointestinal malignancy can produce these findings, peritoneal carcinomatosis is most commonly ascribed to ovarian cancer, even in patients with apparently normal ovaries at the time of laparotomy. Especially if psammoma bodies or a papillary configuration is noted in the pathology examination or if the CA-125 level is elevated, women with adenocarcinoma of the peritoneal cavity without a defined primary should receive maximum surgical cytoreduction followed by cisplatin (or carboplatin) plus paclitaxel. The stage-specific response to such therapy appears to be comparable to that for patients with proven ovarian cancer. About 10% of patients who present in this fashion may remain free of disease 2 years after diagnosis.

Carcinoma in an axillary lymph node in a female Women with adenocarcinoma or poorly differentiated carcinoma in an axillary mass should receive treatment for stage II breast cancer whether or not a careful breast examination or mammography suggests the diagnosis of primary breast cancer and whether or not estrogen or progesterone receptors are detectable in the node. Even if no lesion is found in the breast, a breast recurrence will develop in one-half of these patients if no mastectomy is performed. Modified radical mastectomy or breast irradiation reduces the risk of local recurrence. In addition, adjuvant systemic therapy (chemotherapy and/or tamoxifen, depending on menopausal and estrogen receptor status) should be given to reduce the risk of developing evident metastatic breast cancer (Chap. 89).

Adjuvant systemic therapy may be administered before definitive local radiation treatment. Women with axillary metastases without an obvious breast primary appear to have the same likelihood of prolonged disease-free survival as patients with typical stage II breast cancer.

Bone metastases in males Particularly if the lesions are osteoblastic, the serum PSA level should be measured, as the probability of prostate carcinoma is high. Empirical hormonal therapy (e.g., leuprolide and flutamide) should be strongly considered.

Cervical lymph node metastases Patients who present with a neck mass should be considered to have a primary tumor of the upper aerodigestive tract (*head and neck cancer*) until a different source is proven. Especially if the pathologist diagnoses squamous histology and the node is located in a high or midcervical area, a careful ear, nose, and throat examination including direct laryngoscopy, nasopharyngoscopy, and random blind biopsies should be undertaken. A thyroid examination and scan should be performed to rule out a primary thyroid tumor, especially if the histology is not definitely squamous. Definitive local therapy (external beam radiation or radical neck dissection) combined with platinum-based chemotherapy may lead to prolonged survival in those with head and neck primaries (Chap. 87).

Adenocarcinoma and liver metastases Liver metastases from an adenocarcinoma is not as well characterized as a syndrome as the unrecognized germ cell cancer syndrome (nor as responsive to therapy). However, such patients may have a primary stomach, biliary, or colorectal tumor. Tumors with limited hepatic involvement may be amenable to resection. A flexible sigmoidoscopy or colonoscopy may detect a potentially obstructive colonic lesion. If a tumor is found, resection may be beneficial, depending on the tumor's size; even if none is found, treatment with a combination of 5-fluorouracil plus leucovorin is palliative for some patients with presumed metastatic gastrointestinal malignancy. Given the severe diarrhea that may be a consequence of this regimen and the relative resistance of gastrointestinal tumors to chemotherapy, patients should be informed of the risks before treatment.

Patients not falling into one of the preceding categories should be treated palliatively. In some patients, observation is appropriate. For example, individuals without evidence of additional metastatic disease who have undergone resection of a solitary pulmonary nodule containing malignant cells may actually have undergone definitive therapy for a small primary lung tumor. Radiation therapy may relieve symptoms in patients with bony pain or neurologic compromise. The largest and most poorly responsive subgroup are those with moderate to well-differentiated adenocarcinomas. Combination chemotherapy is frequently employed in such patients; however, response rates to "all-purpose" regimens [e.g., FAM (5-fluorouracil, doxorubicin, mitomycin C), FACP (5-fluorouracil, doxorubicin, cyclophosphamide, cisplatin)], or to ICE (ifosfamide, carboplatin, etoposide) are generally well under 50%, especially if patients with poorly differentiated adenocarcinoma, who have a higher response rate, are excluded; complete responses are rare. Regimens containing mitomycin C are associated with the risk of hemolytic uremic syndrome. In some series, patients with a good performance status whose disease is limited to soft tissue sites or extends only above the diaphragm have shown a better rate of response to therapy. While patients whose disease responds to treatment seem to have better survival than those whose disease does not respond, the difference may be related to inherent characteristics of the tumor rather than to a beneficial effect of chemotherapy.

Before combination chemotherapy is attempted in a patient with CUPS, the potential benefits must be weighed carefully against the certainty of toxicity. While some randomized studies have reported a benefit of one form of therapy over another, these reports are generally plagued by small numbers of patients and inadequate control of potential prognostic variables. Depending on motivation, eligibility, and availability, patients with CUPS may be candidates for evaluation of new (phase I) therapies.

BIBLIOGRAPHY

ABBRUZZESE JL et al: Analysis of a diagnostic strategy for patients with suspected tumors of unknown origin. J Clin Oncol 13:2094, 1995

CALIFANO J et al: Unknown primary head and neck squamous cell carcinoma: Molecular identification of the site or origin. J Natl Cancer Inst 91:599, 1999

DE BRAUD F, AL-SERRAF M: Diagnosis and management of squamous cell carcinoma of unknown primary tumor site of the neck. Semin Oncol 20:273, 1993

ETTINGER DS et al: NCCN practice guidelines for occult primary tumors. Oncology 12:226, 1998

GOLUB TR et al: Molecular classification of cancer: Class discovery and class prediction by gene expression monitoring. Science 256:531, 1999

HESS KR et al: Classification and regression tree analysis of 1000 consecutive patients with unknown primary carcinoma. Clin Cancer Res 5:3403, 1999

HAINSWORTH JD, GRECO FA: Management of patients with cancer of an unknown primary site. Oncology 14:563, 2000

LENZI R et al: Poorly differentiated carcinoma and poorly differentiated adenocarcinoma of unknown origin: Favorable subsets of patients with unknown primary carcinoma? J Clin Oncol 15:2056, 1997

MOTZER RJ et al: Molecular and cytogenetic studies in the diagnosis of patients with poorly differentiated carcinomas of unknown primary site. J Clin Oncol 13:274, 1995

MUGGIA FM, BARANDA J: Management of peritoneal carcinomatosis of unknown primary tumor site. Semin Oncol 20:268, 1993

100 Bruce E. Johnson

PARANEOPLASTIC SYNDROMES

ENDOCRINE SYNDROMES

Paraneoplastic syndromes are caused by factors produced by cancer cells that often act at a distance from both the primary cancer site and its metastases. The accurate documentation of a paraneoplastic endocrine syndrome requires (1) demonstration of mRNA expression and protein production by the tumor tissue, (2) biochemical and clinical resolution of the syndrome following successful surgical resection, (3) elevated levels of the hormone in the peripheral blood, (4) a tenfold or greater concentration gradient in the blood before and after it passes through the cancer, and (5) normal or suppressed endogenous hormone production.

The three major classes of hormones are steroids, monoamines, and peptides/proteins. Production of steroid hormones by malignant tumors is rare; lymphomas may produce 1,25-dihydroxyvitamin D from circulating 1-hydroxyvitamin D, but most other steroid-producing tumors are benign tumors of the glands that normally secrete the steroid. Monoamines such as norepinephrine and epinephrine are secreted by pheochromocytomas (Chap. 332), but they are not secreted ectopically by malignant tumor cells.

Most hormonal syndromes in patients with cancer are related to the production of peptide or protein hormones. The most common of these endocrine syndromes are listed in Table 100-1, together with the protein hormones that mediate them and the tumors that most commonly produce the hormones. A peptide hormone generally is encoded by an mRNA that is translated into a larger prohormone molecule, which undergoes a number of posttranslational modifications, including cleavage, glycosylation, and/or other steps. For example, pro-opiomelanocortin can be cleaved to yield adrenocorticotropic hormone (ACTH), lipotropin, endorphin, melanocyte-stimulating hormone, and/or enkephalin, with different cell types producing different products. In addition, some cells use alternatively spliced forms of the message to produce different proteins (e.g., calcitonin vs. calcitonin gene-related peptide).

Tumor cells of nonendocrine organs often lack certain components of the pathway that leads from prohormone to biologically active hormone to secreted product. Generally, as a result of defects in protein processing or post-translational changes, tumor cells may produce pro-teins that are structurally related to but biologically less active than the normal hormones. Thus, cancer patients may have elevated levels of immunoreactive hormones in plasma in the absence of clinical syndromes of hormone excess.

The severity of paraneoplastic endocrine syndromes often parallels the clinical course of the cancer. However, with some benign or slowly growing tumors, the hormone syndrome can be the major cause of morbidity. Despite their production by tumor cells, hormones are not very good tumor markers. Human chorionic gonadotropin (hCG) is a reliable tumor marker in some forms of testicular cancer, but no other hormone is used to quantitate tumor mass.

Most endocrine cancer syndromes occur with tumors derived from neuroendocrine or neural crest tissue (small cell lung cancer, carcinoid tumors). The genetic mechanisms that account for the production of a hormone by a cell that does not usually produce it are not clear. Oncogenes may activate other cellular genes (including genes that encode hormones) that normally are silent. Alternatively, demethylation of normally methylated inactive genes may permit expression in rapidly dividing cells.

HYPERCALCEMIA OF MALIGNANCY Hypercalcemia of malignancy, the most common paraneoplastic endocrine syndrome, is responsible for approximately 40% of all hypercalcemia (Chap. 341). Hypercalcemia with cancer is classified as humoral hypercalcemia of malignancy (HHM), which is caused by circulating hormones, or local osteolytic hypercalcemia (LOH), which is caused by local paracrine factors secreted by cancers within bone. Parathyroid hormone-related peptide (PTHrP) causes nearly all cases of HHM, while the mediators of LOH in bone are heterogeneous.

Pathogenesis Eighty percent of patients with hypercalcemia of malignancy have HHM. PTHrP is composed of 139 to 173 amino acids; 8 of the first 13 amino acids at the amino-terminal end are identical to the amino-terminal portion of parathyroid hormone (PTH). PTHrP binds to PTH receptors in the bone and kidney and causes increased bone resorption, decreased bone formation, increased renal tubular reabsorption of calcium, increased phosphaturia, and increased urinary levels of cyclic adenosine monophosphate, leading to hypercalcemia. PTHrP is detected in the plasma in ~80% of cancer patients with hypercalcemia. Rare patients have been reported to have hypercalcemia caused by ectopically produced authentic PTH. HHM in lymphoma may be caused by the production of 1,25-dihydroxyvitamin D by the tumor.

Twenty percent of patients with hypercalcemia have LOH, in which hypercalcemia is caused by the local production of hormones or cytokines by cancers that have spread to the bone or bone marrow; such factors increase bone resorption in the area around the cancer. The ectopically produced hormones that may play a role in LOH include transforming growth factors α and β, interleukin (IL)-1, IL-6, prostaglandins, and tumor necrosis factor.

Clinical Manifestations The initial symptoms and signs of hypercalcemia (calcium level ≥ 2.6 mmol/L)[1] include malaise, fatigue, confusion, anorexia, bone pain, polyuria, polydipsia, weakness, constipation, nausea, and vomiting. Neurologic symptoms and signs in profound hypercalcemia (>3.5 mmol/L) include confusion, lethargy, coma, and death. The cancers associated with HHM are non-small cell lung cancer and cancers of the breast, kidney, head and neck, and bladder. HHM is particularly common in patients with cancers of squamous cell histology. Hypercalcemia is uncommon at presentation (<1% of patients) but becomes more common as the cancer progresses and is present in 10 to 20% of patients near the time of death. LOH is responsible for hypercalcemia in patients with breast cancer, myeloma, lymphoma, and leukemia. Among hypercalcemic patients with breast cancer, approximately half have HHM and half have LOH.

---

[1]Calcium measurements given in millimoles per liter can be multiplied by 4 to convert to milligrams per deciliter or by 2 to convert to milliequivalents per liter.

Diagnosis The patient with cancer who develops hypercalcemia should be evaluated for other causes of hypercalcemia, including use of thiazide diuretics, vitamin D, or lithium, hyperthyroidism, and sarcoidosis. If the underlying cancer is controlled, elevation of serum PTH as measured by immunoassay suggests primary hyperparathyroidism, which may be responsible for as many as 10% of cases of hypercalcemia of cancer and which should be treated like other cases of hyperparathyroidism (Chap. 341). A normal PTH level and a low serum phosphorus level in the absence of bone metastases support the diagnosis of HHM, while a normal PTHrP level and normal phosphorus in a patient with bone metastases suggest LOH.

℞ **TREATMENT** The median survival of patients with hypercalcemia of malignancy is only 1 to 3 months. Intervention to reverse hypercalcemia should be undertaken when the cancer is likely to be controlled with appropriate systemic or local treatment.

The treatment of HHM and LOH is similar (Chap. 341). Patients with mild to moderate hypercalcemia (2.7 to 3.5 mmol/L) can be treated with 2 to 4 L of saline hydration per day and furosemide to prevent intravascular volume overload. The bisphosphonate pamidronate (90 mg intravenously) decreases osteoclastic bone resorption. Combined administration of diuretics and pamidronate reduces the serum calcium to normal values in 90% of patients within 7 days. Doses may be repeated as needed. In patients with LOH, glucocorticoids may inhibit the production of cytokines that promote bone resorption. Severe hypercalcemia [3.50 mmol/L (>14 mg/dL)] with alteration of mental status can be treated with all of the above plus salmon calcitonin, 4 to 8 U/kg, administered intramuscularly or subcutaneously every 12 h. Calcitonin administration will decrease the serum calcium within 24 h, and its hypocalcemic effect can be prolonged in patients with LOH by adding glucocorticoids. If these agents are not effective in reducing the serum calcium, plicamycin and gallium nitrate may be added.

HYPONATREMIA OF MALIGNANCY Hyponatremia of malignancy (Na$^+$ level <130 mmol/L) is usually due to the inappropriate secretion of arginine vasopressin (AVP) and is termed the *syndrome of inappropriate antidiuretic hormone secretion* (SIADH). In rare cases, atrial natriuretic peptide produces hyponatremia.

Pathogenesis Small cell lung cancer is the malignancy chiefly responsible for producing ectopic AVP. AVP mRNA is expressed and translated, and the product is processed into the nonapeptide AVP, which is secreted into the circulation. The ectopically produced AVP binds to receptors in the kidney, causing retention of free water with resulting hypoosmolality in the plasma and hyperosmolality in urine (Chap. 329).

About 15% of cancer patients with SIADH do not have evidence of ectopic production of AVP. In some of these patients, tumors secrete atrial natriuretic peptide. This hormone inhibits sodium reabsorption in the proximal tubule and inhibits release of renin and aldosterone. How atrial natriuretic peptide leads to hyponatremia is not clear.

Clinical Manifestations SIADH is commonly recognized as asymptomatic hyponatremia on routine serum chemistry examination. It is present at the time of diagnosis in 15% of patients with small cell lung cancer, 3% of patients with head and neck cancer, and <1% of patients with non-small cell lung cancer. Hyponatremia may also occur with primary brain tumors, hematologic malignancies, melanoma, sarcoma, and gynecologic, gastrointestinal, breast, prostate, and bladder cancers. The symptoms of mild hyponatremia (>120 mmol/L) include difficulty focusing attention, fatigue, nausea, vomiting, anorexia,

Table 100-1   Common Paraneoplastic Endocrine Syndromes

Syndrome	Proteins	Tumors Typically Associated with Syndrome
Hypercalcemia of malignancy	Parathyroid hormone-related peptide (PTHrP) Parathyroid hormone (PTH)	Non-small cell lung cancer Breast cancer Renal cell carcinoma Head and neck cancer Bladder cancer Myeloma
Syndrome of inappropriate antidiuretic hormone secretion (SIADH)	Arginine vasopressin (AVP) Atrial natriuretic peptide	Small cell lung cancer Head and neck cancer Non-small cell lung cancer
Cushing's syndrome	Adrenocorticotropic hormone (ACTH) Corticotropin-releasing hormone (CRH)	Small cell lung cancer Carcinoid tumors
Acromegaly	Growth hormone–releasing hormone (GHRH) Growth hormone (GH)	Carcinoid tumors Small cell lung cancer Pancreatic islet cell tumors
Gynecomastia	Human chorionic gonadotropin (hCG)	Testicular cancer Lung cancer Carcinoid tumors of the lung and gastrointestinal tract
Non-islet cell tumor hypoglycemia	Insulin-like growth factor-2 (IGF-2)	Sarcomas

weakness, and headache. Profound hyponatremia (<120 mmol/L) can cause confusion, lethargy, coma, seizures, and death.

Diagnosis (See also Chap. 329)   SIADH is suspected in patients with hyponatremia (serum sodium <130 mmol/L) and a concentrated urine (osmolality >300 mosm/kg). Patients are euvolemic, are not using diuretics, and have normal thyroid and adrenal function. Polydipsia is excluded by the urine osmolality. Pseudohyponatremia can be present if serum glucose, triglyceride, or protein levels are high. Conditions other than cancer that can cause SIADH include central nervous system disorders, pulmonary infections, positive-pressure breathing, pneumothorax, asthma, and a wide array of drugs, including chemotherapeutic agents (vincristine, vinblastine, cisplatin, cyclophosphamide, melphalan), thiazide diuretics, carbamazepine, antidepressants, nicotine, and narcotics.

℞ **TREATMENT** Treatment should be directed at the underlying cancer. Patients whose tumors have not been or cannot be controlled are candidates for restriction of fluid intake to 500 mL/d. Such restriction corrects hyponatremia within 7 days in most patients, but it is difficult and uncomfortable for patients to maintain fluid restriction for extended periods. Oral demeclocycline (600 to 1200 mg/d) may be useful in blocking the effects of AVP but can cause renal insufficiency. Other agents that may be used for the treatment of hyponatremia include dilantin and lithium.

Rare patients develop profound hyponatremia and altered mental status. These patients should be treated with normal saline hydration and furosemide diuresis. If that is not effective, 3% saline can be administered via a central line together with furosemide diuresis to prevent hypervolemia. Hypertonic saline is rarely required and must be given slowly; fluid balance and electrolytes should be monitored several times per day, and the increase in sodium should be limited to 0.5 mmol/L per hour to prevent pontine lysis (Chap. 329).

ECTOPIC ACTH SYNDROME Ectopic production of ACTH by cancer cells is responsible for ~15% of all cases of Cushing's syndrome and for most cases of Cushing's syndrome that occur in cancer patients (Chaps. 328, 331). In rare patients, Cushing's syndrome is caused by ectopically produced corticotropin-releasing hormone (CRH), which stimulates pituitary ACTH release.

Pathogenesis When pro-opiomelanocortin mRNA is expressed in cancer cells, the 241-amino-acid prohormone is translated and processed into a variety of molecules, including, in some cases, the 39-amino-acid hormone ACTH, which can be secreted into the circulation. The ectopically produced ACTH causes excessive secretion of glucocorticoids and mineralocorticoids by the adrenals.

Clinical Manifestations   Women make up 50% of patients with ectopic ACTH syndrome and 90% of patients with pituitary Cushing's disease. Therefore, Cushing's syndrome in men is more likely to be caused by ectopic ACTH than by a pituitary tumor. Because of mineralocorticoid excess, patients with ectopic Cushing's syndrome usually have hypokalemic alkalosis at presentation, a rare finding in patients with Cushing's disease. Other common manifestations of ectopic ACTH syndrome include weakness, hypertension, and hyperglycemia. Ectopic ACTH syndrome in patients with slow-growing cancers (e.g., carcinoids) may develop typical features of central obesity, moon facies, hyperpigmentation, and hirsutism in addition to the metabolic abnormalities.

Ectopic ACTH syndrome is most commonly due to small cell lung cancer (50% of cases), bronchial carcinoid tumors (10%), thymic carcinoid tumors or thymomas (10%), pancreatic islet cell tumors (10%), pheochromocytoma or other neural crest tumors (5%), or medullary carcinoma of the thyroid (5%). About 2% of patients with small cell lung cancer and bronchial carcinoids have ectopic ACTH syndrome at the time of diagnosis. Patients with small cell lung cancer and ectopic ACTH syndrome have shorter survival rates than patients without the syndrome and are more likely to develop opportunistic infections.

Diagnosis (See also Chaps. 328, 331)   Ectopic ACTH syndrome is usually characterized by elevated levels of urinary free cortisol that do not decrease after administration of high doses of dexamethasone (8 mg/d). However, in 20 to 30% of patients with ectopic ACTH syndrome, urinary cortisol levels decrease by >50% after administration of high-dose dexamethasone. The plasma levels of ACTH are markedly elevated in more than half of patients. If these tests do not provide definitive evidence of ectopic ACTH syndrome, bilateral inferior petrosal vein sampling will show an elevated ACTH level in petrosal vein blood that does not increase after administration of CRH.

℞ TREATMENT   Treatment of the ectopic ACTH syndrome should be directed at the underlying cancer: chemotherapy for small cell lung cancer; surgical resection or radiation therapy for carcinoids. Some patients with ectopic Cushing's syndrome have no evidence of tumor after extensive evaluation. These patients should be treated symptomatically and followed closely with periodic imaging studies, because they may have slow-growing tumors amenable to surgical resection.

Agents that inhibit steroidogenesis in the adrenal gland include ketoconazole (400 to 1200 mg/d), which reduces urinary cortisol excretion by more than half in two-thirds of patients, and metyrapone (1 to 4 g/d), which also reduces urinary cortisol excretion. Patients who are in good condition and whose manifestations are not controlled by drugs may be considered for adrenalectomy.

ECTOPIC ACROMEGALY   Ectopic production of growth hormone-releasing hormone (GHRH) is the predominant cause of ectopic acromegaly (Chap. 328).

Pathogenesis   GHRH is processed into 40- and 44-amino-acid peptides and binds to receptors in the pituitary, increasing production of growth hormone that increases insulin-like growth factor (IGF)-1 production in peripheral tissues. Rare cases of ectopic acromegaly are due to ectopic production of growth hormone itself by tumors.

Clinical Manifestations   The symptoms and signs of ectopic acromegaly develop over several years and include increasing glove and shoe size, facial disfigurement, arthralgias, amenorrhea-galactorrhea or impotence, hypertension, muscle weakness, and diabetes mellitus. Ectopic acromegaly has been reported in fewer than 100 patients and accounts for 1% or less of all cases of acromegaly. The cancers associated with ectopic acromegaly include carcinoid tumors of the bron-

chus, pancreatic islet cell tumors, and cancers of the lung, breast, colon, and adrenal glands.

Diagnosis   If a clinical diagnosis of acromegaly is suspected in a patient with cancer, the serum levels of GHRH and IGF-1 and the glucose-suppressed growth hormone (GH) serum level should be measured (Chap. 328). Patients with elevated GHRH levels and acromegaly have ectopic acromegaly. Patients without evidence of cancer who have elevated GHRH levels should undergo imaging of the central nervous system, chest, and abdomen to look for an occult cancer. Patients with cancer, low GHRH levels, high GH levels, and elevated IGF-1 levels should undergo magnetic resonance imaging of the pituitary and hypothalamus. If no pituitary tumor is detected, GH may be secreted directly by the known tumor. Not all GH -secreting tumors of the pituitary are demonstrable by imaging techniques, however.

℞ TREATMENT   The therapy of ectopic acromegaly should be directed at the underlying cancer and should consist of surgical resection or radiation therapy for patients with carcinoid and islet cell tumors. Medical control of ectopic acromegaly is obtained by using octreotide (100 to 250 μg every 8 h), which inhibits pituitary secretion of growth hormone. Octreotide produces symptomatic improvement in approximately two-thirds of patients.

GYNECOMASTIA   Ectopic production of hCG or estrogens by tumors such as cancers of the lung and testis is responsible for approximately 3% of cases of gynecomastia detected in men (Chap. 337). Ectopic production of hCG is the most common cause of paraneoplastic gynecomastia; the hCG acts by stimulating the Leydig cells of the testis to produce increased amounts of estrogen. Alternatively, on rare occasions, a tumor (such as a hepatoma or a germ cell tumor with choriocarcinoma elements) contains aromatase enzyme activity that converts circulating androgens to estrogen. Leydig cell or Sertoli cell tumors may also secrete estradiol. In all cases, the increased ratio of estrogen to testosterone leads to the proliferation of breast tissue and gynecomastia. Other tumors rarely associated with ectopic gynecomastia include carcinoid tumors of the bronchus, intestine, and small cell lung cancer.

About 5% of men with testicular choriocarcinoma present with an enlarging breast mass. In the absence of an obvious cancer, men presenting with gynecomastia should have a careful examination of the testes and measurement of serum hCG. Patients with a testicular mass should undergo an inguinal orchiectomy for diagnosis and treatment. If no testicular mass is found by physical examination, the testes should be examined with ultrasound. Patients with an elevated hCG level and no testicular mass should undergo evaluation for an extragonadal germ cell tumor.

℞ TREATMENT   The therapy of tumor-associated gynecomastia should be directed at the underlying cancer: chemotherapy is used for testicular cancers, and surgical resection or radiation therapy for carcinoids and islet cell tumors. In patients with successfully treated testicular cancer, gynecomastia completely resolves in three-fourths of cases.

NON-ISLET CELL TUMOR HYPOGLYCEMIA   Hypoglycemia that is not caused by the ectopic production of insulin (as in patients with islet cell tumors of the pancreas) can occur with large, slow-growing sarcomas, mesotheliomas, and hepatomas (Chap. 334). Ectopic production of IGF-2 is responsible for hypoglycemia in most patients with non-islet cell tumors. The ectopically produced IGF-2 inhibits glycogenolysis and gluconeogenesis in the liver, suppresses lipolysis, and increases peripheral glucose utilization, thereby causing hypoglycemia. IGF-2 may also act as an autocrine growth factor for the tumor.

Patients with large sarcomas (1 to 10 kg) may develop hypoglycemia, particularly with fasting. Headache, fatigue, confusion, or seizures may occur. Patients with a large sarcoma and hypoglycemia are likely to have non-islet cell tumor hypoglycemia. Although IGF-2 protein or mRNA is detectable in tumor tissue, the diagnosis is usually made on clinical grounds, because the plasma levels of IGF-2 are typically not elevated. Levels of IGF binding proteins may be increased.

℞ **TREATMENT** The therapy of non-islet cell hypoglycemia should be directed at the underlying cancer: surgical resection or radiation therapy. Patients whose tumors cannot be successfully resected or irradiated can be treated with frequent oral feedings or constant intravenous administration of glucose.

HEMATOLOGIC SYNDROMES

The elevation of granulocyte, platelet, and eosinophil counts in most patients with myeloproliferative disorders is caused by the proliferation of the myeloid elements due to the underlying disease rather than a paraneoplastic syndrome. The paraneoplastic hematologic syndromes in patients with solid tumors are less well characterized than the endocrine syndromes, because the ectopic hormone(s) or cytokines responsible have not been identified in most of these tumors (Table 100-2). The severity of the paraneoplastic syndromes parallels the course of the cancer.

ERYTHROCYTOSIS Ectopic production of erythropoietin by cancer cells causes most paraneoplastic erythrocytosis. The ectopically produced erythropoietin stimulates the production of red blood cells in the bone marrow and raises the hematocrit. Other lymphokines and hormones produced by cancer cells may stimulate erythropoietin release but have not been proven to cause erythrocytosis.

Most patients with erythrocytosis have an elevated hematocrit (>52% in men; 48% in women) that is detected on a routine blood count. Approximately 3% of patients with renal cell cancer, 10% of patients with hepatoma, and 15% of patients with cerebellar hemangioblastomas have erythrocytosis. In most cases the erythrocytosis is asymptomatic.

Patients with erythrocytosis due to a renal cell cancer, hepatoma, or central nervous system cancer should have measurement of red cell mass. If the red cell mass is elevated, the serum erythropoietin level should then be measured. Patients with an appropriate cancer, elevated erythropoietin levels, and no other explanation for erythrocytosis (e.g., a hemoglobinopathy that causes increased O_2 affinity, Chap. 106) have the paraneoplastic syndrome.

Table 100-2 Paraneoplastic Hematologic Syndromes

Syndrome	Proteins	Cancers Typically Associated with Syndrome
Erythrocytosis	Erythropoietin	Renal cancers
		Hepatocarcinoma
		Cerebellar hemangioblastomas
Granulocytosis	G-CSF	Lung cancer
	GM-CSF	Gastrointestinal cancer
	IL-6	Ovarian cancer
		Genitourinary cancer
Thrombocytosis	IL-6	Lung cancer
		Gastrointestinal cancer
		Breast cancer
		Ovarian cancer
		Lymphoma
Eosinophilia	IL-5	Lymphoma
		Leukemia
		Lung cancer
Thrombophlebitis	Unknown	Lung cancer
		Pancreatic cancer
		Gastrointestinal cancer
		Breast cancer
		Genitourinary cancer
		Ovarian cancer
		Prostate cancer
		Lymphoma

℞ **TREATMENT** Successful resection of the cancer usually resolves the erythrocytosis. If the tumor neither can be resected nor treated effectively with radiation therapy or chemotherapy, phlebotomy may control any symptoms related to erythrocytosis.

GRANULOCYTOSIS Approximately 30% of patients with solid tumors have granulocytosis (granulocyte count >8000/μL). In about half of patients with granulocytosis and cancer, the granulocytosis has an identifiable nonparaneoplastic etiology (infection, tumor necrosis, glucocorticoid administration, etc.). The other patients have proteins in urine and serum that stimulate the growth of bone marrow cells. Tumors and tumor cell lines from patients with lung, ovarian, and bladder cancers have been documented to produce granulocyte colony-stimulating factor (G-CSF), granulocyte-macrophage colony-stimulating factor (GM-CSF), and/or IL-6. However, the etiology of granulocytosis has not been characterized in most patients.

Patients with granulocytosis are nearly all asymptomatic, and the differential white blood cell count does not have a shift to immature forms of neutrophils. Granulocytosis occurs in 40% of patients with lung and gastrointestinal cancers, 20% of patients with breast cancer, 30% of patients with brain tumors and ovarian cancers, and 10% of patients with renal cell carcinoma. Patients with advanced-stage disease are more likely to have granulocytosis than those with early-stage disease.

Paraneoplastic granulocytosis does not require treatment. The granulocytosis resolves when the underlying cancer is successfully treated.

THROMBOCYTOSIS Thirty-five percent of patients with thrombocytosis (platelet count >400,000/μL) have an underlying diagnosis of cancer. IL-6, a candidate molecule for the etiology of paraneoplastic thrombocytosis, stimulates the production of platelets in vitro and in vivo. Some patients with cancer and thrombocytosis have elevated levels of IL-6 in plasma. Another candidate molecule is thrombopoietin, a peptide hormone that stimulates megakaryocyte proliferation and platelet production. The etiology of thrombocytosis has not been established in most cases.

Patients with thrombocytosis are nearly all asymptomatic. Thrombocytosis is not clearly linked to thrombosis in patients with cancer. Thrombocytosis is present in 40% of patients with lung and gastrointestinal cancers, 20% of patients with breast, endometrial, and ovarian cancers, and 10% of patients with lymphoma. Patients with thrombocytosis are more likely to have advanced-stage disease and have a poorer prognosis than patients without thrombocytosis. Paraneoplastic thrombocytosis does not require treatment.

EOSINOPHILIA Eosinophilia is present in ~1% of patients with cancer. Tumors and tumor cell lines from patients with lymphomas or leukemia may produce IL-5, which stimulates eosinophil growth. Activation of IL-5 transcription in lymphomas and leukemias may involve translocation of the long arm of chromosome 5, to which the genes for IL-5 and other cytokines map.

Patients with eosinophilia are typically asymptomatic. Eosinophilia is present in 10% of patients with lymphoma, 3% of patients with lung cancer, and occasional patients with cervical, gastrointestinal, renal, and breast cancer. Patients with markedly elevated eosinophil counts (>5000/μL) can develop shortness of breath and wheezing. A chest radiograph may reveal diffuse pulmonary infiltrates from eosinophil infiltration and activation in the lungs.

℞ **TREATMENT** Definitive treatment is directed at the underlying malignancy: tumors should be resected or treated with radiation or chemotherapy. In most patients who develop shortness of breath related to eosinophilia, symptoms resolve with the use of oral or inhaled glucocorticoids.

THROMBOPHLEBITIS Deep venous thrombosis and pulmonary embolism are the most common thrombotic conditions in patients with cancer. Migratory or recurrent thrombophlebitis may be the initial manifestation of cancer. Approximately 15% of patients who develop deep venous thrombosis or pulmonary embolism have a diagnosis of cancer (Chap. 117). The coexistence of peripheral venous thrombosis with visceral carcinoma, particularly pancreatic cancer, is called *Trousseau's syndrome.*

Pathogenesis   Patients with cancer are predisposed to thromboembolism because they are often at bedrest or immobilized, and tumors may obstruct or slow blood flow. In addition, clotting may be promoted by release of procoagulants or cytokines from tumor cells or associated inflammatory cells, or by platelet adhesion or aggregation. The specific molecules that mediate the increased risk of thromboembolism have not been identified.

Clinical Manifestations   Patients with cancer who develop deep venous thrombosis usually develop swelling or pain in the leg, and physical examination reveals tenderness, warmth, and redness. Patients who present with pulmonary embolism develop dyspnea, chest pain, and syncope, and physical examination shows tachycardia, cyanosis, and hypotension. Approximately 5% of patients with no history of cancer who have a diagnosis of deep venous thrombosis or pulmonary embolism will have a diagnosis of cancer within 1 year. The most common cancers associated with thromboembolic episodes include lung, pancreatic, gastrointestinal, breast, ovarian, and genitourinary cancers, lymphomas, and brain tumors. Patients with cancer who undergo surgical procedures requiring general anesthesia have a 20 to 30% risk of deep venous thrombosis.

Diagnosis   The diagnosis of deep venous thrombosis in patients with cancer is made by impedance plethysmography or bilateral compression ultrasonography of the leg veins. Patients with a noncompressible venous segment have deep venous thrombosis. If compression ultrasonography is normal and a high clinical suspicion exists for deep venous thrombosis, venography should be done to look for a luminal filling defect. Elevation of D-dimer is not as predictive of deep venous thrombosis in patients with cancer as in patients without cancer.

Patients with symptoms and signs suggesting a pulmonary embolism should be evaluated with a chest radiograph, electrocardiogram, arterial blood gas analysis, and ventilation–perfusion scan. Patients with mismatched segmental perfusion defects have a pulmonary embolus. Patients with equivocal ventilation–perfusion findings should be evaluated as described above for deep venous thrombosis in their legs. If deep venous thrombosis is detected, they should be anticoagulated. If deep venous thrombosis is not detected, they should be considered for a pulmonary angiogram.

Patients without a diagnosis of cancer who present with an initial episode of thrombophlebitis or pulmonary embolus need no additional tests for cancer other than a careful history and physical exam. In light of the many possible primary sites, diagnostic testing in asymptomatic patients is wasteful. However, if the clot is refractory to standard treatment or is in an unusual site, or if the thrombophlebitis is migratory or recurrent, efforts to find an underlying cancer are indicated.

 TREATMENT   Patients with cancer and a diagnosis of deep venous thrombosis or pulmonary embolism should be treated initially with intravenous unfractionated heparin or low molecular weight heparin for at least 5 days and coumadin started within 1 or 2 days. The coumadin dose should be adjusted so the INR is 2 to 3. Patients with proximal deep venous thrombosis and a relative contraindication to heparin anticoagulation (hemorrhagic brain metastases or pericardial effusion) should be considered for placement of a filter in the inferior vena cava (Greenfield filter) to prevent pulmonary embolism. Coumadin should be administered for 3 to 6 months. Patients with cancer who undergo a major surgical procedure should be considered for heparin prophylaxis or pneumatic boots. Breast cancer patients undergoing chemotherapy and patients with implanted catheters should be considered for prophylaxis (1 mg coumadin per day).

→*Cutaneous paraneoplastic syndromes are discussed in Chap. 57. Neurologic paraneoplastic syndromes are discussed in Chap. 101. More extensive discussion of functional endocrine tumors is given in Chap. 93.*

BIBLIOGRAPHY

BARTTER F, SCHWARTZ W: The syndrome of inappropriate secretion of antidiuretic hormone. Am J Med 42:790, 1967

BODY JJ et al: Current use of bisphosphonates in oncology. International Bone and Cancer Study Group. J Clin Oncol 16:3890, 1998

BRAUNSTEIN GD: Gynecomastia. N Engl J Med 328:490, 1993

EZZAT S: Acromegaly. Endocrinol Metab Clin North Am 26:703, 1997

JOHNSON BE et al: A prospective study of patients with lung cancer and hyponatremia of malignancy. Am J Respir Crit Care Med 156:1669, 1997

LEE AY et al: Clinical utility of a rapid whole-blood D-dimer assay in patients with cancer who present with suspected acute deep venous thrombosis. Ann Intern Med 131:417, 1999

LEVINE MN, LEE AY: Treatment of venous thromboembolism in cancer patients. Semin Thromb Hemost 25:245, 1999

NEWELL-PRICE J et al: The diagnosis and differential diagnosis of Cushing's syndrome and pseudo-Cushing's states. Endocr Rev 19:647, 1998

WINQUIST EW et al: Ketoconazole in the management of paraneoplastic Cushing's syndrome secondary to ectopic adrenocorticotropin production. J Clin Oncol 13:157, 1995

101   *Muhammad T. Al-Lozi, Alan Pestronk*

PARANEOPLASTIC NEUROLOGIC SYNDROMES

GENERAL PRINCIPLES

A paraneoplastic neurologic syndrome (PNNS) is a neurologic disorder that is associated with a neoplasm but lies anatomically remote from it. Paraneoplastic disorders are caused by immune or other mechanisms and are not due to direct effects of the tumor itself, metastases, opportunistic infections, complications of drug or radiation therapy, or malnutrition. Clinical features of a PNNS are often distinctive. Onset can be dramatic, arising subacutely over weeks or even days to produce neurologic symptoms that may be profoundly disabling.

PNNS associated with autoantibodies can be grouped into (1) disorders in which the neoplasm contains a surface antigen or intracellular protein that is the antigenic target, and (2) monoclonal gammopathy syndromes associated with secretion of an antibody by the neoplasm. Each subgroup has typical clinical, pathologic, and immune characteristics (Table 101-1). Some PNNS, including lymphoma-associated motor neuropathy, subacute necrotic myopathy, dermatomyositis, and necrotizing myopathy, have no currently identified antibody or target antigen and are not yet classifiable in this scheme.

The temporal relationship of a PNNS to the associated neoplasm is variable. The PNNS may precede or follow the identification of a neoplasm by weeks, months, or occasionally years. The strength of the association between neoplasms and PNNS varies with different syndromes, different neoplasms, and the clinical context. In some PNNS, such as the sensory neuronopathy associated with anti-Hu antibodies, the association with neoplasm is very strong. By contrast, the Lambert-Eaton myasthenic syndrome (LEMS) is associated with neoplasm in approximately 50% of cases only; the relationship is probably stronger in older individuals who have a history of cigarette smoking. Disorders that are clinically identical to most PNNS also occur in the absence of cancer. Nonetheless, the development of a PNNS in a previously healthy individual should in most circumstances prompt a thorough search for its associated neoplasms.

PNNS-associated neoplasms vary considerably in terms of malignancy. Tumors associated with subacute necrotic myelopathy are often severe and unresponsive to therapy. In other syndromes, the tumor either remains small or can be effectively treated; in such cases, the

Table 101-1 General Features of Paraneoplastic Neurologic Syndromes (PNNS) Associated with Autoantibodies

Features		Tumor Protein is Antigenic Target		Neoplasm Produces Antibody
		Intracellular Antigen	Surface Membrane Antigen	
Clinical	Disease location	Central NS	Nerve or muscle	Peripheral nerve
		Occasionally peripheral NS	Rarely central NS	Occasionally muscle
	Disease course	Subacute onset → plateau	Subacute onset → plateau	Chronic progression
	Treatment	Rarely effective	Immunomodulation, many types	Immunomodulation, cytotoxic
	Disease pathology	Neural cell death	Membrane dysfunction	Damage to axons or myelin
			Focal damage to nerve or muscle cell	
	Typical disorders	Sensory neuronopathy (Hu)	Myasthenia gravis	Motor neuropathy (IgM anti-G_{M1})
		Cerebellar ataxia (Yo)	LEMS	Anti-MAG neuropathy (IgM)
		Limbic encephalitis (Hu; Ma2)	Isaac's neuromyotonia	POEMS (IgG or IgA)
				Cryoglobulinemia
				Amyloidosis
Antigen	Location	PNNS target; neoplasm	PNNS target; neoplasm	PNNS target
		Nuclear or cytoplasmic	Surface membrane	Cell surface
	Type	RNA binding proteins	Transmitter receptor	Glycolipid
		Golgi-related proteins	Ion channel	Glycoprotein
Antibody	Location	Serum	Serum	Serum
		CSF	Usually not CSF	
	Type	Polyclonal IgG	Polyclonal IgG	Monoclonal
				IgM: known target
				IgG or IgA: ? target
	Pathogenic	Rarely	Often	Probably
Neoplasm types		Small cell lung	Small cell lung	MGUS
		Gynecologic	Thymoma	Lymphoma
		Testicular	Lymphoma	
Neoplasm frequency		Nearly always: 80 to 95%	Variable: 10 to 70%	Nearly always

NOTE: NS, nervous system; LEMS, Lambert-Eaton myasthenic syndrome; G_{M1}, G_{M1} ganglioside; MAG, myelin-associated glycoprotein; CSF, cerebrospinal fluid; POEMS, polyneuropathy, organomegaly, endocrinopathy, m-protein, skin changes; MGUS, monoclonal gammopathy of unknown significance.

long-term prognosis is determined by the effectiveness of management of the paraneoplastic syndrome. Thymoma associated with myasthenia gravis is an example of a tumor in this category. In some PNNS, such as those associated with small cell lung cancer (SCLC) and anti-Hu antibodies, it has been suggested that the presence of the autoantibodies may confer a more favorable prognosis by inhibiting tumor growth.

As outlined in Table 101-2, certain syndromes are associated with particular types of tumors, and more than one syndrome may occur with a given neoplasm. For example, SCLCs are associated with a variety of PNNS, including limbic encephalitis, cerebellar ataxia, opsoclonus-myoclonus, necrotic myelopathy, sensory neuronopathy, autonomic neuropathy, and LEMS.

Prevalence estimates vary with the particular syndrome. Tumors that are most often associated with PNNS are cancers of the lung, stomach, breast, ovary, and colon. Some 30% of patients with thymoma also develop myasthenia gravis as a paraneoplastic syndrome. A poorly characterized neuromyopathy with proximal weakness and distal sensory loss is very common in patients who have lost more than 15% of their body weight. In contrast, most of the well-defined PNNS are rare, with estimated prevalence rates of <1% of the population with cancer.

The diagnosis of a PNNS depends primarily on (1) the presence of a recognized clinical paraneoplastic syndrome; (2) careful exclusion of other cancer-related disorders; and (3) appropriate confirmatory studies, including measurement of specific antibodies and neurophysiologic studies to define the anatomic distribution of the disease process.

PNNS OF THE CENTRAL NERVOUS SYSTEM

LIMBIC ENCEPHALITIS Limbic encephalitis is a feature of several paraneoplastic syndromes. It occurs in isolation or overlaps with syndromes that also involve the brainstem, cerebellum, spinal cord, and posterior root ganglia. Patients present with seizures, confusion, psychiatric symptoms (agitation, hallucinations, depression, anxiety, and changes in personality), or severe short-term memory loss. Seizures are commonly complex-partial in type, with or without secondary generalization, and may be intractable and refractory to treatment. Other features can include vertigo, ataxia, nystagmus, numbness/paresthesias, and symmetric or asymmetric weakness. Limbic encephalitis typically progresses over a period of weeks before stabilizing. Exacerbations may occur, and remissions are rare, with or without treatment. The onset of symptoms may precede or follow the discovery of tumor. Limbic encephalitis is most commonly associated with SCLC; less frequently with testicular cancer; and occasionally with thymoma, Hodgkin's disease, non-SCLC, breast, colon, and bladder cancer. Some cases are not associated with cancer.

Magnetic resonance imaging (MRI) suggests that paraneoplastic limbic encephalitis is often a relatively widespread disease of the central nervous system. The T2 signal may be increased not only in the temporal lobes but also in the cortex or brainstem. Approximately 75% of patients show electroencephalographic abnormalities that may include focal slowing and/or paroxysmal sharp waves and spikes. Cerebrospinal fluid (CSF) often shows elevated protein, mild mononuclear pleocytosis, oligoclonal bands, or increased IgG synthesis but may be normal.

Neuropathologic features of limbic encephalitis include neuronal loss in the hippocampus, cingulate gyrus, orbital frontal lobe, brainstem, and posterior root ganglia. Additionally, there may be scattered gliosis, microglial nodules, and/or perivascular lymphocytic cuffing.

Anti-Hu antibodies (Table 101-2) are detected in the serum and CSF in the majority of patients with paraneoplastic limbic encephalitis. Most patients with anti-Hu antibodies have SCLC; however, breast and prostate cancer and neuroblastoma are also described. Approximately 20% of patients with SCLC without neurologic symptoms have low titers of anti-Hu antibodies. Anti-Hu antibodies are strongly (>90%) associated with neoplasms; patients with positive antibody titers but a negative initial malignancy workup should have a search for neoplasm repeated every 6 to 12 months. Immunotherapy [plasma exchange, intravenous immunoglobulin (IVIg), cyclophosphamide, or glucocorticoids] and/or resection of primary tumor are only rarely associated with improvement in the limbic encephalitis.

Patients with limbic and/or brainstem encephalitis and testicular cancer may have serum IgG antibodies that bind to Ma2, a 40-kD cytoplasmic and nuclear protein. Ma2 is expressed in both brain tissue

Table 101-2 Neurologic Paraneoplastic Syndromes

Syndrome	Features	Antibody Target	Neoplasm/Percentage
BRAIN			
Limbic encephalitis	Onset: subacute Confusion Memory loss Temporal lobe seizures	Hu	SCLC, testicular cancer, breast, colon, bladder, lymphoma
Brainstem encephalitis	Vertigo Cerebellar: ataxia, nystagmus Ocular: diplopia, gaze palsies	Hu	SCLC
Cerebellar degeneration	Cerebellar: ataxia, dysarthria	Yo Tr Glutamate receptors	Ovary, uterus, SCLC, Hodgkin's lymphoma
Opsoclonus/myoclonus	Involuntary eye movements: rapid, random directions Ataxia Encephalopathy	Ri (NOVA) Hu Neurofilament	Neuroblastoma, lung, breast
SPINAL CORD			
Necrotizing myelopathy	Weakness: paraplegia or quadriplegia Sensory loss: spinal level Urinary incontinence	Not known	SCLC, lymphoma
PERIPHERAL NERVE			
Neuronopathies			
Sensory neuronopathy	Onset: subacute Sensory loss; diffuse, asymmetric, numbness/paresthesias, dysesthesia/pain Sensory ataxia: pseudoathetosis ± encephalomyelitis	Hu	SCLC (90% of cases), breast, ovary, prostate
Motor neuronopathy	Onset: subacute Weakness: arms > legs Usually asymmetric	Not known	Lymphoma
Axonal neuropathies			
Sensorimotor neuropathy	Distal motor and sensory loss Most common paraneoplastic neuropathy, especially with >15% weight loss Axonal neuropathy	None	Many neoplasms
Mononeuritis multiplex	Weakness and/or sensory loss in the distribution of multiple nerves Onset: acute to subacute	Not known	Cryoglobulinemia, leukemia, lymphoma
Neuromyotonia (Isaacs)	Weakness: distal and proximal Stiffness Fasciculations	Voltage-gated potassium channels	Thymoma
Amyloid neuropathy	Distal symmetric axonal loss: small > large Autonomic symptoms prominent	Not known	Multiple myeloma
Autonomic neuropathies			
Enteric neuropathy	Gastroparesis Intestinal pseudo-obstruction Esophageal achalasia Dysphagia	Hu	Thymoma, SCLC
Demyelinating neuropathies			
Anti-MAG	Sensory > motor Distal, symmetric Gait disorder Tremor Slowly progressive NCV: Long distal latencies, Conduction block uncommon	Myelin-associated glycoprotein (MAG)	MGUS, IgM M-protein in 85%
Multifocal motor neuropathy	Slowly progressive Motor Distal > proximal Asymmetric NCV: Motor conduction block Motor axon loss (late)	G_{M1} ganglioside	MGUS, IgM M-protein in 20%
Anti-sulfatide	Slowly progressive Sensory > motor Distal, symmetric Demyelinating or axonal	Sulfatide	MGUS, IgM M-protein in 90% with demyelinating neuropathy
POEMS	Sensorimotor neuropathy Symmetric Mixed demyelinating and axonal	Not known	Multiple myeloma, IgG or IgA M-protein in 90%
CIDP	Chronic or relapsing Motor > sensory Distal and proximal weakness Usually symmetric NCV: Conduction block, slow sensory and motor conduction velocities	β-Tubulin in 20%	MGUS, IgM or IgG M-protein in 15%, lymphoma

(continued)

Table 101-2—(continued)

Syndrome	Features	Antibody Target	Neoplasm/Percentage
NEUROMUSCULAR JUNCTION			
LEMS	Weakness: proximal and distal Ocular: ptosis May improve with exercise Dry mouth Rapid repetitive stimulation: increment	Voltage-gated P/Q calcium channels	SCLC in 60% of cases, especially older and smoking history

Myasthenia gravis	Weakness
	  Cranial: ocular, face, bulbar
	  Respiratory, limbs, trunk
	Fatigue
	Slow repetitive stimulation: decrement
		Nicotinic acetylcholine receptor	Thymoma in 10%, especially >30 years

MUSCLE			
Necrotizing myopathy	Males > 40 Rapid-onset weakness Necrosis on muscle biopsy May improve with treatment of cancer	Not known	Lung, breast, alimentary tract
Dermatomyositis	Females > 40 Proximal muscle weakness Skin rash	Not known	Ovarian, nasopharyngeal
Type II atrophy	Especially with weight loss > 15% Wasting > weakness	Not known	Many neoplasms
Myopathy with anti-decorin antibodies	> 50 years of age Proximal symmetric weakness Mildly elevated creatine kinase	Decorin	Waldenström's macroglobulinemia, IgM M-protein
Rippling muscle disease	Cramps induced by touching muscle Muscle waves induced by percussion Electrically silent	Not known	Thymoma
Scleromyxedema	Skin papules Raynaud's phenomenon Proximal muscle weakness High creatine kinase Myopathic electromyography	Not known	MGUS, IgG or IgA λ M-protein

NOTE: SCLC, small cell lung cancer; NCV, nerve conduction velocity; MGUS, monoclonal gammopathy of undetermined significance; POEMS, polyneuropathy, organomegaly, endocrinopathy, m-protein, skin changes; CIDP, chronic inflammatory demyelinating polyneuropathy; LEMS, Lambert-Eaton myasthenic syndrome.

and testicular tumors. Occasional patients in this subgroup have improved after treatment of the primary neoplasm.

BRAINSTEM ENCEPHALITIS Paraneoplastic brainstem encephalitis is usually associated with disease elsewhere in the central or peripheral nervous system. Symptoms of brainstem encephalitis relate to the distribution of the disease process. The predominant symptoms are due to medullary involvement producing nausea, vomiting, nystagmus, vertigo, and ataxia. A rare syndrome of marked dysarthria and dysphagia is associated with pontine involvement. Mesencephalic inflammation and neuronal loss result in nuclear or internuclear eye movement abnormalities; diplopia and oscillopsia may be disabling. Rostral midbrain and nigral involvement may cause rigidity. Other rare disorders are deafness and hypoventilation.

PARANEOPLASTIC CEREBELLAR DEGENERATION (PCD) Approximately 90% of PCD occurs with SCLC, Hodgkin's lymphoma, or breast or ovarian cancer. Patients usually present with the subacute onset of a pancerebellar disorder consisting of nystagmus, oculomotor ataxia, dysarthric speech, and limb and gait ataxia (Chaps. 22 and 364). In many patients, especially those with the anti-Yo antibody syndrome, signs are restricted to cerebellar dysfunction. However, symptoms of more widespread central (lethargy, cognitive abnormalities) and peripheral (weakness, sensory changes, and dry mouth) nervous system involvement may be present. Symptoms usually progress over weeks and eventually stabilize, leaving the patient severely disabled.

MRI usually reveals cerebellar atrophy. The CSF may be normal or show mildly elevated protein, mononuclear pleocytosis, increased IgG index, and/or oligoclonal bands. The most consistent neuropathologic feature is a diffuse loss of Purkinje cells. Neuronal loss in the granular cell layer and deep cerebellar nuclei may also occur. Perivascular cuffing has been observed in the cerebellum and leptomeninges.

PCD may be associated with polyclonal IgG anti-Yo, anti-Tr, or anti-glutamate receptor (mGluR1) antibodies in the serum and CSF. Anti-Yo antibodies are commonly associated with breast or ovarian cancer. The Yo autoantigens are proteins that are prominently expressed in Purkinje cell cytoplasm (Golgi) and proximal dendrites but not in the nucleus. Anti-Tr and anti-mGluR1 antibodies occur with Hodgkin's lymphoma. Clinical features in the three antibody groups are similar. PCD syndromes rarely improve after treatment; however, occasional anti-Tr patients improve after treatment of Hodgkin's lymphoma. Reappearance or exacerbation of the PCD may indicate recurrence of the tumor.

PARANEOPLASTIC OPSOCLONUS-MYOCLONUS (POM) This disorder is also known as the "dancing eyes–dancing feet" syndrome. Opsoclonic eye movements are involuntary, high-amplitude, arrhythmic, multidirectional, conjugate saccades. They are often nearly continuous and persist with the eyes closed and during sleep. Opsoclonus is associated with blinking and myoclonus and increases with visual pursuit and voluntary ocular refixation. The syndrome may occur in isolation or as a component of other PNNS, including limbic or brainstem encephalitis. POM occurs in 2% of young children with neuroblastoma and may precede or follow the discovery of the neoplasm; 50% of children with POM harbor neuroblastoma. Patients may also manifest ataxia, irritability, and vomiting. Antibodies directed against neurofilaments have been described. In the pediatric population, POM may improve following treatment with adrenocorticotropic hormone (ACTH), glucocorticoids, or IVIg, but residual central nervous system signs are frequent.

In adults, opsoclonus/myoclonus syndromes may develop in association with neoplasms of the lung (anti-Hu antibodies), breast (anti-Ri antibodies), thymus, lymphoid cells, ovaries, uterus, and bladder. Anti-Ri antibodies bind to neuronal nuclear antigens, including NOVA-1, a protein that regulates RNA splicing or metabolism in a subset of developing neurons. Remissions may occur spontaneously or following treatment of the underlying tumor. Clonazepam and/or valproate may be useful for symptomatic control of opsoclonus and myoclonus.

CARCINOMA-ASSOCIATED RETINOPATHY (CAR) The chief complaint in CAR is unilateral or bilateral, symmetric or asymmetric, loss of vision. Night blindness may be the presenting symptom. The visual loss occurs either gradually or in a stepwise pattern over weeks to months. Other symptoms may include visual shimmering, sparkling, or distortions. Examination shows poor visual acuity, impaired color vision, and an afferent pupillary defect. Visual field defects most commonly consist of central and/or ring scotomas. CAR occurs mainly with SCLC (90%) but may also occur with melanoma and gynecologic neoplasms. CAR visual loss frequently precedes the discovery of SCLC. CAR associated with melanoma usually follows the discovery of cancer, with an interval of up to 10 years. Histologically, there is severe loss of the inner and outer segments of the rods and cones, with widespread degeneration of the outer nuclear layer. The electroretinogram is usually flat due to loss of the rod and cone cells. Polyclonal IgG antibodies in SCLC/CAR are directed against recoverin, a 23-kD retinal photoreceptor–specific calcium-binding protein. Other autoantigens include retinal enolase, the S-antigen, and tubby-like protein 1 (TULP1) which is a molecule expressed in synaptic terminals of photoreceptor cells. Treatment with glucocorticoids (prednisone) produces mild to moderate improvement in most patients.

PARANEOPLASTIC MYELOPATHY Paraneoplastic myelopathy is a rare disorder that presents as acute spinal shock manifest as flaccid paraparesis with a sensory level and sphincter disturbances (Chap. 368). Spinal cord dysfunction is rapidly progressive and ascending. The prognosis is poor. The CSF is often cellular with a high protein. MRI may show T2 signal changes in the spinal cord, with cord swelling and involvement of both white and gray matter structures. The onset of the syndrome may precede or follow detection of a neoplasm, typically lymphoma, leukemia, or lung cancer.

STIFF-PERSON SYNDROME (SPS) SPS is characterized by stiffness and painful spasms, especially in axial and proximal limb muscles, due to hyperexcitability of motor neurons (Chap. 22). The stiffness produces lumbar hyperlordosis. Muscle spasms are triggered by stretching, emotion, and sensory stimulation. A small minority of SPS occurs in association with neoplasms such as breast cancer, SCLC, thymoma, Hodgkin's disease, and colon cancer. IgG polyclonal antibodies directed against amphiphysin, a 125-kD synaptic vesicle–associated protein, have been detected in sera of some SPS patients, primarily those with breast cancer. Some patients respond to glucocorticoids or tumor resection. Treatment with diazepam, clonazepam, lioresal, or sodium valproate may produce symptomatic improvement.

PNNS OF THE NEUROMUSCULAR SYSTEM

Paraneoplastic neuromuscular syndromes may selectively involve nerve cell bodies (anterior horn or dorsal root ganglia), peripheral nerves (myelin or motor, sensory, or autonomic axons), the neuromuscular junction, or muscle. Some neuromuscular PNNS, including sensory neuronopathy with anti-Hu antibodies, are almost always associated with cancer. Other syndromes, such as myasthenia gravis, are statistically associated with neoplasms but in up to 90% of patients a neoplasm is never found. Some neuromuscular PNNS have protean clinical manifestations that are not distinctive; correct diagnosis may rely upon serologic testing for specific autoantibodies (Tables 101-2 and 101-3).

NEURONOPATHIES Neuronopathies, indicating damage to the cell body of the neuron, are typically asymmetric and produce proximal as well as distal involvement early in their clinical course. They are generally poorly responsive to treatment.

Subacute sensory neuronopathy (SSN) presents with numbness and pain that evolves in a progressive fashion over 1 to 8 weeks. A history of smoking is found in >95% of patients. Examination shows asymmetric sensory loss that may involve the face and trunk and proximal as well as distal regions of the upper and lower extremities. All sensory modalities are affected. Patients may become disabled by severe sensory ataxia and pseudoathetosis resulting from the deafferentation. Strength is usually normal. Tendon reflexes are diffusely diminished or absent. Nerve conduction studies show diminished or absent sensory responses with normal motor studies. SSN may occur in isolation but is often associated with central nervous system signs, ranging from mild nystagmus to severe encephalopathy. CSF commonly shows a mild pleocytosis and elevated protein levels. Serum IgG antibodies that bind to the Hu family of 35- to 40-kDa nuclear proteins are characteristic of SSN and are a useful diagnostic test. Hu proteins are neuron-specific but are also found in SCLC cells. Although anti-Hu antibodies have strong specificity for SSN and other PNNS, there is no evidence that the antibodies play a pathogenic role. Morphologically there is neuronal loss with perivascular inflammatory infiltrates in the dorsal root ganglia. SSN with anti-Hu antibodies is almost always associated with a neoplasm, especially SCLC, but neoplasm is found at initial evaluation in only 50% of patients. As noted above, the presence of anti-Hu antibodies is associated with a lower degree of malignancy of the SCLC, suggesting that the antibodies may inhibit tumor growth. The differential diagnosis of SSN includes Sjögren's syndrome and drug toxicity from cisplatin or pyridoxine. Treatment consists of therapy for the associated neoplasm. There is almost never improvement in the SSN itself; however, physical therapy may allow the patient, over time, to partially compensate for the sensory loss.

Motor neuronopathy is a rare syndrome that begins subacutely and then reaches a plateau. Patients have asymmetric weakness that may involve the arms more than the legs. The bulbar muscles are spared. Sensation is normal. Motor neuronopathy often manifests after the detection of a neoplasm, typically lymphoma. CSF shows elevated protein levels and oligoclonal bands in 60% of cases.

PERIPHERAL NEUROPATHY These disorders typically present with distal symptoms and signs in the limbs. They may be axonal, demyelinating, or a combination of the two types. The presence of circulating paraproteins or serologic markers often helps to define paraneoplastic neuropathy syndromes (Table 101-2).

Polyneuropathies associated with circulating paraproteins include: (1) chronic inflammatory demyelinating polyneuropathy (CIDP); (2) demyelinating neuropathy with serum IgM binding to antimyelin-associated glycoprotein (MAG); (3) multifocal motor neuropathy; (4) POEMS syndrome (*p*olyneuropathy, *o*rganomegaly, *e*ndocrinopathy or edema, *M* protein, and *s*kin changes); and (5) primary acquired amyloidosis. →*For further discussion of polyneuropathies associated with circulating paraproteins, see Chap. 378.*

An *axonal sensorimotor neuropathy* is frequently associated with neoplasms. This syndrome is especially common in patients with long-standing cancer and substantial weight loss (>15% of baseline weight). The neuropathy is characterized by distal, symmetric sensory loss and paresthesias, which may be painful, and by weakness and muscle wasting, which is especially prominent in the distal legs. Pathologically there is noninflammatory degeneration of axons and mild myelin loss, presumably secondary to the axonopathy. An accompanying myopathy with atrophy of type II muscle fibers may produce proximal muscle weakness. Axonal loss, with low-amplitude sensory and motor amplitudes and normal conduction velocities, is seen on electrophysiologic studies. This neuromyopathy has been described in association with a variety of solid tumors (lung, breast, stomach), lymphoma, and plasma cell dyscrasia. Successful treatment of the neoplasm may result in improvement or stabilization of the neuromyopathy.

Other axonal neuropathies may be PNNS, but their associations with neoplasms are less clearly established. *Peripheral nerve vasculitis*, producing mononeuritis multiplex or asymmetric sensorimotor polyneuropathy, has been reported with lymphomas or carcinoma of the lung, prostate, kidney, or stomach. *Polyneuropathy*, presenting

Table 101-3 Antibodies Associated with Paraneoplastic Syndromes

Antibody	Antigen Name	Antigen Location	Antigen Function/ Characteristics	Neoplasm	Clinical Syndromes
ANTIBODIES AGAINST INTRACELLULAR ANTIGENS					
Anti-Hu	Hu	Neuronal nuclei, CNS, dorsal root	RNA binding protein	SCLC, neuroblastoma, non-SCLC	Encephalomyelitis Limbic encephalitis Cerebellar ataxia Sensory neuronopathy Autonomic neuropathy
Anti-Yo	CRD 1 CRD 2	Purkinje cells, cytoplasm	Possible c-*myc* binding	Ovary, breast, uterine	Cerebellar degeneration
Anti-Ri	Ri (Nova)	CNS, neuronal nuclei	RNA binding protein	Breast, SCLC	Opsoclonus/myoclonus
Anti-Ma1	Ma1	Nuclei, nucleoli, cytoplasm	Phosphoprotein? Function?	Breast, colon, parotid	Cerebellar ataxia Brainstem encephalitis
Anti-Ma2 (Ta)	Ma2	Normal brain, testicular tumor	Phosphoprotein Function?	Testicular	Limbic encephalitis Brainstem encephalitis
Anti-CV2	CV2	Oligodenodrocyte cytoplasm	?	SCLC, thymoma	Cerebellar ataxia Limbic encephalitis Polyneuropathy
Anti-Tr	Not known	Purkinje cell cytoplasm	?	Hodgkin's	Cerebellar ataxia
ANTIBODIES AGAINST CELL SURFACE ANTIGENS					
Anti-VGCC	P/Q VGCC	Peripheral cholinergic synapses	Control permeability of calcium	SCLC	Lambert-Eaton myasthenic syndrome
Anti-AChR	AChR	Neuromuscular junction	Transmitter receptor	Thymoma	Myasthenia gravis
Anti-VGKC	VGKC	Peripheral nerve	Control permeability of potassium	Thymoma	Neuromyotonia
Anti-amphiphysin	Amphiphysin	Synaptic vesicles	Synaptic vesicles	Breast	Stiff-person syndrome
Anti-mGluR1	Metabotropic glutamate receptor	Cell surface receptors	Excitatory receptor	Hodgkin's	Cerebellar ataxia
Anti-MAG	Myelin-associated glycoprotein	Non-compact myelin	Glycoprotein	MGUS	Demyelinating sensorimotor neuropathy, tremor, gait ataxia
Anti-GM1	G_{M1} ganglioside	Peripheral nerve	Glycolipid	MGUS	Multifocal motor neuropathy
Anti-Sulfatide	Sulfatide	Peripheral nerve	Glycolipid	MGUS	Demyelinating neuropathy

NOTE: CNS, central nervous system; SCLC, small cell lung cancer; VGCC, voltage-gated calcium channel; AChR, acetylcholine receptor; VGKC, voltage-gated potassium channel; MGUS, monoclonal gammopathy of undetermined significance.

with either a subacute mononeuritis multiplex or a slowly progressive distal symmetric sensorimotor polyneuropathy, occurs in approximately 20% of patients with cryoglobulinemia. *Guillain-Barré syndrome* (Chap. 378) may be associated with Hodgkin's disease; it is characterized by subacute motor weakness; sensory loss, which is often mild in comparison with the motor deficits; areflexia; and a characteristic elevation of spinal fluid protein concentration without pleocytosis. *Enteric autonomic neuropathy* with anti-Hu antibodies, commonly presenting as intestinal pseudoobstruction, has been described in association with SCLC.

NEUROMUSCULAR JUNCTION *Lambert-Eaton myasthenic syndrome* is a disorder of the presynaptic component of neuromuscular transmission. Common symptoms in LEMS are weakness, fatigue, and dryness of the mouth. Some patients complain of paresthesias, myalgia, or impotence. Weakness is symmetric, proximal, and most prominent in the lower limbs. Strength can decrease with rest and improve with exercise. Ocular (diplopia and ptosis) and bulbar (dysphagia and dysarthria) symptoms may occur in some patients. Respiratory muscle weakness is rare. Tendon reflexes are either diminished or absent at rest but may increase after exercise. About 50% of patients have an associated neoplasm, most commonly SCLC and less often a lymphoproliferative disorder. About 3% of patients with SCLC have LEMS. Almost all patients with both SCLC and LEMS have a smoking history. LEMS may precede the detection of cancer by 2 to 3 years.

The most useful diagnostic test for LEMS is repetitive nerve stimulation, specifically the finding of compound muscle action potential (CMAP) amplitudes that are small at rest but increase by at least 100% after rapid repetitive nerve stimulation (30 to 50 Hz) or maximal muscle contraction sustained for at least 10 s. LEMS is believed to be an autoimmune disorder associated with diminished quantal release of acetylcholine. IgG antibodies directed against P/Q voltage-gated calcium channels (VGCC) in the motor nerve terminal are found in the sera of ~90% of patients with LEMS and in nearly 100% when LEMS is associated with neoplasm. False-positive findings occur with hypergammaglobulinemia, chronic liver disorders, and (in <3% of normal individuals) infection. Ultrastructurally, the number of active zones, which represent the P/Q VGCC in the presynaptic nerve terminal membrane, is decreased in LEMS. This humoral immune response to P/Q VGCC may be stimulated by similar VGCC expressed by the tumor cells. Edrophonium chloride (Tensilon) generally does not improve strength. Treatment of LEMS is directed at tumor resection, enhancing the release of acetylcholine from the presynaptic terminal, and modulating the autoimmune response. Treatment modalities directed at improving neuromuscular transmission include 3,4-diaminopyridine, guanidine, and pyridostigmine. Immunomodulation may include plasmapheresis, glucocorticoids, azathioprine, and cyclosporine.

Myasthenia gravis (MG) is associated with thymoma in 10 to 15% of patients, especially those who present at ≥30 years. Fatigable weakness may involve the ocular, facial, bulbar, and/or limb muscles. Anti-acetylcholine receptor antibodies are detected in about 85% of cases. Slow repetitive nerve stimulation (5 Hz) of proximal or facial muscles produces a decrement of ≥10% in 70% of patients. Single-fiber electromyography is a sensitive but not specific confirmatory test in difficult cases. →*Myasthenia gravis is discussed in Chap. 380.*

MYOPATHY   Mild proximal muscle weakness with type II muscle fiber atrophy is commonly encountered in patients with cancer, especially when weight loss of >15% is present. Muscle wasting is more prominent than muscle weakness in this syndrome. Inflammatory myopathy, especially dermatomyositis in older females, may occur in association with a variety of neoplasms (Chap. 382).

Necrotizing myopathy presents with a subacute onset of weakness that is typically proximal and ranges from mild to severe. Some patients experience myalgia in addition to muscle weakness. The serum creatine kinase levels are very high. Muscle fiber necrosis is the predominant finding in muscle biopsy. Necrotizing myopathy is most commonly seen with adenocarcinoma and non-small cell cancer of the lung but may also be associated with a variety of other neoplasms. The overall prognosis depends on the malignancy of the associated neoplasm. Weakness may improve following tumor resection or glucocorticoid treatment.

Chronic proximal myopathies have been described with an IgM M-protein binding to decorin; scleromyxedema with IgG or IgA M-proteins; a rippling muscle disease has been reported to occur with thymoma. Hormone-secreting (ACTH or parathyroid hormone–like) tumors may also be associated with proximal myopathies.

BIBLIOGRAPHY

DALMAU J et al: Ma1, a novel neuron- and testis-specific protein, is recognized by the serum of patients with paraneoplastic syndromes. Brain 122:27, 1999

DROPCHO EJ: Neurological paraneoplastic syndromes. J Neurol Sci 153:264, 1998

GIOMETTO B et al: Autoimmunity in paraneoplastic neurological syndromes. Brain Pathol 9:261, 1999

GRISOLD W, DRLICEK M: Paraneoplastic neuropathy. Curr Opin Neurol 12:617, 1999

LEVIN M et al: Paraneoplastic necrotizing myopathy: Clinical and pathological features. Neurology 50:764, 1998

NEWSOM-DAVIS J: Paraneoplastic neurological disorders. J R Coll Physicians Lond 33:225, 1999

PESTRONK A: Chronic immune polyneuropathies and serum autoantibodies, in *Neuroimmunology for the Clinician*, LA Polak, Y Harada (eds). Boston, Butterworth-Heinemann, 1997

———: Paraneoplastic syndromes. Neuromuscular Disease Center at Washington University in Saint Louis. www.neuro.wustl.edu/neuromuscular

REES J: Paraneoplastic syndromes. Curr Opin Neurol 11:633, 1998

SCARAVILLI F et al: The neuropathology of paraneoplastic syndromes. Brain Pathol 9:251, 1999

SMITH PS et al: Paraneoplastic cerebellar ataxia due to autoantibodies against a glutamate receptor. N Engl J Med 342:21, 2000

102   *Rasim Gucalp, Janice Dutcher*

ONCOLOGIC EMERGENCIES

CNS	central nervous system	PTH	parathormone
CSF	cerebrospinal fluid	SVCS	superior vena cava syndrome
CT	computed tomography	SVC	superior vena cava
HUS	hemolytic-uremic syndrome	SIADH	syndrome of inappropriate
MRI	magnetic resonance imaging		secretion of antidiuretic hormone
PTHrP	parathormone-related	TTP	thrombotic thrombocytopenic
	protein		purpura

Emergencies in patients with cancer may be classified into three groups: pressure or obstruction caused by a space-occupying lesion, metabolic or hormonal problems (paraneoplastic syndromes, Chap. 100), and complications arising from the effects of treatment.

STRUCTURAL-OBSTRUCTIVE ONCOLOGIC EMERGENCIES

SUPERIOR VENA CAVA SYNDROME   Superior vena cava syndrome (SVCS) is the clinical manifestation of superior vena cava (SVC) obstruction, with severe reduction in venous return from the head, neck, and upper extremities. Malignant tumors, such as lung cancer, lymphoma, and metastatic tumors, are responsible for more than 90% of all SVCS cases. Lung cancer, particularly of small-cell and squamous-cell histologies, accounts for approximately 85% of all cases of malignant origin. Metastatic cancers to the mediastinum, such as testicular and breast carcinomas, account for a small proportion of cases. Other causes include benign tumors, aortic aneurysm, thyroid enlargement, thrombosis, and fibrosing mediastinitis caused by prior irradiation or histoplasmosis.

Patients with SVCS usually present with neck and facial swelling (especially around the eyes), dyspnea, and cough. Other symptoms include hoarseness, tongue swelling, headaches, nasal congestion, epistaxis, hemoptysis, dysphagia, pain, dizziness, syncope, and lethargy. Bending forward or lying down may aggravate the symptoms. The characteristic physical findings are dilated neck veins, an increased number of collateral veins covering the anterior chest wall, cyanosis, and edema of the face, arms, and chest. More severe cases include proptosis, glossal and laryngeal edema, and obtundation. The clinical picture is milder if the obstruction is located above the azygos vein.

The diagnosis of SVCS is a clinical one. The most significant chest radiographic finding is widening of the superior mediastinum, most commonly on the right side. Pleural effusion occurs in only 25% of patients, often on the right side. However, a normal chest radiograph is still compatible with the diagnosis if other characteristic findings are present. Computed tomography (CT) provides the most reliable view of the mediastinal anatomy. The diagnosis of SVCS requires diminished or absent opacification of central venous structures with prominent collateral venous circulation. Magnetic resonance imaging (MRI) has no advantages over CT. Invasive procedures, including bronchoscopy, percutaneous needle biopsy, mediastinoscopy, and even thoracotomy, can be performed by a skilled clinician without any major risk of bleeding. For patients with a known cancer, a detailed workup usually is not necessary, and appropriate treatment may be started after obtaining a CT scan of the thorax. For those with no history of malignancy, a detailed evaluation is absolutely necessary to rule out benign causes and determine a specific diagnosis to direct the appropriate therapy.

TREATMENT   The one potentially life-threatening complication of a superior mediastinal mass is tracheal obstruction. Upper airway obstruction demands emergent therapy. Diuretics with a low salt diet, head elevation, and oxygen may produce temporary symptomatic relief.

Radiation therapy is the primary treatment for SVCS caused by non-small cell lung cancer and other metastatic solid tumors. Chemotherapy is effective when the underlying cancer is small cell carcinoma of the lung or lymphoma. Recurrent SVCS occurs in 10 to 30% of patients after initial therapy; it may be palliated with the use of intravascular self-expanding stents (Fig. 102-1). Surgery may provide immediate relief for patients in whom a benign process is the cause.

Clinical improvement occurs in most patients, although this improvement may be due to the development of adequate collateral circulation. The mortality associated with SVCS does not relate to caval obstruction, but rather to the underlying cause.

SVCS and Central Venous Catheters in Adults   The use of long-term central venous catheters has become common practice in patients with cancer. Major vessel thrombosis may occur. In these cases, catheter removal should be combined with anticoagulation to

A

B

C

FIGURE 102-1 *A.* Chest radiographs of a 59-year-old man with recurrent SVCS caused by non-small cell lung cancer showing right paratracheal mass with right pleural effusion. *B.* Computed tomography of same patient demonstrating obstruction of SVC with thrombosis (arrow) by the lung cancer (square) and collaterals (arrowheads). *C.* Balloon angioplasty (arrowhead) with walstent (arrow) in same patient.

prevent embolization. SVCS in this setting, if detected early, can be treated successfully by fibrinolytic therapy without sacrificing the catheter. Warfarin (1 mg/d) reduces the incidence of thrombosis without altering coagulation tests.

PERICARDIAL EFFUSION/TAMPONADE Malignant pericardial disease is found at autopsy in 5 to 10% of patients with cancer, most frequently with lung cancer, breast cancer, leukemias, and lymphomas. Cardiac tamponade as the initial presentation of extrathoracic malignancy is rare. The origin is not malignancy in about 50% of cancer patients with symptomatic pericardial disease, but can be related to irradiation, drug-induced pericarditis, hypothyroidism, idiopathic pericarditis, infection, or autoimmune diseases. Two types of radiation pericarditis have been described: an acute inflammatory, effusive pericarditis occurring within months of irradiation, which usually resolves spontaneously, and a chronic effusive pericarditis that may appear up to 20 years after radiotherapy and is accompanied by a thickened pericardium.

Most patients with pericardial metastasis are asymptomatic. However, the common symptoms are dyspnea, cough, chest pain, orthopnea, and weakness. Pleural effusion, sinus tachycardia, jugular venous distension, hepatomegaly, peripheral edema, and cyanosis are the most frequent physical findings. Relatively specific diagnostic findings, such as paradoxical pulse, diminished heart sounds, pulsus alternans (pulse waves alternating between those of greater and lesser amplitude with successive beats), and friction rub are less common than with nonmalignant pericardial disease. Chest radiographs and ECG reveal abnormalities in 90% of patients, but half of these abnormalities are nonspecific. Echocardiography is the most helpful diagnostic test. Pericardial fluid may be serous, serosanguineous, or hemorrhagic, and cytologic examination of pericardial fluid is diagnostic in most patients. False negative cytology may occur in patients with lymphoma and mesothelioma.

℞ TREATMENT Pericardiocentesis with or without the introduction of sclerosing agents, the creation of a pericardial window, complete pericardial stripping, cardiac irradiation, or systemic chemotherapy are effective treatments. Acute pericardial tamponade with life-threatening hemodynamic instability requires immediate drainage of fluid. This can be quickly achieved by pericardiocentesis. Alternatively, subxyphoid pericardiotomy can be performed in 45 min under local anesthesia.

INTESTINAL OBSTRUCTION Intestinal obstruction and reobstruction are common problems in patients with advanced cancer, particularly colorectal or ovarian carcinoma. However, other cancers, such as lung or breast cancer and melanoma, can metastasize within the abdomen, leading to intestinal obstruction. Typically, obstruction occurs at multiple sites. Intestinal pseudoobstruction is caused by infiltration of the mesentery or bowel muscle by tumor, involvement of the celiac plexus, or paraneoplastic neuropathy in patients with small cell lung cancer. Paraneoplastic neuropathy is associated with IgG antibodies reactive to neurons of the myenteric and submucosal plexuses of the jejunum and stomach. Ovarian cancer can lead either to authentic luminal obstruction or to pseudoobstruction that results when circumferential invasion of a bowel segment arrests the forward progression of peristaltic contractions.

The onset of obstruction is usually insidious. Pain is the most common symptom and is usually colicky in nature. Pain can also be due to abdominal distention, tumor masses, or hepatomegaly. Vomiting can be intermittent or continuous. Patients with complete obstruction usually have constipation. Physical examination may reveal abdominal distention with tympany, ascites, visible peristalsis, high-pitched bowel sounds, and tumor masses. Erect plain abdominal films may reveal multiple air-fluid levels and dilation of the small or large bowel. Acute cecal dilation to more than 12 to 14 cm is considered a surgical emergency because of the high likelihood of rupture. The overall prognosis for the patient with cancer who develops intestinal obstruction is poor; median survival is 3 to 4 months. About one-fourth to one-third of patients are found to have intestinal obstruction due to causes other than cancer. Adhesions from previous operations are a common benign cause. Ileus induced by vincristine is another reversible cause.

℞ TREATMENT The management of intestinal obstruction in patients with advanced malignancy depends on the extent of the underlying malignancy and the functional status of the major organs. The initial management should include surgical evaluation. Operation is not always successful and may lead to further complications with a substantial mortality rate (10 to 20%). Self-expanding metal stents placed in the gastric outlet, duodenum, proximal jejunum, colon, or rectum may palliate obstructive symptoms at those sites without major surgery. Patients known to have advanced intraabdominal malignancy should receive a prolonged course of conservative management, including nasogastric decompression. Treatment with antiemetics, antispasmodics, and analgesics may allow patients to remain outside the hospital. The somatostatin analogue octreotide may relieve obstructive symptoms through its inhibitory effect on gastrointestinal secretion.

URINARY OBSTRUCTION Urinary obstruction may occur in patients with prostatic or gynecologic malignancies, particularly cervical carcinoma, or metastatic disease from other primary sites. Radiation therapy to pelvic tumors may cause fibrosis and subsequent ureteral obstruction. Bladder outlet obstruction is usually due to prostate and cervical cancers and may lead to bilateral hydronephrosis and renal failure.

Flank pain is the most common symptom. Persistent urinary tract infection, persistent proteinuria, or hematuria in patients with a cancer should raise suspicion of ureteral obstruction. Total anuria and/or anuria alternating with polyuria may occur. A slow, continuous rise in the serum creatinine level necessitates immediate evaluation in patients with cancer. Renal ultrasound examination is the safest and cheapest way to identify hydronephrosis. The function of an obstructed kidney can be evaluated by a nuclear scan. CT can be helpful in identifying a retroperitoneal mass or retroperitoneal adenopathy.

℞ TREATMENT Obstruction associated with flank pain, sepsis, or fistula formation is an indication for immediate palliative urinary diversion. There are many newer techniques by which internal ureteral stents can be placed under local anesthesia. Percutaneous nephrostomy offers an alternative approach for drainage. In the case of bladder outlet obstruction due to malignancy, a suprapubic cystostomy can be used for urinary drainage.

MALIGNANT BILIARY OBSTRUCTION This common clinical problem can be caused by a primary carcinoma arising in the pancreas, ampulla of Vater, bile duct, or liver or by metastatic disease to the periductal lymph nodes or liver parenchyma. The most common metastatic tumors causing biliary obstruction are gastric, colon, breast, and lung cancers. Jaundice, light-colored stools, dark urine, pruritus, and weight loss due to malabsorption are usual symptoms. Pain and secondary infection are uncommon in malignant biliary obstruction. Ultrasound, CT, or percutaneous transhepatic or endoscopic retrograde cholangiography will identify the site and nature of the biliary obstruction.

℞ TREATMENT Palliative intervention is indicated only in patients with disabling pruritus resistant to medical treatment, severe malabsorption, or infection. Stenting under radiographic control, surgical bypass, or radiation therapy with or without chemotherapy may alleviate the obstruction. The choice of modality should be based on the site of obstruction (proximal versus distal), the type of tumor (sensitive to radiotherapy, chemotherapy, or neither), and the general condition of the patient. In the absence of pruritus, biliary obstruction may be a largely asymptomatic cause of death.

SPINAL CORD COMPRESSION Spinal cord compression occurs in 5 to 10% of patients with cancer. Epidural tumor is the first manifestation of malignancy in about 10% of patients. The underlying cancer is usually identified during the initial evaluation; lung cancer is most commonly the primary malignancy.

Metastatic tumor involves the vertebral column more often than any other part of the bony skeleton. Lung, breast, and prostate cancer are the most frequent offenders. Multiple myeloma also has a high incidence of spine involvement. The thoracic spine is the most common site (70%), followed by the lumbosacral spine (20%) and the cervical spine (10%). Involvement of multiple sites is most frequent in patients with breast and prostatic carcinoma. Cord injury develops when metastases to the vertebral body or pedicle enlarge and compress the underlying dura. Another cause of cord compression is direct extension of a paravertebral lesion through the intervertebral foramen. These cases usually involve a lymphoma, myeloma, or pediatric neoplasm. Parenchymal spinal cord metastasis due to hematogenous spread is rare.

The most common initial symptom in patients with spinal cord compression is localized back pain and tenderness due to involvement of vertebrae by tumor. Pain is usually present for days or months before other neurologic findings appear. It is exacerbated by movement and by coughing or sneezing. It can be differentiated from the pain of disk disease by the fact that it worsens when the patient is supine. Radicular pain is less common than localized back pain and usually develops later. Radicular pain in the cervical or lumbosacral areas may be unilateral or bilateral. Radicular pain from the thoracic roots is often bilateral and is described by patients as a feeling of tight, band-like constriction around the thorax and abdomen. Typical cervical radicular pain radiates down the arm; in the lumbar region, the radiation is down the legs. Loss of bowel or bladder control may be the presenting symptom, but usually occurs late in the course.

On physical examination, pain induced by straight leg raising, neck flexion, or vertebral percussion may help to determine the level of cord compression. Patients develop numbness and paresthesias in the extremities or trunk. Loss of sensibility to pinprick is as common as loss of sensibility to vibration or position. The upper limit of the zone of sensory loss is often one or two vertebrae below the site of compression. Motor findings include weakness, spasticity, and abnormal muscle stretching. The presence of an extensor plantar reflex reflects significant compression. Deep tendon reflexes may be brisk. Motor and sensory loss usually precede sphincter disturbance. Patients with autonomic dysfunction may present with decreased anal tonus, decreased perineal sensibility, and a distended bladder. The absence of the anal wink reflex or the bulbocavernosus reflex confirms cord (conus or cauda equina) involvement. In doubtful cases, evaluation of post-voiding urinary residual volume can be helpful. A residual volume of more than 150 mL suggests bladder dysfunction. Autonomic dysfunction is an unfavorable prognostic factor. Patients with progressive neurologic symptoms should have frequent neurologic examinations and rapid therapeutic intervention.

Patients with cancer who develop back pain should be evaluated for spinal cord compression as quickly as possible (Fig. 102-2). Treatment is more often successful in patients who are ambulatory and still have sphincter control at the time treatment is initiated. Patients should have a neurologic examination and plain films of the spine. Those whose physical examination suggests cord compression should receive dexamethasone (24 mg intravenously every 6 h), starting immediately.

Erosion of the pedicles (the "winking owl" sign) is the earliest radiologic finding of vertebral tumor. Other radiographic changes include increased intrapedicular distance, vertebral destruction, lytic or

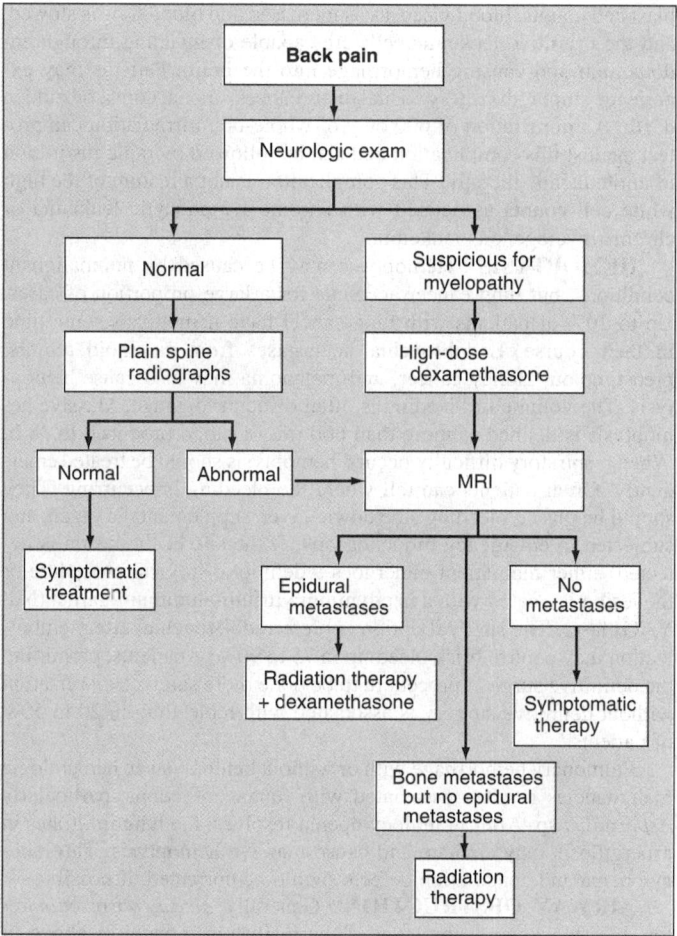

FIGURE 102-2 Management of cancer patients with back pain.

sclerotic lesions, scalloped vertebral bodies, and vertebral body collapse. Vertebral collapse is not a reliable indicator of the presence of tumor; about 20% of cases of vertebral collapse, particularly those in older patients and postmenopausal women, are due not to cancer but to osteoporosis. Also, a normal appearance on plain films of the spine does not exclude the diagnosis of cancer. The role of bone scans in the detection of cord compression is not clear; this method is sensitive but less specific than spinal radiography.

The full-length image of the cord provided by MRI is useful. On T1-weighted images, good contrast is noted between the cord, cerebrospinal fluid, and extradural lesions. Owing to their sensitivity in demonstrating the replacement of bone marrow by tumor, MRI can show which parts of a vertebra are involved by tumor (the body, pedicle, lamina, spinous process). MRI also visualizes intraspinal extradural masses compressing the cord. T2-weighted images are most useful for the demonstration of intramedullary pathology. Gadolinium-enhanced MRI can help to characterize and delineate intramedullary disease. MRI is as good as or better than myelography plus postmyelogram CT in detecting metastatic epidural disease with cord compression. Myelography should be reserved for patients who have poor MR images or who cannot undergo MRI promptly. CT in conjunction with myelography enhances the detection of small areas of spinal destruction.

In patients with spinal cord compression and an unknown primary tumor, a simple workup including chest radiography, mammography, measurement of prostate-specific antigen, and abdominal CT usually reveals the underlying malignancy.

TREATMENT The treatment of patients with spinal cord compression is aimed at relief of pain and restoration of neurologic function (Fig. 102-2).

Radiation therapy plus glucocorticoids is generally the initial treatment of choice for spinal cord compression. Up to 75% of patients treated when still ambulatory remain ambulatory, but only 10% of patients with paraplegia recover walking capacity. Indications for surgical intervention include unknown etiology, failure of radiation therapy, a radioresistant tumor type (e.g., melanoma or renal cell cancer), pathologic fracture dislocation, and rapidly evolving neurologic symptoms. Until recently, laminectomy was the standard operation for metastatic spinal cord compression, although results were poor. At present, laminectomy should be used only for tissue diagnosis and for the removal of posteriorly localized epidural deposits in the absence of vertebral disease. Because most cases of epidural spinal cord compression are due to anterior or anterolateral extradural disease, resection of the anterior vertebral body along with the tumor, followed by spinal stabilization, has achieved good results and low mortality rate. Chemotherapy may have a role in patients with chemosensitive tumors who have had prior radiation therapy to the same region and who are not candidates for surgery.

The histology of the tumor is an important determinant of both recovery and survival. Rapid onset and quick progression are poor prognostic features.

INCREASED INTRACRANIAL PRESSURE About 25% of patients with cancer die with intracranial metastases. The cancers that most often metastasize to the brain are lung and breast cancers and melanoma. Brain metastases often occur in the presence of systemic disease, and they frequently cause major symptoms, disability, and early death.

The signs and symptoms of a metastatic brain tumor are similar to those of other intracranial expanding lesions: headache, nausea, vomiting, behavioral changes, seizures, and focal, progressive neurologic changes. Occasionally the onset is abrupt, resembling a stroke, with the sudden appearance of headache, nausea, vomiting, and neurologic deficits. This picture is usually due to hemorrhage into the metastasis. Melanoma, germ cell tumors, and renal cell cancers have a particularly high incidence of intracranial bleeding. The tumor mass and surrounding edema may cause obstruction of the circulation of cerebrospinal fluid, with resulting hydrocephalus. Patients with increased intracranial pressure may have papilledema with visual disturbances and neck stiffness. As the mass enlarges, brain tissue may be displaced through the fixed cranial openings, producing various herniation syndromes.

CT and MRI are equally effective in the diagnosis of brain metastases. CT with contrast should be used as a screening procedure. The CT scan shows brain metastases as multiple enhancing lesions of various sizes with surrounding areas of low-density edema. If a single lesion or no metastases are visualized by contrast-enhanced CT, MRI of the brain should be performed. Gadolinium-enhanced MRI is more sensitive than CT at revealing small lesions, particularly in the brainstem or cerebellum.

TREATMENT If signs and symptoms of brain herniation (particularly headache, drowsiness, and papilledema) are present, the patient should be intubated and hyperventilated to maintain P_{CO_2} between 25 and 30 mmHg and should receive infusions of mannitol (1 to 1.5 g/kg) every 6 h. Dexamethasone is the best initial treatment for all symptomatic patients with brain metastases (see above). Patients with multiple lesions should receive whole-brain radiation therapy. Patients with a single brain metastasis and with controlled extracranial disease may be treated with surgical excision followed by whole-brain radiation therapy, especially if they are younger than 60 years. Radioresistant tumors should be resected if possible. Stereotactic radiosurgery is an effective treatment for inaccessible or recurrent lesions. With a gamma knife or linear accelerator, multiple small, well-colimated beams of ionizing radiation destroy lesions seen on MRI. Some patients with increased intracranial pressure associated with hydrocephalus may benefit from shunt placement.

NEOPLASTIC MENINGITIS   Tumor involving the leptomeninges is a complication of both primary tumors of the central nervous system (CNS) and tumors that metastasize to the CNS. The incidence is estimated at 3 to 8% of patients with cancer. Melanoma, breast and lung cancer, lymphoma (including AIDS-associated), and acute leukemia are the most common causes.

Patients typically present with multifocal neurologic signs and symptoms including headache, gait abnormality, mental changes, nausea, vomiting, seizures, back or radicular pain, and limb weakness. Signs include cranial nerve palsies, extremity weakness, paresthesia, and decreased deep tendon reflexes.

Diagnosis is made by demonstrating malignant cells in the cerebrospinal fluid (CSF); however, up to 40% of patients may have false negative CSF cytology. An elevated CSF protein level is nearly always present (except in HLTV-1-associated adult T cell leukemia). Patients with neurologic signs and symptoms consistent with neoplastic meningitis who have a negative CSF cytology but an elevated CSF protein level should have the spinal tap repeated at least three times for repeated cytologic examination before the diagnosis is rejected. MRI may show hydrocephalus or smooth or nodular enhancement of the meninges.

The development of neoplastic meningitis usually occurs in the setting of uncontrolled cancer outside the CNS; thus, prognosis is poor (median survival 10 to 12 weeks). However, treatment of the neoplastic meningitis may successfully alleviate symptoms and control the CNS spread.

℞ **TREATMENT**   Intrathecal chemotherapy, usually methotrexate, cytarabine, or thiotepa, is delivered by lumbar puncture or by an intraventricular reservoir (Ommaya) three times a week until the CSF is free of malignant cells. Then injections are given twice a week for a month and then weekly for a month. An extended release preparation of cytarabine (Depocyte) has a longer half-life and is more effective than regular formulations. Among solid tumors, breast cancer responds best to therapy. Patients with neoplastic meningitis from either acute leukemia or lymphoma may be cured of their CNS disease if the systemic disease can be eliminated.

SEIZURES   Seizures occurring in a patient with cancer can be caused by the tumor itself, by metabolic disturbances, by radiation injury, by cerebral infarctions, by chemotherapy-related encephalopathies, or by CNS infections. Metastatic disease to the CNS is the most common cause of seizures in patients with cancer. Seizures are a presenting symptom of CNS metastasis in 6 to 29% of cases. Approximately 10% of patients with CNS metastasis eventually develop seizures. The presence of frontal lesions correlates with early seizures, and the presence of hemispheric symptoms increases the risk for late seizures. Both early and late seizures are uncommon in patients with posterior fossa lesions. Seizures are also common in patients with CNS metastases from melanoma. Very rarely, cytotoxic drugs such as etoposide, busulfan, and chlorambucil cause seizures.

℞ **TREATMENT**   Patients in whom seizures due to CNS metastases have been demonstrated should receive anticonvulsive treatment with diphenylhydantoin. Prophylactic anticonvulsant therapy is not recommended unless the patient is at a high risk for late seizures. In those patients, serum diphenylhydantoin levels should be monitored closely and the dosage adjusted accordingly.

INTRACEREBRAL LEUKOCYTOSTASIS   Intracerebral leukocytostasis (Ball's disease) is a potentially fatal complication of acute leukemia (particularly myelogenous leukemia) that can occur when the peripheral blast cell count is greater than $100,000/\mu L$. At such high blast cell counts, blood viscosity is increased and blood flow is slowed, and the primitive leukemic cells are capable of invading through endothelium and causing hemorrhage into the brain. Patients may experience stupor, dizziness, visual disturbances, ataxia, coma, or sudden death. Administration of 600 cGy of whole-brain irradiation can protect against this complication and can be followed by rapid institution of antileukemic therapy. This complication is not a feature of the high white cell counts associated with chronic lymphocytic leukemia or chronic myelogenous leukemia.

HEMOPTYSIS   Hemoptysis may be caused by nonmalignant conditions, but lung cancer accounts for a large proportion of cases. Up to 20% of patients with lung cancer have hemoptysis some time in their course. Endobronchial metastases from carcinoid tumors, breast, colon, kidney cancer, and melanoma may also cause hemoptysis. The volume of bleeding is often difficult to gauge. Massive hemoptysis is defined as more than 600 mL of blood produced in 48 h. When respiratory difficulty occurs, hemoptysis should be treated emergently. Often patients can tell where the bleeding is occurring. They should be placed bleeding side down, given supplemental oxygen, and subjected to emergency bronchoscopy. If the site of the lesion is detected, either the patient undergoes a definitive surgical procedure or the lesion is treated with a neodymium:yttrium-aluminum-garnet (Nd: YAG) laser. The surgical option is preferred. Bronchial artery embolization may control brisk bleeding in 75 to 90% of patients, permitting the definitive surgical procedure to be done more safely. Embolization without definitive surgery is associated with rebleeding in 20 to 50% of patients.

Pulmonary hemorrhage with or without hemoptysis in hematologic malignancies is often associated with fungal infections, particularly *Aspergillus* sp. After granulocytopenia resolves, the lung infiltrates in aspergillosis may cavitate and cause massive hemoptysis. Thrombocytopenia and coagulation defects should be corrected, if possible.

AIRWAY OBSTRUCTION   Generally, *airway obstruction* refers to a blockage at the level of the mainstem bronchi or above. It may result either from intraluminal tumor growth or from extrinsic compression of the airway. If the obstruction is proximal to the larynx, a tracheostomy may be life-saving. For more distal obstructions, particularly intrinsic lesions incompletely obstucting the airway, bronchoscopy with laser treatment, photodynamic therapy, or stenting can produce immediate relief in most patients. However, radiation therapy (either external-beam irradiation or brachytherapy) given together with glucocorticoids may also open the airway. Symptomatic extrinsic compression may be palliated by stenting.

METABOLIC EMERGENCIES

HYPERCALCEMIA   Hypercalcemia is the most common paraneoplastic syndrome (Chaps. 100 and 341), occurring in about 10% of patients with advanced cancer. It is associated most often with cancers of the lung, breast, head and neck, and kidney and with multiple myeloma and some B and T cell lymphomas.

Increased release of calcium from bone is the main factor leading to hypercalcemia. Bone resorption is increased dramatically through stimulation of the proliferation and activity of osteoclasts, and bone formation is not stimulated in parallel. The kidney may play an important role through an increase in the reabsorption of calcium in the distal tubule. Parathormone-related protein (PTHrP) produced by tumors has a central role as a mediator of hypercalcemia in cancer. PTHrP shares 80% homology with the first 13 amino acids of parathormone (PTH), which are in the region responsible for binding to the PTH receptor. PTHrP acts via the PTH hormone receptors on osteoblasts and renal tubular cells to stimulate bone resorption and renal calcium conservation, leading to hypercalcemia. Elevated plasma PTHrP levels are also found in most hypercalcemic patients with bone metastases, whose hypercalcemia has traditionally been explained by local osteolysis due to the production of osteolytic factors by tumors. Transforming growth factors, cytokines (interleukins 1 and 6), and other unknown factors could play a contributory role. True "ectopic"

PTH production by malignant tumors is rare. In lymphoma, a vitamin D–related product of the tumor may also increase calcium absorption in the gut.

The clinical features of hypercalcemia in patients with cancer are nonspecific and include fatigue, anorexia, constipation, polydipsia, muscle weakness, nausea, and vomiting. They may easily be attributed to the malignancy itself or to its treatment. Laboratory assessment should include measurement of serum electrolytes, calcium, phosphate, and albumin. Hypoalbuminemia is common in malignancy and affects the total serum concentration of calcium. If the ionized calcium level cannot be obtained, then the corrected serum calcium concentration should be calculated with the following formula:

Corrected serum calcium = measured serum calcium
+ 0.8 (4.0 − measured serum albumin)

Most patients with hypercalcemia of malignancy have obvious evidence of malignancy, and their serum PTH levels are suppressed. Measurements of PTHrP and serum 1,25-dihydroxyvitamin D are not indicated. Routine serum chemistry evaluations are not able to distinguish between malignant and nonmalignant causes of hypercalcemia.

℞ TREATMENT Not all patients with moderate to severe hypercalcemia (corrected calcium ≥12 mg/dL) should be treated. The decision to treat will depend on the patient's quality of life, the current symptoms, and the prospect for further cancer treatment. Treatment directed at hypercalcemia only extends life in patients for whom effective cancer treatment is available. Nonetheless, therapy may be indicated to reduce symptoms and improve the quality of life. Treatment of symptomatic hypercalcemia begins with intravenous saline to restore the depleted intravascular volume, which may be 4 to 8 L below normal at presentation. Rehydration usually has little effect on calcium levels, producing a median decrease of only 1 mg/dL. Antiresorptive agents are essential to decrease osteoclastic activity and control hypercalcemia. Bisphosphonates, which are potent inhibitors of bone resorption, are easy to administer, virtually free of side effects, and rapidly effective in lowering the serum calcium level. Pamidronate is the most effective of the commercially available bisphosphonates. The recommended dose of pamidronate is 60 mg for moderate hypercalcemia (corrected calcium 12 to 13.5 mg/dL) and 90 mg for severe hypercalcemia (corrected calcium >13.5 mg/dL). The dose is given as a single infusion over 4 or 24 h.

SYNDROME OF INAPPROPRIATE SECRETION OF ANTIDIURETIC HORMONE (SIADH) SIADH is attributed to production of arginine vasopressin by the tumor cells and is characterized by hyponatremia, urine osmolarity inappropriately higher than plasma osmolarity, and high urinary sodium excretion in the absence of volume depletion. Renal, adrenal, and thyroid insufficiency must be excluded, because these disorders can also present with hyponatremia and impaired urinary dilution. Low serum levels of urea and uric acid are useful in distinguishing SIADH from conditions associated with renal hypoperfusion (Chaps. 100 and 329).

A broad spectrum of malignant tumors have been reported to cause SIADH. Ectopic vasopressin secretion may occur in some 38% of small cell carcinomas of the lung; often adrenocorticotropic hormone is also produced. The presence of hyponatremia in patients with small cell lung cancer confers a poor prognosis. SIADH may also be caused by various other conditions, such as CNS and pulmonary disorders and some surgical procedures. A variety of drugs have also been shown to produce SIADH, including antidepressants, angiotensin converting-enzyme inhibitors, and cytotoxic drugs such as vincristine, vinorelbine, ifosfamide, cyclophosphamide, cisplatin, levamisole, and melphalan.

Most patients with SIADH are asymptomatic. The severity of symptoms and signs is related to the degree of hyponatremia and the rapidity with which it develops. Early changes include anorexia, depression, lethargy, irritability, confusion, muscle weakness, and

marked personality changes. When the plasma sodium level falls below 110 mEq/L, extensor plantar responses, areflexia, and pseudobulbar palsy may be noted; and further reductions may cause coma, convulsions, and death.

℞ TREATMENT The optimal therapy for SIADH is to treat the underlying malignancy. If that is not possible, other therapeutic approaches are available, such as water restriction or the administration of demeclocycline (900 to 1200 mg per os bid), urea, or lithium carbonate (300 mg per os tid). Demeclocycline is usually used first. Demeclocycline and lithium inhibit the effects of vasopressin on the distal renal tubule. Patients with seizure or coma from hyponatremia may require normal saline infusion plus furosemide to enhance free water clearance. The rate of sodium correction should be slow [0.5 to 1 (mEq/L)/h] to prevent rapid fluid shifts and central pontine myelinolysis. The serum calcium level should be monitored closely to avoid hypocalcemia.

LACTIC ACIDOSIS Lactic acidosis is a rare and potentially fatal metabolic complication of cancer. Lactic acidosis associated with sepsis and circulatory failure is a common preterminal event in many malignancies. Lactic acidosis in the absence of hypoxemia may occur in patients with leukemia, lymphoma, or solid tumors. Extensive involvement of the liver by tumor is present in most cases. Alteration of liver function may be responsible for the lactate accumulation. Tachypnea, tachycardia, change of mental status, and hepatomegaly may be seen. The serum level of lactic acid may reach 10 to 20 meq/L (90 to 180 mg/dL). Treatment is aimed at the underlying disease. The danger from lactic acidosis is from the acidosis, not the lactate. Sodium bicarbonate should be added if acidosis is very severe or if hydrogen ion production is very rapid and uncontrolled. The prognosis is poor.

HYPOGLYCEMIA Persistent hypoglycemia occasionally is associated with tumors other than pancreatic islet cell tumors. Usually these tumors are large, and often they are of mesenchymal origin or are hepatomas or adrenocortical tumors. Mesenchymal tumors are usually located in the retroperitoneum or thorax. In these patients, obtundation, confusion, and behavioral aberrations occur in the postabsorptive period and may precede the diagnosis of the tumor. Hypoglycemia is due to tumor overproduction of insulin-like growth factor, a peptide hormone with structural homology to proinsulin but having only about 1% of its biologic effects. Additionally, the development of hepatic dysfunction from liver metastases and increased glucose consumption by the tumor can contribute to hypoglycemia. If the tumor cannot be resected, treatment of the hypoglycemia has generally been relief of symptoms, with the administration of glucose, glucocorticoids, or glucagon.

Hypoglycemia can be artifactual; hyperleukocytosis from leukemia, myeloproliferative diseases, leukemoid reactions, or colony stimulating factor treatment can increase glucose consumption in the test tube after blood is drawn, leading to pseudohypoglycemia.

ADRENAL INSUFFICIENCY In patients with cancer, adrenal insufficiency may go unrecognized because the symptoms, such as nausea, vomiting, anorexia, and orthostatic hypotension, are nonspecific and may be mistakenly attributed to progressive cancer or to cancer therapy. Primary adrenal insufficiency may develop owing to replacement of both glands by metastases (lung, breast, colon, or kidney cancer, lymphoma), to removal of both glands, or to hemorrhagic necrosis in association with sepsis or anticoagulation. Impaired adrenal steroid synthesis occurs in patients being treated for cancer with mitotane, ketoconazole, aminoglutethimide, or the investigational agent suramin or in those undergoing rapid reduction in glucocorticoid therapy. Rarely, metastatic replacement causes primary adrenal insufficiency as the first manifestation of an occult malignancy. Metastasis to the pituitary or hypothalamus is found at autopsy in up to 5% of patients with cancer, but associated secondary adrenal insufficiency is rare. Patients abruptly discontinuing megestrol acetate therapy (for cancer cachexia) may develop Addisonian crisis from central suppression of the pituitary-adrenal axis with decreased serum levels of cortisol and adrenocorticotropic hormone.

Acute adrenal insufficiency is potentially lethal. Treatment of suspected adrenal crisis is initiated after the sampling of serum cortisol and ACTH levels (Chap. 331).

TREATMENT-RELATED EMERGENCIES

TUMOR LYSIS SYNDROME Tumor lysis syndrome is a well-recognized clinical entity that is characterized by various combinations of hyperuricemia, hyperkalemia, hyperphosphatemia, lactic acidosis, and hypocalcemia and is caused by the destruction of a large number of rapidly proliferating neoplastic cells. Frequently, acute renal failure develops as a result of the syndrome.

Tumor lysis syndrome is most frequently associated with the treatment of Burkitt's lymphoma, acute lymphoblastic leukemia, and other high-grade lymphomas, but it also may be seen with chronic leukemias and, rarely, with solid tumors. This syndrome has been seen in patients with chronic lymphocytic leukemia after treatment with fludarabine and cladribine. Tumor lysis syndrome usually occurs during or shortly (1 to 5 days) after chemotherapy. Rarely, spontaneous necrosis of malignancies causes tumor lysis syndrome.

Hyperuricemia may be present at the time of chemotherapy. Effective treatment accelerates the destruction of malignant cells and leads to increased serum uric acid levels from the turnover of nucleic acids. Owing to the acidic local environment, uric acid can precipitate in the tubules, medulla, and collecting ducts of the kidney, leading to renal failure. Lactic acidosis and dehydration may contribute to the precipitation of uric acid in the renal tubules. The finding of uric acid crystals in the urine is strong evidence for uric acid nephropathy. The ratio of urinary uric acid to urinary creatinine is >1 in patients with acute hyperuricemic nephropathy and <1 in patients with renal failure due to other causes.

Hyperphosphatemia, which can be caused by the release of intracellular phosphate pools by tumor cell lysis, produces a reciprocal depression in serum calcium, which causes severe neuromuscular irritability and tetany. Deposition of calcium phosphate in the kidney and hyperphosphatemia may cause renal failure. Potassium is the principal intracellular cation, and massive destruction of malignant cells may lead to hyperkalemia. Hyperkalemia in patients with renal failure may rapidly become life-threatening. Hyperkalemia can cause ventricular arrhythmias and sudden death.

The likelihood that the tumor lysis syndrome will occur in patients with Burkitt's lymphoma is related to the tumor burden and renal function. Hyperuricemia and high serum levels of lactate dehydrogenase LDH (>1500 U/L), both of which correlate with total tumor burden, also correlate with the risk of tumor lysis syndrome. In patients at risk for tumor lysis, pretreatment evaluations should include a complete blood count, serum chemistry evaluation, and urine analysis. High leukocyte and platelet counts may artificially elevate potassium levels ("pseudohyperkalemia") due to lysis of these cells after the blood is drawn. In these cases, plasma potassium instead of serum potassium should be followed. In pseudohyperkalemia, no electrocardiographic abnormalities are present. In patients with abnormal baseline renal function, the kidneys and retroperitoneal area should be evaluated by sonography and/or CT. Urine output should be watched closely.

Recognition of risk and prevention are the most important steps in the management of this syndrome (Fig. 102-3). Despite aggressive prophylaxis, tumor lysis syndrome and/or oliguric or anuric renal failure may occur. Dialysis is often necessary and should be considered early in the course. Hemodialysis is preferred. The prognosis is excellent, and renal function recovers after the uric acid level is lowered to <10 to 20 mg/dL.

FIGURE 102-3 Management of patients at high risk for the tumor lysis syndrome.

HUMAN ANTIBODY INFUSION REACTIONS The initial infusion of human or humanized antibodies (e.g., rituximab) is associated with fever, chills, nausea, asthenia, and headache in up to half of treated patients. Bronchospasm and hypotension occur in 1% of patients. The pathogenesis is thought to be activation of immune effector processes (cells and complement). In the presence of high levels of circulating tumor cells, thrombocytopenia, a rapid fall in circulating tumor cells, and mild tumor lysis syndrome may also occur. Diphenhydramine and acetaminophen can often prevent or suppress the symptoms. If they occur, the infusion should be stopped and restarted at half the initial infusion rate after the symptoms have abated.

HEMOLYTIC-UREMIC SYNDROME Hemolytic-uremic syndrome (HUS) and, less commonly, thrombotic thrombocytopenic purpura (TTP) occurring after treatment with antineoplastic drugs have been described. Mitomycin is by far the most common agent causing this peculiar syndrome. Other chemotherapeutic agents, including cisplatin, bleomycin, and gemcitabine, have also been reported to be associated with this syndrome. It occurs most often in patients with gastric, colorectal, and breast carcinoma. In one series, 35% of patients were without evident cancer at the time this syndrome appeared. Secondary HUS/TTP has also been reported as a rare but sometimes fatal complication of bone marrow transplantation.

HUS usually has its onset 4 to 8 weeks after the last dose of chemotherapy, but it is not rare to detect it several months later. HUS is characterized by microangiopathic hemolytic anemia, thrombocytopenia, and renal failure. Dyspnea, weakness, fatigue, oliguria, and purpura are also common initial symptoms and findings. Systemic hypertension and pulmonary edema frequently occur. Severe hypertension, pulmonary edema, and rapid worsening of hemolysis and renal function may occur after a blood transfusion. Cardiac findings include atrial arrhythmias, pericardial friction rub, and pericardial effusion. Raynaud's phenomenon is part of the syndrome in patients treated with bleomycin.

Laboratory findings include severe to moderate anemia associated with red blood cell fragmentation and numerous schistocytes on peripheral smear. Reticulocytosis, decreased plasma haptoglobin, and an elevated lactic dehydrogenase (LDH) level document hemolysis. The serum bilirubin level is usually normal or slightly elevated. The Coombs test is negative. The white cell count is usually normal, and thrombocytopenia ($<100,000/\mu L$) is almost always present. Most patients have a normal coagulation profile, although some have mild elevations in thrombin time and in level of fibrin degradation products. The serum creatinine level is elevated at presentation and shows a pattern of subacute worsening within weeks of the initial azotemia. The urinalysis reveals hematuria, proteinuria, and granular or hyaline casts; and circulating immune complexes may be present.

The basic pathologic lesion appears to be deposition of fibrin in the walls of capillaries and arterioles, and these deposits are similar to those seen in HUS due to other causes. These microvascular abnormalities involve mainly the kidneys and rarely occur in other organs. The pathogenesis of chemotherapy-related HUS is unknown. Immune complexes have been proposed but not confirmed to be etiologic.

The case fatality rate is high; most patients die within a few months. Plasmapheresis and plasma exchange may normalize the hematologic abnormalities, but renal failure is not reversed in most patients. Immunoperfusion over a staphylococcal protein A column is the most successful treatment. About half of the patients treated with immunoperfusion respond with resolution of thrombocytopenia, improvement in anemia, and stabilization of renal failure. Treatment is well tolerated. It is not clear how the treatment works.

NEUTROPENIA AND INFECTION These remain the most common serious complications of cancer therapy. →*They are covered in detail in Chap. 85.*

PULMONARY INFILTRATES Patients with cancer may present with dyspnea associated with diffuse interstitial infiltrates on chest radiographs. Such infiltrates may be due to progression of the underlying malignancy, treatment-related toxicities, infection, and/or unrelated diseases. The cause may be multifactorial; however, most commonly they occur as a consequence of treatment. Infiltration of the lung by malignancy has been described in patients with leukemia, lymphoma, and breast and other solid cancers. Pulmonary lymphatics may be involved diffusely by neoplasm (pulmonary lymphangitic carcinomatosis), resulting in a diffuse increase in interstitial markings on chest radiographs. The patient is often mildly dyspneic at the onset, but pulmonary failure develops over a period of weeks. In some patients, dyspnea precedes changes on the chest radiographs and is accompanied by a nonproductive cough. This syndrome is characteristic of solid tumors. In patients with leukemia, diffuse microscopic neoplastic peribronchial and peribronchiolar infiltration is frequent but may be asymptomatic. However, some patients present with diffuse interstitial infiltrates, an alveolar capillary block syndrome, and respiratory distress. In these situations, glucocorticoids can provide symptomatic relief, but specific chemotherapy should always be started promptly.

In addition, accumulation of leukemic blasts in the pulmonary capillary system may cause pulmonary distress and failure in patients with acute myelogenous leukemia. This complication is strongly related to high peripheral blast counts ($>100,000/\mu L$) and a short tumor cell doubling time. Some patients with pulmonary leukostasis may have nodular and/or floccular, diffuse infiltrates on chest radiographs. In addition to dyspnea, patients may develop dizziness, confusion, tinnitus, ataxia, visual blurring, and retinal abnormalities due to leukostasis in cerebral vessels. Leukapheresis and/or chemotherapy should be started without delay. Pulmonary irradiation may reduce symptoms.

Several cytotoxic agents, such as bleomycin, methotrexate, busul-

fan, and the nitrosoureas, may cause pulmonary damage. The most frequent presentations are interstitial pneumonitis, alveolitis, and pulmonary fibrosis. Some cytotoxic agents, including methotrexate and procarbazine, may cause an acute hypersensitivity reaction. Cytosine arabinoside has been associated with noncardiogenic pulmonary edema. Administration of multiple cytotoxic drugs, as well as radiation therapy and preexisting lung disease, may potentiate the pulmonary toxicity. Supplemental oxygen may potentiate the effects of drugs and radiation injury. Patients should always be managed with the lowest FI_{O_2} that is sufficient to maintain hemoglobin saturation.

The onset of symptoms may be insidious, with symptoms including dyspnea, nonproductive cough, and tachycardia. Patients may have bibasilar crepitant rales, end-inspiratory crackles, fever, and cyanosis. The chest radiograph generally shows an interstitial and sometimes an intraalveolar pattern that is strongest at the lung bases and may be symmetric. A small effusion may occur. Hypoxemia with decreased carbon monoxide diffusing capacity is always present. Glucocorticoids may be helpful in patients in whom pulmonary toxicity is related to radiation therapy or to chemotherapy. Treatment is otherwise supportive.

Radiation pneumonitis and/or fibrosis is a relatively frequent side effect of thoracic radiation therapy when the dosage exceeds 40 Gy; it may be acute or chronic. It has its onset usually from 2 to 6 months after completion of radiation therapy. The clinical syndrome, which varies in severity, consists of dyspnea, cough with scanty sputum, low-grade fever, and an initial hazy infiltrate on chest radiographs. The infiltrate and tissue damage generally are confined to the radiation field. The patients subsequently may develop a patchy alveolar infiltrate and air bronchograms, which may progress to acute respiratory failure that is sometimes fatal. A lung biopsy may be necessary to make the diagnosis. Asymptomatic infiltrates found incidentally after radiation therapy need not be treated. However, prednisone should be administered to patients with fever or other symptoms. The dosage should be tapered slowly after the resolution of radiation pneumonitis, as abrupt withdrawal of glucocorticoids may cause an exacerbation of pneumonia. Delayed radiation fibrosis may occur years after radiation therapy and is signaled by dyspnea on exertion. Often it is mild, but it can progress to chronic respiratory failure. Therapy is supportive.

Classical radiation pneumonitis that leads to pulmonary fibrosis is due to radiation-induced production of local cytokines such as platelet-derived growth factor β, tumor necrosis factor, and transforming growth factor β in the radiation field. An immunologically mediated sporadic radiation pneumonitis occurs in about 10% of patients; bilateral alveolitis mediated by T cells results in infiltrates outside the radiation field. This form of radiation pneumonitis usually resolves without sequelae.

Pneumonia is a common problem in patients undergoing treatment for cancer. Bacterial pneumonia typically causes a localized infiltrate on chest radiographs. Therapy is tailored to the causative organism. When diffuse interstitial infiltrates appear in a febrile patient, the differential diagnosis is extensive and includes pneumonia due to infection with *Pneumocystis carinii*, cytomegalovirus, or intracellular pathogens such as mycoplasma and *Legionella*; effects of drugs or radiation; tumor progression; nonspecific pneumonitis; and fungal disease. Patients with cancer who are neutropenic and have fever and local infiltrates on chest radiograph should be treated with a third generation cephalosporin perhaps together with an aminoglycoside or imipenem. A new or persistent focal infiltrate not responding to broad spectrum antibiotics argues for initiation of empiric antifungal therapy. When diffuse bilateral infiltrates develop in patients with febrile neutropenia, broad spectrum antibiotics plus trimethoprim-sulfamethoxazole with or without erythromycin should be initiated. The empiric administration of trimethoprim-sulfamethoxazole plus erythromycin to patients without neutropenia and these antibiotics plus ceftazidime to patients with neutropenia covers nearly every treatable diagnosis (except tumor progression) and gives as good overall survival as a strategy based on early invasive intervention with bronchoalveolar lavage or open lung biopsy. If the patient does not improve in 4 days, open lung biopsy is the procedure of choice. Bronchoscopy with bronchoalveolar lavage may be used in patients who are poor candidates for surgery.

In patients with pulmonary infiltrates who are afebrile, heart failure and multiple pulmonary emboli form part of the differential diagnosis.

TYPHLITIS Neutropenic enterocolitis (typhlitis) is a necrosis of the cecum and adjacent colon that may complicate the treatment of acute leukemia. The patient develops right lower quadrant abdominal pain, often with rebound tenderness and a tense, distended abdomen, in a setting of fever and neutropenia. Watery diarrhea (often containing sloughed mucosa) and bacteremia are common, and bleeding may occur. Plain abdominal films are generally of little value in the diagnosis; CT scan may show marked bowel wall thickening, particularly in the cecum, with bowel wall edema. Rapid institution of broad-spectrum antibiotic coverage and nasogastric suction may reverse the disease. Surgical intervention should be considered if there is no improvement by 24 h after the start of antibiotic treatment. If the localized abdominal findings become diffuse, the prognosis is poor.

HEMORRHAGIC CYSTITIS Hemorrhagic cystitis can develop in patients receiving cyclophosphamide or ifosfamide. Both drugs are metabolized to acrolein, which is a strong chemical irritant that is excreted in the urine. Prolonged contact or high concentrations may lead to bladder irritation and hemorrhage. Symptoms include gross hematuria, frequency, dysuria, burning, urgency, incontinence, and nocturia. The best management is prevention. Maintaining a high rate of urine flow minimizes exposure. In addition, 2-mercaptoethanesulfonate (mesna) detoxifies the metabolites and can be coadministered with the instigating drugs. Mesna usually is given three times on the day of ifosfamide administration in doses that are each 20% of the total ifosfamide dose. If hemorrhagic cystitis develops, the maintenance of a high urine flow may be sufficient supportive care. If conservative management is not effective, irrigation of the bladder with an 0.37 to 0.74% formalin solution for 10 min stops the bleeding in most cases. *N*-acetylcysteine may also be an effective irrigant. Prostaglandins (carboprost tromethamine) can inhibit the progress. In extreme cases, ligation of the hypogastric arteries, urinary diversion, or cystectomy may be necessary.

In summary, the diagnosis of cancer and its treatment carry risk of a multitude of medical problems. Knowledge of both the disease process and the potential hazards of the treatment is required to anticipate and treat these emergent complications.

BIBLIOGRAPHY

ALBANELL J, BASELGA J: Systemic therapy emergencies. Semin Oncol 27:347, 2000

ALLEN KB et al: Pericardial effusion: subxiphoid pericardiostomy versus percutaneous catheter drainage. Ann Thorac Surg 67:437, 1999

BOOGERD W et al: Diagnosis and treatment of spinal cord compression in malignant disease. Cancer Treat Rev 19:129, 1993

BOYD TS et al: Radiosurgery for brain metastases. Neurosurg Clin North Am 10:337, 1999

COLLIN BA et al: Pneumonia in the compromised host including cancer patients and transplant patients. Infect Dis Clin North Am 12:781, 1998

DIAZ PL et al: Palliative treatment of malignant colorectal strictures with metallic stents. Cardiovasc Intervent Radiol 22:29, 1999

JONES DP et al: Tumor lysis syndrome: Pathogenesis and management. Pediatr Nephrol 9:206, 1995

LABLAW A et al: Emergency treatment of malignant extradural spinal cord compression. J Clin Oncol 16:1613, 1998

SEBER A et al: Risk factors for severe hemorrhagic cystitis following BMT. Bone Marrow Transplant 23:35, 1999

SNYDER HW et al: Treatment of cancer chemotherapy–associated thrombotic thrombocytopenic/hemolytic uremic syndrome by protein A immunoadsorption of plasma. Cancer 71:1882, 1993

103 *Michael C. Perry, Dan L. Longo*

LATE CONSEQUENCES OF CANCER AND ITS TREATMENT

The 5-year survival rate of all patients diagnosed with cancer is now 59%. This year alone, nearly 700,000 survivors will be added to the 7 million already considered cured. Virtually all of these survivors will bear some mark of their diagnosis and its therapy, and many will experience long-term complications, including medical problems, psychosocial disturbances, sexual dysfunction, and inability to find employment or insurance.

Problems may be related to the cancer itself (for example, patients with primary cancers of the head and neck are at increased risk for subsequent lung cancer) or to the normal aging process (surviving one cancer does not necessarily alter the risk of other common tumors that increase in frequency with age). However, many of the problems affecting cured patients are related to the treatments. Large numbers of individuals carefully followed for periods up to 30 years have taught us the spectrum of problems that can be encountered. Because of heterogeneity in treatment details and in completeness of follow-up, some treatment-related problems went undetected for many years. However, studies of long-term survivors of childhood cancers, acute leukemia, Hodgkin's disease, lymphomas, testicular cancer, and localized solid tumors have identified the features of cancer treatment that are associated with later morbidity and mortality. We have been somewhat slow to act in changing those aspects of primary treatment that contribute to these late problems. This reticence is due to the uncertainty associated with changing a treatment that is known to work before having a replacement that works as well.

The first task is always to eradicate the diagnosed malignancy. Late problems occurring in cured patients reflect the success of treatment. Such problems never develop in those who do not survive the cancer. Morbidity and mortality from iatrogenic disease should be avoided, if possible. However, the risk of late complications should not lead to the failure to apply potentially curative treatment. The challenge is to preserve or augment the cure rate while decreasing the risk of serious treatment-related illness.

The mechanisms of damage vary. Surgical procedures can create abnormal physiology (such as blind loops leading to malabsorption) or interfere with normal organ function (splenectomy leading to impaired immune response). Radiation therapy can damage organ function directly (salivary gland toxicity leading to dry mouth and dental caries), act as a carcinogen (second solid tumors in radiation ports), or promote accelerated aging-associated changes (atherosclerosis). Cancer chemotherapy can produce damage to the bone marrow and immune system and induce a spectrum of organ dysfunctions. Therapy may produce subclinical damage that may only become recognized in the presence of a second inciting factor (such as the increased incidence of melanoma in patients with dysplastic nevus syndrome treated for Hodgkin's disease with radiation therapy). Finally, although the mechanisms are not elucidated, cancer and its treatment are associated with psychosocial problems that can impair the survivor's ability to adapt to life after cancer.

Late effects by treatment modality are shown in Table 103-1. →*Toxicities associated with drugs are discussed in Chap. 84; radiation toxicity is discussed in Chap 394.*

CONSEQUENCES BY ORGAN SYSTEM **Cardiovascular Dysfunction** Most anthracyclines damage the heart muscle. A dose-dependent dropout of myocardial cells is seen on endomyocardial biopsy, and eventually ventricular failure ensues. About 5% of patients who receive >550 mg/m^2 of doxorubicin will develop congestive heart failure (CHF). Coexisting cardiac disease, hypertension, advanced age, and concomitant therapy with thoracic radiation therapy or mitomycin may hasten the onset of CHF. Anthracycline-induced CHF is not readily reversible; mortality is as high as 50%, thus, prevention is the best approach. Mitoxantrone is a related drug that has less cardiac toxicity. Administration of doxorubicin by continuous infusion or encapsulated in liposomes appears to decrease the risk of heart damage. Dexrazoxane, an intracellular iron chelator, may protect the heart against anthracycline toxicity by preventing iron-dependent free-radical generation.

Mediastinal radiation therapy that includes the heart can induce acute pericarditis, chronic constrictive pericarditis, myocardial fibrosis, or accelerated premature coronary atherosclerosis. The incidence of acute pericarditis is 5 to 13%; patients may be asymptomatic or have dyspnea on exertion, fever, chest pain. Onset is insidious with a peak about 9 months after treatment. Pericardial effusion may be present. Chronic constrictive pericarditis can develop 5 to 10 years after treatment and usually presents with dyspnea on exertion. Myocardial fibrosis may present as unexplained CHF with diagnostic evaluation showing restrictive cardiomyopathy. Patients may have aortic insufficiency from valvular thickening or mitral regurgitation from papillary muscle dysfunction. Patients who receive mantle field radiation therapy have a three-fold increased risk of *fatal* myocardial infarction. Similarly, radiation of the carotids is associated with premature atherosclerosis of the carotids and can produce central nervous system (CNS) embolic disease.

At very high doses, cyclophosphamide can produce a hemorrhagic myocarditis. Patients receiving bleomycin may develop Raynaud's phenomenon. The symptoms range from mild to debilitating; up to 40% of patients receiving bleomycin for testicular cancer report this problem.

Pulmonary Dysfunction Pulmonary fibrosis from bleomycin is dose-related, with potential exacerbation by age, preexisting lung disease, thoracic radiation, high concentrations of inhaled oxygen, and the concomitant use of other chemotherapeutic agents. Several other chemotherapy agents and radiation therapy can cause pulmonary fibrosis, and at least five can cause pulmonary venoocclusive disease, especially following high-dose therapy such as that involved in stem cell/bone marrow transplantation.

Liver Dysfunction Clinically significant long-term damage to the liver from standard dose chemotherapy is relatively infrequent, and mostly confined to patients who have received chronic methotrexate for maintenance therapy of acute lymphoblastic leukemia. Radiation doses to the liver exceeding 1500 cGy can produce liver dysfunction. Although rarely seen with standard dose chemotherapy, hepatic venoocclusive disease is more common with high-dose therapy, such as that given to prepare patients for autologous or allogeneic stem cell transplantation. Endothelial damage is probably the inciting event.

Renal/Bladder Dysfunction Reduced renal function may be produced by cisplatin and is usually asymptomatic, but may also render the patient that much more susceptible to other renal insults. Cyclophosphamide cystitis may eventually lead to the development of bladder cancer. Ifosfamide produces cystitis and a proximal tubular defect, a Fanconi-like syndrome that is usually, but not always, reversible.

Endocrine Dysfunction Long-term survivors of childhood cancer who received cranial irradiation are shorter, more likely to be obese, and have reductions in strength, exercise tolerance, and bone mineral density. The obesity may be related to alterations in leptin biology. Growth hormone deficiency is the most common hormone deficiency.

Thyroid disease is common in patients who have received radiation therapy to the neck, such as patients with Hodgkin's disease, with an incidence of up to 62% at 26 years post-therapy. Hypothyroidism is the most common abnormality, followed by Graves' disease, thyroiditis, and cancer. Such patients should have frequent thyroid-stimulating hormone (TSH) levels to detect hypothyroidism early and suppress the TSH drive, which may contribute to thyroid cancer.

Nervous System Dysfunction Although many patients experience peripheral neuropathy during chemotherapy, only a few have chronic problems, perhaps because they have other co-existing diseases such as diabetes mellitus. High doses of cisplatin can produce severe sensorimotor neuropathy. Vincristine may produce permanent numbness and tingling in the fingers and toes.

Neurocognitive sequelae from intrathecal chemotherapy, with or without radiation therapy, are recognized complications of the successful therapy of childhood acute lymphoblastic leukemia. Cognitive decline has been attributed to radiating the brain in the treatment of a variety of tumor types. In addition, cognitive decline can follow the use of adjuvant chemotherapy in women being treated for breast cancer. Because the agents are given at modest doses and are not thought to cross the blood-brain barrier, the mechanism of the cognitive decline is not defined.

Many patients suffer intrusive thoughts about cancer recurrence for many years after successful treatment. Adjustment to normal expectations can be difficult. Cancer survivors may often have more

Table 103-1   Late Effects of Cancer Therapy

Surgical Procedure		Effect
Amputation		Functional loss
Lymph node dissection		Risk of lymphedema
Ostomy		Psychosocial impact
Splenectomy		Risk of sepsis
Adhesions		Risk of obstruction
Bowel anastomoses		Malabsorption syndromes

Radiation Therapy		Effect
Organ		
Bone		Premature termination of growth, osteonecrosis
Soft tissues		Atrophy, fibrosis
Brain		Neuropsychiatric deficits, cognitive dysfunction
Thyroid		Hypothyroidism, Graves' disease, cancer
Salivary glands		Dry mouth, carries, dysgeusia
Eyes		Cataracts
Heart		Pericarditis, myocarditis, coronary artery disease
Lung		Pulmonary fibrosis
Kidney		Decreased function, hypertension
Liver		Decreased function
Intestine		Malabsorption, stricture
Gonads		Infertility, premature menopause
Any		Secondary neoplasia

Chemotherapy		Effect
Organ	Drug	
Bone	Glucocorticoids	Osteoporosis, avascular necrosis
Brain	Methotrexate, ara-C, others	Neuropsychiatric deficits, cognitive decline?
Peripheral nerves	Vincristine, platinum	Neuropathy, hearing loss
Eyes	Glucocorticoids	Cataracts
Heart	Anthracyclines	Cardiomyopathy
Lung	Bleomycin	Pulmonary fibrosis
	Methotrexate	Pulmonary hypersensitivity
Kidney	Platinum, others	Decreased function, hypomagnesemia
Liver	Various	Altered function
Gonads	Alkylating agents, others	Infertility, premature menopause
Bone marrow	Various	Aplasia, myelodysplasia, secondary leukemia

problems holding a job, staying in a stable relationship, and coping with the usual stresses of daily life.

A dose-related hearing loss can occur with the use of cisplatin, usually with doses in excess of 400 mg/m^2. This is irreversible and patients should be screened with audiometric exams periodically during such therapy.

Eyes   Cataracts may be caused by chronic glucocorticoid use, radiation therapy to the head, and, rarely, by tamoxifen.

Sexual and Reproductive Dysfunction   Reversible azoospermia can be caused by many chemotherapy agents. The gonads may also be permanently damaged by radiation therapy or by chemotherapeutic agents, particularly the alkylating agents. The extent of the damage depends upon the patient's age and the total dose administered. As a woman nears menopause, smaller amounts of chemotherapy will produce ovarian failure. In men, chemotherapy may produce infertility, but hormone production is not usually affected. Women, however, commonly lose both fertility and hormone production. The premature induction of menopause in a young woman can have serious medical and psychological consequences. Hormone replacement therapy is controversial, but most evidence supports its use. Paroxetine may be useful in controlling hot flashes.

Musculoskeletal Dysfunction   Late consequences of radiation therapy on the musculoskeletal system occur mostly in children and are related to the radiation dose, volume of tissue irradiated, and the age of the child at the time of therapy. Damage to the microvasculature of the epiphyseal growth zone may result in leg length discrepancy, scoliosis, and short stature.

Oral Complications   Radiation therapy can damage the salivary glands, producing dry mouth. Without saliva, dental caries develop and many patients have poor dentition. In rare patients, taste can be adversely affected and appetite can be suppressed.

SECOND MALIGNANCIES   Second malignancies are a major cause of death for those cured of cancer. Second malignancies can be grouped into three categories: those associated with the primary cancer, those caused by radiation therapy, and those caused by chemotherapy.

Primary cancers increase the risk of secondary cancers in a number of settings. Patients with head and neck cancers are at increased risk of developing a lung cancer, and vice versa, probably because of shared risk factors, especially tobacco abuse. Patients with breast cancer are at increased risk of a second breast cancer in the contralateral breast. Patients with Hodgkin's disease are at increased risk of non-Hodgkin's lymphoma. Patients with genetic syndromes, such as MEN 1 or Lynch syndrome, are at increased risk of second cancers of specific types. In none of these examples does it appear that treatment of primary cancer is the cause of the secondary cancer, but a role for treatment is difficult to exclude. These predispositions should result in heightened surveillance in persons at risk. Patients with head and neck cancer may have a reduced risk of developing lung cancer with retinoic acid treatment. Other cancer preventions have not been proved effective.

Patients treated with radiation therapy have an increasing and apparently life-long risk of developing second solid tumors, usually in or adjacent to the radiation field. The risk is modest in the first decade after treatment but reaches 1% per year in the second decade, such that populations followed for 25 years or more have a ≥25% chance of developing a second treatment-related tumor. Some organs differ in their susceptibility to radiation carcinogenesis with age; women receiving chest radiation therapy after age 30 have a small increased risk of breast cancer, but those under 30 have a 128-fold increased risk. The chances of curing the second malignancies hinge on early diagnosis. Patients who were treated with radiation therapy should be carefully examined on an annual basis and evaluated for any abnormalities in organs and tissues that were in the radiation field. Symptoms in a patient cured of cancer should not be dismissed as they may be an early sign of second cancers.

Chemotherapy produces two clinical syndromes that can be fatal: myelodysplasia and acute myeloid leukemia. Two types of acute leukemia have been described. The first occurs in patients treated with alkylating agents, especially over a protracted period. The malignant cells frequently carry genetic deletions in chromosomes 5 or 7. The lifetime risk is about 2%; the risk is increased by the addition of radiation therapy and is about 3 times higher in people treated over age 40. It peaks in incidence 4 to 6 years after treatment; the risk returns to baseline if no disease has developed within 10 years of treatment. The second type of acute leukemia occurs after exposure to topoisomerase II inhibitors such as doxorubicin or etoposide. It is morphologically indistinguishable from the first but contains a characteristic chromosome translocation involving 10q23. The incidence is <1%, and it usually occurs 1 1/2 to 3 years after treatment. Both forms of acute leukemia are highly refractory to treatment, and no preventive strategy has been developed.

Hormonal manipulations can also cause second tumors. Tamoxifen induces endometrial cancer in about 1 to 2% of women taking it 5 years or longer. Usually these tumors are found at early stage; mortality from endometrial cancer is very low compared to the benefit from tamoxifen use as adjuvant therapy in women with breast cancer.

CONSEQUENCES BY CANCER TYPE   Pediatric Cancers   Quality of life is often excellent, although the majority have at least one late effect. About one-third of long-term survivors have moderate to severe problems. Cognitive function may be impaired. Late effects are worse for those with poor socioeconomic status. Functional impairments in the cardiovascular system due to radiation therapy and anthracyclines, and in the lungs due to radiation therapy, are rare. Scoliosis and/or delayed growth due to radiation of the skeleton is more common. Many have psychosocial and sexual problems. Second malignant neoplasms are a significant cause of death.

Hodgkin's Disease   The patient cured of Hodgkin's disease remains subject to long-term medical problems such as thyroid dysfunction, premature coronary artery disease, gonadal dysfunction, postsplenectomy sepsis, and second malignancies. The second malignancies encountered include myelodysplasia and acute myeloid leukemia, non-Hodgkin's lymphomas, breast cancer, lung cancer, and melanoma. The major risk factor for hematologic malignancies is treatment with alkylating agents, while solid tumors are more likely to be seen with the use of radiation therapy. Patients cured of Hodgkin's disease seem to have greater fatigue, more psychosocial and sexual problems, and report a poorer quality of life than patients cured of acute leukemia.

Non-Hodgkin's Lymphomas   The patient cured of a non-Hodgkin's lymphoma may be at increased risk of myelodysplasia and acute leukemia if high doses or prolonged alkylating agents were used. Chronic exposure to cyclophosphamide increases the risk of bladder cancer. Patients cured of lymphoma report a very good quality of life.

Acute Leukemia   The late effects of anti-leukemic therapy include second malignancies (hematologic and solid tumors), neuropsychiatric difficulties, subnormal growth, thyroid abnormalities, and infertility.

Head and Neck Cancer   Patients frequently have poor dentition, dry mouth, trismus, difficulty in eating, and poor nutrition. Those with nasopharyngeal cancer report the poorest long-term quality of life, possibly related to the volume of disease that is radiated.

Stem Cell Transplantation   Cured patients are at risk of second cancers, especially if radiation therapy was part of the treatment. They are also subject to gonadal damage and infertility. Graft-versus-host disease is the leading factor contributing to the morbidity and mortality from allogeneic bone marrow transplantation, with an immune-mediated attack against the skin, liver, and gut epithelium. About half of patients report psychosexual problems.

Breast Cancer   Patients treated with adjuvant chemotherapy and/or hormonal therapy for breast cancer are at risk for endometrial cancer from the use of tamoxifen. Those patients who have received chemotherapy may be at risk from doxorubicin or radiation-induced cardiomyopathy and acute leukemia. The development of premature ovarian failure from chemotherapy may cause hormone-deficient symptoms (hot flashes, decreased vaginal secretions, dyspareunia) and places women at risk for osteoporosis and cardiovascular deaths. Patients commonly report intrusive thoughts of cancer and psychological distress.

Testicular Cancer Depending on the modalities used for therapy, patients cured of testicular cancer can anticipate Raynaud's phenomena, renal and/or pulmonary damage from chemotherapy, and ejaculatory dysfunction from retroperitoneal lymph node dissection. Sexual dysfunction is reported by 15% of patients cured of testicular cancer.

Colon Cancer To date the major threat to patients with colorectal cancer treated with chemotherapy and or radiation therapy remains the risk of a second colorectal cancer. Quality of life is reported as high in long-term survivors.

Prostate Cancer Radical surgical treatment is often accompanied by impotence and about 10 to 15% develop some urine incontinence. Use of radiation therapy increases the risk of second cancers.

The challenge for the future is to integrate new chemotherapy and biologic agents and newer techniques of delivering radiation therapy in a fashion that increases cure rates and lowers the late effects of treatment. Additional populations at risk for late effects include those with cancers where therapy is becoming more effective, such as ovarian cancer, and cancers where chemotherapy and radiation therapy are used together in an organ-sparing approach, such as bladder cancer, anal cancer, and laryngeal cancer. Patients who have been cured of a cancer represent an important resource for cancer prevention studies.

BIBLIOGRAPHY

BOOKMAN MA et al: Late complications of curative treatment in Hodgkin's disease. JAMA 260:680, 1988

MACKIE E et al: Adult psychosocial outcomes in long-term survivors of acute lymphoblastic leukemia and Wilms' tumor: A controlled study. Lancet 355:1310, 2000

SOCIE G et al: New malignant disease after allogeneic marrow transplantation for childhood acute leukemia. J Clin Oncol 18:348, 2000

VAN LEEUWEN FE et al: Long-term risk of second malignancy in survivors of Hodgkin's disease treated during adolescence or young adulthood. J Clin Oncol 18: 487, 2000

Section 2
DISORDERS OF HEMATOPOIESIS

104

Peter J. Quesenberry, Gerald A. Colvin

HEMATOPOIESIS

Hematopoiesis is the production of blood cells. It is a tightly regulated system exquisitely responsive to functional demands. The level of neutrophils, eosinophils, and basophils are maintained in discrete ranges with rapid adjustments when demands such as bacterial infection, parasitic infection, or allergic reaction are imposed. Similarly, lymphocytes, monocytes, platelets, and red cells, while maintained in normal ranges, respond rapidly to demands—lymphocytes to immune challenge, monocytes to various infections, platelets to hemorrhage or inflammation, and red cells to tissue hypoxia from many causes. Derangements in marrow function can lead to an excess of white cells, such as leukemia or leukemoid reactions, or an inadequate number of cells, such as anemia, thrombocytopenia, or leukopenia. Kinetics of cytopenia induction after marrow injury with drugs, radiation, or infections reflect the life span of these cells in peripheral blood. The first lineage to drop are the neutrophils with a blood life span of 6 to 8 h, followed by platelets with a 10-day life span. Anemia develops over a longer time in the absence of blood loss, reflecting the 120-day life span of red blood cells. All of these cell types are produced by primitive cells termed *stem cells*, which are present in the bone marrow of adult mammals.

The production of all the cell types except lymphocytes is usually very efficient, and production is controlled largely by negative feedback. When demand for production of cells of a particular lineage increases or peripheral levels of the cells fall, stimulatory cytokines are released and generate new cells with a time delay of a few days, or the time required for maturation from stem cell precursors. By contrast, production of lymphocytes is highly inefficient. Each day many more cells are generated than are required in the periphery. Most lymphocytes are destroyed during development; this is due at least in part to the destruction of cells that express antigen receptors specific for self antigens.

HEMATOPOIETIC STEM CELLS Hematopoietic stem cells are characterized by extensive proliferation and differentiation capacity, with the ability to self-renew on a population basis (Fig. 104-1). They also express a variety of cell-surface proteins and have the ability to rapidly "home" to bone marrow after intravenous injection. Human stem cells lack markers of lineage commitment (i.e., lineage-negative) and express c-Kit, c-mpl, and usually cluster of differentiation determinant-34 (CD34); a small subset of stem cells may be CD34-negative. Murine cells are also lineage-negative and express c-Kit, CD34, c-mpl, and Ly6A or Sca. The most primitive cells are characterized by low-level expression of a relatively large number of cytokine receptors and by relative exclusion (or pumping out) of the dyes rhodamine and Hoechst. These cells express a variety of adhesion proteins presumptively involved in marrow homing, including alpha$_4$, alpha$_5$, alpha$_6$, L-selectin, and platelet/endothelial cell adhesion molecule (PECAM) (Fig. 104-2). Another characteristic of the stem cell is a functional plasticity in response to cytokines as it transits the cell cycle (Fig. 104-3). Engraftment capacity is good in G$_1$ but virtually lost in late S and early G$_2$.

The stem cell is also a highly mobile cell with the capacity to evolve rapidly or involute pseudopodial extensions. The gold standard for defining the stem cell has been in vivo repopulation and long-term reconstitution of lethally irradiated mice. In vivo repopulation studies using unique radiation-induced chromosomal abnormalities or retroviral markers have shown that one or, at most, a few stem cells are capable of reconstituting the entire lymphohematopoietic system of a mouse; they also have defined classes of stem cells with short, medium, or long-term repopulating capacity. These are cell types that differ in the kinetics of hematopoietic reconstitution. Short-term cells repopulate in the first few weeks after transplantation but are not long-lasting; long-term cells account for long-lived reconstitution beginning a few months after reconstitution and lasting the entire life span; medium-term cells bridge the time between short- and long-term cells. When relatively small numbers of marked stem cells—obtained by limiting dilution of sorted marrow cells—are transplanted, lymphohematopoiesis may be clonal or oligoclonal, initially. Normal polyclonal lymphohematopoiesis derives from a relatively large number of clones. Both competitive marrow repopulation and mathematical studies support the model of polyclonal hematopoiesis. The most primitive long-term repopulating cells on activation with cytokines can rapidly alter phenotype and become short-term repopulating cells.

FIGURE 104-1 Cellular basis of hematopoiesis. Mature cells are derived from a common multipotent progenitor. Lineage development appears to occur as a consequence of the ordered expression of transcription factors (in blue). Thus, mice in which PU.1 expression has been blocked develop normal erythrocytes and megakaryocytes, but no other cell lineages. Once lineage commitment occurs, cytokines and colony-stimulating factors (in black) regulate development, again through the induction of transcription factors. Abbreviations: HSC, hematopoietic stem cell; GEMML, cell giving rise to granulocyte, erythroid, monocyte, megakaryocyte, and lymphoid cells: GEMM, cell giving rise to granulocytic, erythroid, monocyte, and megakaryocytic cells; GM, cell giving rise to granulocytic and monocyte cells; ME, cell giving rise to megakaryocytic and erythroid cells; L, lymphoid lineage stem cell.

While stable multilineage chimerism has been documented in humans after clinical marrow transplantation, no assay system exists for human stem cell activity. A number of surrogate assays are used for the long-term, multilineage-repopulating cell in both humans and mice. These include the multifactor-responsive, high-proliferative potential colony-forming cells (HPP-CFC) and variations of stromal-based assays including the cobblestone-forming cell, long-term culture-initiating cell (LTC-IC) or LTC-IC–extended (LTC-IC–e). The adequacy of these assays is still the subject of debate. In addition, the NOD-SCID immunodeficient mouse has become a surrogate model for assaying human hematopoietic stem cells, although lineage skewing and variability of engraftment undermine its reliability.

LINEAGE PLASTICITY OF STEM CELLS Tissue stem cells are capable of producing a wide variety of differentiated cell lineages, depending on intrinsic cell programming and the microenvironmental signals. Marrow cells may differentiate into mesenchy-

mal, myocyte, endothelial, hematopoietic, and neural cells. Neural muscle and hepatic stem cells have been reported to give rise to hematopoiesis in transplanted mice. The regulation of stem cell plasticity and life span remains incompletely understood. However, once a particular set of transcription factors has been induced, either through an intrinsic program or from extracellular signals, reversibility is limited. The sequentially ordered activation of transcription factors leads to lineage commitment.

MICROENVIRONMENT Nonhematopoietic tissues exert major influences on hematopoiesis, both short- and long-range. The nonhematopoietic tissues immediately abutting hematopoietic tissue have been termed the hematopoietic microenvironment, and the cells that comprise the environment influence hematopoiesis. For example, a surface location of adoptively transferred murine stem cells in the spleen of lethally irradiated mice favored erythropoiesis, while an intrasplenic trabecular location was biased toward granulocyte production. In both human and murine species, various cell types have been identified in stroma, including hematopoietically derived macrophages and nonhematopoietic preadipocytic fibroblasts, endothelial cells, and vascular smooth muscle. This system appears capable of supporting the most primitive stem cells and controlling their proliferation and self-renewal. Most stem cells are resting under normal physiologic conditions but can be recruited into the cell cycle by demands of increased terminally differentiated hematopoietic cells. Cell-cell contact is critical in determining the microenvironment stimulus. Stem cells and primitive cells bind tightly to the stroma, while maturing precursors and terminally differentiated cells are nonadherent. Blocking interactions between stem cells and stromal cells with antibodies to vascular cell adhesion molecule (VCAM)-1 on stromal cells

FIGURE 104-2 The phenotype of human and murine stem cells.

FIGURE 104-3 The functional plasticity of stem cells in response to cytokines as it transits the cell cycle. The stem cell has the capacity to differentiate into morphologically different phenotypes as it marches through the cell cycle (depicted as Stem Cell A-D). Engraftment capacity is good in G_1 but virtually lost in late S and early G_2.

or its ligand, VLA-4, on stem cells block the interaction. Cytokine receptors binding to membrane-associated cytokines like stem cell factor, or to extracellular matrix-bound ligands, contribute other adhesive interactions.

PROGENITORS Bone marrow stem cells can be induced to proliferate and differentiate into a wide variety of mature cell types in vitro in the presence of an appropriate colony-stimulating factor (CSF). Cells that give rise to mature colonies of granulocytes and macrophages are called granulocyte-macrophage colony-forming units (CFU-GM) (Fig. 104-4). The particular hematopoietic growth factor that stimulates the development of these colonies is called granulocyte-macrophage colony-stimulating factor (GM-CSF). Distinct culture conditions and supplemental growth factors, alone and in combination, are capable of producing a range of cell expansions from multilineage colonies that include lymphocytes to single-lineage clones. The different stem/progenitor clones are summarized in Table 104-1. Progenitor cells in general are found to have a higher proliferative rate and more lineage restriction than stem cells. They are also responsive to smaller numbers of cytokines. Thus, they are defined by expression of a limited variety of cytokine receptors.

The size of the colonies denotes the activity of cells at different stages of differentiation. Terminally acting cytokines produce smaller colonies called CFU (colony-forming units). When progenitors are stimulated with mixtures of early- and late-acting cytokines and are cultured for longer periods of time, the colonies are larger and multiple lineages are represented. Primitive multifactor-responsive erythroid colonies are termed burst-forming unit erythroid (BFU-E) while even more primitive colonies with great proliferative potential are termed HPP-CFC.

CYTOKINES The lymphohematopoietic stem/progenitor populations and their progeny are largely defined by their cytokine responsiveness and cytokine receptor phenotype. Major efforts to define the regulators of granulocyte, erythroid, and platelet production have culminated in the definitions of a variety of glycoproteins. Acting through cell surface receptors at very low concentrations, these glycoproteins control the production of stem cells in vivo. Most prominent have been erythropoietin for red blood cells, GM-CSF for granulocytes and macrophages, granulocyte-CSF (G-CSF) for granulocytes, and thrombopoietin for platelets. In addition, macrophage-CSF or CSF-1, was defined as a primary regulator of macrophage-monocyte production and function. These cytokines exert prominent actions on specific cell lineages, but all exert actions on different cell lineages or on cells that have the potential to differentiate along more than one lineage.

In addition to the more lineage-restricted cytokines, a large number (perhaps up to 70) act broadly on multiple lineages and at multiple stages of lymphohematopoiesis. They exert effects on renewal, proliferation, survival, and differentiation; these effects may be stimulatory or inhibitory, and the cytokines usually show additive or synergistic effects with other cytokines. The cytokines also modulate intrinsic functions of early stem cells (migration and cell adherence) and pro-

Table 104-1 Progenitor Stem Cells

In Vitro Assay	Stem/Progenitor Clones
GM-colony forming unit culture (G-CSF, GM-CSF, CSF-1)	Defined by cytokine regulators Produces colonies of granulocytes, granulocytes/macrophages, or macrophages
CFU-E	Small colonies of red cells; need only erythropoietin
CFU-MEG	Small colonies of megakaryocytes
BFU-E	Large aggregates of red cells; needs erythropoietin plus other cytokines
BFU-MEG	Large colonies of megakaryocytes; needs multiple cytokines
HPP-CFC	Stimulated by multiple factors with great proliferative and differentiative potential Large colonies surrogate for primitive stem cells
Colony-forming unit blast	Small colonies of undifferentiated blasts; needs multiple cytokines
Cobblestone forming or long term culture initiating cell (LTC-IC)	Forms granulocyte/macrophage colonies after culture with adherent stroma Relatively primitive cell
LTC-IC extended	May be a more primitive stem cell Long time growth on stroma produces multipotential lymphomyeloid progenitors

NOTE: CFU, colony-forming unit; BFU, burst-forming unit; HPP-CFC, high-proliferative potential colony-forming cells.

mote the effector functions of their terminally differentiated progeny. G-CSF primes neutrophils to undergo oxidative metabolism in response to formyl-methionyl-leucyl-phenylalanine (fMLF) and enhances cell migration, while interleukin (IL) 3 activates basophils, mast cells, and eosinophils. CSF-1 at low levels supports survival of murine marrow macrophages and at higher levels stimulates protein synthesis, cell division, and various macrophage functions, including antitumor activity, secretion of products of oxygen reduction, and plasminogen activator. CSF-1 also induces secretion of IL-1 from macrophages. Many of the hematopoietically active cytokines induce secretion of other cytokines, either inhibitory or stimulatory, creating multiple cytokine regulatory loops. Transforming growth factor β (TGF-β) is an inhibitory cytokine but also an autocrine factor supporting survival of pluripotent hematopoietic stem cells by blocking G1 to S phase transition. TGF-β conversely shows stimulatory effects on progenitors. Cytokines also modulate adhesion protein and integrin expression on multiple cell types. They exert their effects by interacting with surface-based receptors and initiating second-messenger cascades (see below).

The lymphohematopoietic cytokines can be broadly divided into colony-stimulating factors, erythropoietin, thrombopoietin, the interleukins, the inhibitory cytokines, chemokines that regulate cell migration and activation, and a variety of other hematopoietically active cytokines. A noninclusive overview of these cytokines emphasizing their primary, highlighted, or first-described action is presented in Tables 104-2, 104-3 and 104-4. The general characteristics of cytokines are summarized in Table 104-5.

CYTOKINE RECEPTORS, SIGNAL TRANSDUCTION, AND TRANSCRIPTION FACTORS Cytokines induce their effects through cell-surface membrane receptors. Several cytokine receptor families have been identified. The hematopoietic receptor family includes IL-2, IL-3, IL-4, IL-5, IL-6, IL-7, IL-9, G-CSF, GM-CSF, and erythropoietin. Common characteristics of this family include four conserved cysteine residues and a WSXWS motif (X is a variable, nonconserved amino acid). Some also have immunoglobulin-like structures in their extracellular domains. Receptors frequently consist of multiple chains, and dimerization on cytokine binding is a usual feature of receptor biology. These receptors have no intrinsic signaling capacity and transmit signals by attaching to intracellular signaling molecules, such as the src family and the JAK family kinases. GM-

Marrow cells

CFU-GM (granulocyte and macrophage colonies)

Time 7–14 days

Petri dish—Semi-solid matrix (agar) stimulator (GM-CSF, G-CSF, CSF-1)

Stimulate by GM-CSF and combinations of G-CSF, GM-CSF and CSF-1

FIGURE 104-4 Marrow cells in semi-solid media in the presence of stimulatory factors in conditioned media or serum form colonies of granulocytes and macrophages.

Table 104-2 Lymphohematopoietic Cytokines

Growth Factor	Highlighted and/or Predominant Actions
Erythropoietin	Limited proliferative effects; modulates/stimulates survival and terminal maturation of CFU-E
	Globin synthesis and proliferation of proerythroblasts and basophilic erythroblasts
	Increases in vivo red cell production
GM-CSF	Predominant action on granulocyte/macrophage progenitors
	Action on multipotent neutrophil, macrophage megakaryocyte, eosinophil, erythroid, and dendritic progenitors
	Stimulates function of mature neutrophils and macrophages
	Inhibits neutrophil migration and stimulates cytotoxic and phagocytic activity against yeast, parasites, and antibody-coated tumor cells
	In vivo, increases granulocytes, monocytes, eosinophils, and dendritic cells
	Has a variable effect on the platelet count
G-CSF	Stimulates granulocyte and pre-B cell production in vitro and primes neutrophils for function
	Increases neutrophil levels in vivo
CSF-1	Stimulates a population of progenitors that make macrophages
	Also stimulates function and cell division of mature macrophages
IL-3 or Multi-CSF	Multilineage stimulator with direct megakaryocyte, mast cell/basophil, B cell, and eosinophil stimulatory activity
	Synergizes with EPO to stimulate primitive erythroid stem cells and with multiple factors to stimulate HPP-CFC
	In vivo, increases blood eosinophil, granulocyte, and monocyte levels as well as tissue mast cells
Thrombopoietin	Ligand for C-mpl
	Major regulator of megakaryocyte proliferation, differentiation, and platelet production
	Stimulates and supports survival of primitive stem cells
	In vivo, increases platelet production

NOTE: CFU, colony-forming unit; CSF, colony-stimulating factor; GM-CSF, granulocyte-macrophage colony-stimulating factor; G-CSF, granulocyte-CSF; EPO, erythropoietin.

CSF, IL-3, and IL-5 receptors have low-affinity alpha chains and a common high-affinity beta chain. The common beta chain may play a role in the competitive binding of these ligands.

Receptors for FLT-3 ligand, c-kit, platelet-derived growth factor (PDGF), CSF-1, and thrombopoietin constitute the tyrosine kinase receptor family. These receptors have conserved cysteines in the extracellular domain, with tyrosine kinase activity in the cytoplasmic domain, an immunoglobulin-like structure involved in ligand, and binding. Chemokine receptors are seven-transmembrane (serpin) G-protein linked receptors that signal cell activation and migration.

Cytokines typically cause receptor oligomerization on hematopoietic cells, followed by activation of intrinsic (receptor) or extrinsic tyrosine kinases, phosphorylation of the receptor and recruitment of Src-homology (SH2), and phospho-tyrosine binding (PT3) domain proteins to the receptor. Subsequent steps vary with different cytokines but essentially represent a series of phosphorylation-dephosphorylation events, with the final activation or nuclear translocation of a protein or protein complex that binds specific regions of DNA and initiates various genetic programs (i.e., acts as a transcription factor).

The complexity of these second-messenger signaling systems is illustrated by signaling through the GM-CSF, IL-3, and IL-5 receptors, which share a common beta chain. The beta chain does not have kinase activity but induces tyrosine phosphorylation of itself and a number of cytoplasmic proteins, including kinases, such as P1-3 kinase; adapters illustrated by Grb2; the insulin receptor-substrate 2 Cbl and Shc;

guanine nucleotide exchange factors such as Vav; phosphastases such as SH2-domain protein tyrosine phosphatase-2 and SH2-containing inositol phosphatase; and transcription factors such as STAT 5.

Receptor phosphorylation is mediated by receptor-associated kinases, such as JAK2 (Janus family kinase 2, named Janus for the Roman god who guards the gates and looks in two directions; original Janus kinases were felt to have both tyrosine and serine kinase activity) and Src-family kinases. These sequential protein interactions lead to the evolution of proteins or protein complexes, termed *transcription factors*, that bind to specific regions of DNA to initiate genetic pro-

Table 104-3 Interleukins

Cytokine	Action
IL-1	Regulation immune system, induction fever, acute phase protein, tissue repair and cytotoxicity
	Directly stimulates early stem cells and acts synergistically with many other cytokines to stimulate HPP-CFC
	A prominent inducer of other cytokines from many cell types
IL-2	T cell growth factor
	Increases production of gamma interferon
	Stimulates and activates B cells and natural killer cells
	Inhibits GM colony formation and erythropoiesis
IL-4	Stimulates B cell maturation, immunoglobin synthesis and generation of cytotoxic and helper T lymphocytes
	Synergizes with other cytokines to stimulate GM, mast cell, erythroid, and megakaryocyte proliferation
	Stimulates proliferation and differentiation of dendritic cells
	Inhibits monocyte cytokine production
IL-5	Stimulates B cells and supports the proliferation, maturation and function of eosinophils
IL-6	Stimulates megakaryopoiesis and synergizes with IL-1, 2, 3, 4, GM-CSF, and CSF-1 to stimulate myeloid proliferation
	Plasma cell proliferation-enhanced
	Induces hepatocyte protein synthesis
IL-7	B and T cell stimulation
	Stimulates early hematopoietic stem cells and has activity with kit-ligand in inducing pre-B cells in culture
IL-8	Chemotactic factor for granulocytes
	Mobilizes stem cells into the peripheral blood
IL-9	T cell growth factor
	Supports erythroid burst development and has mast cell growth-promoting activity
IL-10	Inhibits INF-γ production by T cells
	Increases cytotoxic T cell precursors and function
	Synergistically stimulates mast cells
IL-11	Very similar in action to IL-6
IL-12	NK cell stimulatory factor
	In synergy with IL-2 generates cytotoxic T cells
	Induces INF-γ production by NK and T cells
IL-13	Similar in action to IL-4 on B cells and monocytes
	In contrast to IL-4, induces production of IFN-γ by large granular lymphocytes and stimulates T cells
IL-14	Induces B cell proliferation and inhibits immunoglobin synthesis
IL-15	Shares biologic activity with IL-2
	Stimulates proliferation of activated CD4+, CD8+, $\gamma\delta$ subsets of T cells, NK cells, and mast cells
	Costimulator with IL-12 to facilitate production of IFN-γ and TNF-α
IL-16	CD4+ lymphocyte chemoattractant and growth factor stimulator
IL-17	Stimulates adherent cell types, such as macrophage, epithelial, endothelial, keratinocyte, or fibroblast, to secrete a variety of cytokines including: IL-6, IL-8, G-CSF, TNF-α, IL-1 beta, IL-10, IL-12, and IL-1R antagonist
	Induces proliferation of T cells and growth and differentiation of CD34+ human progenitor into neutrophils (with co-culture)
	Stimulates granulopoiesis in vivo
IL-18	Functional properties similar to IL-12
	Augments cell-mediated immunity
	Modulates T, B, and NK cell function
	Induces IFN-γ in type 1 helper T and NK cells

NOTE: GM, granulocyte-macrophage; IFN, interferon; NK, natural killer; TNF, tumor necrosis factor; IL, interleukin.

Table 104-4   Other Lymphohematopoietic Cytokines

Cytokine	Action
Kit ligand	Identical with hematolymphopoietic growth factor
	Synergizes with a large number of cytokines to stimulate HPP-CFC
	With IL-7 stimulates pre-B cell generation
	Multilineage effects in mice and primates with mast cell activation
	Acts on primitive stem/progenitor cells
FLT-3	Acts on relatively primitive progenitor/stem cells showing synergies with G-CSF, GM-CSF, M-CSF, IL-3, and kit-ligand
	Stimulates dendritic cell formation
b-FbF	Pleiotropic growth factor stimulating primitive marrow cells, megakaryocyte progenitors, and marrow stromal cells
LIF	Supports proliferation of IL-3 dependent cell line DA-1 and has multiple non-hematopoietic actions
	Sustains proliferation of embryonic stem cells
TGF-β	Inhibits early stem cells while stimulating progenitors, possibly through modulating surface cytokine receptor expression
	Probable autocrine factor for early stem cell survival
Mip-1α	Blocks stem cell entry into cell cycle and quiesces stem cells
Pentapeptide	Removes stem/progenitor cells from S phase
Tetrapeptide	Blocks entry of stem cells into S phase
Platelet-derived growth factor	Acts on erythroid and granulocytic progenitors and, indirectly, on early multilineage stem cells
Hepatocyte growth factor	Synergizes with other growth factors at the progenitor cell level

grams determining survival, proliferation, differentiation, and function.

As with second messengers, the transcription factor field is complex and evolving, but a number of transcription factors associated with specific stem cell levels or differentiation pathways have been described. Transcription factors that act at the earliest stem cell levels include c-myb, p45-NF-E2, GATA-2, AML-1 and tal-1/SCL, while Ikaros and PU-1 may act at the earliest lymphoid level. GATA-1 influences erythroid, mast cell, and megakaryocyte lineages, while FOG (friend of GATA-1) acts in concert with GATA-1. PU-1 appears to influence granulocyte and monocyte differentiation, P45-NF-E2 affects megakaryocyte lineages, and PAX-5 B lymphoid development. These transcription factors usually act in complexes with specific conformations binding to particular DNA sequences.

MIGRATION HOMING AND ADHESION PROTEINS
The process of stem cell homing to the marrow is complex and involves a number of adhesion proteins. Very late antigen (VLA) 4, VLA-5, VLA-6, PECAM, P- and E-selectin, CD44, CXCR, and a receptor for ligand-bearing galactosyl and mannosyl residues have been shown to be expressed by hematopoietic stem/progenitor cells and

Table 104-5   General Characteristics of Cytokines

Cytokines are glycoproteins acting at very low concentrations

Almost all cytokines are pleiotropic effectors, showing multiple biologic activities

The activity of most cytokines is strictly regulated, addresses multiple target cells, is normally transient, and can be regulated at all levels of gene expression

Factors are usually produced only by activated cells in response to an induction signal

Cell surface receptor is bound to initiate second-messenger cascade

Cytokines play a pivotal role in cell-to-cell communication processes, inducing the synthesis of novel gene products once they have bound to their respective receptors

Frequently act on stem/progenitors and their differentiated progeny to stimulate *or* inhibit renewal, survival, proliferation, differentiation, and function

Usually act on multiple different lineages, activate stimulatory or inhibitory activities, and synergize or antagonize the actions of other factors

Frequently act on neoplastic counterpart of normal target cell

implicated in marrow homing. The integrins α_4 and/or α_5 are expressed on immature blasts, erythroid progenitors, monocytes, and CD34+ cells; in general, expression of α_4 appears to decrease with maturation. Hematopoietic cells also bind differentially to different extracellular matrix components: erythroid cells to fibronectin, CFU-GM and BFU-E to collagen.

Antibody to VLA-4 given in vivo causes mobilization of hematopoietic progenitors in normal or cytokine-treated primates and/or mice. Stem cell mobilization by cytokines involves down regulation of adhesion protein expression on hematopoietic stem cells. The cell-cycle related fluctuations in engraftment appear to be based on alterations on different surface adhesion proteins. The stem cells are highly motile and move in a direction of cytokine or chemokine gradients with steel factor and stromal-derived factor 1 (SDF-1) being active. Adhesion proteins act not only for motility/adhesion, but also serve a regulatory role that is similar in some cases to traditional cytokines.

PHYSIOLOGY OF HEMATOPOIESIS AND SOURCES OF CYTOKINES   Erythropoietin is produced largely by the kidney in response to tissue hypoxia. The regulation of granulocyte and monocyte production is more complex, but appears to be in response to various infectious or noxious agents, such as gram-negative bacteria, the endotoxin in the cell wall of these bacteria, and antigen stimulation. All of these interact with peripheral tissue cells to generate a variety of cytokine messages, resulting in increase production in specific cell types. Parasitic infections appear to elicit IL-5, which modulates the eosinophilia and mast cell lineages. Viral infections have specific effects on lymphocyte classes; typically bacterial infections stimulate granulocyte production. Tuberculosis or other mycobacterial infections predominantly induce increased monocyte production. All of these biologic affects appear to be mediated by the selective evolution of cytokine complexes from tissue endothelial cells, fibroblasts, macrophages, and lymphocytes. Most cells produce a large variety of cytokines, but the key is the relative levels, combinations, and timing of the production of these cytokines (Fig. 104-5).

HEMATOPOIETIC STEM CELL AND CYTOKINE DISEASES   The classic stem cell disease is *chronic myeloid leukemia*. Here a specific genetic translocation between chromosomes 9 and 22 at the stem cell level leads to excess production of granulocytes, monocytes, basophils, frequently platelets, and less frequently red cells. Other lymphohematopoietic clonal stem cell diseases include polycythemia vera, myelofibrosis with myeloid metaplasia, paroxysmal nocturnal hemoglobinuria, and acute myeloid leukemia. Out of the scope of this chapter, but relevant to these discussions, is the fact that many lymphoid neoplasms are clonal diseases at early stages of development, but probably not at the mature stage suggested by the tumor cell-surface phenotype. The vast majority of peripheral B cell and T cell malignancies have genetic lesions associated with receptor gene rearrangements, which occur early in lymphoid cell development. Aplastic anemia appears to be a disease characterized by a defective number of hematopoietic stem cells. Cyclic hematopoiesis is another disease of hematopoietic stem cells. In gray collie dogs with this disorder, levels of platelets, reticulocytes, monocytes, and granulocytes cycle. This disease can be cured or transmitted by marrow transplantation. The human disease, cyclical neutropenia—or cyclic hematopoiesis in which blood cells oscillate with a 21-day period—is caused by missense and splicing mutations in the gene encoding neutrophil elastase, thus implicating this inflammatory chymotryptic serine protease in the oscillatory timing of hematopoiesis. The stem cell diseases are summarized in Table 104-6.

A number of cytokine disorders or diseases have now been defined. The best characterized is the anemia of renal failure, an erythropoietin deficiency state that can be corrected by the administration of erythropoietin. Various tumors, particularly lung cancer, increase peripheral granulocyte counts secondary to the production of G-CSF. The IL-6 family of cytokines appears to be prominently involved in a number of inflammatory states, causes the systemic symptoms associated with

FIGURE 104-5 The cellular and humoral influence on hematopoietic stem cells.

Numbers of cells are sometimes limiting for adult recipients (Chap 115).

Cytokines Demonstration that hematopoietic cytokines could modulate red blood cell and white cell production in humans has been useful in some clinical settings. Erythropoietin treatment improves hematocrit and quality of life in patients with chronic renal failure. Erythropoietin has been tried in myelodysplastic syndromes (MDS), a group of clonal stem cell disorders. Meta-analysis shows an overall response rate of only 13%; the actual overall clinical benefit was exceedingly small. In addition, the best results were seen in patients receiving daily injections. Prohibitive costs and often poor response limits use to those patients with serum EPO levels lower than 500 mU/L, and less than 5% myeloblasts. The utilization of erythropoietin in other settings than renal failure remains controversial and its use may relate more to effective marketing than to the science.

Castleman's disease and atrial myxoma, and may be an etiologic factor in multiple myeloma. IL-6 may also be a major cause of symptoms in various lymphomas. Abnormalities of the c-Kit receptor may underlie a number of mast cell diseases in humans; IL-5 production is the proximate cause of a number of eosinophilic states. A deficiency of IL-1 is a feature of aplastic anemia. Mutations in the G-CSF receptor in chronic congenital neutropenia (Kostmann's syndrome) may be a causative factor in the evolution of acute myeloid leukemia in some of these patients.

THERAPEUTIC IMPLICATIONS OF STEM CELLS AND CYTOKINES Stem Cells Stem cell transplantation was first established as an effective therapy for relapsed acute myeloid leukemia and aplastic anemia. It is now a mainstay of therapy for virtually all leukemias and some relapsed lymphomas. Application of this treatment to a number of solid tumors has been disappointing. Major expectations with regard to its potential in breast cancer have not yet been fulfilled, although it appears to be effective in relapsed testicular cancer. The rationale is the use of very high doses of drugs or radiation designed to kill all tumor cells, but at levels where marrow toxicity would be lethal. Marrow damage is the dose-limiting toxicity for many chemotherapeutic agents. If marrow function is replaced by transplant, it might be possible to increase the dose of chemotherapy substantially before another organ toxicity becomes dose-limiting.

The strategy is somewhat different in intrinsic marrow diseases, such as aplastic anemia, where marrow function is restored without the need for killing tumor cells, or in genetic marrow diseases such as thalassemia and sickle cell anemia, where replacement of the abnormal marrow with normal marrow corrects the disease state. Aggressive autoimmune diseases are also being treated with marrow replacement. Stem cells can come from a related or unrelated allogeneic source or directly from the patient. The sources of the stem cells also vary. Initially, marrow aspirate was the predominant source, but now apheresed peripheral blood stem cells are the most utilized. In addition, umbilical vein cord blood, especially in pediatric patients, appears effective.

These concerns are multiplied for the use of the myeloid growth factors, G-CSF, and GM-CSF. These agents elevate neutrophil and monocyte counts, and under very selective conditions they can result in a reduced toxicity of various chemotherapeutic regimens (Table 104-7). Unfortunately, they save about the same amount of money in hospitalizations for febrile neutropenia as they cost, and their use has not increased survival rate. Virtually all of the G-CSF and GM-CSF trials in cancer patients have been flawed by design; they involve escalation of drugs to toxic levels and reversal of toxicity without addressing the question of whether the patient's survival is affected by the treatment. GM-CSF and G-CSF are grossly overutilized; they are often used in settings where their efficacy has not been shown (e.g., patients with a low probability of neutropenia). Their use should still be considered experimental, and they should continue to be studied in a protocol setting but not used routinely. G-CSF is useful in mobilization of stem cells, and it is also effective in treatment of various chronic neutropenias, in particular cyclic neutropenia and Kostmann's syndrome. G-CSF may be involved in the evolution to acute myeloid leukemia in some patients, but overall it appears to be an effective intervention in these seriously ill patients. G-CSF may also aid in healing of diabetic skin ulcers.

IL-11 and thrombopoietin can elevate platelet counts in experimental animals, but their place in clinical practice is unclear. IL-11 has been approved for use in chemotherapy-induced thrombocytopenia, but its effects are small. Use of pegylated recombinant human megakaryocyte growth and development factor—the truncated version of thrombopoietin—has resulted in production of neutralizing antithrombopoietin antibodies and thrombocytopenia. Recombinant human thrombopoietin does not commonly elicit neutralizing antithrombopoietin antibodies. Clinical benefit (or cost effectiveness) has not yet been shown with thrombopoietin. Surrogate values of platelet counts or number of platelet transfusions are not valid criteria for clinical benefit. Thrombopoietin may eventually find a role as an expander of early stem cells in vitro. Active research in this important area continues.

Gene Therapy Hematopoietic stem cells provide an ideal vehicle for various gene therapy approaches. These cells can be easily induced into the cell cycle for retroviral integration. Long-term expression of introduced genes is currently being obtained in animal models. Initial clinical application has been disappointing, but success has been obtained in Gaucher's disease, suggesting that gene therapy will eventually become a successful approach to a number of hematopoietic diseases.

Table 104-6 Stem Cell Diseases

Chronic myeloid leukemia	Most lymphomas and probably
Most acute leukemias	multiple myeloma
Polycythemia vera	Many chronic neutropenias
Myelofibrosis with myeloid	Pure red cell aplasia and Fanconi's
metaplasia	anemia
Primary thrombocytosis	Cyclic neutropenias
Paroxysmal nocturnal hemoglo-	Shwachman-Diamond syndrome
binuria	Aplastic anemia

Table 104-7 Clinical Cytokine Application

Cytokine	Clinical Indications/New Directions	Clinical Toxicity
G-CSF	Clear use for G-CSF in mobilization of stem cells and perhaps in high dose chemotherapy when expected risk of febrile neutropenia is over 40%. Effective in treatment of various chronic neutropenias, in particular cyclic neutropenia, Kostmann and possible Shwachman-Diamond sydrome. *Routine use* for chemotherapy induced neutropenia is *not warranted* as a survival advantage has not been seen, and there is prohibitive cost vs. benefit ratio. Use in AIDS is FDA-approved, but actual clinical utility also in doubt.	Bone pain, splenomegaly (splenic rupture has been reported), exacerbation of psoriasis and other dermatological conditions, Sweet's syndrome (neutrophilic dermatitis), hair loss, elevation of leukocyte alkaline phosphatase and lactate dehydrogenase, and potential activation of some leukemias.
GM-CSF	FDA-approved for use in treatment of neutropenia in elderly patients undergoing induction for AML, high-dose chemotherapy and bone marrow transplant. Impressive response seen at our institution in use with low-dose ARA-c for treatment of AML arising out of a myelodysplastic syndrome (MDS). Clinical utility in solid tumors limited.	Hyperpyrexia, arthralgias, myalgias, serositis. IV administration can cause dyspnea, tachycardia, hypotension, flushing and myalgias.
Erythropoietin (EPO)	Clear use only in anemia of renal failure where the pathophysiology of that disease is pure EPO deficiency. Used in patients with cancer who are Jehovah's Witnesses (if they agree, as there is a small amount of albumin in product). Studies show improved quality of life in chemotherapy-induced anemia, but the actual benefit is probably small, with prohibitive cost versus benefit ratio. Most benefit from chemotherapy-induced anemia in platinum-treated patients. Limited use in MDS-induced anemia with a 13% overall response rate. HIV-related anemia can respond to EPO with decreased blood transfusions if the serum EPO level <500 U/L.	Hypertension, seizures, exacerbation of porphyria, potentially increased chance of thrombotic event.
IL-2	Well studied in a variety of malignancies as an immune modulator. Used alone or in conjunction with other cytokines or chemotherapy for malignant melanoma, renal cell carcinoma, lymphoma, cutaneous-T cell lymphoma, AML, and post-BMT to enhance graft-versus-tumor effect. Poor toxicity profile and very modest response rates limit clinical use. A 10 to 20% response rate was seen in melanoma and renal cell carcinoma.	Hyperpyrexia, hypotension, vascular leak syndrome, malaise, flulike symptoms, cholestasis, hepatic dysfunction, thyroiditis, vitiligo, inflammatory bowel changes, myocardial infarction, arrhythmia, ARDS, pulmonary edema, cytopenias, renal failure, and other toxicities.
Interferons (IFN-α,-β,-γ)	IFN-α: Clear use in CML, especially early stage, where up to an 80% response rate has been observed. Also quite active in treatment of hairy cell leukemia, with up to a 90% response rate. Clinical utility in treating mycosis fungoides, Sezary syndrome, HTLV-1−associated T cell leukemia/lymphoma, malignant melanoma, and multiple myeloma. IFN-β: Clinical use in relapsed, remitting multiple sclerosis. IFN-γ: May be protective in development of GVHD. May inhibit IL-6 mediated cell growth. Trials with cyclosporine to induce autologous graft-versus-host syndrome are currently being investigated. Has been used in patients with chronic granulomatous disease and idiopathic pulmonary fibrosis.	Hyperpyrexia, flulike symptoms, malaise, fatigue, chills, headache, myalgias, and hyperlipidemia. Neurologic toxicity can be seen with depression, agitation, insomnia, and seizures. Cytopenia, arrhythmia, and elevated transaminases can also be seen.
IL-11	Mild activity in chemotherapy-induced thrombocytopenia. Limited clinical application, no completed studies on use in aplastic anemia, MDS, or immune-related thrombocytopenia. Use of lower dose IL-11 is currently under investigation for use in inflammatory bowel disease and psoriasis.	Myalgias, arthralgias, fatigue, lower extremity edema, treatment-related anemia (secondary to increased plasma volume), and rarely arrhythmia. There is also increased levels of acute phase reactants such as fibrinogen, C-reactive protein, and haptoglobin.
Thrombopoietin (TPO)	Pegylated recombinant human megakaryocyte growth and development factor (truncated TPO) generated neutralizing antibodies causing thrombocytopenia in some patients. Recombinant human TPO in early trials was generally well tolerated with rare and transient antibody formation, but true clinical benefit has yet to be established. May eventually find a role as a research tool to expand early progenitor/stem cells in vitro.	Initial studies of TPO showed the development of neutralizing antibodies to endogenous regulatory proteins worsening thrombocytopenia.
Tumor necrosis factor α (TNF-α)	Remains investigational in humans with severe toxicity when given systemically. Good preliminary results when used via isolated limb perfusion in patients with sarcoma or melanoma, with up to a 51% response rate allowing limb salvage ~80% of time in these patients. Animal studies suggest direct cytotoxicity against malignant cells acting via immune mediation, and vascular changes.	Hyperpyrexia, severe hypotension limiting systemic administration.
Keratinocyte growth factor (KGF)	Exciting murine data show that administration of human recombinant KGF can decrease gut GVHD while preserving graft-versus-leukemia effect. May improve wound healing. Modulation of KGF may be used in the future as a treatment modality in prostate cancer.	Unknown.
Monocyte/Macrophage Colony Stimulating Factor (M-CSF)	Currently being investigated with phase I protocols for effectiveness in renal cell carcinoma, melanoma, other malignancies and severe fungal infections.	Malaise, iritis, periorbital inflammation, thrombocytopenia.
Stem Cell Factor (SCF)	Phase I studies in patients with metastatic lung and breast cancer showed in vitro hematopoietic progenitor stimulation but no clear clinical benefit in blood count recovery. Use of SCF with G-CSF to mobilize stem cells in phase III trials reduced the number of aphereses needed by half when compared with G-CSF alone. Modest trilineage response in phase I trials in patients with aplastic anemia.	Allergy-like reaction including respiratory difficulties and uticarial rash because of mast cell degranulation. Aggressive premedication ameliorates reaction.

(continued)

Table 104-7 Clinical Cytokine Application—(continued)

Cytokine	Clinical Indications/New Directions	Clinical Toxicity
IL-6	Preclinical data held promise as a thrombopoietic factor. Disappointing clinical results secondary to dose limitation below calculated effectiveness because of severe toxicity. No current clinical benefit when used as an anti-tumor agent in phase I-III trials.	Hyperpyrexia, chills, malaise, fatigue, treatment-related anemia (secondary to increased plasma volume), hepatotoxicity, and cardiac arrhythmia. There is also increased levels of acute phase reactants such as fibrinogen. C-reactive protein, and haptoglobin.
IL-12	Phase I study in patients with HIV and malignancy show increased levels of IFN-γ. Anti-tumor effect being studied currently in many types of malignancies with phase II studies.	Oral stomatitis, transient hepatic dysfunction.

NOTE: AML, acute myeloid leukemia; ARA-c, cystosine arabinoside; MDS, myelodysplastic syndrome; IL, interleukin; BMT, bone marrow transplantation; ARDS, acute respiratory distress syndrome; CML, chronic myeloid leukemia; HTLV, human T-cell leukemia; GVHD, graft-versus-host disease.

ACKNOWLEDGMENT

Dr. Francis Ruscetti and Dr. Jonathan Keller contributed this chapter in the 14th edition and portions of their chapter have been retained here.

BIBLIOGRAPHY

BJORNSON CR et al: Turning brain into blood: A hematopoietic fate adopted by adult neural stem cells in vivo. Science 283:534, 1999

ORKIN SH: Hematopoiesis: How does it happen? Curr Opin Cell Biol 7:870, 1995

QUESENBERRY PJ, BECKER PS: Stem cell homing: Rolling, crawling, and nesting. Proc Natl Acad Sci USA 95:15155, 1998

QUESENBERRY P et al: Chiaroscuro hematopoietic stem cell. Trans Am Clin Climatol Assoc 109:19, 1998

SHIVDASANI RA, ORKIN SH: The transcriptional control of hematopoiesis. Blood 87:4025, 1996

WARD AC et al: The Jak-Stat pathway in normal and perturbed hematopoiesis. Blood 95:19, 2000

105 *John W. Adamson*

IRON DEFICIENCY AND OTHER HYPOPROLIFERATIVE ANEMIAS

Anemias associated with normocytic and normochromic red cells and an inappropriately low reticulocyte response (reticulocyte index <2.5) are *hypoproliferative anemias*. This category includes early iron deficiency (before hypochromic microcytic red cells develop), acute and chronic inflammation (including many malignancies), renal disease, hypometabolic states such as protein malnutrition and endocrine deficiencies, and anemias from marrow damage. Marrow damage states are discussed in Chap. 109. Hypoproliferative anemias are the most common anemias and anemia associated with acute and chronic inflammation is the most common of these. The anemia of acute and chronic inflammation, like iron deficiency, is related in part to abnormal iron metabolism. The anemias associated with renal disease, inflammation, cancer, and hypometabolic states are characterized by an abnormal erythropoietin response to anemia.

IRON METABOLISM

Iron is a critical element in the function of all cells, although the amount of iron required by individual tissues varies during development. At the same time, the body must protect itself from free iron, which is highly toxic in that it participates in chemical reactions that generate free radicals such as singlet O_2 or OH^-. Consequently, elaborate mechanisms have evolved that allow iron to be made available for critical physiologic functions while at the same time conserving this element and handling it in such a way that toxicity is avoided.

The major role of iron in mammals is to carry O_2 as part of the heme protein that, in turn, is part of hemoglobin. O_2 also is bound by a heme protein in muscle, myoglobin. Iron also is a critical element in iron-containing enzymes, including the cytochrome system in mitochondria. Iron distribution in the body is shown in Table 105-1. Without iron, cells lose their capacity for electron transport and energy metabolism; in erythroid cells hemoglobin synthesis is impaired, resulting in anemia and reduced O_2 delivery to tissue.

THE IRON CYCLE IN HUMANS Figure 105-1 outlines the major pathways of internal iron exchange in humans. Iron absorbed from the diet or released from stores circulates in the plasma bound to *transferrin*, the iron transport protein. Transferrin is a bilobed glycoprotein with two iron binding sites. Transferrin that carries iron exists in two forms—*monoferric* (one iron atom) or *diferric* (two iron atoms). The turnover (half-clearance time) of transferrin-bound iron is very rapid—typically 60 to 90 min. Because the overwhelming majority of iron transported by transferrin is delivered to the erythroid marrow, the clearance time of transferrin-bound iron from the circulation is affected most by the plasma iron level and the activity of the erythroid marrow. When erythropoiesis is markedly stimulated, the pool of erythroid cells requiring iron increases and the clearance time of iron from the circulation decreases. The half-clearance time of iron in the presence of iron deficiency is as short as 10-15 min; this value reflects the limits of iron delivery as a function of the cardiac output going to the bone marrow. With suppression of the erythroid marrow, the plasma iron level typically is increased and the half-clearance time is prolonged to as much as several hours. Normally, the iron bound to transferrin turns over 10 to 20 times per day. Assuming a normal plasma iron level of 80 to 100 μg/dL, the amount of iron passing through the transferrin pool is 20 to 24 mg/d.

The iron-transferrin complex circulates in the plasma until the iron-carrying transferrin interacts with specific *transferrin receptors* on the surface of marrow erythroid cells. Diferric transferrin has the highest affinity for transferrin receptors; apotransferrin (transferrin not carrying iron) has very little affinity. While transferrin receptors are found on cells in many tissues within the body—and all cells at some time during development will display transferrin receptors—the cell having the greatest number of receptors (300,000 to 400,000/cell) is the developing erythroblast.

Once the iron-bearing transferrin interacts with its receptor, the iron-transferrin-receptor complex is internalized via clathrin-coated pits and transported to an acidic endosome, where the iron is released at the low pH. The iron is then made available for heme synthesis while the transferrin-receptor complex is recycled to the surface of the cell, where the bulk of the transferrin is released back into the circulation and the transferrin receptor reanchors into the cell membrane. At this point a certain amount of the transferrin receptor protein may be released into circulation. Within the erythroid cell, iron that is in excess of the amount needed for hemoglobin synthesis binds to a stor-

Table 105-1 Body Iron Distribution

	Iron Content, mg	
	Adult Male (80 kg)	Adult Female (60 kg)
Hemoglobin	2500	1700
Myoglobin/enzymes	500	300
Transferrin iron	3	3
Iron stores	600–1000	0–300

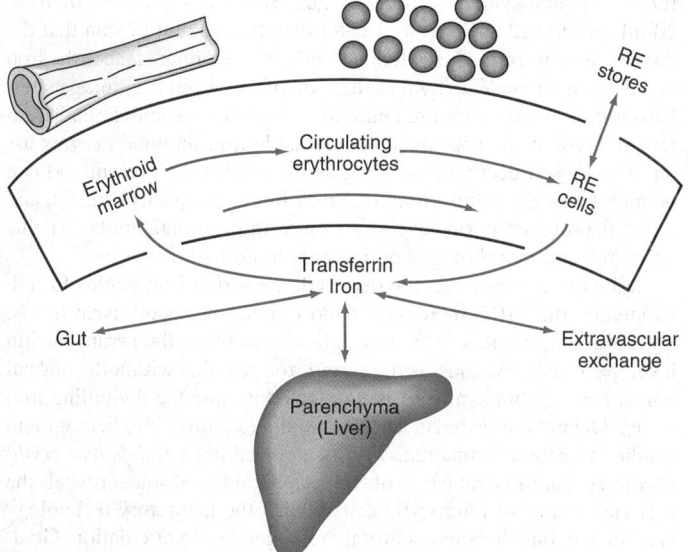

FIGURE 105-1 Internal iron exchange. Normally about 80% of iron passing through the plasma transferrin pool is recycled from broken down red cells. Absorption of about 1 mg/d is required from the diet in men, 1.4 mg/d in women to maintain homeostasis. As long as transferrin saturation is maintained between 20 to 60% and erythropoiesis is not increased, iron stores are not required. However, in the event of blood loss, dietary iron deficiency, or inadequate iron absorption, up to 40 mg/d of iron can be mobilized from stores.

age protein, *apoferritin*, forming *ferritin*. This mechanism of iron exchange also takes place in other cells of the body expressing transferrin receptors, especially liver parenchymal cells where the iron can be incorporated into heme-containing enzymes or stored. The iron incorporated into hemoglobin subsequently enters the circulation as new red cells are released from the bone marrow. The iron is then part of the red cell mass and will not become available for reutilization until the red cell dies.

In a normal individual, the average red cell life span is 120 days. Thus, 0.8 to 1.0% of red cells turn over each day. At the end of its life span, the red cell is recognized as senescent by the cells of the *reticuloendothelial (RE) system*, and the cell undergoes phagocytosis. Once within the RE cell, the hemoglobin from the ingested red cell is broken down, the globin and other proteins are returned to the amino acid pool, and the iron is shuttled back to the surface of the RE cell, where it is presented to circulating transferrin. The "harvesting" of iron from senescent red cells is both efficient and rapid, with newly recycled iron appearing in the circulation within 10 min of ingestion of the red cell. It is the efficient and highly conserved recycling of iron from senescent red cells that supports steady state (and even mildly accelerated) erythropoiesis.

Since each milliliter of red cells contains 1 mg of elemental iron, the amount of iron needed to replace those red cells lost through senescence amounts to 16 to 20 mg/day (assuming an adult with a red cell mass of 2 L). Any additional iron required for daily red cell production comes from the diet. Normally, an adult male will need to absorb at least 1 mg of elemental iron daily to meet needs, while females in the childbearing years will need to absorb an average of 1.4 mg/d. However, to achieve a maximum proliferative erythroid marrow response to anemia, additional iron must be available. With markedly stimulated erythropoiesis, demands for iron are increased by as much as six- to eightfold. With hemolytic anemias, the rate of red cell destruction is increased, but the iron recovered from the red cells is efficiently reutilized for hemoglobin synthesis. In contrast, with blood loss anemia the rate of red cell production is limited by the amount of iron that can be mobilized from ferritin and hemosiderin stores. Typically, the rate of mobilization under these circumstances will not support red cell production more than 2.5 to 3 times normal. If the delivery of iron to the stimulated marrow is suboptimal, the marrow's proliferative response is blunted and normal hemoglobin synthesis is im-

paired. The result is a hypoproliferative marrow accompanied by microcytic, hypochromic anemia.

While blood loss or hemolysis places a demand for iron to be supplied to the erythroid marrow, other conditions such as inflammation interfere with iron release from stores and can result in a rapid decrease in the serum iron (see below).

NUTRITIONAL IRON BALANCE The balance of iron metabolism in the organism is tightly controlled and designed to conserve iron for reutilization. There is no excretory pathway for iron, and the only mechanisms by which iron is lost from the body are blood loss (via gastrointestinal bleeding, menses, or other forms of bleeding) and the loss of epidermal cells from the skin and gut. Normally, the only route by which iron comes into the body is via absorption from food (dietary iron intake) or from medicinal iron taken orally. Iron may also enter the body through red cell transfusions or injection of iron complexes. The margin between the amount of iron available for absorption and the requirement for iron in growing infants and the adult female is narrow. The narrowness of this margin accounts for the great prevalence of iron deficiency worldwide—currently estimated at one-half billion people.

External iron exchange—the amount of iron required from the diet to replace losses—averages about 10% of body iron content a year in the male and 15% in women of childbearing age, equivalent to 1.0 and 1.4 mg of elemental iron daily, respectively. Dietary iron content is closely related to total caloric intake (approximately 6 mg of elemental iron per 1000 calories). Iron bioavailability is affected by the nature of the foodstuff with heme iron (e.g., red meat) being most readily absorbed. In the United States, the average iron intake in an adult male is 15 mg/d with 6% absorption; for the average female, the daily intake is 11 mg/d with 12% absorption. An individual with iron deficiency can increase iron absorption to about 20% of the iron present in a meat-containing diet but only 5 to 10% of the iron in a vegetarian diet. As a result, nearly one-third of the female population in the United States has virtually no iron stores. Vegetarians are at an additional disadvantage because certain foodstuffs that include phytates and phosphates reduce iron absorption by about 50%. When ionizable iron salts are given together with food, the amount of iron absorbed is reduced. This is particularly true with iron in the ferric state. When the percentage of iron absorbed from individual food items is compared with the percentage for an equivalent amount of ferrous salt, iron in vegetables is only about one-twentieth as available, egg iron one-eighth, liver iron one-half, and heme iron one-half to two-thirds. Therefore, liver and heme iron are absorbed nearly as well as iron salt added to food, while the iron in vegetables and eggs is much less available.

Infants, children, and adolescents may be unable to maintain normal iron balance because of the demands of body growth and lower dietary intake of iron. In pregnancy during the last two trimesters, daily iron requirements increase to 5 to 6 mg. That is the reason why iron supplements are almost universally prescribed for pregnant women in developed countries. Enthusiasm for supplementing foods such as bread and cereals with iron has waned in the face of concerns that the very prevalent hemochromatosis gene would result in an unacceptable risk of iron overload.

Iron absorption takes place largely in the proximal small intestine and is a carefully regulated process. For absorption, iron must be taken up by the luminal cell. That process is facilitated by the acidic contents of the stomach, which maintains the iron in solution. At the brush border of the absorptive cell, the ferric iron is converted to the ferrous form by a ferrireductase. Transport across the membrane is accomplished by divalent metal transporter 1 (DMT 1, also known as Nramp 2 or DCT 1). DMT 1 is a general cation transporter. Once iron is inside the gut cell, the iron may be stored as ferritin or transported through the cell to be released at the basolateral surface to plasma transferrin. It is likely another transporter acts here in concert with hephaestin, another ferroxidase. Hephaestin is similar to ceruloplasmin, the copper-carrying protein.

Iron absorption is influenced by a number of physiologic states. Erythroid hyperplasia, for example, stimulates iron absorption, even in the face of normal or increased iron stores. Patients with anemias associated with high levels of ineffective erythropoiesis absorb excess amounts of dietary iron. Over time, this may lead to iron overload and tissue damage. In iron deficiency iron is much more efficiently absorbed from a given diet while the contrary is true in the presence of iron overload. This is possibly mediated through signals that become fixed before the jejunal crypt cell migrates up the villus to become an absorptive cell. The normal individual can reduce iron absorption in situations of excessive intake or medicinal iron intake; however, while the percent of iron absorbed goes down, the absolute amount goes up. This accounts for the acute iron toxicity occasionally seen when children ingest large numbers of iron tablets. Under these circumstances, the amount of iron absorbed exceeds the transferrin binding capacity of the plasma, resulting in free iron that affects critical organs such as cardiac muscle cells.

IRON DEFICIENCY ANEMIA

STAGES OF IRON DEFICIENCY Iron deficiency anemia is the condition in which there is anemia and clear evidence of iron deficiency. However, it is worthwhile to consider the steps by which iron deficiency occurs (Fig. 105-2). These can be divided into three stages. The first stage is *negative iron balance*, in which the demands for (or losses of) iron exceed the body's ability to absorb iron from the diet. This stage can result from a number of physiologic mechanisms including blood loss, pregnancy (in which the demands for red cell production by the fetus outstrip the mother's ability to provide iron), rapid growth spurts in the adolescent, or inadequate dietary iron intake. Most commonly, the growth needs of the fetus or rapidly growing child exceed the individual's ability to absorb the iron necessary

for hemoglobin synthesis from the diet. Blood loss in excess of 10 to 20 mL of red cells per day is greater than the amount of iron that the gut can absorb from a normal diet. Under these circumstances the iron deficit must be made up by mobilization of iron from RE storage sites. During this period measurements of iron stores—such as the serum ferritin level or the appearance of stainable iron on bone marrow aspirations—will decrease. As long as iron stores are present and can be mobilized, the serum iron, total iron-binding capacity (TIBC), and red cell protoporphyrin levels remain within normal limits. At this stage, red cell morphology and indices are normal.

When iron stores become depleted, the serum iron begins to fall. Gradually, the TIBC increases, as do red cell protoporphyrin levels. By definition, marrow iron stores are absent when the serum ferritin level <15 μg/L. As long as the serum iron remains within the normal range, hemoglobin synthesis is unaffected despite the dwindling iron stores. Once the transferrin saturation falls to 15 to 20%, hemoglobin synthesis becomes impaired. This is a period of *iron-deficient erythropoiesis*. Careful evaluation of the peripheral blood smear reveals the first appearance of microcytic cells, and if the laboratory technology is available, one finds hypochromic reticulocytes in circulation. Gradually, the hemoglobin and hematocrit begin to fall, reflecting *iron deficiency anemia*. The transferrin saturation at this point is 10 to 15%.

When moderate anemia is present (hemoglobin 10–13 g/dL), the bone marrow remains hypoproliferative. With more severe anemia (hemoglobin 7–8 g/dL), hypochromia and microcytosis become more prominent, misshapen red cells (poikilocytes) appear on the blood smear as cigar or pencil-shaped forms and target cells, and the erythroid marrow becomes increasingly ineffective. Consequently, with severe prolonged iron deficiency anemia, erythroid hyperplasia of the marrow develops rather than hypoproliferation.

CAUSES OF IRON DEFICIENCY Conditions that increase demand for iron, increase iron loss, or decrease iron intake, absorption, or use can produce iron deficiency (Table 105-2).

CLINICAL PRESENTATION OF IRON DEFICIENCY Certain clinical conditions carry an increased likelihood of iron deficiency. Pregnancy, adolescence, periods of rapid growth, and an intermittent history of blood loss of any kind should alert the clinician to possible iron deficiency. A cardinal rule is that the appearance of iron deficiency in an adult male means gastrointestinal blood loss until proven otherwise. Signs related to iron deficiency depend upon the severity and chronicity of the anemia in addition to the usual signs of anemia—fatigue, pallor, and reduced exercise capacity. *Cheilosis* (fissures at the corners of the mouth) and *koilonychia* (spooning of the fingernails) are signs of advanced tissue iron deficiency. The diagnosis of iron deficiency is typically based on laboratory results.

LABORATORY IRON STUDIES Serum Iron and Total Iron-Binding Capacity The serum iron level represents the amount of circulating iron bound to transferrin. The TIBC is an indirect measure of the circulating transferrin. The normal range for the serum iron is 50 to 150 μg/dL; the normal range for TIBC is 300 to 360 μg/dL. Transferrin saturation, which is normally 25 to 50%, is obtained by

	Normal	Negative iron balance	Iron-deficient erythropoiesis	Iron-deficiency anemia
Iron stores				
Erythron iron				
Marrow iron stores	1-3+	0-1+	0	0
Serum ferritin (μg/L)	50-200	<20	<15	<15
TIBC (μg/dL)	300-360	>360	>380	>400
SI (μg/dL)	50-150	NL	<50	<30
Saturation (%)	30-50	NL	<20	<10
Marrow sideroblasts (%)	40-60	NL	<10	<10
RBC protoporphyrin (μg/dL)	30-50	NL	>100	>200
RBC morphology	NL	NL	NL	Microcytic/ hypochromic

FIGURE 105-2 Laboratory studies in the evolution of iron deficiency. Measurements of marrow iron stores, serum ferritin, and total iron-binding capacity (TIBC) are sensitive to early iron-store depletion. Iron-deficient erythropoiesis is recognized from additional abnormalities in the serum iron (SI), percent transferrin saturation, the pattern of marrow sideroblasts, and the red cell protoporphyrin level. Patients with iron deficiency anemia demonstrate all the same abnormalities plus hypochromic microcytic anemia. *(From Hillman and Finch, with permission)*

Table 105-2 Causes of Iron Deficiency

Increased demand for iron and/or hematopoiesis
  rapid growth in infancy or adolescence
  pregnancy
  erythropoietin therapy
Increased iron loss
  chronic blood loss
  menses
  acute blood loss
  blood donation
  phlebotomy as treatment for polycythemia vera
Decreased iron intake, absorption, or use
  inadequate diet
  malabsorption from disease (sprue, Crohn's disease)
  malabsorption from surgery (post-gastrectomy)
  acute or chronic inflammation

FIGURE 105-3 Serum ferritin levels as a function of sex and age. Iron store depletion and iron deficiency are accompanied by a fall in serum ferritin level below 20 μg/L. *(From Hillman and Ault)*

Table 105-3   Iron Store Measurements

Iron Stores	Marrow Iron Stain, 0–4+	Serum Ferritin, μg/L
0	0	<15
1–300 mg	Trace to 1+	15–30
300–800 mg	2+	30–60
800–1000 mg	3+	60–150
1–2 g	4+	>150
Iron overload	—	>500–1000

the following formula: serum iron × 100 ÷ TIBC. Iron deficiency states are associated with saturation levels below 18%. In evaluating the serum iron, the clinician should be aware that there is a diurnal variation in the value. A transferrin saturation rate of >50% indicates that a disproportionate amount of the iron bound to transferrin is being delivered to nonerythroid tissues. If this condition persists for an extended time, tissue iron overload may occur.

Serum Ferritin   Free iron is toxic to cells, and the body has established an elaborate set of protective mechanisms to bind iron in various tissue compartments. Within cells, iron is stored complexed to protein as ferritin or hemosiderin. Apoferritin binds to free ferrous iron and stores it in the ferric state. As ferritin accumulates within cells of the RE system, protein aggregates are formed as hemosiderin. Iron in ferritin or hemosiderin can be extracted for release by the RE cells although hemosiderin is less readily available. Under steady state conditions, the serum ferritin level correlates with total body iron stores; thus, the serum ferritin level is the most convenient laboratory test to estimate iron stores. The normal value for ferritin varies according to the age and gender of the individual (Fig. 105-3). Adult males have serum ferritin values averaging about 100 μg/L, while adult females have levels averaging 30 μg/L. As iron stores are depleted, the serum ferritin falls to <15 μg/L. Such levels are virtually always diagnostic of absent body iron stores.

Evaluation of Bone Marrow Iron Stores   Although RE cell iron stores can also be estimated from the iron stain of a bone marrow aspirate or biopsy, the measurement of serum ferritin has largely supplanted bone marrow aspirates for determination of storage iron (Table 105-3). The serum ferritin level is a better indicator of iron overload than the marrow iron stain. However, in addition to storage iron the marrow iron stain provides information about the effective delivery of iron to developing erythroblasts. Normally, 40 to 60% of developing erythroblasts—called *sideroblasts*—will have visible ferritin granules in their cytoplasm. This represents iron in excess of that needed for hemoglobin synthesis. In states in which release of iron from storage sites is blocked, RE iron will be detectable, and there will be few or no sideroblasts. In the myelodysplastic syndromes, mitochondrial dysfunction occurs, and accumulation of iron in mitochondria appears in a necklace fashion around the nucleus of the erythroblast. Such cells are referred to as *ringed sideroblasts*.

Red Cell Protoporphyrin Levels   Protoporphyrin is an intermediate in the pathway to heme synthesis. Under conditions in which heme synthesis is impaired, protoporphyrin ac-

cumulates within the red cell. This can reflect an inadequate iron supply to erythroid precursors to support hemoglobin synthesis. Normal values are less than 30 μg/dL of red cells. In iron deficiency, values in excess of 100 μg/dL are seen. The most common causes of increased red cell protoporphyrin levels are absolute or relative iron deficiency and lead poisoning.

Serum Levels of Transferrin Receptor Protein   Because erythroid cells have the highest numbers of transferrin receptors on their surface of any cell in the body, and because transferrin receptor protein (TRP) is released by cells into the circulation, serum levels of TRP reflect the total erythroid marrow mass. Another condition in which TRP levels are elevated is absolute iron deficiency. Normal values are 4 to 9 μg/L determined by immunoassay. This laboratory test is becoming increasingly available and has been proposed to measure the serial expansion of the erythroid marrow in response to recombinant erythropoietin therapy.

DIFFERENTIAL DIAGNOSIS   Other than iron deficiency, only three conditions need to be considered in the differential diagnosis of a hypochromic microcytic anemia (Table 105-4). The first is inherited defects in globin chain synthesis: the thalassemias. These are differentiated from iron deficiency most readily by serum iron values, since it is characteristic to have at least normal—if not increased—serum iron levels and transferrin saturation with the thalassemias.

The second condition is chronic inflammatory disease with inadequate iron supply to the erythroid marrow. The distinction between true iron deficiency anemia and the anemia associated with chronic inflammatory states is among the most common diagnostic problems encountered by clinicians (see below). Usually the anemia of chronic disease is normocytic and normochromic. Again, the iron values usually make the differential diagnosis clear, as the ferritin level is normal or increased and the TIBC is typically below normal.

Finally, the myelodysplastic syndromes comprise the third condition. Some patients with myelodysplasia have impaired hemoglobin synthesis with mitochondrial dysfunction resulting in impaired iron incorporation into heme. The iron values again reveal normal stores and more than an adequate supply to the marrow, despite the microcytosis and hypochromia.

℞ **TREATMENT**   The severity and cause of iron deficiency anemia will determine the appropriate approach to treatment. As an example, symptomatic elderly patients with severe iron deficiency anemia and cardiovascular instability may require red cell transfusions. Younger individuals who have compensated for their anemia can be

Table 105-4   Diagnosis of Microcytic Anemia

Tests	Iron Deficiency	Inflammation	Thalassemia	Sideroblastic Anemia
Smear	Micro/hypo	Normal micro/hypo	Micro/hypo with targeting	Variable
SI	<30	<50	Normal to high	Normal to high
TIBC	>360	<300	Normal	Normal
Percent saturation	<10	10–20	30–80	30–80
Ferritin (μg/L)	<15	30–200	50–300	50–300
Hemoglobin pattern	Normal	Normal	Abnormal	Normal

NOTE: SI, serum iron; TIBC, total iron-binding capacity

treated more conservatively with iron replacement. The foremost issue for the latter patient is the precise identification of the cause of the iron deficiency.

For the majority of cases of iron deficiency (pregnant women, growing children and adolescents, patients with infrequent episodes of bleeding, and those with inadequate dietary intake of iron), oral iron therapy will suffice. For patients with unusual blood loss or malabsorption, specific diagnostic tests and appropriate therapy take priority. Once the diagnosis of iron deficiency anemia and its cause is made, and a therapeutic approach is charted, there are three major approaches.

Red Cell Transfusion Transfusion therapy is reserved for those individuals who have symptoms of anemia, cardiovascular instability, and continued and excessive blood loss from whatever source, and those who require immediate intervention. The management of these patients is less related to the iron deficiency than it is to the consequences of the severe anemia. Not only do transfusions correct the anemia acutely, but the transfused red cells provide a source of iron for reutilization, assuming they are not lost through continued bleeding. Transfusion therapy will stabilize the patient while other options are reviewed.

Oral Iron Therapy In the patient with established iron deficiency anemia who is asymptomatic, treatment with oral iron is usually adequate. Multiple preparations are available ranging from simple iron salts to complex iron compounds designed for sustained release throughout the small intestine (Table 105-5). While the various preparations contain different amounts of iron, they are generally all absorbed well and are effective in treatment. Some come with other compounds designed to enhance iron absorption, such as citric acid. It is not clear whether the benefits of such compounds justify their costs. Typically, for iron replacement therapy up to 300 mg of elemental iron per day is given, usually as three or four iron tablets (each containing 50 to 65 mg elemental iron) given over the course of the day. Ideally, oral iron preparations should be taken on an empty stomach, since foods may inhibit iron absorption. Some patients with gastric disease or prior gastric surgery require special treatment with iron solutions, since the retention capacity of the stomach may be reduced. The retention capacity is necessary for dissolving the shell of the iron tablet before the release of iron. A dose of 200 to 300 mg of elemental iron per day should result in the absorption of up to 50 mg of iron per day. This supports a red cell production level of two to three times normal in an individual with a normally functioning marrow and appropriate erythropoietin stimulus. However, as the hemoglobin level rises, erythropoietin stimulation decreases, and the amount of iron absorbed is reduced. The goal of therapy in individuals with iron deficiency anemia is not only to repair the anemia, but also to provide stores of at least ½ to 1 g of iron. Sustained treatment for a period of 6 to 12 months after correction of the anemia will be necessary to achieve this.

Of the complications of oral iron therapy, gastrointestinal distress is the most prominent and is seen in 15 to 20% of patients. For these patients, abdominal pain, nausea, vomiting, or constipation often lead to noncompliance. Although small doses of iron or iron preparations with delayed release may help somewhat, the gastrointestinal side effects are a major impediment to the effective treatment of a number of patients.

The response to iron therapy varies, depending upon the erythropoietin stimulus and the rate of absorption. Typically, the reticulocyte count should begin to increase within 4 to 7 days after initiation of therapy and peak at 1½ weeks. The absence of a response may be due to poor adsorption, noncompliance (which is common), or a confounding diagnosis. If iron deficiency persists, it may be necessary to switch to parenteral iron therapy.

Parenteral Iron Therapy Intramuscular or intravenous iron can be given to patients who are unable to tolerate oral iron, whose needs are relatively acute, or who need iron on an ongoing basis, usually due to persistent gastrointestinal blood loss. Currently, the intravenous route is used routinely. Parenteral iron use has been rising rapidly in the last several years with the recognition that recombinant erythropoietin therapy induces a large demand for iron—a demand that frequently cannot be met through the physiologic release of iron from RE sources. Concern has been raised about the safety of parenteral iron—particularly iron dextran. The serious adverse reaction rate to intravenous iron dextran is 0.7%. Fortunately, newer iron complexes are becoming available in the United States that are likely to have an even lower rate of adverse effects. The most recently approved preparation is intravenous iron gluconate (Ferrlecit).

There are two approaches to the use of parenteral iron: one is to administer the total dose of iron required to correct the hemoglobin deficit and provide the patient with at least 500 mg of iron stores; the second is to give repeated small doses of parenteral iron over a protracted period. The latter approach is common in dialysis centers, where it is not unusual for 100 mg of elemental iron to be given weekly for 10 weeks to augment the erythropoietic response to recombinant erythropoietin therapy. The amount of iron needed by an individual patient is calculated by the following formula: body weight (kg) $\times$ 2.3 $\times$ (15 $-$ patient's hemoglobin, g/dL) + 500 or 1000 mg (for stores).

In administering intravenous iron, anaphylaxis is always a concern. Anaphylaxis is less common with the newer preparations. The factors that have correlated with a serious anaphylactic-like reaction include a history of multiple allergies or a prior allergic reaction to dextran (in the case of iron dextran). Generalized symptoms appearing several days after the infusion of a large dose of iron can include arthralgias, skin rash, and low-grade fever. This may be dose-related, but it does not preclude the further use of parenteral iron in the patient. To date, patients with sensitivity to iron dextran have been safely treated with iron gluconate. If a large dose of iron dextran is to be given (>100 mg) the iron preparation should be diluted in 5% dextrose in water or 0.9% NaCl solution. The iron solution can then be infused over a 60 to 90 min period (for larger doses) or at a rate convenient for the attending nurse or physician. While a test dose (25 mg) of parenteral iron is recommended, in reality a slow infusion of a larger dose of parenteral iron solution will afford the same kind of early warning as a separately injected test dose. Early in the infusion of iron, if chest pain, wheezing, a fall in blood pressure, or other systemic manifestations occur, the infusion of iron—whether as a large solution or a test dose—should be interrupted immediately.

OTHER HYPOPROLIFERATIVE ANEMIAS

In addition to mild to moderate iron deficiency anemia, the hypoproliferative anemias can be divided into four categories: (1) chronic inflammation/infection; (2) renal disease; (3) endocrine and nutritional deficiencies (hypometabolic states); and (4) marrow damage (Chap. 109). With chronic inflammation, renal disease, or hypometabolism, endogenous erythropoietin production is inadequate for the degree of anemia observed. For the anemia of chronic inflammation (anemia of chronic disease), the erythroid marrow also responds inadequately to stimulation in part due to defects in iron reutilization. As a result of the lack of adequate erythropoietin stimulation, an examination of the peripheral blood smear will disclose only an occasional polychromat-

Table 105-5   Oral Iron Preparations

Generic Name	Tablet (Iron Content), mg	Elixir (Iron Content), mg in 5 mL
Ferrous sulfate	325 (65)	300 (60)
	195 (39)	90 (18)
Extended release	525 (105)	
Ferrous fumarate	325 (107)	
	195 (64)	100 (33)
Ferrous gluconate	325 (39)	300 (35)
Polysaccharide iron	150 (150)	100 (100)
	50 (50)	

FIGURE 105-4 Suppression of erythropoiesis by inflammatory cytokines. Neoplasms and bacterial infections through the release of TNF and IFN-β suppress erythropoietin production, release of iron from reticuloendothelial stores, and the proliferation of erythroid progenitors (BFU/CFU-E). The mediators in patients with vasculitis and rheumatoid arthritis include IL-1 and IFN-γ. The blue arrows indicated sites of inflammatory cytokine inhibitory effects.

ophilic (shift) reticulocyte. In the cases of iron deficiency or marrow damage, appropriate elevations in endogenous erythropoietin levels are typically found, and "shift" reticulocytes will be present on the blood smear.

ANEMIA OF ACUTE AND CHRONIC INFLAMMATION/INFECTION (THE ANEMIA OF CHRONIC DISEASE)

The anemia of chronic disease—which encompasses inflammation, infection, tissue injury, and conditions associated with the release of proinflammatory cytokines (such as cancer)—is one of the most common forms of anemia seen clinically and is probably the most important in the differential diagnosis of iron deficiency, since many of the features of the anemia are brought about by inadequate iron delivery to the marrow, despite the presence of normal or increased iron stores. This is reflected by a low serum iron, increased red cell protoporphyrin, a hypoproliferative marrow, transferrin saturation in the range of 15 to 20%, and a normal or increased serum ferritin. The serum ferritin values are often the most distinguishing feature between true iron deficiency anemia and the iron-deficient erythropoiesis associated with inflammation. Typically, serum ferritin values increase three-fold over basal levels in the face of inflammation. All of these changes are due to the effects of inflammatory cytokines at several levels of erythropoiesis (Fig. 105-4). IL-1 directly decreases erythropoietin production in response to anemia. IL-1, acting through accessory cell release of IFN-γ, suppresses the response of the erythroid marrow to erythropoietin—an effect that can be overcome by increased erythropoietin administration in vitro and in vivo. In addition, tumor necrosis factor (TNF), acting through the release of IFN-β by marrow stromal cells, also suppresses the response to erythropoietin; several of these same cytokines, acting in concert, block the release of iron from RE storage sites. The overall result is a chronic hypoproliferative anemia with classic changes in iron metabolism. The anemia is further compounded by a mild to moderate shortening in red cell survival.

With chronic inflammation/infection, the primary disease will determine the severity and characteristics of the anemia. For instance, many patients with cancer also have anemia that is typically normocytic and normochromic. In contrast, patients with long-standing active rheumatoid arthritis or chronic infections such as tuberculosis will have a microcytic, hypochromic anemia. In both cases, the bone marrow is hypoproliferative, but the differences in red cell indices reflect differences in the availability of iron for hemoglobin synthesis. Occasionally, conditions associated with chronic inflammation are also associated with chronic blood loss. Under these circumstances, a bone marrow aspirate stained for iron may be necessary to rule out absolute iron deficiency. However, the administration of iron in this case will correct the iron deficiency component of the anemia and leave the inflammatory component unaffected.

The anemia associated with acute infection or inflammation is typically mild, but becomes more pronounced over time. Acute infection can produce a fall in hemoglobin levels of 2 to 3 g/dL within 1 or 2 days; this is largely related to the hemolysis of red cells near the end of their natural life span. The fever and cytokines released exert a selective pressure against cells with more limited capacity to maintain the red cell membrane. In most individuals the mild anemia is reasonably well tolerated, and symptoms, if present, are associated with the underlying disease. Occasionally, in patients with preexisting cardiac disease, moderate anemia (hemoglobin 10–11 g/dL) may be associated with angina, exercise intolerance, and shortness of breath. The red cell indices vary from normocytic, normochromic to microcytic, hypochromic. The serum iron values tend to correlate with the red cell indices. The erythropoietic profile that distinguishes the anemia of inflammation from the other causes of hypoproliferative anemias is shown in Table 105-6.

ANEMIA OF RENAL DISEASE

Chronic renal failure is usually associated with a moderate to severe hypoproliferative anemia; the level of the anemia correlates with the severity of the renal failure. Red cells are typically normocytic and normochromic. Reticulocytes are decreased. The anemia is due to a failure to produce adequate amounts of erythropoietin and a reduction in red cell survival. In certain forms of acute renal failure, the correlation between the anemia and renal function is weaker. Patients with the hemolytic-uremic syndrome increase erythropoiesis in response to the hemolysis, despite renal failure requiring dialysis. Polycystic renal disease also shows a smaller degree of erythropoietin deficiency for a given level of renal failure. By contrast, patients with diabetes have more severe erythropoietin deficiency for a given level of renal failure.

Assessment of iron status provides information to distinguish the anemia of renal disease from the other forms of hypoproliferative anemia (Table 105-6) and to guide management. Patients with the anemia of renal disease usually present with normal serum iron, TIBC, and ferritin levels. However, those maintained on chronic hemodialysis may develop iron deficiency from blood loss through the dialysis procedure. Iron must be replenished in these patients to ensure an adequate response to erythropoietin therapy (see below).

ANEMIA IN HYPOMETABOLIC STATES

Patients who are starving, particularly for protein, and those with a variety of endocrine disorders that produce lower metabolic rates may develop a mild to moderate hypoproliferative anemia. The release of erythropoietin from the kidney is sensitive to the need for O_2, not just O_2 levels. Thus, erythropoietin production is triggered at lower levels of O_2 tension in disease states (such as hypothyroidism and starvation) where metabolic activity and thus O_2 demand is decreased.

Table 105-6 Diagnosis of Hypoproliferative Anemias

Tests	Iron Deficiency	Inflammation	Renal Disease	Hypometabolic States
Anemia	Mild to severe	Mild	Mild to severe	Mild
MCV (fL)	70–90	80–90	90	90
Morphology	Normo-microcytic	Normocytic	Normocytic	Normocytic
SI	<30	<50	Normal	Normal
TIBC	>360	<300	Normal	Normal
Saturation (%)	<10	10–20	Normal	Normal
Serum ferritin (μg/L)	<15	30–200	115–150	Normal
Iron stores	0	2–4+	1–4+	Normal

NOTE: MCV, mean corpuscular volume; SI, serum iron; TIBC, total iron-binding capacity

Endocrine Deficiency States   The difference in the levels of hemoglobin between men and women is related to the effects of androgen and estrogen on erythropoiesis. Testosterone and anabolic steroids augment erythropoiesis; castration and estrogen administration to males decrease erythropoiesis. Patients who are hypothyroid or have deficits in pituitary hormones also may develop a mild anemia. Pathogenesis may be complicated by other nutritional deficiencies as iron and folic acid absorption can be affected by these disorders. Usually, correction of the hormone deficiency reverses the anemia.

Anemia may be more severe in Addison's disease, depending on the level of thyroid and androgen hormone dysfunction; however, anemia may be masked by decreases in plasma volume. Once such patients are given cortisol and volume replacement, the hemoglobin level may fall rapidly. Mild anemia complicating hyperparathyroidism may be due to decreased erythropoietin production as a consequence of the renal effects of hypercalcemia or to impaired proliferation of erythroid progenitors.

Protein Starvation   Decreased dietary intake of protein may lead to mild to moderate hypoproliferative anemia; this form of anemia may be prevalent in the elderly. The anemia can be more severe in patients with a greater degree of starvation. In marasmus, where patients are both protein- and calorie-deficient, the release of erythropoietin is impaired in proportion to the reduction in metabolic rate; however, the degree of anemia may be masked by volume depletion and becomes apparent after refeeding. Deficiencies in other nutrients (iron, folate) may also complicate the clinical picture but may not be apparent at diagnosis. Changes in the erythrocyte indices on refeeding should prompt evaluation of iron, folate, and B$_{12}$ status.

Anemia in Liver Disease   A mild hypoproliferative anemia may develop in patients with chronic liver disease from nearly any cause. The peripheral blood smear may show burr cells and stomatocytes from the accumulation of excess cholesterol in the membrane from a deficiency of lecithin cholesterol acyltransferase. Red cell survival is shortened, and the production of erythropoietin is inadequate to compensate. In alcoholic liver disease, nutritional deficiencies can add complexity to the management. Folate deficiency from inadequate intake and iron deficiency from blood loss and inadequate intake can alter the red cell indices.

℞ TREATMENT   Many patients with hypoproliferative anemias experience recovery of normal hemoglobin levels when the underlying disease is appropriately treated. For those in whom such reversals are not possible—such as patients with end-stage renal failure, cancer, and chronic inflammatory diseases—symptomatic anemia requires treatment. The two major forms of treatment are transfusions and erythropoietin.

Transfusions   Thresholds for transfusion should be altered based on the patient's symptoms. In general, patients without serious underlying cardiovascular or pulmonary disease can tolerate hemoglobin levels above 8 g/dL and do not require intervention until the hemoglobin falls below that level. Patients with more physiologic compromise may need to have their hemoglobin levels kept above 11 g/dL. A typical unit of packed red cells increases the hemoglobin level by 1 g/dL. Transfusions are associated with certain infectious risks (Chap. 114) and chronic transfusions can produce iron overload.

Erythropoietin   Erythropoietin is particularly useful in anemias in which endogenous erythropoietin levels are inappropriately low, such as the hypoproliferative anemias. Iron status must be evaluated and iron repleted to obtain optimal effects from erythropoietin. In patients with chronic renal failure, the usual dose of erythropoietin is 50 to 150 U/kg three times a week subcutaneously. The dose needed to correct the anemia in patients with cancer is higher, up to 300 U/kg three times a week. Hemoglobin levels of 10 to 12 g/dL are usually reached within 4 to 6 weeks if iron levels are adequate. Once a target hemoglobin level is reached, the erythropoietin dose can be decreased

to 75 U/kg three times a week. A fall in hemoglobin level occurring in the face of erythropoietin therapy usually signifies the development of an infection or iron depletion. Aluminum toxicity and hyperparathyroidism can also compromise the erythropoietin response. When an infection intervenes, it is best to interrupt the erythropoietin therapy and rely on transfusion to correct the anemia until the infection is adequately treated.

ACKNOWLEDGMENT
Dr. Robert S. Hillman was the author of this chapter in the 14th edition, and material from his chapter has been retained.

BIBLIOGRAPHY

BAILIE GR et al: Parenteral iron use in the management of anemia in end-stage renal disease patients. Am J Kidney Dis 35:1, 2000

HILLMAN RS, AULT KA: *Hematology in Clinical Practice*, 2d ed. New York, McGraw-Hill, 1998

HILLMAN RS, FINCH CA: *Red Cell Manual*, 7th ed. Philadelphia, Davis, 1996

TSAKIRIS D: Morbidity and mortality reduction associated with the use of erythropoietin. Nephron 85 (Suppl S1):2, 2000

---

106   Edward J. Benz, Jr.

HEMOGLOBINOPATHIES

Hemoglobin is critical for normal oxygen delivery to tissues; it is also present in erythrocytes in such high concentrations that it can alter red cell shape, deformability, and viscosity. Hemoglobinopathies are disorders affecting the structure, function, or production of hemoglobin. These disorders are usually inherited and range in severity from asymptomatic laboratory abnormalities to death in utero. Different forms may present as hemolytic anemia, erythrocytosis, cyanosis, or vasoocclusive stigmata.

PROPERTIES OF THE HUMAN HEMOGLOBINS

HEMOGLOBIN STRUCTURE   Different hemoglobins are produced during embryonic, fetal, and adult life (Fig. 106-1). Each consists of a tetramer of globin polypeptide chains: a pair of α-like chains 141 amino acids long and a pair of β-like chains 146 amino acids long. The major adult hemoglobin, HbA, has the structure $\alpha_2\beta_2$. HbF ($\alpha_2\gamma_2$) predominates during most of gestation, and HbA$_2$ ($\alpha_2\delta_2$) is a minor adult hemoglobin.

Each globin chain enfolds a single heme moiety, consisting of a

FIGURE 106-1   The globin genes. The α-like genes (α,ζ) are encoded on chromosome 16; the β-like genes ($\beta,\gamma,\delta,\varepsilon$) are encoded on chromosome 11. The ζ and ε genes encode embryonic globins.

protoporphyrin IX ring complexed with a single iron atom in the ferrous state (Fe^{2+}), positioned in a manner optimal for reversible binding of oxygen. Each heme moiety can bind a single oxygen molecule; every molecule of hemoglobin can thus transport up to four oxygen molecules.

The amino acid sequences of the various globins are highly homologous to one another. Each has a highly helical *secondary structure*. Their globular *tertiary structures* cause the exterior surfaces to be rich in polar (hydrophilic) amino acids that enhance solubility and the interior to be lined with nonpolar groups, forming a hydrophobic "pocket" into which heme is inserted. The tetrameric *quaternary structure* of HbA contains two $\alpha\beta$ dimers. Numerous tight interactions (i.e., $\alpha_1\beta_1$ contacts) hold the α and β chains together. The complete tetramer is held together by interfaces (i.e., $\alpha_1\beta_2$ contacts) between the α-like chain of one dimer and the non-α chain of the other dimer.

The hemoglobin tetramer is highly soluble, but individual globin chains are insoluble. Unpaired globin precipitates, forming inclusions (Heinz bodies) that damage the cell. Normal globin chain synthesis is balanced so that each newly synthesized α or non-α globin chain will have an available partner with which to pair to form hemoglobin.

Solubility and reversible oxygen binding are the key properties deranged in hemoglobinopathies. Both depend most on the hydrophilic surface amino acids, the hydrophobic amino acids lining the heme pocket, a key histidine in the F helix, and the amino acids forming the $\alpha_1\beta_1$ and $\alpha_1\beta_2$ contact points. Mutations in these strategic regions tend to be the ones that alter clinical behavior.

FUNCTION OF HEMOGLOBIN To support oxygen transport, hemoglobin must bind O_2 efficiently at the partial pressure of oxygen (PO_2) of the alveolus, retain it, and release it to tissues at the PO_2 of tissue capillary beds. Oxygen acquisition and delivery over a relatively narrow range of oxygen tensions depend on a property inherent in the tetrameric arrangement of heme and globin subunits within the hemoglobin molecule called *cooperativity* or *heme-heme interaction*.

At low oxygen tensions, the hemoglobin tetramer is fully deoxygenated (Fig. 106-2). Oxygen binding begins slowly as O_2 tension rises. However, as soon as some oxygen has been bound by the tetramer, an abrupt increase occurs in the slope of the curve. Thus, hemoglobin molecules that have bound some oxygen develop a higher oxygen affinity, greatly accelerating their ability to combine with more oxygen. This S-shaped oxygen equilibrium curve, along which substantial amounts of oxygen loading *and unloading* can occur over a narrow range of oxygen tensions, is physiologically more useful than the high-affinity hyperbolic curve of individual monomers.

Oxygen affinity is modulated by several factors. The Bohr effect arises from the stabilizing action of protons on deoxyhemoglobin, which binds protons more readily than oxyhemoglobin because it is a weaker acid. Thus, hemoglobin has a lower oxygen affinity at low pH, facilitating delivery to tissues (Fig. 106-2). The major small molecule that alters oxygen affinity in humans is 2,3-bisphosphoglycerate (2,3-BPG, formerly 2,3-DPG), which lowers oxygen affinity when bound to hemoglobin. HbA has a reasonably high affinity for 2,3-BPG. HbF does not bind 2,3-BPG, so it tends to have a higher oxygen affinity in vivo. Hemoglobin may also bind nitric oxide reversibly, thereby contributing to vascular tone.

FIGURE 106-2 Hemoglobin-oxygen dissociation curve. The hemoglobin tetramer can bind up to four molecules of oxygen in the iron-containing sites of the heme molecules. As oxygen is bound, 2,3-BPG and CO_2 are expelled. Salt bridges are broken, and each of the globin molecules changes its conformation to facilitate oxygen binding. Oxygen release to the tissues is the reverse process, salt bridges being formed and 2,3-BPG and CO_2 bound. Deoxyhemoglobin does not bind oxygen efficiently until the cell returns to conditions of higher pH, the most important modulator of O_2 affinity (Bohr effect). When acid is produced in the tissues, the dissociation curve shifts to the right, facilitating oxygen release and CO_2 binding. Alkalosis has the opposite effect, reducing oxygen delivery.

To understand hemoglobinopathies, it is sufficient to understand that proper oxygen transport depends on the tetrameric structure of the proteins, the proper arrangement of the charged amino acids, and interaction with low-molecular-weight substances such as protons or 2,3-BPG.

DEVELOPMENTAL BIOLOGY Red cells first appearing at about 6 weeks after conception contain the embryonic hemoglobins Hb Portland ($\zeta_2\gamma_2$), Hb Gower I ($\zeta_2\varepsilon_2$), and Hb Gower II ($\alpha_2\varepsilon_2$). At 10 to 11 weeks, fetal hemoglobin (HbF; $\alpha_2\gamma_2$) becomes predominant. The switch to nearly exclusive synthesis of adult hemoglobin (HbA; $\alpha_2\beta_2$) occurs at about 38 weeks (Fig. 106-1). Fetuses and newborns therefore require α-globin but not β-globin for normal gestation. Small amounts of HbF are produced during postnatal life. A few red cell clones called *F cells* are progeny of a small pool of immature committed erythroid precursors (BFU-e) that retain the ability to produce HbF. Profound erythroid stress, such as that seen in severe hemolytic anemias, after bone marrow transplant, or during chemotherapy, cause more of the "F potent" BFU-e to be recruited. HbF levels thus tend to rise in some patients with sickle cell anemia or thalassemia. This phenomenon is also important because it probably explains the ability of hydroxyurea to increase levels of HbF in adults. Fetal globin genes can also be partially activated after birth by agents such as butyrate, which inhibit histone deacetylase and modify the structure of chromatin.

GENETICS AND BIOSYNTHESIS OF HUMAN HEMOGLOBIN The human hemoglobins are encoded in two tightly linked gene clusters; the α-like globin genes are clustered on chromosome 16, and the β-like genes on chromosome 11 (Fig. 106-1). The α-like cluster consists of two α-globin genes and a single copy of the ζ gene. The non-α gene cluster consists of a single ε gene, the Gγ and Aγ fetal globin genes, and the adult δ and β genes.

Important regulatory sequences flank each gene. Immediately upstream are typical promoter elements needed for the assembly of the transcription initiation complex. Sequences in the 5' flanking region of the γ and the β genes appear to be crucial for the correct developmental regulation of these genes, while elements that function like classic enhancers and silencers are in the 3' flanking regions. The locus control region (LCR) elements located far upstream appear to control the overall level of expression of each cluster. These elements achieve their regulatory effects by interacting with *trans*-acting transcription factors. Some of these factors are ubiquitous (e.g., Sp1 and YY1), while others are more or less limited to erythroid cells (e.g., GATA-1, NFE-2, and EKLF). The latter also appear to modulate genes specifically expressed during erythropoiesis, such as the genes that encode the enzymes of the heme biosynthetic pathway. This is relevant since normal red blood cell (RBC) differentiation also requires the coordinated expression of the globin genes with the genes responsible for heme and iron metabolism.

CLASSIFICATION OF HEMOGLOBINOPATHIES

There are five major classes of hemoglobinopathies (Table 106-1). *Structural hemoglobinopathies* occur when mutations alter the amino acid sequence of a globin chain, altering the physiologic properties of the variant hemoglobins and producing the characteristic clinical abnormalities. The variant hemoglobins relevant to this chapter polymerize abnormally, as in sickle cell anemia, or exhibit altered solubility or oxygen-binding affinity. *Thalassemia syndromes* arise from mutations that impair production or translation of globin mRNA, leading to deficient globin chain biosynthesis. Clinical abnormalities are attributable to the inadequate supply of hemoglobin and the imbalances in the production of individual globin chains, leading to premature destruction of erythroblasts and red cells. *Thalassemic hemoglobin variants* combine features of thalassemia (e.g., abnormal globin biosynthesis) and of structural hemoglobinopathies (e.g., an abnormal amino acid sequence). Hereditary persistence of fetal hemoglobin (HPFH) is characterized by synthesis of high levels of fetal hemoglobin in adult life. *Acquired hemoglobinopathies* include modifications of the hemoglobin molecule by toxins (e.g., acquired methemoglobinemia) and abnormal hemoglobin synthesis (e.g., high levels of HbF production in preleukemia and α-thalassemia in myeloproliferative disorders).

EPIDEMIOLOGY Hemoglobinopathies are especially common in areas where malaria is endemic. This clustering of hemoglobinopathies is assumed to reflect a selective survival advantage for the abnormal red cells, which presumably provide a less hospitable environment during the obligate intraerythrocytic stages of the parasitic

Table 106-1 Classification of Hemoglobinopathies

I. Structural hemoglobinopathies—hemoglobins with altered amino acid sequences that result in deranged function or altered physical or chemical properties
   A. Abnormal hemoglobin polymerization—HbS, hemoglobin sickling
   B. Altered O_2 affinity
      1. High affinity—polycythemia
      2. Low affinity—cyanosis, pseudoanemia
   C. Hemoglobins that oxidize readily
      1. Unstable hemoglobins—hemolytic anemia, jaundice
      2. M hemoglobins—methemoglobinemia, cyanosis
II. Thalassemias—defective biosynthesis of globin chains
   A. α Thalassemias
   B. β Thalassemias
   C. $\delta\beta$, $\gamma\delta\beta$, $\alpha\beta$ Thalassemias
III. Thalassemic hemoglobin variants—structurally abnormal Hb associated with coinherited thalassemic phenotype
   A. HbE
   B. Hb Constant Spring
   C. Hb Lepore
IV. Hereditary persistence of fetal hemoglobin—persistence of high levels of HbF in adults
V. Acquired hemoglobinopathies
   A. Methemoglobin due to toxic exposures
   B. Sulfhemoglobin due to toxic exposures
   C. Carboxyhemoglobin
   D. HbH in erythroleukemia
   E. Elevated HbF in states of erythroid stress and bone marrow dysplasia

life cycle. Very young children with α-thalassemia are *more* susceptible to infection with the nonlethal *Plasmodium vivax*. Thalassemia might then favor a natural "vaccination" against infection with the more lethal *P. falciparum*.

Thalassemias are the most common genetic disorders in the world, affecting nearly 200 million people worldwide. About 15% of American blacks are silent carriers for α thalassemia; α-thalassemia trait (minor) occurs in 3% of American blacks and in 1 to 15% of persons of Mediterranean origin. β Thalassemia has a 10 to 15% incidence in individuals from the Mediterranean and Southeast Asia and 0.8% in American blacks. The number of severe cases of thalassemia in the United States is about 1000. Sickle cell disease is the most common structural hemoglobinopathy occurring in heterozygous form in about 8% of American blacks and in homozygous form in 1 in 400. Between 2 and 3% of American blacks carry a hemoglobin C allele.

INHERITANCE AND ONTOGENY Hemoglobinopathies are autosomal "codominant" traits—compound heterozygotes that inherit a different abnormal mutant allele from each parent exhibit composite features of each. For example, patients inheriting sickle β thalassemia exhibit features of β thalassemia and sickle cell anemia. The α-chain is present in HbA, HbA_2, and HbF; α-chain mutations thus cause abnormalities in all three. The α-globin hemoglobinopathies are symptomatic in utero and after birth because normal function of the α-globin gene is required throughout gestation and adult life. In contrast, infants with β-globin hemoglobinopathies tend to be asymptomatic until 3 to 9 months of age, when HbA has largely replaced HbF.

DETECTION AND CHARACTERIZATION OF HEMOGLOBINOPATHIES— GENERAL METHODS

Electrophoretic techniques are used for routine hemoglobin analysis. Electrophoresis at pH-8.6 on cellulose acetate membranes is simple, inexpensive, and reliable for initial screening. Hemoglobins S, G, and D have the same mobility at pH-8.6. Agar gel electrophoresis at pH-6.1 in citrate buffer is often used as a complementary method because it detects different variants (S migration differs from G and D). Comparison of results obtained in each system usually allows unambiguous diagnosis, but some important variants are electrophoretically silent. These mutant hemoglobins can usually be characterized by more specialized techniques such as isoelectric focusing and/or high-pressure liquid chromatography (HPLC).

Quantitation of the hemoglobin profile is often desirable. HbA_2 is frequently elevated in β-thalassemia trait and depressed in iron deficiency. HbF is elevated in HPFH, some β thalassemia syndromes, and occasional periods of erythroid stress or marrow dysplasia. For characterization of sickle cell trait, sickle thalassemia syndromes, or hemoglobin SC disease, and for monitoring the progress of exchange transfusion therapy to lower the percentage of circulating HbS, quantitation of individual hemoglobins is also required. In most laboratories, quantitation is performed only if the test is specifically ordered.

Because some variants can comigrate with HbA or HbS (sickle hemoglobin), electrophoretic assessment should always be regarded as incomplete unless functional assays for hemoglobin sickling, solubility, or oxygen affinity are also performed, as dictated by the clinical presentation. The best sickling assays involve measurement of the degree to which the hemoglobin becomes insoluble, or gelated, as it is deoxygenated (i.e., sickle solubility test). Unstable hemoglobins are detected by their precipitation in isopropanol or after heating to 50°C. High-O_2 affinity and low-O_2 affinity variants are detected by quantitating the partial pressure of oxygen at which the hemoglobin sample becomes 50% saturated with oxygen (P_{50} test). Direct tests for the percentages of carboxyhemoglobin and methemoglobin, employing spectrophotometric techniques, can readily be obtained from most clinical laboratories on an urgent basis.

Complete characterization, including amino acid sequencing or gene cloning and sequencing, is available from several investigational

FIGURE 106-3 Pathophysiology of sickle cell crisis.

laboratories around the world. The advent of the polymerase chain reaction (PCR), allele-specific oligonucleotide hybridization, and automated DNA sequencing has made it possible to identify globin gene mutations in a few days.

Diagnosis is best established by recognition of a characteristic history, physical findings, peripheral blood smear morphology, and abnormalities of the complete blood cell count (e.g., profound microcytosis with minimal anemia in thalassemia trait). Laboratory evaluation identifies the specific hemoglobinopathy suspected clinically.

STRUCTURALLY ABNORMAL HEMOGLOBINS

SICKLE CELL SYNDROMES The sickle cell syndromes are caused by a mutation in the β-globin gene that changes the sixth amino acid from glutamic acid to valine. HbS ($\alpha_2\beta_2^{6Glu\rightarrow Val}$) polymerizes reversibly when deoxygenated to form a gelatinous network of fibrous polymers that stiffen the erythrocyte membrane, increase viscosity, and cause dehydration due to potassium leakage and calcium influx (Fig. 106-3). These changes also produce the characteristic sickle shape. Sickled cells lose the pliability needed to traverse small capillaries. They possess altered "sticky" membranes (especially reticulocytes) that are abnormally adherent to the endothelium of small venules. These abnormalities provoke unpredictable episodes of microvascular vasoocclusion and premature red cell destruction (hemolytic anemia). Hemolysis occurs because the abnormal erythrocytes are destroyed by the spleen. The rigid adherent cells also clog small capillaries and venules, causing tissue ischemia, acute pain, and gradual end-organ damage. This venooclusive component usually dominates the clinical course. Prominent manifestations include episodes of ischemic pain (i.e., painful crises) and ischemic malfunction or frank infarction in the spleen, central nervous system, bones, liver, kidneys, and lungs.

The prototype disease, sickle cell anemia, is the homozygous state for HbS (Table 106-2). Several sickle syndromes occur as the result of inheritance of HbS from one parent and another hemoglobinopathy, such as β thalassemia or HbC ($\alpha_2\beta_2^{6Glu\rightarrow Lys}$) from the other parent.

Clinical Manifestations • Sickle cell anemia Most patients with sickling syndromes suffer from hemolytic anemia, with hematocrits of 15 to 30%, and significant reticulocytosis. Anemia was once thought to exert protective effects against vasoocclusion by reducing blood viscosity. Natural history and drug therapy trials suggest that an *increase* in the hematocrit with feedback inhibition of reticulocytosis might be beneficial, even at the expense of increased blood viscosity. The role of adhesive reticulocytes in vasoocclusion might account for these paradoxical effects.

Granulocytosis is common. The white cell count can fluctuate substantially and unpredictably during and between painful crises, infectious episodes, and other intercurrent illnesses.

Vasoocclusion causes protean manifestations; intermittent episodes in connective and musculoskeletal structures produce painful ischemia manifested by acute pain and tenderness, fever, tachycardia, and anxiety. These recurrent episodes, called *painful crises*, are the most common clinical manifestation. Their frequency and severity vary greatly. Pain can develop almost anywhere in the body and may last from a few hours to 2 weeks. Repeated crises requiring hospitalization (more than three per year) correlate with reduced survival in adult life, suggesting that these episodes are associated with accumulation of chronic end-organ damage. Provocative factors include infection, fever, excessive exercise, anxiety, abrupt changes in temperature, hypoxia, or hypertonic dyes.

Repeated microinfarction can destroy tissues having microvascular beds that promote sickling. Thus, the spleen is frequently infarcted within the first 18 to 36 months of life, causing susceptibility to infection, particularly from pneumococci. Acute venous obstruction of the spleen (*splenic sequestration crisis*), a rare occurrence in early childhood, may require emergency transfusion and/or splenectomy to prevent trapping of the entire arterial output in the obstructed spleen. Occlusion of retinal vessels can produce hemorrhage, neovascularization, and eventual detachments. Renal papillary necrosis invariably produces isosthenuria. More widespread renal necrosis leads to renal failure in adults, a common late cause of death. Bone and joint ischemia can lead to aseptic necrosis (especially of the femoral or humeral heads), chronic arthropathy, and unusual susceptibility to osteomyelitis, which may be caused by organisms such as *Salmonella*, rarely encountered in other settings. The *hand-foot syndrome* is caused by painful infarcts of the digits and dactylitis. Stroke is especially common in children, a small subset of whom tend to suffer repeated episodes; stroke is less common in adults and is often hemorrhagic. A particularly painful complication in males is priapism, due to infarction of the penile venous outflow tracts; permanent impotence is a frequent consequence. Chronic lower leg ulcers probably arise from ischemia and superinfection in the distal circulation.

Acute chest syndrome is a distinctive manifestation characterized

Table 106-2 Clinical Features of Sickle Hemoglobinopathies

Condition	Clinical Abnormalities	Hemoglobin Level g/L (g/dL)	Mean Corpuscular Volume, fL	Hemoglobin Electrophoresis
Sickle cell trait	None; rare painless hematuria	Normal	Normal	Hb S/A:40/60
Sickle cell anemia	Vasoocclusive crises with infarction of spleen, brain, marrow, kidney, lung; aseptic necrosis of bone; gallstones; priapism; ankle ulcers	70–100 (7–10)	80–100	Hb S/A:100/0 Hb F:2–25%
S/β° thalassemia	Vasoocclusive crises; aseptic necrosis of bone	70–100 (7–10)	60–80	Hb S/A:100/0 Hb F:1–10%
S/β^+ thalassemia	Rare crises and aseptic necrosis	100–140 (10–14)	70–80	Hb S/A:60/40
Hemoglobin SC	Rare crises and aseptic necrosis; painless hematuria	100–140 (10–14)	80–100	Hb S/A:50/0 Hb C:50%

by chest pain, tachypnea, fever, cough, and arterial oxygen desaturation. It can mimic pneumonia, pulmonary emboli, bone marrow infarction and embolism, myocardial ischemia, or in situ lung infarction. Acute chest syndrome is thought to reflect in situ sickling within the lung, producing pain and temporary pulmonary dysfunction. Acute chest syndrome may be difficult or impossible to distinguish from other entities. Pulmonary infarction and pneumonia are the most frequent underlying or concomitant conditions in patients with this syndrome. Repeated episodes of acute chest pain correlate with reduced survival. Acutely, reduction in arterial oxygen saturation is especially ominous because it promotes sickling on a massive scale. Repeated acute or subacute pulmonary crises lead to pulmonary hypertension and cor pulmonale, an increasingly common cause of death as patients survive further into adult life.

Sickle cell syndromes are remarkable for their clinical heterogeneity. Some patients remain virtually asymptomatic into or even through adult life, while others suffer repeated crises requiring hospitalization from early childhood. At least five haplotypes of sickle cell disease are recognized based upon their origin: Senegal, Cameroon, Benin, Central African Republic, and India. Among these, patients of the Central African Republic have the worst disease and those of Senegal the least severe. Patients with sickle thalassemia and sickle-HbE tend to have similar, slightly milder, symptoms, perhaps because of the ameliorating effects of production of other hemoglobins within the red cell. Hemoglobin SC disease, one of the more common variants of sickle cell anemia, is frequently marked by lesser degrees of hemolytic anemia and a greater propensity for the development of retinopathy and aseptic necrosis of bones. In most respects, however, the clinical manifestations resemble sickle cell anemia. Some rare hemoglobin variants actually aggravate the sickling phenomenon.

Sickle cell trait   Sickle cell trait is usually asymptomatic. Anemia and painful crises are exceedingly rare. An uncommon, but highly distinctive, symptom is painless hematuria, often occurring in adolescent males, probably due to papillary necrosis. Sloughing of papillae with ureteral obstruction has been reported, as have isolated cases of massive sickling or sudden death due to exposure to high altitudes or extraordinary extremes of exercise and dehydration.

Diagnosis   Sickle cell syndromes are readily suspected on the basis of characteristic hemolytic anemia, red cell morphology (**Plate V-39**), and intermittent episodes of ischemic pain. Diagnosis is confirmed by hemoglobin electrophoresis and sickling tests. Thorough characterization of the exact hemoglobin profile of the patient is important, because sickle thalassemia and hemoglobin SC disease are correlated with alterations in prognosis or clinical features. The diagnosis is usually established in childhood, but occasional patients, often with compound heterozygous states, do not develop symptoms until the onset of puberty, pregnancy, or early adult life. Genotyping of family members and potential parental partners is critical for genetic counseling. Details of the childhood history help to establish prognosis and eligibility for aggressive or experimental therapies. Factors associated with increased morbidity and mortality are more than three crises requiring hospitalization per year, chronic neutrophilia, a history of splenic sequestration or hand-foot syndrome, and second episodes of acute chest syndrome. Patients with a history of cerebrovascular accidents are at higher risk for repeated episodes and require especially close monitoring.

TREATMENT   Patients with sickle cell syndromes require ongoing continuity of care. Familiarity with the pattern of symptoms provides the best safeguard against excessive use of the emergency room, hospitalization, and habituation to addictive narcotics. Additional preventive measures include regular slit-lamp examinations to monitor development of retinopathy; antibiotic prophylaxis appropriate for splenectomized patients during dental or other invasive procedures; vaccination against pneumococci and *Haemophilus influenzae*; and vigorous oral hydration before or during periods of extreme exercise, exposure to heat or cold, emotional stress, or infection.

The management of acute painful crisis includes vigorous hydration, thorough evaluation for underlying causes (such as infection), and aggressive narcotic analgesia administered by a standing order and/or PCA pump. Morphine (0.1 to 0.15 mg/kg every 3 to 4 h) or meperidine (0.75 to 1.5 mg/kg every 2 to 4 h) should control severe pain. Bone pain may respond as well to ketorolac (30 to 60 mg initial dose, then 15 to 30 mg every 6 to 8 h). Many crises can be managed at home with oral hydration and oral analgesia. Use of the emergency room should be reserved for especially severe symptoms or circumstances in which other processes (e.g., infection) are strongly suspected. Nasal oxygen should be employed as appropriate to protect arterial saturation. Most crises resolve in 1 to 7 days. Use of blood transfusion should be reserved for extreme cases; transfusion does not shorten the crisis.

No tests are definitive to diagnose acute painful crisis. Critical to good management is an approach that recognizes that most patients reporting crisis symptoms do indeed have crisis or another significant medical problem. Diligent diagnostic evaluation for underlying causes is imperative, even though these are found infrequently. In adults, the possibility of aseptic necrosis or sickle arthropathy must be considered, especially if pain and immobility become repeated or chronic at a single site. Nonsteroidal anti-inflammatory agents are often effective for sickle cell arthropathy.

Acute chest syndrome is a medical emergency that may require management in an intensive care unit. Hydration should be monitored carefully to avoid the development of pulmonary edema, and oxygen therapy should be especially vigorous for protection of arterial saturation. Diagnostic evaluation for pneumonia and pulmonary embolism should be thorough, since these may occur with atypical symptoms. Critical interventions are transfusion to maintain a hematocrit >30 and emergency exchange transfusion if arterial saturation drops below 90%.

As patients with sickle cell syndromes increasingly survive into their fifth and sixth decades (median age at death is 42 years for men, 48 years for women), end-stage renal failure and pulmonary hypertension are becoming increasingly prominent causes of end-stage morbidity; anecdotal evidence suggests that a sickle cell cardiomyopathy and/or premature coronary artery disease may compromise cardiac function in later years. Sickle cell patients have received kidney transplants, but they often experience an increase in the frequency and severity of crises, possibly due to increased infection as a consequence of immunosuppression.

The most significant advance in the therapy of sickle cell anemia has been the introduction of hydroxyurea as a mainstay of therapy for patients with severe symptoms. Hydroxyurea (10 to 30 mg/kg/per day) increases fetal hemoglobin and may also exert beneficial affects on red cell hydration, vascular wall adherence, and suppression of the granulocyte and reticulocyte counts; indeed, dosage is titrated to maintain a white cell count between 5,000 and 8,000. White cells and reticulocytes may play a major role in the pathogenesis of sickle cell crisis, and their suppression may be an important benefit of hydroxyurea therapy.

Hydroxyurea should be considered in patients experiencing repeated episodes of acute chest syndrome or more than three crises per year requiring hospitalization. The utility of this agent for reducing the incidence of other complications (e.g., priapism, retinopathy) is under evaluation, as are the long-term side effects. Therefore, when possible, treatment should be instituted as part of a clinical trial. Most patients respond within a few months with elevations of fetal hemoglobin.

Bone marrow transplantation can provide definitive cures but is known to be effective and safe only in children. Prognostic features justifying bone marrow transplant are the presence of repeated crises early in life, a high neutrophil count, or the development of hand-foot syndrome. Children at risk for stroke can be identified through the use of Doppler ultrasound techniques. Prophylactic exchange transfusion appears to reduce the risk of stroke substantially in this population. Children who do suffer a cerebrovascular accident should be maintained for at least 3 to 5 years on a program of vigorous exchange transfusion, since the risk of second strokes is extremely high in this population.

Gene therapy for sickle cell anemia is under investigation, but no safe therapy is currently available. Agents blocking red cell hydration or vascular adhesion, such as clotrimazole, may have value as an adjunct to hydroxyurea therapy; trials are ongoing.

UNSTABLE HEMOGLOBINS Amino acid substitutions that reduce solubility or increase susceptibility to oxidation produce "unstable" hemoglobins that precipitate, forming inclusion bodies injurious to the red cell membrane. Representative mutations are those that interfere with contact points between the α and β subunits [e.g., Hb Philly ($\beta^{35Tyr \rightarrow Phe}$)], alter the helical segments [e.g., Hb Genova ($\beta^{28Leu \rightarrow Pro}$)], or disrupt interactions of the hydrophobic pockets of the globin subunits with heme [e.g., Hb Koln ($\beta^{98Val \rightarrow Met}$)] (Table 106-3). The inclusions, called *Heinz bodies*, are clinically detectable by staining with supravital dyes such as crystal violet (Heinz body test). Removal of these inclusions by the spleen generates pitted, rigid cells that have shortened life spans, producing hemolytic anemia of variable severity, sometimes requiring chronic transfusion support. Splenectomy may be needed to correct the anemia. Leg ulcers and premature gallbladder disease due to bilirubin turnover are frequent stigmata.

Unstable hemoglobins occur sporadically, often by spontaneous new mutations. Heterozygotes are often symptomatic because a significant Heinz body burden can develop even when the unstable variant accounts for a portion of the total hemoglobin. Symptomatic unstable hemoglobins tend to be β-globin variants, because sporadic mutations affecting only one of the four α globins would generate only 20 to 30% abnormal hemoglobin.

HEMOGLOBINS WITH ALTERED OXYGEN AFFINITY *High-affinity hemoglobins* [e.g., Hb Yakima ($\beta^{99Asp \rightarrow His}$)] bind oxygen more readily but deliver less O_2 to tissues at normal capillary P_{O_2} levels (Fig. 106-2). Mild tissue hypoxia ensues, stimulating RBC production and erythrocytosis (Table 106-3). In extreme cases, the hematocrit can rise to 60 to 65%, increasing blood viscosity and producing typical symptoms (headache, somnolence, or dizziness). Phlebotomy may be required. Typical mutations alter interactions within the heme pocket or disrupt the Bohr effect or salt-bond site. Mutations that impair the interaction of HbA with 2,3-BPG can increase O_2 affinity, because 2,3-BPG binding lowers O_2 affinity.

Low-affinity hemoglobins [e.g., Hb Kansas ($\beta^{102Asn \rightarrow Thr}$)] bind sufficient oxygen in the lungs, despite their lower oxygen affinity, to achieve nearly full saturation. At capillary oxygen tensions, they lose sufficient amounts of oxygen to maintain homeostasis at a low hematocrit (Fig. 106-2) (pseudoanemia). Capillary hemoglobin desaturation can also be sufficient to produce clinically apparent cyanosis. Despite these findings, patients usually require no specific treatment.

METHEMOGLOBINEMIAS Methemoglobin is generated by oxidation of the heme iron moieties to the ferric state, causing a char-

acteristic bluish-brown, muddy color resembling cyanosis. Methemoglobin has such high oxygen affinity that virtually no oxygen is delivered to tissues. Levels >50 to 60% are often fatal.

Congenital methemoglobinemia arises from globin mutations that stabilize iron in the ferric state [e.g., HbM Iwata ($\alpha^{87His \rightarrow Tyr}$), Table 106-3] or from mutations that impair the enzymes that reduce methemoglobin to hemoglobin (e.g., methemoglobin reductase, NADP diaphorase). Acquired methemoglobinemia is caused by toxins that oxidize heme iron, notably nitrate and nitrite-containing compounds.

DIAGNOSIS AND MANAGEMENT OF PATIENTS WITH UNSTABLE HEMOGLOBINS, HIGH-AFFINITY HEMOGLOBINS, AND METHEMOGLOBINEMIA *Unstable hemoglobin variants* should be suspected in patients with nonimmune hemolytic anemia, jaundice, splenomegaly, or premature biliary tract disease. Severe hemolysis usually presents during infancy as neonatal jaundice or anemia. Milder cases may present in adult life with anemia or only as unexplained reticulocytosis, hepatosplenomegaly, premature biliary tract disease, or leg ulcers. Because spontaneous mutation is common, family history of anemia may be absent. The peripheral blood smear often shows anisocytosis, abundant cells with punctate inclusions, and irregular shapes (i.e., poikilocytosis).

The two best tests for diagnosing unstable hemoglobins are the Heinz body preparation and the isopropanol or heat stability test. Many unstable Hb variants are electrophoretically silent. A normal electrophoresis does not rule out the diagnosis.

Severely affected patients may require transfusion support for the first 3 years of life, because splenectomy before age 3 is associated with a significantly greater immune deficit. Splenectomy is usually effective thereafter, but occasional patients may require lifelong transfusion support. Even after splenectomy, patients can develop cholelithiasis and leg ulcers. Splenectomy can also be considered in patients exhibiting severe secondary complications of chronic hemolysis, even if anemia is absent. Precipitation of unstable hemoglobins is aggravated by oxidative stress, e.g., infection, antimalarial drugs.

High-O_2-affinity hemoglobin variants should be suspected in patients with erythrocytosis. The best test for confirmation is measurement of the P_{50}. A high-O_2-affinity Hb causes a significant left shift (i.e., lower numeric value of the P_{50}); confounding conditions, e.g., tobacco smoking or carbon monoxide exposure, can also lower the P_{50}.

Patients with high-affinity hemoglobin are often asymptomatic; rubor or plethora may be telltale signs. When the hematocrit reaches 55 to 60%, symptoms of high blood viscosity and sluggish flow (headache, lethargy, dizziness, etc.) may be present. These symptoms respond to judicious phlebotomy. Erythrocytosis represents an appropriate attempt to compensate for the impaired oxygen delivery by the abnormal variant. Overzealous phlebotomy may stimulate increased erythropoiesis or aggravate symptoms by thwarting this compensatory mechanism. The guiding principle of phlebotomy should be to improve oxygen delivery by reducing blood viscosity and increasing blood flow rather than restoration of a normal hematocrit. Modest iron deficiency may aid in control.

Low-affinity hemoglobins should be considered in patients with cyanosis or a low hematocrit with no other cause apparent after thorough evaluation. The P_{50} test confirms the diagnosis. Counseling and reassurance are the interventions of choice.

Methemoglobin should be suspected in patients with hypoxic symptoms who appear cyanotic but have a Pa_{O_2} sufficiently high that hemoglobin should be fully saturated with oxygen. A history of nitrite or other oxidant ingestions may not always be available; some exposures may be unapparent to the patient, and others may result from suicide attempts. The characteristic muddy appearance of freshly drawn blood can be a critical clue. The diagnostic test of choice is measurement of the methemoglobin content, which is usually available on an emergency basis.

Methemoglobinemia often causes symptoms of cerebral ischemia

Table 106-3 Representative Abnormal Hemoglobins with Altered Synthesis or Function

Designation	Mutation	Population	Main Clinical Effects[a]
Sickle or S	$\beta^{6Glu \rightarrow Val}$	African	Anemia, ischemic infarcts
C	$\beta^{6Glu \rightarrow Lys}$	African	Mild anemia; interacts with HbS
E	$\beta^{26Glu \rightarrow Lys}$	Southeast Asian	Microcytic anemia, splenomegaly, thalassemic phenotype
Köln	$\beta^{98Val \rightarrow Met}$	Sporadic	Hemolytic anemia, Heinz bodies when splenectomized
Yakima	$\beta^{99Asp \rightarrow His}$	Sporadic	Polycythemia
Kansas	$\beta^{102Asn \rightarrow Lys}$	Sporadic	Mild anemia
M. Iwata	$\alpha^{87His \rightarrow Tyr}$	Sporadic	Methemoglobinemia

[a] See text for details.

Table 106-4   The α Thalassemias

Condition	Hemoglobin A, %	Hemoglobin H (β^4), %	Hemoglobin level, g/L (g/dL)	MCV, fL
Normal	97	0	150 (15)	90
Silent thalassemia: $-\alpha/\alpha\alpha$	98–100	0	150 (15)	90
Thalassemia trait: $-\alpha/-\alpha$ homozygous α-thal-2[a] or $--/\alpha\alpha$ heterozygous α-thal-1[a]	85–95	Rare red blood cell inclusions	120–130 (12–13)	70–80
Hemoglobin H disease: $--/-\alpha$ heterozygous α-thal-1/α-thal-2	70–95	5–30	60–100 (6–10)	60–70
Hydrops fetalis: $--/--$ homozygous α-thal-1	0	5–10[b]	Fatal in utero or at birth	

[a] When both α alleles on one chromosome are deleted, the locus is called α-thal-1; when only a single α allele on one chromosome is deleted, the locus is called α-thal-2.

[b] 90–95% of the hemoglobin is hemoglobin Barts (tetramers of γ chains).

at levels >15%; levels >60% are usually lethal. Intravenous injection of 1 mg/kg of methylene blue is effective emergency therapy. Milder cases and follow-up of severe cases can be treated orally with methylene blue (60 mg three to four times each day) or ascorbic acid (300 to 600 mg/d).

THALASSEMIA SYNDROMES

The thalassemia syndromes are inherited disorders of α- or β-globin biosynthesis. The reduced supply of globin diminishes production of hemoglobin tetramers, causing hypochromia and microcytosis. Unbalanced accumulation of α and β subunits occurs because the synthesis of the unaffected globins proceeds at normal rate. Unbalanced chain accumulation dominates the clinical phenotype. Clinical severity varies widely, depending on the degree to which the synthesis of the affected globin is impaired, altered synthesis of other globin chains, and coinheritance of other abnormal globin alleles.

β-THALASSEMIA SYNDROMES   Mutations causing thalassemia can affect any step in the pathway of globin gene expression: transcription, processing of the mRNA precursor, translation, and post-translational metabolism of the β-globin polypeptide chain. The most common forms arise from mutations that derange splicing of the mRNA precursor or prematurely terminate translation of the mRNA.

Hypochromia and microcytosis due to reduced amounts of hemoglobin tetramers characterize all forms of β thalassemia. In heterozygotes (β-thalassemia trait), this is the only abnormality seen; anemia is minimal. In homozygous states, unbalanced α- and β-globin accumulation causes accumulation of highly insoluble unpaired α chains, which form toxic inclusion bodies that kill developing erythroblasts in the marrow. Few of the proerythroblasts beginning erythroid maturation survive. The few surviving red cells bear a burden of inclusion bodies, detected in the spleen, shortening the red cell life span and producing severe hemolytic anemia. The resulting profound anemia stimulates erythropoietin release and compensatory erythroid hyperplasia, but the marrow response is sabotaged by ineffective erythropoiesis. Anemia persists. Erythroid hyperplasia can become exuberant and produce extramedullary erythropoietic tissue in the liver and spleen.

Massive bone marrow expansion deranges growth and development. Children develop characteristic "chipmunk" facies due to maxillary marrow hyperplasia and frontal bossing, thinning and pathologic fracture of long bones and vertebrae due to cortical invasion by erythroid elements, and profound growth retardation. Hemolytic anemia causes hepatosplenomegaly, leg ulcers, gallstones, and high-output congestive heart failure. The conscription of caloric resources to support erythropoiesis leads to inanition, susceptibility to infection, endocrine dysfunction, and, in the most severe cases, death during the first decade of life. Chronic transfusions with red cells improves oxygen delivery, suppresses the excessive ineffective erythropoiesis, and prolongs life, but the inevitable side effects, notably iron overload, usually prove fatal by age 30. Bone marrow transplantation in childhood is the only curative therapy.

Severity is highly variable. Known modulating factors are those that ameliorate the burden of unpaired α-globin inclusions. Alleles associated with milder synthetic defects and coinheritance of α-thalassemia trait reduce clinical severity by reducing accumulation of excess α globin. HbF persists to various degrees in β thalassemias. γ-Globin gene chains can substitute for β chains, simultaneously generating more hemoglobin and reducing the burden of α-globin inclusions. The terms β-thalassemia major and β-thalassemia intermedia are used to reflect the clinical heterogeneity. Patients with β-thalassemia major require intensive transfusion support to survive. Patients with β-thalassemia intermedia have a somewhat milder phenotype and can survive without transfusion. The terms β-thalassemia minor and β-thalassemia trait describe asymptomatic heterozygotes for β thalassemia.

α-THALASSEMIA SYNDROMES   The four classic α thalassemias, most common in Asians, are α-thalassemia-2 trait, in which one of the four α-globin loci is deleted; α-thalassemia-1 trait, with two deleted loci; HbH disease, with three loci deleted; and hydrops fetalis with Hb Bart's, with all four loci deleted (Table 106-4). Nondeletion forms of α thalassemia also exist.

α-Thalassemia-2 trait is an asymptomatic, silent carrier state. α-Thalassemia-1 trait resembles β-thalassemia minor. Offspring doubly heterozygous for α-thalassemia-2 and α-thalassemia-1 exhibit a more severe phenotype, called HbH disease. Heterozygosity for a deletion that removes both genes from the same chromosome (cis deletion) is common in Asians and Mediterranean individuals, as is homozygosity for α-thalassemia-2 (trans deletion). Both produce asymptomatic hypochromia and microcytosis.

In HbH disease, HbA production is only 25 to 30% of normal. Fetuses accumulate some unpaired β chains. In adults, unpaired β chains accumulate and are soluble enough to form β_4 tetramers called HbH. HbH forms few inclusions in erythroblasts but does precipitate in circulating red cells. Patients with HbH disease have thalassemia intermedia characterized by moderately severe hemolytic anemia but milder ineffective erythropoiesis. Survival into midadult life without transfusions is common.

The homozygous state for the α-thalassemia-1 cis deletion (hydrops fetalis) causes total absence of α-globin synthesis. No physiologically useful hemoglobin is produced beyond the embryonic stage. Excess γ globin forms tetramers called Hb Bart's (γ_4), which has an extraordinarily high oxygen affinity. It delivers almost no O_2 to fetal tissues, causing tissue asphyxia, edema (hydrops fetalis), congestive heart failure, and death in utero. α-Thalassemia-2 trait is common (15 to 20%) among people of African descent. The cis α-thalassemia-1 deletion is almost never seen, however. Thus, α-thalassemia-2 and the trans form of α-thalassemia-1 are very common, but HbH disease and hydrops fetalis are almost never encountered.

DIAGNOSIS AND MANAGEMENT   The diagnosis of β-thalassemia major is readily made during childhood on the basis of severe anemia accompanied by hepatosplenomegaly; profound microcytosis; a characteristic blood smear (**Plate V-2**); and elevated levels of HbF, HbA$_2$, or both. Many patients require chronic hypertransfusion therapy designed to maintain a hematocrit of at least 27 to 30% so that erythropoiesis is suppressed. Splenectomy is required if the annual transfusion requirement (volume of RBCs per kilogram body weight per year) increases by >50%. Folic acid supplements may be useful. Vaccination with pneumococcal vaccine in anticipation of eventual splenectomy is advised, as is close monitoring for infection, leg ulcers, and biliary tract disease. Early endocrine evaluation is required for or secondary sexual characteristics. Many patients develop endocrine deficiencies as a result of iron overload.

Patients with β-thalassemia intermedia exhibit similar stigmata but can survive without chronic hypertransfusion. Management is particularly challenging because a number of factors can aggravate the anemia, including infection, onset of puberty, and development of splenomegaly and hypersplenism. Some patients may eventually benefit from splenectomy. The expanded erythron can cause excess absorption of dietary iron and hemosiderosis, even without transfusion.

β-Thalassemia minor (i.e., thalassemia trait) usually presents as profound microcytosis and hypochromia with target cells but only minimal or mild anemia. The mean corpuscular volume is rarely >75 fL; the hematocrit is rarely <30 to 33%. Hemoglobin electrophoresis classically reveals an elevated HbA_2 (3.5 to 7.5%), but some forms are associated with normal HbA_2 and/or elevated HbF. Genetic counseling and patient education are essential. Patients with β-thalassemia trait should be warned that their blood picture resembles iron deficiency and can be misdiagnosed. They should eschew routine use of iron but know that iron deficiency requiring supplementation can develop, as in other persons, during pregnancy or from chronic bleeding.

Persons with α-thalassemia trait may exhibit mild hypochromia and microcytosis, usually without anemia. HbA_2 and HbF levels are normal. Affected individuals usually require only genetic counseling. HbH disease resembles β-thalassemia intermedia, with the added complication that the HbH molecule behaves like a moderately unstable hemoglobin. Patients with HbH disease should undergo splenectomy if excessive anemia or a transfusion requirement develops. Oxidative drugs should be avoided. Iron overload leading to death can occur in more severely affected patients.

PREVENTION Antenatal diagnosis of thalassemia syndromes is now widely available. DNA diagnosis is based on PCR amplification of fetal DNA, obtained by amniocentesis or chorionic villus biopsy followed by hybridization to allele-specific oligonucleotides probes. The probes can be designed to detect simultaneously the subset of mutations that account for 95 to 99% of the α or β thalassemias that occur in a particular ethnic group.

THALASSEMIC STRUCTURAL VARIANTS

Thalassemic structural variants are characterized by both defective synthesis and abnormal structure.

HEMOGLOBIN LEPORE Hb Lepore [$\alpha_2(\delta\beta)_2$] arises by an unequal crossover and recombination event that fuses the proximal end of the δ gene with the distal end of the closely linked β gene. The resulting chromosome contains only the fused $\delta\beta$ gene. The Lepore ($\delta\beta$) globin is synthesized poorly because the fused gene is under the control of the weak δ-globin promoter. Hb Lepore alleles have a phenotype like β-thalassemia, except for the added presence of 2 to 20% Hb Lepore. Compound heterozygotes for Hb Lepore and a classic β-thalassemia allele may also have severe thalassemia.

HEMOGLOBIN E HbE (i.e., $\alpha_2\beta_2^{26Glu \rightarrow Lys}$) is extremely common in Cambodia, Thailand, and Vietnam. The gene has become far more prevalent in the United States as a result of immigration of Asian persons, especially in California, where HbE is the most common variant detected. HbE is mildly unstable but not enough to affect RBC life span significantly. The high frequency of the HbE gene may be a result of the thalassemia phenotype associated with its inheritance. Heterozygotes resemble individuals with mild β-thalassemia trait. Homozygotes have somewhat more marked abnormalities but are asymptomatic. Compound heterozygotes for HbE and a β-thalassemia gene can have β-thalassemia intermedia or β-thalassemia major, depending on the severity of the coinherited thalassemic gene.

The β^E allele contains only a single base change, in codon 26, that causes the amino acid substitution. However, this mutation activates a cryptic RNA splice site generating a structurally abnormal globin mRNA that cannot be translated from about 50% of the initial pre-

mRNA molecules. The remaining 40 to 50%, which are normally spliced, generate functional mRNA that is translated into β^E globin because the mature mRNA carries the base change that alters codon 26.

Genetic counseling of the persons at risk for HbE should focus on the interaction of HbE with β-thalassemia rather than HbE homozygosity, a condition associated with microcytosis and hypchromia that is usually asymptomatic, with hemoglobin levels rarely <10 gm/dL.

OTHER UNCOMMON HEMOGLOBINOPATHIES

HEREDITARY PERSISTENCE OF FETAL HEMOGLOBIN HPFH is characterized by continued synthesis of high levels of HbF in adult life. No deleterious effects are apparent, even when all of the hemoglobin produced is HbF. These rare patients demonstrate convincingly that prevention or reversal of the fetal to adult hemoglobin switch would provide efficacious therapy for sickle cell anemia and β thalassemia.

ACQUIRED HEMOGLOBINOPATHIES The two most important acquired hemoglobinopathies are carbon monoxide poisoning and methemoglobinemia (see above). Carbon monoxide has a higher affinity for hemoglobin than does oxygen; it can replace oxygen and diminish O_2 delivery. Chronic elevation of carboxyhemoglobin levels to 10 or 15%, as occurs in smokers, can lead to secondary polycythemia. Carboxyhemoglobin is cherry red in color and masks the development of cyanosis usually associated with poor O_2 delivery to tissues.

Abnormalities of hemoglobin biosynthesis have also been described in blood dyscrasias. In some patients with myelodysplastic, erythroleukemic, or myeloproliferative disorders, a mild form of HbH disease may also be seen. The abnormalities are not severe enough to alter the course of the underlying disease.

MANAGEMENT OF TRANSFUSIONAL HEMOSIDEROSIS

Chronic blood transfusion can lead to blood-borne infection, alloimmunization, febrile reactions, and lethal iron overload. A unit of packed RBCs contains 250 to 300 mg iron (1 mg/mL). The iron assimilated by a single transfusion of two units of packed RBCs is thus equal to a 1- to 2-year intake of iron. Iron accumulates in chronically transfused patients because no mechanisms exist for increasing iron excretion; an expanded erythron causes especially rapid development of iron overload because accelerated erythropoiesis promotes excessive absorption of dietary iron. Vitamin C should not be supplemented because it generates free radicals in iron excess states.

Patients who receive >100 units of packed RBCs usually develop hemosiderosis. The ferritin level rises, followed by early endocrine dysfunction (glucose intolerance and delayed puberty), cirrhosis, and cardiomyopathy. Liver biopsy shows both parenchymal and reticuloendothelial iron. Newer methods for assessing hepatic iron such as the superconducting quantum-interference device (SQUID) are accurate but not widely available. Cardiac toxicity is often insidious. Early development of pericarditis is followed by dysrhythmia and pump failure. The onset of heart failure is ominous, often presaging death within a year (Chap. 345).

The decision to start long-term transfusion support should be accompanied by therapy with iron-chelating agents. The only approved and available iron chelator, desferoxamine (Desferal), is expensive and poorly absorbed from the gastrointestinal tract. Its iron-binding kinetics require chronic slow infusion via a metering pump. The constant presence of the drug improves the efficiency of chelation and protects tissues from occasional releases of the most toxic fraction of iron—low-molecular-weight iron—which may not be sequestered by protective proteins. Oral iron-chelating agents such as deferiprone showed initial promise, but long-term trials have raised serious doubts about their efficacy and safety.

Desferoxamine is relatively nontoxic. Occasional cataracts, deafness, and local skin reactions, including urticaria, occur. Skin reactions can usually be managed with antihistamines. Negative iron balance can be achieved, even in the face of a high transfusion requirement, but this alone does not prevent long-term morbidity and mortality in chronically transfused patients. Irreversible end-organ deterioration develops at relatively modest levels of iron overload, even if symptoms do not appear for many years thereafter. To obtain a significant survival advantage, chelation must begin before 5 to 8 years of age.

EXPERIMENTAL THERAPIES

Bone marrow transplantation provides stem cells able to express normal hemoglobin; it has been used in a large number of patients with β thalassemia and a smaller number of patients with sickle cell anemia. Early in the course of disease, before end-organ damage occurs, transplantation is curative in 80 to 90% of patients. In highly experienced centers, the treatment-related mortality is <10%. Since survival into adult life is possible with conventional therapy, the decision to transplant is best made in consultation with specialized centers.

Gene therapy of thalassemia and sickle cell disease has proved to be an elusive goal. Uptake of gene vectors into the nondividing hematopoietic stem cells has been disappointingly inefficient.

Reestablishing high levels of fetal hemoglobin synthesis should ameliorate the symptoms of β thalassemia. Cytotoxic agents such as hydroxyurea and cytarabine promote high levels of HbF synthesis, probably by stimulating proliferation of the primitive HbF-producing progenitor cell population (i.e., F cell progenitors). Unfortunately, no regimen has yet been identified that ameliorates the clinical manifestations of β thalassemia. Butyrates stimulate HbF production, but only transiently. Pulsed or intermittent administration has been found to sustain HbF induction in the majority of patients with sickle cell disease. It is unclear whether butyrate will have similar activity in patients with β thalassemia.

APLASTIC AND HYPOPLASTIC CRISIS IN PATIENTS WITH HEMOGLOBINOPATHIES

Patients with hemolytic anemia sometimes exhibit an alarming decline in hematocrit during and immediately after acute illnesses. Bone marrow suppression occurs in almost everyone during acute inflammatory illnesses. In patients with shortened red cell life spans, suppression can cause anemia. These hypoplastic crises are usually transient and do not require transfusion.

Aplastic crisis refers to a profound cessation of erythroid activity in patients with chronic hemolytic anemia. It is associated with a rapidly falling hematocrit. Episodes are usually self-limited. Aplastic crises are caused by infection with a particular strain of parvovirus (B19A). Children infected with this virus usually develop permanent immunity. Aplastic crises do not often recur and are rarely seen in adults. Management requires close monitoring of the hematocrit and reticulocyte count. If anemia becomes symptomatic, transfusion support is indicated. Most crises resolve spontaneously within 1 to 2 weeks.

ACKNOWLEDGMENT
Some material from Chap. 107 by Dr. Ernest Beutler in the last edition has been retained in this edition. In addition, portions of this chapter describe well-established aspects of this topic and are revised and updated from earlier chapters on this topic by the author.

BIBLIOGRAPHY

BENZ EJ: Hemoglobin variants associated with hemolytic anemia, altered oxygen affinity, and methemoglobinemias, in *Hematology: Basic Principles and Practice*, 3d ed, R Hoffman et al (eds). New York, Churchill Livingstone, 2000, pp 554–561

EMBURY SH, VICHINSKY EP: Sickle cell disease, in *Hematology: Basic Principles and Practice*. 3d ed, R Hoffman et al (eds). New York, Churchill Livingstone, 2000, pp 510–554

FORGET BG: Thalassemia syndromes, in *Hematology: Basic Principles and Practice*, 3d ed, R Hoffman et al (eds). New York, Churchill Livingstone, 2000, pp 485–510

OLIVIERI NF: The beta-thalassemias. N Engl J Med 341:99, 1999

STEINBERG MH: Drug therapy: Management of sickle cell disease. N Engl J Med 340: 1021, 1999

——, BENZ EJ JR: Pathobiology of the human erythrocyte and its hemoglobins, in *Hematology: Basic Principles and Practice*, 3d ed, R Hoffman et al (eds). New York, Churchill Livingstone, 2000, pp 356–367

107   *Bernard M. Babior, H. Franklin Bunn*

MEGALOBLASTIC ANEMIAS

The megaloblastic anemias are disorders caused by impaired DNA synthesis. Cells primarily affected are those having relatively rapid turnover, especially hematopoietic precursors and gastrointestinal epithelial cells. Cell division is sluggish, but cytoplasmic development progresses normally, so megaloblastic cells tend to be large, with an increased ratio of RNA to DNA. Megaloblastic erythroid progenitors tend to be destroyed in the marrow. Thus, marrow cellularity is often increased but production of red blood cells (RBC) is decreased, an abnormality termed *ineffective erythropoiesis* (Chap. 61).

Most megaloblastic anemias are due to a deficiency of cobalamin (vitamin B_{12}) and/or folic acid. The various clinical entities associated with megaloblastic anemia are listed in Table 107-1.

PHYSIOLOGIC AND BIOCHEMICAL CONSIDERATIONS

FOLIC ACID   Folic acid is the common name for pteroylmonoglutamic acid. It is synthesized by many different plants and bacteria. Fruits and vegetables constitute the primary dietary source of the vitamin. Some forms of dietary folic acid are labile and may be destroyed by cooking. The minimum daily requirement is normally about 50 μg, but this may be increased severalfold during periods of enhanced metabolic demand such as pregnancy.

The assimilation of adequate amounts of folic acid depends on the nature of the diet and its means of preparation. Folates in various foodstuffs are largely conjugated to a chain of glutamic acid residues. This highly polar side chain impairs the intestinal absorption of the vitamin. However, conjugases (γ-glutamyl carboxypeptidases) in the lumen of the gut convert polyglutamates to mono- and diglutamates, which are readily absorbed in the proximal jejunum.

Plasma folate is primarily in the form of N^5-methyltetrahydrofolate, a monoglutamate, which is transported into cells by a carrier that is specific for the tetrahydro forms of the vitamin. Once in the cell, the N^5-methyl group is removed in a cobalamin-requiring reaction (see below), and the folate is then reconverted to the polyglutamate form. The polyglutamate form may be useful for retention of folate by the cell.

A folate-binding protein occurs in plasma, milk, and other body fluids. The function of this folate binder and its membrane-bound precursor is unknown. Neither the binder nor its precursor is related to the tetrahydrofolate carrier.

Normal individuals have about 5 to 20 mg folic acid in various body stores, half in the liver. In light of the minimum daily requirement, it is not surprising that a deficiency will occur within months if dietary intake or intestinal absorption is curtailed.

The prime function of folate compounds is to transfer 1-carbon moieties such as methyl and formyl groups to various organic compounds (Fig. 107-1). The sources of these 1-carbon moieties is usually serine, which reacts with tetrahydrofolate to produce glycine and $N^{5,10}$-methylenetetrahydrofolate. An alternative source is formiminoglutamic acid, an intermediate in histidine catabolism, which gives up its formimino group to tetrahydrofolate to yield N^5-formiminotetrahydrofol-

Table 107-1 Classification of the Megaloblastic Anemias

COBALAMIN DEFICIENCY

I. Inadequate intake: vegetarians (rare)
II. Malabsorption
   A. Defective release of cobalamin from food
      1. Gastric achlorhydria
      2. Partial gastrectomy
      3. Drugs that block acid secretion
   B. Inadequate production of intrinsic factor (IF)
      1. Pernicious anemia
      2. Total gastrectomy
      3. Congenital absence or functional abnormality of IF (rare)
   C. Disorders of terminal ileum
      1. Tropical sprue
      2. Nontropical sprue
      3. Regional enteritis
      4. Intestinal resection
      5. Neoplasms and granulomatous disorders (rare)
      6. Selective cobalamin malabsorption (Imerslund's syndrome) (rare)
   D. Competition for cobalamin
      1. Fish tapeworm (Diphyllobothrium latum)
      2. Bacteria: "blind loop" syndrome
   E. Drugs: *p*-aminosalicylic acid, colchicine, neomycin
III. Other
   A. Nitrous oxide
   B. Transcobalamin II deficiency (rare)
   C. Congenital enzyme defects (rare)

FOLIC ACID DEFICIENCY

I. Inadequate intake: unbalanced diet (common in alcoholics, teenagers, some infants)
II. Increased requirements
   A. Pregnancy
   B. Infancy
   C. Malignancy
   D. Increased hematopoiesis (chronic hemolytic anemias)
   E. Chronic exfoliative skin disorders
   F. Hemodialysis
III. Malabsorption
   A. Tropical sprue
   B. Nontropical sprue
   C. Drugs: Phenytoin, barbiturates, (?) ethanol
IV. Impaired metabolism
   A. Inhibitors of dihydrofolate reductase: methotrexate, pyrimethamine, triamterene, pentamidine, trimethoprim
   B. Alcohol
   C. Rare enzyme deficiencies: dihydrofolate reductase, others

OTHER CAUSES

I. Drugs that impair DNA metabolism
   A. Purine antagonists: 6-mercaptopurine, azathioprine, etc.
   B. Pyrimidine antagonists: 5-fluorouracil, cytosine arabinoside, etc.
   C. Others: procarbazine, hydroxyurea, acyclovir, zidovudine
II. Metabolic disorders (rare)
   A. Hereditary orotic aciduria
   B. Lesch-Nyhan syndrome
   C. Others
III. Megaloblastic anemia of unknown etiology
   A. Refractory megaloblastic anemia
   B. Di Guglielmo's syndrome[a]
   C. Congenital dyserythropoietic anemia

[a] A form of acute myeloid leukemia with atypical, dysplastic changes in erythroid series.

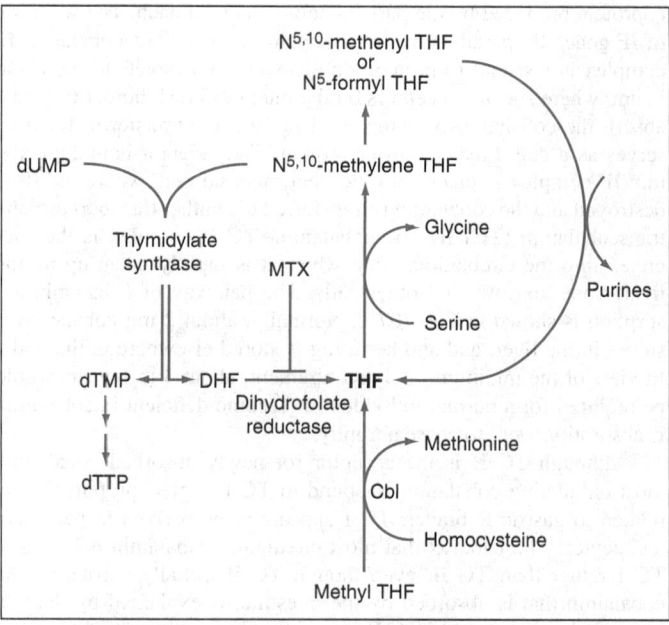

FIGURE 107-1 Folate metabolism. Folate is essential for the de novo synthesis of purines, deoxythymidylate monophosphate (dTMP) and methionine, serving as an intermediate carrier of 1-carbon fragments used in the biosynthesis of these compounds. Its active form is tetrahydrofolate (THF). THF acquires the 1-carbon fragment principally from serine, which is converted to glycine in the course of the reaction. For purine synthesis, the 1-carbon fragment is first oxidized to the level of formic acid, then transferred to substrate. For methionine synthesis, a cobalamin-requiring reaction, the 1-carbon fragment is first reduced to the level of a methyl group, then transferred to homocysteine. In these reactions the cofactor is released as THF, which can immediately participate in another 1-carbon transfer cycle. During the production of dTMP from dUMP, however, the 1-carbon fragment is reduced from formaldehyde to a methyl group in the course of the transfer reaction. The hydrogen atoms used for this reduction come from the cofactor, which is therefore released, not as THF, but as dihydrofolate (DHF). To participate further in the 1-carbon transfer cycle, the DHF has to be re-reduced to THF, a reaction catalyzed by dihydrofolate reductase.

ate and glutamic acid. These derivatives provide entry into an interconvertible donor pool consisting of tetrahydrofolate derivatives carrying various 1-carbon moieties. The constituents of this pool can donate their 1-carbon moieties to appropriate acceptor compounds to form metabolic intermediates, which are ultimately converted to building blocks used in the synthesis of macromolecules. The most important building blocks are (1) purines, in which the C-2 and C-8 atoms are introduced in folate-dependent reactions; (2) deoxythymidylate monophosphate (dTMP), synthesized from $N^{5,10}$-methylenetetrahydrofolate and deoxyuridylate monophosphate (dUMP); and (3) methionine, formed by the transfer of a methyl group from N^5-methyltetrahydrofolate to homocysteine (two of these three reactions are shown in Fig. 107-1).

In all but one of the 1-carbon transfer reactions, tetrahydrofolate is produced. It can immediately accept a 1-carbon moiety and reenter the donor pool. The single exception is the thymidylate synthase reaction (dUMP → dTMP), in which dihydrofolate is the product (Fig. 107-1). This must be reduced to tetrahydrofolate by the enzyme dihydrofolate reductase before it can reenter the donor pool. A number of drugs are able to inhibit dihydrofolate reductase (Table 107-1), thereby diverting folate from the donor pool and producing what amounts to a state of folate deficiency in the face of normal tissue folate concentrations.

COBALAMIN This vitamin is a complex organometallic compound in which a cobalt atom is situated within a corrin ring, a structure similar to the porphyrin from which heme is formed. Unlike heme, however, cobalamin cannot be synthesized in the human body and must be supplied in the diet. The only dietary source of cobalamin is animal products: meat and dairy foods. The minimum daily requirement for cobalamin is about 2.5 μg.

During gastric digestion, cobalamin in food is released and forms a stable complex with gastric R binder, one of a closely related group of glycoproteins of unknown function that are found in secretions (e.g., saliva, milk, gastric juice, bile), phagocytes, and plasma. On entering the duodenum, the cobalamin–R binder complex is digested, releasing the cobalamin, which then binds to intrinsic factor (IF), a 50-kDa glycoprotein produced by the parietal cells of the stomach. The secretion of IF generally parallels that of hydrochloric acid. The cobalamin-IF complex is resistant to proteolytic digestion and travels to the distal ileum, where specific receptors on the mucosal brush border bind and absorb the cobalamin-IF complex. Thus IF, like transferrin for iron, serves as a cell-directed carrier protein. The receptor-bound cobalamin-IF complex is taken into the ileal mucosal cell, where the IF is destroyed and the cobalamin is transferred to another transport protein, transcobalamin (TC) II. The cobalamin–TC II complex is then secreted into the circulation, from which it is rapidly taken up by the liver, bone marrow, and other cells. The pathway of cobalamin absorption is shown in Fig. 107-2. Normally, about 2 mg cobalamin is stored in the liver, and another 2 mg is stored elsewhere in the body. In view of the minimum daily requirement, about 3 to 6 years would be required for a normal individual to become deficient in cobalamin if absorption were to cease abruptly.

Although TC II is the acceptor for newly absorbed cobalamin, most circulating cobalamin is bound to TC I, a glycoprotein closely related to gastric R binder. TC I appears to be derived in part from leukocytes. The paradox that most circulating cobalamin is bound to TC I rather than TC II, even though TC II initially carries all the cobalamin that is absorbed by the intestine, is explained by the fact that cobalamin bound to TC II is rapidly cleared from the blood ($t_{1/2}$ about 1 h), while clearance of cobalamin bound to TC I requires many days. The function of TC I is unknown.

Cobalamin is an essential cofactor for two enzymes in human cells: methionine synthase and methylmalonyl-CoA synthase. Cobalamin exists in two metabolically active forms, identified by the alkyl group attached to the sixth coordination position of the cobalt atom: methylcobalamin and adenosylcobalamin. The vitamin preparation that is used therapeutically is cyanocobalamin (also called vitamin B_{12}). Cyanocobalamin has no known physiologic role and must be converted to a biologically active form before it can be used by tissues.

Methylcobalamin is the form required for methionine synthase, which catalyzes the conversion of homocysteine to methionine (Fig. 107-1). When this reaction is impaired, folate metabolism is deranged, and it is this derangement that underlies the defect in DNA synthesis and the megaloblastic maturation pattern in patients who are deficient in cobalamin. In cobalamin deficiency, the unconjugated N^5-methyltetrahydrofolate newly taken from the bloodstream cannot be converted to other forms of tetrahydrofolate by methyl transfer. This is the so-called folate trap hypothesis. Because N^5-methyltetrahydrofolate is a poor substrate for the conjugating enzyme, it largely remains in the unconjugated form and slowly leaks from the cell. Tissue folate deficiency therefore develops, and this results in megaloblastic hematopoiesis. This hypothesis explains why tissue folate stores in cobalamin deficiency are substantially reduced, with a disproportionate reduction in conjugated, as compared with unconjugated, folates, despite normal or supranormal serum folate levels. It also explains why large doses of folate can produce a partial hematologic remission in patients with cobalamin deficiency.

Megaloblastic changes in both cobalamin and folate deficiency as well as in methotrexate treatment are related to a deficiency in production of dTMP. In addition, the excess deoxyuridylate that accumulates can be phosphorylated and mistakenly incorporated into DNA in place of thymidylate; base pairing can be affected by this U-for-T substitution.

Plasma homocysteine levels are elevated in both folate and cobalamin deficiency, and high levels of plasma homocysteine appear to be a risk factor for thrombosis in both veins and arteries. It is not yet known, however, if hyperhomocysteinemia due to folate or cobalamin deficiency predisposes to thrombosis or alters its response to treatment.

Impairment in the conversion of homocysteine to methionine may also be partly responsible for the neurologic complications of cobalamin deficiency (see below). The methionine formed in this reaction is needed for the production of choline and choline-containing phospholipids. Nervous system damage is postulated to result at least in part from interference with these processes due to decreased methionine production in cobalamin deficiency.

Adenosylcobalamin is required for the conversion of methylmalonyl CoA to succinyl CoA. Lack of this cofactor leads to large increases in the tissue levels of methylmalonyl CoA and its precursor, propionyl CoA. As a consequence, nonphysiologic fatty acids containing an odd number of carbon atoms are synthesized and incorporated into neuronal lipids. This biochemical abnormality may also contribute to the neurologic complications of cobalamin deficiency (see below).

CLINICAL DISORDERS

CLASSIFICATION OF MEGALOBLASTIC ANEMIAS

(Table 107-1) The cause of megaloblastic anemia varies in different parts of the world. In temperate zones, folate deficiency in alcoholics and pernicious anemia are the common types of megaloblastic anemias. In certain areas close to the equator, tropical sprue is endemic and an important cause of megaloblastic anemia, while in Scandinavia, infestations by the fish tapeworm, *Diphyllobothrium latum*, may be a cause.

The dietary intake of cobalamin is more than adequate for the body's requirements, except in true vegetarians and their breast-fed infants. Thus deficiency of cobalamin is almost always due to malabsorption. Malabsorption can occur at several levels. In contrast, the dietary intake of folic acid is marginal in many parts of the world. Furthermore, because the body's stores of folate are relatively low, folic acid deficiency can arise rather suddenly during periods of de-

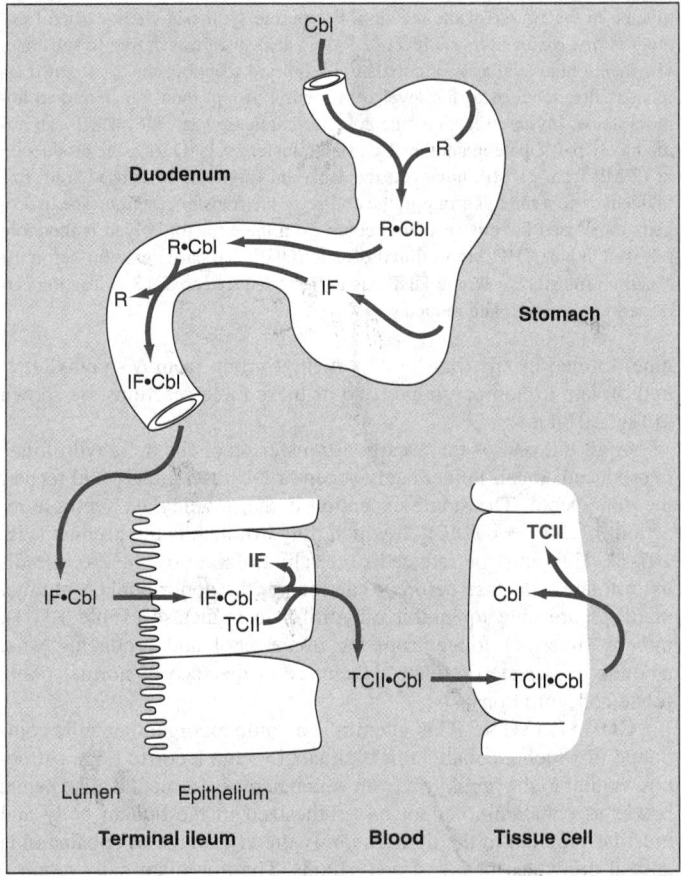

FIGURE 107-2 The assimilation of cobalamin. On entering the stomach, dietary cobalamin (Cbl) forms a complex with R binding protein. As this protein is digested in the small intestine, cobalamin is transferred to intrinsic factor (IF). This complex passes through the intestine until it reaches specific receptors on the mucosa of the distal ileum. The internalized Cbl is then transferred to transcobalamin II (TC II), which circulates in the plasma until it binds to receptors on cells throughout the body and is internalized.

creased dietary intake or increased metabolic demand. Finally, folic acid deficiency may be due to malabsorption. Often two or more of these factors coexist in a given patient.

Combined deficiencies of cobalamin and folic acid are not uncommon. Patients with tropical sprue are often deficient in both vitamins. The biochemical lesion that results in megaloblastic maturation of bone marrow cells also causes structural and functional abnormalities of the rapidly proliferating epithelial cells of the intestinal mucosa. Thus severe deficiency of one vitamin can lead to malabsorption of the other. Furthermore, as discussed above, a deficiency of cobalamin causes a secondary reduction in cellular folic acid.

Finally, megaloblastic anemias may occasionally be induced by factors unrelated to a vitamin deficiency. Most such cases are caused by one or more of the many drugs that interfere with DNA synthesis. Less commonly, megaloblastic maturation is encountered in certain acquired defects of hematopoietic stem cells. Rarest of all are specific congenital enzyme deficiencies.

COBALAMIN DEFICIENCY   The clinical features of cobalamin deficiency involve the blood, the gastrointestinal tract, and the nervous system.

The hematologic manifestations are almost entirely the result of anemia, although very rarely purpura may appear, due to thrombocytopenia. Symptoms of anemia may include weakness, light-headedness, vertigo, and tinnitus, as well as palpitations, angina, and the symptoms of congestive failure. On physical examination, the patient with florid cobalamin deficiency is pale, with slightly icteric skin and eyes. Elevated bilirubin levels are related to high erythroid cell turnover in the marrow. The pulse is rapid, and the heart may be enlarged; auscultation will usually reveal a systolic flow murmur.

The gastrointestinal manifestations reflect the effect of cobalamin deficiency on the rapidly proliferating gastrointestinal epithelium. The patient sometimes complains of a sore tongue, which on inspection will be smooth and beefy red. Anorexia with moderate weight loss may also be evident, possibly accompanied by diarrhea and other gastrointestinal symptoms. These latter manifestations may be caused in part by megaloblastosis of the small intestinal epithelium, which results in malabsorption.

The neurologic manifestations often fail to remit fully on treatment. They begin pathologically with demyelination, followed by axonal degeneration and eventual neuronal death; the final stage, of course, is irreversible. Sites of involvement include peripheral nerves; the spinal cord, where the posterior and lateral columns undergo demyelination; and the cerebrum itself. Signs and symptoms include numbness and paresthesia in the extremities (the earliest neurologic manifestations), weakness, and ataxia. There may be sphincter disturbances. Reflexes may be diminished or increased. The Romberg and Babinski signs may be positive, and position and vibration senses are usually diminished. Disturbances of mentation will vary from mild irritability and forgetfulness to severe dementia or frank psychosis. It should be emphasized that *neurologic disease may occur in a patient with a normal hematocrit* and normal RBC indexes. Although it has many benefits, folate supplementation of food may increase the likelihood of neurologic presentations of cobalamin deficiency.

In the classic patient, in whom hematologic problems predominate, the blood and bone marrow show characteristic megaloblastic changes (described under "Diagnosis," below). The anemia may be very severe—hematocrits of 15 to 20 are not infrequent—but is surprisingly well tolerated by the patient because it develops so slowly.

Defective Release of Cobalamin from Food   Cobalamin in food is tightly bound to enzymes in meat and is split from these enzymes by hydrochloric acid and pepsin in the stomach. People older than 70 years are commonly unable to release cobalamin from food sources but retain the ability to absorb crystalline B_{12}, the form most commonly found in multivitamins. The exact incidence of the defect in cobalamin release from food has not been well defined; estimates vary from 10 to greater than 50% of those over age 70 years. Only a minority of these persons go on to develop frank cobalamin deficiency, but many have biochemical changes, including low levels of cobala-

min bound to TC II and elevated homocysteine levels, that augur cobalamin deficiency (see below).

Similarly, patients on drugs that suppress gastric acid production, such as omeprazole, may also fail to release cobalamin from food.

Pernicious Anemia   Pernicious anemia, considered the most common cause of cobalamin deficiency, is caused by the absence of IF, from either atrophy of the gastric mucosa or autoimmune destruction of parietal cells. It is most frequently seen in individuals of northern European descent and African Americans and is much less common in southern Europeans and Asians. Men and women are equally affected. It is a disease of the elderly, the average patient presenting near age 60; it is rare under age 30, although typical pernicious anemia can be seen in children under age 10 (juvenile pernicious anemia). Inherited conditions in which a histologically normal stomach secretes either an abnormal IF or none at all will induce cobalamin deficiency in infancy or early childhood.

The incidence of pernicious anemia is substantially increased in patients with other diseases thought to be of immunologic origin, including Graves' disease, myxedema, thyroiditis, idiopathic adrenocortical insufficiency, vitiligo, and hypoparathyroidism. Patients with pernicious anemia also have abnormal circulating antibodies related to their disease: 90% have antiparietal cell antibody, which is directed against the H^+,K^+-ATPase, while 60% have anti-IF antibody. Antiparietal cell antibody is also found in 50% of patients with gastric atrophy without pernicious anemia, as well as in 10 to 15% of an unselected patient population, but anti-IF antibody is usually absent from these patients. Relatives of patients with pernicious anemia have an increased incidence of the disease, and even clinically unaffected relatives may have anti-IF antibody in their serum. Finally, treatment with glucocorticoids may reverse the disease.

The destruction of parietal cells in pernicious anemia is thought to be mediated by cytotoxic T cells. Pernicious anemia is unusually common in patients with agammaglobulinemia, suggesting that the cellular immune system plays a role in its pathogenesis. In contrast, *Helicobacter pylori* does not cause parietal cell destruction in pernicious anemia.

The most characteristic finding in pernicious anemia is gastric atrophy affecting the acid- and pepsin-secreting portion of the stomach; the antrum is spared. Other pathologic changes are secondary to the deficiency of cobalamin; these include megaloblastic alterations in the gastric and intestinal epithelium and the neurologic changes described above. The abnormalities in the gastric epithelium appear as cellular atypia in gastric cytology specimens, a finding that must be carefully distinguished from the cytologic abnormalities seen in gastric malignancy.

The *clinical manifestations* are primarily those of cobalamin deficiency, as described above. The disease is of insidious onset and progresses slowly. Laboratory examination will reveal hypergastrinemia and pentagastrin-fast achlorhydria as well as the hematologic and other laboratory abnormalities discussed under "Diagnosis."

Through appropriate replacement therapy, patients with pernicious anemia should experience complete and lifelong correction of all abnormalities that are due to cobalamin deficiency, except to the extent that irreversible changes in the nervous system may have occurred before treatment. These patients, however, are unusually subject to gastric polyps and have about twice the normal incidence of cancer of the stomach. Thus, patients should be followed with frequent stool guaiac examinations and endoscopy when indicated.

Postgastrectomy   Following total gastrectomy or extensive damage to gastric mucosa as, for example, by ingestion of corrosive agents, megaloblastic anemia will develop because the source of IF has been removed. In all such patients, the absorption of orally administered cobalamin is impaired. Megaloblastic anemia may also follow partial gastrectomy, but the incidence is lower than after total gastrectomy. The cause of cobalamin deficiency after partial gastrectomy is not clear; defective release of cobalamin from food and intestinal overgrowth of bacteria have been suggested, but response to antibiotics is not common.

Intestinal Organisms Megaloblastic anemia may occur with intestinal stasis due to anatomic lesions (strictures, diverticula, anastomoses, "blind loops") or pseudoobstruction (diabetes mellitus, scleroderma, amyloid). This anemia is caused by colonization of the small intestine by large masses of bacteria that consume intestinal cobalamin before absorption. Steatorrhea may also be seen under these circumstances because bile salt metabolism is disturbed when the intestine is heavily colonized with bacteria. Hematologic responses have been observed after administration of oral antibiotics such as tetracycline and ampicillin. Megaloblastic anemia is seen in persons harboring the fish tapeworm, *D. latum*, due to competition by the worm for cobalamin. Destruction of the worm eliminates the problem.

Ileal Abnormalities Cobalamin deficiency is common in tropical sprue, while it is an unusual complication of nontropical sprue (gluten-sensitive enteropathy; Chap. 286). Virtually any disorder that compromises the absorptive capacity of the distal ileum can result in cobalamin deficiency. Specific entities include regional enteritis, Whipple's disease, and tuberculosis. Segmental involvement of the distal ileum by disease can cause megaloblastic anemia without any other manifestations of intestinal malabsorption such as steatorrhea. Cobalamin malabsorption is also seen after ileal resection. The Zollinger-Ellison syndrome (intense gastric hyperacidity due to a gastrin-secreting tumor) may cause cobalamin malabsorption by acidifying the small intestine, retarding the transfer of the vitamin from R binder to IF and impairing the binding of the cobalamin-IF complex to the ileal receptors. Chronic pancreatitis may also cause cobalamin malabsorption by impairing the transfer of the vitamin from R binder to IF. This abnormality can be detected by tests of cobalamin absorption (see below, Schilling test), but it is invariably mild and never causes clinical cobalamin deficiency. Finally, there is a rare congenital disorder, Imerslund-Gräsbeck disease, in which a selective defect in cobalamin absorption is accompanied by proteinuria. Affected individuals have a mutation in cubulin, a receptor that mediates intestinal absorption of the cobalamin-IF complex.

Nitrous Oxide Inhalation of nitrous oxide as an anesthetic destroys endogenous cobalamin. As ordinarily used, the magnitude of the effects are not sufficient to cause clinical cobalamin deficiency, but repeated or protracted exposure (>6 h), particularly in older patients with borderline cobalamin stores, can lead to severe megaloblastic anemia and/or acute neurologic deficits.

FOLIC ACID DEFICIENCY Since January, 1998, folic acid has been added to all enriched grain products by order of the U.S. Food and Drug Administration; accordingly, the incidence of folic acid deficiency has fallen markedly. Patients with folic acid deficiency are more often malnourished than those with cobalamin deficiency. The gastrointestinal manifestations are similar to but may be more widespread and more severe than those of pernicious anemia. Diarrhea is often present, and cheilosis and glossitis are also encountered. However, in contrast to cobalamin deficiency, neurologic abnormalities do not occur.

The hematologic manifestations of folic acid deficiency are the same as those of cobalamin deficiency. Folic acid deficiency can generally be attributed to one or more of the following factors: inadequate intake, increased demand, or malabsorption.

Inadequate Intake Alcoholics may become folate deficient because their main source of caloric intake is alcoholic beverages. Distilled spirits are virtually devoid of folic acid, while beer and wine do not contain enough of the vitamin to satisfy the daily requirement. In addition, alcohol may interfere with folate metabolism. Narcotic addicts are also prone to become folate deficient because of malnutrition. Many indigent and elderly individuals who subsist primarily on canned foods or "tea and toast" and occasional teenagers whose diet consists of "junk food" develop folate deficiency. Food folate supplementation has made folate deficiency very rare.

Increased Demand Tissues with a relatively high rate of cell division such as the bone marrow or gut mucosa have a large requirement for folate. Therefore, patients with chronic hemolytic anemias or other causes of very active erythropoiesis may become deficient. Pregnant women formerly were at risk to become deficient in folic acid because of the high demand of the developing fetus. Deficiency in the first weeks of pregnancy can cause neural tube defects in newborns. Often the pregnancy was not detected until the defect had developed; thus, provision of folate supplementation to women after they learned they were pregnant was ineffective. However, folate food supplementation has decreased neural tube defects by more than 50%. Folate deficiency may also occur during the growth spurts of infancy and adolescence. Patients on chronic hemodialysis may require supplementary folate to replace that lost in the dialysate.

Malabsorption Folic acid deficiency is a common accompaniment of tropical sprue. Both the gastrointestinal symptoms and malabsorption are improved by the administration of either folic acid or antibiotics by mouth. Patients with nontropical sprue (gluten-sensitive enteropathy) may also develop significant folic acid deficiency that parallels other parameters of malabsorption. Similarly, folate deficiency in alcoholics may be due in part to malabsorption. In addition, other primary small-bowel disorders are sometimes associated with folate deficiency (Chap. 286).

DRUGS Next to deficiency of folate or cobalamin, the most common cause of megaloblastic anemia is drugs. Agents that cause megaloblastic anemia do so by interfering with DNA synthesis, either directly or by antagonizing the action of folate. They can be classified as follows:

1. *Direct inhibitors of DNA synthesis.* They include purine analogues (6-thioguanine, azathioprine, 6-mercaptopurine), pyrimidine analogues (5-fluorouracil, cytosine arabinoside), and other drugs that interfere with DNA synthesis by a variety of mechanisms (hydroxyurea, procarbazine). The antiviral agent zidovudine (AZT), used for treating HIV, often causes severe megaloblastic anemia.

2. *Folate antagonists.* The most toxic of these is methotrexate, a powerful inhibitor of dihydrofolate reductase which is used in the treatment of certain malignancies. Much less toxic but still capable of inducing a megaloblastic anemia are several weak dihydrofolate reductase inhibitors used to treat a variety of nonmalignant conditions including pentamidine, trimethoprim, triamterene, and pyrimethamine.

3. *Others.* A number of drugs antagonize folate by mechanisms that are poorly understood but are thought to involve an effect on absorption of the vitamin by the intestine. In this category are the anticonvulsants phenytoin, primidone, and phenobarbital. Megaloblastic anemia induced by these agents is mild.

OTHER MECHANISMS Hereditary Megaloblastic anemia may be seen in several hereditary disorders. Orotic aciduria is a deficiency of orotidylic decarboxylase and phosphorylase, leading to a defect in pyrimidine metabolism and characterized by retarded growth and development as well as by the excretion of large amounts of orotic acid. Megaloblastic anemia has been reported in a single case of the Lesch-Nyhan syndrome, a condition resulting from a deficiency of hypoxanthine-guanine phosphoribosyltransferase whose clinical manifestations include gout, mental retardation, and self-mutilation. It has also been described in methylmalonic aciduria due to a combined defect in the biosynthesis of methyl and adenosyl cobalamins, although it is not seen in methylmalonic aciduria due to methylmalonyl CoA mutase deficiency. Congenital folate malabsorption causes megaloblastic anemia, accompanied by ataxia and mental retardation. Megaloblastic anemia has been reported to accompany the congenital deficiency of two other folate-metabolizing enzymes: dihydrofolate reductase and N^5-methyltetrahydrofolate:homocysteine methyltransferase. These deficiencies are less well documented than is congenital folate malabsorption. A thiamine-responsive megaloblastic anemia accompanied by nerve deafness and diabetes mellitus has been reported in several children. Megaloblastic changes as well as multinuclearity of red blood cell precursors are seen in the marrow of certain patients with congenital dyserythropoietic anemia, a group of inherited

TC II deficiency, like the congenital abnormalities in cobalamin absorption described previously, causes pronounced deficiency in cobalamin in infancy or early childhood, with all the accompanying manifestations. Megaloblastic anemia is not seen in hereditary TC I deficiency.

Refractory Megaloblastic Anemia This is a form of myelodysplasia in which megaloblastic erythropoiesis may sometimes be seen. Megaloblastic changes are restricted to the RBC series (see below). As with other forms of myelodysplasia, refractory megaloblastic anemia is associated with an increased incidence of acute leukemia.

Megaloblastic changes are seen in erythremic myelosis and acute erythroleukemia (di Guglielmo), where RBC precursors are prominently involved. Here, the marrow is characterized by bizarre erythroid maturation, with multinuclearity and multipolar mitotic figures in the RBC precursors (Chap. 111).

MEGALOBLASTIC DISEASE WITHOUT ANEMIA Megaloblastic disease is easily overlooked in nonanemic patients. It can present in one of two ways.

Acute Megaloblastic Anemia Occasionally, a full-blown megaloblastic state can develop over the course of just a few days. This is usually seen following nitrous oxide anesthesia but may occur in any patient with a serious illness requiring intensive care, especially a patient receiving multiple transfusions, dialysis, or total parenteral nutrition. An acute megaloblastic state can also be precipitated by the administration of a weak antifolate (e.g., trimethoprim) to a patient with marginal tissue folate stores.

The condition resembles an immune cytopenia, with a rapidly developing thrombocytopenia and/or leukopenia in the absence of anemia. The blood smear may be completely normal, but the marrow is floridly megaloblastic. Acute megaloblastic anemia responds rapidly to treatment with folate plus cobalamin in the usual therapeutic doses.

Cobalamin Deficiency without Anemia Cobalamin deficiency without hematologic abnormalities is surprisingly common, especially in the elderly. The risk of a nonhematologic presentation for cobalamin deficiency is increased by the folate food fortification because folate can mask the hematologic effects of cobalamin deficiency. Between 10 and 30% of persons over age 70 years have metabolic evidence of cobalamin deficiency, either elevated homocysteine levels, low cobalamin-TCII levels, or both. Only 10% of these patients have defective production of IF, and the remainder often have atrophic gastritis and cannot release cobalamin from their food (see above). These patients may present with neuropsychiatric abnormalities, including peripheral neuropathies, gait disturbance, memory loss, and psychiatric symptoms, sometimes with abnormal evoked potentials. Serum cobalamin levels may be normal or low, but serum levels of methylmalonic acid are almost invariably increased due to a deficiency of cobalamin at the tissue level. The neuropsychiatric abnormalities tend to improve and serum methylmalonic acid levels generally return to normal after treatment with cobalamin. Neurologic defects do not always reverse with cobalamin supplementation.

DIAGNOSIS The finding of significant macrocytosis [mean corpuscular volume (MCV) > 100 fL] suggests the presence of a megaloblastic anemia. Other causes of macrocytosis include hemolysis, liver disease, alcoholism, hypothyroidism, and aplastic anemia. If the macrocytosis is marked (MCV > 110 fL), the patient is much more likely to have a megaloblastic anemia. Macrocytosis is less marked with concurrent iron deficiency or thalassemia. The reticulocyte count is low, and the leukocyte and platelet count may also be decreased, particularly in severely anemic patients. The blood smear (**see Plate V-24**) demonstrates marked anisocytosis and poikilocytosis, together with macroovalocytes, which are large, oval, fully hemoglobinized erythrocytes typical of megaloblastic anemias. There is some basophilic stippling, and an occasional nucleated RBC may be seen. In the white blood cell series, the neutrophils show hypersegmentation of the nucleus (**see Plate V-38**). This is such a characteristic finding that a single cell with a nucleus of six lobes or more should raise the im-

mediate suspicion of a megaloblastic anemia. A rare myelocyte may also be seen. Bizarre, misshapen platelets are also observed. The reticulocyte index is low. The bone marrow is hypercellular with a decreased myeloid/erythroid ratio and abundant stainable iron. RBC precursors are abnormally large and have nuclei that appear much less mature than would be expected from the development of the cytoplasm (nuclear-cytoplasmic asynchrony). The nuclear chromatin is more dispersed than expected, and it condenses in a peculiar fenestrated pattern that is very characteristic of megaloblastic erythropoiesis. Abnormal mitoses may be seen. Granulocyte precursors are also affected, many being larger than normal, including giant bands and metamyelocytes. Megakaryocytes are decreased and show abnormal morphology.

Megaloblastic anemias are characterized by ineffective erythropoiesis (Chap. 61). In a severely megaloblastic patient, as many as 90% of the RBC precursors may be destroyed before they are released into the bloodstream, compared with 10 to 15% in normal individuals. Enhanced intramedullary destruction of erythroblasts results in an increase in unconjugated bilirubin and lactic acid dehydrogenase (isoenzyme 1) in plasma. Abnormalities in iron kinetics also attest to the presence of ineffective erythropoiesis, with increased iron turnover but low incorporation of labeled iron into circulating RBCs.

In evaluating a patient with megaloblastic anemia, it is important to determine whether there is a specific vitamin deficiency by measuring serum cobalamin and folate levels. The normal range of cobalamin in serum is 200 to 900 pg/mL; values <100 pg/mL indicate clinically significant deficiency. Measurements of cobalamin bound to TC II would be a more physiologic measure of cobalamin status, but such assays are not yet routinely available. The normal serum concentration of folic acid ranges from 6 to 20 ng/mL; values ≤4 ng/mL are generally considered to be diagnostic of folate deficiency. Unlike serum cobalamin, serum folate levels may reflect recent alterations in dietary intake. Measurement of RBC folate level provides useful information because it is not subject to short-term fluctuations in folate intake and is better than serum folate as an index of folate stores.

Once cobalamin deficiency has been established, its pathogenesis can be delineated by means of a Schilling test. A patient is given radioactive cobalamin by mouth, followed shortly thereafter by an intramuscular injection of unlabeled cobalamin. The proportion of the administered radioactivity excreted in the urine during the next 24 h provides an accurate measure of absorption of cobalamin, assuming that a complete urine sample has been collected. Because cobalamin deficiency is almost always due to malabsorption (Table 107-1), this first stage of the Schilling test should be abnormal (i.e., small amounts of radioactivity in the urine). The patient is then given labeled cobalamin bound to IF. Absorption of the vitamin will now approach normal if the patient has pernicious anemia or some other type of IF deficiency. If cobalamin absorption is still decreased, the patient may have bacterial overgrowth (blind loop syndrome) or ileal disease (including an ileal absorptive defect secondary to the cobalamin deficiency itself). Cobalamin malabsorption due to bacterial overgrowth can frequently be corrected by the administration of antibiotics. The Schilling test can provide equally reliable information after the patient has had adequate therapy with parenteral cobalamin.

A normal Schilling test in a patient with documented cobalamin deficiency may indicate poor absorption of the vitamin when mixed with food. This can be established by repeating the Schilling test with radioactive cobalamin scrambled with an egg.

Serum methylmalonic acid and homocysteine levels are also useful in the diagnosis of megaloblastic anemias. Both are elevated in cobalamin deficiency, while elevated levels of homocysteine but not methylmalonic acid are seen in folate deficiency. These tests measure tissue vitamin stores and may demonstrate a deficiency even when the more traditional but less reliable folate and cobalamin levels are borderline or even normal. Patients (particularly older patients) without anemia and with normal serum cobalamin levels but elevated levels of serum methylmalonic acid may develop neuropsychiatric abnormalities. Treatment of patients with this "subtle" cobalamin deficiency will usually prevent further deterioration and may result in improvement.

℞ **TREATMENT   Cobalamin Deficiency**   Apart from specific therapy related to the underlying disorder (e.g., antibiotics for intestinal overgrowth with bacteria), the mainstay of treatment for cobalamin deficiency is replacement therapy. Because the defect is nearly always malabsorption, patients are generally given parenteral treatment, specifically in the form of intramuscular cyanocobalamin. Parenteral treatment begins with 1000 μg cobalamin per week for 8 weeks, followed by 1000 μg cyanocobalamin intramuscularly every month for the rest of the patient's life. However, cobalamin deficiency can also be managed very effectively by oral replacement therapy with 2 mg crystalline B_{12} per day.

The response to treatment is gratifying. Shortly after treatment is begun, and several days before a hematologic response is evident in the peripheral blood, the patient will experience an increase in strength and an improved sense of well-being. Marrow morphology begins to revert toward normal within a few hours after treatment is initiated. Reticulocytosis begins 4 to 5 days after therapy is started and peaks at about day 7 (Fig. 107-3), with subsequent remission of the anemia over the next several weeks. If a reticulocytosis does not occur, or if it is less brisk than expected from the level of the hematocrit, a search should be made for other factors contributing to the anemia (e.g., infection, coexisting iron and/or folate deficiency, or hypothyroidism). Hypokalemia and salt retention may occur early in the course of therapy. Thrombocytosis may also be seen.

In most cases, replacement therapy is all that is needed for the treatment of cobalamin deficiency. Occasionally, however, a patient with a severe anemia will have such a precarious cardiovascular status that emergency transfusion is necessary. This must be done with great care, because such patients may develop heart failure from fluid overload. Blood must be administered slowly in the form of packed RBCs, with very close observation. A small volume of packed RBCs will frequently be enough to ameliorate the acute cardiovascular problems. If necessary, blood may be administered by exchanging patient blood (mostly plasma) for packed cells.

With lifelong treatment, patients should experience no further manifestations of cobalamin deficiency, although neurologic symptoms may not be fully corrected even by optimal therapy. The potential for late development of gastric carcinoma in pernicious anemia necessitates careful follow-up of the patient.

Folate, particularly in large doses, can correct the megaloblastic anemia of cobalamin deficiency without altering the neurologic abnormalities. The neurologic manifestations may even be aggravated by folate therapy. Cobalamin deficiency can thus be masked in patients who are taking large doses of folate. For this reason, a hematologic response to folate must never be used to rule out cobalamin deficiency in a given patient; cobalamin deficiency can be excluded only by appropriate laboratory evaluation.

In light of the high frequency of defective cobalamin absorption in older people and the possible increased risk that overt cobalamin deficiency will present with neurologic rather than hematologic symptoms (because of folate food fortification), some experts have recommended the use of 0.1 mg oral crystalline cobalamin prophylaxis daily in people over age 65 years.

Folate Deficiency   As for cobalamin deficiency, folate deficiency is treated by replacement therapy. The usual dose of folate is 1 mg/d, by mouth, but higher doses (up to 5 mg/d) may be required for folate deficiency due to malabsorption. Parenteral folate is rarely necessary. The hematologic response is similar to that seen after replacement therapy for cobalamin deficiency, i.e., a brisk reticulocytosis after about 4 days, followed by correction of the anemia over the next 1 to 2 months. The duration of therapy depends on the basis of the deficiency state. Patients with a continuously increased requirement (such as patients with hemolytic anemia) or those with malabsorption or chronic malnutrition should continue to receive oral folic acid indefinitely. In addition, the patient should be encouraged to maintain an optimal diet containing adequate amounts of folate.

Other Causes of Megaloblastic Anemia   Megaloblastic anemia due to drugs can be treated, if necessary, by reducing the dose of the drug or eliminating it altogether. The effects of folate antagonists that inhibit dihydrofolate reductase can be counteracted by folinic acid [5-formyl tetrahydrofolate (THF)] in a dose of 100 to 200 mg/d (Fig. 107-1), which circumvents the block in folate metabolism by providing a form of folate that can be converted to 5,10-methylene THF. For the megaloblastic forms of sideroblastic anemia, pyridoxine in pharmacologic doses (as high as 300 mg/d) should be tried. If this fails, pyridoxal phosphate may work, presumably in part by promoting the conversion of THF to 5,10-methylene THF. Simple supportive measures are all that appear to be in order for treatment of refractory megaloblastic anemia. Acute erythroleukemia (di Guglielmo's disease) is usually treated like other types of acute myeloid leukemia (Chap. 111).

BIBLIOGRAPHY

ALLEN RH et al: Metabolic abnormalities in cobalamin [vitamin B_{12}] and folate deficiencies. FASEB J 7:1344, 1993

BABIOR BM: The megaloblastic anemias, in *Williams' Hematology*, 6th ed, E Beutler et al (eds). New York, McGraw-Hill, 2000

CARMEL R : Prevalence of undiagnosed pernicious anemia in the elderly. Arch Intern Med 156:1097, 1996

————: Cobalamin, the stomach and aging. Am J Clin Nutr 66:750, 1997.

———— et al: The frequently low cobalamin levels in dementia usually signify treatable metabolic, neurologic and electrophysiologic abnormalities. Eur J Haematol 54:245, 1995

COOPER TR, ROSENBLATT DS: Inherited defects of vitamin B_{12} metabolism. Annu Rev Nutr 7:291, 1987

D'ANGELO A, SELHUB J: Homocysteine and thrombotic disease. Blood 90:1, 1997

HSING AW et al: Pernicious anemia and subsequent cancer. Cancer 71:745, 1993

JACQUES PF et al: The effect of folic acid fortification on plasma folate and total homocysteine concentrations. N Engl J Med 340:1449, 1999

JOSTEN E et al: Metabolic evidence that deficiencies of vitamin B_{12}, folate, and vitamin B_6 occur commonly in the elderly. Am J Clin Nutr 58:468, 1993

KUZMINSKI AM et al: Effective treatment of cobalamin deficiency with oral cobalamin. Blood 92:1191, 1998

LINDENBAUM J et al: Neuropsychiatric disorders caused by cobalamin deficiency in the absence of anemia or macrocytosis. N Engl J Med 318:1720, 1988

METZ J et al: The significance of subnormal vitamin B_{12} concentration in older people: A case-control study. J Am Geriatr Soc 44:1355, 1996

SAVAGE DG et al: Sensitivity of serum methylmalonic acid and total homocysteine determinations for diagnosing cobalamin and folate deficiencies. Am J Med 96:239, 1994

SCHILLING RF, WILLIAMS WJ: Vitamin B_{12} deficiency: Underdiagnosed, overtreated? Hosp Pract (Off Ed) 30:47, 1995

TOH BH et al: Pernicious anemia. N Engl J Med 337:1441, 1997

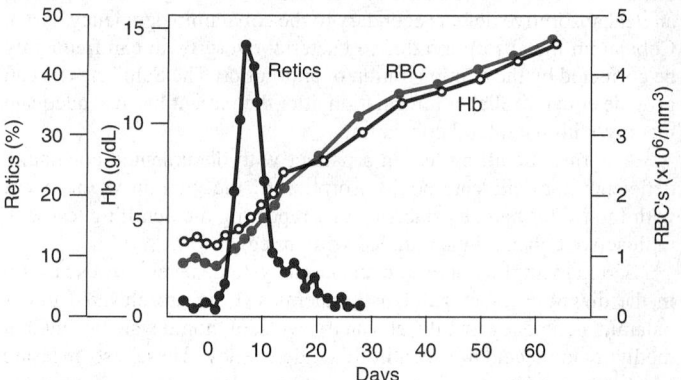

FIGURE 107-3   Hematologic response of a patient with pernicious anemia to an intramuscular injection of 100 μg cobalamin on day 0. (From A Erslev, TG Gabuzda, *Pathophysiology of Blood*, Philadelphia, Saunders, 1975, with permission.)

HEMOLYTIC ANEMIAS AND ACUTE BLOOD LOSS

DIC	disseminated intravascular coagulation	PCH	paroxysmal cold hemoglobinuria
G6PD	glucose-6-phosphate dehydrogenase	PNH	paroxysmal nocturnal hemoglobinuria
LDH	lactate dehydrogenase	PK	pyruvate kinase
MCHC	mean corpuscular hemoglobin concentration	RBC	red blood cells
MCV	mean corpuscular volume	TTP	thrombotic thrombocytopenia purpura

The loss of red cells either through hemorrhage or, less commonly, through premature destruction of the red cells (hemolysis) may cause anemia. Hemolysis or blood loss normally leads to an increase in red cell production, which is clinically manifested by an increase in reticulocytes.

HEMOLYTIC ANEMIAS

Red blood cells (RBC) normally survive 90 to 120 days in the circulation. The life span of RBC may be shortened in a number of disorders, often resulting in anemia if the bone marrow is not able to replenish adequately the prematurely destroyed RBC. The disorders associated with hemolytic anemias are generally identified by the abnormality that brings about the premature destruction of the RBC.

In all patients with hemolytic anemia, a careful history and physical examination provide important clues to the diagnosis. The patient may complain of fatigue and other symptoms of anemia (Chap. 61). Less commonly, jaundice and even red-brown urine (hemoglobinuria) are reported. A complete drug and toxin exposure history and the family history often provide crucial information. The physical examination may show jaundice of skin and mucosae. Splenomegaly is encountered in a variety of hemolytic anemias. A wide array of other historic and physical findings is associated with specific hemolytic anemias (see below).

Laboratory tests may be used initially to demonstrate the presence of hemolysis (Table 108-1) and define its cause. An elevated reticulocyte count in the patient with anemia is the most useful indicator of hemolysis, reflecting erythroid hyperplasia of the bone marrow; biopsy of the bone marrow is often unnecessary. Reticulocytes are also elevated in patients with active blood loss, those with myelophthisis, and those who are recovering from suppression of erythropoiesis (Chap. 61). The morphology of the RBC may provide evidence both of hemolysis and of its cause; the characteristic abnormalities and their associated causes and syndromes are listed in Table 108-2. While the findings on the peripheral blood smear alone are rarely pathognomonic, they may provide important clues to the presence of hemolysis and to diagnosis.

RBC may be prematurely removed from the circulation by macrophages, particularly those of the spleen and liver (extravascular lysis), or, less commonly, by disruption of their membranes during their circulation (intravascular hemolysis). Both mechanisms result in increased heme catabolism and enhanced formation of unconjugated bilirubin, which is normally conjugated by the liver and excreted. The plasma level of unconjugated bilirubin may be high enough to produce readily apparent jaundice (detectable usually when serum bilirubin is >34 μmol/L or 2 mg/dL). The unconjugated (indirect) bilirubin level can be further elevated by a commonly encountered defect in conjugation of bilirubin (Gilbert's syndrome) (Chap. 294). In patients with hemolysis, the level of unconjugated bilirubin never exceeds 70 to 85 μmol/L (4 to 5 mg/dL), unless liver function is impaired.

In the absence of tissue damage in other organs, serum enzyme levels can be useful in the diagnosis and monitoring of patients with hemolysis. Lactate dehydrogenase (LDH), particularly LDH-2, is elevated by accelerated RBC destruction. Serum AST (SGOT) may be somewhat elevated, whereas ALT (SGPT) is not.

Haptoglobin is an α globulin that is present in high concentration (~1.0 g/L) in the plasma (and serum). It binds specifically and tightly to the globin in hemoglobin. The hemoglobin-haptoglobin complex is cleared within minutes by the mononuclear phagocyte system. Thus patients with significant hemolysis, either intravascular or extravascular, have low or absent levels of serum haptoglobin. The fact that haptoglobin synthesis is decreased in patients with hepatocellular disease and increased in inflammatory states must be considered in the interpretation of serum haptoglobin.

Intravascular hemolysis (which is uncommon) results in the release of hemoglobin into the plasma. In these cases, plasma hemoglobin is increased in proportion to the degree of hemolysis. Plasma hemoglobin may be falsely elevated due to lysis of RBC in vitro. If the haptoglobin-binding capacity of the plasma is exceeded, free hemoglobin passes through renal glomeruli. This filtered hemoglobin is reabsorbed by the proximal tubule, where it is catabolized in situ, and the heme iron is incorporated into storage proteins (ferritin and hemosiderin). The presence of hemosiderin in the urine, detected by staining the sediment with Prussian blue, indicates that a significant amount of circulating free hemoglobin has been filtered by the kidneys. Hemosiderin appears 3 to 4 days after the onset of hemoglobinuria and may persist for weeks after its cessation. When the absorptive capacity of the tubular cells is exceeded, hemoglobinuria ensues. Hemoglobinuria indicates severe intravascular hemolysis. Hemoglobinuria must be distinguished from

Table 108-1   Laboratory Evaluation of Hemolysis

	Extravascular	Intravascular
HEMATOLOGIC		
Routine blood film	Polychromatophilia	Polychromatophilia
Reticulocyte count	↑	↑
Bone marrow examination	Erythroid hyperplasia	Erythroid hyperplasia
PLASMA OR SERUM		
Bilirubin	↑ Unconjugated	↑ Unconjugated
Haptoglobin	↓, Absent	Absent
Plasma hemoglobin	N–↑	↑ ↑
Lactate dehydrogenase	↑ (Variable)	↑ ↑ (Variable)
URINE		
Bilirubin	0	0
Hemosiderin	0	+
Hemoglobin	0	+ in severe cases

NOTE: N, normal.

Table 108-2   Red Blood Cell Morphology in the Diagnosis of Hemolytic Anemia

Morphology	Cause	Syndromes
Spherocytes	Loss of membrane	Hereditary spherocytosis, autoimmune hemolytic anemia
Target cells	Increased ratio of RBC surface area to volume	Hemoglobin disorders: thalassemias, hemoglobin S, C, etc.; liver disease
Schistocytes	Traumatic disruption of membrane	Microangiopathy, intravascular prostheses
Sickled cells	Polymerization of hemoglobin S	Sickle cell syndromes
Acanthocytes	?Abnormal membrane lipids	Severe liver disease (spur cell anemia)
Agglutinated cells	Presence of IgM antibody	Cold agglutinin disease
Heinz bodies	Precipitated hemoglobin	Unstable hemoglobin, oxidant stress

hematuria (in which case RBC are seen on urine examination) and from myoglobin due to rhabdomyolysis; in all three cases, the urine is positive with the benzidine reaction, commonly used in analysis of urine. The distinction between hemoglobinuria and myoglobinuria can best be made by specific tests that exploit immunologic differences or differences in solubility. After centrifugation of an anticoagulated blood specimen, the plasma of patients with hemoglobinuria has a reddish-brown color, whereas that of patients with myoglobinuria is normal in color. Because of its higher molecular weight, hemoglobin has lower glomerular permeability than myoglobin and is less rapidly cleared by the kidneys.

CLASSIFICATION   The hemolytic anemias can be grouped in three different ways, shown in Table 108-3. The cause of accelerated RBC destruction can be regarded as (1) a molecular defect (hemoglobinopathy or enzymopathy) inside the red cell, (2) an abnormality in membrane structure and function, or (3) an environmental factor such as mechanical trauma or an autoantibody. In *intracorpuscular types* of hemolysis, the patient's RBC have an abnormally short life span in a normal recipient (with a compatible blood type), while compatible normal RBC survive normally in the patient. The opposite is true in *extracorpuscular types* of hemolysis. Finally, hemolytic disorders can be classified as either inherited or acquired.

INHERITED HEMOLYTIC ANEMIAS   The inherited hemolytic anemias are due to inborn defects in one of three main components of red cells: the membrane, the enzymes, or hemoglobin. These defects are often known at the genomic level, but their identification still largely depends on their clinical and laboratory manifestations.

Red Cell Membrane Disorders   These are usually readily detected by morphologic abnormalities of the RBC on the blood film. There are three types of inherited RBC membrane abnormalities: hereditary spherocytosis, hereditary elliptocytosis (including hereditary pyropoikilocytosis), and hereditary stomatocytosis.

Hereditary spherocytosis   This condition is characterized by spherical RBC due to a molecular defect in one of the proteins in the cytoskeleton of the RBC membrane, leading to a loss of membrane and hence decreased ratio of surface area to volume and consequently spherocytosis. This disorder usually has an autosomal dominant inheritance pattern and an incidence of approximately 1:1000 to 1:4500. In ~20% of patients, the absence of hematologic abnormalities in family members suggests either autosomal recessive inheritance or a spontaneous mutation. The disorder is sometimes clinically apparent in early infancy but often escapes detection until adult life.

CLINICAL MANIFESTATIONS   The major clinical features of hereditary spherocytosis are anemia, splenomegaly, and jaundice. The prominence of jaundice accounts for the disorder's prior designation as "congenital hemolytic jaundice" and is due to an increased concentration of unconjugated (indirect-reacting) bilirubin in plasma. Jaundice may be intermittent and tends to be less pronounced in early childhood. Because of the increased bile pigment production, pigmented gallstones are common, even in childhood. Compensatory erythroid hyperplasia of the bone marrow occurs, with the extension of red marrow into the midshafts of long bones and occasionally with extramedullary erythropoiesis, at times leading to the formation of paravertebral masses visible on chest x-ray. Because the bone marrow's capacity to increase erythropoiesis by six- to eightfold exceeds the usual rate of hemolysis, anemia is usually mild or moderate and may even be absent in an otherwise healthy individual. Compensation may be temporarily interrupted by episodes of relative erythroid hypoplasia precipitated by infections, particularly parvovirus, trauma, surgery, and pregnancy. Splenomegaly is very common. The hemolytic rate may increase transiently during systemic infections, which induce further splenic enlargement. Chronic leg ulcers, similar to those observed in sickle cell anemia, occur occasionally.

The characteristic erythrocyte abnormality is the spherocyte (**Plate V-26**). The mean corpuscular volume (MCV) is usually normal or slightly decreased, and the mean corpuscular hemoglobin concentration (MCHC) is increased to 350 to 400 g/L. Spheroidicity may be quantitatively assessed by measurement of the osmotic fragility of the RBC on exposure to hypoosmotic solutions causing a net influx of water (Fig. 108-1). Because spherocytes have a decreased surface area per unit volume, they are able to take in less water and hence lyse at a higher concentration of saline than normal cells. On microscopic examination, spherocytes are usually detected as small cells without central pallor. They will ordinarily not influence the osmotic fragility test unless they constitute more than 1 or 2% of the total cell population. The autohemolysis test, which measures the amount of spontaneous hemolysis occurring after 48 h of sterile incubation, is also useful.

PATHOGENESIS   The molecular abnormality in hereditary spherocytosis primarily involves the proteins responsible for tethering the lipid bilayer to the underlying cytoskeletal network. Nearly all patients have a significant deficiency of spectrin, which is sometimes secondary to an inherited molecular defect in that protein. About 50% of patients have a defect in ankyrin, the protein that forms a bridge between protein 3 and spectrin (Fig. 108-2). Homozygotes who have a recessive inheritance pattern for ankyrin deficiency have more severe anemia than heterozygotes with the more common dominant form. About 25% of patients have a mutation of protein 3, resulting in a deficiency of that protein and mild anemia with dominant inheritance. Most of the remaining 25% have mutations of spectrin, leading to impaired synthesis or self-association; β-spectrin deficiency is generally mild, with dominant inheritance, while α-spectrin deficiency is severe, with a recessive inheritance pattern. Because the lipid bilayer is not well anchored when these proteins are defective, part of it is lost by vesiculation, resulting in a more spherical and less deformable cell. Because of their shape and rigidity, spherocytes cannot traverse the interstices of the spleen where their increased metabolic rate cannot be sustained, causing a further loss of surface membrane. This "conditioning" produces a subpopulation of hyperspheroidal RBC in the peripheral blood.

Table 108-3   Classification of Hemolytic Anemias

Intracorpuscular	1. Abnormalities of RBC interior
	   a. Enzyme defects
	   b. Hemoglobinopathies
	      (Chap. 106)
	2. RBC membrane abnormalities
	   a. Hereditary spherocytosis etc.
	   b. Paroxysmal nocturnal
	      hemoglobinuria
	   c. Spur cell anemia
		Hereditary

Extracorpuscular	3. Extrinsic factors
	   a. Hypersplenism
	   b. Antibody: immune hemolysis
	   c. Microangiopathic hemolysis
	   d. Infections, toxins, etc.
		Acquired

FIGURE 108-1   Osmotic fragility of RBC in hereditary spherocytosis (HS). The results from two patients are compared to that from a normal individual.

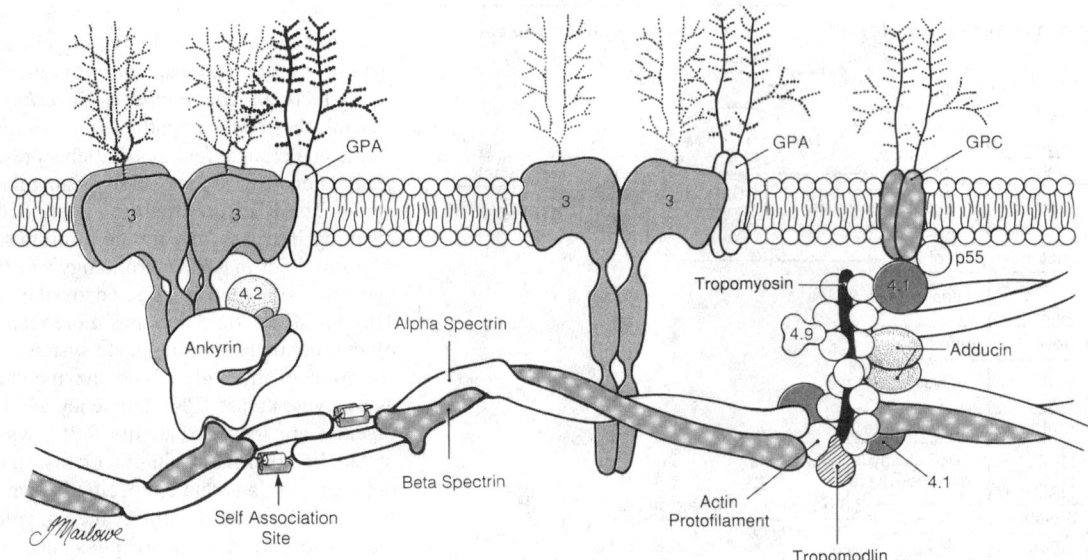

FIGURE 108-2 Diagram of a cross section of the RBC membrane. Spectrin, actin, tropomyosin, adducin, and protein 4.1 form a meshwork that laminates the inner surface of the membrane. In contrast, other proteins such as the glycophorins (GPA and GPC) and protein 3 (anion transport channel) traverse the lipid bilayer. Long polysaccharide chains are covalently attached to these proteins on the outer surface of the cell and also to glycolipid. Ankyrin and protein 4.2 form a bridge between spectrin and a fraction of the anion transport proteins. Protein 4.1 binds to GPC. *(Lux SE, Palek, J, with permission.)*

DIAGNOSIS Hereditary spherocytosis must be distinguished primarily from the spherocytic hemolytic anemias associated with RBC antibodies. The family history of anemia and/or splenectomy is helpful, when present. The diagnosis of immune spherocytosis is usually readily established by a positive direct Coombs test (see below). Spherocytes are also seen in association with hemolysis induced by splenomegaly in patients with cirrhosis, in clostridial infections, and in certain snake envenomations (due to the action of phospholipases on the membrane). A few spherocytes are seen in the course of a wide variety of hemolytic disorders, particularly glucose-6-phosphate dehydrogenase (G6PD) deficiency.

℞ TREATMENT Splenectomy reliably corrects the anemia, although the RBC defect and its consequent morphology persist. The operative risk is low. RBC survival after splenectomy is normal or nearly so; if it is not, an accessory spleen or another diagnosis should be sought. Because of the potential for gallstones and for episodes of bone marrow hypoplasia or hemolytic crises, splenectomy should be performed in symptomatic individuals; cholecystectomy should not be performed without splenectomy, as intrahepatic gallstones may result. Splenectomy in children should be postponed until age 4, if possible, to minimize the risk of severe infections with gram-positive encapsulated organisms. Polyvalent pneumococcal vaccine should be administered at least 2 weeks before splenectomy. In patients with severe hemolysis, folic acid (1 mg/d) should be administered prophylactically.

Hereditary elliptocytosis and hereditary pyropoikilocytosis
Oval or elliptic RBC are normally found in birds, reptiles, camels, and llamas; however, they occur in appreciable numbers in humans only in *hereditary elliptocytosis*, a disorder that is transmitted as an autosomal dominant trait and affects 1 per 4000 to 5000 people, a frequency similar to that of hereditary spherocytosis (rarely, patients with myelodysplastic disorders of the bone marrow may have acquired elliptocytosis). The elliptic shape is acquired as the cell deforms to traverse the microcirculation but does not spring back to its initial biconcave shape. In most affected individuals, a structural abnormality of erythrocyte spectrin that leads to impaired assembly of the cytoskeleton. In some families, affected individuals have a deficiency of erythrocyte membrane protein 4.1, which stabilizes the interaction of spectrin and actin in the cytoskeleton (Fig. 108-2); homozygotes with absence of this protein have more marked hemolysis. In Southeast

Asia, there is a high incidence of hereditary ovalocytosis, in which a small internal deletion of protein 3 makes the membrane rigid and confers resistance against malaria.

The great majority of patients manifest only mild hemolysis, with hemoglobin levels >120 g/L, reticulocytes <4% (0.2 × 10^{12}/L), depressed haptoglobin levels, and RBC survival times just under the normal range. In 10 to 15% of patients with more severe abnormalities, the rate of hemolysis is substantially increased, with median survival times of RBC as short as 5 days and reticulocytes ranging up to 20%. Hemoglobin levels rarely fall below 90 to 100 g/L. RBC destruction occurs predominantly in the spleen, which is enlarged in patients with overt hemolysis. Hemolysis is corrected by splenectomy.

In both the anemic and nonanemic varieties of this disorder, at least 25% and, more commonly, >75% of RBC are elliptic, with an axial ratio (width/length) of <0.78. Patients with hemolysis frequently have microovalocytes, bizarre-shaped RBC, and RBC fragments, all of which increase in number after splenectomy. The degree of hemolysis does not correlate with the percentage of elliptocytes. Osmotic fragility is usually normal but may be increased in patients with overt hemolysis.

Hereditary pyropoikilocytosis is a rare disorder related to hereditary elliptocytosis and is characterized by bizarre-shaped, microcytic RBC that undergo disruption at temperatures of 44 to 45°C (in contrast, normal RBC are stable up to 49°C). This condition results from a deficiency of spectrin and an abnormality of spectrin self-assembly. Hemolysis is usually severe, is recognized in childhood, and is partially responsive to splenectomy.

Hereditary stomatocytosis Stomatocytes are cup-shaped RBC (concave on one face and convex on the other). This formation results in a slitlike central zone of pallor on dried smears. The syndrome of hereditary hemolytic anemia and stomatocytic RBC is inherited in an autosomal dominant pattern. RBC have an increased permeability to sodium and potassium, which is compensated for by an increased active transport of these cations. In some patients, the RBC are swollen with an excess of ions and water and a decreased mean corpuscular hemoglobin concentration (overhydrated stomatocytes, "hydrocytosis"); many of these patients lack the RBC membrane protein 7.2 (stomatin). In other patients, the RBC are shrunken, with a decreased ion and water content and an increased mean corpuscular hemoglobin concentration (dehydrated stomatocytes, "desiccytosis" or "xerocytosis"). Those patients in whom the RBC are overhydrated have true stomatocytes on dried smears. Dehydrated stomatocytes assume the mor-

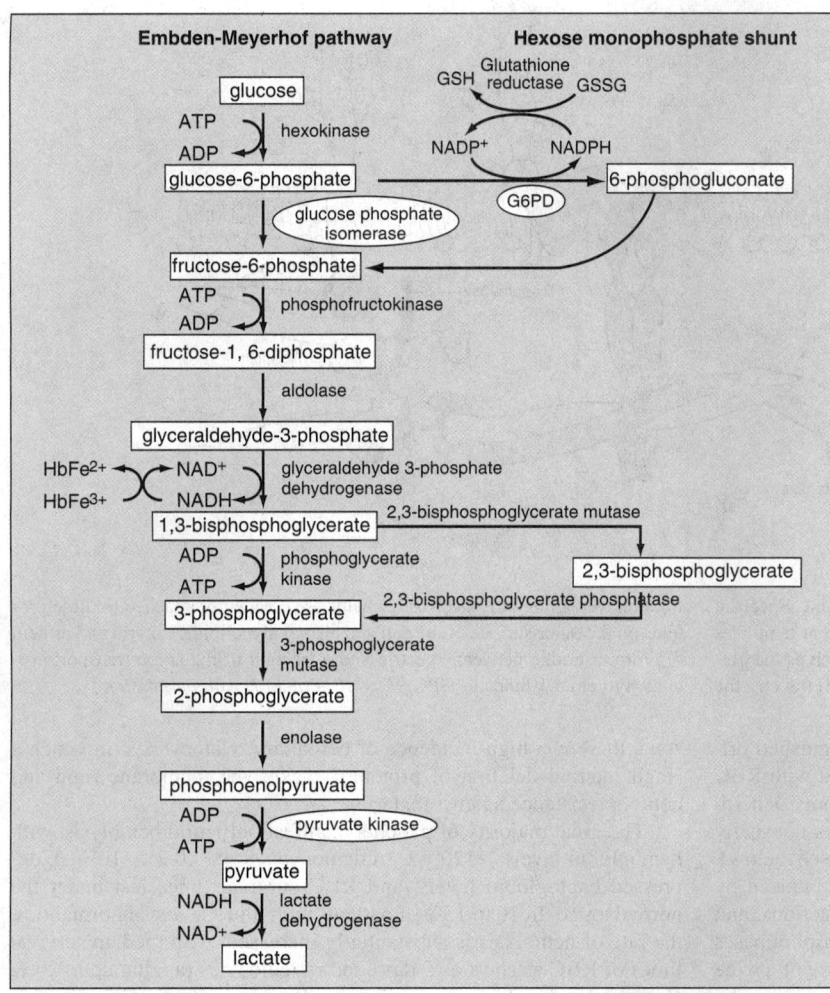

Embden-Meyerhof pathway — **Hexose monophosphate shunt**

FIGURE 108-3 RBC metabolism. The Embden-Meyerhof pathway (glycolysis) generates ATP for energy and membrane maintenance. The generation of NADPH maintains hemoglobin in a reduced state. The hexose monophosphate shunt generates NADPH that is used to reduce glutathione, which protects the red cell against oxidant stress. The Rapaport-Luebering shunt regulates 2,3-bisphosphoglycerate levels, a critical determinant of oxygen affinity of hemoglobin. Enzyme deficiency states in order of prevalence: glucose-6-phosphate dehydrogenase (G6PD) $\gg$ pyruvate kinase > glucose-6-phosphate isomerase > rare deficiencies of other enzymes in the pathway. The more common enzyme deficiencies are encircled.

phology of target cells on dried smears. Osmotic fragility is increased in overhydrated stomatocytes and decreased in underhydrated stomatocytes. RBC lacking Rh proteins (Rh$_{null}$ cells) are stomatocytic and have a shortened life span.

Most patients have splenomegaly and mild anemia. Splenectomy decreases but does not totally correct the hemolytic process.

Red Cell Enzyme Defects During its maturation, the RBC loses its nucleus, ribosomes, and mitochondria and thus its capability for protein synthesis and oxidative phosphorylation. The mature circulating RBC has a relatively simple pattern of intermediary metabolism (Fig. 108-3) in keeping with its modest metabolic obligations. ATP must be generated from the Embden-Meyerhof pathway to drive the cation pump that maintains the ionic milieu in the RBC. Smaller amounts of energy are needed for the preservation of hemoglobin iron in the ferrous (Fe^{2+}) state and perhaps for the renewal of the lipids in the RBC membrane. About 10% of the glucose consumed by the RBC is metabolized via the hexose-monophosphate shunt (Fig. 108-3), which protects both hemoglobin and the membrane from exogenous oxidants, including certain drugs.

Deficiency states have been reported for most of the enzymes shown in Fig. 108-3. Many of these enzyme abnormalities appear to be restricted to RBC. Mutations can result in no protein product, a dysfunctional product, or an unstable product. Mutations resulting in

decreased stability will be detected more readily in RBC compared with other cells having either a shorter life span or the synthetic capability to renew the enzyme.

Defects in the Embden-Meyerhof pathway In general, these enzymopathies have similar pathophysiologic and clinical features. Patients present with a congenital nonspherocytic hemolytic anemia of variable severity. The RBC are often relatively deficient in ATP, resulting in a leak of potassium ion out of these cells. Abnormalities in RBC morphology (see below) indicate that the membrane is affected by the enzyme defect. These RBC are rigid and thus more readily sequestered by the mononuclear phagocyte system.

Some of these glycolytic enzyme deficiencies such as pyruvate kinase (PK) deficiency and hexokinase deficiency are localized to the RBC, with no apparent metabolic abnormality in other cells; in the case of PK deficiency, this is due to specific isozymes confined to the RBC. In other disorders, the enzyme deficiency is more widespread. Glucose phosphate isomerase deficiency and phosphoglycerate kinase deficiency also involve leukocytes, although affected individuals have no apparent abnormalities of leukocyte function. Individuals with deficiency of triose phosphate isomerase have decreased levels of enzyme in leukocytes, muscle cells, and cerebrospinal fluid, and they have a progressive neurologic disorder. Some patients with phosphofructokinase deficiency have a myopathy.

About 95% of the clinically significant defects in the glycolytic pathway are due to PK deficiency, and about 4% are due to glucose phosphate isomerase deficiency. The remainder, shown in Fig. 108-3, are extremely rare. Most have been encountered in isolated families; clinical manifestations are variable. A number of different mutations result in PK deficiency. Some missense mutations in decreased reaction with substrate (phosphoenolpyruvate), an enhancing molecule (fructose 1,6 diphosphate), or ADP. Thus, there is considerable variability in the clinical manifestations and laboratory findings among individuals reported as having PK deficiency. Most of these patients are compound heterozygotes who have inherited a different defective enzyme from each parent.

Most of the glycolytic enzyme defects are inherited in an autosomal recessive pattern. The parents of affected patients are heterozygotes and express half-normal levels of enzyme activity, which are more than adequate for normal metabolic function. Thus, the parents are entirely asymptomatic. Since the gene frequency for this group of enzymopathies is low, true homozygotes are often the offspring of a consanguineous mating. More often, affected individuals are compound heterozygotes. Phosphoglycerate kinase deficiency is inherited as a sex-linked disorder. Affected males have a severe hemolytic anemia, while female carriers may have a mild hemolytic process.

CLINICAL MANIFESTATIONS Patients with severe hemolysis usually present during early childhood with anemia, jaundice, and splenomegaly.

LABORATORY FINDINGS Patients have a normocytic (or slightly macrocytic), normochromic anemia with reticulocytosis. In those with PK deficiency, bizarre erythrocytes, including spiculated cells, are noted on the peripheral smear, especially after splenectomy. Spherocytes are usually absent; hence the term *congenital nonspherocytic hemolytic anemia* has been applied to these disorders. Unlike hereditary spherocytosis, the osmotic fragility of freshly drawn blood is usually normal. Incubation brings out an osmotically fragile population of RBC, an abnormality not corrected by the addition of glucose.

The diagnosis of this group of anemias depends on specific enzymatic assays; care must be taken to provide an appropriate concentration of substrate to detect those variants with a low affinity for substrate or enhancing molecule. An abnormality in enzyme kinetics, differences in electrophoretic mobility, pH optimum, or heat stability may be useful in documenting heterogeneity among enzyme variants.

℞ **TREATMENT** Most patients do not require therapy. Those with severe hemolysis should be given folic acid (1 mg/d). Blood transfusions may be necessary during a hypoplastic crisis. Women with PK deficiency may become very anemic during pregnancy, sometimes leading to the diagnosis for the first time.

Because of their enzymatic defect, the younger cells (reticulocytes) depend on mitochondrial respiration rather than glycolysis for maintenance of ATP. However, in the hypoxic environment of the spleen, aerobic metabolism is curtailed and the ATP-depleted cells are destroyed in situ. Reticulocytes are normally retained in the spleen for 24 to 48 h. Patients with PK deficiency may benefit from splenectomy, which usually leads to a marked increase in circulating reticulocytes. Patients with deficiency of glucose phosphate isomerase also may improve after splenectomy. Splenectomy has not been proven effective in individuals with other glycolytic enzymopathies.

Defects in the hexose-monophosphate shunt The normal RBC is well protected against oxidant stress. When the cell is exposed to a drug or toxin that generates oxygen radicals, glucose metabolism via the hexose-monophosphate shunt is normally increased severalfold. Reduced glutathione is regenerated, protecting the sulfhydryl groups of hemoglobin and the RBC membrane from oxidation. Individuals with an inherited defect in the hexose-monophosphate shunt are unable to maintain an adequate level of reduced glutathione in their RBC, hemoglobin sulfhydryl groups become oxidized, and the hemoglobin precipitates within the RBC, forming Heinz bodies.

G6PD DEFICIENCY This is by far the most common congenital shunt defect, affecting more than 200 million people throughout the world; like hemoglobin S, it partially protects the patient from malaria by providing a defective home for the merozoite. Considerable genetic heterogeneity exists among affected individuals, and over 400 variants of G6PD have been described. In most cases, the alteration is a base substitution, leading to an amino acid replacement rather than a deletion or truncation of the protein. The mutations generate enzymes with differences in electrophoretic mobility, enzyme kinetics, pH optimum, and heat stability. These differences result in great variation of clinical severity, ranging from nonspherocytic hemolytic anemia without demonstrable oxidant stress (particularly shortly after birth), through hemolytic anemia only when stimulated by marked to mild oxidant stress, to no clinically detectable abnormality. The normal G6PD is designated as type B. About 20% of individuals of African descent have a G6PD (designated A+) that differs by a single amino acid and is electrophoretically distinguishable but functionally normal. Among the clinically significant G6PD variants, the most common, the so-called A− type, is due to two base substitutions and is encountered primarily in individuals of central African descent. The A− G6PD has the same electrophoretic mobility as the A+ type, but it is unstable and has abnormal kinetic properties. This variant is found in about 11% of African American males. A second relatively common G6PD variant is encountered among peoples of Mediterranean origin, particularly Sardinians and Sephardic Jews; this variant is more severe than the A− variant and may result in nonspherocytic hemolytic anemia in the absence of known oxidative stress. A third relatively common and slightly less severe variant occurs in southern Chinese populations.

The G6PD gene is located on the X chromosome; thus the deficiency state is a sex-linked trait. Affected males (hemizygotes) inherit the abnormal gene from their mothers who are usually carriers (heterozygotes). Because of inactivation of one of the two X chromosomes (Lyon hypothesis: Chap. 65), the heterozygote has two populations of RBC: normal and deficient in G6PD. Most female carriers are asymptomatic. Those who happen to have a high proportion of deficient cells

resemble the male hemizygotes. G6PD activity normally declines ~50% during the 120-day life span of the RBC. This decay is moderately accelerated in A− RBC and markedly so in RBC containing the Mediterranean variant. Individuals with the A− variant normally have a slightly shortened RBC survival time, but they are not anemic. Clinical problems arise only when the affected individual is subjected to some type of environmental stress. Most often, hemolytic episodes are triggered by viral and bacterial infections. The mechanism is unknown. In addition, drugs or toxins that pose an oxidant threat to the RBC (most commonly sulfa drugs, antimalarials, and nitrofurantoin) cause hemolysis in individuals deficient in G6PD (Table 108-4). Although aspirin is frequently mentioned as a likely offender, it has no deleterious effect in A− individuals. Accidental ingestion of toxic compounds such as naphthalene (moth balls) may cause severe hemolysis. Metabolic acidosis can precipitate an episode of hemolysis in individuals deficient in G6PD.

CLINICAL AND LABORATORY FEATURES The patient may experience an acute hemolytic crisis within hours of exposure to the oxidant stress, leading to hemoglobinuria and peripheral vascular collapse in severe cases. Since only the older population of RBC is rapidly destroyed, the hemolytic crisis is usually self-limited, even if the exposure to the oxidant continues. Among black males with the A− variant, the RBC mass decreases by a maximum of 25 to 30%. During acute hemolysis, a rapid drop in hematocrit is accompanied by a rise in plasma hemoglobin and unconjugated bilirubin and a decrease in plasma haptoglobin. The oxidation of hemoglobin leads to the formation of Heinz bodies, visualized by means of a supravital stain such as crystal violet. However, Heinz bodies are usually not seen after the first day or so, since these inclusions are readily removed by the spleen. Their removal leads to the formation of "bite cells" (RBC that have lost a peripheral portion of the cell). Multiple bites cause the formation of fragments. A few spherocytes also may be present. Individuals with the Mediterranean type G6PD have a more unstable enzyme and, therefore, a much lower overall enzyme activity than individuals with the A− variant. As a result, they have more severe clinical manifestations. A minority of patients are exquisitely sensitive to fava beans and develop a fulminant hemolytic crisis after exposure. The oxidants in *Vicia fava* are two β-glycosides whose aglycones, when autooxidized, produce oxygen free radicals. The incidence of favism is highly variable due to variations in concentration, in absorption, or in metabolism of the aglycones. Favism is not encountered in individuals with the A− variant.

The *diagnosis* of G6PD deficiency should be considered in any individual, particularly a male of African or Mediterranean descent, who experiences an acute hemolytic episode. The patient should be questioned about possible exposure to oxidant agents. The diagnosis can be established by a number of tests that assess either the enzyme activity or the effects of its deficiency. However, the test may yield a false-negative result during a hemolytic episode when the old RBC containing the defective enzyme have already lysed.

℞ **TREATMENT** Since hemolysis in patients deficient in A− G6PD is usually self-limited, no specific treatment is necessary. Splenectomy does not benefit Mediterranean patients with chronic hemolysis. Blood transfusions are rarely indicated. Adequate urine flow should be maintained if hemoglobinuria develops during an acute hemolytic episode.

Table 108-4 Drugs Causing Hemolysis in Subjects Deficient in G6PD

Antimalarials: Primaquine, pamaquine, dapsone
Sulfonamides: Sulfamethoxazole
Nitrofurantoin
Analgesics: Acetanilid
Miscellaneous: Vitamin K (water-soluble form), doxorubicin, methylene blue, nalidixic acid, furazolidone, niridazole, phenazopyridine

Prevention of hemolytic episodes is best. Infections ought to be treated promptly. Patients should be warned about risks posed by oxidant drugs and fava beans. Any patient of African or Mediterranean ancestry about to be given an oxidant drug should be screened for G6PD deficiency.

OTHER DEFECTS OF THE HEXOSE-MONOPHOSPHATE SHUNT   A few kindreds have been found to have congenital deficiency in RBC glutathione due to a defect in either of the two enzymes responsible for the synthesis of this tripeptide. Affected individuals have a hemolytic anemia with Heinz bodies that is aggravated by oxidant drugs. Deficiency of glutathione reductase has been reported, but its relationship to clinically significant hemolysis is not well established. Sometimes the deficiency state can be corrected by the administration of riboflavin (5 mg/d). Deficiencies of glutathione peroxidase and 6-phosphogluconate dehydrogenase have been observed, but their association with hemolysis is uncertain.

Other enzyme defects   Hemolytic anemia may sometimes be caused by abnormalities in enzymes of nucleotide metabolism. Individuals with pyrimidine 5′-nucleotidase deficiency have marked coarse basophilic stippling in their RBC because the mRNA of the cell is not properly metabolized. Hemolytic anemia also has been noted in individuals whose RBC have supranormal levels of adenosine deaminase and relatively low levels of ATP.

Hemoglobinopathies   The sickling disorders constitute an important form of congenital hemolytic anemia. Less commonly, hemolysis may be due to the inheritance of an unstable hemoglobin variant. →*For further discussion, see Chap. 106.*

ACQUIRED HEMOLYTIC ANEMIAS   In most patients with acquired hemolytic anemia, RBC are made normally but are prematurely destroyed because of damage acquired in the circulation. (The exceptions are rare disorders characterized by acquired dysplasia of the cells of the bone marrow and the production of structurally and functionally abnormal RBC.) The damage that occurs may be mediated by antibodies or toxins or may be due to abnormalities in the circulation, including an overactive mononuclear phagocyte system or traumatic lysis by natural or artificial impediments to circulation. The acquired hemolytic anemias can be classified into five categories (Table 108-5).

Hypersplenism   The spleen is particularly efficient in trapping and destroying RBC that have minimal defects. This unique ability of the spleen to filter mildly damaged RBC results from its unusual vascular anatomy (Chap. 63). Almost all the blood circulating through the spleen flows rapidly from arterioles in the white pulp to sinuses in the spleen's red pulp and then into the venous system. In contrast, a small portion of splenic blood flow (normally 1 to 2%) passes into the "marginal zone" of the lymphatic white pulp. Although the cells that occupy this zone are not phagocytic, they serve as a mechanical filter that hinders the progress of severely damaged blood cells. As RBC leave this zone and enter the red pulp, they flow into narrow cords, rich in macrophages, that end blindly but communicate with sinuses through small openings between the lining cells of the sinuses. These openings, averaging 3 μm in diameter, test the ability of RBC (4.5 μm in diameter) to undergo a deformation. RBC that cannot re-enter the vascular sinuses are engulfed by phagocytic cells and destroyed (see Fig. 63-1).

The normal spleen retains reticulocytes for 1 to 2 days but otherwise poses no threat to normal RBC until they become senescent. However, in the face of splenomegaly, increased destruction of the cells of the blood, including the RBC, may take place due to pooling of the blood in a relatively nutrient-poor environment full of phagocytic cells. When splenic sequestration causes cytopenia, hypersplenism is diagnosed. In infiltrative diseases of the spleen, substantial splenomegaly may exist with no apparent hemolysis; inflammatory and congestive splenomegaly is commonly associated with modest shortening of RBC survival time, along with more marked granulocytopenia and thrombocytopenia. Patients with cytopenia(s) sufficient to produce symptoms generally benefit from splenectomy.

Immunologic Causes of Hemolysis   Immune hemolysis in the adult is usually induced by IgG or IgM antibodies with specificity for antigens associated with the patient's RBC (often called "autoantibodies") (Table 108-6); rarely, transfused RBC may be hemolyzed by alloantibodies directed against foreign antigens on those cells (Chap. 114).

The Coombs antiglobulin test is the major tool for diagnosing autoimmune hemolysis. This test relies on the ability of antibodies specific for immunoglobulins (especially IgG) or complement components (especially C3) to agglutinate RBC when these proteins are present on the RBC. The *direct Coombs test* measures the ability of anti-IgG or anti-C3 antisera to agglutinate the patient's RBC. The presence or absence of IgG and/or C3 may help define the origin of the immune hemolytic anemia (Table 108-6). Rarely, neither IgG nor complement may be found on the RBC of the patient (Coombs-negative immune hemolytic anemia).

Antibodies to particular RBC antigens in the serum of the patient can be detected by reacting the serum with normal RBC bearing the antigen. IgM antibodies (usually cold-reacting) may be detected by agglutination of normal or fetal RBC. IgG antibodies may be detected by the *indirect Coombs test*, in which the serum of the patient is incubated with normal RBC and antibody is detected with anti-IgG, as in the direct Coombs test.

"Warm" antibodies   Antibodies that react with protein antigens are nearly always IgG and react at body temperature; occasionally, they are IgA and rarely IgM. Hemolysis due to autologous antibodies is called *autoimmune hemolytic (or immunohemolytic) anemia, warm antibody type.*

Table 108-5   Causes of Acquired Hemolytic Anemia

I. Entrapment
II. Immune
   A. Warm-reactive (IgG) antibody
   B. Cold-reactive IgM antibody (cold agglutinin disease)
   C. Cold-reactive IgG antibody (paroxysmal cold hemoglobinuria)
   D. Drug-dependent antibody
     1. Autoimmune
     2. Haptene
III. Traumatic hemolytic anemia
   A. Impact hemolysis
   B. Macrovascular defects—prostheses
   C. Microvascular causes
     1. Thrombotic thrombocytopenic purpura/hemolytic-uremic syndrome
     2. Other causes of microvascular abnormalities
     3. Disseminated intravascular hemolysis
IV. Hemolytic anemia due to toxic effects on the membrane
   A. Spur cell anemia
   B. External toxins
     1. Animal or spider bites
     2. Metals (e.g., copper)
     3. Organic compounds
V. Paroxysmal nocturnal hemoglobinuria

Table 108-6   Use of the Direct Coombs Test in Diagnosing the Cause of Autoimmune Hemolytic Anemia

Reaction with		
Anti-IgG	**Anti-C3**	**Causes**
Yes	No	Antibodies to Rh proteins, hemolysis caused by α-methyldopa or penicillin
Yes	Yes	Antibodies to glycoprotein antigens, SLE
No	Yes	Cold-reacting antibodies (agglutinins or Donath-Landsteiner antibody), most drug-related antibodies, IgM antibodies, IgG antibodies of low affinity, activation of complement by immune complexes

CLINICAL MANIFESTATIONS Immunohemolytic anemia of the warm antibody type is induced by IgG antibody and occurs at all ages, but it is more common in adults, particularly women. In approximately one-fourth of patients this disorder occurs as a complication of an underlying disease affecting the immune system, especially lymphoid neoplasms (Chap. 112); collagen vascular diseases, especially systemic lupus erythematosus (SLE); and congenital immunodeficiency diseases (Table 108-7). In the initial evaluation of the patient, drugs that are known to cause immunohemolytic anemia must be ruled out (see below). The presentation and course of IgG immunohemolytic anemia are quite variable. In its mildest form, the only manifestation is a positive direct Coombs test. In this instance, insufficient antibody is present on the RBC surface to permit the reticuloendothelial system to recognize the cell as abnormal.

Most symptomatic patients have a moderate to severe anemia [hemoglobin levels 60 to 100 g/L and reticulocyte counts 10 to 30% (200 to $600 \times 10^3/\mu L$)], spherocytosis (**Plate V-8**), and splenomegaly.

Severe immunohemolytic anemia presents with fulminant hemolysis associated with hemoglobinemia, hemoglobinuria, and shock; this syndrome may be rapidly fatal unless aggressively treated.

The direct Coombs test is positive in 98% of patients; usually IgG is detected with or without C3. Rarely, the cells may be agglutinated by the antibody, causing difficulty in analysis by flow cytometry.

Immune thrombocytopenia also may be present (*Evans's syndrome*), a disorder in which separate antibodies are directed against platelets and RBC. Occasionally, venous thrombosis occurs.

PATHOGENESIS IgG antibodies lyse RBC by two mechanisms: (1) immune adherence of RBC to phagocytes mediated by the antibody and by complement components that become fixed to the membrane (by far the more important mechanism of destruction), and (2) complement activation. Upon binding to Fc receptors on macrophages, the antibody-coated red cell is engulfed and destroyed. If internalization is only partial, the RBC membrane is removed, resulting in the formation of spherocytes, which are destroyed in the spleen. Complement-mediated immune adherence involves the interaction of C3b and C4b with receptors on the macrophage; while much less likely to lead to RBC lysis, this mechanism markedly increases the immune adherence due to IgG. Immune adherence, particularly that due to the IgG antibody, is also enhanced by the transit of RBC into the cords and sinuses of the spleen, which brings cells into intimate contact with phagocytic cells.

℞ **TREATMENT** Patients having a mild degree of hemolysis usually do not require therapy. In those with clinically significant hemolysis, initial therapy consists of glucocorticoids (e.g., prednisone, 1.0 mg/kg per day). A rise in hemoglobin is frequently noted within 3 or 4 days and occurs in most patients within 1 to 2 weeks. Prednisone is continued until the hemoglobin level has risen to normal values, and thereafter it is tapered rapidly to about 20 mg/d, then slowly over

Table 108-7 Hemolysis due to Antibodies

WARM-ANTIBODY IMMUNOHEMOLYTIC ANEMIA

1. Idiopathic
2. Lymphomas: Chronic lymphocytic leukemia, non-Hodgkin's lymphomas, Hodgkin's disease (infrequent)
3. SLE and other collagen-vascular diseases
4. Drugs
   a. α-Methyldopa type (autoantibody to Rh antigens)
   b. Penicillin type (stable hapten)
   c. Quinidine type (unstable hapten)
5. Postviral infections
6. Other tumors (rare)

COLD-ANTIBODY IMMUNOHEMOLYTIC ANEMIA

1. Cold agglutinin disease
   a. Acute: *Mycoplasma* infection, infectious mononucleosis
   b. Chronic: Idiopathic, lymphoma
2. Paroxysmal cold hemoglobinuria

the course of several months. An algorithm for this tapering process is given in Fig. 108-4. For chronic therapy with prednisone, alternate-day administration is preferred. More than 75% of patients achieve an initial significant and sustained reduction in hemolysis; however, in half these patients the disease recurs, either during glucocorticoid tapering or after its cessation. Glucocorticoids have two modes of action: an immediate effect due to inhibition of the clearance of IgG-coated RBC by the mononuclear phagocyte system and a later effect due to inhibition of antibody synthesis. Splenectomy is recommended for patients who cannot tolerate or fail to respond to glucocorticoid therapy.

Patients who have been refractory to glucocorticoid therapy and to splenectomy are treated with immunosuppressive drugs such as azathioprine and cyclophosphamide. A success rate of ~50% has been reported with each. Intravenous gamma globulin may cause rapid cessation of hemolysis; however, it is not nearly as effective in this disorder as in immune thrombocytopenia.

Patients with severe anemia may require blood transfusions. Because the antibody in this disease is usually a "panagglutinin," reacting with nearly all normal donor cells, cross-matching is impossible. The goal in selecting blood for transfusion is to avoid administering RBC with antigens to which the patient may have alloantibodies. A common procedure is to adsorb the panagglutinin present in the patient's serum with the patient's own RBC from which antibody has been previously eluted. Serum cleared of autoantibody can then be tested for the presence of alloantibody to donor blood groups. ABO-compatible RBC matched in this fashion are administered slowly, with watchfulness for signs of an immediate-type hemolytic transfusion reaction.

PROGNOSIS In most patients, hemolysis is controlled by glucocorticoid therapy alone, by splenectomy, or by a combination. Fatalities occur among three rare subsets of patients: (1) those with overwhelming hemolysis who die from anemia; (2) those whose host defenses are impaired by glucocorticoids, splenectomy, and/or immunosuppressive agents; and (3) those with major thrombotic events coincident with active hemolysis.

When immunohemolysis develops as a complication of an under-

FIGURE 108-4 Algorithm for the treatment of patients with IgG-mediated immune hemolytic anemia. The patient with minimal disease may be watched carefully. The patient with very severe disease may need all modalities of treatment applied at once. The more common patient with moderate disease may be treated with prednisone at a high dose; if no response is seen, then either splenectomy or chemotherapy is given. If a response is seen, the dose of prednisone is reduced over time. If relapse occurs during this process, splenectomy or chemotherapy may be needed.

lying disorder, the prognosis is often dominated by that of the primary disease.

Immunohemolytic anemia secondary to drugs Drugs cause immunohemolytic anemia by two mechanisms of action: (1) they induce a disorder identical in almost every respect to warm-antibody immunohemolytic anemia (e.g., α-methyldopa (an antihypertensive; Chap. 246), and (2) they become associated as haptenes with the RBC surface and induce the formation of an antibody directed against the RBC-drug complex (e.g., penicillin, quinidine).

A positive direct Coombs test is observed in up to 10% of patients receiving α-methyldopa therapy in doses of 2 g/d or higher. A small minority of these patients develop spherocytosis and hemolysis, which may be severe. α-Methyldopa alters and makes immunogenic the protein(s) of the Rh complex; the resulting antibodies cross-react with the normal Rh protein. Thus the antibody does not react with the drug, and the indirect Coombs test is positive in almost all patients even when the drug is not added to the test. The RBC are coated with IgG but not C3. Hemolysis decreases over the course of several weeks after cessation of drug therapy, although the direct Coombs test may remain positive for more than 1 year.

In most other cases of drug-induced hemolysis, the antibody is directed against the combination of the drug and the membrane glycoprotein to which it is attached. The hemolytic reaction in vivo is dependent on the presence of the drug and usually ceases shortly after the drug has been discontinued. Penicillin and its congeners may cause this type of reaction if the drug is given in very high doses (10 million units per day or more). The drug adheres relatively firmly to the protein of the RBC membrane. Complement is not usually fixed, and the hemolysis in vivo is usually not severe. Since the antibody is usually IgG, spherocytosis and splenic destruction may occur. Most other drugs (such as quinine, quinidine, sulfonamides, sulfonureas, phenacetin, stibophen, and dipyrone) do not adhere as tightly to their glycoproteins, and the drug-antibody complexes are removed during the washing steps of the direct and indirect Coombs reactions. These antibodies (particularly IgM) are usually able to fix complement, and these components remain on the RBC surface; thus the direct Coombs test is positive with anti-C3 but not anti-IgG. The antibody is detected in the *indirect* Coombs test only when the drug is added to the incubation mixture. Hemolysis may be quite severe, sometimes resulting in signs of intravascular hemolysis; resolution is usually prompt after the drug is discontinued.

Immune hemolysis due to cold-reactive antibodies Antibodies that react with polysaccharide antigens are usually IgM and react better at temperatures lower than 37°C, hence the name *cold-reactive antibodies*. Uncommonly, the antibody is IgG (the Donath-Landsteiner antibody of paroxysmal cold hemoglobinuria).

Cold agglutinins arise in two clinical settings: (1) monoclonal antibodies, the product of lymphocytic neoplasia or paraneoplasia, and (2) polyclonal antibodies in response to infection. In many elderly patients, the "neoplasm" is benign monoclonal gammopathy that does not progress, and the paraprotein remains its only manifestation. Occasionally, cold agglutinins are found in patients with nonlymphoid neoplasms.

Transient cold agglutinins occur commonly in two infections: *Mycoplasma pneumoniae* infection and infectious mononucleosis. In both, the titer of antibody is usually too low to cause clinical symptoms, but its presence is of diagnostic value; only occasionally is hemolysis present. Cold agglutinins are less frequently encountered in a number of other viral infections. Their manifestations are usually benign.

The specificity of the antibody may be of diagnostic value. Cold agglutinins reacting more strongly with adult RBC than fetal (cord) RBC are called *anti-I*; these antibodies are seen in benign lymphoproliferation (chronic cold agglutinin monoclonal gammopathy) and in *Mycoplasma* infections. Those reacting more strongly with cord RBC cells are called *anti-i*; these antibodies are seen in aggressive

lymphomas and in infectious mononucleosis. Rarely, the antibody may react with other antigens that are equally expressed on adult and cord RBC. The clinical manifestations elicited by the antibody on exposure to cold are of two sorts: intravascular agglutination (acrocyanosis) and hemolysis. Acrocyanosis is the marked purpling of the extremities, ears, and nose when the blood becomes cold enough to agglutinate in the veins; it clears on warming and does not have the vasospastic characteristics of Raynaud's phenomenon (Chap. 248). Patients may also have symptoms when swallowing cold food or drinks.

The hemolysis is usually not severe and is manifested by a mild reticulocytosis, agglutination on the blood film, and agglutination during analysis of the blood by particle analysis (giving rise to a falsely high mean corpuscular volume). The degree of hemolysis depends on several variables.

1. *Antibody titer.* In general, the titer in symptomatic patients is above 1:2000 dilution of serum and may range to as high as 1:50,000. When collecting samples, great care must be taken that the serum is separated from the cells while the sample is maintained at 37°C so that the antibody will not adsorb onto the patient's own cells.

2. *Thermal amplitude of the antibody* (the highest temperature at which the antibody will react with the RBC). For most antibodies, this is 23 to 30°C. Those with a higher thermal amplitude (up to 37°C) are more hemolytic, since it is more likely that these temperatures will be encountered during RBC circulation.

3. *Environmental temperature.* Since the reaction can occur only at temperatures below body temperature, frequency and degree of exposure to cold are major determinants of the rate of hemolysis.

The hemolysis that occurs is due primarily to the hemolytic action of complement, since there are no functional Fc receptors for the IgM antibody. Complement is readily fixed; a single molecule of IgM is enough to effect binding of C1 and initiate the cascade. However, the normal human RBC is remarkably resistant to the hemolytic action of complement because of several defense mechanisms. Therefore, severe hemolysis with hemoglobinuria occurs only with massive activation of the antibody, such as by sudden cooling. The activation of complement is always marked by the accumulation of a degradation product of C3, C3dg, on the surface; this product is what is detected with appropriate antisera in the direct Coombs test in all patients with significant cold agglutinin disease. The cutaneous manifestations and hemolysis are best treated by maintaining the patient in a warm environment.

Splenectomy is usually not of value in this disorder. Glucocorticoids are of limited value, although patients with the panthermal variety of cold agglutinin disease may respond. Chlorambucil and cyclophosphamide are commonly used to treat patients who have hemolysis associated with monoclonal gammopathy, but their efficacy is usually marginal. Successful treatment of the malignant neoplasm responsible for the cold agglutinin often reduces the titer of antibody and the severity of the hemolysis.

Chronic cold agglutinin disease tends to be unremitting. The overall prognosis is dominated by the underlying lymphoproliferative disease, if present. In those patients in whom cold agglutinin disease appears to arise spontaneously, malignant lymphoma may develop after several years.

Paroxysmal cold hemoglobinuria (PCH) Now a rare disorder, PCH was more frequent when tertiary syphilis was prevalent; now, most cases are either secondary to a viral infection or are autoimmune. PCH results from the formation of the Donath-Landsteiner antibody, an IgG antibody that is directed against the P antigen (Chap. 114) and that can induce complement-mediated lysis. Attacks are precipitated by exposure to cold and are associated with hemoglobinemia and hemoglobinuria; chills and fever; back, leg, and abdominal pain; headache; and malaise. Recovery from the acute episode is prompt, and between episodes patients are usually asymptomatic. When this syndrome accompanies acute viral infections (e.g., measles and mumps in children), it is self-limited but may be severe. Although the direct Coombs test may show complement to be present (seldom IgG), this test may be negative. The diagnosis is made by demonstrating cold-reacting IgG antibodies either by lytic tests (when the titer is very high) or by special antiglobulin tests. When PCH is secondary to syphilis, it responds to therapy for syphilis. Chronic autoimmune PCH may respond to prednisone or cytotoxic therapy (azathioprine or cyclophosphamide) but does not respond to splenectomy. The natural history of this disease often extends over many years.

Hemolysis due to Trauma in the Circulation RBC may be fragmented by mechanical trauma as they circulate; this circumstance leads to intravascular hemolysis and in most cases to RBC fragments called *schistocytes*. Schistocytes are identified by the sharp points that result from the faulty resealing of the fractured membrane (**Plate V-28**). Mechanical trauma leading to hemolysis occurs in three clinical settings: (1) when RBC flow through small vessels over the surface of bony prominences and are subject to external impact during various physical activities, (2) when RBC flow across a pressure gradient created by an abnormal heart valve or valve prosthesis (macrovascular), and (3) when the deposition of fibrin or small platelet thrombi in the microvasculature exposes RBC to a physical impediment that fragments them (microvascular) (Table 108-8).

External impact Hemoglobinemia and hemoglobinuria have been observed in a small proportion of individuals who have undergone a prolonged march or a prolonged run, most typically on a hard surface and while wearing thin-soled shoes. The role of direct external trauma in this process has been demonstrated by the fact that hemolysis can be prevented by the insertion of a soft inner sole in the runner's shoes. Similar types of hemolysis have been described following karate and the playing of bongo drums. No abnormality of RBC has been demonstrated, even during the acute episode. Susceptible individuals will develop hemoglobinemia and hemoglobinuria when exposed to the conditions described above. Muscle damage during some of these activities may produce myoglobinuria, but renal function is preserved. No specific therapy is required except to obtain better running shoes.

Macrovascular traumatic hemolysis Hemolysis associated with fragmented RBC (**Plate V-28**) occurs in approximately 10% of patients with artificial aortic valve prostheses. This incidence is somewhat greater with valves having stellite rather than Silastic occluders, greater with small valves as compared with larger valves, and greater when valves are cloth-covered or when there is a paravalvular leak. Traumatic hemolysis is rare in recipients of porcine valves. Severe hemolysis may occur after repair of ostium primum or endocardial cushion defects with a prosthetic patch. Mitral valve prostheses may produce hemolysis, but since the pressure gradient across these valves is lower than across aortic prostheses, the incidence is lower. A moderately shortened RBC survival time with little or no anemia occurs in some patients with severe calcific aortic stenosis. Indeed, almost any intracardiac lesion that alters hemodynamics may lead to some shortening of RBC survival. Traumatic hemolysis has been observed in patients who have undergone aortofemoral bypass.

Table 108-8   Changes in RBC and Platelets Induced by Intravascular Trauma

Etiology	Fragments	Hemolysis	Thrombocytopenia
Impact: march hemoglobinuria, etc.	0	+	0
Cardiac (turbulence):			
Aortic valve prosthesis	++++	++++	0
Mitral valve prosthesis	++	++	0
Calcific aortic stenoses	+	±	0
Vessel disease[a]	+++	+	+
Thrombotic thrombocytopenic purpura	++++	++++	++++
Hemolytic-uremic syndrome	++++	++++	++++
Adenocarcinoma	++++	++++	++++
Disseminated intravascular coagulation	++	±	++++

[a] Malignant hypertension, eclampsia, renal graft rejection, hemangiomas, immune disease (scleroderma).

CLINICAL MANIFESTATIONS In severe cases, hemoglobin levels fall to 50 to 70 g/L with reticulocytosis, fragmented RBC in the peripheral blood, depressed haptoglobin, elevated serum LDH, and hemoglobinemia and hemoglobinuria. Iron loss (as hemoglobin or hemosiderin) in the urine may lead to iron deficiency. The direct Coombs test may rarely become positive.

PATHOGENESIS A number of factors combine to cause the fragmentation of RBC by prostheses: (1) the shear stress resulting from turbulent blood flow, particularly when blood is forced through a small aperture by high pressure (e.g., a paravalvular leak around an aortic valve); (2) direct mechanical trauma of RBC at the time of seating of the occluder of the prosthetic valve; and (3) the deposition of fibrin across disrupted attachment points.

℞ TREATMENT Iron deficiency should be corrected by the administration of oral iron. The elevated hemoglobin that results may permit a decrease in the cardiac output and a slowing of the hemolytic rate. Limitation in physical activity also lessens the hemolytic rate. When these measures fail, any paravalvular leak must be repaired or the prosthetic valve replaced.

Microvascular traumatic hemolysis If fibrin or platelet microthrombi are deposited in arteriolar sites, RBC may be trapped on the meshwork and fragmented by high shear forces.

ABNORMALITIES OF THE VESSEL WALL Disorders such as malignant hypertension, eclampsia, renal allograft rejection, disseminated cancer, hemangiomas, or disseminated intravascular coagulation (DIC) may cause traumatic hemolysis. The degree of hemolysis induced by this family of disorders is usually quite mild, but a large number of fragments may be seen in the peripheral blood. In some patients, thrombocytopenia may be severe. Therapy is best directed at the primary disease. Thus, reversal of renal graft rejection, treatment of malignant hypertension and eclampsia, control of cancer, and the like, lead to a cessation of hemolysis. The relative importance of the primary vascular abnormality versus fibrin deposition is unclear.

Thrombotic thrombocytopenia purpura (TTP) This disorder is characterized by arteriolar lesions in various organs that contain platelet thrombi and produce thrombocytopenia and hemolytic anemia due to fragmentation of RBC. Tissue hypoxia resulting from vessel occlusion may cause organ dysfunction, most frequently manifest in the nervous system or the kidney. The disease affects individuals of all ages, but primarily young adults and more often women.

CLINICAL MANIFESTATIONS The classic pentad of TTP includes hemolytic anemia with fragmentation of erythrocytes and signs of intravascular hemolysis, thrombocytopenia, diffuse and nonfocal neurologic findings, decreased renal function, and fever. These signs and symptoms occur variably, depending on the number and sites of the arteriolar lesions. The anemia may be very mild to very severe, and the thrombocytopenia often parallels it. The neurologic and renal symptoms are usually seen only when the platelet count is markedly diminished (<20 to $30 \times 10^3/\mu L$). Fever is not reliably present. TTP may be acute in onset, but its course spans days to weeks in most patients and occasionally continues for months. Proteinuria and a moderate elevation of blood urea nitrogen may be found on initial presentation; the latter continues to rise while urine output falls if the patient develops renal failure. Neurologic symptoms develop in $>90\%$ of patients whose disease terminates in death. Initially, changes in mental status such as confusion, delirium, or altered states of consciousness may occur. Focal findings include seizures, hemiparesis, aphasia, and visual field defects. These neurologic symptoms may fluctuate and terminate in coma. Involvement of myocardial blood vessels may be a cause of sudden death. The severity of the disorder can be estimated from the degree of anemia and thrombocytopenia and the serum LDH level. Prothrombin time, partial thromboplastin time, fibrinogen concentration, and the level of fibrin split products are usually normal or only mildly abnormal. If the coagulation tests indicate a major consumption of clotting factors, the diagnosis of TTP is doubtful. A positive antinuclear antibody (ANA) determination is obtained in approximately 20% of patients.

PATHOGENESIS The manifestations of TTP can be explained by *localized* platelet thrombi. The agglutination of platelets is mediated by unusually large multimers of von Willebrand factor. Patients with TTP have acquired an antibody that inhibits a protease that normally cleaves von Willebrand factor. Arterioles are filled with hyalin material, presumably fibrin and platelets, and similar material may be seen beneath the endothelium of otherwise uninvolved vessels. Immunofluorescence studies have shown the presence of immunoglobulin and complement in arterioles. Microaneurysms of arterioles are often present. An association with pregnancy, AIDS, systemic lupus erythematosus (SLE), scleroderma, and Sjögren's syndrome suggests an immunologic origin.

DIAGNOSIS The combination of hemolytic anemia with fragmented RBC, thrombocytopenia, normal coagulation tests, fever, neurologic disorders, and renal dysfunction is virtually pathognomonic of TTP. Although they are not usually required for diagnosis, biopsies of skin and muscle, gingiva, lymph node, or bone marrow may show the typical arteriolar abnormalities. TTP must be distinguished from idiopathic thrombocytopenic purpura or Evans's syndrome (the former plus immunohemolytic anemia) by the finding of fragmented but not spherocytic RBC in the peripheral blood and a negative direct Coombs test.

℞ TREATMENT Plasma exhange permits >90% of patients to survive if therapy is promptly instituted. Many patients require daily or even twice daily plasmapheresis with plasma replacement. If a response is obtained (as indicated by increasing platelet count and decreasing plasma LDH and fragmented RBC), plasmapheresis may be done less frequently but sometimes must be continued for several weeks to months. Most patients also receive high doses of glucocorticoids and some receive platelet-active agents (dipyridamole, sulfinpyrazone, dextran, aspirin), but their efficacy is not proven. Vincristine, cyclophosphamide, or splenectomy has been used to treat patients who do not respond to plasma exchange. Even coma is not a contraindication to therapy, since full neurologic recovery is the rule in patients responding to therapy. Relapses have been noted in ~10% of patients but are usually responsive to retreatment. Platelet transfusions should not be given because they can precipitate thrombotic events.

Hemolytic-uremic syndrome This disorder is similar to TTP and is characterized by the same arteriolar lesions, which may be confined to the kidney, and by similar laboratory findings. It is usually encountered in young children. Often the patient has a prodrome of a gastroenteritic bloody diarrhea caused by *Escherichia coli* 0157:H7, and the lesions are thought to be due to the elaboration of Shiga-like verotoxins that damage renal vascular endothelial cells. This disorder has been associated with eating undercooked meat. Very rarely, the disorder appears to be familial. Patients present with acute hemolytic anemia, thrombocytopenic purpura, and acute oliguric renal failure. Most patients have either hemoglobinuria or anuria. Unlike TTP, neurologic manifestations are uncommon. The peripheral blood and coagulation tests are usually indistinguishable from those of TTP.

Patients are treated with plasmapheresis, dialysis, and transfusions. The efficacy of glucocorticoids, dextran, and heparin is uncertain. The mortality rate in children ranges from 5 to 20% but is considerably higher in adults. A disorder resembling the hemolytic-uremic syndrome has been described in adults treated with the antineoplastic drug mitomycin C, usually in combination with other drugs. It may also occur in patients receiving high-dose chemotherapy with autologous stem cell transplantation.

Disseminated intravascular coagulation Inappropriate activation of the clotting system with deposition of fibrin in small vessels may lead to RBC fragmentation in the microvasculature. RBC fragmentation occurs in about one-fourth of patients with DIC (Chap. 117). The degree of hemolysis is much less in DIC than in either TTP or the hemolytic-uremic syndrome, and anemia with reticulocytosis is rare.

Environmental Alteration of the Red Cell Membrane by "Toxic" Effects A variety of infections may be associated with severe hemolysis. The microbes that cause bartonellosis (Chap. 163), as well as malaria and babesiosis (Chap. 214) directly parasitize RBC. *Clostridium welchii* (Chap. 145) produces a phospholipase that can cleave the phosphoryl bond of lecithin, thereby lysing human RBC. A mild, transient hemolysis frequently accompanies bacteremia with diverse organisms such as pneumococci, staphylococci, and *E. coli*.

Hemolysis may result from the direct action of snake and spider venoms on the RBC. Although cobra venom is directly lytic in vitro, the clinical disease induced by the bite of the cobra is one of moderate hemolysis associated with spherocytosis. Spider bites, particularly the bite of the brown recluse spider, induce acute intravascular hemolysis associated with spherocytosis and fragments of complement components on the RBC. The hemolysis continues for several days up to 1 week.

Copper has a direct hemolytic effect on RBC. Hemolysis has been observed after exposure of individuals to copper salts (such as during hemodialysis). Transient episodes of hemolysis occur in patients with Wilson's disease (Chap. 348).

The RBC membrane is unstable at temperatures above 49°C due to denaturation of the cytoskeletal protein spectrin. The RBC undergoes a process of budding, cleavage, and resealing above this temperature. Patients with extensive burns have prominent spherocytosis, hemoglobinemia, and sometimes hemoglobinuria.

Spur Cell Anemia Hemolytic anemia with bizarre-shaped RBC occurs in about 5% of patients with severe hepatocellular disease, particularly advanced Laennec's cirrhosis.

Clinical manifestations Anemia is more severe than is observed in otherwise uncomplicated cirrhosis. Hematocrit levels range between 15 and 25%. Splenomegaly is always present and is greater than in patients who have cirrhosis without spur cell anemia. Jaundice may be severe because of the hemolysis and liver dysfunction, and hepatic encephalopathy is common. The RBC are irregularly shaped with multiple spicules, and a small number of bizarre-shaped fragments are commonly seen on peripheral blood smears **(Plate V-27)**. Reticulocytosis and other signs of hemolysis are present. The tests of liver function are typical of patients with severe cirrhosis.

RBC half-life is decreased to as short as 6 days (normal being 26 to 32 days); RBC destruction is localized to the spleen. Normal transfused RBC acquire the defect and have a survival time similar to that of the patient's own RBC.

Pathogenesis The surface membrane of a spur cell contains 50 to 70% excess cholesterol, but its total phospholipid content is normal. By contrast, the target-shaped RBC is more common in liver disease and has an excess of both cholesterol and phospholipid. The selective cholesterol excess in the spur cell is due to abnormal low-density lipoprotein with an increased mole ratio of free (unesterified) cholesterol to phospholipid. Cholesterol out of proportion to phospholipid decreases the fluidity of the spur cell membrane, and cell deformability is decreased. These rigid, cholesterol-laden RBC cannot pass through the filtering system of the spleen, further impeded by congestive splenomegaly in cirrhosis.

Diagnosis Patients with spur cell anemia have severe hemolysis and characteristic RBC morphology. Increasing anemia in a patient with chronic cirrhosis most commonly results from blood loss, folic acid deficiency, or iron deficiency.

RBC of similar morphology are seen in patients with abetalipoproteinemia. However, hemolysis is minimal.

Spur cells or acanthocytes have irregular spikes (irregular in length of projections and their spacing) and must be distinguished from regularly spaced, crenated RBC (echinocytes). Echinocytes are a frequent artifact on portions of some blood smears, and they are uniformly present in some patients with uremia ("burr cells") **(Plate V-3)**. Small, dense crenated spheres (spheroechinocytes) are sometimes seen in congenital nonspherocytic hemolytic anemia due to enzyme deficiencies in the Embden-Meyerhof pathway (see above).

℞ TREATMENT Transfusion therapy is of limited benefit. Attempts to influence RBC cholesterol with various lipid-lowering agents have been unsuccessful. Splenectomy has been reported to prevent both the conditioning of RBC in the spleen and their premature destruction. However, splenectomy carries a high risk in patients with severe liver disease complicated by portal hypertension and coagulation defects. It must be reserved for patients in whom hemolysis is a major problem and who are relatively good surgical risks.

Prognosis Spur cell anemia occurs during the late stages of cirrhosis, and >90% of patients succumb to their underlying liver disease within 1 year of the diagnosis of spur cell anemia.

Paroxysmal Nocturnal Hemoglobinuria (PNH) This hemolytic disorder is distinctive because it is an intracorpuscular defect acquired at the stem cell level.

Clinical manifestations The three common manifestations of PNH are: hemolytic anemia, venous thrombosis, and deficient hematopoiesis. Anemia is highly variable with hematocrit values ranging from ≤20% to normal. RBC are normochromic and normocytic unless iron deficiency has occurred from chronic iron loss in the urine.

Granulocytopenia and thrombocytopenia are common and reflect deficient hematopoiesis. Clinical hemoglobinuria is intermittent in most patients and never occurs in some, but hemosiderinuria is usually present. The lack of two proteins, decay-accelerating factor (DAF, CD55) and a membrane inhibitor of reactive lysis (MIRL, CD59) (see below) make the RBC more sensitive to the lytic effect of complement.

DAF normally disrupts the enzyme complexes from either the classical (antibody-driven) pathway or the alternative pathway that activate C3 and C5; CD59 inhibits the conversion of C9 by the membrane attack complex C5b-8 to a polymeric complex capable of penetrating the membrane.

The platelets also lack these proteins, but the life span of the platelet is normal. However, the activation of complement indirectly stimulates platelet aggregation and hypercoagulability; this probably accounts for the tendency to thrombosis seen in PNH.

Venous thrombosis is a common complication of patients of European origin, affecting ~40% at one time or another; it is less common in Asian patients. It occurs primarily in intraabdominal veins (hepatic, portal, mesenteric) and results in the Budd-Chiari syndrome, congestive splenomegaly, and abdominal pain. It may occur in cerebral venous sinuses and is a common cause of death in patients with PNH. The bone marrow may appear normocellular, but in vitro marrow progenitor assays are abnormal. In about 15 to 30% of long-term survivors of aplastic anemia, PNH cells appear in the circulation; in some patients, the manifestations of PNH become dominant. Patients with PNH may have aplastic periods lasting from weeks to years. PNH may be seen in association with other stem cell disorders, including myelofibrosis, and (rarely) other myelodysplastic or myeloproliferative disorders.

Pathogenesis PNH is an acquired clonal disease, arising from an inactivating somatic mutation in a single abnormal stem cell of a gene on the X-chromosome (*pig-A*) important for the biosynthesis of the glycosylphosphatidylinositol (GPI) anchor. This anchor is necessary for the attachment of a number of proteins to the external membrane surface, and its partial or complete absence results in the absence of those proteins; to date, about 20 proteins have been found to be missing on the blood cells of patients with PNH. The normal clone of stem cells does not completely disappear, and the proportion of cells that are abnormal varies among patients and over time in a single patient.

Diagnosis PNH should be suspected in anyone with otherwise unexplained hemolytic anemia, especially with leukopenia and/or thrombocytopenia and with evidence of intravascular hemolysis (hemoglobinemia, hemoglobinuria, hemosiderinuria, elevated LDH). Any-

one recovering from aplastic anemia should be examined at intervals for the appearance of the diagnostic cells. The diagnosis is often delayed because (1) it is not considered, (2) hemoglobinuria is confused with hematuria, (3) elevation of the LDH is attributed to liver disease, and (4) the diagnostic tests (Ham's test and the sucrose lysis test) are not reliable.

For many years, the diagnosis of PNH depended on the demonstration of the lysis of RBC after complement activation either by acid (Ham or acidified serum lysis test) or by reduction in ionic strength (sucrose lysis test). These tests are inferior to the analysis of GPI-linked proteins (e.g., CD59, DAF) on RBC and granulocytes by flow cytometry.

℞ TREATMENT Transfusion therapy is useful in PNH not only for raising the hemoglobin level but also for suppressing the marrow production of RBC during episodes of sustained hemoglobinuria. Washed RBC are the preferred source to prevent exacerbation of hemolysis. Therapy with androgens sometimes results in a rise in hemoglobin level. Glucocorticoids reduce the rate of hemolysis in moderate doses (15 to 30 mg prednisone) on alternate days.

Iron deficiency is common. Iron replacement may exacerbate hemolysis because of the formation of many new RBC, which may be sensitive to complement. This occurrence may be minimized by giving prednisone (60 mg/d) or by suppressing the bone marrow with transfusions.

Acute thrombosis in PNH, particularly the Budd-Chiari syndrome and cerebral thrombosis, should be treated with thrombolytic agents. Heparin therapy should be instituted rapidly and maintained for several days before changing to coumadin therapy. Antithymoctye globulin (total dose of 150 mg/kg over 4 to 10 days) is often of use in treating marrow hypoplasia; prednisone counteracts the immune-complex disease that results from the administration of this foreign protein.

In patients with either hypoplasia or thrombosis who have an appropriate sibling donor, marrow transplantation should be considered early in the course of the disease. The usual conditioning programs are sufficient to eradicate the aberrant clone.

ANEMIA OF ACUTE BLOOD LOSS

The normal capacity to compensate for acute blood loss involves cardiovascular mechanisms, an adjustment in the oxygen affinity of hemoglobin, and an increase in erythropoiesis in the marrow. The signs and symptoms of blood loss relate to the volume of the blood loss and the time frame over which the hemorrhage occurs (Table 108-9). Losses of up to 20% of the blood volume are normally tolerated by redistribution of blood flow mediated by reflex venospasm, but the presence of fever or pain may interfere with this compensation. With larger losses, blood volume redistribution is not adequate to maintain normal blood pressure: initially, hypotension is only seen on standing, but with greater losses progressively greater problems are encountered

Table 108-9 Signs and Symptoms of Acute Blood Loss

Blood Loss			
%,[a]	Volume, mL	Symptoms	Signs
<20	<1000	Restlessness	+/− Vasovagal reaction
20–30	1000–1500	Anxiety, DOE	Orthostatic hypotension, tachycardia on exertion
30–40	1500–2000	Syncope on sitting or standing	Orthostatic hypotension, tachycardia at rest
>40	>2000	Confusion, shortness of breath	Shock, poor perfusion

[a] Based on an estimated total blood volume of 5000 mL (70-kg adult).

in maintaining blood pressure in sitting or supine positions. If the blood loss is more gradual, plasma volume increases, but albumin production usually lags behind the fluid shifts. It may take 2 to 3 days for the liver to generate the albumin lost in a 1500-mL bleed.

The most rapid hematologic adjustment to acute blood loss is an increase in oxygen delivery to the tissues. This is first mediated by the Bohr effect, where the more acidic milieu of the hypoperfused hypoxic tissues shifts the hemoglobin oxygen dissociation curve to the right. Over several hours the RBC increase their production of 2,3-bisphosphoglycerate, which also enhances the unloading of oxygen to tissues. These two mechanisms can substantially increase the capacity of RBC to deliver oxygen to the tissues.

The marrow response to hemorrhage is related to the generation of erythropoietin in the kidney in response to decreased oxygen tensions. A normal response depends on the production of erythropoietin, the presence of normal erythroid progenitors in the marrow, and an adequate supply of iron. If these three elements are normal, reticulocytes begin to increase in number in the first 2 days based on early release of reticulocytes from the marrow. However, it takes 3 to 6 days for erythroid hyperplasia to appear and 7 to 10 days before the erythropoietic response is maximal, producing reticulocyte counts up to 20 to 30%, a reticulocyte index of ≥ 3, and a marked increase in the marrow erythoid/granulocytic ratio.

DIAGNOSIS Usually it is clear that a patient is bleeding; however, in some cases, large volumes of blood loss can occur internally from the gastrointestinal tract (esophageal varicies, cancer in the stomach or colon), a ruptured spleen, fractures and other trauma, or other lesions that can cause massive hemorrhage into the peritoneal cavity, pleural cavity, or the retroperitoneal space. Patients who have bled sufficiently to develop hypotension generally develop anemia, which is apparent only after volume replacement. The granulocyte count may increase to $\geq 20,000$ cells/μL and include immature cell types such as metamyelocytes and myelocytes. Epinephrine-induced demargination of peripheral granulocytes and release of cells from the marrow may account for this change. Nucleated RBC may appear in the circulation, and platelet counts may exceed 1×10^6/μL. The basis for the increased platelet count is unclear. Hemorrhage in an internal cavity is accompanied by a rise in unconjugated bilirubin and a fall in serum haptoglobin.

℞ **TREATMENT** Treatment of the underlying cause of the hemorrhage is of paramount importance. If the patient is severely anemic or sufficiently hypovolemic, packed RBC should be transfused. In less severe cases, if the patient has normal kidneys (and presumably a normal erythropoietin response to anemia), normal bone marrow function, and an adequate supply of iron, no specific therapy for the anemia is required.

BIBLIOGRAPHY

AMIDON TM et al: Mitral and aortic paravalvular leaks with hemolytic anemia. Am Heart J 125:266, 1993

BEUTLER E: Study of glucose-6-phosphate dehydrogenase: History and molecular biology. Am J Hematol 42:53, 1993

FURLAN M et al: Von Willebrand factor-cleaving protease in thrombotic thrombocytopenic purpura and the hemolytic-uremic syndrome. N Engl J Med 339:1578, 1998

HIRONO A et al: Enzymatic diagnosis in non-spherocytic hemolytic anemia. Medicine 67: 110, 1988

LUX SE, PALEK J: Disorders of the red cell membrane, in *Blood: Principles and Practice of Hematology*, RI Handin et al (eds). Philadelphia, Lippincott, 1995

MIWA S, FUJII H: Molecular basis of erythroenzymopathies associated with hemolytic anemia: Tabulation of mutant enzymes. Am J Hematol 51:122, 1996

ROSE M et al: The changing course of thrombotic thrombocytopenic purpura and modern therapy. Blood Rev 7:94, 1993

ROSSE WF: Paroxysmal nocturnal hemoglobinuria as a molecular disease. Medicine 76: 63, 1997

TSAI H-M, LIAN E C-Y: Antibodies to von Willebrand factor-cleaving protease in acute thrombotic thrombocytopenic purpura. N Engl J Med 339:1585, 1998

109

Neal S. Young

APLASTIC ANEMIA, MYELODYSPLASIA, AND RELATED BONE MARROW FAILURE SYNDROMES

The hypoproliferative anemias associated with marrow damage include aplastic anemia, myelodysplasia (MDS), pure red cell aplasia (PRCA), and myelopthisis. Anemia in these disorders, which is normochromic, normocytic, or macrocytic and characterized by low reticulocyte count, is not a solitary or even the major finding in these diseases, which are better described as marrow failure states. In bone marrow failure, pancytopenia—anemia, leukopenia, and thrombocytopenia (sometimes in various combinations)—results from deficient hematopoiesis, as distinguished from blood count depression due to peripheral destruction of red cells (hemolytic anemias), platelets (idiopathic thrombocytopenic purpura or due to splenomegaly), and granulocytes (as in the immune leukopenias).

Hematopoietic failure syndromes are classified by dominant morphologic features of the bone marrow (Table 109-1). While practical distinction among these syndromes is clear in stereotypical cases, they can, of course, occur secondary to other diseases, and are so closely related that the differential diagnosis may be arbitrary, patients may seem to suffer from two or three related diseases simultaneously, or one diagnosis may appear to evolve into another. Finally, there is an important pathophysiologic relationship among these syndromes in their sharing of immune-mediated mechanisms of marrow destruction and some element of genomic instability resulting in a higher rate of malignant transformation.

APLASTIC ANEMIA

DEFINITION Aplastic anemia is pancytopenia with bone marrow hypocellularity. Acquired aplastic anemia is distinguished from iatrogenic marrow aplasia, the common occurrence of marrow hypo-

Table 109-1   Differential Diagnosis of Pancytopenia

Pancytopenia with hypocellular bone marrow
  Acquired aplastic anemia
  Inherited aplastic anemia (Fanconi's anemia)
  Some myelodysplasia syndromes
  Rare aleukemic leukemia (AML)
  Some acute lymphoid leukemia
  Some lymphomas of bone marrow
Pancytopenia with cellular bone marrow
  Primary bone marrow diseases
    Myelodysplasia syndromes
    Paroxysmal nocturnal hemoglobinuria
    Myelofibrosis
    Some aleukemic leukemia
    Myelophthisis
    Bone marrow lymphoma
    Hairy cell leukemia
  Secondary to systemic diseases
    Systemic lupus erythematosus
    Hypersplenism
    B_{12}, folate deficiency
    Overwhelming infection
    Alcohol
    Brucellosis
    Sarcoidosis
    Tuberculosis
    Leishmaniasis
Hypocellular bone marrow ± cytopenia
  Q fever
  Legionnaires' disease
  Anorexia nervosa, starvation
  Mycobacteria

cellularity after intensive cytotoxic chemotherapy for cancer. Aplastic anemia can also be constitutional: the genetic disease Fanconi's anemia, while frequently associated with typical physical anomalies and the development of pancytopenia early in life, can also present as marrow failure in normal-appearing adults. Acquired aplastic anemia is often stereotypical in its manifestations, with the abrupt onset of low blood counts in a previously well young adult; seronegative hepatitis or a course of an incriminated medical drug may precede the onset. The diagnosis in these instances is uncomplicated. Sometimes blood count depression is moderate or incomplete, resulting in anemia, leukopenia, and thrombocytopenia in some combination. Aplastic anemia is related to both paroxysmal nocturnal hemoglobinuria (PNH; Chap. 108) and to MDS, and in some cases a clear distinction among these disorders may not be possible.

EPIDEMIOLOGY The incidence of acquired aplastic anemia in Europe and Israel is 2 cases per million persons annually. In Thailand and China, rates of 5 to 7 per million have been established. In general, men and women are affected with equal frequency, but there is a biphasic age distribution, with the major peak among older children and young adults and a second rise in the elderly.

ETIOLOGY The origins of aplastic anemia have been inferred from several recurring clinical associations (Table 109-2); unfortunately, these relationships are neither a reliable guide in an individual patient nor necessarily etiologic. In addition, while most cases of aplastic anemia are idiopathic, little other than history separates these cases from those with a presumed etiology such as a drug exposure.

Radiation Marrow aplasia is a major acute sequela of radiation. Radiation damages DNA; tissues dependent on active mitosis are par-ticularly susceptible. Nuclear accidents can involve not only power plant workers but also employees of hospitals, laboratories, and industry (food sterilization, metal radiography, etc.), as well as innocents exposed to stolen, misplaced, or misused sources. While the radiation dose can be approximated from the rate and degree of decline in blood counts, dosimetry by reconstruction of the exposure can help to estimate the patient's prognosis and also to protect medical personnel from contact with radioactive tissue and excreta. MDS and leukemia, but probably not aplastic anemia, are late effects of irradiation.

Chemicals Benzene is a notorious cause of bone marrow failure. Vast quantities of epidemiologic, clinical, and laboratory data link benzene to aplastic anemia, acute leukemia, and blood and marrow abnormalities. The occurrence of leukemia is roughly correlated with cumulative exposure, but susceptibility must also be important, as only a minority of even heavily exposed workers develop benzene myelotoxicity. The employment history is important, especially in industries where benzene is used for a secondary purpose, usually as a solvent. Benzene-related blood diseases have declined with regulation of industrial exposure. Although benzene is no longer generally available as a household solvent, exposure to its metabolites occurs in the normal diet and in the use of lead-free gasoline. The association between marrow failure and other chemicals that contain a benzene ring is much less well substantiated; these chemicals may have been contaminated with benzene in manufacture, or petroleum distillates may have been used to dissolve the product.

Drugs (See Table 109-3) Many chemotherapeutic drugs have marrow suppression as a major toxicity; effects are dose-dependent and will occur in all recipients. In contrast, idiosyncratic reactions to

Table 109-2 Classification of Aplastic Anemia and Single Cytopenias

Acquired	Inherited
APLASTIC ANEMIA	
Secondary	Fanconi's anemia
Radiation	Dyskeratosis congenita
Drugs and chemicals	Shwachman-Diamond syndrome
Regular effects	Reticular dysgenesis
Idiosyncratic reactions	Amegakaryocytic thrombocytopenia
Viruses	Familial aplastic anemias
Epstein-Barr virus (infectious mononucleosis)	Preleukemia (monosomy 7, etc.)
Hepatitis (non-A, non-B, non-C hepatitis)	Nonhematologic syndrome (Down's, Dubowitz, Seckel)
Parvovirus B19 (transient aplastic crisis, PRCA)	
HIV-1 (AIDS)	
Immune diseases	
Eosinophilic fasciitis	
Hypoimmunoglobulinemia	
Thymoma/thymic carcinoma	
Graft-versus-host disease in immunodeficiency	
Paroxysmal nocturnal hemoglobinuria	
Pregnancy	
Idiopathic	
CYTOPENIAS	
PRCA (see Table 109-4)	Congenital PRCA (Diamond-Blackfan anemia)
	Transient erythroblastopenia of childhood
Neutropenia/Agranulocytosis	
Idiopathic	Kostmann's Syndrome
Drugs, toxins	Shwachman-Diamond syndrome
Pure white cell aplasia	Reticular dysgenesis
Thrombocytopenia	
Drugs, toxins	Amegakaryocytic thrombocytopenia
Idiopathic amegakaryocytic	Thrombocytopenia with absent radii

NOTE: PRCA, pure red cell aplasia.

Table 109-3 Some Drugs and Chemicals Associated with Aplastic Anemia

Agents that regularly produce marrow depression as major toxicity in commonly employed doses or normal exposures:
  Cytotoxic drugs used in cancer chemotherapy: *alkylating agents*, antimetabolites, antimitotics, some antibiotics

Agents that frequently but not inevitably produce marrow aplasia:
  Benzene (and benzene-containing chemicals such as kerosene, carbon tetrachloride, Stoddard's solvent, chlorophenols)

Agents associated with aplastic anemia but with a relatively low probability:
  Chloramphenicol
  Insecticides
  Antiprotozoals: *quinacrine* and chloroquine, mepacrine
  Nonsteroidal anti-inflammatory drugs (including *phenylbutazone*, indomethacin, ibuprofen, sulindac, aspirin)
  Anticonvulsants (*hydantoins*, *carbamazapine*, phenacemide, felbamate)
  Heavy metals (*gold*, arsenic, bismuth, mercury)
  Sulfonamides: some antibiotics, antithyroid drugs (methimazole, methylthiouracil, propylthiouracil), antidiabetes drugs (tolbutamide, chlorpropamide), carbonic anhydrase inhibitors (acetazolamide and methazolamide)
  Antihistamines (*cimetidine*, chlorpheniramine)
  D-Penicillamine
  Estrogens (in pregnancy and in high doses in animals)

Agents whose association with aplastic anemia is more tenuous:
  Other antibiotics (streptomycin, tetracycline, methicillin, mebendazole, trimethoprim/sulfamethoxazole, flucytosine)
  Sedatives and tranquilizers (chlorpromazine, prochlorperazine, piperacetazine, chlordiazepoxide, meprobamate, methyprylon)
  Allopurinol
  Methyldopa
  Quinidine
  Lithium
  Guanidine
  Potassium perchlorate
  Thiocyanate
  Carbimazole

NOTE: Terms set in italic show the most consistent association with aplastic anemia.

a large and diverse group of drugs may lead to aplastic anemia without a clear dose-response relationship. These associations rest largely on accumulated case reports, but a massive international study in Europe in the 1980s quantitated drug relationships, especially for nonsteroidal analgesics, sulfonamides, thyrostatic drugs, some psychotropics, penicillamine, allopurinol, and gold. Not all associations necessarily reflect causation: a drug may have been used to treat the first symptoms of bone marrow failure (antibiotics for fever or the preceding viral illness) or provoked the first symptom of a preexisting disease (petechiae by nonsteroidal anti-inflammatory agents administered to the thrombocytopenic patient). In the context of total drug use, idiosyncratic reactions, while individually devastating, are exceedingly rare events. Chloramphenicol, the most infamous culprit, reportedly produced aplasia in only about 1/60,000 therapy courses, and even this number is almost certainly an overestimate (risks are almost invariably exaggerated when based on collections of cases; although the introduction of chloramphenicol was perceived to have created an epidemic of aplastic anemia, its diminished use was not followed by a changed frequency of marrow failure). Risk estimates are usually lower when determined in population-based studies; furthermore, the low absolute risk is also made more obvious: even a 10- or 20-fold increase in risk translates, in a rare disease, to but a handful of drug-induced aplastic anemia cases among hundreds of thousands of exposed patients.

Infections   Hepatitis is the most common preceding infection, and posthepatitis marrow failure accounts for about 5% of etiologic associations in most series. Patients are usually young men who have recovered from a mild bout of liver inflammation 1 to 2 months earlier; the subsequent pancytopenia is very severe. The hepatitis is almost invariably seronegative (non-A, non-B, non-C, non-G) and presumably due to a novel, as yet undiscovered, virus. Fulminant liver failure in childhood can follow seronegative hepatitis, and marrow failure occurs at a high rate in these patients as well. Aplastic anemia can rarely follow infectious mononucleosis, and Epstein-Barr virus has been found in the marrow of a few aplastic anemia patients, some without a suggestive preceding history. Parvovirus B19, the cause of transient aplastic crisis in hemolytic anemias and of some pure red cell aplasia (see below), does not usually cause generalized bone marrow failure. Blood count depression is frequent in the course of many viral and bacterial infections but is comparatively moderate and resolves with the infection.

Immunologic Diseases   Aplasia is a major consequence and the cause of death in *transfusion-associated graft-versus-host disease*, which can occur after infusion of unirradiated blood products to an immunodeficient recipient. Aplastic anemia is strongly associated with the rare collagen vascular syndrome called *eosinophilic fasciitis*, which is characterized by painful induration of subcutaneous tissues (Chap. 313). Pancytopenia with marrow hypoplasia can also occur in systemic lupus erythematosus.

Pregnancy   Aplastic anemia very rarely may occur and recur during pregnancy and resolve with delivery or with spontaneous or induced abortion.

Paroxysmal Nocturnal Hemoglobinuria   An acquired mutation in the *PIG-A* gene in a hematopoietic stem cell is required for the development of PNH, but *PIG-A* mutations probably occur commonly in normal individuals. If the PIG-A mutant stem cell proliferates, the result is a clone of progeny deficient in glycosylphosphatidylinositol-linked cell surface membrane proteins (Chap. 108). Such PNH cells are now most accurately enumerated using fluorescence-activated flow cytometry of CD55 or CD59 expression on granulocytes rather than Ham or sucrose lysis tests on red cells. Deficient cells can be detected in about a quarter of patients with aplastic anemia at the time of presentation [and PNH cells are also seen in cases of hypocellular MDS (see below)]. In addition, functional studies of bone marrow from PNH patients, even those with mainly hemolytic manifestations, show evidence of defective hematopoiesis. Patients with an initial clinical di-

agnosis of PNH, especially younger individuals, may later develop frank marrow aplasia and pancytopenia; patients with an initial diagnosis of aplastic anemia may suffer from hemolytic PNH years after recovery of blood counts. One explanation for the aplastic anemia/PNH syndrome is selection of the deficient clones, perhaps because they are favored for proliferation in the peculiar environment of immune-mediated marrow destruction.

Congenital Disorders   Fanconi's anemia, an autosomal recessive disorder, manifests as progressive pancytopenia, increased chromosome fragility, congenital developmental anomalies, and an increased risk of malignancy. Patients with Fanconi's anemia typically have short stature; café au lait spots; and anomalies involving the thumb, radius, and genitourinary tract. At least seven different genetic defects have been defined by complementation analysis. The most common, type A Fanconi's anemia, is due to a mutation in *FANCA*. The function of the four cloned genes so far identified in Fanconi's anemia remains unknown.

Patients with Shwachman-Diamond syndrome may develop pancreatic insufficiency, malabsorption, and neutropenia and are at risk of aplastic anemia. Dyskeratosis congenita is an X-linked disorder characterized by mucous membrane leukoplasia, dystrophic nails, reticular hyperpigmentation, and the later development of aplastic anemia in about half of patients. Mutation in the *DKC1 (dyskerin)* gene has been found in some cases.

PATHOPHYSIOLOGY   Bone marrow failure results from severe damage to the hematopoietic cell compartment. In aplastic anemia, replacement of the bone marrow by fat is apparent in the morphology of the biopsy specimen (Fig. 109-1; **Plate V-13**) and magnetic resonance imaging of the spine; cells bearing the CD34 antigen, a marker of early hematopoietic cells, are greatly diminished; and in functional studies, committed and primitive progenitor cells are virtually absent—in vitro assays have suggested that the stem cell pool is reduced to ≤1% of normal in severe disease at the time of presentation. Qualitative abnormalities, such as limited number of operating stem cell clones or shortened telomere length, may follow from the quantitative deficiency, reflecting the shrunken and stressed state of hematopoiesis. An intrinsic stem cell defect exists for constitutional aplastic anemia, as cells from patients with Fanconi's anemia exhibit chromosome damage and death on exposure to certain chemical agents, but there is no convenient mechanism for the propagation of an *acquired* genetic abnormality that would produce a hypoproliferative (as opposed to neoplastic) disease. Aplastic anemia does not appear to result from defective stroma or growth factor production.

Drug Injury   Extrinsic damage to the marrow follows massive physical or chemical insults such as high doses of radiation and toxic chemicals. For the more common idiosyncratic reaction to modest doses of medical drugs, altered drug metabolism has been invoked as a likely mechanism. The metabolic pathways of many drugs and chemicals, especially if they are polar and have limited water solubility, involve enzymatic degradation to highly reactive electrophilic compounds; these intermediates are toxic because of their propensity to bind to cellular macromolecules. For example, derivative hydroquinones and quinolones are responsible for benzene-induced tissue injury. Excessive generation of toxic intermediates or failure to detoxify the intermediates may be genetically determined and apparent only on specific drug challenge; the complexity and specificity of the pathways imply multiple susceptible loci and would provide an explanation for the rarity of idiosyncratic drug reactions.

Immune-Mediated Injury   The recovery of marrow function in some patients prepared for bone marrow transplantation with antilymphocyte globulin (ALG) first suggested that aplastic anemia might be immune-mediated. Consistent with this hypothesis was the frequent failure of simple bone marrow transplantation from a syngeneic twin, without conditioning cytotoxic chemotherapy, which also argued both *against* simple stem cell absence as the cause and *for* the presence of a host factor producing marrow failure. Laboratory data support an important role for the immune system in aplastic anemia. Blood and bone marrow cells of patients can suppress normal hematopoietic pro-

A

B

C

D

FIGURE 109-1 *A*. Normal bone marrow biopsy. *B*. Normal bone marrow aspirate smear. The marrow is normally 30 to 70% cellular, and there is a heterogeneous mix of myeloid, erythroid, and lymphoid cells. *C*. Aplastic ane-mia biopsy. *D*. Smear in aplastic anemia, showing replacement of hematopoietic tissue by fat and only residual stromal and lymphoid cells.

genitor cell growth, and removal of T cells from aplastic anemia bone marrow improves colony formation in vitro. Increased numbers of activated cytotoxic T cells are observed in aplastic anemia patients and usually decline with successful immunosuppressive therapy; cytokine measurements suggest a predominant T_H1 immune response (interferon γ, interleukin 2, and tumor necrosis factor). Interferon and tumor necrosis factor induce Fas expression on CD34 cells, leading to apoptotic cell death; localization of activated T cells to bone marrow and local production of their soluble factors are probably important in stem cell destruction.

Early immune system events in aplastic anemia are not well understood. Many different exogeneous antigens appear capable of initiating a pathologic immune response, but at least some of the active T cells recognize true self-antigens. The rarity of occurrence of aplastic anemia despite common exposures (medical drugs, hepatitis virus) suggests that genetically determined features of the immune response can convert a normal physiologic response into a sustained abnormal autoimmune process.

CLINICAL FEATURES History Aplastic anemia can appear with seeming abruptness or have a more insidious onset. Bleeding is the most common early symptom; a complaint of days to weeks of easy bruising, oozing from the gums, nose bleeds, heavy menstrual flow, and sometimes petechiae will have been noticed. With thrombocytopenia, massive hemorrhage is unusual, but small amounts of bleeding in the central nervous system can result in catastrophic intracranial or retinal hemorrhage. Symptoms of anemia are also frequent, including lassitude, weakness, shortness of breath, and a pounding sensation in the ears. Infection is an unusual first symptom in aplastic anemia (unlike in agranulocytosis, where pharyngitis, anorectal infection, or frank sepsis occur early). A striking feature of aplastic anemia is the restriction of symptoms to the hematologic system, and patients often feel and look remarkably well despite drastically reduced blood counts. Systemic complaints and weight loss should point to other etiologies of pancytopenia. History of drug use, chemical exposure, and preceding viral illnesses must often be elicited with repeated questioning.

Physical Examination Petechiae and ecchymoses are often present, and retinal hemorrhages may be present. Pelvic and rectal examinations should be performed with great gentleness to avoid trauma; these will often show bleeding from the cervical os and blood in the stool. Pallor of the skin and mucous membranes is common except in the most acute cases or those already transfused. Infection on presentation is unusual but may be present if the patient has been symptomatic for a few weeks. Lymphadenopathy and splenomegaly are highly atypical of aplastic anemia. Café au lait spots and short stature suggest Fanconi's anemia; peculiar nails, dyskeratosis congenita.

LABORATORY STUDIES Blood The smear shows large erythrocytes and a paucity of platelets and granulocytes. Mean corpuscular volume (MCV) is commonly increased. Reticulocytes are absent or few, and lymphocyte numbers may be normal or reduced. The presence of immature myeloid forms suggests leukemia or MDS; nucleated red blood cells suggest marrow fibrosis or tumor invasion; abnormal platelets suggest either peripheral destruction or MDS.

Bone Marrow The bone marrow is usually readily aspirated but appears dilute on smear, and the fatty biopsy specimen may be grossly pale on withdrawal; a "dry tap" suggests fibrosis or myelophthisis. In severe aplasia the smear of the aspirated specimen shows only red cells, residual lymphocytes, and stromal cells; the biopsy, which should be >1 cm in length, is superior for determination of cellularity and shows mainly fat under the microscope, with hematopoietic cells occupying, by definition, <25% of the marrow space. In the most serious cases the biopsy is virtually 100% fat. The correlation between marrow cellularity and disease severity is imperfect. Some patients with moderate disease by blood counts will have empty iliac crest biopsies, while "hot spots" of hematopoiesis may be seen in severe cases. If an iliac crest specimen is inadequate, cells should also be obtained by aspiration from the sternum. Residual hematopoietic cells should have normal morphology, except for mildly megaloblastic erythropoiesis; megakaryocytes are invariably greatly reduced and usually absent. Areas adjacent to the spicule should be searched for myeloblasts. Granulomas (in cellular specimens) may indicate an infectious etiology of the marrow failure.

Ancillary Studies Chromosome breakage studies of peripheral blood using diepoxybutane (DEB) or mitomycin C should be performed on children and younger adults to exclude Fanconi's anemia. Chromosome studies of bone marrow cells are often revealing in MDS and should be negative in typical aplastic anemia. Flow cytometric assays have replaced the Ham test for the diagnosis of PNH. Serologic studies may show evidence of viral infection, especially Epstein-Barr virus and HIV. Posthepatitis aplastic anemia is typically seronegative. The spleen size should be determined by scanning if the physical examination of the abdomen is unsatisfactory. Magnetic resonance imaging may be helpful to assess the fat content on a few vertebrae in order to distinguish aplasia from MDS.

DIAGNOSIS The diagnosis of aplastic anemia is usually straightforward, based on the combination of pancytopenia with a fatty, empty bone marrow. Aplastic anemia is a disease of the young and should be a leading diagnosis in the pancytopenic adolescent or young adult. When pancytopenia is secondary, the primary diagnosis is usually obvious from either history or physical examination: the massive spleen of alcoholic cirrhosis, the history or metastatic cancer or systemic lupus erythematosus, or obvious miliary tuberculosis on chest radiograph (Table 109-1).

Diagnostic problems can occur with atypical presentations and among related hematologic diseases. While pancytopenia is most common, some patients with bone marrow hypocellularity have depression of only one or two of three blood lines, sometimes showing later progression to more recognizable aplastic anemia. The bone marrow in constitutional or Fanconi's anemia is indistinguishable morphologically from the aspirate in acquired disease. The diagnosis can be suggested by family history, abnormal blood counts since childhood, or the presence of associated anomalies of the skeletal and urogenital

systems. Patients with Fanconi's anemia may have no peculiar physical findings and can present with aplastic anemia as adults, in the third and fourth decades and, rarely, even later. Aplastic anemia may be difficult to distinguish from the hypocellular variety of MDS: MDS is favored by finding morphologic abnormalities, particularly of megakaryocytes and myeloid precursor cells, and typical cytogenetic abnormalities (see below).

PROGNOSIS The natural history of severe aplastic anemia is rapid deterioration and death. Provision first of red blood cell and later platelet transfusions and effective antibiotics were of some benefit, but few patients showed spontaneous recovery. The major prognostic determinant is the blood count; severe disease is defined by the presence of two of three parameters: absolute neutrophil count <500/μL, platelet count <20,000/μL, and corrected reticulocyte count <1% (or absolute reticulocyte count <50,000/μL). Survival of patients who fulfill these criteria is about 20% at 1 year after diagnosis; patients with very severe disease, defined by an absolute neutrophil count <200/μL, fare even more poorly. Treatment has markedly improved survival in this disease.

$\boxed{R_x}$ **TREATMENT** Treatment includes therapies that reverse the underlying marrow failure and supportive care of the pancytopenic patient. Severe acquired aplastic anemia can be cured by replacement of the absent hematopoietic cells (and the immune system) by stem cell transplant, or ameliorated by suppression of the immune system to allow recovery of the patient's residual bone marrow function. Hematopoietic growth factors have limited usefulness and glucocorticoids are of no value. Suspect exposures to drugs or chemicals should be discontinued; however, spontaneous recovery of severe blood count depression is rare, and a waiting period before beginning treatment may not be advisable unless the blood counts are only modestly depressed.

Bone Marrow Transplantation This is the best therapy for the young patient with a fully histocompatible sibling donor (Chap. 115). HLA typing should be ordered as soon as the diagnosis of aplastic anemia is established in a child or younger adult. In transplant candidates, transfusion of blood from family members should be avoided so as to prevent sensitization to histocompatability antigens; while transfusions in general should be minimized, limited numbers of blood products probably do not seriously affect outcome.

For allogeneic transplant from fully matched siblings, long-term survival rates for children are about 80%. Transplant morbidity and mortality are increased among adults, due mainly to the increased risk of chronic graft-versus-host disease and serious infections. Graft rejection was historically a major determinant of outcome in bone marrow transplant for aplastic anemia; high rates of primary or secondary graft failure may be related to the pathophysiology of marrow failure as well as to alloimmunization from transfusions.

Most patients do not have a suitable sibling donor. Occasionally, a full phenotypic match can be found within the family and serve as well. Far more available are other alternative donors, either unrelated but histocompatible volunteers, or closely but not perfectly matched family members. Survival using alternative donors is about half that of conventional sibling transplants. These patients will be at risk for late complications, especially a higher rate of cancer, if radiation is used as a component of conditioning. The majority of adults who undergo alternative donor transplants succumb to transplant-related complications.

Immunosuppression Used alone, ALG or antithymocyte globulin (ATG) induces hematologic recovery (independence from transfusion and a leukocyte count adequate to prevent infection) in about 50% of patients. The addition of cyclosporine to either ALG or ATG has further increased response rates to about 70 to 80% and especially improved outcomes for children and for severely neutropenic patients. Combined treatment is now standard for patients with severe disease. Hematologic response strongly correlates with survival. Improvement in granulocyte number is generally apparent within 2 months of treatment. Most recovered patients continue to have some degree of blood cellularity returns towards normal only very slowly, if at all. Relapse (recurrent pancytopenia) is frequent, often occurring as cyclosporine is discontinued; most, but not all, patients respond to reinstitution of immunosuppression, and some responders become dependent on continued cyclosporine administration. Development of MDS, with typical marrow morphologic or cytogenetic abnormalities, occurs in about 15% of treated patients, usually but not invariably associated with a return of pancytopenia, and some patients develop leukemia. Although the laboratory diagnosis of PNH can generally be made at the time of presentation of aplastic anemia by flow cytometry, recovered patients showing frank hemolysis or, less commonly, thrombosis should be retested for PNH. Bone marrow examinations should be performed annually or if there is an unfavorable change in blood counts.

Horse ATG (ATGAM; Upjohn) is given at 40 mg/kg per day for 4 days; rabbit ALG (Thymoglobulin; SangStat), is administered at 3.5 mg/kg per day for 5 days. For ATG, anaphylaxis is a rare but occasionally fatal complication; allergy should be tested by a prick skin test with an undiluted solution and immediate observation; desensitization is feasible. ATG binds to peripheral blood cells, and therefore, platelet and granulocyte numbers may fall further during active treatment. Serum sickness, a flulike illness with a characteristic cutaneous eruption and arthralgia, often develops about 10 days after initiating treatment. Most patients are given methylprednisolone, 1 mg/kg per day for 2 weeks, to ameliorate the immune consequences of heterologous protein infusion. Excessive or extended glucocorticoid therapy is associated with avascular joint necrosis. Cyclosporine is administered orally at an initial dose of 12 mg/kg per day in adults (15 mg/kg per day in children), with subsequent adjustment according to blood levels obtained every 2 weeks. Trough levels should be between 150 and 200 ng/mL. The most important side effects of chronic cyclosporine treatment are nephrotoxicity, hypertension, seizures, and opportunistic infections, especially *Pneumocystis carinii* (prophylactic treatment with monthly inhaled pentamidine is recommended).

Most patients with aplastic anemia lack a suitable marrow donor and immunosuppression is the treatment of choice. Long-term survival is equivalent with transplantation and immunosuppression. However, successful transplant cures marrow failure, while patients who recover adequate blood counts after immunosuppression remain at risk of relapse and malignant evolution. Because of the excellent results in children, allogeneic transplant should always be performed in the pediatric population if a suitable sibling donor is available. Increasing age and the severity of neutropenia are the most important factors weighing in the decision between transplant and immunosuppression in adults who have a matched family donor: older patients do better with ATG and cyclosporine, while transplant is preferred if granulocytopenia is profound. Some reluctant patients may be treated by immunosuppression followed by transplant for failure to recover blood counts or occurrence of late complications.

Outcomes following both transplant and immunosuppression have improved with time. High doses of cyclophosphamide, without stem cell rescue, have been reported to produce durable hematologic recovery, without relapse or evolution to MDS, but this treatment can produce sustained severe neutropenia and response is often delayed. Novel immunosuppressive drugs such as mycophenolate mofetil may further improve outcome.

Other Therapies The effectiveness of androgen therapy has not been verified in controlled trials, but occasional patients will respond or even demonstrate blood count dependence on continued therapy. For patients with moderate disease or those with severe pancytopenia who have failed immunosuppression, a 3- to 4-month trial is appropriate. Hematopoietic growth factors, granulocyte colony stimulating factor (G-CSF), granulocyte-macrophage CSF (GM-CSF), and interleukin 3, are not recommended as initial therapy for severe aplastic anemia, and even their role as adjuncts to immunosuppression is not well defined. Some patients may respond to chronic administration of growth factors in combination after failing immunosuppression. Sple-

nectomy may occasionally increase blood counts in relapsed or refractory cases.

Supportive Care Meticulous medical attention is required so that the patient may survive to benefit from definitive therapy or, having failed treatment, to maintain a reasonable existence in the face of pancytopenia. First and most important, infection in the presence of severe neutropenia must be aggressively treated by prompt institution of parenteral, broad-spectrum antibiotics, usually ceftazadime or a combination of an aminoglycoside, cephalosporin, and semisynthetic penicillin. Therapy is empirical and must not await results of culture, although specific foci of infection such as oropharyngeal or anorectal abscesses, pneumonia, sinusitis, and typhlitis (necrotizing colitis) should be sought on physical examination and with radiographic studies. When indwelling plastic catheters become contaminated, vancomycin should be added. Persistent or recrudescent fever implies fungal disease: *Candida* or *Aspergillus* are common, especially after several courses of antibacterial antibiotics, and a progressive course may be averted by timely initiation of amphotericin. Granulocyte transfusions using G-CSF–mobilized peripheral blood have been effective in the treatment of overwhelming infections in a few patients. Hand washing, the single most effective method of preventing the spread of infection, remains a neglected practice. Nonabsorbed antibiotics for gut decontamination are poorly tolerated and not of proven value. Total reverse isolation is not clearly beneficial in reducing mortality from infections.

Both platelet and erythrocyte numbers can be maintained by transfusion. Alloimmunization limits the usefulness of platelet transfusions and can be avoided or minimized by several strategies, including use of single donors to reduce exposure and physical or chemical methods to diminish leukocytes in the product; HLA-matched platelets are often effective in patients refractory to random donor products. Inhibitors of fibrinolysis such as aminocaproic acid have not been shown to relieve mucosal oozing; the use of low-dose glucocorticoids to induce "vascular stability" is unproven. Whether platelet transfusions are better used prophylactically or only as needed remains unclear. Any rational regimen of prophylaxis requires transfusions once or twice weekly in order to maintain the platelet count $>10,000/\mu L$ (oozing from the gut, and presumably also from other vascular beds, increases precipitously at counts $<5000/\mu L$). Menstruation should be suppressed either by oral estrogens or nasal follicle-stimulating hormone/luteinizing hormone (FSH/LH) antagonists. Aspirin and other nonsteroidal anti-inflammatory agents inhibit platelet function and must be avoided.

Red blood cells should be transfused to maintain a normal level of activity, usually at a hemoglobin value of 70 g/L (90 g/L if there is underlying cardiac or pulmonary disease); a regimen of 2 units every 2 weeks will replace normal losses in a patient without a functioning bone marrow. In chronic anemia, the iron chelator deferoxamine should be added at the time of the fiftieth transfusion in order to avoid secondary hemochromatosis.

PURE RED CELL APLASIA

More restricted forms of marrow failure occur, in which only a single circulating cell type is affected and the aregenerative marrow shows corresponding absence or decreased numbers of specific precursor cells: aregenerative anemia as in PRCA (see below), thrombocytopenia with amegakaryocytosis (Chap. 116), and neutropenia without marrow myeloid cells in agranulocytosis (Chap. 64). In general, and in contrast to aplastic anemia and MDS, the unaffected lineages appear quantitatively and qualitatively normal. Agranulocytosis, the most frequent of these syndromes, is usually a complication of medical drug use (with agents similar to those related to aplastic anemia), either by a mechanism of direct chemical toxicity or by immunologic mediation. Agranulocytosis has an incidence similar to aplastic anemia but is especially frequent among the elderly and in women. The syndrome should resolve with discontinuation of exposure, but significant mortality is attached to neutropenia in the older and often previously unwell patient. Both pure white cell aplasia (agranulocytosis without incriminating drug exposure) and amegakaryocytic thrombocytopenia are exceedingly rare and, like PRCA, appear to be due to destructive antibodies or lymphocytes and can respond to immunosuppressive therapies. In all the single lineage failure syndromes, progression to pancytopenia or leukemia is unusual.

DEFINITION AND DIFFERENTIAL DIAGNOSIS PRCA is characterized by anemia, reticulocytopenia, and absent or rare erythroid precursor cells in the bone marrow. The classification of PRCA is shown in Table 109-4. In adults, PRCA is acquired. An identical syndrome can occur constitutionally: Diamond-Blackfan anemia, or congenital PRCA, is diagnosed at birth or in early childhood and often responds to glucocorticoid treatment. Temporary red cell failure occurs in transient aplastic crisis of hemolytic anemias, due to acute parvovirus infection (Chap. 187), and in transient erythroblastopenia of childhood, which affects normal children.

CLINICAL ASSOCIATIONS AND ETIOLOGY PRCA has important associations with immune system diseases. A small minority of cases occur with a thymoma. More frequently, red cell aplasia can be the major manifestation of large granular lymphocytosis or may occur in chronic lymphocytic leukemia. Some patients may be hypogammaglobulinemic. As with agranulocytosis, PRCA can be due to an idiosyncratic reaction to a drug.

Like aplastic anemia, PRCA results from diverse mechanisms. Antibodies to red blood cell precursors are frequently present in the blood, but T cell inhibition is probably the more common immune mechanism. Cytotoxic lymphocyte activity restricted by histocompatibility locus or specific for human T cell leukemia/lymphoma virus I–infected cells, as well as natural killer cell activity inhibitory of erythropoiesis, have been demonstrated in particularly well-studied individual cases.

Persistent Parvovirus B19 Infection Chronic parvovirus infection is an important, treatable cause of PRCA. This common virus causes a benign exanthem of childhood (fifth disease) and a polyarthralgia syndrome in adults. In patients with underlying hemolysis (or any condition that increases demand for red blood cell production), parvovirus infection can cause a transient aplastic crisis and an abrupt but temporary worsening of the anemia due to failed erythropoiesis. In normal individuals, acute infection is resolved by production of neutralizing antibodies to the virus, but in the setting of congenital, acquired, or iatrogenic immunodeficiency, persistent viral infection

may occur. The bone marrow shows red cell aplasia and the presence of giant pronormoblasts (Fig. 109-2), the cytopathic sign of B19 parvovirus infection and highly suggestive of the diagnosis. Viral tropism for human erythroid progenitor cells is due to its use of erythrocyte P antigen as a cellular receptor for entry. Direct cytotoxicity of virus causes anemia if demands on erythrocyte production are high; in normal individuals, the temporary cessation of red cell production is not clinically apparent, and skin and joint symptoms are mediated by immune complex deposition.

TREATMENT History, physical examination, and routine laboratory studies may disclose an underlying disease or a suspect drug exposure. Thymoma should be sought by radiographic procedures. Tumor excision is indicated, but anemia does not necessarily improve with surgery. The diagnosis of parvovirus infection requires detection of viral DNA sequences in the blood (IgG and IgM antibodies are commonly absent). The presence of erythroid colonies has been considered predictive of response to immunosuppressive therapy in idiopathic PRCA.

Red cell aplasia is compatible with long survival with supportive care alone, a combination of erythrocyte transfusions and iron chelation. For persistent B19 parvovirus infection, almost all patients respond to intravenous immunoglobulin therapy (for example, 0.4 g/kg daily for 5 days), although relapse and retreatment may be expected, especially in patients with AIDS. The majority of patients with idiopathic PRCA respond favorably to immunosuppression. Most first receive a course of glucocorticoids, followed in the absence of a response by cyclosporine, ATG, azathioprine, or cyclophosphamide.

MYELODYSPLASIA

DEFINITION The myelodysplastic syndromes are a heterogeneous group of hematologic disorders broadly characterized by cytopenias associated with a dysmorphic (or abnormal appearing) and usually cellular bone marrow, and consequent ineffective blood cell production (Table 109-5). The current nomenclature was developed by the French-American-British (FAB) Cooperative Group and, while increasing recognition of the syndromes, is not entirely satisfactory: chronic myelomonocytic leukemia, while associated with dysplastic morphology, behaves as a myeloproliferative disease; sideroblastic anemias likely have a distinctive etiology; and the borderline between refractory anemia with excess blasts in transformation and acute myeloid leukemia is so arbitrary as to have been abandoned in the most recent World Health Organization classification. The FAB scheme has been recently supplemented by the International Prognostic Scoring System (IPSS; Table 109-6).

EPIDEMIOLOGY Idiopathic MDS is a disease of the elderly; the mean age at onset is 68 years. There is a slight male preponderance. MDS is a relatively common form of bone marrow failure, with incidence rates reported of 35 to >100 per million persons in the general population and 120 to >500 per million in the aged. MDS is rare in children, but monocytic leukemia can be seen. Therapy-related MDS is not age-related and may occur in as many as 15% of patients within a decade following intensive combined modality treatment for cancer. Rates of MDS have increased over time, due to the recognition of the syndrome by physicians and the aging of the population.

ETIOLOGY AND PATHOPHYSIOLOGY The myelodysplastic syndromes have been convincingly linked to environmental exposures such as radiation and benzene; other risk factors have been reported inconsistently. Secondary MDS occurs as a stereotypical late toxicity of cancer treatment, usually with a combination of radiation and the radiomimetic alkylating agents such as busulfan, nitrosourea, or procarbazine (with a latent period of 5 to 7 years) or the DNA topoisomerase inhibitors (2 years). Both acquired aplastic anemia following immunosuppressive treatment and Fanconi's anemia can evolve into MDS.

MDS is a clonal hematopoietic stem cell disorder leading to impaired cell proliferation and differentiation. Cytogenetic abnormalities

---

Table 109-4 Classification of Pure Red Cell Aplasia

Self-limited
  Transient erythroblastopenia of childhood
  Transient aplastic crisis of hemolysis (B19 parvovirus infection)
Fetal red blood cell aplasia
  Nonimmune hydrops fetalis (in utero B19 parvovirus infection)
Hereditary pure red cell aplasia
  Congenital pure red cell aplasia (Diamond-Blackfan syndrome)
Acquired pure red cell aplasia
  Thymoma and malignancy
    Thymoma
    Lymphoid malignancies (and more rarely other hematologic diseases)
    Paraneoplastic to solid tumors
  Connective tissue disorders with immunologic abnormalities
    Systemic lupus erythematosus, juvenile rheumatoid arthritis, rheumatoid arthritis
    Multiple endocrine gland insufficiency
  Virus
    B19 parvovirus, hepatitis, adult T cell leukemia virus, Epstein-Barr virus
  Pregnancy
  Drugs
    Especially phenytoin, azathioprine, chloramphenicol, procaineamide, isoniazid
  Idiopathic

A

B

C

D

FIGURE 109-2 Pathognomonic cells in marrow failure syndromes. *A.* Giant pronormoblast, the cytopathic effect of B19 parvovirus infection of the erythroid progenitor cell. *B.* Uninuclear megakaryocyte and microblastic erythroid precursors typical of the 5q- myelodysplasia syndrome. *C.* Ringed sideroblast showing perinuclear iron granules. *D.* Tumor cells present on a touch preparation made from the marrow biopsy of a patient with metastatic carcinoma.

are found in about half of patients, and some of the same specific lesions are also seen in frank leukemia; deletions are more frequent than translocations. Both presenting and evolving hematologic manifestations result from the accumulation of multiple genetic lesions, loss of tumor suppressor genes, activating oncogene mutations, or other harmful alterations. Cytogenetic abnormalities are not random (loss of all or part of 5, 7, and 20, trisomy of 8) and may be related to etiology (11q23 following topoisomerase II inhibitors); chronic myelomonocytic leukemia is often associated with t(5;12) that creates a chimeric *tel-PDGFβ* gene. The type and number of cytogenetic abnormalities strongly correlate with the probability of leukemic transformation and survival. Mutations of N-*ras* (an oncogene), *p53* and *IRF-1* (tumor suppressor genes), *Bcl-2* (an antiapoptotic gene), and others have been reported in some patients but may occur relatively late in the sequence leading to leukemic transformation. Apoptosis of marrow cells is increased in MDS, presumably due to these acquired genetic alterations or possibly to an overlaid immune response. Sideroblastic anemia may be related to mutations in mitochondrial genes. Ineffective erythro-poiesis and disordered iron metabolism are the functional consequences of the genetic alterations.

CLINICAL FEATURES Anemia dominates the early course. Most symptomatic patients complain of the gradual onset of fatigue and weakness, dyspnea, and pallor, but at least half the patients are asymptomatic and MDS is discovered only incidentally on routine blood counts. Previous chemotherapy or radiation exposure is an important historic fact. Fever and weight loss should point to a myelo-proliferative rather than myelodysplastic process. Children with Down's syndrome are susceptible to MDS, and a family history may indicate a hereditary form of sideroblastic anemia or Fanconi's anemia.

The physical examination is remarkable for signs of anemia; about 20% of patients have splenomegaly. Some unusual skin lesions, including Sweet's syndrome (febrile neutrophilic dermatosis), have been associated with MDS.

LABORATORY STUDIES Blood Anemia is present in the majority of cases, either alone or as part of bi- or pancytopenia; isolated neutropenia or thrombocytopenia is more unusual. Macrocytosis

Table 109-5 Classification of Myelodysplasia (MDS)

Subtype	Blood	Marrow[a]	% of MDS Cases	Median Survival, Months	Leukemic Evolution, %[b]
Refractory anemia	Blasts <1%	Blasts <5%	27	50	16
Refractory anemia with ringed sidero-blasts	Blasts <1%	Blasts <5%	20	65	15
Refractory anemia with excess blasts	Blasts ≤5%	Blasts 5–20%	26	15	48
Refractory anemia with excess blasts in transformation	Blasts >5%	Blasts 20–30% or Auer rods	13	9	62
Chronic myelomonocytic leukemia	≥1 × 10⁹/L monocytes	Any number	14	23	29

[a] By definition, the bone marrow of acute myeloid leukemia contains >30% blasts.
[b] Leukemic evolution refers to the percentage of cases that transform into acute myeloid leukemia.

is common, and the smear may be dimorphic with a distinctive population of large red blood cells. Platelets are also large and lack granules. In functional studies, they may show marked abnormalities, and patients may have bleeding symptoms despite seemingly adequate numbers. Neutrophils are hypogranulated; have hyposegmented, ringed, or abnormally segmented nuclei; and contain Dohle bodies and may be functionally deficient. Circulating myeloblasts usually correlate with marrow blast numbers, and their quantitation is important for classification and prognosis. The total white blood cell count is usually normal or low, except in chronic myelomonocytic leukemia. As in aplastic anemia, MDS also can be associated with a clonal population of PNH cells.

Bone Marrow The bone marrow is usually normal or hypercellular but in 20% of cases is sufficiently hypocellular to be confused with aplasia. No single characteristic feature of marrow morphology distinguishes MDS, but the following are commonly observed: dyserythropoietic changes (especially nuclear abnormalities) and ringed sideroblasts in the erythroid lineage; hypogranulation and hyposegmentation in granulocytic precursors, with an increase in myeloblasts; and megakaryocytes showing reduced numbers of disorganized nuclei. Prognosis strongly correlates with the proportion of marrow blasts. Cytogenetic analysis also is important. A much more sensitive method to detect infrequent chromosome aberrations is fluorescent in situ hybridization, and gene amplification by polymerase chain reaction can detect known chromosomal translocations.

DIFFERENTIAL DIAGNOSIS Deficiencies of vitamin B$_{12}$ or folate should be suggested by history and excluded by appropriate blood tests; vitamin B$_6$ deficiency can be assessed by a therapeutic trial of pyridoxine if the bone marrow shows ringed sideroblasts. Marrow dysplasia can be observed in acute viral infections, drug reactions, or chemical toxicity but should be transient. More difficult (arbitrary) are the distinctions between hypocellular MDS and aplasia or between refractory anemia with excess blasts in transformation and early acute leukemia.

PROGNOSIS The median survival varies greatly with FAB type and, according to IPSS calculations, ranges from years for patients with 5q- or sideroblastic anemia to a few months in refractory anemia with excess blasts or severe pancytopenia associated with monosomy 7. Most patients die as a result of complications of pancytopenia and not due to leukemic transformation; perhaps one-third will succumb to other diseases unrelated to their MDS. Precipitous worsening of pancytopenia, acquisition of new chromosomal abnormalities on serial cytogenetic determination, and increase in the number of blasts are all poor prognostic indicators. The outlook in therapy-related MDS, regardless of FAB type, is very poor, and most patients will progress within a few months to refractory acute myeloid leukemia.

TREATMENT The therapy of MDS is generally unsatisfactory. Only stem cell transplantation offers cure: survival rates of 40% have been reported, but older patients are particularly prone to develop treatment-related mortality and morbidity. Those with better prognostic features (and a more favorable natural history) have much better outcomes than patients with more malignant subtypes. Surprisingly, results of transplant using matched unrelated donor are comparable, although most series contain younger and more highly selected cases.

MDS has been regarded as particularly refractory to cytotoxic chemotherapy regimens but is probably no more resistant to effective treatment than acute myeloid leukemia in the elderly, in whom drug toxicity is often fatal and remissions, if achieved, are brief. Low doses of cytotoxic drugs have been administered for their "differentiating" potential: responses to cytosine arabinoside did not translate into a survival advantage; etoposide and 5-azacytidine are under active study. Amifostine, an organic thiophosphonate that blocks apoptosis, can improve blood counts but has significant toxicities. Immunosuppressive therapies, including ATG and cyclosporine, that are effective in aplastic anemia may induce sustained remissions in a high proportion of patients with refractory anemia, especially in those with hypocellular marrows or without cytogenetic abnormalities.

Hematopoietic growth factors can improve blood counts but, as in most other marrow failure states, have been most beneficial in patients with the least severe pancytopenia. G-CSF treatment alone failed to improve survival in a controlled trial. The combination of G-CSF and erythropoietin increased blood counts in one-third to one-half of patients, but survival advantage is not yet proven.

The same principles of supportive care described for aplastic anemia apply to MDS. Because many patients will be anemic for years, erythrocyte transfusion support should be accompanied by iron chelation in order to prevent secondary hemochromatosis.

Table 109-6 International Prognostic Scoring System

Prognostic Variable	Score Value				
	0	0.5	1.0	1.5	2.0
Bone marrow blasts (%)	<5%	5–10%		11–20%	21–30%
Karyotype[a]	Good	Intermediate	Poor		
Cytopenia[b] (lineages affected)	0 or 1	2 or 3			
Risk Group Scores	**Score**				
Low	0				
Intermediate-1	0.5–1.0				
Intermediate-2	1.5–2.0				
High	≥2.5				

[a] Good = normal, -Y, del(5q), del (20q); intermediate = all other abnormalities; poor = complex (≥3 abnormalities) or chromosome 7 abnormalities.
[b] Cytopenias defined as Hb <100 g/L, platelet count < 100,000/μL, absolute neutrophil count <1500/μL.

MYELOPHTHISIC ANEMIAS

Fibrosis of the bone marrow (see Plate V-19), usually accompanied by a characteristic blood smear picture called *leukoerythroblastosis*, can occur as a primary hematologic disease, called *myelofibrosis* or *myeloid metaplasia* (Chap. 110), and as a secondary process, called *myelophthisis*. Myelophthisis, or secondary myelofibrosis, is reactive. Fibrosis can be a response to invading tumor cells, usually of an epithelial cancer of breast, lung, and prostate or neuroblastoma. Marrow fibrosis may occur with infection of mycobacteria (both *Mycobacterium tuberculosis* and *M. avium*) fungi, or

HIV, and in sarcoidosis. Intracellular lipid deposition in Gaucher's disease and obliteration of the marrow space related to absence of osteoclast remodeling in congenital osteopetrosis also can produce fibrosis. Secondary myelofibrosis is a late consequence of radiation therapy or treatment with radiomimetic drugs. Usually, the infectious or malignant underlying processes are obvious. Marrow fibrosis can also be a feature of a variety of hematologic syndromes, especially chronic myeloid leukemia, multiple myeloma, lymphomas, myeloma, and hairy cell leukemia.

The pathophysiology has three distinct features: proliferation of fibroblasts in the marrow space (myelofibrosis); the extension of hematopoiesis into the long bones and most particularly into extramedullary sites, usually the spleen, liver, and lymph nodes (myeloid metaplasia); and ineffective erythropoiesis. The etiology of fibrosis is unknown but most likely involves dysregulated production of growth factors: platelet-derived growth factor and transforming growth factor β have been implicated. Abnormal regulation of other hematopoietins would lead to localization of blood-producing cells in nonhematopoietic tissues and uncoupling of the usually balanced processes of stem cell proliferation and differentiation. Myelofibrosis is remarkable for pancytopenia despite extraordinarily large numbers of circulating hematopoietic progenitor cells.

Anemia is dominant in secondary myelofibrosis, usually normocytic and normochromic. The diagnosis is suggested by the characteristic leukoerythroblastic smear (see Plate V-9). Erythrocyte morphology is very abnormal, with circulating nucleated red blood cells, teardrops, and shape distortions. White blood cell numbers are often elevated, sometimes mimicking a leukemoid reaction, with circulating myelocytes, promyelocytes, and myeloblasts. Platelets may be abundant and are often giant size. Inability to aspirate the bone marrow, the characteristic "dry tap," can allow a presumptive diagnosis before the biopsy is decalcified.

The course of secondary myelofibrosis is determined by its cause, usually a metastatic tumor or an advanced hematologic malignancy. Treatable causes must be excluded, especially tuberculosis and fungus. Transfusion support can relieve symptoms.

BIBLIOGRAPHY

BROWN KE, YOUNG NS: Parvovirus B19 in human disease. Annu Rev Med 48:59, 1997

ERSLEV AJ, SOLTAN A: Pure red cell aplasia: A review. Blood Rev 10:20, 1996

GREENBERG P et al: International scoring system for evaluating prognosis in myelodysplastic syndromes. Blood 89:2079, 1997

HEANEY ML, GOLDE DW: Myelodysplasia. N Engl J Med 340:1649, 1999

YOUNG NS: *The Bone Marrow Failure Syndromes.* Philadelphia, Saunders, 2000

————, ALTER BP: *Aplastic Anemia, Acquired and Inherited.* Philadelphia, Saunders, 1994

————, BARRETT AJ: The treatment of severe acquired aplastic anemia. Blood 85:3367, 1995

110   *Jerry L. Spivak*

POLYCYTHEMIA VERA AND OTHER MYELOPROLIFERATIVE DISEASES

Polycythemia vera, idiopathic myelofibrosis, essential thrombocytosis, and chronic myeloid leukemia (CML) are commonly classified together under the rubric *the chronic myeloproliferative disorders*, because their pathophysiology involves the clonal expansion of a multipotent hematopoietic progenitor cell with the overproduction of one or more of the formed elements of the blood. These entities may transform into acute leukemia naturally or as a consequence of mutagenic treatment. However, while polycythemia vera, idiopathic myelofibrosis, essential thrombocytosis, and CML share similar phenotypic characteristics, CML is genotypically distinct from the other three disorders because it alone is associated with translocation of genetic material between the long arms of chromosomes 9 and 22, resulting in the production of the unique fusion protein, bcr-abl. Furthermore, based on its natural history, CML is more appropriately considered as a form of leukemia. →*CML is discussed with the acute myeloid leukemias in Chap. 111.*

POLYCYTHEMIA VERA

Polycythemia vera is a clonal disorder involving a multipotent hematopoietic progenitor cell in which there is accumulation of phenotypically normal red cells, granulocytes, and platelets in the absence of a recognizable physiologic stimulus. Polycythemia vera, the most common of the chronic myeloproliferative disorders, occurs in about 2 per 100,000 people. It spares no adult age group. Vertical transmission has been documented, establishing a genetic basis for the disorder. A slight overall male predominance has been observed, but females predominate within the reproductive age range.

ETIOLOGY The etiology of polycythemia vera is unknown. Although nonrandom chromosome abnormalities such as 20q-, trisomy 8 or 9 have been documented in a small percentage of untreated polycythemia vera patients, no consistent cytogenetic abnormality has been associated with the disorder and no specific genetic defect has yet been identified. Impaired posttranslational processing of the thrombopoietin receptor, Mpl, has been noted in polycythemia vera patients; the extent of the defect correlated with disease duration and splenomegaly. While this defect is specific for polycythemia vera and is not found in secondary polycythemias, its role in the pathophysiology of the disorder is still undefined. In contrast to normal erythroid progenitor cells, polycythemia vera erythroid progenitor cells can grow in vitro in the absence of erythropoietin due to hypersensitivity to insulin-like growth factor I. However, this phenotypic abnormality is not specific for polycythemia vera and has been documented in essential thrombocytosis and secondary polycythemias. Polycythemia vera erythroid progenitor cells are more resistant to apoptosis induced by erythropoietin deprivation, due to upregulation of bcl-X_L, an antiapoptotic protein. The polycythemia vera erythroid progenitors do not divide more rapidly than their normal counterparts, but they accumulate because they do not die normally. Additionally, the transformed hematopoietic progenitor cells in polycythemia vera, as in other neoplastic disorders, exhibit clonal dominance and suppress the proliferation of normal hematopoietic progenitor cells by an unknown mechanism. Consequently, the circulating formed elements of the blood represent only progeny of the transformed clone.

CLINICAL FEATURES Although massive splenomegaly may be the initial presenting sign in polycythemia vera, most often the disorder is first recognized by the discovery of a high hemoglobin or hematocrit, and with the exception of aquagenic pruritus, no symptoms distinguish polycythemia vera from other causes of erythrocytosis.

Uncontrolled erythrocytosis can lead to neurologic symptoms such as vertigo, tinnitus, headache, and visual disturbances. Systolic hypertension also accompanies an elevated red cell mass. In some patients, venous or arterial thrombosis may be the presenting manifestation of polycythemia vera. Intraabdominal venous thrombosis is particularly common and may be catastrophic when there is sudden compromise of the hepatic vein. Polycythemia vera should be suspected in any patient who develops the Budd-Chiari syndrome. Digital ischemia may also occur. Easy bruising, epistaxis, or gastrointestinal hemorrhage may be observed, and polycythemia vera patients are frequently hypermetabolic. Hypercuricemia with secondary gout and uric acid stones and acid-peptic disease also complicate the disorder. Because isolated erythrocytosis is a common initial presentation for polycythemia vera but no clonal marker is available for the disease, the first task of the physician is to distinguish this autonomous clonal form of erythrocytosis from the many other types of erythrocytosis, most of which are correctable (Table 110-1).

Erythropoiesis is normally regulated by the glycoprotein hormone erythropoietin. Erythropoietin, which in adults is produced primarily in the kidneys and to a small extent in the liver, promotes the proliferation of erythroid progenitor cells, maintains their survival, and facilitates their differentiation. Because erythropoietin acts as a survival factor, it is constitutively produced and, like the red cell mass, its level is constant as long as tissue oxygenation is adequate. The plasma erythropoietin level, like the red cell mass, differs among individuals but in adults is not affected by either age or gender. Erythropoietin production is regulated at the level of gene transcription. Hypoxia is the only physiologic stimulus that increases the number of cells producing erythropoietin, and thus the production and metabolism of erythropoietin are independent of its plasma level. In the absence of renal or hepatic disease, plasma erythropoietin levels reflect erythropoietin production, and therefore the assay for plasma erythropoietin is a surrogate assay for tissue hypoxia. Erythropoietin is active at the picomolar level, and its production is tightly regulated. Thus, the plasma erythropoietin level does not rise outside the normal range until the hemoglobin level falls below 105 g/L. This is not meant to imply that an increase in erythropoietin production does not occur as the hemoglobin level falls below normal, but because the normal range for plasma erythropoietin is wide (4 to 26 mU/mL), unless the patient's baseline level is known, any increase will not be recognized until the hemoglobin falls below 105 g/L. Thereafter, there is a log-linear inverse correlation between the levels of plasma erythropoietin and hemoglobin. With erythrocytosis, erythropoietin production is suppressed; this suppression reflects not only the increase in tissue oxygen transport associated with the increase in red cell number but also additional negative-feedback mechanism unrelated to oxygen transport but related to the increase in blood viscosity and an increase in red cell precursors capable of taking up erythropoietin. The summation of these mechanisms accounts for the paradoxical observation that many patients with hypoxic erythrocytosis due to cyanotic congenital heart disease or obstructive lung disease have a "normal" plasma erythropoietin level. The plasma erythropoietin level is a useful diagnostic test in patients with isolated erythrocytosis, because an elevated level essentially excludes polycythemia vera as the cause for the erythrocytosis.

DIAGNOSIS   When confronted with an elevated hemoglobin or hematocrit level, it is important to obtain previous values to determine the duration of this laboratory abnormality. Because the hemoglobin or hematocrit level is affected by the plasma volume, and hematocrit and red cell mass are not linearly related, a red cell mass determination must also be performed to distinguish absolute erythrocytosis from relative erythrocytosis due to a reduction in plasma volume alone (also

known as *stress* or *spurious erythrocytosis* or *Geisböck's syndrome*). Red cell mass determination is important because in polycythemia vera, in contrast to erythropoietin-driven erythrocytosis, the plasma volume is frequently elevated, not only masking the true extent of red cell mass expansion but often its presence. Indeed, a significant proportion of patients with polycythemia vera have a hematocrit within the normal range, particularly in patients with a substantial splenomegaly. Failure to recognize this phenomenon is undoubtedly the basis for many of the reported instances of hepatic or portal vein thrombosis in patients with a so-called undefined myeloproliferative disorder.

Red cell mass is reliably determined by isotope dilution using the patient's ^{51}Cr-tagged red cells; extrapolations made by determining directly only the plasma volume are unacceptable. Furthermore, to allow ample time for equilibration of the labeled red cells, measurements should be made over a period of ≥ 90 min.

Once the presence of absolute erythrocytosis has been established, its cause must be determined. An elevated plasma erythropoietin level suggests either an hypoxic cause for erythrocytosis or autonomous erythropoietin production, in which case assessment of pulmonary function and an abdominal computed tomography scan to evaluate renal and hepatic anatomy are appropriate. A normal erythropoietin level does not exclude an hypoxic cause for erythrocytosis. In polycythemia vera, in contrast to hypoxic erythrocytosis, the arterial oxygen saturation is normal. However, a normal oxygen saturation does not exclude a high-affinity hemoglobin as a cause for erythrocytosis, and it is here that documentation of previous hemoglobin levels and a family study become important. Because there is no clonal marker for polycythemia vera, clinical guidelines have been proposed to define the disease. A modified version is provided in Table 110-2. However, these guidelines do not establish clonality, and in some patients only with time will the underlying disorder become apparent. Diagnostic ambiguity does not preclude the initiation of therapy.

Other laboratory studies that may aid in diagnosis include the red cell count, mean corpuscular volume, and red cell distribution width (RDW). Only three situations cause microcytic erythrocytosis: β-thalassemia trait, hypoxic erythrocytosis, and polycythemia vera. However, with β-thalassemia trait the RDW is normal, whereas with hypoxic erythrocytosis and polycythemia vera, the RDW is usually elevated. A properly made blood smear from a patient with erythrocytosis will be virtually unreadable due to the marked elevation in red cell count, but no specific morphologic abnormalities are seen in the leukocytes or platelets in polycythemia vera. However, when these are also elevated the diagnosis is assured. In many patients, the leukocyte alkaline phosphatase level is also increased, as is the uric acid level. Elevated serum vitamin B_{12} or B_{12}-binding capacity may be present. In patients with associated acid-peptic disease, occult gastrointestinal bleeding may lead to presentation with hypochromic, microcytic anemia.

A bone marrow aspirate and biopsy will provide no specific diagnostic information, and unless there is a need to establish the presence of myelofibrosis or exclude some other disorder, these procedures need not be done. Although the presence of a cytogenetic abnormality such as trisomy 8 or 9 or 20q- in the setting of an expansion of the red cell mass supports the clonal etiology, no specific cytogenetic abnormality is associated with polycythemia vera, and the absence of a cytogenetic marker does not exclude the diagnosis.

COMPLICATIONS   The major clinical complications of polycythemia vera relate directly to the increase in blood viscosity asso-

Table 110-1   Causes of Absolute Erythrocytosis

Hypoxia	Tumors
Carbon monoxide intoxication	Hypernephroma
High altitude	Hepatoma
Pulmonary disease	Cerebellar hemangioblastoma
High-affinity hemoglobin	Adrenal adenoma
Sleep-apnea syndrome	Pheochromocytoma
Respiratory center	Meningioma
dysfunction	Uterine fibromyoma
Supine hypoventilation	Familial (with normal hemoglobin
Right-to-left cardiac shunts	function)
Renal disease	Erythropoietin receptor mutations
Renal cysts	DPG mutase deficiency
Hydronephrosis	Bartter's syndrome
Renal artery stenosis	Androgen therapy
Focal glomerulonephritis	Recombinant erythropoietin therapy
Renal transplantation	Polycythemia vera

NOTE: DPG, diphosphoglycerate

Table 110-2   Suggested Criteria for the Clinical Diagnosis of Polycythemia Vera[a]

Elevated red cell mass
Normal arterial oxygen saturation
Splenomegaly
In the absence of splenomegaly:
   Leukocytosis and thrombocytosis

[a] It must be emphasized that these criteria do not establish clonality.

ciated with elevation of the red cell mass and indirectly to the increased turnover of red cells, leukocytes, and platelets and the attendant increase in uric acid and histamine production. The latter appears to be responsible for the increase in peptic ulcer disease and for the pruritus associated with this disorder, although little formal proof for this has been obtained. A sudden massive increase in spleen size is another problem and can be associated with splenic infarction or progressive cachexia. Myelofibrosis and myeloid metaplasia can also develop with transfusion-dependent anemia, but the frequency is low in those not receiving chemotherapy or irradiation. Although acute nonlymphocytic leukemia is reported to be increased in polycythemia vera, the incidence of acute leukemia in patients not exposed to chemotherapy or radiation is low and the development of leukemia is not related to disease duration, suggesting that the treatment exposure may be a more important risk factor than the disease itself.

Erythromelalgia is a curious syndrome of unknown etiology involving primarily the lower extremities and manifested usually by erythema, warmth, and pain of the affected appendage and occasionally digital infarction. It occurs with a variable frequency in patients with a myeloproliferative disorder and is usually responsive to salicylates. Some of the central nervous system symptoms observed in patients with polycythemia vera may represent a variant of erythromelalgia.

If left uncontrolled, erythrocytosis can lead to intravascular thrombosis involving vital organs such as the liver, heart, brain, or lungs. Patients with massive splenomegaly are particularly prone to thrombotic events because the associated increase in plasma volume masks the true extent of the red cell mass elevation as measured by the hematocrit or hemoglobin level. A "normal" hematocrit or hemoglobin level in a polycythemia vera patient with massive splenomegaly should be considered as indicative of an elevated red cell mass until proven otherwise.

℞ **TREATMENT** Polycythemia vera is generally an indolent disorder whose clinical course can run many decades, and its medical management should reflect the tempo of the disorder. Maintenance of the hemoglobin level at ≤140 g/L in men and ≤120 g/L in women is mandatory to avoid the thrombotic complications. Thrombosis due to erythrocytosis is the most significant complication of this disorder. Phlebotomy serves initially to reduce hyperviscosity by bringing the red cell mass into the normal range. Periodic phlebotomies thereafter serve to maintain the red cell mass within the range of normal and to induce a state of iron deficiency, which prevents an accelerated reexpansion of the red cell mass. In most polycythemia vera patients, once an iron-deficient state is achieved, phlebotomy is usually required only at 3-month intervals. Although both phlebotomy and iron deficiency, in addition to the disease itself, tend to increase the platelet count, thrombocytosis is not correlated with thrombosis in polycythemia vera, in contrast to the strong correlation between erythrocytosis and thrombosis in this disease. The use of salicylates as a tonic against thrombosis in polycythemia vera patients is potentially harmful, and salicylates should be employed only to treat erythromelalgia. Oral anticoagulants are not routinely indicated and are difficult to assess owing to the artifactual imbalance between the test tube anticoagulant and plasma that occurs when blood from these patients is assayed for prothrombin or partial thromboplastin activity. Asymptomatic hyperuricemia requires no therapy, but allopurinol should be administered to avoid further elevation of the uric acid when chemotherapy is employed to reduce splenomegaly or leukocytosis-associated pruritus. Generalized pruritus intractable to antihistamines can be a major problem in polycythemia vera, and hydroxyurea, interferon (IFN)-α, and psoralens with ultraviolet light in the A range (PUVA) therapy may have some palliative effects. Asymptomatic thrombocytosis requires no therapy. Symptomatic thrombocytosis or splenomegaly can be treated with hydroxyurea or IFN-α, although each can be associated with significant side effects. Anagrelide, a quinazolin derivative and platelet antiaggregant that also lowers the platelet count, can control thrombocytosis. A reduction in platelet number may be necessary in the treatment of erythromelalgia if salicylates are not effective or if the thrombocytosis is associated with migraine-like symptoms. However, the highest priority for treatment is reduction of the red cell mass to normal. Alkylating agents and ^{32}P are leukemogenic in polycythemia vera, and their use should be avoided. If a cytotoxic agent must be used, hydroxyurea is preferred, but it also may be leukemogenic with chronic use. Chemotherapy should be used for as short a time as possible. In some patients, massive splenomegaly unresponsive to reduction by hydroxyurea or IFN-α therapy and associated with intractable weight loss will require splenectomy. Allogeneic bone marrow transplantation may be effective in young patients.

Patients with polycythemia vera can be expected to live long and useful lives when their red cell mass is effectively managed with phlebotomy. Chemotherapy is never indicated to control the red cell mass unless venous access is impossible.

IDIOPATHIC MYELOFIBROSIS

Idiopathic myelofibrosis (other designations include *agnogenic myeloid metaplasia* or *myelofibrosis with myeloid metaplasia*) is a clonal disorder of a multipotent hematopoietic progenitor cell of unknown etiology characterized by marrow fibrosis, myeloid metaplasia with extramedullary hematopoiesis, and splenomegaly. Idiopathic myelofibrosis is uncommon; in the absence of a specific clonal marker, establishing this diagnosis is difficult because myelofibrosis and myeloid metaplasia with splenomegaly are also features of both polycythemia vera and CML. Furthermore, myelofibrosis and splenomegaly occur in a variety of benign and malignant disorders (Table 110-3), many of which are amenable to specific therapies not effective in idiopathic myelofibrosis. In contrast to the other chronic myeloproliferative disorders and so-called acute or malignant myelofibrosis, which can occur at any age, idiopathic myelofibrosis primarily afflicts individuals in their sixth decade or later.

ETIOLOGY The etiology of idiopathic myelofibrosis is unknown. Although nonrandom chromosome abnormalities such as 20q-, 13q-, and trisomy 1q are not uncommon, no specific cytogenetic abnormality has been identified. The degree of myelofibrosis and the extent of extramedullary hematopoiesis are not related. This disorder is associated with overproduction of type III collagen, a finding that has been attributed to platelet-derived growth factor or transforming growth factor β, but no proof has been forthcoming. Importantly, fibroblasts in idiopathic myelofibrosis are not part of the neoplastic clone.

CLINICAL FEATURES No specific signs or symptoms are associated with idiopathic myelofibrosis. Most patients are asymptomatic at presentation and are usually detected by the discovery of splenic enlargement and/or abnormal blood counts during a routine examination. A blood smear reveals the characteristic features of extramedullary hematopoiesis: teardrop-shaped red cells, nucleated red cells, myelocytes, and promyelocytes; myeloblasts may also be present but have no prognostic significance. Anemia, usually mild initially, is the rule, while the leukocyte and platelet counts are either normal or increased but either can be depressed. Mild hepatomegaly may accompany the splenomegaly, and both the lactate dehydrogenase and serum alkaline phosphatase levels can be elevated. The level of leukocyte

Table 110-3 Causes of Myelofibrosis

Carcinoma metastatic to the marrow	Chronic myeloid leukemia
	Polycythemia vera
Infection	Idiopathic myelofibrosis
Lymphoma	Systemic mastocytosis
Hodgkin's disease	Thorium dioxide (Thorotrast) exposure
Acute leukemia (lymphoid or myeloid)	Systemic lupus erythematosus
	Renal osteodystrophy
Hairy cell leukemia	
Multiple myeloma	

alkaline phosphatase can be low, normal, or elevated. Marrow may be unaspirable due to the myelofibrosis, and bone x-rays may reveal osteosclerosis. Exuberant extramedullary hematopoiesis can cause ascites, pulmonary hypertension, intestinal or ureteral obstruction, intracranial hypertension, pericardial tamponade, spinal cord compression, or skin nodules. Splenic enlargement can be sufficiently rapid to cause splenic infarctions with fever and pleuritic chest pain. Hyperuricemia and secondary gout may ensue.

DIAGNOSIS While the clinical picture described above is characteristic of idiopathic myelofibrosis, all of the clinical features described can be observed in polycythemia vera or CML. Massive splenomegaly commonly masks erythrocytosis in polycythemia vera, and reports of intraabdominal thromboses in idiopathic myelofibrosis likely represent instances of unrecognized polycythemia vera. Furthermore, many other disorders have features that overlap with idiopathic myelofibrosis but respond to distinctly different therapies. Therefore, the diagnosis of idiopathic myelofibrosis is one of exclusion, which requires that the disorders listed in Table 110-3 be ruled out.

The presence of teardrop-shaped red cells, nucleated red cells, myelocytes, and promyelocytes establishes the presence of extramedullary hematopoiesis; the presence of leukocytosis, thrombocytosis with large and bizarre platelets, as well as circulating myeloblasts suggests the presence of a myeloproliferative disorder as opposed to a secondary form of myelofibrosis (Table 110-3). Marrow is usually not aspirable due to increased marrow reticulin, but marrow biopsy will reveal a hypercellular marrow with trilineage hyperplasia and, in particular, increased megakaryocytes, but there are no characteristic morphologic abnormalities that distinguish idiopathic myelofibrosis from the other chronic myeloproliferative disorders. Splenomegaly due to extramedullary hematopoiesis may be sufficiently massive to cause portal hypertension and variceal formation. In some patients, exuberant extramedullary hematopoiesis can dominate the clinical picture. An intriguing feature of idiopathic myelofibrosis is the occurrence of autoimmune abnormalities such as immune complexes, antinuclear antibodies, rheumatoid factor, or a positive Coombs' test. Whether these represent a host reaction to the disorder or are involved in its pathogenesis is unknown. Cytogenetic analysis of blood or marrow is useful both to exclude CML and for prognostic purposes, because complex karyotype abnormalities portend a poor prognosis in idiopathic myelofibrosis.

COMPLICATIONS Idiopathic myelofibrosis is a chronic disorder but with a median survival of only 5 years (range 1 to 15 years), a duration much shorter than for polycythemia vera or essential thrombocytosis. The natural history of idiopathic myelofibrosis is one of inexorable marrow failure with transfusion-dependent anemia and increasing organomegaly. Patients are prone to deep-seated tissue infections, particularly of the lungs. As with CML, idiopathic myelofibrosis can evolve from a chronic phase to an accelerated phase with constitutional symptoms and increasing marrow failure. About 10% of patients develop an aggressive form of acute leukemia for which therapy is usually ineffective. Important prognostic factors for disease acceleration include anemia; thrombocytopenia; age; the presence of complex cytogenetic abnormalities; and constitutional symptoms such as unexplained fever, night sweats, or weight loss. Any nonrandom cytogenetic abnormality is associated with a shortened life span, and the presence or development of multiple cytogenetic abnormalities is highly indicative of disease acceleration.

℞ **TREATMENT** There is no specific therapy for idiopathic myelofibrosis. Anemia may be exacerbated by deficiency of folic acid or iron, and in rare instances, pyridoxine therapy has been effective. However, anemia is more often due to ineffective erythropoiesis not compensated for by the extramedullary hematopoiesis in the spleen and liver; neither androgens nor erythropoietin has been consistently effective therapy. Erythropoietin may worsen splenomegaly. A red cell

splenic sequestration study can establish the presence of hypersplenism, for which splenectomy is indicated. Splenectomy may also be necessary if splenomegaly impairs alimentation and should be performed before cachexia sets in. In this situation, splenectomy should not be avoided because of concern over rebound thrombocytosis, loss of hematopoietic capacity, or compensatory hepatomegaly. However, for unexplained reasons, splenectomy increases the risk of blastic transformation. Allopurinol can control significant hyperuricemia and hydroxyurea has proved useful for controlling organomegaly. The role of interferon-α is undefined, and its side effects are more pronounced in the older individuals who are affected with this disorder, but reversal of myelofibrosis has been observed. Glucocorticoids are used to control autoimmune complications. Allogeneic bone marrow transplantation should be considered in younger patients.

ESSENTIAL THROMBOCYTOSIS

Essential thrombocytosis (other designations include *essential thrombocythemia, idiopathic thrombocytosis, primary thrombocytosis, hemorrhagic thrombocythemia*) is a clonal disorder of unknown etiology involving a multipotent hematopoietic progenitor cell and is manifested clinically by the overproduction of platelets without a definable cause. Essential thrombocytosis is an uncommon disorder, but its exact frequency is unknown. No clonal marker distinguishes it from the more common nonclonal, reactive forms of thrombocytosis (Table 110-4). Clinical recognition of thrombocytosis is unlikely in the largely asymptomatic persons affected by this disorder. As a consequence, essential thrombocytosis was formerly considered to be a disease of the elderly and to be responsible for significant morbidity due to hemorrhage or thrombosis. However, with the widespread application of platelet counting, it is now clear that essential thrombocytosis can occur at any age in adults and often occurs without symptoms or disturbances of hemostasis. There is an unexplained female predominance, in contrast to the reactive forms of thrombocytosis where no sex bias exists. Because no clonal marker is available for the disorder, clinical criteria have been proposed to distinguish it from the other chronic myeloproliferative disorders, which may also present with thrombocytosis but have distinct prognosis and treatment (Table 110-5). These criteria do not establish clonality; therefore, they are truly useful only in identifying disorders such as CML, polycythemia vera, or myelodysplasia, which can masquerade as essential thrombocytosis, as opposed to establishing the presence of essential thrombocytosis. Furthermore, as with "primary" erythrocytosis, nonclonal, benign forms of thrombocytosis exist (such as hereditary overproduction of thrombopoietin) that are not widely recognized because we currently lack the diagnostic tools to do so.

ETIOLOGY Megakaryocytopoiesis and platelet production depend upon thrombopoietin and its receptor, Mpl. As in the case of early erythroid and myeloid progenitor cells, early megakaryocytic progenitors require the presence of interleukin (IL) 3 and stem cell factor for optimal proliferation, and their subsequent development is enhanced by IL-6 and -11. However, megakaryocyte maturation and differentiation require thrombopoietin.

Megakaryocytes are unique amongst hematopoietic progenitor

Table 110-4   Causes of Thrombocytosis

Iron-deficiency anemia	Idiopathic myelofibrosis
Hyposplenism	Essential thrombocytosis
Postsplenectomy[a]	Chronic myeloid leukemia
Malignancy	Idiopathic sideroblastic anemia
Collagen vascular disease	Myelodysplasia (5q- syndrome)
Inflammatory bowel disease	Postsurgery
Infection	Rebound (cessation of ethanol intake,
Hemolysis	correction of vitamin B_{12} or folate
Hemorrhage	deficiency)
Polycythemia vera	

[a] If the platelet count is greater than $2 \times 10^6/\mu L$, the etiology is most likely a myeloproliferative disorder.

Table 110-5 Suggested Criteria for the Clinical Diagnosis of Essential Thrombocytosis[a]

Platelet count $\geq$ 500,000/μL
Absence of a known cause of reactive thrombocytosis (see Table 110-4)
Absence of the Ph chromosome and the bcr-abl gene rearrangement
Normal red cell mass
Presence of marrow iron
Absence of myelofibrosis
Absence of myelodysplasia clinically and by cytogenetic analysis
Splenomegaly

[a] The concept that a platelet count greater than 1×10^6/μL distinguishes essential thrombocytosis from other causes of thrombocytosis has no clinical validity.

cells because they undergo endomitotic as opposed to mitotic reduplication of their genome. In the absence of thrombopoietin, endomitotic megakaryocytic reduplication and, by extension, the cytoplasmic development necessary for platelet production are impaired. Like erythropoietin, thrombopoietin is produced in both the liver and the kidneys, and an inverse correlation between the platelet count and plasma thrombopoietic activity exists. Like erythropoietin, plasma levels of thrombopoietin are controlled in part by the size of its progenitor cell pool. In contrast to erythropoietin, but like its myeloid counterparts granulocyte and granulocyte-macrophage colony stimulating factors, thrombopoietin not only enhances the proliferation of its target cells but also enhances the reactivity of their end-stage product, the platelet. In addition to its role in thrombopoiesis, thrombopoietin enhances the survival of multipotent hematopoietic stem cells.

The clonality of essential thrombocytosis has been established by the use of the isoenzymes of glucose-6-phosphate dehydrogenase in patients who are hemizygous for this gene, by the use of X-linked DNA polymorphisms, and by the identification of nonrandom, although variable cytogenetic abnormalities. The multipotent hematopoietic progenitor cell involved in this disorder can vary; in some patients lymphocytes contained the same clonal marker as the megakaryocytes, erythrocytes, and myeloid cells, whereas in others the lymphocytes were not involved. Similar observations have been made in polycythemia vera. Furthermore, a number of families have been described in which essential thrombocytosis was inherited, in one instance as an autosomal dominant trait. In one kindred, in addition to essential thrombocytosis, idiopathic myelofibrosis and polycythemia vera were also individually documented.

CLINICAL FEATURES Clinically, essential thrombocytosis is most often identified incidentally when a platelet count is obtained during the course of a routine evaluation. Occasionally, review of previous platelet counts will reveal that an elevation was present but overlooked. No symptoms or signs are specific for essential thrombocytosis, but patients do have hemorrhagic and thrombotic tendencies expressed as easy bruising for the former or microvascular occlusions for the latter, which may be manifested by erythromelalgia, migraine, or transient ischemic attacks. Physical examination is generally unremarkable except for the presence of mild splenomegaly. Massive splenomegaly is more characteristic of the other myeloproliferative disorders, particularly polycythemia vera or idiopathic myelofibrosis.

Anemia is unusual, but a mild neutrophilic leukocytosis is not. The blood smear, however, is most remarkable for the number of platelets present, some of which may be very large. The leukocyte alkaline phosphatase score is either normal or elevated. The large mass of circulating platelets may prevent the accurate measurement of serum potassium due to the release of platelet potassium upon blood clotting. This hyperkalemia is a laboratory artifact and is not associated with any electrocardiographic abnormalities. Similarly, arterial oxygen measurements can be inaccurate unless the blood is collected on ice. The prothrombin and partial thromboplastin times are normal, while abnormalities of platelet function such as a prolonged bleeding time and impaired platelet aggregation can be present. However, in spite of much study, characteristic platelet function abnormalities associated are not defined, and no platelet function test predicts the presence of clinically significant bleeding or thrombosis.

The elevated platelet count may hinder the collection of a marrow aspirate, but marrow biopsy usually reveals both megakaryocyte hyperplasia and hypertrophy, as well as an overall increase in marrow cellularity. An increase in marrow reticulin may be present, but if extensive, another diagnosis should be considered. The absence of stainable iron demands an explanation, because iron deficiency alone can cause thrombocytosis and absent marrow iron is a feature of polycythemia vera.

While nonrandom cytogenetic abnormalities have been identified in essential thrombocytosis, no consistently identifiable abnormality is noted, even involving chromosomes 3 and 1 where the genes for thrombopoietin and its receptor Mpl, respectively, are located.

DIAGNOSIS Thrombocytosis is encountered in a variety of clinical disorders (Table 110-4) in which production of cytokines is increased. Thus, the first obligation when confronted with a high platelet count is to determine if it is a consequence of another disorder. Cytogenetic evaluation is mandatory to determine if the thrombocytosis is due to CML or a myelodysplastic disorder such as the 5q-syndrome. Because the bcr-abl translocation can be present in the absence of the Ph chromosome, polymerase chain reaction analysis for bcr-abl expression should be performed in all patients with thrombocytosis in whom a cytogenetic study is normal. Anemia and ringed sideroblasts are not features of essential thrombocytosis, but they are features of idiopathic refractory sideroblastic anemia, in which thrombocytosis can also occur. The presence of massive splenomegaly should suggest the possibility of another myeloproliferative disorder, and in this setting a red cell mass determination is mandatory because substantial splenomegaly can mask the presence of erythrocytosis. What appears to be essential thrombocytosis can evolve into polycythemia vera, revealing the true nature of the underlying myeloproliferative disorder.

COMPLICATIONS Perhaps no other condition in clinical medicine has caused otherwise astute physicians to intervene inappropriately more often than thrombocytosis, particularly if the platelet count is greater than 1×10^6/μL. It is commonly believed that a high platelet count must cause intravascular stasis and thrombosis; however, no controlled clinical study has ever established either association.

To the contrary, very high platelet counts are associated primarily with hemorrhage, while platelet counts of $<1 \times 10^6$/μL are more often associated with thrombosis. This is not meant to imply that an elevated platelet count cannot cause symptoms in a patient with essential thrombocytosis, but rather that the focus should be on the patient, not the platelet count. For example, some of the most dramatic neurologic problems in essential thrombocytosis are migraine-related but may respond only to lowering of the platelet count; other symptoms may be a manifestation of erythromelalgia and respond simply to platelet cyclooxygenase inhibitors such as aspirin, without a reduction in platelet number. Still others may represent an interaction between an atherosclerotic vascular system and a high platelet count, and others may have no relationship to the platelet count whatsoever. Progress in distinguishing essential thrombocytosis from polycythemia vera and in defining new causes of hypercoagulability (like factor V Leiden) make the older literature on thrombocytosis less reliable.

TREATMENT An elevated platelet count in an asymptomatic patient requires no therapy, and before any therapy is initiated in a patient with thrombocytosis, the cause of symptoms must be clearly identified to be a consequence of the elevated platelet count. Plasmapheresis and cytotoxic therapy have never been proven efficacious and cannot be recommended. Furthermore, patients with essential thrombocytosis treated with ^{32}P, hydroxyurea, or alkylating agents are placed at risk of developed acute leukemia without any proof of benefit from such therapy. If platelet reduction is deemed necessary on the basis of neurologic symptoms refractory to salicylates, IFN-α or anagrelide, a quinazolin derivative, can reduce the platelet count, but neither is uniformly effective nor without significant side effects. Bleeding associated with thrombocytosis usually responds to ϵ-aminocaproic acid, which can be given prophylactically before and after elective surgery. As more clinical experience is acquired, it appears that essential thrombocytosis is more benign than previously thought, and that evolution to acute leukemia is more likely to be a consequence of prior therapy than of the disease itself. In managing patients with thrombocytosis, the physician's first obligation is to do no harm.

BIBLIOGRAPHY

ADAMSON JW et al: Polycythemia vera: Stem cell and probable clonal origin of the disease. N Engl J Med 295:913, 1976

BAROSI G: Myelofibrosis with myeloid metaplasia: Diagnostic definition and prognostic classification for clinical studies and treatment guidelines. J Clin Oncol 17:2954, 1999

BUSS DH et al: The incidence of thrombotic and hemorrhagic disorders in association with extreme thrombocytosis: An analysis of 129 cases. Am J Hematol 20:365, 1985

MOLITERNO AR et al: Posttranslational processing of the thrombopoietin receptor is impaired in polycythemia vera platelets. Blood 94:2555, 1999

REILLY JT et al: Cytogenetic abnormalities and their prognostic significance in idiopathic myelofibrosis: A study of 106 cases. Br J Haematol 98:96, 1997

SCHAFER AI: Bleeding and thrombosis in the myeloproliferative disorders. Blood 64:1, 1984

STERKERS Y et al: Acute myeloid leukemia and myelodysplastic syndromes following essential thrombocythemia treated with hydroxyurea: High proportion of cases with 17p deletion. Blood 91:616, 1998

TARTAGLIA AP et al: Adverse effects of antiaggregating platelet therapy in the treatment of polycythemia vera. Semin Hematol 23:172, 1986

111   *Meir Wetzler, John C. Byrd, Clara D. Bloomfield*

ACUTE AND CHRONIC MYELOID LEUKEMIA

The myeloid leukemias are a heterogeneous group of diseases characterized by infiltration of the blood, bone marrow, and other tissues by neoplastic cells of the hematopoietic system. In 2000, the estimated number of new myeloid leukemia cases in the United States was 10,100. These leukemias comprise a spectrum of malignancies that, untreated, range from rapidly fatal to slowly growing. Based on their untreated course, the myeloid leukemias have traditionally been designated *acute* or *chronic*.

ACUTE MYELOID LEUKEMIA

INCIDENCE   The incidence of acute myeloid leukemia (AML) is approximately 2.3 per 100,000 people per year, and the age-adjusted incidence is higher in men than in women (2.9 versus 1.9). AML incidence increases with age; it is 1.3 in individuals younger than 65 years and 12.2 in those older than 65. No significant change in AML incidence has occurred over the past 20 years.

ETIOLOGY   Heredity, radiation, chemical and other occupational exposures, and drugs have been implicated in the development of AML. No direct evidence suggests a viral etiology.

Heredity   Certain syndromes with somatic cell chromosome aneuploidy, e.g., Down (chromosome 21 trisomy), Klinefelter (XXY and variants), and Patau (chromosome 13 trisomy), are associated with an increased incidence of AML. Inherited diseases with excessive chromatin fragility, e.g., Fanconi anemia, Bloom syndrome, ataxia telangiectasia, and Kostmann syndrome, are also associated with AML.

Radiation   Survivors of the atomic bomb explosions in Japan had an increased incidence of myeloid leukemias that peaked 5 to 7 years after exposure. Therapeutic radiation alone seems to add little risk of AML but can increase the risk in people exposed to alkylating agents (see below).

Chemical and Other Exposures   Exposure to benzene, which is used as a solvent in the chemical, plastic, rubber, and pharmaceutical industries, is associated with an increased incidence of AML. Smoking and exposure to petroleum products, paint, embalming fluids, ethylene oxide, herbicides, and pesticides, have also been associated with an increased risk of AML.

Drugs   Anticancer drugs are the leading cause of treatment-associated AML. Alkylating agent–associated leukemias occur on average 4 to 6 years after exposure, and affected individuals have aberrations in chromosomes 5 and 7. Topoisomerase II inhibitor–associated leukemias occur 1 to 3 years after exposure, and affected individuals usually have aberrations involving chromosome 11q23. Chloramphenicol, phenylbutazone, and, less commonly, chloroquine and methoxypsoralen can result in bone marrow failure that may evolve into AML.

CLASSIFICATION   The categorization of acute leukemia into biologically distinct groups is based on morphology, cytochemistry, and immunophenotype as well as cytogenetic and molecular techniques.

Morphologic and Cytochemical Classification   The diagnosis of AML is established by the presence of >20% myeloblasts in blood and/or bone marrow. Myeloblasts have nuclear chromatin that is uniformly fine or lacelike in appearance and large nucleoli (two to five per cell). If specific cytoplasmic granules, Auer rods, or the nuclear folding and clefting characteristic of monocytoid cells are not present, the morphologic features observed under light microscopy may not be sufficient to clarify the diagnosis. A positive myeloperoxidase reaction in >3% of the blasts may be the only feature distinguishing AML from acute lymphoblastic leukemia (ALL).

AML is classified based on morphology and cytochemistry according to the French, American, and British (FAB) schema, which includes eight major subtypes, M0 to M7 (Table 111-1). The World Health Organization classification incorporates molecular (including cytogenetic), morphologic, and clinical features (such as prior hematologic disorder) in defining disease entities (Table 111-1).

Immunophenotypic Classification   The phenotype of human myeloid leukemia cells can be studied by multiparameter flow cytometry after the cells are labeled with monoclonal antibodies to cell-surface antigens. For example, M0, which is characterized by immature morphology and no lineage-specific cytochemical reactions, is diagnosed by flow cytometric demonstration of the myeloid-specific antigens cluster designation (CD) 13 or 33. Similarly, M7 can often be diagnosed only by expression of the platelet-specific antigen CD41 or by electron-microscopic demonstration of myeloperoxidase.

Chromosomal Classification   Chromosomal analysis of the leukemic cell provides the most important pretreatment prognostic information in AML. Only two cytogenetic abnormalities have been invariably associated with a specific FAB group: t(15;17)(q22;q12) with M3 and inv(16)(p13q22) with M4Eo. However, many chromosomal abnormalities have been associated primarily with one FAB group, including t(8;21)(q22;q22) with M2, and t(9;11)(p22;q23), and other translocations involving 11q23, with M5. Many of the recurring chromosomal abnormalities in AML have been associated with specific clinical characteristics. More commonly associated with younger age are t(8;21) and t(15;17), and with older age, del(5q) and del(7q). Granulocytic sarcomas are associated with t(8;21); disseminated intravascular coagulation (DIC) with t(15;17); and diabetes insipidus, fever, and infection all with monosomy 7. The reasons for most associations of chromosomal abnormalities with specific clinical features are unknown.

Molecular Classification   The many recurring cytogenetic abnormalities led to molecular studies, which have revealed genes that may be involved in leukemogenesis. The 15;17 translocation, characteristic of M3, encodes a chimeric protein, Pml/Rarα, which is formed by the fusion of the retinoic acid receptor-α (*RAR*α) gene from chromosome 17 and the promyelocytic leukemia (*PML*) gene from chromosome 15. The *RAR*α gene encodes a member of the nuclear

French-American-British (FAB) Classification[a]

M0: Minimally differentiated leukemia
M1: Myeloblastic leukemia without maturation
M2: Myeloblastic leukemia with maturation
M3: Hypergranular promyelocytic leukemia
M4Eo: Variant: Increase in abnormal marrow eosinophils
M4: Myelomonocytic leukemia
M5: Moncytic leukemia
M6: Erythroleukemia (DiGuglielmo's disease)
M7: Megakaryoblastic leukemia

World Health Organization Classification[b]

I. AML with recurrent cytogenetic translocations
   AML with t(8;21)(q22;q22);*AML1(CBFα)/ETO*
   Acute promyelocytic leukemia [AML with t(15;17)(q22;q12) and variants; *PML/RARα*]
   AML with abnormal bone marrow eosinophils [inv(16)(p13q22) or t(16;16)(p13;q22) *CBFβ/MYH11*]
   AML with 11q23 (*MLL*) abnormalities
II. AML with multilineage dysplasia
   With prior myelodysplastic syndrome
   Without prior myelodysplastic syndrome
III. AML and myelodysplastic syndrome, therapy-related
   Alkylating agent-related
   Epipodophyllotoxin-related
   Other types
IV. AML not otherwise categorized
   AML minimally differentiated
   AML without maturation
   AML with maturation
   Acute myelomonocytic leukemia
   Acute monocytic leukemia
   Acute erythroid leukemia
   Acute megakaryocytic leukemia
   Acute basophilic leukemia
   Acute panmyelosis with myelofibrosis

[a] JM Bennett et al: Ann Intern Med 103:620, 1985
[b] NL Harris et al: J Clin Oncol 17:3835, 1999

hormone receptor family of transcription factors. After binding retinoic acid, *RARα* can promote expression of a variety of genes. The 15;17 translocation juxtaposes *PML* with *RARα* in a head-to-tail configuration that is under the transcriptional control of *PML*. Three different breakpoints in the *PML* gene lead to various fusion proteins. The Pml-Rarα fusion protein tends to suppress gene transcription and blocks differentiation of the cells. Pharmacologic doses of the Rarα ligand, all-trans-retinoic acid (tretinoin or ATRA), relieve the block and promote differentiation (see below).

The inv(16), characteristic of M4Eo or AML with abnormal bone marrow eosinophils, and the t(8;21) characteristic of M2 both involve subunits of the transcription factor complex core-binding factor (Cbf), also known as polyomavirus enhancer binding protein 2. This transcription factor contains two subunits, an α subunit, the Am11 protein, and a β subunit, the Pebp2 protein, and is involved in the expression of a number of differentiation-dependent genes in myeloid cells. The inv(16) results in a fusion of the core-binding factor β (*CBFB*) gene on the q arm (encodes Pebp2 protein) and the myosin heavy chain (*MYH11*) gene on the p arm. The 8;21 translocation involves the core-binding factor α (*CBFA*) gene on chromosome 21, called the *AML1* gene, joining the *ETO* gene on chromosome 8. Similar to the t(15;17) gene product, the Aml1/Eto protein acts to block transcription of *CBFA-CBFB*-controlled genes.

Most translocations that involve 11q23 rearrange the *MLL* (myeloid-lymphoid or mixed-lineage leukemia) gene. The *MLL* gene has two regions that encompass multiple zinc fingers and has at least two additional potential DNA-binding motifs. Abnormalities in the *MLL* gene are relatively common in patients with AML who do not have 11q23 rearrangements cytogenetically.

These molecular aberrations are increasingly being used for diagnosis and detection of residual disease after treatment.

CLINICAL PRESENTATION   Symptoms   Patients with AML most often present with nonspecific symptoms that begin gradually or abruptly and are the consequence of anemia, leukocytosis, leukopenia or leukocyte dysfunction, or thrombocytopenia. Nearly half have had symptoms for 3 months or more before the leukemia is diagnosed.

Half mention fatigue as the first symptom, but most complain of fatigue or weakness at the time of diagnosis. Anorexia and weight loss are common. Fever with or without an identifiable infection is the initial symptom in ~10% of patients. Signs of abnormal hemostasis (bleeding, easy bruising) are noted first in 5% of patients. On occasion, bone pain, lymphadenopathy, nonspecific cough, headache, or diaphoresis is the presenting symptom.

Rarely patients may present with symptoms from a mass lesion located in the soft tissues, breast, uterus, ovary, cranial or spinal dura, gastrointestinal tract, lung, mediastinum, prostate, bone, or other organs. The mass lesion represents a tumor of leukemic cells and is called a *granulocytic sarcoma*, or *chloroma*. Typical AML may occur simultaneously, later, or not at all in these patients. This rare presentation is more common in patients with 8;21 translocations.

Physical Findings   Fever, splenomegaly, hepatomegaly, lymphadenopathy, sternal tenderness, and evidence of infection and hemorrhage are often found at diagnosis. Significant gastrointestinal bleeding, intrapulmonary hemorrhage, or intracranial hemorrhage occur most often in M3 AML. Bleeding associated with coagulopathies may also occur in M5 AML and with extreme degrees of leukocytosis or thrombocytopenia in other FAB subtypes. Retinal hemorrhages are detected in 15% of patients. Infiltration of the gingivae, skin, soft tissues, or the meninges with leukemic blasts at diagnosis is characteristic of the monocytic subtypes (M4 and M5).

Hematologic Findings   Anemia is usually present at diagnosis and can be severe. The degree varies considerably irrespective of other hematologic findings, splenomegaly, or the duration of symptoms. The anemia is usually normochromic normocytic. Decreased erythropoiesis often results in a reduced reticulocyte count, and erythrocyte survival is decreased by accelerated destruction. Active blood loss also contributes to the anemia.

The median presenting leukocyte count is about 15,000/μL. Twenty-five to 40% of patients have counts <5000/μL, and 20% have counts >100,000/μL. Fewer than 5% have no detectable leukemic cells in the blood. Poor neutrophil function may be noted functionally by impaired phagocytosis and migration and morphologically by abnormal lobulation and deficient granulation.

Platelet counts <100,000/μL are found at diagnosis in ~75% of patients, and about 25% have counts <25,000/μL. Both morphologic and functional platelet abnormalities can be observed, including large and bizarre shapes with abnormal granulation and inability of platelets to aggregate or adhere normally to one another.

Pretreatment Evaluation   Once the diagnosis of AML is suspected, a rapid evaluation and initiation of appropriate therapy should follow (Table 111-2). In addition to clarifying the subtype of leukemia, initial studies should evaluate the overall functional integrity of the major organ systems, including the cardiovascular, pulmonary, hepatic, and renal systems. Factors that have prognostic significance, either for achieving complete remission (CR) or for predicting the duration of CR, should also be assessed before initiating treatment. Leukemic cells should be obtained from all patients and cryopreserved for future use as new tests become available. All patients should be evaluated for infection.

Most patients are anemic and thrombocytopenic at presentation. Replacement of the appropriate blood components, if necessary, should begin promptly. Because qualitative platelet dysfunction or the presence of an infection may increase the likelihood of bleeding, evidence of hemorrhage justifies the immediate use of platelet transfusion, even if the platelet count is only moderately decreased.

About 50% of patients have a mild to moderate elevation of serum

**Table 111-2 Initial Diagnostic Evaluation and Management of Adult
Patients with AML**

History
  Increasing fatigue or decreased exercise tolerance (anemia)
  Excess bleeding or bleeding from unusual sites (DIC, thrombocytopenia)
  Fevers or recurrent infections (granulocytopenia)
  Headache, vision changes, nonfocal neurologic abnormalities (CNS leuke-
    mia or bleed)
  Early satiety (splenomegaly)
  Family history of AML (Fanconi, Bloom or Kostmann syndromes or
    ataxia telangiectasia)
  History of cancer (exposure to alkylating agents, radiation, topoisomerase
    II inhibitors)
  Occupational exposures (radiation, benzene, petroleum products, paint,
    smoking, pesticides
Physical Examination
  Performance status (prognostic factor)
  Ecchymosis and oozing from IV sites (DIC, possible acute promyelocytic
    leukemia)
  Fever and tachycardia (signs of infection)
  Papilledema, retinal infiltrates, cranial nerve abnormalities (CNS leukemia)
  Poor dentition, dental abscesses
  Gum hypertrophy (leukemic infiltration, most common in monocytic leu-
    kemia)
  Skin infiltration or nodules (leukemia infiltration, most common in mono-
    cytic leukemia)
  Lymphadenopathy, splenomegaly, hepatosplenomegaly
  Back pain, lower extremity weakness [spinal granulocytic sarcoma, most
    likely in t(8;21) patients]
Laboratory and Radiologic Studies
  CBC with manual differential cell count
  Chemistry tests (electrolytes, creatinine, hepatic enzymes, BUN, calcium,
    phosphorus, LDH, uric acid, bilirubin, amylase, lipase)
  Clotting studies (prothrombin time, partial thromboplastin time, fibrinogen,
    D-dimer)
  Viral serologies (CMV, HSV-1, Varicella zoster)
  RBC type and screen
  HLA-typing of patient, siblings, and parents for potential allogeneic SCT
  Bone marrow aspirate and biopsy (morphology, cytochemistry, cytogenet-
    ics, flow cytometry, molecular studies)
  Cryopreservation of viable leukemia cells (for later study)
  Echocardiogram
  PA and lateral chest radiograph
  Placement of central venous access device
Interventions for Specific Patients
  Dental evaluation (for those with poor dentition)
  Lumbar puncture (for those with symptoms of CNS involvement)
  Screening spine MRI (for patients with back pain, lower extremity weak-
    ness, paresthesias)
  Social work referral for patient and family psychosocial support
Counseling for All Patients
  Provide patient with disease information, financial information, support
    group information

uric acid at presentation. Only 10% have marked elevations, but renal precipitation of uric acid and the nephropathy that may result is a serious but uncommon complication. The initiation of chemotherapy may aggravate hyperuricemia, and patients are usually immediately started on allopurinol and hydration at diagnosis. Finally, the presence in high concentrations of lysozyme, a marker for monocytic differentiation, may be etiologic in renal tubular dysfunction, which could worsen other renal problems that arise during the initial phases of therapy.

PROGNOSTIC FACTORS The single most important prognostic factor is attainment of CR. CR is defined after examination of both blood and bone marrow and should last $\geq$4 weeks. The blood neutrophil count must be $\geq$1500/μL and the platelet count $\geq$100,000/μL. Hemoglobin concentration or hematocrit are not considered in determining CR. Circulating blasts should be absent. While rare blasts may be detected in the blood during marrow regeneration, they should disappear on successive studies. Bone marrow cellularity should be

$>$20% with trilineage maturation. The bone marrow should contain $<$5% blasts, and Auer rods should be absent. Extramedullary leukemia should not be present. For patients in CR, reverse transcriptase polymerase chain reaction (RT-PCR) to detect AML-associated molecular abnormalities, and fluorescence in situ hybridization (FISH) to detect AML-associated cytogenetic aberrations are currently used to detect residual disease. Such detection of minimal residual disease may become a reliable discriminator between patients in CR who do or do not require additional and/or alternative therapies.

Many factors influence the likelihood of entering CR, the length of CR, and the curability of AML. Prognostic factors are influenced by the treatment used. Age at diagnosis remains among the most important pretreatment risk factors, with $>$60 years being associated with a poorer prognosis primarily because of its influence on the patient's ability to survive induction therapy and thus achieve CR. Chronic and intercurrent diseases impair tolerance to rigorous therapy; acute medical problems at diagnosis reduce the likelihood of survival. Performance status, independent of age, also influences ability to survive induction therapy and thus respond to treatment. Age may also influence outcome because AML in older patients differs biologically. The leukemic cells in elderly patients more commonly express CD34 and the mdr1 efflux pump that conveys resistance to natural product-derived agents such as the anthracyclines (see below). With each successive decade of age, a greater proportion of patients have more resistant disease.

Chromosome findings at diagnosis are an independent prognostic factor. Patients with t(8;21), inv(16), or t(15;17) have extremely good prognoses, while those with no cytogenetic abnormality have a moderately favorable outcome when treated with high-dose cytarabine. Patients with del(5q), -7, and abnormalities involving 12p have a very poor prognosis. Patients with certain abnormalities, such as inv(3), rarely achieve CR with standard induction chemotherapy.

A prolonged symptomatic interval with cytopenias preceding diagnosis or a history of an antecedent hematologic disorder are other pretreatment clinical features that are associated with a lower CR rate and shorter survival time. The CR rate is lower in patients who have had anemia, leukopenia, and/or thrombocytopenia for $>$1 month before the diagnosis of AML when compared to those without such a history. Responsiveness to chemotherapy declines as the duration of the antecedent disorder(s) increases. Secondary AML developing after treatment with cytotoxic agents and/or irradiation for other malignancies is extremely difficult to treat successfully.

A high presenting leukocyte count is an independent prognostic factor; duration of CR is inversely related to the presenting leukocyte count or absolute circulating myeloblast count. Among patients with hyperleukocytosis ($>$100,000/μL), early central nervous system bleeding and pulmonary leukostasis and late relapse contribute to poor outcome.

The FAB classification diagnosis has been found to be an independent prognostic factor in some series. Other characteristics of the leukemic cell have been reported to have prognostic significance, including Auer rods, ultrastructural features, in vitro and in vivo growth characteristics and chemotherapeutic sensitivity, and immunophenotype. Expression of the *MDR1* gene adversely influences outcome. This gene encodes a protein that actively pumps out a variety of lipophilic compounds (e.g., anthracyclines) from the cell.

In addition to pretreatment variables, several treatment factors have been reported to correlate with prognosis in AML, in particular with CR duration. One is the rapidity with which the blast cells disappear from the blood after the institution of therapy. In addition, patients who achieve CR after one induction cycle have longer CR than those requiring multiple cycles.

TREATMENT Treatment of the newly diagnosed patient with AML is usually divided into two phases, induction and postremission management (Fig. 111-1). The initial goal is to quickly induce CR. Once CR is obtained, further therapy must be used to prolong survival.

FIGURE 111-1 Flow chart for the therapy of newly diagnosed AML. For all forms of AML except acute promyelocytic leukemia, standard therapy includes a 7-day continuous infusion of cytarabine (100–200 mg/m² per day) and a 3-day course of daunorubicin (45 mg/m² per day) or idarubicin (12–13 mg/m² per day) with or without 3 days of etoposide. Patients who achieve CR undergo some form of consolidation therapy, including sequential courses of high-dose cytarabine, high-dose combination chemotherapy with allogeneic SCT or novel therapies, based on their predicted risk of relapse (i.e., risk-stratified therapy). Patients with acute promyelocytic leukemia usually receive tretinoin together with combination chemotherapy for remission induction and then receive consolidation chemotherapy (daunorubicin and cytarabine) followed by maintenance tretinoin.

Induction Chemotherapy   The most commonly used CR induction regimens (for patients with all FAB subtypes except M3) consist of combination chemotherapy with cytarabine (cytosine arabinoside) and an anthracycline. Cytarabine is a cell cycle S-phase-specific antimetabolite that becomes phosphorylated to an active triphosphate form that interferes with DNA synthesis. Anthracyclines are DNA intercalaters. Their primary mode of action is thought to be inhibition of topoisomerase II, leading to DNA breaks. Cytarabine is usually administered as a continuous intravenous infusion at 100 to 200 mg/m² per day for 7 days. Anthracycline therapy generally consists of daunorubicin, 45 mg/m² intravenously on days 1, 2, and 3 (*the 7 and 3 regimen*). Treatment with idarubicin at 12 or 13 mg/m² per day for 3 days in conjunction with cytarabine by 7-day continuous infusion is at least as effective and may be superior to daunorubicin in younger patients. The addition of etoposide or other agents does not increase the CR rate but may improve the CR duration.

After induction chemotherapy, the bone marrow is examined to determine if the leukemia has been eliminated. If >5% blasts exist with ≥20% cellularity, the patient has traditionally been retreated with cytarabine and an anthracycline in doses similar to those given initially, but for 5 and 2 days, respectively. Our recommendation, however, is to consider changing therapy in this setting. Patients who fail to attain CR after two induction courses should immediately proceed to an allogeneic stem cell transplant (SCT) if an appropriate donor exists.

With the 7 and 3 cytarabine/daunorubicin regimen outlined above, 65 to 75% of adults with de novo AML achieve CR. Two-thirds

achieve CR after a single course of therapy, and one-third require two courses. About 50% of patients who do not achieve CR have a drug-resistant leukemia, and 50% do not achieve CR because of fatal complications of bone marrow aplasia or impaired recovery of normal stem cells.

High-dose cytarabine-based regimens have very high CR rates after a single cycle of therapy. When given in high doses, more cytarabine may enter the cells, saturate the cytarabine-inactivating enzymes, and increase the intracellular levels of 1-β-D-arabinofuranylcytosine-triphosphate, the active metabolite incorporated into DNA. Thus, higher doses of cytarabine may increase the inhibition of DNA synthesis and thereby overcome resistance to standard-dose cytarabine. In two randomized studies, one by the Southwest Oncology Group (SWOG) and one by the Australian Leukemia Study Group (ALSG), high-dose cytarabine with an anthracycline produced CR rates similar to those achieved with standard 7 and 3 regimens. However, the ALSG demonstrated that the CR duration was much longer after high-dose cytarabine than after standard-dose cytarabine.

The hematologic toxicity of high-dose cytarabine-based induction regimens has typically been greater than that associated with 7 and 3 regimens. Toxicity with high-dose cytarabine includes myelosuppression, pulmonary toxicity, and significant and occasionally irreversible cerebellar toxicity. All patients treated with high-dose cytarabine must be closely monitored for cerebellar toxicity. Full cerebellar testing should be performed before each dose, and further high-dose cytarabine should be withheld if evidence of cerebellar toxicity develops.

Supportive Care   Measures geared to supporting patients through several weeks of granulocytopenia and thrombocytopenia are critical to the success of AML therapy. Patients with AML should be treated in centers expert in providing supportive measures for their management.

Recombinant hematopoietic growth factors have been incorporated into clinical trials in AML. These trials have been designed to lower the infection rate after chemotherapy or to sensitize (prime) the leukemic blasts to chemotherapy, or both. Both granulocyte colony stimulating factor (G-CSF) and granulocyte-macrophage colony stimulating factor (GM-CSF) have reduced the median time to neutrophil recovery by an average of 5 to 7 days. This accelerated rate of neutrophil recovery, however, has not always translated into significant reductions in infection rates. In most randomized studies, both G-CSF and GM-CSF have failed to improve the CR rate, disease-free survival, or overall survival. Although receptors for both G-CSF and GM-CSF are present on AML blasts, therapeutic efficacy is neither enhanced nor inhibited by these agents. The use of growth factors as supportive care for AML patients is controversial. We favor their use in elderly patients, those receiving intensive regimens, patients with uncontrolled infections, or those participating in clinical trials.

Multilumen right atrial catheters should be inserted through a subcutaneous tunnel as soon as patients with newly diagnosed AML have been stabilized. They should be used thereafter for administration of intravenous medications and transfusions, as well as for blood drawing. The separation between the vascular access site and the exit site and the presence of a Dacron cuff in the subcutaneous channel reduce the risk of infection. With meticulous attention to sterile technique in catheter placement and maintenance, catheters may often be left in place for months.

Adequate and prompt blood bank support is critical to therapy of AML. Platelet transfusions should be given as needed to maintain a platelet count >10,000 to 20,000/μL. We believe that the platelet count should be kept at higher levels in febrile patients and during episodes of active bleeding or DIC. Patients with poor posttransfusion platelet count increments may benefit from administration of platelets from human leukocyte antigen (HLA)-matched donors. Red blood cell transfusions should be administered to keep the hemoglobin level >80 g/L (8 g/dL) in the absence of active bleeding or DIC. Blood products leukodepleted by filtration should be used to avert or delay alloimmunization as well as febrile reactions. Blood products should also be irradiated to prevent graft-versus-host disease (GVHD). Cytomegalovirus (CMV)-negative blood products should be used for CMV-seronegative patients who are potential candidates for allogeneic SCT. Leukodepleted products are also effective for these patients if CMV-negative products are not available.

Infectious complications remain the major cause of morbidity and death during induction and postremission chemotherapy for AML. Prophylactic administration of antibiotics in the absence of fever is controversial. Oral nystatin or clotrimazole are recommended to prevent localized candidiasis. For patients who are herpes simplex virus antibody titer–positive, acyclovir prophylaxis is effective in preventing reactivation of latent oral herpes infections.

Fever develops in most patients with AML, but infections are documented in only half of febrile patients. Early initiation of empiric broad-spectrum antibacterial and antifungal antibiotics has significantly reduced the number of patients dying of infectious complications (Chap. 85). An antibiotic regimen adequate to treat gram-negative and gram-positive organisms should be instituted at the onset of fever in a granulocytopenic patient after clinical evaluation, including a detailed physical examination with inspection of the indwelling catheter exit site and a perirectal examination, as well as procurement of cultures and radiographs aimed at documenting the source of fever. Specific antibiotic regimens should be based on antibiotic sensitivity data obtained from the institution at which the patient is being treated. Acceptable regimens include imipenem-cilastin, an antipseudomonal semisynthetic penicillin (e.g., piperacillin) combined with an aminoglycoside, a third-generation cephalosporin with antipseudomonal activity (i.e., ceftazidine or cefapime) or double β-lactam combinations (ceftazidine and piperacillin). Empiric vancomycin is not given initially in the absence of suspected gram-positive infection or mucositis. Aminoglycosides should be avoided if possible in patients with renal insufficiency. For patients with known immediate-type hypersensitivity reactions to penicillin, aztreonam may be substituted for β-lactams. Aztreonam should be combined with an aminoglycoside or a quinolone antibiotic rather than used alone. Empiric vancomycin should be initiated in neutropenic patients who remain febrile for 3 days, and amphotericin B is added at 7 days if fever persists. Liposomal amphotericin is at least equivalent to regular amphotericin for empiric antifungal treatment and has less renal toxicity. Antibacterial and antifungal antibiotics should be continued until patients are no longer neutropenic, regardless of whether a specific source has been found for the fever.

Treatment of Promyelocytic Leukemia　ATRA is an oral drug that induces the differentiation of leukemic cells bearing the t(15;17); it is not effective in other forms of AML. Acute promyelocytic leukemia is responsive to cytarabine and daunarubicin, but about 10% of patients treated with these drugs die from DIC induced by the release of granule components by dying tumor cells. ATRA does not produce DIC but produces another complication called the retinoic acid syndrome. Occurring within the first 3 weeks of treatment, it is characterized by fever, dyspnea, chest pain, pulmonary infiltrates, pleural and pericardial effusions, and hypoxia. The syndrome is related to the adhesion of differentiated neoplastic cells in the pulmonary vasculature. Glucocorticoids, chemotherapy, and/or supportive measures can be effective. About 10% of patients die from this syndrome.

ATRA (45 mg/m^2 per day orally until remission is documented) plus concurrent chemotherapy (7 and 3) appears to be the safest and most effective treatment for acute promyelocytic leukemia. Unlike patients with other types of AML, patients with this subtype may benefit from maintenance therapy with either ATRA or chemotherapy. The optimal regimen is being sought in clinical studies.

Arsenic trioxide produces meaningful responses in patients refractory to ATRA.

The detection of minimal residual disease by RT-PCR amplification of the t(15;17) chimeric gene product appears to predict relapse.

Disappearance of the signal is associated with long-term disease-free survival; its persistence predicts relapse. With increases in the sensitivity of the assay, some patients with persistent abnormal gene product have been found who do not suffer a relapse. It is not known whether there is a critical threshold level of transcripts that predicts for leukemia relapse.

Postremission Therapy　Induction of a durable first CR is critical to long-term disease-free survival in AML. Without further therapy virtually all patients experience relapse. Once relapse has occurred, AML is generally curable only by SCT.

Postremission therapy is designed to eradicate any residual leukemic cells. Therefore, it should prevent relapse and prolong survival. Approaches to postremission therapy in AML include intensive chemotherapy and allogeneic or autologous SCT. In patients older than 65 years, such therapy is of uncertain benefit. High-dose cytarabine is more effective than standard-dose cytarabine. The Cancer and Leukemia Group B, for example, compared the duration of CR in patients randomly assigned postremission to four cycles of high (3 g/m^2 every 12 h on days 1, 3, and 5), intermediate (400 mg/m^2 for 5 days by continuous infusion), or standard (100 mg/m^2 per day for 5 days by continuous infusion) doses of cytarabine. A dose-response effect for cytarabine in patients with AML who were age 60 years or younger was demonstrated. High-dose cytarabine significantly prolonged CR and increased the fraction cured in patients with favorable [t(8;21) and inv(16)] and normal cytogenetics, but it had no significant effect on patients with other abnormal karyotypes.

Allogeneic and autologous SCT in first CR has been studied extensively in younger patients with no major organ dysfunction. Allogeneic SCT is used in patients <55 years with an HLA-compatible donor. Relapse with this therapy occurs in only a small fraction of patients, but toxicity is relatively high from treatment; complications include veno-occlusive disease, GVHD, and infections. Autologous transplantation can be used in young and older patients and uses the same type of high-dose therapy. Patients subsequently receive their own stem cells collected while in remission. The toxicity is lower with autologous SCT (5% mortality rate), but the relapse rate is higher than with allogeneic SCT. The increased relapse rate is due to the absence of the graft-vs-leukemia effect seen with allogeneic SCT and possible contamination of the autologous stem cells with tumor cells. Purging the autologous stem cells does not lower the relapse rate with autologous SCT.

Randomized trials comparing intensive therapy and autologous and allogeneic SCT have shown improved duration of remission with allogeneic SCT compared to autologous SCT or chemotherapy alone. However, overall survival is generally not different; the improved disease control with allogeneic SCT is erased by the increase in fatal toxicity. Prognostic factors may help select patients in first CR for whom transplant is most effective.

Our approach includes strong consideration for allogeneic SCT in first CR for patients with high risk karyotypes. Patients with normal karyotypes who have other poor risk factors (antecedent hematologic disorder, failure to attain remission with a single induction course, hyperleukocytosis, *MLL* gene abnormalities) are also potential candidates. If a suitable HLA donor does not exist, autologous SCT or novel therapeutic approaches are considered. Patients with t(8;21) and inv(16) are treated with repetitive doses of high-dose cytarabine, which offers a high frequency of cure without the morbidity of transplant.

Relapse　Once relapse occurs after the standard induction and postremission chemotherapy approach described above and outlined in Fig. 111-1, patients are rarely cured with further standard-dose chemotherapy. Patients eligible for allogeneic SCT should receive transplants expeditiously at the first sign of relapse. Long-term disease-free survival is approximately the same (30 to 50%) with allogeneic SCT in first relapse or in second remission. Autologous SCT rescues about 20% of relapsed patients with AML who have chemosensitive disease. The most important factors predicting response at relapse are the length of the previous CR, whether initial CR was achieved with one or two courses of chemotherapy, and the type of postremission

Class of Drugs	Example Agent(s)
MDR1 modulator	Cyclosporine analogues, PSC-833
Demethylating agent	Decitabine, 5-azacytidine
Histone deacetylase inhibitor	Phenylbutyrate, depsipeptide
Heavy metals	Arsenic trioxide, antimony
Protein kinase C inhibitor	Bryostatin, UCN-01
Cell cycle inhibitor	Flavopiridol
Humanized antibodies	Anti-CD33 (HuM195)
Toxin-conjugated antibodies	CMA-676 (anti-CD33 linked to calicheamicin)
Radiolabeled antibodies	Yttrium-90-labeled human M195
Cytokines	Recombinant human IL-2 and IL-12

therapy. Because of the poor outcome of patients in early ($<$12 months) first relapse, it is justified (for patients without HLA-compatible donors) to explore innovative approaches, such as new drugs or immunotherapies (Table 111-3). Patients with longer ($>$12 months) first CR generally relapse with drug-sensitive disease and may achieve a second remission with the original induction regimen. However, cure for these patients is uncommon, and treatment with novel approaches should be considered if SCT is not possible. It is not yet clear whether careful monitoring for residual disease by RT-PCR, FISH and quantitative PCR identifies patients destined to relapse who are more readily cured by salvage therapy given before overt clinical relapse.

CHRONIC MYELOID LEUKEMIA

INCIDENCE The incidence of chronic myeloid leukemia (CML) is 1.3 per 100,000 people per year, and the age-adjusted incidence is higher in men than in women (1.7 versus 1.0). CML incidence decreased slightly between 1973 and 1991 (1.5 versus 1.3). The incidence of CML increases slowly with age until the middle forties, when it starts to rise rapidly.

DEFINITION The diagnosis of CML is established by identifying a clonal expansion of a hematopoietic stem cell possessing a reciprocal translocation between chromosomes 9 and 22. This translocation results in the head-to-tail fusion of the breakpoint cluster region (*BCR*) gene on chromosome 22q11 with the *ABL* (named after the abelson murine leukemia virus) gene located on chromosome 9q34. Untreated, the disease is characterized by the inevitable transition from a chronic phase to an accelerated phase and on to blast crisis.

ETIOLOGY No clear correlation with exposure to cytotoxic drugs, such as alkylating agents, has been found, and there is no direct evidence of a viral etiology. Cigarette smoking has been shown to accelerate the progression to blast crisis and therefore has an adverse effect on survival in CML. The effect of radiation was demonstrated in the study of the atomic bomb survivors, where it has been estimated that the development of a CML cell mass of $10,000/\mu L$ takes 6.3 years. No increase in CML incidence was found in the survivors of the Chernobyl accident, suggesting that only large doses of radiation can induce CML.

PATHOPHYSIOLOGY The product of the fusion gene resulting from the t(9;22) plays a central role in the development of CML. This chimeric gene is transcribed into a hybrid *BCR/ABL* mRNA in which exon 1 of ABL is replaced by variable numbers of 5′ BCR exons. Bcr/Abl fusion proteins, p210$^{BCR-ABL}$, are produced that contain NH$_2$-terminal domains of Bcr and the COOH-terminal domains of Abl. Bcr/Abl fusion proteins can transform hematopoietic progenitor cells in vitro. Furthermore, reconstituting lethally irradiated mice with bone marrow cells infected with retrovirus carrying the gene encoding the p210$^{BCR-ABL}$ leads to the development of a myeloproliferative syndrome resembling CML in 50% of the mice. Specific antisense oligomers to the *BCR/ABL* junctions inhibit the growth of t(9;22)-positive leukemic cells without affecting normal colony formation.

The mechanism(s) by which p210$^{BCR-ABL}$ promotes the transition from the benign state to the fully malignant one is still unclear. Messenger RNA for *BCR/ABL* can occasionally be detected in normal individuals. However, attachment of the *BCR* sequences to *ABL* results in three critical functional changes: (1) the Abl protein becomes constitutively active as a tyrosine kinase enzyme, (2) the DNA protein–binding activity of Abl is attenuated, and (3) the binding of Abl to cytoskeletal actin microfilaments is enhanced.

Disease Progression The events associated with transition to the acute phase are poorly understood. Chromosomal instability of the malignant clone, resulting, for example, in the acquisition of an additional t(9;22), trisomy 8, or 17p- (p53 loss), is a fundamental characteristic of CML. Acquisition of these additional genetic and/or molecular abnormalities is critical to the phenotypic transformation. The site of the breakpoint within the *BCR* gene may predict the time to development of blast crisis, but this claim has been refuted by others. Heterogeneous structural alterations of the p53 gene, as well as structural alterations and lack of protein production of the retinoblastoma gene, have been associated with disease progression in a subset of patients. Rare patients show alterations in *RAS*. Sporadic reports also document the presence of an altered *MYC* (named after the myelocytomatosis virus) gene or the appearance of p190$^{BCR-ABL}$, the protein commonly found in adult ALL and occasionally in AML, during the clinical evolution of small numbers of patients with CML. Progressive de novo DNA methylation at the *BCR/ABL* locus has also been shown to herald blastic transformation. Finally, interleukin (IL)-1β may be involved in the progression of CML to the blastic phase. Multiple pathways to disease transformation exist, but the exact timing and relevance of each of these remains unclear.

CLINICAL PRESENTATION Symptoms The clinical onset of the chronic phase is generally insidious. Accordingly, some patients are diagnosed while still asymptomatic, during health screening tests; other patients present with fatigue, malaise, and weight loss or have symptoms resulting from splenic enlargement, such as early satiety and left upper quadrant pain or mass. Less common are features related to granulocyte or platelet dysfunction, such as infections, thrombosis, or bleeding. Occasionally, patients present with leukostatic manifestations due to severe leukocytosis or thrombosis such as vasoocclusive disease, cerebrovascular accidents, myocardial infarction, venous thrombosis, priapism, visual disturbances, and pulmonary insufficiency.

Progression of CML is associated with worsening symptoms. Unexplained fever, significant weight loss, increasing dose requirement of the drugs controlling the disease, bone and joint pain, bleeding, thrombosis, and infections suggest transformation into accelerated or blastic phases. Fewer than 10 to 15% of newly diagnosed patients present with accelerated disease or with de novo blastic phase CML.

Physical Findings In most patients the abnormal finding on physical examination at diagnosis is minimal to moderate splenomegaly; mild hepatomegaly is found occasionally. Persistent splenomegaly despite continued therapy is a sign of disease acceleration. Lymphadenopathy and extramedullary myeloid tumors (granulocytic sarcomas) are unusual except late in the course of the disease; when they are present, the prognosis is poor.

Hematologic Findings Elevated white blood cell counts, with various degrees of immaturity of the granulocytic series, are present at diagnosis. Usually $<$5% circulating blasts and $<$10% blasts and promyelocytes are noted. Cycling of the counts may be observed in patients followed without treatment. Platelet counts are almost always elevated at diagnosis, and a mild degree of normochromic normocytic anemia is present. Leukocyte alkaline phosphatase is characteristically low in CML cells. Serum levels of vitamin B$_{12}$ and vitamin B$_{12}$–binding proteins are generally elevated. Phagocytic functions are usually normal at diagnosis and remain normal during the chronic phase. Histamine production secondary to basophilia is increased in later stages, causing pruritus, diarrhea, and flushing.

At diagnosis, bone marrow cellularity, primarily of the myeloid and megakaryocytic lineages, with a greatly altered myeloid to ery-throid ratio, is increased in almost all patients with CML. The marrow blast percentage is generally normal or slightly elevated. Marrow or blood basophilia, eosinophilia, and monocytosis may be present. While collagen fibrosis in the marrow is unusual at presentation, sig-nificant degrees of reticulin stain–measured fibrosis are noted in about half of the patients.

Disease acceleration is defined by the development of increasing degrees of anemia unaccounted for by bleeding or chemotherapy, cyto-genetic clonal evolution, or blood or marrow blasts between 10 and 20%, blood or marrow basophils ≥20%, or platelet count <100,000/μL. *Blast crisis* is defined as acute leukemia, with blood or marrow blasts ≥20%. Hyposegmented neutrophils may appear (Pelger-Huët anomaly). Blast cells can be classified as myeloid, lymphoid, ery-throid, or undifferentiated, based on morphologic, cytochemical, and immunologic features. About half the cases are myeloid, one-third lymphoid, 10% erythroid, and the rest are undifferentiated.

Chromosomal Findings   The cytogenetic hallmark of CML, found in 90 to 95% of patients, is the t(9;22)(q34;q11). Originally, this was recognized by the presence of a shortened chromosome 22 (22q-), designated as the *Philadelphia chromosome*, that arises from the reciprocal 9;22 translocation. Some patients may have complex translocations (designated as *variant translocations*) involving three, four, or five chromosomes (usually including chromosomes 9 and 22). However, the molecular consequences of these changes appear similar to those resulting from the typical t(9;22).

PROGNOSTIC FACTORS   The clinical outcome of patients with CML is variable. Death is expected in 10% of patients within 2 years and in about 20% yearly thereafter. The median survival time is ~4 years. Therefore, several prognostic models that identify different risk groups in CML have been developed. The most commonly used staging systems have been derived from multivariate analyses of prog-nostic factors. The Sokal index identified percentage of circulating blasts, spleen size, platelet count, cytogenetic clonal evolution, and age as the most important prognostic indicators. Two models, that of Tura and the combined model of Kantarjian, divide patients according to the number of negative prognostic factors. Age ≥60 years, spleen ≥10 cm below the costal margin, blasts ≥3% in blood or ≥5% in marrow, basophils ≥7% in blood or ≥3% in marrow, platelets ≥700,000/μL, or any of the characteristics of accelerated disease are associated with a very poor short-term prognosis and a threefold higher hazard rate, or risk of death per unit of time, in the first year. A prog-nostic scoring system to estimate the survival of CML patients treated with interferon (IFN) α has been developed.

℞ TREATMENT   The goal of therapy in CML is to achieve pro-longed, durable, nonneoplastic, nonclonal hematopoiesis, which entails the eradication of any residual cells containing the BCR/ABL transcript. Hence the goal is complete molecular remission and cure (Table 111-4). A proposed treatment plan for the newly diagnosed patient with CML is presented in Fig. 111-2.

Allogeneic SCT   Allogeneic SCT is the only curative therapy for CML and, when feasible, is the treatment of choice. However, it is complicated by a high early mortality rate owing to the transplant procedure. When the outcome of all patients undergoing allogeneic SCT reported to the International Bone Marrow Transplant Registry was compared with the outcome of all patients treated with hydroxy-urea or interferon (IFN) α by the German CML Study Group, the survival for the former group was statistically better, but only starting 5 years after transplant. When only low-risk patients (by Sokal's cri-teria) were evaluated, the benefit in survival for allogeneic SCT was seen after 6 years. Outcome of SCT depends on multiple factors in-cluding: (1) the patient (i.e., age and phase of disease); (2) the type of donor [i.e., syngeneic (monozygotic twins) or HLA-compatible allo-geneic, related or unrelated]; (3) the preparative regimen; (4) GVHD; and (5) posttransplantation treatment.

Table 111-4   Response Criteria in CML

Hematologic	
Complete response[a]	White blood cell count <10,000/μL, normal morphology
	Normal hemoglobin and platelet counts
Incomplete response	White blood cell count ≥10,000/μL
Cytogenetic	Percentage of bone marrow metaphases with t(9;22)
Complete response	0
Partial response	≤35
Minor response	36–85[b]
No response	85–100
Molecular	Presence of BCR/ABL transcript by RT-PCR
Complete response	None
Incomplete response	Any

[a] Complete hematologic response requires the disappearance of splenomegaly.
[b] Up to 15% normal metaphases are occasionally seen at diagnosis (when 30 metaphases are analyzed).

The patient   As experience has been gained and safety and effi-cacy have been established, it has become clear that patients should be younger than 65 years and have a healthy and histocompatible donor. Furthermore, survival after SCT in the accelerated and blastic phases of the disease is significantly diminished and is associated with a very high rate of relapse. The Seattle data demonstrate that SCT early in the chronic phase (1 to 2 years from diagnosis) is superior to later SCT. While overall survival, disease-free survival, and relapse rates are not influenced by prior IFN-α treatment, incidence and se-verity of acute and chronic GVHD correlate with prior IFN-α treatment in the unrelated donor and possibly also in the related donor setting. Therefore, because early SCT is more effective than late SCT, the decision to perform allogeneic SCT should probably be made within a year of diagnosis when IFN-α is the initial therapy; a 3-month hiatus is recommended between discontinuing IFN-α and initiating SCT.

The donor   Transplantation from a family donor, who is either fully matched or mismatched at only one HLA locus, should be con-sidered standard therapy for any patient with CML who is a candidate for an HLA-related sibling transplant. Syngeneic SCT in patients with chronic phase CML has been reported from the Seattle group to result in 7-year disease-free survival in 55%, with a 30% relapse rate. With HLA-identical sibling SCT in the chronic phase, many groups have reported 5-year disease-free survival in 40 to 70% of patients, with a 25% relapse rate. SCT from an HLA-matched unrelated donor has

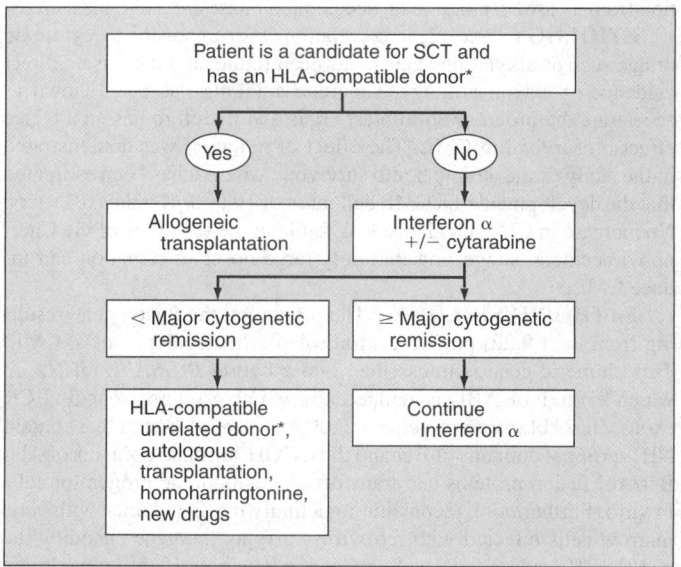

FIGURE 111-2   Flow chart for the therapy of newly diagnosed CML. Please refer to text for details. The asterisk denotes that some centers use an HLA-compatible unrelated donor for SCT at this time and some only use unrelated donors if interferon α fails.

been reported by the Seattle group to result in a 74% probability of surviving 3 years for patients transplanted in chronic phase less than 1 year from diagnosis and younger than 50 years. A 2-year disease-free (based on hematologic analyses) survival of 45% (±21%) for patients receiving SCT from unrelated individuals, matched or mismatched at only one locus, transplanted less than 1 year from diagnosis was reported by the National Marrow Donor Program. Patients age 40 to 50 years fared poorly (15 of 55 survived). The probability of 2-year disease-free (based on cytogenetic analyses) survival in a report on unrelated transplants from the Medical College of Wisconsin, using a standardized conditioning regimen and T cell depletion, was 52% for patients transplanted in chronic phase (regardless of the time from diagnosis). Patients receiving transplants from unrelated individuals have higher rates of graft failure and acute and chronic GVHD and prolonged convalescence after treatment, compared to those who receive allogeneic transplants from related individuals. Peripheral blood is now being studied as a source of hematopoietic progenitor cells; it may offer rapid engraftment and less risk for the donor. Umbilical-cord blood may permit mismatched SCT with notably less GVHD; graft-versus-leukemia (GVL) effects do not appear to be impaired. A problem with cord blood is obtaining an appropriate number of progenitor cells to reconstitute hematopoiesis in an adult.

Preparative regimens These regimens have been studied by several groups. A randomized study by the Seattle group compared cyclophosphamide and total-body irradiation with busulphan and cyclophosphamide. They found no significant differences in the 3-year probabilities of survival, relapse, event-free survival, speed of engraftment, or incidence of venoocclusive disease of the liver. Significantly more patients in the total-body irradiation arm experienced major elevations of creatinine, acute GVHD, longer periods of fever, positive blood cultures, hospital admissions, and longer inpatient hospital stays. However, increased chronic GVHD, obstructive bronchiolitis and alopecia were noted with busulphan. Intravenous busulphan may permit better control of serum levels. Minitransplants in which the preparative regimen is aimed at eliminating host lymphocytes rather than bone marrow are being tested. Reduced toxicity with preserved antitumor efficacy is the goal.

Development and type of GVHD Development of grade I GVHD, as compared to no GVHD, decreases the risk of relapse. A lower relapse rate was observed also in patients with grade II GVHD but was accompanied by a substantially higher transplant-related mortality rate. The decreased relapse rate may be caused by a GVL effect. Depletion of T lymphocytes from donor marrow can prevent GVHD but results in an increased risk of relapse, which exceeds the relapse rate after syngeneic SCT. Thus, T lymphocytes from the donor marrow mediate a significant antileukemic, or GVL, effect, and even syngeneic marrow may exhibit limited GVL activity in CML.

Posttransplantation treatment Further support for the existence of an immunologically mediated GVL effect comes from the observation that donor leukocyte infusions (without prior conditioning or GVHD prophylaxis) can induce hematologic and cytogenetic remissions in patients with CML who have relapsed after allogeneic SCT.

The activity of IFN-α in patients with early chronic-phase CML was the basis for the use of IFN-α after SCT, either to induce cytogenetic remissions in relapsed patients or to prevent relapse after SCT for high-risk patients. The main concern about IFN-α use after allogeneic SCT has been the development or worsening of GVHD, because IFN-α acts as an immunomodulator. However, in published reports encompassing 52 allogeneic recipients who were free of GVHD and were either at high risk for relapse or had already relapsed, only 6 subsequently developed GVHD after IFN-α therapy was initiated. IFN-α has also been combined with mononuclear cells obtained from donor blood to induce cytogenetic remissions in relapsed patients. Cytogenetic remissions have been achieved, but the exact role of IFN-α as opposed to the mononuclear cells is unclear. IL-2, with or without IFN-α, is also being evaluated for its ability to restore complete cytogenetic remission in patients who suffer relapses after SCT.

IFN-α has been used after SCT to prevent relapse in patients with

advanced disease at time of transplant (patients at high risk for relapse). Cytogenetic CR has been maintained for as long as 2 years posttransplantation in small numbers of patients with blast crisis or second chronic phase. Similarly, IL-2 (2.5×10^6 to 6×10^6 units/m^2 per day) has been given to patients after T cell–depleted allogeneic SCT in an effort to induce GVL without GVHD, and thus prevent relapse. Compared with historical control subjects, patients treated with IL-2 have a lower risk of disease relapse. A randomized trial is warranted.

Interferons When allogeneic SCT is not feasible, IFN-α therapy is the treatment of choice. The interferons are a complex group of naturally occurring proteins produced by eukaryotic cells in response to viruses, antigens, and mitogens. Three distinct groups of IFN species have been identified: IFN-α, -β, and -γ. Although various interferons have become available for clinical investigation, most data have been generated with IFN-α preparations.

Interferons have potent, pleiotropic biologic effects, spanning a spectrum of antiviral, microbicidal, immunomodulatory, and antiproliferative properties. While interferons downregulate the expression of several oncogenes and cytokines, they also upregulate the expression of IFN regulatory factor-1 (a transcriptional activator with antioncogenic activity), adhesion molecules, and the histocompatibility genes. Interferons also inhibit angiogenesis and induce a cellular immune response. However, their mode(s) of action are still unknown.

In seven randomized studies comparing IFN-α and chemotherapy, both modalities have been found to be effective in achieving hematologic remissions. However, patients treated with IFN-α survived longer than patients treated with hydroxyurea or busulphan. The 5-year survival rate was 51% with IFN-α and 42% with chemotherapy.

Patients develop both acute and chronic side effects from IFN-α therapy. Acute side effects (flulike symptoms) appear early in the course of the treatment. Most flulike symptoms respond to acetaminophen, and tachyphylaxis develops within 1 to 2 weeks. Chronic reactions, such as fatigue and lethargy, depression, weight loss, myalgias, and arthralgias, occur in about half of the patients and may require dose reduction. Patients also report cough, postnasal drip, and dryness of the skin. Infrequently, immune-mediated thrombocytopenia and anemia develop. In addition, long-term therapy has been associated with late autoimmune side effects, such as hypothyroidism and occasionally generalized autoimmune phenomena.

The most important persistent side effects in patients with CML who are treated with IFN-α are neurologic. All patients treated with IFN-α are subject to some neurologic toxicity, the most common symptom being lethargy. Up to 20% of patients have neurologic side effects that are associated with compromised quality of life and reduced ability to carry out their regular activity, such as full-time work. In addition, at the required doses, impotence in men is not infrequent.

Hematologic remissions are generally achieved within 1 to 2 months of starting IFN-α. However, some patients have a cyclic response pattern with progressively lower peak and nadir counts over a period of months. The increase in counts during the cycling that occurs in the first few months of therapy should not be confused with resistance. Cytogenetic responses generally start at 3 to 12 months, and complete cytogenetic responses may require 6 months to 4 years of therapy. However, most complete cytogenetic responses are achieved within 12 to 18 months; and in single-agent, single-arm studies they have been identified in up to 26% of patients.

The combination of IFN-α with cytarabine has produced better results than those with IFN-α alone; cytogenetic responses occurred earlier, but the influence on survival is not yet known.

Chemotherapy Initial management of patients with chemotherapy is currently reserved for rapid lowering of white blood cell counts, reduction of symptoms, and reversal of symptomatic splenomegaly. Hydroxyurea, a ribonucleotide reductase inhibitor, induces rapid disease control. The initial dose is 1 to 4 g/d, and the dose should be reduced by half with each 50% reduction of the leukocyte count. Unfortunately, cytogenetic remissions with hydroxyurea are uncommon. Busulphan, an alkylating agent that acts on early progenitor cells, has a more prolonged effect. However, we do not recommend its use because of its serious side effects, which include unexpected, and occasionally fatal, myelosuppression in 5 to 10% of patients; pulmonary, endocardial, and marrow fibrosis; and an Addison-like wasting syndrome.

Homoharringtonine (HHT) is a plant alkaloid derived from a tree, *Cephalotaxus fortuneii* sp. *harringtonii*. HHT blocks peptide bond formation after binding of the aminoacyl-transfer RNA to the ribosome. In patients whose disease progressed during treatment with IFN-α or who were in later chronic phase (>1 year from diagnosis), HHT induced 72% complete hematologic responses and 22% complete or major cytogenetic responses. The use of HHT before IFN-α in early chronic phase resulted in a 92% complete hematologic response rate and a 27% major cytogenetic response rate. Toxicity is mainly related to myelosuppression.

Intensive combination chemotherapy has also been used in chronic phase CML, with 30 to 50% of patients achieving complete cytogenetic responses. However these cytogenetic remissions have been short lived. Consequently, intensive combination chemotherapy regimens are being used today only to mobilize normal progenitors in the blood in order to collect circulating stem cells for autologous transplantation.

Autologous SCT   Autologous SCT could potentially cure CML if a means to select the residual normal progenitors, which coexist with their malignant counterparts, could be developed. As a source of autologous hematopoietic stem cells for transplantation, blood offers certain advantages over marrow (e.g., faster engraftment and no general anesthesia). Normal hematopoietic stem cells appear with increased frequency in the blood of patients with CML during the recovery phase after chemotherapy and G-CSF.

A retrospective analysis of >200 autologous SCT performed for CML at eight centers worldwide suggests that autologous SCT prolongs survival in chronic- or accelerated-phase patients when compared with conventional therapy. At transplant 93 patients were in chronic phase, 25 were in accelerated phase, and 114 were in blast crisis or second chronic phase. Patients received autologous bone marrow and/or blood hematopoietic stem cells. In 42 cases the hematopoietic progenitors were subjected to ex vivo manipulation by long-term bone marrow culture, by incubation with recombinant IFN-γ, or by chemotherapy. In 49 cases the hematopoietic progenitors were harvested during the recovery phase after various chemotherapy regimens. After autologous SCT, 29 of 93 (31%) patients in first chronic phase achieved complete cytogenetic remissions. The median duration of cytogenetic remission was 14 months, with a range of 2 to 68 months. Approaches to treat minimal residual disease after autologous transplantation, such as immune modulation, are currently being investigated.

Leukapheresis and Splenectomy   Intensive leukapheresis may control the blood counts in chronic phase CML; however, it is expensive and cumbersome. It is useful in emergencies where leukostasis-related complications such as pulmonary failure or cerebrovascular accidents are likely. It may also have a role in the treatment of pregnant women in whom it is important to avoid potentially teratogenic drugs.

Splenectomy was used in CML in the past because of the suggestion that evolution to the acute phase might occur in the spleen. However, this does not appear to be the case, and splenectomy is now reserved for symptomatic relief of painful splenomegaly unresponsive to chemotherapy or for significant anemia or thrombocytopenia associated with hypersplenism. Splenic radiation is used rarely to reduce the size of the spleen.

Minimal Residual Disease   The correlation between residual cells with the t(9;22) and disease recurrence is not completely understood. In initial studies with RT-PCR used to predict disease recurrence after IFN-α therapy, residual disease was found in all samples tested from patients with complete cytogenetic remissions. Later stud-

ies demonstrated the elimination of the BCR/ABL mRNA transcript after more prolonged IFN-α treatment in some cases. It is now possible to quantitate transcripts, and longer follow-up may indicate whether quantitation of the BCR/ABL transcript is useful for predicting cytogenetic and clinical relapse.

After allogeneic SCT, RT-PCR analysis may be positive for residual disease during the first 6 months in patients who subsequently achieve a long-lasting remission. However, late persistence of RT-PCR positivity appears to indicate a reduced probability of cure. RT-PCR positivity at any single time point is not predictive of imminent relapse. After allogeneic SCT, patients are often divided according to RT-PCR results into one of three groups: (1) persistently positive, (2) intermittently negative, and (3) persistently negative. These three groups have low, intermediate, and high probability of maintaining remission and disease free-survival, respectively. Although these data suggest that patients who are persistently RT-PCR positive more than 6 months after allogeneic SCT need additional therapeutic interventions, this conclusion has not been rigorously established. The studies have used an assortment of techniques for measuring minimal residual disease, the level of sensitivity has been variable, and the follow-up durations of patients are short. Real-time RT-PCR may provide a more sensitive tool to predict relapse in CML and in other cancers. In patients who do not have any evidence for GVHD and are intermittently RT-PCR negative, GVL may be induced by alloreactive donor cells (without the side effects of GVHD) to suppress the proliferation of the leukemic cells.

Future Directions   The synthetic inhibitor of the BCR/ABL kinase, STI571, induces selective inhibition in the growth of t(9;22)-bearing tumor cells in vitro and some responses in patients. Inhibition of *RAS* with a farnesyl transferase inhibitor that blocks its insertion into the membrane may have antitumor activity in CML on the basis of early clinical trials. Preclinical efforts to use BCR/ABL peptides as a tumor vaccine appear promising. The use of BCR/ABL antisense oligonucleotides to purge residual leukemic cells from autologous hematopoietic progenitors before reinfusion, as well as approaches to induce GVL in the setting of minimal residual disease without inducing GVHD, are underway.

Treatment of Blast Crisis   The treatment for all forms of blast crisis is generally ineffective. Treatment is tailored to the phenotype of the blast cell. Myeloid crises and erythroid crisis are treated as for AML, but remissions occur in only a minority of cases and are generally short lived. Patients may present without having had a chronic phase. AML with a t(9;22) is probably blast crisis of CML and carries a poor prognosis.

Lymphoid blast crisis is treated like ALL (Chap. 112) with vincristine (1.4 mg/m^2 weekly) plus prednisone (60 mg/m^2 orally qd) induction therapy with or without an anthracycline. About one-third of patients will reenter chronic phase after 2 to 3 weeks of treatment, but the remissions last only a median of ~4 months. Even SCT is minimally effective during blast crises. Novel treatment approaches are needed.

BIBLIOGRAPHY

BLOOMFIELD CD et al: Frequency of prolonged remission duration following high-dose cytarabine intensification in acute myeloid leukemia varies by cytogenetic subtype. Cancer Res 58:4173, 1998

DRUKER BJ, LYDON NB: Lessons learned from the development of an abl tyrosine kinase inhibitor. Clin Invest 105:3, 2000

FADERL S et al: The biology of chronic myeloid leukemia. N Engl J Med 341:164, 1999

HIDDEMANN W et al: Management of acute myeloid leukemia in elderly patients. J Clin Oncol 17:3569, 1999

LOWENBERG B et al: Acute myeloid leukemia. N Engl J Med 341:1051, 1999

SAWYERS CL: Chronic myeloid leukemia. N Engl J Med 340:1330, 1999

SILVER RT et al: An evidence-based analysis of the effect of busulfan, hydroxyurea, interferon, and allogeneic bone marrow transplantation in treating the chronic phase of chronic myeloid leukemia: Developed for the American Society of Hematology. Blood 94:1517, 1999

SLACK JL: The biology and treatment of acute progranulocytic leukemia. Curr Opin Oncol 11:93, 1999

MALIGNANCIES OF LYMPHOID CELLS

ABVD	doxorubicin, bleomycin, vinblastine, and dacarbazine	EBV	Epstein-Barr virus
ALLs	acute lymphoid leukemias	HTLV	human T cell lymphotropic virus
ATL	adult T cell lymphoma	IPI	International Prognostic Index
CHOP	cyclophosphamide, doxorubicin, vincristine, and prednisone	LDH	lactate dehydrogenase
		MALT	mucosa-associated lymphoid tissue
CLL	chronic lymphoid leukemia	MOPP	mechlorethamine, vincristine, procarbazine, and prednisone
CNS	central nervous system		
CT	computed tomography	NK	natural killer
CVP	cyclophosphamide, vincristine, and prednisone		

Malignancies of lymphoid cells range from the most indolent to the most aggressive human malignancies. These cancers arise from cells of the immune system at different stages of differentiation, resulting in a wide range of morphologic, immunologic, and clinical findings. Advances in our understanding of the normal immune system have allowed a better understanding of these sometimes confusing disorders.

Some malignancies of lymphoid cells almost always present as leukemia (i.e., primary involvement of bone marrow and blood), while others almost always present as lymphomas (i.e., solid tumors of the immune system). However, other malignancies of lymphoid cells can present as either leukemia or lymphoma. In addition, the clinical pattern can change over the course of the illness. This change is more often seen in a patient who seems to have a lymphoma and then develops the manifestations of leukemia over the course of the illness.

BIOLOGY OF LYMPHOID MALIGNANCIES: CONCEPTS OF THE WHO CLASSIFICATION OF LYMPHOID MALIGNANCIES

The classification of lymphoid malignancy evolved steadily throughout the twentieth century. The distinction between leukemia and lymphoma was made early, and separate classification systems were developed for each. Leukemias were first divided into acute and chronic subtypes based on average survival. Chronic leukemias were easily subdivided into those of lymphoid or myeloid origin based on morphologic characteristics. However, in recent years, a spectrum of diseases that were formerly all called chronic lymphoid leukemia has become apparent (Table 112-1). The acute leukemias were usually malignancies of blast cells with few identifying characteristics. When cytochemical stains became available, it was possible to divide these objectively into myeloid malignancies and acute leukemias of lymphoid cells. Acute leukemias of lymphoid cells have been subdivided based on morphologic characteristics by the French-American-British (FAB) group (Table 112-2). Using this system, lymphoid malignancies of small uniform blasts (e.g., typical childhood acute lymphoblastic

Table 112-1 Lymphoid Disorders that Can Present as "Chronic Leukemia" and Be Confused with Typical B Cell Chronic Lymphoid Leukemia.

Follicular lymphoma
Splenic marginal zone lymphoma
Nodal marginal zone lymphoma
Mantle cell lymphoma
Hairy cell leukemia
Prolymphocytic leukemia (B cell or T cell)
Lymphoplasmacytic lymphoma
Sézary syndrome
Smoldering adult T cell leukemia/lymphoma

Table 112-2 Classification of Acute Lymphoid Leukemia (ALL)

Immunologic Subtype	% of Cases	FAB Subtype	Cytogenetic Abnormalities
Pre-B ALL	75	L1, L2	t(9;22), t(4;11), t(1;19)
T cell ALL	20	L1, L2	14q11 or 7q34
B cell ALL	5	L3	t(8;14), t(8;22), t(2;8)

NOTE: FAB, French-American-British classification.

leukemia) were called L1, lymphoid malignancies with larger and more variable size cells were called L2, and lymphoid malignancies of uniform cells with basophilic and sometimes vacuolated cytoplasm were called L3 (e.g., typical Burkitt's lymphoma cells). Acute leukemias of lymphoid cells have also been subdivided based on immunologic (i.e., T vs. B) and cytogenetic abnormalities (Table 112-2). Major cytogenetic subgroups include the t(9;22) (e.g., Philadelphia chromosome–positive acute lymphoblastic leukemia) and the t(8;14) found in the L3 or Burkitt's leukemia.

Non-Hodgkin's lymphomas were separated from Hodgkin's disease by recognition of the Sternberg-Reed cells early in the twentieth century. The first systematic classification for non-Hodgkin's lymphomas was proposed by Gall and Mallory in the first half of the twentieth century and divided non-Hodgkin's lymphomas into giant follicular lymphoma, lymphosarcoma, and reticulum cell sarcoma. Unfortunately, this fairly simple system proved to be imprecise in its definitions and only marginally clinically useful. In the 1950s, Henry Rappaport and colleagues recognized the importance of growth pattern in subdividing non-Hodgkin's lymphomas and used pattern in addition to cell size and shape as the basis for a new classification that proved more clinically relevant. In the 1970s, it was recognized that non-Hodgkin's lymphomas were all tumors of lymphocytes and were derived from either T or B cells. This led to immunologically based classifications of lymphomas such as the Lukes-Collins classification in the United States and the Kiel classification proposed by Lennert and associates in Europe. In an attempt to unify terminology and improve the effectiveness of communication between pathologists and clinicians, the Working Formulation was proposed in 1982. Over the next two decades the Kiel classification dominated clinical practice in Europe, whereas the Working Formulation became the main classification system used in North America.

In the past two decades, increased understanding of the immune system and the genetic abnormalities associated with non-Hodgkin's lymphoma have led to the identification of several previously unrecognized types of lymphoma. The recognition of these new and clinically relevant lymphomas led to proposals for changing existing classifications. A new proposal that is part of the basis of the new World Health Organization classification of lymphoid malignancies takes into account morphologic, clinical, immunologic, and genetic information and attempts to divide non-Hodgkin's lymphomas and other lymphoid malignancies into clinical/pathological entities that have clinical and therapeutic relevance. This system is presented in Table 112-3. Clinical studies have shown that this new system is clinically relevant and has a higher degree of diagnostic accuracy than those used previously. The possibilities for subdividing lymphoid malignancies are extensive. However, Table 112-3 presents in bold those malignancies that occur in at least 1% of patients. Specific lymphoma subtypes will be dealt with in more detail below.

GENERAL ASPECTS OF LYMPHOID MALIGNANCIES

ETIOLOGY AND EPIDEMIOLOGY Chronic lymphoid leukemia (CLL) is the most prevalent form of leukemia in western countries. It occurs most frequently in older adults and is exceedingly rare in children. Approximately 13,000 new cases are diagnosed in the

Table 112-3 WHO Classification of Lymphoid Malignancies

B Cell	T Cell	Hodgkin's Disease
Precursor B cell neoplasm	Precursor T cell neoplasm	Nodular lymphocyte-predominant Hodgkin's disease
Precursor B lymphoblastic leukemia/lymphoma (precursor B cell acute lymphoblastic leukemia)	**Precursor T lymphoblastic lymphoma/leukemia (precursor T cell acute lymphoblastic leukemia)**	
Mature (peripheral) B cell neoplasms	Mature (peripheral) T cell neoplasms	Classical Hodgkin's disease
B cell chronic lymphocytic leukemia/small lymphocytic lymphoma	T cell prolymphocytic leukemia	Nodular sclerosis Hodgkin's disease
B cell prolymphocytic leukemia	T cell granular lymphocytic leukemia	Lymphocyte-rich classical Hodgkin's disease
Lymphoplasmacytic lymphoma	Aggressive NK cell leukemia	Mixed-cellularity Hodgkin's disease
Splenic marginal zone B cell lymphoma (± villous lymphocytes)	Adult T cell lymphoma/leukemia (HTLV-I+)	Lymphocyte-depletion Hodgkin's disease
Hairy cell leukemia	Extranodal NK/T cell lymphoma, nasal type	
Plasma cell myeloma/plasmacytoma	Enteropathy-type T cell lymphoma	
Extranodal marginal zone B cell lymphoma of MALT type	Hepatosplenic γδ T cell lymphoma	
Mantle cell lymphoma	Subcutaneous panniculitis-like T cell lymphoma	
Follicular lymphoma	**Mycosis fungoides/Sézary syndrome**	
Nodal marginal zone B cell lymphoma (± monocytoid B cells)	Anaplastic large cell lymphoma, primary cutaneous type	
Diffuse large B cell lymphoma	**Peripheral T cell lymphoma, not otherwise specified (NOS)**	
Burkitt's lymphoma/Burkitt cell leukemia	**Angioimmunoblastic T cell lymphoma**	
	Anaplastic large cell lymphoma, primary systemic type	

NOTE: HTLV, human T cell lymphotropic virus; MALT, mucosa-associated lymphoid tissue; NK, natural killer; WHO, World Health Organization.
SOURCE: Adapted from Harris et al.

United States each year, but because of the prolonged survival associated with this disorder, the total prevalence is many times higher. CLL is more common in men than in women and more common in whites than in blacks. This is an uncommon malignancy in Asia. The etiologic factors for typical CLL are unknown.

In contrast to CLL, acute lymphoid leukemias (ALLs) are predominantly cancers of children and young adults. The L3 or Burkitt's leukemia occurring in children in developing countries seems to be associated with infection by the Epstein-Barr virus (EBV) in infancy. However, the explanation for the etiology of more common subtypes of ALL is much less certain. Childhood ALL occurs more often in higher socioeconomic subgroups. Children with trisomy 21 (Down's syndrome) have an increased risk for childhood acute lymphoblastic leukemia as well as acute myeloid leukemia. Exposure to high-energy radiation in early childhood increases the risk of developing T cell acute lymphoblastic leukemia.

The etiology of ALL in adults is also uncertain. ALL is unusual in middle-aged adults but increases in incidence in the elderly. However, acute myeloid leukemia is still much more common in these patients. Environmental exposures including certain industrial exposures, exposure to agricultural chemicals, and smoking might increase the risk of developing ALL as an adult.

The cell of origin of Hodgkin's disease has not been determined definitively, but molecular evidence suggests that most are of B cell origin. The incidence of Hodgkin's disease appears fairly stable, with approximately 8000 new cases diagnosed each year in the United States. Hodgkin's disease is more common in whites than in blacks

and more common in males than in females. A bimodal distribution of age at diagnosis has been observed, with one peak incidence occurring in patients in their 20s and the other in those in their 80s. Patients in the younger age groups diagnosed in the United States largely have the nodular sclerosing subtype of Hodgkin's disease. Elderly patients, patients infected with HIV, and patients in third world countries more commonly have mixed-cellularity Hodgkin's disease or lymphocyte-depleted Hodgkin's disease. Infection by HIV is a risk factor for developing Hodgkin's disease. In addition, an association between infection by EBV and Hodgkin's disease has been demonstrated. A monoclonal or oligoclonal proliferation of EBV-infected cells in 20 to 40% of the patients with Hodgkin's disease has led to proposals for this virus having an etiologic role in Hodgkin's disease. However, the matter is not settled definitively.

For unknown reasons, non-Hodgkin's lymphomas have increased in frequency in the United States at the rate of 4% per year since 1950. Almost 60,000 new cases of non-Hodgkin's lymphoma were diagnosed in the United States in the year 2000. Non-Hodgkin's lymphomas are more frequent in the elderly and more frequent in men. Patients with both primary and secondary immunodeficiency states are predisposed to developing non-Hodgkin's lymphomas. These include patients with HIV infection; patients who have undergone organ transplantation; and patients with inherited immune deficiencies, the sicca syndrome, and rheumatoid arthritis.

The incidence of non-Hodgkin's lymphomas and the patterns of expression of the various subtypes differ geographically. T cell lymphomas are more common in Asia than in western countries, while certain subtypes of B cell lymphomas such as follicular lymphoma are more common in western countries. A specific subtype of non-Hodgkin's lymphoma known as the angiocentric nasal T/natural killer (NK) cell lymphoma has a striking geographic occurrence, being most frequent in Southern Asia and parts of Latin America. Another subtype of non-Hodgkin's lymphoma associated with infection by human T cell lymphotropic virus (HTLV) I is seen particularly in southern Japan and the Caribbean.

A number of environmental factors have been implicated in the occurrence of non-Hodgkin's lymphoma, including infectious agents, chemical exposures, and medical treatments. Several studies have demonstrated an association between exposure to agricultural chemicals and an increased incidence in non-Hodgkin's lymphoma. Patients treated for Hodgkin's disease can develop non-Hodgkin's lymphoma; it is unclear whether this is a consequence of the Hodgkin's disease or its treatment. However, the infectious etiology of non-Hodgkin's lymphoma is the area where evidence has been expanding most rapidly in recent years. Table 112-4 illustrates those infectious agents associated with the development of non-Hodgkin's lymphoma. HTLV-I infects T cells and leads directly to the development of adult T cell lymphoma (ATL) in a small percentage of infected patients. The cumulative lifetime risk of developing lymphoma in an infected patient is 2.5%. The virus is transmitted by infected lymphocytes ingested by nursing babies of infected mothers, blood-borne transmission, or sexually. The median age of patients with ATL is about 56 years, emphasizing the long latency.

EBV is associated with the development of Burkitt's lymphoma

Infectious Agent	Lymphoid Malignancy
Epstein-Barr virus	Burkitt's lymphoma
	Post–organ transplant lymphoma
	Primary CNS diffuse large B cell lymphoma
	Hodgkin's disease
	Extranodal NK/T cell lymphoma, nasal type
HTLV-I	Adult T cell leukemia/lymphoma
HIV	Diffuse large B cell lymphoma
	Burkitt's lymphoma
Hepatitis C virus	Lymphoplasmacytic lymphoma
Helicobacter pylori	Gastric MALT lymphoma
Human herpesvirus 8	Primary effusion lymphoma
	Multicentric Castleman's disease

NOTE: CNS, central nervous system; HTLV, human T cell lymphotropic virus; MALT, mucosa-associated lymphoid tissue; NK, natural killer.

in Central Africa and the occurrence of aggressive non-Hodgkin's lymphomas in immunosuppressed patients in western countries. EBV infection is strongly associated with the occurrence of extranodal nasal T/NK cell lymphomas in Asia and South America. Infection with HIV predisposes to the development of aggressive, B cell non-Hodgkin's lymphoma. This may be through overexpression of interleukin 6 by infected macrophages. Infection of the stomach by the bacterium *Helicobacter pylori* induces the development of gastric MALT (mucosa-associated lymphoid tissue) lymphomas. This association is supported by evidence that patients treated with antibiotics to eradicate *H. pylori* have regression of their MALT lymphoma. The bacterium does not transform lymphocytes to produce the lymphoma; instead, a vigorous immune response is made to the bacterium and the chronic antigenic stimulation leads to the neoplasia.

Chronic hepatitis C virus infection has been associated with the development of lymphoplasmacytic lymphoma. Human herpesvirus 8 is associated with primary effusion lymphoma in HIV-infected persons and multicentric Castleman's disease, a diffuse lymphadenopathy associated with systemic symptoms of fever, malaise, and weight loss.

In addition to infectious agents, a number of other diseases or exposures may predispose to developing lymphoma (Table 112-5).

IMMUNOLOGY All lymphoid cells are derived from a common hematopoietic progenitor that gives rise to lymphoid, myeloid, erythroid, monocyte, and megakaryocyte lineages. Through the ordered and sequential activation of a series of transcription factors, the cell first becomes committed to the lymphoid lineage and then gives rise to B and T cells. About 75% of all lymphoid leukemias and 90% of all lymphomas are of B cell origin. A cell becomes committed to B cell development when it begins to rearrange its immunoglobulin genes. The sequence of cellular changes, including changes in cell-surface phenotype, that characterize normal B cell development are shown in Fig. 112-1. A cell becomes committed to T cell differentiation upon migration to the thymus and rearrangement of T cell antigen

Table 112-5 Diseases or Exposures Associated with Increased Risk of Development of Malignant Lymphoma

Inherited immunodeficiency disease	Autoimmune disease
Klinefelter's syndrome	Sjögren's syndrome
Chédiak-Higashi syndrome	Celiac sprue
Ataxia telangiectasia syndrome	Rheumatoid arthritis and systemic lupus erythematosus
Wiscott-Aldrich syndrome	
Common variable immunodeficiency disease	Chemical or drug exposures
	Phenytoin
Acquired immunodeficiency diseases	Dioxin, phenoxyherbicides
Iatrogenic immunosuppression	Radiation
HIV-1 infection	Prior chemotherapy and radiation therapy
Acquired hypogammaglobulinemia	

receptor genes. The sequence of the events that characterize T cell development are depicted in Fig. 112-2.

Although lymphoid malignancies often retain the cell-surface phenotype of lymphoid cells at particular stages of differentiation, this information is of little consequence. The so-called stage of differentiation of a malignant lymphoma does not predict its natural history. For example, the clinically most aggressive lymphoid leukemia is Burkitt's leukemia, which has the phenotype of a mature follicle center IgM-bearing B cell. Leukemias bearing the immunologic cell-surface phenotype of more primitive cells (e.g., pre-B ALL, CD10+) are less aggressive and more amenable to curative therapy than the "more mature" appearing Burkitt's leukemia cells. Furthermore, the apparent stage of differentiation of the malignant cell does not reflect the stage at which the genetic lesions that gave rise to the malignancy developed. For example, follicular lymphoma has the cell-surface phenotype of a follicle center cell, but its characteristic chromosomal translocation, the t(14;18), which involves juxtaposition of the anti-apoptotic *bcl-2* gene next to the immunoglobulin heavy chain gene (see below), had to develop early in ontogeny as an error in the process of immunoglobulin gene rearrangement. Why the subsequent steps that led to transformation became manifest in a cell of follicle center differentiation is not clear.

The major value of cell-surface phenotyping is to aid in the differential diagnosis of lymphoid tumors that appear similar by light microscopy. For example, benign follicular hyperplasia may resemble follicular lymphoma; however, the demonstration that all the cells bear the same immunoglobulin light chain isotype strongly suggests the mass is a clonal proliferation rather than a polyclonal response to an exogenous stimulus.

GENETIC CONSIDERATIONS Malignancies of lymphoid cells are associated with recurring genetic abnormalities. While specific genetic abnormalities have not been identified for all subtypes of lymphoid malignancies, it is presumed that they exist. Genetic abnormalities can be identified at a variety of levels including gross chromosomal changes (i.e., translocations, additions, or deletions); rearrangement of specific genes that may or may not be apparent from cytogenetic studies; and overexpression, underexpression, or mutation of specific oncogenes. Altered expression or mutation of specific proteins is particularly important. Many lymphomas contain balanced chromosomal translocations involving the antigen receptor genes; immunoglobulin genes on chromosomes 2, 14, and 22 in B cells; and T cell antigen receptor genes on chromosomes 7 and 14 in T cells. The rearrangement of chromosome segments to generate mature antigen receptors must create a site of vulnerability to aberrant recombination. B cells are even more susceptible to acquiring mutations during their maturation in germinal centers; the generation of antibody of higher affinity requires the introduction of mutations into the variable region genes in the germinal centers. Other nonimmunoglobulin genes, for example *bcl-6*, may acquire mutations as well.

In the case of diffuse large B cell lymphoma, the translocation t(14;18) occurs in approximately 30% of patients and leads to overexpression of the *bcl-2* gene found on chromosome 18. Some other patients without the translocation also overexpress the BCL-2 protein. This protein is involved in suppressing apoptosis—i.e., the mechanism of cell death most often induced by cytotoxic chemotherapeutic agents. A higher relapse rate has been observed in patients whose tumors overexpress the BCL-2 protein, but not in those patients whose lymphoma cells show only the translocation. Thus, particular genetic mechanisms have clinical ramifications.

Table 112-6 presents the best documented translocations and associated oncogenes for various subtypes of lymphoid malignancies. In some cases, such as the association of the t(14;18) in follicular lymphoma, the t(2;5) in anaplastic large T/null-cell lymphoma, the t(8;14) in Burkitt's lymphoma, and the t(11;14) in mantle cell lymphoma, the great majority of tumors in patients with these diagnoses display these

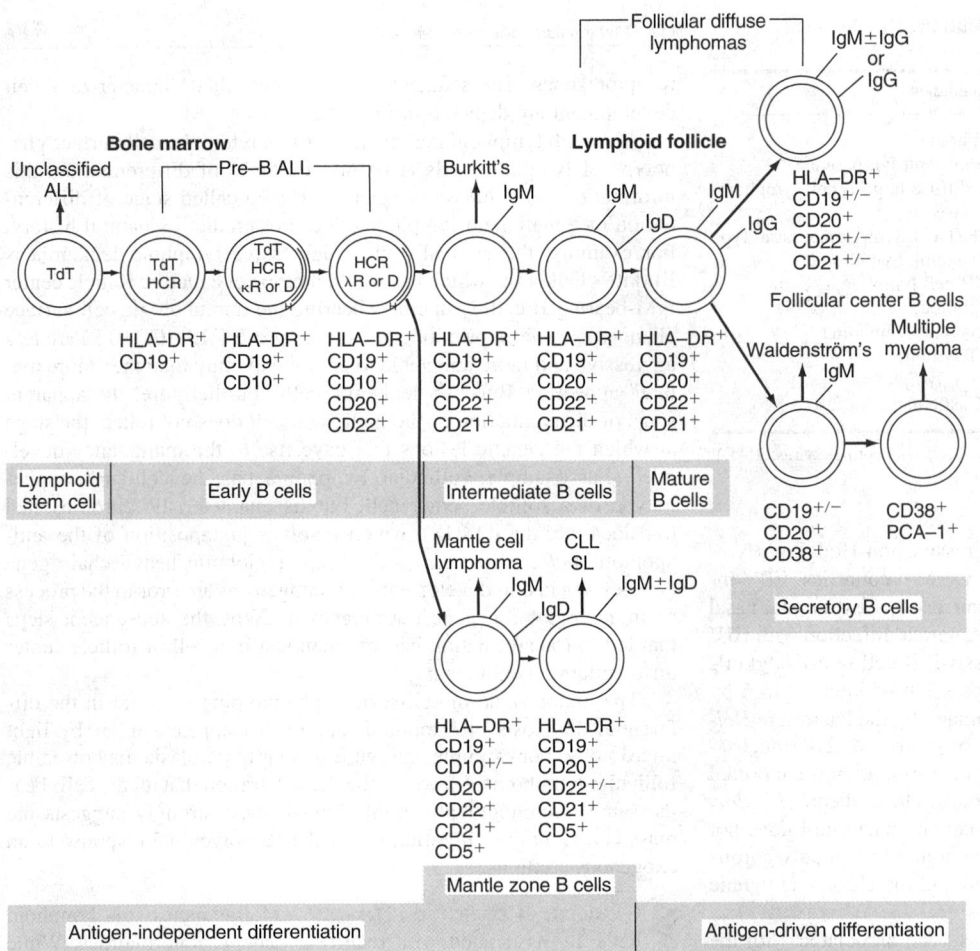

FIGURE 112-1 Pathway of normal B cell differentiation and relationship to B cell lymphomas. HLA-DR, CD10, CD19, CD20, CD21, CD22, CD5, and CD38 are cell markers used to distinguish stages of development. Terminal transferase (TdT) is a cellular enzyme. Immunoglobulin heavy chain gene rearrangement (HCR) and light chain gene rearrangement or deletion (κ R or D, λ R or D) occur early in B cell development. The approximate normal stage of differentiation associated with particular lymphomas is shown. ALL, acute lymphoid leukemia; CLL, chronic lymphoid leukemia; SL, small lymphocytic lymphoma.

abnormalities. In other types of lymphoma where a minority of the patients have tumors expressing specific genetic abnormalities, the defects may have prognostic significance. No specific genetic abnormalities have been identified in Hodgkin's disease.

In typical B cell CLL, trisomy 12 conveys a poorer prognosis. In ALL in both adults and children, genetic abnormalities have important prognostic significance. Patients whose tumor cells display the t(9;22) have a much poorer outlook than patients who do not have this translocation. Other genetic abnormalities that occur frequently in adults with ALL include the t(4;11) and the t(8;14). The t(4;11) is associated with younger age, female predominance, high white cell counts, and L1 morphology. The t(8;14) is associated with older age, male predominance, frequent central nervous system (CNS) involvement, and L3 morphology. Both are associated with a poor prognosis. In childhood ALL, hyperdiploidy has been shown to have a favorable prognosis. ■

Approach to the Patient

Regardless of the type of lymphoid malignancy, the initial evaluation of the patient should include performance of a careful history and physical examination. These will help confirm the diagnosis, identify those manifestations of the disease that might require prompt attention, and aid in the selection of further studies to optimally characterize the patient's status to allow the best choice of therapy. It is difficult to overemphasize the importance of a carefully done history and physical examination. They might provide observations that lead to reconsid-

ering the diagnosis, provide hints at etiology, clarify the stage, and allow the physician to establish rapport with the patient that will make it possible to develop and carry out a therapeutic plan.

For patients with ALL, evaluation is usually completed after a complete blood count, chemistry studies reflecting major organ function, a bone marrow biopsy with genetic and immunologic studies, and a lumbar puncture. The latter is necessary to rule out occult CNS involvement. At this point, most patients would be ready to begin therapy. In ALL, prognosis is dependent upon the genetic characteristics of the tumor, the patient's age, the white cell count, and the patient's overall clinical status and major organ function.

In CLL, the patient evaluation should include a complete blood count, chemistry tests to measure major organ function, serum protein electrophoresis, and a bone marrow biopsy. However, some physicians believe that the diagnosis would not always require a bone marrow biopsy. Patients often have imaging studies of the chest and abdomen looking for pathologic lymphadenopathy. Patients with typical B cell CLL can be subdivided into three major prognostic groups. Those patients with only blood and bone marrow involvement by leukemia but no lymphadenopathy, organomegaly, or signs of bone marrow failure have the best prognosis. Those with lymphadenopathy and organomegaly have an intermediate prognosis, and patients with bone marrow failure, defined as hemoglobin <100 g/L (10 g/dL) or platelet count <100,000/μL, have the worst prognosis. The

pathogenesis of the anemia or thrombocytopenia is important to discern. The prognosis is adversely affected when either or both of these abnormalities are due to progressive marrow infiltration and loss of productive marrow. However, either or both may be due to autoimmune phenomena or to hypersplenism that can develop during the course of the disease. These destructive mechanisms are usually completely reversible (glucocorticoids for autoimmune disease; splenectomy for hypersplenism) and do not influence disease prognosis.

Two popular staging systems have been developed to reflect these prognostic groupings (Table 112-7). Patients with typical B cell CLL can have their course complicated by immunologic abnormalities including autoimmune hemolytic anemia, autoimmune thrombocytopenia, and hypogammaglobulinemia. Patients with hypogammaglobulinemia benefit from regular (monthly) γ globulin administration. Because of expense, γ globulin is often withheld until the patient experiences a significant infection. These abnormalities do not have a clear prognostic significance and should not be used to assign a higher stage.

The initial evaluation of a patient with Hodgkin's disease or non-Hodgkin's lymphoma is similar. In both situations, the determination of an accurate anatomic stage is an important part of the evaluation. The staging system that is utilized is the Ann Arbor staging system originally developed for Hodgkin's disease (Table 112-8).

Evaluation of patients with Hodgkin's disease will typically include a complete blood count; erythrocyte sedimentation rate; chemistry studies reflecting major organ function; computed tomography

T CELL DIFFERENTIATION

THYMUS

T CELL MALIGNANCIES

Stage I
Prothymocyte

CD: 2, 7, 38, 71

Majority of
T cell ALL

Stage II
Thymocyte

CD: 1, 2, 4, 7, 8, 38

Minority of T-ALL
Majority of T-LL

Stage III
Thymocyte

CD: 2, 3, 4/8, 5, 6, 7; TCR

Minority of T-LL
Rare T-ALL

PERIPHERAL BLOOD AND NODES

Mature T Helper
Cell

CD: 2, 3, 4, 5, 6, 7; TCR

Majority of
T-CLL, CTCL,
Sezary Cell, NHL

Mature T Cytotoxic/
Suppressor Cell

CD: 2, 3, 4, 5, 6, 7; TCR

Minority of
T-CLL, NHL

FIGURE 112-2 Pathway of normal T cell differentiation and relationship to T cell lymphomas. CD1, CD2, CD3, CD4, CD5, CD6, CD7, CD8, CD38, and CD71 are cell markers used to distinguish stages of development. T cell antigen receptors (TCR) rearrange in the thymus, and mature T cells emigrate to nodes and peripheral blood. ALL, acute lymphoid leukemia; T-ALL, T cell ALL; T-LL, T cell lymphoblastic lymphoma; T-CLL, T cell chronic lymphoid leukemia; CTCL, cutaneous T cell lymphoma; NHL, non-Hodgkin's lymphoma.

(CT) scans of the chest, abdomen, and pelvis; and a bone marrow biopsy. A gallium scan is not necessary for primary staging, but when it is performed at the completion of therapy it allows evaluation of persistent radiographic abnormalities, particularly the mediastinum. In most cases, these studies will allow assignment of anatomic stage and the development of a therapeutic plan.

In patients with non-Hodgkin's lymphoma, the same evaluation

Table 112-6 Cytogenetic Translocation and Associated Oncogenes Often Seen in Lymphoid Malignancies

Disease	Cytogenetic Abnormality	Oncogene
CLL/small lymphocytic lymphoma	t(14;15)(q32;q13)	—
MALT lymphoma	t(11;18)(q21;q21)	—
Precursor B cell acute lymphoid leukemia	t(9;22)(q34;q11) or variant	BCR/ABL
	t(4;11)(q21;q23)	AF4, ALLI
Precursor acute lymphoid leukemia	t(9;22)	BCR, ABL
	t(1;19)	E2A, PBX
	t(17;19)	HLF, E2A
	t(5;14)	IL3, IGμ
Mantle cell lymphoma	t(11;14)(q13;q32)	BCL-1
Follicular lymphoma	t(14;18)(q32;q21)	BCL-2
Diffuse large-cell lymphoma	t(3;-)(q27;-)[a]	BCL-6
	t(17;-)(p13-)	p53
Burkitt's lymphoma, Burkitt's leukemia	t(8;-)(q24;-)[a]	C-MYC
CD30+ Anaplastic large cell lymphoma	t(2;5)(p23;q35)	ALK
Lymphoplasmacytoid lymphoma	t(9;14)(p13;q32)	—

[a] Numerous sites of translocation may be involved with these genes.
NOTE: CLL, chronic lymphoid leukemia; MALT, mucosa-associated lymphoid tissue.

described for patients with Hodgkin's disease is usually carried out. In addition, serum levels of lactate dehydrogenase (LDH) and β_2-microglobulin and serum protein electrophoresis are often included in the evaluation. Anatomic stage is assigned in the same manner as used for Hodgkin's disease. However, the prognosis of patients with non-Hodgkin's lymphoma is best assigned using the International Prognostic Index (IPI) (Table 112-9). This is a powerful predictor of outcome in all subtypes of non-Hodgkin's lymphoma. Patients are assigned an IPI score based on the presence or absence of five adverse prognostic factors and may have none or all five of these adverse prognostic factors. Figure 112-3 shows the prognostic significance of this score in 1300 patients with all types of non-Hodgkin's lymphoma.

CLINICAL FEATURES, TREATMENT, AND PROGNOSIS OF SPECIFIC LYMPHOID MALIGNANCIES

PRECURSOR CELL B CELL NEOPLASMS   Precursor B Cell Lymphoblastic Leukemia/Lymphoma   The most common cancer in childhood is B cell acute lymphoblastic leukemia (ALL). Although this disorder can also present as a lymphoma in either adults or children, presentation as lymphoma is quite rare.

The malignant cells in patients with precursor B cell lymphoblastic leukemia are most commonly of pre-B cell origin. Patients typically present with signs of bone marrow failure such as pallor, fatigue, bleeding, fever, and infection related to peripheral blood cytopenias. Peripheral blood counts regularly show anemia and thrombocytopenia but might show leukopenia, a normal leukocyte count, or leukocytosis based largely on the number of circulating malignant cells (**see Plate V-24**). Extranodal sites of disease are frequently involved in patients who present with leukemia, which might be manifested by lymphadenopathy, hepato- or splenomegaly, CNS disease, testicular enlargement, and/or cutaneous infiltration.

The diagnosis is usually made by bone marrow biopsy, which shows infiltration by malignant lymphoblasts. Demonstration of a pre-B cell immunophenotype (Fig. 112-1) and, often, characteristic cytogenetic abnormalities (Table 112-6) confirm the diagnosis. An adverse prognosis in patients with precursor B cell ALL is predicted by a very high white cell count, the presence of symptomatic CNS disease, and unfavorable cytogenetic abnormalities. For example, t(9;22) is frequently found in adults with B cell lymphoblastic leukemia and is associated with a very poor outlook.

TREATMENT   The treatment of patients with precursor B cell lymphoblastic leukemia involves remission induction with combination chemotherapy, a consolidation phase that includes administration of high-dose systemic therapy and treatment to eliminate disease in the CNS, and a period of continuing therapy to prevent relapse and effect cure. The overall cure rate in children is 85%, while about 50% of adults are long-term disease-free survivors. This reflects the high proportion of adverse cytogenetic abnormalities seen in adults with precursor B cell lymphoblastic leukemia.

Precursor B cell lymphoblastic lymphoma is a rare presentation of precursor B cell lymphoblastic malignancy. These patients often have a rapid transformation to leukemia, and similar treatment approaches as are used in patients presenting with leukemia are appropriate. In the few patients who present with the disease confined to lymph nodes, a high cure rate has been reported.

MATURE (PERIPHERAL) B CELL NEOPLASMS
B Cell Chronic Lymphoid Leukemia/Small Lymphocytic Lymphoma   B cell CLL/small lymphocytic lymphoma represents by far the most common lymphoid leukemia, and when presenting as a lymphoma, it accounts for ~7% of non-Hodgkin's lymphomas. As the name implies, presentation can be as either leukemia or lymphoma.

Table 112-7   Staging of Typical B Cell Lymphoid Leukemia

Stage	Clinical Features	Median Survival, Years
RAI SYSTEM		
0: Low risk	Lymphocytosis only in blood and marrow	>10
I: Intermediate risk	Lymphocytosis + lymphadenopathy + splenomegaly ± hepatomegaly	7
II		
III: High risk	Lymphocytosis + anemia + thrombocytopenia	1.5
IV		
BINET SYSTEM		
A	Fewer than three areas of clinical lymphadenopathy; no anemia or thrombocytopenia	>10
B	Three or more involved node areas; no anemia or thrombocytopenia	7
C	Hemoglobin ≤10 g/dL and/or platelets <100,000/μl	2

The major clinical characteristics of B cell CLL/small lymphocytic lymphoma are presented in Table 112-10.

The diagnosis of typical B cell CLL is made when an increased number of circulating lymphocytes (i.e., $>4 \times 10^9$/L and usually $>10 \times 10^9$/L) is found (**see Plate V-17**) that are monoclonal B cells and display the CD5 antigen. Confirmation of bone marrow infiltration by the same cells confirms the diagnosis. The peripheral blood smear in such patients typically shows many "smudge" or "basket" cells, nuclear remnants of cells damaged by the physical shear stress of making the blood smear. If cytogenetic studies are performed, trisomy 12 is found in ~25 to 30% of patients. Abnormalities in chromosome 13 are also seen.

If the primary presentation is lymphadenopathy and a lymph node biopsy is performed, pathologists usually have little difficulty in making the diagnosis of small lymphocytic lymphoma based on morphologic findings and immunophenotype. However, even in these patients ~70 to 75% will be found to have bone marrow involvement and the search for circulating monoclonal B lymphocytes is often positive.

The differential diagnosis of typical B cell CLL is extensive and presented in Table 112-1. Immunophenotyping will eliminate the T cell disorders and can often help sort out other B cell malignancies. For example, only mantle cell lymphoma and typical B cell CLL are usually CD5 positive. Typical B cell small lymphocytic lymphoma can be confused with other B cell disorders including lymphoplasmacytic lymphoma (i.e., the tissue manifestation of Waldenström's

Table 112-8   The Ann Arbor Staging System for Hodgkin's Disease

Stage	Definition
I	Involvement of a single lymph node region or lymphoid structure (e.g., spleen, thymus, Waldeyer's ring)
II	Involvement of two or more lymph node regions on the same side of the diaphragm (the mediastinum is a single site; hilar lymph nodes should be considered "lateralized" and, when involved on both sides, constitute stage II disease)
III	Involvement of lymph node regions or lymphoid structures on both sides of the diaphragm
III₁	Subdiaphragmatic involvement limited to spleen, splenic hilar nodes, celiac nodes, or portal nodes
III₂	Subdiaphragmatic involvement includes paraaortic, iliac, or mesenteric nodes plus structures in III₁
IV	Involvement of extranodal site(s) beyond that designated as "E" More than one extranodal deposit at any location Any involvement of liver or bone marrow
A	No symptoms
B	Unexplained weight loss of >10% of the body weight during the 6 months before staging investigation Unexplained, persistent, or recurrent fever with temperatures >38°C during the previous month Recurrent drenching night sweats during the previous month
E	Localized, solitary involvement of extralymphatic tissue, excluding liver and bone marrow

macroglobulinemia), nodal marginal zone B cell lymphoma, and mantle cell lymphoma. In addition, some small lymphocytic lymphomas have areas of large cells that can lead to confusion with diffuse large B cell lymphoma. An expert hematopathologist is vital for making this distinction.

Typical B cell CLL is often found incidentally when a complete blood count is done for another reason. However, complaints that might lead to the diagnosis include fatigue, frequent infections, and new lymphadenopathy. The diagnosis of typical B cell CLL should be considered in a patient presenting with an autoimmune hemolytic anemia or autoimmune thrombocytopenia. B cell CLL has also been associated with red cell aplasia. When this disorder presents as lymphoma, the most common abnormality is asymptomatic new lymphadenopathy, with or without splenomegaly. The staging systems used to predict prognosis in patients with typical B cell CLL are presented in Table 112-7. The IPI for non-Hodgkin's lymphomas, which also predicts prognosis in these patients, is presented in Table 112-9. The evaluation of a new patient with typical B cell CLL/small lymphocytic lymphoma will include many of the studies included in Table 112-11, which describes the initial evaluation of a new patient with non-Hodgkin's lymphoma. In addition, particular attention needs to be given to detecting immune abnormalities such as autoimmune hemolytic anemia, autoimmune thrombocytopenia, hypogammaglobulinemia, and red cell aplasia.

℞ TREATMENT   Patients whose presentation is typical B cell CLL with no manifestations of the disease other than bone marrow involvement and lymphocytosis (i.e., Rai stage O and Binet stage A; Table 112-7) can be followed without specific therapy for their malignancy. These patients have a median survival >10 years, and some will never require therapy for this disorder. If the patient has an adequate number of circulating normal blood cells and is asymptomatic, many physicians would not initiate therapy for patients in the intermediate stage of the disease manifested by lymphadenopathy and/or hepatosplenomegaly. However, the median survival for these patients is ~7 years, and most will require treatment in the first few years of follow-up. Patients who present with bone marrow failure (i.e., Rai stage III or IV or Binet stage C) will require initial therapy in almost all cases. These patients have a serious disorder with a median survival of only 1.5 years. It must be remembered that immune manifestations of typical B cell CLL should be managed independently of specific antileukemia therapy. For example, glucocorticoid therapy for autoimmune cytopenias and γ globulin replacement for patients with hypogammaglobulinanemia should be used whether or not antileukemia therapy is given.

Patients who present primarily with lymphoma and have a low IPI score have a 5-year survival of ~75%, but those with a high IPI score

Table 112-9   International Prognostic Index for Non-Hodgkin's Lymphoma

Five clinical risk factors
  age ≥ 60 years
  serum lactate dehydrogenase levels elevated
  performance status ≥ 2 (ECOG) or ≤ 70 (Karnofsky)
  Ann Arbor stage III or IV
  >1 site of extranodal involvement
Patients are assigned a number for each risk factor they have
Patients are grouped differently based upon the type of lymphoma
For diffuse large B cell lymphoma:

0,1 factor = low risk	35% of cases; 5-year survival, 73%
2 factors = low-intermediate risk	27% of cases; 5-year survival, 51%
3 factors = high-intermediate risk	22% of cases; 5-year survival, 43%
4,5 factors = high risk	16% of cases; 5-year survival, 26%

have a 5-year survival of <40% and are more likely to require early therapy.

The most common treatments for patients with typical B cell CLL/small lymphocytic lymphoma have been the use of single-agent chlorambucil or single-agent fludarabine. Chlorambucil can be administered orally with few immediate side effects, while fludarabine is administered intravenously and is associated with significant immune suppression. However, fludarabine is by far the more active agent and is the only drug associated with a significant incidence of complete remission. For young patients presenting with leukemia requiring therapy, fludarabine is today the treatment of choice. Because fludarabine is an effective second-line agent in patients with tumors unresponsive to chlorambucil, the latter agent is often chosen in elderly patients who require therapy. Many patients who present with lymphoma will receive a combination chemotherapy regimen used in other lymphomas such as CVP (cyclophosphamide, vincristine, and prednisone), or CHOP (cyclophosphamide, doxorubicin, vincristine, and prednisone). Young patients with this disease can be candidates for bone marrow transplantation. Allogeneic bone marrow transplantation can be curative but is associated with a significant treatment-related mortality. The place of autologous transplantation in patients with this disorder remains uncertain.

Molecular analysis of immunoglobulin gene sequences in CLL has demonstrated that about half the patients have tumors expressing mutated immunoglobulin genes and half have tumors expressing unmutated or germ-line immunoglobulin sequences. Patients with unmutated immunoglobulins tend to have a more aggressive clinical course and are less responsive to therapy. Unfortunately, immunoglobulin gene sequencing is not routinely available. CD38 expression is said to be low in the better-prognosis patients expressing mutated immunoglobulin and high in poorer-prognosis patients expressing unmutated immunoglobulin, but this test has not been confirmed as a reliable means of distinguishing the two groups.

Extranodal Marginal Zone B Cell Lymphoma of MALT Type
Extranodal marginal zone B cell lymphoma of MALT type makes up approximately 8% of non-Hodgkin's lymphomas. This small-cell lymphoma presents in extranodal sites. It was previously considered a

FIGURE 112-3 Relationship of International Prognostic Index (IPI) to survival. Kaplan-Meier survival curves for 1300 patients with various kinds of lymphoma stratified according to the IPI.

small lymphocytic lymphoma or sometimes a pseudolymphoma. The recognition that the gastric presentation of this lymphoma was associated with *H. pylori* infection was an important step in recognizing it as a separate entity. The clinical characteristics of extranodal marginal zone B cell lymphoma of MALT type are presented in Table 112-10.

The diagnosis of extranodal marginal zone B cell lymphoma of MALT type can be made accurately by an expert hematopathologist based on a characteristic pattern of infiltration of small lymphocytes that are monoclonal B cells and CD5 negative. In some cases, transformation to diffuse large B cell lymphoma occurs, and both diagnoses may be made in the same biopsy. The differential diagnosis includes benign lymphocytic infiltration of extranodal organs and other small-cell B cell lymphomas.

Extranodal marginal zone B cell lymphoma of MALT type may occur in the stomach, orbit, intestine, lung, thyroid, salivary gland, skin, soft tissues, bladder, kidney, and CNS. It may present as a new mass, be found on routine imaging studies, or be associated with local symptoms such as upper abdominal discomfort in gastric lymphoma. These lymphomas are localized to the organ in question in ~40% of cases and to the organ and regional lymph nodes in ~30% of patients. However, distant metastasis can occur—particularly with transformation to diffuse large B cell lymphoma. Many patients who develop

Table 112-10 Clinical Characteristics of Patients with Common Types of Non-Hodgkin's Lymphomas (NHL)

Disease	Median Age, years	Frequency in Children	% Male	Stage I/II vs III/IV, %	B Symptoms, %	Bone Marrow Involvement, %	Gastrointestinal Tract Involvement, %	% Surviving 5 years
B cell chronic lymphocytic leukemia/small lymphocytic lymphoma	65	Rare	53	9 vs 91	33	72	3	51
Mantle cell lymphoma	63	Rare	74	20 vs 80	28	64	9	27
Extranodal marginal zone B cell lymphoma of MALT type	60	Rare	48	67 vs 33	19	14	50	74
Follicular lymphoma	59	Rare	42	33 vs 67	28	42	4	72
Diffuse large B cell lymphoma	64	~25% of childhood NHL	55	54 vs 46	33	16	18	46
Burkitt's lymphoma	31	~30% of childhood NHL	89	62 vs 38	22	33	11	45
Precursor T cell lymphoblastic lymphoma	28	~40% of childhood NHL	64	11 vs 89	21	50	4	26
Anaplastic large T/null cell lymphoma	34	Common	69	51 vs 49	53	13	9	77
Peripheral T cell non-Hodgkin's lymphoma	61	~5% of childhood NHL	55	20 vs 80	50	36	15	25

NOTE: MALT, mucosa-associated lymphoid tissue.

Table 112-11   Staging Evaluation for Non-Hodgkin's Lymphoma

Physical examination
Documentation of B symptoms
Laboratory evaluation
   Complete blood counts
   Liver function tests
   Uric acid
   Calcium
   Serum protein electrophoresis
   Serum β_2-microglobulin
Chest radiograph
CT scan of abdomen, pelvis, and usually chest
Bone marrow biopsy
Lumbar puncture in lymphoblastic, Burkitt's, and diffuse large B cell
  lymphoma with positive marrow biopsy
Gallium scan (SPECT) in large-cell lymphoma

NOTE: CT, computed tomography; SPECT, single photon emission CT.

this lymphoma will have an autoimmune or inflammatory process such as Sjögren's syndrome (salivary gland MALT), Hashimoto's thyroiditis (thyroid MALT), or *Helicobacter* gastritis (gastric MALT).

Evaluation of patients with extranodal marginal zone B cell lymphoma of MALT type follows the pattern set forth in Table 112-11 for staging a patient with non-Hodgkin's lymphoma. In particular, patients with gastric lymphoma need to have studies performed to document the presence or absence of *H. pylori* infection. Endoscopic studies including ultrasound can help define the extent of gastric involvement. Most patients with extranodal marginal zone B cell lymphoma of MALT type have a good prognosis, with a 5-year survival of ~75%. In patients with a low IPI score, the 5-year survival is ~90%, while it drops to ~40% in patients with a high IPI score.

TREATMENT   Extranodal marginal zone B cell lymphoma of MALT type is curable when localized. Local therapy such as radiation or surgery can effect cure, and this is one of the few times where surgery might be a reasonable primary therapy for a patient with non-Hodgkin's lymphoma. Patients with gastric MALT lymphomas who are infected with *H. pylori* can achieve remission in the majority of cases with eradication of the infection. These remissions can be durable. Patients who present with more extensive disease are most often treated with single-agent chemotherapy such as chlorambucil. Coexistent diffuse large B cell lymphoma must be treated with combination chemotherapy. The additional acquired mutations that mediate the histologic progression also convey *Helicobacter* independence to the growth.

Mantle Cell Lymphoma   Mantle cell lymphoma makes up ~6% of all non-Hodgkin's lymphomas. Recognized as a separate entity only in the past decade, this lymphoma was previously placed in a number of other subtypes. Its existence was confirmed by the recognition that these lymphomas have a characteristic chromosomal translocation, t(11;14) between the immunoglobulin heavy chain gene on chromosome 14 and the *bcl-1* gene on chromosome 11, and regularly overexpress the BCL-1 protein. The clinical characteristics of mantle cell lymphoma are presented in Table 112-10.

The diagnosis of mantle cell lymphoma can be made accurately by an expert hematopathologist based on morphologic findings and proof that the tumor is a B cell lymphoma. As with all subtypes of lymphoma, an adequate biopsy is important. The differential diagnosis of mantle cell lymphoma includes other small-cell B cell lymphomas. In particular, mantle cell lymphoma and small lymphocytic lymphoma share a characteristic expression of CD5. Mantle cell lymphoma usually has a slightly indented nucleus.

The most common presentation of mantle cell lymphoma is with palpable lymphadenopathy, frequently accompanied by systemic symptoms. Approximately 70% of patients will be stage IV at the time of diagnosis, with frequent bone marrow and peripheral blood involvement. Of the extranodal organs that can be involved, gastrointestinal involvement is particularly important to recognize. Patients who present with lymphomatosis polyposis in the large intestine usually have mantle cell lymphoma. The evaluation of patients with mantle cell lymphoma involves the studies presented in Table 112-11 for staging of patients with non-Hodgkin's lymphoma. Patients who present with gastrointestinal tract involvement often have Waldeyer's ring involvement, and vice versa. The 5-year survival for all patients with mantle cell lymphoma is ~25%, with only occasional patients who present with a high IPI score surviving 5 years and ~50% of patients with a low IPI score surviving 5 years.

TREATMENT   Current therapies for mantle cell lymphoma are unsatisfactory. Patients with localized disease might be treated with combination chemotherapy followed by radiotherapy; however, these patients are exceedingly rare. For the usual presentation with disseminated disease, treatments are unsatisfactory, with the minority of patients achieving complete remission. Aggressive combination chemotherapy regimens followed by autologous or allogeneic bone marrow transplantation are frequently offered to younger patients. For the occasional elderly, asymptomatic patient, observation followed by single-agent chemotherapy might be the most practical approach. Combined used of rituximab (anti-CD20 antibody) and chemotherapy may be associated with better response rates.

Follicular Lymphoma   Follicular lymphomas make up 22% of non-Hodgkin's lymphomas worldwide and at least 30% of non-Hodgkin's lymphomas diagnosed in the United States. This type of lymphoma can be diagnosed accurately on morphologic findings alone and has been the diagnosis in the majority of patients in therapeutic trials for "low-grade" lymphoma in the past. The clinical characteristics of follicular lymphoma are presented in Table 112-10.

Evaluation of an adequate biopsy by an expert hematopathologist is sufficient to make a diagnosis of follicular lymphoma. The tumor is composed of small cleaved and large cells in varying proportions organized in a follicular pattern of growth (**see Plate V-30**). Confirmation of B cell immunophenotype and the existence of the t(14;18) and abnormal expression of BCL-2 protein are confirmatory. The major differential diagnosis is between lymphoma and reactive follicular hyperplasia. The coexistence of diffuse large B cell lymphoma must be considered. Patients with follicular lymphoma are often subclassified into those with predominantly small cells, those with a mixture of small and large cells, and those with predominantly large cells. While this distinction cannot be made simply or very accurately, these subdivisions do have prognostic significance. Patients with follicular lymphoma with predominantly large cells have a higher proliferative fraction, progress more rapidly, and have a shorter overall survival with simple chemotherapy regimens.

The most common presentation for follicular lymphoma is with new, painless lymphadenopathy. Multiple sites of lymphoid involvement are typical, and unusual sites such as epitrochlear nodes are sometimes seen. However, essentially any organ can be involved, and extranodal presentations do occur. Most patients do not have fevers, sweats, or weight loss, and an IPI score of 0 or 1 is found in ~50% of patients. Fewer than 10% of patients have a high (i.e., 4 or 5) IPI score. The staging evaluation for patients with follicular lymphoma should include the studies included in Table 112-11 for the staging of patients with non-Hodgkin's lymphoma.

TREATMENT   Follicular lymphoma is one of the malignancies most responsive to chemotherapy and radiotherapy. In addition, as many as 25% of the patients undergo spontaneous regression—usually transient—when followed without therapy. In an asymptomatic patient, no initial treatment and watchful waiting can be an appropriate management strategy and is particularly likely to be adopted for older patients. For patients who do require treatment, single-agent chlorambucil or cyclophosphamide or combination chemotherapy with CVP or CHOP are most frequently used. With adequate treatment, between 50 and 75% of patients will achieve a complete remission. While most patients relapse (median response duration is about 2 years), at least 20% of complete responders will remain in remission for >10 years. For the rare patient with localized follicular lymphoma, involved field radiotherapy produces an excellent treatment result.

A number of new therapies have been shown to be active in the treatment of patients with follicular lymphoma. These include new cytotoxic agents such as fludarabine, interferon α, monoclonal antibodies with or without radionuclides, and lymphoma vaccines. In patients treated with a doxorubicin-containing combination chemotherapy regimen, interferon α given to patients in complete remission seems to prolong survival. The monoclonal antibody rituximab can cause objective responses in 35 to 50% of patients with relapsed follicular lymphoma, and radiolabeled antibodies appear to have response rates well in excess of 50%. Trials with tumor vaccines have been encouraging. Both autologous and allogeneic hematopoietic stem cell transplantation yield high complete response rates in patients with relapsed follicular lymphoma, and long-term remissions can occur.

Patients with follicular lymphoma with a predominance of large cells have a shorter survival when treated with single-agent chemotherapy but seem to benefit from receiving an anthracycline-containing combination chemotherapy regimen. When their disease is treated aggressively, the overall survival for such patients is no lower than for patients with other follicular lymphomas, and the failure-free survival is superior.

Patients with follicular lymphoma have a high rate of histologic transformation to diffuse large B cell lymphoma ($\sim$7% per year). This is recognized $\sim$40% of the time during the course of the illness by repeat biopsy and is present in almost all patients at autopsy. This transformation is usually heralded by rapid growths of lymph nodes—often localized—and the development of systemic symptoms such as fevers, sweats, and weight loss. Although these patients have a poor prognosis, aggressive combination chemotherapy regimens can sometimes cause a complete remission in the diffuse large B cell lymphoma, usually leaving the patient with persisting follicular lymphoma.

Diffuse Large B Cell Lymphoma Diffuse large B cell lymphoma is the most common type of non-Hodgkin's lymphoma, representing approximately one-third of all cases. This lymphoma makes up the majority of cases in previous clinical trials of "aggressive" or "intermediate-grade" lymphoma. The clinical characteristics of diffuse large B cell lymphoma are presented in Table 112-10.

The diagnosis of diffuse large B cell lymphoma can be made accurately by an expert hematopathologist when review of an adequate biopsy and proof of B cell immunophenotype are available (**see Plate V-22**). Cytogenetic and molecular genetic studies are not necessary for diagnosis, but some evidence has accumulated that patients who overexpress the BCL-2 protein might be more likely to relapse than others. Patients with prominent mediastinal involvement are sometimes diagnosed as a separate subgroup having primary mediastinal diffuse large B cell lymphoma. This latter group of patients has a younger median age (i.e., 37 years) and a female predominance (66%). Subtypes of diffuse large B cell lymphoma, including those with an immunoblastic subtype and tumors with extensive fibrosis, are recognized by pathologists but do not appear to have important, independent prognostic significance.

Diffuse large B cell lymphoma can present as either primary lymph node disease or at extranodal sites. More than 50% of patients will have some site of extranodal involvement at diagnosis, with the most common sites being the gastrointestinal tract and bone marrow, each being involved in 15 to 20% of patients. Essentially any organ can be involved, making a diagnostic biopsy imperative. For example, diffuse large B cell lymphoma of the pancreas has a much better prognosis than pancreatic carcinoma but would be missed without biopsy. Primary diffuse large B cell lymphoma of the brain is being diagnosed with increasing frequency.

The initial evaluation of patients with diffuse large B cell lymphoma involves the studies presented in Table 112-11 for staging of patients with non-Hodgkin's lymphoma. After a careful staging evaluation, $\sim$50% of patients will be found to have stage I or II disease and $\sim$50% will have widely disseminated lymphoma. Bone marrow biopsy shows involvement by lymphoma in about 15% of cases, with marrow involvement by small cells more frequent than with large cells.

TREATMENT The initial treatment of all patients with diffuse large B cell lymphoma should be with a combination chemotherapy regimen. The most popular regimen in the United States is CHOP, although a variety of other anthracycline-containing combination chemotherapy regimens appear to be equally efficacious. Patients with stage I or nonbulky stage II can be effectively treated with three to four cycles of combination chemotherapy followed by involved field radiotherapy. The results are at least equal and probably superior to six to eight cycles of combination therapy, and cure rates of 60 to 70% in stage II disease and 80 to 90% in stage I disease can be expected.

For patients with bulky stage II, stage III, or stage IV, six to eight cycles of combination chemotherapy regimen such as CHOP are usually administered. A frequent approach would be to administer four cycles of therapy and then reevaluate. If the patient has achieved a complete remission after four cycles, two more cycles of treatment might be given and then therapy discontinued. Using this approach, $\sim$60 to 70% of patients can be expected to achieve a complete remission, and 50 to 70% of complete responders will be cured. The chances for a favorable response to treatment are predicted by the IPI. In fact, the IPI was developed specifically to predict outcome in patients with diffuse large-cell lymphoma. For the 35% of patients with a low IPI score of 0 to 1, the 5-year survival is >70%, while for the 20% of patients with a high IPI score of 4 to 5, the 5-year survival is $\sim$20%. A number of other factors, including molecular features of the tumor, levels of circulating cytokines and soluble receptors, and other surrogate markers, have been shown to influence prognosis. However, they have not been validated as rigorously as the IPI and have not been uniformly applied clinically.

Because a large number of patients with diffuse large B cell lymphoma are either initially refractory to therapy or relapse after apparently effective chemotherapy, >50% of patients will be candidates for salvage treatment at some point. Alternative combination chemotherapy regimens can induce complete remission in as many as 50% of these patients, but long-term disease-free survival is seen in $\leq$10%. Autologous bone marrow transplantation has been shown to be superior to salvage chemotherapy at usual doses and leads to long-term disease-free survival in $\sim$40% of patients whose lymphomas remain chemotherapy-sensitive after relapse.

Burkitt's Lymphoma/Leukemia Burkitt's lymphoma/leukemia is a rare disease in adults in the United States, making up <1% of non-Hodgkin's lymphomas, but it makes up $\sim$30% of childhood non-Hodgkin's lymphoma. Burkitt's leukemia, or L3 ALL, makes up a small proportion of childhood and adult acute leukemias. The clinical features of Burkitt's lymphoma occurring in adults are presented in Table 112-10.

Burkitt's lymphoma can be diagnosed morphologically by an expert hematopathologist with a high degree of accuracy. The cells are homogeneous in size and shape (**see Plate V-4**). Demonstration of a very high proliferative fraction and the presence of the t(8;14) or one of its variants, t(2;8) (*c-myc* and the λ light chain gene) or t(8;22) (*c-myc* and the κ light chain gene), can be confirmatory. Burkitt's cell leukemia is recognized by the typical medium-sized cells with round nuclei, multiple nucleoli, and basophilic cytoplasm with cytoplasmic vacuoles. Demonstration of a B cell immunophenotype and one of the above-noted cytogenetic abnormalities is confirmatory.

The three distinct clinical forms of Burkitt's lymphoma that are recognized are endemic, sporadic, and immunodeficiency-associated.

Endemic and sporadic Burkitt's lymphomas occur frequently in children in Africa, and the sporadic form in western countries. Immunodeficiency-associated Burkitt's lymphoma is seen in patients with HIV infection.

Pathologists sometimes have difficulty distinguishing between Burkitt's lymphoma and diffuse large B cell lymphoma. In the past, a separate subgroup of non-Hodgkin's lymphoma intermediate between the two was recognized. When tested, this subgroup could not be diagnosed accurately. Distinction between the two major types of B cell aggressive non-Hodgkin's lymphoma can sometimes be made based on the extremely high proliferative fraction seen in patients with Burkitt's lymphoma (i.e., essentially 100% of tumor cells are in cycle) caused by c-myc deregulation.

Most patients in the United States with Burkitt's lymphoma present with peripheral lymphadenopathy or an intraabdominal mass. The disease is typically rapidly progressive and has a propensity to metastasize to the CNS. Initial evaluation should always include an examination of cerebral spinal fluid to rule out metastasis in addition to the other staging evaluations noted in Table 112-11. Once the diagnosis of Burkitt's lymphoma is suspected, a diagnosis must be made promptly and staging evaluation must be accomplished expeditiously. This is the most rapidly progressive human tumor, and any delay in initiating therapy can adversely affect the patient's prognosis.

℞ **TREATMENT** Treatment of Burkitt's lymphoma in both children and adults involves the use of intensive combination chemotherapy regimens incorporating administered high doses of cyclophosphamide. Prophylactic therapy to the CNS is mandatory and incorporated in all modern regimens. Burkitt's lymphoma was one of the first cancers shown to be curable by chemotherapy. Today, cure can be expected in 70% of both children and young adults when effective therapy is administered precisely. Salvage therapy has been generally ineffective in patients failing the initial treatment, emphasizing the importance of the initial treatment approach.

Other B Cell Lymphoid Malignancies *B-cell prolymphocytic leukemia* involves blood and marrow infiltration by large lymphocytes with prominent nucleoli. Patients typically have a high white cell count, splenomegaly, and minimal lymphadenopathy. The chances for a complete response to therapy are poor.

Hairy cell leukemia is a rare disease that presents predominantly in older males. Typical presentation involves pancytopenia, although occasional patients will have a leukemic presentation. Splenomegaly is usual. The malignant cells appear to have "hairy" projections on light and electron microscopy and show a characteristic staining pattern with tartrate-resistant acid phosphatase. Bone marrow is typically not able to be aspirated, and biopsy shows a pattern of fibrosis with diffuse infiltration by the malignant cells. Patients with this disorder are prone to unusual infections including infection by *Mycobacterium avium intracellulare*, and vasculitic syndromes have been described. Hairy cell leukemia is responsive to chemotherapy with interferon α, pentostatin, or cladribine, with the latter being the usually preferred treatment. Clinical complete remissions with cladribine occur in the majority of patients, and long-term disease-free survival is frequent.

Splenic marginal zone lymphoma involves infiltration of the splenic white pulp by small, monoclonal B lymphocytes. This is a rare disorder that can present as leukemia as well as lymphoma. Definitive diagnosis is often made at splenectomy, which is also an effective therapy. This is an extremely indolent disorder, but when chemotherapy is required, the most usual treatment has been chlorambucil.

Lymphoplasmacytic lymphoma is the tissue manifestation of Waldenström's macroglobulinemia (Chap. 113). This type of lymphoma has been associated with chronic hepatitis C virus infection, and an etiologic association has been proposed. Patients typically present with lymphadenopathy, splenomegaly, bone marrow involvement, and occasionally peripheral blood involvement. The tumor cells do not express CD5. Patients often have a monoclonal IgM protein, high levels of which can dominate the clinical picture with the symptoms of hyperviscosity. Treatment of lymphoplasmacytic lymphoma can be aimed primarily at reducing the abnormal protein, if present, but will usually also involve chemotherapy. Chlorambucil, fludarabine, and cladribine have been utilized. The median 5-year survival for patients with this disorder is ~60%.

Nodal marginal zone lymphoma, also known as *monocytoid B cell lymphoma*, represents ~1% of non-Hodgkin's lymphomas. This lymphoma has a slight female predominance and presents with disseminated disease (i.e., stage III or IV) in 75% of patients. Approximately one-third of patients have bone marrow involvement, and a leukemic presentation occasionally occurs. The staging evaluation and therapy should use the same approach as used for patients with follicular lymphoma. Approximately 60% of the patients with nodal marginal zone lymphoma will survive 5 years after diagnosis.

PRECURSOR CELL T CELL MALIGNANCIES **Precursor T Cell Lymphoblastic Leukemia/Lymphoma** Precursor T cell malignancies can present either as ALL or as an aggressive lymphoma. These malignancies are more common in children and young adults, with males more frequently affected than females.

Precursor T cell ALL can present with bone marrow failure, although the severity of anemia, neutropenia, and thrombocytopenia is often less than in precursor B cell ALL. These patients sometimes have very high white cell counts, a mediastinal mass, lymphadenopathy, and hepatosplenomegaly. Precursor T cell lymphoblastic lymphoma is most often found in young men presenting with a large mediastinal mass and pleural effusions. Both presentations have a propensity to metastasize to the CNS, and CNS involvement is often present at diagnosis.

℞ **TREATMENT** Children with precursor T cell ALL seem to benefit from very intensive remission induction and consolidation regimens. The majority of patients treated in this manner can be cured. Older children and young adults with precursor T cell lymphoblastic lymphoma are also often treated with "leukemia-like" regimens. Patients who present with localized disease have an excellent prognosis. However, advanced age is an adverse prognostic factor. Adults with precursor T cell lymphoblastic lymphoma who present with high LDH levels or bone marrow or CNS involvement are often offered bone marrow transplantation as part of their primary therapy.

MATURE (PERIPHERAL) T CELL DISORDERS **Mycosis Fungoides** Mycosis fungoides is also known as *cutaneous T cell lymphoma*. This lymphoma is more often seen by dermatologists than internists. The median age of onset is in the mid-fifties, and the disease is more common in males and in blacks.

Mycosis fungoides is an indolent lymphoma with patients often having several years of eczematous or dermatitic skin lesions before the diagnosis is finally established. The skin lesions progress from patch stage to plaque stage to cutaneous tumors. Early in the disease, biopsies are often difficult to interpret, and the diagnosis may only become apparent by observing the patient over time. In advanced stages, the lymphoma can metastasize to lymph nodes and visceral organs. A particular syndrome in patients with this lymphoma involves erythroderma and circulating tumor cells. This is known as Sézary's syndrome.

Rare patients with localized early stage mycosis fungoides can be cured with radiotherapy, often total-skin electron beam irradiation. More advanced disease has been treated with topical glucocorticoids, topical nitrogen mustard, phototherapy, psoralen with ultraviolet A (PUVA), electron beam radiation, interferon, and systemic cytotoxic therapy. Unfortunately, these treatments are palliative.

Adult T Cell Lymphoma/Leukemia Adult T cell lymphoma/leukemia is one manifestation of infection by the HTLV-I retrovirus. Patients can be infected through transplacental transmission, blood transfusion, and by sexual transmission of the virus. Patients who acquire the virus from their mother through breast milk are most likely to develop lymphoma, but the risk is still only 2.5% and the latency averages 55 years. Tropical spastic paraparesis, another manifestation of HTLV-I infection (Chap. 191), occurs after a shorter latency (1 to 3 years) and is most common in people who acquire the virus during adulthood from transfusion or sex.

The diagnosis of adult T cell lymphoma/leukemia is made when an expert hematopathologist recognizes the typical morphologic picture, a T cell immunophenotype (i.e., CD4 positive) of malignant cells has been demonstrated, and the existence of antibodies to HTLV-I is proven. Examination of the peripheral blood will usually reveal characteristic, pleomorphic abnormal CD4-positive cells with indented nuclei, which have been called "flower" cells (see Plate V-40).

A subset of patients have a smoldering clinical course and long survival, but most patients present with an aggressive disease manifested by lymphadenopathy, hepatosplenomegaly, skin infiltration, hypercalcemia, lytic bone lesions, and elevated LDH levels. The skin lesions can be papules, plaques, tumors, and ulcerations. Bone marrow involvement is not usually extensive, and anemia and thrombocytopenia are not usually prominent. Although treatment by combination chemotherapy regimens can result in objective responses, true complete remissions are unusual, and the median survival of patients is about 7 months.

Anaplastic Large T/Null Cell Lymphoma Anaplastic large T/null cell lymphoma was previously usually diagnosed as undifferentiated carcinoma or malignant histiocytosis. Discovery of the CD30, or Ki-1, antigen and the recognition that some patients with previously unclassified malignancies displayed this antigen led to the identification of a new type of lymphoma. Subsequently, discovery of the t(2;5) and the resultant frequent overexpression of the anaplastic lymphoma kinase (alk) protein confirmed the existence of this entity. This lymphoma accounts for ~2% of all non-Hodgkin's lymphomas. The clinical characteristics of patients with anaplastic large T/null cell lymphoma are presented in Table 112-10.

The diagnosis of anaplastic large T/null cell lymphoma is made when an expert hematopathologist recognizes the typical morphologic picture and a T cell or null cell immunophenotype is demonstrated along with CD30 positivity. Documentation of the t(2;5) and/or overexpression of alk protein confirm the diagnosis. Some diffuse large B cell lymphomas can also have an anaplastic appearance but have the same clinical course or response to therapy as other diffuse large B cell lymphomas.

Patients with anaplastic large T/cell null cell lymphoma are typically young (median age, 33 years) and male (~70%). Some 50% of patients present in stage I/II, and the remainder with more extensive disease. Systemic symptoms and elevated LDH levels are seen in about one-half of patients. Bone marrow and the gastrointestinal tract are rarely involved, but skin involvement is frequent. Some patients with disease confined to the skin have a different and more indolent disorder that has been termed *cutaneous anaplastic large T/null cell lymphoma* and might be related to lymphomatoid papulosis.

℞ **TREATMENT** Treatment regimens appropriate for other aggressive lymphomas, such as diffuse large B cell lymphoma, should be utilized in patients with anaplastic large T/null cell lymphoma. Surprisingly, given the anaplastic appearance, this disorder has the best survival rate of any aggressive lymphoma. The 5-year survival is >75%. While traditional prognostic factors such as the IPI predict treatment outcome, overexpression of the alk protein is an important prognostic factor, with patients overexpressing this protein having a superior treatment outcome.

Peripheral T Cell Lymphoma The peripheral T cell lymphomas make up a heterogenous morphologic group of aggressive neoplasms that share a mature T cell immunophenotype. They represent ~7% of all cases of non-Hodgkin's lymphoma. A number of distinct clinical syndromes are included in this group of disorders. The clinical characteristics of patients with peripheral T cell lymphoma are presented in Table 112-10.

The diagnosis of peripheral T cell lymphoma, or any of its specific subtypes, requires an expert hematopathologist, an adequate biopsy, and immunophenotyping. Most peripheral T cell lymphomas are CD4-positive, but a few will be CD8-positive, both CD4- and CD8-positive, or have an NK-cell immunophenotype. No characteristic genetic abnormalities have yet been identified, but translocations involving the T cell antigen receptor genes on chromosomes 7 or 14 may be detected. The differential diagnosis of patients suspected of having peripheral T cell lymphoma includes reactive T cell infiltrative processes. In some cases, demonstration of a monoclonal T cell population using T cell receptor gene rearrangement studies will be required to make a diagnosis.

The initial evaluation of a patient with a peripheral T cell lymphoma should include the studies in Table 112-11 for staging patients with non-Hodgkin's lymphoma. Unfortunately, patients with peripheral T cell lymphoma usually present with adverse prognostic factors, with >80% of patients having an IPI score ≥2 and >30% having an IPI score ≥4. As this would predict, peripheral T cell lymphomas are associated with a poor outcome, and only 25% of the patients survive 5 years after diagnosis. Treatment regimens are the same as those used for diffuse large B cell lymphoma, but patients with peripheral T cell lymphoma have a poorer response to treatment. Because of this poor treatment outcome, hematopoietic stem cell transplantation is often considered early in the care of young patients.

A number of specific clinical syndromes are seen in the peripheral T cell lymphomas. *Angioimmunoblastic T cell lymphoma* is one of the more common subtypes, making up ~20% of T cell lymphomas. These patients typically present with generalized lymphadenopathy, fever, weight loss, skin rash, and polyclonal hypergammaglobunenemia. In some cases, it is difficult to separate patients with a reactive disorder from those with true lymphoma.

Extranodal T/NK cell lymphoma of nasal type has also been called *angiocentric lymphoma* and was previously termed *lethal midline granuloma*. This disorder is more frequent in Asia and South America than in the United States and Europe. Although most frequent in the upper airway, it can involve other organs. The course is aggressive, and patients frequently have the hemophagocytic syndrome. When marrow and blood involvement occur, distinction between this disease and leukemia might be difficult. Some patients will respond to aggressive combination chemotherapy regimens, but the overall outlook is poor.

Enteropathy-type intestinal T cell lymphoma is a rare disorder that occurs in patients with untreated gluten-sensitive enteropathy. Patients are frequently wasted and sometimes present with intestinal perforation. The prognosis is poor. *Hepatosplenic γδ T cell lymphoma* is a systemic illness that presents with sinusoidal infiltration of the liver, spleen, and bone marrow by malignant T cells. Tumor masses generally do not occur. The disease is associated with systemic symptoms and is often difficult to diagnosis. Treatment outcome is poor. *Subcutaneous panniculitis-like T cell lymphoma* is a rare disorder that is often confused with panniculitis. Patients present with multiple subcutaneous nodules, which progress and can ulcerate. Hemophagocytic syndrome is common. Response to therapy is poor. The development of the hemophagocytic syndrome (profound anemia, ingestion of erythrocytes by monocytes and macrophages) in the course of any peripheral T cell lymphoma is generally associated with a fatal outcome.

HODGKIN'S DISEASE **Nodular Lymphocyte-Predominant Hodgkin's Disease** Nodular lymphocyte predominant Hodgkin's disease is now recognized as an entity distinct from classic Hodgkin's disease. Previous classification systems recognized that biopsies from a subset of patients diagnosed as having Hodgkin's disease contained a predominance of small lymphocytes and rare Sternberg-Reed cells. In recent years, it was recognized that a subset of these patients had a nodular growth pattern and a clinical course that varied from that of patients with classic Hodgkin's disease. This is an unusual clinical entity and represents <5% of cases of Hodgkin's disease.

Nodular lymphocyte-predominant Hodgkin's disease has a number of characteristics that suggest its relationship to non-Hodgkin's lymphoma. These include a clonal proliferation of B cells and a distinctive immunophenotype; tumor cells express J chain and display CD45 and epithelial membrane antigen (ema) and do not express two markers normally found on Sternberg-Reed cells, CD30 and CD15. This lymphoma tends to have a chronic, relapsing course and sometimes transforms to diffuse large B cell lymphoma.

The treatment of patients with nodular lymphocyte-predominant Hodgkin's disease is controversial. Some clinicians favor no treatment and merely close follow-up. In the United States, most physicians will treat localized disease with radiotherapy and disseminated disease with regimens utilized for patients with classic Hodgkin's disease. Regardless of the therapy utilized, most series report a long-term survival of >80%.

Classical Hodgkin's Disease Hodgkin's disease occurs in ~8000 patients in the United States each year, and the disease does not appear to be increasing in frequency. Most patients present with palpable lymphadenopathy that is nontender; in most patients, these lymph nodes are in the neck, supraclavicular area, and axilla. More than half the patients will have mediastinal adenopathy at diagnosis, and this is sometimes the initial manifestation. Subdiaphragmatic presentation of Hodgkin's disease is unusual and more common in older males. Approximately one-third of patients present with fevers, night sweats, and/or weight loss—B symptoms in the Ann Arbor staging classification (Table 112-8). Occasionally, Hodgkin's disease can present as a fever of unknown origin. This is more common in older patients who are found to have mixed-cellularity Hodgkin's disease in an abdominal site. Rarely, the fevers persist for days to weeks, followed by afebrile intervals and then recurrence of the fever. This pattern is known as *Pel-Epstein fever*. Hodgkin's disease can occasionally present with unusual manifestations. These include severe and unexplained itching, cutaneous disorders such as erythema nodosum and ichthyosiform atrophy, paraneoplastic cerebellar degeneration and other distant effects on the CNS, nephrotic syndrome, immune hemolytic anemia and thrombocytopenia, hypercalcemia, and pain in lymph nodes on alcohol ingestion.

The diagnosis of Hodgkin's disease is established by review of an adequate biopsy specimen by an expert hematopathologist. In the United States, most patients would be classified as having nodular sclerosing Hodgkin's disease, with a minority of patients having mixed-cellularity Hodgkin's disease. Lymphocyte-predominant and lymphocyte-depleted Hodgkin's disease are rare. Mixed-cellularity Hodgkin's disease or lymphocyte-depletion Hodgkin's disease are seen more frequently in patients infected by HIV (**see Plate V-18**). The differential diagnosis of a lymph node biopsy suspicious for Hodgkin's disease includes inflammatory processes, mononucleosis, non-Hodgkin's lymphoma, diphenylhydantoin-induced lymphadenopathy, and nonlymphomatous malignancies.

The staging evaluation for a patient with Hodgkin's disease would typically include a careful history and physical examination; complete blood count; erythrocyte sedimentation rate; serum chemistry studies including LDH; chest radiograph; CT scan of the chest, abdomen, and pelvis; and bone marrow biopsy. Many patients would also have a gallium scan. If radiologic expertise is available, a bipedal lymphangiogram can be helpful. Gallium scans are most useful at the completion of therapy to document remission. Staging laparotomies were once popular for most patients with Hodgkin's disease but are now done rarely because of an increased reliance on systemic rather than local therapy.

℞ **TREATMENT** Patients with localized Hodgkin's disease are cured >90% of the time. In patients with good prognostic factors, extended field radiotherapy has a high cure rate. Increasingly, patients with all stages of Hodgkin's disease are treated initially with chemotherapy. Patients with localized or good-prognosis disease receive a brief course of chemotherapy followed by radiotherapy to sites of node involvement. Patients with more extensive disease or those with B symptoms receive a complete course of chemotherapy. The most popular chemotherapy regimens used in the treatment of Hodgkin's disease include doxorubicin, bleomycin, vinblastine, and dacarbazine (ABVD) and mechlorethamine, vincristine, procarbazine, and prednisone (MOPP), or combinations of the drugs in these two regimens. Today, most patients in the United States receive ABVD. Long-term disease-free survival in patients with advanced disease can be achieved in >75% of patients who lack systemic symptoms and in 50 to 70% of patients with systemic symptoms.

Patients who relapse after primary therapy of Hodgkin's disease can frequently still be cured. Patients who relapse after initial treatment only with radiotherapy have an excellent outcome when treated with chemotherapy. Patients who relapse after an effective chemotherapy regimen are usually not curable with subsequent chemotherapy administered at standard doses. However, patients with a long initial remission can be an exception to this rule. Autologous bone marrow transplantation can cure half of patients who fail effective chemotherapy regimens.

Because of the very high cure rate in patients with Hodgkin's disease, long-term complications have become a major focus for clinical research. In fact, in some series of patients with early-stage disease, more patients died from late complications of therapy than from Hodgkin's disease itself. This is particularly true in patients with localized disease. The most serious late side effects include second malignancies and cardiac injury. Patients are at risk for the development of acute leukemia in the first 10 years after treatment with combination chemotherapy regimens that contain alkylating agents. The risk for development of acute leukemia appears to be greater after MOPP-like regimens than with ABVD. The development of carcinomas as a complication of treatment for Hodgkin's disease has become a major problem. These tumors usually occur ≥10 years after treatment and are associated more with radiotherapy than with chemotherapy. For this reason, young women treated with thoracic radiotherapy for Hodgkin's disease should institute screening mammograms 5 to 10 years after treatment, and all patients who receive thoracic radiotherapy for Hodgkin's disease should be discouraged from smoking. Thoracic radiation also accelerates coronary artery disease, and patients should be encouraged to minimize risk factors for coronary artery disease such as smoking and elevated cholesterol levels.

A number of other late side effects from the treatment of Hodgkin's disease are well known. Patients who receive thoracic radiotherapy are at very high risk for the eventual development of hypothyroidism and should be observed for this complication; intermittent measurement of thyrotropin should be made to identify the condition before it becomes symptomatic. Lhermitte's syndrome occurs in ~15% of patients who receive thoracic radiotherapy. This syndrome is manifested by an "electric shock" sensation into the lower extremities on flexion of the neck. Infertility is a concern for all patients undergoing treatment for Hodgkin's disease. In both women and men, the risk of permanent infertility is age-related, with younger patients more likely to recover fertility. In addition, treatment with ABVD rather than MOPP increases the chances to retain fertility.

LYMPHOMA-LIKE DISORDERS

The most common condition that pathologists and clinicians might confuse with lymphoma is reactive, atypical lymphoid hyperplasia. Patients might have localized or disseminated lymphadenopathy and might have the systemic symptoms characteristic of lymphoma. Underlying causes include a drug reaction to diphenylhydantoin or carbamezepine. Immune disorders such as rheumatoid arthritis and lupus erythematosus, viral infections such as cytomegalovirus and EBV, and bacterial infections such as cat-scratch disease may cause adenopathy (Chap. 63). In the absence of a definitive diagnosis after initial biopsy, continued follow-up, further testing, and repeated biopsies, if necessary, are the appropriate approach rather than instituting therapy.

Specific conditions that can be confused with lymphoma include *Castleman's disease*, which can present with localized or disseminated lymphadenopathy; some patients have systemic symptoms. The disseminated form is often accompanied by anemia and polyclonal hypergammaglobulinemia, and the condition seems to be related to an overproduction of interleukin 6, possibly produced by human herpesvirus 8. Patients with localized disease can be treated effectively with local therapy, while the initial treatment for patients with disseminated disease is usually with systemic glucocorticoids.

Sinus histiocytosis with massive lymphadenopathy (Rosai-Dorfman's disease) usually presents with bulky lymphadenopathy in children or young adults. The disease is usually nonprogressive and self-limited, but patients can manifest autoimmune hemolytic anemia.

Lymphomatoid papulosis is a cutaneous lymphoproliferative disorder that is often confused with anaplastic large-cell lymphoma involving the skin. The cells of lymphomatoid papulosis are similar to those seen in lymphoma and stain for CD30, and T cell receptor gene rearrangements are sometimes seen. However, the condition is characterized by waxing and waning skin lesions that usually heal, leaving small scars. In the absence of effective communication between the clinician and the pathologist regarding the clinical course in the patient, this disease will be misdiagnosed. Since the clinical picture is usually benign, misdiagnosis is a serious mistake.

ACKNOWLEDGMENT

Dr. Arnold Freedman and Dr. Lee Nadler contributed this chapter to the 14th edition, and some elements of that chapter were retained here.

BIBLIOGRAPHY

ARMITAGE JO et al: *Text Atlas of Lymphomas*. London, Martin Dunitz, 1999

HARRIS NL et al: World Health Organization classification of neoplastic diseases of the hematopoietic and lymphoid tissues: Report of the Clinical Advisory Committee Meeting, Airlie House, Virginia, November, 1997. J Clin Oncol 17:3835, 1999

HAUKE RJ, ARMITAGE JO: A new approach to non-Hodgkin's lymphoma. Intern Med 39:197, 2000

URBA WJ, LONGO DL: Hodgkin's disease. N Engl J Med 326:678, 1992

113 Dan L. Longo

PLASMA CELL DISORDERS

GENERAL PRINCIPLES The *plasma cell disorders* are monoclonal neoplasms related to each other by virtue of their development from common progenitors in the B lymphocyte lineage. Multiple myeloma, Waldenström's macroglobulinemia, primary amyloidosis (Chap. 319), and the heavy chain diseases comprise this group and may be designated by a variety of synonyms such as *monoclonal gammopathies, paraproteinemias, plasma cell dyscrasias,* and *dysproteinemias.* Mature B lymphocytes destined to produce IgG bear surface immunoglobulin molecules of both M and G heavy chain isotypes with both isotypes having identical idiotypes (variable regions). Under normal circumstances, maturation to antibody-secreting plasma cells is stimulated by exposure to the antigen for which the surface immunoglobulin is specific; however, in the plasma cell disorders the control over this process is lost. The clinical manifestations of all the plasma cell disorders relate to the expansion of the neoplastic cells, to the secretion of cell products (immunoglobulin molecules or subunits, lymphokines), and to some extent to the host's response to the tumor.

→*Normal development of B lymphocytes is discussed in Chap. 305.*

There are three categories of structural variation among immunoglobulin molecules that form antigenic determinants, and these are used to classify immunoglobulins (Chap. 305). *Isotypes* are those determinants that distinguish among the main classes of antibodies of a given species and are the same in all normal individuals of that species.

Therefore, isotypic determinants are, by definition, recognized by antibodies from a distinct species (heterologous sera) but not by antibodies from the same species (homologous sera). There are five heavy chain isotypes (M, G, A, D, E) and two light chain isotypes (κ, λ). *Allotypes* are distinct determinants that reflect regular small differences between individuals of the same species in the amino acid sequences of otherwise similar immunoglobulins. These differences are determined by allelic genes; by definition, they are detected by antibodies made in the same species. *Idiotypes* are the third category of antigenic determinants. They are unique to the molecules produced by a given clone of antibody-producing cells. Idiotypes are formed by the unique structure of the antigen-binding portion of the molecule.

Antibody molecules (Fig. 305-8) are composed of two heavy chains (mol wt ~50,000) and two light chains (mol wt ~25,000). Each chain has a constant portion (limited amino acid sequence variability) and a variable region (extensive sequence variability). The light and heavy chains are linked by disulfide bonds and are aligned so that their variable regions are adjacent to one another. This variable region forms the antigen recognition site of the antibody molecule; its unique structural features form a particular set of determinants, or idiotypes, that are reliable markers for a particular clone of cells because each antibody is formed and secreted by a single clone. Each chain is specified by distinct genes, synthesized separately, and assembled into an intact antibody molecule after translation (Fig. 113-1). Because of the mechanics of the gene rearrangements necessary to specify the immunoglobulin variable regions (VDJ joining for the heavy chain, VJ joining for the light chain), a particular clone rearranges only one of the two chromosomes to produce an immunoglobulin molecule of only one light chain isotype and only one allotype (allelic exclusion). After exposure to antigen, the variable region may become associated with a new heavy chain isotype (class switch). Each clone of cells performs these sequential gene arrangements in a unique way. This results in each clone producing a unique immunoglobulin molecule. In most cells, light chains are synthesized in slight excess, are secreted as free light chains by plasma cells, and are cleared by the kidney, but <10 mg of such light chains is excreted per day.

Electrophoretic analysis of components of the serum proteins permits determination of the amount of immunoglobulin in the serum (Fig. 113-2). The variety of immunoglobulins move heterogeneously in an electric field and form a broad peak in the gamma region. The gamma globulin region of the electrophoretic pattern is usually increased in the sera of patients and animals with plasma cell tumors. There is a sharp spike in this region called an *M component* (M for monoclonal). Less commonly, the M component may appear in the beta$_2$ or alpha$_2$ globulin region. The antibody must be present at a concentration of at least 5 g/L (0.5 g/dL) to be detectable by this method. This corresponds to approximately 10^9 cells producing the antibody. Confirmation that such an M component is truly monoclonal relies on the use of immunoelectrophoresis that shows a single light and heavy chain type. Hence immunoelectrophoresis and electrophoresis provide qualitative and quantitative assessment of the M component, respectively. Once the presence of an M component has been confirmed, electrophoresis provides the more practical information for managing patients with monoclonal gammopathies. In a given patient, the amount of M component in the serum is a reliable measure of the tumor burden. This makes the M component an excellent tumor marker, yet it is not specific enough to be used to screen asymptomatic patients. In addition to the plasma cell disorders, M components may be detected in other lymphoid neoplasms such as chronic lymphocytic leukemia and lymphomas of B or T cell origin; nonlymphoid neoplasms such as chronic myeloid leukemia, breast cancer, and colon cancer; a variety of nonneoplastic conditions such as cirrhosis, sarcoidosis, parasitic diseases, Gaucher's disease, and pyoderma gangrenosum; and a number of autoimmune conditions, including rheumatoid arthritis, myasthenia gravis, and cold agglutinin disease. A very rare skin disease known as lichen myxedematosus or papular muci-

FIGURE 113-1 Immunoglobulin heavy chains are encoded by four distinct genetic elements: variable (Igh-V), diversity (Igh-D), joining (Igh-J), and constant (Igh-C) genes. The variable region of the immunoglobulin heavy chain is encoded by the V, D, and J genes. The same variable region may be associated with any of the 10 heavy chain constant region genes. In the germ-line genome (all cells except B cells) the V, D, and J genes are widely separated and exist in numerous forms. Once a cell becomes committed to B cell differ-entiation, a single V gene and a single D gene translocate to a single J gene, and the intervening genetic material is excised (VDJ joining). The newly formed VDJ gene is transcribed into a single message along with either an M or D isotype C gene. Upon exposure to antigen, another rearrangement may occur so that the VDJ gene may be associated with a G, A, or E isotype C gene. In light chain genes there appear to be no D genes, and thus light chain variable regions are formed by VJ joining.

nosis is associated with a monoclonal gammopathy. Highly cationic IgG is deposited in the dermis of patients with this disease. This organ specificity may reflect the specificity of the antibody for some antigenic component of the dermis.

The nature of the M component is variable in plasma cell disorders. It may be an intact antibody molecule of any heavy chain subclass, or it may be an altered antibody or fragment. Isolated light or heavy chains may be produced. In some plasma cell tumors such as extramedullary or solitary bone plasmacytomas, less than a third of patients will have an M component. In about 20% of myelomas, only light chains are produced and in most cases are secreted in the urine as Bence Jones proteins. The frequency of myelomas of a particular heavy chain class is roughly proportional to the serum concentration, and therefore IgG myelomas are more common than IgA and IgD myelomas.

MULTIPLE MYELOMA **Definition** Multiple myeloma represents a malignant proliferation of plasma cells derived from a single clone. The terms *multiple myeloma* and *myeloma* may be used interchangeably. The tumor, its products, and the host response to it result in a number of organ dysfunctions and symptoms of bone pain or fracture, renal failure, susceptibility to infection, anemia, hypercalcemia, and occasionally clotting abnormalities, neurologic symptoms, and vascular manifestations of hyperviscosity.

Etiology The cause of myeloma is not known. Myeloma occurred with increased frequency in those exposed to the radiation of nuclear warheads in World War II after a 20-year latency. A variety of chromosomal alterations have been found in patients with myeloma; 13q14 deletions, 17p13 deletions, and 11q abnormalities predominate. The most common translocation is t(11;14)(q13;q32), and evidence is strong that errors in switch recombination—the genetic mechanism to change antibody heavy chain isotype—participate in the transformation pathway. Overexpression of *myc* or *ras* genes has been noted in some cases. Mutations in p53 and Rb-1 have also been described, but no common molecular pathogenesis has yet emerged.

Myeloma has been seen more commonly than expected among farmers, wood workers, leather workers, and those exposed to petroleum products. The neoplastic event in myeloma may involve cells earlier in B cell differentiation than the plasma cell. Circulating B cells bearing surface immunoglobulin that share the idiotype of the M component are present in myeloma patients. Interleukin (IL) 6 may play a role in driving myeloma cell proliferation; a large fraction of myeloma cells exposed to IL-6 in vitro respond by proliferating. The IL-6 de-pendency of myeloma is controversial. Infection of marrow macrophages with human herpesvirus 8 has been noted in some cases leading to the hypothesis that viral IL-6 may contribute to the pathogenesis. This notion is also debated. It remains difficult to distinguish benign from malignant plasma cells on the basis of morphologic criteria in all but a few cases (**see Plate V-27**).

Incidence and Prevalence About 13,200 cases of myeloma were diagnosed in 2000, and 11,200 people died from the disease. Myeloma increases in incidence with age. The median age at diagnosis is 68 years; it is rare under age 40. The yearly incidence is around 4 per 100,000 and remarkably similar throughout the world. Males are slightly more commonly affected than females, and blacks have nearly twice the incidence of whites. In the age group over 25 the incidence is 30 per 100,000. Myeloma accounts for about 1% of all malignancies in whites and 2% in blacks; 13% of all hematologic cancers in whites and 33% in blacks.

Pathogenesis and Clinical Manifestations (Table 113-1) Bone pain is the most common symptom in myeloma, affecting nearly 70% of patients. The pain usually involves the back and ribs, and unlike the pain of metastatic carcinoma, which often is worse at night, the pain of myeloma is precipitated by movement. Persistent localized pain in a patient with myeloma usually signifies a pathologic fracture. The bone lesions of myeloma are caused by the proliferation of tumor cells and the activation of osteoclasts that destroy the bone. The osteoclasts respond to osteoclast activating factors (OAF) made by the myeloma cells [OAF activity can be mediated by several cytokines, including IL-1, lymphotoxin, and tumor necrosis factor (TNF)]. However, production of these factors stops following administration of glucocorticoids or interferon (IFN)-α. The bone lesions are lytic in nature and are rarely associated with osteoblastic new bone formation. Therefore, radioisotopic bone scanning is less useful in diagnosis than is plain radiography. The bony lysis results in substantial mobilization of calcium from bone, and serious acute and chronic complications of hypercalcemia may dominate the clinical picture (see below). Localized bone lesions may expand to the point that mass lesions may be palpated, especially on the skull (Fig. 113-3), clavicles, and sternum, and the collapse of vertebrae may lead to spinal cord compression.

The next most common clinical problem in patients with myeloma is susceptibility to bacterial infections. The most common infections are pneumonias and pyelonephritis, and the most frequent pathogens are *Streptococcus pneumoniae*, *Staphylococcus aureus*, and *Klebsiella pneumoniae* in the lungs and *Escherichia coli* and other gram-negative

FIGURE 113-2 Representative patterns of serum electrophoresis. The upper panel illustrates the normal pattern of serum protein on electrophoresis. Since there are many different immunoglobulins in the serum, their differing mobilities in an electric field produce a broad peak. In conditions associated with increases in polyclonal immunoglobulin, the broad peak is more prominent (middle panel). In monoclonal gammopathies, the predominance of a product of a single cell produces a "church spire" sharp peak, usually in the gamma globulin region (bottom panel).

Table 113-1 Pathogenesis and Clinical Manifestations of Multiple Myeloma

Clinical Finding	Underlying Cause	Pathogenic Mechanism
Hypercalcemia, pathologic fractures, cord compression, lytic bone lesions, osteoporosis, bone pain	Skeletal destruction	Tumor expansion; production of osteoclast activating factors (OAF) by tumor cells
Renal failure	Light chain proteinuria, hypercalcemia, urate nephropathy, amyloid glomerulopathy (rare) Pyelonephritis	Toxic effects of tumor products, light chains, OAF, DNA breakdown products Hypogammaglobulinemia
Anemia	Myelophthisis, decreased production, increased destruction	Tumor expansion; production of inhibitory factors and autoantibodies by tumor cells
Infection	Hypogammaglobulinemia, decreased neutrophil migration	Decreased production due to tumor-induced suppression; increased IgG catabolism
Neurologic symptoms	Hyperviscosity, cryoglobulins, amyloid deposits Hypercalcemia, cord compression	Products of tumor; properties of M component; light chains OAF
Bleeding	Interference with clotting factors, amyloid damage of endothelium, platelet dysfunction	Products of tumor; antibodies to clotting factors; light chains; antibody coating of platelets
Mass lesions		Tumor expansion

organisms in the urinary tract. In about 25% of patients, recurrent infections are the presenting features, and over 75% of patients will have a serious infection at some time in their course. The susceptibility to infection has several contributing causes. First, patients with myeloma have diffuse hypogammaglobulinemia if the M component is excluded. The hypogammaglobulinemia is related to both decreased production and increased destruction of normal antibodies. Moreover, some patients generate a population of circulating regulatory cells in response to their myeloma that can suppress normal antibody synthesis. In the case of IgG myeloma, normal IgG antibodies are broken down more rapidly than normal because the catabolic rate for IgG antibodies varies directly with the serum concentration. The large M component results in fractional catabolic rates of 8 to 16% instead of the normal 2%. These patients have very poor antibody responses, especially to polysaccharide antigens such as those on bacterial cell walls. Most measures of T cell function in myeloma are normal, but a subset of CD4+ cells may be decreased. Granulocyte lysozyme content is low, and granulocyte migration is not as rapid as normal in patients with myeloma, probably the result of a tumor product. There are also a variety of abnormalities in complement functions in myeloma patients. All these factors contribute to the immune deficiency of these patients.

Renal failure occurs in nearly 25% of myeloma patients, and some renal pathology is noted in over half. Many factors contribute to this. Hypercalcemia is the most common cause of renal failure. Glomerular deposits of amyloid, hyperuricemia, recurrent infections, and occasional infiltration of the kidney by myeloma cells all may contribute to renal dysfunction. However, tubular damage associated with the

excretion of light chains is almost always present. Normally, light chains are filtered, reabsorbed in the tubules, and catabolized. With the increase in the amount of light chains presented to the tubule, the tubular cells become overloaded with these proteins, and tubular damage results either directly from light chain toxic effects or indirectly from the release of intracellular lysosomal enzymes. The earliest manifestation of this tubular damage is the adult Fanconi syndrome (a type

FIGURE 113-3 Bony lesions in multiple myeloma. The skull demonstrates the typical "punched out" lesions characteristic of multiple myeloma. The lesion represents a purely osteolytic lesion with little or no osteoblastic activity. *(Courtesy of Dr. Geraldine Schechter.)*

2 proximal renal tubular acidosis), with increased loss of glucose, amino acids, and defects in the ability of the kidney to acidify and concentrate the urine. The proteinuria is not accompanied by hypertension, and the protein is nearly all light chains. Generally, very little albumin is in the urine because glomerular function is usually normal. When the glomeruli are involved, the proteinuria is nonselective. Patients with myeloma also have a decreased anion gap [i.e., $Na^+ - (Cl^- + HCO_3^-)$] because the M component is cationic, resulting in retention of chloride. This is often accompanied by hyponatremia that is felt to be artificial (pseudohyponatremia) because each volume of serum has less water as a result of the increased protein. Myeloma patients are susceptible to developing acute renal failure if they become dehydrated.

Anemia occurs in about 80% of myeloma patients. It is usually normocytic and normochromic and related both to the replacement of normal marrow by expanding tumor cells and to the inhibition of hematopoiesis by factors made by the tumor. In addition, mild hemolysis may contribute to the anemia. A larger than expected fraction of patients may have megaloblastic anemia due to either folate or vitamin B_{12} deficiency. Granulocytopenia and thrombocytopenia are very rare. Clotting abnormalities may be seen due to the failure of antibody-coated platelets to function properly or to the interaction of the M component with clotting factors I, II, V, VII, or VIII. Raynaud's phenomenon and impaired circulation may result if the M component forms cryoglobulins, and hyperviscosity syndromes may develop depending on the physical properties of the M component (most common with IgM, IgG3, and IgA paraproteins). Hyperviscosity is defined on the basis of the relative viscosity of serum as compared with water. Normal relative serum viscosity is 1.8 (i.e., serum is normally almost twice as viscous as water). Symptoms of hyperviscosity occur at a level of 5 to 6, a level usually reached at paraprotein concentrations of around 40 g/L (4 g/dL) for IgM, 50 g/L (5 g/dL) for IgG3, and 70 g/L (7 g/dL) for IgA.

Although neurologic symptoms occur in a minority of patients, they may have many causes. Hypercalcemia may produce lethargy, weakness, depression, and confusion. Hyperviscosity may lead to headache, fatigue, visual disturbances, and retinopathy. Bony damage and collapse may lead to cord compression, radicular pain, and loss of bowel and bladder control. Infiltration of peripheral nerves by amyloid can be a cause of carpal tunnel syndrome and other sensorimotor mono- and polyneuropathies.

Many of the clinical features of myeloma, e.g., cord compression, pathologic fractures, hyperviscosity, sepsis, and hypercalcemia, can present as medical emergencies. Despite the widespread distribution of plasma cells in the body, tumor expansion is dominantly within bone and bone marrow, and, for reasons unknown, rarely causes enlargement of spleen, lymph nodes, or gut-associated lymphatic tissue.

Diagnosis and Staging The classic triad of myeloma is marrow plasmacytosis (>10%), lytic bone lesions, and a serum and/or urine M component. The diagnosis may be made in the absence of bone lesions if the plasmacytosis is associated with a progressive increase in the M component over time or if extramedullary mass lesions develop. There are two important variants of myeloma, solitary bone plasmacytoma and extramedullary plasmacytoma. These lesions are associated with an M component in fewer than 30% of the cases, they may affect younger individuals, and both are associated with median survivals of 10 or more years. Solitary bone plasmacytoma is a single lytic bone lesion without marrow plasmacytosis. Extramedullary plasmacytomas usually involve the submucosal lymphoid tissue of the nasopharynx or paranasal sinuses without marrow plasmacytosis. Both tumors are highly responsive to local radiation therapy. If an M component is present, it should disappear after treatment. Solitary bone plasmacytomas may recur in other bony sites or evolve into myeloma. Extramedullary plasmacytomas rarely recur or progress.

The most difficult differential diagnosis in patients with myeloma involves their separation from individuals with benign monoclonal gammopathies or monoclonal gammopathies of uncertain significance (MGUS). MGUS are vastly more common than myeloma, occurring in 1% of the population over age 50 and in up to 10% over age 75. Patients with MGUS usually have <10% bone marrow plasma cells; <30 g/L (3 g/dL) of M components; no urinary Bence Jones protein; and no anemia, renal failure, lytic bone lesions, or hypercalcemia. When bone marrow cells are exposed to radioactive thymidine in order to quantitate dividing cells, patients with MGUS always have a labeling index <1%; patients with myeloma always have a labeling index >1%. Other discriminators include plasma cell acid phosphatase and β-glucuronidase, both of which are low in MGUS patients, and the salmon calcitonin stimulation test, which is positive only in patients with active ongoing bone destruction. With long-term follow-up, about 25% of patients with MGUS go on to develop myeloma. Typically, patients with MGUS require no therapy. Their survival is about 2 years shorter than age-matched controls without MGUS.

The clinical evaluation of patients with myeloma includes a careful physical examination searching for tender bones and masses. It is paradoxical that only a small minority of patients have an enlargement of the spleen and lymph nodes, the physiologic sites of antibody production. Chest and bone radiographs may reveal lytic lesions or diffuse osteopenia. A complete blood count with differential may reveal anemia. Erythrocyte sedimentation rate is elevated. Rare patients (~2%) may have plasma cell leukemia with more than 2000 plasma cells/μL. This may be seen in disproportionate frequency in IgD (12%) and IgE (25%) myelomas. Serum calcium, urea nitrogen, creatinine, and uric acid levels may be elevated. Protein electrophoresis and measurement of serum immunoglobulins are useful for detecting and characterizing M spikes, supplemented by immunoelectrophoresis, which is especially sensitive for identifying low concentrations of M components not detectable by protein electrophoresis. A 24-h urine specimen is necessary to quantitate protein excretion, and a concentrated aliquot is used for electrophoresis and immunologic typing of any M component. Serum alkaline phosphatase is usually normal even with extensive bone involvement because of the absence of osteoblastic activity. It is also important to quantitate serum β_2-microglobulin (see below). Serum soluble IL-6 receptor levels and C-reactive protein may reflect physiologic IL-6 levels in the patient.

The serum M component will be IgG in 53% of patients, IgA in 25%, and IgD in 1%; 20% of patients will have only light chains in serum and urine. Dipsticks for detecting proteinuria are not reliable at identifying light chains, and the heat test for detecting Bence Jones protein is falsely negative in about 50% of patients with light chain myeloma. Fewer than 1% of patients have no identifiable M component; these patients usually have light chain myelomas in which renal catabolism has made the light chains undetectable in the urine. IgD myeloma may also present as light chain myeloma. About two-thirds of patients with serum M components also have urinary light chains. The light chain isotype may have an impact on survival. Patients secreting lambda light chains have a significantly shorter overall survival than those secreting kappa light chains. It is not clear whether this is due to some genetically important determinant of cell proliferation or because lambda light chains are more likely to cause renal damage and form amyloid than are kappa light chains. The heavy chain isotype may have an impact on patient management as well. About half of patients with IgM paraproteins develop hyperviscosity compared with only 2 to 4% of patients with IgA and IgG M components. Among IgG myelomas, it is the IgG3 subclass that has the highest tendency to form both concentration- and temperature-dependent aggregates, leading to hyperviscosity and cold agglutination at lower serum concentrations.

The staging system for patients with myeloma is a functional system for predicting survival and is based on a variety of clinical and laboratory tests, unlike the anatomic staging systems for solid tumors. Details of the staging system are given in Table 113-2. Based on the hemoglobin, calcium, M component, and degree of skeletal involvement, the total-body tumor burden is estimated to be low (stage I, $<0.6 \times 10^{12}$ cells/m²), intermediate (stage II, 0.6 to 1.2×10^{12} cells/

Table 113-2 Myeloma Staging System

Stage	Criteria	Estimated Tumor Burden, $\times 10^{12}$ cells/m^2

I	All of the following:
	1. Hemoglobin >100 g/L (>10 g/dL)
	2. Serum calcium <3 mmol/L (<12 mg/dL)
	3. Normal bone x-ray or solitary lesion
	4. Low M-component production
	   a. IgG level <50 g/L (<5 g/dL)
	   b. IgA level <30 g/L (<3 g/dL)
	   c. Urine light chain <4 g/24 h
		<0.6 (low)

II	Fitting neither I nor III	0.6–1.20 (intermediate)

III	One or more of the following:
	1. Hemoglobin <85 g/L (<8.5 g/dL)
	2. Serum calcium >3 mmol/L (>12 mg/dL)
	3. Advanced lytic bone lesions
	4. High M-component production
	   a. IgG level >70 g/L (>7 g/dL)
	   b. IgA level >50 g/L (>5 g/dL)
	   c. Urine light chains >12 g/24 h
		>1.20 (high)

SUBCLASSIFICATION BASED ON SERUM CREATININE LEVELS

Level	Stage	Median Survival, Months
A < 177 μmol/L (<2 mg/dL)	IA	61
B > 177 μmol/L (>2 mg/dL)	IIA,B	55
	IIIA	30
	IIIB	15

STAGING BASED ON SERUM β_2-MICROGLOBULIN LEVELS

Level	Stage	Median Survival, Months
<0.004 g/L (<4 μg/mL)	I	43
>0.004 g/L (>4 μg/mL)	II	12

m^2), or high (stage III, >1.2 $\times$ 10^{12} cells/m^2), and the stages are further subdivided on the basis of renal function [A if serum creatinine <177 mol/L (<2 mg/dL), B if >177 (>2)]. Patients in stage IA have a median survival of more than 5 years and those in stage IIIB about 15 months. β_2-Microglobulin is a protein of 11,000 mol wt with homologies with the constant region of immunoglobulins that is the light chain of the class I major histocompatibility antigens (HLA-A, -B, -C) on the surface of every cell. Serum β_2-microglobulin is the single most powerful predictor of survival and can substitute for staging. Patients with β_2-microglobulin levels <0.004 g/L have a median survival of 43 months and those with levels >0.004 g/L only 12 months. It is also felt that once the diagnosis of myeloma is firm, histologic features of atypia may also exert an influence on prognosis. IL-6 may be an autocrine and/or paracrine growth factor for myeloma cells; elevated levels are associated with more aggressive disease. High labeling index and high levels of lactate dehydrogenase and thymidine kinase are also associated with poor prognosis.

Other factors that may influence prognosis are the number of cytogenetic abnormalities, % plasma cells in the marrow, performance status, and serum levels of IL-6, soluble IL-6 receptors, C-reactive protein, hepatocyte growth factor, C-terminal cross-linked telopeptide of collagen I, TGF-β, and syndecan-1.

R$_x$ **TREATMENT** About 10% of patients with myeloma will have an indolent course demonstrating only very slow progression of disease over many years. Such patients only require antitumor therapy when the serum myeloma protein level rises above 50 g/L (5 g/dL) or progressive bone lesions develop. Patients with solitary bone plasmacytomas and extramedullary plasmacytomas may be expected to enjoy prolonged disease-free survival after local radiation therapy to a dose of around 40 Gy. There is a low incidence of occult marrow involvement in patients with solitary bone plasmacytoma. Such pa-

tients are usually detected because their serum M component falls slowly or disappears initially only to return after a few months. These patients respond well to systemic chemotherapy.

The vast majority of patients with myeloma require therapeutic intervention. In general such therapy is of two sorts: systemic chemotherapy to control the progression of myeloma, and symptomatic supportive care to prevent serious morbidity from the complications of the disease. All patients with stage II or III disease and stage I patients exhibiting Bence Jones proteinuria, progressive lytic bone lesions, vertebral compression fractures, recurrent infections, or rising serum M component should be treated with systemic combination chemotherapy. Therapy can prolong and improve the quality of life for myeloma patients.

The standard treatment has consisted of intermittent pulses of an alkylating agent [L-phenylalanine mustard (L-PAM, melphalan), cyclophosphamide, or chlorambucil] and prednisone administered for 4 to 7 days every 4 to 6 weeks. The alkylating agents appear to be roughly equally active, but resistance to one agent is often accompanied by resistance to the others. The usual doses are as follows: melphalan, 8 mg/m^2 per day; cyclophosphamide, 200 mg/m^2 per day; chlorambucil, 8 mg/m^2 per day; prednisone, 25 to 60 mg/m^2 per day. Melphalan is used most commonly, but because of their near equivalence in antitumor efficacy, we favor cyclophosphamide as the alkylating agent because it is less toxic to the marrow stem cell compartment and results in a lower incidence of acute myelodysplastic syndromes than do the other alkylating agents. Doses may need adjustment based on marrow tolerance. However, there are few constraints on the dose of the steroid pulse, and it appears that more is better. Patients responding to therapy generally have a prompt and gratifying reduction in bone pain, hypercalcemia, and anemia, and often have fewer infections. The serum M component lags substantially behind the symptomatic improvement, often taking 4 to 6 weeks to fall. This fall depends on the rate of tumor kill and the fractional catabolic rate of immunoglobulin, which in turn depends on the serum concentration (for IgG). Light chain excretion, with a functional half-life of approximately 6 h, may fall within the first week of treatment. However, since urine light chain levels may relate to renal tubular function, they are not a reliable measure of tumor cell kill. Calculations of tumor cell kill are made by extrapolation of the serum M component level and rely heavily on the assumption that every tumor cell produces immunoglobulin at a constant rate. About 60% of patients will achieve at least a 75% reduction in serum M component level and tumor cell mass in response to an alkylating agent and prednisone. Although this is a tumor reduction of less than one log, clinical responses may last many months. The important feature of the level of the M protein is not how far or how fast it falls, but the rate of its increase after therapy. Efforts to improve the fraction of patients responding and the degree of response have involved adding other active chemotherapeutic agents to the treatment program. Patients with more advanced disease may benefit most from such an approach. High-dose therapy with hematopoietic support is also being tested in younger patients. Sequential treatment with combination chemotherapy regimens followed by two successive high-dose melphalan treatments, each supported with peripheral blood stem cell transplants, have achieved complete responses in 50% of patients treated within a year of diagnosis. Complete responses are rare (<10%) with standard therapy. Long-term follow-up is not yet available. Allogeneic transplants may also produce high response rates, but treatment-related mortality may be as high as 40%.

The ideal duration of therapy has not been determined. Most physicians treat every 4 to 6 weeks for 1 or 2 years. Cessation of therapy is followed by relapse, usually within a year. Retreatment may be associated with a second response in up to 80% of patients. Maintenance therapy (e.g., with IFN-α) may prolong the duration of response, but this therapy is toxic and has generally not prolonged survival. The regrowth rate of the tumor during relapse accelerates with each relapse. This observation suggests that kinetic resistance to therapy (i.e., increase in cycling cells) is perhaps more important than drug resistance controlled by mdr-1 expression. Patients often respond to treatment, but the length of the response progressively shortens. Patients primarily resistant to initial therapy have a median survival of less than a year. High-dose pulsed steroids used alone (200 mg prednisone every other day or 1 g/m^2 per day methylprednisolone for 5 days) or VAD combination chemotherapy (vincristine, 0.4 mg/d in a 4-day continuous infusion; doxorubicin, 9 mg/m^2 per day in a 4-day continuous infusion; dexamethasone, 40 mg/d for 4 days per week for 3 weeks) may offer useful palliation in patients resistant to primary therapy. High-dose melphalan has activity in patients with refractory disease. Thalidomide, which inhibits angiogenesis, also produces responses in refractory cases, but at doses that may cause somnolence.

About 15% of patients die within the first 3 months after diagnosis; subsequently, the death rate is about 15% per year. The disease usually follows a chronic course for 2 to 5 years before developing an acute terminal phase, usually marked by the development of pancytopenia with a cellular marrow that is refractory to treatment. Widespread organ infiltration by myeloma cells occurs, and survival is less than 6 months. About 46% of patients die in the chronic phase of disease from progressive myeloma (16%) and renal failure (10%), sepsis (14%), or both (6%). Death in the acute terminal phase (26%) is chiefly from progressive myeloma (13%) and sepsis (9%). Five percent of patients die of acute leukemia, myeloblastic or monocytic. Although it has been debated that this is related to the primary disease, it appears more likely to be the result of chronic therapy with alkylating agents. Nearly 23% of patients die of myocardial infarction, chronic lung disease, diabetes, or stroke, all intercurrent illnesses related more to the age of the patient group than to the tumor.

Supportive care directed at the anticipated complications of the disease may be as important as primary antitumor therapy. The hypercalcemia generally responds well to glucocorticoid therapy, hydration, and natriuresis. Calcitonin may add to the inhibitory effects of steroids on bone resorption. Bisphosphonates (e.g., pamidronate 90 mg once a month) reduce osteoclastic bone resorption and preserve performance status and quality of life; antitumor effects are also possible. Treatments aimed at strengthening the skeleton, such as fluorides, calcium, and vitamin D, with or without androgens, have been suggested but are not of proven efficacy. Iatrogenic worsening of renal function may be prevented by the use of allopurinol during chemotherapy to avoid urate nephropathy and by maintaining a high fluid intake to prevent dehydration and to help excrete light chains and calcium. In the event of acute renal failure, plasmapheresis is approximately 10 times more effective at clearing light chains than peritoneal dialysis, and acutely reducing the protein load may result in functional improvement. Urinary tract infections should be watched for and treated early. Chronic dialysis probably should not be initiated in patients who have failed to respond to antitumor therapy. Plasmapheresis may be the treatment of choice for hyperviscosity syndromes. Although the pneumococcus is a dreaded pathogen in myeloma patients, pneumococcal polysaccharide vaccines may not elicit an antibody response. The advent of intravenous gamma globulin preparations raises some hope that prophylactic administration may prevent some serious infections, but this has not been tested. Chronic oral antibiotic prophylaxis is probably not warranted. Patients developing neurologic symptoms in the lower extremities, severe localized back pain, or problems with bowel and bladder control may need emergency myelography and radiation therapy for palliation. Most bone lesions respond to analgesics and chemotherapy, but certain painful lesions may respond most promptly to localized radiation. The chronic anemia may respond to hematinics (iron, folate, cobalamin), and some have responded to androgens. The pathogenesis of the anemia should be established and specific therapy instituted, where possible.

WALDENSTRÖM'S MACROGLOBULINEMIA   In 1948, Waldenström described a malignancy of lymphoplasmacytoid cells

that secreted IgM. In contrast to myeloma, the disease was associated with lymphadenopathy and hepatosplenomegaly, but the major clinical manifestation was the hyperviscosity syndrome. The disease resembles the related diseases chronic lymphocytic leukemia, myeloma, and lymphocytic lymphoma. Waldenström's macroglobulinemia and IgM myeloma both follow a similar clinical course. The diagnosis of IgM myeloma is usually reserved for patients with lytic bone lesions and is important only because of the hazard of pathologic fractures.

The cause of macroglobulinemia is unknown. The disease is similar to myeloma in being slightly more common in men and occurring with increased incidence with age (median 64 years). There have been reports that the IgM in some patients with macroglobulinemia may have specificity for myelin-associated glycoprotein (MAG), a protein that has been associated with demyelinating disease of the peripheral nervous system and may be lost earlier and to a greater extent than the better known myelin basic protein in patients with multiple sclerosis. Sometimes patients with macroglobulinemia develop a peripheral neuropathy before the appearance of the neoplasm. There is speculation that the whole process begins with a viral infection that may elicit an antibody response that cross-reacts with a normal tissue component.

Like myeloma, the disease involves the bone marrow, but unlike myeloma, it does not cause bone lesions or hypercalcemia. Like myeloma, a serum M component is present in the serum in excess of 30 g/L (3 g/dL), but unlike myeloma, the size of the IgM paraprotein results in little renal excretion and only around 20% of patients excrete light chains. Therefore, renal disease is not common. The light chain isotype is kappa in 80% of the cases. Patients present with weakness, fatigue, and recurrent infections, similar to myeloma patients, but epistaxis, visual disturbances, and neurologic symptoms such as peripheral neuropathy, dizziness, headache, and transient paresis are much more common in macroglobulinemia. Physical examination reveals adenopathy and hepatosplenomegaly, and ophthalmoscopic examination may reveal vascular segmentation and dilatation of the retinal veins characteristic of hyperviscosity states. Patients may have a normocytic, normochromic anemia, but rouleaux formation and a positive Coombs' test are much more common than in myeloma. Malignant lymphocytes are usually present in the peripheral blood. About 10% of macroglobulins are cryoglobulins. These are pure M components and are not the mixed cryoglobulins seen in rheumatoid arthritis and other autoimmune diseases. Mixed cryoglobulins are composed of IgM or IgA complexed with IgG, for which they are specific. In both cases, Raynaud's phenomenon and serious vascular symptoms precipitated by the cold may occur, but mixed cryoglobulins are not commonly associated with malignancy. Patients suspected of having a cryoglobulin based on history and physical examination should have their blood drawn into a warm syringe and delivered to the laboratory in a container of warm water to avoid errors in quantitating the cryoglobulin.

℞ **TREATMENT**   Control of serious hyperviscosity symptoms such as an altered state of consciousness or paresis can be achieved acutely by plasmapheresis because 80% of the IgM paraprotein is intravascular. Fludarabine (25 mg/m^2 per day for 5 days every 4 weeks) or cladribine (0.1 mg/kg per day for 7 days every 4 weeks) are highly effective single agents. About 80% of patients respond to chemotherapy, and their median survival is over 3 years. The absence of other serious organ toxicities results in a longer life span of patients with macroglobulinemia compared with those with myeloma.

POEMS SYNDROME   The features of this syndrome are *p*olyneuropathy, *o*rganomegaly, *e*ndocrinopathy, *m*ultiple myeloma, and *s*kin changes (POEMS). Patients usually have a severe, progressive sensorimotor polyneuropathy associated with sclerotic bone lesions from myeloma. Polyneuropathy occurs in about 1.4% of myelomas, but the POEMS syndrome is only a rare subset of that group. Unlike typical myeloma, hepatomegaly and lymphadenopathy occur in about two-thirds of patients, and splenomegaly is seen in one-third. The lymphadenopathy frequently resembles Castleman's disease histologically, a condition that has been linked to IL-6 overproduction. The endocrine manifestations include amenorrhea in women and impotence and gynecomastia in men. Hyperprolactinemia due to loss of normal inhibitory control by the hypothalamus may be associated with other central nervous system manifestations such as papilledema and elevated cerebrospinal fluid pressure and protein. Type 2 diabetes mellitus occurs in about one-third of patients. Hypothyroidism and adrenal insufficiency are occasionally noted. Skin changes are diverse: hyperpigmentation, hypertrichosis, skin thickening, and digital clubbing. Other manifestations include peripheral edema, ascites, pleural effusions, fever, and thrombocytosis.

The pathogenesis of the disease is unclear, but high circulating levels of the proinflammatory cytokines IL-1, IL-6, and TNF have been documented and levels of the inhibitory cytokine transforming growth factor β (TGF-β) are lower than expected. Treatment of the myeloma may result in an improvement in the other disease manifestations.

HEAVY CHAIN DISEASES The heavy chain diseases are rare lymphoplasmacytic malignancies. Their clinical manifestations vary with the heavy chain isotype. Patients secrete a defective heavy chain that usually has an intact Fc fragment and a deletion in the Fd region. Gamma, alpha, and mu heavy chain diseases have been described, but no reports of delta or epsilon heavy chain diseases have appeared. Molecular biologic analysis of these tumors has revealed structural genetic defects that may account for the aberrant chain secreted.

Gamma Heavy Chain Disease (Franklin's Disease) This disease affects people of widely different age groups and countries of origin. It is characterized by lymphadenopathy, fever, anemia, malaise, hepatosplenomegaly, and weakness. Its most distinctive symptom is palatal edema, resulting from node involvement of Waldeyer's ring, and this may progress to produce respiratory compromise. The diagnosis depends on the demonstration of an anomalous serum M component [often <20 g/L (<2 g/dL)] that reacts with anti-IgG but not anti-light chain reagents. *The M component is typically present in both serum and urine.* Most of the paraproteins have been of the gamma subclass, but other subclasses have been seen. The patients may have thrombocytopenia, eosinophilia, and nondiagnostic bone marrow. Patients usually have a rapid downhill course and die of infection; however, some patients have survived 5 years with chemotherapy.

Alpha Heavy Chain Disease (Seligmann's Disease) This is the most common of the heavy chain diseases. It is closely related to a malignancy known as *Mediterranean lymphoma*, a disease that affects young people in parts of the world where intestinal parasites are common, such as the Mediterranean, Asia, and South America. The disease is characterized by an infiltration of the lamina propria of the small intestine with lymphoplasmacytoid cells that secrete truncated alpha chains. Demonstrating alpha heavy chains is difficult because the alpha chains tend to polymerize and appear as a smear instead of a sharp peak on electrophoretic profiles. Despite the polymerization, hyperviscosity is not a common problem in alpha heavy chain disease. Without J chain–facilitated dimerization, viscosity does not increase dramatically. Light chains are absent from serum and urine. The patients present with chronic diarrhea, weight loss, and malabsorption and have extensive mesenteric and para-aortic adenopathy. Respiratory tract involvement occurs rarely. Patients may vary widely in their clinical course. Some may develop diffuse aggressive histologies of malignant lymphoma. Chemotherapy may produce long-term remissions. Rare patients appear to have responded to antibiotic therapy, raising the question of the etiologic role of antigenic stimulation, perhaps by some chronic intestinal infection. Chemotherapy plus antibiotics may be more effective than chemotherapy alone.

Mu Heavy Chain Disease The secretion of isolated mu heavy chains into the serum appears to occur in a very rare subset of patients with chronic lymphocytic leukemia. The only features that may distinguish patients with mu heavy chain disease are the presence of vacuoles in the malignant lymphocytes and the excretion of kappa light chains in the urine. The diagnosis requires ultracentrifugation or gel filtration to confirm the nonreactivity of the paraprotein with the light chain reagents, because some intact macroglobulins fail to interact with these serums. The tumor cells seem to have a defect in the assembly of light and heavy chains, because they appear to contain both in their cytoplasm. There is no evidence that such patients should be treated differently from other patients with chronic lymphocytic leukemia (Chap. 112).

BIBLIOGRAPHY

BATAILLE R, HAROUSSEAU J-L: Multiple myeloma. N Engl J Med 336:1657, 1997

DIMOPOULOS MA, ALEXANIAN R: Waldenström's macroglobulinemia. Blood 83:1452, 1994

GARCIA-SANZ R et al: Primary plasma cell leukemia: Clinical, immunophenotypic, DNA ploidy, and cytogenetic characteristics. Blood 93:1032, 1999

GHERARDI RK et al: Overproduction of proinflammatory cytokines imbalanced by their antagonists in POEMS syndrome. Blood 87:1458, 1996

HU K, YAHALOM J: Radiotherapy in the management of plasma cell tumors. Oncology 14:101, 2000

KONINGSBERG R et al: Predictive role of interphase cytogenetics for survival of patients with multiple myeloma. J Clin Oncol 18:804, 2000

KYLE RA: "Benign" monoclonal gammopathy—after 20–35 years of follow-up. Mayo Clin Proc 68:26, 1993

———: Plasma cell disorders. Hematol/Oncol Clin North Am 13:1117, 1999

LENHOFF S et al: Impact on survival of high-dose therpy with autologous stem cell support in patients younger than 60 years with newly diagnosed multiple myeloma: A population-based study. Blood 95:7, 2000

SINGHAL S et al: Antitumor activity of thalidomide in refractory myeloma. N Engl J Med 341:1565, 1999

VESOLE DH et al: High-dose melphalan with autotransplantation for refractory multiple myeloma: Results of a Southwest Oncology Group phase II trial. J Clin Oncol 17:2173, 1999

| **114** | *Jeffery S. Dzieczkowski, Kenneth C. Anderson* |

TRANSFUSION BIOLOGY AND THERAPY

ACE	angiotensin-converting enzyme	HBV	hepatitis B virus
CCI	corrected count increment	HCV	hepatitis C virus
CMV	cytomegalovirus	HGV	hepatitis G virus
DAT	direct antiglobulin test	HTLV	human T lymphotropic virus
DHTRs	delayed hemolytic transfusion reactions	PRBC	packed RBC
DIC	disseminated intravascular coagulation	RBC	red blood cell
		RD	random donor
FFP	fresh frozen plasma	SDAP	single-donor apheresis platelets
FNHTR	febrile nonhemolytic transfusion reaction	TA-GVHD	transfusion-associated graft-versus-host disease
GVHD	graft-versus-host disease	vWF	von Willebrand factor

BLOOD GROUP ANTIGENS AND ANTIBODIES

The study of red blood cell (RBC) antigens and antibodies forms the foundation of transfusion medicine. Serologic studies initially characterized these antigens, but now the molecular composition and structure of many are known. Antigens, either carbohydrate or protein, are assigned to a blood group system based upon the structure and the similarity of the determinant epitopes. Other cellular blood elements and plasma proteins are also antigenic and can result in *alloimmunization*, the production of antibodies directed against the blood group antigens of another individual. These antibodies are called *alloantibodies*.

Antibodies directed against RBC antigens may result from "natural" exposure, particularly to carbohydrates that mimic some blood group antigens. Those antibodies that occur via natural stimuli are usually produced by a T cell–independent response (thus, generating no memory) and are IgM isotype. *Autoantibodies* (antibodies against autologous blood group antigens) arise spontaneously or as the result of infectious sequelae (e.g., from *Mycoplasma pneumoniae*) and are also often IgM. These antibodies are often clinically insignificant due to their low affinity for antigen at body temperature. However, IgM antibodies can activate the complement cascade and result in hemolysis. Antibodies that result from allogeneic exposure, such as transfusion or pregnancy, are usually IgG. IgG antibodies commonly bind to antigen at warmer temperatures and may hemolyze RBCs. Unlike IgM antibodies, IgG antibodies can cross the placenta and bind fetal erythrocytes bearing the corresponding antigen, resulting in hemolytic disease of the newborn, or *hydrops fetalis*.

Alloimmunization to leukocytes, platelets, and plasma proteins may also result in transfusion complications such as fevers and urticaria but generally does not cause hemolysis. Assay for these other alloantibodies is not routinely performed; however, they may be detected using special assays.

ABO ANTIGENS AND ANTIBODIES   The first blood group antigen system, recognized in 1900, was ABO, the most important in transfusion medicine. The major blood groups of this system are A, B, AB, and O. O type RBCs lack A or B antigens. These antigens are carbohydrates attached to a precursor backbone, may be found on the cellular membrane either as glycosphingolipids or glycoproteins, and are secreted into plasma and body fluids as glycoproteins. H substance is the immediate precursor upon which the A and B antigens are added. This H substance is formed by the addition of fucose to the glycolipid or glycoprotein backbone. The subsequent addition of *N*-acetylgalactosamine creates the A antigen, while the addition of galactose produces the B antigen.

The genes that determine the A and B phenotypes are found on chromosome 9p and are expressed in a Mendelian codominant manner. The gene products are glycosyl transferases, which confer the enzymatic capability of attaching the specific antigenic carbohydrate. Individuals who lack the "A" and "B" transferases are phenotypically type "O," while those who inherit both transferases are type "AB." Rare individuals lack the H gene, which codes for fucose transferase, and cannot form H substance. These individuals are homozygous for the silent h allele (hh) and have Bombay phenotype (O$_h$).

The ABO blood group system is important because essentially all individuals produce antibodies to the ABH carbohydrate antigen that they lack. The naturally occurring anti-A and anti-B antibodies are termed *isoagglutinins*. Thus, type A individuals produce anti-B, while type B individuals make anti-A. Neither isoagglutinin is found in type AB individuals, while type O individuals produce both anti-A and anti-B. Thus, persons with type AB are "universal recipients" because they do not have antibodies against any ABO phenotype, while persons with type O blood can donate to essentially all recipients because their cells are not recognized by any ABO isoagglutinins. The rare individuals with Bombay phenotype produce antibodies to H substance (which is present on all red cells except those of hh phenotype) as well as to both A and B antigens and are therefore compatible only with other hh donors.

In most people, A and B antigens are secreted by the cells and are present in the circulation. Nonsecretors are susceptible to a variety of infections (e.g., *Candida albicans*, *Neisseria meningitidis*, *Streptococcus pneumoniae*, *Haemophilus influenzae*) as many organisms may bind to polysaccharides on cells. Soluble blood group antigens may block this binding.

Rh SYSTEM   The Rh system is the second most important blood group system in pretransfusion testing. The Rh antigens are found on a 30- to 32-kDa RBC membrane protein, which has no defined function. Although more than 40 different antigens in the Rh system have been described, five determinants account for the vast majority of phenotypes. The presence of the D antigen confers Rh "positivity," while people who lack the D antigen are Rh negative. Two allelic antigen pairs, E/e and C/c, are also found on the Rh protein.

The three Rh genes, E/e, D, and C/c, are arranged in tandem on chromosome 1 and inherited as a haplotype, i.e., cDE or Cde. Two haplotypes can result in the phenotypic expression of two to five Rh antigens.

The D antigen is a potent alloantigen. About 15% of people lack this antigen. Exposure of these Rh-negative people to even small amounts of Rh-positive cells, by either transfusion or pregnancy, can result in the production of anti-D alloantibody.

OTHER BLOOD GROUP SYSTEMS AND ALLOANTIBODIES   More than 100 blood group systems are recognized, composed of more than 500 antigens. The presence or absence of certain antigens has been associated with various diseases and anomalies; antigens also act as receptors for infectious agents. Alloantibodies of importance in routine clinical practice are listed in Table 114-1.

Antibodies to *Lewis system* carbohydrate antigens are the most common cause of incompatibility during pretransfusion screening. The Lewis gene product is a fucosyl transferase and maps to chromosome 19. The antigen is not an integral membrane structure but is adsorbed to the RBC membrane from the plasma. Antibodies to Lewis antigens are usually IgM and cannot cross the placenta. Lewis antigens may be adsorbed onto tumor cells and may be targets of therapy.

I system antigens are also oligosaccharides related to H, A, B, and Le. I and i are not allelic pairs but are carbohydrate antigens that differ only in the extent of branching. The i antigen is an unbranched chain that is converted by the I gene product, a glycosyltransferase, into a branched chain. The branching process affects all the ABH antigens, which become progressively more branched in the first 2 years of life. Some patients with cold agglutinin disease or lymphomas can produce anti-I autoantibodies that cause RBC destruction. Occasional patients with mononucleosis or *Mycoplasma* pneumonia may develop cold agglutinins of either anti-I or anti-i specificity. Most adults lack i expression; thus, finding a donor for patients with anti-i is not difficult. Even though most adults express I antigen, binding is generally low at body temperature. Thus, administration of warm blood prevents isoagglutination.

The *P system* is another group of carbohydrate antigens controlled by specific glycosyltransferases. Its clinical significance is in rare cases of syphilis and viral infection that lead to paroxysmal cold hemoglobinuria. In these cases, an unusual autoantibody to P is produced that binds to RBCs in the cold and fixes complement upon warming. Antibodies with these biphasic properties are called *Donath-Landsteiner antibodies*. The P antigen is also expressed on urothelial cells and may be a receptor for *Escherichia coli* binding.

The *MNSsU system* is regulated by genes on chromosome 4. M and N are determinants on glycophorin A, an RBC membrane protein, and S and s are determinants on glycophorin B. Anti-S and anti-s IgG antibodies may develop after pregnancy or transfusion and lead to hemolysis. Anti-U antibodies are rare but problematic; virtually every donor is incompatible because nearly all persons express U.

The *Kell* protein is very large (720 amino acids) and its secondary structure contains many different antigenic epitopes. The immunoge-

Table 114-1   RBC Blood Group Systems and Alloantigens

Blood Group System	Antigen	Alloantibody	Clinical Significance
Rh (D, C/c, E/e)	RBC protein	IgG	HTR, HDN
Lewis (Le^a, Le^b)	Oligosaccharide	IgM/IgG	Rare HTR
Kell (K/k)	RBC protein	IgG	HTR, HDN
Duffy (Fy^a/Fy^b)	RBC protein	IgG	HTR, HDN
Kidd (Jk^a/Jk^b)	RBC protein	IgG	HTR (often delayed), HDN (mild)
I/i	Carbohydrate	IgM	None
MNSsU	RBC protein	IgM/IgG	Anti-M rare HDN, anti-S, -s, and -U HDN, HTR

NOTE: RBC, red blood cell; HDN, hemolytic disease of the newborn; HTR, hemolytic transfusion reaction.

nicity of Kell is third behind the ABO and Rh systems. The absence of the Kell precursor protein (controlled by a gene on X) is associated with acanthocytosis, shortened RBC survival, and a progressive form of muscular dystrophy that includes cardiac defects. This rare condition is called the *McLeod phenotype*. The K_x gene is linked to the 91-kDa component of the NADPH-oxidase on the X chromosome, deletion or mutation of which accounts for about 60% of cases of chronic granulomatous disease.

The *Duffy* antigens are codominant alleles, Fy^a and Fy^b, that also serve as receptors for *Plasmodium vivax*. More than 70% of persons in malaria-endemic areas lack these antigens, probably from selective influences of the infection on the population.

The *Kidd* antigens, Jk^a and Jk^b, may elicit antibodies transiently. A delayed hemolytic transfusion reaction that occurs with blood tested as compatible is often related to delayed appearance of anti-Jk^a.

PRETRANSFUSION TESTING

Pretransfusion testing of a potential recipient consists of the "type and screen." The "forward type" determines the ABO and Rh phenotype of the recipient's RBC by using antisera directed against the A, B, and D antigens. The "reverse type" detects isoagglutinins in the patient's serum and should correlate with the ABO phenotype, or forward type.

The alloantibody screen identifies antibodies directed against other RBC antigens. The alloantibody screen is performed by mixing patient serum with type O RBCs that contain the major antigens of most blood group systems and whose extended phenotype is known. The specificity of the alloantibody is identified by correlating the presence or absence of antigen with the results of the agglutination.

Cross matching is ordered when there is a high probability that the patient will require a packed RBC (PRBC) transfusion. Blood selected for cross matching must be ABO compatible and lack antigens for which the patient has alloantibodies. Nonreactive cross matching confirms the absence of any major incompatibility and reserves that unit for the patient.

In the case of Rh-negative patients, every attempt must be made to provide Rh-negative blood components to prevent alloimmunization to the D antigen. In an emergency, Rh-positive blood can be safely transfused to a Rh-negative patient who lacks anti-D; however, the recipient is likely to become alloimmunized and produce anti-D. Rh-negative women of child-bearing age who are transfused with products containing Rh-positive RBCs should receive passive immunization with anti-D (RhoGam or WinRho) to reduce or prevent sensitization.

BLOOD COMPONENTS

Blood products intended for transfusion are routinely collected as whole blood (450 mL) in various anticoagulants. Most donated blood is processed into components: PRBCs, platelets, and fresh frozen plasma (FFP) or cryoprecipitate (Table 114-2). Whole blood is first separated into PRBCs and platelet-rich plasma by slow centrifugation. The platelet-rich plasma is then centrifuged at high speed to yield one unit of random donor (RD) platelets and one unit of FFP. Cryoprecipitate is produced by thawing FFP to precipitate the plasma proteins, which are then separated by centrifugation.

Apheresis technology is used for the collection of multiple units of platelets from a single donor. These single-donor apheresis platelets (SDAP) contain the equivalent of at least six units of RD platelets and have fewer contaminating leukocytes than pooled RD platelets.

Table 114-2   Characteristics of Selected Blood Components

Component	Volume, mL	Content	Clinical Response
PRBC	180–200	RBCs with variable leukocyte content and small amount of plasma	Increase hemoglobin 10 g/L and hematocrit 3%
Platelets	50–70	5.5×10^{10}/RD unit	Increase platelet count 5000–10,000/μL
	200–400	$\geq 3.0 \times 10^{11}$/SDAP product	CCI $\geq 10 \times 10^9$/L within 1 h and $\geq 7.5 \times 10^9$/L within 24 h posttransfusion
FFP	200–250	Plasma proteins—coagulation factors, proteins C and S, antithrombin	Increases coagulation factors about 2%
Cryoprecipitate	10–15	Cold-insoluble plasma proteins, fibrinogen, factor VIII, vWF	Topical fibrin glue, also 80 IU factor VIII

NOTE: PRBC, packed red blood cells; RBC, red blood cell; RD, random donor; SDAP, single-donor apheresis platelets; CCI, corrected count increment; FFP, fresh frozen plasma; vWF, von Willebrand factor.

Plasma may also be collected by apheresis. Plasma derivatives such as albumin, intravenous immunoglobulin, antithrombin, and coagulation factor concentrates are prepared from pooled plasma from many donors and are treated to eliminate infectious agents.

WHOLE BLOOD   Whole blood provides both oxygen-carrying capacity and volume expansion. It is the ideal component for patients who have sustained acute hemorrhage of 25% or greater total blood volume loss. Whole blood is stored at 4°C to maintain erythrocyte viability, but platelet dysfunction and degradation of some coagulation factors occurs. In addition, 2,3-BPG levels fall over time, leading to an increase in the oxygen affinity of the hemoglobin and a decreased capacity to deliver oxygen to the tissues, a problem with all red cell storage. Whole blood is not readily available since it is routinely processed into components.

PACKED RED BLOOD CELLS   This product increases oxygen-carrying capacity in the anemic patient. Adequate oxygenation can be maintained with a hemoglobin content of 70 g/L in the normovolemic patient without cardiac disease; however, comorbid factors often necessitate transfusion at a higher threshold. The decision to transfuse should be guided by the clinical situation and not by an arbitrary laboratory value. In the critical care setting, liberal use of transfusions to maintain near normal levels of hemoglobin may have unexpected negative effects on survival. In most patients requiring transfusion, levels of hemoglobin of 100 g/L are sufficient to keep oxygen supply from being critically low.

PRBCs may be modified to prevent certain adverse reactions. Contaminating leukocytes are responsible for inducing fevers and causing alloimmunization to HLA antigens. Leukocytes can be removed by several methods. Bedside filtration is the most popular method and removes 99.9% of donor leukocytes. Leukoreduction may be done in the blood bank before storage of cellular components; this practice results in less cytokine release from the cells. Plasma, which may cause allergic reactions, can be removed from cellular blood components by washing.

PLATELETS   Thrombocytopenia is a risk factor for hemorrhage, and platelet transfusion reduces the incidence of bleeding. The threshold for prophylactic platelet transfusion is 10,000/μL. In patients without fever or infections, a threshold of 5000/μL may be sufficient to prevent spontaneous hemorrhage. For invasive procedures, 50,000/μL platelets is the usual target level.

Platelets are given either as pools prepared from five to eight RDs or as SDAPs from a single donor. In an unsensitized patient without increased platelet consumption [splenomegaly, fever, disseminated intravascular coagulation (DIC)], six to eight units of RD platelets (about 1 unit per 10 kg body weight) are transfused, and each unit is anticipated to increase the platelet count 5000 to 10,000/μL. Patients who have received multiple transfusions may be alloimmunized to many HLA- and platelet-specific antigens and have little or no increase in their posttransfusion platelet counts. Patients who may require multiple transfusions are best served by receiving SDAP and leukocyte-reduced components to lower the risk of alloimmunization.

Refractoriness to platelet transfusion may be evaluated using the corrected count increment (CCI):

$$CCI = \frac{\text{posttransfusion count} - \text{pretransfusion count}}{\text{number of platelets transfused} \times 10^{11}} \times BSA$$

where BSA is body surface area measured in square meters. The platelet count performed 1 h after the transfusion is acceptable if the CCI is 10×10^9/mL, and after 18 to 24 h an increment of 7.5×10^9/mL is expected. Patients who have suboptimal responses are likely to have received multiple transfusions and have antibodies directed against class I HLA antigens. Refractoriness can be investigated by detecting anti-HLA antibodies in the recipient's serum. Patients who are sensitized will often react with 100% of the lymphocytes used for the HLA-antibody screen, and HLA-matched SDAPs should be considered for those patients who require transfusion. Although ABO-identical HLA-matched SDAPs provide the best chance for increasing the platelet count, locating these products is difficult. Platelet cross matching is available in some centers. Additional clinical causes for a low platelet CCI include fever, bleeding, splenomegaly, DIC, or medications in the recipient.

FRESH FROZEN PLASMA FFP contains stable coagulation factors and plasma proteins: fibrinogen, antithrombin, albumin, as well as proteins C and S. Indications for FFP include correction of coagulopathies, including the rapid reversal of coumadin; supplying deficient plasma proteins; and treatment of thrombotic thrombocytopenic purpura. FFP should not be routinely used to expand blood volume. FFP is an acellular component and does not transmit intracellular infections, e.g., cytomegalovirus (CMV). Patients who are IgA-deficient and require plasma support should receive FFP from IgA-deficient donors to prevent anaphylaxis (see below).

CRYOPRECIPITATE Cryoprecipitate is a source of fibrinogen, factor VIII, and von Willebrand factor (vWF). It is ideal for supplying fibrinogen to the volume-sensitive patient. When factor VIII concentrates are not available, cyroprecipitate may be used since each unit contains approximately 80 units of factor VIII. Cryoprecipitate may also be used as a source of vWF for patients with dysfunctional (type II) or absent (type III) von Willebrand disease.

PLASMA DERIVATIVES Plasma from thousands of donors may be pooled to derive specific protein concentrates, including albumin, intravenous immunoglobulin, antithrombin, and coagulation factors. In addition, donors who have high-titer antibodies to specific agents or antigens provide hyperimmune globulins, such as anti-D (RhoGam, WinRho), and antisera to hepatitis B virus (HBV), varicella-zoster virus, CMV, and other infectious agents.

ADVERSE REACTIONS TO BLOOD TRANSFUSION

Adverse reactions to transfused blood components occur despite multiple tests, inspections, and checks. Fortunately, the most common reactions are not life-threatening, although serious reactions can present with mild symptoms and signs. Some reactions can be reduced or prevented by modified (filtered, washed, or irradiated) blood components. When an adverse reaction is suspected, the transfusion should be stopped and reported to the blood bank for investigation.

Transfusion reactions may result from immune and nonimmune mechanisms. Immune-mediated reactions are often due to preformed donor or recipient antibody; however, cellular elements may also cause adverse effects. Nonimmune causes of reactions are due to the chemical and physical properties of the stored blood component and its additives.

Infectious complications of transfusion have become less frequent, although fear of these complications remains a primary concern. The incidence of transfusion-related infections has been reduced substantially due to improved donor screening and testing of collected blood. Infections, like any adverse transfusion reaction, must be brought to the attention of the blood bank for appropriate studies (Table 114-3).

IMMUNE-MEDIATED REACTIONS Acute Hemolytic Transfusion Reactions Immune-mediated hemolysis occurs when the recipient has preformed antibodies that lyse donor erythrocytes. The ABO isoagglutinins are responsible for the majority of these reactions, although alloantibodies directed against other RBC antigens, i.e., Rh, Kell, and Duffy, may result in hemolysis.

Acute hemolytic reactions may present with hypotension, tachypnea, tachycardia, fever, chills, hemoglobinemia, hemoglobinuria, chest and/or flank pain, and discomfort at the infusion site. Monitoring the patient's vital signs before and during the transfusion is important to identify reactions promptly. When acute hemolysis is suspected, the transfusion must be stopped immediately, intravenous access maintained, and the reaction reported to the blood bank. A correctly labeled posttransfusion blood sample and any untransfused blood should be sent to the blood bank for analysis. The laboratory evaluation for hemolysis includes the measurement of serum haptoglobin, lactate dehydrogenase (LDH), and indirect bilirubin levels.

The immune complexes that result in RBC lysis can cause renal dysfunction and failure. Diuresis should be induced with intravenous fluids and furosemide or mannitol. Tissue factor released from the lysed erythrocytes may initiate DIC. Coagulation studies including prothrombin time (PT), activated partial thromboplastin time (aPTT), fibrinogen, and platelet count should be monitored in patients with hemolytic reactions.

Errors at the patient's bedside, such as mislabeling the sample or transfusing the wrong patient, are responsible for the majority of these reactions. The blood bank investigation of these reactions includes examination of the pre- and posttransfusion samples for hemolysis and repeat typing of the patient samples; direct antiglobulin test (DAT), sometimes called the direct Coombs test, of the posttransfusion sample; repeating the cross matching of the blood component; and checking all clerical records for errors. DAT detects the presence of antibody or complement bound to RBCs in vivo.

Delayed Hemolytic and Serologic Transfusion Reactions Delayed hemolytic transfusion reactions (DHTRs) are not completely preventable. These reactions occur in patients previously sensitized to RBC alloantigens who have a negative alloantibody screen due to low antibody levels. When the patient is transfused with antigen-positive blood, an anamnestic response results in the early production of al-

Table 114-3 Risks of Transfusion Complications

	Frequency, Episodes:Unit
Reactions	
Febrile (FNHTR)	1–4:100
Allergic	1–4:100
Delayed hemolytic	1:1,000
TRALI	1:5,000
Acute hemolytic	1:12,000
Fatal hemolytic	1:100,000
Anaphylactic	1:150,000
Infections[a]	
Hepatitis B	1:66,000
Hepatitis C	1:103,000
HIV-1	1:676,000
HIV-2	None reported
HTLV-I and -II	1:641,000
Malaria	1:4,000,000
Other complications	
RBC allosensitization	1:100
HLA allosensitization	1:10
Graft-versus-host disease	Rare

[a] Infectious agents rarely associated with transfusion, theoretically possible or of unknown risk include: Hepatitis A virus, parvovirus B-19, *Babesia microti* (babesiosis), *Borrelia burgdorferi* (Lyme disease), *Trypanosoma cruzi* (Chagas' disease), and *Treponema pallidum*, human herpesvirus-8 and hepatitis G virus.

NOTE: FNHTR, febrile nonhemolytic transfusion reaction; TRALI, transfusion-related acute lung injury; HTLV, human T lymphotropic virus; RBC, red blood cell loantibody that binds donor RBCs. The alloantibody is detectable 1 to 2 weeks following the transfusion, and the posttransfusion DAT may become positive due to circulating donor RBCs coated with antibody or complement. The transfused, alloantibody-coated erythrocytes are cleared by the extravascular reticuloendothelial system. These reactions are detected most commonly in the blood bank when a subsequent patient sample reveals a positive alloantibody screen or a new alloantibody in a recently transfused recipient.

No specific therapy is usually required, although additional RBC transfusions may be necessary. Delayed serologic transfusion reactions (DSTR) are similar to DHTR, as the DAT is positive and alloantibody is detected; however, RBC clearance is not increased.

Febrile Nonhemolytic Transfusion Reaction   The most frequent reaction associated with the transfusion of cellular blood components is a febrile nonhemolytic transfusion reaction (FNHTR). These reactions are characterized by chills and rigors and a 1°C or greater rise in temperature. FNHTR is diagnosed when other causes of fever in the transfused patient are ruled out. Antibodies directed against donor leukocyte and HLA antigens may mediate these reactions; thus, multiply transfused patients and multiparous women are felt to be at increased risk. Although antibodies may be demonstrated in the recipient's serum, investigation is not routinely done because of the mild nature of most FNHTR. The use of leukocyte-reduced blood products may prevent or delay sensitization to leukocyte antigens and thereby reduce the incidence of these febrile episodes. Cytokines released from cells within stored blood components may mediate FNHTR; thus, leukoreduction before storage may prevent these reactions. The incidence and severity of these reactions can be decreased in patients with recurrent reactions by premedicating with acetaminophen or other antipyretic agents.

Allergic Reactions   Urticarial reactions are related to plasma proteins found in transfused components. Mild reactions may be treated symptomatically by temporarily stopping the transfusion and administering antihistamines (diphenhydramine, 50 mg orally or intramuscularly). The transfusion may be completed after the signs and/ or symptoms resolve. Patients with a history of allergic transfusion reaction should be premedicated with an antihistamine. Cellular components can be washed to remove residual plasma for the extremely sensitized patient.

Anaphylactic Reaction   This severe reaction presents after transfusion of only a few milliliters of the blood component. Symptoms and signs include difficulty breathing, coughing, nausea and vomiting, hypotension, bronchospasm, loss of consciousness, respiratory arrest, and shock. Treatment includes stopping the transfusion, maintaining vascular access, and administering epinephrine (0.5 to 1.0 mL of 1:1000 dilution SQ). Glucocorticoids may be required in severe cases.

Patients who are IgA-deficient may be sensitized to this Ig class and are at risk for anaphylactic reactions associated with plasma transfusion. Individuals with severe IgA deficiency should therefore receive only IgA-deficient plasma and washed cellular blood components. Patients who have anaphylactic or repeated allergic reactions to blood components should be tested for IgA deficiency.

Graft-Versus-Host Disease   Graft-versus-host disease (GVHD) is a frequent complication of allogeneic bone marrow transplantation, in which viable lymphocytes from donor marrow attack and cannot be eliminated by an immunodeficient host. Transfusion-related GVHD is mediated by donor T lymphocytes that recognize host HLA antigens as foreign and mount an immune response, which is manifested clinically by the development of fever, a characteristic cutaneous eruption, diarrhea, and liver function abnormalities. GVHD can also occur when blood components that contain viable T lymphocytes are transfused to immunodeficient recipients or to immunocompetent recipients who share HLA antigens with the donor (e.g., a family donor). In addition to the aforementioned clinical features of GVHD, transfusion-associated GVHD (TA-GVHD) is characterized by marrow aplasia and pancytopenia. TA-GVHD is highly resistant to treatment with immunosuppressive therapies, including glucocorticoids, cyclosporine, antithymocyte globulin, and ablative therapy followed by allogeneic bone marrow transplantation. Clinical manifestations appear at 8 to 10 days, and death occurs at 3 to 4 weeks posttransfusion.

TA-GVHD can be prevented by irradiation of cellular components (minimum of 2500 cGy) before transfusion to patients at risk. Patients at risk for TA-GVHD include fetuses receiving intrauterine transfusions, selected immunocompetent (e.g., lymphoma patients) or immunocompromised recipients, recipients of donor units known to be from a blood relative, and recipients who have undergone marrow transplantation. Directed donations by family members should be discouraged (they are not less likely to transmit infection); lacking other options, the blood products from family members should always be irradiated.

Transfusion-Related Acute Lung Injury   This uncommon reaction results from the transfusion of donor plasma that contains high titer anti-HLA antibodies that bind recipient leukocytes. The leukocytes aggregate in the pulmonary vasculature and release mediators that increase capillary permeability. The recipient develops symptoms of respiratory compromise and signs of noncardiogenic pulmonary edema, including bilateral interstitial infiltrates on chest x-ray. Treatment is supportive, and patients usually recover without sequelae. Testing the donor's plasma for anti-HLA antibodies can support this diagnosis. The implicated donors are frequently multiparous women, and transfusion of their plasma component should be avoided.

Posttransfusion Purpura   This reaction presents as thrombocytopenia 7 to 10 days after platelet transfusion and occurs predominantly in women. Platelet-specific antibodies are found in the recipient's serum, and the most frequently recognized antigen is HPA-1a found on the platelet glycoprotein IIIa receptor. The delayed thrombocytopenia is due to the production of antibodies that react to both donor and recipient platelets. Additional platelet transfusions can worsen the thrombocytopenia and should be avoided. Treatment with intravenous immunoglobulin may neutralize the effector antibodies, or plasmapheresis can be used to remove the antibodies.

Alloimmunization   A recipient may become alloimmunized to a number of antigens on cellular blood elements and plasma proteins. Alloantibodies to RBC antigens are detected during pretransfusion testing, and their presence may delay finding antigen-negative crossmatch-compatible products for transfusion. Women of child-bearing age who are sensitized to certain RBC antigens (i.e., D, c, E, Kell, or Duffy) are at risk for bearing a fetus with hemolytic disease of the newborn. Matching for D antigen is the only pretransfusion selection test to prevent RBC alloimmunization.

Alloimmunization to antigens on leukocytes and platelets can result in refractoriness to platelet transfusions. Once alloimmunization has developed, HLA-compatible platelets from donors who share similar antigens with the recipient may be difficult to find. Hence, prudent transfusion practice is directed at preventing sensitization through the use of leukocyte-reduced cellular components, as well as limiting antigenic exposure by the judicious use of transfusions and use of SDAPs.

NONIMMUNOLOGIC REACTIONS   **Fluid Overload**   Blood components are excellent volume expanders, and transfusion may quickly lead to volume overload. Monitoring the rate and volume of the transfusion, along with the use of a diuretic, can minimize this problem.

Hypothermia   Refrigerated (4°C) or frozen (−18°C or below) blood components can result in hypothermia when rapidly infused. Cardiac dysrhythmias can result from exposing the sinoatrial node to cold fluid. Use of an in-line warmer will prevent this complication.

Electrolyte Toxicity   RBC leakage during storage increases the concentration of potassium in the unit. Neonates and patients in renal failure are at risk for hyperkalemia. Preventive measures, such as using fresh or washed RBCs, are warranted for neonatal transfusions because this complication can be fatal.

Citrate, commonly used to anticoagulate blood components, chelates calcium and thereby inhibits the coagulation cascade. Hypocalcemia, manifested by circumoral numbness and/or tingling sensation of the fingers and toes, may result from multiple rapid transfusions. Because citrate is quickly metabolized to bicarbonate, calcium infusion is seldom required in this setting. If calcium or any other intravenous infusion is necessary, it must be given through a separate intravenous line.

Iron Overload Each unit of RBCs contains 200 to 250 mg of iron. Symptoms and signs of iron overload affecting endocrine, hepatic, and cardiac function are common after 100 units of RBCs have been transfused (total body iron load of 20 g). Preventing this complication by using alternative therapies (e.g., erythropoietin) and judicious transfusion is preferable and cost effective. Deferoxamine and other chelating agents are available, but the response is often suboptimal.

Hypotensive Reactions Transient hypotension may be noted among transfused patients who take angiotensin-converting enzyme (ACE) inhibitors. Since blood products contain bradykinin that is normally degraded by ACE, patients on ACE inhibitors may have increased bradykinin levels that cause hypotension. The blood pressure typically returns to normal without intervention.

Immunomodulation Transfusion of allogeneic blood is immunosuppressive. Multiply transfused renal transplant recipients are less likely to reject the graft. However, in postoperative settings and in cancer patients, immune suppression is dangerous. The use of leukocyte-depleted cellular products may reduce the immunosuppression, though controlled data have not been obtained.

INFECTIOUS COMPLICATIONS Viral Infections • *Hepatitis C virus (HCV)* The use of an improved screening test for HCV antibodies has reduced the incidence of posttransfusion HCV infection to 1 in 103,000 transfusions. Infection with HCV may be asymptomatic or lead to chronic active hepatitis, cirrhosis, and liver failure.

Hepatitis B virus Transfusion-associated HBV infection has been reduced with improved donor selection and screening, along with increased vaccination of the donor and recipient population. However, some data suggest that HBV is more commonly transmitted by transfusion than HCV. Vaccination of individuals who require long-term transfusion therapy can prevent this complication.

Hepatitis G virus (HGV) This hepatotropic virus is transmitted by transfusion. Infection with HGV results in no apparent adverse effects. Routine testing is not available and does not appear to be warranted.

Human immunodeficiency virus type 1 Intensive donor screening and testing has dramatically reduced the risk of HIV-1 infection by blood transfusion. Donated blood is tested for HIV-1 p24 antigen. Two antigen-positive seronegative donors have been identified. The risk of HIV-1 infection per transfusion episode is 1 in 676,000. A specific assay to detect antibodies to HIV-2 is also performed on donated blood. No cases of HIV-2 infection have been reported in the United States since 1992, and only three donors have been found to have HIV-2 antibodies.

Cytomegalovirus This ubiquitous virus infects 50% or more of the general population and is transmitted by the infected "passenger" white blood cells found in transfused PRBCs or platelet components. Donated blood is not routinely tested for serologic evidence of donor exposure, but assays can be performed to identify CMV-seronegative donors, if needed. Alternatively, cellular components that are leukocyte-reduced have a decreased risk of transmitting CMV, regardless of the serologic status of the donor. Groups at risk for CMV infections include immunosuppressed patients, CMV-seronegative transplant recipients, and neonates; these patients should receive seronegative or leukocyte-depleted components.

Human T lymphotropic virus (HTLV) type I Assays to detect HTLV-I and -II are used to screen all donated blood. HTLV-1 is associated with adult T cell leukemia/lymphoma and tropical spastic paraparesis in a small percentage of infected persons (Chap. 191). The reported risk of HTLV-I infection via transfusion is 1 in 641,000 transfusion episodes. HTLV-II is not clearly associated with any disease.

Parvovirus B-19 Blood components and products derived from pooled plasma can transmit this virus, the etiologic agent of erythema infectiosum, or fifth disease, in children. Parvovirus B-19 shows tropism for erythroid precursors and inhibits both erythrocyte production and maturation. Pure red cell aplasia, presenting either as acute aplastic crisis or chronic anemia with shortened RBC survival, may occur in individuals with an underlying hematologic disease, such as sickle cell disease or thalassemia. The fetus of a seronegative woman is at risk for developing hydrops if infected with this virus.

Bacterial Contamination Most bacteria do not grow well at cold temperatures; thus, PRBCs and FFP are not common sources of bacterial contamination. However, some gram-negative bacteria, notably *Yersinia* and *Pseudomonas* species, can grow at 1° to 6°C. Platelet concentrates, which are stored at room temperature, are more likely to be contaminated with skin contaminants such as gram-positive organisms, including coagulase-negative staphylococci.

Recipients of transfusions contaminated with bacteria may develop fever and chills, which can progress to septic shock and DIC. These reactions may occur abruptly, within minutes of initiating the transfusion, or after several hours. The onset of symptoms and signs is often sudden and fulminant, which aids in differentiating bacterial contamination from a FNHTR. The reactions, particularly those related to gram-negative contaminants, are the result of infused endotoxins formed within the contaminated stored component.

When contaminated transfusions are suspected (i.e., when there is sudden development of shock), the transfusion must be stopped immediately. Therapy is directed at supporting the recipient's blood pressure, cardiac output, oxygenation, and renal function. The laboratory investigation should include cultures of any untransfused component, along with the routine blood bank clerical checks and serologic studies. Broad-spectrum antibiotic coverage should be started immediately and may be adjusted based on culture and sensitivity.

Parasites Various parasites including those causing malaria, babesiosis, and Chagas' disease can be transmitted by blood transfusion rarely. Geographical migration and travel of donors can shift the incidence of these rare infections. Because these infections can prove fatal, they should be considered in the transfused patient in the appropriate clinical setting.

ALTERNATIVES TO TRANSFUSION

Alternatives to allogeneic blood transfusions that avoid homologous donor exposures with attendant immunologic and infectious risks remain attractive. Autologous blood is the best option when transfusion is anticipated. However, the cost:benefit ratio of autologous transfusion remains high. No transfusion is a zero-risk event; clerical errors and bacterial contamination remain potential complications even with autologous transfusions. Additional methods of autologous transfusion in the surgical patient include preoperative hemodilution, recovery of shed blood from sterile surgical sites, and postoperative drainage collection. Directed or designated donation from friends and family of the potential recipient has not been safer than volunteer donor component transfusions. Such directed donations may in fact place the recipient at higher risk for complications such as GVHD and alloimmunization.

Oxygen-carrying blood substitutes, such as perfluorocarbons and aggregated hemoglobin solution, are presently in various stages of clinical trials. Granulocyte- and granulocyte-macrophage colony stimulating factor (G- or GM-CSF) are clinically useful to hasten leukocyte recovery in patients with leukopenia related to high-dose chemotherapy. Erythropoietin stimulates erythrocyte production in patients with anemia of chronic renal failure and other conditions, thus avoiding or reducing the need for transfusion. This hormone can also stimulate erythropoiesis in the autologous donor to enable additional donation. Thrombopoietin, a cytokine that promotes megakaryocyte proliferation and maturation, is being tested for its ability to reduce the need for platelet transfusion.

ANDERSON KC, NESS PM (eds): *Scientific Basis of Transfusion Medicine, Implications for Clinical Practice*. Philadelphia, Saunders, 1999

CARSON JL et al: Perioperative blood transfusion and postoperative mortality. JAMA 279: 199, 1998

ETCHSON J et al: The cost effectiveness of preoperative autologous blood donations. N Engl J Med 332:719, 1995

GOODNOUGH LT et al: Transfusion medicine (2 parts). N Engl J Med 340:438, 525, 1999

HEBERT PC et al: A multicenter, randomized, controlled clinical trial of transfusion requirements in critical care. N Engl J Med 340:409, 1999

KUTER DJ et al: Platelet growth factors: Potential impact on transfusion medicine. Transfusion 39:321, 1999

MENITOVE JE et al: *The Technical Manual*, 18th ed. Arlington VA, American Association of Blood Banks, 1997

RUBELLA P et al: A multicenter randomized study of the threshold for prophylactic platelet transfusions in adults with acute myeloid leukemia. N Engl J Med 337:1870, 1997

SAGMEISTER M et al: A restrictive platelet transfusion policy allowing long-term support of outpatients with severe aplastic anemia. Blood 93:3124, 1999

SCHREIBER GB et al: The risk of transfusion-transmitted viral infections. N Engl J Med 334:1685, 1996

115

Frederick R. Appelbaum

BONE MARROW AND STEM CELL TRANSPLANTATION

Bone marrow transplantation is the generic term used to describe the collection and transplantation of hematopoietic stem cells. The procedure is usually carried out for one of two purposes: (1) to replace an abnormal but nonmalignant lymphohematopoietic system with one from a normal donor, or (2) to treat malignancy by allowing the administration of higher doses of myelosuppressive therapy than would otherwise be possible. The use of bone marrow transplantation has been steadily increasing, both because of the its demonstrated effectiveness in selected diseases and because of increasing availability of donors. The International Bone Marrow Transplant Registry estimates that about 50,000 transplants were performed during 1999.

THE HEMATOPOIETIC STEM CELL

Several features of the hematopoietic stem cell make bone marrow transplantation clinically feasible, including its remarkable regenerative capacity, its ability to home to the marrow space following intravenous injection, and the ability of the stem cell to be cryopreserved. Transplantation of a single stem cell can replace the entire lymphohematopoietic system of an adult mouse. In humans, transplantation of a few percent of a donor's bone marrow volume regularly results in complete and sustained replacement of the recipient's entire lymphohematopoietic system, including all red cells, granulocytes, B and T lymphocytes, and platelets, as well as cells comprising the fixed macrophage population, including Kupffer cells of the liver, pulmonary alveolar macrophages, osteoclasts, Langerhans cells of the skin, and brain microglial cells. The ability of the hematopoietic stem cell to home to the marrow following intravenous injection is mediated, at least in part, by the interaction of specific cell molecules, termed *selectins*, on bone marrow endothelial cells with their unique ligands, termed *integrins*, on early hematopoietic cells. Human hematopoietic stem cells can survive freezing and thawing with little, if any, damage, making it possible to remove and store a portion of the patient's own bone marrow for later reinfusion following treatment of the patient with high-dose myelotoxic therapy.

CATEGORIES OF BONE MARROW TRANSPLANTATION

Bone marrow transplantation can be described according to the relationship between the patient and the donor and by the anatomic source of stem cells. In approximately 1% of cases, patients have identical twins who can serve as donors. Syngeneic donors represent the best source of stem cells; unlike allogeneic donors, there is no risk of graft-versus-host disease (GVHD) and, unlike use of autologous marrow, there is no risk that the stem cells are contaminated with tumor cells.

Allogeneic transplantation involves a donor and recipient who are not immunologically identical. Following allogeneic transplantation immune cells transplanted with the marrow or developing from it can react against the patient, causing GVHD. Alternatively, if the immunosuppressive preparative regimen used to treat the patient before transplant is inadequate, immunocompetent cells of the patient can cause graft rejection. The risks of these complications are greatly influenced by the degree of matching between donor and recipient for antigens encoded by genes of the major histocompatibility complex.

The human leukocyte antigen (HLA) molecules are responsible for binding antigenic proteins and presenting them to T cells. The antigens presented by HLA molecules may derive from exogenous sources (e.g., during active infections) or may be endogenous proteins produced by the cell. If individuals are not matched for HLA, T cells from one individual will react strongly to the mismatched HLA, or "major antigens," of the second. Even if the individuals are HLA-matched, the T cells of the donor may react to differing endogenous, or "minor antigens," presented by the HLA of the recipient. Reactions to minor antigens tend to be less vigorous. The genes of major relevance to transplantation include HLA-A, -B, -C, and -D; they are closely linked and therefore tend to be inherited as haplotypes, with only rare crossovers between them. Thus, the odds that any one full sibling will match a patient are one in four, and the probability that the patient has an HLA-identical sibling is $1 - (0.75)^n$ where *n* equals the number of siblings.

With current techniques, the risk of graft rejection is 1 to 3%, and the risk of severe, life-threatening acute GVHD is approximately 15% following transplantation between HLA-identical siblings. The incidence of graft rejection and GVHD increases progressively with the use of family member donors mismatched for one, two, or three antigens. While survival following a one-antigen mismatched transplant is not markedly altered, survival following two- or three-antigen mismatched transplants is significantly impaired, and such transplants should only be performed as part of clinical trials.

The formation of the National Marrow Donor Program has allowed for the identification of HLA-matched unrelated donors for many patients. The genes encoding HLA antigens are highly polymorphic, and thus the odds of any two unrelated individuals being HLA-identical are extremely low, somewhat less than 1 in 10,000. However, by identifying and typing >3 million volunteer donors, HLA-matched donors now can found for approximately 50% of patients for whom a search is initiated. It takes, on average, 3 to 4 months to complete a search and schedule and initiate an unrelated donor transplant. Results so far suggest that GVHD is somewhat increased and survival somewhat poorer with such donors than with HLA-matched siblings.

Autologous transplantation involves the removal and storage of the patient's own stem cells with subsequent reinfusion after the patient receives high-dose myeloablative therapy. Unlike allogeneic transplantation, there is no risk of GVHD or graft rejection with autologous transplantation. On the other hand, autologous transplantation lacks a graft-versus-tumor effect, and the autologous stem cell product can be contaminated with tumor cells that could lead to relapse. A variety of techniques have been developed to "purge" autologous products of tumor cells. Some use antibodies directed at tumor-associated antigens plus complement, antibodies linked to toxins, or antibodies conjugated to immunomagnetic beads. In vitro incubation with certain chemotherapeutic agents such as 4-hydroperoxycylophosphamide and long-term culture of bone marrow has also been shown to diminish tumor cell numbers in stem cell products. Another technique is positive selection of stem cells using antibodies to CD34, with subsequent column adherence or flow techniques to select normal stem cells while leaving tumor cells behind. All these approaches can reduce the number of tumor cells from 1000- to 10,000-fold and are clinically feasible; however, no prospective randomized trials have yet shown that any of these approaches results in a decrease in relapse rates or improvements in disease-free or overall survival.

Bone marrow aspirated from the posterior and anterior iliac crests has traditionally been the source of hematopoietic stem cells for transplantation. Typically, anywhere from 1.5 to 5×10^8 nucleated marrow cells per kilogram are collected for allogeneic transplantation. Several recent studies have found improved survival in the settings of both matched sibling and unrelated transplantation by transplanting higher numbers of bone marrow cells.

Hematopoietic stem cells circulate in the peripheral blood but in very low concentrations. Following the administration of certain hematopoietic growth factors, including granulocyte colony stimulating factor (G-CSF) or granulocyte-macrophage colony stimulating factor (GM-CSF), and during recovery from intensive chemotherapy, the concentration of hematopoietic progenitor cells in blood, as measured either by colony forming units or expression of the CD34 antigen, increases markedly. This has made it possible to harvest adequate numbers of stem cells from the peripheral blood for transplantation. Donors are typically treated with 4 or 5 days of hematopoietic growth factor, following which stem cells are collected in one or two 4-h pheresis sessions. In the autologous setting, transplantation of $>2.5 \times 10^6$ CD34 cells per kilogram, a number easily collected in most circumstances, leads to rapid and sustained engraftment in virtually all cases. Compared to the use of autologous marrow, use of peripheral blood stem cells results in more rapid hematopoietic recovery, with granulocytes recovering to $500/\mu L$ by day 12 and platelets recovering to $20,000/\mu L$ by day 14. While this more rapid recovery diminishes the morbidity of transplantation, no studies show an improvement in survival.

Hesitation in studying the use of peripheral blood stem cells for allogeneic transplantation was because peripheral blood stem cell products contain as much as one log more T cells than are contained in the typical marrow harvest; in animal models, the incidence of GVHD is related to the number of T cells transplanted. Nonetheless, phase II and now randomized phase III trials have shown that the use of growth factor–mobilized peripheral blood stem cells from HLA-matched family members leads to faster engraftment without an increase in acute GVHD. Chronic GVHD may be increased with peripheral blood stem cells, but in trials conducted so far, this has been more than balanced by reductions in relapse rates and nonrelapse mortality, with the use of peripheral blood stem cells resulting in improved overall survival.

Umbilical cord blood contains a high concentration of hematopoietic progenitor cells, allowing for its use as a source of stem cells for transplantation. Cord blood transplantation from family members has been explored in the setting where the immediate need for transplantation precludes waiting the 9 or so months generally required for the baby to mature to the point of donating marrow. Use of cord blood in such settings results in somewhat slower engraftment than seen with marrow but a low incidence of GVHD, perhaps reflecting the low number of T cells in cord blood. More recently, several banks have been developed to harvest and store cord blood for possible transplantation to unrelated patients from material that would otherwise be discarded. A summary of the first 272 unrelated cord blood transplants, facilitated by the New York Blood Center, reported engraftment in approximately 90% of patients but at a slower pace than seen with a marrow. Significant GVHD was seen in 40% of patients. The risk of graft failure was related to the dose of cord blood cells per kilogram infused. The low cell content of most cord blood collections has limited the use of this approach as a source of stem cells for adult patients.

THE TRANSPLANT PREPARATIVE REGIMEN

The treatment regimen administered to patients immediately preceding transplantation is designed to eradicate the patient's underlying disease and, in the setting of allogeneic transplantation, immunosuppress the patient adequately to prevent rejection of the transplanted marrow. The appropriate regimen, therefore, depends on the disease setting and source of marrow. For example, when transplantation is performed to treat severe combined immunodeficiency and the donor is a histocompatible sibling, no treatment is required because no host cells require eradication and the patient is already too immunoincompetent to reject the transplanted marrow. For aplastic anemia, there is no large population of cells to eradicate and high-dose cyclophosphamide plus antithymocyte globulin is sufficient to immunosuppress the patient adequately to accept the marrow graft. In the setting of thalassemia and sickle cell anemia, high-dose busulfan is frequently added to cyclophosphamide in order to eradicate the hyperplastic host hematopoiesis. A variety of different regimens have been developed to treat malignant diseases. Most of these regimens included agents that have high activity against the tumor in question at conventional doses and have myelosuppression as their predominant dose-limiting toxicity. Therefore, these regimens commonly include busulfan, cyclophosphamide, melphalan, thiotepa, carmustine, etoposide, and total-body irradiation in various combinations.

THE TRANSPLANT PROCEDURE

Marrow is usually collected from the donor's posterior and sometimes anterior iliac crests with the donor under general or spinal anesthesia. Typically, 10 to 15 mL/kg of marrow is aspirated, placed in heparinized media, and filtered through 0.3- and 0.2-mm screens to remove fat and bony spicules. The collected marrow may undergo further processing depending on the clinical situation, such as the removal of red cells to prevent hemolysis in ABO-incompatible transplants, the removal of donor T cells to prevent GVHD, or attempts to remove possible contaminating tumor cells in autologous transplantation. Marrow donation is a safe procedure, with only very rare complications reported.

Peripheral blood stem cells are collected by leukopheresis after the donor has been treated with hematopoietic growth factors or, in the setting of autologous transplantation, sometimes after treatment with a combination of chemotherapy and growth factors. Stem cells for transplantation are generally infused through a large-bore central venous catheter. Such infusions are usually well tolerated, although occasionally patients develop fever, cough, or shortness of breath. These symptoms usually resolve with slowing of the infusion. When the stem cell product has been cryopreserved using dimethyl sulfoxide, patients more often experience short-lived nausea or vomiting due to the odor and taste of the cryoprotectant.

ENGRAFTMENT

Peripheral blood counts usually reach their nadir several days to a week posttransplant as a consequence of the preparative regimen, then cells produced by the transplanted stem cells begin to appear in the peripheral blood. The rate of recovery depends on the source of stem cells, the use of posttransplant growth factors, and the form of GVHD prophylaxis employed. If marrow is the source of stem cells, recovery to 100 granulocytes per microliter occurs by day 16 and $500/\mu L$ by day 22. Use of G-CSF-mobilized peripheral blood stem cells speeds the rate of recovery by approximately 1 week when compared to marrow. Use of myeloid growth factor (G-CSF or GM-CSF) posttransplant can further accelerate recovery by 3 to 5 days, while use of methotrexate to prevent GVHD delays engraftment by a similar period. Following allogeneic transplantation, engraftment can be documented using fluorescence in situ hybridization of sex chromosomes if donor and recipient are sex-mismatched, HLA-typing if HLA-mismatched, or restriction fragment length polymorphism analysis if sex- and HLA-matched.

COMPLICATIONS FOLLOWING BONE MARROW TRANSPLANT

EARLY DIRECT CHEMORADIO-TOXICITIES The transplant preparative regimens commonly used cause a spectrum of acute toxicities that vary according to the specific regimen but frequently result in nausea, vomiting, and mild skin erythema (Fig. 115-1). Regimens that include high-dose cyclophosphamide can result in hemorrhagic cystitis, which can usually be prevented by bladder irrigation or therapy with the sulfhydryl compound, mercaptoethanesulfonate (MESNA); rarely, acute hemorrhagic carditis is seen. Most preparative regimens will result in oral mucositis, which typically develops approximately 5 to 7 days posttransplant and often requires narcotic analgesia. Use of a patient-controlled analgesic pump provides the greatest patient satisfaction and results in a lower cumulative dose of narcotic. Patients begin losing their hair 5 to 6 days posttransplant and by 1 week are usually profoundly pancytopenic.

Approximately 10% of patients will develop venoocclusive disease of the liver, a syndrome resulting from direct cytotoxic injury to hepatic-venular and sinusoidal endothelium, with subsequent deposition of fibrin and the development of a local hypercoagulable state. This chain of events results in the clinical symptoms of tender hepatomegaly, ascites, jaundice, and fluid retention. These symptoms can develop any time during the first month posttransplant, with the peak incidence at day 16. The mortality of venoocclusive disease is approximately 30%, with progressive hepatic failure culminating in a terminal hepatorenal syndrome. Both thrombolytic and antithrombotic agents, such as tissue plasminogen activator, heparin, and prostaglandin E, have been studied as therapy, but none has proven of consistent major benefit in controlled trials and all have significant toxicity. Early studies with defibrotide, a polydeoxyribonucleotide, seem encouraging.

Although most pneumonias developing posttransplant are caused by infectious agents, in approximately 5% of patients a diffuse interstitial pneumonia will develop that is thought to be the result of direct toxicity of the preparative regimen. Bronchoalveolar lavage typically shows alveolar hemorrhage, and biopsies are typically characterized by diffuse alveolar damage, although some cases may have a more clearly interstitial pattern. High-dose glucocorticoids are often used as treatment, although randomized trials testing their utility have not been reported.

LATE DIRECT CHEMORADIOTOXICITIES Late complications of the preparative regimen include decreased growth velocity in children and delayed development of secondary sex characteristics. These complications can be partly ameliorated with the use of appropriate growth and sex hormone replacement. Most men become azoospermic, and most postpubertal women will develop ovarian failure, which should be treated. Thyroid dysfunction, usually well compensated, is sometimes seen. Cataracts develop in 10 to 20% of patients and are most common in patients treated with total-body irradiation and those who receive glucocorticoid therapy posttransplant for treatment of GVHD. Aseptic necrosis of the femoral head is seen in 10% of patients and is particularly frequent in those receiving chronic glucocorticoid therapy.

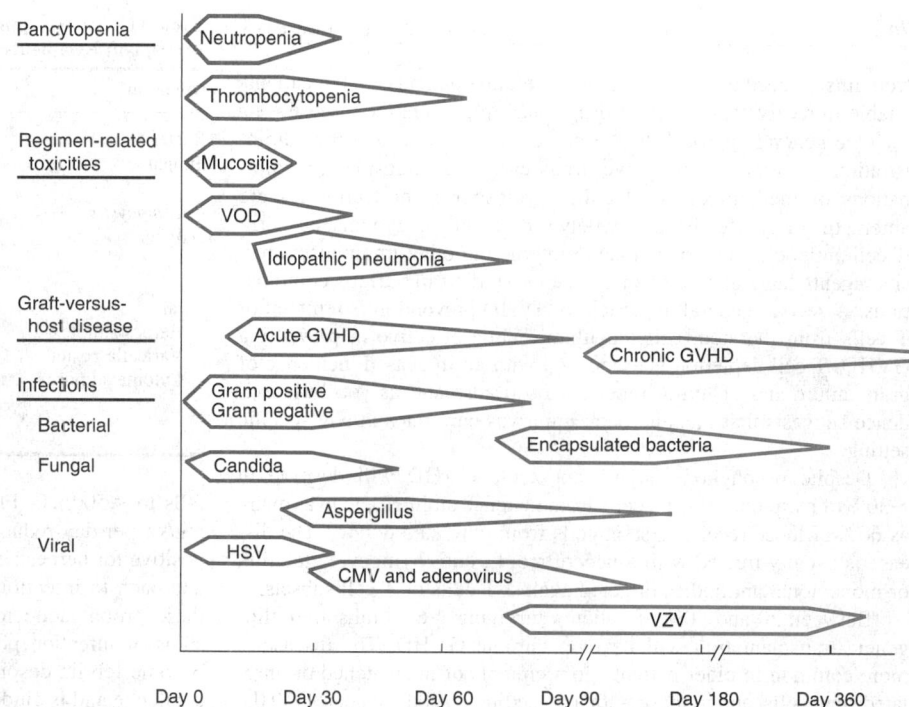

FIGURE 115-1 Major syndromes complicating marrow transplantation. VOD, venocclusive disease; GVHD, graft-versus-host disease; HSV, herpes simplex virus; CMV, cytomegalovirus; VZV, varicella-zoster virus. The size of the box roughly reflects the risk of the complication.

GRAFT-VERSUS-HOST DISEASE GVHD is the result of allogeneic T cells that were either transferred with the donor's stem cell inoculum or develop from it, reacting with antigenic targets on host cells. GVHD developing within the first 3 months posttransplant is termed *acute GVHD*, while GVHD developing or persisting beyond 3 months posttransplant is termed *chronic GVHD*. Acute GVHD most often first becomes apparent between 2 and 4 weeks posttransplant and is characterized by an erythematous maculopapular rash; persistent anorexia or diarrhea, or both; and by liver disease with increased serum levels of bilirubin, alanine and aspartate aminotransferase, and alkaline phosphatase. Since many conditions can mimic acute GVHD, diagnosis usually requires skin, liver, or endoscopic biopsy for confirmation. In all these organs, endothelial damage and lymphocytic infiltrates are seen. In skin, the epidermis and hair follicles are damaged; in liver, the small bile ducts show segmental disruption; and in intestines, destruction of the crypts and mucosal ulceration may be noted. A commonly used rating system for acute GVHD is shown in Table 115-1. Grade I acute GVHD is of little clinical significance, does not affect the likelihood of survival, and does not require treatment. In contrast, grades II to IV GVHD are associated with significant symptoms and a poorer probability of survival and require aggressive therapy. The incidence of acute GVHD is higher in recipients of stem cells

Table 115-1 Clinical Staging and Grading of Acute Graft-Versus-Host Disease

Clinical Stage	Skin	Liver—Bilirubin, μmol/L (mg/dL)	Gut
1	Rash <25% body surface	34–51 (2–3)	Diarrhea 500–1000 mL/d
2	Rash <25–50% body surface	51–103 (3–6)	Diarrhea 1000–1500 mL/d
3	Generalized erythroderma	103–257 (6–15)	Diarrhea > 1500 mL/d
4	Desquamation and bullae	>257 (> 15)	Ileus

OVERALL CLINICAL GRADE	SKIN STAGE	LIVER STAGE	GUT STAGE
I	1–2	0	0
II	1–3	1	1
III	1–3	2–3	2–3
IV	2–4	2–4	2–4

from mismatched or unrelated donors, in older patients, and in patients unable to receive full doses of drugs used to prevent the disease.

One general approach to the prevention of GVHD is the administration of immunosuppressive drugs early after transplant. Combinations of methotrexate and either cyclosporine or tacrolimus are among the most effective and widely used regimens. Prednisone, anti–T cell antibodies, mycophenolate mofetil, and other immunosuppressive agents have also been or are being studied in various combinations. A second general approach to GVHD prevention is removal of T cells from the stem cell inoculum. While effective in preventing GVHD, T cell depletion is associated with an increased incidence of graft failure and of tumor recurrent posttransplant; as yet, little evidence suggests that this approach improves cure rates in any specific setting.

Despite prophylaxis, significant acute GVHD will develop in ~30% of recipients of stem cells from matched siblings and in as many as 60% of those receiving stem cells from unrelated donors. The disease is usually treated with glucocorticoids, anti-thymocyte globulin, or monoclonal antibodies targeted against T cells or T cell subsets.

Between 20 and 50% of patients surviving >6 months after allogeneic transplantation will develop chronic GVHD. The disease is more common in older patients, in recipients of mismatched or unrelated stem cells, and in those with a preceding episode of acute GVHD. The disease resembles an autoimmune disorder with malar rash, sicca syndrome, arthritis, obliterative bronchiolitis, and bile duct degeneration and cholestasis. Single-agent prednisone or cyclosporine is standard treatment at present, although trials of other agents, including thalidomide, are under way. In most patients, chronic GVHD resolves, but it may require 1 to 3 years of immunosuppressive treatment before these agents can be withdrawn without the disease recurring. Because patients with chronic GVHD are susceptible to significant infection, they should receive prophylactic trimethoprim-sulfamethoxazole, and all suspected infections should be investigated and treated aggressively.

GRAFT FAILURE   While complete and sustained engraftment are usually seen posttransplant, occasionally marrow function either does not return or, after a brief period of engraftment, is lost. Graft failure after autologous transplantation can be the result of inadequate numbers of stem cells being transplanted, damage during ex vivo treatment or storage, or exposure of the patient to myelotoxic agents posttransplant. Infections with cytomegalovirus (CMV) or human herpes virus type 6 have also been associated with loss of marrow function. Graft failure after allogeneic transplantation can also be due to immunologic rejection of the graft by immunocompetent host cells. Immunologically based graft rejection is more common following use of less immunosuppressive preparative regimens, in recipients of T cell–depleted stem cell products, and in patients receiving grafts from HLA-mismatched donors.

Treatment of graft failure usually involves removing all potentially myelotoxic agents from the patient's regimen and attempting a short trial of myeloid growth factor. Persistence of lymphocytes of host origin in allogeneic transplant recipients with graft failure indicates immunologic rejection. Reinfusion of donor stem cells in such patients is usually unsuccessful unless preceded by a second immunosuppressive preparative regimen. Standard preparative regimens are generally tolerated poorly if administered within 100 days of a first transplant because of cumulative toxicities. However, use of regimens combining, for example, anti-CD3 antibodies with high-dose glucocorticoids have been successful in achieving engraftment in >50% of patients.

INFECTION   The general problem of infection in the immunocompromised host is discussed in Chap. 136. Posttransplant patients, particularly recipients of allogeneic transplantation, require unique approaches. Early after transplantation, patients are profoundly neutropenic, and because the risk of bacterial infection is so great, most centers initiate antibiotic treatment once the granulocyte count

Table 115-2   An Approach to Infection Prophylaxis in Allogeneic Transplant Recipients

Organism		Approach
Bacterial	Ceftazidime	2 g IV q8h while neutropenic
Fungal	Fluconazole	400 mg PO qd to day 75 posttransplant
Pneumocystis carinii	Trimethoprim-sulfamethoxazole	1 double-strength tablet PO bid 2 days/week until day 180 or off immunosuppression
Viral		
Herpes simplex	Acyclovir	800 mg PO bid to day 30
Varicella zoster	Acyclovir	800 mg PO bid to day 365
Cytomegalovirus	Ganciclovir	5 mg/kg IV bid for 7 days, then 5 (mg/kg)/d 5 days/week to day 100

falls to <500/μL. Fluconazole prophylaxis at a dose of 200 to 400 mg/kg per day reduces the risk of candidal infections. Patients seropositive for herpes simplex should receive acyclovir prophylaxis. One approach to infection prophylaxis is shown in Table 115-2. Despite these prophylactic measures, most patients will develop fever and signs of infection posttransplant. The management of patients who become febrile despite bacterial and fungal prophylaxis is a difficult challenge and is guided by individual aspects of the patient and by the institution's experience.

Once patients engraft, the incidence of bacterial infection diminishes; however, patients, particularly allogeneic transplant recipients, remain at significant risk of infection. During the period from engraftment until about 3 months posttransplant, the most common causes of infection are gram-positive bacteria, fungi (particularly *Aspergillus*) and viruses including CMV. CMV infection, which in the past was frequently seen and often fatal, can be prevented in seronegative patients by the use of seronegative blood products. The use of ganciclovir, either as prophylaxis beginning at the time of engraftment or initiated when CMV first reactivates as evidenced by development of antigenemia, can significantly reduce the risk of CMV disease in seropositive patients. Foscarnet is effective for some patients who develop CMV antigenemia or infection despite the use of ganciclovir or who cannot tolerate the drug.

Pneumocystis carinii pneumonia, once seen in 5 to 10% of patients, can be prevented by treating patients with oral trimethoprim-sulfamethoxazole for 1 week pretransplant and resuming the treatment once patients have engrafted.

The risk of infection diminishes considerably beyond 3 months after transplant unless chronic GVHD develops, requiring continuous immunosuppression. Most transplant centers recommend continuing trimethoprim-sulfamethoxazole prophylaxis while patients are receiving any immunosuppressive drugs and also recommend careful monitoring for late CMV reactivation. In addition, most centers recommend prophylaxis against varicella zoster, using acyclovir for 1 year posttransplant.

TREATMENT OF SPECIFIC DISEASES USING BONE MARROW TRANSPLANTATION

NONMALIGNANT DISEASES   Immunodeficiency Disorders   By replacing abnormal stem cells with cells from a normal donor, marrow transplantation can cure patients of a variety of immunodeficiency disorders including severe combined immunodeficiency, Wiskott-Aldrich syndrome, and Chédiak-Higashi syndrome. The widest experience has been with severe combined immunodeficiency disease, where cure rates of 90% can be expected with HLA-identical donors and success rates of 50 to 70% have been reported using haplotype-mismatched parents as donors (Table 115-3).

Aplastic Anemia   Transplantation from matched siblings after a preparative regimen of high-dose cyclophosphamide and antithymo-

Disease	Allogeneic, %	Autologous, %
Severe combined immunodeficiency	90	N/A
Aplastic anemia	90	N/A
Thalassemia	90	N/A
Acute myeloid leukemia		
First remission	55–60	50
Second remission	40	30
Acute lymphoblastic leukemia		
First remission	50	40
Second remission	40	30
Chronic myeloid leukemia		
Chronic phase	70	ID
Accelerated phase	40	ID
Blast crisis	15	ID
Chronic lymphoblastic leukemia	50	ID
Myelodysplasia	45	ID
Multiple myeloma	30	35
Non-Hodgkin's lymphoma		
First relapse/second remission	40	40
Hodgkin's disease		
First relapse/second remission	40	50
Breast cancer		
High-risk stage II	N/A	70
Stage IV	N/A	15

^a These estimates are generally based on data reported by the International Bone Marrow Transplant Registry. The analysis has not been reviewed by their Advisory Committee.
NOTE: N/A, not applicable; ID, insufficient data.

cyte globulin can cure up to 90% of patients younger than age 40 with severe aplastic anemia. Results in older patients and in recipients of mismatched family member or unrelated marrow are less favorable; therefore, a trial of immunosuppressive therapy is generally recommended for such patients before considering transplantation. Transplantation is effective in all forms of aplastic anemia including, for example, the syndromes associated with paroxysmal nocturnal hemoglobinuria and Fanconi's anemia. Patients with Fanconi's anemia are abnormally sensitive to the toxic effects of alkylating agents and so less intensive preparative regimens must be used in their treatment (Chap. 109).

Hemoglobinopathies   Marrow transplantation from an HLA-identical sibling following a preparative regimen of busulfan and cyclophosphamide can cure 70 to 90% of patients with thalassemia major. The best outcomes can be expected if patients are transplanted before they develop hepatomegaly or portal fibrosis and if they have been given adequate iron chelation therapy. Among such patients, the probabilities of 5-year survival and disease-free survival are 95 and 90%, respectively. Although prolonged survival can be achieved with aggressive chelation therapy, transplantation is the only curative treatment for thalassemia. Transplantation is being studied as a curative approach to patients with sickle cell anemia. Two-year survival and disease-free survival rates of 90 and 80%, respectively, have been reported following matched sibling transplantation. Decisions about patient selection and the timing of transplantation remain difficult, but transplantation seems to represent a reasonable option for younger patients who suffer repeated crises or other significant complications and who have not responded to other interventions (Chap 106).

Other Nonmalignant Diseases   Theoretically, marrow transplantation should be able to cure any disease that results from an inborn error of the lymphohematopoietic system. Transplantation has been used successfully to treat congenital disorders of white blood cells such as Kostmann's syndrome, chronic granulomatous disease, and leukocyte adhesion deficiency. Congenital anemias such as Blackfan-Diamond anemia can also be cured with transplantation. Infantile malignant osteopetrosis is due to an inability of the osteoclast to resorb bone, and since osteoclasts derive from the marrow, transplantation can cure this rare inherited disorder.

Marrow transplantation has been used as treatment for a number

of storage diseases caused by enzymatic deficiencies, such as Gaucher's disease, Hurler's syndrome, Hunter's syndrome, and infantile metachromatic leukodystrophy. Transplantation for these diseases has not been uniformly successful, but treatment early in the course of these diseases, before irreversible damage to extramedullary organs has occurred, increases the chance for success.

Transplantation is being explored as a treatment for severe acquired autoimmune disorders. These trials are based on studies demonstrating that transplantation can reverse autoimmune disorders in animal models and on the observation that occasional patients with coexisting autoimmune disorders and hematologic malignancies have been cured of both with transplantation.

MALIGNANT DISEASES   Acute Leukemia   Allogeneic marrow transplantation cures 15 to 20% of patients who do not achieve complete response from induction chemotherapy for acute myeloid leukemia (AML) and is the only form of therapy that can cure such patients. Cure rates of 30 to 35% are seen when patients are transplanted in second remission or in first relapse. The best results with allogeneic transplantation are achieved when applied during first remission, with disease-free survival rates averaging between 55 and 60%. Chemotherapy alone can cure a portion of AML patients, and so the relative merits of transplanting all patients during first remission versus only transplanting very high risk patients and those who relapse continue to be discussed. Autologous transplantation is also able to cure a portion of patients with AML. The rates of disease recurrence with autologous transplantation are higher than seen after allogeneic transplantation, and cure rates are generally somewhat less.

Similar to patients with AML, adults with acute lymphoblastic leukemia who do not achieve a complete response to induction chemotherapy can be cured in 15 to 20% of cases with immediate marrow transplantation. Cure rates improve to 30 to 50% in second remission, and therefore transplantation can be recommended for adults who have persistent disease after induction chemotherapy or who have subsequently relapsed. Transplantation in first remission results in cure rates around 55%. While transplantation appears to offer a clear advantage over chemotherapy for patients with high-risk disease, such as those with Philadelphia chromosome–positive disease, debate continues about whether adults with standard-risk disease would be transplanted in first remission or whether transplantation should be reserved until relapse. Autologous transplantation is associated with a higher relapse rate but a somewhat lower risk of nonrelapse mortality when compared to allogeneic transplantation. On balance, most experts recommend use of allogeneic stem cells if an appropriate donor is available.

Chronic Leukemia   Allogeneic marrow transplantation is the only therapy shown to cure a substantial portion of patients with chronic myeloid leukemia. Five-year disease-free survival rates are 60 to 70% for patients transplanted during chronic phase, 30 to 40% for patients transplanted during accelerated phase, and 15 to 20% for patients transplanted in blast crisis. Time from diagnosis to transplantation influences outcome, with best results obtained among patients transplanted within 1 year of diagnosis. Use of unrelated donors results in more GVHD and slightly worse survival than seen with matched siblings, although, at some large centers, 3-year disease-free survival rates of 70% have been reported. Autologous transplantation is being studied; however, few data suggest that this approach has curative potential in this disease. Given the excellent results obtained with matched sibling transplantation, most experts recommend early transplantation for younger patients with matched siblings. For older patients or those without matched siblings, it is not unreasonable to consider a trial of an interferon α–containing regimen to see if a major cytogenetic response can be achieved before making a decision about transplantation (Chap. 111).

Allogeneic transplantation has been used to only a limited extent for chronic lymphocytic leukemia, in large part because of the chronic nature of the disease and because of the age profile of patients. With allogeneic transplantation, complete remissions have been achieved in the majority of patients so far reported, with disease-free survival rates of approximately 50% at 3 years. However, treatment-related mortality has been substantial, and further follow-up is needed. There is even less experience with autologous transplantation in this disorder.

Myelodysplasia Between 40 and 50% of patients with myelodysplasia appear to be cured with allogeneic marrow transplantation. Results are better among younger patients and those with less advanced disease. However, some patients with myelodysplasia can live for extended periods without intervention, and so transplantation is generally recommended only for patients with disease categorized as intermediate risk I or greater according to the International Prognostic Scoring System (Chap. 109).

Lymphoma Patients with disseminated intermediate- or high-grade non-Hodgkin's lymphoma who have not been cured by first-line chemotherapy and are transplanted in first relapse or second remission can still be cured in 40 to 50% of cases. This represents a clear advantage over results obtained with salvage chemotherapy. It is unsettled whether patients with high-risk disease benefit from transplantation in first remission. Most experts favor the use of autologous rather than allogeneic transplantation for patients with non-Hodgkin's lymphoma, because fewer complications occur with this approach and survival appears equivalent. The role of transplantation in patients with indolent non-Hodgkin's lymphoma is less well defined. Long-term remissions can be obtained in many patients with acceptable toxicity and results with transplantation in patients with recurrent disease generally appear better than one would expect with conventional-dose chemotherapy. However, late relapses are seen after transplantation, and no randomized study has confirmed its superiority.

The role of transplantation in Hodgkin's disease is similar to that in non-Hodgkin's lymphoma. With transplantation, 5-year disease-free survival ranges from 20 to 30% in patients who never achieve a first remission with standard chemotherapy and up to 60% for those transplanted in second remission. Transplantation has no defined role in first remission in Hodgkin's disease.

Myeloma Patients with myeloma who have progressed on first-line therapy can sometimes benefit from allogeneic or autologous transplantation. Autologous transplantation has been studied as part of the initial therapy of patients, and in randomized trials, both disease-free survival as well as overall survival were improved with this approach.

Solid Tumors Among women with metastatic breast cancer, between 15 and 20% disease-free survival rates at 3 years have been reported, with better results seen in younger patients who have responded completely to standard-dose therapy before undergoing transplantation. Randomized trials have not shown superior survival for patients treated for metastatic disease with high-dose chemotherapy plus stem cell support. Randomized trials evaluating transplantation as treatment for primary breast cancer are being conducted, but final results are not yet available.

Patients with testicular cancer who have failed first-line chemotherapy have been treated with autologous transplantation. Approximately 10 to 20% of such patients apparently have been cured with this approach.

The use of high-dose chemotherapy with autologous stem cell support is being studied for several other solid tumors, including ovarian cancer, small-cell lung cancer, neuroblastoma, and pediatric sarcomas. As in most other settings, the best results have been obtained in patients with limited amounts of disease and where the remaining tumor retains sensitivity to conventional-dose chemotherapy. Few randomized trials of transplantation in these diseases have been completed.

Posttransplant Relapse Patients who relapse following autologous transplantation sometimes respond to further chemotherapy, particularly if the remission following transplantation was long. More options are available for patients who relapse following allogeneic transplantation. Of particular interest are the response rates seen with infusion of unirradiated donor lymphocytes. Complete responses in as many as 75% of patients with chronic myeloid leukemia, 40% in myelodysplasia, 25% in AML, and 15% in myeloma have been reported. Major complications of donor lymphocyte infusions include transient myelosuppression and the development of GVHD. These complications appear to be dependent on the number of donor lymphocytes infused. The impressive responses seen with donor lymphocyte infusions in some patients has encouraged investigation into the use of "nonablative" transplant regimens as treatment for various malignancies. In this approach, preparative regimens and posttransplant immunosuppression are selected that allow for engraftment without regard to their direct antitumor activities. The antitumor effects are the result of a graft-versus-tumor effect arising from the transplanted stem cells or subsequent infusion of donor lymphocytes. While engraftment can be reliably achieved with this approach, with little toxicity, and complete responses are seen, neither the rate of complete responses nor their duration have yet been entirely determined for any specific disease category.

BIBLIOGRAPHY

CURTIS RE et al: Solid cancers after bone marrow transplantation. N Engl J Med 336: 897, 1997

FISCHER A: Thirty years of bone marrow transplantation for severe combined immunodeficiency (Editorial). N Engl J Med 340:559, 1999

GOODMAN JL et al: A controlled trial of fluconazole to prevent fungal infections in patients undergoing bone marrow transplantation. N Engl J Med 326:845, 1992

GOODRICH JM et al: Ganciclovir prophylaxis to prevent cytomegalovirus disease after allogeneic marrow transplant. Ann Intern Med 118:173, 1993

HANSEN JA et al: Bone marrow transplants from unrelated donors for patients with chronic myeloid leukemia. N Engl J Med 338:962, 1998

PHILIP T et al: Autologous bone marrow transplantation as compared with salvage chemotherapy in relapses of chemotherapy-sensitive non-Hodgkin's lymphoma. N Engl J Med 333:1540, 1995

ROWLINGS PA et al: Factors correlated with progression-free survival after high-dose chemotherapy and hematopoietic stem cell transplantation for metastatic breast cancer. JAMA 282:1335, 1999

RUBINSTEIN P et al: Outcomes among 562 recipients of placental-blood transplants from unrelated donors. N Engl J Med 339:1565, 1998

WALTERS MC et al: Bone marrow transplantation for sickle cell disease. N Engl J Med 335:369, 1996

ZITTOUN RA et al: Autologous or allogeneic bone marrow transplantation compared with intensive chemotherapy in acute myelogenous leukemia. N Engl J Med 332:217, 1995

116   *Robert I. Handin*

DISORDERS OF THE PLATELET AND VESSEL WALL

Patients with platelet or vessel wall disorders usually bleed into superficial sites such as the skin, mucous membranes, or genitourinary or gastrointestinal tract. Bleeding begins immediately after trauma and either responds to simple measures such as pressure and packing or requires systemic therapy with glucocorticoids, desmopressin [1-desamino-8-D-arginine vasopressin (DDAVP)], plasma fractions, or platelet concentrates. The most common platelet/vessel wall disorders are (1) various forms of thrombocytopenia, (2) von Willebrand's disease (vWD), and (3) drug-induced platelet dysfunction. This chapter reviews the diagnosis and treatment of quantitative and qualitative platelet disorders as well as vessel wall defects that cause bleeding.→*For further discussion of the physiology of normal hemostasis and the cardinal manifestations of bleeding arising from hemostatic disorders, see Chap. 62.*

PLATELET DISORDERS

Platelets arise from the fragmentation of megakaryocytes, which are very large, polyploid bone marrow cells produced by the process of endomitosis. They undergo from three to five cycles of chromosomal duplication without cytoplasmic division. After leaving the marrow space, about one-third of the platelets are sequestered in the spleen, while the other two-thirds circulate for 7 to 10 days. Normally, only a small fraction of the platelet mass is consumed in the process of hemostasis, so most platelets circulate until they become senescent and are removed by phagocytic cells. The normal blood platelet count is 150,000 to 450,000/μl. A decrease in platelet count stimulates an increase in the number, size, and ploidy of megakaryocytes, releasing additional platelets into the circulation. This process is regulated by thrombopoietin (TPO) binding to its megakaryocyte receptor, a proto-oncogene c-mpl. TPO (c-mpl ligand) is secreted continuously at a low level and binds tightly to circulating platelets. A reduction in platelet count increases the level of free TPO and thereby stimulates megakaryocyte and platelet production.

The platelet count varies during the menstrual cycle, rising following ovulation and falling at the onset of menses. It is also influenced by the patient's nutritional state and can be decreased in severe iron, folic acid, or vitamin B_{12} deficiency. Platelets are *acute-phase reactants*, and patients with systemic inflammation, tumors, bleeding, and mild iron deficiency may have an increased platelet count, a benign condition called *secondary* or *reactive thrombocytosis*. The cytokines interleukin (IL)-3, IL-6, and IL-11 may stimulate platelet production in acute inflammation. In contrast, the increase in platelet count that is characteristic of the myeloproliferative disorders such as polycythemia vera, chronic myelogenous leukemia, myeloid metaplasia, and essential thrombocytosis can cause either severe bleeding or thrombosis. In these patients, unregulated platelet production is secondary to a clonal stem cell abnormality affecting all the bone marrow progenitors.

THROMBOCYTOPENIA Thrombocytopenia is caused by one of three mechanisms—decreased bone marrow production, increased splenic sequestration, or accelerated destruction of platelets. In order to determine the etiology of thrombocytopenia, each patient should have a careful examination of the peripheral blood film, an assessment of marrow morphology by examination of an aspirate or biopsy, and an estimate of splenic size by bedside palpation supplemented, if necessary, by ultrasonography or computed tomographic (CT) scan. Occasional patients have "pseudothrombocytopenia," a benign condition in which platelets agglutinate or adhere to leukocytes when blood is collected with EDTA as anticoagulant. This is a laboratory artifact, and the actual platelet count in vivo is normal. A scheme for classifying patients with thrombocytopenia based on these clinical observations and laboratory tests is outlined in Fig. 116-1.

Impaired Production Disorders that injure stem cells or prevent their proliferation frequently cause thrombocytopenia. They usually affect multiple hematopoietic cell lines so that thrombocytopenia is accompanied by varying degrees of anemia and leukopenia. Diagnosis of a platelet production defect is readily established by examination of a bone marrow aspirate or biopsy, which should show a reduced number of megakaryocytes. The most common causes of decreased platelet production are marrow aplasia, fibrosis, or infiltration with malignant cells, all of which produce highly characteristic marrow abnormalities. Occasionally, thrombocytopenia is the presenting laboratory abnormality in these disorders. Cytotoxic drugs impair megakaryocyte proliferation and maturation and frequently cause thrombocytopenia. Rare marrow disorders such as congenital amegakaryocytic hypoplasia and *t*hrombocytopenia with *a*bsent *r*adii (TAR syndrome), produce a selective decrease in megakaryocyte production.

Splenic Sequestration Since one-third of the platelet mass is normally sequestered in the spleen, splenectomy will increase the platelet count by 30%. Postsplenectomy thrombocytosis is a benign self-limited condition that does not require specific therapy. In contrast, when the spleen enlarges, the fraction of sequestered platelets increases, lowering the platelet count. The most common causes of splenomegaly are portal hypertension secondary to liver disease and splenic infiltration with tumor cells in myeloproliferative or lymphoproliferative disorders (Chap. 63). Isolated splenomegaly is rare, and in most patients it is accompanied by other clinical manifestations of an underlying disease. Many patients with leukemia, lymphoma, or a myeloproliferative syndrome have both marrow infiltration and splenomegaly and develop thrombocytopenia from a combination of impaired marrow production and splenic sequestration of platelets.

Accelerated Destruction Abnormal vessels, fibrin thrombi, and intravascular prostheses can all shorten platelet survival and cause *nonimmunologic thrombocytopenia*. Thrombocytopenia is common in patients with vasculitis, the hemolytic uremic syndrome (HUS), thrombotic thrombocytopenic purpura (TTP), or as a manifestation of disseminated intravascular coagulation (DIC). In addition, platelets coated with antibody, immune complexes, or complement are rapidly cleared by mononuclear phagocytes in the spleen or other tissues, inducing *immunologic thrombocytopenia*. The most common causes of immunologic thrombocytopenia are viral or bacterial infections, drugs, and a chronic autoimmune disorder referred to as *idiopathic thrombocytopenic purpura* (ITP). Patients with immunologic thrombocytopenia do not usually have splenomegaly and have an increased number of bone marrow megakaryocytes.

DRUG-INDUCED THROMBOCYTOPENIA Many common drugs can cause thrombocytopenia (Table 116-1). Cancer chemotherapeutic agents may depress megakaryocyte production. Ingestion of large quantities of alcohol has a marrow-depressing effect leading to transient thrombocytopenia, particularly in binge drinkers. Thiazide diuretics, used to treat hypertension or congestive heart failure, impair megakaryocyte production and can produce mild thrombocytopenia (50,000 to 100,000/μL), which may persist for several months after the drug is discontinued.

Most drugs induce thrombocytopenia by eliciting an immune response in which the platelet is an innocent bystander. The platelet is damaged by complement activation following the formation of drug-antibody complexes. Current laboratory tests can identify the causative agent in 10% of patients with clinical evidence of drug-induced thrombocytopenia. The best proof of a drug-induced etiology is a prompt

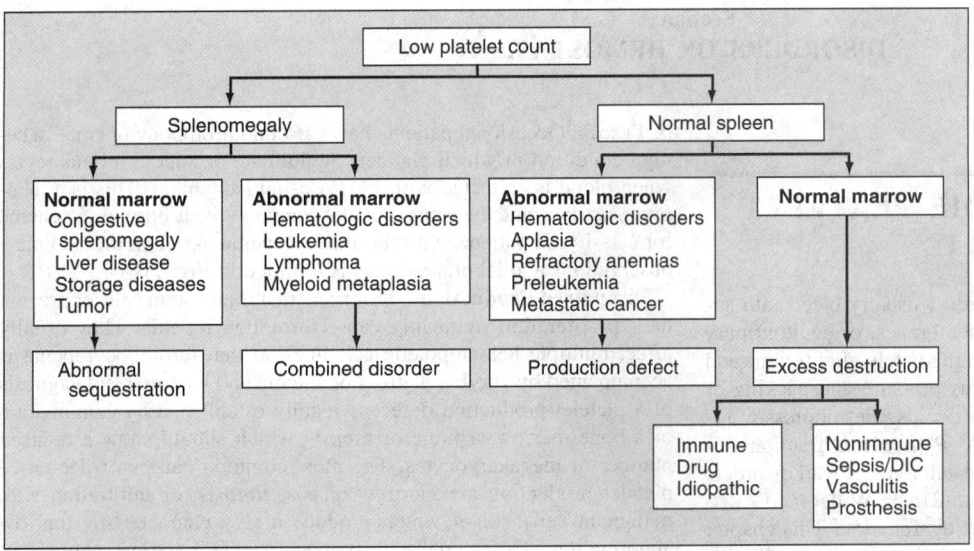

FIGURE 116-1 Clinical evaluation of patients with thrombocytopenia. [*Modified from RI Handin, in W Beck (ed), Hematology, 4th ed. Cambridge, MA, MIT Press, 1985.*]

rise in the platelet count when the suspected drug is discontinued. Patients with drug-induced platelet destruction may also have a secondary increase in megakaryocyte number without other marrow abnormalities.

Although most patients recover within 7 to 10 days and do not require therapy, occasional patients with platelet counts <10,000 to 20,000/μL have severe hemorrhage and may require temporary support with glucocorticoids, plasmapheresis, or platelet transfusions while waiting for the platelet count to rise. A patient who has recovered from drug-induced immunologic thrombocytopenia should be instructed to avoid the offending drug in the future, since only minute amounts of drug are needed to set up subsequent immune reactions. Certain drugs that are cleared from body storage depots quite slowly, such as phenytoin, may induce prolonged thrombocytopenia.

Heparin is a common cause of thrombocytopenia in hospitalized patients. Between 10 and 15% of patients receiving therapeutic doses of heparin develop thrombocytopenia and, occasionally, may have severe bleeding or intravascular platelet aggregation and paradoxical thrombosis. Heparin-induced thrombosis, sometimes called the "white clot syndrome," can be fatal unless recognized promptly. Most cases of heparin thrombocytopenia are due to drug-antibody binding to platelets; some are secondary to direct platelet agglutination by heparin. The offending antigen is a complex formed between heparin and the platelet-derived heparin neutralizing protein, platelet factor 4. Prompt cessation of heparin will reverse both thrombocytopenia and heparin-induced thrombosis. Low-molecular-weight heparin products have reduced the incidence of heparin-induced thrombocytopenia. They are effective antithrombotic agents (Chap. 118) and are less immunogenic. Unfortunately, 80 to 90% of the antibodies generated against conventional heparins cross-react with low-molecular-weight heparins, so only a minority of patients with preformed antibody can be treated with this product.

IDIOPATHIC THROMBOCYTOPENIC PURPURA The immunologic thrombocytopenias can be classified on the basis of the pathologic mechanism, the inciting agent, or the duration of the illness. The explosive onset of severe thrombocytopenia following recovery from a viral exanthem or upper respiratory illness (*acute ITP*) is common in children and accounts for 90% of the pediatric cases of immunologic thrombocytopenia. Of these patients, 60% recover in 4 to 6 weeks and >90% recover within 3 to 6 months. Transient immunologic thrombocytopenia also complicates some cases of infectious mononucleosis, acute toxoplasmosis, or cytomegalovirus infection and can be part of the prodromal phase of viral hepatitis and initial infection with HIV. Acute ITP is rare in adults and accounts for <10% of postpubertal patients with immune thrombocytopenia. Acute ITP is caused by immune complexes containing viral antigens that bind to platelet Fc receptors or by antibodies produced against viral antigens that cross-react with the platelet. In addition to these viral disorders, the differential diagnosis includes atypical presentations of aplastic anemia, acute leukemias, or metastatic tumor. A bone marrow examination is essential to exclude these disorders, which can occasionally mimic acute ITP.

Most adults present with a more indolent form of thrombocytopenia that may persist for many years and is referred to as *chronic ITP*. Women age 20 to 40 are afflicted most commonly and outnumber men by a ratio of 3:1. They may present with an abrupt fall in platelet count and bleeding similar to patients with acute ITP. More often they have a prior history of easy bruising or menometrorrhagia. These patients have an autoimmune disorder with antibodies directed against target antigens on the glycoprotein IIb-IIIa or glycoprotein Ib-IX complex (Fig. 62-2). Although most antibodies function as opsonins and accelerate platelet clearance by phagocytic cells, occasional antibodies bind to epitopes on critical regions of these glycoproteins and impair platelet function. Platelet-associated IgG can be measured but specificity is a problem. High "background" level of IgG on normal platelets and elevations in plasma immunoglobulin levels or in circulating immune complexes will nonspecifically increase platelet-associated IgG. Few clinical situations require platelet-associated IgG testing.

A low platelet count may be the initial manifestation of systemic lupus erythematosus (SLE) or the first sign of a primary hematologic disorder. Thus, patients with chronic ITP should have a bone marrow examination and an antinuclear antibody determination. In addition, patients with hepatic or splenic enlargement, lymphadenopathy, or atypical lymphocytes should have serologic studies for hepatitis viruses, cytomegalovirus, Epstein-Barr virus, toxoplasma, and HIV. HIV infection is a common cause of immunologic thrombocytopenia. Thrombocytopenia can be the initial symptom of HIV infection or a complication of fully developed clinical AIDS.

℞ TREATMENT Treatment of patients with ITP must take into account the age of the patient, the severity of the illness, and the anticipated natural history. Although adults have a higher incidence of intracranial bleeding than children, specific therapy may not be necessary unless the platelet count is <20,000/μL or there is extensive bleeding. Hemorrhage in patients with either acute or chronic ITP can usually be controlled with glucocorticoids but, in rare cases, may require temporary phagocytic blockade with intravenous immunoglobulin (IVIG) or anti-RhD (WinRho). Although antibody preparations are effective, they are expensive and should be reserved for patients with severe thrombocytopenia and clinical bleeding who are refractory to other measures. Emergency splenectomy is usually reserved for patients with acute or chronic ITP who are desperately ill and have not responded to any medical measures. The treatment of symptomatic thrombocytopenia in patients with HIV infection is more complex be-

Table 116-1 Drugs that May Cause Thrombocytopenia

1. Chemotherapeutic agents—especially carboplatin, alkylating agents, anthracyclines, antimetabolites
2. Antibiotics—sulfonamides, penicillins, cephalosporins
3. Heparins—highest incidence is with unfractionated products
4. Cardiovascular agents—thiazide diuretics, rarely angiotensin converting enzyme inhibitors

cause the administration of glucocorticoids or splenectomy may increase susceptibility to opportunistic infections. Splenectomy has been effective in the course of HIV before the onset of symptomatic AIDS. Treatment with zidovudine (AZT) and other antiviral agents that reduce viral load can improve the platelet count in patients with HIV-induced thrombocytopenia.

Symptomatic patients with chronic ITP are usually placed on prednisone, 60 mg/d for 4 to 6 weeks. The drug is then decreased slowly over another few weeks. About 50% of patients with chronic ITP will normalize their platelet count on high doses of prednisone. However, the majority will have a fall in platelet count following steroid withdrawal. Patients with chronic ITP who fail to maintain a normal platelet count after a course of prednisone are eligible for elective splenectomy. These steroid-responsive but steroid-dependent patients are very likely to respond to splenectomy, and 70% will have a normal platelet count within 1 week after surgery. Some patients who do not respond to glucocorticoids may still respond to splenectomy. Occasionally, patients may fail to respond to splenectomy because of the failure to remove an accessory spleen. In other patients, a small, inactive accessory spleen may grow or new splenic foci may develop from splenic cells shed at the time of surgery and cause the late onset of thrombocytopenia. In either case, the presence of splenic tissue can be diagnosed by examination of the blood smear for Howell-Jolly bodies that appear in the red cells of asplenic individuals. Persistent splenic tissue can be confirmed by a radionuclide scan.

Patients still thrombocytopenic after splenectomy or who relapse months to years after initial therapy have received a variety of immunosuppressive drugs including azathioprine, cyclophosphamide, vincristine, vinblastine, and cyclosporine. Danazol has also been used with some success. Although each of these drugs may be beneficial, they have serious side effects and should be used judiciously. IVIG and anti-RhD are only transiently effective and expensive. IVIG can cause meningismus and headache, and some lots have carried hepatitis C virus. Anti-RhD can cause hemolysis. These drugs should be used to raise the platelet count temporarily and to support patients before surgery or labor and delivery; they are not substitutes for splenectomy. If a patient is not bleeding and maintains a platelet count >20,000/μL, consideration should be given to withholding therapy. Patients with severe chronic thrombocytopenia may live with their disease for two or three decades.

FUNCTIONAL PLATELET DISORDERS   As described in Chap. 62, normal hemostasis requires three critical platelet reactions—adhesion, aggregation, and granule release. Clinical bleeding can result from a failure of any of these important functions. Table 116-2 lists the major functional platelet disorders. Table 116-3 lists methods to assess platelet function.

Von Willebrand's Disease   vWD is the most common inherited bleeding disorder, occurring in 1 in 800 to 1000 individuals. The von Willebrand factor (vWF) is a heterogeneous multimeric plasma glycoprotein with two major functions: (1) It facilitates platelet adhesion under conditions of high shear stress by linking platelet membrane receptors to vascular subendothelium; and (2) it serves as the plasma carrier for factor VIII, the antihemophilic factor, a critical blood coagulation protein. Discrete domains in each vWF subunit mediate each of these important functions. The normal plasma vWF level is 10 mg/L. The vWF activity is distributed among a series of plasma multimers with estimated molecular weights ranging from 400,000 to >20 million. A single large vWF precursor subunit is synthesized in endothelial cells and megakaryocytes, where it is cleaved and assembled into the disulfide-linked multimers present in plasma, platelets, and vascular subendothelium. A modest reduction in plasma vWF concentration or a selective loss in the high-molecular-weight multimers decreases platelet adhesion and causes clinical bleeding.

Although vWD is heterogeneous, certain clinical features are common to all the syndromes. With one exception (type III disease), all forms are inherited as autosomal dominant traits, and affected patients are heterozygous with one normal and one abnormal vWF allele. In

Table 116-2   Classification of Functional Platelet Disorders

I. Disorders of adhesion
   A. Inherited
      1. Bernard-Soulier syndrome
      2. von Willebrand's disease (vWD)
   B. Acquired
      1. Uremia
      2. Acquired vWD
II. Disorders of aggregation
   A. Inherited
      1. Glanzmann's thrombasthenia
      2. Afibrinogenemia
   B. Acquired
      1. Fibrin degradation product inhibition
      2. Dysproteinemias
      3. Drugs—e.g., ticlopidine, Gp IIb/IIIa inhibitors
III. Disorders of granule release
   A. Inherited
      1. Oculocutaneous albinism (Hermansky-Pudlak syndrome)
      2. Chédiak-Higashi syndrome
      3. Isolated dense (δ) granule deficiency
      4. Gray-platelet syndrome—combined α and β granule deficiency
   B. Acquired
      1. Cardiopulmonary bypass
      2. Myeloproliferative disorders
      3. Drugs—aspirin and other nonsteroidal anti-inflammatory agents

mild cases, bleeding occurs only after surgery or trauma. More severely affected patients have spontaneous epistaxis or oral mucosal, gastrointestinal, or genitourinary bleeding. The laboratory findings are variable. The most diagnostic pattern is the combination of (1) a prolonged bleeding time, (2) a reduction in plasma vWF concentration, (3) a parallel reduction in biologic activity as measured with the ristocetin cofactor assay, and (4) reduced factor VIII activity. The variability in laboratory tests is related to both the heterogeneous nature of the defects in vWD and the fact that plasma levels are influenced by ABO blood group type, central nervous system disorders, systemic inflammation, and pregnancy. Since vWD is an autosomal dominant disorder, some vWF is produced by the remaining normal allele. Thus patients with mild defects may have laboratory values that fluctuate over time and may occasionally be within the normal range.

There are three major types of vWD. Their mode of inheritance and laboratory findings are shown in Fig. 116-2. Patients with *type I disease*, the most common abnormality, have a mild to moderate de-

Table 116-3   Evaluation of Platelet Function

Bleeding time
   Modified Ivy method
   Skin incision—time to stop bleeding
   Global screen of platelet role in hemostasis
von Willebrand factor assays
   vWF Ag—immunoassay of total vWF protein
   vWF R:Cof—bioassay of vWF that measures ability of patient plasma to support agglutination of normal platelets in the presence of ristocetin
   Factor VIII—coagulation assay of factor VIII bound and carried by plasma vWF
Platelet aggregometry
   Measures platelet aggregation in response to a panel of agonists, usually ADP, collagen, arachidonic acid, and epinephrine
Membrane glycoproteins
   Presence of glycoproteins Ib-IX and IIb-IIIa can be measured using monoclonal antibodies and flow cytometry
Platelet granule content
   Dense granules—electron microscopy or uptake and retention of radiolabeled serotonin
   Alpha granules—electron microscopy and/or immunoassays for platelet-associated proteins—vWF, fibrinogen, platelet factor four

NOTE: vWF, von Willebrand factor; ADP, adenosine diphosphate; Ag, antigen, R:Cof, ristocetin cofactor.

FIGURE 116-2 Pattern of inheritance and laboratory findings in von Willebrand's disease. The assays of platelet function include a coagulation assay of factor VIII bound and carried by von Willebrand factor (vWF), abbreviated as VIII; immunoassay of total vWF protein, abbreviated vWF:Ag; bioassay of the ability of patient plasma to support ristocetin-induced agglutination of normal platelets, abbreviated vWF:RCoF; and ristocetin-induced aggregation of patient platelets, abbreviated RIPA. The multimer pattern illustrates the protein bonds present when plasma is electrophoresed in a polyacrylamide gel. The II-1 and II-2 columns refer to the phenotypes of the second-generation offspring.

crease in plasma vWF. In the milder cases, although hemostasis is impaired, the vWF level is just below normal (50% activity, or 5 mg/L). In type I disease, vWF antigen, factor VIII activity, and ristocetin cofactor activity are decreased with a normal spectrum of multimers detected by sodium dodecyl sulfate (SDS)–agarose gel electrophoresis.

The variant forms of vWD (*type II disease*) are much less common and characterized by normal or near-normal levels of a dysfunctional protein. Patients with the *type IIa variant* of vWD have a deficiency in the high- and medium-molecular-weight forms of vWF multimer detected by SDS-agarose electrophoresis. This is due either to an inability to secrete the high-molecular-weight vWF multimers or to proteolysis of the multimers soon after they leave the endothelial cell and enter the circulation. Mutations in a localized region of the vWF A-2 domain have been identified in families with type IIa vWD (Fig. 116-3). The quantity of vWF antigen and the amount of associated factor VIII are usually normal. In the *type IIb variant*, high-molecular-weight multimers are also decreased; however, the decrease is due to the inappropriate binding of vWF to platelets. Intravascular platelet aggregates form that are rapidly cleared from the circulation, causing mild, variable thrombocytopenia. Mutations in a disulfide-bonded loop in the A-1 domain that binds to glycoprotein Ib-IX are the cause of the type IIb defect (Fig. 116-3). A few patients have a platelet mem-

brane disorder that mimics type IIb vWD—*platelet-type vWD*. It is due to mutations in the portion of glycoprotein Ib-IX that interacts with vWF. Levels of total vWF antigen and factor VIII are normal.

Approximately 1 in 1 million individuals has a very severe form of vWD that is phenotypically recessive (*type III disease*). Type III patients are usually the offspring of two parents (usually asymptomatic) with mild type I disease. Type III patients may inherit a different abnormality from each parent (a doubly heterozygous or compound heterozygous state) or be homozygous for a single defect. Type III patients have severe mucosal bleeding and no detectable vWF antigen or activity and, like patients with mild hemophilia, may have sufficiently low factor VIII that they have occasional hemarthroses. Major deletions in the vWF gene have been found in some type III families. Families with nonsense mutations and the combination of a deleted and nonsense mutant allele have also been described.

Type IIN disease is due to a defect in the factor VIII binding site of vWF. Patients resemble those with mild hemophilia and have low levels of factor VIII. The presence of disease in both males and females in a family is a clue to the role of vWF in this disease.

℞ **TREATMENT** There are two therapeutic options. Factor VIII concentrates retain high-molecular-weight vWF multimers (Humate-P, Alfanate), are highly purified and heat-treated to destroy HIV, and are appropriate treatments for all the inherited forms of vWD. During surgery or after major trauma, patients should receive factor VIII concentrates twice daily for 2 or 3 days to assure optimal hemostasis. Minor bleeding episodes such as prolonged epistaxis or severe menorrhagia may respond to a single infusion. Recurrent menorrhagia, a major problem for women with severe vWD, can be treated effectively with oral contraceptive agents that suppress menses.

A second therapeutic option, which avoids the use of plasma, is the use of DDAVP or desmopressin, a vasopressin analogue that has minimal blood pressure–elevating and fluid-retaining properties and raises the plasma vWF level in both normal individuals and patients with mild vWD. Patients with type I disease are the best candidates for DDAVP therapy. However, they must be tested for an adequate response before anticipated surgery, and vWF levels must be monitored closely during therapy, since the patient may develop tachyphylaxis when therapy is continued for more than 48 h. DDAVP should not be given to patients with variant forms of vWD without prior testing, since it may not improve multimer pattern or hemostasis in type IIa patients and may actually worsen the defect by depleting high-molecular-weight multimers, inducing intravascular platelet aggregation, and lowering the platelet count in type IIb patients. It is ineffective therapy for the severe (type III) form of vWD.

Acquired vWD Although most cases of vWD are inherited, acquired vWD may be caused by antibodies that inhibit vWF function or by lymphoid or other tumors that selectively adsorb vWF multimers onto their surfaces. Anti-vWF antibodies have developed in patients with severe vWD following multiple transfusions, as well as in patients with autoimmune and lymphoproliferative disorders. Adsorption of vWF to tumor surfaces has been documented in patients with Waldenström's macroglobulinemia and Wilms' tumor and inferred in other patients with lymphoma. Treatment of acquired vWD should focus on the underlying disease, since plasma derivatives and DDAVP are often not effective and the disorder can be fatal.

Platelet Membrane Defects Receptors that modulate platelet adhesion and aggregation are located on the two major platelet surface glycoproteins. vWF facilitates platelet adhesion by binding to glycoprotein Ib-IX, while fibrinogen links platelets into aggregates via sites on the glycoprotein IIb-IIIa complex. Two rare platelet defects are characterized by a loss of or a defect in these glycoprotein receptors. Patients with the *Bernard-Soulier syndrome* have markedly reduced platelet adhesion and cannot bind vWF to their platelets due to deficiency or dysfunction of the glycoprotein Ib-IX complex. They also have reduced levels of several other membrane proteins, mild thrombocytopenia, and extremely large, lymphocytoid platelets. Platelets from patients with *Glanzmann's disease* or *thrombasthenia* are deficient or defective in the glycoprotein IIb-IIIa complex. Their platelets do not bind fibrinogen and cannot form aggregates, although the platelets undergo shape change and secretion and are of normal size.

Both these disorders are autosomal recessive traits and are characterized by markedly impaired hemostasis and recurrent episodes of severe mucosal hemorrhage. Bernard-Soulier platelets react normally to all stimuli except ristocetin. In contrast, thrombasthenic platelets adhere normally and will agglutinate with ristocetin but will not aggregate with any of the agonists that require fibrinogen binding, such as adenosine diphosphate (ADP), thrombin, or epinephrine.

FIGURE 116-3 Location of mutations in types IIa and IIb von Willebrand's disease. Mutations in the region of the protein between amino acids 742 and 875 have been identified in patients with type IIa disease. These result in a deficiency in high- and medium-molecular-weight multimers due either to failure to secrete high-molecular-weight forms of vWF or to their proteolytic degradation in the circulation. In type IIb disease, there is also a decrease in high-molecular-weight vWF, but the defect is due to the failure of vWF with mutations in the A-1 domain of the protein (amino acids 509–695) to bind properly to platelet glycoprotein Ib-IX.

The only effective therapy for hemorrhagic episodes in these two disorders is transfusion with normal platelets. Alloimmunization will eventually limit the life span of infused platelets. In addition, a few patients have developed inhibitor antibodies with specificity for the missing protein. These antibodies bind to the protein that is expressed on the transfused normal platelets and impair their function.

Platelet Release Defects The most common mild bleeding disorders arise from the ingestion of aspirin and other nonsteroidal anti-inflammatory drugs (NSAIDs) that inhibit platelet production of thromboxane A_2, an important mediator of platelet secretion and aggregation (Figs. 62-3 and 62-4). These drugs inhibit cyclooxygenase, which converts arachidonic acid to a labile endoperoxide intermediate that is critical for thromboxane formation. Aspirin is the most potent agent, since it irreversibly acetylates the platelet enzyme so that a single dose impairs hemostasis for 5 to 7 days. The other agents are competitive and reversible inhibitors with more transient effects. Blocking thromboxane A_2 synthesis partially inhibits platelet release and aggregation with weak agonists, such as ADP and epinephrine, and produces a mild hemostatic defect. The administration of high doses of certain antibiotics, particularly penicillin, can coat the platelet surface, block platelet release, and impair hemostasis.

Patients generally have minimal symptoms such as easy bruising, and bleeding is usually confined to the skin. Occasional patients will have prolonged oozing after surgery, particularly with procedures involving mucous membranes such as periodontal, oral, or reconstructive plastic surgery. The antiplatelet effect of drugs such as aspirin is more dramatic when they are administered to patients with underlying defects such as vWD or hemophilia. Patients with drug-induced cyclooxygenase deficiency often have a mildly prolonged bleeding time, and their platelets fail to aggregate when incubated with arachidonic acid, epinephrine, or low doses of ADP. Patients who have taken aspirin should be treated as if they have a mild hemostatic defect for the next 5 to 7 days. Platelet responses to collagen and thrombin are impaired at low doses but normal at higher doses. Symptomatic patients should be encouraged to use drugs such as acetaminophen that do not impair platelet function. Although most cases of cyclooxygenase deficiency are drug-induced, occasional patients have inherited disorders in platelet cyclooxygenase activity that impair thromboxane production or receptor level defects that prevent platelets from responding to thromboxane A_2.

Of the metabolic disorders that can perturb hemostasis, uremic platelet dysfunction is clinically the most important. The mechanism by which uremia impairs platelet function is not well understood, and retention of phenolic and guanidinosuccinic acids, excess prostacyclin production, or impaired vWF-platelet interactions have all been implicated. The degree of uremia correlates with bleeding symptoms and anemia. Bleeding can usually be reversed by dialysis and often improves after red cell transfusion or treatment with erythropoietin. In addition, factor VIII concentrate or DDAVP, both of which raise plasma vWF levels, can also improve hemostasis. Conjugated estrogens improve hemostasis and can be used as long-term therapy.

Storage Pool Defects Platelet granules have considerable amounts of adenine nucleotides, calcium, and adhesive glycoproteins such as thrombospondin, fibronectin, and vWF, all of which promote platelet adhesion and aggregation. Patients with defective platelet granules have a mild bleeding disorder. Platelet storage pool defects may be inherited as an isolated disorder or be part of systemic granule packaging defects such as oculocutaneous albinism or the Hermansky-Pudlak or Chédiak-Higashi syndromes. Clinically, these patients cannot be distinguished from those with other functional platelet disorders, since they all have easy bruising, mucosal bleeding, and a prolonged bleeding time. They can be differentiated from patients with the cyclooxygenase defects because their platelets will usually aggregate in response to arachidonic acid. In addition, their platelets have decreased levels of specific granule constituents such as ADP and serotonin and abnormalities in granule morphology that are best visualized by electron microscopy.

Occasionally, patients with acute or chronic leukemia or one of the myeloproliferative disorders develop an acquired storage pool disorder due to dysplastic megakaryocyte development. In addition, patients with liver disease and some patients with SLE or other immune complex–mediated disorders may have circulating platelets that have degranulated prematurely. Platelet degranulation and a transient storage pool disorder may occur after prolonged cardiopulmonary bypass. Fortunately, most patients with storage pool defects have only mildly impaired hemostasis. They can be treated with platelet transfusions. Occasional patients have responded to DDAVP.

VESSEL WALL DISORDERS

Bleeding from vascular disorders (nonthrombocytopenic purpura) is usually mild and confined to the skin and mucous membranes. The pathogenesis of bleeding is poorly defined in many of the syndromes, and classic tests of hemostasis, including the bleeding time and tests of platelet function, are usually normal. Vascular purpura arises from damage to capillary endothelium, abnormalities in the vascular subendothelial matrix or extravascular connective tissues that support blood vessels, or from the formation of abnormal blood vessels. Several idiopathic disorders involve the vessel wall and can cause more severe bleeding and organ dysfunction.

THROMBOTIC THROMBOCYTOPENIC PURPURA TTP is a fulminant, often lethal disorder that may be initiated by endothelial injury and subsequent release of vWF and other procoagulant materials from the endothelial cell. Causes include pregnancy, metastatic cancer, mitomycin C, high-dose chemotherapy, HIV infection, and certain drugs, such as the antiplatelet angent ticlopidine. Characteristic findings include the microvascular deposition of hyaline fibrin thrombi, thrombocytopenia, microangiopathic hemolytic anemia, fever, renal failure, fluctuating levels of consciousness, and evanescent focal neurologic deficits. The presence of hyaline thrombi in arterioles, capillaries, and venules without any inflammatory changes in the vessel wall is diagnostic. The presence of a severe Coombs-negative hemolytic anemia with schistocytes or fragmented red blood cells in the peripheral blood smear, coupled with thrombocytopenia, and minimal activation of the coagulation system help to confirm the clinical suspicion of TTP. This disorder should be distinguished from vasculitis and SLE, which can predispose patients to TTP. Platelet-associated IgG and complement levels are usually normal in TTP.

The treatment of acute TTP has focused on the use of exchange transfusion or intensive plasmapheresis coupled with infusion of fresh frozen plasma. Patients with TTP become transiently deficient in a plasma enzyme that depolymerizes ultra-high-molecular-weight vWF released from endothelial cells. Therapy may remove abnormal forms of vWF and replenish the deficient enzyme. Overall mortality has been markedly reduced, and the majority of patients with TTP recover from this formerly fatal disorder. Most patients surviving the acute illness recover completely, with no residual renal or neurologic disease. Occasional patients with a chronic, relapsing form of TTP require maintenance plasmapheresis and plasma infusion, and a few patients are controlled only with glucocorticoids.

HEMOLYTIC-UREMIC SYNDROME HUS is a disease of infancy and early childhood that closely resembles TTP. Patients present with fever, thrombocytopenia, microangiopathic hemolytic anemia, hypertension, and varying degrees of acute renal failure. In many cases, onset is preceded by a minor febrile or viral illness, and an infectious or immune complex–mediated cause has been proposed. Epidemics related to infection with a specific strain of *Escherichia coli* (O157:H7) have been documented. As in TTP, disseminated intravascular coagulation is not found. In contrast to TTP, the disorder remains localized to the kidney, where hyaline thrombi are seen in the afferent arterioles and glomerular capillaries. Such thrombi are not present in other vessels, and neurologic symptoms, other than those associated with uremia, are uncommon. No therapy is proven effective; however, with dialysis for acute renal failure, the initial mortality is only 5%. Between 10 and 50% of patients have some chronic renal impairment.

HENOCH-SCHÖNLEIN PURPURA Henoch-Schönlein, or anaphylactoid, purpura is a distinct, self-limited type of vasculitis that occurs in children and young adults. Patients have an acute inflammatory reaction in capillaries, mesangial tissues, and small arterioles that leads to increased vascular permeability, exudation, and hemorrhage. Vessel lesions contain IgA and complement components. The syndrome may be preceded by an upper respiratory infection or streptococcal pharyngitis or be associated with food or drug allergies. Patients develop a purpuric or urticarial rash on the extensor surfaces of the arms and legs and on the buttocks as well as polyarthralgias or arthritis, colicky abdominal pain, and hematuria from focal glomerulonephritis. Despite the hemorrhagic features, all coagulation tests are normal. A small number of patients may develop fatal acute renal failure, and 5 to 10% develop chronic nephritis. Glucocorticoids provide symptomatic relief of the joint and abdominal pains but do not alter the course of the illness.

METABOLIC AND INFLAMMATORY DISORDERS Acute febrile illnesses may cause capillary fragility and skin bleeding. Immune complexes containing viral antigens or the viruses themselves may damage endothelial cells. In addition, certain pathogens such as the rickettsiae that cause Rocky Mountain spotted fever replicate in endothelial cells and damage them. Thrombocytopenia is also a frequent finding in acute infectious disorders and may contribute to skin bleeding. In addition, whenever the platelet count is $<10,000/\mu L$, gaps develop between endothelial cells, which allow the diapedesis of red cells into the dermis, forming petechiae. Drugs such as the sulfonamides, penicillin, and allopurinol may cause vascular inflammation, resulting in maculopapular or urticarial rashes. Some of these mechanisms are additive, and drug reactions in thrombocytopenic individuals cause an intensely hemorrhagic rash.

Occasionally, patients with diffuse polyclonal hyperglobulinemia will develop purpuric lesions on the lower limbs—a benign condition referred to as *hyperglobulinemic purpura*. Vascular purpura may occur in patients with various monoclonal gammopathies, including Waldenström's macroglobulinemia, multiple myeloma, and cryoglobulinemia. These proteins markedly increase serum viscosity and may impair blood flow through capillaries and lead to retinal hemorrhage, central nervous system dysfunction, and skin necrosis. In addition, the globulins may impair platelet aggregation and adhesion and interfere with fibrin polymerization. Patients with mixed cryoglobulinemia develop a more extensive maculopapular lesion due to immune complex–mediated damage to the vessel wall. The mixed cryoglobulinemia (usually IgG and anti-IgG) may be associated with arthralgias, diffuse weakness, and unexplained nephritis. Plasmapheresis will temporarily lower the level of globulins, remove immune complexes, and improve symptoms in these patients. However, long-term management must include control of the underlying disease that produces the abnormal globulins or immune complexes.

Patients with *scurvy* (vitamin C deficiency) develop painful episodes of perifollicular skin bleeding as well as bleeding into muscles and, occasionally, into the gastrointestinal and genitourinary tracts. The diagnosis is confirmed by the presence of hyperkeratosis of skin, gum swelling, and low levels of the vitamin in leukocytes. Vitamin C is needed to synthesize hydroxyproline, an essential constituent of collagen. Thus, collagen synthesis is impaired by scurvy. Patients with *Cushing's syndrome*, an excess production of glucocorticoids, or patients on large doses of glucocorticoids develop generalized protein wasting and may show skin bleeding or easy bruising due to atrophy of the supporting connective tissue around blood vessels. Aging causes a similar atrophy of perivascular connective tissue on the extensor surfaces of the hands and arms, leading to *senile purpura*—dark purple, irregularly shaped hemorrhagic areas due to abnormal skin mobility that tears small blood vessels.

Patients with inherited disorders of the connective tissue matrix such as *Marfan's syndrome*, *Ehlers-Danlos syndrome*, and *pseudoxanthoma elasticum* also have easy bruising. In addition to having fragile skin vessels and easy bruising, patients with Ehlers-Danlos syndrome may develop aneurysms in intraabdominal vessels and apoplectic rupture and hemorrhage due to defects in the vascular collagen network. Primary vascular abnormalities can also lead to bleeding. Patients with *Osler-Weber-Rendu disease* (hereditary hemorrhagic telangiectasia), an inherited autosomal dominant disorder, have frequent episodes of nasal and gastrointestinal bleeding from abnormal telangiectatic capillaries. They may develop pulmonary arteriovenous fistulas. Two genetic defects have been identified in these patients both involving proteins that bind to transforming growth factor β (TGF-β); HHT-1 has mutations in endoglin, and HHT-2 has mutations in ALK-1. Patients with *angiodysplasia* of the colon have increased incidence of gastrointestinal bleeding. In the *Kasabach-Merritt syndrome*, patients may have very extensive and progressively enlarging vascular malformation that may involve large portions of their extremities. Bleeding is secondary to disseminated intravascular coagulation triggered by stagnant blood flow through the tortuous vessels.

BIBLIOGRAPHY

AMERICAN SOCIETY OF HEMATOLOGY PRACTICE GUIDELINE PANEL: Diagnosis and treatment of idiopathic thrombocytopenic purpura. Ann Intern Med 126:316, 1997

EWENSTEIN BM, HANDIN RI: von Willebrand's disease, in *Blood: Principles and Practice of Hematology*, RI Handin et al (eds). Philadelphia, Lippincott, 1994, pp 1069–1094

KELTON JG: The clinical management of heparin-induced thrombocytopenia. Semin Hematol 36:17, 1999

WARKENTON TE, KELTON J: The platelet life cycle: Quantitative disorders in blood, in *Blood: Principles and Practice of Hematology*, RI Handin et al (eds). Philadelphia, Lippincott, 1994, pp 973–1049

DISORDERS OF COAGULATION AND THROMBOSIS

Patients with congenital plasma coagulation defects characteristically bleed into muscles, joints, and body cavities hours or days after an injury. Most of the *inherited* plasma coagulation disorders are due to defects in single coagulation proteins, with the two X-linked disorders, factors VIII and IX deficiency, accounting for the majority. These patients may have severe bleeding and chronic disability and require specialized medical therapy. With rare exceptions, the known disorders prolong either the prothrombin time (PT), partial thromboplastin time (PTT), or both. If they are abnormal, quantitative assays of specific coagulation proteins are then carried out using the PT or PTT tests with plasma from congenitally deficient individuals as substrate. The corrective effect of varying concentrations of patient plasma is measured and expressed as a percentage of a normal pooled plasma standard. The interval range for most coagulation factors is from 50 to 150% of this average value, and the minimal level of most individual factors needed for adequate hemostasis is 25%.

Acquired coagulation disorders are both more frequent and more complex, arising from deficiencies of multiple coagulation proteins and simultaneously affecting both primary and secondary hemostasis. The most common acquired hemorrhagic disorders are (1) disseminated intravascular coagulation (DIC), (2) the hemorrhagic diathesis of liver disease, and (3) vitamin K deficiency and complications of anticoagulant therapy.

Although congenital and acquired bleeding disorders are relatively rare, venous and arterial thrombosis and embolism are common medical disorders that have been recognized for >100 years. Although risk factors such as atherosclerotic vascular disease, congestive heart failure, malignancy, and immobility predispose patients to thrombosis, specific coagulation defects have not yet been identified in most patients with thromboembolism. Several inherited coagulation abnormalities induce a hypercoagulable or prethrombotic state and predispose patients to thrombosis. These disorders affect young people, cause recurrent episodes of thromboembolism, and may involve multiple members of a single family. An understanding of the biochemical basis of thromboembolism is also important because anticoagulant and antithrombotic regimens are based on the premise that modifying critical coagulation reactions will reduce the incidence of thrombosis.
→*For further discussion of the physiology of normal hemostasis and the cardinal manifestations of the hemorrhagic and thrombotic disorders, see Chap. 62.*

FACTOR VIII DEFICIENCY—HEMOPHILIA A **Pathogenesis and Clinical Manifestations** The antihemophilic factor (AHF), or factor VIII coagulant protein, is a large (265-kDa), single-chain protein that regulates the activation of factor X by proteases generated in the intrinsic coagulation pathway (Figs. 62-5 and 62-6). It is synthesized in liver and circulates complexed to the von Willebrand factor (vWF) protein. Factor VIII molecule is present in low concentration (10 μg/L) and is susceptible to proteolysis. The gene for factor VIII is on the X chromosome, and carrier detection and prenatal diagnosis are well established.

One in 10,000 males is born with deficiency or dysfunction of the factor VIII molecule. The resulting disorder, *hemophilia A*, is characterized by bleeding into soft tissues, muscles, and weight-bearing joints. Symptomatic patients usually have factor VIII levels <5%, with a close correlation between the clinical severity of hemophilia and plasma AHF level. Patients with <1% factor VIII activity have *severe* disease; they bleed frequently even without discernible trauma. Patients with levels of 1 to 5% have *moderate* disease with less frequent bleeding episodes. Those with levels >5% have *mild* disease with infrequent bleeding that is usually secondary to trauma. Occasional patients with factor VIII levels as high as 25% are discovered when

they bleed after major trauma or surgery. The majority of patients with hemophilia A have factor VIII levels below <5%.

Hemophilic bleeding occurs hours or days after injury, can involve any organ, and, if untreated, may continue for days or weeks. This can result in large collections of partially clotted blood putting pressure on adjacent normal tissues and can cause necrosis of muscle (compartment syndromes), venous congestion (pseudophlebitis), or ischemic damage to nerves. Patients with hemophilia often develop femoral neuropathy due to pressure from an unsuspected retroperitoneal hematoma. They can also develop large calcified masses of blood and inflammatory tissue that are mistaken for cancers (pseudotumor syndrome).

Patients with severe hemophilia are usually diagnosed shortly after birth because of an extensive cephalhematoma or profuse bleeding at circumcision. However, young children with moderate disease may not bleed until they begin to walk or crawl, and individuals with mild hemophilia may not be diagnosed until they are adolescents or young adults. Typically, a hemophilia patient presents with pain followed by swelling in a weight-bearing joint, such as the hip, knee, or ankle. The presence of blood in the joint (*hemarthrosis*) causes synovial inflammation, and repetitive bleeding erodes articular cartilage and causes osteoarthritis, articular fibrosis, joint ankylosis, and eventually muscle atrophy. Bleeding may occur into any joint, but after a joint has been damaged, it may become a site for subsequent bleeding episodes.

Hematuria, without any genitourinary pathology, is also common. It is usually self-limited and may not require specific therapy. The most feared complications of hemophilia are oropharyngeal and central nervous system bleeding. Patients with oropharyngeal bleeding may require emergency intubation to maintain an adequate airway. Central nervous system bleeding can occur without antecedent trauma or without evidence of a specific lesion.

Patients suspected of having hemophilia should have a platelet count, bleeding time, PT, and PTT. Typically, the patient will have a prolonged PTT with all other tests normal. Because of the clinical similarity of factor VIII deficiency and factor IX deficiency, any male with an appropriate bleeding history and a prolonged PTT should have specific assays for factor VIII and factor IX.

℞ **TREATMENT** Tenets regarding the treatment of bleeding in hemophilia patients include the following: (1) Symptoms often precede objective evidence of bleeding. (2) Signs of bleeding may not appear until several days after well-documented trauma. The patients can generally be relied upon to identify early symptoms, usually pain. Early treatment is more effective, less costly, and can be lifesaving. (3) Avoid the use of aspirin or aspirin-containing drugs, which impair platelet function and may cause severe hemorrhage. COX-2 inhibitors can be used, as they do not impair platelet function.

Plasma products enriched in factor VIII have revolutionized the care of hemophilia patients, reduced the degree of orthopedic deformity, and permitted virtually any form of elective and emergency surgery. The widespread use of factor VIII concentrates has also produced serious complications, including viral hepatitis, chronic liver disease, and AIDS. *Cryoprecipitate*, which contains about half the factor VIII activity of fresh-frozen plasma in one-tenth the original volume, is simple to prepare and is produced in hospital or regional blood banks.

Three developments have increased the safety of factor VIII therapy and have changed medical practice. First, heating of lyophilized factor VIII concentrates under carefully controlled conditions can inactivate HIV without destroying factor VIII activity. Second, highly purified factor VIII can be produced by adsorbing and eluting factor VIII from monoclonal antibody columns. Third, recombinant factor VIII is now available. Patients with hemophilia should receive either monoclonal purified or recombinant factor VIII to minimize viral infections and exposure to irrelevant proteins.

Each unit of factor VIII infused, defined as the amount present in 1 mL normal plasma, will raise the plasma level of the recipient by

2%/kg of body weight. Factor VIII has a half-life of 8 to 12 h, making it necessary to infuse it continuously or at least twice daily to sustain a chosen factor VIII level. In patients with mild hemophilia, an alternative treatment is desmopressin (DDAVP), which transiently increases the factor VIII level. DDAVP will increase the factor level two- to threefold. Although generally safe, it occasionally causes hyponatremia or may precipitate thrombosis in elderly patients.

An uncomplicated episode of soft tissue bleeding or an early hemarthrosis can be treated with one infusion of sufficient factor VIII concentrate to raise the factor VIII level to 15 or 20%. A more extensive hemarthrosis or retroperitoneal bleeding requires twice-daily or continuous infusions in order to keep the factor VIII level at 25 to 50% for at least 72 h. Life-threatening bleeding into the central nervous system or major surgery may require therapy for 2 weeks with levels kept at a minimum of 50% normal. Patients also need skilled orthopedic care, with immobilization of inflamed joints to promote healing and to prevent contractures, and physical therapy to strengthen muscles and maintain joint mobility.

Before surgery, every hemophilia patient should be screened for the presence of an inhibitor to factor VIII. Patients with hemophilia who do not have an inhibitor should receive factor VIII infusions just before surgery and will require daily monitoring so that the factor VIII level is maintained >50% for 10 to 14 days after surgery. When patients undergo joint replacement or other major orthopedic surgery, therapy should be continued for 3 weeks to permit wound healing and the institution of physical therapy.

Hemophilia patients also require treatment before dental procedures. Filling of a carious tooth can be managed by a single infusion of factor VIII concentrate coupled with the administration of 4 to 6 g of ε-aminocaproic acid (EACA) four times daily for 3 to 4 days after the dental procedure. EACA is a potent antifibrinolytic agent that inhibits plasminogen activators present in oral secretions and stabilizes clot formation in oral tissue. Alternatives include tranexamic acid, a longer-acting antifibrinolytic. EACA is also effective when used as a mouthwash. For major oral and periodontal surgery and extractions of permanent teeth, patients should probably be hospitalized briefly and also treated with factor VIII concentrates. Therapy should begin just before surgery and continue for at least 2 to 3 days.

Many centers have organized home-care programs so that patients can administer their own factor VIII infusions with the onset of symptoms. Occasional patients with very frequent bleeding receive regularly scheduled infusions. Despite the expense and inconvenience of "prophylactic" infusions, their use in early childhood has reduced or eliminated hemarthroses. Concern about transmission of AIDS has made some patients reluctant to treat themselves, despite the fact that current blood products carry a very low or no risk of transmitting HIV.

The prospects for correcting factor VIII deficiency by gene therapy are promising; some success has been achieved in dogs. Clinical studies in humans are underway.

Complications   Most hemophilia patients have had multiple episodes of hepatitis, and a majority have elevated hepatocellular enzyme levels and abnormalities on liver biopsy. Ten to 20% of patients also have hepatosplenomegaly, and a small number develop chronic active or persistent hepatitis or cirrhosis. A few patients with hemophilia and end-stage liver disease have received liver transplants with cure of both diseases. Along with homosexuals and intravenous drug abusers, hemophilia patients are at high risk for AIDS because they frequently receive blood products; they can also present with the full range of AIDS-related syndromes, including diffuse lymphadenopathy and immune thrombocytopenia. Although up to 50% of multiply transfused hemophiliacs are HIV-positive and many have clinical AIDS, the advances in factor VIII concentrate production should prevent future HIV infection.

Despite frequent bleeding, severe iron-deficiency anemia is uncommon because most of the bleeding is internal and iron is effectively recycled. Mild iron deficiency from chronic epistaxis or gastrointestinal bleeding occurs in some patients. In addition, some patients have developed a mild Coombs-positive hemolytic anemia due to small amounts of anti-A and anti-B antibody that are present in intermediate purity factor VIII concentrates.

Following multiple transfusions, 10 to 20% of patients with severe hemophilia develop inhibitors to factor VIII. Inhibitors are usually IgG antibodies that rapidly neutralize factor VIII activity. Two types of inhibitors are found with different biologic characteristics and different clinical presentations. Patients with type I inhibitors have a typical anamnestic response and raise their antibody titer following exposure to factor VIII. Patients with a type II inhibitor have a low antibody titer that is not stimulated by factor VIII infusion. Patients with the type I inhibitor should not receive factor VIII. Control of bleeding may require the infusion of either porcine factor VIII concentrates, which may not be affected by inhibitors, or prothrombin complex concentrates, which contain trace quantities of activated coagulation factors and can bypass the block in coagulation produced by the inhibitor. Patients with low-titer type II antibodies may respond to higher doses of factor VIII.

Protocols to induce tolerance to human factor VIII use massive doses of the factor coupled with immunosuppression. Tolerance induction is expensive and not always effective; it should be reserved for severely affected patients.

Genetic Counseling and Carrier Detection   It is possible to trace the defective allele in some families by examining the inheritance of restriction fragment length polymorphisms (RFLP) linked to the factor VIII gene. In addition, in families in which a specific mutation has been defined in the factor VIII gene, it can be readily detected by gene amplification and allele-specific oligonucleotide hybridization. For example, 45% of patients with severe hemophilia A have a chromosomal inversion arising from homologous recombination between sequences in intron 22 and an upstream gene. The inversion is readily detected by polymerase chain reaction (PCR) or Southern blotting. Precise diagnosis is possible early in pregnancy from either chorionic villus biopsy or amniocentesis.

Female carriers of hemophilia, who are heterozygotes, usually produce sufficient factor VIII from the factor VIII allele on their normal X chromosome for normal hemostasis. However, occasional hemophilia carriers will have factor VIII levels far below 50% due to random inactivation of normal X chromosomes in tissue producing factor VIII. These symptomatic carriers may bleed with major surgery or bleed occasionally with menses. Rarely, true female hemophiliacs arise from consanguinity within families with hemophilia or from concomitant Turner's syndrome or XO mosaicism in a carrier female.

FACTOR IX DEFICIENCY—HEMOPHILIA B   Factor IX is a single-chain, 55-kDa proenzyme that is converted to an active protease (IXa) by factor XIa or by the tissue factor–VIIa complex. Factor IXa then activates factor X in conjunction with activated factor VIII. Factor IX is one of six proteins synthesized in the liver that require vitamin K for biologic activity. Vitamin K is a cofactor for a unique posttranslational modification that inserts a second carboxyl group onto certain glutamic acid residues on factor IX (Chap. 62). This modification permits calcium binding and adsorption onto phospholipid surfaces. Factor IX gene is on the X chromosome.

Factor IX deficiency or dysfunction (hemophilia B, Christmas disease) occurs in 1 in 100,000 male births. Accurate laboratory diagnosis is critical, since it is indistinguishable clinically from factor VIII deficiency (hemophilia A) but requires different treatment. Either fresh-frozen plasma or a plasma fraction enriched in the prothrombin complex proteins is used. Monoclonally purified or recombinant factor IX preparations are now available. In addition to the expected complications of hepatitis, chronic liver disease, and AIDS, the therapy of factor IX deficiency has a special hazard. Trace quantities of activated coagulation factors in prothrombin complex concentrates may activate the coagulation system and cause thrombosis and embolism. This is particularly common in immobilized surgical patients and patients with liver disease. As a result, some centers have returned to fresh-frozen plasma for factor IX–deficient surgical patients, while others have recommended the addition of small doses of heparin to the concentrate to activate antithrombin III during the infusion and reduce hypercoagulability. The recombinant or monoclonally purified products are less likely to be thrombogenic.

FACTOR XI DEFICIENCY   Factor XI is a 160-kDa dimeric protein activated to an active protease (XIa) by factor XIIa, in conjunction with high-molecular-weight kininogen and kallikrein (Figs. 62-5 and 62-6). Factor XI deficiency is inherited as an autosomal recessive trait and is especially common in Ashkenazi Jews. In contrast to deficiency in factors VIII and IX, the correlation between factor level and propensity to bleed is not as precise, spontaneous bleeding is less, and hemarthroses are rare. Many patients with factor XI deficiency present with posttraumatic bleeding or with bleeding in the perioperative period, and occasional factor XI–deficient women have menorrhagia. Daily infusions of fresh-frozen plasma are sufficient, since the half-life of factor XI is approximately 24 h. The majority of defective factor XI alleles were accounted for by a limited number of mutations.

OTHER FACTOR DEFICIENCIES   Deficiencies in factors V, VII, X, and prothrombin (factor II) are exceedingly rare autosomal recessive disorders. Spontaneous or posttraumatic musculoskeletal bleeding or menorrhagia can occur with these deficiencies, but hemarthroses are uncommon. Fresh-frozen plasma is the appropriate therapy, although prothrombin concentrates may be employed for patients with severe prothrombin deficiency or decreases in factors VII and X as long as the risks of hepatitis and thrombosis are recognized.

Defects in the contact activation pathway involving Hageman factor (factor XII), high-molecular-weight kininogen, and prekallikrein cause laboratory abnormalities but no clinical bleeding. Despite dramatic prolongation of the PTT, often to greater than 100 s, deficient individuals have normal hemostasis and can undergo major surgery without plasma replacement therapy. Direct activation of factor IX by the tissue factor–VIIa complex may bypass this defective step in coagulation (Fig. 62-7). Recognition of these disorders is important because such patients should neither be treated inappropriately with plasma nor denied indicated surgery on the basis of these laboratory abnormalities.

AFIBRINOGENEMIA AND DYSFIBRINOGENEMIA   Fibrinogen is a 340-kDa dimeric molecule made up of two sets of three covalently linked polypeptide chains. Thrombin sequentially cleaves fibrinopeptides A and B from the $A\alpha$ and $B\beta$ chains of fibrinogen to produce fibrin monomer, which then polymerizes to form a fibrin clot. Although fibrinogen is needed for platelet aggregation and fibrin formation, severe fibrinogen deficiency does not usually cause serious bleeding except after surgery. Patients with afibrinogenemia, who have no detectable fibrinogen in plasma or platelets, may have infrequent, mild bleeding episodes. Preliminary genetic analyses do not show any gross deletion or structural changes in the genes encoding the α, β, and γ chains of fibrinogen despite the total absence of plasma fibrinogen.

Fibrinogen is an abundant plasma protein (2.5 g/L). Mutations have been identified that alter the release of fibrinopeptides from the $A\alpha$ and $B\beta$ chains of fibrinogen, the rate of polymerization of fibrin monomers, and the sites for fibrin cross-linking. These dysfibrinogenemias are almost always inherited as autosomal dominant traits, so patients have nearly equal concentrations of normal and mutant fibrinogen in their plasma. Patients with dysfibrinogenemia have a slightly prolonged PT and PTT, a prolonged thrombin time, and a disparity in levels of fibrinogen measured with functional and immunologic assays. Despite these abnormalities, most patients have no symptoms or only moderate bleeding. A few dysfibrinogenemias induce a hypercoagulable state and increase the risk of thrombosis, and others have been associated with an increased incidence of abortion (Chap. 118). Some patients with liver disease, hepatomas, AIDS, and lymphoproliferative disorders develop an acquired form of dysfibrinogenemia.

FACTOR XIII DEFICIENCY AND DEFECTIVE FIBRIN CROSS-LINKING   Factor XIII is a transglutaminase that stabilizes fibrin clots by forming ε-amino–γ-glutamyl cross-links between ad-

jacent α and γ chains of fibrin. Factor XIII deficiency is an extremely rare inherited syndrome. Patients usually bleed in the neonatal period from their umbilical stump or circumcision. In addition to hemorrhage, these patients may have poor wound healing, a high incidence of infertility among males and abortion among affected females, and a high incidence of intracerebral hemorrhage. These observations suggest that the enzyme may be important in other physiologic and pathologic processes beyond hemostasis, including placental implantation, spermatogenesis, and wound healing. Several drugs, including isoniazid, may bind to cross-linking sites on fibrinogen and mimic factor XIII deficiency by blocking enzyme activity. Normal hemostasis requires only 1% of normal enzyme activity, which can be achieved with a single infusion of fresh-frozen plasma or a purified factor XIII–rich product derived from human placenta called Fibrogammin. Factor XIII has a 14-day half-life.

VITAMIN K DEFICIENCY   Vitamin K is a fat-soluble vitamin that plays a critical role in hemostasis. Dietary vitamin K is absorbed in the small intestine and stored in the liver. The vitamin is also synthesized by endogenous bacterial flora in the small intestine and colon; however, the quantity of endogenous vitamin K absorbed from the large intestine is debated. Following absorption and transport, vitamin K is converted to an active epoxide in liver microsomes and serves as a cofactor in the enzymatic carboxylation of glutamic acid residues on prothrombin complex proteins (Fig. 117-1).

The three major causes of vitamin K deficiency are inadequate dietary intake, intestinal malabsorption, and loss of storage sites due to hepatocellular disease. Neonatal vitamin K deficiency, which causes hemorrhagic disease of the newborn, has disappeared from western countries with the routine administration of vitamin K to all newborn infants. Although a 30-day supply of vitamin K is stored in the normal liver, acutely ill patients can become deficient within 7 to 10 days. Acute vitamin K deficiency is particularly common in patients recovering from biliary tract surgery who have no dietary intake of vitamin K, have T-tube drainage of bile, and are on broad-spectrum antibiotics. Vitamin K deficiency is also seen in chronic liver disease, particularly primary biliary cirrhosis, and in some malabsorption states (Chaps. 286 and 298). The cephalosporins inhibit the reduction and recycling of vitamin K, much like coumarin.

With vitamin K deficiency, plasma levels of all the prothrombin complex proteins (factors II, VII, IX, X; proteins C and S) decrease. Factor VII and protein C, which have the shortest half-lives, decrease first. Because of the rapid fall in factor VII, patients with mild vitamin K deficiency may have a prolonged PT and a normal PTT. Later, as the levels of the other factors fall, the PTT will also become prolonged. Parenteral administration of 10 mg vitamin K rapidly restores vitamin K levels in the liver and permits normal production of prothrombin complex proteins within 8 to 10 h. Severe hemorrhage can be treated with fresh-frozen plasma, which immediately corrects the hemostatic

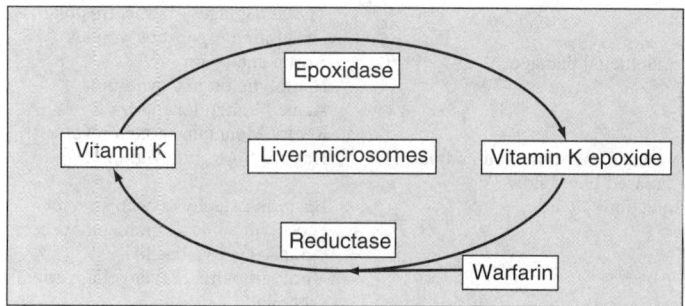

FIGURE 117-1   The mechanism of action of vitamin K, a cofactor in the formation of di-γ-carboxyglutamic acid residues on coagulation proteins, is depicted. Vitamin K is converted to an epoxide in liver microsomes. The epoxide is the active form and is reduced back to vitamin K by a liver membrane reductase. Warfarin blocks the action of the reductase and competitively inhibits the effects of vitamin K.

defect. If the cause of vitamin K deficiency cannot be eliminated, patients may need monthly injections. Purified prothrombin complex concentrates should be avoided because they contain trace quantities of activated forms of the prothrombin complex proteins and can cause thrombosis in patients with liver disease. They also carry an increased risk of hepatitis.

DISSEMINATED INTRAVASCULAR COAGULATION

DIC can be either an explosive and life-threatening bleeding disorder or a relatively mild or subclinical disorder. Although a long list of diseases can be complicated by DIC, it is most frequently associated with obstetric catastrophes, metastatic malignancy, massive trauma, and bacterial sepsis (Table 117-1). In each case, a tentative triggering mechanism has been identified. For example, tumors and traumatized or necrotic tissue release tissue factor into the circulation, while endotoxin from gram-negative bacteria activates several steps in the coagulation cascade. In addition to a direct effect on the activation of Hageman factor (factor XII), endotoxin induces the expression of tissue factor on the surface of monocytes and endothelial cells. These activated cell surfaces then accelerate coagulation reactions. These potent thrombogenic stimuli cause the deposition of small thrombi and emboli throughout the microvasculature. This early thrombotic phase of DIC is then followed by a phase of procoagulant consumption and secondary fibrinolysis. Continued fibrin formation and fibrinolysis lead to hemorrhage from the coagulation factor and platelet depletion and the antihemostatic effects of fibrin degradation products (Fig. 117-2).

The clinical presentation varies with the stage and severity of the syndrome. Most patients have extensive skin and mucous membrane bleeding and hemorrhage from surgical incisions or venipuncture or catheter sites. Less often, patients present with peripheral acrocyanosis, thrombosis, and pregangrenous changes in digits, genitalia, and nose—areas where blood flow is markedly reduced by vasospasm or microthrombi. Some patients, particularly those with chronic DIC secondary to malignancy, have laboratory abnormalities without any evidence of thrombosis or hemorrhage.

The laboratory manifestations include thrombocytopenia and the

FIGURE 117-2 The pathophysiology of disseminated intravascular coagulation (DIC). Shown are the interactions between coagulation and fibrinolytic pathways that result in bleeding in patients with DIC.

presence of schistocytes or fragmented red blood cells that arise from cell trapping and damage within fibrin thrombi; prolonged PT and PTT and thrombin time and a reduced fibrinogen level from depletion of coagulation proteins; and elevated fibrin degradation products (FDP) from intense secondary fibrinolysis. The D dimer immunoassay, which specifically measures cross-linked fibrin derivatives, is a more specific FDP assay. The abnormality in DIC that predicts bleeding is the plasma fibrinogen level; low fibrinogen levels are associated with more bleeding.

TREATMENT   DIC, although sometimes indolent, can cause life-threatening hemorrhage and may require emergency treatment. This should include (1) an attempt to correct any reversible cause of DIC; (2) measures to control the major symptom, either bleeding or thrombosis; and (3) a prophylactic regimen to prevent recurrence in cases of chronic DIC. Treatment will vary with the clinical presentation. In patients with an obstetric complication such as abruptio placentae or acute bacterial sepsis, the underlying disorder is easy to correct, and prompt delivery of the fetus and placenta or treatment with appropriate antibiotics will reverse the DIC syndrome. In patients with metastatic tumor causing DIC, control of the primary disease may not be possible, and long-term prophylaxis may be necessary.

Patients with bleeding as a major symptom should receive fresh-frozen plasma to replace depleted clotting factors and platelet concentrates to correct thrombocytopenia. Those with acrocyanosis and incipient gangrene or other thrombotic problems need immediate anticoagulation with intravenous heparin. The use of heparin in the treatment of bleeding is still controversial. Although it is a logical way to reduce thrombin generation and prevent further consumption of clotting proteins, it should be reserved for patients with thrombosis or who continue to bleed despite vigorous treatment with plasma and platelets.

Patients who initially have mild DIC and may not be symptomatic may begin to bleed following surgery or chemotherapy. For example, mild DIC, without clinical bleeding, has been documented during saline- or prostaglandin-induced midtrimester abortions. Prophylactic treatment of patients with heparin may prevent progression of a mild DIC syndrome and has been used in the treatment of patients with acute promyelocytic leukemia and in some patients with a retained dead fetus who require surgical extraction. However, most patients with low-grade DIC can be managed with plasma and platelet replacement and do not require heparin. Chronic DIC does not respond to oral warfarin anticoagulants, but it can be controlled with long-term heparin infusion. Occasional patients with indolent tumors and severe DIC have been maintained on heparin administered by intermittent subcutaneous injection or continuous infusion with portable pumps.

Despite our detailed understanding of the pathophysiology of DIC and a vigorous approach to therapy, treatment does not change the natural history of the underlying disorder. Therapy will only stabilize the patient, prevent exsanguination or massive thrombosis, and permit institution of definitive therapy.

Table 117-1   Etiologic Factors and Disorders Causing Disseminated Intravascular Coagulation

Liberation of tissue factors	Obstetric syndromes—abruptio placentae, amniotic fluid embolism, retained dead fetus, second trimester abortion
	Hemolysis
	Neoplasms, particularly mucinous adenocarcinomas, acute promyelocytic leukemia
	Intravascular hemolysis
	Fat embolism
	Tissue damage—burns, frostbite, head injury, gunshot wounds
Endothelial damage	Aortic aneurysm
	Hemolytic uremic syndrome
	Acute glomerulonephritis
	Rocky Mountain spotted fever
Vascular malformation and decreased blood flow	Kasabach-Merritt syndrome
Infections	Bacterial: staphylococci, streptococci, pneumococci, meningococci, gram-negative bacilli
	Viral: arboviruses, varicella, variola, rubella
	Parasitic: malaria, kala-azar
	Rickettsial: Rocky Mountain spotted fever
	Mycotic: acute histoplasmosis

SOURCE: Modified from RI Handin, RD Rosenberg, in *Hematology*, 4th ed, WS Beck (ed), Cambridge, MA, MIT Press, 1985.

COAGULATION DISORDERS IN LIVER DISEASE

Liver dysfunction is frequently accompanied by a hemostatic defect. The major causes of hemorrhage in patients with liver disease are shown in Table 117-2. Bleeding is usually due to an anatomic lesion that is exacerbated by a hemostatic defect. Most patients bleed from complications of portal hypertension, esophageal varices, or gastritis and peptic ulcer disease. Portal hypertension also causes splenomegaly, with splenic sequestration of platelets and thrombocytopenia, which contributes to the hemostatic defect (Chap. 298).

Patients with hepatocellular liver disease cannot store vitamin K optimally and may have some degree of vitamin K deficiency. Cholestasis, a frequent feature of liver disease, impairs vitamin K absorption and further decreases liver vitamin K stores. Abnormalities in the γ-carboxylation of prothrombin complex proteins independent of vitamin K and the production of abnormal proteins have also been described. Patients may also have decreased production of other coagulation proteins, including fibrinogen and factor V. The liver also produces inhibitors of coagulation such as antithrombin III and proteins C and S and is the clearance site for activated coagulation factors and fibrinolytic enzymes. Thus patients with liver disease are also "hypercoagulable" and predisposed to developing DIC or systemic fibrinolysis. Coagulation defects in advanced liver failure are often difficult to distinguish from those of DIC.

Each patient with hemorrhage and liver disease should have a PT, PTT, platelet count, and fibrinogen determination, although it is not always possible to determine the major hemostatic abnormality from a single set of laboratory values. It is helpful to have previous laboratory data available for patients with chronic liver disease who develop an acute complication. The degree of prolongation of the PT predicts the risk of bleeding. Most patients present with moderate prolongation of the PT and PTT, mild thrombocytopenia, and a normal fibrinogen level. However, they may also present with a more complex defect combining defective synthesis, abnormal clearance, and active consumption of coagulation proteins. Since vitamin K deficiency is so common, a single parenteral dose of vitamin K is given after initial laboratory studies have been obtained, even though this may only partially correct the laboratory abnormalities. The presence of severe thrombocytopenia or a low fibrinogen level suggests the additional complication of DIC and may require further studies and therapy.

The safest replacement therapy for a patient with liver disease is fresh-frozen plasma, since it supplies all known coagulation factors. However, even this form of therapy has drawbacks, since large quantities of plasma may precipitate hepatic encephalopathy and cause fluid and sodium overload. Prothrombin complex concentrates should be avoided because they replace only the vitamin K–dependent factors, may be contaminated with hepatitis and AIDS virus, and contain trace quantities of activated coagulation proteins. Similarly, fibrinogen concentrates (or cryoprecipitate), rich in factor VIII and fibrinogen, should not be used without additional fresh-frozen plasma. Anticoagulation with heparin has been advocated to control DIC, but this is particularly hazardous and not recommended in cirrhosis because heparin is metabolized erratically and may lead to severe bleeding.

FIBRINOLYTIC DEFECTS Bleeding can also occur from defects in the fibrinolytic system. Patients with α_2 plasmin inhibitor deficiency or plasminogen activator inhibitor (PAI) 1 have rapid fibrinolysis following fibrin deposition after trauma or surgery and may experience recurrent hemorrhage. Similarly, patients with cirrhosis have an impaired clearance of tissue plasminogen activator (tPA) and systemic fibrinolysis that may contribute to their hemorrhagic defect. Rarely, patients with tumors such as metastatic prostatic cancer may develop diffuse bleeding from primary fibrinolysis rather than DIC. Clues to the diagnosis include a disproportionately low fibrinogen level with a relatively normal PT and PTT and the presence of a normal or nearly normal platelet count. With rare exceptions, patients with primary fibrinolysis should have an elevated titer of FDP but a normal D dimer level. However, it is sometimes difficult or impossible to differentiate primary fibrinolysis from the secondary fibrinolysis accompanying DIC. Patients with clearly established primary fibrinolysis should not receive heparin; they require plasma therapy and, occasionally, fibrinolytic inhibitors such as EACA. However, EACA should not be given to patients suspected of having DIC unless they are also receiving heparin, since EACA can cause massive, often fatal, thrombosis in a patient with DIC.

CIRCULATING ANTICOAGULANTS Circulating anticoagulants, or inhibitors, are usually IgG antibodies that interfere with coagulation reactions. Specific inhibitors inactivate individual coagulation proteins and may cause severe hemorrhage. They arise in 15 to 20% of patients with factor VIII or factor IX deficiency who have received plasma infusions. *Specific* inhibitors also occur in previously normal individuals. Although the most common target protein is factor VIII, inhibitors with specificity for each of the coagulation proteins occur. In addition to hemophiliacs, anti-factor VIII antibodies are seen in postpartum females, in patients on various drugs, as part of the spectrum of autoantibodies in systemic lupus erythematosus (SLE) patients, and in normal elderly individuals. Circulating anticoagulants also occur in patients with AIDS.

Nonspecific (lupus-like) inhibitors prolong coagulation tests by binding to phospholipids. They are assayed by their anticoagulant effect [lupus anticoagulant (LA) activity] or their ability to bind to the complex phospholipid cardiolipin [anticardiolipin antibody (ACLA) activity]. While most often encountered in patients with SLE, these nonspecific inhibitors may develop in patients with many other disorders and also in otherwise normal individuals.

The critical laboratory feature that identifies the presence of either type of inhibitor is the failure of normal plasma to correct a prolonged PT, PTT, or both. Plasma from patients with a specific inhibitor will progressively inactivate a coagulation protein and thus prolong whichever of these screening tests requires the participation of that clotting factor. This effect persists after dilution. Nonspecific inhibitors immediately prolong the PT and PTT and, at low dilution, block multiple coagulation reactions. However, these effects can be overcome by altering the quantity or type of phospholipid or by diluting the plasma.

Hemorrhage in patients with specific inhibitors may require treatment with massive plasma or concentrate infusion, the use of activated prothrombin complex concentrates to bypass the antibodies against factors VIII or IX, and plasmapheresis or exchange transfusion to lower antibody titer. Chronic immunosuppressive regimens have been particularly useful in otherwise normal individuals with an acquired factor VIII antibody. Many patients lose their antibody and recover within 6 to 12 months, although the acute mortality rate from uncontrollable bleeding may approach 10%.

Patients with LA activity have normal hemostasis and will not bleed unless they have concomitant thrombocytopenia or prothrombin

Table 117-2 Causes of Bleeding in Liver Disease

Anatomic Factors
  Portal hypertension
    Varices
    Splenomegaly and secondary thrombocytopenia
  Peptic ulceration
  Gastritis
Hepatic Function Abnormalities
  Decreased synthesis of procoagulant proteins: fibrinogen, prothrombin, factors V, VII, IX, X, XI
  Decreased synthesis of coagulation inhibitors: protein C, protein S, antithrombin III
  Impaired absorption and metabolism of vitamin K
  Failure to clear activated coagulation proteins leading to:
    Disseminated intravascular coagulation
    Systemic fibrinolysis
Complications of Therapy
  Dilution of platelets and coagulation proteins from massive transfusions
  Infusion of activated coagulation proteins in prothrombin complex concentrates
  Bleeding from heparin; thrombosis from ε-aminocaproic acid (EACA)

deficiency. Both thrombocytopenia and hypoprothrombinemia are secondary to autoantibodies that bind either to platelets or the prothrombin molecule. While these antibodies have no effect on function, they accelerate clearance of the coated platelets or the antibody-prothrombin complexes.

The presence of LA activity may predispose patients to venous and arterial thromboembolism and may cause midtrimester abortions. However, the risk of thrombosis is difficult to estimate and the appropriate therapy for individual patients difficult to choose. Tests for either LA or ACLA activity are not well standardized, and results vary among and within patients. The best predictor is a consistent prolongation of more than one coagulation test coupled with a high titer of ACLA activity. Second, the risk of thrombosis is increased in patients who have SLE compared with those with idiopathic LA or ACLA activity. Prophylactic therapy is not clearly beneficial, and treatments aimed at reducing the titer of antibody are not superior to conventional antithrombotic therapy.

Therapy should be individualized. Patients with SLE and either LA or ACLA activity who have had a thrombotic episode are at high risk for a recurrence and should receive long-term anticoagulant therapy. Women who have had more than one midtrimester abortion, especially those with SLE, should have a trial of anticoagulant therapy. Patients with a single thrombotic episode (stroke or pulmonary embolus) and no other risk factor except LA or ACLA activity should be treated. No consensus has been reached about treatment after an initial minor event [deep venous thrombosis (DVT)]. Asymptomatic patients with only laboratory abnormalities should not be treated. Glucocorticoids should be administered only in conjunction with antithrombotic agents and are not of proven efficacy.

INHERITED PRETHROMBOTIC DISORDERS Coagulation is carefully regulated by a series of inhibitors that limit thrombin generation and fibrin formation and by the fibrinolytic system, which effectively removes fibrin thrombi (Figs. 62-5 and 62-6). Inherited defects in the natural coagulation inhibitors (i.e., antithrombin, proteins C and S), abnormalities in the fibrinolytic system, and certain dysfibrinogenemias predispose patients to thrombosis (Table 62-5). A single point mutation in the factor V gene (factor V Leiden), which converts arginine 506 to glutamine and makes the molecule resistant to degradation by activated protein C, may account for 25% of inherited prethrombotic states. Antithrombin, protein C, and protein S defects are all autosomal dominant traits, so heterozygous individuals, who have a 50% reduction in protein concentration or a mixture of mutant and normal molecules, will have an increased risk of thrombosis. The patients have similar clinical presentations with a strong family history of thrombosis, episodes of recurrent venous thromboembolism, and symptoms by their early twenties. Any patient with this distinctive history should be tested for specific abnormalities.

ANTITHROMBIN DEFICIENCY Antithrombin complexes with activated coagulation proteins and blocks their biologic activity (Fig. 62-5). The rate of this reaction is enhanced by heparin-like molecules within the vessel wall or on endothelial cells. Plasma antithrombin III content is 5 to 15 mg/L (50 to 150%), with values only slightly below normal increasing the risk of thrombosis. For optimal screening, the antithrombin III concentration is measured by immunoassay and the plasma antithrombin and heparin cofactor activity assessed with functional assays. The most common defect (1 in 2000 indidivuals) is mild (heterozygous) antithrombin deficiency. Dysfunctional antithrombin molecules with mutations affecting either the serine protease or heparin-binding site or activation of inhibitor by heparin have also been described.

Patients with antithrombin deficiency who develop acute thrombosis or embolism can be treated with intravenous heparin, since there is usually sufficient normal antithrombin to act as a heparin cofactor. Following their first episode of thromboembolism, patients should be placed on oral anticoagulants for life to prevent recurrent thrombosis. Family studies should be conducted when an antithrombin-deficient

individual is discovered, since up to half the members of a kindred may be affected. Asymptomatic individuals with antithrombin deficiency should receive prophylactic anticoagulation with heparin or plasma infusions to raise their antithrombin level before medical or surgical procedures that may increase their risk of thrombosis. Chronic oral anticoagulation is not recommended until individuals at risk have a thrombotic episode.

DEFICIENCIES OF PROTEINS C AND S Protein C is a vitamin K–dependent hepatic protein that binds to the endothelial cell surface protein thrombomodulin and is converted to an active protease by thrombin (Fig. 62-5). Activated protein C, in conjunction with protein S, proteolyzes factors Va and VIIIa, which shuts off fibrin formation. Activated protein C may also stimulate fibrinolysis and accelerate clot lysis. Deficiencies of proteins C and S are usually autosomal dominant disorders, and deficiencies in the two proteins cause an identical syndrome of recurrent venous thrombosis and pulmonary embolism. Dysfunctional molecules have also been identified in some patients with thrombosis. Rare patients with homozygous protein C deficiency have fulminant neonatal intravascular coagulation and require prompt diagnosis and treatment.

The correlation between protein C and S levels and the risk of thrombosis is not as precise as for antithrombin III deficiency. In fact, some asymptomatic individuals with protein C "deficiency" have been discovered. In some well-studied protein C–deficient kindreds, asymptomatic individuals may have protein C levels as low as or lower than relatives with recurrent thrombosis. It is possible that an undiscovered cofactor is present in symptomatic patients. Finally, since a fraction of the available protein S is bound to C4b-binding protein and is unavailable for coagulation reactions, both free and total protein S levels or C4b-binding protein levels should be assessed for maximum accuracy.

Heterozygous patients with protein C or S deficiencies who develop acute thrombosis should be heparinized and then placed on oral anticoagulants. There are, however, two potential problems with the use of coumarin anticoagulants in these patients. First, these vitamin K antagonists (Fig. 117-1; Fig. 62-5), which lower the level of the procoagulant factors II, VII, IX, and X, may also reduce the concentration of proteins C and S sufficiently to nullify the desired antithrombotic effect. In addition, patients who are protein C–deficient may develop coumarin-induced skin necrosis; this defect may predispose patients to a rare but serious complication. Patients with homozygous protein C deficiency require periodic plasma infusions rather than oral anticoagulants to prevent recurrent intravascular coagulation and thrombosis.

RESISTANCE TO ACTIVATED PROTEIN C AND THE FACTOR V LEIDEN MUTATION Some patients with familial or recurrent venous thromboembolism were found not to prolong their PTT when activated protein C was added to their plasma. These patients were found to have an identical mutation in which arginine 506 in factor V is converted to glutamine. This amino acid substitution abolishes a protein C cleavage site in factor V and thus prolongs the thrombogenic effect of factor V activation. About 3% of the population worldwide is heterozygous for this mutation. The mutation is absent in certain populations, e.g., Asians, African Americans, and Native Americans. It may account for 25% of patients with recurrent deep venous thrombosis or pulmonary embolism.

Heterozygosity at this allele increases an individual's lifetime risk of venous thromboembolism sevenfold. The risk rises steadily with age. A homozygote has a twentyfold increased risk of thrombosis. Heterozygosity coupled with ingestion of oral contraceptives or pregnancy increases the risk at least fifteenfold. Coinheritance of factor V Leiden and another low-penetrance defect such as protein C or S deficiency is also additive. Many previous studies of risk factors predisposing patients to venous thromboembolism are being reevaluated to take into account this common mutation.

PROTHROMBIN GENE MUTATION A specific point mutation in the prothrombin gene [conversion of G to A at position 20210 (G20210A)] also predisposes to venous thrombosis and embolism.

This mutation is in the 3'-untranslated region of the gene and results in a 30% increase in plasma prothrombin levels, either through more efficient translation or greater stability of the message. Heterozygotes account for ~18% of cases with family histories of venous thrombosis and 6% of patients with first episodes of DVT.

The inheritance of multiple mutations increases the risk of thrombosis. The relationship between known mutations and the type of thrombosis is shown in Table 117-3. The fraction of patients with DVT with known mutations is shown in Table 117-4.

TREATMENT Patients who develop venous thromboembolism without a clear predisposing factor, have a strong family history, present under the age 30, or have more than one episode should have assays for antithrombin III, proteins C and S, and factor V Leiden. Patients who present with DVT or pulmonary embolism during pregnancy or while using oral contraceptives have a 30% chance of having factor V Leiden.

Treatment recommendations for patients with the inherited prethrombotic disorders are still evolving. All patients should receive standard initial therapy with heparin, either conventional or low dose (Chap. 118), followed by 3 months of oral warfarin. This regimen should allow for maximal healing and reendothelialization of the thrombosed vessels and minimize recurrence in the damaged vascular beds. It is not clear which patients should go on to receive long-term (perhaps lifelong) anticoagulation, a judgment that depends on assessing the risk/benefit ratio.

Patients with antithrombin III deficiency who become symptomatic have a high likelihood of recurrent events and should be placed on lifelong anticoagulation. Patients with protein C or S deficiency or heterozygous factor V Leiden and prothrombin G20210A patients have a lower likelihood of recurrent disease. Long-term anticoagulation should be reserved until their second or subsequent episode of thromboembolism. Homozygous factor V Leiden patients should be placed on long-term anticoagulation after their initial episode, and all patients should receive replacement therapy or receive heparin prophylaxis during surgery or after trauma; women with these defects should avoid the use of oral contraceptives. The asymptomatic relatives of patients shown to have these disorders should be screened to determine if they have inherited the defective gene. If so, they should receive appropriate prophylaxis but not start anticoagulation until they are symptomatic. In the absence of a congenital defect predisposing a patient to thrombosis, recurring or migratory thrombophlebitis may indicate an underlying malignancy.

DYSFIBRINOGENEMIAS AND FIBRINOLYTIC DEFECTS Recurrent venous thrombosis and embolism may be due to familial defects in fibrinogen or plasminogen or decreased synthesis or release of tPA. While most dysfibrinogenemias cause bleeding, several variants have excessively rapid release of fibrinopeptides and recurrent thromboembolism. Patients with this disorder and those with an abnormal plasminogen that resists activation by streptokinase and urokinase have been treated successfully with heparin and oral anticoagulants. Defects in tPA content or release have not been completely characterized. One group of patients with recurrent venous thrombosis and embolism failed to increase venous blood fibrinolytic activity

Table 117-3 Relationship Between Coagulation Defect and Site of Thrombosis

Abnormality	Arterial	Venous
Factor V Leiden R506 Q	−	+
Prothrombin G20210A	−	+
Antithrombin III	−	+
Protein C	−	+
Protein S	−	+
Homocysteinemia	+	+
Antiphospholipid antibody[a]	+	+

[a] Anticardiolipin antibody—lupus anticoagulant.

Table 117-4 Prevalence of Coagulation Defects in Patients with Venous Thrombosis

Defect	Prevalence, %
Factor V Leiden (Arg506Gln) R506 Q	12–40
Hyperhomocysteinemia	10–20
Prothrombin G20210A	6–18
Deficiencies of antithrombin III, proteins C and S	5–15
Antiphospholipid antibody syndrome	10–20

when challenged with local ischemia or physical exercise. The other group had impaired fibrinolytic activity in extracts prepared from biopsied veins. Young patients with acute myocardial infarction may have impaired fibrinolysis due to increased plasma levels of PAI, a serine protease inhibitor that binds to tPA and is derived from endothelial cells.

Many common illnesses are associated with an increased risk of thrombosis (Table 62-5). These patients are said to have a "hypercoagulable" or "prethrombotic" state. This increased risk is seen in patients with chronic congestive heart failure and metastatic cancer and in patients undergoing major surgery. The generation of tissue factor activity in damaged or ischemic tissue or metastatic tumor, coupled with venous stasis and endothelial injury, induces the formation of venous and, more rarely, arterial thrombi. Several hematologic disorders, paroxysmal nocturnal hemoglobinuria, essential thrombocythemia, and polycythemia vera predispose patients to venous and arterial thrombosis through diverse mechanisms related to increased blood viscosity and abnormal blood cells. Diseases that affect the endothelial cell, such as Behçet's syndrome, Kawasaki's disease, and homocystinuria, or the administration of drugs such as the oral contraceptives, which lower antithrombin III levels, or L-asparaginase, which inhibits production of multiple coagulation factors, may also predispose patients to thrombosis. Infusion of granulocyte-macrophage colony stimulating factor (GM-CSF) has been associated with thrombosis. Tamoxifen, an estrogen receptor antagonist, can cause venous thrombosis. The mechanism is unclear.

Plasma homocysteine levels influence the risk of both venous and arterial thromboembolism. Individuals with the congenital homocystinuria syndrome have, in addition to their Marfanoid habitus, an increased incidence of strokes and coronary artery disease. These patients have well-recognized enzyme defects (Chap. 352), excrete homocysteine in their urine, and have very high plasma levels of the amino acid. Some patients with early-onset cerebral vascular events have mild homocystinuria that can be brought out by a methionine loading test. Epidemiologic studies show a relationship between homocysteine levels that are nearer to the normal range and coronary artery disease. Although this correlation is not yet definitive, the relationship remains intriguing and of potential clinical relevance. Vitamin B_{12} deficiency occurs in about 30% of people over age 70, produces elevated homocysteine levels, and may be a reversible cause of thrombotic disease.

BIBLIOGRAPHY

ANTONARAKIS SE: Molecular genetics of factor VIII gene and haemophilia A. Haemophilia 4:1, 1998

FEINSTEIN DI: Lupus anticoagulant, anticardiolipin antibodies, fetal loss and systemic lupus erythematosus. Blood 80:859, 1992

GREAVES M: Antiphospholipid antibodies and thrombosis. Lancet 353:1348, 1999

KAY MA, HIGH K: Gene therapy for the hemophilias. Proc Natl Acad Sci USA 96:10379, 1999

LEE C: Recombinant clotting factors in the treatment of hemophilia. Thromb Haemost 82: 516, 1999

LEVI M, TEN CATE H: Current concepts: Disseminated intravascular coagulation. N Engl J Med 341:586, 1999

MANUCC PM, TUDDENHAM EG: The hemophilias: Progress and problems. Semin Hematol 36:104, 1999

118   *Robert I. Handin*

ANTICOAGULANT, FIBRINOLYTIC, AND ANTIPLATELET THERAPY

ANTICOAGULANT AND FIBRINOLYTIC THERAPY

Anticoagulation with heparin, followed by treatment with oral vitamin K antagonists, is the standard treatment for acute venous thrombosis and pulmonary embolism. In addition, chronic oral anticoagulation is used to prevent cerebral arterial embolism from cardiac sources such as ventricular mural thrombi or atrial thrombi or from an atherosclerotic, partially stenosed carotid or vertebral artery. Anticoagulants are also used, less successfully, to treat peripheral or mesenteric arterial thrombosis. These agents retard fibrin deposition on established thrombi and prevent the formation of new thrombi. The induction of a fibrinolytic state by the infusion of plasminogen activators such as recombinant tissue plasminogen activator (rtPA), streptokinase (SK), or urokinase (UK) has become an accepted mode of therapy for some thromboembolic disorders. Fibrinolytic therapy has been proposed for patients with massive pulmonary embolism and systemic hypotension and to restore the patency of acutely occluded peripheral and coronary arteries. Prompt fibrinolytic therapy can reduce both myocardial damage and mortality following acute coronary occlusion (Chap. 243), though mechanical interventions such as angioplasty and stent placement are also effective ways to restore vessel patency. Fibrinolytic therapy may also be effective in acute thrombotic strokes and in venoocclusive disease of the liver.

ACUTE ANTICOAGULATION WITH HEPARIN   Heparin is a naturally occurring mucopolysaccharide polymer with tetrasaccharide sequences that bind to and activate antithrombin III. It can dramatically reduce thrombin generation and fibrin formation in patients with acute venous and arterial thrombosis or embolism (Table 118-1). Heparin is administered to patients with acute thrombosis or embolism by giving an initial loading dose of 5000 to 10,000 units followed by a continuous intravenous infusion at a rate sufficient to keep the activated partial thromboplastin time (APTT) at 1.5 to 2 times the patient's preheparin APTT. This requires infusion of 800 to 1000 U.S.P. units per hour and is continued while patients are begun on oral anticoagulants and achieve appropriate prolongation of the prothrombin time. The usual duration of combined heparin-warfarin therapy is 5 to 7 days. Heparin is then discontinued, and the patient is maintained on warfarin. Alternatives to a continuous infusion include the administration of 5000 U.S.P. units of heparin four times a day either subcutaneously or intravenously. Unfractionated conventional heparin preparations are heterogeneous, with only 20% of the product biologically active. In addition, active heparin fractions may vary considerably in molecular weight. Biologically active, low-molecular-weight heparin (LMWH) preparations, while more expensive than unfractionated heparin, have several advantages: (1) they can be administered subcutaneously once or twice daily, (2) their pharmacokinetics are so predictable that APTT monitoring is not necessary, and (3) they are less immunogenic and less likely to cause thrombocytopenia. Many patients with deep venous thrombosis, a frequent cause for hospitalization, can be given LMWH as outpatients. Given their other advantages and equivalent efficacy, LMWH preparations have largely replaced unfractionated heparin (Table 118-1).

Patients with recurrent thromboembolism refractory to oral anticoagulants, pregnant women with thromboembolism, and patients with chronic disseminated intravascular coagulation (DIC) may be treated with daily injections of LMWH preparations such as enoxaparin or dalteparin. These agents are also effective in prevention of venous thrombosis in high-risk surgical and medical patients, including those with congestive heart failure, myocardial infarction, or cardiomyopathy.

The major complication of unfractionated heparin therapy is bleeding—especially from surgical sites and into the retroperitoneum. Aspirin or aspirin-containing drugs impair platelet function. Thus, intramuscular injections in patients on both heparin and an antiplatelet drug may cause significant bleeding. Heparin's anticoagulant effect can be rapidly reversed by the administration of protamine sulfate. However, this is usually not necessary, since reduction or omission of a heparin dose usually improves hemostasis and stops bleeding. Thrombocytopenia occurs in ~10% of recipients and is usually mild, with the platelet count falling to 50,000 to 100,000/μL. Thrombocytopenia is more common in patients receiving heparin derived from beef lung as opposed to porcine intestinal mucosa. LMWH is less likely to cause either thrombocytopenia or bleeding. However, antibodies arising from exposure to unfractionated heparin often cross-react with LMWH. Thus, LMWH cannot usually be used to treat patients with established thrombocytopenia.

Heparin-induced thrombocytopenia (HIT) results from generation of an autoantibody to a complex of unfractionated heparin with the anti-heparin protein platelet factor 4 (PF-4). Heparin-PF-4-antibody complexes can bind to the platelet Fc receptor and cause platelet activation, agglutination, and arterial thrombosis. Recognition of the rare complication of thrombocytopenia and paradoxical thrombosis is critical, since discontinuing heparin can promptly reverse the syndrome and may be lifesaving. Heparin administration for >5 months also carries a risk of osteoporosis, perhaps through its activation of osteoclasts. LMWH causes less osteoporosis on chronic administration.

Table 118-1   Anticoagulant Therapy with Low-Molecular-Weight and Unfractionated Heparin

Clinical Indication	Heparin Dose and Schedule	Target PTT[a]	LMWH Dose and Schedule[b]
Venous thrombosis pulmonary embolism			
Treatment	5000 U IV bolus; 1000–1500 U/h	2–2.5	100 U/kg SC bid
Prophylaxis	5000 U SC q8–12h	<1.5	100 U/kg SC bid
Acute myocardial infarction			
With thrombolytic therapy	5000 U IV bolus; 1000 U/h	1.5–2.5	100 U/kg SC bid
With mural thrombus	8000 U SC q8h + warfarin	1.5–2.0	100 U /kg SC bid
Unstable angina	5000 U IV bolus; 1000 U/h	1.5–2.5	100 U/kg SC bid
Prophylaxis			
General surgery	5000 U SC bid	<1.5	100 U/kg SC before and bid
Orthopedic surgery	10000 U SC bid	1.5	100 U/kg SC before and bid
Medical patients with CHF, MI	10000 U SC bid	1.5	100 U/kg SC bid

[a] Times normal control; assumes PTT has been standardized to heparin levels so that 1.5–2.5× normal equals 0.2–0.4 U/mL; if PTT is normal (27–35 S), start with 5000 U bolus 1300 U/h infusion monitoring PTT; if PTT at recheck is <50 S, rebolus with 5000 U and increase infusion by 100 U/h; if PTT at recheck is 50–60 s, increase infusion rate by 100 U/h; if PTT at recheck is 60–85 s, no change; if PTT at recheck is 85–100 s, decrease infusion rate 100 U/h; if PTT at recheck is 100–120 s, stop infusion for 30 min and decrease rate 100 U/h at restart; if PTT at recheck is >120 s, stop infusion for 60 min and decrease rate 200 U/h at restart.

[b] LMWH does not affect PTT and PTT is not used to adjust dosage.

NOTE: PTT, partial thromboplastin time; LMWH, low-molecular-weight heparin; CHF, congestive heart failure; MI, myocardial infarction.

The coumarin anticoagulants, which include warfarin and dicumarol (dicoumarol), prevent the reduction of vitamin K epoxides in liver microsomes and induce a state of vitamin K deficiency (see Fig. 117-1). They slow thrombin generation and clot formation by impairing the biologic activity of the prothrombin complex proteins and are used to prevent the recurrence of venous thrombosis and pulmonary embolism. Although regimens employing loading doses of drug have been advocated, the simplest way to induce anticoagulation is to administer a single dose of a coumarin compound and monitor the prothrombin time (PT) until the desired prolongation is achieved. For example, treatment can be initiated with 5 mg/d of warfarin or equivalent, with the goal of prolonging the PT to 1.5 to 2 times the control value. Although the PT may reach this value after a few days of therapy, effective anticoagulation, with stable reduction of all the prothrombin complex proteins, requires at least 1 week of warfarin administration. Most patients require a daily maintenance dose of 2.5 to 7.5 mg of warfarin to remain anticoagulated.

Because commercial thromboplastins have different potencies, the PT can vary widely. In an effort to standardize oral anticoagulation, the International Normalized Ratio (INR) method has been adopted by most hospital laboratories and clinicians. In this reporting method, the ratio of the patient's PT is compared to the mean PT for a group of normal individuals. The ratio is adjusted for the sensitivity of the laboratory's thromboplastin determined by the International Sensitivity Index (ISI). Thus, $INR = (PT_{patient}/PT_{normal})^{ISI}$. Use of the INR permits physicians to obtain the appropriate level of anticoagulation independent of laboratory reagents and to follow published recommendations for intensity of anticoagulation. The intensity of anticoagulation may be varied somewhat depending on the clinical indication (Table 118-2). Patients with chronic indwelling venous catheters have been maintained on 1 mg/d of warfarin to prevent clot formation at the catheter tip; such a dose has no effect on the PT.

Although warfarin anticoagulants reduce the recurrence of deep venous thrombosis and pulmonary or cerebral embolism, they may also cause bleeding. Any patient who takes oral anticoagulants requires frequent monitoring of the PT. Despite the most careful management, fluctuations in PT can occur. Various drugs that alter liver microsomal metabolism of coumarins or compete for albumin-binding sites can increase or decrease the potency of these drugs (Table 118-3).

The risk of bleeding increases and, up to a point, the risk of recurrent thrombosis declines with the duration of anticoagulation. Patients with a single uncomplicated thromboembolic event achieve maximal benefit after 3 to 6 months of anticoagulation. About 10% of patients on an oral anticoagulant for 1 year have a bleeding complication requiring medical supervision, and 0.5 to 1% have a fatal hemorrhage. The anticoagulant effects of coumarins can be reversed by infusion of fresh-frozen plasma or by the administration of vitamin K. Fresh-frozen plasma works immediately, but the effects last only a few hours. Vitamin K takes 8 to 12 h to become effective; after vitamin K administration, vitamin K antagonists are more difficult to use for reinduction of anticoagulation. In many cases, reduction or omission of several doses of warfarin improves hemostasis and stops hemorrhage.

Table 118-2 INR Target Ranges for Oral Anticoagulation

Condition	INR	Duration
Venous thrombosis		
Treatment	2–3	3–6 months
Prevention	1.5–1.5	Chronic
Atrial fibrillation	1.5–2	Chronic
Myocardial infarction	2–3	2–3 months
Lupus-like anticoagulants	3–4	Chronic
Mechanical heart valves		
Tissue valves	2–2.5	Chronic
Mechanical valves	3–4	Chronic
Cardiomyopathy	2–3	Chronic

NOTE: INR, International Normalized Ratio.

Table 118-3 Effect of Drugs and Metabolic Changes on Oral Anticoagulant Potency

I. Factors leading to enhanced potency and increased prothrombin time
  A. Reduced coumarin clearance
    1. Disulfiram
    2. Metronidazole
    3. Trimethoprim-sulfamethoxazole
  B. Reduced albumin binding
    Phenylbutazone
  C. Additive hemostatic effect of certain drugs or disorders
    1. Aspirin
    2. Heparin
    3. Liver disease
    4. Thrombocytopenia
    5. Vitamin K deficiency
  D. Increased turnover of vitamin K
    1. Clofibrate
    2. Hypermetabolism (e.g., hyperthyroidism)
II. Factors leading to diminished potency and decreased prothrombin time
  A. Accelerated coumarin clearance—induction of hepatic metabolizing enzymes
    1. Barbiturates
    2. Rifampin
  B. Reduced absorption
    Cholestyramine
  C. Impaired metabolism
    Genetic coumarin resistance

Despite the risk of bleeding, some patients may require lifelong anticoagulation.

Hemorrhagic skin necrosis is a rare complication. Some patients with this complication are deficient in protein C, an anticoagulant protein whose activity is reduced by vitamin K antagonists. Patients suspected of protein C deficiency should only begin oral anticoagulant therapy when combined with heparin or plasma infusions to restore protein C levels to normal. Patients with an inherited coumarin resistance may require extremely high doses to get an anticoagulant effect. Psychologically disturbed patients may surreptitiously ingest coumarin and present with unexplained bleeding and a prolonged PT. Plasma coumarin levels can be measured to confirm such ingestion.

FIBRINOLYTIC THERAPY Fibrinolysis, an important part of the normal hemostatic process, is initiated by the release of either tissue plasminogen activator (tPA) or pro-urokinase (proUK) from endothelial cells. These agents preferentially activate plasminogen adsorbed onto fibrin clots, a mechanism that localizes the lytic process to sites that contain fibrin thrombi. Although fibrinolysis begins immediately after vascular injury, clot lysis and vessel recanalization may not be complete for 7 to 10 days. The fibrinolytic pathway is important in normal hemostasis; defects can predispose patients to either hemorrhage or recurrent thrombosis (Chap. 117). Activators of the fibrinolytic system are frequently used to accelerate clot lysis in patients with thromboembolism (Fig. 118-1; Table 118-4).

The pharmacologic agents being used to accelerate clot lysis are either derived from natural products or are chemically modified derivatives. They differ with respect to fibrin specificity and some types of complications (Table 118-4). For example, many individuals have antistreptococcal antibodies that react with SK and reduce its potency and cause febrile reactions. All fibrinolytic agents cause hemorrhage. In addition to tPA and proUK, several other agents are relatively "fibrin-specific" and preferentially activate plasminogen in the presence of fibrin. Although this makes it theoretically possible to achieve selective clot lysis, in practice the efficacy and toxicity of the "specific" and "nonspecific" fibrinolytic agents are similar. However, equivalent doses of rtPA cost 10 times more than SK.

Some systemic fibrinolysis always occurs after the infusion of clinically effective doses of fibrin-specific agents. Fibrinogen level falls ~25% after infusion of lytic doses of rtPA. In addition, both the fibrin-specific and -nonspecific agents can cause hemorrhage as they cannot

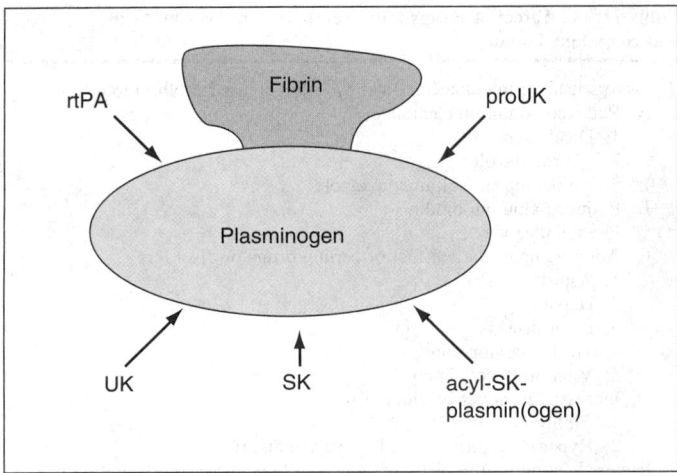

FIGURE 118-1 The mechanism of action of various plasminogen activators used for thrombolytic therapy. Recombinant tissue plasminogen activator (rtPA) and pro-urokinase (proUK) preferentially activate plasminogen bound to fibrin and are called "fibrin-specific" activators. Urokinase (UK), streptokinase (SK), and acylated streptokinase-plasminogen conjugates activate both free and fibrin-bound plasminogen.

differentiate between vital hemostatic plugs and pathologic thrombi. To minimize the risk of bleeding, systemic lytic therapy is not recommended for patients with recent surgery or a history of neurologic lesions, gastrointestinal bleeding, or hypertension.

The current indications for fibrinolytic therapy are listed in Table 118-5. Fibrinolytic therapy is currently recommended for patients with massive pulmonary embolism that is complicated by hypotension, hypoxemia, and right heart strain. It is also used for selected patients with peripheral arterial embolism or occlusion and for patients with extensive iliofemoral thrombophlebitis. While lytic therapy may hasten the resolution of venous thrombi, the long-term benefit still remains unproven, and no firm evidence proves that lytic therapy reduces postphlebitic complications. In contrast, fibrinolytic therapy may be of distinct benefit in patients with axillary vein thrombosis, a condition that does not usually respond to conventional anticoagulation. Fibrinolytic agents are also used to restore the patency of occluded venous catheters and dialysis shunts. For this indication the agents are instilled locally. The extensive literature on the use of fibrinolytic agents to treat patients with coronary artery disease and myocardial infarction is reviewed in Chap. 243. When given within a few hours of infarction, fibrinolytic therapy reduces mortality and myocardial damage.

Although the doses and mode of administration may differ slightly, the general principles and complications are the same for all the fibrinolytic agents. SK and UK are the oldest and most extensively studied

Table 118-5 Possible Indications for Fibrinolytic Therapy

Acute coronary occlusion
Acute peripheral arterial occlusion
Massive pulmonary embolism with severe hypoxemia and hypotension
Axillary vein thrombosis
Massive iliofemoral vein thrombosis—efficacy as yet unproven
Occluded arterial or venous cannulae—low dose, direct infusion into cannula
Venoocclusive disease of the liver

fibrinolytic agents. SK is a bacterial enzyme, and UK is a product of renal tubular epithelial cells. SK is an indirect plasminogen activator that interacts with circulating plasminogen to form an equimolar complex with proteolytic activity. The SK-plasminogen complex then activates additional plasminogen molecules that initiate fibrinolysis. In contrast, UK has intrinsic proteolytic activity and can activate plasminogen directly.

In the case of SK, a loading dose of 250,000 units is usually given irrespective of body weight. Since patients may have antistreptococcal antibodies, the loading dose may need to be repeated. In addition, patients may develop acute allergic symptoms including urticaria and, occasionally, serum sickness reactions. With UK, a loading dose of 4400 units per kilogram body weight is administered over 10 to 30 min. Both regimens induce an intense lytic state as evidenced by a drop in fibrinogen, prolongation of the thrombin time, and a prolongation of the euglobulin lysis time—an in vitro measure of fibrinolytic activity. After the initial loading dose, 100,000 units of SK or 4400 units of UK per kilogram body weight are administered hourly for 24 to 72 h. At the desired time, the lytic state is reversed by discontinuing UK or SK and by administering heparin for 7 to 10 days. Heparin can be started at the same time as the fibrinolytic agent. Fibrinolytic therapy should be initiated as soon as possible after the onset of thrombosis or embolism.

Fibrin-specific agents such as rtPA or proUK are also administered intravenously. Systemic infusion of 100 mg rtPA over 6 h restores coronary artery patency in ~75% of patients. Patients are then maintained on heparin for several days. ProUK given in a similar manner has almost identical effects, but large clinical trials suggest that rtPA is superior to other fibrinolytic agents in maintaining patency of acutely occluded coronary arteries.

ANTIPLATELET DRUG THERAPY

Antiplatelet drugs play a critical role in the management of patients with arterial vascular disease and thromboembolism. Aspirin is the most widely studied of these drugs because of its unique pharmacology. A single dose of aspirin irreversibly acetylates and inactivates the enzyme cyclooxygenase and thereby inhibits platelet production of thromboxane A_2. Although aspirin may also inactivate cyclooxygenase in other tissues, including endothelial cells, such cells recover rapidly by synthesizing new enzyme. Platelets, which are anucleate, cannot synthesize new enzyme and remain inactive for the rest of their life span. As little as one 160-mg tablet of aspirin daily or a 325-mg tablet every other day inhibits platelet thromboxane production and aggregation.

Patients with coronary artery disease who have unstable angina are at high risk for myocardial infarction (Chap. 243). The prompt administration of aspirin dramatically reduces progression to myocardial infarction in this group, although aspirin has no effect on the frequency, intensity, or duration of chronic angina. Aspirin also reduces the incidence of second infarction by 25% when administered to patients who have had a myocardial infarct.

Table 118-4 Fibrinolytic Activators

Product	Source	Molecular Weight	Fibrin-Specific	Complications
Recombinant tissue plasminogen activator (rtPA)	Recombinant	70,000	+	Bleeding
Pro-urokinase (proUK)	Melanoma cell cultures	55,000	+	Bleeding
Urokinase (UK)	Renal tubular cell cultures	33,000	−	Bleeding
Streptokinase (SK)	β-Hemolytic streptococci	47,000	−	Immune reactions—hypotension, fever Bleeding
Acyl-SK-plasmin(ogen)	Chemical synthesis	139,000	+/−	Immune reactions—hypotension, fever Bleeding

Daily aspirin therapy also reduces the incidence of first infarcts. The combination of aspirin and dipyridamole, when begun before surgery, may also increase the patency of coronary bypass grafts; the same combination reduces the incidence of cerebral emboli in patients on warfarin who have prosthetic intracardiac valves. Although dipyridamole has been a popular antithrombotic agent, it has little efficacy when given alone. Aspirin may be the active agent in the combination aspirin-dipyridamole trials.

Aspirin also reduces the frequency of transient ischemic attacks in patients with occlusive cerebrovascular disease. It has largely supplanted anticoagulation with the coumarin compounds in patients with transient ischemia. Aspirin also reduces the incidence of a second stroke by 25% when administered to men following a first stroke. Aspirin is also effective in maintaining the patency of arteriovenous cannulas inserted into patients with renal failure who require hemodialysis. Aspirin plus dipyridamole may also slow the progression of some forms of glomerulonephritis, although these drugs are not widely used in the treatment of renal disease. Aspirin is not effective in maintaining the patency of vessels following percutaneous angioplasty or stent placement.

Although aspirin is clearly the most efficacious antiplatelet agent in clinical use today, a large number of new drugs are being tested that may supplement aspirin therapy. Ticlopidine, a potent inhibitor of platelet function, is effective as an alternative to aspirin in patients with cerebrovascular disease and is superior to aspirin or warfarin in maintaining coronary stent patency. Ticlopidine is more expensive than aspirin and causes some serious side effects, including neutropenia and occasional rare episodes of thrombotic thrombocytopenic purpura (TTP). A related drug, clopidogrel (Plavix), has been proposed as a substitute, but rare cases of TTP have also been noted with its use.

Monoclonal antibodies and both recombinant and chemically synthesized peptides that block either platelet adhesion or aggregation are being tested in clinical trials. A monoclonal antibody Fab fragment that blocks fibrinogen binding to platelet GpIIb/IIIa, thus inhibiting platelet aggregation (abciximab, RheoPro), is used in patients with coronary artery disease who undergo angioplasty. RheoPro is also being evaluated in other settings, e.g., as an adjunct to fibrinolytic therapy in patients with an acute myocardial infarction. A cyclic peptide based on the consensus fibronectin adhesion sequence RGD (arginine, glycine, aspartic acid) called eptifibatide (Integrilin) is as effective as RheoPro for maintaining patency after angioplasty and stent placement as is a small molecule inhibitor (Aggrestat). Orally active GpIIb/IIIa inhibitors have not been proven safe or effective.

The uses of antithrombotic therapy are evolving rapidly. However, aspirin is the current mainstay for chronic therapy and should be used (325 qd or qod) indefinitely in any patient who has had a coronary or cerebral thrombosis. It will reduce ischemic events by 25% or more. Patients undergoing angioplasty or stent placement should receive RheoPro/Integrilin or Aggrestat acutely, followed by 3 weeks of ticlopidine or clopidogrel.

BIBLIOGRAPHY

ANANTHASUBRAMANIAM K et al: Heparin-induced thrombocytopenia and thrombosis. Prog Cardiovasc Dis 42:247, 2000

AWTRY EH, LOSCALZO J: Aspirin. Circulation 101:1206, 2000

BHATT DL, TOPOL EJ: Antiplatelet and anticoagulant therapy in the secondary prevention of ischemic heart disease. Med Clin North Am 84:163, 2000

TCHENG JE: Clinical challenges of platelet glycoprotein IIb/IIIa receptor inhibitor therapy: Bleeding, reversal, thrombocytopenia, and retreatment. Am Heart J 139:538, 2000

NOBEL PRIZE IN PHYSIOLOGY OR MEDICINE, 1930

Karl Landsteiner was born in Vienna, Austria, on June 14, 1868, the only child of Leopold and Fanny Landsteiner. He was only 6 years old when his father died. After *Gymnasium* (German high school), he entered the University of Vienna Medical School at age 17. On graduation from medical school in 1891, he decided on a career in laboratory research rather than the practice of medicine. Landsteiner undertook research with Emil Fischer (a Nobel laureate in 1902) at the University of Würzburg. In 1899 at the age of 31, while working as an assistant in Anton Weichselbaum's laboratory in the Department of Pathology at the University of Vienna, he discovered the blood groups A, B, and O using agglutination techniques. The fourth group, AB, was added a year later by Landsteiner. The original publication of the identification of groups was only three pages, and Landsteiner was the sole author. In the next 8 years little attention was paid to this highly significant discovery. However, in 1910 it was demonstrated that these blood groups were transmitted by Gregor Mendel's laws of inheritance—A, B, and AB were autosomal dominant, and O was recessive. Until Landsteiner's discovery, blood transfusions had been abandoned because of serious complications. Subsequently, blood typing allowed the use of blood transfusions to save millions of lives.

With the devastation of Vienna during World War I, Landsteiner was forced to move to a small hospital in Leiden, Holland, where he worked as a pathologist until he was invited to become a member of the Rockefeller Institute in New York in 1922. In 1930 Landsteiner received the Nobel Prize, some 30 years after his discovery of blood groups. His family only learned that Landsteiner (a modest man) had received the Nobel Prize when a friend arrived at his home to congratulate him. In 1940 at the age of 72, Landsteiner and his co-workers made another important discovery—a new factor in the blood named the rhesus (Rh) factor. This discovery explained the deaths of newborn babies from erythroblastosis fetalis when there was incompatibility between an Rh-negative mother and an Rh-positive baby. This discovery also allowed incompatibilities in blood transfusion due to Rh factor incompatibility to be avoided. At the age of 75 Landsteiner had a fatal heart attack while at his laboratory workbench, with a pipette in his hand, at the Rockefeller Institute. It was written, "Landsteiner belonged to those scholars for whom the aim of science is first of all the honour of the human spirit."

REFERENCES

1. Magill FN (ed): *Nobel Prize Winners: Physiology or Medicine*, vol 1, Pasadena, Salem Press, 1993
2. Schrier RW: *A Salute to Nobel Laureates in Physiology and Medicine*, Proceedings of the Association of American Physicians 108(1): Jan 1996
3. Sourkes TL: *Nobel Prize Winners in Medicine and Physiology 1910–1965*. London, Abelard-Schuman, 1967

Robert W. Schrier, MD

NOBEL PRIZE IN PHYSIOLOGY OR MEDICINE, 1962

Francis Harry Compton Crick was born in Northampton, England, on June 8, 1916. He had his early education in Northampton and then received his B.Sc. degree in physics from University College London. The German bombing in World War II destroyed the physics laboratory at UCL, forcing Crick to abandon his Ph.D. research. Instead, he became a research scientist for the British Admiralty, studying magnetic and acoustic mines. In 1949 Crick decided to change his interests to biology and entered a doctorate program at the Medical Research Council's Cavendish Laboratory at Cambridge. He worked with Nobel Laureates Laurence Bragg and Max Perutz, using x-ray diffraction studies of biological molecules, particularly proteins. At Cambridge he met 23-year-old James D. Watson and began a scientific collaboration that would change the world of science.

James Dewey Watson was born in Chicago, Illinois, on April 6, 1928. He was a brilliant student and received a scholarship to enter the University of Chicago at the age of 15. He received his B.S. degree there in zoology in 1947 and then entered Indiana University to obtain a Ph.D. degree in the same field, writing his thesis on bacteriophage proliferation and the effects of x-rays on the process, under the supervision of Nobel Laureates Salvador Edward Luria and Hermann Joseph Muller. After receiving his Ph.D. he moved to Copenhagen, Denmark, to study phage infection of bacteria. At a meeting in Italy, he met Maurice Wilkins, who presented a paper on x-ray diffraction through crystalline DNA, which indicated that DNA might be helical in nature. This work enhanced Watson's interest in DNA, and he decided in 1952 to move to the Cavendish Laboratory in Cambridge where he met Francis Crick, who was also interested in the structure of DNA. At that time DNA was felt to be the genetic material of heredity; thus an understanding of its structure could lead to the genetic code whereby proteins, cells, and organisms are created.

The challenge of understanding the structure of DNA excited Crick and Watson more than their primary work at the Cavendish—the study of the hemoglobin structure and the genetics of viruses, respectively. With their knowledge of the chemistry of nucleotides and the x-ray diffraction results from Rosalind Franklin and Maurice Wilkins, in 1951 Crick and Watson initially proposed a single structure chain helical model of DNA. Franklin, however, found this proposal incompatible with her x-ray diffraction studies. After this failure, Crick and Watson were ordered by their supervisors at the Cavendish to return to their primary tasks; they assumed that Watson and Crick could not compete with the senior and established Wilkins-Franklin group at King's College in London. Even Wilkins told them: "DNA, you know, is Midas' gold. Everyone who touches it goes mad."

A great coincidence then occurred. Although Linus Pauling, who had described the helix in protein structure, was not allowed to travel outside the United States because of his antinuclear views, his son, Peter Pauling, was working at the Cavendish at the same time as Watson and Crick. Peter Pauling shared with Crick and Watson a paper that had been submitted to the *Proceedings of the National Academy of Science*, purporting to have described the structure of DNA as a triple helix. Crick and Watson immediately recognized the flaws in this proposal and thus were allowed to return to their real passion, the study of the structure of DNA. On this second attempt, however, they were equipped with more knowledge about the molecule. They had seen Franklin's excellent DNA diffraction photographs that suggested that there were two helically arranged polynucleotide chains. Moreover, Erwin Chargaff had shown that in various species, including humans, the amount of thymine equalled the amount of adenine and the amount of guanine equalled the amount of cytosine. Crick and Watson then began to build a cardboard and metal model of DNA. Their structure this time consisted of two polynucleotide chains running in opposite directions in a double helical shape like a right-handed spiral staircase.

This time, the Crick and Watson double-helix structure of DNA was supported by the x-ray diffraction results of Rosalind Franklin. Thus, Crick and Watson quickly published three brief papers in the spring of 1953 that drastically changed genetic research.

Maurice Hugh Frederick Wilkins was born on December 15, 1916, in Pongaroa, New Zealand, to Edgar Henry and Eveline Constance Jane Wilkins, both of Dublin, Ireland. Edgar Wilkins was a school physician who had been interested in research but had little time to pursue it because of his practice. Maurice was sent to England at an early age to pursue his education, first at King Edward's School in Birmingham, and at St. John's College at the University of Cambridge for his B.A. He earned his Ph.D. from Birmingham University with a thesis on the luminescence of solids and the electron trap theory of phosphorescence. During World War II he joined the Manhattan Project team in Berkeley, California, where he was involved in the mass spectrography studies of the separation of uranium isotopes. After the war and the devastating explosion of atomic bombs at Hiroshima and Nagasaki, Wilkins decided to apply his knowledge of physics to biological systems to try to obtain a better understanding of heredity and disease.

Wilkins became quite interested in the structure of DNA. He found that the DNA fibers in gel were particularly amenable to analysis by x-ray diffraction techniques. The results of crystallography studies suggested that the DNA structure was helical in nature. The width of the helix suggested that it was composed of two strands, that is, a double helix. He and Rosalind Franklin shared this information with Crick and Watson, who ultimately published the double-helix structure of DNA. In 1962 Wilkins shared the Nobel Prize in Physiology or Medicine with Crick and Watson. His only disappointment was that Franklin could not share in this deserved honor because in 1957 she had died of cancer at the young age of 37.

The discovery of the structure of DNA has been compared to finding the Rosetta Stone or to splitting the atom, or to the greatest step in understanding genetics since Gregor Mendel illustrated the fundamentals of inheritance in the middle of the nineteenth century.

REFERENCES

1. Aaseng N: *The Disease Fighters*. Minneapolis, Lerner Publications, 1987
2. Magill FN (ed): *Nobel Prize Winners: Physiology and Medicine*, vol 2. Pasadena, Salem Press, 1993
3. Schrier RW: *A Salute to Nobel Laureates in Physiology and Medicine*, Proceedings of the Association of American Physicians 108(1): Jan 1996
4. Sourkes TL: *Nobel Prize Winners in Medicine and Physiology 1901–1965*. London, Abelard-Schuman, 1967
5. Watson JD: *The Double Helix*. New York, Penguin Books, 1968

Robert W. Schrier, MD

Section 1
BASIC CONSIDERATIONS IN INFECTIOUS DISEASES

119

Lawrence C. Madoff, Dennis L. Kasper

INTRODUCTION TO INFECTIOUS DISEASES: HOST–PARASITE INTERACTIONS

Despite decades of dramatic progress in their treatment and prevention, infectious diseases remain a major cause of death and debility and are responsible for worsening the living conditions of many millions of people around the world. Infections frequently challenge the physician's diagnostic skill and must be considered in the differential diagnoses of syndromes affecting every organ system.

CHANGING EPIDEMIOLOGY OF INFECTIOUS DISEASES With the advent of antimicrobial agents, some medical leaders believed that infectious diseases would soon be eliminated and become of historic interest only. Indeed, the hundreds of chemotherapeutic agents developed since World War II, most of which are potent and safe, include drugs effective not only against bacteria but also against viruses, fungi, and parasites. Nevertheless, we now realize that as we developed antimicrobial agents, microbes developed the ability to elude our best weapons and to counterattack with new survival strategies. Antibiotic resistance occurs at an alarming rate among all classes of mammalian pathogens. Pneumococci resistant to penicillin and enterococci resistant to vancomycin have become commonplace. Even *Staphylococcus aureus* with reduced susceptibility to vancomycin has appeared. Such pathogens present real clinical problems in managing infections that were easily treatable just a few years ago. Diseases once thought to have been nearly eradicated from the developed world—tuberculosis, cholera, and rheumatic fever, for example—have rebounded with renewed ferocity. Newly discovered and emerging infectious agents appear to have been brought into contact with humans by changes in the environment and by movements of human and animal populations. An example of the propensity for pathogens to escape from their usual niche is the alarming 1999 outbreak in New York of encephalitis due to a flavivirus similar or identical to West Nile virus, which had never previously been isolated in the Americas.

Many infectious agents have been discovered only in recent decades. Ebola virus, hantavirus, the agent of human granulocytotropic ehrlichiosis, and retroviruses such as HIV humble us despite our deepening understanding of pathogenesis at the most basic molecular level. Even in developed countries, infectious diseases have made a resurgence. Between 1980 and 1996, mortality from infectious diseases in the United States increased by 64% to levels not seen since the 1940s.

The role of infectious agents in the etiology of diseases once believed to be noninfectious is being increasingly recognized. For example, it is now widely accepted that *Helicobacter pylori* is the causative agent of peptic ulcer disease and perhaps of gastric malignancy. Human papillomavirus is likely to be the most important cause of invasive cervical cancer. A new human herpesvirus (HHV-8) is believed to be the cause of most cases of Kaposi's sarcoma. Epstein-Barr virus is a cause of certain lymphomas and may play a role in the genesis of Hodgkin's disease. The possibility certainly exists that other diseases of unknown cause, such as rheumatoid arthritis, sarcoidosis,

or inflammatory bowel disease, have infectious etiologies. There is even evidence that atherosclerosis may have an infectious component.

Medical advances over infectious diseases have been hindered by changes in the patient population. Immunocompromised hosts now constitute a significant proportion of the seriously infected population. Physicians immunosuppress their patients to prevent the rejection of transplants and to treat neoplastic and inflammatory diseases. Some infections, most notably that caused by HIV, immunocompromise the host in and of themselves. Lesser degrees of immunosuppression are associated with other infections, such as influenza and syphilis. Infectious agents that coexist peacefully with immunocompetent hosts wreak havoc in those who lack a complete immune system. AIDS has brought to prominence once-obscure organisms such as *Pneumocystis carinii*, *Cryptosporidium parvum*, and *Mycobacterium avium*.

BIOTERRORISM In recent years, the efforts of some governments and terrorist organizations to use biological weaponry have refocused public concern on the topic. To date, there is little evidence that biological weapons have ever been effectively used; indeed, their ease of use may be overstated. However, the ability of infectious agents to inflict widespread illness and thus to cause societal disruption and panic, together with the relatively low cost of these agents, has led to their being called a "poor man's nuclear arsenal."

Several pathogens have been considered likely candidates for biological warfare. *Bacillus anthracis*, which causes the zoonosis anthrax, is widely viewed as the leading contender. The hardy spores of the bacillus can be distributed by bombardment or other dispersal mechanisms. Inhalation of this pathogen results in severe pneumonia with a mortality rate of 95% in untreated persons. A World Health Organization report estimated that 50 kg of *B. anthracis* released upwind of a city with a population of 500,000 would result in up to 95,000 fatalities, with an additional 125,000 persons incapacitated. Moreover, the attack might go undetected until large numbers of seriously ill individuals presented with overt disease. In 1979, an accidental release from a military microbiology facility near Sverdlovsk in the former Soviet Union caused at least 66 deaths from inhalational anthrax along a 4-km-wide path downwind of the facility. The vast scope of the Soviet Union's biological warfare program, employing 60,000 people at its height, has only recently come to light. This endeavor is thought to be echoed by efforts in many other countries in the world today. In response to the perceived threat of anthrax as a biological weapon, the U.S. military recently decided to vaccinate more than 2 million of its members against this infection.

Smallpox, an ancient scourge caused by variola virus, has also been considered as a bioweapon owing to its contagiousness and high mortality rate and to the declining population of immunized persons. Indeed, one of the earliest accounts of biological warfare involved the distribution of smallpox-infected blankets to Native American tribes by British troops. Debate continues about whether to eradicate the two known existing stocks of the virus in U.S. and Russian government laboratories. Many investigators believe that additional undocumented stockpiles of the virus exist around the world.

Other infectious organisms that combine the virulence and stability necessary for biological weapons include *Yersinia pestis*, the agent of plague, and *Francisella tularensis*, the agent of tularemia. Viral hemorrhagic fever agents such as the Ebola and Marburg viruses as well as toxins such as that from *Clostridium botulinum* have also been considered as biological weapons. While some of the diseases caused by these agents can be effectively treated or prevented if sufficient resources exist to do so, it may also be possible for an aggressor to render organisms resistant to antibiotics or even to vaccines through genetic manipulation or other means.

HOST FACTORS IN INFECTION For any infectious process to occur, the parasite and the host must first encounter each other. Factors such as geography, environment, and behavior thus influence the likelihood of infection. Though the initial encounter between a susceptible host and a virulent organism frequently results in disease, some organisms can be harbored in the host for years before disease becomes clinically evident. For a complete view, individual patients must be considered in the context of the population to which they belong. Infectious diseases do not often occur in isolation; rather, they spread through a group exposed from a point source (e.g., a contaminated water supply) or from individual to individual (e.g., via respiratory droplets). Thus, the clinician must be alert to infections prevalent in the community as a whole. A detailed history, including information on travel, behavioral factors, exposures to animals or potentially contaminated environments, and living and occupational conditions, must be elicited. For example, the likelihood of infection by *Plasmodium falciparum* can be significantly affected by altitude, climate, terrain, season, and even time of day. Antibiotic-resistant strains are localized to specific geographic regions, and a seemingly minor alteration in a travel itinerary can dramatically influence the likelihood of acquiring chloroquine-resistant malaria. If such important details in the history are overlooked, inappropriate treatment may result in the death of the patient. Likewise, the chance of acquiring a sexually transmitted disease can be greatly affected by a relatively minor variation in sexual practices, such as the method used for birth control. Knowledge of the relationship between specific risk factors and disease allows the physician to influence a patient's health even before the development of infection by modification of these risk factors and—when a vaccine is available—by immunization.

Many specific host factors influence the likelihood of acquiring an infectious disease. Age, immunization history, prior illnesses, level of nutrition, pregnancy, coexisting illness, and perhaps emotional state all have some impact on the risk of infection after exposure to a potential pathogen. The importance of individual host defense mechanisms, either specific or nonspecific, becomes apparent in their absence, and our understanding of these immune mechanisms is enhanced by studies of clinical syndromes developing in immunodeficient patients (Table 119-1). For example, the frequent occurrence of meningococcal disease in people with deficiencies in specific complement proteins of the "membrane attack complex" underscores the importance of an intact complement system in the prevention of meningococcal infection.

Medical care itself increases the patient's risk of acquiring an infection in several ways: (1) through contact with pathogens during hospitalization, (2) through breaching of the skin (with intravenous devices or surgical incisions) or mucosal surfaces (with endotracheal tubes or bladder catheters), (3) through introduction of foreign bodies, (4) through alteration of the natural flora with antibiotics, and (5) through treatment with immunosuppressive drugs.

THE IMMUNE RESPONSE Infection involves complicated interactions of parasite and host and inevitably affects both. In most cases, a pathogenic process consisting of several steps is required for the development of infections. Since the competent host has a complex series of barricades in place to prevent infection, the successful parasite must utilize specific strategies at each of these steps. The specific strategies used by bacteria, viruses, and parasites (Chaps. 120 and 180) have some remarkable conceptual similarities, but the strategic details are unique not only for each class of organism but also for individual species within a class.

Once in the bloodstream or a normally sterile body site, the microorganism faces the host's tightly integrated cellular and humoral immune systems. Cellular immunity (Chap. 305), comprising T lym-

phocytes, macrophages, and natural killer cells, primarily recognizes and combats pathogens that proliferate intracellularly. Cellular immune mechanisms are important in immunity to all classes of infectious agents, including most viruses and many bacteria (e.g., *Mycoplasma*, *Chlamydia*, *Listeria*, *Salmonella*, and *Mycobacterium*), parasites (e.g., *Trypanosoma*, *Toxoplasma*, and *Leishmania*), and fungi (e.g., *Histoplasma*, *Cryptococcus*, and *Coccidioides*). Usually, T lymphocytes are activated by macrophages and B lymphocytes, which present foreign antigens along with the host's own major histocompatibility complex antigen. Activated T cells may then act in several ways to fight infection. Cytotoxic T cells may directly attack and lyse host cells that express foreign antigens. Helper T cells stimulate the proliferation of B cells and the production of immunoglobulins. B cells and T cells communicate with each other via a variety of signals, and often more than one signal is employed simultaneously. For example, costimulation through the CD40-CD40 ligand increases B cell responses, and costimulation via the B7-CD28 axis is required for activation of the CD4+ helper T cell. T cells elaborate cytokines (e.g., interferon), which directly inhibit the growth of pathogens or stimulate killing by host macrophages and cytotoxic cells. Cytokines also augment the host's immunity by stimulating the inflammatory response (fever, the production of acute-phase serum components, and the proliferation of leukocytes). Cytokine stimulation does not always result in a favorable response in the host; septic shock (Chap. 124) and toxic shock syndrome (Chaps. 139 and 140) are among the conditions that are mediated by these inflammatory substances.

The reticuloendothelial system comprises monocyte-derived phagocytic cells that are located in the liver (Kupffer cells), lung (alveolar macrophages), spleen, kidney (mesangial cells), brain (microglia), and lymph nodes and that clear circulating microorganisms. Although these tissue macrophages and polymorphonuclear leukocytes (PMNs) are capable of killing microorganisms without help, they function much more efficiently when pathogens are first *opsonized* (Greek, "to prepare for eating") by components of the complement system such as C3b and/or by antibodies.

Extracellular pathogens, including most encapsulated bacteria, are attacked by the humoral immune system, which includes antibodies, the complement cascade, and phagocytic cells. Antibodies are complex glycoproteins (also called immunoglobulins) that are produced by mature B lymphocytes, circulate in body fluids, and are secreted on mucosal surfaces. Antibodies specifically recognize and bind to foreign antigens. One of the most impressive features of the immune system is the ability to generate an incredible diversity of antibodies capable of recognizing virtually every foreign antigen yet not reacting with self. In addition to being exquisitely specific for antigens, antibodies come in different structural and functional classes: IgG predominates in the circulation and persists for many years after exposure; IgM is the earliest specific antibody to appear in response to infection; secretory IgA is important in immunity at mucosal surfaces, while monomeric IgA appears in the serum; and IgE is important in allergic and parasitic diseases. Antibodies may directly impede the function of an invading organism, neutralize secreted toxins and enzymes, or facilitate the removal of the antigen (invading organism) by phagocytic cells. Immunoglobulins participate in cell-mediated immunity by promoting the antibody-dependent cellular cytotoxicity functions of certain T lymphocytes. Antibodies also promote the deposition of complement components on the surface of the invader.

The complement system (Chap. 305) consists of a group of serum proteins functioning as a cooperative, self-regulating cascade of enzymes that adhere to—and in some cases disrupt—the surface of invading organisms. Some of these surface-adherent proteins (e.g., C3b) can then act as opsonins for destruction of microbes by phagocytes. The later, "terminal" components (C7, C8, and C9) can directly kill some bacterial invaders (notably, many of the neisseriae) by forming a "membrane attack complex" and disrupting the integrity of the bacterial membrane, thus causing bacteriolysis. Other complement components, such as C5a, act as chemoattractants for PMNs. Complement activation and deposition occur by either or both of two pathways: the

Table 119-1 Infections Associated with Selected Defects in Immunity

Host Defect	Disease or Therapy Associated with Defect	Common Etiologic Agent of Infection
NONSPECIFIC IMMUNITY		
Impaired cough	Rib fracture, neuromuscular dysfunction	Bacteria causing pneumonia, aerobic and anaerobic oral flora
Loss of gastric acidity	Achlorhydria, histamine blockade	*Salmonella* spp., enteric pathogens
Loss of cutaneous integrity	Penetrating trauma, athlete's foot	*Staphylococcus* spp., *Streptococcus* spp.
	Burn	*Pseudomonas aeruginosa*
	Intravenous catheter	*Staphylococcus* spp., *Streptococcus* spp., gram-negative rods, coagulase-negative staphylococci
Implantable device	Heart valve	*Streptococcus* spp., coagulase-negative staphylococci, *Staphylococcus aureus*
	Artificial joint	*Staphylococcus* spp., *Streptococcus* spp., gram-negative rods
Loss of normal bacterial flora	Antibiotic use	*Clostridium difficile, Candida* spp.
Impaired clearance		
Poor drainage	Urinary tract infection	*Escherichia coli*
Abnormal secretions	Cystic fibrosis	Chronic pulmonary infection with *P. aeruginosa*
INFLAMMATORY RESPONSE		
Neutropenia	Hematologic malignancy, cytotoxic chemotherapy, aplastic anemia, HIV infection	Gram-negative enteric bacilli, *Pseudomonas* spp., *Staphylococcus* spp., *Candida* spp.
Chemotaxis	Chédiak-Higashi syndrome, Job's syndrome, protein-calorie malnutrition	*S. aureus, Streptococcus pyogenes, Haemophilus influenzae,* gram-negative bacilli
	Leukocyte adhesion defects 1 and 2	Bacteria causing skin and systemic infections, gingivitis
Phagocytosis (cellular)	Systemic lupus erythematosus, chronic myelogenous leukemia, megaloblastic anemia	*Streptococcus pneumoniae, H. influenzae*
Splenectomy	—	*H. influenzae, S. pneumoniae,* other streptococci, *Capnocytophaga* spp., *Babesia microti, Salmonella* spp.
Microbicidal defect	Chronic granulomatous disease	Catalase-positive bacteria and fungi: staphylococci, *E. coli, Klebsiella* spp., *P. aeruginosa, Aspergillus* spp., *Nocardia* spp.
	Chédiak-Higashi syndrome	*S. aureus, S. pyogenes*
	Interferon γ receptor defect, interleukin 12 deficiency, interleukin 12 receptor defect	*Mycobacterium* spp., *Salmonella* spp.
COMPLEMENT SYSTEM		
C3	Congenital liver disease, systemic lupus erythematosus, nephrotic syndrome	*S. aureus, S. pneumoniae, Pseudomonas* spp., *Proteus* spp.
C5	Congenital	*Neisseria* spp., gram-negative rods
C6, C7, C8	Congenital, systemic lupus erythematosus	*Neisseria meningitidis, N. gonorrhoeae*
Alternative pathway	Sickle cell disease	*S. pneumoniae, Salmonella* spp.
IMMUNE RESPONSE		
T lymphocyte deficiency/dysfunction	Thymic aplasia, thymic hypoplasia, Hodgkin's disease, sarcoidosis, lepromatous leprosy	*Listeria monocytogenes, Mycobacterium* spp., *Candida* spp., *Aspergillus* spp., *Cryptococcus neoformans,* herpes simplex virus, varicella-zoster virus
	AIDS	*Pneumocystis carinii,* cytomegalovirus, herpes simplex virus, *Mycobacterium avium-intracellulare, C. neoformans, Candida* spp.
	Mucocutaneous candidiasis	*Candida* spp.
	Purine nucleoside phosphorylase deficiency	Fungi, viruses
B cell deficiency/dysfunction	Bruton's X-linked agammaglobulinemia	*S. pneumoniae,* other streptococci
	Agammaglobulinemia, chronic lymphocytic leukemia, multiple myeloma, dysglobulinemia	*H. influenzae, N. meningitidis, S. aureus, Klebsiella pneumoniae, E. coli, Giardia lamblia, P. carinii,* enteroviruses
	Selective IgM deficiency	*S. pneumoniae, H. influenzae, E. coli*
	Selective IgA deficiency	*G. lamblia,* hepatitis virus, *S. pneumoniae, H. influenzae*
Mixed T and B cell deficiency/dysfunction	Common variable hypogammaglobulinemia	*P. carinii,* cytomegalovirus, *S. pneumoniae, H. influenzae,* various other bacteria
	Ataxia-telangiectasia	*S. pneumoniae, H. influenzae, S. aureus,* rubella virus, *G. lamblia*
	Severe combined immunodeficiency	*S. aureus, S. pneumoniae, H. influenzae, Candida albicans, P. carinii,* varicella-zoster virus, rubella virus, cytomegalovirus
	Wiskott-Aldrich syndrome	Agents of infections associated with T and B cell abnormalities
	X-linked hyper-IgM syndrome	*P. carinii,* cytomegalovirus, *Cryptosporidium parvum*

SOURCE: Adapted from H Masur and A Fauci, in *Harrison's Principles of Internal Medicine,* 13th ed, KJ Isselbacher et al (eds), New York, McGraw-Hill, 1994.

classic pathway is activated primarily by immune complexes (i.e., antibody bound to antigen), and the alternative pathway is activated by microbial components, frequently in the absence of antibody. PMNs have receptors for both antibody and C3b, and antibody and complement function together to aid in the clearance of infectious agents.

PMNs, short-lived white blood cells that engulf and kill invading microbes, are first attracted to inflammatory sites by chemoattractants such as C5a, which is a product of complement activation at the site of infection. PMNs localize to the site of infection by adhering to cellular adhesion molecules expressed by endothelial cells. Endothelial cells express these receptors, called *selectins* (CD-62, ELAM-1), in response to inflammatory cytokines such as tumor necrosis factor

(TNF) α and interleukin 1. The binding of these selectin molecules to specific receptors on PMNs results in the adherence of the PMNs to the endothelium. Cytokine-mediated upregulation and expression of intercellular adhesion molecule 1 (ICAM 1) on endothelial cells then take place, and this latter receptor binds to β_2 integrins on PMNs, thereby facilitating diapedesis into the extravascular compartment. Once the PMNs are in the extravascular compartment, various molecules such as arachidonic acids further enhance the inflammatory process.

Approach to the Patient

The clinical manifestations of infectious diseases at presentation are myriad, varying from fulminant life-threatening processes to brief and self-limited conditions to indolent chronic maladies. The clinician must use all the skills of medicine to diagnose the infection and prescribe appropriate treatment. First, a careful history is essential and must include details on underlying chronic diseases; medications; occupation; travel; and risk factors for exposure to certain types of pathogens, such as those associated with sexual contacts, family illnesses, illicit drug use, particular animals, blood transfusions, ingestion of contaminated liquids or foods, or bites of insect vectors. Since infectious diseases may involve many organ systems, a careful review of systems may elicit important clues as to the disease process. The physical examination must be thorough, and attention must be paid to seemingly minor details: a soft heart murmur that might indicate bacterial endocarditis; an evanescent skin rash that suggests rheumatic fever; or a retinal lesion that suggests disseminated candidiasis or cytomegalovirus (CMV) infection.

LABORATORY INVESTIGATIONS   Laboratory studies must be carefully considered and directed toward establishing an etiologic diagnosis in the shortest possible time, at the lowest possible cost, and with the least possible discomfort to the patient. Cultures must be performed in a manner that minimizes the likelihood of contamination with normal flora while maximizing the yield. A sputum sample is far more likely to be valuable when elicited with careful coaching by the clinician than when collected in a container simply left at the bedside with cursory instructions. Gram's stains of specimens should be interpreted carefully and the quality of the specimen assessed. The findings on Gram's staining should correspond to the results of culture; a discrepancy may suggest diagnostic possibilities such as infection due to fastidious or anaerobic bacteria.

The microbiology laboratory must be an ally in the diagnostic endeavor (Chap. 121). Astute laboratory personnel will suggest optimal culture and transport conditions or alternative tests to facilitate diagnosis. If informed about specific potential pathogens, an alert laboratory staff will allow sufficient time for these organisms to become evident in culture, even when present in small numbers or when slow-growing. The parasitology technician who is attuned to the specific diagnostic considerations relevant to a particular case may be able to detect the rare, otherwise-elusive egg or cyst in a stool specimen. In cases where a diagnosis appears difficult, serum should be stored during the early acute phase of the illness so that a diagnostic rise in titer of antibody to a specific pathogen can be detected later. Bacterial and fungal antigens can sometimes be detected in body fluids, even when cultures are negative or are rendered sterile by antibiotic therapy. Techniques such as the polymerase chain reaction allow the amplification of specific DNA sequences so that minute quantities of foreign nucleic acids can be recognized in host specimens.

℞ TREATMENT   Optimal therapy for infectious diseases requires a broad knowledge of medicine and careful clinical judgment. Life-threatening infections such as bacterial meningitis or sepsis, viral encephalitis, or falciparum malaria must be treated immediately, often before a specific causative organism is identified. Antimicrobial agents must be chosen empirically and must be active against the range of potential infectious agents consistent with the clinical scenario. In contrast, good clinical judgment sometimes dictates withholding of antimicrobials in a self-limited process or until a specific diagnosis is made. The dictum *primum non nocere* should be adhered to, and it should be remembered that all antimicrobials carry a risk (and a cost) to the patient. Direct toxicity may be encountered—e.g., ototoxicity due to aminoglycosides, lipodystrophy due to HIV protease inhibitors, and hepatotoxicity due to antituberculous agents such as isoniazid and rifampin. Allergic reactions are common and can be serious. Since superinfection sometimes follows the eradication of the normal flora and colonization by a resistant organism, one invariable principle is that infectious disease therapy should be directed toward as narrow a spectrum of infectious agents as possible. Treatment specific for the pathogen should result in as little perturbation as possible of the host's microflora. With few exceptions, abscesses require surgical or percutaneous drainage for cure. Foreign bodies, including medical devices, must generally be removed in order to eliminate an infection of the device or of the adjacent tissue. Other infections, such as necrotizing fasciitis, peritonitis due to a perforated organ, gas gangrene, and chronic osteomyelitis, require surgery as the primary means of cure; in these conditions, antibiotics play only an adjunctive role.

The role of immunomodulators in the management of infectious diseases has received increasing attention. Glucocorticoids have been shown to be of benefit in the treatment of *Haemophilus influenzae* meningitis in children and in therapy for *P. carinii* pneumonia in patients with AIDS. The use of these agents in other infectious processes remains less clear and in some cases (in cerebral malaria and septic shock, for example) is detrimental. Other agents that modulate the immune response include prostaglandin inhibitors, specific lymphokines, and TNF inhibitors. Specific antibody therapy plays a role in the treatment and prevention of many diseases. Specific immunoglobulins have long been known to prevent the development of symptomatic rabies and tetanus. More recently, CMV immune globulin has been recognized as important not only in preventing the transmission of the virus during organ transplantation but also in treating CMV pneumonia in bone marrow transplant recipients. There is a strong need for well-designed clinical trials to evaluate each new interventional modality.

PERSPECTIVE   The genetic simplicity of many infectious agents allows them to undergo rapid evolution and to develop selective advantages that result in constant variation in the clinical manifestations of infection. Moreover, changes in the environment and the host can predispose new populations to a particular infection. An epidemic of lethal respiratory failure—later identified as hantavirus pulmonary syndrome—on a Navajo reservation in the southwestern United States in 1993 caused nationwide alarm, exemplifying the fear that new plagues induce in the human psyche.

The potential for infectious agents to emerge in novel and unexpected ways requires that physicians and public health officials be knowledgeable, vigilant, and open-minded in their approach to unexplained illness. The emergence of antimicrobial-resistant pathogens (e.g., enterococci that are resistant to all known antimicrobial agents and cause infections that are essentially untreatable) has led some to conclude that we are entering the "postantibiotic era." Others have held to the perception that infectious diseases no longer represent as serious a concern to world health as they once did. The progress that science, medicine, and society as a whole have made in combating these maladies is impressive, and it is ironic that, as we stand on the threshold of an understanding of the most basic biology of the microbe, infectious diseases are posing renewed problems. We are threatened by the appearance of new diseases such as AIDS, hepatitis C, and Ebola virus infection and by the reemergence of old foes such as tuberculosis, cholera, plague, and *Streptococcus pyogenes* infection. True students of infectious diseases were perhaps less surprised than anyone else by these developments. Those who know pathogens are aware of their incredible adaptability and diversity. As ingenious and

767

successful as therapeutic approaches may be, our ability to develop methods to counter infectious agents so far has not matched the myriad strategies employed by the sea of microbes that surrounds us. Their sheer numbers and the rate at which they can evolve are daunting. Moreover, environmental changes, rapid global travel, population movements, and medicine itself—through its use of antibiotics and immunosuppressive agents—all increase the impact of infectious diseases. Although new vaccines, new antibiotics, improved global communication, and new modalities for treating and preventing infection will be developed, pathogenic microbes will continue to develop new strategies of their own, presenting us with an unending and dynamic challenge.

BIBLIOGRAPHY

ARMSTRONG G et al: Trends in infectious disease mortality in the United States during the 20th century. JAMA 281:61, 1999

BERKELMAN RL, HUGHES JM: The conquest of infectious diseases: Who are we kidding? Ann Intern Med 119:426, 1993

BUCKLEY RH: Immunodeficiency diseases. JAMA 268:2797, 1992

DE JONG R et al: Severe mycobacterial and *Salmonella* infections in interleukin-12 receptor-deficient patients. Science 280:1435, 1998

FIELDS BN: Pathogenesis of viral infections, in *Virology*, BN Fields (ed). New York, Raven, 1996, pp 191–239

GOLD HS, EISENSTEIN BI: Introduction to bacterial diseases, in *Principles and Practice of Infectious Diseases*, 5th ed, GL Mandell et al (eds). New York, Churchill Livingstone, 2000, p 2065

GRAYSTON JT, CAMPBELL LA: Editorial response: The role of *Chlamydia pneumoniae* in atherosclerosis. Clin Infect Dis 28:993, 1999

HENDERSON DA: Bioterrorism as a public health threat. Emerg Infect Dis 4:488, 1998

NEWPORT MJ et al: A mutation in the interferon-γ-receptor gene and susceptibility to mycobacterial infection. N Engl J Med 335:1941, 1996

PILE JC et al: Anthrax as a potential biological warfare agent. Arch Intern Med 158:429, 1998

PUCK JM: Primary immunodeficiency diseases. JAMA 278:1835, 1997

QUAGLIARELLO V, SCHELD MW: Bacterial meningitis: Pathogenesis, pathophysiology, and progress. N Engl J Med 327:864, 1992

---

120 *Gerald B. Pier*

MOLECULAR MECHANISMS OF MICROBIAL PATHOGENESIS

Over the past two decades, molecular studies of microbial pathogenesis have yielded an explosion of information about the various microbial and host molecules that contribute to the processes of infection and disease. These processes can be classified into several stages: microbial encounter with and entry into the host; microbial growth after entry; avoidance of innate host defenses; tissue invasion and tropism; tissue damage; and transmission to new hosts. Virulence is the measure of an organism's capacity to cause disease and is a function of the pathogenic factors elaborated by microbes. These factors promote colonization (the simple presence of potentially pathogenic microbes in or on a host), infection (attachment and growth of pathogens and avoidance of host defenses), and disease (often, but not always, the activities of secreted toxins or toxic metabolites). In addition, the host's inflammatory response to infection greatly contributes to disease and its attendant clinical signs and symptoms. Knowledge of the molecular structures of the microbial surface, their interactions with the host, and the host response is critical to an understanding of the basic processes of infection and disease.

MICROBIAL ENTRY AND ADHERENCE

ENTRY SITES A microbial pathogen can potentially enter any part of a host organism. In general, the type of disease produced by a particular microbe is often a direct consequence of its route of entry into the body. The most common sites of entry are body parts in con-

tact with the external environment, including mucosal surfaces (particularly those of the respiratory, alimentary, and urogenital tracts) and the skin. Ingestion, inhalation, and sexual contact are typical routes of microbial entry. Other portals of entry include injuries to the skin (cuts, bites, burns, trauma) along with injection via natural (i.e., vector-borne) or artificial (i.e., needle-stick injury) routes. A few pathogens, such as *Schistosoma* spp., can penetrate unbroken skin. The conjunctiva can serve as an entry point for pathogens of the eye.

Microbial entry usually relies on the organism's biologic characteristics and reflects the presence of specific microbial factors needed for persistence and growth in a tissue. Fecal-oral spread via the alimentary tract requires a biology consistent with survival in the varied environments of the gastrointestinal tract (including the low pH of the stomach and the high bile content of the intestine) as well as in contaminated food or water outside the host. Organisms that gain entry via the respiratory tract are most often those that survive well in small moist droplets produced during sneezing and coughing; most such pathogens do not survive well once they dry out. Pathogens that enter by venereal routes often survive best on the warm moist environment of the urogenital mucosa. Many sexually transmitted human pathogens have restricted host ranges and do not infect other animals (e.g., *Neisseria gonorrhoeae*, *Treponema pallidum*, and HIV).

The biology of microbes entering through the skin is highly varied. Some of these organisms can survive in a broad range of environments, such as the salivary glands or alimentary tracts of arthropod vectors, the mouths of larger animals, soil, and water. A complex biology allows protozoan parasites such as *Plasmodium*, *Leishmania*, and *Trypanosoma* spp. to undergo morphogenic changes that allow the organism to be transmitted to mammalian hosts during insect feeding for blood meals. Plasmodia are injected as infective sporozoites from the salivary glands during mosquito feeding. *Leishmania* parasites are regurgitated as promastigotes from the alimentary tract of sandflies and injected by bite into a susceptible host. Trypanosomes are first ingested from infected hosts by reduviid bugs; the pathogens then multiply in the gastrointestinal tract of the insects and are released in feces onto the host's skin during subsequent feedings. Most microbes that land directly on intact skin are destined to die, as survival on the skin or in hair follicles requires resistance to fatty acids, low pH, and other antimicrobial factors on skin. Once it is damaged (and particularly if it becomes necrotic), the skin can be a major portal of growth and entry for pathogens or their toxic products. Tetanus and burn wound infections are clear examples. After animal bites, pathogens resident in the animal's saliva gain access through the skin to the victim's tissues. Rabies is the paradigm for this pathogenic process; rabies virus grows in striated muscle cells at the site of inoculation.

MICROBIAL ADHERENCE Once in or on a host, most microbes must anchor themselves to a tissue or tissue factor; the possible exceptions are organisms that directly enter the bloodstream and multiply there. Specific microbial ligands or adhesins for host receptors constitute a major area of study in the field of microbial pathogenesis. Adhesins comprise a wide range of surface structures, not only anchoring the microbe to a tissue and promoting cellular entry where appropriate but also eliciting host responses critical to the pathogenic process (Table 120-1). Most microbes produce multiple adhesins specific for multiple host receptors. These adhesins are often redundant, are serologically variable, and act additively or synergistically with other microbial factors to promote microbial sticking to host tissues. In addition, some microbes (such as *Mycobacterium tuberculosis* and *Legionella pneumophila*) adsorb host proteins (such as complement components) onto their surface and utilize the natural host protein receptor for microbial binding and entry into target cells.

All viral pathogens must bind to host cells, enter them, and replicate within them. Viral coat proteins serve as the ligands for cellular entry, and more than one ligand-receptor interaction may be needed; for example, HIV utilizes its envelope glycoprotein (gp) 120 to enter host cells by binding to both CD4 and one of several receptors for

Table 120-1 Examples of Microbial Ligand-Receptor Interactions

Microorganism	Type of Microbial Ligand	Host Receptor
VIRAL PATHOGENS		
Influenza virus	Hemagglutinin	Sialic acid
Measles virus	H glycoprotein	CD46/moesin
Herpes simplex virus	gC protein	Heparin sulfate
Human herpesvirus type 6	?	CD46
HIV	Surface glycoprotein	CD4 and chemokine
Epstein-Barr virus	Envelope protein	CD21 (=CR2)
Adenovirus and coxsackie-virus	Fiber protein	Coxsackie-adenovirus receptor (CAR) and major histocompatibility class I antigens
BACTERIAL PATHOGENS		
Neisseria spp.	Pili	Membrane cofactor protein (CD46)
Pseudomonas aeruginosa	Pili and flagella	Asialo-GM1
	Lipopolysaccharide	Cystic fibrosis transmembrane conductance regulator
Escherichia coli	Pili	Ceramides/mannose and digalactosyl residues
Streptococcus pyogenes	Hyaluronic acid capsule	CD44
Yersinia spp.	Invasin/accessory invasin locus	β_1 Integrins
Bordetella pertussis	Filamentous hemagglutinin	CR3
Legionella pneumophila	Adsorbed C3bi	CR3
Mycobacterium tuberculosis	Adsorbed C3bi	CR3
FUNGAL PATHOGENS		
Blastomyces dermatitidis	WI-1	Possibly matrix proteins and integrins
Candida albicans	int1p	Extracellular matrix proteins
PROTOZOAL PATHOGENS		
Plasmodium vivax	Merozoite form	Duffy Fy antigen
Plasmodium falciparum	EBA-175	Glycophorin A
Entamoeba histolytica	Surface lectin	N-Acetylglucosamine

chemokines. Similarly, the measles virus H glycoprotein binds to both CD46 and the membrane-organizing protein moesin. The gC protein on herpes simplex virus binds to heparin sulfate; this step is followed by attachment to cells mediated by the viral gD (and possibly gH) protein. CD46 has now been shown to be the cellular receptor for human herpesvirus type 6. Eukaryotic parasites use complicated surface glycoproteins as adhesins, some of which are lectins with specificity for carbohydrates on host cells.

Among the microbial adhesins studied in greatest detail are bacterial pili and flagella. *Pili* or *fimbriae* are commonly used by gram-negative bacteria for attachment to host cells and tissues. In electron micrographs, these hairlike projections (up to several hundred per cell) may be confined to one end of the organism (polar pili) or distributed more evenly over the surface. An individual cell may have pili with a variety of functions. Most pili are made up of a major pilin protein subunit (molecular weight, 17,000 to 30,000) that polymerizes to form the pilus. Many strains of *Escherichia coli* express mucus-binding type 1 pili, whose binding to host tissues is inhibited by D-mannose. Other strains produce the Pap (pyelonephritis-associated) or P pilus adhesin that mediates binding to digalactose (gal-gal) residues on globosides of the human P blood groups. These pili have proteins located at the tips of the main pilus unit that are critical to the binding specificity of the whole pilus unit. Immunization with the mannose-binding FimH tip protein of type 1 pili prevents experimental *E. coli* bladder infections in mice and monkeys. *E. coli* cells causing diarrheal disease express pilus-like receptors for enterocytes on the small bowel, along with other receptors termed *colonization factors*.

A common type of pilus found in *Neisseria* spp., *Moraxella* spp., *Vibrio cholerae*, and *Pseudomonas aeruginosa* mediates adherence of these organisms to target surfaces. These pili tend to have a relatively conserved amino-terminal region and a more variable carboxyl-terminal region. For some species such as *N. gonorrhoeae* and *Neisseria*

meningitidis, the pili are critical for attachment to mucosal epithelial cells. For others, such as *P. aeruginosa*, the pili only partially mediate the cells' adherence to host tissues. *V. cholerae* cells appear to use two different types of pili for intestinal colonization. Whereas interference with this stage of colonization would appear to be an effective antibacterial strategy, attempts to develop pilus-based vaccines for human diseases have not been highly successful to date.

Flagella are long appendages attached at either one or both ends of the bacterial cell (polar flagella) or distributed over the entire cell surface (peritrichous flagella). Flagella, like pili, are composed of a polymerized or aggregated basic protein. In flagella, the protein subunits form a tight helical structure and vary serologically with the species. Spirochetes such as *T. pallidum* and *Borrelia burgdorferi* have axial filaments similar to flagella running down the long axis of the center of the cell, and they "swim" by rotation around these filaments. Some bacteria can glide over a surface in the absence of obvious motility structures.

Other bacterial structures involved in adherence to host tissues include specific staphylococcal and streptococcal proteins that bind to human extracellular matrix proteins such as fibrin, fibronectin, laminin, and collagen. Fibronectin appears to be a commonly used receptor for various pathogens; a particular sequence, Arg-Gly-Asp or RGD, is critical for bacterial binding. Surface lipoteichoic acids may also promote streptococcal adherence to mucosal surfaces. The surface lipopolysaccharide (LPS) of *P. aeruginosa* mediates binding to the cystic fibrosis transmembrane conductance regulator (CFTR) on airway epithelial cells. Coagulase-negative staphylococci readily colonize prosthetic devices and catheters commonly used in medical care; the surface capsular polysaccharide of these organisms promotes binding to the prosthetic material. It has been reported that *Staphylococcus aureus* produces the same capsular polysaccharide and may also use this material to colonize prosthetic devices.

FUNGAL ADHESINS Several fungal adhesins have been described that mediate colonization of epithelial surfaces, particularly adherence to structures like fibronectin, laminin, and collagen. The product of the *Candida albicans INT1* gene, int1p, bears similarity to mammalian integrins that bind to extracellular matrix proteins. Transformation of normally nonadherent *Saccharomyces cerevisiae* with this gene allows these yeast cells to adhere to human epithelial cells. Disruption of *INT1* in *C. albicans* diminishes but does not eliminate epithelial cell adhesion; this result indicates that both int1p and other adhesins mediate binding of *C. albicans* to epithelial cells. Moreover, int1p is needed for filamentous growth of *C. albicans*—a phenotype linked to virulence, and particularly to the ability to penetrate keratinized epithelium. *INT1*-deficient *C. albicans* exhibits markedly reduced virulence in a mouse model of infection.

For several fungal pathogens that initiate infections after inhalation of infectious material, the inoculum is ingested by alveolar macrophages, in which the cells transform to pathogenic phenotypes. Like *C. albicans*, *Blastomyces dermatitidis* binds to CD11b/CD18 integrins as well as to CD14 on macrophages. *B. dermatitidis* produces a 120-kDa surface protein, designated WI-1, that mediates this adherence. The binding domain of WI-1 is homologous to the invasin protein of *Yersinia* that binds to the same type of host cell receptor. An unidentified factor on *Histoplasma capsulatum* also mediates binding of this fungal pathogen to the integrin surface proteins.

Host receptors are found both on target cells (such as epithelial cells lining mucosal surfaces) and within the mucus layer covering these cells. Microbial pathogens bind to a wide range of host receptors to establish infection (Table 120-1). Selective loss of host receptors for a pathogen may confer natural resistance to an otherwise susceptible population. For example, *Plasmodium vivax*, one of four *Plasmodium* species causing malaria, binds to the Duffy blood group antigen, Fy, on erythrocytes. In West Africa, 70% of individuals lack Fy antigens and are resistant to *P. vivax* infection. *Salmonella typhi*, the etiologic agent of typhoid fever, uses CFTR to enter the gastrointestinal submucosa after being ingested. As homozygous mutations in *CFTR* are the cause of the life-shortening disease cystic fibrosis, heterozygote carriers (e.g., 4 to 5% of individuals of European ancestry) may have had a selective advantage due to decreased susceptibility to *S. typhi* infection.

Numerous virus–target cell interactions have been described, and it is now clear that different viruses can use similar host cell receptors for entry. The list of certain and likely host receptors for viral pathogens is long. Among the host membrane components that can serve as receptors for viruses are sialic acids, gangliosides, glycosaminoglycans, integrins and other members of the immunoglobulin superfamily, histocompatibility antigens, and regulators and receptors for complement components.

MICROBIAL GROWTH AFTER ENTRY

Once established on a mucosal or skin site, pathogenic microbes must replicate before causing full-blown infection and disease. Within cells, viral particles release their nucleic acids, which may be directly translated into viral proteins (positive-strand RNA viruses), transcribed from a negative strand of RNA into a complementary mRNA (negative-strand RNA viruses), or transcribed into a complementary strand of DNA (retroviruses); for DNA viruses, mRNA may be transcribed directly from viral DNA, either in the cell nucleus or in the cytoplasm. To grow, bacteria must acquire specific nutrients or synthesize them from precursors in host tissues. For example, since aromatic amino acids are not available as nutrients in host tissues, pathogenic bacteria must synthesize them from precursors. Many infectious processes are usually confined to specific epithelial surfaces—influenza to the respiratory mucosa, gonorrhea to the urogenital epithelium, shigellosis to the gastrointestinal epithelium. While there are multiple reasons for this specificity, one important consideration is probably the ability of these pathogens to obtain from these specific environments the nutrients needed for growth and survival.

Temperature restrictions also play a role in limiting certain pathogens to specific tissues. Rhinoviruses, a cause of the common cold, grow best at 33°C and replicate in cooler nasal tissues but not in the lung. Leprosy lesions due to *Mycobacterium leprae* are found in and on relatively cool body sites. Fungal pathogens that infect the skin, hair follicles, and nails (dermatophyte infections) remain confined to the cooler, exterior, keratinous layer of the epithelium.

A topic of major interest is the ability of many bacterial, fungal, and protozoal species to grow in multicellular masses referred to as *biofilms*. These masses are biochemically and morphologically quite distinct from the free-living individual cells referred to as *planktonic cells*. Growth in biofilms leads to altered microbial metabolism, production of extracellular virulence factors, and decreased susceptibility to biocides, antimicrobial agents, and host defense molecules and cells. Regulation of biofilm morphogenesis is controlled by bacterial quorum-sensing systems. Quorum sensing for some organisms involves the production of homoserine lactone molecules such as *N*-(3-oxododecanoyl)homoserine lactone and *N*-butyrylhomoserine lactone, which combine with transcriptional activators to control gene expression. *P. aeruginosa* growing on the bronchial mucosa during chronic infection, staphylococci and other pathogens growing on implanted medical devices, and dental pathogens growing on tooth surfaces to form plaques represent several examples of microbial biofilm growth associated with human disease. Many other pathogens can form biofilms during

in vitro growth, including *Helicobacter pylori*, the cause of stomach ulcers; *E. coli* O157, one cause of the hemolytic-uremic syndrome; and *Gardnerella vaginalis*, an organism associated with bacterial vaginosis.

AVOIDANCE OF INNATE HOST DEFENSES

As microbes have probably interacted with mucosal/epithelial surfaces since the emergence of multicellular organisms, it is not surprising that multicellular hosts have a variety of innate surface defense mechanisms that can sense when pathogens are present and contribute to their elimination. The skin, a formidable physical barrier to microbial entry, is both acidic and bathed with fatty acids toxic to many microbes. Successful skin pathogens such as staphylococci must tolerate these adverse conditions. Mucosal surfaces themselves present a barrier composed of a thick mucus layer that entraps microbes and facilitates their transport out of the body by such processes as mucociliary clearance, coughing, and urination. Mucous secretions, saliva, and tears contain antibacterial factors such as lysozyme and antiviral factors such as interferons. Gastric acidity is inimical to the survival of many ingested pathogens, and many mucosal surfaces—particularly the nasopharynx, the vaginal tract, and the gastrointestinal tract—contain a resident flora of commensal microbes that interfere with the ability of pathogens to colonize and infect a host.

Pathogens that survive these factors must still contend with host endocytic, phagocytic, and inflammatory responses as well as with host genetic factors that determine the degree to which a pathogen can survive and grow. The growth of viral pathogens entering skin or mucosal epithelial cells can be limited by a variety of host genetic factors, including production of interferons, modulation of receptors for viral entry, and age- and hormone-related susceptibility factors; by nutritional status; and even by personal habits such as smoking and exercise.

ENCOUNTERS WITH EPITHELIAL CELLS Over the past decade, many bacterial pathogens have been shown to enter epithelial cells (Fig. 120-1), often using specialized surface structures that bind to receptors for internalization. However, the exact role and the importance of this process in infection and disease are not well defined for most of these pathogens. Bacterial entry into host epithelial cells is seen as a means for dissemination to adjacent or deeper tissues or as a route to sanctuary to avoid ingestion and killing by professional phagocytes. Epithelial cell entry appears, for instance, to be a critical aspect of dysentery induction by *Shigella*.

Curiously, the less virulent strains of many bacterial pathogens are more adept at entering epithelial cells than are more virulent strains; examples include pathogens that lack the surface polysaccharide capsule needed to cause serious disease. Thus, for *Haemophilus influenzae*, *Streptococcus pneumoniae*, *S. agalactiae* (group B *Streptococcus*), and *S. pyogenes*, isogenic mutants or variants lacking capsules enter epithelial cells better than the wild-type, encapsulated parental forms that cause disseminated disease. These observations have led to the proposal that epithelial cell entry may be a manifestation of host defense, resulting in bacterial clearance by both shedding of epithelial cells containing internalized bacteria and initiation of a subclinical inflammatory response. However, a consequence of this process would be the opening of a hole in the epithelium, potentially allowing uningested organisms to enter the submucosa. This scenario has been documented in murine *Salmonella typhimurium* infections and in experimental bladder infections with uropathogenic *E. coli*. In the latter system, bacterial pili mediate cell attachment to integral membrane glycoproteins called uroplakins that coat the host cells, resulting in exfoliation of the cells with attached bacteria. Subsequently, infection is produced by residual bacterial cells that invade the denuded epithelium. Perhaps at low bacterial inocula epithelial cell ingestion and subclinical inflammation are efficient means to eliminate pathogens, while at higher inocula a proportion of surviving bacterial cells enter the host tissue through the damaged mucosal surface and multiply,

FIGURE 120-1   Entry of bacteria into epithelial cells. *A.* Internalization of *P. aeruginosa* by cultured airway epithelial cells expressing wild-type cystic fibrosis transmembrane conductance regulator (CFTR), the cell receptor for bacterial ingestion. *B.* Entry of *P. aeruginosa* into murine tracheal epithelial cells after murine infection by the intranasal route.

producing disease. Alternatively, failure of the appropriate epithelial cell response to a pathogen may allow the organism to survive on a mucosal surface where, if it avoids other host defenses, it can grow and cause a local infection. Along these lines, as noted above, *P. aeruginosa* is taken into epithelial cells by CFTR, a protein missing or nonfunctional in most severe cases of cystic fibrosis. The major clinical consequence of this disease is chronic airway-surface infection with *P. aeruginosa* in 80 to 90% of patients with cystic fibrosis. The failure of airway epithelial cells to ingest and promote the removal of *P. aeruginosa* has been proposed as a key component of the hypersusceptibility of these patients to chronic airway infection.

ENCOUNTERS WITH PHAGOCYTES   Phagocytosis of microbes is a major innate host defense that limits the growth and spread of pathogens. Phagocytes appear rapidly at sites of infection in conjunction with the initiation of inflammation. Ingestion of microbes

by both tissue-fixed macrophages and migrating phagocytes probably accounts for the limited ability of most microbial agents to cause disease. A family of related molecules called *collectins*, *soluble defense collagens*, or *pattern recognition molecules* are found in blood (mannose-binding lectin), in lung (surfactant proteins A and D), and most likely in other tissues as well and bind to carbohydrates on microbial surfaces to promote phagocyte clearance. Bacterial pathogens seem to be ingested principally by polymorphonuclear neutrophils (PMNs), while eosinophils are frequently found at sites of infection by protozoan or multicellular parasites. Successful pathogens, by definition, must avoid being cleared by professional phagocytes. One of several antiphagocytic strategies employed by bacteria and by the fungal pathogen *Cryptococcus neoformans* is to elaborate large-molecular-weight surface polysaccharide antigens, often in the form of a capsule that coats the cell surface. Most pathogenic bacteria produce such antiphagocytic capsules.

As activation of local phagocytes in tissues is a key step in initiating inflammation and migration of additional phagocytes into infected sites, much attention has been paid to microbial factors that initiate inflammation. Encounters with phagocytes are governed largely by the structure of the microbial constituents that elicit inflammation, and detailed knowledge of these structures for bacterial pathogens has contributed greatly to our understanding of molecular mechanisms of microbial pathogenesis (Fig. 120-2). The best-studied system involves the interaction of LPS from gram-negative bacteria and the glycosylphosphatidylinositol (GPI)-anchored membrane protein CD14 found on the surface of professional phagocytes, including migrating and tissue-fixed macrophages and PMNs. A soluble form of CD14 is also found in plasma and on mucosal surfaces. A plasma protein, LPS-binding protein (LBP), transfers LPS to membrane-bound CD14 on myeloid cells and promotes binding of LPS to soluble CD14. Soluble CD14/LPS/LBP complexes bind to many cell types and may be internalized to initiate cellular responses to microbial pathogens. It has been shown that peptidoglycan and lipoteichoic acid from gram-positive bacteria and cell-surface products of mycobacteria and spirochetes can interact with CD14 (Fig. 120-2).

GPI-anchored receptors do not have intracellular signaling domains, and mammalian Toll-like receptors (TLRs) transduce signals for cellular activation due to LPS binding. TLRs initiate cellular activation through a series of signal-transducing molecules (Fig. 120-2) that lead to nuclear translocation of the transcription factor NF-κB, a master-switch for production of important inflammatory cytokines such as tumor necrosis factor α (TNF-α) and interleukin (IL) 1.

The initiation of inflammation can occur not only with LPS and peptidoglycan but also with viral particles and other microbial products such as polysaccharides, enzymes, and toxins.

Bacterial Cell Wall Structure   Gram-positive bacteria have a rigid cell wall that gives the organisms their characteristic shape, differentiates them from eukaryotic cells, and allows them to survive in osmotically unfavorable environments. The cell wall is composed mainly of peptidoglycan (Fig. 120-3, panel *C*; a polymer of *N*-acetylglucosamine and its lactyl ether, *N*-acetylmuramic acid), with peptide side chains covalently bound to the lactyl group (Fig. 120-3, panel *A*). The peptide chains consist of alternating D and L amino acids and are usually linked to each other by a pentaglycine bridge binding a terminal D-alanine on one peptide substituent to the penultimate L-lysine on a neighboring peptide. Variations in this basic structure have been described for a number of bacterial genera. In addition, the cell walls of gram-positive bacteria contain teichoic acids (Fig. 120-3, panel *D*), phosphate-linked polymers of ribitol or glycerol that can have additional compounds linked to available side groups. Lipid tails anchor these acids to the cytoplasmic membrane, giving rise to lipoteichoic acids.

Gram-negative bacteria possess a cytoplasmic membrane and a peptidoglycan layer similar to but reduced from that found in gram-positive organisms, but these organisms also produce an outer membrane that is covalently linked to the tetrapeptides of the peptidoglycan layer by a lipoprotein (Fig. 120-3, panel *B*). Embedded in the outer membrane are special proteins with important functions, including maintaining the outer membrane's integrity, acting as a selective barrier for diffusion of molecules into the cell, serving as receptors for bacteriophages, and binding siderophores that scavenge iron for transport into the bacterial cell. The exterior layer of the outer membrane contains the major surface glycolipid, which can be either a classical bacterial LPS or a lipooligosaccharide (LOS); pathogens such as *Neisseria* and *Haemophilus* spp. express LOS, which contains smaller polysaccharide constituents. Although LPS/LOS was thought to be essential to the viability of gram-negative bacteria, a viable strain of *N. meningitidis* lacking LOS has now been made.

Exterior to the LPS for many, but not all, gram-negative pathogens is a capsular polysaccharide, which (along with LPS for some pathogenic species) confers resistance to phagocytosis by preventing innate host opsonins, such as the complement proteins C3 and C4, from coating the organisms—a process that promotes their uptake by phagocytes. Capsular polysaccharides are also important extracellular components of gram-positive bacteria, serving as critical factors in bacterial resistance to opsonophagocytosis and phagocytic killing. Variation in the expression of the capsule in *S. pneumoniae* accounts for the different morphologies of colonies of this pathogen on agar plates (smooth and rough phenotypes); this property was exploited in studies proving that DNA carries genetic information in a cell.

Lipopolysaccharide   Most of the important biologic properties associated with LPS (endotoxin) are due to the lipid A portion (Fig. 120-3, panel *E*), a relatively conserved, highly acylated di-*N*-acetylglucosamine backbone linked β 1→6 and containing phosphate groups on the reducing 1 and nonreducing 4′ carbons. Attached to carbon 6′ is the inner polysaccharide core, which is usually, but not always, composed of a di- or trisaccharide of 2-keto-3-deoxyoctonate (KDO). Additional sugar substituents are linked to the inner core, forming a complete core. Attached to the complete core are either short polysaccharide side chains (forming LOS) or longer O polysaccharide side chains (forming complete LPS) composed of a variety of monosaccharides, substituted with a variety of components, such as formyl, acetyl, and hydroxybutyryl side chains; amino acids or peptides; and phosphate groups. Further biologic functions of LOS/LPS that are important to the survival of microbes after entry into a host include resistance to the bacteriolytic effects of complement and protection against antimicrobial factors such as defensins and bactericidal permeability-increasing protein, a molecule closely related to LBP in structure and function. Defensins are found in high concentrations in granules of myeloid cells, including platelets, and are usually highly cationic peptides capable of insertion into bacterial cells and killing of these cells.

Additional Interactions of Microbial Pathogens and Phagocytes   Other ways that microbial pathogens avoid destruction by phagocytes include production of factors that are toxic to the phagocytes or that interfere with the chemotactic and ingestion function of phagocytes. Hemolysins, leukocidins, and the like are microbial proteins that can kill phagocytes that are attempting to ingest organisms elaborating these substances. For example, staphylococcal hemolysins

FIGURE 120-2   Cellular signaling pathways for production of inflammatory cytokines in response to microbial products. Various microbial cell-surface constituents interact with CD14, which in turn interacts in a currently unknown fashion with toll-like receptors (TLR). Both CD14 and TLRs contain extracellular leucine-rich domains. The cytoplasmic domains of TLRs are oligomerized for binding to the general adaptor protein MyD88, which also binds to members of the interleukin-1 receptor (IL-1Rc) transmembrane proteins due to homology in the intracellular domain. Oligomerization is followed by activation of signal-transducing molecules such as IRAK-1 (IL-1Rc-associated kinase 1), TRAF-6 (tumor necrosis factor receptor–associated factor 6), TAK-1 (transforming growth factor β–activating kinase 1), and NIK (Nck-interacting kinase). In addition to activating other signaling pathways leading to cytokine production and stress responses, such as the c-Jun *N*-terminal kinase (JNK) pathway and MAP kinase kinase kinase (MEKK1) pathway [via evolutionarily conserved signaling intermediate in Toll pathways (ECSIT)], TLR-mediated signaling leads to activation of the inducible kinase complex, IKK-α, -β, and -γ. These are part of a larger complex that phosphorylates the inhibitory portion (I) of nuclear factor κB (NF-κB), resulting in release of IκB from NF-κB. Phosphorylated (PP) IκB is then degraded and NF-κB translocates to the nucleus, where it binds to transcriptional sites on target genes, many of which encode inflammatory proteins. *(Figure courtesy of Dr. Terry Means and Dr. Douglas Golenbock.)*

inhibit macrophage chemotaxis and kill these phagocytes. Streptolysin O made by *S. pyogenes* binds to cholesterol in phagocyte membranes and initiates a process of internal degranulation, with the release of normally granule-sequestered toxic components into the phagocyte's cytoplasm. *Entamoeba histolytica*, an intestinal protozoan that causes amebic dysentery, can disrupt phagocyte membranes after direct contact via the release of protozoal phospholipase A and pore-forming peptides.

Microbial Survival Inside Phagocytes   Many important microbial pathogens use a variety of strategies to survive inside phagocytes (particularly macrophages) after ingestion. Inhibition of fusion of the phagocytic vacuole (the phagosome) containing the ingested microbe with the lysosomal granules containing antimicrobial substances (the lysosome) allows *M. tuberculosis*, *S. typhi*, and *Toxoplasma gondii* to survive inside macrophages. Some organisms, such as *Listeria monocytogenes*, escape into the phagocyte's cytoplasm to grow and eventually spread to other cells. Resistance to killing within the macrophage and subsequent growth are critical to successful infection by herpes-type viruses, measles virus, poxviruses, *Salmonella*, *Yersinia*, *Legionella*, *Mycobacterium*, *Trypanosoma*, *Nocardia*, *Histoplasma*, *Toxoplasma*, and *Rickettsia*. *Salmonella* spp. use a master regulatory system, in which the *PhoP/PhoQ* genes control other genes, to enter and survive within cells, with intracellular survival entailing structural changes in the cell envelope LPS.

FIGURE 120-3 Schematic representations of bacterial surface structures. *A*. Cytoplasmic membrane and cell wall typical of gram-positive bacteria. *B*. Outer structure of a gram-negative organism (OM = outer membrane). *C*. Detailed structure of peptidoglycan showing backbone of *N*-acetylmuramic acid (MurNAc) and *N*-acetylglucosamine (GlcNAc); tetrapeptide bridges composed of L-alanine (L-ala), D-glutamate (D-glu-N), L-lysine (L-lys), and D-alanine (D-ala); and pentaglycine [Gly(5)] cross-bridges. *D*. Teichoic acid backbone. *E*. Detailed structure of lipopolysaccharide typical of *Salmonella* spp., including the lipid A sugars glucosamine (GlcN) and 4-amino arabinose (AraN) and the core sugars 2-keto-3-deoxyoctonate (KDO), heptose (Hep), glucose (Glc), galactose (Gal), and *N*-acetylglucosamine (GlcNAc). Hexagons depicting the O-specific chain represent variable monosaccharide residues that comprise this structure. *(Drawing courtesy of TJ DiCesare.)*

TISSUE INVASION AND TISSUE TROPISM

TISSUE INVASION Most viral pathogens cause disease by growth at skin or mucosal entry sites, but some pathogens spread from the initial site to deeper tissues. Virus can spread via the nerves (rabies virus) or plasma (picornaviruses) or within migratory blood cells (poliovirus, Epstein-Barr virus, and many others). Specific viral genes determine where and how individual viral strains can spread.

Bacteria may invade deeper layers of mucosal tissue via intracellular uptake by epithelial cells, traversal of epithelial cell junctions, or penetration through denuded epithelial surfaces. Among virulent *Shigella* strains and invasive *E. coli*, outer-membrane proteins are critical to epithelial cell invasion and bacterial multiplication. *Neisseria* and *Haemophilus* spp. penetrate mucosal cells by poorly understood mechanisms before dissemination into the bloodstream. Staphylococci and streptococci elaborate a variety of extracellular enzymes, such as hyaluronidase, lipases, nucleases, and hemolysins, that are probably important in breaking down cellular and matrix structures and allowing the bacteria access to deeper tissues and blood. Organisms that colonize the gastrointestinal tract can often translocate through the mucosa into the blood and, under circumstances in which host defenses are inadequate, cause bacteremia. *Yersinia enterocolitica* can invade the mucosa through the activity of the invasin protein. Some bacteria (e.g., *Brucella*) can be carried from a mucosal site to a distant site by phagocytic cells (e.g., PMNs) that ingest but fail to kill the bacteria.

Fungal pathogens almost always take advantage of host immunocompromise to spread hematogenously to deeper tissues. The AIDS epidemic has resoundingly illustrated this principle: the immunodeficiency of many HIV-infected patients permits the development of life-threatening fungal infections of the lung, blood, and brain. Other than the capsule of *C. neoformans*, specific fungal antigens involved in tissue invasion are not well characterized. Both fungal pathogens and protozoal pathogens (e.g., *Plasmodium* spp. and *E. histolytica*) undergo morphologic changes to spread within a host. Malarial parasites grow in liver cells as merozoites and are released into the blood to invade erythrocytes and become trophozoites. *E. histolytica* is found as both a cyst and a trophozoite in the intestinal lumen, through which this pathogen enters the host, but only the trophozoite form can spread systemically to cause amebic liver abscesses. Other protozoal pathogens, such as *T. gondii*, *Giardia lamblia*, and *Cryptosporidium*, also undergo extensive morphologic changes after initial infection to spread to other tissues.

TISSUE TROPISM The propensity of certain microbes to cause disease by infecting specific tissues has been known since the early days of bacteriology, yet the molecular basis for this propensity is understood somewhat better for viral pathogens than for other agents of infectious disease. Specific receptor-ligand interactions clearly underlie the ability of certain viruses to enter cells within tissues and disrupt normal tissue function, but the mere presence of a receptor for a virus on a target tissue is not sufficient for tissue tropism. Factors in the cell, route of viral entry, viral capacity to penetrate into cells, viral genetic elements that regulate gene expression, and pathways of viral spread in a tissue all affect tissue tropism. Some viral genes are best transcribed in specific target cells, such as hepatitis B genes in liver cells and Epstein-Barr virus genes in B lymphocytes. The route of inoculation of poliovirus determines its neurotropism, although the molecular basis for this circumstance is not understood.

The lesser understanding of the tissue tropism of bacterial and parasitic infections is exemplified by *Neisseria* spp. There is no well-accepted explanation of why *N. gonorrhoeae* colonizes and infects the human genital tract while the closely related species *N. meningitidis* principally colonizes the human oropharynx. *N. meningitidis* expresses a capsular polysaccharide, while *N. gonorrhoeae* does not; however, there is no indication that this property plays a role in the different tissue tropisms displayed by these two bacterial species. *N. gonorrhoeae* can use cytidine monophosphate *N*-acetylneuraminic acid from host tissues to add *N*-acetylneuraminic acid (sialic acid) to its LOS O side chain, and this alteration appears to make the organism resistant to host defenses. Lactate, present at high levels on genital mucosal surfaces, stimulates sialylation of gonococcal LOS. Bacteria with sialic acid sugars in their capsules, such as *N. meningitidis*, *E. coli* K-1, and group B streptococci, have a propensity to cause meningitis, but this generalization has many exceptions. For example, all recognized serotypes of group B streptococci contain sialic acid in their capsules, but only one serotype (III) is responsible for most cases of group B streptococcal meningitis. Moreover, both *H. influenzae* and *S. pneumoniae* can readily cause meningitis, but these organisms do not have sialic acid in their capsules.

TISSUE DAMAGE AND DISEASE

Disease is a complex phenomenon resulting from tissue invasion and destruction, toxin elaboration, and host response. Viruses cause much of their damage by exerting a cytopathic effect on host cells and inhibiting host defenses. The growth of bacterial, fungal, and protozoal parasites in tissue, which may or may not be accompanied by toxin elaboration, can also compromise tissue function and lead to disease. For some bacterial and possibly some fungal pathogens, toxin production is one of the best-characterized molecular mechanisms of pathogenesis, while host factors such as IL-1, TNF-α, kinins, inflammatory proteins, products of complement activation, and mediators derived from arachidonic acid metabolites (leukotrienes) and cellular degranulation (histamines) readily contribute to the severity of disease.

VIRAL DISEASE Viral pathogens are well known to inhibit host immune responses by a variety of mechanisms. Immune responses can be affected by down-regulating production of most major histocompatibility complex (MHC) molecules (adenovirus E3 protein), by diminishing cytotoxic T cell recognition of virus-infected cells (Epstein-Barr virus EBNA1 antigen and cytomegalovirus IE protein), by producing virus-encoded complement receptor proteins (herpesvirus and vaccinia virus) that protect infected cells from complement-mediated lysis, by making proteins that interfere with the action of interferon (influenza virus and poxvirus), and by elaborating superantigen-like proteins (mouse mammary tumor virus and related retroviruses, rabies nucleocapsid, and possibly the Nef protein of HIV). Superantigens activate large populations of T cells that express particular subsets of the T cell receptor β protein, causing massive cytokine release and subsequent host reactions. Another molecular mechanism of viral virulence involves the production of peptide growth factors for host cells, which disrupt normal cellular growth, proliferation, and differentiation. In addition, viral factors can bind to and interfere with the function of host receptors for signaling molecules. Modulation of cytokine production during viral infection can stimulate viral growth inside cells with receptors for the cytokine, and virus-encoded cytokine homologues (e.g., the Epstein-Barr virus BCRF1 protein, which is highly homologous to the immunoinhibitory IL-10 molecule) can potentially prevent immune-mediated clearance

of viral particles. Viruses can cause disease in neural cells by interfering with levels of neurotransmitters without necessarily destroying the cells, or they may induce either programmed cell death (apoptosis) to destroy tissues or inhibitors of apoptosis to allow for prolonged viral infection of cells. Overall, any disruption of normal cellular and tissue function due to viral infection can underlie the resultant clinical disease.

BACTERIAL TOXINS Among the first infectious diseases to be understood were those due to toxin-elaborating bacteria. Diphtheria, botulism, and tetanus toxins are responsible for the diseases associated with local infections due to *Corynebacterium diphtheriae*, *Clostridium botulinum*, and *Clostridium tetani*, respectively. Enterotoxins produced by *E. coli*, *Salmonella*, *Shigella*, *Staphylococcus*, and *V. cholerae* contribute to diarrheal disease caused by these organisms. Staphylococci, streptococci, *P. aeruginosa*, and *Bordetella* elaborate various toxins that cause or contribute to disease, including toxic shock syndrome toxin 1 (TSST-1); erythrogenic toxin; exotoxins A, S, and U; and pertussis toxin. A number of these toxins (e.g., cholera toxin, diphtheria toxin, pertussis toxin, *E. coli* heat-labile toxin, and *P. aeruginosa* exotoxin) have adenosine diphosphate (ADP)-ribosyltransferase activity; i.e., the toxins enzymatically catalyze the transfer of the ADP-ribosyl portion of nicotinamide adenine diphosphate to target proteins and inactivate them. The staphylococcal enterotoxins, TSST-1, and the streptococcal pyogenic exotoxins behave as superantigens, stimulating certain T cells to proliferate without processing of the protein toxin by antigen-presenting cells. Part of this process involves stimulation of the antigen-presenting cells to produce IL-1 and TNF-α, which have been implicated in many of the clinical features of diseases like toxic shock syndrome and scarlet fever. A number of gram-negative pathogens (*Salmonella*, *Yersinia*, and *P. aeruginosa*) possess the ability to inject toxins directly into host target cells by means of a complex set of proteins referred to as the type III secretion system.

ENDOTOXIN The lipid A portion of gram-negative LPS has potent biologic activities that cause many of the clinical manifestations of gram-negative bacterial sepsis, including fever, muscle proteolysis, uncontrolled intravascular coagulation, and shock. The effects of lipid A appear to be mediated by the production of potent cytokines due to LPS binding to CD14 and signal transduction via TLRs, particularly TLR4. Cytokines exhibit potent hypothermic activity through effects on the hypothalamus; they also increase vascular permeability, alter the activity of endothelial cells, and induce endothelial-cell procoagulant activity. Numerous therapeutic strategies aimed at neutralizing the effects of endotoxin are under investigation, but so far the results have been disappointing.

INVASION Many diseases are caused primarily by pathogens growing in tissue sites that are normally sterile. Pneumococcal pneumonia is mostly attributable to the growth of *S. pneumoniae* in the lung and the attendant host inflammatory response, although specific factors that enhance this process (e.g., pneumolysin) may be responsible for some of the pathogenic potential of the pneumococcus. Disease that follows bacteremia and invasion of the meninges by meningitis-producing bacteria such as *N. meningitidis*, *H. influenzae*, *E. coli* K1, and group B streptococci appears to be due solely to the ability of these organisms to gain access to these tissues, multiply in them, and provoke cytokine production leading to tissue-damaging host inflammation.

Specific molecular mechanisms accounting for tissue invasion by fungal and protozoal pathogens are less well described. Except for studies pointing to factors like capsule and melanin production by *C. neoformans* and possibly levels of cell wall glucans in some pathogenic fungi, the molecular basis for fungal invasiveness is not well defined. Melanism has been shown to protect the fungal cell against death caused by phagocyte factors such as nitric oxide, superoxide, and hypochlorite. Morphogenic variation and production of proteases (e.g., the *Candida* aspartyl proteinase) have been implicated in fungal invasion of host tissues.

If pathogens are effectively to invade host tissues (particularly the blood), they must avoid the major host defenses represented by complement and phagocytic cells. Bacteria most often avoid these defenses through their cell surface polysaccharides—either capsular polysaccharides or long O-side-chain antigens characteristic of the smooth LPS of gram-negative bacteria. These molecules can prevent the activation and/or deposition of complement opsonins or limit the access of phagocytic cells with receptors for complement opsonins to these molecules when they are deposited on the bacterial surface below the capsular layer. Another potential mechanism of microbial virulence is the ability of some organisms to present the capsule as an apparent self antigen through molecular mimicry. For example, the polysialic acid capsule of group B *N. meningitidis* is chemically identical to an oligosaccharide found on human brain cells.

Immunochemical studies of capsular polysaccharides have led to an appreciation of the tremendous chemical diversity that can result from the linking of a few monosaccharides. For example, three hexoses can link up in more than 300 different, potentially serologically distinct ways, while three amino acids have only six possible peptide combinations. Capsular polysaccharides have been used as effective vaccines against meningococcal meningitis as well as against pneumococcal and *H. influenzae* infections and may prove to be of value as vaccines against any organisms that express a nontoxic, immunogenic capsular polysaccharide. In addition, most encapsulated pathogens become virtually avirulent when capsule production is interrupted by genetic manipulation; this observation emphasizes the importance of this structure in pathogenesis.

HOST RESPONSE   The inflammatory response of the host is critical for interruption and resolution of the infectious process but also is often responsible for the signs and symptoms of disease. Infection promotes a complex series of host responses involving the complement, kinin, and coagulation pathways. The production of cytokines such as IL-1, TNF-α, and other factors regulated in part by the NF-κB transcription factor leads to fever, muscle proteolysis, and other effects, as noted above. An inability to kill or contain the microbe usually results in further damage due to the progression of inflammation and infection. For example, in many chronic infections, degranulation of host inflammatory cells can lead to release of host proteases, elastases, histamines, and other toxic substances that can degrade host tissues. Chronic inflammation in any tissue can lead to the destruction of that tissue and to clinical disease associated with loss of organ function, such as sterility from pelvic inflammatory disease caused by chronic infection with *N. gonorrhoeae*.

The nature of the host response elicited by the pathogen often determines the pathology of a particular infection. Local inflammation produces local tissue damage, while systemic inflammation, such as that seen during sepsis, can result in the signs and symptoms of septic shock. The severity of septic shock is associated with the degree of production of host effectors. Disease due to intracellular parasitism results from the formation of granulomas, wherein the host attempts to wall off the parasite inside a fibrotic lesion surrounded by fused epithelial cells that make up so-called multinucleated giant cells. A number of pathogens, particularly anaerobic bacteria, staphylococci, and streptococci, provoke the formation of an abscess, probably because of the presence of zwitterionic surface polysaccharides such as the capsular polysaccharide of *Bacteroides fragilis*. The outcome of an infection depends on the balance between an effective host response that eliminates a pathogen and an excessive inflammatory response that is associated with an inability to eliminate a pathogen and with the resultant tissue damage that leads to disease.

TRANSMISSION TO NEW HOSTS

As part of the pathogenic process, most microbes are shed from the host, often in a form infectious for susceptible individuals. However, the rate of transmissibility may not necessarily be high, even if the disease is severe in the infected individual, as these traits are not linked. Most pathogens exit via the same route by which they entered: respiratory pathogens by aerosols from sneezing or coughing or through salivary spread, gastrointestinal pathogens by fecal-oral spread, sexually transmitted diseases by venereal spread, and vector-borne organisms by either direct contact with the vector through a blood meal or indirect contact with organisms shed into environmental sources such as water. Microbial factors that specifically promote transmission are not well characterized. Respiratory shedding is facilitated by overproduction of mucous secretions, with consequently enhanced sneezing and coughing. Diarrheal toxins such as cholera toxin, *E. coli* heat-labile toxins, and *Shigella* toxins probably facilitate fecal-oral spread of microbial cells in the high volumes of diarrheal fluid produced during infection. The ability to produce phenotypic variants that resist hostile environmental factors (e.g., the highly resistant cysts of *E. histolytica* shed in feces) represents another mechanism of pathogenesis relevant to transmission. Blood parasites such as *Plasmodium* spp. change phenotype after ingestion by a mosquito—a prerequisite for the continued transmission of this pathogen. Venereally transmitted pathogens may undergo phenotypic variation due to the production of specific factors to facilitate transmission, but shedding of these pathogens into the environment does not result in the formation of infectious foci.

In summary, the molecular mechanisms used by pathogens to colonize, invade, infect, and disrupt the host are numerous and diverse. Each phase of the infectious process involves a variety of microbial and host factors interacting in a manner that can result in disease. Recognition of the coordinated genetic regulation of virulence factor elaboration when organisms move from their natural environment into the mammalian host emphasizes the complex nature of the host-parasite interaction. Fortunately, the need for diverse factors in successful infection and disease implies that a variety of therapeutic strategies may be developed to interrupt this process and thereby prevent and treat microbial infections.

BIBLIOGRAPHY

ANDERSON DM, SCHNEEWIND O: Type III machines of gram-negative pathogens: Injecting virulence factors into host cells and more. Curr Opin Microbiol 2:18, 1999

BERGER EA et al: Chemokine receptors as HIV-1 coreceptors: Roles in viral entry, tropism, and disease. Annu Rev Immunol 17:657, 1999

BRANDHORST TT: Targeted gene disruption reveals an adhesin indispensable for pathogenicity of *Blastomyces dermatitidis*. J Exp Med 189:1207, 1999

CHOW JC et al: Toll-like receptor-4 mediates lipopolysaccharide-induced signal transduction. J Biol Chem 274:10689, 1999

DAVIES DG et al: The involvement of cell-to-cell signals in the development of a bacterial biofilm. Science 280:295, 1998

ERNST RK et al: How intracellular bacteria survive: Surface modifications that promote resistance to host innate immune responses. J Infect Dis 179(Suppl 2):S326, 1999

GALE CA et al: Linkage of adhesion, filamentous growth, and virulence in *Candida albicans* to a single gene, *INT1*. Science 279:1355, 1998

GARTEN W, KLENK H-D: Understanding influenza virus pathogenicity. Trends Microbiol 7:99, 1999

MULVEY MA et al: Induction and evasion of host defenses by type 1–piliated uropathogenic *Escherichia coli*. Science 282:1494, 1998

PIER GB et al: *Salmonella typhi* uses CFTR to enter intestinal epithelial cells. Nature 392:79, 1998

SCHNEIDER-SCHAULIES S, TER MEULEN V: Pathogenic aspects of measles virus infections. Arch Virol Suppl 15:139, 1999

SOTO GE, HULTGREN SJ: Bacterial adhesins: Common themes and variations in architecture and assembly. J Bacteriol 181:1059, 1999

SVANBORG C et al: Cytokine responses during mucosal infections: Role in disease pathogenesis and host defence. Curr Opin Microbiol 2:99, 1999

LABORATORY DIAGNOSIS OF INFECTIOUS DISEASES

The laboratory diagnosis of infection requires the demonstration, either direct or indirect, of viral, bacterial, fungal, or parasitic agents in tissues, fluids, or excreta of the host. Clinical microbiology laboratories are responsible for processing these specimens and also for determining the antibiotic susceptibility of bacterial pathogens. Traditionally, detection of pathogenic agents has relied largely on either the microscopic visualization of pathogens in clinical material or the growth of microorganisms in the laboratory. Identification is generally based on phenotypic characteristics, such as fermentation profiles for bacteria, cytopathic effects in tissue culture for viral agents, and microscopic morphology for fungi and parasites. These techniques are reliable but are often time-consuming. Increasingly, the use of nucleic acid probes is becoming a standard detection and/or identification method in the clinical microbiology laboratory, gradually replacing phenotypic characterization and microscopic visualization methods.

DETECTION METHODS

Reappraisal of the methods employed in the clinical microbiology laboratory has led to the development of strategies for detection of pathogenic agents through nonvisual biologic signal detection systems. Much of this methodology is based on either computerization of detection systems with relatively inexpensive but sophisticated computers or the use of nucleic acid probes directed at specific DNA or RNA targets. This chapter discusses both the methods that are currently available and those that are being developed.

BIOLOGIC SIGNALS A *biologic signal* is a material that can be reproducibly differentiated from other substances present in the same physical environment. Key issues in the use of a biologic (or electronic) signal are distinguishing it from background noise and translating it into meaningful information. Examples of biologic signals applicable to clinical microbiology include structural components of bacteria, fungi, and viruses; specific antigens; metabolic end products; unique DNA or RNA base sequences; enzymes; toxins or other proteins; and surface polysaccharides.

DETECTION SYSTEMS A detector is used to sense a signal and to discriminate between the signal and background noise. Detection systems range from the trained eyes of a technologist assessing morphologic variations to sensitive electronic instruments, such as gas-liquid chromatographs coupled to computer systems for signal analysis. The sensitivity with which signals can be detected varies widely. It is essential to use a detection system that discerns small amounts of signal even when biologic background noise is present—i.e., that is both sensitive and specific. Common detection systems include immunofluorescence; chemiluminescence for DNA/RNA probes; flame ionization detection of short- or long-chain fatty acids; and detection of substrate utilization or end-product formation as color changes, of enzyme activity as a change in light absorbance, of turbidity changes, of cytopathic effects in cell lines, and of particle agglutination.

AMPLIFICATION Amplification enhances the sensitivity with which weak signals can be detected. The most common microbiologic amplification technique is growth of a single bacterium into a discrete colony on an agar plate or into a suspension containing many identical organisms. The advantage of growth as an amplification method is that it requires only an appropriate growth medium; the disadvantage is the amount of time required for amplification. More rapid specific amplification of biologic signals can be achieved with techniques such as polymerase (ligase) chain reactions (PCRs, for DNA/RNA), enzyme immunoassays (EIAs, for antigens and antibodies), electronic amplification (for gas-liquid chromatography assays), antibody capture methods (for concentration and/or separation), and selective filtration

or centrifugation. Although a variety of methods are available for the amplification and detection of biologic signals in research, thorough testing is required before they are validated as diagnostic assays.

DIRECT DETECTION

MICROSCOPY The field of microbiology has been defined largely by the development and use of the microscope. The examination of specimens by microscopic methods rapidly provides useful diagnostic information. Staining techniques permit organisms to be seen more clearly.

The simplest method for microscopic evaluation is the wet mount, which is used, for example, to examine cerebrospinal fluid (CSF) for the presence of *Cryptococcus neoformans*, with India ink as a background against which to visualize large-capsuled yeast cells. Wet mounts with dark-field illumination are also used to detect spirochetes from genital lesions and to reveal *Borrelia* or *Leptospira* in blood. Skin scrapings and hair samples can be examined with use of either 10% KOH wet-mount preparations or the calcofluor white method and ultraviolet illumination to detect fungal elements as fluorescing structures. Staining of wet mounts—for example, with lactophenol cotton blue stain for fungal elements—is often used for morphologic identification. These techniques enhance signal detection and decrease the background, making it easier to identify specific fungal structures.

STAINING **Gram's Stain** Without staining, bacteria are difficult to see at the magnifications (400 to 1000×) used for their detection. Although simple one-step stains can be used, differential stains are more common. Gram's stain differentiates between organisms with thick peptidoglycan cell walls (gram-positive) and those with outer membranes that can be dissolved with alcohol or acetone (gram-negative).

Gram's stain is particularly useful for examining sputum for polymorphonuclear leukocytes (PMNs) and bacteria. Sputum specimens with 25 or more PMNs and fewer than 10 epithelial cells per low-power field often provide clinically useful information. However, the presence in "sputum" samples of more than 10 epithelial cells per low-power field and of multiple bacterial types suggests contamination with oral microflora. Despite the difficulty of discriminating between normal microflora and pathogens, Gram's stain may prove useful for specimens from areas with a large resident microflora if a useful biologic marker (signal) is available. Gram's staining of vaginal swab specimens can be used to detect epithelial cells covered with gram-positive bacteria in the absence of lactobacilli and the presence of gram-negative rods—a scenario regarded as a sign of bacterial vaginosis. Similarly, examination of stained stool specimens for leukocytes is useful as a screening procedure before testing for *Clostridium difficile* toxin or other enteric pathogens.

The examination of CSF and joint, pleural, or peritoneal fluid with Gram's stain is useful for determining whether bacteria and/or PMNs are present. The sensitivity is such that $>10^4$ bacteria per milliliter should be detected. Centrifugation is often performed before staining to concentrate specimens thought to contain low numbers of organisms. The pellet is examined after staining. This simple method is particularly useful for examination of CSF for bacteria and white blood cells or of sputum for acid-fast bacilli (AFB).

Acid-Fast Stain The acid-fast stain identifies organisms that retain carbol fuchsin dye after acid/organic solvent disruption (e.g., *Mycobacterium* spp.). Modifications of this procedure allow the differentiation of *Actinomyces* from *Nocardia* or other weakly acid-fast organisms. The acid-fast stain is applied to sputum, other fluids, and tissue samples when AFB (e.g., *Mycobacterium* spp.) are suspected. The identification of the pink/red AFB against the blue background of the counterstain requires a trained eye, since few AFB may be detected in an entire smear, even when the specimen has been concentrated by centrifugation. An alternative method is the auramine-rhodamine combination fluorescent dye technique.

Fluorochrome Stains   Fluorochrome stains, such as acridine orange, are used to identify white blood cells, yeasts, and bacteria in body fluids. Other specialized stains, such as Dappe's stain, may be used for the detection of *Mycoplasma* in cell cultures. Capsular, flagellar, and spore stains are used for identification or demonstration of characteristic structures.

Immunofluorescent Stains   The direct immunofluorescent antibody technique uses antibody coupled to a fluorescing compound, such as fluorescein, and directed at a specific antigenic target to visualize organisms or subcellular structures. When samples are examined under appropriate conditions, the fluorescing compound absorbs ultraviolet light and reemits light at a higher (visible) wavelength detectable by the human eye. In the indirect immunofluorescent antibody technique, an unlabeled (target) antibody binds a specific antigen. The specimen is then stained with fluorescein-labeled polyclonal antibody directed at the target antibody. Because each unlabeled target antibody attached to the appropriate antigen has multiple sites for attachment of the second antibody, the visual signal can be intensified (i.e., amplified). This form of staining is called *indirect* because a two-antibody system is used to generate the signal for detection of the antigen. Both direct and indirect methods detect viral inclusions (e.g., cytomegalovirus and herpes simplex virus) within cultured cells as well as many difficult-to-grow bacterial agents (e.g., *Legionella pneumophila*) directly in clinical specimens.

MACROSCOPIC ANTIGEN DETECTION   Latex agglutination assays and EIAs are rapid and inexpensive methods for identifying organisms, extracellular toxins, and viral agents by means of protein and polysaccharide antigens. Such assays may be performed directly on clinical samples or after growth of organisms on agar plates or in viral cell cultures. The biologic signal in each case is the antigen to be detected. Monoclonal or polyclonal antibodies coupled to a reporter (such as latex particles or an enzyme) are used for detection of antibody-antigen binding reactions.

Techniques such as direct agglutination of bacterial cells with specific antibody are simple but relatively insensitive, while latex agglutination and EIAs are more sensitive. Some cell-associated antigens, such as capsular polysaccharides and lipopolysaccharides, can be detected by agglutination of a suspension of bacterial cells when antibody is added; this method is useful for typing of the somatic antigens of *Shigella* and *Salmonella*. In systems such as EIAs, which employ antibodies coupled to an enzyme, an antigen-antibody reaction results in the conversion of a colorless substrate to a colored product. Because the coupling of an enzyme to the antibody can amplify a weak biologic signal, the sensitivity of such assays is often high. In each instance, the basis for antigen detection is antigen-antibody binding, with the detection system changed to accommodate the biologic signal. Most such assays provide information as to whether antigen is present but do not quantify the antigen. EIAs are also useful for detecting bacterial toxins—e.g., *C. difficile* toxins A and B in stool.

DETECTION OF PATHOGENIC AGENTS BY CULTURE

SPECIMEN COLLECTION AND TRANSPORT   To culture bacterial, mycotic, or viral pathogens, an appropriate sample must be placed into the proper medium for growth (amplification). The success of efforts to identify a specific pathogen often depends on the collection and transport process coupled to a laboratory-processing algorithm suitable for the specific sample/agent. In some instances, it is better for specimens to be plated at the time of collection rather than first being transported to the laboratory (e.g., urethral swabs being cultured for *Neisseria gonorrhoeae* or sputum specimens for pneumococci). In general, the more rapidly a specimen is plated onto appropriate media, the better the chance for isolating bacterial pathogens. Appendix B lists procedures for collection and transport of common

specimens. Because there are many pathogen-specific paradigms for these procedures, it is important to seek advice from the microbiology laboratory when in doubt about a particular situation.

ISOLATION OF BACTERIAL PATHOGENS   Isolation of suspect pathogen(s) from clinical material relies on the use of artificial media that support bacterial growth in vitro. Such media are composed of agar, which is not metabolized by bacteria; nutrients to support the growth of the species of interest; and sometimes substances to inhibit the growth of other bacteria. Broth is employed for growth (amplification) of organisms from specimens with few bacteria, such as peritoneal dialysis fluid, CSF, or samples in which anaerobes or other fastidious organisms may be present. The general use of liquid medium for all specimens is not worthwhile.

Two basic strategies are used to isolate pathogenic bacteria. The first is to employ enriched media that support the growth of any bacteria that may be present in a sample such as blood or CSF, which contain no bacteria under normal conditions. Broths that allow the growth of small numbers of organisms may be subcultured to solid media when growth is detected. The second strategy is to isolate (amplify) specific bacterial species from stool, genital tract secretions, or sputum—sites that contain many bacteria under normal conditions. Antimicrobial agents or other inhibitory substances are incorporated into the agar medium to inhibit growth of all but the bacteria of interest. After incubation, organisms that grow on such media are further characterized to determine whether they are pathogens. Selection for organisms that may be pathogens from the normal microflora shortens the time required for diagnosis (Fig. 121-1).

ISOLATION OF VIRAL AGENTS   (See also Chap. 180) Pathogenic viral agents often are cultured when the presence of serum antibody is not a criterion for active infection or when an increase in serum antibody may not be detected during infection. The biologic signal—virus—is amplified to a detectable level. Although a number of techniques are available, an essential element is a monolayer of cultured mammalian cells sensitive to infection with the suspected virus. These cells serve as the amplification system by allowing the proliferation of viral particles. Virus may be detected by direct observation of the cultured cells for cytopathic effects or by immunofluorescent detection of viral antigens following incubation. Culture methods are particularly useful for detection of rapidly propagated agents, such as cytomegalovirus or herpes simplex virus.

AUTOMATION OF MICROBIAL DETECTION IN BLOOD

The detection of microbial pathogens in blood is difficult because the number of organisms present in the sample is often low and the organisms' integrity and ability to replicate may be damaged by humoral defense mechanisms or antimicrobial agents. Over the years, systems that rely on the detection of CO_2 produced by bacteria and yeasts in blood culture medium have allowed the automation of the detection procedure. The most common systems involve either the insertion of a sampling device into each culture bottle at periodic intervals, with drawing off of the head-space gas for analysis by an infrared monitor, or the use of reflectance optics, with a light-emitting diode and photodiode employed to detect a color change in a CO_2-sensitive indicator built into the bottom of the culture bottle. These systems measure CO_2 concentration as indicative of microbial growth. Sophisticated algorithms are used to evaluate the rate at which CO_2 is being produced and then to determine whether the rate of change is consistent with microbial growth. Such methods are no more sensitive than the human eye in detecting a positive culture; however, because the bottles in an automated system are monitored more frequently, a positive culture is often detected more rapidly than by manual techniques, and important information, including the result of Gram's stain and preliminary susceptibility assays, can be obtained sooner. One advantage of reflectance optic systems is that the bottles are scanned continuously in a

FIGURE 121-1 Common specimen-processing algorithms used in clinical microbiology laboratories. Abbreviations: BAP, blood agar plate; CMV, cytomegalovirus; CPE, cytopathic effects; CSF, cerebrospinal fluid; DFA, direct fluorescent antibody; EIA, enzyme immunoassay; ESBL, extended-spectrum β-lactamase; GBS, group B *Streptococcus*; GC, *Neisseria gonorrhoeae*; GLC, gas-liquid chromatography; HACEK, *Haemophilus aphrophilus/parainfluenzae/paraphrophilus*, *Actinobacillus actinomycetemcomitans*, *Cardiobacterium hominis*, *Eikenella corrodens*, and *Kingella kingae*; HE, Hektoen enteric medium; HepC, hepatitis C virus; HIV, human immunodeficiency virus; MRSA, methicillin-resistant *Staphylococcus aureus*; TB, *Mycobacterium tuberculosis*; VREF, vancomycin-resistant *Enterococcus faecium*.

noninvasive monitoring procedure, and thus the likelihood of laboratory contamination is decreased.

Automated systems also have been applied to the detection of microbial growth from specimens other than blood, such as peritoneal and other normally sterile fluids. *Mycobacterium* spp. can be detected in certain automated systems if appropriate liquid media are used for culture.

DETECTION OF PATHOGENIC AGENTS BY SEROLOGIC METHODS

Measurement of serum antibody provides an indirect marker for past or current infection with a specific viral agent or other pathogens, including *Brucella*, *Legionella*, *Rickettsia*, and *Helicobacter pylori*. The biologic signal is usually either IgM or IgG antibody directed at surface-expressed antigen(s). The detection systems include those used for bacterial antigens (agglutination reactions, immunofluorescence, and EIA) and unique systems such as hemolysis inhibition and complement fixation. Serologic methods generally fall into two categories: those that determine protective antibody levels and those that measure changing antibody titers during infection. Determination of an antibody response as a measure of current immunity is important in the case of viral agents for which there are vaccines, such as rubella virus or varicella-zoster virus; assays for this purpose normally use one or two dilutions of serum for a qualitative determination of protective antibody levels. Quantitative serologic assays to detect increases in antibody titers most often employ paired serum samples obtained 10 to 14 days apart (i.e., acute- and convalescent-phase samples). Since the incubation period before symptoms are noted may be long enough for an antibody response to occur, the demonstration of acute-phase antibody alone is often insufficient to establish the diagnosis of active infection as opposed to past exposure. In such circumstances, IgM may be useful as a measure of an early, acute-phase antibody response. A fourfold increase in total antibody titer or in EIA activity between the acute- and convalescent-phase samples is also regarded as evidence for active infection.

For certain viral agents, such as Epstein-Barr virus, the antibodies produced may be directed at different antigens during different phases of the infection. For this reason, most laboratories test for antibody directed at both viral capsid antigens and antigens associated with recently infected host cells to determine the stage of infection.

IDENTIFICATION METHODS

Once bacteria are isolated, traditional methods of phenotypic characterization are often used to identify specific isolates. An organism's phenotypic characteristics include traits that are readily detectable after growth on agar media (colony size, color, hemolytic reactions, odor), use of specific substrates and carbon sources (such as carbohydrates), formation of specific end products during growth, and microscopic appearance. Broth tubes containing specific substrates are commonly employed for phenotypic characterization. While such methods have been used since the time of Pasteur, their simplicity and low cost continue to make them appealing today.

CLASSIC PHENOTYPING Automated systems allow rapid phenotypic identification of bacterial pathogens. Most such systems are based on biotyping techniques, in which isolates are grown on multiple substrates and the reaction pattern is compared with known patterns for various bacterial species. This procedure is relatively fast, and commercially available systems include miniaturized fermentation, coding to simplify recording of results, and probability calculations for the most likely pathogens. If the biotyping approach is automated and the reading process is coupled to computer-based data analysis, rapidly growing organisms, such as Enterobacteriaceae, can be identified within hours of detection on agar plates.

Several systems use preformed enzymes for even speedier identification (within 2 to 3 h). Such systems do not rely on bacterial growth per se to determine whether a substrate has been used or not. They employ a heavy inoculum in which specific bacterial enzymes are present in sufficient quantity to convert substrate to product rapidly. In addition, some systems use fluorogenic substrate/end-product detection methods to increase sensitivity (through signal amplification).

GAS-LIQUID CHROMATOGRAPHY Gas-liquid chromatography is often used to detect metabolic end products of bacterial fermentations. One common application is identification of short-chain fatty acids produced by obligate anaerobes during glucose fermentation. Because the types and relative concentrations of volatile acids differ among the various genera and species that make up this group of organisms, such information serves as a metabolic "fingerprint" for a particular isolate.

Gas-liquid chromatography can be coupled to a sophisticated signal-analysis software system for identification and quantitation of long-chain fatty acids (LCFAs) in the outer membranes and cell walls of bacteria and fungi. For any given species, the types and relative concentrations of LCFAs are distinctive enough to allow identification of even closely related species. An organism may be identified definitively within a few hours after detection of growth on appropriate media. LCFA analysis is one of the most advanced procedures currently available for phenotypic characterization.

NUCLEIC ACID PROBES Techniques for the detection and quantitation of specific DNA and RNA base sequences in clinical specimens have become powerful tools for the diagnosis of bacterial, viral, parasitic, and fungal infections. The basic strategy is to detect a relatively short sequence of bases specific for a particular pathogen on single-stranded DNA or RNA by hybridization of a complementary sequence of bases (probe) coupled to a "reporter" system that serves as the signal for detection. Detection of an organism by nucleic acid probes offers a decided advantage over culture methods for difficult-to-grow organisms. Current technology encompasses a wide array of methods for amplification and signal detection, some of which have been approved by the U.S. Food and Drug Administration (FDA) for clinical diagnosis.

Use of nucleic acid probes generally involves lysis of intact cells and denaturation of the DNA or RNA to render it single-stranded. The probe may be hybridized to the target sequence in a solution or on a solid support, depending on the system employed. In situ hybridization of a probe to a target is also possible and allows the use of probes with agents present in tissue specimens. Once the probe has been hybridized to the target (biologic signal), a variety of strategies may be employed to amplify and/or quantify the target-probe complex (Fig. 121-2).

Probes for Direct Detection of Pathogens in Clinical Specimens Nucleic acid probes are available commercially for direct detection of various bacterial and parasitic pathogens, including *L. pneumophila*, *Chlamydia trachomatis*, *N. gonorrhoeae*, group A *Streptococcus*, *Gardnerella vaginalis*, *Mycoplasma hominis*, and *Giardia lamblia*. In addition, probes for direct detection of human papillomavirus, *Can-*

dida spp., and *Trichomonas vaginalis* have been approved. An assortment of probes for confirming the identity of cultured pathogens, such as *Mycobacterium* and *Salmonella* spp., are also available. Probes for the direct detection of bacterial pathogens are often aimed at highly conserved 16S ribosomal RNA sequences, of which there are many more copies than there are of any single genomic DNA sequence in a bacterial cell. The sensitivity and specificity of probe assays for direct detection are comparable to those of more traditional assays, including EIA and culture. Many laboratories have developed their own probes for pathogens; however, unless a method-validation protocol for diagnostic testing has been performed, the use of such probes is restricted to research by federal law in the United States.

Nucleic Acid Probe Target-Amplification Strategies In theory, a single target nucleic acid sequence can be amplified to detectable levels. There are several strategies for target and/or probe amplification, including PCR, ligase chain reaction, strand displacement amplification, and self-sustaining sequence replication. In each case, a target sequence or hybridized probe is amplified exponentially to obtain sufficient signal for detection, usually by the attachment of chemiluminescent reporter groups to the amplified product. The PCR strategy requires repeated heating of the DNA or RNA to separate the two complementary strands of the double helix, hybridization of a primer sequence to the appropriate target sequence, target amplification using the PCR for complementary strand extension, and signal detection via a labeled probe. The sensitivity of such assays is far greater than that of traditional assay methods such as culture. However, the care with which the assays are performed is important, because cross-contamination of clinical material with DNA or RNA from other sources (even at low levels) can cause false-positive results. An alternative method employs transcription-mediated amplification, in which an RNA target sequence is converted to DNA, which is then exponentially transcribed into RNA target. The advantage of this method is that only a single heating/annealing step is required for amplification. At present, amplification assays for *Mycobacterium tuberculosis*, *N. gonorrhoeae*, *C. trachomatis*, and *M. hominis* are on the market. Again, many laboratories have used commercially available *taq* polymerase, probe sequences, and reagents to develop "in-house" assays for diagnostic use. Issues related to quality control, interpretation of results, sample processing, and regulatory requirements have slowed the commercial development of diagnostic assay kits.

Signal Amplification Strategies Alternative systems for signal amplification have great appeal, particularly for quantitative determination of the amount of target present in a given specimen. With the advent of newer therapeutic regimens for HIV-associated disease, cytomegalovirus infection, and hepatitis C virus infection, the response to therapy has been monitored by determining both genotype and "viral load" at various times after treatment initiation. Target amplification (PCR, transcription-mediated amplification) is difficult to control in a manner that allows accurate determination of the original target (genome) concentration. In other systems, probes attached to complementary target sequences are amplified by the attachment of a second probe and an amplification multimer to the original probe. In one such system, branched-chain DNA (bDNA)-based amplification, bDNA is attached to a site different from the target-binding sequence of the original probe. Chemiluminescent-labeled oligonucleotides can then bind to multiple repeating sequences on the bDNA. The amplified bDNA signal is detected by chemiluminescence. Alternatively, a DNA probe may be attached to an RNA target and the resulting DNA/RNA hybrid captured on a solid support by antibody specific for DNA/RNA hybrids (concentration/amplification) and detected by chemiluminescent-labeled antibody specific for DNA/RNA hybrids. Both methods can be used to determine the approximate number of target copies (virus) in the starting material. The advantage of these systems over PCR is that only a single heating/annealing step is required to hybridize the target-binding probe to the target sequence for amplification.

Application of Nucleic Acid Probe Technology Nucleic acid probe technology is being used to identify difficult-to-grow or non-cultivable bacterial pathogens, such as *Mycobacterium*, *Legionella*,

FIGURE 121-2 Strategies for amplification and/or detection of a target-probe complex. DNA or RNA extracted from microorganisms is heated to create single-stranded (ss) DNA/RNA containing appropriate target sequences. These target sequences may be hybridized directly (direct detection) with probes attached to reporter molecules; they may be amplified by repetitive cycles of complementary strand extension (polymerase chain reaction) before attachment of a reporter probe; or the original target-probe signal may be amplified via hybridization with an additional probe containing multiple copies of a secondary reporter target sequence (branched-chain DNA, or bDNA). DNA/RNA hybrids can also be "captured" on a solid support (hybrid capture), with antibody directed at the DNA/RNA hybrids used to concentrate them and a second antibody coupled to a reporter molecule attached to the captured hybrid.

Ehrlichia, Rickettsia, Babesia, Borrelia, and *Tropheryma whippelii.* Amplification methods are also being used to detect chronic viral infections, such as herpes simplex encephalitis, cytomegalovirus infection, and hepatitis C. The monitoring of therapy with quantitative viral-load testing is a significant new application of nucleic acid technology. Further applications will likely include the replacement of culture for identification of many pathogens with solid-state DNA/RNA chip technology, in which thousands of unique nucleic acid sequences can be detected on a single computer chip. Probe technology also has the potential to detect viral pathogens faster than is possible with current culture techniques. However, if laboratories are to take full advantage of probe technology, the cost of reagents and assay automation must be competitive with the cost of existing methodology. At present, the detection of agents such as *C. trachomatis* or *N. gonorrhoeae* by probe technology is more expensive for most laboratories than detection by traditional culture or EIA. Moreover, because automated processing equipment is just beginning to find its way into the laboratory for these assays, nucleic acid amplification methods are both more labor-intensive and more expensive than other detection systems. In the absence of clear documentation of clinical utility, many laboratories continue to wait for FDA approval of commercially available DNA/RNA probe assays rather than validating in-house assays.

SUSCEPTIBILITY TESTING A principal responsibility of the clinical microbiology laboratory is to determine which antimicrobial agents inhibit a specific bacterial isolate. Such testing is used to screen for infection control problems, such as methicillin-resistant *Staphylococcus aureus*, vancomycin-resistant *Enterococcus faecium*, or extended-spectrum β-lactamase-producing organisms. Two approaches are useful. The first is a qualitative assessment of susceptibility, with responses categorized as susceptible, resistant, or intermediate. This approach can involve either the placement of paper disks containing antibiotics on an agar surface inoculated with the bacterial strain to be tested (Kirby-Bauer or disk/agar diffusion method), with measurement of the zones of growth inhibition following incubation, or the use of broth tubes containing a set concentration of antibiotic (breakpoint method). These methods have been carefully calibrated against quantitative methods and clinical experience with each antibiotic, and zones of inhibition and breakpoints have been calculated on a species-by-species basis.

The second approach is to inoculate the test strain of bacteria into a series of broth tubes (or agar plates) with increasing concentrations of antibiotic. The lowest concentration of antibiotic that inhibits microbial growth in this test system is known as the *minimum inhibitory concentration* (MIC). If tubes in which no growth occurs are subcultured, the minimum concentration of antibiotic required to kill the starting inoculum can also be determined (*minimum bactericidal concentration*, or MBC). Quantitative susceptibility testing by the microbroth dilution technique, a miniaturized version of the broth dilution technique using microwell plates, lends itself to automation and is commonly used in larger clinical laboratories.

A novel version of the disk/agar diffusion method employs a quantitative diffusion gradient, or epsilometer (E-test), and uses an absorbent strip with a known gradient of antibiotic concentrations along its length. When the strip is placed on the surface of an agar plate seeded with a bacterial strain to be tested, antibiotic diffuses into the medium, and bacterial growth is inhibited. The MIC is estimated as the lowest concentration that inhibits growth.

For some organisms, such as obligate anaerobes, routine susceptibility testing generally is not performed because of the difficulty of growing the organisms and the predictable sensitivity of most isolates to specific antibiotics.

BIBLIOGRAPHY

McNicol AM et al: In situ hybridization and its diagnostic applications in pathology. J Pathol 182:250, 1997

Miller JM et al: Specimen collection, transport and storage, in *Manual of Clinical Microbiology*, 6th ed, P Murray et al (eds). Washington, DC, American Society for Microbiology, 1995

Salfinger M et al: Diagnostic tools in tuberculosis. Present and future. Respiration 65: 163, 1998

Sarasini A et al: Diagnostic significance and clinical impact of quantitative assays for diagnosis of human cytomegalovirus infection/disease in immunocompromised patients. New Microbiol 21:293, 1998

Trabaud MA et al: Comparison of HCV RNA assays for the detection and quantification of hepatitis C virus RNA levels in serum of patients with chronic hepatitis C treated with interferon. J Med Virol 52:105, 1997

Yeghiazarian T et al: Quantitation of human immunodeficiency virus type 1 RNA levels in plasma by using small-volume-format branched-DNA assays. J Clin Microbiol 36: 2096, 1998

122 *Gerald T. Keusch, Kenneth J. Bart*

IMMUNIZATION PRINCIPLES AND VACCINE USE

CDC	Centers for Disease Control and Prevention	HBV hepatitis B virus
DTaP	diphtheria/tetanus/acellular pertussis vaccine	Hib *H. influenzae* type b
		IPV inactivated poliovirus vaccine
DTP	diphtheria/tetanus/pertussis	MMR measles/mumps/rubella
FDA	Food and Drug Administration	NCVIA National Childhood Vaccine Injury Act
GMPs	good manufacturing practices	OPV oral poliovirus vaccine
HBsAg	hepatitis B surface antigen	Td tetanus/diphtheria

Most humans live their lives ignoring the certainty of their own mortality. Perhaps this fact explains why the adage "an ounce of prevention is worth a pound of cure" has so little effect on their everyday behavior. Even when it comes to acting to protect their young, parents are capable of ignoring the potential for mortality among their children (in the developed world) and of accepting the certainty of childhood deaths (in the developing world). In both settings, parents all too often fail to seek out and demand the best preventive measures available. Unless mandated by the law in the former setting or provided by benevolent organizations or governments in the latter, universal immunization has invariably remained an unattained goal. Compulsion and benevolence, it seems, are two essential components of immunization.

However, the integration of immunization practices (a major component of primary disease prevention) into routine health care services has provided caregivers with control over a substantial proportion of the disease and mortality that plagued the United States during the first half of the twentieth century (Table 122-1). For society today, immunization represents one of the most cost-effective means of preventing infectious disease. For every dollar spent, diphtheria/tetanus/pertussis (DTP) vaccine saves $29, measles/mumps/rubella (MMR) vaccine saves $21, trivalent oral poliovirus vaccine (OPV) saves $6, varicella vaccine saves $5, and *Haemophilus influenzae* type b vaccine saves $2. At present, >50 biologic products are licensed in the United States, and 6 vaccines (12 antigens) are used for routine immunization in the young, including diphtheria/tetanus/acellular pertussis vaccine (DTaP), inactivated poliovirus vaccine (IPV), MMR, *H. influenzae* type b (Hib) vaccine, hepatitis B virus (HBV) vaccine, and varicella vaccine. Five vaccines are designed for routine use in adults: tetanus/diphtheria (Td) toxoids, adsorbed, for adult use; HBV vaccine; influenza virus vaccine; polyvalent pneumococcal polysaccharide vaccine; and varicella vaccine. Some preparations are designated as special-use vaccines (e.g., hepatitis A vaccine for travelers). Unfortunately, vaccines for eukaryotic pathogens (protozoa and helminths), which affect a large proportion of the world's population, have been difficult to develop and remain only a hope for the future.

IMPACT OF IMMUNIZATION The epidemiologically appropriate use of vaccines has resulted in the global eradication of smallpox and in the potential eradication of poliomyelitis in the next few years and of measles by 2020. Already achieved are the virtual elimination of congenital rubella syndrome, tetanus, and diphtheria as well as a dramatic reduction in pertussis, rubella, measles, and mumps in the United States. The introduction of Hib conjugate vaccines for immunization of infants has all but eliminated invasive *Haemophilus* infections (including meningitis and pneumonia), presumably because these vaccines also reduce nasopharyngeal carriage of Hib and induce protection before the period of greatest vulnerability in infancy. The recently licensed polyvalent pneumococcal polysaccharide conjugate vaccine promises to have the same impact on invasive pneumococcal disease, including otitis media.

DEFINITIONS *Vaccination* and *immunization* are often used as interchangeable terms. However, the former denotes only the administration of a vaccine or toxoid, whereas the latter describes the process of inducing or providing immunity by any means, whether active or passive. Thus, vaccination does not guarantee immunization. *Active immunization* refers to the induction of immune defenses by the administration of antigens in appropriate forms, whereas *passive immunization* involves the provision of temporary protection by the administration of exogenously produced immune substances. Immunizing agents thus include vaccines, toxoids, and antibody-containing immunoglobulin preparations from human or animal donors (Table 122-2).

PRINCIPLES OF IMMUNIZATION Artificial induction of immunity closely follows two well-tested principles of nature. The first, active immunization, can be traced at least as far back as Thucydides, who noted that people surviving epidemics of plague in Athens were spared during later outbreaks of the same disease. The second, passive immunization, is a natural process as well and is exemplified by the transplacental transmission of maternal antibodies to the fetus to provide protection against several diseases during the first months of life. Use of the two measures together may produce a complementary effect (as with HBV vaccine plus hepatitis B immune globulin) or may actually interfere with the development of immunity (as when measles vaccine is administered within 6 weeks of immunoglobulin). Depending on whether there are multiple species or serotypes of an organism and—if so—whether there are common, cross-reactive, protective antigens, a specific vaccine may induce protection against all representative forms of an infectious agent or against the immunizing strain only. One of the intrinsic virtues of whole-organism vaccines is that they potentially contain all protective antigens of the organism. However, this virtue is counterbalanced by an inherent problem with such vaccines: the possibility of adverse responses to reactive but nonprotective antigens present in the mix. Because the immune response to specific antigens is controlled genetically, all individuals cannot be expected to respond identically to the same vaccine.

APPROACHES TO ACTIVE IMMUNIZATION The two standard approaches to active immunization are (1) the use of live, generally attenuated, infectious agents (e.g., measles virus); and (2) the use of inactivated agents or their constituents or products obtained by genetic recombination (e.g., acellular pertussis vaccines). For many diseases (e.g., poliomyelitis, influenza), both approaches have been employed. Live attenuated vaccines are believed to induce an immunologic response more nearly like that resulting from natural infection than the response induced by killed vaccines. Currently available inactivated or killed vaccines consist of inactivated whole organisms (e.g., plague vaccine); detoxified protein exotoxins (e.g., tetanus toxoid); recombinant protein antigens (e.g., HBV vaccine); or carbohydrate antigens, either present as soluble purified capsular material (e.g., *Streptococcus pneumoniae* polysaccharides) or conjugated to a protein carrier (e.g., Hib polysaccharide conjugated to diphtheria or tetanus toxoids).

Table 122-1 Changes in Morbidity due to Vaccine-Preventable Diseases in the United States

Disease	Baseline 20th-Century Annual Morbidity	Year Vaccine Introduced	1998 Provisional Morbidity	Decrease, %
Diphtheria	175,885	1923	1	>99.99
Pertussis	147,271	1926	6279	95.7
Tetanus	1314	1927	34	97.4
Poliomyelitis, paralytic	16,316	1955	0	100
Measles	503,282	1963	89	>99.99
Mumps	152,209	1967	606	99.6
Rubella (congenital)	47,745 (823)	1969	345 (5)	99.3 (99.4)
Haemophilus influenzae type b	20,000	1985	54	99.7

SOURCE: National Vaccine Program Office, Centers for Disease Control and Prevention [MMWR 48(12):243, 1999].

APPROACHES TO PASSIVE IMMUNIZATION Passive immunization is generally used to provide temporary immunity in an unimmunized subject exposed to an infectious disease when active immunization either is unavailable (e.g., for cytomegalovirus infection) or has not been implemented before exposure (e.g., for rabies). Passive immunization is used in the treatment of certain disorders associated with toxins (e.g., diphtheria), in certain bites (those of snakes and spiders), and as a specific or nonspecific immunosuppressant [Rho(D) immune globulin and antilymphocyte globulin, respectively].

Three types of preparations are used in passive immunization: (1) standard human immune serum globulin for general use (e.g., gamma globulin), administered intramuscularly or intravenously; (2) special immune serum globulins with a known content of antibody for specific agents (e.g., HBV or varicella-zoster immune globulin); and (3) animal sera and antitoxins.

ROUTE OF ADMINISTRATION The route of administration in part determines the rapidity and nature of the immune responses to vaccines. Vaccines can be administered orally, intranasally, intradermally, subcutaneously, or intramuscularly. Parenterally administered vaccine may not induce mucosal secretory IgA, and mucosal immunization may not induce good systemic responses. Vaccines must be administered by the licensed route to ensure immunogenicity and safety. For example, administration of HBV vaccine into the gluteal rather than the deltoid muscle often fails to induce an adequate immune response, while subcutaneous rather than intramuscular administration of DTP increases the risk of reactions.

AGE Because age influences the response to vaccines, schedules for immunization are based on age-dependent responses determined empirically from clinical trials. The presence of high levels of maternal antibody and/or the immaturity of the immune system in the early months of life impairs the initial immune response to some vaccines (e.g., measles or Hib polysaccharide but not HBV). In the elderly, vaccine responses may be diminished because of natural waning of the immune system. Hence, larger amounts of an antigen may be required to produce the desired response (e.g., in vaccination against influenza).

ADJUVANT POTENTIATION The immune response to some antigens is potentiated by the addition of adjuvants such as aluminum salts or, in the case of polysaccharides (e.g., the polyribose phosphate oligosaccharide of Hib), by conjugation to a carrier protein. Adjuvants, nonspecific boosters of immune responses, are used with inactivated products such as diphtheria and tetanus toxoids, acellular pertussis (aP) vaccine, and HBV vaccine. The mechanism for adjuvant enhancement of immunogenicity is not well defined but relates in part to the rendering of soluble antigens into a particulate form, the mobilization of phagocytes to the site of antigen deposition, and the slowing down of the release of antigens, which prolongs stimulation of the immune response.

THE IMMUNE RESPONSE While many constituents of infectious microorganisms and their products, such as exotoxins, are or can be made to be immunogenic, only a limited number stimulate a protective immune response. The immune system is complex, and antigen composition and presentation are critical for stimulation of the desired immune responses.

The Primary Response In the primary response to a vaccine antigen, an apparent latent period of several days precedes the detection of humoral and cell-mediated immunity. Although the immune response is turned on by contact with the antigen and the immune system, measurable circulating antibodies do not appear for 7 to 10 days. The immunoglobulin class of the response also changes over time. Early-appearing IgM antibodies generally exhibit only low affinity for the antigen, whereas later-appearing IgG antibodies display high affinity. For "thymus-dependent" antigens, CD4+ T helper lymphocytes control the switch from IgM to IgG. Some individuals do not respond, even when presented repeatedly with a vaccine antigen, often because they lack the major histocompatibility complex determinants required to recognize the antigen. This situation is known as *primary vaccine failure*.

The Secondary Response Heightened humoral or cell-mediated responses are elicited by a second exposure to the same antigen. These secondary responses occur rapidly, usually within 4 or 5 days, and result, for example, in increased titers of IgG antibody. The secondary response depends on immunologic memory after the first exposure and is characterized by a marked proliferation of antibody-producing B lymphocytes and/or effector T cells. Polysaccharide vaccines, such as that for *S. pneumoniae*, evoke immune responses that are independent of T cells and are not enhanced by repeated administration. Covalent linking of polysaccharides to proteins converts the former to T cell–dependent antigens that induce immunologic memory and secondary responses to revaccination. Although levels of vaccine-induced antibodies may decline over time (*secondary vaccine failure*), revaccination or exposure to the organism may elicit a rapid protective secondary response consisting of IgG antibodies with little or no detectable IgM. This *anamnestic response* indicates that immunity has persisted. The lack of measurable antibody does not necessarily mean that the

Table 122-2 Definitions of Immunizing Agents

Term	Definition
Vaccine	A suspension of attenuated live or killed microorganisms or antigenic portions of these agents presented to a potential host to induce immunity and prevent disease
Toxoid	A modified bacterial toxin that has been made nontoxic but retains the capacity to stimulate the formation of antitoxin
Immune globulin	An antibody-containing solution derived from human blood by cold ethanol fractionation of large pools of plasma and used primarily for maintenance of the immunity of immunodeficient persons or for passive immunization; intramuscular and intravenous preparations available
Antitoxin	An antibody derived from the serum of animals after stimulation with specific antigens and used to provide passive immunity

individual is unprotected. Furthermore, the mere presence of detectable antibodies after the administration of some vaccines and toxoids does not ensure clinical protection. A minimal circulating level of antibody is known to be required for protection from some diseases (e.g., 0.01 IU/mL for tetanus antitoxin).

Hypersensitivity Reactions   Independent of antibody production, the stimulation of the immune system by vaccination may elicit unanticipated responses, especially hypersensitivity reactions. In the past, killed measles vaccine induced incomplete humoral immunity and cell-mediated hypersensitivity, resulting in the development of a syndrome of atypical measles in some children after subsequent exposure; thus this type of vaccine is no longer in use.

Mucosal Immunity   Some pathogens are confined to and replicate only at mucosal surfaces (e.g., *Vibrio cholerae*), while others are able to penetrate the mucosa and replicate (e.g., poliovirus, rubella virus, and influenza virus). At the mucosal site, these organisms induce secretory IgA. The induction of secretory IgA by vaccines may be an efficient way to block the essential first steps in pathogenesis, whether the organism is restricted to mucosal surfaces or systemically invades the host across mucosal surfaces.

Measurement of the Immune Response   Immune responses to vaccines are often gauged by the concentration of specific antibody in serum. While seroconversion serves as a dependable indicator of an immune response, it measures only one immunologic parameter and does not necessarily indicate protection. The development of circulating antibodies after immunization often correlates directly with clinical protection (e.g., against measles or rubella). Some responses may not in themselves confer immunity but may be sufficiently associated with protection that they remain useful proxy measures of protective immunity (e.g., vibriocidal serum antibodies in cholera).

HERD IMMUNITY   It is not necessary to immunize every person in order to stop transmission of an infectious agent through a population. For those organisms dependent on person-to-person transmission, there may be a definable prevalence of immunity in the population above which it becomes difficult for the organism to circulate and reach new susceptibles. This prevalence is called *herd immunity*. When herd immunity is operative, the goals of immunization are converted from the immunization of every person in the community to the immunization of a specified minimum percentage of persons at risk. Herd immunity may wane if immunization capacity fails (as in diphtheria in the new independent states of the former Soviet Union) or if a sufficient percentage of individuals refuse to be immunized (as in pertussis in the United Kingdom and Japan in the 1970s because concern about infrequent—albeit severe—vaccine reactions came to exceed the fear of the disease itself). In both situations, loss of herd immunity led to renewed circulation of the organism and increased susceptibility to infection, with subsequent large outbreaks.

TARGET POPULATIONS AND TIMING OF IMMUNIZATION   For common and highly communicable childhood diseases like measles, the target population is the universe of susceptible individuals, and the time to immunize is as early in life as is feasible. Epidemiologic differences in measles in different settings, however, dictate different strategies of immunization. In the industrialized world, immunization with live-virus vaccine at 12 to 15 months of age has been the norm because the vaccine protects >95% of those immunized at this age and there is little measles morbidity/mortality among very young infants. In contrast, in the developing world, measles accounts for a significant proportion of deaths of young infants. Thus it is desirable to immunize children during the first few months of life in order to narrow the window of vulnerability between the rapid decline of maternal antibody after 4 to 6 months and the development of vaccine-induced active immunity.

Hib causes meningitis, epiglottitis, and pneumonia in early childhood, with rates rising sharply after the disappearance of maternally derived antibody. The first Hib vaccines often failed when administered during infancy; this failure was due mainly to an age-related inability to respond to polysaccharide antigens. To overcome this problem, the protective polysaccharide was coupled to protein and converted to a T cell–dependent antigen to which young infants could respond.

In contrast to measles and Hib infection, rubella is primarily a threat to the fetus; young infants and children are not at risk of serious illness. Given the susceptibility of the fetus, immunization of all women of reproductive age before pregnancy would be an ideal strategy. However, it is difficult to systematically vaccinate adolescent and young-adult females. Thus, to assure the protection of as many women as possible, the rubella component is included in a combination vaccine with mumps and measles (MMR) that is administered during infancy.

Some vaccines are now used primarily for adults. For example, influenza virus and polyvalent pneumococcal polysaccharide vaccines are used to prevent pneumonia deaths in the elderly. Unfortunately, these vaccines are underutilized, in part because physicians and otherwise healthy individuals in the target group ignore the indications and in part because there is still a tendency to think about disease prevention with vaccines as a strategy for children. Pneumococcal polysaccharide vaccine is also recommended for children >2 years old who are at risk of severe or even life-threatening pneumococcal infection, such as those with sickle cell disease, asplenia (whether functional or anatomic), renal failure with nephrotic syndrome, cerebrospinal fluid leak, and HIV infection or other immunosuppressive disease states.

THE DEVELOPMENT OF VACCINES

BIOLOGIC IMPEDIMENTS   There are often major technical problems to overcome in vaccine development. Although just one major antigenic type of influenza virus is typically in circulation at any one time, the virus is characterized biologically by its antigenic drift. Thus, a new antigenic version capable of causing a global pandemic emerges periodically, and a new vaccine must be rapidly devised, produced, and distributed. In contrast, many prevalent pneumococcal polysaccharide serotypes circulate at all times. Because immunity to the pneumococcus is serotype specific, an individual is susceptible to all serotypes against which he or she lacks antibody. Serotype-specific protection has made it more difficult to develop an effective pneumococcal vaccine than it was to develop a vaccine against *H. influenzae*, of which one capsular serotype (type b) is associated with nearly all cases of severe disease. To overcome this problem, pneumococcal vaccine currently includes 23 polysaccharides that represent ~80% of the virulent serotypes commonly encountered in the United States. Unfortunately, some serotypes are poorly immunogenic, and immunized individuals remain susceptible to the serotypes not included in the vaccine.

STRATEGY FOR VACCINE DEVELOPMENT   Vaccine development depends on the systematic application of a four-phase strategy: (1) studies in animals to identify protective antigen, (2) determination of how to present this antigen effectively to the immune system, (3) assessment of the safety and immunogenicity of the preparation in small and then in large human populations at various ages, and (4) evaluation of safety and efficacy in the target population. Each of these steps is simple in concept but difficult in execution, not least because of the clinical trials necessary to assess safety and efficacy; failure at any level stops the process. Thus, in 1995, >190 candidate vaccines were under investigation, but just 5 new products were licensed in the United States. Progress in immunology has taught us much about the organization and function of the immune system (Chap. 305); it has also taught us that the immune system is complicated and that details of antigen composition and presentation are critical for stimulating desired immune responses.

Ultimately, vaccines for humans must be tested in humans. After initial animal studies and small phase 1 and 2 human studies to assess immune responses, optimal dosage, and safety, clinical trials of vaccine efficacy are performed, sometimes with informed volunteers who are challenged with a virulent strain. Larger clinical effectiveness trials in the community, typically involving 1000 to 10,000 vaccinees, may lead to application for licensure. Because of their limited size, however, these trials cannot be expected to detect rare adverse effects. Thus, licensing does not guarantee that a new vaccine is completely safe, and postlicensing monitoring is needed to ensure effectiveness and to document the occurrence of adverse events of low frequency. In 1999, the recently licensed rhesus rotavirus vaccine was withdrawn because postmarketing surveillance uncovered an association with a rare event in infants, intussusception of the bowel.

The development of vaccines goes beyond technology and proof of principle to issues such as development costs, manufacturers' liability and indemnity, perceived public health needs, and the likelihood that a product will be used or sold. Given the complex science required, the costs of vaccine development are high and success is uncertain, adding risk to the development decision. It is unfortunate that the one sure implication of uncertainty in vaccine development is increased cost. In addition, a rational assignment of costs for development between the public and private sectors in the United States has never been achieved.

VACCINE FORMULATIONS Studies of clinical immunology have shown that living and dead antigens do not necessarily induce the same immune responses and that the requirements for the development of protective immunity differ with the organism. These insights, together with the refinement of epidemiologic concepts surrounding immunization, have changed the strategy of vaccine development. The goal is not only to select the correct antigens but also to ensure that the vaccines will result in the type of immune response needed for protection, whether the T cell–mediated activation of macrophages or the generation of cytotoxic T cells, B cell–mediated secretory IgA, or a particular IgG subtype response to a specific polysaccharide epitope.

Live vaccines consist of selected or genetically altered organisms that are avirulent or dramatically attenuated yet remain immunogenic. These agents are expected to cause a subclinical illness that mimics natural infection except for the lack of clinically significant disease. They offer the advantage of replication in vivo, which increases the antigenic load presented to the host's immune system; they may confer lifelong protection with one dose; they present all expressed antigens, thus overcoming immunogenetic restrictions in some hosts; they may reach the local sites most relevant to the induction of protective immunity; and they may produce important protective antigens in vivo that are not efficiently expressed in vitro.

Nonviable vaccines may fail to elicit mucosal IgA-mediated immunity, as they lack a delivery system that will effectively transport them to local antigen-processing cells. Moreover, except for pure polysaccharide antigens, these preparations must almost always be given in multiple doses to induce effective responses. However, killed vaccines can be extremely effective. For example, the nonviable hepatitis A vaccine formulation appears to be close to 100% effective in inducing protective immunity. Methods are under development to incorporate vaccine antigens into degradable polymers that may release antigen at predictable times after a single inoculation and simulate multiple injections over time of the same vaccine.

In spite of their advantages, live vaccines are not always to be preferred. For example, live OPV is contraindicated for use in children with immune-deficiency diseases and in their adult contacts. In addition, even though killed poliovirus vaccine does not completely immunize the gut and can neither reduce the circulation of wild-type poliovirus nor immunize contacts of vaccine recipients, the United States has now switched to a four-dose schedule of this vaccine because of the risk of vaccine-associated polio posed by live OPV.

To create a deliverable vaccine, constituents other than the antigens are required (Table 122-3). These constituents can affect the immunogenicity, efficacy, and safety of a vaccine and can render one formulation superior to another.

NEW VACCINE APPROACHES The first generation of vaccines included whole killed—or, more recently, live—attenuated microorganisms or partially purified microbial products, such as teta-

Table 122-3   Constituents of Vaccines

Constituent(s)	Examples/Purpose
Preservatives, stabilizers, antibiotics	These components are used to prevent the vaccine's deterioration before use, to inhibit or prevent bacterial growth, or to stabilize the antigen. Any of these additives may elicit allergic reactions.
Adjuvants	An aluminum salt is used in some vaccines (e.g., toxoids, hepatitis B vaccine) to enhance the immune response.
Suspending fluid	The suspending fluid can be sterile water, saline, buffer, or more complex fluids derived from the growth medium or biologic system in which the agent is produced (e.g., egg antigens, cell culture ingredients, serum proteins).

nus toxoid, that induced protective antibodies. The second generation of vaccines has taken advantage of molecular genetics and protein chemistry to isolate and manipulate purified proteins or components or subunits of organisms or to generate genetically engineered and attenuated live native organisms or cloned antigens expressed by harmless vector organisms. One conceptual leap is the production of transgenic plants expressing protective vaccine antigens (cloned, for example, in potatoes or bananas) that, when ingested orally, induce mucosal and systemic immune responses to homologous infectious challenges. While the practical use of this technique awaits further refinement, the concept that protective immunity can be induced in this manner has been proven in both animals and humans. Ease of production, stability, ease of administration without equipment, and low cost are the obvious advantages.

Another conceptual leap has led to a third generation of vaccines, in which nucleic acids (either DNA or RNA) are used to induce immunity. Development of DNA vaccines is at a more advanced stage. The principle is simple. First, a DNA plasmid containing the gene sequence for the immunogenic protein or fragment of interest is assembled, and the gene is placed under the control of a strong promoter and an appropriate transcription termination sequence. A single immunization with the plasmid (via intramuscular or intradermal injection, helium-accelerated gene gun injection of DNA-coated gold particles, compressed-air pneumatic jet injection of soluble DNA, direct skin application after suitable preparation, or even insertion of biodegradable stents loaded with the DNA of interest) results in DNA uptake into cells where the gene is expressed and processed normally; thus the product stimulates an immune response. Alteration of the DNA construct or of the mode of administration or the coadministration of cytokine genes can determine whether the immune response is humoral or cellular or whether it involves primarily Th1, Th2, or cytotoxic T cells. Such decisions can be used to optimize the protective immunity induced.

This form of immunization offers real advantages and only theoretical and remote disadvantages (Table 122-4). Moreover, DNA vaccines may be useful in inducing tumor immunity, treating allergy (by suppressing IgE production), or even administering genes for gene therapy. RNA vaccines would avoid some of the potential concerns raised by DNA vaccines because RNA is less stable and does not persist or integrate into the chromosome or cause insertional mutagenesis. However, this lack of stability and the likely need for multiple doses, along with the increased cost of producing, storing, and transporting RNA, are significant disadvantages that remain to be overcome. The concept of nucleic acid vaccines—whether based on DNA or RNA—has been validated experimentally, and early human trials have begun. There is great optimism for the future but much to be learned if we are to apply this powerful new immunization technique successfully.

PRODUCTION OF VACCINES As products to be given to healthy individuals to prevent disease, vaccines must not only be ef-

Table 122-4 Advantages and Disadvantages of DNA Vaccines

Advantages	Disadvantages
Safe; cannot cause infection; stable and heat resistant	Potential risk of integration of viral oncogenes from the vector
No need to express or purify antigens in vitro; no need for adjuvants; can be genetically engineered	Tumor promotion from integration near proto-oncogene or tumor suppressor genes
Normal processing of gene product closely resembling native conformation	Possible induction of tolerance or autoimmunity by vaccine persistence causing a persistent immune response
Persistence for prolonged periods; induction of durable immune response	Possible influence of strong promoter on expression of host genes, with adverse consequences
Induction of both humoral and cell-mediated immunity, including cytotoxic T cells	
Likely to be safe in pregnant women, immunosuppressed patients, or infants in the presence of maternal antibodies	

ficacious but also cause no harm. In the United States, quality assurance is the responsibility of vaccine manufacturers. Standards of manufacture of biologics [known as good manufacturing practices (GMPs)] are regulated and supervised by the U.S. Food and Drug Administration (FDA). Proof of the safety, efficacy, sterility, and purity of products is required before licensure, and sterility and purity are continually monitored for all lots of vaccine after licensure. Postmarketing studies of safety (phase IV studies) are part of routine regulatory control. On rare occasions, either GMP or quality assurance is inadequate; for example, the release of incompletely killed Salk polio vaccine in 1955 caused an outbreak of poliomyelitis in nearly 200 vaccine recipients and their contacts. Unregulated and uncontrolled manufacture of vaccines in developing countries has sometimes led to immunization with inactive products that fail to provide the expected protective immunity.

Another problem in the production of vaccines has unexpectedly cropped up in the past decade. For various reasons, including the high costs of vaccine development and the prospect of much higher profitability from investments in other products, the number of vaccine manufacturers in the United States has declined and the cost of some basic childhood vaccines has increased. Concern therefore exists about the future availability of these essential biologics for national use. Furthermore, pricing decisions made within the private-sector pharmaceutical industry can have a major impact on vaccine use. This situation has stimulated an initiative toward increased public involvement in supplying vaccine to individuals for whom price is an issue as well as in oversight of the vaccine supply and of price negotiations with the industry.

ADMINISTRATION OF VACCINES Health care workers administering vaccines must take the precautions necessary to minimize the risk of spreading disease—for example, hand washing between immunizations. They should be immunized against hepatitis B, measles, rubella, influenza, and varicella. Different vaccines should not be mixed in the same syringe unless such a practice is specifically endorsed by licensure. Disposable needles and syringes should be discarded in labeled, puncture-proof containers to prevent inadvertent needlestick injury or reuse.

The addition of new, individually injectable vaccines to the immunization schedule has heightened parental concerns about the administration of up to four injections at a single clinic visit. The development and use of combinations of vaccines are intended to mitigate these concerns. Even when multiple injections are required, providers must make every effort to administer all indicated vaccines at each visit.

Wherever effective primary health care systems ensure access to medical services for the majority and the population is educated about the need for and efficacy of vaccines, coverage rates for basic immunization are usually high, regardless of the route of vaccine administration or the number of doses necessary. However, without systematic attention to the completion of multiple-dose vaccine schedules, coverage rates for second, third, and booster doses may drop off significantly.

USE OF VACCINES

Recommendations for vaccine use in the United States are developed by several different groups. These recommendations are the result of a collaborative process among the recommending groups, the pharmaceutical industry, and the FDA.

Vaccines recommended in 1999 for routine administration to infants, children, and adults are shown in Table 122-5; vaccines recommended for special use are shown in Table 122-6; and schedules for immunization of children and adults are shown in Fig. 122-1 and Table 122-7, respectively. The recommendations on route, site, and dosages for vaccination are derived from theoretical considerations, experimental trials, and clinical experience; deviation from these recommendations can result in inadequate protection. The administration of doses at intervals longer than those recommended does not diminish the ultimate protective response but merely delays it. It is not necessary to restart an interrupted series from the beginning or to add an extra dose. In contrast, giving vaccines at shorter-than-recommended intervals may result in poor responses.

RECORDING AND REPORTING REQUIREMENTS Certain aspects of vaccine use are regulated by the National Childhood Vaccine Injury Act (NCVIA) of 1986 (modified in 1995). The act requires that all mandated childhood vaccinations be recorded by health care providers in the child's permanent medical record, including date of administration, manufacturer and lot number, and name of the provider administering the vaccine. State-based immunization information systems and registries are being developed to help public and private providers manage their immunization activities and particularly to address the problem of assessing immunization coverage when an individual's records are divided among multiple medical facilities.

Parents must be informed about the benefits and risks of immunization and should maintain an up-to-date immunization record on their children. Educational materials providing the required information (Vaccine Information Statements, VISs) are available from the American Academy of Pediatrics (AAP) or the Centers for Disease Control and Prevention (CDC).

VACCINES FOR ROUTINE USE Infants and Children Recommended routine-use vaccines and schedules for their administration to infants and children are shown in Table 122-5 and Fig. 122-1, respectively. It is current practice for all children in the United States to receive DTaP, poliovirus, MMR, Hib, HBV, and varicella vaccines unless there are specific contraindications. Hepatitis A vaccine is currently recommended when there is a special risk of exposure to infection due to residence in communities with elevated rates of hepatitis A or travel to highly endemic countries.

Adults (See Table 122-7) All adults should be immune to diphtheria and tetanus. If not previously immunized, adults require a primary immunizing course of Td. Many individuals remain immune to tetanus into adulthood because they have received tetanus toxoid rather than Td after injuries, but they are commonly at risk of diphtheria because of the decline in titer of diphtheria antitoxin and the lack of boosting against diphtheria. The development of acellular pertussis vaccines that appear to be safe in adults may lead to a recommendation for booster immunization of adults if clinical trials confirm safety and efficacy. Routine immunization against polio is not recommended for adults unless they are at particular risk of exposure (e.g., through travel to endemic regions, as discussed below) or are the parents or guardians of a child with an immunodeficiency disorder. Adults should be pro-

Table 122-5 Routinely Recommended Vaccines for Infants, Children, and Adults

Vaccine	Year Licensed	Type of Immunizing Agent	Protective Antibody	Route of Administration	Efficacy, %	Adverse Events
DT	1949	Toxoid	Diphtheria and tetanus neutralizing antitoxins, ≥ 0.1 IU/mL each	IM	D: 95	Local reactions
Td	1955				T: 95	Hypersensitivity to tetanus toxoid
aP	1993	Inactivated bacterial antigen	Not known	IM	80–90	Reduced local reactions compared with whole-cell vaccines; no serious reactions reported
	1996	Acellular (DTaP)				
Hib	1987	Bacterial polysaccharide-protein conjugate	Antibody to capsular polysaccharide, 0.15 µg/mL	IM	90	Few local, no serious reactions
HBV	1981	Inactivated serum-derived viral antigen	Antibody to surface antigen, 10 mIU/mL	IM	80–95	Few (? Guillain-Barré syndrome)
	1987	Recombinant antigen				
Influenza	1945	Inactivated virus or viral components[a]	Neutralizing antibody	IM	40–60	? Guillain-Barré syndrome with swine influenza vaccine
MMR	1971	Live viruses	Neutralizing measles antibody, ≥ 200 mIU/mL; not known for mumps or rubella	SC	M: 95	Acute encephalopathy (measles)
					Mu: 90	Rare parotitis or orchitis (mumps)
					R: 95	Arthralgia and rare arthropathy (rubella)
Pneumococcus	1983	Bacterial polysaccharide of 23 types	Antibody to capsular polysaccharide	IM or SC	60–80	Local reactions; rare anaphylaxis
Poliomyelitis	1963	OPV, live virus of 3 serotypes	Neutralizing antibody at any detectable titer	Oral	95[b]	Rare vaccine-associated polio
	1967	IPV, inactivated virus of 3 serotypes		SC	95	No significant reactions

[a] Only "split-virus" influenza vaccine should be given to children <13 years old since whole-virus influenza vaccines are associated with higher rates of adverse reactions in young children.

[b] In developing countries, OPV efficacy is only 70 to 90%, presumably because of interfering enteroviruses in the intestinal tract.

NOTE: DT, diphtheria and tetanus toxoids, adsorbed; Td, tetanus and diphtheria toxoids, adsorbed, for adult use; aP, acellular pertussis; Hib, *Haemophilus influenzae* type b; HBV, hepatitis B virus; MMR, measles-mumps-rubella; OPV, trivalent oral poliovirus vaccine; IPV, inactivated poliovirus vaccine; IM, intramuscular; SC, subcutaneous.

SOURCE: Recommendations of the Advisory Committee on Immunization Practices, the American Academy of Pediatrics, and the American College of Physicians.

tected from measles, mumps, and rubella; they should be vaccinated unless they are known to have received vaccine on or after their first birthday or to have had physician-diagnosed disease. Rubella vaccine should be given to all women of childbearing age unless they have documentary proof of immunization after their first birthday or laboratory evidence of immunity. An unsupported history of rubella disease is unreliable and should not be accepted. Adults without a clear history of chickenpox should receive varicella vaccine. College students, particularly freshmen living in a dormitory, are at increased risk of meningococcal meningitis. They should be made aware of the polysaccharide vaccine for serogroups A, C, Y, and W-135 and should be offered the option of immunization.

Current recommendations also include influenza vaccine for routine annual administration to adults ≥ 65 years of age and to individuals with chronic illness at any age. Polyvalent pneumococcal polysaccharide vaccine is similarly recommended for the elderly or chronically ill. HBV vaccine is recommended for individuals at high risk of exposure, including health care workers exposed to potentially infected blood or blood products, homosexuals, injection drug users, individuals living and working in institutions for the mentally retarded, and household contacts of known carriers of hepatitis B surface antigen (HBsAg). A new recombinant outer-surface protein A (rOspA) is licensed for persons 15 to 70 years of age for Lyme disease (LYMErix, SmithKline Beecham Pharmaceuticals), with use based on individual risk (geography and risk of exposure to ticks).

Adverse Events Modern vaccines, while safe and effective, are associated with adverse effects that range from infrequent and very mild to rare and life-threatening. The decision to use a vaccine involves an assessment of the risks of disease, the benefits of vaccination, and the risks associated with vaccination. Because these factors may change over time, continued assessment is essential. Table 122-8 lists valid and invalid contraindications to immunization and describes appropriate precautions in the use of specific vaccines. Antivaccine advocacy groups actively encourage avoidance of immunization because of their unproven belief that vaccines may cause certain disorders (for example, autism). This situation presents a challenge to the physician in educating parents about vaccine benefits and risks.

Vaccine components, including protective antigens, animal proteins introduced during vaccine production, and antibiotics or other preservatives or stabilizers, can cause allergic reactions in some recipients. These reactions may be local or systemic and may include urticaria and serious anaphylaxis. The most common extraneous allergen is egg protein introduced when vaccines such as those for measles, mumps, influenza, and yellow fever are prepared in embryonated eggs. Local or systemic reactions can result from too-frequent administration of vaccines such as Td, diphtheria/tetanus (DT), or rabies; these reactions are probably due to antigen-antibody complexes. In addition, live-virus vaccines can interfere with tuberculin test responses. When a tuberculin skin test is indicated, it should be done either on the day of immunization or 6 weeks later. When influenza vaccine is given to children <13 years old, only "split-virus" preparations should be used since whole-virus vaccines are associated with higher rates of adverse reactions in young children. Cumulative exposure to mercury in thimerosal-preserved vaccines is a concern, and plans are under way to replace current vaccines with thimerosal-free products. In the interim, infants born to HBsAg-negative mothers should not receive the initial dose of HBV vaccine at birth.

All detected adverse events temporally related to vaccination are expected to be reported to both the local health department and the vaccine manufacturer. The NCVIA requires health care providers to report certain suspected adverse events following the receipt of a mandated vaccine to the FDA's Vaccine Adverse Events Reporting System (Table 122-9). Although a temporal relationship does not establish cause and effect, this surveillance system remains the only mechanism for collecting the data needed to form conclusions and make decisions.

USE OF VACCINES IN SPECIAL CIRCUMSTANCES

Pregnancy Because of theoretical risk to the fetus and real risk of litigation to the practitioner, routine immunization of pregnant women

Table 122-6   Special-Use Vaccines

Vaccine	Year Licensed in United States	Type of Immunizing Agent	Route of Administration	Indications	Efficacy	Adverse Events
Anthrax	1970	Inactivated avirulent bacteria	SC (6 doses primary; annual booster)	For high risk of exposure (i.e., persons in contact with or involved in manufacture of animal hides, furs, bone meal, wool, goat hair)	90% antibody response but efficacy uncertain	No serious adverse effects known
Tuberculosis (BCG)	1950	Living bacteria (attenuated *Mycobacterium bovis*)	ID	PPD-negative individuals in prolonged contact with active TB patient	Controversial; reduces disseminated disease in children (0–80% protection against pulmonary TB; 75–86% protection against miliary and meningitic TB)	Regional adenitis, disseminated BCG infection, osteitis
Hepatitis A	1995	Killed virus antigen	IM	Travelers or persons living in high-risk areas	94%	Local reactions
Cholera	1914	Inactivated bacteria	SC or IM	Not recommended for public health use	50% (short-lived)	Frequent fever, local pain, swelling
Meningococcus A, C, Y, W-135	1981	Bacterial polysaccharide of 4 serotypes	SC	Military personnel; principally travelers to epidemic areas	90% for 2- to 3-year-olds	Rare
Plague	1911	Inactivated bacteria	IM	Laboratory workers; foresters in endemic areas; travelers	90% antibody response but efficacy uncertain	10% local reactions; rare sterile abscesses and hypersensitivity
Rabies (human diploid)	1980	Inactivated virus	IM or ID	Travelers; laboratory workers; veterinarians	Virtually 100%	25% local reactions; 6% arthropathy, arthritis, angioedema
Yellow fever	1953	Live virus	SC	Laboratory workers; travelers	High	Encephalitis; encephalopathy
Japanese encephalitis	1993	Inactivated virus	SC	Travelers	80–90%	Anaphylactic/severe delayed allergic reactions common; recipient should be observed for 10 days
Typhoid						
Phenol and heat-killed	1952	Killed whole bacteria	IM	Not routinely recommended in U.S.; used for travelers, contacts of carriers	50–70% (short-lived)	Frequent fever, local swelling, pain
Ty$_{21a}$	1992	Live mutant bacteria	Oral	Travelers, contacts of carriers	50–70%	None
Vi	1995	Vi capsular polysaccharide	IM	Travelers	70–75%	Local reactions
Lyme disease	1999	Recombinant outer-surface protein	IM	For high risk of exposure to infected ticks	76% (3 doses)	Local reactions

NOTE: SC, subcutaneous; BCG, bacille Calmette-Guérin; ID, intradermal; PPD, purified protein derivative; TB, tuberculosis; IM, intramuscular.

SOURCE: Recommendations of the Advisory Committee on Immunization Practices, the American Academy of Pediatrics, and the American College of Physicians.

is best avoided. However, wherever hygienic conditions during delivery cannot be guaranteed, it is essential to ensure that pregnant women are immune to tetanus: the transfer of maternal antitoxin is an important means of preventing neonatal tetanus, and pregnant women can safely receive tetanus as well as diphtheria toxoids. Although live-virus vaccines in general should be withheld during pregnancy, polio and yellow fever vaccines are exceptions and may be administered if the risk of exposure to disease is great. If indicated, some inactivated vaccines (e.g., HBV, influenza, and pneumococcal vaccines) are safe for pregnant women. Known pregnancy is considered a contraindication to the receipt of rubella, measles, mumps, and varicella vaccines. Although of theoretical concern, no cases of congenital rubella syndrome or abnormalities attributable to rubella vaccine virus have been observed in infants born to susceptible mothers who received rubella vaccine during pregnancy.

Breast Feeding   Neither killed nor live vaccine affects the safety of breast feeding for either mother or infant. Breast-fed infants can be immunized on a normal schedule.

Occupational Exposure   Immunization recommendations for most occupational groups remain to be developed. Specific practices are now mandated by the Occupational Safety and Health Administration for the immunization of health care workers against hepatitis B in the United States. Rubella is transmitted to and from health care workers in medical facilities, particularly in pediatric practice. Health care workers who might transmit rubella to pregnant patients should be immune to rubella; it is prudent to screen these employees for antibodies to rubella virus and to immunize susceptible individuals. Persons providing health care are also at greater risk from measles and varicella than the general public, and those who are likely to come into contact with measles- and varicella-infected patients should be immune. Persons employed in caring for patients with chronic diseases can transmit influenza; such workers should be vaccinated annually. Unfortunately, these recommendations often are not fully implemented, even in academic institutions.

HIV Infection and Other Immunocompromised States   Limited studies in HIV-infected individuals have found no increase in the risk of adverse events from live or inactivated vaccines. However, immune responses may not be as vigorous in immunocompromised individuals as in those with a normal immune system. Persons known to be infected with HIV should be immunized with recommended vaccines in the same manner as individuals with a normal immune system and as early in the course of their disease as possible, before immune function becomes significantly impaired. Live attenuated MMR vaccine can be administered to this group, but OPV cannot (Table 122-10). IPV should be used when vaccination against polio is indicated. Household contacts of immunocompromised individuals should be immune to polio; when vaccinated, they should receive IPV. In practice, it is not necessary to test for HIV before making decisions about the immunization of asymptomatic individuals from known HIV risk groups.

Live attenuated vaccines are normally contraindicated in immunocompromised patients, including those with congenital immunodeficiency syndromes and those receiving immunosuppressive therapy. Passive immunization with immunoglobulin preparations or antitoxins can be considered in individual cases, either as postexposure prophylaxis or as part of the treatment of established infection.

Postexposure Immunization
For certain infections, active or passive immunization soon after exposure prevents or attenuates disease expression. Recommended postexposure immunization regimens are compiled in Table 122-11. Measles immune globulin given within 6 days of exposure may prevent or modify infection, and measles vaccine given within the first few days after exposure may prevent symptomatic infection. Although clinical manifestations of rubella in pregnant women are minimized by postexposure passive immunization, this approach may not prevent maternal viremia, fetal infection, and congenital rubella syndrome. Therefore, the administration of immune globulin is recommended only for women developing rubella during pregnancy who will not consider abortion under any circumstances. Tetanus immune globulin can be used in patients with tetanus. Survivors with no history of tetanus immunization should receive a primary series of toxoid injections since disease does not result in the

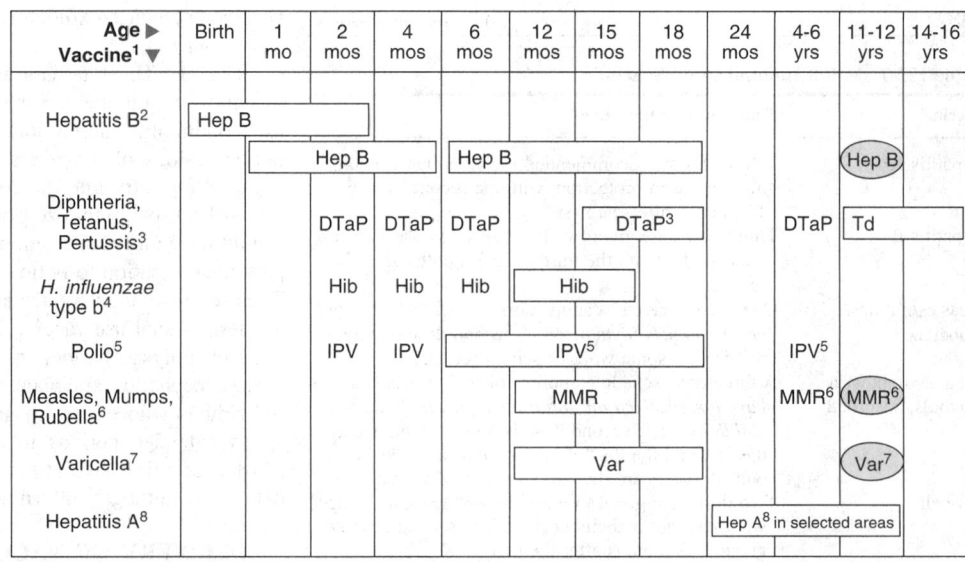

FIGURE 122-1 Recommended childhood immunization schedule in the United States for January through December 2000. Vaccines are listed under the routinely recommended ages. Clear bars indicate a range of acceptable ages for vaccination; shaded ovals indicate timing of catch-up vaccination: at 11 or 12 years of age, hepatitis B vaccine and measles/mumps/rubella vaccine should be administered to children not previously vaccinated, and varicella vaccine should be administered to children not previously vaccinated who lack a reliable history of chickenpox. Vaccine abbreviations: Hep B, hepatitis B; DTaP, diphtheria/tetanus/acellular pertussis; Hib, *Haemophilus influenzae* type b; Td, tetanus/diphtheria toxoids, adsorbed; IPV, inactivated poliovirus vaccine; MMR, measles/mumps/rubella; Var, varicella-zoster; Hep A, hepatitis A. **Key to footnotes:** [1]*This schedule indicates the recommended ages* for routine administration of licensed childhood vaccines as of November 1, 1999. Additional vaccines may subsequently be licensed and recommended. A licensed combination vaccine may be used whenever any of its components is indicated and its other components are not contraindicated. Because clinical studies of infants have demonstrated that some combination products may induce a weaker immune response to the Hib vaccine component, DTaP/Hib combination products should not be used for primary immunization of infants at 2, 4, or 6 months of age unless approved by the FDA for these ages. Providers should consult the manufacturers' package inserts for detailed recommendations. [2]*The hepatitis B surface antigen (HBsAg) status of pregnant women*, if not known, should be determined as soon as possible during pregnancy. *Infants born to HBsAg-negative mothers* should receive the first dose of Hep B vaccine by age 2 months. The second dose should be given at least 1 month after the first dose. The third dose should be administered at least 4 months after the first dose and at least 2 months after the second dose, but not before 6 months of age. In this setting, a licensed combination Hep B/Hib vaccine may be used (e.g., ComVax; Merck) at 2, 4, and 12 to 15 months of age in place of the usual immunization schedule for each vaccine given independently. *Infants born to HBsAg-positive mothers* should receive Hep B vaccine and immunoprophylaxis with 0.5 mL of hepatitis B immune globulin (HBIG)—at separate sites—within 12 h of birth. The second dose is recommended at 1 month of age and the third dose at 6 months of age. *Infants born to mothers whose HBsAg status is unknown* should receive Hep B vaccine within 12 h of birth. Maternal blood should be drawn at delivery and HBsAg status determined; if the mother's HBsAg test is positive, the infant should receive HBIG no later than 1 week of age. All children and adolescents through 18 years of age who have not been immunized against hepatitis B may begin the series during any visit. Special efforts should be made to immunize children who were born in, or whose parents were born in, areas of the world with moderate or high endemicity of hepatitis B virus infection. [3]*DTaP is the preferred vaccine for all doses.* The fourth dose of DTaP may be administered as early as 12 months of age, provided 6 months have elapsed since the third dose and the child is unlikely to return at age 15 to 18 months. Td is recommended at 11 to 12 years of age if at least 5 years have elapsed since the last dose of DTaP, diphtheria/tetanus/pertussis (DTP) vaccine, or diphtheria/tetanus (DT) vaccine. Subsequent routine Td boosters are recommended every 10 years. [4]*Three Hib conjugate vaccines* are licensed for infant use. If PRP-OMP [PedvaxHIB or ComVax (Merck)] is administered at 2 and 4 months of age, a dose at 6 months is not required. [5]*To eliminate the risk of vaccine-associated paralytic polio* (VAPP), an all-IPV schedule is now recommended for routine childhood polio vaccination in the United States. All children should receive four doses of IPV at 2, 4, and 6 to 18 months and 4 to 6 years. If available, trivalent oral poliovirus vaccine (OPV) may be used *only* for mass vaccination campaigns to control outbreaks of paralytic polio, for unvaccinated children who will be traveling in <4 weeks to areas where polio is endemic or epidemic, and for children of parents who do not accept the recommended number of vaccine injections. The latter children may receive OPV only for the third and/or fourth dose; in this situation, health care professionals should administer OPV only after discussing the risk for VAPP with parents or caregivers. [6]The second dose of MMR vaccine is recommended routinely at 4 to 6 years but may be administered during any visit, provided that at least 4 weeks have elapsed since receipt of the first dose and that both doses are administered beginning at or after 12 months of age. Children who have not previously received the second dose should complete the schedule by the 11- to 12-year-old visit. [7]Var vaccine is recommended at any visit on or after the first birthday for susceptible children, i.e., those who lack a reliable history of chickenpox (as judged by a health care professional) and who have not been immunized. Susceptible persons ≥13 years of age should receive two doses at least 4 weeks apart. [8]Hep A vaccine is recommended for use in selected states and/or regions with higher-than-average infection rates. Information may be obtained from local public health departments. *(From the Advisory Committee on Immunization Practices, the American Academy of Pediatrics, and the American Academy of Family Physicians.)*

Table 122-7   Adult Immunization Schedule

Vaccine	Timing of Immunization
Hepatitis A[a]	Two doses are recommended for individuals requiring long-term protection, with the second dose 6–12 months after the first.
Hepatitis B[a]	Three doses are given, with the second dose 1 month after the first and the third dose 5 months after the second.
Measles/mumps/ rubella	One dose is given to adults born in 1957 or later *and not previously immunized*. A second dose may be required in some work or school settings.
Tetanus/diphtheria toxoids, adsorbed	A three-dose schedule applies for individuals who *have not received an initial immunization series in childhood*. The second dose is given 1 month after the first and the third dose 6 months after the second. Boosters are then given every 10 years.
Varicella	Two doses are given to individuals ≥13 years of age who have not had chickenpox. The second dose is given 1–2 months after the first.
Influenza	Vaccine is administered yearly to individuals ≥65 years of age; to younger people with chronic medical problems, such as heart disease and diabetes; and to those who work or live with high-risk persons.
Streptococcus pneumoniae (polysaccharide)	Vaccine is usually given once to individuals ≥65 years of age. A repeat dose may be given 5 years later for those at highest risk. Immunization is also recommended for younger people with chronic medical problems, such as heart disease, diabetes, renal failure, and sickle cell anemia, and for those who work or live with high-risk persons.

[a] For individuals at risk.
SOURCE: National Coalition for Adult Immunization.

development of protective levels of antitoxin. Administration of rabies immune globulin plus rabies vaccine in the immediate postexposure period is highly effective in preventing disease. Similarly, for persons who have not been actively immunized, the use of immune globulin within 2 weeks of exposure to hepatitis A is likely to prevent clinical illness. Good data indicate the efficacy of human hepatitis B immune globulin in preventing disease after exposure. While no high-titer preparation is available for postexposure protection against non-A, non-B hepatitis, standard human immune serum globulin is efficacious.

Simultaneous Administration of Multiple Vaccines   The simultaneous administration of the most widely used live and inactivated vaccines has not resulted in impaired antibody responses or in increased rates of adverse reactions. Simultaneous administration of vaccines is advantageous in that it increases the probability that a child will ultimately be fully immunized; it is also useful in any age group when the potential exists for exposure to multiple infectious diseases during travel to endemic countries. However, combination DTaP/Hib vaccines should not be used for primary immunization of infants because the response to Hib is blunted and suboptimal. Live-virus vaccines not given together on the same day should generally be administered at least 30 days apart.

High doses of immune globulin may inhibit the efficacy of measles and rubella vaccines, and an interval of at least 3 months is recommended between the administration of immune globulin and that of MMR vaccine or its components. Postpartum vaccination of rubella-susceptible women should not be delayed because of the administration of anti-Rho(D) immune globulin or any other blood product during the last trimester or at delivery. Should administration of an immune globulin preparation become necessary after vaccination, it should be postponed, if possible, for at least 14 days to allow time for vaccine-virus replication and development of immunity. In general, there is little interaction of immune globulin with inactivated vaccines, and postexposure passive prophylaxis can be given together with HBV

vaccine or tetanus toxoid, resulting in both immediate and long-lasting protection.

Travel   The International Sanitary Regulations allow countries to impose requirements for yellow fever and killed cholera vaccines as a condition for admission, even though the latter is not an effective public health tool. Travelers should know whether these vaccines are required for entry into the countries on their itinerary to avoid being turned back or immunized on the spot. Infants, children, and adults should have all routine immunizations updated before traveling, with particular attention to polio, measles, and DTP/DTaP or Td vaccines. The use of hepatitis A vaccine may be advisable for travelers to some locales. Special-use vaccines (Table 122-6), including rabies, meningococcal polysaccharide, typhoid (oral live or Vi polysaccharide), Japanese encephalitis, and plague vaccines, should be considered for those individuals who expect to go beyond the usual tourist routes or to spend extended periods in rural areas in disease-endemic regions. Most U.S. cities have at least one travel clinic that maintains up-to-date epidemiologic information and can provide the appropriate vaccines.

DELIVERY OF VACCINES   Over the past 25 years, considerable progress has been made to ensure that every child in the United States is fully immunized by the time of school entry. All 50 states now require immunization for school entry, and most have laws addressing attendance at preschools and day-care centers. The impact of immunization and of other improvements in the health care provided to the American population on the incidence of vaccine-preventable illness is shown in Table 122-1. Nonetheless, many children are not fully immunized, especially in poor and underserved communities. The failure to vaccinate preschool children was largely responsible for the resurgence of measles between 1989 and 1991, with >55,000 cases and >130 measles-related deaths. Outbreaks of pertussis, mumps, and congenital rubella syndrome have occurred for the same reason: low immunization rates among preschool children.

ACCESS TO IMMUNIZATION   Four major barriers to infant and childhood immunization have been identified within the health care system: (1) low public awareness and lack of public demand for immunization, (2) inadequate access to immunization services, (3) missed opportunities to administer vaccines, and (4) inadequate resources for public health and preventive programs. These problems are sources of public concern, and their solution is a priority for national health policy in the United States. In response, the Children's Immunization Initiative was begun in 1990. At the national level, this program includes outreach and educational campaigns to promote parental awareness of the value of vaccination and to encourage health care providers to use every opportunity to vaccinate the children in their care. At the state and local levels, community and business groups, religious and service groups, schools, and the media have joined together in community-based networks. A National Immunization Week each April has been established to focus attention on the vaccination needs of infants and children. To improve the quality and quantity of vaccination services, expanded immunization-clinic hours and computerization of immunization records are being implemented as well.

There has been only modest progress towards the goals for adult immunization in the United States. Adult-immunization goals are important: As many as 60,000 adults die each year of vaccine-preventable diseases for which effective vaccines are not being optimally used. Most persons ≥65 years of age do not receive influenza vaccine each year, and even fewer have ever received pneumococcal vaccine. Health care providers more often miss vaccination opportunities with adults than with infants and children. From 60 to 90% of adults hospitalized for or dying of influenza-associated respiratory disease have received medical care during the previous year and could have been immunized at that time. Medicare reimbursement for excess hospitalization during influenza epidemics ranges from $750 million to $1 billion. Additional efforts are required to ensure that adults receive pneumococcal, Td, and HBV vaccines as well.

A special setting for adult immunization is the administration of

Table 122-8 Immunization Contraindications and Precautions

Vaccine	Contraindication or Precaution[a] Valid	Invalid
General[b]	Anaphylactic reaction to vaccine (contraindication to further doses of that vaccine)	Mild to moderate local reaction (soreness, redness, swelling) following dose of injectable antigen
	Anaphylactic reaction to vaccine constituent (contraindication to use of vaccines containing that substance)	Mild acute illness, with or without low-grade fever
	Moderate or severe illnesses, with or without fever	Current antimicrobial therapy
		Convalescent phase of illness
		Prematurity (same dosage and indications as for normal, full-term infants)
		Recent exposure to an infectious disease
		History of penicillin or other nonspecific allergies or family history of such allergies
DTaP/DTP	Encephalopathy within 72 h after dose	Temperature of <40.5°C (105°F) after dose
	Fever of ≥40.5°C (105°F) within 48 h after dose (P)	Family history of convulsions[c]
	Collapse or shocklike state (hypotonic-hyporesponsive episode) within 48 h after dose (P)	Family history of an adverse event following vaccination
	Seizures within 3 days after dose (P)	Family history of sudden infant death syndrome
	Persistent, inconsolable crying lasting ≥3 h within 48 h after dose (P)	
OPV[d]	Infection with HIV or a household contact infected with HIV	Breast feeding
	Known immunodeficiency (hematologic and solid tumors, congenital immunodeficiency, and long-term immunosuppressive therapy)	Current antimicrobial therapy
	Immunodeficient household contact	Diarrhea
	Pregnancy[e] (P)	
IPV	Anaphylactic reactions to neomycin or streptomycin	—
	Pregnancy[e]	
MMR	Anaphylactic reactions to eggs or to neomycin[f]	Tuberculosis or positive PPD test
	Pregnancy	Simultaneous TB skin testing[g]
	Known immunodeficiency (hematologic and solid tumors, congenital immunodeficiency syndrome, and long-term immunosuppressive therapy)	Breast feeding
		Pregnancy of mother of recipient
		Immunodeficient family member or household contact
	Recent IG administration (P)	Infection with HIV
		Nonanaphylactic reactions to eggs or neomycin
Hib	None identified	History of Hib disease
HBV	None identified	Pregnancy
Influenza	First trimester of pregnancy (vaccination avoided on theoretical grounds)	—
	Anaphylactic reactions to eggs	
Pneumococcus	Has not been evaluated in pregnancy	—
Varicella	Primary acquired immunodeficiency	Contact dermatitis in response to neomycin
	History of anaphylactic reaction to neomycin	
	Pregnancy	

[a] Precautions are followed by "(P)." The events or conditions listed as precautions, although not contraindications, should be carefully reviewed. The benefits and risks of administering a specific vaccine to an individual under the circumstances should be considered. If the risks are believed to outweigh the benefits, the vaccine should be withheld; if the benefits are believed to outweigh the risks (for example, during an outbreak or foreign travel), the vaccine should be administered. Whether and when to administer DTaP to children with proven or suspected underlying neurologic disorders should be decided on an individual basis.
[b] For DTP/ DTaP, OPV, IPV, MMR, Hib, HBV, influenza, pneumococcus, and varicella.
[c] If a child has a precaution to the receipt of a subsequent dose of whole-cell DTP, the child should not routinely receive DTaP. If a child has a contraindication to the receipt of a subsequent dose of whole-cell DTP, the child should not receive DTaP. Acetaminophen given before DTaP and thereafter every 4 h for 24 h should be considered for children with a personal or family (sibling or parent) history of convulsions.
[d] No data exist to substantiate the theoretical risk of a suboptimal immune response when OPV and MMR are given within 30 days of each other.
[e] It is prudent on theoretical grounds to avoid vaccinating pregnant women. However, if immediate protection against poliomyelitis is needed, OPV is preferred, although IPV may be considered if vaccination can be completed before the anticipated imminent exposure.
[f] Persons with a history of anaphylactic reactions following egg ingestion should be vaccinated only with caution. Protocols have been developed for vaccinating such persons and should be consulted (J Pediatr 102:196, 1983; J Pediatr 113:504, 1988).
[g] Measles vaccination may temporarily suppress tuberculin reactivity. If skin testing cannot be done on the day of MMR vaccination, the test should be postponed for 4 to 6 weeks.
NOTE: IPV, inactivated polio vaccine; PPD, purified protein derivative; TB, tuberculosis; IG, immunoglobulin.
SOURCES: This information is based on the recommendations of the Advisory Committee on Immunization Practices (ACIP) and those of the Committee on Infectious Diseases (Red Book Committee) of the American Academy of Pediatrics (AAP). Sometimes these recommendations vary from those contained in the manufacturers' package inserts. For more detailed information, providers should consult the published recommendations of the ACIP (Vaccine side effects, adverse reactions, contraindications, and precautions. MMWR 45:1, 1996) and the AAP as well as the manufacturers' package inserts.

certain vaccines to pregnant women to enhance passive immunity in their offspring (e.g., tetanus toxoid). In most cases the mother herself derives important benefits as well. Immunization of the mother should be undertaken at least 6 weeks before delivery to allow for efficient transplacental transfer of antibody to the fetus.

STANDARDS FOR IMMUNIZATION PRACTICES National standards of immunization for adult and pediatric practice have been established to define common policies and practices for public health clinics and in physicians' private offices (Table 122-12). These guidelines highlight the need to distinguish between valid contraindications and conditions that are often considered but are not in fact contraindications (Table 122-8). Among the valid contraindications applicable to all vaccines are a history of anaphylaxis or other serious allergic reactions to a vaccine or vaccine component and the presence of a moderate or severe illness, with or without fever. Infants who develop encephalopathy within 72 h of a dose of DTP or DTaP should not receive further doses; those who develop a "precaution" (Table 122-8) should not normally receive further doses. Because of theoretical risks to the fetus, pregnant women should not receive MMR or varicella vaccine. Diarrhea, minor respiratory illness with or without fever, mild to moderate local reactions to a previous dose of vaccine, the concurrent or recent use of antimicrobial agents, mild to moderate malnutrition, or the convalescent phase of an acute illness are not valid contraindications to routine immunization. Failure to vaccinate chil-

Table 122-9   Reportable Events Following Vaccination, as Required by the National Childhood Vaccine Injury Act of 1986 (Modified in 1995)[a]

Vaccine/Toxoid	Event	Interval from Vaccination
DTaP; P; DTP-Hib; DT; Td or TT	Anaphylaxis	4 h
	Encephalopathy (or encephalitis)	72 h
MMR, MR, or M	Anaphylaxis	4 h
	Encephalopathy (or encephalitis)	5–15 days
	Residual seizure disorder	5–15 days
Rubella-containing vaccines (MMR, MR, R)	Chronic arthritis	42 days
	Anaphylaxis	4 h
	Encephalopathy (or encephalitis)	5–15 days
	Residual seizure disorder	5–15 days
OPV	Paralytic poliomyelitis	
	In an immunocompetent recipient	30 days
	In an immunocompromised recipient	6 months
	In a vaccine-associated community case	No limits
IPV	Anaphylaxis	4 h

[a] Compensation (under the NCVIA) is effective for claims filed on or after March 10, 1995. Any acute complications or sequelae of an illness, disability, injury, or condition that arose within the prescribed period (including deaths) are also covered.

NOTE: P, pertussis; TT, tetanus toxoid; MR, measles/rubella; M, measles; R, rubella.

dren because of these conditions is increasingly viewed as a missed opportunity for immunization.

BIOTERRORISM   The end of the twentieth century witnessed a rise in the risk of bioterrorism. While smallpox has been eradicated, known stocks of smallpox virus still exist in the United States and Russia, and unknown stocks probably exist in other countries considered likely to engage in terrorism. Global supplies of smallpox vaccine for use in case of deliberate release of smallpox virus are inadequate, and millions of people are likely to become infected and die in the event of such a release. Steps are only now being taken to ensure sufficient stockpiles of vaccine for this eventuality, and it will be several more years before these reach a critical size.

THE NATIONAL VACCINE INJURY COMPENSATION PROGRAM   The use of mandated vaccines benefits society as a whole by reducing morbidity and the cost of care for preventable diseases and by reducing childhood mortality. Thus, in the United States, society has assumed the obligation to care for those injured by the administration of mandated vaccines. The NCVIA of 1986 (modified in 1995) is the instrument in use to ensure fairness to injured persons as well as protection for federal, state, and local immunization programs; private immunization providers; and vaccine manufacturers. The act was designed to implement two vital public policies: (1) to provide prompt and fair compensation to the families of children who have died or have been injured as a result of routine mandated immunization; and (2) to reduce the adverse impact of the tort system on vaccine supply, cost, and innovation/development. The success of immunization programs in the United States depends upon the continued viability of the National Vaccine Injury Compensation Program.

CONTROL OF VACCINE-PREVENTABLE DISEASE

A continuing task of public health practice is to maintain individual and herd immunity. The job is not over once a population is fully vaccinated; rather, it is imperative to immunize each subsequent generation as long as the threat of the disease persists. Ongoing surveillance and prompt reporting of disease to local or state health departments are essential to this goal, ensuring a continuing awareness of the possibility of vaccine-preventable illness. Nearly all vaccine-preventable diseases are now notifiable, and individual case data are routinely forwarded to the CDC. These data are used to detect outbreaks or other unusual events that require investigation and to evaluate prevention and control policies, practices, and strategies.

As a direct consequence of successes in immunization, vaccine-preventable diseases have become less visible; ironically, this situation may foster complacency among parents and health care providers about routine immunization of children. Even among the affluent and educated, immunization levels may be low, reflecting a misunderstanding of the continuing threat of disease with which parents and health care providers have limited experience or perhaps an unjustifiably greater fear of adverse reactions to vaccination than of the potential for illness and death due to vaccine-preventable diseases. Health care workers play an essential role in influencing the attitudes of patients regarding appropriate immunization; therefore, it is essential that these professionals continually update their own knowledge about vaccines and about the epidemiology of vaccine-preventable illnesses.

RESEARCH ON VACCINES AND IMMUNIZATION

The potential to eradicate selected diseases and to build sustainable immunization programs that reach every child is not being fulfilled with existing vaccines and delivery technology. New vaccines or new formulations that will not only improve protective responses but also simplify the immunization schedule are needed. The ideal would be vaccines that can be administered orally early in life, that provide lifelong protection against multiple infections, that can be given as one or only a few doses, and that are less reactive and more heat stable than current vaccines. To attain these ambitious goals may take decades, but progress is already being made in the development of new combinations of current vaccines to facilitate complete immunization. The results will be applicable to immunization programs in both developed and developing countries.

REEMERGENCE OF CONTROLLED DISEASE AND EMERGENCE OF NEW DISEASE   The emergence of new pathogens is fostered

Table 122-10   Recommendations for Routine Immunization of HIV-Infected Persons in the United States

Vaccine	HIV Clinical Status Asymptomatic	Symptomatic	Comments
DTaP/Td	Yes	Yes	No change in usual immunization schedule
OPV	No	No	Increased risk of vaccine virus proliferation and paralytic polio; IPV used for household contacts of HIV-infected persons
IPV	Yes	Yes	Antibody response potentially impaired in symptomatic patients
MMR	Yes	Yes	No change in usual immunization schedule; with high risk of exposure to measles, first dose given at 6–11 months of age, second dose at >12 months of age; with documented infection, measles immune globulin potentially administered (see Table 122-11)
Hib conjugate	Yes	Yes	No change in usual immunization schedule
HBV	Yes	Yes	Antibody response potentially impaired; higher-dose vaccine available, but no data address optimal dose; possibly wise to check antibody titer after immunization and give additional doses if titer is inadequate
Pneumococcus	Yes	Yes	Should be given to all ≥2 years old
Influenza	Yes	Yes	Antibody response potentially impaired in symptomatic patients
Varicella	No	No	Use in asymptomatic HIV-infected persons not studied

SOURCE: Centers for Disease Control and Prevention.

by the genetic potential of microbes to evolve as well as by rapid changes in human demographics and behavior and in a global ecology that creates new or more favorable hosts. Proof of the need for continuing vaccine research is found in the emergence of new infectious diseases such as HIV infection, Lyme borreliosis, hantavirus pulmonary syndrome, and hepatitis C; the appearance of a new epidemic cholera strain (serotype O139 Bengal) that exhibits no cross-immunity with the traditional O1 serotype; and the increase in global incidence and in drug resistance of familiar diseases that were once considered under control, such as tuberculosis and malaria. In addition, some common illnesses without a previously known etiology, such as peptic ulcer disease and cervical and nasopharyngeal cancer, have now been epidemiologically linked to specific infectious agents and have thus become potentially vaccine-preventable conditions.

DEVELOPMENT OF NEW VACCINES For many serious or even life-threatening infectious diseases, no effective vaccines are available. Although many new vaccines are undergoing human trials, the task of developing vaccines is proving very complex. Priorities for the United States currently include research on the following vaccines: HIV, pneumococcus (conjugate), group B *Streptococcus*, respiratory syncytial virus, rotavirus, *Mycobacterium tuberculosis*, herpes simplex virus, influenza A and B viruses, and hepatitis C virus. Also of high priority are vaccines for two virus-associated tumors: cervical cancer (human papillomavirus) and nasopharyngeal cancer (Epstein-Barr virus).

INTERNATIONAL CONSIDERATIONS

Since the establishment of the World Health Organization's Expanded Programme on Immunization in 1981, levels of coverage for the recommended basic children's vaccines (bacille Calmette-Guérin, polio, DTP/DTaP, measles, and HBV) have risen from 5% to ~80% worldwide. Each year, at least 2.7 million deaths from measles, neonatal tetanus, and pertussis and 200,000 cases of paralysis due to polio are prevented by immunization. Despite the successes of this program, many vaccine-preventable diseases remain prevalent in the developing world. Measles, for example, continues to kill an estimated 1.5 million children each year, and cases of diphtheria, whooping cough, polio, and neonatal tetanus still occur at unacceptably high rates. It is estimated that between 20 and 35% of all deaths of children under the age of 5 years are still associated with vaccine-preventable diseases.

In addition to the antigens included in the Expanded Programme for routine use in the developing world, others (Hib, Japanese B encephalitis, yellow fever, group A meningococcus, mumps, and rubella) are used regionally, depending on disease epidemiology and resources. Polio has been targeted for eradication; this disease has already been eliminated in the Americas and Europe and is close to elimination in the Western Pacific.

Table 122-11 Recommended Postexposure Immunization with Immunoglobulin Preparations in the United States

Disease	Indicated	Comments
Measles	Yes	Standard human immune globulin is recommended for exposed infants and adults with normal immunocompetence (but with a contraindication to measles vaccine) and for immunocompromised patients exposed to measles (regardless of immunization status). Patients should be immunized 3–6 months after immunoglobulin administration. Recommended dose: 0.25–0.5 mL/kg (40–80 mg of IgG/kg) IM; 80 mg of IgG/kg for immunocompromised contact; maximum, 15 mL.
Rubella	No	Efficacy is unreliable; therefore, standard human immune globulin is recommended for administration only to antibody-negative pregnant women in the first trimester who have a documented rubella exposure and who will not consider terminating the pregnancy. Recommended dose: 0.55 mL/kg (90 mg of IgG/kg) IM.
Tetanus	Yes	Human tetanus immune globulin (TIG) has replaced equine tetanus antitoxin because of the risk of serum sickness with equine serum. Recommended dose for postexposure prophylaxis: 250–500 units of TIG (10–20 mg of IgG/kg) IM. Recommended dose for treatment of tetanus: 3000–6000 units of TIG IM.
Rabies	Yes	Human rabies immune globulin (RIG) is preferred over equine rabies antiserum because of the risk of serum sickness. RIG or antiserum is recommended for nonimmunized individuals with animal bites in which rabies cannot be ruled out and with other exposures to known rabid animals. Recommended dose of RIG: 20 IU/kg (22 mg of IgG/kg). Recommended dose of antiserum: 40 IU/kg. Rabies vaccine is given as well at 0, 3, 7, 14, and 28 days.
Hepatitis A	Yes	Standard immune serum globulin is given in a single dose of 0.02–0.04 mL/kg or (for continuous exposure) in a dose of up to 0.06 mL/kg every 5 months. Postexposure treatment with hepatitis A immune globulin has not been studied.
Hepatitis B	Yes	Standard immune serum globulin is not reliably effective. Special human hepatitis B immune globulin is useful and is recommended for neonates born to an infected mother and after mucous-membrane or parenteral contact with infected persons or infected blood or serum. Recommended dose for neonates: 0.5 mL IM within 12 h of birth. Recommended dose for percutaneous or mucosal exposure: 0.06 mL/kg (10 mg of IgG/kg) IM.
Non-A, non-B hepatitis	Yes	Standard immune serum globulin may be valuable. Recommended dose: 0.12 mL/kg (10 mg of IgG/kg) IM, up to 10 mL.

Because infectious diseases know no geographic or political boundaries, uncontrolled disease anywhere in the world poses a threat to the United States. Vaccines offer the opportunity to control and even eradicate some diseases, and eradication means that vaccines are no longer needed. Vaccines represent the best hope for stopping the pandemic of HIV infection throughout the world. The experience with smallpox has shown that the eradication of disease is a remarkably good economic investment. The entire sum that the United States spent for the global smallpox eradication campaign has been recouped, in 1968 dollars, every 2.5 months since 1971. The global eradication of polio will save the United States over $300 million a year in vaccine and associated delivery costs and will save over $1.5 billion a year worldwide.

Issues of cost, liability, risk, and profitability limit the interest of the pharmaceutical industry in the development of vaccines (e.g., for malaria) that will be used primarily in poor developing countries. Efforts have been made to create partnerships in public research and privately funded development. Activities of established international organizations (such as the World Health Organization) and some new organizations (such as the Global Alliance for Vaccines and Immunization, the International AIDS Vaccine Initiative, and the Bill and Melinda Gates Foundation) have helped to move the process forward with strategy development and implementation or new funding. New international schemes are being considered by wealthy industrial nations; for example, advance-purchase schemes are being proposed in which the purchase of effective vaccines is guaranteed, ensuring the profitability that the marketplace has provided for industry in the wealthy countries. The effectiveness of such approaches remains to be seen, but they offer much-needed hope for at-risk populations around the world.

Table 122-12 Standards for Immunization Practices

Standard Number	Standard
Pediatric Practice	
1.	Immunization services are readily available.
2.	There are no barriers to or unnecessary prerequisites for the receipt of vaccines.
3.	Immunization services are available free or for a minimal fee.
4.	Providers use all clinical encounters to screen and, when indicated, immunize children.
5.	Providers educate parents and guardians about immunization in general terms.
6.	Providers question parents or guardians about contraindications and, before immunizing a child, inform them in specific terms about the risks and benefits of the immunizations their child is to receive.
7.	Providers follow only true contraindications.
8.	Providers administer simultaneously all vaccine doses for which a child is eligible at the time of each visit.
9.	Providers use accurate and complete recording procedures.
10.	Providers coschedule immunization appointments in conjunction with appointments for other child health services.
11.	Providers report adverse events following immunization promptly, accurately, and completely.
12.	Providers operate a tracking system.
13.	Providers adhere to appropriate procedures for vaccine management.
14.	Providers conduct semiannual audits to assess immunization coverage levels and to review immunization records for the patient populations they serve.
15.	Providers maintain up-to-date, easily retrievable medical protocols at all locations where vaccines are administered.
16.	Providers operate with patient-oriented and community-based approaches.
17.	Vaccines are administered by properly trained individuals.
18.	Providers receive ongoing education and training on current immunization recommendations.
Adult Practice	
1.	Appropriate vaccine use is promoted through information campaigns for health care practitioners and trainees, employers, and the public about the benefits of immunizations.
2.	Providers are completely immunized to protect themselves and prevent transmission to patients.
3.	Providers routinely determine the immunization status of their adult patients, offer vaccines to those for whom they are indicated, and maintain complete immunization records.
4.	Providers identify high-risk patients in need of influenza vaccine and develop a system to recall them for annual immunization.
5.	Providers and institutions identify high-risk adult patients in hospitals and other treatment centers and ensure that appropriate vaccination is considered either before discharge or as part of discharge planning.
6.	Licensing/accreditation agencies support the development by health care institutions of comprehensive immunization programs for staff, trainees, volunteer workers, inpatients, and outpatients.
7.	States establish preenrollment immunization requirements for colleges and other institutions of higher education.
8.	Institutions that train health care professionals, deliver health care, or provide laboratory or other medical support services require appropriate immunizations for persons at risk of contracting or transmitting vaccine-preventable illnesses.
9.	Health care benefit programs, third-party payers, and government health care programs provide coverage for adult immunization services.
10.	A standard personal and institutional immunization record is adopted as a means of verifying the immunization status of patients and staff.

SOURCE: For pediatric standards: Ad Hoc Working Group for the Development of Standards for Pediatric Immunization Practices. JAMA 269:1817, 1993; for adult standards: The National Coalition for Adult Immunization.

SOURCES OF INFORMATION ON IMMUNIZATION

- Official vaccine package circulars and Vaccine Administration Statements from the Centers for Disease Control and Prevention
- Report of the Committee on Infectious Diseases of the American Academy of Pediatrics ("Red Book")
- Recommendations of the Advisory Committee on Immunization Practices, Centers for Disease Control and Prevention
- Guide for Adult Immunization, American College of Physicians
- Health Information for International Travel (published yearly) and Advisory Memoranda on Travel (published periodically), Centers for Disease Control and Prevention
- Control of Communicable Diseases in Man, American Public Health Association
- Technical Bulletin of the College of Obstetrics and Gynecology
- National Network for Immunization Information, Infectious Diseases Society of America/Pediatric Infectious Diseases Society/American Academy of Pediatrics/American Nurses Association

BIBLIOGRAPHY

ADVISORY COMMITTEE ON IMMUNIZATION PRACTICES: Recommended childhood immunization schedule—United States. MMWR 48:12, 1999

ALARCON JB et al: DNA vaccines: Technology and application as anti-parasite and anti-microbial agents. Adv Parasitol 42:343, 1999

CASADEVALL A: Passive antibody therapies: Progress and continuing challenges. Clin Immunol 93:5, 1999

CHAPEL HM: Safety and availability of immunoglobulin replacement therapy in relation to potentially transmissible agents. IUIS Committee on Primary Immunodeficiency Disease. International Union of Immunological Societies. Clin Exp Immunol 118(Suppl 1):29, 1999

CLELAND JL: Single-administration vaccines: Controlled-release technology to mimic repeated immunizations. Trends Biotechnol 17:25, 1999

CUTTS FT et al: Measles elimination: Progress and challenges. Vaccine 17(Suppl 2):S47, 1999

CZERKINSKY C et al: Mucosal immunity and tolerance: Relevance to vaccine development. Immunol Rev 170:197, 1999

GARDNER P: Indications for acellular pertussis vaccines in adults: The case for selective, rather than universal, recommendations. Clin Infect Dis 28(Suppl 2):S131, 1999

GELLIN BG et al: Adult immunization: Principles and practice. Adv Intern Med 44:327, 1999

GLEZEN WP, ALPERS M: Maternal immunization. Clin Infect Dis 28:219, 1999

JONG EC: Travel immunization. Med Clin North Am 83:903, 1999

KEITEL WA: Cellular and acellular pertussis vaccines in adults. Clin Infect Dis 28(Suppl 2):S118, 1999

KILLEEN K et al: Bacterial mucosal vaccines: *Vibrio cholerae* as a live attenuated vaccine/vector paradigm. Curr Top Microbiol Immunol 236:237, 1999

LINDBERG AA: Glycoprotein conjugate vaccines. Vaccine 17(Suppl 2):S28, 1999

MAHONEY RT, MAYNARD JE: The introduction of new vaccines into developing countries. Vaccine 17:646, 1999

MOLRINE DC et al: Normal IgG and impaired IgM responses to polysaccharide vaccines in asplenic patients. J Infect Dis 179:513, 1999

RICHTER L, KIPP B: Transgenic plants as edible vaccines. Curr Top Microbiol Immunol 240:159, 1999

SINGHAL S, MEHTA J: Reimmunization after blood or marrow stem cell transplantation. Bone Marrow Transplant 23:637, 1999

Vaccine-preventable diseases: Improving vaccination coverage in children, adolescents, and adults. A report on recommendations from the Task Force on Community Preventive Services. MMWR 48(RR-8):1, 1999

WEBSITES OF INTEREST

www.cdc.gov/nip
www.idsociety.org/vaccine/resources.html
www.nfid.org/factsheets
www.genweb.com/Dnavax/dnavax.html

123

J.S. Keystone, P.E. Kozarsky

HEALTH ADVICE FOR INTERNATIONAL TRAVEL

In 1991, the World Health Organization estimated that more than 30 million persons traveled from industrialized countries to the developing world. Studies show that between 50 and 75% of short-term travelers to the tropics or subtropics report some health impairment. Most of these health problems are minor, with only 5% requiring medical attention and fewer than 1% requiring hospitalization.

Although infectious agents contribute substantially to morbidity in travelers, these pathogens account for only about 1% of deaths among this population. Cardiovascular disease and injuries are the most frequent causes of death among travelers from the United States, accounting for 49 and 22% of deaths, respectively. Age-specific rates of mortality due to cardiovascular disease are similar to those among nontravelers. In contrast, rates of death due to injury—the majority from motor vehicle, drowning, or aircraft accidents—are several times higher among travelers. Figure 123-1 summarizes the monthly incidence of health problems during travel in developing countries.

GENERAL ADVICE

Staying healthy during travel requires familiarity with the health risks that may be encountered at a given destination. However, health maintenance recommendations are based not only on the traveler's destination but also on risk assessment, which is determined by health status, specific itinerary, and lifestyle during travel. Detailed information regarding country-specific risks and recommendations may be obtained from many sources, including those listed under "Sources of Information on Travel Medicine."

IMMUNIZATIONS FOR TRAVEL Immunizations for travel are generally divided into three categories: routine (childhood/adult boosters that are necessary regardless of travel), required (immunizations that are mandated by international regulations for entry into certain areas or for border crossings), and recommended (immunizations that are desirable because they confer protection against a variety of

illnesses for which travel increases the risk). Vaccines commonly given to travelers are listed in Table 123-1.

Routine Immunizations • *Diphtheria, tetanus, and polio* Diphtheria continues to be a problem worldwide, with large outbreaks in the independent states formerly encompassed by the Soviet Union. Serosurveys show that tetanus antitoxin is lacking in many North Americans, especially those over the age of 50. Although the risk of polio to the international traveler is extremely low and although polio has been eradicated from the western hemisphere, studies in the United States have found varying levels of immunity in the general population; data indicate that 12% of adult American travelers are unprotected against at least one poliovirus serogroup. Foreign travel offers an ideal opportunity to have these immunizations updated.

Measles Measles (rubeola) continues to be a major cause of morbidity and mortality in the developing world (Chap. 194). Several outbreaks of measles in the United States have been linked to imported cases. The group at highest risk consists of persons born after 1956 and vaccinated before 1980, in many of whom primary vaccination failed. Travelers in this group should be reimmunized.

Influenza Influenza occurs year-round in the tropics and during the summer months in the southern hemisphere (which coincide with the winter months in the northern hemisphere). Vaccination should be considered for all travelers to these regions, particularly those who are elderly or chronically ill. The largest outbreak of travel-related influenza occurred in the summer of 1998 in Alaska and the Northwest Territories of Canada among cruise ship passengers and staff (Chap. 190).

Pneumococcal infection Pneumococcal vaccine should be administered routinely to persons at high risk of serious pneumococcal infection, such as individuals with chronic heart, lung, or renal disease and those who have been splenectomized or have sickle cell disease.

Required Immunizations • *Yellow fever* Documentation of yellow fever vaccination may be required for entry into countries of sub-Saharan Africa and equatorial South America, where the disease is endemic or epidemic, or into countries that are at risk of having the infection introduced. This vaccine is given only by state-authorized yellow fever centers, and its administration must be documented on an official International Certificate of Vaccination. The incidence of yellow fever among travelers is extremely low, probably because the vaccine is highly efficacious.

Cholera According to the World Health Organization, cholera vaccine should no longer be required for entry into any country. (However, see *recommended* use below.)

Meningococcal meningitis Meningococcal vaccination is required for entry into Saudi Arabia during the Hajj. (For information on *recommended* use, see below.)

Recommended Immunizations • *Hepatitis A and B* Hepatitis A is the most frequent vaccine-preventable infection of travelers; the incidence of symptomatic infection during a 1-month stay in a developing country ranges from 3 to 6 cases per 1000. The risk is six times greater for those who stray from the usual tourist routes. The mortality rate for hepatitis A increases with age, reaching almost 3% among symptomatic individuals over age 50. Several vaccines are available in North America, each of which has an efficacy rate of >95%. The monthly incidence of hepatitis B infection, both symptomatic and asymptomatic, is 80 to 240 cases per 100,000. For reasons that are not entirely clear, long-stay overseas workers are at considerable risk for hepatitis B infection. In the near future, a combined hepatitis A and B vaccine should become available in the United States.

Typhoid fever The attack rate for typhoid fever is 1 case per 30,000 per month of travel to the developing world (Chap. 156). However, the rates in India, Senegal, and North Africa are tenfold higher, and, within these areas, rates are especially high among travelers to relatively remote destinations and among persons who are returning to their homelands to stay with relatives or friends. Each of the three

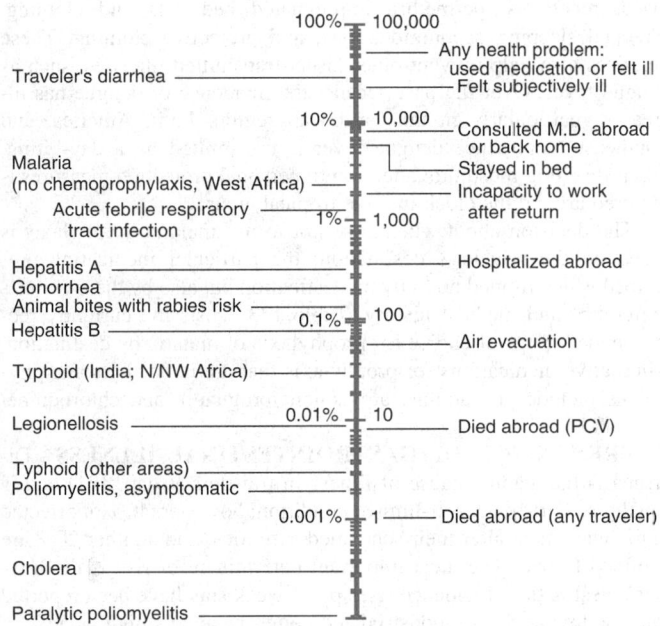

FIGURE 123-1 Incidence rate, per month, of health problems during a stay in developing countries. PCV, Peace Corps volunteer. *(From Steffen and Lobel, with permission from Chapman and Hall, New York.)*

Table 123-1 Vaccines Commonly Used for Travel

Vaccine	Primary Series	Booster Interval
Cholera, parenteral	2 doses, ≥1 week apart, SC or IM	6 months
Cholera, live oral (CVD 103 - HgR)	1 dose	6 months
Hepatitis A (Havrix), 1440 enzyme immunoassay units/mL	2 doses, 6–12 months apart, IM	>10 years
Hepatitis A (VAQTA)[a]	2 doses, 6–12 months apart, IM	>10 years
Hepatitis A/B combined (Twinrix)	3 doses at 0, 1, and 6–12 months, IM	>10 years
Hepatitis B (Engerix B): accelerated schedule	3 doses at 0, 1, and 2 months *or* 0, 7, and 21 days, IM	12 months, once only
Hepatitis B (Engerix B or Recombivax): standard schedule	3 doses at 0, 1, and 6 months, IM	None required
Immune globulin (hepatitis A prevention)	1 dose IM	Intervals of 3–5 months, depending on initial dose
Japanese encephalitis (JEV, Biken)	3 doses, 1 week apart, SC	12–18 months (first booster), then 4 years
Lyme disease (PMC)	3 doses at 0, 1, and 12 months, IM	Optimum booster schedule not yet determined
Meningococcus, quadrivalent	1 dose SC	>3 years (optimum booster schedule not yet determined)
Rabies, human diploid cell vaccine (HDCV)	3 doses at 0, 7, and 21 or 28 days, ID	None required except with exposure
Rabies (HDCV), rabies vaccine absorbed (RVA), or purified chick embryo cell vaccine (PCEC)	3 doses at 0, 7, and 21 or 28 days, IM	None required except with exposure
Typhoid, heat-phenol-inactivated	2 doses, ≥4 weeks apart, SC	3 years
Typhoid Ty21a, oral live attenuated (Vivotif)	1 capsule every other day × 4 doses	5 years
Typhoid Vi capsular polysaccharide, injectable (Typhim Vi)	1 dose IM	2 years
Yellow fever	1 dose SC	10 years

[a] Two new vaccines have been marketed (AVAXIM and EPAXAL).

available vaccines—one oral and two injectable—has an efficacy rate of approximately 70%.

Meningococcal meningitis Although the risk of meningococcal disease among travelers has not been quantified, it is likely to be higher among those who live with poor indigenous populations in overcrowded conditions. The vaccine is recommended for persons traveling to sub-Saharan Africa during the dry season or to areas of the world where there are epidemics. Meningococcal vaccine, which protects against serogroups A/C/Y/W-135, has an efficacy rate of >90%.

Japanese encephalitis The risk of Japanese encephalitis, an infection transmitted by mosquitoes in rural Asia and Southeast Asia, is approximately 1 case per 5000 per month of stay in an endemic area. Most symptomatic infections in U.S. residents have involved military personnel or their families. The vaccine efficacy rate is >80%. Serious allergic reactions sometimes occur; these reactions may be delayed in onset, developing up to 10 days after immunization. The vaccine is recommended for persons staying >1 month in endemic areas.

Cholera The risk of cholera is extremely low, with approximately 1 case per 500,000 journeys to endemic areas. Cholera vaccine is rarely recommended but should be considered for aid workers in refugee camps or in disaster/war-torn areas. The injectable vaccine available in the United States is only 30 to 50% effective, and its protective effect persists for only a short period. A more effective oral cholera vaccine is available in other countries.

Rabies Many cases of rabies have been reported in travelers, but there are no data on the risk of infection. Domestic animals are the major transmitters of rabies in developing countries (Chap. 197). Countries where canine rabies is highly endemic include Mexico, the Philippines, Sri Lanka, India, Thailand, and Vietnam. Each of the three vaccines available in the United States provides >90% protection. Rabies vaccine is recommended for long-stay travelers, particularly children, and persons who may be occupationally exposed in endemic areas.

PREVENTION OF MALARIA AND OTHER INSECT-BORNE DISEASES It is estimated that more than 30,000 American and European travelers develop malaria each year (Chap. 214). Nevertheless, several studies indicate that fewer than 50% of U.S. travelers to malaria-endemic regions adhere to basic recommendations for malaria prevention.

The risk of malaria is highest in sub-Saharan Africa and Oceania (1:50 to 1:1000) and during the past decade has increased by more than fivefold for travelers to Kenya. The risk is intermediate (1:1000 to 1:12,000) for travelers to Haiti and the Indian subcontinent and is low (<1:50,000) for travelers to Asia and to Central and South America. Of the 1000 cases of malaria reported annually in the United States, 90% of those due to *Plasmodium falciparum* occur in travelers returning or immigrating from Africa and Oceania. With the worldwide increase in chloroquine- and multidrug-resistant falciparum malaria, decisions about chemoprophylaxis have become more difficult. Moreover, the spread of malaria due to primaquine- and chloroquine-resistant strains of *P. vivax* has added to the complexity of treatment. The case-fatality rate of falciparum malaria in the United States is 4%; however, in only one-third of patients who die is the diagnosis of malaria considered before death.

Compliance with chemoprophylaxis regimens and use of personal protection measures are keys to the prevention of malaria. Personal protection measures are aimed at preventing mosquito bites, especially between dusk and dawn, and include the use of DEET-containing insect repellents, permethrin-impregnated bed nets and clothing, screened sleeping accommodations, and protective clothing. These practices also help prevent other insect-transmitted illnesses, such as dengue fever. Over the past decade, the incidence of dengue has increased, particularly in the Caribbean region, Latin America, and Southeast Asia. Since dengue fever is transmitted by a day-biting, urban-dwelling mosquito, attention to personal protection measures is required around the clock in most tropical areas.

The decision about whether or not to use malaria prophylaxis is based on the traveler's destination; the particular medication prescribed is determined not only by destination but also by the traveler's preference and medical history. Table 123-2 lists the currently recommended drugs of choice for prophylaxis of malaria by destination. Alternative medications for prophylaxis that are in use by some physicians include primaquine, atovaquone/proguanil, and chloroquine/proguanil.

PREVENTION OF GASTROINTESTINAL ILLNESS Diarrhea is the leading cause of illness in travelers (Chap. 131) and is usually a short-lived, self-limited condition; however, 40% of affected individuals must alter their scheduled activities, and another 20% are confined to bed. The most important determinant of risk is the traveler's destination. Incidence rates per 2-week stay have been reported to be as low as 8% in industrialized countries and as high as 55% in parts of Africa, Central and South America, and Southeast Asia. Infants and young adults are at particularly high risk. The incidence of diarrhea is proportional to the number of dietary indiscretions. Studies of U.S. students in Mexico showed that eating meals in restaurants and cafe-

Geographic Area	Drug of Choice	Alternatives
Central America (north of Panama), Haiti, Dominican Republic, Iraq, Egypt, Turkey, northern Argentina, and Paraguay	Chloroquine	Mefloquine Doxycycline Atovaquone/proguanil
South America including Panama (except northern Argentina and Paraguay); Asia (including Southeast Asia); Africa; and Oceania	Mefloquine	Doxycycline Atovaquone/proguanil
Thai, Myanmar, and Cambodian borders	Doxycycline	Atovaquone/proguanil Primaquine?

[a] See CDC's *Health Information for International Travel 1999–2000.*
NOTE: See also Chap. 214.

terias or consuming food from street vendors was associated with increased risk.

The most frequently identified pathogen causing traveler's diarrhea is toxigenic *Escherichia coli*, although in some parts of the world (notably northern Africa and Southeast Asia) *Campylobacter* infections appear to predominate. Other common causative organisms include *Salmonella, Shigella*, rotavirus, and the Norwalk agent. Except for giardiasis, parasitic infections are uncommon causes of traveler's diarrhea. A growing problem for travelers is the development of antibiotic resistance in many bacterial pathogens, including strains of *Campylobacter* and *Salmonella* resistant to quinolones and strains of *E. coli, Shigella*, and *Salmonella* resistant to trimethoprim-sulfamethoxazole.

Although the mainstay of prevention of traveler's diarrhea involves food and water precautions, the literature has repeatedly documented dietary indiscretions in 98% of travelers within the first 48 h after arrival at their destination. The old maxim "Boil it, cook it, peel it, or forget it!" is easy to remember but appears to be difficult to adhere to. General food and water precautions include eating foods piping hot; avoiding foods that are raw, poorly cooked, or sold by street vendors; and drinking boiled or commercially bottled beverages, particularly those that are carbonated. Heating kills diarrhea-causing organisms, whereas freezing does not; therefore, ice cubes made from unpurified water should be avoided.

As traveler's diarrhea can occur despite rigorous food and water precautions, travelers should carry medications for self-treatment. For mild to moderate diarrhea, loperamide and fluid replacement may be sufficient. An antibiotic is useful in reducing the frequency of bowel movements and duration of illness in moderate to severe diarrhea. The standard regimen is a 3-day course of a quinolone taken twice daily or (in the case of some of the newer agents) once daily. However, studies have shown that a single large dose of a quinolone may be as effective as the 3-day regimen, particularly if infection with a multidrug-resistant organism is not suspected. For diarrhea acquired in areas such as Thailand, where >70% of *Campylobacter* infections are quinolone resistant, azithromycin may be a better choice.

Prophylaxis of traveler's diarrhea with bismuth subsalicylate is widely used but only about 60% effective. For certain individuals (e.g., athletes who must be in peak physical condition to perform, persons with a repeated history of traveler's diarrhea, and some persons with chronic diseases), a single daily dose of a quinolone antibiotic during travel of <1 month's duration is highly effective.

PREVENTION OF OTHER TRAVEL-RELATED PROBLEMS Travelers are at high risk for *sexually transmitted diseases.* Surveys have shown that large numbers engage in casual sex, and there is a reluctance to use condoms consistently. An increasing number of travelers are being diagnosed with *schistosomiasis.* Travelers should be cautioned to avoid bathing, swimming, or wading in freshwater lakes, streams, or rivers in the parts of tropical South America, the Caribbean, Africa, and Southeast Asia where this infection can be acquired. Travelers are cautioned to avoid walking barefoot because of the risk of *hookworm* and *strongyloidiasis* and, at night, *snakebites.* Prevention of *travel-associated injury* depends mostly on commonsense precautions. Riding on motorcycles and overcrowded public vehicles is not recommended; in particular, individuals should not travel by road after dark in rural areas. In addition to its association with motor vehicle accidents, excessive alcohol use has been a significant factor in drownings, assaults, and injuries.

THE TRAVELER'S MEDICAL KIT A traveler's medical kit is strongly advisable, particularly for long-stay travelers. The contents may vary widely, depending on the itinerary, duration of stay, style of travel, and local medical facilities. While many medications are available abroad, often over the counter, directions for their use may be nonexistent or in a foreign language, and, more important, a product may be outdated or counterfeit. Therefore, if possible, a complete supply of medications should accompany the traveler. In the kit, the short-term traveler should consider carrying an analgesic, an antidiarrheal agent, antihistamines, a laxative, oral rehydration salts, sunscreen with a skin protection factor of at least 30, insect repellents (DEET) for the skin, an insecticide for clothing (permethrin), and (if necessary) an antimalarial. To these medications the long-stay traveler might add a broad-spectrum general-purpose antibiotic, an antibacterial eye and skin ointment, and a topical antifungal cream. Regardless of the duration of travel, a first-aid kit containing items such as scissors, tweezers, and bandages should be considered.

TRAVEL AND SPECIAL HOSTS

PREGNANCY AND TRAVEL A woman's medical history and itinerary, the quality of medical care at her destinations, and her degree of flexibility determine whether travel is wise during pregnancy. According to the American College of Obstetrics and Gynecology, the safest part of pregnancy in which to travel is the second trimester (between 18 and 24 weeks), when there is the least danger of spontaneous abortion or premature labor. Some obstetricians prefer that women stay within a few hundred miles of home after the 28th week of pregnancy in case problems arise; in general, however, healthy women may be advised that it is acceptable to travel.

Despite this general recommendation, there are some relative contraindications to international travel during pregnancy, including certain obstetric risk factors: a history of miscarriage, premature labor, incompetent cervix, or toxemia. General medical problems such as diabetes, heart failure, severe anemia, or a history of thromboembolic disease should also prompt the pregnant woman to postpone her travels. Finally, regions in which the pregnant woman and her fetus may be at excessive risk (e.g., those at high altitudes and those where live-virus vaccines are required or where multidrug-resistant malaria is endemic) are not ideal destinations during any trimester.

Malaria Malaria during pregnancy carries a significant risk of morbidity and death. Levels of parasitemia are highest and failure to clear the parasites after chloroquine treatment are most frequent among primigravidae. Severe disease, with complications such as cerebral malaria, massive hemolysis, and renal failure, is especially likely in pregnancy. Fetal sequelae include spontaneous abortion, stillbirth, preterm delivery, and congenital infection.

Traveler's Diarrhea Because dehydration due to traveler's diarrhea can lead to inadequate placental blood flow, pregnant travelers must be extremely cautious regarding their food and beverage intake. The exclusive consumption of bottled (carbonated) or boiled drinks without ice, the eating of well-cooked meats and pasteurized dairy products, and the avoidance of pre-prepared salad items should help protect against traveler's diarrhea due to the usual causes as well as against infections such as toxoplasmosis, hepatitis E, and listeriosis, which can have serious sequelae in pregnancy.

The mainstay of therapy for traveler's diarrhea is rehydration. Kaolin-pectin combinations and loperamide may be used if necessary, but many of the usual antibiotics (e.g., quinolones) are contraindicated during pregnancy. Ampicillin alone or with clavulanic acid may be used, but many strains of *E. coli* and other organisms implicated in traveler's diarrhea are resistant. Azithromycin or an oral third-generation cephalosporin may be the best option.

Because of the major problems encountered when infants are given local foods and beverages, women are strongly encouraged to breast-feed when traveling with a neonate. A nursing mother with traveler's diarrhea should not stop breast-feeding but should increase her fluid intake.

Air Travel and High-Altitude Destinations   Commercial air travel is not a risk to the healthy pregnant woman or to the fetus. Fetal oxygenation is not adversely affected by the decreased cabin pressures because of the fetal hemoglobin dissociation curve; the higher radiation levels reported at altitudes >10,500 m (35,000 ft) should pose no problem to the healthy pregnant traveler. Since each airline has a policy regarding pregnancy and flying, it is best to check with the specific carrier when booking reservations. Domestic air travel is usually permitted until the 36th week, whereas international air travel is generally curtailed after the 32nd week.

There are no known risks for pregnant women who travel to high-altitude destinations and stay for short periods. However, there are likewise no data on the safety of pregnant women at altitudes >4500 m (15,000 ft). Because of the harsh conditions usually associated with such trips, they are generally contraindicated for other reasons.

THE HIV-INFECTED TRAVELER   The traveler infected with HIV is at special risk of serious infections due to a number of pathogens that may be more prevalent at travel destinations than at home. However, the degree of risk depends primarily on the state of the immune system at the time of travel. For persons whose CD4+ cell counts are normal or >500/μL, no data suggest a greater risk during travel than for persons without HIV infection. Individuals with AIDS (CD4+ counts <200/μL) and others who are symptomatic need special counseling and should visit a travel medicine practitioner before departure, especially when traveling to the developing world.

Several countries now routinely deny entry to HIV-positive individuals, even though no data show that these restrictions decrease rates of transmission of the virus. In general, HIV testing is required of those individuals who wish to stay abroad longer than 3 months or who intend to work or study abroad. Some countries will accept an HIV serologic test done within 6 months of departure, whereas others will not accept a blood test done at any time in the traveler's home country. In addition, border officials often have the authority to make inquiries of individuals entering a country and to check the medications they are carrying. If a drug such as zidovudine (AZT) is identified, the person may be barred from entering the country. Information on testing requirements for specific countries is available from consular offices but is subject to frequent change.

Health insurance policies should be checked to make sure they are valid for care in other countries. The HIV-positive traveler should strongly consider obtaining trip cancellation insurance and evacuation insurance in case of illness. It is ideal to have the name of a physician at the travel destination who is familiar with the treatment of patients with AIDS, as the clinical findings associated with infection may be atypical in a patient with AIDS, and several infections may exist simultaneously. The traveler should be encouraged to visit the physician promptly if problems arise.

Immunizations   All of the HIV-infected traveler's routine immunizations should be up to date (Chap. 122). The response to immunization may be impaired at CD4+ cell counts of <200/μL (and in some cases at even higher counts). However, when the risk of illness is high or the sequelae of illness are serious, immunization is recommended. In certain circumstances, it may be prudent to check the adequacy of the serum antibody response before departure (e.g., yellow fever neutralization inhibition if exposure is unavoidable).

Because of the increased risk of infections due to *Streptococcus pneumoniae* and other bacterial pathogens that cause pneumonia following influenza, pneumococcal polysaccharide and influenza vaccines should be administered. The estimated rates of response to influenza vaccine are >80% among persons with asymptomatic HIV infection and <50% among those with AIDS.

In general, live attenuated vaccines are contraindicated for persons with immune dysfunction. Live oral polio vaccine should not be given to HIV-infected patients or to members of their households. Instead, inactivated polio vaccine (eIPV) should be used; most HIV-infected individuals without AIDS will develop protective antibody levels in response to this vaccine.

Because measles (rubeola) can be a severe and lethal infection in HIV-positive patients, the measles vaccine (or the combination measles-mumps-rubella vaccine) should be given to these individuals. Although this is a live vaccine, there have been no reports of serious complications in this population. Between 18 and 58% of symptomatic HIV-infected vaccinees develop adequate antibody titers, and between 50 and 100% of those who are infected but asymptomatic seroconvert.

The decision of whether or not to administer any of the special vaccines to an HIV-infected traveler should be based on the individual's risk. Inactivated vaccines can be administered without concern for safety but with concern about adequate protection. For example, data suggest that HIV-infected persons do not have as strong an antibody response to the meningococcal meningitis vaccine as do uninfected persons. Moreover, few data are available on the efficacy of many of the other vaccines (e.g., those for hepatitis A, typhoid, and cholera).

It is recommended that the live yellow fever vaccine not be given to HIV-infected travelers. Nevertheless, when inadvertently administered to HIV-positive military personnel, this vaccine elicited no adverse reactions. Therefore, if the traveler's CD4+ count is >200/μL and travel in an endemic area is absolutely necessary, the vaccine can probably be administered safely. HIV-infected persons whose CD4+ count is <200/μL should be discouraged from traveling to endemic regions. If the traveler is passing through or traveling to an area where the vaccine is required but the disease risk is low, a physician's waiver should be issued. Bacille Calmette-Guérin vaccine should not be given because of reports of disseminated infection in HIV-infected persons.

A transient (days to weeks) burst of viremia has been demonstrated in HIV-infected individuals following immunization with vaccines for such diseases as influenza, pneumococcal infection, and tetanus (Chap. 309). However, at this point, there is no evidence that this transient increase in viremia is detrimental over time. Furthermore, it is likely that immune activation associated with infection with the live organisms in question would result in increases in viremia of greater magnitude and duration than those associated with vaccination. Therefore, the vaccination recommendations discussed above need not be modified at this time.

Gastrointestinal Illness   Decreased levels of gastric acid, abnormal gastrointestinal mucosal immunity, other complications of HIV infection, and medications taken by HIV-infected patients make traveler's diarrhea especially problematic in these individuals. Traveler's diarrhea is likely to occur more frequently, be more severe, and be more difficult to treat in association with HIV infection. *Salmonella*, *Shigella*, and *Campylobacter* infections are also more protracted and more often accompanied by bacteremia in HIV-infected persons.

Cryptosporidium (Chap. 218), a common cause of diarrhea in tropical countries, produces severe chronic diarrhea and cholecystitis with increased mortality among patients with AIDS. *Isospora belli* causes infections at high rates among AIDS patients in the developing world; this infection is associated with malabsorption, weight loss, and relapses after treatment. Persistent diarrhea due to microsporidiosis has been reported.

Because of these potential problems, the HIV-infected traveler must be careful to consume only appropriately prepared foods and beverages. In addition, this group of individuals may benefit from prophylaxis for traveler's diarrhea, using bismuth subsalicylate or a daily antibiotic (ideally a quinolone derivative) for short-term travel to the developing world. If the traveler is already taking a sulfonamide preparation for prophylaxis of *Pneumocystis* pneumonia, a regimen of self-treatment with a quinolone would be appropriate.

Other Travel-Related Infections Data are lacking on the severity of vector-borne diseases in HIV-infected individuals. Malaria is especially severe in asplenic and certain immunocompromised hosts, although increased severity has not been demonstrated in AIDS. *Babesia* infection is known to cause serious illness and to recur in HIV-infected patients; this tick-transmitted illness occurs in parts of the United States but is not known to be a widespread problem.

Visceral leishmaniasis (Chap. 215) has been reported in numerous HIV-infected travelers. Because the usual signs—splenomegaly and hyperglobulinemia—are nonspecific and may even be lacking, the diagnosis is difficult to make. In addition, serologic results are often negative. This infection is difficult to treat, and its associated mortality is high. Even short-term travelers to southern Europe have developed the illness; thus, the avoidance of sandfly bites is critical.

Certain respiratory illnesses, such as histoplasmosis and coccidioidomycosis, cause greater morbidity and mortality among patients with AIDS than in the general population. Though tuberculosis is common among HIV-infected persons (especially in developing countries), the acquisition of this infection by the short-term traveler is not a major concern. The possibility of acquiring *Legionella* infections from spas should be considered, although no data confirm an increase in the severity of such infections in AIDS.

Finally, the HIV-infected traveler should always be cautioned about safe sexual practices, which may help prevent both the transmission of HIV to others and the acquisition by the traveler of other sexually transmitted diseases that may be drug resistant or may result in serious sequelae (e.g., syphilis).

Medications Adverse events due to medications and drug interactions are common and raise complex issues for HIV-infected persons. In addition, rates of cutaneous reaction are unusually high among patients with AIDS. Physicians advising these travelers need to consider the problems that may arise from the use of agents such as antimalarial drugs, medications for altitude acclimatization, or antidiarrheal compounds; one example is increased cutaneous sensitivity to sulfonamides. Since zidovudine is metabolized by hepatic glucuronidation, inhibitors of this process may elevate serum levels of the drug. Though quinine does not affect levels of zidovudine, there are no relevant data on chloroquine, primaquine, or mefloquine. Furthermore, it is not known whether the antagonistic effect of zidovudine on pyrimethamine has clinical relevance in the treatment or prevention of plasmodial infections.

CHRONIC ILLNESS, DISABILITY, AND TRAVEL Evaluating fitness for travel is a growing issue in view of the increased number of elderly and chronically ill individuals journeying to exotic destinations. Conditions encountered during flight are of particular concern in these cases. Since most commercial aircraft are pressurized to 2500 m (8000 ft) above sea level, corresponding to a Pa_{O_2} of about 55 mmHg, individuals with serious cardiopulmonary problems should be evaluated before travel. In addition, those who have recently had surgery, a myocardial infarction, a cerebrovascular accident, or another medical crisis may be at high risk for adverse events in flight. A summary of current recommendations regarding fitness to fly has been published by the Aerospace Medical Association Air Transport Medical Committee. Chronic health problems should not prevent travel, but special measures can make the journey safer and more comfortable.

Heart Disease Cardiovascular events are the main cause of deaths among travelers and of in-flight emergencies on commercial aircraft. Persons with underlying heart disease should review their itineraries with a physician prior to departure; travel in harsh environments or to remote destinations is not wise. Extra supplies of all medications should be kept in carry-on luggage, along with a recent copy of an electrocardiogram and the name and telephone number of the traveler's physician at home. Pacemakers are not affected by airport security devices, but electronic telephone checks of pacemaker function cannot be transmitted by international satellites. The traveler may benefit from supplemental oxygen, which should be ordered by a physician (since oxygen delivery systems are not standard) 48 to 72 h before flight time. Personal oxygen tanks are not permitted on aircraft. Travelers should request aisle seating and should walk, perform stretching and flexing exercises, and remain hydrated during the flight to prevent venous thrombosis and pulmonary embolism.

Chronic Lung Disease Chronic obstructive pulmonary disease (COPD) is one of the most common diagnoses in patients who require emergency-room evaluation for symptoms occurring during airline flights. Patients with COPD experience dyspnea, edema, wheezing, cyanosis, and chest pain. The best predictor of the development of these symptoms is the sea level Pa_{O_2}. A Pa_{O_2} of at least 72 mmHg corresponds to an in-flight Pa_{O_2} of 55 mmHg when the cabin is pressurized to 2500 m (8000 ft). Therefore, if the traveler's baseline Pa_{O_2} is <72 mmHg, the provision of supplemental oxygen during the flight should be considered. Pulmonary function is also maximized by continuing bronchodilator treatment and the use of glucocorticoids as prescribed. Contraindications to flight include active bronchospasm, lower respiratory infection, phlebitis, pulmonary hypertension, and recent thoracic surgery (within the preceding 3 weeks) or pneumothorax. Consideration should be given to decreasing the amount of outdoor activity at the destination if there is excessive air pollution.

Diabetes Mellitus Alterations in glucose control and changes in insulin requirements are common problems when diabetic patients travel. Changes in time zone, in the amount and timing of food intake, and in physical activity demand more vigilant assessment of metabolic control. The diabetic traveler should pack medication (including a bottle of regular insulin for emergencies), insulin syringes and needles, equipment and supplies for glucose monitoring, and snacks in carry-on luggage. Insulin is stable for about 3 months at room temperature but should be kept as cool as possible. The name and telephone number of the home physician and a card and necklace listing the medical problems and the type and dose of insulin used should accompany the traveler. When six or more time zones are crossed, insulin requirements may be temporarily altered, depending on food intake and physical activity. In traveling eastward (e.g., from the United States to Europe), the morning insulin dose on arrival may need to be decreased. The blood glucose can then be checked during the day to determine whether additional insulin is required. For flights westward, with lengthening of the day, an additional dose of regular insulin may be required. Comfortable footwear is essential for the diabetic traveler.

Other Special Groups Other groups for whom special travel measures are now being encouraged include patients undergoing dialysis, those with transplants, and those with other disabilities. Up to 13% of travelers have some disability, but few advocacy groups and tour companies dedicate themselves to this growing population. The key to safe travel in each case is adequate research ahead of time. Patients undergoing chronic ambulatory peritoneal dialysis may ship their dialysis solutions to their destinations before traveling. They should carry essential medical records as well as antibiotics for self-treatment of presumed peritonitis. Hemodialysis patients need to reserve appointments at dialysis centers prior to their departure from home. Travel by transplant recipients to distant destinations should ideally be scheduled at least 1 year after surgery, as most rejection episodes occur early. Medication interactions are a source of serious concern for these travelers, and appropriate medical information should be carried, along with the home physician's name and telephone number. Some travelers taking glucocorticoids carry stress doses in case they become ill. Immunization of these immunocompromised travelers may result in less than adequate protection against certain diseases. Thus, the traveler and physician must carefully consider which destinations are appropriate.

PROBLEMS AFTER RETURN

The most frequent medical problems encountered by travelers after their return home are diarrhea, fever, respiratory illnesses, and skin diseases. Frequently ignored problems are fatigue and emotional stress, especially in long-stay travelers. The approach to diagnosis requires some knowledge of geographic medicine, in particular the epidemiology and clinical presentation of infectious disorders. A geographic history should focus on the traveler's exact itinerary, including dates of arrival and departure; exposure history (food indiscretions, drinking-water sources, freshwater contact, sexual activity, animal contact, insect bites); location and style of travel (urban vs. rural, first-class hotel accommodation vs. camping); immunization history; and use of antimalarial chemosuppression.

DIARRHEA　Although extremely common, acute traveler's diarrhea is usually self-limited or amenable to antibiotic therapy. Bowel symptoms that persist after the traveler's return home have a less well-defined etiology and may require medical attention from a specialist. Infectious agents appear to be responsible for only a small proportion of cases with persistent bowel symptoms. Of the pathogens detected in these instances, *Giardia lamblia* (Chap. 218) is by far the most common; *Cyclospora cayetanensis*, *Cryptosporidium* spp., and *Entamoeba histolytica* are rare isolates. The most frequent causes of persistent diarrhea after travel are postinfectious sequelae, such as lactose intolerance or an irritable bowel syndrome. When no infectious etiology can be identified, a trial of metronidazole therapy for presumed giardiasis, a strict lactose-free diet for 1 week, or a several-week trial of high-dose hydrophilic mucilloid relieves the symptoms of many patients.

FEVER　Fever in a traveler who has returned from a malarious area should be considered a medical emergency because death from *P. falciparum* malaria can follow an illness of only several days' duration. Although "fever from the tropics" does not always have a tropical cause, malaria should be the first diagnosis considered. The risk of *P. falciparum* malaria is highest among travelers returning from Africa or Oceania and among those who become symptomatic within the first 2 months after return. Other important causes of fever after travel include viral hepatitis (hepatitis A and E), typhoid fever, bacterial enteritis, arbovirus infections (e.g., dengue fever), rickettsial infections (including tick and scrub typhus or Q fever) and—in rare instances—leptospirosis, acute HIV infection, and amebic liver abscess. In at least 25% of cases, no etiology can be found, and the illness resolves spontaneously. Clinicians should keep in mind that no present-day antimalarial agent guarantees protection from malaria and that some immunizations—notably, those against typhoid and cholera—are only partially protective.

As noted above, the approach to the febrile returned traveler begins with a detailed medical and geographic history. Knowing exact dates of arrival and departure from tropical areas enables the physician to ascertain the shortest and longest possible incubation periods for illnesses in the differential diagnosis. For example, a traveler who develops fever <1 week after arrival in a malarious area cannot have malaria because the incubation period is too short, whereas a fever whose onset comes >2 weeks after departure from an endemic area cannot be dengue fever because the incubation period is too long. In the physical examination, particular attention should be given to the skin so as not to miss a subtle rash or eschar.

When no specific diagnosis is forthcoming, the following investigations may be helpful: complete blood count, liver function tests, thick/thin blood films for malaria (repeated twice if necessary), urinalysis, blood cultures (repeated once if necessary), and collection of an acute-phase serum sample to be held for later examination along with a paired convalescent-phase serum sample.

SKIN DISEASES　Pyodermas, sunburn, insect bites, skin ulcers, and cutaneous larva migrans are the most common skin conditions encountered in travelers after their return home. In those with persistent skin ulcers, the diagnoses of cutaneous leishmaniasis, mycobacterial infection, or fungal infection should be considered. Careful, complete inspection of the skin is important in detecting the rickettsial eschar in a febrile patient or the central breathing hole in a "boil" due to myiasis.

EMERGING INFECTIOUS DISEASES　In recent years, travel and commerce have fostered the worldwide spread of HIV infection, led to the reemergence of cholera as a global health threat, and created considerable fear about the possible spread of Ebola virus infection and plague. For travelers, there are more realistic concerns. One of the largest outbreaks of dengue fever ever documented is now raging in Latin America; schistosomiasis is being described in previously unaffected lakes in Africa; and antibiotic-resistant strains of sexually transmitted and enteric pathogens are emerging at an alarming rate in the developing world. As Nobel Laureate Dr. Joshua Lederberg pointed out, "The microbe that felled one child in a distant continent yesterday can reach yours today and seed a global pandemic tomorrow." The vigilant clinician understands that the importance of a thorough travel history cannot be overemphasized.

SOURCES OF INFORMATION ON TRAVEL MEDICINE

- CDC publication *Health Information for International Travel*
- CDC home page: www.cdc.gov
- CDC travel information: www.cdc.gov/travel/travel.html
- Health Canada: www.hwc.ca/hpb/lcdc
- International Society of Travel Medicine: www.istm.org

BIBLIOGRAPHY

AEROSPACE MEDICAL ASSOCIATION, AIR TRANSPORT MEDICINE COMMITTEE: Medical guidelines for air travel. Aviat Space Environ Med 67(Suppl 10):b1, 1996

CAUMES E et al: Dermatoses associated with travel to tropical countries: A prospective study of the diagnosis and management of 269 patients presenting to a tropical disease unit. Clin Infect Dis 20:542, 1995

CENTERS FOR DISEASE CONTROL AND PREVENTION: *Health Information for International Travel 1999–2000*, publication no. (CDC) 92-8280. Washington, DC, Government Printing Office, 1999

ERICSSON CD: Travelers' diarrhea: Epidemiology, prevention and self-treatment. Infect Dis Clin North Am 12:285, 1998

FRADIN MS: Mosquitoes and mosquito repellents: A clinician's guide. Ann Intern Med 128:931, 1998

KEMMERER TP et al: Health problems of corporate travelers: Risk factors and management. J Trav Med 5:184, 1998

MAGILL AJ: Fever in the returned traveler. Infect Dis Clin North Am 12:455, 1998

MILENO MD, BIA FS: The compromised traveler. Infect Dis Clin North Am 12:369, 1998

SAMUEL B, BARRY M: The pregnant traveler. Infect Dis Clin North Am 12:323, 1998

STEFFEN R, LOBEL HO: Epidemiologic basis for the practice of travel medicine. J Wilderness Med 5:56, 1994

WILSON ME: *A World Guide to Infectious Diseases, Distribution, Diagnosis*. New York, Oxford University Press, 1991

124 *Robert S. Munford*

SEPSIS AND SEPTIC SHOCK

ARDS acute respiratory distress syndrome	LPS lipopolysaccharide
	PAF platelet-activating factor
DIC disseminated intravascular coagulation	SIRS systemic inflammatory response syndrome
IL interleukin	TGF-β transforming growth factor β
IL-1Ra IL-1 receptor antagonist	
iNOS inducible nitric oxide synthase	TNF tumor necrosis factor
LBP LPS-binding protein	

DEFINITIONS (See Table 124-1) The host's reaction to invading microbes involves a rapidly amplifying polyphony of signals and responses that may spread beyond the invaded tissue. Fever or hypothermia, tachypnea, and tachycardia often herald the onset of *sepsis*, the systemic response to microbial invasion. When counterregulatory control mechanisms are overwhelmed, homeostasis may fail, and dysfunction of major organs may supervene (*severe sepsis*). Further regulatory imbalance leads to *septic shock*, which is characterized by hypotension as well as organ dysfunction. As sepsis progresses to septic shock, the risk of dying increases substantially. Sepsis is usually reversible, whereas patients with septic shock often succumb despite aggressive therapy.

The *systemic inflammatory response syndrome* (SIRS), as defined in the early 1990s by critical care specialists, may have an infectious or a noninfectious etiology. If infection is suspected or proven, a patient with SIRS is said to have sepsis.

ETIOLOGY Sepsis can be a response to any class of microorganism. Microbial invasion of the bloodstream is not essential for the development of sepsis, since local or systemic spread of microbial

Table 124-1 Definitions Used to Describe the Condition of Patients with Sepsis

Bacteremia	Presence of bacteria in the blood, as evidenced by positive blood cultures
Septicemia	Presence of microbes or their toxins in blood
Systemic inflammatory response syndrome (SIRS)	Two or more of the following conditions: (1) fever (oral temperature >38°C) or hypothermia (<36°C); (2) tachypnea (>24 breaths/min); (3) tachycardia (heart rate >90 beats/min); (4) leukocytosis (>12,000/μL), leukopenia (<4,000/μL), or >10% bands. May have an infectious or a noninfectious etiology
Sepsis	SIRS that has a proven or suspected microbial etiology
Severe sepsis (similar to "sepsis syndrome")	Sepsis with one or more signs of organ dysfunction (such as metabolic acidosis, acute encephalopathy, oliguria, hypoxemia, or disseminated intravascular coagulation) or hypotension
Septic shock	Sepsis with hypotension (arterial blood pressure of <90 mmHg systolic or 40 mmHg less than patient's normal blood pressure) that is unresponsive to fluid resuscitation, along with organ dysfunction (see severe sepsis)
Refractory septic shock	Septic shock that lasts for >1 h and does not respond to fluid or pressor administration
Multiple-organ dysfunction syndrome (MODS)	Dysfunction of more than one organ, requiring intervention to maintain homeostasis

SOURCE: Adapted from American College of Chest Physicians/Society of Critical Care Medicine Consensus Conference Committee.

signal molecules or toxins can also elicit the response. Blood cultures yield bacteria or fungi in ~20 to 40% of cases of severe sepsis and 40 to 70% of cases of septic shock. Individual gram-negative or gram-positive bacteria account for ~70% of these isolates; the remainder are fungi or a mixture of microorganisms (Table 124-2). In patients whose blood cultures are negative, the etiologic agent is often established by culture or microscopic examination of infected material from a local site. In some case series, a majority of patients with a clinical picture of severe sepsis or septic shock have had negative microbiologic data.

Factors that predispose to gram-negative bacillary bacteremia include diabetes mellitus, lymphoproliferative diseases, cirrhosis of the liver, burns, invasive procedures or devices, and treatment with drugs that cause neutropenia. Major risk factors for gram-positive bacteremia include vascular catheterization, the presence of indwelling mechanical devices, burns, and intravenous drug use. Fungemia occurs most often in immunosuppressed patients with neutropenia, often after broad-spectrum antimicrobial therapy. In patients who experience bacteremia, factors that increase the risk of developing severe sepsis include age (>50 years) and a primary pulmonary, abdominal, or neuromeningeal site of infection. Bacteremia that arises from an intravascular catheter or the urinary tract is less likely to induce severe sepsis.

EPIDEMIOLOGY The septic response is now a contributing factor in >100,000 deaths per year in the United States. The incidence of severe sepsis and septic shock has increased over the last 15 years and is now probably between 300,000 and 500,000 cases per year. Approximately two-thirds of cases occur in patients hospitalized for other illnesses. The increasing incidence of severe sepsis in the United States is attributable to the aging of the population, the increasing longevity of patients with chronic diseases, and the relatively high frequency with which sepsis develops in patients with AIDS. The widespread use of antimicrobial agents, glucocorticoids, indwelling catheters and mechanical devices, and mechanical ventilation also plays a role.

PATHOPHYSIOLOGY The septic response is often triggered when microorganisms spread from the gastrointestinal tract or skin into contiguous tissues. Localized tissue infection may then lead to bacteremia or fungemia. Alternatively, microorganisms may be introduced directly into the bloodstream (for example, via intravenous catheters). In general, the septic response occurs when immune defenses fail to contain an invading microbe. Since most cases are triggered by microbes that do not ordinarily cause systemic disease in normal hosts (Table 124-2), deficiencies in nonadaptive host factors may be most important. The septic response may also be induced by microbial ex-

Table 124-2 Microorganisms Involved in Episodes of Severe Sepsis at Eight Academic Medical Centers

Microorganisms	Episodes with Bloodstream Infection, % (n = 436)	Episodes with Documented Infection but No Bloodstream Infection, % (n = 430)	Total Episodes, % (n = 866)
Gram-negative bacteria[a]	35	44	40
Gram-positive bacteria[b]	40	24	31
Fungi	7	5	6
Polymicrobial	11	21	16
Classic pathogens[c]	<5	<5	<5

[a] Enterobacteriaceae, pseudomonads, *Haemophilus* spp., other gram-negative bacteria.

[b] *Staphylococcus aureus*, coagulase-negative staphylococci, enterococci, *Streptococcus pneumoniae*, other streptococci, other gram-positive bacteria.

[c] Such as *Neisseria meningitidis*, *S. pneumoniae*, *H. influenzae*, and *Streptococcus pyogenes*.

SOURCE: Adapted from Sands et al.

otoxins that act as superantigens (e.g., toxic shock syndrome toxin 1; Chap. 139).

Microbial Signals Animals recognize certain microbial molecules as signals that microorganisms have invaded. Lipopolysaccharide (LPS, also called *endotoxin*) is the most potent and best-studied gram-negative bacterial signal molecule. A plasma protein (LPS-binding protein, or LBP) transfers LPS to CD14 on the surfaces of monocytes, macrophages, and neutrophils. This interaction rapidly triggers the production and release of mediators, such as tumor necrosis factor (TNF) α (see below), that amplify the LPS signal and transmit it to other cells and tissues. Soluble CD14 may also bind LPS in plasma and transfer it to cells that lack cell-surface CD14. The peptidoglycan and lipoteichoic acids of gram-positive bacteria, certain polysaccharides, extracellular enzymes, and toxins elicit responses in animals that are similar to those induced by LPS; some of these molecules may also bind CD14. CD14 thus attracts numerous non-self molecules to the surfaces of myeloid cells, greatly increasing the sensitivity with which these molecules can be recognized by the host. Evidence suggests that signal specificity occurs in or on the plasma membrane and is conferred, at least in part, by members of the toll-like receptor family of transmembrane proteins. Other innate immune mechanisms for recognizing microbial molecules include complement (principally the alternative pathway), mannose-binding protein, and C-reactive protein.

Host Responses The septic response involves complex interactions among microbial signal molecules, leukocytes, humoral mediators, and the vascular endothelium.

Cytokines Inflammatory cytokines amplify and diversify the response. These proteins can exert endocrine, paracrine, and autocrine effects (Chap. 305). TNF-α stimulates leukocytes and vascular endothelial cells to release other cytokines (as well as additional TNF-α), to express cell-surface adhesion molecules, and to increase arachidonic acid turnover. Blood levels of TNF-α are high in most patients with severe sepsis or septic shock. Moreover, intravenous infusion of TNF-α can elicit many of the characteristic abnormalities of sepsis, including fever, tachycardia, tachypnea, leukocytosis, myalgias, and somnolence. In animals, larger doses of TNF-α induce shock, disseminated intravascular coagulation (DIC), and death. Specific TNF-α antagonists can abrogate the septic response and prevent the deaths of experimental animals challenged with endotoxin.

Although TNF-α is a central mediator, it is only one of many cytokines that contribute to the septic process. Interleukin (IL) 1β, for example, which exhibits many of the same activities as TNF-α, seems to play an increasingly significant role as sepsis intensifies. TNF-α, IL-1β, interferon-γ, IL-8, and other cytokines probably interact synergistically with each other and with additional mediators. Moreover, some mediators (such as IL-1β and TNF-α) may enhance their own rates of synthesis by positive feedback. As sepsis progresses, the mixture of cytokines and other molecules becomes very complex: elevated blood levels of >50 molecules have been found in patients with septic shock. In animal models, the septic response can be interrupted by early interventions that neutralize one or another of its many components; this observation testifies to the importance of mediator interactions for the overall outcome. It has been much more difficult to rescue animals from severe sepsis and septic shock.

Phospholipid-derived mediators Arachidonic acid, released from membrane phospholipids by phospholipase A$_2$, is converted by the cyclooxygenase pathway into prostaglandins and thromboxanes. Prostaglandin E$_2$ and prostacyclin cause peripheral vasodilatation, whereas thromboxane is a vasoconstrictor and promotes platelet aggregation. Administration of the cyclooxygenase inhibitor ibuprofen for 48 h to patients with severe sepsis suppressed production of these metabolites and decreased body temperature, heart rate, and metabolic acidosis without reducing mortality. Leukotrienes are also potent mediators of ischemia and shock; the fact that the reaction to endotoxin challenge is normal in mice that lack the 5-lipoxygenase gene, however, casts doubt on the role of leukotrienes in the septic response.

Another important phospholipid-derived mediator is platelet-activating factor (PAF; 1-O-alkyl-2-acetyl-sn-glycero-3-phosphorylcholine). PAF potently stimulates neutrophil aggregation and degranulation, promotes platelet aggregation, and may contribute to tissue injury.

Coagulation factors Intravascular fibrin deposition, thrombosis, and DIC are important features of the septic response. IL-6 and other mediators promote intravascular coagulation initially by inducing blood monocytes to express tissue factor (Chap. 62). When tissue factor is expressed on monocytes, it binds to factor VIIa to form an active complex that can convert factors X and IX to enzymatically active forms. The result is activation of both extrinsic and intrinsic clotting pathways, culminating in the generation of fibrin. Clotting is also favored by impaired function of the protein C–protein S inhibitory pathway and depletion of antithrombin, while fibrinolysis is prevented by increased plasma levels of plasminogen activator inhibitor 1. Thus, there may be a striking propensity to intravascular fibrin deposition, thrombosis, and bleeding (Chap. 146). Contact-system activation occurs during sepsis but contributes more to the development of hypotension than to DIC.

Complement C5a and other products of complement activation may promote neutrophil reactions such as chemotaxis, aggregation, degranulation, and oxygen-radical production. When administered to animals, C5a induces hypotension, pulmonary vasoconstriction, neutropenia, and vascular leakiness due in part to endothelial damage.

Activation of the vascular endothelium Many tissues may be damaged by the septic response. The probable underlying mechanism is widespread vascular endothelial injury, with fluid extravasation and microthrombosis that decrease oxygen and substrate utilization by the affected tissues. Leukocyte-derived mediators and platelet-leukocyte-fibrin thrombi contribute to this injury, but the vascular endothelium itself seems to play an active role. Stimuli such as TNF-α induce vascular endothelial cells to produce and release cytokines, procoagulant molecules, PAF, endothelium-derived relaxing factor (nitric oxide), and other mediators. In addition, regulated cell-adhesion molecules promote the adherence of neutrophils to endothelial cells. While these responses may attract phagocytes to infected sites and activate their antimicrobial arsenals, endothelial cell activation can also promote increased vascular permeability, microvascular thrombosis, DIC, and hypotension. Moreover, vascular integrity may be damaged by neutrophil enzymes (such as elastase) and toxic oxygen metabolites so that local hemorrhage ensues. Blocking the adhesion of leukocytes to endothelial cell surfaces, as with monoclonal antibodies to intercellular adhesion molecule 1, can prevent tissue necrosis in response to endotoxin administration in animals.

Septic shock Much evidence now implicates nitric oxide, produced by inducible nitric oxide synthase (iNOS), as a mediator of septic shock in experimental animals and probably in humans. Mice that lack the *iNOS* gene may not be resistant to endotoxic shock, however. Other prominent hypotensive molecules are β-endorphin, bradykinin, PAF, and prostacyclin. Agents that inhibit the synthesis or action of each of these mediators can prevent or reverse endotoxic shock in animals. However, in clinical trials, neither a PAF receptor antagonist nor a bradykinin antagonist improved the survival rate of patients with septic shock, and a NOS inhibitor, L-N^G-methylarginine HCl, actually increased the mortality rate.

Control mechanisms Elaborate host mechanisms regulate both microbial signals and the inflammatory response. While plasma LBP promotes the inflammatory response by facilitating the interaction of LPS with monocyte cell-surface CD14, LBP and other plasma proteins (such as phospholipid transfer protein) also can prevent LPS signaling by transferring LPS molecules into plasma lipoprotein particles. The relative plasma concentrations of LPS, LBP, CD14, and lipoproteins may therefore govern the intensity with which LPS—and probably other microbial molecules—can trigger host responses. The mechanisms that control the inflammatory response are also complex, overlapping, and poorly understood. Glucocorticoids inhibit cytokine synthesis by monocytes in vitro and, when administered with or shortly after an inflammatory stimulus, may protect animals from septic shock. The increase in blood cortisol levels early in the septic response presumably plays a similar inhibitory role. In addition, certain cytokine antagonists may contribute. Blood levels of IL-1 receptor antagonist (IL-1Ra) often greatly exceed those of circulating IL-1β, and this excess may result in inhibition of the binding of IL-1β to its receptors. Transforming growth factor β (TGF-β) and IL-10 can also inhibit LPS-induced responses by human monocytes in vitro and prevent endotoxic death in animals. Blood and tissue levels of prostaglandin E$_2$, TGF-β, α-melanocyte-stimulating hormone, cortisol, IL-1Ra, soluble TNF receptors, and IL-10 increase during the septic response, and these molecules probably act in concert to diminish its intensity. In fact, very high concentrations of many anti-inflammatory molecules are found in the blood of patients with severe sepsis or septic shock, so that the net mediator balance in the blood of these extremely sick patients may actually be anti-inflammatory. In addition, blood leukocytes from patients with severe sepsis are often hyporesponsive to agonists such as LPS. In patients with severe sepsis, persistence of leukocyte hyporesponsiveness has been associated with an increased risk of dying. Research is needed to clarify the role of the anti-inflammatory response in the septic process.

CLINICAL MANIFESTATIONS The manifestations of the septic response are usually superimposed on the symptoms and signs of the patient's underlying illness and primary infection. The systemic response to infection often intensifies over time from mild (sepsis) to extremely severe (septic shock). The rate at which the response increases may differ from patient to patient, and there are striking individual variations in its manifestations. For example, some patients with sepsis are normo- or hypothermic; the absence of fever is most common in neonates, in elderly patients, and in persons with uremia or alcoholism.

Hyperventilation is often an early sign. Disorientation, confusion, and other manifestations of encephalopathy may also develop early in the septic response, particularly in the elderly and in individuals with preexisting neurologic impairment. Focal neurologic signs are uncommon, although preexisting focal deficits may become more prominent.

Hypotension and DIC predispose to acrocyanosis and ischemic necrosis of peripheral tissues, most commonly the digits. Cellulitis, pustules, bullae, or hemorrhagic lesions may develop when hematogenous bacteria or fungi seed the skin or underlying soft tissue. Bacterial toxins may also be distributed hematogenously to elicit diffuse cutaneous reactions. On occasion, skin lesions may suggest specific pathogens. When sepsis is accompanied by cutaneous petechiae or purpura, infection with *Neisseria meningitidis* (or, less commonly, *Haemophilus influenzae*) should be suspected **(Plate IID-44)**; in a patient who has been bitten by a tick while in an endemic area, petechial lesions also suggest Rocky Mountain spotted fever **(Plate IID-45)**. A cutaneous lesion seen almost exclusively in neutropenic patients is ecthyma gangrenosum, usually caused by *Pseudomonas aeruginosa*. It is a bullous lesion, surrounded by edema, that undergoes central hemorrhage and necrosis **(Plate IID-57C)**. Histopathologic examination shows bacteria in and around the wall of a small vessel, with little or no neutrophilic response. Hemorrhagic or bullous lesions in a septic patient who has recently eaten raw oysters suggest *Vibrio vulnificus* bacteremia, while such lesions in a patient who has recently suffered a dog bite may indicate bloodstream infection due to *Capnocytophaga canimorsus* or *C. cynodegmi*. Generalized erythroderma in a septic patient suggests the toxic shock syndrome due to *Staphylococcus aureus* or *Streptococcus pyogenes*.

Gastrointestinal manifestations such as nausea, vomiting, diarrhea, and ileus may suggest acute gastroenteritis. Stress ulceration can lead to upper gastrointestinal bleeding. Cholestatic jaundice, with elevated levels of serum bilirubin (mostly conjugated) and alkaline phosphatase, may precede other signs of sepsis. Hepatocellular or canalicular dysfunction appears to underlie most cases, and the results of hepatic function tests return to normal with resolution of the infection. Prolonged or severe hypotension may induce acute hepatic injury or ischemic bowel necrosis.

Many tissues may be unable to extract oxygen normally from the blood, so that anaerobic metabolism occurs despite near-normal mixed venous oxygen saturation. Blood lactate levels rise early, in part because of increased glycolysis with impaired clearance of the resulting lactate and pyruvate by the liver and kidneys. As hypoperfusion develops, tissue hypoxia generates more lactic acid, contributing to metabolic acidosis. The blood glucose concentration often increases, particularly in patients with diabetes, although impaired gluconeogenesis and excessive insulin release on occasion produce hypoglycemia. The cytokine-driven acute-phase response inhibits the synthesis of albumin and transthyretin while enhancing the production of C-reactive protein, LBP, fibrinogen, and complement components. Protein catabolism is often markedly accelerated.

MAJOR COMPLICATIONS **Cardiopulmonary Complications** Ventilation-perfusion mismatching produces a fall in arterial P$_{O_2}$ early in the course. Increasing alveolar capillary permeability results in an increased pulmonary water content, which decreases pulmonary compliance and interferes with oxygen exchange. Progressive diffuse pulmonary infiltrates and arterial hypoxemia (Pa$_{O_2}$/FI$_{O_2}$, <200 mmHg) indicate the development of the acute respiratory distress syndrome (ARDS). ARDS develops in ~50% of patients with severe sepsis or septic shock. The failure of the respiratory muscles can exacerbate hypoxemia and hypercapnia. An elevated pulmonary capillary wedge pressure (>18 mmHg) suggests fluid volume overload or cardiac failure rather than ARDS. Pneumonia caused by viruses or by *Pneumocystis carinii* may be clinically indistinguishable from ARDS.

Sepsis-induced hypotension usually results from a generalized maldistribution of blood flow and blood volume and from hypovolemia that is due, at least in part, to diffuse capillary leakage of intravascular fluid. Other factors that may decrease effective intravascular volume include dehydration from antecedent disease or insensible fluid losses, vomiting or diarrhea, and polyuria. During early septic shock, systemic vascular resistance is usually elevated and cardiac output may be low. After fluid repletion, in contrast, cardiac output typically increases and systemic vascular resistance falls. Indeed, normal or increased cardiac output and decreased systemic vascular resistance distinguish septic shock from cardiogenic, extracardiac obstructive, and hypovolemic shock; other processes that can produce this combination include anaphylaxis, beriberi, cirrhosis, and overdoses of nitroprusside or narcotics (Chap. 38).

Depression of myocardial function, manifested as increased end-diastolic and systolic ventricular volumes with a decreased ejection fraction, develops within 24 h in most patients with severe sepsis. Cardiac output is maintained despite the low ejection fraction because ventricular dilatation permits a normal stroke volume. In survivors, myocardial function returns to normal over several days. Although myocardial dysfunction may contribute to hypotension, refractory hypotension is usually due to a low systemic vascular resistance, and death results from refractory shock or the failure of multiple organs rather than from cardiac dysfunction per se.

Renal Complications Oliguria, azotemia, proteinuria, and nonspecific urinary casts are frequently found. Many patients are inappropriately polyuric; hyperglycemia may exacerbate this tendency. Most renal failure is due to acute tubular necrosis induced by hypotension or capillary injury, although some patients also have glomerulonephritis, renal cortical necrosis, or interstitial nephritis. Drug-induced renal damage may complicate therapy, particularly when hypotensive patients are given aminoglycoside antibiotics.

Coagulation Although thrombocytopenia occurs in 10 to 30% of patients, the underlying mechanism(s) are not understood. Platelet counts are usually very low (<50,000/μL) in patients with DIC; these low counts typically reflect diffuse endothelial injury or microvascular thrombosis.

Neurologic Complications When the septic illness lasts for weeks to months, "critical-illness" polyneuropathy may prevent weaning from ventilatory support and produce distal motor weakness. Electrophysiologic studies are diagnostic. Guillain-Barré syndrome, metabolic disturbances, and toxin activity must be ruled out.

LABORATORY FINDINGS Abnormalities that occur early in the septic response may include leukocytosis with a left shift, thrombocytopenia, hyperbilirubinemia, and proteinuria. Leukopenia may develop. The neutrophils may contain toxic granulations, Döhle bodies, or cytoplasmic vacuoles. As the septic response becomes more severe, thrombocytopenia worsens (often with prolongation of the thrombin time, decreased fibrinogen, and the presence of D-dimers, suggesting DIC), azotemia and hyperbilirubinemia become more prominent, and levels of aminotransferases rise. Active hemolysis suggests clostridial bacteremia, malaria, a drug reaction, or DIC; in the case of DIC, microangiopathic changes may be seen on a blood smear.

During early sepsis, hyperventilation induces respiratory alkalosis. With respiratory muscle fatigue and the accumulation of lactate, metabolic acidosis (with increased anion gap) typically supervenes. Evaluation of arterial blood gases reveals hypoxemia, which is initially correctable with supplemental oxygen but whose later refractoriness to 100% oxygen inhalation indicates right-to-left shunting. The chest radiograph may be normal or may show evidence of underlying pneumonia, volume overload, or the diffuse infiltrates of ARDS. The electrocardiogram may show only sinus tachycardia or nonspecific ST-T wave abnormalities.

Most diabetic patients with sepsis develop hyperglycemia. Severe infection may precipitate diabetic ketoacidosis, which may exacerbate hypotension (Chap. 333). Hypoglycemia occurs rarely. The serum albumin level, initially within the normal range, declines as sepsis continues. Serum lipid concentrations are often elevated. Hypocalcemia is rare.

DIAGNOSIS There is no specific test. Diagnostically sensitive findings in a patient with suspected or proven infection include fever or hypothermia, tachypnea, tachycardia, and leukocytosis or leukopenia (Table 124-1); acutely altered mental status, thrombocytopenia, or hypotension also suggests the diagnosis. The septic response can be quite variable, however. In one study, 36% of patients with severe sepsis had a normal temperature, 40% had a normal respiratory rate, 10% had a normal pulse rate, and 33% had normal white blood cell counts. Moreover, the systemic responses of uninfected patients with other conditions may be similar to those characteristic of sepsis. Noninfectious etiologies of SIRS (Table 124-1) include pancreatitis, burns, trauma, adrenal insufficiency, pulmonary embolism, dissecting or ruptured aortic aneurysm, myocardial infarction, occult hemorrhage, cardiac tamponade, post-cardiopulmonary bypass syndrome, anaphylaxis, and drug overdose.

Definitive etiologic diagnosis requires isolation of the microorganism from blood or a local site of infection. At least two blood samples (10 mL each) should be obtained (from different venipuncture sites) for culture. Because gram-negative bacteremia is typically low-grade (<10 organisms per milliliter of blood), multiple blood cultures or prolonged incubation of cultures may be necessary; *S. aureus* grows more readily and is detectable in blood cultures within 48 h in most instances. In many cases, blood cultures are negative; this result can reflect prior antibiotic administration, the presence of slow-growing or fastidious organisms, or the absence of microbial invasion of the bloodstream. In these cases, Gram's staining and culture of material from the primary site of infection or of infected cutaneous lesions may help establish the microbial etiology. The skin and mucosae should be examined carefully and repeatedly for lesions that might yield diagnostic information. With overwhelming bacteremia (e.g., pneumococcal sepsis in splenectomized individuals or fulminant meningococcemia), microorganisms are sometimes visible on buffy coat smears of peripheral blood.

Detection of endotoxin in blood by the limulus lysate test may portend a poor outcome, but this assay is not useful for diagnosing gram-negative bacterial infections, including gram-negative bacteremia. Although blood levels of IL-6 also may correlate with prognosis,

cytokine assays are poorly standardized and currently have limited clinical value.

Rx **TREATMENT** Patients in whom sepsis is suspected must be managed expeditiously. This task is best accomplished in an intensive care unit by personnel who are experienced in the care of the critically ill. Successful management requires urgent measures to treat the local site of infection, to provide hemodynamic and respiratory support, and to eliminate the offending microorganism. The outcome is also influenced by the patient's underlying disease, which should be managed aggressively.

Antimicrobial Agents Antimicrobial chemotherapy should be initiated as soon as samples of blood and other relevant sites have been cultured. The choice of initial therapy is based on knowledge of the likely pathogens at specific sites of local infection. Available information about patterns of antimicrobial susceptibility among bacterial isolates from the community, the hospital, and the patient also should be taken into account. It is important, pending culture results, to initiate empirical antimicrobial therapy that is effective against both gram-positive and gram-negative bacteria (Table 124-3). Maximal recommended doses of antimicrobial drugs should be given intravenously, with adjustment for impaired renal function when necessary. When

Table 124-3 Initial Antimicrobial Therapy for Severe Sepsis with No Obvious Source in Adults with Normal Renal Function

Clinical Condition	Antimicrobial Regimens (Intravenous Therapy)
Immunocompetent adult	The many acceptable regimens include (1) ceftriaxone (1 g q12h) *or* ticarcillin-clavulanate (3.1 g q4-6h) *or* piperacillin-tazobactam (3.75 g q4–6h); (2) imipenem-cilastatin (0.5 g q6h) *or* meropenem (1 g q8h). Gentamicin or tobramycin (5 mg/kg q24h) may be *added* to either regimen. If the patient is allergic to β-lactam agents, use ciprofloxacin (400 mg q12h) *plus* clindamycin (600 mg q8h). If the institution has a high incidence of MRSA infections, *add* vancomycin (15 mg/kg q12h) to each of the above regimens.
Neutropenia[a] (<500 neutrophils/μL)	Regimens include (1) ceftazidime (2 g q8h) *or* ticarcillin-clavulanate (3.1 g q4h) *or* piperacillin-tazobactam (3.75 g q4h) *plus* tobramycin (5 mg/kg q24h); (2) imipenem-cilastatin (0.5 g q6h) *or* meropenem (1 g q8h) *or* ceftazidime *or* cefepime (2 g q12h). Vancomycin (15 mg/kg q12h) and ceftazidime should be used if the patient has an infected vascular catheter, if staphylococci are suspected, if the patient has received quinolone prophylaxis, if the patient has received intensive chemotherapy that produces mucosal damage, or if the institution has a high incidence of MRSA infections.
Splenectomy	Cefotaxime (2 g q6–8h) *or* ceftriaxone (2 g q12h) should be used. If the local prevalence of cephalosporin-resistant pneumococci is high, *add* vancomycin. If the patient is allergic to β-lactam drugs, vancomycin (15 mg/kg q12h) *plus* ciprofloxacin (400 mg q12h) *or* aztreonam (2 g q8h) should be used.
IV drug user	Nafcillin *or* oxacillin (2 g q4h) *plus* gentamicin (5 mg/kg q24h). If the local prevalence of MRSA is high or if the patient is allergic to β-lactam drugs, vancomycin (15 mg/kg q12h) with gentamicin should be used.
AIDS	Ceftazidime (2 g q8h), ticarcillin-clavulanate (3.1 g q4h), *or* piperacillin-tazobactam (3.75 g q4h) *plus* tobramycin (5 mg/kg q24h) should be used. If the patient is allergic to β-lactam drugs, ciprofloxacin (400 mg q12h) *plus* vancomycin (15 mg/kg q12h) *plus* tobramycin should be used.

[a] Adapted in part from WT Hughes et al: Clin Infect Dis 25:551, 1997.
NOTE: MRSA, methicillin-resistant *Staphylococcus aureus*.

culture results become available, the regimen can often be simplified, as a single antimicrobial agent is frequently adequate for the treatment of a known pathogen. Most patients require antimicrobial therapy for at least 1 week; the duration of treatment is typically influenced by factors such as the site of tissue infection, the adequacy of surgical drainage, the patient's underlying disease, and the antimicrobial susceptibility of the bacterial isolate(s).

Removal of the Source of Infection Removal or drainage of a focal source of infection is essential. Sites of occult infection should be sought carefully. Indwelling intravenous catheters should be removed, the tip rolled over a blood agar plate for quantitative culture, and a new catheter inserted at a different site. Foley and drainage catheters should be replaced. The possibility of paranasal sinusitis (often caused by gram-negative bacteria) should be considered if the patient has undergone nasal intubation. In the neutropenic patient, cutaneous sites of tenderness and erythema, particularly in the perianal region, must be carefully sought. In patients with sacral or ischial decubitus ulcers, it is important to exclude pelvic or other soft-tissue pus collections (by computed tomography or magnetic resonance imaging, if necessary). In patients with severe sepsis arising from the urinary tract, sonography or computed tomography should be used to rule out ureteral obstruction, perinephric abscess, and renal abscess. These studies are not so urgent in patients with less severe urosepsis, provided that a clinical response is evident within 48 to 72 h.

Hemodynamic, Respiratory, and Metabolic Support (See also Chap. 38) The primary goal is to restore adequate oxygen and substrate delivery to the tissues. Adequate organ perfusion is essential. Effective intravascular volume depletion is common in patients with sepsis, and initial management of hypotension should include the administration of intravenous fluids, typically 1 to 2 L of normal saline over 1 to 2 h. The pulmonary capillary wedge pressure or the central venous pressure must be monitored in patients with refractory shock or underlying cardiac or renal disease. To avoid pulmonary edema, the pulmonary capillary wedge pressure should be maintained between 12 and 16 mmHg or the central venous pressure between 10 and 12 cmH_2O. The urine output rate should be kept above 30 mL/h by continuing fluid administration; a diuretic such as furosemide may be used if needed. In about one-third of patients, hypotension and organ hypoperfusion respond to fluid resuscitation; a reasonable goal is to maintain a mean arterial blood pressure of >60 mmHg (systolic pressure, >90 mmHg) and a cardiac index of ≥ 4 (L/min)/m². If these guidelines cannot be met by volume infusion, inotropic and vasopressor therapy is indicated (Chap. 38). Circulatory adequacy is also assessed by clinical parameters (mentation, urine output, skin perfusion) and, when possible, by measurements of oxygen delivery and consumption.

Adrenal insufficiency should be considered in septic patients with refractory hypotension, fulminant *N. meningitidis* bacteremia, prior glucocorticoid use, disseminated tuberculosis, or AIDS. The cosyntropin (α^{1-24}-ACTH) stimulation test (Chap. 331) may suggest absolute or partial adrenal insufficiency. Supplemental hydrocortisone (50 mg intravenously every 6 h) may be given while the results of the cosyntropin test are awaited.

Ventilator therapy is indicated for progressive hypoxemia, hypercapnia, neurologic deterioration, or respiratory muscle failure. Sustained tachypnea (respiratory rate, >30 breaths/min) is frequently a harbinger of impending respiratory collapse; mechanical ventilation is often initiated to ensure adequate oxygenation, divert blood from the muscles of respiration, prevent aspiration of oropharyngeal contents, and reduce the cardiac afterload. Blood or erythrocyte transfusion is indicated if oxygen delivery is compromised by a low hemoglobin concentration (<8 to 10 g/dL).

Bicarbonate is sometimes administered for severe metabolic acidosis (arterial pH < 7.2). DIC, if complicated by major bleeding, should be treated with transfusion of fresh-frozen plasma and platelets. Successful treatment of the underlying infection is essential to reverse both acidosis and DIC.

These are consensus recommendations; none of these generally accepted components of resuscitative care has been validated in randomized clinical trials.

General Support In patients with prolonged severe sepsis (i.e., that lasting more than 2 or 3 days), nutritional supplementation may reduce the impact of protein hypercatabolism; available evidence favors the enteral delivery route. Recovery is also assisted by preventing skin breakdown, deep venous thrombosis, nosocomial infections, and stress ulcers.

Other Measures Despite aggressive management, many patients with severe sepsis or septic shock die. Two kinds of agents that may help prevent these deaths are being investigated: (1) drugs that neutralize bacterial endotoxin, thereby potentially benefiting the fraction (approximately half) of septic patients who have gram-negative bacterial infection, and (2) drugs that interfere with one or more mediators of the inflammatory response and may benefit all patients with sepsis.

Antiendotoxin agents Lipid A, the toxic moiety of endotoxin, is conserved in the LPS of gram-negative bacteria. Despite much effort to develop drugs that bind lipid A and neutralize endotoxin in vivo, the potential of endotoxin as a target for therapeutic intervention remains controversial. In placebo-controlled clinical trials, two monoclonal antibodies to endotoxin did not prevent the death of patients with severe gram-negative bacterial sepsis. In retrospective studies, these antibodies did not bind to LPS with high affinity, and one was reported to be a polyreactive autoantibody. A theoretically more promising agent is bactericidal permeability-increasing protein, a human neutrophil protein that neutralizes the toxicity of lipid A and may be bactericidal to many gram-negative bacteria. In one clinical trial, this protein decreased morbidity and mortality among children with fulminant meningococcemia. Other investigational drugs include nontoxic lipid A analogs that reduce host responses to endotoxins and lipoproteins (such as high-density lipoprotein) that bind and neutralize endotoxin in the circulation and can remove it from the surfaces of myeloid cells.

Antimediator agents Other adjunctive therapies are intended to control the inflammatory response, regardless of the microbial stimulus. However, numerous agents that directly or indirectly interfere with the actions of inflammatory mediators have not prevented the death of patients with severe sepsis or septic shock. Many factors have probably contributed to the unsuccessful outcomes of these trials, including problems with study design (inappropriate end points, inadequate sample size, population heterogeneity, multiple covariates) and drug administration (wrong dose, time, or duration of administration). Anti-inflammatory drugs tested in clinical trials include methylprednisolone, ibuprofen, recombinant IL-1Ra, genetically engineered soluble receptors for TNF-α, and monoclonal antibodies to TNF-α. Because TNF-α and IL-1β doubtless play key roles in antimicrobial host defense, neutralizing these cytokines could be detrimental in some cases. In addition, studies suggest that many anti-inflammatory molecules, including soluble TNF receptors and IL-1Ra, may already be present at high concentrations in the plasma of patients with septic shock. Identifying beneficial regimens of treatment with drugs that neutralize TNF-α and IL-1β may therefore be very difficult. Clinical trials are testing drugs (antithrombin, activated protein C, tissue factor pathway inhibitor) intended to prevent or reverse microthombosis and evaluating regimens in which low doses of glucocorticoids are administered for prolonged periods.

All of the more recent clinical trials have enrolled patients with severe sepsis or septic shock. Neither the ability of adjunctive agents to prevent severe sepsis or septic shock in high-risk patients nor the value of combination therapy with two or more adjunctive drugs has been tested.

PROGNOSIS Approximately 20 to 35% of patients with severe sepsis and 40 to 60% of patients with septic shock die within 30 days. Others die within the ensuing 6 months. Late deaths often result from poorly controlled infection, complications of intensive care, failure of multiple organs, or the patient's underlying disease.

Several prognostic stratification systems indicate that factoring in the patient's age, underlying condition, and various physiologic variables can yield estimates of the risk of dying of severe sepsis. Of the individual covariates, the severity of underlying disease most strongly influences the risk of dying. Septic shock is also a strong predictor of short- and long-term mortality. Case-fatality rates are similar for culture-positive and culture-negative severe sepsis.

PREVENTION   Prevention offers the best opportunity to reduce morbidity and mortality. Most episodes of severe sepsis and septic shock are nosocomial. These cases might be prevented by reducing the number of invasive procedures undertaken, by limiting the use (and duration of use) of indwelling vascular and bladder catheters, by reducing the incidence and duration of profound neutropenia (<500 neutrophils/μL), and by more aggressively treating localized nosocomial infections. Indiscriminate use of antimicrobial agents and glucocorticoids should be avoided, and optimal infection-control measures (Chap. 134) should be used. In addition, prompt and aggressive management of patients with sepsis is imperative. Studies indicate that 50 to 70% of patients who develop nosocomial severe sepsis or septic shock have experienced a less severe stage of the septic response (e.g., SIRS, sepsis) on at least one previous day in the hospital. Research is needed to identify patients at high risk for severe sepsis and to develop adjunctive agents that can damp the septic response before organ dysfunction or hypotension occurs.

BIBLIOGRAPHY

AMERICAN COLLEGE OF CHEST PHYSICIANS/SOCIETY OF CRITICAL CARE MEDICINE CONSENSUS CONFERENCE COMMITTEE: Definitions for sepsis and organ failure and guidelines for the use of innovative therapies in sepsis. Crit Care Med 20:864, 1992

ASTIZ ME, RACKOW EC: Septic shock. Lancet 351:1501, 1998

BRUN-BUISSON C et al: Bacteremia and severe sepsis in adults: A multicenter prospective survey in ICUs and wards of 24 hospitals. Am J Respir Crit Care Med 154:617, 1996

CAIN BS et al: The physiologic basis for anticytokine clinical trials in the treatment of sepsis. J Am Coll Surg 186:337, 1998

EIDELMAN LA et al: The spectrum of septic encephalopathy. Definitions, etiologies, and mortalities. JAMA 275:470, 1996

JAMES JH et al: Lactate is an unreliable indicator of tissue hypoxia in injury or sepsis. Lancet 354:505, 1999

LEVI M et al: The cytokine-mediated imbalance between coagulant and anticoagulant mechanisms in sepsis and endotoxaemia. Eur J Clin Invest 27:3, 1997

QUARTIN AA et al: Magnitude and duration of the effect of sepsis on survival. JAMA 277:1058, 1997

RANGEL-FRAUSTO MS et al: The natural history of the systemic inflammatory response syndrome (SIRS). A prospective study. JAMA 273:117, 1995

SANDS KE et al: Epidemiology of sepsis syndrome in 8 academic medical centers. JAMA 278:234, 1997

WHEELER AP, BERNARD GR: Treating patients with severe sepsis. N Engl J Med 340:207, 1999

125   *Jeffrey A. Gelfand*

FEVER OF UNKNOWN ORIGIN

CMV cytomegalovirus	MRI magnetic resonance imaging
CSF cerebrospinal fluid	NSAIDs nonsteroidal anti-
CT computed tomography	inflammatory agents
ESR erythrocyte sedimentation rate	PCR polymerase chain reaction
FUO fever of unknown origin	PPD purified protein derivative
IDSA Infectious Diseases Society of America	

DEFINITION AND CLASSIFICATION   *Fever of unknown origin* (FUO) was defined by Petersdorf and Beeson in 1961 as (1)

temperatures >38.3°C (101°F) on several occasions; (2) a duration of fever of >3 weeks; and (3) failure to reach a diagnosis despite 1 week of inpatient investigation. While this classification has stood for more than 30 years, Durack and Street have proposed a new system for classification of FUO: (1) classic FUO; (2) nosocomial FUO; (3) neutropenic FUO; and (4) FUO associated with HIV infection (Table 125-1).

Classic FUO   Classic FUO corresponds closely to the earlier definition of FUO, differing only with regard to the prior requirement for 1 week's study in the hospital. The new definition is broader, stipulating three outpatient visits or 3 days in the hospital without elucidation of a cause or 1 week of "intelligent and invasive" ambulatory investigation.

Nosocomial FUO   In nosocomial FUO, a temperature of ≥38.3°C (101°F) develops on several occasions in a hospitalized patient who is receiving acute care and in whom infection was not manifest or incubating on admission. Three days of investigation, including at least 2 days' incubation of cultures, is the minimum requirement for this diagnosis.

Neutropenic FUO   Neutropenic FUO is defined as a temperature of ≥38.3°C (101°F) on several occasions in a patient whose neutrophil count is <500/μL or is expected to fall to that level in 1 to 2 days. The diagnosis of neutropenic FUO is invoked if a specific cause is not identified after 3 days of investigation, including at least 2 days' incubation of cultures.

HIV-Associated FUO   FUO associated with HIV infection is defined by a temperature of ≥38.3°C (101°F) on several occasions over a period of >4 weeks for outpatients or >3 days for hospitalized patients with HIV infection. This diagnosis is invoked if appropriate investigation over 3 days, including 2 days' incubation of cultures, reveals no source.

Adoption of these categories of FUO on a wide scale in the literature would allow a more rational compilation of data regarding these disparate groups. In the remainder of this chapter, the discussion will focus on classic FUO unless otherwise specified.

CAUSES OF CLASSIC FUO   Table 125-2 summarizes the findings of several large studies of FUO carried out since the advent of the antibiotic era, including a prospective study of 167 adult patients with FUO encompassing all 8 university hospitals in the Netherlands and using a standardized protocol in which the first author reviewed every patient. Coincident with the widespread use of antibiotics, increasingly useful diagnostic technologies—both noninvasive and invasive—have been developed. Newer studies reflect not only changing patterns of disease but also the impact of diagnostic techniques that make it possible to eliminate many patients with specific illness from the FUO category. The ubiquitous use of microbiologic cultures and the widespread use of potent broad-spectrum antibiotics may have decreased the number of infections causing FUO. The wide availability of ultrasonography, computed tomography (CT), and magnetic resonance imaging (MRI) has enhanced the detection of occult neoplasms and lymphomas in patients previously thought to have FUO. Likewise, the widespread availability of highly specific and sensitive immunologic testing has reduced the number of undetected cases of systemic lupus erythematosus and other autoimmune diseases.

Several generalizations can be made. Infections, especially extrapulmonary tuberculosis, remain the leading diagnosable cause of FUO. Prolonged mononucleosis syndromes caused by Epstein-Barr virus, cytomegalovirus (CMV), or HIV are conditions whose consideration as a cause of FUO is sometimes confounded by delayed antibody responses. Intraabdominal abscesses (sometimes poorly localized) and renal, retroperitoneal, and paraspinal abscesses continue to be difficult to diagnose. Renal malacoplakia, with submucosal plaques or nodules involving the urinary tract, may cause FUO and is often fatal if untreated. It is associated with coliform infection, is seen most often in patients with defects of intracellular bacterial killing, and is treated with fluoroquinolones or trimethoprim-sulfamethoxazole. Occasionally, other organs may be involved. Osteomyelitis, especially where prosthetic devices have been implanted, and infective endocarditis

Table 125-1 Categories of FUO[a]

Feature	Category of FUO			
	Nosocomial	**Neutropenic**	**HIV-Associated**	**Classic**
Patient's situation	Hospitalized, acute care, no infection when admitted	Neutrophil count either <500/μL or expected to reach that level in 1–2 days	Confirmed HIV-positive	All others with fevers for ≥3 weeks
Duration of illness while under investigation	3 days[b]	3 days[b]	3 days[b] (or 4 weeks as out-patient)	3 days[b] or three outpatient visits
Examples of cause	Septic thrombophlebitis, sinusitis, *Clostridium difficile* colitis, drug fever	Perianal infection, aspergillosis, candidemia	MAI[c] infection, tuberculosis, non-Hodgkin's lymphoma, drug fever	Infections, malignancy, inflammatory diseases, drug fever

[a] All require temperatures of ≥38.3°C (101°F) on several occasions.
[b] Includes at least 2 days' incubation of microbiology cultures.
[c] *M. avium/M. intracellulare.*

SOURCE: Modified from DT Durack, AC Street, in JS Remington, MN Swartz (eds): *Current Clinical Topics in Infectious Diseases.* Cambridge, MA, Blackwell, 1991.

Table 125-2 Classic FUO in Adults

Authors (Year of Publication)	Years of Study	No. of Cases	Infections (%)	Neoplasms (%)	Noninfectious Inflammatory Diseases (%)	Miscellaneous Causes (%)	Undiagnosed Causes (%)
Petersdorf and Beeson (1961)	1952–1957	100	36	19	19[a]	19[a]	7
Larson and Featherstone (1982)	1970–1980	105	32	20	16[a]	11[a]	7
Knockaert and Vanneste (1992)	1980–1989	199	22.5	7	23[a]	21.5[a]	25.5
DeKleijn et al. (1997, Part I)	1992–1994	167	26	12.5	24	8	30

[a] Authors' raw data retabulated to conform to altered diagnostic categories.

SOURCE: Modified from DeKleijn et al., 1997 (Part I).

must be considered. Although true culture-negative infective endocarditis is rare, one may be misled by slow-growing organisms of the HACEK group (*Haemophilus aphrophilus, Actinobacillus actinomycetemcomitans, Cardiobacterium hominis, Eikenella corrodens,* and *Kingella kingae*; Chap. 150), *Bartonella* spp. (previously *Rochalimaea*), *Legionella* spp., *Coxiella burnetii, Chlamydia psittaci,* and fungi. Prostatitis, dental abscesses, sinusitis, and cholangitis continue to be sources of occult fever.

Fungal disease, most notably histoplasmosis involving the reticuloendothelial system, may cause FUO. FUO with headache should prompt examination of spinal fluid for *Cryptococcus neoformans.* Malaria (which may result from transfusion, the failure to take a prescribed prophylactic agent, or infection with a drug-resistant strain) continues to be a cause, particularly of nonsynchronized FUO. A related protozoan species, *Babesia,* may cause FUO and is increasing in incidence.

In most earlier series, neoplasms were the next most common cause of FUO after infections (Table 125-3). In the two most recent series, a decrease in the percentage of FUO cases due to malignancy was attributed to improvement in diagnostic technologies. This observation does not diminish the importance of considering neoplasia in the initial diagnostic evaluation of a patient with fever. A number of patients in these series had temporal arteritis, adult Still's disease, drug-related fever, and factitious fever. In recent series, approximately 25 to 30% of cases of FUO have remained undiagnosed. The general term *noninfectious inflammatory diseases* applies to systemic rheumatologic or vasculitic diseases such as polymyalgia rheumatica, lupus, and adult Still's disease as well as to granulomatous diseases such as sarcoidosis and Crohn's and granulomatous hepatitis.

In the elderly, multisystem disease is the most frequent cause of FUO, giant cell arteritis being the leading etiologic entity in this category. Tuberculosis is the most common infection causing FUO in the elderly, and colon cancer is an important cause of FUO with malignancy.

Many diseases have been grouped in the various studies as "miscellaneous." On this list are drug fever, pulmonary embolism, factitious fever, familial Mediterranean fever, and Fabry's disease.

A drug-related etiology must be considered in any case of prolonged fever. Any febrile pattern may be elicited by a drug, and both relative bradycardia and hypotension are uncommon. Eosinophilia and/or rash is found in only one-fifth of patients with drug fever, which usually begins 1 to 3 weeks after the start of therapy and remits 2 to 3 days after therapy is stopped. Virtually all classes of drugs cause fever, but antimicrobials (especially β-lactam antibiotics), cardiovascular drugs (e.g., quinidine), antineoplastic drugs, and drugs acting on the central nervous system (e.g., phenytoin) are particularly common causes.

It is axiomatic that, as the duration of fever increases, the likelihood of an infectious cause decreases (Table 125-4). In a series of 347

Table 125-3 Malignancies Commonly Associated with FUO

Hodgkin's disease
Non-Hodgkin's lymphoma
Leukemia (including preleukemic and aleukemic phases)
Renal cell carcinoma
Hepatoma
Colon carcinoma

Table 125-4 Causes of FUO Lasting >6 Months

Cause	Cases (%)
None identified	19
Miscellaneous causes	13
Factitious causes	9
Granulomatous hepatitis	8
Neoplasm	7
Still's disease	6
Infection	6
Collagen vascular disease	4
Familial Mediterranean fever	3
No fever[a]	27

[a] No actual fever observed during 2 to 3 weeks of inpatient observation. Includes patients with exaggerated circadian rhythm.
SOURCE: From a study of 347 patients referred to the National Institutes of Health from 1961 to 1977 with a presumptive diagnosis of FUO of >6 months' duration (Aduan et al.)

patients referred to the National Institutes of Health from 1961 to 1977, only 6% had an infection. A significant proportion (9%) had factitious fevers—i.e., fevers due either to false elevations of temperature or to self-induced disease. A substantial number of these factitious cases were in young women in the health professions. It is worth noting that 8% of the patients with prolonged fevers (some of whom had completely normal liver function studies) had granulomatous hepatitis, and 6% had adult Still's disease. After prolonged investigation, 19% of cases still had no specific diagnosis. A total of 27% of patients either had no actual fever during the weeks of inpatient observation or had an exaggerated circadian temperature rhythm without chills, elevated pulse, or other abnormalities.

The conditions that may be considered in a differential diagnosis of classic FUO in adults are listed in Table 125-5. This list applies strictly to the United States; the frequency of global travel underscores the need for a detailed travel history, and the continuing emergence of new infectious diseases makes this listing potentially incomplete.

SPECIALIZED DIAGNOSTIC STUDIES   Classic FUO Certain specific diagnostic maneuvers become critical in dealing with prolonged fevers. If factitious fever is suspected, electronic thermom-

---

Table 125-5   Causes of FUO in Adults in the United States

Infections
  Localized pyogenic infections
    Appendicitis
    Cat-scratch disease
    Cholangitis
    Cholecystitis
    Dental abscess
    Diverticulitis/abscess
    Lesser sac abscess
    Liver abscess
    Mesenteric lymphadenitis
    Osteomyelitis
    Pancreatic abscess
    Pelvic inflammatory disease
    Perinephric/intrarenal abscess
    Prostatic abscess
    Renal malacoplakia
    Sinusitis
    Subphrenic abscess
    Suppurative thrombophlebitis
    Tuboovarian abscess
  Intravascular infections
    Bacterial aortitis
    Bacterial endocarditis
    Vascular catheter infection
  Systemic bacterial infections
    Bartonellosis
    Brucellosis
    Campylobacter infection
    Cat-scratch disease/bacillary angiomatosis
      (*B. henselae*)
    Gonococcemia
    Legionnaires' disease
    Leptospirosis
    Listeriosis
    Lyme disease
    Melioidosis
    Meningococcemia
    Rat-bite fever
    Relapsing fever
    Salmonellosis
    Syphilis
    Tularemia
    Typhoid fever
    Vibriosis
    Yersinia infection
  Mycobacterial infections
    M. avium/M. intracellulare infections
    Other atypical mycobacterial infections
    Tuberculosis
  Fungal infections
    Aspergillosis
    Blastomycosis
    Candidiasis
    Coccidioidomycosis
    Cryptococcosis
    Histoplasmosis
    Mucormycosis
    Paracoccidioidomycosis
    Sporotrichosis

  Other bacterial infections
    Actinomycosis
    Nocardiosis
    Whipple's disease
  Rickettsial infections
    Ehrlichiosis
    Murine typhus
    Q fever
    Rickettsialpox
    Rocky Mountain spotted fever
  Mycoplasmal infections
  Chlamydial infections
    Lymphogranuloma venereum
    Psittacosis
    TWAR (*C. pneumoniae*) infection
  Viral infections
    Colorado tick fever
    Coxsackievirus group B infection
    Cytomegalovirus infection
    Dengue
    Epstein-Barr virus infection
    Hepatitis A, B, C, D, and E
    Human herpesvirus 6 infection
    Human immunodeficiency virus infection
    Lymphocytic choriomeningitis
    Parvovirus B19 infection
  Parasitic infections
    Amebiasis
    Babesiosis
    Chagas' disease
    Leishmaniasis
    Malaria
    P. carinii infection
    Strongyloidiasis
    Toxocariasis
    Toxoplasmosis
    Trichinosis
  Presumed infections, agent undetermined
    Kawasaki's disease (mucocutaneous lymph
      node syndrome)
    Kikuchi's disease (necrotizing lymphadeni-
      tis)

Neoplasms
  Malignant
    Colon cancer
    Hepatoma
    Hodgkin's lymphoma
    Immunoblastic lymphadenopathy
    Leukemia
    Lymphomatoid granulomatosis
    Malignant histiocytosis
    Nephroma
    Non-Hodgkin's lymphoma
    Pancreatic cancer
    Sarcoma
  Benign
    Atrial myxoma
    Castleman's disease
    Renal angiomyolipoma

Collagen vascular/hypersensitivity diseases
  Adult Still's disease
  Behçet's disease
  Erythema multiforme
  Erythema nodosum
  Giant-cell arteritis/polymyalgia rheumatica
  Hypersensitivity pneumonitis (e.g., "metal fume
    fever," "farmer's lung," "air-conditioner lung")
  Hypersensitivity vasculitis
  Mixed connective-tissue disease
  Polyarteritis nodosa
  Relapsing polychondritis
  Rheumatic fever
  Rheumatoid arthritis
  Schnitzler's syndrome
  Systemic lupus erythematosus
  Takayasu's aortitis
  Weber-Christian disease
  Wegener's granulomatosis
Granulomatous diseases
  Crohn's disease
  Idiopathic granulomatous hepatitis
  Midline granuloma
  Sarcoidosis
Miscellaneous conditions
  Aortic dissection
  Drug fever
  Gout
  Hematomas
  Hemolytic diseases/hemoglobinopathies
  Laennec's cirrhosis
  PFPA syndrome: periodic fever, adenitis, phar-
    yngitis, aphthae
  Postmyocardial infarction syndrome
  Recurrent pulmonary emboli
  Subacute thyroiditis (de Quervain's)
  Tissue infarction/necrosis
Inherited and metabolic diseases
  Adrenal insufficiency
  Cyclic neutropenia
  Deafness, urticaria, and amyloidosis
  Fabry's disease
  Familial Mediterranean fever
  Hyperimmunoglobulinemia D and periodic fever
  Type V hypertriglyceridemia
Thermoregulatory disorders
  Central
    Brain tumor
    Cerebrovascular accident
    Encephalitis
    Hypothalamic dysfunction
  Peripheral
    Hyperthyroidism
    Pheochromocytoma
Factitious fevers
"Afebrile" FUO (<38.3°C)
Habitual hyperthermia (exaggerated circadian
  rhythm)

SOURCE: Modified from RK Root, RG Petersdorf, in JD Wilson et al (eds): *Harrison's Principles of Internal Medicine,* 12th ed. New York, McGraw-Hill, 1991.

eters should be used, temperature-taking should be supervised, and simultaneous urine and body temperatures should be measured. Any tissue removed during prior relevant surgery should be reexamined; slides should be requested, and, if need be, paraffin blocks of fixed pathologic material should be reexamined and additional special studies performed. Relevant x-rays should be reexamined; reviewing of prior radiologic reports may be insufficient. Serum should be set aside in the laboratory as soon as possible and retained for future examination for rising antibody titers. *Febrile agglutinins* is a vague term that in most laboratories refers to serologic studies for salmonellosis, brucellosis, and rickettsial diseases. These studies are seldom useful, having low sensitivity and variable specificity. Rising titers of antibody to *Brucella* (Chap. 160) are usually diagnostic, but false-positive results may be obtained in typhoid fever, tularemia, and yersinial infections. Infection with *Brucella canis* may be missed with standard antibody tests for *Brucella*. *Salmonella* infection (Chap. 156) elevates antibody titers to the H and O antigens. High titers of antibody to the H antigen persist for years and may reflect previous infection or immunization. Serology for *Yersinia enterocolitica* may be useful. The measurement of specific antirickettsial titers should be requested for the diagnosis of Rocky Mountain spotted fever and Q fever. Multiple blood samples (no fewer than three, rarely more than six), including samples for anaerobic culture, should be cultured in the laboratory for at least 2 weeks to ensure that any HACEK-group organisms that may be present have ample time to grow (Chap. 150). Lysis-centrifugation blood culture techniques should be employed in cases where prior antimicrobial therapy or fungal or atypical mycobacterial infection is suspected. Blood culture media should be supplemented with L-cysteine or pyridoxal to assist in the isolation of nutritionally variant streptococci. It should be noted that sequential cultures positive for multiple organisms may reflect self-injection of contaminated substances. Urine cultures, including cultures for mycobacteria, fungi, and CMV, are indicated. Blood, urine, or cerebrospinal fluid (CSF) can now be tested for a variety of pathogens such as CMV or hepatitis C virus by using the polymerase chain reaction (PCR) to amplify and hence detect viral nucleic acid (Chap. 121). Liver biopsy, even when the results of liver function studies are normal, should be considered and pursued if the diagnosis remains elusive. Specimens should be cultured for mycobacteria and fungi. Likewise, bone marrow biopsy (not simple aspiration) should be used to obtain specimens for histology and culture. The blood smear should be examined for *Plasmodium*, *Babesia*, *Trypanosoma*, *Leishmania*, and *Borrelia*.

In an FUO workup, the erythrocyte sedimentation rate (ESR) should be determined. Striking elevation of the ESR and anemia of chronic disease are frequently seen in association with giant cell arteritis or polymyalgia rheumatica, common causes of FUO in patients over 50 years of age. Still's disease is also suggested by elevations of ESR, leukocytosis, and anemia and is often accompanied by arthralgias, polyserositis (pleuritis, pericarditis), lymphadenopathy, splenomegaly, and rash. Antinuclear antibody, antineutrophil cytoplasmic antibody, rheumatoid factor, and serum cryoglobulins should be measured to rule out other collagen vascular diseases and vasculitis. Another cause of an extremely high ESR may be a false-positive value attributable to a cold agglutinin with a broad thermal amplitude. The ESR test is nonspecific, yielding values that depend on certain serum proteins (most notably fibrinogen) known to interfere with the zeta-potential that keeps erythrocytes from clumping. When fibrinogen levels go up, the zeta-potential is inhibited, erythrocytes clump, and the ESR is high. A cold agglutinin, by binding to erythrocytes, can produce a false-positive agglutinin that mimics an acute-phase response; cold agglutinins may be seen in *Mycoplasma* and Epstein-Barr virus infections and in lymphomas.

With rare exceptions, the intermediate-strength purified protein derivative (PPD) skin test should be used to screen for tuberculosis in patients with classic FUO. Concurrent control tests, such as the CMI test (Connaught Labs, Swiftwater, PA), which is especially effective, should be employed. It should be kept in mind that both the PPD skin test and control tests may yield negative results in miliary tuberculosis,

sarcoidosis, Hodgkin's disease, malnutrition, or AIDS. Noninvasive procedures should include an upper gastrointestinal contrast study with small-bowel follow-through and barium enema to include the terminal ileum and cecum. Chest x-rays should be repeated if new symptoms arise. In some cases, pulmonary function studies may be necessary. A diminished carbon monoxide diffusing capacity may indicate a restrictive lung disease such as sarcoidosis, even with a normal chest x-ray. In such cases, transbronchial biopsy may prove diagnostic. Flexible colonoscopy may be advisable, since colon carcinoma is a cause of FUO and easily escapes detection by ultrasound and CT.

CT of the chest and abdomen should be performed. If a spinal or paraspinal lesion is suspected, however, MRI is preferred. MRI may be superior to CT in demonstrating intraabdominal abscesses and aortic dissection, but the relative utility of MRI and CT in the diagnosis of FUO is unknown. At present, it appears that abdominal CT, with oral and intravenous contrast, should be used unless MRI is specifically indicated. Arteriography may be useful for patients in whom systemic necrotizing vasculitis is suspected. Saccular aneurysms may be seen, most commonly in renal or hepatic vessels, and may permit diagnosis of arteritis when biopsy is difficult. Figure 125-1 shows a renal angiogram of a patient with polyarteritis nodosa. Ultrasonography of the abdomen is useful for the investigation of the hepatobiliary tract, kidneys, spleen, and pelvis. Echocardiography may be helpful in an evaluation for bacterial endocarditis, pericarditis, nonbacterial thrombotic endocarditis, and atrial myxomas. Transesophageal echocardiography is especially sensitive for these lesions.

Radionuclide scanning procedures using technetium (Tc) 99m sulfur colloid, gallium (Ga) 67 citrate, or indium (In) 111–labeled leukocytes or immunoglobulin may be useful in identifying and/or localizing inflammatory processes. In a recent study, Ga scintigraphy yielded useful diagnostic information in almost one-third of cases, and it was suggested that this procedure might actually be used before other

FIGURE 125-1 Renal arteriogram from a patient with fever. Arteriography showed a remarkable number of sacculated aneurysms, associated with narrowing and tapering of the arteries, consistent with systemic vasculitis—in this case, polyarteritis nodosa. (Photo courtesy of Dr. Neil Haline.)

imaging techniques if no specific organ is suspected of being abnormal. Tc bone scan should be undertaken to look for osteomyelitis or bony metastases; ^{67}Ga scan may be used to identify sarcoidosis (Chap. 318) or *Pneumocystis carinii* (Chap. 209) in the lungs or Crohn's disease (Chap. 287) in the abdomen. ^{111}In-labeled white blood cell (WBC) scan may be used to locate abscesses; ^{111}In-labeled immunoglobulin scan also shows promise in this regard. With ^{67}Ga, ^{111}In-WBC, and ^{111}In-immunoglobulin scans, false-positive and false-negative findings are common.

Biopsy of the liver and bone marrow should be considered routine in the workup of FUO if the studies mentioned above are unrevealing or if fever is prolonged. It goes without saying that areas of suspected abnormality should be sampled for pathologic examination whenever practical. When possible, a section of the tissue block should be retained for further sections or stains. PCR technology makes it possible to identify and speciate mycobacterial DNA in paraffin-embedded, fixed tissues. Thus, in some cases, it is possible to make a retrospective diagnosis based on studies of long-fixed pathologic tissues. In a patient over age 50 (or occasionally in a younger patient) with the appropriate symptoms and laboratory findings, "blind biopsy" of one or both temporal arteries may yield a diagnosis of arteritis. If noted, tenderness or decreased pulsation should guide the selection of a site for biopsy. Lymph node biopsy may be helpful if nodes are enlarged, but inguinal nodes are often palpable and are seldom diagnostically useful.

Exploratory laparotomy has been performed when all other diagnostic procedures fail but has largely been replaced by modern imaging and guided-biopsy techniques. Laparoscopic biopsy may provide more adequate guided sampling of lymph nodes or liver.

Nosocomial FUO The primary considerations in diagnosing nosocomial FUO are the underlying susceptibility of the patient coupled with the potential complications of hospitalization. The original surgical or procedural field is the place to begin a directed physical and laboratory examination for abscesses, hematomas, or infected foreign bodies. More than 50% of patients with nosocomial FUO are infected, and intravascular lines, septic phlebitis, and prostheses are all suspect. In this setting, the approach is to focus on sites where occult infections may be sequestered, such as the sinuses of intubated patients or a prostatic abscess in a man with a urinary catheter. *Clostridium difficile* colitis may be associated with fever and leukocytosis before the onset of diarrhea. In approximately 25% of patients with nosocomial FUO, the fever has a noninfectious cause. Among these causes are acalculous cholecystitis, deep vein thrombophlebitis, and pulmonary embolism. Drug fever, transfusion reactions, alcohol/drug withdrawal, adrenal insufficiency, thyroiditis, pancreatitis, gout, and pseudogout are among the many possible causes to consider. As in classic FUO, repeated meticulous physical examinations, coupled with focused diagnostic techniques, are imperative. Multiple blood, wound, and fluid cultures are mandatory. The pace of diagnostic tests is accelerated, and the threshold for procedures—CT scans, ultrasonography, ^{111}In-WBC scans, noninvasive venous studies—is low. Even so, 20% of cases of nosocomial FUO may go undiagnosed.

Like diagnostic measures, therapeutic maneuvers must be swift and decisive, as many patients are already critically ill. Intravenous lines must be changed (and cultured), drugs stopped for 72 h, and empirical therapy started if bacteremia is a threat. In many hospital settings, empirical antibiotic coverage for nosocomial FUO now includes vancomycin for methicillin-resistant *Staphylococcus aureus* as well as broad-spectrum gram-negative coverage with piperacillin/tazobactam, ticarcillin/clavulanate, imipenem, or meropenem. Practice guidelines covering many of these issues have been published jointly by the Infectious Diseases Society of America (IDSA) and the Society for Critical Care Medicine and can be accessed on the IDSA website (www.idsociety.org/practice/index.html).

Neutropenic FUO (See also Chap. 85) Neutropenic patients are susceptible to focal bacterial and fungal infections, to bacteremic infections, to infections involving catheters (including septic thrombophlebitis), and to perianal infections. *Candida* and *Aspergillus* infections are common. Infections due to herpes simplex virus or CMV are sometimes causes of FUO in this group. While the duration of illness may be short in these patients, the consequences of untreated infection may be catastrophic, with 50 to 60% infected, and 20% bacteremic. The IDSA has published extensive practice guidelines covering these critically ill neutropenic patients; these guidelines appear on the website cited in the previous section. In these patients, severe mucositis, quinolone prophylaxis, colonization with methicillin-resistant *S. aureus*, obvious catheter-related infection, or hypotension would dictate the use of vancomycin plus ceftazidime or imipenem to provide empirical coverage for bacterial sepsis.

HIV-Associated FUO HIV infection alone may be a cause of fever. Infection due to *Mycobacterium avium* or *Mycobacterium intracellulare*, tuberculosis, toxoplasmosis, CMV infection, *P. carinii* infection, salmonellosis, cryptococcosis, histoplasmosis, non-Hodgkin's lymphoma, and (of particular importance) drug fever are all possible causes of FUO. Mycobacterial infection can be diagnosed by blood cultures and by liver, bone marrow, and lymph node biopsies. Chest CT should be performed to identify enlarged mediastinal nodes. Serologic studies may reveal cryptococcal antigen, and ^{67}Ga scan may help identify *P. carinii* pulmonary infection. More than 80% of HIV patients with FUO are infected, but drug fever and lymphoma remain important considerations. →*Treatment of HIV-associated FUO depends on many factors and is discussed in Chap. 309.*

Rx| **TREATMENT** The emphasis in patients with classic FUO is on continued observation and examination, with the avoidance of "shotgun" empirical therapy. Empirical treatment for endocarditis, for example, should be avoided unless there are specific reasons beyond fever to invoke this diagnosis. Every patient with FUO should undergo an exhaustive examination for tuberculosis. If the PPD skin test is positive or if granulomatous hepatitis or other granulomatous disease is present with anergy (and sarcoid seems unlikely), then a therapeutic trial with isoniazid and rifampin (and possibly a third drug) should be undertaken, with treatment usually continued for up to 6 weeks. A failure of the fever to respond over this period suggests an alternative diagnosis.

The response of rheumatic fever and Still's disease to aspirin and nonsteroidal anti-inflammatory agents (NSAIDs) may be dramatic. The effects of glucocorticoids on temporal arteritis, polymyalgia rheumatica, and granulomatous hepatitis are equally dramatic. Colchicine is highly effective in preventing attacks of familial Mediterranean fever but is of little use once an attack is well under way. The ability of glucocorticoids and NSAIDs to mask fever while permitting the spread of infection dictates that their use be avoided unless infection has been largely ruled out and unless inflammatory disease is both probable and debilitating or threatening.

When no underlying source of FUO is identified after prolonged observation (>6 months), the prognosis is generally good, however vexing the fever may be to the patient. Under such circumstances, debilitating symptoms are treated with NSAIDs, and glucocorticoids are the last resort. The initiation of empirical therapy does not mark the end of the diagnostic workup; rather, it commits the physician to continued thoughtful reexamination and evaluation. Patience, compassion, equanimity, and intellectual flexibility are indispensable attributes for the clinician in dealing successfully with FUO.

ACKNOWLEDGMENT
Sheldon M. Wolff, MD, now deceased, was an author of a previous version of this chapter. It is to his memory that the chapter is dedicated.

BIBLIOGRAPHY

ADUAN R et al: Prolonged fever of unknown origin. Clin Res 26:558A, 1978

DEKLEIJN EMHA et al: Fever of unknown origin (FUO): I. A prospective multicenter study of 167 patients with FUO, using fixed epidemiologic entry criteria. Medicine 76:392, 1997

—— et al: Fever of unknown origin (FUO): II. Diagnostic procedures in a prospective multicenter study of 167 patients. Medicine 76:401, 1997

HIRSCHMANN JV: Fever of unknown origin in adults. Clin Infect Dis 24:291, 1997

HOEN B et al: The Duke criteria for diagnosing infective endocarditis are specific: Analysis of 100 patients with acute fever or fever of unknown origin. Clin Infect Dis 23:298, 1996

HUGHES WT et al: 1997 guidelines for the use of antimicrobial agents in neutropenic patients with unexplained fever. Clin Infect Dis 25:551, 1997

KAZANJIAN PH: Fever of unknown origin: Review of 86 patients treated in community hospitals. Clin Infect Dis 15:968, 1992

KNOCKAERT DC et al: Long-term follow-up of patients with undiagnosed fever of unknown origin. Arch Intern Med 156:618, 1996

——, VANNESTE LJ: Fever of unknown origin in the 1980s. Arch Intern Med 152:51, 1992

——, VANNESTE LJ: Fever of unknown origin in elderly patients. J Am Geriatr Soc 41:1187, 1993

LARSON EB, FEATHERSTONE HJ: Fever of undetermined origin: Diagnosis and follow-up of 105 cases, 1970–80. Medicine 61:269, 1982

MITCHELL MA et al: Bilateral renal parenchymal malacoplakia presenting as fever of unknown origin: Case report and review. Clin Infect Dis 18:704, 1994

O'GRADY NP et al: Practice guidelines for evaluating new fever in critically ill adult patients. Clin Infect Dis 26:1042, 1998

PETERS AM: The use of nuclear medicine in infections. Br J Radiol 71:252, 1998

PETERSDORF RC, BEESON PB: Fever of unexplained origin. Medicine 40:1, 1961

VOLK EE et al: The diagnostic usefulness of bone marrow cultures in patients with fever of unknown origin. Am J Clin Pathol 110:150, 1998

126

Adolf W. Karchmer

INFECTIVE ENDOCARDITIS

The proliferation of microorganisms on the endothelium of the heart results in infective endocarditis. The prototypic lesion at the site of infection, the *vegetation* (see Plate IID-59), is a mass of platelets, fibrin, microcolonies of microorganisms, and scant inflammatory cells. Infection most commonly involves heart valves (either native or prosthetic) but may also occur on the low-pressure side of the ventricular septum at the site of a defect, on the mural endocardium where it is damaged by aberrant jets of blood or foreign bodies, or on intracardiac devices themselves. The analogous process involving arteriovenous shunts, arterioarterial shunts (patent ductus arteriosus), or a coarctation of the aorta is called *infective endarteritis*.

Endocarditis may be classified according to the temporal evolution of disease, the site of infection, the cause of infection, or a predisposing risk factor such as injection drug use. While each classification criterion provides therapeutic and prognostic insight, the methods overlap and none is sufficient alone. The classification of endocarditis as acute and subacute was initially used to describe the illness and the time elapsed until death; presently it is applied to the features and progression of infection until diagnosis. *Acute endocarditis* is a hectically febrile illness, rapidly damages cardiac structures, hematogenously seeds extracardiac sites, and, if untreated, progresses to death within weeks. *Subacute endocarditis* follows an indolent course; causes structural cardiac damage only slowly, if at all; rarely causes metastatic infection; and is gradually progressive unless complicated by a major embolic event or ruptured mycotic aneurysm.

In developed countries, the incidence of endocarditis ranges from 1.5 to 6.2 cases per 100,000 population per year. In the late 1980s in a metropolitan area of the United States (Philadelphia), endocarditis occurred in 9.3 persons per 100,000 population per year. However, half of these cases arose as a consequence of injection drug use. The incidence of endocarditis is notably increased among the elderly. The cumulative rate of prosthetic valve endocarditis is 1.5 to 3.0% at 1 year after valve replacement and 3 to 6% at 5 years; the risk is greatest during the first 6 months after valve replacement.

ETIOLOGY A vast array of microorganisms, including many species of bacteria and fungi, have been reported to cause sporadic episodes of endocarditis. Nevertheless, a small number of bacterial species cause the majority of cases (Table 126-1). The causative microorganisms vary somewhat among the major clinical types of endocarditis, in part because of the different portals of entry. The oral cavity, skin, and upper respiratory tract are the respective primary portals for the viridans streptococci, staphylococci, and HACEK organisms (*Haemophilus, Actinobacillus, Cardiobacterium, Eikenella,* and *Kingella*) causing community-acquired native valve endocarditis. *Streptococcus bovis* originates from the gastrointestinal tract, where it is associated with polyps and colonic tumors, and enterococci enter the bloodstream from the genitourinary tract. Nosocomial native valve endocarditis is largely the consequence of bacteremia arising from intravascular catheters and less commonly from nosocomial wound and urinary tract infection. Endocarditis complicates 6 to 25% of episodes of catheter-associated *Staphylococcus aureus* bacteremia; higher rates are detected by careful transesophageal echocardiography (TEE) screening (see "Echocardiography," below).

Prosthetic valve endocarditis arising within 2 months of valve surgery is generally the result of intraoperative contamination of the prosthesis or a bacteremic postoperative complication. The nosocomial nature of these infections is reflected in their primary microbial causes: coagulase-negative staphylococci, *S. aureus*, facultative gram-negative bacilli, diphtheroids, and fungi. The portals of entry and organisms causing cases beginning >12 months after surgery are similar to those in community-acquired native valve endocarditis. Epidemiologic evidence suggests that prosthetic valve endocarditis due to coagulase-negative staphylococci that presents between 2 and 12 months after surgery is often nosocomial in origin but with a delayed onset. At least 85% of coagulase-negative staphylococci that cause prosthetic valve endocarditis within 12 months of surgery are methicillin-resistant; the rate of methicillin resistance decreases to 25% among coagulase-negative staphylococci causing prosthetic endocarditis that presents >1 year after valve surgery.

Transvenous pacemaker lead and/or implanted defibrillator–associated endocarditis is usually a nosocomial infection. The majority of episodes occur within weeks of implantation or generator change and are caused by *S. aureus* or coagulase-negative staphylococci.

Endocarditis occurring among injection drug users, especially when infection involves the tricuspid valve, is commonly caused by *S. aureus* strains, many of which are methicillin-resistant. The causes of left-sided valve infection in addicts are more varied, and the involved valves have often been damaged by prior episodes of endocarditis. A number of these cases are caused by *Pseudomonas aeruginosa* and *Candida* species, and sporadic cases are due to unusual organisms such as *Bacillus, Lactobacillus,* and *Corynebacterium* species. Polymicrobial endocarditis occurs more frequently in injection drug users than in patients who do not inject drugs. The presence of HIV in this population does not significantly impact the causes of endocarditis.

From 5 to 15% of patients with endocarditis have negative blood cultures; in one-third to one-half of these cases, cultures are negative because of prior antibiotic exposure. The remainder of these patients are infected by fastidious organisms, such as pyridoxal-requiring streptococci (now designated *Abiotrophia* species), the gram-negative coccobacillary HACEK organisms, *Bartonella henselae,* or *Bartonella quintana*. Some fastidious organisms that cause endocarditis have characteristic epidemiologic settings (e.g., *Coxiella burnetii* in Europe, *Brucella* species in the Middle East). *Tropheryma whippelii* causes an indolent, culture-negative, afebrile form of endocarditis.

PATHOGENESIS Unless it is injured, the normal endothelium is resistant to infection by most bacteria and to thrombus formation. Endothelial injury (e.g., at the site of impact of high-velocity jets or on the low-pressure side of a cardiac structural lesion) causes aberrant flow and allows either direct infection by virulent organisms or the development of an uninfected platelet-fibrin thrombus—a condition called *nonbacterial thrombotic endocarditis* (NBTE). The thrombus subsequently serves as a site of bacterial attachment during transient

Table 126-1   Organisms Causing Major Clinical Forms of Endocarditis

| | Percent of Cases | | | | | | | |
| Organism | Native Valve Endocarditis | | Prosthetic Valve Endocarditis at Indicated Time of Onset (Months) After Valve Surgery | | | Endocarditis in Injection Drug Users | | |
	Community-Acquired (*n* = 683)	Nosocomial (*n* = 82)	< 2 (*n* = 144)	2–12 (*n* = 31)	> 12 (*n* = 194)	Right-Sided (*n* = 346)	Left-Sided (*n* = 204)	Total (*n* = 675)
Streptococci[a]	32	7	1	9	31	5	15	12
Pneumococci	1	—	—	—	—	—	—	—
Enterococci	8	16	8	12	11	2	24	9
Staphylococcus aureus	35	55	22	12	18	77	23	57
Coagulase-negative staphylococci	4	10	33	32	11	—	—	—
Fastidious gram-negative coccobacilli (HACEK group)[b]	3	—	—	—	6	—	—	—
Gram-negative bacilli	3	5	13	3	6	5	13	7
Candida spp.	1	4	8	12	1	—	12	4
Polymicrobial/miscellaneous	6	1	3	6	5	8	10	7
Diphtheroids	—	—	6	—	3	—	—	0.1
Culture-negative	5	2	5	6	8	3	3	3

[a] Includes viridans streptococci; *Streptococcus bovis*; other non–group A, groupable streptococci; and *Abiotrophia* spp. (nutritionally variant, pyridoxal-requiring streptococci).
[b] Includes *Haemophilus* spp., *Actinobacillus actinomycetemcomitans*, *Cardiobacterium hominis*, *Eikenella* spp., and *Kingella kingae*.
NOTE: Data are compiled from multiple studies.

bacteremia. The cardiac lesions most commonly resulting in NBTE are mitral regurgitation, aortic stenosis, aortic regurgitation, ventricular septal defects, and complex congenital heart disease. These lesions result from rheumatic heart disease (particularly in the developing world, where rheumatic fever remains prevalent), mitral valve prolapse, degenerative heart disease, and congenital malformations. NBTE also arises as a result of a hypercoagulable state; this phenomenon gives rise to the clinical entity of *marantic endocarditis* (seen in patients with malignancy) and to bland vegetations complicating systemic lupus erythematosus and the antiphospholipid antibody syndrome.

Organisms that cause endocarditis generally enter the bloodstream from mucosal surfaces, the skin, or sites of focal infection. Except for more virulent bacteria (e.g., *S. aureus*) that can adhere directly to intact endothelium or exposed subendothelial tissue, microorganisms in the blood adhere to thrombi. If resistant to the bactericidal activity of serum and the microbicidal peptides released by platelets, the organisms proliferate and either stimulate tissues to produce a procoagulant or themselves exert procoagulant activity leading to further platelet-fibrin deposition and vegetation formation. Although an enormous variety of microorganisms circulate transiently in the bloodstream, only a limited number commonly cause endocarditis. The etiologic organisms of endocarditis bear surface components that facilitate adherence to injured endothelium and host proteins or to thrombi. Experiments suggest that fibronectin receptors present on many gram-positive bacteria, clumping factor (a fibrinogen-binding surface protein) on *S. aureus*, and dextrans on streptococci facilitate adherence. Organisms become enmeshed in the growing platelet-fibrin vegetation and, in the absence of host defenses, proliferate to form dense microcolonies. More than 90% of the organisms in vegetations are metabolically inactive (nongrowing) and thus are relatively resistant to killing by antimicrobial agents. Proliferating surface organisms are shed into the bloodstream continuously, whereupon some are cleared by the reticuloendothelial system and others are redeposited on the vegetation and stimulate further vegetation growth.

The pathophysiologic consequences and clinical manifestations of endocarditis—other than constitutional symptoms, which are probably a result of cytokine production—arise from damage to intracardiac structures; embolization of vegetation fragments, leading to infection or infarction of remote tissues; hematogenous infection of sites during bacteremia; and tissue injury due to the deposition of circulating immune complexes or immune responses to deposited bacterial antigens.

CLINICAL MANIFESTATIONS   The clinical syndrome of infective endocarditis is highly variable, may involve multiple organs, and spans a continuum between acute and subacute presentations. Na-

tive valve endocarditis (whether acquired in the community or nosocomially), prosthetic valve endocarditis, and endocarditis due to injection drug use share clinical and laboratory manifestations (Table 126-2). Although the relationship is not absolute, the causative microorganism is primarily responsible for the temporal course of endocarditis. β-Hemolytic streptococci, *S. aureus*, and pneumococci typically result in an acute course, although *S. aureus* occasionally causes subacute disease. Endocarditis caused by *Staphylococcus lugdunensis* (a coagulase-negative species) or by enterococci may present acutely. Subacute endocarditis is typically caused by viridans streptococci, enterococci, coagulase-negative staphylococci, and the HACEK group. Endocarditis caused by *Bartonella* species and the agent of Q fever, *C. burnetii*, is exceptionally indolent.

The clinical features of endocarditis are nonspecific. However, these symptoms in a febrile patient with valvular abnormalities or a behavior pattern (injection drug use) that predisposes to endocarditis suggest the diagnosis, as do bacteremia with organisms that frequently cause endocarditis, otherwise unexplained arterial emboli, and progressive cardiac valvular incompetence. In patients with subacute presentations, fever is typically low-grade and rarely exceeds 39.4°C (103°F); in contrast, temperatures between 39.4 and 40°C (103 and

Table 126-2   Clinical and Laboratory Features of Infective Endocarditis

Feature	Frequency, %
Fever	80–90
Chills and sweats	40–75
Anorexia, weight loss, malaise	25–50
Myalgias, arthralgias	15–30
Back pain	7–15
Heart murmur	80–85
New/worsened regurgitant murmur	10–40
Arterial emboli	20–50
Splenomegaly	15–50
Clubbing	10–20
Neurologic manifestations	20–40
Peripheral manifestations (Osler's nodes, subungual hemorrhages, Janeway lesions, Roth's spots)	2–15
Petechiae	10–40
Laboratory manifestations	
Anemia	70–90
Leukocytosis	20–30
Microscopic hematuria	30–50
Elevated erythrocyte sedimentation rate	>90
Rheumatoid factor	50
Circulating immune complexes	65–100
Decreased serum complement	5–40

104°F) are often noted in acute endocarditis. Fever may be blunted or absent in patients who are elderly or severely debilitated or who have marked cardiac or renal failure.

Cardiac Manifestations Although heart murmurs are usually indicative of the predisposing cardiac pathology rather than of endocarditis, valvular damage and ruptured chordae may result in new regurgitant murmurs. In acute endocarditis involving a normal valve, murmurs are heard on presentation in only 30 to 45% of patients but ultimately are detected in 85%. Congestive heart failure develops in 30 to 40% of patients; it is usually a consequence of valvular dysfunction but occasionally is due to endocarditis-associated myocarditis or an intracardiac fistula. The temporal progression of heart failure is variable and depends upon the severity of valvular dysfunction; failure due to aortic valve dysfunction progresses more rapidly than that due to mitral valve dysfunction. Extension of infection beyond valve leaflets into adjacent annular or myocardial tissue results in perivalvular abscesses, which in turn may cause fistulae (from the root of the aorta into cardiac chambers or between cardiac chambers) with new murmurs. Abscesses may burrow from the aortic valve annulus through the epicardium, causing pericarditis. Extension of infection into paravalvular tissue adjacent to either the right or the noncoronary cusp of the aortic valve may interrupt the conduction system in the upper interventricular septum, leading to varying degrees of heart block. Although perivalvular abscesses arising from the mitral valve may potentially interrupt conduction pathways near the atrioventricular node or in the proximal bundle of His, such interruption occurs infrequently. Emboli to a coronary artery may result in myocardial infarction; nevertheless, embolic transmural infarcts are rare.

Noncardiac Manifestations The classic nonsuppurative peripheral manifestations of subacute endocarditis are related to the duration of infection and, with early diagnosis and treatment, have become infrequent. In contrast, septic embolization mimicking some of these lesions (subungual hemorrhage, Osler's nodes) is common in patients with acute *S. aureus* endocarditis **(see Plate IID-58)**. Musculoskeletal symptoms, including nonspecific inflammatory arthritis and back pain, usually remit promptly with treatment but must be distinguished from the symptoms of focal metastatic infection. Hematogenously seeded focal infection may involve any organ but most often is clinically evident in the skin, spleen, kidneys, skeletal system, and meninges. Arterial emboli, which may be asymptomatic and discovered only at autopsy, are clinically apparent in up to 50% of patients. Vegetations >10 mm in diameter (as measured by echocardiography) and those located on the mitral valve are more likely to embolize than are smaller or nonmitral vegetations. Embolic events—often with infarction—involving the extremities, spleen, kidneys (Fig. 126-1), bowel, or brain

FIGURE 126-1 Computed tomography of the abdomen showing large embolic infarcts in the spleen and left kidney of a patient with *Bartonella* endocarditis.

are often noted at presentation. With antibiotic treatment, the frequency of embolic events decreases from 13 per 1000 patient-days during the initial week to 1.2 per 1000 patient-days after the third week. Emboli occurring late during or after effective therapy do not in themselves constitute evidence of failed antimicrobial treatment. Neurologic symptoms, most often resulting from embolic strokes, occur in up to 40% of patients. Other neurologic complications include aseptic or purulent meningitis, intracranial hemorrhage due to hemorrhagic infarcts or ruptured mycotic aneurysms, seizures, and encephalopathy. Microabscesses in brain and meninges occur commonly in *S. aureus* endocarditis; surgically drainable abscesses are infrequent.

Immune complex deposition on the glomerular basement membrane causes diffuse hypocomplementemic glomerulonephritis and renal dysfunction, which typically improve with effective antimicrobial therapy. Embolic renal infarcts cause flank pain and hematuria but rarely cause renal dysfunction.

Manifestations of Specific Predisposing Conditions Among injection drug users, infection involving valves on the left side of the heart presents with the typical clinical features of endocarditis. In almost 50% of patients with endocarditis associated with injection drug use, infection is limited to the tricuspid valve. These patients present with fever, faint or no murmur, and (in 75% of cases) prominent pulmonary findings, including cough, pleuritic chest pain, nodular pulmonary infiltrates, and occasionally pyopneumothorax.

Nosocomial endocarditis (defined as that which results from hospital care within the prior month and most commonly presenting as intravascular catheter–associated bacteremia), if not associated with a retained intracardiac device, has typical manifestations. Endocarditis associated with flow-directed pulmonary artery catheters is often cryptic, with symptoms masked by comorbid critical illness, and is commonly diagnosed at autopsy. Transvenous pacemaker lead and/or implanted defibrillator–associated endocarditis commonly follows initial implantation or a generator unit change; may be associated with obvious or cryptic generator pocket infection; and results in fever, minimal murmur, and pulmonary symptoms similar to those encountered in addicts with tricuspid endocarditis.

Prosthetic valve endocarditis presents with typical clinical features. Cases arising within 60 days of valve surgery (early onset) lack peripheral vascular manifestations and may be obscured by comorbidity associated with recent surgery. In both early-onset and more delayed presentations, paravalvular infection is common and often results in partial valve dehiscence, regurgitant murmurs, congestive heart failure, or disruption of the conduction system.

DIAGNOSIS   The Duke Criteria The diagnosis of infective endocarditis is established with certainty only when vegetations obtained at cardiac surgery, at autopsy, or from an artery (an embolus) are examined histologically and microbiologically. Nevertheless, a highly sensitive and specific diagnostic schema—known as the *Duke criteria*—has been developed on the basis of clinical, laboratory, and echocardiographic findings (Table 126-3). Documentation of two major criteria, of one major and three minor criteria, or of five minor criteria allows a clinical diagnosis of definite endocarditis. The diagnosis of endocarditis is rejected if an alternative diagnosis is established, if symptoms resolve and do not recur with ≤4 days of antibiotic therapy, or if surgery or autopsy after ≤4 days of antimicrobial therapy yields no histologic evidence of endocarditis. Illnesses not classified as definite endocarditis or rejected are considered cases of possible infective endocarditis. When pathologically confirmed cases have been scored retrospectively by these criteria, 90% fulfill the definition of definite or possible endocarditis; 10% are rejected (primarily because of an incomplete echocardiographic evaluation). In comparison with expert opinion, the Duke criteria identify cases considered to be endocarditis but also accept a small percentage of cases rejected by the experts. This potential for a false-positive diagnosis is the major deficiency in this schema when used clinically. If all patients with a diagnosis of definite or possible endocarditis are fully treated for en-

Table 126-3   The Duke Criteria for the Clinical Diagnosis of Infective Endocarditis

MAJOR CRITERIA

Positive blood culture

Typical microorganism for infective endocarditis from two separate blood cultures

Viridans streptococci, *Streptococcus bovis*, HACEK group, *or*

Community-acquired *Staphylococcus aureus* or enterococci in the absence of a primary focus, *or*

Persistently positive blood culture, defined as recovery of a microorganism consistent with infective endocarditis from:

Blood cultures drawn >12 h apart; *or*

All of three or a majority of four or more separate blood cultures, with first and last drawn at least 1 h apart

Evidence of endocardial involvement

Positive echocardiogram

Oscillating intracardiac mass on valve or supporting structures or in the path of regurgitant jets or in implanted material, in the absence of an alternative anatomic explanation, *or*

Abscess, *or*

New partial dehiscence of prosthetic valve, *or*

New valvular regurgitation (increase or change in preexisting murmur not sufficient)

MINOR CRITERIA

Predisposition: predisposing heart condition or injection drug use

Fever ≥38.0°C (≥100.4°F)

Vascular phenomena: major arterial emboli, septic pulmonary infarcts, mycotic aneurysm, intracranial hemorrhage, conjunctival hemorrhages, Janeway lesions

Immunologic phenomena: glomerulonephritis, Osler's nodes, Roth's spots, rheumatoid factor

Microbiologic evidence: positive blood culture but not meeting major criterion as noted previously[a] or serologic evidence of active infection with organism consistent with infective endocarditis

Echocardiogram: consistent with infective endocarditis but not meeting major criterion

---

[a] Excluding single positive cultures for coagulase-negative staphylococci and diphtheroids, which are common culture contaminants, and organisms that do not cause endocarditis frequently, such as gram-negative bacilli.

NOTE: HACEK, *Haemophilus* spp., *Actinobacillus actinomycetemcomitans*, *Cardiobacterium hominis*, *Eikenella corrodens*, *Kingella kingae*.

SOURCE: Adapted from Durack et al., with permission from Excerpta Medica, Inc.

docarditis, this reduced specificity results in excess treatment for some patients. A modification of the schema has been proposed in order to increase its specificity without significantly reducing its sensitivity. This modification would require documentation of at least one major or three minor criteria for cases to be categorized as possible endocarditis.

The roles of bacteremia and echocardiographic findings in the diagnosis of endocarditis are appropriately emphasized in the Duke criteria. That multiple blood cultures obtained over time are positive is consistent with the known continuous low-density nature of bacteremia in patients with endocarditis (≤100 organisms per milliliter). Among untreated endocarditis patients who ultimately have a positive blood culture, 95% of all blood cultures are positive, and in 98% of cases one of the initial two sets of cultures yields the microorganism. The diagnostic criteria attach significance to the species of organism isolated from blood cultures. To fulfill a major criterion, the isolation of an organism that causes both endocarditis and bacteremia in the absence of endocarditis (e.g., *S. aureus*, enterococci) must take place repeatedly (i.e., persistent bacteremia) and in the absence of a primary focus of infection. Organisms that rarely cause endocarditis but commonly contaminate blood cultures (e.g., diphtheroids, coagulase-negative species) must be isolated repeatedly if their isolation is to serve as a major criterion.

Blood Cultures   Isolation of the causative microorganism from blood cultures is critical not only for diagnosis but also for determination of antimicrobial susceptibility and planning of treatment. In the absence of prior antibiotic therapy, a total of three blood culture sets, ideally with the first separated from the last by at least 1 h, should be obtained from different venipuncture sites over 24 h. If the cultures remain negative after 48 to 72 h, two or three additional blood cultures, including a lysis-centrifugation culture, should be obtained, and the laboratory should be asked to pursue fastidious microorganisms by prolonging incubation time and performing special subcultures. Empirical antimicrobial therapy should not be administered initially to hemodynamically stable patients with subacute endocarditis, especially those who have received antibiotics within the preceding 2 weeks; thus, if necessary, additional blood cultures can be obtained without the confounding effect of empirical treatment. Patients with acute endocarditis or with deteriorating hemodynamics that may require urgent surgery should be treated empirically immediately after obtaining the initial three sets of blood cultures.

Non-Blood-Culture Tests for the Etiologic Agent   Serologic tests can be used to identify some organisms causing endocarditis that are difficult to recover by blood culture: *Brucella*, *Bartonella*, *Legionella*, and *C. burnetii*. Pathogens can also be identified in vegetations by culture, by microscopic examination with special stains, and by use of polymerase chain reaction to recover unique microbial DNA or 16S rRNA.

Echocardiography   Cardiac imaging with echocardiography allows anatomic confirmation of infective endocarditis, sizing of vegetations, detection of intracardiac complications, and assessment of cardiac function. A two-dimensional study with color flow and continuous as well as pulsed Doppler is optimal. Transthoracic echocardiography (TTE) is noninvasive and exceptionally specific; however, it cannot image vegetations <2 mm in diameter, and in 20% of patients it is technically inadequate because of emphysema or body habitus. Thus, TTE detects vegetations in only 65% of patients with definite clinical endocarditis (i.e., it has a sensitivity of 65%). Moreover, TTE is not adequate for evaluating prosthetic valves or detecting intracardiac complications. Transesophageal echocardiography (TEE) is safe and significantly more sensitive than TTE. It detects vegetations in >90% of patients with definite endocarditis; nevertheless, false-negative studies are noted in 6 to 18% of endocarditis patients. TEE is the optimal method for the diagnosis of prosthetic endocarditis or the detection of myocardial abscess, valve perforation, or intracardiac fistulae.

Experts favor echocardiographic evaluation of all patients with a clinical diagnosis of endocarditis; however, the test should not be used to screen patients with otherwise explained positive blood cultures or patients with unexplained fever. In patients with a low pretest likelihood of endocarditis (<5%), a high-quality TTE that is negative is sufficient to exclude endocarditis. For patients whose habitus makes them difficult to study with TTE and for those who may have prosthetic valve endocarditis or who are at high risk of intracardiac complications, TEE is the preferred imaging modality. For patients with a pretest probability of endocarditis ranging from 5 to 50%, initial evaluation by TEE—in lieu of a sequential strategy of TTE, which, if negative, will be followed by TEE—is cost-effective. A negative TEE when endocarditis is likely does not exclude the diagnosis but rather warrants repetition of the study in 7 to 10 days with optimal multiplanar technique.

Other Studies   Many laboratory studies that do not aid in diagnostic evaluation are nevertheless important in the management of patients with endocarditis; these studies include complete blood counts, creatinine measurement, chest radiography, and electrocardiography. The erythrocyte sedimentation rate, C-reactive protein level, circulating immune complex titer, and rheumatoid factor concentration are commonly increased in endocarditis (Table 126-2). Cardiac catheterization is useful only to assess coronary artery patency in older individuals who are to undergo surgery for endocarditis.

℞ **TREATMENT   Antimicrobial Therapy**   It is difficult to eradicate bacteria from the avascular vegetation in infective endocarditis because this site is relatively inaccessible to host defenses and because the bacteria are nongrowing and metabolically inactive. Since all bacteria in the vegetation must be killed, therapy for endocarditis must be bactericidal and must be given for prolonged periods. Antibiotics are generally given parenterally and must reach high serum concentrations that will, through passive diffusion, lead to effective concentrations in the depths of the vegetation. The choice of effective therapy requires precise knowledge of the susceptibility of the causative microorganisms. The initiation of treatment before a cause is defined must balance the need to establish a microbiologic diagnosis against the potential progression of disease or the need for urgent surgery (see "Blood Cultures" above). The individual vulnerabilities of the patient should be weighed in the selection of therapy—e.g., allergies, end-organ dysfunction, interactions with concomitant medications, and risks of adverse events.

Although given for several weeks longer, the regimens recommended for the treatment of endocarditis involving prosthetic valves (except for staphylococcal infections) are similar to those used to treat native valve infection (Table 126-4). Recommended doses and duration of therapy should be adhered to unless alterations are required by adverse events.

Organism-specific therapies • STREPTOCOCCI Although most strains of viridans streptococci and *S. bovis* that cause endocarditis are susceptible to penicillin [minimum inhibitory concentration (MIC) ≤0.1 μg/mL], recent reports indicate increasing penicillin resistance among viridans streptococci recovered from blood cultures. In the selection of optimal therapy, the penicillin MIC must be determined

Table 126-4 Antibiotic Treatment for Infective Endocarditis Caused by Common Organisms*a*

Organism	Drug, Dose, Duration	Comments
Streptococci		
Penicillin-susceptible*b* streptococci, *S. bovis*	Penicillin G 2–3 million units IV q4h for 4 weeks	—
	Penicillin G 2–3 million units IV q4h *plus* gentamicin*c* 1 mg/kg IM or IV q8h, both for 2 weeks	Avoid penicillin plus gentamicin if risks of aminoglycoside toxicity are increased or case is complicated
	Ceftriaxone 2 g/d IV as single dose for 4 weeks	Can use ceftriaxone in patients with nonimmediate penicillin allergy
	Vancomycin*d* 15 mg/kg IV q12h for 4 weeks	Use vancomycin in patients with severe or immediate β-lactam allergy
Relatively penicillin-resistant*e* streptococci	Penicillin G 3 million units IV q4h for 4–6 weeks *plus* gentamicin*c* 1 mg/kg IV q8h for 2 weeks	Preferred for treatment of prosthetic valve endocarditis caused by penicillin-susceptible streptococci; continue penicillin for 6 weeks in this setting
Penicillin-resistant*f* streptococci, pyridoxal-requiring streptococci (*Abiotrophia* spp.)	Penicillin G 3–4 million units IV q4h *plus* gentamicin*c* 1 mg/kg IV q8h, both for 4–6 weeks	—
Enterococci*g*	Penicillin G 3–4 million units IV q4h *plus* gentamicin*c* 1 mg/kg IV q8h, both for 4–6 weeks	Can use streptomycin 7.5 mg/kg q12h in lieu of gentamicin if there is not high-level resistance to streptomycin
	Ampicillin 2 g IV q4h *plus* gentamicin*c* 1 mg/kg IV q8h, both for 4–6 weeks	Do not use cephalosporins or carbapenems for treatment of enterococcal endocarditis
	Vancomycin*d* 15 mg/kg IV q12h *plus* gentamicin*c* 1 mg/kg IV q8h, both for 4–6 weeks	Use vancomycin plus gentamicin for penicillin-allergic patients or desensitize to penicillin
Staphylococci		
Methicillin-susceptible, infecting native valves (no foreign devices)	Nafcillin or oxacillin 2 g IV q4h for 4–6 weeks *plus* (optional) gentamicin*c* 1 mg/kg IM or IV q8h for 3–5 days	May use penicillin 3–4 million units q6h if isolate is penicillin-susceptible (does not produce β-lactamase)
	Cefazolin 2 g IV q8h for 4–6 weeks *plus* (optional) gentamicin*c* 1 mg/kg IM or IV q8h for 3–5 days	Can use cefazolin regimen for patients with nonimmediate penicillin allergy
	Vancomycin*d* 15 mg/kg IV q12h for 4–6 weeks	Use vancomycin for patients with immediate (urticarial) or severe penicillin allergy
Methicillin-resistant, infecting native valves (no foreign devices)	Vancomycin*d* 15 mg/kg IV q12h for 4–6 weeks	No role for routine use of rifampin
Methicillin-susceptible, infecting prosthetic valves	Nafcillin or oxacillin 2 g IV q4h for 6–8 weeks *plus* gentamicin*c* 1 mg/kg IM or IV q8h for 2 weeks *plus* rifampin*h* 300 mg PO q8h for 6–8 weeks	Use gentamicin during initial 2 weeks; determine susceptibility to gentamicin before initiating rifampin (see text); if patient is highly allergic to penicillin, use regimen for methicillin-resistant staphylococci; if β-lactam allergy is of the minor, nonimmediate type, can substitute cefazolin for oxacillin/nafcillin
Methicillin-resistant, infecting prosthetic valves	Vancomycin*d* 15 mg/kg IV q12h for 6–8 weeks *plus* gentamicin*c* 1 mg/kg IM or IV q8h for 2 weeks *plus* rifampin*h* 300 mg PO q8h for 6–8 weeks	Use gentamicin during initial 2 weeks; determine gentamicin susceptibility before initiating rifampin (see text)
HACEK organisms	Ceftriaxone 2 g/d IV as single dose for 4 weeks	May use another third-generation cephalosporin at comparable dosage
	Ampicillin 2 g IV q4h *plus* gentamicin*c* 1 mg/kg IM or IV q8h, both for 4 weeks	Determine ampicillin susceptibility; do not use ampicillin if β-lactamase is produced

a Doses are for adults with normal renal function. Doses of gentamicin, streptomycin, and vancomycin must be adjusted for reduced renal function. Ideal body weight is used to calculate doses per kilogram (men = 50 kg + 2.3 kg per inch over 5 feet; women = 45.5 kg + 2.3 kg per inch over 5 feet).
b MIC ≤ 0.1 μg/mL.
c Aminoglycosides should not be administered as single daily doses and should be introduced as part of the initial treatment. Target peak and trough serum concentrations of gentamicin 1 h after a 20- to 30-min infusion or IM injection are 3–5 μg/mL and ≤1

μg/mL, respectively; the target peak serum concentration of streptomycin (timing as with gentamicin) is 20–25 μg/mL.
d Desirable peak vancomycin level 1 h after completion of a 1-h infusion is 30–45 μg/mL.
e MIC > 0.1 μg/mL and <0.5 μg/mL.
f MIC ≥ 0.5 μg/mL.
g Antimicrobial susceptibility must be evaluated; see text.
h Rifampin increases warfarin and dicumarol requirements for anticoagulation.

(Table 126-4). The 2-week penicillin/gentamicin regimen should not be used to treat complicated native valve infection or prosthetic valve endocarditis. Although small studies have suggested that a 2-week regimen of single daily doses of ceftriaxone (2 g IV) plus gentamicin (3 mg/kg) or netilmicin (4 mg/kg) is effective for penicillin-susceptible streptococcal endocarditis, the data are not sufficient to support routine use of this regimen. Penicillin/gentamicin is recommended for the treatment of endocarditis caused by group B streptococci.

ENTEROCOCCI Enterococci are resistant to oxacillin, nafcillin, and the cephalosporins and are inhibited only by penicillin, ampicillin, teicoplanin (not available in the United States), and vancomycin. To kill enterococci requires the synergistic interaction of a cell wall–active antibiotic (penicillin, ampicillin, vancomycin, or teicoplanin) that is effective at achievable serum concentrations and an aminoglycoside (gentamicin or streptomycin) to which the isolate does not exhibit high-level resistance. An isolate's resistance to cell wall–active agents or ability to replicate in the presence of gentamicin at $\geq$500 μg/mL or streptomycin at 2000 μg/mL—a phenomenon called *high-level aminoglycoside resistance*—indicates that the ineffective antimicrobial cannot participate in the interaction to produce killing. High-level resistance to gentamicin predicts that tobramycin, netilmicin, amikacin, and kanamycin will also be ineffective. In fact, even when enterococci are not highly resistant to gentamicin, it is difficult to predict the ability of these other aminoglycosides to participate in synergistic killing; consequently, they should not in general be used to treat enterococcal endocarditis.

Clearly, enterococci causing endocarditis must be tested for high-level resistance to streptomycin and gentamicin, β-lactamase production, and susceptibility to penicillin and ampicillin (MIC, $\leq$16 μg/mL) and to vancomycin (MIC, $\leq$8 μg/mL). If the isolate produces β-lactamase, ampicillin/sulbactam or vancomycin can be used as the cell wall–active component; if the penicillin/ampicillin MIC is >16 μg/mL, vancomycin can be considered; and if the vancomycin MIC is >8 μg/mL, penicillin or ampicillin may be considered. Based on the absence of high-level resistance, gentamicin or streptomycin should be used as the aminoglycoside. If there is high-level resistance to both these drugs, no aminoglycoside should be given; instead, an 8- to 12-week course of a single cell wall–active agent is suggested. If single-drug therapy fails or the isolate is resistant to all of the commonly used agents, surgical treatment is advised. The role of newer agents potentially active against multidrug-resistant enterococci (quinupristin/dalfopristin, linezolid, and daptomycin) in the treatment of endocarditis has not been established.

STAPHYLOCOCCI The regimens used to treat staphylococcal endocarditis are not based upon coagulase production but rather upon the presence or absence of a prosthetic valve or foreign device, the native valve(s) involved, and the resistance of the isolate to penicillin and methicillin. Penicillinase is produced by 95% of staphylococci; thus, all isolates should be considered penicillin-resistant until shown not to produce this enzyme. The addition of gentamicin (if the isolate is susceptible) to a β-lactam antibiotic to enhance therapy for native mitral or aortic valve endocarditis is optional. Its addition hastens eradication of bacteremia but does not improve survival rates. If added, gentamicin should be limited to the initial 3 to 5 days of therapy to avoid nephrotoxicity. Gentamicin generally is not added to the vancomycin regimen in this setting.

Methicillin-susceptible *S. aureus* endocarditis that is uncomplicated and limited to the tricuspid or pulmonic valve—a condition occurring almost exclusively in injection drug users—can often be treated with a 2-week course that combines oxacillin or nafcillin (but not vancomycin) with gentamicin. Prolonged fevers ($\geq$ 5 days) during therapy suggest that these patients should receive standard therapy.

Staphylococcal prosthetic valve endocarditis is treated for 6 to 8 weeks with a multidrug regimen. Rifampin is an essential component because it kills staphylococci that are adherent to foreign material. Two other agents (selected on the basis of susceptibility testing) are combined with rifampin to prevent in vivo emergence of resistance. Because many staphylococci, particularly methicillin-resistant *S. aureus* and *S. epidermidis*, are resistant to gentamicin, the utility of gentamicin should be established before rifampin treatment is begun. If the isolate is resistant to gentamicin, another aminoglycoside or a fluoroquinolone (chosen in light of susceptibility results) should be substituted.

OTHER ORGANISMS Although penicillin is the therapy of choice for endocarditis caused by *S. pneumoniae*, therapy should be initiated with ceftriaxone and vancomycin until susceptibility to penicillin is established. *P. aeruginosa* endocarditis is treated with an antipseudomonal penicillin (ticarcillin or piperacillin) and high doses of tobramycin (8 mg/kg per day in three divided doses). Endocarditis caused by Enterobacteriaceae is treated with a potent β-lactam antibiotic plus an aminoglycoside. Corynebacterial endocarditis is treated with penicillin plus an aminoglycoside (if the organism is susceptible to the aminoglycoside) or with vancomycin, which is highly bactericidal for most strains. Therapy for *Candida* endocarditis consists of amphotericin B plus flucytosine and early surgery; long-term (if not indefinite) suppression with fluconazole is used increasingly.

Empirical therapy In designing and executing therapy without culture data (i.e., before culture results are known or when cultures are negative), clinical and epidemiologic clues to etiology must be weighed, and both the pathogens associated with the specific endocarditis syndrome and the hazards of suboptimal therapy must be considered. Thus, empirical therapy for acute endocarditis in an injection drug user should cover methicillin-resistant *S. aureus* and gram-negative bacilli. The initiation of treatment with vancomycin plus gentamicin immediately after blood is obtained for cultures covers these as well as many other potential causes. In treating culture-negative episodes, marantic endocarditis must be excluded and fastidious organisms sought serologically. In the absence of confounding prior antibiotic therapy, it is unlikely that *S. aureus* or enterococcal infection will present with negative blood cultures. Thus, in this situation, these organisms are not the determinants of therapy for subacute endocarditis. Blood culture–negative native valve endocarditis is treated with ceftriaxone (or ampicillin) plus gentamicin; these two antimicrobials plus vancomycin should be used if prosthetic valves are involved.

Outpatient antimicrobial therapy Fully compliant patients who have sterile blood cultures, are afebrile during therapy, and have no clinical or echocardiographic findings that suggest an impending complication may complete therapy as outpatients. Careful follow-up and a stable home setting are necessary, as are predictable intravenous access and selection of antimicrobials that are stable in solution.

Monitoring antimicrobial therapy The serum bactericidal titer—the highest dilution of the patient's serum during therapy that kills 99.9% of the standard inoculum of the infecting organism—is no longer recommended for assessment of patients receiving standard regimens. However, in the treatment of endocarditis caused by unusual organisms, this measurement, although not standardized and difficult to interpret, may provide a patient-specific assessment of in vivo antibiotic effect. Serum concentrations of aminoglycosides and vancomycin should be monitored.

Antibiotic toxicities, including allergic reactions, occur in 25 to 40% of patients and commonly arise during the third week of therapy. Blood tests to detect antibiotic-specific potential end-organ toxicity should be performed periodically.

In most patients effective antibiotic therapy results in subjective improvement and resolution of fever within 5 to 7 days. Blood cultures should be repeated daily until sterile, rechecked if there is recrudescent fever, and performed again 4 to 6 weeks after therapy to document cure. Blood cultures become sterile within 2 days after the start of appropriate therapy when infection is caused by viridans streptococci, enterococci, or HACEK organisms. In *S. aureus* endocarditis, β-lactam therapy results in sterile cultures in 3 to 5 days, whereas positive cultures may persist for 7 to 9 days with vancomycin treatment. When fever persists for 7 days in spite of appropriate antibiotic therapy, patients should be evaluated for paravalvular abscess and for extra-cardiac abscesses (spleen, kidney) or complications (embolic events). Recrudescent fever raises the question of these complications but also of drug reactions or complications of hospitalization. Serologic abnormalities (e.g., erythrocyte sedimentation rate, rheumatoid factor) resolve slowly and do not reflect response to treatment. Vegetations become smaller with effective therapy, but at 3 months after cure half are unchanged and 25% are slightly larger.

Surgical Treatment Intracardiac and central nervous system complications of endocarditis are important causes of the morbidity and mortality associated with this infection. In some cases, effective treatment for these complications requires surgery. Most of the clinical indications for surgical treatment of endocarditis are not absolute (Table 126-5). The risks and benefits as well as the timing of surgical treatment must therefore be individualized.

Intracardiac surgical indications Most surgical interventions are clearly warranted by intracardiac findings, often detected by echocardiography. Because of the highly invasive nature of prosthetic valve endocarditis, as many as 40% of affected patients merit surgical treatment. In many patients, coincident rather than single intracardiac events necessitate surgery.

CONGESTIVE HEART FAILURE Moderate to severe refractory congestive heart failure caused by new or worsening valve dysfunction is the major indication for cardiac surgical treatment of endocarditis. Of patients with moderate to severe heart failure due to valve dysfunction who are treated medically, 60 to 90% die within 6 months. In the setting of similar hemodynamic dysfunction, surgical treatment is associated with mortality rates of 20 to 40% with native valve endocarditis and 35 to 55% with prosthetic valve infection. Surgery may be required to relieve functional stenosis due to large vegetations or to restore competence to damaged regurgitant valves.

PERIVALVULAR INFECTION This complication, which occurs in 10 to 15% of native valve and 45 to 60% of prosthetic valve infections, is suggested by persistent unexplained fever during appropriate therapy, new electrocardiographic conduction disturbances, and pericarditis. Extension can occur from any valve but is most common with aortic valve infection. TEE with color Doppler is the test of choice to detect perivalvular abscesses (sensitivity, ≥85%). Although occasional perivalvular infections are cured medically, surgery is warranted when fever persists, fistulae develop, prostheses are dehisced and unstable, and infection relapses after appropriate treatment. Cardiac rhythm must be monitored since high-grade heart block may require insertion of a pacemaker.

Table 126-5 Indications for Cardiac Surgical Intervention in Patients with Endocarditis

Surgery required for optimal outcome
  Moderate to severe congestive heart failure due to valve dysfunction
  Partially dehisced unstable prosthetic valve
  Persistent bacteremia despite optimal antimicrobial therapy
  Lack of effective microbicidal therapy (e.g., fungal or *Brucella* endocarditis)
  S. aureus prosthetic valve endocarditis with an intracardiac complication
  Relapse of prosthetic valve endocarditis after optimal antimicrobial therapy
  Persistent unexplained fever (≥10 days) in culture-negative prosthetic valve endocarditis
Surgery to be strongly considered for improved outcome[a]
  Perivalvular extension of infection
  Poorly responsive *S. aureus* endocarditis involving the aortic or mitral valve
  Large (>10-mm diameter) hypermobile vegetations with increased risk of embolism
  Persistent unexplained fever (≥10 days) in culture-negative native valve endocarditis
  Poorly responsive or relapsed endocarditis due to highly antibiotic-resistant enterococci or gram-negative bacilli

[a] Surgery must be carefully considered; findings are often combined with other indications to prompt surgery.

UNCONTROLLED INFECTION Continued positive blood cultures or otherwise unexplained persistent fevers (in patients with either blood culture–positive or –negative endocarditis) despite optimal antibiotic therapy may reflect uncontrolled infection and warrant surgery. Surgical treatment is also advised for endocarditis caused by those organisms against which clinical experience indicates that effective antimicrobial therapy is lacking. This category includes infections caused by yeasts, fungi, *P. aeruginosa*, other highly resistant gram-negative bacilli, *Brucella* species, and probably *C. burnetii*.

S. AUREUS ENDOCARDITIS Mortality rates for *S. aureus* prosthetic valve endocarditis exceed 70% with medical treatment but are reduced to 25% with surgical treatment. In patients with intracardiac complications associated with *S. aureus* prosthetic valve infection, surgical treatment reduces mortality by twentyfold. Surgical treatment should be considered for patients with *S. aureus* native aortic or mitral valve infection who have TTE-demonstrable vegetations and remain septic during the initial week of therapy. Isolated tricuspid valve endocarditis, even with persistent fever, rarely requires surgery.

PREVENTION OF SYSTEMIC EMBOLI Mortality and persisting morbidity due to emboli are largely limited to patients suffering occlusion of cerebral or coronary arteries. Echocardiographic determination of vegetation size and anatomy, although predictive of patients at high risk of systemic emboli, does not identify those patients in whom the benefits of surgery to prevent emboli clearly exceed the risks of the surgical procedure. Net benefits favoring surgery are most likely when the risk of embolism is high and other surgical benefits can be achieved simultaneously—e.g., repair of a moderately dysfunctional valve or debridement of a paravalvular abscess.

Timing of cardiac surgery Surgery to correct valvular dysfunction and progressive congestive heart failure should not be delayed simply to permit additional antibiotic therapy, since this course of action increases the risk of mortality. Similarly, surgery should not be delayed when the indication is uncontrolled or perivalvular infection. Delay is justified only when infection is controlled and congestive heart failure is fully compensated with medical therapy. Recrudescent endocarditis involving a prosthetic valve follows surgery in 2% of patients with culture-positive native valve endocarditis and 15% of patients with active prosthetic valve endocarditis. These risks are more acceptable than the high mortality rates that result when surgery is inappropriately delayed or not performed.

Among patients who have experienced a neurologic complication of endocarditis, further neurologic deterioration can occur as a consequence of cardiac surgery. The risk of significant neurologic exacerbation is related to the interval between the complication and surgery. Where feasible, cardiac surgery should be delayed for 2 to 3 weeks after a nonhemorrhagic embolic stroke and for 4 weeks after a hemorrhagic embolic stroke. A ruptured mycotic aneurysm should be clipped and cerebral edema allowed to resolve prior to cardiac surgery.

Extracardiac complications Splenic abscess develops in 3 to 5% of patients with endocarditis. Effective therapy requires either computed tomography–guided percutaneous drainage or splenectomy. Mycotic aneurysms occur in 2 to 15% of endocarditis patients; half of these cases involve the cerebral arteries and present as headaches, focal neurologic symptoms, or hemorrhage. Cerebral aneurysms should be monitored by angiography. Some will resolve, but those that persist, enlarge, or leak should be treated surgically if possible. Extracerebral aneurysms present as local pain, a mass, local ischemia, or bleeding; generally these aneurysms are treated by resection.

OUTCOME The outcome of infective endocarditis is affected by a variety of factors, some of which are interrelated. Factors with an adverse impact include older age, severe comorbid conditions, delayed diagnosis, involvement of prosthetic valves or the aortic valve, an invasive (*S. aureus*) or antibiotic-resistant (*P. aeruginosa*, yeast) pathogen, intracardiac complications, and major neurologic complications. Death and poor outcome often are related not to failure of

Table 126-6   Procedures for Which Endocarditis Prophylaxis Is Advised in Patients at High or Moderate Risk for Endocarditis[a]

Dental procedures
  Extractions
  Periodontal procedures, cleaning causing gingival bleeding
  Implant placement, reimplantation of avulsed teeth
  Endodontic instrumentation (root canal) or surgery beyond the apex
  Subgingival placement of antibiotic fibers or strips
  Placement of orthodontic bands but not brackets
  Intraligamentary injections (anesthetic)
Respiratory procedures
  Operations involving the mucosa
  Bronchoscopy with rigid bronchoscope
Gastrointestinal procedures[b]
  Esophageal: Sclerotherapy of varices, stricture dilation
  Biliary tract: Endoscopic retrograde cholangiography with biliary obstruction, biliary tract surgery
  Intestinal tract: Surgery involving the mucosa
Genitourinary procedures
  Urethral dilation, prostate or urethral surgery
  Cystoscopy

[a] Prophylaxis is optional for high-risk patients undergoing bronchoscopy or gastrointestinal endoscopy with/without biopsy, vaginal delivery, vaginal hysterectomy, or transesophageal echocardiography.
[b] Prophylaxis is recommended for high-risk patients and optional for moderate-risk group (see Table 126-7).
SOURCE: Adapted from Dajani et al.

antibiotic therapy but rather to the interactions of comorbidities and endocarditis-related end-organ complications. The overall survival rate for patients with native valve endocarditis caused by viridans streptococci, HACEK organisms, or enterococci (susceptible to synergistic therapy) ranges from 85 to 90%. For *S. aureus* native valve endocarditis in patients who do not inject drugs, survival rates are 55 to 70%, whereas 85 to 90% of injection drug users survive this infection. Prosthetic valve endocarditis beginning within 2 months of valve replacement results in mortality rates of 40 to 50%, whereas rates are only 10 to 20% in later-onset cases.

PREVENTION   Antibiotics have been administered in conjunction with selected procedures considered to entail a risk for bacteremia and endocarditis. The benefits of antibiotic prophylaxis are not established and in fact may be modest: only 50% of patients with native valve endocarditis knew that they had a valve lesion predisposing to infection, most endocarditis cases do not follow a procedure, and 35% of cases are caused by organisms not targeted by prophylaxis. Dental treatments, the procedures most widely accepted as predisposing to endocarditis, are no more frequent during the 3 months preceding this diagnosis than in uninfected matched controls. Nevertheless, an expert committee of the American Heart Association, along with similar advisory groups in other developed countries, has identified procedures that may precipitate bacteremia with organisms that cause endocarditis (Table 126-6), patients who should receive prophylaxis based on the relative risk for developing endocarditis and the severity of subsequent

Table 126-7   Cardiac Lesions for Which Endocarditis Prophylaxis Is Advised

High Risk	Moderate Risk
Prosthetic heart valves	Congenital cardiac malformations (other than high-/low-risk lesions), ventricular septal defect, bicuspid aortic valve
Prior bacterial endocarditis	
Complex cyanotic congenital heart disease; other complex congenital lesions after correction (see text)	Acquired aortic and mitral valve dysfunction
Patent ductus arteriosus	Hypertrophic cardiomyopathy (asymmetric septal hypertrophy)
Coarctation of the aorta	Mitral valve prolapse with valvular regurgitation and/or thickened leaflets
Surgically constructed systemic-pulmonary shunts	

Table 126-8   Antibiotic Regimens for Prophylaxis of Endocarditis in Adults at Moderate or High Risk[a]

I. Oral cavity, respiratory tract, or esophageal procedures[b]
  A. Standard regimen
    1. Amoxicillin 2.0 g PO 1 h before procedure
  B. Inability to take oral medication
    1. Ampicillin 2.0 g IV or IM within 30 min of procedure
  C. Penicillin allergy
    1. Clarithromycin 500 mg PO 1 h before procedure
    2. Cephalexin[c] or cefadroxil[c] 2.0 g PO 1 h before procedure
    3. Clindamycin 600 mg PO 1 h before procedure or IV 30 min before procedure
  D. Inability to take oral medication
    1. Cefazolin[c] 1.0 g IV or IM 30 min before procedure
II. Genitourinary and gastrointestinal tract[d] procedures
  A. High-risk patients
    1. Ampicillin 2.0 g IV or IM *plus* gentamicin 1.5 mg/kg (not to exceed 120 mg) IV or IM within 30 min of procedure; repeat ampicillin 1.0 g IV or IM or amoxicillin 1.0 g PO 6 h later
  B. High-risk, penicillin-allergic patients
    1. Vancomycin 1.0 g IV over 1-2 h *plus* gentamicin 1.5 mg/kg (not to exceed 120 mg) IV or IM within 30 min before procedure; no second dose recommended
  C. Moderate-risk patients
    1. Amoxicillin 2.0 g PO 1 h before procedure or ampicillin 2.0 g IV or IM within 30 min before procedure
  D. Moderate-risk, penicillin-allergic patients
    1. Vancomycin 1.0 g IV infused over 1-2 h and completed within 30 min of procedure

[a] Dosing for children: for amoxicillin, ampicillin, cephalexin, or cefadroxil, use 50 mg/kg PO; cefazolin, 25 mg/kg IV; clindamycin, 20 mg/kg PO, 25 mg/kg IV; clarithromycin, 15 mg/kg PO; gentamicin, 1.5 mg/kg IV or IM; and vancomycin, 20 mg/kg IV.
[b] For patients at high risk (Table 126-7), administer a half-dose 6 h after the initial dose.
[c] Do not use cephalosporins in patients with immediate hypersensitivity (urticaria, angioedema, anaphylaxis) to penicillin.
[d] Excludes esophageal procedures.
SOURCE: Adapted from Dajani et al.

infection (Table 126-7), and regimens that may be used for prophylaxis (Table 126-8). Except for an isolated secundum atrial septal defect and a totally corrected patent ductus arteriosus, ventricular septal defect, or pulmonary stenosis, patients with congenital heart defects continue to experience high rates of endocarditis despite total surgical correction of the defect. In vulnerable patients, maintaining good dental hygiene and aggressively treating local infections may reduce the risk of endocarditis.

BIBLIOGRAPHY

BAYER AS et al: Diagnosis and management of infective endocarditis and its complications. Circulation 98:2936, 1998

DAJANI AS et al: Prevention of bacterial endocarditis: Recommendations by the American Heart Association, from the Committee on Rheumatic Fever, Endocarditis, and Kawasaki Disease, Council on Cardiovascular Diseases in the Young. JAMA 277:1794, 1997

D'UDEKEM Y et al: Long-term results of operation for paravalvular abscess. Ann Thorac Surg 62:48, 1996

DURACK D et al: New criteria for diagnosis of infective endocarditis: Utilization of specific echocardiographic findings. Am J Med 96:200, 1994

HEIDENREICH PA et al: Echocardiography in patients with suspected endocarditis: A cost-effective analysis. Am J Med 107:198, 1999

KARCHMER AW: Infections of prosthetic valves and intravascular devices, in *Mandell, Douglas, and Bennett's Principles and Practice of Infectious Diseases*, 5th ed, GL Mandell et al (eds). New York, Churchill Livingstone, 2000, pp 903–917

———: Infective endocarditis, in *Heart Disease*, 6th ed, E Braunwald et al (eds). Philadelphia, Saunders, 2000

KAYE D (ed): *Infective Endocarditis*, 2d ed. New York, Raven, 1992

MORRIS CD et al: Thirty-year incidence of infective endocarditis after surgery for congenital heart defect. JAMA 279:599, 1998

RAOULT D et al: Cultivation of the bacillus of Whipple's disease. N Engl J Med 342:620, 2000

STROM BL et al: Dental and cardiac risk factors for infective endocarditis: A population-based, case-control study. Ann Intern Med 129:761, 1998

WILSON WR et al: Antibiotic treatment of adults with infective endocarditis due to viridans streptococci, enterococci, other streptococci, staphylococci, and HACEK microorganisms. JAMA 274:1706, 1995

INFECTIOUS COMPLICATIONS OF BITES AND BURNS

The skin is an essential component of the nonspecific immune system, protecting the host from potential pathogens in the environment. Breaches in this protective barrier thus represent a form of immunocompromise that predisposes the patient to infection. Bites and scratches from animals and humans allow the inoculation of microorganisms past the skin's protective barrier into deeper, susceptible host tissues. Thermal burns may cause massive destruction of the integument as well as derangements in humoral and cellular immunity, enabling environmental opportunists and components of the host's own skin flora to cause infection.

ANIMAL BITES AND SCRATCHES   Each year in the United States, between 1 and 2 million animal-bite wounds are sustained; the vast majority are inflicted by pet dogs and cats, which number more than 100 million. Other bite wounds are a consequence of encounters with animals in the wild or in occupational settings. While many of these wounds require minimal or no therapy, a significant number result in infection, which may be life-threatening. The microbiology of bite-wound infections in general reflects the oropharyngeal flora of the biting animal, although organisms from the soil, the skin of the animal and victim, and the animal's feces may also be involved.

Dog Bites   Dogs are responsible for approximately 80% of bite wounds, an estimated 15 to 20% of which become infected. A study for the period 1992 through 1994 found that dog bites resulted in more than 900 emergency department visits each day in the United States. Most dog bites are provoked and are inflicted by the victim's pet or by a dog known to the victim. These bites frequently occur during efforts to break up a dogfight. Victims tend to be male, and bites most often involve a lower extremity. Infection typically manifests 8 to 24 h after the bite as pain at the site of injury with cellulitis accompanied by purulent, sometimes foul-smelling discharge. Septic arthritis and osteomyelitis may develop if the canine tooth penetrates synovium or bone. Systemic manifestations such as fever, lymphadenopathy, and lymphangitis may also occur. The microbiology of dog-bite wound infections is usually mixed and includes α-hemolytic streptococci, *Pasteurella* spp., *Staphylococcus* spp., *Eikenella corrodens*, and *Capnocytophaga canimorsus* (formerly designated DF-2). Many wounds also include anaerobic bacteria such as *Actinomyces*, *Fusobacterium*, *Prevotella*, and *Porphyromonas* spp.

While most infections resulting from dog-bite injuries are localized to the area of injury, many of the microorganisms involved are capable of causing systemic infection, including bacteremia, meningitis, brain abscess, endocarditis, and chorioamnionitis. These infections are particularly likely in hosts with edema or compromised lymphatic drainage in the involved extremity (e.g., following a bite on the arm after radical or modified radical mastectomy) and in patients who are immunocompromised by medication or disease (e.g., glucocorticoid use, systemic lupus erythematosus, acute leukemia, or hepatic cirrhosis). In addition, dog bites and scratches may result in systemic illnesses such as rabies (Chap. 197) and tetanus (Chap. 143).

Infection with *C. canimorsus* following dog-bite wounds may result in fulminant sepsis, disseminated intravascular coagulation, and renal failure, particularly in hosts who have impaired hepatic function, who have undergone splenectomy, or who are immunosuppressed. This organism is a thin gram-negative rod that is difficult to culture on most solid media but grows in a variety of liquid media. The bacteria are occasionally seen within polymorphonuclear leukocytes on Wright-stained smears of peripheral blood from septic patients.

Cat Bites   Although less common than dog bites, cat bites and scratches result in infection in more than half of all cases. Because the narrow, sharp feline incisors penetrate deeply into tissue, cat bites are more likely than dog bites to cause septic arthritis and osteomyelitis; the development of these conditions is particularly likely when punctures are located over or near a joint, especially in the hand. Women sustain cat bites more frequently than do men. These bites most often involve the hands and arms. Both bites and scratches from cats are prone to infection from organisms in the cat's oropharynx. *Pasteurella multocida*, a normal component of the feline oral flora, is a small gram-negative coccobacillus implicated in the majority of cat-bite wound infections. Like that of dog-bite wound infections, however, the microflora of cat-bite wound infections is usually mixed. Other microorganisms causing infection after cat bites are similar to those causing dog-bite wound infections.

The same risk factors for systemic infection following dog-bite wounds apply to cat-bite wounds. *Pasteurella* infections tend to advance rapidly, often within hours, causing severe inflammation accompanied by purulent drainage; *Pasteurella* may also be spread by respiratory droplets from animals, resulting in pneumonia or bacteremia. Like dog-bite wounds, cat-bite wounds may result in the transmission of rabies or in the development of tetanus. Infection with *Bartonella henselae* causes cat-scratch disease (Chap. 163) and is an important late consequence of cat bites and scratches. Tularemia (Chap. 161) has also been reported to follow cat bites.

Other Animal Bites   Infections have been attributed to bites from many animal species, often as a consequence of occupational exposure (farmers, laboratory workers, veterinarians) or recreational exposure (hunters and trappers, wilderness campers, owners of exotic pets). Generally, the microflora of bite wounds reflects the oral flora of the biting animal. Most members of the cat family, including feral cats, harbor *P. multocida*. Bite wounds from aquatic animals such as alligators or piranhas may contain *Aeromonas hydrophila*. Venomous snakebites (Chap. 397) result in severe inflammatory responses and tissue necrosis—conditions that render these injuries prone to infection. The snake's oral flora includes many species of aerobes and anaerobes, such as *Pseudomonas aeruginosa*, *Proteus* spp., *Staphylococcus epidermidis*, *Bacteroides fragilis*, and *Clostridium* spp. Bites from nonhuman primates are highly susceptible to infection with pathogens similar to those isolated from human bites (which are discussed later in this chapter). Bites from Old World monkeys (*Macaca*) may also result in the transmission of B virus (*Herpesvirus simiae*, cercopithecine herpesvirus), a cause of serious infection of the human central nervous system. Bites of seals, walruses, and polar bears may cause a chronic suppurative infection known as *seal finger*, which is probably due to one or more species of *Mycoplasma* colonizing these animals.

Small rodents, including rats, mice, and gerbils, as well as animals that prey on rodents may transmit *Streptobacillus moniliformis* (a microaerophilic, pleomorphic gram-negative rod) or *Spirillum minor* (a spirochete), which cause a clinical illness known as *rat-bite fever*. The vast majority of cases in the United States are streptobacillary, whereas *Spirillum* infection occurs mainly in Asia.

In the United States, the risk of rodent bite mainly affects laboratory workers or inhabitants of rodent-infested dwellings (particularly children). Rat-bite fever is distinguished from acute bite-wound infection by its typical manifestation after the initial wound has healed. Streptobacillary disease follows an incubation period of 3 to 10 days. Fever, chills, myalgias, headache, and severe migratory arthralgias are usually followed by a maculopapular rash, which characteristically involves the palms and soles and may become confluent or purpuric. Complications include endocarditis, myocarditis, meningitis, pneumonia, and abscesses in many organs. *Haverhill fever* is an *S. moniliformis* infection acquired from contaminated milk or drinking water and has similar manifestations. Streptobacillary rat-bite fever was frequently fatal in the preantibiotic era. The differential diagnosis includes Rocky Mountain spotted fever, Lyme disease, leptospirosis, and secondary syphilis. The diagnosis is made by direct observation of the causative organisms in tissue or blood, by culture on enriched media, or by serologic testing with specific agglutinins.

Spirillum infection (referred to in Japan as *sodoku*) causes pain and purple swelling at the site of the initial bite, with associated lymphangitis and regional lymphadenopathy, after an incubation period of 1 to 4 weeks. The systemic illness includes fever, chills, and headache. The original lesion may eventually progress to an eschar. The infection is diagnosed by direct visualization of the spirochetes in blood or tissue or by animal inoculation.

Human Bites   Human bites may be self-inflicted; may be sustained by medical personnel caring for patients; or may take place during fights, domestic abuse, or sexual activity. Human bites more frequently become infected than do bites inflicted by other animals. These infections reflect the diverse oral microflora of humans, which includes multiple species of aerobic and anaerobic bacteria. Common aerobic isolates include viridans streptococci, *Staphylococcus aureus*, *E. corrodens* (which is particularly common in clenched-fist injury; see below), and *Haemophilus influenzae*. Anaerobic species, including *Fusobacterium nucleatum* and *Prevotella*, *Porphyromonas*, and *Peptostreptococcus* spp., are isolated from 50% of human-bite wound infections; many of these isolates produce β-lactamases. The oral flora of hospitalized and debilitated patients often includes Enterobacteriaceae in addition to the usual organisms. Both HIV and hepatitis B virus have been reported to be transmitted by human bite, but these instances appear to be quite rare.

Human bites are categorized as "occlusional" injuries, which are inflicted by actual biting, and "clenched-fist" injuries, which are sustained when the fist of one individual strikes the teeth of another, causing traumatic laceration of the hand. For several reasons, clenched-fist injuries result in particularly serious infections. The deep spaces of the hand, including the bone, joint, and tendons, are frequently inoculated with organisms in the course of such injuries. The clenched position of the fist during injury, followed by extension of the hand, may further promote the introduction of bacteria as contaminated tendons retract beneath the skin's surface. Moreover, medical attention is often sought only after frank infection develops.

℞ **TREATMENT   Initial Assessment**   A careful history should be elicited, including the type of biting animal, the type of attack (provoked or unprovoked), and the amount of time elapsed since injury. Local and regional authorities should be contacted to determine whether an individual species could be rabid and/or to locate and observe the biting animal when rabies prophylaxis may be indicated (Chap. 197). Suspicious human-bite wounds should provoke careful questioning regarding domestic or child abuse. Details on antibiotic allergies, immunosuppression, splenectomy, liver disease, mastectomy, and immunization history should be obtained. The wound should be inspected carefully for evidence of infection, including redness, exudate, and foul odor. The type of wound (puncture, laceration, or scratch); the depth of penetration; and the possible involvement of joints, tendons, nerves, and bone should be assessed. It is often useful to include a diagram or photograph of the wound in the medical record. In addition, a general physical examination should be conducted and should include an assessment of vital signs as well as an evaluation for evidence of lymphangitis, lymphadenopathy, dermatologic lesions, and functional limitations. Injuries to the hand warrant consultation with a hand surgeon for the assessment of tendon, nerve, and muscular damage. Radiographs should be obtained when the bone may have been penetrated or a tooth fragment may be present. Culture and Gram's staining of all infected wounds are essential; anaerobic cultures should be undertaken if abscesses, devitalized tissue, or foul-smelling exudate is present. A small-tipped swab may be used to culture deep punctures or small lacerations. It is also reasonable to culture samples from uninfected wounds due to bites inflicted by animals other than dogs and cats, since the microorganisms causing disease are less predictable in these cases. A white blood cell count should be determined and blood cultured if systemic infection is suspected.

Wound Management   Wound closure is controversial in bite injuries. Many authorities prefer not to attempt primary closure of wounds that are or may become infected, preferring to irrigate these wounds copiously, debride devitalized tissue, remove foreign bodies, and approximate the wound edges. Delayed primary closure may be undertaken after the risk of infection is over. Small uninfected wounds may be allowed to close by secondary intention. Puncture wounds due to cat bites should be left unsutured because of the high rate at which they become infected. Facial wounds are usually sutured after thorough cleaning and irrigation because of the importance of a good cosmetic result in this area and because anatomic factors such as an excellent blood supply and the absence of dependent edema lessen the risk of infection.

Antibiotic Therapy • *Established infection*   Antibiotics should be administered in all established bite-wound infections and should be chosen in light of the most likely potential pathogens, as indicated by the biting species and by Gram's stain and culture results (Table 127-1). For dog and cat bites, antibiotics should be effective against *S. aureus*, *Pasteurella* spp., *C. canimorsus*, streptococci, and oral anaerobes. For human bites, agents with activity against *S. aureus*, *H. influenzae*, and β-lactamase-positive oral anaerobes should be used. The combination of an extended-spectrum penicillin with a β-lactamase inhibitor (amoxicillin/clavulanic acid, ticarcillin/clavulanic acid, ampicillin/sulbactam) appears to offer the most reliable coverage for these pathogens. Second-generation cephalosporins (cefuroxime, cefoxitin) also offer substantial coverage. The choice of antibiotics in penicillin-allergic patients (particularly those in whom immediate-type hypersensitivity makes the use of cephalosporins hazardous) is more difficult and is based primarily on in vitro sensitivity since data on clinical efficacy are inadequate. The combination of an antibiotic active against gram-positive cocci and anaerobes (such as clindamycin) with trimethoprim-sulfamethoxazole or a fluoroquinolone, which is active against many of the other potential pathogens, would appear reasonable. In vitro data suggest that either trovafloxacin or azithromycin alone provides coverage against most commonly isolated bite-wound pathogens.

Antibiotics are normally given for 10 to 14 days, but the response to therapy must be carefully monitored. Failure to respond should prompt a consideration of diagnostic alternatives and surgical evaluation for possible drainage or debridement. Complications such as osteomyelitis or septic arthritis mandate a longer duration of therapy.

Management of *C. canimorsus* sepsis requires a 2-week course of intravenous penicillin G (2 million units intravenously every 4 h) and supportive measures. Alternative agents for the treatment of *C. canimorsus* infection include cephalosporins and fluoroquinolones. Serious infection with *P. multocida* (e.g., pneumonia, sepsis, or meningitis) should also be treated with intravenous penicillin G. Alternative agents include second- or third-generation cephalosporins or ciprofloxacin.

Bites by venomous snakes may not require antibiotic treatment, but it is often difficult to distinguish signs of infection from tissue damage caused by the envenomation. Thus many authorities continue to recommend treatment directed against the snake's oral flora—i.e., the administration of broadly active agents such as ceftriaxone (1 to 2 g intravenously every 12 to 24 h) or ampicillin/sulbactam (1.5 to 3.0 g intravenously every 6 h).

Seal finger appears to respond to doxycycline (100 mg twice daily for an interval guided by the response to therapy).

Presumptive or prophylactic therapy   The use of antibiotics in patients presenting early after bite injury (within 8 h) is controversial. Although symptomatic infection will not yet be manifest in many of these wounds at this point, many early wounds will harbor pathogens, and many will become infected. Studies of the use of prophylactic antibiotics in wound infections are limited and have often included small numbers of cases in which various types of wounds have been managed according to various protocols. A recent meta-analysis of eight randomized trials of prophylactic antibiotics in patients with dog-bite wounds demonstrated a reduction of the rate of infection by approximately 50% with prophylaxis. However, in the absence of sound

Table 127-1 Management of Wound Infections Following Animal Bites

Biting Species	Commonly Isolated Pathogens	Preferred Antibiotic(s)[a]	Alternative Agent(s) for Penicillin-Allergic Patients	Recommendation for Prophylaxis in Patients with Recent Uninfected Wounds[b]	Other Considerations
Dog	*Staphylococcus aureus, Streptococcus* spp., *Pasteurella* spp., anaerobes, *Capnocytophaga canimorsus*	Amoxicillin/clavulanic acid (250–500 mg PO tid); or ampicillin/sulbactam (1.5–3.0 g IV q6h)	Clindamycin (150–300 mg PO qid) plus either TMP-SMZ (1 double-strength tablet bid) or ciprofloxacin (500 mg PO bid)	Sometimes[c]	Consider rabies prophylaxis.
Cat	*Pasteurella multocida, S. aureus, Streptococcus* spp., anaerobes	Amoxicillin/clavulanic acid or ampicillin/sulbactam, as for dog bite	Clindamycin plus either TMP-SMZ or a fluoroquinolone	Usually	Consider rabies prophylaxis; carefully evaluate for joint/bone penetration.
Human; occlusional bite	Viridans streptococci, *S. aureus, Haemophilus influenzae*, anaerobes	Amoxicillin/clavulanic acid or ampicillin/sulbactam, as for dog bite	Erythromycin, fluoroquinolone	Always	—
Human; clenched-fist injury	As for occlusional bite plus *Eikenella corrodens*	Ampicillin/sulbactam, as for dog bite, or imipenem	Cefoxitin[d] (1.5 g IV q6h)	Always	Examine for tendon/nerve/joint involvement.
Monkey	As for human bite	As for human bite	As for human bite	Always	For macaque monkeys, consider B virus prophylaxis with acyclovir.
Snake	*Pseudomonas aeruginosa, Proteus* spp., *Bacteroides fragilis, Clostridium* spp.	Ceftriaxone (1–2 g IV q12–24h); or ampicillin/sulbactam, as for dog bite	Clindamycin plus either TMP-SMZ or a fluoroquinolone	Sometimes, especially for venomous snakebite	Use antivenin for venomous snakebite.
Rodent	*Streptobacillus moniliformis, Leptospira* spp., *P. multocida*	Penicillin VK (500 mg PO bid)	Doxycycline (100 mg PO qd)	Sometimes[c]	—

[a] Antibiotic choices should be based on culture data, when available. Duration of therapy must be guided by response, but normally a minimum course of 10 to 14 days is required for established soft tissue infection. Osteomyelitis and septic arthritis require longer treatment. These suggestions for empirical therapy need to be tailored to individual circumstances and local conditions. Intravenous regimens should be used for hospitalized patients. When the patient is to be discharged after initial management, a single intravenous dose of antibiotic may be given and followed by oral therapy.

[b] Prophylactic antibiotics are usually given for 3 to 5 days.

[c] Prophylactic antibiotics are suggested for severe or extensive wounds, facial wounds, or crush injuries; when bone or joint may be involved; or when comorbidity exists (see text).

[d] Cefoxitin may be hazardous to patients with immediate-type hypersensitivity to penicillin.

NOTE: TMP-SMZ, trimethoprim-sulfamethoxazole.

clinical trials, many clinicians base the decision to treat bite wounds with empirical antibiotics on the species of the biting animal; the location, severity, and extent of the bite wound; and the existence of comorbid conditions in the host. All human- and monkey-bite wounds should be treated presumptively because of the high rate of infection. Most cat-bite wounds, particularly those involving the hand, should be treated. Other factors favoring treatment for bite wounds include severe injury, as in crush wounds; potential bone or joint involvement; involvement of the hands or genital region; host immunocompromise, including that due to liver disease or splenectomy; and prior mastectomy on the side of an involved upper extremity. When prophylactic antibiotics are administered, they are usually given for 3 to 5 days.

Rabies and Tetanus Prophylaxis Rabies prophylaxis, consisting of both passive administration of rabies immune globulin (with as much of the dose as possible infiltrated in and around the wound) and active immunization with rabies vaccine, should be given in consultation with local and regional public health authorities for many wild-animal (and some domestic-animal) bites and scratches as well as for certain nonbite exposures (Chap. 197). Rabies is endemic in a variety of animals, including dogs and cats in many areas of the world. Many local health authorities require the reporting of all animal bites. A tetanus booster immunization should be given if the patient has undergone primary immunization but has not received a booster dose in the past 5 years. Patients who have not previously completed primary immunization should be immunized and should also receive tetanus immune globulin. Elevation of the site of injury is an important adjunct to antimicrobial therapy. Immobilization of the infected area, especially the hand, is also beneficial.

BURNS Epidemiology More than 2 million burn injuries are brought to medical attention in the United States each year. While many burn injuries are minor and require little or no intervention, approximately 70,000 persons are hospitalized for these injuries, and 20,000 of this number are burned severely enough to require admission to a specialized burn unit. Scalds, structural fires, and flammable liquids and gases are the major causes of burns, but electrical, chemical, and smoking-related sources are also important. Burns predispose to infection by damaging the protective barrier function of the skin, thus facilitating the entry of pathogenic microorganisms, and by inducing systemic immunosuppression. It is therefore not surprising that infectious complications are the major cause of morbidity and mortality in serious burn injury and that as many as 10,000 patients in the United States die of burn-related infections each year.

Pathophysiology Loss of the cutaneous barrier facilitates entry of the patient's own flora and of organisms from the hospital environment into the burn wound. The wound often contains devitalized or frankly necrotic tissue that quickly becomes contaminated with bacteria. Invasive infection—localized and/or systemic—occurs when bacteria penetrate viable tissue, usually below the eschar. Streptococci and staphylococci were the predominant causes of burn-wound infection in the preantibiotic era and remain important pathogens at present. With the advent of antimicrobial agents, *P. aeruginosa* became a major problem in burn-wound management. As antibiotics more effective against *Pseudomonas* have become available, fungi (particularly *Candida albicans*, *Aspergillus* spp., and the agents of mucormycosis) have emerged as increasingly important pathogens in burn-wound patients. Herpes simplex virus infection has also been found in burn wounds, especially on the face.

The frequency of infection parallels the extent and severity of burn injury. Severe burns cause defects in both cellular and humoral immunity that have a major impact on infection. For example, decreases in the number and activity of circulating helper T cells, increases in suppressor T cells, and diminution in levels of immunoglobulin follow major burns. Neutrophil function has also been shown to be impaired after burns. The increased levels of multiple cytokines detected in burn patients are compatible with the widely held belief that the inflammatory response becomes dysregulated in these individuals. Increased permeability of the gut wall to bacteria and their components, such as endotoxin, also contributes to immune dysregulation and sepsis. Thus, the burn patient is predisposed to infection at remote sites (see below) as well as at the sites of burn injury.

Clinical Manifestations   Since clinical indications of wound infection are difficult to interpret, wounds must be monitored carefully for changes that may reflect infection. A margin of erythema frequently surrounds the sites of burns and by itself is not usually indicative of infection. Signs of infection include the conversion of a partial-thickness to a full-thickness burn, color changes (e.g., the appearance of a dark brown or black discoloration of the wound), the new appearance of erythema or violaceous edema in normal tissue at the wound margins, the sudden separation of the eschar from subcutaneous tissues, and the degeneration of the wound with the appearance of a new eschar. The appearance of a green discoloration of the wound or subcutaneous fat or the development of ecthyma gangrenosum at a remote site points to a diagnosis of invasive *P. aeruginosa* infection. Changes in body temperature, hypotension, tachycardia, altered mentation, neutropenia or neutrophilia, thrombocytopenia, and renal failure may result from invasive burn wounds and sepsis. However, because profound alterations in homeostasis occur as a consequence of burns per se and because inflammation without infection is a normal component of these injuries, the assessment of these changes is complicated. Alterations in body temperature, for example, are attributable to thermoregulatory dysfunction; tachycardia and hyperventilation accompany the metabolic changes induced by extensive burn injury and are not necessarily indicative of bacterial sepsis.

Given the difficulty of evaluating burn wounds solely on the basis of clinical observation and laboratory data, wound biopsies are necessary for definitive diagnosis of infection. The timing of these biopsies can be guided by clinical changes, but in some centers burn wounds are routinely biopsied at regular intervals. The biopsy specimen is examined for histologic evidence of bacterial invasion, and quantitative microbiologic cultures are performed. The presence of $>10^5$ viable bacteria per gram of tissue is highly suggestive of invasive infection and of a dramatically increased risk of sepsis. Histopathologic evidence of invasion of viable tissue by microorganisms is a more definitive indicator of infection. A blood culture positive for the same organism seen in large quantities in biopsied tissue is a reliable indicator of burn sepsis. Surface cultures may provide some indication of the microorganisms present in the hospital environment but are not indicative of the etiology of infection.

In addition to infection of the burn wound itself, a number of other infections due to the immunosuppression caused by extensive burns and the manipulations necessary for clinical care put burn patients at risk. Pneumonia, now the most common infectious complication among hospitalized burn patients, is most often nosocomially acquired via the respiratory route; septic pulmonary emboli may also occur. Suppurative thrombophlebitis may complicate the vascular catheterization necessary for fluid and nutritional support in burns. Endocarditis, urinary tract infection, bacterial chondritis (particularly in patients with burned ears), and intraabdominal infection also complicate serious burn injury.

℞   **TREATMENT**   The ultimate goal of burn-wound management is closure and healing of the wound. Early surgical excision of burned tissue, with extensive debridement of necrotic tissue and grafting of skin or skin substitutes, greatly decreases the mortality associated with severe burns. In addition, the three widely used topical antimicrobial agents—silver sulfadiazine cream, mafenide acetate cream, and silver nitrate—dramatically decrease the bacterial burden of burn wounds and reduce the incidence of burn-wound infection; they are routinely applied to partial- and full-thickness burns. All three agents are broadly active against many bacteria and against some fungi and are useful before bacterial colonization is established. Silver sulfadiazine is often used initially, but its value can be limited by bacterial resistance. Mafenide acetate has broader activity; the cream penetrates eschars and thus can prevent or treat infection beneath the eschars. The foremost disadvantages of this agent are that it can inhibit carbonic anhydrase, resulting in metabolic acidosis, and that it elicits hypersensitivity reactions in up to 7% of patients. This agent is most often used when gram-negative bacteria invade the burn wound and when treatment with silver sulfadiazine fails.

When invasive wound infection is diagnosed, topical therapy should be changed to mafenide acetate. Subeschar clysis (the direct instillation of an antibiotic, often piperacillin, under the eschar into wound tissues) is a useful adjunct to surgical and systemic antimicrobial therapy. Systemic treatment with antibiotics active against the pathogens present in the wound should be instituted. In the absence of culture data, treatment is broad and should cover organisms commonly encountered in the particular burn unit. Usually such coverage is achieved with an antibiotic active against gram-positive pathogens, such as oxacillin (2 g intravenously every 4 h), and with antibiotics active against *P. aeruginosa* and other gram-negative rods, such as mezlocillin (3 g intravenously every 4 h) and gentamicin (5 mg/kg intravenously per day). In the penicillin-allergic patient, vancomycin (1 g intravenously every 12 h) may be substituted for oxacillin (and is efficacious when methicillin-resistant *S. aureus* is present), and ciprofloxacin (400 mg intravenously every 12 h) may be substituted for mezlocillin. Patients with burn wounds frequently have alterations in metabolism and renal clearance mechanisms that mandate the monitoring of serum antibiotic levels; the levels achieved with standard doses are often subtherapeutic.

In general, prophylactic systemic antibiotics have no role in the management of burn wounds (except for minor burns in outpatients) and can in fact lead to colonization with resistant microorganisms. An exception involves cases requiring burn-wound manipulation. Since procedures such as debridement, excision, or grafting frequently result in bacteremia, prophylactic systemic antibiotics are administered at the time of burn-wound manipulation; the particular agents used should be chosen on the basis of data obtained by wound culture or data on the hospital's resident flora. All burn-injury patients should undergo tetanus booster immunization if they have completed primary immunization but have not received a booster dose in the past 5 years. Patients without prior immunization should receive tetanus immune globulin and undergo primary immunization. Infection control measures play a major role in preventing burn-wound infection and limiting the spread of antibiotic-resistant nosocomial pathogens.

BIBLIOGRAPHY

BAKER AS et al: Isolation of *Mycoplasma* species from a patient with seal finger. Clin Infect Dis 27:1168, 1998

CUMMINGS P: Antibiotics to prevent infection in patients with dog bite wounds: A meta-analysis of randomized trials. Ann Emerg Med 23:535, 1994

FLEISHER GR: The management of bite wounds. N Engl J Med 340:138, 1999

GOLDSTEIN EJ: Bite wounds and infection. Clin Infect Dis 14:633, 1992

KULLBERG BJ et al: Purpura fulminans and symmetrical peripheral gangrene caused by *Capnocytophaga canimorsus* (formerly DF-2) septicemia—a complication of dog bite. Medicine (Baltimore) 70:287, 1991

PRUITT BJ et al: The changing epidemiology of infection in burn patients. World J Surg 16:57, 1992

TALAN DA et al: Bacteriological analysis of infected dog and cat bites. N Engl J Med 340:85, 1999

WEBER DJ et al: Infections resulting from animal bites. Infect Dis Clin North Am 5:663, 1991

WEISS HB et al: Incidence of dog bite injuries treated in emergency departments. JAMA 279:51, 1998

YURT R: Burns, in *Mandell, Douglas and Bennett's Principles and Practice of Infectious Diseases*, 4th ed, G Mandell et al (eds). New York, Churchill Livingstone, 1995, pp 2761–2765

INFECTIONS OF THE SKIN, MUSCLE, AND SOFT TISSUES

ANATOMIC RELATIONSHIPS: CLUES TO THE DIAGNOSIS OF SOFT TISSUE INFECTIONS Protection against infection of the epidermis is dependent on the mechanical barrier afforded by the stratum corneum, since the epidermis itself is devoid of blood vessels (Fig. 128-1). Disruption of this layer by burns or bites (Chap. 127), abrasions, foreign bodies, primary dermatologic disorders (e.g., herpes simplex, varicella, and ecthyma gangrenosum), surgery, or vascular or pressure ulcer allows penetration of bacteria to the deeper structures. Similarly, the hair follicle can serve as a portal either for components of the normal flora (e.g., *Staphylococcus*) or for extrinsic bacteria (e.g., *Pseudomonas* in hot-tub folliculitis). Intracellular infection of the squamous epithelium with vesicle formation may arise from cutaneous inoculation, as in infection with herpes simplex virus (HSV) type 1; from the dermal capillary plexus, as in varicella and infections due to other viruses associated with viremia; or from cutaneous nerve roots, as in herpes zoster. Bacteria infecting the epidermis, such as *Streptococcus pyogenes*, may be translocated laterally to deeper structures via lymphatics, an event that results in the rapid superficial spread of erysipelas. Later, engorgement or obstruction of lymphatics causes flaccid edema of the epidermis, another characteristic of erysipelas.

The rich plexus of capillaries beneath the dermal papillae provides nutrition to the stratum germinativum, and physiologic responses of this plexus produce important clinical signs and symptoms. For example, infective vasculitis of the plexus results in petechiae, Osler's nodes, Janeway lesions, and palpable purpura, which are important clues to the existence of endocarditis (Chap. 126). In addition, metastatic infection within this plexus can result in cutaneous manifestations of disseminated fungal infection (Chap. 205), gonococcal infection (Chap. 147), *Salmonella* infection (Chap. 156), *Pseudomonas* infection (i.e., ecthyma gangrenosum; Chap. 155), meningococcemia (Chap. 146), and staphylococcal infection (Chap. 139). The plexus also provides access for bacteria to the circulation, thereby facilitating local spread or bacteremia. The postcapillary venules of this plexus are a major site of polymorphonuclear leukocyte sequestration, diapedesis, and chemotaxis to the site of cutaneous infection.

Exaggeration of these physiologic mechanisms by excessive levels of cytokines or bacterial toxins causes leukostasis, venous occlusion, and pitting edema. Edema with purple bullae, ecchymosis, and cutaneous anesthesia suggests loss of vascular integrity and necessitates exploration of the deeper structures for evidence of necrotizing fasciitis or myonecrosis. An early diagnosis requires a high level of suspicion in instances of unexplained fever and of pain and tenderness in the soft tissue, even in the absence of acute cutaneous inflammation.

INFECTIONS ASSOCIATED WITH VESICLES (Table 128-1) Vesicle formation due to infection is caused by viral proliferation within the epidermis. In varicella and variola, viremia precedes the onset of a diffuse centripetal rash that progresses from macules to vesicles, then to pustules, and finally to scabs over the course of 1 to 2 weeks. Vesicles of varicella have a "dewdrop" appearance and develop in crops randomly about the trunk, extremities, and face over 3 to 4 days. Herpes zoster occurs in a single dermatome; the appearance of vesicles is preceded by pain for several days. Zoster may occur in persons of any age but is most common among immunosuppressed individuals and elderly patients, whereas most cases of varicella occur in young children. Vesicles due to HSV are found on or around the lips (HSV-1) or genitals (HSV-2) but may appear on the head and neck of young wrestlers (herpes gladiatorum) or on the digits of health care workers (herpetic whitlow). Coxsackievirus A16 characteristically causes vesicles on the hands, feet, and mouth of children. Orf is caused by a DNA virus related to smallpox virus and infects the fingers of individuals who work around goats and sheep. Molluscum contagiosum virus induces flaccid vesicles on the skin of healthy and immunocompromised individuals.

Rickettsialpox begins following mite-bite inoculation of *Rickettsia akari* into the skin. A papule with a central vesicle evolves to form a 1- to 2.5-cm painless crusted black eschar with an erythematous halo and proximal adenopathy. While more common in the northeastern United States and the Ukraine in 1940–1950, rickettsialpox has recently been described in Ohio, Arizona, and Utah. Blistering dactylitis is a painful, vesicular, localized *Staphylococcus aureus* or group A streptococcal infection of the pulps of the distal digits of the hands.

INFECTIONS ASSOCIATED WITH BULLAE (Table 128-1) Staphylococcal scalded-skin syndrome (SSSS) in neonates is caused by a toxin (exfoliatin) from phage group II *S. aureus*. SSSS must be distinguished from toxic epidermal necrolysis (TEN), which occurs primarily in adults, is drug-induced, and has a higher mortality. Punch biopsy with frozen section is useful in making this distinction since the cleavage plane is the stratum corneum in SSSS (Fig. 128-1) and the stratum germinativum in TEN. Intravenous γ-globulin is a promising treatment for TEN. Necrotizing fasciitis and gas gangrene also induce bulla formation (see "Necrotizing Fasciitis," below). Halophilic vibrio infection can be as aggressive and fulminant as necrotizing fasciitis; a helpful clue in its diagnosis is a history of exposure to waters of the Gulf of Mexico or the Atlantic seaboard or (in a patient with cirrhosis) the ingestion of raw seafood. The etiologic organism (*Vibrio vulnificus*) is highly susceptible to tetracycline.

INFECTIONS ASSOCIATED WITH CRUSTED LESIONS (Table 128-1) Impetigo contagiosa is caused by *S. pyogenes*, and bullous impetigo is due to *S. aureus*. Both skin lesions may have an early bullous stage but then appear as thick crusts with a golden-brown color. Streptococcal lesions are most common among children 2 to 5 years of age, and epidemics may occur in settings of poor hygiene, particularly among children of lower socioeconomic status in tropical climates. It is important to recognize impetigo contagiosa because of its relationship to poststreptococcal glomerulonephritis. Superficial dermatophyte infection (ringworm) can occur on any skin surface, and skin scrapings with KOH staining are diagnostic. Primary infections with dimorphic fungi such as *Blastomyces dermatitidis* and *Sporothrix schenckii* can initially present as crusted skin lesions resembling ringworm. Disseminated infection with *Coccidioides immitis* can also involve the skin, and biopsy and culture should be performed on crusted lesions in patients from endemic areas.

FIGURE 128-1 Structural components of the skin and soft tissue, superficial infections, and infections of the deeper structures. The rich capillary network beneath the dermal papillae plays a key role in the localization of infection and in the development of the acute inflammatory reaction.

Table 128-1 Skin and Soft Tissue Infections

Lesion, Clinical Syndrome	Infectious Agent	Chapter(s)
Vesicles		
Smallpox	Variola virus	186
Chickenpox	Varicella-zoster virus	183
Shingles (herpes zoster)	Varicella-zoster virus	183
Cold sores, herpetic whitlow, herpes gladiatorum	Herpes simplex virus	182
Hand-foot-and-mouth disease	Coxsackievirus A16	193
Orf	Parapoxvirus	186
Molluscum contagiosum	Pox-like virus	186
Rickettsialpox	*Rickettsia akari*	177
Bullae		
Staphylococcal scalded-skin syndrome	*Staphylococcus aureus*	139
Blistering distal dactylitis	*S. aureus* or *Streptococcus pyogenes*	139, 140
Necrotizing fasciitis	*S. pyogenes, Clostridium* spp., mixed aerobes and anaerobes	167
Gas gangrene	*Clostridium* spp.	145
Halophilic vibrio	*Vibrio vulnificus*	159
Crusted lesions		
Bullous impetigo/ecthyma	*S. aureus*	139
Impetigo contagiosa	*S. pyogenes*	140
Ringworm	Superficial dermatophyte fungi	208
Sporotrichosis	*Sporothrix schenckii*	208
Histoplasmosis	*Histoplasma capsulatum*	201
Coccidioidomycosis	*Coccidioides immitis*	202
Blastomycosis	*Blastomyces dermatitidis*	203
Cutaneous leishmaniasis	*Leishmania* spp.	215
Cutaneous tuberculosis	*Mycobacterium tuberculosis*	169
Nocardiosis	*Nocardia asteroides*	165
Folliculitis		
Furunculosis	*S. aureus*	139
Hot-tub folliculitis	*Pseudomonas aeruginosa*	155
Swimmer's itch	*Schistosoma* spp.	222
Acne vulgaris	*Propionibacterium acnes*	56
Papular and nodular lesions		
Fish-tank or swimming-pool granuloma	*Mycobacterium marinum*	171
Creeping eruption (cutaneous larva migrans)	*Ancylostoma braziliense*	219
Dracunculiasis	*Dracunculus medinensis*	221
Cercarial dermatitis	*Schistosoma mansoni*	222
Verruca vulgaris	Human papillomaviruses 1, 2, 4	188
Condylomata acuminata (anogenital warts)	Human papillomaviruses 6, 11, 16, 18	188
Onchocerciasis nodule	*Onchocerca volvulus*	221
Cutaneous myiasis	*Dermatobia hominis*	398
Verruca peruana	*Bartonella bacilliformis*	163
Cat-scratch disease	*Bartonella henselae*	163
Lepromatous leprosy	*Mycobacterium leprae*	170
Secondary syphilis (papulosquamous, nodular, and condylomata lata lesions)	*Treponema pallidum*	172
Tertiary syphilis (nodular gummatous lesions)	*T. pallidum*	172
Ulcers with or without eschars		
Anthrax	*Bacillus anthracis*	141
Ulceroglandular tularemia	*Francisella tularensis*	161
Bubonic plague	*Yersinia pestis*	162
Buruli ulcer	*Mycobacterium ulcerans*	171
Leprosy	*M. leprae*	170
Cutaneous tuberculosis	*M. tuberculosis*	169
Chancroid	*Haemophilus ducreyi*	149
Primary syphilis	*T. pallidum*	172
Erysipelas	*S. pyogenes*	140
Cellulitis	*Staphylococcus* spp., *Streptococcus* spp., various other bacteria	Various
Necrotizing fasciitis		
Streptococcal gangrene	*S. pyogenes*	140
Fournier's gangrene	Mixed aerobic and anaerobic bacteria	167
Myositis and myonecrosis		
Pyomyositis	*S. aureus*	139
Streptococcal necrotizing myositis	*S. pyogenes*	140
Gas gangrene	*Clostridium* spp.	145
Nonclostridial (crepitant) myositis	Mixed aerobic and anaerobic bacteria	167
Synergistic nonclostridial anaerobic myonecrosis	Mixed aerobic and anaerobic bacteria	167

Crusted nodular lesions caused by *Mycobacterium chelonei* have been described in HIV-seropositive patients. Treatment with clarithromycin looks promising.

FOLLICULITIS (Table 128-1) Hair follicles serve as a portal for a number of bacteria, though *S. aureus* is the most common cause of localized folliculitis. Sebaceous glands empty into hair follicles and ducts and, if blocked, form sebaceous cysts, which may resemble staphylococcal abscesses or may become secondarily infected. Infection of sweat glands (hidradenitis suppurativa) can also mimic infection of hair follicles, particularly in the axillae. Chronic folliculitis is uncommon except in acne vulgaris, where constituents of the normal flora (e.g., *Propionibacterium acnes*) may play a role.

Diffuse folliculitis occurs in two settings. "Hot-tub folliculitis" is caused by *Pseudomonas aeruginosa* in waters that are insufficiently chlorinated and maintained at temperatures between 37 and 40°C. Infection is usually self-limited, though bacteremia and shock have been reported. Swimmer's itch occurs when a skin surface is exposed to water infested with freshwater avian schistosomes. Warm water temperatures and alkaline pH are suitable for mollusks that serve as intermediate hosts between birds and humans. Free-swimming schistosomal cercariae readily penetrate human hair follicles or pores but quickly die and elicit a brisk allergic reaction causing intense itching and erythema.

PAPULAR AND NODULAR LESIONS (Table 128-1) Raised lesions of the skin occur in many different forms. *Mycobacterium marinum* infections of the skin may present as cellulitis or as raised erythematous nodules. Erythematous papules are early manifestations of cat-scratch disease (primary site of inoculation) and bacillary angiomatosis (*Bartonella henselae*). Raised serpiginous or linear eruptions are characteristic of cutaneous larva migrans, which is caused by burrowing larvae of dog or cat hookworms (*Ancylostoma braziliense*) and which humans acquire through contact with soil that has been contaminated with dog or cat feces. Similar burrowing raised lesions are present in dracunculiasis caused by migration of the adult female nematode *Dracunculus medinensis*. Nodules caused by *Onchocerca volvulus* may range from 1 to 10 cm in diameter and occur largely in persons bitten by *Simulium* flies in Africa. The nodules contain the adult worm encased in fibrous tissue. Migration of microfilariae into the eyes may result in blindness. Verruca peruana is caused by *Bartonella* *bacilliformis*, which is transmitted to humans by the sandfly *Phlebotomus*. This condition can take the form of single gigantic lesions (several centimeters in diameter) or multiple small lesions (several millimeters in diameter). Numerous subcutaneous nodules may also be present in cysticercosis caused by larvae of *Taenia solium*. Multiple erythematous papules develop in schistosomiasis; each represents a cercarial invasion site. Skin nodules as well as thickened subcutaneous tissue are prominent features of lepromatous leprosy. Large nodules or gummas are features of tertiary syphilis, whereas flat papulosquamous lesions are characteristic of secondary syphilis. Human papillomavirus may cause singular warts (verruca vulgaris) or multiple warts in the anogenital area (condylomata acuminata).

ULCERS WITH OR WITHOUT ESCHARS (Table 128-1) Cutaneous anthrax begins as a pruritic papule, which develops within days into an ulcer with surrounding vesicles and edema and then into an enlarging ulcer with a black eschar. Cutaneous anthrax may cause chronic nonhealing ulcers with an overlying dirty-gray membrane, though lesions may also mimic psoriasis, eczema, or impetigo. Ulceroglandular tularemia may have associated ulcerated skin lesions with painful regional adenopathy. Although buboes are the major cutaneous manifestation of plague, in 25% of cases ulcers with eschars, papules, or pustules are also present.

Mycobacterium ulcerans typically causes chronic skin ulcers on the extremities of individuals living in the tropics. *Mycobacterium leprae* may be associated with cutaneous ulcerations in patients with lepromatous leprosy related to Lucio's phenomenon or during reversal reactions. *Mycobacterium tuberculosis* may also cause ulcerations, papules, or erythematous macular lesions of the skin in both normal and immunocompromised patients.

Decubitus ulcers are due to tissue hypoxia secondary to pressure-induced vascular insufficiency and may become secondarily infected with components of the skin and gastrointestinal flora, including anaerobes. Ulcerative lesions on the anterior shins may be due to pyoderma gangrenosum, which must be distinguished from similar lesions of infectious etiology by histologic evaluation of biopsy sites. Ulcerated lesions on the genitals may be either painful (chancroid) or painless (primary syphilis).

ERYSIPELAS (Table 128-1) Erysipelas is due to *S. pyogenes* and is characterized by an abrupt onset of fiery-red swelling of the face or extremities. The distinctive features of erysipelas are well-defined indurated margins, particularly along the nasolabial fold; rapid progression; and intense pain. Flaccid bullae may develop during the second or third day of illness, but extension to deeper soft tissues is rare. Treatment with penicillin is effective; swelling may progress despite appropriate treatment, though fever, pain, and the intense red color diminish. Desquamation of the involved skin occurs 5 to 10 days into the illness. Infants and elderly adults are most commonly afflicted, and the severity of systemic toxicity varies.

CELLULITIS (Table 128-1) Cellulitis is an acute inflammatory condition of the skin that is characterized by localized pain, erythema, swelling, and heat. Cellulitis may be caused by indigenous flora colonizing the skin and appendages (e.g., *S. aureus* and *S. pyogenes*) or by a wide variety of exogenous bacteria. Because the exogenous bacteria involved in cellulitis occupy unique niches in nature, a thorough history including epidemiologic data provides important clues to etiology. When there is drainage, an open wound, or an obvious portal of entry, Gram's stain and culture provide a definitive diagnosis. In the absence of these findings, the bacterial etiology of cellulitis is difficult to establish, and in some cases staphylococcal and streptococcal cellulitis may have similar features. Even with needle aspiration of the leading edge or a punch biopsy of the cellulitis tissue itself, cultures are positive in only 20% of cases. This observation suggests that relatively low numbers of bacteria may cause cellulitis and that the expanding area of erythema within the skin may be a direct effect of extracellular toxins or of the soluble mediators of inflammation elicited by the host.

Bacteria may gain access to the epidermis through cracks in the skin, abrasions, cuts, burns, insect bites, surgical incisions, and intra-venous catheters. Cellulitis caused by *S. aureus* spreads from a central localized infection, such as an abscess, folliculitis, or an infected foreign body (e.g., a splinter, a prosthetic device, or an intravenous catheter). In contrast, cellulitis due to *Staphylococcus pyogenes* is a more rapidly spreading, diffuse process frequently associated with lymphangitis and fever. Recurrent streptococcal cellulitis of the lower extremities may be caused by organisms of group A, C, or G in association with chronic venous stasis or with saphenous venectomy for coronary artery bypass surgery. Streptococci also cause recurrent cellulitis among patients with chronic lymphedema resulting from elephantiasis, lymph node dissection, or Milroy's disease. Recurrent staphylococcal cutaneous infections are more common among individuals who have eosinophilia and elevated serum levels of IgE (Job's syndrome) and among nasal carriers of staphylococci. Cellulitis caused by *S. agalactiae* (group B streptococci) occurs primarily in elderly patients and those with diabetes mellitus or peripheral vascular disease. *Haemophilus influenzae* typically causes periorbital cellulitis in children in association with sinusitis, otitis media, or epiglottitis. It is unclear whether this form of cellulitis will (like meningitis) become less common as a result of the impressive efficacy of the *H. influenzae* type b vaccine.

Many other bacteria also cause cellulitis. Fortunately, these organisms occur in such characteristic settings that a good history provides useful clues to the diagnosis. Cellulitis associated with cat bites and, to a lesser degree, with dog bites is commonly caused by *Pasteurella multocida*, though in the latter case *Staphylococcus intermedius* and *Capnocytophaga canimorsus* (formerly DF-2) must also be considered. Sites of cellulitis and abscesses associated with dog bites and human bites also contain a variety of anaerobic organisms, including *Fusobacterium*, *Bacteroides*, aerobic and anaerobic streptococci, and *Eikenella corrodens*. *Pasteurella* is notoriously resistant to dicloxacillin and nafcillin but is sensitive to all other β-lactam antimicrobials as well as to quinolones, tetracycline, and erythromycin. Ampicillin/clavulanate, ampicillin/sulbactam, and cefoxitin are good choices for the treatment of animal or human bite infections. *Aeromonas hydrophila* causes aggressive cellulitis in tissues surrounding lacerations sustained in fresh water (lakes, rivers, and streams). This organism remains sensitive to aminoglycosides, fluoroquinolones, chloramphenicol, trimethoprim-sulfamethoxazole, and third-generation cephalosporins; it is resistant to ampicillin, however.

P. aeruginosa causes three types of soft tissue infection: ecthyma gangrenosum in neutropenic patients, hot-tub folliculitis, and cellulitis following penetrating injury. Most commonly, *P. aeruginosa* is introduced into the deep tissues when a person steps on a nail. Treatment includes surgical inspection and drainage, particularly if the injury also involves bone or joint capsule. Choices for empirical treatment while antimicrobial susceptibility data are awaited include an aminoglycoside, a third-generation cephalosporin (ceftazidime, cefoperazone, or cefotaxime), a semisynthetic penicillin (ticarcillin, mezlocillin, or piperacillin), or a fluoroquinolone (though drugs of the last class are not indicated for the treatment of children <13 years old).

Gram-negative bacillary cellulitis, including that due to *P. aeruginosa*, is most common among hospitalized, immunocompromised hosts. Cultures and sensitivity tests are critically important in this setting because of multidrug resistance (Chap. 155).

The gram-positive aerobic rod *Erysipelothrix rhusiopathiae* is most often associated with fish and domestic swine and causes cellulitis primarily in bone renderers and fishmongers. *E. rhusiopathiae* remains susceptible to most β-lactam antibiotics (including penicillin), erythromycin, clindamycin, tetracycline, and cephalosporins but is resistant to sulfonamides, chloramphenicol, and vancomycin. Its resistance to vancomycin, which is unusual among gram-positive bacteria, is of potential clinical significance since this agent is sometimes used in empirical therapy for skin infection. Fish food containing the water flea *Daphnia* is sometimes contaminated with *M. marinum*, which can cause cellulitis or granulomas on skin surfaces exposed to the water in aquariums or injured in swimming pools. Rifampin plus ethambutol has been an effective therapeutic combination in some cases, though no comprehensive studies have been undertaken. In addition, some strains of *M. marinum* are susceptible to tetracycline or to trimethoprim-sulfamethoxazole.

NECROTIZING FASCIITIS (Table 128-1) Necrotizing fasciitis, formerly called streptococcal gangrene, may be associated with group A *Streptococcus* or mixed aerobic-anaerobic bacteria or may occur as part of gas gangrene caused by *Clostridium perfringens*. Early diagnosis may be difficult when pain or unexplained fever is the only presenting manifestation. Swelling then develops and is followed by brawny edema and tenderness. With progression, dark red induration of the epidermis appears along with bullae filled with blue or purple fluid. Later the skin becomes friable and takes on a bluish, maroon, or black color. By this stage, thrombosis of blood vessels in the dermal papillae (Fig. 128-1) is extensive. Extension of infection to the level of the deep fascia causes this tissue to take on a brownish-gray appearance. Rapid spread occurs along fascial planes, through venous channels and lymphatics. Patients in the later stages are toxic and frequently manifest shock and multiorgan failure.

Necrotizing fasciitis caused by mixed aerobic-anaerobic bacteria begins with a breach in the integrity of a mucous membrane barrier, such as the mucosa of the gastrointestinal or genitourinary tract. The portal can be a malignancy, diverticulum, hemorrhoid, anal fissure, or urethral tear. Other predisposing factors include peripheral vascular disease, diabetes mellitus, surgery, and penetrating injury to the abdomen. Leakage into the perineal area results in a syndrome called *Fournier's gangrene*, characterized by massive swelling of the scrotum and penis with extension into the perineum or the abdominal wall and legs.

Necrotizing fasciitis caused by *S. pyogenes* has increased in frequency and severity since 1985. It frequently begins deep at the site of a nonpenetrating minor trauma such as a bruise or a muscle strain. Seeding of the site via transient bacteremia is likely, though most patients deny antecedent streptococcal infection. Alternatively, *S. pyogenes* may reach the deep fascia from a site of cutaneous infection or penetrating trauma. Toxicity is severe, and renal impairment may precede the development of shock. In 20 to 40% of cases, myositis occurs concomitantly, and, as in gas gangrene (see below), serum creatinine phosphokinase values may be markedly elevated. Necrotizing fasciitis due to mixed aerobic-anaerobic bacteria may be associated with gas in the deep tissue, but gas is not usually present when the cause is *S. pyogenes*. Prompt surgical exploration down to the deep fascia and muscle is essential. Necrotic tissue must be surgically removed, and Gram's staining and culture of excised tissue are useful in establishing whether group A streptococci, mixed aerobic-anaerobic bacteria, or *Clostridium* spp. are present (see "Treatment" below).

MYOSITIS/MYONECROSIS (Table 128-1) Muscle involvement can occur with virus infection (e.g., influenza virus, dengue virus, or coxsackievirus B) or parasitic invasion (e.g., trichinosis, cysticercosis, or toxoplasmosis). Although myalgia can occur in most of these infections, severe muscle pain is the hallmark of pleurodynia (cox-

Table 128-2 Treatment of Common Infections of the Skin

Diagnosis/Condition	Primary Treatment	Alternative Treatment	See Also Chap(s).
Animal bite (prophylaxis or early infection)[a]	Amoxicillin/clavulanate, 875/125 mg PO bid	Doxycycline, 100 mg PO bid	127
Animal bite[a] (established infection)	Ampicillin/sulbactam, 1.5 g IV q6h	Clindamycin, 600–900 mg IV q8h, *plus* Ciprofloxacin, 400 mg IV q12H *or* Cefoxitin, 2 g IV q6h	127
Bacillary angiomatosis	Erythromycin, 500 mg PO qid	Doxycycline, 100 mg PO bid	163
Herpes simplex (primary genital)	Acyclovir, 400 mg PO tid for 10 days	Famciclovir, 250 mg PO tid for 5–10 days *or* Valacyclovir, 1000 mg PO bid for 10 days	182
Herpes zoster (immunocompetent host >50 years of age)	Acyclovir, 800 mg PO 5 times daily for 7–10 days	Famciclovir, 500 mg PO tid for 7–10 days *or* Valacyclovir, 1000 mg PO tid for 7 days	183
Cellulitis (staphylococcal or streptococcal[b,c])	Nafcillin or oxacillin, 2 g IV q4–6h	Cefazolin, 1–2 g q8h, *plus* Ampicillin/sulbactam, 1.5–3.0 g IV q6h *or* Erythromycin, 0.5–1.0 g IV q6h *or* Clindamycin, 600–900 mg IV q8h	139, 140
Necrotizing fasciitis (group A streptococcal[b])	Clindamycin, 600–900 mg IV q6–8h, *plus* Penicillin G, 4 million units IV q4h	Clindamycin, 600–900 mg IV q6–8h, *plus* Cephalosporin (first- or second-generation)	140
Necrotizing fasciitis (mixed aerobes and anaerobes)	Ampicillin, 2 g IV q4h, *plus* Clindamycin, 600–900 mg IV q6–8h, *plus* Ciprofloxacin, 400 mg IV q6–8h	Vancomycin, 1 g IV q6h, *plus* Metronidazole, 500 mg IV q6h, *plus* Ciprofloxacin, 400 mg IV q6–8h	167
Gas gangrene	Clindamycin, 600–900 mg IV q6–8h, *plus* Penicillin G, 4 million units IV q4–6h	Clindamycin, 600–900 mg IV q6–8h, *plus* Cefoxitin, 2 g IV q6h	145

[a] *Pasteurella multocida*, a species commonly associated with both dog and cat bites, is resistant to cephalexin, dicloxacillin, clindamycin, and erythromycin. *Eikenella corrodens*, a bacterium commonly associated with human bites, is resistant to clindamycin, penicillinase-resistant penicillins, and metronidazole but is sensitive to trimethoprim-sulfamethoxazole and fluoroquinolones.
[b] The frequency of erythromycin resistance in group A *Streptococcus* is currently about 5% in the United States but has reached 70 to 100% in some other countries. Most, but not all, erythromycin-resistant group A streptococci are susceptible to clindamycin. Approximately 90 to 95% of *Staphylococcus aureus* strains are sensitive to clindamycin.
[c] Severe hospital-acquired *S. aureus* infections or community-acquired *S. aureus* infections that are not responding to the β-lactam antibiotics recommended in this table may be caused by methicillin-resistant strains, requiring a switch to vancomycin.

sackie virus B), trichinosis, and bacterial infection. Acute rhabdomyolysis predictably occurs with clostridial and streptococcal myositis but may also be associated with influenza virus, echovirus, coxsackievirus, Epstein-Barr virus, and *Legionella* infection.

Pyomyositis is usually due to *S. aureus*, is common in tropical areas, and generally has no known portal of entry. Infection remains localized, and shock does not develop unless organisms produce toxic shock syndrome toxin 1 or certain enterotoxins and the patient lacks antibodies to the toxin produced by the infecting organisms. In contrast, *S. pyogenes* may induce primary myositis referred to as *streptococcal necrotizing myositis*, which is associated with severe systemic toxicity. Myonecrosis occurs concomitantly with necrotizing fasciitis in about 50% of cases. Both are part of the streptococcal toxic shock syndrome.

Gas gangrene usually follows severe penetrating injuries that result in interruption of the blood supply and introduction of soil into wounds. Such cases of traumatic gangrene are usually caused by *C. perfringens*, *C. septicum*, or *C. histolyticum*. Rarely, latent or recurrent gangrene can occur years after penetrating trauma, most likely owing to dormant spores that reside at the site of previous injury. Spontaneous nontraumatic gangrene among patients with neutropenia, gastrointestinal malignancy, diverticulosis, or recent radiation therapy to the abdomen is caused by several clostridial species, although *C. septicum* is most common. The tolerance of this anaerobe to oxygen probably explains why it can initiate infection spontaneously in normal tissue anywhere in the body.

Synergistic nonclostridial anaerobic myonecrosis, also known as necrotizing cutaneous myositis and synergistic necrotizing cellulitis, is a variant of necrotizing fasciitis caused by mixed aerobic and anaerobic bacteria with the exclusion of clostridial organisms (see "Necrotizing Fasciitis," above).

DIAGNOSIS   This chapter has emphasized the physical appearance and location of lesions within the soft tissues as important diagnostic clues. The temporal progression of the lesions as well as the patient's travel history, animal exposure or bite history, age, underlying disease status, and lifestyle are also crucial considerations in the formulation of a narrowed differential diagnosis. However, even the astute clinician may find it challenging to diagnose all infections of the soft tissues by history and inspection alone. Soft tissue radiography, computed tomography, and magnetic resonance imaging may be useful in determining the depth of infection and should be performed in patients with rapidly progressing lesions or in those with evidence of systemic inflammatory response syndrome. These tests are particularly valuable for defining a localized abscess or detecting gas in tissue. Unfortunately, they may reveal only soft tissue swelling and thus are not specific for fulminant infections such as necrotizing fasciitis or myonecrosis caused by group A *Streptococcus*, where gas is not found in lesions.

Aspiration of the leading edge or punch biopsy with frozen section may be helpful if the results are positive, but false-negative results occur in approximately 80% of cases. There is some evidence that aspiration alone may be superior to injection and aspiration using normal saline. Frozen sections are especially useful in distinguishing SSSS from TEN and are quite valuable in cases of necrotizing fasciitis. Open surgical inspection with debridement as indicated is clearly the best way to determine the extent and severity of infection and to obtain material for Gram's staining and culture. Such an aggressive approach is important and may be lifesaving if undertaken early in the course of fulminant infections where there is evidence of systemic toxicity.

℞ **TREATMENT**   A full description of the treatment of all the clinical entities described herein is beyond the scope of this chapter. As a guide to the clinician in selecting appropriate treatment, the antimicrobial agents useful in the most common and the most fulminant cutaneous infections are listed in Table 128-2.

Early and aggressive surgical exploration is essential in patients with suspected necrotizing fasciitis, myositis, or gangrene in order to (1) visualize the deep structures, (2) remove necrotic tissue, (3) reduce compartment pressure, and (4) obtain suitable material for Gram's staining and for aerobic and anaerobic cultures. Appropriate empirical antibiotic treatment for mixed aerobic-anaerobic infections could consist of ampicillin/sulbactam, cefoxitin, or the following combination: (1) clindamycin (600 to 900 mg intravenously every 8 h) or metronidazole (750 mg every 6 h) plus (2) ampicillin or ampicillin/sulbactam (2 to 3 g intravenously every 6 h) plus (3) gentamicin (1.0 to 1.5 mg/kg every 8 h). Group A streptococcal and clostridial infection of the fascia and/or muscle carries a mortality rate of 20 to 50% with penicillin treatment. In experimental models of streptococcal and clostridial necrotizing fasciitis/myositis, clindamycin has exhibited markedly superior efficacy, but no comparative trials have been performed in humans. Hyperbaric oxygen treatment may also be useful in gas gangrene due to clostridial species. Antibiotic treatment should be continued until all signs of systemic toxicity have resolved, all devitalized tissue has been removed, and granulation tissue has developed (Chaps. 140, 145, and 167).

In summary, infections of the skin and soft tissues are diverse in presentation and severity and offer a great challenge to the clinician. This chapter provides an approach to diagnosis and understanding of the pathophysiologic mechanisms involved in these infections. More in-depth information is found in chapters on specific infections.

BIBLIOGRAPHY

BISNO AI, STEVENS DL: Streptococcal infections in skin and soft tissues. N Engl J Med 334:240, 1996

FRANCIS JS, NEFF J: Viral infections of the skin and soft tissues, in *Atlas of Infectious Diseases*, DL Stevens (ed). Philadelphia, Churchill Livingstone, 1994

GARDAM MA et al: Group B streptococcal necrotizing fasciitis and streptococcal toxic shock–like syndrome in adults. Arch Intern Med 158:1704, 1998

GOLDSTEIN EJC: Bite wounds and infection. Clin Infect Dis 14:633, 1992

HOOK EW et al: Microbiologic evaluation of cutaneous cellulitis in adults. Arch Intern Med 146:295, 1986

NORRBY-TEGLUND A, STEVENS DL: Novel therapies in streptococcal toxic shock syndrome: Attenuation of virulence factor expression and modulation of host response. Curr Opin Infect Dis 11:285, 1998

SIMMONS RL, AHRENHOLZ DH: Infections of the skin and soft tissue, in *Surgical Infectious Diseases*, 2d ed, RJ Howard, RL Simmons (eds). Norwalk, CT, Appleton & Lange, 1988, p 377

STEVENS DL: Invasive group A streptococcus infections. Clin Infect Dis 14:2, 1992

———: Necrotizing infections of the skin and soft tissues, in *Atlas of Infectious Diseases*, DL Stevens (ed). Philadelphia, Churchill Livingstone, 1994

———: Streptococcal toxic shock syndrome: Spectrum of disease, pathogenesis and new concepts in treatment. Emerging Infect Dis 1:69, 1995

———: The flesh-eating bacterium: What's next? J Infect Dis 179:S366, 1999

——— et al: Effect of antibiotics on toxin production and viability of *Clostridium perfringens*. Antimicrob Agents Chemother 31:213, 1987

——— et al: Spontaneous, nontraumatic gangrene due to *Clostridium septicum*. Rev Infect Dis 12:286, 1990

——— et al: Penicillin binding protein expression at different growth stages determines penicillin efficacy in vitro and in vivo: An explanation for the inoculum effect. J Infect Dis 167:1401, 1993

TRAYLOR KK, TODD JK: Needle aspirate culture method in soft tissue infections: Injection of saline vs. direct aspiration. Pediatr Infect Dis J 17:840, 1998

WALLACE RJ et al: Clinical trial of clarithromycin for cutaneous (disseminated) infection due to *Mycobacterium chelonae*. Ann Intern Med 119:482, 1993

129   *James H. Maguire*

OSTEOMYELITIS

Osteomyelitis, an infection of bone, is caused most commonly by pyogenic bacteria and mycobacteria. Classification of cases on the basis of the causative agent; the route, duration, and anatomic location of infection; and local and systemic host factors provides a useful framework for evaluating the patient and planning treatment.

PATHOGENESIS AND PATHOLOGY Microorganisms enter bone by the hematogenous route, by direct introduction from a contiguous focus of infection, or by a penetrating wound. Trauma, ischemia, and foreign bodies enhance the susceptibility of bone to microbial invasion by exposing sites to which bacteria can bind. Phagocytes attempt to contain the infections and, in the process, release enzymes that lyse bone. Pus spreads into vascular channels, raising intraosseous pressure and impairing the flow of blood; as the untreated infection becomes chronic, ischemic necrosis of bone results in the separation of large devascularized fragments (*sequestra*). When pus breaks through the cortex, subperiosteal or soft tissue abscesses form, and the elevated periosteum deposits new bone (the *involucrum*) around the sequestrum. Bacteria escape host defenses by adhering tightly to damaged bone, by entering and persisting within osteoblasts, and by coating themselves and underlying surfaces with a protective polysaccharide-rich biofilm.

Microorganisms, infiltrates of neutrophils, and congested or thrombosed blood vessels are the principal histologic findings of acute osteomyelitis. The distinguishing feature of chronic osteomyelitis is necrotic bone, which is characterized by the absence of living osteocytes. Mononuclear cells predominate in chronic infections, and granulation and fibrous tissues replace bone that has been resorbed by osteoclasts. In the chronic stage, organisms may be too few to be seen.

HEMATOGENOUS OSTEOMYELITIS Hematogenous infection accounts for ~20% of cases of osteomyelitis and primarily affects children, in whom the long bones are infected, and older adults and intravenous drug users, in whom the spine is the usual site of infection.

Acute Hematogenous Osteomyelitis Infection usually involves a single bone, most commonly the tibia, femur, or humerus. Bacteria settle in the well-perfused metaphysis, where functioning phagocytes are scarce, a network of venous sinusoids slows the flow of blood, and fenestrations in capillaries allow organisms to escape into the extravascular space. Because vascular anatomy changes with age, hematogenous infection of long bones is uncommon during adulthood and, when it occurs, usually involves the diaphysis.

In children, the source of bacteremia is often inapparent, although there may have been recent blunt trauma to the extremity leading to a small intraosseous hematoma or vascular obstruction. On presentation, the child usually appears acutely ill, with high fever, chills, localized pain and tenderness, and leukocytosis. Cutaneous erythema and swelling indicate extension of pus through the cortex. During infancy and after puberty, infection may spread through the epiphysis into the joint space. In children of other ages (i.e., between infancy and puberty), extension of infection through the cortex results in involvement of joints if the metaphysis is intracapsular. Thus, septic arthritis of the elbow, shoulder, and hip may complicate osteomyelitis of the proximal radius, humerus, and femur, respectively.

Plain radiographs initially show soft tissue swelling, but the first change in bone—a periosteal reaction—is not evident until at least 10 days after the onset of infection. Lytic changes can be detected after 2 to 6 weeks, when 50 to 75% of bone density has been lost. Rarely, a well-circumscribed lytic lesion, or *Brodie's abscess*, is seen in a child who has been in pain for several months but has had no fever.

Chronic Hematogenous Osteomyelitis With prompt treatment, <5% of cases of acute hematogenous osteomyelitis progress to chronic osteomyelitis. On average, 10 days are required for the formation of necrotic bone, but plain radiographs are unable to detect sequestra or sclerotic new bone for many weeks.

A protracted clinical course, long periods of quiescence, and recurrent exacerbations are characteristic of chronic osteomyelitis. Sinus tracts between bone and skin may drain purulent material and occasionally pieces of necrotic bone. An increase in drainage, pain, or the erythrocyte sedimentation rate (ESR) signals an exacerbation. Fever is unusual except when obstruction of a sinus tract leads to soft tissue

infection. Rare late complications include pathologic fractures, squamous cell carcinoma of the sinus tract, and amyloidosis.

Vertebral Osteomyelitis Organisms reach the well-perfused vertebral body of adults via spinal arteries and quickly spread from the end plate into the disk space and then to the adjacent vertebral body. The infection may originate in the urinary tract, and it does so particularly often among elderly men. Other sources of bacteremia include endocarditis, soft tissue infection, and a contaminated intravenous line; these sources are usually obvious. Diabetes mellitus, hemodialysis, and intravenous drug use carry an increased risk of spinal infection. Penetrating injuries and surgical procedures to the spine may cause nonhematogenous vertebral osteomyelitis or infection localized to the disk.

Most patients with vertebral osteomyelitis report neck or back pain; 15% describe atypical pain in the chest, the abdomen, or an extremity that is due to irritation of nerve roots. Symptoms are localized to the lumbar spine more often than to the thoracic spine (>50% vs. 35% of cases) or the cervical spine in pyogenic infections, but the thoracic spine is involved most commonly in tuberculous spondylitis (Pott's disease). Percussion over the involved vertebra elicits tenderness, and physical examination may reveal spasm of the paraspinal muscles and a limitation of motion. More than 50% of patients experience a subacute illness in which a vague, dull pain gradually intensifies over 2 to 3 months; fever is low grade or absent, and the white blood cell count is normal. An acute presentation with high fever and toxicity is less common and suggests ongoing bacteremia.

Usually, by the time the patient seeks medical attention, the ESR is elevated, and plain radiographs show irregular erosions in the end plates of adjacent vertebral bodies and narrowing of the intervening disk space. This radiographic pattern is virtually diagnostic of bacterial infection because tumors and other diseases of the spine rarely cross the disk space. Computed tomography (CT) or magnetic resonance imaging (MRI) may demonstrate epidural, paraspinal, retropharyngeal, mediastinal, retroperitoneal, or psoas abscesses that originate in the spine. An epidural abscess may evolve suddenly or over several weeks; irreversible paralysis may result from failure to recognize the classic clinical presentation of a spinal epidural abscess: spinal pain progressing to radicular pain and weakness.

Microbiology More than 95% of cases of hematogenous osteomyelitis are caused by a single organism. *Staphylococcus aureus* accounts for 50% of isolates. Other common pathogens include group B streptococci and *Escherichia coli* during the newborn period and group A streptococci and *Haemophilus influenzae* in early childhood. Vertebral osteomyelitis is due to *E. coli* and other enteric bacilli in ~25% of cases. *S. aureus*, *Pseudomonas aeruginosa*, and *Serratia* infections are associated with intravenous drug use in some parts of the United States and may involve the sacroiliac, sternoclavicular, or pubic joints as well as the spine. *Salmonella* spp. and *S. aureus* are the major causes of long-bone osteomyelitis complicating sickle cell anemia and other hemoglobinopathies. Tuberculosis and brucellosis affect the spine more often than other bones. Other common sites of tuberculous osteomyelitis include the small bones of the hands and feet, the metaphyses of long bones, the ribs, and the sternum.

Unusual causes of hematogenous osteomyelitis include disseminated histoplasmosis, coccidioidomycosis, and blastomycosis in endemic areas. Immunocompromised persons on rare occasions develop osteomyelitis due to atypical mycobacteria, *Bartonella henselae*, or *Pneumocystis carinii* or to species of *Candida*, *Cryptococcus*, or *Aspergillus*. Syphilis, yaws, varicella, and vaccinia may involve bone. The etiology of chronic relapsing multifocal osteomyelitis, an inflammatory condition of children that is characterized by recurrent episodes of painful lytic lesions in multiple bones, has not yet been identified.

OSTEOMYELITIS SECONDARY TO A CONTIGUOUS FOCUS OF INFECTION   Clinical Features This broad category of osteomyelitis includes infections introduced by penetrating injuries and surgical procedures and by direct extension of infection from adjacent soft tissues. It accounts for the greatest number of cases of osteomyelitis and occurs most commonly in adults.

Frequently, the diagnosis is not made until the infection has already become chronic. The pain, fever, and inflammatory signs due to acute osteomyelitis may be attributed to the original injury or soft tissue infection. An indolent infection may become apparent only weeks or months later, when a sinus tract develops, a surgical wound breaks down, or a fracture fails to heal. It may be impossible to distinguish radiographic abnormalities due to osteomyelitis from those due to the precipitating condition.

A special type of contiguous-focus osteomyelitis occurs in the setting of peripheral vascular disease and nearly always involves the small bones of the feet of adult diabetic patients. Diabetic neuropathy exposes the foot to frequent trauma and pressure sores, and the patient may be unaware of infection as it spreads into bone. Poor tissue perfusion impairs normal inflammatory responses and wound healing and creates a milieu that is conducive to anaerobic infections. It is often during the evaluation of a nonhealing ulcer, a swollen toe, or acute cellulitis that a radiograph provides the first evidence of osteomyelitis. If bone is palpable during examination of the base of an ulcer with a blunt surgical probe, osteomyelitis is likely.

Microbiology   S. aureus is a pathogen in more than half of cases of contiguous-focus osteomyelitis. However, in contrast to hematogenous osteomyelitis, these infections are often polymicrobial and are more likely to involve gram-negative and anaerobic bacteria. Hence a mixture of staphylococci, streptococci, enteric organisms, and anaerobic bacteria may be isolated from a diabetic foot infection or pelvic osteomyelitis underlying a decubitus ulcer. Aerobic and anaerobic bacteria cause osteomyelitis following surgery or soft tissue infection of the oropharynx, paranasal sinuses, gastrointestinal tract, or female genital tract. S. aureus is the principal cause of postoperative infections; coagulase-negative staphylococci are common pathogens after implantation of orthopedic appliances; and these organisms as well as gram-negative enteric bacilli, atypical mycobacteria, and Mycoplasma may cause sternal osteomyelitis after cardiac surgery. Infection with P. aeruginosa is frequently associated with puncture wounds of the foot or with thermal burns, and Pasteurella multocida infection commonly follows cat bites (Chap. 127).

DIAGNOSIS   Early diagnosis of acute osteomyelitis is critical because prompt antibiotic therapy may prevent the necrosis of bone. The evaluation usually begins with plain radiographs because of their ready availability, although they frequently show no abnormalities during early infection. The ESR and C-reactive protein levels are elevated in most cases of active osteomyelitis, including those in which constitutional symptoms and leukocytosis are lacking. These findings are not specific to osteomyelitis, however, and the ESR is occasionally normal in early infections. In 95% of cases, the technetium radionuclide scan using ^{99m}Tc diphosphonate is positive within 24 h of the onset of symptoms. Falsely negative scans usually indicate obstruction of blood flow to the bone. Because the uptake of technetium reflects osteoblastic activity and skeletal vascularity, the bone scan cannot differentiate osteomyelitis from fractures, tumors, infarction, or neuropathic osteopathy. ^{67}Ga citrate– and ^{111}In-labeled leukocyte or immunoglobulin scans, which have greater specificity for inflammation, may help distinguish infectious from noninfectious processes and indicate inflammatory changes within bones that for other reasons are already abnormal on radiography and technetium scanning. Ultrasound can be used to diagnose osteomyelitis by the detection of subperiosteal fluid collections, soft tissue abscesses adjacent to bone, and periosteal thickening and elevation.

MRI is as sensitive as the bone scan for the diagnosis of acute osteomyelitis because it is able to detect changes in the water content of marrow. MRI yields better anatomic resolution of epidural abscesses and other soft tissue processes than CT and is currently the imaging technique of choice for vertebral osteomyelitis (Fig. 129-1).

The role of diagnostic imaging in chronic osteomyelitis is to determine the presence of active infection and delineate the extent of debridement necessary to remove necrotic bone and abnormal soft tissues. Although plain films accurately reflect chronic changes, the

FIGURE 129-1   Osteomyelitis of the lumbar spine demonstrated on a sagittal T1-weighted magnetic resonance image after the administration of intravenous gadolinium. At L2–L3 there is involvement of the adjacent vertebral bodies and intervening disk. An epidural abscess compresses the thecal sac (open arrow), and the inflammatory process extends into the anterior prevertebral space (closed arrows).

CT scan is more sensitive for the detection of sequestra, sinus tracts, and soft tissue abscesses. Both CT and ultrasound are useful for guiding percutaneous aspiration of subperiosteal and soft tissue fluid collections. Sequential technetium and gallium or indium scans may help determine whether infection is active and may distinguish infection from noninflammatory bone changes; these methods do not, however, provide good anatomic detail. MRI provides detailed information about the activity and the anatomic extent of infection but does not always distinguish osteomyelitis from healing fractures and tumors. MRI is particularly useful in distinguishing cellulitis from osteomyelitis in the diabetic foot; however, no imaging modality consistently distinguishes infection from neuropathic osteopathy.

Appropriate samples for microbiologic studies should be obtained in all cases of suspected osteomyelitis before the initiation of antimicrobial therapy. Blood cultures are indicated in acute cases and are positive in more than one-third of cases of hematogenous osteomyelitis in children and in 25% of cases of vertebral osteomyelitis in adults. If the clinical picture demands immediate antibiotic therapy or if blood cultures are negative, samples from needle aspiration of pus in bone or soft tissues or from a bone biopsy should be obtained for culture.

The results of culture of specimens obtained by swabbing of a sinus tract or the base of an ulcer correlate poorly with the organisms infecting the bone. For this reason, in cases of chronic osteomyelitis and contiguous-focus osteomyelitis, samples for aerobic and anaerobic culture should be obtained from several sites by percutaneous needle aspiration, percutaneous biopsy, or intraoperative biopsy at the time of debridement. Isolates of coagulase-negative staphylococci and other organisms of low virulence should not automatically be disregarded as contaminants, especially in the presence of prosthetic materials. Special culture media may be necessary for the isolation of mycobacteria, fungi, and less common pathogens. In some cases, histopathologic examination of biopsy specimens may be the only way to make a diagnosis.

R̲x̲ **TREATMENT** **Antibiotic Therapy** Antibiotics are administered only after appropriate specimens have been obtained for culture. The antibiotics selected should be bactericidal and, at least initially, should be given intravenously. When necessary, empirical therapy is guided by findings on Gram's staining of a specimen from the bone or abscess or is chosen to cover the most likely pathogens. Empirical therapy in most cases should include high doses of an agent active against *S. aureus* (such as oxacillin, nafcillin, a cephalosporin, or vancomycin) and, if gram-negative organisms are likely to be involved, a third-generation cephalosporin, an aminoglycoside, or a fluoroquinolone.

Specific intravenous therapy is based on the in vitro susceptibility of the organism(s) isolated from bone or blood. Penicillin G (3 to 4 million units every 4 h) is the drug of choice for the treatment of infections due to penicillin-sensitive staphylococci and streptococci; nafcillin or oxacillin (2 g every 4 h) is preferred for penicillin-resistant, methicillin-sensitive staphylococci. Cefazolin (1 to 2 g every 8 h) or vancomycin [15 mg/kg (up to 1 g) every 12 h] is an alternative for persons allergic to penicillins. Infections due to methicillin-resistant staphylococci are treated with vancomycin. Regimens for infections due to susceptible gram-negative rods include ampicillin (2 g every 4 h), cefazolin, a second-generation cephalosporin such as cefuroxime (1.5 g every 8 h), or a fluoroquinolone such as ciprofloxacin (400 mg every 12 h) or levofloxacin (500 mg every 24 h). Initial therapy for osteomyelitis due to *P. aeruginosa* or *Enterobacter* spp. should not consist of a β-lactam antibiotic alone because of the potential for these organisms to develop resistance during therapy. Appropriate intravenous therapies for *P. aeruginosa* infections include tobramycin (1.7 mg/kg every 8 h, or 5 to 7 mg/kg every 24 h) and a broad-spectrum β-lactam compound such as ticarcillin (3 g every 4 h), ceftazidime (1 to 2 g every 8 h), or aztreonam (1 to 2 g every 8 h); a fluoroquinolone may be substituted for one of the latter. *Enterobacter* infections can be treated with a fluoroquinolone alone or with combinations of a broad-spectrum β-lactam antibiotic and gentamicin in the same doses as tobramycin. Serum levels of aminoglycosides should be monitored closely to avoid toxicity.

The duration of therapy is typically 4 to 6 weeks; at-home intravenous administration of antibiotics or oral therapy is appropriate for motivated and medically stable patients. Antibiotics that require infrequent dosing, such as ceftriaxone and vancomycin, facilitate home therapy. Children with acute hematogenous osteomyelitis routinely receive oral antibiotics after 5 to 10 days of parenteral therapy if signs of active infection have resolved; such treatment has been as successful as standard parenteral therapy. The doses of oral penicillins or cephalosporins required for the treatment of osteomyelitis are several times higher than the doses of these drugs given for common infections. Adults may not tolerate these high doses as well as children, and, except in the case of the fluoroquinolones, few data support the use of oral antibiotics by adults. For treatment of osteomyelitis due to Enterobacteriaceae, oral administration of an agent such as ciprofloxacin (750 mg every 12 h) or levofloxacin (500 mg every 24 h) has been as successful as intravenous administration of β-lactam antibiotics. Caution should be exercised in the use of fluoroquinolones as the sole agents for treatment of infection due to *S. aureus* or *P. aeruginosa* because resistance may develop during therapy. Addition of rifampin to a quinolone has yielded encouraging results in infections due to *S. aureus*, but further studies are necessary to confirm these findings. Oral administration of clindamycin (300 to 450 mg every 6 h) or metronidazole (500 mg every 8 h) results in high drug levels in serum and can take the place of intravenous regimens for the treatment of *Bacteroides* infections. Oral clindamycin has produced good results in therapy for osteomyelitis due to *S. aureus*, especially in children. There are few data to support the routine use of the serum minimal bactericidal concentration (MBC) other than to document adherence to treatment.

Acute Osteomyelitis Early treatment of acute hematogenous osteomyelitis of childhood with 4 to 6 weeks of an appropriate antibiotic is usually successful; treatment for <3 weeks has resulted in a 10-fold greater rate of failure. Surgical intervention in childhood cases is indicated for intraosseous or subperiosteal abscesses, concomitant septic arthritis, and failure of the acute signs of infection to improve in 24 to 48 h. Acute hematogenous osteomyelitis of bones other than the spine in adults often requires surgical debridement.

Vertebral Osteomyelitis A 4- to 6-week course of treatment with an appropriate antibiotic is usually sufficient to cure vertebral osteomyelitis. Failure of the ESR to drop by two-thirds or more of its pretreatment level is an indication for longer treatment. Surgery is seldom necessary, even in cases of many months' duration, except in instances of spinal instability, new or progressive neurologic deficits, large soft tissue abscesses that cannot be drained percutaneously, or a failure of medical treatment. Patients should maintain bed rest until back pain has declined to the point at which ambulation is possible. Body casts are no longer used. Spontaneous fusion of involved vertebrae occurs in the majority of cases after successful treatment.

Contiguous-Focus Osteomyelitis Even when diagnosed early, contiguous-focus osteomyelitis usually requires surgery in addition to 4 to 6 weeks of appropriate antibiotic therapy because of underlying soft tissue infection or damage to bone from an injury or surgery. A 2-week course of antibiotics following thorough debridement and soft tissue coverage has yielded excellent results in treatment of superficial osteomyelitis involving only the outer cortex of bone.

Chronic Osteomyelitis The risks and benefits of aggressive therapy for chronic osteomyelitis should be weighed before any attempt is made to eradicate the infection. Some patients with extensive disease prefer to live with their infections rather than undergo multiple surgical procedures, take prolonged courses of antimicrobial therapy, and face the risk of loss of an extremity. Such persons often benefit from intermittent courses of oral antibiotics to suppress acute exacerbations.

Once the decision has been made to treat chronic osteomyelitis aggressively, the patient's nutritional and metabolic status should be optimized to expedite healing of soft tissues and bone. Antibiotic administration should be started several days before surgery to reduce inflammation if the etiology of the infection is known preoperatively. If not, antibiotic therapy should be withheld until surgical debridement. An empirical antibiotic regimen is started intraoperatively after culture specimens are obtained. A 4- to 6-week course of appropriate antibiotic therapy is given postoperatively on the basis of the susceptibility pattern of organisms isolated from the bone. The benefit of prolonged oral antibiotic therapy after 4 to 6 weeks of parenteral therapy remains unproven. There is insufficient information to recommend the routine use of hyperbaric oxygen to enhance the killing of microorganisms by phagocytes or of instillation pumps and antibiotic-impregnated methacrylate beads to deliver high levels of antibiotics to the bone.

The success of therapy for chronic osteomyelitis rests largely on the complete surgical removal of necrotic bone and abnormal soft tissues. Modern imaging techniques allow accurate preoperative delineation of tissues to be debrided, but it remains difficult for the surgeon to determine intraoperatively whether all necrotic and infected tissue has been removed. In the past, the inability to repair large defects in bone and soft tissue limited the extent of debridement. Muscle flaps and skin grafts are now used routinely to cover large soft tissue defects and fill dead space, and bone grafts and vascularized bone transfer may restore a seriously compromised bone to a functional state.

In infections of recent fractures, internal fixators are often left in place, and the infection is controlled by limited debridement and suppressive antibiotic therapy. Definitive surgical/antimicrobial therapy is delayed until after bony union of the fracture is achieved. If there is nonunion of the fracture or loosening of the fixator, the appliance should be removed, the bone debrided, and an external fixator or a new internal fixator applied.

Osteomyelitis of the small bones of the feet in persons with vascular disease also requires surgical treatment. The effectiveness of the surgery is limited by the blood supply to the site and the body's ability to heal the wound. Revascularization of the extremity is indicated if the vascular disease involves large arteries. In cases of decreased perfusion due to small-vessel disease, foot-sparing surgery may fail, and the best option is suppressive therapy or amputation. The duration of antibiotic therapy depends on the surgical procedure performed. When the infected bone is removed entirely but residual infection of soft tissues remains, antibiotic therapy should be given for 2 weeks; if amputation eliminates infected bone and soft tissue, standard surgical prophylaxis is given; otherwise, postoperative antibiotics must be given for 4 to 6 weeks.

BIBLIOGRAPHY

LEW DP, WALDVOGEL FA: Osteomyelitis. N Engl J Med 336:999, 1997

——, ——: Use of quinolones in osteomyelitis and infected orthopaedic prosthesis. Drugs 58(Suppl 2):85, 1999

LIPSKY BA: Osteomyelitis of the foot in diabetic patients. Clin Infect Dis 25:1318, 1997

MADER JT et al: Staging and staging application in osteomyelitis. Clin Infect Dis 25:1303, 1997

NORDEN C et al: Infections in Bones and Joints. Boston, Blackwell Scientific, 1994

REZAI AR et al: Contemporary management of spinal osteomyelitis. Neurosurgery 44:1018, 1999

SAMMAK B et al: Osteomyelitis: A review of currently used imaging techniques. Eur Radiol 9:894, 1999

SWIONTKOWSKI MF et al: A comparison of short- and long-term intravenous antibiotic therapy in the postoperative management of adult osteomyelitis. J Bone Joint Surg (Br) 81:1046, 1999

TICE AD: Outpatient parenteral antimicrobial therapy for osteomyelitis. Infect Dis Clin North Am 12:903, 1998

TSUKAYAMA DT: Pathophysiology of posttraumatic osteomyelitis. Clin Orthop 360:22, 1999

130 Dori F. Zaleznik, Dennis L. Kasper

INTRAABDOMINAL INFECTIONS AND ABSCESSES

CAPD continuous ambulatory peritoneal dialysis	SBP spontaneous bacterial peritonitis
CPC capsular polysaccharide complex	TNF-α tumor necrosis factor α
CT computed tomography	VISA vancomycin-intermediate
FUO fever of unknown origin	S. aureus
ICAM-1 intercellular adhesion molecule 1	VRE vancomycin-resistant enterococci
PMNs polymorphonuclear leukocytes	WBCs white blood cells
PS A surface polysaccharide A	

Intraperitoneal infections generally arise because a normal anatomic barrier is disrupted. This disruption may occur when the appendix, a diverticulum, or an ulcer ruptures; when the bowel wall is weakened by ischemia, tumor, or inflammation (e.g., in inflammatory bowel disease); or with adjacent inflammatory processes, such as pancreatitis or pelvic inflammatory disease, in which enzymes (in the former case) or organisms (in the latter) may leak into the peritoneal cavity. Whatever the inciting event, once inflammation develops and organisms usually contained within the bowel or another organ enter the normally sterile peritoneal space, a predictable series of events takes place. Intraabdominal infections occur in two stages: peritonitis and—if it goes untreated—abscess formation. The types of microorganisms predominating in each stage of infection are responsible for the pathogenesis of disease.

PERITONITIS

The peritoneal cavity is large but is divided into compartments. The upper and lower peritoneal cavities are divided by the transverse mesocolon; the greater omentum extends from the transverse mesocolon and from the lower pole of the stomach to line the lower peritoneal cavity. The pancreas, duodenum, and ascending and descending colon are located in the anterior retroperitoneal space; the kidneys, ureters, and adrenals are found in the posterior retroperitoneal space. The other organs, including liver, stomach, gallbladder, spleen, jejunum, ileum, transverse and sigmoid colon, cecum, and appendix, are found within the peritoneal cavity itself. Normally the cavity is lined with a serous membrane that can serve as a conduit for fluids—a property utilized in peritoneal dialysis. A small amount of fluid, sufficient to allow movement of organs, is normally present in the peritoneal space. This fluid is serous, with a protein content (consisting mainly of albumin) of <30 g/L and fewer than 300 white blood cells (WBCs, generally mononuclear cells) per microliter. In the presence of infection, some of these compartments collect fluid or pus more often than others. These compartments include the pelvis (the lowest portion), the subphrenic spaces on the right and left sides, and Morrison's pouch, which is a posterosuperior extension of the subhepatic spaces and is the lowest part of the paravertebral groove when a patient is recumbent. The falciform ligament separating the right and left subphrenic spaces appears to act as a barrier to the spread of infection; consequently, it is unusual to find bilateral subphrenic collections.

SPONTANEOUS BACTERIAL PERITONITIS Peritonitis is either primary (without an apparent source of contamination) or secondary. The types of organisms found and the clinical presentation of these two processes are different. In adults, primary or spontaneous bacterial peritonitis (SBP) occurs most commonly in conjunction with cirrhosis of the liver (frequently the result of alcoholism). It virtually always develops in patients with ascites. Nevertheless, it is not a common event, occurring in ≤10% of cirrhotic patients. The cause of SBP has not been established definitively but is believed to involve hematogenous spread of organisms in a patient in whom a diseased liver and altered portal circulation result in a defect in the usual filtration function. Organisms are able to multiply in ascites, a good medium for growth. The proteins of the complement cascade have been found in peritoneal fluid, with lower levels in cirrhotic patients than in patients with ascites of other etiologies. The opsonic and phagocytic properties of neutrophils are decreased in patients with advanced liver disease.

The presentation of SBP differs from that of secondary peritonitis. The most common manifestation is fever, which is reported in as many as 80% of patients. Ascites is found but virtually always predates infection. Abdominal pain, an acute onset of symptoms, and peritoneal irritation detected during physical examination can be helpful diagnostically, but the absence of any of these findings does not exclude this often-subtle diagnosis. It is vital to sample the peritoneal fluid of any cirrhotic patient with ascites and fever. The finding of >300 polymorphonuclear leukocytes (PMNs) per microliter is diagnostic for SBP, according to Conn. The microbiology of SBP is also distinctive. While enteric gram-negative bacilli such as Escherichia coli are most commonly encountered, gram-positive organisms such as streptococci, enterococci, or even pneumococci are sometimes found. In SBP, a single organism is typically isolated; anaerobes are found less frequently in SBP than in secondary peritonitis, in which a mixed flora including anaerobes is the rule. In fact, if SBP is suspected and multiple organisms including anaerobes are recovered from the peritoneal fluid, the diagnosis must be reconsidered and a source of secondary peritonitis sought.

The diagnosis of SBP is not easy. It depends on the exclusion of a primary intraabdominal source of infection. Contrast-enhanced computed tomography (CT) is very useful in identifying an intraabdominal source for infection. It may be difficult to recover organisms from cultures of peritoneal fluid, presumably because the burden of organisms is low. However, the yield can be improved if 10 mL of peritoneal fluid is placed directly into a blood culture bottle. Bacteremia frequently accompanies SBP; therefore, blood should be cultured simultaneously. No specific radiographic studies are helpful in the diagnosis of SBP. A plain film of the abdomen would be expected to show ascites. Chest and abdominal radiography should be performed in patients with abdominal pain to exclude free air, which signals a perforation.

℞ **TREATMENT** Treatment for SBP is directed at the isolate from blood or peritoneal fluid. Gram's staining of peritoneal fluid often gives negative results in primary peritonitis; therefore, until culture results become available, empirical therapy should cover gram-negative aerobic bacilli and gram-positive cocci. Ampicillin plus gentamicin is a reasonable initial regimen. Third-generation cephalosporins, carbapenems, or broad-spectrum penicillin/β-lactamase inhibitor combinations are also options. Empirical coverage for anaerobes is not necessary. After the infecting organism is identified, therapy should be narrowed to target that specific pathogen. Patients with SBP usually respond within 72 h to appropriate antibiotic therapy.

SECONDARY PERITONITIS Secondary peritonitis develops when bacteria contaminate the peritoneum as a result of spillage from an intraabdominal viscus. The organisms found almost always constitute a mixed flora in which facultative gram-negative bacilli and anaerobes predominate, especially when the contaminating source is colonic. Early in the course of infection, when the host response is directed toward containment of the infection, exudate containing fibrin and PMNs is found. Early death in this setting is attributable to gram-negative bacillary sepsis and to potent endotoxins circulating in the bloodstream (Chap. 124). Gram-negative bacilli, particularly *E. coli*, are common bloodstream isolates, but *Bacteroides fragilis* bacteremia occurs as well. The severity of abdominal pain and the clinical course depend on the inciting process. The species of organisms isolated from the peritoneum also vary with the source of the initial process and the normal flora present at that site. Peritonitis can result primarily from chemical irritation or bacterial contamination. For example, as long as the patient is not achlorhydric, a ruptured gastric ulcer will release low-pH gastric contents that will serve as a chemical irritant. The normal flora of the stomach comprises the same organisms found in the oropharynx (Chap. 167) but in lower numbers. The surfaces of teeth contain $\sim 10^7$ aerobic and 10^7 anaerobic organisms per milliliter of saliva; the normally acidic stomach contains an equal ratio of aerobic and anaerobic species, but in concentrations more in the range of 10^5/mL. After meals, when gastric acidity is highest, this number may fall to 10^3/mL. Thus, the bacterial burden in a ruptured gastric ulcer—or even a duodenal ulcer—is negligible compared with that in a ruptured appendix. The normal flora of the colon below the ligament of Treitz contains $\sim 10^{11}$ anaerobic organisms per gram of feces but only 10^8 aerobes per gram; therefore, anaerobic species account for 99% of the bacteria. Leakage of colonic contents (pH 7 to 8) does not cause significant chemical peritonitis, but infection is intense because of the heavy bacterial load.

Depending on the inciting event, local symptoms may initially be found in secondary peritonitis—for example, epigastric pain from a ruptured gastric ulcer. In appendicitis (Chap. 291), the initial presenting symptoms are often vague, with periumbilical discomfort and nausea followed in a number of hours by pain more localized to the right lower quadrant. Unusual locations of the appendix (including a retrocecal position) can complicate this presentation further. Once infection has spread to the peritoneal cavity, however, pain increases, particularly with infection involving the parietal peritoneum, which is innervated extensively. Patients usually lie motionless, often with knees drawn up to avoid stretching the nerve fibers of the peritoneal cavity.

Coughing and sneezing, which increase pressure within the peritoneal cavity, are associated with sharp pain. There may or may not be pain localized to the infected or diseased organ from which secondary peritonitis has arisen. Patients with secondary peritonitis generally have abnormal findings on abdominal examination, with marked voluntary and involuntary guarding of the anterior abdominal musculature. Later findings include tenderness, especially rebound tenderness. In addition, there may be localized findings in the area of the inciting event. In general, patients are febrile, with marked leukocytosis and a left shift of the WBCs to earlier granulocyte forms.

While recovery of organisms from peritoneal fluid is easier in secondary than in primary peritonitis, a tap of the abdomen is rarely the procedure of choice in secondary peritonitis. An exception is in cases involving trauma, where the possibility of a hemoperitoneum may need to be excluded early.

℞ **TREATMENT** Treatment for secondary peritonitis includes early administration of antibiotics aimed particularly at aerobic gram-negative bacilli and anaerobes (see below) as well as etiologic studies. Secondary peritonitis usually requires both surgical intervention to address the inciting process and antibiotic administration to treat early bacteremia, to decrease the incidence of abscess formation and wound infection, and to prevent more distant spread of infection. In SBP in adults, surgery is rarely indicated. In secondary peritonitis, surgery may be life-saving.

PERITONITIS IN PATIENTS UNDERGOING CAPD A third type of peritonitis arises in patients who are undergoing continuous ambulatory peritoneal dialysis (CAPD). Unlike primary and secondary peritonitis, which are caused by endogenous bacteria, peritonitis in CAPD patients usually involves skin organisms. The pathogenesis of infection is similar to that of intravascular-device infection, in which skin organisms migrate along the catheter, which both serves as an entry point and exerts the effects of a foreign body. Exit-site or tunnel infection may or may not accompany CAPD peritonitis. Like primary peritonitis, CAPD peritonitis is usually caused by a single organism. Peritonitis is, in fact, the most common reason for discontinuation of CAPD. Improvements in equipment design, especially that of the Y-set connector, have resulted in a decrease from one case of peritonitis per 9 months of CAPD to one case per 15 months.

The clinical presentation of CAPD peritonitis resembles that of secondary peritonitis in that diffuse pain and peritoneal signs are common. The dialysate is usually cloudy and contains >100 WBCs per microliter, >50% of which are neutrophils. The most common etiologic organism is coagulase-negative *Staphylococcus*, which accounts for $\sim 30\%$ of cases. *S. aureus* causes $\sim 10\%$ of cases, is more commonly identified among patients who are nasal carriers of the organism, and is the most frequent pathogen in those with an overt exit-site infection. Gram-negative bacilli and fungi such as *Candida* species are also found. Vancomycin-resistant enterococci (VRE) and vancomycin-intermediate *S. aureus* (VISA) have been reported to produce peritonitis in CAPD patients. The finding of more than one organism in dialysate culture should prompt a search for a cause of secondary peritonitis. As with primary peritonitis, culture of dialysate fluid in blood culture bottles improves the yield.

℞ **TREATMENT** Empirical therapy for CAPD peritonitis should be directed at coagulase-negative *Staphylococcus*, *S. aureus*, and gram-negative bacilli until the results of cultures are available. Since the advent of VRE and VISA, recommended treatment has changed from vancomycin and an aminoglycoside to a first-generation cephalosporin such as cefazolin and an aminoglycoside, which can be administered together in the same bag. A loading dose of cefazolin (500 mg/L) is administered intraperitoneally, with a maintenance dose of 125 mg/L in each bag. Ototoxicity is a significant concern in patients receiving aminoglycosides; some data suggest that administration of a single daily dose lessens this risk. Thus, gentamicin is usually administered at a dose of 20 mg/L once a day. If methicillin-resistant *S.*

aureus is a relatively common isolate in a community, vancomycin may still be a reasonable first choice for empirical therapy, especially in a toxic-appearing patient or a patient with an overt exit-site infection. The dose (2 g) is allowed to remain in the peritoneal cavity for 6 h. The clinical response to an empirical treatment regimen should be rapid; if the patient has not responded after 48 h of treatment, catheter removal should be considered.

INTRAPERITONEAL ABSCESSES

Abscess formation is common in untreated peritonitis if overt gram-negative sepsis either does not develop or develops but is not fatal. In experimental models of abscess formation, mixed aerobic and anaerobic organisms have been implanted intraperitoneally. Without therapy directed at anaerobes, animals develop intraabdominal abscesses. As in humans, these experimental abscesses may stud the peritoneal cavity, lie within the omentum or mesentery, or even develop on the surface of or within viscera such as the liver.

PATHOGENESIS AND IMMUNITY There is often disagreement about whether an abscess represents a disease state or a host response. In a sense, it represents both: While an abscess is an infection in which viable infecting organisms and PMNs are contained in a fibrous capsule, it is also a process by which the host confines microbes to a limited space, thereby preventing further spread of infection. Experimental work has helped to define both the host cells and the bacterial virulence factors responsible—most notably, in the case of *B. fragilis*. This organism, although accounting for only 0.5% of the normal colonic flora, is the anaerobe most frequently isolated from intraabdominal infections and is the most common anaerobic bloodstream isolate. On clinical grounds, therefore, *B. fragilis* appears to be uniquely virulent. Moreover, *B. fragilis* causes abscesses in animal models of intraabdominal infection, whereas most other *Bacteroides* species must act synergistically with a facultative organism to induce abscess formation.

Of the several virulence factors identified in *B. fragilis*, one is critical—the capsular polysaccharide complex (CPC) found on the bacterial surface. The CPC comprises several distinct surface polysaccharides. Structural analysis of the polysaccharides in the CPC has shown an unusual motif of oppositely charged sugars. Polysaccharides having these *zwitterionic* characteristics evoke a host response in the peritoneal cavity that localizes bacteria into abscesses. *B. fragilis* and the CPC have been found to adhere to primary mesothelial cells in vitro; this adherence, in turn, stimulates the production of tumor necrosis factor α (TNF-α) and intercellular adhesion molecule 1 (ICAM-1) by peritoneal macrophages. Mice treated with antibodies to TNF-α or ICAM-1 did not develop abscesses in the mouse peritonitis model. Although abscesses characteristically contain PMNs, the process of abscess induction depends on the stimulation of T lymphocytes by these unique polysaccharides. Experimentally, the essential role of T cells in initiating abscess formation has been proven following blockage of the CD28-B7 costimulatory pathway. The alternative pathways of complement and fibrinogen also participate in abscess formation.

While antibodies to the CPC are not critical in immunity to abscesses, they enhance bloodstream clearance of *B. fragilis*. When administered subcutaneously, *B. fragilis* surface polysaccharide A (PS A) has immunomodulatory characteristics and stimulates T cells via an interleukin-2-dependent mechanism to inhibit the host response of abscess formation to intraperitoneal challenge with *B. fragilis*. Treatment of experimental animals with PS A or other zwitterionic molecules reduces abscess development and can be administered after bacterial contamination of the peritoneal cavity.

CLINICAL PRESENTATION Most intraperitoneal abscesses result from fecal spillage from a colonic source, such as an inflamed appendix. Of all intraabdominal abscesses, 74% are intraperitoneal or retroperitoneal and are not visceral. Abscesses can also arise from a number of other processes. They usually form within weeks of the development of peritonitis and may be found in a variety of locations, from omentum to mesentery, pelvis to psoas muscles, and subphrenic

space to a visceral organ such as the liver, where they may develop either on the surface of the organ or within it. Periappendiceal and diverticular abscesses have traditionally been frequent. Diverticular abscesses are least likely to rupture. Infections of the female genital tract and pancreatitis are also among the more common causative events. When abscesses occur in the female genital tract—either as a primary infection (e.g., tuboovarian abscess) or as an infection extending into the pelvic cavity or peritoneum—*B. fragilis* figures prominently among the organisms isolated. *B. fragilis* is not found in large numbers in the normal vaginal flora. It is encountered less commonly in pelvic inflammatory disease and endometritis, for example, without an associated abscess. In pancreatitis with leakage of damaging pancreatic enzymes, inflammation is prominent. Therefore, clinical findings such as fever, leukocytosis, and even abdominal pain do not distinguish pancreatitis itself from complications such as pancreatic pseudocyst, pancreatic abscess (Chap. 304), or intraabdominal collections of pus. Especially in cases of necrotizing pancreatitis, in which the incidence of local pancreatic infection may be as high as 30%, needle aspiration under CT guidance is performed as often as once a week to sample fluid for culture. Many centers prescribe prophylactic antibiotics to prevent infection in patients with necrotizing pancreatitis. Imipenem is the most frequently used drug for this purpose since it achieves high tissue levels in the pancreas, although it is not unique in this regard. If infected fluid is removed during needle aspiration, most experts agree that surgery is superior to percutaneous drainage.

The psoas muscle of the anterior back is another location in which abscesses are encountered. These abscesses may arise from a presumed hematogenous source, by contiguous spread from an intraabdominal or pelvic process, or by contiguous spread from nearby bony structures such as vertebral bodies. Associated osteomyelitis due to spread from bone to muscle or from muscle to bone is common in psoas abscesses. When Pott's disease was common, *Mycobacterium tuberculosis* was a frequent cause of psoas abscess. Currently in the United States, the usual isolates from psoas abscesses are either *S. aureus* or a mixture of enteric organisms including aerobic gram-negative bacilli. *S. aureus* is most likely to be isolated when a psoas abscess arises from hematogenous spread or a contiguous focus of osteomyelitis; a mixed enteric flora is most likely when the abscess has an intraabdominal or pelvic source.

DIAGNOSIS A variety of scanning procedures have considerably facilitated the diagnosis of intraabdominal abscesses. Abdominal CT probably has the highest yield, although ultrasonography is particularly useful for the right upper quadrant, kidneys, and pelvis. Both indium-labeled WBCs and gallium tend to localize in abscesses and may be useful in finding a collection. Since gallium is taken up in the bowel, indium-labeled WBCs may have a slightly greater yield for abscesses near the bowel. Neither indium-labeled WBC nor gallium scans serve as a basis for a definitive diagnosis, however; both need to be followed by other, more specific studies, such as CT, if an area of possible abnormality is identified. Abscesses contiguous with or contained within outpouchings of bowel are particularly difficult to diagnose with scanning procedures. Occasionally, a barium enema may detect a diverticular abscess not diagnosed by other procedures, although barium should not be injected if a free perforation is suspected. If one study is negative, a second study sometimes reveals a collection. On occasion, exploratory laparotomy still must be undertaken if an abscess is strongly suspected on clinical grounds, although this procedure has been less commonly used since the advent of CT.

℞ **TREATMENT** An algorithm for the management of patients with intraabdominal abcesses is presented in Fig. 130-1. The treatment of intraabdominal infections involves the determination of the initial focus of infection, the administration of broad-spectrum antibiotics targeted at organisms involved in the associated infection, and the performance of a drainage procedure if one or more definitive abscesses have formed already. It cannot be overemphasized that an-

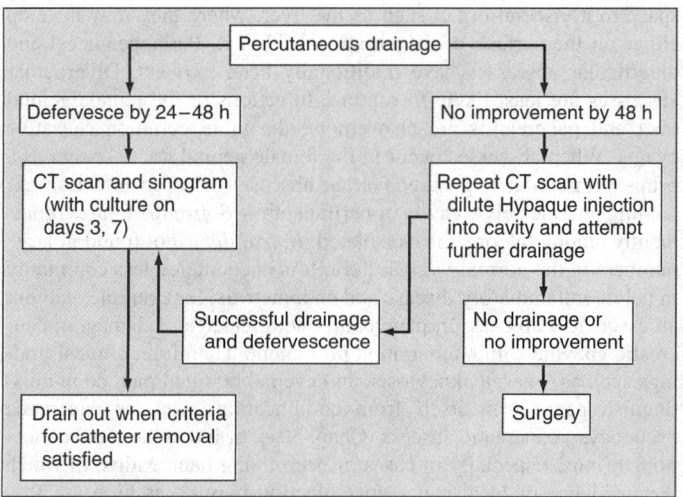

FIGURE 130-1 Algorithm for the management of patients with intraabdominal abscesses using percutaneous drainage. Antimicrobial therapy should be administered concomitantly. CT, computed tomography. *[Reprinted with permission from Lorber B (ed): Atlas of Infectious Diseases, vol VII: Intra-abdominal Infections, Hepatitis, and Gastroenteritis. Philadelphia, Current Medicine, 1995, pp 1–101, as adapted from OD Rotstein, RL Simmons, Intraabdominal abscesses, in SL Gorbach et al (eds): Infectious Diseases, Philadelphia, Saunders, 1992, p. 668.]*

timicrobial therapy, in general, is adjunctive to drainage and/or surgical correction of an underlying lesion or process in intraabdominal abscesses. Unlike the intraabdominal abscesses precipitated by most infections, for which drainage of some kind is generally required, abscesses associated with diverticulitis usually wall off locally after rupture of a diverticulum, so that surgical intervention is not routinely required.

A number of antimicrobial agents exhibit excellent activity against aerobic gram-negative bacilli. Since mortality in intraabdominal sepsis is linked to gram-negative bacteremia, empirical therapy for intraabdominal infection always needs to include adequate coverage of gram-negative aerobic and facultative organisms. Aminoglycosides and second- and third-generation cephalosporins are the agents most widely tested and used in intraabdominal processes. Newer antibiotics, such as aztreonam, imipenem, ticarcillin/clavulanic acid, piperacillin/tazobactam, and quinolones (e.g., ciprofloxacin), cover these organisms as well, although at a higher cost. Second-generation cephalosporins, such as cefoxitin or cefotetan, are not as uniformly active as the other agents against all of the aerobic gram-negative species. Aztreonam, ciprofloxacin, aminoglycosides, and most of the third-generation cephalosporins are not active against anaerobes; for the treatment of intraabdominal infections, these drugs need to be used in combination with another antibiotic. Since a number of antibiotics highly effective against anaerobes are available, third-generation cephalosporins generally should not be considered for use against the anaerobic bacteria involved in intraabdominal sepsis.

The most active and cost-effective antibiotic for anaerobic coverage currently is metronidazole (Chap. 167). Only rare isolates of *B. fragilis* have been reported to be resistant to this drug. In a study of 3177 anaerobic isolates from eight centers in the United States over a 5-year period, no strains resistant to metronidazole were documented among *B. fragilis* isolates, and resistance to imipenem, ampicillin/sulbactam, and piperacillin/tazobactam was exceedingly rare. In contrast, resistance to cefotetan, ceftizoxime, and clindamycin increased during this interval, and resistance to cefoxitin was measurable but unchanged during the study. Despite increasing reports of in vitro resistance of *B. fragilis* to a number of agents, clinical failures are still limited to case reports; therefore, the clinical significance of antimicrobial resistance in anaerobes is uncertain. One report describes a bloodstream isolate of *B. fragilis* with resistance to metronidazole and with reduced susceptibility to imipenem and amoxicillin/clavulanic acid that became resistant to both of the latter two drugs after treatment of the patient with imipenem. Among newer agents, imipenem, ticarcillin/clavulanic acid, piperacillin/tazobactam, meropenem, and ampicillin/sulbactam are highly active against anaerobes. Chloramphenicol, which exhibits strong activity against *B. fragilis* in vitro, nevertheless should probably not be considered a first-line drug for use against anaerobes, since failures of treatment have been documented in both experimental and clinical intraabdominal infections. Neither metronidazole nor clindamycin covers aerobic gram-negative bacilli; thus, these drugs must be combined with other agents for use in this setting. Metronidazole is also less active against gram-positive than against gram-negative anaerobic species.

VISCERAL ABSCESSES Liver Abscesses The liver is the organ most subject to the development of abscesses. Altemeier and associates studied 540 intraabdominal abscesses over a 12-year period. Of these abscesses 26% were visceral. Liver abscesses made up 13% of the total number of abscesses, or 48% of all visceral abscesses. Liver abscesses may be solitary or multiple; they may arise from hematogenous spread of bacteria or from local spread from contiguous sites of infection within the peritoneal cavity. In the past, appendicitis with rupture and subsequent spread of infection was the most common route for the development of a liver abscess. Currently, associated disease of the biliary tract is most often the etiology. Suppurative pylephlebitis (suppurative thrombosis of the portal vein), usually arising from infection in the pelvis but sometimes from infection elsewhere in the peritoneal cavity, is another common source for bacterial seeding of the liver.

Fever is the most common presenting sign of liver abscess. Some patients, particularly those with active associated disease of the biliary tract, have symptoms and signs localized to the right upper quadrant, including pain, guarding, punch tenderness, and even rebound tenderness. Nonspecific symptoms, such as chills, anorexia, weight loss, nausea, and vomiting, may also develop. Only 50% of patients with liver abscesses, however, have hepatomegaly, right-upper-quadrant tenderness, or jaundice; thus, half of patients have no symptoms or signs that would direct attention to the liver. Fever of unknown origin (FUO) may be the only presenting manifestation of liver abscess, especially in the elderly. Diagnostic studies of the abdomen, especially the right upper quadrant, should be a part of any FUO workup. The single most reliable laboratory finding is an elevated serum concentration of alkaline phosphatase, which is documented in 70% of patients with liver abscesses. Other tests of liver function may yield normal results, but 50% of patients have elevated serum levels of bilirubin, and 48% have elevated concentrations of aspartate aminotransferase. Other associated laboratory findings include leukocytosis in 77% of patients, anemia (usually normochromic, normocytic) in 50%, and hypoalbuminemia in 33%. Concomitant bacteremia is found in one-third of patients. A liver abscess is sometimes suggested by chest radiography, especially if a new elevation of the right hemidiaphragm is seen; other suggestive findings include a right basilar infiltrate and a right pleural effusion.

Imaging studies are the most reliable methods for diagnosing liver abscesses. These studies include ultrasonography, CT, indium-labeled WBC or gallium scans, and even magnetic resonance imaging. In an occasional case, more than one such study may be required. Organisms recovered from liver abscesses vary with the etiology. In liver infection arising from the biliary tree, enteric gram-negative aerobic bacilli and enterococci are common isolates. Unless previous surgery has been performed, anaerobes are not generally involved in liver abscesses arising from biliary infections. In contrast, in liver abscesses arising from pelvic and other intraperitoneal sources, a mixed flora including aerobic and anaerobic species (especially *B. fragilis*) is common. With hematogenous spread of infection, usually only a single organism is encountered; this species may be *S. aureus* or a streptococcal species such as *S. milleri*.

Liver abscesses may also be caused by *Candida* species; such abscesses usually follow fungemia in patients receiving chemotherapy for cancer and often present when neutrophils return after a period of neutropenia. Amebic liver abscesses are not an uncommon problem (Chap. 213). Amebic serologic testing gives positive results in >95% of cases; thus, a negative result helps to exclude this diagnosis.

℞ **TREATMENT** While drainage—either percutaneous (with a pigtail catheter kept in place) or surgical—remains the mainstay of therapy for intraabdominal abscesses (including liver abscesses), there is growing interest in medical management alone for pyogenic liver abscesses. The drugs used in empirical broad-spectrum antibiotic therapy include the same ones used in intraabdominal sepsis. Usually, a diagnostic aspirate of abscess contents should be obtained before the initiation of empirical therapy, with antibiotic choices adjusted when the results of Gram's staining and culture become available. Cases treated without definitive drainage generally require longer courses of antibiotic therapy. When percutaneous drainage was compared with open surgical drainage, the average length of hospital stay for the former was almost twice that for the latter, although both the time required for fever to resolve and mortality were the same for the two procedures. Mortality was appreciable despite treatment, averaging 15%. Several factors may predict the failure of percutaneous drainage and therefore may favor primary surgical intervention. These factors include the presence of multiple, sizable abscesses; viscous abscess contents that tend to plug the catheter; associated disease (e.g., disease of the biliary tract) that requires surgery; or the lack of a clinical response to percutaneous drainage in 4 to 7 days.

Treatment of candidal liver abscesses usually entails lengthy administration of amphotericin B, although reports have described successful maintenance therapy with fluconazole after an initial course of amphotericin (Chap. 205).

Splenic Abscesses Splenic abscesses are much less common than liver abscesses. In fact, no splenic abscesses were observed in Altemeier's series of 540 intraabdominal abscesses. The incidence of splenic abscesses has ranged from 0.14 to 0.7% in various autopsy series. The clinical setting and the organisms isolated usually differ from those for liver abscesses. The degree of clinical suspicion for splenic abscess needs to be high, as this condition is frequently fatal if left untreated. Even in the most recently published series, diagnosis was made only at autopsy in 37% of cases. While splenic abscesses may arise occasionally from contiguous spread of infection or from direct trauma to the spleen, hematogenous spread of infection is the usual mode of development. Bacterial endocarditis is the most common associated infection. Splenic abscesses can develop in patients who have received extensive immunosuppressive therapy (particularly those with malignancy involving the spleen) and in patients with hemoglobinopathies or other hematologic disorders (especially sickle cell anemia).

While ~50% of patients with splenic abscesses have abdominal pain, the pain is localized to the left upper quadrant in only half of these cases. Splenomegaly is found in ~50% of cases. Fever and leukocytosis are generally present; the development of fever preceded diagnosis by an average of 20 days in one series. Left-sided chest findings may include abnormalities to auscultation, and chest radiographic findings may include an infiltrate or a left-sided pleural effusion. When splenic abscesses are being considered in a differential diagnosis, CT scan of the abdomen has been the most sensitive diagnostic tool. Ultrasonography can yield the diagnosis, but cases have been missed with this modality. Liver-spleen scan or gallium scan may also be useful. Streptococcal species are the most common bacterial isolates from splenic abscesses, and *S. aureus* is the next most common; presumably these prevalences reflect the bacterial cause of the associated endocarditis. An increase in the frequency of isolation of gram-negative aerobic organisms from splenic abscesses has been reported; these organisms often derive from a urinary tract focus, with associated bacteremia, or from another intraabdominal source. *Sal-*

monella species are seen fairly commonly, especially in patients with sickle cell hemoglobinopathy. Anaerobic species accounted for only 5% of isolates in the largest collected series, but the reporting of a number of "sterile abscesses" may indicate that optimal techniques for the isolation of anaerobes were not employed.

℞ **TREATMENT** Because of the high mortality figures reported for splenic abscesses, the treatment of choice is splenectomy with adjunctive antibiotics. However, percutaneous drainage has been successful. The most important factor in successful treatment of splenic abscesses is early consideration of the diagnosis.

Perinephric and Renal Abscesses Perinephric and renal abscesses are not common: The former accounted for only ~0.02% of hospital admissions and the latter for ~0.2% in Altemeier's series of 540 intraabdominal abscesses. While liver abscesses generally arise from contiguous foci of infection or track from other intraabdominal sources and splenic abscesses usually arise from hematogenous spread (e.g., spread from bacterial endocarditis), perinephric and renal abscesses have a different pathogenesis. Before antibiotics became available, most renal and perinephric abscesses were hematogenous in origin, with *S. aureus* most commonly recovered. Now, in contrast, >75% of perinephric and renal abscesses arise from an initial urinary tract infection. Infection ascends from the bladder to the kidney, with pyelonephritis occurring first. Bacteria may directly invade the renal parenchyma from medulla to cortex. Local vascular channels within the kidney may also facilitate the transport of organisms. Areas of abscess developing within the parenchyma may rupture into the perinephric space. The kidneys and adrenal glands are surrounded by a layer of perirenal fat that, in turn, is surrounded by Gerota's fascia, which extends superiorly to the diaphragm and inferiorly to the pelvic fat. When abscesses extend into the perinephric space, tracking may occur through Gerota's fascia into the psoas or transversalis muscles, into the anterior peritoneal cavity, superiorly to the subdiaphragmatic space, or inferiorly to the pelvis. Of the several risk factors that have been associated with the development of perinephric abscesses, the most important is the presence of concomitant nephrolithiasis producing local obstruction to urinary flow. Of patients with perinephric abscess, 20 to 60% have renal stones. In addition, other structural abnormalities of the urinary tract, a history of urologic surgery, trauma, and diabetes mellitus have all been identified as risk factors.

The organisms most frequently encountered in perinephric and renal abscesses are *E. coli*, *Proteus* species, and *Klebsiella* species. *E. coli*, the aerobic species most commonly found in colonic flora, seems to have unique virulence properties in the urinary tract, including factors promoting adherence to uroepithelial cells. The urease of *Proteus* species splits urea, thereby creating a more alkaline and hospitable environment for bacterial proliferation. *Proteus* species are frequently found in association with large struvite stones caused by the precipitation of magnesium ammonium sulfate in an alkaline environment. These stones serve as a nidus for recurrent urinary tract infection. While a single bacterial species is usually recovered from a perinephric or renal abscess, multiple species may also be found. If a urine culture is not contaminated with periurethral flora and is found to contain more than one organism, a perinephric abscess or renal abscess should be considered in the differential diagnosis. Urine cultures may also be polymicrobial in cases of bladder diverticulum.

Candida species should be considered in the etiology of renal abscesses. This fungus may spread to the kidney via the hematogenous route or by ascension from the bladder. The hallmark of the latter route of infection is ureteral obstruction with large fungal balls.

The presentation of perinephric and renal abscesses is quite nonspecific. Flank pain and abdominal pain are common. At least 50% of patients are febrile. Pain may be referred to the groin or leg, particularly with extension of infection. The diagnosis of perinephric abscess, like that of splenic abscess, is frequently delayed, and mortality in some series is appreciable, although lower than in the past. Perinephric or renal abscess should be most seriously considered when a patient presents with symptoms and signs of pyelonephritis and remains febrile after 4 or 5 days, by which time the fever should have resolved. Moreover, when a urine culture yields a polymicrobial flora, when a patient is known to have renal stone disease, or when fever and pyuria coexist with a sterile urine culture, the diagnosis of perinephric or renal abscess should be entertained.

Renal ultrasonography and abdominal CT are the most useful diagnostic modalities. If a renal abscess or perinephric abscess is diagnosed, nephrolithiasis should be excluded, especially when a high urinary pH suggests the presence of a urea-splitting organism.

℞ **TREATMENT** Treatment for perinephric or renal abscesses, like that for other intraabdominal abscesses, includes drainage of pus and antibiotic therapy directed at the organism(s) recovered. For perinephric abscesses, percutaneous drainage is usually successful.

Pancreatic Abscesses →*See Chap. 304.*

BIBLIOGRAPHY

ALTEMEIER WA et al: Intra-abdominal abscesses. Am J Surg 125:70, 1973

BASSI C et al: Controlled clinical trial of pefloxacin versus imipenem in severe acute pancreatitis. Gastroenterology 115:1513, 1998

CHOU YH et al: Ultrasound-guided interventional procedures in splenic abscesses. Eur J Radiol 28:167, 1998

FINEGOLD SM: Anaerobic bacteria: General concepts, in *Principles and Practice of Infectious Diseases*, 5th ed, GL Mandell et al (eds). New York, Churchill Livingstone, 2000, pp 2519–2537

GIBSON FC III et al: Cellular mechanism of intraabdominal abscess formation by *Bacteroides fragilis*. J Immunol 160:5000, 1998

HUTCHISON FN, KAYSEN GA: Perinephric abscess: The missed diagnosis. Med Clin North Am 72:993, 1988

LEVISON ME, BUSH LM: Peritonitis and other intra-abdominal infections, in *Principles and Practice of Infectious Diseases*, 5th ed, GL Mandell et al (eds). New York, Churchill Livingstone, 2000, pp 821–856

SNYDMAN DR et al: Analysis of trends in antimicrobial resistance patterns among clinical isolates of *Bacteroides fragilis* group species from 1990 to 1994. Clin Infect Dis 23: S54, 1996

SOLOMKIN JS et al: Results of a randomized trial comparing sequential intravenous/oral treatment with ciprofloxacin plus metronidazole to imipenem/cilastatin for intra-abdominal infections. Ann Surg 223:303, 1996

—— et al: Polysaccharide-mediated protection against abscess formation in experimental intra-abdominal sepsis. J Clin Invest 96:2727, 1995

—— et al: T cells activated by zwitterionic molecules prevent abscesses induced by pathogenic bacteria. J Biol Chem 275:6733, 2000

131 *Joan R. Butterton, Stephen B. Calderwood*

ACUTE INFECTIOUS DIARRHEAL DISEASES AND BACTERIAL FOOD POISONING

Ranging from mild annoyances during vacations to devastating dehydrating illnesses that can kill within hours, acute gastrointestinal illnesses rank second only to acute upper respiratory illnesses as the most common diseases worldwide. In children <5 years old, attack rates range from 2 to 3 illnesses per child per year in developed countries to as high as 10 to 18 illnesses per child per year in developing countries. In Asia, Africa, and Latin America, acute diarrheal illnesses are not only a leading cause of morbidity in children—with an estimated 1 billion cases per year—but also the major cause of mortality, being responsible for 4 to 6 million deaths per year, or a sobering total of 12,600 deaths per day. In some areas, more than 50% of childhood

deaths are directly attributable to acute diarrheal illnesses. In addition, by contributing to malnutrition and thereby reducing resistance to other infectious agents, gastrointestinal illnesses may be indirect factors in a far greater burden of disease.

The wide range of clinical manifestations of acute gastrointestinal illnesses is matched by the wide variety of infectious agents involved, including viruses, bacteria, and parasitic pathogens (Table 131-1). This chapter will discuss factors that enable gastrointestinal pathogens to cause disease, will review host defense mechanisms, and will delineate an approach to the evaluation and treatment of patients presenting with acute diarrhea. Individual organisms causing acute gastrointestinal illnesses are discussed in detail in subsequent chapters.

PATHOGENIC MECHANISMS Enteric pathogens have developed a variety of tactics to overcome host defenses. Understanding the virulence factors employed by these organisms is important in the diagnosis and treatment of clinical disease.

Inoculum Size The number of microorganisms that must be ingested to cause disease varies considerably from species to species. For *Shigella*, enterohemorrhagic *Escherichia coli*, *Giardia lamblia*, or *Entamoeba*, as few as 10 to 100 bacteria or cysts can produce infection, while 10^5 to 10^8 *Vibrio cholerae* organisms must be ingested orally to cause disease. The infective dose of *Salmonella* varies widely, depending on the species, host, and food vehicle. The ability of organisms to overcome host defenses has important implications for transmission; *Shigella*, enterohemorrhagic *E. coli*, *Entamoeba*, and *Giardia* can spread by person-to-person contact, whereas under some circumstances *Salmonella* may have to grow in food for several hours before reaching an effective infectious dose.

Adherence Many organisms must adhere to the gastrointestinal mucosa as an initial step in the pathogenic process; thus, organisms that can compete with the normal bowel flora and colonize the mucosa have an important advantage in causing disease. Specific cell-surface proteins involved in attachment of bacteria to intestinal cells are important virulence determinants. *V. cholerae*, for example, adheres to the brush border of small-intestinal enterocytes via specific surface adhesins, including the toxin-coregulated pilus and other accessory colonization factors. Enterotoxigenic *E. coli* produces an adherence protein called *colonization factor antigen* that is necessary for colonization of the upper small intestine by the organism prior to the production of enterotoxin. Enteropathogenic and enterohemorrhagic strains of *E. coli* produce virulence determinants that allow these organisms to attach to and efface the brush border of the intestinal epithelium.

Toxin Production The production of one or more exotoxins is important in the pathogenesis of numerous enteric organisms. Such toxins include *enterotoxins*, which cause watery diarrhea by acting directly on secretory mechanisms in the intestinal mucosa; *cytotoxins*, which cause destruction of mucosal cells and associated inflammatory diarrhea; and *neurotoxins*, which act directly on the central or peripheral nervous system. Some exotoxins act by more than one mechanism; *Shigella dysenteriae* type 1, for example, produces an exotoxin that has both enterotoxic and cytotoxic activities.

The prototypical enterotoxin is cholera toxin, a heterodimeric protein composed of one A and five B subunits. The A subunit contains the enzymatic activity of the toxin, while the B subunit pentamer binds holotoxin to the enterocyte surface receptor, the ganglioside G_{M1}. After the binding of holotoxin, a fragment of the A subunit is translocated across the eukaryotic cell membrane into the cytoplasm, where it catalyzes the ADP-ribosylation of a GTP-binding protein and causes persistent activation of adenylate cyclase. The end result is an increase of cyclic AMP in the intestinal mucosa, which increases Cl^- secretion and decreases Na^+ absorption, leading to loss of fluid and the production of diarrhea.

Enterotoxigenic strains of *E. coli* may produce a protein called *heat-labile enterotoxin* (LT) that is similar to cholera toxin and causes secretory diarrhea by the same mechanism. Alternatively, enterotoxigenic strains of *E. coli* may produce *heat-stable enterotoxin* (ST), one form of which causes diarrhea by activation of guanylate cyclase and elevation of intracellular cyclic GMP. Some enterotoxigenic strains produce both LT and ST.

Bacterial cytotoxins, in contrast, destroy intestinal mucosal cells and produce the syndrome of dysentery, with bloody stools containing inflammatory cells. Enteric pathogens that produce such cytotoxins include *S. dysenteriae* type 1, *Vibrio parahaemolyticus*, and *Clostridium difficile*. Shiga toxin–producing strains of *E. coli*, most commonly serotype O157:H7 in the United States, produce potent cytotoxins that are highly related to the Shiga toxin of *S. dysenteriae* type 1. Such strains of *E. coli* have been associated with outbreaks of hemorrhagic colitis and hemolyticuremic syndrome.

Neurotoxins usually are produced by the responsible organism outside the host and therefore cause symptoms soon after ingestion. Included are the staphylococcal and *Bacillus cereus* toxins, which act on the central nervous system to produce vomiting.

Invasion Dysentery may result not only from the production of cytotoxins but also from bacterial invasion and destruction of intestinal mucosal cells. Infections due to *Shigella* and enteroinvasive *E. coli*, for example, are characterized by the organisms' invasion of mucosal epithelial cells, intraepithelial multiplication, and subsequent spread to adjacent cells. *Salmonella*, on the other hand, causes inflammatory diarrhea by invasion of the bowel mucosa but generally is not associated with the destruction of enterocytes or the full clinical syndrome of dysentery. *Salmonella typhi* and *Yersinia enterocolitica* can penetrate intact intestinal mucosa, multiply intracellularly in Peyer's patches and intestinal lymph nodes, and then disseminate through the bloodstream to cause enteric fever, a syndrome characterized by fever, headache, relative bradycardia, abdominal pain, splenomegaly, and leukopenia.

HOST DEFENSES Given the enormous number of microorganisms ingested with every meal, the normal host must possess effective defense mechanisms to combat a constant influx of potential enteric pathogens. Studies of infections in patients with alterations in these defenses have led to a greater understanding of the variety of ways in which the normal host can protect itself against disease.

Normal Flora The large numbers of bacteria that normally inhabit the intestine act as an important host defense by preventing colonization by potential enteric pathogens. Persons with fewer intestinal bacteria, such as infants who have not yet developed normal enteric colonization or patients receiving antibiotics, are at significantly greater risk of developing infections with enteric pathogens. The composition of the intestinal flora is as important as the number of organisms present. More than 99% of the normal colonic flora is made up of anaerobic bacteria, and the acidic pH and volatile fatty acids produced by these organisms appear to be critical elements in resistance to colonization.

Gastric Acid The acidic pH of the stomach is an important barrier to enteric pathogens, and an increased frequency of infections due to *Salmonella*, *G. lamblia*, and a variety of helminths has been reported among patients who have undergone gastric surgery or are achlorhydric for some other reason. Neutralization of gastric acid with antacids or H_2 blockers—common among hospitalized patients—similarly increases the risk of enteric colonization. Some microorganisms, however, can survive the extreme acidity of the gastric environment; rotavirus, for example, is highly stable to acidity.

Table 131-1   Gastrointestinal Pathogens Causing Acute Diarrhea

Mechanism	Location	Illness	Stool Findings	Examples of Pathogens Involved
Noninflammatory (enterotoxin)	Proximal small bowel	Watery diarrhea	No fecal leukocytes	*Vibrio cholerae*, enterotoxigenic *Escherichia coli* (LT and/or ST), *Clostridium perfringens*, *Bacillus cereus*, *Staphylococcus aureus*, *Aeromonas hydrophila*, *Plesiomonas shigelloides*, rotavirus, Norwalk-like viruses, enteric adenoviruses, *Giardia lamblia*, *Cryptosporidium* spp., *Cyclospora* spp.
Inflammatory (invasion or cytotoxin)	Colon or distal small bowel	Dysentery or inflammatory diarrhea	Fecal polymorphonuclear leukocytes	*Shigella* spp., *Salmonella* spp., *Campylobacter jejuni*, enterohemorrhagic *E. coli*, enteroinvasive *E. coli*, *Yersinia enterocolitica*, *Vibrio parahaemolyticus*, *Clostridium difficile*, ? *A. hydrophila*, ? *P. shigelloides*, *Entamoeba histolytica*
Penetrating	Distal small bowel	Enteric fever	Fecal mononuclear leukocytes	*Salmonella typhi*, *Y. enterocolitica*

SOURCE: After Guerrant.

Intestinal Motility Normal peristalsis is the major mechanism for clearance of bacteria from the proximal small intestine, although gastric acidity and secreted immunoglobulins also play a role in limiting the number of organisms present. When intestinal motility is impaired—for example, by treatment with opiates or other antimotility drugs, anatomic abnormalities (diverticula, fistulas, or afferent-loop stasis following surgery), or hypomotility states (as in diabetes mellitus or scleroderma)—the frequency of bacterial overgrowth and infection of the small bowel with enteric pathogens is much increased. Some patients in whom *Shigella* infection is treated with diphenoxylate hydrochloride with atropine (Lomotil) experience prolonged fever and shedding of organisms, while patients treated with opiates for mild *Salmonella* gastroenteritis have a higher frequency of bacteremia than those not treated with opiates.

Immunity Both cellular immune responses and antibody production play important roles in protecting susceptible hosts from enteric infections. The wide spectrum of viral, bacterial, parasitic, and fungal gastrointestinal infections in patients with AIDS highlights the significance of cell-mediated immunity in protecting the normal host from these pathogens. Humoral immunity is also important and consists of systemic IgG and IgM as well as secretory IgA. Growing evidence supports the concept of a mucosal immune system for secretory IgA in which binding of bacterial antigens to the luminal surface of M cells in the distal small bowel and subsequent presentation of the antigens to subepithelial lymphoid tissue lead to the proliferation of sensitized lymphocytes. These lymphocytes circulate and populate all of the mucosal tissues of the body as IgA-secreting plasma cells.

Approach to the Patient

The approach to the patient with possible infectious diarrhea or bacterial food poisoning is shown in Fig. 131-1.

History The answers to questions with high discriminating value can quickly narrow the range of potential causes of diarrhea and help determine whether treatment is needed. Important elements of the narrative history are detailed in Fig. 131-1.

Physical Examination The examination of patients for signs of dehydration provides essential information about the severity of the diarrheal illness and the need for rapid therapy. Mild dehydration is indicated by thirst, dry mouth, decreased axillary sweat, decreased urine output, and slight weight loss. Signs of moderate dehydration include an orthostatic fall in blood pressure, skin tenting, and sunken eyes (or, in infants, a sunken fontanelle). Signs of severe dehydration range from hypotension and tachycardia to confusion and frank shock.

Diagnostic Approach After the severity of illness is assessed, the most important distinction that the clinician must make is between *inflammatory* and *noninflammatory* disease. Using the history and epidemiologic features of the case as guides in making this distinction, the clinician can rapidly evaluate the need for further efforts to define a specific etiology and for therapeutic intervention. Examination of a stool sample is an important supplement to the narrative history. Grossly bloody or mucoid stool suggests an inflammatory process, but all stools should be examined for fecal leukocytes; the latter task is accomplished by the preparation of a thin smear of the stool on a glass slide, the addition of a drop of methylene blue, and examination of the wet mount. Causes of acute infectious diarrhea, categorized as inflammatory and noninflammatory, are listed in Table 131-1.

EPIDEMIOLOGY **Travel History** Of the 12 to 20 million people who travel from temperate industrialized countries to tropical regions of Asia, Africa, and Central and South America each year, 20 to 50% experience a sudden onset of abdominal cramps, anorexia, and watery diarrhea; thus *traveler's diarrhea* is the most common travel-related illness (Chap. 123). The time of onset is usually 3 days to 2 weeks after the traveler's arrival in a tropical area; most cases begin within the first 3 to 5 days. The illness is generally self-limited, lasting 1 to 5 days. The high rate of diarrhea among travelers to underdeveloped areas is related to the ingestion of contaminated food or water.

The organisms that cause traveler's diarrhea vary considerably with location. In all areas, enterotoxigenic *E. coli* is the most common isolate from persons with the classic secretory traveler's diarrhea syndrome; the proportion of cases accounted for by this organism ranges from a high of approximately 50% in Latin America to a low of 15% in Asia. *Shigella*, *Salmonella*, and *Campylobacter* spp. are classically considered to cause more invasive dysenteric disease than enterotoxigenic *E. coli*, but clinical differentiation of infections attributable to these organisms can be difficult. *Shigella*, *Salmonella*, and *Campylobacter* are isolated in 1 to 15% of cases, with different organisms being more common in different locations. *Vibrio* spp. are most common in Asia, although *V. cholerae* O1 reached epidemic proportions in parts of Central and South America in 1991 and remains a significant source of concern to travelers to these regions. Epidemic *V. cholerae* O139 Bengal has spread throughout India and Southeast Asia since 1992. Less frequently isolated bacteria are *Aeromonas hydrophila* and *Plesiomonas shigelloides*, which are more common among travelers to Thailand. Parasitic causes of traveler's diarrhea include *Entamoeba histolytica*, which is responsible for up to 5% of cases in Mexico and Thailand, and *G. lamblia*, which has been associated with contaminated freshwater supplies in many areas of the world. *Giardia* is found in association with zoonotic reservoirs in the northern United States and poses a risk to hikers and campers who drink from freshwater streams. A striking association of *Giardia* with contaminated water supplies has likewise been noted in Russia. *Cryptosporidium* has been recognized as a problem in travelers to the former Soviet Republics, Mexico, and Africa and has caused large-scale urban outbreaks of infection in the United States. Disease due to *Cyclospora* and microsporidia has recently been recognized. Viruses such as rotavirus and Norwalk-like viruses have been isolated from as many as 10 to 40% of visitors to areas of Latin America, Asia, and Africa who develop traveler's diarrhea.

Location Day-care centers are sites of particularly high attack rates of enteric infections. Rotavirus is most common among children <2 years old, with attack rates of 75 to 100% among those exposed.

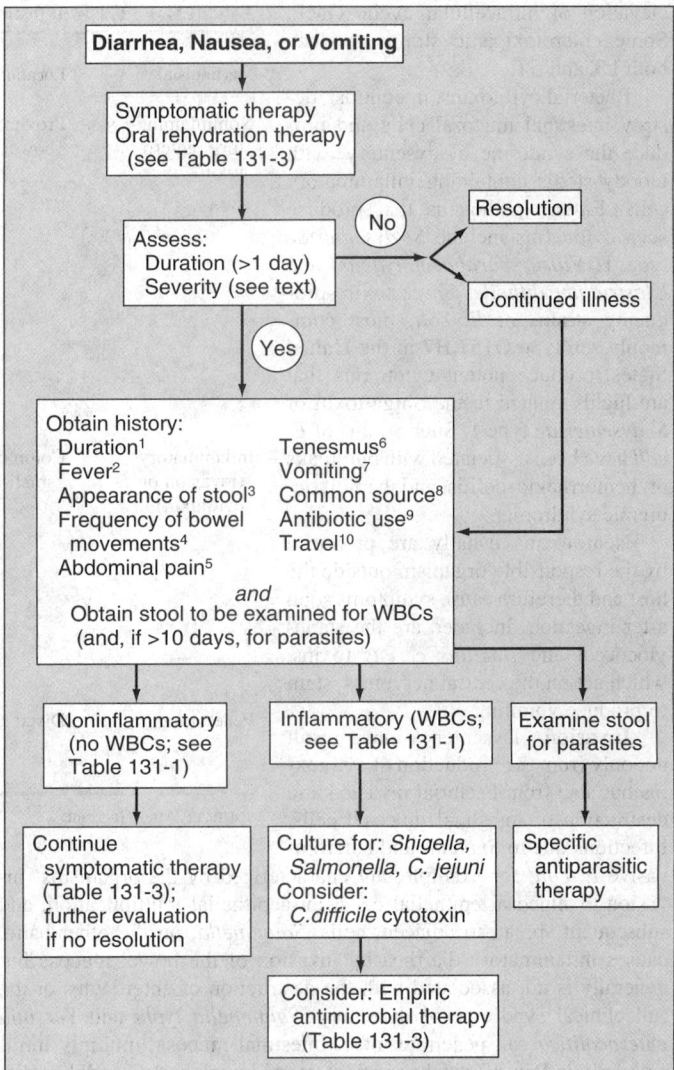

FIGURE 131-1 Clinical algorithm for the approach to patients with community-acquired infectious diarrhea or bacterial food poisoning. Key to superscripts: 1. Diarrhea lasting more than 2 weeks generally is defined as chronic; in such cases, many of the causes of acute diarrhea are much less likely, and a new spectrum of causes needs to be considered. 2. Fever often implies invasive disease, although fever and diarrhea also may result from infection outside the gastrointestinal tract, as in malaria. 3. Stools that contain blood or mucus indicate ulceration of the large bowel. Bloody stools without fecal leukocytes should alert the laboratory to the possibility of infection with Shiga toxin–producing enterohemorrhagic *Escherichia coli*. Bulky white stools suggest a small-intestinal process that is causing malabsorption. Profuse "rice-water" stools suggest cholera or a similar toxigenic process. 4. Frequent stools over a given period can provide the first warning of impending dehydration. 5. Abdominal pain may be most severe in inflammatory processes like those due to *Shigella*, *Campylobacter*, and necrotizing toxins. Painful abdominal muscle cramps, caused by electrolyte loss, can develop in severe cases of cholera. Bloating is common in giardiasis. An appendicitis-like syndrome should prompt a culture for *Yersinia enterocolitica* with cold enrichment. 6. Tenesmus (cramps in the rectum felt after a bowel movement) may be a feature of cases with inflammation of the rectum, as in shigellosis. 7. Vomiting implies an acute infection (e.g., a toxin-mediated illness or food poisoning) but can also be prominent in a variety of systemic illnesses (e.g., malaria) and in intestinal obstruction. 8. Asking patients whether anyone else they know is sick is a more efficient means of identifying a common source than is constructing a list of recently eaten foods. If a common source seems likely, specific foods can be investigated. See text for a discussion of bacterial food poisoning. 9. Stop antibiotic treatment if possible and consider culture for cytotoxigenic *Clostridium difficile*. Antibiotic use may increase the risk of other infections, such as salmonellosis. 10. See text for a discussion of traveler's diarrhea. (*After Guerrant and Guerrant and Bobak.*)

G. lamblia is more common among older children, with somewhat lower attack rates. Other common organisms, often spread by fecal-oral contact, are *Shigella*, *Campylobacter jejuni*, and *Cryptosporidium*. A characteristic feature of infection in day-care centers is the high rate of secondary cases among family members.

Similarly, hospitals are sites for concentrations of enteric infections. In medical intensive-care units and pediatric wards, diarrhea is among the most common nosocomial infections. *C. difficile* is the predominant cause of nosocomial diarrhea among adults in the United States; viral pathogens, especially rotavirus, can spread rapidly in pediatric wards. Enteropathogenic *E. coli* has been associated with outbreaks of diarrhea in nurseries for newborns. One-third of elderly patients in chronic-care institutions develop a significant diarrheal illness each year. Surveillance stool cultures suggest that 25% of the residents of these institutions harbor cytotoxin-producing *C. difficile*, which causes more than half of all cases of diarrhea in this population. Antimicrobial therapy can predispose to pseudomembranous colitis by altering the normal colonic flora and allowing the multiplication of *C. difficile*.

Age Most of the morbidity and mortality from enteric pathogens involves children <5 years of age. Breast-fed infants are protected from contaminated food and water and derive some protection from maternal antibodies, but their risk of infection rises dramatically when they begin to eat solid foods. Infants and younger children are more likely than adults to develop rotaviral disease, while older children and adults are more commonly infected with Norwalk-like viruses. Other organisms with higher attack rates among children than among adults include enterotoxigenic, enteropathogenic, and enterohemorrhagic *E. coli*; *C. jejuni*; and *G. lamblia*. In children, the incidence of *Salmonella* infections is highest among infants <1 year of age, while the attack rate for *Shigella* infections is greatest among children aged 6 months to 4 years.

Bacterial Food Poisoning If the history and the stool examination indicate a noninflammatory etiology of diarrhea and there is evidence of a common-source outbreak, questions concerning the ingestion of specific foods and the time of onset of the diarrhea after a meal can provide clues to the bacterial cause of the illness. Potential causes of bacterial food poisoning are shown in Table 131-2.

Bacterial disease caused by an enterotoxin elaborated outside the host, such as that due to *Staphylococcus aureus* or *B. cereus*, has the shortest incubation period (1 to 6 h) and generally lasts <12 h. Most cases of staphylococcal food poisoning are caused by contamination from infected human carriers. Staphylococci can multiply at a wide range of temperatures; thus, if food is left to cool slowly and remains at room temperature after cooking, the organisms will have the opportunity to form enterotoxin. Outbreaks following picnics where potato salad, mayonnaise, and cream pastries have been served offer classic examples of staphylococcal food poisoning. Diarrhea, nausea, vomiting, and abdominal cramping are common, while fever is less so.

B. cereus can produce either a syndrome with a short incubation period—the *emetic* form, mediated by a staphylococcal type of enterotoxin—or one with a longer incubation period (8 to 16 h)—the *diarrheal* form, caused by an enterotoxin resembling *E. coli* LT, in which diarrhea and abdominal cramps are characteristic but vomiting is uncommon. The emetic form of *B. cereus* food poisoning is associated with contaminated fried rice; the organism is common in uncooked rice, and its heat-resistant spores survive boiling. If cooked rice is not refrigerated, the spores can germinate and produce toxin. Frying before serving may not destroy the preformed, heat-stable toxin.

Food poisoning due to *C. perfringens* also has a slightly longer incubation period (8 to 14 h) and results from the survival of heat-resistant spores in inadequately cooked meat, poultry, or legumes. After ingestion, toxin is produced in the intestinal tract, causing moderately severe abdominal cramps and diarrhea; vomiting is rare, as is fever. The illness is self-limited, rarely lasting for more than 24 h.

Not all food poisoning has a bacterial cause. Diagnostic confusion

Table 131-2 Bacterial Food Poisoning

Incubation Period, Organisms	Symptoms	Common Food Sources
1 TO 6 H		
Staphylococcus aureus	Nausea, vomiting, diarrhea	Ham, poultry, potato or egg salad, mayonnaise, cream pastries
Bacillus cereus	Nausea, vomiting, diarrhea	Fried rice
8 TO 16 H		
Clostridium perfringens	Abdominal cramps, diarrhea (vomiting rare)	Beef, poultry, legumes, gravies
B. cereus	Abdominal cramps, diarrhea (vomiting rare)	Meats, vegetables, dried beans, cereals
>16 H		
Vibrio cholerae	Watery diarrhea	Shellfish
Enterotoxigenic *Escherichia coli*	Watery diarrhea	Salads, cheese, meats, water
Enterohemorrhagic *E. coli*	Bloody diarrhea	Ground beef, roast beef, salami, raw milk, raw vegetables, apple juice
Salmonella spp.	Inflammatory diarrhea	Beef, poultry, eggs, dairy products
Shigella spp.	Dysentery	Potato or egg salad, lettuce, raw vegetables
Vibrio parahaemolyticus	Dysentery	Mollusks, crustaceans

can result from diarrhea caused by nonbacterial agents of short-incubation food poisoning, including capsaicin, which is found in hot peppers, and a variety of toxins found in fish and shellfish (Chap. 397).

LABORATORY EVALUATION Many cases of noninflammatory diarrhea are self-limited or can be treated empirically, and in these instances the clinician may not need to determine a specific etiology. Potentially pathogenic *E. coli* cannot be distinguished from normal fecal flora by routine culture. Special tests to detect LT and ST are not available in most clinical laboratories. In situations in which cholera is a concern, stool should be cultured on thiosulfate-citrate-bile salts-sucrose (TCBS) agar. A latex agglutination test has made the rapid detection of rotavirus in stool practical for many laboratories, while reverse transcriptase polymerase chain reaction and specific antigen enzyme immunoassays have been developed for the identification of Norwalk-like viruses. At least three stool specimens should be examined for *Giardia* cysts or stained for *Cryptosporidium* if the level of clinical suspicion regarding the involvement of these organisms is high.

All patients with fever and evidence of inflammatory disease acquired outside the hospital should have stool cultured for *Salmonella*, *Shigella*, and *Campylobacter*. *Salmonella* and *Shigella* can be selected on MacConkey's agar as non-lactose-fermenting (colorless) colonies or can be grown on *Salmonella-Shigella* agar or in selenite enrichment broth, both of which inhibit most organisms except these pathogens. Evaluation of nosocomial diarrhea should initially focus on *C. difficile*; stool culture for other pathogens in this setting has an extremely low yield and is not cost-effective. Pathogenic strains of *C. difficile* generally produce two toxins, A and B. Toxin B can be detected with a cytotoxin assay; if the toxin is present, a monolayer culture of fibroblasts will show cytopathic effects within 6 to 24 h. Rapid enzyme immunoassays and latex agglutination tests for both toxin A and toxin B have recently been developed (Chap. 145). Isolation of *C. jejuni* requires inoculation of fresh stool onto selective growth medium and incubation at 42°C in a microaerophilic atmosphere. In many laboratories in the United States, *E. coli* O157:H7 is among the most common pathogens isolated from visible bloody stools. Strains of this enterohemorrhagic serotype can be identified in specialized laboratories by serotyping but also can be identified presumptively as lactose-fermenting, indole-positive colonies of sorbitol nonfermenters (white colonies) on sorbitol MacConkey plates. Fresh stools should be examined for amebic cysts and trophozoites.

℞ **TREATMENT**   In many cases, a specific diagnosis is not necessary or not available to guide treatment. The clinician can proceed with the information obtained from the history, stool examination, and evaluation of the severity of dehydration. Empirical regimens for the treatment of traveler's diarrhea are listed in Table 131-3.

The mainstay of treatment is adequate rehydration. The treatment of cholera and other dehydrating diarrheal diseases was revolutionized by the promotion of oral rehydration solutions, the efficacy of which depends on the fact that glucose-facilitated absorption of sodium and water in the small intestine remains intact in the presence of cholera toxin. The use of oral rehydration solutions has reduced mortality due to cholera from >50% (in untreated cases) to <1%. The World Health Organization recommends a solution containing 3.5 g sodium chloride, 2.5 g sodium bicarbonate, 1.5 g potassium chloride, and 20 g glucose (or 40 g sucrose) per liter of water. Patients who are severely dehydrated or in whom vomiting precludes the use of oral therapy should receive intravenous solutions such as Ringer's lactate.

Although most secretory forms of traveler's diarrhea—usually due to enterotoxigenic *E. coli*—can be treated effectively with rehydration, bismuth subsalicylate, or antiperistaltic agents, antimicrobial agents can shorten the duration of illness from between 3 and 4 days to between 24 and 36 h.

PROPHYLAXIS   Improvements in hygiene to limit fecal-oral spread of enteric pathogens will be necessary if the prevalence of diarrheal diseases is to be significantly reduced in developing countries. Travelers can reduce their risk of diarrhea by eating only hot, freshly cooked food; by avoiding raw vegetables, salads, and unpeeled fruit; and by drinking only boiled or treated water and avoiding ice. In one cross-sectional epidemiologic survey, fewer than 3% of all European and North American travelers to Jamaica adhered to prescribed dietary restrictions, and travel health advice had no impact on the incidence of traveler's diarrhea; overall, the diarrhea attack rate among these travelers was 23.6%, with classic traveler's diarrhea in 11.7%.

Bismuth subsalicylate is an inexpensive agent for the prophylaxis of traveler's diarrhea; it is taken at a dosage of 2 tablets (525 mg) four times a day. Treatment appears to be effective and safe for up to 3 weeks. Prophylactic antimicrobial agents, although effective, are not generally recommended for the prevention of traveler's diarrhea, except when travelers are immunosuppressed or have other underlying illnesses that place them at high risk for morbidity from gastrointestinal infection. The risk of side effects and the possibility of developing an infection with a drug-resistant organism or with more harmful, invasive bacteria make it more reasonable to institute a short course of treatment once symptoms have developed.

The possibility of exerting a major impact on the worldwide morbidity and mortality associated with diarrheal diseases has led to intense efforts to develop effective vaccines against the common bacterial and viral enteric pathogens. Recent research has shown promising advances in the development of vaccines against rotavirus, *Shigella*, *V. cholerae*, *S. typhi*, and enterotoxigenic *E. coli*.

Table 131-3   Treatment of Traveler's Diarrhea on the Basis of Clinical Features

Clinical Syndrome	Suggested Therapy
Watery diarrhea (no blood in stool, no fever), 1 or 2 unformed stools per day without distressing enteric symptoms	Oral fluids (Pedialyte, Lytren, or flavored mineral water) and saltine crackers
Watery diarrhea (no blood in stool, no fever), 1 or 2 unformed stools per day with distressing enteric symptoms	Bismuth subsalicylate (for adults): 30 mL or 2 tablets (262 mg/tablet) every 30 min for 8 doses; or loperamide[a]: 4 mg initially followed by 2 mg after passage of each unformed stool, not to exceed 8 tablets (16 mg) per day (prescription dose) or 4 caplets (8 mg) per day (over-the-counter dose); drugs can be taken for 2 days
Watery diarrhea (no blood in stool, no distressing abdominal pain, no fever), >2 unformed stools per day	Antibacterial drug[b] plus (for adults) loperamide[a] (see dose above)
Dysentery (passage of bloody stools) or fever (>37.8°C)	Antibacterial drug[b]
Vomiting, minimal diarrhea	Bismuth subsalicylate (for adults; see dose above)
Diarrhea in infants (<2 y old)	Fluids and electrolytes (Pedialyte, Lytren); continue feeding, especially with breast milk; seek medical attention for moderate dehydration, fever lasting >24 h, bloody stools, or diarrhea lasting more than several days
Diarrhea in pregnant women	Fluids and electrolytes; can consider attapulgite, 3 g initially, with dose repeated after passage of each unformed stool or every 2 h (whichever is earlier), for a total dosage of 9 g/d; seek medical attention for persistent or severe symptoms
Diarrhea despite trimethoprim-sulfamethoxazole prophylaxis	Fluoroquinolone—with loperamide[a] (see dose above) if no fever and no blood in stool, alone in cases of fever/dysentery
Diarrhea despite fluoroquinolone prophylaxis	Bismuth subsalicylate (see dose above) for mild to moderate disease; consult physician for moderate to severe disease or if disease persists

[a] Loperamide should not be used by patients with fever or dysentery; its use may prolong diarrhea in patients with infection due to *Shigella* or other invasive organisms.
[b] The recommended antibacterial drugs are as follows:
  Travel to Mexican interior, summer: *Adults:* Trimethoprim-sulfamethoxazole (TMP-SMZ), 160 mg/800 mg bid for 3 days
   Children: TMP-SMZ, 4/20 mg/kg per day, given bid for 3 days
  Travel to other areas in other seasons: *Adults:* A quinolone, such as norfloxacin, 400 mg bid; ciprofloxacin, 500 mg bid; ofloxacin, 400 mg bid; or levofloxacin, 500 mg/d, for 3 days

Children: TMP-SMZ (above dose) plus erythromycin at dose based on weight (<11 kg, 250 mg/d; 11–18 kg, 375 mg/d; 18.5–25 kg, 500 mg/d; 25.5–36 kg, 750 mg/d; and >36 kg, 1000 mg/d) in four divided doses for 5 days. Alternative single agents: azithromycin, 10 mg/kg per day for 3 days; or furazolidone, 7.5 mg/kg per day in four divided doses for 5 days
All patients should take oral fluids (Pedialyte, Lytren, or flavored mineral water) plus saltine crackers. If diarrhea becomes moderate or severe, if fever persists, or if bloody stools or dehydration develops, the patient should seek medical attention.
SOURCE: After Dupont.

BLASER MJ: Epidemiologic and clinical features of *Campylobacter jejuni* infections. J Infect Dis 176(Suppl 2):S103, 1997

DUPONT HL: Travelers' diarrhea, in *Infections of the Gastrointestinal Tract*, MJ Blaser et al (eds). New York, Raven, 1995, chap 22

GLYNN KM et al: Emergence of multidrug-resistant *Salmonella enterica* serotype typhimurium DT104 infections in the United States. N Engl J Med 338:1333, 1998

GUERRANT RL: Principles and syndromes of enteric infection, in *Mandell, Douglas and Bennett's Principles and Practice of Infectious Diseases*, 4th ed, GL Mandell et al (eds). New York, Churchill Livingstone, 1995, chap 75

————, BOBAK DA: Bacterial and protozoal gastroenteritis. N Engl J Med 325:327, 1991

MEAD PS, GRIFFIN PM: *Escherichia coli* O157:H7. Lancet 352:1207, 1998

PASSARO DJ, PARSONNET J: Advances in the prevention and management of traveler's diarrhea. Curr Clin Top Infect Dis 18:217, 1998

SLUTSKER L et al: A nationwide case-control study of *Escherichia coli* O157:H7 infection in the United States. J Infect Dis 177:962, 1998

STEFFEN R et al: Epidemiology, etiology, and impact of traveler's diarrhea in Jamaica. JAMA 281:811, 1999

TAUXE RV, HUGHES JM: Food-borne disease, in *Mandell, Douglas and Bennett's Principles and Practice of Infectious Diseases*, 4th ed, GL Mandell et al (eds). New York, Churchill Livingstone, 1995, chap 81

132 *King K. Holmes*

SEXUALLY TRANSMITTED DISEASES: OVERVIEW AND CLINICAL APPROACH

HBV	hepatitis B virus	PCR	polymerase chain reaction
HPV	human papillomavirus	PID	pelvic inflammatory disease
HSV	herpes simplex virus	STDs	sexually transmitted diseases
LGV	lymphogranuloma venereum	STI	sexually transmitted infection
MPC	mucopurulent cervicitis	UTI	urinary tract infection
NGU	nongonococcal urethritis		

In all societies, sexually transmitted diseases (STDs) rank among the most common of all infectious diseases, with over 30 infections now classified as predominantly sexually transmitted or as frequently sexually transmissible (Table 132-1). The many new sexually transmitted pathogens recognized and characterized since 1980 include HIV types 1 and 2, human T cell lymphotropic virus (HTLV) types I and II, many genital types of human papillomavirus (HPV), *Mycoplasma genitalium*, two species of *Mobiluncus* (associated with bacterial vaginosis), two species of *Helicobacter* (initially associated with proctocolitis in homosexual men and later, during the AIDS era, with bacteremia, dermatitis, and fever among immunosuppressed individuals), and the Kaposi's sarcoma–associated herpesvirus (human herpesvirus type 8, or HHV-8).

In developing countries, with three-quarters of the world's population and 90% of the world's STDs, such factors as population growth (especially in adolescent and young-adult age groups), rural-to-urban migration, wars, and poverty create exceptional vulnerability to disease resulting from risky sexual behaviors. This situation leads to the spread of STD, with the emergence of new pathogens and new variants of old pathogens. During the 1990s, in China, Russia, the states of the former Soviet Union, and South Africa, internal social structures changed rapidly as borders opened to the West, unleashing enormous new epidemics of HIV infection and other STDs. HIV has become the leading cause of death in some developing countries, and HPV and hepatitis B virus (HBV) remain important causes of cervical and hepatocellular carcinoma, respectively—two of the commonest malignancies in the developing world. Sexually transmitted herpes simplex virus (HSV) infections now cause most genital ulcer disease throughout the world and an increasing proportion of cases of genital herpes in developing countries with generalized HIV epidemics, where the positive feedback loop between HSV and HIV transmission is a growing, intractable problem. Globally, the agents of curable STDs—gonorrhea, chlamydial infections, syphilis, chancroid, and trichomoniasis—caused ~350 million new infections annually in the mid-1990s. Bacterial vaginosis (arguably acquired sexually) occurs in up to 50% of women of reproductive age in developing countries. Thus, there are probably close to 1 billion cases of these curable infections annually, all six of which are associated with increased risk of HIV transmission or acquisition.

In the industrialized countries, fear of HIV infection since the mid-1980s, coupled with widespread behavioral interventions and better-organized systems of care for the curable STDs, have helped curb the transmission of the latter diseases. Nonetheless, viral STDs, such as genital herpes and HPV infection, had not obviously decreased in incidence at the turn of the millennium, and infection with HIV remains a leading cause of death in persons 25 to 44 years of age in the United States, as in developing countries, despite the advent of potent antiretroviral therapy.

Although rates of the bacterial STDs have fallen in all industrialized countries over the past 20 years, foci of hyperendemic transmission persist in the southeastern United States and in most large U.S. cities. Rates of gonorrhea and syphilis remain higher in the United States than in any other Western industrialized country. The reemergence of syphilis and gonorrhea epidemics in Russia and the former Soviet states has created similar foci for reintroduction of these STDs into western Europe. The remarkable return of high rates of gonorrhea and syphilis among homosexual and bisexual men in many parts of the United States reflects increased risk-taking since the advent of potent antiretroviral therapy and may portend resurgent transmission of HIV in this group.

CLASSIFICATION AND EPIDEMIOLOGY

Sexually transmitted infection (STI) may or may not result in disease (STD). Some prefer the term *reproductive tract infection* to destigmatize the diagnosis and treatment of STIs and to encompass conditions such as bacterial vaginosis, whose designation as an STD is debated.

Certain STDs (such as syphilis, gonorrhea, HIV infection, hepatitis B, and chancroid) are most concentrated within "core populations" having high rates of partner change, concurrent partners, or "dense" sexual networks—for example, prostitutes and their clients and persons involved in the use of illicit drugs, particularly crack cocaine. Poor access to or low motivation for obtaining early treatment also fosters spread of the curable STIs. In most of the United States, groups most vulnerable to STDs, including HIV infection, consist predominantly of young unmarried individuals of low socioeconomic status who often reside within crowded urban neighborhoods, although some rural areas (e.g., in the southeastern United States) also have high rates of STIs. Other STDs are distributed more evenly in society. For example, chlamydial infections can persist for many months, often asymptomatically, and can propagate widely in populations that do not share all of the characteristics of core groups described above. Similarly, genital HPV infections and genital herpes persist and spread efficiently in relatively low-risk populations.

In general, the product of three factors determines the initial rate of spread of any STI within a population: rate of exposure, efficiency of transmission per exposure, and duration of infectivity of those infected. Efforts to prevent and control STIs attempt to decrease the duration of infectivity (through early diagnosis and curative or suppressive treatment), to decrease the efficiency of transmission (e.g., through promotion of condom use and safer sexual practices), and to decrease the rate of exposure of susceptibles to infected persons (e.g., through provision of information, health education, and counseling and efforts to change the norms of sexual behavior).

Table 132-1 Sexually Transmitted and Sexually Transmissible Microorganisms

Bacteria	Viruses	Other[a]
TRANSMITTED IN ADULTS PREDOMINANTLY BY SEXUAL INTERCOURSE		
Neisseria gonorrhoeae	HIV (types 1 and 2)	*Trichomonas vaginalis*
Chlamydia trachomatis	Human T cell lymphotropic virus	*Phthirus pubis*
Treponema pallidum	type I	
Haemophilus ducreyi	Herpes simplex virus type 2	
Calymmatobacterium granulomatis	Human papillomavirus (multiple	
Ureaplasma urealyticum	genotypes)	
	Hepatitis B virus[b]	
	Molluscum contagiosum virus	
SEXUAL TRANSMISSION REPEATEDLY DESCRIBED BUT NOT WELL DEFINED OR NOT THE PREDOMINANT MODE		
Mycoplasma hominis	Cytomegalovirus	*Candida albicans*
Mycoplasma genitalium	Human T cell lymphotropic virus	*Sarcoptes scabiei*
Gardnerella vaginalis and other	type II	
vaginal bacteria	(?) Hepatitis C, D viruses	
Group B *Streptococcus*	Herpes simplex virus type 1	
Mobiluncus spp.	(?) Epstein-Barr virus	
Helicobacter cinaedi	Kaposi's sarcoma–associated	
Helicobacter fennelliae	herpesvirus[c]	
	Transfusion-transmitted virus	
TRANSMITTED BY SEXUAL CONTACT INVOLVING ORAL-FECAL EXPOSURE; OF DECLINING IMPORTANCE IN HOMOSEXUAL MEN		
Shigella spp.	Hepatitis A virus	*Giardia lamblia*
Campylobacter spp.		*Entamoeba histolytica*

[a] Includes protozoa, ectoparasites, and fungi.
[b] Among U.S. patients for whom a risk factor can be ascertained, most hepatitis B virus infections are transmitted sexually or by injection drug use.
[c] Human herpesvirus type 8.

MANAGEMENT OF COMMON STD SYNDROMES

Although other chapters discuss management of specific STIs, delineating treatment based on diagnosis of a specific infection, most patients are actually managed (at least initially) on the basis of presenting symptoms and signs and associated risk factors, even in industrialized countries. Table 132-2 lists some of the most common clinical STD syndromes and their microbial etiologies. Strategies for their management are outlined below. Chaps. 191 and 309 address the management of infections with human retroviruses.

RISK ASSESSMENT Routine patient care begins with risk assessment (e.g., for heart disease, cancer). An overall risk assessment interview should include STD/HIV in primary care, urgent care, and emergency care settings as well as in specialty clinics providing adolescent, prenatal, and family planning services. STD/HIV risk assessment guides interpretation of symptoms that could reflect an STD; decisions on screening or prophylactic/preventive treatment; risk reduction counseling and intervention (e.g., hepatitis B vaccination); and notification of partners of patients with known infections. Consideration of routine demographic data (e.g., gender, age, marital status, area of residence) is a simple first step in STD/HIV risk assessment. For example, national guidelines recommend routine screening of sexually active females ≤25 years of age for *C. trachomatis* infection. Table 132-3 provides a set of 10 STD/HIV risk assessment questions that clinicians can pose verbally or that health care systems can adapt (with yes/no responses) into a routine self-administered questionnaire for use in clinics. The initial framing statement gives permission to discuss taboo topics.

Risk assessment is followed by clinical assessment (elicitation of information on specific current symptoms and signs of STDs). Confirmatory diagnostic tests (for those with symptoms or signs) or screening tests (for those without symptoms or signs) may involve microscopic examination, culture, antigen detection tests, genetic probe or amplification tests, or serology. Initial syndrome-based treatment should cover the most likely causes. For certain syndromes, results of rapid tests can narrow the spectrum of this initial therapy (e.g., wet mount of vaginal fluid for women with vaginal discharge, Gram's stain of urethral discharge for men with urethral discharge, rapid plasma reagin test for genital ulcer). After the institution of treatment, STD management proceeds to the "4 C's" of prevention and control: contact tracing (see "Prevention and Control of STDs," below), ensuring compliance with therapy, and counseling on risk reduction, including condom promotion and provision.

URETHRITIS IN MEN The incidence of reported gonococcal urethritis in the United States has fallen to the lowest level since reporting began, while that of nongonococcal urethritis (NGU) remains high—a pattern typical of all industrialized countries. Until recently, *Chlamydia trachomatis* caused ~30 to 40% of NGU cases, but the proportion of cases due to this organism may have declined in some populations served by effective chlamydial control programs. HSV and *Trichomonas vaginalis* each cause a small proportion of NGU cases in the United States. Case-control studies have also implicated *Ureaplasma urealyticum* and *M. genitalium* as probable causes of many *Chlamydia*-negative cases, and coliform bacteria can cause urethritis in men who practice insertive anal intercourse. The initial diagnosis of urethritis in men currently includes specific tests only for *Neisseria gonorrhoeae* and *C. trachomatis*. Table 132-4 summarizes the steps in management of sexually active men with symptoms of urethral discharge and/or dysuria.

1. *Establish the presence of urethritis.* If proximal-to-distal "milking" of the urethra does not express a purulent or mucopurulent discharge, even after the patient has not voided for several hours or preferably overnight, the centrifuged sediment of the first 20 to 30 mL of voided urine can be examined for inflammatory cells, either by microscopy or by the leukocyte esterase test. In urethral gonococcal or chlamydial infection, a Gram's-stained smear of overt discharge or of an anterior urethral specimen obtained by passage of a small urethrogenital swab 2 to 3 cm into the urethra usually reveals ≥5 neutrophils per 1000× field in areas containing cells; in gonococcal infection, such a smear also usually reveals gram-negative intracellular diplococci. Patients with symptoms who lack objective evidence of urethritis may have functional rather than organic problems and generally do not benefit from repeated courses of antibiotics.

2. *Evaluate for complications or alternative diagnoses.* A brief history and examination will exclude epididymitis and systemic complications, such as disseminated gonococcal infection and Reiter's syndrome. Although digital examination of the prostate gland seldom contributes to the evaluation of sexually active young men with urethritis, men with dysuria who lack evidence of urethritis as well as sexually inactive men with urethritis should undergo prostate palpation, urinalysis, and urine culture to exclude bacterial prostatitis and cystitis.

3. *Evaluate for gonococcal and chlamydial infection.* An absence of typical gram-negative diplococci on Gram's-stained smear of urethral exudate containing inflammatory cells warrants a preliminary diagnosis of NGU and should lead to testing of the urethral specimen for *C. trachomatis*. Culture or DNA detection tests for *N. gonorrhoeae* may be positive when Gram's staining is negative; certain strains of *N. gonorrhoeae* reportedly can result in negative urethral Gram's stains in up to 30% of cases of urethritis. Results of tests for gonococcal and chlamydial infection predict the patient's prognosis (with greater risk for recurrent NGU if neither

Syndrome	ST Microbial Etiologies
AIDS	HIV types 1 and 2
Urethritis: males	*Neisseria gonorrhoeae, Chlamydia trachomatis, Ureaplasma urealyticum, Trichomonas vaginalis,* HSV
Epididymitis	*C. trachomatis, N. gonorrhoeae*
Lower genital tract infections: females	
Cystitis/urethritis	*C. trachomatis, N. gonorrhoeae,* HSV
Mucopurulent cervicitis	*C. trachomatis, N. gonorrhoeae*
Vulvitis	*Candida albicans,* HSV
Vulvovaginitis	*C. albicans, T. vaginalis*
Bacterial vaginosis (BV)	BV-associated bacteria (see text)
Acute pelvic inflammatory disease	*N. gonorrhoeae, C. trachomatis,* BV-associated bacteria, group B streptococci
Infertility	*N. gonorrhoeae, C. trachomatis,* BV-associated bacteria
Ulcerative lesions of the genitalia	HSV-1, HSV-2, *Treponema pallidum, Haemophilus ducreyi, C. trachomatis* (LGV strains), *Calymmatobacterium granulomatis*
Complications of pregnancy/puerperium	Several agents implicated
Intestinal infections	
Proctitis	*C. trachomatis, N. gonorrhoeae,* HSV, *T. pallidum*
Proctocolitis or enterocolitis	*Campylobacter* spp., *Shigella* spp., *Entamoeba histolytica,* other enteric pathogens
Enteritis	*Giardia lamblia*
Acute arthritis with urogenital infection or viremia	*N. gonorrhoeae* (e.g., DGI), *C. trachomatis* (e.g., Reiter's syndrome), HBV
Genital and anal warts	HPV (30 genital types)
Mononucleosis syndrome	CMV, HIV, EBV
Hepatitis	Hepatitis viruses, *T. pallidum* , CMV, EBV
Neoplasias	
Squamous cell dysplasias and cancers of the cervix, anus, vulva, vagina, or penis	HPV (especially types 16, 18, 31, 45)
Kaposi's sarcoma, body-cavity lymphomas	HHV-8
T cell leukemia	HTLV-I
Hepatocellular carcinoma	HBV
Tropical spastic paraparesis	HTLV-I
Scabies	*Sarcoptes scabiei*
Pubic lice	*Phthirus pubis*

NOTE: HSV, herpes simplex virus; LGV, lymphogranuloma venereum; DGI, disseminated gonococcal infection; HPV, human papillomavirus; CMV, cytomegalovirus; EBV, Epstein-Barr virus; HBV, hepatitis B virus; HTLV, human T cell lymphotropic virus; HHV-8, human herpesvirus type 8.

chlamydiae nor gonococci are found than if either is detected) and can guide both the counseling given to the patient and the management of the patient's sexual partner(s).

4. *Treat urethritis.*

℞ **TREATMENT** In practice, if Gram's stain does not reveal gonococci, urethritis is treated with a regimen effective for NGU, such as azithromycin (1.0 g orally in a single dose). If gonococci are demonstrated by Gram's stain or if no diagnostic tests are performed to definitively exclude gonorrhea, treatment should also include a single-dose regimen for gonorrhea (Chap. 147). Sexual partners should be tested for gonorrhea and chlamydial infection and should receive the same regimen given to the male index case.

EPIDIDYMITIS Acute epididymitis, almost always unilateral, must be differentiated from testicular torsion, tumor, and trauma. Torsion, a surgical emergency, usually occurs in the second or third decade of life and produces a sudden onset of pain, elevation of the testicle

Table 132-3 Ten-Question STD/HIV Risk Assessment

Framing Statement:
In order to provide the best care for you today and to understand your risk for certain infections, it is necessary for us to talk about your sexual behavior.

Screening Questions:
1) Do you have any reason to think you might have an STD? If so, what reason?
2) For all adolescents <18 years old: Have you begun having any kind of sex yet?

STD History:
3) Have you ever had any sexually transmitted diseases or any genital infections? If so, which ones?

Sexual Preference:
4) Have you had sex with men, women, or both?

Injection Drug Use:
5) Have you ever injected yourself ("shot up") with drugs? (If yes, have you ever shared needles or injection equipment?)
6) Have you ever had sex with a gay or bisexual man or with anyone who had ever injected drugs?

Characteristics of Partner(s):
7) Has your sex partner(s) had any sexually transmitted infections? If so, which ones?

STD Symptoms Checklist:
8) Have you recently developed any of these symptoms?

For Men	For Women
a) Discharge of pus (drip) from the penis	a) Abnormal vaginal discharge (increased amount, abnormal odor, abnormal yellow color)
b) Genital sores (ulcers) or rash	b) Genital sores (ulcers), rash, or itching

Sexual Practices, Past 2 Months (for patients answering yes to any of the above questions, to guide examination and testing):
9) Now I'd like to ask what parts of your body may have been sexually exposed to an STD (e.g., your penis, mouth, vagina, anus)?

Query about Interest in STD Screening Tests (for patients answering no to all of the above questions):
10) Would you like to be tested for HIV or any other STDs today? (If yes, clinician can explore which STD and why.)

SOURCE: Adapted from JR Curtis and KK Holmes. Individual-level risk assessment for STD/HIV infections. In KK Holmes et al (eds): *Sexually Transmitted Diseases,* 3rd ed. New York, McGraw-Hill, 1999, pp 669–683.

within the scrotal sac, rotation of the epididymis from a posterior to an anterior position, and absence of blood flow on Doppler examination or ^{99m}Tc scan. Persistence of symptoms after a course of therapy for epididymitis suggests the possibility of testicular tumor. In sexually active men under age 35, acute epididymitis is caused most frequently by *C. trachomatis* and less commonly by *N. gonorrhoeae* and is usually associated with overt or subclinical urethritis. Acute epididymitis in older men or following urinary tract instrumentation is usually caused by urinary pathogens. Similarly, epididymitis in men who have practiced insertive rectal intercourse is often caused by Enterobacteriaceae. These men usually have no urethritis but do have bacteriuria.

℞ **TREATMENT** Ofloxacin (300 mg orally bid for 10 days) is an optimal agent for syndrome-based treatment of epididymitis because of its effectiveness against *N. gonorrhoeae, C. trachomatis,* and Enterobacteriaceae. Alternatively, ceftriaxone (250 mg intramuscularly) followed by doxycycline (100 mg orally bid for 10 days) is effective for epididymitis caused by *N. gonorrhoeae* or *C. trachomatis.*

URETHRITIS AND THE URETHRAL SYNDROME IN WOMEN *C. trachomatis, N. gonorrhoeae,* and occasionally HSV cause symptomatic urethritis—known as the urethral syndrome in women—characterized by "internal" dysuria (usually without urinary urgency or frequency) and pyuria, with *Escherichia coli* or other uropathogens not present in urine at counts of $\geq 10^2$/mL. In contrast, the

Table 132-4   Management of Urethral Discharge in Men

Usual causes	Usual initial evaluation
Chlamydia trachomatis	Demonstration of urethral discharge or
Neisseria gonorrhoeae	pyuria
Ureaplasma urealyticum	Exclusion of local or systemic complications
Trichomonas vaginalis	Urethral Gram's stain to confirm urethritis,
Herpes simplex virus	detect gram-negative diplococci
Mycoplasma genitalium	Test for *N. gonorrhoeae, C. trachomatis*

INITIAL TREATMENT FOR PATIENT AND PARTNERS

Treat gonorrhea (unless excluded):	plus	Treat chlamydial infection:
Cefixime, 400 mg PO; *or*		Azithromycin, 1 g PO; *or*
Ceftriaxone, 125 mg IM; *or*		Doxycycline, 100 mg bid for
Fluoroquinolone (e.g., cipro-		7 days
floxacin, 500 mg PO)		

MANAGEMENT OF RECURRENCE

Confirm objective evidence of urethritis. If patient was reexposed to untreated or new partner, repeat treatment of patient and partner.

If patient was not reexposed, consider infection with *T. vaginalis*[a] or doxycycline-resistant *Ureaplasma*, and consider treatment with metronidazole or azithromycin.

[a] In men, the diagnosis of *T. vaginalis* infection requires culture of early-morning first-voided urine sediment or of a urethral swab specimen obtained before voiding.

dysuria associated with vulvar herpes or vulvovaginal candidiasis (and perhaps with trichomoniasis) is often described as "external," being caused by painful contact of urine with the inflamed or ulcerated labia or introitus. Acute onset, association with urinary urgency or frequency, hematuria, or suprapubic bladder tenderness suggests bacterial cystitis. Among women with symptoms of acute bacterial cystitis, costovertebral pain and tenderness or fever suggests acute pyelonephritis. The management of bacterial urinary tract infection (UTI) is discussed in Chap. 280.

Signs of vulvovaginitis, coupled with symptoms of external dysuria, suggest vulvar infection (e.g., with HSV or *Candida albicans*). Among dysuric women without signs of vulvovaginitis, bacterial UTI must be differentiated from the urethral syndrome by assessment of risk, evaluation of the pattern of symptoms and signs, and specific microbiologic testing. An STD etiology of the urethral syndrome is suggested by young age, more than one current sexual partner or a new partner within the past month, or coexisting mucopurulent cervicitis (MPC; see below). The finding of a single urinary pathogen, such as *E. coli* or *Staphylococcus saprophyticus*, at a concentration of $\geq 10^2$/mL in a properly collected specimen of midstream urine from a dysuric woman with pyuria indicates probable bacterial UTI, whereas pyuria with $< 10^2$ conventional uropathogens per milliliter of urine ("sterile" pyuria) suggests acute urethral syndrome due to *C. trachomatis* or *N. gonorrhoeae*. Gonorrhea and chlamydial infection should be sought by specific tests. Among women with sterile pyuria caused by chlamydial infection, treatment with doxycycline (100 mg bid for 7 days) alleviates dysuria.

VULVOVAGINAL INFECTIONS   Abnormal Vaginal Discharge   If directly questioned during routine health checkups, many women acknowledge having nonspecific symptoms of vaginal discharge that do not correlate with objective signs of inflammation or with actual infection. However, unsolicited reporting of abnormal vaginal discharge does suggest bacterial vaginosis or trichomoniasis. Specifically, an abnormally increased amount, an abnormal odor, and an abnormal yellow color of the discharge are associated with one or both of these conditions. Cervical infection with *N. gonorrhoeae* or *C. trachomatis* does not appear to cause an increased amount or abnormal odor of discharge, but cervicitis, like trichomoniasis, can include the production of an increased number of neutrophils in vaginal fluid, resulting in a yellow color. Vulvar conditions such as genital herpes or vulvovaginal candidiasis can cause vulvar pruritus, burning,

irritation, or lesions as well as external dysuria (as urine passes over the inflamed vulva) or vulvar dyspareunia.

Certain vulvovaginal infections may have serious sequelae. Trichomoniasis, bacterial vaginosis, and vulvovaginal candidiasis have all been associated with increased risk of acquisition of HIV infection. Vaginal trichomoniasis and bacterial vaginosis early in pregnancy independently predict premature onset of labor. Bacterial vaginosis can also lead to anaerobic bacterial infection of the endometrium and salpinges. Vaginitis may be an early and prominent feature of toxic shock syndrome, and recurrent or chronic vulvovaginal candidiasis develops with increased frequency among women with systemic illnesses, such as diabetes mellitus or HIV-related immunosuppression (although only a very small proportion of women with recurrent vulvovaginal candidiasis in the United States actually have a serious predisposing illness).

Thus vulvovaginal symptoms or signs warrant careful evaluation, including pelvic examination, simple rapid diagnostic tests, and appropriate therapy specific for the anatomic site and type of infection. Unfortunately, a recent survey in the United States indicated that clinicians seldom perform the tests required to establish the cause of such symptoms. The diagnosis and treatment of the three most common types of vaginal infection are summarized in Table 132-5.

Inspection of the vulva and perineum may reveal tender genital ulcerations (typically due to HSV infection, occasionally to chancroid) or fissures (typically due to vulvovaginal candidiasis) or discharge visible at the introitus before insertion of a speculum (suggestive of bacterial vaginosis or trichomoniasis). Speculum examination permits the clinician to discern whether the discharge in fact looks abnormal and whether any abnormal discharge in the vagina emanates from the cervical os (mucoid and, if abnormal, yellow) or from the vagina (not mucoid, since the vaginal epithelium does not produce mucus). Symptoms or signs of abnormal vaginal discharge should prompt testing of vaginal fluid for pH, odor when mixed with 10% KOH, and microscopic features when mixed with saline and with 10% KOH. Additional objective laboratory tests useful for establishing the cause of abnormal vaginal discharge include Gram's staining to detect alterations in the vaginal flora; new card and dipstick tests for bacterial vaginosis, as described below; and a new DNA probe test purported to detect *T. vaginalis* and *C. albicans* as well as the increased concentrations of *Gardnerella vaginalis* associated with bacterial vaginosis.

℞ **TREATMENT**   Patterns of treatment for vaginal discharge vary widely. In developing countries, where clinics or pharmacies often dispense treatment based on symptoms alone without examination or testing, oral treatment with metronidazole, either as a 2-g single dose or as a 7-day regimen, provides reasonable coverage against both trichomoniasis and bacterial vaginosis, the usual causes of symptoms of vaginal discharge; metronidazole treatment of sex partners would prevent reinfection of women with trichomoniasis even if it does not help prevent the recurrence of bacterial vaginosis. Guidelines promulgated during the 1990s by the World Health Organization suggested treatment for cervical infection and for vulvovaginal candidiasis in women with symptoms of abnormal vaginal discharge; in retrospect, these recommendations were faulty, since these conditions seldom produce such symptoms.

In industrialized countries, clinicians treating symptoms and signs of abnormal vaginal discharge should at least differentiate between bacterial vaginosis and trichomoniasis, because optimal management of patients and partners differs for these two conditions, as discussed briefly below.

Vaginal Trichomoniasis (See also Chap. 218)   Symptomatic trichomoniasis characteristically produces a profuse, yellow, purulent, homogeneous vaginal discharge and vulvar irritation, often with visible inflammation of the vaginal and vulvar epithelium and petechial lesions on the cervix (the so-called strawberry cervix, usually evident only by colposcopy). The pH of vaginal fluid usually rises to ≥ 5.0. In women with typical symptoms and signs of trichomoniasis, micro-

Table 132-5 Diagnostic Features and Management of Vaginal Infection

Feature	Normal Vaginal Examination	Vulvovaginal Candidiasis	Trichomonal Vaginitis	Bacterial Vaginosis
Etiology	Uninfected; lactobacilli predominant	*Candida albicans*	*Trichomonas vaginalis*	Associated with *Gardnerella vaginalis*, various anaerobic bacteria, and mycoplasmas
Typical symptoms	None	Vulvar itching and/or irritation	Profuse purulent discharge; vulvar itching	Malodorous, slightly increased discharge
Discharge				
Amount	Variable; usually scant	Scant	Profuse	Moderate
Color[a]	Clear or white	White	Yellow	White or gray
Consistency	Nonhomogeneous, floccular	Clumped; adherent plaques	Homogeneous	Homogeneous, low viscosity; uniformly coats vaginal walls
Inflammation of vulvar or vaginal epithelium	None	Erythema of vaginal epithelium, introitus; vulvar dermatitis common	Erythema of vaginal and vulvar epithelium; colpitis macularis	None
pH of vaginal fluid[b]	Usually ≤4.5	Usually ≤4.5	Usually ≥5.0	Usually >4.5
Amine ("fishy") odor with 10% KOH	None	None	May be present	Present
Microscopy[c]	Normal epithelial cells; lactobacilli predominant	Leukocytes, epithelial cells; mycelia or pseudomycelia in up to 80% of *C. albicans* culture-positive persons with typical symptoms	Leukocytes; motile trichomonads seen in 80 to 90% of symptomatic patients, less often in the absence of symptoms	Clue cells; few leukocytes; no lactobacilli or only a few outnumbered by profuse mixed flora, nearly always including *G. vaginalis* plus anaerobic species on Gram's stain
Usual treatment	None	Azole cream, tablet, or suppository—e.g., miconazole 100-mg vaginal suppository or clotrimazole 100-mg vaginal tablet, once daily for 7 days. Fluconazole, 150 mg orally (single dose)	Metronidazole, 2 g orally (single dose) Metronidazole, 500 mg PO bid for 7 days	Metronidazole, 500 mg PO bid for 7 days Clindamycin, 2% cream, one full applicator vaginally each night for 7 days Metronidazole gel, 0.75%, one full applicator vaginally twice daily for 5 days Metronidazole, 2 g PO (single dose)[d]
Usual management of sexual partner	None	None; topical treatment if candidal dermatitis of penis is detected	Examination for STD; treatment with metronidazole, 2 g PO (single dose)	Examination for STD; no treatment if normal

[a] Color of discharge is best determined by examination against the white background of a swab.
[b] pH determination is not useful if blood is present.
[c] To detect fungal elements, vaginal fluid is digested with 10% KOH prior to microscopic examination; to examine for other features, fluid is mixed (1:1) with physiologic saline.

Gram's stain is also excellent for detecting yeasts and pseudomycelia and for distinguishing normal flora from the mixed flora seen in bacterial vaginosis, but it is less sensitive than the saline preparation for detection of *T. vaginalis*.
[d] Single-dose regimen is less effective than 7-day metronidazole regimen.

scopic examination of vaginal discharge mixed with saline reveals motile trichomonads in at least 80% of culture-positive cases. However, in the absence of symptoms or signs, culture is often required for detection of the organism. Treatment of asymptomatic as well as symptomatic cases reduces rates of transmission and prevents later development of symptoms.

℞ **TREATMENT** Only nitroimidazoles consistently cure trichomoniasis. Tinidazole and ornidazole have longer half-lives than metronidazole but do not give better results than a single 2-g oral dose of metronidazole, the treatment of choice. Treatment of male sexual partners—often facilitated by dispensing metronidazole to the female patient to give to her partner(s), with a warning about avoiding the concurrent use of alcohol—reduces both the risk of reinfection and the reservoir of infection. Treatment with 0.75% metronidazole gel intravaginally, although effective for bacterial vaginosis, is not reliable for vaginal trichomoniasis. Systemic use of metronidazole is not recommended during the first trimester of pregnancy but is considered safe thereafter.

Bacterial Vaginosis This syndrome (formerly termed *nonspecific vaginitis*, *Haemophilus vaginitis*, *anaerobic vaginitis*, or *Gardnerella-associated vaginal discharge*) is characterized by symptoms of vaginal malodor and a slightly to moderately increased white discharge, which appears homogeneous, is low in viscosity, and smoothly coats the vaginal mucosa. Risk factors include multiple sexual partners and recent intercourse with a new partner, but antibiotic treatment of male partners has not reduced the rate of recurrence among affected women.

The vaginal fluid of women with bacterial vaginosis is characterized by markedly increased prevalences and concentrations of *G. vaginalis*, *Mycoplasma hominis*, and several anaerobic bacteria [e.g., *Mobiluncus* spp., *Prevotella* spp. (formerly *Bacteroides* spp.), and some *Peptostreptococcus* spp.]. The vaginal fluid usually lacks hydrogen peroxide–producing *Lactobacillus* spp., which constitute most of the normal vaginal flora and perhaps help protect against certain cervical and vaginal infections. Vaginal douching, use of intravaginal nonoxynol-9 spermicide, and new sexual partners can all result in loss of vaginal colonization by hydrogen peroxide–producing lactobacilli.

Bacterial vaginosis is conventionally diagnosed clinically with the *Amsel criteria*, which include any three of the following four clinical abnormalities: (1) objective signs of increased white homogeneous vaginal discharge; (2) a vaginal discharge pH of >4.5; (3) liberation of a distinct fishy odor (attributable to volatile amines such as trimethylamine) immediately after vaginal secretions are mixed with a 10% solution of KOH; and (4) microscopic demonstration of "clue cells" (vaginal epithelial cells coated with coccobacillary organisms giving them a granular appearance and indistinct borders; Fig. 132-1) on a wet mount prepared by mixing vaginal secretions with normal

FIGURE 132-1 *A.* Vaginal epithelial "clue cells." Note granular appearance due to adherent *G. vaginalis* and indistinct cell margins (400×). *B.* Normal vaginal epithelial cells. The cell margins are distinct and lack granularity.

saline in a ratio of ~1:1. A new card test now facilitates screening of vaginal fluid for pH >4.5 and trimethylamine, and a new dipstick test detects proline aminopeptidase, an enzyme associated with this syndrome.

Alternatively, the microbiology laboratory can determine the *Nugent score* by examining a Gram-stained smear of vaginal discharge. A score of 7 to 10, based on reduced numbers or the absence of large gram-positive rods (lactobacilli) and the presence of small gram-negative or variable rods (*Gardnerella* and anaerobic rods) and of curved gram-negative or variable rods (*Mobiluncus*), has high sensitivity and specificity for the diagnosis of bacterial vaginosis. Attempts to isolate *G. vaginalis*, genital mycoplasmas, or anaerobic bacteria do not aid in the diagnosis of bacterial vaginosis because these organisms occur (albeit in much lower concentrations) in the vaginal flora of many women without the syndrome.

TREATMENT The standard dosage of metronidazole for the treatment of bacterial vaginosis is 500 mg orally bid for 7 days. Alternatively, the single 2-g oral dose of metronidazole recommended for trichomoniasis produces short-term rates of recurrence of bacterial vaginosis somewhat higher than those obtained with the 7-day regimen. Intravaginal treatment with 2% clindamycin cream [one full applicator (5 g containing 100 mg of clindamycin phosphate) each night for 7 nights] or with 0.75% metronidazole gel [one full applicator (5 g containing 37.5 mg of metronidazole) twice daily for 5 days] is also effective and does not elicit systemic adverse reactions. Nonetheless, long-term recurrence (i.e., after several months) is distressingly common after either oral or intravaginal treatment. Treatment of male

partners with metronidazole does not prevent recurrence of bacterial vaginosis, even though new sexual partners have been implicated as a risk factor for recurrence.

No controlled data support the use of currently available vaginal or oral preparations of lactobacilli for the treatment or prevention of recurrence of bacterial vaginosis. Clinical trials are evaluating prevention of recurrence by repeated intravaginal inoculation of a vaginal *Lactobacillus* species that produces hydrogen peroxide and adheres to vaginal epithelium.

Vulvovaginal Pruritus, Burning, or Irritation Vulvovaginal candidiasis produces vulvar pruritus, burning, or irritation, generally without symptoms of increased vaginal discharge or malodor. Genital herpes can produce similar symptoms, with lesions sometimes difficult to distinguish from the fissures caused by candidiasis. Signs of vulvovaginal candidiasis include vulvar erythema, edema, fissures, and tenderness. With candidiasis, a white scanty vaginal discharge sometimes takes the form of white thrushlike plaques or cottage cheese–like curds adhering loosely to the vaginal mucosa. *C. albicans* accounts for nearly all cases of symptomatic vulvovaginal candidiasis, which probably arise from endogenous strains of *C. albicans* that have colonized the vagina or the intestinal tract.

The diagnosis of vulvovaginal candidiasis usually involves the demonstration of pseudohyphae or hyphae by microscopic examination of vaginal fluid mixed with saline or 10% KOH or subjected to Gram's staining. Microscopic examination is less sensitive than culture but correlates better with symptoms.

TREATMENT Symptoms and signs of vulvovaginal candidiasis warrant treatment, usually intravaginal administration of any of several imidazole antibiotics (e.g., miconazole or clotrimazole) for 3 to 7 days. Over-the-counter marketing of such preparations has reduced the cost of care and made treatment more convenient for many women with recurrent yeast vulvovaginitis. However, most women who purchase these preparations do not have vulvovaginal candidiasis, while many do have other vaginal infections that require different treatment. Therefore, only women with classic symptoms of vulvar pruritus and a history of previous episodes of yeast vulvovaginitis documented by an experienced clinician should self-treat. Single-dose oral treatment with fluconazole (150 mg) is also effective and is preferred by many patients. Prolonged or periodic oral therapy may benefit women with severe or frequently recurrent vulvovaginal candidiasis and those who do not respond to intravaginal or single-dose oral therapy. Such patients probably should be evaluated for diabetes and HIV infection, although such systemic illnesses seldom explain recurrent vulvovaginal candidiasis. Treatment of sexual partners is not routinely indicated.

Other Causes of Vaginal Discharge or Vaginitis In the ulcerative vaginitis associated with staphylococcal toxic shock syndrome, *Staphylococcus aureus* should be promptly identified in vaginal fluid by Gram's stain and by culture. In desquamative inflammatory vaginitis, smears of vaginal fluid reveal neutrophils, massive vaginal epithelial cell exfoliation with increased numbers of parabasal cells, and gram-positive cocci; this syndrome responds to treatment with 2% clindamycin cream. Additional causes of vaginitis and vulvovaginal symptoms in women include retained foreign bodies (e.g., tampons), cervical caps, vaginal spermicides, vaginal antiseptic preparations or douches, vaginal epithelial atrophy in postmenopausal women or in the postpartum period during prolonged breast-feeding, allergic reactions to latex condoms, vaginal aphthae associated with HIV infection or Behçet's syndrome, and vestibulitis (a poorly understood syndrome).

MUCOPURULENT CERVICITIS MPC refers to inflammation of the columnar epithelium and subepithelium of the endocervix and of any contiguous columnar epithelium that lies exposed in an ectopic position on the exocervix. MPC in women represents the "silent partner" of urethritis in men, being equally common and often caused by the same agents (*N. gonorrhoeae* or *C. trachomatis*) but more difficult to recognize. As the most common manifestation of these serious bacterial infections in women, MPC can be a harbinger or sign of pelvic inflammatory disease (PID) and—in pregnant women—can lead to obstetric complications. More than half of all cases of this syndrome in the United States today remain idiopathic.

The diagnosis of MPC rests on the detection of yellow mucopurulent discharge from the cervical os or of increased numbers of polymorphonuclear leukocytes in Gram-stained or Papanicolaou-stained smears of endocervical mucus. MPC due to *C. trachomatis* can also produce edematous cervical ectopy (see below) and endocervical bleeding upon gentle swabbing. Unlike the endocervicitis produced by gonococcal or chlamydial infection, cervicitis caused by HSV produces ulcerative lesions on the stratified squamous epithelium of the exocervix as well as on the columnar epithelium. Yellow cervical mucus on a white swab removed from the endocervix indicates the presence of polymorphonuclear leukocytes. The mucus should be rolled thinly on a slide for Gram's staining. The presence of ≥20 polymorphonuclear cells per 1000× microscopic field within strands of cervical mucus not contaminated by vaginal squamous epithelial cells or vaginal bacteria indicates endocervicitis (Fig. 132-2). Detection of intracellular gram-negative diplococci in carefully collected endocervical mucus is quite specific but ≤50% sensitive for gonorrhea. Therefore, specific and sensitive tests for *N. gonorrhoeae* as well as *C. trachomatis* are also indicated in evaluation of MPC.

℞ **TREATMENT** Although the above criteria for MPC are neither highly specific nor highly predictive of gonococcal or chlamydial infection in many settings, current guidelines of the Centers for Disease Control and Prevention call for consideration of empirical treatment for MPC, pending test results, "for a patient who has suspected gonorrhea or chlamydial infection, if the prevalences of these infections are high in the patient population, and the patient might be difficult to locate after treatment." In this situation, therapy should

FIGURE 132-2 Gram's stain of cervical mucus, showing a strand of cervical mucus containing many polymorphonuclear leukocytes. This picture is typical of mucopurulent cervicitis. Note that leukocytes are not seen in areas of the slide containing vaginal epithelial cells, adjacent to the mucus strands. *[(From KK Holmes and WE Stamm: Lower genital tract infection in women, in KK Holmes et al (eds). Sexually Transmitted Diseases, 3d ed. New York, McGraw-Hill, 1999, pp 761–781.)]*

include a single-dose regimen effective for gonorrhea plus treatment for chlamydial infection, as outlined in Table 132-4 for treatment of urethritis. In settings where gonorrhea is much less common than chlamydial infection, initial therapy for chlamydial infection alone suffices. The etiology and potential benefit of treatment of endocervicitis not associated with gonorrhea or chlamydial infection remain undefined. Sexual partner(s) of a woman with MPC should be examined and given a regimen similar to that chosen for the woman unless results of tests for gonorrhea or chlamydial infection in either partner warrant different therapy or no therapy.

CERVICAL ECTOPY Cervical ectopy, often mislabeled "cervical erosion," is easily confused with infectious endocervicitis. Ectopy represents the presence of the one-cell-thick columnar epithelium extending from the endocervix out onto the visible ectocervix. In ectopy, the cervical os may contain clear or slightly cloudy mucus but usually not yellow mucopus. Colposcopy shows intact epithelium. Normally found during adolescence and early adulthood, ectopy gradually recedes through the second and third decades of life, as squamous metaplasia replaces the ectopic columnar epithelium. Oral contraceptive use favors the persistence or reappearance of ectopy, while smoking apparently accelerates squamous metaplasia. Cauterization for the elimination of ectopy is not warranted. Ectopy may render the cervix more susceptible to infection with *N. gonorrhoeae*, *C. trachomatis*, or HIV by exposing a larger area of susceptible columnar epithelium on the exocervix.

PELVIC INFLAMMATORY DISEASE See Chap. 133.

ULCERATIVE GENITAL LESIONS Genital ulceration reflects a set of important STIs, most of which also sharply increase the risk of sexual acquisition and shedding of HIV. Accurate diagnosis, treatment, and prevention of these infections are high priorities. In a study of genital ulcers carried out in 1996 in 10 of the U.S. cities with the highest rates of primary syphilis, polymerase chain reaction (PCR) testing of ulcer specimens demonstrated HSV in 62% of patients, *Treponema pallidum* in 13%, and *Haemophilus ducreyi* in 12 to 20%.

In Asia and Africa, chancroid was once considered the most common type of genital ulcer, followed by primary syphilis and then genital herpes. With increased efforts to control chancroid and syphilis, together with more frequent recurrences or persistence of genital herpes attributable to the growing numbers of immunosuppressed persons with HIV infection, PCR testing of genital ulcers now clearly implicates genital herpes as the most common cause of genital ulceration in some developing countries. Lymphogranuloma venereum (LGV) and donovanosis (granuloma inguinale) continue to cause genital ulceration in developing countries but rarely occur today in North America or Europe. Other causes of genital ulcer include (1) candidiasis and traumatized genital warts—both readily recognized; (2) lesions due to genital involvement of more widespread dermatoses; and (3) cutaneous manifestations of systemic diseases, such as genital mucosal ulceration in Stevens-Johnson syndrome.

Although most genital ulcerations cannot be diagnosed confidently on clinical grounds alone, clinical findings plus epidemiologic considerations (Table 132-6) can usually guide initial management (Table 132-7) pending results of further tests. Clinicians should order a rapid serologic test for syphilis in all cases of genital ulcer and a dark-field, direct immunofluorescence, or PCR test for *T. pallidum* from all lesions except those highly characteristic of infection with HSV (i.e., those with herpetic vesicles).

Typical vesicles or pustules or a cluster of painful ulcers preceded by vesiculopustular lesions suggests genital herpes. These typical clinical presentations make detection of the virus optional; however, many patients want confirmation of the diagnosis, and differentiation of HSV-1 from HSV-2 has prognostic implications, since the latter causes more frequent recurrences.

Painless, nontender, indurated ulcers with firm, nontender inguinal adenopathy suggest primary syphilis. If the results of dark-field ex-

Table 132-6 Clinical Features of Genital Ulcers

Feature	Syphilis	Herpes	Chancroid	Lymphogranuloma Venereum	Donovanosis
Incubation period	9–90 days	2–7 days	1–14 days	3 days–6 weeks	1–4 weeks (up to 6 months)
Early primary lesions	Papule	Vesicle	Pustule	Papule, pustule, or vesicle	Papule
No. of lesions	Usually one	Multiple, may coalesce	Usually multiple, may coalesce	Usually one	Variable
Diameter	5–15 mm	1–2 mm	Variable	2–10 mm	Variable
Edges	Sharply demarcated, elevated, round, or oval	Erythematous	Undermined, ragged, irregular	Elevated, round, or oval	Elevated, irregular
Depth	Superficial or deep	Superficial	Excavated	Superficial or deep	Elevated
Base	Smooth, nonpurulent, relatively nonvascular	Serous, erythematous, nonvascular	Purulent, bleeds easily	Variable, nonvascular	Red and velvety, bleeds readily
Induration	Firm	None	Soft	Occasionally firm	Firm
Pain	Uncommon	Frequently tender	Usually very tender	Variable	Uncommon
Lymphadenopathy	Firm, nontender, bilateral	Firm, tender, often bilateral with initial episode	Tender, may suppurate, loculated, usually unilateral	Tender, may suppurate, loculated, usually unilateral	None; pseudobuboes

SOURCE: From RM Ballard, KK Holmes et al (eds): *Sexually Transmitted Diseases*, 3rd ed. New York, McGraw-Hill, 1999.

amination and a rapid serologic test for syphilis are initially negative and the patient will comply with follow-up and sexual abstinence, the performance of two more dark-field examinations on successive days before treatment is begun will improve the sensitivity of diagnosis of syphilis, as will repeated serologic testing for syphilis 1 or 2 weeks later.

"Atypical" or clinically trivial ulcers may be more common manifestations of genital herpes than classic vesiculopustular lesions. Specific tests for HSV in the lesions are therefore indicated (Chap. 182). Type-specific serologic tests for serum antibody to HSV-2, now commercially available, may give negative results, especially when patients present early with the initial episode of genital herpes or when HSV-1 is the cause of genital herpes (as in 15 to 30% of cases today). Furthermore, a positive test for HSV-2 antibody does not prove that the current lesions are herpetic, since nearly one-fourth of the general population of the United States becomes seropositive for HSV-2 during early adulthood. Nonetheless, a positive HSV-2 serology does enable the clinician to tell the patient that he or she has had genital herpes, should learn to recognize symptoms, should avoid sex during recurrences, and should consider use of condoms at other times.

Demonstration of *H. ducreyi* by culture (or by PCR test, when available) is most useful when ulcers are painful and purulent, especially when inguinal lymphadenopathy with fluctuance or overlying erythema is noted; if chancroid is prevalent in the community; or if the patient has recently had a sexual exposure in a chancroid-endemic area (e.g., a developing country or certain North American cities). Enlarged, fluctuant lymph nodes should be aspirated for culture or PCR tests to detect *H. ducreyi* as well as for Gram's staining and culture to rule out the presence of other pyogenic bacteria.

When genital ulcers persist beyond the natural history of initial episodes of herpes (2 to 3 weeks) or of chancroid or syphilis (up to 6 weeks) and do not resolve with syndrome-based antimicrobial therapy, then—in addition to the usual tests for herpes, syphilis, and chancroid—biopsy is indicated to exclude donovanosis, carcinoma, and other nonvenereal dermatoses. HIV serology should also be undertaken, since chronic, persistent genital herpes is common in AIDS.

Immediate syndrome-based treatment for acute genital ulcerations (after collection of all necessary diagnostic specimens) is often appropriate. Patients with typical initial or recurrent episodes of genital or anorectal herpes can benefit from prompt oral antiviral therapy (Chap. 182). The patient with nonvesicular ulcerative lesions who may not return for follow-up or may continue sexual activity should receive initial treatment for syphilis, together with empirical therapy for chancroid if exposed in an area where chancroid occurs or if regional lymph node suppuration is evident. In resource-poor settings lacking ready access to diagnostic tests, this approach to syndromic treatment for syphilis and chancroid has helped bring these two diseases under better control. Finally, empirical antimicrobial therapy may be indicated if ulcers persist and the diagnosis remains unclear after a week of observation despite attempts to diagnose herpes, syphilis, and chancroid.

PROCTITIS, PROCTOCOLITIS, ENTEROCOLITIS, AND ENTERITIS Sexually acquired proctitis, with inflammation limited to the rectal mucosa, results from direct rectal inoculation of typical STD pathogens. In contrast, inflammation extending from the rectum to the colon (proctocolitis), involving both the small and the large bowel (enterocolitis), or involving the small bowel alone (enteritis) can result from ingestion of typical intestinal pathogens through oral-anal exposure during sexual contact. Anorectal pain and mucopurulent, bloody rectal discharge suggest proctitis or protocolitis. Proctitis commonly produces tenesmus (causing frequent attempts to defecate, but not true diarrhea) and constipation, whereas proctocolitis and enterocolitis more often cause true diarrhea. In all three conditions, anoscopy usually shows mucosal exudate and easily induced mucosal bleeding (i.e., a positive "wipe test"), sometimes with petechiae or mucosal ulcers. Exudate should be sampled for Gram's staining and

Table 132-7 Initial Management of Genital Ulcer

Usual causes
Herpes simplex virus (HSV)
Treponema pallidum (primary syphilis)
Haemophilus ducreyi (chancroid)
Usual initial laboratory evaluation
Dark-field exam, direct FA, or PCR for *T. pallidum*; RPR test (if negative but primary syphilis suspected, repeat RPR in 1 week); culture, direct FA, ELISA, or PCR for HSV. In endemic area: PCR or culture for *H. ducreyi*

INITIAL TREATMENT

Herpes confirmed or suspected (history or sign of vesicles):
Treat for genital herpes with acyclovir, valacyclovir, or famciclovir
Syphilis confirmed (dark-field, FA, or PCR showing *T. pallidum*, or RPR reactive):
Benzathine penicillin 2.4 million units IM once to patient, recent (e.g., within 3 months) seronegative partner(s), and all seropositive partner(s)
Chancroid confirmed or suspected (diagnostic test positive, or HSV and syphilis excluded, and lesion persists):
Ciprofloxacin 500 mg PO as single dose
or
Ceftriaxone 250 mg IM as single dose

NOTE: FA, fluorescent antibody; PCR, polymerase chain reaction; RPR, rapid plasma reagin; ELISA, enzyme-linked immunosorbent assay; HSV, herpes simplex virus.

other microbiologic studies. Sigmoidoscopy or colonoscopy shows inflammation limited to the rectum in proctitis or disease extending at least into the sigmoid colon in proctocolitis.

The AIDS era has brought an extraordinary shift in the clinical and etiologic spectrum of intestinal infections among homosexual men. The number of cases of the acute intestinal STIs described above has fallen as high-risk sexual behaviors have become less common in this group. At the same time, the number of AIDS-related opportunistic intestinal infections has risen rapidly, many associated with chronic or recurrent symptoms. Acquisition of *N. gonorrhoeae*, HSV, or *C. trachomatis* during receptive anorectal intercourse causes most cases of infectious proctitis. Primary and secondary syphilis can also produce anal or anorectal lesions, with or without symptoms. Gonococcal or chlamydial proctitis typically involves the most distal rectal mucosa and the anal crypts and is clinically mild, without systemic manifestations. In contrast, primary proctitis due to HSV and proctocolitis due to the strains of *C. trachomatis* that cause LGV usually produce severe anorectal pain and often cause fever. Perianal ulcers and inguinal lymphadenopathy, most commonly due to HSV, can also occur in LGV or syphilis. Sacral nerve root radiculopathies, usually presenting as urinary retention, laxity of the anal sphincter, or constipation, may complicate primary herpetic proctitis. In LGV, rectal biopsy typically shows crypt abscesses, granulomas, and giant cells—findings resembling those in Crohn's disease; such findings should always prompt rectal culture and serology for LGV, which is a curable infection. Syphilis can also produce rectal granulomas, usually in association with infiltration by plasma cells or other mononuclear cells.

Diarrhea and abdominal bloating or cramping pain without anorectal symptoms and with normal findings on anoscopy and sigmoidoscopy occur with inflammation of the small intestine (enteritis) or with proximal colitis. In homosexual men without HIV infection, enteritis is often attributable to *Giardia lamblia*. Sexually acquired proctocolitis is most often due to *Campylobacter* or *Shigella* spp.

PREVENTION AND CONTROL OF STDS

Although rates of all curable STDs fell in the United States throughout the 1990s, all other industrialized countries of comparable economic development have made greater progress. For example, Sweden has virtually eliminated the transmission of gonorrhea, syphilis, and chancroid and has achieved very low rates of HIV transmission. Elimination of syphilis as an endemic disease is now a national goal in the United States, but stronger efforts toward prevention and control of all STDs are necessary.

Prevention and control of STDs require (1) reduction of the average rate of sexual exposure through alteration of behaviors and behavioral norms among both susceptible and infected persons in all population groups; (2) reduction of the efficiency of transmission through the promotion of safer sexual practices, the use of condoms during casual or commercial sex, hepatitis B immunization, and many other approaches (e.g., early detection and treatment of other STIs to reduce the efficiency of sexual transmission of HIV); and (3) shortening of the duration of infectivity of STDs through early detection and curative or suppressive treatment of patients and their sexual partners.

Primary care physicians usually do not screen for illicit drug use or sexual risk behaviors, even when typical patients have classic presentations for HIV infection or another STD. In fact, clinicians often focus only on detection and treatment of curable STDs to reduce the duration of infectivity. They generally have relatively little training or experience in risk assessment, counseling on risk reduction, tracing and treatment of sexual contacts, or condom promotion. Financial and time constraints imposed by managed-care practice patterns may further curtail screening and prevention services. As outlined in Fig. 132-3, the efforts of clinicians simply to detect and treat STDs depend in part on societal efforts to teach young people how to recognize symptoms of STDs; to motivate those with symptoms to seek care promptly; and to make such care accessible, affordable, and acceptable, especially to the young indigent patients most likely to acquire an STD.

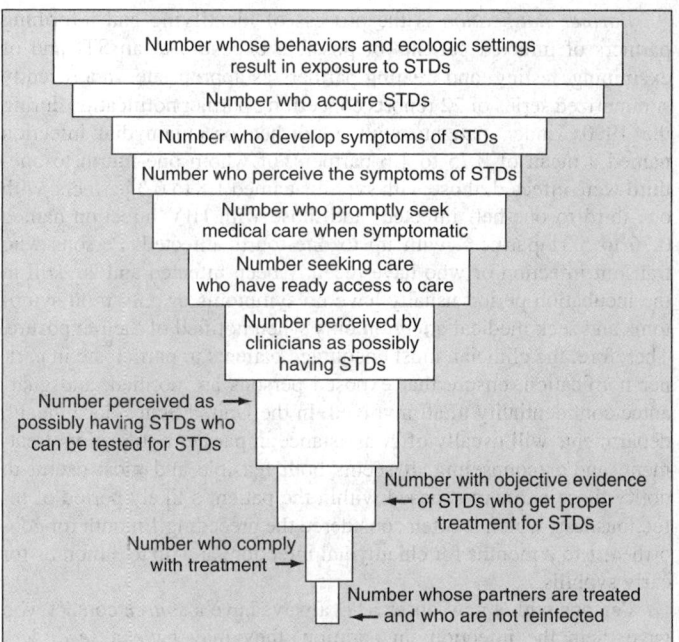

FIGURE 132-3 Critical control points for preventive and clinical interventions against sexually transmitted diseases (STDs). *(Adapted from HT Waller and MA Piot: Bull World Health Organ 41:75, 1969 and 43:1, 1970; and from "Resource allocation model for public health planning—a case study of tuberculosis control," Bull World Health Organ 84(Suppl) 1973.)*

Since many infected individuals develop no symptoms or fail to recognize and report symptoms, clinicians should routinely perform an STI risk assessment for teenagers and young adults as a selective screen. U.S. Preventive Services Task Force Guidelines recommend screening sexually active females ≤25 years of age for *C. trachomatis* whenever they present for health care (at least once a year); older women should be tested if they have more than one sexual partner, have begun a new sexual relationship since the previous test, or have another STD diagnosed. In the United States, widespread selective screening of young women for cervical *C. trachomatis* infection in some regions has been associated with a 50 to 60% drop in prevalence, and such screening also protects the individual woman from PID. Sensitive urine-based genetic amplification tests permit expansion of screening to men and teenage boys and to women in settings where a pelvic examination is not planned or is impractical.

Although gonorrhea is now substantially less common than chlamydial infection in industrialized countries, screening tests for *N. gonorrhoeae* are still appropriate for women and teenage girls attending STD clinics and for sexually active teens and young women from areas of high gonorrhea prevalence. Routine screening of asymptomatic men for urethral gonorrhea has a very low yield in the primary care setting. However, genetic amplification tests that combine screening for *N. gonorrhoeae* and *C. trachomatis* in a single low-cost assay may facilitate the prevention and control of both infections in populations at high risk.

All patients with newly detected STIs or at high risk for STIs according to routine risk assessment as well as all pregnant women should be encouraged to undergo serologic testing for syphilis and HIV infection, with appropriate HIV counseling before and after testing. Several randomized trials have shown that *risk reduction counseling* of patients with STDs significantly lowers subsequent risk of acquiring an STD. Preimmunization serologic testing for antibody to HBV is indicated for unvaccinated persons who are known to be at high risk, such as homosexually active men and injection drug users. In most young persons, however, it is more cost-effective to vaccinate against HBV without serologic screening.

Partner notification is the process of identifying and informing partners of infected patients of possible exposure to an STI and of examining, testing, and treating partners as appropriate. In a recently summarized series of 22 reports concerning partner notification during the 1990s, index patients with gonorrhea or chlamydial infection named a mean of 0.75 to 1.6 partners, of whom one-fourth to one-third were infected; those with syphilis named 1.8 to 6.3 partners, with one-third to one-half infected; and those with HIV infection named 0.76 to 5.31 partners, with up to one-fourth infected. Persons who transmit infection or who have recently been infected and are still in the incubation period usually have no symptoms or only mild symptoms and seek medical attention only when notified of their exposure. Therefore, the clinician must encourage patients to participate in partner notification, ensure that exposed persons are notified, and guarantee confidentiality to all involved. In the United States, local health departments will usually offer assistance in partner notification, treatment, and/or counseling. It seems both feasible and most useful to notify those partners exposed within the patient's likely period of infectiousness, which is often considered the preceding 1 month for gonorrhea, 1 to 2 months for chlamydial infection, and up to 3 months for early syphilis.

Persons with a new-onset STD always have a *source* contact who gave them the infection; in addition, they may have a *secondary* (*spread* or *exposed*) contact with whom they had sex after becoming infected. The identification and treatment of these two types of contacts have different objectives. Treatment of the source contact (often a casual contact) benefits the community by preventing further transmission; treatment of the recently exposed secondary contact (typically a spouse or another steady sexual partner) prevents both the development of serious complications (such as PID) in the partner and reinfection of the index patient.

In summary, clinicians and public health agencies share responsibility for the prevention and control of STDs. In the managed-care era, the role of primary care clinicians has become increasingly important in prevention as well as in diagnosis and treatment.

BIBLIOGRAPHY

CENTERS FOR DISEASE CONTROL AND PREVENTION: 1998 Guidelines for treatment of sexually transmitted diseases. MMWR 47(RR-1):1, 1998

CHERNESKY MA: Nucleic acid tests for the diagnosis of sexually transmitted diseases. FEMS Immunol Med Microbiol 24:437, 1999

CURTIS R, HOLMES KK: Individual-level risk assessment for STD/HIV, in *Sexually Transmitted Diseases*, 3d ed, KK Holmes et al (eds). New York, McGraw-Hill, 1999, pp 669–683

DALABETTA G et al (eds): Syndromic management of sexually transmitted diseases. Sex Transm Dis 74(Suppl 1):S1, 1998

DIVISION OF STD PREVENTION: *Sexually Transmitted Disease Surveillance, 1998*. Atlanta, Centers for Disease Control and Prevention, 1999

ECKERT LO et al: Vulvovaginal candidiasis: Clinical manifestations, risk factors, and algorithm for case management. Obstet Gynecol 92:757, 1998

HOLMES KK et al (eds): *Sexually Transmitted Diseases*, 3d ed. New York, McGraw-Hill, 1999

INSTITUTE OF MEDICINE: *The Hidden Epidemic: Confronting Sexually Transmitted Diseases*, TR Eng, WT Butler (eds). Washington, DC, National Academy Press, 1997

JOINT UNITED NATIONS PROGRAMME ON HIV/AIDS (UNAIDS) AND WORLD HEALTH ORGANIZATION (WHO): *Sexually Transmitted Diseases: Policies and Principles for Prevention and Care*. UNAIDS/97.6, Geneva, 1999

KAMB ML et al: Efficacy of risk-reduction counseling to prevent human immunodeficiency virus and sexually transmitted diseases: A randomized controlled trial. Project RESPECT Study Group. JAMA 280:1161, 1998

MERTZ KJ et al: Etiology of genital ulcers and prevalence of human immunodeficiency virus coinfection in 10 US cities. The Genital Ulcer Disease Surveillance Group. J Infect Dis 178:1795, 1998

ROTHENBERG R, POTTERAT J: Partner notification for sexually transmitted diseases and HIV infection, in *Sexually Transmitted Diseases*, 3d ed, KK Holmes et al (eds). New York, McGraw-Hill, 1999

TAO G et al: Missed opportunities to assess sexually transmitted diseases in U.S. adults during routine medical checkups. Am J Prev Med 18:109, 2000

VAN DYCK E et al (eds): *Laboratory Diagnosis of Sexually Transmitted Diseases*. Albany, NY, World Health Organization, 1999

133   *King K. Holmes, Robert C. Brunham*

PELVIC INFLAMMATORY DISEASE

DEFINITION   The term *pelvic inflammatory disease* (PID) usually refers to infection that ascends from the cervix or vagina to involve the endometrium and/or fallopian tubes. Infection can extend beyond the reproductive tract to cause pelvic peritonitis, generalized peritonitis, perihepatitis, or pelvic abscess. In rare instances, infection extends secondarily to the pelvic organs from adjacent foci of inflammation (e.g., sites of appendicitis, regional ileitis, or diverticulitis), as a result of hematogenous dissemination (e.g., of tuberculosis), or as a rare complication of certain tropical diseases (e.g., schistosomiasis). Intrauterine infection can be primary (spontaneously occurring and usually sexually transmitted) or secondary to invasive intrauterine surgical procedures (e.g., dilatation and curettage, termination of pregnancy, insertion of an intrauterine device, or hysterosalpingography) or to parturition. Endometritis or endomyometritis is particularly common following delivery by emergency cesarean section when antibiotic prophylaxis is not used.

PID is uncommon during pregnancy itself. The uterotubal junction is closed as early as the seventh week of pregnancy, and the chorioamnion becomes approximated to the endocervical os, sealing off the intrauterine cavity, at the twelfth to fifteenth week of gestation. As a consequence, ascending intrauterine infection prior to the twelfth week of gestation may be associated (as either cause or effect) with endometritis and spontaneous abortion, while ascending infection after the twelfth week may be associated with chorioamnionitis.

Spontaneously occurring PID can be of the chronic or the acute type. Chronic PID due to *Mycobacterium tuberculosis* has become uncommon in industrialized countries. However, subacute or chronic PID caused by persistent or repeated infection with *Chlamydia trachomatis* is thought to be common.

Although the clinical diagnosis of PID is imprecise, the use of endometrial biopsy together with laparoscopy provides objective evidence of a continuum progressing from cervicitis alone to endometritis, to salpingitis, and to peritonitis. In this chapter, *PID* is used to refer to the clinical syndrome that includes these conditions, while the term *salpingitis* is restricted to cases of visually or histopathologically confirmed inflammation of the fallopian tubes. The distinction between endometritis and salpingitis may be important, because long-term sequelae are much more common after salpingitis. These sequelae include infertility due to bilateral tubal occlusion, peritubal adhesions, ectopic pregnancy due to tubal damage without occlusion, chronic pelvic pain, and recurrent PID.

ETIOLOGY   The etiology of PID has varied greatly among studies for reasons related to the selection of patients, the prevalence of sexually transmitted disease (STD) pathogens at the time and place of the study, and methodology. As is summarized in Table 133-1, the agents most often implicated in acute PID include those that are primary causes of cervicitis (*Neisseria gonorrhoeae* and *C. trachomatis*) and those that can be regarded as components of an altered vaginal flora.

Table 133-1   Cervical and Vaginal Organisms Most Often Implicated in Acute PID

Cervical Pathogens	Vaginal Flora Components
Neisseria gonorrhoeae *Chlamydia trachomatis*	Anaerobic bacteria
	Prevotella, Peptostreptococcus, Mobiluncus, and *Actinomyces*
	Facultative bacteria
	Enterobacteriaceae, *Haemophilus influenzae, Gardnerella vaginalis,* group B *Streptococcus*
	Mycoplasmas
	Mycoplasma hominis, Ureaplasma urealyticum, ?Mycoplasma genitalium

found in 65% of women with a clinical diagnosis of PID at San Francisco General Hospital and in 85% of patients with proven salpingitis and endometritis in Seattle; in both studies, gonorrhea was nearly twice as common as chlamydial infection and dual infection was common. However, in Western Europe and parts of the United States, as gonococcal infection has come under much better control, endocervical gonococcal infection has been found in a declining proportion of women with PID, and the microbial etiology cannot be defined in a substantial proportion of cases. In general, PID is most often associated with gonorrhea where there is a high incidence of gonorrhea—e.g., in developing countries and in indigent, inner-city populations in the United States. In several studies of women with PID, up to two-thirds of women with endocervical cultures positive for *N. gonorrhoeae* have also had endometrial, peritoneal, or tubal cultures positive for this organism. Similarly, studies of women with proven PID have shown that *C. trachomatis* can be demonstrated by culture or immunofluorescent staining in the endometrium or tubes of the majority of those who have endocervical chlamydial infection.

Anaerobic and facultative anaerobic organisms (especially *Prevotella* species, peptostreptococci, *Escherichia coli*, and group B streptococci) and genital mycoplasmas have been isolated from specimens obtained at laparoscopy from the peritoneal fluid or fallopian tubes in a varying proportion—typically one-fourth to one-third—of women with PID studied in the United States. These vaginal organisms can be found in association with chlamydial or gonococcal infection as well as in the absence of such infection. The importance of vaginal organisms in salpingitis has probably been overestimated in some studies in which specimens were obtained for cultures by culdocentesis or endometrial aspiration, procedures in which contamination of the aspirated specimen by vaginal flora is possible. However, specimens obtained by laparoscopy from some patients with PID have also contained anaerobic and facultative species. A compilation of seven studies of the microbial etiology of PID showed that 5 to 78% of patients had anaerobes and facultative bacteria isolated from the upper genital tract. It is extremely difficult to determine the exact microbial etiology of an individual case of PID because of the frequency of mixed infection, the difficulty in sampling the fallopian tube itself, and the complexity of the microbiologic techniques required to detect the various fastidious pathogens involved. This situation has implications for the approach to empirical antimicrobial treatment of PID.

In general, first episodes of acute PID are particularly likely to be caused by *N. gonorrhoeae* and/or *C. trachomatis*. These sexually transmitted pathogens are implicated somewhat less often in recurrent bouts of acute PID, in episodes occurring in women with intrauterine devices (IUDs), in episodes precipitated by invasive intrauterine diagnostic or therapeutic procedures (which are often associated with ascending infection caused by endogenous vaginal flora), and perhaps in HIV-associated PID.

EPIDEMIOLOGY It has been estimated that about 850,000 cases of PID occurred in the United States each year during the mid-1970s. PID is not a reportable disease in the United States; surveillance of physicians in private practice and of hospital discharges suggests that the incidence of PID increased from the mid-1960s through the mid-1970s and may then have decreased. Hospitalization for acute PID declined steadily from 1982 through 1997, and initial visits to physicians' offices for PID have been declining since the mid-1980s. Furthermore, the number of hospitalizations for ectopic pregnancy in the United States fell by about two-thirds from 1989 to 1997.

Acute PID is almost exclusively a disease of sexually active women. Important risk factors include a history of salpingitis or of recent vaginal douching; the use of an IUD, particularly the Dalkon shield, has also been a risk factor. In most studies, the relative risk of PID among IUD users is higher in nulliparous than in parous women and is greatest during the first few months after IUD insertion. The increased risk of PID among IUD users is evident mainly among those with multiple sex partners. In contrast, women using oral contraceptives appear to be at decreased risk of PID. Barrier methods of contraception also make PID less likely by reducing the risk of chlamydial and gonococcal infection. Tubal sterilization reduces (but does not completely eliminate) the risk of salpingitis by preventing intraluminal spread of infection into the tubes.

PATHOGENESIS Factors cited as possibly contributing to the upward spread of gonococci and chlamydiae from the endocervix to the endometrium and endosalpinx include estrogen-dominated (thin) cervical mucus, attachment to sperm that migrate upward into the tubes, use of an IUD, vaginal douching, menstruation, and subendometrial myometrial contractions, which move particulate matter from the cervix to the fundus of the uterus between days 5 and 14 of the menstrual cycle. It is important that the onset of symptoms of *N. gonorrhoeae*–associated and *C. trachomatis*–associated PID often occurs during or soon after the menstrual period. In fallopian tube organ cultures in vitro, gonococci attach to the surface of the secretory columnar cells (but not the ciliated cells) of the endosalpinx. Gonococcal pili and perhaps other surface proteins are important in this attachment. Gonococci are then taken into the secretory cells by endocytosis. They pass through the cells—and perhaps between cells—and are extruded through the base of the cell into the submucosal connective tissue. Ciliary motion ceases, and then ciliated cells, although not directly invaded by gonococci, are sloughed from the mucosa—a factor that may render the tubes more susceptible to superinfection by other organisms. It is uncertain whether this loss of ciliated cells is irreversible in vivo. Gonococcal endotoxin and peptidoglycan as well as certain cytokines (such as tumor necrosis factor α) appear to be responsible for these cytotoxic effects.

C. trachomatis also infects the columnar cells of the fallopian tube but produces little damage in tubal organ cultures, perhaps because the host response is more important than directly toxic effects of bacterial products in the pathogenesis of chlamydial salpingitis. *Chlamydia*-infected epithelial cells secrete a number of proinflammatory cytokines, which are chemotactic for neutrophils and mononuclear cells. Routine endometrial biopsies from women with chlamydial mucopurulent cervicitis (MPC) show endometritis in approximately one-half of cases. Endometritis detected in this way is sometimes but not always associated with symptoms of severe abdominal pain, presentation during days 1 through 7 of the menstrual cycle, signs of uterine tenderness, and an erythrocyte sedimentation rate (ESR) of ≥ 20 mm/h. Adnexal tenderness, cervical motion tenderness, and rebound tenderness as well as leukocytosis and elevated C-reactive protein levels are all more common in women with laparoscopic evidence of salpingitis than in those with endometritis alone. Chlamydial inclusions are demonstrable by direct immunofluorescence in columnar epithelial cells of the endometrium and endosalpinx. The endometrial biopsies usually show neutrophils infiltrating the epithelium and plasma cells infiltrating the stroma, findings also seen in gonococcal endometritis but not in the uninfected endometrium. Experimental inoculation of the fallopian tubes of lower primates with *C. trachomatis* has shown that repeated exposure to *C. trachomatis* leads to the greatest degree of tissue inflammation and damage; this finding suggests that immunopathology also underlies the pathogenesis of chlamydial disease.

The pathogenesis of PID attributable to mycoplasmas or other vaginal anaerobic or facultative organisms is less well studied. It is possible that other vaginal organisms implicated in PID often cause tubal infection in women whose tubes have already been damaged by a primary sexually transmitted pathogen (i.e., *N. gonorrhoeae* or *C. trachomatis*). The vaginal organisms implicated in PID are found in the vagina most often and in greatest concentration in bacterial vaginosis, and there is epidemiologic evidence that bacterial vaginosis itself is a predisposing factor for PID (just as poor oral hygiene is a risk factor for aspiration pneumonia).

Certain other iatrogenic factors, such as dilatation and curettage or cesarean section, can increase the risk of PID in women with endocervical gonococcal or chlamydial infection. Evidence indicates that among women undergoing cesarean section, the presence of bacterial vaginosis increases the risk of postpartum endometritis.

CLINICAL MANIFESTATIONS **Tuberculous Salpingitis** Unlike nontuberculous salpingitis, genital tuberculosis often occurs in older women, many of whom are postmenopausal. Presenting symptoms include abnormal vaginal bleeding, pain (including dysmenorrhea), and infertility. Bimanual pelvic examination may be normal, though about one-quarter of these women have had adnexal masses. Endometrial biopsy shows tuberculous granulomas and provides optimal specimens for culture.

Nontuberculous Salpingitis Symptoms of nontuberculous salpingitis classically evolve from a yellow or malodorous vaginal discharge caused by MPC and/or bacterial vaginosis to midline abdominal pain and abnormal vaginal bleeding caused by endometritis and then to bilateral lower abdominal and pelvic pain caused by salpingitis, with nausea and vomiting and increased abdominal tenderness caused by peritonitis. Some patients have diffuse abdominal pain caused by generalized peritonitis or pleuritic right upper quadrant pain caused by perihepatitis. The pattern in which symptoms evolve varies from patient to patient and is also related to the etiology of the PID.

The onset of IUD-associated PID is typically gradual and may be preceded by the malodorous vaginal discharge characteristic of bacterial vaginosis. The onset of gonococcal PID may be more acute than that of chlamydial PID, and PID of either etiology usually presents during the first half of the menstrual cycle.

The abdominal pain in nontuberculous salpingitis is usually described as dull or aching. In some cases, pain is lacking or is atypical, and active inflammatory changes are found in the course of an unrelated evaluation or procedure, such as a tubal ligation or a laparoscopic evaluation for infertility. Abnormal uterine bleeding precedes or coincides with the onset of pain in ~40% of women with PID, symptoms of urethritis (dysuria) occur in 20%, and symptoms of proctitis (anorectal pain, tenesmus, and rectal discharge or bleeding) are occasionally seen in women with gonococcal or chlamydial infection.

Speculum examination shows evidence of MPC (yellow endocervical discharge, easily induced endocervical bleeding) in the majority of women with gonococcal or chlamydial PID. Cervical motion tenderness is produced by stretching of the adnexal attachments on the side toward which the cervix is pushed. Bimanual examination reveals uterine fundal tenderness due to endometritis and abnormal adnexal tenderness due to salpingitis that is usually, but not necessarily, bilateral. Adnexal swelling is palpable in about one-half of women with acute salpingitis, but evaluation of the adnexae in a patient with marked tenderness—even by an experienced examiner—is not reliable. The initial temperature is >38°C in only about one-third of patients with acute salpingitis; thus fever is not required for the diagnosis. Laboratory findings include elevation of the ESR in 75% of patients with acute salpingitis and elevation of the peripheral white blood cell count in up to 60%.

Certain clinical manifestations of acute PID have been correlated with microbial etiology. For example, the onset of salpingitis is related to menses in women with gonococcal or chlamydial infection. Women with *N. gonorrhoeae*– or *C. trachomatis*–associated salpingitis are significantly younger than women with salpingitis of other etiologies. In a Swedish study, women with *Chlamydia*-associated salpingitis had more indolent disease, with mild symptoms of significantly longer duration and less fever, than women with gonorrhea-associated salpingitis. Women with polymicrobial PID more often have tubal or pelvic abscess formation. It is suspected that, for all recognized cases of symptomatic acute chlamydial salpingitis, there is a comparable number of unrecognized cases of indolent or mildly symptomatic chlamydial salpingitis. Furthermore, it is thought that subclinical chronic or recurrent chlamydial salpingitis may be a major cause of female infertility.

Perihepatitis and Periappendicitis Symptoms of perihepatitis, including pleuritic upper abdominal pain and tenderness (usually localized to the right upper quadrant), develop in 3 to 10% of women with acute PID. The onset of symptoms of perihepatitis takes place during or after the onset of symptoms of PID and may overshadow lower abdominal symptoms, thereby leading to a mistaken diagnosis of cholecystitis. In perhaps 5% of cases of acute salpingitis, early laparoscopy reveals inflammation ranging from edema and erythema of the liver capsule to exudate with fibrinous adhesions between the visceral and parietal peritoneum. When treatment is delayed and laparoscopy is performed late, dense "violin-string" adhesions are seen over the liver; chronic exertional or positional right upper quadrant pain ensues when traction is placed on the adhesions. Although perihepatitis, also known as the *Fitz-Hugh–Curtis syndrome*, was for many years specifically attributed to gonococcal PID, most cases are now attributed to chlamydial salpingitis. In patients with chlamydial salpingitis, serum titers of microimmunofluorescent antibody to *C. trachomatis* are typically much higher when perihepatitis is present than when it is absent, and it has been suggested that repeated chlamydial infections are responsible for perihepatitis.

Physical findings include right upper quadrant tenderness and usually include adnexal tenderness and cervicitis, even in patients whose symptoms are not suggestive of salpingitis. Liver function tests are nearly always normal, since inflammation is largely limited to the liver capsule and usually spares the parenchyma. Ultrasonography of the right upper quadrant is normal. The presence of MPC and pelvic tenderness in a young woman with subacute pleuritic right upper quadrant pain and normal ultrasonography of the gallbladder points to a diagnosis of perihepatitis.

Periappendicitis (appendiceal serositis without involvement of the intestinal mucosa) has been found in ~5% of patients undergoing appendectomy for suspected appendicitis and can occur as a complication of gonococcal or chlamydial salpingitis.

Influence of HIV Infection HIV infection with immunosuppression increases the risk of repeated gonococcal and chlamydial infections among repeatedly exposed female sex workers, presumably by attenuating the immune response to repeated infection. Further, among women who acquire gonococcal or chlamydial infection of the cervix, HIV infection with immunosuppression increases the likelihood of developing clinical manifestations of salpingitis. Finally, among women with salpingitis, HIV infection is associated with increased severity of salpingitis and with tuboovarian abscess requiring hospitalization and surgical drainage. However, among African women with confirmed PID, those with HIV infection appear less likely to have gonorrhea or chlamydial infection than those without HIV infection, a difference suggesting that other etiologies are especially important in the immunosuppressed patient. Nonetheless, among women with HIV infection and salpingitis, the clinical reponse to conventional antimicrobial therapy (coupled with drainage of tuboovarian abscess, when found) has been satisfactory.

DIAGNOSIS Early diagnosis and initiation of therapy are essential to minimize tubal scarring. A reanalysis of Weström's cohort of Swedish women with proven salpingitis showed that those who delayed seeking care were three times more likely than those who sought care promptly to experience subsequent infertility or ectopic pregnancy. Appropriate treatment must not be withheld from patients who have an equivocal diagnosis; it is better to err on the side of overdiagnosis and overtreatment. On the other hand, it is essential to differentiate between salpingitis and other pelvic pathology, particularly surgical emergencies such as appendicitis and ectopic pregnancy.

No readily available clinical finding or laboratory test, short of laparoscopy, definitively identifies salpingitis, and routine laparoscopy to confirm suspected salpingitis is generally impractical. Most patients with acute PID have lower abdominal pain of <3 weeks' duration, pelvic tenderness on bimanual pelvic examination, and evidence of lower genital tract infection (e.g., MPC). Approximately 60% of such patients have salpingitis at laparoscopy. Among the patients with these findings, a rectal temperature >38°C, a palpable adnexal mass, and elevation of the ESR over 15 mm/h also raise the probability of salpingitis, which has been found at laparoscopy in 68% of patients with one of these additional findings, 90% of patients with two, and 96% of patients with three. However, only 17% of all patients with laparoscopy-confirmed salpingitis have had all three additional findings.

MPC is probably responsible for the presence of neutrophils in vaginal fluid in PID. In a woman with pelvic pain and tenderness, demonstration of an increased number of neutrophils (30 per 1000× microscopic field in strands of cervical mucus) increases the predictive value of a clinical diagnosis of acute PID.

Several clinical features other than the presence of cervicitis also favor the diagnosis of acute PID. These include onset with menses, history of recent abnormal menstrual bleeding, presence of an IUD, history of salpingitis, and sexual exposure to a male with urethritis. Detection of polymorphonuclear leukocytes in pelvic peritoneal fluid aspirated by culdocentesis supports a diagnosis of suspected salpingitis. Urethritis or proctitis may occur in chlamydial or gonococcal infection but may also represent a urinary tract source or an intestinal source, respectively. Appendicitis or another disorder of the gut is favored by the early onset of anorexia, nausea, or vomiting; the onset of pain later than day 14 of the menstrual cycle; or unilateral pain limited to the right or left lower quadrant. All women in whom the diagnosis of PID is being considered should be evaluated for ectopic pregnancy. The more sensitive serum assays for human β-chorionic gonadotropin are usually positive when ectopic pregnancy is the diagnosis. Ultrasonography and magnetic resonance imaging (MRI) can be useful for the identification of tuboovarian or pelvic abscess. MRI or intravaginal ultrasound assessment of the tubes has been reported to show increased tubal diameter, intratubal fluid, or tubal wall thickening in cases of salpingitis.

Laparoscopy is the most specific method for diagnosis of acute salpingitis. Although laparoscopic findings may be normal if inflammation is limited to the endosalpinx or the endometrium, patients with suspected PID who have a normal laparoscopy have a better prognosis (with no sequelae at all or fewer sequelae) than patients who have abnormal laparoscopic findings. The primary and uncontested value of laparoscopy in women with lower abdominal pain is for the exclusion of other surgical problems. Some of the most common or serious problems that may be confused with salpingitis (e.g., acute appendicitis, ectopic pregnancy, corpus luteum bleeding, ovarian tumor) are unilateral. Unilateral pain or pelvic mass, though not incompatible with PID, is a strong indication for laparoscopy unless the clinical picture warrants laparotomy instead. Atypical clinical findings, such as the absence of lower genital tract infection, a missed menstrual period, a positive pregnancy test, or failure to respond to appropriate therapy, are other frequent indications for laparoscopy.

Laparoscopic criteria used for the diagnosis of salpingitis include (1) erythema of the fallopian tube, (2) edema of the fallopian tube, and (3) seropurulent exudate or fresh, easily lysed adhesions at the fimbriated end or on the serosal surface of a fallopian tube.

Endometrial biopsy is relatively sensitive and specific for the diagnosis of endometritis when the endometrial changes described above are found, and the presence of endometritis correlates well with the presence of salpingitis. Endometritis is found in at least three-fourths of women with laparoscopically confirmed salpingitis and is not found in women without PID.

The etiologic diagnosis of PID can be further studied by culture or other testing of specimens obtained by endocervical swab, endometrial aspiration, or culdocentesis or by laparoscopy or laparotomy. Endocervical swab specimens should be examined by Gram's staining for neutrophils and gram-negative diplococci and by culture or DNA amplification test for *N. gonorrhoeae*. Compared with culture, the sensitivity of Gram's staining is ~60% and the specificity is >95%. The endocervical swab specimen should also be tested for *C. trachomatis* by culture or amplification assays for chlamydial DNA or RNA. Although detection of either *N. gonorrhoeae* or *C. trachomatis* in the endocervix does not prove that either agent is also present in the upper genital tract, this finding strongly supports the diagnosis of PID. The clinical diagnosis of PID made by expert gynecologists is confirmed by laparoscopy or endometrial biopsy in only ~60% of patients but

in ~90% of those who also have cultures positive for *N. gonorrhoeae* or *C. trachomatis*. There is no evidence that the isolation of anaerobes or facultative aerobes from the cervix or vagina correlates with the presence of these organisms in the upper genital tract in acute PID, but this point has not been well studied. In one study, the isolation of *Haemophilus influenzae* from the endocervix was highly correlated with this organism's recovery from the fallopian tube in cases of salpingitis. Despite the risk of contamination of endometrial specimens with components of the vaginal flora, one study showed a 2.6-fold increase in the rate of recovery of anaerobic gram-negative rods (especially *Prevotella*, black-pigmented rods, and *Fusobacterium*) by endometrial biopsy in women with endometritis compared with control women. When laparoscopy is performed, material can be obtained directly from the cul-de-sac or the fimbriated opening of the tube or by tubal aspiration if pyosalpinx is present. Such specimens should be cultured for anaerobic and facultative pathogens as well as for *N. gonorrhoeae* and *C. trachomatis*.

TREATMENT Women with PID can be treated as either outpatients or inpatients. Over the past decade, the costs of PID treatment have declined considerably because of the increased management of patients in the ambulatory setting, with use of highly active, well-absorbed antimicrobial agents. Nonetheless, hospitalization may be necessary and should be considered when (1) the diagnosis is uncertain and surgical emergencies such as appendicitis and ectopic pregnancy cannot be excluded, (2) pelvic abscess is suspected, (3) severe illness or nausea and vomiting preclude outpatient management, (4) the patient has HIV infection, (5) the patient is assessed as unable to follow or tolerate an outpatient regimen, or (6) the patient has failed to respond to outpatient therapy. If outpatient treatment is embarked on, clinical follow-up after 48 to 72 h of antibiotic treatment should be arranged. Treatment should cover *N. gonorrhoeae*, *C. trachomatis*, gram-negative facultative bacteria (especially *E. coli* and *H. influenzae*), vaginal anaerobes, and group B streptococci. Several antimicrobial combinations do provide a broad spectrum of activity against the major pathogens in vitro, but many have not been adequately evaluated for clinical efficacy in PID (Table 133-2).

Examples of Combination Regimens with Broad Activity Against Major Pathogens in PID Recommended combination regimens for ambulatory or parenteral management of PID are presented in Table 133-3.

Women managed as outpatients should receive a combined regimen with broad activity, such as ceftriaxone [250 mg intramuscularly (IM)] followed by doxycycline (100 mg by mouth, twice a day for 14 days). Metronidazole (500 mg by mouth twice daily) can be added, if tolerated, to enhance activity against anaerobes. Alternatively, ofloxacin (400 mg twice daily) plus metronidazole (500 mg twice daily), both continued for 14 days, provide good coverage of the major pathogens.

The following two parenteral regimens have given nearly identical results in a multicenter randomized trial:

1. Doxycycline [100 mg twice a day, given intravenously (IV) or orally] plus cefotetan (2.0 g IV every 12 h) or cefoxitin (2.0 g IV every 6 h). These drugs should be continued by the IV route for at least 48 h after the patient's condition improves, then followed with doxycycline (100 mg by mouth, twice a day) to complete 14 days of therapy.

2. Clindamycin (900 mg IV every 8 h) plus gentamicin (2.0 mg/kg IV or IM followed by 1.5 mg/kg every 8 h) in patients with normal renal function. Once-daily dosing of gentamicin (with combination of the total daily dose into a single daily dose) has not been evaluated in PID but has been efficacious in other serious infections and could be substituted. Treatment with these drugs should be continued for at least 48 h after the patient's condition improves, then followed with doxycycline (100 mg orally twice a day) or with clindamycin (450 mg orally four times a day) to complete 14 days of therapy. In cases with

Agent	Relative Activity Against Indicated Pathogen[a]					
			Vaginal Anaerobes		PID-Associated Facultative	
	N. gonorrhoeae	C. trachomatis	GPC[b]	GNR[c]	GNR	M. hominis
Ampicillin/amoxicillin	2+	2+	4+	2+	2+	0
Doxycycline	2+	4+	2+	1+	1+	2+
Cefoxitin, cefotetan	3+	0	4+	3+	3+	0
Ceftriaxone	4+	0	3+	2+	4+	0
Gentamicin/tobramycin	2+	0	1+	0	4+	2+?
Ciprofloxacin	4+	0	1+	0	3+	2+
Ofloxacin	4+	3+	1+	1+	4+	1+
Levofloxacin	4+	3+	2+	1+	4+	3+
Azithromycin	2+	4+	2+	?+	2+	?
Clindamycin	1+	3+	4+	4+	0	3+
Metronidazole	0	0	4+	4+	0	0

[a] No single antimicrobial agent offers optimal activity against all of these pathogens, but certain combinations (e.g., cefoxitin plus doxycycline, gentamicin plus clindamycin, and ofloxacin plus metronidazole) have complementary activity. Relative activity is indicated on a scale of 0 to 4+.

[b] GPC, gram-positive cocci (peptostreptococci).

[c] GNR, gram-negative rods. Anaerobic GNR include *Prevotella*; facultative GNR include Enterobacteriaceae and *Haemophilus influenzae*.

SOURCE: Adapted from Kato N et al: Clin Infect Dis 23(Suppl 1):S31, 1996; and Waites KB et al: Antimicrob Agents Chemother 43:2571, 1999.

tuboovarian abscess, many experts use oral clindamycin rather than doxycycline for continued therapy to provide better coverage for anaerobic infection.

Management of Sexual Partners Sexual partners of patients with acute PID—particularly those who have been partners within the 1 to 2 months before the onset of symptoms of PID—should be examined for STDs and promptly treated with a regimen effective against uncomplicated gonococcal and chlamydial infection. An important point is that ≥50% of the sexual partners of women with gonococcal and/or chlamydial PID have subclinical urethral infection and may be unaware of their infection status. Treatment of PID should be considered inadequate until sexual partners have been properly evaluated and treated.

Follow-Up Hospitalized patients should show substantial clinical improvement within 3 to 5 days. Women treated as outpatients should be clinically reevaluated within 72 h. A follow-up telephone survey of women seen in an emergency room and given a prescription

Table 133-3 Combination Antimicrobial Regimens Recommended for Outpatient Treatment or for Parenteral Treatment of PID

Outpatient Regimens	Parenteral Regimens
Regimen A	**Regimen A**
Ofloxacin 400 mg PO bid for 14 days	Initiate parenteral therapy with either of the following regimens;
plus	continue parenteral therapy until 48 h after clinical improvement;
Metronidazole 500 mg PO bid for 14 days	then change to outpatient therapy, as described in text.
Regimen B	Cefotetan 2 g IV q12h
Ceftriaxone 250 mg IM once	*or*
plus	Cefoxitin 2 g IV q6h
Doxycycline 100 mg PO bid for 14 days	*plus*
plus[a]	Doxycycline 100 mg IV or PO q12h
Metronidazole 500 mg PO bid for 14 days	**Regimen B**
	Clindamycin 900 mg IV q8h
	plus
	Gentamicin, loading dose of 2 mg/kg IV or IM, then maintenance dose of 1.5 mg/kg q8h

[a] The addition of metronidazole is recommended by some experts.

SOURCE: Adapted from Centers for Disease Control and Prevention: MMWR 47:1, 1998.

for 10 days of oral doxycycline for PID found that 28% never filled the prescription and 41% stopped taking medication early (after an average of 4.1 days), often because of persistent symptoms, lack of symptoms, or side effects. Women not responding favorably to ambulatory therapy should be hospitalized. After completion of treatment, tests for persistent or recurrent infection with *N. gonorrhoeae* or *C. trachomatis* should be performed if symptoms persist or recur or if the patient has not complied with therapy or has been reexposed to an untreated sex partner.

Removal of an IUD Although a beneficial impact of IUD removal on the response of acute salpingitis to antimicrobial therapy and on the risk of recurrent salpingitis has not been proven, removal of the IUD 2 or 3 days after the initiation of antimicrobial therapy seems reasonable. When an IUD is removed, contraceptive counseling is essential.

Surgery Surgery is necessary for the treatment of salpingitis only in the face of life-threatening infection (such as rupture or threatened rupture of a tuboovarian abscess) or for drainage of an abscess. Ultrasonography and MRI are useful for diagnosing and monitoring pelvic abscesses. Conservative surgical procedures are usually sufficient. Pelvic abscesses can often be drained by posterior colpotomy, and peritoneal lavage can be used if there is generalized peritonitis.

PROGNOSIS Among 900 women who underwent long-term follow-up for a mean period of 8 years after successful treatment of an acute episode of PID with various regimens in Sweden, late sequelae included infertility due to bilateral tubal occlusion, ectopic pregnancy due to tubal scarring without occlusion, chronic pelvic pain, and recurrent salpingitis. Chronic pain lasting >6 months was seen in 18% of patients, and infertility due to tubal occlusion in 17%; 4% of the pregnancies that did occur were ectopic, representing approximately a sixfold increase over the expected rate of ectopic pregnancies. The rate of infertility after salpingitis was found to be related to the age of the patient, the duration of symptoms when treatment was started, the severity of salpingitis (as determined by laparoscopy) at the time of diagnosis, and the number of episodes of salpingitis. The postsalpingitis risk of infertility due to tubal occlusion among sexually active women not using contraceptives was 14% at 15 to 24 years of age and 26% at 25 to 34 years of age; the risk for women of all ages combined was 11% after one episode of salpingitis, 23% after two episodes, and 54% after three or more episodes. Women with chlamydial salpingitis who developed more severe inflammatory damage to the reproductive tract had significantly increased titers of antibody to the chlamydial heat-shock protein HSP60, as did women with infertility or ectopic pregnancy following chlamydial salpingitis. The risk of infertility after treated gonococcal salpingitis appeared lower than that after chlamydial salpingitis or polymicrobial PID. A study of outcomes of PID at the University of Washington found a sevenfold increase in the risk of ectopic pregnancy and an eightfold increase in the rate of hysterectomy after PID.

In several countries, a striking relationship has also been found between infertility due to tubal occlusion and the prevalence and titer of antibody to *C. trachomatis*. Recurrent salpingitis has been seen in ~15 to 25% of women treated for salpingitis in various studies.

PREVENTION Prevention of PID depends first on the effective control of gonococcal and chlamydial infection in the general population. Effective methods include the promotion of changes in sexual behavior and the use of barrier contraceptives together with ensuring ready access to modern methods of diagnosis of these infections and effective treatment of sex partners to control further spread. The decline in popularity of the IUD, particularly among nulliparous women, has undoubtedly helped to reduce the incidence of PID. It is also possible, but not proven, that the use of oral contraceptives and the declining proportion of women who have practiced vaginal douching since the link between douching and PID became known have contributed to lower rates of PID. A randomized controlled trial designed to determine whether selective screening for chlamydial infection reduced the risk of subsequent PID showed that women randomized to undergo screening had a 56% lower rate of PID over the following year than did women receiving the usual care without screening. This report strongly supports risk-based screening for *Chlamydia* as a highly effective way to reduce the incidence of PID and the prevalence of post-PID sequelae.

The complications and sequelae of salpingitis are minimized by early diagnosis and prompt effective treatment. It seems logical, but is unproven, that broad-spectrum therapy effective against all of the common causes of PID offers the best outcome. Although few methodologically sound clinical trials (especially with prolonged follow-up) have been conducted, one meta-analysis showed a benefit of providing good coverage against anaerobes. One placebo-controlled study showed that concurrent anti-inflammatory therapy with prednisolone hastened the reduction of acute inflammatory changes but did not improve the end results, as measured by fertility, hysterosalpingographic findings, or chronic pain. The potential value of anti-inflammatory therapy remains to be evaluated adequately.

BIBLIOGRAPHY

CENTERS FOR DISEASE CONTROL AND PREVENTION: 1998 Guidelines for treatment of sexually transmitted diseases. MMWR 47(RR-1):1, 1998

COHEN CR et al: Effect of human immunodeficiency virus type 1 infection upon acute salpingitis: A laparoscopic study. J Infect Dis 178:1352, 1998

HILLIER SL et al: Role of bacterial vaginosis–associated microorganisms in endometritis. Am J Obstet Gynecol 175:435, 1996

KIVIAT N et al: Endometrial histopathology in patients with culture-proven upper genital tract infection and laparoscopically diagnosed acute salpingitis. Am J Surg Pathol 14:167, 1990

RASMUSSEN SJ et al: Secretion of proinflammatory cytokines by epithelial cells in response to chlamydial infection suggests a central role for chlamydial pathogenesis. J Clin Invest 99:77, 1997

SCHOLES D et al: Prevention of pelvic inflammatory disease by screening for cervical chlamydial infection. N Engl J Med 334:1362, 1996

WALKER CK et al: Pelvic inflammatory disease: Meta-analysis of antimicrobial regimen efficacy. J Infect Dis 168:969, 1993

——— et al: Anaerobes in pelvic inflammatory disease: Implications for the Centers for Disease Control and Prevention's guidelines for the treatment of sexually transmitted diseases. Clin Infect Dis 28(Suppl 1):S29, 1999

WASSERHEIT JN et al: Microbial causes of proven pelvic inflammatory disease and efficacy of clindamycin with tobramycin. Ann Intern Med 104:187, 1986

WØLNER-HANSSEN P: Silent pelvic inflammatory disease: Is it overstated? Obstet Gynecol 86:321, 1995

Section 3
CLINICAL SYNDROMES: NOSOCOMIAL INFECTIONS

134

Robert A. Weinstein

INFECTION CONTROL IN THE HOSPITAL

The costs of nosocomial (hospital-acquired) infections are great. It is estimated that nosocomial infections cost $4.5 billion and contribute to 88,000 deaths annually. Although infection-control and hospital epidemiology activities have been the subjects of increasing scientific study over the past 30 years, efforts to lower infection risks have been continually challenged by the growing numbers of immunocompromised patients, antibiotic-resistant bacteria, fungal and viral superinfections, and invasive devices and procedures. Four international decennial conferences on infection control, organized by the Centers for Disease Control and Prevention (CDC), have clearly documented these formidable trends. This chapter reviews the basic surveillance and prevention activities that have been developed to deal with these problems and that form the foundation for current hospital epidemiology programs.

ORGANIZATION AND RESPONSIBILITIES OF INFECTION-CONTROL PROGRAMS The standards of the Joint Commission on Accreditation of Healthcare Organizations require all accredited hospitals to have an active program for surveillance, prevention, and control of nosocomial infections; a multidisciplinary infection-control committee usually oversees the program. The agents of the committee are the chairperson, who is preferably an infectious disease physician, and the infection-control practitioners, who are usually trained in nursing or medical technology and in epidemiology and public health. Education of physicians in infection control and hospital epidemiology is required in infectious disease fellowship programs and is available in courses provided by professional societies, primarily the Society for Healthcare Epidemiology of America.

In the 1970s, the CDC's extensive Study on the Efficacy of Nosocomial Infection Control found that nosocomial infection rates fell by 32% in hospitals that established programs with organized surveillance and control activities; a trained, effectual infection-control physician; and one infection-control practitioner per 250 beds. In contrast, rates in hospitals without effective programs increased by 18%. Since that study, the responsibilities and roles of hospital epidemiology programs have expanded in several directions. Diagnosis-related reimbursement has led hospital administrators to place increased emphasis on cost containment and on documentation of the cost-effectiveness of infection control. The quality-improvement movements and the Joint Commission have redirected infection-control attention, in part, beyond the mere writing of policies and procedures to improvement of the actual processes and optimization of outcomes. In a few hospitals, epidemiology programs have taken on additional pharmacoepidemiologic and antibiotic-use review responsibilities. Finally, all programs must now respond to increasing governmental regulation of hospital waste and to standards mandated by the Occupational Safety and Health Administration for protecting health care workers from occupational exposure to bloodborne pathogens and tuberculosis.

SURVEILLANCE Traditionally, infection-control practitioners survey inpatients for nosocomial infections (defined as those neither present nor incubating at the time of admission). Surveillance involves a review of microbiology laboratory results, "shoe-leather" epidemiology on the nursing wards, application of standardized definitions of infection, ongoing dialogue with hospital workers, and common sense. Some innovative infection-control programs have taken advantage of the increased use of computerized pharmacy, microbiology, and other databases in hospitals to create algorithm-driven surveillance activities.

Most hospitals aim surveillance at infections that (1) are associated with a high level of morbidity, e.g., intensive care unit (ICU)–related infections and nosocomial pneumonia; (2) are costly, e.g., cardiac surgical wound infections; (3) are difficult to treat, e.g., infections due to antibiotic-resistant bacteria; (4) pose recurring epidemic problems, e.g., *Clostridium difficile*–related diarrhea; and (5) are potentially preventable, e.g., vascular access–related infections. Quality-assurance activities in infection control have led to increased surveillance of the compliance of personnel with infection-control policies (e.g., monitoring of actual adherence to hand-washing recommendations).

The results of surveillance are expressed as rates; for example, 5 to 10% of patients develop nosocomial infections. Although such overall statistics are often requested of hospitals by administrators or surveyors, they have little value unless qualified by site of infection, by patient population, and by exposure to risk factors. Meaningful denominators for infection rates include the number of patients exposed to a specific risk (e.g., rates of pneumonia among patients using mechanical ventilators) and the number of intervention days (e.g., rates of pneumonia per 1000 patient-days on a ventilator).

Temporal trends in rates should be reviewed, and rates should be compared with regional and national norms. However, even comparison rates generated by the CDC's ongoing National Nosocomial Infections Surveillance System, which collects data from more than 270 hospitals that use standardized definitions of nosocomial infections, have not been validated independently and represent a nonrandom sample of hospitals. Interhospital comparisons are easily confounded by the wide range in risk factors and in severity of underlying illnesses; unless rates are adjusted for these factors, comparisons may be misleading. Unfortunately, systems for making such adjustments either are rudimentary or have not been well validated.

The ongoing analysis of an individual hospital's infection rates helps to determine whether control efforts are succeeding and where increased education and control measures should be focused. Knowledge of infection rates is also useful in discussions with the hospital administration regarding areas to which additional resources should be directed.

PREVENTION AND CONTROL MEASURES Epidemiologic Basis and General Measures Nosocomial infections follow basic epidemiologic patterns that can help to direct prevention and control measures. Nosocomial pathogens have reservoirs, are transmitted by predictable routes, and require susceptible hosts. Reservoirs and sources exist in the inanimate environment (e.g., tap water contaminated with *Legionella*) and in the animate environment (e.g., infected or colonized health care workers, patients, and hospital visitors). The mode of transmission most often is either cross-infection (e.g., indirect spread of pathogens from one patient to another on the inadequately washed hands of hospital personnel) or autoinoculation (e.g., aspiration of oropharyngeal flora into the lung along an endotracheal tube). Occasionally, pathogens (e.g., group A streptococci and many respiratory viruses) are spread indirectly from person to person via infectious droplets released by coughing or sneezing. Much less common—but often devastating in terms of epidemic risk—is true airborne spread of droplet nuclei (as in nosocomial chickenpox) or common-source spread by contaminated materials (e.g., iodophors contaminated with *Pseudomonas*). Factors that increase host susceptibility include underlying conditions and the many medical-surgical interventions and procedures that bypass or compromise normal host defenses.

Through its program, the hospital's infection-control committee must determine the general and specific measures used to control infections and must review and recommend specific antiseptics and disinfectants for hospital use. Given the prominence of cross-infection, hand washing is the single most important preventive measure in hospitals. Many studies have examined the antimicrobial activity of a wide variety of antiseptic-containing hand-washing agents. The use of such medicated agents is important before invasive procedures and possibly in ICU settings. In light of the poor general compliance with hand-washing recommendations, the importance of using any hand cleanser between patient contacts cannot be overemphasized (Table 134-1).

Table 134-1 Examples of Ways in Which Physicians Can Contribute to Infection-Control Efforts

- Act as role models for other personnel by paying careful attention to hand-washing recommendations and barrier precautions during contact with patients and by observing posted isolation precautions.
- Give corrective feedback to caregivers who do not adhere to hand-washing recommendations or isolation precautions.
- Place invasive devices based on clinical need (not just on convenience).
- Remove invasive devices promptly when they are no longer needed clinically.
- Limit surgical antimicrobial prophylaxis to the perioperative period.
- Exercise care in initial empirical antibiotic selection (avoid "shotgun" approaches).
- Narrow the spectrum of antibiotic therapy once a pathogen is recovered.
- Discontinue antibiotic therapy in a timely fashion.
- Become familiar with the hospital's bloodborne pathogen and tuberculosis control plans.
- Order appropriate isolation precautions promptly for infected patients.
- During patient rounds, alert nursing staff to lapses in asepsis (e.g., soiled dressings at sites of intravascular catheters) and to infection-predisposing situations (e.g., aspiration-prone positioning of patients).
- Notify infection-control practitioners of potential infection-control problems (e.g., surgical wound infections that manifest after a patient's discharge).

The fact that 25 to 50% of nosocomial infections are due to the combined effect of the patient's own flora and invasive devices highlights the importance of improvements in the use and design of such devices (Chap. 135). Intensive educational programs can be associated with at least a temporary reduction in infection rates through improved asepsis in handling and earlier removal of invasive devices, but the maintenance of such gains is often difficult. Epidemiologic studies are used increasingly to assess the value of newer devices and site-specific control measures and to debunk some traditional yet ineffective and costly measures, such as routine culturing of the environment and personnel for "pathogens."

Urinary Tract Infections Approaches to the prevention of urinary tract infections have included the use of topical meatal antimicrobials, drainage bag disinfectants, antimicrobial-coated catheters, and sealed catheter–drainage tube junctions to eliminate inadvertent breaks in the system. Because of conflicting study results, none of these measures is considered routine. Systemic antimicrobials given for other purposes decrease the risk of urinary tract infection during the first 4 days of catheterization, after which resistant bacteria or yeasts emerge as pathogens. Selective decontamination of the gut is also associated with a reduced risk. Again, however, neither approach is routine. Irrigation of catheters, with or without antimicrobials, may actually increase the risk of infection.

Pneumonia Control measures for pneumonia are aimed at the remediation of risk factors in general patient care (e.g., minimizing aspiration-prone supine positioning) and at meticulous aseptic care of respirator equipment (e.g., disinfecting or sterilizing all in-line reusable components such as nebulizers, replacing tubing circuits at intervals of >48 h—rather than more frequently—to lessen the number of breaks in the system, and teaching aseptic technique for suctioning). In a large multicenter trial, sucralfate, which provides stress-ulcer prophylaxis without altering gastric pH, did not reduce the risk of ventilator-associated pneumonia, despite the theoretical advantage of lessened risk for gastric colonization by gram-negative bacilli. The benefit of selective decontamination of the oropharynx and gut with nonabsorbable antimicrobials has been controversial.

Surgical Wound Infections The most important control measures for surgical wound infections include the use of antimicrobial prophylaxis at the start of high-risk procedures, attention to technical surgical issues and operating-room asepsis (e.g., not shaving the operative site until surgery and avoiding open or prophylactic drains), and preoperative therapy for active infection. In one study, rates of postoperative infection were lower among patients who had normothermia maintained during colorectal surgery. Reporting of surveillance results to surgeons has been associated with reductions in infection rates. The increasingly extensive review of infection rates by regulatory agencies and third-party payers emphasizes the importance of stratifying rates by patient-related risk factors and of developing meaningful systems for interhospital comparisons and for wound surveillance after the patient's discharge from the hospital or clinic (when more than 50% of infections first become apparent).

Infections Related to Vascular Access and Monitoring (See also Chap. 135)   Control measures for infections associated with vascular access and monitoring include the moving of peripheral or arterial catheters to a new site at specified intervals (e.g., every 72 h for peripheral intravenous catheters), which may be facilitated by use of an intravenous team; application of disposable transducers and aseptic technique for the accessing of transducers or other vascular ports; removal of "idle" catheters; and consideration of use of central venous catheters impregnated with anti-infective agents. Unresolved issues include the best frequency for the rotation of central venous catheter sites (guidewire-assisted catheter changes at the same site do not lessen infection risk); the best antiseptics for site preparation and for catheter dressing; the appropriate role for mupirocin ointment, a topical antibiotic with excellent antistaphylococcal activity, in site care; and the relative degrees of risk posed by percutaneous central catheters and by newer designs—tunneled, totally implanted, or peripherally inserted central catheters (PICC lines). Improvements in composition of semitransparent access-site dressings and potential nursing benefits (ease of bathing and site inspection and protection of the site from secretions) favor use of such coverings.

Isolation Techniques   Written policies for the isolation of infectious patients are a standard component of infection-control programs. In 1996, the CDC revised its isolation guidelines to be simpler; to recognize the importance of all body fluids, secretions, and excretions in the transmission of nosocomial pathogens; and to focus precautions on the major routes of infection transmission.

The revised guidelines contain two tiers of precautions. *Standard precautions* are designed for the care of all patients in hospitals to reduce the risk of transmission of microorganisms from both recognized and unrecognized sources of infection. These precautions include gloving, as well as hand washing, for potential contact with blood; with all other body fluids, secretions, and excretions, regardless of whether they contain visible blood; with nonintact skin; and with mucous membranes. Depending on exposure risks, standard precautions also include use of masks, eye protection, and gowns.

In the second tier are precautions for the care of patients with suspected or diagnosed colonization or infection with transmissible pathogens. These transmission-based guidelines collapse the older category- and disease-specific isolation guidelines into three sets of precautions based on probable routes of transmission: *airborne precautions, droplet precautions,* and *contact precautions.* Sets of precautions may be combined for diseases that have more than one route of transmission (e.g., varicella). Potentially contagious clinical syndromes, such as acute diarrhea, are included in the revised guidelines.

Because some prevalent antibiotic-resistant pathogens, particularly vancomycin-resistant enterococci (VRE), may be present on *intact* skin of patients in hospitals, some experts recommend gloving for all contact with patients who are acutely ill and/or from high-risk units, such as ICUs. In recent trials, wearing gloves did not replace the need for hand washing because hands occasionally became contaminated during wearing or removal of gloves. Some studies have suggested that use of gowns and gloves compared with routine care of patients (i.e., using neither of these barriers) decreases the risk of nosocomial infection; however, more recent evaluation suggests that gowning by personnel does not add benefit beyond that conferred by gloving and hand washing. Nevertheless, requiring increased precaution levels can improve the compliance of health care workers with isolation recommendations by 30%.

EPIDEMIC PROBLEMS   Outbreaks are always big news but probably account for fewer than 5% of nosocomial infections. The investigation and control of epidemics in hospitals require that infection-control personnel develop a case definition, confirm that an outbreak really exists (since many apparent epidemics are actually pseudo-outbreaks due to surveillance or laboratory artifacts), review aseptic practices and disinfectant use, determine the extent of the outbreak, perform an epidemiologic investigation to determine modes of transmission, work closely with microbiology personnel to culture for common sources or personnel carriers as appropriate and to type epidemiologically important isolates, and heighten surveillance to judge the effect of control measures. Control measures generally include the early reinforcement of routine aseptic practices during a search for compliance problems that may have fostered the outbreak, the ensuring of the appropriate isolation of cases (and the institution of cohort isolation and nursing if needed), and the implementation of further controls on the basis of the findings of the investigation. Examples of some potential epidemic problems follow.

Chickenpox   When health care workers are exposed to chickenpox in the community or through patients with initially unrecognized infections, or when these employees work during the 24 h before developing chickenpox, infection-control practitioners institute a varicella exposure investigation and control plan. The names of exposed workers and patients are obtained; medical histories are reviewed, and (if necessary) serologic tests for immunity are conducted; physicians are notified of susceptible exposed patients; postexposure prophylaxis with varicella-zoster immune globulin (VZIG) is considered for immunocompromised or pregnant contacts (see Table 183-1); preemptive use of acyclovir is considered as an alternative strategy in some susceptible persons; and susceptible exposed employees are furloughed during the at-risk period for disease (8 to 21 days, or 28 days if VZIG has been administered). Preexposure varicella vaccination can markedly decrease risk for susceptible employees.

Tuberculosis   The resurgence of pulmonary tuberculosis in the United States since 1987 and a series of nosocomial outbreaks of infection with multidrug-resistant strains—primarily involving patients with AIDS and their caregivers—have led to a reevaluation of tuberculosis control. Important control measures include prompt recognition, isolation, and treatment of cases; recognition of atypical presentations (e.g., lower-lobe infiltrates without cavitation); use of negative pressure, 100% exhaust, private isolation rooms with closed doors, and six air changes per hour; use of face masks (approved by the National Institute for Occupational Safety and Health) by caregivers entering isolation rooms; possible use of high-efficiency particulate air filter units and/or ultraviolet lights for disinfecting air when other engineering controls are not feasible or reliable; and follow-up skin-testing of susceptible personnel who have been exposed to infectious patients before isolation.

Group A Streptococci   The potential for a group A streptococcal outbreak should be considered when even a single nosocomial case occurs. Most outbreaks involve surgical wounds and are due to the presence of an asymptomatic carrier in the operating room. Investigation can be confounded by carriage at extrapharyngeal sites such as the rectum and vagina. Health care workers in whom carriage has been linked to nosocomial transmission of group A streptococci are removed from the patient-care setting and are not permitted to return until carriage has been eliminated by antimicrobial therapy.

Aspergillus   *Aspergillus* spores are common in the environment, particularly on dusty surfaces. When hospital ceiling tiles are removed to provide access for electrical wiring or plumbing or when dusty areas are disturbed during hospital renovation, the spores become airborne. Inhalation of spores by immunosuppressed (particularly neutropenic) patients creates a risk of pulmonary and/or paranasal sinus infection and disseminated aspergillosis. Routine surveillance among neutropenic patients for infections with filamentous fungi, such as *Aspergillus* and *Fusarium*, helps hospitals to determine whether they have unduly large environmental loads of these organisms. To lower the risk, hospitals should inspect and clean air-handling equipment on a routine schedule, review all planned hospital renovations with infection-control personnel and subsequently construct appropriate barriers, remove immunosuppressed patients from renovation sites, and consider the use of high-efficiency particulate air filters for rooms housing immunosuppressed patients.

Legionella Sporadic and epidemic cases of nosocomial *Legionella* pneumonia are most often due to the contamination of potable water and predominantly affect immunosuppressed patients, particularly those receiving glucocorticoid medication. The risk varies greatly within and among geographic regions, depending on the extent of hospital hot-water contamination, on the presence or absence of high-risk patient populations, and on specific hospital practices (e.g., inappropriate use of nonsterile water in respiratory therapy equipment). Laboratory-based surveillance for nosocomial *Legionella* should be performed, and a diagnosis of legionellosis should probably be considered more often than it is. If cases are detected, environmental samples (e.g., tap water) should be cultured. If cultures yield *Legionella* and if typing of clinical and environmental isolates reveals a correlation, eradication measures should be pursued (Chap. 151). An alternative approach is to periodically culture tap water on wards housing high-risk patients. If *Legionella* is found, a concerted effort should be made to culture samples from all patients with nosocomial pneumonia for *Legionella*.

Antibiotic-Resistant Bacteria Outbreaks of antibiotic resistance can depend on any of the following events: Darwinian selection of bacterial chromosomal mutations, spread of plasmid- and/or transposon-borne resistance among bacterial species, and (re)admission to the hospital of patients chronically infected with resistant bacteria. After the introduction of resistant strains, dissemination occurs by cross-infection on unwashed hands of caregivers or, occasionally, via personnel carriage and/or environmental contamination. Outbreak control depends on close laboratory surveillance, with early detection of problems; on the reinforcement of routine asepsis (e.g., hand washing); on the implementation of barrier precautions for all colonized and/or infected patients; on the use of patient-surveillance cultures to more fully ascertain the extent of patient colonization; and on the timely initiation of an epidemiologic investigation when rates increase. Colonized personnel who are implicated in nosocomial transmission and patients who pose a threat may be decontaminated; for example, colonization with methicillin-resistant *Staphylococcus aureus* may be controlled with oral antibiotics, including trimethoprim-sulfamethoxazole and rifampin, and with topical agents, including hexachlorophene or chlorhexidine and mupirocin. In a few ICUs, selective decontamination has been used successfully as a temporary emergency control measure for outbreaks of infection due to gram-negative bacilli.

The most recent bacterial-resistance problem to plague hospitals is the emergence of VRE. Initially an ICU problem, VRE have now spread onto general wards in many hospitals. VRE are particularly problematic because of a substantial "iceberg" effect (i.e., the fact that, for each individual with a clinical infection, many other patients are colonized); the occurrence of both gastrointestinal and skin colonization (reflecting fecal contamination on the skin of ill, hospitalized patients); and the propensity for these organisms to contaminate the patient's environment, which may increase the risk of cross-infection. Control of VRE requires strict attention to hand washing by personnel, concerted use of barrier precautions or cohort nursing for patients known to be colonized or infected, and emphasis on thorough cleaning of the rooms of these patients.

Spread of vancomycin resistance to *S. aureus* is a major concern. Clinical infections with methicillin-resistant *S. aureus* strains that exhibit reduced susceptibility to vancomycin have been reported in a few patients, usually in the setting of prolonged or repeated treatment with vancomycin. The detection of these strains requires augmented laboratory activities, and their identification should trigger an aggressive epidemiologic investigation and aggressive infection-control measures.

Because the excessive use of broad-spectrum antibiotics underlies many resistance problems, antibiotic-control policies (Table 134-2)

Table 134-2 Elements of an Antibiotic-Control Program

- Review antimicrobial agents and select a basic formulary.
- Establish prophylactic, empirical, and therapeutic guidelines.
- Restrict the use of agents that have special limited indications, cause excessive toxicity, or are costly.
- Release restricted agents for use in predetermined circumstances or after prospective approval.
- Ensure that the antibiotics on the formulary are the same as those being used for susceptibility testing by the microbiology laboratory.
- Monitor patterns of antibiotic susceptibility and trends in antibiotic use, providing regular feedback to the medical staff.
- Audit the use of specific antibiotics.
- Conduct ongoing educational programs.
- Regulate in-hospital promotional efforts of pharmaceutical companies.

SOURCE: After JP Flaherty, RA Weinstein, Infect Control Hosp Epidemiol 17:236, 1996.

must be considered a cornerstone of resistance-control efforts. Although the efficacy of antibiotic-control measures in reducing rates of antimicrobial resistance has not been proved in prospective controlled trials, it seems worthwhile to restrict the use of particular agents to narrowly defined indications or possibly to cycle the use of antibiotic classes to limit selective pressure on the nosocomial flora.

EMPLOYEE HEALTH SERVICE ISSUES An institution's employee health service is a critical component of its infection-control efforts. New employees should be processed through the service, where a contagious-disease history can be taken; evidence of immunity to a variety of diseases, such as hepatitis B, chickenpox, measles, and rubella, can be sought; immunizations for hepatitis B, measles, rubella, and varicella can be given as needed and a reminder about the need for yearly influenza immunization can be imparted; baseline and "booster" purified protein derivative of tuberculin skin-testing can be performed; and education about personal responsibility for infection control can be initiated. Evaluations of employees should be codified to meet the requirements of accrediting and regulatory agencies.

The employee health service must have protocols for dealing with workers who have been exposed to contagious diseases, such as those percutaneously or mucosally exposed to the blood of patients infected with HIV. Postexposure HIV prophylaxis with a combination of antiretroviral agents (e.g., zidovudine and lamivudine, with or without indinavir or nelfinavir) is recommended. Protocols are also needed for dealing with caregivers who have common contagious diseases, such as chickenpox, group A streptococcal infections, respiratory infections, and infectious diarrhea, and for those who have less common but high-visibility public health problems, such as chronic hepatitis B or C or HIV infection, for which exposure-control guidelines have been published by the CDC and by the Society for Healthcare Epidemiology of America.

BIBLIOGRAPHY

BENNETT JV, BRACHMAN PS (eds): *Hospital Infections*, 5th ed. Philadelphia, Lippincott-Raven, 1998

BOLYARD EA et al: Guideline for infection control in healthcare personnel, 1998. Infect Control Hosp Epidemiol 19:411, 1998

CENTERS FOR DISEASE CONTROL: Report of the National Nosocomial Infections Surveillance (NNIS) System: Nosocomial infection rates for interhospital comparison: Limitations and possible solutions. Infect Control Hosp Epidemiol 12:609, 1991

GARNER JS, INFECTION CONTROL PRACTICES ADVISORY COMMITTEE: Guideline for isolation precautions in hospitals. Infect Control Hosp Epidemiol 17:53, 1996

GOLDMANN DA et al: Strategies to prevent and control the emergence and spread of antimicrobial-resistant microorganisms in hospitals—a challenge to hospital leadership. JAMA 275:234, 1996

KLEMPNER MS (ed): Hospital infections and health-care epidemiology, in *Infectious Diseases Medical Knowledge Self-Assessment Program*, 2d ed. Philadelphia, American College of Physicians, 1998

MAYHALL CG (ed): *Hospital Epidemiology and Infection Control*, 2d ed. New York, Lippincott Williams & Wilkins, 1999

SCHECKLER WE et al: Requirements for infrastructure and essential activities of infection control and epidemiology in hospitals: A consensus panel report. Infect Control Hosp Epidemiol 19:114, 1998

WEINSTEIN RA: Nosocomial infection update. Emerg Infect Dis 4:416, 1998

HOSPITAL-ACQUIRED AND INTRAVASCULAR DEVICE–RELATED INFECTIONS

Nosocomial infections are defined as infections acquired during or as a result of hospitalization. Generally, a patient who has been in the hospital for <48 h and develops an infection is considered to have been incubating the infection before hospital admission. Most infections that become manifest after 48 h are considered to be nosocomial. A patient may develop a nosocomial infection after being discharged from the hospital if the organism apparently was acquired in the hospital. Surgical wound infection developing in the weeks after hospital discharge is an example of such nosocomial infection.

INCIDENCE AND COSTS   Nosocomial infections contribute significantly to morbidity and mortality as well as to excess costs for hospitalized patients. It is estimated that 5% of patients admitted to an acute care hospital in the United States acquire a new infection, with >2 million nosocomial infections per year and an annual cost of >$2 billion. Some authorities estimate that the odds of death are doubled for patients who develop a nosocomial infection, although clearly such factors as underlying disease and severity of illness also play an important role in outcome.

Although immunosuppressed hosts are especially vulnerable to infections acquired in a hospital, common nosocomial infections occur even in immunocompetent hosts. The National Nosocomial Infections Surveillance (NNIS) Registry has been monitoring nosocomial infection rates since 1970. Its most recent report covers the period from October 1996 through April 1998 and includes both teaching and nonteaching hospitals and both small and large facilities. The most common nosocomial infections have remained the same. Urinary tract infections (UTIs), pneumonia, and surgical-site infections (SSIs, formerly termed wound infections) are most frequent. However, primary bloodstream infections, especially those associated with intravascular devices, have increased in frequency, as have infections in medical and surgical intensive care units (ICUs) and infections caused by antimicrobial-resistant pathogens.

The potential impact of nosocomial infections is considerable when assessed in terms of incidence, morbidity, mortality, and financial burden. Analyses of these factors examine nosocomial infections as both medical and economic issues. The clinical problem facing the physician is the development of a new fever in a patient in the hospital. In the evaluation of such a patient, information about the most common categories of infection may not be sufficient. Rather, the clinician must also use clinical clues from the patient's presentation and hospitalization to diagnose a nosocomial infection.

Approach to the Patient

The evaluation of a hospitalized patient with new fever should include a careful history (Chap. 17). Particular attention should be paid to symptoms of headache, cough, abdominal pain, diarrhea, flank pain, dysuria, urinary frequency, and leg pain. Other features related to the patient's hospitalization are also important, such as the presence and type of intravenous devices, the past or current use of a urinary catheter, the surgical procedure conducted (if any), and the new medications administered, including those for surgical prophylaxis. The physical examination should be directed at possible sources of infection and should focus particularly on the skin (with a search for rash or embolic lesions); the lungs; the abdomen (especially the right upper quadrant); the costovertebral angles; surgical wounds; the calves; and current and old intravenous access sites (for signs of phlebitis). The laboratory evaluation of all hospitalized patients with new fever should include a complete blood count with differential, a chest radiograph, and blood and urine cultures. Other diagnostic tests to consider include liver function tests, plain-film or other studies of the abdomen, routine aerobic cultures of sputum or other relevant body fluids, and (in cases of diarrhea) testing of stool for *Clostridium difficile* toxin.

CATEGORIES OF INFECTION   **Pneumonia**   Certainly the astute clinician will question the patient thoroughly and perform a rapid comprehensive physical examination. One way to continue the approach to the hospitalized patient with a new fever is to consider potential infections that may be life-threatening, such as pneumonia. Most at risk for developing nosocomial pneumonia are patients in an ICU, especially those who are intubated; patients with an altered level of consciousness, especially those with nasogastric tubes; elderly patients; patients with chronic lung disease; postoperative patients; and any of the above patients taking H_2 blockers or antacids. Nosocomial pneumonia in the NNIS Registry is diagnosed 4 to 7 times per 1000 hospitalizations. Among patients on ventilators, the occurrence of pneumonia is estimated at 15 cases per 1000 ventilator days in medical and surgical ICUs. Mortality figures for nosocomial pneumonia are as high as 50%.

Oropharyngeal and gastric colonization plays a critical role in the pathogenesis of pneumonia in hospitalized patients. The oropharynx can become colonized by many species of aerobic gram-negative organisms within 48 h of the patient's hospitalization; aspiration occurs commonly during sleep and is increased by such factors as a nasogastric tube, altered consciousness, decreased gag reflex, or delayed gastric emptying. As for gastric colonization, bacterial counts in the stomach rise in the presence of medications that raise gastric pH, such as H_2 blockers and antacids, as well as in malnourished, achlorhydric, and some elderly patients. The prevalence of pneumonia is reportedly two to three times higher among intubated patients receiving H_2 blockers or antacids for stress-ulcer prophylaxis than among intubated patients receiving sucralfate, a medication that heals ulcers without altering gastric pH. Gastric colonization is believed to influence the development of pneumonia by retrograde colonization of the oropharynx. Ventilated patients are also at risk of developing pneumonia by exposure to bacteria leaking around the cuff of the endotracheal tube or to bacteria from nebulizers, condensate within ventilator circuits, or humidifiers.

Outside the ICU, pneumonia should be suspected when a patient develops a new cough, fever, leukocytosis, sputum production, and a new infiltrate on chest x-ray. Diagnosis can be complicated in patients with congestive heart failure who have concomitant chest x-ray abnormalities or in patients with chronic sputum production. Some organisms, such as *Legionella* spp., may not be associated with peripheral leukocytosis.

In ICU patients, especially those who are intubated, the signs of pneumonia are relatively subtle, and thus the diagnosis is often relatively complex. In particular, the chest x-rays are difficult to interpret, because fluid overload, congestive heart failure, and acute respiratory distress syndrome (ARDS) are all common findings in intubated patients. Polymorphonuclear leukocytes (PMNs) are often present on Gram-stained preparations of purulent secretions from these patients. An important clue to pneumonia is a change in the output or character of these secretions. If their volume or thickness increases or their color changes, a sputum Gram's stain should be performed and pneumonia seriously considered in the differential diagnosis. Serial Gram's stains are useful, as the number of PMNs may increase substantially and the type(s) of organisms may shift with the development of pneumonia. For example, the baseline sputum sample from an intubated patient may contain about 25 PMNs per high-power field and have mixed gram-positive and gram-negative organisms of several morphologic types in moderate numbers. On the day of a new fever, the same patient may have copious amounts of more tenacious sputum with more PMNs and a predominance of enteric-appearing gram-negative rods. Even without distinct changes in the chest x-ray, this patient would be considered to have developed pneumonia. Another subtle sign of pneumonia in the intubated patient is a requirement for change in ventilator settings in the absence of fluid overload, a mechanical alteration (e.g., a shift in endotracheal tube placement), or a pneumothorax.

The major organisms of concern in nosocomial pneumonia are gram-negative aerobic bacteria. *Pseudomonas aeruginosa* was the most common isolate in the NNIS survey of ICUs, with a frequency of 21%; *Staphylococcus aureus* was next most common at 20%. *Acinetobacter* has become a more common pathogen in ventilator-associated pneumonia. While surveys of organisms are useful, it is essential to know which pathogens are common in a given institution, as hospitals and especially ICUs differ in their resident flora. In some institutions, methicillin-resistant *S. aureus*, *Stenotrophomonas* (formerly *Xanthomonas*) *maltophilia*, *Flavobacterium* spp., and even *Legionella* spp. may be of particular concern. Viruses such as respiratory syncytial virus and adenovirus are receiving increased attention as etiologic agents of nosocomial pneumonia in both adults and children. In the past, viruses have been underrepresented in statistics on the agents of nosocomial pneumonia because the diagnosis of viral infection is more difficult and because many microbiology laboratories do not have the capability to isolate viruses.

Antibiotic resistance is another important issue to address in the management of a hospitalized patient. An outgrowth of the NNIS surveys is Project ICARE, which tracks antibiotic usage patterns and resistance rates in a subset of NNIS institutions. Rates of resistance are generally higher in ICUs and track with increased use of antibiotics. *P. aeruginosa*, *Enterobacter* spp., and enterococci are the pathogens of greatest concern in the development of antibiotic resistance. In addition to knowing the sensitivity patterns of the hospital flora, one must consider whether a patient has received continuous or multiple courses of antibiotic therapy. To reduce the likelihood of altering the sensitivity patterns of the patient's flora, antibiotic courses for pneumonia should be kept as short as possible, with coverage as narrow as possible for the organism(s) involved.

Bacteremia   Another potentially life-threatening nosocomial infection to consider in the evaluation of the patient with a new fever is bacteremia, which is usually related to the presence of an intravascular device (Chap. 134). While many common nosocomial infections such as pneumonia or UTI can be accompanied by bacteremia, primary bacteremia is defined by isolation of a recognized pathogen from the blood without an infection at another site. One carefully controlled study reported bloodstream infection in 2.7% of admissions to a surgical ICU, with 50% mortality and a prolongation of hospitalization by 24 days in survivors.

One difficulty in assessing the significance of bacteremia is to distinguish true pathogens from contaminating skin flora. This distinction is especially important in establishing an infection of an indwelling intravascular catheter because organisms that inhabit the skin, such as coagulase-negative staphylococci, also frequently cause infection. The most common point of entry for infection related to intravascular devices is the insertion site, with spread of the infection along the outside of the device initially. Other means of entry for infecting organisms include introduction via contaminated infusates or tubing, ports, or leaking connections and hematogenous seeding of a catheter during bacteremia. While gram-negative aerobic bacilli are probably the most feared nosocomial bloodstream pathogens, the NNIS data for 1980 through 1989 showed that the isolation of these organisms had not increased in frequency over the decade. The frequency of bloodstream isolation increased the most for coagulase-negative staphylococci, with the next highest increase for *Candida* spp. Other leading causes of line-related bacteremia were *S. aureus* and enterococci. Subsequent studies confirmed these findings. Nosocomial endocarditis is an important, newly recognized entity that develops largely as a complication of invasive procedures or intravascular devices and may account for as many as 10% of cases of infective endocarditis.

Establishing an infection of an intravascular device or primary bacteremia as the cause of fever in a hospitalized patient is a diagnosis of exclusion. If a patient has a fever and signs of cutaneous involvement (erythema, induration, tenderness, or purulent drainage) at the insertion site of a catheter, full cultures should be performed, the vascular-access line removed, and the catheter tip sent for quantitative culture. Studies have correlated the growth of ≥15 colonies from a catheter tip with infection of the line. More commonly, the exit site does not show signs of infection, and there is considerable debate about the necessity of removing a line from a febrile patient at that point. Although line changes over a guidewire have been shown to be safe, unless another site of infection is obvious, it is generally advisable to remove the line and to change the site when a patient develops a new fever. The traditional teaching is that an infected intravenous device should be removed. In current practice, however, especially with surgically implanted intravenous catheters, a decision may be made to attempt treatment with antibiotics while leaving the catheter in place. This practice is often successful when the infecting organism is a coagulase-negative *Staphylococcus* species but is less often effective with other organisms, particularly *Candida* spp. and gram-negative bacilli. Salvage of catheters used for hemodialysis is especially important and has been successfully accomplished with infections caused by a variety of organisms.

Another controversial management issue is whether to draw blood for culture through a line. While some studies report a correlation in the 90% range between culture results for blood drawn through vascular-access lines and those for peripheral blood, the former cultures can be either false-positive or false-negative. If the line culture is positive and no peripheral blood has been drawn, it is impossible to determine whether the patient has true bacteremia or the culture merely reflects bacteria associated with the line. Whether bacteremia is high- or low-grade and whether it is sustained or transient may influence the duration of antibiotic therapy and cannot be determined from cultures of blood specimens obtained through a line.

An area of considerable interest and controversy is the prevention of catheter-related infections through the use of intravenous devices impregnated with chlorhexidine/silver sulfadiazine or minocycline/rifampin. A meta-analysis of 11 studies found a decrease in both catheter colonization and catheter-related bacteremia with chlorhexidine/silver sulfadiazine–impregnated catheters, with associated cost savings. One multicenter prospective randomized trial directly compared the two types of catheters and found the minocycline/rifampin-impregnated catheter to be superior. Antibiotic-resistant strains were not recovered in this trial, although concern has been raised that antibiotic impregnation may increase the development of resistance. The several other studies that do not support these findings include one in which the incidence of bacteremia did not decrease with the use of chlorhexidine/silver sulfadiazine–impregnated catheters.

Surgical-Site Infection   Evaluation of fever in the postoperative patient must include careful evaluation of the surgical wound. Although SSI reportedly accounts for 19% of nosocomial infections, the true incidence of postoperative wound infection is difficult to assess, particularly at a time when many patients are hospitalized for relatively short periods. In a number of studies, careful follow-up for the development of SSI after discharge—especially observation of the wound by a trained observer, such as a nurse—has shown the actual rates of SSI in all categories of surgery to be greater than the reported rates. SSI rates vary from 4.6 to 8.2% for nonteaching and large teaching hospitals, respectively. Rates also vary by procedure, with abdominal surgery resulting in the highest rates.

Risk factors for the development of postoperative wound infection include the presence of a drain; a long preoperative length of stay, with the rates doubling for each week of preoperative hospitalization; preoperative shaving of the field, especially if performed ≥24 h beforehand; a long duration of surgery; and the presence of an untreated remote infection. Infection rates also vary with the surgeon. Perioperative antibiotic prophylaxis has been shown to decrease rates of wound infection in a number of careful studies, including those of

A surgical wound should be examined for localized tenderness and induration, fluctuance, drainage of purulent material, and dehiscence of sutures. Mechanical factors, as well as infection, can cause wound dehiscence. Sternal wounds following cardiac surgery are of special concern because the consequences of infection can be severe. The surface of the wound may not present an obvious cause for concern, but ongoing fevers, serous drainage, and especially the development of rocking or instability of the sternum may be sufficient cause for surgical exploration of the wound in some cases. Mediastinitis or sternal osteomyelitis is a severe complication of cardiac surgery. Wounds associated with the placement of prosthetic devices, such as mechanical joints, are also of special concern. Infection of these wounds can lead to infection of the prosthesis, and clearance of prosthetic joint infections generally requires surgical removal of the device.

The most common pathogens causing SSI are coagulase-negative *Staphylococcus* and *S. aureus*, but antibiotic-resistant bacteria and fungi are also becoming more frequent etiologies. Early infections may be associated with organisms that produce rapid, progressive skin infection, such as group A *Streptococcus* and *Clostridium* spp. Group A *Streptococcus* has been identified in some cases of recurrent infection of saphenous-vein graft harvest sites.

Urinary Tract Infection UTI, the most common type of nosocomial infection, is generally the easiest to treat and has the least severe sequelae. Four principal risk factors have been associated repeatedly with the development of UTI in hospitalized patients: female sex, prolonged urinary catheterization, lack of systemic antibiotic therapy, and breach of appropriate catheter care. The administration of systemic antibiotics to patients with urinary catheters in place for 1 to 5 days has been associated with a decrease in rates of bacteriuria. For patients with catheters in place for ≥ 6 days, however, this benefit is not observed.

The pathogenesis of catheter-associated UTI appears to differ in men and women. In women, the typical mechanism involves periurethral colonization with fecal flora and tracking of organisms up the catheter to the bladder; thus the pathogenesis resembles that of UTI in noncatheterized female patients, in whom bacteria track up the short female urethra. In contrast, periurethral colonization often cannot be demonstrated in men; most infections seem to arise from intraluminal spread of organisms to the bladder. Some organisms, such as *Proteus* and *Pseudomonas* spp., appear to facilitate the growth along the inside of the urinary catheter of a biofilm that encrusts and obstructs the flow of urine.

UTI is certainly an extremely common nosocomial infection; however, it is important to define this type of infection precisely. Especially in the evaluation of a febrile hospitalized patient, it is crucial to think carefully about all possible sources of infection and not to assume that UTI is the probable cause. In patients who have had urinary catheters in place for a number of days, fever, dysuria, frequency, leukocytosis, and especially flank pain or costovertebral angle tenderness are highly suggestive of bladder infection or pyelonephritis. In patients with fever but no other symptoms or signs referable to the urinary tract, one should look for ancillary findings suggestive of urinary tract involvement, such as white blood cells without epithelial cells in the urine sediment or leukocyte esterase or nitrite on urinalysis. A urine culture positive for a single organism should not be accepted as definitive evidence of UTI in an asymptomatic patient. While one might treat the febrile patient who has a positive urine culture with antibiotics, it is prudent to repeat the culture before the institution of therapy. Inability to recover any organism or the same organism on repeat culture, particularly if the patient does not respond to antibiotics, should raise questions about the validity of the diagnosis of UTI. In addition, isolation of two or more bacteria from a single specimen is most likely due to contamination unless there is reason to suspect a bladder diverticulum or a perinephric abscess.

Other Infectious Sources of Fever Several other types of infection may cause fever in the hospitalized patient and should be considered in the differential diagnosis of new fever. In patients who have received antibiotics (even a single dose as surgical prophylaxis), antibiotic-associated diarrhea may develop. This condition is usually caused by the spore-forming organism *C. difficile*, which produces toxins that cause diarrhea. Some patients may appear quite toxic with this infection, with high fevers, leukocytosis, and profuse diarrhea. The organism is quite hardy and is difficult to eradicate from the hospital environment. The hands of hospital personnel have been implicated as a mode of transmission of this organism, as have electronic rectal thermometers. The colon may become colonized with *C. difficile* while the patient is in the hospital, but—particularly if the patient is still taking antibiotics when sent home—diarrhea may not develop until after discharge.

Unless patients are consuming foods from outside the hospital, food-borne diarrheal illness is uncommon among hospitalized patients. Thus, an extensive stool evaluation is generally not cost-effective in the management of these patients.

Other infections to consider in the hospitalized patient include decubitus ulcers, particularly in patients in chronic-care wards or confined to bed rest for prolonged periods, and sinusitis, especially in intubated patients.

NONINFECTIOUS SOURCES OF FEVER A consideration of several common noninfectious causes of fever in hospitalized patients is part of a thorough evaluation of new fever. Drug treatment is the foremost noninfectious cause of fever. Drug fever may occur with or without an accompanying rash or eosinophilia and can be caused by a new medication or by medications the patient has been receiving for some time. Particular agents associated with drug fever include phenytoin, H_2 blockers, procainamide, and antibiotics, most notably sulfonamides. Even drug-associated fevers can be quite high in some patients and may take up to 5 days to resolve after discontinuation of treatment with the offending agent. Other noninfectious causes of fever include phlebitis, often at the site of an old intravenous line and sometimes followed by suppurative thrombophlebitis with clots or septic emboli, and pulmonary emboli, especially in patients undergoing prolonged bed rest; prophylactic heparin or mechanical boots are often used to reduce the risk of pulmonary embolism in the latter patients. Other entities to consider include tissue necrosis following surgery, trauma, or burns; hematomas; pancreatitis; atelectasis; and acalculous cholecystitis.

CONCLUSION The range of possibilities for the etiology of a new fever in a hospitalized patient is quite broad. An attention to detail, a careful history and physical examination, and a knowledge of the infections and organisms likely to cause nosocomial problems usually lead to an accurate diagnosis.

BIBLIOGRAPHY

DAROUICHE RO et al: A comparison of two antimicrobial-impregnated central venous catheters. N Engl J Med 340:1, 1999

FRIDKIN SK et al: Surveillance of antimicrobial use and antimicrobial resistance in United States hospitals: Project ICARE phase 2. Project Intensive Care Antimicrobial Resistance Epidemiology (ICARE) hospitals. Clin Infect Dis 29:245, 1999

GARROUSTE-OREGEAS M et al: Oropharyngeal or gastric colonization and nosocomial pneumonia in adult intensive care unit patients. Am J Respir Crit Care Med 156:1647, 1997

GOLUB R et al: Laparoscopic versus open appendectomy: A meta-analysis. J Am Coll Surg 186:545, 1998

MARR KA et al: Catheter-related bacteremia and outcome of attempted catheter salvage in patients undergoing hemodialysis. Ann Intern Med 127:275, 1997

NATIONAL NOSOCOMIAL INFECTIONS SURVEILLANCE (NNIS) SYSTEM: Report, data summary from October 1986–April 1998, issued June 1998. Am J Infect Control 26: 522, 1998

RICHARDS MJ et al: Nosocomial infections in medical intensive care units in the United States. National Nosocomial Infections Surveillance System. Crit Care Med 27:887, 1999

VEENSTRA D et al: Efficacy of antiseptic-impregnated central venous catheters in preventing catheter-related bloodstream infection. A meta-analysis. JAMA 281:261, 1999

136 *Robert Finberg, Joyce Fingeroth*

INFECTIONS IN TRANSPLANT RECIPIENTS

BMT	bone marrow transplant	HSCT	hematopoietic stem cell
CMV	cytomegalovirus		transplant
CNS	central nervous system	HSV	herpes simplex virus
CSF	cerebrospinal fluid	IVIG	intravenous immune globulin
EBV	Epstein-Barr virus	LPD	lymphoproliferative disease
GVHD	graft-versus-host disease	MMR	measles/mumps/rubella
HHV	human herpesvirus	RSV	respiratory syncytial virus
HPVs	human papillomaviruses	VZV	varicella-zoster virus

The evaluation of infections in transplant recipients involves consideration of both the donor and the recipient of the transplanted organ. Infections following transplantation are complicated by the use of drugs that are necessary to enhance the likelihood of survival of the transplanted organ but that also cause the host to be immunocompromised. Thus what might have been a latent or asymptomatic infection in an immunocompetent donor or in the recipient prior to therapy becomes a life-threatening problem when the recipient becomes immunosuppressed.

A variety of organisms have been transmitted by organ transplantation (Table 136-1). Careful attention to the sterility of the medium used to process the organ combined with meticulous microbiologic evaluation reduces rates of transmission of bacteria that may be present or grow in the organ culture medium. From 2% to >20% of donor kidneys are estimated to be contaminated with bacteria—in most cases, with the organisms that colonize the skin or grow in the tissue culture medium used to bathe the donor kidney while it awaits implantation. The reported rate of bacterial contamination of transplanted

Table 136-1 Organisms Transmitted by Organ Transplantation and Common Sites of Reactivation Disease

	Site					
Organism	Blood	Lungs	Heart	Brain	Liver	Skin
Viruses						
Cytomegalovirus[a]	+	+	+/−	+	+	+
Epstein-Barr virus[b]	+	+	+	+	+	+
Herpes simplex virus		+			+	+
Human herpesvirus 6	+	+		+		+
Human herpesvirus 8	+					+
Hepatitis B and C viruses					+	
Fungi						
Candida albicans	+	+			+	+
Histoplasma capsulatum	+	+			+	
Cryptococcus	+	+		+		+
Parasites						
Toxoplasma gondii[c]		+	+	+		
Strongyloides stercoralis[d,e]		+				
Trypanosoma cruzi[e]			+			
Plasmodium falciparum[e]	+					

[a] Cytomegalovirus reactivation is prone to occur in the transplanted organ.
[b] Epstein-Barr virus reactivation usually presents as a proliferation of transformed B cells and can either be a diffuse disease or produce a mass lesion in a single organ.
[c] *T. gondii* usually causes disease in the brain. In bone marrow transplant recipients, acute pulmonary disease may also occur.
[d] *Strongyloides* "hyperinfection" may present with pulmonary disease—often associated with bacterial pneumonia.
[e] While transmission with organs has been described, it is unusual.

bone marrow is as high as 17% but is most commonly ~1%. The use of enrichment columns and monoclonal-antibody depletion procedures results in a higher incidence of contamination. Approximately 2% of cryopreserved marrow and peripheral blood stem cells transfused as part of treatment for cancer are contaminated. In one series of patients receiving contaminated products, 14% had fever or bacteremia, but none died. Results of cultures performed at the time of cryopreservation and at the time of thawing were helpful in guiding therapy for the recipient.

In many transplantation centers, transmission of infections that may be latent or clinically inapparent in the donor organ has resulted in the development of specific donor-screening protocols. In addition to ordering serologic studies focusing on viruses such as herpes-group viruses [herpes simplex virus (HSV) 1, HSV-2], varicella-zoster virus (VZV), cytomegalovirus (CMV), human herpesvirus (HHV) 6, Epstein-Barr virus (EBV), HHV-8, hepatitis B and C viruses, and HIV and on parasites such as *Toxoplasma gondii*, clinicians caring for organ donors should consider assessing stool (for parasites) and skin testing for *Mycobacterium tuberculosis*. It is expected that the recipient will have been likewise assessed. This chapter considers aspects of infection unique to various transplantation settings.

INFECTIONS IN BONE MARROW AND HEMATOPOIETIC STEM CELL TRANSPLANT RECIPIENTS

Bone marrow or hematopoietic stem cell transplantation for either immunodeficiency or cancer results in a transient state of complete immune incompetence. Immediately after transplantation, both phagocytes and immune cells (T and B cells) are absent, and the host is extremely susceptible to infection. The reconstitution that follows transplantation has been likened to maturation of the immune system in neonates. The analogy does not entirely predict infections seen in bone marrow transplant (BMT) and hematopoietic stem cell transplant (HSCT) recipients, however, because the new marrow matures in an old host who has several latent infections already.

TIMING OF INFECTIONS In the first month after bone marrow or hematopoietic stem cell transplantation, infectious complications are similar to those in granulocytopenic patients receiving chemotherapy for acute leukemia (Chap. 85). Because of the anticipated 1- to 4-week duration of neutropenia in this population, many centers give prophylactic antibiotics to patients upon initiation of chemotherapy. Prophylactic trimethoprim-sulfamethoxazole or ciprofloxacin decreases the incidence of gram-negative bacteremia among these patients.

In the second month after transplantation, a major concern (particularly in allogeneic BMT/HSCT recipients) is CMV disease (Chap. 185), which rarely has its onset earlier than 14 days after transplantation and may become evident up to 4 months after the procedure (most commonly at 1 to 3 months). In cases in which the donor marrow is depleted of T cells [to prevent graft-versus-host disease (GVHD) or eliminate a T cell tumor], the disease may be manifested earlier. Patients who receive ganciclovir (for prophylaxis, preemptive treatment, or treatment; see below) may develop CMV infection even later than 4 months after transplantation; treatment appears to delay the development of the normal immune response to CMV infection. Although CMV disease may present as isolated fever, cytopenia, or gastrointestinal disease, the foremost cause of death from CMV infection in this setting is pneumonia.

The diagnosis of pneumonia in BMT/HSCT recipients poses some special problems (Table 85-5). Because patients have undergone treatment with multiple chemotherapeutic agents and sometimes radiation, their differential diagnosis should include—in addition to bacterial pneumonia—CMV pneumonitis, pneumonia of other viral or fungal etiology, parasitic pneumonia, diffuse alveolar hemorrhage, and chemical- or radiation-associated pneumonitis. Since fungal disease and viruses such as respiratory syncytial virus (RSV), parainfluenza virus (types 1, 2, and 3), influenza A and B viruses, and adenovirus are also causes of pneumonia in this setting, it is important to diagnose CMV specifically (see below). *M. tuberculosis* has been an uncommon cause of pneumonia among BMT/HSCT recipients in western countries (<0.1 to 0.2%) but is common in Hong Kong (5.5%) and in countries where the prevalence of tuberculosis is high. The exposure history of the recipient is clearly critical in an assessment of posttransplantation infections.

Episodes of bacteremia due to encapsulated organisms and reactivation of VZV mark the late posttransplantation period (6 months after bone marrow reconstitution). Because of the high and prolonged risk of *Pneumocystis carinii* pneumonia (especially among patients being treated for hematologic malignancies), most patients should be maintained on prophylactic doses of trimethoprim-sulfamethoxazole starting 1 month after engraftment and continuing for at least 1 year. Such prophylaxis may also protect patients seropositive for *T. gondii*, which may cause pneumonia as well as central nervous system (CNS) lesions. The advantages of maintaining patients on daily trimethoprim-sulfamethoxazole for 1 year after transplantation include protection against *Listeria monocytogenes* and nocardial disease as well as late bacterial infections with pneumococci and *Haemophilus influenzae*, which are a consequence of the inability of the immature bone marrow to respond to polysaccharide antigens. In patients with GVHD who require prolonged or indefinite courses of steroids and other immunosuppressive agents (e.g., cyclosporine, tacrolimus), there is a high risk of fungal infections (usually with *Candida* or *Aspergillus*), even after engraftment and resolution of neutropenia.

VIRAL INFECTIONS   BMT/HSCT recipients are susceptible to infection with a variety of viruses, including reactivation syndromes caused by most HHVs (Table 136-2) and infections caused by viruses that circulate in the community.

Herpes Simplex Virus   Within the first 2 weeks after transplantation, most patients who are seropositive for HSV-1 excrete the virus in the oropharynx. The ability to isolate HSV declines with time. Administration of prophylactic acyclovir to seropositive BMT/HSCT recipients has been shown to reduce mucositis and prevent HSV pneumonia (a rare condition reported almost exclusively in BMT recipients). Both esophagitis (usually due to HSV-1) and anogenital disease (commonly induced by HSV-2) may be prevented with acyclovir prophylaxis. →*For further discussion, see Chap. 182.*

Varicella-Zoster Virus   Reactivation of herpes zoster may occur within the first month but more commonly occurs several months after transplantation (**see Plate IID-37**). Reactivation rates are ~40% for allogeneic recipients and 25% for autologous recipients. Localized zoster can spread in an immunosuppressed patient. Fortunately, disseminated disease can usually be controlled with high doses of acyclovir. Because of the high incidence of dissemination of herpes zoster among patients with skin lesions, acyclovir is given prophylactically in some centers to prevent severe disease. Low doses of acyclovir (400 mg orally, three times daily) appear to be effective in preventing reactivation of VZV. However, acyclovir also inhibits the development of VZV-specific immunity. Thus, its administration for only 6 months after transplantation does not prevent zoster from occurring when treatment is stopped. Some data suggest that administration of low doses of acyclovir for an entire year after transplantation is effective and may eliminate most cases of posttransplantation zoster. →*For further discussion, see Chap. 183.*

Cytomegalovirus   The onset of CMV disease usually comes between 30 and 90 days after transplantation, when the granulocyte count is adequate but immunologic reconstitution has not occurred. CMV may cause interstitial pneumonia, bone marrow suppression, or graft failure. With the standard use of CMV-negative or filtered blood products, primary CMV infection should be a risk in allogeneic transplantation only when the donor is CMV-seropositive and the recipient is CMV-seronegative. Reactivation disease or superinfection with another strain from the donor is also common in CMV-positive recipients, and most seropositive patients who undergo bone marrow transplantation excrete CMV, with or without clinical findings. Serious CMV disease is much more common among allogeneic recipients and is often associated with GVHD. In addition to pneumonia and marrow suppression (and, less often, graft failure), manifestations of CMV disease in BMT/HSCT recipients include fever with or without arthralgias, myalgias, and esophagitis. CMV ulcerations occur in both the lower and upper gastrointestinal tract, and it may be difficult to distinguish diarrhea due to GVHD from that due to CMV infection. The finding of CMV in the liver of a patient with GVHD does not necessarily mean that CMV is responsible for hepatic enzyme abnormalities.

Management of CMV disease in BMT/HSCT recipients includes strategies directed at prophylaxis, suppression, preemptive therapy, or treatment. Prophylaxis results in a lower incidence of disease at the cost of treating many patients who otherwise would not require therapy. Because of the high fatality rate associated with CMV pneumonia in these patients and the difficulty of early diagnosis of CMV infection, prophylactic ganciclovir has been used in some centers and has been shown to abort CMV disease during the period of maximal vulnerability (from engraftment to day 120 after transplantation). The foremost problem with the administration of this drug relates to adverse effects, which include dose-related bone marrow suppression (thrombocytopenia, leukopenia, anemia, and pancytopenia). Because the frequency of CMV pneumonia is lower among autologous BMT recipients (2 to 7%) than among allogeneic BMT recipients (10 to 40%), prophylaxis in the former group will not become the rule until a less toxic antiviral agent becomes available.

Like prophylaxis, suppressive treatment, which targets patients with polymerase chain reaction evidence of CMV or CMV-positive urine cultures, entails the unnecessary treatment of many individuals (on the basis of a laboratory test that is not highly predictive of disease) with drugs that have adverse effects. Currently, because of the neutropenia associated with ganciclovir in BMT/HSCT recipients, a preemptive approach—treatment of those patients in whose blood CMV is detected by an antigen or DNA test—is used at most centers. This approach is almost as effective as prophylaxis or suppression and causes less toxicity. The use of the leukocyte antigen test for CMV disease (fluorescent staining of leukocytes for CMV antigens) allows earlier diagnosis but leads to treatment of more patients than would be treated on the basis of blood cultures, with a consequent increase in very late disease (>120 days after transplantation). The use of quantitative viral load assays, which are not dependent on circulating polymorphonuclear leukocytes, should permit early accurate diagnosis in the future.

Table 136-2   Herpes-Group Virus Syndromes in Transplant Recipients

Virus	Reactivation Disease
Herpes simplex virus type 1	Oral lesions, sometimes with spread Pneumonia, described only in BMT patients Hepatitis
Herpes simplex virus type 2	Severe and/or persistent anogenital lesions Hepatitis
Varicella-zoster virus	Zoster (dissemination may occur)
Cytomegalovirus	Associated with graft rejection, fever, bone marrow failure, pneumonitis, gastrointestinal disease
Epstein-Barr virus	B cell lymphoproliferative disease (EBV-LPD) Oral hairy leukoplakia (rare)
Human herpesvirus 6	Fever, rash,[a] pneumonitis, bone marrow suppression, encephalitis (manifestations are controversial)
Human herpesvirus 7	Undefined
Kaposi's sarcoma–associated virus/human herpesvirus 8	Kaposi's sarcoma Primary effusion lymphoma (rare) Multicentric Castleman's disease (rare)

[a] A rash may be seen with primary infections, but it is difficult to distinguish from other rashes seen in these patients.
NOTE: BMT, bone marrow transplant.

Treatment of CMV pneumonia in BMT/HSCT recipients requires both intravenous immune globulin (IVIG) and ganciclovir. In patients who cannot tolerate ganciclovir, foscarnet is a useful alternative, although it may produce nephrotoxicity and electrolyte imbalance. Transfusion of CMV-specific T cells from the donor decreased viral load in a small series of patients; this result suggests that immunotherapy may play a role in the treatment of this disease in the future. →*For further discussion, see Chap. 185.*

Human Herpesviruses 6 and 7 HHV-6, the cause of exanthem subitum in children (Chap. 185), is a ubiquitous herpesvirus that reactivates (as determined by culture of the virus from the blood) in ~50% of transplant recipients between 2 and 4 weeks after surgery. In some cases, reactivation of HHV-6 appears to be associated with neutropenia; since, like CMV, this virus can be found in marrow cells, it is possible that HHV-6 reactivation is responsible for some of the neutropenia that follows bone marrow transplantation. Although encephalitis developing after transplantation has been associated with HHV-6 in cerebrospinal fluid (CSF), the causality of the association is not well defined. HHV-6 DNA is sometimes found in lung samples after transplantation. However, its role in pneumonitis is unclear. While HHV-6 has been shown to be sensitive to foscarnet (and in some instances to ganciclovir) in vitro, the efficacy of antiviral treatment has not been well studied. Little is known about the related herpesvirus HHV-7 or its role in posttransplantation infection. →*For further discussion, see Chap. 185.*

Epstein-Barr Virus Primary EBV infection can be fatal to transplant recipients; EBV reactivation can cause EBV–B cell lymphoproliferative disease (LPD), which may also be fatal to patients taking immunosuppressive drugs. The localization of EBV to B cells leads to several interesting phenomena in BMT/HSCT recipients. The marrow ablation that occurs as part of the BMT/HSCT procedure may eliminate latent EBV from the host. Infection can then be reacquired immediately after transplantation by transfer of infected donor B cells. Alternatively, transplantation from a seronegative donor may result in cure. The recipient is then at risk for a second primary infection.

EBV-LPD can develop in the recipient's B cells (if any should survive marrow ablation) but is more likely to be a consequence of outgrowth of infected donor cells. Both lytic and latent EBV replication are more likely during immunosuppression (e.g., they are associated with GVHD and the use of antibodies to T cells). Although less likely in autologous transplantation, reactivation can occur in T cell–depleted autologous recipients (e.g., patients being treated for a T cell lymphoma with marrow depletion using antibodies to T cells). EBV-LPD, which usually becomes apparent 1 to 3 months after engraftment, can cause high fevers and cervical adenopathy resembling the symptoms of infectious mononucleosis but more commonly presents as an extranodal mass. The incidence of 0.6% among allogeneic BMT/HSCT recipients contrasts with figures of ~5% for renal transplant recipients and up to 20% for cardiac transplant patients. In all cases, EBV-LPD is more likely to occur with continued immunosuppression (especially that caused by the use of antibodies to T cells and cyclosporine or tacrolimus).

EBV-specific T cells generated from the donor have been used experimentally to prevent and to treat EBV-LPD in the allogeneic recipient. Some studies indicate that EBV-LPD can be treated with antibodies to B cell surface antigens. Use of an anti-CD20 monoclonal antibody (Rituximab) to treat B cell lymphomas that express this surface protein has elicited some dramatic responses. Studies are in progress to assess efficacy in EBV-LPD, in which the involved B cells commonly bear CD20. The role of antivirals is uncertain because no available agents have been documented to have activity against latent EBV infection. Ganciclovir has been postulated to have activity on the basis of its ability to inhibit proliferation of B cells, but this activity is associated with toxicity. Both interferon α and retinoic acid have been used in the treatment of EBV-LPD, as has IVIG, but no large studies have assessed the efficacy of these agents. Chemotherapeutic regimens have been used as a last resort, even though patients' tolerance and long-term results have been disappointing in this setting. →*For further discussion, see Chap. 184.*

Human Herpesvirus 8 The EBV-related gamma herpesvirus HHV-8, which is causally associated with Kaposi's sarcoma, with primary effusion lymphoma, and sometimes with multicentric Castleman's disease, has rarely resulted in disease in BMT/HSCT recipients. The reasons may be a relatively low seroprevalence in the population and the limited duration of profound T cell suppression after bone marrow/hematopoietic stem cell transplantation. →*For further discussion, see Chap. 185.*

Other (Nonherpes) Viruses Both RSV and parainfluenza viruses, particularly type 3, can cause severe or even fatal pneumonia in BMT recipients. Infections with both of these agents sometimes occur as disastrous nosocomial epidemics. Therapy with aerosolized ribavirin as well as RSV immunoglobulin or monoclonal antibody to RSV (Palivizumab) has been reported to lessen the severity of RSV disease, but there are no large studies to prove efficacy. Influenza is also seen in BMT recipients and generally mirrors the presence of infection in the community. Several drugs are available for the treatment of influenza (amantadine/rimantadine, ribavirin?) but have limited effects, primarily reducing symptoms and shortening the duration of illness. The newly approved neuraminidase inhibitors are active against both influenza A virus and influenza B virus. Their role in ameliorating disease in this patient population is unknown. Adenovirus can be isolated from BMT recipients at rates varying from 5 to 18%. Although hemorrhagic cystitis, pneumonia, and fatal disseminated infection have been reported, adenovirus infection, which (like CMV infection) usually occurs in the first or second month after transplantation, is often asymptomatic. Therapy with intravenous ribavirin is questionably effective. Cidofovir has proved effective in animal models and in case reports. Infections with parvovirus B19 (presenting as anemia or occasionally pancytopenia) and enteroviruses (sometimes fatal) can occur. Pleconaril, a newly developed capsid-binding agent, is being studied for treatment of enterovirus infection. Rotaviruses are a common cause of gastroenteritis in BMT/HSCT recipients. BK and, to a lesser extent, JC virus (polyomavirus hominis 1 and 2, respectively) are found in the urine of some transplant recipients. BK viruria may be associated with hemorrhagic cystitis. Progressive multifocal leukoencephalopathy caused by JC virus is rare among BMT/HSCT recipients compared with the rate among patients with impaired T cell function due to HIV infection. There is no known treatment for this disease; however, cidofovir and other agents are under study.

INFECTIONS IN SOLID ORGAN TRANSPLANT RECIPIENTS

Morbidity and mortality among solid organ transplant recipients have been reduced by the use of more effective antibiotics. The organisms that cause infections in recipients of solid organ transplants are different from those that infect BMT/HSCT recipients because solid organ recipients do not go through a period of neutropenia. As the transplantation procedure involves surgery, however, solid organ recipients are subject to infections at anastomotic sites and to wound infections. Compared with BMT/HSCT recipients, organ transplant patients are immunosuppressed for more prolonged periods (often permanently). Thus they are susceptible to the same organisms as patients with chronically impaired T cell immunity (Chap. 85, especially Table 85-1).

During the early period (<1 month after transplantation), infections are most often caused by extracellular bacteria (staphylococci, streptococci, *Escherichia coli*, other gram-negative organisms), which often originate in surgical wound or anastomotic sites. The spectrum of infection is largely determined by the type of transplant.

In subsequent weeks, the consequences of the administration of agents that suppress cell-mediated immunity and of the acquisition or reactivation (from the transplanted organ) of viruses and parasites become apparent. CMV infection is often a problem in the first 6 months after transplantation and may present as severe systemic disease or as an infection of the transplanted organ. HHV-6 reactivation (assessed by blood culture) occurs within the first 2 to 4 weeks after transplantation and may be associated with fever and granulocytopenia.

CMV is associated not only with generalized immunosuppression but also with organ-specific, rejection-related syndromes: glomerulopathy in kidney transplant recipients, bronchiolitis obliterans in lung transplant recipients, vasculopathy in heart transplant recipients, and the vanishing bile duct syndrome in liver transplant recipients. A complex interplay between increased CMV replication and enhanced graft rejection is well established: Increasing immunosuppression leads to increased CMV replication, which is associated with graft rejection. For this reason, considerable attention has been focused on the diagnosis, treatment, and prophylaxis of CMV infection in organ transplant recipients.

Beyond 6 months after transplantation, infections characteristic of patients with defects in cell-mediated immunity—e.g., infections with *Listeria*, *Nocardia*, various fungi, and other intracellular pathogens—may be a problem. Elimination of these late infections will not be possible until specific tolerance to the transplanted organ can be achieved without the administration of drugs that lead to generalized immunosuppression. Meanwhile, vigilance, prophylaxis/preemptive therapy (when indicated), and rapid diagnosis and treatment of infections can be lifesaving in solid organ transplant recipients, who, unlike most BMT recipients, continue to be immunosuppressed.

Solid organ transplant recipients are susceptible to EBV-LPD from as early as 2 months to many years after transplantation. The prevalence of this complication is increased by potent and prolonged use of T cell–suppressive drugs. The condition may be reversed (in some cases) by decreasing the degree of immunosuppression. Among organ transplant patients, those with heart and lung transplants—who receive the most intensive immunosuppressive regimens—are most likely to develop EBV-LPD, particularly in the lungs. Although disease usually originates in recipient B cells, several cases of donor origin have been reported. There is a notable tendency for EBV-LPD to develop in the transplanted organ. High organ-specific content of B lymphoid tissues (i.e., bronchial-associated lymphoid tissue in the lung), anatomic factors (i.e., lack of access of host T cells to the transplanted organ because of disturbed lymphatics), and differences in major histocompatibility loci between the host T cells and the organ (i.e., lack of cell migration or lack of effective T cell/macrophage cooperation) may result in defective elimination of EBV-infected B cells.

INFECTIOUS COMPLICATIONS OF KIDNEY TRANSPLANTATION (See Table 136-3) **Early Infections** Infections developing soon after kidney transplantation are often caused by bacteria associated with skin or wound infections. Some data indicate a role for perioperative antibiotic prophylaxis, and many centers give cephalosporins or a penicillin with an aminoglycoside to decrease the risk of postoperative complications. Urinary tract infections developing soon after transplantation are usually related to anatomic alterations resulting from surgery. Such early infections may require prolonged treatment (e.g., 6 weeks of antibiotic administration for pyelonephritis). Urinary tract infections that occur >6 months after transplantation do not seem to be associated with the high rate of pyelo-

nephritis or relapse seen with infections that occur in the first 3 months and may be treated for shorter periods.

Prophylaxis with trimethoprim-sulfamethoxazole [1 double-strength tablet (800 mg sulfamethoxazole, 160 mg trimethoprim) per day] for the first 4 months after transplantation decreases the incidence of early and middle-period infections (see below and Table 136-4).

Middle-Period Infections Because of continuing immunosuppression, kidney transplant recipients are predisposed to lung infections characteristic of those in patients with T cell deficiency (i.e., infections with intracellular bacteria, mycobacteria, nocardiae, fungi, viruses, and parasites). The high mortality associated with *Legionella pneumophila* infection (Chap. 151) led to the closing of renal transplant units in hospitals with endemic legionellosis.

About 50% of all renal transplant recipients presenting with fever 1 to 4 months after transplantation have evidence of CMV disease; CMV itself accounts for the fever in over two-thirds of cases and thus is the predominant pathogen during this period. CMV infection (Chap. 185) may also present as arthralgias or myalgias. During this period, this infection may represent primary disease (in the case of a seronegative recipient of a kidney from a seropositive donor) or may present as reactivation disease or superinfection. Patients may have atypical lymphocytosis. Unlike immunocompetent patients, however, they often do not have lymphadenopathy or splenomegaly. Therefore, clinical suspicion and laboratory confirmation are necessary for diagnosis. The clinical syndrome may be accompanied by bone marrow suppression

Table 136-3 Infections After Kidney Transplantation

Site	Period After Transplantation		
	Early (<1 month)	Middle (1–4 months)	Late (>6 months)
Urinary tract	Bacteria (*Escherichia coli*, *Klebsiella*, Enterobacteriaceae, *Pseudomonas*, *Enterococcus*) associated with bacteremia and pyelonephritis, *Candida*	CMV (fever alone is common)	Bacteria; late UTIs usually not associated with bacteremia
Lungs	Bacteria (*Legionella* in endemic settings)	CMV diffuse interstitial pneumonitis, *Pneumocystis carinii*, *Aspergillus*, *Legionella*	*Nocardia, Aspergillus, Mucor*
Central nervous system	—	*Listeria* meningitis, CMV encephalitis, toxoplasmosis	CMV retinitis, *Listeria* meningitis, cryptococcal meningitis, *Aspergillus, Nocardia*

NOTE: CMV, cytomegalovirus; UTIs, urinary tract infections.

Table 136-4 Prophylaxis of Infections in Transplant Recipients

Risk Factor	Infection or Organism	Prophylactic Antibiotics	Examinations
Travel or residence in area with known risk of fungal infection	Coccidioidomycosis, histoplasmosis, blastomycosis	Imidazoles[a] or amphotericin B	Chest radiography
Latent viruses	HSV, VZV, EBV, CMV	Acyclovir after BMT for HSV and VZV; ganciclovir in some settings	Serologic testing for HSV, VZV, CMV, HHV-6, EBV, HHV-8
Latent fungi/parasites	*Pneumocystis carinii, Toxoplasma gondii*	Trimethoprim-sulfamethoxazole or dapsone plus pyrimethamine	Serologic testing for *Toxoplasma*
History of exposure to tuberculosis	*Mycobacterium tuberculosis*	Isoniazid in cases with recent conversion of PPD to positive and no previous treatment	PPD skin testing and chest radiography

[a] The use of imidazoles in this setting is under study.

NOTE: HSV, herpes simplex virus; VZV, varicella-zoster virus; EBV, Epstein-Barr virus; CMV, cytomegalovirus; BMT, bone marrow transplantation; HHV, human herpesvirus; PPD, purified protein derivative.

(particularly leukopenia). CMV also causes glomerulopathy and is associated with an increased incidence of other opportunistic infections. Because of the frequency and severity of CMV disease, a considerable effort has been made to prevent and treat it in renal transplant recipients. Administration of an immune globulin preparation enriched with antibodies to CMV (CMV-Ig) decreases the incidence in the group at highest risk for severe infections (seronegative recipients of seropositive kidneys). Ganciclovir is useful for the treatment of serious CMV disease. One study showed a significant (50%) reduction in CMV disease and rejection at 6 months in patients who received prophylactic valacyclovir (an acyclovir congener) for the first 90 days after renal transplantation. If confirmed, these results will likely change practice.

Infection with the other herpes-group viruses may become evident within 6 months after transplantation or later. Early after transplantation, HSV may cause either oral or anogenital lesions that are usually responsive to acyclovir. Large ulcerating lesions in the anogenital area may lead to bladder and rectal dysfunction as well as predisposing to bacterial infection. VZV may cause fatal disseminated infection in nonimmune kidney transplant recipients, but in immune patients reactivation zoster usually does not disseminate outside the dermatome; thus disseminated VZV infection is a less fearsome complication in kidney transplantation than in bone marrow transplantation. HHV-6 may reactivate and (although usually asymptomatic) may be associated with fever, rash, marrow suppression, or encephalitis.

EBV reactivation disease is more serious; it may present as an extranodal proliferation of B cells that invade the CNS, nasopharynx, liver, small bowel, heart, and transplanted kidney. The disease is diagnosed by the finding of a proliferation of EBV-positive B cells. The incidence of EBV-LPD is higher among patients given high doses of cyclosporine, tacrolimus, or other immunosuppressive agents (including anti-T cell antibodies). Fortunately, disease often regresses once immunocompetence is restored. HHV-8 infection can be transmitted with the donor kidney and is associated with the development of Kaposi's sarcoma in the recipient. Kaposi's sarcoma (primary vs. reactivation of HHV-8) often appears within 1 year after transplantation, although the range of onset times is wide (1 month to ~20 years).

The papovaviruses BK and JC (polyomaviruses hominis 1 and 2) have been cultured from the urine of kidney transplant recipients (as they have from that of BMT recipients). The excretion of BK virus is associated with ureteral strictures and that of JC virus with progressive multifocal leukoencephalopathy (rare). Adenoviruses may persist with continued immunosuppression in these patients.

Kidney transplant recipients are also subject to infections with other intracellular organisms. These patients may develop pulmonary infections with *Nocardia*, *Aspergillus*, and *Mucor* as well as infections with other pathogens in which the T cell/macrophage axis plays an important role. In patients without intravenous catheters, *L. monocytogenes* is the most common cause of bacteremia ≥1 month after renal transplantation. Kidney transplant recipients may develop *Salmonella* bacteremia, which can lead to endovascular infections and require prolonged therapy. Pulmonary infections with *P. carinii* are common unless the patient is maintained on trimethoprim-sulfamethoxazole prophylaxis. *Nocardia* infection (Chap. 165) may present in the skin, bones, lungs, or CNS (where it usually takes the form of single or multiple brain abscesses). *Nocardia* infection generally occurs ≥1 month after transplantation and may follow immunosuppressive treatment for an episode of rejection. Pulmonary findings are nonspecific: localized disease with or without cavities is most common, but the disease may disseminate. The diagnosis is made by culture of the organism from sputum or from the involved nodule. As with *P. carinii*, prophylaxis with trimethoprim-sulfamethoxazole appears to be efficacious in the prevention of disease. The occurrence of *Nocardia* infections >2 years after transplantation suggests that a long-term prophylactic regimen may be justified.

Toxoplasmosis can occur in seropositive patients, usually developing in the first few months after kidney transplantation. Again, trimethoprim-sulfamethoxazole is helpful in prevention. In endemic areas, histoplasmosis, coccidioidomycosis, and blastomycosis may cause pulmonary infiltrates or disseminated disease.

Late Infections Late infections (>6 months after kidney transplantation) include CMV retinitis and a variety of CNS complications. Patients (particularly those whose immunosuppression has been increased) are at risk for subacute meningitis due to *Cryptococcus neoformans*. Cryptococcal disease may present in an insidious manner (sometimes as a skin infection before the development of clear CNS findings). *Listeria* meningitis may have an acute presentation and requires prompt therapy to avoid a fatal outcome.

Patients who continue to take glucocorticoids are predisposed to infection. "Transplant elbow" is a recurrent bacterial infection in and around the elbow that is thought to result from a combination of poor tensile strength of the skin of steroid-treated patients and steroid-induced proximal myopathy that requires patients to push themselves up with their elbows to get out of chairs. Bouts of cellulitis (usually caused by *Staphylococcus aureus*) recur until patients are provided with elbow protection.

Kidney transplant recipients are susceptible to invasive fungal infections—such as those due to *Aspergillus* and *Rhizopus*, which may present as superficial lesions before dissemination. Mycobacterial infection (particularly that with *M. marinum*) can be diagnosed by skin examination. Infection with *Prototheca wickerhamii* (an achlorophyllic alga) has been diagnosed by skin biopsy. Warts caused by human papillomaviruses (HPVs) are a late consequence of persistent immunosuppression; local therapy is usually satisfactory.

HEART TRANSPLANTATION **Early Infections** Sternal wound infection and mediastinitis are early complications of heart transplantation. An indolent course is common, with fever or a mildly elevated white blood cell count preceding the development of site tenderness or drainage. Clinical suspicion based on evidence of sternal instability and failure to heal may lead to the diagnosis. Although common residents of the skin (e.g., *S. aureus* and *S. epidermidis*) as well as gram-negative organisms (e.g., *Pseudomonas aeruginosa*) and fungi (e.g., *Candida*) are often involved, mediastinitis in these patients (in rare cases) can also be due to *Mycoplasma hominis* (Chap. 178). Since this organism requires an anaerobic environment for growth and may be difficult to see on conventional medium, the laboratory should be alerted that *M. hominis* infection is suspected. *M. hominis* mediastinitis has been cured with a combination of surgical debridement (sometimes requiring muscle-flap placement) plus clindamycin and tetracycline. Organisms associated with mediastinitis may be cultured from accompanying pericardial fluid.

Middle-Period Infections *T. gondii* (Chap. 217) resident in the heart of a seropositive donor may be transmitted to a seronegative recipient. Thus serologic screening for *T. gondii* infection is important before and in the months after cardiac transplantation. Rarely, active disease can be introduced at the time of transplantation. The overall incidence of toxoplasmosis is so high in this setting that some prophylaxis is warranted. Although alternatives are available, the most frequently used agent is trimethoprim-sulfamethoxazole, which prevents infection with *Pneumocystis*, *Nocardia*, and other bacterial pathogens. CMV has also been transmitted by heart transplantation. CNS infections can be caused by *Toxoplasma*, *Nocardia*, and *Aspergillus*. *L. monocytogenes* meningitis should be considered in heart transplant recipients with fever and headache.

CMV infection is associated with poor outcomes after heart transplantation. The virus is usually cultivable 1 to 2 months after transplantation, causes manifestations (usually fever and atypical lymphocytosis, often associated with leukopenia and thrombocytopenia) at 2 to 3 months, and produces severe disease (e.g., pneumonia) at 3 to 4 months. Seropositive recipients usually develop cultivable virus faster than patients whose primary CMV infection is a consequence of transplantation. Between 40 and 70% of patients develop symptomatic CMV disease in the form of (1) CMV pneumonia, the most likely form of CMV disease to be fatal; (2) CMV esophagitis and gastritis, sometimes accompanied by abdominal pain with or without ulcerations and bleeding; and (3) the CMV syndrome consisting of CMV in the blood with fever, leukopenia, thrombocytopenia, and hepatic enzyme abnormalities. Ganciclovir is efficacious in the treatment of CMV infection; prophylaxis with ganciclovir or possibly with other antivirals, as described for renal transplantation, may reduce the incidence of CMV-related disease.

Late Infections EBV infection usually presents as a lymphoma-like proliferation of B cells late after heart transplantation, particularly in patients maintained on heavy immunosuppression. A subset of heart and heart-lung transplant recipients may develop early (within 2 months) fulminant EBV-LPD. Treatment includes the reduction of immunosuppression if possible and the consideration of B cell antibodies (Rituximab), immunomodulatory agents, or chemotherapy, as discussed earlier under bone marrow/hematopoietic stem cell transplantation. HHV-8-associated disease, including primary effusion lymphoma, has been reported in heart transplant recipients. Prophylaxis for *P. carinii* infection is required for these patients (see below).

LUNG TRANSPLANTATION **Early Infections** It is not surprising that lung transplants are predisposed to the development of pneumonia. The combination of ischemia and the resulting mucosal damage together with accompanying denervation and lack of lymph drainage probably contributes to the high rate of pneumonia (66% in one series). The prophylactic use of high doses of broad-spectrum antibiotics for the first 3 or 4 days after surgery decreases the incidence of pneumonia. Gram-negative pathogens (Enterobacteriaceae and *Pseudomonas* species) are troublesome in the first 2 weeks after surgery (the period of maximal vulnerability). Pneumonia can also be caused by *Candida* (possibly as a result of colonization of the donor lung), *Aspergillus*, and *Cryptococcus*.

Mediastinitis may occur at an even higher rate among lung transplant recipients than among heart transplant recipients and most commonly develops within 2 weeks of surgery. Pneumonitis due to CMV (which may be transmitted as a consequence of transplantation) usually presents between 2 weeks and 3 months after surgery, with primary disease occurring later than reactivation disease.

Middle-Period Infections The incidence of CMV infection, either reactivated or primary, is between 75 and 100% if either the donor or the recipient is seropositive for CMV. CMV-induced disease appears to be most severe in recipients of lung and heart-lung transplants. Whether this severity relates to the mismatch in lung antigen-presenting and host immune cells or is attributable to other (nonimmune) factors is not known. More than half of lung transplant recipients with symptomatic CMV disease have pneumonia. Difficulty in distinguishing the radiographic picture of CMV infection from organ rejection further complicates therapy. CMV can also cause bronchiolitis obliterans in lung transplants. The development of pneumonitis related to HSV has led to the prophylactic use of acyclovir. Such prophylaxis may also decrease rates of CMV disease, but ganciclovir is more active against CMV and is also active against HSV. Ganciclovir prophylaxis for CMV disease in lung transplant recipients is recommended.

Late Infections The incidence of *P. carinii* infection (which may present with a paucity of findings) is high among lung and heart-lung transplant recipients. Some form of prophylaxis for *P. carinii* pneumonia is indicated in all organ transplant situations (Tables 136-4 and 136-5). Trimethoprim-sulfamethoxazole prophylaxis for 12 months after transplantation may be sufficient to prevent *P. carinii* disease in patients whose degree of immunosuppression is not increased.

As in other transplant recipients, infection with EBV may cause either a mononucleosis-like syndrome or LPD. The tendency of the B cell blasts to present in the lung appears to be greater after lung transplantation than after the transplantation of other organs. Reduction of immunosuppression causes remission in some cases, but airway compression can be fatal and more rapid intervention may therefore become necessary. The approach to EBV-LPD is similar to that described in other sections.

LIVER TRANSPLANTATION **Early Infections** As in other types of transplantation, early bacterial infections are a major problem after liver transplantation. Many centers administer systemic

Table 136-5 Prophylactic Antibiotics or Vaccination for Immunocompromised Patients

Underlying Problem	Therapy
Splenectomy	Vaccination against pneumococci, *Haemophilus influenzae*, meningococci[a]
T cell defects (e.g., solid organ transplantation)	Prophylaxis for *P. carinii* while patient is immunosuppressed
Antibody defects (bone marrow/hematopoietic stem cell transplantation)	Vaccination for pneumococcus, *H. influenzae*, meningococci; intravenous immune globulin in some settings

[a] Patients should be advised of the importance of seeking immediate medical attention for suspected infections; it may be advisable for patients to have antibiotics (e.g., amoxicillin or amoxicillin/clavulanate) at home.

broad-spectrum antibiotics for the first 5 days after surgery, even in the absence of documented infection. However, despite prophylaxis, infectious complications are common and are correlated with the duration of the surgical procedure and the type of biliary drainage. An operation lasting >12 h is associated with an increased likelihood of infection. Patients who have a choledochojejunostomy with drainage of the biliary duct to a Roux-en-Y jejunal bowel loop have more fungal infections than those whose bile is drained via a choledochocholedochostomy with anastomosis of the donor common bile duct to the recipient common bile duct.

Peritonitis and intraabdominal abscesses are common complications of liver transplantation. Bacterial peritonitis may result from biliary leaks and primary or secondary infection after leakage of bile. Peritonitis in liver transplant recipients is often polymicrobial, commonly involving enterococci, aerobic gram-negative bacteria, staphylococci, anaerobes, or *Candida*. Only one-third of patients with intraabdominal abscesses have bacteremia. Abscesses within the first month after surgery may occur not only over the liver but also in the spleen, pericolic area, and pelvis. Treatment includes antibiotic administration and drainage as necessary.

Liver transplant patients have a high incidence of fungal infections, and the occurrence of fungal infection (often candidiasis) correlates with preoperative use of glucocorticoids, a long duration of treatment with antibacterial agents, and posttransplantation use of immunosuppressive agents.

Middle-Period Infections The development of postsurgical biliary stricture predisposes patients to cholangitis. These patients may lack the characteristic signs and symptoms of cholangitis: fever, abdominal pain, and jaundice. Alternatively, these findings may be present but may suggest graft rejection. The diagnosis of cholangitis in liver transplant recipients therefore requires documentation of bacteremia or demonstration of aggregated neutrophils in bile duct biopsy specimens. Unfortunately, invasive studies of the biliary tract (either T-tube cholangiography or endoscopic retrograde cholangiopancreatography) may themselves lead to cholangitis. For this reason, many clinicians recommend prophylaxis with antibiotics covering gram-negative organisms and anaerobes when these procedures are performed in liver transplant recipients.

Viral hepatitis is a common complication of liver transplantation (Chap. 295). Reactivation of hepatitis B and C infections, for which transplantation may be performed, is problematic. To prevent hepatitis B infection, high-dose intravenous hepatitis B immune globulin is often administered. The long-term efficacy of lamivudine (3TC) in inhibiting hepatitis B viral replication after transplantation is being studied. A combination of interferon α and ribavirin is being tested for treatment/prophylaxis of hepatitis C infection.

As in other transplantation settings, reactivation disease with herpes-group viruses is common (Table 136-2). Herpesviruses can be transmitted in donor organs. Although CMV hepatitis occurs in ~4% of liver transplant recipients, it is usually not so severe as to require retransplantation. CMV disease develops in the majority of seronegative recipients of organs from CMV-positive donors, but fatality rates are lower in liver transplant recipients than in lung or heart-lung transplant recipients. Disease due to CMV is associated with the vanishing bile duct syndrome after liver transplantation. Patients respond to treatment with ganciclovir; prophylaxis with CMV immune globulin and acyclovir or oral ganciclovir may modify disease. A role for HHV-6 in posttransplantation fever and leukopenia has been proposed. EBV-LPD after liver transplantation shows a propensity for involvement of the liver, and such disease may be of donor origin.

PANCREAS TRANSPLANTATION Transplantation of the pancreas is complicated by early abdominal infection in ~20 to 40% of cases. To prevent contamination of the allograft with enteric bacteria and yeasts, some surgeons, instead of draining the pancreas through the bowel, drain secretions into the urinary tract or bladder. A cuff of duodenum is often used in the anastomosis between the pancreatic graft and the bladder. In addition to bicarbonate loss, this technique causes a high rate of urinary tract infection (30 to 40%) and sterile cystitis. Over the long term, bowel drainage is better tolerated. An alternative method—the transplantation of islet cells only—may eliminate the problems characteristically posed by wound and urinary tract sepsis in pancreas transplant recipients.

Issues related to the development of CMV infection, EBV-LPD, and infections with opportunistic pathogens in patients receiving a pancreas are similar to those in other solid organ transplant recipients.

MISCELLANEOUS INFECTIONS IN SOLID ORGAN TRANSPLANTATION Indwelling Intravenous Catheter Infections The prolonged use of indwelling intravenous catheters for administration of medication, blood products, and nutrition is common in diverse transplantation settings and poses a risk of local and bloodstream infection. Significant insertion-site infection is most commonly caused by *S. aureus*. Bloodstream infection most frequently develops within a week of catheter placement or in patients who become neutropenic. Coagulase-negative staphylococci are the most common isolates from the blood. →*For further discussion of differential diagnosis and therapeutic options, see Chap. 85.*

Tuberculosis The incidence of tuberculosis occurring within 12 months after solid organ transplantation ranges broadly worldwide (0.35 to 15%), reflecting prevalences in local populations. Nonrenal transplantation, GVHD within 6 months, and intensity of immunosuppression are predictive of tuberculosis reactivation and development of disseminated disease in a host with latent disease. Tuberculosis has rarely been transmitted from the donor organ. In contrast to the low mortality in BMT/HSCT recipients, mortality in solid organ transplant patients is reported to be 29%. Isoniazid toxicity has not been a significant problem except in the liver transplantation setting.

Virus-Associated Malignancies In addition to malignancy associated with gammaherpesvirus infection (EBV, HHV-8) and simple warts (HPV), transplant recipients, particularly those who require long-term immunosuppression, are more likely than the general population to develop tumors that are virus-associated or suspected of being virus-associated. The interval to tumor development is usually >1 year. Transplant recipients develop nonmelanoma skin or lip cancers that, in contrast to de novo skin cancers, have a high squamous cell-to-basal cell ratio. Whether HPV plays a major role in these lesions is being investigated. Cervical and vulvar carcinomas, quite clearly associated with HPV, develop with increased frequency in female transplant recipients. In renal transplant recipients, rates of melanoma are modestly increased and rates of cancers of the kidney and bladder are increased.

VACCINATION OF TRANSPLANT RECIPIENTS

In addition to receiving antibiotic prophylaxis, transplant recipients should be vaccinated against likely pathogens (Table 136-6). In the

Table 136-6 Vaccination for Bone Marrow or Solid Organ Transplant Recipients

Vaccine	Use with Indicated Type of Transplantation	
	Bone Marrow	Solid Organ
Pneumococcal, *Haemophilus influenzae*, meningococcal infections	Immunize after transplantation (optimal timing not established); preimmunize[a]	Immunize before transplantation and every 5 years for Pneumovax (others not established)
Seasonal influenza	Vaccinate in the fall Vaccinate close contacts	Vaccinate before transplantation if possible
Poliomyelitis	Administer inactivated vaccine	Administer inactivated vaccine
Measles/mumps/rubella	Immunize 24 months after transplantation if graft-versus-host disease does not develop	Immunize before transplantation
Tetanus, diphtheria	Reimmunize after transplantation	Immunize before transplantation; give boosters at 10 years or as required; new primary series not required

[a] Studies indicate that it is possible to "immunize the graft" before transplantation.

case of BMT recipients, optimal responses cannot be achieved until after reconstitution, despite previous immunization of both donor and recipient. Recipients of allogeneic BMTs must be reimmunized if they are to be protected against pathogens. The situation is less clear-cut in the case of autologous transplantation. T and B cells in the peripheral blood may reconstitute the response if they are transferred in adequate numbers. However, cancer patients (particularly those with Hodgkin's disease, in whom vaccination has been extensively studied) who are undergoing chemotherapy do not respond normally to immunization, and titers of antibodies to infectious agents fall more rapidly than in healthy individuals. Therefore, even immunosuppressed patients who have not had marrow transplants may need booster vaccine injections. If memory cells are specifically eliminated as part of a marrow "cleanup" procedure, it will be necessary to reimmunize the recipient with a new primary series. Optimal times for immunizations of different transplant populations are being evaluated. Immunization of household and other contacts (including health care personnel) against influenza every season is likely to benefit the patient by preventing local spread.

In the absence of compelling data as to optimal timing, it is reasonable to administer the pneumococcal and *H. influenzae* type b conjugate vaccines to both autologous and allogeneic BMT recipients 12 months after transplantation and again 12 months later (since the response to the initial vaccine dose is weak in the early posttransplantation period). These two vaccines are particularly important for patients who have undergone splenectomy. In addition, *Neisseria meningitidis* polysaccharide vaccine, diphtheria vaccine, tetanus vaccine, and inactivated polio vaccine can all be given at these same intervals (12 and 24 months after transplantation). Some authorities recommend a new primary series for tetanus/diphtheria and inactivated polio vaccine (vaccination 12, 14, and 16 months after transplantation). Because of the risk of spread, household contacts of BMT recipients (or of patients immunosuppressed as a result of chemotherapy) should receive only inactivated polio vaccine. Live-virus measles/mumps/rubella (MMR) vaccine can be given to autologous BMT recipients 24 months after transplantation and to most allogeneic BMT recipients at the same point if they are not receiving maintenance therapy with immunosuppressive drugs and do not have ongoing GVHD. The risk of spread from a household contact is lower for MMR than for polio vaccine. In patients who have active GVHD and/or are taking high maintenance doses of glucocorticoids, it may be prudent to avoid all live-virus vaccines. In the absence of detectable antibody titers, vaccination to prevent hepatitis B and hepatitis A also seems advisable.

In the case of solid organ transplant recipients, administration of all the usual vaccines and of the indicated booster doses should be completed before immunosuppression, if possible, to maximize responses. For patients taking immunosuppressive agents, the administration of pneumococcal vaccine should be repeated every 5 years. No data are available for meningococcal polysaccharide vaccine, but it is probably reasonable to administer it along with the pneumococcal vaccine or more frequently (every 3 years for persons with significant exposure risk). *H. influenzae* conjugate vaccine is safe and should be efficacious in this population; therefore, its administration before transplantation is recommended. Booster doses of this vaccine are not recommended for adults. Solid organ transplant recipients who continue to receive immunosuppressive drugs (glucocorticoids, cyclosporine) should not receive live-virus vaccines. A person in this group exposed to measles should be given immune globulin. Similarly, an immunocompromised patient who is seronegative for varicella and who comes into contact with a person who has chickenpox should be given varicella-zoster immune globulin as soon as possible (and certainly within 96 h) or, if this is not possible, started immediately on a 10- to 14-day course of acyclovir therapy. Susceptible household contacts of transplant recipients should receive live attenuated VZV vaccine, but vaccinees should avoid direct contact with the patient if a rash develops.

Immunocompromised patients who travel may benefit from some but not all vaccines. In general, they should receive any killed or inactivated vaccine preparation appropriate to the area they are visiting; this recommendation includes the vaccines for Japanese encephalitis, hepatitis A and B, poliomyelitis, meningococcal infection, and typhoid. The live typhoid vaccines are not recommended for use in most immunocompromised patients, but inactivated typhoid or the purified polysaccharide vaccine can be used. Live yellow fever vaccine should not be administered. Phenol-inactivated cholera vaccine is probably of little use in this setting. On the other hand, immunization with the purified-protein hepatitis B vaccine is indicated if patients are likely to be exposed. Patients who will reside for >6 months in areas where hepatitis B is common (Africa, Southeast Asia, the Middle East, Eastern Europe, parts of South America, and the Caribbean) should receive hepatitis B vaccine. Inactivated hepatitis A vaccine should be used in the appropriate setting (Chap. 122). If hepatitis A vaccine is not administered, travelers should consider receiving passive protection with immune globulin (the dose depending on the duration of travel in the high-risk area).

BIBLIOGRAPHY

CHANG FY et al: Fever in liver transplant recipients: Changing spectrum of etiologic agents. Clin Infect Dis 26:59, 1998

CONE RW et al: Human herpesvirus 6 infections after bone marrow transplantation: Clinical and virologic manifestations. J Infect Dis 179:311, 1999

DE OTERO J et al: Cytomegalovirus disease as a risk factor for graft loss and death after orthotopic liver transplantation. Clin Infect Dis 26:865, 1998

ENGELS EA et al: Early infection in bone marrow transplantation: Quantitative study of clinical factors that affect risk. Clin Infect Dis 28:256, 1999

FISHMAN JA, RUBIN RH: Infection in organ-transplant recipients. N Engl J Med 338: 1741, 1998

MUELLER N: Overview of the epidemiology of malignancy in immune-deficiency. J AIDS 21 (Suppl 1):S5, 1999

PRENTICE HG, KHO P: Clinical strategies for the management of cytomegalovirus infection and disease in allogeneic bone marrow transplant. Bone Marrow Transplant 19: 135, 1997

REGAMEY N et al: Transmission of human herpesvirus 8 infections from renal-transplant donors to recipients. N Engl J Med 339:1358, 1998

ROONEY CM et al: Use of gene-modified virus-specific T lymphocytes to control Epstein-Barr-virus related lymphoproliferation. Lancet 345:9, 1995

SOMANI J, LARSON RA: Reimmunization after allogeneic bone marrow transplantation. Am J Med 98:389, 1995

WEBB IJ et al: Sources and sequelae of bacterial contamination of hematopoietic stem cell products: Implications for safety and hematotherapy and graft engineering. Transfusion 36:782, 1996

Section 4
APPROACH TO THERAPY FOR BACTERIAL DISEASES

137

Gordon L. Archer, Ronald E. Polk

TREATMENT AND PROPHYLAXIS OF BACTERIAL INFECTIONS

The development of drugs that prevent and cure bacterial infections is one of the twentieth century's major contributions to human longevity and quality of life. Antibacterial agents are among the most commonly prescribed drugs of any kind worldwide. Used appropriately, these drugs are lifesaving. However, their indiscriminate use drives up the cost of health care, leads to a plethora of side effects and drug interactions, and fosters the emergence of bacterial resistance, rendering previously valuable drugs useless. The rational use of antibacterial agents depends on an understanding of their mechanisms of action, pharmacokinetics, toxicities, and interactions; bacterial strategies for resistance; and bacterial susceptibility in vitro. In addition, patient-associated parameters, such as the site of infection and the immune and excretory status of the host, are critically important to appropriate therapeutic decisions. This chapter provides specific data required for making an informed choice of antibacterial agent.

MECHANISMS OF ACTION

Antibacterial agents, like all antimicrobial drugs, are directed against unique targets not present in mammalian cells. The goal is to limit toxicity to the host and maximize chemotherapeutic activity affecting invading microbes only. The mechanisms of action of the antibacterial agents to be discussed in this section are summarized in Table 137-1 and are depicted in Fig. 137-1.

INHIBITION OF CELL-WALL SYNTHESIS One major difference between bacterial and mammalian cells is the presence in bacteria of a rigid wall external to the cell membrane. The wall protects bacterial cells from osmotic rupture, which would result from the cell's usual marked hyperosmolarity (by up to 20 atm) relative to the host environment. The structure conferring cell-wall rigidity and resistance to osmotic lysis in both gram-positive and -negative bacteria is peptidoglycan, a large, covalently linked sacculus that surrounds the bacterium. In gram-positive bacteria, peptidoglycan is the only layered structure external to the cell membrane and is thick (20 to 80 nm); in gram-negative bacteria, there is an outer membrane external to a very thin (1-nm) peptidoglycan layer.

Chemotherapeutic agents directed at any stage of the synthesis, export, assembly, or cross-linking of peptidoglycan lead to inhibition

Table 137-1 Mechanisms of Action of and Resistance to Major Classes of Antibacterial Agents

Letter for Fig. 137-1	Antibacterial Agent[a]	Major Cellular Target	Mechanism of Action	Major Mechanisms of Resistance
A	β-Lactams (penicillins and cephalosporins)	Cell wall	Inhibit cell-wall cross-linking	1. Drug inactivation (β-lactamase) 2. Insensitivity of target (altered penicillin-binding proteins) 3. Decreased permeability (altered gram-negative outer-membrane porins) 4. Active efflux
B	Vancomycin	Cell wall	Interferes with addition of new cell-wall subunits (muramyl pentapeptides)	Alteration of target (substitution of terminal amino acid of peptidoglycan subunit)
	Bacitracin	Cell wall	Prevents addition of cell-wall subunits by inhibiting recycling of membrane lipid carrier	Not defined
C	Macrolides (erythromycin)	Protein synthesis	Bind to 50S ribosomal subunit	1. Alteration of target (ribosomal methylation) 2. Active efflux
	Lincosamides (clindamycin)	Protein synthesis	Bind to 50S ribosomal subunit	Alteration of target (ribosomal methylation)
D	Chloramphenicol	Protein synthesis	Binds to 50S ribosomal subunit	1. Drug inactivation (chloramphenicol acetyltransferase) 2. Active efflux
E	Tetracycline	Protein synthesis	Binds to 30S ribosomal subunit	1. Decreased intracellular drug accumulation (active efflux) 2. Insensitivity of target
F	Aminoglycosides (gentamicin)	Protein synthesis	Bind to 30S ribosomal subunit	1. Drug inactivation (aminoglycoside-modifying enzyme) 2. Decreased permeability through gram-negative outer membrane 3. Active efflux
G	Mupirocin	Protein synthesis	Inhibits isoleucine tRNA synthetase	Mutation of gene for target protein or acquisition of new gene for drug-insensitive target
H	Sulfonamides and trimethoprim	Cell metabolism	Competitively inhibit enzymes involved in two steps of folic acid biosynthesis	Production of insensitive targets [dihydropteroate synthetase (sulfonamides) and dihydrofolate reductase (trimethoprim)] that bypass metabolic block
I	Rifampin	Nucleic acid synthesis	Inhibits DNA-dependent RNA polymerase	Insensitivity of target (mutation of polymerase gene)
J	Metronidazole	Nucleic acid synthesis	Intracellularly generates short-lived reactive intermediates by electron transfer system	Not defined
K	Quinolones (ciprofloxacin)	DNA synthesis	Inhibit DNA gyrase (A subunit) and topoisomerase IV	1. Insensitivity of target (mutation of gyrase genes) 2. Decreased intracellular drug accumulation (active efflux)
	Novobiocin	DNA synthesis	Inhibits DNA gyrase (B subunit)	Not defined
L	Polymyxins (polymyxin B)	Cell membrane	Disrupt membrane permeability by charge alteration	Not defined
	Gramicidin	Cell membrane	Forms pores	Not defined

[a] Compounds in parentheses are major representatives for the class.

of bacterial cell growth and, in most cases, to cell death. Peptidoglycan is composed of (1) a backbone of two alternating sugars, N-acetylglucosamine and N-acetylmuramic acid; (2) a chain of four amino acids that extends down from the backbone (stem peptides); and (3) a peptide bridge that cross-links the peptide chains. Peptidoglycan is formed by the addition of subunits (a sugar with its five attached amino acids) that are assembled in the cytoplasm and transported through the cytoplasmic membrane to the cell surface. Subsequent cross-linking is driven by cleavage of the terminal stem-peptide amino acid. Antibacterial agents act to inhibit cell-wall synthesis in several ways, as described below.

Bacitracin, a cyclic peptide antibiotic, inhibits the conversion to its active form of the lipid carrier that moves the water-soluble cytoplasmic peptidoglycan subunits through the cell membrane to the cell exterior. Cell-wall subunits accumulate in the cytoplasm and cannot be added to the growing peptidoglycan chain.

Glycopeptides (vancomycin and teicoplanin) are high-molecular-weight antibiotics that bind to the terminal D-alanine–D-alanine component of the stem peptide while the subunits are external to the cell membrane but still linked to the lipid carrier. This binding sterically inhibits the addition of subunits to the peptidoglycan backbone.

β-Lactam antibiotics (penicillins, cephalosporins, carbapenems,

and monobactams; Table 137-2), characterized by a four-membered β-lactam ring, prevent the cross-linking reaction called *transpeptidation*. The energy for attaching a peptide cross-bridge from the stem peptide of one peptidoglycan subunit to another is derived from the cleavage of a terminal D-alanine residue from the subunit stem peptide. The cross-bridge amino acid is then attached to the penultimate D-alanine by transpeptidase enzymes. The β-lactam ring of the antibiotic forms an irreversible covalent acyl bond with the transpeptidase enzyme (probably because of the antibiotic's steric similarity to the enzyme's D-alanine–D-alanine target), preventing the cross-linking reaction. Transpeptidases and similar enzymes involved in cross-linking are called *penicillin-binding proteins* (PBPs) because they all have active sites that bind β-lactam antibiotics.

Virtually all the antibiotics that inhibit bacterial cell-wall synthesis are bactericidal. That is, they eventually result in the cell's death due to osmotic lysis. However, much of the loss of cell-wall integrity following treatment with cell wall–active agents is due to the bacteria's own cell-wall remodeling enzymes (autolysins) that cleave peptidoglycan bonds in the normal course of cell growth. In the presence of antibacterial agents that inhibit cell-wall growth, autolysis proceeds without normal cell-wall repair; weakness and eventual cellular lysis occur.

Mechanisms of Action

GRAM NEGATIVE | **GRAM POSITIVE**

Mechanisms of Resistance

GRAM NEGATIVE | **GRAM POSITIVE**

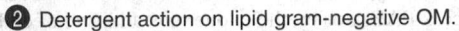

② Detergent action on lipid gram-negative OM.

③ Penetration of hydrophilic drugs through porin channels in gram-negative OM.

④ Free diffusion through gram-positive cell envelope with binding to cell-wall PG *or*

⑤ Binding to cell-membrane PBP. Drug confined to space external to IM.

⑥ Diffusion or transport of drugs with intracellular target through IM.

⑦ Binding to ribosomal target for protein synthesis inhibition.

⑧ Antibiotic interaction with target protein leading to metabolic (DHFR, DHPS), protein synthetic (tRNA synthetase), or nucleic acid (DNA gyrase, RNA polymerase) abnormalities.

⑨ Direct interaction of reactive intermediates with nucleic acid.

① *Intrinsic resistance*: Inability of antibiotic to penetrate gram-negative envelope (e.g., vancomycin).

③ Mutant porin channels *decrease* antimicrobial *penetration*.

④ *Production of insensitive target* by acquired gene mediating production of altered PG.

⑤ₐ *Production of β-lactam-insensitive PBP target* by mutation of gene or acquisition of new gene.

⑤ᵦ *Inactivation* of β-lactam antibiotic by β-lactamases in periplasm (gram-negative) or surrounding medium (gram-positive).

⑥ *Active efflux* of drugs from cytoplasm or from gram-negative periplasm.

⑦ₐ Decreased ribosomal binding due to *target site alteration*.

⑦ᵦ *Inactivation* of drug by chemical modification leading to decreased ribosomal interaction.

⑧ Mutation of target gene or acquisition of new gene producing a *drug-insensitive target* protein.

FIGURE 137-1 Mechanisms of action of and resistance to antibacterial agents. Blue lines trace the routes of drug interaction with bacterial cells, from entry to target site. The letters in each figure indicate specific antibacterial agents or classes of agents, as shown in Table 137-1. The numbers correspond to mechanisms listed beneath each panel. Abbreviations: LPS, lipopolysaccha-ride; OM, outer membrane; PG, peptidoglycan; PBP, penicillin-binding protein; IM, inner (cytoplasmic) membrane; 50s and 30s, large and small ribosome subunits; DHFR, dihydrofolate reductase; DHPS, dihydropteroate synthetase; Ac, acetylation; Ad, adenylation; P, phosphorylation.

INHIBITION OF PROTEIN SYNTHESIS

Most of the antibacterial agents that inhibit protein synthesis interact with the bacterial ribosome. The difference between the composition of bacterial and mammalian ribosomes gives these compounds their selectivity.

Aminoglycosides (gentamicin, kanamycin, tobramycin, streptomycin, netilmicin, neomycin, and amikacin) are a group of structurally related compounds containing three linked hexose sugars. They exert a bactericidal effect by binding irreversibly to the 30S subunit of the bacterial ribosome and blocking initiation of protein synthesis. The reason for the lethal effect of aminoglycosides (as opposed to the largely bacteriostatic effect of other protein synthesis–inhibiting antibacterial drugs, including the macrolides, the lincosamides, chloramphenicol, and tetracycline) is not completely understood. Uptake of aminoglycosides and their penetration through the cell membrane constitute an aerobic, energy-dependent process. Thus, aminoglycoside activity is markedly reduced in an anaerobic environment. *Spectinomycin*, an aminocyclitol antibiotic, also acts on the 30S ribosomal

Table 137-2 Classification of β-Lactam Antibiotics

Class	Route of Administration	
	Parenteral	Oral
Penicillins		
β-Lactamase–susceptible		
Narrow-spectrum	Penicillin G	Penicillin V
Enteric-active	Ampicillin	Amoxicillin, ampicillin
Enteric-active and antipseudomonal	Carbenicillin, ticarcillin, mezlocillin, azlocillin, piperacillin	Indanyl carbenicillin
β-Lactamase–resistant		
Antistaphylococcal	Methicillin, oxacillin, nafcillin	Cloxacillin, dicloxacillin
Combined with β-lactamase inhibitors	Ticarcillin plus clavulanic acid, ampicillin plus sulbactam, piperacillin plus tazobactam	Amoxicillin plus clavulanic acid
Cephalosporins		
First-generation	Cefazolin, cephalothin, cephapirin	Cephalexin, cephradine, cefadroxil
Second-generation		
Haemophilus-active	Cefamandole, cefuroxime, cefonicid, ceforanide	Cefaclor, cefuroxime axetil, ceftibuten, cefdinir, cefixime,[a] cefprozil, cefpodoxime,[a] loracarbef
Bacteroides-active	Cefoxitin, cefotetan, cefmetazole	None
Third-generation		
Extended-spectrum	Ceftriaxone, cefotaxime, ceftizoxime	None
Extended-spectrum and antipseudomonal	Ceftazidime, cefoperazone, cefepime	None
Carbapenems	Imipenem-cilastatin, meropenem	None
Monobactams	Aztreonam	None

[a] Some sources classify cefixime and cefpodoxime as third-generation oral agents because of a marginally broader spectrum.

subunit but has a different mechanism of action from the aminoglycosides and is bacteriostatic rather than bactericidal.

Macrolides (erythromycin, clarithromycin, and azithromycin) consist of a large lactone ring to which sugars are attached. They bind specifically to the 50S portion of the bacterial ribosome. After attachment of mRNA to the initiation site of the 30S ribosomal subunit (the process blocked by aminoglycosides), the 50S subunit becomes bound to the 30S component to form the 70S ribosomal complex, and protein chain elongation proceeds. Binding of macrolides to the 50S ribosomal subunit inhibits protein chain elongation.

Lincosamides (clindamycin and lincomycin), although structurally unrelated to macrolides, bind to a site on the 50S ribosome nearly identical to the binding site for macrolides. Although the mechanism and site of action of macrolides and lincosamides are similar, the number and types of bacteria against which these two groups of agents are active differ.

Chloramphenicol consists of a single aromatic ring and a short side chain. This antibiotic binds reversibly to the 50S portion of the bacterial ribosome at a site close to but not identical with the binding sites of the macrolides and lincosamides. The ribosomal binding of chloramphenicol inhibits peptide bond formation.

Tetracyclines (tetracycline, doxycycline, and minocycline) consist of four aromatic rings with various substituent groups. They interact reversibly with the bacterial 30S ribosomal subunit, blocking the binding of aminoacyl tRNA to the mRNA-ribosome complex. This mechanism is markedly different from that of the aminoglycosides, which also bind to the 30S subunit. The specificity of tetracyclines for bacteria depends both on their selectivity for bacterial ribosomes and on their requirement for active, energy-dependent transport into the bacterial cell by a system not found in mammalian cell membranes.

Mupirocin (pseudomonic acid) is produced by the bacterium *Pseudomonas fluorescens*. Its mechanism of action is unique in that it inhibits the enzyme isoleucine tRNA synthetase by competing with bacterial isoleucine for its binding site on the enzyme. Inhibition of this enzyme depletes cellular stores of isoleucine-charged tRNA and therefore leads to a cessation of protein synthesis. The antibiotic is selective for bacteria because mammalian isoleucine tRNA synthetase lacks affinity for the compound.

INHIBITION OF BACTERIAL METABOLISM The *antimetabolites* are all synthetic compounds that interfere with bacterial synthesis of folic acid. Products of the folic acid synthesis pathway function as coenzymes for the one-carbon transfer reactions that are essential for the synthesis of thymidine, all purines, and several amino acids. Inhibition of folate synthesis leads to cessation of bacterial cell growth and, in some cases, to bacterial cell death. The principal antibacterial antimetabolites are sulfonamides (sulfisoxazole, sulfadiazine, and sulfamethoxazole) and trimethoprim.

Sulfonamides are structural analogues of *p*-aminobenzoic acid (PABA), one of the three structural components of folic acid (the other two being pteridine and glutamate). The first step in the synthesis of folic acid is the addition of PABA to pteridine by the enzyme dihydropteroic acid synthetase. Sulfonamides compete with PABA as substrates for the enzyme. The selective effect of sulfonamides is due to the fact that bacteria synthesize folic acid, while mammalian cells cannot synthesize the cofactor and must have exogenous supplies. However, the activity of sulfonamides can be greatly reduced by the presence of excess PABA or by the exogenous addition of end products of one-carbon transfer reactions (e.g., thymidine and purines). High concentrations of the latter substances may be present in some infections as a result of tissue and white cell breakdown, compromising sulfonamide activity.

Trimethoprim is a diaminopyrimidine, a structural analogue of the pteridine moiety of folic acid. It is a competitive inhibitor of dihydrofolate reductase; this enzyme is responsible for reduction of dihydrofolic acid to tetrahydrofolic acid, the essential final component in the folic acid synthesis pathway that is necessary for all one-carbon transfer reactions. Like the sulfonamides, trimethoprim is bactericidal in the absence of thymine but is only bacteriostatic when this pyrimidine is present in high concentration. The selective antibacterial activity of trimethoprim is based on the extreme sensitivity of bacterial dihydrofolate reductase to inhibition by this drug in comparison with the mammalian enzyme. The bacterial enzyme is approximately 50,000 times more sensitive to such inhibition.

INHIBITION OF NUCLEIC ACID SYNTHESIS OR ACTIVITY Numerous antibacterial compounds have disparate effects on nucleic acids. The *quinolones*, including nalidixic acid and its fluorinated derivatives (norfloxacin, ciprofloxacin, ofloxacin, levofloxacin, sparfloxacin, grepafloxacin, and trovafloxacin), are synthetic compounds that inhibit the activity of the A subunit of the bacterial enzyme DNA gyrase as well as topoisomerase IV. DNA gyrase and topoisomerases are responsible for negative supercoiling of DNA, an essential conformation for DNA replication in the intact cell. Inhibition of the activity of DNA gyrase and topoisomerase IV is lethal to bacterial cells. The antibiotic *novobiocin* also interferes with the activity of DNA gyrase, but it interferes with the B subunit.

Rifampin, used primarily against *Mycobacterium tuberculosis*, is also active against a variety of other bacteria. Rifampin binds tightly to the B subunit of bacterial DNA-dependent RNA polymerase, thus inhibiting transcription of DNA into RNA. Mammalian-cell RNA polymerase is not sensitive to the compound.

Nitrofurantoin, a synthetic compound, causes DNA damage. The nitrofurans, compounds containing a single five-membered ring, are reduced by a bacterial enzyme to highly reactive, short-lived intermediates that are thought to cause DNA strand breakage, either directly or indirectly.

Metronidazole, a synthetic imidazole, is active against a wide range of anaerobic bacteria and protozoa. This activity is totally dependent on the organism's anaerobic electron-transport system for energy production. In the presence of this system, the nitro group of metronidazole is reduced to a series of transiently produced, reactive intermediates that are thought to cause DNA damage. The unique redox system of anaerobes accounts for the selective antibacterial activity of metronidazole. This compound is also a mutagen and a radiosensitizer of hypoxic mammalian cells.

ALTERATION OF CELL-MEMBRANE PERMEABILITY
The *polymyxins* (polymyxin B and colistin, or polymyxin E) are cyclic, basic polypeptides. They behave as cationic, surface-active compounds that disrupt the permeability of both the outer and the cytoplasmic membranes of gram-negative bacteria.

Gramicidin A is a polypeptide of 15 amino acids that acts as an ionophore, forming pores or channels in lipid bilayers.

MECHANISMS OF RESISTANCE

Some bacteria have *intrinsic resistance* to certain classes of antibacterial agents (e.g., obligate anaerobic bacteria to aminoglycosides and gram-negative bacteria to vancomycin). Clearly these agents can never be used alone in the treatment of infections caused by resistant bacteria. In addition, bacteria that are ordinarily susceptible to antibacterial agents can acquire resistance. *Acquired resistance* is one of the major limitations to effective antibacterial chemotherapy. Resistance can develop by mutation of resident genes or by acquisition of new genes. New genes mediating resistance are usually spread from cell to cell by way of mobile genetic elements such as plasmids, transposons, and bacteriophages. The resistant bacterial populations flourish in areas of high antimicrobial use, where they enjoy a selective advantage over susceptible populations.

The major mechanisms used by bacteria to resist the action of antimicrobial agents are inactivation of the compound, alteration or overproduction of the antibacterial target through mutation of the target protein's gene, acquisition of a new gene that encodes a drug-insensitive target, decreased permeability of the cell envelope to the agent, and active elimination of the compound from the periplasm or interior of the cell. Specific mechanisms of bacterial resistance to the major antibacterial agents are outlined below, summarized in Table 137-1, and depicted in Fig. 137-1.

β-LACTAMS Bacteria develop resistance to β-lactam antibiotics by a variety of mechanisms. Most common is the destruction of the drug by β-lactamases. The β-lactamases of gram-negative bacteria are confined to the periplasm, between the inner and outer membranes, while gram-positive bacteria secrete their β-lactamases into the surrounding medium. These enzymes have a higher affinity for the antibiotic than the antibiotic has for its target. Binding results in hydrolysis of the β-lactam ring. Genes encoding β-lactamases have been found in both chromosomal and extrachromosomal locations and in both gram-positive and -negative bacteria; these genes are often on mobile genetic elements. One strategy that has been devised for circumventing resistance mediated by β-lactamases is to combine the susceptible β-lactam with an inhibitor that avidly binds the inactivating enzyme, preventing its attack on the antibiotic. Unfortunately, the inhibitors (e.g., clavulanic acid, sulbactam, and tazobactam) do not bind all classes of β-lactamase and thus cannot be depended on to prevent the inactivation of β-lactam antibiotics by such enzymes. No β-lactam antibiotic or inhibitor has been produced that can resist all of the many β-lactamases that have been identified.

A second mechanism of bacterial resistance to β-lactam antibiotics is an alteration in PBP targets so that the PBPs have a markedly re-

duced affinity for the drug. While this alteration may occur by mutation of existing genes, the acquisition of new PBP genes (as in staphylococcal resistance to methicillin) or of new pieces of PBP genes (as in streptococcal, gonococcal, and meningococcal resistance to penicillin) is more important.

A final resistance mechanism is the coupling, in gram-negative bacteria, of a decrease in outer-membrane permeability with rapid efflux of the antibiotic from the periplasm to the cell exterior. Mutations of genes encoding outer-membrane proteins called *porins* decrease the entry of β-lactam antibiotics into the cell, while additional proteins form channels that actively pump β-lactams out of the cell. Resistance of Enterobacteriaceae to some cephalosporins and resistance of *Pseudomonas* spp. to cephalosporins and ureidopenicillins are the best examples of this mechanism.

VANCOMYCIN Clinically important resistance to vancomycin was first described among enterococci in France in 1988. Vancomycin-resistant enterococci have subsequently become disseminated worldwide. The genes encoding resistance are carried on plasmids that can transfer themselves from cell to cell. Resistance is mediated by enzymes that substitute D-lactate for D-alanine on the peptidoglycan stem peptide so that there is no longer an appropriate target for vancomycin binding. This alteration does not appear to affect cell-wall integrity, however. This type of acquired vancomycin resistance is so far confined to enterococci and is seen in *Enterococcus faecium* rather than in the more common pathogen *E. faecalis*. Most clinically important staphylococci (i.e., *Staphylococcus aureus* and *S. epidermidis*) remain susceptible. However, in 1996, an isolate of *S. aureus* recovered from an infected patient in Japan was shown to be eight times less susceptible to vancomycin than were usual isolates. Since that report, an additional three *S. aureus* isolates with intermediate susceptibility to vancomycin have been recovered from infected patients in the United States, as have numerous coagulase-negative staphylococci with reduced vancomycin susceptibility. These isolates have not acquired the genes that mediate vancomycin resistance in enterococci but are mutant bacteria with markedly thickened cell walls. These mutants were apparently selected in patients who were undergoing prolonged vancomycin therapy.

AMINOGLYCOSIDES The most common aminoglycoside resistance mechanism is inactivation of the antibiotic. Aminoglycoside-modifying enzymes, usually encoded on plasmids, transfer phosphate, adenyl, or acetyl residues from intracellular molecules to hydroxyl or amino side groups on the antibiotic. The modified antibiotic is less active because of diminished binding to its ribosomal target. Modifying enzymes that can inactivate any of the available aminoglycosides have been found in both gram-positive and -negative bacteria.

A second aminoglycoside resistance mechanism that has been identified predominantly in clinical isolates of *Pseudomonas aeruginosa* is decreased antibiotic uptake, presumably due to alterations in the bacterial outer membrane.

MACROLIDES AND LINCOSAMIDES Resistance in gram-positive bacteria, the usual target organisms for macrolides and lincosamides, is due to the production of an enzyme—most commonly plasmid-encoded—that methylates ribosomal RNA, interfering with binding of the antibiotics to their target. Methylation mediates resistance to erythromycin, clarithromycin, azithromycin, and clindamycin. Streptococci can also actively efflux these compounds.

CHLORAMPHENICOL Most bacteria resistant to chloramphenicol produce a plasmid-encoded enzyme, chloramphenicol acetyltransferase, that inactivates the compound by acetylation.

TETRACYCLINES The most common mechanism of tetracycline resistance in gram-negative bacteria is a plasmid-encoded active-efflux pump that is inserted into the cytoplasmic membrane and extrudes antibiotic from the cell. Resistance in gram-positive bacteria is due either to active efflux or to ribosomal alterations that diminish binding of the antibiotic to its target. Genes involved in ribosomal protection are found on mobile genetic elements.

MUPIROCIN Although the topical compound mupirocin was relatively recently introduced into clinical use, resistance is already becoming widespread in some areas. The mechanism appears to be either mutation of the target isoleucine tRNA synthetase so that it is no longer inhibited by the antibiotic or plasmid-encoded production of a form of the target enzyme that binds mupirocin poorly.

TRIMETHOPRIM AND SULFONAMIDES The most prevalent mechanism of resistance to trimethoprim and the sulfonamides in both gram-positive and -negative bacteria is the acquisition of plasmid-encoded genes that produce a new, drug-insensitive target—specifically, an insensitive dihydrofolate reductase for trimethoprim and an altered dihydropteroate synthetase for sulfonamides.

QUINOLONES Resistance to the newer fluoroquinolones emerged rapidly among *Staphylococcus* and *Pseudomonas* spp. after the introduction of these agents. The most common mechanism is the development of one or more mutations in target DNA gyrases and topoisomerase IV that prevent the antibacterial agent from interfering with the activity of the enzyme. Some gram-negative bacteria develop mutations that both decrease outer-membrane porin permeability and cause active drug efflux from the cytoplasm. Mutations that result in active quinolone efflux are also found in gram-positive bacteria.

RIFAMPIN Bacteria rapidly become resistant to rifampin by developing mutations in the B subunit of RNA polymerase that render the enzyme unable to bind the antibiotic. The rapid selection of resistant mutants is the major limitation to the use of this antibiotic against otherwise-susceptible staphylococci and requires that it be used in combination with another antistaphylococcal agent.

MULTIPLE ANTIBIOTIC RESISTANCE The acquisition by one bacterium of resistance to multiple antibacterial agents is becoming increasingly common. The two major mechanisms are the acquisition of multiple unrelated resistance genes and the development of mutations in a single gene or gene complex that mediate resistance to a series of unrelated compounds. The construction of multiresistant strains by acquisition of multiple genes occurs by sequential steps of gene transfer and environmental selection in areas of high-level antimicrobial use. In contrast, mutations in a single gene can conceivably be selected in a single step. Bacteria that are multiresistant by virtue of the acquisition of new genes include hospital-associated gram-negative bacteria, enterococci, and staphylococci and community-acquired strains of salmonellae, gonococci, and pneumococci. Mutations that confer resistance to multiple unrelated antimicrobial agents occur in the genes encoding outer-membrane porins and efflux proteins in gram-negative bacteria. These mutations decrease bacterial intracellular and periplasmic accumulation of β-lactams, quinolones, tetracycline, chloramphenicol, and trimethoprim. Multiresistant bacterial isolates pose increasing problems in U.S. hospitals; strains resistant to all available antibacterial chemotherapy have already been identified.

PHARMACOKINETICS

The *pharmacokinetic profile* of an antibacterial agent refers to concentrations in serum and tissue versus time and reflects the processes of absorption, distribution, metabolism, and excretion. Important characteristics include peak and trough serum concentrations and mathematically derived parameters such as half-life, clearance, and distribution volume. Pharmacokinetic information is useful for estimating the appropriate antibacterial dose and frequency of administration, for adjusting dosages in patients with impaired excretory capacity, and for comparing one drug with another. →*For further discussion of basic pharmacokinetic principles, see Chap. 70.*

ABSORPTION Data on absorption can refer to oral, intramuscular, or intravenous administration.

Oral Administration Most patients with infection are treated with oral antibacterial agents in the outpatient setting. Advantages of oral therapy over parenteral therapy include lower cost, generally fewer adverse effects (including complications of indwelling lines), and greater acceptance by patients. The percentage of an orally administered antibacterial agent that is absorbed (i.e., the agent's *bioavailability*) ranges from as little as 10 to 20% (erythromycin and penicillin G) to nearly 100% (clindamycin, metronidazole, doxycycline, and trimethoprim-sulfamethoxazole). These differences in bioavailability are not clinically important as long as concentrations at the site of infection are sufficient to inhibit or kill the pathogen. However, therapeutic efficacy may be compromised when absorption is reduced as a result of physiologic or pathologic conditions (such as the presence of food for some drugs or the shunting of blood away from the gastrointestinal tract in patients with hypotension), drug interactions (such as that of quinolones and metal cations), or noncompliance. The oral route is usually used for patients with relatively mild infections in whom absorption is not thought to be compromised by the preceding conditions. In addition, the oral route can be used in more severely ill patients after they have responded to parenteral therapy.

Intramuscular Administration Although the intramuscular route of administration usually results in 100% bioavailability, it is not as widely used in the United States as the oral and intravenous routes, in part because of the pain often associated with intramuscular injections and the relative ease of intravenous access in the hospitalized patient. Intramuscular injection may be suitable for specific indications requiring an "immediate" and reliable effect (e.g., with long-acting forms of penicillin, including benzathine and procaine, and with single doses of ceftriaxone for uncomplicated gonococcal infection).

Intravenous Administration The intravenous route is appropriate when oral antibacterial agents are not effective against a particular pathogen, when bioavailability is uncertain, or when larger doses are required than are feasible with the oral route. After intravenous administration, bioavailability is 100%; serum concentrations are maximal at the end of the infusion. For many patients requiring long-term antimicrobial therapy, outpatient intravenous administration with the use of convenient portable pumps may be cost-effective and safe when oral therapy is not feasible. Alternatively, some oral antibacterial drugs such as fluoroquinolones are sufficiently active against Enterobacteriaceae to rival parenteral therapy; their use may allow the patient to return home from the hospital earlier or to avoid hospitalization entirely.

DISTRIBUTION To be effective, an antibacterial agent must exceed the minimal concentration required to inhibit bacterial growth (MIC; Chap. 121). Serum concentrations usually exceed the MIC for susceptible bacteria, but since most infections are extravascular, the antibiotic must also distribute to the site of the infection. Concentrations of most antibacterials in interstitial fluid are similar to free drug concentrations in serum. However, when the infection is located in a "protected" site where penetration is poor, such as cerebrospinal fluid (CSF), the eye, the prostate, or infected cardiac vegetations, high parenteral doses or local administration for prolonged periods may be required for cure. In addition, even though an antibacterial agent may penetrate to the site of infection, its activity may be antagonized by factors in the local environment, such as an unfavorable pH or inactivation by cellular degradation products. For example, since the activity of aminoglycosides is reduced at acidic pH, the acidic environment in many infected tissues may be partly responsible for the relatively poor efficacy of aminoglycoside monotherapy. In addition, the abscess milieu reduces the activity of many antibacterial compounds, so that surgical drainage may be required for cure.

Most bacteria that cause human infections are located extracellularly. Intracellular pathogens such as *Legionella*, *Chlamydia*, *Brucella*, and *Salmonella* may persist or cause relapse if the antibacterial agent does not enter the cell. In general, β-lactams, vancomycin, and aminoglycosides penetrate cells poorly, whereas macrolides, tetracyclines, metronidazole, chloramphenicol, rifampin, trimethoprim-sulfamethoxazole, and quinolones penetrate cells well.

METABOLISM AND ELIMINATION Like other drugs, antibacterial agents are disposed of by hepatic elimination (metabolism or biliary elimination), by renal excretion in unchanged or metabolized form, or by a combination of the two processes. For most antibacterial drugs, metabolism leads to loss of in vitro activity, although some agents, such as cefotaxime, rifampin, and clarithromycin, have bioactive metabolites that may contribute to their overall efficacy.

The most practical application of knowing the mode of excretion of an antibacterial agent is adjustment of the dosage when elimination capability is impaired. Direct, nonidiosyncratic toxicity from antibacterial drugs most often results from failure to reduce the dosage appropriately in a patient with impaired elimination. For agents that are primarily cleared intact by glomerular filtration, drug clearance is linearly correlated with creatinine clearance. Unfortunately, for drugs whose elimination is primarily hepatic, no simple marker (such as serum creatinine) is useful for dosage adjustment in subjects with liver disease. Even in patients with severe hepatic disease, residual metabolic capability is usually sufficient to preclude accumulation and toxic effects. However, for drugs that undergo hepatic metabolism and have a narrow therapeutic index (such as chloramphenicol), alternative therapy may be warranted in patients with liver disease, since the technology for the monitoring of serum levels is not widely available.

PRINCIPLES OF ANTIBACTERIAL CHEMOTHERAPY

The choice of an antibacterial compound for a particular patient and a specific infection involves more than just a knowledge of the agent's mechanism of action and pharmacokinetic profile. The basic tenets of chemotherapy, to be elaborated below, include the following: First, material containing the infecting organism(s) should be obtained before the start of treatment so that presumptive identification can be made by microscopic examination of stained specimens and the organism can be grown for definitive identification and susceptibility testing. Second, once the organism is identified and its susceptibility to antibacterial agents is determined, the regimen with the narrowest effective spectrum should be chosen. Third, the choice of antibacterial agent is guided by the pharmacokinetic and adverse-reaction profile of active compounds, the site of infection, the immune status of the host, and evidence of efficacy from well-performed clinical trials. Finally, if all other factors are equal, the least expensive antibacterial regimen should be chosen.

SUSCEPTIBILITY OF BACTERIA TO ANTIBACTERIAL DRUGS IN VITRO The determination of the susceptibility of the patient's infecting organism to a panel of appropriate antibacterial agents is an essential first step in devising a chemotherapeutic regimen. The details of susceptibility testing are discussed elsewhere (Chap. 121). Such testing is designed to estimate the susceptibility of a bacterial isolate to an antibacterial drug under standardized conditions that favor rapidly growing aerobic or facultative organisms and to assess bacteriostasis only. Specialized testing is required for the assessment of bactericidal antimicrobial activity; for the detection of resistance among such fastidious organisms as obligate anaerobes, *Haemophilus* spp., and pneumococci; and for the determination of resistance phenotypes with variable expression, such as resistance to methicillin or oxacillin among staphylococci.

RELATIONSHIP OF PHARMACOKINETICS AND IN VITRO SUSCEPTIBILITY TO CLINICAL RESPONSE The relationship between the report of susceptibility in vitro and the clinical pharmacokinetics of the antibacterial agent helps predict clinical response. Bacteria are usually considered to be *susceptible* to a drug if the achievable peak serum concentration exceeds the MIC by at least fourfold. The *breakpoint* is the concentration of the antibiotic that separates susceptible from resistant bacteria (Fig. 137-2). When a majority of the isolates of a given bacterial species are inhibited at concentrations below the breakpoint, the species is considered to be within the spectrum of the antibiotic (see "Choice of Antibacterial Therapy," below).

The pharmacodynamic profile of an antibiotic is the quantitative relationship among the time course of antibiotic concentrations in se-

FIGURE 137-2 Relationship between pharmacokinetics of an antibiotic and susceptibility. Organism A is resistant, organism B is moderately susceptible, and organism C is very susceptible.

rum and tissue, in vitro susceptibility, and microbial response. Three pharmacodynamic parameters quantify these relationships: the ratio of the area under the curve (AUC) for the plasma concentration vs. time curve to MIC (AUC/MIC), the ratio of the maximal serum concentration to the MIC (C_{max}/MIC), and the time during a dosing interval that plasma concentrations exceed the MIC ($t > MIC$). The pharmacodynamic profile of an antibiotic class is characterized as either concentration dependent (fluoroquinolones, aminoglycosides), such that the increase in antibiotic concentration leads to a more rapid rate of bacterial death, or time dependent (β-lactams, vancomycin), such that the reduction in bacterial density is proportional to the time that concentrations exceed the MIC. For concentration-dependent antibiotics, the C_{max}/MIC or AUC/MIC ratio correlates best with the reduction in microbial density in vitro and in animal investigations. Dosing strategies attempt to maximize these ratios by the administration of a "large" dose relative to the MIC for anticipated pathogens, often at "long" intervals (relative to the serum half-life). Once-daily dosing of aminoglycoside antibiotics is the practical consequence of these relationships. In contrast, dosage strategies for time-dependent antibiotics emphasize the administration of sufficient doses at appropriate intervals to maintain serum concentrations above the MIC, typically for at least 40 to 50% of the dosing interval. The clinical implications of these relationships are in the early stages of investigation, but their elucidation should eventually result in more rational antibacterial regimens.

STATUS OF THE HOST Various host factors must be considered in the devising of antibacterial chemotherapy. The host's antibacterial *immune function* is of importance, particularly as it relates to opsonophagocytic function. Since the major host defense against acute, overwhelming bacterial infection is the polymorphonuclear leukocyte, patients with neutropenia must be treated aggressively and empirically with bactericidal drugs for suspected infection (Chap. 85). Likewise, patients who have deficient humoral immunity (e.g., those with chronic lymphocytic leukemia and multiple myeloma) and individuals with surgical or functional asplenia (e.g., those with sickle cell disease) should be treated empirically for infections with encapsulated organisms, especially the pneumococcus.

Pregnancy increases the risk of toxicity of certain antibacterial drugs for the mother (e.g., the hepatic toxicity of tetracycline), affects drug disposition and pharmacokinetics, and—because of the risk of fetal toxicity—severely limits the choice of agents for treating infections. Certain antibacterials are contraindicated in pregnancy either because their safety has not been established or because they are known to be toxic. These agents include all fluoroquinolones, clarithromycin, erythromycin estolate (but not erythromycin base), and tetracyclines. Data on the safety of many other antibacterial drugs are limited, but these drugs may be used cautiously when there is no suitable alternative and the perceived benefit outweighs the risk. These agents include the aminoglycosides, azithromycin, clindamycin, imipenem, metronidazole, trimethoprim, and vancomycin. Chloramphenicol, nitrofurantoin, and the sulfonamides are contraindicated in the third trimester but can be used cautiously in the first two trimesters.

In patients with *concomitant viral infections*, the incidence of adverse reactions to antibacterial drugs may be unusually high. For example, persons with infectious mononucleosis and those infected with HIV may react more often to ampicillin and folic acid synthesis inhibitors, respectively.

In addition, the patient's age, sex, racial heritage, and excretory status all determine the incidence and type of side effects that can be expected with certain antibacterial agents.

SITE OF INFECTION The location of the infected site may play a major role in the choice and dose of antimicrobial drug. Patients with suspected *meningitis* should receive drugs that can cross the blood-CSF barrier; in addition, because of the relative paucity of phagocytes and opsonins at the site of infection, the agents should be bactericidal. Chloramphenicol, one of the standard drugs used in the treatment of meningitis, is bactericidal for common organisms causing meningitis (i.e., meningococci, pneumococci, and *Haemophilus influenzae*, but *not* enteric gram-negative bacilli), is highly lipid-soluble, and enters the CSF well. However, β-lactams, the mainstay of therapy for most of these infections, do not normally reach high levels in CSF. Their efficacy is based on the increased permeability of the blood-brain and blood-CSF barriers to hydrophilic molecules during inflammation and the extreme susceptibility of most infectious organisms to even small amounts of β-lactam drug.

The vegetation, which is the major site of infection in *bacterial endocarditis*, is also a focus that is protected from normal host-defense mechanisms. Antibacterial therapy needs to be bactericidal, with the selected agent administered parenterally over a long period and at a dose that produces serum levels at least eight times higher than the minimal bactericidal concentration (MBC) for the infecting organism. Likewise, *osteomyelitis* involves a site that is somewhat resistant to opsonophagocytic removal of infecting bacteria; furthermore, avascular bone (sequestrum) represents a foreign body that thwarts normal host-defense mechanisms. *Chronic prostatitis* is exceedingly difficult to cure because most antibiotics do not penetrate the nonfenestrated capillaries serving the prostate, especially when acute inflammation is absent. Drugs that are "ion trapped" after entering prostatic tissue, such as trimethoprim and fluoroquinolones, may be uniquely effective because of this mechanism. *Intraocular infections*, especially endophthalmitis, are difficult to treat because drug penetration into the vitreous from blood is hindered by retinal capillaries lacking fenestration. Inflammation does little to disrupt this barrier. Thus, direct injection into the vitreous is necessary in many cases. Antibiotic penetration into *abscesses* is usually poor. Even when an antibiotic does penetrate into the abscess, local conditions, such as low pH or the presence of enzymes that hydrolyze the drug, may antagonize its activity.

In contrast, *urinary tract infections*, when confined to the bladder, are relatively easy to cure, in part because of the higher concentration of most antibiotics in urine than in blood. Since blood is the usual reference fluid in defining susceptibility, even organisms found to be "resistant" to achievable serum concentrations may be susceptible to achievable urine concentrations. For drugs that are used only for the treatment of urinary tract infections, such as nitrofurantoin and methenamine salts, achievable urine concentrations are used to determine susceptibility.

COMBINATION CHEMOTHERAPY One of the tenets of antibacterial chemotherapy is that if the infecting bacterium has been identified, the most specific chemotherapy possible should be used. The use of a single agent with a narrow spectrum of activity against the pathogen diminishes the alteration of normal flora and thus limits the overgrowth of resistant nosocomial organisms (e.g., *Candida albicans*, enterococci, *Clostridium difficile*, or methicillin-resistant

staphylococci), avoids the potential toxicity of multiple-drug regimens, and reduces cost. However, certain circumstances call for the use of more than one antibacterial agent. These are summarized below.

1. *Prevention of the emergence of resistant mutants*. Spontaneous mutations occur at a detectable frequency in certain genes encoding the target proteins for some antibacterial agents. The use of these agents can eliminate the susceptible population, select out resistant mutants at the site of infection, and result in the failure of chemotherapy. Resistant mutants are usually selected when the MIC of the antibacterial agent for the infecting bacterium is close to achievable levels in serum or tissues and/or when the site of infection limits the access or activity of the agent. Among the most common examples are rifampin for staphylococci, imipenem for *Pseudomonas*, and ciprofloxacin for staphylococci and *Pseudomonas*. Small-colony variants of staphylococci resistant to aminoglycosides also emerge during monotherapy with these antibiotics. A second antibacterial agent with a mechanism of action different from that of the first is added to prevent the emergence of these resistant mutants (e.g., imipenem plus an aminoglycoside for systemic *Pseudomonas* infections). However, since resistant mutants have emerged following combination chemotherapy, this approach is not uniformly successful.

2. *Synergistic or additive activity*. Against some bacteria, two or more agents are clearly more active than one; whether or not this is the case is usually judged on the basis of testing in vitro. Synergistic or additive activity involves a lowering of the MIC or MBC of each or all of the drugs tested in combination against a specific bacterium. In *synergy*, *each* agent is more active when combined with a second drug than it would be alone, and the drugs' combined activity is therefore greater than the sum of the individual activities of each drug. In an *additive relationship*, the combined activity of the drugs is equal to the sum of their individual activities. Among the best examples of a synergistic or additive effect, confirmed both in vitro and by animal studies, are the enhanced bactericidal activities of certain β-lactam/aminoglycoside combinations against enterococci, viridans streptococci, and *P. aeruginosa*. The synergistic or additive activity of these combinations has also been demonstrated for selected isolates of enteric gram-negative bacteria and staphylococci. The combination of trimethoprim and sulfamethoxazole has synergistic or additive activity against many enteric gram-negative bacteria. Most other antimicrobial combinations display indifferent activity (i.e., the combination is *no better* than the more active of the two agents alone), and some combinations (e.g., penicillin plus tetracycline against pneumococci) may be antagonistic (i.e., the combination is *worse* than either drug alone).

3. *Therapy directed against multiple potential pathogens*. For certain infections, either a mixture of pathogens is suspected or the patient is desperately ill with an as-yet-unidentified infection (see "Empirical Therapy," below). In these situations, the most important of the likely infecting bacteria must be covered by therapy until culture and susceptibility results become available. Examples of the former infections are intraabdominal or brain abscesses and infections of limbs in diabetic patients with microvascular disease. The latter situations include fevers in neutropenic patients, acute pneumonia from aspiration of oral flora by hospitalized patients, and septic shock or sepsis syndrome.

EMPIRICAL THERAPY In certain situations, antibacterial therapy is begun before a specific bacterial pathogen has been identified. The choice of agent is guided by the results of studies identifying the usual pathogens at that site or in that clinical setting, by pharmacodynamic considerations, and by the resistance profile of the expected pathogens in a particular hospital or geographic area. Situations in which empirical therapy is appropriate include the following:

1. *Life-threatening infection*. Any suspected bacterial infection in a patient with a life-threatening illness should be treated presumptively. Therapy is usually begun with more than one agent and is later tailored to a specific pathogen if one is eventually identified.

2. *Treatment of infections in unhospitalized patients with no cultures performed*. In many situations, it is appropriate to treat non-life-threatening infections without obtaining cultures. These situations in-

clude outpatient infections such as community-acquired cases of pneumonia, cystitis, cellulitis or local wound infection, sinusitis, otitis, urethritis, and prostatitis. However, if any of these infections recurs or fails to respond to initial therapy, every effort should be made to obtain cultures to guide re-treatment.

CHOICE OF ANTIBACTERIAL THERAPY

The antibacterial spectrum of specific agents and the infections for which they represent the treatment of choice are detailed below. No attempt has been made to include all the potential situations in which antibacterial agents may be used. A more detailed discussion of specific bacteria and infections that they cause can be found elsewhere in this volume.

β-LACTAMS (Table 137-2) All *penicillins* (except for the semisynthetic, penicillinase-resistant antistaphylococcal agents) are hydrolyzed by *β*-lactamases and are ineffective against isolates that produce these enzymes. Penicillin G has a spectrum that includes spirochetes (*Treponema pallidum*, *Borrelia*, and *Leptospira*), streptococci (groups A and B, viridans, and *Streptococcus pneumoniae*), enterococci, most *Neisseria* spp., a few staphylococci, many fastidious oral bacteria (including many *Porphyromonas* and *Prevotella* spp., streptococci, *Actinomyces*, and *Fusobacterium*), *Clostridium* spp. (except *C. difficile*), *Pasteurella multocida*, *Erysipelothrix rhusiopathiae*, and *Streptobacillus moniliformis*. However, penicillin G resistance is widespread among staphylococci; is increasing rapidly among gonococci, enterococci, and pneumococci; and is emerging among meningococci, viridans streptococci, and oral anaerobes such as *Porphyromonas* and *Prevotella*. Penicillin G is the *drug of choice* for syphilis, yaws, leptospirosis, group A and B streptococcal infections, actinomycosis, oral and periodontal infections, meningococcal meningitis and meningococcemia, viridans streptococcal endocarditis, clostridial myonecrosis, tetanus, anthrax, rat-bite fever, *P. multocida* infections, and erysipeloid (*E. rhusiopathiae*).

Ampicillin extends the spectrum of penicillin G to some gram-negative rods. It is active against some isolates of *Escherichia coli*, *Proteus mirabilis*, *Salmonella*, *Shigella*, and *H. influenzae* and is one of the *drugs of choice* for susceptible organisms causing urinary tract infections, salmonellosis, *H. influenzae* meningitis and epiglottitis, and *Listeria monocytogenes* meningitis. High rates of resistance have lessened its value as empirical therapy in some situations. For example, more than 80% of isolates of *E. coli* and *P. mirabilis* are resistant in some hospitals, as are 10 to 30% of isolates of *H. influenzae*; moreover, in some outbreaks of infection due to salmonellae, all isolates are ampicillin-resistant.

The *penicillinase-resistant penicillins* are used solely for the treatment of staphylococcal infections and are the *drugs of choice* for systemic or deep staphylococcal infections caused by susceptible organisms. Unfortunately, on average, approximately 30% of *S. aureus* isolates and more than 60% of coagulase-negative staphylococcal isolates acquired in U.S. hospitals are resistant to these agents (i.e., methicillin-resistant). The spectrum of these agents also includes most of the same gram-positive bacteria that are susceptible to penicillin G.

The spectrum of the *antipseudomonal penicillins* includes the bacteria covered by ampicillin as well as some additional nonpseudomonal enteric gram-negative bacilli. For example, piperacillin is active against many indole-positive *Proteus*, *Enterobacter*, *Klebsiella*, *Providencia*, and *Serratia* spp. However, the susceptibility of these penicillins to *β*-lactamase markedly limits their utility as empirical therapy when infections caused by gram-negative enteric organisms are suspected. The major use of these compounds is in the treatment of proven or suspected infections with *P. aeruginosa* and *Acinetobacter*, for which they are among the *drugs of choice*. Their relative antipseudomonal activities can be ranked as follows: piperacillin > mezlocillin/ticarcillin > carbenicillin.

The addition of *β-lactamase inhibitors* (clavulanic acid, sulbactam, or tazobactam) to ampicillin, amoxicillin, ticarcillin, or piperacillin extends the spectrum of these agents to include many organisms that are resistant by virtue of *β*-lactamase production. These organisms include *E. coli*, *Klebsiella* spp., all *Proteus* spp., *H. influenzae*, *Moraxella catarrhalis*, *Providencia* spp., and *Bacteroides* spp. Such combinations are also active against staphylococci that produce *β*-lactamase but are not methicillin-resistant. However, the efficacy of these combinations in serious staphylococcal infections has not been adequately proven. Furthermore, *Enterobacter*, *Pseudomonas*, *Acinetobacter*, and various enteric gram-negative isolates either produce *β*-lactamases not inhibited by these compounds or develop resistance attributable to non-*β*-lactamase-mediated mechanisms.

The *first-generation cephalosporins* have a spectrum that includes penicillinase-producing, methicillin-susceptible staphylococci and streptococci. While these drugs may be used when infections with gram-positive bacteria are suspected, they are *not* the drugs of choice for such infections. They have excellent activity against many isolates of *E. coli*, *Klebsiella pneumoniae*, and *P. mirabilis* and are among the *drugs of choice* in presumptive therapy for community-acquired urinary tract infections. They have no activity against *Bacteroides fragilis*, enterococci, methicillin-resistant staphylococci, *Pseudomonas*, *Acinetobacter*, *Enterobacter*, indole-positive *Proteus*, and *Serratia* and poor activity against *H. influenzae*.

The *parenteral second-generation cephalosporins* extend the gram-negative spectrum of first-generation compounds. The various second-generation agents have differing activities. Cefuroxime and cefamandole retain activity against gram-positive cocci and are also active against *H. influenzae*, *Neisseria*, some *Enterobacter* isolates, and indole-positive *Proteus* but exhibit poor activity against *B. fragilis*. Cefoxitin and cefotetan have reasonably good activity against *B. fragilis*, but cefotetan is less effective against some other *Bacteroides* spp. (Chaps. 130 and 167). Both of the latter drugs display poor activity against gram-positive cocci and *Enterobacter*. No second-generation cephalosporin is active against *Pseudomonas* or *Acinetobacter*.

Oral second-generation cephalosporins have fair activity against gram-positive cocci and *H. influenzae* and are widely used in outpatient therapy for otitis media, sinusitis, and lower respiratory tract infections, although cheaper agents that are equally effective are preferable. Cefixime, cefuroxime axetil, and cefpodoxime are among the *drugs of choice* for single-dose treatment of gonococcal urethritis.

Third-generation cephalosporins all have a broad spectrum of activity against enteric gram-negative rods and are especially useful for treating hospital-acquired infections caused by multiresistant organisms. In addition, ceftazidime and cefepime have excellent antipseudomonal activity. The other third-generation cephalosporins have poor antipseudomonal activity. Since resistance to third-generation cephalosporins is increasing among all nosocomial gram-negative rods, the use of these agents should be guided by susceptibility testing. The gram-positive spectrum of the third-generation cephalosporins is variable. All are less active than first-generation cephalosporins against methicillin-susceptible staphylococci; ceftazidime has the least antistaphylococcal activity of this group. However, ceftriaxone, ceftizoxime, and cefotaxime have excellent activity against streptococci, especially *S. pneumoniae*. Ceftazidime is not recommended for treatment of streptococcal infections.

Because of its excellent gram-negative spectrum; its activity against *Haemophilus*, many *S. pneumoniae* strains, and penicillin-resistant *Neisseria*; its long serum half-life; and its high serum and CSF levels, ceftriaxone has become one of the *drugs of choice* for empirical therapy for bacterial meningitis (except that caused by *Listeria* and by highly penicillin-resistant pneumococcal strains), all gonococcal infections, salmonellosis, and typhoid fever. The third-generation cephalosporins are among the *drugs of choice* for nonpseudomonal hospital-acquired pneumonia. Cefepime is more resistant to chromosomal *β*-lactamase produced by *Enterobacter* spp. than are other third-generation cephalosporins. Third-generation cephalosporins have poor activity against *Bacteroides* and no activity against methicillin-resistant staphylococci, *Enterococcus*, *Acinetobacter*, or *Stenotrophomonas*.

The *carbapenems* currently available in the United States are imipenem and meropenem. Imipenem is marketed in combination with the renal dipeptidase inhibitor cilastatin, which enables imipenem to escape renal inactivation and thus to reach higher urinary levels. Imipenem and meropenem have excellent activity in vitro against virtually all bacterial pathogens except *Stenotrophomonas*, methicillin-resistant staphylococci, and *E. faecium*. Limitations to their use are their relatively low blood levels, short serum half-life, and high cost. Imipenem has dose-related central nervous system side effects that appear to be less frequent with meropenem. Resistance to imipenem and meropenem is a problem only among nosocomial isolates of *P. aeruginosa*, approximately 20% of which are resistant. Because of their broad spectrum, carbapenems can be used as empirical therapy for serious nosocomial infections thought to be caused by multiple bacterial species or multiresistant organisms. Imipenem and meropenem are often used to treat hospital-acquired infections caused by *Enterobacter* spp. because these organisms produce inducible β-lactamases that inactivate third-generation cephalosporins but not the carbapenems. The latter antibiotics are often held in reserve as therapy for nosocomial infections due to gram-negative pathogens resistant to third-generation cephalosporins.

The only *monobactam* currently available is aztreonam. This antibiotic has a spectrum limited to facultative gram-negative enteric bacilli. It has no activity against any gram-positive or anaerobic bacterium. Its gram-negative spectrum is similar to that of ceftazidime, with equally good activity against *Pseudomonas*. Its primary advantages are its theoretical ability to preserve the normal gram-positive and anaerobic flora and the lack of cross-reactive immediate hypersensitivity in patients who have had this type of reaction to other β-lactam antibiotics.

VANCOMYCIN The spectrum of vancomycin is limited to gram-positive cocci, especially enterococci, streptococci, and staphylococci. Vancomycin serves as second-line therapy for most gram-positive bacterial infections but is the *drug of choice* for infections caused by methicillin-resistant staphylococci or *Corynebacterium jeikeium* and for serious infections in penicillin-allergic patients. Given orally (a route by which it is not absorbed), vancomycin can be used to treat antibiotic-associated pseudomembranous colitis caused by *C. difficile* in patients who have failed to respond to metronidazole, the *drug of choice*. Vancomycin has also been recommended as initial empirical therapy for presumed pneumococcal meningitis because of increasing pneumococcal resistance to penicillins and cephalosporins. Resistance to vancomycin is increasing rapidly among isolates of *E. faecium* in large hospitals, particularly in areas of high vancomycin use. In addition, *S. aureus* isolates with reduced susceptibility to vancomycin have now been detected. Because of the growing threat of vancomycin-resistant enterococci and the potential for increasing resistance among staphylococci, a national advisory committee has established guidelines for appropriate and limited use of this antibiotic.

AMINOGLYCOSIDES The aminoglycosides are rapidly bactericidal in vitro at low concentrations, with activity limited to facultative gram-negative bacteria and staphylococci. They have no activity against anaerobic bacteria and are not effective in environments that are acidic or have a low oxygen tension. However, their spectrum includes virtually all gram-negative bacteria that are not strict anaerobes, and they are among the *drugs of choice* for any suspected gram-negative bacteremic infection, particularly in neutropenic patients. Aminoglycosides are synergistically bactericidal in combination with a penicillin for the treatment of staphylococcal, enterococcal, or viridans streptococcal endocarditis and are usually combined with a β-lactam antibiotic for the treatment of gram-negative bacteremia. Aminoglycosides are also among the *drugs of choice* for severe infections of the upper urinary tract. The major limitations to use of aminoglycosides are their renal and otic toxicity, their diminished activity at certain sites of infection (e.g., abscesses and the central nervous system), and the resistance of target bacteria. Among the available agents, gentamicin is generally preferred because of its low cost; however, tobramycin has slightly greater activity against *P. aeruginosa*, and amikacin retains activity against many tobramycin- and gentamicin-resistant gram-negative bacteria because it is inactivated by fewer aminoglycoside-modifying enzymes. Streptomycin is still one of the *drugs of choice* in initial therapy for tularemia, plague, glanders, and brucellosis and is a second-line agent for the treatment of tuberculosis.

MACROLIDES Erythromycin has broad-spectrum activity against gram-positive bacteria, with additional activity against *Legionella*, *Mycoplasma*, *Campylobacter*, and some *Chlamydia* isolates. It is the *drug of choice* for infections due to *Legionella*, *Campylobacter*, and *Mycoplasma* and is among the *drugs of choice* for community-acquired pneumococcal pneumonia and group A streptococcal pharyngitis in penicillin-allergic patients. However, resistance to erythromycin among group A streptococci and pneumococci is increasing dramatically in some areas. Erythromycin also appears to be one of the *drugs of choice* for infections caused by the agent of bacillary angiomatosis (*Bartonella henselae*) in immunocompromised patients. The newer macrolides clarithromycin and azithromycin have an antibacterial spectrum similar to that of erythromycin in vitro. However, azithromycin has greater activity against *Chlamydia*. Clarithromycin, in combination with a proton pump inhibitor, has been designated a *drug of choice* for the treatment of gastric infections due to *Helicobacter pylori* (gastritis, gastric and duodenal ulcers). Both azithromycin and clarithromycin are active against nontuberculous mycobacteria, and both appear to have fewer gastrointestinal side effects than does erythromycin.

LINCOSAMIDES The only lincosamide used in the United States is clindamycin. It shares the gram-positive coccal spectrum of erythromycin but is more active, in some cases showing bactericidal activity, against susceptible staphylococci. However, resistance among staphylococci and some streptococci, mediated by the same genes responsible for macrolide resistance, limits clindamycin's usefulness against gram-positive cocci. In general, all staphylococci resistant to erythromycin should be considered resistant to clindamycin regardless of the results of in vitro susceptibility testing. However, at least half of the streptococci resistant to erythromycin are truly susceptible to clindamycin. In these bacteria, resistance is mediated by a drug-efflux pump that removes macrolides but not lincosamides. Despite increasing resistance, clindamycin remains useful for most anaerobic infections because of its broad spectrum of activity against both gram-positive and -negative strict anaerobes. It is also a *drug of choice* for the treatment of severe, invasive group A streptococcal infections. In contrast, clindamycin, like erythromycin, has no clinically significant activity against facultative gram-negative enteric bacilli. Appropriate use is limited only by resistance or the development of pseudomembranous colitis, the major serious side effect of this drug.

CHLORAMPHENICOL Chloramphenicol has a broad spectrum of activity against gram-positive and -negative bacteria, although plasmid-mediated resistance has diminished its effective spectrum. This antibiotic is rarely used in adult infections because of the rare idiosyncratic side effect of irreversible bone-marrow aplasia and the availability of other agents with similar activity. It remains one of the *drugs of choice* for the treatment of typhoid fever and plague and is still useful for the treatment of brucellosis and both pneumococcal and meningococcal meningitis in penicillin-allergic patients.

TETRACYCLINES Tetracyclines have a broad spectrum of bacteriostatic activity against gram-positive and -negative bacteria and are widely used in a variety of community-acquired infections. These agents are among the *drugs of choice* for chronic bronchitis, granuloma inguinale, brucellosis (with streptomycin), tularemia, glanders, melioidosis, spirochetal infections caused by *Borrelia* (Lyme disease and relapsing fever; doxycycline), infections caused by *Vibrio vulnificus*, some *Aeromonas* infections, infections due to *Stenotrophomonas* (minocycline), plague, and ehrlichiosis (doxycycline). The tetracyclines are also used in penicillin-allergic patients for the treatment of leptospirosis, syphilis, actinomycosis, and skin and soft-tissue infections caused by gram-positive cocci. They are among the *drugs of* *choice* for infections due to chlamydiae (doxycycline), rickettsiae, and ehrlichiae and for granulomatous skin infection due to *Mycobacterium marinum* (minocycline). Doxycycline is also among the drugs recommended for the treatment of community-acquired pneumonia.

SULFONAMIDES AND TRIMETHOPRIM The folic acid synthesis inhibitors have a broad spectrum of bacteriostatic activity individually; in combination, they can be bactericidal against facultative gram-negative bacteria and staphylococci. The fixed combination of sulfamethoxazole and trimethoprim, the major folic acid synthesis inhibitors used in therapy for bacterial infections, has modest activity against some streptococci and no activity against strict anaerobes. However, resistance to the combination of sulfamethoxazole and trimethoprim is common among methicillin-resistant staphylococci and penicillin-resistant pneumococci and is increasing among *E. coli* strains that cause urinary tract infections. The individual sulfonamides are rarely used in the treatment of bacterial infections but are among the *drugs of choice* for the treatment of nocardial infections, leprosy (dapsone, a sulfone), and toxoplasmosis (sulfadiazine). Although increasing resistance has been reported among gram-negative organisms, trimethoprim-sulfamethoxazole remains one of the *drugs of choice* for the treatment of uncomplicated urinary tract infections (except for those caused by enterococci) and is widely used in the treatment of otitis media. It can be used in therapy for upper respiratory tract infections in which *S. pneumoniae*, *H. influenzae*, or *M. catarrhalis* is suspected; for gonococcal and meningococcal infections; for chancroid; and for infections thought to be caused by *Aeromonas*, *Stenotrophomonas*, *Burkholderia cepacia*, *Acinetobacter*, and *Yersinia enterocolitica*. For nosocomial infections due to *Stenotrophomonas*, trimethoprim-sulfamethoxazole is the *drug of choice*.

FLUOROQUINOLONES The fluoroquinolones have excellent activity against most facultative gram-negative rods and variable activity against gram-positive cocci; only trovafloxacin is active against obligate anaerobes. The quinolones are the oral agents with greatest activity against *P. aeruginosa*; ciprofloxacin is the most active against this species. All the quinolones except norfloxacin are well absorbed orally; ciprofloxacin, levofloxacin, trovafloxacin, and ofloxacin are also administered as intravenous formulations. The quinolones are among the *drugs of choice* for urinary tract infections, bacterial gastroenteritis, community-acquired pneumonia, and enteric fever and may be useful in therapy for serious hospital-acquired infections caused by gram-negative organisms. While older quinolones (ciprofloxacin, ofloxacin, and norfloxacin) have limited activity against gram-positive bacteria, the newer quinolones have an expanded spectrum of activity against gram-positive cocci, including staphylococci (both methicillin-susceptible and methicillin-resistant) and streptococci (especially *S. pneumoniae*). However, because of the potential for development of severe liver toxicity, it has been recommended that trovafloxacin use be limited to hospitalized patients with serious or life-threatening infections. Quinolones can also be used as prophylaxis for persons at risk for meningococcal meningitis. However, rapid expansion in the use of quinolones should be coupled with a consideration of the potential for development of resistance among all bacteria targeted by these drugs.

RIFAMPIN Rifampin has been used in combinations for the treatment of serious infections due to methicillin-resistant staphylococci (e.g., coagulase-negative staphylococcal foreign-body infections). Because the spontaneous selection of rifampin-resistant mutants occurs rapidly, rifampin should never be used alone in the treatment of staphylococcal infections. Rifampin is also used for chemoprophylaxis in persons at risk of meningococcal meningitis and for the treatment of *Legionella* pneumonia.

METRONIDAZOLE Metronidazole has a spectrum limited to anaerobic bacteria. It is one of the *drugs of choice* for the treatment of any abscess in which the involvement of obligate anaerobes is suspected (e.g., lung, brain, or intraabdominal abscesses) because of its spectrum and its ability to penetrate into the area of infection. Other antibacterial agents should be used in combination with metronidazole if facultative and aerobic pathogens are also thought to be involved.

Metronidazole is the *drug of choice* for the treatment of bacterial vaginosis and antibiotic-associated pseudomembranous colitis.

URINARY TRACT ANTISEPTICS Urinary tract antiseptics are active only in the lower urinary tract and cannot be used for the treatment of upper urinary tract or systemic infections. Their activity is limited to susceptible gram-negative enteric bacteria. The available agents in this category include nitrofurantoin and methenamine salts.

TOPICAL ANTIBACTERIAL AGENTS Mupirocin is available only as a topical preparation for use against staphylococci and streptococci. Its major applications are for impetigo and eradication of the staphylococcal carrier state. It is the *drug of choice* for the elimination of nasal carriage of both methicillin-susceptible and methicillin-resistant staphylococci. Unfortunately, the emergence of resistance is limiting its usefulness in some hospitals.

Although their efficacy has never been well documented, topical preparations that include sulfonamides, polymyxin B, neomycin, bacitracin, gramicidin, and novobiocin in a variety of combinations are widely used as eye drops, irrigation solutions, and ointments for superficial skin infections.

ADVERSE REACTIONS

Adverse drug reactions are frequently classified by mechanism as either dose-related ("toxic") effects or unpredictable reactions. Unpredictable reactions are further categorized as either idiosyncratic or allergic. Dose-related reactions include aminoglycoside-induced nephrotoxicity, penicillin-induced seizures, and vancomycin-induced anaphylactoid reactions. Many of these reactions can be avoided by reducing dosage, limiting the duration of therapy, or reducing the frequency or rate of administration. Adverse reactions to antibacterial agents are a common cause of morbidity, requiring alteration in therapy and additional expense, and they occasionally result in death. The elderly, often those with the more severe infections, may be especially prone to certain adverse reactions. →*For further discussion of adverse drug reactions, see Chap. 71.*

β-LACTAMS The therapeutic index for β-lactam antibiotics is broad, and dose-related adverse reactions are uncommon and largely preventable. The greatest concern is allergic reactions. All types can occur, including anaphylaxis (type 1, hypersensitivity reactions), nephritis and Coombs-positive hemolytic anemia (type 2, cytotoxic reactions), drug fever and serum sickness (type 3, immune-complex formation), contact dermatitis (type 4, cell-mediated effects), and maculopapular eruption (type 5, idiopathic reactions). Approximately 1 to 4% of treatment courses result in an allergic reaction, and approximately 0.004 to 0.015% of treatment courses result in anaphylaxis. Fewer than half the patients who claim an allergy to penicillin react to skin testing with the major and minor determinants (penicilloyl-polylysine and benzylpenicillin degradation products, respectively); those with negative skin tests only rarely react adversely to subsequent therapeutic doses. Generally, a suitable alternative to β-lactams is available for patients who have a severe allergy, and penicillin desensitization can be carefully undertaken if there is no suitable alternative. A small proportion (<2%) of persons who are allergic to penicillin react similarly when a cephalosporin is administered; thus, cephalosporins are contraindicated in patients with a history of an immediate reaction to penicillin, although they are often used in patients with a history of mild reactions. The same precaution applies to imipenem, but aztreonam is antigenically distinct and can be administered safely to the penicillin-allergic patient.

Other reactions thought to have an allergic basis include nephritis (associated with methicillin and occasionally nafcillin), hepatitis (related to oxacillin), leukopenia (following high doses of most β-lactams administered for prolonged periods), and severe skin rashes (toxic epidermal necrolysis and Stevens-Johnson syndrome). These reactions are not IgE-mediated, and skin testing is not predictive of their occurrence. For unclear reasons, most patients who have infectious mononucleosis develop a rash when given ampicillin or amoxicillin.

Miscellaneous reactions to β-lactams include gastrointestinal side effects ranging in severity from mild diarrhea (5 to 10%) to pseudomembranous colitis (<1%). Although the probability of antibiotic-associated colitis is low, a large number of cases occur because β-lactams are so commonly prescribed. Drugs excreted to a large extent through the bile, such as ampicillin and ceftriaxone, may be especially prone to cause diarrhea. The addition of clavulanic acid to amoxicillin further increases the frequency of diarrhea. Ceftriaxone, because of extremely high concentrations in bile, can cause "sludging" in the gallbladder and occasionally produces symptoms compatible with acute cholecystitis.

In high doses—and most often in patients with renal impairment who receive an excessive dose—penicillins (especially ticarcillin and penicillin G) can cause bleeding from impaired platelet aggregation. Ticarcillin is a disodium salt and in high doses can cause hypokalemia and fluid overload.

Seizures are occasionally observed with β-lactams, especially penicillin G and imipenem. This reaction is most common when excessive doses relative to renal function are administered or when the patient has a history of seizures.

VANCOMYCIN When vancomycin was first used clinically in 1956, local intolerance at the infusion site was common, as were systemic reactions, including ototoxicity and nephrotoxicity. Current formulations are of higher purity and, when proper dosage guidelines are followed, are very safe, although phlebitis can still be troublesome. The most common adverse reaction is called *red man syndrome* and is characterized by pruritus, flushing, and erythema of the head and upper torso. This anaphylactoid reaction usually follows the first dose, is dependent on dose size and infusion time, and results from vancomycin-induced release of histamine. The reaction is usually mild in adult patients who receive 1 g over 60 min and diminishes with repeated doses. If vancomycin is mistakenly given as a bolus, severe hypotension may result. In unusually sensitive patients, extending the infusion time or administering H_1 receptor antagonists is usually effective in preventing this reaction or reducing its severity. Patients with this reaction must not be mislabeled as having an allergy to vancomycin, since vancomycin may be the only effective treatment for certain infections, such as those due to methicillin-resistant staphylococci.

Nephrotoxicity from vancomycin is mild and occurs in fewer than 5% of patients. Although some data suggest that aminoglycosides and vancomycin are synergistically nephrotoxic, this point is difficult to prove, and the simultaneous use of these agents should not be avoided if clinically indicated, as in the treatment of enterococcal endocarditis in penicillin-allergic patients.

Ototoxicity from vancomycin is rare as long as doses are appropriately reduced in patients with renal insufficiency. Other uncommon adverse reactions include leukopenia, skin rashes, and true allergy. Serum concentrations of vancomycin are of little use in predicting toxicity but may be of value in selecting dosages for patients with unstable renal function.

AMINOGLYCOSIDES Aminoglycoside antibiotics have a narrow therapeutic index. The two most common adverse reactions are nephrotoxicity and ototoxicity. Rarely, respiratory depression is observed. Nephrotoxicity results from accumulation of the aminoglycoside in the peritubular space, with damage to the proximal tubule and a corresponding reduction in the glomerular filtration rate. The incidence of nephrotoxicity, defined as a >0.5% increase over baseline in the serum creatinine level, is approximately 5 to 10% among adult patients who receive therapy for 10 to 14 days. However, many cofactors also influence the frequency of toxicity, such as extremes of age (toxicity is uncommon among children, more common among the elderly), concomitant drug therapy, and hydration status. Nephrotoxicity is manifested clinically by a gradual rise in serum creatinine levels after a few days of therapy and is reversible if the dosage is reduced

or treatment is discontinued. Serum creatinine levels should be monitored every 3 to 5 days or more often if changes are seen. There is not an important difference among the most useful agents (gentamicin, tobramycin, and amikacin) in terms of the frequency of nephrotoxicity; streptomycin is a rare cause of nephrotoxicity. Some data suggest that once-daily administration may cause less nephrotoxicity.

Ototoxicity from aminoglycoside therapy presents as either auditory or vestibular damage. Since the aminoglycosides can destroy hair cells in the inner ear, ototoxicity may be permanent. The risk of ototoxicity increases with prolonged therapy, higher serum concentrations (especially in patients with renal impairment), hypovolemia, and concurrent treatment with other ototoxins, especially ethacrynic acid. Clinically apparent ototoxicity, manifested by diminished acuity or vestibular imbalance, is uncommon (probably occurring in <1% of cases) when the duration of therapy is kept to a minimum. With more sensitive monitoring (e.g., audiograms), asymptomatic high-tone hearing loss is more commonly noted. There are no clinically important differences among the aminoglycosides in the overall frequency of ototoxicity.

Neuromuscular depression from aminoglycosides is caused by reduced acetylcholine activity at postsynaptic membranes and can result in rare but severe respiratory depression. Risk factors include hypocalcemia, peritoneal administration, use of neuromuscular blockers, and preexisting respiratory depression. This complication can be largely avoided if the aminoglycoside is administered intravenously over 30 min or by intramuscular injection; if respiratory depression occurs, it is reversed by the administration of calcium.

Fear of toxicity should not prevent the use of aminoglycosides for a legitimate indication, since toxicity is usually mild and reversible. The value of measuring serum concentrations is controversial; these measurements are usually unnecessary when the patient is receiving once-daily therapy.

MACROLIDES Serious adverse reactions to the macrolide antibiotics are very rare. Gastrointestinal effects, such as burning, nausea, and vomiting, are the most common adverse reactions to the macrolides; depending on dosage, these reactions may occur in up to 50% of patients, occasionally requiring early discontinuation of therapy. The mechanism is thought to be the binding of erythromycin to motilin receptors, with a consequent increase in gastrointestinal motility. Gastrointestinal side effects appear equally common for all the oral formulations and also occur with intravenous administration. Clarithromycin and azithromycin are better tolerated than erythromycin, although gastrointestinal distress is still their most common adverse effect.

Less common reactions include hepatotoxicity and ototoxicity. Hepatotoxicity is a rare, nonfatal complication that is usually associated with erythromycin estolate and presents as an allergic cholestatic jaundice. Ototoxicity is rare after oral administration but may occur in a dose-dependent pattern in up to 20% of adults who receive intravenous erythromycin (4 g/d) and have audiograms performed. Ototoxicity is usually reversible and mild. Allergic cutaneous reactions are observed in rare cases.

LINCOSAMIDES The most common adverse effect of clindamycin is gastrointestinal distress. Diarrhea has been reported in up to 20% of patients and pseudomembranous colitis in 0.01 to 10%. The mechanism of pseudomembranous colitis is production of a toxin by *C. difficile* (Chap. 145). *C. difficile* colonizes the gastrointestinal tract and may produce a toxin when the normal flora is suppressed by clindamycin and other antibiotics, especially β-lactams. This toxin causes mucosal damage that results in cramps, pain, and diarrhea that may be bloody. Pseudomembranous colitis may follow both intravenous and oral administration and may not become manifest until after completion of therapy. Oral metronidazole or oral vancomycin is effective in treating symptomatic patients with toxin-positive stools, but some spores may survive, and relapse is frequent. Metronidazole is the *drug of choice* since oral treatment with vancomycin can select for vancomycin-resistant enterococci. Although diarrhea and pseudomembranous colitis can be caused by most antibacterial agents, the incidence in relation to the amount used appears to be highest for clindamycin. Allergic reactions (such as rashes and fever), hepatotoxicity, and neutropenia are observed only rarely.

CHLORAMPHENICOL Chloramphenicol causes two types of bone marrow suppression: a dose-related, reversible suppression of all elements, which occurs commonly during therapy at the maximal recommended doses (4 g/d in adults), and an idiosyncratic, irreversible aplastic anemia, which occurs in approximately 1 in every 25,000 to 40,000 exposures. The irreversible form has been reported to follow all types of chloramphenicol treatment, including ocular administration, and often develops months after therapy is discontinued.

In premature neonates and infants, chloramphenicol can cause a dose-related "gray syndrome" that is characterized by cyanosis, hypotension, and death and that results from an inability of the newborn to metabolize the drug. These potentially serious toxicities and the availability of newer drugs have substantially reduced the indications for chloramphenicol.

TETRACYCLINES Gastrointestinal effects are the most common adverse reactions to the tetracyclines. These problems may be related to a direct irritant effect, since tetracyclines can also cause esophageal ulceration when they dissolve before reaching the stomach. It is important that nighttime doses be taken with sufficient fluid. Concurrent food intake may improve tolerance, but absorption of tetracycline HCl is impaired when the drug is taken with food.

Hepatotoxicity has been reported after administration of >2 g of tetracycline intravenously and at lower doses during pregnancy. There are currently no indications for intravenous tetracycline treatment in pregnancy. All tetracyclines can cause phototoxic skin reactions; these reactions are most common with doxycycline. Other dermal reactions, including rash, are uncommon. Tetracyclines are contraindicated in children <8 years of age because of mottling of the permanent teeth; doxycycline may be less likely than the other tetracyclines to cause this problem. Worsening of renal function in patients with preexisting renal dysfunction has been reported with use of tetracycline, although some of the increased azotemia may be due to amino acid catabolism. Doxycycline and perhaps minocycline appear to be free from these renal side effects. Alternative effective agents are nearly always available for use in patients with renal dysfunction. Minocycline can cause vertigo in up to 70% of women receiving therapeutic doses and in a lower percentage of men.

SULFONAMIDES AND TRIMETHOPRIM The sulfonamides are generally safe, but the list of possible adverse reactions is very long. These compounds occasionally cause a number of allergic reactions, from relatively minor skin rashes (including maculopapular rashes and urticarial reactions typically appearing after a week of therapy) to severe or even life-threatening reactions such as erythema multiforme, Stevens-Johnson syndrome, and toxic epidermal necrolysis. The severe hypersensitivity reactions have occurred most commonly after treatment with the long-acting sulfonamides, such as sulfamethoxypyridazine, which are no longer used. Pyrimethamine plus sulfadoxine (Fansidar), used for malaria prophylaxis, may cause severe allergic reactions, including hepatic and hematologic toxicities, in addition to dermatologic toxicity. Photosensitivity reactions are also relatively common with sulfonamides.

Many patients infected with HIV who receive trimethoprim-sulfamethoxazole have adverse dermatologic reactions. These reactions are usually not life-threatening and appear to regress in many cases despite continuation of therapy. In high doses, trimethoprim interferes with the renal secretion of potassium. Hyperkalemia is relatively common among HIV-positive patients and is most often found after 7 days of trimethoprim-sulfamethoxazole therapy for pneumonia caused by *Pneumocystis carinii*.

Sulfonamides and trimethoprim may also cause severe hematologic complications, including agranulocytosis, hemolytic and megaloblastic anemia, and thrombocytopenia. These dose-related side effects may be greater in patients with renal insufficiency. Hemolytic anemia is most common in patients with glucose-6-phosphate dehydrogenase deficiency who take long-acting compounds; trimethoprim-

sulfamethoxazole rarely causes hemolysis in such subjects. Granulocytopenia from trimethoprim-sulfamethoxazole is especially common in HIV-infected patients, occurring in 10 to 50% of this group.

Renal insufficiency, caused by crystals of the relatively insoluble acetyl metabolite, is observed primarily with the long-acting sulfonamides. Many cases of crystalluria in HIV-infected patients taking sulfadiazine for toxoplasmosis have been reported. A high level of fluid intake may prevent this complication.

It is recommended that sulfonamides not be administered to the newborn because of concerns that bilirubin may be displaced from protein-binding sites, with subsequent jaundice and kernicterus.

In addition to the preceding problems, sulfonamides may occasionally cause drug fever with serum sickness, hepatic toxicity (including necrosis), and systemic lupus erythematosus.

FLUOROQUINOLONES Fluoroquinolones are relatively safe; adverse reactions rarely require discontinuation of therapy. The most common reactions include gastrointestinal distress, such as nausea or diarrhea (<5%), and central nervous system effects, including insomnia and dizziness (<5%). Trovafloxacin is prone to causing dizziness, especially among women. However, of more serious concern is the report of more than 100 cases of symptomatic liver toxicity in patients receiving trovafloxacin, including 14 cases of acute liver failure strongly associated with trovafloxacin exposure. As a result, the Food and Drug Administration has recommended that this quinolone be used only in hospitalized patients with serious or life-threatening conditions in which the benefits offered by the drug outweigh its potential risks. Phototoxicity can be severe, especially with sparfloxacin. Rarely, hepatic and renal dysfunction and anaphylactoid and allergic reactions are observed. Tendon rupture has also been associated with quinolone use in rare instances. The use of these drugs is contraindicated in patients <18 years of age because of evidence in animals of cartilage damage in developing joints. In carefully selected situations in which the perceived benefits outweigh the risks (e.g., in adolescent patients with cystic fibrosis who have pulmonary exacerbations), fluoroquinolones may be useful for short-term therapy. They are contraindicated in pregnancy because of concern for the developing fetus.

RIFAMPIN Rifampin is generally well tolerated but has several important side effects. Some patients have transient rises in hepatic aminotransferases, but these levels usually return to normal without discontinuation of the drug. Although hepatitis from rifampin itself develops only rarely, the drug is thought by some investigators to potentiate the hepatic toxicity of concomitantly administered isoniazid. Intermittent administration of rifampin (usually fewer than three times per week) has been associated with symptoms that seem to have an immunologic basis. These include flulike symptoms and (rarely) hemolysis, thrombocytopenia, shock, and renal failure. Minor gastrointestinal side effects, skin rashes, and interstitial nephritis have also been reported. Patients should be warned that rifampin and its metabolites cause secretions such as urine, tears, sweat, and saliva to turn orange and that contact lenses may be stained.

METRONIDAZOLE Serious adverse reactions to metronidazole are uncommon. Gastrointestinal side effects such as nausea are most frequent but rarely necessitate discontinuation of therapy. Pseudomembranous colitis in association with metronidazole has been reported but is very rare. A metallic taste is relatively common, and stomatitis and glossitis are occasionally reported. Disulfiram-like reactions can occur if ethanol is ingested concurrently. Peripheral neuropathy develops in some patients, and seizures and encephalopathy have been reported after high doses and in patients with hepatic failure.

Concerns about mutagenicity and carcinogenicity from metronidazole have led to recommendations that it not be used in pregnancy (especially during the first trimester) when alternative agents are available. Although retrospective studies have found no association between metronidazole and carcinogenesis, long-term administration of high doses should be avoided when therapeutic alternatives exist.

Table 137-3   Interactions of Antibacterial Agents with Other Drugs

Antibiotic	Interacts with	Potential Consequence (Clinical Significance[a])
Erythromycin/ clarithromycin	Theophylline	Theophylline toxicity—e.g., seizures (1)
	Carbamazepine	Central nervous system depression (1)
	Digoxin	Digoxin toxicity (3)
	Triazolam/midazolam	Central nervous system depression (2)
	Ergotamine	Ergotism (1)
	Warfarin	Bleeding (2)
	Cyclosporine/tacrolimus	Nephrotoxicity (1)
	Astemizole, terfenadine, cisapride, pimozide	Cardiac arrhythmias (1)
	"Statins"	Rhabdomyolysis (2)
	Valproate	Valproate toxicity (2)
Fluoroquinolones[b]	Theophylline	Theophylline toxicity (2)
	Antacids/sucralfate	Subtherapeutic antibiotic levels (1)
Tetracycline	Antacids/sucralfate	Subtherapeutic antibiotic levels (1)
Trimethoprim- sulfamethoxazole	Phenytoin	Phenytoin toxicity (2)
	Oral hypoglycemics	Hypoglycemia (2)
	Digoxin	Digoxin toxicity (3)
	Warfarin	Bleeding (2)
Metronidazole	Ethanol	Disulfiram-like reactions (2)
	Fluorouracil	Bone marrow suppression (1)
	Warfarin	Bleeding (2)
Rifampin	Warfarin	Clot formation (1)
	Oral contraceptives	Pregnancy (1)
	Cyclosporine/tacrolimus	Rejection (1)
	HIV-1 protease inhibitors	Increased viral load, resistance (1)
	Nonnucleoside reverse transcriptase inhibitors	Increased viral load, resistance (1)
	Glucocorticoids	
	Methadone	Loss of steroid effect (1)
	Digoxin	Withdrawal (1)
	Itraconazole	Subtherapeutic digoxin levels (1)
	Phenytoin	Subtherapeutic itraconazole levels (1)
	"Statins"	Loss of seizure control (1)
	Diltiazem	Hypercholesterolemia (1)
	Verapamil	Subtherapeutic diltiazem levels (1)
		Subtherapeutic verapamil levels (1)

[a] 1, a well-documented interaction with clinically important consequences; 2, an interaction of uncertain frequency but of potential clinical importance; 3, an unusual interaction of possible clinical importance.

[b] Ciprofloxacin, grepafloxacin > levofloxacin, trovafloxacin.

DRUG INTERACTIONS

Historically, clinically important interactions involving antibacterial drugs were generally of little concern, since β-lactams were the most widely used agents and rarely interacted with other drugs in a manner that affected the patient adversely. However, fluoroquinolones, macrolides, and rifampin are now more widely used, and interactions are of increasing concern. Table 137-3 lists the most common and best-documented interactions of antibacterial agents with other drugs and characterizes the clinical relevance of these interactions. Coadministration of drugs paired in Table 137-3 does not necessarily have clinically important adverse consequences. The result depends on the timing of administration, the dose and duration of therapy, the baseline serum concentration of the non-antibacterial drug administered, the patient's susceptibility to the pharmacologic effect of the non-antibacterial drug, and other, less-well-described cofactors. Recognition of the potential for an interaction before the administration of an antibacterial agent is crucial to the rational use of these drugs, since adverse consequences can often be prevented if the interaction is anticipated. Table 137-3 is intended only to heighten awareness of the potential for an interaction. Additional sources should be consulted to identify appropriate options. →*For further discussion of drug interactions, see Chap. 70.*

MACROLIDES   Erythromycin and clarithromycin can inhibit the P450 enzyme CYP3A and thus the metabolism of many concurrently administered drugs, such as cisapride, theophylline, carbamazepine, terfenadine, astemizole, warfarin, and ergot alkaloids. The magnitude of the theophylline interaction is highly variable and is proportional to the dose and duration of erythromycin treatment. In contrast, cyclosporine levels predictably increase when erythromycin is administered, since CYP3A is responsible for cyclosporine metabolism. Decreased metabolism of terfenadine, astemizole, cisapride, and pimozide has been reported to cause severe cardiac dysfunction. Azithromycin has little effect on the metabolism of other drugs. In approximately 10% of patients receiving digoxin, concentrations increase when erythromycin is also given.

TETRACYCLINES   The most important interaction involving tetracyclines is the reduction in absorption when these drugs are coadministered with di- and trivalent cations, such as antacids, iron compounds, or dairy products. A similar interaction is seen with quinolones (see below). Food also adversely affects absorption of most tetracyclines. Inducers of hepatic isoenzymes, such as phenytoin and barbiturates, increase the clearance of doxycycline; although the clinical significance of this effect is unknown, use of an alternative antibiotic may be appropriate.

SULFONAMIDES   Sulfonamides may increase the hypoprothrombinemic effect of warfarin by inhibition of its metabolism and possibly by protein-binding displacement. Sulfonamides may also potentiate the effects of oral hypoglycemic agents and phenytoin through reduction in metabolism or displacement from serum protein.

FLUOROQUINOLONES   There are two clinically important drug interactions involving fluoroquinolones. First, like tetracyclines, all fluoroquinolones are chelated by divalent and trivalent cations, which prevent most of the dose from being absorbed. Second, certain fluoroquinolones (grepafloxacin, ciprofloxacin, and—to a much lesser extent—levofloxacin and trovafloxacin) can inhibit hepatic enzymes that metabolize theophylline, with resultant theophylline toxicity. The same mechanism accounts for increases in serum caffeine concentrations, but the clinical significance of this interaction is unknown. Scattered reports indicate that quinolones can also potentiate the nephrotoxicity of cyclosporine, exaggerate the effects of warfarin, and increase neurotoxicity when coadministered with nonsteroidal anti-inflammatory agents. However, these interactions have not been confirmed by controlled trials.

RIFAMPIN   Rifampin is an excellent inducer of many cytochrome P450 enzymes and increases the hepatic clearance of a number of drugs, including the following (with the indicated predictable outcomes): HIV-1 protease inhibitors (loss of viral suppression), oral contraceptives (pregnancy), warfarin (decreased prothrombin times), cyclosporine and prednisone (organ rejection or exacerbations of any underlying inflammatory condition), and verapamil and diltiazem (increased dosage requirements). Before rifampin is prescribed for any patient, a review of concomitant drug therapy is essential.

METRONIDAZOLE   Metronidazole can cause a disulfiram-like syndrome when alcohol is ingested; thus, patients taking metronidazole should be instructed to avoid alcohol. Inhibition of the metabolism of warfarin by metronidazole leads to significant rises in prothrombin times.

PROPHYLAXIS OF BACTERIAL INFECTIONS

Antibacterial agents are occasionally indicated for use in patients who have no evidence of infection but who have been or are expected to be exposed to bacterial pathogens under circumstances that constitute a major risk of infection. The basic tenets of antimicrobial prophylaxis are as follows: First, the risk or potential severity of infection should be greater than the risk of side effects from the antibacterial agent. Second, the antibacterial agent should be given for the shortest period necessary to prevent target infections. Third, the antibacterial agent should be given before the expected period of risk (e.g., surgical prophylaxis) or as soon as possible after contact with an infected individual (e.g., prophylaxis for meningococcal meningitis).

Table 137-4 lists the major indications for antibacterial prophylaxis in adults. (The use of antibacterial agents in children to prevent rheumatic fever and otitis media under certain circumstances is also common practice.) The table includes only those indications that are widely accepted, supported by well-designed studies, or recommended by expert panels. Prophylaxis is also used but is less widely accepted for recurrent cellulitis in conjunction with lymphedema, recurrent pneumococcal meningitis in conjunction with deficiencies in humoral immunity or CSF leaks, traveler's diarrhea, gram-negative sepsis in conjunction with neutropenia, and spontaneous bacterial peritonitis in conjunction with ascites.

The major use of antibacterial prophylaxis in the United States is for infections following surgical procedures. Antibacterial agents are administered just before the surgical procedure—and, for long operations, during the procedure as well—to ensure high levels in serum and tissues during surgery. The objective is to eradicate bacteria originating from the air of the operating suite, the skin of the surgical team, or the patient's own flora that may contaminate the wound. In all but colorectal surgical procedures, prophylaxis is predominantly directed against staphylococci. Prophylaxis is intended to prevent wound infection or infection of implanted devices, not all infections that may occur during the postoperative period (e.g., urinary tract infections or pneumonia). Prolonged prophylaxis merely alters the normal flora and favors infections with organisms resistant to the antibacterial agents used.

ANTIBACTERIAL COSTS AND INAPPROPRIATE USE

Use of antibacterial agents in hospitals in the United States accounts for an important percentage of all drug costs and may represent the largest expenditure for any pharmacologic class. In the outpatient setting, the costs of antibacterial drugs are second only to those of cardiovascular agents. A survey of office-based physicians found that between 1980 and 1992 there was a marked increase in the use of expensive broad-spectrum antimicrobials. It is not unusual for the purchase cost (in 2000 dollars) of a newer parenteral antibiotic to be $1000 to $2000 for a 10- to 14-day course of treatment. Therapy with a new oral antibiotic can easily cost $50 to $75. Administration costs, monitoring costs, and pharmacy charges must be added to these figures. While some newer antibacterial agents undeniably represent important

Table 137-4   Prophylaxis of Bacterial Infections in Adults

Condition	Antibacterial Agent	Timing or Duration of Prophylaxis
Nonsurgical		
Cardiac lesions susceptible to bacterial endocarditis	Amoxicillin[a]	Before and after procedures causing bacteremia
Recurrent *S. aureus* infections	Mupirocin	5 days (intranasal)
Contact with patient with meningococcal meningitis	Rifampin Ciprofloxacin or ofloxacin	2 days Single dose
Bite wounds[b]	Penicillin V or amoxicillin/ clavulanic acid	3–5 days
Recurrent cystitis	Trimethoprim-sulfamethoxazole or a quinolone or nitrofurantoin	3 times per week for up to 1 year or after sexual intercourse
Surgical		
Clean (cardiac, vascular, neurologic, or orthopedic surgery)	Cefazolin (vancomycin)[c]	Before and during procedure
Ocular	Topical combinations and subconjunctival cefazolin	During and at end of procedure
Clean-contaminated (head and neck, high-risk gastroduodenal or biliary tract surgery; high-risk cesarean section; hysterectomy)	Cefazolin (or clindamycin for head and neck)	Before and during procedure
Clean-contaminated (vaginal or abdominal hysterectomy)	Cefazolin or cefoxitin or cefotetan	Before and during procedure
Clean-contaminated (high-risk genitourinary surgery)	Ciprofloxacin	Before and during procedure
Clean-contaminated (colorectal surgery or appendectomy)	Cefoxitin or cefotetan (add oral neomycin + erythromycin for colorectal)	Before and during procedure
Dirty[b] (ruptured viscus)	Cefoxitin or cefotetan ± gentamicin (clindamycin + gentamicin) or another appropriate regimen directed at anaerobes and gram-negative aerobes	Before and for 3–5 days after procedure
Dirty[b] (traumatic wound)	Cefazolin	Before and for 3–5 days after trauma

[a] Gentamicin should be added to the amoxicillin regimen for high-risk gastrointestinal and genitourinary procedures; vancomycin should be used in penicillin-allergic patients.
[b] In these cases, use of antibacterial agents actually constitutes treatment of infection rather than prophylaxis.
[c] Vancomycin is recommended only in institutions that have a high incidence of infection with methicillin-resistant staphylococci.

advances in therapy, many newer drugs offer no advantage over older, less expensive agents.

Clinicians are understandably confused by the bewildering array of available drugs. Numerous surveys have reported that approximately 50% of antibiotic use is in some way "inappropriate." Aside from the monetary cost of unnecessary antibiotics, there are the costs of excess morbidity from adverse effects and drug interactions and the eventual costs of treating more resistant organisms. The following suggestions are intended to provide guidance through the antibiotic maze.

First, objective evidence regarding the merits of newer drugs is available through publications such as *The Medical Letter*, including the annual update of *Drugs of Choice*. Second, clinicians should become comfortable using a few drugs recommended by independent experts and should resist the temptation to use a new drug unless the merits are clear. A new antibacterial agent with a "broader spectrum and greater potency" or a "longer half-life and higher tissue levels" does not necessarily mean greater clinical efficacy. Third, the clinician must become familiar with local bacterial susceptibility profiles. It may not be necessary to use a new drug with "improved activity against *P. aeruginosa*" if that pathogen is rarely encountered or if it retains full susceptibility to older drugs. Finally, with regard to inpatient use of antibacterial drugs, appropriate empirical treatment with one or more broad-spectrum agents may often be simplified, with use of a narrower-spectrum agent or even an oral drug, once the results of cultures and susceptibility tests become available. While there is an understandable temptation not to alter effective therapy, switching to a more specific agent, once the patient has improved clinically, does not compromise eventual outcome. If these guidelines are followed, the care

881

of patients will not be undermined, many unnecessary complications and expenses will be avoided, and the useful life of valuable drugs will be extended.

BIBLIOGRAPHY

ANNÉ S, REISMAN RE: Risk of administering cephalosporin antibiotics to patients with histories of penicillin allergy. Ann Allergy Asthma Immunol 74:167, 1995

Antimicrobial prophylaxis in surgery. Med Lett Drugs Ther 39:97, 1997

BARTLETT JG et al: Community-acquired pneumonia in adults: Guidelines for management. Clin Infect Dis 26:811, 1998

CRAIG WA: Pharmacokinetic/pharmacodynamic parameters: Rationale for antibacterial dosing of mice and men. Clin Infect Dis 26:1, 1998

GONZALES R et al: Antibiotic prescribing for adults with colds, upper respiratory tract infections, and bronchitis by ambulatory care physicians. JAMA 278:901, 1997

HOSPITAL INFECTION CONTROL PRACTICES ADVISORY COMMITTEE: Recommendations for preventing the spread of vancomycin resistance. Infect Control Hosp Epidemiol 16:105, 1995

POLK R: Optimal use of modern antibiotics: Emerging trends. Clin Infect Dis 29:264, 1999

SEPPALA H et al: The effects of changes in the consumption of macrolide antibiotics on erythromycin resistance in group A streptococci in Finland. N Engl J Med 337:441, 1997

SHLAES DM et al: Guidelines for the prevention of antimicrobial resistance in hospitals. Clin Infect Dis 25:584, 1997

SMITH T et al: Emergence of vancomycin resistance in *Staphylococcus aureus*. N Engl J Med 340:493, 1999

The choice of antibacterial drugs. Med Lett Drugs Ther 40:33, 1998

Section 5
DISEASES CAUSED BY GRAM-POSITIVE BACTERIA

138　　*Daniel M. Musher*

PNEUMOCOCCAL INFECTIONS

Streptococcus pneumoniae (the pneumococcus) was recognized as a major cause of pneumonia in the 1880s and has been a central focus of study leading to the modern understanding of humoral immunity. The name *Diplococcus pneumoniae* was assigned to the organism in 1926 on the basis of its appearance in Gram-stained sputum. In 1974, the organism was renamed *Streptococcus pneumoniae* because of its growth in chains in liquid medium. Around 1900, pneumococcal serotypes were recognized when the injection of killed organisms into a rabbit stimulated the production of serum antibody that agglutinated and caused increased capsular density of the immunizing strain as well as of some but not all other pneumococcal isolates. Ninety serotypes have now been identified, each possessing a unique polysaccharide capsule.

MICROBIOLOGY　Pneumococci are identified in the clinical laboratory as gram-positive cocci that grow in chains and are catalase-negative. They produce pneumolysin, a toxin that breaks down hemoglobin into a greenish degeneration product, thereby causing α hemolysis on blood agar. More than 98% of pneumococcal isolates are susceptible to ethylhydrocupreine (optochin), and virtually all pneumococcal colonies are dissolved by bile salts.

Peptidoglycan and teichoic acid are the principal constituents of the pneumococcal cell wall. The cell wall's integrity depends on the presence of numerous peptide side chains cross-linked by the activity of enzymes such as trans- and carboxypeptidases. β-Lactam antibiotics inactivate these enzymes by covalently binding their active site. Unique to *S. pneumoniae* and present in all strains is C (for "cell-wall") substance, a polysaccharide consisting of teichoic acid with a phosphorylcholine residue. Surface-exposed choline-binding proteins serve as a site of attachment for potential virulence factors, such as PspA, which may prevent phagocytosis. Nearly every clinical isolate of *S. pneumoniae* has a polysaccharide capsule.

There are two systems for numbering the 90 known distinct capsules of *S. pneumoniae*. In the American system, serotypes are numbered in the order in which they were identified. The strains that most frequently cause human disease were generally the earliest to be identified and thus tend to have lower numbers. The more widely accepted Danish system places serotypes into groups based on antigenic similarities; for example, Danish group 19 includes types 19F ("first recognized"), 19A, 19B, and 19C, which in the American system would be types 19, 57, 58, and 59, respectively. Serotyping was clinically relevant in the 1930s, when type-specific antisera were administered as therapy, and (although genetic typing is more specific) it has again become important for epidemiologic studies of the spread of antibiotic-resistant isolates in communities and among countries. Capsule switching has been documented and to some extent limits the epidemiologic reliability of serotyping.

EPIDEMIOLOGY　*S. pneumoniae* colonizes the nasopharynx and can be isolated from 5 to 10% of healthy adults and from 20 to 40% of healthy children. Once the organisms have colonized an adult, they are likely to persist for 2 to 4 weeks but may persist for as long as 6 months. Pneumococci spread from one individual to another as a result of extensive close contact; transmission may be enhanced by poor ventilation. Day-care centers have been a site of spread, especially of penicillin-resistant strains of serotypes 6B, 14, 19F, and 23F. Outbreaks occur among adults in crowded living conditions—e.g., in military barracks, prisons, and shelters for the homeless—as well as among susceptible populations in settings such as nursing homes. The risk of pneumococcal pneumonia is not increased by contact in schools or workplaces (including hospitals).

The incidence of pneumococcal bacteremia is relatively high among infants up to 2 years of age and low among teenagers and young adults; rates increase beginning at around age 55. A surveillance study in South Carolina showed the incidences of pneumococcal bacteremia among infants, young adults, and persons ≥ 70 years of age to be 160, 5, and 70 cases per 100,000 population, respectively. Most cases of pneumococcal bacteremia in adults are due to pneumonia, and there are three to four cases of nonbacteremic pneumonia for every bacteremic case. Thus, it is estimated that there are 20 cases of pneumococcal pneumonia annually per 100,000 young adults and 280 cases annually per 100,000 persons over the age of 70. The incidence of pneumococcal bacteremia among adults exhibits a distinct midwinter peak and a striking dip in summer. In children, the incidence of bacteremia is relatively constant throughout the year except for a marked dip in midsummer. For reasons that are unclear, certain populations, including Native Americans, Native Alaskans, and African Americans, appear to be unusually susceptible to invasive pneumococcal disease. This enhanced susceptibility, not unlike that to infection with *Haemophilus influenzae*, is thought to have a genetic basic that thus far remains unelucidated.

PATHOGENETIC MECHANISMS　*S. pneumoniae* attaches to human nasopharyngeal cells through the specific interaction of bacterial surface adhesins, such as pneumococcal surface antigen A or choline-binding proteins, with epithelial cell receptors. Epithelial cell glycoconjugates containing the disaccharide GlcNAcβ1-4Gal or asialo-GM1 glycolipid are possible binding sites. Pneumococcal phase variation, in which organisms switch between transparent and opaque, may also play a role in adherence. Upon culture, a mixed population of transparent and opaque pneumococcal colonies can be identified. Organisms from opaque colonies have relatively little peptidoglycan and relatively large capsules; those from transparent colonies have much more phosphorylcholine (which contributes to their capacity to adhere to mammalian cells) and less capsular polysaccharide. When an opaque colony is inoculated intranasally into an experimental animal, only those organisms that form transparent colonies persist. In contrast, after intraperitoneal inoculation, organisms that yield transparent colonies are rapidly cleared from the blood, while those that make opaque colonies resist clearance.

Once the nasopharynx has been colonized, infection results if the organisms are carried into anatomically contiguous areas such as the eustachian tubes or the nasal sinuses and if their clearance is hindered, for example, by mucosal edema due to allergy or viral infection. Similarly, pneumonia ensues if organisms are inhaled or aspirated into the bronchioles or alveoli and then are not cleared—in many cases, because viral infection or cigarette smoke or other toxic substances have increased mucus production and/or damaged ciliary action. A mechanism by which pneumococci may bind to pneumocytes after viral infection has been suggested. Pneumocytes activated by cytokines have been shown to express the receptor for platelet-activating factor. This receptor binds the phosphorylcholine residue on pneumococcal C substance, facilitating the adherence of pneumococci. Studies suggest that pneumococci may invade tissues by penetrating mucosal layers; the clinical significance of this finding remains to be determined.

Once pneumococci reach an area where they do not naturally belong, they activate complement by classic and alternative pathways and stimulate cytokine production, which leads to the attraction of polymorphonuclear neutrophils (PMNs). The polysaccharide capsule, however, renders the organisms resistant to phagocytosis. In the absence of anticapsular antibody, phagocytic cells such as alveolar macrophages have a limited capacity to ingest and kill pneumococci; a large bacterial inoculum and/or the compromise of phagocytic function allows the initiation of lung infection. Infection of the meninges, joint spaces, bones, and peritoneal cavity results from the spread of pneumococci through the bloodstream, usually but not always from a recognized focus of infection in the respiratory tract.

The capacity to cause disease reflects the ability of pneumococci to escape ingestion and killing by host phagocytic cells, on the one hand, and to stimulate an inflammatory response and damage tissues, on the other. Encapsulated pneumococci are poorly ingested and killed in vivo in the immunologically naive host or in vitro by mammalian phagocytic cells in the absence of anticapsular antibody and complement. Unencapsulated pneumococci virtually never cause invasive disease (although they can cause conjunctivitis), and mutants lacking a capsule are essentially avirulent in experimental animals. Symptoms of disease are largely attributable to the generation of an inflammatory response that may cause pain by increasing pressure (as in otitis media) or may interfere with vital bodily functions, such as oxygenation of blood (as in pneumonia) or cerebral function (as in meningitis). Cell-wall constituents of *S. pneumoniae*, including teichoic acid, C substance, and (in particular) peptidoglycan, activate complement by the alternative pathway; the reaction between cell-wall structures and antibody also activates the classic complement pathway. The result is the release of C5a, a potent attractant for PMNs, into the surrounding medium. Inflammation is also facilitated by the ability of peptidoglycan to stimulate cytokine production, which activates endothelial cells to express selectin and integrin receptors for inflammatory cells. Inflammation in the central nervous system (CNS) during meningitis is a major contributor to neuronal cell injury. Pneumolysin, a thiol-activated toxin, exerts a variety of effects on ciliary cells and PMNs and also activates the classic complement pathway by direct binding of Clq. Injection of pneumolysin into the lungs of experimental animals produces the histologic features of pneumonia; in mice, immunization with this substance or challenge with genetically engineered mutants that do not produce pneumolysin is associated with a significant reduction in virulence. Autolysin may contribute to the pathogenesis of pneumococcal disease by lysing bacteria, thereby releasing their constituents and heightening the reaction with human tissues. The release of excitatory amino acids in neuronal tissue may contribute to damage caused by meningitis.

HOST DEFENSE MECHANISMS Mechanisms of host defense may be immunologically nonspecific or specific. Nonspecific mechanisms include laminar airflow across mucous layers that filter inspired air, the glottal reflex, laryngeal closure, the cough reflex, the clearance of organisms from the lower airways by ciliated cells, and the ingestion by pulmonary macrophages and PMNs of small bacterial inocula that manage to reach alveolar spaces. Respiratory virus infection, chronic pulmonary disease, or heart failure compromises these mechanisms, predisposing to the development of pneumococcal pneumonia. Antibody to PspA and other pneumococcal constituents such as pneumolysin may be prevalent in the population and may contribute to immunity that is immunologically specific but not type specific.

Anticapsular antibody provides serotype-specific protection against pneumococcal infection. However, most healthy adults lack IgG antibody to most pneumococcal capsular polysaccharides. Antibody appears after colonization, infection, or vaccination. In the first few weeks after colonization, nonspecific mechanisms probably protect the host from infection. Thereafter, newly developed anticapsular antibody provides a high degree of specific protection. In contrast to this normal situation, adults who are at risk of aspirating pharyngeal contents and/or who have diminished mechanisms of lower airway clearance are at risk of developing pneumonia before antibody is produced. Similarly, children whose nasal mucosal membranes become acutely congested around the time of colonization are at risk of developing otitis media. Persons with a diminished capacity to form antibody remain susceptible for as long as they are colonized.

The risk of serious pneumococcal infection is greatly increased in persons with conditions that compromise IgG synthesis and/or the phagocytic function of PMNs and macrophages; this risk is also elevated in the presence of conditions associated with debilitation or malnutrition. Nearly all adults who are hospitalized for pneumococcal pneumonia have at least one of the conditions listed in Table 138-1 and/or fall into one of the groups known to be at high risk on epidemiologic grounds. Prior hospitalization either predisposes to or serves as a strong marker for pneumococcal infection. The susceptibility of elderly individuals to pneumococcal pneumonia may reflect diminished clearance mechanisms as well as debilitation, malnutrition, and comorbid diseases. Although IgG responses to capsular polysaccharides, as measured by enzyme-linked immunosorbent assay (ELISA), are more or less normal in elderly persons, the functional capacity of the antibody appears to be decreased. The remarkably high incidence of pneumococcal infection—perhaps 100-fold above baseline—among persons with AIDS is noteworthy.

Once a pneumococcal infection has been initiated, the absence of a spleen predisposes to fulminant disease. The liver is able to remove opsonized (antibody-coated) pneumococci from the circulation; in the absence of antibody, however, only the slow passage of blood through the splenic sinuses and prolonged contact with reticuloendothelial cells in the cords of Billroth allow time for bacterial clearance. Patients without spleens may die of pneumococcal pneumonia and sepsis at such an early stage of the illness that pulmonary consolidation is not evident on x-ray before death but rather is found only at autopsy.

SPECIFIC INFECTIONS CAUSED BY *S. PNEUMONIAE* *S. pneumoniae* causes infections of the middle ear, sinuses, trachea, bronchi, and lungs (Table 138-2) by direct spread from the nasopharyngeal site of colonization. Infections of the CNS, heart valves, bones, joints, and peritoneal cavity usually arise by hematogenous spread; in rare cases peritoneal infection develops via ascent through the fallo-

Table 138-1   Conditions That Commonly Predispose to Pneumococcal Infection

Defective antibody formation
   Common variable hypogammaglobulinemia
   Selective IgG-subclass deficiency
   Multiple myeloma
   Chronic lymphocytic leukemia
   Lymphoma
Defective complement function
Defective clearance of pneumococcal bacteremia[a]
   Congenital asplenia, hyposplenia
   Splenectomy
   Sickle cell disease
Multifactorial conditions
   Infancy and aging
   Chronic disease, hospitalization
   Glucocorticoid treatment
   Malnutrition
   Infection with HIV
   Alcoholism
   Cirrhosis of the liver
   Renal insufficiency
   Diabetes mellitus
   Fatigue, stress, and/or exposure to cold
Increased risk of exposure
   Day-care centers
   Military training camps
   Prisons
   Shelters for the homeless
Respiratory infection, inflammation[b]
   Influenza, other viral respiratory infections
   Air pollution
   Allergies
   Cigarette smoking
   Chronic obstructive pulmonary disease
   Other causes of chronic pulmonary inflammation or obstruction
Anatomic disruption of meninges (dural tear)[c]

[a] The absence of a spleen predisposes to more fulminant infection (see text).
[b] Predisposes specifically to infections of the upper or lower respiratory tract.
[c] Predisposes to recurrent bacterial meningitis.

pian tubes. The CNS may also be infected by contiguous spread of organisms, as in patients who have a tear in the dura. Primary bacteremia—i.e., the presence of pneumococci in the blood with no apparent source—occurs commonly in children under 2 years of age and as a small percentage of all pneumococcal bacteremias in adults; if no therapy is given, a source may become apparent. Pleural infection results either from direct extension of pneumonia to the visceral pleura or from hematogenous spread of bacteria from a pulmonary or extrapulmonary focus; the route cannot be determined in any individual case.

Otitis Media and Sinusitis   When fluid from the middle ear is cultured during acute otitis media or fluid from a paranasal sinus is cultured during acute sinusitis, *S. pneumoniae* is the most common isolate or is second only to nontypable *H. influenzae*. Whether in adults or in children, pneumococci are identified in about 40 to 50% of cases of otitis in which an etiologic agent is isolated. Prior infection by a

Table 138-2   Most Common Infections Caused by *Streptococcus pneumoniae*

Acute sinusitis	Osteomyelitis
Pneumonia	Septic arthritis
Acute purulent tracheobronchitis	Peritonitis
Otitis media	Endocarditis
Empyema	Pericarditis
Meningitis	Endometritis
Primary bacteremia	Cellulitis
	Brain abscess

NOTE: The order of the list very roughly approximates the order of frequency among adults, from most to least common.

respiratory virus or allergy is thought to contribute significantly to these pneumococcal infections by causing congestion of the openings to the eustachian tubes or the paranasal sinuses. Prospective studies of young children have shown that colonization precedes infection in most cases. For reasons that are unclear, serotypes 6B, 14, 19F, and 23F predominate both as colonizing and as infecting organisms of children; therefore, these serotypes are currently being studied most intensively for use in vaccines to be administered to young children.

Meningitis   Except during outbreaks of meningococcal infection, *S. pneumoniae* is the most common etiologic agent of bacterial meningitis in adults. Because of the remarkable success of *H. influenzae* type b vaccine, *S. pneumoniae* now predominates among cases in infants and toddlers as well (but not among those in newborns). Meningitis develops either by the direct extension of infection from the sinuses or the middle ear or as a result of bacteremia with seeding of the choroid plexus. Favoring the former possibility are the association between acute otitis media and meningitis as well as the documented role of *S. pneumoniae* as the most common cause of recurrent bacterial meningitis associated with head trauma, cerebrospinal fluid (CSF) leak, and/or dural tear. Favoring the latter are the association between pneumococcal bacteremia from any source and meningitis as well as an autopsy study of temporal bone from children who died of bacterial meningitis, which yielded no evidence of extension from the middle ear.

In the meninges and subarachnoid space, pneumococcal peptidoglycan stimulates an intense inflammatory response mediated by the release of interleukin (IL)1, IL-6, C5a, tumor necrosis factor (TNF), and other proinflammatory cytokines. This inflammatory response results in raised intracranial pressure, brain edema, and decreased blood flow leading to meningismus, drowsiness, or coma. Focal neurologic signs may result from vasculitis with venous or arterial thrombosis, from cranial neuropathy due to entrapment or infarction, from local cerebritis, from subdural effusion, or from brain herniation (Chap. 372).

No distinctive clinical or laboratory feature differentiates meningitis due to *S. pneumoniae* from that due to other bacteria. Patients note the sudden onset of fever, headache, and stiffness or pain in the neck. Without treatment, there is a progression over 24 to 48 h to confusion and then obtundation. On physical examination, the patient looks acutely ill and has a rigid neck. In such cases lumbar puncture should not be delayed for computed tomography (CT) of the head unless papilledema or focal neurologic signs are evident. Typical CSF findings consist of pleocytosis (500 to 10,000 cells/μL) with a predominance of PMNs, an elevated protein level (100 to 500 mg/dL), and a decrease in glucose content. If antibiotics have not been given, large numbers of pneumococci can be seen in a Gram-stained specimen of CSF in nearly all cases, and specific therapy can be administered, although *Listeria* may be misidentified as the pneumococcus. If an effective antibiotic has already been given, the number of bacteria may be greatly decreased and microscopic examination of a Gram-stained specimen may yield negative results. In this situation, immunologic methods for the detection of pneumococcal capsule in the CSF may identify an etiologic agent in up to two-thirds of cases, although these methods have fallen out of favor. Most physicians prefer to use empirical broad-spectrum antibiotic therapy until the etiologic agent has been definitively identified and its susceptibility has been reported.

Pneumonia   The distinctive symptoms and signs of pneumococcal pneumonia are (1) cough and sputum production, which reflect the proliferation of bacteria and the resulting inflammatory response in the alveoli; (2) fever; and (3) radiographic detection of an infiltrate.

Predisposing conditions   Pneumococcal pneumonia is most common at the extremes of age. Despite the undisputed role of *S. pneumoniae* as a major pathogenic bacterium for humans, the great majority of adults with pneumococcal pneumonia have underlying diseases that predispose them to infection. Otherwise-healthy military recruits involved in outbreaks of infection may be an exception to this rule; however, many of those affected have an antecedent viral-type illness that may reduce normal host resistance. In addition to prior viral respiratory illness, the most common predisposing conditions are alcoholism, malnutrition, chronic pulmonary disease of any kind, cigarette smoking, infection with HIV, diabetes mellitus, cirrhosis of the liver, anemia, prior hospitalization for any reason, renal insufficiency, and coronary artery disease (with or without recognized congestive heart failure). HIV infection is such an important predisposing factor that some authorities recommend that any young adult with pneumococcal pneumonia be tested for antibody to HIV.

Presenting symptoms Patients often present with a preexisting respiratory condition that has distinctly deteriorated. If a viral upper respiratory illness is the predisposing factor, the patient may have felt unwell for several days, with coryza or a nonproductive cough and low-grade fever; at the time of onset of pneumonia, the temperature may rise to 38.9 to 39.4°C (102 to 103°F), and sputum production becomes prominent. In a patient who has chronic bronchitis, the sputum may increase in volume, become yellow or green and thicker than usual, and be associated with a fever that becomes progressively higher over 48 to 72 h. In a small proportion of cases, the onset of disease follows a hyperacute pattern in which the patient suddenly has a single episode of shaking chills followed by sustained fever and a cough productive of blood-tinged sputum. This clinical picture is unfortunately called "classic," a vague term that is best avoided because many physicians believe that it means "most common," which is clearly not the case. In elderly subjects, the onset of disease may be especially insidious and may not suggest pneumonia at all. Persons in their eighties may have minimal cough, no sputum production, and no fever, instead appearing tired or confused. For the reasons noted above, the most abrupt progression of pneumococcal disease is seen in patients who have previously undergone splenectomy; these individuals may go from apparent good health to death in as little as 24 h. In pneumonia, pleuritic chest pain may result from extension of the inflammatory process to the visceral pleura; persistence of this pain, especially after the first day or two of treatment, raises concern about empyema (see "Complications," below). Nausea and vomiting or diarrhea, sometimes quite prominent, occur in up to 20% of cases. Clearly, the range of symptoms is sufficiently broad that there is no characteristic presentation to distinguish pneumococcal from other types of bacterial pneumonia (or from some types of nonbacterial pneumonia).

Physical findings Patients with pneumococcal pneumonia usually appear ill and have a grayish, anxious appearance that differs from that of persons with viral or mycoplasmal pneumonia. Typically, the temperature is 38.9 to 39.4°C (102 to 103°F), the pulse 90 to 110 beats per minute, and the respiratory rate >20 breaths per minute. Elderly patients may have only a slight temperature elevation or be afebrile. Hypothermia is associated with increased morbidity and mortality. Herpes labialis appears in a small percentage of cases. Pain may cause diminished respiratory excursion (splinting) on the affected side. Dullness to percussion is noted in about half of cases, and vocal fremitus is increased. Breath sounds may be bronchial or tubular, and crackles are heard in most cases if enough air is being moved to generate them. Flatness to percussion at the lung base and inability to detect the expected degree of diaphragmatic motion suggest the presence of pleural fluid, which raises the possibility of empyema; the failure to assess fremitus, to distinguish dullness from flatness by percussion, or to examine for diaphragmatic excursion may leave the physician at the mercy of often ambiguous radiologic interpretations. The finding of a heart murmur, certainly if new, raises concern about endocarditis, a rare but serious complication. Hypoxia or the generalized response to pneumonia may cause the patient to be confused, but the appearance of confusion should raise concern about meningitis. Obtundation or neck stiffness should lead to an immediate consideration of this complication.

Radiographic findings Pneumococcal pneumonia involves only one lung segment or a portion thereof in one-fourth of cases; it involves more than one segment but only one lobe or a portion thereof in another one-fourth of instances. Thus multilobar disease is seen in half of cases. Air-space consolidation is the predominant finding and

is detected in 80% of cases. Air bronchogram (visualization of the air-filled bronchus against a background of consolidation in the alveoli) is evident in fewer than half of cases and is more common in bacteremic than in nonbacteremic disease. In rare instances, pneumococcal pneumonia leads to a lung abscess; a malignancy or a mixture of anaerobic and microaerophilic organisms is likely to be implicated as well. Although some pleural fluid may actually be present in half of cases, no more than 20% of patients have a sufficient volume of fluid to allow aspiration, and in only a minority of these patients is empyema documented.

General laboratory findings The peripheral-blood white blood cell (WBC) count exceeds 12,000/μL in the great majority of patients with pneumococcal pneumonia. However, the count is <6000/μL in 5 to 10% of persons hospitalized for pneumococcal pneumonia. Such a low count is strongly associated with lethal disease and is often but not always associated with bone marrow suppression due to alcohol ingestion. The serum bilirubin level may be modestly elevated; hypoxia, inflammatory changes in the liver, and breakdown of red blood cells in the lung are all thought to contribute to this increase. Levels of lactate dehydrogenase may be elevated. A variety of other abnormalities may be present, reflecting the contributory role of underlying diseases. →*Abnormalities of pleural fluid in empyema are reviewed in Chap. 255.*

Differential diagnosis Patients who present with community-acquired pneumonia may actually have infection of the lungs due to one of many organisms. The extensive list includes the following: *H. influenzae* or *Moraxella catarrhalis* in persons with little to predispose them other than chronic or acute inflammation of the airways; *Staphylococcus aureus* in persons who take glucocorticoids or who have major anatomic disruption of the airways; *Streptococcus pyogenes*; *Neisseria meningitidis*; anaerobic species in persons who have seizures or may have aspirated oropharyngeal or gastric secretions for some other reason; *Legionella*; *Pasteurella multocida* in dog or cat owners; gram-negative bacilli, especially in persons with severely damaged lungs who are taking glucocorticoids; viruses, especially influenza virus (in season), adenovirus, or respiratory syncytial virus; *Mycobacterium tuberculosis*; fungi, including *Pneumocystis carinii* (depending upon epidemiologic factors and the possible presence of HIV infection); *Mycoplasma*; *Chlamydia pneumoniae*, especially in older adults; and *Chlamydia psittaci* in bird owners. Many older men with lung cancer present with pneumonia, as do persons who have acute-onset inflammatory pulmonary conditions of uncertain etiology or those with pulmonary embolus and infarction. The breadth of this list vividly illustrates the difficulty of using empirical therapy for community-acquired pneumonia. Many of these diseases require evaluation, and specific therapy is available for an increasing number. Moreover, pneumococci—perhaps the most common cause of community-acquired pneumonia—are increasingly resistant to available antibiotics. Taken together, these factors favor precise determination of the etiology of a pneumonia syndrome whenever possible.

Diagnostic microbiology An etiologic role for the pneumococcus in pneumonia is strongly suggested by the microscopic demonstration of large numbers of PMNs and slightly elongated gram-positive cocci in pairs and chains in the sputum (**Plate VI-2**). Capsules may be seen surrounding the bacterial forms. Examined areas of the slide must be free of buccal epithelial cells, which indicate the admixture of saliva with sputum; saliva may contain 10^7 viridans streptococci per milliliter. When characteristic microscopic findings are noted, the identification of *S. pneumoniae* in sputum culture strongly indicates pneumococcal infection of the lower respiratory tract. In the absence of such microscopic findings, the identification of pneumococci by culture may be nonspecific, reflecting colonization of the upper airways. Culture is also less sensitive than microscopic examination for identifying pneumococci. Since most pneumococci do not produce distinctively mucoid colonies, their identification in the laboratory depends on the ability to select putative pneumococcal colonies for further study from among α-hemolytic streptococci of the mouth. In short, laboratory diagnosis by sputum culture relies on the quality of the specimen provided, the care with which the relevant purulent component is separated for culture, and the assiduity with which α-hemolytic colonies are studied. These factors need to be considered when sputum cultures from patients who appear to have pneumococcal pneumonia are said to yield only "normal mouth flora" and when the medical literature describes what appear to be poor results of sputum culture. Because of the central role of microscopic examination in diagnosis, physicians may wish to view the slides with the microbiologist. Blood cultures yield *S. pneumoniae* in about 25% of cases of pneumococcal pneumonia. Modern, automated systems often yield positive blood cultures within 12 h after the sample is obtained.

Complications Empyema is the most common complication of pneumococcal pneumonia, occurring in about 2% of cases. As noted above, some fluid appears in the pleural space in a substantial proportion of cases of pneumococcal pneumonia, but this parapneumonic effusion usually reflects an inflammatory response to infection that has been contained within the lung, and its presence is self-limited. When bacteria reach the pleural space—either hematogenously or as a result of contiguous spread, possibly across lymphatics of the visceral pleura—empyema results. The finding of frank pus, a positive result on Gram's staining, or the presence of fluid with a pH of ≤7.1 indicates the need for aggressive and complete drainage, preferably by prompt insertion of a chest tube, with verification by CT that fluid has been removed. If there is no response, thoracotomy is indicated. Persistence of fever (even if low-grade) and leukocytosis after 4 or 5 days of appropriate antibiotic treatment for pneumococcal pneumonia suggests empyema. In this setting, the diagnosis is exceedingly likely if the x-ray shows the persistence of pleural fluid. At this stage, thoracotomy is often needed for cure. Aggressive drainage is likely to reduce morbidity and mortality from empyema (Chap. 262).

Other Syndromes The appearance of pneumococcal infection at other, usually sterile body sites indicates hematogenous spread, either during frank pneumonia or, in a smaller proportion of cases, from an inapparent focus of infection. A case of pneumococcal endocarditis is seen every few years at large tertiary-care hospitals. Purulent pericarditis due to this organism, occurring as a separate entity or together with endocarditis, is even rarer. Most cases of spontaneous bacterial peritonitis in children and some cases in adults are caused by *S. pneumoniae*. Peritonitis in women may be related to the use of an intrauterine contraceptive device, and pneumococcal infections of the female reproductive organs continue to be described. Septic arthritis can arise spontaneously in a natural or prosthetic joint or as a complication of rheumatoid arthritis. Osteomyelitis in adults tends to involve vertebral bones. Epidural and brain abscesses are rarely described. Cellulitis can develop and does so most often in persons who have connective tissue diseases or HIV infection. The appearance of any of these unusual pneumococcal infections in a young adult may suggest that tests for HIV infection should be undertaken.

℞ TREATMENT **Antibiotic Susceptibility** β-Lactam antibiotics, the cornerstone of therapy for serious pneumococcal infection, bind covalently to the active site and thereby block the action of

the cell-membrane enzymes (endo-, trans-, and carboxypeptidases) that are responsible for cell-wall synthesis. These enzymes were identified by their reaction with radiolabeled penicillin and thus are called *penicillin-binding proteins*. In the 1960s, virtually all clinical isolates of *S. pneumoniae* were susceptible to penicillin (i.e., were inhibited in vitro by concentrations of <0.06 μg/mL). During the past 20 years in Europe and the past 10 years or so in the United States, a steadily increasing number of pneumococcal isolates have shown some degree of resistance to penicillin. Resistance results when spontaneous mutation or acquisition of new genetic material alters penicillin-binding proteins in a manner that reduces their affinity for penicillin, thereby necessitating a higher concentration of penicillin for their saturation. The genetic information acquired also conveys resistance to other antibiotics. Mutation and selection of strains in communities in the United States—especially in areas of high antibiotic use, such as daycare centers—and spread of identifiable strains from other countries where antibiotics are available without prescription have contributed to the prevalence of resistance.

For most of the antibiotic era, pneumococcal susceptibility was not studied in vitro because of the organism's high degree of susceptibility to virtually all recommended antibiotics. Clearly, the situation has changed, and it seems important to study pneumococcal isolates, especially those causing invasive disease, for antibiotic susceptibility. In 1997, about 20% of pneumococcal isolates in the United States were intermediately susceptible to penicillin [minimal inhibitory concentration (MIC), 0.1 to 1.0 μg/mL] and 15% were resistant (MIC, ≥ 2.0 μg/mL; Table 138-3). The clinical significance of the MIC varies with the infection being treated. An intermediately resistant strain (e.g., MIC = 0.5 μg/mL) behaves as a susceptible organism when it causes pneumonia, but probably not when it causes otitis and certainly not when it causes meningitis. As a result, susceptibility may eventually be redefined on the basis of the site infected—a concept supported by pharmacokinetic considerations and validated by outcome studies. Amoxicillin, with two- and fourfold lower MICs, appears to be more active against *S. pneumoniae* than penicillin—thus the emerging preference for amoxicillin. Penicillin-susceptible pneumococci are susceptible to all commonly used cephalosporins. Penicillin-intermediate strains are resistant to all first- and many second-generation cephalosporins (of which cefuroxime retains the best efficacy) but are susceptible to some third-generation cephalosporins, including cefotaxime, ceftriaxone, cefepime, and cefpodoxime. One-half of highly penicillin-resistant pneumococci are also resistant to cefotaxime and ceftriaxone, a higher proportion are resistant to cefepime, and nearly all are resistant to cefpodoxime. Pneumonia caused by intermediately penicillin-resistant strains responds well to β-lactam antibiotics. Pneumonia due to fully resistant strains also responds, but probably not as reliably; data that address this issue are currently being examined. Sinusitis and otitis media caused by intermediately resistant *S. pneumoniae* do not reliably respond to therapy, and failure of therapy may be common when these conditions are caused by highly resistant pneumococcal strains.

Resistance to erythromycin extends to the new macrolides, including azithromycin and clarithromycin. This resistance will certainly affect empirical therapy for bronchitis, sinusitis, and pneumonia. In the United States, the majority of macrolide-resistant pneumococci bear the so-called M phenotype (erythromycin MIC = 1 to 8 μg/mL) and

Table 138-3 Antibiotic Susceptibility of Pneumococci Stratified According to Penicillin Susceptibility

| Status of Strain | Percentage of Isolates Susceptible to Indicated Agent | | | | | | | | | |
	Tet	Em	TMP-SMZ	Cfur	Ctax or Ctri	Clin	Newer Mac	Quin	Imi	Vm
Pen-S	90	95	90	100	100	100	95	98	100	100
Pen-I	80	80	70	75	95	90	80	98	90	100
Pen-R	60	50	23	25	50	85	50	98	80	100

Abbreviations: Pen-S, sensitive to penicillin; Pen-I, intermediately resistant to penicillin; Pen-R, resistant to penicillin; Tet, tetracycline; Em, erythromycin; TMP-SMZ, trimethoprim-sulfamethoxazole; Cfur, cefuroxime; Ctax, cefotaxime; Ctri, ceftriaxone; Clin, clin- damycin; Mac, macrolides; Quin, quinolones; Imi, imipenem; Vm, vancomycin. NOTE: These percentages reflect a composite of the data available in March 1999; actual results vary with the time and locale.

are susceptible to clindamycin. In this case, resistance is mediated by an efflux pump mechanism; it is not yet known whether M-type resistance can be overcome by clinically achievable levels of macrolides. In Europe, most macrolide resistance is due to a mutation in *ermB*, which confers high-level resistance not only to macrolides but also to clindamycin. Rates of resistance to doxycycline among pneumococci of varying susceptibility to penicillin are similar to those observed for macrolides, whereas the overall rate of pneumococcal resistance to trimethoprim-sulfamethoxazole (25%) is sufficiently high to discourage therapy with this agent unless an isolate is known to be susceptible.

The newer fluoroquinolones remain highly effective against pneumococci, with equal efficacy against penicillin-susceptible and -resistant strains. All pneumococci are susceptible to vancomycin, although it is feared that the acquisition of vancomycin resistance by enterococci and other gram-positive bacteria may eventually lead to pneumococcal transformation to resistance. Of drugs under study, the oxazolidinones and glycopeptides appear to be most promising, with MICs for drug-resistant *S. pneumoniae* strains no higher than for penicillin-susceptible strains. Resistance to streptogramins parallels that to macrolides and limits the usefulness of these drugs for the treatment of pneumonia.

Pneumococcal susceptibility patterns vary greatly between and even within individual communities and the data are in a state of flux. It does appear, however, that the constant trend is toward more widespread resistance.

General Therapy There has been increased emphasis on outpatient therapy in patients who are at low risk (as determined by PORT score according to criteria described by the Pneumonia Outcomes Research Team; Chap. 255). This approach appears to be safe. However, if the physician is in doubt about the severity of illness, the social circumstances, or the likelihood of compliance with the prescribed antibiotic regimen, it may be best to hospitalize the patient, at least briefly.

Specific Antibiotic Therapy • *Pneumonia* This section will deal primarily with the treatment of pneumonia that is known to be due to *S. pneumoniae*. The broader issue of empirical therapy for community-acquired pneumonia is covered in detail elsewhere (Chap. 255). However, a few general comments on empirical therapy apply. An important problem in treating pneumonia is that, without a good sputum sample that can be Gram-stained and examined microscopically, the etiologic agent is not known at the time when treatment needs to be initiated and is not likely to become known later. Empirical therapy in such cases must be effective against *S. pneumoniae*, which remains the most likely causative agent of community-acquired pneumonia, unless epidemiologic, clinical, and radiologic findings strongly favor another etiologic entity. If a good sputum sample is obtained and only *S. pneumoniae* is visible, therapy can be focused on this organism, although additional treatment may be added for organisms that are not visualized microscopically—e.g., influenza virus in a patient hospitalized during an influenza outbreak. Even if the pneumococcus is suspected, a certain degree of empiricism is required, because the antibiotic susceptibility of the strain involved will not be known for 1 or 2 days.

OUTPATIENT THERAPY Amoxicillin (500 mg four times daily) effectively treats all cases of pneumococcal pneumonia except those caused by the most highly penicillin-resistant isolates. Neither cefuroxime nor cefpodoxime offers any advantages over amoxicillin since these drugs are less likely, even at high dosages, to be active against highly resistant pneumococcal strains. One of the newer fluoroquinolones in an accepted dosage for pneumonia is highly likely to be effective. Doxycycline, azithromycin, or clarithromycin will be effective in 85 to 90% of cases and clindamycin in a higher proportion. The trend toward increasing resistance to all these drugs is worrisome. Because one-fourth of all isolates are now resistant to trimethoprim-sulfamethoxazole, this agent can no longer be recommended. Since none of these therapies ensures the kind of antibiotic coverage that it would have in the past, patients should be instructed to remain in close contact with the prescribing physician, especially if there is any de-

terioration in their condition. It is worth noting that an outcomes study using data from the mid-1990s, when the rate of resistance was lower, showed that treatment with any of the above-mentioned antibiotics was associated with a good outcome; the majority of cases in which an etiologic agent was identified were due to *S. pneumoniae*.

INPATIENT THERAPY Pneumonia caused by penicillin-susceptible or intermediately penicillin-resistant pneumococcal isolates is readily treatable with penicillin. The dosages that follow are acceptable against intermediately resistant strains and against many or most fully resistant isolates, although they are excessive for use against susceptible isolates. Lower doses, however, cannot be recommended initially because susceptibility is not known until 24 to 72 h after treatment is begun. Patients who are sick enough to be hospitalized should be treated promptly. Most physicians favor parenteral antibiotics, although oral administration of well-absorbed drugs may be acceptable if the patient is not vomiting or hypotensive. Recommended regimens include ceftriaxone (1 to 2 g/d) or cefotaxime (1 to 2 g every 6 to 8 h). Ampicillin (1 to 2 g every 6 h) is also widely used. A quinolone or azithromycin can be given parenterally or orally. About 10 to 15% of all pneumococci are resistant to macrolides, and 1 to 2% are resistant to quinolones. Much of the resistance to macrolides among pneumococcal isolates may be overcome by the administration of azithromycin at a dosage of 500 mg on the first day and 250 mg/d thereafter. Clindamycin is effective against a higher proportion of resistant pneumococci than are the macrolides. Vancomycin is uniformly effective against pneumococci and should be used for initial therapy if there is reason to believe that a patient is infected with a strain that is resistant to the drugs listed above. As antimicrobial resistance among pneumococci evolves, updated recommendations will be issued by the Infectious Diseases Society of America, the American Thoracic Society, and the Centers for Disease Control and Prevention (CDC).

Patients with severe allergic reactions to β-lactam antibiotics should receive vancomycin (500 mg intravenously every 6 h) or a quinolone. As noted above, there have always been treatment failures unrelated to the antimicrobial susceptibility of the organism; nevertheless, the failure of a patient to respond promptly should raise the question of resistance, and vancomycin should be given until the susceptibility of the infecting strain to other drugs has been documented. Of course, evidence for loculated infections (such as empyema) and/or other causes of fever should be sought.

DURATION OF THERAPY The optimal duration of treatment for pneumococcal pneumonia is uncertain. Penicillin-susceptible strains disappear from the sputum within several hours of the first dose of penicillin, and a single dose of procaine penicillin, which results in the maintenance of an effective antimicrobial level for 24 h, was said to cure pneumococcal pneumonia in otherwise-healthy young adults at the time when all isolates were susceptible. Most older physicians treat pneumococcal pneumonia for 5 to 10 days. In the absence of reports of therapy failure, younger physicians have tended to treat the infection for 10 to 14 days. Prolongation of therapy is a two-edged sword, especially in debilitated patients, because the risk of complications increases with each day of antibiotic treatment, particularly in the hospital setting. A few days of close observation and parenteral therapy followed by an oral antibiotic—with the entire course of treatment continuing for no more than 5 days after the patient becomes afebrile—may be the best approach.

Otitis media and acute sinusitis Current treatment recommendations for otitis media and acute sinusitis—conditions whose pathogenesis and microbial etiology are similar—are based on the following points: (1) Acute otitis media is the most common infection for which antibiotics are prescribed in the United States. (2) As noted above, *S. pneumoniae* is the most likely treatable cause; taken together, *H. influenzae* and *M. catarrhalis*, many strains of which produce β-lactamases, are implicated nearly as frequently as pneumococci. (3) In the absence of diagnostic tympanocentesis, the etiologic diagnosis is nearly always presumptive. (4) Because penetration into a closed space is required, high serum levels of an effective antibiotic are required to treat otitis caused by intermediately or fully resistant pneumococci. (5) Otitis due to *S. pneumoniae* is more likely to fail to respond and to produce complications without specific therapy. (6) Antibiotics that are effective against pneumococci and yet resist β-lactamases tend to be very expensive compared with amoxicillin.

As a result of these considerations, the CDC's Otitis Media Working Group recommends that initial therapy be amoxicillin in a high dosage—e.g., 80 mg/kg for infants and toddlers or 500 mg four times daily for adults. If this regimen fails, highly penicillin-resistant pneumococci or β-lactamase-producing bacteria may be responsible, and a course of cefpodoxime, perhaps preceded by a single parenteral dose of ceftriaxone, is recommended. Once therapy has begun, patients must be monitored closely for a response. Despite the detection (by molecular analysis) of pneumococcal DNA in middle-ear fluid, chronic serous otitis ("glue ear") is probably not due to active infection and does not require antibiotic therapy.

Meningitis A reasonable recommendation is that pneumococcal meningitis be treated initially with cefotaxime (2 g every 6 h) or ceftriaxone (1 to 2 g every 12 h) plus vancomycin (500 mg every 6 h or 1 g every 12 h). Two drugs are given initially because the cephalosporin is likely to be effective against most isolates and readily penetrates the blood-brain barrier, whereas vancomycin is uniformly effective but has a somewhat unpredictable capacity to cross the blood-brain barrier. If the isolate is shown to be penicillin-susceptible, treatment can be continued with 24 million units of penicillin every 24 h, given every 4 h in divided doses or continuously. If the isolate exhibits reduced susceptibility to penicillin but is susceptible to cefotaxime or ceftriaxone, the administration of vancomycin may be discontinued. Rifampin inhibits the bactericidal activity of β-lactam antibiotics and probably should not be added to the regimen. The total duration of therapy for pneumococcal meningitis is 10 to 14 days. Despite the central pathogenic role of inflammation in meningitis, the use of glucocorticoids or other anti-inflammatory agents is controversial, even in children, in whom most of the relevant studies have been done. Data simply do not exist on which to base an informed decision regarding the administration of glucocorticoids or cyclooxygenase inhibitors to adults with pneumococcal meningitis (Chap. 372). Meningitis should be treated in an intensive care unit and with the participation of appropriate consultants, generally including a neurologist and a specialist in infectious diseases.

Endocarditis Pneumococcal endocarditis is associated with rapid destruction of heart valves. Vancomycin should be given pending assays for the minimal bactericidal concentrations of β-lactam antibiotics. There is no clear evidence that the addition of another antibiotic to the regimen is beneficial; aminoglycosides are somewhat synergistic and rifampin or quinolones are antagonistic with β-lactams. Endocarditis and meningitis should be treated initially in an intensive care unit, with the participation of appropriate consultants. Patients with endocarditis should probably be treated in collaboration with an infectious disease consultant, a cardiologist, and a cardiovascular surgeon.

Other Therapeutic Modalities A variety of agents that block the action of TNF-α, IL-1, or platelet-activating factor have conferred no benefit in and may have had a detrimental effect on pneumococcal sepsis. Similar results have been obtained with glucocorticoids.

PREVENTION Pneumococcal vaccine contains 25 μg of capsular polysaccharide from the 23 most prevalent serotypes of *S. pneumoniae*; vaccination stimulates antibody to most serotypes in most recipients. In adults under 55 years old, protection rates are at least 85%, even 5 years or longer after vaccination. The level and duration of protection decrease with advancing age, perhaps because of a diminished avidity of the antibody for the capsular polysaccharide. As a result, persons in their eighties have 50% protection for 3 years and very little or no protection thereafter. In subgroups of the population at high risk (e.g., debilitated elderly persons and individuals with severe chronic lung disease), vaccine has not been shown conclusively to be effective. Persons who most need the vaccine because of poor IgG responses are not likely to respond to immunization with significant increases in antibody level. Nevertheless, the poor average rate of response should not deter the physician from administering vaccine to individual patients who are at increased risk of pneumococcal infection. In light of the safety, low cost, and efficacy of vaccine and the emergence of antibiotic-resistant strains, the failure to vaccinate elderly persons and individuals who have conditions predisposing to pneumococcal disease is viewed by some authorities as a missed opportunity in public health policy.

The CDC's Immunization Practices Advisory Committee has broadened its recommendations for pneumococcal vaccination to include all persons over the age of 2 years who are at substantially increased risk of developing pneumococcal infection and/or a serious complication of such an infection. General categories included within these recommendations are as follows: (1) persons over the age of 65; (2) persons with anatomic or functional asplenia, CSF leak, diabetes mellitus, alcoholism, cirrhosis, chronic renal insufficiency, chronic pulmonary disease, or advanced cardiovascular disease; (3) persons who have an immunocompromising condition associated with increased risk of pneumococcal disease, such as multiple myeloma, lymphoma, Hodgkin's disease, HIV infection, organ transplantation, or chronic use of glucocorticoids; (4) persons who are genetically at increased risk, such as Native Americans and Alaskans; and (5) persons who live in special environments where outbreaks are particularly likely to occur, such as nursing homes. This list should not be regarded as all-inclusive.

Recommendations regarding revaccination seem to be somewhat inconsistent. A single revaccination is advocated for persons over the age of 65. Since antibody levels decline and there is no anamnestic response, it seems more reasonable simply to recommend revaccination at 5-year intervals, especially in persons over the age of 65, who tend to have almost no local reaction, and in splenectomized patients, who are most in need. If penicillin-resistant pneumococci continue to increase in prevalence, routine immunization of children over the age of 2 years should be considered. Pneumococcal vaccine has not been useful in children <2 years of age, who do not respond well to polysaccharide antigens. In a recent field trial, a heptavalent protein-conjugate pneumococcal polysaccharide vaccine protected infants and children against pneumococcal pneumonia, bacteremia, and meningitis; this vaccine is likely to be released for administration to young children in the next few years.

BIBLIOGRAPHY

AFESSA B et al: Pneumococcal bacteremia in adults: A 14-year experience in an inner-city university hospital. Clin Infect Dis 21:345, 1995

BARTLETT JG et al: Community-acquired pneumonia in adults: Guidelines for management. Clin Infect Dis 26:811, 1998

DAGAN R et al: Bacteriologic response to oral cephalosporins: Are established susceptibility breakpoints appropriate in the case of acute otitis media? J Infect Dis 176:1253, 1997

DOERN GV et al: Prevalence of antimicrobial resistance among respiratory tract isolates of *Streptococcus pneumoniae* in North America: 1997 results from the SENTRY antimicrobial surveillance program. Clin Infect Dis 27:111, 1998

——— et al: Antimicrobial resistance with *Streptococcus pneumoniae* in the United States, 1997–98. Emerg Infect Dis 5:757, 1999

DOWELL SF et al: Otitis media—management and surveillance in the era of pneumococcal resistance: A report from the Drug-Resistant *Streptococcus pneumoniae* Therapeutic Working Group. Pediatr Infect Dis J 18:1, 1999

FEDSON DS, MUSHER DM: Pneumococcal vaccine, in *Vaccines*, 3d ed, SA Plotkin, EA Mortimer Jr (eds). Philadelphia, Saunders, 1998

HAUSDORFF WP et al: The contribution of specific pneumococcal serogroups to different disease manifestations: Implications for conjugate vaccine formulation and use, part II. Clin Infect Dis 30:122, 2000

HEFFRON R: *Pneumonia: With Special Reference to Pneumococcus Lobar Pneumonia.* A Commonwealth Fund Book, © 1939. Reprinted by Harvard University Press, Cambridge, MA, 1979

MUSHER DM: *Streptococcus pneumoniae,* in *Principles and Practice of Infectious Diseases,* 5th ed, GL Mandell et al (eds). New York, Churchill Livingstone, 1999

———— et al: Antibody to capsular polysaccharides of *Streptococcus pneumoniae* in adults: Prevalence, persistence, relation to carriage, and resistance to infection. Clin Infect Dis 17:66, 1993

PASTOR P et al: Invasive pneumococcal disease in Dallas County, Texas: Results from population-based surveillance in 1995. Clin Infect Dis 26:590, 1998

PATON JC et al: Molecular analysis of putative pneumococcal virulence proteins. Microb Drug Resist 3:1, 1997

PLOUFFE JF et al: Bacteremia with *Streptococcus pneumoniae*: Implications for therapy and prevention. Franklin County Pneumonia Study Group. JAMA 275:194, 1996

RAHAV G et al: Invasive pneumococcal infections: A comparison between adults and children. Medicine 76:295, 1997

RODRIGUEZ MC et al: Unusual manifestations of pneumococcal infection in HIV-infected individuals: The past revisited. Clin Infect Dis 14:192, 1992

SHAPIRO ED et al: The protective efficacy of polyvalent pneumococcal polysaccharide vaccine. N Engl J Med 325:1453, 1991

TUOMANEN EI et al: Pathogenesis of pneumococcal infection. N Engl J Med 332:1280, 1995

WATANAKUNAKORN C et al: Adult bacteremic pneumococcal pneumonia in a community teaching hospital, 1992–1996. A detailed analyis of 108 cases. Arch Intern Med 157: 1965, 1997

139

Jeffrey Parsonnet, Robert L. Deresiewicz

STAFFYLOCOCCAL INFECTIONS

STAPHYLOCOCCAL INFECTIONS

CoNS coagulase-negative staphylococci	TEE transesophageal echocardiography
CSF cerebrospinal fluid	TEN toxic epidermal necrolysis
CT computed tomography	TSS toxic shock syndrome
ETs exfoliative toxins	TSST-1 toxic shock syndrome toxin 1
MICs minimum inhibitory concentrations	TTE transthoracic echocardiography
MRI magnetic resonance imaging	VISA vancomycin-intermediate *S. aureus*
MRSA methicillin-resistant *S. aureus*	
PBPs penicillin-binding proteins	VRE vancomycin-resistant enterococci
SCVs small-colony variants	
SEs staphylococcal enterotoxins	

The staphylococci are hardy and ubiquitous colonizers of human skin and mucous membranes and were among the first human pathogens identified. They cause a variety of syndromes, including superficial and deep pyogenic infections, systemic intoxications, and urinary tract infections. Staphylococci are the leading cause of bacteremia, surgical wound infections, and infections of bioprosthetic materials in the United States; in addition, they are the second leading cause of nosocomial infections. Organisms of this genus are also a significant cause of bacterial food poisoning.

Staphylococcus aureus is the most important human pathogen in the genus. It remains a major public health concern due to its tenacity, potential destructiveness, and increasing resistance to antimicrobial agents. Although less virulent, the coagulase-negative staphylococci (CoNS), especially *S. epidermidis*, adhere avidly to prosthetic materials and are important nosocomial pathogens, especially of compromised hosts. Another CoNS species, *S. saprophyticus*, is a common cause of urinary tract infections.

TAXONOMY AND MICROBIOLOGY   Members of the genus *Staphylococcus* are nonmotile, nonsporulating gram-positive cocci, 0.5 to 1.5 μm in diameter, that occur singly and in pairs, short chains, and the irregular three-dimensional clusters from which their name is derived (Greek *staphulé,* "grape-like"). Staphylococci can grow over a wide range of environmental conditions, but they grow best at temperatures between 30°C and 37°C and at a pH around neutrality. They are resistant to desiccation and to chemical disinfectants, and they tolerate NaCl concentrations up to 12%. With rare exceptions, the staphylococci are facultatively anaerobic. The more virulent staphylococci can clot plasma (coagulase-positive), while the less virulent cannot (coagulase-negative). Of the six recognized coagulase-positive

staphylococcal species, the only important human pathogen is *S. aureus*, whose colonies are larger than those of *S. epidermidis*, are often pigmented (golden yellow), and are usually β-hemolytic on sheep blood agar. Twenty-eight species of CoNS are recognized. Of these, *S. epidermidis* is by far the most common nonurinary human isolate. Strains of *S. epidermidis* are typically white and nonhemolytic and may be tenaciously adherent as a result of their production of polysaccharide adhesin. *S. epidermidis* is followed in frequency by *S. hominis*, *S. haemolyticus*, and *S. warneri*. *S. lugdunensis* is increasingly recognized as a cause of serious human infection. *S. saprophyticus* is the most common staphylococcal urinary isolate.

STAPHYLOCOCCUS AUREUS

EPIDEMIOLOGY   Humans constitute the major reservoir of *S. aureus* in nature. The mucous membranes of the anterior nasopharynx are the principal site of carriage, with roughly 30% of healthy adults being so colonized at any point in time. Other common sites of colonization include the axillae, the vagina, damaged skin, and the perineum. Among postmenarcheal U.S. women, the rate of vaginal colonization by *S. aureus* ranges from 5 to 15% but rises to 30% during menses—a change that is relevant to the pathogenesis of the toxic shock syndrome (TSS). Most adults are colonized by *S. aureus* intermittently, whereas 10 to 20% have persistent colonization and about the same percentage are never found to harbor the organism. Colonization is influenced by both microbial and host factors as well as by the nature of the competing nonstaphylococcal flora. Carriage is more common among persons with frequent staphylococcal exposure and those with habitual or chronic disruption of cutaneous epithelial integrity. Thus, colonization rates are higher among health care workers, dialysis patients, patients with type 1 diabetes, injection drug users, persons infected with HIV, and individuals with chronic dermatologic conditions. After 2 weeks in a hospital, colonization rates rise to 30 to 50%, and colonizing strains are more likely to be resistant to antibiotics.

Colonization of mucocutaneous sites is an important risk factor for staphylococcal infection. For example, surgical wound infection following cardiothoracic surgery is up to 10 times more likely among patients who harbor *S. aureus* in the nares preoperatively than among those who do not. The vast majority of postoperative wound infections of all types are caused by a strain of *S. aureus* that was present in the nares before surgery. Furthermore, presurgical clearance of carriage with topical and systemic antibiotics decreases the incidence of postoperative staphylococcal infection, but it is not yet standard practice to screen and treat patients before surgery.

PATHOGENESIS AND HOST DEFENSE   *S. aureus* causes two types of syndrome: *intoxications* and *infections*. The clinical manifestations of intoxications are attributable to the action of one or a few secreted products of the microorganism (toxins), and these clinical features can be reproduced by administration of the toxin(s) in the absence of the microorganism. The toxin can be produced either in vivo (as in TSS or staphylococcal scalded skin syndrome) or in a suitable vector that subsequently delivers it to the host (as in staphylococcal food poisoning). Infections, in contrast, involve bacterial proliferation, invasion or destruction of host tissues, and—in most cases—local and systemic inflammatory responses by the host to these events. The ability of a microorganism to infect is predicated on its ability to produce certain products that enable it to survive and prosper in the host (*virulence factors*), and *S. aureus* is particularly well-armed in this regard.

Steps in Pathogenesis   The pathogenesis of staphylococcal intoxications is straightforward and involves four steps: colonization by a toxigenic strain of the bacterium, toxin production, toxin absorption, and intoxication. The pathogenesis of invasive infections is more complex and the steps are less discrete. They include colonization, invasion of the bacterium across epithelial or mucosal barriers, adherence to materials in the extracellular matrix, evasion or neutralization of host defenses, and destruction of host tissues. For both intoxications and infections, the entire process is carefully orchestrated by the bacterium in response to specific environmental conditions.

Physical preservation of cellular integrity Staphylococci are robust and adaptable organisms that can survive under relatively harsh environmental conditions. A rigid cell wall confers shape and strength to the organisms. The major component of the cell wall, *peptidoglycan*, is responsible for its physical properties. Disruption of peptidoglycan cross-linking by cell wall–active antibiotics (β-lactams or glycopeptides) renders staphylococci susceptible to lysis mediated by endogenous peptidoglycan hydrolases (*autolysins*). The osmotolerance exhibited by *S. aureus* enables the organism to grow without microbial competition in foods of low water activity and so sets the stage for contamination of food by staphylococcal enterotoxins (SEs), which cause food poisoning.

Colonization Staphylococcal colonization of the nasal mucosa is mediated by adherence of cell-surface components to host molecules (e.g., mucin carbohydrate). Factors contributing to colonization of other surfaces, such as the vaginal mucosa, are poorly understood. After colonization, the production of certain staphylococcal toxins [toxic shock syndrome toxin 1 (TSST-1), exfoliative toxins, or SEs] can ensue under the appropriate environmental conditions. Colonization may be transient or persistent; the latter condition increases the likelihood that organisms will gain access to deeper tissues, beginning the process of infection.

Invasion and adherence to the extracellular matrix Staphylococci generally cannot invade through intact epithelial surfaces, which represent the primary line of antistaphylococcal defense. Invasion is facilitated by a mechanical break in the epithelium or by plugging of a gland or hair follicle. Once the epithelial barrier is breached, colonization of host tissues is facilitated by adherence of *S. aureus* to molecules present either on host cell surfaces or in the extracellular matrix. Several staphylococcal surface proteins, including protein A, function as adhesins by binding extracellular matrix molecules. These proteins have been designated "microbial-surface components recognizing adhesive matrix molecules" and may adhere to fibrinogen, fibronectin, collagen, elastin, and other serum constituents.

Destruction of host cells and alteration of the host microenvironment A number of products of *S. aureus* alter the host environment in a way that benefits the bacterium. *Coagulase* is a secreted enzyme that binds prothrombin and thereby causes the conversion of fibrinogen to fibrin; it may aid in the establishment of an environment within host tissues that is protected from cells of the immune system or from antibiotics. *S. aureus* produces a number of *lipases*, which may enhance the organism's survival in sebaceous areas of the human body. *Hyaluronidase* hydrolyzes hyaluronic acid, a mucopolysaccharide present in extracellular ground substance; its action may facilitate the spread of the organism through the extracellular matrix to adjoining tissues. *Staphylokinase*, *thermonuclease*, and *serine protease* are other extracellular enzymatic products that may play roles in pathogenesis.

S. aureus produces a number of membrane-active toxins that probably contribute to pathogenesis by damaging host cells, although their exact role in pathogenesis remains uncertain. These toxins include α-, β-, and δ-hemolysins and the synergohymenotropic toxins (γ-hemolysin and Panton-Valentine leukocidin). *α-Hemolysin* (α-toxin) is the prototypic pore-forming toxin; it inserts into the cell membrane, creating ion-conductive channels that destroy membrane integrity. The toxin is dermonecrotic on subcutaneous injection, induces proinflammatory changes in mammalian cells, and—in animal models—induces many findings seen in sepsis, including hypotension and thrombocytopenia. The *synergohymenotropic toxins* are a family of bicomponent toxins. Their name derives from the fact that their two components are tropic for cell membranes and are synergistically active against them. Like α-toxin, the synergohymenotropic toxins are

pore-forming toxins. *Panton-Valentine leukocidin* is most active against polymorphonuclear cells, monocytes, and macrophages. It is dermonecrotic to rabbit skin, and strains producing it are strongly associated with human furunculosis.

Evasion of host defense Once staphylococci have breached mucosal or epithelial barriers, the host's immune response is directed at containing and eliminating them, principally by polymorphonuclear recruitment and phagocytic killing. The bacteria fight back by cloaking antigenic determinants on their surface, by interfering with the function of opsonins, by directly killing the phagocytes, and by developing strategies to survive within them. The pyogenic abscess, the histologic hallmark of staphylococcal infection, represents the battlefield for this encounter, in which the microorganism survives in an environment in which leukocyte function is impaired and into which antibiotics penetrate poorly. Although the abscess may contain the spread of the bacteria, patients with abscesses are symptomatic and usually require surgical drainage for relief.

Some staphylococcal components and products are direct chemoattractants for polymorphonuclear leukocytes; others provoke the release of chemoattractant cytokines that recruit phagocytic cells to the infected area. Histologic sections of early lesions typically reveal a central focus of organisms surrounded by a zone of necrotic debris, which in turn is surrounded by a zone of viable inflammatory cells. The toxic action of staphylococcal leukocidin may in part explain the zone of necrosis. After several days, fibroblasts populate the margin of the abscess and there elaborate collagen, which creates a true capsule around the abscess.

Staphylococcal cell-wall peptidoglycan activates complement, which is an important opsonin in persons lacking antibody to staphylococcal surface components. Peptidoglycan also acts as a general stimulator of inflammatory cytokine release and may thereby contribute to sepsis, but it is weaker in this regard than gram-negative lipopolysaccharide. Opsonic antibodies specific for peptidoglycan or capsule mediate phagocytosis by polymorphonuclear leukocytes and macrophages in vitro, although the role of antibody in vivo is less certain. There is considerable interstrain variation in susceptibility to opsonization, and acquired protective immunity to staphylococcal infection is generally thought *not* to develop. (In contrast, acquired antibody-mediated immunity to systemic staphylococcal intoxications does occur; e.g., >90% of healthy adults have protective antibody to the most common TSS toxin, TSST-1.) Mitigating against opsonization is *protein A*, an important cell-surface component; protein A binds the Fc portion of IgG subclasses 1, 2, and 4 and thereby interferes with antibody-mediated opsonization. Polysaccharide capsule, which is produced by most clinical isolates, may also interfere with opsonization.

S. aureus has numerous defenses against killing after phagocytosis. Intracellular bacteria are usually killed rapidly by the oxidative burst within the phagosome, but staphylococcal catalase, which converts hydrogen peroxide to oxygen and water, detoxifies oxygen radicals and potentiates intracellular survival. Staphylococci are also taken up by nondedicated phagocytes, such as endothelial cells and osteoblasts, and may survive within them. One strategy for intracellular survival is the genesis of small-colony variants (SCVs). These slow-growing cells exhibit alterations in electron transport and generally produce reduced amounts of virulence determinants such as α-toxin and coagulase. They are relatively resistant to cell wall–active antibiotics and aminoglycosides and are capable of persisting intracellularly for extended periods, thereby evading host defenses. Their slow growth also makes them less likely to be recovered in the clinical laboratory and then targeted for treatment. Their existence may in part explain the startling capacity of certain *S. aureus* infections (e.g., chronic osteomyelitis) to recrudesce after years of dormancy and the difficulty of curing infections in intravascular sites and bone. Prolonged exposure to aminoglycosides or to trimethoprim-sulfamethoxazole appears to be a risk factor for the development of SCVs.

Hosts at particular risk for staphylococcal infection include those with frequent or chronic disruptions in epithelial or mucosal integrity;

those with disordered leukocyte chemotaxis, such as patients with the Chédiak-Higashi or Wiskott-Aldrich syndrome; those whose phagocytes are defective in oxidative killing, as in chronic granulomatous disease; those with neutropenia or acquired functional deficiencies (e.g., deficiencies induced by exogenous glucocorticoids); and those with indwelling foreign bodies, which provide a matrix for staphylococcal adherence and biofilm formation and seriously impair phagocytic function. Patients with disorders of immunoglobulin or complement (especially C1–C4 deficiencies) are also at increased risk for *S. aureus* infection.

Superantigens The superantigens are V_β-restricted T cell mitogens: they bind directly and without prior processing to major histocompatibility class II molecules on the surface of antigen-presenting cells, thereby stimulating T cells on the basis of the sequence of the variable region of the β chain of the T cell

FIGURE 139-1 Cutaneous manifestations of toxic shock syndrome. The patient was a 7-year-old child with osteomyelitis and nonmenstrual TSS. *Left:* Diffuse erythroderma. The rubor was intense on the chest wall of this patient and is accurately represented in this photograph. Circumoral pallor is evident. *Right:* Desquamation of the fingers during convalescence. *(From Deresiewicz, with permission.)*

receptor rather than on the basis of the epitope specified by this receptor. Accordingly, a superantigen may be able to stimulate >10% of the T cells in a given individual—a percentage much higher than the ~1 in 10^6 cells stimulated by conventional antigens. This massive T cell stimulation provokes an exuberant and dysregulated immune response characterized by the release of the cytokines interleukins 1 and 2, tumor necrosis factor, and interferon γ. TSS is a manifestation of this process, as some aspects of septic shock may be as well. *S. aureus* produces a number of superantigens, including the SEs, TSST-1, and possibly the exfoliative toxins (ETs). Ten SEs have been identified to date, several of which are common causative agents of staphylococcal food poisoning. The mechanism by which the SEs cause vomiting is uncertain but may involve direct neural stimulation of the autonomic nervous system rather than a local effect on the gastrointestinal mucosa. The superantigenic properties of TSST-1 and the SEs are thought to explain their ability to cause TSS, although the exact mechanism by which they craft the various clinical manifestations of TSS is uncertain. There is conflicting evidence as to whether the ETs, which cause scalded skin syndrome, are superantigens; structural data suggest that they may instead be related to the serine proteases.

Genetic Regulation of Virulence Genes The production of virulence factors by bacteria is typically tightly and coordinately regulated by genetic apparatuses that sense and respond to environmental cues. Such coordinate regulation enables an organism to rapidly tailor its repertoire of proteins to suit its changing needs, either as it passes between microenvironments or as the environment evolves around it. Many of the staphylococcal exoproteins are typical virulence factors in this regard. For example, α-, β-, and δ-hemolysins, TSST-1, staphylococcal enterotoxin B, serine protease, and thermonuclease are all produced during the late logarithmic phase of growth in batch culture, at a time when nutrients become scarce and cell density reaches saturation. Their production is coordinately regulated and occurs reciprocally to that of the cell wall–associated staphylococcal proteins protein A and coagulase. Several genetic regulatory loci modulate these events, as do specific environmental conditions that presumably operate through those genetic loci. Foreign materials that increase the risk of TSS and conditions in food that predispose to staphylococcal food poisoning probably do so by presenting microenvironments that stimulate production of the relevant toxins. Similar events are undoubtedly operative within the environment of host tissues during infection, even in the absence of a foreign body.

Several distinct genetic loci regulate exoprotein production in *S. aureus*, the best-studied of which are *agr* (accessory gene regulator)

and *sar* (staphylococcal accessory regulator). Both affect gene expression primarily at the level of transcription, and both activate the expression of secreted proteins and diminish the expression of cell wall–associated proteins during the late logarithmic phase of bacterial growth. Data suggest that *agr* may function primarily as a "quorum sensor," an apparatus that informs the bacterium of the density of staphylococci in its environment. Exoprotein regulation in *S. aureus* apparently results from a complex interplay of environmental factors and gene products.

STAPHYLOCOCCAL INTOXICATIONS **Toxic Shock Syndrome** TSS is an acute, life-threatening intoxication characterized by fever, hypotension, rash, multiorgan dysfunction, and desquamation during the early convalescent period (Fig. 139-1). The disease was first characterized in 1978 but gained notoriety in 1980 upon the recognition of many cases among menstruating women. It is a relatively uncommon illness, with a reported annual incidence (among menstruating women) of 1 case per 100,000; it is likely, however, that the disease is substantially underreported, especially nonmenstrual cases. About half of all cases occur in settings other than menstruation and are distributed among individuals of both sexes and all ages. Menstrual and nonmenstrual cases are clinically indistinguishable. Among cases reported to the Centers for Disease Control and Prevention between 1985 and 1994, the minimum case-fatality rate was 2.5% for menstrual cases and 6.4% for nonmenstrual cases.

TSS is caused by any of several related exoproteins produced by *S. aureus*. TSST-1 is the toxin most frequently implicated (causing virtually all menstrual cases), and staphylococcal enterotoxin B is the second most frequent. For illness to develop, an individual must be colonized or infected with a toxigenic strain of *S. aureus* and must lack a protective level of antibody to the toxin made by that strain. That TSS is primarily a disease of the young reflects the fact that >90% of adults have antibodies to TSS toxins.

Menstruation remains the most common setting for TSS, but the disease can also complicate the use of barrier contraceptives and childbirth. Moreover, nonmenstrual TSS can ensue after superinfection of skin lesions of many types, including burns, insect bites, varicella lesions, and surgical wounds. Postoperative disease can develop from hours to weeks after any surgical procedure. Staphylococcal superinfection after influenza is a common setting for TSS, as is acute sinusitis. Overt infection with *S. aureus* is not required for the development of TSS; mere colonization with a toxigenic strain may suffice. Accordingly, the primary site of toxin production in TSS may appear entirely benign.

TSS remains a clinically defined syndrome (Table 139-1). Patients

Table 139-1 Staphylococcal Toxic Shock Syndrome: Case Definition

1. Fever: temperature of ≥38.9°C (≥102°F)
2. Rash: diffuse macular erythroderma ("sunburn" rash)
3. Hypotension: systolic blood pressure of ≤90 mmHg (adults) or <5th percentile for age (children <16 years of age); or orthostatic hypotension (orthostatic drop in diastolic blood pressure by ≥15 mmHg, orthostatic dizziness, or orthostatic syncope)
4. Involvement of at least three of the following organ systems:
   a. Gastrointestinal: vomiting or diarrhea at onset of illness
   b. Muscular: severe myalgias or serum creatine phosphokinase level at least twice the upper limit of normal
   c. Mucous membranes: vaginal, oropharyngeal, or conjunctival hyperemia
   d. Renal: blood urea nitrogen or creatinine level at least twice the upper limit of normal; or pyuria (≥5 leukocytes per high-power field) in the absence of urinary tract infection
   e. Hepatic: total serum bilirubin or aminotransferase (alanine or aspartate) level at least twice the upper limit of normal
   f. Hematologic: thrombocytopenia (platelet count ≤100,000/μL)
   g. Central nervous: disorientation or alteration in consciousness but no focal neurologic signs at a time when fever and hypotension are absent
5. Desquamation: 1 to 2 weeks after the onset of illness (typically palms and soles)
6. Evidence against an alternative diagnosis: negative results of cultures of blood, throat, or CSF (if performed);[a] no rise in titers of antibody to the agents of Rocky Mountain spotted fever, leptospirosis, and rubeola (if obtained)

[a] Blood culture may be positive for *S. aureus*. CSF, cerebrospinal fluid.
SOURCE: AL Reingold et al, Ann Intern Med 96(part 2):875, 1982.

meeting the case definition are severely ill, although milder forms of "staphylococcal toxin-mediated disease" do occur. The illness usually begins precipitously, with high fever and a complex of symptoms that may include nausea, vomiting, abdominal pain, diarrhea, muscular pain, sore throat, and headache. Dizziness is common as a manifestation of orthostatic or frank hypotension. The characteristic macular erythroderma develops over the first 2 days of illness. It is usually generalized but is sometimes locally confined; it can be evanescent or persistent. The patient's mental status is often abnormal to a degree that is out of proportion to the degree of hypotension. Conjunctival suffusion, pharyngeal injection, and peripheral edema are evident in many cases; a so-called strawberry tongue develops in up to half of patients. In menstrual disease, the vaginal mucosa may be erythematous and a purulent vaginal discharge may be present, but these findings are not universal. Common laboratory abnormalities include azotemia, hypoalbuminemia, hypocalcemia, hypophosphatemia, creatine phosphokinase elevation, leukocytosis or leukopenia with a left shift, thrombocytopenia, and pyuria.

The early signs and symptoms of TSS resolve within the first few days of illness, after which complications of organ hypoperfusion, such as renal and myocardial dysfunction, fluid overload, and adult respiratory distress syndrome, dominate the picture. After about a week of illness, desquamation begins with superficial flaking of the skin of the torso, face, and extremities, which may be followed by full-thickness desquamation of the palms, soles, and digits. Common late sequelae include peripheral gangrene, reversible nail and hair loss, muscle weakness, and lingering asthenia and neuropsychiatric dysfunction.

The differential diagnosis of TSS is that of a severe febrile exanthem with hypotension. In the setting of menstruation accompanied by purulent vaginal discharge, the diagnosis may be obvious. The challenge is to recognize the less obvious cases, in which the exanthem may be fleeting, multiorgan dysfunction may be subtle, or (in nonmenstrual cases) a primary site of infection may be inapparent. Recovery of *S. aureus* supports the diagnosis, as does demonstration of toxin production by the strain and serologic susceptibility to the toxin. Other diagnoses to consider include streptococcal TSS, staphylococcal scalded skin syndrome, Kawasaki syndrome, Rocky Mountain spotted fever, leptospirosis, meningococcemia, gram-negative sepsis, exan-

thematous viral syndromes, and severe drug reactions. Staphylococcal TSS and streptococcal TSS (Chap. 140) can be clinically indistinguishable.

Treatment of TSS involves drainage of the site of toxin production, aggressive fluid resuscitation, and administration of antistaphylococcal antibiotics. Recent surgical wounds should be explored and irrigated, even when signs of inflammation are lacking; foreign bodies should be removed. Pressors should be used for sustained hypotension that is unresponsive to fluids. Electrolyte abnormalities, particularly hypocalcemia and hypomagnesemia, must be corrected. Penicillinase-resistant penicillins (nafcillin, oxacillin) and first-generation cephalosporins have been widely used in TSS. A growing body of clinical and laboratory evidence indicates, however, that a protein synthesis inhibitor, such as clindamycin, might be superior to β-lactam agents. The authors recommend therapy with clindamycin (900 mg intravenously every 8 h), either alone or in combination with a β-lactam antibiotic [or vancomycin for patients perceived to be at risk for infection with methicillin-resistant *S. aureus* (MRSA)]. For a seriously ill patient in whom the diagnosis of TSS is uncertain, broad-spectrum antibiotics may be appropriate until the diagnosis is confirmed. A 14-day course of therapy—some of which may be administered perorally—is reasonable. Patients whose illness is severe enough to warrant vasopressors, who require mechanical ventilation, who have worsening renal function, or who have an undrainable focus of infection should be treated with intravenous immunoglobulin, which contains high levels of neutralizing antibody to TSS toxins. A single infusion of 400 mg/kg generates a protective level of antibody to TSST-1 that persists for weeks. Glucocorticoids have not been shown to be of significant benefit.

Because vaginal staphylococcal carriage can be persistent or recurrent and because in more than half of all cases TSS does not elicit immunity, recurrent menstrual TSS is a concern; recurrent nonmenstrual TSS has also been reported. The risk of recurrent illness can be assessed by tests for seroconversion to TSST-1. Women who do not seroconvert after acute illness (or who are not tested for antibody) should refrain indefinitely from using tampons or barrier contraceptives.

Staphylococcal Scalded Skin Syndrome This syndrome encompasses a range of cutaneous diseases of varying severity caused by ET-producing strains of *S. aureus*. The most severe form of staphylococcal scalded skin syndrome is termed *Ritter's disease* in newborns and *toxic epidermal necrolysis* (TEN) in older individuals. Milder and more common forms include *pemphigus neonatorum* and (in children and adults) *bullous impetigo* (see "Skin and Soft Tissue Infections," below). Persons >5 years old rarely develop staphylococcal TEN; those who do almost invariably have underlying disease (renal insufficiency, systemic immunosuppression). The rarity of the syndrome in adults has been ascribed to acquired immunity to the inciting toxins, to enhanced renal clearance of the toxins, and perhaps to diminished sensitivity to the action of the toxins.

Staphylococcal TEN, or Ritter's disease, often begins with a nonspecific prodrome. The acute phase starts with the onset of an erythematous rash. The erythema begins in the periorbital and perioral areas and spreads to the trunk and centrifugally to the limbs. Pastia's lines may be apparent. The skin has a sandpaper texture and is often tender. Periorbital edema is common. In infants and children, fever and irritability or lethargy are common, but systemic toxicity is not. Within hours or days, wrinkling and sloughing of the epidermis begin; sloughing can be provoked by gentle stroking of the skin (Nikolsky's sign), even in areas that appear uninvolved. The denuded areas are red and glistening but not purulent, and staphylococci are not present. Exfoliation may continue in large sheets or in ragged snippets of tissue. Large, flaccid bullae may develop. As in thermal burns, significant fluid and electrolyte loss can occur at this stage, as can secondary infection. Within about 48 h, the exfoliated areas dry and secondary desquamation begins. The entire illness resolves within about 10 days. Mortality (from hypovolemia or sepsis) is ~3% among children but approaches 50% among adults. Treatment includes the administration of antistaphylococcal agents, fluid and electrolyte management, and local care to the denuded skin.

Staphylococcal Food Poisoning Between 2 and 6 h after ingestion of contaminated food, staphylococcal food poisoning begins abruptly with nausea, vomiting, crampy abdominal pain, and diarrhea. The diarrhea is usually noninflammatory and is of lower volume than that in cholera or toxigenic *Escherichia coli* infection. Fever and rash are absent, and the patient is neurologically normal. The majority of cases are self-limited and resolve between 8 and 24 h after onset. In severe cases, hypovolemia and hypotension can develop. Although most cases probably do not come to medical attention and are not diagnosed, staphylococcal intoxication is the second or third leading cause of diagnosed food poisoning in the United States.

Food poisoning is caused by the ingestion of any of the SEs, which are produced by *S. aureus* in contaminated food before it is eaten. The presence of SEs in the food vector before its consumption accounts for the short incubation period of this illness. The SEs are heat stable, thus tolerating cooking conditions that kill the organisms that produced them. The disease has a high attack rate and is somewhat more common during the summer than at other times of the year. Processed meats and custard-filled baked goods are common food vectors, perhaps because staphylococci can tolerate conditions of high protein, salt, or sugar and so grow without competition in these environments. The most important epidemiologic risk factor in outbreaks of this disease is the ingestion of food that has been left at warm temperatures for prolonged periods, thereby allowing toxin production to occur before consumption. Contaminated preparation equipment and poor personal hygiene of food handlers are frequently implicated as well.

STAPHYLOCOCCAL INFECTIONS *S. aureus* causes invasive disease by breaching host defense barriers, often after disruption or dysfunction of such barriers. The most common portals of entry leading to staphylococcal invasion are the skin and associated structures. A nidus for staphylococcal colonization and subsequent invasion is provided by chronic skin conditions, such as eczema and psoriasis; acute breaks in the skin, such as puncture wounds, abrasions, and lacerations; and abnormalities of skin appendages, such as hair follicles and nails. Colonization of the nasopharynx predisposes to respiratory tract infection after aspiration, obstruction (e.g., of a bronchus by carcinoma or of sinus ostia by trauma, edema, or polyps), or impaired ciliary function (e.g., in chronic bronchitis or acute viral infection). Intubation of the trachea provides a conduit by which upper respiratory flora, including pathogens such as *S. aureus*, can reach the lower respiratory tract.

Skin and Soft Tissue Infections *S. aureus* is the most common etiologic agent of skin and soft tissue infections (Chap. 128). Such infections are usually caused by endogenous flora—i.e., strains of *S. aureus* that are harbored in the nares or other sites of colonization. Infection may represent a primary pathologic process, with direct invasion of skin and adjacent tissues, or a secondary process complicating preexisting lesions.

Staphylococcal infections originating in hair follicles range in severity from trivial to life-threatening. *Folliculitis* is an infection of follicular ostia; the appearance is that of a domed yellow pustule with a narrow red margin. Infection is often self-limited, although healing may be hastened by topical antiseptics and more severe cases may benefit from topical or systemic antibiotics. A *furuncle* (often called a *boil*) is a deep-seated necrotic infection of a hair follicle, most often located on the buttocks, face, or neck. Furuncles are painful and tender, and their appearance is often accompanied by fever and constitutional symptoms. Surgical drainage and systemic antibiotic treatment may hasten recovery and limit scar formation. Deep infection of a group of contiguous follicles is called a *carbuncle*. This type of painful necrotic lesion occurs most commonly on the back of the neck, shoulders, hips, and thighs, typically in middle-aged or elderly men. There is intense inflammation of surrounding and underlying connective tissue, and the infection may be complicated by bacteremia. Surgical drainage and systemic antibiotic administration are indicated. *S. aureus* is also the

most common cause of acute *paronychia*, infection of the lateral nail folds.

S. aureus causes *bullous impetigo*, a superficial cutaneous disorder occurring predominantly in children. An epidermal split caused by ET results in the formation of 1- to 2-cm bullae containing neutrophils and organisms. *Nonbullous impetigo* is most often caused by β-hemolytic streptococci, but *S. aureus* can secondarily infect impetiginous lesions. Treatment of impetigo with a topical antibiotic, such as mupirocin, may suffice for mild and localized infection, whereas systemic therapy is indicated for widespread or severe disease or for infection accompanied by lymphadenopathy.

Cellulitis, a spreading infection of subcutaneous tissue, is occasionally caused by *S. aureus*, but β-hemolytic streptococci are more common agents of this disease (Chap. 140). Secondary infection of surgical and traumatic wounds is more likely to be staphylococcal in etiology than is cellulitis arising from minor or inapparent breaks in the skin, and empiric treatment directed against both *S. aureus* and streptococci is reasonable in these settings. *Erysipelas*, the hallmark of which is a well-demarcated raised border, is a more superficial infection of the dermis and subcutaneous tissue; it is usually caused by group A streptococci and only rarely, if ever, by *S. aureus*.

Respiratory Tract Infections *S. aureus* can gain access to the lung parenchyma by two routes: aspiration of upper respiratory flora and hematogenous spread. Staphylococcal pneumonia is a relatively uncommon but severe infection, characterized clinically by chest pain, systemic toxicity, and dyspnea and pathologically by intense neutrophilic infiltration, necrosis, and abscess formation. *Pleural empyema* is a common complication and increases the already-considerable morbidity associated with this infection. Only rarely does *S. aureus* cause pneumonia without predisposing epidemiologic or host factors that favor colonization of the respiratory tract and/or that impair defense mechanisms. Residence in a chronic care facility, recent use of antibiotics, and hospitalization favor colonization—and hence respiratory tract infection—with *S. aureus*. Staphylococcal pneumonia most commonly follows tracheal intubation of a hospitalized patient or viral infection of the respiratory tract. Influenza virus is known both to increase respiratory colonization by *S. aureus* and to impair ciliary function (and therefore clearance of staphylococci). In a classic scenario, a patient (often elderly and/or institutionalized) develops a flu-like respiratory illness and then, after several days, deteriorates rapidly, with high fever, dyspnea, productive cough, and obtundation. The diagnosis of staphylococcal pneumonia is readily established by Gram's staining of expectorated sputum, which reveals abundant clusters of gram-positive cocci.

Hematogenous seeding of the lungs with *S. aureus* follows embolization from an intravascular nidus of infection. Common settings for septic pulmonary embolization are right-sided endocarditis (especially common among injection drug users) and septic thrombophlebitis, which is most often a complication of an indwelling venous catheter. Pneumonia is heralded by the acute onset of pleuritic chest pain and dyspnea; although diagnostic sputum may be lacking, a chest radiograph typically shows multiple nodular infiltrates, providing an important clue to both the diagnosis and the pathogenesis of disease.

Although not typically considered in the differential diagnosis of sore throat, *S. aureus* is occasionally isolated as the dominant organism from patients (especially children) with exudative *pharyngitis*. The illness may be accompanied by a scarlatiniform rash and may result in systemic toxicity (like that seen in TSS). Staphylococcal *tracheitis* may be diagnosed in children who have systemic toxicity and positive respiratory cultures but who lack pulmonary infiltrates. *S. aureus* is a prominent cause of *chronic sinusitis*, typically following the selection pressure of antimicrobial regimens that lack activity against this organism. Finally, *S. aureus* is a major etiologic agent of *sphenoid sinusitis*.

Infections of the Central Nervous System *S. aureus* gains access to structures of the central nervous system by hematogenous spread or by direct extension from contiguous structures. This organism is a prominent cause of *brain abscess*, especially as a result of embolization during mitral or aortic valve endocarditis. Such abscesses are often multiple, small, and scattered diffusely throughout the brain. Brain abscess can also develop by direct extension from frontoethmoid or sphenoid sinuses or from infected soft tissue after surgery or penetrating trauma. Patients with staphylococcal brain abscesses are more likely to have fever, meningismus, and other signs of infection than are patients with anaerobic bacterial or mixed-etiology brain abscesses. Purulent *meningitis* may accompany staphylococcal brain abscess or may develop during bacteremia in the absence of demonstrable abscesses.

S. aureus is the organism most likely to cause a variety of other space-occupying, suppurative intracranial infections. *Subdural empyema* usually develops by direct extension of osteomyelitis of the skull, after surgery or trauma, or in the setting of sinusitis. This condition may be accompanied by meningitis, epidural abscess, or intracranial phlebitis. The cardinal features of subdural empyema are fever, headache, vomiting, and signs of meningeal irritation. As the infection progresses, cerebral edema, often with infarction, may ensue and may be accompanied by alteration in mental status, seizures, and focal neurologic signs, which sometimes progress rapidly. The diagnosis should be suspected in any patient with meningeal signs and focal neurologic findings. Magnetic resonance imaging (MRI) is the diagnostic procedure of choice; lumbar puncture is contraindicated because of the danger of brainstem herniation. Early surgical drainage and treatment with an antibiotic that penetrates well into the central nervous system may be curative, although neurologic sequelae are not uncommon.

S. aureus is the most common cause of *spinal epidural abscess*, which develops most often in association with vertebral osteomyelitis or diskitis. The diagnosis is suggested by some combination of fever, back pain, radicular pain, lower-extremity weakness, and bowel or bladder dysfunction, but the presentation is often subtle, resulting in delayed diagnosis. Patients may report only difficulty in walking or weakness, and objective findings may initially be lacking. The principal danger is the potential for necrosis of the spinal cord by compression and/or venous involvement. Early recognition of this condition is critical if long-term sequelae, such as paraplegia, are to be averted. An MRI scan of the spine establishes whether or not an epidural collection is present. Fluoroscopy- or computed tomography (CT)-guided needle aspiration may confirm the diagnosis, but an open procedure offers a higher yield. Prompt surgical decompression by laminectomy is often required for preservation of neurologic function, although a trial of antibiotic therapy alone may be considered if no focal neurologic deficits are detected at the time of diagnosis. Any deterioration in neurologic status should prompt urgent surgical intervention. The pathogenesis of *intracerebral epidural abscess* is similar to that of subdural empyema, with staphylococcal infection usually following sinusitis, craniotomy, or trauma. Clinical manifestations reflect the anatomy of the underlying osteomyelitis plus the mass effect of the abscess, cerebral edema, and (often) secondary involvement of the subdural space. Emergent surgical drainage is usually required for cure.

Finally, *S. aureus* is the most common cause of *septic intracranial thrombophlebitis*, typically following sinusitis, mastoiditis, or soft tissue infection of the face. Clinical manifestations reflect the underlying condition and the anatomic structures in contiguity with the infected vein or sinus. Focal neurologic deficits, particularly of cranial nerve function, are characteristic of cavernous sinus thrombosis. Sagittal sinus thrombosis may be manifested by leg and arm weakness and by altered mental status; infections of the lateral and petrosal sinuses also produce characteristic clinical syndromes. Intracranial phlebitis may accompany epidural abscess, subdural empyema, and meningitis and is sometimes clinically indistinguishable from other types of intracranial infection. MRI is the diagnostic procedure of choice.

Urinary Tract Infections   *S. aureus* is an uncommon cause of urinary tract infection. Ascending infection almost exclusively follows instrumentation of the bladder (e.g., cystoscopy or placement of an indwelling catheter). Under other circumstances, the presence of *S. aureus* in the urine, even in low numbers, suggests staphylococcal bacteremia and hematogenous seeding of the kidneys, with or without abscess formation; staphylococcal endocarditis should be considered in this setting.

Endovascular Infections   *S. aureus* is the most common cause of acute bacterial *endocarditis* of both native and prosthetic valves (Chap. 126). The organism may infect previously normal valves. Staphylococcal endocarditis presents as an acute febrile illness, rarely of more than a few weeks' duration; complications such as meningitis, brain or visceral abscess, peripheral vascular embolization, valvular incompetence with heart failure, myocardial abscess, and purulent pericarditis have often developed by the time a patient seeks medical attention. The valves most commonly involved are the mitral and/or the aortic except among injection drug users, in whom infection of the tricuspid valve is most common.

The diagnosis of endocarditis is suggested by a heart murmur and the presence of conjunctival hemorrhages, subungual petechiae, or purpuric lesions on the distal extremities; it is readily confirmed by demonstration of high-grade bacteremia and echocardiography showing valvular vegetations. Echocardiography also helps establish which valve(s) are infected, the degree of valvular dysfunction or destruction, the quality of left ventricular function, and the presence or absence of annular or myocardial abscess. Transesophageal echocardiography (TEE) is more sensitive than transthoracic echocardiography (TTE) in detecting vegetations and abscesses, but it is also more invasive. TEE need not be performed in all cases of proven or suspected endocarditis. This approach is useful, however, in the setting of persistent bacteremia or fever (to evaluate for abscess) and in anticipation of surgery if TTE has not been sufficiently informative.

Native valve staphylococcal endocarditis carries a high mortality rate (on the order of 40%) and mandates prompt initiation of antimicrobial therapy. In addition to blood cultures and echocardiography, evaluation may include CT of the head and lumbar puncture if brain abscess or meningitis is suspected; a radionucleotide study if osteomyelitis is suspected; and abdominal CT if visceral abscess is suggested by abdominal pain or persistent fever or bacteremia. Indications for valve replacement are the same as those in endocarditis caused by other organisms: persistent bacteremia (beyond 5 to 7 days of therapy), valvular dysfunction resulting in heart failure, perivalvular or myocardial abscess, or recurrent embolization. Early consultation with a cardiothoracic surgeon is advisable in all cases because of the high proportion of patients with *S. aureus* endocarditis (around half) who develop one of these complications and therefore require valve replacement, often urgently. Once there is an indication for removal of an infected valve, nothing is gained and much can be lost by delaying surgery. *S. aureus* infection of a prosthetic valve (as an early or a late complication of valve replacement) almost always requires surgery for one of the above indications.

Right-sided endocarditis, which most often develops in association with injection drug use or venous catheterization, is frequently complicated by septic pulmonary emboli but otherwise carries a lower rate of serious complications than left-sided disease. Surgery is rarely required for right-sided infection. A relatively short course of parenteral combination therapy (2 weeks) may be curative, and the prognosis is relatively good.

The propensity of *S. aureus* to adhere to and infect damaged tissues makes it the foremost cause of endovascular infections other than endocarditis. Vascular infection is a consequence of hematogenous seeding of damaged vessels, especially large arteries with atheromatous plaques, resulting in the development of a mycotic aneurysm. It may also develop by spread from a contiguous focus of infection (e.g., after vascular surgery), often resulting in an infected pseudoaneurysm, or by contamination of an intravascular device, resulting in septic phlebitis. Staphylococcal infection of an atherosclerotic artery (most commonly the abdominal aorta or iliac arteries), which may be aneurysmal to begin with, is a potentially catastrophic event. Such infections are associated with high-grade bacteremia, may result in rupture and massive hemorrhage, and require surgical resection and bypass of the infected vessel. Septic phlebitis is also associated with high-grade bacteremia and systemic toxicity but is less likely than arteritis to result in rupture. Persistent bacteremia suggests the need for surgical removal of infected thrombus or vein, but the technical difficulty of such surgery may warrant an attempt at cure with antibiotics and anticoagulants alone.

Bacteremia A classic clinical scenario is that of a patient presenting with *S. aureus* bacteremia but without a demonstrable primary site of infection. Even in the absence of a changing murmur, peripheral embolic lesions, or a diagnostic echocardiogram, the possibility of endocarditis must be considered carefully in this situation. It is often hard to differentiate between endocarditis and bacteremia arising from another primary site; in addition, *S. aureus* may secondarily seed endovascular sites, such as heart valves or atheromatous plaques. Several criteria increase the likelihood that a patient has endocarditis as opposed to simple bacteremia: community (vs. nosocomial) acquisition of infection, absence of an apparent primary site of infection, and evidence of metastatic infection. The evaluation of a bacteremic patient should be tailored to the individual but may include an abdominal CT scan and a bone scan or gallium scan to detect an occult visceral abscess or osteomyelitis. TEE has demonstrated valvular abnormalities suggestive of endocarditis in up to one-fourth of bacteremic patients who lack clinical or TTE evidence of endocarditis. This finding has prompted some authorities to recommend TEE for all patients with staphylococcal bacteremia. The authors favor performance of this test for patients with persistent fever or bacteremia.

Complications of *S. aureus* bacteremia include abscesses of abdominal viscera, brain abscess, meningitis, septic arthritis, osteomyelitis, epidural abscess, and mycotic aneurysm. High-grade or persistent bacteremia mandates a thorough evaluation for these complications, even if a primary site of infection has been identified. The reported mortality rate for staphylococcal bacteremia ranges from 11 to 43%, with catheter-related infections carrying lower rates of complications and mortality than noncatheter infections.

Musculoskeletal Infections *S. aureus* is the most common cause of *acute osteomyelitis* (Chap. 129) in adults and one of the leading causes in children. Acute osteomyelitis develops as a result of either hematogenous seeding of bone (especially damaged bone) or direct extension from a contiguous focus of infection. The most common sites of hematogenous staphylococcal osteomyelitis in adults are the vertebral bodies; in children, the highly vascular metaphyses of long bones are most often affected. Acute osteomyelitis in adults usually presents with constitutional symptoms and pain over the affected area, often developing over several weeks or months. Leukocytosis and an elevated erythrocyte sedimentation rate or C-reactive protein level are laboratory clues to the diagnosis. Bacteremia may or may not be demonstrable. Four weeks of parenteral antibiotic therapy is usually curative.

S. aureus is also a prominent cause of *chronic osteomyelitis*, which develops at sites of previous surgery, trauma, or devascularization. In light of the hectic pace of many infections caused by *S. aureus*, chronic staphylococcal osteomyelitis can be impressively indolent; the infection may be asymptomatic for years or even decades, only to reawaken spontaneously and cause pain, sinus tract formation, and purulent drainage. A plain film of the affected area reveals bony destruction. The staphylococcal etiology of infection is best established by biopsy and culture of bone, as cultures of superficial or sinus tract drainage may yield misleading results. Cure requires surgical debridement of necrotic bone followed by a prolonged course of antibiotics. →*For consensus definitions of acute and chronic osteomyelitis, see Chap. 129.*

A special form of osteomyelitis is that associated with prosthetic joints or with internal or external fixation devices. Pain, fever, swelling, and decreased range of motion are cardinal features of an infected prosthesis. A plain film may suggest loosening of the prosthesis, often as radiolucency at the interface between bone and cement. *S. aureus* osteomyelitis associated with a prosthesis is infrequently cured by antibiotics alone. Persistent sepsis, persistent bacteremia, and clinical or radiologic evidence of loosening are absolute indications for removal of the prosthesis. *S. aureus* infection of fixation devices requires their removal, although this procedure may occasionally be delayed long enough to allow healing of the underlying fracture. Late relapses after apparent medical cure are not uncommon. A strategy of microbial suppression with oral antibiotics after a course of high-dose parenteral therapy is occasionally employed when removal of hardware is deemed too aggressive a measure for a particular patient.

S. aureus is a major cause of *septic arthritis* in adults (Chap. 323). Predisposing factors include injection drug use, rheumatoid arthritis, use of systemic or intraarticular steroids, penetrating trauma, and joints previously damaged by trauma or disease. Knees, hips, and sacroiliac joints are most frequently infected. In addition to parenteral antibiotics, cure requires either repeated joint aspirations—the end points being sterilization of the joint space, a decrease in the number of leukocytes in the joint aspirate, and no reaccumulation of fluid—or open or arthroscopic debridement and drainage. Failure to adequately drain joints infected with *S. aureus* poses a risk of permanent loss of function. *S. aureus* is also the most common cause of *septic bursitis* (Chap. 325), which most often involves bursae of the elbows, knees, and shoulders. As in arthritis, adequate drainage (via repeat aspiration, placement of a drain, or open debridement) hastens recovery and minimizes loss of function.

S. aureus infection of muscle (*pyomyositis*; Chap. 128) is relatively uncommon in temperate climates; *psoas abscess* is the most common such infection. The psoas muscle is seeded either hematogenously or by direct extension from the site of vertebral osteomyelitis; the results are pain upon extension of the hip and fever. Although formerly a cause of fever of unknown origin, psoas abscess is now relatively easy to diagnose by abdominal CT or MRI. Psoas abscesses are occasionally amenable to drainage via a percutaneous catheter; if not, then surgical drainage is indicated. For reasons that are not well understood, most other cases of staphylococcal pyomyositis occur in the tropics (tropical pyomyositis); in the United States, pyomyositis is seen most often in patients with underlying conditions such as diabetes mellitus, alcoholism, immunosuppressive therapy, and hematologic malignancy.

DIAGNOSIS The diagnosis of *S. aureus* infection is generally straightforward and is based on the isolation of the organism either from purulent material or from a normally sterile body fluid. Rarely should *S. aureus* growing from even a single blood culture be considered a contaminant. Clinical samples require no special transport media to preserve the viability of the organisms. Gram's staining of purulent material from a staphylococcal abscess invariably reveals abundant neutrophils and intra- and extracellular gram-positive cocci, which may be found singly or in pairs, tetrads, or clusters. *S. aureus* grows readily on standard laboratory media. Colonies that are catalase-positive and coagulase- or thermonuclease-positive are identified presumptively as *S. aureus*. Commercial kits are also available for the identification of gram-positive cocci and are generally reliable for identification of *S. aureus*.

The diagnosis of staphylococcal intoxications (such as TSS) may be more difficult and may in fact rely entirely on clinical data. The contribution of the laboratory may be confirmatory—for example, the demonstration of seroconversion to TSST-1 following a compatible illness, the demonstration of toxin production in vitro by a strain isolated from a patient, or the detection of SE in a food sample.

℞ TREATMENT The essential elements of therapy for staphylococcal infections are drainage of purulent collections of pus, debridement of necrotic tissue, removal of foreign bodies, and administration of antimicrobial agents. The importance of adequate drainage cannot be overemphasized; all but the smallest of staphylococcal abscesses require drainage for cure. In skin and soft tissue infections, surgical drainage is occasionally all that is required for cure. It is very difficult to eradicate *S. aureus* infection in the presence of a foreign body, such as a piece of orthopedic hardware, an intravascular catheter or other device, or a pacemaker. For example, patients with catheter-associated bacteremia who are treated with antibiotics but do not have their catheters removed have been found to be six times more likely to experience a relapse or to die of their infection than are patients whose catheters are removed. Only under extraordinary circumstances should an attempt be made to cure such infections without removal of foreign material or debridement of necrotic tissue.

Antimicrobial resistance   The relentless spread of antibiotic resistance among strains of *S. aureus* is one of the great challenges facing clinicians today. Within 4 years of the introduction of penicillin G into clinical practice in 1941, β-lactamase-mediated resistance to penicillin was reported. As additional antibiotics became available in the 1950s, resistance rapidly emerged to them as well. Bacterial killing by β-lactam antibiotics depends on binding of the drugs to penicillin-binding proteins (PBPs), a group of transpeptidases that catalyze the terminal steps in peptidoglycan assembly. *S. aureus* normally produces four PBPs, all of which are inhibited by β-lactam antibiotics and several of which are essential for bacterial integrity and multiplication. Penicillin resistance in *S. aureus* is largely due to bacterial production of β-lactamase, a serine peptidase that enzymatically degrades the β-lactam ring of penicillin, thereby inactivating the drug before it can interact with the PBPs. In most communities, >90% of *S. aureus* strains produce β-lactamase and hence are resistant to penicillin.

Methicillin, the first β-lactamase-stable semisynthetic penicillin, was introduced in 1960; it took only 1 year, however, for an MRSA strain to be isolated. Classic methicillin resistance is encoded by the methicillin resistance determinant (*mec*), a 30- to 50-kb transposon-like segment of DNA that is present in MRSA strains and absent from sensitive strains. The *mecA* gene encodes a variant PBP called *PBP2′* or *PBP2a*. PBP2′ has reduced affinity for β-lactam antibiotics and can substitute for the essential PBPs if they have been inactivated by β-lactams. MRSA strains are resistant to the action of all β-lactam antibiotics, including penicillins, cephalosporins, and carbapenems. Since the early 1980s, these strains have tended to be resistant to most other antibiotics as well, including chloramphenicol, tetracyclines, and macrolides, through other resistance mechanisms. Nosocomial (as opposed to community-acquired) isolates of MRSA are especially likely to be multidrug-resistant. Classic methicillin resistance can be detected readily in the clinical microbiology laboratory by a variety of techniques. An additional mechanism of relative resistance to methicillin—hyperproduction of β-lactamase—has been described, but the clinical significance of this form of resistance is uncertain.

Until recently, all strains of MRSA remained susceptible to vancomycin (if nothing else), making this the drug of choice for the treatment of infections caused by suspected or proven MRSA. Unfortunately, the efficacy of vancomycin for serious *S. aureus* infections, regardless of susceptibility to other agents, is suboptimal (see "Selection of Antibiotics," below). Furthermore, resistance of *S. aureus* to vancomycin has now emerged as well (see below), making the search for new antistaphylococcal agents all the more urgent. If isolates are shown to be susceptible to clindamycin or trimethoprim-sulfamethoxazole, these agents can be effective for treatment of MRSA infection—but again, many strains are resistant. Two newly licensed antibiotics, representing the vanguard of two new classes of drugs, may prove to be useful for treatment of infections caused by MRSA. A new antibiotic that combines two streptogramins, quinupristin and dalfopristin, blocks protein synthesis at two ribosomal sites, resulting in a synergistic bactericidal effect on *S. aureus* and other gram-positive cocci. Linezolid, the first representative of the new oxazolidinone class of antibiotics, also demonstrates excellent activity against *S. aureus*, including multidrug-resistant strains of MRSA. Oxazolidinones are

bacteriostatic, but resistance to them is unusual and there is no cross-resistance with other classes of compounds. Until data reveal the relative efficacies and toxicities of vancomycin and these new compounds, however, vancomycin remains the drug of choice for treatment of MRSA infections.

In 1996, a long-predicted monster—*S. aureus* with decreased susceptibility to vancomycin—finally emerged from the theoretical nightmares of microbiologists into the clinical realm. The term *vancomycin-intermediate S. aureus* (VISA) has been widely used to describe these strains, whose minimum inhibitory concentrations (MICs) of vancomycin (8 to 16 μg/mL) should theoretically confer only intermediate resistance to this agent. The clinical experience has been one of treatment failure, however. In 1997, four patients with VISA infection were reported from Japan and the United States; all died, although only one death was a direct result of the VISA infection. As of this writing, about a dozen additional cases have been reported from Asia, North America, and Europe, and the VISA genotype is already widespread in Japan. The risk factors for infection with VISA are uncertain because of the small number of reported cases, but they appear to include a history of dialysis, multiple prior courses of antibiotics (including vancomycin), admission to an intensive care unit, and prior infection with MRSA.

The mechanism for decreased susceptibility to vancomycin in *S. aureus* appears to be novel and unrelated to the mechanism of resistance of vancomycin-resistant enterococci (VRE). VISA strains have unusually thick extracellular matrices that make it more difficult for vancomycin to reach its binding site at the level of the murein monomer of the cell wall. In addition, peptidoglycan from VISA appears to bind more vancomycin than does peptidoglycan from susceptible strains of *S. aureus*. These two factors create a "vancomycin sink," resulting in an increase in the MIC of vancomycin. VISA strains may also be characterized by increased expression of PBPs, slower growth, and decreased autolysis, all potentially contributing to antimicrobial resistance. Vancomycin resistance within a population of organisms is expressed in a heterogeneous manner, which may lead to difficulty in detection of the phenotype by usual susceptibility testing and may explain the failure of antimicrobial therapy in some cases. Therefore, infection with VISA should be suspected in any patient for whom seemingly appropriate therapy with vancomycin is ineffective. Removal of prosthetic material associated with infection is even more critical than usual in treating a patient infected with MRSA or VISA. Antimicrobial therapy for infections caused by VISA is discussed below (see "Selection of antibiotics").

In recent years, the percentage of staphylococcal isolates that are methicillin-resistant has risen substantially in U.S. hospitals; this trend has been driven by widespread (and often indiscriminate) antibiotic use. In some tertiary care institutions, up to 40% of *S. aureus* isolates are now resistant to methicillin, although rates of 5 to 15% are more typical. This situation is problematic for several reasons. Hospitalized patients colonized with MRSA are at increased risk (up to fourfold higher) of developing staphylococcal bacteremia than are patients colonized with methicillin-sensitive strains. The extent to which this difference reflects differences in bacterial virulence (as opposed to host factors or appropriateness of therapy) remains unclear; MRSA strains have not been shown consistently to be more virulent than sensitive strains, but the breadth of their resistance renders colonization more persistent, which in turn increases the rate of infection. In addition, higher rates of MRSA infection within an institution cause increased use of vancomycin, which contributes to the emergence of VRE and apparently puts additional pressure on MRSA to develop resistance to vancomycin as well.

A second development over the past decade has been an apparent increase in the incidence in some communities of MRSA infection among individuals without apparent risk factors for MRSA. Previously identified risk factors for MRSA include residence in a long-term-care facility; hospitalization; chronic liver, lung, or vascular disease; dialysis; malignancy; and prolonged exposure to antibiotics. An increase in community-acquired cases of MRSA infection has been reported in several locations in the United States and suggests a change in the epidemiology of infection with this organism. It is hypothesized that strains of MRSA spread from the hospital to the community, where continued exposure to antibiotics (both appropriate and unnecessary) leads to their survival advantage and persistence. These reports have been based on retrospective observations, however, and have not yet been confirmed by prospective studies. The obvious question is whether β-lactam antibiotics should continue to be used as the empirical agents of choice for community-acquired staphylococcal infections. For the time being, the incidence of MRSA infection in the community seems too low to justify more widespread use of vancomycin in this setting. There are situations, however, in which empirical use of vancomycin for community-acquired infections is justifiable and even advisable, as discussed below.

Selection of antibiotics (Table 139-2)   Although most pathogenic strains of *S. aureus* are resistant to penicillin, the development of penicillins and cephalosporins that are resistant to β-lactamase has allowed these classes of antibiotics to remain useful for treatment of most *S. aureus* infections. Nafcillin and oxacillin, both of which are β-lactamase-resistant penicillins, are the drugs of choice for parenteral treatment of serious staphylococcal infections. Penicillin remains the drug of choice for infections caused by susceptible organisms. Drug combinations consisting of a penicillin plus a β-lactamase inhibitor are also effective but are best reserved for treatment of polymicrobial infections. Penicillin-allergic patients can usually be given a cephalosporin, although caution should be exercised if the prior adverse reaction to penicillin was anaphylaxis. Of the cephalosporins, the first-generation agents (e.g., cefazolin) are preferred for reasons related to cost and breadth of spectrum. For patients who are intolerant of all β-lactam agents, the best alternatives for parenteral administration are vancomycin and clindamycin. Dicloxacillin and cephalexin are recommended for oral treatment of minor infections or for continuation therapy; clindamycin is an alternative oral agent for most strains. Routine use of quinolones is not recommended because of the possibility of emergent resistance during therapy.

Use of vancomycin has increased dramatically over the past 20 years in response to the emergence of MRSA, for which it has often been the sole therapeutic option, and the increasing number of infections caused by CoNS and other gram-positive cocci. Vancomycin's favorable pharmacokinetic properties and relatively low toxicity profile have also contributed to its widespread use. Unfortunately, increased use of vancomycin has resulted in the emergence of both VRE and VISA, which are now poised to be the microbial scourges of the next decade. Equally important, however, is the fact—often not recognized by practitioners—that vancomycin is *less effective* than numerous other agents at our disposal. Vancomycin is generally only weakly bactericidal or even bacteriostatic for many strains of *S. aureus*. Studies of animal models have repeatedly shown vancomycin to be inferior to β-lactam agents for treatment of serious staphylococcal infections. Bacteremia is cleared more slowly in patients treated with vancomycin than in those treated with β-lactams, and clinical cure rates with vancomycin are significantly lower than with β-lactams as well. For all of these reasons, use of vancomycin should be reserved for situations in which there are no suitable alternative agents. It should not be used routinely for prophylaxis of staphylococcal infections, for empirical therapy in patients with fever and neutropenia (unless staphylococcal infection is especially likely), for decontamination of the digestive tract, for clearance of MRSA colonization, or for treatment of established gram-positive infections not due to resistant organisms. It is hoped that judicious use of vancomycin will help limit the spread of VRE and VISA and ensure that patients receive the most potent therapeutic agents.

Vancomycin remains the drug of choice for treatment of infections caused by MRSA, although sensitive strains may be amenable to therapy with clindamycin or trimethoprim-sulfamethoxazole. As discussed above, two new agents, quinupristin/dalfopristin and linezolid, offer promise for treatment of MRSA, but further studies are needed before they can be recommended for routine or preferential use. Optimal ther-

apy for infections caused by VISA is unknown. To date, all isolates of VISA have been susceptible to alternative agents. Therapeutic options include the combination of vancomycin plus a β-lactam (based largely on in vitro data), quinupristin/dalfopristin, linezolid, or one of the new quinolone antibiotics, although the potential for development of resistance to the quinolones during therapy makes their use a questionable approach for infections requiring a prolonged course of antibiotic.

In most clinical settings, no significant benefit is attained by treating *S. aureus* infections with more than one drug to which the organism is known to be susceptible. Synergy has been demonstrated in vitro for β-lactam/aminoglycoside combinations, which hasten sterilization of the blood in endocarditis. Accordingly, therapy for *S. aureus* bacteremia is often initiated with such a combination for a brief period (e.g., 5 to 7 days)—a strategy that seems reasonable when rapid clearance of bacteremia is deemed to be critical, as in prosthetic valve endocarditis. Thereafter, the toxicity of an aminoglycoside cannot be justified. Use of rifampin in conjunction with a β-lactam antibiotic (or vancomycin) occasionally results in microbial eradication and clinical cure of otherwise refractory infections, particularly those involving foreign bodies that are judged to be unremovable or those involving avascular tissue. These successes may relate to the high level of activity of rifampin against intracellular organisms, including SCVs. Chronic osteomyelitis, parameningeal infections, and septic phlebitis have all been successfully treated with rifampin plus a cell wall–active agent. Nevertheless, routine use of rifampin for serious *S. aureus* infections is not recommended because of potential added toxicity, drug interactions, and theoretical antimicrobial antagonism. Rifampin should be reserved for refractory, relapsing, or inoperable infections and should never be administered as monotherapy, which rapidly leads to resistance.

Route and duration of therapy   Because of poor bioavailability of most oral antistaphylococcal agents, parenteral therapy should be used for infections that require high concentrations of antibiotic, such as endovascular infections, infections of poorly vascularized tissue (including abscesses), and infections of the central nervous system. Given the propensity of *S. aureus* to adhere to endovascular and devitalized or damaged tissues, high doses of antibiotics (e.g., 12 g/d of nafcillin) should be used for bacteremic infections. When high serum levels of antibiotic are required to produce adequate tissue levels (e.g., in endocarditis or osteomyelitis), the parenteral route should be used for the duration of therapy. Oral agents may suffice for the treatment of nonbacteremic infections in which high serum levels of antibiotic are not requisite (e.g., skin, soft tissue, and upper respiratory tract infections).

With the notable exceptions of bacteremia (including endocarditis) and osteomyelitis, the duration of therapy for *S. aureus* infections can be tailored to the severity of illness, the immunologic status of the host, and the response to treatment. Because antibiotics penetrate bone poorly, treatment of acute osteomyelitis in adults requires at least 4 weeks of parenteral therapy. Chronic osteomyelitis is often treated with 6 to 8 weeks of parenterally administered antibiotics followed by several months of oral therapy, especially if the adequacy of debridement is uncertain.

Acute endocarditis and other endovascular infections caused by *S. aureus* should be treated with parenteral antibiotics for 4 weeks (6 weeks in the case of prosthetic valves). Simple bacteremia, as might occur with a removable or drainable focus of infection, is curable with a shorter duration of therapy, but a 2-week course of *parenteral* therapy has traditionally been recommended *for all patients* with *S. aureus* bacteremia, even under these circumstances. The costs and effort implicit in this recommendation are apparent, but shorter courses of therapy are associated with an unacceptable rate of secondary complications. Data suggest that a 7-day course of parenteral therapy may be adequate for simple bacteremia if the clinical response to therapy is prompt, if cultures of blood obtained after 2 days of therapy are neg-

Table 139-2   Antimicrobial Therapy for Infections Caused by *Staphylococcus aureus*

Infection	Antibiotic of Choice and Dose	Alternative Agents	Duration of Therapy
INTOXICATIONS			
Toxic shock syndrome	Clindamycin 900 mg IV q8h[a] or nafcillin 2 g IV q4h[a] *plus* IVIG 400 mg/kg once for severe illness (see text)	Cefazolin 1 g IV q8h for penicillin-allergic patients (instead of nafcillin);[a] vancomycin 1 g IV q12h for suspected MRSA	Total of 14 days; conversion from IV to PO therapy after resolution of fever, hypotension, and gastrointestinal symptoms; oral agents: dicloxacillin 500 mg qid, cephalexin 500 mg qid, clindamycin 300 mg qid
Scalded skin syndrome	Nafcillin or clindamycin IV at high doses, adjusted for age in children	Cefazolin	Total of 10–14 days, parenteral followed by oral therapy
Food poisoning	None	—	—
INVASIVE INFECTIONS			
Skin and soft tissue			
Folliculitis	Topical agent (e.g., mupirocin) or oral antibiotic: dicloxacillin or cephalexin 250 mg qid	Clindamycin 150–300 mg PO tid, TMP-SMZ DS 1 tablet bid, tetracycline 250 mg qid	Until resolution of infection, often 5–7 days
Furuncle/carbuncle	For severe infections (e.g., with systemic toxicity): nafcillin 1–2 g IV q4h; for mild infections: dicloxacillin or cephalexin 250–500 mg PO qid	Cefazolin 1 g IV q8h, clindamycin 600 mg IV q8h or 300 mg PO tid, vancomycin 1 g IV q12h (for severe penicillin allergy or suspected MRSA)	Until resolution of infection, often 7–10 days
Paronychia	Dicloxacillin or cephalexin 250 mg PO qid	Clindamycin 150–300 mg PO tid, TMP-SMZ DS 1 tablet bid, tetracycline 250 mg qid	Until resolution of infection, often 5–7 days
Cellulitis	Nafcillin 2 g IV q4–6h	Cefazolin 1 g IV q8h, clindamycin 600 mg IV q8h; vancomycin 1 g IV q12h for suspected infection with MRSA	Total of 10–14 days; conversion from IV to PO agent (as for TSS) after erythema and systemic symptoms have resolved
Respiratory tract			
Sinusitis	Dicloxacillin or cephalexin 500 mg PO qid or amoxicillin/clavulanate 875 mg PO bid	TMP-SMZ DS 1 tablet bid, clindamycin 300 mg PO tid, clarithromycin 500 mg PO bid	Generally 14–21 days, in accordance with severity of illness and response to therapy
Pneumonia	Nafcillin 2 g IV q4h[b]	Cefazolin 1 g IV q8h[b] or cefuroxime 1.5 g IV q8h or clindamycin 900 mg IV q8h;[b] vancomycin 1 g IV q12h for suspected MRSA	Prolonged course of parenteral therapy, often 14–21 days, as dictated by severity of illness and response to therapy; longer course of therapy in pneumonia caused by hematogenous seeding of lung parenchyma
Empyema	Nafcillin 2 g IV q4h;[b] possible addition of rifampin 300 mg PO bid for loculated empyema or persistent systemic toxicity	Cefazolin 1 g IV q8h[b] or clindamycin 900 mg IV q8h;[b] vancomycin 1 g IV q12h for suspected MRSA	Prolonged course of parenteral therapy, as dictated by clinical and radiographic response to therapy
Central nervous system			
Meningitis	Nafcillin 2 g IV q4h[a]	Vancomycin 1 g IV q12h (for severe penicillin allergy or MRSA)	Prolonged course of parenteral therapy, at least 14–21 days, depending on pathogenesis of infection and clinical response to therapy
Subdural empyema, septic phlebitis, brain abscess	Nafcillin 2 g IV q4h;[a] possible addition of rifampin 300 mg PO bid for infections not amenable to drainage	Vancomycin 1 g IV q12h (for severe penicillin allergy or MRSA)	Prolonged course of parenteral therapy, at least 4 weeks, as dictated by clinical and radiographic response to therapy
Epidural abscess (without meningitis)	Nafcillin 2 g IV q4h[b]	Cefazolin 1 g IV q8h[b] or clindamycin 900 mg IV q8h;[b] vancomycin 1 g IV q12h for MRSA	Prolonged course of parenteral therapy, at least 4 weeks
Endovascular			
Native valve endocarditis, left-sided	Nafcillin 2 g IV q4h,[b] ± gentamicin 1 mg/kg q8h for first 5–7 days	Cephalothin 2 g IV q4h or cefazolin 1 g IV q8h[b] (penicillin allergy) or vancomycin 1 g IV q12h (for MRSA or severe penicillin allergy), ± gentamicin	4 weeks of parenteral therapy
Native valve endocarditis, right-sided	Nafcillin 2 g IV q4h; or nafcillin plus gentamicin 1 mg/kg q8h for short-course therapy	Cefazolin 1 g IV q8h or vancomycin 1 g IV q12h, plus gentamicin; ciprofloxacin 750 mg PO bid plus rifampin 300 mg PO bid	4 weeks of parenteral monotherapy or oral combination therapy; 2 weeks of combination parenteral therapy

(continued)

Table 139-2—(continued)

Infection	Antibiotic of Choice and Dose	Alternative Agents	Duration of Therapy
Prosthetic valve endocarditis	Nafcillin 2 g IV q4h[b] plus rifampin 300 mg PO tid plus gentamicin 1 mg/kg q8h for first 2 weeks	Cephalothin 2 g IV q4h or cefazolin 1 g IV q8h,[b] or vancomycin 1 g IV q12h (as above) plus gentamicin, ± rifampin	6 weeks
Simple bacteremia	Nafcillin 2 g IV q4h[b]	Cefazolin 1 g IV q8h or vancomycin 1 g IV q12h (as above)	14 days of parenteral therapy; 7 days probably adequate under some circumstances (see text)
Complicated bacteremia	Nafcillin 2 g IV q4h[b]	Cefazolin 1 g IV q8h or vancomycin 1 g IV q12h (as above)	4 weeks of parenteral therapy
Mycotic aneurysm, pseudoaneurysm	Nafcillin 2 g IV q4h[b]	Cefazolin 1 g IV q8h[b] or vancomycin 1 g IV q12h (as above)	4 weeks of parenteral therapy
Musculoskeletal			
Acute osteomyelitis	Nafcillin 2 g IV q4h	Cefazolin 1 g IV q8h, clindamycin 900 mg IV q8h, or vancomycin 1 g IV q12h (for MRSA)	4 weeks of parenteral therapy
Chronic osteomyelitis	Nafcillin 2 g IV q4h, ± rifampin 300 mg PO bid	Cefazolin 1 g IV q8h, clindamycin 900 mg IV q8h, or vancomycin 1 g IV q12h (for MRSA), ± rifampin	6 to 8 weeks of parenteral therapy, often followed by several months of oral therapy (dicloxacillin or cephalexin 500 mg qid, clindamycin 300 mg qid, TMP-SMZ DS 1 tablet bid)
Septic arthritis, native joint	Nafcillin 2 g IV q4h	Cefazolin 1 g IV q8h or vancomycin 1 g IV q12h (for severe penicillin allergy or MRSA)	At least 3 weeks of parenteral therapy, as indicated by cultures and clinical course
Septic arthritis, prosthetic joint	Nafcillin 2 g IV q4h; add rifampin 300 mg PO bid if retention of prosthesis is to be attempted	Cefazolin 1 g IV q8h or vancomycin 1 g IV q12h (for severe penicillin allergy or MRSA)	4 weeks
Septic bursitis	Nafcillin 2 g IV q4h	Cefazolin 1 g IV q8h (penicillin allergy), vancomycin 1 g IV q12h (MRSA)	Parenteral therapy until resolution of systemic and local signs and symptoms, followed by several weeks of oral therapy (dicloxacillin, cephalexin, or clindamycin, as above)
Pyomyositis	Nafcillin 2 g IV q4h	Cefazolin 1 g IV q8h (penicillin allergy), vancomycin 1 g IV q12h (MRSA)	Usually 4 weeks of parenteral therapy, assuming hematogenous route of infection

[a] Vancomycin 1 g IV q12h should be given in addition to the antibiotic listed as part of initial therapy when the risk of infection with MRSA is thought to be significant (see text) or in life-threatening illness; vancomycin should be discontinued when susceptibilities are known, as appropriate.

[b] Vancomycin may be substituted for the antibiotic shown when the risk of infection with MRSA is thought to be significant (see text) or in life-threatening illness; switch to alternative agent if possible when susceptibilities are known.

ABBREVIATIONS: IVIG, intravenous immunoglobulin; MRSA, methicillin-resistant *S. aureus*; TMP-SMZ, trimethoprim-sulfamethoxazole; DS, double-strength.

COMMENTS: A. Penicillin is the β-lactam antibiotic of choice for strains of *S. aureus* that are shown to be susceptible. Penicillin should not be used before results of sensitivity testing are known, however, because of the high prevalence of resistance.
B. Patients with a history of hypersensitivity reactions to penicillin *other than anaphylaxis* may generally be treated with cephalosporins. Patients with a history of anaphylaxis to penicillin should be treated with non-β-lactam agents until hypersensitivity testing can be performed.
C. Oxacillin may be substituted for nafcillin, at the same dosages, for all indications.
D. Additional agents with excellent antistaphylococcal activity in vitro are linezolid (available in peroral and parenteral formulations), quinupristin/dalfopristin (parenteral only), and new quinolones. Until additional experience is gained with these agents, however, they should be reserved for situations in which antibiotics with established efficacies cannot be used for reasons of tolerability or antimicrobial resistance.

ative, and if TEE is negative for vegetations. These data require confirmation, however. One of the more challenging aspects of treating staphylococcal bacteremia is deciding whether to administer parenteral therapy for 2 or 4 weeks. A conservative approach (one that is supported by numerous studies) dictates that *4 weeks* should be standard unless specific criteria are met (Fig. 139-2).

PREVENTION AND CONTROL Nosocomial staphylococcal outbreaks and the spread of resistant strains of *S. aureus* are serious global problems. Within an institution, the most important vector of transmission of *S. aureus* is the hands of health care workers. Patients with exposed wounds or with nasal colonization are important reservoirs of the organisms. Transmission of *S. aureus*—and hence the incidence of staphylococcal infection within an institution—can be reduced most effectively by meticulous hand washing before and after contact with patients. The incidence of postoperative staphylococcal infection can be reduced by perioperative administration of an antibiotic with a favorable spectrum of activity and favorable pharmacokinetic properties, such as cefazolin, cefuroxime, or vancomycin. Elimination of nasal carriage before surgery (see below) may also prove to be effective in this regard.

More stringent infection-control measures must be taken to prevent the nosocomial spread of MRSA. Such measures include assigning patients colonized or infected with MRSA to private rooms, wearing gloves for contact with contaminated wounds and mucous membranes as well as a gown if contamination of clothing is likely, and hand washing with an antiseptic soap after patient contact. Patients who are colonized but not infected with MRSA should not be treated with vancomycin merely for the sake of eliminating carriage of this organism.

Staphylococcal skin and soft tissue infections may recur once a person has been colonized with a virulent strain. In this context, therapy directed at the elimination of staphylococcal colonization may be warranted, especially for patients at particular risk for complications of infection. Use of an oral β-lactam antibiotic alone is ineffective, but combination therapy for 10 to 14 days with dicloxacillin or cephalexin (500 mg four times a day) plus rifampin (300 mg twice a day) plus mupirocin (2% ointment applied topically to both nares twice a day) is usually effective at clearing the carrier state, at least for a period of months.

COAGULASE-NEGATIVE STAPHYLOCOCCI

CoNS are a major cause of nosocomial infection and are the organisms most frequently isolated from the blood of hospitalized patients. The

899

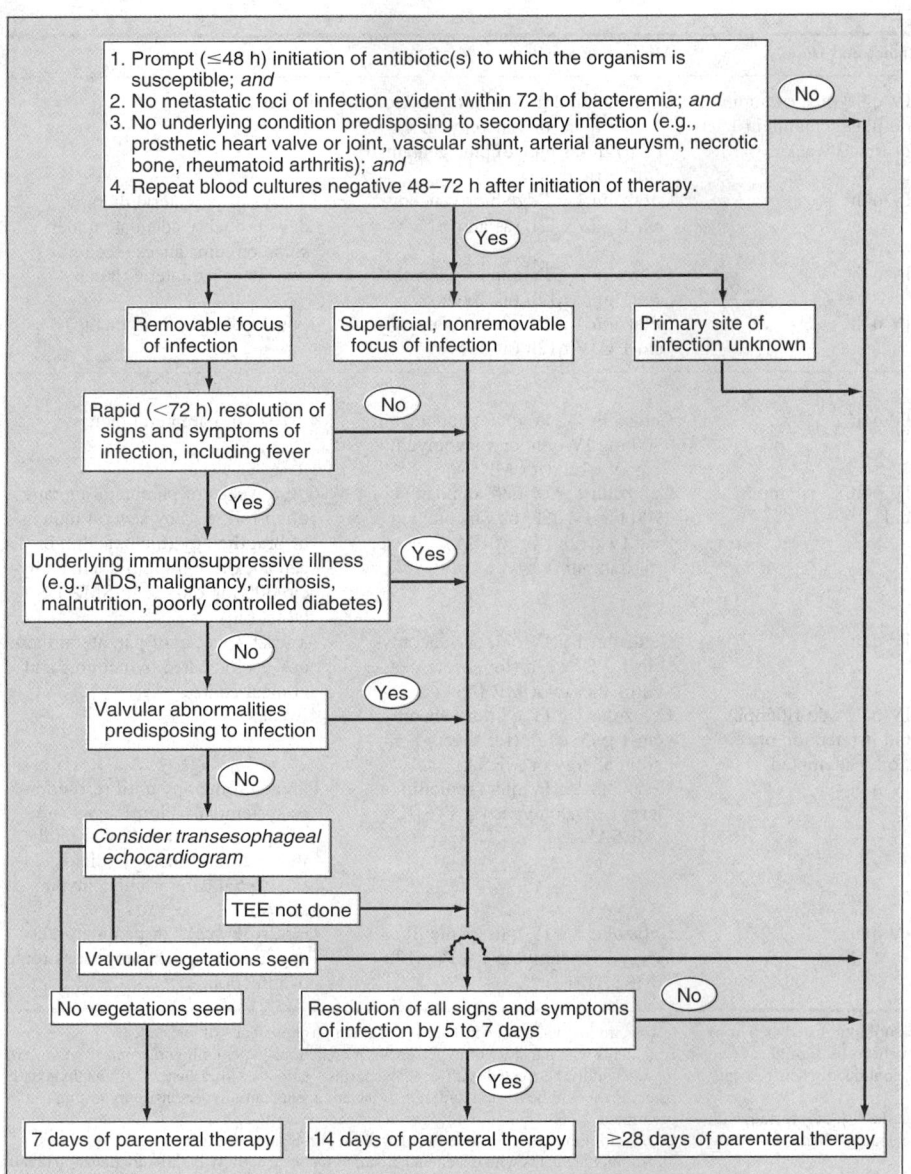

1. Prompt (≤48 h) initiation of antibiotic(s) to which the organism is susceptible; *and*
2. No metastatic foci of infection evident within 72 h of bacteremia; *and*
3. No underlying condition predisposing to secondary infection (e.g., prosthetic heart valve or joint, vascular shunt, arterial aneurysm, necrotic bone, rheumatoid arthritis); *and*
4. Repeat blood cultures negative 48–72 h after initiation of therapy.

No

Yes

Removable focus of infection

Superficial, nonremovable focus of infection

Primary site of infection unknown

Rapid (<72 h) resolution of signs and symptoms of infection, including fever   No

Yes

Underlying immunosuppressive illness (e.g., AIDS, malignancy, cirrhosis, malnutrition, poorly controlled diabetes)   Yes

No

Valvular abnormalities predisposing to infection   Yes

No

Consider transesophageal echocardiogram

TEE not done

Valvular vegetations seen

No vegetations seen

Resolution of all signs and symptoms of infection by 5 to 7 days   No

Yes

7 days of parenteral therapy

14 days of parenteral therapy

≥28 days of parenteral therapy

FIGURE 139-2 Factors to be considered in determining the duration of therapy for *S. aureus* bacteremia. *(Modified from Fowler VG Jr et al: Outcome of Staphylococcus aureus bacteremia according to compliance with recommendations of infectious disease specialists: Experience with 244 patients. Clin Infect Dis 27:478, 1998.)*

EPIDEMIOLOGY AND PATHOGENESIS

CoNS, particularly *S. epidermidis*, are invariable and prominent constituents of the normal human skin flora. Infection most often results from direct inoculation of a foreign body at the time it is inserted, although hematogenous seeding can also occur.

CoNS are the quintessential pathogens of medical devices. The array of virulence factors produced by CoNS is meager compared with that of the virulence factors produced by *S. aureus*, but among these few factors are substances that promote bacterial adherence to and persistence on foreign bodies. A variety of surface antigens that promote colonization of medical devices by CoNS (particularly *S. epidermidis*) have been proposed; the best-studied of these is capsular polysaccharide adhesin, which serves as the organism's capsule and promotes the initial interaction of the bacteria and a foreign body. This polysaccharide is a major component of the *S. epidermidis* biofilm, which is important in the persistence of infection; the biofilm thwarts host defenses by coating staphylococcal cells onto foreign materials and impairing phagocytic killing. CoNS appear not to make toxic exoproteins or toxins; rather, they cause disease by tenaciously persisting on foreign materials, resulting in a local and occasionally a systemic inflammatory response.

The most important risk factor for infection with CoNS is the presence of a foreign body, especially an indwelling catheter. A second major risk factor for infection is deficient phagocyte function—especially neutropenia, which is most often an iatrogenic complication of chemotherapy for cancer but may also reflect an underlying disease process (such as leukemia). The likelihood of catheter-related infection depends upon a number of variables, including the experience and skill of the person who inserts the catheter, the length of time that a catheter is left in place, and the quality of postinsertion care of the catheter site. CoNS only rarely cause infections (other than urinary tract infections) in immunologically normal hosts and typically do so only under extenuating circumstances.

CLINICAL SYNDROMES

Because CoNS can adhere to a variety of materials, virtually all *foreign bodies* are susceptible to colonization by these organisms. CoNS are the most common pathogens complicating the use of intravenous catheters, hemodialysis shunts and grafts, cerebrospinal fluid (CSF) shunts, peritoneal dialysis catheters, pacemaker wires and electrodes, prosthetic joints, vascular grafts, and prosthetic valves. CoNS infection of intravenous catheters may or may not be accompanied by signs of inflammation at the site of catheter insertion, and the degree of systemic toxicity (including fever) ranges from minimal to moderately severe. The diagnosis can be established by the culturing of blood drawn from the catheter and by venipuncture. Infection of CSF shunts is usually evident within several weeks of implantation. Signs of meningitis are sometimes readily apparent but more often are subtle or absent; malfunction of the shunt may be the only manifestation of shunt infection. CoNS infection of a prosthetic joint often does not become evident until long after implantation, although the inciting contamination usually occurs at the time of implantation. Infection of vascular grafts may result in the development of an aneurysm or a pseudoaneurysm, with catastrophic consequences.

frequency with which they cause opportunistic infection in immunocompromised hosts attests more to the increased vulnerability of such hosts in modern medical practice than to the intrinsic virulence of the organisms. Despite the weak pathogenicity of these bacteria, the global impact of CoNS infection is considerable, including increased length and cost of hospital stay; increased use of antibiotics in general; and increased use of vancomycin in particular, which has contributed to the recent emergence of vancomycin-resistant gram-positive bacteria.

Although the variety of clinical syndromes caused by CoNS is impressive, several characteristics apply to most such infections. First, they tend to be *indolent*. There is often a long latent period between the time of contamination (e.g., of a medical device) and the onset of clinical illness; bacteremia in neutropenic patients can be an exception to this rule. Second, most CoNS infections are nosocomial in origin; important exceptions are prosthetic valve endocarditis and *S. saprophyticus* infections of the urinary tract. Third, most clinically significant infections are caused by strains of CoNS that are resistant to multiple antibiotics, including penicillins and cephalosporins. Finally, most CoNS infections are associated with a medical device of some kind, and removal of such devices is often required for cure.

CoNS are a prominent cause of *bacteremia* in immunosuppressed patients. While such infections in immunocompetent hosts are relatively benign, patients with neutropenia may have high-grade bacteremia that results in significant systemic toxicity. A serious consequence of bacteremia is the seeding of a secondary foreign body, such as a prosthetic heart valve or joint or a pacemaker.

CoNS are the organisms most commonly responsible for *prosthetic valve endocarditis*, causing the majority of infections that develop within several months of implantation as well as a substantial percentage of late infections. The syndrome is one of subacute endocarditis (thus contrasting with the syndrome produced by *S. aureus*), with an illness that is clinically indistinguishable from that caused by viridans streptococci. Infection of prosthetic valves is often complicated by valvular dysfunction secondary either to dehiscence of the sewing ring or obstruction of the valve's orifice by bulky vegetations. CoNS are a less frequent but important cause of *native valve endocarditis*, accounting for <5% of such infections and usually affecting abnormal valves.

S. saprophyticus is a common cause of *urinary tract infection* among sexually active young women, in whom it is second only to *E. coli* in frequency. Exposure to spermicide-coated condoms may increase the incidence of infection. *S. saprophyticus* produces a syndrome indistinguishable from that caused by other etiologic agents, with pyuria and symptoms of dysuria, frequency, and abdominal pain. Infection with *S. saprophyticus* is readily amenable to therapy with most agents commonly used to treat urinary tract infections. CoNS can also cause urinary tract infection in hospitalized patients who have undergone invasive procedures; such infections are especially likely to be asymptomatic and may be difficult to treat because of antimicrobial resistance.

DIAGNOSIS Although CoNS are the most common cause of nosocomial bacteremia, they are also the most common contaminants of blood cultures; differentiation between infection and contamination often poses a challenge, with major therapeutic implications. Positive blood cultures are more likely to be "true positives" when there is a clinical illness suggestive of infection, when there is an indwelling catheter or some other risk factor for CoNS infection, and when cultures of blood drawn from multiple sites are positive for phenotypically identical organisms with the same antimicrobial susceptibility patterns. Except in the setting of neutropenia, physicians often have the luxury of awaiting the results of repeat cultures when the significance of CoNS growing from a blood culture is questionable.

℞ **TREATMENT** Removal of the foreign body (especially when it is an intravenous catheter) often constitutes adequate therapy for CoNS infection related to that device. Most infections involving a foreign body require the removal of the device—whether a prosthetic valve, prosthetic joint, CSF shunt, vascular graft, pacemaker or defibrillator and associated hardware, or hemodialysis shunt. Cures of all such infections with antibiotics alone have been reported, however, and a patient's poor medical condition or the hazards of surgery occasionally warrant an attempt at medical cure without extirpation of the device (see below). Infections of peritoneal dialysis catheters can be cured with antibiotics alone often enough that an attempt should be made to do so. CoNS infections of central venous catheters are also amenable to medical therapy, although relapses are common. Persistent bacteremia during therapy is an absolute indication for removal of a catheter, and bacteremia after a catheter's removal suggests seeding of a secondary site.

It is difficult to make generalizations about the optimal duration of therapy for CoNS infections. In general, the duration of treatment is the same as for infection syndromes caused by other bacteria. For example, native valve endocarditis should be treated for 4 weeks, prosthetic valve endocarditis for 6. Transient bacteremia in an immunocompetent host may require no antimicrobial therapy after removal of an offending catheter. The efficacy of therapy can occasionally be enhanced by the delivery of antibiotics directly to the site of infection—e.g., by intraventricular administration of vancomycin for cen-

tral nervous system infections or by intraperitoneal administration of antibiotic for infections of peritoneal dialysis catheters.

Despite the low degree of pathogenicity of CoNS, treatment of serious infections due to these organisms is often problematic because of the high percentage of strains that are resistant to commonly used antibiotics, including most oral agents. Most strains of CoNS isolated from patients in U.S. hospitals are resistant not only to penicillin but also to the penicillinase-resistant penicillins and cephalosporins. Nosocomial isolates are usually resistant to other classes of antibiotics as well. Vancomycin, to which the vast majority of CoNS remain susceptible, is of necessity the drug of choice for *empirical* therapy for serious CoNS infections. Strains proved to be susceptible to nafcillin (oxacillin) or penicillin should be treated with one of these agents or with a first-generation cephalosporin.

Synergistic combinations of antibiotics are often useful in the treatment of CoNS infections. Rifampin plays a unique role in this endeavor by virtue of its potency against most staphylococci, its excellent penetration into tissues (including those that are poorly vascularized), and the high levels it reaches within human cells and biofilm. Rifampin must be used in combination with other antibiotics because of the frequent and rapid emergence of microbial resistance to the drug when it is used alone. If an effort must be made to eradicate infection of a medical device without its removal, the concomitant use of a β-lactam antibiotic to which the organism is susceptible plus rifampin (300 mg twice daily by mouth) plus gentamicin affords the best chance for success. Vancomycin can be substituted for the β-lactam agent if so dictated by an organism's susceptibility pattern or by a patient's drug allergy.

BIBLIOGRAPHY

CHAMBERS HF: Methicillin resistance in staphylococci: Molecular and biochemical basis and clinical implications. Clin Microbiol Rev 10:781, 1997

DERESIEWICZ RL: Staphylococcal toxic shock syndrome, in *Superantigens: Molecular Biology, Immunology, and Relevance to Human Disease,* DYM Leung et al (eds). New York, Marcel Dekker, 1997, pp 435–479

FOWLER VG JR et al: Role of echocardiography in evaluation of patients with *Staphylococcus aureus* bacteremia: Experience in 103 patients. J Am Coll Cardiol 30:1072, 1997

HEROLD BC et al: Community-acquired methicillin-resistant *Staphylococcus aureus* in children with no identified predisposing risk. JAMA 279:593, 1998

JERNIGAN JA, FARR BM: Short-course therapy of catheter-related *Staphylococcus aureus* bacteremia: A meta-analysis. Ann Intern Med 119:304, 1993

MARRACK P, KAPPLER J: The staphylococcal enterotoxins and their relatives. Science 248:705, 1990

MUSHER DM et al: The current spectrum of *Staphylococcus aureus* infection in a tertiary care hospital. Medicine 73:186, 1994

PROCTOR RA, PETERS G: Small colony variants in staphylococcal infections: Diagnostic and therapeutic implications. Clin Infect Dis 27:419, 1998

RUPP ME, ARCHER GL: Coagulase-negative staphylococci: Pathogens associated with medical progress. Clin Infect Dis 19:231, 1994

SMITH TL et al: Emergence of vancomycin resistance in *Staphylococcus aureus*. N Engl J Med 340:493, 1999

140 *Michael R. Wessels*

STREPTOCOCCAL AND ENTEROCOCCAL INFECTIONS

Many varieties of streptococci are found as part of the normal human flora colonizing the respiratory, gastrointestinal, and genitourinary tracts. Several species are important causes of human disease. Group A *Streptococcus*, or *S. pyogenes*, is responsible for streptococcal pharyngitis, one of the most common bacterial infections of school-age-

Table 140-1   Classification of Streptococci Responsible for Human Infections

Lancefield Group	Representative Species	Hemolysis	Typical Infections
A	S. pyogenes	β	Pharyngitis, impetigo, cellulitis, scarlet fever
B	S. agalactiae	β	Neonatal sepsis and meningitis, puerperal infection, UTI, diabetic ulcer infection, endocarditis
C	S. equisimilis	β	Cellulitis, bacteremia, endocarditis
D	Enterococci: E. faecalis; E. faecium	Usually nonhemolytic	UTI, nosocomial bacteremia, endocarditis
	Nonenterococci: S. bovis	Usually nonhemolytic	Bacteremia, endocarditis
G	S. canis	β	Cellulitis, bacteremia, endocarditis, septic arthritis
Variable or nongroupable	Viridans streptococci: S. sanguis; S. mitis	α	Endocarditis, dental abscess, brain abscess
	Intermedius, milleri or anginosus group S. intermedius; S. anginosus; S. constellatus	Variable	Brain abscess, visceral abscess
	Anaerobic streptococci: Peptostreptococcus magnus	Usually nonhemolytic	Sinusitis, pneumonia, empyema, brain abscess, liver abscess

children, and for the postinfectious syndromes of acute rheumatic fever and poststreptococcal glomerulonephritis. Group B *Streptococcus*, or *S. agalactiae*, is the leading cause of bacterial sepsis and meningitis in newborns and a major cause of endometritis and fever in parturient women. Enterococci are important causes of urinary tract infection, nosocomial bacteremia, and endocarditis. Viridans streptococci are the most common cause of bacterial endocarditis.

Streptococci are gram-positive bacteria of spherical to ovoid shape that characteristically form chains when grown in liquid media. Most streptococci that cause human infections are facultative anaerobes, although some are strict anaerobes. Streptococci are relatively fastidious organisms, requiring enriched media for growth in the laboratory. No single scheme for classification of streptococci is entirely satisfactory. Consequently, clinicians and clinical microbiologists often identify streptococci by any of several classification systems, including hemolytic pattern, Lancefield group, species name, and common or trivial name. Many of the streptococci associated with human infection produce a zone of complete hemolysis around the bacterial colony when cultured on blood agar, a pattern known as β hemolysis. The β-hemolytic streptococci can be classified by the Lancefield system, a serologic grouping based on the reaction of specific antisera with cell-wall carbohydrate antigens of the bacteria. With rare exceptions, organisms belonging to Lancefield groups A, B, C, and G are all β-hemolytic streptococci, and each is associated with characteristic patterns of human infection. Other streptococci produce a zone of partial (α) hemolysis, often imparting a greenish appearance to the agar. These α-hemolytic streptococci are further identified by biochemical testing and include *S. pneumoniae*, an important cause of pneumonia, meningitis, and other infections, and several species of streptococci referred to collectively as the *viridans streptococci*, which are part of the normal oral flora and are important as agents of subacute bacterial endocarditis. Finally, some streptococci are nonhemolytic, a pattern sometimes called γ hemolysis. The classification of the major groups of streptococci responsible for human infections is outlined in Table 140-1. Among the organisms classified serologically as group D streptococci, the enterococci are now considered to constitute a separate genus on the basis of DNA homology studies. Thus, species previously designated as *S. faecalis* and *S. faecium* have been renamed *Enterococcus faecalis* and *E. faecium*, respectively. →*For further discussion of pneumococcal infections, see Chap. 138.*

Lancefield's group A consists of a single species, *S. pyogenes*. As its species name implies, this organism is associated with a variety of suppurative infections. In addition, group A streptococci can trigger the postinfectious syndromes of acute rheumatic fever (which is uniquely associated with *S. pyogenes* infection; Chap. 235) and poststreptococcal glomerulonephritis (Chap. 274).

PATHOGENESIS   Group A streptococci elaborate a number of cell-surface components and extracellular products important both in the pathogenesis of infection and in the immune response of the human host. The cell wall contains a carbohydrate antigen that may be released by treatment with acid. The reaction of such acid extracts with group A–specific antiserum is the basis for the definitive identification of a streptococcal strain as *S. pyogenes*. The major surface protein of group A streptococci is M protein, which occurs in more than 100 antigenically distinct types and is the basis for the serotyping of strains with specific antisera. The M protein molecules are fibrillar structures anchored in the cell wall of the organism and extending as hairlike projections away from the cell surface. The amino acid sequence of the distal or amino-terminal portion of the M protein molecule is quite variable, accounting for the antigenic variation of the different M types, while more proximal regions of the protein are relatively conserved. A newer technique for assignment of M type to group A streptococcal isolates uses the polymerase chain reaction to amplify the variable region of the M protein gene. DNA sequence analysis of the amplified gene segment can be compared with an extensive data base [developed at the Centers for Disease Control and Prevention (CDC)] for assignment of M type. This method eliminates the need for typing sera, which are available in only a few reference laboratories. The presence of M protein on a group A streptococcal isolate correlates with its capacity to resist phagocytic killing in fresh human blood; this phenomenon appears to be due, at least in part, to the binding of plasma fibrinogen to M protein molecules on the streptococcal surface, which interferes with complement activation and deposition of opsonic complement fragments on the bacterial cell. This resistance to phagocytosis may be overcome by M protein–specific antibodies, and thus individuals with antibodies to a given M type acquired as a result of prior infection are protected against subsequent infection with organisms of the same M type but not against that with different M types.

Group A streptococci also elaborate, to varying degrees, a polysaccharide capsule composed of hyaluronic acid. The production of large amounts of hyaluronic acid capsule by certain strains lends a characteristic mucoid appearance to the bacterial colonies. The capsular polysaccharide also plays an important role in protecting the organisms from ingestion and killing by phagocytes. In contrast to M protein, the hyaluronic acid capsule is a weak immunogen, and antibodies to hyaluronate have not been shown to be important in protective immunity; the presumed explanation is the apparent structural identity between streptococcal hyaluronic acid and the hyaluronic acid of mammalian connective tissues. The capsular polysaccharide may also play a role in group A streptococcal colonization of the pharynx by binding to CD44, a hyaluronic acid–binding protein expressed on human pharyngeal epithelial cells.

Group A streptococci produce a large number of extracellular products that may be important in local and systemic toxicity and in the spread of infection through tissues. These products include streptolysins S and O, toxins that damage cell membranes and account for the hemolysis produced by the organisms; streptokinase; DNases; protease; and pyrogenic exotoxins A, B, and C. The pyrogenic exotoxins, previously known as erythrogenic toxins, cause the rash of scarlet fever. Since the mid-1980s, pyrogenic exotoxin-producing strains of group A *Streptococcus* have been linked to unusually severe invasive infections, including necrotizing fasciitis and a systemic syndrome termed the *streptococcal toxic shock syndrome*. Several extracellular products stimulate specific antibody responses useful in the serodiagnosis of recent streptococcal infection. Tests for these antibodies are used primarily for the detection of preceding streptococcal infection in cases of suspected acute rheumatic fever or poststreptococcal glomerulonephritis.

CLINICAL MANIFESTATIONS **Pharyngitis** Although seen in patients of all ages, group A streptococcal pharyngitis is one of the most common bacterial infections of childhood, accounting for 20 to 40% of all cases of exudative pharyngitis in children. It is rare among those under the age of 3. Younger children may manifest streptococcal infection with a syndrome of fever, malaise, and lymphadenopathy without exudative pharyngitis. Infection is acquired through contact with another individual carrying the organism. Respiratory droplets are the usual mechanism of spread, although other routes, including food-borne outbreaks, have been well described.

The incubation period is 1 to 4 days. Symptoms include sore throat, fever and chills, malaise, and sometimes abdominal complaints and vomiting, particularly in children. Both symptoms and signs are quite variable, ranging from mild throat discomfort with minimal physical findings to high fever and severe sore throat associated with intense erythema and swelling of the pharyngeal mucosa and the presence of purulent exudate over the posterior pharyngeal wall and tonsillar pillars. Enlarged, tender anterior cervical lymph nodes commonly accompany exudative pharyngitis.

The differential diagnosis of streptococcal pharyngitis includes the many other bacterial and viral causes of pharyngitis. Streptococcal infection is unlikely to be the cause of pharyngitis when symptoms and signs suggestive of viral infection are prominent (conjunctivitis, coryza, cough, hoarseness, or discrete ulcerative lesions of the buccal or pharyngeal mucosa). Other infections commonly producing exudative pharyngitis include infectious mononucleosis and adenovirus infection. Now rare in the United States, the pseudomembrane of diphtheria may give a similar appearance. The coryneform organism *Arcanobacterium haemolyticum* may cause pharyngitis, often in association with a scarlet fever–like rash (Chap. 141). Other causes of pharyngitis, usually without a purulent exudate, include coxsackievirus, influenza virus, mycoplasmas, and *Neisseria gonorrhoeae* and acute infection with HIV. Because of the range of clinical presentations of streptococcal pharyngitis and the large number of other agents that can produce the same clinical picture, diagnosis of streptococcal pharyngitis on clinical grounds alone is not reliable.

The throat culture remains the diagnostic "gold standard." Culture of a throat specimen that is properly collected (i.e., by vigorous rubbing of a sterile swab over both tonsillar pillars) and properly processed is the most sensitive and specific means available to make a definitive diagnosis. A rapid diagnostic kit using latex agglutination or enzyme immunoassay of swab specimens can serve as a useful adjunct to the throat culture. While precise figures on sensitivity and specificity vary among studies, the rapid diagnostic kits generally are >95% specific. Thus a positive result can be relied upon for definitive diagnosis and eliminates the need for a throat culture. However, because the rapid diagnostic tests are less sensitive than throat culture (with a relative sensitivity ranging from 55 to 90% in comparative studies), a negative result should be confirmed with a throat culture.

Ɍx **TREATMENT** In the usual course of uncomplicated streptococcal pharyngitis, symptoms resolve after 3 to 5 days. The course is shortened little by treatment, which is given primarily to prevent suppurative complications and rheumatic fever. Prevention of rheumatic fever depends on eradication of the organism from the pharynx,

not simply on resolution of symptoms, and requires 10 days of penicillin treatment—either a single intramuscular dose of benzathine penicillin G or a 10-day course of oral penicillin (Table 140-2). Erythromycin may be substituted for penicillin in the treatment of individuals allergic to penicillin. Follow-up culture after treatment is no longer routinely recommended but may be warranted in selected cases, such as those involving patients or families with frequent streptococcal infections or those occurring in situations in which the risk of rheumatic fever is thought to be high (e.g., when cases of rheumatic fever have recently been reported in the community).

Complications Suppurative complications of streptococcal pharyngitis have become uncommon with the widespread use of antibiotics for most cases of symptomatic streptococcal infection. The complications result from the spread of infection from the pharyngeal mucosa to deeper tissues by direct extension or by the hematogenous or lymphatic route and may include cervical lymphadenitis, peritonsillar or retropharyngeal abscess, sinusitis, otitis media, meningitis, bacteremia, endocarditis, and pneumonia. Local complications, such as abscess formation in the peritonsillar or parapharyngeal space, should be considered in a patient with unusually severe or prolonged symptoms or localized pain associated with high fever and a toxic appearance.

Asymptomatic Carrier State Surveillance cultures have shown that up to 20% of individuals in certain populations may have asymptomatic pharyngeal colonization with group A streptococci. There are no definitive guidelines for management of these asymptomatic carriers or of asymptomatic individuals who still have a positive throat culture after a full course of treatment for symptomatic pharyngitis. A reasonable course of action is to give a single 10-day course of penicillin for symptomatic pharyngitis and, if positive cultures persist, not to re-treat unless symptoms recur. Studies of the natural history of streptococcal carriage and infection have shown that the risk both of developing rheumatic fever and of transmitting infection to others is substantially lower among asymptomatic carriers than among individuals with symptomatic pharyngitis. Therefore, overly aggressive attempts to eradicate carriage are probably not justified under most circumstances. An exception is the situation in which an asymptomatic carrier is a potential source of infection to others. Outbreaks of food-borne infection and nosocomial puerperal infection have been traced to asymptomatic carriers who may harbor the organisms in the throat, on the skin, or in the vagina or anus.

Ɍx **TREATMENT** In cases in which a carrier is transmitting infection to others, attempts to eradicate carriage are warranted, although data are limited on the best regimen to use to clear the organism after penicillin alone has failed. The combination of penicillin

Table 140-2   Treatment of Group A Streptococcal Infections

Infection	Treatment[a]
Pharyngitis	Benzathine penicillin G, 1.2 mU IM; or penicillin V, 250 mg PO qid × 10 days
	(Children <27 kg: Benzathine penicillin G, 600,000 units IM; or penicillin V, 125 mg PO qid × 10 days)
Impetigo	Same as pharyngitis
Erysipelas/cellulitis	Severe: Penicillin G, 1–2 mU IV q4h
	Mild to moderate: Procaine penicillin, 1.2 mU IM bid
Necrotizing fasciitis/myositis	Surgical debridement plus penicillin G, 2–4 mU IV q4h
Pneumonia/empyema	Penicillin G, 2–4 mU IV q4h plus drainage of empyema

[a] Penicillin allergy: Erythromycin (10 mg/kg PO qid up to maximum of 250 mg per dose) may be substituted for oral penicillin. Alternative agents for parenteral therapy include first-generation cephalosporins—if the allergy does not manifest as immediate hypersensitivity (anaphylaxis or urticaria) or as another potentially life-threatening reaction (e.g., severe rash and fever)—or vancomycin.

V (500 mg four times daily for 10 days) and rifampin (600 mg twice daily for the last 4 days) has been used to eliminate pharyngeal carriage. A 10-day course of oral vancomycin (250 mg four times daily) and rifampin (600 mg twice daily) has eradicated rectal colonization. However, experience is not extensive with any regimen.

Scarlet Fever   Scarlet fever consists of streptococcal infection, usually pharyngitis, accompanied by a characteristic rash. The rash arises from the effects of one of three toxins, currently designated streptococcal pyrogenic exotoxins A, B, and C and previously known as erythrogenic or scarlet fever toxins. In the past, scarlet fever was thought to reflect infection of an individual lacking toxin-specific immunity with a toxin-producing strain of group A *Streptococcus*. Susceptibility to scarlet fever was correlated with results of the Dick test. A small amount of erythrogenic toxin injected intradermally produced local erythema in susceptible individuals but elicited no reaction in those with specific immunity. Subsequent studies have suggested that development of the scarlet fever rash may reflect a hypersensitivity reaction requiring prior exposure to the toxin. For reasons that are not clear, scarlet fever has become less common in recent years, although strains of group A streptococci that produce pyrogenic exotoxins continue to be prevalent in the population.

The symptoms of scarlet fever are the same as those of pharyngitis alone. The rash typically begins on the first or second day of illness over the upper trunk, spreading to involve the extremities but sparing the palms and soles. The rash is made up of minute papules, giving a characteristic "sandpaper" feel to the skin. Associated findings include circumoral pallor, "strawberry tongue" (enlarged papillae on a coated tongue, which later may become denuded), and accentuation of the rash in the skin folds (Pastia's lines). Subsidence of the rash in 6 to 9 days is followed after several days by desquamation of the palms and soles. The differential diagnosis of scarlet fever includes other causes of fever and generalized rash, such as measles and other viral exanthems, Kawasaki disease, toxic shock syndrome, and systemic allergic reactions (e.g., drug eruptions).

Skin and Soft Tissue Infections   Group A streptococci—and occasionally other streptococcal species—cause a variety of infections involving the skin, subcutaneous tissues, muscles, and fascia. While several clinical syndromes, recognized according to the tissues involved, offer a useful means for classification of skin and soft tissue infections, not all cases fit exactly into a single category. The classic syndromes should be considered as general guides to predicting the level of tissue involvement in a particular patient, the probable clinical course, and the likelihood that surgical intervention or aggressive life-support will be required.

Impetigo (pyoderma)   Impetigo is a superficial infection of the skin caused primarily by group A streptococci and occasionally by other streptococci or by *Staphylococcus aureus*. Impetigo is seen most often in young children, tends to occur during the warmer months, and is more common in semitropical or tropical climates than in cooler regions. Infection is more common among children living under conditions of poor hygiene. Prospective studies have shown that colonization of unbroken skin with group A streptococci precedes the development of clinical infection. Minor trauma, such as a scratch or an insect bite, may then serve to inoculate organisms into the skin. Impetigo is best prevented, therefore, by attention to adequate hygiene. The usual sites of involvement are the face (particularly around the nose and mouth) and the legs, although lesions may occur at other locations. Individual lesions begin as red papules, which evolve quickly into vesicular and then pustular lesions that break down and coalesce to form characteristic honeycomb-like crusts (**Plate IID-38**). Lesions are generally not painful, and patients do not appear ill. Fever is not a feature of impetigo and, if present, suggests either infection extending to deeper tissues or another diagnosis.

The classic presentation of impetigo usually poses little diagnostic difficulty. Cultures of impetiginous lesions often yield *S. aureus* as well as group A streptococci, but longitudinal studies have shown that, in almost all cases, streptococci can be isolated initially, with staphylococci appearing later, presumably as secondary colonizing flora. In the past, penicillin was nearly always effective against these infections; in recent years, however, penicillin treatment failures have become more common, an observation suggesting that *S. aureus* infection may have become more prominent as a cause of impetigo. *Bullous impetigo* due to *S. aureus* is distinguished from typical streptococcal infection by the presence of more extensive, bullous lesions that break down and leave thin paper-like crusts instead of the thick amber crusts of streptococcal impetigo. Other skin lesions that may be confused with impetigo include herpetic lesions—either those of orolabial herpes simplex or those of chickenpox or zoster. Herpetic lesions can generally be distinguished by their appearance as more discrete, grouped vesicles and by a positive Tzanck test. In difficult cases, cultures of vesicular fluid should yield group A streptococci in impetigo and the responsible virus in *Herpesvirus* infections.

℞ TREATMENT   Treatment of streptococcal impetigo is the same as that for streptococcal pharyngitis. In view of evidence that *S. aureus* has become a relatively frequent cause of impetigo, empirical regimens should cover both streptococci and *S. aureus*. For example, either dicloxacillin or cephalexin can be given at a dose of 250 mg four times daily for 10 days. Topical mupirocin ointment is also effective. Rheumatic fever (unlike pharyngitis) is not a sequela to streptococcal skin infections, although poststreptococcal glomerulonephritis may follow either skin or throat infection. The reason for this difference is not known. One hypothesis is that the immune response necessary for development of rheumatic fever occurs only after infection of the pharyngeal mucosa. In addition, the strains of group A streptococci that cause pharyngitis are generally of different M protein types than those associated with skin infections; thus the strains that cause pharyngitis may have rheumatogenic potential, while the skin-infecting strains may not.

Cellulitis   Inoculation of organisms into the skin may lead to infection involving the skin and subcutaneous tissues, or *cellulitis*. The portal of entry may be a traumatic or surgical wound, an insect bite, or any other break in skin integrity. Often, no entry site is apparent.

One form of streptococcal cellulitis, *erysipelas*, is characterized by a bright red appearance of the involved skin, which forms a plateau sharply demarcated from surrounding normal skin (**Plate IID-34**). The lesion is warm to the touch, may be tender, and appears shiny and swollen. The skin often has a *peau d'orange* texture, which is thought to reflect involvement of superficial lymphatics; superficial blebs or bullae may form, usually 2 or 3 days after onset. The lesion typically develops over a few hours and is associated with fever and chills. Erysipelas tends to occur in certain characteristic locations: the malar area of the face (often with extension over the bridge of the nose to the contralateral malar region) and the lower extremities. After one episode, recurrence at the same site—sometimes years later—is not uncommon.

Classic cases of erysipelas, with the typical features described above, are almost always due to β-hemolytic streptococci, usually those of group A and occasionally those of group C or G. Often, however, the appearance of streptococcal cellulitis is not sufficiently distinctive to permit a specific diagnosis on clinical grounds. The area of involvement may not be one of the typical sites for erysipelas, the lesion may be less intensely red than usual and may fade into surrounding skin, and/or the patient may appear only mildly ill. In such cases, it is prudent to broaden the spectrum of empiric antimicrobial therapy to include other pathogens, particularly *S. aureus*, that can produce cellulitis with the same appearance. Staphylococcal infection should be suspected if cellulitis develops around a wound or ulcer.

Streptococcal cellulitis tends to develop at anatomic sites in which normal lymphatic drainage has been disrupted, such as sites of prior episodes of cellulitis, the arm ipsilateral to a mastectomy and axillary lymph node dissection, a lower extremity previously involved in deep venous thrombosis or chronic lymphedema, and the leg from which a saphenous vein has been harvested for coronary artery bypass grafting. The organism may enter via a breach in the dermal barrier at a location some distance from the eventual site of clinical cellulitis. For example, some patients with recurrent episodes of leg cellulitis following saphenous vein removal stop having recurrent episodes only after treatment of tinea pedis on the affected extremity, fissures in the skin presumably having served as a portal of entry for streptococci, which then produced infection more proximally in the leg at the site of previous injury. Streptococcal cellulitis may also involve recent surgical wounds. Group A streptococci are among the few bacterial pathogens that typically produce signs of wound infection and surrounding cellulitis within the first 24 h after surgery. These wound infections are usually associated with a thin exudate and may spread rapidly, either as cellulitis in the skin and subcutaneous tissue or as a deeper tissue infection (see below). Streptococcal wound infection or localized cellulitis may also be associated with *lymphangitis*, manifested by red streaks extending proximally along superficial lymphatics from the site of infection.

℞ TREATMENT   See Table 140-2 and Chap. 128.

Deep soft tissue infections   *Necrotizing fasciitis*, also referred to as *hemolytic streptococcal gangrene*, is an infection involving the superficial and/or deep fascia investing the muscles of an extremity or the trunk. The source of the infection is either the skin, with organisms introduced into the tissue as a result of trauma (sometimes trivial), or the bowel flora, with organisms released during abdominal surgery or from an occult enteric source, such as a diverticular or appendiceal abscess. The site of inoculation in both forms of necrotizing fasciitis may be inapparent and is often some distance from the site of clinical involvement; e.g., the introduction of organisms via minor trauma to the hand may be associated with clinical infection of the tissues overlying the shoulder or chest. In cases associated with the bowel flora, the infection is usually polymicrobial, involving a mixture of anaerobic bacteria (such as *Bacteroides fragilis* or anaerobic streptococci) and facultative organisms (usually gram-negative bacilli). Cases unrelated to contamination from bowel organisms are most commonly caused by group A streptococci, either alone or in combination with other organisms (most often *S. aureus*). Overall, group A streptococci are implicated in about 60% of cases of necrotizing fasciitis. The onset of symptoms is usually quite acute and is marked by severe pain at the site of involvement, malaise, fever, chills, and a toxic appearance. The physical findings, particularly early in the illness, may not be striking, with only minimal erythema of the overlying skin. Pain and tenderness are usually severe; in contrast, in more superficial cellulitis, the skin appearance is more abnormal, but pain and tenderness are only mild or moderate. As the infection progresses (often in a matter of several hours), the severity and extent of symptoms worsen, and skin changes become more evident, with the appearance of dusky or mottled erythema and edema. The marked tenderness of the involved area may evolve into anesthesia as the spreading inflammatory process produces infarction of cutaneous nerves.

Although myositis is more commonly due to *S. aureus* infection, group A streptococci occasionally produce abscesses in skeletal muscles (*streptococcal myositis*), with little or no involvement of the surrounding fascia or overlying skin. The presentation is usually subacute, but a fulminant form has been described in association with severe systemic toxicity, bacteremia, and a high mortality rate. The fulminant form may reflect the same basic disease process as that seen in necrotizing fasciitis, but with the necrotizing inflammatory process extending into the muscles themselves rather than remaining limited to the fascial layers.

℞ TREATMENT   Once necrotizing fasciitis is suspected, early surgical exploration is both diagnostically and therapeutically indicated. Surgery reveals necrosis and inflammatory fluid tracking along the fascial planes above and between muscle groups, without involvement of the muscles themselves. The process usually extends beyond the area of clinical involvement, and extensive debridement is required. Drainage and debridement are central to the management of necrotizing fasciitis; antibiotic treatment is a useful adjunct (Table 140-2), but surgery is life-saving.

Treatment for streptococcal myositis consists of surgical drainage—usually by an open procedure that permits evaluation of the extent of the infection and ensures adequate debridement of involved tissues—and high-dose penicillin (Table 140-2).

Pneumonia and Empyema   Group A streptococci are an occasional cause of pneumonia, generally in previously healthy individuals. The onset of symptoms may be abrupt or gradual. Pleuritic chest pain, fever, chills, and dyspnea are the characteristic symptoms. Cough is usually present but may not be prominent. Approximately one-half of patients with group A streptococcal pneumonia have an accompanying pleural effusion. In contrast to the sterile parapneumonic effusions typical of pneumococcal pneumonia, those complicating streptococcal pneumonia are almost always infected. The empyema fluid is usually visible by chest radiography on initial presentation and may enlarge rapidly. These pleural collections should be drained early, as they tend to become loculated rapidly, resulting in a chronic fibrotic reaction that may require thoracotomy for removal.

Bacteremia, Puerperal Sepsis, and Streptococcal Toxic Shock Syndrome   Group A streptococcal bacteremia is usually associated with an identifiable local infection. Bacteremia occurs rarely with otherwise uncomplicated pharyngitis, occasionally with cellulitis or pneumonia, and relatively frequently with necrotizing fasciitis. Bacteremia without an identified source raises the possibility of endocarditis, an occult abscess, or osteomyelitis. A variety of focal infections may arise secondarily from streptococcal bacteremia, including endocarditis, meningitis, septic arthritis, osteomyelitis, peritonitis, and visceral abscesses.

Group A streptococci are occasionally implicated in infectious complications of childbirth, usually endometritis and associated bacteremia. In the preantibiotic era, puerperal sepsis was commonly caused by group A streptococci, but currently it is more often caused by group B streptococci. Several nosocomial outbreaks of puerperal infection due to group A streptococci have been traced to an asymptomatic carrier, usually an individual present at the delivery of the infant. The site of carriage may be the skin, throat, anus, or vagina.

Beginning in the late 1980s, several reports described patients who had group A streptococcal infections associated with shock and multisystem organ failure. This syndrome has been called the streptococcal toxic shock syndrome because it shares certain features with staphylococcal toxic shock syndrome. In 1993, a case definition for group A streptococcal toxic shock syndrome was formulated by a group of clinicians, microbiologists, and epidemiologists in conjunction with the CDC (Table 140-3). The general features of the illness include fever, hypotension, renal impairment, and respiratory distress syndrome. Various types of rash have been described, but rash usually does not develop. Laboratory abnormalities include a marked shift to the left in the white blood cell differential, with many immature granulocytes; hypocalcemia; hypoalbuminemia; and thrombocytopenia, which usually becomes more pronounced on the second or third day of illness. In contrast to those with staphylococcal toxic shock, the majority of patients with the streptococcal syndrome are bacteremic. The most common associated infection is a soft tissue infection—necrotizing fasciitis, myositis, or cellulitis—although a variety of other associated local infections have been described, including pneumonia, peritonitis, osteomyelitis, and myometritis. Streptococcal toxic shock syndrome is associated with a mortality rate of 30%, with most deaths secondary to shock and respiratory failure. Because of its rapidly progressive and lethal course, early recognition of the syndrome is essential. Patients should be given aggressive supportive care in the

Table 140-3 Proposed Case Definition for the Streptococcal Toxic Shock Syndrome[a]

I. Isolation of group A streptococci (*S. pyogenes*)
  A. From a normally sterile site (e.g., blood, cerebrospinal fluid, pleural or peritoneal fluid, tissue biopsy, surgical wound)
  B. From a nonsterile site (e.g., throat, sputum, vagina, superficial skin lesion)
II. Clinical signs of severity
  A. Hypotension: Systolic blood pressure of ≤90 mmHg in adults or in the 5th percentile for age in children **and**
  B. Two or more of the following signs:
    1. Renal impairment: Serum creatinine level of ≥177 μmol/L (≥2 mg/dL) for adults or at least twice the upper limit of normal for age; in patients with preexisting renal disease, an elevation over the baseline level by a factor of 2 or more
    2. Coagulopathy: Platelet count of ≤100 × 10⁹/L (100,000/μL) or disseminated intravascular coagulation, defined by prolonged clotting times, low fibrinogen level, and the presence of fibrin degradation products
    3. Liver involvement: Alanine aminotransferase (SGOT), aspartate aminotransferase (SGPT), or total bilirubin level at least twice the upper limit of normal for age; in patients with preexisting liver disease, an elevation over the baseline level by a factor of 2 or more
    4. Adult respiratory distress syndrome, defined by acute onset of diffuse pulmonary infiltrates and hypoxemia in the absence of cardiac failure; or evidence of diffuse capillary leakage manifested by acute onset of generalized edema; or pleural or peritoneal effusions with hypoalbuminemia
    5. Generalized erythematous macular rash that may desquamate
    6. Soft tissue necrosis, including necrotizing fasciitis or myositis, or gangrene

[a] An illness fulfilling criteria IA, IIA, and IIB is defined as a *definite* case. An illness fulfilling criteria IB, IIA, and IIB is defined as a *probable* case if no other etiology is identified.
SOURCE: Working Group.

form of fluid resuscitation, pressors, and mechanical ventilation in addition to antimicrobial therapy and, in cases associated with necrotizing fasciitis, surgical debridement. Exactly why certain patients develop this fulminant syndrome is not known; however, early studies of the streptococcal strains isolated from these patients demonstrated a strong association with the production of pyrogenic exotoxin A. In subsequent case series, particularly from Europe, the syndrome was also associated with strains producing exotoxin B or C.

TREATMENT In light of the possible role of exotoxins or other streptococcal toxins in streptococcal toxic shock syndrome, treatment of the affected patients with clindamycin has been advocated by some authorities, who argue that, through its direct action on protein synthesis, clindamycin is more effective in rapidly terminating toxin production than penicillin—a cell-wall agent. Support for this view comes from studies of an experimental model of streptococcal myositis, in which mice treated with clindamycin had a higher rate of survival than those given penicillin. Comparable data on the treatment of human infections are not available. Although clindamycin resistance in group A streptococci is uncommon (<2% among U.S. isolates), it has been documented. Thus, if clindamycin is used for initial treatment of a critically ill patient, penicillin should be given as well until the antibiotic susceptibility of the streptococcal isolate is known.

Intravenous immunoglobulin has been suggested as adjunctive therapy for streptococcal toxic shock; pooled immunoglobulin preparations are likely to contain antibodies capable of neutralizing the effects of streptococcal toxins. Anecdotal reports have suggested favorable clinical responses to intravenous immunoglobulin, but no controlled trials of this modality of therapy have yet been reported.

STREPTOCOCCI OF GROUPS C AND G

Group C and group G streptococci are β-hemolytic bacteria that occasionally cause human infections similar to those caused by group A streptococci, including pharyngitis, cellulitis and soft-tissue infections, pneumonia, bacteremia, endocarditis, and septic arthritis. Puerperal sepsis, meningitis, epidural abscess, intraabdominal abscess, urinary tract infection, and neonatal sepsis have also been reported. Group C streptococci are a common cause of infection in domesticated animals, especially horses and cattle, and some human infections have been acquired through contact with animals or through consumption of unpasteurized milk. Bacteremia and septic arthritis more frequently involve group G than group C streptococci. Group C or G streptococcal bacteremia occurs most often in patients who are elderly or chronically ill and, in the absence of an obvious local infection, is likely to reflect endocarditis. Septic arthritis, sometimes involving multiple joints, may complicate endocarditis or develop in its absence.

TREATMENT Penicillin is the drug of choice for therapy of infections due to group C or G streptococci. Antibiotic treatment is the same as for patients with similar syndromes due to group A *Streptococcus* (Table 140-2). Patients with bacteremia or septic arthritis should receive intravenous penicillin (2 to 4 mU every 4 h). All group C and G streptococci are sensitive to penicillin; nearly all are inhibited in vitro by concentrations of ≤0.03 μg/mL. Occasional isolates exhibit tolerance: although inhibited by low concentrations of penicillin, they are killed only by significantly higher concentrations. The clinical significance of tolerance is unknown. Because of the poor clinical response of some patients to penicillin alone, the addition of gentamicin (1 mg/kg every 8 h for patients with normal renal function) is recommended by some authors for treatment of endocarditis or septic arthritis due to group C or G streptococci; however, combination therapy has not been shown to be superior to treatment with penicillin alone.

Patients with joint infections often require repeated aspiration or open drainage and debridement for cure; the response to treatment may be slow, particularly in debilitated patients and those with involvement of more than one joint. Infection of prosthetic joints almost always requires removal of the prosthesis in addition to antibiotic therapy.

GROUP B STREPTOCOCCI

Identified first as a cause of mastitis in cows, streptococci belonging to Lancefield's group B have since been recognized as a major cause of sepsis and meningitis in human neonates. Group B streptococci are also a frequent cause of peripartum fever in women and an occasional cause of serious infection in nonpregnant adults. Lancefield group B consists of a single species, *S. agalactiae*, which is definitively identified with specific antiserum to the group B cell wall–associated carbohydrate antigen. A streptococcal isolate can be classified presumptively as belonging to group B on the basis of biochemical tests, including hydrolysis of sodium hippurate (in which 99% of isolates are positive), hydrolysis of bile esculin agar (in which 99 to 100% are negative), bacitracin susceptibility (in which 92% are resistant), and production of CAMP factor (in which 98 to 100% are positive). CAMP factor is a phospholipase produced by group B streptococci that results in synergistic hemolysis with β lysin produced by certain strains of *S. aureus*. Its presence can be demonstrated by cross-streaking of the test isolate and an appropriate staphylococcal strain on a blood agar plate. Group B streptococci causing human infections are encapsulated by one of nine antigenically distinct polysaccharides. The capsular polysaccharide has been shown experimentally to be important in the virulence of the organism. Antibodies to the capsular polysaccharide afford protection against group B streptococci of the same (but not of a different) capsular type.

INFECTION IN NEONATES Two general types of group B streptococcal infection in infants are defined by the age of the patient at presentation. *Early-onset infections* occur within the first week of life, with a median age of 20 h at the onset of illness. Approximately half of these infants have signs of group B streptococcal disease at birth. The infection is acquired during or shortly before birth from organisms colonizing the maternal genital tract. Surveillance studies have shown that 5 to 40% of women are vaginal or rectal carriers of group B streptococci. Approximately 50% of infants delivered vaginally by carrier mothers become colonized, although only 1 to 2% of those colonized develop clinically evident infection. Prematurity and maternal risk factors (prolonged labor, obstetric complications, and maternal fever) are often involved. The presentation of early-onset infection is the same as that of other forms of neonatal sepsis. Typical findings include respiratory distress, lethargy, and hypotension. Essentially all infants with early-onset disease are bacteremic, one-third to one-half have pneumonia and/or respiratory distress syndrome, and one-third have meningitis.

Late-onset infections occur in infants between 1 week and 3 months of age, with a mean age at onset of 3 to 4 weeks. The infecting organism may be acquired during delivery (as in early-onset cases) or during later contact with a colonized mother, nursery personnel, or another source. Meningitis is the most common manifestation of late-onset infection and in most cases is associated with a strain of capsular type III. Infants present with fever, lethargy or irritability, poor feeding, and seizures. The various other types of late-onset infection include bacteremia without an identified source, osteomyelitis, septic arthritis, and facial cellulitis associated with submandibular or preauricular adenitis.

TREATMENT Penicillin is the treatment of choice for all group B streptococcal infections. Empirical broad-spectrum therapy for suspected bacterial sepsis, consisting of ampicillin and gentamicin, is generally administered until culture results become available. If cultures yield group B streptococci, many pediatricians continue to administer gentamicin, along with ampicillin or penicillin, for a few days until clinical improvement becomes evident. Infants with bacteremia or soft-tissue infection should receive penicillin at a dosage of 200,000 units/kg per day in divided doses; those with meningitis should receive 400,000 units/kg per day. Meningitis should be treated for at least 14 days because of the risk of relapse with shorter courses.

Prevention The incidence of group B streptococcal infection is unusually high among infants of women with risk factors: preterm delivery, early rupture of membranes (>24 h before delivery), prolonged labor, fever, or chorioamnionitis. Because the usual source of the organisms infecting a neonate is the mother's birth canal, efforts have been made to prevent group B streptococcal infections by the identification of high-risk carrier mothers and their treatment with various forms of antibiotic or immunoprophylaxis. Prophylactic administration of ampicillin or penicillin to such patients during delivery has been shown to reduce the risk of infection in the newborn. This approach has been hampered by the logistical difficulties of identifying colonized women before delivery, since the results of vaginal cultures early in pregnancy are poor predictors of carrier status at delivery. The CDC has suggested two alternative approaches to the prevention of neonatal group B streptococcal infection: In the first approach, women are screened for anogenital colonization at 35 to 37 weeks of pregnancy by means of a swab culture of the lower vagina and anorectum; intrapartum chemoprophylaxis is offered to carriers and is *recommended* for those carriers with any of the risk factors noted above, those anticipating multiple births, and those who have previously given birth to an infant with group B streptococcal infection. In the second approach, screening cultures need not be performed, but intrapartum chemoprophylaxis is recommended for *all* women with one or more of the risk factors noted above. The recommended regimen for chemoprophylaxis is 5 million units of penicillin G followed by 2.5 million units every 4 h until delivery. Clindamycin or erythromycin may be substituted in women allergic to penicillin.

Treatment of all pregnant women who are colonized or who have risk factors for neonatal infection will result in exposure of 15 to 25% of pregnant women and newborns to antibiotics, with the attendant risks of allergic reactions and selection for resistant organisms. Al-

though still in the developmental stages, a group B streptococcal vaccine may ultimately offer a better solution to prevention. Because transplacental passage of maternal antibodies produces protective antibody levels in the newborn, efforts are under way to develop a vaccine against group B streptococci that can be given to childbearing women before or during pregnancy. Results of phase 1 clinical trials of group B streptococcal capsular polysaccharide–protein conjugate vaccines suggest that a multivalent conjugate vaccine would be safe and highly immunogenic.

INFECTION IN ADULTS The majority of group B streptococcal infections in adults are related to pregnancy and parturition. Peripartum fever, the most common manifestation, is sometimes accompanied by symptoms and signs of endometritis or chorioamnionitis (abdominal distention and uterine or adnexal tenderness). Blood cultures are often positive, as are cultures of vaginal swabs. Bacteremia is usually transitory but occasionally results in meningitis or endocarditis. Infections in adults that are not associated with the peripartum period generally involve individuals who are elderly or have some underlying chronic illness, such as diabetes mellitus or a malignancy. Among the infections that develop with some frequency in adults are cellulitis and soft tissue infection (including infected diabetic skin ulcers), urinary tract infection, pneumonia, endocarditis, and septic arthritis. Other reported infections include meningitis, osteomyelitis, and intraabdominal or pelvic abscesses.

TREATMENT Group B streptococci are less sensitive to penicillin than group A organisms, requiring somewhat higher doses. Adults with serious localized infections (pneumonia, pyelonephritis, abscess) should receive doses in the range of 12 million units of penicillin G daily, while patients with endocarditis or meningitis should receive 18 to 24 million units per day in divided doses. Vancomycin is an acceptable alternative for patients allergic to penicillin.

ENTEROCOCCI, GROUP D STREPTOCOCCI

ENTEROCOCCI Lancefield group D includes the enterococci, organisms now classified in a separate genus from other streptococci, and nonenterococcal group D streptococci. Enterococci are distinguished from nonenterococcal group D streptococci by their ability to grow in the presence of 6.5% sodium chloride and by the results of other biochemical tests. The enterococcal species that are significant pathogens for humans are *E. faecalis* and *E. faecium*. These organisms tend to produce infection in patients who are elderly or debilitated or in whom mucosal or epithelial barriers have been disrupted or the balance of the normal flora altered by antibiotic treatment. Urinary tract infections due to enterococci are quite common, particularly among patients who have received antibiotic treatment or undergone instrumentation of the urinary tract. Enterococci are a frequent cause of nosocomial bacteremia in patients with intravascular catheters. These organisms account for 10 to 20% of cases of bacterial endocarditis on both native and prosthetic valves. The presentation of enterococcal endocarditis is usually subacute but may be acute, with rapidly progressive valve destruction. Enterococci are frequently cultured from bile and are involved in infectious complications of biliary surgery and in liver abscesses. Moreover, enterococci are often isolated from polymicrobial infections arising from the bowel flora (e.g., intraabdominal abscesses), from abdominal surgical wounds, and from diabetic foot ulcers. While such mixed infections are frequently cured by antimicrobials not active against enterococci, specific therapy directed against enterococci is warranted when these organisms are the predominant species or are isolated from blood cultures.

TREATMENT Unlike other streptococci, enterococci are not reliably killed by penicillin or ampicillin alone at concentrations achieved clinically in the blood or tissues. Ampicillin reaches sufficiently high urinary concentrations to constitute adequate monotherapy for uncomplicated urinary tract infections. Because in vitro testing has shown evidence of synergistic killing of most enterococcal strains by the combination of penicillin or ampicillin with an aminoglycoside, combined therapy is recommended for enterococcal endocarditis and meningitis; the regimen is penicillin (3 to 4 million units every 4 h) or ampicillin (2 g every 4 h) plus moderate-dose gentamicin (1 mg/kg every 8 h for patients with normal renal function). Enterococcal endocarditis should be treated for a minimum of 4 weeks and for 6 weeks if symptoms have been present for ≥3 months or if the infection involves a prosthetic heart valve. For nonendocarditis bacteremia and other serious enterococcal infections, it is not known whether the efficacy of single-agent β-lactam therapy is improved by the addition of gentamicin, but many infectious disease specialists use combination therapy for such infections, especially in critically ill patients. Vancomycin, in combination with gentamicin, may be substituted for penicillin in allergic patients. Enterococci are resistant to all cephalosporins; therefore, this class of antibiotics should not be used for treatment of enterococcal infections.

Antimicrobial susceptibility testing should be performed routinely on enterococcal isolates from patients with serious infections, and therapy should be adjusted according to the results (Table 140-4). Most enterococci are resistant to streptomycin, and this drug should not be used for treatment of enterococcal infection unless in vitro testing of the strain indicates susceptibility. Though less widespread than streptomycin resistance, high-level resistance to gentamicin—with a minimum inhibitory concentration (MIC) of >2000 μg/mL—has become common. Gentamicin-resistant enterococci should be tested for susceptibility to streptomycin; occasional gentamicin-resistant enterococci are sensitive to streptomycin. If the isolate is resistant to all aminoglycosides, treatment with penicillin or ampicillin alone may be successful. The prolonged administration (i.e., for at least 6 weeks) of high-dose ampicillin (e.g., 12 g/d) is recommended for endocarditis due to these highly resistant enterococci.

Enterococci may be resistant to penicillins via two distinct mechanisms. The first is the production of β-lactamase (mediating resistance to penicillin and ampicillin), which has been reported for *E. faecalis* isolates from several locations in the United States and other countries. Because the amount of β-lactamase produced by enterococci may be insufficient for detection by routine antibiotic susceptibility testing, isolates from serious infections should be screened specifically for β-lactamase production with use of a chromogenic cephalosporin or by another method. For the treatment of β-lactamase-producing strains, vancomycin, ampicillin/sulbactam, amoxicillin/clavulanate, or imipenem may be used in combination with gentamicin.

The second mechanism of penicillin resistance is not mediated by β-lactamase and may be due to altered penicillin-binding proteins. This intrinsic penicillin resistance is common among *E. faecium* isolates, which routinely are more resistant to β-lactam antibiotics than

are isolates of *E. faecalis*. Moderately resistant enterococci (MICs of penicillin and ampicillin, 16 to 64 μg/mL) may be susceptible to high-dose penicillin or ampicillin plus gentamicin, but strains with MICs of ≥200 μg/mL must be considered resistant to clinically achievable levels of β-lactam antibiotics, including imipenem. Vancomycin plus gentamicin is the recommended regimen for infections due to enterococci with high-level intrinsic resistance to β-lactams.

Vancomycin-resistant enterococci, first reported from clinical sources in the late 1980s, have become common in many hospitals. Three major vancomycin resistance phenotypes have been described: VanA, VanB, and VanC. The VanA phenotype is associated with high-level resistance to vancomycin and to teicoplanin, a related glycopeptide antibiotic not currently available in the United States. VanB and VanC strains are resistant to vancomycin but susceptible to teicoplanin, although teicoplanin resistance may develop during treatment in VanB strains. For enterococci resistant to both vancomycin and β-lactams, there are no established therapies. Regimens that have been tried with some success in individual cases or experimentally include ciprofloxacin plus rifampin plus gentamicin; ampicillin plus vancomycin (particularly if in vitro testing shows synergistic bacteriostatic activity); and chloramphenicol or tetracycline (if the strain is susceptible in vitro). Quinupristin/dalfopristin (Synercid) is a streptogramin combination with in vitro activity against *E. faecium*, including vancomycin-resistant isolates, but not against *E. faecalis* or other enterococcal species. The evidence for clinical efficacy of this agent in serious enterococcal infections is limited, and, as of this writing, quinupristin/dalfopristin is not yet licensed for use in the United States.

OTHER GROUP D STREPTOCOCCI   The main nonenterococcal group D streptococcal species that causes human infections is *S. bovis*. *S. bovis* endocarditis is often associated with neoplasms of the gastrointestinal tract—most frequently a colon carcinoma or polyp—but is also reported in association with other bowel lesions. When occult gastrointestinal lesions are carefully sought, abnormalities are found in ≥60% of patients with *S. bovis* endocarditis. In contrast to the enterococci, nonenterococcal group D streptococci like *S. bovis* are reliably killed by penicillin as a single agent, and penicillin is the treatment of choice for *S. bovis* infections.

VIRIDANS AND OTHER STREPTOCOCCI

VIRIDANS STREPTOCOCCI   Consisting of multiple species of α-hemolytic streptococci, the viridans streptococci are a heterogeneous group of organisms that are important as agents of bacterial endocarditis (Chap. 126). Several species of viridans streptococci, including *S. salivarius*, *S. mitis*, *S. sanguis*, and *S. mutans*, are part of the normal flora of the mouth, where they live in close association with the teeth and gingiva. Some species contribute to the development of dental caries. The transient viridans streptococcal bacteremia induced by eating, tooth-brushing, flossing, and other sources of minor trauma, together with adherence to biologic surfaces, is thought to account for the predilection of these organisms to cause endocarditis. Viridans streptococci are also isolated, often as part of a mixed flora, from sites of sinusitis, brain abscess, and liver abscess.

Viridans streptococcal bacteremia occurs relatively frequently in neutropenic patients, particularly after bone marrow transplantation or high-dose chemotherapy for cancer. Some of these patients develop a sepsis syndrome with high fever and shock. Risk factors for viridans streptococcal bacteremia include chemotherapy with high-dose cytosine arabinoside, prior treatment with trimethoprim-sulfamethoxazole or a fluoroquinolone, treatment with antacids or histamine antagonists, mucositis, and profound neutropenia.

The *S. milleri* group (also referred to as the *S. intermedius* or *S. anginosus* group) includes three species that cause human disease: *S. intermedius*, *S. anginosus*, and *S. constellatus*. These organisms are often are considered viridans streptococci, although they differ somewhat from other viridans streptococci in both their hemolytic pattern (they may be α-, β-, or nonhemolytic) and the disease syndromes they

Table 140-4   Treatment Options for Antibiotic-Resistant Enterococcal Infections

Resistance Pattern	Recommended Therapy
β-Lactamase production	Gentamicin plus ampicillin/sulbactam, amoxicillin/clavulanate, imipenem, or vancomycin
β-Lactam resistance, but no β-lactamase production	Gentamicin plus vancomycin
High-level gentamicin resistance	Streptomycin-sensitive isolate: Streptomycin plus ampicillin or vancomycin Streptomycin-resistant isolate: No proven therapy (continuous-infusion ampicillin, prolonged treatment)
Vancomycin resistance	Ampicillin plus gentamicin
Vancomycin and β-lactam resistance	Unknown; teicoplanin active against strains with low-level vancomycin resistance (VanB or VanC phenotype, but not VanA)

cause. This group commonly produces suppurative infections, particularly abscesses of brain and abdominal viscera, and infections related to the oral cavity or respiratory tract, such as peritonsillar abscess, lung abscess, and empyema.

℞ **TREATMENT**   Isolates from neutropenic patients with bacteremia often are resistant to penicillin; thus these patients should be treated presumptively with vancomycin until the results of susceptibility testing become available. Viridans streptococci isolated in other clinical settings usually are sensitive to penicillin.

NUTRITIONALLY VARIANT STREPTOCOCCI   Occasional isolates cultured from the blood of patients with endocarditis fail to grow when subcultured on solid media. These *nutritionally variant streptococci* require supplemental thiol compounds or active forms of vitamin B_6 (pyridoxal or pyridoxamine) for growth in the laboratory. The nutritionally variant streptococci are generally grouped with the viridans streptococci because they cause similar types of infections. However, they have been reclassified on the basis of 16S RNA sequence comparisons into a separate genus, *Abiotrophia*, with two species: *A. defectivus* and *A. adjacens*.

℞ **TREATMENT**   Because treatment failure and relapse appear to be more common for cases of endocarditis due to nutritionally variant streptococci than for usual viridans streptococci, the addition of gentamicin (1 mg/kg every 8 h for patients with normal renal function) to the penicillin regimen is recommended in therapy for endocarditis due to these organisms.

OTHER STREPTOCOCCI   *S. suis* is an important pathogen in swine and has been reported to cause meningitis in humans, usually in individuals with occupational exposure to pigs. Strains of *S. suis* associated with human infections have generally reacted with Lancefield group R typing serum and sometimes with group D typing serum as well. Isolates may be α- or β-hemolytic and are sensitive to penicillin. *S. iniae*, a pathogen of fish, has been associated with infections in humans who have handled live or freshly killed fish. Cellulitis of the hand is the most common form of human infection, although bacteremia and endocarditis have been reported. *Anaerobic streptococci*, or *peptostreptococci*, are part of the normal flora of the oral cavity, bowel, and vagina. Infections caused by the anaerobic streptococci are discussed in Chap. 167.

BIBLIOGRAPHY

BISNO AL, STEVENS DL: Streptococcal infections of skin and soft tissues. N Engl J Med 334:240, 1996

———— et al: Diagnosis and management of group A streptococcal pharyngitis: A practice guideline. Clin Infect Dis 25:574, 1997

BRADLEY SF et al: Group C streptococcal bacteremia: Analysis of 88 cases. Rev Infect Dis 13:270, 1991

CENTERS FOR DISEASE CONTROL AND PREVENTION: Prevention of perinatal group B streptococcal disease: A public health perspective. MMWR 45(RR-7):1, 1996

EDWARDS MS, BAKER CJ: *Streptococcus agalactiae* (group B *Streptococcus*), in *Principles and Practice of Infectious Diseases*, 4th ed, GL Mandell et al (eds). New York, Churchill Livingstone, 1995

ELIOPOULOS GM: Vancomycin-resistant enterococci. Mechanism and clinical relevance. Infect Dis Clin North Am 11:851, 1997

JACKSON LA et al: Risk factors for group B streptococcal disease in adults. Ann Intern Med 123:415, 1995

MOELLERING RC JR: Emergence of *Enterococcus* as a significant pathogen. Clin Infect Dis 14:1173, 1992

RICHARD P et al: Viridans streptococcal bacteraemia in patients with neutropenia. Lancet 345:1607, 1995

VARTIAN C et al: Infections due to Lancefield group G streptococci. Medicine 6:75, 1985

WEINSTEIN MR et al: Invasive infections due to a fish pathogen, *Streptococcus iniae*. *S. iniae* Study Group. N Engl J Med 337:589, 1997

WORKING GROUP ON SEVERE STREPTOCOCCAL INFECTIONS: Defining the group A streptococcal toxic shock syndrome: Rationale and consensus definitions. JAMA 269:390, 1993

ZURAWSKI CA et al: Invasive group A streptococcal disease in metropolitan Atlanta: A population-based assessment. Clin Infect Dis 27:150, 1998

141   *Randall K. Holmes*

DIPHTHERIA, OTHER CORYNEBACTERIAL INFECTIONS, AND ANTHRAX

DIPHTHERIA

DEFINITION   Diphtheria is a localized infection of mucous membranes or skin caused by *Corynebacterium diphtheriae*. A characteristic pseudomembrane may be present at the site of infection. Some strains of *C. diphtheriae* produce diphtheria toxin, a protein that can cause myocarditis, polyneuritis, and other systemic toxic effects. Respiratory diphtheria is usually caused by toxinogenic (tox^+) *C. diphtheriae*, but cutaneous diphtheria is frequently caused by nontoxinogenic (tox^-) strains.

ETIOLOGY   *C. diphtheriae* is an aerobic, nonmotile, nonsporulating, irregularly staining, gram-positive rod. The bacteria are club-shaped and are often arranged in clusters (*Chinese letters*) or parallel arrays (*palisades*). *C. diphtheriae* forms gray to black colonies on selective media containing tellurite. The gravis, mitis, and intermedius biotypes are distinguished by colonial morphology and laboratory tests. Both tox^+ and tox^- strains cause infections, and tox^+ strains of all three biotypes can cause severe disease. The gene for diphtheria toxin is present in specific corynephages, and tox^- *C. diphtheriae* can acquire the ability to produce diphtheria toxin by infection with tox^+ phages (*phage conversion*). Growth of *C. diphtheriae* under low-iron conditions that mimic the environment of host tissues induces production of diphtheria toxin and expression of systems for siderophore-dependent iron uptake and utilization of iron from heme.

IMMUNOLOGY   Treatment of diphtheria toxin with formaldehyde converts it to a nontoxic but immunogenic product (*diphtheria toxoid*). Immunization with toxoid elicits antibody (*antitoxin*) that neutralizes the toxin and prevents diphtheria. The attack rate and mortality rate for diphtheria are low in immune individuals with antitoxin titers of >0.01 unit per milliliter. Antitoxin neither prevents colonization by *C. diphtheriae* nor eradicates the *carrier state*. When most individuals in a population have protective levels of antitoxin (*herd immunity*), the carrier rate for tox^+ strains of *C. diphtheriae* falls to a low level, and the risk that susceptible individuals will be exposed to tox^+ *C. diphtheriae* decreases dramatically. Susceptible individuals may contract diphtheria if they travel to regions where the disease is present or if tox^+ strains of *C. diphtheriae* are introduced into their community.

EPIDEMIOLOGY AND IMMUNITY   Humans are the principal reservoir for *C. diphtheriae*. Transmission occurs primarily by close personal contact. The risk is greater that *C. diphtheriae* will be transmitted to susceptible individuals from patients with diphtheria than from carriers. The incubation period for respiratory diphtheria is typically 2 to 5 days and rarely up to 8 days. Cutaneous diphtheria is usually a secondary infection whose signs develop an average of 7 days (range, 1 to >21 days) after the appearance of primary dermatologic lesions of other etiologies.

In temperate climates, diphtheria primarily involves the respiratory tract; occurs throughout the year, with a peak incidence in colder months; and is usually caused by tox^+ *C. diphtheriae*. Before immunization was introduced, diphtheria was primarily a disease of children; it affected up to 10% of individuals in this group and sometimes caused devastating epidemics. Most young infants were immune because of transplacental transfer of maternal IgG antitoxin, but children became susceptible by 6 to 12 months of age. Approximately 75% of individuals became immune by age 10 as a result of contact with *C. diphtheriae*. Mortality rates of 30 to 40% were common in untreated disease and were sometimes >50% in epidemics. Treatment with antitoxin reduced the case-fatality rate to 5 to 10%.

Routine immunization of children in the United States resulted in a progressive decrease of diphtheria from the peak of 206,939 cases (incidence rate, 191 cases per 100,000 population) in 1921 to <5 cases per year since 1980. Concomitantly, circulation of tox+ strains of C. diphtheriae among the population decreased dramatically, although an endemic focus for transmission of tox+ and tox− strains without clinical disease was recently identified in North Dakota. As the incidence rate of diphtheria decreased, a higher proportion of cases occurred in older persons (who were never immunized or whose immunity waned because it was not boosted by either booster doses of vaccine or contact with C. diphtheriae), but the case-fatality ratio remained unchanged at 5 to 10%. High rates of immunization are currently achieved by school entry (>96%), but immunization rates for younger children are substantially lower. Among adults >20 years of age, 19 to 77% are susceptible as a consequence of failure to receive periodic booster immunizations and lack of contact with C. diphtheriae. The most recent large diphtheria outbreak in the United States (about 1100 cases) occurred in Seattle, Washington, between 1972 and 1982. Alcoholism, low socioeconomic status, crowded living conditions, and Native-American ethnic background were significant risk factors in this outbreak.

A massive diphtheria epidemic (>157,000 cases and 5000 deaths) occurred recently in the states of the former Soviet Union and accounted for >80% of diphtheria cases reported worldwide during that interval. The epidemic began in 1990 with 1436 cases (0.49 per 100,000 population), peaked in 1995 with 50,425 cases (17.29 per 100,000 population), and waned by 1998 with 2720 cases (0.93 per 100,000 population) as the result of a mass immunization program. The progression of the epidemic was associated with emergence of a previously uncommon clonal group of tox+ C. diphtheriae strains that accounted for >80% of isolates by 1994; molecular analysis of the tox gene from these strains demonstrated that the existing diphtheria toxoid vaccine remained appropriate for control of the epidemic by vaccination.

A majority of cases throughout this epidemic occurred in persons ≥15 years old, and adults from 40 to 49 years old had very high incidence and death rates. In 1994, case-fatality rates varied from 2.8% in the Russian Federation to 23% in Lithuania and Turkmenistan. Factors that facilitated the spread of this epidemic included large-scale population movements, socioeconomic instability, deteriorating health infrastructure, delayed implementation of aggressive control measures in response to the epidemic, inadequate information for physicians and the public, and frequent shortages of supplies for prevention and treatment of the disease. The most important risk factor for diphtheria in the Republic of Georgia was lack of vaccination (matched odds ratio, 19.2), but household diphtheria exposure, exposure to skin lesions, the presence of tonsils, a history of eczema, preceding fever with myalgia, sharing a bed, sharing glasses and cups, and taking a bath less often than weekly were also significant risk factors. Although small numbers of imported cases from this epidemic occurred in western European countries, none resulted in secondary transmission of diphtheria, notwithstanding a high proportion of susceptible adults in countries with imported cases. Inadequate primary immunization of children in the states of the former Soviet Union in the years preceding the epidemic, along with failure to maintain adequate immunity in adults by booster immunization, may have synergistically facilitated transmission of diphtheria and emergence of the massive epidemic in this region.

In the tropics, cutaneous diphtheria is more common than respiratory diphtheria, occurs throughout the year, and often develops as a secondary infection complicating other dermatoses. Isolates of C. diphtheriae from skin lesions are more often tox− than tox+. Cutaneous diphtheria is increasingly recognized in temperate climates and accounted for 86% of the 1100 cases in the Seattle epidemic of 1972 to 1982. Since 1980, cutaneous diphtheria has not been a reportable disease in the United States, and recent health statistics include only respiratory diphtheria.

During the 1990s, tox− strains of C. diphtheriae were associated with new types of infections. In the United Kingdom, these strains caused symptomatic pharyngitis, predominantly among homosexual men, that was sometimes accompanied by tonsillar exudate. In Switzerland, strains with a high potential for invasiveness were isolated from 38 intravenous drug users and shown by ribotyping to be clonally related. The latter strains caused infections of the skin (15 cases), respiratory tract (10 cases), and blood (13 cases). Among the patients with bloodstream infections, 9 had endocarditis, and 4 of these 9 patients died.

PATHOLOGY AND PATHOGENESIS C. diphtheriae infects mucous membranes, most commonly in the respiratory tract, and also invades open skin lesions resulting from insect bites or trauma. In infections caused by tox+ C. diphtheriae, initial edema and hyperemia are often followed by epithelial necrosis and acute inflammation. Coagulation of the dense fibrinopurulent exudate produces a pseudomembrane, and the inflammatory reaction accompanied by vascular congestion extends into the underlying tissues. The pseudomembrane contains large numbers of C. diphtheriae organisms, but the bacteria are rarely isolated from the blood or internal organs.

Diphtheria toxin acts both locally and systemically, and the lethal dose for humans is ~0.1 μg/kg. Toxin contributes locally to pseudomembrane formation; systemically, it can cause myocarditis, neuritis, and focal necrosis in various organs, including the kidneys, liver, and adrenal glands. Changes in the myocardium include cloudy swelling of muscle fibers and interstitial edema. These changes are followed within weeks by hyaline and granular degeneration (sometimes with fatty degeneration), progressing to myolysis and finally to the replacement of lost muscle by fibrosis. Thus, diphtheria can cause permanent cardiac damage. In diphtheritic polyneuritis, pathologic changes include patchy breakdown of myelin sheaths in peripheral and autonomic nerves, but recovery of nerve damage is the rule if the patient survives.

Diphtheria toxin is produced by C. diphtheriae as an extracellular polypeptide. Proteolytic cleavage forms nicked toxin consisting of fragments A and B. Fragment B binds to a plasma-membrane receptor (a precursor of a heparin-binding growth factor resembling epidermal growth factor), and the bound toxin is internalized by receptor-mediated endocytosis. Fragment A is translocated across the endosomal membrane and released into the cytoplasm, where it catalyzes the transfer of the adenosine diphosphate ribose moiety from nicotinamide adenine dinucleotide (NAD) to a modified histidine residue (diphthamide) on elongation factor 2 (EF-2), thereby inactivating EF-2 and inhibiting protein synthesis. One molecule of fragment A in the cytoplasm can kill a cell. Other metabolic alterations are secondary to inhibition of protein synthesis.

CLINICAL MANIFESTATIONS Patients with C. diphtheriae in the respiratory tract are classified as diphtheria cases if pseudomembranes are present and as diphtheria carriers if pseudomembranes are absent. The disease is graded as tonsillar if pseudomembranes are localized to the tonsils, as combined types or delayed diagnosis if more extensive pseudomembranes are present, and as severe if cervical adenopathy or cervical edema is also present. Onset is often gradual, but most patients seek medical care within a few days of becoming ill. Fever of 37.8° to 38.9°C (100° to 102°F), sore throat, and weakness are the most common symptoms, while dysphagia, headache, and change of voice occur in fewer than half of patients. Neck edema and difficulty breathing are noted in ≤10% of patients and are associated with an increased risk of death. Systemic manifestations are due primarily to toxic effects of diphtheria toxin. Patients without toxicity exhibit discomfort and malaise associated with local infection, whereas severely toxic patients may develop listlessness, pallor, and tachycardia that can progress rapidly to vascular collapse.

Primary infection in the respiratory tract is most often tonsillopharyngeal but may also be (in decreasing order) laryngeal, nasal, and tracheobronchial. Multiple sites are frequently involved, and secondary spread of pharyngeal infection upward to the nasal mucosa or downward to the larynx and tracheobronchial tree is much more common than primary infection at those sites. Systemic toxicity is usually most severe when extensive pseudomembrane extends from the tonsils and pharynx into contiguous regions. A small percentage of patients present with malignant or "bull-neck" diphtheria, with extensive pseudomembrane formation, foul breath, massive swelling of the tonsils and uvula, thick speech, cervical lymphadenopathy, striking edematous swelling of the submandibular region and anterior neck, and severe toxicity.

In tonsillopharyngeal diphtheria, isolated spots of gray or white exudate may appear first. These spots often extend and coalesce within a day to form a confluent, sharply demarcated pseudomembrane that becomes progressively thicker, more tightly adherent to the underlying tissue, and darker gray in color. Unlike the exudate in streptococcal pharyngitis, the diphtheritic pseudomembrane often extends beyond the margin of the tonsils onto the tonsillar pillars, palate, or uvula. Dislodging the membrane is likely to cause bleeding. Laryngeal diphtheria often presents as hoarseness and cough. Demonstration of laryngeal pseudomembrane by laryngoscopy helps distinguish diphtheria from other infectious forms of laryngitis. Patients with nasal diphtheria may present with unilateral or bilateral serosanguineous nasal discharge associated with irritation of the nares or lip. Primary or secondary diphtheritic infection occasionally involves other mucous membranes, including the conjunctiva and the membranes of the genitourinary and gastrointestinal tracts.

Cutaneous diphtheria usually presents as an infection by *C. diphtheriae* of preexisting dermatoses involving the lower extremities, upper extremities, head, or trunk. The clinical features are similar to those of other secondary cutaneous bacterial infections. In the tropics, cutaneous diphtheria may present as a primary cutaneous lesion, typically with morphologically distinct "punched-out" ulcers that are covered by necrotic slough or membrane and have well-demarcated edges.

C. diphtheriae is an occasional cause of invasive infections, including endocarditis and septic arthritis. Risk factors for such infections include preexisting cardiac abnormalities, abuse of intravenous drugs, and alcoholic cirrhosis.

COMPLICATIONS Obstruction of the respiratory tract can be caused by extensive pseudomembrane formation and swelling early in the disease or by sloughed pseudomembrane that becomes lodged in the airways later in the disease. The risk is greater when infection involves the larynx or the tracheobronchial tree and in children because of the small size of the airways.

Myocarditis and polyneuritis are the most prominent toxic manifestations of diphtheria. The risk of each is proportional to the severity of local disease. Myocarditis occurred in 22% and neuritis in 5% of 656 hospitalized patients (54% female, 70% ≥15 years old) with diphtheria in the Kyrgyz Republic in 1995; 7% of patients with myocarditis and 2% of patients without myocarditis died. The median interval from hospitalization to death was 4.5 days (range, 0 to 13 days).

Bulbar dysfunction in diphtheritic neuritis typically develops during the first 2 weeks. Palatal and pharyngeal paralysis usually develops first. Swallowing is difficult, the voice is nasal, and ingested fluids may be regurgitated through the nose. Additional bulbar signs may develop over several weeks, with oculomotor and ciliary paralysis more common than facial or laryngeal paralysis. Peripheral polyneuritis typically begins from 1 to 3 months after the onset of diphtheria with proximal weakness of the extremities, which spreads distally. Paresthesia may occur, most often in a glove-and-stocking distribution. Polyneuritis usually resolves completely, with the time needed for improvement approximately equal to that elapsing from exposure to the development of symptoms.

Pneumonia occurs in more than one-half of fatal cases of diphtheria. Less common complications include renal failure, encephalitis, cerebral infarction, pulmonary embolism, and bacteremia or endocarditis due to invasive infection by *C. diphtheriae*. Serum sickness may result from antitoxin therapy.

COURSE AND PROGNOSIS Most cases of diphtheria develop in nonimmunized patients. The attack rate, severity of disease,

and risk of complications are much lower in immunized patients. The pseudomembrane may continue to increase in size during the first day after administration of antitoxin. During the next several days to a week, it becomes softer, less adherent, and nonconfluent and eventually disappears. In the preantibiotic era, *C. diphtheriae* persisted in the throat for ~2 weeks in one-half of patients and for ≥1 month in about one-fifth. Mortality increases with the severity of local disease, the extent of pseudomembrane formation, and the delay between onset of local disease and administration of antitoxin. The death rate is highest during the first week of illness; among patients with bull-neck diphtheria; among patients with myocarditis who develop ventricular tachycardia, atrial fibrillation, or complete heart block; among patients with laryngeal or tracheobronchial involvement; among infants and patients >60 years of age; and among alcoholics. Both the mortality rate and the risk of myocarditis or peripheral neuropathy are significantly lower in cutaneous diphtheria than in respiratory diphtheria.

DIAGNOSIS A characteristic pseudomembrane on the mucosa of the tonsils, palate, oropharynx, nasopharynx, nose, or larynx suggests diphtheria but is not uniformly present. Diphtheritic pseudomembrane must be distinguished from other pharyngeal exudates, including those of group A β-hemolytic streptococcal infections, infectious mononucleosis, viral pharyngitis, fusospirochetal infection, and candidiasis. Diphtheria should be considered in patients with sore throat, cervical adenopathy or swelling, and low-grade fever, especially when these manifestations are accompanied by systemic toxicity, hoarseness, stridor, palatal paralysis, or serosanguineous nasal discharge with or without demonstrable pseudomembrane. Treatment with diphtheria antitoxin should begin as soon as the clinical diagnosis of diphtheria is made.

Definitive diagnosis of diphtheria depends on the isolation of *C. diphtheriae* from local lesions. The laboratory should be notified that diphtheria is suspected to ensure the use of selective tellurite medium appropriate for the isolation of *C. diphtheriae*. All isolates of *C. diphtheriae* should be subjected to toxicity testing. Primary isolates can be screened rapidly for the presence of the *tox* gene by the polymerase chain reaction, although occasional strains of *C. diphtheriae* that carry an inactive toxin gene give false-positive results. Biochemical tests needed to differentiate *C. diphtheriae* from corynebacteria of the normal flora (diphtheroids) require several days. Group A β-hemolytic streptococci and *Staphylococcus aureus* are also isolated frequently from patients with diphtheria.

Cutaneous diphtheria may present as a characteristic "punched-out" ulcer with a membrane, but it is more often indistinguishable from other inflammatory dermatoses. Diagnosis depends on a high degree of suspicion and on culture of cutaneous lesions on laboratory media appropriate for isolation of *C. diphtheriae*. Throat samples from all patients with cutaneous diphtheria should be cultured for *C. diphtheriae*.

℞ TREATMENT The decision to administer diphtheria antitoxin must be based on the clinical diagnosis of diphtheria without definitive laboratory confirmation, since each day of delay in treatment is associated with increased mortality. Because diphtheria antitoxin is produced in horses, it is necessary to inquire about possible allergy to horse serum and to perform a conjunctival or intracutaneous test with diluted antitoxin for immediate hypersensitivity. Epinephrine must be available for immediate administration to patients with severe allergic reactions. Patients with immediate hypersensitivity should be desensitized before a full therapeutic dose of antitoxin is given. The dose of diphtheria antitoxin currently recommended by the Committee on Infectious Diseases of the American Academy of Pediatrics is based on the site of the primary infection and the duration and severity of disease: 20,000 to 40,000 units for disease that has been present for ≤48 h and involves the pharynx or larynx; 40,000 to 60,000 units for nasopharyngeal infections; and 80,000 to 100,000 units for disease that is extensive, has been present for ≥3 days, or is accompanied by diffuse swelling of the neck. Antitoxin is administered intravenously by infusion in saline over 60 min to neutralize unbound toxin rapidly. The ~10% risk of serum sickness is acceptable because of the established therapeutic value of antitoxin in decreasing mortality from respiratory diphtheria. The risk of systemic toxicity is lower in cutaneous diphtheria than in respiratory diphtheria and must be weighed against the potential adverse effects of antitoxin treatment; authorities are not unanimous in recommending antitoxin therapy for cutaneous diphtheria.

Antibiotics have little demonstrated effect on the healing of local infection in diphtheria patients treated with antitoxin. The primary goal of antibiotic therapy for patients or carriers is therefore to eradicate *C. diphtheriae* and prevent its transmission from the patient to susceptible contacts. Erythromycin, penicillin G, rifampin, or clindamycin is recommended by most authorities. Commonly recommended regimens for the treatment of adults with respiratory diphtheria are erythromycin (500 mg four times daily, given parenterally or orally) or intramuscular procaine penicillin G (600,000 units at 12-h intervals) for 14 days. Patients with cutaneous diphtheria and carriers can be treated orally with erythromycin (500 mg four times daily) or rifampin (600 mg once daily) for 7 days. If compliance is in question, a single dose of benzathine penicillin G (1.2 to 2.4 million units intramuscularly) can be substituted. Eradication of *C. diphtheriae* should be documented by negative cultures of samples taken on two or three successive days, beginning at least 24 h after the completion of antibiotic therapy. Some authorities also recommend a repeat throat culture 2 weeks later. The small percentage of patients who continue to be infected with *C. diphtheriae* after treatment should receive an additional 10-day course of oral erythromycin or rifampin. Plasmid-mediated resistance to erythromycin of the MLS type emerged transiently in *C. diphtheriae* during the Seattle epidemic, but its frequency declined dramatically after the routine use of erythromycin was discontinued.

Patients with respiratory or cutaneous diphtheria caused by tox$^+$ *C. diphtheriae* or by strains of unknown toxinogenicity should be hospitalized, kept in bed initially, handled with isolation procedures appropriate for the site of infection, and given supportive care as needed. Respiratory and cardiac function must be monitored closely. Early intubation or tracheostomy is recommended when the larynx is involved or signs of impending airway obstruction are detected. Tracheobronchial membrane can sometimes be removed mechanically via the endotracheal tube or tracheostomy. Primary or secondary pneumonia should be diagnosed and treated promptly. Sedative or hypnotic drugs that may mask respiratory symptoms are contraindicated. Close electrocardiographic monitoring, treatment of arrhythmias, and electrical pacing for heart block are essential. Congestive heart failure should be treated as described in Chap. 232. Glucocorticoids do not reduce the risk of diphtheritic myocarditis or polyneuritis. Ulcerative or ecthymatous cutaneous lesions should be treated with Burow's solution applied on wet compresses after debridement of necrotic areas, and treatment for associated conditions such as pediculosis, scabies, or underlying dermatoses should be instituted. Recovery from diphtheria does not always confer active immunity, and initiation of an immunization regimen for diphtheria that is appropriate for the patient's age should be an integral part of the treatment plan.

PREVENTION Vaccines available in the United States for immunization against diphtheria include diphtheria and tetanus toxoids and pertussis vaccine adsorbed (DTP), diphtheria and tetanus toxoids and acellular pertussis vaccine adsorbed (DTaP), diphtheria and tetanus toxoids adsorbed (DT; for pediatric use), and tetanus and diphtheria toxoids adsorbed (Td; for adult use). DTaP is preferred over DTP for primary immunization of children without contraindications, and use of DTP is no longer recommended. Td contains less diphtheria toxoid than DTP, DTaP, or DT and causes fewer adverse reactions in adults. Current guidelines for primary immunization of children and

adults against diphtheria and for maintaining immunity by periodic booster doses of appropriate vaccines throughout life are summarized in Chap. 122.

Close contacts of diphtheria patients should be cultured for *C. diphtheriae*, kept under surveillance for 1 week, and treated with appropriate antibiotics if cultures are positive. Previously immunized close contacts should receive an appropriate booster containing diphtheria toxoid if their last booster was given >5 years previously. If immunization status is uncertain, close contacts should receive an antibiotic regimen appropriate for carriers and a primary immunization series appropriate for their age.

OTHER CORYNEBACTERIAL INFECTIONS

DEFINITION Medically important coryneform bacteria (formerly called *diphtheroids*) include members of the normal flora that cause opportunistic infections, human pathogens of relatively low virulence, and animal pathogens that cause occasional zoonotic infections. Reported infections caused by coryneform bacteria have increased substantially in number over the past two decades. Isolates of *C. jeikeium* and *C. urealyticum* are often resistant to multiple antibiotics.

ETIOLOGY AND LABORATORY DIAGNOSIS Because coryneform bacteria are potential pathogens, it is important not to dismiss them as constituents of the normal flora or as contaminants when they are found in clinical specimens. Laboratory differentiation of coryneform bacteria is important when they are isolated repeatedly, when they are recovered in pure culture or in large numbers, or when they form pigmented or hemolytic colonies.

The coryneform bacteria are a large, heterogeneous group of gram-positive, pleomorphic, irregularly staining bacilli or coccobacilli that superficially resemble *C. diphtheriae* and are difficult to identify and classify. The genus *Corynebacterium* is currently divided into three groups of species: the nonlipophilic, fermentative corynebacteria (including *C. diphtheriae*, *C. xerosis*, *C. striatum*, *C. minutissimum*, and others); the nonlipophilic, nonfermentative corynebacteria (including *C. pseudodiphtheriticum* and others); and the lipophilic corynebacteria (including *C. jeikeium*, *C. urealyticum*, and others). Coryneform bacteria also belong to many other genera (including *Actinomyces*, *Arcanobacterium*, and *Rhodococcus*) as well as to several groups that have not yet been assigned to genera and species by the U.S. Centers for Disease Control and Prevention (CDC).

ECOLOGY AND EPIDEMIOLOGY Humans are the probable natural reservoir for *C. xerosis*, *C. pseudodiphtheriticum* (formerly *C. hofmannii*), *C. striatum*, *C. minutissimum*, *C. jeikeium* (formerly CDC group JK), *C. urealyticum* (formerly CDC group D2), and *Arcanobacterium haemolyticum* (formerly *C. haemolyticum*). Animals are the probable natural reservoir for *Actinomyces pyogenes* (formerly *C. pyogenes*; cows, sheep, pigs), *C. ulcerans* (cows, horses), and *C. pseudotuberculosis* (sheep, horses, goats, cattle). The natural reservoir for *Rhodococcus equi* (formerly *C. equi*) is soil. The ecologic niches for many other coryneform bacteria of medical importance are not well defined.

The coryneform bacteria found most frequently as components of the normal flora include *C. pseudodiphtheriticum* (pharynx, skin), *C. xerosis* (conjunctival sac, nasopharynx, skin), and *C. striatum* (anterior nares, skin). Coryneform bacteria that commonly colonize the skin of hospitalized patients include *C. jeikeium* (axilla, groin, perineum) and *C. urealyticum*. *C. jeikeium* most often colonizes patients with malignancies or severe immunodeficiency; it is also isolated from environmental sources (surfaces, air) in hospitals and from the hands of ward staff. *C. ulcerans* infections are acquired by consumption of raw milk. *C. pseudotuberculosis* infections are acquired by contact with animals or animal products or by consumption of raw milk.

PATHOGENESIS AND CLINICAL MANIFESTATIONS *C. jeikeium* was recognized in 1976 as a cause of infections in immunocompromised hosts. This organism also causes infections in immunocompetent hosts, but severe infections continue to be most frequent in patients with hematologic malignancies and neutropenia. Skin colonization precedes clinical infection. Additional risk factors for nosocomial *C. jeikeium* sepsis include prolonged hospitalization, breaks in the integument, chronic intravascular catheterization, and prior treatment with broad-spectrum antibiotics. Other presentations of *C. jeikeium* infection include endocarditis, device-related infections, pulmonary infiltrates, cutaneous septic emboli, soft tissue infections, and rashes. Endocarditis due to *C. jeikeium* occurs primarily in patients with prosthetic heart valves. *C. jeikeium* is a rare cause of central nervous system infections in patients with ventricular shunts.

C. urealyticum (formerly CDC group D2) was identified in 1985 as a significant cause of nosocomial urinary tract infections, including acute and chronic cystitis and pyelonephritis. The organism closely resembles *C. jeikeium* but differs from the latter by producing urease and failing to convert glucose to acidic metabolites. Hydrolysis of urea by urease causes alkalinization of the urine and formation of ammonium magnesium phosphate (struvite) stones. *C. urealyticum* is a cause of alkaline-encrusted cystitis in patients with preexisting bladder lesions that serve as foci for precipitation of struvite crystals. Risk factors associated with symptomatic urinary tract infections include preexisting immunosuppression, recent urologic procedures (including renal transplantation), underlying disorders of the genitourinary tract, and a history of urinary tract infections.

A. haemolyticum causes pharyngitis and chronic skin ulcers; less frequently, it causes a variety of deep tissue infections, septicemia, and endocarditis. Some 90% of *A. haemolyticum* infections occur in patients between 10 and 30 years old. *A. haemolyticum* pharyngitis in this age group is 5 to 13% as frequent as *Streptococcus pyogenes* pharyngitis. An erythematous rash is present in 30 to 67% of cases. The rash is usually scarlatiniform and most pronounced on the trunk and proximal extremities, but it sometimes resembles urticaria or erythema multiforme. Because rash is more frequent in *A. haemolyticum* infections than in *S. pyogenes* infections, *A. haemolyticum* should be considered as a possible etiology in older children and adults who present with the scarlet fever syndrome. Infection due to *A. haemolyticum* can also present as extensive pharyngeal exudate and can mimic diphtheria. *A. haemolyticum* occasionally causes peritonsillar abscess, sepsis, endocarditis, or meningitis.

C. minutissimum is frequently isolated from the lesions of erythrasma, a common superficial skin infection characterized by the presence in intertriginous areas of reddish-brown, scaly, pruritic, macular patches that exhibit coral-red fluorescence under a Wood's light. The etiology of erythrasma appears to be polymicrobial; infection of the skin by *C. minutissimum* has been shown to follow the onset of maceration and scaling. Deep infections caused by *C. minutissimum* are rare and include abscesses, bacteremia, endocarditis, peritonitis, pyelonephritis, and infection of central venous catheters.

Among coryneform bacteria that cause disease in animals and occasionally in humans, *R. equi* has emerged as an important intracellular opportunistic pathogen in immunocompromised patients. Most reported cases are necrotizing pulmonary infections that resemble tuberculosis or nocardiosis in patients with severely defective cell-mediated immunity. Cases of *R. equi* infection are being diagnosed with increasing frequency in patients with AIDS.

A. pyogenes causes bovine mastitis, a disease transmitted by flies. Yearly epidemics of leg ulcers infected with *A. pyogenes* occurred among schoolchildren in Thailand between 1979 and 1984 and were postulated to have resulted from introduction of the organism into traumatic skin lesions by flies. Reported *A. pyogenes* infections in adults in Denmark have included abscesses, cystitis, intraabdominal infections, and mastoiditis with bacteremia.

C. ulcerans infections in humans usually present as pharyngitis and can mimic respiratory diphtheria, whereas infections caused by *C. pseudotuberculosis* typically present as suppurative granulomatous lymphadenitis. Some strains of *C. ulcerans* and *C. pseudotuberculosis* produce diphtheria toxin. Human infections by *tox*⁺ strains of *C. ul-*

cerans—but not by *tox*⁺ strains of *C. pseudotuberculosis*—have been reported, and administration of diphtheria antitoxin is therefore warranted in infections by *C. ulcerans* that are presumed on clinical grounds to be caused by toxinogenic strains.

C. pseudodiphtheriticum, a commensal of low virulence, is an uncommon cause of pneumonia in men with AIDS and of endocarditis, necrotizing tracheitis, tracheobronchitis, and urinary tract infection in patients without known immune deficiencies. Likewise, *C. xerosis* and *C. striatum* only occasionally cause human infections.

DIAGNOSIS The clinical features of *C. jeikeium* infections are not pathognomonic. The diagnosis of these infections is based on a high index of suspicion, identification of the organism by culture in appropriate clinical specimens, and exclusion of other likely causes of infection.

C. urealyticum often goes undetected by routine urine cultures; rather, it is necessary to incubate the cultures for 24 to 48 h on blood agar or on special media. Cultivation should be prolonged in selected cases—i.e., those involving patients (especially elderly men with preexisting genitourinary abnormalities) with alkaline urine, ammonium magnesium phosphate stones, gram-positive bacilli in the urine, or negative standard urine cultures despite clinical evidence of bacteriuria. Other microbes that can cause urinary tract infections with alkaline urine include *Proteus*, *Ureaplasma*, and some staphylococci and streptococci. Alkaline-encrusted cystitis is an anatomic diagnosis made by cystoscopy.

The differential diagnosis of *A. haemolyticum* pharyngitis with rash includes scarlet fever; rubella; staphylococcal and streptococcal toxic shock syndromes; infections caused by Epstein-Barr virus, cytomegalovirus, and enteroviruses (especially coxsackieviruses); disseminated gonococcal infection; secondary syphilis; and drug allergy. Routine diagnostic methods for throat cultures are not ideal for the detection of *A. haemolyticum*, nor is this organism detected by the rapid tests for *S. pyogenes* that are sometimes substituted for throat cultures. Pharyngitis caused by *A. haemolyticum* in adolescents and adults is likely to be underdiagnosed until improved tests for the organism are used by diagnostic laboratories.

Erythrasma is diagnosed clinically. Because of uncertainty about the etiologic role of *C. minutissimum*, culture of erythrasma lesions is not currently recommended. Pharyngitis caused by *tox*⁺ strains of *C. ulcerans* may be clinically indistinguishable from diphtheria. The presentations of infections caused by other coryneform bacteria are not usually diagnostic; cultures are required for identification of the causal organisms.

TREATMENT Strains of *C. jeikeium* are typically resistant to most antibiotics. Vancomycin is the drug of choice for empirical treatment of infections caused by this organism, although antimicrobial susceptibility testing may reveal other antibiotic options for some isolates. For device-related *C. jeikeium* infections, removal of the infected device is usually required in addition to appropriate antibiotic therapy.

C. urealyticum is often resistant to the antibiotics used commonly for the treatment of urinary tract infections. Empirical treatment with vancomycin is appropriate pending the results of antimicrobial susceptibility testing. Several courses of antibiotic therapy may be necessary for bacteriologic cure. Patients with alkaline-encrusted cystitis require resection of the encrusted lesions in addition to antibiotic therapy.

No controlled trials of treatment for *A. haemolyticum* infections have been performed. In vitro tests usually demonstrate susceptibility to penicillins, erythromycin, azithromycin, clindamycin, doxycycline, ciprofloxacin, and vancomycin, but treatment failures have been reported with appropriate doses of penicillins. Limited data suggest that the clinical course of *A. haemolyticum* pharyngitis may be shortened by treatment with erythromycin.

Infections with *C. ulcerans* that present like diphtheria or are known to be caused by *tox*⁺ strains should be treated like diphtheria. Oral erythromycin is usually effective for treatment of erythrasma. For infections caused by *R. equi*, vancomycin is the drug of choice. Possible alternatives include erythromycin, rifampin, aminoglycosides, and chloramphenicol; the combination of erythromycin and rifampin is attractive because of possible synergy. Penicillins should not be used, because *R. equi* rapidly develops resistance. Many weeks of antibiotic treatment, sometimes supplemented by surgical intervention, are often needed for infections caused by *R. equi*. Suppressive therapy with antibiotics should be continued indefinitely in patients with AIDS after initial treatment of infections caused by *R. equi*. Initial treatment of infections caused by other coryneform bacteria should be based on the identity of the organism and published data regarding antibiotic susceptibility. Therapy should be modified, when necessary, in light of the results of antibiotic susceptibility tests.

ANTHRAX

DEFINITION Anthrax is an infection caused by *Bacillus anthracis* that occurs primarily in herbivores. Humans become infected when *B. anthracis* spores are introduced into the body by contact with infected animals or contaminated animal products, insect bites, ingestion, or inhalation. Aerosolized spores of *B. anthracis* have the potential for use in biological warfare or bioterrorism. Cutaneous anthrax is most common and is characterized by the development of a localized skin lesion with a central eschar surrounded by marked nonpitting edema. Inhalation anthrax (woolsorters' disease) typically involves hemorrhagic mediastinitis, rapidly progressive systemic infection, and a very high mortality rate. Gastrointestinal anthrax is rare and is associated with a high mortality rate.

ETIOLOGIC AGENT AND EPIDEMIOLOGY *B. anthracis* is a large, aerobic, spore-forming, gram-positive rod that is encapsulated and nonmotile and grows in chains. Sporulation does not take place in living animals. The rectangular shape of the individual bacteria gives chains of *B. anthracis* a boxcar-like appearance. Virulent strains of *B. anthracis* are pathogenic for animals, including mice and guinea pigs. Spores of *B. anthracis* can survive for years in dry earth but are destroyed by boiling for 10 min, by treatment with oxidizing agents such as potassium permanganate or hydrogen peroxide, or by dilute formaldehyde. Most strains of *B. anthracis* are susceptible to penicillin.

Anthrax occurs worldwide and is most prevalent among domestic herbivores (including cattle, sheep, horses, and goats) and wild herbivores. Grazing animals become infected when they forage for food in areas contaminated with spores of *B. anthracis*. Anthrax in herbivores tends to be severe, with high mortality. Terminally ill animals with overwhelming bacteremic infections often bleed from the nose, mouth, and bowel, thereby contaminating soil or water with vegetative *B. anthracis* that can sporulate and persist in the environment. The carcasses of infected animals provide additional potential foci of contamination.

Humans are more resistant to anthrax than are herbivorous animals. The estimated number of human cases worldwide is 20,000 to 100,000 per year. Human cases are classified as agricultural or industrial. Agricultural cases result most often from contact with animals that have anthrax (e.g., during skinning, butchering, or dissecting), from bites of contaminated or infected flies, and (in rare instances) from consumption of contaminated meat. Industrial cases are associated with exposure to contaminated hides, goat hair, wool, or bones. Only three cases of cutaneous anthrax were reported to the CDC from 1984 through 1993, and gastrointestinal anthrax has never been documented in the United States. In an epidemic in the former Soviet Union at Sverdlovsk in 1979, cases were initially reported as cutaneous and gastrointestinal anthrax associated with contaminated meat; however, subsequent analysis of epidemiologic data and autopsy findings for most of the fatal cases established that the disease was inhalational anthrax associated with accidental airborne release of *B. anthracis* from a nearby military biological weapons facility. A massive outbreak in Zimbabwe between 1978 and the early 1980s involved more than 9700 cases of agricultural anthrax in humans. This outbreak occurred during wartime and was associated with disruption of the veterinary and medical infrastructure and cessation of veterinary anthrax vaccination programs.

PATHOGENESIS *B. anthracis* can evade phagocytosis, invade the bloodstream, multiply rapidly to a high population density in vivo, and kill quickly. The poly-D-glutamic acid capsule of *B. anthracis* confers resistance to phagocytosis. Anthrax toxin consists of three different proteins called *protective antigen* (PA), *edema factor* (EF), and *lethal factor* (LF). The toxin was discovered in studies demonstrating that transfer of sterile blood from guinea pigs dying of anthrax to uninfected guinea pigs killed the recipients. PA binds to plasma membranes of target cells and is cleaved by a cellular protease into two fragments. The larger fragment remains on the cell surface, displays a binding site for a domain that is present in both EF and LF, and serves as a specific receptor that mediates endocytic entry of EF or LF into the target cells. The catalytic activity of EF, a calmodulin-dependent adenylate cyclase, is expressed in the cytoplasm of human or animal cells that contain both calmodulin and ATP. The biologic effects of EF, which include formation of edema in anthrax lesions and inhibition of polymorphonuclear leukocyte functions, are mediated by the intracellular cyclic AMP that is produced by the enzymatic action of EF. In contrast, LF is a highly specific endopeptidase that cleaves several members of the MAP-kinase-kinase protein family and inactivates their functions in signal transduction pathways. Macrophages appear to be the principal targets of LF in animals, and intoxication of macrophages by LF is associated with production of reactive oxygen species, release of cytokines (including tumor necrosis factor α and interleukin 1β), shock, and death.

Cutaneous anthrax is initiated when spores of *B. anthracis* are introduced into the skin through cuts or abrasions or by biting flies. The spores germinate within hours, and the vegetative cells multiply and produce anthrax toxin. The cutaneous anthrax lesion is characterized by necrosis, vascular congestion, hemorrhage, and gelatinous edema, but few leukocytes are present.

In inhalational anthrax, *B. anthracis* spores in airborne particles <5 μm in diameter are deposited directly into the alveoli or alveolar ducts. The spores are phagocytized by alveolar macrophages, and some are carried to and germinate in mediastinal nodes. Hemorrhagic necrosis of the nodes, associated with hemorrhagic mediastinitis and overwhelming *B. anthracis* bacteremia, may develop rapidly. Secondary pneumonia sometimes occurs.

Gastrointestinal anthrax usually results from ingestion of inadequately cooked meat from animals with anthrax. Primary infection can be initiated in the intestine by organisms that survive passage through the stomach. An oropharyngeal form of the disease has also been described. Lesions in the throat or intestine are usually accompanied by hemorrhagic lymphadenitis.

B. anthracis bacteremia occurs in almost all cases of anthrax that progress to a fatal outcome.

CLINICAL MANIFESTATIONS Approximately 95% of human cases of anthrax are the cutaneous form, and ~5% are the inhalational form. Gastrointestinal anthrax is very rare. Anthrax meningitis can occur as a complication of overwhelming *B. anthracis* bacteremia.

Cutaneous Anthrax The cutaneous lesion in anthrax is most often found on exposed areas of skin. A small red macule develops within days after inoculation of *B. anthracis* spores into skin. During the next week, the lesion typically progresses through papular and vesicular or pustular stages to the formation of an ulcer with a blackened necrotic eschar surrounded by a highly characteristic expanding zone of brawny edema. The early lesion may be pruritic, and the fully developed lesion is painless. Small satellite vesicles may surround the original lesion, and painful nonspecific regional lymphadenitis is common. Most patients are afebrile, with mild or no constitutional symptoms; in severe cases, edema may be extensive and associated with shock. Spontaneous healing occurs in 80 to 90% of untreated cases, but edema may persist for weeks. In the 10 to 20% of untreated patients who have progressive infection, bacteremia develops and is often associated with high fever and rapid death. The differential diagnosis includes staphylococcal skin infections, tularemia, plague, and orf. Cutaneous anthrax should be considered when patients have painless ulcers associated with vesicles and edema and have had contact with animals or animal products.

Inhalational Anthrax   The presenting symptoms of inhalational anthrax (woolsorters' disease) resemble those of severe viral respiratory diseases. Early diagnosis of inhalational anthrax that occurs naturally or as a consequence of biological warfare or bioterrorism is difficult. After 1 to 3 days, an acute phase supervenes, with increasing fever, dyspnea, stridor, hypoxia, and hypotension usually leading to death within 24 h. Occasionally, patients present with fulminant disease. A characteristic radiologic finding associated with hemorrhagic mediastinitis is symmetric mediastinal widening, which may provide an early clue to the diagnosis of inhalational anthrax.

Gastrointestinal Anthrax   Symptoms of gastrointestinal anthrax are variable and include fever, nausea and vomiting, abdominal pain, bloody diarrhea, and sometimes rapidly developing ascites. Diarrhea is occasionally massive in volume. The major features of oropharyngeal anthrax are fever, sore throat, dysphagia, painful regional lymphadenopathy, and toxemia; respiratory distress may be evident. The primary lesion is most often located on the tonsils.

LABORATORY DIAGNOSIS   *B. anthracis* is present in large numbers in cutaneous lesions of anthrax and can be demonstrated by Gram's staining, direct fluorescent antibody staining, or culture unless the patient has been treated with antibiotics. A small proportion of patients with anthrax have bacteremia. Patients with anthrax meningitis have bloody spinal fluid containing large numbers of *B. anthracis* demonstrable by staining or culture. Patients with mild disease usually have normal leukocyte counts, but those with disseminated disease typically have polymorphonuclear leukocytosis. Tests for antibody to *B. anthracis* are useful in confirming the diagnosis of anthrax.

R̲x̲ **TREATMENT**   Viable *B. anthracis* disappears from the lesions of cutaneous anthrax within 5 h of the initiation of treatment with parenteral penicillin G. The recommended regimen for adults is 2 million units of penicillin G at intervals of 6 h until edema subsides, with the subsequent administration of oral penicillin to complete a 7- to 10-day course. For penicillin-sensitive adults, treatment with ciprofloxacin, erythromycin, tetracycline, or chloramphenicol can be substituted. Antibiotics decrease local edema and systemic toxicity in cutaneous anthrax but do not prevent eschar formation. Cutaneous lesions should be cleaned and covered, and used dressings should be decontaminated. For inhalational or gastrointestinal anthrax, high-dose penicillin (8 to 12 million units per day in divided doses at intervals of 4 to 6 h) is recommended. A rational case can be made for passive immunization with anthrax antitoxin in addition to antibiotic therapy in severely ill patients with anthrax, but no appropriate antitoxin is commercially available.

PREVENTION   Inhalational anthrax was essentially eliminated in England before 1940 through the development of methods to decontaminate wool and goat hair and the improvement of working conditions for handlers of animal products.

Nonliving vaccines consisting of alum-precipitated or aluminum hydroxide–adsorbed extracellular components of unencapsulated *B. anthracis* are used in the United States for military personnel, agricultural workers, veterinary personnel, and others at risk of exposure to anthrax. The major active component of these vaccines is protective antigen. Live attenuated vaccines containing spores of *B. anthracis* are used in both developed and developing countries to immunize domestic herbivores; these preparations are also used to immunize humans in Russia but not in the United States. The probable basis for attenuation of the original Pasteur spore vaccine is partial loss of a plasmid that encodes anthrax toxin. The basis for attenuation of the current Sterne spore vaccine is loss of a plasmid that encodes capsular polypeptide.

Improved anthrax vaccines for humans are needed because the current vaccines are impure and chemically complex, elicit only slow onset of protective immunity, provide incomplete protection, and cause significant adverse reactions. In addition to agricultural and industrial anthrax, the possible use of *B. anthracis* as an agent of biological warfare or bioterrorism is a stimulus for the development of an improved vaccine. Current strategies for vaccine development include purification of candidate protective antigens, expression of protective antigens in recombinant microbial vaccines, and construction of improved live attenuated strains of *B. anthracis*.

Carcasses of animals that succumb to anthrax should be buried intact or cremated. Necropsy or butchering of infected animals should be avoided because sporulation of *B. anthracis* occurs only in the presence of oxygen.

PROGNOSIS   The mortality rate is 10 to 20% for untreated cutaneous anthrax but is very low with appropriate antibiotic therapy. In contrast, the mortality rate for inhalational anthrax approaches 100%, and therapy is usually unsuccessful. The mortality rate in treated gastrointestinal anthrax is ~50%. Anthrax meningitis is usually fatal.

BIBLIOGRAPHY

BROWN AE: Other corynebacteria and *Rhodococcus*, in *Mandell, Douglas, and Bennett's Principles and Practice of Infectious Diseases*, vol 2, 5th ed, GL Mandell et al (eds). Philadelphia, Churchill Livingstone, 2000, pp 2198–2208

DITTMAN S et al: Successful control of epidemic diphtheria in the states of the former Union of Soviet Socialist Republics: Lessons learned. J Infect Dis 181(Suppl 1):S10, 2000

DIXON TC et al: Anthrax. N Engl J Med 341:815, 1999

DUESBERY NS, VANDE WOUDE GF: Anthrax toxins. Cell Mol Life Sci 55:1599, 1999

FRIEDLANDER AM et al: Anthrax vaccine: Evidence for safety and efficacy against inhalational anthrax. JAMA 282:2104, 1999

FUNKE G et al: Clinical microbiology of coryneform bacteria. Clin Microbiol Rev 10:125, 1997

GUBLER J et al: An outbreak of nontoxigenic *Corynebacterium diphtheriae* infection: Single bacterial clone causing invasive infection among Swiss drug users. Clin Infect Dis 27:1295, 1998

HADFIELD TL: The pathology of diphtheria. J Infect Dis 181(Suppl 1):S116, 2000

HOLMES RK: Biology and molecular epidemiology of diphtheria toxin and the *tox* gene. J Infect Dis 181(Suppl 1):S156, 2000

KADIROVA R et al: Clinical characteristics and management of 676 hospitalized diphtheria cases, Kyrgyz Republic, 1995. J Infect Dis 181(Suppl 1):S110, 2000

LITTLE SE, IVINS BE: Molecular pathogenesis of *Bacillus anthracis* infection. Microbes and Infection 2:131, 1999

PILE JC et al: Anthrax as a potential biological warfare agent. Arch Intern Med 158:429, 1998

POPOVIC T et al: Use of molecular subtyping to document long-term persistence of *Corynebacterium diphtheriae* in South Dakota. J Clin Microbiol 37:1092, 1999

QUICK ML et al: Risk factors for diphtheria: A prospective case-control study in the Republic of Georgia, 1995–1996. J Infect Dis 181(Suppl 1):S121, 2000

142

Anne Schuchat, Claire V. Broome

INFECTIONS CAUSED BY *LISTERIA MONOCYTOGENES*

Listeria monocytogenes is a gram-positive rod that can be isolated from soil, vegetation, and many animal reservoirs. Human disease due to *L. monocytogenes* generally occurs in the setting of pregnancy or of immunosuppression caused by illness or medication. Increasing evidence suggests that a substantial portion of cases of human listeriosis are attributable to the food-borne transmission of *L. monocytogenes*. Unlike most food-borne pathogens, which cause primarily gastrointestinal illness, *L. monocytogenes* causes invasive syndromes, such as meningitis, sepsis, chorioamnionitis, and stillbirth.

ETIOLOGY   Listeriae are aerobic or facultatively anaerobic nonsporulating bacilli that grow at 1 to 45°C and typically have tumbling motility when cultured at 20 to 25°C. Characteristics that help distinguish *L. monocytogenes* from other *Listeria* spp. include the formation of a narrow zone of β hemolysis on sheep blood agar and the production of acid from glucose, maltose, L-rhamnose, and α-methyl-D-mannoside but not from D-xylose. Determination of the serotype of *L. monocytogenes* is based on somatic (O) and flagellar (H) antigens. Most cases of human disease are caused by serotypes 1/2a, 1/2b, and 4b. Molecular subtyping techniques have made it easier to discriminate among strains of *Listeria* and thus to link environmental or food isolates with clinical infections.

PATHOGENESIS   *L. monocytogenes* is an intracellular pathogen—a characteristic consistent with its predilection for causing illness in persons with deficient cell-mediated immunity. The organism can be found as part of the gastrointestinal flora in healthy individuals. Lack of gastric acidity and abnormal gastrointestinal functioning may increase the risk of invasive disease following exposure to the organism in the gastrointestinal tract. The increased risk of *L. monocytogenes* infection in pregnant women may be due to both systemic and local immunologic changes associated with pregnancy. For example, local immunosuppression at the maternal-fetal interface of the placenta may facilitate intrauterine infection following transient maternal bacteremia.

The molecular pathogenesis of *L. monocytogenes* has recently been elucidated. The cell-surface protein internalin interacts with specific receptors to induce phagocytosis. Both listeriolysin O and phospholipases permit the organism to escape from the phagosome into the cytosol while avoiding intracellular killing. Through the surface protein Act A, *L. monocytogenes* uses actin-based motility to move to the cell membrane. Efficient cell-to-cell spread is accomplished by both actin filament formation and phospholipase production. Genetic determinants of these proteins have been characterized. Because the organism is adapted for both intracellular survival and direct cell-to-cell spread, it is not eliminated by antibodies.

EPIDEMIOLOGY   Long recognized as a veterinary pathogen, *L. monocytogenes* causes basilar meningitis ("circling disease") and stillbirth in sheep and cattle. The occurrence of listeriosis among humans has received increasing attention as the role of contaminated foods in the pathogenesis of epidemic listeriosis has been recognized and reports of disease associated with the expanding immunosuppressed population have accumulated.

Invasive listeriosis—confirmed by culture of blood or cerebrospinal fluid (CSF)—occurs in approximately 5 individuals per million population annually in the United States, for an estimated 1400 cases per year. Perinatal listeriosis complicates 9 births per 100,000. A 40% decline in incidence since the period from 1986 through 1990 may be attributable to aggressive food regulation and industrial clean-up efforts. Multistate surveillance for sporadic listeriosis suggests that 20% of infections are fatal or result in stillbirth, although higher case-fatality rates have been reported during listeriosis epidemics and were described in early series. Most cases of disease due to *L. monocytogenes* are sporadic; however, investigation of several outbreaks of listeriosis during the 1980s and 1990s demonstrated common-source food-borne transmission as a cause of human illness and showed that the incubation period for disease following consumption of contaminated food can be 2 to 6 weeks. The largest North American outbreak, which took place in Los Angeles in 1985, involved more than 100 cases and 48 deaths or stillbirths. A nationwide outbreak in France in 1992 involved 279 cases and 63 deaths. Foods implicated in outbreaks

of listeriosis include contaminated coleslaw, pasteurized milk, soft cheeses, pâté, ready-to-eat pork products, and hot dogs, while epidemiologic studies have implicated undercooked chicken, uncooked hot dogs, soft cheeses, and food from store delicatessen counters in sporadic disease. Listerial contamination of foods is relatively common. Among foods contaminated with the organism, those that are purchased ready to eat, are contaminated with serotype 4b, and are contaminated at a relatively high level may be the most likely to cause illness. The long incubation period associated with listeriosis contributes to the difficulty of implicating specific foods as the cause of either common-source outbreaks or sporadic cases.

Although food-borne transmission appears to be the foremost cause of epidemic and sporadic disease, several clusters of late-onset neonatal infection suggest nosocomial transmission of *L. monocytogenes*. Contaminated multiuse materials and equipment have been suggested as causes of some nosocomial clusters. Listeriosis has been reported in veterinarians and other persons in close contact with infected animals.

CLINICAL PRESENTATION   *Pregnancy-associated listeriosis* may occur during any stage of pregnancy, although most infections are detected during the third trimester, possibly because of failure to obtain specimens for bacterial culture earlier during gestation in instances of abortion and stillbirth. One-half to two-thirds of pregnant women with perinatal listeriosis experience a mild illness characterized by fever, myalgias, malaise, and backache, which sometimes are accompanied by diarrhea, abdominal pain, nausea, and/or vomiting during the bacteremic phase. Blood cultures should be used for diagnosis. Transplacental spread of the organism results in intrauterine infection, which can lead to chorioamnionitis, premature labor, intrauterine fetal demise, or early-onset disease of the newborn. Women with listeriosis diagnosed during pregnancy have a favorable clinical outcome after antibiotic therapy or delivery. Although often included in the differential diagnosis of recurrent spontaneous abortion, infection with *L. monocytogenes* appears to cause fewer than 2% of stillbirths.

Neonatal listeriosis can be classified under the same categories used for group B streptococcal infection (Chap. 140), with early-onset disease evident during the first week of life and late-onset disease developing thereafter. Infants may be symptomatic at birth; most infants with early-onset disease are symptomatic by the second day of life. Aspiration of infected amniotic fluid contributes to pathogenesis. Early-onset disease may include sepsis, respiratory distress, skin lesions, and the syndrome called *granulomatosis infantisepticum*, which is characterized by disseminated abscesses involving the liver, spleen, adrenal glands, lungs, and other sites. Infants with late-onset neonatal disease are more likely than those with early-onset disease to develop meningitis. While early-onset disease is often associated with obstetric complications such as premature delivery and chorioamnionitis, late-onset disease typically affects infants born at term by uncomplicated deliveries. Infants may acquire *L. monocytogenes* during passage through the birth canal; except in several clusters of late-onset neonatal infections linked to nosocomial transmission, the pathogenesis of late-onset disease is not well understood.

Listeriosis not associated with pregnancy usually affects persons with immunosuppressive conditions, although invasive disease can also affect immunocompetent adults, particularly elderly persons. The most common underlying conditions in nonpregnant adults with listeriosis are chronic glucocorticoid therapy, solid or hematologic malignancies, diabetes mellitus, renal disease, liver disease, and AIDS. Although the prevalence of listeriosis among persons infected with HIV is much higher than that in the general population, listeriosis is a relatively uncommon opportunistic infection in AIDS.

Sepsis   Clinical studies have shown that bacteremic infection without an evident focus is the most common clinical manifestation of listeriosis among immunocompromised hosts, while infection of the central nervous system (CNS) ranks second in frequency. Listerial sepsis cannot be distinguished clinically from bacteremia involving other organisms. Patients are usually febrile, often appear extremely ill, and may have prodromal symptoms including myalgia, nausea, vomiting, and diarrhea. Immunocompromised patients with listeriosis are less likely than other adults to present with CNS infection, possibly because they are more likely to have blood cultured during febrile episodes and thus to have transient listerial bacteremia recognized.

CNS Infection The most common presentation of CNS infection due to *L. monocytogenes* is meningitis, which can present as either an acute or (less often) a subacute illness. Presenting symptoms include fever, headache, and an altered level of consciousness. Examination of CSF usually reveals pleocytosis, increased protein concentrations, and normal glucose levels, although other patterns are sometimes found. Gram's stain is often unrevealing. The diagnosis is made when *L. monocytogenes* is identified on culture. Despite its name, *L. monocytogenes* is rarely associated with monocytosis of either CSF or blood. Other syndromes seen in CNS infection include meningoencephalitis; cerebritis; and brainstem, spinal cord, or intracranial abscesses. The unusual syndrome of rhombencephalitis includes asymmetric cranial-nerve palsies, altered consciousness, cerebellar signs, and motor or sensory loss. Symptoms of other nonmeningitic CNS infections include fever, ataxia, seizures, personality changes, and coma. Nuchal rigidity is rare in nonmeningitic infections. CSF cultures may be sterile; blood cultures are usually diagnostic.

Endocarditis Like most forms of bacterial endocarditis, listerial endocarditis typically occurs in patients with prosthetic or previously damaged valves. The organism has a predilection for the left side of the heart. Endocarditis due to *L. monocytogenes* is often associated with systemic embolization.

Focal Infections Other focal infections that can follow unrecognized bacteremia include endophthalmitis, peritonitis, osteomyelitis, visceral abscess, pleuropulmonary infection, and cholecystitis. Cutaneous lesions may develop without systemic involvement and have been reported in veterinarians and poultry workers.

Recurrences Recurrent infection with *L. monocytogenes* has been reported but is rare. Many recurrences are due to the subtype responsible for the initial infection. The implication is that such recurrences result either from insufficient treatment of a focus of primary infection or from repeated exposure to a persistently contaminated source.

Gastrointestinal Illness Several common-source outbreaks of acute gastroenteritis suggest that *L. monocytogenes* can cause an acute diarrheal syndrome in persons without immunocompromising conditions. The importance of *L. monocytogenes* in sporadic diarrheal illness is unclear. Although the organism is not identified by the culture methods routinely used for stool specimens, studies using selective enrichment media for evaluation of consecutive specimens from patients hospitalized with acute diarrhea have suggested that *L. monocytogenes* is not a major cause of sporadic diarrhea.

DIAGNOSIS Invasive listeriosis is diagnosed when the organism is cultured from a site that is usually sterile, such as blood, CSF, or amniotic fluid. The organism grows readily within 36 h on routine culture media, but morphologic similarities between *Listeria* and both diphtheroids and streptococci make it necessary to use biochemical tests to identify the species. Serologic assays with whole-cell antigens have not been useful for the diagnosis of listeriosis, both because exposure to the organism (and thus the presence of antibody) may be common and because infected individuals may not produce antibody. Assays for antibody to listeriolysin O have been applied in epidemiologic investigations and, retrospectively, in the diagnosis of culture-negative CNS infection. Culture of the organism from nonsterile sites such as the vagina and rectum is not useful for clinical diagnosis, as the organism may be carried at these sites by approximately 5% of healthy individuals.

Differential diagnosis of prematurity, spontaneous abortion, or stillbirth includes infectious diseases such as group B streptococcal infection, congenital syphilis, and toxoplasmosis; pathogens such as group B streptococci and *Escherichia coli* are more common than *L. monocytogenes* as causes of meningitis and sepsis in the newborn period. Listerial infection should always be considered in the differential diagnosis of meningitis in immunosuppressed persons, particularly transplant recipients and others undergoing glucocorticoid treatment, patients with hematologic malignancy, and HIV-infected patients. Among healthy adults, meningitis is much more likely to be caused by *Neisseria meningitidis*, *Streptococcus pneumoniae*, or viral pathogens than by *L. monocytogenes*.

℞ TREATMENT The treatment of choice for listeriosis is intravenous administration of either ampicillin or penicillin, often in combination with an aminoglycoside for synergy. Trimethoprim-sulfamethoxazole is bactericidal against *L. monocytogenes* and has been used successfully in the treatment of patients with penicillin allergy. *L. monocytogenes* is susceptible in vitro to penicillin G, ampicillin, erythromycin, trimethoprim-sulfamethoxazole, chloramphenicol, rifampin, tetracyclines, aminoglycosides, and imipenem. However, chloramphenicol and rifampin may antagonize the bactericidal effect of penicillins. Because *L. monocytogenes* is not sensitive to cephalosporins, these agents should not be used for single-agent empirical treatment of neonatal sepsis or of meningitis in newborns or immunocompromised hosts.

Dosages and durations of therapy have not been subjected to controlled trials. For nonpregnant adults with listeriosis, the regimen of choice is either ampicillin (12 g intravenously per day in six divided doses) or penicillin G (15 to 20 million units intravenously per day in six divided doses); for immunosuppressed patients with meningitis, some experts add gentamicin (1.3 mg/kg intravenously every 8 h) for synergy. Penicillin-allergic patients may be treated with trimethoprim-sulfamethoxazole (15/75 mg/kg intravenously per day in three equal portions every 8 h). Meningitis in an immunocompetent patient may require 2 to 3 weeks of antibiotic therapy after defervescence. Meningitis, bacteremia, endocarditis, and nonmeningitic listeriosis in immunosuppressed patients should be treated longer, probably for 4 to 6 weeks. Neonatal listeriosis can be treated with a 2-week course of ampicillin. Infants weighing <2000 g should receive 100 mg/kg per day in two equal doses during the first week of life and 150 mg/kg per day during the second week. Infants weighing ≥2000 g should receive 150 mg/kg per day in three equal doses during the first week of life and 200 mg/kg per day during the second week. The addition of an aminoglycoside should be considered for neonatal infection (gentamicin, 5 mg/kg per day in two divided doses during the first week of life; 7.5 mg/kg per day in three equal doses during the second week). For listeriosis in pregnant women, a 2-week course of ampicillin (4 to 6 g per day in four equal doses) is recommended. During the last month of pregnancy, infected women with serious penicillin allergies may be treated with erythromycin.

PROGNOSIS Treatment of maternal bacteremia during pregnancy can prevent neonatal infection. Antibiotic therapy for the newborn can limit sequelae, although the widely disseminated disease characteristic of granulomatosis infantisepticum is frequently fatal regardless of treatment. Early-onset disease carries a higher mortality risk than late-onset infection, and immunocompromised hosts have a worse prognosis than do otherwise healthy adults with listeriosis.

PREVENTION *L. monocytogenes* is frequently isolated from food; the Food and Drug Administration, the U.S. Department of Agriculture, and manufacturers are pursuing further measures to reduce *L. monocytogenes* contamination of foods that have been subjected to listericidal processing. Prevention of listeriosis requires dietary counseling of persons at increased risk of disease (Table 142-1). There is no role for the administration of prophylaxis to contacts of patients with listeriosis. Clinicians are encouraged to report cases of listeriosis to local or state health departments. Case reporting and subtyping of clinical isolates can facilitate early recognition of outbreaks and prevention of subsequent cases.

Table 142-1 Dietary Recommendations for the Prevention of Food-Borne Listeriosis

Recommendations to all individuals
1. Thoroughly cook raw food from animal sources, such as beef, pork, and poultry.
2. Wash raw vegetables thoroughly before eating them.
3. Keep uncooked meats separate from vegetables and from cooked and ready-to-eat foods.
4. Avoid raw (unpasteurized) milk or foods made from raw milk.
5. Wash hands, knives, and cutting boards after handling uncooked foods.

Additional recommendations to high-risk individuals[a]
- Avoid soft cheeses such as Mexican-style, feta, Brie, Camembert, and blue-veined cheese. There is no need to avoid hard cheeses, cream cheese, cottage cheese, or yogurt.
- Leftover foods or ready-to-eat foods, such as hot dogs, should be reheated until steaming hot before being eaten.
- Although the risk of listeriosis associated with foods from delicatessen counters is relatively low and poorly characterized, pregnant women and immunosuppressed persons may choose to avoid these foods or to thoroughly reheat cold cuts before eating them.

[a] Persons immunocompromised by illness or medications; pregnant women.

BIBLIOGRAPHY

DALTON CB et al: Listeriosis from chocolate milk: Linking of an outbreak of febrile gastroenteritis and "sporadic" invasive disease. N Engl J Med 336:100, 1997

LORBER B: Listeriosis. Clin Infect Dis 24:1, 1997

PINNER RW et al: Role of foods in sporadic listeriosis: II. Microbiologic and epidemiologic investigation. JAMA 267:2046, 1992

RYSER ET, MARTH EH (eds): Listeria, Listeriosis, and Food Safety, 2d ed. New York, Marcel Dekker, 1999

SCHLECH WF et al: Epidemic listeriosis—evidence for transmission by food. N Engl J Med 308:203, 1983

SCHUCHAT A et al: Role of foods in sporadic listeriosis: I. Case-control study of dietary risk factors. JAMA 267:2041, 1992

——— et al: Epidemiology of human listeriosis. Clin Microbiol Rev 4:169, 1991

SOUTHWICK FS, PURICH DL: Intracellular pathogenesis of listeriosis. N Engl J Med 334:770, 1996

SWAMINATHAN B et al: Listeria, in Manual of Clinical Microbiology, PR Murray et al (eds). Washington, DC, ASM Press, 1995, p 341

TAPPERO JW et al: Reduction in the incidence of human listeriosis in the United States—effectiveness of prevention efforts? JAMA 273:1118, 1995

143 Elias Abrutyn

TETANUS

DEFINITION Tetanus is a neurologic disorder, characterized by increased muscle tone and spasms, that is caused by tetanospasmin, a powerful protein toxin elaborated by *Clostridium tetani*. Tetanus occurs in several clinical forms, including generalized, neonatal, and localized disease.

ETIOLOGIC AGENT *C. tetani* is an anaerobic, motile gram-positive rod that forms an oval, colorless, terminal spore and thus assumes a shape resembling a tennis racket or drumstick. The organism is found worldwide in soil, in the inanimate environment, in animal feces, and occasionally in human feces. Spores may survive for years in some environments and are resistant to various disinfectants and to boiling for 20 min. Vegetative cells, however, are easily inactivated and are susceptible to several antibiotics (metronidazole, penicillin, and others).

Tetanospasmin is formed in vegetative cells under plasmid control. It is a single-polypeptide chain. With autolysis, the single-chain toxin is released and cleaved to form a heterodimer consisting of a heavy chain (100 kDa), which mediates binding to nerve-cell receptors and entry into these cells, and a light chain (50 kDa), which acts to block neurotransmitter release. The amino acid structures of the two most powerful toxins known, botulinum toxin and tetanus toxin, are partially homologous.

EPIDEMIOLOGY Tetanus occurs sporadically and almost always affects nonimmunized persons, partially immunized persons, or fully immunized individuals who fail to maintain adequate immunity with booster doses of vaccine. Although tetanus is entirely preventable by immunization, the burden of disease is large worldwide. The disease is common in areas where soil is cultivated, in rural areas, in warm climates, during summer months, and among males. In countries without a comprehensive immunization program, tetanus occurs predominantly in neonates and other young children; an estimated 490,000 neonates died of tetanus worldwide in 1994—a reduction from 550,000 in 1993. In the United States and other nations with successful immunization programs, neonatal tetanus is rare and the disease affects other age groups and groups inadequately covered by immunization (such as nonwhites). The risk for the development of tetanus and for the most severe illness is highest among the elderly. Only 27% of persons aged 70 or older—as opposed to 88% of 6- to 11-year-olds—have protective antibody levels. During the years 1995 through 1997, a total of 124 cases were reported to the Centers for Disease Control and Prevention; both the overall incidence (0.15 cases per 100,000 population) and the annual average (41 cases) were the lowest ever reported in the United States. The actual burden of illness, however, was greater, because reporting is incomplete. Although the elderly customarily account for the highest proportion of cases, in 1995 through 1997 individuals ≥60 years of age accounted for only 35% of cases, whereas those 20 to 59 years of age accounted for 60% and those under 20 for 5% (with one case of neonatal tetanus). The change is attributed to a decrease in incidence in both the ≥60 and the <20 age groups, along with an increase among persons 20 to 59 years of age, particularly injection drug users.

In the United States, most cases of tetanus follow an acute injury, such as a puncture wound, laceration, or abrasion. Tetanus is acquired indoors or during farming, gardening, and other outdoor activities. The injury may be major but often is trivial, so that medical attention is not sought; in some instances no injury can be identified. The disease may complicate chronic conditions such as skin ulcers, abscesses, and gangrene. Tetanus is also associated with burns, frostbite, middle-ear infection, surgery, abortion, childbirth, and drug abuse, notably "skin popping." In some patients no portal of entry for the organism can be identified.

PATHOGENESIS Contamination of wounds with spores of *C. tetani* is probably frequent. Germination and toxin production, however, take place only in wounds with low oxidation-reduction potential, such as those with devitalized tissue, foreign bodies, or active infection. *C. tetani* does not itself evoke inflammation, and the portal of entry retains a benign appearance unless infection with other organisms is present.

Toxin released in the wound binds to peripheral motor neuron terminals, enters the axon, and is transported to the nerve-cell body in the brainstem and spinal cord by retrograde intraneuronal transport. The toxin then migrates across the synapse to presynaptic terminals, where it blocks release of the inhibitory neurotransmitters glycine and γ-aminobutyric acid (GABA). The blocking of neurotransmitter release by tetanospasmin, a zinc metalloprotease, involves the cleavage of protein(s) critical to proper function of the synaptic vesicle release apparatus. With diminished inhibition, the resting firing rate of the α motor neuron increases, producing rigidity. With lessened activity of reflexes that limit polysynaptic spread of impulses (a glycinergic activity), agonists and antagonists may be recruited rather than inhibited, with the consequent production of spasms. Loss of inhibition may also affect preganglionic sympathetic neurons in the lateral gray matter of the spinal cord and produce sympathetic hyperactivity and high circulating catecholamine levels. Tetanospasmin, like botulinum toxin, may block neurotransmitter release at the neuromuscular junction and produce weakness or paralysis; recovery requires sprouting of new nerve terminals.

In local tetanus, only the nerves supplying the affected muscles are involved. Generalized tetanus occurs when toxin released in the wound enters the lymphatics and bloodstream and is spread widely to distant nerve terminals; the blood-brain barrier blocks direct entry into the central nervous system. If it is assumed that intraneuronal transport times are equal for all nerves, short nerves are affected before long nerves: this fact explains the sequential involvement of nerves of the head, trunk, and extremities in generalized tetanus.

CLINICAL MANIFESTATIONS *Generalized tetanus*, the most common form of the disease, is characterized by increased muscle tone and generalized spasms. The median time of onset after injury is 7 days; 15% of cases occur within 3 days and 10% after 14 days.

Typically, the patient first notices increased tone in the masseter muscles (trismus, or lockjaw). Dysphagia or stiffness or pain in the neck, shoulder, and back muscles appears concurrently or soon thereafter. The subsequent involvement of other muscles produces a rigid abdomen and stiff proximal limb muscles; the hands and feet are relatively spared. Sustained contraction of the facial muscles results in a grimace or sneer (risus sardonicus), and contraction of the back muscles produces an arched back (opisthotonos). Some patients develop paroxysmal, violent, painful, generalized muscle spasms that may cause cyanosis and threaten ventilation. These spasms occur repetitively and may be spontaneous or provoked by even the slightest stimulation. A constant threat during generalized spasms is reduced ventilation or apnea or laryngospasm. The severity of illness may be mild (muscle rigidity and few or no spasms), moderate (trismus, dysphagia, rigidity, and spasms), or severe (frequent explosive paroxysms). The patient may be febrile, although many have no fever; mentation is unimpaired. Deep tendon reflexes may be increased. Dysphagia or ileus may preclude oral feeding.

Autonomic dysfunction commonly complicates severe cases and is characterized by labile or sustained hypertension, tachycardia, dysrhythmia, hyperpyrexia, profuse sweating, peripheral vasoconstriction, and increased plasma and urinary catecholamine levels. Periods of bradycardia and hypotension may also be documented. Sudden cardiac arrest sometimes occurs, but its basis is unknown. Other complications include aspiration pneumonia, fractures, muscle rupture, deep vein thrombophlebitis, pulmonary emboli, decubitus ulcer, and rhabdomyolysis.

Neonatal tetanus usually occurs as the generalized form and is usually fatal if left untreated. It develops in children born to inadequately immunized mothers, frequently after unsterile treatment of the umbilical cord stump. Its onset generally comes during the first 2 weeks of life. Poor feeding, rigidity, and spasms are typical features of neonatal tetanus.

Local tetanus is an uncommon form in which manifestations are restricted to muscles near the wound. The prognosis is excellent.

Cephalic tetanus, a rare form of local tetanus, follows head injury or ear infection. Trismus and dysfunction of one or more cranial nerves, often the seventh nerve, are found. The incubation period is a few days and the mortality is high.

DIAGNOSIS The diagnosis of tetanus is based entirely on clinical findings. Tetanus is unlikely if a reliable history indicates the completion of a primary vaccination series and the receipt of appropriate booster doses. Wounds should be cultured in suspected cases. However, *C. tetani* can be isolated from wounds of patients without tetanus and frequently cannot be recovered from wounds of those with tetanus. The leukocyte count may be elevated. Cerebrospinal fluid examination yields normal results. Electromyograms may show continuous discharge of motor units and shortening or absence of the silent interval normally seen after an action potential. Nonspecific changes may be evident on the electrocardiogram. Muscle enzyme levels may be raised. Serum antitoxin levels of ≥ 0.01 U/mL are considered protective and make tetanus unlikely, although cases developing despite protective antitoxin levels have been reported.

The differential diagnosis includes local conditions also producing trismus, such as alveolar abscess, strychnine poisoning, dystonic drug reactions (e.g., to phenothiazines and metoclopramide), and hypocalcemic tetany. Other conditions sometimes confused with tetanus include meningitis/encephalitis, rabies, and an acute intraabdominal process (because of the rigid abdomen). Markedly increased tone in central muscles (face, neck, chest, back, and abdomen) with superimposed generalized spasms and relative sparing of the hands and feet strongly suggests tetanus.

TREATMENT **General Measures** The goals of therapy are to eliminate the source of toxin, neutralize unbound toxin, and prevent muscle spasms, monitoring the patient's condition and providing support—especially respiratory support—until recovery. Patients should be admitted to a quiet room in an intensive care unit, where observation and cardiopulmonary monitoring can be maintained continuously but stimulation can be minimized. Protection of the airway is vital. Wounds should be explored, carefully cleansed, and thoroughly debrided.

Antibiotic Therapy Although of unproven value, antibiotic therapy is administered to eradicate vegetative cells—the source of toxin. The use of penicillin (10 to 12 million units intravenously, given daily for 10 days) has been recommended, but metronidazole (500 mg every 6 h or 1 g every 12 h) is preferred by some experts on the basis of this drug's excellent antimicrobial activity, a survival rate higher than that obtained with penicillin in one nonrandomized trial, and the absence of the GABA antagonistic activity seen with penicillin. Clindamycin and erythromycin are also alternatives for the treatment of penicillin-allergic patients. Additional specific antimicrobial therapy should be given for active infection with other organisms.

Antitoxin Given to neutralize circulating toxin and unbound toxin in the wound, antitoxin effectively lowers mortality; toxin already bound to neural tissue is unaffected. Human tetanus immune globulin (TIG) is the preparation of choice and should be given promptly. The dose is 3000 to 6000 units intramuscularly, usually in divided doses because the volume is large. The optimal dose is not known, however, and results from one study indicated that a 500-unit dose was as effective as higher doses. Pooled intravenous immunoglobulin may be an alternative to TIG, but the specific antitoxin concentration in this formulation is not standardized. It may be best to administer antitoxin before manipulating the wound; the value of injecting a dose proximal to the wound or infiltrating the wound is unclear. Additional doses are unnecessary because the half-life of antitoxin is long. Antibody does not penetrate the blood-brain barrier. Intrathecal administration should be considered experimental. Equine tetanus antitoxin (TAT) is not available in the United States but is used elsewhere. It is cheaper than human antitoxin, but its half-life is shorter and its administration commonly elicits hypersensitivity and serum sickness.

Control of Muscle Spasms Many agents, alone and in combination, have been used to treat the muscle spasms of tetanus, which are painful and can threaten ventilation by causing laryngospasm or sustained contraction of ventilatory muscles. The ideal therapeutic regimen would abolish spasmodic activity without causing oversedation and hypoventilation. Diazepam, a benzodiazepine and GABA agonist, is in wide use. The dose is titrated, and large doses (≥ 250 mg/d) may be required. Lorazepam, with a longer duration of action, and midazolam, with a short half-life, are other options. Barbiturates and chlorpromazine are considered second-line agents. Therapeutic paralysis with a nondepolarizing neuromuscular blocking agent and mechanical ventilation may be required for the treatment of spasms unresponsive to medication or spasms that threaten ventilation. However, prolonged paralysis after the discontinuation of therapy with such agents has been described, and both the need for continued paralysis and the occurrence of complications should be assessed daily. Alternative agents include propofol, which is expensive, and dantrolene and baclofen, which are being investigated in the hope of shortening the period of therapeutic paralysis.

Respiratory Care Intubation or tracheostomy, with or without mechanical ventilation, may be required for hypoventilation due to oversedation or laryngospasm or for the avoidance of aspiration by patients with trismus, disordered swallowing, or dysphagia. The need for these procedures should be anticipated, and they should be undertaken electively and early.

Autonomic Dysfunction The optimal therapy for sympathetic overactivity has not been defined. Agents that have been considered include labetalol (an α- and β-adrenergic blocking agent that is recommended by some experts but that reportedly has caused sudden death), esmolol administered by continuous infusion (a beta blocker whose short half-life may be advantageous in the event of severe hypertension from unopposed α-adrenergic activity), clonidine (a central-acting antiadrenergic drug), and morphine sulfate. Parenteral magnesium sulfate and continuous spinal or epidural anesthesia have been used but may be more difficult to administer and monitor. The relative efficacy of these modalities has yet to be determined. Hypotension or bradycardia may require volume expansion, use of vasopressors or chronotropic agents, or pacemaker insertion.

Vaccine Patients recovering from tetanus should be actively immunized (see below) because immunity is not induced by the small amount of toxin that produces disease.

Additional Measures Additional therapeutic measures include hydration to control insensible and other fluid losses, which may be significant; the meeting of the patient's increased nutritional requirements by enteral or parenteral means; physiotherapy to prevent contractures; and administration of heparin or another anticoagulant to prevent pulmonary emboli. Bowel, bladder, and renal function must be monitored. Gastrointestinal bleeding and decubitus ulcers must be prevented, and intercurrent infection should be treated.

PREVENTION **Active Immunization** All partially immunized and unimmunized adults should receive vaccine, as should those recovering from tetanus. The primary series for adults consists of three doses: the first and second doses are given 4 to 8 weeks apart, and the third dose is given 6 to 12 months after the second. A booster dose is required every 10 years and may be given at mid-decade ages—35, 45, and so on. Combined tetanus and diphtheria toxoid (Td) adsorbed (for adult use), rather than single-antigen tetanus toxoid, is preferred for persons >7 years of age.

Wound Management Proper wound management requires consideration of the need for (1) passive immunization with TIG and (2) active immunization with vaccine, preferably Td in persons over age 7. For clean minor wounds, Td is administered to persons who (1) have unknown tetanus immunization histories; (2) have received fewer than three doses of adsorbed tetanus toxoid; (3) have received three or more doses of adsorbed vaccine, with the last dose given >10 years previously; and (4) have received three doses of *fluid* (nonadsorbed) vaccine. The recommendations for contaminated or severe wounds are identical, except that vaccine should be given to those who have received three or more doses of adsorbed tetanus toxoid if >5 years have elapsed since the last dose. Passive immunization with TIG is not recommended for clean minor wounds but is given for all other wounds if the patient's vaccination history indicates unknown or partial immunization. The dose of TIG for passive immunization of persons with wounds of average severity is 250 units intramuscularly, which produces a protective antibody level in the serum for at least 4 to 6 weeks; the appropriate dose of TAT is 3000 to 6000 units. Vaccine and tetanus antitoxin should be administered at separate sites in separate syringes.

Neonatal Tetanus Measures aimed at preventing neonatal tetanus include maternal vaccination, even during pregnancy; efforts to increase the proportion of births that take place in the hospital; and the provision of training for nonmedical birth attendants.

PROGNOSIS The application of methods to monitor and support oxygenation has markedly improved the prognosis in tetanus;

mortality rates as low as 10% have been reported from units accustomed to handling such cases. In the United States during the period 1995 through 1997, the case-fatality rate was 11%; 11 deaths from tetanus were reported in 1990, 11 in 1991, and 9 in 1992. The outcome is poor in neonates and the elderly and in patients with a short incubation period, a short interval from the onset of symptoms to admission, or a short period from onset of symptoms to the first spasm (period of onset). Outcome is also related to the extent of prior vaccination.

The course of tetanus extends over 4 to 6 weeks, and patients may require ventilatory support for 3 weeks during this period. Increased tone and minor spasms can last for months, but recovery is usually complete.

BIBLIOGRAPHY

ABRUTYN E, BERLIN JA: Intrathecal therapy of tetanus: A meta-analysis. JAMA 266: 2262, 1991

AHMADSYAH I, SALIM A: Treatment of tetanus: An open study to compare the efficacy of procaine penicillin and metronidazole. BMJ 291:648, 1985

BARDENHEIER B et al: Tetanus surveillance—United States, 1995–1997. MMWR 47:1, 1998

BLECK TP: *Clostridium tetani* (tetanus), in *Principles and Practice of Infectious Diseases*, 5th ed, GL Mandell et al (eds). New York, Churchill Livingstone, 2000, pp 2537–2543

CENTERS FOR DISEASE CONTROL AND PREVENTION: Tetanus among injecting-drug users—California, 1997. MMWR 47:149, 1998

TOBIAS JD: Anesthetic implications of tetanus. South Med J 91:384, 1998

---

144   *Elias Abrutyn*

BOTULISM

DEFINITION Botulism is a paralytic disease that begins with cranial nerve involvement and progresses caudally to involve the extremities. It is caused by potent protein neurotoxins elaborated by *Clostridium botulinum*. The toxins' high potency has led to consideration of their use in bioterrorism or biological warfare. Cases may be classified as (1) *food-borne botulism*, from ingestion of preformed toxin in food contaminated with *C. botulinum*; (2) *wound botulism*, from toxin produced in wounds contaminated with the organism; (3) *infant botulism*, from ingestion of spores and production of toxin in the intestine of infants; or (4) *adult infectious botulism*, a group that includes some cases in older children and adults in which disease is produced by a mechanism similar to that described for infant botulism.

ETIOLOGIC AGENT *C. botulinum*, a species encompassing a heterogeneous group of anaerobic gram-positive organisms that form subterminal spores, is found in soil and marine environments throughout the world and elaborates the most potent bacterial toxin known. Organisms of types A through G have been distinguished by the antigenic specificities of their toxins; a classification system based on physiologic characteristics has also been described. Rare strains of other clostridial species—*C. butyricum* and *C. baratii*—have also been found to produce toxin. *C. botulinum* strains with proteolytic activity can digest food and produce a spoiled appearance; nonproteolytic types leave the appearance of food unchanged.

Of the eight distinct toxin types described (A, B, C_1, C_2, D, E, F, and G), all except C_2 are neurotoxins; C_2 is a cytotoxin of unknown clinical significance. Botulinum neurotoxin, whether ingested or produced in the intestine or a wound, enters the vascular system and is transported to peripheral cholinergic nerve terminals, including neuromuscular junctions, postganglionic parasympathetic nerve endings, and peripheral ganglia. The central nervous system is not involved. Active neurotoxin (150 kDa) is composed of a heavy chain (a 100-kDa fragment responsible for neurospecific binding and translocation into the nerve cell) and a light chain (a 50-kDa fragment responsible for intracellular catalytic activity). The steps involved in neurotoxin activity include (1) specific binding to presynaptic nerve cells at the myoneural junction, (2) internalization of the toxin inside the nerve cell in endocytic vesicles, (3) translocation of the toxin into the cytosol, and (4) proteolysis by toxin (a zinc endopeptidase) of components of the neuroexocytosis apparatus curtailing release of the neurotransmitter acetylcholine. Cure follows sprouting of new nerve terminals.

Toxin is heat-labile, but spores are highly heat-resistant; both can be inactivated under appropriate conditions (see "Prevention," below). In the gastrointestinal tract, toxin is complexed with nontoxin proteins and resists degradation.

Toxin types A, B, E, and (in rare instances) F cause human disease; type G (now called *C. argentinense*) has been associated with sudden death, but not with neuroparalytic illness, in a few patients in Switzerland; and types C and D cause animal disease.

EPIDEMIOLOGY Human botulism occurs worldwide. In the United States, the geographic distribution of cases by toxin type parallels the distribution of organism types found in the environment. Type A predominates west of the Rocky Mountains; type B is generally distributed but is more common in the East; and type E is found in the Pacific Northwest, Alaska, and the Great Lakes area. In the United States, food-borne botulism has been associated primarily with home-canned food, particularly vegetables, fruit, and condiments, and less commonly with meat and fish. Type E outbreaks are frequently associated with fish products. Commercial products occasionally cause outbreaks, but some of these outbreaks have resulted from improper handling after purchase. Outbreaks in restaurants, schools, and private homes have been traced to uncommon sources (commercial potpies, beef stew, turkey loaf, sauteed onions, baked potatoes, and chopped garlic in oil). Food-borne botulism can occur when (1) a food to be preserved is contaminated with spores, (2) preservation does not inactivate the spores but kills other putrefactive bacteria that might inhibit the growth of *C. botulinum* and provides anaerobic conditions at a pH and temperature that allow germination and toxin production, and (3) food is not heated to a temperature that destroys toxin before being eaten.

CLINICAL MANIFESTATIONS **Food-Borne Botulism** Following ingestion of food containing toxin, illness varies from a mild condition for which no medical advice is sought to very severe disease that can result in death within 24 h. The incubation period is usually 18 to 36 h but, depending on toxin dose, can extend from a few hours to several days. Symmetric descending paralysis is characteristic and can lead to respiratory failure and death. Cranial nerve involvement, which almost always marks the onset of symptoms, usually produces diplopia, dysarthria, and/or dysphagia. Weakness progresses, often rapidly, from the head to involve the neck, arms, thorax, and legs; the weakness is occasionally asymmetric. Nausea, vomiting, and abdominal pain may precede or follow the onset of paralysis. Dizziness, blurred vision, dry mouth, and very dry, occasionally sore throat are common. Patients are generally alert and oriented, but they may be drowsy, agitated, and anxious. Typically, they have no fever. Ptosis is frequent; the pupillary reflexes may be depressed, and fixed or dilated pupils are noted in half of patients. The gag reflex may be suppressed, and deep tendon reflexes may be normal or decreased. Paralytic ileus, severe constipation, and urinary retention are common.

Wound Botulism When wounds are contaminated with *C. botulinum* spores, the spores may germinate into vegetative organisms that produce toxin. This rare condition resembles food-borne illness except that the incubation period is longer, averaging about 10 days, and gastrointestinal symptoms are lacking. Wound botulism has been documented after traumatic injury involving contamination with soil; in injection drug users, for whom black-tar heroin use has been identified as a risk factor; and after cesarean delivery. The illness has occurred even after antibiotics have been given to prevent wound infection. When present, fever is probably attributable to concurrent infection with other bacteria. The wound may appear benign.

Infant Botulism In infant botulism, the most common form of the disease, toxin is produced in and absorbed from the intestine after the germination of ingested spores. The severity ranges from mild illness with failure to thrive to fulminant severe paralysis with respiratory failure and may be one cause of sudden infant death. The identification of contaminated honey as one source of spores has led to the recommendation that honey not be fed to children <12 months of age. Most cases cannot be attributed to a particular food source. The factors permitting intestinal colonization with *C. botulinum* are not fully defined, but cases usually involve infants <6 months of age; susceptibility may decrease as the normal intestinal flora develops.

Adult Infectious Botulism Rarely, botulism in adults is produced by a mechanism similar to that operative in infant botulism: intestinal colonization and toxin production. The patient may have a history of gastrointestinal disease, surgery, or recent antibiotic therapy. Toxin and organisms may be identified in the stool.

DIAGNOSIS A diagnosis of botulism must be considered in afebrile, mentally intact patients who have symmetric descending paralysis without sensory findings. The diagnosis must be suspected on clinical grounds in the context of an appropriate history. Conditions often confused with botulism include myasthenia gravis, which may be ruled out by electromyography and antibody studies, and Guillain-Barré syndrome, which is characterized by ascending paralysis, sensory abnormalities, and elevation of the protein concentration in cerebrospinal fluid. The Fisher variant of Guillain-Barré—a descending paralysis—can indeed be difficult to differentiate from botulism. Other conditions that may resemble botulism include Lambert-Eaton syndrome, poliomyelitis, tick paralysis, diphtheria, and intoxications from mushrooms, medications, or chemicals. Hypermagnesemia should be considered.

The demonstration of toxin in serum by bioassay in mice is definitive, but this test may be negative, particularly in wound and infant botulism. It is performed only by specific laboratories, which can be identified through regional public health authorities. Other assays are being developed and remain experimental. The demonstration of the organism or its toxin in vomitus, gastric fluid, or stool is strongly suggestive of the diagnosis, because intestinal carriage is rare. Isolation of the organism from food without toxin is insufficient grounds for the diagnosis. Wound cultures yielding the organism are suggestive of botulism. The edrophonium chloride (Tensilon) test for myasthenia gravis may be falsely positive in botulism but is usually less dramatically positive than in the former condition. Nerve conduction velocity is normal, but compound muscle action potentials on routine nerve stimulation studies are decreased with a supramaximal stimulus, and facilitation is evident after repetitive stimulation at high frequency. Single-fiber electromyography may be helpful. The white blood cell count and erythrocyte sedimentation rate are normal.

℞ TREATMENT Patients should be hospitalized and monitored closely, both clinically and by spirometry, pulse oximetry, and measurement of arterial blood gases for incipient respiratory failure. Intubation and mechanical ventilation should be strongly considered when the vital capacity is <30% of predicted, especially when paralysis is progressing rapidly and hypoxemia with absolute or relative hypercarbia is documented (Chap. 266). Serial measurements of the maximal static inspiratory pressure may be useful in predicting respiratory failure.

In food-borne illness, trivalent (types A, B, and E) equine antitoxin should be administered as soon as possible after specimens are obtained for laboratory analysis. The initiation of treatment should not await laboratory confirmation, which may take days. After testing for hypersensitivity to horse serum, a vial of antitoxin is given; repeated doses are not considered necessary. Anaphylaxis and serum sickness are risks inherent in use of the equine product, and desensitization of allergic patients may be required. If there is no ileus, cathartics and enemas may be given to purge the gut of toxin; emetics or gastric lavage can also be used if the time since ingestion is brief (only a few hours). Use of antibiotics to eliminate an intestinal source for possible continued toxin production and of guanidine hydrochloride and other drugs to reverse paralysis is of unproven value. In the United States, antitoxin as well as help in clinical management and laboratory confirmation are available at *any* time from state health departments or from the Centers for Disease Control and Prevention [at (404)639-2206; emergency number: (404)639-2888].

Treatment of infant botulism requires supportive care. Neither equine antitoxin nor antibiotics have been shown to be beneficial, and the value of human botulism immune globulin, an experimental preparation, is still being evaluated. In wound botulism, equine antitoxin is administered. The wound should be thoroughly explored and debrided, and an antibiotic such as penicillin should be given to eradicate *C. botulinum* from the site, even though the benefit of this therapy is unproven. Results of wound cultures should guide the use of other antibiotics.

Botulinum toxin is being used as therapy for strabismus, blepharospasm, and other dystonias and appears safe and effective. Generalized botulism-like weakness complicating therapy has been reported.

PROGNOSIS Type A disease is generally more severe than type B, and mortality from botulism is higher among patients above age 60 than among younger patients. With improved respiratory and intensive care, the case-fatality rate in food-borne illness has been reduced to ~7.5% and is low in infant botulism as well. Artificial respiratory support may be required for months in severe cases. Some patients experience residual weakness and autonomic dysfunction for as long as a year after disease onset.

PREVENTION A pentavalent vaccine (A–E) is available for use in highly exposed individuals. Spores can be inactivated by exposure to a temperature of 116° to 121°C (e.g., in steam sterilizers or pressure cookers). Toxin can be inactivated by exposure to a temperature of 100°C for 10 min. Newly identified cases should be reported immediately to public health authorities.

BIBLIOGRAPHY

Angulo FJ et al: Large outbreak of botulism: The hazardous baked potato. Clin Infect Dis 178:172, 1998

Bhatia KP et al: Generalised muscular weakness after botulinum toxin injection for dystonia: A report of three cases. J Neurol Neurosurg Psychiatry 67:90, 1999

Cherington M: Clinical spectrum of botulism. Muscle Nerve 21:701, 1998

Hatheway CL: Botulism: The present status of disease. Curr Top Microbiol Immunol 195:55, 1995

Montecucco C et al: Botulinum neurotoxins: Mechanism of action and therapeutic implications. Mol Med Today 2:418, 1996

Passaro DJ et al: Wound botulism associated with black tar heroin among injecting drug users. JAMA 279:859, 1998

Shapiro RL et al: Botulism in the United States: A clinical and epidemiologic review. Ann Intern Med 129:221, 1998

145 *Dennis L. Kasper, Dori F. Zaleznik*

GAS GANGRENE, ANTIBIOTIC-ASSOCIATED COLITIS, AND OTHER CLOSTRIDIAL INFECTIONS

DEFINITION Bacteria of the genus *Clostridium* are gram-positive, spore-forming, obligate anaerobes that are ubiquitous in nature. There are more than 60 recognized species of clostridia, many of which are generally considered saprophytic. Some of these species are pathogenic for humans and animals, particularly under conditions of lowered oxidation-reduction potential. Infections associated with these organisms range from localized wound contamination to overwhelming

systemic disease. The four major disease categories for which clostridia are responsible are intestinal disorders, deep tissue suppurative infections, skin and soft tissue infections, and bacteremia (Table 145-1). Toxins play a major role in some of these syndromes.

ETIOLOGY In humans, clostridia normally reside in the gastrointestinal tract and in the female genital tract, although they occasionally are isolated from the skin or the mouth. Of the known species of the genus *Clostridium*, at least 30 have been isolated from human infections. Like several other pathogenic anaerobic bacterial species, clostridia are quite aerotolerant, but they do not grow on artificial media in the presence of oxygen. Clostridia characteristically produce abundant gas in artificial media and form subterminal endospores. *C. perfringens*, one of the most important species, is encapsulated and nonmotile and rarely sporulates in artificial media; the spores can usually be destroyed by boiling. *C. tetani* and *C. botulinum* are discussed in detail in Chaps. 143 and 144, respectively.

Clostridia are present in the normal colonic flora at concentrations of 10^9 to 10^{10} per gram. Of the 30 or more species that normally colonize humans, *C. ramosum* is the most common and is followed in frequency by *C. perfringens*. These organisms are universally present in soil at concentrations of up to 10^4 per gram. Although clostridia are gram-positive organisms, many species may appear to be gram-negative in clinical specimens or stationary-phase cultures. Therefore, the results of Gram's staining of cultures or clinical material should be interpreted with great care.

C. perfringens is the most common of the clostridial species isolated from tissue infections and bacteremias; next in frequency are *C. novyi* and *C. septicum*. In the category of enteric infections, *C. difficile* is an important cause of antibiotic-associated colitis, and *C. perfringens* is associated with food poisoning (type A) and enteritis necroticans (type C).

PATHOGENESIS Despite the isolation of clostridial species from many serious traumatic wounds, the prevalence of severe infections due to these organisms is low. Two factors that appear to be essential to the development of severe disease are tissue necrosis and a low oxidation-reduction potential. *C. perfringens* requires about 14 amino acids and at least 6 additional growth factors for optimal growth. These nutrients are not found in appreciable concentrations in normal body fluids but are present in necrotic tissue. When *C. perfringens* grows in necrotic tissue, a zone of tissue damage due to the toxins elaborated by the organism allows progressive growth. In contrast, when only a few bacteria leak into the bloodstream from a small defect in the intestinal wall, the organisms do not have the opportunity to multiply rapidly because blood as a medium for growth is relatively deficient in certain amino acids and growth factors. Therefore, in a patient without tissue necrosis, bacteremia is usually benign.

C. perfringens possesses at least 17 possible virulence factors, including 12 active tissue toxins and enterotoxins. This species has been divided into five types (A through E) on the basis of four major lethal toxins: α, β, ϵ, and ι. The α toxin is a phospholipase C (lecithinase) that splits lecithin into phosphorylcholine and diglyceride. This α toxin has been associated with gas gangrene and is known to be hemolytic, to destroy platelets and polymorphonuclear leukocytes (PMNs), and to cause widespread capillary damage. When injected intravenously, it causes massive intravascular hemolysis and damages liver mitochondria. The α toxin may be important in the initiation of muscle

Table 145-1 Classification of Diseases Caused by Clostridia

1. Intestinal disorders
   a. Food poisoning
   b. Enteritis necroticans
   c. Antibiotic-associated colitis
2. Suppurative deep tissue infections
   a. Mixed bacterial infections
   b. Monobacterial infections
3. Skin and soft tissue infections
   a. Simple contamination
   b. Local infection without systemic signs
   c. Spreading cellulitis and fasciitis
   d. Myonecrosis (gas gangrene)
4. Bacteremia
   a. Transient bacteremia
   b. Sepsis

infections that may progress to gas gangrene. Experimentally, the higher the concentration of α toxin in the culture fluid, the smaller the dose of *C. perfringens* required to produce infection. The protective effect of antiserum is directly proportional to its content of α antitoxin. Studies suggest that θ toxin may also play an important role in pathogenesis by promoting vascular leukostasis, endothelial cell injury, and regional tissue hypoxia. The resulting perfusion defects extend the anaerobic environment and contribute to rapidly advancing tissue destruction. A characteristic pathologic finding in gas gangrene is the near absence of PMNs despite extensive tissue destruction. Experimental data indicate that both α and θ toxins are essential in the leukocyte aggregation that occurs at the margins of tissue injury instead of the expected infiltration of these cells into the area of damage. Genetically altered strains induce less leukocyte aggregation when α toxin is absent and none when θ toxin is missing. The other major toxins, β, ϵ, and ι, are known to increase capillary permeability.

C. difficile produces two major toxins, designated A and B. Both toxins appear to act by the same mechanism, but toxin B is 1000 times more potent. These toxins exert their effect by binding to small guanosine triphosphate–binding proteins in the Rho family within target cells. The toxins are uridine diphosphoglucose hydrolases and glucosyltransferases that glycosylate the guanosine triphosphatases, inactivating these proteins and resulting in disruption of actin. Once the actin filaments are destroyed, the cell is unable to function. Toxin B has 100-fold greater enzymatic activity than toxin A.

Diarrheal disease due to *C. difficile* is toxin-mediated. Earlier teaching about the pathogenesis of this disease centered on the overgrowth of *C. difficile* when antibiotics suppress the normal bowel flora. Actually, the mechanism is probably more complex, since many of the antibiotics that cause this disease are active against *C. difficile* as well as other members of the bowel flora and since many patients who become colonized with *C. difficile* do not develop diarrhea. Critical features in the pathogenesis of this disease include mechanisms of toxin production and the interaction of *C. difficile* with other components of the bowel flora. Some antibiotics may actually trigger toxin production by the organism. In turn, other constituents of the bowel flora may suppress or inhibit toxin production. *C. sordellii*, for example, neutralizes cytotoxin B in vitro. In addition, when antibiotics eliminate more sensitive members of the bowel flora, more resistant organisms may produce enzymes such as β-lactamases that can inactivate antibiotics and thereby facilitate the growth of *C. difficile*.

CLINICAL MANIFESTATIONS **Intestinal Disorders** •
Food poisoning *C. perfringens*, primarily type A, is the second or third most common cause of food poisoning in the United States (Chap. 131). The responsible toxin is thought to be a cytotoxin produced by more than 75% of strains isolated from cases of foodborne disease. The cytotoxin binds to a receptor on the small-bowel brush border and induces a calcium ion–dependent alteration in permeability. The associated loss of ions alters intracellular metabolism, resulting in cell death. Outbreaks generally have resulted from problems in the cooling and storage of food cooked in bulk. The food sources primarily involved are meat, meat products, and poultry. Generally, the implicated meats have been cooked, allowed to cool, and then recooked the following day, often in a stew or hash. Strains of *C. perfringens* that contaminate meat manage to survive initial cooking. During reheating, the organisms sporulate and germinate. The disease is associated with an attack rate that is often as high as 70%. Symptoms of food poisoning from type A strains develop 8 to 24 h after ingestion of foods heavily contaminated with the organism. The primary symptoms include epigastric pain, nausea, and watery diarrhea usually lasting 12 to 24 h. Fever and vomiting are uncommon. Molecular methods including ribotyping and pulsed-field gel electrophoresis have been used to detect fecal cytotoxin in outbreaks of food poisoning caused by *C. perfringens*.

C. perfringens has also been implicated in a more severe form of diarrhea than that of classic food poisoning. This more severe disease tends to occur in the elderly and has been associated with antibiotic use in hospitalized populations. In this form of disease, diarrhea is generally more profuse, of longer duration, and accompanied by abdominal pain. Blood and mucus have been detected in the feces of the affected patients. In one hospital-based study of a cluster of cases, widespread environmental contamination with *C. perfringens* spores was documented.

Enteritis necroticans Necrotizing enteritis (enteritis necroticans, or *pigbel*) is caused by β toxin produced by type C strains of *C. perfringens* following ingestion of a high-protein meal in conjunction with trypsin inhibitors (e.g., in sweet potatoes) by a susceptible host who has limited intestinal proteolytic activity. This disease has been reported among children and adults in New Guinea. A similar disease, *darmbrand*, was epidemic in Germany after World War II. Clinical features of pigbel include acute abdominal pain, bloody diarrhea, vomiting, shock, and peritonitis; 40% of patients die. Pathologic studies reveal an acute ulcerative process of the bowel restricted to the small intestine. The mucosa is lifted off the submucosa, with the formation of large denuded areas. Pseudomembranes composed of sloughed epithelium are common, and gas may dissect into the submucosa. The source of the organisms may be the patient's own intestinal flora; cultures of ingested pork have failed to yield the organism. Antibodies to the β toxin of *C. perfringens* have been of considerable benefit in changing the course of established disease. In a large-scale trial, children immunized with *C. perfringens* β toxoid were protected.

Neutropenic enterocolitis (typhlitis) See Chaps. 85 and 167.

Antibiotic-associated colitis Strains of *C. difficile* that produce toxins detectable in the stool are the only identified cause of colitis induced by antibiotic use. The diagnosis of this type of colitis requires that there be no other identifiable cause of diarrhea and that the onset of symptoms occur either during antimicrobial administration or within 4 weeks after treatment with the implicated agent has been discontinued. Essentially any antibiotic can cause this syndrome; even metronidazole and vancomycin, which are used to treat the disease, have been implicated as etiologic agents in some cases. On a per-use basis, clindamycin, which was the first antibiotic described to cause this entity, is the most commonly implicated antibiotic. However, since other antibiotics are prescribed more often than clindamycin in the United States, cephalosporins are currently the antibiotics that most commonly cause *C. difficile* enterocolitis, and penicillins rank next in frequency. Diarrhea due to *C. difficile* has been reported in patients with some forms of malignancy or renal transplantation who have received tacrolimus without concomitant or previous antibiotic administration.

Antimicrobial-associated diarrhea can be divided into four categories based on the appearance of the colon: (1) normal colonic mucosa; (2) mild erythema with some edema; (3) granular, friable, or hemorrhagic mucosa; and (4) pseudomembrane formation. Most patients with antibiotic-associated diarrhea have a normal, minimally erythematous colonic mucosa with some edema. Occasionally, colitis is more severe and is characterized by a granular, friable, or hemorrhagic mucosa. Examination of stool from the affected patients may reveal large numbers of red blood cells and some leukocytes. Biopsy shows subepithelial edema with round cell infiltration of the lamina propria and focal extravasation of erythrocytes. *C. difficile* cytotoxin B has been found in 15 to 75% of stools from patients in the first three categories, which suggests that other factors are involved in the pathogenesis of antibiotic-associated diarrhea.

The most characteristic form of antibiotic-associated colitis caused by *C. difficile* is pseudomembranous colitis (PMC). More than 95% of patients with documented PMC have positive stool toxin assays. Close inspection of pseudomembranes reveals exudative, punctate, raised plaques with skip areas or edematous hyperemic mucosa. These plaques can enlarge and coalesce over large segments of intestine in the later stages of disease. The clinical spectrum of antibiotic-associated PMC is diverse. Diarrhea is the key feature; stools are usually watery, voluminous, and without gross blood or mucus. Most patients have abdominal cramps and tenderness, fever, and leukocytosis. However, the symptoms vary considerably. At one end of the spectrum are many patients with annoying diarrhea but no systemic signs or symptoms, while at the other end are those with severe systemic toxicity, fever (40° to 40.6°C, or 104° to 105°F), and peripheral white blood cell counts of up to 50,000/μL with a marked left shift. Fecal examination frequently reveals leukocytes. Without specific therapy, the course is highly variable. Some patients, particularly those with clinically mild disease, experience prompt resolution of symptoms with discontinuation of drug treatment, while others have protracted diarrhea with large stool volumes for up to 8 weeks, with resultant hypoalbuminemia and electrolyte imbalance. Severely ill patients with toxic megacolon and colonic perforation have been reported. Among patients who are severely ill mortality rates may be as high as 30%, while in most of those with minimal symptoms disease may resolve with the discontinuation of antibiotic treatment alone. In the majority of patients, symptoms begin 4 to 10 days after antibiotic therapy is initiated. However, ~25% of patients do not develop symptoms until use of the implicated antimicrobial has been discontinued, in some instances as long as 4 weeks afterward. Some cases have been reported within hours after initiation of antibiotic therapy or after a single dose of antibiotic administered for surgical prophylaxis.

Suppurative Deep Tissue Infections Clostridia are frequently recovered from various suppurative conditions in conjunction with other anaerobic and aerobic bacteria but can also be the only organisms isolated. These suppurative conditions, which exist with severe local inflammation but usually without the characteristic systemic signs induced by clostridial toxins, include intraabdominal sepsis, empyema, pelvic abscess, subcutaneous abscess, frostbite with gas gangrene, infection of a stump in an amputee, brain abscess, prostatic abscess, perianal abscess, conjunctivitis, infection of a renal cell carcinoma, and infection of an aortic graft.

Clostridia are isolated from approximately two-thirds of patients with intraabdominal infections resulting from intestinal perforation. *C. ramosum*, *C. perfringens*, and *C. bifermentans* are the most commonly isolated species. The presence of clostridial species does not affect the clinical presentation or outcome of these infections (Chap. 167).

An association has been made between malignancy and the isolation of *C. septicum* in the absence of grossly contaminated deep traumatic wounds. A major site for such a malignancy is the gastrointestinal tract, particularly the colon. An association with leukemia or with other solid tumors has also been noted, and one case of fatal myonecrosis has been reported in a patient with ovarian cancer. Some of these patients present with *C. septicum* bacteremia; these cases have a fulminant clinical course (discussed below). Others develop localized suppurative infection in the abdomen or the abdominal wall without bacteremia. Presumably, this infection arises from a silent perforation that leads to intraabdominal abscess formation.

Clostridia have been isolated from suppurative infections of the female genital tract, particularly tuboovarian and pelvic abscesses. The major species involved has been *C. perfringens*. Most of these are mild suppurative infections without evidence of uterine gangrene. *C. perfringens* has been isolated from as many as 20% of diseased gallbladders at surgery. One clinical syndrome, emphysematous cholecystitis, is caused by clostridial species at least 50% of the time. In this syndrome, gas forms in the biliary radicles and the wall of the gallbladder. It is seen most often in diabetic patients. Although the mortality rate in this entity is higher than in more common forms of cholecystitis, there is no evidence of myonecrosis.

Clostridia are among the many organisms found in empyema fluid or isolated by transtracheal aspiration from patients with lung abscesses. There is no unique clinical clue to the presence of clostridia (as opposed to other organisms) in these infections. *C. perfringens* has been reported as a cause of empyema arising from aspiration pneumonia, pulmonary emboli, and infarction. However, the majority of cases of clostridial empyema are secondary to trauma.

Skin and Soft Tissue Infections Various categories of traumatic wound infections due to clostridia have been described: simple contamination, anaerobic cellulitis, fasciitis with or without systemic manifestations, and anaerobic myonecrosis.

Simple contamination Clostridia are cultured most often from wounds in the absence of clinical signs of sepsis. As many as 30% of battle wounds are contaminated by clostridia without signs of suppuration, and 16% of penetrating abdominal wounds yield clostridia on culture despite treatment with cephalothin and kanamycin. In cases of trauma, clostridia are isolated with equal frequency from suppurative and well-healing wounds. Thus the diagnosis of clostridial infection should be based on clinical rather than bacteriologic criteria.

Localized infection of the skin and soft tissue without systemic signs This condition, originally referred to as *anaerobic cellulitis*, is a localized infection involving the skin and soft tissue and is due to clostridia alone or with other bacteria. There are no systemic signs of toxicity, although the infection may invade locally, producing necrosis. These infections tend to be relatively indolent, spreading slowly to contiguous areas. Localized infections are relatively free of pain and edema. Perhaps because of the lack of edema, gas that is limited to the wound and the immediately surrounding tissue may be more evident than in gas gangrene. In these localized infections, gas is never found intramuscularly. Cellulitis, perirectal abscesses, and diabetic foot ulcers are typical infections from which clostridial species can be isolated. If inadequately treated, these localized infections advance by extension through subcutaneous tissue and fascial planes into muscle and may produce severe systemic disease with signs of toxemia.

A localized form of suppurative myositis has been described in heroin addicts. These patients develop local pain and tenderness in discrete areas (particularly the thigh and forearm), with the subsequent appearance of fluctuance and crepitance that require surgical drainage. The unusual aspect of these infections is that they remain localized without systemic signs of toxicity. Moreover, the affected local areas are not necessarily sites of trauma or heroin injection. Pathologic examination reveals subcutaneous abscesses, purulent myositis, and fasciitis from which clostridia are recovered in pure culture; on occasion, mixed infections involving aerobes and anaerobes are found. Wound botulism has been reported in association with the injection of black tar heroin.

Spreading cellulitis and fasciitis with systemic toxicity This condition involves diffuse spreading cellulitis and fasciitis, without myonecrosis and with only mild inflammation in muscle. Patients present with the abrupt onset of a syndrome that progresses rapidly (within hours) through the fascial planes. In cases with suppuration and gas in soft tissues as well as overwhelming toxemia, the infection is rapidly fatal. On physical examination there is subcutaneous crepitation but little localized pain. Surgery is of no proven value because there are no discretely involved tissues amenable to resection, as may be the case in myonecrosis. However, in rapidly advancing fasciitis, incision of the affected area is still the cornerstone of therapy. The initial local lesion may be quite innocuous and arises from an area involved by tumor or other infection and not by injury. The systemic toxic effects include hemolysis and injury of capillary membranes. Usually, this infection is uniformly fatal within 48 h, despite intensive therapy involving antitoxin and exchange transfusion. This syndrome is seen most commonly in patients with carcinoma, especially of the sigmoid or the cecum. Presumably, the tumor invades the fascia, and colonic contents leak into the abdominal wall. Patients present with extreme toxicity and occasionally with total-body crepitation. The syndrome differs from necrotizing fasciitis caused by other organisms in three respects: (1) rapid mortality, (2) rapid tissue invasion, and (3) the systemic effects of the toxin, typified by massive hemolysis.

Clostridial myonecrosis (gas gangrene) Clostridial myonecrosis occurs when bacteria invade healthy muscle from adjacent traumatized muscle or soft tissue. The infection originates in a wound contaminated with clostridia. Although >30% of deep wounds are infected with clostridia, the incidence of clostridial myonecrosis is quite low. These infections occur in both military and civilian settings. An essential factor in the genesis of gas gangrene appears to be trauma, particularly involving deep muscle laceration. The entity of clostridial myonecrosis is relatively uncommon after simple, through-and-through bullet wounds without shattering of bone and is relatively common following shrapnel fragmentation wounds, particularly when deep muscle is involved. In civilian cases, gas gangrene can follow trauma, surgery, or intramuscular injection. The trauma need not be severe; however, the wound must be deep, necrotic, and without communication to the surface.

The incubation period of gas gangrene is usually short: almost always <3 days and frequently <24 h. Some 80% of cases are caused by *C. perfringens*, while *C. novyi*, *C. septicum*, and *C. histolyticum* cause most of the other cases. Typically, gas gangrene begins with the sudden onset of pain in the region of the wound, which helps to differentiate it from spreading cellulitis. Once established, the pain increases steadily in severity but remains localized to the infected area and spreads only if the infection spreads. Soon after pain develops, local swelling and edema—ac-

FIGURE 145-1 Spontaneous gas gangrene. Radiographs of the elbow (*A*) and shoulder (*B*) show gas in tissue. The patient developed spontaneous gas gangrene of the hand, which spread rapidly up the arm and onto the thorax. *C. septicum* was grown from blood and necrotic tissue of the arm. *[Reprinted with permission from DL Stevens (ed): Atlas of Infecticus Diseases, vol II: Skin, Soft Tissue, Bone and Joint Infections. Philadelphia, Current Medicine, 1995.]*

companied by a thin, often hemorrhagic exudate—appear. Patients frequently develop marked tachycardia, but elevation in temperature may be only minimal. Gas is usually not obvious at this early stage and may be completely absent. Frothiness of the wound exudate may be noted. The skin is tense, white, often marbled with blue, and cooler than normal. The symptoms progress rapidly; swelling, edema, and toxemia increase, and a profuse serous discharge, which may have a peculiar sweetish smell, appears. Gram's staining of the wound exudate shows many gram-positive rods with relatively few inflammatory cells.

At surgery, muscle may appear pale because of the intensity of edema, but it does not contract when probed with a scalpel. When dissected, the muscle is beefy red and nonviable and can progress to become black, friable, and gangrenous. It is important to establish a diagnosis early, preferably by frozen-section biopsy of muscle.

Despite hypotension, renal failure, and (often) body crepitation, patients with myonecrosis frequently have a heightened awareness of their surroundings until just before death, when they lapse into toxic delirium and coma. In untreated cases, as the local wounds progress, the skin becomes bronzed; bullae appear, become filled with dark red fluid, and are accompanied by dark patches of cutaneous gangrene. Gas appears in later phases (Fig. 145-1) but may not be as obvious as in anaerobic cellulitis. Jaundice is rare in wound gas gangrene (in contrast to uterine infections) and, when it does appear, is almost invariably associated with hemoglobinuria, hemoglobinemia, and septicemia. Cases of clostridial myonecrosis without a history of trauma have been reported. These patients have bullous lesions and crepitation of the skin; they present with a rapidly worsening course that includes myonecrosis, especially of the extremities.

Bacteremia and Clostridial Sepsis The relatively common entity of transient clostridial bacteremia can arise in any hospitalized patient but is most common with a predisposing focus in the gastrointestinal tract, biliary tract, or uterus. Fever frequently resolves within 24 to 48 h without therapy. Despite the finding of clostridial bacteremia following septic abortions and the frequent isolation of clostridia from the lochia, most of the patients involved do not have evidence of sepsis. In one series of 60 patients with clostridial bacteremia, half had an infected site that could be associated with the bacteremia, while

the other half had a totally unrelated illness, such as tuberculous pneumonia, meningitis, or benign gastroenteritis. By the time blood culture reports are returned, patients frequently are completely well and sometimes have been discharged. Therefore, when a blood culture is positive for clostridia, the patient must be assessed clinically rather than simply treated on the basis of the culture result.

Clostridial sepsis is an uncommon but almost invariably fatal illness following clostridial infection—primarily that of the uterus, colon, or biliary tract. This entity must be differentiated from transient clostridial bacteremia which is much more common. *C. perfringens* causes the majority of cases of sepsis as well as the majority of cases of transient bacteremia. *C. septicum, C. sordellii,* and *C. novyi* account for most of the remainder of cases. Clostridia account for 1 to 2.5% of all positive blood cultures in major hospital centers.

The majority of cases of clostridial sepsis originate from the female genital tract and follow septic abortion. Introduction of a foreign body is a common antecedent event. In the uterus, residual necrotic fetal and placental tissues and traumatized endometrium may allow the growth of clostridia. Only a small fraction of cases of septic abortion (1%) are followed by serious sepsis. In these patients, sepsis, fever, and chills begin from 1 to 3 days after the attempted abortion. The initial signs are malaise, headache, severe myalgias, abdominal pain, nausea, vomiting, and occasionally diarrhea. Frequently, a bloody or brown vaginal discharge is noted. Patients may rapidly develop oliguria, hypotension, jaundice, and hemoglobinuria. The hemolysis, which is secondary to *C. perfringens* α toxin, causes a characteristic bronzing of the skin. As in myonecrosis, the mental status of severely ill patients is characterized by increased alertness and apprehension. Local examination of the pelvis reveals foul cervical discharge, occasionally with gas. Frequently, laceration marks around the cervix or perforation of the cervical segment is evident. If the infection involves the myometrium or has spread to the adnexa, extreme tenderness, guarding, and an adnexal mass may be found.

Laboratory studies in patients with sepsis reveal an elevated white blood cell count and may show pink, hemoglobin-tinged plasma. Anemia is proportional to the degree of hemolysis, and the hematocrit may be extremely low. Platelet counts may be reduced, and there is often evidence of disseminated intravascular coagulation. Oliguria or anuria, increasingly refractory hypotension, and hemorrhage and bruising may develop.

Clostridia may enter the bloodstream from the gastrointestinal or biliary tract. This occurrence is associated with ulcerative lesions or obstruction of the small or large intestine, necrotic or infiltrating malignancy, bowel surgery, or various abdominal catastrophes. The patient may present with an acute febrile illness, with chills and fever but no other signs of localized infection. Intravascular hemolysis occurs in as many as half of such cases. Biliary or gastrointestinal symptoms, if present, may be the only clue to the etiology. Positive blood cultures provide the definitive clue to the diagnosis.

Patients with malignant disease can also develop rapidly fatal clostridial sepsis, particularly from a gastrointestinal focus. The most common species in this setting is *C. septicum*. Characteristic signs and symptoms include fever, tachycardia, hypotension, abdominal pain or tenderness, nausea, vomiting, and (preterminally) coma. The tachycardia may be out of proportion to the fever. Only ~20 to 30% of patients develop hemolysis. A striking feature of this syndrome is the rapidity of death, which frequently occurs in <12 h.

DIAGNOSIS The diagnosis of clostridial disease, in association with positive cultures, must be based primarily on clinical findings. Because of the presence of clostridia in many wounds, their mere isolation from any site, including the blood, does not necessarily indicate severe disease. Smears of wound exudates, uterine scrapings, or cervical discharge may show abundant large gram-positive rods as well as other organisms. Cultures should be placed in selective media and incubated anaerobically for identification of clostridia. The diagnosis of clostridial myonecrosis can be established by frozen-section biopsy of muscle.

The urine of patients with severe clostridial sepsis may contain protein and casts, and some patients may develop severe uremia. Profound alterations of circulating erythrocytes are seen in severely toxemic patients. Patients have hemolytic anemia, which develops extremely rapidly, along with hemoglobinemia, hemoglobinuria, and elevated levels of serum bilirubin. Spherocytosis, increased osmotic and mechanical red blood cell fragility, erythrophagocytosis, and methemoglobinemia have been described. Disseminated intravascular coagulation may develop in patients with severe infection. In patients with severe sepsis, Wright's or Gram's staining of a smear of peripheral blood or buffy coat may demonstrate clostridia.

X-ray examination sometimes provides an important clue to the diagnosis by revealing gas in muscles, subcutaneous tissue, or the uterus. However, the finding of gas is not pathognomonic for clostridial infection. Other anaerobic bacteria, frequently mixed with aerobic organisms, may produce gas.

The diagnosis of *C. difficile*–associated colitis is most often made by an enzyme-linked immunosorbent assay (ELISA) for toxin A. Compared with the "gold standard" tissue culture assay used primarily for the detection of toxin B, the ELISA exhibits comparable specificity and only slightly lower sensitivity (70 to 90%). The cytotoxicity assay requires a tissue culture facility, skilled laboratory technicians, and time (usually 48 h), since neutralization of the cytopathic effect with *C. sordellii* or *C. difficile* antitoxin is required before the test can be labeled positive. ELISA is more rapid and easier to perform. However, in difficult situations where the clinical diagnosis remains a possibility and ELISA results are negative, consideration should be given to requesting the cytotoxicity assay since it may detect 5 to 10% more cases. Repeat stool testing with the same assay generally does not increase the diagnostic yield for this entity. Endoscopy, although useful in establishing the presence of PMC, does not establish the etiology and should be reserved for cases with more serious disease manifestations, in which it can be used to exclude alternative diagnoses. Isolation of *C. difficile* from stool cultures is difficult. This approach should be reserved for epidemiologic studies of outbreaks since asymptomatic persons may harbor the pathogen, but production of toxin is the hallmark of disease.

TREATMENT Traumatic wounds should be thoroughly cleansed and debrided. Traditionally, the antibiotic treatment of choice for severe clostridial infection has been penicillin G (20 million units a day in adults). Penicillin G treatment of gas gangrene has become more controversial because of increasing resistance to this drug and data obtained from animal models of infection. In a mouse model of gas gangrene, antibiotics inhibiting toxin synthesis appeared to be preferable to cell wall–active drugs; clindamycin treatment enhanced survival more than therapy with penicillin; and the combination of clindamycin and penicillin was superior to penicillin alone. For severe clostridial sepsis, clindamycin may be used at a dose of 600 mg every 6 h in combination with high-dose penicillin (3 to 4 million units every 4 h). Although no clinical trials validate this choice, it is gaining acceptance in the infectious disease community.

In cases of penicillin sensitivity or allergy, other antibiotics should be considered, but all should be tested for in vitro activity because of the occasional isolation of resistant strains. Clostridia are frequently, but not universally, susceptible in vitro to cefoxitin, carbenicillin, chloramphenicol, clindamycin, metronidazole, doxycycline, imipenem, minocycline, tetracycline, third-generation cephalosporins, and vancomycin. For severe clostridial infections, sensitivity testing should be done before an antimicrobial with unpredictable activity is used. Simple contamination of a wound with clostridia should not be treated with antibiotics. Localized skin and soft tissue infection can be managed by debridement rather than with systemic antibiotics. Drugs are required when the process extends into adjacent tissue or when fever and systemic signs of sepsis are present. Surgery is a mainstay of therapy for clostridial myonecrosis or gas gangrene. Amputation may be required for rapidly spreading infection involving a limb. Hysterectomy is required for uterine myonecrosis. Abdominal wall myonecrosis usually continues despite initial aggressive surgery and antibiotic therapy and requires repeated surgical debridement of all involved muscle.

Suppurative infections should be treated with antibiotics. Frequently, broad-spectrum antibiotics must be used because of the mixed flora involved in these infections. Aminoglycosides can be used for the aerobic gram-negative bacteria involved in mixed infections.

The use of a polyvalent gas gangrene antitoxin is still recommended by some authorities. At present, no such antitoxin is produced in the United States, and most centers have discontinued its use in the management of patients with suspected gas gangrene or clostridial postabortion sepsis because of questionable efficacy and the substantial risk of hypersensitivity to horse serum, from which the antitoxin is derived.

The use of hyperbaric oxygen in the treatment of gas gangrene is also controversial. Studies in humans are not well designed to answer questions on efficacy, but several knowledgeable authors believe that hyperbaric oxygen therapy has contributed to dramatic clinical improvement. Such therapy may, however, be associated with untoward effects due to oxygen toxicity and high atmospheric pressure. Some centers without hyperbaric chambers have reported acceptable mortality rates; thus expert surgical and medical management and control of complications are probably the most important factors in the treatment of gas gangrene. Fasciotomy should not be delayed for hyperbaric oxygen therapy.

The treatment of *C. difficile*–associated colitis requires discontinuation of therapy with the offending antimicrobial agent. In some patients, symptoms will resolve over a period of 2 weeks if the infection is left untreated. However, specific therapy shortens the duration of symptoms.

Diarrhea due to *C. difficile* should be treated with metronidazole (500 mg orally tid for 10 to 14 days). A randomized trial comparing metronidazole (250 mg qid) with oral vancomycin showed equal efficacy and relapse rates of ~9% for both regimens. Since both treatment regimens are effective, metronidazole is preferred because it is far less costly and has not been linked to the development of vancomycin-resistant enterococci. When a patient relapses, antibiotic resistance should not be inferred since it is rare; a repeat course of metronidazole is appropriate. When a patient with *C. difficile*–associated diarrhea requires continued antibiotic treatment for a serious infection such as infective endocarditis, it is often reasonable to continue therapy against *C. difficile* for the duration of the offending antibiotic treatment course and for a full 10 to 14 days following its completion. When vancomycin is used for the treatment of *C. difficile*–associated diarrhea, the starting dose should be 125 mg orally qid, although doses as high as 500 mg qid can be used if needed. When a patient requires parenteral therapy for antibiotic-associated diarrhea, intravenous metronidazole can be administered. Vancomycin is effective only if used orally; the drug is poorly absorbed after oral administration. If patients continue to have diarrhea and have signs of systemic toxicity (e.g., fever and/or leukocytosis) after 48 h of treatment with metronidazole, it is reasonable to switch to vancomycin. For especially severe disease, some experts advocate treatment with both oral vancomycin and metronidazole, although there are no trials to support this regimen.

A number of patients who respond to initial therapy present with a relapse of symptoms and a repeat positive toxin assay. Relapses following therapy are much more frequent than failures to respond to initial therapy. Most relapses occur 3 to 10 days after discontinuation of treatment. Most relapsing patients respond to a second course of antibiotics, but some go on to suffer multiple relapses. A number of options are available in this situation. Some authors report success with tapering regimens of vancomycin given daily or every other day for 1 to 2 months to avoid relapse. The resin cholestyramine binds the cytotoxin of *C. difficile* and has been used with some success to treat severe cases. Since cholestyramine also binds vancomycin, the two agents should not be used in combination. Repopulation of the normal colonic flora has also been tried in relapsing disease. Ingestion of capsules of the yeast *Saccharomyces boulardii* showed some promise in one trial; oral lactobacilli have also been used in uncontrolled studies. The administration of intravenous immunoglobulin has been tried with

success in a few children and adults with relapsing infection, although this approach is not yet considered to be recommended therapy.

BIBLIOGRAPHY

BORRIELLO SP: Clostridial disease of the gut. Clin Infect Dis 20:S242, 1995

CASTAGLIUOLO I et al: *Clostridium difficile* toxin A stimulates macrophage-inflammatory protein-2 production in rat intestinal epithelial cells. J Immunol 160:6039, 1998

CHAVES-OLARTE E et al: Toxins A and B from *Clostridium difficile* differ with respect to enzymatic potencies, cellular substrate specificities, and surface binding to cultured cells. J Clin Invest 100:1734, 1997

CLEARY RK: *Clostridium difficile*–associated diarrhea and colitis: Clinical manifestations, diagnosis, and treatment. Dis Colon Rectum 41:1435, 1998

ELLEMOR DM et al: Use of genetically manipulated strains of *Clostridium perfringens* reveals that both alpha-toxin and theta-toxin are required for vascular leukostasis to occur in experimental gas gangrene. Infect Immun 67:4902, 1999

GERDING DN et al: *Clostridium difficile*–associated diarrhea and colitis. Infect Control Hosp Epidemiol 16:459, 1995

JOHNSON S et al: Epidemics of diarrhea caused by a clindamycin-resistant strain of *Clostridium difficile* in four hospitals. N Engl J Med 341:1645, 1999

JUST I et al: Glucosylation of Rho proteins by *Clostridium difficile* toxin B. Nature 375:500, 1995

KYNE L et al: Asymptomatic carriage of *Clostridium difficile* and serum levels of IgG antibody against toxin A. N Engl J Med 342:390, 2000

LORBER B: Gas gangrene and other *Clostridium*-associated diseases, in *Principles and Practice of Infectious Diseases*, 5th ed, GL Mandell et al (eds). New York, Churchill Livingstone, 2000, pp 2549–2560

PRINSSEN HM et al: *Clostridium septicum* myonecrosis and ovarian cancer: A case report and review of literature. Gynecol Oncol 72:116, 1999

ROOD JI: Virulence genes of *Clostridium perfringens*. Annu Rev Microbiol 52:333, 1998

SCHALCH B et al: Molecular methods for the analysis of *Clostridium perfringens* relevant to food hygiene. FEMS Immunol Med Microbiol 24:281, 1999

SHARMA AK, HOLDER FE: *Clostridium difficile* diarrhea after use of tacrolimus following renal transplantation. Clin Infect Dis 27:1540, 1998

TIBBLES PM, EDELSBERG JS: Medical progress: Hyperbaric-oxygen therapy. N Engl J Med 334:1642, 1996

Section 6
DISEASES CAUSED BY GRAM-NEGATIVE BACTERIA

146

Robert S. Munford

MENINGOCOCCAL INFECTIONS

DEFINITION *Neisseria meningitidis* is the etiologic agent of two life-threatening diseases: meningococcal meningitis and fulminant meningococcemia. Meningococci also cause pneumonia, septic arthritis, pericarditis, urethritis, and conjunctivitis. Most cases are potentially preventable by vaccination.

ETIOLOGIC AGENT *N. meningitidis* bacteria are gram-negative aerobic diplococci. Unlike the other neisseriae, they have a polysaccharide capsule. They are transmitted among humans, their only known habitat, via respiratory secretions. Colonization of the nasopharynx or pharynx is much more common than invasive disease.

EPIDEMIOLOGY Meningococcal disease occurs worldwide as isolated (sporadic) cases, institution- or community-based outbreaks, and large epidemics.

Meningococci are classified into serogroups based on the antigenicity of their capsular polysaccharides. Antigenicity reflects structural differences in these polysaccharides. Five serogroups (A, B, C, Y, and W-135) are responsible for >90% of cases of meningococcal disease worldwide. Serogroup A strains, which caused most of the large epidemics of meningococcal disease during the first half of the twentieth

century, are now associated with recurring epidemics in sub-Saharan Africa and other locales in the developing world. Serogroups B, C, and Y cause most cases of sporadic and epidemic meningococcal disease in industrialized countries. In the United States and Canada during the 1990s, serogroup B was the most common cause of sporadic disease, while serogroup C was a more frequent cause of outbreaks. Serogroup Y has recently been isolated from almost one-third of cases of meningococcal disease in the United States. In general, patients with serogroup Y disease are older and more likely to have a chronic underlying illness than are patients with disease caused by other serogroups. Serogroups Y and W-135 are isolated more often than the other serogroups from patients with pneumonia.

One limitation of the serogroup classification is that the genes for capsule biosynthesis can be transferred from one strain to another, with consequent changes in the capsule structure of the recipient strain and therefore in its serogroup. Other methods for tracking meningococcal strains have thus become increasingly useful. Meningococcal serotypes and subtypes are defined by antigenic differences in specific outer-membrane proteins (OMPs), whereas multilocus enzyme electrophoresis classifies bacteria into electrophoretic types (ETs). Other techniques for establishing strain identity or nonidentity are pulsed-field gel electrophoresis and amplification of bacterial genomic sequences by polymerase chain reaction. The virulent III-1 clonal complex of serogroup A was first recognized in Nepal in 1983 to 1984; it spread to Mecca, then to sub-Saharan Africa, and subsequently to temperate Africa. Increased virulence and epidemic potential have also been ascribed to the serogroup B ET-5 complex, which was first identified in Norway in the 1970s and later caused outbreaks in Europe, Cuba, and South and North America (most recently, in the Pacific Northwest). Serogroup C ET-24 (the ET-37 complex) has caused sporadic cases and outbreaks in Canada and the United States and in some analyses has been associated with high mortality and morbidity.

Meningococcal colonization of the nasopharynx (asymptomatic carriage) can persist for months. In nonepidemic periods, ~10% of healthy individuals are colonized. Factors that predispose individuals to colonization with N. meningitidis include residence in the same household with a person who has meningococcal disease or is a carrier, household or institutional crowding, active or passive exposure to tobacco smoke, and a recent history of a viral upper respiratory infection. These factors have also been associated with an increased risk of meningococcal disease.

In countries with temperate climates, the attack rate for sporadic meningococcal disease is ~1 case per 100,000 persons per year. Peak disease incidence coincides with the winter peak of respiratory viral illnesses. Disease attack rates are highest among infants 3 to 9 months of age (10 to 15 cases per 100,000 infants per year). Children also have higher attack rates than adults, and there is a second peak of incidence among teenagers, in whom outbreaks have often been tied to residence in barracks, dormitories, or other crowded conditions. Although the age-specific incidence is much lower among adults (<1 case per 100,000 persons per year), approximately one-third of all cases of sporadic meningococcal disease occur in individuals ≥18 years of age. During epidemics, disease incidence increases disproportionately among teenagers and young adults and during the summer and autumn.

Meningococcal disease occurs more commonly in the household contacts of primary cases. The secondary attack rate is 400 to 1000 per 100,000 household members. School-based clusters of cases have also been described; the attack rate among school contacts of cases has been estimated at 2 to 4 cases per 100,000 exposed individuals. In outbreaks on college campuses, attack rates have been highest among students living in dormitories. Most secondary cases occur within 2 weeks of the primary case, although some may develop as long as several months later. Secondary cases account for <2% of all cases reported each year in the United States.

In an outbreak, the case isolates of N. meningitidis are identical when they are assessed by molecular typing methods. Recent outbreaks of meningococcal disease have occurred among persons whose common exposure took place in military barracks, schools, a university campus tavern, a jail, a school bus, a disco bar, a sports club, and a hotel.

PATHOGENESIS Meningococci that colonize the upper respiratory tract are internalized by nonciliated mucosal cells and may traverse them to enter the submucosa, from which they can make their way into the bloodstream. While meningococcal colonization occurs often in healthy humans, bloodstream infection is an infrequent event that is not essential for the organisms' survival and spread; as is often the case, the production of human disease has no obvious evolutionary advantage for either pathogen or host. Although some strains of N. meningitidis are thought to cause more severe disease in humans than do other strains, the basis for this difference is not understood. Meningococci may undergo important phenotypic changes when they adapt to growth in vivo; presumed virulence traits include the antiphagocytic capsular polysaccharide, an ability to sialylate the cell wall lipooligosaccharide (LOS) so that it mimics host cell carbohydrate moieties, the secretion of IgA protease, and mechanisms for iron acquisition. The ET-5 strain of serogroup B N. meningitidis has been associated with high case-fatality rates in some populations but not in others, however, suggesting that host factors also contribute importantly to disease pathogenesis.

A meningococcus that enters the blood from the nasopharynx and survives host defenses generally has one of two fates. If multiplication occurs slowly, the bacteria eventually seed local sites, such as the meninges, joints, or pericardium. More rapid multiplication in the blood is associated with disseminated intravascular coagulation (DIC) and shock, which usually cause symptoms before local sites become infected. There is thus a remarkable compartmentalization of bacterial growth and host inflammation in either the blood or a local site, usually the meninges.

Fulminant Meningococcemia (Purpura Fulminans) Fulminant meningococcemia is perhaps the most rapidly lethal form of septic shock experienced by humans. It differs from most other forms of septic shock by the prominence of hemorrhagic skin lesions (petechiae, purpura) and the consistent development of DIC.

The dominant proinflammatory molecule in the meningococcal cell wall is the endotoxin or LOS, and the outer membrane that contains it is poorly tethered to the underlying peptidoglycan. This structural peculiarity seems to account for the fact that meningococci shed LOS-containing membrane blebs as they grow. The bacteria can multiply to very high concentrations in the blood. The concentrations of endotoxin detected in the blood of patients with fulminant meningococcemia are 10- to 1000-fold greater than those found in the blood of patients with bacteremia due to other gram-negative bacteria. The bacteria and endotoxin-containing blebs stimulate monocytes, neutrophils, and endothelial cells, which then release cytokines and other mediators that can activate many distant targets, including other leukocytes and endothelial cells. In addition, meningococci can invade the vascular endothelium. When activated, the endothelium produces molecules that can be procoagulant as well as adhesive for leukocytes.

Patients with fulminant meningococcemia usually have extremely high blood levels of both proinflammatory mediators—i.e., tumor necrosis factor (TNF) α, interleukin (IL) 1, interferon γ, and IL-8—and anti-inflammatory mediators—i.e., IL-1 receptor antagonist (IL-1Ra), soluble IL-1 receptors, soluble TNF receptors, and IL-10. The plasma of patients with meningococcal shock can decrease the responses of normal leukocytes to stimuli such as LOS; the implication is that anti-inflammatory mediators predominate in the blood.

Procoagulant, antifibrinolytic forces are predominant in the blood of patients with fulminant meningococcemia (Fig. 146-1). Monocytes express large amounts of tissue factor. Fibrinopeptide A and thrombin-antithrombin levels are high, reflecting active clotting, while antithrombin and fibrinogen levels are low. Although the tissue factor–regulated ("extrinsic") arm of coagulation predominates, the contact system (factors XII and XI, prekallikrein, high-molecular-weight kininogen) is also activated. Striking deficiencies of antithrombin and proteins C and S can occur; studies have found a strong negative correlation between protein C activity and both the size of purpuric skin lesions and mortality. Plasminogen levels are decreased, while plas-

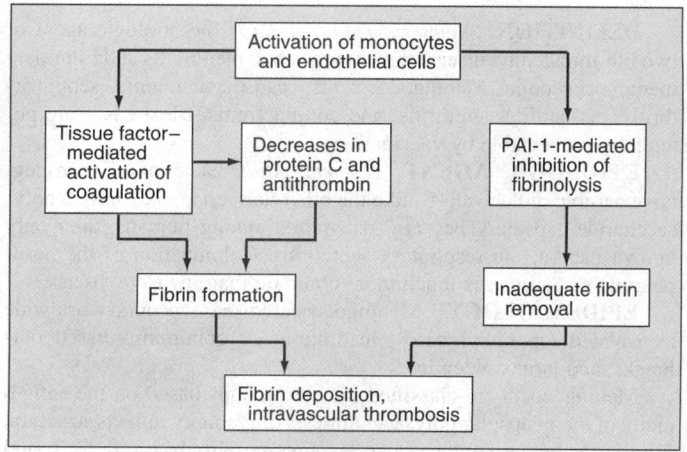

FIGURE 146-1 The pathogenesis of fibrin deposition in patients with fulminant meningococcemia. PAI-1, plasminogen activator inhibitor 1. (*Adapted from M Levi et al: Eur J Clin Invest 27:3, 1997.*)

min-antiplasmin complexes and plasminogen activator inhibitor 1 (PAI-1) levels in the blood are very high. PAI-1 levels have been correlated with mortality risk, as has a function-related polymorphism in the promoter of the PAI-1 gene.

Fibrin deposition is therefore favored both by the *procoagulant* tendency, promoted through activation of tissue factor and deficiencies of proteins C and S and antithrombin, and by an *antifibrinolytic* tendency, favored by excessive PAI-1. Both platelets and leukocytes doubtless contribute to the formation of microthrombi and to the vascular injury that ensues. Thrombosis of larger vessels leads to peripheral necrosis and gangrene that may require limb or digit amputation.

None of the candidate mediators of septic shock has proven primacy (Chaps. 38 and 124). Numerous studies have suggested that shock and DIC are not intimately linked and that the contact arm of clotting, which is of secondary importance in the pathogenesis of DIC, plays at least a contributory role in the pathogenesis of shock. The independence of DIC and shock suggests that therapies that prevent or reverse DIC may not be helpful for patients with septic shock.

Meningitis *N. meningitidis* has a striking tropism for the meninges. Infection of the central nervous system begins in the choroid plexus or in the ependyma that lines the cerebral ventricles. Meningococci adhere to cerebral capillary endothelial cells and then enter the subarachnoid space. A vigorous local inflammatory response ensues, probably triggered by endotoxin-containing meningococcal membranes. Both bacterial growth and the inflammatory response occur within the cerebrospinal fluid (CSF), where levels of endotoxin, IL-6, TNF-α, IL-1β, IL-1Ra, and IL-10 exceed the concentrations found in plasma by 100- to 1000-fold. The inflammatory response is largely confined to the subarachnoid space and contiguous structures.

Patients who develop meningitis may be individuals in whom meningococci do not grow rapidly in the blood; they may have a more vigorous initial inflammatory response to invading meningococci, may have antibodies or phagocytes that slow meningococcal growth, or may lack the (unknown) factors that allow *N. meningitidis* to multiply rapidly in vivo. The prognosis of patients with meningococcal meningitis is substantially better than that of patients with fulminant meningococcemia (Table 146-1).

HOST DEFENSE MECHANISMS Preventing meningococcal growth in blood requires bactericidal and opsonic antibodies, complement, and phagocytes (Fig. 146-2). The major bactericidal antibodies are IgM and IgG, which bind to the capsular polysaccharide. Immunity to meningococci is therefore serogroup specific. Antibodies to other surface (subcapsular) antigens may confer cross-serogroup protection. Infants are protected from meningococcal disease during the first months of life by passively transferred maternal IgG antibodies. As maternal antibody levels wane, the attack rate increases, peaking

FIGURE 146-2 Protection from meningococcal disease involves both antimeningococcal immunoglobulins and complement. Activation of complement by antimeningococcal IgM or IgG promotes bacterial lysis via the membrane attack complex (C5–C9), while C3b (produced by either alternative or classic pathway activation) and antimeningococcal IgG$_2$ cooperate to produce effective opsonophagocytosis. A neutrophil defect in binding IgG$_2$ (the FcγRIIA R131 allele) has been associated with more severe meningococcal disease. CR1, complement receptor 1; LOS, lipooligosaccharide.

from 3 to 9 months of age. Disease incidence declines as protective antibodies are induced by colonization with nonpathogenic bacteria that have cross-reactive antigens. In addition to *N. lactamica*, which frequently colonizes young children, some enteric bacteria have antigens that cross-react with those of meningococci. One theory relates the occurrence of meningococcal disease to the presence of high levels of IgA antibodies to meningococci, since these antibodies can block the bactericidal activity of IgM.

Complement is required for bactericidal activity and for efficient opsonophagocytosis. Individuals deficient in any of the late complement components (C5 to C9) cannot assemble the membrane attack complex needed to kill *Neisseria*. These persons typically develop less severe meningococcal disease than complement-sufficient individuals, do so at an older age, and tend to have disease due to uncommon serogroups (W-135, X, Y, Z, and 29E). Although only one-half of individuals with known late-complement-component deficiency ever experience meningococcal disease, some affected persons have several episodes. Deficiency of each of the terminal complement components is inherited in an autosomal recessive fashion. Properdin deficiency, in contrast, is X-linked; some affected males develop overwhelming meningococcal disease, an observation indicating that the alternative complement pathway is also needed for antimeningococcal host defense. The age of disease onset in properdin-deficient individuals is typically in the teens or twenties.

Activation of the classic pathway of complement by antigen-antibody complexes or of the alternative pathway by LOS or capsular polysaccharide is important for producing and maintaining C3b (Fig. 146-2). Without C3b, neither bactericidal lysis nor phagocytosis can proceed effectively. When C3b is generated, meningococcal growth is probably checked by the membrane attack complex, which produces bacterial lysis, and by robust phagocytosis. Most IgG antibodies to the meningococcal polysaccharide are of the IgG$_2$ isotype; a phagocytic cell defect (the FcγRIIA R131 allele) that impairs the phagocytosis of IgG$_2$-coated particles has been associated with more severe meningococcal disease. This allele has also been associated with a more severe clinical course in patients with late-complement-component deficiency; thus effective phagocytosis may contribute to the relatively mild meningococcal disease usually observed in these individuals.

Indirect evidence indicates that persons who mount a vigorous inflammatory response to meningococcal LOS may experience less severe disease than those whose initial response is anti-inflammatory. This observation suggests that the inflammatory response may be critical for restraining meningococcal growth. Attempts to identify dis-

Table 146-1   Clinical Spectrum of Meningococcal Meningitis and Fulminant Meningococcemia

Feature	Fulminant Meningococcemia	Meningococcal Meningitis
Interval from onset of symptoms to presentation for medical care	Short (median, 12 h)	Longer ($\geq$1 day)
Symptoms, signs	Prostration, petechiae/purpura, fever	Fever, headache, meningismus, altered mental status, seizures
CSF culture	Often negative	Usually positive
CSF endotoxin, cytokine levels	Low	High
Blood endotoxin, cytokine levels	High	Low
Case-fatality rate	20–40%	3–10%
Fraction of total cases	~10–30%	~30–40%

NOTE: CSF, cerebrospinal fluid.

ease- or severity-associated polymorphisms in cytokine genes have had inconclusive results, however.

CLINICAL MANIFESTATIONS **Upper Respiratory Tract Infections** Although many patients who develop meningococcal meningitis or meningococcemia report having had throat soreness or other upper respiratory symptoms during the preceding week, it is uncertain whether these symptoms are due to infection with meningococci. Meningococcal pharyngitis is rarely diagnosed. Adult patients with *N. meningitidis* bacteremia more often have clinically apparent disease of the respiratory tract (pneumonia, sinusitis, tracheobronchitis, conjunctivitis) than do younger patients.

Meningococcemia Most patients with meningococcal disease have both meningococcemia *and* meningitis. These conditions have a wide clinical spectrum, with many overlapping features (Table 146-1).

Approximately 10 to 30% of patients with meningococcal disease have meningococcemia without clinically apparent meningitis. Although meningococcemia is occasionally transient and asymptomatic, in most individuals it is associated with fever, chills, nausea, vomiting, and myalgias. Prostration is common. The most distinctive feature is rash. Erythematous macules rapidly become petechial and, in severe cases, purpuric. Although the lesions are typically found on the trunk and lower extremities, they may also occur on the face, arms, and mucous membranes. The petechiae may coalesce into hemorrhagic bullae or may undergo necrosis and ulcerate. Patients with severe coagulopathy may develop ischemic extremities or digits, often with a sharp line of demarcation between normal and ischemic tissue.

In many patients with fulminant meningococcemia, the CSF is normal and the CSF culture is negative. Indeed, the absence of meningitis in a patient with meningococcemia is a poor prognostic sign; it suggests that the bacteria have multiplied so rapidly in the blood that meningeal seeding has not yet had time to elicit inflammation in the CSF. Most of these patients also lack evidence of an acute-phase response; i.e., the erythrocyte sedimentation rate is normal, and the C-reactive protein concentration in blood is low.

The Waterhouse-Friderichsen syndrome is a dramatic example of DIC-induced microthrombosis, hemorrhage, and tissue injury. Although overt adrenal failure is infrequently documented in patients with fulminant meningococcemia, patients may have partial adrenal insufficiency and be unable to mount the normal hypercortisolemic response to severe stress or cosyntropin stimulation. Almost all patients who die from fulminant meningococcemia have adrenal hemorrhages at autopsy.

Chronic meningococcemia is a rare syndrome of episodic fever, rash, and arthralgias that can last for weeks to months. The rash may be maculopapular; it is occasionally petechial. Splenomegaly may develop. If untreated or if treated with glucocorticoids, chronic meningococcemia may evolve into meningitis, fulminant meningococcemia, or (rarely) endocarditis.

Meningitis (See also Chap. 372) Patients with meningococcal meningitis have usually been sick for ≥24 h before they seek medical attention. Common presenting symptoms include nausea and vomiting, headache, neck stiffness, lethargy, and confusion. The symptoms and signs of meningococcal meningitis cannot be distinguished from those elicited by other meningeal pathogens. Many patients with meningococcal meningitis have concurrent meningococcemia, however, and petechial or purpuric skin lesions may suggest the correct diagnosis. CSF findings are consistent with those of purulent meningitis: hypoglycorrhachia, an elevated protein concentration, and a neutrophilic leukocytosis. A Gram's stain of CSF is usually positive (see "Diagnosis," below); when this finding is unaccompanied by CSF leukocytosis, the prognosis for normal recovery is often poor.

Other Manifestations Arthritis occurs in ~10% of patients with meningococcal disease. When arthritis develops during the first few days of the patient's illness, it usually reflects direct meningococcal invasion of the joint. Arthritis that begins later in the course is thought to be due to immune complex deposition. Primary meningococcal pneumonia occurs principally in adults, often in military populations, and is most often due to serogroup Y. While meningococcal pericarditis is occasionally seen, endocarditis due to *N. meningitidis* is now exceedingly rare. Primary meningococcal conjunctivitis can be complicated by meningococcemia; systemic therapy is therefore warranted when this condition is diagnosed. Meningococcal urethritis has been reported in individuals who practice oral sex.

Complications Patients with meningococcal meningitis may develop cranial nerve palsies, cortical venous thrombophlebitis, and cerebral edema. In children subdural effusions may occur. Permanent sequelae can include mental retardation, deafness, and hemiparesis. The major long-term morbidity of fulminant meningococcemia is the loss of skin, limbs, or digits that results from ischemic necrosis and infarction.

DIAGNOSIS Few clinical clues help the physician distinguish the patient with early meningococcal disease from patients with other acute systemic infections. The most useful clinical finding is the petechial or purpuric rash **(see Plate IID-44)**, but it must be differentiated from the petechial lesions seen with gonococcemia **(see Plate IID-60)**, Rocky Mountain spotted fever **(see Plate IID-45)**, hypersensitivity vasculitis **(see Plate IIE-71)**, endemic typhus, and some viruses. In one case series, one-half of the adults with meningococcal bacteremia had neither meningitis nor a rash.

The definitive diagnosis is established by recovering *N. meningitidis*, its antigens, or its DNA from normally sterile body fluids, such as blood, CSF, or synovial fluid, or from skin lesions. Meningococci grow best on Mueller-Hinton or chocolate blood agar at 35°C in an atmosphere that contains 5 to 10% CO_2. Specimens should be plated without delay. *N. meningitidis* bacteria are oxidase-positive, gram-negative diplococci that typically utilize maltose and glucose.

A Gram's stain of CSF reveals intra- or extracellular organisms in ~85% of patients with meningococcal meningitis. The latex agglutination test for meningococcal polysaccharides is somewhat less sensitive. Reports suggest that polymerase chain reaction amplification of DNA in buffy coat or CSF samples may be more sensitive than either of these tests, and, like the latex agglutination test, this method is not affected by prior antibiotic therapy.

Throat or nasopharyngeal specimens should be cultured on Thayer-Martin medium, which suppresses the competing oral flora. Throat or nasopharyngeal cultures are recommended only for research or epidemiologic purposes, since a positive result merely confirms the carrier state and does not establish the existence of systemic disease.

℞ **TREATMENT** A second-generation cephalosporin, such as cefotaxime (2 g intravenously every 8 h) or ceftriaxone (1 g intravenously every 12 h), is preferred for initial therapy, as it may cover other bacteria (such as *Streptococcus pneumoniae* and *Haemophilus influenzae*) that can cause the same syndromes (Chap. 372). Penicillin G (4 million units intravenously every 4 h) remains an acceptable alternative in most countries; high-level penicillin resistance has been reported from Spain. In the patient who is allergic to β-lactam drugs, chloramphenicol (75 to 100 mg/kg every 6 h) is a suitable alternative; chloramphenicol-resistant meningococci have been reported from Vietnam and France, however. Although some cases of mild disease may be cured with only 2 days of treatment, most patients with meningococcal meningitis should be given antimicrobial therapy for at least 5 days. While glucocorticoid therapy for meningitis in adults is controversial, many experts administer dexamethasone, beginning if possible before antibiotic therapy is initiated (Chap. 372).

Patients with fulminant meningococcemia often experience diffuse leakage of fluid into extravascular spaces, shock, and multiple-organ dysfunction (Chaps. 38 and 124). Myocardial depression may be prominent. Supportive therapy has never been studied in randomized, placebo-controlled trials. Standard measures include vigorous fluid resuscitation (often requiring several liters over the first 24 h), elective ventilation, and pressors (epinephrine or dopamine). Some authorities recommend early hemodialysis or hemofiltration. Fresh frozen plasma is often given to patients who are bleeding extensively or who have severely deranged clotting parameters. Many European experts prefer to administer antithrombin to such patients. Patients with fulminant meningococcemia in whom shock persists despite vigorous fluid resuscitation should receive supplemental glucocorticoid treatment (hydrocortisone, 1 mg/kg every 6 h) pending tests of adrenal reserve. Investigational drugs for fulminant meningococcemia include bactericidal permeability-increasing (BPI) protein—a bactericidal neutrophil protein that binds and neutralizes meningococcal LOS—as well as several anticoagulants (activated protein C, antithrombin, and tissue factor pathway inhibitor). In a recent clinical trial, recombinant BPI protein reduced long-term complications in children with fulminant meningococcemia without definitely reducing mortality.

PROGNOSIS When patients are first evaluated, the clinical features most strongly associated with a fatal outcome are shock, a purpuric or ecchymotic rash, a low or normal blood leukocyte count, an age ≥60 years, and coma. The absence of meningitis, the presence of thrombocytopenia, low blood concentrations of antithrombin or proteins S and C, high blood levels of PAI-1, and a low erythrocyte sedimentation rate (or C-reactive protein level) have also been associated with increased mortality from meningococcal disease. In contrast, having received antibiotics prior to hospital admission has been associated with lower mortality in some studies.

PREVENTION **Meningococcal Polysaccharide Vaccines** A single injection of quadrivalent meningococcal polysaccharide vaccine (serogroups A, C, W-135, and Y) immunizes ~80 to 95% of immunocompetent adults. Children ≥3 months of age can be vaccinated to prevent serogroup A disease, but multiple doses are required; the vaccine is otherwise ineffective in children <2 years old. The duration of vaccine-induced immunity in adults is probably <5 years. There is currently no vaccine for serogroup B; its polysaccharide is a sialic acid homopolymer that is poorly immunogenic in humans. In addition to individuals with late-complement-component or properdin deficiency, persons with sickle cell anemia, asplenia, or splenectomy should receive the quadrivalent vaccine. Vaccination is also recommended for military recruits and for individuals traveling to sub-Saharan Africa during the dry months (June to December) or to other areas with epidemic meningococcal disease. Some authorities recommend vaccination of incoming college freshmen who will live in dormitories. In general, the vaccine should be given only to persons ≥2 years of age. Investigational polysaccharide-protein conjugate meningococcal vaccines appear promising; a serogroup C conjugate vaccine was licensed for use in the United Kingdom in 1999.

Screening tests for late-complement-component deficiency should be done in family members of patients who have a family history of meningococcal disease, in patients who have a recurrence, in those whose first case occurs at ≥15 years of age, and in those with cases caused by serogroups other than A, B, or C.

Antimicrobial Chemoprophylaxis The attack rate for meningococcal disease among household contacts of cases is ~500-fold greater than that in the population as a whole. Close contacts of cases should receive chemoprophylaxis with rifampin (adult dosage, 600 mg orally every 12 h for four doses), ciprofloxacin (a single oral dose of 500 mg), or ofloxacin (a single oral dose of 400 mg). A single intramuscular injection of ceftriaxone (250 mg) is also effective. Close contacts include persons who live in the same household, day-care center contacts, and anyone directly exposed to the patient's oral secretions. Casual contacts are not at increased risk. Chemoprophylaxis should be administered as soon as possible after the case is identified.

Isolation Precautions The Centers for Disease Control and Prevention recommend that patients with meningococcal disease who are hospitalized be placed in respiratory isolation for the first 24 h.

Outbreak Control An organization- or community-based outbreak of meningococcal disease is defined as the occurrence of three or more cases within ≤3 months in persons who have a common affiliation or reside in the same area but who are not close contacts of one another; in addition, the primary disease attack rate must exceed

10 cases per 100,000 persons, and the case strains of *N. meningitidis* must be of the same molecular type. Mass vaccination should be considered when such outbreaks occur, and mass chemoprophylaxis may be used to control school- or other institution-based outbreaks. Consultation with public health authorities is recommended when such campaigns are contemplated.

BIBLIOGRAPHY

BRANDTZAEG P et al: Net inflammatory capacity of human septic shock plasma evaluated by a monocyte-based target cell assay: Identification of interleukin-10 as a major functional deactivator of human monocytes. J Exp Med 184:51, 1996

CENTERS FOR DISEASE CONTROL AND PREVENTION: Control and prevention of meningococcal disease. MMWR 46 (RR-5), 1997

FIJEN CA et al: Assessment of complement deficiency in patients with meningococcal disease in the Netherlands. Clin Infect Dis 28:98, 1999

KIRSCH EA et al: Pathophysiology, treatment and outcome of meningococcemia: A review and recent experience. Pediatr Infect Dis J 15:967, 1996

LEVIN P et al: Recombinant bactericidal/permeability-increasing protein (rBPI21) as adjunctive treatment for children with severe meningococcal sepsis: A randomised trial. Lancet 356:961, 2000

MACDONALD NE et al: Induction of immunologic memory by conjugated vs plain meningococcal C polysaccharide vaccine in toddlers—a randomized controlled trial. JAMA 280:1685, 1998

PLATONOV AE et al: Meningococcal disease and polymorphism of FcγRllA (CD32) in late complement component–deficient individuals. Clin Exp Immunol 111:97, 1998

ROSENSTEIN N et al: Efficacy of meningococcal vaccine and barriers to vaccination. JAMA 279:435, 1998

——— et al: The changing epidemiology of meningococcal disease in the United States, 1992–1996. J Infect Dis 180:1894, 1999

STEPHENS DS et al: Sporadic meningococcal disease in adults: Results of a 5-year population-based study. Ann Intern Med 123:937, 1995

WESTENDORP RGJ et al: Genetic influence on cytokine production and fatal meningococcal disease. Lancet 349:170, 1997

147 *Sanjay Ram, Peter A. Rice*

GONOCOCCAL INFECTIONS

DEFINITION Gonorrhea is a sexually transmitted infection of epithelium and commonly manifests as cervicitis, urethritis, proctitis, and conjunctivitis. If untreated, infections at these sites can lead to local complications such as endometritis, salpingitis, tuboovarian abscess, bartholinitis, peritonitis, and perihepatitis in the female; periurethritis and epididymitis in the male; and ophthalmia neonatorum in the newborn. Disseminated gonococcemia is an uncommon event whose manifestations include skin lesions, tenosynovitis, arthritis, and (in rare cases) endocarditis or meningitis.

Neisseria gonorrhoeae is a gram-negative, nonmotile, non-spore-forming organism that grows in pairs (diplococci). Each individual organism is shaped like a coffee bean, with adjacent concave sides seen on Gram's stain. Gonococci, like all other *Neisseria* spp., are oxidase positive. They are distinguished from other *Neisseria* by their ability to grow on selective media and to utilize glucose but not maltose, sucrose, or lactose.

EPIDEMIOLOGY The incidence of gonorrhea has declined significantly in the United States, but there are still ~315,000 newly reported cases each year. Gonorrhea remains a major public health problem worldwide, is a significant cause of morbidity in developing countries, and may play a role in enhancing transmission of HIV.

Gonorrhea predominantly affects young, nonwhite, unmarried, less educated members of urban populations. The number of reported cases probably represents half of the true number of cases—a discrepancy resulting from underreporting, self-treatment, and nonspecific treatment without a culture-proven diagnosis. The number of reported cases of gonorrhea in the United States rose from ~250,000 in the early 1960s to a high of 1.01 million in 1978. The peak recorded incidence of gonorrhea in modern times was noted in 1975, with 468 cases per 100,000 population in the United States. This peak was attributable to the interaction of several variables, including improved accuracy of diagnosis, changes in patterns of contraceptive use, and changes in sexual behavior. The incidence of the disease has since gradually declined and is currently estimated at 120 cases per 100,000, a figure that is still the highest among industrialized countries. A further decline in the overall incidence of gonorrhea in the United States over the past decade may reflect increased condom use resulting from public health efforts to curtail HIV transmission. Presently, the attack rate in the United States is highest in the 20- to 24-year age group, in which 75% of all cases occur. With adjustment for sexual experience, the risk is highest among sexually active 15- to 19-year-old women. In terms of ethnicity, rates are highest among African-Americans and lowest among persons of Asian or Pacific Island descent.

The highest incidence of gonorrhea occurs in developing countries. The exact incidence of any of the sexually transmitted diseases (STDs) is difficult to ascertain in developing countries because of limited surveillance and variable diagnostic criteria. For example, in Kenya, it was estimated in 1987 that 10% of all live births were adversely affected by STDs, and gonococcal ophthalmia neonatorum reportedly affected 4% of all live-born infants. The median prevalence of gonorrhea in unselected populations of pregnant women has been estimated at 10% in Africa, 5% in Latin America, and 4% in Asia. Studies in Africa have clearly demonstrated that nonulcerative STDs such as gonorrhea are an independent risk factor for the transmission of HIV (Chap. 309).

Gonorrhea is transmitted from males to females more efficiently than in the opposite direction. The rate of transmission to a woman following a single unprotected sexual encounter with an infected man is on the order of 40 to 60%. Oropharyngeal gonorrhea occurs in ~20% of women who practice fellatio with infected partners. Transmission in either direction by cunnilingus is rare.

There exists in any population a small minority of individuals who have high rates of new partner acquisition. These "core-group members" or "high-frequency transmitters" are vital in sustaining STD transmission at the population level. Another instrumental factor in sustaining gonorrhea in the population is the large number of infected individuals who are asymptomatic or have minor symptoms that are ignored. These persons, unlike symptomatic individuals, do not cease sexual activity and therefore continue to transmit the disease. This situation underscores the importance of contact tracing and empirical treatment of sex partners of index cases.

PATHOGENESIS AND IMMUNOLOGY **Outer-Membrane Proteins • Pili** Fresh clinical isolates of *N. gonorrhoeae* initially form piliated (fimbriated) colonies distinguishable on translucent agar. Pilus expression is rapidly switched off with unselected subculture because of rearrangements in pilus genes. This change is a basis for phase variation of gonococci. Piliated strains adhere better to cells derived from human mucosal surfaces and are more virulent in organ culture models and human inoculation experiments than nonpiliated variants. In a fallopian tube explant model, pili mediate gonococcal attachment to nonciliated columnar epithelial cells. This event initiates gonococcal phagocytosis and transport through these cells to intercellular spaces near the basement membrane or directly into the subepithelial tissue. Damage to nearby ciliated columnar epithelial cells, which is caused by the release of cytokines, results in loss of cilia and sloughing of ciliated cells and diminishes the integrity of the fallopian tube. Nonpiliated gonococci cause epithelial damage at a much slower rate. CD46 (membrane cofactor protein) is present on urogenital epithelial cells in both men and women and has been determined to be a receptor for PilC; this subunit is located at the tip of the pilus molecule and is critical in mediating adherence. Pili are also essential for genetic competence and transformation of *N. gonorrhoeae*, which permits horizontal transfer of genetic material between different gonococcal lineages in vivo.

Opacity-associated protein Another gonococcal surface protein that is important in adherence to epithelial cells is opacity-associated protein (Opa, formerly called protein II). Opa contributes to intergonococcal adhesion, which is responsible for the opaque nature of gonococcal colonies on translucent agar and the organism's adherence to a variety of eukaryotic cells, including polymorphonuclear leukocytes (PMNs). Certain Opa variants promote invasion of epithelial cells, and this effect has been linked with the ability of Opa to bind vitronectin, glycosaminoglycans, and several members of the carcinoembryonic antigen family (CD66). Each strain of *N. gonorrhoeae* possesses as many as 11 different *opa* genes, but usually only up to 3 types are expressed at any given time. Isolates from normally sterile sites such as the fallopian tube and synovial fluid usually fail to express Opa, while isolates from mucosal sites usually form opaque colonies. Female commercial sex workers with antibodies to Opa may be less likely to develop pelvic inflammatory disease (PID) than women without such antibodies.

Porin Porin (previously designated protein I) is the most abundant gonococcal surface protein, accounting for >50% of the organism's total outer-membrane protein. Porin molecules exist as trimers that provide anion aqueous channels through the otherwise hydrophobic outer membrane. Porin shows stable interstrain antigenic variation and forms the basis for gonococcal serotyping. Two main serotypes have been identified: Por1A strains are often associated with disseminated gonococcal infection (DGI), while Por1B strains usually cause local genital infections only. DGI strains are generally resistant to the killing action of normal human serum, do not incite a significant local inflammatory response, and therefore may not cause symptoms at genital sites. These characteristics may be related to the ability of Por1A strains to bind to complement-downregulatory molecules, resulting in a diminished inflammatory response. Porin can translocate to the cytoplasmic membrane of host cells—a process that could initiate gonococcal endocytosis and invasion. In addition, porin is an immunologic target of bactericidal and opsonophagocytic antibodies that may arise in response to immune stimulation resulting from infection or immunization with porin-containing vaccine candidates.

Other outer-membrane proteins Other notable outer-membrane proteins include H.8, a lipoprotein that is present on the surface of all gonococcal strains in high concentration and is an excellent target for antibody-based diagnostic testing, as well as transferrin-binding proteins (Tbp1 and Tbp2) and lactoferrin-binding protein, which are required for scavenging iron from transferrin and lactoferrin in vivo. Transferrin and iron have been shown to increase attachment of iron-deprived *N. gonorrhoeae* to human endometrial cells. Gonococci deficient in transferrin- and lactoferrin-binding proteins cannot establish infection in male volunteers. IgA1 protease is produced by *N. gonorrhoeae* and may protect the organism from the action of mucosal IgA.

Lipooligosaccharide Gonococcal lipooligosaccharide (LOS) consists of a lipid A and a core oligosaccharide that lacks the repeating O-carbohydrate antigenic side chain seen in other gram-negative bacteria (Chap. 120). Gonococcal LOS possesses marked endotoxic activity and contributes to the local cytotoxic effect in the fallopian tube model. LOS core sugars undergo a high degree of antigenic variation under different conditions of growth; this variation reflects genetic regulation and expression of glycotransferase genes that dictate the carbohydrate structure of LOS. These phenotypic changes may affect interactions of *N. gonorrhoeae* with elements of the humoral immune system (antibodies and complement) and may also influence direct binding of organisms to both professional and nonprofessional phagocytes (epithelial cells). For example, gonococci that are sialylated at their LOS sites bind complement factor H and downregulate the alternative pathway of complement. LOS sialylation may also mask bactericidal antibody–binding epitopes on LOS and porin and may decrease opsonophagocytosis and inhibit the oxidative burst in PMNs. While sialylation of LOS confers on the bacteria the ability to attenuate the inflammatory response and evade the innate immune system, experiments in male volunteers suggest that sialylated gonococci may be less capable of establishing infection than their unsialylated counterparts. This difference could be explained by the observation that the unsialylated terminal lactosamine residue of LOS binds to an asialoglycoprotein receptor on epithelial cells that would otherwise facilitate binding and subsequent gonococcal invasion of these cells.

Host Factors In addition to gonococcal structures that interact with epithelial cells, host factors seem to be important in mediating entry of gonococci into nonphagocytic cells. Activation of phosphatidylcholine-specific phospholipase C and acidic sphingomyelinase by *N. gonorrhoeae*, which results in the release of diacylglycerol and ceramide, is an essential requirement for the entry of *N. gonorrhoeae* into epithelial cells. Ceramide accumulation within cells leads to apoptosis, which may disrupt epithelial integrity and facilitate entry of gonococci into subepithelial tissue. Release of chemotactic factors as a result of complement activation contributes to inflammation, as does the toxic effect of LOS in provoking the release of inflammatory cytokines.

The importance of humoral immunity in host defenses against neisserial infections is best illustrated by the predisposition of persons deficient in terminal complement components (C5 through C9) to recurrent bacteremic gonococcal infections and to recurrent meningococcal meningitis or meningococcemia. Gonococcal porin induces T cell proliferative responses in persons with urogenital gonococcal disease. A significant increase in porin-specific interleukin (IL) 4–producing CD4+ as well as CD8+ lymphocytes is seen in individuals with mucosal gonococcal disease. A portion of these lymphocytes that show a porin-specific T_H2-type response could traffic to mucosal surfaces and play a role in immune protection against the disease. Few data clearly indicate that protective immunity is acquired from a previous gonococcal infection, although bactericidal and opsonophagocytic antibodies to porin and LOS may offer partial protection. On the other hand, women who are infected and acquire high levels of antibody to another outer-membrane protein, Rmp (reduction modifiable protein, formerly called protein III), may be especially likely to become reinfected with *N. gonorrhoeae* because Rmp antibodies block the effect of bactericidal antibodies to porin and LOS. Rmp shows little, if any, interstrain antigenic variation; therefore, Rmp antibodies potentially may block antibody-mediated killing of all gonococci. The mechanism of blocking has not been fully characterized, but Rmp antibodies noncompetitively inhibit binding of porin and LOS antibodies because of the proximity of these structures in the gonococcal outer membrane. Less well understood is how blocking antibody may divert complement binding to the gonococcal surface or otherwise hasten inactivation of complement. In male volunteers who have no history of gonorrhea, the net effect of these events may influence the outcome of experimental challenge with *N. gonorrhoeae*. Because Rmp bears extensive homology to enterobacterial OmpA and meningococcal class 4 proteins, it is possible that these blocking antibodies result from prior exposure to cross-reacting proteins from these species and also play a role in first-time infection with *N. gonorrhoeae*.

CLINICAL MANIFESTATIONS **Gonococcal Infection in Males** Acute urethritis is the most common clinical manifestation of gonorrhea in males. The usual incubation period following exposure is 2 to 7 days, although the interval can be longer and some men remain asymptomatic. Strains of the Por1A serotype, with nutritional requirements for arginine, hypoxanthine, and uracil (i.e., the AHU auxotype), tend to cause a greater proportion of cases of mild and asymptomatic urethritis than Por1B strains. Urethral discharge and dysuria, usually without urinary frequency or urgency, are the major symptoms. The discharge initially is scant and mucoid but becomes profuse and purulent within a day or two. The clinical manifestations of gonococcal urethritis are usually more severe and overt than those of nongonococcal urethritis, including urethritis caused by *Chlamydia trachomatis* (Chap. 179); however, exceptions are common, and it is often impossible to differentiate the causes of urethritis on clinical grounds alone. Most symptomatic males seek treatment and cease to be infectious. The remaining men, who are largely asymptomatic, accumulate in number over time and constitute about two-thirds of all infected men

at any point in time. Together with men incubating the organism (who shed the organism but are asymptomatic), they serve as the source of spread of infection. Prior to the antibiotic era, symptoms of urethritis persisted for about 8 weeks. Epididymitis is now an uncommon complication, and gonococcal prostatitis occurs rarely, if at all. Other unusual local complications of gonococcal urethritis include edema of the penis due to dorsal lymphangitis or thrombophlebitis, submucous inflammatory "soft" infiltration of the urethral wall, periurethral abscess or fistulae, inflammation or abscess of Cowper's gland, and seminal vesiculitis. Balanitis may develop in uncircumcised men. After a decline in gonococcal infections among homosexual men early in the era of AIDS, a disturbing increase in gonorrhea was observed among young homosexual men in the 1990s, probably related to decreased condom use. The clinical features of anorectal and pharyngeal gonorrhea are discussed below.

Gonococcal Infections in Females • *Gonococcal cervicitis* Mucopurulent cervicitis is the most common STD diagnosis in American women and may be caused by *N. gonorrhoeae*, *C. trachomatis*, and other organisms. Cervicitis may coexist with candidal or trichomonal vaginitis. *N. gonorrhoeae* primarily infects the cervical os but can also infect more peripheral areas of the cervix where columnar epithelium meets stratified squamous epithelium. Except in rare instances, the vaginal mucosa, which is lined by stratified squamous epithelium, does not become infected. Bartholin's glands occasionally become infected.

Women infected with *N. gonorrhoeae* usually develop symptoms. However, the women who either remain asymptomatic or have only minor symptoms may delay in seeking medical attention. Increased vaginal discharge and dysuria (often without urgency or frequency) are the most common symptoms. Although the incubation period of gonorrhea is less well defined in women than in men, symptoms usually develop within 10 days of infection and are more acute and intense than those of chlamydial cervicitis.

The physical examination may reveal a mucopurulent discharge (mucopus) issuing from the cervical os. The examiner may check for mucopurulent discharge by swabbing a sample of mucus from the endocervix and observing its color against the white background of the swab; yellow or green mucus suggests mucopus. However, only 35% of women with gonococcal cervicitis actually have a mucopurulent discharge defined by these criteria. Since Gram's stain is not sensitive for the diagnosis of gonorrhea in women, specimens should be submitted for culture or a nonculture assay (see below). Edematous and friable cervical ectopy as well as endocervical bleeding induced by gentle swabbing are more often seen in chlamydial infection.

N. gonorrhoeae may be recovered from the urethra and rectum of women with cervicitis, but these are rarely the sole infected sites. Urethritis in women may produce symptoms of internal dysuria, which is often attributed to "cystitis." Pyuria in the absence of bacteriuria seen on Gram's stain of unspun urine, accompanied by urine cultures that fail to yield $>10^5$ colonies of bacteria usually associated with urinary tract infection, signifies the possibility of urethritis due to *C. trachomatis*. Urethral infection with *N. gonorrhoeae* may also occur in this context, but in this instance urethral cultures will usually be positive. Compression of the urethra through the anterior vaginal wall against the symphysis pubis may express urethral exudate.

Complications of gonococcal cervicitis Gonococcal infection may extend deep enough to produce dyspareunia and lower abdominal or back pain. In such cases, it is imperative to consider a diagnosis of PID and to administer treatment for that disease (Chap. 133). Ascending infection of the genital tract follows ~20% of cases of gonococcal cervicitis and may result in acute endometritis accompanied by abnormal menstrual bleeding, midline lower abdominal pain and tenderness, and dyspareunia. Spread to the fallopian tubes results in acute salpingitis, whose symptoms may be accompanied by signs of cervical motion tenderness and abnormal adnexal mass on pelvic examination. Patients may be febrile, and leukocytosis and an elevated erythrocyte sedimentation rate or C-reactive protein level may be detected. Co-infection with *C. trachomatis* may increase the risk of PID, which is the clinical counterpart of endometritis and salpingitis. Tubal scarring leading to infertility is the most devastating sequela of salpingitis; the increased risk of ectopic pregnancy is also significant. Prompt and appropriate antibiotic therapy for gonococcal salpingitis (prior to the development of an adnexal mass) can prevent tubal infertility in nearly all cases. Bilateral tubal damage occurs in ~20% of women with an adnexal mass. More than half of women with tubal infertility give no history of PID. These women with "silent salpingitis" may report abdominal or pelvic discomfort (such as dysmenorrhea or dyspareunia) that may be attributed to other diagnoses (such as endometriosis). Spread of infection to the pelvis may result in pelvic peritonitis characterized by nausea and vomiting. Spread of gonococci—or, more commonly, of chlamydiae—via the peritoneal cavity to the upper abdomen may cause perihepatitis (Fitz-Hugh–Curtis syndrome; Chap. 133).

Gonococcal vaginitis   The vaginal mucosa of healthy women is lined by stratified squamous epithelium and is usually not infected by *N. gonorrhoeae*. However, gonococcal vaginitis can occur in anestrogenic women (e.g., prepubertal girls and postmenopausal women), in whom the vaginal stratified squamous epithelial layers are often thinned down to the basilar layer, which can be infected by *N. gonorrhoeae*. The intense inflammation of the vagina makes the physical (speculum and bimanual) examination extremely painful. The vaginal mucosa is red and edematous, and an abundant purulent discharge is present. Infection in the urethra and in Skene's and Bartholin's glands often accompanies gonococcal vaginitis. Inflamed cervical erosion or abscesses in nabothian cysts may also occur. Coexisting cervicitis may result in pus in the cervical os.

Anorectal Gonorrhea   Because the female anatomy permits the spread of cervical exudate to the rectum, *N. gonorrhoeae* is sometimes recovered from the rectum of women with uncomplicated gonococcal cervicitis. The rectum is the sole site of infection in only 5% of women with gonorrhea. Such women are usually asymptomatic but occasionally have acute proctitis manifested by anorectal pain or pruritus, tenesmus, purulent rectal discharge, and rectal bleeding. Among homosexual men, the frequency of gonococcal infection, including rectal infection, fell by ≥90% throughout the United States in the early 1980s, but a resurgence of gonorrhea among homosexual men was documented in several cities during the 1990s. Gonococcal isolates from the rectum of homosexual men tend to be more resistant than other gonococcal isolates to antimicrobials. Gonococci with multidrug resistance (*mtr*) are more resistant to bile salts and fatty acids in feces and thus are found with increased frequency in homosexual men. The *mtr* mutation involves a DNA-binding protein and results in the derepression of genes encoding an efflux mechanism of resistance. This situation may have been responsible for higher rates of treatment failure for rectal gonorrhea with older regimens consisting of penicillin or tetracyclines.

Pharyngeal Gonorrhea   Pharyngeal gonorrhea is usually mild or asymptomatic, although symptomatic pharyngitis does occasionally occur with cervical lymphadenitis. The mode of acquisition is oral-genital sexual exposure, with fellatio being a more efficient means of transmission than cunnilingus. Most cases resolve spontaneously, and transmission from the pharynx to sexual contacts is rare. Pharyngeal infection almost always coexists with genital infection. Swabs from the pharynx should be plated directly onto gonococcal selective media. Because pharyngeal colonization with *N. meningitidis* needs to be differentiated from that with other *Neisseria* species, the diagnosis of pharyngeal gonorrhea is more expensive and difficult than that of anogenital gonorrhea.

Ocular Gonorrhea in Adults   Ocular gonorrhea in an adult usually results from autoinoculation from an infected genital site. As in genital infection, the manifestations range from severe to occasionally mild or asymptomatic disease. The variability in clinical manifestations may result from differences in the ability of the infecting strain to elicit an inflammatory response.

Infection may result in a markedly swollen eyelid, severe hyperemia and chemosis, and a profuse purulent discharge. The massively inflamed conjunctiva may be draped over the cornea and limbus. Lytic enzymes from the infiltrating PMNs occasionally cause corneal ulceration and rarely cause perforation.

Prompt recognition and treatment of this condition are of paramount importance. Gram's stain and culture of the purulent discharge establish the diagnosis. Genital cultures should also be performed.

Gonorrhea in Pregnant Women, Neonates, and Children Gonorrhea in pregnancy can have serious consequences for both the mother and the infant. Therefore, early detection and eradication of the disease in the mother are extremely important. Recognition of gonorrhea early in pregnancy also identifies a population at risk for other STDs, particularly *Chlamydia* infection and syphilis. These women should be monitored closely for these infections throughout pregnancy. The incidence of gonorrhea in pregnancy ranges from rare to ~10%, depending upon the population surveyed. Salpingitis and PID can occur during the first trimester and are associated with a high rate of fetal loss. In the second and third trimesters, the relative impermeability of the cervical mucus (under the influence of progesterone) and the obliteration of the intrauterine cavity (resulting from the attachment of the chorion to the endometrial decidua by around the twelfth week of gestation) pose physical barriers that usually prevent ascending infection. Pharyngeal infection, most often asymptomatic, may be more common during pregnancy because of altered sexual practices. Acquisition of gonococcal infection late in pregnancy can adversely affect labor and delivery as well as the well-being of the fetus. Prolonged rupture of the membranes, premature delivery, chorioamnionitis, funisitis (infection of the umbilical cord stump), and sepsis in the infant (with *N. gonorrhoeae* detected in the gastric aspirate of the newborn during delivery) are common complications of maternal gonococcal infection at term. Hazards to the fetus include spontaneous abortion, perinatal death, premature delivery, perinatal distress, and premature rupture of membranes. Other microorganisms and conditions, including *Mycoplasma hominis*, *Ureaplasma urealyticum*, *C. trachomatis*, and bacterial vaginosis, have been associated with similar complications.

The most common form of gonorrhea in neonates is *ophthalmia neonatorum*, which results from exposure to infected cervical secretions during parturition. Ocular neonatal instillation of a prophylactic agent (e.g., 1% silver nitrate eyedrops or ophthalmic preparations containing erythromycin or tetracycline) is a cost-effective measure for the prevention of ophthalmia neonatorum but is not effective for its treatment, which requires systemic antibiotics. The clinical manifestations are acute and begin 2 to 5 days after birth. A small inoculum of organisms, low virulence of the infecting strain, or partial suppression by ophthalmic prophylaxis can result in a more indolent course. Therefore, gonococcal infection must be ruled out by culture in every case of conjunctivitis in infants. An initial nonspecific conjunctivitis with a serosanguineous discharge is followed by tense edema of both eyelids, chemosis, and a profuse, thick, purulent discharge. Corneal ulcerations that result in nebulae or perforation may lead to anterior synechiae, anterior staphyloma, panophthalmitis, and blindness. Infections described at other mucosal sites in infants, including vaginitis, rhinitis, and anorectal infection, are likely to be asymptomatic. Pharyngeal colonization has been demonstrated in 35% of infants with gonococcal ophthalmia, and coughing is the most prominent symptom in these cases. Septic arthritis is the most common manifestation of systemic gonococcal infection in the newborn. The primary focus of DGI in most of these cases is uncertain. The onset usually comes at 3 to 21 days of age, and polyarticular involvement is common. Sepsis, meningitis, and pneumonia are seen in rare instances.

Any STD in children beyond the neonatal period raises the possibility of sexual abuse. In most cases of abuse, the perpetrator is a male assailant known to the child. Gonococcal vulvovaginitis is the most common manifestation of gonococcal infection in children beyond infancy. Anorectal and pharyngeal infections are common in these children and are frequently asymptomatic. The urethra, Bartholin's and Skene's glands, and the upper genital tract are rarely involved. All children with gonococcal infection should also be evaluated for *Chlamydia* infection, syphilis, and possibly HIV infection. All cases of suspected and confirmed child abuse should be reported to the appropriate social service agency in the county where the child resides.

Disseminated Gonococcal Infection DGI results from gonococcal bacteremia. In the 1970s, DGI occurred in ~0.5% to 3% of persons with untreated gonococcal mucosal infection. The lower incidence at present is probably attributable to a decline in the prevalence of particular strains that are likely to disseminate. DGI strains resist the bactericidal action of human serum and generally do not incite inflammation at genital sites, probably because of limited generation of chemotactic factors. These strains are often of the Por1A serotype, are highly susceptible to penicillin, and have special nutritional requirements (i.e., the AHU auxotype). Menstruation is a risk factor for dissemination, and approximately two-thirds of cases of DGI are in women. In about half of affected women, symptoms of DGI begin within 7 days of onset of menses. Complement deficiencies, especially of the components involved in the assembly of the membrane attack complex (C5 through C9), predispose to neisserial bacteremia. Up to 13% of patients with DGI have complement deficiencies, and persons with more than one episode of DGI should be screened with an assay for total hemolytic complement activity.

The clinical manifestations of DGI have sometimes been classified into two stages: a bacteremic stage and a joint-localized stage with suppurative arthritis. A clear-cut progression usually is not evident. Patients in the bacteremic stage have higher temperatures, and their fever is more frequently accompanied by chills. Painful joints are common and often occur in conjunction with tenosynovitis and skin lesions.

Polyarthralgias usually include the knees, elbows, and more distal joints; the axial skeleton is generally spared. Skin lesions are seen in ~75% of patients and include papules and pustules, often with a hemorrhagic component (**see Plate IID-60**). These lesions are usually on the extremities and number between 5 and 40. Frank arthritis, when it develops, involves one or two joints, most often (in decreasing order of frequency) the knees, wrists, ankles, and elbows. The occurrence of arthritis in the absence of signs and symptoms of the bacteremic stage has led to the suggestion that these are separate syndromes. Other joints, such as the small joints of the hands and feet and the sternoclavicular and temporomandibular joints, are occasionally involved. Most patients who develop gonococcal septic arthritis do so without prior polyarthralgias or skin lesions; in the absence of symptomatic genital infection, this disease cannot be distinguished from septic arthritis caused by other pathogens. Rarely, osteomyelitis complicates septic arthritis involving small joints.

Although it has been postulated that the initial arthritis and skin lesions are due to direct tissue invasion by *N. gonorrhoeae*, the organism has been recovered from fewer than 5% of skin lesions cultured. This low isolation rate has been attributed to either a small inoculum of infecting organisms or the fastidious growth requirements of *N. gonorrhoeae* strains that disseminate. Gonococcal antigens have been identified in "sterile" skin lesions by immunofluorescent staining techniques. There is also evidence that immune-mediated or hypersensitivity phenomena caused by gonococcal antigens account for skin lesions. Other manifestations of noninfectious dermatitis, such as nodular lesions, urticaria, and erythema multiforme, have been described. Gonococcal endocarditis, although rare today, was relatively common in the preantibiotic era, causing about one-quarter of reported cases of endocarditis. Another unusual complication of DGI is meningitis.

Gonococcal Infection in HIV-Infected Persons The association between gonorrhea and the acquisition of HIV has been demonstrated in several well-controlled studies, mainly in Kenya and Zaire. The nonulcerative STDs enhance the transmission of HIV by three- to fivefold, possibly because of increased viral shedding in persons with urethritis or cervicitis (Chap. 309). HIV has been detected by polymerase chain reaction (PCR) more commonly in ejaculates from HIV-positive men with gonococcal urethritis than in those from HIV-positive men with nongonococcal urethritis. PCR positivity diminishes by twofold following appropriate therapy for urethritis. Not only does gonorrhea enhance the transmission of HIV; it may also increase the individual's risk for acquisition of HIV. A proposed mechanism is the significantly greater number of CD4+ lymphocytes and dendritic cells that can be infected by HIV in endocervical secretions of women with nonulcerative STDs than in those of women with ulcerative STDs.

DIFFERENTIAL DIAGNOSIS The clinical features of uncomplicated gonococcal infections closely resemble those of genital infections caused by *C. trachomatis*. Although the symptoms produced by chlamydial infections tend to be milder, the two infections are often indistinguishable on clinical grounds alone. Co-infection with *N. gonorrhoeae* and *C. trachomatis* is seen in up to 40% of cases. The differential diagnosis of urethritis, epididymitis, and proctitis in men, of cervicitis in women, and of vaginitis in prepubertal girls is discussed in Chap. 132; that of PID in Chap. 133; and that of acute arthritis in young adults in Chap. 323. The differential diagnosis of the bacteremic stage of DGI includes acute rheumatoid arthritis, sarcoidosis, erythema nodosum, drug-induced arthritis, and viral infections (e.g., hepatitis B and acute HIV infection).

LABORATORY DIAGNOSIS A rapid diagnosis of gonococcal infection in men may be obtained by Gram's staining of urethral exudates. The detection of gram-negative intracellular diplococci (GNID) is usually highly specific and sensitive in diagnosing gonococcal urethritis in symptomatic males but is only ~50% sensitive in diagnosing gonococcal cervicitis. Samples should be collected with Dacron or rayon swabs. Part of the sample should be inoculated onto a plate of modified Thayer-Martin or other gonococcal selective medium for culture. It is important to process all samples immediately because gonococci do not tolerate drying. If plates cannot be incubated immediately, they can be held safely for several hours at room temperature in candle extinction jars prior to incubation. If processing is to occur within 6 h, transport of specimens may be facilitated by the use of nonnutritive swab transport systems such as Stuart or Amies medium. For longer holding periods (e.g., when specimens for culture are to be mailed), culture media with self-contained CO_2-generating systems (such as the JEMBEC or Gono-Pak systems) may be used. Specimens should also be obtained for the diagnosis of chlamydial infection.

PMNs are often seen in the endocervix on a Gram's stain, and an abnormally increased number ($\geq$30 PMNs per field in five 1000$\times$ oil-immersion fields) establishes the presence of an inflammatory discharge (mucopurulent cervicitis). Unfortunately, the presence or absence of GNID in cervical smears does not accurately predict which patients have gonorrhea, and the diagnosis in this setting should be made by culture. The sensitivity of a single endocervical culture is ~80 to 90%, with the precise figure depending on the quality of the medium and the adequacy of the clinical specimen. The yield can be enhanced by culture of a second cervical specimen. If a history of rectal sex is elicited, a rectal wall swab (uncontaminated with feces) should be cultured. A presumptive diagnosis of gonorrhea cannot be made on the basis of gram-negative diplococci in smears from the pharynx, where other *Neisseria* species are components of the normal flora.

Nucleic acid probe tests are now widely used for the direct detection of *N. gonorrhoeae* in urogenital specimens. A common assay employs a nonisotopic chemiluminescent DNA probe that hybridizes specifically with gonococcal 16S ribosomal RNA. Studies assessing the utility of the nucleic acid probe system in high-risk outpatients undergoing screening for STDs have revealed that it is at least as sensitive as conventional culture techniques and may be a cost-effective alternative to culture, especially in high-risk males. A disadvantage of non-culture-based assays in general is that specimens submitted in probe-transport systems cannot be cultured subsequently. Therefore, a culture-confirmatory test is not possible, and formal antimicrobial susceptibility testing, if needed, cannot be performed. Low-cost point-of-care tests are under development for use in resource-poor settings, where specific diagnosis often gives way to syndromic management. DNA amplification techniques such as PCR may eventually prove to be equivalent to or more sensitive than culture methods.

Because of the legal implications, gonococcal infection in children must be diagnosed only with standard culture systems. Nonculture tests for gonococcal infection should not be used alone and have not been approved by the U.S. Food and Drug Administration for use with specimens obtained from the genital tract, pharynx, and rectum of infected children. Cultures should be obtained from the pharynx and anus of both girls and boys, the vagina of girls, and the urethra of boys. Cervical specimens are not recommended for prepubertal girls. For boys with a urethral discharge, a meatal specimen of the discharge is adequate for culture. Presumptive colonies of *N. gonorrhoeae* should be identified definitively by at least two independent methods (e.g., biochemical, enzyme substrate, or serologic).

Blood should be cultured in suspected cases of DGI. The use of Isolator blood culture tubes may enhance the yield. The probability of positive blood cultures decreases after 48 h of illness. Synovial fluid should be inoculated into blood culture broth medium and plated onto chocolate agar rather than selective medium because this fluid is not likely to be contaminated with commensal bacteria. Gonococci are infrequently recovered from early joint effusions containing <20,000 leukocytes/μL but may be recovered from effusions containing >80,000 leukocytes/μL. The organisms are seldom recovered from blood and synovial fluid of the same patient.

℞ **TREATMENT** It is no surprise that *N. gonorrhoeae*, with its remarkable capacity to alter its antigenic structure and adapt to changes in the microenvironment, has become resistant to numerous antibiotics. The first effective agents against gonorrhea were the sulfonamides, which were introduced in the 1930s. Within a decade, antibiotic resistance emerged, resulting in treatment failures in one-third of patients. Penicillin was then employed as the drug of choice for the treatment of gonorrhea. By 1965, 42% of gonococcal isolates had developed low-level resistance to penicillin G. To prevent treatment failures, the Centers for Disease Control and Prevention (CDC) at that time recommended doubling the dose of penicillin for the treatment of gonorrhea. Resistance due to the production of penicillinase arose later.

Gonococci become fully resistant to antibiotics either by chromosomal mutations or by acquisition of R factors (plasmids). Two types of chromosomal mutations have been described. The first type, which is drug specific, is a single-step mutation leading to high-level resistance. The second type involves mutations at several chromosomal loci that combine to determine the level as well as the pattern of resistance. Strains with mutations in chromosomal genes were first observed in the late 1950s. As recently as 1997, strains with chromosomal resistance (CMRNG) accounted for resistance to penicillin, tetracycline, or both in ~20% of strains surveyed in the United States.

β-Lactamase (penicillinase)–producing strains of *N. gonorrhoeae* (PPNG) carrying plasmids with the Pc^r determinant were seen almost simultaneously in the United States, England, western Africa, and the Philippines in the late 1970s. PPNG strains have since spread worldwide and by the early 1980s accounted for >50% of all gonococcal isolates in some parts of the developing world. The average prevalence of PPNG in the United States dropped by two-thirds after most penicillin use was discontinued and is now on the order of 4%, with higher rates reported from certain areas. *N. gonorrhoeae* strains with plasmid-borne tetracycline resistance (TRNG) can mobilize some β-lactamase plasmids, and PPNG and TRNG occur together, sometimes along with CMRNG. Penicillin, ampicillin, and tetracycline are no longer reliable agents for the treatment of gonorrhea and should not be used. Third-generation cephalosporins have remained highly effective as single-

dose therapy for gonorrhea. Even though the minimal inhibitory concentrations (MICs) of ceftriaxone for certain strains may reach 0.015 to 0.125 mg/L [higher than MICs for fully susceptible strains (0.0001 to 0.008 mg/L)], these levels are greatly exceeded in blood, the urethra, and the cervix when the routinely recommended ceftriaxone and cefixime regimens are administered (see below). These regimens almost always result in an effective cure.

Quinolone-containing regimens are also recommended for treatment of gonococcal infections; the fluoroquinolones offer the advantage of antichlamydial activity when administered for 7 days. Serum concentrations following therapeutic dosages of the quinolones exceed the MIC for *N. gonorrhoeae* by ~100-fold. However, quinolone-resistant *N. gonorrhoeae* (QRNG) appeared soon after these agents were first used to treat gonorrhea, particularly in Southeast Asia. QRNG strains have been reported recently in the United States, mostly in the far western states. Alterations in DNA gyrase and topoisomerase IV have been implicated as mechanisms of fluoroquinolone resistance.

Resistance to spectinomycin, which is used as an alternative agent, has been reported, but resistance to this agent is usually not associated with resistance to other antibiotics. Therefore, spectinomycin can be reserved for use against multiresistant strains of *N. gonorrhoeae*. Nevertheless, outbreaks caused by strains resistant to spectinomycin have been documented in Korea and England when the drug was used as a primary agent to treat gonorrhea.

Although clinical isolates of *N. gonorrhoeae* vary in their antimicrobial susceptibility patterns in different parts of the world, they remain susceptible to a wide variety of agents. Because failure of treatment can lead to continued transmission and the emergence of antibiotic resistance, the importance of adequate treatment with a regimen that the patient will adhere to cannot be overemphasized. Thus highly effective single-dose regimens have been developed for the treatment of uncomplicated gonococcal infections. The 1998 CDC treatment guidelines for gonococcal infections are summarized in Table 147-1; the recommendations for uncomplicated gonorrhea apply to HIV-infected as well as HIV-uninfected patients. The third-generation cephalosporins cefixime and ceftriaxone are the mainstay of therapy for uncomplicated gonococcal infection of the urethra, cervix, rectum, or pharynx. Single doses of ciprofloxacin or ofloxacin are also effective first-line regimens. Because of resistance to fluoroquinolones in several parts of Southeast Asia, these agents can no longer be considered effective in that region. Because co-infection with *C. trachomatis* occurs frequently, initial treatment regimens must incorporate an agent (e.g., azithromycin or doxycycline) effective against chlamydial infection. Pregnant women with gonorrhea should receive concurrent treatment with a macrolide antibiotic for possible *Chlamydia* infection; doxycycline should not be used during pregnancy. A single 1-g dose of azithromycin, which is effective therapy for uncomplicated chlamydial infections, results in an unacceptably low cure rate (93%) for gonococcal infections and should not be used alone. Uncomplicated gonococcal infections in penicillin-allergic persons who cannot tolerate quinolones may be treated with a single dose of spectinomycin. Persons with uncomplicated infections who receive a recommended regimen need not return for a test of cure. Cultures for *N. gonorrhoeae* should be performed if symptoms persist after therapy with an established regimen, and any gonococci isolated should be tested for antimicrobial susceptibility.

Symptomatic gonococcal pharyngitis is more difficult to eradicate than genital infection. Few regimens result in cure rates of >90%. Persons who cannot tolerate cephalosporins or quinolones can be treated with spectinomycin, but this agent results in a cure rate of ≤52%. Therefore, persons given spectinomycin should have a pharyngeal culture performed 3 to 5 days after treatment as a test of cure.

Treatments for gonococcal epididymitis and PID are discussed in Chaps. 132 and 133, respectively. Ocular gonococcal infections in older children and adults should be managed with a single dose of ceftriaxone combined with saline irrigation of the conjunctivae (both undertaken expeditiously), and patients should undergo a careful ophthalmologic evaluation that includes a slit-lamp examination.

Table 147-1   Recommended Treatment for Gonococcal Infections: 1998 Guidelines of the Centers for Disease Control and Prevention

Diagnosis	Treatment of Choice
Uncomplicated gonococcal infection of the cervix, urethra, pharynx, or rectum[a]	
First-line regimens	Cefixime (400 mg PO, single dose) *or* Ceftriaxone (125 mg IM, single dose) *or* Ciprofloxacin (500 mg PO, single dose) *or* Ofloxacin (400 mg PO, single dose) *plus* A regimen effective against possible *Chlamydia* co-infection, such as: Azithromycin (1 g PO, single dose) *or* Doxycycline (100 mg PO bid for 7 days)
Alternative regimens	Spectinomycin (2 g IM, single dose) *or* Ceftizoxime (500 mg IM, single dose) *or* Cefotaxime (500 mg IM, single dose) *or* Cefotetan (1 g IM, single dose) *or* Cefoxitin (2 g IM, single dose) *plus* probenecid (1 g PO, single dose)
Epididymitis	See Chap. 132
Pelvic inflammatory disease	See Chap. 133
Gonococcal conjunctivitis in an adult	Ceftriaxone (1 g IM, single dose)[b]
Ophthalmia neonatorum[c]	Ceftriaxone (25–50 mg/kg IV or IM, single dose, not to exceed 125 mg)
Disseminated gonococcal infection[d]	
Initial therapy[e]	
Patients tolerant of β-lactam drugs	Ceftriaxone (1 g IM or IV q24h; *recommended*) *or* Cefotaxime (1 g IV q8h) *or* Ceftizoxime (1 g IV q8h)
Patients allergic to β-lactam drugs	Ciprofloxacin (500 mg IV q12h) *or* Ofloxacin (400 mg IV q12h) *or* Spectinomycin (2 g IM q12h)
Continuation therapy	Cefixime (400 mg PO bid) *or* Ciprofloxacin (500 mg PO bid) *or* Ofloxacin (400 mg PO bid)
Meningitis or endocarditis	See text[f]

[a] True failure of treatment with a recommended regimen is rare and should prompt an evaluation for reinfection or consideration of an alternative diagnosis. In cases of quinolone failure, the isolate should be tested for drug resistance if possible.

[b] Plus lavage of the infected eye with saline solution (once).

[c] Prophylactic regimens are discussed in the text.

[d] Hospitalization is indicated if the diagnosis is uncertain, if the patient has frank arthritis with an effusion, or if the patient cannot be relied on to comply with treatment.

[e] All initial regimens should be continued for 24–48 h after clinical improvement begins, at which time therapy may be switched to one of the continuation regimens to complete a full week of antimicrobial treatment.

[f] Hospitalization is recommended to exclude suspected meningitis or endocarditis.

DGI may require higher dosages and longer durations of therapy (Table 147-1). Hospitalization is indicated if the diagnosis is uncertain, if the patient has localized joint disease that requires aspiration, or if the patient cannot be relied on to comply with treatment. Open drainage is necessary only occasionally, e.g., for management of hip infections that may be difficult to drain percutaneously. Nonsteroidal anti-inflammatory agents may be indicated to alleviate pain and hasten improvement of affected joints. Gonococcal meningitis and endocarditis should be treated in the hospital with high-dose intravenous ceftriaxone (1 to 2 g every 12 h); therapy should continue for 10 to 14 days for meningitis and for at least 4 weeks for endocarditis. All persons who experience more than one episode of DGI should be evaluated for complement deficiency.

PREVENTION AND CONTROL Condoms, if properly used, provide effective protection against the transmission and acquisition of gonorrhea as well as other infections that are transmitted to and from genital mucosal surfaces. Spermicidal preparations used with a diaphragm or cervical sponges impregnated with nonoxynol 9 offer some protection against gonorrhea and chlamydial infection. However, the frequent use of preparations that contain nonoxynol 9 is associated with mucosal disruption that paradoxically may enhance the risk of HIV infection in the event of exposure. All patients should be instructed to refer sex partners for evaluation and treatment. All sex partners of persons with gonorrhea should be evaluated and treated for *N. gonorrhoeae* and *C. trachomatis* infections if their last contact with the patient took place within 60 days before the onset of symptoms or the diagnosis of infection in the patient. If the patient's last sexual encounter was >60 days before onset of symptoms or diagnosis, the patient's most recent sex partner should be treated. Patients should be instructed to abstain from sexual intercourse until therapy is completed and until they and their sex partners no longer have symptoms. Greater emphasis must be placed on prevention by public health education, individual patient counseling, and behavior modification. Preventing the spread of gonorrhea may help reduce the transmission of HIV. No effective vaccine for gonorrhea is yet available, but efforts to test a porin vaccine candidate are under way.

ACKNOWLEDGMENT
The authors acknowledge the contributions of Dr. King K. Holmes and Dr. Stephen A. Morse to the chapter on this subject in the earlier editions.

BIBLIOGRAPHY

BLAKE MS, WETZLER LM: Vaccines for gonorrhea: Where are we on the curve? Trends Microbiol 3:469, 1995

CENTERS FOR DISEASE CONTROL AND PREVENTION: Annual Report; Gonococcal Isolate Surveillance Project (GISP); www.cdc.gov/ncidod/dastlr/gcdir/Resist/gisp.html

———: 1998 Guidelines for treatment of sexually transmitted diseases. MMWR 47 (RR-1):1, 1998

COHEN MS, CANNON JG: Human experimentation with *Neisseria gonorrhoeae*: Progress and goals. J Infect Dis 179:S375, 1999

HOOK EW III, HOLMES KK: Gonococcal infections. Ann Intern Med 102:229, 1985

JERSE AE, REST RF: Adhesion and invasion by the pathogenic *Neisseria*. Trends Microbiol 5:217, 1997

LAGA M et al: Non-ulcerative sexually transmitted diseases as risk factors for HIV-1 transmission in women: Results from a cohort study. AIDS 7:95, 1993

McQUILLEN DP et al: Complement processing and immunoglobulin binding to *Neisseria gonorrhoeae* determined in vitro simulates in vivo effects. J Infect Dis 179:124, 1999

O'BRIEN JP et al: Disseminated gonococcal infection: A prospective analysis of 49 patients and a review of pathophysiology and immune mechanisms. Medicine (Baltimore) 62:395, 1983

US DEPARTMENT OF HEALTH AND HUMAN SERVICES: Sexually transmitted disease surveillance 1997:1, 1998

148 *Daniel M. Musher*

MORAXELLA CATARRHALIS AND OTHER MORAXELLA SPECIES

MORAXELLA CATARRHALIS

The gram-negative coccus now known as *Moraxella catarrhalis* has undergone three changes of name in as many decades. Originally called *Micrococcus catarrhalis*, it was renamed *Neisseria catarrhalis* in the 1960s because of its morphologic similarity to *Neisseria* spp. Then, in 1970, it was elevated to the status of a distinct genus, *Branhamella*, on the basis of DNA homology. In 1979 this organism was placed into the genus *Moraxella*, of which *Branhamella* may be a subgenus. A component of the normal bacterial flora of the upper airways, *M. catarrhalis* has been increasingly recognized as a cause of otitis media, sinusitis, and bronchopulmonary infection.

BACTERIOLOGY AND IMMUNITY On Gram's staining, *M. catarrhalis* organisms appear as gram-negative cocci, sometimes occurring in pairs and retaining the side-by-side kidney-bean configuration of *Neisseria* (**Plate VI-1**). These cocci tend to retain crystal violet during the decolorizing step and may be confused with *Staphylococcus aureus*. *Moraxella* colonies grow well on blood or chocolate agar but may be overlooked because of their resemblance to *Neisseria* spp. (a major component of the normal pharyngeal flora). *Moraxella* is readily distinguishable from *Neisseria* spp. by biochemical tests.

Strains of *M. catarrhalis* show a surprising degree of homogeneity in terms of their outer-membrane proteins. Antibody to some of these proteins is generally present in serum of children over the age of 4 years; however, colonizing or disease-causing isolates may survive in serum despite this naturally present antibody and complement. Bactericidal antibody emerges following natural infection and may be directed against one or more conserved outer-membrane proteins—a property of potential value in vaccine development. The presence of certain outer-membrane proteins is associated with virulence in mice, and antibody may be protective. These proteins are under investigation for use as vaccines.

EPIDEMIOLOGY With repeated cultures and the use of selective media, *M. catarrhalis* can be isolated from the upper respiratory tract or saliva of 50% of healthy schoolchildren and of up to 7% of healthy adults. When conventional microbiologic techniques are used, *Moraxella* can be isolated from sputum of about 10% of persons who have chronic bronchitis and 25% of those who have bronchiectasis in the absence of acute infection. Investigators in both the northern and southern hemispheres have reported a striking seasonal variation in the isolation of this organism from clinical specimens, with a peak in late winter/early spring and a nadir in late summer/early fall. Direct contact has not been shown to contribute to community-acquired infection, but nosocomial spread of infection has been documented occasionally.

OTITIS MEDIA AND SINUSITIS *M. catarrhalis* has repeatedly been shown to be the third most common bacterial isolate from middle-ear fluid of children who have otitis media, being surpassed only by *Streptococcus pneumoniae* and nontypable *Haemophilus influenzae*. Recent studies have shown that this organism is also a prominent isolate from sinus cavities in acute and chronic sinusitis.

PURULENT TRACHEOBRONCHITIS AND PNEUMONIA *M. catarrhalis* causes acute exacerbations of chronic bronchitis (increased production and/or purulence of sputum), purulent tracheobronchitis (the latter also involving fever and leukocytosis), and pneumonia. The great majority of infected persons are >50 years old and have a long history of cigarette smoking and underlying chronic obstructive pulmonary disease (COPD); many have lung cancer as well. In one study, 76% of affected persons had COPD (severe in many cases), and one-third of those with COPD had lung cancer; most patients also had clinical evidence of malnutrition. In one extensive series of cases, *M. catarrhalis* pneumonia did not occur in otherwise-healthy hosts.

Symptoms of *M. catarrhalis* infection have been regarded as modest in severity. Both cough and the amount and purulence of sputum are usually increased above baseline. Chills are reported in one-quarter of patients, pleuritic pain in one-third, and malaise in 40%. Most patients have peak temperatures of <38.3°C (<101°F), and peripheral white blood cell counts are <10,000/μL in nearly one-quarter of cases. Microscopic examination of a good sputum specimen following Gram's staining regularly reveals profuse organisms, and quantitative culture yields ~ 2 × 10^8 colony-forming units per milliliter (**Plate VI-1**). The radiologic appearance is variable; in one study, 43% of subjects had segmental or lobar infiltrates, and the remainder had a mixed pattern of subsegmental, segmental, interstitial, and diffuse involvement. These clinical, laboratory, and radiographic findings do not differ from those of pneumococcal or *Haemophilus* pneumonia in an older patient population. However, a far lesser degree of bloodstream invasion occurs in *M. catarrhalis* infection; in one series, none of 25 patients with *M. catarrhalis* pneumonia had bacteremia. Nevertheless, pneumonia due to *M. catarrhalis* is a marker for severe underlying disease: nearly half of patients die within 3 months of onset.

OTHER SYNDROMES Local extension causing empyema is very uncommon, and, as might be inferred from the low rate of bacteremia, metastatic complications of *M. catarrhalis* pneumonia, such as septic arthritis, are exceedingly rare. As of 1995, 58 cases of bacteremic infection due to *M. catarrhalis* had been reported, mainly in children <10 years old or adults >60 years old; most of these patients were immunocompromised. The syndromes reported have included bacteremia with no apparent focus, pneumonia, endocarditis, and meningitis. A petechial or purpuric rash, reminiscent of that observed in meningococcal sepsis and associated with disseminated intravascular coagulation, has been described in a few cases.

R_X **TREATMENT** Treatment of *M. catarrhalis* infection with a penicillin/clavulanic acid combination seems highly appropriate. Penicillin resistance first appeared in *Branhamella* isolates in the mid-1970s and is now found in 85% of clinical isolates. Resistance is mediated by two closely related β-lactamases, BRO-1 and BRO-2, which are present in 90% and 10% of resistant isolates, respectively. These enzymes are active against penicillin, ampicillin, and amoxicillin but less so against cephalosporins, especially third-generation cephalosporins, and they bind avidly to clavulanic acid and sulbactam.

Cephalosporins, especially those of the second and third generations, are effective alternatives. Isolates in the United States are also nearly uniformly susceptible to tetracycline, erythromycin, trimethoprim-sulfamethoxazole, quinolones, and chloramphenicol, although tetracycline resistance—perhaps due to TetB determinants—is increasing in Europe and Asia and has been documented in the United States. A 5-day course of therapy has been shown to cure respiratory infection, although a slightly longer course may be required in sinusitis.

During the period between the identification of gram-negative cocci in a Gram-stained specimen and the final identification of the organisms by culture, the severity of the condition and the potential presence of other infecting organisms should guide antibiotic selection. For example, an exacerbation of bronchitis caused by *M. catarrhalis* might be treated with tetracycline or trimethoprim-sulfamethoxazole; however, in a patient with pneumonia, the possibility that pneumococci resistant to these agents also might be present dictates the choice of ampicillin/sulbactam or a third-generation cephalosporin, at least until culture results become available.

OTHER MORAXELLA SPECIES

Other *Moraxella* species cause a wide range of infections, including bronchitis, pneumonia, empyema, endocarditis, meningitis, conjunctivitis, urinary tract infection, septic arthritis, and wound infection. In a report on all *Moraxella* isolates submitted to the Centers for Disease

Table 148-1   *Moraxella* Species

Moraxella Species	Number of Isolates	Common Sites/ Clinical Association	Number (Percent) for Each Site
M. osloensis[a]	199	Blood	44 (22)
		CSF	18 (9)
		Urine	17 (9)
		Respiratory tract	24 (12)
M. nonliquefaciens	356	Blood	27 (8)
		CSF	6 (2)
		Respiratory tract	196 (55)
M. canis	74	Dog-bite wound	53 (72)
M-6	47	Blood, bone	15 (32)
M. lacunata	33	Conjunctivitis, keratitis	23 (70)
M. urethralis	28	Urine	16 (57)
		Genital tract	3 (11)
M. phenylpyruvica	73	Blood	19 (26)
		CSF	8 (11)
		Urine	12 (16)
M. atlantae	44	Blood	20 (45)
		CSF	5 (11)

[a] Some of these isolates would now be distinguished as a new species, *Moraxella lincolnii*.

NOTE: CSF, cerebrospinal fluid.

SOURCE: Adapted from a summary of CDC experience (Graham et al).

Control and Prevention between 1953 and 1980, certain clinical associations were apparent (Table 148-1). *M. osloensis* and *M. nonliquefaciens*, the most commonly isolated species, were cultured from a wide range of normally sterile body sites, including blood, cerebrospinal fluid, and joints. *M. osloensis* was the *Moraxella* species most frequently isolated from blood; *M. nonliquefaciens* tended to be isolated from the ears, nose, or throat (47%) or the sputum (8%) and has since been implicated as a cause of conjunctivitis and keratitis. *M. urethralis* was isolated most often from urine and the genital tract and probably represents the *Moraxella* species implicated previously in urethritis. More than half of isolates of *M. phenylpyruvica* and *M. atlantae* were obtained from normally sterile sites. A recent study found *Moraxella* spp., including *M. catarrhalis*, in 35% of infected wounds following cat bites and in 10% of those following dog bites. The clinical features of infections due to *Moraxella* spp. other than *M. catarrhalis* and the nature of the hosts in which they occur have not been fully characterized.

BIBLIOGRAPHY

GRAHAM D et al: Infections caused by *Moraxella, Moraxella urethralis, Moraxella*-like groups M-5 and M-6, and *Kingella kingae* in the United States, 1953–1980. Rev Infect Dis 12:423, 1990

IOANNIDIS JPA et al: Spectrum and significance of bacteremia due to *Moraxella catarrhalis*. Clin Infect Dis 21:390, 1995

MURPHY TF: *Branhamella catarrhalis*: Epidemiology, surface antigenic structure and immune response. Microbiol Rev 60:267, 1996

TALAN DA et al: Bacteriologic analysis of infected dog and cat bites. N Engl J Med 340:85, 1999

WRIGHT PW et al: A descriptive study of 42 cases of *Branhamella catarrhalis* pneumonia. Am J Med 88(Suppl 5A):2S, 1990

149   *Timothy F. Murphy*

HAEMOPHILUS INFECTIONS

HAEMOPHILUS INFLUENZAE

MICROBIOLOGY   *Haemophilus influenzae* was first recognized in 1892 by Pfeiffer, who erroneously concluded that the bacterium was the cause of influenza. The bacterium is a small (1- by 0.3-μm) gram-negative organism of variable shape; hence, it is often described as a pleomorphic coccobacillus. In clinical specimens such

as cerebrospinal fluid (CSF) and sputum, it frequently stains only faintly with phenosafranin and therefore can easily be overlooked.

H. influenzae grows both aerobically and anaerobically. Its aerobic growth requires two factors: hemin (X factor) and nicotinamide adenine dinucleotide (V factor). These requirements are used in the clinical laboratory to identify the bacterium. Six major serotypes of *H. influenzae* have been identified; designated *a* through *f*, they are based on antigenically distinct polysaccharide capsules. In addition, some strains lack a polysaccharide capsule and are referred to as *nontypable* strains. Type b and nontypable strains are the most relevant strains clinically, although encapsulated strains other than type b can cause disease. *H. influenzae* was the first free-living organism to have its entire genome sequenced.

The antigenically distinct type b capsule is a linear polymer composed of ribosyl-ribitol phosphate. Strains of *H. influenzae* type b (Hib) cause disease primarily in infants and children under the age of 6 years. Nontypable strains are primarily mucosal pathogens, although the incidence of invasive disease caused by these strains is increasing.

EPIDEMIOLOGY AND TRANSMISSION   *H. influenzae* is an exclusively human pathogen. The organism is spread by airborne droplets or by direct contact with secretions or fomites. Nontypable strains colonize the upper respiratory tract of up to three-fourths of healthy adults. Colonization with nontypable *H. influenzae* is a dynamic process; new strains are acquired and other strains are replaced periodically.

Hib strains colonize the nasopharynx of children at a rate of 3 to 5%; before the introduction of type b vaccine, higher rates were seen in day-care centers. The widespread use of conjugate vaccines has resulted in a striking decrease not only in the rate of nasopharyngeal colonization by Hib but also in the incidence of meningitis due to Hib. Studies in selected populations suggest the reemergence of invasive Hib infections and higher than expected rates of nasopharyngeal colonization by Hib in vaccinated children. Continued surveillance of Hib disease and colonization rates will be important in evaluating the success of current vaccination strategies.

Certain population groups have a higher incidence of invasive Hib disease than the general population. The incidence of meningitis due to Hib has been three to four times higher among black children than among white children in several studies. In some Native American groups, the incidence of invasive Hib disease is 10 times higher than that in the general population. Although this increased incidence has not yet been accounted for, several factors may be relevant, including age at exposure to the bacterium, socioeconomic conditions, and genetic differences in the ability to mount an immune response.

PATHOGENESIS   Hib strains cause systemic disease by invasion and hematogenous spread to distant sites such as the meninges, bones, and joints. The type b polysaccharide capsule is an important virulence factor affecting the bacterium's ability to avoid opsonization and cause systemic disease.

Nontypable strains cause disease by local invasion of mucosal surfaces. Otitis media results when bacteria reach the middle ear by way of the eustachian tube. Adults with chronic bronchitis experience recurrent lower respiratory tract infection due to nontypable strains. The incidence of invasive disease caused by nontypable strains is low but increasing.

IMMUNE RESPONSE   Antibody to capsule is important in protection from infection by Hib strains. The level of (maternally acquired) serum antibody to the capsular polysaccharide, which is a polymer of polyribitol ribose phosphate (PRP), declines from birth to 6 months of age and, in the absence of vaccination, remains low until around 2 or 3 years of age. The age at the antibody nadir correlates with that of the peak incidence of type b disease. Antibody to PRP then appears partly as a result of exposure to Hib or cross-reacting antigens. Systemic Hib disease is unusual after the age of 6 years because of the presence of protective antibody. Vaccines in which PRP is conjugated to protein carrier molecules have been developed and are now used widely. These vaccines generate an antibody response to PRP in infants and are effective in preventing invasive infections in infants and children.

Since nontypable strains lack a capsule, the immune response to infection is directed at noncapsular antigens. These noncapsular antigens of *H. influenzae* have generated considerable interest as targets of the human immune response and as potential vaccine components.

CLINICAL MANIFESTATIONS Hib The most serious manifestation of infection with Hib is meningitis. The age of peak incidence varies somewhat among populations, depending in part on the use of vaccine, but this infection primarily affects infants under 2 years of age. The clinical manifestations of meningitis caused by Hib are similar to those of meningitis caused by other bacterial pathogens. Fever and altered central nervous system function are the most common features at presentation. Nuchal rigidity may or may not be evident. Subdural effusion, the most common complication, is suspected when, despite 2 or 3 days of appropriate antibiotic therapy, the infant has seizures, hemiparesis, or continued obtundation. The overall mortality from meningitis caused by Hib is approximately 5%, and the rate of morbidity is high. Of survivors, 6% have permanent sensorineural hearing loss, and about one-fourth have a significant handicap of some type. If more subtle handicaps are sought, up to half of survivors are found to have some neurologic sequelae, such as partial hearing loss and delay in language development.

Epiglottitis is a life-threatening infection involving cellulitis of the epiglottis and supraglottic tissues. It can lead to acute upper airway obstruction. Its unique epidemiologic features are its occurrence in an older age group (2 to 7 years old) than other Hib infections and its absence among Navajo Indians and Alaskan Eskimos. Sore throat and fever rapidly progress to dysphagia, drooling, and airway obstruction.

Cellulitis due to Hib occurs in young children. The most common location is on the head or neck, and the involved area sometimes takes on a characteristic bluish-red color. Most patients have bacteremia, and 10% have an additional focus of infection.

Hib causes *pneumonia* in infants. The infection is clinically indistinguishable from other types of bacterial pneumonia (e.g., pneumococcal pneumonia) except that Hib is more likely to involve the pleura.

Several less common invasive conditions can be important clinical manifestations of Hib infection in children. These include osteomyelitis, septic arthritis, pericarditis, orbital cellulitis, endophthalmitis, urinary tract infection, abscesses, and bacteremia without an identifiable focus. As has already been mentioned, infections due to Hib are unusual among patients older than 6 years.

Nontypable *H. influenzae* Nontypable *H. influenzae* is the second most common cause (after *Streptococcus pneumoniae*) of community-acquired bacterial pneumonia in adults. Nontypable *H. influenzae* pneumonia is especially common among patients with chronic obstructive pulmonary disease (COPD) or AIDS. The clinical features of pneumonia due to *H. influenzae* are similar to those of other types of bacterial pneumonia (including pneumococcal pneumonia). Patients present with fever, cough, and purulent sputum, usually of several days' duration. Chest radiography reveals alveolar infiltrates in a patchy or lobar distribution. Gram-stained sputum contains a predominance of small, pleomorphic, coccobacillary gram-negative bacteria.

Exacerbations of COPD caused by nontypable *H. influenzae* are characterized by increased cough, sputum production, and shortness of breath. Fever is low-grade, and no infiltrates are evident on chest x-ray.

Nontypable *H. influenzae* is one of the three most common causes of childhood otitis media (the other two being *S. pneumoniae* and *Moraxella catarrhalis*). Infants are febrile and irritable, while older children report ear pain. Symptoms of viral upper respiratory infection often precede otitis media. The diagnosis is made by pneumatic otoscopy. An etiologic diagnosis, although not routinely sought, can be established by tympanocentesis and culture of middle-ear fluid.

Nontypable *H. influenzae* also causes puerperal sepsis and is an important cause of neonatal bacteremia. These nontypable strains tend to be of biotype IV and cause invasive disease after colonizing the female genital tract.

Nontypable *H. influenzae* causes sinusitis in adults and children. In addition, the bacterium is a less common cause of various invasive infections that are reported primarily as small-series descriptions and case reports. These infections include empyema, adult epiglottitis, pericarditis, cellulitis, septic arthritis, osteomyelitis, endocarditis, cholecystitis, intraabdominal infections, urinary tract infections, mastoiditis, aortic graft infection, and bacteremia without a detectable focus.

DIAGNOSIS The most reliable method for establishing a diagnosis of Hib infection is recovery of the organism in culture. The CSF of a patient in whom meningitis is suspected should be subjected to Gram's staining and culture. The presence of gram-negative coccobacilli in Gram-stained CSF is strong evidence for Hib meningitis. Recovery of the organism from CSF confirms the diagnosis. Cultures of other normally sterile body fluids, such as blood, joint fluid, pleural fluid, pericardial fluid, and subdural effusion, are confirmatory in other infections.

Detection of PRP is an important adjunct to culture in rapid diagnosis. Immunoelectrophoresis, latex agglutination, coagglutination, and enzyme-linked immunosorbent assay are effective in detecting PRP. These assays are particularly helpful when patients have received prior antimicrobial therapy and thus are especially likely to have negative cultures.

Before the early 1980s, nontypable strains of *H. influenzae* were frequently misidentified as Hib because of their autoagglutination when serotypes were determined in agglutination assays. Since nontypable *H. influenzae* is primarily a mucosal pathogen, it is a component of a mixed flora; this situation makes etiologic diagnosis challenging. Nontypable *H. influenzae* infection is strongly suggested by the predominance of gram-negative coccobacilli among abundant polymorphonuclear leukocytes in a Gram-stained sputum specimen from a patient in whom pneumonia or tracheobronchitis is suspected. A sputum culture is helpful when interpreted along with the results of Gram's staining. Although bacteremia is detectable in a small proportion of patients with pneumonia due to nontypable *H. influenzae*, most such patients have negative blood cultures.

A diagnosis of otitis media is based on the detection by pneumatic otoscopy of fluid in the middle ear. An etiologic diagnosis requires tympanocentesis but is not routinely sought. An invasive procedure is also required to determine the etiology of sinusitis; thus, treatment is often empirical once the diagnosis is suspected in light of clinical symptoms and sinus radiographs.

℞ **TREATMENT** Initial therapy for meningitis due to Hib should consist of a cephalosporin such as ceftriaxone or cefotaxime. For children, the dose of ceftriaxone is 75 to 100 mg/kg daily given in two doses 12 h apart. The pediatric dose of cefotaxime is 200 mg/kg daily given in four doses 6 h apart. Adult doses are 2 g every 12 h for ceftriaxone and 2 g every 4 to 6 h for cefotaxime. An alternative regimen for initial therapy is ampicillin (200 to 300 mg/kg daily in four divided doses) plus chloramphenicol (75 to 100 mg/kg daily in four divided doses). Therapy should continue for a total of 1 to 2 weeks.

Administration of glucocorticoids to patients with Hib meningitis reduces the incidence of neurologic sequelae. The presumed mechanism is reduction of the inflammation induced by bacterial cell-wall mediators of inflammation when cells are killed by antimicrobial agents. Dexamethasone (0.6 mg/kg per day intravenously in four divided doses for 2 days) is recommended for the treatment of Hib meningitis in children over 2 months of age.

Invasive infections other than meningitis are treated with the same antimicrobial agents. For epiglottitis, the dose of ceftriaxone is 50 mg/kg daily, and the dose of cefotaxime is 150 mg/kg daily, given in three divided doses 8 h apart. Epiglottitis constitutes a medical emergency, and maintenance of an airway is critical. The duration of therapy is determined by the clinical response. A course of 1 to 2 weeks is usually appropriate.

Many infections caused by nontypable strains of *H. influenzae*, such as otitis media, sinusitis, and exacerbations of COPD, can be treated with oral antimicrobial agents. Approximately 25% of nontypable strains produce β-lactamase and are resistant to ampicillin. Infections caused by ampicillin-resistant strains can be treated with a variety of agents, including trimethoprim-sulfamethoxazole, amoxicillin/clavulanic acid, various extended-spectrum cephalosporins, and newer macrolides (azithromycin and clarithromycin). Fluoroquinolones are highly active against *H. influenzae* but are not currently recommended for the treatment of children or pregnant women because of possible effects on articular cartilage.

PREVENTION Vaccination The development of conjugate vaccines that prevent invasive infections with Hib in infants and children has been a dramatic success. Four such vaccines are licensed in the United States. In addition to eliciting protective antibody, these vaccines prevent disease by reducing pharyngeal colonization with Hib.

All children should be immunized with an Hib conjugate vaccine, receiving the first dose at approximately 2 months of age, the rest of the primary series between 2 and 6 months of age, and a booster dose at 12 to 15 months of age. Specific recommendations vary for the different conjugate vaccines. The reader is referred to the recommendations of the American Academy of Pediatrics. Currently, no vaccines are available for the prevention of disease caused by nontypable *H. influenzae*.

Chemoprophylaxis The risk of secondary disease is greater than normal among household contacts of patients with Hib disease. The attack rate is as high as 4% among susceptible infants. Therefore, all children and adults in households where there are contacts <4 years old should receive prophylaxis with oral rifampin. (This rule does not apply when all household contacts under the age of 4 years have been completely immunized with conjugate vaccine.) Children <12 years old should receive rifampin at a dose of 20 mg/kg once daily for 4 days, and adults should receive 600 mg daily for 4 days. The index case should receive rifampin before or at the time of discharge from the hospital because antimicrobial agents used for the treatment of meningitis do not reliably eradicate Hib from the nasopharynx.

When two or more cases of invasive Hib disease have occurred within 60 days at a child-care facility attended by incompletely vaccinated children, administration of rifampin to all attendees and personnel is indicated, as is recommended for household contacts. The data on secondary cases among contacts in child-care facilities following a single case are less clear. The administration of rifampin prophylaxis to contacts should be considered, but each decision should be individualized and in part based on the contacts' immunization history, the size of the center, and the extent of contact.

HAEMOPHILUS INFLUENZAE BIOGROUP AEGYPTIUS

H. influenzae biogroup aegyptius was formerly called *Haemophilus aegyptius* because of phenotypic characteristics distinct from those of *H. influenzae*. However, later studies involving DNA hybridization and DNA transformation demonstrated that *H. aegyptius* and *H. influenzae* are members of the same species.

H. influenzae biogroup aegyptius has long been associated with conjunctivitis. Moreover, this strain is now known to be the cause of Brazilian purpuric fever (BPF), which was first recognized in 1984 in the rural Brazilian town of Promissao. The sharing of many phenotypic and genotypic characteristics by the various strains of *H. influenzae* biogroup aegyptius that cause BPF indicates that these strains represent a clone of *H. influenzae*. The age of peak incidence of BPF is 1 to 4 years, with a range of 3 months to 8 years. The illness can occur sporadically or in outbreaks. Typically, after an episode of purulent conjunctivitis, high fever occurs in association with vomiting and abdominal pain. Within 12 to 48 h after onset, the patient develops petechiae, purpura, and peripheral necrosis and experiences vascular collapse. The characteristic laboratory features are thrombocytopenia, prolonged prothrombin time, uniformly unrevealing CSF findings, and blood cultures positive for *H. influenzae* biogroup aegyptius. Initial reports cited high mortality (70%), but subsequent studies have indicated that milder forms of the illness exist. Most patients have resolved or resolving purulent conjunctivitis, and culture of the conjunctiva is positive in approximately one-third of cases. BPF has been seen in several towns in Brazil and on two occasions in Australia.

HAEMOPHILUS DUCREYI

Haemophilus ducreyi is the etiologic agent of chancroid, a sexually transmitted disease characterized by genital ulceration and inguinal adenitis. *H. ducreyi* poses a significant health problem in developing countries. Although this infection is less common in the United States, its incidence has increased dramatically in the past several years. In addition to being a cause of morbidity in itself, chancroid is associated with infection with HIV because of the role of genital ulceration in the transmission of HIV.

MICROBIOLOGY *H. ducreyi* is a highly fastidious coccobacillary gram-negative bacterium whose growth requires X factor (hemin). Although, in light of this requirement, the bacterium has been classified in the genus *Haemophilus*, DNA homology and chemotaxonomic studies have established substantial differences between *H. ducreyi* and other *Haemophilus* species. Taxonomic reclassification of the organism is likely in the future but awaits further study.

The histology of the genital ulcer of chancroid is characterized by perivascular and interstitial infiltrates of macrophages and of CD4+ and CD8+ lymphocytes. The appearance is consistent with a delayed-type hypersensitivity, cell-mediated immune response. The presence of CD4+ cells and macrophages in the ulcer may explain, in part, the facilitation of transmission of HIV in patients with chancroid.

EPIDEMIOLOGY AND PREVALENCE (See also Chap. 132) Chancroid is a common cause of genital ulcers in developing countries. In the United States, chancroid is now endemic in some regions, and several large outbreaks have occurred since 1981. Recurring epidemiologic themes have been apparent in these outbreaks: (1) transmission has been predominantly heterosexual; (2) males have outnumbered females by ratios of 3:1 to 25:1; (3) prostitutes have been important in transmission of the infection; and (4) chancroid has been strongly associated with illicit drug use. The incidence of chancroid in the United States will undoubtedly increase in the coming years, and the genital ulcers associated with this infection will continue to play a role in the transmission of HIV.

CLINICAL MANIFESTATIONS Infection is acquired as the result of a break in the epithelium during sexual contact with an infected individual. After an incubation period of 4 to 7 days, the initial lesion—a papule with surrounding erythema—appears (**Plate IID-54**). In 2 to 3 days, the papule evolves into a pustule, which spontaneously ruptures and forms a sharply circumscribed ulcer that is generally not indurated. The ulcers are painful and bleed easily; little or no inflammation of the surrounding skin is evident. Approximately half of patients develop enlarged, tender inguinal lymph nodes, which frequently become fluctuant and spontaneously rupture.

The presentation of chancroid does not usually include all of the typical clinical features and is sometimes atypical. Multiple ulcers can coalesce to form giant ulcers. Ulcers can appear and then resolve, with inguinal adenitis and suppuration following 1 to 3 weeks later; this clinical picture can be confused with that of lymphogranuloma venereum. Multiple small ulcers can resemble folliculitis. Other differential diagnostic considerations include the various infections causing genital ulceration, such as primary syphilis, condyloma latum of secondary syphilis, genital herpes, and donovanosis. In rare cases chancroid lesions become secondarily infected with bacteria; the result is extensive inflammation.

DIAGNOSIS Clinical diagnosis of chancroid is often inaccurate, and laboratory confirmation should be attempted in suspected cases. Gram's staining of a swab of the lesion may reveal a predominance of characteristic gram-negative coccobacilli, but the presence of other bacteria often makes it difficult to interpret this result. An accurate diagnosis of chancroid relies on cultures of *H. ducreyi* from the lesion. In addition, aspiration and culture of suppurative lymph nodes should be considered. Since the organism can be difficult to grow, the use of selective and supplemented media is necessary.

℞ **TREATMENT** Clinical isolates of *H. ducreyi* often exhibit plasmid-mediated resistance to ampicillin, chloramphenicol, tetracyclines, and sulfonamides. Nevertheless, chancroid can be treated effectively with several regimens, including (1) ceftriaxone, 250 mg intramuscularly as a single dose; (2) azithromycin, 1 g orally as a single dose; (3) erythromycin, 500 mg orally four times daily for 7 days; and (4) ciprofloxacin, 500 mg orally twice daily for 3 days. Ciprofloxacin should not be administered to pregnant or lactating women or to persons <18 years old. Any therapeutic regimen may fail; single-dose ceftriaxone has a high failure rate in HIV-positive individuals. Isolates from patients who do not respond promptly to treatment should be tested for antimicrobial susceptibility. In patients with HIV infection, healing may be slow and longer courses of treatment may be necessary. Contacts of patients with chancroid should be identified and treated whenever possible.

OTHER *HAEMOPHILUS* SPECIES

Haemophilus species are often recovered as components of the flora of the normal human upper respiratory tract. However, these bacteria are infrequent causes of infection because of their low pathogenic potential. *Haemophilus* species have fastidious growth requirements and are generally rather slow-growing. The species implicated in human infections include *H. parainfluenzae*, *H. aphrophilus*, and *H. paraphrophilus* (Chap. 150); *H. parahaemolyticus*; *H. haemolyticus*; and *H. segnis*. *Haemophilus* species are differentiated from one another by several characteristics, primarily their requirements for X and V factors. Species designated *para-* require V factor but not X factor for growth, whereas the others require either X and V or X only.

A variety of infections involving almost all organ systems can be caused by *Haemophilus* species. Most of these unusual manifestations have been reported as single cases and small series.

The antimicrobial susceptibility characteristics of other *Haemophilus* species are similar to those of *H. influenzae*. Some strains produce β-lactamase and are thereby resistant to ampicillin. Other strains are sensitive to ampicillin, and this agent has been used successfully to treat many infections. Alternative agents with good activity against most *Haemophilus* species include trimethoprim-sulfamethoxazole, third-generation cephalosporins, tetracycline, chloramphenicol, and aminoglycosides. Endocarditis caused by ampicillin-sensitive strains should be treated with ampicillin plus an aminoglycoside.

BIBLIOGRAPHY

COMMITTEE ON INFECTIOUS DISEASES: *Haemophilus influenzae* infections, in *1997 Red Book, Report of the Committee on Infectious Diseases*, G Peter et al (eds). Elk Grove Village, IL, American Academy of Pediatrics, 1997

DOERN GV et al: *Haemophilus influenzae* and *Moraxella catarrhalis* from patients with community-acquired respiratory tract infections: Antimicrobial susceptibility patterns from the SENTRY Antimicrobial Surveillance Program (United States and Canada, 1997). Antimicrob Agents Chemother 43:385, 1999

FADEN H et al: Relationship between nasopharyngeal colonization and the development of otitis media in children. J Infect Dis 175:1440, 1997

FOXWELL AR et al: Nontypeable *Haemophilus influenzae*: Pathogenesis and prevention. Microbiol Mol Biol Rev 62:294, 1998

GALIL K et al: Reemergence of invasive *Haemophilus influenzae* type b disease in a well-vaccinated population in remote Alaska. J Infect Dis 179:101, 1999

KING R et al: An immunohistochemical analysis of naturally occurring chancroid. J Infect Dis 174:427, 1996

KLEIN JO: Clinical implications of antibiotic resistance for management of acute otitis media. Pediatr Infect Dis J 17:1084, 1998

MERTZ KJ et al: An investigation of genital ulcers in Jackson, Mississippi, with use of a multiplex polymerase chain reaction assay: High prevalence of chancroid and human immunodeficiency virus infection. J Infect Dis 178:1060, 1998

PELTOLA H et al: Perspective: A five-country analysis of the impact of four different *Haemophilus influenzae* type b conjugates and vaccination strategies in Scandinavia. J Infect Dis 179:223, 1999

QUAGLIARELLO VJ, SCHELD WM: Treatment of bacterial meningitis. N Engl J Med 336:708, 1997

SCHMID GP: Treatment of chancroid, 1997. Clin Infect Dis 28(Suppl 1):S14, 1999

YI K et al: Human immune response to nontypeable *Haemophilus influenzae* in chronic bronchitis. J Infect Dis 176:1247, 1997

150 *Dennis L. Kasper, Tamar F. Barlam*

INFECTIONS DUE TO THE HACEK GROUP AND MISCELLANEOUS GRAM-NEGATIVE BACTERIA

HACEK GROUP ORGANISMS

HACEK organisms are a group of fastidious, slow-growing, gram-negative bacteria whose growth requires an atmosphere of carbon dioxide. Species belonging to this group include several *Haemophilus* species, *Actinobacillus actinomycetemcomitans*, *Cardiobacterium hominis*, *Eikenella corrodens*, and *Kingella kingae*. HACEK bacteria normally reside in the oral cavity and have been associated with local infections in the mouth. They are also known to cause severe systemic infections, most often bacterial endocarditis (Chap. 126).

Of the HACEK group, the *Haemophilus* species, *A. actinomycetemcomitans*, and *C. hominis* are most frequently associated with endocarditis, which can develop on either native or prosthetic valves. In large series, up to 3% of cases of infective endocarditis are attributable to HACEK organisms. The clinical course of HACEK endocarditis tends to be subacute; however, embolization is common. The overall prevalence of major emboli associated with HACEK endocarditis ranges from 28 to 60% in different series. Cultures of blood from patients with suspected HACEK endocarditis may require up to 30 days to become positive, although most are positive within the first week. Because of this slow growth, antimicrobial testing may be difficult, and strains producing β-lactamase may not be identified accurately. This factor should be considered when choosing a therapeutic regimen.

The cure rates for HACEK prosthetic valve endocarditis appear to be high. Unlike prosthetic valve endocarditis caused by other gram-negative organisms, HACEK endocarditis is often cured with antibiotic treatment alone—i.e., without surgical intervention.

Haemophilus **Species** *Haemophilus* species cause over half of all cases of HACEK endocarditis. *H. parainfluenzae* is most common, with *H. aphrophilus* and *H. paraphrophilus* less common. Up to 50% of patients with native valve endocarditis due to *Haemophilus* species report a history of cardiac valvular disease, 60% have been ill for <2 months before presentation, and 50% are anemic at presentation. Some 19% of these patients develop congestive heart failure. Mortality rates of up to 30% have been reported, with most deaths attributed to cerebral embolism; however, recent studies have documented mortality rates of <5%. In rare cases, *H. parainfluenzae* has been isolated from other infections, such as meningitis; brain, dental, and liver abscess; pneumonia; and septicemia.

℞ **TREATMENT** Therapy for endocarditis due to *Haemophilus* species should be based on antibiotic sensitivity testing. Empirical combination therapy with ampicillin and gentamicin, successful in prior studies, is no longer recommended because of increasing β-lactamase production by these strains. Treatment with ceftriaxone (2 g/d) is a reasonable initial approach.

Actinobacillus actinomycetemcomitans *A. actinomycetemcomitans*, another slow-growing inhabitant of the oral cavity, can be isolated from soft tissue infections and abscesses in association with *Actinomyces israelii*. About 30% of actinomycotic lesions also yield *A. actinomycetemcomitans* on culture. *A. actinomycetemcomitans* has been associated with severe destructive periodontal disease, characterized by loss of alveolar bone of the molars and incisors, in both children and adults. Patients who develop endocarditis with this organism typically have severe periodontal disease and underlying cardiac valvular damage as well as high rates of embolic phenomena. *A. actinomycetemcomitans* has been isolated from patients with brain abscess, meningitis, parotitis, osteomyelitis, urinary tract infection, pneumonia, and empyema, among other infections.

℞ **TREATMENT** Most isolates are susceptible to third-generation cephalosporins such as ceftriaxone (2 g/d), semisynthetic penicillins such as mezlocillin, trimethoprim-sulfamethoxazole, quinolones, and azithromycin. However, because of the variability among strains, susceptibility testing should be undertaken. Endocarditis should normally be treated for 4 weeks; however, prosthetic valve infections or infections in patients with complications such as embolization justify 6 weeks of therapy.

Cardiobacterium hominis *C. hominis* primarily causes endocarditis in patients with underlying valvular heart disease or with prosthetic valves. Many patients have signs and symptoms of long-standing infection before diagnosis and have evidence of arterial embolization, vasculitis, cerebrovascular accidents, immune complex glomerulonephritis, or arthritis at presentation. As in endocarditis due to other HACEK organisms, embolization, mycotic aneurysms, and congestive heart failure are frequent.

℞ **TREATMENT** Antibiotic sensitivity testing of *C. hominis* is difficult. Most cases of infection due to *C. hominis* are treated with penicillin (16 to 18 million units per day in 6 divided doses), either alone or in combination with an aminoglycoside (e.g., gentamicin, 5 to 6 mg/kg per day in 3 divided doses). The value of the aminoglycoside in this situation has not been established.

Eikenella corrodens *E. corrodens*, a fastidious, facultative gram-negative organism, is part of the endogenous flora of the mouth and nasopharynx. It is most frequently recovered from sites of infection in conjunction with other bacterial species. Clinical sources of *E. corrodens* include sites of human bite wounds (clenched-fist injuries), endocarditis, soft tissue infections of the head and neck, soft tissue infections in injection drug users, osteomyelitis, respiratory infections, chorioamnionitis, gynecologic infections associated with intrauterine devices, meningitis and brain abscesses, and visceral abscesses.

℞ **TREATMENT** *E. corrodens*–associated infections can be treated with ampicillin (2 g every 4 h) or with second- or third-generation cephalosporins. The organism is susceptible to the fluoroquinolones in vitro but is resistant to metronidazole and clindamycin.

Kingella kingae *K. kingae* is a β-hemolytic, fastidious, non-motile gram-negative rod. Because of improved microbiologic methodology, isolation of this organism is increasingly common. In young children, *K. kingae* causes septic arthritis and osteomyelitis. In several series, *K. kingae* has been the third most common cause of septic arthritis in children <24 months of age; staphylococcal and strepto-

coccal species remain most prevalent. In children <4 years of age, there is evidence for prolonged nasopharyngeal colonization, with carriage rates of 10%. Invasive *K. kingae* infections with bacteremia are associated with stomatitis. Both *K. kingae* colonization and primary herpes—a major cause of stomatitis—peak in children 6 to 48 months of age. *K. kingae* bacteremia can present with a petechial rash similar to that seen with *Neisseria meningitidis* sepsis.

Infective endocarditis, unlike other infections with *K. kingae*, occurs in older children and adults. The majority of patients have pre-existing valvular disease. As in endocarditis caused by the other HACEK organisms, there is a high incidence of complications, including arterial emboli, cerebrovascular accidents, tricuspid insufficiency, and congestive heart failure with cardiovascular collapse.

℞ **TREATMENT** *K. kingae* can be susceptible to ampicillin, second- and third-generation cephalosporins, fluoroquinolones, vancomycin, clindamycin, macrolides, and trimethoprim-sulfamethoxazole. Because of increasing β-lactamase production in *K. kingae* strains, susceptibility testing should be performed to guide therapy. Ceftriaxone (2 g/d) or ampicillin-sulbactam (3 g of ampicillin every 6 h) are both appropriate choices for initial therapy.

OTHER GRAM-NEGATIVE BACTERIA

***Acinetobacter* Species** See Chap. 153.

Achromobacter xylosoxidans Previously known as *Alcaligenes xylosoxidans*, the gram-negative bacillus *Achromobacter xylosoxidans* is probably part of the endogenous intestinal flora and has been isolated from water sources. Immunocompromised hosts appear to be at increased risk for infection with this organism. Nosocomial sources to which outbreaks of infection with *A. xylosoxidans* have been attributed include contaminated intravenous fluids, pressure transducers, and disinfectants. Clinical illness has been associated with isolates from many sites, including blood (often in the setting of infected intravascular devices), urine, respiratory secretions, cerebrospinal fluid, peritoneal and pleural fluids, and endocarditic prosthetic valves. Community-acquired bacteremia with *A. xylosoxidans* usually occurs in the setting of pneumonia. Metastatic skin lesions are present in one-fifth of cases. The reported mortality rate is 67%, similar to rates for other bacteremic gram-negative pneumonias.

℞ **TREATMENT** In vitro susceptibility testing of all clinically relevant isolates is essential to the selection of appropriate therapy.

Agrobacterium radiobacter (tumefaciens) This organism has been associated with intravascular catheter–related infections in immunocompromised hosts, especially individuals infected with HIV. Clinically important infections associated with *A. radiobacter* include prosthetic joint and prosthetic valve infections, bacteremia, peritonitis, and urinary tract infections.

℞ **TREATMENT** Antibiotic sensitivity testing is essential in the choice of therapy.

***Capnocytophaga* Species** This genus of fusiform, long, thin, gram-negative coccobacilli is facultatively anaerobic and requires an atmosphere enriched in carbon dioxide for optimal growth. *C. ochracea*, *C. gingivalis*, and *C. sputigena* are inhabitants of the healthy human oral cavity and have been isolated from the female genital tract. Their isolation has also been reported from blood, cerebrospinal fluid, and respiratory fluids (including pleural collections). These organisms have been associated with sepsis in immunocompromised hosts; particularly at risk are patients with acute myelogenous leukemia or acute lymphocytic leukemia. In the immunocompetent host, these three species probably play a role in localized juvenile periodontitis; however, they have been isolated from many other sites as well, usually as part of a polymicrobial infection. In vitro sensitivity testing of these organisms is difficult because they are slow-growing and fastidious.

C. canimorsus and *C. cynodegmi* are endogenous to the canine mouth. Patients infected with these species frequently have a history of dog bites or of exposure to dogs without scratches or bites. Asplenia, glucocorticoid therapy, and alcohol abuse are predisposing conditions and are associated with relatively fulminant infections. The interval from dog bite to presentation averages 5 days but ranges from 1 day to 1 month. *C. canimorsus* causes a wide range of infections, including severe sepsis with shock and disseminated intravascular coagulation, meningitis, endocarditis, cellulitis, and septic arthritis. In the asplenic individual who has recently sustained a dog bite, infection with this organism must be considered early because of a potentially rapid progression to death.

TREATMENT   Although penicillin has been considered first-line therapy for infections due to *C. ochracea*, *C. gingivalis*, and *C. sputigena*, an increasing number of isolates reportedly produce β-lactamase. Clindamycin (600 to 900 mg every 6 to 8 h) or drug combinations including a penicillin derivative plus a β-lactamase inhibitor—such as ampicillin/sulbactam (1.5 to 3.0 g of ampicillin every 6 h)—are currently recommended for empirical therapy. Penicillin (12 to 18 million units daily in 6 divided doses) is the drug of choice for infections with *C. canimorsus*. This regimen should also be given prophylactically to asplenic patients sustaining dog-bite injuries. Patients with suspected infection due to *C. canimorsus* should be treated empirically, because identification of this organism and determination of its antibiotic sensitivity can take many days. Other drugs to which *C. canimorsus* is reportedly susceptible include clindamycin, imipenem, quinolones, and third-generation cephalosporins.

Chromobacterium violaceum   This organism is rarely a human pathogen but reportedly has been responsible for life-threatening infections with severe sepsis and metastatic abscesses. A slender, slightly curved, gram-negative rod that is facultatively anaerobic, *C. violaceum* inhabits tropical water and soil and causes infection after contamination of skin wounds. Patients with defective neutrophil function (e.g., those with chronic granulomatous disease) are infected by this organism with unusual frequency. The mortality rate in the United States from infection with *C. violaceum* has been reported at >60%.

TREATMENT   *C. violaceum* is generally susceptible to ciprofloxacin (500 mg every 12 h orally or 400 mg every 12 h intravenously), trimethoprim-sulfamethoxazole, gentamicin, and chloramphenicol.

***Chryseobacterium* Species**   *C. meningosepticum* and *C. indologenes* were previously classified as *Flavobacterium* species. *C. meningosepticum* is a ubiquitous organism and an important cause of nosocomial infections. It has been associated with outbreaks due to contaminated fluids, such as disinfectants, arterial catheter flush solutions, and aerosolized antibiotics, and with sporadic infections due to indwelling devices, vials, sink traps, feeding tubes, and other fluid-associated apparatus. Patients with nosocomial *C. meningosepticum* infection usually have underlying immunosuppression (e.g., related to malignancy). *C. meningosepticum* has been reported to cause meningitis (primarily in neonates), sepsis, endocarditis, bacteremia, soft tissue infections, and pneumonia. *C. indologenes* has caused bacteremia, sepsis, and pneumonia, typically in immunocompromised patients with indwelling devices.

TREATMENT   Antibiotic treatment should be based on susceptibility results because of the high likelihood that *C. meningosepticum* will produce β-lactamase. Early reports suggested that vancomycin might be efficacious, but more recent data refute this conclusion.

Plesiomonas shigelloides   This freshwater organism is a cause of acute diarrhea (Chap. 131) and occasionally of serious extraintestinal disease. *P. shigelloides* is transmitted to humans via contaminated water or food. This motile, facultatively anaerobic gram-negative rod most often produces mild diarrhea with mucoid, bloody feces containing leukocytes. Severe extraintestinal infections have been reported, most commonly in immunocompromised hosts, and include bacteremia, cellulitis, neonatal sepsis and meningitis, and septic arthritis.

TREATMENT   There is great variability among strains in terms of antibiotic sensitivity patterns, and isolates must be tested before appropriate therapy can be selected.

***Aeromonas* Species**   Five species of *Aeromonas* are known to be associated with disease in humans, but >85% of these infections are caused by *A. hydrophila*, *A. caviae*, and *A. veronii* biovar. *sobria*. *Aeromonas* proliferates in potable and fresh water and in soil. It remains controversial whether *Aeromonas* is a cause of bacterial gastroenteritis. Although many case reports have associated *Aeromonas* with gastroenteritis, no clear outbreaks with a single isolate have been documented, no conclusive animal model exists, and asymptomatic colonization of the intestinal tract with *Aeromonas* occurs frequently. However, rare cases of hemolytic-uremic syndrome occurring after bloody diarrhea have been shown to be secondary to the presence of *Aeromonas*. In addition, identification of an enterotoxin (different from the Shiga-like toxin produced by *Escherichia coli* O157:H7) in these cases supports the hypothesis that *Aeromonas* causes gastroenteritis.

Aeromonas causes sepsis and bacteremia in infants with multiple medical problems and in immunocompromised hosts, particularly those with cancer or hepatobiliary disease. *Aeromonas* infection and sepsis can occur in trauma patients with myonecrosis or in burn patients exposed to *Aeromonas* by environmental contamination of their wounds from fresh water or soil sources. Mortality ranges from 25% for sepsis in immunocompromised adults to >90% in patients with myonecrosis. *Aeromonas* can produce skin lesions resembling the ecthyma gangrenosum lesions seen in *Pseudomonas aeruginosa* infection. These lesions are hemorrhagic vesicles surrounded by a rim of erythema with central necrosis and ulceration.

Aeromonas wound infections can occur in healthy adults who sustain minor trauma with environmental contamination, usually water-related; after severe trauma and crush injuries with sepsis and environmental exposure, usually to soil; and in nosocomial infections related to catheters, surgical incisions, or use of leeches. Other clinical manifestations include meningitis, peritonitis, pneumonia, and ocular infections.

TREATMENT   Treatment should be guided by antimicrobial susceptibility testing. *Aeromonas* species are generally susceptible to fluoroquinolones (e.g., ciprofloxacin at a dosage of 500 mg every 12 h orally or 400 mg every 12 h intravenously), trimethoprim-sulfamethoxazole at a trimethoprim dosage of 10 mg/kg per day in 3 or 4 divided doses, third-generation cephalosporins, and aminoglycosides. However, resistance is increasing.

Miscellaneous Organisms   Many other gram-negative rods have been reported to cause occasional infections in hosts who are immunologically unprepared to deal with relatively avirulent organisms or who are unfortunate enough to encounter an exceptionally large inoculum. Such organisms include *Weeksella* species; various CDC groups, such as EF-4, Ve-2 (*Flavimonas* species), IVc-2, NO-1, WO-1, and Gilardi Group WO-1; *Sphingobacterium* species; *Protomonas* species; *Ochrobactrum anthropi*; *Oligella urethralis*; and *Shewanella putrefaciens*. The reader is advised to consult subspecialty texts and references for further guidance on these organisms.

BILGRAMI S et al: *Capnocytophaga* bacteremia in a patient with Hodgkin's disease following bone marrow transplantation: Case report and review. Clin Infect Dis 14:10–5, 1992

BLOCK KC et al: *Chryseobacterium meningosepticum*: An emerging pathogen among immunocompromised adults. Medicine 76:30, 1997

DARRAS-JOLY C et al: *Haemophilus* endocarditis: Report of 42 cases in adults and review. Clin Infect Dis 24:1087, 1997

DAS M et al: Infective endocarditis caused by HACEK microorganisms. Annu Rev Med 48:25, 1997

HULSE M et al: *Agrobacterium* infection in humans: Experience at one hospital and review. Clin Infect Dis 16:112, 1993

JANDA JM et al: Evolving concepts regarding the genus *Aeromonas*: An expanding panorama of species, disease presentations, and unanswered questions. Clin Infect Dis 27:332, 1998

KUGLER KC et al: Determination of the antimicrobial activity of 29 clinically important compounds tested against fastidious HACEK group organisms. Diagn Microbiol Infect Dis 34:73, 1999

KULLBERG JB et al: Purpura fulminans and symmetrical peripheral gangrene caused by *Capnocytophaga canimorsus* (formerly DF-2) septicemia—a complication of dog bite. Medicine 70:287, 1991

MAURY S et al: Bacteremia due to *Capnocytophaga* species in patients with neutropenia: High frequency of beta-lactamase producing strains. Clin Infect Dis 28:1172, 1999

PAJU S et al: Heterogeneity of *Actinobacillus actinomycetemcomitans* strains in various human infections and relationships between serotype, genotype and antimicrobial susceptibility. J Clin Microbiol 38:79, 2000

PATRICK WD et al: Infective endocarditis due to *Eikenella corrodens*: Case report and review of the literature. Can J Infect Dis 1:139, 1990

TI T-Y et al: Nonfatal and fatal infections caused by *Chromobacterium violaceum*. Clin Infect Dis 17:505, 1993

WALSH RD et al: *Achromobacter xylosoxidans* osteomyelitis. Clin Infect Dis 16:176, 1993

WILSON ME: Prosthetic valve endocarditis and paravalvular abscess caused by *Actinobacillus actinomycetemcomitans*. Rev Infect Dis 11:665, 1989

YAGUPSKY P et al: *Kingella kingae*: An emerging cause of invasive infections in young children. Clin Infect Dis 24:86, 1997

151 *Feng-Yee Chang, Victor L. Yu*

LEGIONELLA INFECTION

DEFINITION *Legionellosis* refers to the two clinical syndromes caused by bacteria of the genus *Legionella*. *Pontiac fever* is an acute, febrile, self-limited illness that has been serologically linked to *Legionella* species, whereas *Legionnaires' disease* is the designation for pneumonia caused by these species.

HISTORY Legionnaires' disease was first recognized in 1976, when an outbreak of pneumonia took place at a hotel in Philadelphia during the American Legion Convention. Investigators from the Centers for Disease Control and Prevention (CDC) identified the causative aerobic gram-negative bacterium in lung specimens obtained from the victims at autopsy and named this organism *L. pneumophila*. Retrospective studies of stored serum samples revealed that an epidemic of Legionnaires' disease had occurred in 1957 in Austin, Minnesota. In this epidemic 78 persons were hospitalized with acute respiratory infection. Antibody determinations showed seroconversion to *L. pneumophila* in most cases.

MICROBIOLOGY At present, the family Legionellaceae comprises 41 species with 64 serogroups. The species *L. pneumophila* causes 80 to 90% of human infections and includes at least 14 serogroups; serogroups 1, 4, and 6 are most commonly implicated in human infections. To date, 17 species other than *L. pneumophila* have been associated with human infections, among which *L. micdadei*

(Pittsburgh pneumonia agent), *L. bozemanii*, *L. dumoffii*, and *L. longbeachae* are the most common.

Members of the Legionellaceae are aerobic, thin, gram-negative bacilli that do not grow on routine microbiologic media. Buffered charcoal yeast extract (BCYE) agar is the medium used to grow *Legionella*. This highly enhanced medium contains the amino acid L-cysteine, which is an absolute growth requirement for *Legionella*. Growth of the organism on BCYE medium is usually visible in 3 to 5 days at 35 to 37°C. *L. micdadei* and *L. maceachernii* produce blue colonies on BCYE medium containing bromocresol purple and bromothymol blue dyes, while the other species produce green colonies.

Antimicrobial agents, including polymyxin B, cefamandole, and vancomycin, are used in *Legionella*-selective media to suppress competing components of the microflora. Although *L. pneumophila* is relatively tolerant to these antibiotics, the drugs may inhibit the growth of other legionellae; for example, cefamandole-containing media suppress the growth of *L. micdadei*.

Traditional biochemical tests are not particularly helpful in distinguishing one *Legionella* species from another. Fatty-acid profile determination by gas-liquid chromatography and ubiquinone analysis allow identification to the genus level. The direct fluorescent antibody (DFA) test can definitively identify a number of individual species. In *L. pneumophila*, lipopolysaccharide is a prominent constituent of the outer membrane, and the serogroup-specific antigen and antibodies detected by immunofluorescence are directed primarily at the lipopolysaccharide. Both polyclonal and monoclonal DFA reagents are commercially available. The monoclonal antibody reagent is less cross-reactive but is specific for *L. pneumophila*. Genetic analysis has been considered the definitive arbiter for the identification of individual species, with the degree of DNA sequence homology the most common criterion employed. A nucleic-acid hybridization probe reactive to *Legionella* ribosomal RNA, used with a single reagent, can identify a member of the genus within hours.

ECOLOGY AND TRANSMISSION The natural habitats for *L. pneumophila* are aquatic bodies, including lakes and streams; *L. longbeachae* has been isolated from soil. Legionellae can survive under a wide range of environmental conditions; for example, the organisms can live for years in refrigerated water samples. Natural bodies of water contain only small numbers of legionellae. However, once the organisms enter human-constructed aquatic reservoirs (such as cooling towers or water-distribution systems), they can grow and proliferate. Factors known to enhance colonization by and amplification of legionellae include warm temperatures (25° to 42°C), stagnation, and scale and sediment. The presence of symbiotic microorganisms, including algae, amebas, ciliated protozoa, and other water-dwelling bacteria, likewise promotes growth of *L. pneumophila*.

Hot-water tanks colonized with *L. pneumophila* are significantly more likely than uncolonized tanks to be cooler (<60°C), to have a vertical configuration, to be older, and to have higher concentrations of calcium and magnesium. Vertical tanks, especially those that are electric coil-heated rather than gas-heated, have a pronounced temperature stratification and thick sediment accumulation at the bottom. Studies have shown that neither a high degree of outward cleanliness nor routine application of maintenance measures decreases the frequency or intensity of *Legionella* colonization. Thus, engineering guidelines and building codes, although often advocated as preventive measures, have relatively little impact on *Legionella* colonization.

The source of *Legionella* is water, but the mode of transmission from the environmental reservoir to the patient remains controversial. Early investigations that implicated cooling towers antedated the discovery that the organism could also exist in potable water distribution systems. It is now known that, in many outbreaks, cases of Legionnaires' disease continued to occur despite disinfection of cooling towers and the potable water supply was the actual source. Koch's postulates have been fulfilled in epidemiologic studies using molecular fingerprinting methods to link potable water sources (rather than cooling towers) to *Legionella* infection in humans. Community-acquired Legionnaires' disease has been linked to colonization of residential and industrial water supplies.

Multiple modes of transmission of *Legionella* to humans exist, including aerosolization, aspiration, and direct instillation into the lung during respiratory tract manipulations. Aspiration may be the predominant mode of transmission, but it is unclear whether *Legionella* enters the lung via oropharyngeal colonization or directly via the drinking of contaminated water. Nasogastric tubes have been linked to nosocomial Legionnaires' disease in several reports; microaspiration of contaminated water was the hypothesized mode of transmission. Surgery with general anesthesia is a known risk factor that is consistent with aspiration. Especially compelling is the reported 30% incidence of postoperative *Legionella* pneumonia among patients undergoing head and neck surgery in a hospital with a contaminated water supply; aspiration is a recognized sequela in such cases. Studies of patients with hospital-acquired Legionnaires' disease showed that these individuals underwent endotracheal intubation significantly more often and for a significantly longer duration than patients with nosocomial pneumonia of other etiologies.

Aerosolization of legionellae by devices filled with tap water, including nebulizers and humidifiers, has caused cases of Legionnaires' disease. An ultrasonic mist machine in the produce section of a grocery store was implicated in a community outbreak. Pontiac fever has been linked to *Legionella*-containing aerosols from water-using machinery, a cooling tower, air-conditioners, and whirlpools.

EPIDEMIOLOGY   The incidence of Legionnaires' disease depends on the degree of contamination of the aquatic reservoir, the susceptibility and immune status of the persons exposed to the water from that reservoir, the intensity of exposure, and the availability of specialized laboratory tests on which the correct diagnosis can be based.

Numerous prospective studies have found *Legionella* to rank among the top four microbial causes of community-acquired pneumonia (*Streptococcus pneumoniae*, *Haemophilus influenzae*, and *Chlamydia pneumoniae* usually ranking first, second, and third), accounting for 3 to 15% of cases. On the basis of a multihospital study of community-acquired pneumonia in Ohio, the CDC has estimated that only 3% of sporadic cases of Legionnaires' disease are correctly diagnosed. Legionellae are responsible for 10 to 50% of nosocomial pneumonias when a hospital's water system is colonized with the organisms. One situation in which the diagnosis of Legionnaires' disease should be considered is that in which the presenting patient has been hospitalized within 10 days before the onset of symptoms. In one study, a number of patients had been discharged from the hospital and readmitted with Legionnaires' disease; molecular fingerprinting showed that the isolates obtained from patients and the isolate from the hospital's water supply were similar.

The most common risk factors for Legionnaires' disease are cigarette smoking, chronic lung disease, advanced age, and immunosuppression. The disease most often develops in elderly men; this predilection is probably related to cigarette smoking. Surgery is a prominent predisposing factor in nosocomial infection, with transplant recipients at highest risk. Nosocomial cases are now being recognized among neonates and among children with immunosuppression or underlying pulmonary disease.

Pontiac fever occurs in epidemics. The high attack rate (>90%) reflects airborne transmission.

PATHOGENESIS   Legionellae enter the lungs through aspiration or direct inhalation. The organisms possess pili that may mediate adherence to respiratory tract epithelial cells. Thus, conditions that impair mucociliary clearance, including cigarette smoking, lung disease, or alcoholism, predispose to Legionnaires' disease.

Cell-mediated immunity is the primary mechanism of host defense against *Legionella*, as it is against other intracellular pathogens, including *Mycobacterium tuberculosis*, *Listeria*, and *Toxoplasma*. Al-

veolar macrophages readily phagocytose legionellae. The attachment of the bacteria to phagocytes is mediated via complement receptors, which attach to the bacterial major outer-membrane protein. Binding to these receptors promotes phagocytosis but fails to trigger an oxidative burst. Although many legionellae are killed, some proliferate intracellularly until the cells rupture; the bacteria are then phagocytosed again by newly recruited phagocytes, and the cycle begins anew. Legionnaires' disease is more common and the disease manifestations are more severe in patients with depressed cell-mediated immunity, including transplant recipients, patients infected with HIV, and patients receiving glucocorticoids. The disease also occurs with unusual frequency among patients with hairy cell leukemia (which is characterized by monocyte deficiency and dysfunction) but not among patients with other types of leukemia.

The role of neutrophils in immunity appears to be minimal: neutropenic patients are not predisposed to Legionnaires' disease. Although *L. pneumophila* is susceptible to oxygen-dependent microbiologic systems in vitro, it resists killing by neutrophils.

The humoral immune system is active against *Legionella*. Type-specific IgM and IgG antibodies are measurable within weeks of infection. In vitro, antibodies promote killing of legionellae by phagocytes (neutrophils, monocytes, and alveolar macrophages). However, antibodies neither enhance lysis by complement nor inhibit intracellular multiplication within phagocytes. Immunized animals develop a specific antibody response, with subsequent resistance to *Legionella* challenge.

Some *L. pneumophila* strains are clearly more virulent than others, although the precise factors mediating virulence remain uncertain. For example, although multiple strains may colonize water-distribution systems, only a few cause disease in patients exposed to that water. At least one surface epitope of *L. pneumophila* serogroup 1 is associated with virulence. *L. pneumophila* serogroup 6 is more commonly involved in nosocomial Legionnaires' disease and is more likely to be associated with a poor outcome.

PATHOLOGY   The consistent pathologic features of Legionnaires' disease are confined to the lungs. Findings in infected lung tissue range from multifocal pneumonia with patchy lobular inflammation to extensive multilobar consolidation. Visible abscesses with central necrosis were seen in 20% of autopsied cases in one study. On histologic examination, fibrinopurulent pneumonia with intensive alveolitis and bronchiolitis is evident. Lesions of longer standing can have a nodular appearance with a central area of necrosis surrounded by macrophages and other cells. The alveoli are filled with fibrin, neutrophils, and alveolar macrophages.

Usual tissue stains, including Gram's, hematoxylin and eosin, Brown-Brenn, and methenamine silver, do not reveal the organism. Giminez stain can be used for imprints on fresh or fixed tissue. Dieterle's silver stain or modified Giminez stain, although nonspecific and relatively insensitive, can be used for paraffin-fixed specimens. The DFA stain is not only specific but also the most sensitive option for visualization of the organism in tissues. Polyvalent DFA stains but not monoclonal DFA stain can be used for formalinized specimens. Because the DFA stains are species and serogroup specific, false-negative results can be obtained if the incorrect reagent is used. Thus, culture is the preferred method for diagnosis based on clinical specimens.

CLINICAL AND LABORATORY FEATURES   **Pontiac Fever**   Pontiac fever is an acute, self-limiting, flulike illness with a 24- to 48-h incubation period. Pneumonia does not develop in Pontiac fever. Malaise, fatigue, and myalgias are the most frequent symptoms, occurring in 97% of cases. Fever (usually with chills) develops in 80 to 90% of cases and headache in 80%. Other symptoms (seen in fewer than 50% of cases) include arthralgias, nausea, cough, abdominal pain, and diarrhea. Modest leukocytosis with a neutrophilic predominance is sometimes detected. Complete recovery takes place within only a few days without antibiotic therapy; a few patients may experience lassitude for many weeks thereafter. The diagnosis is established by antibody seroconversion.

Legionnaires' Disease (Pneumonia) Clinical findings that raise the possibility of Legionnaires' disease are summarized in Table 151-1. Although these manifestations may provide clues to the diagnosis, prospective comparative studies have shown that they are generally nonspecific and do not serve to distinguish Legionnaires' disease from pneumonia of other etiologies. Legionnaires' disease is often included in the differential diagnosis of "atypical pneumonia," along with infection due to *Chlamydia pneumoniae, C. psittaci, Mycoplasma pneumoniae, Coxiella burnetii*, and some viruses. The clinical similarities among these types of pneumonia include a relatively nonproductive cough and a low incidence of grossly purulent sputum. However, the clinical manifestations of Legionnaires' disease are usually more severe than those of most "atypical" pneumonias, and the course and prognosis of *Legionella* pneumonia more resemble those of bacteremic pneumococcal pneumonia than those of pneumonia due to other "atypical" pathogens. Patients with community-acquired Legionnaires' disease are significantly more likely than patients with pneumonia of other etiologies to be admitted to an intensive care unit on presentation.

The incubation period for Legionnaires' disease is 2 to 10 days. The symptoms and signs may range from a mild cough and a slight fever to stupor with widespread pulmonary infiltrates and multisystem failure. Nonspecific symptoms—malaise, fatigue, anorexia, and headache—are seen early in the illness. Myalgias and arthralgias are uncommon but are unusually marked in a few patients. Upper respiratory symptoms, including coryza, are rare.

The mild cough of Legionnaires' disease is only slightly productive. Sometimes the sputum is streaked with blood. Chest pain—either pleuritic or nonpleuritic—can be a prominent feature and, when coupled with hemoptysis, can lead to an incorrect diagnosis of pulmonary embolism. Shortness of breath is reported by one-third to one-half of patients.

Gastrointestinal difficulties are often pronounced; abdominal pain, nausea, and vomiting affect 10 to 20% of patients. Diarrhea (watery rather than bloody) is reported in 25 to 50% of cases. The most common neurologic abnormalities are confusion or changes in mental status; however, the multitudinous neurologic symptoms reported range from headache and lethargy to encephalopathy.

Patients with Legionnaires' disease virtually always have fever. Temperatures in excess of 40.5°C (104.9°F) were recorded in 20% of the cases in one series. Relative bradycardia has been overemphasized as a useful diagnostic finding; it occurs infrequently, primarily affecting older patients with severe pneumonia. Chest examination reveals rales early in the course and evidence of consolidations as the disease progresses. Abdominal examination may reveal generalized or local tenderness.

Diarrhea and hyponatremia occur significantly more often in Legionnaires' disease than in other forms of pneumonia. Hyponatremia is most common in severe cases. The mechanism of hyponatremia does not appear to be related to inappropriate secretion of antidiuretic hormone but instead to salt and water loss. Besides hyponatremia, other laboratory abnormalities include abnormal liver function tests, hypophosphatemia, hematuria, hematologic abnormalities, and thrombocytopenia; although common, these abnormalities are not found significantly more frequently in Legionnaires' disease than in pneumonias of other etiologies.

Table 151-1 Clinical Clues Suggestive of Legionnaires' Disease

Diarrhea
High fever (>40°C or >104°F))
Numerous neutrophils but no organisms revealed by Gram's staining of respiratory secretions
Hyponatremia (serum sodium level of <131 meq/L)
Failure to respond to β-lactam drugs (penicillins or cephalosporins) and aminoglycoside antibiotics
Occurrence of illness in an environment in which the potable water supply is known to be contaminated with *Legionella*
Onset of symptoms within 10 days after discharge from the hospital

Extrapulmonary Legionellosis Since the portal of entry for legionellae is the lung in virtually all cases, extrapulmonary manifestations usually result from bloodborne dissemination from the lung. In a prospective survey of patients with Legionnaires' disease diagnosed by isolation of the organism from sputum, legionellae were isolated from the blood by a special culture method in 38% of cases.

Legionella has been identified in the spleen, liver, or kidneys in 50% of autopsied cases of Legionnaires' disease. The organism has also been isolated from intrathoracic and inguinal lymph nodes—a finding suggesting dissemination by lymphatic pathways. Extrapulmonary involvement, including sinusitis, peritonitis, pyelonephritis, cellulitis, and pancreatitis, has been documented predominantly in immunosuppressed patients.

The most common extrapulmonary site of legionellosis is the heart; numerous reports have described myocarditis, pericarditis, postcardiotomy syndrome, and prosthetic-valve endocarditis. Most cases have been hospital-acquired. Since many of the patients involved have not had overt pneumonia, the lung may not have been the portal of entry. Rather, in these cardiac infections, the organisms may have gained entry through a postoperative sternal wound exposed to contaminated tap water or through a mediastinal-tube insertion site.

Various other sources of or factors promoting *Legionella* infection at various extrapulmonary sites have been postulated, including the presence of foreign bodies, such as sutures and draining tubes (wound infection after cardiothoracic surgery); immersion in a Hubbard tank (superinfection of a hip wound); bloodborne dissemination from a pulmonary infection site (perirectal abscess); and ingestion of contaminated water (peritonitis).

Chest Radiographic Abnormalities Virtually all patients with Legionnaires' disease have abnormal chest radiographs showing pulmonary infiltrates at the time of clinical presentation. In a few cases of nosocomial disease, fever and respiratory tract symptoms have preceded the appearance of the infiltrate on chest radiography. Findings on chest radiography are nonspecific and do not serve to distinguish Legionnaires' disease from pneumonias of other etiologies. Pleural effusion is evident in one-third of cases, and the diagnosis is often based on culture and antigen testing (by the method designed for use with urine) of pleural fluid obtained by thoracentesis.

In immunosuppressed patients, especially those receiving glucocorticoids, distinctive rounded nodular opacities may be seen; these lesions may expand and cavitate (Fig. 151-1). Likewise, pulmonary abscesses can occur in immunosuppressed hosts. The progression of infiltrates on chest radiography despite appropriate antibiotic therapy is common, and radiographic improvement lags behind clinical improvement by several days. Complete clearing of infiltrates requires 1 to 4 months.

DIAGNOSIS The diagnosis of Legionnaires' disease requires special microbiologic tests (Table 151-2). The sensitivity of bronchoscopy specimens is approximately the same as that of sputum samples; if sputum is not available, bronchoscopy specimens may yield the organism. Bronchoalveolar lavage fluid gives higher yields than bronchial wash specimens. Thoracentesis should be performed if pleural effusion is found, and the fluid should be evaluated by DFA staining, culture, and the antigen test designed for use with urine.

Staining Gram's staining of material from normally sterile sites, such as pleural fluid or lung tissue, occasionally suggests the diagnosis; efforts to detect legionellae in sputum by Gram's staining typically reveal numerous leukocytes, but no organisms. When they are visualized, the organisms appear as small, pleomorphic, faint, gram-negative bacilli. *L. micdadei* organisms can be detected as weakly or partially acid-fast bacilli in clinical specimens. Modified acid-fast staining substitutes 1% sulfuric acid for the traditional 3% hydrochloric acid; the less aggressive decolorizer increases the yield of *L. micdadei*. *Legionella*-infected patients have often been treated empirically with antituberculosis medications because of false-positive acid-fast smears.

The DFA test is rapid and highly specific but is less sensitive than

FIGURE 151-1 Chest radiographic findings in a 52-year-old man who presented with pneumonia subsequently diagnosed as Legionnaires' disease. The patient was a cigarette smoker with chronic obstructive pulmonary disease and alcoholic cardiomyopathy; he had received glucocorticoids. *L. pneumophila* was identified by DFA staining and culture of sputum. *Left:* Baseline chest radiograph showing long-standing cardiomegaly. *Center:* Admission chest radiograph showing new rounded opacities. *Right:* Chest radiograph taken 3 days after admission, during treatment with erythromycin.

culture because large numbers of organisms are required for microscopic visualization. This test is more likely to be positive in advanced than in early disease.

Culture The definitive method for diagnosis of *Legionella* infection is isolation of the organism from respiratory secretions or other specimens. As has been mentioned, BCYE agar supplemented with antibiotics and dyes is the most sensitive medium, and colonies grow slowly, requiring 3 to 5 days to become grossly visible. When culture plates are overgrown with other microflora, pretreatment of the specimen with acid or heat can markedly improve the yield. *L. pneumophila* is often isolated from sputum that is not grossly or microscopically purulent; sputum containing more than 25 epithelial cells per high-power field (a finding that classically suggests contamination) may still yield *L. pneumophila*.

Antibody Detection Antibody testing of both acute- and convalescent-phase sera may be necessary. A fourfold rise in titer is diagnostic; 4 to 12 weeks are often required for the detection of an antibody response, and some patients never seroconvert. A single titer of 1:128 in a patient with pneumonia constitutes presumptive (but not definitive) evidence for Legionnaires' disease. Serology is of use primarily in epidemiologic studies. The specificity of serology for the non–*L. pneumophila* species is uncertain; there is cross-reactivity with *L. pneumophila* and some gram-negative bacilli.

Urinary Antigen The assay for *Legionella* soluble antigen in urine (Binax, Portland, ME) is rapid, relative inexpensive, easy to perform, second only to culture in terms of sensitivity, and highly specific. Its use in every clinical laboratory is recommended. The test is available only for *L. pneumophila* serogroup 1, which, as has been mentioned, causes about 80% of *Legionella* infections. Antigen in urine is detectable 3 days after the onset of clinical disease, even if specific therapy has been started; furthermore, urinary antigen persists for several weeks.

Molecular Methods Polymerase chain reaction (PCR) with DNA probes is theoretically more sensitive and specific than other methods, but results have been disappointing to date. PCR has proved useful in the identification of legionellae from environmental water specimens.

℞ TREATMENT Controlled evaluations of antibiotic therapy for Legionnaires' disease have never been conducted. In the 1976 American Legion outbreak, patients treated with erythromycin and tetracycline appeared to have a better outcome than those treated with other agents. These two antibiotics also exhibited intracellular activity against legionellae and were effective in animal models. The fact that *Legionella* is an intracellular pathogen provided the biologic basis for the success of erythromycin and tetracycline, given that relatively high intracellular penetration. Antibiotics capable of achieving intracellular concentrations higher than the minimal inhibitory concentration are the most likely to be efficacious in the clinical setting. The dosages for various drugs used in the treatment of *Legionella* infection are listed in Table 151-3.

The newer macrolides (especially azithromycin) and quinolones are now the antibiotics of choice, displacing erythromycin. Compared with erythromycin, the newer agents azithromycin, clarithromycin, and roxithromycin have superior in vitro activity, display greater intracellular activity, and reach higher concentrations in respiratory secretions and in lung tissue. The pharmacokinetics of the newer macrolides and quinolones also allow once- or twice-daily dosing, in

Table 151-2 Utility of Special Laboratory Tests for the Diagnosis of Legionnaires' Disease

Test	Sensitivity, %	Specificity, %
Culture		
Sputum[a]	80	100
Transtracheal aspirate	90	100
DFA staining of sputum	50–70	96–99
Urinary antigen testing[b]	70	100
Antibody serology[c]	40–60	96–99

[a] Use of multiple selective media with dyes.
[b] Serogroup 1 only.
[c] IgG and IgM testing of both acute- and convalescent-phase sera. A single titer of ≥1:128 is considered presumptive, while a single titer of ≥1:256 or fourfold seroconversion is considered definitive.

Table 151-3 Antibiotic Therapy for *Legionella* Infection[a]

Antimicrobial Agent	Dose, mg[b]	Route[c]	Frequency
Azithromycin	500[d]	PO, IV	q24h
Clarithromycin	500	PO, IV[e]	q12h
Roxithromycin	300[e]	PO	q12h
Erythromycin[f]	1000 (1 g)	IV	q6h
	500	PO	q6h
Ciprofloxacin	400	IV	q8h
	750	PO	q12h
Levofloxacin	500[d]	PO, IV	q24h
Ofloxacin	400	PO, IV	q12h
Doxycycline	100[d]	PO, IV	q12h
Minocycline	100[d]	PO, IV	q12h
Tetracycline	500	PO, IV	q6h
Trimethoprim-sulfamethoxazole	160/800	IV	q8h
	160/800	PO	q12h
Rifampin	300–600	PO, IV	q12h

[a] Total duration of therapy should be 10 to 14 days in immunocompetent hosts and 3 weeks in immunosuppressed patients and in those with advanced disease.
[b] Except as indicated.
[c] Intravenous therapy should be used until the patient's clinical condition improves, after which oral therapy can be substituted.
[d] Doubling of the first dose is recommended.
[e] Investigational in the United States.
[f] Now replaced by newer macrolides (see text).

contrast to the four-times-daily dosing required for erythromycin. Finally, the large fluid volume required for intravenous administration, symptomatic ototoxicity, and gastrointestinal side effects have rendered erythromycin obsolete for the treatment of *Legionella* infection.

The quinolones (levofloxacin, ciprofloxacin, pefloxacin, gemifloxacin, and moxifloxacin) are more active than any of the macrolides against *Legionella* in in vitro dilution susceptibility tests, intracellular models, and animal models. Furthermore, in open noncomparative studies of pneumonia, numerous cases of Legionnaires' disease have been successfully treated with quinolones. Quinolones are the preferred antibiotics for transplant recipients because both macrolides (except azithromycin) and rifampin interact pharmacologically with cyclosporine and tacrolimus.

Alternative agents include tetracycline and its analogues doxycycline and minocycline. Anecdotal reports have described both successes and failures with trimethoprim-sulfamethoxazole, imipenem, and clindamycin. For severely ill patients with Legionnaires' disease, the combination of rifampin plus a macrolide or a quinolone can be used for initial treatment.

Initial therapy should be given by the intravenous route. Usually, a clinical response occurs within 3 to 5 days, after which oral therapy can be substituted. The total duration of therapy in the immunocompetent host is 10 to 14 days; a longer course (3 weeks) may be appropriate for immunosuppressed patients and those with advanced disease. In the oral phase, 5 to 10 days of azithromycin is therapy sufficient.

Mortality rates for Legionnaires' disease vary, depending on the patient's underlying disease and its severity, the patient's immune status, the severity of pneumonia, and the timing of administration of appropriate antimicrobial therapy. Mortality rates are highest (80%) among immunosuppressed patients who do not receive appropriate antimicrobial therapy. With appropriate and timely antibiotic treatment, mortality from community-acquired Legionnaires' disease among immunocompetent patients ranges from 0 to 11%; without treatment, the figure may be as high as 31%. Pontiac fever requires only symptom-based treatment, not antimicrobial therapy.

PREVENTION Routine environmental culture of the hospital water supply is recommended as an approach to the prevention of hospital-acquired Legionnaires' disease. Positive cultures from the water supply mandate the use of specialized laboratory tests (especially culture on selective media and urinary antigen assay) for patients with hospital-acquired pneumonia.

Disinfection of the water supply is now feasible. Two methods have proven reliable and cost-effective. The superheat and flush method requires heating of the water so that the distal-outlet temperature is 70 to 80°C and flushing of the distal outlets with hot water for at least 30 min. This method is ideal for emergency situations. A commercial copper and silver ionization method has proved effective in numerous hospitals. Hyperchlorination is no longer recommended because of its expense, carcinogenicity, corrosive effects on piping, and unreliable efficacy.

BIBLIOGRAPHY

BARBAREE JM et al (eds): *Legionella—Current Status and Emerging Perspectives.* Washington, DC, American Society for Microbiology, 1993

CUNHA B et al: Legionnaires' disease: A symposium. Semin Resp Infect 13:83, 1998

FANG GD et al: Disease due to Legionellaceae (other than *Legionella pneumophila*): Historical, microbiological, clinical and epidemiologic review. Medicine 68:116, 1989

FIORE AE et al: A survey of methods used to detect nosocomial legionellosis among participants in the NNIS system. Infect Control Hosp Epidemiol 20:412, 1999

LIEBERMAN D et al: *Legionella* species community-acquired pneumonia: A review of 56 hospitalized adult patients. Chest 109:1243, 1996

LOWRY PW, TOMPKINS LS: Nosocomial legionellosis: A review of pulmonary and extrapulmonary syndromes. Am J Infect Control 21:21, 1993

SHUMAN HA et al: Intracellular multiplication of *Legionella pneumophila*: Human pathogen or accidental tourist? Curr Top Microbiol Immunol 225:99, 1998

STOUT JE, YU VL: Current concepts: Legionellosis. N Engl J Med 337:682, 1997

YU VL: Could aspiration be the major mode of transmission for *Legionella*? Am J Med 95:13, 1993

————: Resolving the controversy on environmental cultures for *Legionella*. Infect Control Hosp Epidemiol 19:393, 1998

152   *Scott A. Halperin*

PERTUSSIS AND OTHER *BORDETELLA* INFECTIONS

Pertussis is an acute infection of the respiratory tract caused by *Bordetella pertussis*. The name *pertussis* means "violent cough," which aptly describes the most consistent and prominent feature of the illness. The inspiratory sound made at the end of an episode of paroxysmal coughing gives rise to the common name for the illness, "whooping cough"; however, this feature is variable, being uncommon in infants ≤6 months of age and frequently absent in older children and adults. The Chinese name for pertussis is "the 100-day cough," which accurately describes the clinical course of the illness. The identification of *B. pertussis* was first reported by Bordet and Gengou in 1906, and vaccines were produced over the following two decades.

MICROBIOLOGY Six species have been identified in the genus *Bordetella*: *B. pertussis*. *B. parapertussis*, *B. bronchiseptica*, *B. avium*, *B. holmesii*, and *B. hinzii*. *B. pertussis* infects only humans and is the most important *Bordetella* species causing human disease. *B. parapertussis* causes an illness in humans that is similar to pertussis but is typically milder; co-infections with *B. parapertussis* and *B. pertussis* have been documented. *B. bronchiseptica* is an important pathogen of domestic animals that causes kennel cough in dogs, atrophic rhinitis and pneumonia in pigs, and pneumonia in cats. Both respiratory infection and opportunistic infection are occasionally reported in humans. *B. avium* is an important cause of respiratory illness in turkeys. The remaining two species, *B. hinzii* and *B. holmesii*, have been recognized as unusual causes of bacteremia. Both of these species have been isolated from patients with sepsis, most often from those who are immunocompromised.

Bordetella species are gram-negative pleomorphic aerobic bacilli that share common genotypic characteristics. *B. pertussis* and *B. parapertussis* are the most similar of the species but differ in that *B. parapertussis* does not express the gene coding for pertussis toxin. *B. pertussis* is a slow-growing fastidious organism that requires selective medium and forms small glistening bifurcated colonies. Suspicious colonies are presumptively identified as *B. pertussis* by direct fluorescent antibody testing or by agglutination with species-specific antiserum. *B. pertussis* is further differentiated from other *Bordetella* species by biochemical and motility characteristics.

B. pertussis produces a wide array of toxins and biologically active products that are important in its pathogenesis and in immunity. Most of these virulence factors are under the control of a single genetic locus that regulates their production, resulting in antigenic modulation and phase variation. Although these processes occur both in vitro and in vivo, their importance in the pathobiology of the organism is unknown; they may play a role in intracellular persistence and person-to-person spread. The organism's most important virulence factor is *pertussis toxin*, which is composed of a B oligomer-binding subunit and an enzymatically active A protomer that ADP-ribosylates a guanine nucleotide-binding regulatory protein (G protein) in target cells, producing a variety of biologic effects. Pertussis toxin has important mitogenic activity, affects the circulation of lymphocytes, and serves as an adhesin for bacterial binding to respiratory ciliated cells. In animal models, the toxin's effects include histamine sensitization, lymphocytosis promotion, and insulin secretion. Another virulence factor is *filamentous hemagglutinin*, a component of the cell wall and a bacterial adhesin. *Pertactin* is an outer-membrane protein and another important adhesin. *Fimbriae* are bacterial appendages that also play a role in bacterial attachment; they are the major antigens against which agglutinating antibodies are directed. These agglutinating antibodies have historically been the primary means of serotyping *B. pertussis* strains. Other virulence factors include tracheal cytotoxin, which causes respiratory epithelial damage; adenylate cyclase toxin, which impairs host immune cell function; dermonecrotic toxin, which may contribute to respiratory mucosal damage; and lipo-oligosaccharide, which has properties similar to those of other gram-negative bacterial endotoxins.

PATHOGENESIS　Infection with *B. pertussis* is initiated by attachment of the organism to the ciliated epithelial cells of the nasopharynx. Attachment is mediated by surface adhesins (e.g., pertactin and filamentous hemagglutinin), which bind to the integrin family of cell-surface proteins, probably in conjunction with pertussis toxin. The role of fimbriae in adhesion or maintenance of infection has not been fully delineated. At the site of attachment, the organism multiplies, producing a variety of other toxins that cause local mucosal damage (tracheal cytotoxin, dermatonecrotic toxin). Impairment of host defense by *B. pertussis* is mediated by pertussis toxin and adenylate cyclase toxin. There is local cellular invasion, with intracellular bacterial persistence; however, systemic dissemination does not occur. Systemic manifestations (lymphocytosis) result from the effects of the toxins.

The pathogenesis of the clinical manifestations of pertussis is poorly understood. It is not known what causes the paroxysmal cough that is the hallmark of pertussis. A pivotal role for pertussis toxin has been proposed. Proponents of this position point to the efficacy of preventing clinical symptoms with a vaccine containing only pertussis toxoid. Detractors counter that pertussis toxin is not the critical factor because paroxysmal cough also occurs in patients infected with *B. parapertussis*, which does not produce pertussis toxin. It is thought that the neurologic events observed in pertussis, such as seizures and encephalopathy, are due to hypoxia from coughing paroxysms or apnea rather than to the effects of specific bacterial products. *B. pertussis* pneumonia, which occurs in up to 10% of infants with pertussis, is usually a diffuse bilateral primary infection. In older children and adults with pertussis, pneumonia is often due to secondary bacterial infection with streptococci or staphylococci.

IMMUNITY　Both humoral and cell-mediated immunity are thought to be important in pertussis. Antibodies to pertussis toxin, filamentous hemagglutinin, pertactin, and fimbriae are all protective in animal models. Pertussis agglutinins were correlated with protection in early studies of whole-cell pertussis vaccines. Serologic correlates of protection conferred by acellular pertussis vaccines have not been established, although antibody to pertactin, fimbriae, and (to a lesser degree) pertussis toxin correlated best with protection in two acellular pertussis vaccine efficacy trials. The duration of immunity after whole-cell pertussis vaccination is short-lived, with little protection remaining after 10 to 12 years. Data on the duration of protection after acellular pertussis vaccination are still being collected. Although immunity after natural infection has been said to be lifelong, seroepidemiologic evidence suggests that it may not be and that subsequent episodes of clinical pertussis are prevented by intermittent subclinical infection.

EPIDEMIOLOGY　Pertussis is a highly communicable disease, with attack rates of 80 to 100% among unimmunized household contacts and 20% within households in well-immunized populations. The infection has a worldwide distribution, with cyclical outbreaks every 3 to 5 years (a pattern that has persisted despite widespread immunization). Pertussis occurs in all months; however, in North America, pertussis activity peaks in the summer and autumn.

Before the institution of widespread immunization programs, pertussis was one of the most common infectious causes of morbidity and death. In the United States prior to the 1940s, between 115,000 and 270,000 cases of pertussis were reported annually, with an average yearly rate of 150 cases per 100,000 population. With universal childhood immunization, the number of reported cases fell by >95%, with even more dramatic decreases in mortality. Only 1010 cases of pertussis were reported in 1976. Since that time, however, rates have slowly increased. In 1994, over 15,000 cases of pertussis were reported in the United States.

Although thought of as a disease of childhood, pertussis can affect people of all ages and is increasingly being identified as a cause of prolonged coughing illness in adolescents and adults. In unimmunized populations, pertussis incidence peaks in the preschool years, and well over half of children have the disease before reaching adulthood. In highly immunized populations such as those in North America, the peak incidence is in infants <1 year of age who have not completed the three-dose primary immunization series. Recent trends, however, show an increasing incidence of pertussis in adolescents and adults. In the United States in 1997, ~30% of patients were ≤6 months of age, 25% were adolescents, and 20% were adults. The figures for adolescents and adults are probably underestimates because of a greater degree of underrecognition and underreporting in these age groups. A number of studies of prolonged coughing illness suggest that pertussis may be the etiologic agent in 12 to 30% of adults with cough that does not improve within 2 weeks. A seroprevalence study in the United States estimated an annual incidence of pertussis of 176 cases per 100,000 healthy adults. This high incidence undoubtedly includes subclinical and mild cases that would not be readily identified as pertussis; this fact accounts for infection rates similar to those reported before the introduction of routine immunization.

Severe morbidity and mortality, however, are virtually restricted to infants. In Canada, there were 10 deaths from pertussis between 1991 and 1998; all those who died were infants ≤6 months of age. Although school-age children are the source of infection for most households, adults are the likely source for high-risk infants and may serve as the reservoir of infection between epidemic years. In developing countries, pertussis remains an important cause of infant morbidity and mortality. The World Health Organization estimated that in 1995 over 40 million people worldwide were infected by *B. pertussis* and that 355,000 children died of pertussis.

CLINICAL MANIFESTATIONS　Pertussis is a prolonged coughing illness with clinical manifestations that vary by age (Table 152-1). Classic pertussis is most often seen in preschool and school-age children, although it is not uncommon among adolescents and adults. After an incubation period averaging 7 to 10 days, an illness develops that is indistinguishable from the common cold and is characterized by coryza, lacrimation, mild cough, low-grade fever, and malaise. After 1 to 2 weeks, this *catarrhal phase* evolves into the *paroxysmal phase*: the cough becomes more frequent and spasmodic with repetitive bursts of 5 to 10 coughs, often within a single expiration. Posttussive vomiting is frequent, with a mucous plug occasionally expelled at the end of an episode. The episode may be terminated by an audible whoop, which occurs upon rapid inspiration against a closed glottis at the end of a paroxysm. During a spasm, there may be

Table 152-1　Clinical Features of Pertussis, by Age Group and Diagnostic Status

	Percentage of Patients		
	Adolescents and Adults		
Feature	Laboratory Confirmation	No Laboratory Confirmation	Children
Cough	95–100	95–100	95–100
Prolonged	60–80	60–80	60–95
Paroxysmal	60–90	50–90	80–95
Sleep-disturbing	50–80	50–80	90–100
Whoop	10–40	5–30	40–80
Posttussive vomiting	20–50	5–30	80–90

cyanosis. Paroxysms may be precipitated by noise, eating, or physical contact. Between attacks, the patient's appearance is normal but increasing fatigue is evident. The frequency of paroxysmal episodes varies widely, from several per hour to 5 to 10 per day. Episodes are often worse at night and interfere with sleep. Weight loss is not uncommon as a result of interference with eating. Most complications occur during the paroxysmal stage. Fever is uncommon and suggests bacterial superinfection.

After 2 to 4 weeks, the coughing episodes become less frequent and less severe—changes heralding the onset of the *convalescent phase*. This phase can last from 1 to 3 months and is characterized by a gradual resolution of the coughing episodes. For 6 months to a year, intercurrent viral infections may be associated with a recrudescence of paroxysmal cough.

Not all children who develop pertussis have classic disease. Although cough (typically paroxysmal) is nearly always present, whoop may occur in only half of cases. In infants, the illness may be atypical; often apnea and cyanosis are the only symptoms at presentation. Seizures, encephalopathy, and pneumonia are all more common in infants ≤6 months old. Pertussis-associated infant deaths due to apnea may be confused with sudden infant death syndrome. The clinical manifestations in adolescents and adults may be classic but are more often atypical. In a German study of pertussis in adults, over two-thirds had paroxysmal cough and over one-third had whoop. Adult illness in North America differs from this experience: the cough may be severe and prolonged but is less frequently paroxysmal, and a whoop is uncommon. Vomiting with cough is the best predictor of pertussis as the cause of a prolonged cough in adults. Other features predictive of the disease are a cough at night and exposure to other individuals with a prolonged coughing illness.

COMPLICATIONS Complications are frequently associated with pertussis and are more common among infants than among older children or adults. Subconjunctival hemorrhages, abdominal and inguinal hernias, pneumothoraces, and facial and truncal petechiae can result from increased intrathoracic pressure generated by severe fits of coughing. Weight loss can follow decreased caloric intake. In a series of over 1100 children <2 years of age who were hospitalized with pertussis, 27.1% had apnea, 9.4% had pneumonia, 2.6% had seizures, and 0.4% had encephalopathy; 10 children (0.9%) died. Pneumonia is reported in fewer than 5% of adolescents and adults and is usually caused by encapsulated organisms such as *Streptococcus pneumoniae* or *Haemophilus influenzae*; in contrast, infants develop primary *B. pertussis* pneumonia. Pneumothorax, severe weight loss, inguinal hernia, rib fracture, and cough syncope have all been reported in adolescents and adults with pertussis.

DIAGNOSIS If the classic symptoms of pertussis are present, clinical diagnosis is not difficult. However, particularly in older children and adults, it is difficult to differentiate infections caused by *B. pertussis* and *B. parapertussis* from other respiratory tract infections on clinical grounds. Therefore, laboratory confirmation should be attempted in all cases. Lymphocytosis (absolute neutrophil count, >10 × 10⁹/L) is common among young children (in whom it is unusual with other infections) but not among adolescents and adults. Culture of nasopharyngeal secretions remains the "gold standard" of diagnosis; the best specimen is collected by nasopharyngeal aspiration, in which a fine flexible plastic catheter attached to a 10-mL syringe is passed into the nasopharynx and withdrawn while gentle suction is applied. Since *B. pertussis* is highly sensitive to drying, secretions should be inoculated without delay onto appropriate media (Bordet-Gengou or Regan-Lowe) or the catheter should be flushed with a phosphate-buffered saline solution. An alternative is a nasopharyngeal culture with a calcium alginate swab; again, inoculation of culture plates should be immediate or an appropriate transport medium (such as Regan-Lowe charcoal medium) should be used. Cultures become positive by day 5 of incubation, and *B. pertussis* and *B. parapertussis* can be differentiated by agglutination with specific antisera or by direct immunofluorescence.

Nasopharyngeal cultures in untreated pertussis remain positive for a mean of 3 weeks after the onset of illness; these cultures become negative within 5 days of the institution of appropriate antimicrobial therapy. Since much of the period during which the organism can be recovered from the nasopharynx falls in the catarrhal phase, when the etiology of the infection is not suspected, there is only a small window of opportunity for culture-proven diagnosis. Cultures from infants and young children are more frequently positive than those from older children and adults; this difference may reflect earlier presentation of the former age group for medical care. The increasing availability of the polymerase chain reaction for pertussis in diagnostic laboratories is enhancing the sensitivity of the organism's detection. This method may further laboratory confirmation but does not solve problems related to the long delays in specimen procurement that often are encountered in pertussis cases. Direct fluorescent antibody tests of nasopharyngeal secretions for direct diagnosis may still be available in some laboratories but should not be used because of poor sensitivity and specificity.

As a result of the difficulties with laboratory diagnosis of pertussis in adolescents, adults, and any patient who has been symptomatic for >4 weeks, increasing attention is being given to serologic diagnosis. Enzyme immunoassays detecting IgA and IgG antibodies to pertussis toxin, filamentous hemagglutinin, pertactin, and fimbriae have been developed and assessed for their reproducibility. Two- or fourfold increases in antibody are suggestive of pertussis, although cross-reactivity of some antigens (such as filamentous hemagglutinin) among *Bordetella* species makes it difficult to depend diagnostically on seroconversion involving a single type of antibody. Late presentation for medical care and prior immunization also complicate serologic diagnosis because the first sample obtained may in fact be a convalescent-phase specimen. Proposed criteria for serologic diagnosis based on a single serum specimen call for comparison of the patient's antibody levels with established population values; for example, a patient with serologically confirmed pertussis might be required to have a titer greater than two or three standard deviations above the mean titer for a normal population. However, at present, no antibody test is widely or commercially available, and no specific serologic criteria are universally accepted.

DIFFERENTIAL DIAGNOSIS A child presenting with paroxysmal cough, posttussive vomiting, and whoop is likely to have an infection caused by *B. pertussis* or *B. parapertussis*; lymphocytosis increases the likelihood of a *B. pertussis* etiology. Viruses such as respiratory syncytial virus and adenovirus have been isolated from patients with clinical pertussis but probably represent co-infection. In adolescents and adults, among whom paroxysmal cough and whoop are frequently absent, the differential diagnosis of a prolonged coughing illness is more extensive. Pertussis should be suspected in anyone with a cough that does not improve within 14 days, a paroxysmal cough of any duration, or any respiratory symptoms after contact with a laboratory-confirmed case of pertussis. Other etiologies to consider include infections caused by *Mycoplasma pneumoniae*, *Chlamydia pneumoniae*, adenovirus, influenza virus, and other respiratory viruses. Use of angiotensin-converting enzyme (ACE) inhibitors, reactive airway disease, and gastroesophageal reflux disease are well-described noninfectious causes of prolonged cough in adults.

TREATMENT **Antibiotics** The purpose of antibiotic therapy for pertussis is to eradicate the infecting bacteria from the nasopharynx; therapy does not substantially alter the clinical course unless given early in the catarrhal phase. Erythromycin (preferably the estolate form) is recommended at a dose of 50 mg/kg (maximum, 2 g/d) in three divided doses and reliably clears *B. pertussis* from the nasopharynx after 5 days. A dose of 1 g/d has also been shown to be effective and may be better tolerated. Although a 14-day course of therapy has been recommended to prevent relapse, one study showed that a 7-day course was equally effective. Erythromycin is also effective against other pathogens implicated in cough illness, such as *Mycoplasma* and *Chlamydia*.

Other macrolide antibiotics, such as azithromycin and clarithromycin, are active against *B. pertussis* in vitro, but data on their clinical efficacy are limited; clinical trials are under way. Trimethoprim-sulfamethoxazole (8/40 mg/kg per day in two divided doses) is recommended as an alternative for individuals who cannot use erythromycin, although good clinical data to support this recommendation are lacking. A macrolide-resistant *B. pertussis* strain has been reported from a single case in an outbreak in Arizona.

Immune Globulin Although immune globulin was used widely to treat pertussis in the preantibiotic era, evidence for its effectiveness was lacking and the commercially available product was removed from the market. There is renewed interest in the therapeutic use of immune globulin, particularly for infants who develop pertussis while still too young to have completed their primary immunization series. A high-titer pertussis toxin immune globulin for intravenous use is undergoing clinical trials.

Supportive Care Infants have the highest rates of complication and death from pertussis; therefore, most infants and older children with severe disease should be hospitalized. Monitoring for apnea and cyanosis, administration of supplemental oxygen, management of secretions, hydration, and nutritional support are the mainstays of care. A quiet environment may decrease the stimulation that can trigger paroxysmal episodes. Assisted ventilation may be required for management of apnea or pneumonia. Use of β-adrenergic agonists and/or glucocorticoids has been advocated by some but has not been proved to be effective. Cough suppressants are not effective and play no role in the management of pertussis.

Infection Control Measures Hospitalized patients with pertussis should be placed in respiratory isolation, with the use of precautions appropriate for pathogens spread by large respiratory droplets. Isolation should continue for 5 days after initiation of erythromycin therapy or for 3 weeks (i.e., until nasopharyngeal cultures are consistently negative) in those individuals unable to tolerate antimicrobial therapy.

PREVENTION **Chemoprophylaxis** Because the risk of transmission of *B. pertussis* within households is high, chemoprophylaxis is widely recommended for household contacts of pertussis cases. The effectiveness of chemoprophylaxis, although unproven, is supported by several epidemiologic studies of institutional and community outbreaks of pertussis. In the only randomized placebo-controlled study, erythromycin estolate (50 mg/kg per day in three divided doses; maximum dose, 1 g/d) was effective in reducing bacteriologically confirmed pertussis by 67%; however, there was no decrease in the incidence of clinical disease. Despite these disappointing results, many authorities continue to recommend chemoprophylaxis, particularly in households with members at high risk of severe disease (children <1 year of age). Data are not yet available on use of the newer macrolides for chemoprophylaxis.

Immunization (See also Chap. 122) The mainstay of pertussis prevention is active immunization. Pertussis vaccine has been available for over 70 years and became widely used in North America after 1940; reported cases of pertussis have since fallen by >90%. Whole-cell pertussis vaccines are prepared through the heating, chemical inactivation, and purification of whole *B. pertussis* organisms. Although effective (average efficacy estimate, 85%, with results in various studies of different products ranging from 30 to 100%), whole-cell pertussis vaccines are associated with adverse events—both common (fever; injection site pain, erythema, and swelling; irritability) and uncommon (febrile seizures, hypotonic hyporesponsive episodes). Alleged associations of whole-cell pertussis vaccine with encephalopathy, sudden infant death syndrome, and autism, although not substantiated, have spawned an active anti-immunization lobby. The development of acellular pertussis vaccines, which are effective but less reactogenic, has greatly alleviated concerns about the inclusion of

pertussis vaccine in the combined infant immunization series. In some countries (Canada, Sweden, Germany), acellular pertussis vaccines are used exclusively for childhood immunization; in the United States, acellular pertussis vaccines are now the preferred product but whole-cell vaccine is still considered acceptable. In North America, both whole-cell and acellular pertussis vaccines are given as a three-dose primary series at 2, 4, and 6 months of age, with a reinforcing dose between 15 and 18 months of age and a booster dose at 4 to 6 years of age.

A wide variety of acellular pertussis vaccines have been developed, although not all are available in every country. All acellular pertussis vaccines currently available contain pertussis toxoid. Only one monovalent pertussis toxoid vaccine has been licensed in the United States; the remainder of the fully developed vaccines contain filamentous hemagglutinin as well as toxoid. At least four acellular pertussis vaccines also contain pertactin, and two products also contain one or more types of fimbriae. All of the licensed acellular pertussis vaccines have undergone phase 3 efficacy testing. Although differences in study design make direct comparisons difficult, an effort to standardize case definitions and the similarity of some of the studies, which used common vaccine arms to allow "bridging" of the data between studies, have permitted some general conclusions. Even though some would still disagree, most experts have concluded that two-component acellular pertussis vaccines are more effective than monocomponent vaccines and that the addition of pertactin further increases efficacy. The further addition of fimbriae appears to provide some additional protective efficacy against milder disease. In two studies, protection against pertussis by vaccines correlated best with the production of antibody to pertactin, fimbriae, and pertussis toxin.

The development of acellular pertussis vaccines has sparked interest in the potential for control of pertussis in adolescents and adults and in the possibility that pertussis control in those groups will enhance the protection of infants too young to be immunized. Whole-cell pertussis vaccine is contraindicated in individuals ≥ 7 years of age because of their poor toleration of possible adverse events. However, adult formulations of acellular pertussis vaccines, both alone and in combination with adult-formulation diphtheria-tetanus toxoid, have been demonstrated to be safe and immunogenic in clinical trials in adolescents and adults. Further epidemiologic studies and an efficacy study are under way to better delineate the scope of pertussis illness in adolescents and adults as well as the efficacy of a single dose of acellular pertussis vaccine. These data, along with the results of other studies characterizing the spectrum of pertussis disease in adolescents and adults, will help public health authorities and advisory committees to determine the role of adolescent and adult pertussis immunization.

BIBLIOGRAPHY

CHERRY JD et al: A search for serologic correlates of immunity to *Bordetella pertussis* cough illnesses. Vaccine 16:1901, 1998

GRECO D et al: A controlled trial of two acellular vaccines and one whole-cell vaccine against pertussis. Progetto Pertosse Working Group. N Engl J Med 334:341, 1996

GUSTAFSSON L et al: A controlled trial of a two-component acellular, a five-component acellular, and a whole-cell pertussis vaccine. N Engl J Med 334:349, 1996 (published erratum appears in N Engl J Med 334:1207, 1996)

HALPERIN SA et al: Seven days of erythromycin estolate is as effective as fourteen days for the treatment of *Bordetella pertussis* infections. Pediatrics 100:65, 1997

——— et al: A randomized, placebo-controlled trial of erythromycin estolate chemoprophylaxis for household contacts of children with culture-positive *Bordetella pertussis* infection. Pediatrics 104:4, 1999

——— et al: Epidemiological features of hospitalized pertussis cases in Canada, 1991–1997: A report of the immunization monitoring program, Active (IMPACT). Clin Infect Dis 28:1238, 1999

SCHMITT-GROHÉ S et al: Pertussis in German adults. Clin Infect Dis 21:860, 1995

TROLLFORS B et al: A placebo-controlled trial of a pertussis-toxoid vaccine. N Engl J Med 333:1045, 1995

WIRSING VON KÖNIG CH et al: Pertussis in adults: Frequency of transmission after household exposure. Lancet 346:1326, 1995

WRIGHT SW et al: Pertussis infection in adults with persistent cough. JAMA 273:1044, 1995

153   *Thomas A. Russo*

DISEASES CAUSED BY GRAM-NEGATIVE ENTERIC BACILLI

DAEC	diffusely adherent *E. coli*	GNB	gram-negative bacilli
EAEC	enteroaggregative *E. coli*	HUS	hemolytic-uremic syndrome
EHEC	enterohemorrhagic *E. coli*	ICUs	intensive care units
EIEC	enteroinvasive *E. coli*	LPS	lipopolysaccharide
EPEC	enteropathogenic *E. coli*	NNIS	National Nosocomial
ESBLs	extended-spectrum β-lactamases		Infections Study
		STEC	Shiga toxin–producing *E. coli*
ETEC	enterotoxigenic *E. coli*	TMP-SMZ	trimethoprim-sulfamethoxazole
ExPEC	extraintestinal pathogenic strains of *E. coli*		
		UTI	urinary tract infection

GENERAL FEATURES AND PRINCIPLES

EPIDEMIOLOGY This chapter discusses gram-negative bacilli (GNB) belonging to the medically important genera of the family Enterobacteriaceae (*Escherichia, Klebsiella, Proteus, Enterobacter, Serratia, Citrobacter, Morganella, Providencia,* and *Edwardsiella*) as well as the genus *Actinetobacter* from the family Neisseriaceae. These bacteria are members of normal animal and human colonic flora and/or residents of a variety of environmental habitats, including long-term-care facilities and hospitals. In healthy humans, *Escherichia coli* is the predominant species of GNB in the colonic flora. GNB (primarily *E. coli, Klebsiella,* and *Proteus*) only transiently colonize the oropharynx and skin. In contrast, in the long-term-care and hospital settings, a variety of GNB emerge as the dominant components of the colonizing flora of both mucosal and skin surfaces, particularly with antimicrobial use and increasing severity of disease. Acquisition of these GNB from a variety of reservoirs leads to infection.

STRUCTURE AND FUNCTION Structurally, these organisms possess an extracytoplasmic outer membrane, a feature shared among gram-negative bacteria. The outer membrane consists of a lipid bilayer and associated proteins, lipoproteins, and polysaccharides [capsule, lipopolysaccharide (LPS)]. This structure interfaces with the environment, including the human host. A variety of components of the outer membrane are critical determinants in mediating the pathogenesis of infection and antimicrobial resistance.

INFECTIOUS SYNDROMES Depending on both the host and the pathogen, nearly every organ and body cavity can be infected with GNB. *Escherichia* and, to a lesser degree, *Klebsiella* and *Proteus* account for the majority of infections and are the most virulent pathogens of this group. However, the other genera are becoming increasingly important, particularly in long-term-care or hospitalized patients, in large part because of the organisms' innate or acquired resistance to antimicrobial agents and the increasing number of immunocompromised hosts. The mortality rate is significant in many GNB infections and correlates with the severity of illness. Especially problematic are pneumonitis and bacteremia from any source complicated by shock, which have associated mortality rates of 20 to 50%.

DIAGNOSIS Isolation of GNB from sterile sites almost always implies infection. Their isolation from nonsterile sites, particularly from soft tissue and respiratory cultures, requires clinical correlation to differentiate colonization from infection.

TREATMENT AND PREVENTION The antimicrobial resistance of GNB is variable and is influenced by both location and regional antibiotic use. Empirical antimicrobial choices should be based on local susceptibility patterns, but it is critical to be cognizant of emerging resistance. The acquisition of transferable plasmids that possess genes for extended-spectrum β-lactamases (ESBLs) is increasing. To date, these plasmids are most prevalent in *Klebsiella* and *E. coli,* but they have also been described (albeit less frequently) in most of the enteric GNB. The plasmids confer resistance to third-generation cephalosporins and aztreonam and frequently contain linked resistance determinants for aminoglycosides, tetracyclines, and trimethoprim-sulfamethoxazole (TMP-SMZ). In some outbreaks, strains with ESBLs also exhibit associated fluoroquinolone resistance. Derepression of inducible chromosomal β-lactamases, another important resistance mechanism, may be preexisting or may develop during therapy. This determinant confers resistance to second- and third-generation cephalosporins, to aztreonam, and often to β-lactam/β-lactamase inhibitor combinations. Of the enteric GNB, *Enterobacter, Serratia, Citrobacter, Proteus vulgaris, Proteus penneri, Providencia,* and *Morganella* possess this determinant. Although relevant data are suboptimal or conflicting, combination therapy may increase antimicrobial efficacy (particularly in serious infections, such as pneumonitis) and diminish the emergence of resistance. Further, drainage of abscesses and removal of infected foreign bodies are often needed for cure. GNB are commonly part of a polymicrobial infection in which it is difficult to determine the role of each specific pathogen. Although some species are more pathogenic than others, it is usually prudent, if possible, to design an antimicrobial regimen that includes activity against all of the GNB identified, since each is capable of pathogenicity in its own right. Diligent hand washing by health care personnel and avoidance of inappropriate antimicrobial use are the two most important measures for the prevention of infection.

PATHOGENESIS Multiple bacterial traits are required for various aspects of the pathogenesis of GNB. The possession of specialized virulence genes is what defines pathogens and enables them to infect the host efficiently. As more is learned about these genes, it is becoming clear that hosts and their cognate pathogens have been coadapting throughout evolutionary history. In fact, it has been speculated that infection is just a point on the spectrum of evolutionary development between microbes and the host. At one end of this spectrum is a commensal/symbiotic interaction (e.g., mitochondria—formerly bacteria—within eukaryotic cells); at the other is a lethal outcome that results in a "dead-end relationship" (e.g., Ebola virus). During this host-pathogen "chess match" over time, a variety and redundancy of solutions have emerged in both pathogens and hosts that enable the partners to maintain their coexistence (Table 153-1).

Intestinal Infection Intestinal pathogenic strains of *E. coli* cause gastroenteritis by a variety of unique pathogenic mechanisms. Their virulence traits are for the most part distinct from those of *E. coli* strains that cause disease outside the bowel. This difference is not

Table 153-1 Interactions of Extraintestinal Pathogenic *E. coli* and Humans: A Paradigm for Extracellular, Extraintestinal Gram-Negative Bacterial Pathogens

Bacterial Goal	Host Obstacle	Bacterial Solution
Extraintestinal attachment	Flow of urine Mucociliary blanket	Multiple adhesins (e.g., type I, Sfa/Foc, P pili)
Nutrient acquisition for growth	Nutrient sequestration (e.g., iron via intracellular storage and extracellular scavenging via lactoferrin and transferrin)	Cellular lysis (e.g., hemolysin); multiple mechanisms for competing for extracellular iron (e.g., siderophores) and other nutrients
Initial avoidance of host bactericidal activity	Complement Phagocytic cells Defensins	Capsular polysaccharide, lipopolysaccharide
Transmission	Hygiene Infection control Public health measures	Irritant tissue damage resulting in increased excretion (e.g., toxins such as hemolysin)
Late avoidance of host bactericidal activity	Acquired immunity (e.g., specific antibodies) Treatment with antibiotics	? Cell entry Acquisition of antimicrobial resistance

surprising in light of site-dependent differences in host environments and defense mechanisms.

Extraintestinal Infection Extraintestinal pathogenic strains of *E. coli* (ExPEC) and the other genera discussed in this chapter cause infection outside the bowel. All are extracellular pathogens and therefore share certain pathogenic features. Innate defense systems (complement, phagocytes) and humoral immunity are the most critical host defense components. As a result, both susceptibility to and severity of infection are increased with dysfunction or deficiencies of these components (e.g., neutrophils). A given pathogen usually possesses multiple adhesins for binding to a variety of host cells (e.g., in *E. coli*: type I, Sfa/Foc, P pili). Nutrient acquisition (e.g., iron via siderophores) requires many genes that are necessary but not sufficient for pathogenesis. The ability to resist the bactericidal activity of complement and professional phagocytes in the absence of antibody (e.g., conferred by capsule or O antigen of LPS) is one of the defining traits of an extracellular pathogen. Tissue damage (e.g., hemolysis in the case of *E. coli*) may facilitate spread. However, many important virulence genes await identification, and our understanding of many aspects of the pathogenesis of GNB is in its infancy (Chap. 120). The ability to induce septic shock is another defining feature of these genera. GNB are the most common cause of this dangerous complication. The lipid A moiety of LPS and probably other bacterial factors as well (e.g., capsule) stimulate a proinflammatory host response, which, if overexuberant, results in shock (Chap. 124). Lastly, a large number of serotypes (e.g., in *E. coli*, >100 O-specific and >80 capsular antigens) exist within most genera of GNB. This antigenic variability enables immune evasion and successful recurrent infection by strains of the same species and has also impeded vaccine development (Chap. 122).

ESCHERICHIA COLI INFECTIONS

From a clinical perspective, *E. coli* can be divided into three categories: commensal strains, intestinal pathogenic (enteric or diarrheagenic) strains, and ExPEC.

ETIOLOGY, EPIDEMIOLOGY, AND MANIFESTATIONS **Commensal Strains** Commensal strains of *E. coli* constitute the bulk of the facultative fecal flora in most healthy humans. Such strains appear to be adapted for peaceful coexistence with the host and appear not to cause disease within the intestinal tract. Further, in humans, these microorganisms do not usually cause disease outside the intestinal tract except in the presence of precipitating factors, such as an indwelling foreign body or an impairment of host defenses. Commensal *E. coli* strains typically lack the specialized virulence traits of intestinal and ExPEC strains.

Intestinal Pathogenic Strains In contrast to commensal *E. coli*, intestinal pathogenic strains of *E. coli* are rarely encountered in the fecal flora of healthy hosts and instead appear to be essentially obligate pathogens, causing gastroenteritis or colitis whenever ingested in sufficient quantities by a naive host. At least six distinct "pathotypes" of intestinal pathogenic *E. coli* exist: (1) enterotoxigenic *E. coli* (ETEC); (2) Shiga toxin–producing *E. coli* (STEC)/enterohemorrhagic *E. coli* (EHEC); (3) enteropathogenic *E. coli* (EPEC); (4) enteroinvasive *E. coli* (EIEC); (5) enteroaggregative *E. coli* (EAEC); and (6) diffusely adherent *E. coli* (DAEC). Organisms of these pathotypes are acquired via the fecal-oral route. Transmission occurs predominantly via contaminated food and water for ETEC, STEC, EIEC, EAEC, and DAEC and by person-to-person spread for EPEC (and occasionally STEC). Humans appear to be the major reservoir (except for STEC), since the host range appears to be dictated by species-specific attachment factors. Although there is some overlap, each pathotype possesses a unique combination of virulence traits that results in a distinctive intestinal pathogenic mechanism; however, these strains are largely incapable of causing disease outside the intestinal tract.

ETEC In tropical or developing countries, several separate episodes of ETEC infection occur in children over the first 3 years of life.

The incidence of disease diminishes with age, a pattern suggesting the development of immunity. In industrialized countries, infection usually follows travel to endemic areas. ETEC is the most common cause of traveler's diarrhea (Chap. 123), being responsible for 25 to 75% of cases. Cases usually develop within the first few weeks of travel. The incidence of infection is decreased by the prudent avoidance of potentially contaminated fluids and foods. ETEC infection is uncommon in the United States, but outbreaks have taken place secondary to contamination of domestic food products. A high inoculum (10^6 to 10^{10} CFU) is needed to cause disease. After ingestion of contaminated water or food (particularly items poorly cooked, unpeeled, or unrefrigerated), the small bowel is colonized during a 1- to 7-day incubation period. Disease is mediated in part by heat-labile (LT) and/or heat-stable (STa) toxin encoded by genes present on transferable plasmids. These toxins stimulate fluid secretion via activation of adenylate cyclase (LT) and/or guanylate cyclase (STa); the result is watery diarrhea accompanied by cramps. Characteristically absent are histopathologic changes of the small bowel; mucus, blood, and inflammatory cells in stool; and fever. The disease spectrum ranges from mild illness to a life-threatening cholera-like illness. Although symptoms are usually self-limited (2 to 6 days), infection may result in significant morbidity and mortality when health care is poor and small and/or undernourished children are affected.

STEC/EHEC STEC strains constitute an emerging group of pathogens that have received substantial media attention as a result of several large outbreaks attributable to the consumption of undercooked ground beef and other foods. Serotype O157:H7 is the most prominent of the more than 30 serotypes associated with the STEC syndrome (see below). Other common serogroups include O26, O39, O103, O104, and O111. The ability to produce Shiga-like toxin (Stx2 and/or Stx1) or related toxins is the critical factor dictating whether a bacterium can cause the clinical syndrome associated with STEC. *Citrobacter* isolates that produce Stx2 and *Shigella* strains that produce related toxins can cause the same syndrome.

A combination of factors are responsible for the emergence of STEC disease. A number of animals, including cattle and young calves, serve as a major reservoir for these strains. Ground beef, the most common food source, is frequently contaminated during processing. Further, cattle or other animal manure used as fertilizer can contaminate produce (potatoes, lettuce, sprouts, fallen apples) and water (fecal runoff). It is estimated that $<10^3$ CFU of STEC can cause disease. Therefore, not only can low levels of food or environmental contamination (e.g., water swallowed when swimming) result in disease, but person-to-person transmission becomes an important vehicle for secondary spread (e.g., at day-care centers and in institutions). Because of the low infective dose (which is similar to that of *Shigella*), laboratory-associated infections also take place. Both outbreaks and sporadic disease occur with this group of pathogens, with a seasonal peak in the summer.

In contrast to infection with the other five pathotypes, infection with STEC occurs more frequently in developed countries, where consumption of processed foods is more common than in developing regions. FoodNet data indicate that O157 strains are the fourth most common reported cause of bacterial diarrhea in the United States (behind *Campylobacter*, *Salmonella*, and *Shigella*). Colonization of the colon and perhaps of the ileum results in symptoms after an incubation period of 3 or 4 days. Maximal disease expression requires Stx2 (produced by most O157 isolates) and/or Stx1 (more commonly produced by non-O157 isolates) as well as other virulence genes (e.g., *eaeA*). Colonic edema and an initial secretory diarrhea may develop into the syndrome's hallmark trait of grossly bloody diarrhea (detected by history or examination) in >90% of cases. Significant abdominal pain and fecal leukocytes are commonly present (70% of cases), but fever is usually absent. Occasionally, *Clostridium difficile*, *Campylobacter*, and *Salmonella* infection present in a similar fashion, as do noninfectious diseases (e.g., appendicitis, inflammatory bowel disease). STEC disease is usually self-limited, lasting 5 to 10 days. This infection can be complicated by the hemolytic-uremic syndrome (HUS), which oc-very young and the elderly. An estimated 50% of all cases of HUS in the United States are caused by STEC infection. This complication is probably mediated by the systemic translocation of Shiga-like toxins and subsequent cellular damage, particularly to endothelial cells in the renal and cerebral microvasculature. HUS is characterized by microangiopathic hemolytic anemia, thrombocytopenia, and renal failure. Neurologic symptoms, with or without fever, can also occur. Although mortality with dialysis support is <10%, residual renal dysfunction and neurologic sequelae may persist.

EPEC   EPEC causes disease primarily in young children, including neonates. This *E. coli* group was recognized as a cause of diarrheal disease when it was found in outbreaks of infantile diarrhea (some in hospital nurseries) in industrialized countries in the 1940s and 1950s. Presently, however, infection due to EPEC is uncommon in developed countries. In contrast, EPEC is an important cause of infant diarrhea (both sporadic and epidemic) in developing countries. Breast-feeding diminishes the incidence of infection. Rapid person-to-person spread may occur. Upon colonization of the small bowel, symptoms develop after an incubation period of 1 or 2 days. Disease is not toxin-mediated. Studies have identified a variety of virulence traits responsible for adherence and a characteristic effacement of microvilli with formation of cuplike, actin-rich pedestals to which the bacteria attach. Diarrheal stool often contains mucus but not blood. Although usually self-limiting, EPEC diarrhea may persist for weeks.

EIEC   EIEC is a relatively uncommon cause of diarrhea and is rarely identified in the United States, although a few food-related outbreaks have been described. In less developed countries, sporadic disease is infrequently recognized in children and travelers. EIEC shares many features with *Shigella* infection; however, unlike *Shigella*, EIEC causes disease only at a high inoculum (10^8 to 10^{10} CFU). Invasion of and replication within the colonic mucosa result in the development of symptoms after an incubation period of 1 to 3 days. Secretory diarrhea may evolve into inflammatory colitis characterized by fever, abdominal pain, tenesmus, and scant stool containing mucus, blood, and inflammatory cells. Symptoms are usually self-limited, lasting 7 to 10 days.

EAEC and DAEC   These pathotypes have been described primarily in developing countries and mostly affect young children. These strains may also cause some cases of traveler's diarrhea. A high inoculum is required for infection. In vitro, the organisms exhibit a diffuse or "stacked-brick" adherence pattern. Clinical disease has been associated with persistent diarrhea.

DIAGNOSIS   A practical approach in evaluating diarrhea is to distinguish noninflammatory from inflammatory cases (Chap. 131). ETEC, EPEC, EAEC, and DAEC are uncommon causes of noninflammatory diarrhea in the United States. Their diagnosis requires specialized assays that are not routinely available and whose use is rarely indicated since these diseases are self-limiting. ETEC causes the majority of cases of noninflammatory traveler's diarrhea; EAEC and DAEC cause a minority of these cases. Definitive diagnosis generally is not necessary, and empirical antimicrobial treatment is a reasonable approach. If diarrhea persists with treatment, *Giardia* or *Cryptosporidium* should be sought. The diagnosis of infection with EIEC, a rare cause of inflammatory diarrhea in the United States, also requires specialized assays. However, evaluation for STEC, particularly when bloody diarrhea is reported or observed, is appropriate. Although screening for *E. coli* strains that do not ferment sorbitol and subsequent serotyping for O157 constitute the most common method presently used to detect STEC, testing for Shiga-like toxins or toxin genes is more sensitive, specific, and rapid. The latter approach offers another advantage: it detects both non-O157 strains and sorbitol-fermenting strains of O157, which otherwise are difficult to identify. DNA-based, enzyme-linked immunosorbent, and cytotoxicity assays are in various stages of development and will probably become the diagnostic standards in time.

Extraintestinal Pathogenic Strains   From both pathogenic and clinical viewpoints, ExPEC strains are distinct from commensal and intestinal pathogenic strains of *E. coli*. ExPEC strains also make up part of the normal human fecal flora, but, in contrast to commensal strains, possess specialized genes that encode virulence factors enabling the organisms to cause extraintestinal infections (Table 153-1). ExPEC (as opposed to commensal *E. coli*) causes the majority of cases of urinary tract infection (UTI), bacteremia, and neonatal meningitis. It is likely that ExPEC also causes the majority of other extraintestinal infections due to *E. coli*. Entry into an extraintestinal site (e.g., the urinary tract or the peritoneum)—not acquisition—is the limiting factor for infection. All age groups, all types of hosts, and nearly every organ and site are susceptible to infection by ExPEC. Normal, previously healthy hosts infected with ExPEC can become severely ill and die. However, adverse outcomes are more prevalent in the presence of coincidental disease and abnormalities in host defenses. Typical extraintestinal infections include UTI, diverse intraabdominal infections, pneumonia (particularly in hospitalized and institutionalized patients), meningitis (mainly in neonates and patients who have undergone neurosurgery), intravascular device infection, osteomyelitis, and soft tissue infection (which usually occurs in the setting of tissue compromise). Bacteremia can accompany infection at any of these sites. Although *E. coli* is considered to be primarily a community-acquired pathogen, it is the most frequently isolated of the GNB in the ambulatory, long-term-care, and hospital settings. The scope and magnitude of infection caused by ExPEC are as great as for any other invasive bacterial pathogen. Although these isolates do not make headlines, billions of health care dollars, millions of workdays, and thousands of lives are lost to this group of pathogens each year.

Infectious syndromes • URINARY TRACT INFECTION (UTI)   The urinary tract is the site most frequently infected by ExPEC. About 90% of ambulatory UTIs and 25 to 35% of long-term-care and hospital UTIs are due to *E. coli*. The majority of UTIs occur in seven epidemiologically defined groups: children <1 year of age, school-age girls, premenopausal women, men with prostatic or other causes of urinary tract obstruction, postmenopausal women, individuals with neurogenic bladders, and patients with indwelling urinary catheters. In premenopausal women, diaphragm-spermicide use, sexual activity, and a history of UTI are risk factors for infection; 20% of women with an initial infection have frequent recurrences (0.3 to >20 per year). In postmenopausal women, estrogen replacement decreases the incidence of UTI. Acceptance of the diagnosis of UTI in males (beyond the first year of life) requires clear documentation since this infection is unusual in the absence of a history of instrumentation or anal intercourse. UTI in premenopausal women alone accounts for an estimated 7 million office visits and >$1 billion in direct medical costs annually. UTI is the second most common infection (behind lower respiratory tract infection) responsible for hospitalization.

Uncomplicated urethritis or cystitis occurs most commonly and is characterized by symptoms of dysuria, frequency, and suprapubic pain. Fever and/or back pain suggests progression to pyelonephritis. Pregnant women are at unusually high risk for this complication, which can adversely affect the outcome of pregnancy. As a result, prenatal screening for bacteriuria, with treatment when the results are positive, is the standard of care. Fever may take 5 to 7 days to resolve completely in appropriately treated patients with pyelonephritis but should fall over time. Persistently elevated or increasing fever and neutrophil counts should prompt evaluation for intrarenal or perinephric abscess and/or obstruction. Renal parenchymal damage and loss of renal function occur primarily in the setting of obstruction. Prostatic infection is generally a complication of UTI in men with a history of instrumentation and/or prostatic hypertrophy. The diagnosis and treatment of UTI are detailed in Chap. 280 and are tailored according to the host, the nature and site of infection, and the local pattern of antimicrobial susceptibility.

ABDOMINAL INFECTION   The abdomen is the second most frequent site of extraintestinal infection due to *E. coli*. The majority of abdominal *E. coli* infections develop outside the hospital. Any inciting event that results in disruption of the bowel mucosa (particularly the colonic mucosa) often leads to acute peritonitis (secondary peritonitis; Chap. 130). This process is usually polymicrobial, but *E. coli* is isolated in most cases. Bacteremia often complicates this acute stage of infection. Abscess formation within the peritoneum may follow the acute stage or may develop as a consequence of subclinical fecal spillage (e.g., diverticulitis, chronic appendicitis). Intraperitoneal abscesses are almost always polymicrobial, with *E. coli* as the most common GNB isolated. *E. coli* is also the GNB most often responsible for primary hepatic abscesses, hepatic abscesses in the setting of biliary disease and obstruction, septic cholangitis/cholecystitis, pancreatic abscesses, and infected pancreatic pseudocysts. This organism is the leading cause of spontaneous bacterial peritonitis, usually seen in patients who have ascites associated with cirrhosis or occasionally with malignancy. *E. coli* occasionally causes splenic abscesses and peritoneal dialysis–associated peritonitis (Chap. 130).

PNEUMONIA   *E. coli* is not usually considered a cause of pneumonia (Chap. 255). Enteric GNB are responsible for only 2 to 5% of cases of community-acquired pneumonia, in part because these organisms only transiently colonize the oropharynx in a minority of healthy individuals. In contrast, oral colonization with *E. coli* and other GNB increases with the severity of illness and with antibiotic use. Thus, GNB are a common cause of pneumonia acquired by residents of long-term-care institutions and are the most frequent cause of hospital-acquired pneumonia (Chap. 135), particularly in postoperative and intensive care patients. Despite significant institutional variation, *E. coli* is generally the third or fourth most commonly isolated GNB in these settings, behind *Pseudomonas* and *Klebsiella*. Regardless of the host, severe disease and high mortality rates (20 to 60%) are usually seen when GNB cause pneumonia. Tissue necrosis, probably due to cytotoxins produced by GNB, is common. Infection is usually acquired by small-volume aspiration but occasionally occurs via hematogenous spread, in which case multifocal nodular infiltrates can be seen.

MENINGITIS (See Chap. 372)   ExPEC are a leading cause of meningitis in the first month of life. The majority of responsible strains possess the K1 capsular serotype. Outside this setting, meningitis due to *E. coli* is uncommon, occurring predominantly with cirrhosis (Chap. 299) or disruption of the meninges due to surgery or trauma.

CELLULITIS/MUSCULOSKELETAL INFECTION   Infections of decubitus ulcers and the lower extremities in diabetic patients (or other hosts with neurovascular compromise) are usually polymicrobial. *E. coli* frequently contributes to infection of decubiti and occasionally to lower-extremity infections in these patients. It may occasionally cause cellulitis or burn site or surgical wound infection, particularly when the infection originates close to the perineum. Osteomyelitis secondary to contiguous spread can occur in these settings. Hematogenously acquired osteomyelitis, particularly of vertebral bodies, is more common than is appreciated, accounting for 10% of cases in some series (Chap. 129). *E. coli* occasionally causes orthopedic device–associated infection and is a rare cause of hematogenously acquired myositis. Myositis or fasciitis of the upper leg should prompt an evaluation for an abdominal source with contiguous spread.

ENDOVASCULAR INFECTION   Extraintestinal isolates of *E. coli* cause a significant minority of intravascular device–associated infections (Chap. 135). Despite being one of the most common causes of bacteremia, however, *E. coli* rarely seeds native heart valves and is an uncommon cause of prosthetic valve endocarditis. Likewise, *E. coli* infections of aneurysms and vascular grafts are uncommon.

MISCELLANEOUS INFECTIONS   *E. coli* can cause infection in nearly every organ and site. This organism causes a minority—but still a significant number—of surgical site infections (e.g., mediastinitis) and cases of complicated sinusitis. It uncommonly causes endophthalmitis.

BACTEREMIA   *E. coli* bacteremia can result from extraintestinal infection of any site. The incidences of community-acquired and long-term-care/hospital-acquired bacteremia are roughly equal. Overall, it has been amply documented that *E. coli* and *Staphylococcus aureus* are the most common blood isolates (range for *E. coli*, 16 to 37%). *E. coli* is the GNB most frequently isolated from blood in the ambulatory setting and in most long-term-care and hospital settings. When *E. coli* is isolated from the blood, it is almost always clinically significant. Approximately 15% of bacteremias are complicated by septic shock. Two-thirds of bacteremias arise from the urinary tract; these infections are particularly common in the setting of pyelonephritis or obstruction (including kinked urinary catheters) or instrumentation of the urinary tract in the presence of *E. coli*. However, one should be cautious in identifying the urinary tract as the source of *E. coli* bacteremia in the absence of appropriate symptoms, despite a positive urine culture. Asymptomatic bacteriuria is common, particularly in women, even in the absence of an indwelling bladder catheter, with a prevalence of 15 to 25% after the age of 60. Therefore, occult abdominal or other sources should be considered. The abdomen is the second most common source, accounting for 25% of episodes. Although obstructive biliary tract disease (stones, tumor) and overt disruption of the bowel are responsible for many cases of *E. coli* bacteremia, some abdominal sources, such as abscesses, are remarkably silent clinically and require identification via imaging studies (e.g., computed tomography). Soft tissue, bone, and pulmonary infection are the next most frequent sources for bacteremia. As stated above, endocarditis is uncommon, occurring in only 2 of 861 bacteremias in a recent series. In the setting of chemotherapy-induced fever and neutropenia, *E. coli* is a common cause of bacteremia, usually secondary to intestinal mucositis. It is prudent in this situation, however, to exclude perirectal infection or typhlitis (Chap. 89). ExPEC strains are among the most common causes of sepsis in neonates.

Diagnosis   Strains of *E. coli* that cause extraintestinal infections usually grow both aerobically and anaerobically within 24 h on standard diagnostic media and are easily identified by the clinical microbiology laboratory using standard biochemical criteria (Chap. 121). More than 90% of these strains are rapid lactose fermenters.

℞ TREATMENT   Although *E. coli* is generally perceived as an "antibiotic-friendly" pathogen, resistance has increased over the past decade. In general, the frequency of ampicillin resistance precludes its empirical use, even in community-acquired infections. Rates of resistance to first-generation cephalosporins and TMP-SMZ in community-acquired strains are increasing in the United States (5 to 25%) and are even higher in Europe and developing countries. Not surprisingly, long-term-care and hospital isolates are more resistant than community isolates. Significant resistance (30 to 40%) to amoxicillin/clavulanic acid and piperacillin has been increasingly reported. Fortunately, resistance to second- and third-generation cephalosporins [mean rate, 3.2% according to 1998 National Nosocomial Infections Study (NNIS) data], fourth-generation cephalosporins, quinolones, monobactams (e.g., aztreonam), carbapenems (e.g., imipenem), and aminoglycosides is generally found in <10% of strains. An exception is in settings where quinolone prophylaxis is used extensively (patients with leukemia, transplant recipients); in these settings, significant quinolone resistance has emerged. Acquisition of plasmids containing ESBLs and other resistance determinants is likely to increase.

The mainstay of treatment for all diarrheal syndromes is the appropriate replacement of water and electrolytes (Chap. 159). The use of prophylactic antibiotics to prevent traveler's diarrhea should be discouraged, especially in light of high rates of antibiotic resistance. When diarrhea is free of mucus and blood, early patient-initiated treatment with a quinolone significantly decreases the duration of illness, and the use of loperamide may halt symptoms in a few hours (Chap. 123). Treatment of STEC is controversial since antibiotics may increase the incidence of HUS, perhaps via increased release of Shiga-like toxin.

KLEBSIELLA INFECTIONS *K. pneumoniae* is the most important *Klebsiella* species medically, causing community-acquired, long-term-care, and hospital infections. *K. oxytoca* is primarily a pathogen in long-term-care and hospital settings. *K. rhinoscleromatis* and *K. ozaenae* are usually isolated from patients in tropical climates. *Klebsiella* species are broadly prevalent in the environment and colonize mucosal surfaces of mammals. In healthy humans, *K. pneumoniae* colonization rates range from 5 to 35% in the colon and from 1 to 5% in the oropharynx; the skin is usually colonized only transiently. In long-term-care facilities and hospitals, colonization occurs with *K. oxytoxa* as well, and carriage rates are significant among both workers and patients. Person-to-person spread is thought to be the predominant mode of acquisition. Classically, *Klebsiella* is associated with community-acquired pneumonia, primarily in alcoholics. However, the majority of *Klebsiella* infections now occur in long-term-care facilities and hospitals. *Klebsiella* causes a spectrum of extraintestinal infections similar to that caused by *E. coli*. However, extraintestinal infections due to *Klebsiella* occur at a lower incidence in all sites except the respiratory tract. These variances in infection rates are probably due to differences in colonization and site-specific virulence traits. Antibiotic-resistant strains have been responsible for a number of nosocomial outbreaks of infection in intensive care units (ICUs) and neonatal nurseries. The most common clinical syndromes are pneumonia, UTI, abdominal infection, surgical site infection, soft tissue infection, and subsequent bacteremia. *K. rhinoscleromatis* is the causative agent of rhinoscleroma, a slowly progressive (months to years) mucosal upper respiratory infection that causes necrosis and occasional obstruction of the nasal passages. *K. ozaenae* has been implicated as a cause of chronic atrophic rhinitis.

Infectious Syndromes • Pneumonia *K. pneumoniae* causes only a small proportion of cases of community-acquired pneumonia (Chap. 255). This infection occurs primarily in hosts with underlying disease, such as alcoholics, diabetics, and individuals with chronic lung disease. As in all pneumonias due to enteric GNB, purulent sputum production and "airspace" disease on x-ray are typical. Presentation with earlier, less extensive infection is more common than that with the classic lobar infiltrate with a bulging fissure. Pulmonary necrosis, pleural effusion, and empyema occur with progression. Pulmonary infection in residents of long-term-care facilities and in hospitalized patients is especially frequent because of increased oropharyngeal colonization rates. Mechanical ventilation is an important risk factor.

UTI The incidence of *K. pneumoniae* UTI among healthy adults is only 1 to 2%. However, in complicated UTIs (including those associated with indwelling bladder catheters), the incidence of *Klebsiella* infection increases to 5 to 17%.

Abdominal infection *Klebsiella* causes a spectrum of abdominal infections similar to that caused by *E. coli* but is less frequently isolated from these infections.

Other infections *Klebsiella* cellulitis or soft tissue infection occurs most frequently in devitalized tissue (e.g., decubitus ulcers, diabetes, burn sites) or in immunocompromised hosts. *Klebsiella* causes a significant minority of surgical site infections and nosocomial sinusitis cases as well as occasional cases of osteomyelitis contiguous to soft tissue infection, temperate myositis, and neonatal meningitis or meningitis associated with neurosurgery.

Bacteremia *Klebsiella* infection at any site can result in bacteremia. Infections of the urinary tract, respiratory tract, and abdomen each account for 15 to 30% of *Klebsiella* bacteremias. Intravascular device–related infection is another important source (5 to 15%). Surgical site infection and other miscellaneous infections account for the rest. *Klebsiella* is one of the agents that causes sepsis neonatorum and bacteremia with fever and neutropenia. Like enteric GNB in general, *Klebsiella* rarely causes endocarditis or endovascular infection.

Diagnosis Except for *K. rhinoscleromatis* and *K. ozaenae*, klebsiellae are readily isolated and identified by the laboratory and usually ferment lactose.

℞ **TREATMENT** *K. pneumoniae* and *K. oxytoca* have similar antibiotic resistance profiles. They are intrinsically resistant to ampicillin and ticarcillin. NNIS data from 1998 indicated that 10.7% of ICU patients were infected with strains resistant to third-generation cephalosporins. This increasing degree of resistance is primarily mediated by transferable plasmids containing genes that encode ESBLs. In addition, these plasmids usually possess linked resistance determinants for aminoglycosides, tetracyclines, and TMP-SMZ. Resistance to β-lactam/β-lactamase inhibitor combinations and second-generation cephalosporins independent of ESBL-containing plasmids has also been increasingly described. In some outbreaks, ESBL-containing strains have displayed associated fluoroquinolone resistance. At this time, resistance to quinolones, cephamycins (e.g., cefoxitin), fourth-generation cephalosporins (e.g., cefepime), and amikacin is generally <10% but will probably increase. Carbapenems (e.g., imipenem) remain the most active antibiotic class against *Klebsiella*.

PROTEUS INFECTIONS *P. mirabilis* causes 90% of *Proteus* infections. These infections occur in the community, in long-term-care facilities, and in hospitals. *P. vulgaris* and *P. penneri* are isolated primarily from infections contracted in long-term-care facilities or hospitals. *Proteus* species are part of the colonic flora of a wide variety of mammals, birds, fish, and reptiles. Their ability to generate histamine from contaminated fish has implicated these GNB in the pathogenesis of scombroid (fish) poisoning (Chap. 131). *P. mirabilis* colonizes healthy humans (prevalence, 50%), but *P. vulgaris* and *P. penneri* are isolated primarily from individuals with underlying disease. The urinary tract is overwhelmingly the favored site of *Proteus* infection, in part because of unique pathogenic properties of the organisms. However, *Proteus* less commonly causes infection in a variety of extraintestinal sites.

Infectious Syndromes • UTI *P. mirabilis* causes only 1 to 2% of cases of UTI in healthy women, and *Proteus* species cause only 5% of cases of hospital-acquired UTI. However, *Proteus* is responsible for 10 to 15% of cases of complicated UTI, primarily those associated with catheterization; in the setting of long-term catheterization, their prevalence rate ranges from 20 to 45%. This high prevalence is due to the ability of *Proteus* to produce high levels of urease, which hydrolyzes urea to ammonia and results in alkalization of the urine. This situation, in turn, leads to precipitation of organic and inorganic compounds, with the formation of struvite and carbonate-apatite crystals, biofilm formation on catheters, and/or the development of calculi. *Proteus* becomes associated with the stones and usually can be eradicated only by complete stone removal. Over time, staghorn calculi may form and lead to obstruction and renal failure. Therefore, an unexplained alkaline urine should be cultured for *Proteus*, and identification of a *Proteus* species should prompt an evaluation for calculi.

Other infections Although the majority of *Proteus* infections arise from the urinary tract, these bacteria occasionally cause pneumonia (primarily in long-term-care or hospitalized patients), nosocomial sinusitis, intraabdominal abscesses, biliary tract infection, surgical site infection, soft tissue infection (especially decubitus and diabetic ulcers), and osteomyelitis (primarily contiguous); they rarely cause temperate myositis. In addition, *Proteus* occasionally causes neonatal meningitis (with the umbilicus often implicated as the source), and cerebral abscess is a common complication.

Bacteremia The majority of *Proteus* bacteremias originate from the urinary tract; however, any of the less common sites of infection are also potential sources. Infection of intravascular devices should also be considered. Endovascular infection is rare. *Proteus* species are occasional agents of sepsis neonatorum and bacteremia with fever and neutropenia.

Diagnosis *Proteus* is readily isolated and identified by the laboratory. The majority of strains are lactose negative, and most demonstrate characteristic "swarming" motility on agar plates.

℞ **TREATMENT** *P. mirabilis* remains susceptible to most antimicrobial agents except tetracycline. Resistance to ampicillin and first-generation cephalosporins has been acquired by 10 to 20% of strains. Acquisition of ESBLs remains uncommon. *P. vulgaris* and *P. penneri* are more resistant. Resistance to ampicillin and first-generation cephalosporins is the rule for these species. Derepression of an inducible chromosomal β-lactamase (not present in *P. mirabilis*) occurs in up to 30% of strains. Imipenem, fourth-generation cephalosporins (e.g., cefepime), aminoglycosides, TMP-SMZ, and quinolones have excellent activity (90 to 100%).

ENTEROBACTER INFECTIONS *E. cloacae* and *E. aerogenes* are responsible for most *Enterobacter* infections (65 to 75% and 15 to 25%, respectively); *E. agglomerans*, *E. sakazakii*, and *E. gergoviae* are less commonly isolated (5%, 1%, and <1%, respectively). These organisms cause primarily health care– or hospital-related infections. They are prevalent in foods, environmental sources (including health care facility equipment), and a wide variety of animals. Only a minority of healthy humans are colonized, but the percentage increases significantly in the setting of long-term care or hospitalization. Although colonization is an important prelude to infection, direct introduction via intravenous lines (e.g., contaminated intravenous fluids, pressure monitors) also occurs. Significant antibiotic resistance has developed in *Enterobacter* species and has contributed to their emergence as prominent nosocomial pathogens. Individuals who have received prior antibiotic treatment, who have comorbid disease, and who are patients in ICUs are at greatest risk for infection. *Enterobacter* causes a spectrum of extraintestinal infections similar to that described for other GNB in this chapter.

Infectious Syndromes Pneumonitis, UTI (particularly catheter-related), intravascular device–related infection, surgical wound/site infection, and abdominal infection (primarily postoperative or device-related—e.g., biliary stents) are the most common syndromes encountered. Nosocomial sinusitis, meningitis related to neurosurgical procedures (including use of pressure monitors), osteomyelitis, and endophthalmitis after eye surgery are less frequent. *E. sakazakii* is commonly responsible for neonatal meningitis/sepsis (particularly in premature infants), and contaminated formula has been implicated as a source of this infection. Neonatal meningitis is frequently associated with brain abscesses. Bacteremia can result from infection at any of these sites. In the setting of *Enterobacter* bacteremia, contamination of intravenous fluids, blood products, catheter-flushing fluids, pressure monitors, and dialysis equipment should always be considered, particularly with epidemic infection. *Enterobacter* can also cause bacteremia in patients with fever and neutropenia. *Enterobacter* endocarditis is rare, primarily affecting abnormal native or prosthetic valves.

Diagnosis *Enterobacter* is readily isolated and identified by the laboratory. Most strains are lactose positive.

℞ **TREATMENT** Significant antimicrobial resistance exists among *Enterobacter* strains. Ampicillin and the first- and second-generation cephalosporins have little or no activity. The extensive use of third-generation cephalosporins has resulted in the selection of strains that produce high levels of β-lactamase (i.e., derepression of β-lactamase), which confers resistance to second- and third-generation cephalosporins, monobactams (e.g., aztreonam), and (frequently) β-lactam/β-lactamase inhibitor combinations. Resistant isolates may emerge during therapy; their presence should be considered a possibility when clinical deterioration follows several days of improvement. A 34% resistance rate to third-generation cephalosporins was reported

in ICU isolates in 1998 (NNIS data). Imipenem, fourth-generation cephalosporins (e.g., cefepime), aminoglycosides (amikacin > gentamicin), TMP-SMZ, and quinolones have retained excellent activity (90 to 99%). However, increasing resistance to quinolones, in conjunction with the increased use of these agents, is a concern.

ACINETOBACTER INFECTIONS *A. baumannii* is responsible for the majority of *Acinetobacter* infections; a minority are due to *A. calcoaceticus* and *Acinetobacter* genospecies 3 and 13TU. *Acinetobacter* is highly prevalent in the environment. It is found in most water and soil samples and has a wide habitat. *Acinetobacter* has been cultured from the moist skin of healthy humans; increased colonization of the skin and the respiratory and gastrointestinal tracts occurs in individuals in long-term-care facilities and hospitals. Reservoirs for acquisition in these settings include health care personnel, medical equipment, food, and the surrounding environment. Infections in healthy people in the community are unusual, but a few reports of pneumonia have been published. The overwhelming majority of infections are acquired in the hospital and long-term-care facilities. The spectrum of extraintestinal infections caused by *Acinetobacter* is similar to that caused by other GNB. *Acinetobacter* species account for 1 to 3% of hospital-acquired infections and affect primarily immunocompromised hosts and patients with comorbid disease. ICUs are a prominent site of *Acinetobacter* infection. In some centers, the incidence of *Acinetobacter* infections, particularly those due to antibiotic-resistant strains, is increasing. Both sporadic and epidemic infection occurs, usually after the first week of hospitalization.

Infectious Syndromes The respiratory tract (particularly in ventilated patients) and intravascular devices (particularly for non–*A. baumannii* species) are the favored sites of infection. A catheterized urinary tract, postoperative sites, burn sites, biliary stents, sinuses (with tube-related ostial obstruction), and neurosurgical infections (site- or device-associated—e.g., pressure monitors) are less common. Uncommon infections include contiguous osteomyelitis, peritonitis associated with continuous ambulatory peritoneal dialysis, and ophthalmic infection. The respiratory tract and intravascular devices are the most common sources for bacteremia.

Diagnosis On Gram's stain, *Acinetobacter* organisms usually appear as short GNB or coccobacilli. They are strictly aerobic, nonfermenting, and readily isolated and identified.

℞ **TREATMENT** Many strains of *Acinetobacter* are highly resistant to antimicrobial agents. Empirical combination therapy is prudent pending susceptibility studies. Ampicillin, aztreonam, and the first- and second-generation cephalosporins possess little or no activity against these species. The activity of mezlocillin, piperacillin, quinolones, third- and fourth-generation cephalosporins, aminoglycosides, and β-lactam/β-lactamase inhibitor combinations is variable. Imipenem is presently the most active antimicrobial (>95% sensitivity), and β-lactam/sulbactam combinations are often active. Amikacin, third- and fourth-generation cephalosporins, quinolones, and combinations consisting of a β-lactam other than sulbactam plus a β-lactamase inhibitor retain significant activity in some centers, while highly resistant strains are more common in other centers.

SERRATIA INFECTIONS *S. marcescens* causes the majority of *Serratia* infections (>90%), and *S. liquefaciens* is occasionally isolated. Serratiae are found primarily in the environment, including health care institutions and particularly in moist foci. Although strains have been isolated from a variety of animals, healthy humans are rarely colonized. In long-term-care facilities or hospitals, diverse reservoirs for the organisms include the hands of health care personnel, food, sinks, respiratory and other hospital equipment, intravenous solutions, blood products (e.g., platelets), lotions, irrigation solutions, and even disinfectants. Infection results from either direct inoculation (e.g., via intravenous fluid) or colonization (primarily of the respiratory tract) and subsequent infection. Sporadic infection is most common, but occasional epidemics and common-source outbreaks occur. The spectrum of extraintestinal infections caused by *Serratia* is similar to that for other GNB. *Serratia* species account for 1 to 3% of hospital-acquired infections.

Infectious Syndromes The respiratory tract, the genitourinary tract, intravascular devices, and surgical wounds and sites are the most common sites of *Serratia* infection and sources of *Serratia* bacteremia. Soft tissue infections, including myositis, osteomyelitis, abdominal and biliary tract infection (postprocedural), contact lens–associated infection, endophthalmitis, septic arthritis (primarily with intraarticular injections), and infusion-related bacteremias occur less commonly. Serratiae are uncommon causes of neonatal or postsurgical meningitis and bacteremia associated with fever and neutropenia. Endocarditis is rare.

Diagnosis Serratiae are readily cultured and identified by the laboratory and are usually lactose negative. A minority of *S. marcescens* strains are red-pigmented.

℞ **TREATMENT** A high proportion of *Serratia* strains (>80%) are resistant to ampicillin and the first-generation cephalosporins. Significant resistance to ticarcillin, piperacillin, gentamicin, second- and third-generation cephalosporins, β-lactam/β-lactamase inhibitor combinations, and aztreonam has developed and may evolve during therapy. Imipenem, amikacin, cefepime, and quinolones are the most active agents, with >90% of strains susceptible.

***CITROBACTER* INFECTIONS** *C. freundii* and *C. koseri* (formerly *C. diversus*) cause the majority of human *Citrobacter* infections, which are similar epidemiologically and clinically to *Enterobacter* and *Acinetobacter* infections. *Citrobacter* organisms are commonly present in water, food, soil, and the intestinal tracts of animals. *Citrobacter* is part of the normal fecal flora in a minority of healthy humans, but colonization rates increase in long-term care facilities and hospitals—the settings in which nearly all infections occur. *Citrobacter* species account for 1 to 2% of nosocomial infections. The affected hosts are usually immunocompromised or have comorbid disease. *Citrobacter* causes extraintestinal infections whose spectrum is similar to that described for other GNB.

Infectious Syndromes The urinary tract is the site of 40 to 50% of infections due to *Citrobacter*. Less commonly infected sites include the biliary tree (particularly with stones or obstruction), the respiratory tract, surgical sites, soft tissue (e.g., decubitus ulcers), the peritoneum, and intravascular devices. Osteomyelitis (usually contiguous), neurosurgery-related infection, and myositis occur rarely. *Citrobacter* is also an uncommon cause of neonatal meningitis; *C. koseri* accounts for 90% of cases due to this genus. A frequent and devastating complication of this infection (occurring in 50 to 80% of cases) is the development of brain abscesses. Bacteremia is most commonly due to UTI, biliary or abdominal infection, or intravascular devices. *Citrobacter* is an uncommon cause of bacteremia in the setting of fever and neutropenia. Endocarditis or endovascular infection is rare.

Diagnosis *Citrobacter* species are readily isolated and identified, often as part of a polymicrobial culture; 35 to 50% of isolates are lactose positive.

℞ **TREATMENT** *C. freundii* is generally more resistant to antibiotics than *C. koseri*. Ampicillin and the first- and second-generation cephalosporins display poor activity against *Citrobacter*. Resistance is variable but increasing to ticarcillin, mezlocillin, piperacillin, aztreonam, quinolones, gentamicin, and third-generation cephalosporins; such resistance may evolve during therapy. The β-lactamase inhibitors usually do not improve susceptibility to β-lactam agents. Imipenem, amikacin, and the fourth-generation cephalosporins are most active, with >90% of strains sensitive.

***MORGANELLA* AND *PROVIDENCIA* INFECTIONS** *M. morganii* (formerly *Proteus morganii*), *P. stuartii*, and (to a lesser degree) *P. rettgeri* (formerly *Proteus rettgeri*) are the members of these genera that are responsible for human infections. The epidemiologic,

pathogenic, and clinical manifestations of these organisms are similar to those of *Proteus* species; however, *Morganella* and *Providencia* are almost exclusively pathogens of persons in long-term-care facilities and, to a lesser degree, hospitalized patients.

Infectious Syndromes These species are primarily urinary tract pathogens, most often associated with long-term (>30-day) catheterization. UTI in uncatheterized or short-term-catheterized individuals is uncommon. Biofilm formation or encrustation of the catheter usually develops and may lead to catheter obstruction. Likewise, infection may result in the development of struvite bladder or renal stones, which, in turn, may lead to renal obstruction and serve as foci for relapse. Other infectious syndromes occur less commonly but include surgical wound/site infections, soft tissue infection (primarily decubitus and diabetic ulcers), burn site infection, pneumonia (particularly ventilator-associated), intravascular device infection, and intraabdominal infection. Rarely, the other extraintestinal infections described for GNB also occur. Bacteremia is uncommon; although any infected site can serve as the source, the urinary tract accounts for the majority of cases, with surgical wound/site and soft tissue infections less frequently responsible.

Diagnosis *M. morganii* and *Providencia* are readily isolated and identified. Nearly all isolates are unable to ferment lactose.

℞ **TREATMENT** *Morganella* and *Providencia* may be highly resistant to antimicrobial agents. Ampicillin and the first-generation cephalosporins exhibit poor activity against these organisms. Variable resistance is emerging (and may evolve during therapy) against ticarcillin, mezlocillin, piperacillin, aztreonam, gentamicin, TMP-SMZ, and the second- and third-generation cephalosporins and quinolones. The β-lactamase inhibitor tazobactam (but not sulbactam or clavulanic acid) improves susceptibility to β-lactam agents somewhat. Imipenem, amikacin, and the fourth-generation cephalosporins are most active, with >90% of strains susceptible. Removal of an infected catheter or stones is critical for eradication of the organisms from the urinary tract.

***EDWARDSIELLA* INFECTION** *E. tarda* is the only member of this genus associated with human disease. This organism is found predominantly in both freshwater and marine environments and in the animals that live in these environments. Human acquisition occurs primarily during interaction with these reservoirs. *E. tarda* infection is rare in the United States; most recently reported cases are from Southeast Asia. This pathogen shares some of the clinical features of both *Salmonella* species and *Vibrio vulnificus*.

Infectious Syndromes Gastroenteritis is the predominant infectious syndrome reported (50 to 80% of infections). Self-limiting watery diarrhea is most frequent; however, cases of severe colitis responding to therapy have also been described. The most common extraintestinal infection is wound infection due to direct inoculation, which is often associated with freshwater, marine, or snake-related injuries. Other infectious syndromes appear to be due to invasion of the gastrointestinal tract and subsequent bacteremia. The majority of afflicted hosts have either liver disease or an iron-overload state (e.g., sickle cell disease). A primary bacteremic syndrome, sometimes complicated by meningitis, has been described and has a 40% case-fatality rate. Visceral (primarily hepatic) or intraperitoneal abscesses have also been reported.

Diagnosis Although *E. tarda* can readily be isolated and identified, most laboratories do not routinely identify it from stool.

℞ **TREATMENT** *E. tarda* is sensitive to most GNB-appropriate antimicrobial agents. Gastroenteritis is generally self-limiting, but treatment with TMP-SMZ or a quinolone may expedite its resolution. In the setting of overwhelming sepsis, quinolones, third- or fourth-generation cephalosporins, imipenem, and aminoglycosides—alone or in combination—are the safest choices pending susceptibility information.

INFECTIONS CAUSED BY MISCELLANEOUS GENERA Species from genera of GNB such as *Hafnia, Kluyvera, Cedecea, Pantoea,* and *Ewingella* are occasionally isolated from a variety of clinical specimens, including blood, sputum, cerebrospinal fluid, joint fluid, biliary drainage, wounds, and sputum. Although their role in disease has not always been defined, these strains appear to be rare and usually opportunistic human pathogens. The primary medical literature should be consulted for details on their potential role as infectious agents.

BIBLIOGRAPHY

BERGOGNE-BEREZIN E, TOWNER KJ: *Acinetobacter* spp. as nosocomial pathogens: Microbiological, clinical, and epidemiological features. Clin Microbiol Rev 9:148, 1996

GRANSDEN WR et al: Bacteremia due to *Escherichia coli*: A study of 861 episodes. Rev Infect Dis 12:1008, 1990

HEJAZI A, FALKINER FR: *Serratia marcescens*. J Med Microbiol 46:903, 1997

HUSNI RN et al: Risk factors for an outbreak of multi-drug-resistant *Acinetobacter* nosocomial pneumonia among intubated patients. Chest 115:1378, 1999

JANDA JM, ABBOTT SL: Infections associated with the genus *Edwardsiella*: The role of *Edwardsiella tarda* in human disease. Clin Infect Dis 17:742, 1993

NATARO JP, KAPER JB: Diarrheagenic *Escherichia coli*. Clin Microbiol Rev 11:142, 1998 [erratum appears in Clin Microbiol Rev 11:403, 1998]

PODSCHUN R, ULLMANN U: *Klebsiella* spp. as nosocomial pathogens: Epidemiology, taxonomy, typing methods, and pathogenicity factors. Clin Microbiol Rev 11:589, 1998

SANDERS WE JR, SANDERS CC: *Enterobacter* spp.: Pathogens poised to flourish at the turn of the century. Clin Microbiol Rev 10:220, 1997

SHIH CC et al: Bacteremia due to *Citrobacter* species: Significance of primary intraabdominal infection. Clin Infect Dis 23:543, 1996

STAMM WE: Catheter-associated urinary tract infections: Epidemiology, pathogenesis, and prevention. Am J Med 91:65S, 1991

VILLERS D et al: Nosocomial *Acinetobacter baumannii* infections: Microbiological and clinical epidemiology. Ann Intern Med 129:182, 1998

WATANAKUNAKORN C, PERNI SC: *Proteus mirabilis* bacteremia: A review of 176 cases during 1980–1992. Scand J Infect Dis 26:361, 1994

WOODS TD, WATANAKUNAKORN C: Bacteremia due to *Providencia stuartii*: Review of 49 episodes. South Med J 89:221, 1996

154

John C. Atherton, Martin J. Blaser

HELICOBACTER PYLORI INFECTIONS

DEFINITION *Helicobacter pylori* colonizes the human stomach and is of etiologic importance in peptic ulcer disease and gastric malignancy. Other gastric *Helicobacter* species colonize animals, some with a narrow range and others with a broad range of host species specificity. Those with broad specificity are occasionally found in humans, possibly as zoonoses. It is unclear whether *Helicobacter heilmanii* (formerly known as *Gastrospirillum hominis*), the most common of these species among isolates from humans, is associated with human disease. Numerous species of nongastric helicobacters are found in animals, and some have been isolated from human stool and gall bladder; whether these species cause disease is unknown.

ETIOLOGIC AGENT *H. pylori* is a gram-negative, spiral, flagellate bacillus that naturally colonizes humans and monkeys. It is noninvasive, living in gastric mucus; a small proportion of the bacterial cells are adherent to the mucosa. Its spiral shape and flagellae render *H. pylori* motile in the mucous environment, and its efficient urease protects it against acid by catalyzing urea hydrolysis to produce buffering ammonia. In vitro, *H. pylori* is microaerophilic and slow-growing and requires complex growth media. In 1997, the complete genomic sequence of *H. pylori* was published, and this information has greatly advanced the understanding of metabolic pathways and other aspects of the organism's biology. *H. heilmanii* is a longer, more tightly coiled spiral than *H. pylori* and cannot easily be cultured in vitro at present.

EPIDEMIOLOGY The prevalence of *H. pylori* colonization is about 30% in the United States and other developed countries as opposed to >80% in most developing countries. In the United States, prevalence varies with age; around 50% of 60-year-old persons as opposed to 25% of 30-year-old persons are colonized. Spontaneous acquisition or loss of the bacterium in adulthood is uncommon. *H. pylori* is usually acquired in childhood. (The age association is mostly due to a birth-cohort effect.) Other than age, the main risk factor for colonization is low socioeconomic status; crowding and low family income in childhood are especially strong correlates of colonization.

Humans are the only important reservoir of *H. pylori*. Members of a family may carry the same strain, and colonization is particularly common in childhood institutions. These findings imply direct person-to-person spread, but whether transmission takes place by the fecal-oral or oral-oral route is unknown. *H. pylori* DNA has been found in water sources, and indirect epidemiological evidence indicates that contaminated water may lead to human colonization in developing countries. Much research is focused on determining which of these possible routes of acquisition is most important.

CLINICAL MANIFESTATIONS Essentially all *H. pylori*–colonized persons have gastric inflammation, but this condition in itself is asymptomatic (Fig. 154-1). Symptoms are due to illnesses such as peptic ulceration or gastric malignancy, which develop in fewer than 10% of individuals colonized with *H. pylori*. More than 80% of peptic ulcers are related to *H. pylori* colonization, most of the remainder being due to damage caused by aspirin or nonsteroidal anti-inflammatory drugs (NSAIDs). The main lines of evidence for an ulcer-promoting role of *H. pylori* are (1) that the presence of the organism is a risk factor for the development of ulcers, (2) that (non-NSAID-induced) ulcers rarely develop in the absence of *H. pylori*, (3) that eradication of *H. pylori* results in a dramatic drop in the rate of ulcer relapse (from about 80% to 15% in the first year), and (4) that experimental infection of gerbils and mice causes gastroduodenal injury.

Prospective case-control studies have shown that *H. pylori* colonization is a risk factor for adenocarcinomas of the stomach (other than those arising in the gastric cardia). However, persons who have had documented duodenal ulcers are less likely than other persons to develop gastric adenocarcinoma later in life; the implication is that, whereas *H. pylori* colonization increases risk for both duodenal ulcerogenesis and gastric carcinogenesis, other factors determine which disease path is taken. The presence of *H. pylori* is strongly associated with gastric lymphoma. Low-grade B-cell mucosa-associated lymphoid tissue (MALT) lymphomas, which are antigen driven, often regress following *H. pylori* eradication. Whether all such diagnosed cases represent true malignancies remains to be determined.

Most *H. pylori* colonization is asymptomatic. Whether colonization occasionally causes symptoms (nonulcer dyspepsia) in the absence of ulcers or malignancy is controversial. Some but not all trials of *H. pylori* eradication in nonulcer dyspepsia have shown a reduction of symptoms in a small proportion of patients. As there is no prospective method for identifying this small group, eradication of *H. pylori* in patients with nonulcer dyspepsia is not currently indicated.

Much interest has focused on a possible protective role for *H. pylori* in gastroesophageal reflux disease (GERD) and adenocarcinoma of the esophagus and gastric cardia. The main lines of evidence for this role are that (1) there is a temporal relationship between a falling prevalence of *H. pylori* colonization and a rising incidence of these conditions; (2) in most studies, the prevalence of *H. pylori* colonization, especially with *cagA*+ strains, is lower among patients with these esophageal diseases than among control subjects; and (3) eradication of *H. pylori* often leads to the development or worsening of GERD or its symptoms. Although there are plausible mechanisms for a protective effect of *H. pylori* against these diseases, none has yet been definitively identified. Thus a causal link remains probable but unproven.

Several extra-gastrointestinal pathologies have been linked epidemiologically with *H. pylori* colonization. The most notable are ischemic heart disease and cerebrovascular disease. The associations have been found more commonly in small than in large studies, and most authorities consider them to be noncausal and due to confounding factors.

PATHOLOGY AND PATHOGENESIS *H. pylori* colonization induces chronic superficial gastritis, which includes both mononuclear and polymorphonuclear cell infiltration of the mucosa. (The term *gastritis* should be used specifically to describe histologic features; it also has been used to describe endoscopic appearances and even symptoms, neither of which have been linked to microscopic findings or to the presence of *H. pylori*.) The immune response to *H. pylori* includes both the production of antibody (local and systemic) and a cell-mediated response but is ineffective in clearing the bacterium. *H. pylori* and associated inflammation are most evident in the stomach but are also found in areas of gastric metaplasia and heterotopia (e.g., the duodenal bulb).The pattern of gastric inflammation is associated with disease risk: antral-predominant gastritis is most closely linked with duodenal ulceration and is common in the United States and other developed countries, whereas the predominant form in developing countries is pangastritis, which is epidemiologically linked with gastric ulceration and adenocarcinoma. Longitudinal analyses of gastric biopsy specimens taken years apart from the same patient show that inflammation may progress to atrophy, intestinal metaplasia, and dysplasia and then (by implication) to carcinoma. Patients with atrophic gastritis are at risk for vitamin B_{12} deficiency and its associated hematologic and neurologic sequelae. Continuous omeprazole therapy (for example, for GERD) may speed progression to atrophy when *H. pylori* is present.

Most *H. pylori*–colonized persons do not develop clinical sequelae. That some persons develop overt disease whereas others do not is probably due to a combination of bacterial strain differences, host susceptibility to disease, and environmental factors; of these, bacterial factors are best studied.

The two major disease-associated *H. pylori* virulence factors described so far are a vacuolating cytotoxin, VacA, and a group of genes termed the *cag* pathogenicity island (*cag* PaI). VacA occurs in several forms, and its level of production varies between strains; thus, although all strains have the gene (*vacA*) encoding the protein, not all exhibit vacuolating activity in vitro. Cytotoxic strains are more commonly isolated from patients with peptic ulcer disease than from persons without ulcers. The *cag* PaI includes genes that confer enhanced virulence on *H. pylori* strains, at least partly by inducing epithelial cells to produce proinflammatory cytokines. The gene *cagA*, an imperfect marker for the *cag* PaI, is useful for epidemiologic studies because it encodes a highly immunogenic protein, CagA. Patients with peptic ulcers or gastric adenocarcinoma are more likely to have CagA antibodies than persons without these conditions. However, patients with esophageal dysplasia or adenocarcinoma or with the premalignant condition Barrett's esophagus are less likely to harbor *cagA*⁺ strains than are *H. pylori*–positive controls. Thus, eradication of *cagA*⁺ strains from asymptomatic persons to prevent disease is not recommended.

How does gastric *H. pylori* colonization increase risk for duodenal ulceration? One explanation is that antral *H. pylori* colonization diminishes the number of somatostatin-producing cells; somatostatin-mediated inhibition of gastrin release leads to hypergastrinemia. Individuals with antral-predominant gastritis (and thus a normally functioning acid-producing gastric corpus) develop increased acid secretion, which may increase the risk of duodenal ulceration per se or may induce gastric metaplasia in the duodenum, which becomes col-

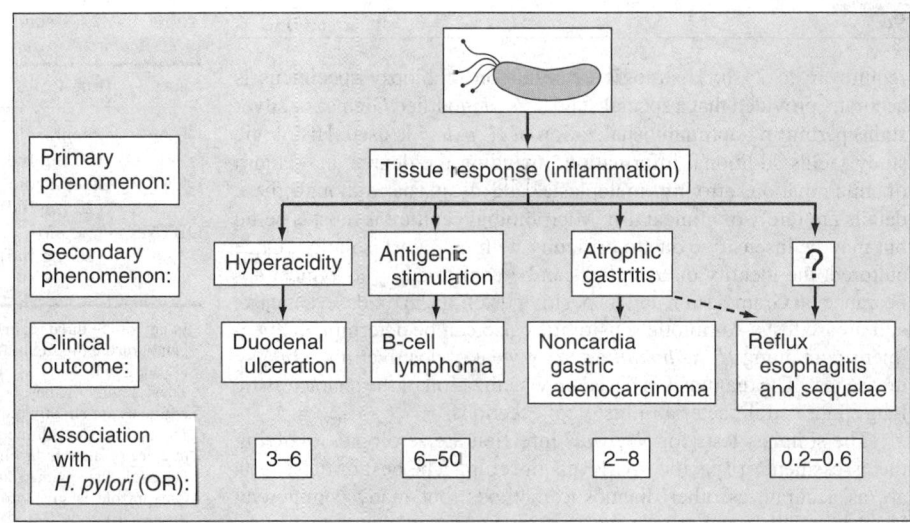

FIGURE 154-1 Schematic of the relationships between colonization with *Helicobacter pylori* and diseases of the upper gastrointestinal tract among persons in developed countries. Essentially all persons colonized with *H. pylori* develop a host response, which is generally termed *chronic gastritis*. The nature of the interaction of the host with the particular bacterial population determines the clinical outcome. *H. pylori* colonization increases the lifetime risk of peptic ulcer disease, noncardia gastric cancer, and B-cell non-Hodgkin's gastric lymphoma [odds ratios (ORs) for all, >1]. In contrast, a growing body of evidence indicates that *H. pylori* colonization protects against adenocarcinoma of the esophagus (and the related gastric cardia) and premalignant lesions such as Barrett's esophagus (OR, <1). While the incidences of peptic ulcer disease (cases not due to nonsteroidal anti-inflammatory drugs) and noncardia gastric cancer are declining in developed countries, the incidence of adenocarcinoma of the esophagus is rapidly increasing. *(Adapted from Blaser 1999, with permission.)*

onized by *H. pylori*, then inflamed, and finally ulcerated. After eradication of *H. pylori* from patients with duodenal ulcer disease, the level of acid secretion often falls.

DIAGNOSIS Tests for *H. pylori* can be divided into two groups: invasive tests, which require upper gastrointestinal endoscopy and are based on the analysis of gastric biopsy specimens, and noninvasive tests (Table 154-1). Invasive tests are preferred for (1) the initial management of dyspeptic patients, because the decision of whether or not to eradicate *H. pylori* depends on ulcer disease status, and (2) follow-up after treatment of patients with gastric ulceration to be certain that the ulcer was not malignant. Follow-up endoscopy should be performed at least 4 weeks after cessation of all anti-*Helicobacter* drugs, since at earlier points the *H. pylori* load may be low and tests may be falsely negative. The most convenient endoscopy-based test is the biopsy urease test, in which two antral biopsy specimens are put into a gel containing urea and an indicator. The presence of *H. pylori* urease elicits a color change, which often takes place within minutes but can

Table 154-1 Commonly Used Tests to Detect *Helicobacter pylori* Infection

Test	Advantages	Disadvantages
INVASIVE (ENDOSCOPIC BIOPSY–BASED)		
Biopsy urease test	Quick, simple	Rapid test not fully sensitive, 24-h test not fully specific
Histology	Widely available; may give additional histologic information	Sensitivity dependent on experience
Culture	Permits determination of antibiotic susceptibilities	Sensitivity dependent on experience
NONINVASIVE		
Serology	Cheap and convenient	Cannot be used for early follow-up
¹³C or ¹⁴C urea breath test	Safer and cheaper than endoscopy	Low-dose irradiation in ¹⁴C test

require up to 24 h. Histologic examination of biopsy specimens is accurate, provided that a special stain (e.g., a modified Giemsa or silver stain) permitting optimal visualization of *H. pylori* is used. Histologic study yields additional information, including the degree and pattern of inflammation, atrophy, metaplasia, and dysplasia, although these details are rarely of clinical use. Microbiologic culture is most specific but may be insensitive due to difficulty with *H. pylori* isolation. Once cultured, the identity of *H. pylori* can be confirmed by its typical appearance on Gram's stain and its positive reactions in oxidase, catalase, and urease tests. Antibiotic sensitivities also can be determined. Specimens containing *H. heilmanii* are only weakly positive in the biopsy urease test. The diagnosis is based on visualization of the characteristic long, tight spiral bacteria in histologic sections.

The simplest tests for *H. pylori* infection are serologic, involving the assessment of specific IgG levels in serum. The best of these tests are as accurate as other diagnostic methods, but many commercial tests, especially rapid office tests, perform poorly. In quantitative tests, a defined drop in antibody titer between matched serum samples taken before and 6 months after treatment (no sooner because of the slow decline in antibody titer) accurately indicates that *H. pylori* infection has been eradicated. The other major noninvasive tests are the ^{13}C and ^{14}C urea breath tests. In these simple tests, the patient drinks a labeled urea solution and then blows into a tube. The urea is labeled with either the nonradioactive isotope ^{13}C or a minute dose of the radioactive isotope ^{14}C (which exposes the patient to less radiation than a standard chest x-ray). If *H. pylori* urease is present, the urea is hydrolyzed and labeled carbon dioxide is detected in breath samples. Unlike serologic tests, urea breath tests can be used to assess the outcome of treatment 1 month after its completion and thus may replace endoscopy for this purpose in the follow-up of duodenal ulcer patients. As for endoscopic tests, all anti-*Helicobacter* drugs should be avoided in this period or the test may be falsely negative.

℞ **TREATMENT** At present, the only clear indications for treatment are *H. pylori*–related duodenal and gastric ulceration and the rare low-grade B-cell MALT lymphoma. *H. pylori* should be eradicated in patients with documented ulcer disease, whether or not the ulcers are currently active, to reduce the likelihood of relapse. At present, treatment is not recommended for nonulcer dyspepsia or for prophylaxis against ulcers or gastric adenocarcinoma (although it may be reasonable to eradicate *H. pylori* in persons with a strong family history of gastric cancer). Reasons for avoiding treatment for these other potential indications include the expense, the induction of morbidity in otherwise healthy people, the risk of inducing widespread antibiotic resistance in *H. pylori* and in other colonizing bacteria, and the risk of inducing or worsening GERD.

H. pylori is susceptible to a wide range of antibiotics in vitro, but monotherapy has been disappointing in vivo, probably because of inadequate antibiotic delivery to the full locus of colonization. Failure of monotherapy has led to the development of multidrug regimens, the most successful of which are triple and quadruple combinations that achieve *H. pylori* eradication rates of >90% in many trials and >75% in clinical practice. Current 7- to 14-day drug regimens consisting of a proton pump inhibitor and two or three antimicrobial agents often require only twice-daily dosing (Table 154-2).

The two most important goals in *H. pylori* eradication are to obtain the patient's compliance with the dosing regimen and to use drugs to which *H. pylori* has not acquired resistance. Treatment failure following minor lapses in compliance is common and often leads to acquired resistance to metronidazole or clarithromycin. To stress the importance of compliance, written instructions should be given to the patient, and minor side effects of the regimen should be explained. Resistance to metronidazole and clarithromycin is of growing concern; however, in multidrug regimens, the clinical significance of single-drug resistance is diminished. Assessment of antibiotic susceptibilities before treatment would be optimal but is not usually undertaken. In the absence

Table 154-2 Recommended 7- to 14-Day Regimens for the Eradication of *Helicobacter pylori*

Name	Drug 1[a]	Drug 2	Drug 3	Drug 4
OCA[b]	Omeprazole (20 mg bid)	Clarithromycin (500 mg bid)	Amoxicillin (1 g bid)	—
OCM[b]	Omeprazole (20 mg bid)	Clarithromycin (250 mg bid)	Metronidazole[c] (500 mg bid)	—
OBTM[d]	Omeprazole (20 mg bid)	Bismuth subsalicylate (2 tabs qid)	Tetracycline HCl (500 mg qid)	Metronidazole[c] (500 mg tid)

[a] In any of the three regimens, omeprazole may be replaced by lansoprazole (30 mg bid), pantoprazole (40 mg bid), ranitidine bismuth citrate (400 mg bid), or possibly ranitidine (150 mg bid). Most available data are for omeprazole.

[b] These regimens may be given for 7 to 14 days; meta-analysis suggests that 14-day regimens are slightly more effective.

[c] The optimal dose of metronidazole is not known. Tinidazole (500 mg bid) can be used in place of metronidazole.

[d] Data for this regimen are mainly from Europe and are based on bismuth subcitrate. Omeprazole is given for 10 days, and the other three agents are given on days 4 through 10.

of susceptibility information, a history of antibiotic use should be obtained, and, if resistance is likely, metronidazole-containing regimens should be avoided. Metronidazole resistance is common among persons who have taken the agent previously, even years earlier, for other conditions such as giardiasis or trichomoniasis. If initial *H. pylori* treatment fails, compliance should be checked and re-treatment should be based on known antibiotic susceptibilities. When this information cannot be obtained, the recommended course is quadruple therapy without clarithromycin (if a clarithromycin-containing regimen was given first) or triple therapy with omeprazole/clarithromycin/amoxicillin (if clarithromycin has not been used) (Table 154-2).

Given the high efficacy of treatment regimens, it is unclear whether the success of attempted *H. pylori* eradication should be checked. For gastric ulceration, the opportunity to retest for *H. pylori* is present at the repeat endoscopy, which is performed to evaluate healing. For duodenal ulceration, although many clinicians prefer to retest only if symptoms recur, a urea breath test or endoscopy should be performed no sooner than 1 month after treatment. This test will provide reassurance if treatment has been successful and will prompt re-treatment in cases of persistence.

Clearance of *H. heilmanii* has been described following the use of bismuth compounds alone or triple-therapy regimens. However, in the absence of trials, it is unclear whether this result represents successful treatment or natural clearance of the bacterium.

PREVENTION Carriage of *H. pylori* has public health significance in developing countries, where gastric adenocarcinoma is a common cause of cancer death. However, *H. pylori* has co-evolved with its human host over millennia, and there may be disadvantages in preventing or eliminating colonization. For example, as has been mentioned, the absence of *H. pylori* appears to increase the risk of developing GERD and esophageal adenocarcinoma. If mass prevention were contemplated, vaccination would be preferred, and experimental immunization of animals has given promising results. However, in the United States and other developed countries, the incidences of *H. pylori* carriage, peptic ulceration, and gastric adenocarcinoma are dropping. Thus, prevention of colonization in these countries may be unnecessary or even unwise.

BIBLIOGRAPHY

ATHERTON JC: *H. pylori* virulence factors. Br Med Bull 54:105, 1998

BLASER MJ: The changing relationships of *Helicobacter pylori* and humans: Implications for health and disease. J Infect Dis 179:1523, 1999

HANSSON L-E et al: The risk of stomach cancer in patients with gastric or duodenal ulcer disease. N Engl J Med 335:242, 1996

KUIPERS E et al: Atrophic gastritis and *Helicobacter pylori* infection in patients with reflux esophagitis treated with omeprazole or fundoplication. N Engl J Med 334:1018, 1996

MARSHALL BJ, WARREN JR: Unidentified curved bacilli in the stomach of patients with gastritis and peptic ulceration. Lancet 1:1311, 1984

NIH CONSENSUS DEVELOPMENT PANEL: *Helicobacter pylori* and peptic ulcer disease. JAMA 272:65, 1994

NOMURA A et al: *Helicobacter pylori* infection and gastric carcinoma in a population of Japanese-Americans in Hawaii. N Engl J Med 325:1132, 1991

PARSONNET J et al: *Helicobacter pylori* infection and gastric lymphoma. N Engl J Med 330:1267, 1994

TOMB JF et al: The complete genome sequence of the gastric pathogen *Helicobacter pylori*. Nature 338:539, 1997

ZUCCA E et al:Molecular analysis of the progression from *Helicobacter pylori*–associated chronic gastritis to mucosa-associated lymphoid-tissue lymphoma of the stomach. N Engl J Med 328:804, 1998

155

Christopher A. Ohl, Matthew Pollack

INFECTIONS DUE TO *PSEUDOMONAS* SPECIES AND RELATED ORGANISMS

Pseudomonas species and phylogenetically related bacteria are ubiquitous, free-living, opportunistic gram-negative pathogens. *P. aeruginosa*, the most common human pathogen in this group, is the primary subject of this chapter. Also discussed are two pathogens of increasing importance: *Burkholderia cepacia* (formerly *P. cepacia*), primarily an opportunistic pathogen, and *Stenotrophomonas maltophilia* (formerly *Xanthomonas maltophilia*), which principally infects hospitalized patients. In addition, melioidosis, a tropical systemic disease with acute and chronic manifestations caused by *B. pseudomallei* (formerly *P. pseudomallei*), will be considered.

INFECTIONS DUE TO *P. AERUGINOSA*

P. aeruginosa is a small, nonsporulating, aerobic gram-negative rod belonging to the family Pseudomonadaceae. It is motile by virtue of its single polar flagellum. More than half of all clinical isolates produce the blue-green pigment pyocyanin; this pigment is helpful in the identification of the organism and accounts for the species name *aeruginosa*, which refers to the distinctive color of copper oxide.

EPIDEMIOLOGY   *P. aeruginosa* is widespread in nature, inhabiting soil, water, plants, and animals (including humans). It has a predilection for moist environments. This organism occasionally colonizes the skin, external ear, upper respiratory tract, or large bowel of healthy humans. Rates of carriage are relatively low, however, except among patients who have serious underlying disease, whose host defenses have been naturally or iatrogenically compromised, who have previously received antibiotic therapy, and/or who have been exposed to the hospital environment. Under these circumstances, colonization with *P. aeruginosa* frequently precedes infection, and factors that predispose to the former also increase the likelihood of the latter.

Most *P. aeruginosa* infections are acquired in the hospital, where intensive care units account for the highest rates of infection. According to the National Nosocomial Infections Surveillance (NNIS) system, between 1992 and 1999, *P. aeruginosa* was the second most common cause of pneumonia, the fourth most common cause of urinary tract infection, and the sixth most frequent bloodstream isolate in intensive care units. Many potential reservoirs of infection have been identified in the hospital environment, including respiratory equipment, cleaning solutions, disinfectants, sinks, vegetables, flowers, endoscopes, and physiotherapy pools. Most reservoirs are associated with moisture. It is assumed that the organism is transmitted to patients via the hands of hospital personnel or via fomites. While some infecting strains of *P. aeruginosa* appear to be endemic within the hospital, others are traced to a common source associated with a specific outbreak or epidemic. Epidemiologic investigation is facilitated by serotyping (immunotyping) of strains on the basis of differences in lipopolysaccharide (LPS) structure and by the use of molecular techniques such as pulsed-field gel electrophoresis.

PATHOGENESIS   That the pathogenesis of infections due to *P. aeruginosa* is complex is evidenced by the clinical diversity of the diseases related to this organism and by the multiplicity of virulence factors it produces. *P. aeruginosa* rarely causes disease in the healthy host. Relative risk for infection is greatly increased, however, when normal cutaneous or mucosal barriers have been breached or bypassed, when immunologic defense mechanisms have been compromised, or when the protective function of the normal bacterial flora has been disrupted (Table 155-1). The ubiquity of the organism, its flexible nutritional and metabolic requirements, its environmental resiliency, and its relative resistance to antibiotics help account for the frequency and success with which it acts as an opportunistic pathogen.

Infections caused by *P. aeruginosa* usually begin with bacterial attachment and superficial colonization of cutaneous or mucosal surfaces and progress to localized bacterial invasion and damage to underlying tissues. The infection may remain anatomically localized or may spread by direct extension to contiguous structures. This process may continue with bloodstream invasion, dissemination, the systemic inflammatory-response syndrome (SIRS), multiple-organ dysfunction, and ultimately death. Not only is local infection more likely to occur in immunocompromised hosts, such as those with profound neutropenia, but it is more likely to culminate in bloodstream invasion and dissemination. LPS (endotoxin), which is a structural component of the bacterial outer membrane, is thought to play a pivotal role in the pathogenesis of the sepsis syndrome or SIRS.

The initial attachment of *P. aeruginosa* to the respiratory epithelium and other epithelial surfaces appears to be mediated by bacterial organelles called *pili* or *fimbriae* and facilitated by *alginate*, a mucoid exopolysaccharide produced by most strains of the bacterium under appropriate environmental conditions. Alginate plays an important role in colonization and infection of the respiratory tract in patients with cystic fibrosis and in the formation of biofilms within which sessile colonies of *P. aeruginosa* enjoy relative protection from host defenses and antimicrobial agents.

P. aeruginosa produces a number of extracellular virulence factors, including alkaline protease, elastase, phospholipase, cytotoxin, and exoenzymes (or exotoxins) A and S. The breakdown of host tissues by these bacterial products creates conditions conducive to enhanced bacterial proliferation, invasion, and tissue injury. Production and secretion of many of these extracellular virulence factors are under the regulatory control of a cell-to-cell signaling system that has been termed *quorum sensing*. Through lactones and other signal molecules secreted by individual *P. aeruginosa* bacteria, the entire bacterial population is able to sense its environment, communicate, and discern its own cell density. This regulatory system conceivably allows *P. aeruginosa* to produce extracellular virulence factors in a coordinated

Table 155-1   Factors Associated with *Pseudomonas aeruginosa* Infections

Disruption of cutaneous or mucosal barriers	Immunosuppression
Burn injury	Neutropenia
Dermatitis	Qualitative white blood cell defects
Penetrating trauma	Hypogammaglobulinemia
Surgery	Defective cell-mediated immunity
Endotracheal intubation	Extremes of age
Indwelling central venous catheterization	Diabetes mellitus
Urinary bladder catheterization	Steroid therapy
Injection drug use	Cystic fibrosis
Disruption of normal bacterial flora	Cancer
Broad-spectrum antibiotic therapy	AIDS
Exposure to the hospital environment	

manner dependent on cell density and may give the pathogen an appreciable advantage over host defense mechanisms.

The extracellular enzyme exotoxin A—a diphtheria-like toxin—is produced by most clinical isolates of *P. aeruginosa*. Exotoxin A inhibits mammalian protein synthesis by transferring the adenosine diphosphate (ADP) ribose moiety of the nicotinamide adenine dinucleotide into covalent linkage with elongation factor 2, inactivating this factor's ability to catalyze the elongation step in polypeptide assembly. Another extracellular cytotoxin, exoenzyme S, is also an adenosine diphosphate ribosyltransferase but, unlike exotoxin A, preferentially ribosylates guanosine triphosphate–binding proteins, resulting in disruption of host cell actin cytoskeletons. Exoenzyme S is one of several extracellular virulence factors of *P. aeruginosa* that is directly introduced from the bacterial cytosol into the host cell cytoplasm via a complex array of transmembrane proteins termed the *type III secretion apparatus*. This process requires direct cell contact and allows the injection of virulence factors from the bacterium into host cells without interference from humoral immune defenses.

CLINICAL MANIFESTATIONS AND DIAGNOSIS Respiratory Tract Infections

Primary pneumonia, or *nonbacteremic pneumonia*, results from aspiration of upper respiratory tract secretions; often develops in patients with chronic lung disease, congestive heart failure, or AIDS; and is most common in an intensive care setting in association with mechanical ventilator use. Fever, chills, severe dyspnea, cyanosis, productive cough, apprehension, confusion, and other signs of severe systemic toxicity characterize this acute, often life-threatening infection. Chest roentgenograms typically show bilateral bronchopneumonia with nodular infiltrates and small areas of radiolucency; pleural effusions are common; empyema is relatively uncommon; and lobar consolidation is occasionally seen. Cavitary lesions are particularly common in AIDS patients with *P. aeruginosa* pneumonia. Pathologic lesions include alveolar necrosis, focal hemorrhages, and microabscesses.

Bacteremic pneumonia due to *P. aeruginosa* begins as a respiratory infection but, in contrast to primary pneumonia, is typically associated with neutropenia, subsequent bloodstream invasion, and metastatic spread that produces characteristic lesions in the lungs and other viscera. Alveolar hemorrhage and necrosis are common. The signs and symptoms of this fulminant disease include those described for nonbacteremic pneumonia caused by this organism as well as those associated with gram-negative sepsis. Chest roentgenograms characteristically demonstrate a rapid progression from pulmonary vascular congestion to interstitial edema, then to pulmonary edema, and finally to diffuse necrotizing bronchopneumonia with cavity formation. The patient typically dies 3 or 4 days after initial presentation.

Chronic infection of the lower respiratory tract with *P. aeruginosa* is caused almost exclusively by mucoid strains, which produce alginate. Such infection is prevalent among older children and young adults with cystic fibrosis and also develops in some patients with AIDS. In patients with cystic fibrosis, mucoid strains invariably colonize and infect patients with increasing prevalence over time, contributing to the acute exacerbations and chronic progression that characterize pulmonary disease in these individuals. Airway obstruction appears to begin with bronchiolitis, which causes mucus plugging and predisposes to *P. aeruginosa* infection. The infection produces more mucus plugging, chronic suppuration, bronchiectasis, atelectasis, and ultimately fibrosis. This process progresses to pulmonary insufficiency, hypoxemia, and alterations in cardiopulmonary dynamics resulting in pulmonary hypertension and cor pulmonale.

Clinical manifestations of lower respiratory tract infections due to *P. aeruginosa* in patients with cystic fibrosis vary with the severity and duration of underlying lung disease, the frequency and intensity of acute episodes, and the presence of coinfecting pathogens such as *B. cepacia* (Chap. 257). Soon after colonization, patients may experience recurrent upper respiratory symptoms followed by a lingering cough. Episodes of pneumonia develop later, with persistent cough between acute episodes. Eventually, patients exhibit a chronic productive cough, wheezing, diminished appetite, weight loss, growth retardation, and decreased activity. Acute exacerbations are typically accompanied by low-grade fever and heightened respiratory symptoms. Physical signs include evidence of malnutrition, an increase in anteroposterior diameter, intercostal retractions, cyanosis, inspiratory and expiratory wheezing, rhonchi, moist rales, abdominal distention, and clubbing of the fingers and toes. Laboratory abnormalities include leukocytosis with a left shift and hypoxemia with or without hypercarbia. Tests of pulmonary function demonstrate obstructive and restrictive defects. Chest roentgenograms reveal overaeration, patchy atelectasis, peribronchial fibrosis, and patchy infiltrates associated with pneumonia. In more advanced disease, there may be evidence of severe overaeration, depressed diaphragm, further increased anteroposterior diameter, extensive peribronchial infiltration, generalized bronchiectasis, and cyst formation.

Bacteremia *P. aeruginosa* remains an important cause of life-threatening bloodstream infection in immunocompromised patients. Bacteremia is frequently iatrogenic and is usually seen in hospitalized patients with various comorbid conditions (Table 155-1). Bloodstream infection can be either primary (with no identifiable source) or secondary to a discrete focus of infection.

The clinical features of *P. aeruginosa* bacteremia are similar to those of other forms of bacteremia. Common primary sites of infection include the urinary tract, gastrointestinal tract, lungs, skin and soft tissues, and intravascular foci, including indwelling central venous catheters. Fever, tachypnea, tachycardia, and prostration are common. Disorientation, confusion, or obtundation may be evident. Hypotension can progress to refractory shock. Renal failure, adult respiratory distress syndrome, and disseminated intravascular coagulation occur as complications.

Pathognomonic skin lesions termed *ecthyma gangrenosum* develop in a relatively small minority of patients with *P. aeruginosa* bacteremia. The lesions begin as small hemorrhagic vesicles surrounded by a rim of erythema and undergo central necrosis with subsequent ulceration (**see Plate IID-57C**). They occur singly or in small numbers on the perineum, buttocks, and extremities; in the axillae; or elsewhere. Histologically, these lesions contain numerous bacteria invading blood vessels but few inflammatory cells. Bacteria are readily visible on Gram's staining and may be cultured from aspirated material.

Endocarditis *P. aeruginosa* infects native heart valves in injection drug users as well as prosthetic heart valves. The source of *P. aeruginosa* strains infecting drug users appears to be standing water contaminating drug paraphernalia. Foreign materials mixed with heroin may cause injury to valve leaflets or mural endocardium, with resulting fibrosis and an increased risk for valve infection. Exposure of the tricuspid valve to both trauma and bacteria apparently accounts for the high incidence of tricuspid involvement in association with injection drug use.

The pulmonic, mitral, or aortic valve and the mural endocardium of either atrium may be affected in *P. aeruginosa* endocarditis. Multiple-valve infections are common. Tricuspid or right-sided involvement is often associated with septic pulmonary emboli. Right-sided *P. aeruginosa* endocarditis usually presents subacutely, while the appearance of left-sided disease is likely to be more acute or even fulminant. Fever is virtually invariable, and murmurs are usually detectable at initial presentation or shortly thereafter. Septic pulmonary emboli associated with right-sided disease result in cough, pleuritic chest pain, sputum production, pulmonary infiltration (with or without abscess formation), and pleural effusion. Left-sided infections may present as intractable heart failure or large systemic emboli. Mycotic aneurysms, cerebritis, or brain abscess may occur; septic infarcts are occasionally found in the spleen. Skin and soft tissue manifestations, including Janeway lesions, Osler's nodes, and ecthyma gangrenosum, are relatively uncommon.

The diagnosis of *P. aeruginosa* endocarditis is based on positive blood culture in the absence of an extracardiac source; an indication of valvular dysfunction or vegetation on an echocardiogram; evidence of septic pulmonary lesions on a chest roentgenogram (in right-sided disease); and the actual demonstration of infected heart valves at the time of surgery.

Central Nervous System Infections   *P. aeruginosa* infections of the central nervous system include meningitis and brain abscess. These infections follow extension from a contiguous parameningeal structure such as the ear, mastoid, or paranasal sinus; direct inoculation into the subarachnoid space or brain through head trauma, surgery, or diagnostic procedures; or bacteremic spread from infection at a distant site. Like *P. aeruginosa* infections at other anatomic sites, central nervous system infections are documented almost exclusively in patients with compromised local or systemic immune-defense mechanisms.

The clinical signs of *P. aeruginosa* meningitis, like those of other forms of acute bacterial meningitis, include fever, headache, stiff neck, confusion, and obtundation. The onset of illness may be acute or even fulminant, particularly in bacteremic patients, with a precipitous downhill course, shock, coma, and early death. In nonbacteremic patients, *P. aeruginosa* meningitis or brain abscess may present more insidiously, with a paucity of systemic symptoms. This presentation is especially common in infections resulting from recent neurosurgery, cancer of the head and neck, or direct extension from a parameningeal focus of chronic infection. Occasionally, *P. aeruginosa* meningitis runs a subacute or relapsing course that is thought to be related to the intermittent release of bacteria from a loculated site of infection.

Ear Infections   *P. aeruginosa* is often found in the external auditory canal, particularly under moist conditions and in the presence of inflammation or maceration (as in "swimmer's ear"). Moreover, this organism is the predominant pathogen associated with external otitis, a usually benign inflammatory process affecting the external auditory canal. The ear is painful or merely itchy, there is a purulent discharge, and pain is elicited by pulling on the pinna. The external canal appears edematous and is filled with detritus that often prevents visualization of the tympanic membrane.

P. aeruginosa occasionally penetrates the epithelium overlying the floor of the external auditory canal at the junction between bone and cartilage and invades underlying soft tissue. The ensuing invasive process, which involves soft tissue, cartilage, and cortical bone, is typically slow but destructive. Termed *malignant external otitis*, this condition occurs predominantly in elderly diabetic patients but is reported occasionally in infants with other underlying diseases and rarely in elderly nondiabetic patients. Virtually all cases of malignant external otitis are caused by *P. aeruginosa*. From the external ear, the infection advances to the retromandibular area or parotid space and enters the mastoid air cells and temporal bone. Advancing osteomyelitis at the base of the skull often involves the seventh, ninth, tenth, and eleventh cranial nerves. The cavernous sinus can become involved, as can the contralateral petrous apex. The middle ear is commonly spared; meningitis and brain abscess are relatively rare complications.

Otorrhea and severe otalgia are common presenting symptoms of malignant external otitis. Facial-nerve paralysis tends to occur early, while other cranial-nerve palsies appear later. There may be a loss of hearing. Constitutional symptoms such as fever and weight loss are relatively uncommon. Physical examination almost always reveals remarkable tenderness of the pinna of the ear and abnormalities of the external auditory canal, including swelling, erythema, purulent discharge, debris, and granulation tissue in the canal wall. The tympanic membrane is often hidden from view and is sometimes perforated. Inflammation may involve the pinna as well as the periauricular, retromandibular, and mastoid areas.

Peripheral leukocytosis is relatively infrequent in malignant external otitis, while the erythrocyte sedimentation rate is usually markedly elevated. Cerebrospinal fluid occasionally exhibits pleocytosis and an elevation in the protein level. Computed tomography (CT) or magnetic resonance imaging (MRI) of the mastoid or temporal bone typically reveals bony erosions and new bone formation, while the floor of the skull may have soft tissue densities associated with areas of cellulitis. In addition, technetium 99m bone scans and gallium 67 scans fre-

quently give positive results. Cultures of samples from the external auditory canal and of surgical specimens are almost always positive for *P. aeruginosa*.

Eye Infections (See also Chap. 28)   *P. aeruginosa* causes bacterial keratitis or corneal ulcer and endophthalmitis in the human eye. Keratitis due to *P. aeruginosa* may result from even minor corneal injury, which interrupts the integrity of the superficial epithelial surface and permits bacterial access to the underlying stroma. Corneal ulcer may complicate contact lens use, particularly when extended-wear soft contact lenses are involved. Contact lens solutions or the lenses themselves may be the source of the organism, which is probably inoculated into the eye at sites of minor lens-induced corneal damage. Patients who have sustained serious burns, have undergone ocular irradiation or tracheostomy, have been exposed to the intensive care environment, and/or are in a coma are also susceptible to *P. aeruginosa*–associated corneal ulcers. *P. aeruginosa* keratitis usually starts as a small central ulcer; spreads concentrically to involve a large portion of the cornea, sclera, and underlying stroma; and in some cases progresses to posterior corneal perforation.

The clinical manifestations of *P. aeruginosa* keratitis include a rapidly expanding, necrotic stromal infiltrate in the bed of an epithelial injury; surrounding epithelial edema; an anterior chamber reaction; and mucopurulent discharge adherent to the ulcer's surface. Corneal ulcer due to *P. aeruginosa* may advance rapidly to involve the entire cornea in ≤2 days or may evolve subacutely over several days. Systemic symptoms are uncommon. Complications include corneal perforation, anterior chamber involvement, and endophthalmitis.

P. aeruginosa endophthalmitis is typically a rapidly progressive, sight-threatening condition that demands immediate therapeutic intervention. It may complicate penetrating injuries of the eye, intraocular surgery, hematogenous spread from other sites of *Pseudomonas* infection, or posterior perforation of corneal ulcers. Clinical manifestations may include eye pain, conjunctival hyperemia, chemosis, lid edema, decreased visual acuity, hypopyon, severe anterior uveitis, and signs of possible vitreous involvement. Panophthalmitis may result from this intraocular infection.

Bone and Joint Infections   Vertebral osteomyelitis due to *P. aeruginosa* is associated with complicated urinary tract infection, genitourinary instrumentation or surgery, and injection drug use. Vertebral infections that are associated with a urinary tract source most often develop in the elderly and usually affect the lumbosacral spine. Presumably the route of infection in these patients is a shared venous plexus between the pelvis and spine. Injection drug use–related infections typically occur in younger patients and may affect the cervical or lumbosacral spine. *P. aeruginosa* vertebral osteomyelitis is usually an indolent disease. Accordingly, symptoms may develop weeks or even months before diagnosis. Back or neck pain is generally reported, while fever and systemic symptoms are relatively uncommon. Local tenderness and decreased range of motion of the affected spine are typical. Leukocytosis may be noted, the erythrocyte sedimentation rate is almost always markedly elevated, and blood cultures are sometimes positive. Roentgenograms reveal loss of bone density, narrowed intervertebral space, destruction of vertebral end plates, lytic lesions of vertebral bodies, sclerosis, and occasionally osteophyte formation. CT and MRI are the most sensitive and specific means of defining lesions. Technetium bone scans and gallium scans usually yield positive results. An etiologic diagnosis requires the culture of material obtained by needle aspiration or biopsy of the affected spine under fluoroscopic guidance; open biopsy is sometimes needed.

Sternoclavicular pyarthrosis caused by *P. aeruginosa* is another complication of injection drug use; in some cases it is associated with *P. aeruginosa* endocarditis, but more often it is not. Joint involvement is usually monoarticular, with the sternoclavicular joint more often affected than sternochondral joints. Patients present with acute or chronic pain in the anterior chest wall, often associated with fever and restricted movement of the homolateral shoulder. Physical examination reveals tenderness, erythema, and swelling over the affected joint. Leukocytosis is common, and the erythrocyte sedimentation rate is almost invariably elevated. Roentgenograms show soft tissue edema; bone demineralization; lytic lesions; and periosteal elevation of the clavicular head, rib, or sternum. Material obtained by arthrocentesis or synovial biopsy yields *P. aeruginosa* in culture.

P. aeruginosa infections of the symphysis pubis are associated with pelvic surgery and injection drug use. The symphysis pubis, like other fibrocartilaginous joints, exhibits a peculiar susceptibility to bloodborne infection with *P. aeruginosa*. Affected patients report pain in the groin, hip, thigh, and/or lower abdomen that is made worse by walking. Fever is variable, and the duration of symptoms before diagnosis ranges from days to months. The erythrocyte sedimentation rate is markedly elevated. Roentgenography or CT shows irregularities of the pubic margins, separation of the symphysis pubis, and osteomyelitic abnormalities of the pubic rami that may be extensive. Bone scans are usually positive. Needle aspiration or biopsy is necessary to obtain material for culture. A positive culture is particularly important for the discrimination of *P. aeruginosa* infections and other pyogenic infections from osteitis pubis, which is thought to be a noninfectious condition complicating pelvic surgery, childbirth, or trauma.

P. aeruginosa osteochondritis of the foot follows puncture wounds of the foot, primarily in children. The organism infects the small joints and bones, including the proximal phalanges, metatarsals, metatarsophalangeal joints, tarsal bones, and calcaneus. On average, local pain and swelling last for several weeks, and systemic symptoms are usually lacking. There may be plantar cellulitis over the involved area or tenderness upon deep palpation. Results of roentgenograms and bone scans are generally positive. Aspiration of the affected joint frequently yields purulent material in which *P. aeruginosa* can be demonstrated by Gram's staining and by culture.

P. aeruginosa is one of the most common causative agents in a variety of other, less specific syndromes involving nonhematogenous infections of bones and joints and collectively referred to as *chronic contiguous osteomyelitis*. These infections may result, for example, from compound fractures, contamination associated with open reduction and fixation of closed fractures, sternotomy performed in conjunction with cardiac surgery, contiguous spread from infected ischemic ulcers related to peripheral vascular disease or diabetes mellitus, and cellulitis in general. The chronicity, indolence, and heterogeneity of these infections explain their varied clinical manifestations and the frequent need for complicated long-term management.

Urinary Tract Infections   *P. aeruginosa* is one of the most common causes of complicated and nosocomial infections of the urinary tract. These infections may result from urinary tract catheterization, instrumentation, surgery, or obstruction; they may arise from persistent foci (e.g., the prostate or stones) and may be chronic or recurrent. The urinary tract may be a target for bloodborne infection in patients with *P. aeruginosa* bacteremia but more often is the source of bacteremia. Chronic *P. aeruginosa* infections of the urinary tract are relatively common among patients with indwelling urinary catheters, altered urinary tract anatomy secondary to diversionary procedures, and paraplegia.

The clinical features of urinary tract infections due to *P. aeruginosa* are usually indistinguishable from those of other bacterial infections. However, *P. aeruginosa* infections exhibit a propensity for persistence, chronicity, resistance to antibiotic therapy, and recurrence. More unusual forms of urinary tract involvement peculiar to *P. aeruginosa* include (1) ulcerative lesions of the renal pelvis, ureters, and bladder that cause sloughing of vesical membranes in the urine; and (2) ecthyma-like lesions of the renal cortex that are seen in association with *Pseudomonas* sepsis.

Skin and Soft Tissue Infections   As indicated above, *P. aeruginosa* bacteremia may be associated with the disseminated skin lesions of ecthyma gangrenosum (**see Plate IID-57C**). Less common skin manifestations of *P. aeruginosa* sepsis include vesicular or pus-

tular lesions, bullae, subcutaneous nodules, deep abscesses, and cellulitis. Metastatic lesions of the skin or mucous membranes complicate *Pseudomonas* sepsis and occasionally produce massive necrosis or gangrene of the extremities, perineum, face, or oropharynx.

Primary *P. aeruginosa* pyoderma occurs when the skin breaks down secondary to trauma, burn injury, dermatitis, or ulcers related to peripheral vascular disease or pressure sores. Moist conditions and neutropenia may predispose to this condition. The clinical appearance of primary *P. aeruginosa* pyoderma, which frequently includes hemorrhage and necrosis, resembles that of metastatic *P. aeruginosa* skin lesions. Histologic studies document vascular invasion by bacteria in both diseases. A rare distinguishing feature of *P. aeruginosa* pyoderma is its association with a blue-green exudate and a characteristic fruity odor.

P. aeruginosa wound sepsis complicating extensive third-degree burn injuries is associated with an extremely high mortality rate. This infection results from colonization of the burn site or burn eschar, invasion of the subeschar space and underlying dermis, vascular invasion, and systemic spread. The development and progression of *P. aeruginosa* burn wound sepsis are facilitated by the injury-associated breakdown of normal skin, selection of empirical antibiotics with inadequate coverage for this pathogen, and burn-related immune defects. Local manifestations include black, dark brown, or violaceous discoloration of the burn eschar; degeneration of underlying granulation tissue, hemorrhage, and premature eschar separation; edema, hemorrhage, and necrosis of skin adjacent to the burn site; and erythematous nodular lesions in unburned skin. Systemic manifestations include fever or hypothermia and other signs of sepsis, SIRS, or multiple-organ system failure. The diagnosis of *P. aeruginosa* burn sepsis is based on these local and systemic clinical manifestations and on a burn wound biopsy that reveals both $>10^5$ colony-forming units of *P. aeruginosa* per gram of tissue and histologic evidence of bacterial invasion of unburned tissue, vasculitis, or intense inflammation at the burn margin.

P. aeruginosa causes diffuse pruritic maculopapular and vesiculopustular rashes associated with exposure to contaminated hot tubs, spas, whirlpools, and swimming pools. Many cases of *P. aeruginosa* dermatitis have occurred in conjunction with a common-source outbreak. At least two nosocomial common-source outbreaks—one related to a physiotherapy pool—have been reported. Skin rashes may be limited to areas covered by swimsuits or may be more diffuse, sparing only the head and neck. Low-grade fever or other associated symptoms are uncommon. The illness is usually self-limited, and the rash resolves without specific therapy after cessation of exposure.

P. aeruginosa Infections in Patients with AIDS   During the 1980s and 1990s, *P. aeruginosa* infections were increasingly associated with AIDS. The vast majority of these infections are currently seen in patients with advanced AIDS, previous opportunistic infections, and CD4+ lymphocyte counts $<100/\mu L$ (often $<50/\mu L$). The specific immunologic factors that lead to *P. aeruginosa* infections in patients with AIDS are not well understood but are speculated to be a loss of mucosal integrity, defects in cellular and humoral immunity, and qualitative leukocyte abnormalities. Of note is that the majority of *P. aeruginosa* infections in this population are community-acquired, in contrast to the nosocomial transmission documented for most *P. aeruginosa* infections in non-AIDS patients.

Pneumonia accounts for a substantial proportion of the *P. aeruginosa* infections in patients with AIDS. In most instances, pneumonia presents as a necrotizing infection of the pulmonary parenchyma, frequently with cavitary lesions, or as a chronic relapsing bronchopulmonary infection reminiscent of the bronchopulmonary disease seen in patients with cystic fibrosis. Also frequent are bloodstream infections, including those associated with indwelling central venous catheters, and infections of the paranasal sinuses, skin and soft tissue, and urinary tract. Bacteremia, either primary or secondary to infection at a remote site, is often recurrent, associated with high mortality, and occasionally accompanied by skin manifestations similar to those seen in non-AIDS patients.

Because *P. aeruginosa* infections occur in patients with advanced

AIDS, survival after recovery from the initial infection may be limited to a few months. However, with the widespread use of highly active antiretroviral therapy and the consequent increase in CD4+ cell counts, the incidence of *P. aeruginosa* infection in patients with AIDS is likely to decline and the natural history of infection to change. For example, a few patients with recalcitrant, relapsing *P. aeruginosa* bronchopulmonary infections have reportedly experienced the resolution of infection soon after initiation of intensive antiretroviral therapy.

℞ **TREATMENT** Table 155-2 lists antimicrobial agents available in the United States that are generally active against *P. aeruginosa*. Table 155-3 outlines suggested antibiotic choices and an approach to therapy for selected sites of infection. The initial antibiotic selection should take into account the local patterns of antimicrobial susceptibility, while the susceptibilities of the isolate from a particular case should guide definitive antibiotic therapy.

In most severe or life-threatening infections due to *P. aeruginosa*, two antipseudomonal antibiotics to which the infecting strain is (or is likely to be) sensitive should be administered together. The benefits of this combined therapy, as determined by in vitro studies, are to increase efficacy, to achieve additive or synergistic killing, and to prevent the emergence of antibiotic resistance. Despite widespread acceptance of combination therapy for *P. aeruginosa* infections, there are few clinical data since the advent of newer β-lactam antibiotics documenting that combination therapy is more efficacious than monotherapy or that it actually forestalls the acquisition of antimicrobial resistance. Nevertheless, combination therapy continues to be recommended for most acute or fulminant infections, as outlined in Table 155-3.

The appropriate duration of antibiotic therapy for disease caused by *P. aeruginosa* depends on the type, location, and severity of infection. In general, chronic infections associated with extensive tissue injury, disruption of normal anatomy, foreign or prosthetic material, or suboptimal antibiotic accessibility require therapy for weeks or even months rather than days. More acute infections may be treated aggressively but for shorter periods.

P. aeruginosa infections of the lower respiratory tract in cystic fibrosis pose a special challenge because of their long-standing nature. In general, antibiotic therapy for acute exacerbations results in short-term clinical improvement, while periodic expectant courses of antimicrobial therapy may limit disease progression. A more novel approach utilizing intermittent, cyclical administration of inhaled tobramycin has been shown to improve pulmonary function, decrease the risk of hospitalization, and reduce the density of *P. aeruginosa* in sputum of older patients with cystic fibrosis. Lung transplantation has also been employed with good results in selected cystic fibrosis patients with severe, progressive lower respiratory tract infections due to *P. aeruginosa*.

Table 155-2 Antimicrobials Available in the United States with Activity Against *Pseudomonas aeruginosa*

Antimicrobial	Dose[a], Route	Comments
Antipseudomonal penicillins		Class is listed in order of decreasing in vitro activity. Piperacillin/tazobactam or ticarcillin/clavulanate has no more activity against *P. aeruginosa* than piperacillin or ticarcillin alone. Monotherapy should not be used for serious infections.
Piperacillin	3–4 g q4–6h IV	
Piperacillin/tazobactam	3.375 g q4h IV	
Mezlocillin	3 g q4h IV	
Ticarcillin	3 g q3–4h IV	
Ticarcillin/clavulanate	3.1 g q4h IV	
Antipseudomonal cephalosporins		Use higher indicated doses for neutropenic or severely immunocompromised patients. Ceftazidime reaches the highest CSF levels of the antipseudomonals (use higher indicated dose). Cefepime has less potential for β-lactamase induction than ceftazidime.
Ceftazidime[b]	2 g q8–12h IV	
Cefoperazone[b]	2 g q6h IV	
Cefepime	2 g q8–12h IV	
Carbapenems[b]		Class is active against strains producing β-lactamases. Imipenem may cause seizures in patients with renal failure (avoid by reducing dose) or with CNS infections or lesions. Meropenem is slightly more active in vitro against *P. aeruginosa* than imipenem.
Imipenem/cilastatin	0.5 g q6h IV	
Meropenem	1 g q8h IV	
Monobactams		Drug can usually be administered to patients with β-lactam hypersensitivity.
Aztreonam	2 g q6–8h IV	
Aminoglycosides[b]		Tobramycin has greater in vitro activity against *P. aeruginosa* than gentamicin, but the drugs' clinical efficacies are probably equivalent. Some *P. aeruginosa* isolates that are resistant to tobramycin or gentamicin may be susceptible to amikacin. Except for UTI, this class should not be used for monotherapy. ODD may reduce adverse effects. Serum levels must be monitored for MD and ODD.
Tobramycin	MD: 2 mg/kg load, then 1.7 mg/kg q8h IV ODD: 5–7 mg/kg q24h IV Aerosolized for CF: 300 mg TOBI q12h via jet nebulizer	
Gentamicin	MD: Same as tobramycin ODD: Same as tobramycin	
Amikacin	MD: 7.5 mg/kg load, then 7.5 mg/kg q12h IV ODD: 15 mg/kg q24h IV	
Fluoroquinolones[b,c]		Of the available fluoroquinolones, ciprofloxacin is the most active against *P. aeruginosa*. Serum levels achieved with oral therapy approximate those obtained with IV therapy; thus oral dosing is useful for long-term therapy in selected patients.
Ciprofloxacin	0.4 g q12h IV 0.5–0.75 g bid PO	
Levofloxacin	0.5 g q24h IV or PO	

[a] Indicated dosages are for the treatment of *P. aeruginosa* infections in adults. Doses should be adjusted for renal insufficiency. Higher doses may be required in patients with cystic fibrosis, and lower doses may be adequate for the treatment of uncomplicated urinary tract infections.
[b] Some strains of *P. aeruginosa* may develop resistance to these agents during therapy.
[c] Trovafloxacin, an additional fluoroquinolone with antipseudomonal activity, has been associated with hepatotoxicity. Although gatifloxacin and moxifloxacin have in vitro activity against *P. aeruginosa*, there are no clinical studies to support their use in *Pseudomonas* or nosocomial infections.
NOTE: CSF, cerebrospinal fluid; CF, cystic fibrosis; MD, multidose; ODD, once-daily dosing; CNS, central nervous system; TOBI, tobramycin inhalation solution; UTI, urinary tract infection.

ANTIMICROBIAL RESISTANCE Antibiotic resistance in *P. aeruginosa* is both intrinsic, as reflected by the relative paucity of antibiotics with inherent antimicrobial activity against wild-type strains, and acquired, as defined by high-level resistance to agents that would be expected to exhibit antimicrobial activity. Acquired resistance is rapidly increasing among *P. aeruginosa* isolates, particularly those associated with cystic fibrosis and with intensive care units. Escalating resistance among intensive care unit isolates is especially

Table 155-3 Recommended Antimicrobial Therapy for Selected Infections due to *Pseudomonas aeruginosa*

Anatomic Site or Diagnosis	Preferred Therapy[a,b]	Alternative Therapy[a,b]	Comments
Bacteremia, endocarditis, wound infections, or pneumonia	Antipseudomonal penicillin *plus* aminoglycoside	Antipseudomonal penicillin *plus* ciprofloxacin (IV) *or* Antipseudomonal cephalosporin *or* aztreonam *or* carbapenem *plus* aminoglycoside *or* ciprofloxacin (IV)	*Bacteremia*: Bacteremia due to infection of an indwelling central venous catheter usually necessitates catheter removal. Monotherapy is often acceptable if the catheter is removed. *Endocarditis*: Use highest indicated doses from Table 155-2. MD is preferable to ODD for aminoglycosides. Serum aminoglycoside levels should be 10X the MBC for the isolate. Valve replacement is often required. *Wounds*: Debridement is required. *Pneumonia*: Combination therapy should be employed initially for severe pneumonia if *P. aeruginosa* is highly suspected or confirmed by culture. Repeated or prolonged therapy may be required in patients with AIDS.
Central nervous system	Ceftazidime *plus or minus* aminoglycoside	Ciprofloxacin (IV)[c] *or* aztreonam[c] *or* meropenem[c]	Aminoglycosides should be administered intrathecally for CNS infections not responding to initial IV therapy. Brain abscesses >2 cm in diameter require drainage.
Bones and joints	Antipseudomonal penicillin *plus* aminoglycoside	Antipseudomonal cephalosporin *or* aztreonam *or* fluoroquinolone *or* carbapenem[c]	A 4- to 6-week course of therapy is often suggested. Limited data suggest that prolonged therapy with an oral fluoroquinolone may be as effective as IV administration. Surgical debridement is often required for osteomyelitis that is chronic or associated with trauma, direct inoculation of bone, or extension from adjacent tissues.
Malignant external otitis	Antipseudomonal cephalosporin *or* carbapenem *or* ciprofloxacin (IV or PO)	Antipseudomonal penicillin or cephalosporin *plus* aminoglycoside	Surgical debridement is usually required. At least 4–6 weeks of therapy is suggested. Oral ciprofloxacin can be used with close follow-up for limited disease or after initial IV therapy.
Eye Keratitis and corneal ulcer	Tobramycin 14 mg/mL topical solution[d] *plus or minus* piperacillin or ticarcillin 6–12 mg/mL topical solution[d]	Ciprofloxacin *or* ofloxacin 0.3% topical solution[d]	Fortified aminoglycoside eye drops require pharmacy preparation. Systemic antibiotics are reserved for severe infections with impending perforation or extension beyond the cornea (see endophthalmitis). If combination therapy is used, the second agent should be administered at least 5 minutes after the first.
Endophthalmitis	Same as for corneal ulcer above *plus* intravitreal amikacin 0.4 mg in 0.1 mL *or* ceftazidime 2.25 mg in 0.1 mL	Same as for corneal ulcer above *plus* intravitreal amikacin 0.4 mg in 0.1 mL *or* ceftazidime 2.25 mg in 0.1 mL	Surgical vitrectomy is usually indicated. Addition of systemic therapy with ceftazidime or an antipseudomonal penicillin plus ciprofloxacin or an aminoglycoside and subconjunctival injection of an intravitreal agent may be beneficial.
Urinary tract	Ciprofloxacin (PO or IV)	Aminoglycoside *or* antipseudomonal penicillin *or* cephalosporin *or* carbapenem	Obstructions (e.g., stones) should be relieved and foreign bodies (e.g., chronic urinary catheters) removed. Monotherapy is usually sufficient.
Dermatitis or folliculitis	None	None	Diffuse folliculitis related to spas, whirlpools, or hot tubs does not require therapy in immunocompetent hosts.

[a] Susceptibility testing should be performed on all significant *Pseudomonas* isolates in order to direct definitive therapy. Empirical antibiotic therapy for suspected *Pseudomonas* infections should take into account the institution's antimicrobial susceptibility patterns.
[b] Dosages for individual agents from each antimicrobial class are listed in Table 155-2.
[c] Clinical experience is limited for treatment of this infection with this agent. Addition of a second antipseudomonal agent is advised.
[d] 1 qqts q5min for 1 h, then q15–30min for 24–48 h; frequency can then be gradually decreased.
NOTE: MD, multidose; ODD, once-daily dosing; CNS, central nervous system; MBC, minimal bactericidal concentration.

alarming. Data from the NNIS system show an increase in rates of resistance to imipenem and fluoroquinolones from 12% during previous years to 18.5% and 23.0%, respectively, during 1999. Factors responsible for this increase may include expanding use of immunosuppressive therapies, increased severity of illness in hospitalized patients, inadequate infection control procedures, and growing antibiotic use. Resistant organisms can be transmitted directly to patients from the hospital staff, other patients, or the environment, or they may arise de novo during therapy with any given agent. Emergence of multidrug-resistant strains has been associated with increases in secondary bacteremia and mortality and has led in some cases to longer hospital stays and increased hospitalization costs. Therapy for patients with resistant *P. aeruginosa* infections should consist of antimicrobial agents selected on the basis of extended susceptibility testing. Increased treatment duration and surgical drainage or removal of infected tissues may be necessary.

INFECTIONS CAUSED BY OTHER *PSEUDOMONAS* SPECIES OR RELATED BACTERIA

Burkholderia cepacia   *B. cepacia*, like *P. aeruginosa*, is primarily an opportunistic pathogen that is implicated in both sporadic endemic infections and occasional nosocomial outbreaks. Hospital epidemics are most frequently associated with a liquid reservoir or a moist environmental surface. Colonization by *B. cepacia* precedes infection, and distinction between the two is often difficult. *B. cepacia* has been reported to cause pneumonia, urinary tract infections, meningitis, peritonitis, surgical and burn wound infections, bacteremia, and endocarditis related to injection drug use. In addition, *B. cepacia* has been implicated as a cause of chronic lower respiratory tract infections in patients with chronic granulomatous disease, in patients with sickle cell hemoglobinopathies, and—together with *P. aeruginosa*—in patients with cystic fibrosis. In some patients with cystic fibrosis, the appearance of *B. cepacia* has been associated with fulminant necrotizing pneumonia, bacteremia, and a rapid downhill course.

℞ **TREATMENT** The treatment of *B. cepacia* infections is complicated by intrinsic resistance of the organism to aminoglycosides and many β-lactam agents. Although trimethoprim-sulfamethoxazole and chloramphenicol have been used successfully in the treatment of *B. cepacia* infections, resistance to these two antimicrobial agents has been reported. Carbapenems, third-generation cephalosporins, and fluoroquinolones may offer activity against sensitive strains, but relevant clinical experience is limited. Some but not all cystic fibrosis centers segregate patients infected with *B. cepacia* in an attempt to reduce horizontal transmission to uninfected patients. In addition, many centers consider lung transplantation contraindicated in these patients because of an unacceptably high mortality rate after surgery.

Stenotrophomonas maltophilia *S. maltophilia* is a ubiquitous, free-living opportunistic bacterium that has emerged as an important pathogen in hospitalized patients, particularly in cancer centers and intensive care units. Factors that lead to colonization and infection include prolonged hospitalization, malignancy, instrumentation (including urinary, peritoneal, and central venous catheterization), and prior administration of broad-spectrum antibiotics. This organism has most commonly been associated with pneumonia but also causes bacteremia, urinary tract infection, wound infection, peritonitis, cholangitis, meningitis, and (rarely) endocarditis. Acute *S. maltophilia* pneumonia—an often devastating disease associated with bacteremia—is being seen with increasing frequency in debilitated patients on intensive care units. Antibiotic resistance in *S. maltophilia*, based on both low outer-membrane permeability and inducible β-lactamases, is at least partly responsible for the emergence of this organism as a nosocomial pathogen under the selective pressure of antibiotic treatment.

℞ **TREATMENT** Trimethoprim-sulfamethoxazole (at a trimethoprim dose of 15 to 20 mg/kg per day for patients with normal renal function) is the drug of choice for treatment of most *S. maltophilia* infections. Alternative agents include ticarcillin/clavulanate, minocycline, and doxycycline. The third-generation cephalosporins cefoperazone and ceftazidime are occasionally active against *S. maltophilia*, but in vitro susceptibilities may not reflect clinical efficacy. The aminoglycosides and imipenem are almost always inactive. Indwelling catheters or appliances that are associated with infection should be removed.

Melioidosis Infections caused by *B. pseudomallei* constitute a broad spectrum of acute and chronic, local and systemic, clinical and subclinical disease processes collectively called *melioidosis*. *B. pseudomallei* and the infections it causes are found mainly in the tropics and are endemic in Southeast Asia and surrounding areas. *B. pseudomallei* is a free-living, small, motile, aerobic, gram-negative bacillary saprophyte normally found in soil, ponds, and rice paddies and on produce from endemic areas. It is occasionally a pathogen for animals. Humans contract the disease through soil contamination of abrasions, ingestion, or inhalation. In contrast to *B. cepacia*, *B. pseudomallei* does not establish colonization without causing infection and is rarely transmitted from person to person.

Melioidosis presents in different forms. High rates of seropositivity in endemic areas such as Vietnam, Thailand, and Malaysia suggest that many infections are clinically inapparent. The occasional diagnosis based solely on abnormal routine chest roentgenograms represents asymptomatic pneumonitis. Acute pulmonary infections may originate in the respiratory tract or result from hematogenous spread, their severity varying from mild bronchitis to extensive necrotizing pneumonia. Onset may be sudden or gradual. Fever, productive cough, and marked tachypnea are frequent. Chest roentgenograms typically reveal upper-lobe infiltrates or thin-walled cavities that may mimic

tuberculosis. Acute, localized, suppurative skin infections associated with nodular lymphangitis and regional lymphadenitis result from direct inoculation at sites of minor skin trauma. Recrudescent disease arising from inactive sites of infection and perhaps triggered by intercurrent illness or other events may present in an acute or chronic form.

Either acute suppurative infections or pulmonary disease may give rise to hematogenous dissemination and the acute septicemic form of melioidosis. This progression is more likely in chronically debilitated patients, such as those with diabetes mellitus or alcoholism. Septicemic patients may present with severe tachypnea, confusion, headache, pharyngitis, diarrhea, and pustular lesions of the head, trunk, and extremities. The skin may be flushed or cyanotic, signs of meningitis or arthritis may be apparent, the liver and spleen may be enlarged, and muscle tenderness may be striking. Chest roentgenograms show diffuse nodular densities that may expand, coalesce, and finally cavitate. The acute septicemic form of melioidosis usually follows a rapid downhill course, ending in early death. Mortality remains high despite optimal therapy.

The diagnosis of melioidosis should be entertained when a febrile patient who has been in an endemic area presents with an acute lower respiratory tract illness associated with tachypnea, exhibits unusual skin or subcutaneous lesions, or has a chest roentgenogram suggesting tuberculosis in the absence of sputum-associated tubercle bacilli. An etiologic diagnosis may be made by microscopic demonstration of small, irregularly staining, gram-negative rods in exudate material; by characteristic bipolar ("safety-pin") staining of organisms with methylene blue; and by a culture positive for *B. pseudomallei* and/or a fourfold or greater rise in the titer of serum antibody to the organism.

℞ **TREATMENT** The mainstay of treatment for melioidosis is antibiotic administration combined with appropriate surgical drainage of abscesses and aggressive support for patients with septicemic forms of the disease. The guidelines for antibiotic therapy are somewhat imprecise. Subclinical infection or mere seropositivity does not usually require specific therapy. Ceftazidime or imipenem appears to be the agent of choice for clinical disease, including severe infections, while trimethoprim-sulfamethoxazole, cefotaxime, and amoxicillin/clavulanate are possible alternatives. Combination therapy with ceftazidime or imipenem plus trimethoprim-sulfamethoxazole may be indicated in severe forms of melioidosis, including septicemia. Unfortunately, increasing resistance of many strains of *B. pseudomallei* to trimethoprim-sulfamethoxazole, particularly in Southeast Asia, is of concern. Patients with acute pulmonary infections who are treated with either ceftazidime or imipenem should receive antibiotics until they show definite evidence of clinical improvement (often after 10 to 30 days), at which time therapy can be switched to an oral maintenance regimen—a combination of chloramphenicol, trimethoprim-sulfamethoxazole, and doxycycline or the single agent amoxicillin/clavulanate—and continued for 12 to 20 weeks. Chronic disease associated with persistently positive sputum cultures and extrapulmonary suppurative disease may require treatment for up to 1 year.

Other Species *Pseudomonas fluorescens* occasionally causes human disease; it is implicated particularly often in infections related to the administration of contaminated (stored) blood products and in pseudoinfections. Additional species that are associated only rarely with human infections include *P. putida*, *P. stutzeri*, *P. pseudoalcaligenes*, and (all formerly *Pseudomonas* species) *Burkholderia gladioli*, *B. pickettii*, *Comamonas acidovorans*, *C. testosteroni*, *Brevundimonas diminuta*, and *B. vesicularis*.

BIBLIOGRAPHY

P. AERUGINOSA INFECTIONS

BALTCH AL, SMITH RP (eds): *Pseudomonas aeruginosa Infections and Treatment.* New York, Marcel Dekker, 1994

CARMELLI Y et al: Health and economic outcomes of antibiotic resistance in *Pseudomonas aeruginosa*. Arch Intern Med 159:1127, 1999

KORVICK JA, YU VL: Antimicrobial agent therapy for *Pseudomonas aeruginosa*. Antimicrob Agents Chemother 35:2167, 1991

MORRISON AF, WENZEL RP: Epidemiology of infections due to *Pseudomonas aeruginosa*. Rev Infect Dis 6(Suppl):S267, 1984

POLLACK M: The virulence of *Pseudomonas aeruginosa*. Rev Infect Dis 6(Suppl):S617, 1984

————: *Pseudomonas aeruginosa*, in *Mandell, Douglas, and Bennett's Principles and Practice of Infectious Diseases*, 5th ed, GL Mandell et al (eds). New York, Churchill Livingstone, 2000, pp 2310–2335

SHEPP DH et al: Serious *Pseudomonas aeruginosa* infection in AIDS. J Acquir Immun Defic Syndr 7:823, 1994

VAN DELDEN C, IGLEWSKI BH: Cell-to-cell signaling and *Pseudomonas aeruginosa* infections. Emerg Infect Dis 4:551, 1998

INFECTIONS DUE TO RELATED ORGANISMS

SIMPSON AJ et al: Comparison of imipenem and ceftazidime as therapy for severe melioidosis. Clin Infect Dis 29:381, 1999

VARTIVARIAN S, ANAISSIE E: *Stenotrophomonas maltophilia* and *Burkholderia cepacia*, in *Mandell, Douglas, and Bennett's Principles and Practice of Infectious Diseases*, 5th ed, GL Mandell et al (eds). New York, Churchill Livingstone, 2000, pp 2335–2339

WHITE NJ: Melioidosis, in *Hunter's Tropical Medicine and Emerging Infectious Diseases*, 8th ed, GT Strickland et al (eds). Philadelphia, Saunders, 2000, pp 313–316

156　　*Cammie F. Lesser, Samuel I. Miller*

SALMONELLOSIS

The salmonellae constitute a genus of over 2300 serotypes that are highly adapted for growth in both human and animal hosts and cause a wide spectrum of disease. A subset of *Salmonella* serotypes that includes *S. typhi* and *S. paratyphi* causes enteric (typhoid) fever and is restricted to growth in human hosts. The remainder of *Salmonella* serotypes, referred to as nontyphoidal *Salmonella*, are prevalent in the gastrointestinal tracts of a broad range of animals, including mammals, reptiles, birds, and insects. Over 200 of these serotypes are pathogenic to humans; these pathogenic serotypes cause gastroenteritis and can be associated with localized infections and/or bacteremia.

ETIOLOGY　　*Salmonella* is a large genus of gram-negative bacilli within the family Enterobacteriaceae. The nomenclature and classification of these bacteria have undergone numerous revisions, most recently in 1983 when—on the basis of a high degree of DNA similarity between the bacterial genomes—over 2000 bacterial strains were grouped into one species, *S. choleraesuis*. This species was further divided into seven subgroups based on host range specificity and additional DNA similarity. Almost all the strains pathogenic for humans are in subgroup 1 (*enterica* or *choleraesuis*) except for those causing rare infections (subgroups 3a and 3b). The nomenclature of this large species is quite complex. For example, the correct taxonomic name for the organism that causes enteric fever is *Salmonella choleraesuis* ssp. *choleraesuis* (or subgroup 1), serovar *typhi*. Given the cumbersome nature of this nomenclature system, a simplified system is in widespread use, in which the common species name that existed before the reclassification of the species is accepted. For example, *S. choleraesuis* ssp. *choleraesuis*, serovar *typhi*, is referred to by its common name, *S. typhi*.

The initial identification of this genus in the clinical laboratory relies on growth characteristics. Like other Enterobacteriaceae, salmonellae produce acid on glucose fermentation, reduce nitrates, and do not produce cytochrome oxidase. They are non-spore-forming and facultatively anaerobic. With few exceptions, salmonellae are motile by means of peritrichous flagella (exception: *S. gallinarum-pullorum*) and produce gas (H_2S) on sugar fermentation (exception: *S. typhi*).

Since 99% of clinical isolates are lactose nonfermenters, rare clinical isolates may not be detected if a high level of suspicion is not maintained.

Salmonella can be further divided into serovars based on the detection of three major antigenic determinants: the somatic O antigen [lipopolysaccharide (LPS) cell-wall components], the surface Vi antigen (restricted to *S. typhi* and *S. paratyphi* C), and the flagellar H antigen. In general, clinical laboratories initially divide *Salmonella* into serogroups (A, B, C_1, C_2, D, and E) based on reactivity to somatic O-antigen antisera. These initial groupings provide only limited clinical information, given their high degree of cross-reactivity. Thus, additional biochemical and serologic tests are needed to determine serotype. For the epidemiologic evaluation of *Salmonella* outbreaks, specific *Salmonella* strains within serovars can be distinguished by bacteriophage typing, plasmid profile determination, and restriction length polymorphism analysis.

PATHOGENESIS　　Salmonellae are transmitted to humans orally by contaminated food or water. The bacteria traverse the gastrointestinal tract, including the acidic environment of the stomach, to colonize the small intestines. In the case of enteric fever (a systemic illness), salmonellae cross the intestinal barrier, where phagocytosis by macrophages results in their dissemination throughout the reticuloendothelial system. In nontyphoidal salmonellosis, the bacteria generally cause a localized infection resulting in an influx of neutrophils to the intestines and self-limited gastroenteritis.

Numerous attempts have been made to determine the infectious dose (ID_{50}) of *Salmonella*, both in the laboratory and in the field. Controlled experiments, in which healthy volunteers were exposed to laboratory-grown strains of *S. typhi*, concluded that the ID_{50} was 10^6 colony-forming units (CFU); increases in the ID_{50} corresponded to decreases in incubation time. However, analyses of salmonellosis outbreaks with a known source indicate that the ID_{50} can be as low as 10^3 CFU. Host defenses, the most important of which appears to be the acidity of the stomach, most likely account for variations in the ID_{50}. Conditions that decrease stomach acidity (an age of <1 year, antacid ingestion, or achlorhydric disease) increase susceptibility to *Salmonella* infection, as do conditions that decrease intestinal integrity (inflammatory bowel disease, history of gastrointestinal surgery, or alteration of the intestinal flora by antibiotic administration).

Once salmonellae reach the small intestine, the bacteria resist a variety of innate immune factors (including bile salts, lysozyme, complement, and cationic antimicrobial peptides) before penetrating the mucus layer. The organisms enter the intestines through phagocytic microfold or M cells overlying the Peyer's patches. Salmonellae also enter normally nonphagocytic epithelial cells by a process known as *bacteria-mediated endocytosis*, whose mechanism is not entirely clear but depends on the direct translocation of *Salmonella* proteins into the host cell cytoplasm by a specialized secretion apparatus (type III secretion).

In enteric (typhoid) fever, salmonellae (*S. typhi* or *S. paratyphi*) undergo phagocytosis by macrophages after crossing the epithelial layer of the small intestine. Once phagocytosed, the bacteria are protected from polymorphonuclear leukocytes (PMNs), the complement system, and the acquired immune response (antibodies). Salmonellae have evolved mechanisms to avoid or delay killing by macrophages. Upon phagocytosis, the bacteria form a "spacious phagosome" and alter the regulation of ~200 bacterial proteins. The best-characterized regulatory system is PhoP/PhoQ, a two-component regulon that senses changes in bacterial location and alters bacterial protein expression. The alterations mediated by PhoP/PhoQ include modifications in LPS and in the synthesis of outer-membrane proteins; these changes presumably remodel the bacteria's outer surface such that the organisms can resist microbicidal activities and possibly alter host cell signaling. PhoP/PhoQ also mediates the synthesis of divalent cationic transporters that scavenge magnesium. By a second type III secretion mechanism, salmonellae can directly translocate bacterial proteins into the macrophage, a phenomenon that is believed to promote survival within phagocytes.

After phagocytosis, salmonellae disseminate throughout the body in macrophages via the lymphatics and colonize reticuloendothelial tissues (liver, spleen, lymph nodes, and bone marrow). During this initial incubation stage, patients are relatively asymptomatic. Signs and symptoms, including fever and abdominal pain, probably result from secretion of cytokines by macrophages when a critical number of organisms have replicated. For example, the observed hepatosplenomegaly is likely to be related to the recruitment of mononuclear cells and the development of a cell-mediated immune response to *S. typhi* colonization. The recruitment of additional mononuclear cells and lymphocytes to Peyer's patches during the several weeks after initial colonization/infection can result in marked enlargement and necrosis of the Peyer's patches, with right-lower-quadrant abdominal pain.

It is not known why *S. typhi* and *S. paratyphi* cause systemic disease while the vast majority of pathogenic *Salmonella* strains cause gastroenteritis. In contrast to enteric fever, which is characterized by an infiltration of mononuclear cells into the small-bowel mucosa, nontyphoidal *Salmonella* gastroenteritis is characterized by massive PMN infiltration into both the large- and the small-bowel mucosa. This response appears to depend on the induction of interleukin (IL) 8, a strong neutrophil chemotactic factor, which is secreted by intestinal cells. The degranulation and release of toxic substances by neutrophils may result in damage to the intestinal mucosa, causing inflammatory diarrhea.

ENTERIC (TYPHOID) FEVER

Typhoid fever is a systemic disease characterized by fever and abdominal pain caused by dissemination of *S. typhi* or *S. paratyphi*. The disease was initially called *typhoid fever* because of its clinical similarity to typhus. However, in the early 1800s, typhoid fever was clearly defined pathologically as a unique illness on the basis of its association with enlarged Peyer's patches and mesenteric lymph nodes. In 1869, given the anatomic site of infection, the term *enteric fever* was proposed as an alternative designation to distinguish typhoid fever from typhus. However, to this day, the two designations are used interchangeably.

EPIDEMIOLOGY In contrast to other *Salmonella* serotypes, the etiologic agents of enteric fever—*S. typhi* and *S. paratyphi*—have no known hosts other than humans. Thus, enteric fever is transmitted only through close contact with acutely infected individuals or chronic carriers. While direct person-to-person transmission through the fecal-oral route has been documented, it is quite rare. Rather, most cases of disease result from ingestion of contaminated food or water. Health care workers occasionally acquire enteric fever after exposure to infected patients, while laboratory workers can acquire the disease after laboratory accidents.

Over the past four decades, with the advent of improvements in food handling and water/sewage treatment, enteric fever has become a rare occurrence in developed nations. Over the past 10 years, ~400 cases of typhoid fever and even fewer cases of paratyphoid fever have been reported annually in the United States. In contrast, enteric fever continues to be a global health problem, with an estimated 13 to 17 million cases worldwide resulting in ~600,000 deaths per year. Children <1 year of age appear to be most susceptible to initial infection and to the development of severe disease.

Enteric fever is endemic in most developing regions, especially the Indian subcontinent, South and Central America, and Asia, and is related to rapid population growth, increased urbanization, inadequate human waste treatment, limited water supply, and overburdened health care systems. These conditions most likely account for the recent epidemics of typhoid fever in eastern Europe. Antibiotic resistance among salmonellae is also a rising concern and has recently been linked to antibiotic use in livestock. Many *S. typhi* strains contain plasmids encoding resistance to chloramphenicol, ampicillin, and trimethoprim—the antibiotics that have long been used to treat enteric fever. In addition, resistance to ciprofloxacin, either chromosomally or plasmid encoded, has been observed in Asia. Morbidity and mortality are increased in outbreaks associated with antibiotic-resistant strains, presumably because of inadequate or delayed appropriate treatment.

The high worldwide prevalence of enteric fever serves as a reservoir for cases in the United States. Over 70% of U.S. cases are related to international travel within 30 days before onset. Only 3% of travelers diagnosed with enteric fever give a history of vaccination against *S. typhi* within the previous 2 years. Of U.S. cases of internationally acquired enteric fever, 80% can be linked to travel in six countries: Mexico (28%), India (25%), the Philippines (10%), Pakistan (8%), El Salvador (5%), and Haiti (4%). While the percentage of cases associated with travel to Mexico is declining, travel to the Indian subcontinent is becoming much riskier, with an incidence 18 times higher than for any other area. The recent trend toward an increased incidence of multidrug-resistant (MDR) *Salmonella* (see "Treatment," below) in developing countries is reflected by the increase in the proportion of U.S. cases caused by MDR strains from 0.6% in 1985–1989 to 12% in 1990–1994.

Almost 30% of the reported cases of enteric fever in the United States are domestically acquired. Although the majority of these cases (80%) are sporadic, large outbreaks do occur. In the most notable outbreak in the past 15 years, 47 culture-proven and 24 potential cases were linked to contaminated orange juice at a resort in New York. Evaluation of this outbreak led to the identification of a previously unknown chronic carrier. Similarly, evaluation of 25% of the 571 cases of domestically acquired enteric fever reported between 1985 and 1994 led to the identification of previously unknown chronic carriers.

CLINICAL COURSE Enteric fever is a misnomer, in that the hallmark features of this disease—fever and abdominal pain—are variable. While fever is documented at presentation in >75% of cases, abdominal pain is reported in only 20 to 40%. Thus, a high index of suspicion for this potentially lethal systemic illness is necessary when a person presents with fever and a history of recent travel to a developing country.

The incubation period for *S. typhi* ranges from 3 to 21 days. This variability is most likely related to the size of the initial inoculum and the health and immune status of the host. The most prominent symptom of this systemic infection is prolonged fever (38.8° to 40.5°C, or 101.8° to 104.9°F). A prodrome of nonspecific symptoms often precedes fever and includes chills, headache, anorexia, cough, weakness, sore throat, dizziness, and muscle pains. Gastrointestinal symptoms are quite variable. Patients can present with either diarrhea or constipation; diarrhea is more common among patients with AIDS and among children <1 year of age. As stated above, only 20 to 40% of patients present with abdominal pain, although the majority have abdominal tenderness over the course of the disease. In general, the symptoms associated with *S. typhi* are more severe than those associated with *S. paratyphi*.

Early physical findings of enteric fever include rash ("rose spots"), hepatosplenomegaly, epistaxis, and relative bradycardia. Rose spots make up a faint, salmon-colored, blanching, maculopapular rash located primarily on the trunk and chest. The rash is evident in ~30% of patients at the end of the first week and resolves after 2 to 5 days without leaving a trace. Patients can have two or three crops of lesions, and *Salmonella* can be cultured from punch biopsies of these lesions. The faintness of the rash makes it difficult to detect in dark-skinned patients. On occasion, patients who remain toxic manifest neuropsychiatric symptoms described as a "muttering delirium" or "coma vigil," with picking at bedclothes or imaginary objects.

Late complications, occurring in the third and fourth weeks of infection, are most common in untreated adults and include intestinal perforation and/or gastrointestinal hemorrhage. These complications can develop despite clinical improvement and presumably result from necrosis at the initial site of *Salmonella* infiltration in the Peyer's patches of the small intestine. Both complications are life-threatening and require immediate medical and surgical interventions, with broadened antibiotic coverage for polymicrobial peritonitis (Chap. 130) and treatment of gastrointestinal hemorrhages, including bowel resection.

Rare complications whose incidences are reduced by prompt antibiotic treatment include pancreatitis, hepatic and splenic abscesses, endocarditis, pericarditis, orchitis, hepatitis, meningitis, nephritis, myocarditis, pneumonia, arthritis, osteomyelitis, and parotitis. Despite prompt antibiotic treatment, relapse rates remain at ~10% in immunocompetent hosts.

Approximately 1 to 5% of patients with enteric fever become long-term, asymptomatic, chronic carriers who shed *S. typhi* in either urine or stool for >1 year. The incidence of chronic carriage is higher among women and among persons with biliary abnormalities (e.g., gallstones, carcinoma of the gallbladder) and gastrointestinal malignancies. The anatomic abnormalities associated with these conditions presumably allow prolonged colonization.

DIAGNOSIS   Other than a positive culture, no specific laboratory test is diagnostic for enteric fever. In 15 to 25% of cases, leukopenia and neutropenia are detectable. In the majority of cases, the white blood cell count is normal despite high fever. However, leukocytosis can develop in typhoid fever (especially in children) during the first 10 days of the illness, or later if the disease course is complicated by intestinal perforation or secondary infection. Other nonspecific laboratory results include moderately elevated values in liver function tests (aminotransferases, alkaline phosphatase, and lactate dehydrogenase). In addition, nonspecific ST and T wave abnormalities can be seen on electrocardiograms.

The diagnostic "gold standard" is a culture positive for *S. typhi* or *S. paratyphi*. The yield of blood cultures is quite variable: it can be as high as 90% during the first week of infection and decrease to 50% by the third week. A low yield is related to low numbers of *Salmonella* (<15 organisms per milliliter) in infected patients and/or to recent antibiotic treatment. Centrifugation to isolate and culture the buffy coat, which contains abundant blood mononuclear cells associated with the bacteria, decreases time to isolation but does not affect culture sensitivity.

A diagnosis can also be based on positive cultures of stool, urine, rose spots, bone marrow, and gastric or intestinal secretions. Unlike blood cultures, bone marrow cultures remain highly (90%) sensitive despite ≤5 days of antibiotic therapy. Culture of intestinal secretions (best obtained by a noninvasive duodenal string test) can be positive despite a negative bone marrow culture. If blood, bone marrow, and intestinal secretions are all cultured, the yield of a positive culture is >90%. Stool cultures, while negative in 60 to 70% of cases during the first week, can become positive during the third week of infection in untreated patients. Although the majority of patients (90%) clear bacteria from the stool by the eighth week, a small percentage become chronic carriers and continue to have positive stool cultures for at least 1 year.

Several serologic tests, including the classic Widal test for "febrile agglutinins," are available; however, given high rates of false-positivity and false-negativity, these tests are not clinically useful. Polymerase chain reaction and DNA probe assays are being developed.

℞ TREATMENT   In the preantibiotic era, the mortality rate from typhoid fever was as high as 15%. The introduction of treatment with chloramphenicol in 1948 greatly altered the disease course, decreasing mortality to <1% and the duration of fever from 14–28 days to 3–5 days. Chloramphenicol remained the standard treatment for enteric fever until the emergence of plasmid-mediated resistance to this drug in the 1970s. Given the increased mortality associated with resistance to chloramphenicol and the rare chloramphenicol-induced bone marrow toxicity, ampicillin (1 g orally every 6 h) and trimethoprim-sulfamethoxazole (TMP-SMZ; one double-strength tablet twice daily) became the mainstays of treatment.

In 1989, MDR *S. typhi* emerged. These bacteria are resistant to chloramphenicol, ampicillin, trimethoprim, streptomycin, sulfona-

mides, and tetracycline. Like chloramphenicol resistance, resistance to ampicillin and trimethoprim is plasmid-encoded. In 1994, 12% of *S. typhi* isolates in the United States were MDR. Thus either quinolones or third-generation cephalosporins are currently recommended for empirical antibiotic treatment. Despite efficient in vitro killing of *Salmonella*, first- and second-generation cephalosporins as well as aminoglycosides are ineffective in treating clinical infections.

Ceftriaxone (1 to 2 g intravenously or intramuscularly) for 10 to 14 days is equivalent to oral or intravenous chloramphenicol in the treatment of susceptible strains. Preliminary studies indicate that a 5- to 7-day course of ceftriaxone is likely to be sufficient for treatment of uncomplicated cases. However, one recent report describes a ceftriaxone-resistant *Salmonella* strain isolated from a child with diarrhea and apparently acquired from antibiotic-treated cattle.

Quinolones are the only available oral antibiotics for the treatment of MDR *S. typhi* infections. The greatest experience has been gained for ciprofloxacin (500 mg orally twice a day for 10 days). Shorter courses of ofloxacin (10 to 15 mg/kg in divided doses twice daily for 2 to 3 days) have also been successful. However, quinolone resistance is emerging. In 1993, an outbreak of nalidixic acid–resistant *S. typhi* (NARST) infections in Vietnam was linked to chromosomal mutations in the gene encoding DNA gyrase (the target of the quinolones). NARST strains have also been isolated in India. Thus, all strains of *S. typhi* must be screened for resistance to nalidixic acid and tested for sensitivity to a clinically appropriate quinolone. Patients infected with NARST strains need to be treated with higher doses of ciprofloxacin (10 mg/kg twice a day for 10 days) or longer courses of ofloxacin (10 to 15 mg/kg in divided doses twice daily for 7 to 10 days) or with other antibiotics to which the strains are sensitive.

In cases of severe typhoid fever (fever; an abnormal state of consciousness—i.e., delirium, obtundation, stupor, or coma—or septic shock; and a positive culture for *S. typhi* or *S. paratyphi* A), dexamethasone treatment should be considered. In a single trial in Jakarta in the early 1980s in chloramphenicol-treated patients, treatment with dexamethasone (a single dose of 3 mg/kg followed by eight doses of 1 mg/kg, given every 6 h) decreased mortality from 56% to 10%.

The 1 to 4% of patients who develop chronic carriage of *Salmonella* can be treated for 6 weeks with an appropriate antibiotic. Treatment with oral amoxicillin, TMP-SMZ, ciprofloxacin, or norfloxacin has been shown to be ~80% effective in eradicating chronic carriage of susceptible organisms. However, in cases of anatomic abnormality (e.g., biliary or kidney stones), eradication of the infection often cannot be achieved by antibiotic therapy alone but also requires surgical correction of the abnormalities.

PREVENTION AND CONTROL   Theoretically, it is possible to eliminate salmonellae that cause enteric fever since the bacteria survive only in human hosts and are spread by contaminated food and water. However, given the high prevalence of the disease in developing countries that lack good facilities for sewage disposal and water treatment, this goal is currently unrealistic. Thus, travelers to developing countries should be advised to monitor their food and water intake carefully and to consider vaccination.

Three vaccine alternatives are available: (1) a heat-killed, phenol-extracted, whole-cell vaccine (two parenteral doses); (2) Ty21a, an attenuated *S. typhi* vaccine (four oral doses); and (3) ViCPS, consisting of purified Vi polysaccharide from the bacterial capsule (one parenteral dose). In addition, an acetone-killed whole-cell vaccine is available only for use by the U.S. military. The minimal ages for vaccination with the whole-cell, Ty21a, and ViCPS vaccines are 6 years, 2 years, and 6 months, respectively. A large-scale meta-analysis of vaccine trials in populations of endemic areas indicates that, while all three vaccines have similar efficacy for the first year, the 3-year cumulative efficacy of the whole-cell vaccine (73%) exceeds that of both Ty21a (51%) and purified Vi (55%). In addition, the heat-killed whole-cell vaccine maintains its efficacy for 5 years, while Ty21a and ViCPS most likely maintain their efficacy for 4 and 2 years, respectively. However, the whole-cell vaccine is associated with a much higher incidence of side effects than the other two vaccines: 16% of whole-cell vaccine recipients develop fever and 10% miss a day of work or school, while only 1 to 2% of persons receiving the alternative vaccines have any fever.

Although data on typhoid vaccines in travelers are limited, some evidence suggests that efficacy may be substantially lower than those for populations in endemic areas. The Centers for Disease Control and Prevention (CDC) currently recommends vaccination for persons traveling to developing countries who will have prolonged exposure to contaminated food and water or close contact with indigenous populations in rural areas. The only recommendations for domestic vaccination include people who have intimate or household contact with a chronic carrier or laboratory workers who frequently work with *S. typhi*. Given the decreased incidence of side effects and the similar short-term efficacy, the current bias is toward vaccination of travelers with either Ty21a or ViCPS.

Enteric fever is a reportable disease in the United States. This reporting system enables public health departments to track down potential source patients and thus to identify and treat chronic carriers in order to prevent further outbreaks. In addition, since 1 to 4% of patients with *S. typhi* infection become chronic carriers, it is important to monitor patients (especially those employed in child care or food handling) for chronic carriage and to treat this condition if indicated.

NONTYPHOIDAL SALMONELLOSIS

EPIDEMIOLOGY The incidence of nontyphoidal salmonellosis has doubled in the United States over the past two decades. Currently, the CDC estimates that there are 2 million cases annually, with 500 to 2000 deaths. Although over 200 serovars of *Salmonella* are considered to be human pathogens, the majority of the reported cases in the United States is caused by *S. typhimurium* or *S. enteritidis*. The incidence of salmonellosis is highest during the rainy season in tropical climates and during the warmer months in temperate climates, coinciding with the peak in food-borne outbreaks. Morbidity and mortality associated with salmonellosis are highest among the elderly, infants, and immunocompromised individuals, including those with hemoglobinopathies and those infected with HIV or with pathogens that cause blockade of the reticuloendothelial system (e.g., patients with bartonellosis, malaria, schistosomiasis, or histoplasmosis).

Unlike *S. typhi* and *S. paratyphi*, whose only reservoir is humans, nontyphoidal salmonellosis is acquired from multiple animal reservoirs. The main mode of transmission is from food products contaminated with animal products or waste—most commonly eggs and poultry but also undercooked meat, unpasteurized dairy products, seafood, and fresh produce.

S. enteritidis associated with chicken eggs is emerging as a major cause of food-borne disease. *S. enteritidis* causes infection of the ovaries and upper oviduct tissue of hens, resulting in contamination of the contents of eggs prior to shell deposition. Approximately 1 in 20,000 eggs is thought to be infected with *S. enteritidis*. Between 1974 and 1994, there was a fivefold increase (from 5% to 25%) in the isolation of *S. enteritidis* from eggs in the United States; in 1998, the U.S. Department of Agriculture estimated that 80% of all salmonellosis cases were caused by infected eggs. Eradication of *S. enteritidis* from hens has proven difficult, given that infection is spread to egg-laying hens both vertically from breeding flocks and horizontally through contact with rodents and manure. Transmission via contaminated eggs can be prevented by cooking of eggs such that the liquid yolk is solidified or through pasteurization of egg products.

Another factor in the increasing incidence of nontyphoidal salmonellosis in developed countries, including the United States, is related to the centralization of food processing and widespread distribution. For example, a 1994 outbreak of ~250,000 cases was linked to a pasteurized ice-cream premix most likely contaminated in tanker trucks that had previously carried unpasteurized eggs. Similar outbreaks have been traced to manufactured foods including pasteurized milk, infant formula, powdered-milk products, paprika-powdered potato chips, and a ready-to-eat savory snack. In addition, large outbreaks have been linked to fresh produce, including alfalfa sprouts, cantaloupe, fresh-squeezed orange juice, and sliced tomatoes, contaminated by manure or water at a single site and then broadly distributed.

A less common source of nontyphoidal *Salmonella* infections is exposure to exotic pets, especially reptiles. Fecal carriage rates in reptiles can be >90%. In the 1970s, 14% of cases of salmonellosis were attributed to small turtles; the distribution of these pets was subsequently prohibited by the U.S. Food and Drug Administration, with a resultant decline in rates of reptile-associated salmonellosis. However, since 1986, an increase in the popularity of nonbanned reptiles, including iguanas, has been followed by increases in rates of *Salmonella* infections. Other pets, including African hedgehogs, snakes, birds, rodents, baby chicks, ducklings, dogs, and cats, can also serve as potential vectors.

Antibiotic resistance is an increasing phenomenon among nontyphoidal *Salmonella* serovars. In particular, *S. typhimurium* of definitive phage type 104 (DT104)—a serotype resistant to ampicillin, chloramphenicol, streptomycin, sulfonamides, and tetracyclines—has become prominent in the United Kingdom. This serotype is associated with greater mortality and morbidity than other nontyphoidal *Salmonella* serotypes. Its acquisition is associated with exposure to ill farm animals and to a variety of meat products. The prevalence of *S. typhimurium* DT104 in the United States increased from 0.6% in 1979–1980 to 34% in 1996. Of concern is the isolation in the United Kingdom in 1996 of *S. typhimurium* DT104 strains resistant to ciprofloxacin (14%) or trimethoprim (24%).

CLINICAL MANIFESTATIONS Gastroenteritis Infection with nontyphoidal *Salmonella* most often results in gastroenteritis indistinguishable from that caused by other bacterial and viral pathogens. Nausea, vomiting, and diarrhea occur 6 to 48 h after the ingestion of contaminated food or water. Patients often experience abdominal cramping and fever (38 to 39°C, or 100.5 to 102.2°F). The diarrhea is usually characterized as loose, nonbloody stools of moderate volume. However, large-volume watery stools, bloody stools, or symptoms of dysentery do not rule out the diagnosis. Rarely, *Salmonella* causes a syndrome of pseudoappendicitis or an illness that mimics inflammatory bowel disease.

Gastroenteritis caused by nontyphoidal *Salmonella* is usually self-limited. Diarrhea resolves within 3 to 7 days and fever within 72 h. Stool cultures remain positive for 4 to 5 weeks after infection and—in rare cases of chronic carriage (<1%)—remain positive for >1 year. Antibiotic treatment is usually not recommended and in some studies has prolonged carriage of *Salmonella*. Neonates, the elderly, and the immunosuppressed (e.g., HIV-infected patients) with nontyphoidal *Salmonella* gastroenteritis are especially susceptible to dehydration and dissemination and may require hospitalization and antibiotic therapy.

Bacteremia and Endovascular Infections Up to 5% of patients with nontyphoidal *Salmonella* gastroenteritis have positive blood cultures, and 5 to 10% of these bacteremic persons develop localized infections. Bacteremia is particularly common and persistent among infants, the elderly, and patients with severe underlying infection or immunosuppression (e.g., transplant recipients, HIV-infected patients). Salmonellae have a propensity for infection of vascular sites; if >50% of three or more blood cultures are positive, an endovascular infection should be suspected. Preexisting valvular heart disease is a strong risk factor for the development of endocarditis, while atherosclerotic plaque, prosthetic grafts, and aortic aneurysms are associated with arteritis. Arteritis should be suspected in elderly patients who have a history of prolonged fever with associated back, chest, or abdominal pain preceded by gastroenteritis. Endocarditis and arteritis are rare (<1% of cases) but are associated with potentially morbid complications. Endocarditis can be complicated by cardiac valve perforation or by ring or septal abscesses, while arteritis can be associated with mycotic aneurysms, ruptured aneurysms, or vertebral osteomyelitis.

Unlike most nontyphoidal *Salmonella* serotypes, *S. choleraesuis* and *S. dublin* are frequently associated with sustained bacteremia and fever, often in the absence of a history of gastroenteritis. Similarly, these serotypes appear to be especially invasive and are often associated with metastatic infection.

Localized Infections • *Intraabdominal infections* Intraabdominal infections due to nontyphoidal *Salmonella* are rare and usually manifest as hepatic or splenic abscesses or as cholecystitis. Involvement of the pancreas and adrenals and even an infected pheochromocytoma have been reported. Risk factors include anatomic abnormalities of the hepatobiliary system, including gallstones; abdominal malignancy; and sickle cell disease (especially with splenic abscesses). Eradication of the infection often requires surgical correction of anatomic abnormalities and drainage of abscesses.

Central nervous system infections *Salmonella* infections of the central nervous system usually manifest as meningitis, although cerebral abscesses have been found. Meningitis is usually seen in neonates (<4 months old) and is associated with severe sequelae, including residual seizures, hydrocephalus, ventriculitis, abscess formation, subdural empyema, and permanent disability (e.g., mental retardation and paralysis).

Pulmonary infections Nontyphoidal *Salmonella* pulmonary infections usually present as lobar pneumonia, sometimes complicated by lung abscesses, empyemas, pleural effusions, and bronchopleural fistulas. The majority of cases occur in patients with a preexisting abnormality of lung or pleura, including malignancy. Additional risk factors include sickle cell disease and glucocorticoid use. It is important to determine whether the pulmonary infection is in fact due to *Salmonella* or whether it is a secondary infection.

Urinary and genital tract infections Urinary tract infections caused by nontyphoidal salmonellae present as either cystitis or pyelonephritis, usually in association with malignancy, urolithiasis, structural abnormalities, or immunosuppression (HIV infection, renal transplantation). Genital infections due to these bacteria are rare and present as ovarian and testicular abscesses, prostatitis, or epididymitis. Like other focal infections, both genital and urinary tract infections can be complicated by abscess formation.

Bone, joint, and soft tissue infections *Salmonella* osteomyelitis most commonly affects the femur, tibia, humerus, or lumbar vertebrae and is most often seen in association with sickle cell disease, hemoglobinopathies, or preexisting bone disease (e.g., fractures). Prolonged antibiotic treatment is recommended to decrease the incidence of relapse and chronic osteomyelitis. Septic arthritis occurs in the same patient population as osteomyelitis and usually presents in the knee, hip, or shoulder joints. Reactive arthritis (Reiter's syndrome) can follow *Salmonella* gastroenteritis and is seen most frequently in persons with the HLA-B27 histocompatibility antigen. *Salmonella* can cause rare soft tissue infections, usually at sites of local trauma in immunosuppressed patients.

DIAGNOSIS Nontyphoidal *Salmonella* gastroenteritis is diagnosed when *Salmonella* is cultured from stool. All salmonellae isolated in clinical laboratories should be sent to local public health departments. In cases where there is concern about bacteremia (i.e., those including prolonged or recurrent fever), blood cultures are indicated. Once bacteremia is documented, it is important to determine whether it is high-grade (>50% of three or more blood cultures positive); if so, endovascular infection is possible and further evaluation to identify the source is indicated. In addition, depending on clinical symptoms and on whether metastatic disease is suspected, other body fluids, such as joint fluid or cerebrospinal fluid, should be cultured.

℞ TREATMENT Antibiotic treatment is not generally recommended for *Salmonella* gastroenteritis. The symptoms are usually self-limited and have not been demonstrated to be altered by short courses of antibiotics. In addition, in case-control and double-blind placebo-controlled trials, antibiotic treatment has been associated with increased rates of relapse and prolonged gastrointestinal carriage. Dehydration secondary to diarrhea should be treated with fluid and electrolyte replacement.

However, preemptive antibiotic treatment should be considered in patients at increased risk for metastatic infection. These patients include neonates (probably up to 3 months of age); persons >50 years old (because of the high risk of atherosclerotic plaque or aneurysm); transplant recipients; and patients with lymphoproliferative disease, HIV infection, prosthetic joints, vascular grafts, significant joint disease, or underlying sickle cell disease. This group should receive a course of oral or intravenous antibiotics lasting for 2 or 3 days or until defervescence. Longer courses of antibiotics are not recommended because they have been associated with higher rates of chronic carriage and relapse. Rare cases of chronic nontyphoidal *Salmonella* carriage should be treated with a prolonged antibiotic course, as described above for chronic carriage of *S. typhi*.

Focal infections or life-threatening bacteremia with nontyphoidal *Salmonella* should be treated with antibiotics (at the same doses used for enteric fever). Given the increasing prevalence of antibiotic resistance, empirical therapy should include a third-generation cephalosporin and/or a quinolone. If the bacteremia is low-grade (<50% of blood cultures positive), the patient should be treated for 7 to 14 days. Patients with AIDS and *Salmonella* bacteremia should receive 1 to 2 weeks of intravenous antibiotic therapy followed by 4 weeks of oral therapy with quinolones. Patients who relapse after this regimen should receive long-term suppressive therapy with a quinolone or TMP-SMZ, as indicated by bacterial sensitivities.

If the patient has an endovascular infection or endocarditis, treatment for 6 weeks with intravenous β-lactam antibiotics is indicated. Chloramphenicol treatment has been associated with high failure rates and is not recommended. Limited case reports have described the successful treatment of *Salmonella* endovascular infections with quinolones, which may prove an alternative approach in cases caused by sensitive strains. However, concern remains about the development of quinolone resistance during prolonged therapy. Surgical resection of infected aneurysms or other infected endovascular sites is often required. If surgical resection is not possible, lifelong suppressive antibiotic therapy may be indicated. For extraintestinal nonvascular infections, 2 to 4 weeks of antibiotic therapy (depending on the site) are usually recommended. In cases of chronic osteomyelitis, abscesses, and urinary or biliary tract abnormality, surgical interventions may be required in addition to prolonged antibiotic therapy to eradicate infection.

PREVENTION AND CONTROL The incidence of nontyphoidal salmonellosis continues to rise along with rates of emergence of antibiotic-resistant strains. The increased centralization of food production plays a prominent role in the growing incidence, as one oversight can result in rapid, widespread distribution of contaminated food. Thus, it is important to monitor every step of food production, from handling of raw products to preparation of finished foods. In particular, with the increasing prevalence of *S. enteritidis* in egg-laying hens, it is recommended that pasteurized eggs be substituted for bulk-pooled eggs at all nursing homes, hospitals, and commercial food-service establishments. All cases of nontyphoidal salmonellosis should be reported to public health departments, since tracking and monitoring of these cases result in the identification of the sources of local outbreaks and help authorities anticipate large-scale international outbreaks. Lastly, the prudent use of antimicrobial agents in both humans and animals is necessary to minimize the further emergence of antibiotic-resistant strains.

BIBLIOGRAPHY

COHEN JI et al: Extra-manifestations of *Salmonella* infections. Medicine 66:349, 1987

ENGELS EA et al: Typhoid fever vaccines: A meta-analysis of studies on efficacy and toxicity. BMJ 316:110, 1998

FEY PD et al: Ceftriaxone-resistant *Salmonella* infection acquired by a child from cattle. N Engl J Med 342:1242, 2000

GLYNN MK et al: Emergence of multidrug-resistant *Salmonella enterica* serotype typhimurium DT104 infections in the United States. N Engl J Med 338:1333, 1998

HOFFMAN SL et al: Reduction in mortality in chloramphenicol-treated severe typhoid fever by high-dose dexamethasone. N Engl J Med 310:82, 1984

HOFFMAN TA et al: Waterborne typhoid fever in Dade County, Florida: Clinical and therapeutic evaluation of 105 bacteremic patients. Am J Med 59:481, 1975

MERMIN JH et al: Typhoid fever in the United States, 1985–1994: Changing risks of international travel and increasing antimicrobial resistance. Arch Intern Med 158:633, 1998

SCHERER CA, MILLER SI: Molecular pathogenesis of salmonellae, in *Molecular Pathogenesis of Salmonellae*, EA Groisman (ed). San Diego, Academic Press, 2000, in press

STUART BM, PULLEN RL: Typhoid: Clinical analysis of three hundred and sixty cases. Arch Intern Med 78:629, 1946

TAUXE RV: Emerging foodborne diseases: An evolving public health challenge. Emerg Infect Dis 3:425, 1997

157

Gerald T. Keusch

SHIGELLOSIS

DEFINITION *Shigellosis* is an acute infectious inflammatory colitis due to one of the members of the genus *Shigella*. Although the disease is often referred to as "bacillary dysentery," many patients have only mild watery diarrhea and never develop dysenteric symptoms. Less severe illness predominates in industrialized countries such as the United States, whereas more severe, often fatal dysentery occurs in patients in developing countries.

ETIOLOGIC AGENT Shigellae are slender, gram-negative, nonmotile bacilli and are members of the family Enterobacteriaceae and the tribe Escherichieae. They are so closely related to *Escherichia coli* that the two genera cannot be distinguished by DNA hybridization methods. In fact, *Shigella* can be thought of as a differentiated pathogenic *E. coli*. The four *Shigella* species (*S. dysenteriae*, *S. flexneri*, *S. boydii*, and *S. sonnei*) are defined on the basis of surface somatic O antigens and carbohydrate fermentation patterns. Most are lactose-negative (*S. sonnei* is a late lactose fermenter) and produce acid but not gas from glucose, resulting in a typical acid butt and alkaline slant in triple sugar iron agar without H_2S production. The genus is characterized by its ability to invade intestinal epithelial cells and to cause infection and illness in humans, even when the inoculum is small (a few hundred to a few thousand organisms).

EPIDEMIOLOGY Worldwide, it is estimated that at least 140 million cases of shigellosis and almost 600,000 deaths due to shigellosis occur annually among children under the age of 5 years, primarily in developing countries. The organism is found everywhere in the world but is most common where poor environmental sanitation and crowding facilitate transmission from person to person. A major outbreak took place in the makeshift camps for refugees fleeing the Rwandan civil war in 1994, with thousands of cases and high mortality.

Data collected by the Centers for Disease Control and Prevention in the United States from 1967 through 1988 suggest an average annual incidence of 6 *Shigella* infections per 100,000 population, with periodic hyperendemic increases (primarily due to large outbreaks of *S. sonnei* infection) raising the rate to between 9 and 10 per 100,000. On the basis of these data, the annual number of episodes of shigellosis in the United States is estimated at 25,000 to 30,000. Incidence rates approximate 27 per 100,000 among children 1 to 4 years of age but are only 2.6 per 100,000 among persons 20 years of age or older. Cases are detected most commonly in counties with a relatively high proportion of low-income minority-group residents, including African Americans, Hispanics, and Native Americans; rates are especially high in poor urban communities, in day-care centers, and among retarded children in custodial care.

A comparison with rates among rural Guatemalan Indian children during the same period puts this disease burden into perspective. A prospective surveillance study among 321 such children revealed an annual incidence of nearly 10,000 per 100,000.

Since the description of the genus *Shigella*, major global shifts in the prevalence of its four species have been noted. Until World War I, *S. dysenteriae* type 1 was the predominant isolate, frequently causing devastating epidemics with high mortality until it was replaced by *S. flexneri*. Since World War II, however, *S. flexneri* has been steadily replaced by *S. sonnei* in the industrialized countries. The reasons for these shifts are not clear. *S. boydii*, the fourth species, has remained largely confined to the Indian subcontinent.

Shigella is highly host-adapted and is a natural pathogen only of humans and a few other primates. Transmission from person to person takes place by the fecal-oral route, generally via direct contact but sometimes through contaminated vectors such as food, water, flies, and fomites. Contaminated imported parsley from Mexico was responsible for one multistate outbreak of *S. sonnei* diarrhea. The organism can even be transmitted during participation in recreational water sports in fecally contaminated pools or lakes and can spread rapidly among confined populations in close contact—for example, in day-care centers, in institutions for the mentally retarded, on cruise ships, or among military personnel. *Shigella* can be transmitted by anal-oral sexual practices among gay men; these cases are almost always due to *S. flexneri*. Rates of *Shigella* infection among HIV-infected individuals greatly exceed those in the non-HIV-infected population (Chap. 309).

Shigellosis is associated with a high rate of secondary household transmission. As many as 40% of children and 20% of adults who are household contacts of a case (generally a preschool child) will develop *Shigella* infection; the infection is often symptomatic in children but asymptomatic in adults, who seem to have an acquired immunity. In contrast, epidemic disease affects all ages, with clusters of severe and fatal cases in the very young and the very old. Since 1969, epidemic *S. dysenteriae* type 1 has reappeared in Latin America, in the Indian subcontinent and elsewhere in Asia, and in central and southern Africa and has been associated with relatively high mortality rates due to antimicrobial resistance and inadequate diagnosis and case management. Prolonged asymptomatic carriage is uncommon; unless there is underlying malnutrition, the organisms are generally cleared in a few weeks.

PATHOGENESIS AND PATHOLOGY Shigellae are orally ingested and, because they survive low pH more easily than other enteric pathogens (a genetically regulated property), seem to have little difficulty in passing the gastric acid barrier. An essential step in pathogenesis is invasion of colonic epithelial cells and cell-to-cell spread of infection. This step involves initial attachment of the organism to colonic cells, entry by an endocytic mechanism in which organisms are initially encased in and then escape from plasma membrane–enclosed vesicles, and a jet propulsion–like movement to the cell membrane, from which the organism can invade the adjacent cell. This sequence of events not only provides the organism with a means to evade host defenses but also allows its effective local spread. Although invasion is initially innocuous, subsequent intracellular multiplication causes cell damage and death, ultimately resulting in characteristic mucosal ulcerations.

These events are extremely complicated and require the functions of multiple genes and regulatory elements encoded on both the chromosome and a large 120- to 140-MDa plasmid present in all virulent shigellae as well as enteroinvasive *E. coli* (EIEC), which can cause a *Shigella*-like disease. The number of structural and regulatory genes known to be involved in pathogenesis continues to increase as the process continues to be dissected. Some of these gene products induce the phagocytosis-like uptake of the organism by causing rearrangements of the host cell's cytoskeleton. Once a single *Shigella* organism has invaded a single host cell, the entire process of bacterial escape from the phagocytic vesicle into the host cell's cytoplasm, multiplication, and cell-to-cell spread can take place without exposure of the bacterium to the extracellular milieu and to the host's defenses.

It was originally thought that shigellae invade the host across the intestinal epithelial cells; however, studies using cell culture or a rabbit-ileum in vivo model have suggested that the initial invasion may occur via the antigen-sampling M cell. The resulting limited penetration by organisms initiates an inflammatory response with neutrophil infiltration of the lamina propria, which alters the functional integrity of tight junctions between epithelial cells. These changes allow more organisms to breach the mucosal barrier at intercellular junctions and are essential for the development of illness. If neutrophil migration is directly inhibited by the treatment of animals with antibody to CD18, the escalating invasion by microorganisms does not take place.

Escape from the phagocytic vesicle is necessary for the virulence of shigellae and permits multiplication of the organisms in the cytoplasm. The multiplying organisms spread within the cytoplasm to the plasma membrane of the host cell and then from cell to cell. This spread is achieved by the polymerization of actin at the back end of the dividing bacteria (defined relative to the subsequent direction of motion). Binding and cross-linking by the host protein plastin result in a sphincter-like contraction that provides a forward propulsive force. This so-called actin motor is energized by ATP generated by a microbial-encoded ATPase called *IcsA*, which is, at the same time, phosphorylated and regulated by cyclic nucleotide-dependent protein kinases of the host. Phosphorylation may serve as a molecular host-defense mechanism to modulate virulence, limiting microbial spread.

Another important host protein involved in pathogenesis of shigellosis is the cadherin L-CAM, which is essential in the cell-to-cell spread of infection. Mutations in L-CAM alter the long finger-like protrusions induced by shigellae when they reach the plasma membrane and impair their subsequent fusion with the plasma membrane of the adjacent cell, thus inhibiting the transfer of the bacterium from one cell to another. Ultimately, the invaded host cell dies, possibly as a result of apoptosis induced by or during the process of microbial invasion.

Another property of apparent importance in virulence for *S. dysenteriae* type 1 is the ability to produce Shiga toxin, which is encoded by the iron-regulated chromosomal gene *stx*. Shiga toxin is composed of two distinct peptide subunits, each with highly conserved active regions. The first, located on the larger A subunit, is an *N*-glycosidase that hydrolyzes adenine from specific sites of ribosomal RNA of the mammalian 60S ribosomal subunit, irreversibly inhibiting protein synthesis. The second common region is a binding site on the B subunit that recognizes glycolipids of target cell membranes that terminate in a galactose $\alpha 1 \rightarrow 4$-galactose disaccharide. The glycolipid Gb3, containing a gal-gal-glu trisaccharide, is a specific receptor present on toxin-sensitive rabbit intestinal villus cells but not crypt cells, and toxin action is specific for the former.

Wild-type toxigenic *S. dysenteriae* causes more severe illness in primates than does an isogenic toxin-negative mutant. The toxin of this organism, the prototype of a family of related toxin proteins produced by enterohemorrhagic *E. coli* (EHEC), appears to play a role in the pathogenesis of microangiopathic complications, hemolytic-uremic syndrome (HUS), and thrombotic thrombocytopenic purpura: only toxin-producing shigellae and *E. coli* are associated with these systemic illnesses. Two new *Shigella* enterotoxins, ShET-1 and -2, have been described; the former is restricted almost exclusively to *S. flexneri* 2a, whereas the latter is distributed more widely (e.g., in the physiologically similar EIEC). The two enterotoxins are encoded by chromosomal and plasmid genes, respectively. Both toxins alter electrolyte transport by segments of gut in vitro and cause net fluid secretion in vivo in ligated rabbit ileal loops. Moreover, both toxins induce antibody in infected humans. However, their role (if any) in the pathogenesis of the watery diarrhea phase of shigellosis remains uncertain.

In shigellosis, the epithelial surface of the human colon shows extensive ulcerations, with an exudate consisting of desquamated colonic cells, polymorphonuclear leukocytes, and erythrocytes; the ulcerations may resemble a pseudomembrane in severely affected areas. Marked mucus depletion and increased mitotic activity are evident in the crypt regions and presumably reflect a response to the loss of surface colonic cells. The lamina propria is edematous and hemorrhagic and is infiltrated by neutrophils and plasma cells. There is also swelling of capillary and venular endothelial cells, with margination of neutrophils. At the ultrastructural level, bacteria can be seen within vesicles as well as free in the cytoplasm. Histologic examination of colon from dysenteric humans shows an alteration of mucosal endothelial cells similar to that induced by endotoxin [lipopolysaccharide (LPS)]. Shiga toxin (protein) targets endothelial cells as well, especially when toxin receptor expression is upregulated by exposure to LPS or proinflammatory cytokines. Levels of circulating LPS are high in *S. dysenteriae* type 1 infection and somewhat lower in *S. flexneri* infection, even without bacteremia. The frequency of endotoxemia in shigellosis suggests a broader role for LPS in the pathogenesis of the disease. One likely mechanism is related to the ability of LPS to induce cytokine gene transcription and the strong association of cytokine secretion and inflammation. However, bacterial invasion of the mucosa itself activates the transcription factor NF-κB, which is involved in regulation of cytokine synthesis. Cytokine-producing cells are present in the mucosa of patients infected with *S. dysenteriae* or *S. flexneri* and in their stools as well. In fact, the number of cells producing interleukin 1, interleukin 6, interferon α, and transforming growth factor β is directly related to the severity of the inflammation. Inflammatory changes in *Shigella* infection thus appear to be components of the pathogenesis of dysentery as much as they are a consequence of the bacterial invasive process.

Epidemiologic evidence indicates that immunity develops and is serotype-specific. The precise nature of this immunity is not known. Common surface outer-membrane proteins involved in invasion elicit serum antibodies; although these are cross-reactive among *Shigella* species and serotypes, they do not seem to be protective. The serotype-specific determinants are likely to be somatic antigens, as serum antibody to LPS predicts resistance to infection, and there is evidence of IgA-mediated mucosal responses to LPS during convalescence from shigellosis.

CLINICAL MANIFESTATIONS Shigellosis in the United States, due primarily to *S. sonnei*, is typically an ambulatory disease, presenting as a self-limited nonbloody watery diarrhea chock full of neutrophils. The spectrum of clinical shigellosis was shown in a study in which adult volunteers ingested 10,000 organisms of *S. flexneri* type 2a. While approximately one-quarter of the volunteers never became ill, over the first 24 to 48 h ~25% developed transient fever, another 25% had fever and self-limited watery diarrhea, and the remaining 25% had fever and watery diarrhea that progressed to bloody diarrhea and dysentery. In young children in particular, the temperature can rise rapidly to 40° to 41°C and sometimes results in generalized seizures. These seizures rarely recur or result in serious sequelae. Dysentery is characterized by frequent passage (usually 10 to 30 times per day) of small-volume stools consisting of blood, mucus, and pus; this diarrhea is accompanied by abdominal cramps and tenesmus—the painful straining with stooling that may lead to rectal prolapse, especially in young children. Severe dysentery is most likely in infection due to *S. dysenteriae* type 1, occurs less commonly with *S. flexneri*, and is least likely in *S. sonnei* infection. Patients with mild disease generally recover without specific therapy in a few days to a week. Severe shigellosis can progress to toxic dilatation and colonic perforation, which may be fatal.

Endoscopy shows the mucosa to be hemorrhagic, with mucous discharge and focal ulcerations and sometimes with overlying exudate. The majority of lesions are in the distal colon and progressively diminish in the more proximal segments of large bowel. Mild dehydration is common among patients with watery diarrhea; severe dehydration is very rare. With extensive colonic involvement, protein-losing enteropathy can occur and can have important adverse nutritional consequences, especially for already poorly nourished children.

A variety of *extraintestinal complications* of shigellosis have been described. The majority arise in patients in developing countries and are related both to the prevalence of infections due to *S. dysenteriae* type 1 and *S. flexneri* and to the poor nutritional state of the host. For example, bacteremia, thought to be relatively infrequent in the United States, develops in up to 8% of patients hospitalized for shigellosis in Dacca, Bangladesh. The causative *Shigella* species is isolated from half the patients; other Enterobacteriaceae are found in the remainder. Bacteremia is associated with higher-than-usual mortality and is more common among infants <1 year of age and among persons with protein-energy malnutrition. Persistent and clinically severe *Shigella* bacteremia has been encountered in the United States in patients with AIDS (Chap. 309).

HUS may occur with *S. dysenteriae* type 1 infection. In the United States, the more likely cause of HUS is one of the hemorrhagic colitis–causing strains of *E. coli* (such as *E. coli* O157:H7) that produce high levels of Shiga-family toxins. HUS usually develops toward the end of the first week of shigellosis, when dysentery is already resolving. Oliguria and a marked drop in hematocrit (by as much as 10% within 24 h) are the first signs and may progress to anuria with renal failure and to severe anemia with congestive heart failure, respectively. Even with advanced therapy, 5 to 10% of patients with HUS die of the acute illness. In addition, renal damage progresses slowly over several decades in survivors, an estimated 50% of whom develop significant renal failure and most of whom require long-term dialysis or renal transplantation. Leukemoid reactions, with leukocyte counts of >50,000/μL, may occur along with HUS; thrombocytopenia (with 30,000 to 100,000 platelets/μL) is common. Profound hyponatremia and severe hypoglycemia may be documented. Central nervous system abnormalities include encephalopathic symptoms, seizures, altered consciousness, and bizarre posturing.

Less common extraintestinal manifestations include seizures in some patients and reactive arthritis in others; both of these manifestations are usually due to infection with *S. flexneri* strains. In patients expressing histocompatibility antigen HLA-B27, the full triad of Reiter's syndrome sometimes develops (Chap. 315). Pneumonia, meningitis, vaginitis (in prepubertal girls), keratoconjunctivitis, and "rose spot" rashes are rare events.

DIAGNOSIS AND LABORATORY FINDINGS Shigellosis is the principal bacterial cause of dysentery and should be considered whenever a patient presents with bloody diarrhea. However, in the United States, because *S. sonnei* is the most common species, most patients present with fever and nonbloody watery diarrhea indistinguishable from signs caused by other bacterial or viral agents of mild to moderate diarrhea, while many patients with bloody diarrhea have EHEC as the cause. The specific diagnosis is based on culture of *Shigella* from the stool; however, diagnosis by the polymerase chain reaction is possible, and a commercial enzyme immunoassay to detect Shiga-family toxins in stool can identify most patients infected with *S. dysenteriae* type 1 or EHEC within 3 h. The yield of *Shigella* is increased if the organism is sought by stool culture when the patient has fecal leukocytes or bloody diarrhea. The organism is very labile and must be transferred quickly to plates or holding media (such as buffered glycerol saline) if it is to survive. Stool samples are preferable to swabs; when the latter are used, a rectal sample should be obtained. More than one selective medium should be used for culture—i.e., MacConkey and one other, such as Hektoen enteric or xylose-lysine-deoxycholate. Stool cultures to diagnose nonbloody watery diarrhea have a very low yield of positives and are not cost-effective.

Serologic tests can be performed, since antibodies to somatic antigens develop early in the acute phase of disease. However, the resources for such tests are not generally available, and serologic assessments usually are used only for epidemiologic studies.

The differential diagnosis includes inflammatory colitis due to other microbial agents: EHEC, EIEC, *Campylobacter jejuni*, *Salmonella enteritidis*, *Yersinia enterocolitica*, *Clostridium difficile*, and the protozoan *Entamoeba histolytica*. Ulcerative colitis and Crohn's colitis are among the "noninfectious" conditions that should be considered (Chap. 287). All these infections except that due to *E. histolytica* are associated with the presence of large numbers of fecal leukocytes. Amebiasis can be diagnosed by the detection of erythrophagocytic trophozoites in the stool (Chap. 213).

Other laboratory studies are nonspecific and may disclose neutrophilic leukocytosis, anemia due to blood loss with hemorrhagic diarrhea, prerenal azotemia, or (if watery diarrhea has been pronounced) hyperchloremic acidosis. Laboratory findings in shigellosis complicated by HUS are discussed above.

TREATMENT The mild to moderate dehydration in shigellosis is readily corrected with oral rehydration solutions (Chap. 159). The role of antibiotic therapy is variable and depends on the organism and the severity of disease. Since *S. sonnei* infection is usually self-limited, culture results generally do not become available until the patient is better and there is little clinical need for further therapy. The use of antibiotics in severe cases with bloody diarrhea or dysentery reduces the duration of illness and can shorten the carriage state. Resistance to sulfonamides, streptomycin, chloramphenicol, and tetracyclines is almost universal, and many shigellae are now resistant to ampicillin and trimethoprim-sulfamethoxazole as well. Knowledge of the pattern of resistance in a given population, which can change with time, is useful. In the United States, multiresistant strains are most likely to be acquired during travel abroad; either ampicillin (50 to 100 mg/kg per day in children or 2 g/d in adults, in divided doses) or trimethoprim-sulfamethoxazole (8/40 mg/kg per day in children or 2 regular-strength tablets twice a day in adults, given for 5 days) is generally recommended for domestically acquired infection. Short courses of treatment (1 or 3 days) or even single doses of drugs like tetracycline and ciprofloxacin have been employed with success and may soon become the standard. Amoxicillin should *not* be substituted for ampicillin because it is not effective against shigellosis. In developing countries, where resistance to both of these drugs is commonplace, the drug of choice for the treatment of multiresistant *S. dysenteriae* type 1 infections has been nalidixic acid (55 mg/kg per day for 5 days); however, resistance to the latter agent is increasing in prevalence. The 4-fluoroquinolones (e.g., ciprofloxacin) are highly effective against all strains (Chap. 137) but are currently too costly in the developing world and are not yet approved for use in children under 17 in the United States; these drugs have caused cartilage damage in young rodents during toxicity tests, although there is no evidence for a similar effect of therapeutic doses in humans. Alternative drugs shown to be effective include oral pivamdinocillin (amdinocillin, pivoxil, pivmecillinam; still not available in the United States), azithromycin, and intravenous ceftriaxone (50 mg/kg per day for 5 days). In small-scale clinical trials, cephalexin has had no effect in limiting symptoms; single doses of ceftriaxone may be effective, but more information is needed. No antibiotic treatment is recommended for the convalescent carrier state, which usually lasts no more than several weeks. Patients with AIDS may develop chronic carriage of *Shigella* and may be subject to relapsing infection with bacteremia (Chap. 309). This cycle may be interrupted by prolonged (several weeks') treatment with a quinolone.

The role of antimotility agents such as atropine sulfate and diphenoxylate (Lomotil) and loperamide (Imodium) in the early phases of shigellosis is controversial. Loperamide, in particular, may reduce diarrhea and in one study was highly effective in combination with antimicrobials. However, these antimotility drugs are suspected of enhancing the severity of disease by delaying excretion of organisms and thus facilitating further invasion of the mucosa and complicating toxic megacolon. Therefore, they are contraindicated in infants and young children. In adults, these agents are contraindicated for use in the dysenteric phase of disease.

Treatment of complications of shigellosis often differs in developed and developing countries. For example, antibiotic-unresponsive toxic megacolon, with or without perforation, is often managed by colectomy in the United States. Surgery is less often employed in developing countries because of a lack of availability or difficulties in ileostomy management. HUS often requires dialysis. In developing countries, dialysis may be needed relatively infrequently because azotemia is slow to develop and the risk of significant hyperkalemia is often diminished by a preexisting deficiency in total-body potassium, with malnutrition and wasting of lean body mass. The management of hyponatremia, usually caused by inappropriate secretion of antidiuretic hormone (vasopressin), is governed by the severity of the condition and the symptomatic state of the patient, as outlined in Chap. 49. Infusion of glucose can reverse clinical manifestations caused by hypoglycemia, and responses can be monitored by finger-stick blood glucose tests if no biochemistry laboratory is available. Optimal nutritional management is needed to correct deficiencies due to underlying malnutrition as well as the superimposed catabolic stress and protein-losing enteropathy of shigellosis. Nutritional support should begin during the acute illness and may be required for months thereafter (Chap. 76).

PREVENTION   Direct-contact transmission of shigellosis can be prevented by appropriate environmental and personal hygiene. Hand washing with soap and water, decontamination of water supplies, use of sanitary latrines or toilets, and precautions in the preparation and storage of food can all reduce the primary and secondary transmission of *Shigella* infection. In highly endemic developing countries, infants are protected during the period of exclusive breast feeding, which should be encouraged. Any measures that reduce the burden of malnutrition will also reduce the burden of shigellosis in the population. Stool precautions should be instituted for hospitalized infected patients to ensure safe disposal of infected excreta and linens, and hospital personnel must wash their hands and medical instruments (such as stethoscopes) after each contact with an infected patient. Cohorting of asymptomatic infected children, use of antibiotics to reduce infectiousness, and scrupulous attention to hygiene are usually successful in nosocomial outbreaks. Children in day care must be kept at home while clinically ill and ideally should have a negative stool culture before returning to the day-care facility. Likewise, food handlers who develop shigellosis should be culture-negative before returning to work. Antibiotic treatment is not indicated for the asymptomatic carrier state. No effective vaccine is available, although promising initial results have been reported with an *S. sonnei* LPS-protein conjugate vaccine.

BIBLIOGRAPHY

BAER JT et al: HIV infection as a risk factor for shigellosis. Emerg Infect Dis 5:820, 1999

FARUQUE AS et al: Shigellosis in children: A clinico-epidemiological comparison between *Shigella dysenteriae* type I and *Shigella flexneri*. Ann Trop Paediatr 18:197, 1998

KEUSCH GT: The rediscovery of Shiga toxin and its role in clinical disease. Jpn J Med Sci Biol 51(Suppl):S5, 1998

KHAN WA et al: Treatment of shigellosis: V. Comparison of azithromycin and ciprofloxacin. A double-blind, randomized, controlled trial. Ann Intern Med 126:697, 1997

——— et al: Central nervous system manifestations of childhood shigellosis: Prevalence, risk factors, and outcome. Pediatrics 103:E18, 1999

KOTLOFF KL et al: Global burden of *Shigella* infection: Implications for vaccine development and implementation of control strategies. Bull World Health Organ 77:651, 1999

LINDBERG AA: Vaccination against enteric pathogens: From science to vaccine trials. Curr Opin Microbiol 1:116, 1998

Outbreaks of *Shigella sonnei* infection associated with eating fresh parsley—United States and Canada, July–August 1998. MMWR 48:285, 1999

SACK RB et al: Antimicrobial resistance in organisms causing diarrheal disease. Clin Infect Dis 24(Suppl 1):S102, 1997

SALAM MA et al: Randomised comparison of ciprofloxacin suspension and pivmecillinam for childhood shigellosis. Lancet 352:522, 1998

SANSONETTI PJ et al: Rupture of the intestinal epithelial barrier and mucosal invasion by *Shigella flexneri*. Clin Infect Dis 28:466, 1999

158

Martin J. Blaser

INFECTIONS DUE TO *CAMPYLOBACTER* AND RELATED SPECIES

DEFINITION   Bacteria of the genus *Campylobacter* and of the related genera *Arcobacter* and *Helicobacter* (Chap. 154) cause a variety of pyogenic infections. Although acute diarrheal illnesses are most common, these organisms may cause infections in virtually all parts of the body, especially in compromised hosts, and these infections may have late nonsuppurative sequelae. The designation *Campylobacter* comes from the Greek for "curved rod" and refers to the organism's vibrio-like morphology.

ETIOLOGY   Campylobacters are motile, non-spore-forming, curved gram-negative rods. Originally known as *Vibrio fetus*, these bacilli were reclassified as a new genus in 1973, after it was recognized that they were quite dissimilar to other vibrios. Since then, more than 15 species have been identified. These species are currently divided into three genera: *Campylobacter*, *Arcobacter*, and *Helicobacter*. Not all of the species are pathogens of humans. The human pathogens can be divided into two major groups: those that primarily cause diarrheal disease and those that cause extraintestinal infection. The principal diarrheal pathogen is *C. jejuni*, which accounts for 80 to 90% of all cases of recognized illness due to campylobacters. Other organisms that cause diarrheal disease include *C. coli*, *C. upsaliensis*, *C. lari*, and *C. fetus*. The major species causing extraintestinal illnesses is *C. fetus*; however, any of the diarrheal agents may cause systemic or localized infection as well. Neither aerobes nor strict anaerobes, these microaerophilic organisms are adapted for survival in the gastrointestinal mucous layer. This chapter will focus on *C. jejuni* and *C. fetus* as the major pathogens and prototypes for their groups; the key features of infection are listed by species (excluding *C. jejuni*, described in detail in the text below) in Table 158-1.

EPIDEMIOLOGY   Campylobacters are found in the gastrointestinal tract of many animals used for food (including poultry, cattle, sheep, and swine) and of many household pets (including birds, dogs, and cats). These microorganisms usually do not cause illness in their animal hosts. In most cases, campylobacters are transmitted to humans in raw or undercooked food products or through direct contact with infected animals. In the United States and other developed countries, ingestion of contaminated poultry that has not been sufficiently cooked is the most common means of acquiring infection (50 to 70% of cases). Other modes of transmission include ingestion of raw (unpasteurized) milk or untreated water, contact with infected household pets, travel to developing countries (campylobacters being among the causes of traveler's diarrhea; Chap. 131), and (occasionally) contact with an index case who is incontinent of stool.

Campylobacter infections are not rare. Several studies indicate that, in the United States, diarrheal disease due to campylobacters is more common than that due to *Salmonella* and *Shigella* combined. Infections occur throughout the year, but their incidence peaks during summer and early autumn. Persons of all ages are affected; however, attack rates for *C. jejuni* are highest among young children and young adults, while those for *C. fetus* are highest at the extremes of age. Systemic infections due to *C. fetus* (and to other *Campylobacter* and related species) are most common in compromised hosts. Persons at increased risk include those with AIDS, hypogammaglobulinemia, neoplasia, liver disease, diabetes mellitus, and generalized atherosclerosis as well as pregnant women. However, apparently healthy nonpregnant persons occasionally develop transient *Campylobacter* bacteremia as part of a gastrointestinal illness.

In developing countries, *C. jejuni* infections are hyperendemic, with the highest rates among children <2 years old. Infection rates fall with age, as does the illness-to-infection ratio; these observations suggest that frequent exposure to *C. jejuni* leads to the acquisition of immunity.

Table 158-1 Clinical Features Associated with Infection due to "Atypical" *Campylobacter* and Related Species Implicated as Causes of Human Illness

Species	Common Clinical Features	Less Common Clinical Features	Additional Information
Campylobacter coli	Fever, diarrhea, abdominal pain	Bacteremia[a]	Clinically indistinguishable from *C. jejuni*
Campylobacter fetus	Bacteremia,[a] sepsis, meningitis, vascular infections	Diarrhea, relapsing fevers	Not usually isolated from media containing cephalothin or incubated at 42°C
Campylobacter upsaliensis	Watery diarrhea, low-grade fever, abdominal pain	Bacteremia, abscesses	Difficult to isolate because of cephalothin susceptibility
Campylobacter lari	Abdominal pain, diarrhea	Colitis, appendicitis	Seagulls frequently colonized; organism often transmitted to humans via contaminated water
Campylobacter hyointestinalis	Watery or bloody diarrhea, vomiting, abdominal pain	Bacteremia	Causes proliferative enteritis in swine
Helicobacter fennelliae	Chronic mild diarrhea, abdominal cramps, proctitis	Bacteremia[a]	Best treated with fluoroquinolones
Helicobacter cinaedi	Chronic mild diarrhea, abdominal cramps, proctitis	Bacteremia[a]	Best treated with fluoroquinolones; identified in healthy hamsters
Campylobacter jejuni subspecies *doylei*	Diarrhea	Chronic gastritis, bacteremia[b]	Uncertain role as human pathogen
Arcobacter cryaerophila	Diarrhea	Bacteremia	Cultured under aerobic conditions
Arcobacter butzleri	Fever, diarrhea, abdominal pain, nausea	Bacteremia, appendicitis	Cultured under aerobic conditions; enzootic in nonhuman primates
Campylobacter sputorum	Pulmonary, perianal, groin, and axillary abscesses	Bacteremia	Three clinically relevant biovars: *C. sputorum* subspecies *sputorum*, *C. sputorum* subspecies *bubulus*, and *Campylobacter mucosalis*

[a] In immunocompromised hosts, especially HIV-infected persons.
[b] In children.

SOURCE: Adapted from Allos and Blaser.

PATHOLOGY AND PATHOGENESIS Many *C. jejuni* infections are subclinical, especially in partially immune hosts. Most illnesses occur within 2 to 4 days (range, 1 to 7 days) of exposure to the organism in food or water. The sites of tissue injury include the jejunum, ileum, and colon. Biopsies show an acute nonspecific inflammatory reaction, with neutrophils, monocytes, and eosinophils in the lamina propria, as well as damage to the epithelium, including loss of mucus, glandular degeneration, and crypt abscesses. Biopsy findings may be consistent with Crohn's disease or ulcerative colitis, but these "idiopathic" chronic inflammatory diseases should not be diagnosed unless infectious colitis, *specifically including* that due to infection with *Campylobacter*, has been ruled out.

The high frequency of *C. jejuni* infections and their severity and recurrence among hypogammaglobulinemic patients suggest that antibodies are important in protective immunity. The pathogenesis of infection is uncertain. Both the motility of the strain and its capacity to adhere to host tissues appear to favor disease, but classic enterotoxins and cytotoxins (although described) appear not to play any substantial role in tissue injury or disease production. The organisms have been visualized in the epithelium, albeit in low numbers. The documentation of a significant tissue response and occasionally of *C. jejuni* bacteremia further suggests that tissue invasion is clinically significant.

The pathogenesis of *C. fetus* infections is better defined. Virtually all clinical isolates of *C. fetus* possess a proteinaceous capsule-like structure (an S-layer) that renders the organism resistant to complement-mediated killing and opsonization. As a result, *C. fetus* can cause bacteremia and can seed sites beyond the intestinal tract. The ability of the organism to switch the S-layer proteins expressed, a phenomenon that results in antigenic variability, may contribute to the chronicity and high rate of recurrence of these infections in compromised hosts.

CLINICAL MANIFESTATIONS OF *C. JEJUNI* AND *C. FETUS* INFECTIONS The clinical features of infections due to all of the *Campylobacter* and related species causing enteric disease appear to be highly similar. There is often a prodrome, with fever, headache, myalgia, and/or malaise, 12 to 48 h before the onset of diarrheal symptoms. The most common symptoms of the intestinal phase are diarrhea, abdominal pain, and fever. The degree of diarrhea varies from several loose stools to grossly bloody stools; most patients presenting for medical attention have 10 or more bowel movements on the worst day of illness. Abdominal pain usually consists of cramp-

ing and may be the most prominent symptom. Pain usually is generalized but may become localized; *C. jejuni* infection may cause pseudoappendicitis. Fever may be the only initial manifestation of *C. jejuni* infection, a situation mimicking the early stages of typhoid fever. Febrile young children may develop convulsions. *Campylobacter* enteritis generally is self-limited; however, symptoms persist for longer than 1 week in 10 to 20% of patients seeking medical attention, and relapses occur in 5 to 10% of untreated patients.

C. fetus may cause a diarrheal illness similar to that due to *C. jejuni*, especially in normal hosts, or may cause either intermittent diarrhea or nonspecific abdominal pain without localizing signs. Sequelae are uncommon, and outcome is benign. *C. fetus* also may cause a prolonged relapsing systemic illness (with fever, chills, and myalgias) that has no obvious primary source; this manifestation is especially common in compromised hosts. Secondary seeding of an organ (e.g., meninges, brain, bone, urinary tract, or soft tissue) complicates the course, which may be fulminant. *C. fetus* infections have a tropism for vascular sites: endocarditis, mycotic aneurysm, and septic thrombophlebitis all may occur. Infection during pregnancy often leads to fetal death. *H. cinaedi* causes recurrent cellulitis with fever and bacteremia in immunocompromised hosts.

COMPLICATIONS Except in the case of infection with *C. fetus*, bacteremia is uncommon, developing most often in immunocompromised hosts and at the extremes of age. Three patterns of extraintestinal infection have been noted: (1) transient bacteremia in a normal host with enteritis (benign course, no specific treatment needed); (2) sustained bacteremia or focal infection in a normal host (bacteremia originating from enteritis, with patients responding well to antimicrobial therapy); and (3) sustained bacteremia or focal infection in a compromised host. Enteritis may not be clinically apparent. Antimicrobial therapy, possibly prolonged, is necessary for suppression or cure of the infection.

Campylobacter infections in patients with AIDS or hypogammaglobulinemia may be severe, persistent, and extraintestinal; relapse after cessation of therapy is common. Hypogammaglobulinemic patients also may develop osteomyelitis and an erysipelas-like rash.

Local suppurative complications of infection include cholecystitis, pancreatitis, and cystitis; distant complications include meningitis, endocarditis, arthritis, peritonitis, cellulitis, and septic abortion. All are rare. Hepatitis, interstitial nephritis, and the hemolytic-uremic syndrome occasionally complicate acute infection. Reactive arthritis and other rheumatologic complaints may develop several weeks after infection, especially in persons with the HLA-B27 phenotype. Guillain-Barré syndrome follows *Campylobacter* infections uncommonly (i.e., in 1 of every 1000 to 2000 cases). For certain *C. jejuni* serotypes, such as O19, Guillain-Barré syndrome may follow 1 in every 100 to 200 cases. Because of their high incidence, it is now estimated that *Campylobacter* infections may trigger 20 to 40% of all cases of Guillain-Barré syndrome.

LABORATORY FINDINGS   In patients with *Campylobacter* enteritis, peripheral leukocyte counts reflect the severity of the inflammatory process. However, stools from nearly all *Campylobacter*-infected patients presenting for medical attention in the United States contain leukocytes or erythrocytes. Fecal smears should be treated with Gram's or Wright's stain and examined in all suspected cases. When the diagnosis of *Campylobacter* enteritis is suspected on the basis of findings indicating inflammatory diarrhea (fever, fecal leukocytes), clinicians can ask the laboratory to attempt the visualization of organisms with characteristic vibrioid morphology by direct microscopic examination of stools with Gram's staining or to use phase-contrast or dark-field microscopy to identify the organisms' characteristic "darting" motility. Confirmation of the diagnosis of *Campylobacter* infection is based on identification of an isolate from cultures of stool, blood, or another site. *Campylobacter*-specific media should be used to culture stools from all patients with inflammatory or bloody diarrhea. Since all *Campylobacter* species are fastidious, they will not be isolated unless selective media or other selective techniques are used. Not all media are equally useful for isolation of the broad array of campylobacters; therefore, failure to isolate campylobacters from stool does not entirely rule out their presence. The detection of the organisms in stool almost always implies infection; there is a brief period of postconvalescent fecal carriage and no commensalism in humans. In contrast, *C. sputorum* and related organisms found in the oral cavity are commensals with rare pathogenic significance.

DIFFERENTIAL DIAGNOSIS   The symptoms of *Campylobacter* enteritis are not sufficiently unusual to distinguish this illness from that due to *Salmonella*, *Shigella*, or *Yersinia*, among other pathogens. The combination of fever and fecal leukocytes or erythrocytes is indicative of inflammatory diarrhea, and definitive diagnosis is based on culture or demonstration of the characteristic organisms on stained fecal smears. Similarly, extraintestinal *Campylobacter* illness is diagnosed by culture. Infection due to *Campylobacter* should be suspected in the setting of septic abortion and that due to *C. fetus* specifically in the setting of septic thrombophlebitis. It is important to reiterate that the presentation of *Campylobacter* enteritis may mimic that of ulcerative colitis or Crohn's disease, that *Campylobacter* enteritis is much more common than either of the latter (especially among young adults), and that biopsy may not distinguish among these entities. Thus a diagnosis of inflammatory bowel disease should not be made until *Campylobacter* infection has been ruled out, especially in persons with a history of foreign travel, significant animal contact, immunodeficiency, or practices incurring a high risk of transmission.

℞ **TREATMENT**   Fluid and electrolyte replacement is central to the treatment of diarrheal illnesses (Chap. 131). Even among patients presenting for medical attention with *Campylobacter* enteritis, fewer than half will clearly benefit from specific antimicrobial therapy. Indications for such therapy include high fever, bloody diarrhea, severe diarrhea, persistence for more than 1 week, and worsening of symptoms. A 5- to 7-day course of erythromycin (250 mg orally four times daily or—for children—30 to 50 mg/kg per day, in divided doses) is the regimen of choice. Although no relevant clinical trials have been conducted, the in vitro susceptibility of *Campylobacter* species to macrolides such as clarithromycin and azithromycin suggests that these antibiotics also would be useful therapeutic agents. An alternative regimen for adults is ciprofloxacin (500 mg orally twice daily) or another fluoroquinolone for 5 to 7 days, but resistance to this class of agents

is increasing. Other alternatives include tetracycline and furazolidone. Use of antimotility agents, which may prolong the duration of symptoms and has been associated with toxic megacolon and with death, is not recommended.

For systemic infections, treatment with gentamicin (1.7 mg/kg intravenously every 8 h after a loading dose of 2 mg/kg), imipenem (500 mg intravenously every 6 h), or chloramphenicol (50 mg/kg intravenously each day in three or four divided doses) should be started empirically, but susceptibility testing should then be performed. Ciprofloxacin and amoxicillin/clavulanate are alternative agents for susceptible strains. In the absence of immunocompromise or endovascular infections, therapy should be administered for 14 days. For immunocompromised patients with systemic infections due to *C. fetus* and for patients with endovascular infections, prolonged therapy (for up to 4 weeks) is usually necessary.

PROGNOSIS   Nearly all patients recover fully from *Campylobacter* enteritis, either spontaneously or after antimicrobial therapy. Volume depletion likely contributes to the few deaths that are reported. As stated above, occasional patients develop reactive arthritis or Guillain-Barré syndrome. Systemic infection with *C. fetus* is much more often fatal than that due to related species; this higher mortality reflects in part the population affected. Prognosis is dependent on the rapidity with which appropriate therapy is begun. Otherwise healthy hosts usually survive *C. fetus* infections without sequelae. Compromised hosts often have recurrent infections.

BIBLIOGRAPHY

ALLOS BM, BLASER MJ: *Campylobacter jejuni* and the expanding spectrum of related infections. Clin Infect Dis 20:1092, 1995

BLASER MJ et al: *Campylobacter* enteritis in the United States: A multicenter study. Ann Intern Med 98:360, 1983

LANG DR et al (eds): Development of Guillain-Barré syndrome following *Campylobacter* infection. J Infect Dis 176 (Suppl 2):S91, 1997

NACHAMKIN I et al (eds): *Campylobacter jejuni: Current Strategy and Future Trends.* Washington, American Society for Microbiology, 1992, pp 1–300

---

159   *Gerald T. Keusch, Matthew K. Waldor*

CHOLERA AND OTHER VIBRIOSES

Members of the genus *Vibrio* cause a number of important infectious syndromes. Classic among them is cholera, a devastating diarrheal disease caused by *V. cholerae* that has been responsible for seven global pandemics and much suffering over the past two centuries. Epidemic cholera remains a major public health concern and is dealt with at length in this chapter. Other vibrioses have also been described, including syndromes of diarrhea, soft tissue infection, or primary sepsis caused by additional named species in the genus *Vibrio*. These, too, are considered below.

All members of the genus are highly motile, facultatively anaerobic, curved gram-negative rods with one or more polar flagella. Except for *V. cholerae* and *V. mimicus*, all require salt for growth ("halophilic vibrios"). In nature, vibrios most commonly reside in tidal rivers and bays under conditions of moderate salinity. They proliferate in the summer months when water temperatures exceed 20°C. As might be expected, the illnesses they cause also increase in frequency during the warm months.

CHOLERA

DEFINITION   Cholera is an acute diarrheal disease that can, in a matter of hours, result in profound, rapidly progressive dehydration and death. Accordingly, cholera gravis (the severe form of cholera) is a much-feared disease, particularly in its epidemic presentation. Fortunately, prompt aggressive fluid repletion and supportive care can obviate the high mortality that it has historically wrought. While the term *cholera* has occasionally been applied to any severely dehydrating secretory diarrheal illness, whether infectious in etiology or not, it has generally referred to disease caused by *V. cholerae* serogroup O1. In 1992, however, a new epidemic serogroup (O139) that causes epidemic cholera emerged on the Indian subcontinent and has since killed many thousands of people.

ETIOLOGY AND EPIDEMIOLOGY The species *V. cholerae* comprises a host of organisms classified on the basis of the carbohydrate determinants of their lipopolysaccharide (LPS) O antigens. Some 155 serogroups have now been recognized. They are divided into those that agglutinate in antisera to the O1 group antigen (*V. cholerae* O1) and those that do not (non-O1 *V. cholerae*). Although some non-O1 *V. cholerae* serogroups have occasionally caused sporadic outbreaks of diarrhea, serogroup O1 was, until the emergence of serogroup O139, the exclusive cause of epidemic cholera. *V. cholerae* O139 (also called *V. cholerae* Bengal) is discussed in greater detail below.

V. cholerae O1 exists in two biotypes, *classical* and *El Tor*, that are distinguished on the basis of a number of characteristics, including phage susceptibility and hemolysin production. Each biotype is further subdivided into two serotypes, termed *Inaba* and *Ogawa*. Serotyping is a useful tool in field epidemiologic studies. Newer molecular epidemiologic techniques, such as ribotyping and other gene-based methods, now make it possible to trace the source and origin of cholera strains from around the world.

The natural habitat of *V. cholerae* is coastal salt water and brackish estuaries, where the organism lives in close relation to plankton and where it may survive in a viable but nonculturable form. Humans become infected incidentally but, once infected, can act as vehicles for spread. Ingestion of water contaminated by human feces is the most common means of acquisition of *V. cholerae*. Consumption of contaminated food in the home, in restaurants, or from street vendors can also contribute to spread. There is no known animal reservoir. While the infectious dose is relatively high, it is markedly reduced in hypochlorhydric persons, in those using antacids, and when gastric acidity is buffered by a meal. Cholera is predominantly a pediatric disease in endemic areas, but it affects adults and children equally when newly introduced into a population. In endemic areas, the disease is more common in the summer and fall months. While this seasonality has not been explained fully, it may be due to environmental conditions that affect the multiplication of vibrios or to seasonal alterations in human behavior that affect contact with water. Asymptomatic infections are frequent and more common with the El Tor than the classical biotype. In endemic areas, children <2 years of age are less likely to develop severe cholera than are older children, perhaps because of passive immunity acquired from breast milk. For unexplained reasons, susceptibility to cholera is significantly influenced by ABO blood group status; those with type O blood are at greatest risk, while those with type AB are at least risk.

Cholera is native to the Ganges delta in the Indian subcontinent. Since 1817, seven global pandemics have occurred. The current (seventh) pandemic—the first due to the El Tor biotype—began in Indonesia in 1961 and spread throughout Asia as *V. cholerae* El Tor displaced the endemic classical strain in many areas. It briefly invaded Europe, but effective public health measures and the high level of sanitation combined to limit its impact. In the early 1970s, El Tor cholera exploded in Africa, causing major epidemics before becoming a persistent endemic problem. Its recent history in Africa has been punctuated by severe outbreaks, often fed by the chaos of war and genocide. Such was the case in the camps for Rwandan refugees set up in 1994 around Goma, Zaire. Tens of thousands of cases occurred and mortality was high. In 1995, the occurrence of hundreds of cases in Romania and the Black Sea states of the former Soviet Union demonstrated the potential of this organism to cause epidemics whenever public health measures break down.

Since 1973, sporadic endemic infections due to vibrios related to the seventh-pandemic strain have been recognized along the U.S. Gulf Coast of Louisiana and Texas. These infections are typically associated with the consumption of contaminated, locally harvested shellfish. Occasionally, cases in U S. locations remote from the Gulf Coast have been linked to shipped-in Gulf Coast seafood.

Although the event was long expected, it was not until 1991 that the current cholera pandemic reached Latin America. Beginning along the Peruvian coast in January 1991, the disease was carried by fishermen to Ecuador and Colombia. It then spread in an explosive epidemic to virtually all of South and Central America and to Mexico (Fig. 159-1). About 400,000 cases were reported in the first year of the outbreak, and >1 million had been reported by the end of 1994. While the cumulative mortality rate has been <1%, the mortality rate approached 30% in the communities first affected, where a lack of familiarity with the disease led initially to the deployment of wholly ineffective treatment. Intensive education of health care providers and of the community at large has enhanced awareness of the disease and its appropriate management and has greatly diminished mortality. As it did in Africa two decades earlier, the epidemic El Tor strain proved capable of establishing itself in inland waters rather than in its classic niche of coastal salt waters; the organism has already become endemic in many of the Latin American countries into which it was recently introduced.

Cases linked to the Latin American epidemic have occurred in the United States. For example, 11 people in New York and New Jersey were infected in two separate outbreaks in 1991 after eating boiled crabmeat illegally transported by travelers from Ecuador. Although secondary spread of this strain has not taken place in the United States, these events underscore the need for vigilance among health care professionals, even in locations remote from an epidemic.

In October 1992, a large-scale outbreak of clinical cholera occurred in the port city of Madras and surrounding towns in southern India.

★ Initial Epidemics
January 1991

----- August 1991

—— February 1992

▬▬ November 1994

FIGURE 159-1 Spread of *Vibrio cholerae* O1 in the Americas, 1991–1994. (*Courtesy of Dr. Robert V. Tauxe, Centers for Disease Control and Prevention, Atlanta.*)

FIGURE 159-2 Spread of *Vibrio cholerae* O139 in the Indian subcontinent and elsewhere in Asia, 1992–1994. *(Courtesy of Dr. Robert V. Tauxe, Centers for Disease Control and Prevention, Atlanta.)*

Legend:
- ✳ Initial Epidemic, October 92
- —— March 1993
- —— October 1994

PATHOGENESIS In the final analysis, cholera is a toxin-mediated disease. Its characteristic watery diarrhea is due to the action of cholera toxin (CTX), a potent protein enterotoxin elaborated by the organism following its colonization of the small intestine. The bacterial properties that facilitate intestinal colonization are incompletely understood. For *V. cholerae* to colonize the small intestine and produce CTX, it must first recognize, contend with, and traverse several hostile environments. The first of these is the acidic milieu of the stomach. To elude the bactericidal effects of gastric acidity, *V. cholerae* relies, at least in part, on a relatively large inoculum size (compared to that needed for colonization by *Shigella*, for instance). The organism must next traverse the mucous layer lining the small bowel. *V. cholerae* chemotaxis and motility and a variety of proteases may allow the organism to traverse this gel covering the intestinal epithelium. Adherence to the intestinal epithelium is believed to be mediated by the toxin-coregulated pilus (TCP), so named because its synthesis is regulated in parallel with that of CTX. Studies of volunteers have established that TCP is essential for *V. cholerae* intestinal colonization. Other *V. cholerae* gene products known to be important in intestinal colonization of experimental animals include accessory colonization factors ABCD, a cell-associated hemagglutinin, iron and magnesium transport proteins, and purine and biotin biosynthesis enzymes.

CTX, TCP, and several other virulence factors, including accessory colonization factors and various outer-membrane proteins, are coordinately regulated by the *toxR* gene product. ToxR protein is a "master switch" that modulates the expression of virulence genes in response to signals that it senses within the environment of the host via a cascade of regulatory proteins. Coordinate regulation of virulence factor expression presumably enables the organism to tailor its repertoire of proteins to suit its needs as it passes from one microenvi-

The etiologic agent proved to be a novel strain of *V. cholerae* belonging neither to the O1 serogroup that typically causes epidemic cholera nor to any of the 137 other serogroups known at the time. This strain spread rapidly up and down the coast of the Bay of Bengal, reaching Bangladesh in December 1992. There alone, it caused more than 100,000 cases of cholera in the first 3 months of 1993. It subsequently spread across the Indian subcontinent and to neighboring countries, affecting Pakistan, Nepal, western China, Thailand, and Malaysia by the end of 1994 (Fig. 159-2). The organism has since been designated *V. cholerae* O139 Bengal in recognition of its novel O antigen and its geographic origin.

The clinical manifestations and epidemiologic features of the disease caused by *V. cholerae* O139 Bengal are indistinguishable from those of O1 cholera. Immunity to the latter, however, is not protective against the former. Thus, although O139 Bengal cholera has been restricted almost exclusively to O1-endemic areas, it has affected patients of all ages, with most cases in adults. Moreover, populations into which *V. cholerae* O139 Bengal has been introduced have responded as virgin populations with respect to severe, lethal cholera. Because naturally acquired immunity to *V. cholerae* O1 does not cross-protect against *V. cholerae* O139 Bengal, vaccines being developed against the former are unlikely to be effective against the latter.

Like the O1 epidemics in cholera-naive areas before it, the O139 epidemic was initially devastating. Some authorities believed that the emergence of *V. cholerae* O139 signaled the beginning of the eighth global cholera pandemic. Indeed, just as O1 El Tor replaced the classical biotype that preceded it, O139 Bengal in 1993 rapidly replaced O1 El Tor as the most common environmental isolate and the predominant cause of clinical cholera in the areas in which it had appeared (Fig. 159-3). However, by the beginning of 1994, O1 El Tor had unexpectedly resumed its dominance in Bangladesh, relegating O139 Bengal cholera to the status of a background endemic infection. In some locales O1 *V. cholerae* remains dominant; in others O139 periodically reemerges. Nevertheless, the potential for global spread of O139 Bengal was underscored by an intercontinental food-borne outbreak that occurred in early 1994 among American and British passengers on a cruise ship in Southeast Asia. Six of the 630 travelers became ill, their symptoms beginning only after they returned home.

FIGURE 159-3 Isolations of *Vibrio cholerae* O1 and *V. cholerae* O139 in Bangladesh, 1993–1994, by month. *(Courtesy of Dr. John Albert and Dr. A.S.G. Faruque, International Centre for Diarrhoeal Disease Research, Bangladesh.)*

ronment to another. Coordinate regulation of virulence gene expression by a central sensor-effect protein like ToxR has become a paradigm for similar systems that have been discovered in a wide range of pathogenic bacteria.

Once established in the human small bowel, the organism produces CTX, which consists of a monomeric enzymatic moiety (the A subunit) and a pentameric binding moiety (the B subunit). The B pentamer binds to G_{M1} ganglioside, a glycolipid on the surface of jejunal epithelial cells that serves as the toxin receptor and makes possible the delivery of the A subunit to its cytosolic target. The activated A subunit (A_1) irreversibly transfers ADP-ribose from nicotinamide adenine dinucleotide to its specific target protein, the GTP-binding regulatory component of adenylate cyclase in intestinal epithelial cells. In this configuration, this G protein permanently upregulates the cyclase catalytic subunit; the result is the intracellular accumulation of high levels of cyclic AMP. In intestinal epithelial cells, cyclic AMP inhibits the absorptive sodium transport system in villus cells and activates the excretory chloride transport system in crypt cells, and these events lead to the accumulation of sodium chloride in the intestinal lumen. Since water moves passively to maintain osmolality, isotonic fluid accumulates in the lumen. When the volume of that fluid exceeds the capacity of the rest of the gut to resorb it, watery diarrhea results. Unless the wasted fluid and electrolytes are adequately replaced, shock (due to profound dehydration) and acidosis (due to loss of bicarbonate) follow.

Although perturbation of the adenylate cyclase pathway is the primary mechanism by which CTX causes excess fluid secretion, it is not the only one. Increasing evidence indicates that CTX also enhances intestinal secretion via prostaglandins and/or neural histamine receptors. It is possible that the redundancy of secretory mechanisms activated by CTX accounts for the profound diarrhea and dehydration characteristic of severe cholera.

The genes encoding CTX (*ctxAB*) are part of the genome of a bacteriophage designated CTXΦ. The receptor for this phage on the *V. cholerae* surface is the essential *V. cholerae* intestinal colonization factor TCP. Following infection of TCP+ *ctxAB*− *V. cholerae* cells, the CTXΦ genome stably integrates at a specific site on the *V. cholerae* chromosome. Since *ctxAB* is part of a mobile genetic element (CTXΦ), horizontal transfer of this bacteriophage may account for the emergence of new toxigenic *V. cholerae* serogroups. In addition, since the CTXΦ receptor TCP is a *V. cholerae* host colonization factor, it is possible that CTXΦ infection of TCP+ *ctxAB*− *V. cholerae* strains occurs primarily within the human intestine. Many of the other genes important for *V. cholerae* pathogenicity, including the genes encoding the biosynthesis of TCP, those encoding accessory colonization factors, and those regulating virulence gene expression, are clustered together on one of the two *V. cholerae* chromosomes. This cluster of virulence genes is referred to as the *V. cholerae pathogenicity island*. Similar clustering of virulence genes is found in other bacterial pathogens. It is believed that these pathogenicity islands have been acquired by horizontal gene transfer.

Molecular analysis of *V. cholerae* O139 Bengal has suggested the basis of its origin and the reasons it was able to cause an explosive epidemic of cholera. Both phenotypically and genotypically, O139 Bengal is closely related to the O1 El Tor strains of the seventh pandemic, and it seems to have arisen from them by horizontal gene transfer. It shares the virulence attributes and general pathogenic mechanisms of O1 vibrios, including possession of the same CTX prophage and the same TCP. *V. cholerae* O139 Bengal is in fact virtually identical to the seventh-pandemic strains of *V. cholerae* O1 El Tor except for two important differences: production of the novel O139 LPS and of an immunologically related O-antigen polysaccharide capsule. Both of these molecules are putative virulence factors, independently enhancing colonization in a murine infection model. The ability to produce the O139 LPS is due to a replacement of a 22-kb DNA segment encoding O1 antigen biosynthesis with a 35-kb segment containing the genes encoding O139 LPS and capsule biosynthesis. Encapsulation is not a feature of O1 strains and may explain the resistance of O139

strains to human serum in vitro as well as the occasional development of O139 bacteremia.

CLINICAL MANIFESTATIONS After a 24- to 48-h incubation period, cholera begins with the sudden onset of painless watery diarrhea that may quickly become voluminous and is often followed shortly by vomiting. In severe cases, stool volume can exceed 250 mL/kg in the first 24 h. If fluids and electrolytes are not replaced, hypovolemic shock and death ensue. Fever is usually absent. Muscle cramps due to electrolyte disturbances are common. The stool has a characteristic appearance: a nonbilious, gray, slightly cloudy fluid with flecks of mucus, no blood, and a somewhat sweet, inoffensive odor. It has been called "rice-water" stool because of its resemblance to the water in which rice has been washed. Clinical symptoms parallel volume contraction: At losses of 3 to 5% of normal body weight, thirst develops; at 5 to 8%, postural hypotension, weakness, tachycardia, and decreased skin turgor are documented; and at >10%, oliguria, weak or absent pulses, sunken eyes (and, in infants, sunken fontanelles), wrinkled ("washerwoman") skin, somnolence, and coma are characteristic. Complications derive exclusively from the effects of volume and electrolyte depletion and include renal failure due to acute tubular necrosis. Thus, if the patient is adequately treated with fluid and salt, complications are averted and the process is self-limited, resolving in a few days.

Laboratory data usually reveal an elevated hematocrit (due to hemoconcentration) in nonanemic patients; mild neutrophilic leukocytosis; elevated levels of blood urea nitrogen and creatinine consistent with prerenal azotemia; normal sodium, potassium, and chloride levels; a markedly reduced bicarbonate level (<15 mmol/L); and an elevated anion gap (due to increases in serum lactate, protein, and phosphate). Arterial pH is usually low (about 7.2).

DIAGNOSIS The clinical suspicion of cholera can be confirmed by the identification of *V. cholerae* in stool; however, the organism must be specifically sought. In experienced hands, it can be detected directly by dark-field microscopy on a wet mount of fresh stool, and its serotype can be discerned by immobilization with Inaba- or Ogawa-specific antiserum. Laboratory isolation of the organism requires the use of a selective medium. The best of these is thiosulfate–citrate–bile salts–sucrose (TCBS) agar, on which the organism grows as a flat yellow colony. If a delay in sample processing is expected, Carey-Blair transport medium and/or alkaline-peptone water-enrichment medium should be inoculated as well. In endemic areas there is little need for biochemical confirmation and characterization, although these tasks may be worthwhile in places where *V. cholerae* is an uncommon isolate. Standard microbiologic biochemical testing for Enterobacteriaceae will suffice for identification of *V. cholerae*. All vibrios are oxidase-positive. *V. cholerae* can be distinguished from the otherwise similar *V. mimicus* by its ability to ferment sucrose.

The yield of stool cultures for the diagnosis of *V. cholerae* infection declines late in the course of the illness or when effective antibacterial therapy is initiated. Although not generally evaluable in clinical laboratories, serum vibriocidal antibody titers can be used to confirm the diagnosis in non-cholera-endemic regions of the world. Monoclonal antibody–based diagnostic kits and methods based on the polymerase chain reaction and on DNA probes have been developed for *V. cholerae* O1 and O139 but are unlikely to become available in U.S. clinical laboratories.

TREATMENT Cholera is simple to treat; only the rapid and adequate replacement of fluids, electrolytes, and base is required. The mortality rate for appropriately treated disease is usually <1%. However, analysis of a large outbreak of cholera among airline travelers from an endemic country to the United States revealed frequent misdiagnoses by U.S. health professionals and poor appreciation on their part of the principles of management. Compounding these problems was the general unavailability of appropriate oral fluids. Even intravenous fluid therapy typically was not optimal.

It has been proved conclusively that fluid may be given orally. This approach takes advantage of the hexose-Na⁺ cotransport mechanism to move Na⁺ across the gut mucosa together with an actively transported molecule such as glucose. Since Na⁺ losses in the stool are high, a fluid containing Na⁺ at 90 mmol/L has been recommended by the World Health Organization (WHO) (Table 159-1). This amount of Na⁺ is higher than that needed to treat diarrhea due to most other causes. The solution is safe, even for infants, if its intake is alternated with the consumption of sodium-free fluids such as breast milk or water. For the sake of simplicity, WHO advises routine use of this single solution for diarrheal disease rather than attempts to choose among multiple formulations according to etiology.

Cereal-based formulations are receiving increased attention as alternative oral rehydration solutions. Because of their lower osmolarity, they may reduce stool output. A mixture with a lower sugar and salt content has also been evaluated in cholera patients, with favorable results. However, concerns have been raised over the safety of its use—in particular, whether it could cause significant hyponatremia in patients with moderate or severe diarrhea. Because commercial oral rehydration solutions also contain concentrations of glucose and sodium lower than those of the WHO formulation, they should not yet be used routinely to treat cholera.

For initial management of severely dehydrated patients, intravenous fluid replacement is preferable, if available. Because profound acidosis (pH < 7.2) is common in this group, Ringer's lactate is the best choice among commercial products (Table 159-2). It must be used with additional potassium supplements, preferably given by mouth. The total fluid deficit in severely dehydrated patients (≥10% of body weight) can be replaced safely within the first 4 h of therapy, half within the first hour. Thereafter, oral therapy can usually be initiated, with the goal of maintaining fluid intake equal to fluid output. However, patients with continued large-volume diarrhea may require prolonged intravenous treatment to keep up with gastrointestinal fluid losses. Severe hypokalemia can develop but will respond to potassium given either intravenously or orally. In the absence of adequate staff to monitor the patient's progress, the oral route of rehydration and potassium replacement is safer than the intravenous route and is physiologically regulated by thirst and urine output.

Although not necessary for cure, the use of an antibiotic to which the organism is susceptible will diminish the duration and volume of fluid loss and will hasten clearance of the organism from the stool. Single-dose tetracycline (2 g) or doxycycline (300 mg) is effective in adults but is not recommended for children under 8 years of age because of possible deposition in bone and developing teeth. Emerging drug resistance is an ever-present concern. For adults with cholera in areas where tetracycline resistance is prevalent, ciprofloxacin—either in a single dose (30 mg/kg, not to exceed a total dose of 1 g) or in a short course (15 mg/kg bid for 3 days, not to exceed a total daily dose of 1 g)—or erythromycin (a total of 40 mg/kg daily in three divided doses for 3 days) is a clinically effective substitute. Both drugs are highly effective in reducing total stool output, and each is significantly better than trimethoprim-sulfamethoxazole. Because of the high cost of quinolones, WHO recommends erythromycin as the first alternative to tetracycline. For children, furazolidone has been the recommended agent and trimethoprim-sulfamethoxazole the second choice. It is of note that *V. cholerae* O139 is often resistant to both of these drugs but is susceptible to quinolones, erythromycin, tetracycline, and ampicillin (among others). Because of cost and/or toxicity issues related to the other drugs, erythromycin is a good choice for pediatric cholera, especially where O139 Bengal is present. The efficacy of single-dose erythromycin therapy for cholera has not been demonstrated.

CONTROL In outbreaks, efforts should first be made to identify case contacts and to treat incubating carriers. Next, epidemiologic studies should be undertaken to establish the modes of transmission to define the best strategy to interrupt them. Both the establishment of rehydration centers and instruction in rehydration techniques are essential to the reduction of mortality. Immunization in these circumstances is not an effective means of control.

PREVENTION Provision of safe water and facilities for sanitary disposal of feces, improved nutrition, and attention to food preparation and storage in the household could significantly reduce the incidence of cholera. Much effort has been devoted to the development of an effective cholera vaccine over the past two decades, with a particular focus on oral vaccine strains. Traditional killed cholera vaccine given intramuscularly provides little protection to nonimmune subjects and predictably causes adverse effects, including pain at the injection site, malaise, and fever. The vaccine's limited efficacy is at least partially due to its failure to induce a local immune response at the intestinal mucosal surface.

Two types of oral cholera vaccines are under development. The first is a killed whole-cell (WC) vaccine. Two formulations of the killed WC vaccine have been prepared: one that also contains the nontoxic B subunit of CTX (WC/BS) and one composed solely of killed bacteria. In field trials in Bangladesh, both of the killed vaccines were compared with placebo and conferred ~50% protection over a 3-year evaluation period. The protective efficacy of WC/BS was superior to that of WC during the initial 8 months of follow-up (69 versus 41%) but equivalent or inferior thereafter. Immunity was relatively sustained in persons vaccinated at an age of >5 years but was not well sustained in younger vaccinees.

The second approach is that of a live attenuated vaccine strain developed, for example, by the isolation or creation of mutants lacking active CTX. Three criteria must be met in live vaccine design: The vaccine strain must induce protective immunity, it must be safe to administer, and it must be minimally reactogenic. *Safety criteria* include the vaccine strain's potential to regain virulence, either spontaneously or via horizontal gene transfer from environmental strains, as well as its potential to donate virulence genes to other strains. *Reactogenicity* refers to its potential to cause symptoms such as fever or diarrhea in vaccinees.

Strain CVD 103-HgR, an oral live cholera vaccine licensed for immunization of travelers in Europe, is derived from a classical biotype strain of *V. cholerae* by the deletion of the CTX A subunit gene and the insertion in the hemolysin gene of a mercury resistance marker.

Table 159-2 Electrolyte Composition of Cholera Stool and of Intravenous Rehydration Solution

Substance	Concentration, mmol/L			
	Na⁺	K⁺	Cl⁻	Base
Stool				
Adult	135	15	90	30
Child	100	25	90	30
Ringer's lactate	130	4[a]	109	28

[a] Potassium supplements, preferably administered by mouth, are required to replace the usual potassium losses from stool.

Table 159-1 Composition of World Health Organization Oral Rehydration Solution (ORS)[a,b]

Constituent	Concentration, mmol/L
Na⁺	90
K⁺	20
Cl⁻	80
Citrate[c]	10
Glucose	110

[a] Contains (per package, to be added to 1 L of drinking water): NaCl, 3.5 g; Na₃C₆H₅O₇·2H₂O, 2.9 g; KCl, 1.5 g; and glucose, 20 g.

[b] If prepackaged ORS is unavailable, a simple homemade alternative can be prepared by combining 5 g NaCl (about 1 level teaspoon) with either 50 g precooked rice cereal or 40 g sucrose in 1 L of drinking water. In that case, potassium must be supplied separately (e.g., in orange juice or coconut water).

[c] 10 mmol citrate per liter, which supplies 30 mmol HCO₃/L.

This strain has been extensively tested in volunteers; although it is poorly excreted in the stool of human vaccinees, a single dose produces a significant increase in the titer of vibriocidal antibody in ~75% of recipients, including children between the ages of 2 and 4 years, with almost no reactogenicity. Studies in volunteers demonstrate that this vaccine is more effective against classical than against El Tor cholera. Unfortunately, in a large field trial in Indonesian children, this vaccine failed to induce protection against clinical cholera.

Other live attenuated vaccine candidate strains have been prepared from El Tor and O139 *V. cholerae*. In studies in volunteers, these vaccine strains have often exhibited significant reactogenicity whose cause (given the absence of active CTX) is unclear. Reactogenicity may result from the production of another toxic moiety (e.g., the hemagglutinin/protease or the RTX toxin) by the live attenuated strain. Alternatively, intestinal colonization itself may result in reactogenicity. These El Tor– and O139-derived live vaccine strains are therefore at least several years away from potential licensing. Because of the minimal efficacy of existing parenteral vaccines, cholera immunization is recommended for U.S. travelers only if it is mandated by the countries they plan to visit.

OTHER *VIBRIO* SPECIES

In recent years, the taxonomic, epidemiologic, pathophysiologic, and clinical features of vibrios that do not cause clinical cholera have become increasingly well understood. Ten human pathogens are currently recognized in the genus *Vibrio*. Included are species associated primarily with gastrointestinal illness (*V. parahaemolyticus*, non-O1 *V. cholerae*, *V. mimicus*, *V. fluvialis*, *V. hollisae*, and *V. furnissii*) and species associated primarily with soft tissue infections (*V. vulnificus*, *V. alginolyticus*, and *V. damsela*). In addition, *V. vulnificus* has emerged as a cause of primary sepsis in certain compromised hosts. Vibrios are abundant in coastal waters the world over and tend to concentrate in the tissues of filter-feeding mollusks. Under optimal conditions, some can double in number in as little as 9 min. Consequently, seawater and raw or undercooked shellfish are important sources of human infection (Table 159-3). Vibrios grow best at temperatures of 28°C to 44°C but not at all below 4°C or above 60°C. Most can be cultured on blood or MacConkey agar, each of which contains enough salt to support the growth of the halophilic organisms (≥0.5%). As with *V. cholerae*, TCBS is the best selective medium. The species can be differentiated in the laboratory by standard biochemical tests. The most important members of the group are *V. parahaemolyticus* and *V. vulnificus*. These and selected other species are considered below in greater detail.

SPECIES ASSOCIATED PRIMARILY WITH GASTROINTESTINAL ILLNESS *V. parahaemolyticus* First implicated as a cause of enteritis by Japanese workers in 1953, *V. parahaemolyticus* is now recognized as an important intestinal pathogen in many parts of the world. In one study from Japan, 24% of reported cases of food poisoning were attributed to this organism, presumably owing to the widespread consumption of raw seafood there. In the United States, *V. parahaemolyticus* has been responsible for several well-documented common-source outbreaks of diarrhea, typically linked to ingestion of undercooked or improperly handled seafood or of other foods that have been contaminated by seawater. Most reports have come from the Atlantic Coast, the Gulf of Mexico, and Hawaii. The organism is ubiquitous in marine environments and is able to grow in saline concentrations as high as 8 to 10%. The ability to cause hemolysis on Wagatsuma agar (known as the *Kanagawa phenomenon*) is closely linked to enteropathogenicity. In one study, 96.5% of isolates from patients with diarrhea were hemolytic versus only ~1% of iso-

Table 159-3 Features of Selected Noncholera Vibrioses

Organism	Vehicle or Activity	Host at Risk	Syndrome
V. parahaemolyticus	Shellfish, seawater	Normal	Gastroenteritis
	Seawater	Normal	Wound infection
Non-O1 *V. cholerae*	Shellfish, travel	Normal	Gastroenteritis
	Seawater	Normal	Wound infection, otitis media
V. vulnificus	Shellfish	Immunosuppressed[a]	Sepsis, secondary cellulitis
	Seawater	Normal	Wound infection, cellulitis
V. alginolyticus	Seawater	Normal	Wound infection, cellulitis, otitis
	Seawater	Burned, other immunosuppressed	Sepsis

[a] Especially with liver disease or hemochromatosis.

lates from seawater. Hemolysis is attributed to a 42-kDa heat-stable protein, the exact pathophysiologic role of which is uncertain. The mechanism by which *V. parahaemolyticus* causes diarrhea is not clear.

V. parahaemolyticus has been associated with two distinct gastrointestinal presentations. The more common is a syndrome of watery diarrhea, accompanied in most cases by abdominal cramps, nausea, and vomiting and in about one-quarter of cases by fever and chills. The incubation period ranges from 4 h to 4 days, and the symptomatic period lasts for a median of 3 days. The vast majority of North American cases have been of this type. The less common syndrome is one of dysentery, described in India and Bangladesh and characterized by severe abdominal cramps, nausea, vomiting, and bloody or mucoid stools. Most cases of either type are self-limited and require neither antimicrobial treatment nor hospitalization. Severe infections are associated with underlying diseases, including diabetes, preexisting liver disease, iron-overload states, or immunosuppression. The occasional severe case should be treated with fluid replacement and antibiotics, as described above for cholera. Death is very rare. There are no reliable differential diagnostic features. *V. parahaemolyticus* should be considered as a possible cause in all cases of diarrhea that can be epidemiologically linked to seafood consumption or to the sea itself.

In addition to gastrointestinal disease, *V. parahaemolyticus* is a rare cause of extraintestinal infections, including wound infections, otitis, and—very rarely—sepsis.

Non-O1 *V. cholerae* The heterogeneous non-O1 *V. cholerae* organisms are biochemically indistinguishable from *V. cholerae* O1 on routine testing but fail to agglutinate in O1 antiserum. While technically a non-O1 vibrio, *V. cholerae* O139 Bengal is not grouped with these pathogens because of its potential to cause epidemic cholera, as detailed above. Non-O1 *V. cholerae* strains have been responsible for several well-described food-borne outbreaks of gastroenteritis as well as for sporadic cases of otitis media, wound infection, and bacteremia. About half of all U.S. isolates are obtained from stool specimens. Like other vibrios, non-O1 *V. cholerae* organisms are widely distributed in marine environments; unlike most other vibrios, however, they require only trace amounts of NaCl to survive (i.e., they are nonhalophilic). Recognized U.S. cases invariably have been associated either with the consumption of raw oysters or with recent travel, typically to Mexico. The clinical spectrum of diarrheal disease caused by non-O1 *V. cholerae* is broad and likely reflects the heterogeneous virulence attributes of the group. Occasional isolates make a protein enterotoxin very similar to CTX. Others produce cytotoxins, hemolysins, or invasins.

Gastroenteritis due to non-O1 *V. cholerae* typically has an incubation period of <2 days. Stools may be copious and watery. On occasion, diarrhea may leave the patient severely dehydrated, as in cholera. Alternatively, the stools may be partly formed, less voluminous, and bloody or mucoid. Abdominal cramps, nausea, vomiting, and fever are often reported. In one series, 11% of patients were hospitalized; in another, the figure was 50%. The duration of illness ranges from about 2 to 7 days. As in cholera, patients with significant dehydration should be treated with oral or intravenous fluids. The role of antibiotics is uncertain.

Wound infection and otitis media each account for ~10% of non-O1 *V. cholerae* isolates. Bacteremia accounts for another 20%. Patients with extraintestinal infection often have a history of occupational or recreational exposure to seawater. Bacteremia is more likely to develop in the presence of liver disease. Extraintestinal infections should be treated with antibiotics. There is a paucity of information to guide the choice of a specific agent and schedule. Most strains are sensitive in vitro to tetracycline, chloramphenicol, and other agents.

SPECIES ASSOCIATED PRIMARILY WITH SOFT TISSUE INFECTION OR BACTEREMIA *V. vulnificus* Though it represents only a small minority of the *Vibrio* species found in nature (4% of Atlantic Coast isolates in one study), *V. vulnificus* is perhaps the most important cause of severe *Vibrio* infections in the United States (0.8 cases per 100,000 population in one study from Louisiana). Formerly included in the species *V. parahaemolyticus*, *V. vulnificus* was distinguished in the 1970s by its ability to ferment lactose and to cause distinct clinical syndromes. Like most vibrios, it proliferates in the warm summer months. It requires a saline environment for growth but prefers concentrations lower than those preferred by *V. parahaemolyticus* and *V. alginolyticus* (range, up to ~8%; optimal, ~1%). Infections in humans typically occur in coastal states between May and October and most often involve men over age 40. *V. vulnificus* has been linked unequivocally to two distinct syndromes: primary sepsis, typically in patients with antecedent liver disease, and primary wound infections, usually in people without underlying disease. Some authors have suggested that this organism causes gastroenteritis, but the evidence for this association is tenuous.

V. vulnificus is remarkably invasive in animal models. It is endowed with a number of virulence attributes, including an antiphagocytic capsule, serum resistance, a cytotoxin/hemolysin (the organism is Kanagawa-positive), collagenase, elastolytic protease, phospholipase, and siderophores. Its virulence, as measured by the 50% lethal dose in mice, is markedly enhanced under conditions of iron overload, a fact consonant with its propensity to infect patients with hemochromatosis.

Primary sepsis occurs most commonly in patients with cirrhosis or hemochromatosis but has also developed in patients with hematopoietic disorders or chronic renal insufficiency, in persons using immunosuppressive medications or alcohol, and (rarely) in individuals without apparent underlying disease. Most of those affected have ingested raw oysters within 2 days of onset (median incubation period, 16 h). The process begins precipitously with malaise, chills, fever (mean temperature, 39.8°C), and prostration. Hypotension develops in one-third of cases, often by the time of admission. Cutaneous manifestations, which develop in three-quarters of cases (usually by 36 h after onset), typically involve the extremities—lower more often than upper. A common sequence is the evolution of erythematous patches followed by ecchymoses, vesicles, and bullae. (Indeed, the presence of sepsis and bullous skin lesions suggests the diagnosis in an appropriate setting.) Necrosis and sloughing may occur. Laboratory study reveals leukopenia more often than leukocytosis, thrombocytopenia, and (occasionally) elevated levels of fibrin split products. *V. vulnificus* can be cultured from blood or cutaneous lesions.

Mortality approaches 50%, with most deaths due to uncontrolled sepsis. Accordingly, prompt treatment is critical and should include empirical antibiotic administration, aggressive debridement, and general supportive care. *V. vulnificus* is sensitive to a number of antimicrobials in vitro, including tetracycline, gentamicin, and third-generation cephalosporins. No compelling clinical data from studies of humans support the preferential use of any one of these agents. Tetracycline is demonstrably superior in a murine model and on that basis is considered the drug of choice (0.5 to 1 g intravenously every 12 h), either alone or in combination with gentamicin. The duration of therapy is guided by the clinical response.

Wound infections with *V. vulnificus* can develop in patients with or without underlying disease and invariably follow contact of seawater with either a prior or a fresh wound. The incubation period is brief (4 h to 4 days; mean, 12 h). The disease begins with swelling, erythema, and—in many cases—intense pain around the wound. Rapidly spreading cellulitis follows, with vesicular, bullous, or necrotic lesions developing in some instances. Metastatic events do not generally occur. Fever (median temperature, 38.9°C) and leukocytosis are demonstrable in most cases. The organism can be cultured from skin lesions and occasionally from blood. Prompt antibiotic therapy and debridement are usually curative.

V. alginolyticus This species was first recognized as a human pathogen in 1973 and is now known to cause occasional wound, ear, and eye infections. It is the most salt-tolerant of the vibrios, able to grow in concentrations >10%. Most clinical isolates come from superinfected wounds, which presumably became contaminated at the beach. Infection varies in severity but is generally not serious and responds well to antibiotic therapy and drainage. A few reports have described otitis externa, otitis media, or conjunctivitis. Therapy with tetracycline is usually curative. *V. alginolyticus* is a rare cause of bacteremia in immunocompromised hosts.

BIBLIOGRAPHY

ALI A et al: *Vibrio vulnificus* sepsis in solid organ transplantation: A medical nemesis. J Heart Lung Transplant 14:598, 1995

BESSER RE et al: Diagnosis and treatment of cholera in the United States. Are we prepared? JAMA 272:1203, 1994

COLWELL RR: Global climate and infectious disease: The cholera paradigm. Science 274:2025, 1996

FYFE M et al: Outbreak of *Vibrio parahaemolyticus* infections associated with eating raw oysters. MMWR 47:457, 1998

KAROLIS DK et al: A *Vibrio cholerae* pathogenicity island associated with epidemic and pandemic strains. Proc Natl Acad Sci USA 95:3134, 1998

KHAN WA et al: Comparative trial of five antimicrobial compounds in the treatment of cholera in adults. Trans R Soc Trop Med Hyg 89:103, 1995

LACEY SW: Cholera: Calamitous past, ominous future. Clin Infect Dis 20:1409, 1995

LIN W et al: Identification of a *Vibrio cholerae* RTX toxin gene cluster that is tightly linked to the cholera toxin prophage. Proc Natl Acad Sci USA 96:1071, 1999

MEKALANOS JJ, SADOFF JC: Cholera vaccines: Fighting an ancient scourge. Science 265:1387, 1994

MORRIS JG JR: Non-O1 *V. cholerae*: A look at the epidemiology of an occasional pathogen. Epidemiol Rev 12:179, 1990

NAFICY A et al: Treatment and vaccination strategies to control cholera in sub-Saharan refugee settings: A cost-effectiveness analysis. JAMA 279:521, 1998

RAUFMAN JP: Cholera. Am J Med 104:386, 1998

SHAPIRO R et al: The role of Gulf Coast oysters harvested in warmer months in *Vibrio vulnificus* infections in the United States, 1988–1996. J Infect Dis 178:752, 1998

TAYLOR DN et al: Cholera among Americans living in Peru. Clin Infect Dis 22:1108, 1996

WALDOR MK, MEKALANOS JJ: Lysogenic conversion by a filamentous phage encoding cholera toxin. Science 272:1910, 1996

—— et al: Emergence of a new cholera pandemic: Molecular analysis of virulence determinants in *Vibrio cholerae* O139 and development of a live vaccine prototype. J Infect Dis 170:278, 1994

—— et al: The *Vibrio cholerae* O139 serogroup antigen includes an O-antigen capsule and lipopolysaccharide virulence determinants. Proc Natl Acad Sci USA 91:11388, 1994

160 *M. Monir Madkour, Dennis L. Kasper*

BRUCELLOSIS

DEFINITION Brucellosis is a zoonosis transmitted to humans from infected animals. Its clinical features are not disease specific. *Brucellosis* has many synonyms derived from the geographical regions in which the disease occurs (e.g., Mediterranean fever, Malta fever, Gibraltar fever, Cyprus fever); from the remittent character of its fever (e.g., undulant fever); or from its resemblance to malaria and typhoid (e.g., typhomalarial fever, intermittent typhoid).

ETIOLOGY Human brucellosis can be caused by any of four species: *Brucella melitensis* (the most common and most virulent cause of brucellosis worldwide) is acquired primarily from goats, sheep, and camels; *B. abortus* from cattle; *B. suis* from hogs; and *B. canis* from dogs. These small aerobic gram-negative bacilli are unencapsulated, nonmotile, non-spore-forming, facultative intracellular parasites that cause lifelong infection in animals. Brucellae are killed by boiling or pasteurization of milk and milk products. They survive for up to 8 weeks in unpasteurized, white, soft cheese made from goat's milk and are not killed by freezing. The organisms remain viable for up to 40 days in dried soil contaminated with infected-animal urine, stool, vaginal discharge, and products of conception and for longer periods in damp soil.

EPIDEMIOLOGY The global incidence of human brucellosis is not known because of the variable quality of disease reporting and notification systems in many countries. Worldwide, the only countries believed to be free of brucellosis are Norway, Sweden, Finland, Denmark, Iceland, Switzerland, the Czech and Slovak republics, Romania, the United Kingdom (including the Channel Islands), the Netherlands, Japan, Luxembourg, Cyprus, and Bulgaria; the U.S. Virgin Islands are also free of the disease. Reports indicate that, even in developed nations, the true incidence of brucellosis may be up to 26 times higher than official figures suggest. In the United States, about 200 new cases are reported every year; however, it is estimated that only 4 to 10% of cases are recognized and reported. Consumption of imported cheese, travel abroad, and occupation-related exposures are the most frequently identified sources of infection. In communities where brucellosis is endemic, the disease occurs in children and the family members of infected persons are at risk. Even in countries where animal brucellosis is controlled, the disease occasionally develops among farmers, meat-processing workers, veterinarians, and laboratory workers.

The *Brucella* organism is transmitted most commonly through the ingestion of untreated milk or milk products; raw meat (i.e., blood) and bone marrow have also been implicated. However, the organism can be contracted via inhalation during contact with animals, especially by children and by slaughterhouse, farm, and laboratory workers. Other routes of infection for at-risk workers include skin abrasion, autoinoculation, and conjunctival splashing. The organism has occasionally been transmitted from person to person through the placenta, during breast-feeding, and during sexual activity. Aerosolized *B. melitensis* is a classic agent of biological warfare.

PATHOGENESIS AND IMMUNITY Serum opsonizes *Brucella* organisms for ingestion by polymorphonuclear leukocytes and activated macrophages. Brucellae resist intracellular phagocytic killing by mechanisms such as the suppression of the myeloperoxide–hydrogen peroxide–halide system and the production of superoxide dismutase. The pathogen-phagocyte interaction plays a key role in determining the severity and outcome of brucellosis. The organisms surviving within and escaping from the phagocytes multiply and reach the bloodstream via the lymphatics, subsequently localizing in the liver, spleen, bones, kidneys, lymph nodes, heart valves, nervous system, and testes. In these organs, the bacteria are ingested by macrophages and survive by inhibition of phagosome-lysosome fusion. In infected tissues, inflammatory responses or noncaseating granulomas typically develop, and caseating granulomas and abscesses have been described.

Cytokines, including interleukin (IL) 1, IL-12, and tumor necrosis factor, appear to be important in host defense against *Brucella* infection. The smooth lipopolysaccharide (LPS) of *Brucella* is the major known virulence factor. Strains with rough LPS are more likely than those with smooth LPS to be lysed by nonimmune serum. In virulent strains, the foremost target for specific antibodies is the LPS. Serum IgM antibodies to LPS appear within 1 week after infection and are followed later by IgG and IgA. Titers of both IgM and IgG antibody fall after treatment, and failure of these titers to decline should prompt an evaluation for relapse or persistent infection.

CLASSIFICATION Brucellosis is classified according to whether or not the disease is active (i.e., symptoms or progressive tissue damage and significantly raised *Brucella* agglutinin levels with or without positive cultures) and whether or not there is localized infection. The state of activity and the site of localization have a significant impact on recommended treatment. Classification of brucellosis as acute, subacute, serologic, bacteremic, or of mixed types serves no purpose in diagnosis and management.

CLINICAL MANIFESTATIONS AND COMPLICATIONS Brucellosis is a systemic disease with protean manifestations. Its features may mimic those of other febrile illnesses. The incubation period lasts for about 1 to 3 weeks but may be as long as several months, depending on the virulence of the organisms, their route of entry, the infecting dose, and the host's preexisting health status. The onset of symptoms may be either abrupt (over 1 to 2 days) or gradual (≥1 week). The most common symptoms are fever, chills, diaphoresis, headaches, myalgia, fatigue, anorexia, joint and low-back pain, weight loss, constipation, sore throat, and dry cough. Physical examination often reveals no abnormalities, and patients can look deceptively well. Some patients, in contrast, are acutely ill, with pallor, lymphadenopathy, hepatosplenomegaly, arthritis, spinal tenderness, epididymoorchitis, rash, meningitis, cardiac murmurs, or pneumonia. The fever of brucellosis has no distinctive pattern but may exhibit diurnal variation, with normal temperatures in the morning and high temperatures in the afternoon and evening. Localization to an organ or a system may be evident at the onset of the disease. Table 160-1 lists the frequencies of key historic features, symptoms, and signs among 500 patients with brucellosis due to *B. melitensis*.

Bones and Joints Although monarticular septic arthritis occurs, 30 to 40% of patients have reactive asymmetric polyarthritis involving the knees, hips, shoulders, and sacroiliac and sternoclavicular joints.

Table 160-1 Relevant Historical Features, Symptoms, and Signs in 500 Patients with Brucellosis due to *Brucella melitensis*

Feature	No. of Patients (%)
History	
Animal contact	368 (74)
Raw milk/cheese ingestion	350 (70)
Raw liver ingestion	147 (29)
Family history of brucellosis	188 (38)
Symptom/Sign	
Fever	464 (93)
Chills	410 (82)
Sweats	437 (87)
Aches	457 (91)
Lack of energy	473 (95)
Joint and back pain	431 (86)
Arthritis	202 (40)
Spinal tenderness	241 (48)
Headache	403 (81)
Loss of appetite	388 (78)
Weight loss	326 (65)
Constipation	234 (47)
Abdominal pain	225 (45)
Diarrhea	34 (7)
Cough	122 (24)
Testicular pain/epididymoorchitis	62 (21[a])
Rash	72 (14)
Sleep disturbances	185 (37)
Ill appearance	127 (25)
Pallor	110 (22)
Lymphadenopathy	160 (32)
Splenomegaly	125 (25)
Hepatomegaly	97 (19)
Jaundice	6 (1)
Central nervous system abnormalities	20 (4)
Cardiac murmur	17 (3)
Pneumonia	7 (1)

[a] Among 290 males.

The total white cell count in synovial fluid ranges from 4000 to 40,000/mL, typically with about 60% polymorphonuclear leukocytes. The synovial fluid glucose concentration may be reduced and the protein concentration elevated; cultures of synovial fluid are positive in about 50% of cases.

Infection with *Brucella* organisms commonly causes osteomyelitis of the lumbar vertebrae, starting at the superior end plate (an area with a rich blood supply) and occasionally progressing to involve the entire vertebra, disk space, and adjacent vertebrae. Extraspinal *Brucella* osteomyelitis is rare. In *Brucella* septic arthritis and osteomyelitis, the peripheral white cell count is typically normal, while the erythrocyte sedimentation rate may be either normal or elevated.

Heart Cardiovascular complications of brucellosis include endocarditis, myocarditis, pericarditis, aortic root abscess, mycotic aneurysms, thrombophlebitis with pulmonary aneurysm, and pulmonary embolism. *Brucella* endocarditis may develop on valves previously damaged by rheumatic fever or congenital malformation but also occurs on previously normal valves. The clinical features are indistinguishable from those of endocarditis caused by other organisms (Chap. 126). Endocarditis is the leading cause of death in brucellosis, although the outcome of *Brucella* endocarditis has been more favorable in recent years because of advances in early diagnosis, antibiotic treatment, and cardiac surgery. Physicians who suspect brucellae as a cause of culture-negative endocarditis in patients with possible environmental exposure should notify the bacteriology laboratory performing the blood culture so that extended incubation, specific media, and biohazard precautions can be employed.

Respiratory Tract Brucellae can produce respiratory symptoms. A flulike illness with sore throat, tonsillitis, and dry cough is common and usually mild. Hilar and paratracheal lymphadenopathy, pneumonia, solitary or multiple pulmonary nodules, lung abscess, and empyema have been reported.

Gastrointestinal Tract and Hepatobiliary System Gastrointestinal manifestations of *Brucella* infection are generally mild and may include nausea, vomiting, constipation, acute abdominal pain, and/or diarrhea. Pathologic examination of the liver may reveal any of several changes, including noncaseating granulomas, suppurative abscesses, mononuclear cell infiltration, or hyperemia of the intestinal mucosa. Acute ileitis with inflammation of Peyer's patches and colitis have been reported. Hepatic and splenic enlargement may be documented in 15 to 20% of cases, and abscesses may develop in the liver and spleen. Infected ascites, pancreatitis, and cholecystitis have been reported. Mild jaundice may be evident, with elevated levels of bilirubin and hepatic enzymes.

Genitourinary Tract The various genitourinary infections attributed to brucellae include unilateral or bilateral epididymoorchitis, which is rarely associated with testicular abscess. Prostatitis, seminal vesiculitis, dysmenorrhea, amenorrhea, tuboovarian abscess, salpingitis, cervicitis, acute pyelonephritis, glomerulonephritis, and massive proteinuria have also been documented. *Brucella* organisms have been cultured from the urine in up to 50% of cases of genitourinary tract infection.

Central Nervous System Neurobrucellosis is uncommon but serious and includes meningitis, meningoencephalitis, multiple cerebral or cerebellar abscesses, ruptured mycotic aneurysms, myelitis, Guillain-Barré syndrome, cranial nerve lesions, hemiplegia, sciatica, myositis, and rhabdomyolysis. Papillitis, papilledema, retrobulbar neuritis, optic atrophy, and ophthalmoplegia due to lesions in cranial nerves III, IV, and VI may occur in *Brucella* meningoencephalitis. Cerebrospinal fluid (CSF) pressure is usually elevated; the fluid may appear clear, turbid, or hemorrhagic; the protein concentration and cell count (predominantly lymphocytes) are elevated; and the glucose concentration may be either reduced or normal. In *Brucella* meningitis, which can occur at any time during the course of the disease, the organism may be cultured from the CSF.

Other Manifestations Conjunctival splashing with live attenuated *B. abortus* vaccine (S19) during animal vaccination may cause conjunctivitis, keratitis, and corneal ulcers, with progression to systemic disease in some cases. Uveitis, optic neuritis, retinopathy, retinal detachment, and endophthalmitis may result from hematogenous spread.

Skin manifestations of brucellosis are uncommon. They include maculopapular eruptions, purpura and petechiae, chronic ulcerations, multiple cutaneous and subcutaneous abscesses, discharging sinuses, superficial thrombophlebitis, erythema nodosum, and pemphigus.

Brucellosis during human pregnancy can cause abortion or intrauterine fetal death. Brucellae have been isolated from the human placenta, fetus, and newborn.

The bone marrow of *Brucella*-infected patients frequently contains noncaseating granulomas. Among the hematologic complications of brucellosis are anemia, leukopenia, and thrombocytopenia.

Endocrinologic findings reported in brucellosis include thyroiditis with abscess formation, adrenal insufficiency, and the syndrome of inappropriate secretion of antidiuretic hormone.

DIAGNOSIS The combination of potential exposure, consistent clinical features, and significantly raised levels of *Brucella* agglutinin (with or without positive cultures of blood, body fluid, or tissues) confirms the diagnosis of active brucellosis. The organism's identity is confirmed by phage typing, DNA characterization, or metabolic profiling. Use of a CO_2 detection system (such as BACTEC; Becton Dickinson, Sparks, MD) for blood culture provides a more sensitive and rapid culture result than standard methods, with positivity usually apparent after only 2 to 5 days of incubation. Serum antibodies to *Brucella* can be detected by several methods, including standard tube agglutinins (STA), the 2-mercaptoethanol agglutination test, Coombs' test, enzyme-linked immunosorbent assay, and polymerase chain reaction (PCR). *B. abortus* antigens, which are commonly used for serologic tests, cross-react with *B. melitensis* and *B. suis* but not with *B. canis*. The specific antigen required for assay of antibodies to *B. canis* is not commercially available. *B. canis* antibody titers can be determined in the United States at the Centers for Disease Control and Prevention in Atlanta. A false-negative result in the STA may be obtained because of the prozone phenomenon, which can be avoided by testing of sera at both low and high dilutions.

In endemic areas a *Brucella* antibody titer of 1:320 or 1:640 is significant, while in nonendemic areas an antibody titer of 1:160 is considered significant. Detection of elevated levels of antibody to *Brucella* organisms in the absence of symptoms during the screening of potential blood donors is common in endemic areas. To establish a diagnosis in these regions, clinical and serologic evaluation should be repeated after 2 to 4 weeks and a further rise in titer sought. A high titer of specific IgM suggests recent exposure, while a high titer of specific IgG suggests active disease. Lower titers of IgG may indicate past exposure or treated infection.

Cooperation and consultation with a clinical microbiology laboratory are important when brucellosis is suspected. It may be necessary to observe culture bottles for up to 6 weeks before organisms become detectable. Subcultures should be prepared on duplicate blood agar plates (with and without an atmosphere of 10% CO_2) and special media (such as a blood- or serum-enriched peptone-based medium) or with a rapid CO_2 detection system. Patients whose blood or bone marrow is cultured are positive at one site or the other in 50 to 70% of cases. The peripheral white cell count is usually normal but may be low, with relative lymphocytosis. Thrombocytopenia and disseminated intravascular coagulation may be documented. Levels of hepatic enzymes and serum bilirubin may be raised.

Radiologic investigations aimed at detecting skeletal involvement include plain radiography, bone scintigraphy, computed tomography (CT), and magnetic resonance imaging (MRI). Bone scintigraphy is more sensitive than conventional radiography in detecting areas of spinal and extraspinal involvement, particularly in the early stage of infection. CT is useful for further evaluation of spinal lesions and of the extension of infection into the spinal canal. MRI is the modality of choice for the assessment of *Brucella* spondylitis and is more sensitive than scintigraphy or CT for demonstration of the extent of disease.

Plain lateral radiography of the spine may reveal bone sclerosis, with destruction and erosion of the superior end plate anteriorly. As the disease progresses, healing with osteophyte formation and reduction of disk space may take place. In *Brucella* septic monarthritis, plain radiography may show effusion and soft tissue swelling without bone or joint destruction. Scintigraphy may document increased uptake in sacroiliac joints or lumbar vertebrae, even when plain radiography gives normal results. MRI shows diffuse high-signal intensity of the affected vertebrae and may reveal narrowing of the spinal canal as well as loss of definition of the posterior aspect of the vertebrae.

℞ TREATMENT Single-agent therapy for brucellosis has now been abandoned because of the high rates of failure and relapse and the potential development of antibiotic resistance. Relatively short courses (<8 weeks) of treatment with antibiotic combinations have similarly been associated with high rates of relapse. The combination of doxycycline and an aminoglycoside (gentamicin, streptomycin, or netilmicin) for 4 weeks followed by the combination of doxycycline and rifampin for 4 to 8 weeks is the most effective regimen. Doxycycline (which is preferred over tetracycline) is given orally in a dose of 100 mg twice daily. Gentamicin is given intramuscularly or as a slow intravenous infusion (3 to 5 mg/kg per day in divided doses every 8 h). Netilmicin (which is preferred to streptomycin) is given (intramuscularly to outpatients, intravenously to inpatients) in a dose of 2 mg/kg every 12 h; trough levels in plasma should be monitored regularly and maintained at ≤2 μg/mL. Streptomycin is given intramuscularly in a dose of 1 g once daily to patients under 45 years of age and in a dose of 0.5 to 0.75 g/d to older patients. Tetracycline is given orally in a dose of 250 mg every 6 h and rifampin as a single daily dose of 600 to 900 mg. An alternative regimen consists of the doxycycline/rifampin combination given for 8 to 12 weeks. The doxycycline/aminoglycoside combination is more effective than the doxycycline/rifampin combination in that rifampin reduces levels of doxycycline in plasma.

Patients with serious complications of brucellosis require urgent surgical and medical treatment. These complications include endocarditis, aortic root abscesses, mycotic aortic aneurysms, meningitis, cerebral or cerebellar abscesses, spinal or extraspinal osteomyelitis, and liver or splenic abscess. These patients should be hospitalized and given first a three-drug regimen—i.e., oral doxycycline with intravenous aminoglycoside and rifampin—for 4 weeks and then a two-drug regimen—i.e., doxycycline and rifampin—for 8 to 12 weeks. In instances of renal failure, doxycycline (at adjusted doses) can be used safely. In contrast, the use of aminoglycosides requires facilities for the monitoring of plasma levels; if such facilities are not available, then the doxycycline/rifampin combination should be administered for 8 to 12 weeks.

When used alone, fluoroquinolones (which exhibit good intracellular penetration and efficacy against *Brucella* organisms in vitro) have been associated with the development of quinolone resistance and with high rates of failure and relapse. At present, clinical data are inadequate for the formulation of recommendations regarding the combination of fluoroquinolones with doxycycline, rifampin, or streptomycin.

Third-generation cephalosporins (e.g., ceftriaxone), although active in vitro against brucellae when used alone, have also been associated with a high incidence of clinical failure and relapse. These agents may be useful in combination with other drugs for the treatment of *Brucella* meningitis.

In pregnancy, trimethoprim-sulfamethoxazole (TMP-SMZ) can be given in combination with rifampin for 8 to 12 weeks. The TMP-SMZ dosage appropriate for pregnant women is two or three tablets every 12 h (each tablet contains 80 mg of TMP and 400 mg of SMZ). Children below the age of 8 years can also be treated with rifampin and TMP-SMZ for 8 to 12 weeks, while older children should receive the same antibiotics as adults in the following doses: doxycycline, 100 mg/d orally; an aminoglycoside (gentamicin, 2 mg/kg per day in divided doses every 8 h); and rifampin, 15 mg/kg per day orally or by slow intravenous infusion. TMP-SMZ is given orally every 12 h in a dose that depends on the patient's age (birth to 6 months, 120 mg; 6 months to 6 years, 240 mg).

Within 4 to 14 days after the initiation of therapy, patients become afebrile and constitutional symptoms disappear. The enlarged liver and spleen return to their normal size within 2 to 4 weeks. An acute, intense flare-up of symptoms may follow the start of treatment, especially that with tetracyclines. This reaction is transient and does not necessitate the discontinuation of therapy. In endemic areas the coexistence of brucellosis and tuberculous spondylitis may result in a failure to respond to appropriate treatment. Treated patients whose infections are apparently cured should be followed clinically and serologically, with repeat blood cultures, every 3 to 6 months for 2 years.

PREVENTION Efforts at prevention should be aimed at the source of infection. Immunization of animals and boiling or pasteurization of milk and milk products are important. Workers in the meat and dairy industries in the former Soviet Union, China, and France have been vaccinated; the vaccine (two injections given 2 weeks apart, each containing 1 mg of an insoluble fraction of phenol-extracted bacteria) markedly reduces the rate of infection. However, the vaccine induces fever in 6% of recipients and severe pain at the injection site in 16%. Moreover, immunity is short-lived, and vaccination should be repeated every 2 years. This vaccine is not used in the United States.

PROGNOSIS Deaths attributable to brucellosis should be avoidable. Even before the discovery of antibiotics, the mortality rate was <2% and endocarditis was most frequently the cause of death. Morbidity due to brucellosis remains significant; its severity depends on the infecting *Brucella* species and is greatest with *B. melitensis*. Spinal damage, paraplegia, and other neurologic deficits may occur. Nerve deafness due to meningitis or secondary to treatment with streptomycin has been documented.

BIBLIOGRAPHY

BANNATYNE RM et al: Rapid diagnosis of *Brucella* bacteremia by using BACTEC 9240 system. J Clin Microbiol 35:673, 1997

CORBEL MJ: Recent advances in brucellosis. J Med Microbiol 46:101, 1997

FRANZ DR et al: Clinical recognition and management of patients exposed to biological warfare agents. JAMA 278:399, 1997

JIANG X, BALDWIN CL: Effect of cytokines on intracellular growth of *Brucella abortus*. Infect Immun 61:124, 1993

LIAUTARD JP et al: Interaction between professional phagocytes and *Brucella* spp. Microbiologia 12:197, 1996

MADKOUR MM: *Brucellosis*. London, Butterworths, 1989

——— et al: Osteoarticular brucellosis: Results of bone scintigraphy in 140 patients. Am J Roentgenol 150:1101, 1988

SIFUENTES RICON AM et al: Detection and differentiation of six *Brucella* species by PCR. Mol Med 3:734, 1997

SOLERA J et al: Doxycycline-rifampin versus doxycycline-streptomycin in treatment of human brucellosis due to *Brucella melitensis*. Antimicrob Agents Chemother 39:2061, 1995

SOLERA L et al: Multivariate model for predicting relapse in human brucellosis. J Infect 36:85, 1998

161   *Richard F. Jacobs*

TULAREMIA

DEFINITION   Tularemia is a zoonosis caused by *Francisella tularensis*, so named in 1974 in recognition of the contributions of Edward Francis. Humans of any age, sex, or race are universally susceptible to this systemic infection. Tularemia is primarily a disease of wild animals and persists in contaminated environments, ectoparasites, and animal carriers. Human infection is incidental and usually results from interaction with biting or blood-sucking insects, wild or domestic animals, or the environment. Tularemia is common in Arkansas, Oklahoma, and Missouri, where more than 50% of the cases in the United States occur. An increasing number of cases of tularemia have been reported from the Scandinavian countries, eastern Europe, and Siberia. The illness is characterized by various clinical syndromes, the most common of which consists of an ulcerative lesion at the site of inoculation, with regional lymphadenopathy and lymphadenitis. Systemic manifestations, including pneumonia, typhoidal tularemia, and fever without localizing findings, pose a greater diagnostic challenge.

ETIOLOGY AND EPIDEMIOLOGY   *F. tularensis* is the etiologic agent of tularemia, which, with rare exceptions, is the only disease produced by this genus. The organism is a small, gram-negative, pleomorphic, nonmotile, non-spore-forming bacillus measuring 0.2 μm by 0.2 to 0.7 μm. Bipolar staining results in a coccoid appearance. The organism is a thinly encapsulated, nonpiliated strict aerobe that invades host cells.

In nature, *F. tularensis* is a hardy organism that persists for weeks or months in mud, water, and decaying animal carcasses. Dozens of biting and blood-sucking insects, especially ticks and tabanid flies, serve as vectors. Ticks and wild rabbits are the source for most of the human cases in the endemic areas of the southeastern United States and the Rocky Mountain states. In Utah, Nevada, and California, tabanid flies are the most common vectors. Animal reservoirs include wild rabbits, squirrels, birds, sheep, beavers, muskrats, and domestic dogs and cats.

The two main biovars of *F. tularensis*—*tularensis* (type A) and *palearctica* (type B)—are both found in the United States. Type A produces more serious disease in humans; without treatment, the associated fatality rate is approximately 5%. Type B produces a milder, often subclinical infection that is usually contracted from water or marine mammals. Although all strains appear serologically identical, individual strains may possess varying degrees of virulence. *F. tularensis* does not produce an exotoxin, but an endotoxin similar to that of other gram-negative bacilli has been identified. The progression of illness depends upon the organism's virulence, the inoculum size, the portal of entry, and the host's immune status.

Ticks pass the organism to their offspring via a transovarian route. The organism is found in tick feces but not in large quantities in tick salivary glands. In the United States, the disease can be carried by *Dermacentor andersoni* (Rocky Mountain wood tick), *D. variabilis* (American dog tick), *D. occidentalis* (Pacific coast dog tick), and *Amblyomma americanum* (Lone Star tick). *F. tularensis* is transmitted frequently during blood meals taken by embedded ticks following hours of attachment. It is the taking of a blood meal through a fecally contaminated field that transmits the organism. Tularemia is more common among men than among women. Person-to-person transmission is rare or nonexistent. Transmission of the organism by ticks and tabanid flies takes place mainly in the spring and summer. However, continued transmission in the winter months by trapped or hunted animals has been documented. The organism is extremely infectious. Biosafety level 2 is recommended for clinical laboratory work with material whose contamination is suspected, and biosafety level 3 is required for culture of the organism in large quantities.

PATHOGENESIS AND PATHOLOGY   The most common portal of entry for human infection is through skin or mucous membranes, either directly—through the bite of ticks, other arthropods, or other animals—or via inapparent abrasions. Inhalation or ingestion of *F. tularensis* can also result in infection. Although more than 10^8 organisms are usually required to produce infection via the oral route (oropharyngeal or gastrointestinal tularemia), fewer than 50 organisms will result in infection when injected into the skin (ulceroglandular/glandular tularemia) or inhaled (pneumonia). After inoculation into the skin, the organism multiplies locally; within 2 to 5 days (range, 1 to 10 days), it produces an erythematous, tender, or pruritic papule. The papule rapidly enlarges and forms an ulcer with a black base (chancriform lesion). The bacteria spread to regional lymph nodes, producing lymphadenopathy (buboes), and, with bacteremia, may spread to distant organs.

Tularemia is characterized by mononuclear cell infiltration with pyogranulomatous pathology. The histopathologic findings can be quite similar to those in tuberculosis, although tularemia develops more rapidly. As a facultatively intracellular bacterium, *F. tularensis* can parasitize both phagocytic and nonphagocytic host cells and survive intracellularly for prolonged periods. In the acute phase of infection, the primary organs affected (skin, lymph nodes, liver, and spleen) include areas of focal necrosis, initially surrounded by polymorphonuclear leukocytes (PMNs). Subsequently, granulomas form, with epithelioid cells, lymphocytes, and multinucleated giant cells surrounded by areas of necrosis. These areas may resemble caseation necrosis but later coalesce to form abscesses.

Conjunctival inoculation can result in infection of the eye, with regional lymph node enlargement (preauricular lymphadenopathy, Parinaud's complex). Aerosolization and inhalation or hematogenous spread of organisms can result in pneumonia. In the lung, an inflammatory reaction—including foci of alveolar necrosis and cell infiltration (initially polymorphonuclear and later mononuclear) with granulomas—develops. Chest roentgenograms usually reveal bilateral patchy infiltrates rather than large areas of consolidation. Pleural effusions are common and may contain blood. Lymphadenopathy occurs in regions draining infected organs. Therefore, in pulmonary infection, mediastinal adenopathy may be evident, while patients with oropharyngeal tularemia develop cervical lymphadenopathy. In gastrointestinal or typhoidal tularemia, mesenteric lymphadenopathy may follow the ingestion of large numbers of organisms. The term *typhoidal tularemia* may be used to describe severe bacteremic disease, irrespective of the mode of transmission or portal of entry. Meningitis has been reported as a primary or secondary manifestation of bacteremia. Patients may also present with fever and no localizing signs.

IMMUNOLOGY   Infection with *F. tularensis* stimulates the host to produce antibodies. However, this antibody response probably plays only a minor role in the containment of infection. In contrast, cell-mediated immunity, which develops over 2 to 4 weeks, plays a major role in containment and eradication of the infection. Macrophages, once activated, are capable of killing *F. tularensis*.

Immunospecific protection against tularemia can be afforded either by natural infection or by vaccination with live attenuated strains of *F. tularensis*. Killed vaccines, on the other hand, induce no protection against virulent *F. tularensis*. After natural infection or vaccination, serum antibodies to surface-exposed carbohydrate antigens predominate, whereas T cell determinants are located on membrane proteins beneath the bacterial capsule. T cell responses are thought to be due to priming by the organism. The anamnestic T cell response to *F. tularensis* seems to involve a multitude of microbial proteins, each with a distinct set of T cell determinants. A predominant role for CD4+ T cells is supported by the results of experiments in mice, which indicated that resistance to infection was restricted at the level of the MHC class II determinants. Humans primed to *F. tularensis* (like those primed to *Mycobacterium tuberculosis*) show a T_H1-like response. T cell proliferation is associated with the production of interleukin (IL) 2 and interferon γ but with little or no production of IL-4.

Investigations of neutrophils in cases of tularemia have suggested that PMNs are needed for defense against primary infection. PMNs may restrict the growth of *F. tularensis* before the organism becomes intracellular.

CLINICAL MANIFESTATIONS Tularemia often starts with a sudden onset of fever, chills, headache, and generalized myalgias and arthralgias (Table 161-1). This onset takes place when the organism penetrates the skin, is ingested, or is inhaled. An incubation period of 2 to 10 days is followed by the formation of an ulcer at the site of penetration, with local inflammation. The ulcer may persist for several months as organisms are transported via the lymphatics to the regional lymph nodes. These nodes enlarge and may become necrotic and suppurative. If the organism enters the bloodstream, widespread dissemination as well as signs and symptoms of endotoxemia may result.

In the United States, most patients with tularemia (75 to 85%) acquire the infection by inoculation of the skin. In adults, the most common localized form is inguinal/femoral lymphadenopathy; in children, it is cervical lymphadenopathy. About 20% of patients develop a generalized maculopapular rash, which occasionally becomes pustular. Erythema nodosum occurs infrequently. The clinical manifestations of tularemia have been divided into various syndromes, which are listed in Table 161-2.

Ulceroglandular/Glandular Tularemia These two forms of tularemia account for approximately 75 to 85% of cases. The predominant form in children involves cervical or posterior auricular lymphadenopathy and is usually related to tick bites on the head and neck. In adults, the most common form is inguinal/femoral lymphadenopathy resulting from insect and tick exposures on the lower limbs. In cases related to wild game, the usual portal of entry for *F. tularensis* is either an injury sustained while skinning or cleaning an animal carcass or a bite (usually on the hand). Epitrochlear lymphadenopathy/lymphadenitis is common in patients with bite-related injuries.

In ulceroglandular tularemia, the ulcer is erythematous, indurated, and nonhealing, with a punched-out appearance that lasts from 1 to 3 weeks. The papule may begin as an erythematous lesion that is tender or pruritic; it evolves over several days into an ulcer with sharply demarcated edges and a yellow exudate. The ulcer gradually develops a black base, and simultaneously the regional lymph nodes become tender and severely enlarged (Fig. 161-1). The affected lymph nodes may become fluctuant and drain spontaneously, but usually the con-

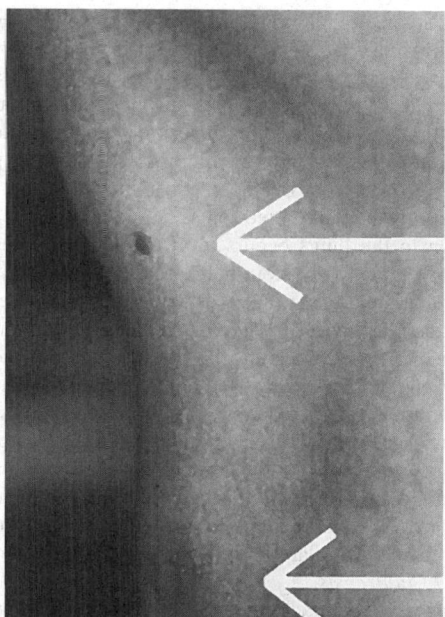

FIGURE 161-1 An ulcerative lesion *(lower arrow)* with adjacent lymphadenitis *(upper arrow)* on the lateral chest wall of a patient with ulceroglandular tularemia.

dition resolves with effective treatment. Late suppuration of lymph nodes has been described in up to 25% of patients with ulceroglandular/glandular tularemia. Examination of material taken from these late fluctuant nodes after successful antimicrobial treatment has revealed sterile necrotic tissue. In 5 to 10% of patients, the skin lesion may be inapparent, with lymphadenopathy plus systemic signs and symptoms the only physical findings. This clinical syndrome is designated *glandular tularemia.* Conversely, a tick or deerfly bite on the trunk may result in an ulcer without evident lymphadenopathy.

Oculoglandular Tularemia In about 1% of patients, the portal of entry for *F. tularensis* is the conjunctiva. Usually, the organism reaches the conjunctiva through contact with contaminated fingers. The inflamed conjunctiva is painful, with numerous yellowish nodules and pinpoint ulcers. Purulent conjunctivitis with regional lymphadenopathy (preauricular, submandibular, or cervical) is evident. Because of debilitating pain, the patient may seek medical attention before regional lymphadenopathy develops. Painful preauricular lymphadenopathy is unique to tularemia and distinguishes it from cat-scratch disease, tuberculosis, sporotrichosis, and syphilis. Corneal perforation may occur.

Oropharyngeal and Gastrointestinal Tularemia Rarely, tularemia follows the ingestion of contaminated undercooked meat, the oral inoculation of *F. tularensis* from the hands in association with the skinning and cleaning of animal carcasses, or the consumption of contaminated food or water. Oral inoculation may result in acute, exudative, or membranous pharyngitis associated with cervical lymphadenopathy or in ulcerative intestinal lesions associated with mesenteric lymphadenopathy, diarrhea, abdominal pain, nausea, vomiting, and gastrointestinal bleeding. Infected tonsils become enlarged and develop a yellowish-white pseudomembrane, which can be confused with that of diphtheria. The clinical severity of gastrointestinal tularemia varies from mild, unexplained, persistent diarrhea with no other symptoms to a rapidly fulminant, fatal disease. In fatal cases, the extensive intestinal ulceration found at autopsy suggests an enormous inoculum.

Pulmonary Tularemia Tularemia pneumonia presents as variable parenchymal infiltrates that are unresponsive to treatment with β-lactam antibiotics. Tularemia must be considered in the differential

Table 161-1 Clinical Presentation of Tularemia

Sign or Symptom	Rate of Occurrence, %	
	Children	Adults
Lymphadenopathy	96	65
Fever (≥38.3°C or ≥101°F)	87	21
Ulcer/eschar/papule	45	51
Myalgias/arthralgias	39	2
Headache	9	5
Cough	9	5
Pharyngitis	43	—
Diarrhea	43	—

SOURCE: Adapted from Jacobs and Narain (1985).

Table 161-2 Clinical Syndromes of Tularemia

Syndrome	Rate of Occurrence, %	
	Children	Adults
Ulceroglandular	45	51
Glandular	25	12
Pulmonary (pneumonia)	14	18
Oropharyngeal	4	—
Oculoglandular	2	—
Typhoidal	2	12
Unclassified	6	11

SOURCE: Adapted from Jacobs and Narain (1985).

diagnosis of atypical pneumonia in a patient with a history of travel to an endemic area. The disease can result from either inhalation of an infectious aerosol or spread to the lungs and pleura after bloodstream dissemination. Inhalation-related pneumonia has been described in laboratory workers after exposure to contaminated materials and is associated with a relatively high mortality rate. Exposure to *F. tularensis* in aerosols from live domestic animals or dead wildlife (including birds) has been reported to cause pneumonia. Hematogenous dissemination to the lungs occurs in 10 to 15% of cases of ulceroglandular tularemia and in about half of cases of typhoidal tularemia. Previously, tularemia pneumonia was thought to be a disease of older patients, but as many as 10 to 15% of children with clinical manifestations of tularemia have parenchymal infiltrates detected by chest roentgenography. Patients with pneumonia usually have a nonproductive cough and may have dyspnea or pleuritic chest pain. Roentgenograms of the chest usually reveal bilateral patchy infiltrates (described as ovoid or lobar densities), lobar parenchymal infiltrates, and cavitary lesions. Pleural effusions may have a predominance of mononuclear leukocytes or PMNs and sometimes red blood cells. Empyema may develop. Patients with tularemia pneumonia can have blood cultures positive for *F. tularensis*.

Typhoidal Tularemia   Once thought to represent up to 10% of all cases of tularemia, the typhoidal presentation is now considered rare in the United States. In this presentation, fever develops without apparent skin lesions or lymphadenopathy. In the absence of a history of possible contact with a vector, diagnosis can be extremely difficult. Blood cultures may be positive and patients may present with classic sepsis or septic shock in this acute systemic form of the infection. Typhoidal tularemia is usually associated with a huge inoculum or with a preexisting compromising condition. High continuous fevers, signs of endotoxemia, and severe headache are common findings. The patient may be delirious and may develop prostration and shock. If presumptive antibiotic therapy in culture-negative cases does not include an aminoglycoside, the mortality rate can approach 30%.

Other Manifestations   *F. tularensis* infection has been associated with meningitis, pericarditis, hepatitis, peritonitis, endocarditis, osteomyelitis, and sepsis and septic shock with rhabdomyolysis and acute renal failure. In the rare cases of tularemia meningitis, a predominantly lymphocytic response is demonstrated in cerebrospinal fluid.

DIFFERENTIAL DIAGNOSIS   When patients in endemic areas present with fever, chronic ulcerative skin lesions, and large tender lymph nodes, a diagnosis of tularemia should be made presumptively, and confirmatory diagnostic testing and appropriate therapy should be undertaken. When the possibility of tularemia is considered in a patient with this presentation in a nonendemic area, an attempt should be made to determine whether the individual has come into contact with a potential animal vector. The level of suspicion of tularemia should be especially high in hunters, trappers, game wardens, veterinarians, laboratory workers, and individuals with a history of exposure to an insect or another animal vector. However, up to 40% of patients with tularemia have no known history of epidemiologic contact with an animal vector.

The characteristic presentation of ulceroglandular tularemia does not pose a diagnostic problem, but a less classic progression of regional lymphadenopathy or glandular tularemia must be differentiated from other diseases. The skin lesion may resemble those seen in sporotrichosis; skin infection with *Staphylococcus aureus*, *Streptococcus pyogenes*, or *Mycobacterium marinum*; syphilis; anthrax; rat-bite fever (due to *Spirillum minus*); or rickettsiosis (scrub typhus). In the latter infections, regional lymphadenopathy is usually not as impressive as in tularemia. The lymphadenopathy of tularemia (especially glandular tularemia) must be differentiated from that of plague, lymphogranuloma venereum, and cat-scratch disease. In children, the differentiation from cat-scratch disease is made more difficult by the chronic papulovesicular lesion associated with *Bartonella henselae* infection (Chap. 163).

Oropharyngeal tularemia can resemble and must be differentiated from pharyngitis due to group A β-hemolytic streptococci, *Arcanobacterium haemolyticum*, or *Corynebacterium diphtheriae* as well as from infectious mononucleosis. Tularemia pneumonia may resemble any of the atypical pneumonias, including those due to various viruses, *Mycoplasma pneumoniae*, *Chlamydia pneumoniae*, *C. psittaci*, *Legionella pneumophila*, *Coxiella burnetii*, and (occasionally) *Histoplasma capsulatum*. Typhoidal tularemia may resemble typhoid fever, other *Salmonella* bacteremias, rickettsial infections (Rocky Mountain spotted fever, ehrlichiosis), brucellosis, infectious mononucleosis, acquired toxoplasmosis, miliary tuberculosis, sarcoidosis, and hematologic or reticuloendothelial malignancies.

LABORATORY DIAGNOSIS   Direct microscopic examination of polychromatically stained tissue smears or clinical specimens reveals *F. tularensis* organisms, singly and in groups, both intra- and extracellularly. Gram's staining of clinical or biopsy material is of little value, as the small, weakly staining organisms cannot be readily distinguished from the background. An indirect fluorescent antibody test with commercially available antisera can be useful, although false-positive results due to *Legionella* spp. have been reported.

The diagnosis of tularemia is most frequently confirmed by serologic testing. In the standard tube agglutination test, a single titer of ≥1:160 is interpreted as a presumptive positive result. A fourfold increase in titer between paired serum samples collected 2 to 3 weeks apart is considered diagnostic. False-negative serologic responses are obtained early in infection; up to 30% of patients infected for 3 weeks have sera that test negative. Late in infection, titers into the thousands are common, and titers of 1:20 to 1:80 may persist for years. A microagglutination test that may be as much as 100-fold more sensitive than the standard tube agglutination test has been described and is currently being used in many clinical microbiology laboratories. Enzyme-linked immunosorbent assays have proven useful for the detection of both antibodies and antigens. Analysis of urine for *F. tularensis* antigen has yielded promising results in clinical trials, but facilities for this type of analysis are not widely available. A skin test for delayed hypersensitivity to *F. tularensis* turns positive during the first week of illness and remains positive for years. The skin-test antigen, which is not commercially available, can boost titers of agglutinating antibody.

Culture and isolation of *F. tularensis* are difficult. In one study the organism was isolated in only 10% of more than 1000 human cases, 84% of which were confirmed by serology. The medium of choice is cysteine-glucose-blood agar. *F. tularensis* can be isolated directly from infected ulcer scrapings, lymph-node biopsy specimens, gastric washings, sputum, and blood cultures. Colonies are blue-gray, round, smooth, and slightly mucoid. On media containing blood, a small zone of α hemolysis usually surrounds the colony. Slide agglutination tests or direct fluorescent antibody tests with commercially available antisera can be applied directly to culture suspensions for identification.

The polymerase chain reaction (PCR) has been used to detect *F. tularensis* DNA. During a recent outbreak, a multiplex PCR was used to target 16S rRNA and to diagnose ulceroglandular tularemia with DNA extracted from wound swabs; the PCR result was positive in 29 (73%) of 40 serologically confirmed cases. However, this test has not been shown to be more sensitive than direct culture and at present remains a research tool.

TREATMENT   *F. tularensis* cannot be subjected to standardized antimicrobial susceptibility testing because the organism will not grow on the media used. A wide variety of antibiotics, including all β-lactam antibiotics and the newer cephalosporins, are ineffective for the treatment of this infection. Several studies indicated that third-generation cephalosporins were active against *F. tularensis* in vitro, but clinical case reports suggested a nearly universal failure rate of ceftriaxone in pediatric patients with tularemia. Although in vitro data indicate that imipenem may be active, therapy with imipenem, sulfanilamides, and macrolides is not presently recommended because of the lack of relevant clinical data. Fluoroquinolones have shown promise in terms of their relatively low toxicity and their potential for oral administration. Chloramphenicol and tetracycline have been used successfully for treatment of the acute stages of tularemia but have been associated with higher relapse rates (up to 20%) than conventionally used agents.

Streptomycin, given intramuscularly at a dose of 7.5 to 10 mg/kg every 12 h, is considered the drug of choice for adults. In severe cases, 15 mg/kg every 12 h may be used for the first 48 to 72 h. Streptomycin is also considered the drug of choice for children; the appropriate dose is 30 to 40 mg/kg daily in two divided doses administered intramuscularly. In children, after a clinical response is demonstrated at 3 to 5 days, the dose can be reduced to 10 to 15 mg/kg daily in two divided doses. Therapy is typically continued for 7 to 10 days; however, in mild to moderate cases of tularemia in which the patient becomes afebrile within the first 48 to 72 h of streptomycin treatment, a 5- to 7-day course has been successful.

Gentamicin, at a dose of 1.7 mg/kg given intravenously or intramuscularly every 8 h, is also effective. The published experience in adults consists of two reports describing, respectively, nine and eight patients who were treated effectively with gentamicin. The eight patients in one of the reports all had fever before treatment, and all eight became afebrile within 24 to 72 h. In a recent pediatric study, other symptoms, such as tender lymphadenitis and pharyngitis, also responded within 24 to 72 h of the start of gentamicin therapy.

Virtually all strains of *F. tularensis* are susceptible to streptomycin and gentamicin. In successfully treated patients, defervescence usually occurs within 2 days, but skin lesions and lymph nodes may take 1 to 2 weeks to heal. When therapy is not initiated within the first several days of illness, defervescence may be delayed. Relapses are uncommon with streptomycin or gentamicin therapy. Late lymph-node suppuration, however, occurs in approximately 40% of children, regardless of the treatment received. These nodes have typically been found to contain sterile necrotic tissue without evidence of active infection. Patients with fluctuant nodes should receive several days of antibiotic therapy before drainage to minimize the risk to hospital personnel. Unlike streptomycin and gentamicin, tobramycin is ineffective in the treatment of tularemia and should not be used.

PROGNOSIS If tularemia goes untreated, symptoms usually last 1 to 4 weeks but may continue for months. The mortality rate from severe untreated infection (including all cases of untreated tularemia pneumonia and typhoidal tularemia) can be as high as 30%. However, the overall mortality rate for untreated tularemia is <8%. Mortality is <1% with appropriate treatment. Poor outcomes are often associated with long delays in diagnosis and treatment. Lifelong immunity usually follows tularemia.

PREVENTION The prevention of tularemia is based on avoidance of exposure to biting and blood-sucking insects, especially ticks and deerflies. An intradermal vaccine made from live attenuated *F. tularensis* is available from the Centers for Disease Control and Prevention. This vaccine is effective in reducing the frequency and severity of infection. Vaccination of high-risk individuals working with large quantities of cultured organisms is recommended. Others who come into contact with the organisms, such as veterinarians, hunters, or game wardens, should consider vaccination, particularly if they live in endemic areas. The avoidance of skinning wild animals, especially rabbits, and the wearing of gloves while handling animal carcasses decrease the risk of transmission. Use of insect repellents and preparations that prevent tick attachment as well as prompt removal of ticks can be helpful. Prophylaxis of tularemia has not proved effective in patients with embedded ticks or insect bites. However, in patients who are known to have been exposed to large quantities of organisms (e.g., in the laboratory) and who have incubating infection with *F. tularensis*, early treatment can prevent the development of significant clinical disease.

BIBLIOGRAPHY

CROSS JT, JACOBS RF: Tularemia: Treatment failures with outpatient use of ceftriaxone. Clin Infect Dis 17:976, 1993

ENDERLIN G et al: Streptomycin and alternative agents for the treatment of tularemia: Review of the literature. Clin Infect Dis 19:42, 1994

JACOBS RF, NARAIN JP: Tularemia in children. Pediatr Infect Dis J 2:487, 1983

———, ———: Tularemia in adults and children: A changing presentation. Pediatrics 76:818, 1985

LONG GW et al: Detection of *Francisella tularensis* in blood by polymerase chain reaction. J Clin Microbiol 31:152, 1993

SCHEEL O et al: Treatment of tularemia with ciprofloxacin. Eur J Microbiol Infect Dis 11:447, 1992

SJOSTEDT A et al: Detection of *Francisella tularensis* in ulcers of patients with tularemia by PCR. J Clin Microbiol 35:1045, 1997

TAYLOR JP et al: Epidemiologic characteristics of human tularemia in the southwest-central states, 1981–1987. Am J Epidemiol 133:1032, 1991

162   *Grant L. Campbell, David T. Dennis*

PLAGUE AND OTHER *YERSINIA* INFECTIONS

PLAGUE

DEFINITION Plague is an acute, febrile, zoonotic disease caused by infection with *Yersinia pestis*. Although human cases are infrequent and are curable with antibiotics, plague is one of the most virulent and potentially lethal bacterial diseases known. The plague bacterium occurs in widely scattered foci in Asia, Africa, and the Americas, where its usual hosts are wild and peridomestic rodents. It is transmitted to humans typically by flea bite and less commonly by direct contact with infected animal tissues or by airborne droplet. The principal clinical forms of plague are bubonic, septicemic, and pneumonic. Although most cases are now sporadic, occurring singly or in small clusters, the potential for epidemic spread remains.

ETIOLOGIC AGENT *Y. pestis* is a gram-negative coccobacillus in the family Enterobacteriaceae. It is microaerophilic, nonmotile, nonsporulating, oxidase and urease negative, and biochemically unreactive. The organism is nonfastidious and infective for laboratory rodents. It grows well, if slowly, on routinely used microbiologic media (e.g., sheep blood agar, brain-heart infusion broth, and MacConkey agar). *Y. pestis* can multiply within a wide range of temperatures ($-2°C$ to $45°C$) and pH values (5.0 to 9.6), but optimal growth occurs at $28°C$ and at pH ~7.4. When incubated on agar plates at $37°C$, colonies are pinpoint in size at 24 h and 1 to 2 mm in diameter at 48 h. The colonies are gray-white with irregular surfaces, described as having a "hammered-metal" appearance when viewed microscopically. In broth culture, *Y. pestis* grows without turbidity in clumps clinging to the sides of tubes. When stained with a polychromatic stain (e.g., Wayson or Giemsa), *Y. pestis* isolated from clinical specimens exhibits a characteristic bipolar appearance, often resembling closed safety pins. The bacterium is nonencapsulated but when grown at $\geq30°C$ produces a plasmid-expressed immunogenic envelope glycoprotein, fraction 1 (F1).

HISTORIC BACKGROUND Plague's deadly epidemic potential is notorious and well documented. The Justinian pandemic (542 to 767 A.D.) spread from central Africa to the Mediterranean littoral and thence to Asia Minor, causing an estimated 40 million deaths. The second pandemic began in central Asia, was carried to Sicily by ship from Constantinople in 1347, and swept through Europe and the British Isles in successive waves over the next four centuries. At its height, it killed as many as a quarter of the affected population and became known as the Black Death. In the third (modern) pandemic, plague appeared in Yunnan, China, in the latter half of the nineteenth century; established itself in Hong Kong in 1894; and spread by ship to Bombay in 1896 and subsequently to major port cities throughout the world, including San Francisco and several other West Coast and Gulf Coast ports in the United States. The plague bacillus was first cultured by

Alexandre Yersin in Hong Kong in 1894. In 1898, Paul-Louis Simond, a French scientist sent to investigate epidemic bubonic plague in Bombay, identified the bacillus in the tissues of dead rats and proposed transmission by rat fleas. Waldemar Haffkine, also in Bombay at that time, developed a crude vaccine.

By 1910, plague had circled the globe and established itself in rodent populations on all inhabited continents other than Australia. After 1920, however, the spread of plague was largely halted by international regulations that mandated control of rats in harbors and inspection and rat-proofing of ships. Before the third pandemic subsided, it resulted in an estimated 26 million plague cases and more than 12 million deaths, the vast majority in India. By 1950, plague outbreaks around the world had become isolated, sporadic, and manageable with modern techniques of surveillance, flea and rat control, and antimicrobial treatment of patients. Plague has nearly disappeared from cities and now occurs mostly in rural and semirural areas, where it is maintained in various rodents and their fleas. In the United States, the last outbreak of urban plague occurred in Los Angeles in 1924 and 1925, and human cases since then have resulted from animal plague exposures in rural areas of western states.

Because of its pandemic history, plague remains one of three quarantinable diseases subject to international health regulations (the other two being cholera and yellow fever). The alarm that plague is still able to evoke was highlighted by the public panic over an exaggerated international response to purported outbreaks of bubonic and pneumonic plague in India in 1994. The plague bacillus is considered to have a high potential for use in biologic terrorism; the agent is available around the world, has been "weaponized" for airborne delivery, and would be expected to cause a high primary fatality rate as well as secondary spread among an affected population.

EPIDEMIOLOGY *Y. pestis* is maintained in enzootic cycles involving relatively resistant wild rodents and their fleas in mostly remote, lightly populated areas of Asia, Africa, and the Americas and in limited rural foci in extreme southeastern Europe near the Caspian Sea. Humans and other nonrodent mammals are incidental hosts. Enzootic transmission places humans at low risk, and cases are typically infrequent and sporadic. Epizootic transmission involving susceptible rodents and efficient flea vectors (both are amplifying hosts) results in local or even widespread depopulation of susceptible rodents and poses a more serious threat to humans than does enzootic transmission. In the United States, the principal epizootic hosts are various ground squirrels, prairie dogs, and chipmunks; a variety of burrowing rodents act as epizootic hosts in rural areas elsewhere in the world. *Y. pestis* occasionally spills over from wild rodents to rat species that inhabit cultivated fields and adjacent homes, villages, and towns. The organism can then be transported from towns to cities by these highly adaptable rats and their fleas. Urban plague is currently reported sporadically from a few countries such as Vietnam, Myanmar, and Madagascar.

Plague in populated areas is most likely to develop when sanitation is poor and rats are numerous—especially the common black or roof rat (*Rattus rattus*), its close relatives, and the larger brown sewer or Norway rat (*R. norvegicus*). A high mortality rate from plague in these susceptible rat populations forces their fleas to seek alternative hosts, including humans. The cosmopolitan oriental rat flea *Xenopsylla cheopis* and (in southern Africa and Brazil) the related species *X. brasiliensis* are efficient vectors of the plague bacillus among rats and are also efficient vectors to humans. *Y. pestis* can multiply to enormous numbers in the foregut (proventriculus) of these fleas, resulting in a bolus of organisms and clotted blood that blocks the passage of subsequent blood meals. This situation occurs only at temperatures of ≤28°C and depends on a single protease expressed by the plasminogen activator (*pla*) gene of a 9.5-kb plasmid of *Y. pestis*. Regurgitation by a "blocked" flea while it feeds facilitates transmission of the plague bacillus to the new host.

Except for large outbreaks of pneumonic plague in Manchuria in the early part of the twentieth century, person-to-person respiratory transmission of plague during and since the third pandemic has occurred only sporadically and has been limited to clusters of close contacts of pneumonic plague patients, such as household members and caregivers. The 1994 outbreak of pneumonic plague in the city of Surat, India, although reported to be extensive, most likely involved fewer than 100 cases and 50 deaths; in 1998, a small outbreak of pneumonic plague occurred in the Ecuadoran Andes.

International health regulations require that national health authorities immediately report plague cases to the World Health Organization. From 1982 through 1996, 23,904 human plague cases and 2105 deaths (mortality, 9%) were reported by 24 countries. In the same 15-year period, the United States reported 212 plague cases (mean, 14 cases per year) and 27 deaths (mortality, 13%). Cases reported by the United States are confirmed by the plague laboratory of the Centers for Disease Control and Prevention (CDC). Animal plague occurs in 17 contiguous western states, extending from the Great Plains states and eastern Texas to the Pacific Coast; around 80% of human cases in this country now occur in New Mexico, Arizona, and Colorado and around 10% in California. Although plague in the United States is a rural disease, more than 50% of cases are thought to be caused by peridomestic exposures, especially in the southwestern states, where homes are often situated in natural surroundings that provide a favorable habitat for plague-susceptible animals (such as rock squirrels and wood rats) and their fleas. In the Sierra Nevadas of California and Nevada, epizootic plague in chipmunks and ground squirrels poses a risk to visitors in public parks. Hikers, campers, and hunters in natural areas throughout the western states are at a small but finite risk of exposure to plague, especially in the summer months.

Plague can be transmitted during the skinning and handling of carcasses of wild animals such as rabbits and hares, prairie dogs, wildcats, and coyotes. Such direct inoculation of mammal-adapted organisms is associated with primary septicemia and high mortality. Oropharyngeal plague can result from the ingestion of undercooked contaminated meat and perhaps from the manual transfer of infected fluids to the mouth during the handling of infected animal tissues.

Carnivores, including dogs and cats, can become infected with *Y. pestis* by eating infected rodents and perhaps by being bitten by fleas from infected rodents. Although clinical plague commonly develops in infected cats, it rarely does so in infected dogs, which thus do not directly expose humans to infection. However, both dogs and cats may transport infected fleas from rodent-infested areas to the home environment.

From 1950 through 1996, 387 plague cases were reported in the United States. Of the 376 evaluable cases, 322 cases (86%) presented as primary lymphadenitic (bubonic) plague, almost all of them thought to be associated with flea bites; 46 cases (12%) presented as primary septicemic plague, many of them following direct animal exposures; and 8 cases (2%) presented as primary pneumonic plague, 6 resulting from the inhalation of respiratory droplets released by infected cats and 2 from unknown sources. The last case of human-to-human plague transmission in the United States occurred in the Los Angeles outbreak of 1924/1925.

PATHOGENESIS AND PATHOLOGY *Y. pestis* is highly invasive and pathogenic. The mechanisms by which the organism causes disease are incompletely understood, but both chromosome- and plasmid-encoded gene products as well as altered cell-mediated immune responses are probably involved. Three plasmids encode for a variety of known or presumed virulence factors, including the F1 envelope antigen, which confers bacterial resistance to phagocytosis by polymorphonuclear leukocytes (PMNs) in vitro; a murine exotoxin; the V antigen, which is essential for virulence, may immunocompromise the host by suppressing the synthesis of interferon γ and tumor necrosis factor α, and stimulates protective immunity in laboratory animals; pesticin, a bactericidal protein of unknown function and importance; a protease that can activate plasminogen and degrade serum complement and that is thought to play a role in the dissemination of *Y. pestis* from peripheral sites of infection; a coagulase; and a fibrinolysin. A lipopolysaccharide endotoxin, believed to be chromosomally encoded, is probably important in triggering the systemic inflammatory response syndrome and its complications.

Y. pestis organisms inoculated through the skin or mucous membranes usually invade superficial lymphatic vessels and are carried to regional lymph nodes, although direct bloodstream inoculation may take place. Mononuclear phagocytes, which can phagocytize *Y. pestis* organisms without destroying them, may play a role in dissemination of the infection to distant sites. Plague can involve almost any organ, and untreated plague generally results in widespread and massive tissue destruction. In the early stages, infected lymph nodes (buboes, Fig. 162-1) are characterized by edema and congestion without inflammatory infiltrates or apparent vascular injury. Fully developed buboes contain huge numbers of infectious plague organisms and show distorted or obliterated lymph node architecture with vascular destruction and hemorrhage, serosanguineous effusion, necrosis, and a mild neutrophilic infiltration. At this stage, the effusion often involves perinodal tissues. If several adjacent lymph nodes are involved, a boggy edematous mass can result.

Primary septicemic plague results from the direct inoculation of bacteria from infected fluids or tissues or from an infective flea bite in the apparent absence of a bubo; secondary septicemic plague occurs when lymphatic and other host defenses are breached and the plague bacillus multiplies within the bloodstream. In fatal septicemic plague, multifocal hepatic and splenic necrosis is common. Diffuse interstitial myocarditis with cardiac dilatation is sometimes found. If disseminated intravascular coagulation (DIC) ensues, vascular necrosis may lead to widespread cutaneous, mucosal, and serosal ecchymoses and petechiae. Acral gangrene sometimes develops.

Primary plague pneumonia generally begins as a lobular process and then extends by confluence, becoming lobar and then multilobar (Fig. 162-2). Plague organisms are typically most numerous in the alveoli. Secondary plague pneumonia begins more diffusely, with organisms usually most numerous in the interstitium. In untreated cases of both primary and secondary plague pneumonia, diffuse pulmonary hemorrhage, necrosis, and neutrophilic infiltration develop.

MANIFESTATIONS Plague is characterized by a rapid onset of fever and other systemic manifestations of gram-negative bacterial infection. If it is not quickly and correctly treated, plague can follow a toxic course, resulting in shock, multiple-organ failure, and death. In humans, the three principal forms of plague are bubonic, septicemic, and pneumonic. Bubonic plague, the most common form, is almost always caused by the bite of an infected flea but occasionally results

FIGURE 162-1 Left inguinal and femoral buboes, with surrounding edema and overlying desquamation.

from direct inoculation of infectious fluids. Septicemic and pneumonic plague can be either primary or secondary to metastatic spread. Unusual secondary forms include plague meningitis, endophthalmitis, and lymphadenitis at multiple sites. Primary plague pharyngitis has been documented by culture of organisms from throat swabs and can result from respiratory exposure or ingestion of contaminated meat.

Bubonic plague usually has an incubation period of 2 to 6 days, occasionally longer. Typically, the patient experiences chills; fever, with temperatures that rise within hours to ≥38°C; myalgias; arthralgias; headache; and a feeling of weakness. Soon—usually within 24 h—the patient notices tenderness and pain in one or more regional lymph nodes proximal to the site of inoculation of the plague bacillus (Fig. 162-1). Because fleas often bite the legs, femoral and inguinal nodes are most commonly involved; axillary and cervical nodes are next most commonly affected. The enlarging bubo becomes progressively painful and tender, sometimes exquisitely so. The patient usually guards against palpation and limits movement, pressure, and stretch around the bubo. The surrounding tissue often becomes edematous, sometimes markedly so, and the overlying skin may be erythematous, warm, and tense. Inspection of the skin surrounding or distal to the bubo sometimes reveals the site of a flea bite marked by a small papule, pustule, eschar, or ulcer. A list of lymphadenitic conditions that could be confused with a plague bubo would include *Staphylococcus aureus* and group A β-hemolytic streptococcal infections, cat-scratch disease, and tularemia. The bubo of plague is distinguishable from lymphadenitis of most other causes, however, by its rapid onset, its extreme tenderness, the accompanying signs of toxemia, and the absence of cellulitis or obvious ascending lymphangitis.

Treated in the uncomplicated state with an appropriate antibiotic, bubonic plague usually responds quickly, with defervescence and alleviation of other systemic manifestations over 2 to 5 days. Buboes often remain enlarged and tender for a week or more after the initiation of treatment and can become fluctuant. Without effective antimicrobial treatment, patients with typical bubonic plague manifest an increasingly toxic state of fever, tachycardia, lethargy leading to prostration, agitation and confusion, and (occasionally) convulsions and delirium. Secondary plague sepsis may result in an alarmingly rapid and refractory cascade of DIC, bleeding, shock, and organ failure. Mild forms of bubonic plague, called *pestis minor*, have been described in South America and elsewhere; in these cases, the patients are ambulatory, are only mildly febrile, and have subacute buboes.

Septicemic plague is a progressive, overwhelming bacterial infection. Primary septicemia develops in the absence of apparent regional lymphadenitis, and the diagnosis of plague is often not suspected until preliminary blood culture results are reported to be positive by the laboratory. *Y. pestis*, however, can also be cultured from the blood of most bubonic plague patients, and bacteremia should be distinguished from septicemia, in which the patient is desperately ill and requires aggressive care. Patients with septicemic plague often present with gastrointestinal symptoms of nausea, vomiting, diarrhea, and abdominal pain, which may further confound the correct diagnosis. If not treated early with appropriate antibiotics, septicemic plague can be fulminant and fatal. In the United States in 1950 through 1996, 66 cases of septicemic plague and 18 deaths were reported, for a case-fatality rate of 27%. Petechiae, ecchymoses, bleeding from puncture wounds and orifices, and gangrene of acral parts are manifestations of DIC; refractory hypotension, renal shutdown, obtundation, and other signs of shock are preterminal events. Adult respiratory distress syndrome (ARDS), which can occur at any stage of septicemic plague, is sometimes confused with other conditions, such as hantavirus pulmonary syndrome.

Of all forms of the disease, pneumonic plague develops most rapidly and is most frequently fatal. The incubation period for primary pneumonic plague is rarely longer than 1 to 4 days. The onset is most often sudden, with chills, fever, headache, myalgias, weakness, and

FIGURE 162-2 Sequential chest radiographs of a patient with fatal primary plague pneumonia. *Left:* Upright posteroanterior film taken at admission to hospital emergency department on third day of illness, showing segmental consolidation of right upper lobe. *Center:* Portable anteroposterior film taken 8 h after admission, showing extension of pneumonia to right middle and right lower lobes. *Right:* Portable anteroposterior film taken 13 h after admission (when patient had clinical adult respiratory distress syndrome), showing diffuse infiltration throughout right lung and patchy infiltration of left lower lung. A cavity later developed at the site of initial right upper lobe consolidation.

dizziness. Pulmonary signs, including cough, sputum production, chest pain, tachypnea, and dyspnea, typically arise on the second day of illness and may be accompanied by hemoptysis, increasing respiratory distress, cardiopulmonary insufficiency, and circulatory collapse. In primary plague pneumonia, the sputum is most often watery or mucoid, frothy, and blood-tinged, but it may become frankly bloody. Pulmonary signs in primary pneumonic plague may indicate involvement of a single lobe in the early stage, with rapidly developing segmental consolidation before bronchopneumonic spread to other lobes of the same and opposite lungs. Liquefaction necrosis and cavitation may occur early in areas of consolidation and may or may not leave significant residual scarring.

Secondary plague pneumonia manifests first as diffuse interstitial pneumonitis in which sputum production is scant; since the sputum is more likely to be inspissated and tenacious in character than the sputum found in primary pneumonia, it may be less infectious. In the United States in 1950 through 1996, 39 cases of secondary pneumonic plague and 8 cases of primary pneumonic plague were reported, with no known transmission to contacts and an overall case-fatality rate of 41%. Observers in the early twentieth century remarked on the relative lack of auscultatory findings, the usual presence of toxemia, and the frequency of sudden death in patients with pneumonic plague as compared to patients with other bacterial pneumonias.

Meningitis is an unusual manifestation of plague. In the United States, there were 12 meningitis cases among the 376 evaluable plague cases reported in 1950 through 1996. All cases of meningitis were complications of bubonic plague, and all patients survived. Although meningitis may be a part of the initial presentation of plague, its onset is often delayed and is a manifestation of insufficient treatment. Recent cases in the United States have occurred during the first and second weeks of antibiotic treatment for bubonic plague. Chronic relapsing meningeal plague over periods of weeks or even months was described in the preantibiotic era. The affected patients typically presented with fever, headache, meningismus, and pleocytosis.

Plague pharyngitis presents as fever, sore throat, cervical lymphadenitis, and headache and is often indistinguishable clinically from pharyngitis of other infectious etiologies. Caregivers working in plague-endemic areas must be alert to the possibility of plague to avoid misdiagnosis leading to delayed and/or inappropriate treatment.

LABORATORY FINDINGS AND DIAGNOSIS Since plague is a rare disease in the United States, a high index of clinical suspicion as well as the elicitation of a thorough clinical and epidemiologic history and a careful physical examination are required for timely diagnosis and prompt institution of specific therapy. When the diagnosis of plague is delayed or missed altogether, a high case-fatality rate results; infected travelers who seek medical care after they have left endemic areas (peripatetic plague cases) are at especially high risk. Plague must be considered in the differential diagnosis of sepsis in an otherwise-healthy person who has a history of recent travel to or res-

idence in the rural western United States. When the diagnosis of plague is being considered, close communication between clinicians and the diagnostic laboratory and between the diagnostic laboratory and a qualified reference laboratory is essential. Tests for plague are highly reliable when conducted by laboratory personnel experienced with *Y. pestis*, but such expertise is usually limited to selected reference laboratories, including state health department laboratories in some plague-endemic states and the CDC plague laboratory (Fort Collins, Colorado; tel. 970-221-6400).

When plague is suspected, specimens should be collected promptly for laboratory studies, chest roentgenograms should be obtained, and specific antimicrobial therapy should be initiated pending confirmation. Appropriate diagnostic specimens for smear and culture include citrated or heparinized whole blood from all patients with suspected plague, bubo aspirates from those with suspected buboes, sputum samples or tracheal aspirates from those with suspected pneumonic plague, and cerebrospinal fluid (CSF) from those with suspected plague meningitis. Since early buboes are often exquisitely tender and are seldom fluctuant or necrotic, these lesions usually require aspiration under local anesthesia following the injection of 1 to 2 mL of normal saline (sterile but nonbacteriostatic) into the bubo with a 20- to 22-gauge needle. A variety of appropriate culture media (including brain-heart infusion broth, sheep blood agar, and MacConkey agar) should be inoculated with a portion of each specimen. Moreover, for each specimen, at least one smear should be examined immediately with Wayson or Giemsa stain and at least one with Gram's stain; a smear should also be submitted for direct fluorescent antibody testing. An acute-phase serum specimen should be tested for antibody to *Y. pestis*; whenever possible, a convalescent-phase serum specimen collected 3 to 4 weeks later should also be tested. When a patient dies and plague is suspected, appropriate autopsy tissues for culture, direct fluorescent antibody testing, and immunohistochemical staining include buboes, all solid organs (especially liver, spleen, and lung), and bone marrow. If culture of such specimens is to be attempted, they should be sent to the laboratory either fresh or frozen on dry ice, not in preservatives or fixatives. If necessary, Cary-Blair or a similar medium can be used to transport *Y. pestis*–infected tissues.

Laboratory confirmation of plague depends on the isolation of *Y. pestis* from cultures of body fluids or tissues. Cultures of three blood samples taken over a 45-min period before treatment will usually result in isolation of the bacterium. *Y. pestis* strains are readily distinguished from those of the closely related species *Y. pseudotuberculosis* by differences in biochemical profile, temperature-dependent susceptibility to lysis by a *Y. pestis*–specific bacteriophage, and motility. Automated bacteriologic test systems can be used to assist in the identification of isolates as *Y. pestis*, but *Y. pestis* can be misidentified (e.g., as *Y. pseudotuberculosis*) or overlooked if these systems are improperly programmed.

In the absence of *Y. pestis* isolation, plague cases can be confirmed

FIGURE 162-3 Peripheral blood smear from a patient with fatal plague septicemia and shock, showing characteristic bipolar-staining *Y. pestis* bacilli (Wright's stain, oil immersion).

either by the demonstration of seroconversion (a fourfold or greater titer rise) to *Y. pestis* F1 antigen in passive hemagglutination tests of acute- and convalescent-phase serum specimens or by detection of an antibody titer of >128 in a single serum sample from a patient with a plague-compatible illness who has not received plague vaccine. The specificity of a positive passive-hemagglutination test requires confirmation with the F1 antigen hemagglutination-inhibition test. A few plague patients seroconvert to F1 antigen as early as 5 days after the onset of illness. Most seroconvert between 1 and 2 weeks after onset; a few seroconvert 3 weeks or more after onset; and a few (<5%) fail to seroconvert at all. Early, specific antibiotic treatment may delay seroconversion by several weeks. After seroconversion, positive serologic titers diminish gradually over months to years. Enzyme-linked immunosorbent assays (ELISAs) for IgM and IgG antibodies to *Y. pestis* are replacing hemagglutination tests in some laboratories. Other new test methods include IgM antibody capture and competitive blocking for detection of antibody to F1.

Detection of F1 antigen in tissues or fluids by direct fluorescent antibody testing or by antigen capture is presumptive evidence of plague, as is an F1 antibody titer of >10 in a single serum sample from a patient with a plague-compatible illness who has not received plague vaccine. Visualization of characteristic bipolar bacilli in a Giemsa- or Wayson-stained smear constitutes supportive evidence of plague. Tularemia, especially the glandular, typhoidal, and pneumonic forms, can sometimes be confused clinically and epidemiologically with plague, but the results of microbiologic and serologic tests should readily distinguish these two diseases.

Patients with plague typically have white blood cell (WBC) counts of 15,000 to 25,000/μL, with a predominance of PMNs and a left shift. Leukemoid reactions with WBC counts as high as 100,000/μL can occur. Modest thrombocytopenia is usually documented, and fibrin-fibrinogen split products are often detected even in patients without frank DIC. Serum levels of aminotransferases and bilirubin may be elevated. Chest roentgenograms of patients with pneumonic plague usually show patchy bronchopneumonic infiltrates as well as lobar or segmental consolidation with or without confluence (Fig. 162-2); they occasionally show cavitation. Stained sputum samples usually contain PMNs and characteristic bipolar-staining bacilli. In *Y. pestis* septicemia, visualization of the characteristic bacilli in a routine blood smear or a buffy-coat smear is an uncommon but grave prognostic sign (Fig. 162-3). In patients with plague meningitis, pleocytosis with a predominance of PMNs is the rule, and the characteristic bacilli are usually visible in stained CSF smears.

℞ **TREATMENT** Left untreated, plague is fatal in more than 50% of cases of bubonic disease and in nearly all cases of septicemic and pneumonic disease. The overall mortality rate for plague cases in the United States since 1950 has been ~16%; deaths are almost always due to delays in seeking treatment, misdiagnosis, delays in the institution of treatment, or incorrect treatment. Rapid diagnosis and appropriate antimicrobial therapy are essential.

Guidelines for the treatment of plague are given in Table 162-1. Although streptomycin is the drug of choice, gentamicin is increasingly used for the treatment of plague in the United States because of its ready availability; it is probably as effective as streptomycin, although results of controlled studies in humans have not been published. Alternative antibiotics include the tetracyclines and chloramphenicol; these agents are usually given orally with initial loading doses but may be given intravenously to critically ill patients and to patients unable to tolerate oral medication. Penicillins, cephalosporins, and macrolides are suboptimal and should not be used. Doxycycline may be as effective as other tetracyclines or even more so, but comparative evaluations have not been made. Trimethoprim-sulfamethoxazole has been used successfully to treat bubonic plague but is not considered a first-line choice. Chloramphenicol is indicated for the treatment of plague meningitis, pleuritis, endophthalmitis, and myocarditis because of its superior tissue penetration; it is used alone or in combination with streptomycin. In general, antimicrobial treatment should be continued for 10 days or for at least 3 days after the patient has become afebrile and has made a clinical recovery. Patients initially given intravenous antibiotics may be switched to oral regimens upon clinical improvement. Such improvement is usually evident 2 or 3 days after the start of treatment, even though fever may continue for several days.

Consequences of delayed treatment of plague include DIC, ARDS, and other complications of gram-negative sepsis. Patients with these disorders require intensive monitoring and close physiologic support, as outlined elsewhere (Chaps. 117 and 265). Buboes may require surgical drainage. Abscessed nodes can cause recurrent fever in patients who have apparently recovered; this relation may be occult if intrathoracic or intraabdominal nodes are involved. Although *Y. pestis* is considered to be genetically stable, a multidrug-resistant strain was isolated from a plague patient in Madagascar. This strain exhibited resistance (mediated by a transferable plasmid) to all first-line antibiotics used for treatment of plague and to the principal alternatives used for treatment and prophylaxis.

PREVENTION AND CONTROL Persons at greatest risk for plague in the United States are those who live, work, and participate in outdoor recreational activities in areas of those western states in which plague is enzootic. Surveillance, education, and environmental management are the cornerstones of prevention and control. A network

Table 162-1 Guidelines for the Treatment of Plague

Drug	Daily Dosage	Interval, h	Route(s) of Administration
Streptomycin			
Adults	2 g	12	IM
Children	30 mg/kg	12	IM
Gentamicin			
Adults	3–5 mg/kg[a]	8	IM or IV
Children	6.0–7.5 mg/kg	8	IM or IV
Infants/neonates	7.5 mg/kg	8	IM or IV
Tetracycline			
Adults	2 g	6	PO or IV
Children ≥8 y	25–50 mg/kg	6	PO or IV
Doxycycline			
Adults	200 mg	12 or 24	PO or IV
Children ≥8 y	4 mg/kg	12 or 24	PO or IV
Oxytetracycline			
Adults	250–300 mg	8, 12, or 24	PO or IM
Children ≥8 y	15–25 mg/kg[b]	8, 12, or 24	PO or IM
Chloramphenicol			
Adults	50 mg/kg[c]	6	PO or IV
Children ≥1 y	50 mg/kg[c]	6	PO or IV

[a] Dosage should be reduced to 3 mg/kg daily as soon as clinically indicated.
[b] Maximum, 250 mg IM in a single daily dose.
[c] For meningitis, up to 100 (mg/kg)/d initially.

of biologists and public health specialists coordinates these activities through local and state health departments and the CDC. Personal protective measures include the avoidance of areas with known epizootic plague (which may be posted) and of sick or dead animals; the use of repellents, insecticides, and protective clothing when at risk of exposure to rodents' fleas; and the wearing of gloves when handling animal carcasses. Short-term antibiotic prophylaxis (Table 162-2) is recommended for persons known to have had direct contact with a patient with suspected or confirmed pneumonic plague and occasionally for persons who are unable to avoid an area where a plague outbreak is in progress or who may be caring for patients with plague. Patients in whom plague is suspected should be managed under isolation precautions for respiratory droplet transmission until pneumonia has been ruled out or until 48 h of specific antimicrobial therapy has been administered, after which universal precautions are adequate.

Rodent food (garbage, pet food) and habitats (brush piles, junk heaps, woodpiles) should be eliminated in domestic, peridomestic, and working environments; buildings and food stores should be rodent-proofed. The control of fleas with insecticides is a key public health measure in situations where epizootic plague activity places humans at high risk; this effort includes dusting and spraying of rodent burrows, rodent runs, and other sites where rodents and their fleas are found. In plague-endemic areas of the western United States, persons should keep their dogs and cats free of fleas and restrained. The decision to control plague by killing rodents should be left to public health authorities, and such a program should be carried out only in conjunction with effective flea control. Killing of rodents has no lasting benefit without environmental sanitation.

The previously used killed, whole-cell plague vaccine is no longer manufactured in the United States. Efforts are being made to develop improved vaccines in which the production of specific immunoprotective antibodies to *Y. pestis* is induced by recombinant antigens. In the United States, the indications for use of these newer vaccines would probably be similar to those for the previously available killed vaccine, which was mostly limited to protecting laboratory personnel who routinely worked with *Y. pestis* and some persons whose vocations brought them into regular contact with wild rodents and their fleas in areas with enzootic or epizootic plague. In addition, a vaccine might be useful in protecting selected military personnel and in responding to the possible use of *Y. pestis* as a weapon of bioterrorism.

OTHER *YERSINIA* INFECTIONS

DEFINITION Yersiniosis is an uncommon bacterial zoonosis caused by infection with either of the two enteropathogenic *Yersinia* species: *Y. enterocolitica* or *Y. pseudotuberculosis*. Reservoir hosts of these bacteria include swine and other wild and domestic animals.

Table 162-2 Guidelines for Plague Prophylaxis

Drug	Daily Dosage	Interval, h	Route of Administration
Tetracycline			
Adults	1–2 g	6 or 12	PO
Children ≥8 y	25–50 mg/kg	6 or 12	PO
Doxycycline			
Adults	100–200 mg	12 or 24	PO
Children ≥8 y	2–4 mg/kg	12 or 24	PO
Trimethoprim-sulfamethoxazole			
Adults	320 mg[a]	12	PO
Children ≥2 mo	8 mg/kg[a]	12	PO

[a] Trimethoprim component.

These yersiniae are transmitted to humans predominantly via the oral route. Both sporadic cases and common-source outbreaks occur. The most frequent acute clinical manifestations are (1) enteritis or enterocolitis with self-limited diarrhea (especially with *Y. enterocolitica*), and (2) mesenteric adenitis and terminal ileitis (especially with *Y. pseudotuberculosis*), which can be difficult to distinguish from acute appendicitis. Septicemia and metastatic focal infections are less common. Some cases of yersiniosis are complicated by nonsuppurative, extraintestinal, inflammatory sequelae—e.g., reactive arthritis (Chap. 315) and erythema nodosum (Chap. 18).

ETIOLOGIC AGENTS *Y. enterocolitica* and *Y. pseudotuberculosis* are pleomorphic gram-negative bacilli in the family Enterobacteriaceae. They are aerobic or facultatively anaerobic, motile at 25°C, nonmotile at 37°C, oxidase negative, urease positive, able to ferment glucose, unable to ferment lactose, and usually able to reduce nitrates. They grow well, if slowly, on nonselective media (e.g., blood agar) and on most of the routine media used to select for enteric bacteria (e.g., MacConkey agar). They can multiply within a wide temperature range (−1°C to 45°C). The most clinically and epidemiologically useful methods for identifying pathogenic *Y. enterocolitica* isolates are biotyping based on biochemical profiles and serotyping according to somatic O and H antigens. Six biotypes and more than 60 serotypes of *Y. enterocolitica* are recognized. A separate serotyping system for *Y. pseudotuberculosis* (also based on somatic antigens) has distinguished six major serotypes (I through VI) and their subtypes.

EPIDEMIOLOGY *Y. enterocolitica* is distributed worldwide and has been isolated from soil, fresh water, contaminated foodstuffs (e.g., meat, milk, and vegetables), and a wide variety of wild and domestic animals, including mammals, birds, amphibians, fish, and shellfish. Many serotypes isolated from environmental sources, however, evidently are not human pathogens. Most human infections have been caused by *Y. enterocolitica* serotypes O:3, O:5, O:8, and O:9, which are primarily associated with wild and domestic mammals. The incidence of these infections and their sequelae is highest in Scandinavia and some other northern European countries, but this observation may be in part an artifact of underrecognition in other countries. Because many individuals with enteric *Y. enterocolitica* infection are asymptomatic or minimally symptomatic and do not seek medical attention, reliable population-based estimates of incidence are unavailable. However, in many clinical microbiology laboratories in recent decades, *Y. enterocolitica* has been the fourth most common bacterial pathogen isolated from patients' fecal specimens, trailing *Salmonella* (the most frequently isolated), *Campylobacter*, and *Shigella* species.

All age groups are susceptible to *Y. enterocolitica* infections, but the majority of cases of enterocolitis are in children aged 1 to 4. Moreover, these infections show a modest predilection for males. Mesenteric adenitis and terminal ileitis are most common among older children and young adults. Risk factors for *Y. enterocolitica* septicemia and metastatic focal infections include chronic liver disease, malignancy, diabetes mellitus, immunosuppressive therapy, alcoholism, malnutrition, advanced age, iron overload (see below), and hemolytic anemias (including the thalassemias). The nonsuppurative sequelae of yersiniosis are most common among adults. HLA-B27 is expressed in 70 to 80% of patients who develop reactive arthritis associated with yersiniosis. HLA-B27 is not a risk factor for *Yersinia*-induced erythema nodosum; females with this condition outnumber males by 2 to 1. In Europe, *Y. enterocolitica* infections are more common in the cooler months than in warmer weather. In North America, no consistent seasonal pattern has been documented.

For several decades, serotypes O:3 and O:9 have predominated among *Y. enterocolitica* isolates from patients in Europe. Serotype O:3 has also predominated in Canada and Japan. In the United States, serotype O:3 emerged in the 1980s to surpass serotype O:8 in frequency of isolation from patients. The incidence of *Yersinia*-induced nonsuppurative sequelae reportedly is 10 to 30% in Scandinavia and much lower in most other countries, including the United States. No convincing explanation for this observation has been confirmed, but reasonable possibilities include population genetic factors and geographic strain variation.

Common-source outbreaks of *Y. enterocolitica* enteritis have been traced to such vehicles as raw milk, contaminated pasteurized milk, and foods prepared with contaminated fresh water. In Belgium, the ingestion of ground raw pork (a regional custom) is a significant risk factor for sporadic infection with *Y. enterocolitica* serotypes O:3 and O:9. These serotypes commonly colonize the oral cavity and intestines of European swine, and *Y. enterocolitica* infection is an occupational risk of swine butchers in Europe. In the United States, sporadic cases and one outbreak of *Y. enterocolitica* O:3 infection have been associated with the preparation or ingestion of raw pork intestines (chitterlings). In some cases of yersiniosis, circumstantial evidence suggests transmission via contact with dogs and cats or their feces. Several nosocomial outbreaks of *Y. enterocolitica* infection have been described; fecal-oral transmission from person to person was suspected. Fecal-oral transmission among family members may also explain occasional secondary cases in households. In a prospective study of 50 children with *Y. enterocolitica* enteritis, fecal excretion of the organism persisted for an average of 27 days (range, 4 to 79 days) after the cessation of symptoms. A chronic carrier state, however, has not been demonstrated. *Y. enterocolitica* is a rare but often lethal cause of transfusion-associated septicemia. The explanation is that blood donors occasionally have transient, occult *Y. enterocolitica* bacteremia and that this organism can slowly multiply to high concentrations in blood refrigerated for at least 10 to 20 days.

The ecology of *Y. pseudotuberculosis* seems to parallel that of *Y. enterocolitica* closely. *Y. pseudotuberculosis* is also widespread in wild and domestic animals and is isolated from many environmental sources. Human infections with *Y. pseudotuberculosis*, however, appear to be rare. In North America and Europe, most such infections have been with serotype I, but outbreaks involving other serotypes have occurred in Japan and Scandinavia. Swine appear to be an important reservoir for pathogenic strains of *Y. pseudotuberculosis*.

PATHOGENESIS AND PATHOLOGY Except in rare instances of transmission via contaminated blood products or direct cutaneous inoculation, the enteropathogenic yersiniae are thought to enter the host via the oral route. The 50% infectious dose in humans is uncertain but may be $\geq 10^9$. The incubation period averages 5 days (range, 1 to 11 days). Studies of animals have shown that the organisms initially invade the ileal epithelium, then are translocated via M cells into the lamina propria, and finally enter Peyer's patches, where they are able to replicate. They subsequently drain into the mesenteric lymph nodes, which undergo hyperplasia and from which the bacteria can be distributed systemically. The mesenteric lymph nodes can become intensely swollen and matted and are occasionally detected on physical examination as a tender right lower quadrant mass. Intestinal inflammation (most commonly of the distal ileum and less commonly of the ascending colon) develops and may be accompanied by mucosal ulcerations and by the shedding of PMNs and red blood cells into the intestinal lumen. In relatively severe cases, thrombosis of mesenteric blood vessels, intestinal hemorrhage, and necrosis can occur. In patients with enteropathogenic yersinial infections who undergo exploratory laparotomy, the appendix usually is histologically normal or shows only lymphoid hyperplasia, but frank suppuration is sometimes evident.

A plasmid of ~70 kb is essential for virulence of the enteropathogenic yersiniae because it encodes at least six *Yersinia* outer-membrane proteins, some of which confer to bacterial strains such properties as cytotoxicity; resistance to phagocytosis by PMNs; and the abilities to cause monocyte apoptosis (programmed cell death), to suppress the host's expression of tumor necrosis factor α, to interfere with platelet aggregation and host complement activation, and to dephosphorylate host proteins. A chromosomal gene (*inv*) encodes for the

surface protein invasin, which is necessary for yersinial invasion of nonphagocytic host cells (e.g., epithelial cells) in vitro and which facilitates the translocation of bacteria across the intestinal epithelium. Both *Y. enterocolitica* and *Y. pseudotuberculosis* can express at least one protein superantigen that selectively stimulates the proliferation of T cells. Many strains of *Y. enterocolitica* produce a heat-stable enterotoxin that is similar to *Escherichia coli* enterotoxin. The cell walls of *Y. enterocolitica* and *Y. pseudotuberculosis* contain a lipopolysaccharide (endotoxin). The roles of superantigens, enterotoxin, and endotoxin in the pathogenesis of yersiniosis are unclear. Some *Yersinia* strains are unable to synthesize bacterial iron chelators called *siderophores*. However, they can exploit host-chelated iron stores and the drug deferoxamine (a siderophore produced by *Streptomyces pilosus*). Therefore, iron overload (e.g., caused by hemodialysis or multiple transfusions) and deferoxamine therapy appear to be independent risk factors for *Y. enterocolitica* bacteremia (especially that involving serotypes O:3 and O:9) and to a lesser degree for *Y. pseudotuberculosis* bacteremia.

Immunogenetic factors and cell-mediated immune responses are clearly involved in the pathogenesis of reactive arthritis following infection with the enteropathogenic yersiniae. As noted above, most patients with *Yersinia*-induced reactive arthritis express HLA-B27. In addition, *Y. pseudotuberculosis* shares at least one cross-reactive epitope with HLA-B27, and *Y. enterocolitica* infection alters the expression of serologic HLA-B27 epitopes on lymphocytes and monocytes. In patients with reactive arthritis following *Y. enterocolitica* infection, yersinial antigens are commonly detectable in synovial fluid cells in the apparent absence of whole organisms. Thus, it is unknown whether the arthritis results from occult bacterial persistence through self-tolerance of HLA-B27 with a failure of cross-reactive immune responses to yersiniae, from an immune response to common antigenic determinants shared by the bacteria and host HLA-B27 (i.e., molecular mimicry), or from other mechanisms. The pathogenesis of *Yersinia*-induced erythema nodosum is obscure.

In some assays, patients with Graves' disease have an increased prevalence of serum antibodies to *Y. enterocolitica*, and the immunoglobulins of patients recovering from *Y. enterocolitica* infections react with the human thyroid-stimulating hormone receptor. However, a link between *Y. enterocolitica* infection and the subsequent development of autoimmune thyroiditis has not been convincingly demonstrated.

MANIFESTATIONS The principal clinical manifestations of *Y. enterocolitica* infection are enteritis, enterocolitis, mesenteric adenitis, and terminal ileitis. Less common manifestations include exudative pharyngitis, septicemia, metastatic focal infections, reactive polyarthritis, and erythema nodosum. When age groups are combined, the most common presentation of *Y. enterocolitica* infection is acute diarrhea from enteritis or enterocolitis. Low-grade fever and cramping abdominal pain occur in most cases, nausea and vomiting in 15 to 40%, hematochezia in up to 30%, and a generalized maculopapular skin rash in a few cases. Diarrhea persists for an average of 2 weeks (range, 1 day to many months), during which the frequency of bowel movements diminishes. Uncommonly, enteritis or enterocolitis can be complicated by severe abdominal pain and high fever. Rare (and sometimes fatal) complications include diffuse inflammation, ulceration, hemorrhage, and necrosis of the small bowel and colon; intestinal perforation; peritonitis; ascending cholangitis; mesenteric vein thrombosis; diverticulitis; toxic megacolon; and ileocecal intussusception.

The syndrome of mesenteric adenitis and terminal ileitis without diarrhea is easily confused with appendicitis. Low-grade fever and right lower quadrant pain, tenderness, guarding, and rebound tenderness are common. During six recognized common-source outbreaks in the United States, 10% of 444 patients with symptomatic undiagnosed *Y. enterocolitica* infections underwent laparotomy for suspected appendicitis; surgical incisions became infected with *Y. enterocolitica* in a few of these cases.

Acute pharyngitis and pharyngotonsillitis, with or without cervical adenitis or intestinal illness, are less common but potentially lethal manifestations of *Y. enterocolitica* infection, particularly in adults. *Y. enterocolitica* septicemia generally presents as a severe illness with fever and leukocytosis, often with abdominal pain and jaundice and without localized signs of infection. Metastatic focal *Y. enterocolitica* infections can occur with or without clinically apparent bacteremia and can affect almost any organ system. Examples include abscess formation (e.g., in liver, spleen, kidney, lung, skeletal muscle, lymph node, or cutaneous tissue), osteomyelitis, meningitis, peritonitis, urinary tract infection, pneumonia, empyema, endocarditis, pericarditis, mycotic aneurysm, septic arthritis, suppurative conjunctivitis, panophthalmitis, Parinaud's oculoglandular syndrome, and cutaneous pustules or bullae.

In Scandinavia, the incidence of reactive arthritis following *Y. enterocolitica* infection among adults is estimated to be at least 10%. About 80% of these patients have preceding symptoms such as fever, diarrhea, or abdominal pain. Typically, these symptoms precede the arthritis by 1 week and are of short duration. The most commonly affected joints are the knees and ankles, but other joints can be involved. Typically, multiple (two to eight) joints become involved sequentially and asymmetrically over a period of a few days to 2 weeks, after which no additional joints are affected. Monoarticular arthritis occurs less commonly. In two-thirds of cases, the acute arthritis remits spontaneously within 1 to 3 months. Chronic joint disease is documented in a minority of cases. A few HLA-B27-positive patients with *Y. enterocolitica*–induced arthritis have subsequent ankylosing spondylitis, but this development is best explained by the fact that HLA-B27 is a major risk factor for each of these diseases. Mild, self-limited myocarditis accompanies about 10% of cases of *Yersinia*-induced arthritis and can occur independently. Typical manifestations include cardiac murmurs and transient electrocardiographic abnormalities, such as prolongation of the PR interval and nonspecific ST-segment and T-wave changes. The syndrome of *Yersinia*-induced arthritis and carditis can be confused with acute rheumatic fever. In Scandinavia, erythema nodosum occurs in 15 to 20% of patients with yersiniosis, usually within a few days to 3 weeks after the onset of intestinal illness. Lesions typically are located on the lower extremities and resolve within 1 month. Less commonly reported nonsuppurative sequelae of *Y. enterocolitica* infections include reactive uveitis, iritis, conjunctivitis, urethritis, and glomerulonephritis. The complete triad of Reiter's syndrome (arthritis, conjunctivitis, and urethritis) is seen in 5 to 10% of patients with *Yersinia*-induced arthritis.

The most common clinical presentation of *Y. pseudotuberculosis* infection is fever and abdominal pain caused by mesenteric adenitis; diarrheal illness is less common than in *Y. enterocolitica* infection. Systemic manifestations, including septicemia, focal infections, reactive arthritis, and erythema nodosum, are generally similar to those associated with *Y. enterocolitica* infection. In addition, *Y. pseudotuberculosis* has been associated with a scarlet fever–like syndrome, acute interstitial nephritis, and hemolytic-uremic syndrome.

LABORATORY FINDINGS AND DIAGNOSIS Results of routine laboratory tests in most patients with yersiniosis are nonspecific. Leukocyte counts are usually normal or slightly elevated, often with a modest left shift. Standard microbiologic methods are sufficient to isolate *Y. enterocolitica* and *Y. pseudotuberculosis* from otherwise-sterile sites, such as blood, CSF, lymph node tissue, and peritoneal fluid, and from abscesses. Isolation of these organisms from feces is impeded by their slow growth and the overgrowth of normal fecal flora on culture media routinely used to select for enteric bacteria. When routine enteric media are used, the yield of yersinial isolates from feces is increased by incubation at 22 to 25°C for 48 h. The yield from feces and other grossly contaminated specimens can be further increased by the use of *Yersinia*-selective cefsulodin-Irgasan-novobiocin (CIN) agar

and by cold enrichment (i.e., inoculation of feces into buffered saline and incubation at 4°C for 2 to 4 weeks, with periodic plating onto enteric media). Because bacteriologic procedures designed to isolate yersiniae from feces are not considered cost-effective, many laboratories undertake them by special request only.

The results of serologic tests can be used to support a diagnosis of yersiniosis. Agglutination tests or ELISAs are used most commonly; immunoblotting has also been used. The existence of multiple serotypes makes routine serologic tests laborious; thus these tests are generally conducted only in research laboratories or large commercial laboratories. Since these tests are experimental and are neither standardized nor well validated, and since some strains of *Yersinia* cross-react with other bacteria (e.g., *Brucella*, *Salmonella*, and *Vibrio*) and with serum from some patients with thyroiditis, results should be interpreted with caution. In typical uncomplicated cases of yersiniosis, agglutinin titers begin to rise within the first week of illness, peak in the second week, and then gradually diminish and return to normal within 3 to 6 months, although agglutinating antibody may remain detectable for several years in some cases. Because an initial serum specimen is often collected a week or more after the onset of illness, when agglutinin titers are already high, it is usually impossible to document a fourfold or greater rise in titer between paired specimens (although a fourfold or greater fall in titer may be found). Immunohistologic techniques and polymerase chain reaction tests to detect yersinial antigens and DNA, respectively, in clinical specimens are experimental at this time.

In patients with *Yersinia*-induced reactive arthritis, synovial fluid is sterile and the leukocyte count ranges from a few hundred to 60,000/μL, with a majority of PMNs. The erythrocyte sedimentation rate is often >100 mm/h. Rheumatoid factor and antinuclear antibodies are usually absent. The diagnosis of *Yersinia*-induced reactive arthritis or other nonsuppurative inflammatory sequelae can be difficult, especially when triggering infections are asymptomatic or clinically mild or occur several weeks before the diagnosis is attempted. Because the isolation of a pathogenic *Yersinia* strain from feces is the most specific diagnostic test in such cases, it should be attempted. Since culture is of limited sensitivity in this clinical setting, a high index of suspicion and positive results of serologic tests for *Y. enterocolitica* or *Y. pseudotuberculosis* are usually required for diagnosis.

℞ TREATMENT The effectiveness of antimicrobial agents in the treatment of yersinial enteritis, enterocolitis, mesenteric adenitis, or terminal ileitis has not been established. These conditions are usually self-limited, and their treatment is symptom-based and supportive. In uncomplicated cases, diarrhea should be treated with fluid and electrolyte replacement, with the route of delivery dependent on clinical severity. Enteric precautions are advisable for patients hospitalized with yersinial diarrhea. In general, antimicrobial treatment should be reserved for patients with septicemia, metastatic focal infections, or immunosuppression and enterocolitis. Controlled clinical comparisons of antimicrobial agents in the treatment of severe cases of yersiniosis have not yet been conducted. In such cases, drug selection should ultimately be guided by clinical response and bacterial sensitivity patterns. Clinical isolates of *Y. enterocolitica* and *Y. pseudotuberculosis* are usually susceptible in vitro to aminoglycosides, third-generation cephalosporins, chloramphenicol, quinolones, tetracyclines, and trimethoprim-sulfamethoxazole. In laboratory animals infected with enteropathogenic yersiniae, the fluoroquinolones have exerted the strongest bactericidal effects in vivo; clinical experience with these drugs against these pathogens in humans is promising but limited. Because they produce β-lactamases, isolates typically are resistant to penicillin, ampicillin, carbenicillin, and first-generation and most second-generation cephalosporins. Optimal dosages and durations of therapy have not been established. Mortality from *Y. enterocolitica* septicemia currently is ~10% despite treatment. Focal extraintestinal infections may require at least 3 weeks of therapy. No role for antimicrobial agents in the management of the nonsuppurative inflammatory manifestations of yersiniosis has been established. Patients with reactive arthritis may benefit from treatment with nonsteroidal anti-inflammatory drugs, intraarticular steroid injections, and physical therapy.

PREVENTION AND CONTROL   The importance of safe food-handling and food-preparation practices in the prevention of yersiniosis cannot be overemphasized. Caution is particularly warranted in the case of pork and other animal products. The consumption of raw or undercooked meats, especially pork, should be avoided. Increased efforts to prevent the spread of enteric pathogens in household, pet-care, day-care, and hospital settings and in the food industry would be likely to decrease the incidence of yersiniosis. Current regulations of the U.S. Food and Drug Administration require visual inspection of packed red cell units before transfusion, with the discarding of units in which bacterial contamination is suspected on the basis of darkening (reflecting decreased oxygen saturation and hemolysis). Since the risk is minimal, more specific measures to further decrease the likelihood of transfusion of *Y. enterocolitica*–contaminated blood products (e.g., limiting the period for which red cells can be stored before transfusion) are not considered cost-effective.

Yersiniosis is not routinely reportable to public health authorities in most jurisdictions. However, clinicians who suspect a common-source outbreak (e.g., because they have documented a familial case cluster or have diagnosed the disease in several apparently unrelated patients over a short period) or some other public health threat (e.g., because they have found occult *Y. enterocolitica* bacteremia in a recent blood donor) should consult promptly with local public health officials.

BIBLIOGRAPHY

PLAGUE

CENTERS FOR DISEASE CONTROL AND PREVENTION: Fatal human plague—Arizona and Colorado, 1996. MMWR 46:617, 1997

CORNELIS GR et al: The virulence plasmid of *Yersinia*, an antihost genome. Microbiol Mol Biol Rev 62:1315, 1998

DENNIS DT: Plague as an emerging disease, in *Emerging Infections 2*, WM Scheld et al (eds). Washington, DC, ASM Press, 1998, pp 169–183

GALIMAND M et al: Multidrug resistance in *Yersinia pestis* mediated by a transferable plasmid. N Engl J Med 337:677, 1997

INGLESBY TV et al: Plague as a biological weapon: Medical and public health management. Consensus statement of the Working Group on Civilian Biodefense. JAMA, 1999 (in press)

OTHER *YERSINIA* INFECTIONS

BOTTONE EJ: *Yersinia enterocolitica*: The charisma continues. Clin Microbiol Rev 10: 257, 1997

RATSITORAHINA M et al: Epidemiological and diagnostic aspects of the outbreak of pneumonic plague in Madagascar. Lancet 355:111, 2000

STOLK-ENGELAAR VM, HOOGKAMP-KORSTANJE JA: Clinical presentation and diagnosis of gastrointestinal infections by *Yersinia enterocolitica* in 261 Dutch patients. Scand J Infect Dis 28:571, 1996

——— et al: In-vitro antimicrobial susceptibility of *Yersinia enterocolitica* isolates from stools of patients in the Netherlands from 1982–1991. J Antimicrob Chemother 36: 839, 1995

WUORELA M et al: Monocytes that have ingested *Yersinia enterocolitica* serotype O:3 acquire enhanced capacity to bind to nonstimulated vascular endothelial cells via P-selectin. Infect Immun 67:726, 1999

YLI-KERTTULA T et al: Ten-year follow up study of patients from a *Yersinia pseudotuberculosis* III outbreak. Clin Exp Rheumatol 13:333, 1995

163   *Lucy Stuart Tompkins*

BARTONELLA INFECTIONS, INCLUDING CAT-SCRATCH DISEASE

Bartonella spp., including *B. bacilliformis*, *B. henselae*, *B. quintana*, and *B. clarridgeiae*, are tiny gram-negative bacilli that can adhere to and invade mammalian cells, including endothelial cells and erythro-

cytes. Previously classified as *Rochalimaea* spp. within the rickettsia group, *Bartonella* spp. have now been removed from the order Rickettsiales on the grounds that they are not obligate intracellular parasites. These agents cause a wide spectrum of clinical illnesses, including trench fever, cat-scratch disease (CSD), bacillary angiomatosis, endocarditis, Oroya fever, and verruga peruana. The pathologic manifestations of *Bartonella* disease vary with the immune status of the host.

OROYA FEVER AND VERRUGA PERUANA

DEFINITION AND ETIOLOGY   Oroya fever and verruga peruana are caused by *B. bacilliformis*. Oroya fever is characterized by fever, profound anemia, and—unless antibiotic treatment is given—high mortality. The lesions referred to as verruga peruana may develop during the convalescent phase of Oroya fever or during chronic infection with *B. bacilliformis*. In 1885 Daniel Carrión, a Peruvian medical student, inoculated himself with blood from a patient with verruga peruana and subsequently died of Oroya fever, thus proving that both diseases are caused by a single agent.

EPIDEMIOLOGY   Infection with *B. bacilliformis* follows the bite of the sandfly vector *Phlebotomus*, an insect found in the river valleys of the Andes Mountains at altitudes of 600 to 2500 m. Oroya fever develops in nonimmune individuals who are not residents of the endemic region, whereas verruga peruana occurs in persons who apparently have been exposed in the past, including those who have recently had Oroya fever. The infection has not been acquired in the United States.

PATHOLOGY   During initial infection in the nonimmune host, *B. bacilliformis* cells adhere to erythrocytes and produce indentations in the cell membrane; the bacteria subsequently enter the erythrocytes and cause persistent deformation of the cytoskeleton. The parasitized erythrocytes are ultimately phagocytosed and destroyed. Although the life span of infected erythrocytes is markedly shortened, not all of this change can be attributed to the mechanical fragility induced by the internalization of bacteria. Decreased bone marrow erythropoiesis also contributes to anemia.

CLINICAL MANIFESTATIONS   The onset of symptoms in Oroya fever may be either insidious or abrupt, after an incubation period of approximately 3 weeks. The subacute presentation may include low-grade fever, malaise, headache, and anorexia. Sudden-onset disease commences with high fever, chills, diaphoresis, headaches, and changes in mental status. These manifestations are followed by the sudden development of profound anemia, which is due to a marked decrease in erythrocyte numbers and is associated with macrocytic changes, poikilocytosis, Howell-Jolly bodies, nucleated erythrocytes, and immature myeloid cells. The leukocyte differential usually shifts to the left, although the total leukocyte count may be normal. The erythrocyte count may fall to extremely low levels. In eosin/thiazine-stained peripheral-blood smears, numerous microorganisms can be seen adhering to most erythrocytes.

During the acute phase, muscle and joint pain and headache may be severe; central nervous system changes include insomnia, delirium, and a decreased level of consciousness. Thrombocytopenic purpura may develop. If the patient survives, a convalescent phase ensues, characterized by the sudden disappearance of bacteria from blood smears, declining fever, and an increase in the erythrocyte count. Although much of the mortality associated with Oroya fever is due to profound anemia and toxicity, secondary bacterial infections (including salmonellosis and other enteric infections, malaria, and tuberculosis) are often an important contributing factor.

After convalescence from acute Oroya fever, verrugas may develop. These red or purple cutaneous lesions may be either tiny and sessile or large, pedunculated, and nodular. They bear a marked resemblance to the lesions of bacillary angiomatosis and to Kaposi's sarcoma.

DIAGNOSIS   During acute infection, bacteria can be cultured from the blood on agar containing rabbit blood, with incubation at 28°C. The hallmark of verruga peruana is the formation of new blood vessels (angiogenesis) at the sites of bacterial replication.

℞ TREATMENT   Oroya fever responds to a variety of antimicrobial agents, including chloramphenicol, tetracyclines, penicillin, and streptomycin. Chloramphenicol is used most often because of its efficacy against most *Salmonella* infections (as salmonellosis may develop intercurrently). Verruga peruana may respond similarly; however, failure to respond to therapy and relapse are common and require the reinstitution of prolonged therapy.

BACILLARY ANGIOMATOSIS

DEFINITION AND ETIOLOGY   Bacillary angiomatosis was initially described as a condition occurring primarily in patients with AIDS and characterized by vascular cutaneous lesions resembling Kaposi's sarcoma. The disease can disseminate to involve virtually any organ system. Immunocompromised individuals, especially those infected with HIV, are at particularly high risk for bacillary angiomatosis, although in rare instances the patient is not obviously immunosuppressed. Both *B. henselae* and *B. quintana* (the infectious agent initially associated with trench fever) produce bacillary angiomatosis in persons with immunodeficiency.

EPIDEMIOLOGY   Acquisition of *B. henselae* has been significantly associated with exposure to young cats infested with fleas (*Ctenocephalides felis*). Because a high percentage of cats are seropositive, it has been suggested that patients with HIV infection avoid exposure to these animals. The finding that a large proportion of cats with fleas have persistent asymptomatic *B. henselae* bacteremia suggests that the domestic cat is the animal reservoir of this microorganism. The flea may serve as a transmitting vector in the cross-infection of cats, but its role in human infection is not clear. Tick-associated cases of *B. henselae* bacteremia have been reported in healthy immunocompetent individuals.

Person-to-person transmission of *B. quintana* by the human body louse (*Pediculus humanis corporis*) was documented during World War I under conditions of poor personal hygiene and sanitation. Although lice are suspected of transmission, the reservoir of *B. quintana* has not been identified.

A case-control study revealed that *B. henselae* and *B. quintana* differ significantly in terms of epidemiologic risk factors. All cases of *B. henselae* infection were associated with exposure to cats and their fleas and occurred sporadically, whereas the cases of *B. quintana* infection occurred in clusters and were associated with low socioeconomic status, homelessness, and exposure to body lice. Direct transmission of *B. henselae* from cats to their owners, presumably through cutaneous trauma, was supported by the matching DNA fingerprint patterns of isolates from the two sources.

MICROBIOLOGY   *B. henselae* can be demonstrated in tissue by Warthin-Starry staining. Clumps and clusters of pleomorphic bacilli appear as purple deposits in tissue stained with hematoxylin and eosin. Although the bacteria may be difficult to cultivate in the laboratory, they can eventually be isolated from cultures of blood and of material from other sites. Colonies develop after prolonged incubation (1 to 4 weeks) on blood-containing media and pit the agar; bacterial cells are gram-negative. *B. quintana* grows as a smooth, nonpitting colony on solid agar after prolonged incubation.

Classification of *B. henselae* was first accomplished when molecular techniques were used to analyze bacterial ribosomal genes extracted from tissue samples. Definitive identification of *Bartonella* spp. is based on sequence analysis of 16S ribosomal DNA.

PATHOGENESIS AND PATHOLOGY   Bacillary angiomatosis is characterized by a lobular proliferation of new blood vessels (angiogenesis) and a neutrophilic inflammatory response to myriad bacilli located within collagen-rich microscopic and macroscopic nodules. The endothelial cells lining the vascular spaces have a typical epithelioid appearance, and the lesions may resemble Kaposi's sarcoma histopathologically, although the characteristic spindle cell of the latter disease is usually absent. The bacterial and eukaryotic host factors that elicit the pathologic response are unknown.

CLINICAL MANIFESTATIONS   The skin lesions of bacillary angiomatosis (also called *epithelioid angiomatosis*) are vascular nodules, papules, or tumors that range from tiny lesions resembling cherry angiomas or pyogenic granulomas to large, pedunculated, exophytic masses (Fig. 163-1). Characteristically, the lesions are red or purple, resembling Kaposi's sarcoma; they may be surrounded by an epithelial collarette, may be located anywhere on the skin, and may involve mucous membranes. The overlying epidermis may be focally ulcerated, and the underlying bone may be invaded and destroyed.

Dissemination of *B. henselae* infection occurs primarily in patients with cellular immune defects. Clinical manifestations accompanying dissemination are often nonspecific and include persistent fever, abdominal pain, weight loss, and malaise. Although the liver, spleen, bone marrow, and lymph nodes are primarily affected, HIV-infected patients may also develop central nervous system abnormalities (including psychiatric disorders and brain lesions), which are responsive to antibiotic therapy. Skin lesions usually are not evident in disseminated infection. Involvement of the liver or spleen may produce bacillary peliosis hepatis. Patients with the latter condition may report localized pain on palpation of the abdomen. Nodular lesions of variable size can be demonstrated by computed tomography or magnetic resonance imaging, with or without contrast agents.

In a case-control study of bacillary angiomatosis (see "Epidemiology" above), only *B. henselae* was associated with hepatosplenic disease (peliosis hepatis) and displayed a predilection for the lymph nodes. *B. quintana*, in contrast, was associated with osseous and subcutaneous infection.

DIAGNOSIS   The diagnosis of bacillary angiomatosis is based primarily on the typical histopathologic findings of angiomas in association with clumps of tiny bacilli revealed by Warthin-Starry silver stain. Infection due to *B. henselae* can also be established by culture or by identification of specific DNA sequences. *B. henselae* is most easily isolated from blood through a lysis-centrifugation system. Colonies may be detected on blood-containing agar (rabbit blood is preferred) incubated with 5 to 10% CO_2 at 37°C for 2 to 4 weeks. *B. quintana* may be isolated from BACTEC (Becton Dickinson, Sparks, MD) aerobic bottles containing resin. Isolation from skin lesions and other tissues is more difficult but should be attempted when feasible. Initial reports suggested that cocultivation with endothelial cell monolayers was necessary; however, isolation by direct plating onto freshly prepared agar media has also been successful. Bacilli picked from new colonies but not subcultured may not stain, even with acridine orange; they stain weakly with safranin. Identification of *B.*

FIGURE 163-1 Characteristic skin lesion of bacillary angiomatosis in an HIV-positive young woman. This large, pedunculated tumor exhibits the typical angiomatous appearance. The patient was treated with oral erythromycin, with nearly complete resolution of the lesion; however, on discontinuation of antibiotic therapy after a 4-week course, the lesion recurred.

henselae and *B. quintana* is based primarily on cellular fatty-acid analysis and polymerase chain reaction (PCR)–based restriction fragment length polymorphism analysis. Definitive identification of *Bartonella* spp. depends on DNA sequence analysis of 16S ribosomal RNA genes. The diagnosis of CSD (see next section) can be made by specific serologic testing that detects *B. henselae*–specific antibodies, but the sensitivity and specificity of this method in patients with cutaneous and disseminated bacillary angiomatosis have not been determined.

DIFFERENTIAL DIAGNOSIS The differential diagnosis of cutaneous bacillary angiomatosis includes Kaposi's sarcoma, angiomas, and pyogenic granulomas. These conditions can be distinguished by histopathologic examination of biopsied material.

Cutaneous bacillary angiomatosis caused by *B. henselae* or *B. quintana* resembles verruga peruana, which is not seen outside of South America. In patients with AIDS, Kaposi's sarcoma lesions and bacillary angiomatosis may coexist.

℞ TREATMENT Cutaneous lesions have been treated with a wide variety of antimicrobial drugs, including macrolides, tetracyclines, and antituberculous agents; *B. henselae* is susceptible to most antibiotics in vitro. Erythromycin (2 g/d), given orally for 3 weeks, is usually effective, as are newer macrolides; however, relapse may require prolonged therapy (3 weeks to 2 months) with an antibiotic that reaches an intracellular compartment, such as a macrolide or doxycycline (200 mg/d). Patients with peliosis hepatis should be treated with intravenous antibiotics, and those with disseminated disease or bacteremia should be treated with a prolonged course (3 weeks to 2 months) of systemic antibiotic, such as a macrolide (e.g., erythromycin, 2 g/d). In a case-control study of bacillary angiomatosis, treatment with a macrolide was associated with a therapeutic response and sterile tissue samples and may have been protective, whereas treatment with trimethoprim-sulfamethoxazole, ciprofloxacin, penicillins, or cephalosporins had no protective effect. Cutaneous lesions may or may not regress spontaneously, perhaps depending on the status of the host's immunity. The safety of ciprofloxacin in pregnant or lactating women has not been established. No antimicrobial has been studied prospectively, and information on efficacy comes only from case reports.

CAT-SCRATCH DISEASE

DEFINITION AND ETIOLOGY Typical CSD is manifested by painful regional lymphadenopathy persisting for several weeks or months after a cat scratch. Occasionally, infection may disseminate and produce more generalized lymphadenopathy and systemic manifestations, which may be confused with the manifestations of lymphoma. *B. henselae* is the causative agent of CSD. There is no evidence that *B. quintana* causes CSD, and this microbe is not carried by cats. The role of *Afipia felis* (originally proposed as the agent of CSD) is unclear inasmuch as only a few cases are associated with its isolation. *B. henselae* remains the predominant species causing typical CSD. Several reports suggest that *B. clarridgeiae* may also cause feline lymphadenopathy.

EPIDEMIOLOGY Approximately 60% of cases of CSD in the United States occur in children. Exposure to bacteremic young cats that either are flea-infested or have been in contact with another cat carrying fleas poses a significant risk of infection. Most infections are caused by a scratch and only rare cases by a bite or by licking. Most cases occur in the warmer months, when fleas are active. Regions of the United States where fleas are endemic have higher rates of infection. The flea may serve to transmit infection between cats; it is not known whether humans can be infected through the bite of an infected flea.

CLINICAL MANIFESTATIONS A localized papule, progressing to a pustule that often crusts over, develops 3 to 5 days after a cat scratch. Tender regional lymphadenopathy develops within 1 to 2 weeks after inoculation; by this time, the papule may have healed spontaneously. Scratches are most often sustained on the hands or face, producing epitrochlear, axillary, pectoral, and cervical lymph node in-

volvement. The involved nodes occasionally become suppurative; bacterial superinfection with staphylococci or other cutaneous pathogens may develop. Although most patients do not have fever, systemic symptoms are frequent and include malaise, anorexia, and weight loss. Without treatment, lymphadenopathy persists for weeks or even months and may be confused with lymphatic malignancy. Other manifestations in apparently immunocompetent patients include encephalitis, seizures and coma (especially in children), meningitis, transverse myelitis, granulomatous hepatitis and splenitis, osteomyelitis, and disseminated infection. Conjunctival inoculation may cause Parinaud's oculoglandular syndrome, with conjunctivitis and preauricular lymphadenopathy.

PATHOLOGY The histopathologic hallmark of CSD is granulomatous inflammation with stellate necrosis but no evidence of angiogenesis. Thus, infection by *B. henselae* can produce two entirely different pathologic reactions, depending on the immune status of the host: CSD or bacillary angiomatosis.

DIAGNOSIS CSD should be suspected if the patient has a history of exposure to cats and develops lymphadenopathy and a skin lesion. The diagnosis can be confirmed by pathologic examination of the involved nodes. Tiny bacilli in clusters can sometimes be seen in biopsy samples stained with Warthin-Starry silver. The CSD skin test, in which lymph node material obtained from patients with CSD serves as an antigen, is no longer used for diagnosis because of concerns about the transmission of viral agents. A specific serologic test has been developed and may produce a positive result in 70 to 90% of patients with intact immunity. The identification of *B. henselae* 16S ribosomal RNA genes in biopsy material by PCR amplification with specific oligonucleotide primers can also be diagnostically useful; however, these methods are not yet commercially available. Cultures of lymph nodes, cerebrospinal fluid, or other tissues are rarely positive.

℞ TREATMENT Although CSD is generally self-limited, tender regional lymphadenopathy and systemic symptoms may be debilitating. Patients with encephalitis or other serious manifestations should be treated with antibiotics. A randomized, double-blind, placebo-controlled trial demonstrated significant clinical benefit of treatment with oral azithromycin for 5 days in cases of typical CSD (regimen for adults weighing >100 lb: one dose of 500 mg on day 1, 250 mg on days 2 through 5). Several reports suggest that aminoglycoside treatment (e.g., intravenous gentamicin at standard doses calculated to result in therapeutic levels) is effective in patients with encephalitis and other systemic infections. The oral agents that appear to be useful are those that also are most effective for the treatment of bacillary angiomatosis; they include ciprofloxacin, doxycycline, and azithromycin. Unlike bacillary angiomatosis, CSD responds to treatment with ciprofloxacin. The necessary duration of therapy is variable.

TRENCH FEVER

DEFINITION AND ETIOLOGY Trench fever was first described as a debilitating febrile illness associated with prolonged *B. quintana* bacteremia in soldiers fighting in Europe during World War I. Although not usually fatal, the illness accounted for substantial morbidity. In recent years, trench fever has reemerged in the United States and has been caused by either *B. henselae*—the agent of CSD and bacillary angiomatosis—or *B. quintana*.

EPIDEMIOLOGY Although trench fever was thought to have disappeared from the United States, recent cases have been diagnosed in homeless persons (*B. quintana*) and in persons bitten by ticks (*B. henselae*). During World War I, trench fever was transmitted from person to person by the human body louse. Transmission by ectoparasites is suspected in the recent cases of *B. quintana* infection but has not been firmly documented. Patients with trench fever have apparently normal immune defenses.

CLINICAL MANIFESTATIONS Trench fever is characterized by the sudden onset of headache, aseptic meningitis, persistent fever (which can be high-grade and is commonly paroxysmal), malaise, weight loss, and other nonspecific symptoms. Severe musculoskeletal pain is more common among immunocompetent than among immunocompromised patients. Bacteremia can persist for days or weeks, and relapses have followed short courses of antibiotic therapy. Localized findings are uncommon.

DIAGNOSIS Trench fever is diagnosed by the finding of sustained bacteremia. *B. henselae* and *B. quintana* grow slowly. Colonies develop on rabbit blood agar after 1 to 4 weeks of incubation under conditions of increased CO_2. Serologic tests for this disease have not yet been standardized.

℞ TREATMENT A prolonged course (4 weeks) of antimicrobial therapy may be required. Agents that can cross the mammalian cell membrane are most effective, including erythromycin (2 g/d) or azithromycin (500 mg/d). Data on the efficacy of these agents come from a limited number of case reports.

OTHER *BARTONELLA* INFECTIONS, INCLUDING CULTURE-NEGATIVE ENDOCARDITIS

The application of molecular methods to the detection of microorganisms that are difficult to cultivate in the laboratory has revealed new *Bartonella* spp. and has established *Bartonella* spp. as a cause of endocarditis cases previously classified as being of unknown etiology. *B. quintana* is the most frequently isolated *Bartonella* species in these cases. Two new species, *B. elizabethae* and *B. clarridgeiae*, as well as *B. henselae* have also been identified as agents of subacute and chronic endocarditis.

The diagnosis of *Bartonella* endocarditis is confirmed by blood cultures. Specific antibodies are produced; however, *B. quintana* infection may produce antibodies that cross-react with *Chlamydia pneumoniae*.

BIBLIOGRAPHY

ANDERSON BE, NEUMAN MA: *Bartonella* spp. as emerging human pathogens. Clin Microbiol Rev 10:203, 1997

BASS JW et al: Prospective randomized double blind placebo-controlled evaluation of azithromycin for treatment of cat-scratch disease. Pediatr Infect Dis J 17:447, 1998

BROUQUI P et al: Chronic *Bartonella quintana* bacteremia in homeless patients. N Engl J Med 340:184, 1999

CARITHERS HA: Cat scratch disease: An overview based on a study of 1,200 patients. Am J Dis Child 139:1124, 1985

COCKERELL DJ, LEBOIT PE: Bacillary angiomatosis: A newly characterized, pseudoneoplastic, infectious, cutaneous vascular disorder. J Am Acad Dermatol 22:501, 1990

KOEHLER JE, TAPPERO JW: *Rochalimaea henselae* infection: A new zoonosis with the domestic cat as reservoir. JAMA 271:531, 1994

———— et al: Molecular epidemiology of *Bartonella* infections in patients with bacillary angiomatosis. N Engl J Med 337:1876, 1997

PERKOCHA LA et al: Clinical and pathological features of bacillary peliosis hepatis in association with human immunodeficiency virus infection. N Engl J Med 323:148, 1990

REGNERY RL et al: Characterization of a novel *Rochalimaea* species, *R. henselae*, sp.nov., isolated from blood of a febrile, human immunodeficiency virus–positive patient. J Clin Microbiol 30:265, 1992

SPACH DH et al: *Bartonella (Rochalimaea) quintana* bacteremia in inner-city patients with chronic alcoholism. N Engl J Med 332:425, 1995

ZANGWILL KM et al: Cat scratch disease in Connecticut: Epidemiology, risk factors, and evaluation of a new diagnostic test. N Engl J Med 329:8, 1993

164 *Gavin Hart*

DONOVANOSIS

Donovanosis is a chronic, progressively destructive bacterial infection of the genital region that is generally regarded as sexually transmitted. The disease has been known by many other names, the most common of which are granuloma inguinale and granuloma venereum.

ETIOLOGY Donovanosis is caused by *Calymmatobacterium granulomatis*, an intracellular, gram-negative, pleomorphic, encapsulated (when mature) bacterium measuring 1.5 by 0.7 μm. *C. granulomatis* shares many morphologic and serologic characteristics and >99% homology at the nucleotide level with *Klebsiella* species that are pathogenic to humans. Polymerase chain reaction amplification of the *phoE* gene shows it to be closely related to that in *Klebsiella pneumoniae*, *K. rhinoscleromatis*, and *K. ozaenae*. Electron microscopy shows typical gram-negative morphology and a large capsule but no flagella. Filiform or vesicular protrusions occur on a corrugated cell wall.

EPIDEMIOLOGY Donovanosis is endemic among Aborigines in central Australia as well as in Papua New Guinea, southeastern India, southern Africa, and the Caribbean and adjacent areas of South America. In the first half of the twentieth century, the disease was endemic in parts of the United States (with an estimated 5000 to 10,000 cases in 1947); small epidemics still occur in this country and in other developed countries. Over 70% of cases involve persons 20 to 40 years of age. The infection is predominantly sexually transmitted, but extragenital skin lesions can follow transmission from concurrent genital lesions via the fingers or through other nonsexual contact, and autoinoculation may produce new lesions from contact with adjacent skin ("kissing" lesions). Infants born to infected mothers have acquired infection at birth.

The classification of donovanosis as a sexually transmitted disease (STD) has been disputed because of cases in young children and occasionally in sexually inactive individuals, transmission by direct body contact and via inanimate intermediaries, and the low and variable prevalence of donovanosis among sexual partners (0.4 to 52%). The dominance of sexual transmission is suggested by the combined factors of lesions predominantly affecting the genitalia, the highest prevalence among persons in age and socioeconomic groups that are most often affected by STDs, and the predictable occurrence of disease in visitors to areas of endemicity following sexual exposure.

CLINICAL MANIFESTATIONS The incubation period is usually 1 to 4 weeks but may extend to 1 year. Skin lesions have been detected in infants 6 weeks to 6 months after birth. The disease begins as one or more subcutaneous nodules that erode through the skin to produce clean, granulomatous, sharply defined, usually painless lesions (Fig. 164-1). These lesions, which bleed readily on contact, slowly enlarge. The genitalia are involved in 90% of cases, the inguinal region in 10%, and the anal region in 5 to 10%. Genital swelling, particularly of the labia, is a common feature and occasionally progresses to pseudoelephantiasis. Phimosis and paraphimosis are common local complications, and progressive erosion of affected tissues may completely destroy the penis or other organs. Less common clinical variants include a hypertrophic form (cauliflower- or wartlike lesions), a necrotic form (destructive lesions with foul-smelling exudate, often resembling amebiasis), and a sclerotic or cicatricial form, which has a dry base with extensive scar tissue.

Extragenital lesions occur in at least 6% of cases. Oral donovanosis, the most common extragenital manifestation, presents as pain or bleeding in the mouth, lesions on the lips, or extensive swelling of the gums and palate. Donovanosis may affect most bones, and sometimes many bones are affected at the same time; the tibia is involved in over 50% of such cases. Bony lesions are associated with constitutional symptoms (weight loss, fever, night sweats, and malaise) and

FIGURE 164-1 Multiple granulomatous lesions of the penis in a patient with donovanosis.

Table 164-1   The Most Effective Antibiotic Regimens for Treatment of Donovanosis[a]

Antibiotic	Oral Dosage
Tetracycline	500 mg qid
Doxycycline	100 mg bid
Trimethoprim-sulfamethoxazole	1 double-strength tablet (160 mg/800 mg) bid
Erythromycin	500 mg qid
Azithromycin	1 g weekly
Chloramphenicol	500 mg tid

[a] Patients should be examined weekly, and therapy should be continued until lesions have healed (3 to 5 weeks, except in severe cases).

are usually found in women. More than 50% of women have primary lesions on the cervix. Prompt pelvic examinations and early diagnosis are likely to substantially decrease the morbidity and mortality (a likely outcome in misdiagnosed spinal lesions) associated with extragenital donovanosis in women.

DIAGNOSIS   Laboratory Diagnosis   The preferred method involves demonstration of typical intracellular Donovan bodies within large mononuclear cells visualized in smears prepared from lesions or biopsy specimens. With typical beefy lesions, a small piece of tissue is removed with forceps and scalpel, and a crush impression of the deep surface is made on a glass slide. The smear is air-dried, heat-fixed, and stained with Giemsa, Leishman's, or Wright's stain. For dry, flat, or necrotic lesions, a punch-biopsy specimen should be obtained from the advancing edge. This specimen can be used to prepare a smear or embedded for histologic examination (with a silver stain). Histologic examination shows epithelial proliferation, often simulating neoplasia, with a heavy inflammatory infiltrate of plasma cells, some neutrophils, and few if any lymphocytes. The large mononuclear cells are 25 to 90 μm in diameter, with a vesicular or pyknotic nucleus. Up to 20 intracytoplasmic vacuoles contain pleomorphic Donovan bodies in either young uncapsulated forms (which often resemble closed safety pins) or mature capsulated forms. *C. granulomatis* has never been grown on artificial solid media but has been cultured in chicken embryonic yolk sacs, on human monocytes, and on human epithelial (HEp-2) cells. A sensitive and specific serologic test, based on indirect immunofluorescence, has been developed.

Differential Diagnosis   Condylomata lata of secondary syphilis may be confused with donovanosis; however, these lesions usually appear as white or pale moist plaques in the anogenital area, whereas the lesions of donovanosis are usually bright red. Syphilis and donovanosis frequently coexist because syphilis is usually highly prevalent in areas where donovanosis is endemic; thus positive syphilis serology does not exclude a diagnosis of donovanosis. Condylomata lata subside within 1 week of treatment with benzathine penicillin (2.4 million units), whereas donovanosis lesions remain unchanged.

The necrotic form of donovanosis may resemble squamous cell carcinoma; likewise, cervical and vulvar lesions may closely resemble carcinoma. Penile amebiasis may resemble necrotic donovanosis but usually follows anal intercourse and is much less common than donovanosis in areas where the latter is endemic. Atypical clinical variants of chancroid, referred to as *pseudogranuloma inguinale*, have been described in patients seen at clinics in Atlanta. Disseminated donovanosis lesions of bones, particularly in the spine, can mimic tuberculosis. Lesions that produce draining sinuses near the jaw may simulate actinomycosis. The histologic findings of donovanosis must be distinguished from those of rhinoscleroma, leishmaniasis, and histoplasmosis. Genital ulcers are a risk factor for HIV acquisition in developing countries, and patients with donovanosis should be tested for HIV infection.

℞ **TREATMENT**   Table 164-1 shows the most effective regimens for treating donovanosis. Doxycycline is the first choice for therapy in developed countries. Erythromycin provides an effective option for pregnant patients, and azithromycin is an effective alternative that is more convenient to administer. Extensive lesions have been cured with oral azithromycin at a dosage of 500 mg/d, but the more convenient dose of 1 g weekly is also effective. Although chloramphenicol is the drug of choice in some developing countries, it is unlikely to be acceptable in developed countries because of bone marrow toxicity. Penicillin is not effective for treating donovanosis. Patients should be examined weekly, and therapy should be continued until lesions have healed (3 to 5 weeks, except in severe cases). If antibiotic therapy is stopped earlier, lesions often continue to heal, but the relapse rate is higher. If the lesions are unchanged after 2 weeks of treatment, an alternative antibiotic regimen should be used.

The treatment regimens just described are usually adequate in HIV-infected patients without immunosuppression, but an increasing failure rate has been reported in immunosuppressed patients, for whom daily administration of azithromycin is recommended if other regimens fail to elicit a response.

BIBLIOGRAPHY

CARTER J et al: Culture of the causative organism of donovanosis (*Calymmatobacterium granulomatis*) in HEp-2 cells. J Clin Microbiol 35:2915, 1997

HART G: Donovanosis (granuloma inguinale), in *Atlas of Infectious Diseases*, vol V: *Sexually Transmitted Diseases*, MF Rein (ed). Philadelphia, Churchill Livingstone, 1996, pp 17.1–17.10

———: Donovanosis. Clin Infect Dis 25:24, 1997

PATERSON DL: Disseminated donovanosis (granuloma inguinale) causing spinal cord compression: Case report and review of donovanosis involving bone. Clin Infect Dis 26:379, 1998

165 *Gregory A. Filice*

NOCARDIOSIS

The term *nocardiosis* refers to invasive disease associated with members of the genus *Nocardia*. Of the several distinctive syndromes, pneumonia and disseminated disease are most common. Others include cellulitis, lymphocutaneous syndrome, actinomycetoma, and keratitis.

MICROBIOLOGY   Nocardiae are saprophytic aerobic actinomycetes that are common worldwide in soil, where they contribute to decay of organic matter. Nocardial taxonomy is complex and incompletely understood. Seven species have been associated with human disease: *N. asteroides*, *N. brasiliensis*, *N. otitidis-caviarum* (formerly *N. caviae*), *N. farcinica*, *N. nova*, *N. transvalensis*, and *N. pseudobrasiliensis*. *N. asteroides* is the species most commonly associated with invasive disease. *N. farcinica* is less common but tends to be virulent and prone to dissemination. The new species *N. pseudobrasiliensis* accounts for most cases of invasive disease previously attributed to *N. brasiliensis*. True *N. brasiliensis* isolates are usually associated with disease limited to the skin. *N. transvalensis* is generally associated with mycetoma or, in immunosuppressed persons, with pulmonary or systemic disease.

EPIDEMIOLOGY   Approximately 1000 cases of nocardial infection are diagnosed annually in the United States, 85% of them pulmonary and/or systemic. The disease is more common among adults and males. Outbreaks, which are rare, have been associated with contamination of the hospital environment, solutions, or drug injection equipment. Person-to-person spread is not well documented. There is no known seasonality.

The risk of pulmonary or disseminated disease is greater than usual among people with deficient cell-mediated immunity, especially that associated with lymphoma, transplantation, or AIDS. In persons with AIDS, nocardiosis usually presents at a CD4+ lymphocyte concentration of <250/μL. Prophylaxis with sulfamethoxazole and trimethoprim appears to reduce the risk of nocardiosis in persons with AIDS or transplanted organs. Nocardiosis has also been associated with pulmonary alveolar proteinosis, tuberculosis and other mycobacterial diseases, and chronic granulomatous disease.

N. brasiliensis, *N. asteroides*, *N. otitidis-caviarum*, and *N. transvalensis* are associated with actinomycetoma. Cases occur mainly in tropical and subtropical regions, especially those of Mexico, Central and South America, Africa, and India. The most important risk factor is frequent contact with soil or vegetable matter.

PATHOLOGY AND PATHOGENESIS   Pneumonia and disseminated disease are both thought to follow inhalation of fragmented bacterial mycelia. The characteristic histologic feature of nocardiosis is an abscess with extensive infiltration by neutrophils and prominent necrosis. Granulation tissue usually surrounds the lesions, but extensive fibrosis or encapsulation is uncommon. Actinomycetoma is characterized by suppurative inflammation with sinus tract formation. Granules—microcolonies composed of dense masses of bacterial filaments extending radially from a central core—are occasionally observed in histologic preparations. They are frequently found in discharges from lesions of actinomycetoma but almost never from lesions in other forms of nocardiosis.

Nocardiae have evolved a number of properties that enable them to survive within phagocytes, including neutralization of oxidants, prevention of phagosome-lysosome fusion, and prevention of phagosome acidification. Neutrophils phagocytose the organisms and limit their growth but do not kill them efficiently. Cell-mediated immunity is important for definitive control and elimination of nocardiae.

CLINICAL MANIFESTATIONS   Respiratory Tract Disease   Pneumonia is by far the most common respiratory tract nocardial disease. Nocardial pneumonia is typically subacute; symptoms have usually been present for days or weeks at presentation. The onset may be more acute in immunosuppressed patients. Cough is prominent and produces small amounts of thick, purulent sputum that is not malodorous. Fever, anorexia, weight loss, and malaise are common; dyspnea, pleuritic pain, and hemoptysis are less common. Remissions and exacerbations over several weeks are frequent.

Roentgenographic patterns are variable, but some characteristics are highly suggestive. Infiltrates vary in size and are typically of at least moderate density. Single or multiple nodules are common, sometimes suggesting metastatic tumors. Infiltrates and nodules tend to cavitate. Empyema is present in one-third of cases.

Nocardiosis may spread directly from the lungs to adjacent tissues. Pericarditis, mediastinitis, and the superior vena cava syndrome have all been reported. Spread through the chest wall is rare.

Nocardial laryngitis, tracheitis, and bronchitis are much less common than pneumonia. In the major airways, disease often presents as a nodular or granulomatous mass. A few cases of sinusitis have been reported.

Nocardiae are sometimes isolated from respiratory secretions of patients without apparent nocardial disease. Most of these patients have chronic pulmonary disease with abnormal airways or parenchyma.

Extrapulmonary Dissemination   In half of all cases of pulmonary nocardiosis, disease appears outside the lungs. In one-fifth of cases of disseminated disease, lung disease is not apparent. The most common site of dissemination is the brain. Other common sites include the skin and supporting structures, kidneys, bone, and muscle, but almost any organ can be involved. Peritonitis and endocarditis have been reported. The typical manifestation of extrapulmonary dissemination is a subacute abscess. A minority of abscesses outside the lungs or central nervous system (CNS) form fistulae and discharge small amounts of pus. Nocardiae have been recovered from blood in a few cases of pneumonia or disseminated disease.

In CNS infections, brain abscesses are usually supratentorial, are often multiloculated, and may be single or multiple (Fig. 165-1). Brain abscesses tend to burrow into the ventricles or extend out into the subarachnoid space. The symptoms and signs are somewhat more indolent than those of other types of bacterial brain abscess. Meningitis is uncommon and is usually due to spread from a nearby brain abscess. Nocardiae are not easily recovered from cerebrospinal fluid (CSF).

Disease Following Transcutaneous Inoculation   Disease following transcutaneous nocardial inoculation usually takes one of three forms: cellulitis, lymphocutaneous syndrome, or actinomycetoma. Cellulitis generally begins 1 to 3 weeks after a recognized breach of the skin, often with soil contamination. Subacute cellulitis with pain, swelling, erythema, and warmth develops over days to weeks. The lesions are usually firm and nonfluctuant. Disease may progress to involve underlying muscle, tendon, bones, or joints. Dissemination is rare. *N. asteroides* is common in colder climates, while *N. brasiliensis* predominates in warmer climates.

In the lymphocutaneous syndrome, there is typically a pyodermatous lesion at the site of inoculation, with central ulceration and purulent or honey-colored drainage. Subcutaneous nodules often appear along lymphatics that drain the primary lesion. The lymphangitic form closely resembles lymphocutaneous sporotrichosis (Chap. 208). Most cases of the lymphocutaneous syndrome are associated with *N. brasiliensis*.

FIGURE 165-1 Nocardial abscesses in the right cerebellum. The appearance suggests one large abscess and multiple daughter abscesses.

Actinomycetoma usually begins with a nodular swelling, sometimes at a site of local trauma. Lesions typically develop on the feet or hands but may involve the posterior part of the neck, the upper back, the head, and other sites. The nodule eventually breaks down and a fistula appears. This fistula is soon accompanied by others. The fistulas tend to come and go, with new ones forming as old ones disappear. The discharge is serous or purulent, may be bloody, and often contains 0.1- to 2-mm white granules consisting of masses of mycelia. The lesions spread slowly along fascial planes to involve adjacent areas of skin, subcutaneous tissue, and bone. Over months or years, there may be extensive deformation of the affected part. Lesions involving soft tissues are only mildly painful; those affecting bones or joints are more so. Systemic symptoms are absent or minimal. Infection rarely disseminates from actinomycetoma, and lesions on the hands and feet usually cause only local disability. Lesions on the head, neck, and trunk can invade locally to involve deep organs and result in severe disability or death.

Keratitis *Nocardia* spp., usually *N. asteroides*, are uncommon causes of subacute keratitis. The infection usually follows eye trauma. Nocardial infection of lacrimal glands has been reported. Disease involving deeper eye structures is usually a manifestation of dissemination.

DIAGNOSIS The first step in diagnosis is examination of sputum or pus for crooked, branching, beaded, gram-positive filaments 1 μm wide and up to 50 μm long. Most nocardiae are acid-fast in direct smears if a weak acid is used for decolorization (e.g., in the modified Kinyoun, Ziehl-Neelsen, and Fite-Faraco methods). The organisms often take up silver stains. Nocardiae grow relatively slowly; colonies may take up to 2 weeks to appear and may not develop their characteristic appearance for up to 4 weeks. Several blood culture systems support nocardial growth. Yield is enhanced when blood cultures are incubated aerobically for up to 4 weeks and when blind subcultures are performed. Nocardial growth is so different from that of more common pathogens that the laboratory should be alerted when nocardiosis is suspected to maximize the likelihood of isolation. Since nocardiae are among the few aerobic microorganisms that use paraffin as a carbon source, paraffin baiting can be useful in isolating the organisms from mixed cultures.

In cases of pneumonia, sputum smears are often negative. Unless the diagnosis can be made in these cases by sampling lesions in other,

more accessible sites, bronchoscopy or lung aspiration is usually necessary. Transtracheal aspiration should be avoided, as it frequently leads to nocardial cellulitis in tissues around the puncture wound.

In patients with nocardial pneumonia, a careful history should be obtained and a thorough physical examination performed to evaluate the possibility of dissemination. Suggestive symptoms or signs should be pursued with further diagnostic tests. Computed tomography or magnetic resonance imaging of the head, with and without contrast material, should be undertaken if signs or symptoms suggest brain involvement. Many authorities recommend brain imaging in all cases of pulmonary or disseminated disease.

When clinically indicated, CSF or urine should be concentrated and then cultured. In actinomycetoma cases, granules should be sought in the discharge. Suspect particles should be washed in saline, examined microscopically, and cultured.

Isolation of nocardiae from sputum or blood occasionally represents colonization, transient infection, or contamination. In typical cases of respiratory tract colonization, Gram-stained specimens are negative and cultures are only intermittently positive. A positive sputum culture in an immunosuppressed patient usually reflects disease. When nocardiae are isolated from an immunocompetent patient without apparent nocardial disease, the patient should be observed carefully without treatment. A patient with a host-defense defect that increases the risk of nocardiosis should usually receive antimicrobial treatment.

Nocardia spp. are difficult to differentiate from one another with standard biochemical tests, and isolates from patients with systemic or severe disease should be sent to a reference laboratory for definitive identification and antimicrobial susceptibility testing. Susceptibility results, which help differentiate species, are of less certain clinical value but sometimes guide therapy in difficult cases.

In vitro, strains of *N. farcinica* differ from most in that they are usually resistant to cephalosporins and in one-fifth of cases are resistant to imipenem. *N. pseudobrasiliensis* strains often exhibit resistance to minocycline or amoxicillin/clavulanic acid and susceptibility to ciprofloxacin or clarithromycin. *N. transvalensis* displays increased resistance to many antimicrobial agents, including amikacin, tobramycin, cefotaxime, ceftriaxone, and amoxicillin/clavulanic acid. *N. nova* isolates appear to be susceptible to ampicillin and erythromycin in vitro but also produce β-lactamase constitutively or in the presence of a β-lactam.

Several presumptive diagnostic tests for nocardial infection have been studied, including tests for antibodies, nocardial metabolites, and nocardial DNA. None is ready for clinical use at this time.

℞ **TREATMENT** Sulfonamides are the drugs of choice for nocardiosis (Table 165-1). Initially, 6 to 8 g of sulfadiazine or sulfisoxazole per day in four divided doses should be used. After disease is controlled, 4 g/d can be used to complete therapy. In difficult cases, sulfonamide levels should be measured and dosages adjusted to keep serum levels between 100 and 150 μg/mL. The combination of sulfamethoxazole (SMZ) and trimethoprim (TMP) is probably equivalent to sulfonamides; some authorities believe that the combination may in fact be more effective, but it also poses a modestly greater risk of hematologic toxicity. At the outset, 10 to 20 mg of TMP per kg and 50 to 100 mg of SMZ per kg should be given each day in two divided doses. Later, the daily doses can be decreased to as little as 5 mg/kg and 25 mg/kg, respectively. In persons with sulfonamide allergies, desensitization usually allows continuation of therapy with these effective and inexpensive drugs.

Minocycline is the best-established alternative oral drug and should be given in doses of 100 to 200 mg twice a day. Other tetracyclines are usually ineffective. *N. nova* infections can be treated with erythromycin (500 to 750 mg four times a day) and/or ampicillin (1 g four times a day), but other *Nocardia* spp. are often resistant to both drugs. Amoxicillin (500 mg) combined with clavulanic acid (125 mg), given three times a day, has been effective in a few cases but should

Table 165-1 Treatment for Nocardiosis

Disease	Duration	Drugs (Daily Dose)[a]
Pulmonary or systemic		**Systemic therapy**
Intact host defenses	6–12 mo	**Oral**
Deficient host defenses	12 mo[b]	1. Sulfonamides (6–8 g) or combination of
CNS disease	12 mo[c]	trimethoprim (10–20 mg/kg) and
Cellulitis, lympho-		sulfamethoxazole (50–100 mg/kg)
cutaneous syndrome	2 mo	2. Minocycline (200–400 mg)
Osteomyelitis, arthritis,		**Parenteral**
laryngitis, sinusitis	4 mo	1. Amikacin (10–15 mg/kg)
Actinomycetoma	6–12 mo after	2. Cefotaxime (6 g), ceftizoxime (6 g),
	clinical cure	ceftriaxone (2 g), imipenem (2 g)
Keratitis	**Topical:** Until apparent cure	1. Sulfonamide drops
		2. Amikacin drops
	Systemic: Until 2–4 mo after apparent cure	Drugs for systemic therapy as listed above

[a] For each category, choices are numbered in order of preference.
[b] In some patients with AIDS or chronic granulomatous disease, therapy for pulmonary or systemic disease must be continued indefinitely.
[c] If all apparent CNS disease has been excised, the duration of therapy may be reduced to 6 months.

be avoided in cases due to *N. nova*, in which clavulanate induces β-lactamase production. Ofloxacin (400 mg twice a day) and clarithromycin (500 mg twice a day) have each been successful in a few cases.

Amikacin, the best-established parenteral drug, is given in doses of 5 to 7.5 mg/kg every 12 h. Serum levels should be monitored with prolonged therapy in patients with diminished renal function and in the elderly. Newer β-lactam antibiotics, including cefotaxime, ceftizoxime, ceftriaxone, and imipenem, are usually effective. They may be less effective in some cases caused by *N. farcinica*.

In patients receiving immunosuppressive therapy, the regimen should be continued if necessary for treatment of an underlying disease or prevention of transplant rejection. In many cases, two or more antimicrobial agents have been used to treat nocardiosis, often in combinations including a sulfonamide or minocycline. Whether such therapy is better than monotherapy is not known, and combination therapy increases the risk of toxicity.

Surgical management of nocardial disease is similar to that of other bacterial diseases. Brain abscesses should be aspirated, drained, or excised if the diagnosis is unclear, if an abscess is large and accessible, or if an abscess fails to respond to chemotherapy. Abscesses that are small or inaccessible should be treated medically; in these cases, clinical improvement should be noticeable within 1 to 2 weeks. Brain imaging should be repeated to document the resolution of lesions, although abatement on images often lags behind clinical improvement.

Antimicrobial therapy usually suffices for nocardial actinomycetoma. In deep or extensive cases, drainage or excision of heavily involved tissue may facilitate healing, but structure and function should be preserved whenever possible.

Nocardial infections tend to relapse (particularly in patients with chronic granulomatous disease), and long courses of antimicrobial therapy are necessary. If disease is unusually extensive, if the patient is immunosuppressed, or if the response to therapy is slow, the recommendations in Table 165-1 should be exceeded.

The mortality rate for pulmonary or disseminated nocardiosis outside the CNS should be <5%. CNS disease carries a higher mortality rate. Patients should be followed carefully for at least 6 months after therapy has ended. Any child with nocardiosis and no known cause of immunosuppression should undergo tests to determine the adequacy of the phagocytic respiratory burst.

BIBLIOGRAPHY

BERKEY P, BODEY GP: Nocardial infection in patients with neoplastic disease. Rev Infect Dis 11:407, 1989

BROWN BA et al: Disseminated *Nocardia pesudobrasiliensis* infection in a patient with AIDS in Brazil. Clin Infect Dis 28:144, 1999

CHOUCIÑO C et al: Nocardial infections in bone marrow transplant recipients. Clin Infect Dis 23:1012, 1996

FILICE GA, NIEWOEHNER DE: Contribution of neutrophils and cell-mediated immunity to control of *Nocardia asteroides* in murine lungs. J Infect Dis 156:113, 1987

———, SIMPSON GL: Management of *Nocardia* infections, in *Current Clinical Topics in Infectious Diseases*, vol 5, JS Remington et al (eds). New York, McGraw-Hill, 1984

KONTOYIANNIS DP et al: *Nocardia* bacteremia. Report of 4 cases and review of the literature. Medicine 77:255, 1998

MINAMOTO GY, SORDILLO EM: Disseminated nocardiosis in a patient with AIDS: Diagnosis by blood and cerebrospinal fluid cultures. Clin Infect Dis 26:242, 1998

PALMER DL et al: Diagnostic and therapeutic considerations in *Nocardia asteroides* infection. Medicine 53:391, 1974

SATTERWHITE TK, WALLACE RJ JR: Primary cutaneous nocardiosis. JAMA 242:333, 1979

SMEGO RA Jr et al: Lymphocutaneous syndrome. A review of non-sporothrix causes. Medicine 78:38, 1999

TIGHT RR, BARTLETT MS: Actinomycetoma in the United States. Rev Infect Dis 3:1139, 1981

UTTAMCHANDANI RB et al: Nocardiosis in 30 patients with advanced human immunodeficiency virus infection: Clinical features and outcome. Clin Infect Dis 18:348, 1994

166

Thomas A. Russo

ACTINOMYCOSIS

Actinomycosis is an indolent, slowly progressive infection caused by anaerobic or microaerophilic bacteria, primarily of the genus *Actinomyces*, that colonize the mouth, colon, and vagina. Mucosal disruption may lead to infection at virtually any site in the body. The clinical presentations of actinomycosis are myriad; however, classic features include purulent foci surrounded by dense fibrosis that, over time, cross natural anatomic boundaries into contiguous structures, with the formation of fistulae and sinus tracts in some cases. In vivo growth of actinomycetes usually results in the formation of clumps called *grains* or *sulfur granules*. This infection is commonly confused with a neoplasm. Common in the preantibiotic era, actinomycosis has diminished in incidence, as has its timely recognition. Actinomycosis has been called "the most misdiagnosed disease," and it has been said that "no disease is so often missed by experienced clinicians." Thus this entity remains a diagnostic challenge. An awareness of the full spectrum of the disease will expedite its diagnosis and treatment and will minimize the unnecessary surgical interventions, morbidity, and mortality that are reported all too often.

ETIOLOGIC AGENTS Actinomycosis is most commonly caused by *A. israelii. A. naeslundii, A. odontolyticus, A. viscosus, A. meyeri, A. gerencseriae*, and *Propionibacterium propionicum* are established but less common causes of the disease. Most if not all actinomycotic infections are polymicrobial. *Actinobacillus actinomycetemcomitans, Eikenella corrodens*, Enterobacteriaceae, and species of *Fusobacterium, Bacteroides, Capnocytophaga, Staphylococcus*, and *Streptococcus* are commonly isolated with actinomycetes in various combinations, depending on the site of infection. The contribution of these other species to the pathogenesis of actinomycosis is uncertain.

An increasing number of bacterial species isolated from human clinical specimens have recently been classified as *Actinomyces*. Although their role in disease has not always been defined, *A. europaeus, A. neuii* subspecies *neuii, A. neuii* subspecies *anitratus, A. radingae*,

A. *graevenitzii*, and A. *turicensis* appear to be infrequent and often opportunistic human pathogens. The nature of the infections described to date does not clearly establish these agents as causes of the typical syndrome of actinomycosis.

EPIDEMIOLOGY The agents of actinomycosis are members of the normal oral flora and are often cultured from the bronchi, the gastrointestinal tract, and the female genital tract. Infection occurs throughout life, with a peak incidence in the middle decades. Males have a threefold higher incidence of infection, possibly because of poorer dental hygiene and/or more frequent trauma. Likely contributing factors to the decrease in the incidence of actinomycosis since the preantibiotic era include improved dental hygiene and the initiation of antimicrobial treatment early on—before the full development of the disease. Individuals who do not seek or have access to health care are undoubtedly at higher risk.

PATHOGENESIS AND PATHOLOGY A vital step in the development of actinomycosis is disruption of the mucosal barrier, which allows the actinomycetes to invade beyond their endogenous habitat in the mouth, lower gastrointestinal tract, and female genitourinary tract. Local infection, subsequent extension, and (in rare instances) distant hematogenous seeding may ensue. Initial acute inflammation is followed by the characteristic chronic, indolent phase. Lesions usually appear as single or multiple indurations. Central fluctuance, with pus containing neutrophils and sulfur granules, is virtually diagnostic of this disease (Fig. 166-1). The fibrous walls of the mass are typically described as "woody." The responsible bacterial and/or host factors have not yet been identified. Once established, actinomycosis spreads contiguously in a slow progressive manner, ignoring tissue planes. Given time, sinus tracts, which can spontaneously close and reopen, will form and extend to skin, adjacent organs, or bone. These unique features of actinomycosis mimic malignancy, with which it is often confused.

Foreign bodies appear to facilitate infection. This association most frequently involves intrauterine contraceptive devices (IUCDs). In addition, an increasing number of reports have described an association of actinomycosis with HIV infection, transplantation, and chemotherapy. Ulcerative mucosal infections (e.g., by herpes simplex virus or cytomegalovirus) and abnormalities in host defenses may facilitate the development of actinomycosis in the latter settings.

FIGURE 166-1 Actinomycotic sulfur granule surrounded by inflammatory cells. The delicate branched filaments of *Actinomyces* are surrounded by the proteinaceous eosinophilic coating of the granule (Slendore-Hoeppli phenomenon).

CLINICAL MANIFESTATIONS **Oral-Cervicofacial Disease** Actinomycosis occurs most frequently at an oral, cervical, or facial site, usually as a soft tissue swelling, abscess, or mass lesion that is often mistaken for a neoplasm. The angle of the jaw is generally involved, but a diagnosis of actinomycosis should be considered with any mass lesion or relapsing infection in the head and neck. Otitis, sinusitis, and canaliculitis can also develop. Pain, fever, and leukocytosis are variably reported. Contiguous extension to the cranium, cervical spine, or thorax is a potential sequela.

Thoracic Disease Thoracic actinomycosis usually follows an indolent progressive course, with involvement of the pulmonary parenchyma and/or the pleural space. Chest pain, fever, and weight loss are common. A cough, when present, is variably productive. The usual radiographic appearance is either a mass lesion or pneumonitis. Cavitary disease or hilar adenopathy may develop. More than 50% of cases include pleural thickening, effusion, or empyema. Rarely, pulmonary nodules or endobronchial lesions occur. Pulmonary lesions suggestive of actinomycosis may cross fissures or pleura; may involve the mediastinum, contiguous bone, or chest wall; or may be associated with a sinus tract. In the absence of these findings, thoracic actinomycosis is usually mistaken for a neoplasm or for pneumonitis due to more usual causes.

Mediastinal infection is uncommon, usually arising from thoracic extension but rarely resulting from perforation of the esophagus, from trauma, or from head and neck or abdominal disease. The structures within the mediastinum and the heart can be involved in various combinations; consequently, the possible presentations are diverse. Isolated disease of the breast has been described.

Abdominal Disease Abdominal actinomycosis poses a great diagnostic challenge. Months or years usually pass from the inciting event (e.g., appendicitis, diverticulitis, peptic ulcer disease, foreign-body perforation, bowel surgery, or ascension from IUCD-associated pelvic disease) to clinical recognition. Because of the flow of peritoneal fluid and/or the direct extension of primary disease, virtually any abdominal organ, region, or space can be involved. The disease usually presents as an abscess or a mass lesion that is often fixed to underlying tissue and mistaken for a tumor. Infiltrative disease with irregular contrast enhancement may be seen on computed tomography (CT). Sinus tracts to the abdominal wall or perianal region may develop. Recurrent disease or a wound or fistula that fails to heal (in the absence of inflammatory bowel disease) suggests actinomycosis.

Hepatic infection usually presents as single or multiple abscesses or masses. Isolated disease presumably develops via hematogenous seeding from cryptic foci. Presently available imaging and percutaneous techniques have resulted in improved diagnosis and treatment.

All levels of the urogenital tract can be infected. Renal disease usually presents as pyelonephritis and/or renal and perinephric abscess. Bladder involvement, usually due to extension of pelvic disease, may result in ureteral obstruction or fistulas to bowel, skin, or uterus.

Pelvic Disease Actinomycotic involvement of the pelvis occurs most commonly in association with an IUCD. Pelvic symptoms when an IUCD is in place or has recently been removed should prompt consideration of actinomycosis. Although the risk has not yet been quantified, it appears to be small. The disease rarely develops when the IUCD has been in place for <1 year, but the risk increases with time. Actinomycosis can also present months after the removal of the device. Symptoms are typically indolent; fever, weight loss, abdominal pain, and abnormal vaginal bleeding or discharge are the most common. The earliest stage of disease—often endometritis—commonly progresses to pelvic masses or a tuboovarian abscess (Fig. 166-2). Unfortunately, because the diagnosis is often delayed, a "frozen pelvis" mimicking malignancy or endometriosis can develop by the time of recognition.

An unresolved issue is whether the isolation of *Actinomyces*-like organisms (ALOs) from cultures of cervical or endometrial specimens

FIGURE 166-2 Computed tomogram showing pelvic actinomycosis associated with an intrauterine contraceptive device. The device is encased by endometrial fibrosis (*solid arrowhead*); also visible are paraendometrial fibrosis (*open arrow*) and an area of suppuration (*open arrowhead*).

or the detection of ALOs by immunofluorescence is correlated with IUCD-associated disease. A Papanicolaou smear may fail to detect ALOs even in the presence of active actinomycosis. Although the risk appears to be small, the consequences of infection are significant. Therefore, until more quantitative data become available, detection of ALOs or immunofluorescence-positive organisms in conjunction with symptoms that cannot be accounted for appears to warrant removal of the IUCD and—if advanced disease is excluded—initiation of a 14-day course of empirical treatment for possible early pelvic actinomycosis. The detection of ALOs or immunofluorescence-positive organisms in the absence of symptoms warrants education of the patient and close follow-up but not removal of the IUCD.

Central Nervous System Disease Actinomycosis of the central nervous system is rare. Single or multiple brain abscesses are most common. An abscess usually appears on CT as a ring-enhancing lesion with a thick wall that may be irregular or nodular. Meningitis, epidural or subdural space infection, and cavernous sinus syndrome have also been described.

Musculoskeletal Infection Actinomycotic infection of the bone is usually due to adjacent soft tissue infection but may be associated with trauma (e.g., fracture of the mandible) or hematogenous spread. Because of slow disease progression, new bone formation and bone destruction are seen concomitantly. Infection of an extremity is uncommon and is usually a result of trauma. Skin, subcutaneous tissue, muscle, and bone (with periostitis or acute or chronic osteomyelitis) are involved alone or in various combinations. Cutaneous sinus tracts frequently develop.

Disseminated Disease Hematogenous dissemination of disease from any location rarely results in multiple organ involvement. The lungs and liver are most commonly affected, with the presentation of multiple nodules mimicking disseminated malignancy. The clinical presentation may be surprisingly indolent given the extent of disease.

DIAGNOSIS The diagnosis of actinomycosis, particularly when it mimics malignancy, is rarely considered. All too often, the first mention of actinomycosis is by the pathologist after extensive surgery has been performed. Since medical therapy alone is often sufficient for cure, the challenge for the clinician is to consider the possibility of actinomycosis in time to diagnose it in the least invasive fashion and to avoid unnecessary surgery. Both fine-needle aspiration and biopsy are being used successfully to obtain clinical material for diagnosis,

as are CT- and ultrasound-guided aspirations or biopsies. The diagnosis is most commonly made by microscopic identification of sulfur granules; occasionally these granules, if sought, can be grossly identified from draining sinus tracts or other purulent material. Although sulfur granules are a defining characteristic of actinomycosis, granules are also found in mycetoma and botryomycosis; however, these entities can easily be differentiated from actinomycosis with appropriate histopathologic and microbiologic studies. Microbiologic identification of actinomycetes is possible in only a minority of cases and is often precluded by prior antimicrobial therapy. Therefore, for optimal yield, the avoidance of even a single dose of antibiotics is mandatory. Primary isolation usually requires 5 to 7 days but may take as long as 2 to 4 weeks. Immunofluorescence testing for *A. israelii*, *A. naeslundii*, and *P. propionicum* (available through the Centers for Disease Control and Prevention in Atlanta) has become a useful diagnostic alternative. Because these organisms are components of the normal oral and genital-tract flora, their identification in sputum, bronchial washings, and cervicovaginal secretions is of little significance in the absence of sulfur granules. *Actinomyces* can be detected in urine by means of appropriate staining and culture.

TREATMENT Actinomycosis must be treated with high doses of antimicrobials for a prolonged period. Although therapy needs to be individualized, the intravenous administration of 18 to 24 million units of penicillin for 2 to 6 weeks, followed by oral therapy with penicillin or amoxicillin for 6 to 12 months, is a reasonable guideline for serious infections. Less extensive disease, particularly that involving the oral-cervicofacial region, may require less intensive therapy. If therapy is extended beyond the point of resolution of measurable disease, the risk of relapse—a clinical hallmark of this infection—will be minimized. A similar approach is reasonable for immunocompromised patients, although refractory disease has been described in HIV-infected individuals. Antimicrobial agents whose use is supported by extensive clinical experience are listed in Table 166-1. Although the role played by "companion" microbes in actinomycosis is unclear, many isolates are pathogens in their own right, and a regimen covering these organisms during the initial treatment course is reasonable. Agents whose success has been reported anecdotally are ceftriaxone, ceftizoxime, imipenem, and ciprofloxacin. Drugs that should be avoided are metronidazole, aminoglycosides, oxacillin, dicloxacillin, and cephalexin.

Combined medical-surgical therapy is still advocated by some authorities. However, an increasing body of literature now supports an initial attempt at cure with medical therapy alone, even in extensive disease. CT and magnetic resonance imaging should be used to monitor the response to therapy. Percutaneous drainage is an additional option. When a critical location is involved (e.g., the epidural space, the central nervous system) or when suitable medical therapy fails, surgical intervention may be appropriate.

Table 166-1 Antibiotic Therapy for Actinomycosis: Regimens Supported by Extensive Clinical Experience

Agent	Dosage
Penicillin	18–24 million units/d IV q4h
	1–2 g/d PO q6h
Erythromycin	2–4 g/d IV q6h
	1–2 g/d PO q6h
Tetracycline	1–2 g/d PO q6h
Doxycycline	200 mg/d IV or PO q12–24h
Minocycline	200 mg/d IV or PO q12h
Clindamycin	2.7 g/d IV q8h
	1.2–1.8 g/d PO q6–8h

NOTE: Additional coverage for concomitant "companion" bacteria may be required. Controlled evaluations have not been performed. Regimens must be individualized according to the site and extent of infection. As a general rule, a maximal antimicrobial dose given parenterally for 2 to 6 weeks, followed by oral therapy, with a total duration of 6 to 12 months, optimizes the likelihood of cure.

FIORINO AS: Intrauterine contraceptive device–associated actinomycotic abscess and *Actinomyces* detection on cervical smear. Obstet Gynecol 87:142, 1996

GOODMAN HM, CENTENO BA: Case records of the Massachusetts General Hospital, case 10-1992. N Engl J Med 326:692, 1992

RUSSO TA: Actinomycosis, in *Principles and Practice of Infectious Diseases*, 5th ed, GL Mandell et al (eds). New York, Churchill Livingstone, 1999

SMEGO RA, FOGLIA G: Actinomycosis. Clin Infect Dis 26:1255, 1998

167 Dennis L. Kasper

INFECTIONS DUE TO MIXED ANAEROBIC ORGANISMS

DEFINITIONS *Anaerobic* bacteria are organisms that require reduced oxygen tension for growth, failing to grow on the surface of solid media in 10% CO_2 in air. (In contrast, *microaerophilic* bacteria can grow in 10% CO_2 in air or under anaerobic or aerobic conditions, although they grow best in the presence of only a small amount of atmospheric oxygen, and *facultative* bacteria can grow in the presence or absence of air.) This chapter describes infections caused by nonsporulating anaerobic bacteria. In general, anaerobes associated with human infections are relatively aerotolerant. They can survive for as long as 72 h in the presence of oxygen, although generally they will not multiply in this environment. A far smaller number of pathogenic anaerobic bacteria (which are also part of the normal flora) die after brief contact with oxygen, even in low concentrations.

The nonsporulating anaerobic bacteria exist as components of the normal flora on the mucosal surfaces of humans and animals. The major reservoirs of these bacteria are the mouth, lower gastrointestinal tract, skin, and female genital tract. Among the constituents of the oral flora, anaerobes are the predominant commensal organisms, ranging in concentration from 10^9/mL in saliva to 10^{12}/mL in gingival scrapings. In the oral cavity, the ratio of anaerobic to aerobic bacteria ranges from 1:1 on the surface of a tooth to 1000:1 in the gingival crevice. Anaerobic bacteria are not found in appreciable numbers in the normal upper intestine until the distal ileum. In the colon, the proportion of anaerobes increases significantly, as does the overall bacterial count. For example, in the colon there are 10^{11} to 10^{12} organisms per gram of stool, with a ratio of anaerobes to aerobes of approximately 1000:1. In the female genital tract, there are approximately 10^9 organisms per milliliter of secretions, with a ratio of anaerobes to aerobes of approximately 10:1.

Hundreds of species of anaerobic bacteria have been identified as part of the normal flora of humans. Identification of as many as 500 different anaerobic species in fecal specimens reflects the diversity of the anaerobic flora. Despite the complex array of bacteria in the normal flora, relatively few species are isolated commonly from human infection.

Anaerobic infections occur when the harmonious relationship between the host and the bacteria is disrupted. Any site in the body is susceptible to infection with these indigenous organisms when a mucosal barrier or the skin is compromised by surgery, trauma, tumor, or ischemia or necrosis, which reduce local tissue redox potentials. Because the sites that are colonized by anaerobes contain many species of bacteria, disruption of anatomic barriers allows penetration of many organisms, resulting in mixed infections involving multiple species of anaerobes combined with facultative or microaerophilic organisms. Such mixed infections are seen in the head and neck (chronic sinusitis, chronic otitis media, Ludwig's angina, and periodontal abscesses). Brain abscesses and subdural empyema are the most frequent anaerobic infections of the central nervous system. Anaerobes are responsible for pleuropulmonary diseases such as aspiration pneumonia, necrotizing pneumonia, lung abscess, and empyema. These organisms also play an important role in various intraabdominal infections, such as peritonitis and intraabdominal and liver abscesses (Chap. 130). They are isolated frequently in female genital tract infections, such as salpingitis, pelvic peritonitis, tuboovarian abscess, vulvovaginal abscess, septic abortion, and endometritis (Chaps. 132 and 133). Anaerobic bacteria also are frequently found in infections of the skin, soft tissues, and bones and in bacteremia.

ETIOLOGY The major anaerobic gram-positive cocci that produce disease are *Peptostreptococcus* spp. The major species involved in infections are *Peptostreptococcus intermedius*, *P. micros*, *P. magnus*, *P. asaccharolyticus*, *P. anaerobius*, and *P. prevotii*. Clostridia are gram-positive rods that are isolated from wounds, abscesses, sites of abdominal infection, and blood; they are discussed in Chap. 145. The principal anaerobic gram-negative bacilli found in human infections are the members of the *Bacteroides* "family," which includes the *Bacteroides fragilis* group as well as *Fusobacterium*, *Prevotella*, and *Porphyromonas* spp. Another gram-negative rod, *Bilophila wadsworthia*, has been isolated from infected sites. Gram-positive anaerobic nonspore-forming bacilli are uncommon as etiologic agents of human infections. *Propionibacterium acnes*, a rare cause of foreign body infections, is one of the few non-clostridial gram-positive rods associated with infections.

The *B. fragilis* group contains the anaerobic pathogens most frequently isolated from clinical infections. Members of this group are part of the normal bowel flora; they include several distinct species, such as *B. fragilis*, *B. thetaiotaomicron*, *B. distasonis*, *B. vulgatus*, *B. uniformis*, and *B. ovatus*. (Ribosomal RNA analysis has shown that *B. distasonis* is more closely related to the genus *Porphyromonas* than it is to other *Bacteroides*.) Of this group, *B. fragilis* is the most important clinical isolate. However, *B. fragilis* is isolated from the normal fecal flora in lower numbers than other *Bacteroides* spp.

A second major group of phenotypically similar organisms is part of the indigenous oral flora. Thus these organisms are found at infected sites that can be seeded with oral microflora. Many of these species are pigment-producing bacteria previously classified as *Bacteroides melaninogenicus*. The nomenclature of this group has changed so that two distinct genera, *Prevotella* and *Porphyromonas*, are now recognized; these genera comprise several pathogenic species, including *Porphyromonas gingivalis*, *Porphyromonas asaccharolytica*, and *Prevotella oralis*. *Porphyromonas* and *Prevotella* spp. cause localized infections that can spread contiguously.

In female genital tract infections, organisms normally colonizing the vagina, such as *Prevotella bivia* and *Prevotella disiens*, are the most frequent isolates, although *B. fragilis* is not uncommon. The *Fusobacterium* species *Fusobacterium necrophorum*, *F. nucleatum*, and *F. varium*, which reside primarily in the oral cavity and the gastrointestinal tract, are also isolated from clinical infections, including necrotizing pneumonia and abscesses. *Bilophila wadsworthia* has been reported to cause serious infections, including bacteremia, necrotizing fasciitis, and abscesses; this organism is frequently resistant to several antimicrobials, including imipenem, cefoxitin, and other β-lactam agents.

Infections caused by anaerobic bacteria most frequently are due to more than one organism. These polymicrobial infections may be caused by one or several anaerobic species or by a combination of anaerobic organisms and microaerophilic or facultative bacteria acting synergistically.

Approach to the Patient

The physician must consider several points when approaching the patient with presumptive infection due to anaerobic bacteria.

1. Most of the organisms colonizing mucosal sites are harmless commensals; very few cause disease.
2. For anaerobes to cause tissue infection, they must spread beyond the normal mucosal barriers.

3. Conditions favoring the propagation of these bacteria, particularly a lowered oxidation-reduction potential, are necessary. These conditions exist at sites of trauma, tissue destruction, compromised vascular supply, and complications of preexisting infection, which produce necrosis.

4. There is a complex array of infecting flora. For example, as many as 12 different types of organisms can be isolated from a suppurative site.

5. Anaerobic organisms tend to be found in abscess cavities or in necrotic tissue. The failure of an abscess to yield organisms on routine culture is a clue that the abscess is likely to contain anaerobic bacteria. Often smears of this "sterile pus" are found to be teeming with bacteria when Gram's stain is applied. Malodorous pus suggests anaerobic infection. Although some facultative organisms, such as *Staphylococcus aureus*, are also capable of causing abscesses, abscesses in organs or deeper body tissues should call to mind anaerobic infection.

6. Gas is found in many anaerobic infections of deep tissues.

7. Some species (the best example being the *B. fragilis* group) require specific therapy. However, many synergistic infections can be cured with antibiotics directed at some but not all of the organisms involved. Antibiotic therapy, combined with debridement and drainage, disrupts the interdependent relationship among the bacteria, and some species that are resistant to the antibiotic do not survive without the coinfecting organisms.

8. Manifestations of disseminated intravascular coagulation are unusual in patients with purely anaerobic infection.

EPIDEMIOLOGY   Difficulties in the performance of appropriate cultures, contamination of cultures by aerobic bacteria or components of the normal flora, and the lack of readily available, reliable culture techniques have made it impossible to obtain accurate incidence or prevalence data. However, anaerobic infections are encountered frequently in hospitals with active surgical, trauma, and obstetric and gynecologic services. In some centers, anaerobic bacteria, particularly *B. fragilis*, account for approximately 4% of positive blood cultures.

PATHOGENESIS   Anaerobic bacterial infections usually occur when an anatomic barrier becomes disrupted and constituents of the local flora enter a site that was previously sterile. Because of the specific growth requirements of anaerobic organisms and their presence as commensals on mucosal surfaces, conditions must arise that allow these organisms to penetrate mucosal barriers and enter tissue with a lowered oxidation-reduction potential. Therefore, tissue ischemia, trauma, surgery, perforated viscus, shock, and aspiration provide environments conducive to the proliferation of anaerobes. In the case of a perforated viscus, hundreds of species of anaerobic bacteria are spilled into the peritoneal cavity, but many of these organisms are unable to survive because the highly vascularized tissue provides a sufficiently high redox potential. The entry of oxygen into the environment results in the selection of the more aerotolerant anaerobic organisms.

The ability of an organism to adhere to host tissues is important to the establishment of infection. Some oral species adhere to crevicular epithelium in the oral cavity. *Prevotella melaninogenica* actually attaches to other microorganisms; *P. gingivalis* is a common isolate in periodontal disease. These organisms have fimbriae that facilitate attachment. Some unencapsulated *Bacteroides* strains appear to be piliated, a characteristic that may account for their ability to adhere.

The most extensively studied virulence factor of the nonsporulating anaerobes is the polysaccharide capsule of *B. fragilis*. This polysaccharide possesses distinct biologic properties, such as the ability (owing to a unique zwitterionic motif of charged sugars) to promote abscess formation. Intraabdominal abscess induction is related to the capacity of the polysaccharide to stimulate the release of cytokines, in particular interleukin 8 (IL-8) and tumor necrosis factor α (TNF-α), from resident peritoneal cells. IL-8 results in the chemotaxis of polymorphonuclear neutrophils (PMNs) into the peritoneum, where they adhere to mesothelial cells induced by TNF-α to upregulate their expression of intercellular adhesion molecule 1 (ICAM-1). PMNs adherent to ICAM-1-expressing cells probably represent the nidus for an abscess. Prophylactic or therapeutic administration of the polysaccharide or a zwitterionic mimetic to experimental animals confers protection against abscess induction following challenge with intestinal microorganisms capable of inducing abscesses. This protection is mediated by T cells controlling cytokine release, which blocks the tissue response of abscess formation. Although abscesses constitute a host response that localizes and contains infecting bacteria, abscess formation in patients with sepsis often results in severe and chronic illness that requires surgical drainage in combination with antimicrobial therapy.

Anaerobic bacteria produce a number of exoproteins that are capable of enhancing the organisms' virulence. The collagenase produced by *P. gingivalis* may enhance tissue destruction. An enterotoxin has been identified in *B. fragilis* strains associated with diarrheal disease in animals and young children. This 20-kDa zinc-dependent metalloprotease reversibly alters the morphology of the tight junctional complexes of intestinal epithelial cells. Both *B. fragilis* and *P. melaninogenica* possess lipopolysaccharides (endotoxins) that are less biologically potent than endotoxins associated with aerobic gram-negative bacteria. This relative biologic inactivity may account for the lower frequency of disseminated intravascular coagulation and purpura in *Bacteroides* bacteremia than in facultative and aerobic gram-negative bacillary bacteremia.

CLINICAL MANIFESTATIONS   **Anaerobic Infections of the Mouth, Head, and Neck** (See also Chap. 30)   Infections of the mouth can arise from either the supragingival or the subgingival dental plaque. Supragingival plaque formation begins with the adherence of gram-positive bacteria to the tooth surface. This form of plaque is influenced by salivary and dietary components, oral hygiene, and local host factors. Once the supragingival plaque is established, the acquisition of pathogenic bacteria and an increase in the amount of plaque are responsible for the ultimate development of gingivitis. Early bacteriologic changes in the supragingival plaque initiate an inflammatory response in the gingiva, including edema, swelling, and increased gingival fluid, and cause the development of caries and endodontic (pulp) infections. In addition, these changes contribute to the subsequent pathogenic alteration in the subgingival plaque that arises from poor or inadequate oral hygiene.

Subgingival plaque is associated with periodontal disease and disseminated infection arising from the oral cavity. Bacteria that colonize the subgingival area are primarily anaerobic. The black-pigmented gram-negative anaerobic bacilli, principally *P. gingivalis* and *P. melaninogenica*, are the most important. Infections in this area are frequently mixed and involve both anaerobic and aerobic bacteria. After establishment of local infection either in root canals or in the periodontal area, infection may extend into the mandible, causing osteomyelitis to the maxillary sinuses; or to local tissues in the submandibular or submental spaces, depending on which teeth are involved. Periodontitis also may result in spreading infection that can involve adjacent bone or soft tissues.

Gingivitis   Gingivitis may become a necrotizing infection (trench mouth, Vincent's stomatitis). The onset of disease is usually sudden and is associated with tender bleeding gums, foul breath, and a bad taste. The gingival mucosa, especially the papillae between the teeth, becomes ulcerated and may be covered by a gray exudate, which is removable with gentle pressure. Patients may become systemically ill, developing fever, cervical lymphadenopathy, and leukocytosis. Occasionally, ulcerative gingivitis can spread to the buccal mucosa, the teeth, and the mandible or maxilla, resulting in widespread destruction of bone and soft tissue. This infection is termed *acute necrotizing ulcerative mucositis* (cancrum oris, noma). It destroys tissue rapidly, causing the teeth to fall out and large areas of bone—or even the whole mandible—to be sloughed. A strong putrid odor is frequently detected, although the lesions are not painful. The gangrenous lesions eventually heal, leaving large disfiguring defects. This infection is seen most commonly following a debilitating illness or in severely malnourished children. It has been known to complicate leukemia or to develop in individuals with a genetic deficiency of catalase.

Acute necrotizing infections of the pharynx These infections usually occur in association with ulcerative gingivitis. Symptoms include an extremely sore throat, foul breath, and a bad taste accompanied by fever and a sensation of choking. Examination of the pharynx demonstrates that the tonsillar pillars are swollen, red, ulcerated, and covered with a grayish membrane that peels easily. Lymphadenopathy and leukocytosis are common. The disease may last for only a few days or, if not treated, may persist for weeks. Lesions begin unilaterally but may spread to the other side of the pharynx or the larynx. Aspiration of the infected material by the patient can result in lung abscesses. Soft tissue infection of the oral-facial area may or may not be odontogenic. *Ludwig's angina*, a periodontal infection usually arising from the tissues surrounding the third molar, may produce submandibular cellulitis that results in marked local swelling of tissues, with pain, trismus, and superior and posterior displacement of the tongue. Submandibular swelling of the neck can impair swallowing and cause respiratory obstruction. In some cases, tracheotomy may be lifesaving.

Fascial infections These infections arise from the spread of organisms originating in the upper airways to potential spaces formed by the fascial planes of the head and neck. Perimandibular space infection most commonly involves the submandibular, peritonsillar, and parapharyngeal spaces. Peritonsillar abscesses occur in association with pharyngitis. Complicated dental infections spread to the submandibular and buccal spaces. Entry of organisms by either portal can result in parapharyngeal space infections. Although there are few well-documented reports on the microbiology of these syndromes, anaerobes from the oral flora have been implicated in many cases. Fascial infections associated with *S. aureus* or *Streptococcus pyogenes* may arise from boils or impetigo, whereas anaerobes are associated with space infections either occurring spontaneously or arising from diseases of the mucous membranes or from dental manipulations.

Sinusitis and otitis The role of anaerobic bacteria in acute sinusitis may be underestimated because of improper collection of specimens. In a study of chronic sinusitis, anaerobic bacteria were found in 52% of specimens collected during external frontoethmoidotomy or radical antrotomy. Anaerobic bacteria are much more easily implicated in chronic suppurative otitis media than in acute otitis media. Purulent exudate from chronically draining ears has been found to contain anaerobes, particularly *Bacteroides* spp., in up to 50% of cases. *B. fragilis* has been isolated from up to 28% of patients with chronic otitis media.

Complications of anaerobic head and neck infections Contiguous craniad spread of these infections may result in osteomyelitis of the skull or mandible or in intracranial infections such as brain abscess and subdural empyema. Caudad spread can produce mediastinitis or pleuropulmonary infection. Hematogenous complications may also result from anaerobic infections of the head and neck. Bacteremia, which occasionally is polymicrobial, can lead to endocarditis or other distant infections. When infections spread to produce suppurative thrombophlebitis of the internal jugular vein, a destructive syndrome (*Lemierre's*)—with prolonged fever, bacteremia, septic emboli to both the lung and the brain, and multiple metastatic foci of suppurative infection—may develop. This syndrome has been reported with fusobacterial septicemia following exudative pharyngitis but has been uncommon in the antimicrobial era.

Central Nervous System Infections Brain abscesses are frequently associated with anaerobic bacteria (Chap. 372). If optimal bacteriologic techniques are employed, as many as 85% of brain abscesses yield anaerobic bacteria—most often anaerobic gram-positive cocci (especially peptostreptococci), which are followed in frequency by *Fusobacterium* and *Bacteroides* spp. Facultative or microaerophilic strep-

tococci and coliforms often are part of a mixed infecting flora in brain abscesses.

Pleuropulmonary Infections Anaerobic pleuropulmonary infections result from the aspiration of oropharyngeal contents, often in the context of an altered state of consciousness or an absent gag reflex. Four clinical syndromes are associated with anaerobic pleuropulmonary infection produced by aspiration: simple aspiration pneumonia, necrotizing pneumonia, lung abscess, and empyema.

Aspiration pneumonitis Aspiration pneumonitis must be distinguished from two other clinical syndromes associated with aspiration that are not of bacterial etiology. One syndrome results from aspiration of solids, usually food. Obstruction of major airways typically results in atelectasis and moderate nonspecific inflammation. Therapy consists of removal of the foreign body.

The second aspiration syndrome is more easily confused with bacterial aspiration. *Mendelson's* syndrome results from regurgitation of stomach contents and aspiration of chemical material, usually gastric juices. Pulmonary inflammation—including the destruction of the alveolar lining, with transudation of fluid into the alveolar space—occurs with remarkable rapidity. Typically this syndrome develops within hours, often following anesthesia when the gag reflex is depressed. The patient becomes tachypneic, hypoxic, and febrile. The leukocyte count may rise, and the chest x-ray may evolve suddenly from normal to a complete bilateral "whiteout" within 8 to 24 h. Sputum production is minimal. The pulmonary signs and symptoms can resolve quickly with symptom-based therapy or can culminate in respiratory failure, with the subsequent development of bacterial superinfection over a period of days. Antibiotic therapy is not indicated unless bacterial infection supervenes. The signs of bacterial infection include sputum production, persistent fever, leukocytosis, and clinical evidence of sepsis.

In contrast to these syndromes, bacterial aspiration pneumonia develops more slowly. It is seen in patients who are hospitalized and have a depressed gag reflex, impaired swallowing, or a tracheal or nasogastric tube; elderly patients; or those with transiently impaired consciousness in the wake of seizures, cerebrovascular accidents, or alcoholic blackouts. Patients who enter the hospital with this syndrome typically have been ill for several days and generally report low-grade fever, malaise, and sputum production. Usually the history reveals factors predisposing to aspiration, such as alcohol overdose or residence in a nursing home. Sputum characteristically is not malodorous unless the process has been under way for at least a week. A mixed bacterial flora with many PMNs is evident on Gram's staining; cultures are reliable only if contamination with the normal oral flora is avoided—that is, if specimens are obtained by transtracheal aspiration. In general, this procedure is not indicated in the evaluation of these patients. The most commonly encountered anaerobes in these infections are pigmented and nonpigmented *Prevotella* spp., *F. nucleatum*, *Peptostreptococcus* spp., and *Bacteroides* spp. Chest x-rays show consolidation in dependent pulmonary segments: in the basilar segments of the lower lobes if the patient has aspirated while upright and in either the posterior segment of the upper lobe (usually on the right side) or the superior segment of the lower lobe if the patient has aspirated while supine. The organisms isolated reflect the pharyngeal flora; *P. melaninogenica, Fusobacterium* spp., and anaerobic cocci are the most frequent isolates. The patient who aspirates in the hospital also may have a mixed infection involving enteric gram-negative rods.

Necrotizing pneumonitis This form of anaerobic pneumonitis is characterized by numerous small abscesses that spread to involve several pulmonary segments. The process can be indolent or fulminating. This syndrome is less common than either aspiration pneumonia or lung abscess and includes features of both types of infection.

Anaerobic lung abscesses These abscesses result from subacute anaerobic pulmonary infection. The clinical syndrome typically involves a history of constitutional symptoms, including malaise, weight loss, fever, chills, and foul-smelling sputum, perhaps over a period of weeks (Chap. 255). Patients who develop lung abscesses characteristically have dental infection and periodontitis, but lung abscesses in edentulous patients have been reported. Abscess cavities may be single or multiple and generally occur in dependent pulmonary segments. Anaerobic abscesses must be distinguished from those associated with tuberculosis, neoplasia, and other conditions. Oral anaerobes predominate, although *B. fragilis* is isolated in up to 10% of cases. *S. aureus* may be found as well.

Empyema Empyema is a manifestation of long-standing anaerobic pulmonary infection. The clinical presentation, which includes the presence of foul-smelling sputum, resembles that of other anaerobic pulmonary infections. Patients may report pleuritic chest pain and marked chest-wall tenderness.

Empyema may be masked by overlying pneumonitis and should be considered especially in cases of persistent fever despite antibiotic therapy. Diligent physical examination and the use of ultrasound to localize a loculated empyema are important diagnostic tools. The collection of a foul-smelling exudate by thoracentesis is typical. Cultures of infected pleural fluid yield an average of 3.5 anaerobes and 0.6 facultative or aerobic bacterial species. Drainage is required. Defervescence, a return to a feeling of well-being, and resolution of the process may require several months.

Extension from a subdiaphragmatic infection also may result in anaerobic empyema. Septic pulmonary emboli may originate from intraabdominal or female genital tract infections and can produce anaerobic pneumonia.

Intraabdominal Infections Enterotoxigenic *B. fragilis* has been associated with watery diarrhea in a small number of young children and adults. In case-control studies of children with undiagnosed diarrheal disease, enterotoxigenic *B. fragilis* was isolated from significantly more children with diarrhea than children in the control group. This organism may play a role in a small proportion of childhood diarrhea cases. Neutropenic enterocolitis (typhlitis) has been associated with anaerobic infection of the cecum but—in the setting of neutropenia (Chap. 85)—may involve the entire bowel. Patients usually present with fever; abdominal pain, tenderness, and distension; and watery diarrhea. The bowel wall is edematous with hemorrhage and necrosis. The primary pathogen is thought by some authorities to be *C. septicum*, but other clostridia and mixed anaerobic infections have also been implicated. More than 50% of patients developing early clinical signs can benefit from antibiotic therapy and bowel rest. Surgery is sometimes required to remove gangrenous bowel. →*See Chap. 130 for a complete discussion of intraabdominal infections.*

Pelvic Infections The vagina of a healthy woman is one of the major reservoirs of anaerobic and aerobic bacteria. In the normal flora of the female genital tract, anaerobes outnumber aerobes by a ratio of approximately 10:1 and include anaerobic gram-positive cocci and *Bacteroides* spp. Anaerobes are isolated from most patients with genital tract infections not caused by a sexually transmitted pathogen. The major anaerobic pathogens are *B. fragilis*, *P. bivia*, *P. disiens*, *P. melaninogenica*, anaerobic cocci, and *Clostridium* spp. Anaerobes frequently are encountered in tuboovarian abscess, septic abortion, pelvic abscess, endometritis, and postoperative wound infection, particularly following hysterectomy. Although these infections are frequently mixed, involving both anaerobes and coliforms, pure anaerobic infections without coliform or other facultative bacterial species occur more often in pelvic than in intraabdominal sites and are characterized by drainage of foul-smelling pus or blood from the uterus, generalized uterine or local pelvic tenderness, and continued fever and chills. Suppurative thrombophlebitis of the pelvic veins may complicate the infections and lead to repeated episodes of septic pulmonary emboli.

Anaerobic bacteria have been thought to be contributing factors in the etiology of *bacterial vaginosis*. This syndrome of unknown etiology is characterized by a profuse malodorous discharge and an increase in the number of bacteria in the vagina, including *Gardnerella vaginalis*, *Prevotella* spp., *Mobiluncus* spp., peptostreptococci, and

genital mycoplasmas. Anaerobic bacteria are thought to play a role in the etiology of pelvic inflammatory disease (Chap. 133), and several investigations have shown an association between bacterial vaginosis and the development of pelvic inflammatory disease.

Pelvic infections due to *Actinomyces* spp. have been associated with use of intrauterine devices (Chap. 166).

Skin and Soft Tissue Infections Injury to skin, bone, or soft tissue by trauma, ischemia, or surgery creates a suitable environment for anaerobic infections. These infections are most frequently found in sites prone to contamination with feces or with upper airway secretions—for example, wounds associated with intestinal surgery, decubitus ulcers, or human bites. Anaerobic bacteria can be isolated in cases of crepitant cellulitis, synergistic cellulitis, or gangrene and necrotizing fasciitis (Chaps. 128 and 145). Moreover, these organisms have been isolated from cutaneous abscesses, rectal abscesses, and axillary sweat gland infections (hydradenitis suppurativa). Anaerobes are frequently cultured from foot ulcers in diabetic patients.

These soft tissue or skin infections are usually polymicrobial. A mean of 4.8 bacterial species are isolated, with a roughly 3:2 ratio of anaerobes to aerobes. The most frequently isolated organisms include *Bacteroides* spp., *Peptostreptococcus* spp., enterococci, *Clostridium* spp., and *Proteus* spp. The involvement of anaerobes in these types of infections is associated with a higher frequency of fever, foul-smelling lesions, gas in the tissues, or visible foot ulcer.

Anaerobic bacterial *synergistic gangrene (Meleney's gangrene)* is characterized by exquisite pain, redness, and swelling followed by induration. Erythema surrounds a central zone of necrosis. A granulating ulcer forms at the original center as necrosis and erythema extend outward. Symptoms are limited to pain; fever is not typical. These infections usually involve a combination of *Peptostreptococcus* spp. and *S. aureus*; the usual site of infection is an abdominal surgical wound or the area surrounding an ulcer on an extremity. Treatment includes surgical removal of necrotic tissue and antimicrobial administration.

Necrotizing fasciitis, a rapidly spreading destructive disease of the fascia, is usually attributed to group A streptococci but can also be caused by anaerobic bacteria, including *Peptostreptococcus* and *Bacteroides* spp. Gas may be found in the tissues. Similarly, myonecrosis can be associated with mixed anaerobic infection. *Fournier's gangrene* consists of cellulitis involving the scrotum, perineum, and anterior abdominal wall, with mixed anaerobic organisms spreading along deep external fascial planes and causing extensive loss of skin.

Bone and Joint Infections Although *actinomycosis* (Chap. 166) accounts on a worldwide basis for most anaerobic infections in bone, organisms including *Peptostreptococcus* spp. or microaerophilic cocci, *Bacteroides* spp., *Fusobacterium* spp., and *Clostridium* spp. can also be found. These infections frequently arise adjacent to soft tissue infections. Hematogenous seeding of bone is uncommon. *Prevotella* and *Porphyromonas* spp. are detected in infections involving the maxilla and mandible, whereas *Clostridium* spp. have been reported as anaerobic pathogens in cases of osteomyelitis of the long bones following fracture or trauma. Fusobacteria have been isolated in pure culture from sites of osteomyelitis adjacent to the perinasal sinuses. *Peptostreptococcus* spp. and microaerophilic cocci have been reported as significant pathogens in infections involving the skull, mastoid, and prosthetic implants placed in bone. In patients with osteomyelitis (Chap. 129), the most reliable culture specimen is a bone biopsy sample free of normal uninfected skin and subcutaneous tissue. In patients with anaerobic osteomyelitis, a mixed flora is frequently isolated from a bone biopsy specimen.

In cases of anaerobic septic arthritis, the most common isolates are *Fusobacterium* spp. Most of the patients involved have uncontrolled peritonsillar infections progressing to septic cervical venous thrombophlebitis and resulting in hematogenous dissemination with a predilection for the joints. Unlike anaerobic osteomyelitis, anaerobic pyoarthritis in most cases is not polymicrobial and may be acquired hematogenously. Anaerobes are important pathogens in infections involving prosthetic joints; in these infections, the causative organisms (such as *Peptostreptococcus* spp. and *P. acnes*) are part of the normal skin flora.

167   Infections due to Anaerobic Organisms   **1015**

Bacteremia Transient bacteremia is a well-known event in healthy people whose anatomic mucosal barriers have been injured (e.g., during dental extractions or dental scaling). These bacteremic episodes, which are often due to anaerobes, have no pathologic consequences. However, anaerobic bacteria are found in cultures of blood from clinically ill patients when proper culture techniques are used. *B. fragilis* is the single most common anaerobic isolate from the bloodstream.

In recent years, the rate of isolation of anaerobic bacteria from blood cultures has been decreasing. Studies from the 1970s and early 1980s found that 10 to 15% of positive blood cultures yielded anaerobes, while more recent surveys have found rates as low as 4%. The cause of this change is unknown but may be related to the administration of antibiotic prophylaxis before intestinal surgery, the earlier recognition of localized infections, and the empirical use of broad-spectrum antibiotics for presumed infection.

Once the organism has been identified, both the portal of bloodstream entry and the underlying problem that probably led to seeding of the bloodstream can often be deduced from an understanding of the organism's normal site of residence. For example, mixed anaerobic bacteremia including *B. fragilis* usually implies colonic pathology with mucosal disruption from neoplasia, diverticulitis, or some other inflammatory lesion. The initial manifestations are determined by the portal of entry and reflect the localized condition. When bloodstream invasion occurs, patients can become extremely ill, with rigors and hectic fevers ranging up to 40.6°C (105°F). The clinical picture may be quite similar to that seen in sepsis involving aerobic gram-negative bacilli. Although other complications of anaerobic bacteremia, such as septic thrombophlebitis and septic shock, have been reported, the incidence of these complications in association with anaerobic bacteremia is low. Anaerobic bacteremia is potentially fatal and requires rapid diagnosis and appropriate therapy. Mortality appears to increase with the age of the patient (with reported rates of more than 66% among patients over 60 years old), with the isolation of multiple species from the bloodstream, and with the failure to surgically remove a focus of infection.

Endocarditis and Pericarditis (See also Chap. 126) Endocarditis due to anaerobes is uncommon. However, anaerobic streptococci, which are often classified incorrectly, are responsible for this disease more frequently than is generally appreciated. Gram-negative anaerobes are unusual causes of endocarditis. Anaerobes, particularly *B. fragilis* and *Peptostreptococcus* spp., are uncommonly found in infected pericardial fluids. Anaerobic pericarditis is associated with a mortality rate of >50%.

DIAGNOSIS Because of the time and difficulty involved in the isolation of anaerobic bacteria, diagnosis of anaerobic infections must frequently be based on presumptive evidence. Certain sites (such as avascular necrotic tissues) with lowered oxidation-reduction potential favor the diagnosis of an anaerobic infection. When infections occur in proximity to mucosal surfaces normally harboring an anaerobic flora, such as the gastrointestinal tract, female genital tract, or oropharynx, anaerobes should be considered as potential etiologic agents. A foul odor is often indicative of anaerobes, which produce certain organic acids as they proliferate in necrotic tissue. Although these odors are nearly pathognomonic for anaerobic infection, the absence of odor does not exclude an anaerobic etiology. Because anaerobes often coexist with other bacteria to cause mixed or synergistic infection, Gram's staining of exudate frequently reveals numerous pleomorphic cocci and bacilli suggestive of anaerobes. Sometimes these organisms have morphologic characteristics associated with specific species.

The presence of gas in tissues is highly suggestive, but not diagnostic, of anaerobic infection. When cultures of obviously infected sites yield no growth, streptococci only, or a single aerobic species (such as *Escherichia coli*) and Gram's staining reveals a mixed flora, the implication is that the anaerobic microorganisms failed to grow because of inadequate transport and/or culture techniques. Failure of a patient to respond to antibiotics that are not active against anaerobes—for example, aminoglycosides and in some circumstances penicillin, cephalosporins, or tetracyclines—suggests anaerobic infection.

There are three critical steps in the diagnosis of anaerobic infection: (1) proper specimen collection; (2) rapid transport of the specimens to the microbiology laboratory, preferably in anaerobic transport media; and (3) proper handling of the specimens by the laboratory. Specimens must be collected by meticulous sampling of infected sites, with avoidance of contamination by the normal flora. When such contamination is likely, the specimen is unacceptable. Examples of specimens unacceptable for anaerobic culture include sputum collected by expectoration or nasal tracheal suction, bronchoscopy specimens, samples collected directly through the vaginal vault, urine collected by voiding, and feces. Specimens that can be cultured for anaerobes include blood, pleural fluid, transtracheal aspirates, pus obtained by direct aspiration from an abscess cavity, fluid obtained by culdocentesis, suprapubic bladder aspirates, cerebrospinal fluid, and lung puncture specimens.

Because even brief exposure to oxygen may kill some anaerobic organisms and result in failure to isolate them in the laboratory, air must be expelled from the syringe used to aspirate the abscess cavity, and the needle must be capped with a sterile rubber stopper. Proper precautions should be used in the handling of contaminated needles. Specimens can be injected into transport bottles containing a reduced medium or taken immediately in syringes to the laboratory for direct culture on anaerobic media. In general, swabs should not be used. If a swab must be used, it should be placed in a reduced semisolid carrying medium before transport to the laboratory. Delays in transport may lead to a failure to isolate anaerobes due to exposure to oxygen or overgrowth of facultative organisms, which may eliminate or obscure any anaerobes that are present. All clinical specimens from suspected anaerobic infections should be Gram-stained and examined for organisms with characteristic morphology. It is not unusual for organisms to be observed on Gram's staining but not isolated in culture. If purulent materials are found to be sterile or organisms are seen on Gram's staining but do not grow in the culture, the involvement of anaerobes should be suspected.

R_x **TREATMENT** Successful therapy for anaerobic infections requires the administration of a combination of appropriate antibiotics, surgical resection, debridement of devitalized tissues, and drainage. Perforations must be closed promptly, closed spaces drained, tissue compartments decompressed, and an adequate blood supply established. Abscess cavities should be drained as soon as fluctuation or localization occurs. Surgery was formerly required to establish drainage; however, computed tomography (CT), magnetic resonance imaging (MRI), and ultrasound now allow diagnostic radiologists to drain many abscess sites percutaneously.

Antibiotic Therapy and Resistance Decisions about the treatment of anaerobic infections with antibiotics are usually based on known resistance patterns in certain species, on the likelihood of encountering a given species in the case at hand, and on Gram's stain findings. Antibiotics active against *Bacteroides* spp., penicillin-resistant *Prevotella* and *Porphyromonas* spp., and *Fusobacterium* spp. can be grouped into four categories on the basis of their predicted activity against anaerobes (Table 167-1). (Nearly all the drugs listed have toxic side effects, which are described in detail in Chap. 137.) In many infections, anaerobes are mixed with coliforms and other facultative organisms. The best therapeutic regimens, therefore, are usually those active against both aerobic and anaerobic bacteria. The choice of empirical antibiotics for the anaerobes in mixed infections can nearly always be made reliably, since patterns of antimicrobial susceptibility are usually predictable (Chap. 137 and Table 167-1).

Antibiotic susceptibility testing of anaerobic bacteria has been difficult and controversial. Owing to the slow growth rate of many an-

Table 167-1   Antimicrobial Therapy for Infections Involving Commonly Encountered Anaerobic Gram-Negative Rods

Group 1 (<1% Resistance)	Group 2 (<15% Resistance)	Group 3 (Variable Resistance)	Group 4 (Resistance)
Metronidazole[a]	Clindamycin	Penicillin	Aminoglycosides
Ampicillin/ sulbactam	Cefoxitin	Cephalosporins	Quinolones
Ticarcillin/ clavulanic acid	High-dose antipseudomonal penicillins	Tetracycline	Monobactams
Piperacillin/ tazobactam		Vancomycin	
Imipenem		Erythromycin	
Meropenem			
Chloramphenicol[b]			
Clinafloxacin			

[a] Usually needs to be given in combination with aerobic bacterial coverage. For infections originating below the diaphragm, aerobic gram-negative coverage is essential. For infections from an oral source, aerobic gram-positive coverage is added. Metronidazole also is not active against *Actinomyces*, *Propionibacterium*, or other gram-positive non-spore-forming bacilli (e.g., *Eubacterium*, *Bifidobacterium*) and is unreliable against peptostreptococci.

[b] Chloramphenicol is probably not as effective as other group 1 antimicrobials in treating anaerobic infections.

aerobes, the lack of standardized testing methods and of clinically relevant standards for resistance, and the generally good results obtained with empirical therapy, susceptibility testing has been recommended only for the study of local or regional resistance patterns, for the prediction of the efficacy of new antibiotics, and for the management of selected patients.

Anaerobic gram-negative rods that are frequently resistant to penicillin are listed in Table 167-2. Clinically important *Bacteroides* spp. are essentially all resistant to penicillin. Failures of therapy are common when documented *Bacteroides* (especially *B. fragilis*) infection is treated with penicillin or first-generation cephalosporins. The number of antimicrobial agents effective against *Bacteroides* spp. has expanded, and there are currently several useful choices (Table 167-1). In general, cure rates of >80% can be attained in patients with *Bacteroides* infection by means of appropriate antimicrobial therapy and drainage.

Resistance to metronidazole has been reported only rarely in *Bacteroides* spp. This well-tolerated drug, which reaches significant levels in serum and also can be found at high concentrations in abscess cavities, should be considered first-line therapy against *Bacteroides* infection. However, if metronidazole is used to treat mixed anaerobic and aerobic infections, it is imperative that other appropriate antibiotics be used in conjunction. Metronidazole is inactive against aerobic and facultative bacteria, *Actinomyces* spp., and *Propionibacterium* spp.

Table 167-2   Frequency of Penicillin Resistance among Commonly Encountered Anaerobic Gram-Negative Rods

Organism	Frequency of Penicillin Resistance[a]
Bacteroides fragilis	High
Bacteroides thetaiotaomicron	High
Bacteroides ovatus	High
Bacteroides distasonis	High
Bacteroides vulgatus	High
Bilophila wadsworthia	High
Fusobacterium nucleatum	Low
Fusobacterium necrophorum	Low
Fusobacterium mortiferum	Low
Fusobacterium varium	Low
Prevotella spp.	Moderate
Porphyromonas spp.	Low

[a] High, >90% of strains; moderate, 5 to 90% of strains; low, <5% of strains.

The sensitivity of peptostreptococci to metronidazole is unpredictable, and penicillin remains the drug of choice.

If a patient fails to respond to one of the group 1 or group 2 drugs (Table 167-1), consideration should be given to alternative therapy and to determination of the resistance patterns among *Bacteroides* isolates. Although in vitro resistance of *Bacteroides* spp. to chloramphenicol has not been reported, this drug may not be as effective as other group 1 drugs. Ampicillin/sulbactam, ticarcillin/clavulanic acid, piperacillin/tazobactam, imipenem, and meropenem have been effective in the treatment of *B. fragilis* infection. Some newer fluoroquinolones, such as clinafloxacin, appear to be highly active against most anaerobes, including *B. fragilis*; however, ciprofloxacin and other earlier-generation quinolones should not be used as primary agents.

Treatment of Infections at Specific Sites   In clinical situations, specific regimens must be tailored to the initial site of infection. The duration of therapy also depends on the infection site; the reader is referred to specific chapters on sites of infection for recommendations.

β-Lactamase production has been reported in anaerobic strains that are usually isolated from infections originating above the diaphragm. Up to 60% of clinical isolates classified as *Prevotella* or *Porphyromonas* spp., non-*B. fragilis* species of *Bacteroides*, or *Fusobacterium* spp. reportedly produce β-lactamase (Table 167-2). The clinical significance of resistance in these organisms has been suggested by studies showing clindamycin to be superior to penicillin (which for many years was considered the therapeutic gold standard) for the treatment of lung abscesses. Presumably, the success of clindamycin is attributable to a broader spectrum of activity against oral anaerobes; thus, a combination of penicillin and metronidazole or another antibiotic combination that is active against both oral anaerobes and aerobes is likely to be as effective as clindamycin. Bronchoscopy in lung abscess is indicated only to rule out airway obstruction and does not enhance drainage; in any event, it should be delayed until the antimicrobial regimen has begun to affect the disease process so that the procedure does not spread the infection. Surgery is almost never indicated because of the danger of spilling the abscess contents into the lungs.

Although most oral anaerobic infections and most cases of anaerobic pneumonia still respond to penicillin therapy, some infections due to oral organisms fail to respond to this drug, and in these cases the use of a drug that is effective against penicillin-resistant anaerobes is recommended (Table 167-1). Life-threatening infections involving the anaerobic flora of the mouth, such as space infections of the head and neck, should be treated empirically as if penicillin-resistant anaerobes are involved. Less serious infections involving the oral microflora can be treated with penicillin alone; metronidazole can be added (or clindamycin can be substituted) if the patient responds poorly to penicillin therapy. Combinations of antibiotics used to treat mixed infections of oral origin must include drugs active against the gram-positive aerobic flora of the mouth.

Chloramphenicol has been used successfully against anaerobic central nervous system infections at doses of 30 to 60 mg/kg per day, with the exact dose depending on the severity of illness. However, penicillin G and metronidazole also cross the blood-brain barrier and are bactericidal for many anaerobic organisms (Chap. 372).

Anaerobic infections arising below the diaphragm (e.g., colonic and intraabdominal infections) must be treated specifically with agents active against *Bacteroides* spp. (see Table 167-1). In intraabdominal sepsis (Chap. 130), the use of antibiotics effective against penicillin-resistant anaerobes has clearly reduced the incidence of postoperative infections and serious infectious complications. Specifically, a drug from group 1 (Table 167-1) must be included for broad-spectrum coverage. Recommended doses for commonly used group 1 drugs are given in Table 167-3. Therapy for intraabdominal sepsis also must include drugs active against the gram-negative aerobic flora of the bowel. If the involvement of gram-positive bacteria such as enterococci is suspected, either ampicillin or vancomycin should be added.

Cases of anaerobic osteomyelitis in which a mixed flora is isolated from a bone biopsy specimen should be treated with a regimen that covers all the isolates. When an anaerobic organism is recognized as

Table 167-3 Doses and Schedules for Treatment of Serious Infections due to Commonly Encountered Anaerobic Gram-Negative Rods

First-Line Therapy	Dose	Schedule[a]
Metronidazole[b]	7.5 mg/kg	q6h
Ticarcillin/clavulanic acid	3.1 g	q4h
Piperacillin/tazobactam	3.375 g	q6h
Imipenem	0.5 g	q6h
Meropenem	1.0 g	q8h

[a] See disease-specific chapters for recommendations on duration of therapy.
[b] Should generally be used in conjunction with drugs active against aerobic or facultative organisms.
NOTE: All drugs are given by the intravenous route.

a major or sole pathogen infecting a joint, the duration of treatment should be similar to that used for arthritis caused by aerobic bacteria (Chap. 323). Therapy includes the management of underlying disease states, the administration of appropriate antimicrobial agents, temporary joint immobilization, percutaneous drainage of effusions, and usually the removal of infected prostheses or internal fixation devices. Surgical drainage and debridement procedures such as sequestrectomy are essential for the removal of necrotic tissue that can sustain anaerobic infections.

The outcome of anaerobic bacteremia has been shown to be significantly better in patients either initially given or switched to appropriate therapy based on known antibiotic susceptibilities.

Failure of Therapy Anaerobic infections that fail to respond to treatment or that relapse should be reassessed. Consideration should be given to additional surgical drainage or debridement. Superinfections with resistant gram-negative facultative or aerobic bacteria should be ruled out. The possibility of drug resistance must be entertained; if resistance is involved, repeated cultures may yield the pathogenic organism.

Supportive Measures Other supportive measures in the management of anaerobic infections include careful attention to fluid and electrolyte balance (since extensive local edema may lead to hypoalbuminemia); hemodynamic support for septic shock; immobilization of infected extremities; maintenance of adequate nutrition during chronic infections by parenteral hyperalimentation; relief of pain; and anticoagulation with heparin for thrombophlebitis. For patients with severe anaerobic infections of soft tissues, hyperbaric oxygen therapy is advocated by some experts, but its value has not been proven in controlled trials.

BIBLIOGRAPHY

APPELBAUM PC et al: β-Lactamase production and susceptibilities to amoxicillin, amoxicillin-clavulanate, ticarcillin, ticarcillin-clavulanate, cefoxitin, imipenem, and metronidazole of 320 non–*Bacteroides fragilis Bacteroides* isolates and 129 fusobacteria from 28 US centers. Antimicrob Agents Chemother 34:1546, 1990

FINEGOLD SM: Anaerobic bacteria: General concepts, in *Principles and Practice of Infectious Diseases*, 4th ed, GL Mandell et al (eds). New York, Churchill Livingstone, 1995

———: Overview of clinically important anaerobes. Clin Infect Dis 20:S205, 1995

FUCHS PC et al: In vitro activities of clinafloxacin against contemporary clinical bacterial isolates from 10 North American centers. Antimicrob Agents Chemother 42:1274, 1998

NICHOLS RL: Surgical infections: Prevention and treatment—1965 to 1995. Am J Surg 172:68, 1996

SALONEN JH et al: Clinical significance and outcome of anaerobic bacteremia. Clin Infect Dis 26:1413, 1998

SEARS CL et al: Enterotoxigenic *Bacteroides fragilis*. Clin Infect Dis 20:S142, 1995

SUMMANEN PH et al: *Bilophila wadsworthia* isolates from clinical specimens. Clin Infect Dis 20:S210, 1995

TZIANABOS AO et al: Structural features of polysaccharides that induce intra-abdominal abscesses. Science 262:416, 1993

Section 8
MYCOBACTERIAL DISEASES

168

Paul W. Wright, Richard J. Wallace, Jr.

ANTIMYCOBACTERIAL AGENTS

The physician is greatly challenged to provide optimal therapy for mycobacterial illnesses because of the advent of AIDS, the increase in both drug-susceptible and multidrug-resistant tuberculosis, and the plethora of new antibiotics with antimycobacterial potential. This chapter reviews the agents used for the treatment of tuberculosis, leprosy (Hansen's disease), and diseases caused by pathogenic nontuberculous mycobacteria, including *Mycobacterium avium-intracellulare*, *M. kansasii*, the rapidly growing mycobacteria, and *M. marinum*. The use of antimycobacterial agents in patients with renal or hepatic disease and in pregnant women is summarized in Table 168-1. The effects of major antimycobacterial agents on the levels, activity, and toxicity of other commonly used drugs are summarized in Table 168-2.

TUBERCULOSIS

Drugs used to treat tuberculosis are classified as first-line and second-line agents. *First-line essential* antituberculous agents are the most effective and are a necessary component of any short-course therapeutic regimen. The three drugs in this category are rifampin, isoniazid,

and pyrazinamide. The *first-line supplemental* agents, which are highly effective and infrequently toxic, include ethambutol and streptomycin. *Second-line* antituberculous drugs are clinically much less effective than first-line agents and much more frequently elicit severe reactions. These drugs are rarely used in therapy and then only by caregivers experienced with their use. They include para-aminosalicylic acid (PAS), ethionamide, cycloserine, kanamycin, amikacin, capreomycin, viomycin, and thiacetazone. *Newer* antituberculous drugs, which have not yet been placed in the above categories, include rifapentine, rifabutin, and the quinolones, especially ciprofloxacin, ofloxacin, and sparfloxacin.

FIRST-LINE ESSENTIAL DRUGS Rifampin Rifampin, a semisynthetic derivative of *Streptomyces mediterranei*, is considered the most important and potent antituberculous agent. It is also active against a wide spectrum of other organisms, including some gram-positive and gram-negative bacteria, *Legionella* spp., *M. kansasii*, and *M. marinum*.

Pharmacology Rifampin is a fat-soluble complex macrocyclic antibiotic that is absorbed readily after either oral or intravenous administration. Serum levels of 10 to 20 μg/mL follow a standard oral dose of 600 mg. Rifampin distributes well throughout most body tissues, including inflamed meninges. The fact that rifampin turns body fluids (urine, saliva, sputum, tears) to a red-orange color makes it simple and inexpensive to check on a patient's compliance with therapy. Rifampin is excreted primarily through the bile and the enterohepatic circulation, while 30 to 40% of a dose is excreted via the kidneys. The

Table 168-1 Use of Antimycobacterial Agents in Patients with Renal or Hepatic Disease and in Pregnant Women

| | | Use in Indicated Circumstances | | |
| | | Renal Disease: Creatinine Clearance Rate | | |
Agent	Severe Hepatic Disease	>30 mL/min	≤30 mL/min	Pregnancy[a]
Azithromycin	No change	No change	?Decrease dose	No evidence of risk (B)
Clarithromycin	No change	No change	Decrease dose	Risk cannot be ruled out (C)
Ethambutol	No change	No change	Decrease dose	Risk cannot be ruled out (C)
Isoniazid	Avoid use or decrease dose	No change	Decrease dose	Risk cannot be ruled out (C)
Pyrazinamide	Avoid use or decrease dose	No change	Decrease dose[b]	Risk cannot be ruled out (C)[c]
Rifabutin	No change	No change	No change	No evidence of risk (B)
Rifampin	Avoid use or decrease dose	No change	No change	Risk cannot be ruled out (C)
Rifapentine	Avoid use or decrease dose	No change	No change	Risk cannot be ruled out (C)
Streptomycin	No change	Decrease dose	Decrease dose and frequency	Definite evidence of risk (D)

[a] Based on Food and Drug Administration pregnancy categories of A–D, X.
[b] Prudent but not absolutely necessary.

[c] Use in pregnancy is recommended by international organizations outside the United States.

drug is administered either twice weekly or daily at a dose of 600 mg for adults (10 mg/kg) and 10 to 20 mg/kg for children.

Mechanism of action Rifampin has both intracellular and extracellular bactericidal activity. It blocks RNA synthesis by specifically binding and inhibiting DNA-dependent RNA polymerase. Susceptible strains of *M. tuberculosis* as well as *M. kansasii* and *M. marinum* are inhibited by ≤1 μg/mL.

Adverse effects (Table 168-3) Rifampin is generally well tolerated; the most common adverse event is gastrointestinal upset. Patients with chronic liver disease, especially those with alcoholism and the elderly, appear to be at unusually high risk for the most serious adverse reaction: hepatitis. Other adverse effects of rifampin include rash (0.8%), hemolytic anemia (<1%), thrombocytopenia, and immunosuppression of unknown clinical importance. Rifampin is a potent inducer of the hepatic microsomal enzymes and thereby decreases the half-life of a number of drugs, including digoxin, warfarin, prednisone,

Table 168-2 Effects of Major Antimycobacterial Agents on Levels/Activity/Toxicity of Other Commonly Used Drugs[a]

Rifampin/rifapentine[b]	Isoniazid
Acetaminophen (↓)	Alcohol (↑ in risk of hepatitis)
Antiarrhythmics (↓)	Carbamazepine (↑)
Anticonvulsants (↓)	Diphenylhydantoin (↑)
Azole antifungals (↓)	Enflurane (↑ in risk of renal failure)
Barbiturates (↓)	Warfarin (↑)
β Blockers (↓)	**Clarithromycin**
Calcium channel blockers (↓)	Astemizole (↑)
Chloramphenicol (↓)	Carbamazepine (↑)
Clarithromycin (↓)	Digoxin (↑)
Cyclosporine (↓)	Rifabutin (↑)
Dapsone (↓)	Ritonavir (↓)
Delavirdine (↓)	Terfenadine (↑)
Diazepam (↓)	Zidovudine (↓)
Digoxin (↓)	
Doxycycline (↓)	
Fluoroquinolones (↓)	
Glucocorticoids (↓)	
Halothane (↓)	
Hormonal contraceptives (↓)	
Narcotics (↓)	
Oral hypoglycemics (↓)	
Probenecid (↓)	
Protease inhibitors (↓)	
Quinidine (↓)	
Theophylline (↓)	
Tricyclic antidepressants (↓)	
Warfarin (↓)	
Zidovudine (↓)	

[a] The following antimycobacterial agents have no or minimal effects on other drugs: amikacin, azithromycin, capreomycin, ethambutol, streptomycin, pyrazinamide.
[b] Rifabutin, which induces the cytochrome P450 system, has the same effects (↓) as rifampin but to a lesser degree. All drugs whose half-life is decreased by rifampin induction of hepatic microsomal enzymes may be subject to the same effect when coadministered with rifabutin; however, this point has not yet been studied.

cyclosporine, methadone, oral contraceptives, clarithromycin, the HIV protease inhibitors, and quinidine (Table 168-2).

Resistance Resistance to rifampin results from spontaneous point mutations that alter the β subunit of the RNA polymerase (*rpoB*) gene. Studies have shown that 96% of rifampin-resistant strains have a missense mutation within a 91-bp central core region of the gene. Rifampin-resistant strains of *M. leprae* have similar mutations that alter a single serine residue (Ser-425) in the same core region of the *rpoB* gene.

Isoniazid Now considered the best antituberculous drug available after rifampin, isoniazid should be included in all tuberculosis treatment regimens unless the organism is resistant. Isoniazid is inexpensive, readily synthesized, available worldwide, highly selective for mycobacteria, and well tolerated, with only 5% of patients exhibiting adverse effects.

Mechanism of action Isoniazid is the hydrazide of isonicotinic acid, a small water-soluble molecule that easily penetrates the cell. Its mechanism of action involves inhibition of mycolic acid cell-wall synthesis via oxygen-dependent pathways such as the catalase-peroxidase reaction. Isoniazid is bacteriostatic against resting bacilli and bactericidal against rapidly multiplying organisms, both extracellularly and intracellularly. The minimal inhibitory concentrations (MICs) of isoniazid for wild-type (untreated) strains of *M. tuberculosis* are <0.1 μg/mL, while those for *M. kansasii* are usually 0.5 to 2.0 μg/mL. The MICs of this drug for other mycobacteria are much higher.

Pharmacology Both oral and intramuscular preparations of isoniazid are readily absorbed. A 300-mg oral dose generally produces peak serum levels of 3 to 5 μg/mL. Isoniazid diffuses well throughout the body and reaches therapeutic concentrations in serum, cerebrospinal fluid (CSF), and infected tissue, including caseous granulomas. Isoniazid is metabolized in the liver via acetylation and hydrolysis; its metabolites are excreted into the urine. The rate of acetylation is genetically controlled. The recommended daily dose for the treatment of tuberculosis in the United States is 5 mg/kg for adults and 10 to 20 mg/kg for children, with a maximal daily dose of 300 mg for both groups. (Tuberculosis organizations outside the United States have recommended 5 mg/kg daily for both groups.) For intermittent therapy (usually directly observed), a maximal dose of 900 mg twice or thrice weekly is used. Even in moderate or severe renal failure, the adult dose rarely needs to be reduced below 200 mg/d.

Adverse effects (Table 168-3) The two most important adverse effects of isoniazid therapy are hepatotoxicity and peripheral neuropathy. Other adverse reactions are either rare or less significant and include rash (2%), fever (1.2%), anemia, acne, arthritic symptoms, a systemic lupus erythematosus–like syndrome, optic atrophy, seizures, and psychiatric symptoms. Isoniazid-associated hepatitis is idiosyncratic and increases in incidence with age. It occurs in 0.3% of treated persons under 35 years of age, 1.2% of those under 49 years of age, and 2.3% of those over 50 years of age. The risk of isoniazid-associated hepatitis is increased by daily alcohol consumption, concomitant

Table 168-3   Monitoring Side Effects of Common Antituberculous Drugs

Drug	Side Effect	Management
Rifampin	Rash	Observe patient
	Liver dysfunction	Monitor AST/limit alcohol consumption/monitor for hepatitis symptoms
	Flulike syndrome	Administer at least twice weekly/limit dose to 10 mg/kg (adults)
	Red-orange urine	Reassure patient
	Drug interactions	Consider monitoring drug levels when possible, especially with contraceptives, anticoagulants, and digoxin/avoid use with protease inhibitors
Isoniazid	Hepatitis	Monitor AST/limit alcohol consumption/monitor for hepatitis symptoms/educate patient/stop drug at first symptoms of hepatitis (nausea, vomiting, anorexia, flulike syndrome)
	Peripheral neuritis	Administer vitamin B_6
	Optic neuritis	Administer vitamin B_6
	Seizures	Administer vitamin B_6
Pyrazinamide	Hepatitis	Monitor AST/limit daily dosage to 15–30 mg/kg
	Hyperuricemia	Monitor uric acid level only in cases of gout or renal failure
Ethambutol	Optic neuritis	Use lower daily dose (15 mg/kg) when possible/monitor visual acuity (eye chart) and red-green color vision (Ishihara Color Book) monthly and with any visual complaint/educate patient/stop drug at first change in vision
Streptomycin, amikacin, capreomycin	Ototoxicity, renal toxicity	Limit dose and duration of therapy as much as possible/avoid daily therapy in patients >50 years old/monitor BUN and serum creatinine levels and possibly conduct audiometry before and as needed during therapy/question patient regularly about tinnitus, dizziness, vertigo, and decreased hearing/measure serum drug levels if possible/educate patient/stop drug at first development of adverse effect

NOTE: AST, aspartate aminotransferase; BUN, blood urea nitrogen.

rifampin administration, and slow isoniazid acetylation. Mortality rates from isoniazid-induced hepatitis have been reported to be 6 to 12%, but the real risk is certainly much lower: the reported rates were documented in high-risk patients who continued to take the drug despite progressive symptoms of hepatitis and without monitoring of liver enzyme levels. Liver enzymes are monitored in most settings among high-risk patients, and administration of the drug is discontinued at the onset of hepatitis. The American Thoracic Society (ATS) recommends that serum concentrations of aspartate aminotransferase (AST) or alanine aminotransferase (ALT) be determined at baseline in patients over 35 years of age who are receiving isoniazid for chemoprophylaxis, with monthly determinations thereafter. The benefit of such routine monitoring remains controversial, however. Measurement of the ALT or AST level is certainly mandatory whenever a patient notices the onset of symptoms suggestive of isoniazid-associated hepatitis (e.g., fever, anorexia, nausea, vomiting, and/or a flulike syndrome including fever and myalgias), and treatment should be discontinued until the relationship between therapy and symptoms is ascertained. Several studies have demonstrated that many patients with isoniazid intolerance can be desensitized. The ATS also recommends that discontinuation of isoniazid be strongly considered whenever an asymptomatic AST or ALT level exceeds 150 to 200 IU (three to five times the upper limit of normal) in high-risk patients whose baseline values were normal. In one study, only 11 (0.1%) of 11,141 patients had hepatotoxic reactions to isoniazid during preventive treatment.

Peripheral neuritis associated with isoniazid develops at a dose-dependent rate of 2 to 20% and probably relates to interference with pyridoxine (vitamin B_6) metabolism. This rate can be reduced to 0.2% with the prophylactic administration of 10 to 50 mg of pyridoxine daily.

Resistance   Isoniazid-resistant mutants of *M. tuberculosis* occur spontaneously at a rate of 1 in 10^5 to 10^6 organisms. The molecular sites of isoniazid resistance have been detailed. Almost all isoniazid-resistant strains have amino acid changes in the catalase-peroxidase gene (*katG*) or a two-gene locus known as *inhA*. Missense mutations or deletion of *katG* is also associated with reduced catalase and peroxidase activity. Primary isoniazid resistance is detected in 7% of untreated patients in native U.S. populations, but the percentage is much higher in many immigrant populations.

Pyrazinamide   A derivative of nicotinic acid, pyrazinamide is an important bactericidal drug used in short-course therapy for tuberculosis.

Pharmacology   Pyrazinamide is well absorbed after oral administration, with a plasma concentration range of 20 to 60 μg/mL 1 to 2 h after oral ingestion of 15 to 30 mg/kg, and is well distributed throughout the body. Levels in CSF are excellent, reaching 50 to 100% of levels in serum. The serum half-life of the drug is 9 to 11 h. Pyrazinamide is metabolized by at least two major pathways and one minor pathway in the liver; its several metabolites include pyrazinoic acid, 5-hydroxypyrazinamide, and 5-hydroxypyrazinoic acid.

Mechanism of action   Pyrazinamide is similar to isoniazid in its narrow spectrum of antibacterial activity, which essentially includes only *M. tuberculosis*. The drug is bactericidal to slowly metabolizing organisms located within the acidic environment of the phagocyte or caseous granuloma; it is active only at a pH of <6.0. Pyrazinamide is considered a prodrug and is converted by the tubercle bacillus to the active form pyrazinoic acid. The target for this compound, however, remains unknown. Susceptible strains of *M. tuberculosis* are inhibited by 20 μg/mL.

Adverse effects (Table 168-3)   At the high dosages used in the past, hepatotoxicity was a prominent complication of pyrazinamide therapy. However, at the currently recommended daily dosage of 15 to 30 mg/kg, with a maximum of 2 g (which can be given in one dose), the frequency of hepatotoxicity is no higher than that for concomitant isoniazid and rifampin therapy. Although pyrazinamide is recommended by international tuberculosis organizations for routine use in pregnancy, it is not recommended in the United States because of inadequate teratogenicity data. Hyperuricemia is a common adverse effect of pyrazinamide therapy whose incidence is probably reduced by concurrent rifampin therapy. Clinical gout is seen only rarely. Polyarthralgias are encountered fairly commonly but are not related to hyperuricemia.

Resistance   Resistance to pyrazinamide is associated with loss of pyrazinamidase activity such that pyrazinamide is no longer converted to pyrazinoic acid. More than 90% of isolates with MICs of >100 μg/mL have mutations in the *pncA* gene, which encodes for pyrazinamidase. All strains of *M. bovis* are naturally resistant to pyrazinamide and have a point mutation within the *pncA* gene.

FIRST-LINE SUPPLEMENTAL DRUGS   Ethambutol   A derivative of ethylenediamine, ethambutol is a water-soluble compound that is active only against mycobacteria. Susceptible species include *M. tuberculosis*, *M. marinum*, *M. kansasii*, and *M. avium-intracellulare* (MAI). Among first-line drugs, ethambutol is the least potent against *M. tuberculosis*. It is used most often with rifampin for the treatment of tuberculosis in patients who cannot tolerate isoniazid or who are thought or known to be infected with isoniazid-resistant organisms.

Mechanism of action   Ethambutol is bacteriostatic against rapidly growing mycobacteria. Its primary mechanism of action appears to be inhibition of arabinosyltransferases that mediate the polymerization of arabinose into arabinogalactan within the cell wall.

Pharmacology   After oral administration, 75 to 80% of a dose of ethambutol is absorbed from the gastrointestinal tract. Serum levels peak at 2 to 4 μg/mL 2 to 4 h after a dose of 15 mg/kg. The drug's distribution throughout the body is adequate except in the CSF, where it reaches only low levels. However, ethambutol can reach CSF levels up to 50% as high as peak plasma levels when administered at a daily dose of 25 mg/kg to a patient with inflamed meninges. Almost all of the dose is excreted by the kidneys within 24 h of ingestion, either unchanged or as metabolites. The usual daily adult dosage of ethambutol is 25 mg/kg (which may be given in one dose) for the first 2 months, with a subsequent reduction to 15 mg/kg. In cases where pretreatment is necessary, the higher dose may be given for the duration. For intermittent therapy, the dosage is 50 mg/kg twice weekly or 30 mg/kg three times weekly. The dosage must be lowered for patients with renal insufficiency (a creatinine clearance rate of <25 mL/min) to prevent drug accumulation and toxicity.

Adverse effects (Table 168-3)   Ethambutol is usually well tolerated. Retrobulbar optic neuritis is the most serious adverse effect; axial or central neuritis—the only form reported in patients taking daily doses of <30 mg/kg—involves the papillomacular bundle of fibers and results in reduced visual acuity, central scotoma, and loss of the ability to see green. Symptoms of ocular toxicity typically develop several months after the initiation of therapy, but rapid-onset optic neuritis has been reported. The risk of optic neuritis depends on the dose and duration of therapy: this reaction develops in 5% of patients receiving a daily dose of 25 mg/kg but in fewer than 1% of patients given a daily dose of 15 mg/kg. Patients taking the lower dose should be tested at baseline and whenever there is a subjective visual change for visual acuity and red-green color discrimination. Patients taking the higher dose should be tested at baseline, monthly thereafter, and whenever there is a subjective visual change. Optic neuritis with associated visual loss is usually reversible, but recovery may take 6 months or longer.

Other adverse effects of ethambutol are infrequent. Hyperuricemia occurs but is usually asymptomatic. Optic neuritis is rare at the low dose in children; however, the use of ethambutol in very young children is problematic because visual complications are difficult to monitor.

Resistance   Resistance in *M. tuberculosis* relates to missense mutations in the *embB* gene that encodes for arabinosyltransferase. Such mutations have been found in 70% of resistant strains and involve amino acid residue 306 in approximately 90% of cases. Species of nontuberculous mycobacteria that are intrinsically resistant to ethambutol have variant amino acids in this region of the gene, while susceptible species have the same amino acid sequences as *M. tuberculosis*.

Streptomycin   An aminoglycoside isolated from *Streptomyces griseus*, streptomycin is available for intramuscular and intravenous administration only. In the United States, it is the least-used first-line supplemental drug for tuberculosis because of its toxicity, the difficulty in obtaining adequate CSF levels, and the inconvenience of its parenteral administration. In developing countries, however, streptomycin is frequently used because of its low cost. The drug is active against untreated strains of *M. tuberculosis*, *M. kansasii*, and *M. marinum* and against some strains of MAI at readily achievable serum levels.

Pharmacology   Serum levels of streptomycin peak at 25 to 40 μg/mL after a 1.0-g dose. Streptomycin is bactericidal for rapidly dividing extracellular mycobacteria but is ineffective in the acidic environment within the macrophage. It diffuses poorly into the meninges

and, in patients with meningitis, reaches CSF levels that are only 20% of serum levels.

The usual adult dose of streptomycin is 0.5 to 1.0 g (10 to 15 mg/kg) daily or five times per week; the pediatric dose is 20 to 40 mg/kg daily, with a maximum of 1 g/d. Because streptomycin is eliminated almost exclusively by the kidneys, the dosage must be lowered and the frequency of administration reduced (to only two or three times per week) in most patients over 50 years of age and in any patient with renal impairment.

Mechanism of action   Streptomycin inhibits protein synthesis by disruption of ribosomal function.

Adverse effects (Table 168-3)   Adverse reactions to streptomycin therapy occur in 10 to 20% of patients. Ototoxicity and renal toxicity are the most common and the most serious. Renal toxicity, usually manifested as nonoliguric renal failure, is less common with streptomycin than with other frequently used aminoglycosides, such as gentamicin. Ototoxicity involves both hearing loss and vestibular dysfunction. The latter is more common and includes loss of balance, vertigo, and tinnitus. Patients receiving streptomycin must be monitored carefully for these adverse effects. Less serious reactions include perioral paresthesia, eosinophilia, rash, and drug fever.

Resistance   Spontaneous resistance to streptomycin occurs in 1 in 10^5 to 10^7 organisms. In two-thirds of streptomycin-resistant strains of *M. tuberculosis*, mutations have been identified in one of two targets: a 16S rRNA gene (*rrs*) and the gene encoding ribosomal protein S12 (*rpsL*). Both targets are believed to be involved in streptomycin ribosomal binding. No mutational change has been identified in the other one-third of resistant isolates. Strains of *M. tuberculosis* that are resistant to streptomycin are not cross-resistant to capreomycin or amikacin.

SECOND-LINE DRUGS   Second-line and/or newer antituberculous agents are used either when tuberculosis is drug resistant or when first-line supplemental drugs are not available. The most important second-line drugs are discussed below in the general (descending) order of usefulness.

Capreomycin   Capreomycin, a complex cyclic polypeptide antibiotic derived from *Streptomyces capreolus*, is similar to streptomycin in terms of dosing, mechanism of action, pharmacology, and toxicity. It is administered only by the intramuscular route in doses of 10 to 15 mg/kg daily or five times per week (maximal daily dose, 1 g), with peak blood levels of 20 to 40 μg/mL. After 2 to 4 months, the dosage should be reduced to 1 g two or three times a week. Cross-resistance to kanamycin and amikacin—but not to streptomycin—is common. After streptomycin, capreomycin is the injectable drug of choice for tuberculosis.

Amikacin and Kanamycin   These well-known aminoglycosides are bactericidal to extracellular organisms. Kanamycin is rarely used because of its toxicity. Amikacin is active against *M. tuberculosis* and several of the nontuberculous species, including the rapidly growing mycobacteria, *M. scrofulaceum*, *M. leprae*, and MAI. The usual adult dosage is 10 to 15 mg/kg intramuscularly or intravenously three to five times per week. Resistance to both drugs relates to a single-base-pair change at position 1408 in the 16S ribosomal RNA gene.

Para-Aminosalicylic Acid   PAS, a calcium or sodium salt that inhibits the growth of *M. tuberculosis* by impairing folate synthesis, is rarely indicated for the treatment of tuberculosis because of its low level of antituberculous activity and its high level of gastrointestinal toxicity (manifesting as nausea, vomiting, and diarrhea). Enteric-coated PAS granules (4 g every 8 h) may be better tolerated than other formulations and produce higher therapeutic blood levels. PAS is well absorbed after oral administration but reaches only low concentrations in the CSF. The drug has a short half-life (1 h), and 80% of the dose is excreted in the urine.

Thiacetazone   Also called amithiozone, thiacetazone is not available in the United States but—because it is inexpensive and readily available—is widely used in the developing world as a single-tablet combination with isoniazid to treat tuberculosis. The usual daily dosage is 150 mg. Thiacetazone is structurally related to isoniazid but is bacteriostatic and more toxic. The World Health Organization advises against the use of thiacetazone by HIV-infected patients because of an unacceptably high rate of severe adverse (gastrointestinal) and fatal (skin) reactions.

Viomycin A complex basic polypeptide antibiotic, viomycin has properties similar to those of capreomycin, amikacin, and kanamycin and must be administered by intramuscular injection. Ninety percent of strains of multidrug-resistant *M. tuberculosis* are inhibited by viomycin levels of 1 to 10 μg/mL. Toxic effects are more common and severe than with other polypeptide antibiotics. This drug is not available in the United States.

Ethionamide Like isoniazid and pyrazinamide, ethionamide is a derivative of isonicotinic acid. This agent is bacteriostatic against metabolizing *M. tuberculosis* and some nontuberculous mycobacteria. It is most useful in therapy for multidrug-resistant tuberculosis. However, its use is severely limited by its toxicity and frequent side effects, which include intense gastrointestinal intolerance (anorexia, vomiting, and dysgeusia), serious neurologic reactions, reversible hepatitis (5% of cases), hypersensitivity reactions, and hypothyroidism. Ethionamide is well absorbed orally and is widely distributed throughout the body at sites including the CSF.

Cycloserine Cycloserine (D-4-amino-3-isoxazolidinone) is produced by *Streptomyces orchidaceus* and is active against a broad spectrum of bacteria, including *M. tuberculosis*. Cycloserine is well absorbed after oral administration and is widely distributed throughout the body fluids, including the CSF. Serious side effects limit the use of this drug and include psychosis (with suicide in some cases), seizures, peripheral neuropathy, headaches, somnolence, and allergic reactions. Cycloserine should not be given to patients with epilepsy, active alcohol abuse, severe renal insufficiency, or a history of depression or psychosis.

Newer Antituberculous Drugs A number of other drugs are being evaluated for their antituberculous activity. This group includes rifabutin, rifapentine, the newer fluorinated quinolones, amoxicillin/clavulanic acid, clofazimine, clarithromycin, and rifamycins not yet approved by the U.S. Food and Drug Administration (FDA), such as KRM-1648 (benzoxazinorifamycin).

Rifabutin Rifabutin, a semisynthetic rifamycin spiropiperidyl derivative, shares many characteristics with rifampin, including activity against *M. tuberculosis*. Rifabutin is also active against some strains of rifampin-resistant *M. tuberculosis* and is more active than rifampin against MAI and other nontuberculous mycobacteria. To date, rifabutin has been most useful in the prophylaxis of disseminated MAI infection and in the treatment of drug-resistant tuberculosis. Because it seems to exhibit more antituberculous activity than rifampin in vitro and in animals, its possible clinical advantages over rifampin are being evaluated. In a multinational trial in which either rifampin (600 mg/d) or rifabutin (150 mg/d) was administered in combination with isoniazid plus a 2-month regimen of pyrazinamide and ethambutol, the two rifamycins were equally effective and well tolerated in the treatment of newly diagnosed pulmonary tuberculosis. Rifabutin is recommended in place of rifampin for the treatment of HIV-positive individuals who are also taking a protease inhibitor.

PHARMACOLOGY The pharmacology of rifabutin is dramatically different from that of rifampin. Rifabutin is readily absorbed after a single oral dose of 300 mg and reaches peak serum levels (0.35 μg/mL) in 2 to 4 h. This lipophilic drug distributes best to tissues: tissue levels are 5 to 10 times higher than plasma levels. CSF concentrations are 30 to 70% of plasma levels in HIV-infected patients who have meningitis. The drug's slow clearance via hepatic metabolism and renal excretion results in a mean serum half-life of 45 h, which is much longer than the 3- to 5-h half-life of rifampin. Clarithromycin (but not azithromycin) and fluconazole appear to block the hepatic metabolism of rifabutin, with consequent increases in serum levels. When rifabutin is administered orally with food, its rate of absorption is slowed, but the extent of its absorption is unchanged. Adjustment of dosage is usually unnecessary in elderly patients and in patients with reduced hepatic or renal function.

MECHANISM OF ACTION In *Escherichia coli* and *Bacillus subtilis*, rifabutin inhibits DNA-dependent RNA polymerase in the same manner as rifampin. Its mode of action against mycobacteria is believed to be the same.

ADVERSE EFFECTS Most adverse effects of rifabutin are dose related and occur most frequently in patients receiving >300 mg/d. Discontinuation of therapy because of adverse drug reactions is reported in 16% of patients receiving rifabutin as opposed to 8% of those receiving a placebo. The most common symptoms are gastrointestinal; other reactions include rash, headache, asthenia, chest pain, myalgia, and insomnia. Like those taking rifampin, most patients taking rifabutin have discolored (orange to tan) urine and other body fluids. Less common adverse reactions include fever, chills, a flulike syndrome, hepatitis, *Clostridium difficile*–associated diarrhea, and a yellow skin discoloration ("pseudojaundice"). After a rifabutin dose of 450 to 600 mg in combination with clarithromycin, anterior uveitis is reported in up to 40% of patients; also common at these high doses are hyperpigmentation and the polymyalgia/arthralgia syndrome. All of these conditions are reversible when treatment is discontinued. Laboratory abnormalities include neutropenia, leukopenia, thrombocytopenia, and increased levels of liver enzymes.

Rifabutin induces the hepatic cytochrome P450 enzymes but does so much less strongly than rifampin. Drugs whose metabolism is enhanced by rifabutin include anticoagulants, quinidine, oral contraceptives, sulfonylureas, analgesics, dapsone, narcotics, glucocorticoids, clarithromycin, zidovudine, and cardiac glycosides.

RESISTANCE Resistance to rifabutin is attributable to the same mechanism as that to rifampin—i.e., mutations involving the *rpoB* gene. However, of the 14 mutant *rpoB* alleles that confer resistance to rifampin, only nine confer high-level resistance to rifabutin, while the remaining five result in only small changes in rifabutin MICs, which remain ≤0.5 μg/mL. The MIC of rifabutin for susceptible strains of *M. tuberculosis* is low (<0.06 μg/mL), and the drug is considered clinically active against partially resistant strains that are inhibited by plasma levels of ≤0.5 μg/mL. Thus rifabutin inhibits about one-quarter of rifampin-resistant strains of *M. tuberculosis*.

Rifapentine A semisynthetic cyclopentyl rifamycin antibiotic, rifapentine has received accelerated approval from the FDA for the treatment of tuberculosis. It is the first new drug approved for tuberculosis in 25 years in the United States. While similar to rifampin, rifapentine is lipophilic and longer acting—characteristics that enhance patient compliance; the drug can be administered at a dose of 600 mg once or twice weekly. It has antibacterial activity against *M. tuberculosis* but has undergone only minimal testing against nontuberculous mycobacteria. Rifapentine has not yet been approved for the treatment of patients with HIV disease because rifapentine/rifampin monoresistance frequently develops in HIV-positive patients receiving isoniazid plus rifapentine. Like rifampin, rifapentine is active against many nonmycobacterial organisms, including *Haemophilus influenzae*, *Bordetella pertussis*, *B. parapertussis*, *Brucella* spp., *Legionella* spp., *Neisseria* spp., streptococci, and staphylococci.

In a randomized comparative study, 672 Chinese patients received isoniazid plus either rifapentine or rifampin. The isoniazid/rifapentine group had a higher relapse rate (10% versus 5%) than the isoniazid/rifampin group. Nevertheless, this disadvantage was considered acceptable in light of the lower rate of adverse effects and less frequent administration in the isoniazid/rifapentine group.

PHARMACOLOGY Food enhances the oral absorption of rifapentine, while antacids impair its absorption. After oral administration with food, this drug reaches peak serum concentrations in 5 to 6 h and achieves a steady state in 10 days. The half-life of rifapentine and its active metabolite 25-desacetyl rifapentine is approximately 13 h. The drug is highly bound to serum protein (93 to 97%), and most of the administered dose is excreted via the liver (70%). Oral clearance is more rapid in males than in females (2.51 vs 1.69 L/h), but the clinical significance of this difference is unknown.

MECHANISM OF ACTION   Rifapentine exerts its bactericidal effect by inhibiting DNA-dependent RNA polymerase in susceptible bacteria. The MICs of rifapentine for rifampin-susceptible strains of *M. tuberculosis* range from 0.03 to 0.12 μg/mL.

ADVERSE EFFECTS   Rifapentine demonstrates an adverse-event pattern similar to that of rifampin. Both drugs are frequently associated with hyperuricemia when administered with pyrazinamide and with elevated hepatocellular enzyme levels in 3 to 4% of patients when administered with other antituberculous agents. Liver enzyme levels should be monitored in patients receiving rifapentine who already have elevated liver enzyme concentrations or known liver disease. Like rifampin, rifapentine causes an orange-red discoloration of body fluids, including urine, saliva, and tears, and stains contact lenses.

Rifapentine induces the hepatic cytochrome P450 enzymes CYP3A4 and 2C8/9. Current induction studies suggest that its potential for drug-drug interaction may be less than that of rifampin but greater than that of rifabutin. Other drugs potentially affected by concomitant administration of rifapentine are listed in Table 168-2.

Rifapentine is in category C for use in pregnancy (Table 168-1) because of its teratogenesis in rats and rabbits. There are insufficient data concerning use of this drug in pregnant and breast-feeding patients.

RESISTANCE   Strains of *M. tuberculosis* resistant to rifapentine, rifampin, and rifabutin all involve spontaneous point mutations in the *rpoB* gene. All strains resistant to rifampin are also resistant to rifapentine.

Quinolones   A surprisingly large number of fluorinated quinolones are being developed and studied as inhibitors of mycobacteria. Their mode of action presumably is the prevention of DNA synthesis through the inhibition of DNA gyrase. Ofloxacin, ciprofloxacin, sparfloxacin, and pefloxacin are active against many mycobacteria, including *M. tuberculosis*, *M. leprae*, *M. marinum*, *M. kansasii*, and *M. fortuitum*. These drugs are well absorbed orally, reach high serum levels, and distribute well to body tissues and fluids. While not approved for antituberculous therapy in the United States, ofloxacin—used in combination with isoniazid and rifampin for the treatment of pulmonary tuberculosis—has been as active and safe as ethambutol in initial trials. Adverse effects are relatively uncommon, occurring in 0.5 to 10% of cases and consisting mostly of benign reactions such as gastrointestinal intolerance, rashes, dizziness, and headache. However, more serious adverse effects are being reported and include confusion, seizures, interstitial nephritis, skin vasculitis, and acute renal failure.

Mycobacterial resistance to the fluoroquinolones develops rapidly. Its molecular basis is complex; only some strains exhibit missense mutations in the A subunit (*gyrA* gene) of DNA gyrase. Fluoroquinolone-resistant tuberculosis is a source of growing concern: 22 such cases were reported recently from New York City. Antituberculous therapy with quinolones should be reserved for patients with multidrug resistance or those who cannot tolerate first-line drugs.

LEPROSY (HANSEN'S DISEASE)

Therapy for leprosy remains difficult, especially in developing countries, because of the long course required, the high cost and low availability of most drugs, the frequency of adverse reactions to drugs, the acquisition of drug resistance, the difficulty of determining a disease end point or cure, and (given that *M. leprae* still cannot be grown in vitro) the difficulty of conducting susceptibility testing. While many drugs are active against *M. leprae*, efficacy in the treatment of leprosy has been established only for dapsone, rifampin, clofazimine, and ethionamide.

Rifampin   Rifampin is considered the most active agent for the treatment of leprosy. Its worldwide use is limited only by its cost. This drug is markedly bactericidal against *M. leprae* and reduces the number of viable bacilli in the patient's tissues faster than any other avail-

able agent. Rifampin must be combined with other antileprosy drugs to forestall resistance. For cost reasons, the drug is given at a dose of 600 mg once a month (supervised) outside the United States, but it is given daily in the United States. For details on pharmacology, adverse events, and resistance, see relevant sections under "Tuberculosis."

Dapsone   Dapsone (4,4'-diaminodiphenylsulfone) inhibits bacterial folic acid synthesis. It is now considered the second drug of choice (after rifampin) in most cases of Hansen's disease because of its ready availability, low cost, and low toxicity and the susceptibility of untreated strains of *M. leprae* to very low concentrations.

Pharmacology   Dapsone is well absorbed orally and distributes well throughout the body. The usual daily dosage is 100 mg for adults and 0.9 to 1.4 mg/kg for children. Plasma concentrations peak within 1 to 3 h. The median elimination half-life is 22 h. Dapsone is cleared by acetylation in the liver, with genetic variation similar to that documented for the acetylation of isoniazid. The drug is 70% bound to plasma protein. Usual daily doses produce serum concentrations of 10 to 15 μg/mL, which far exceed the MIC for *M. leprae* (0.01 to 0.001 μg/mL).

Adverse effects   Hemolysis and methemoglobinemia are common untoward reactions to dapsone. Patients should be screened for glucose-6-phosphate dehydrogenase deficiency to prevent drug-induced hemolysis. However, most patients tolerate dapsone therapy well with adequate clinical and laboratory supervision. Other side effects include gastrointestinal intolerance, headache, pruritus, peripheral neuropathies, nephritic syndrome, fever, and rash. In lepromatous and borderline lepromatous leprosy, erythema nodosum leprosum (ENL) may occur. This reaction may be difficult to distinguish from reactions of leprosy, including drug reactions and the infectious mononucleosis–like dapsone syndrome.

Clofazimine   A phenazine iminoquinone dye, clofazimine is weakly bactericidal against *M. leprae*. It is useful in treating dapsone-resistant leprosy and may lessen the severity of ENL. Clofazimine's mode of action is not well understood, but the drug may inhibit DNA binding. It is absorbed orally and distributed to the fatty tissues and the reticuloendothelial system. Its serum half-life is about 60 to 70 days; only a small proportion of the dose is excreted daily into the urine or bile. Bactericidal activity is very slow and is evident for about 50 days after administration. The usual adult dosage is 50 to 100 mg/d, 100 mg three times a week, or (for treatment of ENL) 300 mg/d. Untoward effects include skin discoloration and, less commonly, gastrointestinal intolerance. Clofazimine was reported to be responsible for a case of cardiotoxicity induced via ventricular arrhythmia. Even though clofazimine-resistant disease has been reported only rarely when this agent is used alone, it should be used with other effective antibiotics. Clofazimine is active in vitro against some nontuberculous mycobacterial species, including MAI, *M. kansasii*, *M. simiae*, and *M. abscessus*.

Ethionamide   While ethionamide (250 mg/d) has not been approved by the FDA for the treatment of leprosy, it is sometimes used in the United States in combination with rifampin (600 mg/d) to treat dapsone-resistant leprosy in patients who cannot accept the skin-depigmentation effect of clofazimine. Because resistance to ethionamide develops quickly when the drug is used alone, it must be used with other effective agents. Patients should be monitored closely for hepatotoxicity when taking ethionamide (especially in combination with rifampin), and treatment should be discontinued if the patient's ALT levels exceed 2.5 times the normal value. Prothionamide, a congener of ethionamide that is not available in the United States, has pharmacologic properties similar to those of ethionamide and is widely used throughout the world.

Other Agents   A number of other drugs exhibit significant activity against *M. leprae*, but clinical experience with these agents is lacking. Thalidomide is now approved by the FDA for treatment of ENL. Although this drug may be useful in suppressing ENL, it acts as a tranquilizer, is extremely teratogenic, and should *never* be taken by anyone who is or may become pregnant. Physicians wishing to prescribe thalidomide must register with the System for Thalidomide Education and Prescription Safety (S.T.E.P.S.) at 1-888-423-5436 (Celgese Corporation).

The newer macrolide antibiotics (particularly clarithromycin), minocycline (a long-acting tetracycline), and a number of fluoroquinolones (including ofloxacin, sparfloxacin, and pefloxacin) have shown promising bactericidal activity against *M. leprae*. Ofloxacin and minocycline are being investigated with rifampin in short-course regimens for lepromatous disease. All of these newer leprosy drugs have low toxicity profiles, modes of action different from those of the established agents, and powerful bactericidal activity against *M. leprae*. However, their levels of bactericidal activity are lower than that of rifampin.

NONTUBERCULOUS MYCOBACTERIA

Although less pathogenic than *M. tuberculosis*, the nontuberculous mycobacteria can cause pulmonary, skin, bone and joint, lymph node, and soft tissue infection as well as disseminated disease in immunocompromised hosts, including patients with AIDS. MAI and *M. kansasii* are the two most common causes of nontuberculous mycobacterial pulmonary infection. Up to 40% of AIDS patients develop disseminated disease due to MAI.

Clarithromycin Clarithromycin (6-*O*-methylerythromycin) is a new macrolide that is similar to erythromycin in its mechanism of action. However, unlike erythromycin, it is well absorbed with or without meals and elicits little gastrointestinal intolerance at low doses. Clarithromycin distributes well into body tissues and fluids and is highly concentrated in macrophages. The drug is metabolized in the liver, and approximately 30% of a given dose is excreted in the urine. The dosage should be reduced if the creatinine clearance rate is ≤30 mL/min. Like erythromycin, clarithromycin binds with plasma proteins (65 to 70%) and can raise the levels of drugs such as theophylline and carbamazepine. As noted earlier, serum levels of clarithromycin are reduced by the concomitant administration of rifampin and to a lesser degree by that of rifabutin; clarithromycin treatment increases serum levels of rifabutin and some antihistamines (e.g., terfenadine), thus increasing their toxicity. Clarithromycin and (probably) azithromycin are the most active agents for the treatment of MAI infections; one of these drugs is considered an essential component of any regimens for this purpose. However, because of mutational drug resistance, clarithromycin should be given in combination with other agents, such as ethambutol and rifampin or rifabutin. The drug is also highly active against almost all other nontuberculous mycobacteria, including *M. marinum*, *M. kansasii*, *M. haemophilum*, *M. genavense*, *M. xenopi*, *M. abscessus*, *M. chelonae*, and most isolates of *M. fortuitum*. Standard antimycobacterial doses have been 500 mg twice daily; doses of 1000 mg twice daily have been associated with increased mortality among patients with AIDS and disseminated MAI disease. The more common side effects of high doses include nausea, vomiting, a bitter taste, and (occasionally) abnormal liver-function tests. Most side effects can be minimized by reducing the dose, usually by 50%. Clarithromycin is teratogenic in laboratory animals and is in category C for use in pregnancy (Table 168-1). Mutational resistance occurs in one in 10^8 to 10^9 organisms and develops rapidly with monotherapy, especially that for disseminated MAI disease. Resistance results from point mutations involving adenine at positions 2058 or 2059 in the 23S ribosomal binding site.

Azithromycin Azithromycin is a macrolide that belongs to the family of azalides. It reaches much lower serum levels than clarithromycin (usually ≤0.5 μg/mL) but attains high tissue and macrophage concentrations and has a longer half-life, which suggests the feasibility of intermittent therapy. It is involved in few drug interactions since it does not affect the cytochrome P450 system. The usual dose is 250 to 500 mg/d. No alteration in dose is required in renal failure. The most common side effects are gastrointestinal symptoms and reversible hearing loss. Azithromycin appears to be less active than clarithromycin for both pulmonary and disseminated MAI disease. Resistance

to azithromycin develops by the same mechanism as that to clarithromycin, with cross-resistance between the two macrolides.

THERAPY FOR SPECIFIC NONTUBERCULOUS MYCOBACTERIA MAI First-line antituberculous drugs are much less active against MAI than against *M. tuberculosis*. Therapy for MAI is controversial because of the lack of controlled clinical trials. In 1990 the ATS recommended the following four-drug regimen for MAI lung disease in HIV-negative patients: 18 to 24 months of isoniazid (300 mg), rifampin (600 mg), and ethambutol (25 mg/kg, then 15 mg/kg beginning in the third month), with intermittent streptomycin. However, two subsequent events—the demonstration of the dramatic activity of clarithromycin against both pulmonary and disseminated MAI infection and the introduction of rifabutin—have altered the therapeutic approach to MAI infection. In the 1997 ATS recommendations for MAI lung disease, clarithromycin (500 mg twice daily) now replaces isoniazid, and rifabutin (300 mg/d) is often used in place of rifampin. Therapy for pulmonary disease is generally given until cultures have been negative for 12 months.

For disseminated disease in AIDS, one of the newer macrolides (clarithromycin or azithromycin) and ethambutol (15 mg/kg) are considered essential components of any treatment regimen, with rifabutin (300 mg) a commonly used third drug in patients not taking a protease inhibitor for their HIV infection. Other alternative drugs include ciprofloxacin, streptomycin, and amikacin. Clofazimine appears to increase mortality and should be avoided. For the prophylaxis of disseminated MAI disease, rifabutin (300 mg/d), clarithromycin (500 mg twice daily), and azithromycin (1200 mg once weekly) have all been demonstrated to be effective in controlled or comparative clinical trials.

Mycobacterium kansasii *M. kansasii* is usually susceptible to most antituberculous drugs except for pyrazinamide. Current ATS recommendations for the treatment of *M. kansasii* pulmonary disease are 18 to 24 months of daily isoniazid (300 mg), rifampin (600 mg), and ethambutol (15 mg/kg). In patients taking protease inhibitors, rifabutin (150 mg) or clarithromycin (500 mg) twice daily should be substituted for rifampin. The potential advantages of the highly active rifabutin and the newer macrolides in immunocompetent patients have not been studied.

Rapidly Growing Mycobacteria *M. fortuitum*, *M. abscessus*, and *M. chelonae* account for more than 80% of cases of clinical disease due to rapidly growing mycobacteria. These organisms are resistant to antituberculous agents other than amikacin but are variably susceptible to several other antibiotics. Clarithromycin has dramatically changed the approach to therapy for infection with these organisms, as it inhibits all rapidly growing mycobacteria—except for 20% of *M. fortuitum* strains and most *M. smegmatis* strains—at concentrations of ≤4 μg/mL. Other drugs with good activity include amikacin (which inhibits 80 to 100% of strains), cefoxitin (80% of *M. abscessus* and *M. fortuitum* strains), doxycycline (50% of *M. fortuitum* strains), imipenem (100% of *M. fortuitum* strains, 70% of *M. chelonae* strains, and 70% of *M. abscessus* strains), the fluorinated quinolones ciprofloxacin and ofloxacin (100% of *M. fortuitum* strains), and sulfonamides (90% of *M. fortuitum* strains).

Mycobacterium marinum *M. marinum*, a photochromogen, is typically susceptible to minocycline, rifampin, ethambutol, clarithromycin, and trimethoprim-sulfamethoxazole and is resistant to isoniazid.

Mycobacterium haemophilum Infection due to *M. haemophilum* occurs most commonly as disseminated disease in immunocompromised patients with or without AIDS. This organism can cause bone and joint infection and skin infection. Isolates typically show in vitro resistance to most drugs but may be susceptible to rifampin, rifabutin, quinolones, and clarithromycin.

Mycobacterium xenopi In the United States, *M. xenopi* most often causes nosocomial infections; these infections most commonly occur in the environment of the hospital's hot-water system. In one study from Brooklyn, NY, *M. xenopi* was the second most common pathogenic nontuberculous mycobacterial species; of the 86 hospitalized patients from whom it was isolated, 41% were HIV-positive. Drug therapy for *M. xenopi* infection is difficult because in vitro drug sensitivity tests do not reliably predict clinical results. *M. xenopi* is often resistant to first-line antituberculous agents but susceptible to the newer macrolides, quinolones, streptomycin, and ethionamide.

Mycobacterium genavense   *M. genavense* is a newly recognized organism that grows only in liquid media, such as Bactec 12B or 13A. This organism almost exclusively infects AIDS patients, causing disseminated disease and being isolated from blood, bone marrow, liver, lymph node, spleen, and intestinal cultures. The in vitro susceptibility profile of *M. genavense* has not been well established. Some isolates are susceptible to amikacin, clarithromycin, ofloxacin, rifampin, and rifabutin.

BIBLIOGRAPHY

ALANGADEN GJ, LERNER SA: The clinical use of fluoroquinolones for the treatment of mycobacterial disease. Clin Infect Dis 25:1213, 1997

ALCAIDE F et al: Role of *embB* in natural and acquired resistance to ethambutol in mycobacteria. Antimicrob Agents Chemother 41:2270, 1997

BROGDEN RN, FITTON A: Rifabutin: A review of its antimicrobial activity, pharmacokinetic properties and therapeutic efficacy. Drugs 47:983, 1994

KEUNG A et al: Single and multiple dose pharmacokinetics of rifapentine in man: Part II. Int J Tuberc Lung Dis 3:437, 1999

MCEVOY GK (ed): *AHFS Drug Information 1999*. Bethesda, MD, American Society of Health-System Pharmacists, 1999, pp 464–502

MUSSER JM: Antimicrobial agent resistance in mycobacteria: Molecular genetic insights. Clin Microbiol Rev 8:496, 1995

NOLAN CM et al: Hepatotoxicity associated with isoniazid preventive therapy: A 7-year survey from a public health tuberculosis clinic. JAMA 281:1014, 1999

SREEVATSAN S et al: Mutations associated with pyrazinamide resistance in *pncA* of *Mycobacterium tuberculosis* complex organisms. Antimicrob Agents Chemother 41:636, 1997

WALLACE RJ JR et al: American Thoracic Society statement: Diagnosis and treatment of disease caused by nontuberculous mycobacteria. Am J Respir Crit Care Med 156: S1, 1997

WHO EXPERT COMMITTEE ON LEPROSY: Seventh report. Geneva, World Health Organization, 1998, Technical Report Series, No. 874

169   *Mario C. Raviglione, Richard J. O'Brien*

TUBERCULOSIS

AFB acid-fast bacilli	MDR multidrug-resistant
ARDS adult respiratory distress syndrome	MRI magnetic resonance imaging
	NK natural killer
BCG bacille Calmette-Guérin	OT "old tuberculin"
CDC Centers for Disease Control and Prevention	PAS para-aminosalicylic acid
	PCR polymerase chain reaction
CSF cerebrospinal fluid	PPD purified protein derivative
CT Computed tomography	SIADH syndrome of inappropriate secretion of antidiuretic hormone
DTH delayed-type hypersensitivity	
IFN-γ interferon γ	TNF-α tumor necrosis factor α
IL interleukin	WHO World Health Organization

DEFINITION   Tuberculosis, one of the oldest diseases known to affect humans, is caused by bacteria belonging to the *Mycobacterium tuberculosis* complex. The disease usually affects the lungs, although in up to one-third of cases other organs are involved. If properly treated, tuberculosis caused by drug-susceptible strains is curable in virtually all cases. If untreated, the disease may be fatal within 5 years in more than half of cases. Transmission usually takes place through the airborne spread of droplet nuclei produced by patients with infectious pulmonary tuberculosis.

ETIOLOGIC AGENT   Mycobacteria belong to the family Mycobacteriaceae and the order Actinomycetales. Of the pathogenic species belonging to the *M. tuberculosis* complex, the most frequent and important agent of human disease is *M. tuberculosis* itself. The complex includes *M. bovis* (the bovine tubercle bacillus, once an important cause of tuberculosis transmitted by unpasteurized milk and currently the cause of a small percentage of cases in developing countries), *M. africanum* (isolated in a small proportion of cases in West and Central Africa), and *M. microti* (the "vole" bacillus, a closely related but rarely encountered organism).

M. tuberculosis is a rod-shaped, non-spore-forming, thin aerobic bacterium measuring about 0.5 μm by 3 μm. Mycobacteria, including *M. tuberculosis*, do not stain readily and are often neutral on Gram's staining. However, once stained, the bacilli cannot be decolorized by acid alcohol, a characteristic justifying their classification as acid-fast bacilli (AFB). Acid fastness is due mainly to the organisms' high content of mycolic acids, long-chain cross-linked fatty acids, and other cell-wall lipids. Microorganisms other than mycobacteria that display some acid fastness include species of *Nocardia* and *Rhodococcus*, *Legionella micdadei*, and the protozoa *Isospora* and *Cryptosporidium*. In the mycobacterial cell wall, lipids (e.g., mycolic acids) are linked to underlying arabinogalactan and peptidoglycan. This structure is responsible for the very low permeability of the cell wall and thus for the ineffectiveness of most antibiotics against the organism. Another molecule in the mycobacterial cell wall, lipoarabinomannan, is involved in the pathogen-host interaction and facilitates the survival of *M. tuberculosis* within macrophages. The several proteins characteristic of *M. tuberculosis* include those in purified protein derivative (PPD) tuberculin, a precipitate of non-species-specific molecules obtained from filtrates of heat-sterilized, concentrated broth cultures. The complete genome sequence of *M. tuberculosis* comprises about 4000 genes and has a high guanine-plus-cytosine content. A large proportion of the genes are devoted to the production of enzymes involved in lipogenesis and lipolysis and of glycine-rich proteins that are probably responsible for antigenic variations.

EPIDEMIOLOGY   Between 3.5 and 4 million new cases of tuberculosis—all forms (pulmonary and extrapulmonary), 90% of them from developing countries—were reported annually to the World Health Organization (WHO) in the late 1990s. However, because of a low level of case detection and incomplete notifications in many national programs, reported cases represent only a fraction of the total. It is estimated that 8 million new cases of tuberculosis occurred worldwide in 1997, 95% of them in developing countries of Asia (5 million), Africa (1.6 million), the Middle East (0.6 million), and Latin America (0.4 million). It is also estimated that nearly 2 million deaths from tuberculosis occurred in 1997, 98% of them in developing countries.

Beginning in the mid-1980s in many industrialized countries, the number of tuberculosis case notifications, which had been falling steadily, stabilized or even began to increase. This phenomenon was first noted in the United States but was soon observed in many European countries as well. A number of factors were implicated in the resurgence of tuberculosis in the United States in 1986 through 1992—most notably, immigration from countries with a high prevalence of tuberculosis; infection with HIV; emergence of multidrug-resistant (MDR) tuberculosis due to strains resistant at least to isoniazid and rifampin; and social problems such as poverty, homelessness, and drug abuse. In some areas (e.g., New York City), deterioration in the public health system and dismantling of tuberculosis management services also contributed to the worsening situation. With the implementation of stronger control programs, cases began to decrease in 1993. In 1998, 18,361 cases of tuberculosis (6.8 per 100,000 population) were reported to the U.S. Centers for Disease Control and Prevention (CDC)—a 31% decrease from the 1992 peak.

In the United States, tuberculosis is uncommon among young adults of European descent, who have only rarely been exposed to *M. tuberculosis* infection during recent decades. In contrast, because of a high risk in the past, the prevalence of *M. tuberculosis* infection is relatively high among elderly Caucasians, who remain at increased

169 Tuberculosis   **1025**

In developing countries of Africa and Asia, tuberculosis trends over the past several decades are not entirely clear. However, in sub-Saharan African countries with reliable reporting systems, the recent spread of the HIV epidemic has been accompanied by doubling or tripling of the number of reported cases of tuberculosis during a period as short as 10 years. The growing number of young adults with *M. tuberculosis* infection has fueled the rates of active tuberculosis in many developing countries. Without greater control efforts, the annual incident cases of tuberculosis globally may increase by 40% between now and 2020.

From Exposure to Infection   *M. tuberculosis* is most commonly transmitted from a patient with infectious pulmonary tuberculosis to other persons by droplet nuclei, which are aerosolized by coughing, sneezing, or speaking. The tiny droplets dry rapidly; the smallest (<5 to 10 μm in diameter) may remain suspended in the air for several hours and may gain direct access to the terminal air passages when inhaled. There may be as many as 3000 infectious nuclei per cough. In the past, a frequent source of infection was raw milk containing *M. bovis* from tuberculous cows. Other routes of transmission of tubercle bacilli, such as through the skin or the placenta, are uncommon and of no epidemiologic significance.

The probability of contact with a case of tuberculosis, the intimacy and duration of that contact, the degree of infectiousness of the case, and the shared environment of the contact are all important determinants of transmission. Several studies of close contacts have clearly demonstrated that tuberculosis patients whose sputum contains AFB visible by microscopy play the greatest role in the spread of infection. These patients often have cavitary pulmonary disease or tuberculosis of the respiratory tract (endobronchial or laryngeal tuberculosis) and produce sputa containing as many as 10^5 AFB/mL. Patients with sputum smear–negative/culture-positive tuberculosis are less infectious, and those with culture-negative pulmonary disease and extrapulmonary tuberculosis are essentially noninfectious. Crowding in poorly ventilated rooms is one of the most important factors in the transmission of tubercle bacilli, since it increases the intensity of contact with a case.

In short, the risk of acquiring *M. tuberculosis* infection is determined mainly by exogenous factors. Because of delays in seeking care and in diagnosis, it is estimated that up to 20 contacts will usually be infected by each AFB-positive case before detection in high-prevalence countries.

From Infection to Disease   Unlike the risk of acquiring infection with *M. tuberculosis*, the risk of developing disease after being infected depends largely on endogenous factors, such as the individual's innate susceptibility to disease and level of function of cell-mediated immunity. Clinical illness directly following infection is classified as *primary tuberculosis* and is common among children up to 4 years of age. Although this form may be severe and disseminated, it is usually not transmissible. When infection is acquired later in life, the chance is greater that the immune system will contain it, at least temporarily. The majority of infected individuals who ultimately develop tuberculosis do so within the first year or two after infection. Dormant bacilli, however, may persist for years before being reactivated to produce *secondary* (or *postprimary*) *tuberculosis*, which is often infectious. Overall, it is estimated that about 10% of infected persons will eventually develop active tuberculosis. *Reinfection* of a previously infected individual, which is probably common in areas with high rates of tuberculosis transmission, may also favor the development of disease. Molecular typing and comparison of strains of *M. tuberculosis* have suggested that up to one-third of cases of active tuberculosis in U.S. inner-city communities are due to recent transmission rather than to reactivation of latent infection.

Age is an important determinant of the risk of disease after infection. Among infected persons, the incidence of tuberculosis is highest during late adolescence and early adulthood; the reasons are unclear. The incidence among women peaks at 25 to 34 years of age. In this age group rates among women are usually higher than those among men, while at older ages the opposite is true. The risk may increase in the elderly, possibly because of waning immunity and comorbidity.

A variety of diseases favor the development of active tuberculosis. The most potent risk factor for tuberculosis among infected individuals is clearly HIV co-infection, which suppresses cellular immunity. The risk that latent *M. tuberculosis* infection will proceed to active disease is directly related to the patient's degree of immunosuppression. In a study of HIV-infected, PPD-positive persons, this risk varied from 2.6 to 13.3 cases per 100 person-years and depended upon the CD4+ cell count. The risk of developing tuberculosis is significantly greater among HIV-infected than among HIV-uninfected hosts. Other conditions known to increase the risk of active tuberculosis among persons infected with tubercle bacilli include silicosis; lymphoma, leukemia, and other malignant neoplasms; hemophilia; chronic renal failure and hemodialysis; insulin-dependent diabetes mellitus; immunosuppressive treatment, including that administered for solid-organ transplantation; and conditions associated with malnutrition, such as gastrectomy and jejunoileal bypass surgery. Finally, the presence of old, self-healed, fibrotic tuberculous lesions constitutes a serious risk of active disease.

NATURAL HISTORY OF DISEASE   Studies conducted in various countries before the advent of chemotherapy clearly showed that untreated tuberculosis is often fatal. About one-third of patients died within 1 year after diagnosis, and one-half within 5 years. Five-year mortality among sputum smear–positive cases was 65%. Of the survivors at 5 years, about 60% had undergone spontaneous remission, while the remainder were still excreting tubercle bacilli.

The introduction of effective chemotherapy has markedly affected the natural history of tuberculosis. With proper treatment, patients have a high chance of being cured. However, improper use of antituberculosis drugs, while reducing mortality, may also result in large numbers of chronic infectious cases, often with drug-resistant bacilli.

PATHOGENESIS AND IMMUNITY   The interaction of *M. tuberculosis* with the human host begins when droplet nuclei containing microorganisms from infectious patients are inhaled. While the majority of inhaled bacilli are trapped in the upper airways and expelled by ciliated mucosal cells, a fraction (usually fewer than 10%) reach the alveoli. There, nonspecifically activated alveolar macrophages ingest the bacilli. Invasion of macrophages by mycobacteria may result in part from association of C2a with the bacterial cell wall followed by C3b opsonization of the bacteria and recognition by the macrophages. The balance between the bactericidal activity of the macrophage and the virulence of the bacillus (the latter being partially linked to the bacterium's lipid-rich cell wall and to its glycolipid capsule, both of which confer resistance to complement and free radicals of the phagocyte) determines the events following phagocytosis. The number of invading bacilli is also important.

Several genes thought to confer virulence to *M. tuberculosis* have been identified. *katG* encodes for catalase, an enzyme protective against oxidative stress; *rpoV* is the main sigma factor initiating transcription of several genes. Defects in these two genes result in loss of virulence. The *erp* gene, encoding a protein required for multiplication, also contributes to virulence. The effects of a highly virulent strain are exemplified by an outbreak of tuberculosis in two rural counties in Tennessee and Kentucky in 1994 through 1996. In this outbreak, both epidemiologic evidence of enhanced transmission with high rates of disease and accelerated growth of the strain in mice were documented.

Several observations suggest that genetic factors play a key role in innate nonimmune resistance to infection with *M. tuberculosis*. The existence of this resistance is suggested by the differing degrees of susceptibility to tuberculosis in different populations. In mice, a gene called *Nramp1* (natural resistance–associated macrophage protein 1) has a regulatory role in resistance/susceptibility to mycobacteria. The human homologue NRAMP1, cloned to chromosome 2q, may have a role in determining susceptibility to tuberculosis. In a study among West Africans, subjects heterozygous for two polymorphisms of NRAMP1 (INT4 and 3′UTR) had an apparently increased risk of tuberculosis, a finding suggesting that the susceptibility allele behaves as dominant.

In the initial stage of host-bacterium interaction, either the host's macrophages contain bacillary multiplication by producing proteolytic enzymes and cytokines or the bacilli begin to multiply. If the bacilli multiply, their growth quickly kills the macrophages, which lyse. Nonactivated monocytes attracted from the bloodstream to the site by various chemotactic factors ingest the bacilli released from the lysed macrophages. These initial stages of infection are usually asymptomatic.

About 2 to 4 weeks after infection, two additional host responses to *M. tuberculosis* develop: a tissue-damaging response and a macrophage-activating response. The *tissue-damaging response* is the result of a delayed-type hypersensitivity (DTH) reaction to various bacillary antigens; it destroys nonactivated macrophages that contain multiplying bacilli. The *macrophage-activating response* is a cell-mediated phenomenon resulting in the activation of macrophages that are capable of killing and digesting tubercle bacilli. Although both of these responses can inhibit mycobacterial growth, it is the balance between the two that determines the form of tuberculosis that will develop subsequently.

With the development of specific immunity and the accumulation of large numbers of activated macrophages at the site of the primary lesion, granulomatous lesions (tubercles) are formed. These lesions consist of lymphocytes and activated macrophages, such as epithelioid cells and giant cells. Initially, the newly developed tissue-damaging response is the only event capable of limiting mycobacterial growth within macrophages. This response, mediated by various bacterial products, not only destroys macrophages but also produces early solid necrosis in the center of the tubercle. Although *M. tuberculosis* can survive, its growth is inhibited within this necrotic environment by low oxygen tension and low pH. At this point, some lesions may heal by fibrosis and calcification, while others undergo further evolution.

Cell-mediated immunity is critical at this early stage. In the majority of infected individuals, local macrophages are activated when bacillary antigens processed by macrophages stimulate T lymphocytes to release a variety of lymphokines. These activated cells aggregate around the lesion's center and effectively neutralize tubercle bacilli without causing further tissue destruction. In the central part of the lesion, the necrotic material resembles soft cheese (*caseous necrosis*). Even when healing takes place, viable bacilli may remain dormant within macrophages or in the necrotic material for years or even throughout the patient's lifetime. These "healed" lesions in the lung parenchyma and hilar lymph nodes may later undergo calcification (*Ranke complex*).

In a minority of cases, the macrophage-activating response is weak, and mycobacterial growth can be inhibited only by intensified DTH reactions, which lead to tissue destruction. The lesion tends to enlarge further, and the surrounding tissue is progressively damaged. At the center of the lesion, the caseous material liquefies. Bronchial walls as well as blood vessels are invaded and destroyed, and cavities are formed. The liquefied caseous material, containing large numbers of bacilli, is drained through bronchi. Within the cavity, tubercle bacilli multiply well and spread into the airways and the environment through expectorated sputum.

In the early stages of infection, bacilli are usually transported by macrophages to regional lymph nodes, from which they disseminate widely to many organs and tissues. The resulting lesions may undergo the same evolution as those in the lungs, although most tend to heal. In young children with poor natural immunity, hematogenous dissemination may result in fatal miliary tuberculosis or tuberculous meningitis.

Cell-mediated immunity confers partial protection against *M. tuberculosis*, while humoral immunity has no defined role in protection. Two types of cells are essential: macrophages, which directly phagocytize tubercle bacilli, and T cells (mainly CD4+ lymphocytes), which induce protection through the production of lymphokines.

After infection with *M. tuberculosis*, alveolar macrophages secrete a number of cytokines: interleukin (IL) 1 contributes to fever; IL-6 contributes to hyperglobulinemia; and tumor necrosis factor α (TNF-α) contributes to the killing of mycobacteria, the formation of granulomas, and a number of systemic effects, such as fever and weight loss. Macrophages are also critical in processing and presenting antigens to T lymphocytes; the result is a proliferation of CD4+ lymphocytes, which are crucial to the host's defense against M. *tuberculosis*. Qualitative and quantitative defects of CD4+ T cells explain the inability of HIV-infected individuals to contain mycobacterial proliferation. Reactive CD4+ lymphocytes produce cytokines of the T$_H$1 pattern and participate in MHC class II–restricted killing of cells infected with *M. tuberculosis*. T$_H$1 CD4+ cells produce interferon γ (IFN-γ) and IL-2 and promote cell-mediated immunity. T$_H$2 cells produce IL-4, IL-5, and IL-10 and promote humoral immunity. The interplay of these various cytokines and their cross-regulation determine the host's response. The role of cytokines in promoting intracellular killing of mycobacteria has not been entirely elucidated. IFN-γ may induce release of nitric oxide, and TNF-α seems also to be important. Finally, the role of other cells, such as natural killer (NK) cells, "double-negative" CD4−CD8− cells, and γ/δ T cells, in protective immunity remains unclear.

M. tuberculosis possesses various protein antigens. Some are present in the cytoplasm and cell wall; others are secreted. That the latter are more important in eliciting a T lymphocyte response is suggested by experiments documenting the appearance of protective immunity in animals after immunization with live, protein-secreting mycobacteria. Among the antigens with a potential protective role are the 30-kDa (or 85B) and the ESAT-6 antigens. Protective immunity is probably the result of reactivity to a large number of different mycobacterial antigens.

Coincident with the appearance of immunity, DTH to *M. tuberculosis* develops. This reactivity is the basis of the PPD skin test, currently the only test that reliably detects *M. tuberculosis* infection in persons without symptoms. The cellular mechanisms responsible for PPD reactivity are related mainly to previously sensitized CD4+ lymphocytes, which are attracted to the skin-test site. There, they proliferate and produce cytokines.

In 1891, Robert Koch discovered components of *M. tuberculosis* in a concentrated liquid culture medium. Subsequently named "old tuberculin" (OT), this material was initially believed to be useful in the treatment of tuberculosis (although this idea was later disproved). It soon became clear that OT was capable of eliciting a skin reaction when injected subcutaneously into patients with tuberculosis. In 1932, Seibert and Munday purified this product by ammonium sulfate precipitation. The result was an active protein fraction known as tuberculin PPD. However, the complexity and diversity of the constituents of PPD rendered its standardization difficult. PPD-S, developed by Seibert and Glenn in 1941, was chosen as the international standard. Later, the WHO and UNICEF sponsored large-scale production of a master batch of PPD, termed RT23, and made it available for general use. The greatest limitation of PPD is its lack of mycobacterial species specificity, a property that is due to the large number of proteins in this product that are highly conserved in the various species of mycobacteria.

While DTH is associated with protective immunity (PPD-positive persons being less susceptible to a new *M. tuberculosis* infection than PPD-negative persons), it by no means guarantees protection against reactivation. In fact, severe cases of active tuberculosis are often accompanied by strongly positive skin-test reactions.

CLINICAL MANIFESTATIONS Tuberculosis is usually classified as pulmonary or extrapulmonary. Before the recognition of HIV infection, more than 80% of all cases of tuberculosis were limited to the lungs. However, up to two-thirds of HIV-infected patients with tuberculosis may have both pulmonary and extrapulmonary disease or extrapulmonary disease alone.

Pulmonary Tuberculosis Pulmonary tuberculosis can be categorized as primary or postprimary (secondary).

Primary disease Primary pulmonary tuberculosis results from an initial infection with tubercle bacilli. In areas of high tuberculosis prevalence, this form of disease is often seen in children and is frequently localized to the middle and lower lung zones. The lesion forming after infection is usually peripheral and accompanied by hilar or paratracheal lymphadenopathy, which may not be detectable on chest radiography. In the majority of cases, the lesion heals spontaneously and may later be evident as a small calcified nodule (*Ghon lesion*).

In children and in persons with impaired immunity, such as those with malnutrition or HIV infection, primary pulmonary tuberculosis may progress rapidly to clinical illness. The initial lesion increases in size and can evolve in different ways. Pleural effusion, a frequent finding, results from the penetration of bacilli into the pleural space from an adjacent subpleural focus. In severe cases, the primary site rapidly enlarges, its central portion undergoes necrosis, and acute cavitation develops (progressive primary tuberculosis). Tuberculosis in young children is almost invariably accompanied by hilar or mediastinal lymphadenopathy due to the spread of bacilli from the lung parenchyma through lymphatic vessels. Enlarged lymph nodes may compress bronchi, causing obstruction and subsequent segmental or lobar collapse. Partial obstruction may cause obstructive emphysema, and bronchiectasis may also develop. Hematogenous dissemination, which is common and is often asymptomatic, may result in the most severe manifestations of primary *M. tuberculosis* infection. Bacilli reach the bloodstream from the pulmonary lesion or the lymph nodes and disseminate into various organs, where they may produce granulomatous lesions. Although healing frequently takes place, immunocompromised persons (e.g., patients with HIV infection and those recovering from measles) may develop miliary tuberculosis and/or tuberculous meningitis.

Postprimary disease Also called adult-type, reactivation, or secondary tuberculosis, postprimary disease results from endogenous reactivation of latent infection and is usually localized to the apical and posterior segments of the upper lobes, where the high oxygen concentration favors mycobacterial growth. In addition, the superior segments of the lower lobes are frequently involved. The extent of lung parenchymal involvement varies greatly, from small infiltrates to extensive cavitary disease. With cavity formation, liquefied necrotic contents are ultimately discharged into the airways, resulting in satellite lesions within the lungs that may in turn undergo cavitation. Massive involvement of pulmonary segments or lobes, with coalescence of lesions, produces tuberculous pneumonia. While up to one-third of untreated patients reportedly succumb to severe pulmonary tuberculosis within a few weeks or months after onset, others undergo a process of spontaneous remission or proceed along a chronic, progressively debilitating course ("consumption"). Under these circumstances, some pulmonary lesions become fibrotic and may later calcify, but cavities persist in other parts of the lungs. Individuals with such chronic disease continue to discharge tubercle bacilli into the environment. Most patients respond to treatment, with defervescence, decreasing cough, weight gain, and a general improvement in well-being within several weeks.

Early in the course of disease, symptoms and signs are often nonspecific and insidious, consisting mainly of fever and night sweats, weight loss, anorexia, general malaise, and weakness. However, in the majority of cases, cough eventually develops—perhaps initially nonproductive and subsequently accompanied by the production of purulent sputum. Blood streaking of the sputum is frequently documented. Massive hemoptysis may ensue as a consequence of the erosion of a fully patent vessel located in the wall of a cavity. Hemoptysis, however, may also result from rupture of a dilated vessel in a cavity (*Rasmussen's aneurysm*) or from aspergilloma formation in an old cavity. Pleuritic chest pain sometimes develops in patients with

subpleural parenchymal lesions but can also result from muscle strain due to persistent coughing. Extensive disease may produce dyspnea and (occasionally) adult respiratory distress syndrome (ARDS).

Physical findings are of limited use in pulmonary tuberculosis. Many patients have no abnormalities detectable by chest examination, while others have detectable rales in the involved areas during inspiration, especially after coughing. Occasionally, rhonchi due to partial bronchial obstruction and classic amphoric breath sounds in areas with large cavities may be heard. Systemic features include fever (often low-grade and intermittent) and wasting. In some cases, pallor and finger clubbing develop. The most common hematologic findings are mild anemia and leukocytosis. Hyponatremia due to the syndrome of inappropriate secretion of antidiuretic hormone (SIADH) has also been reported.

Extrapulmonary Tuberculosis In order of frequency, the extrapulmonary sites most commonly involved in tuberculosis are the lymph nodes, pleura, genitourinary tract, bones and joints, meninges, and peritoneum. However, virtually all organ systems may be affected. As a result of hematogenous dissemination in HIV-infected individuals, extrapulmonary tuberculosis is seen more commonly today than in the past.

Lymph-node tuberculosis (tuberculous lymphadenitis) The commonest presentation of extrapulmonary tuberculosis (being documented in more than 25% of cases), lymph-node disease is particularly frequent among HIV-infected patients. In the United States, children and women (particularly non-Caucasians) also seem to be especially susceptible. Lymph-node tuberculosis presents as painless swelling of the lymph nodes, most commonly at cervical and supraclavicular sites. Lymph nodes are usually discrete in early disease but may be inflamed and have a fistulous tract draining caseous material. Systemic symptoms are usually limited to HIV-infected patients, and concomitant lung disease may or may not be present. The diagnosis is established by fine-needle aspiration or surgical biopsy. AFB are seen in up to 50% of cases, cultures are positive in 70 to 80%, and histologic examination shows granulomatous lesions. Among HIV-infected patients, granulomas are usually not seen. Differential diagnosis includes a variety of infectious conditions as well as neoplastic diseases such as lymphomas or metastatic carcinomas (Chap. 63).

Pleural tuberculosis Involvement of the pleura is common in primary tuberculosis and results from penetration by a few tubercle bacilli into the pleural space. Depending on the extent of reactivity, the effusion may be small, remain unnoticed, and resolve spontaneously or may be sufficiently large to cause symptoms such as fever, pleuritic chest pain, and dyspnea. Physical findings are those of pleural effusion: dullness to percussion and absence of breath sounds. A chest radiograph reveals the effusion and, in no more than one-third of cases, also shows a parenchymal lesion. Thoracentesis is required to ascertain the nature of the effusion. The fluid is straw colored and at times hemorrhagic; it is an exudate with a protein concentration >50% of that in serum, a normal to low glucose concentration, a pH that is generally <7.2, and detectable white blood cells (usually 500 to 2500/mL). Neutrophils may predominate in the early stage, while mononuclear cells are the typical finding later. Mesothelial cells are generally rare or absent. AFB are very rarely seen on direct smear, but cultures may be positive for *M. tuberculosis* in up to one-third of cases. Needle biopsy of the pleura is often required for diagnosis and reveals granulomas and/or yields a positive culture in up to 70% of cases. This form of pleural tuberculosis responds well to chemotherapy and may resolve spontaneously.

Tuberculous empyema is a less common complication of pulmonary tuberculosis. It is usually the result of the rupture of a cavity, with delivery of a large number of organisms into the pleural space, or of a bronchopleural fistula from a pulmonary lesion. A chest radiograph may show pyopneumothorax with an air-fluid level. The effusion is purulent and thick and contains large numbers of lymphocytes. An acid-fast smear of pleural fluid is often found to be positive when examined by microscopy, as is culture of the pleural fluid. Surgical drainage is usually required as an adjunct to chemotherapy. Tuberculous empyema may result in severe pleural fibrosis and restrictive lung disease.

Tuberculosis of the upper airways   Nearly always a complication of advanced cavitary pulmonary tuberculosis, tuberculosis of the upper airways may involve the larynx, pharynx, and epiglottis. Symptoms include hoarseness and dysphagia in addition to chronic productive cough. Findings depend on the site of involvement, and ulcerations may be seen on laryngoscopy. Acid-fast smear of the sputum is often positive, but biopsy may be necessary in some cases to establish the diagnosis. Cancer may have similar features but is usually painless.

Genitourinary tuberculosis   Genitourinary tuberculosis accounts for about 15% of all extrapulmonary cases, may involve any portion of the genitourinary tract, and is usually due to hematogenous seeding following primary infection. Local symptoms predominate. Urinary frequency, dysuria, hematuria, and flank pain are common presentations. However, patients may be asymptomatic and the disease discovered only after severe destructive lesions of the kidneys have developed. Urinalysis gives abnormal results in 90% of cases, revealing pyuria and hematuria. The documentation of culture-negative pyuria in acidic urine raises the suspicion of tuberculosis. An intravenous pyelogram helps in diagnosis. Calcifications and ureteral strictures are suggestive findings. Culture of three morning urine specimens yields a definitive diagnosis in nearly 90% of cases. Severe ureteral strictures may lead to hydronephrosis and renal damage.

Genital tuberculosis is diagnosed more commonly in females than in males. In females, it affects the fallopian tubes and the endometrium and may cause infertility, pelvic pain, and menstrual abnormalities. Diagnosis requires biopsy or culture of specimens obtained by dilatation and curettage. In males, tuberculosis preferentially affects the epididymis, producing a slightly tender mass that may drain externally through a fistulous tract; orchitis and prostatitis may also develop. In almost half of cases of genitourinary tuberculosis, urinary tract disease is also present. Genitourinary tuberculosis responds well to chemotherapy.

Skeletal tuberculosis   In the United States, tuberculosis of the bones and joints is responsible for about 10% of extrapulmonary cases. In bone and joint disease, pathogenesis is related to reactivation of hematogenous foci or to spread from adjacent paravertebral lymph nodes. Weight-bearing joints (spine, hips, and knees—in that order) are affected most commonly. Spinal tuberculosis (Pott's disease or tuberculous spondylitis) often involves two or more adjacent vertebral bodies. While the upper thoracic spine is the most common site of spinal tuberculosis in children, the lower thoracic and upper lumbar vertebrae are usually affected in adults. From the anterior superior or inferior angle of the vertebral body, the lesion reaches the adjacent body, also destroying the intervertebral disk. With advanced disease, collapse of vertebral bodies results in kyphosis (*gibbus*). A paravertebral "cold" abscess may also form. In the upper spine, this abscess may track to the chest wall as a mass; in the lower spine, it may reach the inguinal ligaments or present as a psoas abscess. Computed tomography (CT) or magnetic resonance imaging (MRI) reveals the characteristic lesion and suggests its etiology, although the differential diagnosis includes other infections and tumors. Aspiration of the abscess or bone biopsy confirms the tuberculous etiology, as cultures are usually positive and histologic findings highly typical. A catastrophic complication of Pott's disease is paraplegia, which is usually due to an abscess or a lesion compressing the spinal cord. Paraparesis due to a large abscess is a medical emergency and requires abscess drainage. Tuberculosis of the hip joints causes pain and limping; tuberculosis of the knee produces pain and swelling and sometimes follows trauma. If the disease goes unrecognized, the joints may be destroyed. Skeletal tuberculosis responds to chemotherapy, but severe cases may require surgery.

Tuberculous meningitis and tuberculoma   Tuberculosis of the central nervous system accounts for about 5% of extrapulmonary cases. It is seen most often in young children but also develops in adults, especially those who are infected with HIV. Tuberculous meningitis results from the hematogenous spread of primary or postprimary pulmonary disease or from the rupture of a subependymal tubercle into the subarachnoid space. In more than half of cases, evidence of old pulmonary lesions or a miliary pattern is found on chest radiography. The disease may present subtly as headache and mental changes or acutely as confusion, lethargy, altered sensorium, and neck rigidity. Typically, the disease evolves over 1 or 2 weeks, a course longer than that of bacterial meningitis. Paresis of cranial nerves (ocular nerves in particular) is a frequent finding, and the involvement of cerebral arteries may produce focal ischemia. Hydrocephalus is common. Lumbar puncture is the cornerstone of diagnosis. In general, examination of the cerebrospinal fluid (CSF) reveals a high leukocyte count (usually with a predominance of lymphocytes but often with a predominance of neutrophils in the early stage), a protein content of 1 to 8 g/L (100 to 800 mg/dL), and a low glucose concentration; however, any of these three parameters can be within the normal range. AFB are seen on direct smear of CSF sediment in only 20% of cases, but repeated lumbar punctures increase the yield. Culture of CSF is diagnostic in up to 80% of cases. Imaging studies (CT and MRI) may show hydrocephalus and abnormal enhancement of basal cisterns or ependyma. If unrecognized, tuberculous meningitis is uniformly fatal. This disease responds to chemotherapy; however, neurologic sequelae are documented in 25% of treated cases, in most of which the diagnosis has been delayed. Clinical trials have demonstrated that patients treated with adjunctive glucocorticoids experience a significantly faster resolution of CSF abnormalities and elevated CSF pressure. Adjunctive glucocorticoids enhance survival and reduce the frequency of neurologic sequelae.

Tuberculoma, an uncommon manifestation of tuberculosis, presents as one or more space-occupying lesions and usually causes seizures and focal signs. CT or MRI reveals contrast-enhanced ring lesions, but biopsy is necessary to establish the diagnosis.

Gastrointestinal tuberculosis   Any portion of the gastrointestinal tract may be affected by tuberculosis. Various pathogenetic mechanisms are involved: swallowing of sputum with direct seeding, hematogenous spread, or (although rarely today) ingestion of milk from cows affected by bovine tuberculosis. The terminal ileum and the cecum are the sites most commonly involved. Abdominal pain (at times similar to that associated with appendicitis), diarrhea, obstruction, hematochezia, and a palpable mass in the abdomen are common findings at presentation. Fever, weight loss, and night sweats are also frequent. With intestinal-wall involvement, ulcerations and fistulae may simulate Crohn's disease. Anal fistulae should prompt an evaluation for rectal tuberculosis. As surgery is required in most cases, the diagnosis can be established by histologic examination and culture of specimens obtained intraoperatively.

Tuberculous peritonitis follows either the direct spread of tubercle bacilli from ruptured lymph nodes and intraabdominal organs or hematogenous seeding. Nonspecific abdominal pain, fever, and ascites should raise the suspicion of tuberculous peritonitis. The coexistence of cirrhosis (Chap. 298) in patients with tuberculous peritonitis complicates the diagnosis. In tuberculous peritonitis, paracentesis reveals an exudative fluid with a high protein content and leukocytosis that is usually lymphocytic (although neutrophils occasionally predominate). The yield of direct smear and culture is relatively low; culture of a large volume of ascitic fluid can increase the yield, but peritoneal biopsy is often needed to establish the diagnosis.

Pericardial tuberculosis (tuberculous pericarditis)   Due to direct progression of a primary focus within the pericardium, to reactivation of a latent focus, or to rupture of an adjacent lymph node, pericardial tuberculosis has often been a disease of the elderly in countries with low tuberculosis prevalence but develops frequently in HIV-infected patients. Case-fatality rates are as high as 40% in some series. The onset may be subacute, although an acute presentation, with fever, dull retrosternal pain, and a friction rub, is possible. An effusion eventually develops in many cases; cardiovascular symptoms and signs of cardiac tamponade may ultimately appear (Chap. 239). In the presence of effusion detected on chest radiography, tuberculosis must be suspected if the patient belongs to a high-risk population (HIV-infected, originating in a high-prevalence country), if there is evidence of previous tuberculosis or disease in other organs, or if echocardiography shows thick strands crossing the pericardial space. Diagnosis can be facilitated by pericardiocentesis under echocardiographic guidance. The pericardial fluid must be submitted for biochemical, cytologic, and microbiologic study. The effusion is exudative in nature, with a high count of leukocytes (predominantly mononuclear cells). Hemorrhagic effusion is frequent. Culture of the fluid reveals *M. tuberculosis* in about 30% of cases, while biopsy has a higher yield. Without treatment, pericardial tuberculosis is usually fatal. Even with treatment, complications may develop, including chronic constrictive pericarditis with thickening of the pericardium, fibrosis, and sometimes calcification, which may be visible on a chest radiograph. A course of glucocorticoid treatment is useful in the management of acute disease, reducing effusion, facilitating hemodynamic recovery, and thus decreasing mortality. Progression to chronic constrictive pericarditis, however, seems unaffected by such therapy.

Miliary or disseminated tuberculosis Miliary tuberculosis is due to hematogenous spread of tubercle bacilli. Although in children it is often the consequence of a recent primary infection, in adults it may be due to either recent infection or reactivation of old disseminated foci. Lesions are usually yellowish granulomas 1 to 2 mm in diameter that resemble millet seeds (thus the term *miliary*, coined by nineteenth-century pathologists).

Clinical manifestations are nonspecific and protean, depending on the predominant site of involvement. Fever, night sweats, anorexia, weakness, and weight loss are presenting symptoms in the majority of cases. At times, patients have a cough and other respiratory symptoms due to pulmonary involvement as well as abdominal symptoms. Physical findings include hepatomegaly, splenomegaly, and lymphadenopathy. Eye examination may reveal choroidal tubercles, which are pathognomonic of miliary tuberculosis, in up to 30% of cases. Meningismus occurs in fewer than 10% of cases.

A high index of suspicion is required for the diagnosis of miliary tuberculosis. Frequently, chest radiography reveals a miliary reticulonodular pattern (more easily seen on underpenetrated film), although no radiographic abnormality may be evident early in the course and among HIV-infected patients. Other radiologic findings include large infiltrates, interstitial infiltrates (especially in HIV-infected patients), and pleural effusion. A sputum smear is negative in 80% of cases. Various hematologic abnormalities may be seen, including anemia with leukopenia, neutrophilic leukocytosis and leukemoid reactions, and polycythemia. Disseminated intravascular coagulation has been reported. Elevation of alkaline phosphatase levels and other abnormal values in liver function tests are detected in patients with severe hepatic involvement. The PPD test may be negative in up to half of cases, but reactivity may be restored during chemotherapy. Bronchoalveolar lavage and transbronchial biopsy are more likely to permit bacteriologic confirmation, and granulomas are evident in liver or bone-marrow biopsy specimens from many patients. If it goes unrecognized, miliary tuberculosis is lethal; with proper treatment, however, it is amenable to cure.

A rare presentation seen in the elderly is *cryptic miliary tuberculosis*, which has a chronic course characterized by mild intermittent fever, anemia, and—ultimately—meningeal involvement preceding death. An acute septicemic form, *nonreactive miliary tuberculosis*, occurs very rarely and is due to massive hematogenous dissemination of tubercle bacilli. Pancytopenia is common in this form of disease, which is rapidly fatal. At postmortem examination, multiple necrotic but nongranulomatous ("nonreactive") lesions are detected.

Less common extrapulmonary forms Tuberculosis may cause chorioretinitis, uveitis, panophthalmitis, and painful hypersensitivity-related phlyctenular conjunctivitis. Tuberculous otitis is rare and presents as hearing loss, otorrhea, and tympanic membrane perforation. In the nasopharynx, tuberculosis may simulate Wegener's granulom-

atosis. Cutaneous manifestations of tuberculosis include primary infection due to direct inoculation, abscesses and chronic ulcers, scrofuloderma, lupus vulgaris, miliary lesions, and erythema nodosum. Adrenal tuberculosis is a manifestation of advanced disease presenting as signs of adrenal insufficiency. Finally, congenital tuberculosis results from transplacental spread of tubercle bacilli to the fetus or from ingestion of contaminated amniotic fluid. This rare disease affects the liver, spleen, lymph nodes, and various other organs.

HIV-Associated Tuberculosis Tuberculosis is an important opportunistic disease among HIV-infected persons worldwide. In developing countries of Africa, Southeast Asia, and Latin America, an estimated 10 million persons were coinfected as of 1997. In the United States, coinfection with HIV and *M. tuberculosis* is common in certain segments of the population, including drug users and some minorities. A person with skin test–documented *M. tuberculosis* infection who acquires HIV infection has a 3 to 15% annual risk of developing active tuberculosis.

The association between tuberculosis and HIV infection is supported by other epidemiologic observations. First, the rate of HIV seropositivity among patients with tuberculosis is several times higher than that among the general population: in African countries it reaches 60 to 70%. Second, marked increases in numbers of tuberculosis cases have been reported at locations hard hit by the HIV epidemic, such as large parts of Africa (including Kenya, Tanzania, and Malawi), northern Thailand, and New York City. Globally, the proportion of tuberculosis cases associated with HIV infection reached 8% in 1997.

HIV directly attacks the critical immune mechanisms involved in protection against tuberculosis. Tuberculosis can appear at any stage of HIV infection, but its presentation varies with the stage. When cell-mediated immunity is only partially compromised, pulmonary tuberculosis presents as a typical pattern of upper lobe infiltrates and cavitation, without significant lymphadenopathy or pleural effusion. In late stages of HIV infection, a primary tuberculosis–like pattern, with diffuse interstitial or miliary infiltrates, little or no cavitation, and intrathoracic lymphadenopathy, is more common. Overall, sputum smears may be positive less frequently among tuberculosis patients with HIV infection than among those without; thus the diagnosis of tuberculosis may be unusually difficult, especially in view of the variety of HIV-related pulmonary conditions mimicking tuberculosis.

As has been mentioned, extrapulmonary tuberculosis is common among HIV-infected patients. In various series studied in the United States and many developing countries, extrapulmonary tuberculosis—alone or in association with pulmonary disease—has been documented in 40 to 60% of all cases in HIV co-infected individuals. The most common forms are lymphatic, disseminated, pleural, and pericardial. Mycobacteremia and meningitis are also frequent, particularly in advanced HIV disease.

The diagnosis of tuberculosis in HIV-infected patients may be difficult not only because of the increased frequency of sputum-smear negativity (up to 40% in culture-proven pulmonary cases) but also because of atypical radiographic findings, a lack of classic granuloma formation in the late stages, and negative results in PPD skin tests. Delays in treatment may prove fatal. The response to short-course chemotherapy is similar to that in HIV-seronegative patients. However, adverse effects may be more pronounced, including severe or even fatal skin reactions to amithiozone (thiacetazone).

Exacerbations in symptoms, signs, and laboratory or radiographic manifestations of tuberculosis—termed *paradoxical reactions*—have been associated with the administration of highly active antiretroviral treatment (HAART) regimens. The presumed pathogenesis of paradoxical reactions is an immune response to antigens released as bacilli are killed by effective chemotherapy. In patients in whom antiretroviral therapy has recently been started, paradoxical reactions may be due to improving immune function. The first priority in the management of a possible paradoxical reaction is to ensure that the clinical syndrome does not represent a failure of tuberculosis treatment or the development of another infection. Mild paradoxical reactions can be managed with symptom-based treatment. More severe manifestations may necessitate discontinuation of antiretroviral therapy. Immunomodulators, such as glucocorticoids, have been used to treat severe paradoxical reactions, although this practice has not been formally evaluated in clinical trials.

Recommendations for the prevention and treatment of tuberculosis in HIV-infected individuals have been published by the CDC.

DIAGNOSIS　The key to the diagnosis of tuberculosis is a high index of suspicion. Diagnosis is not difficult with a high-risk patient—e.g., a homeless alcoholic who presents with typical symptoms and a classic chest radiograph showing upper lobe infiltrates with cavities. On the other hand, the diagnosis can easily be missed in an elderly nursing-home resident or a teenager with a focal infiltrate.

Often, the diagnosis is first entertained when the chest radiograph of a patient being evaluated for respiratory symptoms is abnormal. If the patient has no complicating medical conditions that favor immunosuppression, the chest radiograph may show the typical picture of upper lobe infiltrates with cavitation. The longer the delay between the onset of symptoms and the diagnosis, the more likely is the finding of cavitary disease. In contrast, immunosuppressed patients, including those with HIV infection, may have "atypical" findings on chest radiography—e.g., lower zone infiltrates without cavity formation.

AFB Microscopy　A presumptive diagnosis is commonly based on the finding of AFB on microscopic examination of a diagnostic specimen such as a smear of expectorated sputum or of tissue (for example, a lymph node biopsy). Most modern laboratories processing large numbers of diagnostic specimens use auramine-rhodamine staining and fluorescence microscopy. The more traditional method—light microscopy of specimens stained with Kinyoun or Ziehl-Neelsen basic fuchsin dyes—is satisfactory, although more time-consuming. For patients with suspected pulmonary tuberculosis, three sputum specimens, preferably collected early in the morning, should be submitted to the laboratory for AFB smear and mycobacteriology culture. If tissue is obtained, it is critical that the portion of the specimen intended for culture not be put in formaldehyde. The use of AFB microscopy on urine or gastric lavage fluid is limited by the presence of mycobacterial commensals, which can cause false-positive results.

Mycobacterial Culture　Definitive diagnosis depends on the isolation and identification of *M. tuberculosis* from a diagnostic specimen—in most cases, a sputum specimen obtained from a patient with a productive cough. Specimens may be inoculated onto egg- or agar-based medium (e.g., Löwenstein-Jensen or Middlebrook 7H10) and incubated at 37°C under 5% CO_2. Because most species of mycobacteria, including *M. tuberculosis*, grow slowly, 4 to 8 weeks may be required before growth is detected. Although *M. tuberculosis* may be presumptively identified on the basis of growth time and colony pigmentation and morphology, a variety of biochemical tests have traditionally been used to speciate mycobacterial isolates. In today's laboratories, the use of liquid media with radiometric growth detection (e.g., BACTEC-460) and the identification of isolates by nucleic acid probes or high-pressure liquid chromatography of mycolic acids have replaced the traditional methods of isolation on solid media and identification by biochemical tests. These new methods have decreased the time required for isolation and speciation to 2 to 3 weeks. Other systems for culture on liquid media with nonradiometric detection have become available.

Nucleic Acid Amplification　Several test systems based on amplification of mycobacterial nucleic acid are available. These systems permit the diagnosis of tuberculosis in as short a period as several hours. However, their applicability is limited by low sensitivity (lower than culture) and high cost. At present, these tests are approved by the U.S. Food and Drug Administration only for species identification on AFB-positive sputa. With further improvements in performance, these tests may also be useful for the diagnosis of patients with AFB-negative pulmonary and extrapulmonary tuberculosis.

Radiographic Procedures　As noted above, the initial suspicion of pulmonary tuberculosis is often based on abnormal chest radiographic findings in a patient with respiratory symptoms. Although the "classic" picture is that of upper lobe disease with infiltrates and cavities, virtually any radiographic pattern—from a normal film or a solitary pulmonary nodule to diffuse alveolar infiltrates in a patient with ARDS—may be seen. In the era of AIDS, no radiographic pattern can be considered pathognomonic.

PPD Skin Testing　Skin testing with PPD is most widely used in screening for *M. tuberculosis* infection (see below). The test is of limited value in the diagnosis of active tuberculosis because of its low sensitivity and specificity. False-negative reactions are common in immunosuppressed patients and in those with overwhelming tuberculosis. Positive reactions are obtained when patients have been infected with *M. tuberculosis* but do not have active disease and when persons have been sensitized by nontuberculous mycobacteria (Chap. 171) or bacille Calmette-Guérin (BCG) vaccination. Although BCG vaccine is not commonly used in the United States, many immigrants will have received it. In the absence of a history of BCG vaccination, a positive skin test may provide additional support for the diagnosis of tuberculosis in culture-negative cases.

Drug Susceptibility Testing　In general, the initial isolate of *M. tuberculosis* should be tested for susceptibility to the primary drugs used for treatment: isoniazid, rifampin, ethambutol, pyrazinamide, and streptomycin. In addition, drug susceptibility tests are mandatory when patients fail to respond to initial therapy or experience a relapse after the completion of treatment (see below). Susceptibility testing may be conducted directly (with the clinical specimen) or indirectly (with mycobacterial cultures) on solid or liquid medium. Results are obtained most rapidly by direct susceptibility testing on liquid medium, with an average reporting time of 3 weeks. With indirect testing on solid media, results may not be available for 8 weeks or longer. Molecular methods for the rapid identification of drug resistance are becoming available. One of the most promising uses polymerase chain reaction (PCR) for the *rpoB* gene to detect resistance to rifampin.

Additional Diagnostic Procedures　Other diagnostic tests may be used when pulmonary tuberculosis is suspected. Sputum induction by ultrasonic nebulization of hypertonic saline may be useful for patients unable to produce a sputum specimen spontaneously. Frequently, patients with radiographic abnormalities that are consistent with other diagnoses (e.g., bronchogenic carcinoma) undergo fiberoptic bronchoscopy with bronchial brushings or transbronchial biopsy of the lesion. Bronchoalveolar lavage of a lung segment containing an abnormality may also be performed. In all cases, it is essential that specimens be submitted for AFB smear and mycobacterial culture. For the diagnosis of primary pulmonary tuberculosis in children, who often do not expectorate sputum, specimens from early-morning gastric lavage may yield positive cultures.

Invasive diagnostic procedures are indicated for patients with suspected extrapulmonary tuberculosis. In addition to specimens of involved sites (e.g., CSF for tuberculous meningitis, pleural fluid and biopsy samples for pleural disease), bone marrow and liver biopsy and culture have a good diagnostic yield in disseminated (miliary) tuberculosis, particularly in HIV-infected patients, who also have a high frequency of positive blood cultures.

In some cases, cultures will be negative, but a clinical diagnosis of tuberculosis will be supported by consistent epidemiologic evidence (e.g., a history of close contact with an infectious patient), a positive PPD skin test, and a compatible clinical and radiographic response to treatment. In the United States and other industrialized countries with low rates of tuberculosis, some patients with limited abnormalities on chest radiographs and sputum positive for AFB are infected with organisms of the *M. avium* complex or *M. kansasii* (Chap. 171). Factors favoring the diagnosis of nontuberculous mycobacterial disease over tuberculosis include an absence of risk factors for tuberculosis, a negative PPD skin test, and underlying chronic obstructive pulmonary disease.

Patients with HIV-associated tuberculosis pose several diagnostic problems, as noted above in the description of clinical manifestations. Moreover, HIV-infected patients with sputum culture–positive and AFB-positive tuberculosis may present with a normal chest radiograph. Thus, in a patient with HIV infection, the finding of a normal chest radiograph does not rule out the diagnosis of pulmonary tuberculosis. An additional consideration is that, among relatively severely immunosuppressed AIDS patients in Europe and North America, *M. avium* complex disease is more common than tuberculosis, usually presenting as a disseminated disease without pulmonary parenchymal involvement.

Adjunctive Diagnostic Tests A number of methods have been evaluated as adjuncts to standard laboratory diagnosis. The most thoroughly investigated is serologic diagnosis based on detection of antibody to a variety of mycobacterial antigens. However, tests with most of the target antigens have a low predictive value when used in a population with a presumably low probability of disease. Tests aimed at detection of mycobacterial antigen by serologic methods have generally not been sufficiently sensitive to be useful. Nonspecific tests, such as the measurement of adenine deaminase in pleural fluid, have been evaluated but have not gained acceptance.

℞ **TREATMENT** Chemotherapy for tuberculosis became possible with the discovery of streptomycin in the mid-1940s. Randomized clinical trials clearly indicated that the administration of streptomycin to patients with chronic tuberculosis reduced mortality and led to cure in the majority of cases. However, monotherapy with streptomycin was frequently associated with the development of resistance to streptomycin and the attendant failure of treatment. With the discovery of para-aminosalicylic acid (PAS) and isoniazid, it became axiomatic that cure of tuberculosis required the concomitant administration of at least two agents to which the organism was susceptible. Furthermore, early clinical trials demonstrated that a long period of treatment—i.e., 12 to 24 months—was required to prevent the recurrence of tuberculosis.

The introduction of rifampin in the early 1970s heralded the era of effective short-course chemotherapy, with a treatment duration of <12 months. The discovery that pyrazinamide, which was first used in the 1950s, augmented the potency of isoniazid/rifampin regimens led to the use of a 6-month course of this triple-drug regimen as standard therapy.

Drugs Five major drugs are considered the first-line agents for the treatment of tuberculosis: isoniazid, rifampin, pyrazinamide, ethambutol, and streptomycin (Table 169-1). The first four, which are usually given orally, are well absorbed, with peak serum levels at 2 to 4 h and nearly complete elimination within 24 h. These agents are recommended on the basis of their bactericidal activity (ability to rapidly reduce the number of viable organisms), their sterilizing activity (ability to kill all bacilli and thus sterilize the affected organ, measured in terms of the ability to prevent relapses), and their low rate of induction of drug resistance. Rifapentine and rifabutin, two drugs related to rifampin, are also available in the United States. →*For a detailed discussion of the drugs used for the treatment of tuberculosis, see Chap. 168.*

Because of a lower degree of efficacy and a higher degree of intolerability and toxicity, a number of second-line drugs are used only for the treatment of patients with tuberculosis resistant to first-line drugs. Included in this group are the injectable drugs kanamycin, amikacin, and capreomycin and the oral agents ethionamide, cycloserine, and PAS. Recently, quinolone antibiotics have become the most commonly used second-line drugs. Of available agents, ofloxacin is the most widely used, but levofloxacin and sparfloxacin are the most active, although the latter drug is associated with high rates of photosensitization. Other second-line drugs include clofazimine, amithiozone (thiacetazone, widely used with isoniazid in less wealthy countries but not marketed in North America or Europe), and amoxicillin/clavulanic acid.

Regimens Short-course regimens are divided into an initial or bactericidal phase and a continuation or sterilizing phase. During the initial phase, the majority of the tubercle bacilli are killed, symptoms resolve, and the patient becomes noninfectious. The continuation phase is required to eliminate semidormant "persisters."

The treatment regimen of choice for virtually all forms of tuberculosis in both adults and children consists of a 2-month initial phase of isoniazid, rifampin, and pyrazinamide followed by a 4-month continuation phase of isoniazid and rifampin (Table 169-2). Except for patients who seem unlikely on epidemiologic grounds to be initially infected with a drug-resistant strain, ethambutol (or streptomycin)

Table 169-1 Dosage Recommendations for Initial Treatment of Tuberculosis in Adults[a]

Drug	Dosage	
	Daily	Thrice Weekly[b]
Isoniazid	5 mg/kg, max. 300 mg	15 mg/kg, max. 900 mg
Rifampin	10 mg/kg, max. 600 mg	10 mg/kg, max. 600 mg
Pyrazinamide	15–30 mg/kg, max. 2 g	50–70 mg/kg, max. 3 g
Ethambutol	15–25 mg/kg	25–30 mg/kg
Streptomycin	15 mg/kg, max. 1 g	25–30 mg/kg, max. 1.5 g

[a] Dosages for children are similar, except that some authorities recommend higher doses of isoniazid (10–20 mg/kg daily; 20–40 mg/kg intermittent) and rifampin (10–20 mg/kg).
[b] Dosages for twice-weekly administration are the same, except for pyrazinamide (maximum, 4 g/d) and ethambutol (50 mg/kg).
SOURCE: Based on recommendations of the American Thoracic Society, Am J Respir Crit Care Med 149:1359, 1994, and the Centers for Disease Control, 1994.

Table 169-2 Recommended Regimens for the Treatment of Tuberculosis

Indication	Initial Phase		Continuation Phase	
	Duration, Months	Drugs	Duration, Months	Drugs
New smear- or culture-positive case	2	HRZE[a]	4	HR[a]
New culture-negative case	2	HRZE[a]	2 (or 4)	HR[a]
Pregnancy[b]	2	HRE	7	HR
Failure and relapse[c]	—	—	—	—
Standardized re-treatment (susceptibility testing unavailable)	3	HRZES[d]	5	HRE
Resistance to H + R	Throughout (12–18)	ZE + Q + S (or another injectable agent[e])	—	—
Resistance to all first-line drugs	Throughout (24)	1 injectable agent[e] + 3 of these 4: ethionamide, cycloserine, Q, PAS	—	—
Intolerance or resistance to H	2[f]	RZE[f]	7	RE
Intolerance to R	2	HES(Z)	16	HE
Intolerance to Z	2	HRE	7	HR

[a] All drugs can be given daily or intermittently (three times weekly throughout or twice weekly after an initial phase of daily therapy).
[b] See also Table 168-1.
[c] Regimen is tailored according to the results of drug susceptibility tests.
[d] Streptomycin treatment should be discontinued after 2 months.
[e] Amikacin, kanamycin, or capreomycin. Treatment with all of these agents should be discontinued after 2 to 6 months, depending upon the patient's tolerance and response.
[f] RZE can be used throughout (for 6 months).
NOTE: H, isoniazid; R, rifampin; Z, pyrazinamide; E, ethambutol; S, streptomycin; Q, quinolone; PAS, para-aminosalicylic acid.

should be included in the regimen for the first 2 months or until the results of drug susceptibility testing become available. Treatment may be given daily throughout the course or intermittently (either three times weekly throughout the course or twice weekly following an initial phase of daily therapy). A continuation phase of once-weekly rifapentine and isoniazid appears to be effective for patients who have adhered to the initial-phase treatment and have negative sputum cultures at 2 months. Intermittent treatment is especially useful for patients whose therapy is being directly observed (see below). For patients with sputum culture–negative pulmonary tuberculosis, the duration of treatment may be reduced to a total of 4 months. Pyridoxine (10 to 25 mg/d) should be added to the regimen given to persons at high risk of vitamin deficiency (e.g., alcoholics; malnourished persons; pregnant and lactating women; and patients with conditions such as chronic renal failure, diabetes, and HIV infection or AIDS, which are also associated with neuropathy).

Lack of adherence to treatment regimens is recognized worldwide as the most important impediment to cure. Moreover, the mycobacterial strains infecting patients who do not adhere to the prescribed regimen are especially likely to develop acquired drug resistance. Both patient- and provider-related factors may affect compliance. Patient-related factors include a lack of belief that the illness is significant and/or that treatment will have a beneficial effect; the existence of concomitant medical conditions (notably substance abuse); lack of social support; and poverty, with attendant joblessness and homelessness. Provider-related factors that may promote compliance include the education and encouragement of patients, the offering of convenient clinic hours, and the provision of incentives such as bus tokens.

In addition to specific measures addressing noncompliance, two other strategic approaches are used: direct observation of treatment and provision of drugs in combined formulations. Because it is difficult to predict which patients will adhere to the recommended treatment, all patients should have their therapy directly supervised, especially during the initial phase. In the United States, personnel to supervise therapy are usually available through tuberculosis control programs of local public health departments. Supervision increases the proportion of patients completing treatment and greatly lessens the chances of relapse and acquired drug resistance. Combination products (e.g., isoniazid/rifampin and isoniazid/rifampin/pyrazinamide) are available and are strongly recommended as a means of minimizing the likelihood of prescription error and of the development of drug resistance (as the result of treatment with only one agent). In some formulations of these combination products, the bioavailability of rifampin has been found to be substandard. In North America and Europe, regulatory authorities ensure that combination products are of good quality; however, this type of monitoring cannot be assumed to take place in less affluent countries. Alternative regimens for patients who exhibit drug intolerance or adverse reactions are listed in Table 169-2. However, severe side effects prompting discontinuation of any of the first-line drugs and use of these alternative regimens are uncommon.

Monitoring the Response to Treatment Bacteriologic evaluation is the preferred method of monitoring the response to treatment for tuberculosis. Patients with pulmonary disease should have their sputum examined monthly until cultures become negative. With the recommended 6-month regimen, more than 80% of patients will have negative sputum cultures at the end of the second month of treatment. By the end of the third month, virtually all patients should be culture-negative. In some patients, especially those with extensive cavitary disease and large numbers of organisms, AFB smear conversion may follow culture conversion. This phenomenon is presumably due to the expectoration and microscopic visualization of dead bacilli. When a patient's sputum cultures remain positive at or beyond 3 months, treatment failure and drug resistance should be suspected (see below). A sputum specimen should be collected at the end of treatment to document cure. If mycobacterial cultures are not practical, then monitoring by AFB smear examination should be undertaken at 2, 5, and 6

months. Smears positive after 5 months are indicative of treatment failure.

Bacteriologic monitoring of patients with extrapulmonary tuberculosis is more difficult and often is not feasible. In these cases, the response to treatment must be assessed clinically.

Monitoring of the response to treatment during chemotherapy by serial chest radiographs is not recommended, as radiographic changes may lag behind bacteriologic response and are not highly sensitive. After the completion of treatment, neither sputum examination nor chest radiography is recommended for follow-up purposes. However, a chest radiograph may be obtained at the end of treatment and used for comparative purposes should the patient develop symptoms of recurrent tuberculosis months or years later. Patients should be instructed to report promptly for medical assessment should they develop any such symptoms.

During treatment, patients should be monitored for drug toxicity (see also Table 168-3). The most common adverse reaction of significance is hepatitis. Patients should be carefully educated about the signs and symptoms of drug-induced hepatitis (e.g., dark urine, loss of appetite) and should be instructed to discontinue treatment promptly and see their health care provider should these symptoms occur. Although biochemical monitoring is not routinely recommended, all adult patients should undergo baseline assessment of liver function (e.g., measurement of levels of hepatic aminotransferases and serum bilirubin). Older patients, those with histories of hepatic disease, and those using alcohol daily should be monitored especially closely (i.e., monthly), with repeated measurements of aminotransferases, during the initial phase of treatment. Up to 20% of patients have small increases in aspartate aminotransferase (up to three times the upper limit of normal) that are accompanied by no symptoms and are of no consequence. For patients with symptomatic hepatitis and those with marked (five- to sixfold) elevations in aspartate aminotransferase, treatment should be stopped and drugs reintroduced one at a time after liver function has returned to normal.

Hypersensitivity reactions usually require the discontinuation of all drugs and rechallenge to determine which agent is the culprit. Because of the variety of regimens available, it is usually not necessary—although it is possible—to desensitize patients. Hyperuricemia and arthralgia caused by pyrazinamide can usually be managed by the administration of acetylsalicylic acid; however, pyrazinamide treatment should be stopped if the patient develops gouty arthritis. Individuals who develop autoimmune thrombocytopenia secondary to rifampin therapy should not receive the drug thereafter. Similarly, the occurrence of optic neuritis with ethambutol and the development of eighth-nerve damage with streptomycin are indications for permanent discontinuation of these respective drugs. Other common manifestations of drug intolerance, such as pruritus and gastrointestinal upset, can generally be managed without the interruption of therapy.

Treatment Failure and Relapse As stated above, treatment failure should be suspected when a patient's sputum cultures remain positive after 3 months or when AFB smears remain positive after 5 months. In the management of such patients, it is imperative that the current isolate be tested for susceptibility to first- and second-line agents. When the results of susceptibility testing are expected to become available within a few weeks, changes in the regimen can be postponed until that time. However, if the patient's clinical condition is deteriorating, an earlier change in regimen may be indicated. A cardinal rule in the latter situation is always to add more than one drug at a time to a failing regimen: at least two and preferably three drugs that have never been used should be added. The patient may continue to take isoniazid and rifampin along with these new agents pending the results of susceptibility tests.

The mycobacterial strains infecting patients who experience a relapse after apparently successful treatment are less likely to have acquired drug resistance (see below) than are strains from patients in whom treatment has failed. However, if the regimen administered initially does not contain rifampin (and thus is not a short-course regimen), the probability of isoniazid resistance is high. Acquired resistance is uncommon among strains from patients who relapse after completing a short course of therapy. However, it is prudent to begin the treatment of all relapses with all five first-line drugs pending the results of susceptibility testing. In less affluent countries and other settings where facilities for culture and drug susceptibility testing are not available, a standard regimen should be used in all instances of relapse and treatment failure (Table 169-2).

Adjunctive Glucocorticoid Therapy The use of glucocorticoids for adjunctive treatment of tuberculosis is justified by their potent anti-inflammatory activity in a disease where host response plays a major role. There is a sound basis for using glucocorticoids in tuberculous meningitis and pericarditis to hasten clinical improvement (see above). Long-term benefits are limited to reduced mortality in effusive-constrictive pericarditis and decreased neurologic sequelae in meningitis. Studies have indicated that the usefulness of these agents in pleuritis may be less important than previously thought. There is not yet conclusive evidence that glucocorticoids produce benefits in patients with acute life-threatening pulmonary tuberculosis, including ARDS. In general, depending upon the urgency and severity of clinical conditions, prednisone may be administered at a daily dose of 20 to 60 mg for up to 6 weeks. In meningitis, dexamethasone (up to 12 mg/d) is the preferred drug; therapy continues for 4 to 6 weeks, with gradual tapering of the dose after the first 2 weeks. Rifampin interaction with glucocorticoids, resulting in accelerated metabolism and potential adrenal crisis, must be taken into account. Caution should be exercised in the use of glucocorticoids in HIV-infected patients.

Drug-Resistant Tuberculosis Strains of *M. tuberculosis* resistant to individual drugs arise by spontaneous point mutations in the mycobacterial genome, which occur at low but predictable rates. Because there is no cross-resistance among the commonly used drugs, the probability that a strain will be resistant to two drugs is the product of the probabilities of resistance to each drug and thus is low. The development of drug-resistant tuberculosis is invariably the result of monotherapy—i.e., the failure of the health care provider to prescribe at least two drugs to which tubercle bacilli are susceptible or of the patient to take properly prescribed therapy.

Drug-resistant tuberculosis may be either primary or acquired. *Primary* drug resistance is that in a strain infecting a patient who has not previously been treated. *Acquired* resistance develops during treatment with an inappropriate regimen. In North America and Europe, rates of primary resistance are generally low, and isoniazid resistance is most common. In the United States, while isoniazid resistance was stable at about 8% in 1993 through 1996, rates of MDR tuberculosis were declining. Resistance rates are higher among foreign-born and HIV-infected patients. Worldwide, MDR tuberculosis is a serious problem in some regions, especially in the former USSR and parts of Asia. As noted above, drug-resistant tuberculosis can be prevented by adherence to the principles of sound therapy: the inclusion of at least two bactericidal drugs to which the organism is susceptible (in practice, four drugs are commonly given in the initial phase) and the verification that patients complete the prescribed course.

Although the 6-month regimen described in Table 169-2 is highly effective for patients with initial isoniazid-resistant disease, it is prudent to extend treatment to 9 months and to include ethambutol throughout. Alternatively, rifampin, pyrazinamide, and ethambutol may be given for 6 months. For disease with high-level isoniazid resistance, isoniazid probably does not contribute to a successful outcome and can be omitted. MDR tuberculosis is more difficult to manage than is disease caused by a drug-susceptible organism, especially because resistance to other first-line drugs as well as to isoniazid and rifampin is common. For strains resistant to isoniazid and rifampin, combinations of ethambutol, pyrazinamide, and streptomycin (or, for those resistant to streptomycin as well, another injectable agent such as amikacin), given for 12 to 18 months in all and for at least 9 months after sputum culture conversion, may be effective. Many authorities would add a quinolone antibiotic to this regimen. For patients with bacilli resistant to all of the first-line agents, cure may be attained with a combination of four second-line drugs, including one injectable agent

(Table 169-2). The optimal duration of treatment in this situation is not known; however, a duration of up to 24 months is recommended. For patients with localized disease and sufficient pulmonary reserve, lobectomy or pneumonectomy may be helpful. Because the management of patients with MDR tuberculosis is complicated by both social and medical factors, care of these patients should be restricted to specialists and tuberculosis control programs.

Special Clinical Situations Although comparative clinical trials of treatment for extrapulmonary tuberculosis are limited, the available evidence indicates that most forms of disease can be treated with the 6-month regimen recommended for patients with pulmonary disease. The American Academy of Pediatrics recommends that children with bone and joint tuberculosis, tuberculous meningitis, or miliary tuberculosis receive a minimum of 12 months of treatment.

Treatment for tuberculosis may be complicated by underlying medical problems that require special consideration (see also Table 168-1). As a rule, patients with chronic renal failure should not receive aminoglycosides and should receive ethambutol only if serum levels can be monitored. Isoniazid, rifampin, and pyrazinamide may be given in the usual doses in cases of mild to moderate renal failure, but the dosages of isoniazid and pyrazinamide should be reduced for all patients with severe renal failure except those undergoing hemodialysis. Patients with hepatic disease pose a special problem because of the hepatotoxicity of isoniazid, rifampin, and pyrazinamide. Patients with severe hepatic disease may be treated with ethambutol and streptomycin and, if required, with isoniazid and rifampin under close supervision. The use of pyrazinamide by patients with liver failure should be avoided. Silicotuberculosis necessitates the extension of therapy by at least 2 months. Patients with HIV infection or AIDS appear to respond well to standard 6-month therapy, although treatment may need to be prolonged if the response is suboptimal. Rifampin, a powerful inducer of hepatic microsomal enzymes, shortens the half-life of HIV protease inhibitors and therefore is contraindicated for patients receiving these drugs; instead, these individuals should be given rifabutin (150 mg/d or 300 mg twice weekly) with either indinavir or nelfinavir. Studies have shown that total systemic drug exposure, especially for rifampin, is reduced in HIV-infected patients because of decreased bioavailability secondary to malabsorption. The clinical importance of this phenomenon remains unclear.

The regimen of choice for pregnant women (see also Table 168-1) is 9 months of treatment with isoniazid and rifampin supplemented by ethambutol for the first 2 months. When required, pyrazinamide may be given, although there are no data concerning its safety in pregnancy. Streptomycin is contraindicated because it is known to cause eighth-cranial-nerve damage in the fetus. Treatment for tuberculosis is not a contraindication to breast feeding; most of the drugs administered will be present in small quantities in breast milk, albeit at concentrations far too low to provide any therapeutic or prophylactic benefit to the child.

PREVENTION By far the best way to prevent tuberculosis is to diagnose infectious cases rapidly and administer appropriate treatment until cure. Additional strategies include BCG vaccination and preventive chemotherapy.

BCG Vaccination BCG was derived from an attenuated strain of *M. bovis* and was first administered to humans in 1921. Many BCG vaccines are available worldwide; all are derived from the original strain, but the vaccines vary in efficacy. In fact, estimates of efficacy from randomized, placebo-controlled trials have ranged from 80% to nil. A similar range of efficacy was found in recent observational studies (case-control, historic cohort, and cross-sectional) in areas where infants are vaccinated at birth. These studies also found higher rates of efficacy in the protection of infants and young children from relatively serious forms of tuberculosis, such as tuberculous meningitis and miliary tuberculosis.

BCG vaccine is safe and rarely causes serious complications. The local tissue response begins 2 to 3 weeks after vaccination, with scar formation and healing within 3 months. Side effects—most commonly, ulceration at the vaccination site and regional lymphadenitis—occur in 1 to 10% of vaccinated persons. Some vaccine strains have caused osteomyelitis in approximately one case per million doses administered. Disseminated BCG infection and death have occurred in 1 to 10 cases per 10 million doses administered, although this problem is restricted almost exclusively to persons with impaired immunity, such as children with severe combined immunodeficiency syndrome (SCIDS) or adults with HIV infection. BCG vaccination induces PPD reactivity, which tends to wane with time. The presence or size of PPD skin-test reactions after vaccination does not predict the degree of protection afforded.

BCG vaccine is recommended for routine use at birth in countries with high tuberculosis prevalence. However, because of the low risk of transmission of tuberculosis in the United States and the unreliable protection afforded by BCG, the vaccine has never been recommended for general use in the United States. Currently, vaccination should be considered for PPD-negative infants and children who reside in settings where the likelihood of *M. tuberculosis* transmission and subsequent infection is high, provided no other measures can be implemented (e.g., removing the child from the source of infection). BCG vaccination may also be considered for health care workers who are employed in settings where the risk of infection by MDR strains is high despite implementation of comprehensive tuberculosis control measures. The CDC has recommended that HIV-infected adults and children not receive BCG vaccine, although the WHO has recommended that asymptomatic HIV-infected children residing in tuberculosis-endemic areas receive BCG.

Treatment of Latent Tuberculosis Infection A major component of tuberculosis control in the United States is the treatment of selected persons with latent tuberculosis infection to prevent active disease. This intervention (formerly called preventive chemotherapy or chemoprophylaxis) is based on the results of a large number of randomized, placebo-controlled clinical trials demonstrating that a 6- to 12-month course of isoniazid reduces the risk of active tuberculosis in infected people by $\geq$90%. Analysis of available data indicates that the optimal duration of treatment is 9 to 10 months. In the absence of reinfection, the protective effect is believed to be lifelong. Clinical trials have also shown that isoniazid reduces rates of tuberculosis among PPD-positive persons with HIV infection. Studies in HIV-infected patients have demonstrated the effectiveness of a shorter course of rifampin-based treatment.

In most cases, candidates for treatment of latent tuberculosis (Table 169-3) are identified by PPD skin testing of persons in defined high-risk groups. For skin testing, 5 tuberculin units of polysorbate-stabilized PPD should be injected intradermally into the volar surface of the forearm (Mantoux method). Multipuncture tests, which may be useful for screening large populations, are not recommended for this purpose; any positive reaction to a multipuncture test must be confirmed by Mantoux testing. Reactions are read at 48 to 72 h as the transverse diameter in millimeters of induration; the diameter of erythema is not considered. In some persons, PPD reactivity wanes with time but can be recalled by a second skin test administered 1 week or more after the first (i.e., two-step testing). For persons undergoing periodic PPD skin testing, such as health care workers and individuals admitted to long-term-care institutions, initial two-step testing may preclude subsequent misclassification of persons with boosted reactions as PPD converters.

The cutoff for a positive skin test (and thus for treatment) is related both to the probability that the reaction represents true infection and to the likelihood that the individual, if truly infected, will develop tuberculosis (Table 169-3). Thus positive reactions for close contacts of infectious cases, persons with HIV infection, and previously untreated persons whose chest radiograph is consistent with healed tuberculosis are defined as an area of induration 5 mm in diameter. A

Table 169-3 Tuberculin Reaction Size and Treatment of Latent Tuberculosis Infection

Risk Group	Tuberculin Reaction, mm
HIV-infected persons	$\geq$5
Close contacts of tuberculosis patients	$\geq$5[a]
Persons with fibrotic lesions on chest radiography	$\geq$5
Recently infected persons ($\leq$2 years)	$\geq$10
Persons with high-risk medical conditions[b]	$\geq$10
High-risk group, <35 years of age[c]	$\geq$10
Low-risk group, <35 years of age[d]	$\geq$15

[a] Tuberculin-negative contacts, especially children, should receive prophylaxis for 2 to 3 months after contact ends and should then be retested with PPD. Those whose results remain negative should discontinue prophylaxis. HIV-infected contacts should receive a full course of treatment regardless of PPD results.

[b] Includes diabetes mellitus, prolonged therapy with systemic glucocorticoids, other immunosuppressive therapy, some hematologic and reticuloendothelial diseases, injection drug use (with HIV seronegativity), end-stage renal disease, and clinical situations associated with rapid weight loss.

[c] Includes persons born in high-prevalence countries, members of medically underserved low-income populations, and residents of long-term-care facilities.

[d] Decision to treat should be based on individual considerations of risk/benefit.

10-mm cutoff is used to define positive reactions in most other at-risk persons. For persons with a very low risk of developing tuberculosis if infected, a cutoff of 15 mm is used. Persons with a history of BCG vaccination may receive treatment, especially if BCG was given many years before.

Some PPD-negative individuals are also candidates for treatment. Infants and children who have come into contact with infectious cases should be treated and should have a repeat skin test 2 or 3 months after contact ends. Those whose test results remain negative should discontinue treatment. HIV-infected persons who have been exposed to an infectious tuberculosis patient should receive treatment regardless of the PPD test result.

Isoniazid is administered at a daily dose of 5 mg/kg (up to 300 mg/d) for 9 months. On the basis of cost-benefit analyses, a 6-month period of treatment has been recommended in the past and may be considered for HIV-negative adults with normal chest radiographs when financial considerations are important. When supervised treatment is desirable and feasible, isoniazid may be given at a dose of 15 mg/kg (up to 900 mg) twice weekly. There are two recommended alternative regimens for adults: 2 months of daily rifampin plus pyrazinamide and 4 months of daily rifampin. Although the 2-month regimen may be associated with increased drug intolerance, it may be useful in situations where long courses of isoniazid have not been feasible (e.g., jails). Either regimen should be considered for persons who are likely to have been infected with an isoniazid-resistant strain.

Contraindications to treatment with isoniazid and pyrazinamide include active liver disease. Since the major adverse reaction to these drugs is hepatitis, persons at increased risk of toxicity (e.g., those abusing alcohol daily and those with a history of liver disease) should undergo baseline and then monthly assessment of liver function during treatment. All patients should be carefully educated about hepatitis and instructed to discontinue use of the drug immediately should any symptoms develop. Moreover, patients should be seen and questioned monthly during therapy about adverse reactions and should be given no more than 1 month's supply of drug at each visit.

It may be more difficult to ensure compliance when treating persons with latent infection than when treating those with active tuberculosis. If family members of active cases are being treated, compliance and monitoring may be easier. When feasible, twice-weekly supervised therapy may increase the likelihood of completion. As in active cases, the provision of incentives may also be helpful.

BASICS OF CONTROL The highest priority in any tuberculosis control program is the prompt detection of cases and the provision of directly observed short-course chemotherapy to all tuberculosis patients, with emphasis on the cure of sputum smear–positive cases. In addition, in low-prevalence countries with adequate resources, screening of high-risk groups (such as immigrants from high-prevalence countries and HIV-seropositive persons) is recommended. Identification of active cases of tuberculosis should be followed by treatment. PPD-positive high-risk persons should be treated for latent infection. Contact investigation is an important component of efficient tuberculosis control. In the United States, a great deal of attention has been given to the transmission of tuberculosis (particularly in association with HIV infection) in institutional settings such as hospitals, homeless shelters, and prisons. Measures to limit such transmission include respiratory isolation of persons with suspected tuberculosis until they are proven to be noninfectious (i.e., by sputum AFB smear negativity), proper ventilation in rooms of patients with infectious tuberculosis, use of ultraviolet lights in areas of increased risk of tuberculosis transmission, and periodic screening of personnel who may come into contact with known or unsuspected cases of tuberculosis. In the past, radiographic surveys, especially those conducted with portable equipment and miniature films, were advocated for case finding. Today, however, the prevalence of tuberculosis in industrialized countries is sufficiently low that "mass miniature radiography" is not cost-effective. As mentioned above, current recommendations for the prevention and treatment of tuberculosis in HIV-infected individuals have been published by the CDC.

In high-prevalence countries, tuberculosis control programs should be based on the following key elements: (1) case detection through microscopic examination of sputum from patients who present to health care facilities with cough of >3 weeks' duration; (2) administration of standard short-course chemotherapy to all sputum smear–positive patients, with direct observation of drug ingestion; (3) establishment and maintenance of a system of regular drug supply; and (4) establishment and maintenance of an effective surveillance and treatment-monitoring system allowing an analysis of treatment outcomes (e.g., cure, completion of treatment without bacteriologic proof of cure, death, treatment failure, and default) in all cases registered.

BIBLIOGRAPHY

BERTHET FX et al: Attenuation of virulence by disruption of the *Mycobacterium tuberculosis erp* gene. Science 282:759, 1998

BREIMAN RF et al: Proceedings of the International Symposium on Tuberculosis Vaccine Development and Evaluation. Clin Infect Dis 30(Suppl 3):S199-322, 2000

CENTERS FOR DISEASE CONTROL AND PREVENTION: Guidelines for preventing the transmission of *Mycobacterium tuberculosis* in health-care facilities. MMWR 43(RR-13):1, 1994

———: Prevention and treatment of tuberculosis among patients infected with human immunodeficiency virus: Principles of therapy and revised recommendations. MMWR 47(RR-20):1, 1998

COLE ST et al: Deciphering the biology of *Mycobacterium tuberculosis* from the complete genome sequence. Nature 392:537, 1998

COLLINS DM: In search of tuberculosis virulence genes. Trends Microbiol 4:426, 1996

CROFTON J et al: *Guidelines for the Management of Drug-Resistant Tuberculosis*. Geneva, World Health Organization, 1997

DOOLEY DP et al: Adjunctive corticosteroid therapy for tuberculosis: A critical reappraisal of the literature. Clin Infect Dis 25:872, 1997

DYE C et al: Global burden of tuberculosis: Estimated incidence, prevalence, and mortality by country. JAMA 282:677, 1999

ELLNER JJ: The immune response in human tuberculosis—implications for tuberculosis control. J Infect Dis 176:1351, 1997

MOORE MM et al: Trends in drug-resistant tuberculosis in the United States, 1993–1996. JAMA 278:833, 1997

O'BRIEN RJ: Preventive therapy, in *Clinical Tuberculosis*, 2d ed, PDO Davies (ed). London, Chapman & Hall, 1998, pp 397–416

PABLOS-MÉNDEZ A et al: Global surveillance for antituberculosis-drug resistance, 1994–1997. N Engl J Med 338:1641, 1998

RAVIGLIONE MC et al: Assessment of worldwide tuberculosis control. Lancet 350:624, 1997

SCHLOSSBERG D: *Tuberculosis and Nontuberculous Mycobacterial Infections*, 4th ed. Philadelphia, Saunders, 1999

SCHOREY JS et al: A macrophage invasion mechanism of pathogenic mycobacteria. Science 277:1091, 1997

VALWAY SE et al: An outbreak involving extensive transmission of a virulent strain of *Mycobacterium tuberculosis*. N Engl J Med 338:633, 1998

WORLD HEALTH ORGANIZATION: *Treatment of Tuberculosis. Guidelines for National Programmes*. Geneva, World Health Organization, 1997

170

Robert H. Gelber

LEPROSY (HANSEN'S DISEASE)

Leprosy, first described in ancient Indian texts from the sixth century B.C., is a nonfatal, chronic infectious disease caused by *Mycobacterium leprae*, whose clinical manifestations are largely confined to the skin, peripheral nervous system, upper respiratory tract, eyes, and testes. The unique tropism of *M. leprae* for peripheral nerves (from large nerve trunks to microscopic dermal nerves) and certain immunologically mediated reactional states are the major causes of morbidity in leprosy. The propensity of the disease, when untreated, to result in certain characteristic deformities and the recognition in most cultures that the disease is communicable from person to person have resulted historically in a profound social stigma. Today, with early diagnosis and the institution of appropriate and effective antimicrobial therapy, patients can lead productive lives in the community, and deformities and other visible manifestations can largely be prevented.

ETIOLOGY *M. leprae* is an obligate intracellular bacillus (0.3 to 1 μm wide and 1 to 8 μm long) that is acid-fast, indistinguishable microscopically from other mycobacteria, ideally detected in tissue sections by a modified Fite stain, and without demonstrable strain variability. *M. leprae* produces no known toxins and is well adapted to penetrate and reside within macrophages, yet it may survive outside the body for 7 to 10 days. In untreated patients, only ~1% of *M. leprae* organisms are viable. The morphologic index, a measure of the number of acid-fast bacilli (AFB) in skin scrapings that stain uniformly bright, correlates with viability. The bacteriologic index, a logarithmic-scaled measure of the density of *M. leprae* in the dermis, may be as high as 4+ to 6+ in untreated patients, falling by one unit per year during effective therapy; the rate of fall is independent of the relative potency of effective antimicrobial therapy. A rising bacteriologic or morphologic index suggests relapse and perhaps—if the patient is being treated—drug resistance; the latter possibility can be confirmed or excluded in the mouse model.

The genome of *M. leprae* is only 3 million base pairs, two-thirds as large as that of *M. tuberculosis*. The bacterium's complex cell wall has a peptidoglycan backbone, which is linked to arabinogalactan and mycolic acids. Lipoarabinomannan is a key component of the cell membrane, and the outer capsule contains large amounts of an *M. leprae*–specific phenolic glycolipid (PGL-1), which is detected in serologic tests. In addition, highly conserved, usually immunogenic heat-shock proteins containing *M. leprae*–specific and mycobacterial cross-reactive epitopes are found in the cytoplasm and cell wall.

Among the mycobacteria, *M. leprae* is unique in exhibiting dopa oxidase activity and an acid-fastness that is pyridine-extractable. Although it was the first bacterium to be etiologically associated with human disease, *M. leprae* remains one of the few bacterial species that still has not been cultivated on artificial medium or tissue culture. The multiplication of *M. leprae* in mouse footpads (albeit limited, with a doubling time of ~2 weeks) has provided a means to evaluate antimicrobial agents, monitor clinical trials, and screen vaccines. *M. leprae* grows best in cooler tissues (the skin, peripheral nerves, anterior chamber of the eye, upper respiratory tract, and testes), sparing warmer areas of the skin (the axilla, groin, scalp, and midline of the back).

EPIDEMIOLOGY **Demographics** Leprosy is almost exclusively a disease of the developing world, affecting areas of Asia, Africa, Latin America, and the Pacific. While Africa has the highest disease prevalence, Asia has the most cases. More than 80% of the world's cases occur in a few countries: India, China, Myanmar, Indonesia, Brazil, and Nigeria. Within endemic locales, the distribution of leprosy is quite uneven, with areas of high prevalence bordering on areas with little or no disease. In Brazil the majority of cases occur in the Amazon basin, while in Mexico leprosy is mostly confined to western states. Except as imported cases, leprosy is largely absent from the United States, Canada, and northwestern Europe. In the United States, ~4000 persons have leprosy and 100 to 200 new cases are reported annually, most of them in California, Texas, New York, and Hawaii among immigrants from Mexico, Southeast Asia, the Philippines, and the Caribbean.

The global prevalence of leprosy is difficult to assess, given that many of the locales with high prevalence lack a significant medical or public health infrastructure. Estimates range from 1.5 to 8 million affected individuals. The lower estimate includes only persons who have not completed chemotherapy, excluding those who may be physically or psychologically damaged from leprosy and who may yet relapse or develop certain immune-mediated reactions; the higher figure includes patients whose infections probably are already cured and many who have no leprosy-related deformity or disability. Although the figures on the worldwide prevalence of leprosy are debatable, it is generally agreed that the annual incidence of new cases is stable and approximates 600,000.

Leprosy is associated with poverty and rural residence. It appears not to be associated with AIDS, perhaps because of leprosy's long incubation period. Most people appear to be naturally immune to leprosy and do not develop disease manifestations following exposure. The time of peak onset is in the second and third decades of life. The most severe form, lepromatous leprosy, is twice as common among men as among women and is rarely encountered in children. The frequency of the polar forms of leprosy (see "Clinical, Histologic, and Immunologic Spectrum," below) in different countries varies widely and may in part be genetically determined; certain HLA associations are known for both lepromatous and tuberculoid leprosy (see below). In India and Africa, 90% of cases are tuberculoid; in Southeast Asia, 50% are lepromatous and 50% tuberculoid; and in Mexico, 90% are lepromatous.

Transmission   *M. leprae* causes disease primarily in humans. However, in Texas and Louisiana, 15% of nine-banded armadillos are infected, and armadillo contact occasionally results in human disease. Following intravenous experimental inoculation of *M. leprae*, 60% of armadillos develop a heavy disseminated infection of the liver, spleen, lymph nodes, and skin; these experimental animals have been the source of vast quantities of *M. leprae* organisms for laboratory and clinical research.

The route of transmission of leprosy remains uncertain and may be multiple; nasal droplet infection, contact with infected soil, and even insect vectors have been considered the prime candidates. Aerosolized *M. leprae* can cause infection in immunosuppressed mice, and a sneeze from an untreated lepromatous patient may contain $>10^{10}$ AFB. Furthermore, both IgA antibody to *M. leprae* and genes of *M. leprae*—demonstrable by polymerase chain reaction (PCR)—have been found in the nose of individuals without signs of leprosy from endemic areas and in 19% of occupational contacts of lepromatous patients.

Several lines of evidence implicate soil transmission of leprosy. (1) In endemic countries such as India, leprosy is primarily a rural and not an urban disease. (2) *M. leprae* products have been demonstrated to be resident in soil in endemic locales. (3) Direct dermal inoculation (e.g., during tattooing) may transmit *M. leprae*, and common sites of leprosy in children are the buttocks and thighs, suggesting that microinoculation of infected soil may transmit the disease.

Evidence for insect vectors of leprosy includes the demonstration that bedbugs and mosquitoes in the vicinity of leprosaria regularly harbor *M. leprae* and that experimentally infected mosquitoes can transmit infection to mice. Skin-to-skin contact is generally not considered an important route of transmission.

In endemic countries, ~50% of leprosy patients have a history of intimate contact with an infected person (often a household member),

while, for unknown reasons, leprosy patients in nonendemic locales can identify such contact only 10% of the time. Moreover, household contact with an infected lepromatous case carries an eventual risk of disease acquisition of ~10% in endemic areas as opposed to only 1% in nonendemic locales. Contact with a tuberculoid case carries a very low risk. Physicians and nurses caring for leprosy patients and the co-workers of these patients are not at risk for leprosy.

CLINICAL,   HISTOLOGIC,   AND   IMMUNOLOGIC SPECTRUM   The incubation period prior to manifestation of clinical disease can vary between 2 and 40 years, although it is generally 5 to 7 years in duration. Leprosy presents as a spectrum of clinical manifestations that have pathologic and immunologic counterparts. The spectrum from polar tuberculoid (TT) to borderline tuberculoid (BT) to borderline lepromatous (BL) to polar lepromatous (LL) disease is associated with an evolution from localized to more generalized disease manifestations, an increasing bacterial load, and loss of *M. leprae*–specific cellular immunity. Where a patient presents on the clinical spectrum largely determines prognosis, complications, reactional states, and the intensity of antimicrobial therapy required.

Tuberculoid Leprosy   At the less severe end of the spectrum is tuberculoid leprosy, which encompasses TT and BT disease. In general, these forms of leprosy result in symptoms confined to the skin and peripheral nerves. The initial lesion of tuberculoid leprosy is often a hypopigmented macule that is sharply demarcated and hypesthetic. Later, the lesions enlarge by peripheral spread, and the margins become elevated and circinate or gyrate. The central area in turn becomes atrophic and depressed. Fully developed lesions are densely anesthetic and devoid of the normal skin organs (sweat glands and hair follicles). Patients eventually have one or more asymmetrically distributed, hypopigmented, anesthetic, nonpruritic, well-defined macules, often with an erythematous or raised border (Fig. 170-1). Skin lesions of tuberculoid leprosy vary in diameter from one to several centimeters and are often dry, scaly, and anhidrotic. Tuberculoid leprosy patients may also have asymmetric enlargement of one or a few peripheral nerves. Indeed, leprosy and certain rare hereditary neuropathies are the only human diseases associated with peripheral-nerve enlargement. Although any peripheral nerve may be enlarged (including small digital and supraclavicular nerves), those most commonly affected are the ulnar, posterior auricular, peroneal, and posttibial nerves, with associated hypesthesia and myopathy. At times, tuberculoid leprosy may present with only nerve-trunk involvement with no skin lesions; in such cases it is termed *neural leprosy*. TT leprosy may resolve spontaneously and is not associated with lepra reactions (see "Reactional States," below). BT leprosy does not heal spontaneously and may be associated with type 1 lepra reactions but not with erythema nodosum leprosum (ENL). TT leprosy is the most common form of the disease encountered in India and Africa but is virtually absent in Southeast Asia, where BT leprosy is frequent.

In TT leprosy the epidermis may be involved histologically, while

FIGURE 170-1   A skin lesion of tuberculoid leprosy: a well-demarcated, hypopigmented macule with an erythematous, slightly elevated border.

in all other forms of leprosy the epidermis and the superficial dermis are spared, with pathology confined to the deeper dermis. On hematoxylin and eosin staining, TT and BT lesions appear as well-defined noncaseating granulomas with many lymphocytes and Langhans' giant cells. In tuberculoid leprosy, T cells breach the perineurium, and destruction of Schwann cells and axons may be evident, resulting in fibrosis of the epineurium, replacement of the endoneurium with epithelial granulomas, and occasionally caseous necrosis. AFB are generally absent or few in number. Such invasion and destruction of nerves in the dermis by T cells are pathognomonic for leprosy.

Circulating lymphocytes from patients with tuberculoid leprosy readily recognize *M. leprae* and its constituent proteins, and patients have positive lepromin skin tests (see "Diagnosis" below). In tuberculoid leprosy tissue, there is a 2:1 predominance of helper CD4+ over CD8+ T lymphocytes. Tuberculoid tissues are rich in the mRNAs of the proinflammatory T_H1 family of cytokines: interleukin (IL) 2, interferon γ (IFN-γ), and IL-12; in contrast, IL-4, IL-5, and IL-10 mRNAs are scarce.

Lepromatous Leprosy At the more severe end of the leprosy spectrum is lepromatous disease, which encompasses the LL and BL forms. The initial skin lesions of lepromatous leprosy are skin-colored or slightly erythematous papules or nodules. In time, individual lesions grow in diameter up to 2 cm; new papules and nodules then appear and may coalesce. Patients later present with symmetrically distributed skin nodules, raised plaques, or diffuse dermal infiltration, which, when on the face, results in leonine facies. Late manifestations include loss of eyebrows (initially the lateral margins only; **see Plate IID-56**) and eyelashes, pendulous earlobes, and dry scaling skin, particularly on the feet. Almost exclusively found in western Mexico and the Caribbean is a form of lepromatous leprosy without visible skin lesions but with diffuse dermal infiltration and a demonstrably thickened dermis, termed *diffuse lepromatosis*. In lepromatous leprosy, nerve enlargement and damage tend to be symmetric, result from actual bacillary invasion, and are more insidious but ultimately more extensive than in tuberculoid leprosy. Patients with LL leprosy have symmetric acral distal peripheral neuropathy and a tendency toward symmetric nerve-trunk enlargement. They may also have signs and symptoms related to involvement of the upper respiratory tract, the anterior chamber of the eye, and the testes.

Dermatopathology in lepromatous leprosy is confined to the dermis and particularly affects the dermal appendages. Histologically, the dermis characteristically contains highly vacuolated cells (*foam cells*) otherwise found only in certain lipid-storage disorders. Indeed, on fat staining, these vacuoles are highly positive and are seen to include large amounts of *M. leprae*–associated cell wall lipids and the *M. leprae*–specific PGL-1. The dermis in lepromatous leprosy contains few lymphocytes and giant cells, and granulomas are absent. In LL leprosy, bacilli are numerous in the skin (as many as $10^9/g$), where they are often found in large clumps (*globi*), and in peripheral nerves, where they initially invade Schwann cells, resulting in foamy degenerative myelination and axonal degeneration and later in Wallerian degeneration. In addition, bacilli are plentiful in circulating blood and in all organ systems except the lungs and the central nervous system. Nevertheless, patients are afebrile, and there is no evidence of major organ system dysfunction. The dermis contains more lymphocytes and fewer AFB and exhibits less vacuolization in BL than in LL leprosy.

In untreated LL patients, lymphocytes regularly fail to recognize either *M. leprae* or its protein constituents, and lepromin skin tests are negative (see "Diagnosis," below). This loss of protective cellular immunity appears to be antigen-specific, as patients are not unusually susceptible to opportunistic infections, cancer, or AIDS and maintain delayed-type hypersensitivity to *Candida, Trichophyton*, mumps, tetanus toxoid, and even purified protein derivative of tuberculin. At times, *M. leprae*–specific anergy is reversible with effective chemotherapy. In LL tissues, there is a 2:1 ratio of CD8+ to CD4+ T lymphocytes. LL tissues demonstrate a T_H2 cytokine profile, being rich in mRNAs for IL-4, IL-5, and IL-10 and poor in those for IL-2, IFN-γ, and IL-12. It appears that cytokines mediate a protective tissue response in leprosy, as injection of IFN-γ or IL-2 into lepromatous lesions causes a loss of AFB and histopathologic conversion toward a tuberculoid pattern. Macrophages of lepromatous leprosy patients appear to be functionally intact; circulating monocytes exhibit normal microbicidal function and responsiveness to IFN-γ.

LL and BL patients may develop type 2 lepra reactions (ENL; see "Reactional States," below), while BL patients (but not LL patients) can have type 1 lepra reactions.

Reactional States Lepra reactions comprise several common immunologically mediated inflammatory states that cause considerable morbidity. Some of these reactions precede diagnosis and the institution of effective antimicrobial therapy. Indeed, these reactions may precipitate presentation for medical attention and diagnosis; others occur after the initiation of appropriate chemotherapy. In the latter circumstances, patients often lose confidence in conventional therapy, perceiving that their leprosy is worsening. Only by warning patients of the potential for these reactions and describing their manifestations can physicians treating leprosy patients ensure continued credibility.

Type 1 lepra reactions (downgrading and reversal reactions) These reactions occur in almost half of patients with borderline forms of leprosy but not in patients with polar disease. Manifestations include classic signs of inflammation within previously involved macules, papules, and plaques and, on occasion, the appearance of new skin lesions, neuritis, and (less commonly) fever—generally low-grade. The nerve trunk most commonly involved in this process is the ulnar nerve at the elbow, which may be painful and exquisitely tender. If patients with affected nerves are not treated promptly with glucocorticoids (see below), irreversible nerve damage may result in as little as 24 h. The most dramatic manifestation is footdrop, which occurs when the peroneal nerve is involved.

When type 1 lepra reactions precede the initiation of appropriate antimicrobial therapy, they are termed *downgrading reactions*, and the case becomes histologically more lepromatous; when they occur after the initiation of therapy, they are termed *reversal reactions*, and the case becomes more tuberculoid. Reversal reactions often occur in the first months or years after the initiation of therapy but may also develop several years thereafter.

Edema is the most characteristic microscopic feature of type 1 lepra lesions, whose diagnosis is primarily clinical. Reversal reactions are typified by a T_H1 cytokine profile, with an influx of CD4+ helper cells and increased levels of IFN-γ and IL-2. In addition, type 1 reactions are associated with large numbers of T cells bearing γ/∂ receptors—a unique feature of leprosy.

Type 1 lepra reactions are best treated with glucocorticoids (e.g., prednisone, initially at doses of 40 to 60 mg/d). As the inflammation subsides, the glucocorticoid dose can be tapered, but steroid therapy must be continued for at least 3 months lest recurrence supervene. Because of the myriad toxicities of prolonged glucocorticoid therapy, the indications for its initiation are strictly limited to lesions whose intense inflammation poses a threat of ulceration; lesions at cosmetically important sites, such as the face; and the presence of neuritis. Mild to moderate lepra reactions that do not meet these criteria should be tolerated and glucocorticoid treatment withheld. Thalidomide is ineffective against type 1 lepra reactions; clofazimine (200 to 300 mg/d) is of questionable benefit but in any event is far less efficacious than glucocorticoids.

Type 2 lepra reactions (ENL) ENL occurs exclusively in patients near the lepromatous end of the leprosy spectrum, affecting nearly 50% of this group. Although ENL may precede leprosy diagnosis and initiation of therapy—sometimes, in fact, prompting the diagnosis—in 90% of cases it follows the institution of chemotherapy, generally within 2 years. The most common features of ENL are crops of painful erythematous papules that resolve spontaneously in a few days to a week but may recur; malaise; and fever that can be profound. However, patients may also experience symptoms of neuritis, lymphadenitis, uveitis, orchitis, and glomerulonephritis and may develop anemia, leukocytosis, and abnormal liver function tests, particularly increased aminotransferase levels. Individual patients may have either a single bout of ENL or chronic recurrent manifestations. Bouts may be either mild or severe and generalized; in rare instances, ENL results in death.

Skin biopsy of ENL papules reveals vasculitis or panniculitis, sometimes with many lymphocytes but characteristically with polymorphonuclear leukocytes as well.

Elevated levels of circulating tumor necrosis factor (TNF) have been demonstrated in ENL; thus TNF may play a central role in the pathobiology of this syndrome. ENL is thought to be a consequence of immune complex deposition, given its T_H2 cytokine profile and its high levels of IL-6 and IL-8. However, in ENL tissue, the presence of HLA Dr framework antigen of epidermal cells—considered a marker for a delayed-type hypersensitivity response—and evidence for higher levels of IL-2 and IFN-γ than are usually seen in polar lepromatous disease suggest an alternative mechanism.

Treatment must be individualized. If ENL is mild (i.e., without fever or other organ involvement, with occasional crops of only a few skin papules), it may be treated with antipyretics alone. However, in cases with many skin lesions, fever, malaise, and other tissue involvement, brief courses (1 to 2 weeks) of glucocorticoids (initially 40 to 60 mg/d) are often effective. With or without therapy, individual inflamed papules last for ≤1 week. Successful therapy is defined by the cessation of skin lesion development and the disappearance of other systemic signs and symptoms. If, despite two courses of glucocorticoid therapy, ENL appears to be recurring and persisting, treatment with thalidomide (100 to 300 mg nightly) should be initiated, with the dose depending on the initial severity of the reaction. Because even a single dose of thalidomide administered early in pregnancy may result in severe birth defects, including phocomelia, the use of this drug in the United States for the treatment of fertile females is tightly regulated and requires informed consent, prior pregnancy testing, and maintenance of birth control measures. Although the mechanism of thalidomide's dramatic action against ENL is not entirely clear, the drug's efficacy is probably attributable to its reduction of TNF levels and IgM synthesis and its slowing of polymorphonuclear leukocyte migration. After the reaction is controlled, lower doses of thalidomide (50 to 200 mg nightly) are effective in preventing relapses of ENL. Clofazimine in high doses (300 mg nightly) has some efficacy against ENL, but its use permits only a modest reduction of the glucocorticoid dose necessary for ENL control.

Lucio's phenomenon This unusual reaction is seen exclusively in patients from the Caribbean and Mexico who have the diffuse lepromatosis form of lepromatous leprosy, most often those who are untreated. Patients with this reaction develop recurrent crops of large, sharply marginated, ulcerative lesions—particularly on the lower extremities—that may be generalized and, when so, are frequently fatal as a result of secondary infection and consequent septic bacteremia. Histologically, the lesions are characterized by ischemic necrosis of the epidermis and superficial dermis, heavy parasitism of endothelial cells with AFB, and endothelial proliferation and thrombus formation in the larger vessels of the deeper dermis. Like ENL, the Lucio reaction is probably mediated by the immune complex. Neither glucocorticoids nor thalidomide is effective against this syndrome. Optimal wound care and therapy for bacteremia are indicated. Ulcers tend to be chronic and heal poorly. In severe cases, exchange transfusion may prove useful.

Nerve abscesses Patients with various forms of leprosy, but particularly those with the BT form, may develop abscesses of nerves (most commonly the ulnar) with an adjacent cellulitic appearance of the skin. In such conditions, the affected nerve is swollen and exquisitely tender. Although glucocorticoids may reduce signs of inflammation, rapid surgical decompression is necessary to prevent irreversible sequelae.

Complications • ***The extremities*** Complications of the extremities in leprosy patients are primarily a consequence of neuropathy leading to insensitivity and myopathy. Insensitivity affects fine touch, pain, and heat receptors but generally spares position and vibration appreciation. The most commonly affected nerve trunk is the ulnar nerve at the elbow, whose involvement results in clawing of the fourth and fifth fingers, loss of dorsal interosseous musculature in the affected hand, and loss of sensation in these distributions. Median nerve involvement in leprosy impairs thumb opposition and grasp, while radial nerve dysfunction, though rare in leprosy, leads to wristdrop. Tendon transfers can restore hand function but should not be performed until 6 months after the initiation of antimicrobial therapy and the conclusion of episodes of acute neuritis.

Plantar ulceration, particularly at the metatarsal heads, is probably the most frequent complication of leprous neuropathy. Plantar ulcers may become secondarily infected and lead to adjacent cellulitis and osteomyelitis. Because of the importance and critical integrity of the normal plantar fat pad, recurrent ulceration is unfortunately common once initial ulceration has occurred and the pad has been replaced by thin and less resilient fibrous scar tissue. The treatment of plantar ulceration includes debridement of devitalized and undermined tissue; discontinuation of weight-bearing, which may be accomplished by means of a total-contact cast or bed rest; and vigorous treatment of secondary infection, which most commonly is due to *Staphylococcus aureus*. Once healing takes place, walking must be limited, especially during the first week, with slow and progressive increases thereafter. Extra-depth shoes or individually fitted shoes with specially molded inserts are required to prevent recurrence.

Peroneal nerve palsies may result from leprosy itself or from one of its reactional states; the consequence is partial or complete footdrop, which causes an uneven distribution of weight on the plantar surface and hence a predilection to ulceration. Simple nonmetallic braces within the shoe may be useful, while tendon transfers can actually correct footdrop. Although uncommon, Charcot's joints, particularly of the foot and ankle, may result from leprosy.

The loss of distal digits in leprosy is a consequence of insensitivity, trauma, secondary infection, and—in lepromatous patients—a poorly understood and sometimes profound osteolytic process. Conscientious protection of the extremities during cooking and work and the early institution of therapy have substantially reduced the frequency and severity of distal digit loss in recent times.

The nose In lepromatous leprosy, bacillary invasion of the nasal mucosa can result in chronic nasal congestion and epistaxis. Saline nosedrops may relieve these symptoms. Long-untreated LL leprosy may further result in destruction of the nasal cartilage, with consequent saddle-nose deformity or anosmia (more common in the preantibiotic era than at present). Nasal reconstructive procedures can ameliorate significant cosmetic defects.

The eye Owing to cranial nerve palsies, lagophthalmus and corneal insensitivity may complicate leprosy, resulting in trauma, secondary infection, and (without treatment) corneal ulcerations and opacities. For patients with these conditions, eyedrops during the day and ointments at night provide some protection from such consequences. Furthermore, in LL leprosy, the anterior chamber of the eye is invaded by bacilli, and ENL may result in uveitis, with consequent cataracts and glaucoma. Thus leprosy is a major cause of blindness in the developing world. Slit-lamp evaluation of LL patients often reveals "corneal beading," representing globi of *M. leprae*.

The testes *M. leprae* invades the testes, while ENL may cause orchitis. Thus males with lepromatous leprosy often manifest mild to severe testicular dysfunction, with an elevation of luteinizing and follicle-stimulating hormones, decreased testosterone, and aspermia or hypospermia in 85% of LL patients but in only 25% of BL patients. LL patients may become impotent and infertile. Impotence is sometimes responsive to testosterone replacement.

Amyloidosis Secondary amyloidosis is a complication of LL leprosy and ENL that is encountered infrequently in the antibiotic era.

This complication may result in abnormalities of hepatic and particularly renal function.

DIAGNOSIS Leprosy most commonly presents with both characteristic skin lesions and skin histopathology. Thus the disease should be suspected when a patient from an endemic area has suggestive skin lesions or peripheral neuropathy; the diagnosis should be confirmed by histopathology. In tuberculoid leprosy, lesional areas—preferably the advancing edge—must be biopsied because normal-appearing skin does not have pathologic features. In lepromatous leprosy, nodules, plaques, and indurated areas are optimal biopsy sites, but biopsies of normal-appearing skin are also generally diagnostic. Lepromatous leprosy is associated with diffuse hyperglobulinemia, which may result in false-positive serologic tests (e.g., VDRL, RA, ANA) and therefore can cause diagnostic confusion. On occasion, tuberculoid lesions may not (1) appear typical, (2) be hypesthetic, and (3) contain granulomas but only nonspecific lymphocytic infiltrates. In such instances, two of these three characteristics are considered sufficient for a diagnosis. It is preferable to overdiagnose leprosy rather than to allow a patient to remain untreated.

IgM antibodies to PGL-1 are found in 95% of untreated lepromatous leprosy patients; the titer decreases with effective therapy. However, in tuberculoid leprosy—the form of disease most often associated with diagnostic uncertainty owing to the absence of AFB—patients have significant antibodies to PGL-1 only 60% of the time; moreover, in endemic locales, exposed individuals without clinical leprosy may harbor antibodies to PGL-1. Thus PGL-1 serology is of little diagnostic utility in tuberculoid leprosy. Heat-killed *M. leprae* (lepromin) has been used as a skin test reagent. It generally elicits a reaction in tuberculoid leprosy patients, may do so in individuals without leprosy, and gives negative results in lepromatous leprosy patients; consequently, it is likewise of little diagnostic value. Unfortunately, PCR of skin for *M. leprae*, although positive in LL and BL leprosy, yields negative results in 50% of tuberculoid leprosy cases, again offering little diagnostic assistance.

Included in the differential diagnosis of lesions that resemble leprosy are sarcoidosis, leishmaniasis, lupus vulgaris, lymphoma, syphilis, yaws, granuloma annulare, and various other disorders causing hypopigmentation. Sarcoidosis may result in perineural inflammation, but actual granuloma formation within dermal nerves is pathognomonic for leprosy. In lepromatous leprosy, sputum specimens may be loaded with AFB—a finding that can be inappropriately interpreted as representing pulmonary tuberculosis.

℞ **TREATMENT** **Active Agents** Established agents used to treat leprosy include dapsone (50 to 100 mg/d), clofazimine (50 to 100 mg/d, 100 mg three times weekly, or 300 mg monthly), and rifampin (600 mg daily or monthly). Of these drugs, only rifampin is bactericidal. The sulfones (folate antagonists), the foremost of which is dapsone, were the first antimicrobials found to be effective for the treatment of leprosy and are still the mainstay of therapy. With sulfone treatment, skin lesions resolve and numbers of viable bacilli in the skin are reduced. Although primarily bacteriostatic, dapsone monotherapy results in only a 10% resistance-related relapse rate; after ≥18 years of therapy and subsequent discontinuation, only another 10% of patients relapse, developing new, usually asymptomatic, shiny, "histoid" nodules. Dapsone is generally safe and inexpensive. Individuals with glucose-6-phosphate dehydrogenase deficiency who are treated with dapsone may develop severe hemolysis; those without this deficiency also have reduced red cell survival and a hemoglobin decrease averaging 1 g/dL. Dapsone's usefulness is limited occasionally by allergic dermatitis and rarely by the sulfone syndrome (including high fever, anemia, exfoliative dermatitis, and a mononucleosis-type blood picture). It must be remembered that rifampin induces microsomal enzymes, necessitating increased doses of medications such as glucocorticoids and oral birth control regimens. Clofazimine is often cosmetically unacceptable to light-skinned leprosy patients because it causes a red-black skin discoloration that accumulates, particularly in

lesional areas, and makes the patient's diagnosis obvious to members of the community.

Other antimicrobial agents active against *M. leprae* in animal models and at the usual daily doses used in clinical trials include ethionamide/prothionamide; the aminoglycosides streptomycin, kanamycin, and amikacin (but not gentamicin or tobramycin); minocycline; clarithromycin; and several fluoroquinolones, particularly ofloxacin. Next to rifampin, minocycline, clarithromycin, and ofloxacin appear to be most bactericidal for *M. leprae*, but these drugs have not been used extensively in leprosy control programs.

Choice of Regimens Antimicrobial therapy for leprosy must be individualized, depending on the clinical/pathologic form of the disease encountered. Tuberculoid leprosy, which is associated with a low bacterial burden and a protective cellular immune response, is the easier form to treat and can be reliably cured with a finite course of chemotherapy. In contrast, lepromatous leprosy may have a higher bacillary load than any other human bacterial disease, and the absence of a salutary T cell repertoire requires prolonged or even lifelong chemotherapy. Hence, careful classification of disease prior to therapy is important. In developed countries, clinical experience with leprosy classification is limited; fortunately, however, the resources needed for skin biopsy are highly accessible and pathologic interpretation is readily available. In developing countries, clinical expertise is greater, but it may now be waning as the care of leprosy patients is integrated into general health services. In addition, access to dermatopathology services is often limited. In such instances, skin smears may prove useful, but in many locales access to the resources needed for their preparation and interpretation may also be unavailable.

A reasoned approach to the treatment of leprosy is confounded by these and several other issues:

1. Even without therapy, TT leprosy may heal spontaneously, and prolonged dapsone monotherapy (even for LL leprosy) is generally curative in 80% of cases.
2. In tuberculoid disease, there are often no bacilli found in the skin prior to therapy, and thus there is no objective measure of therapeutic success. Furthermore, despite adequate treatment, TT and particularly BT lesions often resolve little or incompletely, while relapse and late type 1 lepra reactions can be difficult to distinguish.
3. LL leprosy patients commonly harbor viable persistent *M. leprae* organisms after prolonged intensive therapy; the propensity of these organisms to initiate clinical relapse is unclear. Because relapse in LL patients after discontinuation of rifampin-containing regimens usually begins only after 7 to 10 years, follow-up over the very long term is necessary to assess ultimate clinical outcomes.
4. Even though primary dapsone resistance is exceedingly rare and multidrug therapy is generally recommended (at least for lepromatous leprosy), there is a paucity of information from experimental animals and clinical trials on the optimal combination of antimicrobials, dosing schedule, or duration of therapy.

In 1982, the World Health Organization (WHO) made recommendations for "the chemotherapy of leprosy for control programs." These recommendations came on the heels of the demonstration of the relative success of long-term dapsone monotherapy and in the context of concerns about dapsone resistance. Other complicating considerations included the limited resources available for leprosy care in the very areas where it is most prevalent and the frustration and discouragement of patients and program managers with the previous requirement for lifelong therapy for many leprosy patients. The WHO delineated for the first time a finite duration of therapy for all forms of leprosy, and—given the prohibitive cost of daily rifampin treatment in developing countries—encouraged the monthly administration of this agent as part of a multidrug regimen.

Over the ensuing years, these WHO recommendations have been broadly implemented, and the duration of therapy required, particularly for lepromatous leprosy, has been progressively shortened. For treatment purposes, the WHO classifies patients as paucibacillary and multibacillary. Previously, patients without demonstrable AFB in the dermis were classified as paucibacillary and those with AFB as multibacillary. Currently, owing to the perceived unreliability of skin smears in the field, patients are classified as multibacillary if they have five or more skin lesions and as paucibacillary if they have fewer than five skin lesions. The WHO recommends that paucibacillary adults be treated with 100 mg of dapsone daily and 600 mg of rifampin monthly (supervised) for 6 months (Table 170-1). Multibacillary adults should be treated with 100 mg of dapsone plus 50 mg of clofazimine daily (unsupervised) and with 600 mg of rifampin plus 300 mg of clofazimine monthly (supervised). Originally, the WHO recommended that lepromatous patients be treated for 2 years or until smears became negative (generally in ~5 years); subsequently, the acceptable course was reduced to 1 year—a change that remains controversial in the absence of clinical trials.

Several factors, including an improved economic climate, the high relapse rates (20 to 40%, depending on the initial bacterial burden) among patients with lepromatous leprosy after WHO-recommended treatment, and the demonstrable lesional activity in fully half of tuberculoid leprosy patients after the completion of therapy, have caused many authorities to question the WHO recommendations and to favor a more intensive approach. This approach (Table 170-1) calls for tuberculoid leprosy to be treated with dapsone (100 mg/d) for 5 years and for lepromatous leprosy to be treated with rifampin (600 mg/d) for 3 years and with dapsone (100 mg/d) throughout life.

On effective antimicrobial therapy, new skin lesions and signs and symptoms of peripheral neuropathy cease appearing. Nodules and plaques of lepromatous leprosy noticeably flatten in 1 to 2 months and resolve in 1 or a few years, while tuberculoid skin lesions may disappear, improve, or remain relatively unchanged. Though the peripheral neuropathy of leprosy may improve somewhat in the first few months of therapy, rarely is it significantly ameliorated by treatment.

PREVENTION AND CONTROL   Vaccination at birth with bacille Calmette-Guérin (BCG) has proved variably effective in preventing leprosy, ranging from totally ineffective to 80% efficacious. The addition of heat-killed *M. leprae* to BCG does not increase vaccine efficacy. Because whole mycobacteria contain large amounts of lipids and carbohydrates that have proven in vitro to be immunosuppressive for lymphocytes and macrophages, *M. leprae* proteins may prove to be superior vaccines. Data from a mouse model support this possibility. Chemoprophylaxis with dapsone may reduce the number of cases of tuberculoid leprosy but not of lepromatous leprosy and hence is not recommended, even for household contacts. Because leprosy transmission appears to require close prolonged household contact, hospitalized patients need not be isolated.

BIBLIOGRAPHY

GELBER RH : Chemotherapy of lepromatous leprosy: Recent developments and prospects for the future. Eur J Clin Microbiol Infect Dis 13:942, 1994

———— et al: Vaccination of mice with a soluble protein fraction of *Mycobacterium leprae* provides consistent and long-term protection against *M. leprae* infection. Infect Immun 60:1840, 1992

JAMET P et al: Marchoux Chemotherapy Study Group. Relapse after long-term follow up of multibacillary patients treated by WHO multidrug regimen. Int J Lepr 63:195, 1995

MARCHOUX CHEMOTHERAPY STUDY GROUP: Relapses in multibacillary leprosy patients after stopping treatment with rifampicin-containing combined regimens. Int J Lepr 60:525, 1992

MODLIN RL, REA TH: Immunology of leprosy granulomas. Springer Semin Immunopathol 10:359, 1998

RIDLEY DS: Histological classification and the immunological spectrum of leprosy. Bull World Health Organ 51:451, 1974

SAMPAIO EP et al: Influence of thalidomide on the clinical and immunologic manifestations of erythema nodosum leprosum. J Infect Dis 168:408, 1993

SHEPARD CC: The experimental disease that follows injection of human leprosy bacilli into foot pads of mice. J Exp Med 112:445, 1960

WHO EXPERT COMMITTEE ON LEPROSY: Seventh Report. WHO Technical Report Series No. 874. Geneva, World Health Organization, 1998

Table 170-1   Antimicrobial Regimens Recommended for the Treatment of Leprosy in Adults

Form of Leprosy	More Intensive Regimen	WHO Recommended Regimen (1982)
Tuberculoid (paucibacillary)	Dapsone (100 mg/d) for 5 years	Dapsone (100 mg/d, unsupervised) *plus* rifampin (600 mg/month, supervised) for 6 months
Lepromatous (multibacillary)	Rifampin (600 mg/d) for 3 years *plus* dapsone (100 mg/d) indefinitely	Dapsone (100 mg/d) *plus* clofazimine (50 mg/d), unsupervised; *and* rifampin (600 mg) *plus* clofazimine (300 mg) monthly (supervised) for 1 year

NOTE: See text for discussion and comparison of WHO recommendations and more intensive approach.

| **171** | *Bernard Hirschel* |

INFECTIONS DUE TO NONTUBERCULOUS MYCOBACTERIA

Mycobacteria are slightly curved or straight, rod-shaped or coccoid bacilli traditionally identified by the property of acid-fastness: once stained, the organisms are not easily decolorized, even with acid-alcohol, because of the composition of their cell walls. The genetic relation of mycobacteria with one another is evidenced by their ribosomal RNA sequence homology, which can be used for diagnostic purposes.

Because of the overwhelming clinical importance of tuberculosis, mycobacteriologists have distinguished the *Mycobacterium tuberculosis* complex (consisting of *M. tuberculosis*, *M. bovis*, and *M. africanum*) from all other mycobacteria. Except for *M. leprae* (Chap. 170), the other mycobacteria are referred to as atypical mycobacteria, mycobacteria other than tuberculosis (MOTT), or nontuberculous mycobacteria (NTM). The most clinically important NTM are listed and described in Table 171-1. The isolation of NTM—or the lack thereof—from an individual patient or laboratory specimen must be interpreted with the following facts in mind:

1. Some NTM require special media and/or growth conditions. The laboratory must be alerted and cultures for acid-fast bacilli requested if the diagnosis of these infections is not to be missed.

2. NTM grow slowly. Even the so-called rapid growers take 3 to 7 days to form visible colonies on solid media, whereas slow-growing mycobacteria take weeks or do not grow at all on artificial media.

3. The slow growth of mycobacteria complicates antibiotic susceptibility testing. During prolonged incubation, antibiotics may be degraded and disappear from the culture medium. Long delays reduce the clinical usefulness of whatever results are eventually obtained.

4. Data on in vitro susceptibility correlate poorly with clinical results. For example, clarithromycin and azithromycin are highly and variably concentrated in tissues; consequently, the concentrations necessary for determining resistance are difficult to establish in vitro. Sensitivity testing, based on achievable serum levels, would have predicted that these drugs would have little efficacy in vivo; in fact, the opposite is true, both in animal models and in humans.

5. In contrast to *M. tuberculosis*, NTM are ubiquitous in the en-

Table 171-1 The Most Important Nontuberculous Mycobacteria

| Mycobacterial Species | Disseminated Infections | Localized Infections | | Skin and Soft Tissue | Contaminant/ Commensal | Recommended Therapy | Percentage of Strains |
		Lung	Lymphadenitis				
M. abscessus	—	—	—	Typical, linked to surgery	Typical	Debridement; clarithromycin, clofazimine, amikacin	<1
M. avium	Typical in AIDS with CD4+ count of <50/μL; rare in other immunode-ficiencies	See M. intracel-lulare	In children (rare)	In disseminated infection (rare)	Typical in sputum and feces	Clarithromycin,[a] ethambutol, rifabutin	30–50
M. celatum	AIDS (rare)	Rare	—	—	—	See M. avium	<1
M. chelonae	Rare	—	—	Typical, linked to surgery	Typical	See M. abscessus	<1
M. fortuitum	Rare	Rare	—	Typical	Typical	Amikacin, ciprofloxacin, sulfonamides, clofazimine, clarithromycin	1
M. genavense	Typical in AIDS	—	Rare	—	—	See M. avium	5
M. gordonae	Rare	—	—	Rare	Typical	—	10–30
M. haemophilum	Typical in AIDS and other immunode-ficiencies	—	—	Typical in AIDS	—	See M. avium	<1
M. intracellulare	See M. avium	Cavities in CF or COPD[b]; lingular infection in normal hosts	In children (rare)	See M. avium	Possible in sputum	See M. avium	4–8
M. kansasii	In AIDS (rare)	Typical, resembling tuberculosis	Rare	Rare	Possible in sputum	Rifampin, isoniazid, etham-butol, clarithromycin, sulfonamides	2–4
M. malmoense	Rare	Rare	—	—	—	See M. avium	1–4
M. marinum	Rare	—	—	Typical	—	Trimethoprim-sulfamethoxazole[c]	1
M. scrofulaceum	Rare	Rare	Typical	—	—	See M. avium	1
M. simiae	In AIDS (rare)	Rare	—	—	Possible	See M. avium	1
M. szulgai	—	Rare	—	Typical	—	Rifampin, isoniazid, ethambutol	<1
M. xenopi	Rare	Rare	—	—	Typical	See M. avium	10–20

[a] Or azithromycin.
[b] CF, cystic fibrosis; COPD, chronic obstructive pulmonary disease.
[c] Or minocycline.

SOURCE: Data are from J Clin Microbiol 31:1882, 1993 (335 strains) and the Mycobac-teriology Laboratory of the University Hospital in Geneva (1993–1994, 313 strains, Dr. P. Rohner).

vironment. Therefore, isolation of NTM from a site that is not normally sterile (such as sputum, urine, skin, or feces) does not constitute proof of disease. In Switzerland between 1983 and 1988, for example, only 23 of 513 HIV-negative patients with NTM isolates had clinically significant disease. Clusters of unusual isolates are more likely to sug-gest contamination—e.g., from tap water or bronchoscopy equip-ment—than to represent an epidemic of disease.

The original method for the classification of NTM, developed be-tween 1950 and 1980, depends on speed of growth, morphology, and pigmentation of colonies on solid media as well as biochemical re-actions. Although reliable and inexpensive, these procedures take a long time; a period of 12 weeks is often required for definitive iden-tification. Of course, such delayed results are of little use in the care of patients.

The isolation of NTM from blood cultures requires the use of a special medium for lysis-centrifugation or broth culture. The lysis-centrifugation method (lysis of blood cells followed by centrifugation and plating of the pellet with the bacteria on solid medium) permits quantification of bacteremia; however, some mycobacteria (e.g., M. genavense) do not grow well on solid medium and will not be detected by this method. Culture in liquid broth, such as that used in the radio-metric Bactec system, shortens the time needed to identify a positive culture but also precludes the study of colonial morphology and pig-mentation. Molecular probes are now used for rapid identification of the most important species (M. avium, M. intracellulare, M. gordonae, M. kansasii, and the M. tuberculosis complex) in a positive culture; a color is produced upon hybridization of the probe to specific sequences of the mycobacterial ribosome.

Twenty years ago, the field of mycobacteriology was something of a backwater. Tuberculosis was incorrectly perceived as a disap-pearing problem, and NTM were causing only rare and chronic dis-eases. AIDS, however, has brought mycobacterial infections to the forefront of clinical medicine once more. HIV and M. tuberculosis make a volatile mixture, and disseminated infections with NTM are extremely frequent in the advanced stages of AIDS (Chap. 309). In this setting, it is fortunate that new molecular techniques based on DNA amplification accelerate diagnosis, identify common sources of infection, and reveal new types of NTM, while new antibiotics, such as the macrolides, the rifamycins, and the fluoroquinolones, offer im-proved options for treatment and prevention. In addition, highly active antiretroviral therapy (HAART) has had a dramatic impact. By pre-venting and reversing immunodeficiency, HAART (Chap. 309) also prevents and reverses NTM infections.

NTM INFECTIONS IN AIDS AND OTHER IMMUNODEFICIENCIES

DISSEMINATED INFECTIONS Etiology The majority of mycobacterial infections in immunocompromised hosts are caused by organisms belonging to the group referred to as the M. avium complex (MAC). This group has always been considered to include M. avium and M. intracellulare (designated by the abbreviation MAI) and in the past encompassed M. scrofulaceum as well (hence the abbreviation MAIS). With the development and marketing of diagnostic probes that distinguish M. avium from M. intracellulare, it has become clear that the vast majority of disseminated "MAC" infections in AIDS are ac-tually caused by M. avium. Thus, from a microbiologic standpoint, this designation is now obsolete. However, it is still used in clinical practice and will be employed in that context herein.

M. genavense causes systemic infections similar to those caused by MAC organisms. *M. genavense* does not grow well in culture and may therefore be missed in some instances. However, in a series of nearly 200 disseminated NTM infections from Switzerland, 13% of cases were due to *M. genavense*. Other NTM, including *M. xenopi*, *M. simiae*, *M. scrofulaceum*, *M. malmoense*, and *M. celatum*, may also be involved in such cases. In addition, AIDS patients with localized NTM diseases (see "Localized Infections," below) often have positive blood cultures (e.g., patients with skin disease due to *M. haemophilum* or with lung disease due to *M. kansasii*).

Epidemiology and Host Factors Because gastrointestinal symptoms often predominate in NTM infection and because the intestinal submucosa is intensely involved, ingestion seems logical as a primary route of infection. Many environments and animals teem with NTM (especially MAC organisms), including swamps in the southeastern United States, swine almost everywhere, piped water in New England and in Finland, and soil from potted plants in San Francisco. Birds are frequently infected with *M. genavense*. Skin-test data and humoral antibody patterns point to widespread exposure. However, a direct connection of the environment to the patient is often lacking, and it is not always clear whether strains found in the environment are pathogenic in humans. In an exhaustive study of dietary factors, patients with NTM were found to have consumed more hard cheese than controls without NTM, but no NTM could be found in samples of cheese. At present, the epidemiologic evidence is not strong enough to serve as a basis for dietary recommendations in persons at high risk of NTM infection. There is no evidence for nosocomial spread of NTM from patient to patient; however, hospital hot-water systems have been suspected as the source of isolated clusters of cases. Whereas regional variations in the environmental frequency of NTM are striking, it is difficult to correlate these variations with the frequency of NTM infection among HIV-infected patients.

Disseminated infections with NTM occur almost exclusively in severely immunosuppressed patients, usually those with AIDS. Rarely, such infections are found in patients immunosuppressed for other reasons, including transplant recipients, and patients with leukemia (in particular, hairy cell leukemia) or lymphoma. Cases in children may suggest the presence of a congenital immunodeficiency disease, such as a deficiency in the receptors for interferon γ (IFN-γ) or interleukin (IL) 12. Finally, rare cases of dissemination occur in immunocompetent patients who have extensive pulmonary disease (see "NTM Infections in Immunocompetent Patients," below).

In patients with AIDS, the risk of NTM infection correlates well with the degree of depletion of CD4+ lymphocytes. Disseminated NTM disease is rare among patients with >100 CD4+ cells per microliter; however, among patients with <10 CD4+ lymphocytes per microliter, the actuarial probability of having a blood culture positive for NTM reaches 40% after 1 year. HAART has greatly diminished the overall incidence of NTM disease in AIDS. Current treatment recommendations suggest starting HAART when the CD4+ count falls below 500/μL. At these levels, NTM disease does not occur. In extremely immunosuppressed patients who start HAART, the CD4+ count typically rises above 100/μL within a few months; such patients are again unlikely to develop NTM disease.

Clinical Manifestations As has already been mentioned, disseminated infection with NTM is essentially a disease of advanced immunodeficiency. In HIV-infected patients, the median CD4+ lymphocyte count at the time of diagnosis is ~10/μL. Certainly, other diagnoses should be considered first when a patient with symptoms suggestive of NTM infection has >100 CD4+ cells per microliter. Prospective monthly blood cultures have shown that NTM bacteremia often causes few or no symptoms. In clinical practice, however, cultures are not performed if the patient is asymptomatic.

Disseminated NTM infection should be suspected on the basis of prolonged fever (sometimes of varying intensity—particularly at first—and accompanied by night sweats) and weight loss. Signs of abdominal involvement that may be evident on computed tomography or ultrasonography include enlargement of the liver and spleen and swelling of abdominal lymph nodes, which may result in diarrhea and/or abdominal pain. Anemia and leukopenia are frequently documented; although it is tempting to relate these abnormalities to infection of bone marrow by NTM, multiple factors are usually involved.

In short, the clinical picture of infection with NTM is not distinctive. Many other conditions, including abdominal lymphoma, the HIV wasting syndrome, *Salmonella* or *Campylobacter* infection, cryptosporidiosis, or microsporidiosis, may mimic (and coexist with) disseminated NTM infection. As stated earlier, suspicion of such infection should prompt a request for blood cultures.

Diagnosis Blood cultures on special media are the cornerstone of the diagnosis of NTM infection, both in patients with organ involvement and in those without. In most symptomatic patients, the intensity of mycobacteremia is such that most or all blood cultures are positive. Therefore, the performance of multiple, repetitive cultures at short intervals is not worthwhile. Rather, in clinical practice, two or three blood cultures are sufficient. In one study, the results of prospective cultures varied, and these variations (positive followed by negative or vice versa) were unrelated to symptom status. As mentioned above, liquid cultures (e.g., the Bactec system) are likely to become positive earlier (within 7 to 14 days) and are therefore preferred to cultures on solid medium. In patients infected with *M. genavense* or *M. xenopi* and in patients being treated for MAC infection, the interval to culture positivity may be much longer. In rare cases, organ involvement in NTM infection may be found to be widespread at autopsy despite multiple negative blood cultures during life.

Because the liver and bone marrow are often involved in disseminated NTM infection, the bacteria may be visible in acid-fast–stained biopsy samples from these sites. Presumptive diagnosis by examination of a biopsied liver specimen saves time. The yield has been as high as 50% in patients with clearly abnormal values in liver function tests. However, the yield of this method has been disappointing in patients with suspected NTM infection, negative blood cultures, and normal or nearly normal results in liver function tests.

℞ TREATMENT Compared with *M. tuberculosis*, NTM are of low virulence. NTM tend to affect severely immunosuppressed patients, who usually have many other medical problems. Treatment is complex, relies on the use of multiple drugs with numerous adverse effects, and may interfere with antiretroviral therapy.

The drugs used for the treatment of disseminated NTM infection are different from those used against tuberculosis (Table 171-1; Chaps. 168 and 169). In particular, isoniazid has little effect on MAC organisms. The best method for antibiotic sensitivity testing of NTM is controversial, and the question of what relation—if any—exists between in vitro resistance and treatment failure remains unanswered. From the clinician's viewpoint, growth inhibition in liquid cultures is preferred to other methods of sensitivity testing because the results become available within 7 days.

The agents most active against MAC organisms are the macrolides clarithromycin and azithromycin. Both of these drugs are well absorbed from the gastrointestinal tract and well concentrated in macrophages and tissues, where their levels exceed those in plasma by more than 10-fold. Given alone, either drug can render blood cultures negative in a substantial proportion of cases. However, resistance (due to a single point mutation in the gene coding for the large ribosomal subunit) invariably develops, and NTM reappear in the bloodstream.

A majority of MAC strains are sensitive to ethambutol, ciprofloxacin, clofazimine, amikacin, rifampin, and rifabutin; that is, the concentrations of these drugs attainable in serum are inhibitory in vitro. However, none of these drugs consistently reduces the intensity of mycobacteremia when used alone. The preferred regimen for treatment of disseminated NTM infections is the combination of rifabutin (300 to 600 mg/d), clarithromycin (1 g twice daily), and ethambutol (900 mg/d). In a randomized trial, this regimen was superior to the combination of rifampin, clofazimine, ciprofloxacin, and ethambutol, with more rapid resolution of bacteremia and increased survival. The higher dose of rifabutin was more effective but frequently caused uveitis. This side effect is of special concern when rifabutin is used in combination with ritonavir, which increases the concentration of a toxic metabolite. Among the HIV protease inhibitors, indinavir and nelfinavir may be used in combination with rifabutin.

The inclusion of intravenous amikacin in multidrug regimens has not conferred additional benefit. Nonetheless, this drug may be useful in certain cases—e.g., when resistance to clarithromycin develops or when severe gastrointestinal symptoms interfere with oral therapy. In addition, amikacin may prevent the emergence of resistance to clarithromycin when the two drugs are used concurrently.

It is not clear how long therapy needs to be administered. Older regimens did not eradicate MAC, and many experts recommended lifelong treatment. Unfortunately, multidrug regimens are often poorly tolerated. In patients whose symptoms have lessened, whose blood cultures have become negative, and whose CD4+ counts have recovered to >100/μL with HAART, it is reasonable to discontinue antimycobacterial treatment.

In vitro and in experimental animals, cytokines such as IL-12, granulocyte-macrophage colony-stimulating factor, and IFN-γ act synergistically with antibiotics against MAC. In a small-scale pilot trial including seven HIV-negative patients, IFN-γ was beneficial.

Encapsulation of many drugs into liposomes enhances their effect in animal models because both liposomes and MAC are ingested by macrophages. Relevant data from studies of humans are still scarce, however.

Disseminated infections caused by NTM other than MAC have been too rare for therapy to be evaluated in controlled trials. The presently recommended treatment for these infections is the same as that for disseminated MAC infections. In particular, *M. genavense* seems to be sensitive to clarithromycin and rifabutin.

Prevention As has been discussed, disseminated infection with MAC occurs almost exclusively in persons severely immunocompromised by HIV infection. Therefore, the best approach to the prevention of MAC infections is the prevention and reversal of immunodeficiency by HAART. In patients whose HIV is resistant to HAART and who are severely immunosuppressed, with CD4+ counts <100/μL, prophylaxis with rifabutin (300 mg/d), clarithromycin (500 mg once or twice daily), or azithromycin (1200 mg weekly) is likely to decrease the incidence of positive blood cultures by ~60%. Patients receiving prophylaxis have also had less fever, experienced less fatigue, and survived longer than patients not receiving prophylaxis. Although breakthrough bacteremia involving resistant organisms is a concern, this condition has not developed with rifabutin prophylaxis and is rare with clarithromycin. However, it is standard practice to rule out preexisting disseminated NTM infection (by blood culture) before starting prophylaxis.

LOCALIZED INFECTIONS **Pulmonary Disease** The significance of isolation of NTM from the airways of AIDS patients merits special discussion. In general, HIV-infected patients who have NTM in sputum or bronchoalveolar lavage fluid but have little evidence of lung damage require no treatment. *M. avium* only rarely causes significant pulmonary disease in AIDS; its isolation from sputum in the absence of radiographic changes is usually without clinical significance. In contrast, the isolation of *M. kansasii* from the lung is clinically significant: this organism causes a disease—often predominant in the upper lobes—that resembles pulmonary tuberculosis, with fever, cough, infiltrates, and cavities. Blood cultures are often positive. Drugs active against *M. tuberculosis*, such as rifampin (600 mg/d) and isoniazid (300 mg/d), are also effective against *M. kansasii*; treatment is generally continued for 18 to 24 months, although some data suggest that 12 months may be adequate.

Skin Disease MAC organisms, which frequently cause disseminated disease with positive blood cultures in AIDS, are also rarely associated with heterogeneous skin manifestations, such as nodules, ulcers, areas of erythema, pustules, abscesses, or panniculitis. Skin biopsies and blood cultures establish the diagnosis.

M. haemophilum In contrast to MAC organisms, *M. haemophilum* has a tendency to involve the skin, bones, joints, and lungs, although most patients also have positive blood cultures. Skin lesions are nodular, may ulcerate, and are disseminated. In the absence of specific data, treatment should follow the guidelines for MAC infection.

NTM INFECTIONS IN IMMUNOCOMPETENT PATIENTS

PULMONARY DISEASE **Etiology** The NTM most frequently causing pulmonary infections are *M. intracellulare*, *M. avium*, and *M. kansasii*. Many other species, such as *M. xenopi*, *M. malmoense*, and *M. interjectum*, can also be involved in these infections. Identification of the specific pathogen is important in the choice among the various therapeutic strategies. For example, *M. kansasii* responds to antituberculosis drugs, including isoniazid.

Epidemiology and Host Factors As has already been noted, NTM are ubiquitous in the environment, but their pathogenicity is low. Preexisting lung disease (e.g., chronic obstructive airway disease, cancer, previous tuberculosis, bronchiectasis, cystic fibrosis, and silicosis, with cavities and bronchiectases) is the main predisposing factor for pulmonary disease due to NTM.

Anecdotal evidence suggests that the proportion of patients without underlying lung pathology who are developing pulmonary disease due to NTM is increasing. These patients are usually elderly; many are women with pectus excavatum or scoliosis. In the latter elderly women, the lingula and the right middle lobes are particularly involved. Somewhat whimsically, the disease in these patients has been called "Lady Windermere syndrome" after the main character in Oscar Wilde's play *Lady Windermere's Fan*, who went to extremes to refrain from coughing.

Clinical Manifestations Most immunocompetent patients with pulmonary NTM infection present with chronic cough, low-grade fever, and malaise; some present with hemoptysis. These symptoms may be masked by those of the underlying disease process.

Diagnosis In contrast to the isolation of *M. tuberculosis*, of which even a single colony—whatever its origin—is clinically significant, the isolation of NTM from the sputum never in itself proves the existence of disease. NTM are frequently commensals and colonize both diseased and normal airways. Because treatment of NTM infection is complicated, it is important that the diagnosis be certain. The American Thoracic Society has formulated the following minimal guidelines for the diagnosis of pulmonary NTM disease: "evidence, such as an infiltrate visible on a chest roentgenogram, of disease, the cause of which has not been determined by careful clinical and laboratory studies, and . . . isolation of multiple colonies of the same strain of mycobacteria repeatedly, usually in the absence of other pathogens." For patients who have pulmonary infiltrates but not cavities, these criteria may not be specific enough; some patients are found to have cleared NTM after a 1-month trial of bronchial hygiene alone (inhalation of saline and bronchodilators to induce cough and sputum production). The detection by computed tomography of bronchiectases and nodular infiltrates in the same lobe may be particularly suggestive of NTM infection.

TREATMENT Lung disease due to NTM may be managed by follow-up without treatment, by resection, or by drug therapy. No randomized trial has determined which is the best option. In retrospectively analyzed case series, patients undergoing surgery have had a better outcome than those treated only with drugs. However, selection bias has probably influenced these results since patients with extensive lung disease are poor candidates for surgery.

As in HIV-infected patients, immunocompetent patients with minimal disease do not need treatment at all. Likewise, NTM disease may present as a solitary pulmonary nodule that, once resected (to confirm or exclude a diagnosis of cancer), requires no further drug treatment.

Most other patients with pulmonary NTM disease are treated with antimicrobials; in addition, they may or may not undergo surgery. The drugs available for the treatment of infection with *M. avium* or *M. intracellulare* have already been discussed. The regimens recommended for disseminated MAC infection are preferred, although large doses of clarithromycin are often poorly tolerated by elderly patients. *M. intracellulare* may be easier to treat and eradicate than *M. avium*. In two small open studies, single-agent treatment with clarithromycin (500 mg twice daily) led to improvements detected by chest radiography and sputum culture.

Indications for surgery are difficult to establish but include a disappointing response to antibiotics, the presence of localized disease, and the absence of contraindications (especially impaired respiratory functions). Ideally, drug treatment should begin before surgery and should render the sputum negative by the time of the operation.

In contrast to MAC organisms, *M. kansasii* is predictably sensitive to antituberculosis agents. Treatment should consist of isoniazid (300 mg/d), rifampin (600 mg/d), and ethambutol (15 to 25 mg/kg per day). The optimal duration of therapy is unknown, but most patients have been treated for 18 to 24 months; 12 months may suffice. Sulfamethoxazole is recommended for the occasional patient whose infection relapses after *M. kansasii* becomes resistant to rifampin.

LYMPHADENITIS NTM are among the causes of localized lymphadenitis. This disease occurs mostly in children between the ages of 1 and 5 years. Painless swelling of one node or a group of nodes usually affects the anterior cervical chain. Nodes may rapidly increase in size, with the formation of fistulas to the skin. *M. scrofulaceum* or MAC organisms most commonly cause NTM lymphadenitis, although many other species may be involved. Once tuberculosis has been excluded, the treatment of choice is excision without chemotherapy. When excision is dangerous because of proximity to the facial nerve, aspiration combined with chemotherapy may be effective.

SKIN DISEASE DUE TO NTM   **Swimming-Pool and Fish-Tank Granuloma** Between 1 week and 2 months (usually 2 to 3 weeks) after contact with contaminated tropical fish tanks, swimming pools, or saltwater fish, a small violet nodule or pustule may appear at a site of minor trauma. This lesion may evolve to form a crusted ulcer or small abscess or may remain warty. Lesions are multiple and disseminated on occasion—particularly, but not exclusively, in immunosuppressed patients. The causative organism is *M. marinum*. The patient's clinical history, combined with the isolation of *M. marinum* after biopsy and culture, establishes the diagnosis. Lesions often heal spontaneously. In cases of persistence or dissemination, rifampin (300 to 600 mg/d) in combination with ethambutol (15 to 25 mg/kg per day), trimethoprim-sulfamethoxazole (160/800 mg twice daily), or minocycline (100 mg/d) may be tried for a period of at least 3 months.

Very rarely, a similar clinical picture is produced by *M. gordonae*, a frequently isolated but usually nonpathogenic species.

Buruli Ulcer In many tropical areas throughout the world, *M. ulcerans* may cause an itching nodule on the arms or legs, which then breaks down to form a shallow ulcer of variable size. The course of this condition is usually prolonged. *M. ulcerans* is difficult to culture; plates need to be incubated at low temperature. Excision constitutes the usual therapy. Treatment with rifampin, clofazimine, or trimethoprim-sulfamethoxazole has met with variable success.

NTM INFECTIONS OF SOFT TISSUE, TENDONS, BONES, AND JOINTS   Infections Linked to Injections and Surgery Occasionally, mycobacteria are isolated from nodular skin lesions of hospitalized patients, particularly those who are immunosuppressed; in some instances there is associated lymphatic spread. Many cases are linked to injection; diabetic patients are at especially high risk. In ophthalmology, mycobacteria may cause keratitis and corneal ulceration after surgery or injury. Epidemics of mycobacterial infection following cardiac surgery have been linked to contaminated ice packs and contaminated porcine heart valves. These infections are usually due to *M. fortuitum*, *M. chelonae*, or *M. abscessus*, which are referred to collectively as the *M. fortuitum* complex. These are the so-called rapidly growing mycobacteria: colonies on solid medium appear 3 to 7 days after inoculation. As organisms may fail to grow at 37°C, incubation at 30 to 33°C is recommended. These mycobacteria are notoriously resistant to most antituberculosis drugs. Debridement is best combined with administration of two or three of the antibiotics mentioned in Table 171-1.

Infections of Tendons, Joints, and Bones In rare cases, mycobacteria invade deep tissues after direct inoculation, via contiguous spread from superficial sites of infection, or through the bloodstream. MAC organisms and *M. ulcerans* are most often cited in these instances. *M. szulgai* seems to be involved particularly frequently in olecranon bursitis.

BIBLIOGRAPHY

ABERG JA et al: Eradication of AIDS-related disseminated *Mycobacterium avium* complex infection after 12 months of antimycobacterial therapy combined with highly active antiretroviral therapy. J Infect Dis 178:1446, 1998

Diagnosis and treatment of disease caused by nontuberculous mycobacteria. Am Rev Respir Dis 142:940, 1990

NEWPORT MJ et al: A mutation in the interferon-gamma-receptor gene and susceptibility to mycobacterial infection. N Engl J Med 335:1941, 1996

SHAFRAN SD et al: A comparison of two regimens for the treatment of *Mycobacterium avium* complex bacteremia in AIDS: Rifabutin, ethambutol, and clarithromycin versus rifampin, ethambutol, clofazimine, and ciprofloxacin. Canadian HIV Trials Network Protocol 010 Study Group. N Engl J Med 335:377, 1996

TANAKA E et al: Effect of clarithromycin regimen for *Mycobacterium avium* complex pulmonary disease. Am J Respir Crit Care Med 160:866, 1999

VAN DER WERF TS et al: *Mycobacterium ulcerans* infection. Lancet 354:1013, 1999

WOLINSKY E: Mycobacterial lymphadenitis in children: A prospective study of 105 nontuberculous cases with long-term follow-up. Clin Infect Dis 20:954, 1995

YAMAZAKI Y et al: Markers indicating deterioration of pulmonary *Mycobacterium avium-intracellulare* infection. Am J Respir Crit Care Med 160:1851, 1999

Section 9
SPIROCHETAL DISEASES

172   *Sheila A. Lukehart*

SYPHILIS

DEFINITION Syphilis, a chronic systemic infection caused by *Treponema pallidum* subspecies *pallidum*, is usually sexually transmitted and is characterized by episodes of active disease interrupted by periods of latency. After an incubation period averaging 2 to 6 weeks, a primary lesion appears, often associated with regional lymphadenopathy. A secondary bacteremic stage, associated with generalized mucocutaneous lesions and generalized lymphadenopathy, is followed by a latent period of subclinical infection lasting many years. In about one-third of untreated cases, the tertiary stage is characterized by progressive destructive mucocutaneous, musculoskeletal, or parenchymal lesions; aortitis; or symptomatic central nervous system (CNS) disease.

ETIOLOGY The Spirochaetales include three genera that are pathogenic for humans and for a variety of other animals: *Leptospira*, which causes human leptospirosis; *Borrelia*, which causes relapsing fever and Lyme disease; and *Treponema*, which causes the diseases known as treponematoses. The genus *Treponema* includes *T. pallidum* subspecies *pallidum*, which causes venereal syphilis; *T. pallidum* subspecies *pertenue*, which causes yaws; *T. pallidum* subspecies *endemicum*, which causes endemic syphilis or bejel; and *T. carateum*, which causes pinta (Chap. 173). Other *Treponema* species found in the human mouth, genital mucosa, and gastrointestinal tract have no proven pathogenic role in human disease. These spirochetes can be confused with *T. pallidum* on dark-field examination. An oral treponeme that is very closely related to *T. pallidum* antigenically has been found to be significantly associated with periodontitis and acute necrotizing ulcerative gingivitis; its etiologic role in these gum diseases is unknown. None of the four pathogenic treponemes has yet been cultured in quantity. Until recently, the subspecies were distinguished primarily by the clinical syndromes they produce. Recent studies have identified molecular signatures that can differentiate *T. pallidum* subspecies *pallidum* from the other pathogenic *T. pallidum* subspecies by culture-independent, polymerase chain reaction (PCR)–based methods.

T. pallidum subspecies *pallidum* (hereafter referred to simply as *T. pallidum*), a thin delicate organism with 6 to 14 spirals and tapered ends, measures 6 to 15 μm in total length and 0.2 μm in width. The cytoplasm is surrounded by a trilaminar cytoplasmic membrane, which in turn is surrounded by a delicate peptidoglycan layer providing some structural rigidity. This layer is surrounded by a lipid-rich outer membrane that contains relatively few integral membrane proteins. Six endoflagella wind around the cell body in a space between the inner cell wall and the outer membrane and may be the elements responsible for motility.

The sequencing of the genome of *T. pallidum* has yielded information about the organism's metabolic capabilities. *T. pallidum* lacks the genes required to synthesize enzyme cofactors, fatty acids, and nucleotides de novo. In addition, it lacks genes encoding the enzymes of the Krebs cycle and oxidative phosphorylation. To compensate, the organism contains numerous genes predicted to code for transporters of amino acids, carbohydrates, and cations. In addition, the genome analyses and other studies have revealed the existence of a 12-member gene family (called *tpr*) that bears similarities to variable outer-membrane antigens of other spirochetes. Although the role of these encoded molecules has not yet been defined, the TprK antigen appears to be preferentially expressed and serves as a target of opsonic antibody.

The only known natural host for *T. pallidum* is the human. *T. pallidum* can infect many mammals, but only humans, higher apes, and a few laboratory animals regularly develop syphilitic lesions. Virulent strains of *T. pallidum* are grown and maintained in rabbits.

EPIDEMIOLOGY Nearly all cases of syphilis are acquired by sexual contact with infectious lesions (i.e., the chancre, mucous patch, skin rash, or condyloma latum). Less common modes of transmission include nonsexual personal contact and infection in utero or following blood transfusions.

The total number of cases of syphilis reported annually in the United States fell steadily from 575,593 in 1943 to a low of 64,621 in 1987—an 88% decrease—but then increased to 134,255 in 1990. The number of new cases of infectious syphilis reached a peak in 1947 and then fell to approximately 6000 in 1956; since then, a rather steady increase in infectious syphilis has been punctuated by four cycles of 7 to 10 years, each with a rapid rise and fall in incidence (with peaks in 1965, 1975, 1982, and 1990). Since 1990, the number of reported cases of infectious syphilis has again declined by >80%. In 1997, there were 8550 reported cases of primary and secondary syphilis and 46,540 cases of all stages.

The populations at highest risk for acquiring syphilis have changed. Between 1977 and 1982, approximately half of all patients with early syphilis in the United States were homosexual or bisexual men. Largely because of changing sexual practices in this population due to the AIDS epidemic, this proportion has decreased. The most recent epidemic of syphilis predominantly involved African-American heterosexual men and women and occurred largely in urban areas, where infectious syphilis has been correlated significantly with the exchange of sex for "crack" cocaine. The incidence of syphilis peaks at 15 to 34 years of age. The reported incidence is much higher among African Americans than in other ethnic groups and is higher in urban than in rural areas; 80% of infectious syphilis cases are reported from 15% of the counties in the United States.

The incidence of congenital syphilis roughly parallels that of infectious syphilis in females. The number of reported cases of congenital syphilis in infants ≤1 year of age was lowest (107 cases) in 1978, when infectious syphilis was most prevalent among homosexual and bisexual men. The dramatic increase in the incidence of primary and secondary syphilis among women from 1986 to 1990 resulted in a proportionate increase in the number of infants born with congenital syphilis—to 3275 infants in 1991. The incidence of early syphilis among men and women has declined since 1991, as has the number of reported cases of congenital syphilis in infants (with 1049 cases in 1997). It is important to note, however, that the case definition for congenital syphilis was broadened in 1989 and now includes all live or stillborn infants delivered to women with untreated or inadequately treated syphilis at delivery.

Approximately one of every two individuals named as sexual contacts of persons with infectious syphilis becomes infected. Many sexual contacts will already have developed manifestations of syphilis when they are first seen, and about 30% of apparently uninfected contacts who are examined within 30 days of exposure actually have incubating infection and will later develop infectious syphilis if not treated. Thus, the identification and "epidemiologic" treatment of all recently exposed sexual contacts constitute an important aspect of syphilis control. Also important is the identification of infected persons by serologic testing of pregnant women, persons admitted to hospitals, military inductees, and persons undergoing examination in physicians' offices. Still controversial are laws and regulations requiring routine premarital serologic testing for syphilis, where—though national data are not available—the yield is undoubtedly lower.

NATURAL COURSE AND PATHOGENESIS OF UNTREATED SYPHILIS *T. pallidum* rapidly penetrates intact mucous membranes or microscopic abrasions in skin and within a few hours enters the lymphatics and blood to produce systemic infection and metastatic foci long before the appearance of a primary lesion. Blood from a patient with incubating or early syphilis is infectious. The generation time of *T. pallidum* during early active disease in vivo is estimated to be 30 to 33 h, and the incubation period of syphilis is inversely proportional to the number of organisms inoculated. The concentration of treponemes generally reaches at least 10^7 per gram of tissue before the appearance of a clinical lesion. On the basis of intradermal injection of graded doses of *T. pallidum* into eight volunteers, the 50% infectious dose was calculated to be 57 organisms. The median incubation period in humans (about 21 days) suggests an average inoculum of 500 to 1000 infectious organisms for naturally acquired disease. The incubation period (from inoculation until the primary lesion becomes discernible) rarely exceeds 6 weeks. Subcurative therapy during the incubation period may delay the onset of the primary lesion, but it is not certain that such treatment reduces the probability that symptomatic disease will ultimately develop.

The primary lesion appears at the site of inoculation, usually persists for 4 to 6 weeks, and then heals spontaneously. Histopathologic examination of primary lesions shows perivascular infiltration, chiefly by lymphocytes (including CD8+ and CD4+ cells), plasma cells, and macrophages, with capillary endothelial proliferation and subsequent obliteration of small blood vessels. The CD4+ infiltration displays a T_H1-type cytokine profile consistent with the activation of macrophages. At this time *T. pallidum* is demonstrable in the chancre in spaces between epithelial cells; within invaginations or phagosomes of epithelial cells, fibroblasts, plasma cells, and the endothelial cells of small capillaries; within lymphatic channels; and in the regional lymph nodes. Phagocytosis of organisms by activated macrophages ultimately causes their destruction, which results in spontaneous resolution of the chancre.

The generalized parenchymal, constitutional, and mucocutaneous manifestations of secondary syphilis usually appear about 6 to 8 weeks after healing of the chancre, although 15% of patients with secondary syphilis still have persisting or healing chancres. In other patients, secondary lesions may appear several months after the chancre has healed, and some patients may enter the latent stage without ever recognizing secondary lesions. The histopathologic features of secondary maculopapular skin lesions are hyperkeratosis of the epidermis; capillary proliferation with endothelial swelling in the superficial corium; and dermal papillae with transmigration of polymorphonuclear leukocytes and, in the deeper corium, perivascular infiltration by monocytes, plasma cells, and lymphocytes. Treponemes are found in many tissues, including the aqueous humor of the eye and the cerebrospinal fluid (CSF). Invasion of the CNS by *T. pallidum* occurs during the first weeks or months of infection, and CSF abnormalities are detected in as many as 40% of patients during the secondary stage. Clinical hepatitis and immune complex–induced membranous glomerulonephritis are relatively rare but recognized manifestations of secondary syphilis; liver function tests may yield abnormal results in up to a quarter of patients with early syphilis. Generalized nontender lymphadenopathy is noted in 85% of patients with secondary syphilis. The paradoxical appearance of secondary manifestations despite high titers of antibody (including immobilizing antibody) to *T. pallidum* is unexplained but may result from changes in expression of surface antigens. Secondary lesions subside within 2 to 6 weeks, and the infection enters the latent stage, which is detectable only by serologic testing. In the preantibiotic era, up to 25% of untreated patients experienced at least one generalized or localized mucocutaneous relapse, usually during the first year; therefore, identification and examination of sexual contacts are most important for patients with syphilis of <1 year's duration. Recurrent generalized rash is now rare.

In the preantibiotic era, about one-third of patients with untreated latent syphilis developed clinically apparent tertiary disease; today, in industrialized countries, specific treatment and coincidental therapy for early and latent syphilis have all but eliminated tertiary disease except for sporadic cases of neurosyphilis in persons infected with HIV. In the past, the most common type of tertiary disease was the gumma, a usually benign granulomatous lesion. Today, gummas are very uncommon. Cardiovascular syphilis, now also rare, is caused by obliterative small-vessel endarteritis, usually involving the vasa vasorum of the ascending aorta and resulting in aneurysm. Asymptomatic CNS involvement is demonstrable in up to 25% of patients with late latent syphilis. The factors that contribute to the development and progression of tertiary disease are unknown.

The course of untreated syphilis was studied retrospectively in a group of nearly 2000 patients with primary or secondary disease diagnosed clinically (the Oslo Study, 1891–1951) and prospectively in 431 African-American men with seropositive latent syphilis of 3 or more years' duration (the notorious Tuskegee Study, 1932–1972). In the Oslo Study, 24% of patients developed relapsing secondary lesions within 4 years, and 28% eventually developed one or more manifestations of tertiary syphilis. Cardiovascular syphilis, including aortitis, was detected in 10% of patients, none of whom had been infected before age 15; 7% of patients developed symptomatic neurosyphilis, and 16% developed benign tertiary syphilis (gummas of the skin, mucous membranes, and skeleton). Syphilis was the primary cause of death in 15% of men and 8% of women. Cardiovascular syphilis was documented in 35% of men and 22% of women who eventually came to autopsy. In general, serious late complications were nearly twice as common among men as among women.

The Tuskegee Study showed that the death rate among untreated African-American men with syphilis (25 to 50 years old) was 17% higher than that among uninfected subjects and that 30% of all deaths were attributable to cardiovascular or CNS syphilis. By far the most important factor in increased mortality was cardiovascular syphilis. Anatomic evidence of aortitis was found in 40 to 60% of autopsied subjects with syphilis (versus 15% of control subjects), while CNS syphilis was found in only 4%. Rates of hypertension were also higher among the infected subjects. The ethical issues eventually raised by this study, begun in the preantibiotic era but continuing into the early 1970s, had a major influence on the development of current guidelines for human medical experimentation, and the history of the study may still contribute to a reluctance of some African Americans to participate as subjects in clinical research.

These two studies both showed that about one-third of patients with untreated syphilis develop clinical or pathologic evidence of tertiary syphilis, that about one-fourth die as a direct result of tertiary syphilis, and that there is additional excess mortality not directly attributable to tertiary syphilis.

MANIFESTATIONS   **Primary Syphilis**   The typical primary chancre usually begins as a single painless papule that rapidly becomes eroded and usually becomes indurated, with a characteristic cartilaginous consistency on palpation of the edge and base of the ulcer (**see Plate IID-47**). In heterosexual men the chancre is usually located on the penis, whereas in homosexual men it is often found in the anal canal or rectum, in the mouth, or on the external genitalia. In women, common primary sites are the cervix and labia. Consequently, primary syphilis goes unrecognized in women and homosexual men more often than in heterosexual men.

Atypical primary lesions are common. The clinical appearance depends on the number of treponemes inoculated and on the immunologic status of the patient. A large inoculum produces a dark-field-positive ulcerative lesion in nonimmune volunteers but may produce a small dark-field-negative papule, an asymptomatic but seropositive latent infection, or no response at all in individuals with a history of syphilis. A small inoculum may produce only a papular lesion, even in nonimmune individuals. Therefore, syphilis should be considered even in the evaluation of trivial or atypical dark-field-negative genital lesions. The genital lesions that most commonly must be differentiated from those of primary syphilis include traumatic superinfected lesions, lesions of herpes simplex virus infection (Chap. 182), and lesions of chancroid (Chap. 149). *Primary genital herpes* may produce inguinal adenopathy, but the nodes are tender and the lesions consist of multiple painful vesicles, which later ulcerate and are often accompanied by systemic symptoms, including fever. *Recurrent genital herpes* typically begins with a unilateral cluster of painful vesicles, usually without associated adenopathy. *Chancroid* produces painful, superficial, exudative, nonindurated ulcers, more often multiple than in syphilis (**see Plate IID-54**); adenopathy is common, can be either unilateral or bilateral, is tender, and may be suppurative.

Regional lymphadenopathy usually accompanies the primary syphilitic lesion, appearing within 1 week of the onset of the lesion. The nodes are firm, nonsuppurative, and painless. Inguinal lymphadenopathy is bilateral and may occur with anal as well as with external genital chancres. Rectal chancres result in perirectal lymphadenopathy, while chancres of the cervix and vagina result in iliac or perirectal adenopathy. The chancre generally heals within 4 to 6 weeks (range, 2 to 12 weeks), but lymphadenopathy may persist for months.

Secondary Syphilis   The protean manifestations of the secondary stage usually include localized or diffuse symmetric mucocutaneous lesions and generalized nontender lymphadenopathy. The healing primary chancre is still present in 15% of cases. The skin rash consists of macular, papular, papulosquamous, and occasionally pustular syphilides; often more than one form is present simultaneously. The eruption may be very subtle. Approximately 25% of patients with a discernible rash of secondary syphilis may be unaware that they have dermatologic manifestations. Initial lesions are bilaterally symmetric, pale red or pink, nonpruritic, discrete, round macules that measure 5 to 10 mm in diameter and are distributed on the trunk and proximal extremities (see **Plate IID-50**). After several days or weeks, red papular lesions 3 to 10 mm in diameter also appear. These lesions, which may progress to necrotic lesions (resembling pustules) in association with increasing endarteritis and perivascular mononuclear infiltration, are distributed widely, frequently involve the palms and soles (see **Plate IID-48**), and may occur on the face and scalp. Tiny papular *follicular syphilides* involving hair follicles may result in patchy alopecia (alopecia areata), with loss of scalp hair, eyebrows, or beard in up to 5% of cases. Progressive endarteritis obliterans and ischemia result in superficial scaling of papules (*papulosquamous syphilides*) and eventually may lead to central necrosis (*pustular syphilides*).

In warm, moist, intertriginous body areas, including the perianal area, vulva, scrotum, inner thighs, axillae, and skin under pendulous breasts, papules can enlarge and become eroded to produce broad, moist, pink or gray-white, highly infectious lesions called *condylomata lata* (see **Plate IID-49**); these lesions develop in 10% of patients with secondary syphilis. Superficial mucosal erosions, called *mucous patches*, occur in 10 to 15% of patients and may involve the lips, oral mucosa, tongue (Fig. 172-1), palate, pharynx, vulva and vagina, glans penis, or inner prepuce. The typical mucous patch is a painless silver-gray erosion surrounded by a red periphery. During relapses of secondary syphilis, condylomata lata are particularly common, and skin lesions tend to be asymmetrically distributed and more infiltrated, resembling skin lesions of late syphilis. These characteristics may reflect increasing cellular immunity.

Constitutional symptoms that may accompany or precede secondary syphilis include sore throat (15 to 30%), fever (5 to 8%), weight loss (2 to 20%), malaise (25%), anorexia (2 to 10%), headache (10%), and meningismus (5%). *Acute meningitis* occurs in only 1 to 2% of cases, but numbers of cells and levels of protein in CSF are increased in ≥30% of cases. *T. pallidum* has been recovered from CSF during primary and secondary syphilis in 30% of cases; this finding is often but not always associated with other CSF abnormalities.

Less common complications of secondary syphilis include hepatitis, nephropathy, gastrointestinal involvement (hypertrophic gastritis, patchy proctitis, ulcerative colitis, or a rectosigmoid mass), arthritis, and periostitis. Ocular findings that suggest secondary syphilis include otherwise-unexplained pupillary abnormalities, optic neuritis, and a retinitis pigmentosa syndrome as well as the classic iritis (especially granulomatous iritis) or uveitis. The diagnosis of secondary syphilis is often considered only after the patient fails to respond to steroid therapy. Anterior uveitis has been reported in 5 to 10% of patients with secondary syphilis, and *T. pallidum* has been demonstrated in the aqueous humor from these patients. *Syphilitic hepatitis* is distinguished by an unusually high serum level of alkaline phosphatase and by a nonspecific histologic appearance that is unlike that of viral hepatitis

and includes moderate inflammation with polymorphonuclear leukocytes and lymphocytes, some hepatocellular damage, and no cholestasis. *Renal involvement* produces proteinuria associated with an acute nephrotic syndrome (or rarely with hemorrhagic glomerulonephritis) and is characterized by subepithelial electron-dense deposits and glomerular immune complexes—findings suggesting immune-complex glomerulonephritis.

Latent Syphilis Positive serologic tests for syphilis, together with a normal CSF examination and the absence of clinical manifestations of syphilis, indicate a diagnosis of latent syphilis. The diagnosis is often suspected on the basis of a history of primary or secondary lesions, a history of exposure to syphilis, or the delivery of an infant with congenital syphilis. A previous negative serologic test or a history of lesions or exposure may help establish the duration of latent infection. *Early latent* syphilis encompasses the first year after infection, while *late latent* syphilis (beginning ≥1 year after infection in the untreated patient) is associated with relative immunity to infectious relapse and with increasing resistance to reinfection. *T. pallidum* may still seed the bloodstream intermittently during this stage. Pregnant women with latent syphilis may infect the fetus in utero. Moreover, syphilis has been transmitted through the transfusion of blood from patients with latent syphilis of many years' duration. It was previously thought that untreated late latent syphilis had three possible outcomes: (1) it could persist throughout the lifetime of the infected individual, (2) it could end in the development of late syphilis, or (3) it could end with the spontaneous cure of infection, with reversion of serologic tests to negative. It is now apparent, however, that the more sensitive treponemal antibody tests rarely, if ever, become negative without treatment. About 70% of untreated patients with latent syphilis never develop clinically evident late syphilis, but the occurrence of spontaneous cure is in doubt.

Late Syphilis The slowly progressive inflammatory disease leading to tertiary manifestations begins early during the pathogenesis of syphilis, although these manifestations may not become clinically apparent for years. Early syphilitic aortitis becomes evident soon after secondary lesions subside, and patients who develop CSF abnormalities during the early stages of syphilis appear to be at highest risk of late neurologic complications.

Asymptomatic neurosyphilis CNS syphilis represents a continuum comprising early invasion, usually within the first weeks or months of infection, and asymptomatic involvement, which may or may not lead to neurologic manifestations. Traditionally, the diagnosis of asymptomatic neurosyphilis has been made in patients who lack neurologic symptoms and signs and who have CSF abnormalities including mononuclear pleocytosis, increased protein concentrations, or a reactive Venereal Disease Research Laboratory (VDRL) slide test. Such abnormalities are found in up to one-quarter of patients with untreated late latent syphilis, and it is these patients who are known to be at risk for neurologic complications. However, in primary and secondary syphilis, *T. pallidum* can be isolated from CSF of 40% of patients even in the absence of other CSF abnormalities. Although the therapeutic implications of these findings in early syphilis are uncertain, it seems appropriate to conclude that even patients with early syphilis who have such findings do indeed have asymptomatic neurosyphilis and should be treated for neurosyphilis. In patients with untreated asymptomatic neurosyphilis, the overall cumulative probability of progression to clinical neurosyphilis is about 20% in the first 10 years but increases with time; the likelihood is highest among patients with the greatest degree of pleocytosis or protein elevation. Patients with untreated latent syphilis and normal CSF probably run no risk of subsequent neurosyphilis.

Symptomatic neurosyphilis Although mixed features are common, the major clinical categories of symptomatic neurosyphilis include meningeal, meningovascular, and parenchymatous syphilis. The last category includes general paresis and tabes dorsalis. The onset of symptoms usually comes <1 year after infection for meningeal syph-

FIGURE 172-1 Mucous patches on the tongue of a patient with secondary syphilis. (*Courtesy of Ron Roddy.*)

ilis, at 5 to 10 years for meningovascular syphilis, at 20 years for general paresis, and at 25 to 30 years for tabes dorsalis. However, symptomatic neurosyphilis, particularly in the antibiotic era, often presents not as a classic picture but rather as mixed and subtle or incomplete syndromes.

Meningeal syphilis may involve either the brain or the spinal cord, and patients may present with headache, nausea, vomiting, neck stiffness, cranial nerve palsies, seizures, and changes in mental status. *Meningovascular syphilis* reflects diffuse inflammation of the pia and arachnoid together with evidence of focal or widespread arterial involvement of small, medium, or large vessels. The most common presentation is a stroke syndrome involving the middle cerebral artery of a relatively young adult; however, unlike the usual thrombotic or embolic stroke syndrome of sudden onset, meningovascular syphilis often becomes manifest after a subacute encephalitic prodrome (with headaches, vertigo, insomnia, and psychological abnormalities), which is followed by a gradually progressive vascular syndrome.

The manifestations of *general paresis* reflect widespread parenchymal damage and include abnormalities corresponding to the mnemonic *paresis*: *p*ersonality, *a*ffect, *r*eflexes (hyperactive), *e*ye (e.g., Argyll Robertson pupils), *s*ensorium (illusions, delusions, hallucinations), *i*ntellect (a decrease in recent memory and in the capacity for orientation, calculations, judgment, and insight), and *s*peech. *Tabes dorsalis* presents as symptoms and signs of demyelination of the posterior columns, dorsal roots, and dorsal root ganglia. Symptoms include ataxic wide-based gait and footslap; paresthesia; bladder disturbances; impotence; areflexia; and loss of position, deep pain, and temperature sensations. Trophic joint degeneration (Charcot's joints) and perforating ulceration of the feet can result from loss of pain sensation. The small, irregular Argyll Robertson pupil, a feature of both tabes dorsalis and paresis, reacts to accommodation but not to light. *Optic atrophy* also occurs frequently in association with tabes.

Cardiovascular syphilis   Cardiovascular manifestations are attributable to endarteritis obliterans of the vasa vasorum, which provide the blood supply to large vessels. This condition produces medial necrosis with destruction of elastic tissue, particularly in the ascending and transverse segments of the aortic arch, resulting in uncomplicated aortitis, aortic regurgitation, saccular aneurysm, or coronary ostial stenosis. Symptoms appear from 10 to 40 years after infection. Cardiovascular complications occur more often and at an earlier age among men than among women and may be more common among African Americans than among whites. In the preantibiotic era, symptomatic cardiovascular complications developed in about 10% of persons with late untreated syphilis, and aortic regurgitation was two to four times as common as aneurysm. However, syphilitic aortitis was demonstrated at autopsy in about one-half of African-American men with untreated syphilis.

Linear calcification of the ascending aorta on chest x-ray films suggests asymptomatic syphilitic aortitis, as arteriosclerosis seldom produces this sign. Aortic dilation and a tambour quality to the sound of aortic closure are unreliable signs of aortitis. Syphilitic aneurysms—usually saccular, occasionally fusiform—do not lead to dissection. Approximately 1 in 10 aortic aneurysms of syphilitic origin involves the abdominal aorta, but these aneurysms tend to occur above the renal arteries, whereas arteriosclerotic abdominal aneurysms are usually found below the renal arteries. With increasing age, the nervous system is also affected in up to 40% of patients with cardiovascular syphilis.

Late lesions of the eyes   Iritis associated with pain, photophobia, and dimness of vision or chorioretinitis occurs not only during secondary syphilis but also as a relatively common manifestation of late syphilis. Adhesions of the iris to the anterior lens may produce a fixed pupil, not to be confused with Argyll Robertson pupil.

Late benign syphilis (gumma)   Gummas may be multiple or diffuse but are usually solitary lesions that range from microscopic size to several centimeters in diameter. From a histologic perspective, gum-

mas consist of a granulomatous inflammation with a central area of necrosis surrounded by mononuclear, epithelioid, and fibroblastic cells; occasional giant cells; and perivasculitis. Although rarely demonstrated microscopically, *T. pallidum* has reportedly been recovered from these lesions. The most commonly involved sites include the skin and skeletal system, the mouth and upper respiratory tract, the larynx, the liver, and the stomach; however, any organ may be involved. Gummas of the skin produce painless and indurated nodular, papulosquamous, or ulcerative lesions that form characteristic circles or arcs, with peripheral hyperpigmentation. Gummas are usually indolent and may heal spontaneously with scarring, but they may also be explosive in onset and are often destructive. These lesions may resemble those of many other chronic granulomatous conditions, including tuberculosis and sarcoidosis, leprosy, and deep fungal infections. Skeletal gummas most frequently involve the long bones of the legs, although any bone may be affected. Trauma may predispose a specific site to involvement. Presenting symptoms usually include focal pain and tenderness. Radiographic abnormalities with advanced gummas of bone include periostitis or destructive or sclerosing osteitis. Upper respiratory gummas can lead to perforation of the nasal septum or palate. Gummatous hepatitis may produce epigastric pain and tenderness as well as low-grade fever and may be associated with splenomegaly and anemia.

The histopathology and extensive tissue necrosis associated with gummas suggest delayed hypersensitivity to *T. pallidum*. Certain individuals appear to develop an exaggerated delayed-hypersensitivity response to *T. pallidum*, which presumably is mediated by sensitized T lymphocytes and macrophages. Because the histologic changes may be suggestive but are nonspecific, the diagnosis of late benign syphilis is confirmed by serologic testing and by therapeutic trial. Treatment with penicillin results in rapid healing of active gummatous lesions.

Congenital Syphilis   Transmission of *T. pallidum* from a syphilitic woman to her fetus across the placenta may occur at any stage of pregnancy, but the lesions of congenital syphilis generally develop after the fourth month of gestation, when fetal immunologic competence begins to develop. This timing suggests that the pathogenesis of congenital syphilis depends on the immune response of the host rather than on a direct toxic effect of *T. pallidum*. The risk of infection of the fetus during untreated early maternal syphilis is estimated to be 75 to 95%, decreasing to about 35% for maternal syphilis of >2 years' duration. Adequate treatment of the mother before the 16th week of pregnancy should prevent fetal damage. Untreated maternal infection may result in a rate of fetal loss of up to 40% (with stillbirth more common than abortion because of the late onset of fetal pathology), prematurity, neonatal death, or nonfatal congenital syphilis. Among infants born alive, only fulminant congenital syphilis is clinically apparent at birth, and these babies have a very poor prognosis. The most common clinical problem is the healthy-appearing baby born to a mother with a positive serologic test. Routine serologic testing in early pregnancy is considered cost-effective in virtually all populations, even in areas with a low prenatal prevalence of syphilis. Where the prevalence of syphilis is high and when the patient is at high risk, syphilis serology should be repeated in the third trimester and at delivery.

The manifestations of congenital syphilis can be divided into three types according to their timing: (1) early manifestations, which appear within the first 2 years of life (often between 2 and 10 weeks of age), are infectious and resemble the manifestations of severe secondary syphilis in the adult; (2) late manifestations, which appear after 2 years and are noninfectious; and (3) residual stigmata. The earliest sign of congenital syphilis is usually rhinitis, or "snuffles" (23%), which is soon followed by other mucocutaneous lesions (35 to 41%). These may include bullae (syphilitic pemphigus), vesicles, superficial desquamation, petechiae, and (later) papulosquamous lesions, mucous patches, and condylomata lata. The most common early manifestations are bone changes (61%), including osteochondritis, osteitis, and periostitis. Hepatosplenomegaly (50%), lymphadenopathy (32%), anemia (34%), jaundice (30%), thrombocytopenia, and leukocytosis are common.

Neonatal congenital syphilis must be differentiated from other generalized congenital infections, including rubella, cytomegalovirus or herpes simplex virus infection, and toxoplasmosis, as well as from erythroblastosis fetalis. Neonatal death is usually due to pulmonary hemorrhage, secondary bacterial infection, or severe hepatitis.

Late congenital syphilis is that which remains untreated after 2 years of age. In perhaps 60% of cases, the infection remains subclinical; the clinical spectrum in the remainder of cases differs in certain respects from that of acquired late syphilis in the adult. For example, cardiovascular syphilis rarely develops in late congenital syphilis, whereas interstitial keratitis is much more common and occurs between the ages of 5 and 25. Other manifestations associated with interstitial keratitis are eighth-nerve deafness and recurrent arthropathy. Bilateral knee effusions are known as *Clutton's joints*. Asymptomatic neurosyphilis is present in about one-third of untreated patients, and clinical neurosyphilis occurs in one-quarter of untreated individuals over 6 years of age. Gummatous periostitis occurs between the ages of 5 and 20 and, as in nonvenereal endemic syphilis, tends to cause destructive lesions of the palate and nasal septum.

Characteristic stigmata include *Hutchinson's teeth*—centrally notched, widely spaced, peg-shaped upper central incisors—and "mulberry" molars—sixth-year molars with multiple, poorly developed cusps. The abnormal facies of patients with congenital syphilis include frontal bossing, saddle nose, and poorly developed maxillae. Saber shins, characterized by anterior tibial bowing, are rare. *Rhagades* are linear scars at the angles of the mouth and nose that are caused by secondary bacterial infection of the early facial eruption. Other stigmata include unexplained nerve deafness, old chorioretinitis, optic atrophy, and corneal opacities due to past interstitial keratitis.

LABORATORY EXAMINATIONS   Demonstration of the Organism   Dark-field microscopic examination of lesion exudate is useful in evaluating moist cutaneous lesions, such as the chancre of primary syphilis or the condylomata lata of secondary syphilis. The identification of a single characteristic motile organism by a trained observer is sufficient for diagnosis. Examination of oral lesions and anal ulcers by this method is not recommended, as it is difficult to differentiate *T. pallidum* from other spirochetes that may be present.

Most syphilis is diagnosed in settings where dark-field microscopy is not available. The direct fluorescent antibody *T. pallidum* (DFA-TP) test, an alternative available at central laboratories, uses fluorescein-conjugated polyclonal antitreponemal antibody for the detection of *T. pallidum* in fixed smears prepared from suspect lesions. More sensitive PCR tests have been developed but are available only in research laboratories.

T. pallidum can be found in tissue with appropriate silver stains, although these results should be interpreted with caution because artifacts resembling *T. pallidum* are often seen. Treponemes can be demonstrated more reliably in tissue by immunofluorescent or immunohistochemical methods using specific monoclonal or polyclonal antibodies to *T. pallidum*.

Serologic Tests for Syphilis   There are two types of serologic tests for syphilis: nontreponemal and treponemal. Both types of tests are reactive in persons with any treponemal infection, including yaws, pinta, and endemic syphilis.

The nontreponemal tests measure IgG and IgM directed against a cardiolipin-lecithin-cholesterol antigen complex. The most widely used nontreponemal antibody tests for syphilis are the rapid plasma reagin (RPR) test, which can be automated (ART), and the VDRL slide test. In these tests, antibody is detected by the microscopic or macroscopic flocculation of the antigen suspension. The RPR test may be more expensive than the VDRL test, but it is easier to perform and uses unheated serum; it is the test of choice for rapid serologic diagnosis in a clinic or office setting. The VDRL test, however, remains the standard for use with CSF.

The RPR and VDRL tests are equally sensitive and may be used for initial screening or for quantitation of serum antibody. The titer reflects the activity of the disease. A fourfold or greater rise in titer may be seen during the evolution of early syphilis. VDRL titers usually

reach 1:32 or higher in secondary syphilis. A persistent fall of two dilutions (fourfold) or greater following treatment of early syphilis provides essential evidence of an adequate response to therapy. VDRL titers do not correspond directly to RPR titers, and sequential quantitative testing (as for response to therapy) must employ a single test.

Two standard treponemal tests are used for confirmation of reactive nontreponemal results: the fluorescent treponemal antibody–absorbed (FTA-ABS) test and the agglutination assays for antibodies to *T. pallidum*. The microhemagglutination assay for *T. pallidum* (MHA-TP) has been replaced by the Serodia TP-PA test (Fujirebio, Tokyo), which is more sensitive for primary syphilis. The *T. pallidum* hemagglutination test (TPHA) is widely used in Europe but is not available in the United States. Both the agglutination assays and the FTA-ABS tests are very specific and, when used for confirmation of positive nontreponemal tests, have a very high positive predictive value for the diagnosis of syphilis. However, even these tests give false-positive results at rates as high as 1 to 2% when used for the screening of normal populations. New enzyme-linked immunosorbent assays have also been approved as confirmatory tests.

The relative sensitivities of the VDRL test, the FTA-ABS test, and the MHA-TP in the various stages of untreated syphilis are shown in Table 172-1. The nontreponemal tests are nonreactive in about one-quarter of patients presenting with primary syphilis. In early primary syphilis, the detection of antibody can be maximized either by the performance of an FTA-ABS test or simply by repetition of a VDRL test after 1 to 2 weeks if the initial VDRL result is negative. All treponemal and nontreponemal tests are reactive during secondary syphilis, and a nonreactive result virtually excludes syphilis in a patient with otherwise-compatible mucocutaneous lesions. (Fewer than 1% of patients with secondary syphilis have a VDRL test that is nonreactive or weakly reactive with undiluted serum but is positive at higher serum dilutions—the *prozone phenomenon*.) While the nontreponemal tests will become nonreactive or will be reactive in lower titers following therapy for early syphilis, the treponemal tests often remain reactive after therapy and therefore are not helpful in determining the infection status of persons with past syphilis.

For practical purposes, most clinicians need to be familiar with the three uses of serologic tests for syphilis: (1) testing of large numbers of sera for screening or diagnostic purposes (e.g., the RPR or VDRL test), (2) quantitative measurement of the antibody titer to assess the clinical activity of syphilis or to monitor the response to therapy (e.g., the VDRL or RPR test), and (3) confirmation of the diagnosis of syphilis in a patient with a positive nontreponemal antibody test or with a suspected clinical diagnosis of syphilis (e.g., the FTA-ABS test or Serodia TP-PA).

For measurement of IgM in neonates in whom congenital syphilis is suspected, the syphilis Captia-M test (Trinity Biotech, Jamestown, NY) and the 19S IgM FTA-ABS test are available.

False-Positive Serologic Tests for Syphilis   Because the antigen used in nontreponemal tests is found in other tissues, the tests may be reactive in persons without treponemal infection, although rarely do titers exceed 1:8 in such patients. In a population selected for screening because of clinical suspicion, history of exposure, or increased risk for

Table 172-1   Sensitivity of Serodiagnostic Tests in Untreated Syphilis

Test[a]	Mean Percentage Positive (Range) at Indicated Stage of Disease[b]			
	Primary	Secondary	Latent	Tertiary
VDRL	78 (74–87)	100	95 (88–100)	71 (37–94)
FTA-ABS	84 (70–100)	100	100	96
MHA-TP[c]	76 (69–90)	100	100	94

[a] The specificity for each of these tests is 97 to 99%.
[b] In CDC studies.
[c] The MHA-TP has recently been replaced by the Serodia TP-PA test. Early evaluations suggest that the TP-PA test is more sensitive than the MHA-TP in primary syphilis.
SOURCE: Modified from SA Larsen et al: Clin Microbiol Rev 8:1, 1995.

sexually transmitted infections, fewer than 1% of reactive tests are falsely positive. The modern VDRL and RPR tests are 97 to 99% specific, and false-positive reactions are now limited largely to those conditions listed in Table 172-2. False positivity is common among persons with autoimmune disorders. The prevalence of false-positive nontreponemal tests increases with advancing age; 10% of people over 70 years of age have false-positive reactions. In the patient with a false-positive nontreponemal test, syphilis is excluded by a nonreactive treponemal test.

Evaluation for Neurosyphilis Asymptomatic involvement of the CNS is detected by examination of CSF for pleocytosis, increased protein concentration, and VDRL activity. CSF abnormalities can be demonstrated in up to 40% of cases of primary or secondary syphilis and in 25% of cases of latent syphilis. In older asymptomatic seropositive individuals, the yield of lumbar puncture is relatively low. *T. pallidum* has been recovered by CSF inoculation into rabbits from up to 30% of patients with primary or secondary syphilis but rarely from those with latent syphilis. The demonstration of *T. pallidum* in CSF is often associated with other CSF abnormalities; however, organisms can be recovered from patients with otherwise-normal CSF. Before the advent of penicillin, the risk of developing clinical neurosyphilis was roughly proportional to the intensity of CSF changes in early syphilis. CSF examination is essential in the evaluation of any seropositive patient with neurologic signs and symptoms and is recommended for all patients with untreated syphilis of unknown duration or of >1 year's duration. The possibility of asymptomatic neurosyphilis in some patients with early disease is not addressed by these recommendations. Because standard therapy with penicillin G benzathine (benzathine benzylpenicillin) for early syphilis fails to result in treponemicidal levels in the CSF, some experts advise lumbar puncture in secondary and early latent syphilis, particularly in patients with HIV infection.

In short, lumbar puncture should be performed in the evaluation of latent syphilis of >1 year's duration, in suspected neurosyphilis, and in late complications other than symptomatic neurosyphilis (since asymptomatic neurosyphilis may coexist with other late complications). CSF examination is most clearly indicated in the following situations: neurologic signs or symptoms, treatment failure, a serum reagin titer ≥ 1:32, HIV antibody positivity, other evidence of active syphilis (e.g., aortitis, gumma, visual or hearing changes), or plans to administer nonpenicillin therapy.

The CSF VDRL test is highly specific but relatively insensitive and may be nonreactive even in cases of progressive symptomatic neurosyphilis. The degree of sensitivity is highest in meningovascular syphilis and paresis and is lower in asymptomatic neurosyphilis and tabes dorsalis. The unabsorbed FTA test on CSF is reactive far more often than the CSF VDRL test in all stages of syphilis, but FTA reactivity may reflect passive transfer of serum antibody into the CSF.

Table 172-2   Causes of False-Positive Reactions in Nontreponemal Serologic Tests for Syphilis

Cause	Rate of False-Positive Reactions, %[a]
ACUTE FALSE-POSITIVE REACTION (<6 MONTHS)	
Recent viral illness or immunization	1–2
Genital herpes	4.4
Human immunodeficiency virus infection	1–4
Malaria	11
Parenteral drug use	20–25
CHRONIC FALSE-POSITIVE REACTION (≥6 MONTHS)	
Aging	9–11
Autoimmune disorders	1–20
Systemic lupus erythematosus	11–20
Rheumatoid arthritis	5
Parenteral drug use	20–25

[a] Data were collected from a variety of published reports.

A nonreactive CSF FTA test, however, may be used to rule out neurosyphilis.

Evaluation for Syphilis in Patients Infected with HIV Because persons at highest risk for syphilis (inner-city populations, homosexually active men, and people in many developing countries) are also at increased risk for HIV infection, these two infections frequently coexist in the same patient. There is evidence that syphilis and other genital-ulcer diseases may be important risk factors for the acquisition and transmission of HIV infection.

The manifestations of syphilis may be altered in patients with concurrent HIV infection, and multiple cases of neurologic relapse following standard therapy have been reported in HIV-infected patients. *T. pallidum* has been isolated from the CSF of several patients after therapy for early syphilis with penicillin G benzathine. A recent multicenter U.S. study of early syphilis found similar therapeutic responses in persons with and without concurrent HIV infection, although the study lacked sufficient statistical power to exclude an effect of HIV and 41% of subjects were lost to follow-up. This investigation confirmed the high rate of CNS invasion in early syphilis and the persistence of *T. pallidum* after standard therapy: 11 of 43 HIV-infected patients and 21 of 88 HIV-uninfected patients had *T. pallidum* detectable in CSF before therapy; 7 of the 35 patients who underwent lumbar puncture after therapy (some HIV-infected and others uninfected) still had *T. pallidum* detectable in CSF.

The frequency of unusual clinical and laboratory manifestations of syphilis among patients co-infected with HIV is unknown. Such changes may be dependent on the stage of HIV infection and the degree of immunosuppression. There is no clear evidence that the sensitivity of serologic tests for syphilis or the serologic response to therapy in the vast majority of HIV-infected patients with early syphilis differs from the corresponding findings in patients not infected with HIV. Interpretation of serologic results should be the same for the two groups.

Persons with newly diagnosed HIV infection should be tested for syphilis. Some authorities, persuaded by reports of the persistence of *T. pallidum* in the CSF of HIV-infected persons after standard penicillin benzathine therapy for early syphilis, recommend examination of CSF for evidence of neurosyphilis for all co-infected patients, regardless of the clinical stage of syphilis, with treatment for neurosyphilis if CSF abnormalities are found or if CSF examination is not performed. Others do not recommend routine CSF examination for HIV-co-infected patients with early syphilis and believe that standard therapy is sufficient. Serologic testing after treatment is important for all patients with syphilis, particularly those also infected with HIV.

℞ TREATMENT   Treatment of Acquired Syphilis Penicillin G is the drug of choice for all stages of syphilis. *T. pallidum* is killed by very low concentrations of penicillin G, although a long period of exposure to penicillin is required because of the unusually slow rate of multiplication of the organism. The efficacy of penicillin for syphilis remains undiminished after 50 years of use. Other antibiotics effective in syphilis include the tetracyclines, erythromycin, and the cephalosporins. Aminoglycosides and spectinomycin inhibit *T. pallidum* only in very large doses, and the sulfonamides and the quinolones are inactive.

Serum levels of penicillin G of ≥0.03 µg/mL for at least 7 days are considered necessary for the cure of early syphilis. Recurrence rates for a given regimen increase as infection progresses from incubating to seronegative primary to seropositive primary to secondary to late syphilis. Therefore, it is probable, but unproven, that a longer duration of therapy is required to effect cure as the infection progresses. For these reasons, some authorities use more prolonged penicillin therapy than that recommended by the U.S. Public Health Service when treating secondary, latent, or late syphilis.

The treatment regimens recommended for syphilis are summarized in Table 172-3 and are discussed below.

Early syphilis Preventive (abortive, "epidemiologic") treatment is recommended for seronegative individuals without signs of syphilis who have been exposed to infectious syphilis within the previous 3 months. Before treatment is given, every effort should be made to establish a diagnosis by examination and serologic testing. *The regimens recommended for prevention are the same as those recommended for early syphilis.*

Penicillin G benzathine is the most widely used agent for the treatment of early syphilis (including primary, secondary, and early latent syphilis), although it is more painful on injection than penicillin G procaine. A single dose of 2.4 million units cures more than 95% of cases of primary syphilis. Because the drug's efficacy in secondary syphilis may be slightly lower, some physicians administer a second dose of 2.4 million units 1 week after the initial dose at this stage of disease. Clinical relapse can follow treatment with penicillin G benzathine in patients with both HIV infection and early syphilis. Because the risk of neurorelapse may be higher in HIV-infected patients, examination of CSF from HIV-seropositive individuals with syphilis of any stage is recommended by some experts; therapy appropriate for neurosyphilis should be given if there is any evidence of CNS syphilis.

For penicillin-allergic patients with early syphilis, a 2-week course of therapy with doxycycline or tetracycline is recommended. These regimens appear to be effective, although no well-controlled studies have been performed and poor compliance may be problematic. Although ceftriaxone and azithromycin have shown activity against *T. pallidum* in animals, human trials have not been of sufficient scope to permit the recommendation of either drug for any stage of syphilis.

Late latent and late syphilis (normal CSF) If CSF abnormalities are found, the patient should be treated for neurosyphilis. The recommended treatment for late latent syphilis with normal CSF, for cardiovascular syphilis, and for late benign syphilis (gumma) is penicillin G benzathine, 2.4 million units intramuscularly once a week for 3 successive weeks (7.2 million units total). Doxycycline or tetracycline (given for 1 month) offers an untested alternative for penicillin-allergic patients with latent or late syphilis and normal CSF. The clinical response to treatment for benign tertiary syphilis is usually impressive; however, responses to therapy for cardiovascular syphilis are not dramatic because aortic aneurysm and aortic regurgitation cannot be reversed by antibiotic treatment.

Neurosyphilis The 1998 neurosyphilis treatment guidelines of the Centers for Disease Control and Prevention (CDC) are presented in Table 172-3. Penicillin G benzathine, given in total doses of up to 7.2 million units to adults or 50,000 units per kilogram to infants, does not produce detectable concentrations of penicillin G in CSF, and asymptomatic neurosyphilis may relapse in patients treated with 2.4 million units; the risk may be higher in HIV-infected patients. Therefore, the use of penicillin G benzathine alone for the treatment of neurosyphilis is not recommended. On the other hand, administration of intravenous penicillin G in doses of ≥12 million units per day for 10 days or longer is thought to ensure treponemicidal concentrations of penicillin G in CSF and occasionally cures infection in patients who fail to respond to other therapy. The clinical response to penicillin therapy for meningeal syphilis is dramatic, but the response to treatment for parenchymal neurosyphilis is variable. In general, treatment of neurosyphilis in which damage has already been done may produce no clinical change but may arrest disease progression.

Table 172-3 Recommendations for the Treatment of Syphilis[a]

Stage of Syphilis	Patients without Penicillin Allergy	Patients with Confirmed Penicillin Allergy
Primary, secondary, or early latent	Penicillin G benzathine (single dose of 2.4 million units IM, 1.2 million units in each buttock)	Tetracycline hydrochloride (500 mg PO qid) or doxycycline (100 mg PO bid) for 2 weeks

Late latent (or latent of uncertain duration), cardiovascular, or benign tertiary	Lumbar puncture
	  CSF normal: Penicillin G benzathine (2.4 million units IM weekly for 3 weeks)
	  CSF abnormal: Treat as neurosyphilis
		Lumbar puncture
		  CSF normal: Tetracycline hydrochloride (500 mg PO qid) or doxycycline (100 mg PO bid) for 4 weeks
		  CSF abnormal: Treat as neurosyphilis

Neurosyphilis (asymptomatic or symptomatic)	Aqueous penicillin G (18–24 million units/d IV, given in divided doses every 4 h) for 10–14 days *or* Aqueous penicillin G procaine (2.4 million units/d IM) plus oral probenecid (500 mg qid), both for 10–14 days	Desensitization and treatment with penicillin if allergy is confirmed by skin testing
Syphilis in pregnancy	According to stage	Desensitization and treatment with penicillin if allergy is confirmed by skin testing

[a] See text for discussion of syphilis therapy in HIV-infected individuals.
SOURCE: These recommendations are modified from those issued by the Centers for Disease Control and Prevention in 1998.

Several recent publications have reported neurologic relapse after high-dose intravenous penicillin therapy for neurosyphilis in HIV-infected patients. No alternative therapies have been explored, but careful follow-up is essential, and re-treatment is warranted in such patients.

No data support the use of antibiotics other than penicillin G for the treatment of neurosyphilis; however, some of the third-generation cephalosporins may deserve further evaluation. In patients with penicillin allergy demonstrated by skin testing, desensitization may be the best course (Chap. 126).

Management of syphilis in pregnancy Every pregnant woman should undergo a nontreponemal test at her first prenatal visit, and women at high risk of exposure should have a repeat test in the third trimester and at delivery. In the pregnant patient with presumed syphilis (evidenced by a reactive serology, with or without clinical manifestations) and with no history of treatment for syphilis, expeditious evaluation and initiation of treatment are essential. Therapy should be administered according to the stage of the disease, as for nonpregnant patients. Patients should be warned of the risk of a Jarisch-Herxheimer reaction, which may be associated with mild premature contractions but rarely results in premature delivery.

Penicillin is the only recommended therapy for syphilis in pregnancy. If the patient has a well-documented penicillin allergy, desensitization and penicillin treatment should be undertaken in a hospital according to the 1998 sexually transmitted diseases treatment guidelines issued by the CDC. After treatment, a quantitative nontreponemal test should be repeated monthly throughout pregnancy. Treated women whose titers rise fourfold or who do not show a fourfold decrease in titer in a 3-month period should be re-treated.

Evaluation and Management of Congenital Syphilis Newborn infants of mothers with reactive VDRL or FTA-ABS tests may themselves have reactive tests, whether or not they have become infected, because of transplacental transfer of maternal IgG antibody. Rising or persistent titers indicate infection, and the infant should be treated. Neonatal IgM antibody can be detected in cord or neonatal serum with the syphilis Captia-M or 19S IgM FTA-ABS test. Alternatively, monthly quantitative nontreponemal tests may be performed on asymptomatic infants born to women treated adequately with penicillin during pregnancy.

An infant should be treated at birth if the seropositive mother has received penicillin therapy in the third trimester, inadequate penicillin treatment, or therapy with a drug other than penicillin; if her treatment status is unknown; or if the infant may be difficult to follow. It is unwise to require proof of diagnosis before treatment in such cases. The CSF should be examined to obtain baseline values before treatment. Penicillin is the only recommended drug for syphilis in infants. The penicillin dosage used for the treatment of the patient with late congenital syphilis is calculated in the same way as for the infant, until dosage based on weight reaches that used for adult neurosyphilis. Specific recommendations for the treatment of infants are included in the CDC's 1998 guidelines.

Jarisch-Herxheimer Reaction A dramatic though usually mild reaction consisting of fever (average temperature elevation, 1.5°C), chills, myalgias, headache, tachycardia, increased respiratory rate, increased circulating neutrophil count, and vasodilation with mild hypotension may follow the initiation of treatment for syphilis. This reaction occurs in approximately 50% of patients with primary syphilis, 90% of those with secondary syphilis, and 25% of those with early latent syphilis. The onset comes within 2 h of treatment, the temperature peaks at about 7 h, and defervescence takes place within 12 to 24 h. The reaction is more delayed in neurosyphilis, with fever peaking after 12 to 14 h. In patients with secondary syphilis, erythema and edema of the mucocutaneous lesions increase; occasionally, subclinical or early mucocutaneous lesions may first become apparent during the reaction. The pathogenesis of this reaction is undefined, although recent studies have demonstrated the induction of inflammatory mediators such as tumor necrosis factor by treponemal lipoproteins. Patients should be warned to expect such symptoms, which can be managed by bed rest and aspirin. Steroid and other anti-inflammatory therapy is not required for this mild transient reaction.

Follow-Up Evaluation of Responses to Therapy The response of early syphilis to treatment should be determined by monitoring of the quantitative VDRL or RPR titer 1, 3, 6, and 12 months after treatment. More frequent serologic examination (1, 2, 3, 6, 9, and 12 months) is recommended for patients concurrently infected with HIV. Because the FTA-ABS and agglutination tests remain positive in most patients treated for seropositive syphilis, these tests are not useful in following the response to therapy. After successful treatment of seropositive first-episode primary or secondary syphilis, the VDRL titer progressively declines, becoming negative by 12 months in 40 to 75% of seropositive primary cases and in 20 to 40% of secondary cases. Patients with a history of syphilis have less rapid declines in titer and are less likely to become VDRL- or RPR-negative. If the VDRL test becomes negative or if VDRL titers drop to a fixed low value within 1 or 2 years, lumbar puncture is unnecessary since the CSF examination is almost invariably normal and there is little risk of subsequent neurosyphilis. However, if a VDRL titer $\geq$1:8 fails to fall by at least fourfold within 12 months, if the VDRL titer rises by fourfold, or if clinical symptoms persist or recur, re-treatment is indicated. Every effort should be made to differentiate treatment failure from reinfection, and the CSF should be examined. Patients in whom treatment failure is suspected, especially those with abnormal CSF, should be treated for neurosyphilis. If the patient remains seropositive but asymptomatic after such re-treatment, no further therapy is necessary. Patients treated for late latent syphilis frequently have low initial VDRL titers and may not have a fourfold drop after therapy with penicillin; about half of these patients remain seropositive (with low titers) for years after therapy. Re-treatment is not warranted unless the titer rises or signs or symptoms of syphilis appear.

The activity of neurosyphilis correlates best with the degree of CSF pleocytosis, and this measure provides the most sensitive index of response to treatment. CSF should be examined every 6 months for 3 years after the treatment of asymptomatic or symptomatic neurosyphilis or until CSF findings return to normal. An elevated CSF cell count falls to $\leq$10/μL in 3 to 12 months in 95% of adequately treated cases and becomes normal in all cases within 2 to 4 years. Elevated levels of CSF protein fall more slowly, and the CSF VDRL titer declines gradually over a period of several years.

Persistence of *T. pallidum* The persistence of *T. pallidum* in the aqueous humor, CSF, lymph nodes, brain, inflamed temporal arteries, and other tissues after "adequate" penicillin treatment has been suggested by dark-field microscopy, immunofluorescent antibody and silver staining techniques, rabbit inoculation, and PCR. Because the data on persisting treponemes are scanty, no modification of the treatment recommendations seems warranted for HIV-uninfected persons. Adherence to recommendations regarding CSF examination before the selection of therapy should minimize the possibility that *T. pallidum* will persist in the CSF.

IMMUNITY TO AND PREVENTION OF SYPHILIS About 60% of contacts of patients with primary and secondary syphilis become infected, with lower risk in contacts exposed to early latent syphilis. The rate of development of acquired resistance to *T. pallidum* after natural or experimental infection is related to the size of the antigenic stimulus, which depends on both the size of the infecting inoculum and the duration of infection before treatment. The role of serum antibody in conferring immunity to syphilis remains controversial. Passively administered antibody prevents or delays the appearance of clinical manifestations of syphilis in the rabbit model; it does not prevent infection. Cellular immunity is considered to be of major importance in the healing of early lesions and the control of syphilitic infection. The cellular infiltration of early lesions predominantly involves T lymphocytes and macrophages. The cytokine milieu of primary and secondary lesions is of the T_H1 type, consistent with the clearance of organisms by activated macrophages. Specific antibody enhances phagocytosis and is required for macrophage-mediated killing of *T. pallidum*.

Inability to cultivate pathogenic treponemes in vitro has hindered the analysis of treponemal antigens. Attempts to induce immunity to syphilis by vaccination have shown limited promise, although repeated injection of rabbits with γ-irradiated motile treponemes has conferred immunity to rechallenge. The outer membrane of *T. pallidum* contains few integral membrane proteins, and none has been definitively identified. Several newly described antigens of *T. pallidum*, including TprK, have induced partial immunity to challenge in the rabbit model, and syphilis vaccine development is being actively pursued.

ACKNOWLEDGMENT
The author wishes to acknowledge the substantive contributions of the former coauthor, Dr. King K. Holmes, to the content and organization of this chapter. His original framework continues to serve as the structure for this revision.

BIBLIOGRAPHY

CENTERS FOR DISEASE CONTROL AND PREVENTION : 1998 sexually transmitted diseases treatment guidelines. MMWR 47(RR-11):1, 1998

CENTURION-LARA A et al: The flanking region sequences of the 15-kDa lipoprotein gene differentiate pathogenic treponemes. J Infect Dis 177:1036, 1998

FLOOD JM et al: Neurosyphilis during the AIDS epidemic, San Francisco, 1985–1992. J Infect Dis 177:931, 1998

FRASER CM et al: Complete genome sequence of *Treponema pallidum*, the syphilis pirochete. Science 281:375, 1998

GORDON SM et al: The response of symptomatic neurosyphilis to high-dose intravenous penicillin G in patients with human immunodeficiency virus infection. N Engl J Med 331:1469, 1994

LUKEHART SA et al: Invasion of the central nervous system by *Treponema pallidum*: Implications for diagnosis and treatment. Ann Intern Med 109:855, 1988

MARRA CM et al: Resolution of serum and cerebrospinal fluid abnormalities after treatment of neurosyphilis: Influence of concomitant human immunodeficiency virus infection. Sex Transm Dis 23:184, 1996

MUSHER DM et al: Effect of human immunodeficiency virus infection on the course of syphilis and on the response to treatment. Ann Intern Med 113:872, 1990

RADOLF JD et al: Outer membrane ultrastructure explains the limited antigenicity of virulent *Treponema pallidum*. Proc Natl Acad Sci USA 86:2051, 1989

ROLFS RT et al: A randomized trial of enhanced therapy for early syphilis in patients with and without human immunodeficiency virus infection. N Engl J Med 337:307, 1997

ROMANOWSKI B et al: Serologic response to treatment of infectious syphilis. Ann Intern Med 114:1005, 1991

THOMAS JC et al: Syphilis in the South: Rural rates surpass urban rates in North Carolina. Am J Public Health 85:1119, 1995

WENDEL GD et al: Penicillin allergy and desensitization in serious infections during pregnancy. N Engl J Med 312:1229, 1985

ENDEMIC TREPONEMATOSES

The endemic, or nonvenereal, treponematoses are bacterial infections that are caused by close relatives of *Treponema pallidum* subspecies *pallidum*, the etiologic agent of venereal syphilis (Chap. 172). Yaws, pinta, and endemic syphilis are distinguished from venereal syphilis by mode of transmission, age of acquisition, geographic distribution, and clinical features. These infections are limited primarily to rural areas of developing nations and are seen in the United States and Europe only in recent immigrants from endemic regions. Much of our "knowledge" about the endemic treponematoses is based upon impressions and observations of health care workers who have visited endemic areas; virtually no well-designed studies of the natural history, diagnosis, or treatment of these infections have been conducted. A comparison of the treponemal infections is shown in Table 173-1.

EPIDEMIOLOGY The endemic treponematoses are chronic diseases acquired during childhood and, like syphilis, can cause severe late manifestations years after initial infection. These infections were very common in Africa, Asia, and South America when the World Health Organization (WHO) and UNICEF embarked on a highly successful mass eradication campaign. From 1952 to 1969, it is estimated that over 160 million people were examined for treponemal infections and over 50 million cases, contacts, and latent infections were treated. This categorical program is one of WHO's outstanding successes in that the prevalence of active yaws was reduced from >20% to <1% in many rural areas and endemic syphilis was eradicated in Bosnia. In the decades since the eradication programs, lack of focused surveillance and diversion of resources to other pressing needs have resulted in a resurgence of these infections in some regions, particularly in Africa. The estimated geographic distribution of the endemic treponematoses in the 1990s is shown in Fig. 173-1. In the early 1980s, WHO sponsored a series of regional meetings on the endemic treponematoses, and areas of resurgent yaws morbidity were identified in West Africa (Ivory Coast, Ghana, Togo, Benin) and extending into the Central African Republic and rural Democratic Republic of Congo (formerly Zaire). The prevalence of endemic syphilis is estimated to be >10% in some regions of Mali, Niger, Burkina Faso, and Senegal. In Asia and the western Pacific, yaws is still prevalent in Indonesia, Papua New Guinea, and the Solomon Islands; cases have also been identified in Laos and Kampuchea. In the Americas, foci of yaws persist in Haiti and other Caribbean islands, Peru, Colombia, Ecuador, Brazil, Guyana, and Surinam. Pinta is limited to Central America and northern South America, where it is found rarely and only in remote villages.

MICROBIOLOGY The etiologic agents of the endemic treponematoses are *T. pallidum* subspecies *pertenue* (yaws), *T. pallidum* subspecies *endemicum* (endemic syphilis), and *T. carateum* (pinta). These little-studied organisms are morphologically identical to *T. pallidum* subspecies *pallidum*, and no antigenic differences among the pathogenic treponemes have been identified to date. A controversy has existed about whether the treponematoses are caused by different organisms or by the same organism, with clinical manifestations and routes of transmission being defined by the climate of the region and the culture of the population. Three of the four organisms have been placed in the same species because of their genetic similarity; the fourth (*T. carateum*) remains a separate species simply because no organisms have been available for genetic studies. However, a molecular signature has been defined that can be used to differentiate *T. pallidum* subspecies *pallidum* from *T. pallidum* subspecies *pertenue* and *T. pallidum* subspecies *endemicum*, and unpublished studies have identified a number of distinct differences in the *tpr* gene family between venereal and nonvenereal treponemes. Whether these differ-

ences are related to the different clinical courses has not yet been determined.

CLINICAL FEATURES All of the treponemal infections are characterized by defined disease stages, with a localized primary lesion, disseminated secondary lesions, periods of latency, and possible late lesions. The stages are most clearly defined in venereal syphilis, while the primary and secondary manifestations are more frequently overlapping in yaws and endemic syphilis; the late manifestations of pinta are very mild relative to the destructive lesions of the other treponematoses. The current preference is to divide the clinical course of the endemic treponematoses into "early" and "late" stages.

The major clinical features that are thought to differ between venereal syphilis and the nonvenereal infections are the lack of congenital transmission and lack of central nervous system (CNS) involvement in the nonvenereal infections. It is not known whether these distinctions are accurate. Because of the high degree of genetic relatedness among the organisms, there is little biologic reason to think that *T. pallidum* subspecies *endemicum* and *T. pallidum* subspecies *pertenue* would be unable to cross the blood-brain barrier or to invade the placenta. These organisms obviously can disseminate from the site of primary infection to other tissues, and they can persist for decades. In this respect, they are like *T. pallidum* subspecies *pallidum*. Even if invasion of the placenta or the CNS occurs in endemic treponemal infection, there are a number of reasons that these manifestations might not have been recognized. The lack of recognized congenital infection may be due to the fact that the nonvenereal treponematoses are usually acquired during childhood. The degree of spirochetemia (the presumed source of placental and fetal infection) is greatly diminished during the latent stage, and by the time an infected girl becomes sexually mature, she would be at low risk for transplacental transmission. Neurologic involvement may not have been recognized in nonvenereal treponemal infection because of the lack of trained medical personnel in endemic regions, the lag of years to decades between acquisition of infection and possible CNS manifestations, or a low rate of symptomatic CNS disease. The lack of longitudinal studies in endemic areas makes conclusions about the natural history of these infections tenuous.

Some published evidence supports congenital transmission as well as cardiovascular, ophthalmologic, and CNS involvement in yaws. Although the case is strong, particularly for CNS involvement, most studies that have shown a relatively high incidence (average, 24.9%) of cerebrospinal fluid (CSF) abnormalities in patients with yaws were not controlled for other possible causes of CSF abnormalities, did not include treponeme-specific tests, or did not follow patients for resolution of abnormalities after antitreponemal therapy. Thus, while no firm conclusions can be drawn about the invasion of the CNS and placenta by the non-*pallidum* treponemes, it may be erroneous to accept unquestioningly the frequently repeated belief that these organisms fail to cause such manifestations.

Yaws Also known as *pian*, *framboesia*, or *bouba*, yaws is a chronic infection that is usually acquired in childhood and is caused by *T. pallidum* subspecies *pertenue*. The disease is characterized by the development of one or several primary lesions (called the "mother yaw"), followed by the appearance of multiple disseminated skin lesions. The early lesions may persist for many months, are infectious, and usually recur several times within the early years of infection. Late manifestations are destructive and can involve skin, bone, and joints.

The infection is transmitted by direct contact with infectious lesions, and transmission may be enhanced by disruption of the skin by insect bites or abrasions. Children with open lesions and without covering clothing are most likely to transmit infection during play or group sleeping. After an average incubation period estimated at 3 to 4 weeks, the first lesion begins as a papule, usually on an extremity, and then enlarges (particularly during moist warm weather) to become papillomatous or "raspberry-like" (thus the name "framboesia") (Fig. 173-2). Regional lymphadenopathy develops, and the lesion usually

Table 173-1 Comparison of the Treponemes and the Diseases They Cause

Feature	Venereal Syphilis	Yaws	Endemic Syphilis	Pinta
Organism	*T. pallidum* subspecies *pallidum*	*T. pallidum* subspecies *pertenue*	*T. pallidum* subspecies *endemicum*	*T. carateum*
Mode of transmission	Sexual, transplacental[a]	Skin-to-skin	Household contacts: mouth-to-mouth or via shared drinking/eating utensils; insect vector?	Skin-to-skin
Usual age of acquisition	Adulthood	Early childhood	Early childhood	Late childhood
Primary lesion	Cutaneous ulcer (chancre)	Papilloma, often ulcerative	Rarely seen	Nonulcerating papule with satellites, pruritic
Location	Genital, oral, anal	Extremities	Oral	Extremities, face
Secondary lesions	Mucocutaneous lesions; condylomata lata	Cutaneous papulosquamous lesions; osteoperiostitis	Florid mucocutaneous lesions (mucous patch, split papule, condyloma latum); osteoperiostitis	Pintides, pigmented, pruritic
Infectious relapses	~25%	Common	Unknown	None
Late complications	Gummas, cardiovascular and CNS involvement[b]	Destructive gummas of skin, bone, cartilage	Destructive gummas of skin, bone, cartilage	Nondestructive, dyschromic, achromic macules

[a] Because the nonvenereal treponematoses are usually acquired in childhood and treponemal bacteremia ceases with time, only in adult-onset venereal syphilis is there a reasonable likelihood that a woman will give birth to an infected child (see text).

[b] CNS involvement in the endemic treponematoses has been postulated by some investigators (see text).

heals within 6 months; dissemination is thought to occur during the early weeks and months of infection. A generalized secondary eruption, accompanied by generalized lymphadenopathy, appears either concurrent with or following the primary lesion, may take several forms (macular, papular, or papillomatous), and may become secondarily infected with other bacteria. Painful papillomatous lesions on the soles of the feet result in a painful crablike gait ("crab yaws"), and periostitis may result in nocturnal bone pain and polydactylitis. All early skin lesions are infectious, and cutaneous relapses are common during the first 5 years. Late yaws is recognized in ~10% of untreated

patients and is manifested by gummas of the skin and long bone, hyperkeratoses of the palms and soles, osteitis and periostitis, and hydrarthrosis. The late gummatous lesions are characteristically very destructive and extensive. Destruction of the nose, maxilla, palate, and pharynx is termed *gangosa* and is similar to the destructive lesions seen in leprosy and leishmaniasis.

Endemic Syphilis Endemic syphilis, also called *bejel, siti, dichuchwa, njovera,* or *skerljevo,* is a chronic infection caused by *T. pallidum* subspecies *endemicum.* Like other endemic treponematoses, endemic syphilis is chronic and is acquired in childhood. The early lesions are primarily localized to the mucocutaneous and mucosal surfaces, and the infection may be transmitted by direct contact or by shared drinking and eating uten-

sils. A role for insects in transmission has been suggested but is unproved. The initial lesion often goes unrecognized, and the first noticeable lesion is usually an intraoral mucous patch or a mucocutaneous lesion resembling the condylomata lata of secondary syphilis (Fig. 173-2). This eruption may last for months or even years, and treponemes can readily be demonstrated in early lesions. Periostitis and regional lymphadenopathy are common. After a variable period of latency, late manifestations may appear, including osseous and cutaneous gummas. Destructive gummas, osteitis, and gangosa are more common in endemic syphilis than in late yaws. Gummas of the

Pinta
Yaws–Pian
Endemic syphilis–Syphillis endémique

WHO 92522

FIGURE 173-1 Geographic distribution of endemic treponematoses in the 1990s. (*Courtesy of World Health Organization.*)

1054

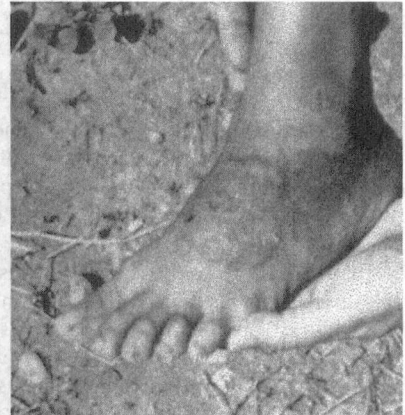

FIGURE 173-2 Clinical manifestations of endemic treponematoses. *Left*: Papillomatous primary lesions of yaws. *Center*: Split papules of early endemic syphilis. *Right*: Pigmented macules of pinta. *(From PL Perine et al.)*

nipples develop in women who have previously had endemic syphilis and who breast-feed infants with oral lesions. Thus, it appears that the late lesion may result from repeated exposure of a sensitized host.

Pinta Pinta (also called *mal del pinto, carate, azul,* or *purupuru*) is the most benign of the treponemal infections and is caused by *T. carateum.* This disease has three stages that are characterized by marked changes in skin color, but it does not appear to cause destructive lesions or to involve other tissues. Transmission occurs by direct contact, usually during late childhood. The initial papule is most often located on the extremities or face and is pruritic. After one to many months of infection, numerous disseminated secondary lesions (*pintides*) appear. These lesions are initially red but become deeply pigmented, ultimately turning a dark slate blue. The secondary lesions are infectious and highly pruritic and may persist for years. Late pigmented lesions are called *dyschromic macules* and contain treponemes. Over time, most pigmented lesions show varying degrees of depigmentation, becoming brown and eventually white and giving the skin a mottled appearance. The white achromic lesions are characteristic of the late stage.

DIAGNOSIS Diagnosis of the endemic treponematoses is based upon clinical manifestations and, when available, serologic testing. The same tests that are used for venereal syphilis (Chap. 172) become reactive during all treponemal infections, and there is no serologic test than can discriminate among the different infections. The nonvenereal treponemal infections should be considered in the evaluation of a reactive syphilis serology in any person who has immigrated from an endemic area.

℞ TREATMENT The recommended therapy for patients and their contacts is benzathine penicillin at a dose of 1.2 million units intramuscularly; that for children under 10 years of age is 600,000 units. This is half the dose recommended for patients and contacts with early venereal syphilis. There have been no controlled studies to show that the lower dose is effective in stopping relapse or progression to late disease. Definitive evidence of resistance to penicillin is lacking. However, because failure to heal existing lesions and frequent relapse following treatment for yaws have been described in Papua New Guinea, some health workers have suggested doubling the recommended dose of benzathine penicillin. Solely on the basis of experience with venereal syphilis, it is thought that doxycycline, tetracycline, and erythromycin (at doses appropriate for syphilis; Chap. 172) are therapeutic alternatives for patients allergic to penicillin. A Jarisch-Herxheimer reaction (Chap. 172) may follow treatment of endemic treponematoses.

CONTROL The endemic treponematoses can be controlled with inexpensive therapy. However, the often-remote locations of the affected populations limit availability of medical care. Although the mass treatment programs of three decades ago were widely successful,

time has shown that sustained control requires vigilance in regular screening and in the investigation of outbreaks—luxuries that are often impossible in countries with more pressing medical needs. There is concern that, as HIV spreads throughout developing countries, it may markedly affect the manifestations and transmission of the endemic treponematoses.

ACKNOWLEDGMENT
The author gratefully acknowledges the substantial contributions of Dr. Peter Perine, the author of previous editions of this chapter, to the framework of the current chapter and to our insight into these little-studied infections.

BIBLIOGRAPHY

BACKHOUSE JL et al: Failure of penicillin treatment of yaws on Karkar Island, Papua New Guinea. Am J Trop Med 59:388, 1998

CENTURION-LARA A et al: The flanking region sequences of the 15 kD lipoprotein gene differentiate pathogenic treponemes. J Infect Dis 177:1036, 1998

ENGELKENS HJH et al: Early yaws: A light microscopic study. Genitourin Med 66:264, 1990

—— et al: Endemic treponematosis. Part 1. Yaws. Int J Dermatol 30:77, 1991

PERINE PL et al: *Handbook of Endemic Treponematoses.* Geneva, World Health Organization, 1984

ROMÁN GC, ROMÁN LN: Occurrence of congenital, cardiovascular, visceral, neurologic, and neuro-ophthalmologic complications in late yaws: A theme for future research. Rev Infect Dis 8:760, 1986

174 *Peter Speelman*

LEPTOSPIROSIS

Leptospirosis is an infectious disease caused by pathogenic leptospires and characterized by a broad spectrum of clinical manifestations, varying from inapparent infection to fulminant, fatal disease. In its mild form, leptospirosis may present as an influenza-like illness with headache and myalgias. Severe leptospirosis, characterized by jaundice, renal dysfunction, and hemorrhagic diathesis, is referred to as *Weil's syndrome.*

ETIOLOGIC AGENTS Leptospires are spirochetes belonging to the order Spirochaetales and the family Leptospiraceae. Traditionally, the genus *Leptospira* comprised two species: the pathogenic *L. interrogans* and the free-living *L. biflexa.* Although seven species of pathogenic leptospires are now recognized on the basis of their DNA relatedness, it is more practical clinically and epidemiologically to use a classification based on serologic differences. The pathogenic leptospires are divided into serovars according to their antigenic composition. More than 200 serovars make up the 23 serogroups.

Leptospires are coiled, thin, highly motile organisms with hooked ends and two periplasmic flagella that permit burrowing into tissue. These organisms are 6 to 20 μm long and about 0.1 μm wide; they stain poorly but can be seen microscopically by dark-field examination and after silver impregnation staining. Leptospires require special media and conditions for growth; it may take weeks for cultures to become positive.

EPIDEMIOLOGY Leptospirosis is a zoonosis with a worldwide distribution that affects at least 160 mammalian species. Rodents, especially rats, are the most important reservoir, although other wild mammals, dogs, fish, and birds may also harbor these microorganisms. Leptospires establish a symbiotic relationship with their host and can persist in the renal tubules for years. Some serovars are associated with particular animals—e.g., icterohaemorrhagiae/copenhageni with rats, grippotyphosa with voles, hardjo with cattle, canicola with dogs, and pomona with pigs.

Transmission of leptospires may follow direct contact with urine, blood, or tissue from an infected animal or exposure to a contaminated environment; human-to-human transmission is rare. Since leptospires are excreted in the urine and can survive in water for many months, water is an important vehicle in their transmission. Epidemics of leptospirosis may result from exposure to flood waters contaminated by urine from infected animals, as has been reported from Nicaragua. Leptospirosis occurs most commonly in the tropics because the climate as well as the sometimes poor working and hygienic conditions favor the pathogen's survival.

Humans are not commonly infected with leptospires. However, in the United States, the 40 to 120 cases reported annually to the Centers for Disease Control and Prevention certainly represent a significant underestimation of the total number. Certain occupational groups are at especially high risk; included are veterinarians, agricultural workers, sewage workers, slaughterhouse employees, and workers in the fishing industry. Such individuals may acquire leptospirosis through direct exposure to or contact with contaminated water and soil. Leptospirosis has also been recognized in deteriorating inner cities where rat populations are expanding. One report described leptospirosis in urban residents of Baltimore who were sporadically exposed to rat urine.

In western countries, recreational exposure and domestic animal contact are also prominent sources of leptospirosis. Recreational water activities, such as canoeing, windsurfing, swimming, and waterskiing, place persons at risk for leptospirosis. Sometimes the infection is acquired during travel abroad. In a recent study in the Netherlands, 14% of patients with confirmed leptospirosis had acquired the infection while traveling in tropical countries, mostly in Southeast Asia. Transmission via laboratory accidents has been reported but is rare. Occasionally, leptospirosis develops after unanticipated immersion in contaminated water (e.g., in an automobile accident). Most cases occur in men, with a peak incidence during the summer and fall in western countries and during the rainy season in the tropics.

PATHOGENESIS The pathogenesis of leptospirosis is incompletely understood. Leptospires may enter the host through abrasions in the skin or through intact mucous membranes, especially the conjunctiva and the lining of the oro- and nasopharynx. Drinking of contaminated water may introduce leptospires through the mouth, throat, or esophagus. After entry of the organisms, leptospiremia develops, with subsequent spread to all organs. Multiplication takes place in blood and in tissues, and leptospires can be isolated from blood and cerebrospinal fluid (CSF) during the first 4 to 10 days of illness. It is not clear why the presence of leptospires in the CSF does not cause damage. All forms of leptospires can damage the wall of small blood vessels; this damage leads to vasculitis with leakage and extravasation of cells, including hemorrhages. The most important known pathogenic properties of leptospires are adhesion to cell surfaces and cellular toxicity.

Vasculitis is responsible for the most important manifestations of

the disease. Although leptospires mainly infect the kidneys and liver, any organ may be affected. In the kidney, leptospires migrate to the interstitium, renal tubules, and tubular lumen, causing interstitial nephritis and tubular necrosis. Hypovolemia due to dehydration or altered capillary permeability may contribute to the development of renal failure. In the liver, centrilobular necrosis with proliferation of Kupffer cells may be found. However, severe hepatocellular necrosis is not a feature of leptospirosis. Pulmonary involvement is the result of hemorrhage and not of inflammation. Invasion of skeletal muscle by leptospires results in swelling, vacuolation of the myofibrils, and focal necrosis. In severe leptospirosis, vasculitis may ultimately impair the microcirculation and increase capillary permeability, resulting in fluid leakage and hypovolemia.

When antibodies are formed, leptospires are eliminated from all sites in the host except the eye, the proximal renal tubules, and perhaps the brain, where they may persist for weeks or months. The persistence of leptospires in the aqueous humor occasionally causes chronic or recurrent uveitis. The systemic immune response is effective in eliminating the organism but may also produce symptomatic inflammatory reactions. A rise in antibody titer coincides with the development of meningitis; this association suggests that an immunologic mechanism is responsible.

After the start of antimicrobial treatment for leptospirosis, a Jarisch-Herxheimer reaction similar to that seen in other spirochetal diseases may develop. Although frequently described in older publications, this reaction seems to be a rare event in leptospirosis and is certainly less frequent in this infection than in other spirochetal diseases.

CLINICAL MANIFESTATIONS It is important to try to obtain a history of exposure to contaminated materials. Serologic evidence of past inapparent infection is found in 15 to 40% of persons who have been exposed but have not become ill. In symptomatic cases of leptospirosis, clinical manifestations vary from mild to serious or even fatal. More than 90% of symptomatic persons have the relatively mild and usually anicteric form of leptospirosis, with or without meningitis. Severe leptospirosis with profound jaundice (Weil's syndrome) develops in 5 to 10% of infected individuals.

The incubation period is usually 1 to 2 weeks but ranges from 2 to 26 days. Typically, an acute leptospiremic phase is followed by an immune leptospiruric phase. The distinction between the first and second phases is not always clear, and milder cases do not always include the second phase.

Anicteric Leptospirosis Leptospirosis may present as an acute influenza-like illness, with fever, chills, severe headache, nausea, vomiting, and myalgias. Muscle pain, which especially affects the calves, back, and abdomen, is an important feature of leptospiral infection. Less common features include sore throat and rash. The patient usually has an intense headache (frontal or retroorbital) and sometimes develops photophobia. Mental confusion may be evident. Pulmonary involvement, manifested in most cases by cough and chest pain and in a few cases by hemoptysis, is not uncommon.

The most common finding on physical examination is fever with conjunctival suffusion. Less common findings include muscle tenderness, lymphadenopathy, pharyngeal injection, rash, hepatomegaly, and splenomegaly. The rash may be macular, maculopapular, erythematous, urticarial, or hemorrhagic. Mild jaundice may be present.

Most patients become asymptomatic within 1 week. After an interval of 1 to 3 days, the illness recurs in a number of cases. The start of this second (immune) phase coincides with the development of antibodies. Symptoms are more variable than during the first (leptospiremic) phase. Usually the symptoms last for only a few days, but occasionally they persist for weeks. Often the fever is less pronounced and the myalgias are less severe than in the leptospiremic phase. An important event during the immune phase is the development of aseptic meningitis. Although no more than 15% of all patients have symptoms and signs of meningitis, many patients may have CSF pleocytosis. Meningeal symptoms usually disappear within a few days but may persist for weeks. Similarly, pleocytosis generally disappears within 2 weeks but occasionally persists for months. Iritis, iridocyclitis, and chorioretinitis—late complications that may persist for years—can become apparent as early as the third week but often present several months after the initial illness. One epidemic of uveitis among patients with leptospirosis has been reported.

Severe Leptospirosis (Weil's Syndrome) Weil's syndrome, the most severe form of leptospirosis, is characterized by jaundice, renal dysfunction, hemorrhagic diathesis, and high mortality. This syndrome is frequently but not exclusively associated with infection due to serovar icterohaemorrhagiae/copenhageni. The onset of illness is no different from that of less severe leptospirosis; however, after 4 to 9 days, jaundice as well as renal and vascular dysfunction generally develop. Although some degree of defervescence may be noted after the first week of illness, a biphasic disease pattern like that seen in anicteric leptospirosis is lacking. The jaundice of Weil's syndrome, which can be profound and give an orange cast to the skin, is usually not associated with severe hepatic necrosis. Death is rarely due to liver failure. Hepatomegaly and tenderness in the right upper quadrant are usually detected. Splenomegaly is found in 20% of cases.

Renal failure may develop, often during the second week of illness. Hypovolemia and decreased renal perfusion contribute to the development of acute tubular necrosis with oliguria or anuria. Dialysis is sometimes required, although a fair number of cases can be managed without dialysis. Renal function may be completely regained.

Pulmonary involvement occurs frequently, resulting in cough, dyspnea, chest pain, and blood-stained sputum, and sometimes in hemoptysis or even respiratory failure. Hemorrhagic manifestations are seen in Weil's syndrome: epistaxis, petechiae, purpura, and ecchymoses are found commonly, while severe gastrointestinal bleeding and adrenal or subarachnoid hemorrhage are detected rarely.

Rhabdomyolysis, hemolysis, myocarditis, pericarditis, congestive heart failure, cardiogenic shock, adult respiratory distress syndrome, and multiorgan failure have all been described during severe leptospirosis.

LABORATORY AND RADIOLOGIC FINDINGS The kidneys are invariably involved in leptospirosis. Related findings range from urinary sediment changes (leukocytes, erythrocytes, and hyaline or granular casts) and mild proteinuria in anicteric leptospirosis to renal failure and azotemia in severe disease.

The erythrocyte sedimentation rate is usually elevated. In anicteric leptospirosis, peripheral leukocyte counts range from 3000 to 26,000/μL, with a left shift; in Weil's syndrome, leukocytosis is often marked. Mild thrombocytopenia occurs in up to 50% of patients and is associated with renal failure.

In contrast to patients with acute viral hepatitis, those with leptospirosis typically have elevated serum levels of bilirubin and alkaline phosphatase as well as mild increases (up to 200 U/L) in serum levels of aminotransferases. In Weil's syndrome, the prothrombin time may be prolonged but can be corrected with vitamin K. Levels of creatine phosphokinase, which are elevated in up to 50% of patients with leptospirosis during the first week of illness, may help to differentiate this infection from viral hepatitis.

When a meningeal reaction develops, polymorphonuclear leukocytes predominate initially and the number of mononuclear cells increases later. The protein concentration in the CSF may be elevated; CSF glucose levels are normal.

In severe leptospirosis, pulmonary radiographic abnormalities are more common than would be expected on the basis of physical examination. These abnormalities most frequently develop 3 to 9 days after the onset of illness. The most common radiographic finding is a patchy alveolar pattern that corresponds to scattered alveolar hemorrhage. Radiographic abnormalities most often affect the lower lobes in the periphery of the lung fields.

DIAGNOSIS A definite diagnosis of leptospirosis is based either on isolation of the organism from the patient or on seroconversion or a rise in antibody titer in the microscopic agglutination test (MAT).

For a presumptive diagnosis of leptospirosis, an antibody titer of $\geq$1:100 in the MAT or a positive macroscopic slide agglutination test in the presence of a compatible clinical illness is required. Antibodies generally do not reach detectable levels until the second week of illness. The antibody response can be affected by early treatment.

The macroscopic slide agglutination test with killed antigen is useful for screening but is not specific. The MAT, which uses a battery of live leptospiral strains, and the enzyme-linked immunosorbent assay (ELISA), which uses a broadly reacting antigen, are the standard serologic procedures. These tests usually are available only in specialized laboratories and are used for the determination of the antibody titer and for the tentative identification of the serovar involved (thus the importance of using antigens representative of the serovars prevalent in the particular geographic area). Since cross-reactions occur frequently, however, it is often impossible to identify the infecting serovar. Serologic testing cannot be used as the basis for a decision about whether to start treatment.

In addition to the MAT and the ELISA, various other tests with diagnostic value have been developed. Some tests, such as an indirect hemagglutination test, a microcapsule agglutination test, and an IgM ELISA, are commercially available. Dot-ELISA, gold immunoblot, and polymerase chain reaction techniques have been developed but are not yet used for routine diagnosis.

Leptospires can be isolated from blood and/or CSF during the first 10 days of illness and from urine for several weeks beginning at around 1 week. Cultures may become positive after 2 to 4 weeks, with a range of 1 week to 4 months. Sometimes urine cultures remain positive for months or years after the start of illness. For isolation of leptospires from body fluids or tissues, Ellinghausen-McCullough-Johnson-Harris (EMJH) medium is useful; other possibilities are Fletcher medium and Korthoff medium. Specimens can be mailed to a reference laboratory for culture, since leptospires remain viable in anticoagulated blood (heparin, EDTA, or citrate) for up to 11 days. Isolation of leptospires is important since it is the only way the infecting serovar can be correctly identified. Dark-field examination of blood or urine frequently results in misdiagnosis and should not be used.

DIFFERENTIAL DIAGNOSIS Leptospirosis should be differentiated from other febrile illnesses associated with headache and muscle pain, such as malaria, enteric fever, viral hepatitis, dengue, *Hantavirus* infections, and rickettsial diseases. In light of the strong similarity in epidemiology and clinical presentation between leptospirosis and *Hantavirus* infections and given the reported occurrence of dual infections, it is advisable to conduct serologic testing for *Hantavirus* in cases of suspected leptospirosis. When patients have a flulike disease with disproportionately severe myalgia or aseptic meningitis, a diagnosis of leptospirosis should be considered.

℞ TREATMENT The effectiveness of antimicrobial therapy for the mild febrile form of leptospirosis is controversial, but such treatment is indicated for more severe forms. Treatment should be initiated as early as possible; nevertheless, contrary to previous reports, treatment started after the first 4 days of illness is effective.

For severe cases of leptospirosis, intravenous administration of penicillin G, amoxicillin, ampicillin, or erythromycin is recommended (Table 174-1). In milder cases, oral treatment with tetracycline, doxycycline, ampicillin, or amoxicillin should be considered. Although several other antibiotics, including newer cephalosporins, are highly active against leptospires in vitro, no clinical experience has yet been gained with these drugs.

In rare cases, a Jarisch-Herxheimer reaction develops within hours after the start of antimicrobial therapy (see "Pathogenesis" above). Although so far the only effective mode of management is supportive, the role of antibodies to tumor necrosis factor in the treatment of this reaction deserves further study. A beneficial effect of the use of such antibodies for the modulation of the reaction has been demonstrated

Table 174-1   Treatment and Chemoprophylaxis of Leptospirosis

Purpose of Drug Administration	Regimen
Treatment	
Mild leptospirosis	Doxycycline, 100 mg orally bid
	or
	Ampicillin, 500–750 mg orally qid
	or
	Amoxicillin, 500 mg orally qid
Moderate/severe leptospirosis	Penicillin G, 1.5 million units IV qid
	or
	Ampicillin, 1 g IV qid
	or
	Amoxicillin, 1 g IV qid
	or
	Erythromycin, 500 mg IV qid
Chemoprophylaxis	Doxycycline, 200 mg orally once a week

NOTE: All regimens used for treatment are administered for 7 days.

in patients with louse-borne relapsing fever. Patients with severe leptospirosis and renal failure may require dialysis. Those with Weil's syndrome may need transfusions of whole blood and/or platelets. Intensive care may be necessary.

PROGNOSIS   Most patients with leptospirosis recover. Mortality is highest among patients who are elderly and those who have Weil's syndrome. Leptospirosis during pregnancy is associated with high fetal mortality. Long-term follow-up of patients with renal failure and hepatic dysfunction has documented good recovery of renal and hepatic function.

PREVENTION   Individuals who may be exposed to leptospires through their occupations or their involvement in recreational water activities should be informed about the risks. Measures for controlling leptospirosis include avoidance of exposure to urine and tissues from infected animals, vaccination of animals, and rodent control. The animal vaccine used in a given area should contain the serovars known to be present in that area. Unfortunately, some vaccinated animals still excrete leptospires in their urine. Vaccination of humans against a specific serovar prevalent in an area has been undertaken in some European and Asian countries and has proved effective. Chemoprophylaxis with doxycycline (200 mg once a week) has appeared to be efficacious in military personnel but is indicated only in rare instances of sustained short-term exposure.

BIBLIOGRAPHY

CHU KM et al: Identification of *Leptospira* species in the pathogenesis of uveitis and determination of clinical ocular characteristics in south India. J Infect Dis 177:1314, 1998

DUPONT H et al: Leptospirosis: Prognostic factors associated with mortality. Clin Infect Dis 25:720, 1997

FARR RW: Leptospirosis. Clin Infect Dis 21:1, 1995

O'NEILL KM et al: Pulmonary manifestations of leptospirosis. Rev Infect Dis 13:705, 1991

TREVEJO RT et al: Epidemic leptospirosis associated with pulmonary hemorrhage—Nicaragua. J Infect Dis 178:1457, 1998

VAN CREVEL R et al: Leptospirosis in travelers. Clin Infect Dis 19:132, 1994

VINETZ JM et al: Sporadic urban leptospirosis. Ann Intern Med 125:794, 1996

WATT G et al: Placebo-controlled trial of intravenous penicillin for severe and late leptospirosis. Lancet 1:433, 1988

——— et al: Skeletal and cardiac muscle involvement in severe, late leptospirosis. J Infect Dis 162:266, 1990

175   *David T. Dennis, Grant L. Campbell*

RELAPSING FEVER

DEFINITION   The term *relapsing fever* describes two distinct borrelial disease entities: louse-borne relapsing fever (LBRF) and tick-borne relapsing fever (TBRF). Both are characterized by recurrent acute episodes of spirochetemia and fever alternating with spirochetal clearance and apyrexia.

ETIOLOGY   The worldwide distribution of relapsing spirochetal fevers was recognized in the early part of the twentieth century, and the causative agents were shown to be transmitted by lice and ticks. *Borrelia recurrentis* was identified as the cause of LBRF; differing strains of borreliae causing TBRF were usually named according to the species of *Ornithodoros* tick responsible for their transmission (Table 175-1). Sequencing of both flagellin and 16S ribosomal RNA genes reveals homogeneity among LBRF strains and considerable heterogeneity between Old World and New World TBRF strains.

Relapsing-fever borreliae are gram-negative bacteria that belong to the family Spirochaetaceae. They are helical in shape and average 0.2 to 0.5 μm in width and 5 to 20 μm in length. They comprise an outer membrane, an intermediate peptidoglycan layer, and an inner cytoplasmic membrane, which encloses the protoplasmic cylinder. Periplasmic flagella (variable numbers have been described) are situated beneath the outer membrane. Relapsing-fever borreliae are slow-growing and microaerophilic; they grow best at 30 to 35°C. Both TBRF and LBRF spirochetes grow well in Barbour-Stoenner-Kelly (BSK II) medium.

Relapsing-fever borreliae are distinguished by remarkable antigenic variability and strain heterogeneity. New *Borrelia* serotypes spontaneously emerge at a high rate, resulting from a unique process of DNA rearrangement within genes located on linear plasmids. These genes code for variable major proteins (VMPs) found on the spirochete's outer-membrane surface. This antigenic variation, generated by sequential expression of previously silent *vmp* genes for serotype-specific VMPs, allows the borreliae to escape the immune response of the host and results in the relapse phenomenon characteristic of infection with these organisms. Borrelial *vmp* gene expression also varies between mammalian and arthropod hosts.

EPIDEMIOLOGY   **Louse-Borne Relapsing Fever**   Body lice (*Pediculus humanus* var. *corporis*) become infected with *B. recurrentis* by feeding on spirochetemic humans, the only reservoirs of infection. In lice, *B. recurrentis* spirochetes are found almost exclusively in the hemolymph; humans acquire infection when infected body lice are crushed and their fluids contaminate mucous membranes or breaks in the skin (such as abrasions caused by scratching of pruritic louse bites). Spirochetes are not transmitted directly by the bite of a louse (anterior station transmission) or by inoculation of louse feces (posterior station transmission). Lice have a life span of only a few weeks, feed at frequent intervals, and survive only a few days off the human host.

LBRF has severely affected military and civilian populations disrupted by war and other disasters. During the Industrial Revolution, the disease was common among slum dwellers, prisoners, and others living in impoverished, overcrowded, and unhygienic conditions. In the first half of the twentieth century, during periods of war and famine, both LBRF and louse-borne typhus were epidemic in eastern Europe, the Balkans, and the former Soviet Union. LBRF has disappeared from its former global range as improvements have been made in standards of living, sanitation, and hygiene; it is now an important disease only in northeastern Africa, especially the highlands of Ethiopia, where an estimated 10,000 cases occur annually. In Ethiopia, the disease affects mostly homeless men crowded together in unhygienic circumstances, especially during the cool rainy season, when it is more difficult for them to change and wash their clothing. LBRF has repeatedly spilled out of Ethiopia into neighboring Somalia and Sudan, especially affecting displaced persons. LBRF does not pose a significant risk to tourists or other casual visitors but can be acquired from lice by persons (such as relief workers) in intimate contact with those affected as well as through accidental needle stick or mucocutaneous contact with infected blood.

Tick-Borne Relapsing Fever Soft ticks (Argasidae, *Ornithodoros* spp.) transmit TBRF. The ticks become infected by feeding on spirochetemic hosts. Except for *B. duttoni* (a prominent cause of TBRF in sub-Saharan Africa), TBRF borreliae are zoonotic disease agents found naturally in rodents (rats, mice, chipmunks, and squirrels) and in lagomorphs (rabbits and hares). The spirochetes are transmitted by ticks to humans and animals via saliva and excretory fluids when the tick feeds. Infection in ticks is transmitted vertically from one stage to the next; in some species, infection is transmitted transovarially over several generations. Soft ticks are hardy and can survive for 10 years or more with only an occasional blood meal. These ticks feed painlessly, relatively quickly (for 20 to 45 min), and usually at night while hosts are sleeping. Thus patients with TBRF are often unaware of tick exposures.

TBRF borreliae are widely distributed throughout the world. Human infection with these organisms is generally underrecognized and underreported. TBRF is most highly endemic in sub-Saharan Africa but is also found in countries of the Mediterranean littoral, Middle Eastern states, southern Russia, the Indian subcontinent, and China. In the United States, this disease occurs west of the Mississippi River, especially in mountainous areas, where *B. hermsii* is the causative agent. TBRF is reported at low frequency throughout Latin America. The disease typically occurs sporadically or in small—often familial—clusters. Infected soft ticks may cause repeated infections among persons living or sleeping in the same dwelling. In sub-Saharan Africa, *O. moubata*, the vector of *B. duttoni*, infests native huts and rest houses, hiding in crevices of floors and walls during the day and emerging at night to feed on sleeping inhabitants. In the United States, *B. hermsii* infections most often occur during spring and summer months among persons sleeping in rustic mountain cabins. Infections of humans are sometimes precipitated by the disappearance of rodents (e.g., as a result of epizootic plague) that nest in foundations, wall spaces, and attics and that serve as the usual maintenance hosts for *O. hermsi* ticks. Outbreaks caused by *B. hermsii* have taken place among persons staying in cabins along the north rim of the Grand Canyon and in the mountains of California, Idaho, and Colorado. Rodent-infested caves in southwestern states are associated with occasional cases of relapsing fever caused by *B. turicatae*.

PATHOGENESIS AND PATHOLOGY In humans, relapsing-fever borreliae penetrate the skin or mucous membranes, multiply in the blood, and circulate in great numbers during febrile periods. The organisms also may be found in the liver, spleen, central nervous sys-

Table 175-1 Characteristics and Distribution of Louse-Borne and Tick-Borne Borreliae

Borrelia Species	Arthropod Vector	Animal Reservoir	Disease Distribution	Type(s) of Relapsing Fever
B. recurrentis[a]	*Pediculus humanus* var. *corporis*	Humans	Northeastern Africa	Louse-borne, epidemic
B. duttoni	*Ornithodoros moubata*	Humans	Central, eastern, southern Africa	East African tick-borne, endemic
B. hispanica	*O. erraticus* (large variety)	Rodents	Spain, Portugal, Morocco, Algeria, Tunisia	Hispano-African tick-borne
B. crocidurae, *B. merionesi,* *B. microti,* *B. dipodilli*	*O. erraticus* (small variety)	Rodents	Morocco, Libya, Egypt, Iran, Turkey, Senegal, Kenya	North African tick-borne
B. persica	*O. tholozani*[b]	Rodents	From western China and Kashmir to Iraq and Egypt, former USSR, India	Asiatic-African tick-borne
B. caucasica	*O. verrucosus*	Rodents	Caucasus to Iraq	Caucasian tick-borne
B. latyschewii	*O. tartakovskyi*	Rodents	Iran, Central Asia	Caucasian tick-borne
B. hermsii	*O. hermsi*	Rodents	Western United States	American tick-borne
B. turicatae	*O. turicata*	Rodents	Southwestern United States	American tick-borne
B. parkeri	*O. parkeri*	Rodents	Western United States	American tick-borne
B. mazzotti	*O. talaje*[c]	Rodents	Southern United States, Mexico, Central and South America	American tick-borne
B. venezuelensis	*O. rudis*[d]	Rodents	Central and South America	American tick-borne

[a] Synonyms: *B. obermeyeri, B. novyi.*
[b] Synonyms: *O. papillipes, O. crossi?*
[c] Synonym: *O. dugesi?*
[d] Synonym: *O. venezuelensis.*
SOURCE: From Burgdorfer and Schwan.

tem, bone marrow, and other tissues and may be sequestered at these sites during periods of remission. The severity of disease is positively related to spirochete density in the blood. Even though the pathophysiologic manifestations of the disease resemble responses to endotoxin, and although plasma from some patients with relapsing fever coagulates *Limulus* amebocyte lysates, borreliae and other spirochetes have not been shown to express a true lipopolysaccharide (endotoxin) molecule. Infection with *B. recurrentis* does, however, activate protein mediators of inflammation, such as Hageman factor, prekallikrein, and proteins of the complement system; furthermore, a spirochetal heat-stable pyrogenic factor stimulates mononuclear phagocytes to express increased amounts of leukocyte pyrogen and thromboplastin.

The Jarisch-Herxheimer reaction in patients with LBRF is associated with a release of various cytokines into the plasma, including interleukin 6, interleukin 8, C-reactive protein, and enormous amounts of tumor necrosis factor α (TNF-α). Pretreatment of LBRF patients with antibody to TNF-α suppresses the Jarisch-Herxheimer reactions that follow penicillin treatment and reduces the plasma concentrations of certain other cytokines.

Findings at autopsy of patients with relapsing fever most often include hepatosplenomegaly and variable edema and swelling of other organs, such as the brain, lungs, and kidneys. On microscopic examination, the spleen is congested and contains multiple microabscesses composed of mononuclear cells that replace the white pulp, the myocardium displays diffuse histiocytic inflammation and interstitial edema, and the liver has areas of midzonal necrosis. Petechial hemorrhages are commonly evident over the surfaces of the meninges, pleura, heart, spleen, liver, kidneys, and mesentery. Subcapsular and parenchymal hemorrhagic infarcts of the spleen, heart, liver, and brain are sometimes grossly visible. Icterus is a common finding in severe and fatal cases of relapsing fever.

CLINICAL MANIFESTATIONS The clinical manifestations of LBRF and TBRF are similar. The mean incubation period is 7 days (range, 2 to 18 days), and the onset of illness is sudden, with fever, headache, shaking chills, sweats, myalgias, and arthralgias. The arthralgia of relapsing fever can be severe, involving small and large joints, but there is no evidence of arthritis. Dizziness, nausea, and vomiting are common. Sleep may be difficult and is sometimes accompanied by disturbing dreams. The patient is coherent but withdrawn, thirsty, and disinterested in food and other outside stimuli. The fever is high from the first, with a usual temperature of $\geq 40°C$ ($\geq 104°F$); fever is most often irregular in pattern and is sometimes accompanied by delirium. Patients become progressively prostrate as the disease advances. The pulse is rapid and the patient is mildly tachypneic. Meningism may be found. The conjunctivae are often injected, and the patient usually exhibits photophobia. The sclerae are sometimes icteric, most commonly in the later stages of illness. The mucous membranes are often dry, and the patient is usually dehydrated. Scattered petechiae develop on the trunk, extremities, and mucous membranes in one-third or more of patients with LBRF and in fewer patients with TBRF. A nonproductive cough is common, but chest sounds are usually normal; pleuritic pain and an accompanying pleuritic rub are sometimes noted. Cardiac findings are compatible with a high-output state; tachycardia and summation gallop are common. Tender enlargement of the spleen and liver frequently characterizes the acute phase of illness.

Epistaxis and blood-tinged sputum are common complications, and gastrointestinal and central nervous system hemorrhage can occur. Because of this coagulopathy, one LBRF outbreak in southern Sudan was thought to be viral hemorrhagic fever. Other complications of variable incidence include iridocyclitis, optic neuritis, meningitis, coma, isolated cranial-nerve palsy, pneumonitis, myocarditis, and rupture of the spleen. Infection during pregnancy can result in spontaneous abortion, stillbirth, or neonatal infection. Life-threatening complications are unusual in otherwise healthy persons given supportive care, especially if the illness is diagnosed and treated early.

Without treatment, symptoms intensify over a 2- to 7-day period (average, 5 days in LBRF and 3 days in TBRF), ending in a spontaneous crisis during which spirochetes disappear from the circulation. Treatment with one of the rapidly acting antibiotics, such as erythromycin, a tetracycline, or chloramphenicol, regularly precipitates a Jarisch-Herxheimer reaction within 1 to 4 h. The severity of this reaction is positively correlated with the density of spirochetes in the blood at the time of treatment. In the first phase of the crisis or reaction (the *chill phase*), rigors and rising fever are accompanied by an increasing metabolic rate, alveolar hyperventilation, high cardiac output, increasing peripheral vascular resistance, and decreased pulmonary arterial pressure. The body temperature commonly rises to $\geq 41°C$ ($\geq 105.8°F$). This high fever is accompanied often by agitation and confusion and sometimes by delirium. Fever can be partially controlled by the use of a cooling blanket and ice packs and by sponging of the patient with tepid water and alcohol. The chill phase terminates after 10 to 30 min, giving way to a *flush phase* characterized by a fall in body temperature, drenching sweats, and sometimes (more commonly in LBRF) a potentially dangerous fall in systemic arterial pressure and rise in pulmonary arterial pressure. Although cardiac output is maintained at high levels, the effective circulating blood volume decreases as peripheral vascular resistance falls. Vital signs must be monitored carefully during this period of the reaction, which usually lasts ≤ 8 h. Clinical and electrocardiographic evidence of myocarditis and myocardial dysfunction includes a prolonged QT_c interval, a third heart sound (S_3), elevated central venous pressure, arterial hypotension, and pulmonary edema.

The crisis is followed by a period of exhaustion, sleep, and an uneventful recovery. Not uncommonly, in the first week of convalescence, patients experience 1 or 2 days of mild fever unassociated with detectable spirochetemia. In untreated patients, spirochetemia and symptoms may recur after a period of several days or weeks (average

interval to first relapse, 9 days in LBRF and 7 days in TBRF). Only one or two relapses characteristically occur in untreated patients with LBRF, whereas as many as 10 (average, three) can occur in untreated patients with TBRF. In most cases, the illness becomes shorter and milder and the afebrile intervals longer with each relapse. Because of the great antigenic variation among *Borrelia* strains, infection confers only partial immunity, and repeated infections of the same individual have been recorded.

Diseases that should be considered in the differential diagnosis of relapsing fever or that may complicate relapsing fever include typhus fever, typhoid, nontyphoid salmonellosis, malaria, dengue and other arboviral illnesses, tuberculosis, leptospirosis, and viral hemorrhagic fevers. In the United States, the geographic distribution of Colorado tick fever overlaps that of TBRF, and the two diseases have similar manifestations early in their courses.

LABORATORY FINDINGS AND DIAGNOSIS   The diagnosis of relapsing fever is confirmed most easily by the detection of spirochetes in blood, bone marrow aspirates, or cerebrospinal fluid. Motile spirochetes can be seen when fresh blood is examined by darkfield microscopy; and fixed organisms are clearly visible in Wright-, Giemsa-, or acridine orange-stained preparations of thin or dehemoglobinized thick smears of peripheral blood or buffy-coat preparations (Fig. 175-1). Organisms are found in blood taken during periods of fever preceding the crisis; smears from $\geq 70\%$ of patients with LBRF and from fewer patients with TBRF are positive. In reference laboratories, relapsing-fever spirochetes are cultured from blood by the inoculation of BSK II medium or by the intraperitoneal inoculation of immature laboratory mice. The detection of agglutinins against *Proteus* OX-K (Weil-Felix reaction) in convalescent-phase serum supports the diagnosis. Serum antibodies to *Borrelia* can be detected by enzyme immunoassays, but these tests are unstandardized and subject to insensitivity due to antigenic variations among strains. Serologic cross-reactions occur with other spirochetes, including *B. burgdorferi* (the agent of Lyme disease) and *Treponema pallidum*.

Other laboratory findings in relapsing fever are generally nonspecific. The leukocyte count is normal or moderately elevated, with an unremarkable cell differential. Serum bilirubin levels are generally only slightly elevated. Thrombocytopenia (mean platelet count, about $50,000/\mu L$) is evident in patients with LBRF during the acute phase of the illness; platelet counts rebound during early convalescence. Prothrombin and partial thromboplastin times are moderately prolonged during acute illness, as are standardized bleeding times. Fibrinogen concentrations in the blood are normal, and fibrinolysis is mild or absent. Results of the Rumpel-Leede tourniquet test are negative, despite the presence of petechiae.

TREATMENT   Relapsing-fever borreliae are exquisitely sensitive to antibiotics. Treatment with erythromycin, a tetracycline, chloramphenicol, or penicillin produces rapid clearance of spirochetes and a remission of symptoms (Table 175-2). Although a single dose of erythromycin, a tetracycline, or chloramphenicol is highly effective in the treatment of LBRF, less is known about the efficacy of single-dose treatment of TBRF. Empirical treatment of TBRF for 7 days is therefore recommended to reduce the risk of persisting or relapsing borreliosis. For children <8 years of age and for pregnant women, erythromycin and penicillin are the preferred drugs.

The use of delayed-release intramuscular penicillin may prolong or delay the clearance of spirochetes and thereby attenuate the accompanying Jarisch-Herxheimer reaction, but this response is not predictable; furthermore, single-dose penicillin treatment sometimes results in relapse of spirochetemia and symptoms. Glucocorticoids and nonsteroidal anti-inflammatory agents do not prevent or significantly modify the cardiopulmonary disturbances of the Jarisch-Herxheimer reaction, although hydrocortisone and acetaminophen given at the same time as antibiotics reduce peak body temperature. Although pretreatment with antibody to TNF-α may moderate the Jarisch-Herxheimer reaction in treated patients with LBRF, its widespread use in LBRF is

FIGURE 175-1 Photomicrograph of tick-borne relapsing fever spirochete (*B. hermsii*) in Wright's-Giemsa-stained peripheral blood film.

impractical and its use in TBRF (whose treatment is associated with a relatively mild Jarisch-Herxheimer reaction) is not warranted. Close monitoring of fluid balance, arterial and venous pressures, and myocardial function is advised in supportive management of the Jarisch-Herxheimer reaction in patients with LBRF.

The management of patients with myocardial dysfunction requires caution in the administration of intravenous fluids and, in some cases, rapid digitalization. Bleeding is not controlled by heparin, and clinical studies do not suggest that disseminated intravascular coagulopathy is important. Vitamin K and other soluble vitamins are sometimes given to counter dietary deficiencies in patients with LBRF. Because postural hypotension is often pronounced during the acute phase of relapsing fever and in the early stage of recovery, patients should be assisted when arising from bed.

Untreated LBRF has a high case-fatality rate, especially among persons in otherwise poor health, such as those in famine-affected populations. The fatality rate among treated persons is usually <5%. In general, TBRF is a milder disease than LBRF: the spontaneous crisis and the Jarisch-Herxheimer reactions are less pronounced and the case-fatality rates are lower for TBRF than for LBRF.

PREVENTION AND CONTROL   LBRF can be prevented by elimination of circumstances that promote louse infestation (crowding, poverty, homelessness, poor personal hygiene), by use of practices that eliminate or reduce numbers of body lice (washing clothes, drying clothes in direct sunlight, changing clothes at frequent intervals), and by application of acaricides. Secondary complications and the spread of infection can be prevented by early case detection and treatment of

Table 175-2   Antibiotic Treatment of Louse-Borne and Tick-Borne Relapsing Fever in Adults

Medication	Louse-Borne Relapsing Fever (Single Dose)	Tick-Borne Relapsing Fever (7-Day Schedule)
Oral		
Erythromycin	500 mg	500 mg q6h
Tetracycline	500 mg	500 mg q6h
Doxycycline	100 mg	100 mg q12h
Chloramphenicol	500 mg	500 mg q6h
Parenteral[a]		
Erythromycin	500 mg	500 mg q6h
Tetracycline	250 mg	250 mg q6h
Doxycycline	100 mg	100 mg q12h
Chloramphenicol	500 mg	500 mg q6h
Penicillin G (procaine)	600,000 IU	600,000 IU daily

[a] For tick-borne relapsing fever, parenteral therapy is used only until oral treatment is tolerated.

infected persons and close contacts. Historically, outbreaks of LBRF have been controlled by mass delousing. In situations like those in refugee camps, individuals, their clothes, and their bedding should be deloused with appropriate acaricides, such as 0.5% permethrin dust. Impregnation of clothing with liquid permethrin, a residual acaricide, can provide long-term protection against infestation. In outbreaks of fever that involve louse-infested populations, empirical single-dose treatment with doxycycline will be effective against typhus as well as LBRF. *B. recurrentis* has a fragile life cycle and is eradicable.

TBRF can be prevented by the avoidance of rodent- and tick-infested dwellings and infested natural sites. Limiting rodent access to the foundations and attics of homes and vacation cabins and eliminating harborage for rodents in and around these dwellings reduce the potential for tick exposure. Rodents and rodent nests should be removed from infested buildings and their surroundings. Tick harborages of infested buildings or other circumscribed sites, such as rodent burrows and nests in hollow logs surrounding dwellings and in rodent-infested caves, can be chemically treated by pest-control specialists using various acaricides, such as carbaryl, diazinon, chlorpyrifos, pyrethrins, and malathion. Persons who enter tick-infested sites can protect themselves by wearing clothing that denies ticks access to the skin, by applying repellents to exposed skin and to clothing, and by applying an acaricide containing permethrin to clothing. Reporting of suspected cases of relapsing fever to public health authorities is important so that an epidemiologic investigation and control measures can be initiated promptly.

BIBLIOGRAPHY

BARBOUR AG: Antigenic variation of relapsing fever *Borrelia* species. Annu Rev Microbiol 44:155, 1990

BURGDORFER W, SCHWAN TG: *Borrelia*, in *Manual of Clinical Microbiology* 6, PR Murray et al (eds). Washington, DC, American Society for Microbiology, 1995, pp 626–635

CADAVID D, BARBOUR AG: Neuroborreliosis during relapsing fever: Review of clinical manifestations, pathology, and treatment of infections in humans and experimental animals. Clin Infect Dis 26:151, 1998

CUTLER SJ et al: *Borrelia recurrentis* characterization and comparison with relapsing fever, Lyme-associated, and other *Borrelia* spp. Int J Syst Bacteriol 47:958, 1997

DWORKIN MS et al: Tick-borne relapsing fever in the northwestern United States and southwestern Canada. Clin Infect Dis 26:122, 1998

FEKADE D et al: Prevention of Jarisch-Herxheimer reactions by treatment with antibodies against tumor necrosis factor α. N Engl J Med 335:311, 1996

HORTON JM, BLASER MJ: The spectrum of relapsing fever in the Rocky Mountains. Arch Intern Med 145:871, 1985

PERINE PL, TEKLU B: Antibiotic treatment of louse-borne relapsing fever in Ethiopia: A report of 377 cases. Am J Trop Med Hyg 32:1096, 1983

SPACH DH et al: Tick-borne diseases in the United States. N Engl J Med 329:936, 1993

176   *Allen C. Steere*

LYME BORRELIOSIS

DEFINITION   Lyme borreliosis, a tick-transmitted spirochetal illness, usually begins with a characteristic expanding skin lesion, erythema migrans (EM; stage 1, localized infection). After several days or weeks, the spirochete may spread hematogenously to many different sites (stage 2, disseminated infection). Possible manifestations of disseminated infection include secondary annular skin lesions, meningitis, cranial or peripheral neuritis, carditis, atrioventricular nodal block, or migratory musculoskeletal pain. Months to years later (usually after periods of latent infection), intermittent or chronic arthritis, chronic encephalopathy or polyneuropathy, or acrodermatitis may develop (stage 3, persistent infection). Most patients experience early symptoms of the illness during the summer, but the infection may not become symptomatic until it progresses to stage 2 or 3. Despite regional variations, the basic stages of the illness are similar worldwide.

ETIOLOGIC AGENT   *Borrelia burgdorferi*, the causative agent of the disease, is a fastidious, microaerophilic bacterium. The organism contains many immunogenic proteins, including a number of differentially expressed lipoproteins, most of which are encoded by plasmid DNA. The spirochete grows best at 33°C in a complex liquid medium called Barbour, Stoenner, Kelly (BSK) medium. Culture of the organism from clinical specimens (except for biopsy samples of skin at sites of EM or acrodermatitis) has been difficult. Three groups of pathogenic *B. burgdorferi* organisms, together referred to as *B. burgdorferi sensu lato*, have been identified, and more groups surely exist. To date, North American strains have belonged to the first group, *B. burgdorferi sensu stricto*. Although all three of the identified groups have been found in Europe and Asia, most isolates there have been strains of group 2 (*B. garinii*) or group 3 (*B. afzelii*). These differences may well account for the clinical variations in the disease in different geographic regions.

EPIDEMIOLOGY   The distribution of Lyme borreliosis correlates closely with the geographic ranges of ticks of the *Ixodes ricinus* complex: *I. scapularis* (also called *I. dammini*), *I. pacificus*, *I. ricinus*, and *I. persulcatus*. *I. scapularis* is the principal vector in the northeastern United States from Massachusetts to Maryland and in the midwestern states of Wisconsin and Minnesota. Surveys in these regions have documented infection in at least 20% of *I. scapularis* ticks; most cases of Lyme disease in the United States have occurred in these areas. *I. pacificus* is the vector in the western states of California and Oregon. The disease is acquired throughout Europe (from Great Britain to Scandinavia to European Russia), where *I. ricinus* is the vector, and in Asian Russia, China, and Japan, where *I. persulcatus* is the vector. These ticks transmit other diseases that may have similar symptoms. In the United States, *I. scapularis* also transmits babesiosis and ehrlichiosis; in Europe and Asia, *I. ricinus* and *I. persulcatus* also transmit tick-borne encephalitis.

Ticks of the *I. ricinus* complex feed once during each of the three stages of their usual 2-year life cycle. Typically, larval ticks take one blood meal in the late summer, nymphs feed during the following spring and early summer, and adults feed during autumn. For *I. scapularis* in the northeast, the white-footed mouse is the preferred host of the immature larval and nymphal ticks. It is critical that both of the tick's immature stages feed on the same host, because the life cycle of the spirochete depends on horizontal transmission: in early summer from infected nymphs to mice and in late summer from infected mice to larvae, which then molt to become the infected nymphs that will begin the cycle again the following year. It is the tiny nymphal tick that is primarily responsible for transmission of the disease to humans during the early summer months. White-tailed deer, which are not involved in the life cycle of the spirochete, are the preferred host for the adult stage of *I. scapularis* and seem to be critical to the tick's survival. The adult tick occasionally transmits the spirochete to humans during the fall, but at this stage the tick is considerably larger and easier to recognize.

Lyme disease is now the most common vector-borne infection in the United States. Since surveillance was begun in 1982, more than 100,000 cases have been reported to the Centers for Disease Control and Prevention (CDC); during the 1990s, more than 10,000 new cases have been reported each summer. Cases have been noted in 48 states, but the life cycle of *B. burgdorferi* has been identified in only 19 states. Cases have occurred in association with hiking, camping, or hunting trips and with residence in wooded or rural areas. Persons of all ages and both sexes are affected.

PATHOGENESIS   To maintain its complex enzootic cycle, *B. burgdorferi* must adapt to two markedly different environments: the tick and the mammalian host. The spirochete expresses outer-surface proteins A and B (OspA and OspB) in the midgut of the tick, whereas OspC is upregulated as the organism travels to the tick's salivary gland and thence to the mammalian host.

After injection into the human skin, *B. burgdorferi* may migrate outward, producing EM, and may spread hematogenously to other organs. Spread within the human host is probably facilitated through binding to the spirochete's surface by human plasminogen and urokinase-type plasminogen activator, which activates plasmin, a potent protease. The spirochete can adhere to many types of mammalian cells; it binds specifically to certain ubiquitous host integrin receptors in the extracellular matrix, to vitronectin and fibronectin, and to matrix glycosaminoglycans. *B. burgdorferi* seems to have a particular tropism for tissues of the skin, nervous system, atrioventricular node, and joints, from all of which it has been cultured, seen in histologic sections, or (more commonly) detected (via its DNA) by the polymerase chain reaction (PCR). These findings and the response of all stages of the disease to antibiotic therapy suggest that the organism persists in affected tissues throughout the illness, but the mechanisms of persistent infection are not yet clear.

The immune response in Lyme disease develops gradually. After the first several weeks of infection, mononuclear cells generally exhibit heightened responsiveness to *B. burgdorferi* antigens, and evidence of B cell hyperactivity is found, including elevated total serum IgM levels, cryoprecipitates, and circulating immune complexes. Titers of specific IgM antibody to *B. burgdorferi* peak between the third and sixth week after disease onset. The specific IgG response develops gradually over months, with response to an increasing array of 12 or more spirochetal polypeptides and maximal expansion during the period of arthritis. The spirochete is a potent inducer of proinflammatory cytokines, including tumor necrosis factor α and interleukin 1β. Histologic examination of all affected tissues reveals an infiltration of lymphocytes and plasma cells with some degree of vascular damage (including mild vasculitis or hypervascular occlusion), suggesting that the spirochete may have been present in or around blood vessels.

CLINICAL MANIFESTATIONS   **Early Infection: Stage 1 (Localized Infection)**   After an incubation period of 3 to 32 days, EM, which occurs at the site of the tick bite, usually begins as a red macule or papule that expands slowly to form a large annular lesion, most often with a bright red outer border and partial central clearing **(Plate IID-46)**. Because of the small size of ixodid ticks, most patients do not remember the preceding tick bite. The center of the lesion sometimes becomes intensely erythematous and indurated, vesicular, or necrotic. In other instances, the expanding lesion remains an even, intense red; several red rings are found within an outside ring; or the central area turns blue before the lesion clears. Although EM can be located anywhere, the thigh, groin, and axilla are particularly common sites. The lesion is warm but not often painful. Perhaps as many as 25% of patients do not exhibit this characteristic skin manifestation.

Early Infection: Stage 2 (Disseminated Infection)   Within days or weeks after the onset of EM, the organism often spreads hematogenously to many sites. In these cases patients frequently develop secondary annular skin lesions similar in appearance to the initial lesion. Skin involvement is commonly accompanied by severe headache, mild stiffness of the neck, fever, chills, migratory musculoskeletal pain, arthralgias, and profound malaise and fatigue. Less common manifestations include generalized lymphadenopathy or splenomegaly, hepatitis, sore throat, nonproductive cough, conjunctivitis, iritis, or testicular swelling. Except for fatigue and lethargy, which are often constant, the early signs and symptoms of Lyme disease are typically intermittent and changing. Even in untreated patients, the early symptoms usually become less severe or disappear within several weeks.

Symptoms suggestive of meningeal irritation may develop early in Lyme disease when EM is present but usually are not associated with cerebrospinal fluid (CSF) pleocytosis or an objective neurologic deficit. After several weeks or months, about 15% of untreated patients develop frank neurologic abnormalities, including meningitis, subtle encephalitic signs, cranial neuritis (including bilateral facial palsy), motor or sensory radiculoneuropathy, mononeuritis multiplex, or myelitis—alone or in various combinations. In the United States, the usual pattern consists of fluctuating symptoms of meningitis accompanied by facial palsy and peripheral radiculoneuropathy. Lymphocytic pleocytosis (about 100 cells per microliter) is found in CSF, often along with elevated protein levels and normal or slightly low glucose concentrations. In Europe and Asia, the first neurologic sign is characteristically radicular pain, which is followed by the development of CSF pleocytosis (called *Bannwarth's syndrome*), but meningeal or encephalitic signs are frequently absent. These early neurologic abnormalities usually resolve completely within months, but chronic neurologic disease may occur later.

Within several weeks after the onset of illness, about 8% of patients develop cardiac involvement. The most common abnormality is a fluctuating degree of atrioventricular block (first-degree, Wenckebach, or complete heart block). Some patients have more diffuse cardiac involvement, including electrocardiographic changes indicative of acute myopericarditis, left ventricular dysfunction evident on radionuclide scans, or (in rare cases) cardiomegaly or pancarditis. Cardiac involvement usually lasts for only a few weeks but may recur. Chronic cardiomyopathy caused by *B. burgdorferi* has been reported in Europe.

During this stage, musculoskeletal pain is common. The typical pattern consists of migratory pain in joints, tendons, bursae, muscles, or bones (usually without joint swelling) lasting for hours or days and affecting one or two locations at a time.

Late Infection: Stage 3 (Persistent Infection) Months after the onset of infection, about 60% of patients in the United States who have received no antibiotic treatment develop frank arthritis. The typical pattern comprises intermittent attacks of oligoarticular arthritis in large joints (especially the knees), lasting for weeks to months in a given joint. Small joints and periarticular sites also may be affected, primarily during early attacks. The number of patients who continue to have recurrent attacks decreases each year. However, in a small percentage of cases, involvement of large joints—usually one or both knees—becomes chronic and may lead to erosion of cartilage and bone. These patients have a higher frequency of the class II major histocompatibility complex alleles associated with rheumatoid arthritis, particularly HLA-DRBI*0401 or *0101 alleles, than patients with brief Lyme arthritis or normal control subjects. Moreover, they may have persistent arthritis for months or even several years after the apparent eradication of spirochetes from the joints with antibiotic therapy. In these genetically susceptible individuals, autoimmunity may develop within the proinflammatory milieu of the joints because of molecular mimicry between the dominant T cell epitope of OspA and human lymphocyte function–associated antigen 1 (hLFA-1).

White cell counts in joint fluid range from 500 to 110,000/μL (average, 25,000/μL); most of these cells are polymorphonuclear leukocytes. Tests for rheumatoid factor or antinuclear antibodies usually give negative results. Examination of synovial biopsy samples reveals fibrin deposits, villous hypertrophy, vascular proliferation, microangiopathic lesions, and a heavy infiltration of lymphocytes and plasma cells.

Although less common, chronic neurologic involvement may also become apparent months or years after the onset of infection, sometimes following long periods of latent infection. The most common form of chronic central nervous system involvement is subtle encephalopathy affecting memory, mood, or sleep and often accompanied by axonal polyneuropathy manifested as either distal paresthesia or spinal radicular pain. Patients with encephalopathy frequently have evidence of memory impairment in neuropsychological tests and abnormal results in CSF analyses. In cases with polyneuropathy, electromyography generally shows extensive abnormalities of proximal and distal nerve segments. Encephalomyelitis or leukoencephalitis, a rare manifestation of Lyme borreliosis reported primarily in Europe, is a severe neurologic disorder that may include spastic paraparesis, upper motor-neuron bladder dysfunction, and lesions in the periventricular white matter. The prolonged course of chronic neuroborreliosis following periods of latent infection is reminiscent of tertiary neurosyphilis.

Acrodermatitis chronica atrophicans, the late skin manifestation of the disorder, has been associated primarily with *B. afzelii* infection in Europe and Asia. It has been observed primarily in elderly women. The skin lesions, which are usually found on the acral surface of an arm or leg, begin insidiously with reddish-violaceous discoloration; they become sclerotic or atrophic over a period of years.

DIAGNOSIS Lyme disease is usually diagnosed by the recognition of a characteristic clinical picture with serologic confirmation. Although serologic testing may yield negative results during the first several weeks of infection, most patients have a positive antibody response to *B. burgdorferi* after that time. The limitation of serologic tests is that they do not clearly distinguish between active and inactive infection. Patients with previous Lyme disease—particularly in cases progressing to late stages—often remain seropositive for years, even after adequate antibiotic treatment. In addition, some patients are seropositive because of asymptomatic infection. If these individuals subsequently develop another illness, the positive serologic test for Lyme disease may cause diagnostic confusion. On the other hand, a few patients who receive inadequate antibiotic therapy during the first several weeks of infection develop subtle joint or neurologic symptoms but are seronegative. The important point is that seronegative Lyme disease is usually a mild, attenuated illness.

For serologic analysis in Lyme disease, the CDC recommends a two-step approach in which samples are first tested by enzyme-linked immunosorbent assay (ELISA) and equivocal or positive results are then tested by western blotting. During the first month of infection, both IgM and IgG responses to the spirochete should be determined, preferably in both acute- and convalescent-phase serum samples. Approximately 20 to 30% of patients have a positive response detectable in acute-phase samples, whereas about 70 to 80% have a positive response during convalescence (2 to 4 weeks later). After that time, the great majority of patients continue to have a positive IgG antibody response, and a single test (that for IgG) is usually sufficient. In persons with illness of longer than 1 month's duration, a positive IgM test result alone is likely to be false-positive; therefore, a positive IgM test should not be used to support the diagnosis in such patients. According to current criteria adopted by the CDC, an IgM western blot is considered positive if two of the following three bands are present: 23, 39, and 41 kDa. However, the combination of the 23- and 41-kDa bands may still represent a false-positive result. An IgG blot is considered positive if 5 of the following 10 bands are present: 18, 23, 28, 30, 39, 41, 45, 58, 66, and 93 kDa.

Because serologic tests do not distinguish between active and inactive infection, tests that detect the spirochete directly are being researched. *B. burgdorferi* may be cultured from skin lesions of patients with the disorder, but its culture from other sites has been a low-yield proposition. Detection of spirochetal DNA by PCR may serve as a substitute for culture in cases of Lyme arthritis. In one study, *B. burgdorferi* DNA was detected in synovial fluid samples from 75 (85%) of 88 patients and in none of 64 control samples. However, the sensitivity of PCR determinations in CSF from patients with neuroborreliosis has been much lower. There seems to be little if any role for PCR in the detection of *B. burgdorferi* DNA in blood or urine samples.

DIFFERENTIAL DIAGNOSIS Classic EM is a slowly expanding erythema with partial central clearing. If the lesion expands little, it may represent the red papule of an uninfected tick bite. If the lesion expands rapidly, it may represent cellulitis (e.g., streptococcal cellulitis) or an allergic reaction, perhaps to tick saliva. Patients with secondary annular lesions may be thought to have erythema multiforme, but neither the development of blistering mucosal lesions nor the involvement of the palms or soles is a feature of *B. burgdorferi* infection. In the southeastern United States, an EM-like skin lesion, sometimes with mild systemic symptoms, may be associated with *Am-*

blyomma americanum tick bites, but the cause of this illness has not yet been identified.

Later in the infection, the most common problem in diagnosis is to mistake Lyme disease for chronic fatigue syndrome or fibromyalgia. This difficulty is compounded by the fact that a small percentage of patients do in fact develop these chronic pain or fatigue syndromes in association with or soon after Lyme disease. Compared with Lyme disease, chronic fatigue syndrome (Chap. 384) or fibromyalgia tends to produce more generalized and disabling symptoms, including marked fatigue, severe headache, diffuse musculoskeletal pain, multiple symmetric tender points in characteristic locations, pain and stiffness in many joints, diffuse dysesthesia, difficulty with concentration, and sleep disturbances. Patients with chronic fatigue syndrome or fibromyalgia lack evidence of joint inflammation; they have normal results in neurologic tests; and they usually have a greater degree of anxiety and depression than patients with chronic neuroborreliosis.

℞ **TREATMENT**   As outlined in the algorithm in Fig. 176-1, the various manifestations of Lyme disease can usually be treated successfully with orally administered antibiotics; the exceptions are objective neurologic abnormalities and third-degree atrioventricular heart block, which seem to require intravenous therapy. For early Lyme disease, doxycycline is effective in men and in nonpregnant women. An advantage of this regimen is that it is also effective against the agent of human granulocytic ehrlichiosis, which is transmitted by the same tick that transmits the Lyme disease agent. Amoxicillin, cefuroxime axetil, and erythromycin or its congeners are second-, third-, and fourth-choice alternatives, respectively. In children, amoxicillin is effective (not more than 2 g/d); in cases of penicillin allergy, cefuroxime axetil or erythromycin may be used. For patients with infection localized to the skin, a 20-day course of therapy is generally sufficient;

in contrast, for patients with disseminated infection, a 30-day course is recommended. Approximately 15% of patients experience a Jarisch-Herxheimer-like reaction during the first 24 h of therapy.

These oral antibiotic regimens, when given for 30 to 60 days, are effective for the treatment of Lyme arthritis. However, the response to oral therapy may be slower than that to intravenous therapy. In the small percentage of patients with arthritis in whom arthritic symptoms persist for months or even years after the apparent eradication of spirochetes from the joints with antimicrobial therapy, treatment with anti-inflammatory agents or synovectomy may be successful.

For objective neurologic abnormalities (with the possible exception of facial palsy alone), parenteral antibiotic therapy seems to be necessary. Intravenous ceftriaxone, given for 4 weeks, is most commonly used for this purpose, but intravenous cefotaxime or intravenous penicillin G for the same duration may also be effective. In patients with high-degree atrioventricular block or a PR interval of greater than 0.3 s, intravenous therapy for at least part of the course and cardiac monitoring are recommended. Prior to the use of antibiotics for the treatment of Lyme disease, the degree of heart block was found to decrease rapidly with prednisone (40 to 60 mg/d). Although rarely used today, glucocorticoids may be of benefit in patients with complete heart block or congestive heart failure if antimicrobial therapy alone does not result in improvement within 24 h.

It is unclear how and whether asymptomatic infection should be treated, but patients with such infection are often given a course of oral antibiotics. The appropriate treatment for Lyme disease during pregnancy is also unclear. Because the risk of maternal-fetal transmission seems to be very low, standard therapy for the documented stage and manifestation of the illness may be sufficient. Relapse may follow the use of any of the antibiotic regimens for Lyme disease, and a second course of therapy may be necessary. On the other hand, in patients who develop chronic fatigue syndrome or fibromyalgia after Lyme disease, further antibiotic therapy does not seem to be of benefit.

The risk of infection with *B. burgdorferi* after a recognized tick bite is so low that antibiotic prophylaxis is not routinely indicated. However, if the tick is engorged, if follow-up is difficult, or if the patient is quite anxious, therapy with amoxicillin or doxycycline for 10 days is likely to prevent Lyme disease.

PROGNOSIS   The response to treatment is best early in the disease. Later treatment of Lyme borreliosis is still effective, but convalescence may be longer. Eventually, most patients recover with minimal or no residual deficits.

ALGORITHM FOR TESTING AND THERAPY   According to guidelines recently published by the American College of Physicians, empirical antibiotic therapy without serologic testing is recommended for patients with a high pretest probability of Lyme disease (such as those with EM); two-step testing (by ELISA and, if positive, by western blot) is recommended for patients with an intermediate pretest probability (such as those with recurrent oligoarticular arthritis); and neither testing nor treatment is recommended for patients with a low pretest probability (such as those with nonspecific symptoms of myalgias, arthralgias, or fatigue).

REINFECTION   Reinfection may occur after EM when patients are treated with antimicrobial agents. In such cases, the immune response is not adequate to provide protection from subsequent infection. However, patients who develop an expanded immune response to the spirochete over a period of months (such as those with Lyme arthritis) have protective immunity for a period of years and do not acquire the infection again.

VACCINATION   A vaccine is now available for the prevention of Lyme disease in the United States. It consists of a recombinant outer-surface lipoprotein A (L-OspA) with adjuvant. High-titered antibody to OspA is necessary for protection. In a phase 3 efficacy trial in which subjects were given three doses of vaccine or placebo on a 0-, 1-, and 12-month schedule, vaccine efficacy in preventing definite cases of Lyme disease was 49% during the first year (after two doses)

FIGURE 176-1   Algorithm for the treatment of the various acute or chronic manifestations of Lyme borreliosis. Relapse may occur with any of these regimens, and a second course of treatment may be necessary. AV, atrioventricular.

and 76% in year 2 (after three doses). Equivalent antibody titers may be obtained if the three doses are given on a 0-, 1-, and 2-month schedule. The third dose should be given in April so that the vaccine recipient will have peak antibody titers during the summer tick-transmission season. Although long-term data are not yet available, yearly booster injections may be necessary. Vaccine injection may cause a mild to moderate local or systemic reaction usually lasting for only a few days. Vaccination should be considered for individuals who live in areas that are highly endemic for the infection and who have frequent exposure to tick habitats.

BIBLIOGRAPHY

BARBOUR AG, HAYES SF: Biology of *Borrelia* species. Microbiol Rev 50:381, 1986

DATTWYLER RJ et al: Ceftriaxone compared with doxycycline for the treatment of acute disseminated Lyme disease. N Engl J Med 337:289, 1997

DRESSLER F et al: Western blotting in the serodiagnosis of Lyme disease. J Infect Dis 167:392, 1993

LOGIGIAN EL et al: Chronic neurologic manifestations of Lyme disease. N Engl J Med 323:1438, 1990

NOCTON JJ et al: Detection of *Borrelia burgdorferi* DNA by polymerase chain reaction in synovial fluid in Lyme arthritis. N Engl J Med 330:229, 1994

RAHN DW, MALAWISTA SE: Lyme disease: Recommendations for diagnosis and treatment. Ann Intern Med 114:472, 1991

STEERE AC: Lyme disease. N Engl J Med 321:586, 1989

———— et al: Vaccination against Lyme disease with recombinant *Borrelia burgdorferi* outer-surface lipoprotein A with adjuvant. N Engl J Med 339:209, 1998

Section 10
RICKETTSIA, MYCOPLASMA, AND *CHLAMYDIA*

177 David Walker, Didier Raoult, J. Stephen Dumler, Thomas Marrie

RICKETTSIAL DISEASES

The rickettsiae make up a family of gram-negative coccobacilli and short bacilli that grow strictly in eukaryotic cells. Characteristics of these organisms include their obligately intracellular location and persistence. The pathogenic rickettsiae move through mammalian reservoirs; they are transmitted by insect or tick vectors. Except for louse-borne typhus, humans are incidental hosts. Among rickettsiae, *Coxiella burnetii* (the agent of Q fever) is notorious for its ability to survive for an extended period outside of the reservoir or vector and for its extreme infectiousness: inhalation of a single microorganism can cause pneumonia. Clinical infections with rickettsiae can be classified into five general groups: (1) tick- and gamasid mite–borne, spotted fever group (SFG) rickettsial diseases; (2) flea- and louse-borne typhus group rickettsial diseases; (3) chigger-borne scrub typhus; (4) ehrlichioses; and (5) Q fever. The rickettsiae that cause spotted fevers, typhus, and scrub typhus are listed along with their vectors, geographic ranges, and associated diseases in Table 177-1.

TICK- AND MITE-BORNE SPOTTED FEVERS

ROCKY MOUNTAIN SPOTTED FEVER Rocky Mountain spotted fever (RMSF), the most severe of the rickettsial diseases, is caused by *Rickettsia rickettsii*. This organism possesses two major immunodominant surface-exposed proteins, rOmpA and rOmpB, which have species-specific conformational epitopes. rOmpA functions as an adhesin for the host cell; rOmpB, the most abundant outer-membrane protein, shares genetic sequences and limited antigens with typhus group rickettsiae. This small (0.3 μm by 1.0 μm) bacillus has a gram-negative cell wall structure; its lipopolysaccharide shares antigens mainly within the SFG and is not endotoxic in the quantities found in human infections.

Discovered in the American West in the late nineteenth century, RMSF is at present documented in 48 states, Canada, Mexico, Costa Rica, Panama, Colombia, and Brazil. It is transmitted by *Dermacentor variabilis,* the American dog tick, in the eastern two-thirds of the United States and California; by *D. andersoni,* the Rocky Mountain wood tick, in the western United States; by *Rhipicephalus sanguineus*

in Mexico; and by *Amblyomma cajennense* in Central and South America. Maintained principally by transovarian transmission from one generation of ticks to the next, *R. rickettsii* can be acquired by uninfected ticks through the ingestion of a blood meal from rickettsemic small mammals.

Humans become infected during the active season of the vector tick species. In northern areas, cases occur mainly in the spring; in warmer southern states, most cases occur from May to September, although some cases are reported in the winter. Although 4% of *D. variabilis* ticks contain rickettsiae, the vast majority of these are nonpathogenic species such as *R. montana* and *R. bellii.* The likelihood of an individual tick's containing *R. rickettsii* is remote. From 1988 to 1997, the reported incidence of RMSF has been in the range of 0.16 to 0.26 cases per 100,000 population in the United States. This rate is probably an underestimate, since the diagnosis is difficult and reporting incomplete. The 5- to 9-year-old age group has the highest incidence. The mortality rate was 20 to 25% in the preantibiotic era and now remains at about 5% because of delayed diagnosis and treatment. The case-fatality ratio is higher for males than females and increases with each decade of life above age 20.

Pathogenesis *R. rickettsii* organisms are inoculated into the dermis along with secretions of the tick's salivary glands after ≥6 h of feeding. Rickettsiae spread lymphohematogenously throughout the body, attach via rOmpA to the endothelial cell membrane, and induce their own engulfment. Once intracellularly located, they escape rapidly from the phagosome, replicate in the cytosol by binary fission, and spread from cell to cell, propelled by polar polymerization of the host cell's actin. The result is numerous foci of contiguous infected endothelial cells that are extensive enough to manifest clinically after a dose-dependent incubation period of approximately 1 week (range, 2 to 14 days). *R. rickettsii* is more invasive than other rickettsiae, routinely spreading to infect vascular smooth-muscle cells. Despite frequent statements to the contrary, occlusive thrombosis and ischemic necrosis are not the fundamental pathologic basis for tissue and organ injury in RMSF. Instead, increased vascular permeability, with resulting edema, hypovolemia, and ischemia, is responsible. Indeed, immunohistologic studies of severely infected humans and animals have demonstrated numerous zones of infected endothelium, only a small proportion of which contain thrombi. The thrombi are usually located to one side of the lumen, which is not occluded. These hemostatic plugs appear to be an appropriate host response rather than a pathogenic process. Consumption of platelets results in thrombocytopenia

Table 177-1 Features of Selected Rickettsial Infections

Disease	Organism	Vector(s)	Geographic Range	Incubation Period	Duration
Rocky Mountain spotted fever	*Rickettsia rickettsii*	*Dermacentor andersoni* *D. variabilis* *Amblyomma cajennense* *Rhipicephalus sanguineus*	United States United States Central/South America Mexico	2–14 days	10–20 days
Mediterranean spotted fever[a]	*R. conorii*	*R. sanguineus*	Southern Europe, Africa, Middle East, Central Asia	5–7 days	7–14 days
Rickettsialpox[a]	*R. akari*	*Liponyssoides sanguineus*	United States, Ukraine, Slovenia	10–17 days	3–11 days
Epidemic typhus	*R. prowazekii*	*Pediculus humanus corporis*	Worldwide	7–14 days	10–18 days
Brill-Zinsser disease	*R. prowazekii*	—[b]	Worldwide	Years	7–11 days
Murine typhus	*R. typhi*	*Xenopsylla cheopis*	Worldwide	8–16 days	8–16 days
Murine typhus	*R. felis*	*Ctenocephalides felis*	Southern Texas, California, Mexico	8–16 days	8–16 days
Scrub typhus[a]	*Orientia tsutsugamushi*	*Leptotrombidium deliense*	Asia, Australia, New Guinea, Pacific Islands	9–18 days	6–21 days

[a] Eschar is usually present at the bite site.
[b] Brill-Zinsser disease represents a recrudescence of latent epidemic typhus.
NOTE: Rocky mountain spotted fever and epidemic typhus often manifest as severe illness, while scrub typhus sometimes does so; murine typhus and Mediterranean spotted fever cause moderately severe illness; and Brill-Zinsser disease and rickettsialpox usually cause mild illness. The rash in Rocky Mountain spotted fever spreads from the extremities to the trunk and face; palms and soles may also be involved. All other rickettsial diseases listed above have a rash that starts on the trunk and spreads to the extremities. The palms and soles are also involved in Mediterranean spotted fever.

in 32 to 52% of patients, but disseminated intravascular coagulation with hypofibrinogenemia is rare. Activation of platelets, generation of thrombin, and activation of the fibrinolytic system all appear to be homeostatic physiologic responses to endothelial injury.

Clinical Manifestations Early in the illness, when medical attention usually is first sought, RMSF is difficult to distinguish from many self-limiting viral illnesses. Fever, headache, malaise, myalgia, nausea, vomiting, and anorexia are the most frequent symptoms during the first 3 days. The patient becomes progressively more ill as vascular infection and injury advance. In one large series, only one-third of patients were diagnosed with presumptive RMSF early in the clinical course and treated appropriately as outpatients. In the tertiary care setting, RMSF is all too often recognized only when its late severe manifestations, developing at the end of the first week or in the second week of illness in patients without appropriate treatment, prompt admission to the intensive care unit.

The progressive nature of the infection is clearly manifested in the skin. Rash is evident in only 14% of patients on the first day of illness and in only 49% during the first 3 days. Macules (1 to 5 mm) appear first on the wrists and ankles and then on the remainder of the extremities and the trunk. Later, more severe vascular damage results in frank hemorrhage at the center of the maculopapule, a petechia that does not disappear upon compression (**Plate IID-45**). This sequence of events is sometimes delayed or aborted by effective treatment. In fact, rash appears on day 6 or later in 20% of cases and does not appear at all in 9 to 16% of cases, including some with severe visceral lesions that result in death. Petechiae occur in 41 to 59% of cases, appearing on or after day 6 in 74% of cases that include a rash. Involvement of the palms and soles, often considered diagnostically important, usually occurs relatively late in the course (after day 5 in 43% of cases) and does not occur at all in 18 to 64% of cases.

The microcirculation, both systemic and pulmonary, is the target of intracellular rickettsial infection, and the clinical manifestations reflect the ensuing vascular changes. Widespread increased vascular permeability results in edema, decreased plasma volume, hypoalbuminemia, reduced serum oncotic pressure, and prerenal azotemia. Hypotension occurs in 17% of cases. Extensive infection of the pulmonary microcirculation is associated with noncardiogenic pulmonary edema. Cardiac involvement is most frequently manifested as dysrhythmia, which is detected in 7 to 16% of cases. Pulmonary involvement, often a major factor in fatal cases, is observed in 17% of cases, of which 12% are considered to represent severe respiratory disease and 8% require mechanical ventilation.

Central nervous system (CNS) involvement is the other important determinant of the outcome of RMSF. Encephalitis, presenting as confusion or lethargy, is apparent in 26 to 28% of cases. Progressively severe encephalitis manifests as stupor or delirium in 21 to 26% of cases, as ataxia in 18%, as coma in 9 to 10%, and as seizures in 8%. Cranial nerve palsy, hearing loss, severe vertigo, nystagmus, dysarthria, aphasia, unilateral corticospinal signs, ankle clonus, extensor toe signs, hyperreflexia, spasticity, fasciculations, athetosis, neurogenic bladder, hemiplegia, paraplegia, and complete paralysis have been reported. Meningoencephalitis results in cerebrospinal fluid (CSF) pleocytosis in 34 to 38% of cases; usually there are 10 to 100 cells per microliter with a mononuclear predominance, but occasionally there are more than 100 cells per microliter and a polymorphonuclear predominance. The CSF protein concentration is increased in 30 to 35% of cases, but the CSF glucose concentration is usually normal.

Renal failure, which occurs in more severely ill patients, is often reversible with rehydration. However, in the most severe cases, shock results in acute tubular necrosis–induced renal failure, which often requires hemodialysis.

Hepatic injury is manifested in 38% of cases as mildly or moderately increased serum aminotransferase concentrations and is due to focal death of individual hepatocytes, but hepatic failure does not occur. Jaundice is recognized in 8 to 9% of cases and an elevated serum bilirubin concentration in 18 to 30%. Marked hyperbilirubinemia occasionally occurs, probably as a consequence of both hemolysis and hepatocytic injury.

Bleeding is a potentially life-threatening effect of severe vascular damage. Anemia develops in 30% of cases and is severe enough to require red blood cell transfusions in 11%. Blood is detected in the stools or vomitus of 10% of patients, and death has followed massive upper gastrointestinal hemorrhage.

Other characteristic clinical laboratory findings include a normal white blood cell count with increased numbers of immature myeloid cells, increased plasma levels of proteins of the acute-phase response (C-reactive protein, fibrinogen, ferritin, and others), and hyponatremia (in 56% of cases) due to the appropriate secretion of antidiuretic hormone in response to the hypovolemic state. Skeletal muscle injury, clinically manifested as myositis, has been documented in several individual cases by the detection of marked elevations in serum creatine kinase or of histopathologic evidence of vascular injury in skeletal muscle and multifocal rhabdomyonecrosis. Ocular involvement includes conjunctivitis in 30% of cases and retinal vein engorgement, flame hemorrhages, arterial occlusion, and papilledema with normal CSF pressure in some instances.

In untreated cases, death usually occurs 8 to 15 days after the onset of illness. A rare presentation, fulminant RMSF, is fatal within 5 days after onset. This fulminant presentation has been associated with RMSF in black males who have glucose-6-phosphate dehydrogenase (G6PD) deficiency and is thought to be related to an undefined effect of hemolysis on the rickettsial infection. Although survivors of RMSF usually appear to return to their previous state of health, permanent sequelae, including neurologic deficits and amputation of gangrenous extremities, may follow severe illness.

Diagnosis The diagnosis of RMSF during the acute stage is more difficult than is generally appreciated. Clinical and epidemiologic considerations are more important than laboratory features early in the illness. The most important epidemiologic factor is a history of exposure within the 12 days preceding disease onset to a potentially tick-infested environment during a season of possible tick activity. However, only 60% of patients actually recall being bitten by a tick during the incubation period.

The differential diagnosis for early clinical manifestations of RMSF (fever, headache, and myalgia without a rash) includes influenza, enteroviral infection, infectious mononucleosis, viral hepatitis, leptospirosis, typhoid fever, gram-negative or -positive bacterial sepsis, human monocytic or granulocytic ehrlichiosis, murine typhus, sylvatic flying-squirrel typhus, and rickettsialpox. Enterocolitis may be suggested by nausea, vomiting, and abdominal pain; prominence of abdominal tenderness has resulted in exploratory laparotomy. CNS involvement may masquerade as bacterial and viral meningoencephalitis, with seizures, coma, neurologic signs, and CSF abnormalities. Cough, pulmonary signs, and chest roentgenographic opacities may lead to a diagnostic consideration of bronchitis or pneumonia.

During the first 3 days of illness, only 3% of patients exhibit the classic triad of fever, rash, and history of tick exposure. When a rash appears, a diagnosis of RMSF should certainly be considered. However, many illnesses considered in the differential diagnosis may also be associated with a rash, including rubeola, rubella, meningococcemia, disseminated gonococcal infection, secondary syphilis, toxic shock syndrome, drug hypersensitivity, idiopathic thrombocytopenic purpura, thrombotic thrombocytopenic purpura, Kawasaki syndrome, and immune complex vasculitis. The converse is also true: any person in an endemic area with a provisional diagnosis of one of the above illnesses may have RMSF.

The most common serologic test for confirmation of the diagnosis is the indirect immunofluorescence assay. Between 7 and 10 days after onset, a diagnostic titer of ≥1:64 is usually detectable. Latex agglutination and a solid-state enzyme immunoassay are also available commercially. Latex agglutination usually yields a diagnostic titer of ≥1: 128 at 7 to 9 days after onset. The sensitivity and specificity of the indirect immunofluorescence assay are 94 to 100% and 100%, respectively, and the latex agglutination test has a sensitivity of 71 to 94% and a specificity of 96 to 99%. The performance of the solid-state immunoassay has not been reported. It is important to understand that serologic tests for RMSF are usually negative at the time of presentation for medical care and that treatment should not be delayed while a positive serologic result is awaited.

The only diagnostic test that is useful during the acute illness is immunohistologic examination (immunofluorescence or immunoenzyme staining) of a cutaneous biopsy of a rash lesion for *R. rickettsii*. Examination of a 3-mm punch biopsy of such a lesion is 70% sensitive

and 100% specific. Polymerase chain reaction (PCR) amplification and detection of *R. rickettsii* DNA in peripheral blood is an insensitive approach except in the preterminal state; rickettsiae are present in large quantities in heavily infected foci of endothelial cells but in relatively low quantities in the circulation. Cultivation of rickettsiae in cell culture is technically feasible but is seldom undertaken because of biohazard and technologic concerns.

℞ **TREATMENT** The drug of choice for the treatment of both children and adults with RMSF is doxycycline, except when the patient is pregnant or allergic to the drug. Doxycycline is administered orally (or, in the presence of coma or vomiting, intravenously) at 200 mg/d in two divided doses. For children with RMSF reinfection, up to five courses of doxycycline may be administered with minimal risk of dental staining. Other regimens include oral tetracycline (25 to 50 mg/kg per day) in four divided doses. β-Lactam antibiotics, erythromycin, and aminoglycosides have no role in the treatment of RMSF, and sulfa-containing drugs are likely to exacerbate this infection. There is not enough clinical experience to comment on the use of fluoroquinolones in this setting. The most seriously ill patients are managed in intensive care units, with careful administration of fluids to achieve optimal tissue perfusion without precipitating noncardiogenic pulmonary edema. In some severely ill patients, hypoxemia requires intubation and mechanical ventilation; oliguric or anuric acute renal failure requires hemodialysis; seizures necessitate the use of antiseizure medication; anemia or severe hemorrhage necessitates transfusions of packed red blood cells; and bleeding with severe thrombocytopenia requires platelet transfusions. Heparin is not a useful component of treatment, and there is no evidence that glucocorticoids, although frequently administered, affect outcome.

Prevention Avoidance of tick bites is the only available preventive approach. Protective clothing and tick repellents, which could reduce the risk, are seldom actually used. After possible tick exposure, it is wise to inspect the body once or twice a day and remove ticks before they can inoculate rickettsiae.

MEDITERRANEAN SPOTTED FEVER (BOUTONNEUSE FEVER) AND OTHER SPOTTED FEVERS The etiologic agent of Mediterranean spotted fever, *R. conorii*, is prevalent in southern Europe (below the 45th parallel), all of Africa, and southwestern and south-central Asia. The tick vector and reservoir is *R. sanguineus*, the dog brown tick. The name of this disease varies with the region in which it occurs; examples include Kenya tick typhus, Indian tick typhus, Israeli spotted fever, and Astrakhan spotted fever. Whatever the designation, the disease is characterized by a high fever, rash, and—in most geographic locales—an inoculation eschar (*tâche noire*) at the site of the tick bite. A severe form of the disease, associated with a 50% mortality rate, has been observed in patients with diabetes, alcoholism, or heart failure.

African tick-bite fever, which is caused by *R. africae* and has been recognized since the beginning of the twentieth century, was first documented in the modern era in Zimbabwe in 1992. The disease occurs in rural areas and follows bites by ticks of cattle and wild animals. *R. africae* is prevalent in *Amblyomma hebraeum* and *A. variegatum* ticks, which readily feed on humans. Cases have been confirmed not only in Zimbabwe but also in Tanzania and South Africa, and the disease is prevalent in the Caribbean islands of Guadeloupe. The incubation period is 7 days. The illness is mild and consists of headache, fever, eschar at the tick bite site, and regional lymphadenopathy. *Amblyomma* ticks often feed in groups, and several ticks may be found on one patient, with the subsequent development of multiple eschars. Rash is frequently lacking or transient and may be vesicular. African tick-bite fever is the most prevalent rickettsiosis worldwide, and, as tourism to sub-Saharan Africa increases, it is expected that more cases will be seen in non-African countries.

Rickettsia japonica causes *Japanese spotted fever* or *Oriental spot-*

Table 177-2 Laboratory Diagnosis and Treatment of Selected Rickettsial Diseases

Disease	Laboratory Diagnosis	Treatment
Mediterranean spotted fever Japanese or Oriental spotted fever Queensland tick typhus Flinders Island spotted fever African tick-bite fever	Isolation of rickettsiae by shell-vial culture; serology, IFA[a] (IgM, ≥1:64; or IgG, ≥1:128); PCR[a] amplification of DNA from tissue specimens (especially for *R. japonica*)	Doxycycline (100 mg bid PO for 1–5 days) *or* Ciprofloxacin (750 mg bid PO for 5 days) *or* Chloramphenicol (500 mg qid PO for 7–10 days) *or* (in pregnancy) Josamycin[b] (3 g/d PO for 5 days)
Rickettsialpox	IFA: seroconversion to a titer of ≥1:64 or a single titer of ≥1:128; cross-adsorption to eliminate antibodies to shared antigens necessary for a specific diagnosis of the spotted fever rickettsial species	Doxycycline (100 mg bid PO for 1–5 days) *or* Ciprofloxacin (750 mg bid PO for 5 days) *or* Chloramphenicol (500 mg qid PO for 7–10 days) *or* (in pregnancy) Josamycin[b] (3 g/d PO for 5 days)
Endemic (murine) typhus	IFA: fourfold rise to a titer of ≥1:64 or a single titer of ≥1:128; immunohistology: skin biopsy; PCR amplification of *R. typhi* or *R. felis* DNA from blood; dot ELISA[a] and immunoperoxidase methods also available	Doxycycline (100 mg bid PO for 7–15 days) *or* Chloramphenicol (500 mg qid PO for 7–15 days)
Epidemic typhus	IFA: titer of ≥1:128; necessary to use clinical and epidemiologic data to distinguish among louse-borne epidemic typhus, flying-squirrel typhus, and Brill-Zinsser disease	Doxycycline (200 mg PO as a single dose or until patient is afebrile for 24 h)
Scrub typhus	IFA: titer of ≥1:200; PCR amplification of *O. tsutsugamushi* DNA from blood of febrile patients	Doxycycline (100 mg bid PO for 7–15 days)[c] *or* Chloramphenicol (500 mg qid PO for 7–15 days *or* (for children) Chloramphenicol (150 mg/kg per day for 5 days)

[a] IFA, indirect immunofluorescence assay; PCR, polymerase chain reaction; ELISA, enzyme-linked immunosorbent assay.
[b] Not approved by the U.S. Food and Drug Administration.
[c] Azithromycin is more effective than doxycycline in vitro against both doxycycline-susceptible and doxycycline-resistant strains of *O. tsutsugamushi*.

ted fever. Patients present with fever, cutaneous eruption, and an inoculation eschar. In Australia, two spotted fevers have been described. *Queensland tick typhus* is due to *R. australis* and is transmitted by *Ixodes holocyclus*. The skin rash in this disease is usually maculopapular but is sometimes vesicular, and there is an inoculation eschar. *Flinders Island spotted fever*, observed on an island close to Tasmania, is due to *R. honei*. In France, a case of *atypical Lyme disease* caused by *R. slovaca* and two cases of infection with *R. mongolotimonae* have been reported.

Diagnosis The diagnosis of these tick-borne spotted fevers is based on clinical and epidemiologic findings and is confirmed by cell-culture isolation of rickettsiae, by PCR of skin biopsies (a method not available in most laboratories), or by serology. The identification of specific species requires cross-adsorption (Table 177-2). In an endemic area, patients presenting with fever, rash, and/or a skin lesion consisting of a black necrotic area or a crust surrounded by erythema should be considered to have one of these rickettsial spotted fevers.

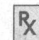 **TREATMENT** See Table 177-2.

RICKETTSIALPOX Rickettsialpox was first described in 1946 by a general practitioner in New York City and soon afterwards

was shown to be caused by a distinct species, *R. akari*. This organism was isolated from mice and their mites (*Liponyssoides sanguineus*), which maintain the organisms by transovarian transmission. *R. akari* shares lipopolysaccharide antigens with other members of the SFG.

Epidemiology More than 100 cases of rickettsialpox were diagnosed annually in the northeastern United States in the late 1940s and the 1950s, and outbreaks occurred in the Ukraine in the 1950s. However, few cases are diagnosed currently. Recently, a culture-confirmed case of rickettsialpox was documented in southern Europe. This case was initially misdiagnosed as Mediterranean spotted fever on the basis of the development of serum antibodies cross-reactive with *R. conorii*. Cases have also been reported in Arizona, Utah, and Ohio.

Clinical Manifestations A papule forms at the site of the mite bite. This lesion develops a central vesicle that becomes a 1- to 2.5-cm painless black crusted eschar surrounded by an erythematous halo. Enlargement of the lymph nodes draining the region of the eschar suggests initial lymphogenous spread. After a 10-day incubation period, during which the eschar and regional lymphadenopathy frequently go unnoticed, the onset of illness is marked by malaise, chills, fever, headache, and myalgia. A macular rash appears 2 to 6 days after onset and evolves sequentially into papules, vesicles, and crusts that heal without scarring. In some cases the rash remains macular or maculopapular. Some patients suffer nausea, vomiting, abdominal pain, cough, conjunctivitis, or photophobia. Untreated rickettsialpox is not fatal, with fever lasting 6 to 10 days.

Diagnosis and Treatment See Table 177-2.

FLEA- AND LOUSE-BORNE RICKETTSIAL DISEASES

ENDEMIC MURINE TYPHUS (FLEA-BORNE) Murine typhus was postulated to be a distinct disease, with rats as the reservoir and fleas as the vector, by Maxcy in 1926. Dyer isolated the etiologic agent, *R. typhi*, from rats and fleas in 1931. By the end of World War II, murine typhus was known to be a global disease. A novel typhus group *Rickettsia* has now been shown to be maintained vertically in cat fleas and to cause human infection. This flea-transmitted species, *R. felis*, reportedly contains antigens most closely resembling typhus group rickettsiae but genetically is an SFG organism. *R. felis* has been found in 4% of cat fleas and in 33% of opossums collected in the vicinity of human murine typhus–like cases in southern Texas.

Epidemiology *R. typhi* is maintained in mammalian host/flea cycles, with rats (*Rattus rattus* and *R. norvegicus*) and the Oriental rat flea (*Xenopsylla cheopis*) as the classic zoonotic niche. Fleas acquire *R. typhi* from rickettsemic rats and carry the organism throughout the rest of their lifespan. Nonimmune rats and humans are infected when rickettsia-laden flea feces are "scratched" into pruritic bite lesions; less frequently, the flea bite itself transmits the organisms. Yet another possible route of transmission is the inhalation of aerosolized flea feces. Infected rats appear healthy, although they are rickettsemic for approximately 2 weeks.

Currently, fewer than 100 cases of endemic typhus are reported annually in the United States. These cases occur mainly in southern Texas and southern California, where the classic rat-flea cycle is absent and an opossum–cat flea (*Ctenocephalides felis*) cycle is prominent. Although *X. cheopis* fleas are inefficient at the transovarian maintenance of *R. felis*, cat fleas are highly effective at vertical transmission of this organism, whose natural occurrence has been detected in fleas in California, Texas, and Oklahoma. Infected opossums and cat fleas as well as a case of human infection were reported from Corpus Christi, Texas, in the same environment where humans, opossums, and cat fleas are infected with *R. typhi*. Cases of endemic typhus occur year-round, mainly in warm (often coastal) areas. This infection has also been reported from Greece, Spain, and Indonesia. The peak prevalence in southern Texas is from April through June and elsewhere is during the warm months of summer and early fall. Patients seldom recall a flea bite or exposure to fleas, although exposure to animals such as cats, opossums, raccoons, skunks, and rats is reported by nearly 40% of those who are questioned.

Clinical Manifestations The incubation period of experimental murine typhus in volunteers averages 11 days, with a range of 8 to 16 days. Close observation during this period reveals prodromal symptoms of headache, myalgia, arthralgia, nausea, and malaise developing 1 to 3 days before the abrupt onset of chills and fever. Nearly all patients experience nausea and vomiting early in the illness.

The duration of untreated illness averages 12 days, with a range of 9 to 18 days. Rash is present in only 13% of patients at the time of presentation for medical care (usually about 4 days after onset of symptoms), appearing an average of 2 days later in half of the remaining patients and never appearing in the other half. The initial macular rash is often detected by careful inspection of the axilla or the inner surface of the arm. Subsequently, the rash becomes maculopapular, involving the trunk more often than the extremities; it is seldom petechial and rarely involves the face, palms, or soles. A rash is detected in only 20% of patients with dark brown or black skin.

Pulmonary involvement is frequently prominent in murine typhus; 35% of patients have a hacking, nonproductive cough, and 23% of patients who undergo chest radiography have pulmonary densities due to interstitial pneumonia, pulmonary edema, and pleural effusions. Bibasilar rales are the most common pulmonary sign. Less common clinical symptoms and signs include abdominal pain, confusion, stupor, seizures, ataxia, coma, and jaundice. Clinical laboratory studies frequently reveal anemia and leukopenia early in the course, leukocytosis late in the course, thrombocytopenia, hyponatremia, hypoalbuminemia, mildly increased serum levels of hepatic aminotransferases, and prerenal azotemia. Complications may include respiratory failure requiring intubation and mechanical ventilation, hematemesis, cerebral hemorrhage, and hemolysis (in patients with G6PD deficiency and some hemoglobinopathies). The illness is severe enough to necessitate the admission of 10% of hospitalized patients to an intensive care unit. Greater severity is generally associated with old age, underlying disease, and treatment with a sulfa drug; the case-fatality rate is 1%. In a study of children with murine typhus, 50% suffered only nocturnal fevers, feeling well enough for active daytime play.

Diagnosis and Treatment See Table 177-2.
EPIDEMIC TYPHUS (LOUSE-BORNE) Epidemic typhus due to infection with *R. prowazekii* is transmitted by the human body louse (*Pediculus humanus corporis*), which lives on clothes and is found in poor hygienic conditions (especially in jails, where the disease it causes is called *jail fever*) and usually in cold areas. Lice acquire *R. prowazekii* when they ingest a blood meal from a rickettsemic patient. The rickettsiae multiply in the midgut epithelial cells of the louse and spill over into the louse feces. The infected louse defecates during its blood meal, and the patient autoinoculates the organisms by scratching. The fact that the louse abandons dead hosts and patients with high fever (>40°C) improves its efficiency as a vector. Since the louse does not pass *R. prowazekii* to its offspring, the disease is usually spread from person to person by the louse-borne route. Lice die within 1 to 2 weeks after infection, turning red just prior to death—hence the name *red louse disease*. This epidemic form of typhus is related to poverty, cold weather, war, and disasters and is currently prevalent in mountainous areas of Africa, South America, and Asia. A large outbreak involving 100,000 people in refugee camps in Burundi occurred in 1997, a small focus was reported in Russia for the first time in 1998, and sporadic cases have been reported from Algeria and from Peru. The global reemergence of the disease is due to proliferation of body lice. In the United States, sporadic cases of epidemic typhus are transmitted by flying-squirrel fleas. Eastern flying-squirrel (*Glaucomys volans*) lice and fleas have been found to be infected with *R. prowazekii*. The flying-squirrel fleas occasionally bite humans.

Brill-Zinsser disease is a recrudescent, mild form of epidemic typhus occurring years after the acute disease, probably as a result of immunosuppression or old age. Nathan Brill first identified recrudescent typhus in New York in 1898. In 1933 Hans Zinsser noted that more than 90% of patients with recrudescent typhus had emigrated from typhus-endemic areas of Europe. Strains of *R. prowazekii* indistinguishable from classic strains were isolated from patients with recrudescent typhus. Furthermore, *R. prowazekii* was isolated from the lymph nodes of patients undergoing elective surgery who had had typhus years earlier. Thus the typhus rickettsiae can remain dormant for years and can reactivate with waning immunity.

Clinical Manifestations After an incubation period of 1 week, the onset of illness is abrupt, with prostration, severe headache, and rapidly rising fever of 38.8 to 40.0°C (102 to 104°F). Cough is frequently prominent, occurring in 70% of patients. Myalgias are usually severe. In the outbreak in Burundi, the disease was referred to as *sutama* ("crouching"), the myalgias being so severe that patients crouched in an attempt to alleviate the pain. A rash begins on the upper trunk, usually on the fifth day, and then becomes generalized, involving all of the body except the face, palms, and soles. Initially, this rash is macular; without treatment, it becomes maculopapular, petechial, and confluent. The rash is frequently absent or not detected on black skin in Africa, where 60% of patients have *spotless epidemic typhus*. Photophobia, with considerable conjunctival injection and eye pain, is frequent. The tongue may be dry, brown, and furred. Confusion and coma are common. Skin necrosis and gangrene of the digits as well as interstitial pneumonia have been noted in severe cases. Untreated disease is fatal in 7 to 40% of cases, with outcome depending primarily on the condition of the host. Patients with untreated infections develop renal insufficiency and multiorgan involvement in which neurologic manifestations are frequently prominent. Overall, 12% of patients with epidemic typhus have neurologic involvement. North American *R. prowazekii* infection transmitted by flying-squirrel ectoparasites is a milder illness; whether this milder disease is due to host factors (e.g., better health status) or organism factors (e.g., attenuated virulence) is unknown.

Prevention Prevention of epidemic typhus involves control of body lice. Clothes should be changed regularly, and insecticides should be used every 6 weeks to control the louse population.

Diagnosis and Treatment See Table 177-2. Epidemic typhus is sometimes misdiagnosed as typhoid fever in tropical countries.

SCRUB TYPHUS

The etiologic agent of scrub typhus is a small, obligately intracellular bacterium of the family Rickettsiaceae that differs substantially from other family members in its genetic makeup and in the composition of its cell wall (which, for example, lacks lipopolysaccharide and peptidoglycan). Consequently, this organism has been classified as a species in a separate genus, *Orientia tsutsugamushi*.

O. tsutsugamushi is maintained in nature by transovarian transmission in trombiculid mites, mainly of the genus *Leptotrombidium*. After hatching, infected larval mites (chiggers, the only stage that feeds on an animal host) inoculate organisms into the skin while feeding. Scrub typhus is found in environments that harbor the infected chiggers, particularly areas of heavy scrub vegetation—e.g., where the forest is regrowing after being cleared and along riverbanks. Infections occur during the wet season, when the mites lay their eggs. The disease is endemic in eastern and southern Asia, northern Australia, and islands of the western Pacific Ocean. Scrub typhus is also found in tropical areas of India, Sri Lanka, Bangladesh, Myanmar, Thailand, Malaysia, Laos, Vietnam, Kampuchea, China, Taiwan, the Philippines, Indonesia, Papua New Guinea, northern Australia, and islands of the South Pacific Ocean; in temperate areas of Japan, Korea, far-eastern Russia, Tadzhikistan, the mountains of northern India, Pakistan, and Nepal; and in nontropical areas of China, such as Tibet and Shangdong Province. Those infected include indigenous rural workers, residents of suburban areas, and westerners visiting endemic areas for professional or recreational purposes. Infections are more prevalent than the number of clinical diagnoses would suggest; in some areas more than 3% of the population is infected or reinfected each month. Immunity wanes over 1 to 3 years, and there is remarkable antigenic diversity.

Clinical Manifestations The illness varies in severity from mild and self-limiting to fatal. After an incubation period of 6 to 21 days (usually 8 to 10 days), the onset of disease is characterized by fever, headache, myalgia, cough, and gastrointestinal symptoms. Some patients develop no further signs or symptoms and recover spontaneously after a few days. The classic case description includes an eschar at the site of chigger feeding, regional lymphadenopathy, and a maculopapular rash—signs that are seldom observed in indigenous patients. Fewer than 50% of westerners develop an eschar, and fewer than 40% develop a rash (on day 4 to 6 of illness). Severe cases typically include prominent encephalitis and interstitial pneumonia as key features of vascular injury. Severe illness in persons with G6PD deficiency has been accompanied by hemolysis. The case-fatality rate for untreated classic cases is 7% but would probably be lower if all relatively mild cases (which are underdiagnosed) were included.

Diagnosis and Treatment See Table 177-2. One report has described cases of scrub typhus in Thailand that do not respond to treatment with doxycycline or chloramphenicol.

EHRLICHIOSES

Ehrlichiae are small, obligately intracellular bacteria with a gram-negative-type cell wall that grow in cytoplasmic vacuoles to form clusters called *morulae* (Fig. 177-1). Two distinct *Ehrlichia* species cause human infections that can be severe and frequent (Table 177-3). *E. chaffeensis*, the agent of human monocytotropic ehrlichiosis (HME), infects predominantly mononuclear phagocytic cells in tissues and blood monocytes. A member of the *E. phagocytophila* group that infects cells of myeloid lineage is the agent of human granulocytotropic ehrlichiosis (HGE). Both *E. chaffeensis* and *E. phagocytophila* are tick-borne but are transmitted by distinct vectors with little geographic overlap. *E. ewingii* is a newly recognized agent of human ehrlichiosis. Identified in four patients to date by means of a broad-range PCR assay, *E. ewingii* has previously been reported as a cause of granulocytotropic ehrlichiosis in dogs.

FIGURE 177-1 *Ehrlichia chaffeensis* microcolonies (morulae) within cytoplasmic vacuoles manifest as two morphologic forms: reticulate cells (r) and dense-core cells (d). Bar = 1 μm. *(Courtesy of Dr. Vsevolod L. Popov.)*

Ehrlichiae were discovered by veterinarians during the investigation of hemolytic anemia of cattle before 1910. Researchers thereafter discerned that "marginal points" within erythrocytes were infectious and named the agent *Anaplasma marginale*. Subsequently, several other species now known as ehrlichiae were detected as veterinary infectious agents, including *Cowdria ruminantium*, *E. canis*, *E. phagocytophila*, and *E. risticii*. In 1953, *E. sennetsu* was identified in humans with mononucleosis-like syndromes in Japan.

The current taxonomic positions are determined by nucleic acid sequences of conserved and unique genes among these species. By analysis of 16S ribosomal RNA sequences, the genus and related organisms can be divided into two major clades: the *E. canis* group (including *E. chaffeensis*) and the *E. phagocytophila* group (including *E. equi* and the agent of HGE). The *E. sennetsu* group is as distantly related to both of these clades as it is to the genus *Rickettsia* and is not tick-borne. Given the lack of transovarian transmission in ticks, the natural maintenance of the tick-borne ehrlichiae clearly depends in part upon transient or persistent infections in wild and feral mam-

Table 177-3 Comparison of Two Human Ehrlichioses: Human Monocytotropic Ehrlichiosis (HME) and Human Granulocytotropic Ehrlichiosis (HGE)

Variable	HME	HGE
Etiologic agent	*E. chaffeensis*	*E. phagocytophila* group
Tick vector(s)	*Amblyomma americanum*, *Dermacentor variabilis* (dog tick)	*Ixodes scapularis* (deer tick), *I. ricinus*, *I. pacificus*
Seasonality	April through September	Year-round (peak: May, June, and July
Major target cell	Monocyte	Granulocyte
Morulae seen	Rarely	Frequently
Antigen used in IFA test	*E. chaffeensis*	HGE strains
Diagnostic titer	Fourfold rise or a single titer of ≥1:128; cutoff for negative titer, 1:64	Fourfold rise; cutoff for negative titer, 1:80
Treatment of choice	Doxycycline	Doxycycline
Mortality	2–3%	<1%

NOTE: IFA, indirect immunofluorescence assay.

malian reservoirs. Thus, these bacteria are propagated by horizontal transmission that relies upon a tick-mammal-tick cycle; humans are inadvertently infected when they impinge upon the natural habitats occupied by the ticks and the reservoir hosts.

HUMAN MONOCYTOTROPIC EHRLICHIOSIS **Epidemiology** Infections caused by *E. chaffeensis* have been documented in more than 500 cases reported to the Centers for Disease Control and Prevention (CDC). However, since HME is not a reportable disease in most states, this figure is a gross underestimate. Most infections have been identified in the south-central, southeastern, and mid-Atlantic states, but cases have also been recognized in California, the Pacific northwest, New England, Europe, and Africa. The vector is the Lone Star tick (*Amblyomma americanum*), which in all its life stages feeds upon white-tailed deer, a major reservoir host. Dogs have been discovered to be subclinically infected and may also be an important reservoir. Tick bites and exposures are reported by patients, frequently in rural areas and especially in the months May through July. The median age of HME patients is 44 years, and 75% of the affected individuals are male; however, severe and fatal infections in children are also well recognized.

Clinical Manifestations *E. chaffeensis* is inoculated into the dermal blood pool created by the feeding tick and subsequently disseminates via the blood to tissues. After a median incubation period of 8 days, illness develops; only about one-third of individuals who seroconvert develop a consistent clinical illness. The classic clinical manifestations are not specific and include fever (97% of cases), headache (81%), myalgia (68%), and malaise (84%); less frequently observed are gastrointestinal involvement (nausea, vomiting, diarrhea; 25 to 68%), cough (25%), rash (36% overall, 6% at presentation), and confusion (20%). HME may be severe: 62% of patients with documented cases are hospitalized, and about 2% die. Severe complications include a toxic shock–like or septic shock–like syndrome, respiratory insufficiency and adult respiratory distress, meningoencephalitis, fulminant infection (in immunocompromised patients), severe opportunistic and nosocomial infections, and hemorrhage. Laboratory findings may be of value in the differential diagnosis; 60 to 74% of patients with HME have leukopenia (initially lymphopenia, later neutropenia), 72% have thrombocytopenia, and nearly 90% have elevations in serum levels of hepatic aminotransferases. With effective therapy, rebound lymphocytosis is common. In spite of abnormal blood counts, examinations reveal hypercellular bone marrow, and noncaseating granulomas may be present. Vasculitis is not a component of HME.

Diagnosis Because HME can be rapidly fatal, empirical antibiotic therapy should be instituted on the basis of a clinical diagnosis. This diagnosis may be suggested by fever in the setting of known tick exposure during the preceding 3 weeks, leukopenia and/or thrombocytopenia, and increased aminotransferase concentrations in serum. Morulae are rarely demonstrated in peripheral blood smears unless an intensive examination is performed; even then, an experienced microscopist is required. The active phase of HME may be diagnosed by PCR amplification of *E. chaffeensis* nucleic acids from EDTA-anticoagulated blood obtained before the start of doxycycline therapy. Retrospective serologic diagnosis requires a consistent clinical picture and detection of a fourfold increase in *E. chaffeensis* antibody titer (to ≥1:64) by indirect immunofluorescence in paired serum samples obtained approximately 30 days apart. It must be underscored that separate specific diagnostic tests for HME and HGE are necessary.

℞ **TREATMENT** Tetracycline is effective therapy for HME. Either tetracycline (250 to 500 mg given orally every 6 h) or doxycycline (100 mg given orally or intravenously twice daily) is associated with a lowered rate of hospitalization and a shortened duration of fever. The use of chloramphenicol is controversial, and *E. chaffeensis* is not susceptible to this drug in vitro. While a few reports document the persistence of *E. chaffeensis* in humans after the acute phase of illness, such persistence is very infrequent; most patients are cured after rel-

atively short courses of tetracycline therapy (continuing for 3 to 5 days after defervescence).

Prevention HME is prevented by the avoidance of ticks in endemic areas. The use of protective clothing and tick repellents, careful tick searches after exposures, and prompt removal of attached ticks markedly diminish risk.

HUMAN GRANULOCYTOTROPIC EHRLICHIOSIS **Epidemiology** As of 1995, approximately 150 cases of HGE had been documented in 11 states (mostly in the upper midwest and the northeast), with a distribution similar to that of Lyme disease. Most cases have been identified within the range of various *I. ricinus*–complex ticks, particularly *I. scapularis*. White-footed deer mice in the United States and red deer in Europe appear to play a role in maintaining HGE in nature. The incidence of HGE peaks in May, June, and July, but the disease may occur throughout the year in conjunction with human exposure to *Ixodes* ticks. HGE affects predominantly males (79%) and older persons (median age, 58 years).

Clinical Manifestations Because of high seroprevalence rates in endemic regions, it seems likely that only a minority of infected individuals develop clinical manifestations. The incubation period for HGE varies between 4 and 8 days, and the disease manifests as fever (94 to 100% of cases), myalgia (78 to 98%), headache (61 to 85%), and malaise (98%)—findings suggestive of an influenza-like illness. A minority of patients develop gastrointestinal involvement, including nausea, vomiting, or diarrhea (22 to 39%); rash (2 to 11%); cough (27%); and confusion (17%). Severe complications occur most often in the elderly, but even children may be severely affected. Respiratory insufficiency, with adult respiratory distress syndrome, a toxic shock–like syndrome, and life-threatening opportunistic infections, are the most worrisome complications. Meningoencephalitis has not yet been conclusively recognized with HGE. The case-fatality rate is probably <1%, but nearly 7% of ill patients may require intensive care. As in HME, laboratory findings are of great assistance; most patients develop leukopenia and/or thrombocytopenia with increased serum levels of hepatic aminotransferases. The pancytopenia observed in HGE presumably relates to sequestration or destruction of platelets and leukocytes, since the bone marrow is ordinarily normo- or hypercellular. Vasculitis is not a component of HGE. Unlike HME, HGE is not associated with granulomas. While clear evidence exists for co-infections with *Borrelia burgdorferi* and *Babesia microti*, which are transmitted by the same tick vector(s), there is little evidence of comorbidity or of a persistent or chronic phase for HGE.

Diagnosis HGE should be included in the differential diagnosis for patients who have been exposed to ticks and who develop an influenza-like illness during the season of *Ixodes* tick activity (May through December). The concurrent detection of thrombocytopenia, leukopenia, and/or elevations in serum aminotransferase activities further increases the likelihood of HGE. A substantial proportion of patients with HGE develop serologic reactions considered diagnostic of Lyme disease in the absence of clear clinical findings consistent with that diagnosis. Thus, HGE should be considered in the differential diagnosis of atypical severe presentations of Lyme disease. Although not highly sensitive, a thorough peripheral blood film examination for morulae in neutrophils may identify 20 to 75% of infections. PCR on EDTA-anticoagulated blood collected before initiation of tetracycline therapy from patients with active disease is a sensitive and specific method for early confirmation. Serodiagnosis is based mostly upon the retrospective demonstration of a fourfold increase in *E. phagocytophila* group antibody titer to a minimum of 1:80 in paired sera obtained approximately 1 month apart. IgM antibodies may be detected in many patients within the first 1.5 months after illness. Approximately 15 to 40% of infected persons have a detectable antibody titer at presentation, but, in regions where seroprevalence is high, a single acute-phase polyvalent titer may be misleading.

℞ **TREATMENT**   Doxycycline (100 mg given orally twice daily) is an effective therapeutic agent, while rifampin has been associated with clinical improvement in pregnant patients with HGE. In vitro studies suggest a role for trovafloxacin, but no prospective studies of any therapy for HGE have been conducted. Most treated patients defervesce within 24 to 48 h.

Prevention   Prevention of HGE requires tick avoidance. The Lyme disease vaccine offers no protection against HGE, and no other vaccine is available.

Q FEVER

Q fever results from infection with *C. burnetii*. This small gram-negative microorganism (0.2 μm by 0.7 μm) exists in two antigenic forms: phase I and phase II. When *C. burnetii* is passaged in cell cultures or embryonated eggs, its lipopolysaccharide undergoes truncation that results in an antigenic change called *phase variation*. The phase I form is extremely infectious and exists in humans and other animals. Passage in cell culture or embryonated eggs results in a shift to the phase II form, which is avirulent. The ability of *C. burnetii* to form spores allows the organism to survive in harsh environments. Indeed, it can survive for more than 40 months in skim milk at room temperature and is readily recovered from soil up to 1 month after contamination. Three different plasmids have been described in various isolates of *C. burnetii*. Q fever encompasses two broad clinical syndromes: acute and chronic infection. It is likely that the host's immune response (rather than characteristics of the infecting strain) determines whether or not chronic Q fever develops.

Epidemiology   Q fever is a zoonosis. The primary sources of human infection are infected cattle, sheep, and goats. However, infected cats, rabbits, and dogs have also been shown to transmit *C. burnetii* to humans. The extensive wildlife reservoir for *C. burnetii* includes mammals, birds, and ticks. In the infected female mammal, *C. burnetii* localizes to the uterus and the mammary glands. Infection is reactivated during pregnancy, and high concentrations of *C. burnetii* are found in the placenta. At parturition, *C. burnetii* is dispersed as an aerosol, and infection follows inhalation of aerosolized organisms by a susceptible host. Infected female animals shed the organism in milk for weeks to months after parturition. In rare instances, human-to-human transmission has followed delivery of an infant to an infected woman or autopsy on an infected individual. *C. burnetii* has been transmitted via blood transfusion. Those at risk for Q fever are abattoir workers, veterinarians, and other individuals who vocationally or avocationally come into contact with infected animals. Exposure to infected newborn animals or to infected products of conception poses the highest risk. Sexual transmission has been demonstrated experimentally in mice, as has transmission during artificial insemination in cattle. Whether *C. burnetii* is sexually transmitted among humans is not yet known. While the experimental evidence on this point is contradictory, the ingestion of contaminated milk in some areas is probably a major route of transmission to humans.

Infections due to *C. burnetii* occur in most countries. Indeed, the only areas known to be free of *C. burnetii* are New Zealand and Antarctica. The primary manifestation of acute Q fever differs from place to place: It is pneumonia in Nova Scotia (Canada) and granulomatous hepatitis in Marseille (France), while both of these manifestations are seen in the Basque country of Spain. These differences may reflect the route of infection; i.e., the ingestion of contaminated milk may result in hepatitis and the inhalation of contaminated aerosols in pneumonia.

Clinical Manifestations • *Acute Q fever*   The incubation period for acute Q fever ranges from 3 to 30 days. The clinical presentations include flulike syndromes, prolonged fever, pneumonia, hepatitis, pericarditis, myocarditis, meningoencephalitis, and infection during pregnancy. The symptoms of acute Q fever are nonspecific; common

among them are fever, extreme fatigue, and severe headache. Other symptoms include chills, sweats, nausea, vomiting, and diarrhea, which occur in 5 to 20% of patients. Cough develops in about half of patients with Q fever pneumonia. Neurologic manifestations of acute Q fever are uncommon; however, in one outbreak in the West Midlands, United Kingdom, 23% of 102 patients had neurologic signs and symptoms as the major manifestation. A nonspecific rash may be evident in 4 to 18% of patients. The white blood cell count is usually normal. Thrombocytopenia is detected in about 25% of patients, and reactive thrombocytosis [with platelet counts of up to 1 million/μL (1×10^{12}/L)] frequently develops during recovery. This thrombocytosis may account for cases of deep vein thrombophlebitis complicating acute Q fever in some series. Uncommon manifestations of acute Q fever include optic neuritis, extrapyramidal neurologic disease, Guillain-Barré syndrome, inappropriate secretion of antidiuretic hormone, epididymitis, orchitis, priapism, hemolytic anemia, mediastinal lymphadenopathy mimicking lymphoma, pancreatitis, erythema nodosum, and mesenteric panniculitis. Chest radiography may show an opacity that is indistinguishable from those seen in pneumonia of other etiologies. Multiple rounded opacities are common; in the appropriate epidemiologic setting, they are highly suggestive of Q fever pneumonia. However, right-sided endocarditis resulting in septic pulmonary emboli can produce the same radiographic appearance.

Chronic Q fever   Chronic Q fever, which is uncommon, almost always implies endocarditis. This infection usually occurs in patients with previous valvular heart disease, immunosuppression, or chronic renal insufficiency. Fever is usually absent or low grade. Patients may have nonspecific symptoms for up to 1 year before diagnosis. Valvular vegetations have been seen in only 12% of patients with transthoracic echocardiograms, but the rate of detection may be higher with the use of transesophageal echocardiography. A high index of suspicion is necessary for a correct diagnosis. The disease should be suspected in all patients with culture-negative endocarditis. In addition, all patients with valvular heart disease and an unexplained purpuric eruption, renal insufficiency, stroke, and/or progressive heart failure should be tested for *C. burnetii* infection. Patients with chronic Q fever have hepatomegaly and/or splenomegaly. These two findings, especially in combination with positive rheumatoid factor, high erythrocyte sedimentation rate, high C-reactive protein level, and/or increased γ-globulin concentrations (up to 60 to 70 g/L), suggest this diagnosis. Other manifestations of chronic Q fever include infection of vascular prostheses, aneurysms, and bone.

Diagnosis   *C. burnetii* can be isolated from buffy-coat blood samples or tissue specimens by a shell-vial technique; however, most laboratories are not permitted to attempt the isolation of *C. burnetii* since it is considered highly infectious. PCR can be used to amplify *C. burnetii* DNA from tissue or biopsy specimens. This technique can also be used on paraffin-embedded tissues. Serology, however, is the most commonly used diagnostic tool. Three techniques are available: complement fixation, indirect immunofluorescence, and enzyme-linked immunosorbent assay. Indirect immunofluorescence is sensitive and specific and is the method of choice. Rheumatoid factor should be adsorbed from the specimen before testing. An IgG titer of ≥1:800 to phase I antigen is suggestive of chronic Q fever. In almost all instances of chronic Q fever, the antibody titer to phase I antigen is much higher than that to phase II antigen. The reverse is true in acute Q fever. In addition, in acute Q fever, it is usually possible to demonstrate a fourfold rise in titer between acute- and convalescent-phase serum samples.

℞ **TREATMENT**   Treatment of acute Q fever with doxycycline (100 mg twice daily for 14 days) is usually successful. Quinolones are also effective. Treatment of chronic Q fever should include at least two antibiotics active against *C. burnetii*. The combination of rifampin and doxycycline has been used with success. For chronic infection, doxycycline should be given as 100 mg twice daily and rifampin as 300 mg once daily. The optimal duration of antibiotic therapy for chronic Q fever remains undetermined. We recommend a minimum of 3 years of treatment, with discontinuation only if the phase I IgA antibody titer is ≤1:50 and the IgG phase I titer is ≤1:200. Another therapeutic option under investigation is the combination of doxycycline (100 mg twice daily) with hydroxychloroquine (600 mg once daily). With this combination, therapy can be completed in 18 months. It is necessary to monitor hydroxychloroquine levels and to adjust the dosage to maintain a plasma concentration of 0.8 to 1.2 μg/mL. In vitro, the addition of 1 mg of hydroxychloroquine/mL renders doxycycline bactericidal for *C. burnetii.*

Prevention   A vaccine has been shown to be effective in preventing Q fever in abattoir workers in Australia.

BIBLIOGRAPHY

ARCHIBALD LK, SEXTON DJ: Long-term sequelae of Rocky Mountain spotted fever. Clin Infect Dis 20:1122, 1995

BAKKEN JS et al: Human granulocytic ehrlichiosis in the upper midwest United States. A new species emerging? JAMA 272:212, 1994

BULLER RS et al: *Ehrlichia ewingii,* a newly recognized agent of human ehrlichiosis. N Engl J Med 341:148, 1999

DALTON MJ et al: National surveillance for Rocky Mountain spotted fever, 1981–1982: Epidemiologic summary and evaluation of risk factors for fatal outcome. Am J Trop Med Hyg 52:405, 1995

DUMLER JS, BAKKEN JS: Human ehrlichioses. Newly recognized infections transmitted by ticks. Annu Rev Med 49:201, 1998

——— et al: Clinical and laboratory features of murine typhus in south Texas, 1980 through 1987. JAMA 266:1365, 1991

FOURNIER PE et al: Outbreak of *Rickettsia africae* infections in participants of an adventure race from South Africa. Clin Infect Dis 27:316, 1998

HELMICK CG et al: Rocky Mountain spotted fever: Clinical, laboratory, and epidemiological features of 262 cases. J Infect Dis 150:480, 1984

KASS EM et al: Rickettsial pox in a New York City hospital, 1980–1989. N Engl J Med 331:1612, 1994

RAOULT D et al: Outbreak of epidemic typhus associated with trench fever in Burundi. Lancet 352:353, 1998

——— et al: Treatment of Q fever endocarditis. Comparisons of 2 regimens containing doxycycline and ofloxacin or hydroxychloroquine. Arch Intern Med 159:167, 1999

RIKIHISA Y: The tribe *Ehrlichieae* and ehrlichial diseases. Clin Microbiol Rev 4:286, 1991

STRICKMAN D et al: In vitro effectiveness of azithromycin against doxycycline-resistant and -susceptible strains of *Rickettsia tsutsugamushi,* etiologic agent of scrub typhus. Antimicrob Agents Chemother 39:2406, 1995

178   William M. McCormack

MYCOPLASMA INFECTIONS

Mycoplasmas, the smallest free-living organisms known, are prokaryotes that are bounded only by a plasma membrane. Their lack of a cell wall is associated with cellular pleomorphism and resistance to cell wall–active antimicrobial agents, such as penicillins and cephalosporins. The organisms' small genome limits biosynthesis and explains the difficulties encountered with in vitro cultivation. Mycoplasmas typically colonize mucosal surfaces of the respiratory and urogenital tracts of many animal species. Sixteen species of mycoplasmas have been recovered from humans. Most are commensals. *Mycoplasma pneumoniae* causes upper and lower respiratory tract infections. *M. genitalium* and *Ureaplasma urealyticum* are established causes of urethritis and have been implicated in other genital conditions. *M. hominis* and *U. urealyticum* are part of the complex microbial flora of bacterial vaginosis.

MECHANISMS OF PATHOGENICITY

Adherence of mycoplasmas to the surface of the host cell is necessary for colonization and infection. Some pathogenic mycoplasmas are flask-shaped, with specialized tips that enhance adherence. *M. pneumoniae* adheres via a network of interactive adhesins and accessory proteins and produces hydrogen peroxide, which may cause injury to host cells. *M. hominis* metabolizes arginine, with the production of potentially cytotoxic amounts of ammonia. Ureaplasmas have been placed in a separate genus because of their unique urease activity; the metabolism of urea also produces ammonia. *M. pneumoniae* may evoke IgM autoantibodies that agglutinate human erythrocytes at 4°C. These cold agglutinins can cause anemia and other complications.

MYCOPLASMA PNEUMONIAE

EPIDEMIOLOGY   *M. pneumoniae* causes upper and lower respiratory tract symptoms in all age groups, with the highest attack rates in 5- to 20-year-olds. The infection is acquired by inhalation of aerosols. The incubation period is 2 to 3 weeks, considerably longer than that of most other respiratory infections. Although epidemics have taken place in closed populations, such as schools and military installations, most cases occur sporadically or in families. In families, cases typically occur serially, with 2- to 3-week intervals between cases. Infections in adults are often the result of contact with children.

Infection with *M. pneumoniae* is worldwide. Cases occur throughout the year, with epidemics every few years. Some studies have noted an increase in the number of cases during the autumn months in temperate climates. Although pneumonia is the classic presentation, nonpneumonic infection is considerably more common. In very young children, most infections result only in upper respiratory symptoms, whereas children >5 and adults may have bronchitis and pneumonia.

CLINICAL PRESENTATION   After a prolonged incubation period, fever and constitutional symptoms develop along with headache and cough, both of which can be prominent and distressing. Symptoms typically progress less rapidly than those of viral respiratory tract infections. In the minority (perhaps 5 to 10%) of infected individuals who develop tracheobronchitis or pneumonia, cough becomes more prominent. Sputum, if produced at all, is usually white and may be tinged with blood. The temperature seldom rises above 38.9 to 39.4°C (102 to 103°F). Shaking chills, myalgias, and gastrointestinal symptoms (e.g., nausea, vomiting, and diarrhea) are unusual. Chest muscle soreness may result from frequent and prolonged coughing, but true pleuritic pain is uncommon.

Pharyngeal injection is often noted. Cervical lymph node enlargement is unusual. Bullous myringitis is a unique but uncommon manifestation. As in other "atypical" pneumonias, findings on auscultation of the lung may be normal or nearly normal despite striking radiographic abnormalities. Pleural effusions develop in <20% of patients.

M. pneumoniae infection may be particularly severe in patients who have sickle cell disease and other hemoglobin S–related hemoglobinopathies. The functional asplenia seen in sickle cell disease may contribute to severe mycoplasmal disease as it does in pneumococcal infection. Severe respiratory distress and large pleural effusions may occur. Digital necrosis has been seen in patients with sickle cell disease who develop very high titers of cold agglutinins.

EXTRAPULMONARY MANIFESTATIONS   A broad array of extrapulmonary abnormalities have been associated with *M. pneumoniae* infection. Although these events are unusual, they complicate other respiratory diseases even more rarely and often provide the only clue that an otherwise unremarkable respiratory infection may be mycoplasmal.

Erythema multiforme (Stevens-Johnson syndrome; **see Plate IIE-67**) typically occurs in young male patients with *M. pneumoniae* infection. Other dermatologic manifestations, such as maculopapular and vesicular exanthems, erythema nodosum, and urticaria, have been reported, but none is as clearly linked to *M. pneumoniae* as is erythema multiforme.

Cardiac abnormalities reported in conjunction with *M. pneumoniae* infection include myocarditis and pericarditis, which may result in abnormalities of conduction. Of the wide variety of neurologic conditions associated with *M. pneumoniae*, most have been documented in case reports, where establishment of a cause-and-effect relationship is problematic. Central nervous system abnormalities that have been associated with *M. pneumoniae* include encephalitis, cerebellar ataxia, Guillain-Barré syndrome, transverse myelitis, and peripheral neuropathies. Arthralgias are not unusual in patients who have mycoplasmal pneumonia; mycoplasmal arthritis is rare except in patients who have hypogammaglobulinemia. Hematologic abnormalities associated with *M. pneumoniae* include hemolytic anemia and coagulopathies.

The pathogenesis of the extrapulmonary manifestations of *M. pneumoniae* infection is controversial. Occasional reports have described the identification of *M. pneumoniae* or its nucleic acids in involved tissues. The fact that most attempts at detection have been negative, however, suggests that these extrapulmonary complications have an immunologic basis. Mycoplasmas, including *M. pneumoniae*, can nonspecifically stimulate B lymphocytes. *M. pneumoniae*–infected individuals can develop autoantibodies, including those reactive with brain, heart, and muscle.

DIAGNOSIS Most infections with *M. pneumoniae* are not diagnosed, as they are indistinguishable from upper and lower respiratory tract infections caused by myriad other viral and bacterial pathogens. When the diagnosis is suspected, it is usually because illness is prolonged or extrapulmonary manifestations develop. The white blood cell count is generally somewhat elevated, with few immature cells. Gram's stain of sputum shows leukocytes without a predominance of any bacterial morphologic type. Since *M. pneumoniae* lacks a cell wall, it cannot be detected on Gram's stain. In patients who have pneumonia, the chest radiograph may show reticulonodular or interstitial infiltration, primarily in the lower lobes. As in other "atypical" pneumonias, radiographic abnormalities may be more prominent than would be predicted by auscultation of the chest.

M. pneumoniae can be grown on artificial media, but the process is exacting, requires special media, and takes upwards of 2 weeks. Thus, mycoplasmal cultures do not provide timely information to aid in patient management. The same, unfortunately, is true of serologic diagnosis. Specific antibodies can be detected by enzyme-linked immunoassays, indirect immunofluorescence, or complement fixation but do not develop early enough to guide decisions regarding treatment. As with most serologic tests, examination of paired acute- and convalescent-phase serum specimens is required for good sensitivity and specificity.

Cold agglutinins are nonspecific but develop within the first 7 to 10 days in more than half of patients with *M. pneumoniae* pneumonia and may be detectable when the patient presents to a health care provider. In a patient with a compatible clinical picture, a cold agglutinin titer of ≥1:32 supports the diagnosis of mycoplasmal pneumonia. Cold agglutinin determinations are readily available from diagnostic laboratories. The test can also be performed at the bedside by the addition of 1 mL of the patient's blood to a tube containing anticoagulant (e.g., a tube used to collect blood for determination of prothrombin activity). Before cooling, the nonaggregated red blood cells coat the sides of the inverted tube. The blood is cooled to 4°C when the tube is placed in an ice bath for 3 to 5 min or in a standard refrigerator. In a positive test, clumps of red blood cells can be observed when the tube is inverted. Rewarming of the sample to 37°C in an incubator or by exposure to body heat should reverse the agglutination. A positive "bedside" cold agglutinin test is equivalent to a laboratory titer of ≥1:64.

The lack of sensitive, specific, and timely diagnostic tests has prompted the development of a variety of antigen detection tests that do not involve serology or the cultivation of live organisms. Such tests include antigen capture, indirect enzyme immunoassays, DNA probing, and nucleic acid amplification. Since many viral and bacterial infections result in clinical presentations similar to that caused by *M. pneumoniae*, examination of specimens for single antigens is unlikely to be useful. Rather, tests that examine an individual specimen for

multiple antigens are needed. Multiplex nucleic acid amplification tests that examine a single throat swab or sputum sample for all of the most likely causative microorganisms are feasible with current technology. Prototype multiplex polymerase chain reaction (PCR) assays have already been developed. If such tests become available clinically, more precise etiologic diagnosis of upper and lower respiratory tract infections will be possible.

℞ TREATMENT Because most mycoplasmal infections are not specifically diagnosed, management is directed at one of two syndromes: upper respiratory tract infection or community-acquired pneumonia. Upper respiratory infections, whether caused by viruses or by *M. pneumoniae*, do not require antimicrobial treatment. Community-acquired pneumonia (Chap. 255) may be caused by bacteria such as *Streptococcus pneumoniae* and *Haemophilus influenzae* or by "atypical" agents such as *Chlamydia pneumoniae*, *Legionella pneumophila*, and *M. pneumoniae*. Recommended treatment regimens include a third-generation cephalosporin, such as intravenous ceftriaxone (1.0 g/d) or cefotaxime (1.0 g every 8 h), that is active against the conventional bacterial pathogens plus intravenous or oral erythromycin (500 mg four times a day) to cover atypical microorganisms. Newer agents that have antimicrobial activity against both conventional and atypical causes of community-acquired pneumonia may be prescribed as monotherapy. These drugs include oral clarithromycin (500 mg twice a day), intravenous or oral azithromycin (500 mg once daily), and intravenous or oral levofloxacin (500 mg once daily). Treatment of documented *M. pneumoniae* pneumonia is usually continued for 14 to 21 days.

Pneumonia due to *M. pneumoniae* is usually self-limited and is seldom life-threatening. Effective antimicrobial agents do shorten the duration of illness and, by reducing coughing, may conceivably render the patient less infectious. Although symptoms are alleviated by antimicrobial treatment, the organism usually is not eradicated. Cultures positive for *M. pneumoniae* may persist for months despite effective antimicrobial treatment. The beneficial effects, if any, of such treatment on extrapulmonary manifestations of *M. pneumoniae* infection are unknown.

GENITAL MYCOPLASMAS (See also Chap. 132)

EPIDEMIOLOGY *M. hominis* and *U. urealyticum* are the most prevalent genital mycoplasmas. Infants may become colonized with one or both of these organisms during passage through a colonized birth canal. Neonatal colonization tends not to persist. Only about 10% of prepubertal girls and even fewer prepubertal boys are colonized with ureaplasmas. After puberty, colonization occurs mainly as a result of sexual activity. Among adults, disadvantaged populations have higher colonization rates. Ureaplasmas can be cultured from the vaginas of ~80% of women cared for in public clinics and about half of women cared for by private obstetricians and gynecologists. Similarly, vaginal *M. hominis* is found in 50% of women attending public clinics and in ~20% of private patients. Men have somewhat lower rates of genital colonization than women. Nonetheless, both *U. urealyticum* and *M. hominis* are frequently detected in genital specimens from healthy, sexually experienced adults. Evaluation of the role of these organisms in human disease must take into account their high prevalence among healthy people.

M. fermentans colonizes both the respiratory and genital tracts in >20% of adults. There is no convincing evidence that *M. fermentans* causes human disease; although it had been implicated as a possible determinant of HIV-1 disease progression, more recent data do not support such a role. *M. genitalium* is a fastidious organism that is difficult to cultivate. PCR studies have identified the organism more successfully. Little is known about the epidemiology of *M. genitalium*.

ASSOCIATION WITH HUMAN DISEASE **Nongonococcal Urethritis** *Chlamydia trachomatis* is the organism most firmly implicated in the etiology of nongonococcal urethritis (NGU). There is no doubt that both *U. urealyticum* and *M. genitalium* also cause some cases of NGU. The ubiquity of ureaplasmas among men who do not have urethritis and the difficulty of identifying *M. genitalium* do not allow precise estimation of the proportion of cases of NGU caused by each of these mycoplasmas. *U. urealyticum* and *M. genitalium* do, however, appear to cause most of the nonchlamydial cases.

Epididymitis and Prostatitis Ureaplasmas may be an occasional cause of epididymitis. *M. hominis* has not been implicated in this disease. Neither organism has been convincingly associated with prostatitis.

Pelvic Inflammatory Disease (PID) (See also Chap. 133) *M. hominis* and *U. urealyticum* are both prominent components of the complex microbial flora of bacterial vaginosis. Since bacterial vaginosis is associated with PID, it is difficult to determine whether either organism plays an independent role in this condition. Although *M. genitalium* is not associated with bacterial vaginosis, preliminary studies have linked it to PID in women who are not infected with either *Neisseria gonorrhoeae* or *C. trachomatis*.

Disorders of Reproduction Ureaplasmas have been considered as causes of involuntary infertility in both men and women, but there is no convincing evidence for such an association. These organisms have been associated with chorioamnionitis and late abortion. Given the close association of ureaplasmas with bacterial vaginosis, a condition that is strongly associated with chorioamnionitis and late abortion, it is difficult to define an independent role for ureaplasmas in this condition. In infants of very low birthweight, ureaplasmas have been shown to cause pneumonia and chronic lung disease.

Extragenital Infections Sexually acquired reactive arthritis and Reiter's disease may be triggered by ureaplasmas, although *C. trachomatis* is the usual triggering agent. Patients who have hypogammaglobulinemia may develop chronic arthritis due to ureaplasmas and some other mycoplasmal species. *M. hominis* has been identified in patients with postthoracotomy sternal wound infection and in rare instances of prosthetic heart valve and prosthetic joint infection.

DIAGNOSIS There is seldom any reason to examine specimens from the lower genital tract (vagina, male urethra) for mycoplasmas. The ubiquity of the organisms among healthy individuals makes a positive result uninterpretable. The organisms should be sought only in specimens from normally sterile areas, such as joint fluid with evidence of inflammation and cultures negative for conventional microorganisms.

M. hominis can replicate in many routine blood culture media without changing the appearance of the media. *M. hominis* forms nonhemolytic pinpoint colonies on blood agar; organisms cannot be visualized in gram-stained smears of these colonies. Neither *U. urealyticum* nor *M. genitalium* will grow in ordinary microbiologic media.

Microbiologic diagnosis of genital mycoplasmal infection requires specially prepared media and is beyond the capability of all but reference and research laboratories. Nucleic acid amplification tests such as PCR have been developed and may become commercially available.

℞ **TREATMENT** Ureaplasmas, *M. genitalium*, and *M. hominis* are usually susceptible to tetracyclines (e.g., doxycycline). Tetracycline-resistant ureaplasmas can be treated with erythromycin, while tetracycline-resistant strains of *M. hominis* respond to treatment with clindamycin. As noted above, a specific microbiologic diagnosis of mycoplasmal infection is seldom made. Appropriate treatment provides antimicrobial coverage for the organisms that cause the particular syndrome. Accordingly, NGU is treated with doxycycline (100 mg orally twice a day for 7 days) or azithromycin (1.0 g as a single oral dose) to provide activity against *C. trachomatis*, *U. urealyticum*, and *M. genitalium*. Recommended regimens for the treatment of PID provide antimicrobial activity against gonococci, chlamydiae, and anaerobes as well as genital mycoplasmas.

BIBLIOGRAPHY

ALEXANDER ER et al: Pneumonia due to *Mycoplasma pneumoniae*. N Engl J Med 275: 131, 1966

BASEMAN JB, TULLY JG: Mycoplasmas: Sophisticated, reemerging, and burdened by their notoriety. Emerg Infect Dis 3:21, 1997

GRONDAHL B et al: Rapid identification of nine microorganisms causing acute respiratory tract infections by single-tube multiplex reverse transcription-PCR: Feasibility study. J Clin Microbiol 37:1, 1999

MURRAY HW et al: The protean manifestations of *Mycoplasma pneumoniae* in adults. Am J Med 58:229, 1975

TAYLOR-ROBINSON D, FURR PM: Update on sexually transmitted mycoplasmas. Lancet 351(Suppl 3):12, 1998

179   *Walter E. Stamm*

CHLAMYDIAL INFECTIONS

DFA	direct immunofluorescent antibody	MPC	mucopurulent cervicitis
ELISA	enzyme-linked immunosorbent assay	NGU	nongonococcal urethritis
		PCR	polymerase chain reaction
HSV	herpes simplex virus	PGU	postgonococcal urethritis
LGV	lymphogranuloma venereum	PID	pelvic inflammatory disease
micro-IF	microimmunofluorescence	STDs	sexually transmitted diseases

The genus *Chlamydia* contains three species that infect humans: *Chlamydia psittaci*, *C. trachomatis*, and *C. pneumoniae* (formerly the TWAR agent). *C. psittaci* is widely distributed in nature, producing genital, conjunctival, intestinal, or respiratory infections in many mammalian and avian species. Genital infections with *C. psittaci* have been well characterized in several species and cause abortion and infertility. Although mammalian strains of *C. psittaci* are not known to infect humans, avian strains occasionally do so, causing pneumonia and the systemic illness known as *psittacosis*.

C. pneumoniae is a fastidious chlamydial species that appears to be a common cause of upper respiratory tract infection and pneumonia, primarily in children and young adults, and is a cause of recurrent respiratory infections in older adults. Studies have also linked *C. pneumoniae* infection to atherosclerotic cardiovascular disease and perhaps to asthma and sarcoidosis. No animal reservoir has been identified for *C. pneumoniae*; it appears to be an exclusively human pathogen spread via the respiratory route through close personal contact. To date, all strains of *C. pneumoniae* studied have been serologically homologous.

C. trachomatis is also an exclusively human pathogen and was identified as the cause of trachoma in the 1940s. Since then, *C. trachomatis* has been recognized as a major cause of sexually transmitted and perinatal infection.

Chlamydiae are obligate intracellular bacteria that are classified in their own order (Chlamydiales). They possess both DNA and RNA, have a cell wall and ribosomes similar to those of gram-negative bacteria, and are inhibited by antibiotics such as tetracycline.

A unique feature of all chlamydiae is their complex reproductive cycle. Two forms of the microorganism—the extracellular elementary body and the intracellular reticulate body—participate in this cycle. The elementary body is adapted for extracellular survival and is the infective form transmitted from one person to another. Elementary bodies attach to susceptible target cells (usually columnar or transitional epithelial cells) and enter the cells inside a phagosome. Within 8 h of cell entry, the elementary bodies reorganize into reticulate bodies, which are adapted to intracellular survival and multiplication. They undergo binary fission, eventually producing numerous replicates contained within the intracellular membrane-bound "inclusion body," which occupies much of the infected host cell. Chlamydial inclusions resist lysosomal fusion until late in the developmental cycle. After 24 h, the reticulate bodies condense and form elementary bodies still contained within the inclusion. The inclusion then ruptures, releasing elementary bodies from the cell to initiate infection of adjacent cells or transmission to another person.

Studies with monoclonal antibodies to and nucleotide sequencing of the major outer-membrane protein have delineated at least 20 serotypes of *C. trachomatis*. According to the classification of Wang and Grayston, strains associated with trachoma have generally been those of the A, B, Ba, and C serovars, while serovars D through K have largely been associated with sexually transmitted and perinatally acquired infections. Serovars L_1, L_2, and L_3 produce lymphogranuloma venereum (LGV) and hemorrhagic proctocolitis. The LGV strains demonstrate unique biologic behavior in that they are more invasive than the other serovars, produce disease in lymphatic tissue, grow readily in cell culture systems and macrophages, and are fatal when inoculated intracerebrally into mice and monkeys. Non-LGV strains of *C. trachomatis* characteristically produce infections involving the superficial columnar epithelium of the eye, genitalia, and respiratory tract.

C. trachomatis has been reported as an infrequent cause of endocarditis, peritonitis, pleuritis, and possibly periappendicitis and may occasionally cause respiratory infections in older children and adults. Some immunosuppressed patients with pneumonia have had either serologic or cultural evidence of *C. trachomatis* infection, but more data are necessary to define a pathogenic role for *Chlamydia* in these patients.

SEXUALLY TRANSMITTED AND PERINATAL INFECTIONS DUE TO *C. TRACHOMATIS*

SPECTRUM OF *C. TRACHOMATIS* GENITAL INFECTIONS   Genital infections caused by *C. trachomatis* represent the most common bacterial sexually transmitted diseases (STDs) in the United States. An estimated 4 million cases occur each year. In adults, the clinical spectrum of sexually transmitted *C. trachomatis* infections parallels that of gonococcal infection. Both infections have been associated with urethritis, proctitis, and conjunctivitis in both sexes; with epididymitis in men; and with mucopurulent cervicitis (MPC), acute salpingitis, bartholinitis, and the Fitz-Hugh–Curtis syndrome (perihepatitis) in women. Moreover, both types of infection can be associated with septic arthritis. In general, however, chlamydial infections produce fewer symptoms and signs than corresponding gonococcal infections at the same anatomic site; in fact, chlamydial infections are often totally asymptomatic. Increasing evidence suggests that many chlamydial infections of the genital tract, especially in women, persist for months without producing symptoms. Simultaneous infection with *C. trachomatis* often occurs in women with cervical gonococcal infection and in heterosexual men with gonococcal urethritis.

EPIDEMIOLOGY   Infections due to *C. trachomatis* are now reportable in the United States, and national incidence data show steadily rising numbers of reported infections, undoubtedly reflecting both increased testing and increased reporting. Most testing has focused upon women to date, and thus the reported incidence is severalfold greater in women than in men; this difference likely represents a surveillance artifact.

The age of peak incidence of genital *C. trachomatis* infections, as of other sexually transmitted infections, is the late teens and early twenties. The prevalence of chlamydial urethral infection among young men is at least 3 to 5% for those seen in general medical settings or in urban high schools, >10% for asymptomatic soldiers undergoing routine physical examination, and 15 to 20% for heterosexual men seen in STD clinics. In areas where chlamydial control programs have been implemented, prevalence may be markedly reduced. In short, prevalence varies widely with the population group studied and with the geographic locale. The ratio of chlamydial to gonococcal urethritis is highest for heterosexual men and for those of high socioeconomic status and is lowest for homosexual men and indigent populations.

The prevalence of cervical infection among women is approximately 5% for asymptomatic college students and prenatal patients in the United States, >10% for women seen in family planning clinics, and >20% for women seen in STD clinics. As in men, prevalence varies substantially by geographic locale. However, substantial prevalences (~8%) of asymptomatic chlamydial infection were recently demonstrated in young female military recruits from all parts of the United States. In this country, the prevalence of *C. trachomatis* in the cervix of pregnant women is 5 to 10 times higher than that of *Neisseria gonorrhoeae*. The prevalence of genital infection with either agent is highest among individuals who are between the ages of 18 and 24, single, and non-Caucasian (e.g., black or hispanic). Recurrent chlamydial infections occur frequently in these same risk groups, often acquired from untreated sexual partners. Oral contraceptive pill use and the presence of cervical ectopy also confer an increased risk of chlamydial infection. The proportion of infections that are asymptomatic appears to be higher for *C. trachomatis* than for *N. gonorrhoeae*, and symptomatic *C. trachomatis* infections are clinically less severe. Mild or asymptomatic chlamydial infections of the fallopian tubes nonetheless cause ongoing tubal damage and infertility. Furthermore, because the total number of *C. trachomatis* infections exceeds the total number of *N. gonorrhoeae* infections in industrialized countries, the total morbidity caused by *C. trachomatis* genital infections in these countries equals or exceeds that caused by *N. gonorrhoeae*. The prevalence of *C. trachomatis* is higher than that of *N. gonorrhoeae* in industrialized countries, in part because measures such as treatment of sex partners and routine cultures for case detection in asymptomatic individuals have been applied much more effectively to the control of gonorrhea than to the control of *C. trachomatis* infection.

PATHOGENESIS   *C. trachomatis* preferentially infects the columnar epithelium of the eye and the respiratory and genital tracts. The infection induces an immune response but often persists for months or years in the absence of antimicrobial therapy. Serious sequelae often occur in association with repeated or persistent infections. The precise mechanism through which repeated infection elicits an inflammatory response that leads to tubal scarring and damage in the female upper genital tract is not yet clear. One antigen, the chlamydial 60-kDa heat-shock protein, may be involved in inducing the pathologic immune response or may elicit antibodies that cross-react with human heat-shock proteins. The recent sequencing of the chlamydial genome may soon offer further insights into the pathogenic mechanisms of *C. trachomatis*.

CLINICAL MANIFESTATIONS   Nongonococcal and Postgonococcal Urethritis   Nongonococcal urethritis (NGU) is a diagnosis of exclusion that is applied to men with symptoms and/or signs of urethritis who do not have gonorrhea. Postgonococcal urethritis (PGU) refers to nongonococcal urethritis developing in men 2 to 3 weeks after treatment of gonococcal urethritis with single doses of agents such as amoxicillin or cephalosporins that lack sufficient activity against chlamydiae. Since current treatment regimens for gonorrhea also include tetracycline, doxycycline, or azithromycin for possible concomitant chlamydial infection, both the incidence of PGU and the causative role of chlamydiae in this syndrome have declined. *C. trachomatis* causes 20 to 40% of cases of NGU in heterosexual men but is less commonly isolated from homosexual men with this syndrome. The cause of most of the remaining cases is uncertain; considerable evidence suggests that *Ureaplasma urealyticum* causes many cases of NGU, while *Trichomonas vaginalis* and herpes simplex virus (HSV) cause some cases.

NGU is diagnosed by documentation of a leukocytic urethral exudate and by exclusion of gonorrhea by Gram's staining or culture. *C. trachomatis* urethritis is generally less severe than gonococcal urethritis, although in an individual patient these two forms of urethritis cannot be reliably differentiated solely on clinical grounds. Symptoms include urethral discharge (often whitish and mucoid rather than frankly purulent), dysuria, and urethral itching. Physical examination may reveal meatal erythema and tenderness and a urethral exudate that is often demonstrable only by stripping of the urethra.

At least one-third of males with *C. trachomatis* urethral infection have no demonstrable signs or symptoms of urethritis. Use of nucleic acid amplification assays on first-void urine specimens to diagnose chlamydial infections in men has facilitated more broadly based testing for asymptomatic infection in males. As a result, asymptomatic chlamydial urethritis has been demonstrated in 5 to 10% of sexually active adolescent males screened in school-based clinics or community centers. Such patients generally have first-glass pyuria ($\geq$15 leukocytes per 400$\times$ microscopic field in the sediment of first-void urine), a positive leukocyte esterase test, or an increased number of leukocytes on Gram-stained smear prepared from a urogenital swab inserted 1 to 2 cm into the anterior urethra. For the enumeration of leukocytes, the smear is first scanned at low power to identify areas of the slide containing the highest concentration of leukocytes. These areas are then examined under oil immersion (1000$\times$). An average of four or more leukocytes in at least three of five 1000$\times$ (oil-immersion) fields is indicative of urethritis and correlates with the recovery of *C. trachomatis*. To differentiate between true urethritis and functional symptoms among symptomatic patients or to make a presumptive diagnosis of *C. trachomatis* infection in a "high-risk" but asymptomatic man (e.g., male patients in STD clinics, sex partners of women with nongonococcal salpingitis or MPC, fathers of children with inclusion conjunctivitis), the examination of an endourethral specimen for increased leukocytes is useful if specific diagnostic tests for chlamydiae are not available. Alternatively, noninvasive screening for urethritis can be accomplished by testing of a first-void urine sample for pyuria, either by microscopy or by the leukocyte esterase test. Urine can also be directly tested for chlamydiae or gonococci by DNA amplification methods, as described below.

Epididymitis   *C. trachomatis* is the foremost cause of epididymitis in sexually active heterosexual men under 35 years of age, accounting for about 70% of cases. *N. gonorrhoeae* causes most of the remaining cases, and some men have simultaneous infections with both pathogens, usually accompanied by asymptomatic urethritis as defined above. In homosexual men, sexually transmitted coliform infection acquired via rectal intercourse may cause epididymitis. Coliform bacteria and *Pseudomonas aeruginosa*, usually in association with preceding urologic instrumentation or surgery, are the most common causes of epididymitis in men over 35. Men with epididymitis typically present with unilateral scrotal pain, fever, and epididymal tenderness or swelling on examination. The illness may be mild enough to treat on an outpatient basis with oral antibiotics or severe enough to require hospitalization and parenteral therapy. Testicular torsion should be excluded promptly by radionuclide scan, Doppler flow study, or surgical exploration in a teenager or young adult who presents with acute unilateral testicular pain without urethritis. The possibility of testicular tumor or chronic infection (e.g., tuberculosis) should be excluded when a patient with unilateral intrascrotal pain and swelling does not respond to appropriate antimicrobial therapy.

Reiter's Syndrome   Reiter's syndrome consists of conjunctivitis, urethritis (or cervicitis in females), arthritis, and characteristic mucocutaneous lesions (Chap. 315). *C. trachomatis* has been recovered from the urethra of up to 70% of men with untreated nondiarrheal Reiter's syndrome and associated urethritis. In the absence of overt urethritis, it is important to exclude subclinical urethritis in the men in whom this diagnosis is suspected.

The pathogenesis of Reiter's syndrome remains obscure. However, since more than 80% of affected patients have the HLA-B27 phenotype and since other mucosal infections (with *Salmonella*, *Shigella*, or *Campylobacter*, for example) produce an identical syndrome, chlamydial infection is thought to initiate an aberrant and hyperactive immune response that produces inflammation at the involved target organs in these genetically predisposed individuals. Evidence of exaggerated cell-mediated and humoral immune responses to chlamydial antigens in Reiter's syndrome supports this hypothesis. The presumptive demonstration of chlamydial elementary bodies and chlamydial DNA in the joint fluid and synovial tissue of patients with Reiter's syndrome suggests that chlamydiae may actually spread from genital to joint tissues in these patients, perhaps in macrophages.

Proctitis   *C. trachomatis* strains of either the genital immunotypes D through K or the LGV immunotypes cause proctitis in homosexual men who practice receptive anorectal intercourse. In the United States, the vast majority of cases are due to immunotypes D through K and present either as asymptomatic infection or as mild proctitis not unlike gonococcal proctitis. These infections may develop in heterosexual women as well. Patients present with mild rectal pain, mucous discharge, tenesmus, and (occasionally) bleeding. Nearly all have neutrophils in their rectal Gram's stain. Anoscopy in these non-LGV cases of chlamydial proctitis reveals mild, patchy mucosal friability and mucopurulent discharge, and the disease process is limited to the distal rectum. LGV strains produce more severe ulcerative proctitis or proctocolitis that can be confused clinically with HSV proctitis (severe rectal pain, bleeding, discharge, and tenesmus) and that histologically resembles Crohn's disease in that giant cell formation and granulomas can be seen (Chap. 287). In the United States, these cases occur almost exclusively in homosexual men.

Mucopurulent Cervicitis   Although many women with *C. trachomatis* infection of the cervix have no symptoms or signs, a careful speculum examination reveals evidence of MPC in 30 to 50% of cases. As is discussed more fully in Chap. 133, MPC is associated with yellow mucopurulent discharge from the endocervical columnar epithelium and with $\geq$20 neutrophils per 1000$\times$ microscopic field within strands of cervical mucus on a thinly smeared, Gram-stained preparation of endocervical exudate. Other characteristic findings include edema of the zone of cervical ectopy and a propensity of the mucosa to bleed on minor trauma—e.g., when specimens are collected with a swab. A Pap smear shows increased numbers of neutrophils as well as a characteristic pattern of mononuclear inflammatory cells, including plasma cells, transformed lymphocytes, and histiocytes. Cervical biopsy shows a predominantly mononuclear cell infiltrate of the subepithelial stroma, often with follicular cervicitis.

Pelvic Inflammatory Disease (PID)   (See also Chap. 133)   *C. trachomatis* plays an important causative role in salpingitis. Infection with *C. trachomatis* has been demonstrated in laparoscopically verified salpingitis, the organism has been recovered from the fallopian tubes in the absence of other pathogens, and serologic evidence of recent *C. trachomatis* infection has been found in women with PID. In the United States, *C. trachomatis* has been identified in the fallopian tubes or endometrium of up to 50% of women with PID, and its role as an important etiologic agent in this syndrome is well accepted.

PID occurs via ascending intraluminal spread of *C. trachomatis* from the lower genital tract. MPC is thus followed by endometritis, endosalpingitis, and finally pelvic peritonitis. Evidence of MPC is usually found in women with laparoscopically verified salpingitis. Similarly, endometritis, demonstrated by endometrial biopsy showing plasma cell infiltration of the endometrial epithelium, is documented in most women with laparoscopically verified chlamydial (or gonococcal) salpingitis. Chlamydial endometritis can also occur in the absence of clinical evidence of salpingitis: approximately 40 to 50% of women with MPC have plasma cell endometritis. Histologic evidence of endometritis has been correlated with an "endometritis syndrome" consisting of vaginal bleeding, lower abdominal pain, and uterine tenderness in the absence of adnexal tenderness. It is not known what proportion of women who have chlamydial endometritis without adnexal tenderness also have salpingitis. However, chlamydial salpingitis produces milder symptoms than does gonococcal salpingitis and may be associated with less marked adnexal tenderness. Mild adnexal or uterine tenderness in sexually active women with cervicitis suggests PID.

Infertility associated with fallopian-tube scarring has been strongly linked to antecedent *C. trachomatis* infection in serologic studies. Since many infertile women with tubal scarring and antichlamydial antibody have no history of PID, it appears that subclinical tubal infection ("silent salpingitis") may produce scarring. Studies in animals and humans with salpingitis and tubal scarring suggest the continuing presence of persistent, slowly replicating chlamydial infection in tubal tissue. Ectopic pregnancy, which occurs in more than 70,000 women in the United States annually, is also thought to be related to *Chlamydia*-induced tubal scarring in many cases. While the pathogenesis of *Chlamydia*-induced tubal scarring remains poorly understood, antibodies to the chlamydial 60-kDa heat-shock protein have been correlated with tubal infertility, ectopic pregnancy, and Fitz-Hugh–Curtis syndrome (see below). Thus this antigen may initiate an immune-mediated process that ultimately damages the fallopian tube. Host genetic susceptibility, as defined by HLA type, may also play an important role.

Perihepatitis, or the Fitz-Hugh–Curtis syndrome, was originally described as a complication of gonococcal PID. However, cultural and/or serologic evidence of *C. trachomatis* infection is found in three-quarters of women with this syndrome. *C. trachomatis* has also been cultured from exudate on the hepatic capsule in laparoscopically verified cases. This syndrome should be suspected whenever a young, sexually active woman presents with an illness resembling cholecystitis (fever and right-upper-quadrant pain of subacute or acute onset). Symptoms and signs of salpingitis may be minimal. High titers of antibodies to *C. trachomatis* are generally present.

Urethral Syndrome in Women   In the absence of infection with uropathogens such as coliforms or *Staphylococcus saprophyticus*, *C. trachomatis* is the pathogen most commonly isolated from college women with dysuria, frequency, and pyuria (Chap. 280). *Chlamydia* can also be isolated from the urethra of women without symptoms of urethritis, and up to 25% of female STD clinic patients with chlamydial urogenital infection have cultures positive for *C. trachomatis* from the urethra only.

C. trachomatis Infection in Pregnancy   *C. trachomatis* in pregnancy has been associated in some studies (but not in others) with premature delivery and with postpartum endometritis. Whether these complications are in part attributable to *C. trachomatis* is not clear.

PERINATAL INFECTIONS: INCLUSION CONJUNCTIVITIS AND PNEUMONIA   **Epidemiology**   Studies in the United States have demonstrated that 5 to 25% of pregnant women have *C. trachomatis* infections of the cervix. In these studies, approximately one-half to two-thirds of children exposed during birth have acquired *C. trachomatis* infection. Roughly half of the infected infants (or 25% of the group exposed) have developed clinical evidence of inclusion conjunctivitis. In addition to infecting the eye, *C. trachomatis* has been isolated frequently and persistently from the nasopharynx, rectum, and vagina of such infants, occasionally for periods exceeding 1 year in the absence of treatment. Pneumonia develops in about 10% of children infected perinatally, and otitis media may in some cases result from perinatally acquired chlamydial infection.

Inclusion Conjunctivitis of the Newborn (Neonatal Chlamydial Conjunctivitis)   Neonatal chlamydial conjunctivitis has an acute onset 5 to 14 days after birth and often produces a profuse mucopurulent discharge. However, it is impossible to differentiate chlamydial conjunctivitis from other forms of neonatal conjunctivitis (such as that due to *N. gonorrhoeae*, *Haemophilus influenzae*, *Streptococcus pneumoniae*, or HSV) on clinical grounds; instead, laboratory diagnosis is required. Inclusions within epithelial cells are often detected in Giemsa-stained conjunctival smears, but these smears are considerably less sensitive than cultures, antigen detection tests, or nucleic acid hybridization tests for chlamydiae. Gram-stained smears may show gonococci or occasional small gram-negative coccobacilli in *Haemophilus* conjunctivitis, but smears should be accompanied by cultures for these agents.

Infant Pneumonia   *C. trachomatis* causes a distinctive pneumonia syndrome in infants. Recent epidemiologic studies have linked chlamydial pulmonary infection in infants with increased occurrence of subacute lung disease (bronchitis, asthma, wheezing) in later childhood.

LYMPHOGRANULOMA VENEREUM   **Definition**   LGV is a sexually transmitted infection caused by *C. trachomatis* strains of the L_1, L_2, and L_3 serovars. In the United States, most cases are caused by L_2 organisms. Acute LGV in heterosexual men is characterized by a transient primary genital lesion followed by multilocular suppurative regional lymphadenopathy. Women, homosexual men, and—in occasional instances—heterosexual men may develop hemorrhagic proctitis with regional lymphadenitis. Acute LGV is almost always associated with systemic symptoms such as fever and leukocytosis but is rarely associated with systemic complications such as meningoencephalitis. After a latent period of years, late complications include genital elephantiasis due to lymphatic involvement; strictures; and fistulas of the penis, urethra, and rectum.

Epidemiology   LGV is usually sexually transmitted, but occasional transmission by nonsexual personal contact, fomites, or laboratory accidents has been documented. Laboratory work involving the creation of aerosols of LGV organisms (e.g., sonication, homogenization) must be conducted only with appropriate measures for biologic containment.

The peak incidence of LGV corresponds to the age of greatest sexual activity: the second and third decades of life. The worldwide incidence of LGV is falling, but the disease is still endemic and a major cause of morbidity in Asia, Africa, South America, and parts of the Caribbean. In the Bahamas, an apparent outbreak of LGV has been described in association with a concurrent increase in heterosexual infection with HIV. However, only 186 cases were reported in the United States in 1995, for a rate of 0.1 case per 100,000 population.

The frequency of infection following exposure is believed to be much lower than that for gonorrhea and syphilis. Early manifestations are recognized far more often in men than in women, who usually present with late complications. In the United States, where the reported male-to-female ratio of cases is 3.4:1, most cases have involved homosexually active men and persons returning from abroad (travelers, sailors, and military personnel). The main reservoir of infection, although it has not been directly demonstrated, is presumed to be asymptomatically infected individuals.

Clinical Manifestations   In heterosexuals, a *primary genital lesion* develops from 3 days to 3 weeks after exposure. It is a small, painless vesicle or nonindurated ulcer or papule located on the penis in men and on the labia, posterior vagina, or fourchette in women. The primary lesion is noticed by fewer than one-third of men with LGV and only rarely by women. It heals in a few days without scarring and, even when noticed, is usually recognized as LGV only in retrospect. LGV strains of *C. trachomatis* have occasionally been recovered from genital ulcers and from the urethra of men and the endocervix of women who present with inguinal adenopathy; these areas may be the primary site of infection in some cases.

In women and homosexual men, *primary anal* or *rectal infection* develops after receptive anorectal intercourse. In women, rectal infection with LGV (or non-LGV) strains of *C. trachomatis* presumably can also arise by the contiguous spread of infected secretions along the perineum (as in rectal gonococcal infections in women) or perhaps by spread to the rectum via the pelvic lymphatics.

From the site of the primary urethral, genital, anal, or rectal infection, the organism spreads via the regional lymphatics. Penile, vulvar, or anal infection can lead to inguinal and femoral lymphadenitis. Rectal infection produces hypogastric and deep iliac lymphadenitis. Upper vaginal or cervical infection results in enlargement of the obturator and iliac nodes.

The most common presenting picture in heterosexual men is the *inguinal syndrome*, which is characterized by painful inguinal lymphadenopathy beginning 2 to 6 weeks after presumed exposure; in rare instances, the onset comes after a few months. The inguinal adenopathy is unilateral in two-thirds of cases, and palpable enlargement of the iliac and femoral nodes is often evident on the same side as the enlarged inguinal nodes. The nodes are initially discrete, but progressive periadenitis results in a matted mass of nodes that becomes fluctuant and suppurative. The overlying skin becomes fixed, inflamed, and thin and finally develops multiple draining fistulas. Extensive enlargement of chains of inguinal nodes above and below the inguinal ligament ("the sign of the groove") is not specific and, although not uncommon, is documented in only a minority of cases. On histologic examination, infected nodes are initially found to have characteristic small stellate abscesses surrounded by histiocytes. These abscesses coalesce to form large, necrotic, suppurative foci. Spontaneous healing usually takes place after several months; inguinal scars or granulomatous masses of various sizes persist for life. Massive pelvic lymphadenopathy in women or homosexual men may lead to exploratory laparotomy.

As cultures and serologic tests for *C. trachomatis* are being used more often, increasing numbers of cases of LGV proctitis are being recognized in homosexual men. Such patients present with anorectal pain and mucopurulent, bloody rectal discharge. Although these patients may complain of diarrhea, they are often referring not to diarrhea but rather to frequent, painful, unsuccessful attempts at defecation (tenesmus). Sigmoidoscopy reveals ulcerative proctitis or proctocolitis, with purulent exudate and mucosal bleeding. The histopathologic findings in the rectal mucosa include granulomas with giant cells, crypt abscesses, and extensive inflammation. These clinical, sigmoidoscopic, and histopathologic findings may closely resemble those of Crohn's disease of the rectum.

Constitutional symptoms are common during the stage of regional lymphadenopathy and, in cases of proctitis, may include fever, chills, headache, meningismus, anorexia, myalgias, and arthralgias. These findings in the presence of lymphadenopathy are sometimes mistakenly interpreted as representing malignant lymphoma. Other systemic complications are infrequent but include arthritis with sterile effusion, aseptic meningitis, meningoencephalitis, conjunctivitis, hepatitis, and erythema nodosum. Chlamydiae have been recovered from the cerebrospinal fluid and in one case were isolated from the blood of a patient with severe constitutional symptoms—a result indicating the dissemination of infection. Laboratory-acquired infections suspected of being due to the inhalation of aerosols have been associated with mediastinal lymphadenitis, pneumonitis, and pleural effusion.

Complications of untreated anorectal infection include perirectal abscess; fistula in ano; and rectovaginal, rectovesical, and ischiorectal fistulas. Secondary bacterial infection probably contributes to these complications. Rectal stricture is a late complication of anorectal infection and usually develops 2 to 6 cm from the anal orifice—i.e., at a site within reach on digital rectal examination. Proximal extension of the stricture for several centimeters may lead to a mistaken clinical and radiographic diagnosis of carcinoma.

A small percentage of cases of LGV in men present as chronic progressive infiltrative, ulcerative, or fistular lesions of the penis, urethra, or scrotum. Associated lymphatic obstruction may produce elephantiasis. When urethral stricture occurs, it usually involves the posterior urethra and causes incontinence or difficulty with urination.

APPROACH TO THE DIAGNOSIS AND TREATMENT OF *C. TRACHOMATIS* GENITAL INFECTIONS

Four types of laboratory procedure are available to confirm *C. trachomatis* infection: direct microscopic examination of tissue scrapings for typical intracytoplasmic inclusions or elementary bodies; isolation of the organism in cell culture; detection of chlamydial antigens or nucleic acid by immunologic or hybridization methods; and detection of antibody in serum or in local secretions.

Except in conjunctivitis, direct microscopic examination of Giemsa-stained cell scrapings for typical inclusions has an unacceptably low degree of sensitivity, and false-positive interpretations by inexperienced observers are common. Even for conjunctivitis, this approach has been replaced by direct fluorescent antibody staining of conjunctival smears to identify chlamydial elementary bodies with specific monoclonal antibodies (see below).

Cell culture techniques for isolation of *C. trachomatis* are available in most large medical centers but not in other clinical settings. In addition to limited availability, other disadvantages of cell culture include its low and variable level of sensitivity (60 to 80%), its requirement for rigorous transport conditions, and its high cost and technically demanding nature. Therefore, nonculture alternatives involving antigen detection or nucleic acid hybridization have been developed. In the direct immunofluorescent antibody (DFA) slide test, potentially infected genital or ocular secretions are smeared onto a slide, fixed, and stained with fluorescein-conjugated monoclonal antibody specific for chlamydial antigens. The observation of fluorescing elementary bodies confirms the diagnosis. Compared with culture, this test is 70 to 85% sensitive, and it is quite specific when used for confirmation of urethral, cervical, or ocular infection in high-risk patients with suspected *C. trachomatis* infection. The sensitivity and specificity of the test depend directly upon the skill of the microscopist. The apparently lower sensitivity of the test in low-risk populations, along with its relatively labor-intensive nature, limits its value as a screening tool.

Enzyme-linked immunosorbent assay (ELISA) techniques for the detection of chlamydial antigens provide another alternative to culture. The reported sensitivity and specificity of these tests for genital infections (as compared with culture) have been 60 to 80% and 97 to 99%, respectively, in high-risk populations. Sensitivities have generally been higher in cervical infection and lower in urethritis among males. Like the DFA slide test, the ELISA is less sensitive and less specific in low-prevalence populations and largely asymptomatic patients. ELISAs are better suited to screening than is DFA because large numbers of specimens can easily be processed.

Assays with nucleic acid probes have also been developed for chlamydial diagnosis. One such test uses DNA-RNA hybridization and appears to be approximately equal to the best ELISAs in terms of sensitivity and specificity. Nucleic acid probes have also been developed for use in amplification assays such as ligase chain reaction and polymerase chain reaction (PCR). These tests are now the most sensitive chlamydial diagnostic methods available, being the first nonculture assays actually to surpass culture itself in sensitivity. In addition, the ability of these tests to detect chlamydial genes in urine with a high degree of sensitivity and specificity allows their use with urine specimens rather than with conventional urethral and cervical swabs for the first time. The use of urine specimens is particularly appealing for public-health chlamydial screening programs because of the ease of sample collection, even in community-based settings.

Serologic tests are of limited usefulness in the diagnosis of chlamydial oculogenital infections. The complement fixation test with heat-stable, genus-specific antigen has been used with some success to diagnose LGV but is insensitive in infections due to non-LGV strains of *C. trachomatis*. The microimmunofluorescence (micro-IF) test with *C. trachomatis* antigens is more sensitive but is generally available only in research laboratories. The test measures antibodies by serovar specificity and by immunoglobulin class (IgM, IgG, IgA, secretory IgA) in both serum and local secretions. Serologic diagnosis by the micro-IF test may be useful in infant pneumonia (in which high-titer IgM antibody and/or fourfold rises in titer are often demonstrated), in chlamydial salpingitis (especially Fitz-Hugh–Curtis syndrome), and in LGV. In all of these more invasive syndromes, high antibody levels are present.

Table 179-1 summarizes the diagnostic tests of choice for patients with suspected *C. trachomatis* infection. With few exceptions, the most suitable method for diagnosis is demonstration of the agent by either cell culture or one of the newer nonculture techniques. Selection of the most appropriate of these tests often depends upon local availability and expertise. However, it is clear that, in most settings and for most purposes, sensitivity and specificity will be greatest with nucleic acid amplification techniques. For patients to whom medicolegal considerations may apply (victims of sexual or child abuse), cultures or nucleic acid amplification methods should always be used. Since *C. trachomatis* is an intracellular pathogen, adequate specimens for chlamydial diagnostic testing must include epithelial cells. Cultures or

Table 179-1 Diagnostic Tests for Sexually Transmitted and Perinatal *Chlamydia trachomatis* Infection

Infection	Suggestive Signs/Symptoms	Presumptive Diagnosis[a]	Confirmatory Test of Choice
MEN			
NGU, PGU	Discharge, dysuria	Gram's stain with >4 neutrophils per oil-immersion field; no gonococci	Urethral culture or nonculture test for *C. trachomatis*; urine PCR or LCR for *C. trachomatis*
Epididymitis	Unilateral intrascrotal swelling, pain, tenderness; fever; NGU	Gram's stain with >4 neutrophils per oil-immersion field; no gonococci; urinalysis with pyuria	Urethral culture or nonculture test for *C. trachomatis*; urine PCR or LCR for *C. trachomatis*
WOMEN			
Cervicitis	Mucopurulent cervical discharge, bleeding and edema of the zone of cervical ectopy	Cervical Gram's stain with ≥20 neutrophils per oil-immersion field in cervical mucus	Cervical culture or nonculture test for *C. trachomatis*; urine PCR or LCR for *C. trachomatis*
Salpingitis	Lower abdominal pain, cervical motion tenderness, adnexal tenderness or masses	*C. trachomatis* always potentially present in salpingitis	Cervical culture or nonculture test for *C. trachomatis*; urine PCR or LCR for *C. trachomatis*
Urethritis	Dysuria and frequency without urgency or hematuria	MPC; sterile pyuria; negative routine urine culture	Urethral and cervical cultures or nonculture test for *C. trachomatis*; urine PCR or LCR for *C. trachomatis*
ADULTS OF EITHER SEX			
Proctitis	Rectal pain, discharge, tenesmus, bleeding; history of receptive anorectal intercourse	Negative gonococcal culture and Gram's stain; at least 1 neutrophil per oil-immersion field in rectal Gram's stain	Rectal culture or direct immunofluorescence test for *C. trachomatis*
Reiter's syndrome	NGU, arthritis, conjunctivitis, typical skin lesions	Gram's stain with >4 neutrophils per oil-immersion field; lack of gonococci indicative of NGU	Urethral culture or nonculture test for *C. trachomatis*
LGV	Regional adenopathy, primary lesion, proctitis, systemic symptoms	None	Isolation of LGV strain from node or rectum, occasionally from urethra or cervix; LGV CF titer, ≥1:64; micro-IF titer, ≥1:512
NEONATES			
Conjunctivitis	Purulent conjunctival discharge 6 to 18 days postdelivery	Negative culture and Gram's stain for gonococci, *Haemophilus* spp., pneumococci, staphylococci	Conjunctival culture or nonculture test for *C. trachomatis*; Giemsa-stained scraping of conjunctival material capable of providing more rapid diagnosis but less sensitive
Infant pneumonia	Afebrile, staccato cough, diffuse rales, bilateral hyperinflation, interstitial infiltrates	None	Chlamydial culture of sputum, pharynx, eye, rectum; micro-IF antibody to *C. trachomatis*—fourfold change in IgG or IgM antibody titer

[a] A presumptive diagnosis of chlamydial infection is often made in the syndromes listed when gonococci are not found. A positive test for *Neisseria gonorrhoeae* does not exclude the involvement of *C. trachomatis*, which often is present in patients with gonorrhea.

NOTE: CF, complement-fixing; LCR, ligase chain reaction; LGV, lymphogranuloma venereum; micro-IF, microimmunofluorescence; MPC, mucopurulent cervicitis; NGU, nongonococcal urethritis; PCR, polymerase chain reaction; PGU, postgonococcal urethritis.

nonculture tests of pus are less often positive. In urethritis, a thin-shafted urogenital swab should be inserted at least 2 cm into the urethra to obtain an appropriate specimen. Although cultures of urine for chlamydiae are less sensitive than urethral cultures, studies suggest that nucleic acid amplification testing of a first-void urine specimen from men is a more sensitive and less painful diagnostic alternative to the more invasive urethral swab–based tests, culture, or antigen detection tests. The first 30 mL of voided urine should be collected for testing. When a cervical sample is collected, the external os should first be cleaned of debris and purulent material; a plastic-shafted swab should then be inserted into the cervix, rotated slowly several times, and withdrawn. For the diagnosis of urogenital (cervical or urethral) infections in women, testing of a first-void urine specimen by nucleic acid amplification methods is at least as sensitive as testing of a cervical swab. When conjunctival specimens are sought, the epithelium should be swabbed to remove cells rather than just purulent material. All specimens for chlamydial culture should be placed immediately into transport medium and then either refrigerated (if they will reach the laboratory within 12 to 18 h) or frozen at −70°C (if longer storage is anticipated). A major advantage of the nonculture diagnostic techniques is their less rigid transport requirements; neither refrigeration nor rapid transport is needed.

From a public health viewpoint, the most effective use of chlamydial diagnostic testing has not been unequivocally established and varies with the clinical population, local resources, and laboratory expertise. Since chlamydial diagnostic testing has become more widely available and is now more sensitive and specific than in the past, its use for specific diagnosis in patients with suspected chlamydial syndromes (such as MPC, NGU, and PID) and their partners should be promoted. High priority should be given to the screening of asymptomatic high-risk women who would not otherwise receive treatment for presumptive chlamydial infection, especially those seen in high-risk settings (e.g., STD clinics or abortion clinics) and those with a high-risk profile (e.g., sexually active and ≤21 years of age, new sex partner within the preceding 2 months, or more than one current sex partner). Similar screening programs should be used to detect and treat asymptomatic urethritis in high-risk adolescent males. Where implemented, screening programs of this type have been associated with reductions in the prevalence of chlamydial infection and of its complications, such as PID.

ANTIMICROBIAL SUSCEPTIBILITY In laboratory tests that evaluate the growth of chlamydiae in cell cultures, the tetracyclines, erythromycin, rifampin, certain fluoroquinolones (especially ofloxacin), and the macrolide azithromycin are all highly active against these organisms. Sulfonamides and clindamycin are also active against *C. trachomatis*, but to a lesser degree. Penicillin and ampicillin suppress chlamydial multiplication but do not eradicate the organism in vitro. The cephalosporins appear to be relatively ineffective against *C. trachomatis*. Streptomycin, gentamicin, neomycin, kanamycin, vancomycin, ristocetin, spectinomycin, and nystatin are not effective at concentrations inhibitory for most bacteria and fungi. There does not appear to be much strain-to-strain variation in susceptibility to antibiotics, and no clinically significant antimicrobial resistance in chlamydiae has been described. Thus antimicrobial susceptibility testing is not needed in the routine management of patients with chlamydial infection, even recurrent infection.

℞ TREATMENT Until the introduction of azithromycin, chlamydial infections could not be eradicated by single-dose or short-term antimicrobial regimens. In most uncomplicated infections in adults, 7 days of treatment with doxycycline or tetracycline have to be given for genital infections, but a 2-week course of therapy is recommended for complicated chlamydial infections (e.g., PID, epididymitis) and at least a 3-week course for LGV. Failure of treatment of genital infections with a tetracycline usually indicates poor compliance or reinfection rather than the involvement of a drug-resistant strain.

Therapy for *C. trachomatis* urethritis is more efficacious than therapy for nonchlamydial NGU. *C. trachomatis* is eradicated from the urethra in nearly all cases by treatment with tetracycline hydrochloride (500 mg qid for 7 days) or doxycycline (100 mg by mouth bid for 7 days).

Eradication of *C. trachomatis* from the cervix by tetracycline, doxycycline, and erythromycin, with doses and durations similar to those specified above for urethritis, has been demonstrated. Erythromycin base (500 mg qid for 10 to 14 days) is the regimen of choice for pregnant women with *C. trachomatis* infection. Amoxicillin (500 mg tid for 10 days) has also been used successfully in pregnant women. Tetracycline hydrochloride (500 mg qid) or doxycycline (100 mg bid) for 14 days produces clinical and microbiologic cure of epididymitis and PID associated with *C. trachomatis* infection, but in this situation a tetracycline should always be used together with a drug that is highly effective against gonorrhea.

Azithromycin is highly active against *C. trachomatis*, exhibits prolonged bioavailability, is concentrated intracellularly, and has offered the prospect of single-dose therapy for chlamydial infection for the first time. In comparative trials, a 1-g single dose of azithromycin has been as effective as 7 days of doxycycline for uncomplicated chlamydial infection. Azithromycin causes fewer adverse gastrointestinal reactions than do older macrolides such as erythromycin. The single-dose regimen of azithromycin has great appeal for the treatment of patients with uncomplicated chlamydial infection (especially those without symptoms and those with a likelihood of poor compliance) and of sexual partners of infected patients. These advantages must be weighed against the considerably greater cost of azithromycin than of doxycycline. Whenever possible, the single 1-g dose should be given as directly observed therapy. Although not approved by the U.S. Food and Drug Administration, the 1-g single-dose regimen of azithromycin appears to be safe and effective in the treatment of pregnant women.

Of the newer fluoroquinolones, ofloxacin (300 mg by mouth bid for 7 days) has been shown to be as effective as doxycycline for the treatment of chlamydial infection and appears to be safe and well tolerated. It cannot be used in pregnancy.

Treatment of Sex Partners The continued high prevalence of chlamydial infections in most parts of the United States is due primarily to the failure to diagnose—and therefore treat—patients with symptomatic or asymptomatic infection and their sex partners. *C. trachomatis* urethral or cervical infection has been well documented in a high proportion of the sex partners of patients with NGU, epididymitis, Reiter's syndrome, salpingitis, or endocervicitis. If possible, confirmatory laboratory tests for *Chlamydia* should be undertaken in these individuals, but even those without evidence of clinical disease who have recently been exposed to proven or possible chlamydial infection (e.g., NGU) should be offered therapy.

Treatment of Neonates and Infants In neonates with conjunctivitis or infants with pneumonia, erythromycin ethylsuccinate or estolate can be given orally in a dose of 50 mg/kg per day, preferably in four divided doses, for 2 weeks. Careful attention must be given to compliance with therapy—a frequent problem. Relapses of eye infection are common following treatment with topical erythromycin or tetracycline ophthalmic ointment and may also occur after oral erythromycin therapy. Thus follow-up cultures should be performed after treatment. Both parents should be examined for *C. trachomatis* infection and, if diagnostic testing is not readily available, should be treated with doxycycline or azithromycin.

PREVENTION Efforts to develop a vaccine for chlamydial infection have not yet been successful. Early diagnosis and treatment shorten the duration of infectiousness of the carrier and therefore constitute primary prevention of chlamydial infection. By the early 1990s, one of the 10 regions of the United States (Region X, the Pacific Northwest) had formally undertaken a chlamydial control program involving widespread screening of women attending family planning clinics. Approximately 500,000 tests per year were conducted at 150 such clinics throughout the region in women meeting the criteria for high risk. Within 5 years, the prevalence of chlamydial infection had been reduced by >30% in this population. While other regions of the United States have now initiated similar programs, many family planning and STD clinics still do not offer chlamydial testing. The availability of highly sensitive and specific diagnostic tests that can be done with urine specimens and of single-dose therapy makes it feasible to mount an effective chlamydial control program nationwide, with screening of high-risk persons both in traditional health care settings and in novel community- and school-based settings.

TRACHOMA AND ADULT INCLUSION CONJUNCTIVITIS

DEFINITION Trachoma is a chronic conjunctivitis associated with infection by *C. trachomatis* serovar A, B, Ba, or C. It has been responsible for an estimated 20 million cases of blindness throughout the world and remains an important cause of preventable blindness. Inclusion conjunctivitis is an acute ocular infection caused by sexually transmitted *C. trachomatis* strains (usually serovars D through K) in adults exposed to infected genital secretions and in their newborn offspring.

EPIDEMIOLOGY Epidemiologically, two types of eye disease are caused by *C. trachomatis*. In trachoma-endemic areas where the classic eye disease is seen, transmission is from eye to eye via hands, flies, towels, and other fomites and usually involves serovar A, B, Ba, or C. In nonendemic areas, organisms of serovars D through K can be transmitted from the genital tract to the eye, usually causing only the inclusion conjunctivitis syndrome, occasionally with keratitis. Rarely, the eye disease acquired in this way progresses, with the development of pannus and scars similar to those seen in endemic trachoma. These cases may be referred to as paratrachoma to differentiate them epidemiologically from eye-to-eye-transmitted endemic trachoma.

The worldwide incidence and severity of trachoma have decreased dramatically during the past 35 years, mainly as a result of improving hygienic and economic conditions. Endemic trachoma is still the major cause of preventable blindness in northern Africa, sub-Saharan Africa, the Middle East, and parts of Asia. The endemic disease is transmitted primarily through close personal contact, particularly among young children in rural communities with limited water supplies. In endemic areas, trachoma is associated with repeated exposure and reinfection, but the infection can also become chronic and persistent. In the United States a mild form of endemic trachoma still occurs in Mexican Americans as well as in immigrants from areas where trachoma is endemic. Acute relapse of old trachoma occasionally follows treatment with cortisone eye ointment or develops in very old persons who were exposed in their youth.

CLINICAL MANIFESTATIONS Both endemic trachoma and adult inclusion conjunctivitis present initially as a conjunctivitis characterized by small lymphoid follicles in the conjunctiva. In regions with hyperendemic classic blinding trachoma, the disease usually starts insidiously before the age of 2 years. Reinfection is common and probably contributes to the pathogenesis of trachoma. Studies using PCR techniques indicate that chlamydial DNA is often present in the ocular secretions of patients with trachoma, even in the absence of positive cultures. Thus persistent infection may be more common than was previously thought.

The cornea becomes involved, with inflammatory leukocytic infiltrations and superficial vascularization (pannus formation). As the inflammation continues, conjunctival scarring eventually distorts the eyelids, causing them to turn inward so that the inturned lashes constantly abrade the eyeball (trichiasis and entropion); eventually the corneal epithelium is abraded and may ulcerate, with subsequent corneal scarring and blindness. Destruction of the conjunctival goblet cells, lacrimal ducts, and lacrimal gland may produce a "dry-eye" syndrome, with resultant corneal opacity due to drying (xerosis) or secondary bacterial corneal ulcers.

Communities with blinding trachoma often experience seasonal epidemics of conjunctivitis due to *H. influenzae* that contribute to the intensity of the inflammatory process. In such areas the active infectious process usually resolves spontaneously in affected persons between 10 and 15 years of age, but the conjunctival scars continue to shrink, producing trichiasis and entropion and subsequent corneal scarring in adults. In areas with milder and less prevalent disease, the process may be much slower, with active disease continuing into adulthood; blindness is rare in these cases.

Eye infection with genital *C. trachomatis* strains in sexually active young adults presents as the acute onset of unilateral follicular conjunctivitis and preauricular lymphadenopathy similar to that seen in acute adenovirus or herpesvirus conjunctivitis. If untreated, the disease may persist for 6 weeks to 2 years. It is frequently associated with corneal inflammation in the form of discrete opacities ("infiltrates"), punctate epithelial erosions, and minor degrees of superficial corneal vascularization. Very rarely, conjunctival scarring and eyelid distortion occur, particularly in patients treated for many months with topical glucocorticoids. Recurrent eye infections develop most often in patients whose sexual consorts are not treated with antimicrobials.

DIAGNOSIS   The clinical diagnosis of classic trachoma can be made if two of the following signs are present:

1. Lymphoid follicles on the upper tarsal conjunctiva
2. Typical conjunctival scarring
3. Vascular pannus
4. Limbal follicles or their sequelae, Herbert's pits

The clinical diagnosis of endemic trachoma should be confirmed by laboratory tests in children with more marked degrees of inflammation. Intracytoplasmic chlamydial inclusions are found in 10 to 60% of Giemsa-stained conjunctival smears in such populations, but isolation in cell cultures, newer antigen detection testing, or chlamydial PCR is more sensitive. Follicular conjunctivitis in adult Europeans or Americans living in trachomatous regions is rarely due to trachoma.

Sporadic cases of adult inclusion conjunctivitis must be differentiated from keratoconjunctivitis due to adenovirus or HSV and from bacterial conjunctivitis during the first 15 days after onset; later, they must be distinguished from other forms of chronic follicular conjunctivitis. Demonstration of chlamydiae by Giemsa- or immunofluorescent-stained smears, by isolation in cell cultures, or by newer nonculture tests constitutes definitive evidence of infection. Genital examination and tests for genital chlamydial infection are indicated. Serum antibody does not constitute evidence of chlamydial eye infection since many sexually active adults have acquired serum antibody from genital infection.

℞ **TREATMENT**   Public health control programs for endemic trachoma have consisted of the mass application of tetracycline or erythromycin ointment to the eyes of all children in affected communities for 21 to 60 days or on an intermittent schedule. These programs also include surgical correction of inturned eyelids by a mobile surgical team that visits each locale. Single-dose azithromycin therapy

is now being evaluated as an alternative method of mass antibiotic treatment for trachoma in young children and pregnant women.

Adult inclusion conjunctivitis responds well to treatment with full doses of systemic tetracycline or erythromycin for 3 weeks. Treatment of all sexual consorts of the patient simultaneously is also necessary to prevent ocular reinfection and to avoid genital disease due to chlamydial infection. Topical antibiotic treatment is not required for patients who receive systemic antibiotics.

PREVENTION   Efforts to develop a trachoma vaccine have not yet been successful. General hygienic measures associated with improved living standards are effective in the elimination of endemic trachoma. An adequate water supply for personal cleanliness may be a key factor. In some areas the reduction of numbers of flies in the household is important.

PSITTACOSIS

DEFINITION   Psittacosis is primarily an infectious disease of birds and mammals that is caused by *C. psittaci*. Transmission of infection from birds to humans results in a febrile illness characterized by pneumonitis and systemic manifestations. Inapparent infections or mild influenza-like illnesses may also occur. The term *ornithosis* is sometimes applied to infections contracted from birds other than parrots or parakeets, but *psittacosis* is the preferred generic term for all forms of the disease.

EPIDEMIOLOGY   Almost any avian species can harbor *C. psittaci*. Psittacine birds (parrots, parakeets, budgerigars) are most commonly infected, but human cases have been traced to contact with pigeons, ducks, turkeys, chickens, and many other birds. Psittacosis may be considered an occupational disease of pet-shop owners, poultry workers, pigeon fanciers, taxidermists, veterinarians, and zoo attendants. During the past 20 years, there has been an increase in incidence, with cases and outbreaks occurring primarily among employees of poultry-processing plants. It is suspected that many cases go undiagnosed and unreported. The disease appears to be especially common in England, where budgerigars are popular household pets and where restrictions on the importation of these birds have been eased.

The agent is present in nasal secretions, excreta, tissues, and feathers of infected birds. Although the disease can be fatal, infected birds frequently show only minor evidence of illness, such as ruffled feathers, lethargy, and anorexia. Asymptomatic avian carriers are common, and complete recovery may be followed by continued shedding of the organism for many months.

Psittacosis is almost always transmitted to humans by the respiratory route. On rare occasions the disease may be acquired from the bite of a pet bird. Prolonged contact is not essential for transmission of the disease; a few minutes spent in an environment previously occupied by an infected bird has resulted in human infection. In one outbreak, gardening rather than direct exposure to birds was associated with infection. A psittacosis-like agent has been transmitted among hospital personnel, with severe and sometimes fatal infections. There is evidence that these "human" strains are more virulent than avian organisms. There is no record of infection acquired by the ingestion of poultry products.

PATHOGENESIS   The psittacosis agent gains entrance to the body through the upper part of the respiratory tract, spreads via the bloodstream, and eventually localizes in the pulmonary alveoli and in the reticuloendothelial cells of the spleen and liver. Invasion of the lung probably takes place by way of the bloodstream rather than by direct extension from the upper air passages. A lymphocytic inflammatory response occurs on both the interstitial and the respiratory surfaces of the alveoli as well as in the perivascular spaces. The alveolar walls and interstitial tissues of the lung are thickened, edematous, necrotic, and occasionally hemorrhagic. Histologic examination of the affected areas reveals alveolar spaces filled with fluid, erythrocytes, and lymphocytes. The picture is not pathognomonic of psittacosis unless macrophages containing characteristic cytoplasmic inclusion bodies (Levinthal-Coles-Lillie bodies) can be identified. The respiratory

179 Chlamydial Infections **1083**

epithelium of the bronchi and bronchioles usually remains intact.

CLINICAL MANIFESTATIONS The clinical manifestations and course of psittacosis are extremely variable. After an incubation period of 7 to 14 days or longer, the disease may start abruptly with shaking chills and fever, with temperatures ranging as high as 40.5°C (105°F); however, the onset is often gradual, with fever increasing over a 3- to 4-day period. Headache is almost always a prominent symptom; it is usually diffuse and excruciating and is often the patient's chief complaint.

Many patients present with a dry hacking cough that is usually nonproductive, but small amounts of mucoid or bloody sputum may be raised as the disease progresses. Cough may begin early in the course of the disease or as late as 5 days after the onset of fever. Chest pain, pleurisy with effusion, or a friction rub may all occur but are rare. Pericarditis and myocarditis have been reported. Most patients have a normal or slightly increased respiratory rate; marked dyspnea with cyanosis occurs only in severe psittacosis with extensive pulmonary involvement. In psittacosis, as in mycoplasmal pneumonias, the physical signs of pneumonitis tend to be less prominent than symptoms and x-ray findings would suggest. The initial examination may reveal fine sibilant rales, or clinical evidence of pneumonia may be completely lacking. Rales usually become audible and more numerous as the illness progresses. Signs of frank pulmonary consolidation are usually absent. Symptoms of upper respiratory tract infection are not prominent, although mild sore throat, pharyngitis, and cervical adenopathy are often documented; on occasion, the last may be the only manifestation of illness. Epistaxis is encountered early in the course of nearly one-fourth of cases. Photophobia is also a common complaint.

Patients often report generalized myalgia, and spasm and stiffness of the muscles of the back and neck may lead to an erroneous diagnosis of meningitis. Lethargy, mental depression, agitation, insomnia, and disorientation have been prominent features of the illness in some epidemics but not in others; delirium and stupor develop near the end of the first week in severe cases. Occasional patients are comatose when first seen, and the diagnosis of psittacosis may be elusive in these cases. Gastrointestinal manifestations such as abdominal pain, nausea, vomiting, or diarrhea are noted in some cases; constipation and abdominal distention sometimes occur as late complications. Icterus, the result of severe hepatic involvement, is a rare and ominous finding. A faint macular rash (Horder's spots) resembling the rose spots of typhoid fever has been described.

Patients without cough or other clinical evidence of respiratory involvement present with fever of unknown origin (Chap. 125). The pulse rate is slow in relation to the fever. When splenomegaly is noted in a patient with acute pneumonitis, psittacosis should be considered; the reported incidence of splenomegaly in this disease ranges from 10 to 70%. Nontender hepatic enlargement also occurs, but jaundice is rare. Thrombophlebitis is not unusual during convalescence; indeed, pulmonary infarction is sometimes a late complication and may be fatal.

In untreated cases of psittacosis, sustained or mildly remittent fever persists for 10 days to 3 weeks or occasionally for as long as 3 months. Over this period, the respiratory manifestations gradually abate. Psittacosis contracted from parrots or parakeets is more likely to be a severe, prolonged illness than infection acquired from pigeons or barnyard fowl. Relapses occur but are rare. Occasional patients develop endocarditis, and *C. psittaci* infection should be considered in cases of culture-negative endocarditis. Secondary bacterial infections are uncommon. Immunity to reinfection is probably permanent.

LABORATORY FINDINGS The chest x-ray in psittacosis is nonspecific and may show pneumonic lesions that are usually patchy in appearance but can be hazy, diffuse, homogeneous, lobar, atelectatic, wedge-shaped, nodular, or miliary. The white blood cell count is normal or moderately decreased in the acute phase of the disease but may rise in convalescence. The erythrocyte sedimentation rate frequently is not elevated. Transient proteinuria is common. The cerebrospinal fluid sometimes contains a few mononuclear cells but is otherwise normal. Despite hepatomegaly, the results of liver function tests are generally normal or mildly elevated.

The diagnosis can be confirmed only by isolation of the causative microorganism or by serologic studies. The agent is present in the blood during the acute phase of the disease and in the bronchial secretions for weeks or sometimes years after infection, but it is difficult to isolate. Further, the organism is hazardous to work with in the laboratory, and most clinical laboratories do not offer culture for *C. psittaci*. Thus psittacosis is most readily diagnosed by the demonstration of a rising titer of complement fixation antibody in the serum of a patient with a compatible clinical syndrome. Both an acute-phase and a convalescent-phase specimen should always be tested. *C. trachomatis*, *C. psittaci*, and *C. pneumoniae* all share a genus-specific "group" antigen, which is the basis of the complement fixation test. Thus acute infections with *C. trachomatis* or *C. pneumoniae* can also produce titer rises in this test. However, these three species have different major outer-membrane proteins that are the principal antigens in the micro-IF test. If there is doubt as to the interpretation of the complement fixation test, the micro-IF test can be used to differentiate among these antigens. The prompt initiation of treatment with tetracycline has been shown to delay an antibody rise in convalescence for several weeks or months.

DIFFERENTIAL DIAGNOSIS A history of exposure to birds may be the only clinical basis for differentiating psittacosis from a variety of infectious and noninfectious febrile disorders. The list of pulmonary diseases that may be confused with psittacosis includes *Mycoplasma* pneumonia, *C. pneumoniae* pneumonia, legionellosis, viral pneumonia, Q fever, coccidioidomycosis, tuberculosis, enterovirus infection, carcinoma of the lung with bronchial obstruction, and common bacterial pneumonias. In the early stages, before pneumonitis appears, psittacosis may be mistaken for influenza, typhoid fever, miliary tuberculosis, or infectious mononucleosis.

℞ TREATMENT The tetracyclines are consistently effective in the treatment of psittacosis. Defervescence and alleviation of symptoms usually take place within 24 to 48 h after the institution of therapy with 2 g daily in four divided doses. To avoid relapse, treatment should probably be continued for at least 7 to 14 days after defervescence. In severe cases, hospitalization and pulmonary intensive care may be indicated. Sulfonamides are not active against *C. psittaci*. Erythromycin can be used in patients allergic to or intolerant of tetracyclines.

C. PNEUMONIAE INFECTIONS

A third chlamydial species that causes disease in humans, *C. pneumoniae*, has been described in the past two decades. *C. pneumoniae* can be distinguished from the other two species on the basis of DNA hybridization and elementary body morphology. Although *C. pneumoniae* can be grown in a variety of cell cultures, it is considerably more difficult to culture than other chlamydiae, especially from clinical specimens. HL cells appear to be the most effective cell line for isolation of *C. pneumoniae*.

Knowledge of the epidemiology of *C. pneumoniae* infections has been derived primarily from serologic studies. Infections begin to occur in late childhood, achieve peak incidence in young adults, but continue throughout adult life. Seroprevalence in the many adult populations that have been tested throughout the world exceeds 40%—a figure suggesting that *C. pneumoniae* infections are ubiquitous. Secondary episodes (reinfections) appear to occur commonly in older adults throughout life. *C. pneumoniae* also produces epidemics of pneumonia and respiratory illness, especially in close residential quarters such as military barracks. The incidence of infections outside of epidemics remains poorly defined. Transmission appears to be from person to person, probably primarily in schools and family units.

Little is known about the pathogenesis of *C. pneumoniae* infection. The infection begins in the upper respiratory tract and in many persons is a long-lived asymptomatic condition of the upper respiratory mucosal surfaces. However, in at least some individuals, the organism is transported to distant sites—perhaps within macrophages—since evidence exists for replication within arteries and synovial membranes of joints. A *C. pneumoniae* outer-membrane protein may induce host immune responses whose cross-reaction with human proteins results in an autoimmune reaction.

The clinical spectrum of *C. pneumoniae* infection includes acute pharyngitis, sinusitis, bronchitis, and pneumonitis, primarily in young adults. The clinical manifestations of primary infection appear to be more severe and prolonged than those of reinfection. The pneumonitis resembles that of *M. pneumoniae* pneumonia in that leukocytosis is frequently lacking and patients often have prominent antecedent upper respiratory tract symptoms, fever, nonproductive cough, a mild to moderate degree of illness, minimal findings on chest auscultation, and small segmental infiltrates on chest x-ray. In elderly patients, pneumonia due to *C. pneumoniae* can be especially severe and may necessitate hospitalization and respiratory support.

Epidemiologic studies have demonstrated an association between serologic evidence of *C. pneumoniae* infection and atherosclerotic disease of the coronary and other arteries. In addition, *C. pneumoniae* has been identified in atherosclerotic plaques by electron microscopy, DNA hybridization, and immunocytochemistry. Recently, the organism has been recovered in culture from atheromatous plaque—a result indicating the presence of viable replicating bacteria in vessels. Evidence from animal models supports the hypothesis that *C. pneumoniae* infection of the upper respiratory tract is followed by recovery of the organism from atheromatous lesions in the aorta and that the infection accelerates the process of atherosclerosis, especially in hypercholesterolemic animals. Antimicrobial treatment of the infected animals reverses the increased risk of atherosclerosis. In humans, two small trials in patients with unstable angina or recent myocardial infarction also suggested that antibiotics reduce subsequent untoward cardiac events. Larger trials have been initiated to determine more definitively whether antibiotics affect the risk of atherosclerosis.

Diagnosis of *C. pneumoniae* infection is currently difficult because cell culture techniques are not available for routine clinical use and nonculture tests using antigen detection methods or DNA probes have not been developed for commercial use. Acute- and convalescent-phase sera can be tested for chlamydial complement fixation antibody to make a retrospective diagnosis. However, this test does not distinguish *C. pneumoniae* infection from infection due to *C. trachomatis* or *C. psittaci*. Although controlled treatment trials have not been conducted, *C. pneumoniae* is inhibited in vitro by erythromycin and tetracycline. Recommended therapy consists of 2 g per day of either agent for 10 to 14 days. Other macrolides, such as azithromycin, and some fluoroquinolones, such as levofloxacin, also appear to be effective.

BIBLIOGRAPHY

BACHMAIER K et al: *Chlamydia* infections and heart disease linked through antigenic mimicry. Science 283:1335, 1999

CENTERS FOR DISEASE CONTROL AND PREVENTION: Recommendations for the prevention and management of *Chlamydia trachomatis* infections, 1993. MMWR 42(RR-12):1, 1993

COULTS II et al: Clinical and radiographic features of psittacosis infection. Thorax 40:530, 1985

GILBERT DN, GRAYSTON JT (eds): The potential etiologic role of *Chlamydia pneumoniae* in atherosclerosis: A multidisciplinary meeting to promote collaborative research. J Infect Dis 181(Suppl 3):S383, 2000

GRAYSTON JT: Infections caused by *Chlamydia pneumoniae*, strain TWAR. Clin Infect Dis 15:757, 1992

HOLMES KK, STAMM WE: Lower genital tract infections in women: Cystitis, urethritis, vulvovaginitis, and cervicitis, in *Sexually Transmitted Diseases*, 3d ed, KK Holmes et al (eds). New York, McGraw-Hill, 1999

MARRAZZO JM, STAMM WE: New approaches to the diagnosis, treatment, and prevention of chlamydial infection. Curr Clin Top Infect Dis 18:37, 1998

——— et al: Community-based urine screening for *Chlamydia trachomatis* with a ligase chain reaction assay. Ann Intern Med 127:796, 1997

MUHLESTEIN JB: Bacterial infections and atherosclerosis. J Investig Med 46:396, 1998

SCHOLES D et al: Prevention of pelvic inflammatory disease by screening for cervical chlamydial infection. N Engl J Med 334:1362, 1996

STAMM WE: Expanding efforts to prevent chlamydial infection. N Engl J Med 339:768, 1998

———: *Chlamydia trachomatis* infections in adults, in *Sexually Transmitted Diseases*, 3d ed, KK Holmes et al (eds). New York, McGraw-Hill, 1999

——— et al: Azithromycin for empirical treatment of the nongonococcal urethritis syndrome in men. A randomized double-blind study. JAMA 274:545, 1995

Section 11
VIRAL DISEASES

180

Fred Wang, Elliott Kieff

MEDICAL VIROLOGY

AAV	adeno-associated virus	HSV	herpes simplex virus
CMV	cytomegalovirus	HTLV	human T-lymphotropic virus
CSF	cerebrospinal fluid	IFN	interferon
EBV	Epstein-Barr virus	IL	interleukin
ELISAs	enzyme-linked immunosorbent assays	KSHV	Kaposi's sarcoma–associated herpesvirus
HBV	hepatitis B virus	MHC	major histocompatibility complex
HCV	hepatitis C virus		
HDV	hepatitis D virus	NK	natural killer
HHV	human herpesvirus	TNF	tumor necrosis factor
HPVs	human papillomaviruses	VZV	varicella-zoster virus

DEFINING A VIRUS

Viruses consist of a nucleic acid surrounded by one or more proteins. Some viruses also have an outer-membrane envelope. Viruses differ from other replicating organisms in that they do not have ribosomes or enzymes for high-energy phosphate generation or for protein, carbohydrate, or lipid metabolism. Viruses are obligate intracellular parasites—that is, they require cells in order to replicate. Typically, viral nucleic acids encode proteins necessary for replicating and packaging the nucleic acids into new viral particles.

Viruses differ from viroids, prions, and virusoids. *Virusoids* are nucleic acids that depend on helper viruses to package the nucleic acids into virus-like particles. *Viroids* are simply molecules of naked, cyclical, mostly double-stranded, small RNAs and appear to be restricted to plants, in which they spread from cell to cell and are replicated by cellular RNA polymerase II. *Prions* (Chap. 375) are protein molecules that can spread from cell to cell and effect changes in the structure of their normal counterparts (cellular proteins). Prions have been implicated in neurodegenerative conditions such as Creutzfeldt-Jakob disease, kuru, and Gerstmann-Straüssler disease. Prions have also been implicated in neurodegeneration associated with human infection with bovine spongiform encephalopathy ("mad cow disease").

VIRAL STRUCTURE

Viruses have from a few to 200 genes. These genes may be embodied in a single-strand or double-strand DNA genome or in a single-strand sense, a single-strand or segmented antisense, or a double-strand segmented RNA genome. Sense-strand RNA genomes can be translated directly into protein. Sense and antisense genomes are also referred to as positive-strand and negative-strand genomes, respectively. The viral nucleic acid is usually associated with one or more virus-encoded nucleoproteins in the core of the viral particle. The viral nucleic acid is almost always enclosed in a protein shell called a *capsid*. Because of the limited genetic complexity of viruses, their capsids are usually composed of multimers of identical capsomers. Capsomers are in turn composed of one or a few proteins. Capsids have icosahedral or helical symmetry. Icosahedral structures approximate spheres but have two-, three-, and fivefold axes of symmetry, while helical structures have only a twofold axis of symmetry. The entire structural unit of nucleic acid, nucleoprotein(s), and capsid is called a *nucleocapsid*. Many human viruses have a simple nucleocapsid structure. For these viruses, the outer surface of the capsid mediates contact with uninfected cells. Other viruses are more complex and have an outer envelope that is derived from membranes of the infected cell. The piece of infected cell membrane that becomes the viral envelope has usually been modified during infection by the insertion of virus-encoded glycoproteins. These glycoproteins usually mediate contact of enveloped viruses with uninfected cells. Enveloped viruses frequently have matrix or tegument proteins that fill the space between the nucleocapsid and the envelope. In general, enveloped viruses are sensitive to solvents and nonionic detergents that can disrupt the envelope, while viruses that consist only of nucleocapsids are usually more resistant. The schematic diagram of a large and complex herpesvirus shown in Fig. 180-1 illustrates the components of a complicated DNA virus. Prototypical pathogenic human viruses are listed in Table 180-1. The relative sizes and structures of typical pathogenic human viruses are shown in Fig. 180-2.

TAXONOMY OF PATHOGENIC HUMAN VIRUSES

As is apparent from Table 180-1 and Fig. 180-2, the classification of viruses into orders and families is based on nucleic acid composition, nucleocapsid size and symmetry, and envelopment status. Viruses of a single family have similar types of genomes and are morphologically similar in electron micrographs. Further subclassification into genus is dependent on similarities in epidemiology and biologic effects and on the degree of colinear nucleic acid sequence homology. In general, each human virus has a common name related to its pathologic effects or the circumstances of its discovery and a formal species name assigned by the International Committee on Taxonomy of Viruses. The latter designation consists of the name of the host followed by the family or genus of the virus and a number. This dual terminology has created a confusing situation in which viruses are referred to and referenced by either name—e.g., varicella-zoster virus (VZV) or human herpesvirus (HHV) 3.

VIRAL INFECTION IN VITRO

STAGES OF INFECTION At the cellular level, viral infection proceeds in stages.

Viral Interactions at the Cell Surface First, virus adsorbs to a receptor on the cell surface. Adsorption is the consequence of a molecular interaction of a viral surface protein with a molecule on the

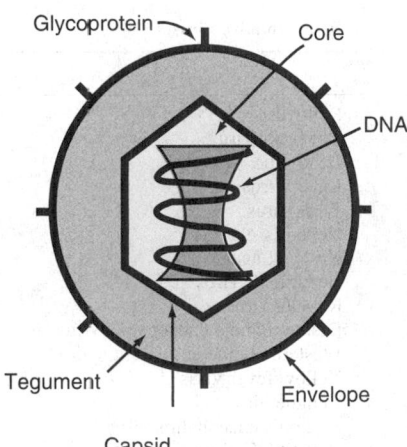

FIGURE 180-1   Schematic diagram of an enveloped herpesvirus with an icosahedral nucleocapsid. The approximate respective dimensions of the nucleocapsid and the enveloped particles are 110 nm and 180 nm. The capsid is composed of 162 capsomeres: 150 with sixfold and 12 with fivefold axes of symmetry.

cell's plasma membrane. For example, a poliovirus capsid protein binds to a cell plasma-membrane protein of the immunoglobulin superfamily type; a rhinovirus capsid protein binds to intracellular adhesion molecule 1; an echovirus capsid protein binds to an integrin; the influenza A virus envelope hemagglutinin protein binds to sialic acid; the HIV envelope glycoprotein binds to CD4 and then engages one of several chemokine receptors that function as coreceptors for the virus; the herpes simplex virus (HSV) envelope glycoproteins bind to heparan sulfate on cell surfaces and then engage one of several immunoglobulin superfamily or tumor necrosis factor (TNF) receptors; and an Epstein-Barr virus (EBV) glycoprotein binds to the B lymphocyte complement receptor CD21. Adsorption characteristically proceeds almost as well at 4°C as at 37°C, and adsorbed virus can still be neutralized by antibody. Adsorption frequently initiates changes in virion surface proteins that result in destabilization and preparation for the next stage of entry into the cell.

After adsorption, viruses penetrate through or fuse with the cell membrane, lose their sensitivity to neutralizing antibody, and become uncoated as they enter the cytoplasm. For all viruses, penetration and uncoating result in viral nucleocapsid or nucleoprotein entry into the cytoplasm. Penetration and uncoating as well as subsequent steps in viral replication depend on the cell's energy metabolism and on biochemical changes in the cell's plasma membrane and cytoskeleton. Therefore, penetration proceeds slowly at temperatures <37°C. Viruses use various strategies to penetrate and enter cells. Interaction of the viral surface protein with a cellular receptor can induce changes in viral glycoproteins or capsid proteins and in cell-surface proteins, with consequent penetration. The interaction of multiple protein molecules on the viral surface with multiple molecules on the cell-surface receptor may induce receptor aggregation at the site of viral adsorption. Receptor aggregation can trigger signaling events within the cytoplasm and changes in the plasma membrane. The cell frequently misperceives that the receptor has encountered its "normal ligand," and the aggregated receptor is internalized with the attached virus through an endocytic process that involves clathrin-coated pits. Endocytosis is important in the entry of viruses as diverse as picornaviruses, influenza viruses, HIV, adenoviruses, and herpesviruses. In many cases, entry of the virus into the cytoplasm depends on acidification of the viral endosome.

One of the best-studied examples of the effect of low pH on viral penetration is influenza virus. Influenza hemagglutinin mediates adsorption, receptor aggregation, and endocytosis. In low-pH endosomes, changes in the conformation of the hemagglutinin expose am-

Table 180-1   Virus Families Pathogenic for Humans

Family	Representative Viruses	Type of RNA/DNA	Lipid Envelope
RNA VIRUSES			
Picornaviridae	Poliovirus Coxsackievirus Echovirus Enterovirus Rhinovirus Hepatitis A virus	(+) RNA	No
Caliciviridae	Norwalk agent Hepatitis E virus	(+) RNA	No
Togaviridae	Rubella virus Eastern equine encephalitis virus Western equine encephalitis virus	(+) RNA	Yes
Flaviviridae	Yellow fever virus Dengue virus St. Louis encephalitis virus Hepatitis C virus Hepatitis G virus	(+) RNA	Yes
Coronaviridae	Coronavirus	(+) RNA	Yes
Rhabdoviridae	Rabies virus Vesicular stomatitis virus	(−) RNA	Yes
Filoviridae	Marburg virus Ebola virus	(−) RNA	Yes
Paramyxoviridae	Parainfluenza virus Respiratory syncytial virus Newcastle disease virus Mumps virus Rubeola (measles) virus	(−) RNA	Yes
Orthomyxoviridae	Influenza A, B, and C viruses	(−) RNA, 8 segments	Yes
Bunyaviridae	Hantavirus California encephalitis virus Sandfly fever virus	(−) RNA, 3 circular segments	Yes
Arenaviridae	Lymphocytic choriomeningitis virus Lassa fever virus South American hemorrhagic fever virus	(−) RNA, 2 circular segments	Yes
Reoviridae	Rotavirus Reovirus Colorado tick fever virus	ds RNA, 10–12 segments	No
Retroviridae	Human T-lymphotropic virus types I and II Human immunodeficiency virus types 1 and 2	(+) RNA, 2 identical segments	Yes
DNA VIRUSES			
Hepadnaviridae	Hepatitis B virus	ds DNA with ss portions	Yes
Parvoviridae	Parvovirus B19	ss DNA	No
Papovaviridae	Human papillomavirus JC virus BK virus	ds DNA	No
Adenoviridae	Human adenovirus	ds DNA	No
Herpesviridae	Herpes simplex virus types 1 and 2[a] Varicella-zoster virus[b] Epstein-Barr virus[c] Cytomegalovirus[d] Human herpesvirus 6 Human herpesvirus 7 Kaposi's sarcoma−associated herpesvirus[e]	ds DNA	Yes
Poxviridae	Variola (smallpox) virus Orf virus Molluscum contagiosum virus	ds DNA	Yes

[a] Also called human herpesvirus (HHV) 1 and 2, respectively.
[b] Also called HHV-3.
[c] Also called HHV-4.
[d] Also called HHV-5.
[e] Also called HHV-8.
ABBREVIATIONS: ds, double-strand; ss, single-strand.

phipathic domains that interact chemically with the cell membrane and initiate fusion of the viral and cellular membranes. Data indicate that the HIV envelope glycoprotein undergoes similar conformational changes after interaction with CD4 and chemokine receptors. For influenza virus, the M2 membrane protein also plays a key role in the uncoating of the viral envelope by providing an ion channel in the envelope. Fusion of viral and cell membranes results in the mixture of viral envelope lipids and proteins with cell membrane lipids and proteins and the penetration of the influenza nucleocapsid into the cytoplasm. Little is known about the details of the fusion processes or the subsequent biochemical interactions. With more complex viruses, such as herpesviruses, different glycoproteins interact with different receptors on different cell types or on different surfaces of polarized epithelial cells. Viral glycoproteins other than the protein that mediates initial adsorption may be critical in mediating envelope fusion with cell membranes.

Viral Gene Expression and Replication
After uncoating and release of viral nucleoprotein into the cytoplasm, the viral genome is transported to a site for expression and replication. In order to produce infectious progeny, viruses must (1) replicate their nucleic acid, (2) produce structural proteins, and (3) assemble the nucleic acid and proteins into progeny virions. Different viruses use different strategies and gene repertoires to accomplish these goals. DNA viruses (except for poxviruses) replicate their nucleic acid and assemble into nucleocapsid complexes in the cell nucleus. RNA viruses (except for influenza viruses) transcribe and replicate their nucleic acid and assemble entirely in the cytoplasm. Thus, the replication strategies of DNA and RNA viruses are presented separately below. Positive-strand and negative-strand RNA viruses are discussed separately. Medically important viruses of each group are used for illustrative purposes.

Positive-strand RNA viruses Medically important positive-strand RNA viruses include picornaviruses, flaviviruses, togaviruses, and caliciviruses. Genomic RNA from positive-strand RNA viruses is released into the cytoplasm without associated enzymes. Cell ribosomes recognize and associate with an internal ribosome entry sequence in the viral genomic RNA and translate a polyprotein that is a fusion of many or all of the viral proteins. The viral RNA polymerase and other viral proteins are cleaved from the polyprotein by protease components of the polyprotein. Antigenomic RNA is then transcribed from the genomic RNA template. Positive-strand genomes and mRNAs are next transcribed from the antigenomic RNA by the viral RNA polymerase. Positive-strand genomic RNA is encapsidated in the cytoplasm.

Negative-strand RNA viruses Medically important negative-strand RNA viruses include rhabdoviruses, filoviruses, paramyxoviruses, and bunyaviruses. Negative-strand RNA virus genomes are released into the cytoplasm with an associated RNA polymerase and one or more accessory proteins. Except for influenza viruses, negative-strand RNA viruses replicate entirely in the cytoplasm. The viral RNA polymerase transcribes messenger RNAs (mRNAs) as well as full-length antigenomic RNA, which is the template for replication of genomic RNA. The mRNAs encode for RNA polymerase and accessory factors as well as for viral structural proteins. Influenza virus is an unusual negative-strand RNA virus that transcribes its mRNAs and antigenomic RNAs in the cell's nucleus. The influenza genome RNA snatches cellular mRNA cap sequences to enhance translation of viral mRNAs and uses cell splicing machinery to encode additional viral mRNAs. All negative-strand RNA viruses, including influenza viruses, assemble in the cytoplasm.

Double-strand segmented RNA viruses These viruses, which are taxonomically grouped in the reovirus family, have 10 to 12 RNA segments that make up their genome. The medically important viruses in this group are rotaviruses and Colorado tick fever virus. Reovirus virions include an RNA polymerase complex. Reoviruses replicate and assemble in the cytoplasm.

DNA viruses Medically important DNA viruses include parvoviruses, papovaviruses, human papillomaviruses (HPVs), adenoviruses, herpesviruses, and poxviruses. Other than poxviruses, most DNA viruses must get to the cell's nucleus for DNA transcription by cellular RNA polymerase II. For example, after receptor binding and fusion, herpesvirus nucleocapsids are released into the cytoplasm along with tegument proteins. The complex is then transported along microtubules to nuclear pores, and the DNA is released into the nucleus.

Transcriptional regulation and mRNA processing for nuclear DNA viruses depend on both viral and cellular proteins. For herpesviruses, the viral tegument protein can activate transcription of viral immediate-early genes, a class of genes expressed immediately after infection. Transcription of immediate-early genes requires the virus tegument protein and preexisting cellular transcription factors. One of the key preexisting cellular factors for HSV-1 immediate-early gene transcription is docked in the cytoplasm in neurons; this fact may explain why HSV-1 goes into a latent state in neurons.

Transcription is often regulated into an organized cascade of viral gene expression. Herpesvirus immediate-early genes turn on the promoters for early genes. Other DNA viruses are not as dependent on transactivators encoded from the viral genome for early-gene transcription. Most early genes encode proteins that are necessary for viral DNA synthesis and for the turn-on of late-gene transcription. Late genes encode mostly viral structural proteins or viral proteins necessary for the assembly and egress of the virus from the infected cell. Late-gene transcription is continuously dependent on DNA replication. Therefore, inhibitors of DNA replication also stop late-gene transcription.

Each DNA virus family uses unique mechanisms for replicating its DNA. Herpesvirus DNAs are linear in the virion but circularize in the infected cell. In lytic virus infection, circular herpesvirus genomes are replicated into linear concatemers through a "rolling-circle" mechanism. Herpesviruses encode a DNA polymerase and at least six other viral proteins necessary for viral DNA replication; these viruses also encode several enzymes that increase the pool of precursor deoxyrucleotide triphosphates. Adenovirus genomes are linear in the virion and are replicated into complementary linear copies by a virus-encoded DNA polymerase and an initiator protein complex. The double-strand circular papovavirus genomes are replicated into progeny circular DNA molecules by cellular DNA replication enzymes. Two viral early proteins contribute to viral DNA replication and to the persistence of papovavirus DNA in latently infected cells. Other early papovavirus proteins stimulate cells to remain in cycle, thus facilitating viral DNA replication. Occasionally, HPVs integrate into the host chromosome; overexpression of viral early proteins and excessive stimulation of cellular growth result. Sometimes the consequence is the development of malignancies such as cervical cancer (see "Persistent Viral Infections and Cancer," below). Parvoviruses are the smallest DNA viruses:

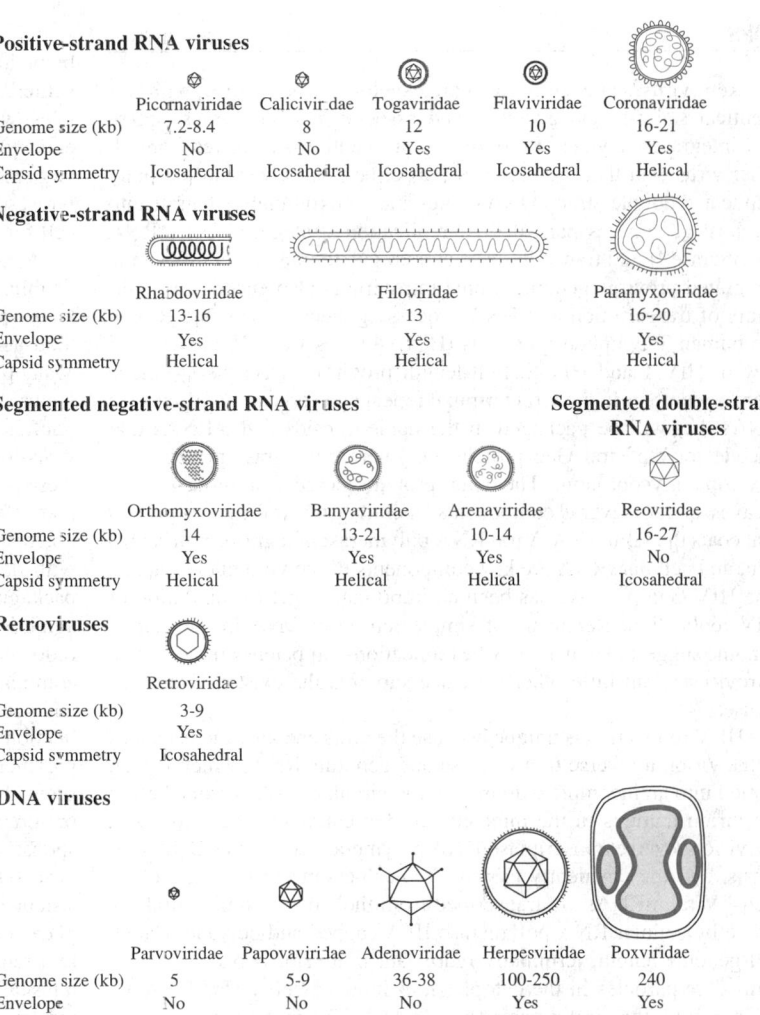

Positive-strand RNA viruses

	Picornaviridae	Caliciviridae	Togaviridae	Flaviviridae	Coronaviridae
Genome size (kb)	7.2–8.4	8	12	10	16–21
Envelope	No	No	Yes	Yes	Yes
Capsid symmetry	Icosahedral	Icosahedral	Icosahedral	Icosahedral	Helical

Negative-strand RNA viruses

	Rhabdoviridae	Filoviridae	Paramyxoviridae
Genome size (kb)	13–16	13	16–20
Envelope	Yes	Yes	Yes
Capsid symmetry	Helical	Helical	Helical

Segmented negative-strand RNA viruses / **Segmented double-strand RNA viruses**

	Orthomyxoviridae	Bunyaviridae	Arenaviridae	Reoviridae
Genome size (kb)	14	13–21	10–14	16–27
Envelope	Yes	Yes	Yes	No
Capsid symmetry	Helical	Helical	Helical	Icosahedral

Retroviruses

	Retroviridae
Genome size (kb)	3–9
Envelope	Yes
Capsid symmetry	Icosahedral

DNA viruses

	Parvoviridae	Papovaviridae	Adenoviridae	Herpesviridae	Poxviridae
Genome size (kb)	5	5–9	36–38	100–250	240
Envelope	No	No	No	Yes	Yes
Capsid symmetry	Icosahedral	Icosahedral	Icosahedral	Icosahedral	Complex

|———| 100 nm

FIGURE 180-2 Schematic diagrams of the major virus families including species that infect humans. The viruses are grouped by genome type and are drawn approximately to scale. Prototype viruses of each family that cause human disease are listed in Table 180-1.

their genomes are half the size of the papovavirus genomes and include only two genes. Parvoviruses have negative single-strand DNA genomes. The replication of autonomous parvoviruses, such as B19, depends on cellular DNA replication and requires the virus-encoded Rep protein. Other parvoviruses, such as adeno-associated virus (AAV), are not autonomous and require helper viruses of the adenovirus or herpesvirus family for their replication. AAV has been touted as a potentially safe human gene vector because its Rep protein causes its integration at a single chromosomal site.

Poxviruses are the largest DNA viruses and are unique among these viruses in replicating and assembling in the cytoplasm. Poxviruses encode transcription factors and an RNA polymerase as well as enzymes for RNA capping and polyadenylation and for DNA synthesis. Poxvirus DNA also has a unique structure. The two strands of the double-strand linear DNA are covalently linked at the ends so that the genome is also a covalently closed single-strand circle. In addition, there are inverted repeats at the ends of the DNA. During DNA replication, the genome is cleaved within the terminal inverted repeat, and the inverted repeats self-prime complementary-strand synthesis by the virus-encoded DNA polymerase. Like herpesviruses, poxviruses encode several enzymes that increase deoxynucleotide triphosphate precursor levels and thus facilitate viral DNA synthesis.

Viruses with both RNA and DNA genomes Retroviruses, lentiviruses, and hepatitis B virus (HBV) are not purely RNA or DNA viruses.

Retroviruses and lentiviruses are enveloped RNA viruses with two identical sense-strand genomes and associated reverse transcriptase and integrase enzymes. Retroviruses and lentiviruses differ from all other viruses in that they reverse-transcribe themselves into partially duplicated double-strand DNA copies and then routinely integrate into the host genome as part of their replication strategy. Cellular RNA polymerase II and transcription factors regulate transcription from the integrated provirus genome. Some retroviruses also encode for regulators of transcription and RNA processing, such as Tax and Rex in the human T-lymphotropic virus (HTLV) types I and II and Tat and Rev in HIV-1 and HIV-2. Full-length proviral transcripts are made from a promoter in the viral terminal repeat and serve as both genomic RNAs that will be packaged in the nucleocapsids and mRNAs that encode for the viral Gag protein, polymerase/integrase protein, and envelope glycoprotein. The Gag protein includes a protease that cleaves it into several components, including a viral matrix protein that coats the viral RNA. Viral RNA polymerase/integrase, matrix protein, and cellular tRNA are key components of the viral nucleocapsid. The HIV Gag protease has been an important target for inhibition of HIV replication. Remnants of simple retroviral DNA in the human genome suggest that there may be replication-competent simple human retroviruses, but little other evidence supports the existence of these viruses.

HBV replication is unique because the virus encodes and packages in the virion a reverse transcriptase and genomic RNA, which is then copied into an incomplete double-strand circular DNA genome before the virion matures in the infected cell. On entry into the cytoplasm, the virion reverse transcriptase/DNA polymerase completes DNA synthesis, and the covalently closed circular genome resides in the nucleus. Viral mRNAs are transcribed from the closed circular viral episome by cellular RNA polymerase II. A capped and polyadenylated, full-genome-length, terminally redundant transcript is packaged into virus core particles in the cytoplasm of infected cells. This RNA associates with the viral reverse transcriptase. The reverse transcriptase converts the full-length, terminally redundant, core-particle, encapsidated RNA genome into partially double-strand DNA. HBV is believed to mature by budding through the cell's plasma membrane, which has been modified by the insertion of viral surface antigen protein.

Viral Assembly and Egress For most viruses, nucleic acid and structural protein synthesis are accompanied by the assembly of protein and nucleic acid complexes. The assembly and egress of mature infectious virus mark the end of the eclipse phase of infection, during which infectious virus cannot be recovered from the infected cell. Nucleic acids from RNA viruses and poxviruses assemble into nucleocapsids in the cytoplasm. For all DNA viruses except poxviruses, viral DNA assembles into nucleocapsids in the nucleus. In general, the capsid proteins of viruses with icosahedral nucleocapsids can self-assemble into densely packed and highly ordered capsid structures. Herpesviruses require an assemblin protein as a scaffold for capsid assembly. Viral nucleic acid then spools into the assembled capsid. For herpesviruses, a full unit of the viral DNA genome is packaged into the capsid, and a capsid-associated nuclease cleaves the viral DNA at both ends. In the case of viruses with helical nucleocapsids, the protein component appears to assemble around the nucleic acid, which contributes to capsid organization.

Viruses must egress from the infected cell and not bind back to its plasma membrane. In many cases, enveloped viruses simply egress and acquire their envelope by budding through the cell's plasma membrane. Excess viral membrane glycoproteins are synthesized to saturate cell receptors and facilitate viral egress. Some viruses encode membrane proteins with enzymatic activity for receptor destruction. Influenza virus, for example, encodes a glycoprotein with neuraminidase activity, which destroys sialic acid on the infected cell's plasma membrane. Herpesvirus nucleocapsids acquire their initial envelope by as-

sembling in the nucleus and then budding through the nuclear membrane into the endoplasmic reticular space. The enveloped herpesvirus is then released from the cell either by maturation in cytoplasmic vesicles, which fuse with the plasma membrane and release the virus by exocytosis, or by "de-envelopment" into the cytoplasm and "re-envelopment" at the plasma membrane. In most instances, nonenveloped viruses appear to depend on the death and dissolution of the infected cell for their release.

FIDELITY OF VIRAL REPLICATION Cells grow by doubling their genome and dividing, whereas viruses typically make large quantities of viral nucleic acid and structural proteins, and thousands of progeny may be produced from a single infected cell. Many particles partially assemble and never mature into virions. Many mature-appearing virions are imperfect and have only incomplete or nonfunctional genomes. Despite the inefficiency of assembly, a typical virus-infected cell releases 10 to 1000 infectious progeny. Some of these progeny may contain genomes that differ from those of the virus that infected the cell. Smaller, "defective" virus genomes have been noted with the replication of many RNA and DNA viruses. Virions with defective genomes can be produced in large numbers through packaging of incompletely synthesized nucleic acid. Adenovirus packaging is notoriously inefficient, and a high particle-to-infectious virus ratio may limit the amount of recombinant adenovirus that can be administered for gene therapy. Mutant viral genomes are also produced and can be of medical significance. In general, viral nucleic acid replication is more error-prone than cellular nucleic acid replication. RNA polymerases and reverse transcriptases are intrinsically more error-prone than DNA polymerases. Mutant viruses can be virulent and may preferentially cause disease through evasion of the host immune response or through resistance to antiviral drugs. Persistent hepatitis C virus (HCV) infection appears to be due to genome mutation and persistent immune escape. Changes in viral nucleic acid can also take place through infection by and recombination or reassortment between two related viruses in a single cell. While this occurrence is highly unusual, the changes could be substantial and could significantly alter virulence or epidemiology. Reassortment of an avian or mammalian influenza A hemagglutinin gene into a human influenza background is believed to play a role in the emergence of new epidemic influenza A strains.

VIRAL GENES NOT REQUIRED FOR VIRAL REPLICATION Viruses frequently have genes encoding proteins that are not directly involved in replication or packaging of the viral nucleic acid, in virion assembly, or in regulation of the transcription of viral genes involved in those processes. Most of these proteins fall into four classes: (1) proteins that directly or indirectly alter cell growth; (2) proteins that inhibit cellular DNA, RNA, or protein synthesis so that viral mRNA can be efficiently transcribed or translated; (3) proteins that promote the cell's survival or inhibit apoptosis so that progeny virus can mature and escape from the infected cell; and (4) proteins that downregulate host inflammatory or immune responses so that virus infection can proceed in an infected person to the maximum extent consistent with virus survival and efficient transmission to a new host. More complex viruses of the poxvirus or herpesvirus family encode many proteins that serve these functions. Some of these viral proteins have motifs similar to those of cell proteins, while others are quite novel. Virology has increasingly focused on these more sophisticated strategies evolved by viruses to permit the establishment of long-term infection in humans and other animals. These strategies often provide unique insights into the control of cell growth, cell survival, macromolecular synthesis, proteolytic processing, immune or inflammatory suppression, immune resistance, cytokine mimicry, or cytokine blockade.

HOST RANGE The concept of host range was originally based on the cell types in which a virus replicated in tissue culture. For the most part, the host range is limited by specific cell-surface proteins required for viral adsorption or penetration. Another common basis for host-range limitation is transcription from viral promoters. Most

DNA viruses depend not only on cellular RNA polymerase II and the basal components of the cellular transcription complex but also on activated components and transcriptional accessory factors, both of which differ among differentiated tissues, among cells at various phases of the cell cycle, and between resting and cycling cells.

The concept of host range for virus infection in humans includes these factors and others since (1) most viruses infect more than one cell type in vivo and (2) the virus life cycle and extent of viral replication can be affected by the differentiation and activated state of a given cell type. This point is particularly relevant for human papovavirus, herpesvirus, and lentivirus infections, in which vigorous replication during initial infection may be followed by quiescent or latent infection—a situation that allows the virus to persist.

VIRAL CYTOPATHIC EFFECTS AND INHIBITORS OF APOPTOSIS The replication of almost all viruses has adverse effects on the infected cell, inhibiting cellular synthesis of DNA, RNA, or proteins. This inhibitory effect probably stems from the viruses' need to prevent or limit nonspecific, innate host resistance factors, including interferon (IFN). Most commonly, viruses specifically inhibit host protein synthesis by attacking a component of the translational initiation complex—frequently, a component that is not required for efficient translation of viral RNAs. Poliovirus protease 2A, for example, cleaves a cellular component of the complex that ordinarily facilitates translation of cell mRNAs by interacting with their 5' cap structure. Poliovirus RNA is efficiently translated without a 5' cap since it has an internal ribosome entry sequence. Influenza virus inhibits the processing of mRNA by snatching 5' cap structures from nascent cellular RNAs and using them as primers in the synthesis of viral mRNA. HSV has a virion tegument protein that inhibits cellular mRNA translation.

Apoptosis is the expected consequence of virus-induced inhibition of cellular macromolecular synthesis and viral nucleic acid replication. While the induction of apoptosis may be important for the release of some viruses (particularly nonenveloped viruses), many viruses have acquired genes or parts of genes that enable them to forestall infected-cell apoptosis. This delay may be advantageous in allowing the completion of viral replication. Adenoviruses and herpesviruses encode analogues of the cellular Bc12 protein, which blocks mitochondrial enhancement of proapoptotic stimuli. Poxviruses and some herpesviruses encode caspase inhibitors. Many viruses, including HPVs and adenoviruses, encode proteins that inhibit p53 or its downstream proapoptotic effects.

VIRAL INFECTION IN VIVO

The capsid and envelope of a virus protect its genome and permit its transmission from cell to cell and to prospective hosts. Most common viral infections are spread by aerosolized particles, by ingestion of contaminated water or food, or by direct contact. In all these situations, infection begins on an epithelial or mucosal surface and spreads along it or from it to deeper tissues. Infection may then spread through the body via the bloodstream, lymphatics, or neural circuits. Parenteral inoculation also serves to transmit some viral infections among humans or from animals (including insects) to humans.

PRIMARY INFECTION The first (primary) episode of viral infection usually lasts from several days to several weeks. During this period, the concentration of virus at sites of infection rises and then falls, usually to unmeasurable levels. The rate at which the intensity of viral infection rises and falls at a given site depends on the accessibility of that organ or tissue to both the virus and systemic immune effectors, the intrinsic ability of the virus to replicate at that site, and endogenous nonspecific and specific resistance. Typically, infections with enterovirus, mumps virus, measles virus, rubella virus, rotavirus, influenza virus, adenovirus, HSV, and VZV are cleared from almost all sites within 3 to 4 weeks. Some of these viruses are especially proficient in altering or evading the innate and acquired immune responses; thus primary infection with these viruses can last for several

months. Characteristically extending beyond several weeks are primary infections due to HBV, HCV, hepatitis D virus (HDV), EBV, cytomegalovirus (CMV), HIV, HPV, and molluscum contagiosum virus. For some of these viruses (e.g., HPV, HBV, HCV, HDV, and molluscum contagiosum virus), the primary phase of infection is almost indistinguishable from the persistent phase.

Disease manifestations usually arise as a consequence of viral replication at a specific site but do not necessarily correlate with levels of replication at that site. For example, the clinical manifestations of limited infection with poliovirus, enterovirus, rabies virus, measles virus, mumps virus, or HSV in neural cells are severe relative to the level of viral replication at mucosal surfaces. Similarly, significant morbidity may accompany in utero fetal infection with rubella virus or CMV.

Primary infections are cleared by specific and nonspecific immune responses. Thereafter, an immunocompetent host is usually immune to the disease manifestations of reinfection by the same virus. Immunity may not prevent transient surface colonization on reexposure, or even persistent colonization.

PERSISTENT AND LATENT INFECTIONS Relatively few viruses cause persistent or latent infections. HBV, HCV, rabies virus, measles virus, HIV, HTLV, HPV, herpesviruses, and some poxviruses are notable exceptions. The mechanisms for persistent infection vary widely. In persistent HCV infection and to a lesser extent in HIV infection, the high mutation rates in viral genome replication significantly facilitate persistent infection, continuously yielding mutant viruses that have lost antigenic determinants to which the host has developed effective immune responses. HIV is directly immunosuppressive, depleting CD4+ T lymphocytes and compromising CD8+ cytotoxic T cell immune responsiveness. Moreover, HIV encodes a Nef protein that downmodulates major histocompatibility complex (MHC) class I expression, rendering HIV-infected cells partially resistant to immune CD8+ cytolysis. The high mutation rate and the magnitude of virus load conspire to promote persistent infection with drug-resistant HIV mutants.

In contrast, herpesviruses and papovaviruses have much lower mutation rates. Their persistence is due to their ability to establish latent infection and to reactivate from latency. In this instance, *latency* is defined as a state of infection with a full viral genome replicated by cellular DNA polymerase in conjunction with the cell genome; there is no expression of viral genes associated with lytic infection and therefore no production of infectious virus. For HPVs, latently infected basal epithelial cells replicate. Some of the progeny cells provide a stable supply of latently infected basal cells, while others go on to squamous differentiation and in the process become permissive for lytic virus infection. For herpesviruses, latent infection is established in nonreplicating neural cells (HSV and VZV) and in replicating cells of early hematopoietic lineages [EBV and probably CMV, HHV-6, HHV-7, and Kaposi's sarcoma–associated herpesvirus (KSHV, also known as HHV-8)]. Reactivation from neural latency appears to be an intermittent process provoked by external stimuli, whereas reactivation from hematopoietic precursors appears to be a more continuous process. In their latent stage, HPV and herpesvirus genomes are hidden from the normal immune response. It is still not fully understood how latent and reactivated HPV and herpesvirus infections escape immediate and effective immune responses in highly immune hosts. HPV, HSV, and VZV may be somewhat protected because of their replication in middle and upper layers of the squamous epithelium. HSV and CMV are also known to encode proteins that downregulate MHC class I expression and antigenic peptide presentation on infected cells, thereby enabling these cells to escape CD8+ T lymphocyte cytotoxicity. Latent infection and intermittent reactivation perpetuate HPV and herpesvirus infections in human populations by allowing the viruses to persist in immune hosts and to be transmitted to the next generation of naive hosts.

Like other poxviruses, molluscum contagiosum virus cannot establish latent infection but rather causes persistent infection in hypertrophic lesions that last for months or years. This virus encodes a chemokine homologue that probably blocks inflammatory responses and an MHC class I analogue that may block cytotoxic T lymphocyte attack.

PERSISTENT VIRAL INFECTIONS AND CANCER Persistent viral infection is estimated to be the root cause of as many as 20% of human malignancies. For the most part, cancer is an accidental and highly unusual or long-term effect of infection with oncogenic human viruses. In these malignancies, viral infection is a critical and ultimately determinative early step, and an unusual virus-infected cell undergoes the subsequent genetic changes that permit the enhanced autonomous growth and survival characteristic of a malignant cell. Most hepatocellular carcinoma is now believed to be caused by chronic inflammatory, immune, and regenerative responses to HBV or HCV infection. Epidemiologic data firmly link HBV and HCV infection to hepatocellular carcinoma, and studies in murine experimental models indicate that chronic liver injury and repair induced by virus-encoded proteins can result in hepatocellular cancer. In rare instances, HBV DNA integrates into cellular DNA—an event that probably contributes to the development of some tumors.

Almost all cervical carcinoma is caused by long-term persistent replication of "high-risk" genital HPV strains. An infrequent consequence of persistent HPV replication is the integration of a small fragment of the HPV genome encoding the HPV E6 and E7 proteins into chromosomal DNA. Overexpression of these proteins of HPV type 16 or 18 eliminates at least two major tumor-suppressive mechanisms in the infected cell and causes profound changes in cellular growth and survival. Nevertheless, subsequent chromosomal changes must occur over ensuing cycles of cell growth if a sufficiently malignant cell is to invade the surrounding tissues.

Similarly, long-term EBV infection and expression of the EBV oncogene LMP1 in a clone of latently infected epithelial cells appears to be a critical early step in the evolution of anaplastic nasopharyngeal carcinoma, a common malignancy in Chinese and North African populations. High-level LMP1 expression is a hallmark of many cases of Hodgkin's disease. Among younger age groups, >50% of Hodgkin's disease tumors are clonally derived from an EBV-infected cell. The HTLV-I Tax and Rex proteins appear to be critical to the initiation of cutaneous adult T cell lymphoma/leukemias that may occur long after primary HTLV-I infection.

A new EBV-related herpesvirus, KSHV, was identified in a search for the postulated sexually transmitted etiologic agent of Kaposi's sarcoma in HIV-infected individuals. Molecular data confirm the presence of KSHV DNA in all Kaposi's tumors, including those associated with HIV infection, transplantation, and familial transmission.

Evidence supporting a causal role of viral infection in these malignancies includes epidemiologic data, the presence of viral DNA in all tumor cells, the ability of the viruses to transform human cells in culture, the results of in vitro assays for transforming effects of specific viral genes on cell growth, and pathologic data indicating the expression of transforming viral genes in premalignant or malignant cells in vivo.

EBV is a unique example of a human virus that relies on the normal immune response to contain the potentially unrestrained growth of infected B lymphocytes. In the initial stages of normal primary EBV infection, EBV "latently" infects B lymphocytes and expresses at least eight viral proteins that cause continuous cell proliferation. The infected cells grow indefinitely in vitro or in T cell–deficient mice. Most of the viral proteins are highly antigenic, and these virus-infected cells, which can transiently constitute 10% of the circulating B lymphocyte population, are met with an overwhelming helper and cytotoxic T cell response during primary infection. The number of virus-infected cells then falls rapidly, and the one EBV-infected cell in a million that persists does not express most of the viral proteins that cause B cell proliferation. These persisting cells are the site of normal latent infec-

tion. Breakthrough growth of the EBV-infected B lymphocytes almost never occurs in immunocompetent hosts. However, in immunosuppressed AIDS patients or organ transplant recipients, EBV-infected B lymphocytes expressing the full set of growth-transforming genes may grow, uncontrolled by the immune system, and cause self-sustained and potentially fatal lymphoproliferative disease. Clinical investigation has resulted in novel strategies for treating these virus-induced malignancies by increasing T cell responsiveness through ex vivo expansion and readministration of EBV-specific T cells and by attacking the proliferating B cells with antibody coupled to toxins.

RESISTANCE TO VIRAL INFECTIONS Resistance to viral infection is initially provided by factors that are not virus-specific. Physical protection is afforded by the cornified layers of the skin and by mucous secretions that continuously sweep over mucosal surfaces. Once the first cell is infected, viral infection induces IFNs, which are important local resistance factors. Viral infection may also cause the release of other cytokines from infected cells. Viral protein epitopes expressed on the cell surface in the context of MHC class I and II HLA proteins attract T cells with appropriate receptors. Cytokines, inflammatory agents, and antigens released by virus-induced cell death attract inflammatory cells, dendritic cells, granulocytes, natural killer (NK) cells, and B lymphocytes to the sites of initial infection. IFNs and NK cells are particularly important in containing viral infection for the first several days. Granulocytes and macrophages are also important in the phagocytosis and degradation of viruses, especially after an initial antibody response.

Some 7 to 10 days after infection, virus-specific antibody responses, virus-specific HLA class II–restricted CD4+ helper T lymphocyte responses, and virus-specific HLA class I–restricted CD8+ cytotoxic T lymphocyte responses are detected. These responses, whose magnitude typically increases over the second and third weeks of infection, are important in rapid recovery. Between the second and third weeks of infection, the antibody type usually changes from IgM to IgG, and IgA antibody is detected at initially infected mucosal surfaces. Antibody may directly neutralize virus by binding to its surface and preventing its adsorption or penetration. Complement usually enhances virus neutralization. Antibody and complement can also lyse virus-infected cells that express viral proteins on their surface. A cell infected with an enveloped virus usually expresses viral envelope glycoprotein components on its surface and is thus rendered subject to destruction by antibodies and complement.

The antibody and CD4+/CD8+ T lymphocyte responses tend to persist for several months after primary infection. Antibody-producing lymphocytes persist in small numbers as memory cells and begin to proliferate rapidly in response to a second infection, providing an early barrier to reinfection with the same virus. Immunologic memory for T cell responses appears to be less long-lived, and redevelopment of T cell immunity may take longer than secondary antibody responses, particularly when many years have elapsed between primary infection and reexposure.

Some viruses have genes that alter innate and acquired host defenses. Adenoviruses encode small RNAs that inhibit IFN shutoff of infected-cell protein synthesis. Adenovirus E1A inhibits IFN-mediated changes in cell gene transcription. Adenovirus E3 proteins prevent TNF-induced cytolysis and block HLA class I antigen synthesis by the infected cell. HSV ICP47 and CMV US11 block class I antigen presentation. EBV encodes an interleukin (IL) 10 homologue that inhibits NK and T cell responses. Vaccinia virus B15R is an IL-1 receptor decoy. Vaccinia virus B8R is a soluble TNF receptor that blocks the effects of TNF. Vaccinia virus CrmA inhibits the ability of CD8+ cytotoxic cells to kill virus-infected cells. Some poxviruses and herpesviruses encode blockers of chemokines and thereby inhibit cellular inflammatory responses. The adoption of these strategies by viruses highlights the importance of these host resistance factors in containing viral infection as well as that of redundancy in host resistance. The ultimate success of a virus requires a live host to help it disseminate.

Much has been written about the role of specific aspects of the host immune response in containment of specific virus infections. Certainly, T lymphocyte disorders are associated with severe primary and reactivated herpesvirus infections, and antibody responses are important in resistance to many RNA virus infections. However, antibody responses are also important in resistance to herpesvirus infections, as is exemplified by the utility of immunoglobulin therapy in early amelioration of these infections. T lymphocyte responses play a significant role in resistance to RNA virus infections, as is illustrated by the presence of cytotoxic T cells specific for influenza virus nucleoprotein.

Host resistance does not come without a price. Clearly, aspects of the host response contribute to the pathophysiologic manifestations and symptoms of viral infection. Inflammation at sites of viral infection can increase rates of local cell death. Immune responses to viral infection can target related epitopes on normal cells. While such effects have been demonstrated in experimental models, their role in the autoimmune manifestations of primary or recurrent human viral infections is uncertain.

INTERFERONS All human cells can synthesize IFN-α or -β in response to viral infection. The IFN response is usually induced by the presence of double-strand viral RNA, which can be made by both RNA and DNA viruses. IFN-γ is not directly related to IFN-α or -β and is produced mainly by NK cells and by immune T lymphocytes responding to IL-12. IFN-α and -β bind to the IFN-α receptor, while IFN-γ binds to a different but related receptor. Both receptors signal through receptor-associated JAK kinases and other cytoplasmic proteins, including "STAT" proteins. These proteins are tyrosine phosphorylated by JAK kinases, translocate to the nucleus, and transactivate promoters for specific cell genes. Three types of antiviral effects are induced by IFN at the transcriptional level. The first effect is attributable to the induction of 2'-5' oligo(A) synthetases, which require double-strand RNA for their activation. Activated synthetase polymerizes oligo(A) and thereby activates RNAse L, which in turn degrades single-strand RNA. The second effect takes place through the induction of PKR, a serine and threonine kinase that is also activated by double-strand RNA. PKR phosphorylates and negatively regulates the translational initiation factor eIF2-α, shutting down protein synthesis in the infected cell. A third effect is initiated through the induction of Mx proteins, a family of GTPases that is particularly important in inhibiting influenza virus and vesicular stomatitis virus replication. None of these IFN effects is directed specifically against the virus; infected-cell RNA and protein synthesis are globally inhibited. IFN probably contributes to the death of the infected cell.

DIAGNOSTIC VIROLOGY A wide variety of methods are now used to diagnose viral infection, but serology and viral isolation in tissue culture remain the backbone of diagnostic virology. Acute- and convalescent-phase sera with rising antibody titers to virus-specific antigens and a shift from IgM to IgG antibodies are generally accepted as diagnostic of acute viral infection. Traditionally, virus-specific antibodies have been detected by hemadsorption, hemagglutination, or indirect immunofluorescence. Immunofluorescence assays use fixed virus-infected cells as a target for serum antibodies. Hemadsorption and hemagglutination assays measure the ability of serum antibodies to the hemagglutinin proteins of RNA viruses to inhibit virus-induced adsorption or agglutination. Serologic diagnosis is based on a greater-than-fourfold rise in IgG antibody concentration when acute- and convalescent-phase serum samples are analyzed at the same time. A simultaneous fall in IgM antibody confirms recent primary viral infection. Immunofluorescence, hemadsorption, and hemagglutination assays are labor-intensive and are being replaced by enzyme-linked immunosorbent assays (ELISAs). ELISAs generally use specific viral proteins purified from virus-infected cells or produced by recombinant DNA technology. These viral antigens are attached to a solid phase, where they can be incubated with serum, washed to eliminate nonspecific antibodies, and reacted with an enzyme-linked reagent to detect human IgG or IgM antibody specifically adhering to the viral antigen on the solid phase. The amount of antibody can then be quantitated by the intensity of a color reaction mediated by the linked enzyme. ELISAs can be automated and can have enhanced sensitivity. Western blots measure antibody to multiple viral proteins

simultaneously. The proteins are separated by size and transferred to an inert membrane, where they are incubated with serum antibodies. Western blots have an internal specificity control, since the level of reactivity for viral proteins can be compared with that for cellular proteins in the same sample. Western blots are a useful confirmatory test but require individual evaluation and are inherently difficult to quantitate.

Viral isolation in tissue culture is dependent on the infection of susceptible cells and amplification through viral replication in infected cells. Virus growing in tissue culture cells can frequently be identified by its effect under light microscopy. For example, HSV produces a typical cytopathic effect in rabbit kidney cells within 3 days. Other viral cytopathic effects may not be as diagnostically useful. Identification may require confirmation by staining with virus-specific monoclonal antibodies. Viruses growing in tissue culture can also be identified by hemadsorption, by interference (e.g., rubella virus–infected cells resist lysis by echovirus), or by electron microscopy (assuming that the specimen has altered cell morphology, as observed by ordinary light microscopy).

The efficiency and speed of virus identification can be enhanced by combining short-term culture with immune detection. In assays with "shell vials" of tissue culture cells growing on a coverslip, viral infection can be detected by staining of the culture with a monoclonal antibody to a specific viral protein expressed early in viral replication. Thus, virus-infected cells can be detected within hours or days of inoculation—before the several rounds of infection that would be required to produce a visible cytopathic effect.

The sensitivity of virus isolation depends on the collection of specimens from the appropriate site and the rapid transport of these specimens in the appropriate medium to the virology laboratory. Rapid transport maintains viral viability and limits bacterial and fungal overgrowth. Lipid-enveloped viruses are generally much more sensitive to freezing and thawing than nonenveloped viruses. The most appropriate site for culture depends on the pathogenesis of the virus in question. Nasopharyngeal, tracheal, or endobronchial aspirates are most appropriate for the identification of respiratory viruses. Sputum cultures generally are not appropriate because bacterial contamination and viscosity threaten tissue-culture cell viability. Aspirates of vesicular fluid are useful for isolation of HSV and VZV. Nasopharyngeal aspirates and stool specimens may be useful when the patient has fever and a rash and an enteroviral infection is suspected. Adenoviruses can be cultured from the urine of patients with hemorrhagic cystitis. CMV can frequently be isolated from cultures of urine or buffy coat. Biopsy material can be effectively cultured when viruses infect major organs, as in HSV encephalitis or adenovirus pneumonia. Unlike serology, the isolation of a virus does not establish the time of primary infection. Many viruses persistently or intermittently colonize normal human mucosal surfaces. Saliva is not infrequently positive for herpesviruses, and 1% of normal urine samples are positive for CMV. Isolations from blood, cerebrospinal fluid (CSF), or biopsy specimens are more often diagnostic of significant virus infection.

Another method aimed at increasing the speed of viral diagnosis is direct antigen testing. Virus-infected cells obtained directly from the patient are detected by staining with virus-specific monoclonal antibodies; for example, epithelial cells obtained by nasopharyngeal aspiration can be stained with a variety of monoclonal antibodies to respiratory viruses. The Tzanck preparation used to detect multinucleated giant cells in HSV- or VSV-induced lesions was the predecessor of these direct antigen tests and can be enhanced by the use of HSV- or VZV-specific monoclonal antibodies. Similarly, monoclonal antibodies can be applied to histopathology specimens to identify virus-infected cells.

Advances in nucleic acid technology are revolutionizing diagnostic virology. The speed and sensitivity of tests that directly amplify minute amounts of viral nucleic acids present in specimens mean that detection no longer depends on viable virus and its replication. For example, amplification and detection of HSV nucleic acids leaking into the CSF of patients with HSV encephalitis can be more sensitive than culture of virus from CSF. The extreme sensitivity of these tests can be a problem, since trivial amounts of contamination can lead to false-positive results. In addition, detection of viral nucleic acids does not necessarily indicate virus-induced disease, especially in cases where viruses (e.g., herpesviruses) can cause persistent asymptomatic infection.

Measurement of the amount of viral RNA or DNA in peripheral blood is becoming an important means for determining which patients are at increased risk for virus-induced disease and for evaluating clinical responses to antiviral chemotherapy. Direct staining with CMV-specific monoclonal antibodies to quantitate virus-infected cells in the peripheral blood or CMV antigenemia can be useful in identifying which immunosuppressed patients may be at risk for CMV-induced disease. New CMV assays using nucleic acid technologies for the same purpose have been approved for clinical use. RNA viral-load measurements by nucleic acid technologies are now routinely used in AIDS patients to evaluate responses to an increasing number of antiviral agents. Viral-load measurements may also be useful for evaluating the treatment of patients with HBV and HCV infections.

The use of antiviral agents for the treatment of herpesvirus and HIV infections has been highly effective. However, the emergence of drug-resistant HIV strains in treated patients can limit efficacy in some cases. The increased number of antiviral agents and drug classes with different viral targets has made the identification of drug-resistant viruses clinically relevant, especially for HIV infection. Drug resistance in herpesviruses is a more unusual problem.

Viral genotyping is a new and faster method for the identification of drug-resistant viruses. Rising viral loads despite antiviral chemotherapy may indicate emergence of resistant HIV strains. Resistance to reverse transcriptase or protease inhibitors has been associated with specific mutations in the reverse transcriptase or protease genes. Identification of these mutations by polymerase chain reaction amplification and nucleic acid sequencing can be clinically useful for determining which antiviral agents may still be effective. Genotyping of HCV may also help identify patients who can benefit from combination chemotherapy.

Viral phenotyping may also be useful for identifying resistant viruses associated with new or unrecognized genetic mutations. These labor-intensive assays are not routinely available, but technical advances and continued evolution of drug-resistant viruses may make these tests more clinically relevant in the near future.

IMMUNIZATION FOR THE PREVENTION OF VIRAL INFECTIONS Viral vaccines were among the outstanding accomplishments of twentieth-century science. The scourge of smallpox has been eradicated. Poliovirus eradication may soon follow. Rabies and measles can be contained or eliminated. Excess mortality due to influenza virus epidemics can be contained, and the threat of influenza pandemics has decreased. Widespread HBV vaccination has dramatically lessened the frequency of acute and chronic hepatitis and is expected to lead to a dramatic decrease in the incidence of hepatocellular carcinoma. The ease with which some viruses are attenuated in tissue culture has led to widespread immunization against rubella, measles, mumps, and chickenpox. Recombinant DNA-based strategies will make it possible to prevent severe infections with many other viruses by using purified proteins or genetically engineered live virus vaccines. Unfortunately, there are limits to these prospects. The evolutionary divergence of HIV and HCV, for example, complicates the development of highly effective immunogens for the prevention of infection with these agents. Modestly effective immunogens that incorporate multiple B and T cell epitopes may prove useful for low-level exposures.

BIBLIOGRAPHY

DURANT J et al: Drug resistance genotyping in HIV-1 therapy: The VIRADAPT randomised controlled trial. Lancet 353:2195, 1999

FIELDS BN et al (eds): Virology, 3d ed. New York, Raven, 1996

LENNETTE EH, SMITH TF (eds): Laboratory Diagnosis of Viral Infections. New York, Marcel Dekker, 1999

PLOEGH HL: Viral strategies of immune evasion. Science 280:248, 1998

ROULSTON A et al: Viruses and apoptosis. Annu Rev Microbiol 53:577, 1999

SENKEVICH T et al: Genome sequence of a human tumorigenic poxvirus: Prediction of specific host response-evasion genes. Science 273:813, 1996

181 *Raphael Dolin*

ANTIVIRAL CHEMOTHERAPY, EXCLUDING ANTIRETROVIRAL DRUGS

ALT	alanine aminotransferase	HCV	hepatitis C virus
CMV	cytomegalovirus	HHV	human herpesvirus
CSF	cerebrospinal fluid	HSV	herpes simplex virus
EBV	Epstein-Barr virus	IFN	interferon
FDA	Food and Drug Administration	RSV	respiratory syncytial virus
HBeAg	hepatitis B e antigen	VZV	varicella-zoster virus
HBV	hepatitis B virus		

The development of drugs for antiviral chemotherapy and chemoprophylaxis is a relatively recent but now very active area of biomedical research. Significant progress has been made in recent years on new drugs for several viral infections. Despite these advances, the field of antiviral therapy—both the number of antiviral drugs and our understanding of their optimal use—continues to lag behind the field of antibacterial drug treatment, in which more than 60 years of experience have now been accumulated.

The development of antiviral drugs poses several challenges. Viruses replicate intracellularly and often employ host cell enzymes, macromolecules, and organelles for synthesis of viral particles. Therefore, useful antiviral compounds must discriminate between host and viral functions with a high degree of specificity; agents without such selectivity are likely to be too toxic for clinical use.

The development of laboratory assays to assist clinicians in the appropriate use of antiviral drugs is also in its infancy. Phenotypic and genotypic assays for resistance to antiviral drugs are becoming more widely available, and correlations of laboratory results with clinical outcomes in various settings are beginning to be defined. Of particular note has been the development of highly sensitive and specific methods to measure the concentration of virus in blood (*virus load*), which permit direct assessment of the antiviral effect of a given drug regimen in the host. Virus load measurements have been useful in recognizing the risk of disease progression in patients with certain viral infections and in identifying patients in whom antiviral chemotherapy might be of greatest benefit. Like any in vitro laboratory test, these tests yield results that are highly dependent on (and likely to vary with) the laboratory techniques employed.

Information regarding the pharmacokinetics of some antiviral drugs, particularly in diverse clinical settings, is limited. Assays to measure the concentrations of these drugs, especially of their active moieties within cells, are not widely available. Thus, there are relatively few guidelines for adjusting dosages of antiviral agents to maximize antiviral activity and minimize toxicity. Clinical use of antiviral drugs must therefore be accompanied by particular vigilance with regard to unanticipated adverse effects.

Like that of other infections, the course of viral infections is profoundly affected by an interplay of the pathogen with a complex set of host defenses. The presence or absence of preexisting immunity and the ability to mount humoral and/or cell-mediated immune responses are important determinants of the outcome of viral infections. The state of the host's defenses needs to be considered when antiviral agents are utilized or evaluated.

As with any therapy, the optimal use of antiviral compounds requires a specific and timely diagnosis. For some viral infections, such as herpes zoster, the clinical manifestations are so characteristic that a diagnosis can be made on clinical grounds alone. For other viral infections, such as influenza A, epidemiologic information (e.g., the documentation of a community-wide outbreak) can be used to make a presumptive diagnosis with a high degree of accuracy. However, for most other viral infections, including herpes simplex encephalitis, cytomegaloviral infections other than retinitis, and enteroviral infections, diagnosis on clinical grounds alone cannot be accomplished with certainty. For such infections, rapid viral diagnostic techniques are of great importance. Considerable progress has been made in recent years in the development of such tests, which are now widely available for a number of viral infections.

Despite these complexities, the efficacy of a number of antiviral compounds has been clearly established in rigorously conducted and controlled studies. As summarized in Table 181-1, this chapter reviews the antiviral drugs that are currently approved or are likely to be considered for approval in the near future for use against viral infections other than those caused by HIV. Antiretroviral drugs are reviewed in Chap. 309.

ANTIVIRAL DRUGS ACTIVE AGAINST RESPIRATORY INFECTIONS

AMANTADINE AND RIMANTADINE Amantadine and the closely related compound rimantadine are primary symmetric amines. Their antiviral activity is limited to influenza A viruses, whose replication they inhibit by interfering with the uncoating of virus after infection of the cell. This interference is attributable to the agents' interaction with the influenza A M2 matrix protein, during which the ion channel function of M2 is inhibited. A substitution of a single amino acid in the M2 protein can result in a virus that is resistant to amantadine and rimantadine.

Amantadine and rimantadine have been demonstrated to be effective in the prophylaxis of influenza A in large-scale studies of young adults and in less extensive studies of children and elderly subjects. In such studies, efficacy rates of 55 to 80% in the prevention of influenza-like illness were noted, and even higher rates were reported when virus-specific attack rates were calculated. Amantadine and rimantadine have also been demonstrated to be effective in the treatment of influenza A infection in studies involving predominantly young adults and, to a lesser extent, children. Administration of these compounds within 24 to 72 h after the onset of illness has resulted in a reduction of the duration of signs and symptoms by ~50% from that in a placebo-treated group. The effect on signs and symptoms of illness is superior to that of commonly used antipyretic-analgesics. Only anecdotal reports are available concerning the efficacy of amantadine or rimantadine in the prevention or treatment of complications of influenza (e.g., pneumonia).

Amantadine and rimantadine are available only in oral formulations and are ordinarily administered to adults once or twice daily in a dose of 100 to 200 mg/d. Despite their structural similarities, the pharmacokinetics of the two compounds are different. Amantadine is not metabolized and is excreted almost entirely by the kidney, with a half-life of 12 to 17 h and peak plasma concentrations of 0.4 μg/mL. Rimantadine is extensively metabolized to hydroxylated derivatives and has a half-life of 30 h. Only 30 to 40% of an orally administered dose is recovered in the urine. The peak plasma levels of rimantadine are approximately half those of amantadine, but rimantadine is concentrated in respiratory secretions to a greater extent than amantadine. For prophylaxis, the compounds must be administered daily for the period at risk (i.e., the peak duration of the outbreak). For therapy, amantadine or rimantadine is generally administered for 5 to 7 days.

Although these compounds are generally well tolerated, 5 to 10% of amantadine recipients experience mild central nervous system side effects consisting primarily of dizziness, anxiety, insomnia, and dif-

ficulty in concentrating. These effects are rapidly reversible upon cessation of the drug's administration. At a dose of 200 mg/d, rimantadine is better tolerated than amantadine; in a large-scale study of young adults, adverse effects were no more frequent among rimantadine recipients than among placebo recipients. Seizures and worsening of congestive heart failure have also been reported in patients treated with amantadine, although a causal relationship has not been established. The dosage of amantadine should be reduced to ≤100 mg/d in patients with renal insufficiency [i.e., a creatinine clearance (Cr_{Cl}) rate of <50 mL/min] and in the elderly. A rimantadine dose of 100 mg/d should be used for patients with a Cr_{Cl} of <10 mL/min and in the elderly. Resistance to amantadine and rimantadine can be induced readily in vitro. The emergence and probable transmission of virus resistant to these drugs have also been noted in vivo after their use for the treatment of children or adults. In the United States, both amantadine and rimantadine are approved for the prophylaxis and treatment of influenza A in adults and for prophylaxis in children. Amantadine is also approved for the treatment of influenza A in children.

RIBAVIRIN Ribavirin is a synthetic nucleoside analogue that inhibits a wide range of RNA and DNA viruses. The mechanism of action of ribavirin is not completely defined and may be different for different groups of viruses. Ribavirin-5'-monophosphate blocks the conversion of inosine-5'-monophosphate to xanthosine-5'-monophosphate and interferes with the synthesis of guanine nucleotides as well as that of both RNA and DNA. Ribavirin-5'-monophosphate also inhibits capping of virus-specific messenger RNA in certain viral systems. In studies demonstrating the effectiveness of ribavirin, the compound has been administered as a small-particle aerosol. It has been used to treat respiratory syncytial virus (RSV) infections in infants and—less extensively—to treat parainfluenza virus infections in children and influenza A and B virus infections in young adults. In infants with RSV infection who were given ribavirin by continuous aerosol for 3 to 6 days, illness and lower respiratory tract signs resolved more rapidly and arterial oxygen desaturation was less pronounced than in placebo-treated groups. Ribavirin has also had a beneficial clinical effect in infants with RSV infection who require mechanical ventilation. Aerosolized ribavirin has been administered to older children and adults with severe RSV and parainfluenza virus infections (including immunosuppressed patients), but the benefit of this treatment, if any, is unclear. In RSV infections, ribavirin is often given in combination with immunoglobulins.

Orally administered ribavirin has not been effective in the treatment of influenza A virus infections. Intravenous or oral ribavirin has reduced mortality among patients with Lassa fever; it has been particularly effective in this regard when given within the first 6 days of illness. Intravenous ribavirin has been reported to be of clinical benefit in the treatment of hemorrhagic fever with renal syndrome caused by Hantaan virus and as therapy for Argentinian hemorrhagic fever. Moreover, oral ribavirin has been recommended for the treatment and prophylaxis of Congo-Crimean hemorrhagic fever. Intravenous ribavirin is being evaluated as therapy for the hemorrhagic fever with pulmonary syndrome caused by newly described hantaviruses in the United States. Oral administration of ribavirin reduces serum aminotransferase levels in patients with chronic hepatitis C virus (HCV) infection; since it appears not to reduce serum HCV RNA levels, the mechanism of this effect is unclear. Given in doses of 1000 to 1200 mg/d in combination with interferon (IFN) α (see below), ribavirin has been approved for the treatment of patients with chronic HCV infection.

Large doses of ribavirin administered orally (800 to 1000 mg/d) have been associated with reversible hematopoietic toxicity. This effect has not been observed with aerosolized ribavirin, apparently because little drug is absorbed systemically. Aerosolized administration of ribavirin is generally well tolerated but occasionally is associated with bronchospasm, rash, or conjunctival irritation. Aerosolized ribavirin has been licensed for treatment of RSV infection in infants and

Table 181-1 Antiviral Chemotherapy and Chemoprophylaxis

Infection	Drug	Route	Dosage	Comment
Influenza A and B Prophylaxis	Amantadine or rimantadine (influenza A only)	Oral	Adults: 200 mg/d for period at risk Children ≤9 yrs: 5 mg/kg per day (maximum, 150 mg/d)	Therapy must continue for duration of outbreak. Dosage should be reduced (more for amantadine) in patients with renal failure and the elderly. Drugs can be administered along with vaccine.
Treatment	Zanamivir	Inhaled orally	10 mg q12h for 5 days in adults and children ≥7 years old	Zanamivir and oseltamivir reduce symptoms by 1.0–1.5 and 1.3 days, respectively, in uncomplicated disease when started within 2 days of onset and are under study in complicated disease. Zanamivir may exacerbate bronchospasm in patients with asthma. Oseltamivir's side effects of nausea and vomiting can be reduced in frequency by administration with food. Both amantadine and rimantadine are effective in uncomplicated influenza. Neither has been thoroughly studied in complicated cases (e.g., pneumonia).
	Oseltamivir	Oral	75 mg bid for 5 days in adults	
	Amantadine (influenza A only)	Oral	100–200 mg/d in adults and dosage for children as above for 5–7 days	
	Rimantadine (influenza A only)	Oral	100–200 mg/d for 5–7 days in adults	
RSV infection	Ribavirin	Small-particle aerosol	Administered continuously from reservoir containing 20 mg/mL for 3–6 days	Ribavirin is used for treatment of infants and young children hospitalized with RSV pneumonia and bronchiolitis.
CMV retinitis in immunocompromised host	Ganciclovir	IV	5 mg/kg bid for 14–21 days; then 5 mg/kg per day as maintenance dose	Both ganciclovir and foscarnet are licensed for treatment of CMV retinitis in immunosuppressed patients, including those with AIDS. They are also used for colitis, pneumonia, or "wasting" syndromes associated with CMV and for prevention of CMV disease in transplant recipients. Foscarnet is not myelosuppressive and is active against acyclovir- and ganciclovir-resistant herpesviruses.
		Oral	1 g tid as maintenance dose	
	Foscarnet	IV	60 mg/kg q8h for 14–21 days; then 90–120 mg/kg per day as maintenance dose	
	Cidofovir	IV	5 mg/kg twice weekly for 2 weeks, then once weekly; given with probenecid	
Varicella Immunocompetent host	Acyclovir	Oral	20 mg/kg (maximum, 800 mg) 4 or 5 times daily for 5 days	Treatment confers modest clinical benefit when administered within 24 h of rash onset.
Immunocompromised host	Acyclovir	IV	500 mg/m² q8h for 7 days	A change to oral valacyclovir can be considered once fever has subsided and there is no evidence of visceral involvement.
Herpes simplex encephalitis	Acyclovir	IV	10 mg/kg q8h for 10–14 days	Results are optimal when therapy is initiated early. Some authorities treat for 21 days to prevent relapses.
Neonatal herpes simplex	Acyclovir	IV	10 mg/kg q8h for 14–21 days	Serious morbidity is frequent despite therapy. Prolonged oral administration of acyclovir after initial IV therapy has been suggested because of long-term sequelae associated with cutaneous recurrences of HSV infection.
Genital herpes simplex Primary (treatment)	Acyclovir	IV	5 mg/kg q8h for 5–10 days	The IV route is preferred for infections severe enough to warrant hospitalization or with neurologic complications.
		Oral	200 mg 5 times daily for 10 days	The oral route is preferred for patients whose condition does not warrant hospitalization. Adequate hydration must be maintained.
		Topical	5% ointment; 4–6 applications daily for 7–10 days	Topical use—largely supplemented by oral therapy—may obviate systemic administration to pregnant women. Systemic symptoms and untreated areas are not affected.
	Valacyclovir	Oral	1 g bid for 10 days	Valacyclovir appears to be as effective as acyclovir but can be administered less frequently.
	Famciclovir	Oral	250 mg bid for 5–10 days[a]	Famciclovir appears to be similar in effectiveness to acyclovir.
Recurrent (treatment)	Acyclovir	Oral	200 mg 5 times daily for 5 days	Clinical effect is modest and is enhanced if therapy is initiated early. Treatment does not affect recurrence rates.
	Famciclovir	Oral	125 mg bid for 5 days	
	Valacyclovir	Oral	500 mg bid for 5 days	

(continued)

Table 181-1—*(continued)*

Infection	Drug	Route	Dosage	Comment
Recurrent (suppression)	Acyclovir Valacyclovir Famciclovir	Oral Oral Oral	400 mg bid for ≥12 months 500–1000 mg daily 125–250 mg bid	Suppressive therapy is recommended only for patients with at least 6–10 recurrences per year. "Breakthrough" occasionally takes place, and asymptomatic shedding of virus occurs. The need for suppressive therapy should be reevaluated after 1 year. Experience with >1 year of valacyclovir or famciclovir therapy is limited.
Mucocutaneous herpes simplex in immunocompromised host Treatment	Acyclovir Valacyclovir Famciclovir	IV Oral Topical Oral Oral	250 mg/m² q8h for 7 days 400 mg 5 times daily for 10 days 5% ointment; 4–6 applications daily for 7 days or until healed 1 g tid for 7 days^a 500 mg bid for 4 days^a	Choice of IV or oral route depends on severity of infection and patient's ability to take oral medication. Oral or IV treatment has supplanted topical therapy except for small, easily accessible lesions. Foscarnet is used for acyclovir-resistant viruses.
Prevention of recurrences during intense immunosuppression	Acyclovir Valacyclovir Famciclovir	Oral IV Oral Oral	200 mg qid 5 mg/kg q12h 1 g tid^a 500 mg bid^a	Treatment is administered during periods when intense immunosuppression is expected—e.g., during antitumor chemotherapy or after transplantation—and is usually continued for 2–3 months.
Herpes simplex orolabialis (recurrent)	Penciclovir	Topical	1.0% cream applied q2h during waking hours for 4 days	Treatment shortens healing time and symptoms by 0.5–1.0 day (compared with placebo).
Herpes simplex keratitis	Trifluridine Vidarabine	Topical Topical	1 drop of 1% ophthalmic solution q2h while awake (maximum, 9 drops daily) 0.5-in. ribbon of 3% ophthalmic ointment 5 times daily	Therapy should be undertaken in consultation with an ophthalmologist.
Herpes zoster Immunocompromised host	Acyclovir Famciclovir	IV Oral Oral	500 mg/m² q8h for 7 days 800 mg 5 times daily for 7 days 500 mg tid for 10 days^a	Effectiveness in localized zoster is most marked when treatment is given early. Foscarnet may be used for VZV infections that are resistant to acyclovir.
Immunocompetent host	Valacyclovir	Oral	1 g tid for 7 days	Valacyclovir may be more effective than acyclovir for pain relief; otherwise, it has a similar effect on cutaneous lesions and should be given within 72 h of rash onset.
	Famciclovir	Oral	500 mg q8h for 7 days	The duration of postherpetic neuralgia is shorter than with placebo. Famciclovir showed overall efficacy similar to that of acyclovir in a comparative trial. It should be given ≤72 h of rash onset.
	Acyclovir	Oral	800 mg 5 times daily for 7–10 days	Acyclovir causes faster resolution of skin lesions than placebo and provides some relief of acute symptoms if given within 72 h of rash onset. Combined with tapering doses of prednisone, acyclovir improves quality-of-life outcomes.
Herpes zoster ophthalmicus	Acyclovir	Oral	600 mg 5 times daily for 10 days	Treatment reduces ocular complications, including ocular keratitis and uveitis.
Condyloma acuminatum	IFN-α2b IFN-αn3	Intralesional Intralesional	1 million units per wart (maximum of 5) thrice weekly for 3 weeks) 250,000 units per wart (maximum of 10) twice weekly for up to 8 weeks	Intralesional treatment frequently results in regression of warts, but lesions often recur. Parenteral administration may be useful if lesions are numerous.
Chronic hepatitis B	IFN-α2b Lamivudine	SC or IM Oral	5 million units daily or 10 million units thrice weekly for 24 weeks 100 mg/d for 1 year	Hepatitis B e antigen and DNA are eliminated in 33–37% of cases. Histopathologic improvement is also seen. Resistance develops in 15–36% of recipients.
Chronic hepatitis C	IFN-α2a or -α2b	SC or IM	3 million units thrice weekly for 12–18 months	A return of alanine aminotransferase levels to normal is documented in 54% of recipients but is sustained in only 28%. Improvement in liver histopathology is seen.

(continued)

Table 181-1 Antiviral Chemotherapy and Chemoprophylaxis—*(continued)*

Infection	Drug	Route	Dosage	Comment
	IFN-α2b/ribavirin	SC or IM/oral	3 million units thrice weekly/ 1000–1200 mg daily for 6–12 months	Combination therapy results in an increase in sustained responses (to 40–50% of recipients).
	IFN alfacon	SC	9–15 μg thrice weekly for 6–12 months	Doses of 9 and 15 μg are equivalent to IFN-α2a or -α2b doses of 3 million units and 5 million units, respectively.
Chronic hepatitis D	IFN-α2a or -α2b	SC or IM	5 million units daily or 10 million units thrice weekly for 6–12 months	The optimal regimen and duration of therapy have not been established. Responses are usually not sustained when therapy is stopped.

[a] Not approved for this indication by the U.S. Food and Drug Administration.

NOTE: CMV, cytomegalovirus; HSV, herpes simplex virus; IFN, interferon; RSV, respiratory syncytial virus; VZV, varicella-zoster virus.

should be administered under close supervision—particularly in the setting of mechanical ventilation, where precipitation of the drug is possible. Health care workers exposed to the drug have experienced minor toxicity, including eye and respiratory tract irritation. Because ribavirin is mutagenic, teratogenic, and embryotoxic, its use is generally contraindicated in pregnancy. Its administration as an aerosol poses a risk to pregnant health care workers.

ZANAMIVIR AND OSELTAMIVIR Influenza viral neuraminidase is essential for release of the virus from infected cells and for its subsequent spread throughout the respiratory tract of the infected host. The enzyme cleaves terminal sialic acid residues, thus destroying the cellular receptors recognized by the viral hemagglutinin. Zanamivir, a sialic acid analogue, is a highly active and specific inhibitor of the neuraminidases of influenza A and B viruses. Oseltamivir is another neuraminidase inhibitor that is a transition-state analogue of sialic acid cleavage. Its antineuraminidase activity is similar to that of zanamivir. Oseltamivir phosphate is an ethyl ester prodrug that is converted to oseltamivir carboxylate by esterases in the liver. Both zanamivir and oseltamivir act through competitive and reversible inhibition of the active site of influenza A and B viral neuraminidases and have relatively little effect on mammalian cell enzymes. As would be expected from their different mechanisms of action, zanamivir and oseltamivir are active against strains of influenza A virus that are resistant to amantadine and rimantadine.

Zanamivir has low oral bioavailability. It is inhaled orally via a hand-held inhaler. By this route, ~15% of the dose is deposited in the lower respiratory tract, and low plasma levels of the drug are detected. Orally administered oseltamivir has an oral bioavailability of >60% and a plasma half-life of 7 to 9 h. The drug is excreted unmetabolized, primarily by the kidney.

Intranasal inhaled zanamivir is generally well tolerated. The most frequent toxicities encountered with orally administered oseltamivir are nausea, gastrointestinal discomfort, and (less commonly) vomiting. Gastrointestinal discomfort is usually transient and is less likely if the drug is administered with food. No serious clinical or laboratory toxicities have yet been reported with zanamivir or oseltamivir in clinical trials.

Inhaled zanamivir and orally administered oseltamivir have been effective in the treatment of naturally occurring influenza A or B in otherwise healthy adults. In placebo-controlled studies, illness has been shortened by 1 to 1.5 days of therapy with either of these drugs. Once-daily inhaled zanamivir or orally administered oseltamivir provides effective prophylaxis against laboratory-documented influenza A–associated illness. The emergence of viruses resistant to zanamivir or oseltamivir appears to be infrequent in clinical studies carried out thus far.

As of this writing, zanamivir and oseltamivir have been approved by the U.S. Food and Drug Administration (FDA) for treatment of influenza in adults (and—in the case of zanamivir—in children ≥7 years of age) who have been symptomatic for ≤2 days. Indications for prophylactic use are under review.

ANTIVIRAL DRUGS ACTIVE AGAINST HERPESVIRUS INFECTIONS

ACYCLOVIR AND VALACYCLOVIR Acyclovir is a highly potent and selective inhibitor of the replication of certain herpesviruses, including herpes simplex virus (HSV) types 1 and 2, varicella-zoster virus (VZV), and Epstein-Barr virus (EBV). It is relatively ineffective in the treatment of human cytomegalovirus (CMV) infections; however, some studies have indicated its effectiveness in the prevention of CMV-associated disease in immunosuppressed patients. Valacyclovir, the L-valyl ester of acyclovir, is converted almost entirely to acyclovir after oral administration. Valacyclovir has pharmacokinetic advantages over orally administered acyclovir: it exhibits significantly greater oral bioavailability, results in higher blood levels, and can be given less frequently than acyclovir.

The high degree of selectivity of acyclovir is related to its mechanism of action, which requires that the compound first be phosphorylated to acyclovir monophosphate. This phosphorylation occurs efficiently in herpesvirus-infected cells by means of a virus-coded thymidine kinase. In uninfected mammalian cells, little phosphorylation of acyclovir occurs, and the drug is therefore concentrated in herpesvirus-infected cells. Acyclovir monophosphate is subsequently converted by host cell kinases to a triphosphate that is a potent inhibitor of virus-induced DNA polymerase but has relatively little effect on host cell DNA polymerase. Acyclovir triphosphate can also be incorporated into viral DNA, with early chain termination.

Acyclovir is available in intravenous, oral, and topical forms, while valacyclovir is available in an oral formulation. Intravenous acyclovir is markedly effective in the treatment of mucocutaneous HSV infections in immunocompromised hosts, reducing time to healing, duration of pain, and virus shedding. When administered prophylactically during periods of intense immunosuppression (e.g., related to chemotherapy for leukemia or transplantation) and before the development of lesions, intravenous acyclovir reduces the frequency of HSV-associated disease. After prophylaxis is discontinued, HSV lesions recur. Intravenous acyclovir is also effective in the treatment of HSV encephalitis; two comparative trials have indicated that acyclovir is more effective than vidarabine for this indication (see below). Because VZV is generally less sensitive to acyclovir than is HSV, higher doses of acyclovir must be used to treat VZV infections. In immunocompromised patients with herpes zoster, intravenous acyclovir reduces the frequency of cutaneous dissemination and visceral complications and—in one comparative trial—was more effective than vidarabine. Acyclovir, administered orally at doses of 800 mg five times a day, had a modest beneficial effect on localized herpes zoster lesions in both immunocompromised and immunocompetent patients. Combination of acyclovir with a tapering regimen of prednisone appeared to be more effective than acyclovir alone in terms of quality-of-life outcomes in immunocompetent herpes zoster patients over age 50. A comparative study of acyclovir (800 mg orally five times daily) and valacyclovir (1 g orally tid) in immunocompetent patients with herpes zoster indicated that the latter drug may be more effective in eliciting the resolution of zoster-associated pain. Orally administered acyclovir (600 mg five times a day) reduced complications of herpes zoster ophthalmicus in a placebo-controlled trial.

In normal children with chickenpox, acyclovir—administered at 20 mg/kg qid, up to a maximum of 800 mg qid, within 24 h of the onset of rash—resulted in a modest overall clinical benefit. Intravenous acyclovir has also been reported to be effective in the treatment of immunocompromised children with chickenpox.

The most widespread use of acyclovir is in the treatment of genital HSV infections. Intravenous or oral acyclovir or oral valacyclovir has shortened the duration of symptoms, reduced virus shedding, and accelerated healing when employed for the treatment of primary genital HSV infections. Oral acyclovir and valacyclovir have also had a modest effect in treatment of recurrent genital HSV infections. However, the failure of treatment of either primary or recurrent disease to reduce the frequency of subsequent recurrences has indicated that acyclovir is ineffective in eliminating latent infection. Chronic oral administration of acyclovir for periods of 1 to 6 years or longer or of valacyclovir for up to 1 year has reduced the frequency of recurrences markedly during therapy; once the drug is discontinued, lesions recur. In AIDS patients, chronic or intermittent administration of acyclovir has been associated with the development of HSV and VZV strains resistant to the action of the drug and with clinical failures. The most common mechanism of resistance is a deficiency of the virus-induced thymidine kinase. Patients with HSV or VZV infections resistant to acyclovir have frequently responded to foscarnet.

With the availability of the oral and intravenous forms, there are few indications for topical acyclovir, although treatment with this formulation has been modestly beneficial in primary genital HSV infections and in mucocutaneous HSV infections in immunocompromised hosts.

Overall, acyclovir is remarkably well tolerated and is generally free of toxicity. The most frequently encountered form of toxicity is renal dysfunction, particularly after rapid intravenous administration or with inadequate hydration. Central nervous system changes, including lethargy and tremors, are occasionally reported, primarily in immunosuppressed patients. However, whether these changes are related to acyclovir, to concurrent administration of other therapy, or to underlying infection remains unclear. Acyclovir is excreted primarily unmetabolized by the kidney, via both glomerular filtration and tubular secretion. Approximately 15% of a dose of acyclovir is metabolized to 9-[(carboxymethoxy)methyl]guanine or other minor metabolites. Reduction in dosage is indicated in patients with a Cr_{Cl} of <50 mL/min per 1.73 m². The half-life of acyclovir is ~3 h in normal adults, and the peak plasma concentration after a 1-h infusion of a dose of 5 mg/kg is 9.8 μg/mL. Approximately 22% of an orally administered acyclovir dose is absorbed, and peak plasma concentrations of 0.3 to 0.9 μg/mL are attained after administration of a 200-mg dose. Acyclovir penetrates relatively well into the cerebrospinal fluid (CSF), with concentrations approaching half of those found in plasma.

Acyclovir causes chromosomal breakage at high doses, but its administration to pregnant women has not been associated with fetal abnormalities. Nonetheless, the potential risks and benefits of acyclovir should be carefully assessed before the drug is used in pregnancy.

Valacyclovir exhibits three to five times greater bioavailability than acyclovir. The concentration-time curve for valacyclovir, given as 1 g orally tid, is similar to that for acyclovir, given as 5 mg/kg intravenously every 8 h. The safety profiles of valacyclovir and acyclovir are similar, although thrombotic thrombocytopenic purpura/hemolytic-uremic syndrome has been reported in immunocompromised patients who have received high doses of valacyclovir. Valacyclovir is approved for the treatment of herpes zoster and for initial and recurrent episodes of genital HSV infections in immunocompetent adults as well as for suppressive treatment of genital herpes. It is being studied for use against other herpesvirus infections in various clinical settings.

CIDOFOVIR Cidofovir is a phosphonate nucleotide analogue of cytosine. Its major use is in CMV infections, particularly retinitis, but it is active against a broad range of herpesviruses, including HSV, human herpesvirus (HHV) type 6, HHV-8, and certain other DNA viruses such as polyomaviruses, papillomaviruses, and adenoviruses. Cidofovir does not require initial phosphorylation by virus-induced kinases; the drug is phosphorylated by host cell enzymes to cidofovir diphosphate, which is a competitive inhibitor of viral DNA polymerases and, to a lesser extent, of host cell DNA polymerases. Incorporation of cidofovir diphosphate slows or terminates nascent DNA chain elongation. Cidofovir is active against HSV isolates that are resistant to acyclovir because of absent or altered thymidine kinase and against CMV isolates that are resistant to ganciclovir because of UL97 mutations. Cidofovir is usually active against foscarnet-resistant CMV, although cross-resistance to foscarnet as well as to ganciclovir has been described.

Cidofovir has poor oral availability and is administered intravenously. It is excreted primarily by the kidney and has a plasma half-life of 2.6 h. Cidofovir diphosphate's intracellular half-life of >48 h is the basis for the recommended dosing regimen of 5 mg/kg twice a week for the initial 2 weeks and then 5 mg/kg once a week. The major toxic effect of cidofovir is proximal renal tubular injury, as manifested by elevated serum creatinine levels and proteinuria. The risk of nephrotoxicity can be reduced by vigorous saline hydration and by concomitant oral administration of probenecid. Neutropenia, rashes, and gastrointestinal tolerance may also occur.

Intravenous cidofovir has been approved for the treatment of CMV retinitis in AIDS patients who are intolerant of ganciclovir or foscarnet or in whom those drugs have failed. In a controlled study, a maintenance dosage of 5 mg/kg a week administered to AIDS patients reduced the progression of CMV retinitis from that seen at 3 mg/kg. Intravenous cidofovir has been reported anecdotally to be effective therapy for acyclovir-resistant mucocutaneous HSV infections. Likewise, topically administered cidofovir is reportedly beneficial against these infections in HIV patients; it is also being studied for the treatment of anogenital warts. Intravenous cidofovir is being evaluated as therapy for progressive multifocal leukoencephalopathy and for Kaposi's sarcoma. An ophthalmic formulation is being studied as treatment for adenoviral keratoconjunctivitis. Intravitreal cidofovir has been used to treat CMV retinitis but has been associated with significant toxicity.

FOMIVIRSEN Fomivirsen is the first antisense oligonucleotide approved by the U.S. Food and Drug Administration (FDA) for therapy in humans. This phosphorothioate oligonucleotide, 21 nucleotides in length, inhibits CMV replication through interaction with CMV messenger RNA. Fomivirsen is complementary to messenger transcripts of the major immediate early region 2 (IE2) of CMV, which codes for proteins regulating viral gene expression. In addition to its antisense mechanism of action, fomivirsen may exert activity against CMV through inhibition of viral adsorption to cells as well as direct inhibition of viral replication. Because of its different mechanism of action, fomivirsen is active against CMV isolates that are resistant to nucleoside or nucleotide analogues, such as ganciclovir, foscarnet, or cidofovir.

Fomivirsen has been approved for intravitreal administration in the treatment of CMV retinitis in AIDS patients who have failed to respond to other treatments or cannot tolerate them. Injections of 330 mg every 2 weeks have resulted in significant reductions in the rate of progression of CMV retinitis. The major toxicity is ocular inflammation, including vitritis and iritis, which usually responds to topically administered glucocorticoids.

GANCICLOVIR An analogue of acyclovir, ganciclovir is active against HSV and VZV and is markedly more active than acyclovir against CMV. Ganciclovir triphosphate inhibits CMV DNA polymerase and can be incorporated into CMV DNA, whose elongation it eventually terminates. In HSV- and VZV-infected cells, ganciclovir is phosphorylated by virus-encoded thymidine kinases; in CMV-infected cells, it is phosphorylated by a viral kinase encoded by the UL97 gene. Ganciclovir triphosphate is present in tenfold higher concentrations in CMV-infected cells than in uninfected cells. Ganciclovir is approved for the treatment of CMV retinitis in immunosuppressed patients and for the prevention of CMV disease in transplant recipients. It is widely used for the treatment of other CMV-associated syndromes, including pneumonia, esophagogastrointestinal infections, hepatitis, and "wasting" illness.

Ganciclovir is available for intravenous or oral administration. Because its oral bioavailability is low (5 to 9%), relatively large doses (1 g tid) must be administered by this route. Oral bioavailability is enhanced if the drug is administered with food, as recommended. The serum half-life of ganciclovir is 3.5 h after intravenous administration and 4.5 h after oral administration. The drug is excreted primarily by the kidney in unmetabolized form, and its dosage should be reduced in cases of renal failure. The most commonly employed dosage for initial therapy—5 mg/kg intravenously every 12 h for 14 to 21 days— is followed by a maintenance dose of 5 mg/kg intravenously per day or 5 times per week, possibly for as long as immunosuppression persists. Oral ganciclovir is approved as an alternative to the intravenous preparation in maintenance therapy for CMV retinitis, where it appears to be somewhat less effective although more convenient than intravenous therapy. Intraocular ganciclovir, given by either intravitreal injection or intraocular implantation, has also been used to treat CMV retinitis.

Ganciclovir is effective as prophylaxis against CMV-associated disease in organ and bone marrow transplant recipients. Oral ganciclovir administered prophylactically to AIDS patients with CD4+ counts of <100/μL provided protection against the development of CMV retinitis in one large-scale study and was subsequently approved for that indication. However, the long-term benefits of this approach to prophylaxis are unestablished, and most experts do not recommend the use of oral ganciclovir for that purpose.

The administration of ganciclovir has been associated with profound bone marrow suppression, particularly neutropenia, which significantly limits the drug's use in many patients. Bone marrow toxicity is potentiated when other bone marrow suppressants, such as zidovudine, are used concomitantly.

Resistance has been noted in CMV isolates obtained after therapy with ganciclovir, especially in patients with AIDS. Such resistance may develop through a mutation in either the viral UL97 gene or the viral DNA polymerase. Ganciclovir-resistant isolates are usually sensitive to foscarnet (see below).

FAMCICLOVIR AND PENCICLOVIR Famciclovir is the diacetyl 6-deoxyester of the guanosine analogue penciclovir. Famciclovir is well absorbed orally, with a bioavailability of 77%, and is rapidly converted by deacetylation and oxidation to penciclovir. Penciclovir's spectrum of activity and mechanism of action are similar to those of acyclovir; thus penciclovir is not active against acyclovir-resistant viruses. Penciclovir is phosphorylated initially by a virus-encoded thymidine kinase and subsequently by cellular kinases to penciclovir triphosphate, which inhibits HSV-1, HSV-2, and VZV DNA polymerases as well as hepatitis B virus (HBV). The serum half-life of penciclovir is 2 h, but the intracellular half-life of penciclovir triphosphate is 7 to 20 h—markedly longer than that of acyclovir triphosphate. Penciclovir is eliminated primarily in the urine by both glomerular filtration and tubular secretion. The usually recommended dosage interval should be adjusted for renal insufficiency.

Clinical trials involving immunocompetent adults with herpes zoster showed that famciclovir was superior to placebo in eliciting the resolution of skin lesions and virus shedding and in shortening the duration of postherpetic neuralgia; moreover, it was at least as effective as acyclovir administered orally at a dose of 800 mg five times daily. Famciclovir was also effective in the treatment of herpes zoster in

immunosuppressed patients. Clinical trials have demonstrated its effectiveness in suppression of genital HSV infections for up to 1 year and in the treatment of initial and recurrent episodes of genital herpes. Famciclovir is effective as therapy for mucocutaneous HSV infections in HIV-infected patients. Application of a 1% penciclovir cream reduces the duration of signs and symptoms of herpes labialis in immunocompetent patients (by 0.5 to 1.0 day) and has been approved for that purpose by the FDA. Famciclovir is generally well tolerated, with occasional headache, nausea, and diarrhea reported in frequencies similar to those among placebo recipients. The administration of high doses of famciclovir for 2 years was associated with an increased incidence of mammary adenocarcinomas in female rats, but the clinical significance of this effect is unknown. Intravenous penciclovir is being investigated for the treatment of mucocutaneous HSV infections in immunosuppressed patients.

FOSCARNET Foscarnet (phosphonoformic acid) is a pyrophosphate-containing compound that potently inhibits herpesviruses, including CMV. This drug inhibits DNA polymerases at the pyrophosphate binding site at concentrations that have relatively little effect on cellular polymerases. Foscarnet does not require phosphorylation to exert its antiviral activity and is therefore active against HSV and VZV isolates that are resistant to acyclovir because of deficiencies in thymidine kinase as well as against most ganciclovir-resistant strains of CMV. Foscarnet also inhibits the reverse transcriptase of HIV and is active against HIV in vivo.

Foscarnet is poorly soluble and must be administered intravenously via an infusion pump in a dilute solution over 1 to 2 h. The plasma half-life of foscarnet is 3 to 5 h and increases with decreasing renal function, since the drug is eliminated primarily by the kidneys. It has been estimated that 10 to 28% of a dose may be deposited in bone, where it can persist for months. The most common initial dosage of foscarnet—60 mg/kg every 8 h for 14 to 21 days—is followed by a maintenance dose of 90 to 120 mg/kg once a day.

Foscarnet is approved for the treatment of CMV retinitis in patients with AIDS and of acyclovir-resistant mucocutaneous HSV infections. In a comparative clinical trial, the drug appeared to be about as efficacious as ganciclovir against CMV retinitis but was associated with a longer survival period, possibly because of its anti-HIV activity. Intraocular foscarnet has been used to treat CMV retinitis. Foscarnet has also been employed to treat acyclovir-resistant HSV and VZV infections as well as ganciclovir-resistant CMV infections, although resistance to foscarnet has been reported in CMV isolates obtained during therapy.

The major form of toxicity associated with foscarnet is renal impairment. Thus renal function should be monitored closely, particularly during the initial phase of therapy. Since foscarnet binds divalent metal ions, hypocalcemia, hypomagnesemia, hypokalemia, and hypo- or hyperphosphatemia can develop. Saline hydration and slow infusion appear to protect the patient against nephrotoxicity and electrolyte disturbances. Although hematologic abnormalities have been documented (most commonly anemia), foscarnet is not generally myelosuppressive and may be administered concomitantly with myelosuppressive medications such as zidovudine.

IDOXURIDINE Idoxuridine inhibits the replication of herpesviruses and poxviruses. It was formerly used systemically to treat herpesvirus infections, but, because of associated toxicity and lack of proven efficacy, its systemic use has largely been abandoned. Topical idoxuridine is effective in the treatment of HSV keratitis, particularly in superficial infections, but has been supplanted by topically applied trifluridine and vidarabine (see below).

TRIFLURIDINE Trifluridine is a pyrimidine nucleoside active against HSV-1, HSV-2, and CMV. Trifluridine monophosphate irreversibly inhibits thymidylate synthetase, and trifluridine triphosphate inhibits viral and, to a lesser extent, cellular DNA polymerases. Because of systemic toxicity, its use is limited to topical therapy. Trifluridine is approved for treatment of HSV keratitis, for which trials have shown that it is more effective than topical idoxuridine but similarly effective to topical vidarabine. The drug has benefited some patients with HSV keratitis who have failed to respond to idoxuridine or vidarabine. Topical application of trifluridine to sites of acyclovir-resistant HSV mucocutaneous infections has also been beneficial in some cases.

VIDARABINE Vidarabine is a purine nucleoside analogue with activity against HSV-1, HSV-2, VZV, and EBV. Vidarabine inhibits viral DNA synthesis through its 5′-triphosphorylated metabolite, although its precise molecular mechanisms of action are not completely understood. Intravenously administered vidarabine has been shown to be effective in the treatment of herpes simplex encephalitis, mucocutaneous HSV infections and herpes zoster in immunocompromised patients and of neonatal HSV infections. Its use has been supplanted by intravenous acyclovir, which is more effective and easier to administer. Production of the intravenous preparation has been discontinued by the manufacturer, but vidarabine is available as an ophthalmic ointment, which is effective in the treatment of HSV keratitis.

OTHER ANTIVIRAL DRUGS *Lamivudine* is a pyrimidine nucleoside analogue that is used primarily in combination therapy against HIV infection (Chap. 309). It is also active against HBV through inhibition of the viral DNA polymerase and has been approved for the treatment of chronic HBV infection. In one study, at doses of 100 mg/d for ≥1 year, lamivudine was well tolerated and resulted in suppression of HBV DNA levels, normalization of serum aminotransferase levels in most patients, and reduction of hepatic inflammation and fibrosis. Loss of hepatitis B e antigen (HBeAg) occurred in a minority of patients. Resistance to lamivudine developed in 15 to 36% of patients treated for 1 year and was associated with changes in the YMDD motif of HBV DNA polymerase. This is an important limitation of monotherapy with the drug. Studies of lamivudine as a component of combination therapy for hepatitis B are under way. Lamivudine also appears to be useful in the prevention or suppression of HBV infection associated with liver transplantation.

Lobucavir is a synthetic cyclobutane nucleoside analogue with activity against a broad range of herpesviruses, HIV, and HBV. It is currently under investigation in clinical trials. Its mechanism of action is through inhibition of viral DNA synthesis. Lobucavir is initially phosphorylated by virus-induced kinases, and lobucavir triphosphate is a potent inhibitor of HSV, CMV, and HBV DNA polymerases. Lobucavir can be administered orally or intravenously. It is excreted largely unmetabolized via the kidney and has a plasma half-life of 2 h after intravenous administration. Its oral availability is dose-dependent, ranging from 25 to 40% at doses of ≤200 mg and decreasing at higher doses. The preclinical toxicity profile of lobucavir appears to be similar to that of ganciclovir. However, neutropenia has been uncommonly encountered in studies in humans. Aminotransferase elevations have been documented after intravenous and (less commonly) oral administration. The most frequent adverse effects after oral administration are headache, insomnia, and gastrointestinal discomfort. In clinical trials to date, oral lobucavir has demonstrated antiviral effects in CMV- and HBV-infected patients as well as clinical benefits against HSV infections in immunocompetent patients. Short-term (1-month) oral administration of 200 mg of lobucavir bid or qid reduced serum HBV DNA levels in chronically infected patients. HBV DNA levels returned to pretreatment values when the drug was stopped, and studies of longer-term administration are under way. Lobucavir is under clinical investigation for use in HIV infection and in several herpesvirus infections.

Pleconaril is an investigational drug active in vitro against picornavirus replication, including over 90% of the most commonly isolated enterovirus types and 80% of rhinovirus serotypes. Its mechanism of action is through binding to a specific hydrophobic pocket in the viral capsid, which prevents attachment and/or uncoating of the virus. Pleconaril is poorly water soluble and is formulated as an oral suspension. After oral administration of 200- and 400-mg doses to adults, peak plasma concentrations are 1.1 and 2.4 μg/mL, respectively, and the terminal plasma half-life is 25 h. Pleconaril is generally well tolerated; the most frequently reported adverse effects are headache, nausea, diarrhea, and gastrointestinal discomfort, which have occurred at rates

similar to those among placebo recipients. Orally administered pleconaril, given before and after experimental infection of healthy volunteers with coxsackievirus A21, reduced peak viral titers by >100-fold and decreased the subsequent rate of development of illness. Pleconaril treatment of adults with enteroviral meningitis decreased the overall duration of illness and headache and reduced the use of analgesics from that by placebo recipients. Clinical studies of pleconaril in other enterovirus-induced diseases are in progress.

INTERFERONS

Interferons are cytokines that exhibit a broad spectrum of antiviral activities as well as immunomodulating and antiproliferative properties. The IFNs are not available for oral administration but must be given intramuscularly, subcutaneously, or intravenously. Early studies with human leukocyte IFN demonstrated an effect in the prophylaxis of experimentally induced rhinovirus infections in humans and in the treatment of VZV infections in immunosuppressed patients. DNA recombinant technology has made available highly purified α, β, and γ IFNs that have been evaluated in a variety of viral infections. Results of such trials have confirmed the effectiveness of intranasally administered IFN in the prophylaxis of rhinovirus infections, although its use has been associated with nasal mucosal irritation. Studies have also demonstrated a beneficial effect of intralesionally or systemically administered IFNs on genital warts. The effect of systemic administration consists primarily of a reduction in the size of lesions, and this mode of therapy may be useful in individuals who have numerous warts that cannot easily be treated by individual intralesional injection. However, lesions frequently recur after intralesional or systemic IFN therapy is discontinued.

Interferons have undergone extensive study in the treatment of chronic HBV infection. The administration of IFN-α2b (5 million units daily for 16 weeks) to patients with stable chronic HBV infection resulted in loss of markers of HBV replication, such as HBeAg and HBV DNA, in 33 to 37% of cases; 10 to 20% of patients also became negative for hepatitis B surface antigen. In >80% of patients who lose HBeAg and HBV DNA markers, serum aminotransferases return to normal levels, and both short- and long-term improvements in liver histopathology have been described. Predictors of a favorable response to therapy include low pretherapy levels of HBV DNA, high pretherapy serum levels of alanine aminotransferase (ALT), a short duration of chronic HBV infection, and active liver histopathology. Poor responses are seen in immunosuppressed patients, including those with HIV infection. Adverse effects of the above dose of IFN are common and include fever, chills, myalgia, fatigue, neurotoxicity (primarily manifested as somnolence and confusion), and leukopenia. Approximately 25% of patients receiving a daily dose of 5 million units require dose reduction, but fewer than 5% require discontinuation of therapy.

Several IFN preparations, including α2a, α2b, alfacon-1, and αm1 (lymphoblastoid), have been studied as therapy for chronic HCV infections. A variety of regimens have been employed, of which the most common is IFN-α2b or -α2a at 3 million units three times per week for 12 months. A complete biochemical response, defined as a return to normal serum ALT values at the end of treatment, has been documented in ~54% of patients. In addition, liver biopsies have shown decreases in lobular and periportal inflammation. However, relapse has occurred in approximately half of all cases upon discontinuation of therapy, so that sustained responses were documented in 28% of cases. The addition of oral ribavirin to IFN-α2b—either as initial therapy or after failure of interferon therapy alone—resulted in significantly higher rates of sustained response (40 to 50%) than were obtained with monotherapy. Prognostic factors for a favorable response include an age of <45 years, a short duration of disease, low levels of HCV RNA, and infection with HCV genotypes other than 1. IFN alfacon, a synthetic "consensus" α interferon, appears to produce response rates similar to those elicited by IFN-α2a or -α2b and has recently been approved in the United States for the treatment of chronic hepatitis C.

Treatment of chronic hepatitis D with IFN-α apparently requires higher doses (5 million units daily or 10 million units three times per week) and is less effective than treatment of chronic hepatitis B or C. After 12 months of therapy, biochemical and virologic responses were detected in $\geq$50% of patients, but few responses were sustained once therapy was stopped.

BIBLIOGRAPHY

BALFOUR HH: Antiviral drugs. N Engl J Med 340:1255, 1999

CRUMPACKER CS: Ganciclovir. N Engl J Med 335:721, 1996

DOLIN R et al: A controlled trial of amantadine and rimantadine in the prophylaxis of influenza A infection. N Engl J Med 307:580, 1982

HALL CB et al: Aerosolized ribavirin treatment of infants with respiratory syncytial viral infection: A randomized double-blind study. N Engl J Med 308:1443, 1983

LALEZARI JP et al: Randomized controlled study of the safety and efficacy of intravenous cidofovir for the treatment of relapsing cytomegalovirus retinitis in patients with AIDS. J AIDS 17:339, 1998

POYNARD T et al: Meta-analysis of interferon randomized trials in the treatment of viral hepatitis C: Effect of dose and duration. Hepatology 24:778, 1996

REICHMAN RC et al: Treatment of condyloma acuminatum with three different interferons administered intralesionally: A double-blind, placebo-controlled trial. Ann Intern Med 108:675, 1988

WHITLEY RJ et al: Herpes simplex encephalitis: Adenine arabinoside versus acyclovir therapies. N Engl J Med 314:144, 1986

WONG DKH et al: Effect of alpha-interferon treatment in patients with hepatitis B e antigen–positive chronic hepatitis B. Ann Intern Med 119:312, 1993

Section 12
DNA VIRUSES

182   *Lawrence Corey*

HERPES SIMPLEX VIRUSES

DEFINITION   Herpes simplex viruses (HSV-1, HSV-2; *Herpesvirus hominis*) produce a variety of infections involving mucocutaneous surfaces, the central nervous system (CNS), and—on occasion—visceral organs. The advent of effective chemotherapy for HSV infections has made prompt recognition of these syndromes even more clinically important than in the past.

ETIOLOGIC AGENT   The genome of HSV is a linear, double-stranded DNA molecule (molecular weight, ~100 $\times$ 10^6) that encodes more than 75 gene products. The genomic structures of the two HSV subtypes are similar, and the overall sequence homology between HSV-1 and HSV-2 is ~50%. The homologous sequences are distributed over the entire genome map, and most of the polypeptides specified by one viral type are antigenically related to polypeptides of the other viral type. Many type-specific regions unique to HSV-1 and HSV-2 proteins do exist, however, and a number of them appear to be important in host immunity. These type-specific regions have been used to develop serologic assays that distinguish between the two viral subtypes. Restriction endonuclease analysis of viral DNA can be used to distinguish between the two subtypes and among strains of each subtype. The variability of nucleotide sequences from clinical strains of HSV-1 and HSV-2 is such that HSV isolates obtained from two individuals can be differentiated by restriction enzyme patterns unless the isolates are from epidemiologically related sources, such as sexual partners, mother-infant pairs, or persons involved in a common-source outbreak.

The viral genome is packaged in a regular icosahedral protein shell (capsid) composed of 162 capsomers. The outer covering of the virus is a lipid-containing membrane (envelope) derived from modified cell membrane and acquired as the DNA-containing capsid buds through the inner nuclear membrane of the host cell. Between the capsid and lipid bilayer of the envelope is the tegument. Viral replication has both nuclear and cytoplasmic phases. The initial steps of replication include attachment, fusion between the viral envelope and the cell membrane to liberate the nucleocapsid into the cytoplasm of the cell, and disassembly of the nucleocapsid to release the viral DNA. Replication of HSV is highly regulated. After fusion of the virion envelope with the host cell membrane, several viral proteins are released from the HSV virion. Some shut off host protein synthesis (by increasing cellular RNA degradation), while others "turn on" transcription of early genes of HSV replication. These early gene products, designated α genes, are required for synthesis of the subsequent polypeptide group, the β polypeptides, many of which are regulatory proteins and enzymes required for DNA replication. Most current antiviral drugs interfere with β proteins, such as the viral DNA polymerase enzyme. The third (γ) class of HSV genes requires viral DNA replication for expression and constitutes most of the structural proteins specified by the virus.

After replication of the viral genome and synthesis of structural proteins, nucleocapsids are assembled in the nucleus of the cell. Envelopment occurs as the nucleocapsids bud through the inner nuclear membrane into the perinuclear space. In some cells, viral replication in the nucleus forms two types of inclusion bodies: type A basophilic Feulgen-positive bodies that contain viral DNA and an eosinophilic inclusion body that is devoid of viral nucleic acid or protein and represents a "scar" of viral infection. Virions are then transported via the endoplasmic reticulum and the Golgi apparatus to the cell surface.

HSV infection of some neuronal cells does not result in cell death. Instead, viral genomes are maintained by the cell in a repressed state compatible with survival and normal activities of the cell, a condition called *latency*. Latency is associated with transcription of only a limited number of virus-encoded proteins. Subsequently, the viral genome may become activated, resulting in the normal pattern of regulated viral gene expression, replication, and release of HSV. The release of virus from the neuron and its subsequent entry into epithelial cells result in viral replication. This process is termed *reactivation*. Whereas infectious virus rarely can be recovered from sensory or autonomic nervous system ganglia dissected from cadavers, maintenance and growth of the neural cells in tissue culture result in production of infectious virions (*explantation*) and in subsequent permissive infection of susceptible cells (*cocultivation*). The fact that HSV replication was first detected in neurons during reactivation in vitro suggested that the neuron harbors the latent virus in vivo. Viral DNA and RNA have since been found in neural tissue at times when infectious virus cannot be isolated. Two RNA "latency-associated" transcripts that overlap the immediate early (α) gene products, called ICP-O, are found in abundance in the nuclei of latently infected neurons. These latency-associated transcripts code proteins in an antisense direction. Deletion mutants of this region that can become latent have been made. However, the efficiency of their later reactivation is reduced; thus, the antisense transcripts may play a role in maintaining rather than in establishing latency. At present, the molecular mechanisms of the latency of HSV-1 and HSV-2 are not well understood, and strategies to interrupt latency or to maintain molecular latency in neurons are not available.

Exposure to HSV at mucosal surfaces or abraded skin sites permits entry of the virus and initiation of its replication in cells of the epidermis and dermis. Investigators have identified several cell receptors that are ligands for HSV attachment proteins. Studies to define how these receptors influence viral replication and pathogenesis are under way. Initial HSV infection is often subclinical—i.e., without clinically apparent lesions. Both clinical acquisition and subclinical acquisition are associated with sufficient viral replication to permit infection of either sensory or autonomic nerve endings. On entry into the neuronal cell, the virus—or, more likely, the nucleocapsid—is transported intraaxonally to the nerve cell bodies in ganglia. In humans, the interval from inoculation of virus in peripheral tissue to spread to the ganglia is unknown. During the initial phase of infection, viral replication occurs in ganglia and contiguous neural tissue. Virus then spreads to other mucosal skin surfaces through centrifugal migration of infectious virions via peripheral sensory nerves. This mode of spread helps explain the large surface area involved, the high frequency of new lesions distant from the initial crop of vesicles that is characteristic in patients with primary genital or oral-labial HSV infection, and the recovery of virus from neural tissue distant from neurons innervating the inoculation site. Contiguous spread of locally inoculated virus also may take place and allow further mucosal extension of disease.

After the resolution of primary disease, infectious HSV can no longer be recovered in the ganglia. However, viral DNA can be found in 10 to 50% of ganglion cells in the anatomic region of the initial infection. Only ~1% of such cells express latency-associated transcripts of RNA detectable by current techniques. The mechanisms controlling the reactivation of HSV infection are unknown. Alterations in cellular transcripts that "maintain" latency are suspected, and several cellular protein kinases are under investigation. Experimentally, ultraviolet light, systemic and local immunosuppression, and trauma to the skin or ganglia are associated with reactivation.

Analysis of the DNA from sequentially isolated strains of HSV or from isolates from multiple infected ganglia in any one individual has revealed identical restriction endonuclease patterns in most persons. Occasionally (most frequently in immunocompromised persons), multiple strains of the same viral subtype are detected in one individual. This finding suggests that exogenous infection with different strains of the same subtype is possible although very uncommon.

IMMUNITY Host responses to infection with HSV influence the acquisition of disease, the severity of infection, resistance to the development of latency, the maintenance of latency, and the frequency of recurrences. Both antibody-mediated and cell-mediated reactions are clinically important. Immunocompromised patients with defects in cell-mediated immunity experience more severe and more extensive HSV infections than those with deficits in humoral immunity, such as agammaglobulinemia. Experimental ablation of lymphocytes indicates that T cells play a major role in preventing lethal disseminated disease, although antibodies help reduce virus titers in neural tissue. Some of the clinical manifestations of HSV disease appear to be related to the host immune response (e.g., stromal opacities associated with recurrent herpetic keratitis). The surface viral glycoproteins have been shown to be antigens recognized by antibodies mediating neutralization and immune-mediated cytolysis (antibody-dependent cell-mediated cytotoxicity). Monoclonal antibodies specific for each of the known viral glycoproteins have, in experimental infections, conferred protection against subsequent neurologic disease or ganglionic latency. However, the use of subunit glycoprotein vaccines in humans has not been successful in reducing acquisition of infection, despite high titers of type-specific antibodies. Multiple cell populations, including natural killer cells, macrophages, a variety of T lymphocytes, and lymphokines generated by these cells, play a role in host defenses against HSV infections. In animals, passive transfer of primed lymphocytes confers protection from subsequent challenge. Maximum protection usually requires the activation of multiple T cell subpopulations, including cytotoxic T cells and T cells responsible for delayed hypersensitivity. The latter cells may confer protection by the antigen-stim-

ulated release of lymphokines (e.g., interferons), which may have a direct antiviral effect and may activate and enhance a variety of specific and nonspecific effector cells. Increasing evidence suggests that HSV-specific CD8+ T cell responses are critical for clearance of virus from lesions. In addition, immunosuppressed patients with frequent and prolonged HSV lesions have fewer functional CD8+ T cells directed at HSV. The HSV virion contains a gene called unique long gene no. 12 (UL-12) that can bind to the cellular transporter-activating protein TAP-1 and reduce the ability of this protein to bind HSV peptides to HLA class I, thereby reducing recognition of viral proteins by cytotoxic T cells of the host. This effect can be overcome by the addition of interferon γ, but this requires 24 to 48 h; thus, the virus has time to replicate and invade other host cells. Prior HSV-1 infection does not appear to reduce the frequency of acquisition of HSV-2 as measured by seroconversion. However, persons with prior HSV-1 infection who acquire HSV-2 appear to have a greater frequency of subclinical acquisition. These data suggest that type-specific immune responses are central to the control of HSV infection.

EPIDEMIOLOGY Seroepidemiologic studies have documented HSV infections worldwide. Much of the humoral immune response to HSV is to type-common antigenic determinants. Serologic assays with whole-virus antigen preparations, such as complement fixation, neutralization, indirect immunofluorescence, passive hemagglutination, radioimmunoassay, and enzyme-linked immunosorbent assay, do not reliably distinguish between the two viral subtypes. Such assays are useful for differentiating uninfected (seronegative) persons from those with past HSV-1 or HSV-2 infection, but they do not reliably distinguish between the two subtypes. Serologic assays that identify antibodies to type-specific surface proteins of the two subtypes have been developed. These assays, which are based on the demonstration of antibodies to type-specific epitopes of the virus, can reliably distinguish between the human antibody responses to HSV-1 and HSV-2. The most commonly used assays are those that measure antibodies to glycoprotein G of HSV-1 (gG1) and HSV-2 (gG2). A western blot assay that can detect several HSV type-specific proteins can also be used.

Infection with HSV-1 is acquired more frequently and earlier than infection with HSV-2. More than 90% of adults have antibodies to HSV-1 by the fifth decade of life. In populations of low socioeconomic status, most persons acquire HSV-1 infection before the third decade of life.

Antibodies to HSV-2 are not detected routinely until puberty. Antibody prevalence rates correlate with past sexual activity and vary greatly among different population groups. Serosurveys indicate that nearly 22% of the United States population has antibodies to HSV-2—a 30% increase in the past 12 years. In most routine obstetric and family planning clinics, 25% of women have HSV-2 antibodies, although only 10% report a history of genital lesions. As many as 50% of heterosexual adults attending sexually transmitted disease clinics have antibodies to HSV-2. Antibody prevalence rates average about 5% higher among women than among men. Several studies suggest that much of this "asymptomatic" infection is largely unrecognized in that when "asymptomatic" seropositive persons are shown pictures of genital lesions, >60% subsequently identify episodes of symptomatic reactivation. Most important, these asymptomatic seropositive persons with reactivation shed virus on mucosal surfaces as frequently as those with symptomatic disease. The large reservoir of unidentified carriers of HSV-2 and the frequent asymptomatic reactivation of virus from the genital tract have fostered the continued spread of genital herpes throughout the world. HSV-2 infection is an independent risk factor for the acquisition and transmission of infection with HIV type 1. Among coinfected persons, HIV-1 virions can be shed from herpetic lesions of the genital region. This shedding may facilitate the spread of HIV through sexual contact.

HSV infections occur throughout the year. The incubation period ranges from 1 to 26 days (median, 6 to 8 days). Transmission can result from contact with persons with active ulcerative lesions or with persons without clinical manifestations of infection who are shedding HSV or on whose mucosal surfaces the virus is replicating. Studies using the polymerase chain reaction (PCR) have shown that HSV reactivation on mucosal surfaces is much more frequent than previously recognized. Among immunocompetent adults, HSV-2 can be isolated from the genital tract on 2 to 3% of days, and HSV DNA can be detected on 20 to 30% of days. Corresponding figures for HSV-1 in oral secretions are similar. Shedding rates are highest during the initial years of acquisition and may be as high as 30 to 50% of days during this period. Immunosuppressed patients shed HSV on mucosal sites at even higher frequency (20 to 50% of days). Daily antiviral chemotherapy can markedly reduce shedding rates. These data indicate that potential exposure to HSV from sexual or other close contact (kissing, sharing of glasses or silverware) is more common than has been thought. These shedding-rate data are consistent with the high seroprevalence of HSV infections worldwide.

CLINICAL SPECTRUM HSV has been isolated from nearly all visceral or mucocutaneous sites. The clinical manifestations and course of HSV infection depend on the anatomic site involved, the age and immune status of the host, and the antigenic type of the virus. Primary HSV infections (i.e., first infections with either HSV-1 or HSV-2 in which the host lacks HSV antibodies in acute-phase serum) are frequently accompanied by systemic signs and symptoms, involve both mucosal and extramucosal sites, and have a longer duration of symptoms, a longer duration of virus isolation from lesions, and a higher rate of complications than recurrent episodes of disease. Both viral subtypes can cause genital and oral-facial infections, and the infections caused by the two subtypes are clinically indistinguishable. However, the frequency of reactivation of infection is influenced by anatomic site and virus type. Genital HSV-2 infection is twice as likely to reactivate and recurs 8 to 10 times more frequently than genital HSV-1 infection. Conversely, oral-labial HSV-1 infection recurs more frequently than oral-labial HSV-2 infection. Asymptomatic shedding rates follow the same pattern.

Oral-Facial Infections Gingivostomatitis and pharyngitis are the most frequent clinical manifestations of first-episode HSV-1 infection, while recurrent herpes labialis is the most frequent clinical manifestation of reactivation HSV infection. HSV pharyngitis and gingivostomatitis usually result from primary infection and are most commonly seen in children and young adults. Clinical symptoms and signs, which include fever, malaise, myalgias, inability to eat, irritability, and cervical adenopathy, may last from 3 to 14 days. Lesions may involve the hard and soft palate, gingiva, tongue, lip, and facial area. HSV-1 or HSV-2 infection of the pharynx usually results in exudative or ulcerative lesions of the posterior pharynx and/or tonsillar pillars. Lesions of the tongue, buccal mucosa, or gingiva may occur later in the course in one-third of cases. Fever lasting from 2 to 7 days and cervical adenopathy are common. It can be difficult to differentiate HSV pharyngitis clinically from bacterial pharyngitis, *Mycoplasma pneumoniae* infections, and pharyngeal ulcerations of noninfectious etiologies (e.g., Stevens-Johnson syndrome). No substantial evidence suggests that reactivation oral-labial HSV infection is associated with symptomatic recurrent pharyngitis.

Reactivation of HSV from the trigeminal ganglia may be associated with asymptomatic virus excretion in the saliva, development of intraoral mucosal ulcerations, or herpetic ulcerations on the vermilion border of the lip or external facial skin. About 50 to 70% of seropositive patients undergoing trigeminal nerve root decompression and 10 to 15% of those undergoing dental extraction develop oral-labial HSV infection a median of 3 days after these procedures.

In immunosuppressed patients, infection may extend into mucosal and deep cutaneous layers. Friability, necrosis, bleeding, severe pain, and inability to eat or drink may result. The lesions of HSV mucositis are clinically similar to mucosal lesions caused by cytotoxic drug therapy, trauma, or fungal or bacterial infections. Persistent ulcerative

HSV infections are among the most common infections in patients with AIDS. HSV and *Candida* infections often occur concurrently. Systemic antiviral therapy speeds the rate of healing and relieves the pain of mucosal HSV infections in immunosuppressed patients. The frequency of HSV reactivation during the early phases of transplantation or induction chemotherapy is high (50 to 90%), and prophylactic systemic antivirals such as intravenous acyclovir or penciclovir are used to reduce reactivation rates. Patients with atopic eczema also may develop severe oral-facial HSV infections (eczema herpeticum), which may rapidly come to involve extensive areas of skin and occasionally disseminate to visceral organs. Extensive eczema herpeticum has resolved promptly with the administration of intravenous acyclovir. Erythema multiforme (EM) also may be associated with HSV infections (**Plate IIE-67**); some evidence suggests that HSV infection is the precipitating event in ~75% of cases of cutaneous EM. HSV antigen has been demonstrated both in circulatory immune complexes and in skin lesion biopsy samples from these patients. Patients with severe HSV-associated EM are candidates for chronic suppressive oral antiviral therapy.

HSV-1 has been implicated in the etiology of Bell's palsy (flaccid paralysis of the mandibular portion of the facial nerve). Whether antiviral chemotherapy can alter the clinical course and complications of this infection is unclear.

Genital Infections First-episode primary genital herpes is characterized by fever, headache, malaise, and myalgias. Pain, itching, dysuria, vaginal and urethral discharge, and tender inguinal lymphadenopathy are the predominant local symptoms. Widely spaced bilateral lesions of the external genitalia are characteristic. Lesions may be present in varying stages, including vesicles, pustules, or painful erythematous ulcers. The cervix and urethra are involved in >80% of women with first-episode infections. First episodes of genital herpes in patients who have had prior HSV-1 infection are associated with less frequent systemic symptoms and faster healing than primary genital herpes. The clinical courses of acute first-episode genital herpes among patients with HSV-1 and HSV-2 infections are similar. However, the recurrence rates of genital disease differ with the viral subtype: the 12-month recurrence rates among patients with first-episode HSV-2 and HSV-1 infections are ~90% and ~55%, respectively (median number of recurrences, 4 and <1, respectively). Recurrence rates for genital HSV-2 infections vary greatly among individuals and over time within the same individual. HSV has been isolated from the urethra and urine of men and women without external genital lesions. A clear mucoid discharge and dysuria are characteristics of symptomatic HSV urethritis. HSV has been isolated from the urethra of 5% of women with the dysuria-frequency syndrome. Occasionally, HSV genital tract disease is manifested by endometritis and salpingitis in women and by prostatitis in men. About 15% of cases of HSV-2 acquisition are associated with these nonlesional clinical syndromes, such as aseptic meningitis, cervicitis, or urethritis.

Both HSV-1 and HSV-2 can cause symptomatic or asymptomatic rectal and perianal infections. HSV proctitis is usually associated with rectal intercourse. However, subclinical perianal shedding of HSV is detected both in heterosexual men and in women who report no rectal intercourse. This phenomenon is due to the establishment of latency in the sacral dermatome from prior genital tract infection, with subsequent reactivation in epithelial cells in the perianal region. Such reactivations are often subclinical. Symptoms of HSV proctitis include anorectal pain, anorectal discharge, tenesmus, and constipation. Sigmoidoscopy reveals ulcerative lesions of the distal 10 cm of the rectal mucosa. Rectal biopsies show mucosal ulceration, necrosis, polymorphonuclear and lymphocytic infiltration of the lamina propria, and (in occasional cases) multinucleated intranuclear inclusion–bearing cells. Perianal herpetic lesions are also found in immunosuppressed patients receiving cytotoxic therapy. Extensive perianal herpetic lesions and/ or HSV proctitis is common among patients with HIV infection.

Herpetic Whitlow Herpetic whitlow—HSV infection of the finger—may occur as a complication of primary oral or genital herpes by inoculation of virus through a break in the epidermal surface or by direct introduction of virus into the hand through occupational or some other type of exposure. Clinical signs and symptoms include the abrupt onset of edema, erythema, and localized tenderness of the infected finger. Vesicular or pustular lesions of the fingertip that are indistinguishable from lesions of pyogenic bacterial infection are seen. Fever, lymphadenitis, and epitrochlear and axillary lymphadenopathy are common. The infection may recur. Prompt diagnosis (to avoid unnecessary and potentially exacerbating surgical therapy and/or transmission) is essential. Antiviral chemotherapy (to speed the healing of the process) is usually recommended (see below).

Herpes Gladiatorum HSV may infect almost any area of skin. Mucocutaneous HSV infections of the thorax, ears, face, and hands have been described among wrestlers. Transmission of these infections is facilitated by trauma to the skin sustained during wrestling. Prompt diagnosis and therapy are required to contain the spread of this infection.

Eye Infections HSV infection of the eye is the most frequent cause of corneal blindness in the United States. HSV keratitis presents with an acute onset of pain, blurring of vision, chemosis, conjunctivitis, and characteristic dendritic lesions of the cornea. Use of topical glucocorticoids may exacerbate symptoms and lead to involvement of deep structures of the eye. Debridement, topical antiviral treatment, and/or interferon therapy hastens healing. However, recurrences are common, and the deeper structures of the eye may sustain immunopathologic injury. Stromal keratitis due to HSV appears to be related to T cell–dependent destruction of deep corneal tissue. An HSV-1 epitope that is autoreactive with T cell–targeting corneal antigens has been postulated to be a factor in this infection. Chorioretinitis, usually a manifestation of disseminated HSV infection, may occur in neonates or in patients with HIV infection. HSV and varicella-zoster virus can cause acute necrotizing retinitis as an uncommon but severe manifestation.

Central and Peripheral Nervous System Infections HSV accounts for 10 to 20% of all cases of sporadic viral encephalitis in the United States. The estimated incidence is about 2.3 cases per million persons per year. Cases are distributed throughout the year, and the age distribution appears to be biphasic, with peaks at 5 to 30 and >50 years of age. Subtype 1 virus causes >95% of cases of HSV encephalitis.

The pathogenesis of HSV encephalitis varies. In children and young adults, primary HSV infection may result in encephalitis; presumably, exogenously acquired virus enters the CNS by neurotropic spread from the periphery via the olfactory bulb. However, most adults with HSV encephalitis have clinical or serologic evidence of mucocutaneous HSV-1 infection before the onset of the CNS symptoms. In ~25% of the cases examined, the HSV-1 strains from the oropharynx and brain tissue of the same patient differ; thus some cases may result from reinfection with another strain of HSV-1 that reaches the CNS. Two theories have been proposed to explain the development of actively replicating HSV in localized areas of the CNS in persons whose ganglionic and CNS isolates are similar. Reactivation of latent HSV-1 infection in trigeminal or autonomic nerve roots may be associated with extension of virus into the CNS via nerves innervating the middle cranial fossa. HSV DNA has been demonstrated by DNA hybridization in brain tissue obtained at autopsy—even from healthy adults. Thus, reactivation of long-standing latent CNS infection may be another mechanism for the development of HSV encephalitis.

The clinical hallmark of HSV encephalitis has been the acute onset of fever and focal neurologic (especially temporal-lobe) symptoms. Clinical differentiation of HSV encephalitis from other viral encephalitides, focal infections, or noninfectious processes is difficult. The most sensitive noninvasive method for early diagnosis of HSV encephalitis is the demonstration of HSV DNA in cerebrospinal fluid (CSF) by PCR. Although titers of CSF and serum antibodies to HSV increase in most cases of HSV encephalitis, they rarely do so earlier than 10 days into the illness and therefore, while useful retrospectively, are generally not helpful in establishing an early clinical diagnosis. Demonstration of HSV antigen, HSV DNA, or HSV replication in

brain tissue obtained by biopsy is highly sensitive and has a low complication rate; examination of such tissue also provides the best opportunity to identify alternative, potentially treatable causes of encephalitis. Antiviral chemotherapy reduces the rate of death from HSV encephalitis. Intravenous acyclovir is more effective than vidarabine. Even with therapy, however, neurologic sequelae are frequent, especially in persons over 35 years of age. Most authorities recommend the administration of intravenous acyclovir to patients with presumed HSV encephalitis until the diagnosis is confirmed or an alternative diagnosis is made.

HSV has been isolated from the CSF of 0.5 to 3% of patients presenting to the hospital with aseptic meningitis. HSV meningitis, which is usually seen in association with primary genital HSV infection, is an acute, self-limited disease manifested by headache, fever, and mild photophobia and lasting from 2 to 7 days. Lymphocytic pleocytosis in the CSF is characteristic. Neurologic sequelae of HSV meningitis are rare. HSV is the most commonly identified cause of recurrent lymphocytic meningitis (Mollaret's meningitis). Demonstration of HSV antibodies in CSF or persistence of HSV DNA in CSF can establish the diagnosis. Daily administration of antiviral therapy aimed at reducing the likelihood of clinical HSV reactivation has been successful in such cases.

Autonomic nervous system dysfunction, especially of the sacral region, has been reported in association with both HSV and varicella-zoster virus infections. Numbness, tingling of the buttocks or perineal areas, urinary retention, constipation, CSF pleocytosis, and (in males) impotence may occur. Symptoms appear to resolve slowly over days to weeks. Occasionally, hypesthesia and/or weakness of the lower extremities may persist for many months. Rarely, transverse myelitis manifested by a rapidly progressive symmetric paralysis of the lower extremities or a Guillain-Barré syndrome may follow HSV infection. Similarly, peripheral nervous system involvement (Bell's palsy) or cranial polyneuritis also may be related to reactivation of HSV-1 infection. Transitory hypesthesia of the area of skin innervated by the trigeminal nerve and vestibular system dysfunction as measured by electronystagmography are the predominant signs of disease. Studies to determine whether antiviral chemotherapy may abort these signs or reduce their frequency and severity are unavailable.

Visceral Infections HSV infection of visceral organs usually results from viremia, and multiple-organ involvement is common. Occasionally, however, the clinical manifestations of HSV infection involve only the esophagus, lung, or liver. HSV esophagitis may result from direct extension of oral-pharyngeal HSV infection into the esophagus or may occur de novo by reactivation and spread of HSV to the esophageal mucosa via the vagus nerve. The predominant symptoms of HSV esophagitis are odynophagia, dysphagia, substernal pain, and weight loss. There are multiple oval ulcerations on an erythematous base with or without a patchy white pseudomembrane. The distal esophagus is most commonly involved. With extensive disease, diffuse friability may spread to the entire esophagus. Neither endoscopic nor barium examination can differentiate HSV esophagitis from *Candida* esophagitis or from esophageal ulcerations due to thermal injury, radiation, or corrosives. Endoscopically obtained secretions for cytologic examination and culture provide the most useful material for diagnosis. Systemic antiviral chemotherapy usually reduces symptoms and heals esophageal ulcerations.

HSV pneumonitis is uncommon except in severely immunosuppressed patients and may result from extension of herpetic tracheobronchitis into lung parenchyma. Focal necrotizing pneumonitis usually ensues. Hematogenous dissemination of virus from sites of oral or genital mucocutaneous disease also may occur and produce bilateral interstitial pneumonitis. Bacterial, fungal, and parasitic pathogens are commonly present in HSV pneumonitis. The mortality rate from untreated HSV pneumonia in immunosuppressed patients is high (>80%). HSV has also been isolated from the lower respiratory tract of persons with adult respiratory distress syndrome (ARDS). However, the relationship between the isolation of HSV and the pathogenesis of ARDS is unclear.

HSV is an uncommon cause of hepatitis in immunocompetent patients. HSV infection of the liver is associated with fever, abrupt elevations of bilirubin and serum aminotransferase levels, and leukopenia (<4000 white blood cells per microliter). Disseminated intravascular coagulation also may develop.

Other reported complications of HSV infection include monarticular arthritis, adrenal necrosis, idiopathic thrombocytopenia, and glomerulonephritis. Disseminated HSV infection in immunocompetent patients is rare. In immunocompromised, burned, or malnourished patients, HSV occasionally disseminates to other visceral organs, such as the adrenal glands, pancreas, small and large intestines, and bone marrow. Rarely, primary HSV infection in pregnancy disseminates and may be associated with the death of both mother and fetus. This uncommon event is usually related to the acquisition of primary infection in the third trimester.

Neonatal HSV Infection Neonates (infants younger than 6 weeks) have the highest frequency of visceral and/or CNS infection of any HSV-infected patient population. Without therapy, the overall rate of death from neonatal herpes is 65%; fewer than 10% of neonates with CNS infection develop normally. Although skin lesions are the most commonly recognized features of disease, many infants do not develop lesions until well into the course of disease. Neonatal infection is usually acquired perinatally from contact with infected genital secretions at the time of delivery. Congenitally infected infants have been reported. In most series, 30% of neonatal HSV infections are due to HSV-1 and 70% to HSV-2. The risk of developing neonatal HSV infection is 10 times higher for an infant born to a mother who has recently acquired HSV than for other infants. Guidelines to evaluate routine serologic testing for HSV in pregnancy are being drafted and will serve as a basis on which to counsel "susceptible" (HSV-2-uninfected) women regarding the dangers of unprotected coitus and HSV-2 infection near term. Neonatal HSV-1 infections may also be acquired through postnatal contact with immediate family members who have symptomatic or asymptomatic oral-labial HSV-1 infection or through nosocomial transmission within the hospital. Antiviral chemotherapy has reduced the rate of death from neonatal herpes to 25%. However, the rate of morbidity, especially in infants with HSV-2 infection involving the CNS, is still very high.

DIAGNOSIS Both clinical and laboratory criteria are useful for establishing the diagnosis of HSV infections. A clinical diagnosis can be made accurately when characteristic multiple vesicular lesions on an erythematous base are present. However, it is increasingly being recognized that herpetic ulcerations may clinically resemble skin ulcerations of other etiologies. Mucosal HSV infections may also present as urethritis or pharyngitis without cutaneous lesions. Thus, laboratory studies to confirm the diagnosis and to guide therapy are recommended. Staining of scrapings from the base of the lesions with Wright's, Giemsa's (Tzanck preparation), or Papanicolaou's stain demonstrates characteristic giant cells or intranuclear inclusions of herpesvirus infection. These cytologic techniques are often useful as quick office procedures to confirm the diagnosis. Limitations of the cytologic method are that it does not differentiate between HSV and varicella-zoster virus infections, that it is relatively insensitive, and that the correct identification of giant cells requires experience.

HSV infection is best confirmed in the laboratory by isolation of virus in tissue culture or by demonstration of HSV antigens or DNA in scrapings from lesions. HSV causes a discernible cytopathic effect in a variety of cell culture systems, and most specimens can be identified within 48 to 96 h after inoculation. Spin-amplified culture with subsequent staining for HSV antigen has shortened the time needed to identify HSV to <24 h. The sensitivity of viral isolation depends on the stage of lesions (with higher sensitivity in vesicular than in ulcerative lesions), on whether the patient has a first or a recurrent episode of the disease (with higher sensitivity in first than in recurrent epi-

sodes), and on whether the sample is from an immunosuppressed or an immunocompetent patient (with more antigen in immunosuppressed patients). Antigen detection procedures have approached viral isolation in terms of sensitivity in detecting HSV in genital or oral-labial lesions; however, antigen detection appears to be only ~50% as sensitive as viral isolation for the identification of HSV in cervical or salivary secretions of asymptomatic patients. PCR techniques appear to be more sensitive for HSV than viral isolation, especially for the diagnosis of CNS infections and for the detection of HSV as a cause of late-stage ulcerative lesions. Laboratory confirmation permits subtyping of the virus; information on subtype may be useful epidemiologically and may help to predict the frequency of reactivation after first-episode oral-labial or genital HSV infection.

Acute- and convalescent-phase serum can be useful in demonstrating seroconversion during primary HSV-1 or HSV-2 infection. However, only 5% of patients with recurrent mucocutaneous HSV infections have a fourfold or greater rise in titer of antibody to HSV in the interval between the collection of the first and second samples. Serologic assays, especially type-specific assays, should be used to identify asymptomatic carriers of HSV-1 or HSV-2 infection.

Several studies have shown that persons seropositive for HSV-2 to whom the clinical manifestations of HSV have been explained are able to identify symptomatic reactivations. Individuals seropositive for HSV-2 should be told about the high frequency of subclinical reactivation in mucosal surfaces not visible to the eye (e.g., cervix, urethra, perianal skin) or in microscopic ulcerations that may not be clinically symptomatic. Transmission of infection during such episodes is well established. HSV-2-seropositive persons should be educated about the high likelihood of subclinical shedding and the role condoms (male or female) may play in reducing transmission. Chronic antiviral therapy is being studied as a means of reducing the transmission of infection.

TREATMENT Many aspects of mucocutaneous and visceral HSV infections are amenable to antiviral chemotherapy. For mucocutaneous infections, acyclovir and its congeners famciclovir and valacyclovir have been the mainstay of therapy. Several antiviral agents are available for topical use in HSV eye infections: idoxuridine, trifluorothymidine, topical vidarabine, and cidofovir. For HSV encephalitis and neonatal herpes, intravenous acyclovir is the treatment of choice.

All licensed antivirals for HSV inhibit the viral DNA polymerase. One class of drugs, typified by the drug acyclovir, is made up of substrates for the HSV enzyme thymidine kinase. Acyclovir, ganciclovir, famciclovir, and valacyclovir are all selectively phosphorylated to the monophosphate form in virus-infected cells. Cellular enzymes convert the monophosphate form of the drug to the triphosphate, which is then incorporated into the viral DNA chain.

Acyclovir is the most frequently used agent for the treatment of HSV infections and is available in intravenous, oral, and topical formulations. Famciclovir, the oral formulation of penciclovir, is clinically effective in the treatment of a variety of HSV-1 and HSV-2 infections. Intravenous penciclovir is also available. Valacyclovir is the valyl ester of acyclovir and has greater bioavailability than acyclovir. Ganciclovir has activity against both HSV-1 and HSV-2; however, it is more toxic than acyclovir, valacyclovir, and famciclovir and is generally not recommended for the treatment of HSV infections.

All three compounds—acyclovir, valacyclovir, and famciclovir—have proven effective in shortening the duration of symptoms and lesions of mucocutaneous HSV infections in both immunocompromised and immunocompetent patients (Table 182-1). Intravenous and oral formulations prevent reactivation of HSV in seropositive immunocompromised patients during induction chemotherapy or in the period immediately after bone marrow or solid organ transplantation. Chronic daily suppressive therapy reduces the frequency of reactivation disease among patients with frequent genital or oral-labial herpes.

Intravenous acyclovir (30 mg/kg per day, given as a 10-mg/kg infusion over 1 h at 8-h intervals) is effective in reducing rates of death and morbidity from HSV encephalitis. Early initiation of therapy is a

Mucocutaneous HSV infections

Infections in immunosuppressed patients

   Acute symptomatic first or recurrent episodes: IV acyclovir (5 mg/kg q8h) or oral acyclovir (400 mg qid for 7–10 days) relieves pain and speeds healing.

   Suppression of reactivation disease: IV acyclovir (5 mg/kg q12h) or oral acyclovir (400–800 mg 3–5 times per day) prevents recurrences during high-risk periods, e.g., the immediate posttransplantation period. In HIV-infected persons, oral famciclovir (500 mg bid) or valacyclovir (500 mg bid) is also effective.

Genital herpes

   First episodes: Oral acyclovir (200 mg 5 times per day or 400 mg tid) is given. Oral valacyclovir (1000 mg bid) or famciclovir (250 mg tid) for 10–14 days is effective. IV acyclovir (5 mg/kg q8h for 5 days) is given for severe disease or neurologic complications such as aseptic meningitis.

   Symptomatic recurrent genital herpes: Oral acyclovir (200 mg 5 times per day or 400 mg tid for 5 days), valacyclovir (500 mg bid), or famciclovir (125 mg bid) is effective in shortening lesion duration and viral excretion time.

   Suppression of recurrent genital herpes: Oral acyclovir (200-mg capsules; 400 mg bid or 800 mg qd), famciclovir (250 mg bid), or valacyclovir (250 or 500 mg bid or 1000 mg qd) prevents symptomatic reactivation.

Oral-labial HSV infections

   First episode: Oral acyclovir (200 mg) is given 4 or 5 times per day. Famciclovir (250 mg bid) or valacyclovir (1000 mg bid) has been used clinically.

   Recurrent episodes: Topical penciclovir cream is effective in speeding the healing of oral-labial HSV. Topical acyclovir cream is licensed in Europe. The ointment formulation of acyclovir available in the U.S. has no clinical benefit. Oral valacyclovir has some benefit. Oral acyclovir has minimal benefit.

   Suppression of reactivation of oral-labial HSV: Oral acyclovir (400 mg bid), if started before exposure and continued for the duration of exposure (usually 5–10 days), prevents reactivation of recurrent oral-labial HSV infection associated with severe sun exposure.

Herpetic whitlow: Oral acyclovir (200 mg) is given 5 times daily for 7–10 days.

HSV proctitis: Oral acyclovir (400 mg 5 times per day) is useful in shortening the course of infection. In immunosuppressed patients or in patients with severe infection, IV acyclovir (5 mg/kg q8h) may be useful.

Herpetic eye infections: In acute keratitis, topical trifluorothymidine, vidarabine, idoxuridine, acyclovir, penciclovir, and interferon are all beneficial. Debridement may be required; topical steroids may worsen disease.

CNS HSV infections

HSV encephalitis: Intravenous acyclovir (10 mg/kg q8h; 30 mg/kg per day) for 10 days is preferred.

HSV aseptic meningitis: No studies of systemic antiviral chemotherapy exist. If therapy is to be given, IV acyclovir (15–30 mg/kg per day) should be used.

Autonomic radiculopathy: No studies are available.

Neonatal HSV infections: Acyclovir (60 mg/kg per day, divided into 3 doses) is given. The recommended duration of treatment is 21 days.

Visceral HSV infections

HSV esophagitis: IV acyclovir (5 mg/kg q8h) is given. In some patients with milder forms of immunosuppression, oral therapy with valacyclovir or famciclovir is effective.

HSV pneumonitis: No controlled studies exist. IV acyclovir (15 mg/kg per day) should be considered.

Surgical prophylaxis: IV acyclovir (5 mg/kg q12h) or oral acyclovir (800 mg bid), famciclovir (250 mg bid), or valacyclovir (500 mg bid) is given 2–3 days before laser resurfacing or other neurologic procedures.

Disseminated HSV infections: No controlled studies exist. Intravenous acyclovir nevertheless should be tried. No definite evidence indicates that therapy decreases the risk of death.

Erythema multiforme associated with HSV: Anecdotal observations suggest that oral acyclovir (400 mg bid or tid) suppresses erythema multiforme.

Infections due to acyclovir-resistant HSV: Foscarnet (40 mg/kg IV q8h) should be given until lesions heal. The optimal duration of therapy and the usefulness of its continuation to suppress lesions are unclear. Some patients may benefit from cutaneous application of trifluorothymidine or 5% cidofovir gel.

---

critical factor in outcome. The major side effect associated with intravenous acyclovir is transient renal insufficiency, usually due to crystallization of the compound in the renal parenchyma. This adverse reaction can be avoided if the medication is given slowly over 1 h and the patient is well hydrated. Because CSF levels of acyclovir average only 30 to 50% of plasma levels, the dosage of acyclovir used for treatment of CNS infection (30 mg/kg per day) is double that used for treatment of mucocutaneous or visceral disease (15 mg/kg per day).

Acyclovir-resistant strains of HSV have been identified. Most of these strains have an altered substrate specificity for phosphorylating acyclovir. Thus, cross-resistance to famciclovir and valacyclovir is usually found. Occasionally, an isolate with altered thymidine kinase (TK) specificity arises and is sensitive to famciclovir but not to acyclovir. In some patients infected with TK-deficient virus, higher doses of acyclovir are associated with clearing of lesions. In others, clinical disease progresses despite high-dose therapy. Almost all clinically significant acyclovir resistance has been seen in immunocompromised patients, and HSV-2 isolates are more often resistant than HSV-1 strains. A study by the Centers for Disease Control and Prevention indicated that ~5% of isolates from HIV-positive persons exhibit some degree of in vitro resistance to acyclovir. Isolation of HSV from persisting lesions despite adequate dosages and blood levels of acyclovir should raise the suspicion of acyclovir resistance. Therapy with the antiviral drug foscarnet is useful (Chap. 181). Because of its toxicity and cost, this drug is usually reserved for patients with extensive mucocutaneous infections. Cidofovir is a nucleotide analogue and exists as a phosphonate or monophosphate form. Most TK-deficient strains of HSV are sensitive to cidofovir. Cidofovir ointment speeds healing of acyclovir-resistant lesions. No well-controlled trials of systemic cidofovir have been reported. True TK-negative variants of HSV appear to have a reduced capacity to spread because of altered neurovirulence—a feature important in the relatively infrequent presence of such strains in immunocompetent populations, even with increasing use of antivirals.

PREVENTION The large reservoir of persons with asymptomatic HSV-1 and HSV-2 infections indicates that the success of efforts to control HSV disease through suppressive antiviral chemotherapy and/or educational programs will be limited. Rather, control of HSV infection will require the prevention of infection—a goal most likely to be attained by vaccination. Several candidate vaccines are under investigation, and the prevention of HSV infection has been assigned a high public health priority.

Barrier forms of contraception, especially condoms, decrease the likelihood of transmission of HSV infection, especially during periods of asymptomatic viral excretion. When lesions are present, HSV infection may be transmitted by skin-to-skin contact despite the use of a condom. Nevertheless, the available data suggest that consistent condom use is an effective means of reducing the risk of genital HSV-2 transmission. Prevention of neonatal HSV requires the prevention of acquisition of HSV in the third trimester of pregnancy. Identification of women or couples susceptible to acquisition of HSV in pregnancy through serologic screening is receiving increasing attention, and such screening is being used with increasing frequency.

BIBLIOGRAPHY

BENEDETTI J et al: Clinical reactivation of genital herpes simplex virus infection decreases in frequency over time. Ann Intern Med 131:14, 1999

BLOWER SM et al: Predicting and preventing the emergence of antiviral drug resistance in HSV-2. Nat Med 4:673, 1998

BROWN ZA et al: The acquisition of herpes simplex virus during pregnancy. N Engl J Med 337:509, 1997

COREY L, SPEAR P: Infections with herpes simplex viruses. N Engl J Med 314:686, 1986

FLEMING DT et al: Herpes simplex virus type 2 in the United States, 1976 to 1994. N Engl J Med 337:1105, 1997

LANGENBERG AGM et al: A prospective study of new infections with herpes simplex virus type 1 and herpes simplex virus type 2. N Engl J Med 341:1532, 1999

MERTZ GJ et al: Oral famciclovir for the suppression of recurrent genital herpes simplex virus infection in women. Arch Intern Med 157:334, 1997

REITANO M et al: Valaciclovir for the suppression of recurrent genital herpes simplex virus infection: A large-scale dose range–finding study. J Infect Dis 178:602, 1998

SCHACKER T et al: Frequent recovery of HIV-1 from genital herpes simplex virus lesions in HIV-1-infected men. JAMA 280:61, 1998

WALD A et al: Suppression of subclinical shedding of herpes simplex virus type 2 with acyclovir. Ann Intern Med 124:8, 1996

—— et al: Frequent genital herpes simplex virus 2 shedding in immunocompetent women: Effect of acyclovir treatment. J Clin Invest 99:1092, 1997

WHITLEY RJ et al: Herpes simplex virus infections of the central nervous system: Therapeutic and diagnostic considerations. Clin Infect Dis 20:414, 1995

—— et al: Herpes simplex viruses. Clin Infect Dis 26:541, 1998

ZHAO ZS et al: Molecular mimicry by herpes simplex virus-type 1: Autoimmune disease after viral infection. Science 279:1344, 1998

183 *Richard J. Whitley*

VARICELLA-ZOSTER VIRUS INFECTIONS

DEFINITION Varicella-zoster virus (VZV) causes two distinct clinical entities: varicella (chickenpox) and herpes zoster (shingles). Chickenpox, a ubiquitous and extremely contagious infection, is usually a benign illness of childhood characterized by an exanthematous vesicular rash. With reactivation of latent VZV (which is most common after the sixth decade of life), herpes zoster presents as a dermatomal vesicular rash, usually associated with severe pain.

ETIOLOGY A clinical association between varicella and herpes zoster has been recognized for nearly 100 years. Early in the twentieth century, similarities in the histopathologic features of skin lesions resulting from varicella and herpes zoster were demonstrated. Viral isolates from patients with chickenpox and herpes zoster produced similar alterations in tissue culture—specifically, the appearance of eosinophilic intranuclear inclusions and multinucleated giant cells. These results suggested that the viruses were biologically similar. Restriction endonuclease analyses of viral DNA from a patient with chickenpox who subsequently developed herpes zoster verified the molecular identity of the two viruses responsible for these different clinical presentations.

VZV is a member of the family Herpesviridae, sharing with other members such structural characteristics as a lipid envelope surrounding a nucleocapsid with icosahedral symmetry, a total diameter of approximately 180 to 200 nm, and centrally located double-stranded DNA that is about 125,000 bp in length.

PATHOGENESIS AND PATHOLOGY **Primary Infection** Transmission is most likely to take place by the respiratory route; the subsequent localized replication of the virus at an undefined site (presumably the nasopharynx) leads to seeding of the reticuloendothelial system and ultimately to the development of viremia. Viremia in patients with chickenpox is reflected in the diffuse and scattered nature of the skin lesions and can be verified in selected cases by the recovery of VZV from the blood. Vesicles involve the corium and dermis, with degenerative changes characterized by ballooning, the presence of multinucleated giant cells, and eosinophilic intranuclear inclusions. Infection may involve localized blood vessels of the skin, resulting in necrosis and epidermal hemorrhage. With the evolution of disease, the vesicular fluid becomes cloudy because of the recruitment of polymorphonuclear leukocytes and the presence of degenerated cells and fibrin. Ultimately, the vesicles either rupture and release their fluid (which includes infectious virus) or are gradually reabsorbed.

Recurrent Infection The mechanism of reactivation of VZV that results in herpes zoster is unknown. Presumably, the virus infects the dorsal root ganglia during chickenpox, where it remains latent until

reactivated. Histopathologic examination of representative dorsal root ganglia during active herpes zoster demonstrates hemorrhage, edema, and lymphocytic infiltration.

Active replication of VZV in other organs, such as the lung or the brain, can occur during either chickenpox or herpes zoster but is uncommon in the immunocompetent host. Pulmonary involvement is characterized by interstitial pneumonitis, multinucleated giant cell formation, intranuclear inclusions, and pulmonary hemorrhage. Central nervous system (CNS) infection leads to histopathologic evidence of perivascular cuffing similar to that encountered in measles and other viral encephalitides. Focal hemorrhagic necrosis of the brain, characteristic of herpes simplex virus encephalitis, is uncommon in VZV infection.

EPIDEMIOLOGY AND CLINICAL MANIFESTATIONS **Chickenpox** Humans are the only known reservoir for VZV. Chickenpox is highly contagious, with an attack rate of at least 90% among susceptible (seronegative) individuals. Persons of both sexes and all races are infected equally often. The virus is endemic in the population at large; however, it becomes epidemic among susceptible individuals during seasonal peaks—namely, late winter and early spring in the temperate zone. Children between the ages of 5 and 9 are most commonly affected and account for 50% of all cases. Most other cases involve children aged 1 to 4 and those aged 10 to 14. Approximately 10% of the population of the United States over the age of 15 is susceptible to infection.

The incubation period of chickenpox ranges between 10 and 21 days but is usually between 14 and 17 days. Secondary attack rates in susceptible siblings within a household are between 70 and 90%. Patients are infectious approximately 48 h prior to the onset of the vesicular rash, during the period of vesicle formation (which generally lasts 4 to 5 days), and until all vesicles are crusted.

Clinically, chickenpox presents as a rash, low-grade fever, and malaise, although a few patients develop a prodrome 1 to 2 days before onset of the exanthem. In the immunocompetent patient, this is usually a benign illness that is associated with lassitude and with body temperatures of 37.8 to 39.4°C (100 to 103°F) of 3 to 5 days' duration. The skin lesions—the hallmark of the infection—include maculopapules, vesicles, and scabs in various stages of evolution (**Plate IID-36**). These lesions, which evolve from maculopapules to vesicles over hours to days, appear on the trunk and face and rapidly spread to involve other areas of the body. Most are small and have an erythematous base with a diameter of 5 to 10 mm. Successive crops appear over a 2- to 4-day period. Lesions also can be found on the mucosa of the pharynx and/or the vagina. Their severity varies from one person to another. Some individuals have very few lesions, while others have as many as 2000. Younger children tend to have fewer vesicles than older individuals. Secondary and tertiary cases within families are associated with a relatively large number of vesicles. Immunocompromised patients—both children and adults, particularly those with leukemia—have lesions (often with a hemorrhagic base) that are more numerous and take longer to heal than those of immunocompetent patients. Immunocompromised individuals are also at greater risk for visceral complications, which occur in 30 to 50% of cases and are fatal 15% of the time.

The most common infectious complication of varicella is secondary bacterial superinfection of the skin, which is usually caused by *Streptococcus pyogenes* or *Staphylococcus aureus*. This complication may result from excoriation of skin lesions after scratching. Gram's staining of skin lesions should help clarify the etiology of unusually erythematous and pustulated lesions.

The most common extracutaneous site of involvement in children is the CNS. The syndrome of acute cerebellar ataxia and meningeal irritation generally appears around 21 days after the onset of the rash and rarely develops in the preeruptive phase. The cerebrospinal fluid (CSF) contains lymphocytes and elevated levels of protein. CNS involvement is a benign complication of VZV infection in children and generally does not require hospitalization. Aseptic meningitis, encephalitis, transverse myelitis, Guillain-Barré syndrome, and Reye's syndrome also can occur. Encephalitis is reported in 0.1 to 0.2% of children with chickenpox. Other than supportive care, no specific therapy is available for patients with CNS involvement.

Varicella pneumonia is the most serious complication following chickenpox, developing more commonly in adults (up to 20% of cases) than in children. It usually has its onset 3 to 5 days into the illness and is associated with tachypnea, cough, dyspnea, and fever. Cyanosis, pleuritic chest pain, and hemoptysis are frequent. Roentgenographic evidence of disease consists of nodular infiltrates and interstitial pneumonitis. Resolution of pneumonitis parallels improvement of the skin rash; however, patients may have persistent fever and compromised pulmonary function for weeks.

Other complications of chickenpox include myocarditis, corneal lesions, nephritis, arthritis, bleeding diatheses, acute glomerulonephritis, and hepatitis. Hepatic involvement, distinct from Reye's syndrome and usually asymptomatic, is common in chickenpox and is usually characterized by elevated levels of liver enzymes, particularly aspartate and alanine aminotransferases.

Perinatal varicella is associated with a high mortality rate when maternal disease develops within 5 days before delivery or within 48 h thereafter. Because the newborn does not receive protective transplacental antibodies and has an immature immune system, the illness may be unusually severe. The reported mortality rate has been as high as 30% in this group. Congenital varicella, with clinical manifestations of limb hypoplasia, cicatricial skin lesions, and microcephaly at birth, is extremely uncommon.

Herpes Zoster Herpes zoster, a sporadic disease, is the consequence of reactivation of latent VZV from the dorsal root ganglia. Most patients have no history of recent exposure to other individuals with VZV infection. Herpes zoster occurs at all ages, but its incidence is highest (5 to 10 cases per 1000 persons) among individuals in the sixth through the eighth decades of life. Recurrent herpes zoster is exceedingly rare except in immunocompromised hosts, especially those with AIDS.

Herpes zoster, also called shingles, is characterized by a unilateral vesicular eruption within a dermatome, often associated with severe pain. The dermatomes from T3 to L3 are most frequently involved. If the ophthalmic branch of the trigeminal nerve is involved, zoster ophthalmicus results. The factors responsible for the reactivation of VZV are not known. In children reactivation is usually benign, whereas in adults it can be debilitating. The continuum of pain from onset to resolution is known as *zoster-associated pain*. The onset of disease is heralded by pain within the dermatome that may precede lesions by 48 to 72 h; an erythematous maculopapular rash evolves rapidly into vesicular lesions. In the normal host, these lesions may remain few in number and continue to form only for a period of 3 to 5 days. The total duration of disease is generally between 7 and 10 days; however, it may take as long as 2 to 4 weeks for the skin to return to normal. In a few patients, characteristic localization of pain to a dermatome with serologic evidence of herpes zoster has been reported in the absence of skin lesions. When branches of the trigeminal nerve are involved, lesions may appear on the face, in the mouth, in the eye, or on the tongue. In the Ramsay Hunt syndrome (**Plate IID-35**), pain and vesicles appear in the external auditory canal, and patients lose their sense of taste in the anterior two-thirds of the tongue while developing ipsilateral facial palsy. The geniculate ganglion of the sensory branch of the facial nerve is involved.

The most debilitating complication of herpes zoster, in both the normal and the immunocompromised host, is pain associated with acute neuritis and postherpetic neuralgia. Postherpetic neuralgia is uncommon in young individuals; however, at least 50% of patients over age 50 with zoster report some degree of pain in the involved dermatome months after the resolution of cutaneous disease. Changes in sensation in the dermatome, resulting in either hypo- or hyperesthesia, are common.

CNS involvement may follow localized herpes zoster. Many patients without signs of meningeal irritation have CSF pleocytosis and moderately elevated levels of CSF protein. Symptomatic meningoencephalitis is characterized by headache, fever, photophobia, meningitis, and vomiting. A rare manifestation of CNS involvement is granulomatous angiitis with contralateral hemiplegia, which can be diagnosed by cerebral arteriography. Other neurologic manifestations include transverse myelitis with or without motor paralysis.

Like chickenpox, herpes zoster is more severe in the immunocompromised host than in the normal individual. Lesions continue to form for over a week, and scabbing is not complete in most cases until 3 weeks into the illness. Patients with Hodgkin's disease and non-Hodgkin's lymphoma are at greatest risk for progressive herpes zoster. Cutaneous dissemination (**Plate IID-37**) develops in about 40% of these patients. Among patients with cutaneous dissemination, the risk of pneumonitis, meningoencephalitis, hepatitis, and other serious complications is increased by 5 to 10%. However, even in immunocompromised patients, disseminated zoster is rarely fatal.

Patients who have received a bone marrow transplant are at particularly high risk of VZV infection. Thirty percent of cases of posttransplantation VZV infection occur within 1 year (50% of these within 9 months); 45% of the patients involved have cutaneous or visceral dissemination. The mortality rate in this situation is 10%. Postherpetic neuralgia, scarring, and bacterial superinfection are especially frequent in VZV infections occurring within 9 months of transplantation. Among infected patients, concomitant graft-versus-host disease increases the chance of dissemination and/or death.

DIFFERENTIAL DIAGNOSIS The diagnosis of chickenpox is not difficult. The characteristic rash and a history of recent exposure should lead to a prompt diagnosis. Other viral infections that can mimic chickenpox include disseminated herpes simplex virus infection in patients with atopic dermatitis and the disseminated vesiculopapular lesions sometimes associated with coxsackievirus infection, echovirus infection, or atypical measles. However, these rashes are more commonly morbilliform with a hemorrhagic component rather than vesicular or vesiculopustular. Rickettsialpox can be confused with chickenpox; however, it can be distinguished easily by detection of the "herald spot" at the site of the mite bite and the development of a more pronounced headache. Serologic testing is also useful in differentiating rickettsialpox from varicella.

Unilateral vesicular lesions in a dermatomal pattern should lead rapidly to the diagnosis of herpes zoster, although the occurrence of shingles without a rash has been reported. Both herpes simplex virus infections and coxsackievirus infections can cause dermatomal vesicular lesions. Supportive diagnostic virology and fluorescent staining of skin scrapings with monoclonal antibodies are helpful in ensuring the proper diagnosis. In the prodromal stage of herpes zoster, the diagnosis can be exceedingly difficult and may be made only after lesions have appeared or by retrospective serologic assessment.

LABORATORY FINDINGS Unequivocal confirmation of the diagnosis is possible only through the isolation of VZV in susceptible tissue-culture cell lines, the demonstration of either seroconversion or a fourfold or greater rise in antibody titer between convalescent- and acute-phase serum specimens, or the detection of VZV DNA by polymerase chain reaction (PCR). A rapid impression can be obtained by a Tzanck smear, with scraping of the base of the lesions in an attempt to demonstrate multinucleated giant cells, although the sensitivity of this method is low (about 60%). PCR technology for the detection of viral DNA in vesicular fluid is available in a limited number of diagnostic laboratories. Direct immunofluorescent staining of cells from the lesion base or detection of viral antigens by other assays (such as the immunoperoxidase assay) is also useful, although these tests are not commercially available. The most frequently employed serologic tools for assessing host response are the immunofluorescent detection of antibodies to VZV membrane antigens, the fluorescent antibody to membrane antigen (FAMA) test, immune adherence hemagglutination, and enzyme-linked immunosorbent assay (ELISA). The FAMA test and the ELISA appear to be the most sensitive.

PROPHYLAXIS   While chickenpox in the otherwise healthy host is relatively benign, it can cause morbidity and death. Furthermore, the parents of a child with chickenpox often lose a significant amount of time from work. A live attenuated varicella vaccine has been licensed and is recommended for administration to all immunocompetent children and adults at risk of infection.

The immunocompromised individual is at significant risk for developing progressive varicella; modalities of prevention include passive immunization or experimental administration of the same live attenuated vaccine used in the immunocompetent child. Immune prophylaxis can consist of the administration of specific zoster immune globulin (ZIG) derived from patients with herpes zoster, varicella-zoster immune globulin (VZIG), or the intravenous formulation of zoster immune plasma (ZIP). Both ZIG and VZIG should be given within 96 h (preferably within 72 h) of exposure to ensure efficacy. It is likely that ZIP can be given somewhat later. Indications for the administration of VZIG are summarized in Table 183-1.

Rx   **TREATMENT**   Medical management of chickenpox in the immunologically normal host is directed toward the prevention of avoidable complications. Obviously, good hygiene includes daily bathing and soaks. Secondary bacterial infection of the skin can be avoided by meticulous skin care, particularly with close cropping of fingernails. Pruritus can be decreased with topical dressings or the administration of antipruritic drugs. Tepid water baths and wet compresses are better than drying lotions for the relief of itching. Aluminum acetate soaks for the management of herpes zoster can be both soothing and cleansing. Administration of aspirin to children with chickenpox should be avoided because of the association of aspirin derivatives with the development of Reye's syndrome. Acyclovir therapy (800 mg by mouth five times daily for 5 to 7 days) is recommended for adolescents and adults with chickenpox of ≤24 h duration. Likewise, acyclovir therapy may be of benefit to children <12 years of age if initiated early in the disease (<24 h) at a dose of 20 mg/kg every 6 h.

Patients with herpes zoster benefit from oral antiviral therapy, as evidenced by accelerated healing of lesions and resolution of zoster-associated pain with acyclovir, valacyclovir, or famciclovir. Acyclovir, now off patent, is administered at a dosage of 800 mg five times daily for 7 to 10 days. Famciclovir, the prodrug of penciclovir, is at least as effective as acyclovir and perhaps more so. One study showed twofold faster resolution of postherpetic neuralgia in famciclovir-treated patients with zoster than in recipients of placebo. The dose is 500 mg by mouth three times daily for 7 days. Valacyclovir, the prodrug of acyclovir, accelerates healing and resolution of zoster-associated pain more promptly than acyclovir. The dose is 1 g by mouth three times daily for 5 to 7 days. Both famciclovir and valacyclovir offer the advantage of a lower dosing frequency than acyclovir.

In the immunocompromised host, both chickenpox and herpes zoster (including disseminated disease) should be treated with intravenous acyclovir, which reduces the occurrence of visceral complications but has no effect on healing of skin lesions or pain. The dose is 10 to 12.5 mg/kg every 8 h for 7 days. Oral acyclovir therapy is not recommended for the treatment of VZV infections in immunocompromised patients. Concomitant with the administration of intravenous acyclovir, it is desirable to attempt to wean these patients from immunosuppressive treatment.

Patients with varicella pneumonia may require removal of bronchial secretions and ventilatory support. Persons with zoster ophthalmicus should be referred immediately to an ophthalmologist. Therapy for this condition consists of the administration of analgesics for severe pain and the use of atropine. Acyclovir accelerates healing.

The management of acute neuritis and/or postherpetic neuralgia can be particularly difficult. In addition to the judicious use of analgesics, ranging from nonnarcotics to narcotic derivatives, drugs such as gabapentin, amitriptyline hydrochloride, and fluphenazine hydrochloride have been reported to be beneficial for pain relief. In one study, glucocorticoid therapy administered early in the course of localized herpes zoster significantly accelerated such quality-of-life improvements as a return to usual activity and termination of analgesia. The dose of prednisone administered orally was 60 mg/d on days 1 through 7, 30 mg/d on days 8 through 14, and 15 mg/d on days 15 through 21. This regimen is appropriate only for relatively healthy elderly persons who have moderate or severe pain at presentation. Patients with osteoporosis, diabetes mellitus, glycosuria, or hypertension may not be appropriate candidates. Glucocorticoids should not be used without concomitant antiviral therapy.

Table 183-1   Recommendations for VZIG Administration

Exposure criteria
1. Both exposure to person with chickenpox or zoster as
   a. Continuous household contact
   b. Playmate for >1 h indoors
   c. Hospital contact (same room or prolonged face-to-face)
   d. Mother (see 3 below)
2. And time elapsed ≤96 h (preferably ≤72 h)

Candidates (provided they have significant exposure) include
1. Immunocompromised susceptible children
2. Immunocompetent susceptible adolescents (≥15 years old) and adults, especially pregnant women
3. Newborn infants of mothers with onset of chickenpox <5 days before or <2 days after delivery
4. Hospitalized premature infants
   a. ≥28 weeks of gestation when mother has no history of chickenpox
   b. <28 weeks of gestation and/or birth weight of ≤1000 g, regardless of maternal history

SOURCE: Adapted from American Academy of Pediatrics, in Red Book, Report of the Committee on Infectious Diseases, G Peter (ed), Elk Grove Village, IL, American Academy of Pediatrics, 1997.

BIBLIOGRAPHY

BEUTNER KR et al: Valacyclovir compared with acyclovir for improved therapy for herpes zoster in immunocompetent adults. Antimicrob Agents Chemother 39:1547, 1995

DUNKLE LM et al: A controlled trial of acyclovir for chickenpox in normal children. N Engl J Med 325:1539, 1991

IZURIETA HS et al: Postlicensure effectiveness of varicella vaccine during an outbreak in a child care center. JAMA 278:1495, 1997

LOCKSLEY RM et al: Infection with varicella-zoster virus after marrow transplantation. J Infect Dis 152:1172, 1985

ROWBOTHAM M et al: Gabapentin for the treatment of postherpetic neuralgia. A randomized controlled trial. JAMA 280:1837, 1998

SHEPP D et al: Treatment of varicella-zoster virus in severely immunocompromised patients: A randomized comparison of acyclovir and vidarabine. N Engl J Med 314:208, 1987

TYRING S et al: Famciclovir for the treatment of acute herpes zoster. Effects on acute disease and postherpetic neuralgia: A randomized, double-blind, placebo-controlled trial. Ann Intern Med 123:89, 1995

WEIBEL RE et al: Live attenuated varicella virus vaccine: Efficacy trial in healthy children. N Engl J Med 310:1409, 1984

WHITLEY RJ et al: Early vidarabine therapy to control the complications of herpes zoster in immunosuppressed patients. N Engl J Med 307:971, 1982

——— et al: Disseminated herpes zoster in the immunocompromised host: A comparative trial of acyclovir and vidarabine. J Infect Dis 165:450, 1992

——— et al: Acyclovir with and without prednisone for the treatment of herpes zoster: A randomized, placebo-controlled trial. Ann Intern Med 125:376, 1996

WOOD MJ et al: A randomized trial of acyclovir for 7 days or 21 days with and without prednisolone for treatment of acute herpes zoster. N Engl J Med 330:896, 1994

184

Jeffrey I. Cohen

EPSTEIN-BARR VIRUS INFECTIONS, INCLUDING INFECTIOUS MONONUCLEOSIS

DEFINITION Epstein-Barr virus (EBV) is the cause of heterophile-positive infectious mononucleosis (IM), which is characterized by fever, sore throat, lymphadenopathy, and atypical lymphocytosis. EBV is also associated with several human tumors, including nasopharyngeal carcinoma, Burkitt's lymphoma, Hodgkin's disease, and—in patients with immunodeficiencies (including AIDS)—B cell lymphoma. The virus, a member of the family Herpesviridae, consists of a linear, double-stranded DNA core surrounded by an icosahedral nucleocapsid and by the viral envelope, which contains glycoproteins. The two types of EBV that are widely prevalent in nature are not distinguishable by conventional serologic tests.

EPIDEMIOLOGY EBV infections occur worldwide. These infections are most common in early childhood, with a second peak during late adolescence. By adulthood, more than 90% of individuals have been infected and have antibodies to the virus. IM is usually a disease of young adults. In lower socioeconomic groups and in areas of the world with lower standards of hygiene (e.g., developing countries), EBV tends to infect children at an early age, and symptomatic IM is uncommon. In areas with higher standards of hygiene (e.g., the United States), infection with EBV is often delayed until adulthood, and IM is more prevalent.

EBV is spread by contact with oral secretions. The virus is frequently transmitted from asymptomatic adults to infants and among young adults by transfer of saliva during kissing. Transmission by less intimate contact is rare. EBV has been transmitted by blood transfusion and by bone marrow transplantation. Studies indicate that more than 90% of asymptomatic seropositive individuals shed the virus in oropharyngeal secretions.

PATHOGENESIS EBV is transmitted by salivary secretions. The virus infects the epithelium of the oropharynx and the salivary glands and is shed from these cells. While B cells may become infected after contact with epithelial cells, studies suggest that lymphocytes in the tonsillar crypts can be infected directly. The virus then spreads through the bloodstream. The proliferation and expansion of EBV-infected B cells along with reactive T cells during IM result in enlargement of lymphoid tissue. Polyclonal activation of B cells leads to the production of antibodies to host-cell and viral proteins. During the acute phase of IM, up to 1 in every 100 B cells in the peripheral blood is infected by EBV, while after recovery, about 1 in every million B cells is infected. During IM there is an inverted CD4+/CD8+ T cell ratio. The percentage of CD4+ T cells decreases, while there are large clonal expansions of CD8+ T cells; up to 40% of CD8+ T cells are directed against EBV antigens during acute infection. Data suggest that memory B cells, not epithelial cells, are the reservoir for EBV in the body: Shedding of EBV from the oropharynx stops but the virus persists in B cells when patients are treated with acyclovir.

The EBV receptor (CD21), present on the surface of B cells and epithelial cells, is also the receptor for the C3d component of complement. EBV infection of epithelial cells results in viral replication and production of virions. When B cells are infected by EBV in vitro, they become transformed and can proliferate indefinitely. During latent infection of B cells, only the EBV nuclear antigens (EBNAs), latent membrane proteins (LMPs), and small EBV RNAs are expressed in vitro. EBV-transformed B cells secrete immunoglobulin; only a small fraction of cells produce virus.

Cellular immunity is more important than humoral immunity in controlling EBV infection. In the initial phase of infection, suppressor T cells, natural killer cells, and nonspecific cytotoxic T cells are important in controlling the proliferation of EBV-infected B cells. Levels of markers of T cell activation and serum interferon γ are elevated.

Later in infection, HLA-restricted cytotoxic T cells that recognize EBNAs and LMPs and destroy EBV-infected cells are generated. Studies have shown that one of the late genes expressed during EBV replication, *BCRF1*, is a homologue of interleukin 10 and can inhibit the production of interferon γ by mononuclear cells in vitro. In addition, EBNA-1 inhibits antigen processing.

If T cell immunity is compromised, EBV-infected B cells may begin to proliferate. When EBV is associated with lymphoma, virus-induced proliferation is but one step in a multistep process of neoplastic transformation. In many EBV-containing tumors, LMP-1 mimics members of the tumor necrosis factor receptor family (e.g., CD40), transmitting growth-proliferating signals.

CLINICAL MANIFESTATIONS Most EBV infections in infants and young children either are asymptomatic or present as mild pharyngitis with or without tonsillitis. In contrast, up to 75% of infections in adolescents present as IM.

Signs and Symptoms The incubation period for IM in young adults is about 4 to 6 weeks. A prodrome of fatigue, malaise, and myalgia may last for 1 to 2 weeks before the onset of fever, sore throat, and lymphadenopathy. Fever is usually low-grade and is most common in the first 2 weeks of the illness; however, it may persist for over a month. Common signs and symptoms are listed along with their frequencies in Table 184-1. Lymphadenopathy and pharyngitis are most prominent during the first 2 weeks of the illness, while splenomegaly is more prominent during the second and third weeks. Lymphadenopathy most often affects the posterior cervical nodes but may be generalized. Enlarged lymph nodes are frequently tender and symmetric but are not fixed in place. Pharyngitis, often the most prominent sign, can be accompanied by enlargement of the tonsils with an exudate resembling that of streptococcal pharyngitis. A morbilliform or papular rash, usually on the arms or trunk, develops in about 5% of cases. Most patients treated with ampicillin develop a macular rash; this rash is not predictive of future adverse reactions to penicillins. Erythema nodosum and erythema multiforme have also been described (Chap. 57). Most patients have symptoms for 2 to 4 weeks, but malaise and difficulty concentrating can persist for months.

Symptomatic IM is uncommon in infants and young children. IM in the elderly presents relatively often as nonspecific symptoms, including prolonged fever, fatigue, myalgia, and malaise; in contrast, pharyngitis, lymphadenopathy, splenomegaly, and atypical lymphocytes are relatively rare in elderly patients.

Laboratory Findings The white blood cell count is usually elevated and peaks at 10,000 to 20,000/μL during the second or third week of illness. Lymphocytosis is usually demonstrable, with more than 10% atypical lymphocytes. The latter cells are enlarged lympho-

Table 184-1 Signs and Symptoms of Infectious Mononucleosis

Manifestation	Median Percentage of Patients (Range)
Symptoms	
Sore throat	75 (50–87)
Malaise	47 (42–76)
Headache	38 (22–67)
Abdominal pain, nausea, or vomiting	17 (5–25)
Chills	10 (9–11)
Signs	
Lymphadenopathy	95 (83–100)
Fever	93 (60–100)
Pharyngitis or tonsillitis	82 (68–90)
Splenomegaly	51 (43–64)
Hepatomegaly	11 (6–15)
Rash	10 (0–25)
Periorbital edema	13 (2–34)
Palatal enanthem	7 (3–13)
Jaundice	5 (2–10)

Table 184-2   Serologic Features of EBV-Associated Diseases

Condition	Heterophile	Anti-VCA		Anti-EA		Anti-EBNA
		IgM	IgG	EA-D	EA-R	
Acute infectious mononucleosis	+	+	++	+	−	−
Convalescence	±	−	+	−	±	+
Past infection	−	−	+	−	−	+
Reactivation with immunodeficiency	−	−	++	+	+	±
Burkitt's lymphoma	−	−	+++	±	++	+
Nasopharyngeal carcinoma	−	−	+++	++	±	+

[a] VCA, viral capsid antigen; EA, early antigen; EA-D antibody, antibody to early antigen, diffuse pattern in nucleus and cytoplasm of infected cells; EA-R antibody, antibody to early antigen, restricted to the cytoplasm; and EBNA, Epstein-Barr nuclear antigen.
SOURCE: Adapted from Okano, 1988.

cytes that have abundant cytoplasm, vacuoles, and indentations of the cell membrane. CD8+ cells predominate among the atypical lymphocytes. Low-grade neutropenia and thrombocytopenia are common during the first month of illness. Liver function is abnormal in more than 90% of cases. Serum levels of aminotransferases and alkaline phosphatase are usually mildly elevated; the serum concentration of bilirubin is elevated in about 40% of cases.

Complications   Most cases of IM are self-limited. Deaths are very rare and most often are due to central nervous system (CNS) complications, splenic rupture, upper airway obstruction, or bacterial superinfection.

When CNS complications develop, they usually do so during the first 2 weeks of EBV infection; in some patients, especially children, they are the only clinical manifestations of IM. Heterophile antibodies and atypical lymphocytes may be absent. Meningitis and encephalitis are the most common neurologic abnormalities, and patients may present with headache, meningismus, or cerebellar ataxia; acute hemiplegia and psychosis have also been described. The cerebrospinal fluid (CSF) contains mainly lymphocytes, with occasional atypical lymphocytes. Most cases resolve without neurologic sequelae. Acute EBV infection has also been associated with cranial nerve palsies (especially ones involving cranial nerve VII), Guillain-Barré syndrome, acute transverse myelitis, and peripheral neuritis.

Autoimmune hemolytic anemia occurs in about 2% of cases during the first 2 weeks. In most cases the anemia is Coombs'-test positive, with cold agglutinins directed against the i red blood cell antigen. Most patients with hemolysis have mild anemia that lasts for 1 or 2 months, but some patients have severe disease with hemoglobinuria and jaundice. Nonspecific antibody responses may also include rheumatoid factor, antinuclear antibodies, anti–smooth muscle antibodies, antiplatelet antibodies, and cryoglobulins. IM has been associated with red-cell aplasia, severe granulocytopenia, thrombocytopenia, pancytopenia, and hemophagocytic syndrome. The spleen ruptures in fewer than 0.5% of cases. Splenic rupture is more common among males than among females and may be manifest as abdominal pain, referred shoulder pain, or hemodynamic compromise.

Hypertrophy of lymphoid tissue in the tonsils or adenoids can result in upper airway obstruction, as can inflammation and edema of the epiglottis, pharynx, or uvula. About 10% of patients with IM develop streptococcal pharyngitis after their initial sore throat resolves.

Other rare complications associated with acute EBV infection include hepatitis (which can be fulminant), myocarditis or pericarditis with electrocardiographic changes, pneumonia with pleural effusion, interstitial nephritis, genital ulcerations, and vasculitis.

OTHER DISEASES ASSOCIATED WITH EBV INFECTION   EBV-associated lymphoproliferative disease has been described in patients with congenital or acquired immunodeficiency, including those with severe combined immunodeficiency or AIDS, recipients of bone marrow transplants, and recipients of organ transplants who are receiving immunosuppressive drugs (especially cyclosporine). Proliferating EBV-infected B cells infiltrate lymph nodes and multiple organs, and patients present with fever and lymphadenopathy or gastrointestinal symptoms. Pathologic studies show B cell hyperplasia or poly- or monoclonal lymphoma. The X-linked lymphoproliferative syndrome (Duncan's disease) is a recessive disorder of young boys who have a normal response to childhood infections but develop fatal lymphoproliferative disorders after infection with EBV. The gene mutated in this syndrome, SAP or SH2D1A, has been identified; its product binds to a protein that mediates interactions of B and T cells. Most patients with this syndrome die of acute IM; others develop hypogammaglobulinemia, malignant B cell lymphomas, aplastic anemia, or agranulocytosis. IM has also proved fatal to some patients with no obvious preexisting immune abnormality.

Oral hairy leukoplakia (**Plate IID-42**) is an early manifestation of infection with HIV in adults (Chap. 309). Most patients present with raised, white corrugated lesions on the tongue (and occasionally on the buccal mucosa) that contain EBV DNA. Children infected with HIV can develop lymphoid interstitial pneumonitis; EBV DNA is often found in lung tissue from these patients.

Patients with the chronic fatigue syndrome may have titers of antibody to EBV that are elevated but are not significantly different from those in healthy EBV-seropositive adults. While some patients have malaise and fatigue that persist for weeks or months after IM, persistent EBV infection is not a cause of the chronic fatigue syndrome. Chronic active EBV infection is very rare and is distinct from the chronic fatigue syndrome. The affected patients have an illness lasting more than 6 months with markedly elevated titers of antibody to EBV and evidence of organ involvement, including hepatosplenomegaly, lymphadenopathy, and pneumonitis, uveitis, or neurologic disease.

EBV is associated with several malignancies. About 15% of cases of Burkitt's lymphoma in the United States and about 90% of those in Africa are associated with EBV (Chap. 112). African patients with Burkitt's lymphoma have high levels of antibody to EBV, and their tumor tissue usually contains viral DNA. EBV-containing Burkitt's lymphoma also occurs in patients with AIDS. Anaplastic nasopharyngeal carcinoma is uniformly associated with EBV; the affected tissues contain viral DNA and antigens. Patients with nasopharyngeal carcinoma often have elevated titers of antibody to EBV (Chap. 87).

EBV has been associated with Hodgkin's disease, especially the mixed-cellularity type (Chap. 112). Patients with Hodgkin's disease often have elevated titers of antibody to EBV, and in about half of cases viral DNA and antigens are found in Reed-Sternberg cells. In some cases, EBV DNA has been detected in tonsillar carcinoma, angioimmunoblastic lymphadenopathy, angiocentric nasal NK/T cell immunoproliferative lesions, T cell lymphoma, thymoma, gastric carcinoma, and CNS lymphoma from patients with no underlying immunodeficiency. Studies have demonstrated viral DNA in leiomyosarcomas from AIDS patients and in smooth-muscle tumors from organ transplant recipients. Virtually all CNS lymphomas in AIDS patients are associated with EBV.

DIAGNOSIS   Serologic Testing   The heterophile test is used for the diagnosis of IM in children and adults (Table 184-2). Heterophile antibody is an IgM antibody that does not bind EBV proteins. In the test for this antibody, human serum is absorbed with guinea pig kidney, and the heterophile titer is defined as the greatest serum dilution that agglutinates sheep, horse, or cow erythrocytes. A titer of 40-fold or greater is diagnostic of acute EBV infection in a patient who has symptoms compatible with IM and atypical lymphocytes. Tests for heterophile antibodies are positive in 40% of patients with IM during the first week of illness and in 80 to 90% during the third week. Therefore, repeated testing may be necessary, especially if the initial test is performed early. Tests usually remain positive for 3 months after the onset of illness, but heterophile antibodies can persist for up to 1 year. These antibodies usually are not detectable in children <5 years of age, in the elderly, or in patients presenting with symptoms not typical of IM. The commercially available monospot test for heterophile antibodies is somewhat more sensitive than the classic heterophile test. False-positive results in the monospot test are more common in children and in patients with other viral infections.

EBV-specific antibody testing is used for patients with suspected acute EBV infection who lack heterophile antibodies and for patients with atypical infections. Serologic tests are particularly useful in young children, who often do not develop heterophile antibodies. Titers of IgM and IgG antibodies to viral capsid antigen (VCA) are elevated in the serum of more than 90% of patients at the onset of disease. IgM antibody to VCA is useful for the diagnosis of acute IM because it is present at elevated titers only during the first 2 months of the disease; in contrast, IgG antibody to VCA is often used to assess exposure to EBV in the past because it persists for life.

Antibodies to early antigens (EAs) are found either in a diffuse pattern in the nucleus and cytoplasm of infected cells (EA-D antibody) or restricted to the cytoplasm (EA-R antibody). These antibodies are detectable 3 to 4 weeks after the onset of symptoms in patients with IM. About 70% of individuals with IM, especially those with relatively severe disease, have EA-D antibodies during the course of their illness. These antibodies usually persist for only 3 to 6 months. Levels of EA-D antibodies are also elevated in patients with nasopharyngeal carcinoma or chronic active EBV infection. EA-R antibodies are only occasionally detected in patients with IM but are often found at elevated titers in patients with African Burkitt's lymphoma or chronic active EBV infection.

IgA antibodies to EBV antigens have proved useful for the identification of patients with nasopharyngeal carcinoma and of persons at high risk for the disease. Seroconversion to EBNA positivity is also useful for the diagnosis of acute infection with EBV. Antibodies to EBNA are detectable relatively late (3 to 6 weeks after the onset of symptoms) in nearly all cases of acute EBV infection and persist for the lifetime of the patient. These antibodies may be lacking in immunodeficient patients and in those with chronic active EBV infection.

Other Studies   Detection of EBV DNA, RNA, or proteins has been valuable in demonstrating the association of the virus with various malignancies. The polymerase chain reaction has been used to detect EBV DNA in the CSF of some AIDS patients with lymphomas and to monitor the amount of EBV DNA in the blood of patients with lymphoproliferative disease. Culture of EBV from throat washings or blood is not helpful in the diagnosis of acute infection, since EBV commonly persists in the oropharynx and in B cells for the lifetime of the infected individual.

Differential Diagnosis   The differential diagnosis of IM and atypical lymphocytosis includes acute infection with cytomegalovirus, *Toxoplasma*, HIV, human herpesvirus 6, and hepatitis viruses as well as drug hypersensitivity reactions. Cytomegalovirus is the most common cause of heterophile-negative mononucleosis, usually involves older patients, and is associated with a lower frequency of sore throat, splenomegaly, and lymphadenopathy than IM due to EBV. Other diseases that share some of the features of IM include rubella, acute infectious lymphocytosis in children, and lymphoma or leukemia.

TREATMENT   Therapy for IM consists of supportive measures, with rest and analgesia. Excessive physical activity during the first month should be avoided to reduce the possibility of splenic rupture. If splenic rupture occurs, splenectomy is required. Glucocorticoid therapy is not indicated for uncomplicated IM and in fact may predispose to bacterial superinfection. Prednisone (40 to 60 mg/d for 2 to 3 days, with subsequent tapering of the dose over 1 to 2 weeks) has been used for the prevention of airway obstruction in patients with severe tonsillar hypertrophy, for autoimmune hemolytic anemia, and for severe thrombocytopenia. Glucocorticoids have also been used in

a few selected patients with severe malaise and fever and in patients with severe CNS or cardiac disease.

Acyclovir has had no significant clinical impact on IM in controlled trials. In one study, the combination of acyclovir and prednisolone had no significant effect on the duration of symptoms of IM. Acyclovir, at a dosage of 400 to 800 mg five times daily, has been effective for the treatment of oral hairy leukoplakia (despite common relapses) and some cases of chronic active EBV disease. This agent generally has not been beneficial for patients with lymphoproliferative syndromes. When possible, therapy for EBV lymphoproliferative disease should be directed toward the reduction of immunosuppressive medication. New therapies, including the use of interferon α and the infusion of donor T cells or EBV-specific cytotoxic T cells, are being studied.

The isolation of patients with IM is unnecessary. Vaccines directed against the major EBV glycoprotein have been effective in animal studies and are currently undergoing small-scale clinical trials.

BIBLIOGRAPHY

AUWAERTER PG: Infectious mononucleosis in middle age. JAMA 281:454, 1999

COHEN JI: Epstein-Barr virus and the immune system—hide and seek. JAMA 278:510, 1997

————: Epstein-Barr virus lymphoproliferative disease associated with acquired immunodeficiency. Medicine 70:137, 1991

HESLOP HE et al: Long-term restoration of immunity against Epstein-Barr virus infection by adoptive transfer of gene-modified virus-specific T lymphocytes. Nat Med 2:551, 1996

LIEBOWITZ D: Epstein-Barr virus and a cellular signaling pathway in lymphomas from immunosuppressed patients. N Engl J Med 338:1413, 1998

OKANO M et al: Epstein-Barr virus and human diseases: Recent advances in diagnosis. Clin Microbiol Rev 1:300, 1988

PAPADOPOULOS EB et al: Infusions of donor leukocytes to treat Epstein-Barr virus-associated lymphoproliferative disorders after allogeneic bone marrow transplantation. N Engl J Med 330:1185, 1994

PATHMANATHAN R et al: Clonal proliferations of cells infected with Epstein-Barr virus in proliferative lesions related to nasopharyngeal carcinoma. N Engl J Med 333:693, 1995

RICKINSON AB, KIEFF E: Epstein-Barr virus, in *Fields Virology,* 3d ed, BN Fields et al (eds). Philadelphia, Lippincott-Raven, 1996

SAYOS J et al: The X-linked lymphoproliferative-disease gene product SAP regulates signals induced through the co-receptor SLAM. Nature 395:462, 1998

STRAUS SE: Epstein-Barr virus infections: Biology, pathogenesis, and management. Ann Intern Med 118:45, 1993

TYNELL E et al: Acyclovir and prednisolone treatment of acute infectious mononucleosis: A multicenter, double blind, placebo-controlled study. J Infect Dis 174:324, 1996

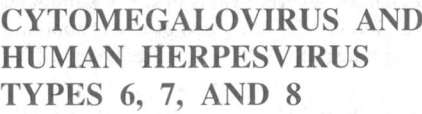

185   *Martin S. Hirsch*

CYTOMEGALOVIRUS AND HUMAN HERPESVIRUS TYPES 6, 7, AND 8

CYTOMEGALOVIRUS

DEFINITION   Cytomegalovirus (CMV), which was initially isolated from patients with congenital cytomegalic inclusion disease, is now recognized as an important pathogen in all age groups. In addition to inducing severe birth defects, CMV causes a wide spectrum of disorders in older children and adults, ranging from an asymptomatic, subclinical infection to a mononucleosis syndrome in healthy individuals to disseminated disease in immunocompromised patients. Human CMV is one of several related species-specific viruses that cause similar diseases in various animals. All are associated with the production of characteristic enlarged cells—hence the name *cytomegalovirus.*

CMV is a member of the β-herpesvirus group and has double-

Table 185-1 CMV in the Immunocompromised Host

Population	Risk Factors	Principal Syndromes	Treatment	Prevention
Fetus	Primary maternal infection/early pregnancy	Cytomegalic inclusion disease	None	Avoidance of exposure
Organ transplant recipient	Seropositive donor, seronegative recipient; intensive immunosuppression, particularly with antilymphocyte globulins, cyclosporine	Febrile leukopenia; pneumonia; gastrointestinal disease	Ganciclovir	Donor matching; CMV immunoglobulin; ganciclovir or high-dose acyclovir
Bone marrow transplant recipient	Graft-vs.-host disease; older age; seropositive recipient; viremia	Pneumonia; gastrointestinal disease	Ganciclovir plus CMV immunoglobulin	Ganciclovir or high-dose acyclovir
Person with AIDS	<100 CD4+ cells per microliter; CMV seropositivity	Retinitis; gastrointestinal disease; neurologic disease	Foscarnet, ganciclovir, or cidofovir	Oral ganciclovir

stranded DNA, a protein capsid, and a lipoprotein envelope. Like other herpesviruses, CMV demonstrates icosahedral symmetry, replicates in the cell nucleus, and can cause either a lytic and productive or a latent infection. CMV can be distinguished from other herpesviruses by certain biologic properties, such as host range and type of cytopathology induced. Viral replication is associated with the production of large intranuclear inclusions and smaller cytoplasmic inclusions. The virus appears to replicate in a variety of cell types in vivo; in tissue culture it grows preferentially in fibroblasts. Although there is little evidence that CMV is oncogenic in vivo, the virus does transform fibroblasts in rare instances, and genomic transforming fragments have been identified.

EPIDEMIOLOGY CMV has a worldwide distribution. Approximately 1% of newborns in the United States are infected with CMV, and the percentage is higher in many less developed countries. Communal living and poor personal hygiene facilitate early spread. Perinatal and early childhood infections are common. Virus may be present in milk, saliva, feces, and urine. Transmission of CMV has been identified among young children in day-care centers and has been traced from infected toddler to pregnant mother to developing fetus. When an infected child introduces CMV into a household, 50% of susceptible family members seroconvert within 6 months.

The virus is not readily spread by casual contact but requires repeated or prolonged intimate exposure for transmission. In late adolescence and young adulthood, CMV is often transmitted sexually, and asymptomatic viral carriage in semen or cervical secretions is common. CMV antibody is present at detectable levels in nearly 100% of female prostitutes and sexually active homosexual men. Sexually active adults may harbor several strains of CMV simultaneously. Transfusion of whole blood or certain blood products containing viable leukocytes may also transmit CMV, with a frequency of 0.14 to 10% per unit transfused.

Once infected, an individual probably carries CMV for life. The infection usually remains latent. However, CMV reactivation syndromes develop frequently when T lymphocyte–mediated immunity is compromised—for example, after organ transplantation or in association with lymphoid neoplasms and certain acquired immunodeficiencies (in particular, infection with HIV; Chap. 309). Most primary CMV infections in organ transplant recipients (Chap. 136) result from transmission of the virus in the graft itself. In CMV-seropositive transplant recipients, infection results from reactivation of latent virus or, less commonly, from reinfection by a new strain of CMV. CMV infection may be associated with coronary artery stenosis following heart transplantation or coronary angioplasty, but this association requires further validation.

PATHOGENESIS Congenital CMV infection can result from either primary or reactivation infection of the mother. However, clinical disease in the fetus or newborn is almost exclusively related to primary maternal infection (Table 185-1). The factors determining the severity of congenital infection are unknown; a deficient capacity to produce precipitating antibodies and to mount T cell responses to CMV is associated with relatively severe disease.

Primary infection in late childhood or adulthood is often associated with a vigorous T lymphocyte response that may contribute to the development of a mononucleosis syndrome similar to that observed following Epstein-Barr virus (EBV) infection (Chap. 184). The hallmark of such infection is the appearance of atypical lymphocytes in the peripheral blood; these cells are predominantly activated CD8+ T lymphocytes. Polyclonal activation of B cells by the virus contributes to the development of rheumatoid factors and other autoantibodies during CMV mononucleosis.

Once acquired by symptomatic or asymptomatic primary infection, CMV persists indefinitely in tissues of the host. The sites of persistent or latent infection are unclear but probably include multiple cell types and various organs. Transmission following blood transfusion or organ transplantation is due to silent infections in these tissues. Autopsy studies suggest that salivary glands and bowel may be areas of latent infection.

If the host's T cell responses become compromised by disease or by iatrogenic immunosuppression, latent virus can be reactivated to cause a variety of syndromes. Chronic antigenic stimulation in the presence of immunosuppression (for example, following tissue transplantation) appears to be an ideal setting for CMV activation and CMV-induced disease. Certain particularly potent suppressants of T cell immunity, such as antithymocyte globulin, are associated with a high rate of clinical CMV syndromes, which may follow either primary or reactivation infection. CMV may itself contribute to further T lymphocyte hyporesponsiveness, which often precedes superinfection with other opportunistic pathogens, such as *Pneumocystis carinii*. CMV and *P. carinii* are frequently found together in immunosuppressed patients with severe interstitial pneumonia. CMV may function as a cofactor to activate latent HIV infection.

PATHOLOGY Cytomegalic cells in vivo (presumed to be infected epithelial cells) are two to four times larger than surrounding cells and often contain an 8- to 10-μm intranuclear inclusion that is eccentrically placed and is surrounded by a clear halo, producing an "owl's eye" appearance. Smaller granular cytoplasmic inclusions are demonstrated occasionally. Cytomegalic cells are found in a wide variety of organs, including salivary gland, lung, liver, kidney, intestine, pancreas, adrenal gland, and the central nervous system.

The cellular inflammatory response to infection consists of plasma cells, lymphocytes, and monocyte-macrophages. Granulomatous reactions occasionally develop, particularly in the liver. Immunopathologic reactions may contribute to CMV disease. Immune complexes have been detected in infected infants, sometimes in association with CMV-related glomerulopathies. Immune-complex glomerulopathy has been observed in some CMV-infected patients after renal transplantation.

CLINICAL MANIFESTATIONS **Congenital CMV Infection** Fetal infections range from inapparent to severe and disseminated. Cytomegalic inclusion disease develops in approximately 5% of infected fetuses and is seen almost exclusively in infants born to mothers who develop primary infections during pregnancy. Petechiae, hepatosplenomegaly, and jaundice are the most common presenting features (60 to 80% of cases). Microcephaly with or without cerebral calcifications, intrauterine growth retardation, and prematurity are reported in 30 to 50% of cases. Inguinal hernias and chorioretinitis are less common. Laboratory abnormalities include elevated alanine aminotransferase levels, thrombocytopenia, conjugated hyperbilirubinemia, hemolysis, and elevated cerebrospinal fluid protein levels. The prognosis for severely infected infants is poor; the mortality rate is 20 to 30%, and few of the patients who survive escape intellectual or hearing difficulties in later years. The differential diagnosis of cytomegalic inclusion disease in infants includes syphilis, rubella, toxoplasmosis, infection with herpes simplex virus or enterovirus, and bacterial sepsis.

Most congenital CMV infections are clinically inapparent at birth. Between 5 and 25% of asymptomatically infected infants develop significant psychomotor, hearing, ocular, or dental abnormalities over the next several years.

Perinatal CMV Infection The newborn may acquire CMV at the time of delivery by passage through an infected birth canal or by postnatal contact with maternal milk or other secretions. Approximately 40 to 60% of infants who are breast-fed for longer than 1 month by seropositive mothers become infected. Iatrogenic transmission also can result from neonatal blood transfusion. Screening of blood products before they are transfused into low-birth-weight seronegative infants or into seronegative pregnant women decreases the risk of infection.

The great majority of infants infected at or after delivery remain asymptomatic. However, protracted interstitial pneumonitis has been associated with perinatally acquired CMV infection, particularly in premature infants, and occasionally has been accompanied by infection with *Chlamydia trachomatis*, *P. carinii*, or *Ureaplasma urealyticum*. Poor weight gain, adenopathy, rash, hepatitis, anemia, and atypical lymphocytosis may also be found, and CMV excretion often persists for months or years.

CMV Mononucleosis The most common clinical manifestation of CMV infection in normal hosts beyond the neonatal period is a heterophil antibody–negative mononucleosis syndrome. This manifestation may develop spontaneously or may follow the transfusion of leukocyte-containing blood products. Although the syndrome occurs at all ages, it most often involves sexually active young adults. Incubation periods range from 20 to 60 days, and the illness generally lasts for 2 to 6 weeks. Prolonged high fevers, sometimes accompanied by chills, profound fatigue, and malaise, characterize this disorder. Myalgias, headache, and splenomegaly are frequent, but in CMV mononucleosis (as opposed to infectious mononucleosis caused by EBV), exudative pharyngitis and cervical lymphadenopathy are rare. Occasional patients develop rubelliform rashes, often after exposure to ampicillin. Less commonly observed are interstitial or segmental pneumonia, myocarditis, pleuritis, arthritis, and encephalitis. In rare cases, Guillain-Barré syndrome complicates CMV mononucleosis. The characteristic laboratory abnormality is relative lymphocytosis in peripheral blood, with more than 10% atypical lymphocytes. Total leukocyte counts may be low, normal, or markedly elevated. Although significant jaundice is uncommon, serum aminotransferase and alkaline phosphatase levels are often moderately elevated. Heterophil antibodies are absent; however, transient immunologic abnormalities are common and may include the presence of cryoglobulins, rheumatoid factors, cold agglutinins, and antinuclear antibodies. Hemolytic anemia, thrombocytopenia, and granulocytopenia complicate recovery in rare instances.

Most patients recover without sequelae, although postviral asthenia may persist for months. The excretion of CMV in urine, genital secretions, and/or saliva often continues for months or years. Rarely, CMV infection is fatal in immunocompetent hosts; even when such patients survive, they can have recurrent episodes of fever and malaise that are sometimes associated with autonomic nervous system dysfunction (e.g., attacks of sweating or flushing).

CMV Infection in the Immunocompromised Host (See also Table 185-1) CMV appears to be the most common and important viral pathogen complicating organ transplantation (Chap. 136). In recipients of kidney, heart, lung, and liver transplants, CMV induces a variety of syndromes, including fever and leukopenia, hepatitis, pneumonitis, esophagitis, gastritis, colitis, and retinitis. CMV disease may be an independent risk factor for both graft loss and death. The period of maximal risk is between 1 and 4 months after transplantation, although retinitis may be a later complication. The risk of disease appears to be greater after primary infection than after reactivation. In addition, molecular studies indicate that seropositive transplant recipients are susceptible to reinfection with donor-derived, genotypically variant CMV, and such infection often results in disease. Reactivation infection, although frequent, is less likely than primary infection to be important clinically. Clinical disease is related to various factors, such as the degree of immunosuppression; patients receiving certain immunosuppressive agents, such as antithymocyte globulin, appear to be more likely to have severe infections than those receiving other agents, such as cyclosporine. The transplanted organ is particularly vulnerable as a target for CMV infection; thus, there is a tendency for CMV hepatitis to follow liver transplantation and for CMV pneumonitis to follow lung transplantation.

CMV pneumonia occurs in 15 to 20% of bone marrow transplant recipients, with a case-fatality rate of 84 to 88%. The risk is greatest between 5 and 13 weeks after transplantation, and the several risk factors identified include certain types of immunosuppressive therapy, acute graft-versus-host disease, older age, viremia, and seropositivity before transplantation.

CMV is recognized as an important pathogen in patients with advanced HIV infection (Chap. 309), in whom it often causes retinitis or disseminated disease, particularly when peripheral-blood CD4+ cell counts fall below 50 to 100/μL. As treatment for underlying HIV infection has improved, the incidence of serious CMV infections (e.g., retinitis) has decreased. However, institution of highly active antiretroviral regimens sometimes leads to acute flare-ups of CMV retinitis during the first few weeks of therapy.

Syndromes produced by CMV in the immunocompromised host often begin with prolonged fever, malaise, anorexia, fatigue, night sweats, and arthralgias or myalgias. Liver function abnormalities, leukopenia, thrombocytopenia, and atypical lymphocytosis may be observed during these episodes. The development of tachypnea, hypoxia, and unproductive cough signals respiratory involvement. Radiologic examination of the lung often demonstrates bilateral interstitial or reticulonodular infiltrates, which begin in the periphery of the lower lobes and spread centrally and superiorly; localized segmental, nodular, or alveolar patterns are less common. The differential diagnosis includes infection with *P. carinii*; infections due to other viral, bacterial, or fungal pathogens; pulmonary hemorrhage; and injury secondary to irradiation or to treatment with cytotoxic drugs.

Gastrointestinal CMV involvement may be localized or extensive and almost exclusively affects compromised hosts. Ulcers of the esophagus, stomach, small intestine, or colon may result in bleeding or perforation. CMV infection may lead to exacerbations of underlying ulcerative colitis. Hepatitis occurs frequently, particularly following liver transplantation, and CMV-associated acalculous cholecystitis and adrenalitis have been described.

CMV rarely causes meningoencephalitis in otherwise healthy individuals. Two forms of CMV encephalitis are seen in patients with AIDS. One resembles HIV encephalitis and presents as progressive dementia; the other is a ventriculoencephalitis characterized by cranial-nerve deficits, nystagmus, disorientation, lethargy, and ventriculomegaly. In immunocompromised patients, CMV can also cause subacute progressive polyradiculopathy, which is often reversible if recognized and treated promptly.

CMV retinitis is an important cause of blindness in immunocompromised patients, particularly patients with advanced AIDS (Chap. 309). Early lesions consist of small, opaque, white areas of granular retinal necrosis that spread in a centrifugal manner and are later accompanied by hemorrhages, vessel sheathing, and retinal edema (see **Plate IV-2**). CMV retinopathy must be distinguished from that due to other conditions, including toxoplasmosis, candidiasis, and herpes simplex virus infection.

Fatal CMV infections are often associated with persistent viremia and the involvement of multiple organ systems. Progressive pulmonary infiltrates, pancytopenia, hyperamylasemia, and hypotension are characteristic features that are frequently found in conjunction with a terminal bacterial, fungal, or protozoan superinfection. Extensive adrenal necrosis with CMV inclusions is often documented at autopsy, as is CMV involvement of many other organs.

DIAGNOSIS   The diagnosis of CMV infection usually cannot be made reliably on clinical grounds alone. Isolation of the virus or detection of CMV antigens or DNA from appropriate clinical specimens, together with demonstration of a fourfold or greater rise in antibody titers or persistently elevated antibody titers, is the preferred diagnostic approach. Virus excretion or viremia is readily detected by culture of appropriate specimens on human fibroblast monolayers. If viral titers are high, as is frequently the case in congenital disseminated infection or in patients with AIDS, characteristic cytopathic effects may be detected within a few days. However, in some situations—such as CMV mononucleosis—viral titers are low, and cytopathic effects may take several weeks to appear. Many laboratories expedite diagnosis with an overnight tissue-culture method (shell vial assay) involving centrifugation and an immunocytochemical detection technique employing monoclonal antibodies to an immediate-early CMV antigen. Isolation of virus from urine or saliva does not, by itself, constitute proof of acute infection, since excretion from these sites may continue for months or years after illness. Detection of CMV viremia is a better predictor of acute infection.

Detection of CMV antigens (pp65) in peripheral-blood leukocytes or of CMV DNA in blood or tissues may hasten the diagnosis of CMV disease in certain populations, including organ transplant recipients and persons with AIDS. Such assays may yield a positive result several days earlier than culture methods. The detection of CMV DNA in cerebrospinal fluid by the polymerase chain reaction is useful in the diagnosis of CMV encephalitis or polyradiculopathy.

A variety of serologic assays are available to detect increases in titers of antibody to CMV antigens. An increased antibody level may not be detectable for up to 4 weeks after primary infection, and titers often remain high for years after infection. For this reason, single-sample antibody determinations are of no value in assessing the acuteness of infection. Detection of CMV-specific IgM is sometimes useful in the diagnosis of recent or active infection; circulating rheumatoid factors may result in occasional false-positive IgM tests.

℞ **TREATMENT**   Several prophylactic measures are useful for the prevention of CMV infection in patients at high risk. The use of blood from seronegative donors or of blood that has been frozen, thawed, and deglycerolized greatly decreases the rate of transfusion-associated transmission of CMV. Similarly, matching of organ or bone marrow transplants by CMV serology, using organs only from seronegative donors for seronegative recipients, reduces rates of primary infection following transplantation. Both live attenuated and CMV subunit vaccines have been evaluated, but neither is close to approval for general use.

CMV immune globulin has been reported to reduce rates of occurrence of CMV-associated syndromes and of fungal or parasitic superinfections among seronegative renal transplant recipients. Studies in bone marrow transplant recipients have produced conflicting results. Prophylactic acyclovir has been demonstrated to reduce rates of CMV infection and disease in certain seronegative renal transplant recipients; acyclovir is not effective in the treatment of active CMV disease, however.

Ganciclovir is a guanosine derivative that has considerably more activity against CMV than its congener acyclovir. After intracellular conversion by a viral phosphotransferase encoded by CMV gene region UL97, ganciclovir triphosphate is a selective inhibitor of CMV DNA polymerase. Several clinical studies have indicated response rates of 70 to 90% among patients with AIDS given ganciclovir for the treatment of CMV retinitis or colitis. In bone marrow transplant recipients with CMV pneumonia, ganciclovir is less effective when given alone, but it elicits a favorable clinical response 50 to 70% of the time when it is combined with CMV immune globulin. Prophylactic or suppressive ganciclovir may be useful in high-risk bone marrow or organ transplant recipients (e.g., those who are CMV-seropositive before transplantation or who are CMV culture–positive afterward). In many patients with AIDS, persistently low CD4+ cell counts, and CMV disease, clinical and virologic relapses occur promptly if treatment with ganciclovir is discontinued. Therefore, prolonged maintenance regimens are recommended for such patients. Resistance to ganciclovir is common among patients treated for more than 3 months and is usually related to mutations in the CMV UL97 gene.

Ganciclovir therapy for CMV retinitis consists of a 14- to 21-day induction course (5 mg/kg intravenously twice a day) followed by a prolonged intravenous or oral maintenance regimen. For parenteral maintenance, the dose is 5 mg/kg daily or 6 mg/kg 5 days per week. Peripheral-blood neutropenia develops in 16 to 29% of treated patients but is often ameliorated by granulocyte or granulocyte-macrophage colony-stimulating factor. Oral ganciclovir at a high dose (3 g/d) can also be used for maintenance, although the blood levels achieved are insufficient for acute induction regimens. Although progression (as assessed by funduscopy) is more rapid with oral than with intravenous ganciclovir maintenance (mean time to progression, 68 vs. 96 days; $p = .03$), the ease of administration and reduced toxicity of the oral preparation may make it an acceptable alternative for some patients who do not have sight-threatening central retinitis. The use of oral ganciclovir as prophylaxis in high-risk AIDS patients (i.e., those with CD4+ cell counts of $<100/\mu L$) has been studied in two placebo-controlled trials, with somewhat contradictory results.

Foscarnet (sodium phosphonoformate) also acts against CMV infection by inhibiting viral DNA polymerase. Because this agent does not require phosphorylation to be active, it is also effective against most ganciclovir-resistant CMV isolates. A comparative trial of foscarnet and ganciclovir in 234 patients with AIDS and CMV retinitis demonstrated equivalent activity against retinitis but longer survival (12.6 vs. 8.5 months) in the foscarnet group. Although the reasons for the latter difference are unclear, the antiretroviral activity of foscarnet and the greater use of zidovudine by foscarnet recipients are strong possibilities. Foscarnet is less well tolerated than ganciclovir and causes considerable toxicity, including renal dysfunction, hypomagnesemia, hypokalemia, hypocalcemia, genital ulcers, dysuria, nausea, and paresthesia. Moreover, foscarnet administration requires the use of an infusion pump and close clinical monitoring. With aggressive hydration and dose adjustments for renal dysfunction, the toxicity of foscarnet can be reduced. The use of foscarnet should be avoided when a saline load cannot be tolerated (e.g., in cardiomyopathy). The approved induction regimen is 60 mg/kg every 8 h for 2 weeks, although 90 mg/kg every 12 h is equally effective and no more toxic. Maintenance infusions should deliver 90 to 120 mg/kg once daily; no oral preparation is available. Foscarnet-resistant viruses may emerge during extended therapy.

Ganciclovir may also be administered via a slow-release pellet sutured into the eye. Although this intraocular device provides good local protection, contralateral eye disease and disseminated disease are not affected, and early retinal detachment is possible. A combination of intraocular and systemic therapy may be better than the intraocular implant alone.

Cidofovir is a nucleotide analogue with a long intracellular half-life that allows intermittent intravenous administration. Induction regimens of 5 mg/kg weekly for 2 weeks are followed by maintenance regimens of 3 to 5 mg/kg every 2 weeks. Cidofovir can cause severe nephrotoxicity through dose-dependent proximal tubular cell injury;

however, this adverse effect can be ameliorated somewhat by saline hydration and probenecid.

HUMAN HERPESVIRUS TYPES 6, 7, AND 8

Human herpesvirus (HHV) type 6 was first isolated in 1986 from peripheral-blood leukocytes of six persons with various lymphoproliferative disorders. The virus has a worldwide distribution, and two genetically distinct variants (HHV-6A and HHV-6B) are now recognized.

Infection with HHV-6 frequently develops during infancy as maternal antibody wanes. Congenital infections have also been described. HHV-6 (mostly variant B) can cause exanthem subitum (roseola infantum), a common illness characterized by fever with subsequent rash. HHV-6 is also a major cause of febrile seizures without rash during infancy. In older age groups, HHV-6 has been associated with mononucleosis syndromes, focal encephalitis, and (in immunocompromised hosts) pneumonitis and disseminated disease. In transplant recipients, HHV-6 infection may be associated with graft dysfunction. As many as 80% of adults are seropositive for HHV-6. The virus may be transmitted by saliva and possibly by genital secretions. There is no established treatment or vaccine.

HHV-7 was isolated in 1990 from T lymphocytes from the peripheral blood of a healthy 26-year-old man. Other isolates have since been obtained. It appears that the virus is frequently acquired during childhood and is frequently present in the saliva of healthy adults. No human disease has yet been definitively linked to HHV-7, although some cases of exanthem subitum and other childhood febrile illnesses have been associated with HHV-7 infection. An association has been made between HHV-7 and pityriasis rosea, but further studies must confirm this relationship.

Unique herpesvirus-like DNA sequences were reported during 1994 and 1995 in tissues derived from Kaposi's sarcoma and body cavity–based lymphoma occurring in patients with AIDS. When subjected to representational-difference analyses, more than 90% of Kaposi's sarcoma tissue samples were found to contain these sequences, whereas appropriate control tissues did not. The same herpesvirus-like DNA sequences have been reported in Kaposi's sarcoma tissue from non-AIDS patients, in a subgroup of AIDS-related B-cell body cavity–based lymphomas, and in lymph nodes from patients with multicentric Castleman's disease (a condition also known as angiofollicular lymph node hyperplasia, giant lymph node hyperplasia, lymphoid hamartoma, and follicular lymphoreticuloma, which is especially aggressive and frequently fatal). Approximately 15% of non–Kaposi's sarcoma tissue specimens from patients with AIDS contain these herpesvirus-like sequences, which have also been found in semen from both AIDS and non-AIDS patients. The virus has been propagated in cell culture and named HHV-8; it is also referred to as Kaposi's sarcoma–associated herpesvirus. Several serologic assays suggest a low rate of background positivity (0 to 29%) among HIV-negative blood donors but a high rate of positivity (>80%) among patients with Kaposi's sarcoma. The etiologic role of HHV-8 in Kaposi's sarcoma and other diseases remains to be established, although HHV-8 seroconversion during HIV infection appears to be highly predictive of the development of Kaposi's sarcoma.

BIBLIOGRAPHY

ADAMS O et al: Congenital infection with human herpesvirus 6. J Infect Dis 178:544, 1998

ADLER SP et al: Prior infection with cytomegalovirus is not a major risk factor for angiographically demonstrated coronary artery atherosclerosis. J Infect Dis 177:209, 1998

ANDERS HJ, GOEBEL F: Cytomegalovirus polyradiculopathy in patients with AIDS. Clin Infect Dis 27:345, 1998

CESARMAN E et al: Kaposi's sarcoma–associated herpesvirus-like DNA sequences in AIDS-related body-cavity-based lymphomas. N Engl J Med 332:1186, 1995

CONE RU et al: Human herpesvirus 6 infections after bone marrow transplantation: Clinical and virologic manifestations. J Infect Dis 179:311, 1999

DE OTERO J et al: Cytomegalovirus disease as a risk factor for graft loss and death after orthotopic liver transplantation. Clin Infect Dis 26:865, 1998

DRAGO F et al: Human herpesvirus 7 in patients with pityriasis rosea. Electron microscopy investigations and polymerase chain reaction in mononuclear cells, plasma and skin. Dermatology 196:275, 1997

EDDLESTON M et al: Severe cytomegalovirus infection in immunocompetent patients. Clin Infect Dis 24:52, 1997

JABS DA et al: Cytomegalovirus retinitis and viral resistance: Ganciclovir resistance. J Infect Dis 177:770, 1998

JACOBSON MA: Treatment of cytomegalovirus retinitis in patients with the acquired immunodeficiency syndrome. N Engl J Med 337:105, 1997

LAUTENSCHLAGER I et al: Human herpesvirus-6 infection after liver transplantation. Clin Infect Dis 26:702, 1998

MCCUTCHAN JA: Cytomegalovirus infections of the nervous system in patients with AIDS. Clin Infect Dis 20:747, 1995

RENWICK N et al: Seroconversion for human herpesvirus 8 during HIV infection is highly predictive of Kaposi's sarcoma. AIDS 12:2481, 1998

SPECTOR SA et al: Plasma cytomegalovirus (CMV) DNA load predicts CMV disease and survival in AIDS patients. J Clin Invest 101:497, 1998

WALMSLEY S et al: Predictive value of cytomegalovirus (CMV) antigenemia and digene hybrid capture DNA assays for CMV disease in human immunodeficiency virus–infected patients. Clin Infect Dis 27:573, 1998

WALSH JC et al: Increasing survival in AIDS patients with cytomegalovirus retinitis treated with combination antiretroviral therapy including protease inhibitors. AIDS 12:613, 1998

WHITLEY RJ et al: Guidelines for the treatment of cytomegalovirus diseases in patients with AIDS in the era of potent antiretroviral therapy. Recommendations of an international panel. Arch Intern Med 158:957, 1998

186 *Fred Wang*

SMALLPOX, VACCINIA, AND OTHER POXVIRUSES

Two poxviruses, smallpox virus and molluscum contagiosum virus, cause natural disease in humans, and other poxviruses are associated with zoonotic infections. Monkeypox virus and smallpox virus typically cause systemic disease with rash, whereas the other poxviruses cause localized skin lesions. Poxviruses are the only DNA viruses that replicate in the cytoplasm, where accumulated viral particles form eosinophilic inclusions, or Guarnieri bodies, visible by light microscopy. Many poxvirus genes interfere with different aspects of the host immune response and provide important insights into the pathogenesis and virulence of viral infection. Genetically engineered vaccinia and avipoxviruses offer great promise as potential vectors for vaccination against other diseases.

SMALLPOX

The last case of endemic smallpox was reported in 1977 from Somalia. In 1980 the World Health Organization officially declared that smallpox had been eliminated worldwide as a result of a global vaccination and eradication program. Important features that contributed to the unique success of this vaccine program included (1) universal interest in eliminating this costly disease with high morbidity and mortality, (2) the infection's long incubation period and low level of communicability, (3) the ease of diagnosis of skin lesions by characteristic histology or antigen detection, (4) the fact that humans were the sole reservoir of the infection, (5) the absence of a carrier state, and (6) the availability of an effective live-virus vaccine that could readily be delivered to less developed countries because of its resistance to chemicals, temperature changes, and drying. The only known remaining repositories of smallpox virus reside in two research laboratories (located in the United States and Russia), and the issue of whether these last samples should be maintained or destroyed remains controversial.

Before the eradication of smallpox, variola virus existed as two related strains: *variola major* (smallpox), with a case-mortality rate of 20 to 50%, and *variola minor* (alastrim), which caused a clinically milder form of smallpox with a mortality of <1%. The clinical presentation of smallpox is now primarily of historic note. However, the threat of biologic terrorism means that smallpox remains a remote possibility in the differential diagnosis of a vesicular exanthem. Fever and macular rash appear after an average incubation period of 12 days, with a progression to typical vesicular and pustular lesions over 1 to 2 weeks. Rash generally appears first on the face, oral mucosa, and arms, with relative sparing of the trunk. Smallpox lesions may be confused with common chickenpox (varicella-zoster) infection but tend to be more diffuse, peripheral, and uniform in their stage of development. Polymerase chain reaction promises to be more useful than traditional electron microscopy or virus isolation for confirming variola or other poxvirus infections.

VACCINIA

The origin of vaccinia virus—the virus used for vaccination against smallpox—is uncertain, but it was probably derived from cowpox virus, variola virus, or a hybrid of the two. It is now a laboratory virus with no natural host. Experience has proven the effectiveness of live vaccinia virus vaccine, although its efficacy and safety were not established in controlled studies. Percutaneous administration of vaccinia virus vaccine results in protective cellular and humoral immune responses in >95% of primary vaccinees. Formation of a pustule and scab at the site of inoculation is indicative of immunity; because immunity wanes after 10 to 20 years, revaccination every 10 years is recommended for continued protection. Routine smallpox vaccination was discontinued in 1971 and has not been required for international travel since 1982. However, the development of recombinant vaccinia viruses for potential use in vaccines against other infectious agents or as immunotherapy against malignant diseases has led to the recommendation that laboratory and health care employees working directly with vaccinia virus vectors be considered for vaccination. Selected groups that may be exposed to poxviruses (e.g., some military personnel and individuals who work with animals) are also vaccinated.

The most frequent adverse complication of vaccination is inadvertent inoculation (usually autoinoculation) at other sites. More serious complications, which are more common among primary vaccinees and infants than among revaccinees and adults, include (1) generalized vaccinia in otherwise healthy individuals, which is generally self-limited; (2) eczema vaccinatum, which consists of disseminated cutaneous lesions in highly susceptible patients with eczema or other chronic skin diseases and is occasionally severe or even fatal; (3) progressive vaccinia (vaccinia necrosum), which is a severe, potentially fatal illness occurring in patients with immunodeficiency, whether congenital, acquired (e.g., via leukemia or lymphoma), iatrogenic (e.g., via chemotherapy or glucocorticoid treatment), or HIV induced; and (4) postinfectious encephalitis, which is rare (3 cases per million primary vaccinees) but can be fatal in 15 to 25% of cases and can leave 25% of patients with permanent neurologic sequelae. Since vaccinees can transmit vaccinia virus to susceptible individuals, vaccination is contraindicated if the proposed recipient or his or her household contacts have eczema, are immunocompromised, or are pregnant. Vaccinia immune globulin (0.6 mL/kg) derived from the plasma of vaccinated persons may be useful for the treatment of severe generalized vaccinia, eczema vaccinatum, progressive vaccinia, and ocular vaccinia resulting from inadvertent inoculation but is of no value for the treatment of postinfectious encephalitis.

MOLLUSCUM CONTAGIOSUM

Molluscum contagiosum is generally a benign disease characterized by pearly, flesh-colored, umbilicated skin lesions 2 to 5 mm in diameter (**Plate IID-41**). A relative lack of inflammation and necrosis distinguishes these proliferative lesions from other poxvirus lesions. The infection can be transmitted by close contact, including sexual intercourse. Swimming pools are a common vector for transmission. Atopy and compromise of skin integrity can increase the risk of infection. Lesions can be found anywhere on the body except the palms and soles and may be associated with an eczematous rash. In most cases the disease is self-limited and has no systemic complications. Molluscum contagiosum develops especially often in association with the advanced stages of HIV infection, with a prevalence of 5 to 18% among HIV-infected patients (Chap. 309). The disease is often more generalized, severe, and persistent in AIDS patients than in other groups, frequently involving the face and upper body. Extensive molluscum contagiosum has also been reported in conjunction with other types of immunodeficiency.

The diagnosis of molluscum contagiosum can be made by histologic demonstration of cytoplasmic eosinophilic inclusions characteristic of poxvirus replication. This virus cannot be propagated in vitro, but electron microscopy and molecular studies can be used for its identification.

There is no specific systemic treatment for molluscum contagiosum, but a variety of techniques for physical ablation have been used. Molluscum contagiosum may respond to effective control of HIV infection with highly active antiretroviral therapy. Cidofovir is also being investigated for potential clinical use against molluscum contagiosum.

MONKEYPOX VIRUS AND OTHER POXVIRUSES

Monkeypox virus naturally infects nonhuman primates in the tropical rain forests of western and central Africa and can infect humans who come into direct contact with infected animals. Human disease is rare and is characterized by a systemic illness and vesicular rash similar to those of variola. A large outbreak of monkeypox occurred between February 1996 and October 1997 in central Africa, with a case-fatality ratio of 3%; a prolonged period of active cases, suggesting a potential for sustained person-to-person transmission; and a high proportion of younger patients, suggesting the possible consequences of discontinued smallpox vaccination. Clinical presentations were occasionally confused with the more common varicella-zoster virus infection.

Other poxviruses can cause localized vesicular lesions when humans come into direct contact with infected animals. These viruses include cowpox virus (rodents, cats); milkers' node virus (cows); buffalopox virus (buffaloes); bovine papular stomatitis virus (cows); and orf virus, which is also known as contagious pustular dermatitis virus (sheep, goats).

BIBLIOGRAPHY

BERTHISTLE K, CARRINGTON D: Molluscum contagiosum virus. J Infect 34:21, 1997

BREMAN JG, HENDERSON D: Poxvirus dilemmas—monkeypox, smallpox, and biologic terrorism. N Engl J Med 339:556, 1998

CATTELAN AM et al: A complete remission of recalcitrant molluscum contagiosum in an AIDS patient following highly active antiretroviral therapy. J Infect 38:58, 1999

FRANZ DR et al: Clinical recognition and management of patients exposed to biological warfare agents. JAMA 278:399, 1997

Human monkeypox—Kasai Oriental, Zaire, 1996–1997. MMWR 46:304, 1997

PAOLETTI E: Applications of pox virus vectors to vaccination: An update. Proc Natl Acad Sci USA 93:11349, 1996

SENKEVICH TG et al: Genome sequence of a human tumorigenic poxvirus: Prediction of specific host response-evasion genes. Science 273:813, 1996

SMITH GL et al: Vaccinia virus immune evasion. Immunol Rev 159:137, 1997

TARTAGLIA J et al: Canarypox virus–based vaccines: Prime-boost strategies to induce cell-mediated and humoral immunity against HIV. AIDS Res Hum Retroviruses 3: S291, 1998

Vaccinia (smallpox) vaccine. Recommendations of the Immunization Practices Advisory Committee (ACIP). MMWR 40:1, 1991

ZABAWSKI EJ, COCKERELL CJ: Topical and intralesional cidofovir: A review of pharmacology and therapeutic effects. J Am Acad Dermatol 39:741, 1998

PARVOVIRUS

DEFINITION The parvovirus group includes several species-specific viruses of animals. One parvovirus, designated B19, is known to be a human pathogen. B19 is a small (diameter, 20 to 25 nm), icosahedral, nonenveloped, single-stranded DNA virus with an outer capsid formed by two structural proteins. Individual virus particles contain DNA strands of positive or negative polarity. The virus is stable and retains infectivity after incubation at 60°C for 16 h. It has failed to grow in conventional cell culture lines and animal model systems but does replicate in vitro in erythroid progenitor cells derived from human bone marrow, umbilical cord, peripheral blood, or fetal liver sources.

During the 1980s, it was discovered that B19 causes a variety of disorders ranging from erythema infectiosum and acute arthropathy in otherwise healthy hosts to transient aplastic crisis and chronic anemia in compromised patients to fetal infection manifested by death or hydrops fetalis. Many of the severe manifestations of B19 viremia relate to the propensity of the virus to infect and lyse erythroid precursor cells in the bone marrow. The name B19 is derived from the code number of the human serum in which the virus was discovered.

PATHOGENESIS Two studies of adult volunteers have provided a basis for understanding the pathogenesis of B19 infection, which has two phases. The first phase is characterized by viremia that develops approximately 6 days after intranasal inoculation of B19 into susceptible individuals who lack serum antibodies to the virus. The viremia lasts about 1 week; its clearance is correlated with the development of IgM antibodies to B19, which remain detectable for up to a few months. IgG antibodies develop several days later and persist indefinitely. Nonspecific systemic symptoms lasting 2 or 3 days occur early during the viremic phase; these symptoms include headache, malaise, myalgia, fever, chills, and pruritus and are accompanied by reticulocytopenia and excretion of the virus from the respiratory tract. Several days after the onset of symptoms, a clinically insignificant decline in hemoglobin concentration is noted; the decreased level is maintained for 7 to 10 days, during which time examination of bone marrow samples reveals a marked depletion of erythroid precursor cells. Transient mild lymphopenia, neutropenia, and a drop in platelet count also may be found. A second phase of illness begins around 17 or 18 days after virus inoculation (after the clearance of viremia, the cessation of viral shedding in throat secretions, and the resolution of reticulocytopenia). This illness mimics erythema infectiosum in adults, with 2 or 3 days of fine maculopapular rash accompanied by arthralgias and arthritis that last another 1 or 2 days. This phase occurs in the presence of rising serum titers of antibody to B19.

The studies just described indicate that B19 disease in the otherwise *healthy host*, manifested by self-limited erythema infectiosum and/or arthropathy, is almost certainly an immune-complex disorder. This concept is supported by the induction of erythema infectiosum through the infusion of immunoglobulins into chronically viremic patients. In contrast, B19 disease in the *compromised host* (chronic hemolytic disease or immunodeficiency syndromes) is often serious, resulting from the destruction by B19 of erythroid precursor cells. Normal hosts can tolerate 7 to 10 days of shutoff of erythropoiesis; however, patients with hemolytic disease who require increased production of erythrocytes do not tolerate erythroid cell destruction and thus usually develop severe transient aplastic crisis. Patients who are immunodeficient may fail to clear B19 viremia, the results being persistent infection of red blood cells and chronic severe anemia. The fetus requires a higher level of red cell production than do adults and has an immature immune system; both these factors could explain B19-induced hydrops fetalis.

B19 binds specifically to a cellular receptor, erythrocyte P antigen; this specific binding explains the tropism of B19 for erythroid progenitor cells, particularly pronormoblasts and normoblasts. The few persons who lack P antigen cannot be infected with B19.

EPIDEMIOLOGY Although B19 infections occur year-round, they appear most commonly as outbreaks of erythema infectiosum in schools during winter and spring months. Between 20 and 60% of children in outbreaks are symptomatic, and many are asymptomatically infected. Seroepidemiologic studies indicate that approximately half of adults possess serum antibodies to B19. Antibody prevalence (reflecting prior exposure and probable immunity to the virus) rises rapidly between the ages of 5 and 18 years and continues to increase with age—a pattern probably indicating ongoing exposure during adulthood. B19 can be detected in throat swabbings, respiratory tract secretions, and serum, and its detection at these sites probably correlates with infectiousness. Thus, patients with transient aplastic crisis are highly infectious. Their infectivity has been firmly documented as the source of one well-defined nosocomial outbreak of erythema infectiosum among nurses. In contrast, individuals with erythema infectiosum are much less infectious. The usual route of viral transmission under natural conditions is unknown but may be respiratory or through direct contact. B19 can be transmitted during therapy with clotting factor concentrate, even after exposure to detergent, steam, or dry heat.

CLINICAL MANIFESTATIONS   **Erythema Infectiosum** Erythema infectiosum is the most common manifestation of B19 infection and occurs predominantly in children. This entity is also called *fifth disease* because it was classified in the late nineteenth century as the fifth in a series of six exanthems of childhood. Normally a mild illness, erythema infectiosum typically presents as a facial rash with a "slapped-cheek" appearance that is sometimes preceded by low-grade fever. The rash may develop quickly on the arms and legs and usually has a lacy, reticular, erythematous appearance (**Plate IID-40**). The trunk, palms, and soles are less commonly involved. Occasionally, the rash appears with maculopapular, morbilliform, vesicular, purpuric, or pruritic characteristics. The typical rash resolves in about a week but can recur intermittently for several weeks, particularly after stress, exercise, exposure to sunlight, bathing, or change in environmental temperature. Arthralgia and arthritis are uncommon among children but are frequent among adults, in whom the rash is often absent or nonspecific, with a lack of the characteristic facial erythema.

Arthropathy B19 infection in adults most commonly presents as acute arthralgias and arthritis, sometimes accompanied by rash. The arthritis is characteristically symmetric and peripheral, involving the wrists, hands, and knees most frequently. It normally resolves in about 3 weeks and is nondestructive. However, a small percentage of patients have arthritis persisting for months or even (in rare cases) for years. It is not known whether these individuals have persistent infection or an abnormal immune response to the virus.

Transient Aplastic Crisis B19 infection is the cause in most instances of transient aplastic crisis developing suddenly in patients with chronic hemolytic disease. Nearly all hemolytic conditions can be affected by B19 infection, including sickle cell disease, erythrocyte enzyme deficiencies, hereditary spherocytosis, thalassemias, paroxysmal nocturnal hemoglobinuria, and autoimmune hemolysis. B19-induced aplastic crisis also can occur in the setting of acute blood loss. Patients present with weakness, lethargy, pallor, and severe anemia, a syndrome often preceded by a few days of nonspecific symptoms. These patients have intense reticulocytopenia lasting 7 to 10 days, and their bone marrow contains no erythroid precursor cells despite a normal myeloid series. Transient aplastic crisis can produce life-threatening anemia and may require urgent transfusion therapy. Unlike patients with erythema infectiosum or arthropathy, those with transient aplastic crisis are viremic and can readily transmit B19 infection to other people.

Chronic Anemia in Immunodeficient Patients　Immunodeficient patients may be unable to eliminate B19 infection, probably because they cannot produce adequate levels of virus-specific IgG antibodies. The result is persistent infection with destruction of erythroid precursor cells in the bone marrow and chronic transfusion-dependent anemia. This condition has been described occasionally in patients with immunodeficiency related to infection with HIV, congenital immunodeficiencies, and acute lymphoblastic leukemia during maintenance chemotherapy as well as in recipients of bone marrow, heart, liver, and renal transplants. In addition, some cases of idiopathic pure red-cell aplasia probably are caused by persistent B19 infection. B19-induced chronic anemia may be the presenting finding of an otherwise unrecognized immunodeficiency. Chronic anemia may fluctuate in intensity over time and may be cured or controlled by immunoglobulin therapy. Both the spectrum of immunodeficiencies associated with B19-induced chronic anemia and the frequency of the association remain to be determined.

Fetal and Congenital Infection　Maternal B19 infections usually do not adversely affect the fetus. More often than not, in fact, the fetus remains uninfected. Therefore, couples in which the pregnant woman is infected should be counseled as to the relatively low risk of fetal infection. It is estimated that fewer than 10% of maternal B19 infections in the first 20 weeks of pregnancy lead to fetal death; when fetal death does occur, it is usually attributable to the development of nonimmune hydrops fetalis, wherein the fetus succumbs to severe anemia and congestive heart failure. In these instances, B19 can be detected in fetal tissues, with predominant infection of erythroblasts. Pregnant women with known exposure to B19 should have their serum monitored for IgM antibodies to the virus and for elevated levels of α-fetoprotein and human chorionic gonadotropin; ultrasonic examinations of the fetus for hydrops should also be conducted. Some hydropic fetuses survive B19 infection and appear normal at delivery. Rarely, fetal infection with hydrops results in congenital anemia and hypogammaglobulinemia that is unresponsive to immunoglobulin therapy.

Possible Clinical Associations　Case studies suggest a link—as yet inconclusive—between B19 and several rheumatic diseases, most notably rheumatoid arthritis but also vasculitis (including polyarteritis, Wegener's granulomatosis, and giant cell arteritis), lupus erythematosus, dermatomyositis, and juvenile rheumatoid arthritis. Other unproven associations include those involving multiple systems: cardiac (myocarditis), hematologic (hemophagocytic syndrome, idiopathic thrombocytopenic purpura), hepatic (fulminant hepatitis), neurologic (meningoencephalitis), and respiratory (pneumonia).

DIAGNOSIS　Diagnosis most commonly relies on measurements of B19-specific IgM and IgG antibodies, which can be detected with commercially available immunoassay kits. The virus, its DNA, or its antigens are also detected in the serum or infected tissues of some patients. Acute infection can be proven by B19-compatible symptoms and the presence of IgM antibodies or virus itself, whereas past infection is documented by IgG antibodies. Individuals with erythema infectiosum and acute arthropathy usually have IgM antibodies without detectable virus in serum. Those with transient aplastic crisis may have IgM antibodies but typically possess high titers of virus and its DNA in serum; the bone marrow of these patients shows characteristic giant pronormoblasts and hypoplasia. Immunodeficient patients with anemia often lack readily detectable antibodies but have viral particles and DNA in serum. Fetal infection may be recognized by hydrops fetalis and the presence of B19 DNA in amniotic fluid or fetal blood in association with maternal IgM antibodies to B19.

℞　**TREATMENT**　Erythema infectiosum usually requires no treatment; the same is true for many cases of arthropathy. More severe cases of arthritis, particularly those involving chronic symptoms, can be treated with nonsteroidal anti-inflammatory agents. Transient aplastic crisis is usually treated with erythrocyte transfusions. In immunodeficient anemic patients, B19 infection should be treated with commercial intravenous immunoglobulin, which is known to contain IgG antibodies to B19. This therapy controls and may cure B19 infection.

PROPHYLAXIS　Prophylaxis of B19 infection with immunoglobulin should be considered for patients with chronic hemolysis or immunodeficiency and for pregnant women. The risk of infection for these persons may be reduced by hand washing before eating or after contact with respiratory or other secretions when B19 is known to be present in a community. Patients with transient aplastic crisis or chronic B19 infection (but not those with erythema infectiosum or arthropathy) pose a serious risk for nosocomial transmission of infection. They should be hospitalized in a private room with contact and respiratory isolation precautions. It is not known whether pre- or postexposure administration of immunoglobulin prevents infection. No vaccine for B19 is currently available; however, a baculovirus-infected insect cell line that expresses noninfectious immunogenic B19 capsid proteins is being evaluated to determine an optimal regimen for use as a vaccine.

BIBLIOGRAPHY

ABKOWITZ JL et al: Clinical relevance of parvovirus B19 as a cause of anemia in patients with human immunodeficiency virus infection. J Infect Dis 176:269, 1997

ANDERSON LJ, YOUNG NS (eds): *Monographs in Virology,* vol 20: *Human Parvovirus B19.* Basel, Karger, 1997

ANDERSON MJ et al: Experimental parvoviral infection in humans. J Infect Dis 152:257, 1985

BROWN KE et al: Resistance to parvovirus B19 infection due to lack of virus receptor (erythrocyte P antigen). N Engl J Med 330:1192, 1994

CENTERS FOR DISEASE CONTROL AND PREVENTION: Risks associated with human parvovirus B19 infection. MMWR 38:81, 1989

KURTZMAN G et al: Pure red-cell aplasia of 10 years' duration due to persistent parvovirus B19 infection and its cure with immunoglobulin therapy. N Engl J Med 321:519, 1989

MILLER E et al: Immediate and long term outcome of human parvovirus B19 infection in pregnancy. Br J Obstet Gynaecol 105:174, 1998

NAIDES SJ et al: Rheumatologic manifestations of human parvovirus B19 infection in adults: Initial two-year clinical experience. Arthritis Rheum 33:1297, 1990

PLUMMER FA et al: An erythema infectiosum–like illness caused by human parvovirus infection. N Engl J Med 313:74, 1985

SOKAL EM et al: Acute parvovirus B19 infection associated with fulminant hepatitis of favourable prognosis in young children. Lancet 352:1739, 1998

TAKAHASHI Y et al: Human parvovirus B19 as a causative agent for rheumatoid arthritis. Proc Natl Acad Sci USA 95:8227, 1998

188　*Richard C. Reichman*

HUMAN PAPILLOMAVIRUSES

DEFINITION　Human papillomaviruses (HPVs) selectively infect the epithelium of the skin and mucous membranes. These infections may be asymptomatic, produce warts, or be associated with a variety of benign and malignant neoplasias.

ETIOLOGIC AGENT　Papillomaviruses are members of the *Papillomavirus* genus of the family Papovaviridae. They are nonenveloped, measure 50 to 55 nm in diameter, have icosahedral capsids composed of 72 capsomeres, and contain a double-stranded circular DNA genome of about 7900 base pairs. The genomic organization of all papillomaviruses is similar and consists of an early (E) region, a late (L) region, and a noncoding upstream regulatory region. Oncogenic HPV types can immortalize human keratinocytes, and this activity has been mapped to products of early genes E6 and E7. E6 protein facilitates the degradation of the p53 tumor suppressor protein, and E7 protein binds the retinoblastoma gene product and related proteins. The E1 and E2 proteins modulate viral DNA replication and regulate gene expression. The L1 gene codes for the major capsid protein, which makes up 80% of the virion mass. L2 codes for a minor capsid protein. Type-specific conformational antigenic determinants are located on the virion surface. Papillomavirus types are distinguished from one another by the degree of nucleic acid sequence homology. Distinct types share fewer than 90% of their DNA sequences in L1. More than 80 types of HPV are recognized, and individual types are associated with specific clinical manifestations (Table 188-1). HPVs are species-specific and have not been propagated in tissue culture or in common experimental animals. However, HPV types 1, 6, 11, 16, 40, and 83 have been produced in human tissues implanted in immunodeficient mice.

EPIDEMIOLOGY There are few good studies of the incidence or prevalence of warts in well-defined human populations. Common warts (verruca vulgaris) are found in as many as 25% of some groups and are most prevalent among young children. Plantar warts (verruca plantaris) are also widely prevalent; they occur most often among adolescents and young adults. Condyloma acuminatum (anogenital warts) is one of the most common sexually transmitted diseases in the United States. HPV infection of the uterine cervix produces the squamous cell abnormalities most frequently detected on Papanicolaou smears.

Most genital HPV infections are transmitted through direct contact with infectious lesions. Close personal contact is also assumed to play a role in the transmission of most cutaneous warts; the importance of fomites in this setting is not clear. Minor trauma at the site of inoculation may facilitate transmission. Recurrent respiratory papillomatosis in young children is an uncommon disease that is acquired from maternal genital tract infection; in adults, the disease may be transmitted through orogenital sexual contact.

HPV infection has been strongly associated with the development of dysplasia and cancer of the uterine cervix. More than 95% of cervical cancers contain DNA of oncogenic (high-risk) HPV types, such as 16, 18, and 31. HPV DNA is also present in the precursor lesions of cervical cancer, known as cervical intraepithelial neoplasias. Such lesions containing DNA of oncogenic HPV types are more likely to progress than those associated with low-risk types, such as 6 and 11. HPV DNA is transcribed in tumor tissues; many epidemiologic studies

have confirmed a relation between HPV infection (with or without cofactors) and the development of cervical cancer, although most cervical HPV infections are self-limited. Infection with specific HPV types has also been associated with squamous cell carcinomas and dysplasias of the penis, anus, vagina, and vulva. In patients with epidermodysplasia verruciformis, squamous cell cancers develop frequently at sites infected with specific HPV types, including 5 and 8.

Serologic studies with virus-like particles as antigens have demonstrated type-specific antibodies in most patients with HPV genital tract infections.

CLINICAL MANIFESTATIONS The clinical manifestations of HPV infection depend on the location of the lesions and the type of virus. Common warts usually occur on the hands as flesh-colored to brown, exophytic, hyperkeratotic papules. Plantar warts may be quite painful; they can be differentiated from calluses by paring of the surface to reveal thrombosed capillaries. Flat warts (verruca plana) are most common among children and occur on the face, neck, chest, and flexor surfaces of the forearms and legs.

Anogenital warts develop on the skin and mucosal surfaces of the external genitalia and perianal areas (**Plate IID-55**). Among circumcised men, warts are most commonly found on the penile shaft. Lesions commonly occur at the urethral meatus and may extend proximally. Perianal warts are common among homosexual men but develop in heterosexual men as well. In women, warts appear first at the posterior introitus and adjacent labia. They then spread to other parts of the vulva and commonly involve the vagina and cervix. These lesions may be present without external warts. The differential diagnosis of anogenital warts includes condylomata lata of secondary syphilis, molluscum contagiosum, hirsutoid papillomatosis (pearly penile papules), fibroepitheliomas, and a variety of benign and malignant mucocutaneous neoplasms. Respiratory papillomatosis in young children may be life-threatening and presents as hoarseness, stridor, or respiratory distress. The disease in adults is usually milder.

Immunosuppressed patients, particularly those undergoing organ transplantation, often develop pityriasis versicolor–like lesions, from which DNA of several HPV types has been extracted. Occasionally, such lesions appear to undergo malignant transformation. Patients infected with HIV frequently have severe clinical manifestations of HPV infection and appear to be at unusually high risk for cervical and anal malignancies. HPV disease in patients with HIV infection is difficult to treat and often recurs.

Epidermodysplasia verruciformis is a rare autosomal recessive disease characterized by the inability to control HPV infection. Patients are often infected with unusual HPV types and frequently develop cutaneous squamous cell malignancies, particularly in sun-exposed areas. The lesions resemble flat warts or macules similar to those of pityriasis versicolor.

The complications of warts include itching and occasionally bleeding. In rare cases warts become secondarily infected with bacteria or fungi. Large masses of warts may cause mechanical problems, such as obstruction of the birth canal. Dysplasias of the uterine cervix are generally asymptomatic until frank carcinoma develops. Patients with anogenital HPV disease may develop serious psychological symptoms due to anxiety or depression over this condition.

PATHOGENESIS The incubation period of HPV disease is usually 3 to 4 months, with a range of 1 month to 2 years. All types of squamous epithelium can be infected by HPV, and the gross and histologic appearances of individual lesions vary with the site of infection and the type of virus. The replication of HPV begins with the infection of basal cells. As cellular differentiation proceeds, HPV DNA replicates and is transcribed. Ultimately, virions are assembled in the nucleus and released when keratinocytes are shed. This process is associated with proliferation of all epidermal layers except the basal layer and produces acanthosis, parakeratosis, and hyperkeratosis. Koilocytes, large round cells with pyknotic nuclei, appear in the granular layer. Histologically normal epithelium may contain HPV DNA,

Table 188-1 Correlation of Human Papillomavirus Type with Disease

Disease	Associated HPV Types
Plantar warts	1,[a] 2,[a] 4, 63
Common warts	1,[a] 2,[a] 4, 26, 27, 29, 41,[b] 57, 65, 77
Common warts of meat handlers	1, 2,[a] 3, 4, 7,[a] 10, 28
Flat warts	3,[a] 10,[a] 27, 38, 41,[b] 49, 75, 76
Intermediate warts	10,[a] 26, 28
Epidermodysplasia verruciformis	2,[a] 3,[a] 5,[ab] 8,[ab] 9,[a] 10,[a] 12,[a] 14,[ab] 15,[a] 17,[ab] 19, 20,[b] 21, 22, 23, 24, 25, 36, 37, 38,[b] 47, 50
Condyloma acuminatum	6,[a] 11,[a] 30,[b] 42, 43, 44, 45,[b] 51,[b] 54, 55, 70
Intraepithelial neoplasias	
Unspecified	30,[b] 34, 39,[b] 40, 53, 57, 59, 61, 62, 64, 66,[b] 67, 69, 71
Low-grade	6,[a] 11,[a] 16,[b] 18,[b] 31,[b] 33,[b] 35,[b] 42, 43, 44, 45,[b] 51,[b] 52,[b] 74
High-grade	6, 11, 16,[ab] 18,[ab] 31,[b] 33,[b] 34, 35,[b] 39,[b] 42, 44, 45,[b] 51,[b] 52,[b] 56,[b] 58,[b] 66[b]
Bowen's disease	16,[ab] 31,[b] 34
Bowenoid papulosis	16,[ab] 34, 39,[b] 42, 45,[b] 55
Cervical carcinoma	16,[ab] 18,[ab] 31,[b] 33,[b] 35,[b] 39,[b] 45,[b] 51,[b] 52,[b] 56,[b] 58,[b] 66,[b] 68, 70
Laryngeal papillomas	6,[a] 11[a]
Focal epithelial hyperplasia of Heck	13,[a] 32[a]
Conjunctival papillomas	6,[a] 11,[a] 16[ab]
Others	6, 11, 16,[b] 30,[b] 33,[b] 36, 37 38,[b] 41,[b] 48,[b] 60, 72, 73

[a] Most common associations.
[b] High malignant potential.
NOTE: Additional information on new HPV types can be found on the HPV Sequence Data Base through the Internet (hpv-web.lanl.gov).

and residual DNA after treatment can be associated with recurrent disease.

Episomal HPV DNA is present in the nuclei of infected cells in benign lesions caused by the virus. However, in severe dysplasias and cancers, HPV DNA is generally integrated, with disruption of the E1/E2 open reading frames. This disruption leads to upregulation of E6 and E7 and subsequent interference with cellular tumor suppressor proteins.

Host defense responses to HPV infection are incompletely understood, and immune correlates of protection from infection and resolution of disease have not been established. Because patients with defects in cell-mediated immune responses, including transplant recipients and patients with HIV infection, frequently develop severe HPV disease, such responses are probably important for the control of virus replication. Histologic studies demonstrating an epidermal lymphomonocytic infiltrate in resolving warts suggest that local immunity may be of particular importance in the resolution of disease. HPV infection can also elicit a serologic response, and antibodies to the viral capsid have been found in sera from patients with anogenital warts, cutaneous warts, and respiratory papillomatosis. Antibodies to E-region proteins, most notably E7, have been detected among patients with cervical carcinoma. Vaccine studies in animals have shown that production of neutralizing antibodies can be associated with protection from papillomavirus infection.

DIAGNOSIS Most warts that are visible to the naked eye can be diagnosed correctly by history and physical examination alone. The use of a colposcope is invaluable in assessing vaginal and cervical lesions and is helpful in the diagnosis of oral and cutaneous HPV disease as well. Papanicolaou smears prepared from cervical scrapings often show cytologic evidence of HPV infection. Persistent or atypical lesions should be biopsied and examined by routine histologic methods. The most sensitive and specific methods of virologic diagnosis entail the use of techniques such as the polymerase chain reaction or the hybrid capture assay to detect HPV nucleic acids and to identify specific virus types. Serologic techniques to diagnose HPV infection are not helpful in individual cases and are not widely available.

℞ TREATMENT Decisions regarding the initiation of therapy should be made with the knowledge that currently available modes of treatment are not completely effective and some have significant side effects. In addition, treatment may be expensive, and many HPV lesions resolve spontaneously. Frequently used therapies include cryosurgery, application of caustic agents, electrodesiccation, surgical excision, and ablation with a laser. Topical antimetabolites such as 5-fluorouracil also have been used. Both failure and recurrence have been well documented with all of these methods of treatment. Cryosurgery is the initial treatment of choice for condyloma acuminatum. Topically applied podophyllum preparations as well as podofilox may also be used. Various interferon preparations have been used with modest success in the treatment of respiratory papillomatosis and condyloma acuminatum. A topically applied interferon inducer, imiquimod, is also of benefit in the treatment of condyloma acuminatum. The diagnosis and management of anogenital dysplasias and of internal anogenital warts require special skills and resources, and patients with such lesions should be referred to a qualified specialist.

No effective methods for the prevention of HPV infections are available at present other than the avoidance of contact with infectious lesions. Barrier methods of contraception may be helpful in preventing the transmission of condyloma acuminatum and other HPV-associated diseases of the genital tract. Vaccines consisting of virus-like particles can prevent papillomavirus disease in some animal models and have been shown to induce neutralizing antibodies in phase 1 studies in humans. More extensive clinical trials of these preparations are under way.

BIBLIOGRAPHY

BONNEZ W, REICHMAN RC: Papillomaviruses, in *Principles and Practice of Infectious Diseases*, 5th ed, GL Mandell et al (eds). Churchill Livingstone, New York, 2000

—— et al: Isolation and propagation of human papillomavirus type 16 in human xenografts implanted in the severe combined immunodeficiency mouse. J Virol 72: 5256, 1998

BROWN DR et al: Nucleotide sequence and characterization of human papillomavirus type 83, a novel genital papillomavirus. Virology 260:165, 1999

FRISCH M et al: Sexually transmitted infection as a cause of anal cancer. N Engl J Med 337:1350, 1997

GALLOWAY DA: Is vaccination against human papillomavirus a possibility? Lancet 351(Suppl 3):22, 1998

HAGENSEE ME et al: Seroprevalence of human papillomavirus types 6 and 16 capsid antibodies in homosexual men. J Infect Dis 176:625, 1997

HO GY et al: Natural history of cervicovaginal papillomavirus infection in young women. N Engl J Med 338:423, 1998

LUQUE AE et al: Association of human papillomavirus infection and disease with magnitude of human immunodeficiency virus type 1 (HIV-1) RNA plasma level among women with HIV-1 infection. J Infect Dis 179:1405, 1999

NOBBENHUIS MAE et al: Relation of human papillomavirus status to cervical lesions and consequences for cervical-cancer screening: A prospective study. Lancet 354:20, 1999

NORTHFELT DW et al: Anal neoplasia. Pathogenesis, diagnosis, and management. Hematol Oncol Clin North Am 10:1177, 1996

REICHMAN RC et al: A phase I study of a recombinant virus-like particle vaccine against human papillomavirus type 11 in healthy adult volunteers, in *Proceedings of the 38th Interscience Conference on Antimicrobial Agents and Chemotherapy*. Washington, DC, American Society of Microbiology, 1998, abstract 330

WIDEROFF L et al: Epidemiologic determinants of seroreactivity to human papillomavirus (HPV) type 16 virus-like particles in cervical HPV-16 DNA-positive and -negative women. J Infect Dis 174:937, 1996

Section 13
DNA AND RNA RESPIRATORY VIRUSES

189 *Raphael Dolin*

COMMON VIRAL RESPIRATORY INFECTIONS

GENERAL CONSIDERATIONS Acute viral respiratory illnesses are among the most common of human diseases, accounting for one-half or more of all acute illnesses. The incidence of acute respiratory disease in the United States is from 3 to 5.6 cases per person per year. The rates are highest among children under 1 year old (6.1 to 8.3 cases per year) and remain high until age 6, when a progressive decrease begins. Adults have 3 to 4 cases per person per year. Morbidity from acute respiratory illnesses accounts for 30 to 50% of time lost from work by adults and for 60 to 80% of time lost from school by children. The use of antibacterial agents to treat viral respiratory infections represents a major source of abuse of that category of drugs.

It has been estimated that two-thirds to three-fourths of cases of acute respiratory illnesses are caused by viruses. More than 200 antigenically distinct viruses from 8 different genera have been reported to cause acute respiratory illness, and it is likely that additional agents will be described in the future. The vast majority of these viral infections involve the upper respiratory tract, but lower respiratory tract disease can also develop, particularly in younger age groups and in certain epidemiologic settings.

The illnesses caused by respiratory viruses traditionally have been divided into multiple distinct syndromes, such as the "common cold," pharyngitis, croup (laryngotracheobronchitis), tracheitis, bronchiolitis, bronchitis, and pneumonia. Each of these general categories of illnesses has a certain epidemiologic and clinical profile; for example, croup occurs exclusively in very young children and has a characteristic clinical course. Some types of respiratory illnesses are more likely to be associated with certain viruses (e.g., the common cold with rhinoviruses), while others occupy characteristic epidemiologic niches (e.g., adenovirus infections in military re-

Table 189-1 Illnesses Associated with Respiratory Viruses

| Virus | Frequency of Respiratory Syndromes | | |
	Most Frequent	Occasional	Infrequent
Rhinoviruses	Common cold	Exacerbation of chronic bronchitis and asthma	Pneumonia in children
Coronaviruses	Common cold	Exacerbation of chronic bronchitis and asthma	Pneumonia and bronchiolitis
Respiratory syncytial virus	Pneumonia and bronchiolitis in young children	Common cold in adults	Pneumonia in elderly and immunosuppressed patients
Parainfluenza viruses	Croup and lower respiratory tract disease in young children	Pharyngitis and common cold	Tracheobronchitis in adults; lower respiratory tract disease in immunosuppressed patients
Adenoviruses	Common cold and pharyngitis in children	Outbreaks of acute respiratory disease in military recruits[a]	Pneumonia in children; lower respiratory tract and disseminated disease in immunosuppressed patients
Influenza A viruses	Influenza[b]	Pneumonia and excess mortality in high-risk patients	Pneumonia in healthy individuals
Influenza B viruses	Influenza[b]	Rhinitis and pharyngitis alone	Pneumonia
Enteroviruses	Acute undifferentiated febrile illnesses[c]	Rhinitis and pharyngitis	Pneumonia
Herpes simplex viruses	Gingivostomatitis in children; pharyngotonsillitis in adults	Tracheitis and pneumonia in immunocompromised patients	Disseminated infection in immunocompromised patients

[a] Serotypes 4 and 7.
[b] Fever, cough, myalgia, malaise.
[c] May or may not have a respiratory component.

cruits). The syndromes most commonly associated with infections with the major respiratory virus groups are summarized in Table 189-1. Most respiratory viruses clearly have the potential to cause more than one type of respiratory illness, and frequently features of several types of illness are found in the same patient. Moreover, the clinical illnesses induced by these viruses are rarely sufficiently distinctive to permit an etiologic diagnosis on clinical grounds alone, although the epidemiologic setting increases the likelihood that one group of viruses rather than another is involved. In general, laboratory methods must be relied on to establish a specific viral diagnosis.

This chapter reviews viral infections caused by five of the major groups of respiratory viruses: rhinoviruses, coronaviruses, respiratory syncytial viruses, parainfluenza viruses, and adenoviruses. Influenza viruses, which are a major cause of mortality as well as morbidity, are reviewed in Chap. 190. Herpesviruses, which occasionally cause pharyngitis and which also cause lower respiratory tract disease in immunosuppressed patients, are reviewed in Chap. 182. Enteroviruses, which account for occasional respiratory illnesses during the summer months, are reviewed in Chap. 193.

RHINOVIRUS INFECTIONS

ETIOLOGIC AGENT Rhinoviruses are members of the Picornaviridae family, small (15 to 30 nm) nonenveloped viruses that contain a single-stranded RNA genome. In contrast to other members of the picornavirus family, such as enteroviruses, rhinoviruses are acid-labile and are almost completely inactivated at pH ≤ 3. Rhinoviruses grow preferentially at 33° to 34°C—the temperature of the human nasal passages—rather than at the higher temperature (37°C) of the lower respiratory tract. One hundred distinct serotypes and one subtype of rhinovirus are recognized.

EPIDEMIOLOGY Rhinoviruses are a major cause of the common cold and have been isolated from 15 to 40% of adults with common cold–like illnesses. Overall rates of infection with rhinoviruses are higher among infants and young children and decrease with increasing age. Rhinovirus infections occur throughout the year, with seasonal peaks in early fall and spring in temperate climates. Rhino-

virus infections are most often introduced into families by preschool or grade-school children younger than 6 years old. Between 25 and 70% of initial illnesses in family settings are followed by secondary cases, with the highest attack rates among the youngest siblings at home. Attack rates also increase with family size.

Rhinoviruses appear to spread through direct contact with infected secretions, usually respiratory droplets. In some studies of volunteers, transmission was most efficient by hand-to-hand contact, with subsequent self-inoculation of the conjunctival or nasal mucosa. In other studies, transmission by large- or small-particle aerosol was demonstrated. Virus also can be recovered from plastic surfaces inoculated 1 to 3 h previously; this observation suggests that environmental surfaces contribute to transmission. In studies of married couples in which neither partner had detectable serum antibody, transmission was associated with prolonged contact (122 h or more) during a 7-day period. Transmission was infrequent unless virus was recoverable from the donor's hands and nasal mucosa, at least 1000 $TCID_{50}$ of virus was present in nasal washes from the donor, and the donor was at least moderately symptomatic with the "cold." Despite anecdotal observations, exposure to cold temperatures, fatigue, or sleep deprivation has not been associated with increased rates of rhinovirus-induced illness in volunteers.

Infection with rhinoviruses is worldwide in distribution. By the time they reach adulthood, nearly all individuals have neutralizing antibodies to multiple serotypes, although the prevalence of antibody to any one serotype varies widely. Multiple serotypes circulate simultaneously, and generally no single serotype or group of serotypes has been more prevalent than the others.

PATHOGENESIS Rhinoviruses infect cells through attachment to specific cellular receptors; most serotypes attach to intercellular adhesion molecule 1, while a few use low-density lipoprotein as the cellular receptor. Relatively limited information is available on the histopathology and pathogenesis of acute rhinovirus infections in humans. Examination of biopsy specimens obtained during experimentally induced and naturally occurring illness indicates that the nasal mucosa is edematous, is often hyperemic, and—during acute illness—is covered by a mucoid discharge. There is a mild infiltrate with inflammatory cells, including neutrophils, lymphocytes, plasma cells, and eosinophils. Mucus-secreting glands in the submucosa appear hyperactive; the nasal turbinates are engorged, a condition that may lead to obstruction of nearby openings of sinus cavities. Several mediators, such as bradykinin, lysylbradykinin, prostaglandins, histamine, and interleukins 1, 6, and 8, have been linked to the development of signs and symptoms in rhinovirus-induced colds.

The incubation period for rhinovirus illness is short, generally 1 or 2 days. Virus shedding coincides with the onset of illness or may begin shortly before symptoms develop. The mechanisms of immunity to rhinovirus are not well worked out. In some studies, the presence of homotypic antibody has been associated with significantly reduced rates of subsequent infection and illness, but data conflict regarding the relative importance of serum and local antibody in protection from rhinovirus infection.

CLINICAL MANIFESTATIONS   The most common clinical manifestations of rhinovirus infections are those of the common cold. Illness usually begins with rhinorrhea and sneezing accompanied by nasal congestion. The throat is frequently sore, and in some cases sore throat is the initial complaint. Systemic signs and symptoms, such as malaise and headache, are mild or absent, and fever is unusual. Illness generally lasts for 4 to 9 days and resolves spontaneously without sequelae. In children, bronchitis, bronchiolitis, and bronchopneumonia have been reported; nevertheless, it appears that rhinoviruses are not major causes of lower respiratory tract disease in children. Rhinoviruses may cause exacerbations of asthma and chronic pulmonary disease in adults. The vast majority of rhinovirus infections resolve without sequelae, but complications related to obstruction of the eustachian tubes or sinus ostia, including otitis media or acute sinusitis, can develop.

DIAGNOSIS   Although rhinoviruses are the most frequently recognized cause of the common cold, similar illnesses are caused by a variety of other viruses, and the etiologic diagnosis cannot be made on clinical grounds alone. Rather, rhinovirus infection is diagnosed by isolation of the virus from nasal washes or nasal secretions in tissue culture. In practice, this procedure is rarely undertaken because of the benign, self-limited nature of the illness. Given the many serotypes of rhinovirus, diagnosis by serum antibody tests is currently impractical. Likewise, common laboratory tests, such as white cell count and sedimentation rate, are not helpful.

℞ TREATMENT   Rhinovirus infections are generally mild and self-limited, so treatment is not usually necessary. Therapy in the form of antihistamines and nonsteroidal anti-inflammatory drugs may be beneficial in patients with particularly pronounced symptoms, and reduction of activity is prudent in instances of significant discomfort or fatigability. Antibacterial agents should be used only if bacterial complications such as otitis media or sinusitis develop. Specific antiviral therapy is not available. Application of interferon sprays intranasally has been effective in the prophylaxis of rhinovirus infections but is also associated with local irritation of the nasal mucosa. Prevention of rhinovirus infection by antibodies directed against rhinovirus receptors or by the soluble purified receptors themselves is under study. Experimental vaccines to certain rhinovirus serotypes have been prepared, but their usefulness is questionable because of the myriad serotypes and the uncertainty about mechanisms of immunity. Thorough hand washing, environmental decontamination, and protection against autoinoculation may help to reduce rates of transmission of infection.

CORONAVIRUS INFECTIONS

ETIOLOGIC AGENT   Coronaviruses are pleomorphic, single-stranded RNA viruses that measure 80 to 160 nm in diameter. The name derives from the crownlike appearance produced by the club-shaped projections that stud the viral envelope. Coronaviruses that infect humans fall into two distinct antigenic groups (I and II), which are represented by prototype isolates 229E and OC43. Coronaviruses are fastidious and are difficult to culture in vitro. Some strains will grow only in human tracheal organ cultures rather than in tissue culture.

EPIDEMIOLOGY   Only limited seroepidemiologic studies of coronavirus infections have been conducted. Seroprevalence studies of strains 229E and OC43 have demonstrated the presence of serum antibodies at rates ranging from 12% to >80% in various populations. Overall, coronaviruses account for 10 to 20% of common colds. Coronavirus infections appear to be particularly prevalent in late fall, winter, and early spring—times when rhinovirus infections are less common. A cyclical pattern has been suggested for outbreaks of infection with strains OC43 and 229E, with outbreaks occurring every 2 to 4 years.

CLINICAL MANIFESTATIONS   The clinical features of illness caused by coronaviruses are similar to those of illness caused by rhinoviruses. In studies of volunteers, the mean incubation period of illness induced by coronaviruses (3 days) is somewhat longer than that of illness caused by rhinoviruses, and the duration of illness is somewhat shorter (mean, 6 to 7 days). In some studies, the amount of nasal discharge was somewhat greater in colds induced by coronaviruses than in those induced by rhinoviruses. Coronaviruses have been recovered from infants with pneumonia and from military recruits with lower respiratory tract disease and have been associated with worsening of chronic bronchitis. However, the overall significance of coronaviruses in lower respiratory tract disease in humans remains unclear.

℞ TREATMENT   The approach to the treatment of common colds caused by coronaviruses is similar to that discussed above for rhinovirus-induced illnesses. Because of uncertainty regarding the number and relative importance of coronavirus subgroups and the mechanisms of immunity, vaccines against coronaviruses have not been developed.

RESPIRATORY SYNCYTIAL VIRUS INFECTIONS

ETIOLOGIC AGENT   Respiratory syncytial virus (RSV) is a member of the Paramyxoviridae family and comprises the genus *Pneumovirus*. RSV, an enveloped virus approximately 150 to 300 nm in diameter, is so named because its replication in vitro leads to the fusion of neighboring cells into large multinucleated syncytia. The single-stranded RNA genome codes for 10 virus-specific proteins. Viral RNA is contained in a helical nucleocapsid surrounded by a lipid envelope bearing two glycoproteins: the G protein, by which the virus attaches to cells, and the F (fusion) protein, which facilitates entry of the virus into the cell by fusing host and viral membranes. RSV was once considered to be of a single antigenic type, but two distinct groups (A and B) and multiple subtypes within each group have now been described. Antigenic diversity is reflected by differences in the G protein, while the F protein is highly conserved. The epidemiologic significance of the antigenic diversity is under investigation. Both antigenic groups can circulate simultaneously in outbreaks, although the relative proportions of each vary.

EPIDEMIOLOGY   RSV is the major respiratory pathogen of young children and the foremost cause of lower respiratory disease in infants. Infection with RSV is seen throughout the world in annual epidemics that occur in late fall, winter, or spring and last up to 5 months. The virus is rarely encountered during the summer. Rates of illness are highest among infants between 1 and 6 months of age, peaking between 2 and 3 months of age. The attack rates among susceptible infants and children are extraordinarily high, approaching 100% in settings such as day-care centers where large numbers of susceptible infants are present. RSV accounts for 20 to 25% of hospital admissions of young infants and children for pneumonia and for up to 75% of cases of bronchiolitis in this age group. It has been estimated that more than half of infants who are at risk will become infected during an RSV epidemic.

189 Common Viral Respiratory Infections **1123**

In older children and adults, reinfection with RSV is frequent but disease is milder than in infancy. A common cold–like syndrome is the illness most commonly associated with RSV infection in adults. Severe lower respiratory tract disease with pneumonitis can occur in elderly (often institutionalized) adults and in patients with immuno-compromising disorders or treatment, including recipients of bone-marrow and solid-organ transplants. RSV is also an important noso-comial pathogen; during an outbreak, it can infect pediatric patients and up to 25 to 50% of the staff on pediatric wards. The spread of virus among families is efficient: up to 40% of siblings may become infected when RSV is introduced into the family setting.

RSV is transmitted primarily by close contact with contaminated fingers or fomites and by self-inoculation of the conjunctiva or anterior nares. Virus also may be spread by coarse aerosols produced by coughing or sneezing, but it is inefficiently spread by fine-particle aerosols. The incubation period is ~4 to 6 days, and virus shedding may last for ≥2 weeks in children and for shorter periods in adults.

PATHOGENESIS Little is known about the histopathology of minor RSV infection. Severe bronchiolitis or pneumonia is character-ized by necrosis of the bronchiolar epithelium and a peribronchiolar infiltrate of lymphocytes and mononuclear cells. Interalveolar thick-ening and filling of alveolar spaces with fluid can also be found. The characteristics of the immune response to RSV are not well elucidated. Because reinfection occurs frequently and is often associated with ill-ness, the immunity that develops after single episodes of infection clearly is not complete or long-lasting. However, the cumulative effect of multiple reinfections is to temper subsequent disease and to provide some temporary measure of protection against infection. Studies of experimentally induced disease in healthy volunteers indicate that the presence of nasal IgA neutralizing antibody correlates more closely with protection than does the presence of serum antibody. Studies in infants, however, suggest that maternally acquired antibody provides some protection from lower respiratory tract disease, although illness can be severe even in infants who have moderate levels of maternally derived serum antibody. The relatively severe disease observed in im-munosuppressed patients and experimental animal models indicates that cell-mediated immunity is an important mechanism of host de-fense against RSV. Evidence suggests that class I MHC-restricted cy-totoxic T cells may be particularly important in this regard.

CLINICAL MANIFESTATIONS RSV infection leads to a wide spectrum of respiratory illnesses. In infants, 25 to 40% of infec-tions result in lower respiratory tract involvement, including pneu-monia, bronchiolitis, and tracheobronchitis. In this age group, illness begins most frequently with rhinorrhea, low-grade fever, and mild sys-temic symptoms, often accompanied by cough and wheezing. Most patients recover gradually over 1 to 2 weeks. In more severe illness, tachypnea and dyspnea develop, and eventually frank hypoxia, cya-nosis, and apnea can ensue. Physical examination may reveal diffuse wheezing, rhonchi, and rales. Chest radiography shows hyperexpan-sion, peribronchial thickening, and variable infiltrates ranging from diffuse interstitial infiltrates to segmental or lobar consolidation. Ill-ness may be particularly severe in children born prematurely and in those with congenital cardiac disease, bronchopulmonary dysplasia, nephrotic syndrome, or immunosuppression. One study documented a 37% mortality rate for infants with RSV pneumonia and congenital cardiac disease.

In adults, the most common symptoms of RSV infection are those of the common cold, with rhinorrhea, sore throat, and cough. Illness is occasionally associated with moderate systemic symptoms such as malaise, headache, and fever. RSV also has been reported to cause lower respiratory tract disease with fever in adults, including severe pneumonia in the elderly. RSV pneumonia can be a significant cause of morbidity and mortality in patients (particularly children) under-going bone-marrow and solid-organ transplantation.

LABORATORY FINDINGS AND DIAGNOSIS The diag-nosis of RSV infection can be suspected on the basis of a suggestive epidemiologic setting—that is, severe illness among infants during an outbreak of RSV in the community. Infections in older children and adults cannot be differentiated with certainty from those caused by other respiratory viruses. The specific diagnosis is established by iso-lation of RSV from respiratory secretions, including sputum, throat swabs, or nasopharyngeal washes. Virus is detected in tissue culture and is identified specifically through immunologic reactions detected by immunofluorescence, enzyme-linked immunosorbent assay (ELISA), or other techniques. Immunofluorescence microscopy of na-sal scrapings or washings provides a rapid diagnosis. Serologic tests that depend on fourfold or greater rises in complement-fixing or neu-tralizing antibody titers are useful for diagnosis in older children and adults but are less sensitive in children under 4 months of age. ELISA is more sensitive than complement-fixation or neutralization tests in the detection of serum antibody. Serologic diagnosis requires com-parison of acute- and convalescent-phase serum specimens and is therefore not useful during acute illness.

℞ TREATMENT Treatment of upper respiratory tract RSV in-fection is aimed primarily at the alleviation of symptoms and is similar to that for other viral infections of the upper respiratory tract. For lower respiratory tract infections, respiratory therapy, including hydration, suctioning of secretions, and administration of humidified oxygen and antibronchospastic agents, is given as needed. In severe hypoxia, intubation and ventilatory assistance may be required. Stud-ies of infants with RSV infection who were given aerosolized ribavirin, a nucleoside analogue active in vitro against RSV, have demonstrated a beneficial effect on the resolution of lower respiratory tract illness, including alleviation of blood-gas abnormalities. Treatment with ri-bavirin is recommended for infants who are severely ill or who are at high risk for complications of RSV infection; included are premature infants and those with bronchopulmonary dysplasia, congenital heart disease, or immunosuppression. The effects of ribavirin in adults with RSV pneumonia have not been established. The monthly administra-tion of human immunoglobulin with high titers of antibody to RSV (RSVIG) or of a chimeric mouse-human IgG antibody to RSV (palivizumab) has been approved as prophylaxis against RSV for chil-dren younger than 2 years of age who have bronchopulmonary dys-plasia or were born prematurely.

Considerable interest exists in the development of vaccines against RSV. Inactivated whole-virus vaccines have been ineffective; in one study, they actually potentiated the disease in infants. Other ap-proaches include immunization with purified F and G surface glyco-proteins of RSV or generation of stable, live attenuated virus vaccines. In settings such as pediatric wards where rates of transmission are high, barrier methods for the protection of hands and conjunctivae may be useful in reducing the spread of virus.

PARAINFLUENZA VIRUS INFECTIONS

ETIOLOGIC AGENT Parainfluenza viruses belong to the Paramyxoviridae family, are 150 to 250 nm in diameter, are enveloped, and contain a single-stranded RNA genome. The envelope is studded with two glycoproteins: one possesses both hemagglutinin and neu-raminidase activity and the other contains fusion activity. The viral RNA genome is enclosed in a helical nucleocapsid and codes for seven or eight virus-specific proteins. All four distinct serotypes of parain-fluenza viruses share certain antigens with other members of the Paramyxoviridae family, including mumps and Newcastle disease viruses.

EPIDEMIOLOGY Parainfluenza viruses are distributed throughout the world; infection with type 4 (subtypes 4A and 4B) has been reported less widely, probably because type 4 is more difficult to grow in tissue culture. Infection is acquired in early childhood, so that by 8 years of age most children have antibodies to serotypes 1, 2, and 3. Types 1 and 2 cause epidemics during the fall, primarily in odd-numbered years. Type 3 infection has been detected during all seasons of the year, but epidemics have occurred annually in the spring.

The contribution of parainfluenza infections to respiratory disease varies with both the location and the year. In studies conducted in the United States, parainfluenza virus infections have accounted for 4.3 to 22% of respiratory illnesses in children. In adults, parainfluenza infections are generally mild and account for fewer than 5% of respiratory illnesses. The major importance of parainfluenza viruses is as a cause of respiratory illness in young children, in whom they rank second only to RSV as causes of lower respiratory tract illness. Parainfluenza virus type 1 is the most frequent cause of croup (laryngotracheobronchitis) in children, while serotype 2 causes similar, although generally less severe, disease. Type 3 is an important cause of bronchiolitis and pneumonia in infants, while illnesses associated with type 4 have generally been mild. Unlike types 1 and 2, type 3 frequently causes illness during the first month of life, when passively acquired maternal antibody is still present. Parainfluenza viruses are spread through infected respiratory secretions, primarily by person-to-person contact and/or by large droplets. The incubation period has varied from 3 to 6 days in experimental infections but may be somewhat shorter for naturally occurring disease in children.

PATHOGENESIS Immunity to parainfluenza viruses is incompletely understood, but evidence suggests that immunity to infections with serotypes 1 and 2 is mediated by local IgA antibodies in the respiratory tract. Passively acquired serum neutralizing antibodies also confer some protection against infection with types 1, 2, and—to a lesser degree—3. Studies in experimental animal models and in immunosuppressed patients suggest that cell-mediated immunity may also be important in parainfluenza virus infections.

CLINICAL MANIFESTATIONS Parainfluenza virus infections occur most frequently among children, in whom initial infection with serotype 1, 2, or 3 is associated with an acute febrile illness 50 to 80% of the time. Children may present with coryza, sore throat, hoarseness, and cough that may or may not be croupy. In severe croup, fever persists, with worsening coryza and sore throat. A brassy or barking cough may progress to frank stridor. Most children recover over the next 1 or 2 days, although progressive airway obstruction and hypoxia ensue occasionally. If bronchiolitis or pneumonia develops, progressive cough accompanied by wheezing, tachypnea, and intercostal retractions may occur. In this setting, sputum production increases modestly. Physical examination shows nasopharyngeal discharge and oropharyngeal injection, along with rhonchi, wheezes, or coarse breath sounds. Chest x-rays can show air trapping and occasionally interstitial infiltrates.

In older children and adults, parainfluenza infections tend to be milder, presenting most frequently as a common cold or as hoarseness, with or without cough. Lower respiratory tract involvement in older children and adults is uncommon, but tracheobronchitis in adults has been reported. Severe, prolonged, and even fatal parainfluenza infection has been reported in children and adults with severe immunosuppression, including bone-marrow and solid-organ transplant recipients.

LABORATORY FINDINGS AND DIAGNOSIS The clinical syndromes caused by parainfluenza viruses (with the possible exception of croup in young children) are not sufficiently distinctive to be diagnosed on clinical grounds alone. A specific diagnosis is established by detection of virus in respiratory tract secretions, throat swabs, or nasopharyngeal washings. Virus is detected by growth in tissue culture (either by hemagglutination or by a cytopathic effect), by immunofluorescence of viral antigens in exfoliated cells from the respiratory tract, or by ELISA. Polymerase chain reaction assays have also been developed. Serologic diagnosis is based on a fourfold or greater rise in antibody titer, as detected by hemagglutination inhibition or by complement-fixation or neutralization tests in acute- and convalescent-phase specimens. However, as frequent heterotypic responses occur among the parainfluenza serotypes, the serotype causing illness often cannot be identified by serologic techniques alone.

Acute epiglottitis caused by *Haemophilus influenzae* type b must be differentiated from viral croup. Influenza A virus also is a common cause of croup during epidemic periods.

℞ TREATMENT For upper respiratory tract illness, symptoms can be treated as discussed for other viral respiratory tract illnesses. If complications such as sinusitis, otitis, or superimposed bacterial bronchitis develop, appropriate antibiotics should be administered. Mild cases of croup should be treated with bed rest and moist air generated by vaporizers. More severe cases require hospitalization and close observation for the development of respiratory distress. If acute respiratory distress develops, humidified oxygen and intermittent racemic epinephrine are usually administered. Aerosolized or systemically administered glucocorticoids are beneficial; the latter have a more profound effect. No specific antiviral therapy is available, although ribavirin is active against parainfluenza viruses in vitro and anecdotal reports describe its use clinically. Effective vaccines against parainfluenza viruses have not been developed.

ADENOVIRUS INFECTIONS

ETIOLOGIC AGENT Adenoviruses are complex DNA viruses that measure 70 to 80 nm in diameter. Human adenoviruses belong to the genus *Mastadenovirus*, which includes at least 47 serotypes. Adenoviruses have a characteristic morphology consisting of an icosahedral shell composed of 20 equilateral triangular faces and 12 vertices. The protein coat (capsid) consists of hexon subunits with group-specific and type-specific antigenic determinants and penton subunits at each vertex primarily containing group-specific antigens. A fiber with a knob at the end projects from each penton; this fiber contains type-specific and some group-specific antigens. Human adenoviruses have been divided into six subgenera (A through F) on the basis of the homology of DNA genomes and other properties. The adenovirus genome is a linear double-stranded DNA that codes for structural and nonstructural polypeptides. The replicative cycle of adenovirus may result either in lytic infection of cells or in the establishment of a latent infection (primarily involving lymphoid cells). Some adenovirus types can induce oncogenic transformation, and tumor formation has been observed in rodents; however, despite intensive investigation, adenoviruses have not been associated with tumors in humans.

EPIDEMIOLOGY Adenovirus infections most frequently affect infants and children. Infections occur throughout the year but are most common from fall to spring. Adenoviruses account for 3 to 5% of acute respiratory infections in children but for fewer than 2% of respiratory illnesses in civilian adults. Nearly 100% of adults have serum antibody to multiple serotypes—a finding indicating that infection is common in childhood. Types 1, 2, 3, and 5 are the most frequent isolates from children. Certain adenovirus serotypes—particularly 4 and 7 but also 3, 14, and 21—are associated with outbreaks of acute respiratory disease in military recruits in winter and spring. Adenovirus infection can be transmitted by inhalation of aerosolized virus, by inoculation of virus into conjunctival sacs, and probably by the fecal-oral route as well. Type-specific antibody generally develops after infection and is associated with protection against infection with the same serotype.

CLINICAL MANIFESTATIONS In children, adenoviruses cause a variety of clinical syndromes. The most common is an acute upper respiratory tract infection, with prominent rhinitis. On occasion, lower respiratory tract disease, including bronchiolitis and pneumonia, also develops. Adenoviruses, particularly types 3 and 7, cause pharyngoconjunctival fever, a characteristic acute febrile illness of children that occurs in outbreaks, most often in summer camps. The syndrome is marked by bilateral conjunctivitis in which the bulbar and palpebral conjunctivae have a granular appearance. Low-grade fever is frequently present for the first 3 to 5 days, and rhinitis, sore throat, and cervical adenopathy develop. The illness generally lasts for 1 to 2 weeks and resolves spontaneously. Febrile pharyngitis without conjunctivitis also has been associated with adenovirus infection. Adenoviruses have been isolated from cases of whooping cough with or without *Bordetella pertussis;* the significance of adenovirus in that disease is unknown.

In adults, the most frequently reported illness has been acute respiratory disease caused by adenovirus types 4 and 7 in military recruits. This illness is marked by a prominent sore throat and the gradual onset of fever, which often reaches 39°C (102.2°F) on the second or third day of illness. Cough is almost always present, and coryza and regional lymphadenopathy are frequently seen. Physical examination may show pharyngeal edema, injection, and tonsillar enlargement with little or no exudate. If pneumonia has developed, auscultation and x-ray of the chest may indicate areas of patchy infiltration.

Adenoviruses have been associated with a number of non–respiratory tract diseases, including acute diarrheal illness caused by types 40 and 41 in young children and hemorrhagic cystitis caused by types 11 and 21. Epidemic keratoconjunctivitis, caused most frequently by types 8, 19, and 37, has been associated with contaminated common sources such as ophthalmic solutions and roller towels. Adenoviruses also have been implicated in disseminated disease and pneumonia in immunosuppressed patients, including recipients of solid-organ or bone-marrow transplants and patients with AIDS. In the latter group, high-numbered and intermediate serotypes have been isolated, usually in the setting of low CD4+ counts, but their isolation frequently has not been clearly linked to disease manifestations. Adenovirus nucleic acids have been detected in myocardial cells from patients with "idiopathic" myocardiopathies, and adenoviruses have been suggested as causative agents in some cases.

LABORATORY FINDINGS AND DIAGNOSIS Adenovirus infection should be suspected in the epidemiologic setting of acute respiratory disease in military recruits and in certain of the clinical syndromes (such as pharyngoconjunctival fever or epidemic keratoconjunctivitis) in which outbreaks of characteristic illnesses occur. In most cases, however, illnesses caused by adenovirus infection cannot be differentiated from those caused by a number of other viral respiratory agents and *Mycoplasma pneumoniae*. A definitive diagnosis of adenovirus infection is established by culture or detection of the virus by means of ELISA or nucleic acid hybridization from sites such as the conjunctiva and oropharynx or from sputum, urine, or stool. Virus may be detected in tissue culture by cytopathic changes and specifically identified by immunofluorescence or other immunologic techniques. Adenovirus types 40 and 41, which have been associated with diarrheal disease in children, require special tissue-culture cells for isolation, and these serotypes are most commonly detected by direct ELISA of stool. Serum antibody rises can be demonstrated by complement-fixation or neutralization tests, ELISA, radioimmunoassay, or (for those adenoviruses that hemagglutinate red cells) hemagglutination inhibition tests.

℞ **TREATMENT** Only symptom-based treatment and supportive therapy are available for adenovirus infections, and no clinically useful antiviral compounds have been identified. Live vaccines have been developed against adenovirus types 4 and 7 and have been used to control illness in military recruits. These vaccines consist of live, unattenuated virus administered in enteric-coated capsules. Infection of the gastrointestinal tract with types 4 and 7 does not cause disease but stimulates local and systemic antibodies that are protective against subsequent acute respiratory disease due to those serotypes. Vaccines prepared from purified subunits of adenovirus are being investigated. Adenoviruses are also being studied as live-virus vectors for the delivery of vaccine antigens and for gene therapy.

BIBLIOGRAPHY

RHINOVIRUSES

GWALTNEY JM: Rhinoviruses, in *Principles and Practice of Infectious Diseases*, 5th ed, GF Mandell et al (eds). New York, Saunders, 2000, pp 1940–1948
MAKELA MJ et al: Viruses and bacteria in the etiology of the common cold. J Clin Microbiol 36:539, 1998

ROSSMAN MG et al: Structure of a human common cold virus and functional relationships to other picornaviruses. Nature 317:145, 1985
TYRRELL DAJ: A view from the Common Cold Unit. Antiviral Res 18:105, 1992

CORONAVIRUSES

LAI MMC: Coronavirus: Organization, replication, and expression of genome. Annu Rev Microbiol 44:303, 1990
LARSON HE et al: Isolation of rhinoviruses and coronaviruses from 38 colds in adults. J Med Virol 5:221, 1980
McINTOSH K: Coronaviruses, in *Virology*, 3d ed, BN Fields (ed). New York, Raven, 1995, pp 1095–1103

RESPIRATORY SYNCYTIAL VIRUS

ANDERSON LJ et al: Multicenter study of strains of respiratory syncytial virus. J Infect Dis 163:687, 1991
CANE PA et al: Molecular epidemiology of human respiratory syncytial virus. Semin Virol 6:371, 1995
CHANOCK RM et al: Serious respiratory tract disease caused by respiratory syncytial virus: Prospects for improved therapy and effective immunization. Pediatrics 90:137, 1992
COMMITTEE ON INFECTIOUS DISEASES: Use of ribavirin in the treatment of respiratory syncytial virus infection. Pediatrics 92:501, 1993
ENGLUND JA et al: Respiratory syncytial virus infection in immunocompromised adults. Ann Intern Med 109:203, 1988
GLEZEN WP et al: Risk of primary infection and reinfection with respiratory syncytial virus. Am J Dis Child 140:543, 1986

PARAINFLUENZA VIRUSES

DENNY FW et al: Croup: An 11 year study in a pediatric practice. Pediatrics 71:871, 1983
REED G et al: Epidemiology and clinical impact of parainfluenza virus infections in otherwise healthy infants and young children <5 years old. J Infect Dis 175:807, 1997
WRIGHT PF: Parainfluenza viruses, in *Viral Infections of the Respiratory Tract*, R Dolin, PF Wright (eds). New York, Marcel Dekker, 1999

ADENOVIRUSES

BAUM SG: Adenoviruses, in *Principles and Practice of Infectious Diseases*, 5th ed, GF Mandell et al (eds). New York, Saunders, 2000, pp 1624–1629
CRAWFORD-MIKSZU XX et al: Seroepidemiology of new AIDS-associated adenoviruses among the San Francisco Men's Health Study. J Med Virol 50:230, 1996
HIERHOLZER JC: Adenoviruses in the immunocompromised host. Clin Microbiol Rev 5: 262, 1992
ROSE HM et al: Adenoviral infection in military recruits. Arch Environ Health 21:356, 1970

190 *Raphael Dolin*

INFLUENZA

DEFINITION Influenza is an acute respiratory illness caused by infection with influenza viruses. The illness affects the upper and/or lower respiratory tract and is often accompanied by systemic signs and symptoms such as fever, headache, myalgia, and weakness. Outbreaks of illness of variable extent and severity occur nearly every winter. Such outbreaks result in significant morbidity in the general population and in increased mortality rates among certain high-risk patients, mainly as a result of pulmonary complications.

ETIOLOGIC AGENT Influenza viruses are members of the Orthomyxoviridae family. Influenza A and B viruses constitute one genus, and influenza C viruses make up the other. The designation of influenza viruses as type A, B, or C is based on antigenic characteristics of the nucleoprotein (NP) and matrix (M) protein antigens. Influenza A viruses are further subdivided (subtyped) on the basis of the surface hemagglutinin (H) and neuraminidase (N) antigens (see below); individual strains are designated according to the site of origin, isolate number, year of isolation, and subtype—for example, influenza A/Sydney/5/97 (H3N2). Influenza B and C viruses are similarly designated, but H and N antigens from these viruses do not receive subtype designations, since intratypic variations in influenza B antigens are less extensive than those in influenza A viruses and may not occur with influenza C virus.

Most of the information on the molecular biology of influenza viruses has come from studies of influenza A viruses; less is known about the replicative cycle of influenza B and C viruses. Morphologically, influenza viruses A, B, and C are similar. The virions are irregularly shaped spherical particles, 80 to 120 nm in diameter, and have a lipid envelope from the surface of which the H and N glycoproteins project (Fig. 190-1). The hemagglutinin is the site by which virus binds to cell receptors, whereas the neuraminidase degrades the receptor and probably plays a role in the release of virus from infected cells after replication has taken place. Influenza viruses enter cells by receptor-mediated endocytosis, forming a virus-containing endosome. The viral hemagglutinin mediates fusion of the endosomal membrane with the virus envelope, and viral nucleocapsids are subsequently released into the cytoplasm. Antibodies to the H antigen are the major determinants of immunity to influenza virus, while those to the N antigen limit viral spread and contribute to reduction of the infection. The inner surface of the lipid envelope contains the M proteins M1 and M2, the functions of which are incompletely understood but which may be involved in virus assembly and in stabilization of the lipid envelope. The virion also contains the NP antigen, which is associated with the viral genome, as well as three polymerase (P) proteins that are essential for transcription and synthesis of viral RNA. Two nonstructural (NS) proteins of unknown function are also present in infected cells.

The genomes of influenza A and B viruses consist of eight single-stranded RNA segments, which code for the structural and nonstructural proteins. Because the genome is segmented, the opportunity for reassortment of genes during infection is high, and reassortment occurs frequently during infection of cells with more than one influenza A virus.

EPIDEMIOLOGY Influenza outbreaks are recorded virtually every year, although their extent and severity vary widely. Localized outbreaks take place at variable intervals, usually every 1 to 3 years. Except for the past two decades, global epidemics or pandemics have occurred approximately every 10 to 15 years since the 1918–1919 pandemic (Table 190-1).

The most extensive and severe outbreaks are caused by influenza A viruses. In part, this predominance is a result of the remarkable propensity of the H and N antigens of influenza A virus to undergo periodic antigenic variation. Major antigenic variations are referred to as *antigenic shifts*, which may be associated with pandemics and are restricted to influenza A viruses. Minor variations are called *antigenic drifts*. These antigenic changes may involve the hemagglutinin alone or both the hemagglutinin and the neuraminidase. In human infections,

Table 190-1 Emergence of Antigenic Subtypes of Influenza A Virus Associated with Pandemic or Epidemic Disease

Years	Subtype	Extent of Outbreak
1889–90	H2N8[a]	Severe pandemic
1900–03	H3N8[a]	?Moderate epidemic
1918–19	H1N1[b] (formerly HswN1)	Severe pandemic
1933–35	H1N1[b] (formerly H0N1)	Mild epidemic
1946–47	H1N1	Mild epidemic
1957–58	H2N2	Severe pandemic
1968–69	H3N2	Moderate pandemic
1977–78[c]	H1N1	Mild pandemic

[a] As determined by retrospective serologic survey of individuals alive during those years ("seroarcheology").

[b] Hemagglutinins formerly designated as Hsw and H0 are now classified as variants of H1.

[c] From this time until the present (1999–2000), viruses of the H1N1 and H3N2 subtypes have circulated either in alternating years or concurrently.

three major antigenic subtypes of hemagglutinins (H1, H2, and H3) and two of neuraminidases (N1 and N2) have been recognized. The hemagglutinins formerly designated as H0 and Hsw are now classified as variants of H1. An example of an antigenic shift involving both the hemagglutinin and the neuraminidase is that of 1957, when the predominant influenza A virus subtype shifted from H1N1 to H2N2; this shift resulted in a severe pandemic, with an estimated 70,000 excess deaths (i.e., deaths in excess of the number expected without an influenza epidemic) in the United States alone. In 1968, an antigenic shift involving only the hemagglutinin occurred (H2N2 to H3N2); the subsequent pandemic was less severe than that of 1957. In 1977, an H1N1 virus emerged and caused a pandemic that primarily affected younger individuals (i.e., those born after 1957). As can be seen in Table 190-1, H1N1 viruses circulated from 1918 to 1956; thus, individuals born prior to 1957 would be expected to have some degree of immunity to H1N1 viruses. During most outbreaks of influenza A, a single subtype has circulated at a time. However, since 1977, H1N1 and H3N2 viruses have circulated simultaneously, resulting in outbreaks of varying severity. In some outbreaks, influenza B viruses have also circulated simultaneously with influenza A viruses.

The origin of pandemic strains is unknown. Given the marked differences between the primary structures of the hemagglutinins of different subtypes of influenza A viruses (H1, H2, and H3), it seems unlikely that antigenic shifts result from spontaneous mutations in the hemagglutinin gene. Because the segmented genome of influenza viruses may result in high rates of reassortment, it has been suggested that pandemic strains may emerge by reassortment of genes between human and animal viruses. There was concern that such reassortment might have occurred in 1997 in Hong Kong, where cases of infection caused by influenza virus A/H5N1 were detected in humans during an extensive outbreak of avian influenza A/H5N1 in poultry. However, only a few cases of A/H5N1 influenza in humans were documented, and the infection did not spread into the community. Influenza B viruses do not have an animal reservoir and do not undergo antigenic shifts, although they do undergo antigenic drift.

Pandemics provide the most dramatic evidence of the impact of influenza. However, illnesses that occur between pandemics account for greater total mortality and morbidity, albeit over a longer period. From 1972 through the present, influenza has been associated with at least 20,000 excess deaths during more than half of the interpandemic epidemics in the United States; more than 40,000 influenza-associated deaths occurred in each of three of these epidemics. Influenza A viruses that circulate between pandemics demonstrate antigenic drifts in the H antigen. These antigenic drifts apparently result from point mutations involving the RNA segment that codes for the hemagglutinin. Epidemiologically significant strains—that is, those with the potential to cause widespread outbreaks—exhibit changes in amino acids in at least two of the major antigenic sites in the hemagglutinin molecule. Since two point mutations are unlikely to occur simultaneously, it is believed that antigenic drifts result from point mutations occurring sequentially during the spread of virus from person to person. Anti-

FIGURE 190-1 An electron micrograph of influenza virus (×143,000). *(From R Dolin, Am Fam Phys 14:74, 1976.)*

genic drifts have been reported nearly annually since 1977 for H1N1 viruses and since 1968 for H3N2 viruses.

Influenza A epidemics begin abruptly, peak over a 2- to 3-week period, generally last for 2 to 3 months, and often subside almost as rapidly as they began. The first indication of influenza activity in a community is an increase in the number of children with febrile respiratory illnesses who present for medical attention. This increase is followed by increases in rates of influenza-like illnesses among adults and eventually by an increase in hospital admissions for patients with pneumonia, worsening of congestive heart failure, and exacerbations of chronic pulmonary disease. Rates of absence from work and school also rise at this time. An increase in the number of deaths caused by pneumonia and influenza is generally a late observation in an outbreak. Attack rates have been highly variable from outbreak to outbreak but most commonly are in the range of 10 to 20% of the general population. During the pandemic of 1957, it was estimated that the attack rate of clinical influenza exceeded 50% in urban populations and that an additional 25% or more of individuals in these populations may have been subclinically infected with influenza A virus. Among institutionalized populations and in semiclosed settings with a large number of susceptible individuals, even higher attack rates have been reported.

Epidemics of influenza occur almost exclusively during the winter months in the temperate zones of the northern and southern hemispheres. In those locations, it is highly unusual to detect influenza A virus at other times, although serologic rises or even outbreaks have been noted rarely during warm-weather months. In contrast, influenza virus infections occur throughout the year in the tropics. Where or how influenza A virus persists between outbreaks in temperate zones is unknown. It is possible that influenza A viruses are maintained in the human population on a worldwide basis by person-to-person transmission and that large population clusters support a low level of interepidemic transmission. Alternatively, human strains may persist in animal reservoirs. Convincing evidence to support either explanation is not available. In the modern era, rapid transportation may contribute to the transmission of viruses among widespread geographic locales.

The factors that result in the inception and termination of outbreaks of influenza are incompletely understood. A major determinant of the extent and severity of an outbreak is the level of immunity in the population at risk. With the emergence of an antigenically novel influenza virus to which little or no antibody is present in a community, extensive outbreaks may occur. When the absence of antibody is worldwide, epidemic disease may spread around the globe, resulting in a pandemic. Such pandemic waves can continue for several years, until immunity in the population reaches a high level. In the years following pandemic influenza, antigenic drifts among influenza viruses result in outbreaks of variable severity in populations with high levels of immunity to the pandemic strain that circulated earlier. This situation persists until another antigenically novel pandemic strain emerges. On the other hand, outbreaks sometimes end despite the persistence of a large pool of susceptible individuals in the population.

Occasionally, the emergence of a significantly different antigenic variant will result only in a localized outbreak. The swine influenza outbreak of 1976 in the United States, caused by an A/H1N1 virus antigenically similar to the virus that circulated in 1918–1919, may be an example, although this outbreak may have represented simply the introduction of a swine influenza virus into a crowded human population without spread beyond that setting. The cluster of human infections with influenza A/H5N1 in Hong Kong in 1997 may also be an example of this phenomenon. It has been suggested that certain viruses, such as recently circulating A/H1N1 strains, may be intrinsically less virulent and cause less severe disease than other variants, even in immunologically virgin subjects. If so, then other (undefined) factors besides the level of preexisting immunity must play a role in the epidemiology of influenza.

Influenza B virus causes outbreaks that are generally less extensive and are associated with less severe disease than those caused by influenza A virus. The hemagglutinin and neuraminidase of influenza B virus undergo less frequent and less extensive variation than those of influenza A viruses; this characteristic may account, in part, for the lesser extent of disease. Influenza B outbreaks are seen most frequently in schools and military camps, although outbreaks in institutions in which elderly individuals reside have also been noted on occasion. The most serious complication of influenza B virus infection is Reye's syndrome (Chap. 300). Influenza C virus has only infrequently been associated with human disease, although the wide prevalence of serum antibody to this virus indicates that asymptomatic infection may be common.

The morbidity and mortality caused by influenza outbreaks continue to be substantial. Most individuals who die in this setting have underlying diseases that place them at high risk for complications of influenza. Excess hospitalizations for adults with high-risk medical conditions have ranged from 20 to 1000 per 100,000 during recent outbreaks of influenza. The most prominent high-risk conditions are chronic cardiac and pulmonary diseases as well as old age. Mortality among individuals with chronic metabolic, renal, and certain immunosuppressive diseases has also been elevated, although lower than that among patients with chronic cardiopulmonary diseases. The morbidity attributable to influenza in the general population is considerable. For each of three outbreaks in the United States that were studied during the 1960s, estimated direct and indirect economic costs ranged from $1.5 to $3.5 billion; today such costs would obviously be much greater.

PATHOGENESIS The initial event in influenza is infection of the respiratory epithelium with influenza virus acquired from respiratory secretions of acutely infected individuals. In all likelihood, transmission occurs via aerosols generated by coughs and sneezes, although hand-to-hand contact, other personal contact, and even fomite transmission may take place. Experimental evidence suggests that infection by a small-particle aerosol (particle diameter, $<10\ \mu m$) is more efficient than that by larger droplets. Initially, viral infection involves the ciliated columnar epithelial cells, but it also may involve other respiratory tract cells, including alveolar cells, mucous gland cells, and macrophages. In infected cells, virus replicates within 4 to 6 h, after which infectious virus is released to infect adjacent or nearby cells. In this way, infection spreads from a few foci to a large number of respiratory cells over several hours. In experimentally induced infection, the incubation period of illness has ranged from 18 to 72 h, depending on the size of the virus inoculum. Histopathologic study reveals degenerative changes, including granulation, vacuolization, swelling, and pyknotic nuclei, in infected ciliated cells. The cells eventually become necrotic and desquamate; in some areas, previously columnar epithelium is replaced by flattened and metaplastic epithelial cells. The severity of illness is correlated with the quantity of virus shed in secretions; thus, the degree of viral replication itself may be an important factor in pathogenesis. Despite the frequent development of systemic signs and symptoms such as fever, headache, and myalgias, influenza virus has only rarely been detected in extrapulmonary sites (including the bloodstream). Evidence suggests that the pathogenesis of systemic symptoms in influenza may be related to the induction of certain cytokines, particularly tumor necrosis factor α and interleukin 6.

The host response to influenza infections involves a complex interplay of humoral antibody, local antibody, cell-mediated immunity, interferon, and other host defenses. Serum antibody responses, which can be detected by the second week after primary infection, are measured by a variety of techniques: hemagglutination inhibition (HI), complement fixation (CF), neutralization, enzyme-linked immunosorbent assay (ELISA), and antineuraminidase antibody assay. Antibodies directed against the hemagglutinin appear to be the most important mediators of immunity; in several studies, HI titers of ≥ 40 have been associated with protection from infection. Secretory antibodies produced in the respiratory tract are predominantly of the IgA class and also play a major role in protection against infection. Secretory antibody neutralization titers of ≥ 4 have also been associated with protection. A variety of cell-mediated immune responses, both antigen-specific and antigen-nonspecific, can be detected early after infection and depend on the prior immune status of the host. These responses include T-cell proliferative, T-cell cytotoxic, and natural killer cell activity. Interferons have been detected in respiratory secretions shortly after the shedding of virus has begun, and rises in interferon titers coincide with decreases in virus shedding.

The host defense factors responsible for cessation of virus shedding and resolution of illness have not been defined specifically. Virus shedding generally stops within 2 to 5 days after symptoms first appear, at a time when serum and local antibody responses often are not detectable by conventional techniques (although antibody rises may be detected earlier by use of highly sensitive techniques, particularly in individuals with previous immunity to the virus). It has been suggested that interferon, cell-mediated immune responses, and/or nonspecific inflammatory responses are important in the resolution of illness.

MANIFESTATIONS Influenza has most frequently been described as an illness characterized by the abrupt onset of systemic symptoms, such as headache, feverishness, chills, myalgia, or malaise, and accompanying respiratory tract signs, particularly cough and sore throat. In many cases, the onset is so abrupt that patients can recall the precise time they became ill. A typical case of naturally occurring influenza is depicted in Fig. 190-2. However, the spectrum of clinical presentations is wide, ranging from a mild, afebrile respiratory illness similar to the common cold (with either a gradual or an abrupt onset) to severe prostration with relatively few respiratory signs and symptoms. In most of the cases that come to a physician's attention, the patient has a fever, with temperatures of 38° to 41°C (100.4° to 105.8°F). A rapid temperature rise within the first 24 h of illness is generally followed by a gradual defervescence over a 2- to 3-day period, although, on occasion, fever may last for as long as a week. Patients report a feverish feeling and chilliness, but true rigors are rare. Headache, either generalized or frontal, is often particularly troublesome. Myalgias may involve any part of the body but are most common in the legs and lumbosacral area. Arthralgias may also develop.

Respiratory complaints often become more prominent as systemic

FIGURE 190-2 Clinical characteristics of a naturally occurring case of influenza A in an otherwise healthy 28-year-old man. *(From R Dolin, Am Fam Phys 14:74, 1976.)*

symptoms subside. Many patients have a sore throat or persistent cough, which may last for a week or more and which is often accompanied by substernal discomfort. Ocular signs and symptoms include pain on motion of the eyes, photophobia, and burning of the eyes.

Physical findings are usually minimal in cases of uncomplicated influenza. Early in the illness, the patient appears flushed and the skin is hot and dry, although diaphoresis and mottled extremities are sometimes evident, particularly in older patients. Examination of the pharynx may yield surprisingly unremarkable results despite a severe sore throat, but injection of the mucous membranes and postnasal discharge are apparent in some cases. Mild cervical lymphadenopathy may be noted, especially in younger individuals. The results of chest examination are largely negative in uncomplicated influenza, although rhonchi, wheezes, and scattered rales have been reported with variable frequency in different outbreaks. Frank dyspnea, hyperpnea, cyanosis, diffuse rales, and signs of consolidation are indicative of pulmonary complications. Patients with apparently uncomplicated influenza have been reported to have a variety of mild ventilatory defects and increased alveolar-capillary diffusion gradients; thus, subclinical pulmonary involvement may be more frequent than is appreciated.

In uncomplicated influenza, the acute illness generally resolves over a 2- to 5-day period, and most patients have largely recovered in 1 week. In a significant minority (particularly the elderly), however, symptoms of weakness or lassitude (postinfluenzal asthenia) may persist for several weeks and may prove troublesome for persons who wish to resume their full level of activity promptly. The pathogenetic basis for this asthenia is unknown, although pulmonary function abnormalities may persist for several weeks after uncomplicated influenza.

COMPLICATIONS The most common complication of influenza is pneumonia: "primary" influenza viral pneumonia, secondary bacterial pneumonia, or mixed viral and bacterial pneumonia. Primary influenza viral pneumonia is the least common but most severe of the pneumonic complications. It presents as acute influenza that does not resolve but instead progresses relentlessly, with persistent fever, dyspnea, and eventual cyanosis. Sputum production is generally scanty, but the sputum can contain blood. Few physical signs may be evident early in the illness. In more advanced cases, diffuse rales may be noted, and chest x-ray findings consistent with diffuse interstitial infiltrates and/or acute respiratory distress syndrome may be present. In such cases, arterial blood-gas determinations show marked hypoxia. Viral cultures of respiratory secretions and lung parenchyma, especially if samples are taken early in illness, yield high titers of virus. In fatal cases of primary viral pneumonia, histopathologic examination reveals a marked inflammatory reaction in the alveolar septa, with edema and infiltration by lymphocytes, macrophages, occasional plasma cells, and variable numbers of neutrophils. Fibrin thrombi in alveolar capillaries, along with necrosis and hemorrhage, have also been noted. Eosinophilic hyaline membranes can be found lining alveoli and alveolar ducts.

Primary influenza viral pneumonia has a predilection for individuals with cardiac disease, particularly those with mitral stenosis, but has also been reported in otherwise healthy young adults as well as in older individuals with chronic pulmonary disorders. In some epidemics of influenza (notably those of 1918 and 1957), pregnancy increased the risk of primary influenza pneumonia.

Secondary bacterial pneumonia follows acute influenza. Improvement of the patient's condition over 2 to 3 days is followed by a reappearance of fever along with clinical signs and symptoms of bacterial pneumonia, including cough, production of purulent sputum, and physical and x-ray signs of consolidation. The most common bacterial pathogens in this setting are *Streptococcus pneumoniae, Staphylococcus aureus*, and *Haemophilus influenzae*—organisms that can colonize the nasopharynx and that cause infection in the wake of changes in bronchopulmonary defenses. The etiology can often be determined by Gram's staining and culture of an appropriately obtained sputum specimen. Secondary bacterial pneumonia occurs most frequently in high-risk individuals with chronic pulmonary and cardiac disease and in elderly individuals. Patients with secondary bacterial pneumonia often respond to antibiotic therapy when it is instituted promptly.

Perhaps the most common pneumonic complications during outbreaks of influenza have mixed features of viral and bacterial pneumonia. Patients may experience a gradual progression of their acute illness or may show transient improvement followed by clinical exacerbation, with eventual manifestation of the clinical features of bacterial pneumonia. Sputum cultures may contain both influenza A virus and one of the bacterial pathogens described above. Patchy infiltrates or areas of consolidation may be detected by physical examination and chest x-ray. Patients with mixed viral and bacterial pneumonia generally have less widespread involvement of the lung than those with primary viral pneumonia, and their bacterial infections may respond to appropriate antibiotics. Mixed viral and bacterial pneumonia occurs primarily in patients with chronic cardiovascular and pulmonary diseases.

Other pulmonary complications associated with influenza include worsening of chronic obstructive pulmonary disease and exacerbation of chronic bronchitis and asthma. In children, influenza infection may present as croup.

In addition to the pulmonary complications of influenza, a number of extrapulmonary complications may occur. These include *Reye's syndrome*, a serious complication in children that is associated with influenza B and to a lesser extent with influenza A virus infection as well as with varicella-zoster virus infection. An epidemiologic association between Reye's syndrome and aspirin therapy for the antecedent viral infection has been noted, and the incidence of Reye's syndrome has decreased markedly with widespread warnings regarding the use of aspirin by children with acute viral respiratory infections. A detailed description of Reye's syndrome is found in Chap. 300.

Myositis, rhabdomyolysis, and myoglobinuria are occasional complications of influenza infection. Although myalgias are exceedingly common in influenza, true myositis is rare. Patients with acute myositis have exquisite tenderness of the affected muscles, most commonly in the legs, and may not be able to tolerate even the slightest pressure, such as the touch of bedsheets. In the most severe cases, there is frank swelling and bogginess of muscles. Serum levels of creatine phosphokinase and aldolase are markedly elevated, and an occasional patient has developed renal failure from myoglobinuria. The pathogenesis of influenza-associated myositis is also unclear, although the presence of influenza virus in affected muscles has been reported.

Myocarditis and pericarditis were reported in association with influenza virus infection during the 1918–1919 pandemic; these reports were based largely on histopathologic findings, and these complications have been reported only infrequently since that time. Electrocardiographic changes during acute influenza are common among patients who have cardiac disease but have been ascribed most often to exacerbations of the underlying cardiac disease rather than to direct involvement of the myocardium with influenza virus.

Central nervous system (CNS) diseases, including encephalitis, transverse myelitis, and Guillain-Barré syndrome, have been reported during influenza. The etiologic relationship of influenza virus to such CNS illnesses remains unestablished. Toxic shock syndrome caused by *S. aureus* infection following acute influenza infection has also been reported (Chap. 139).

In addition to complications involving the specific organ systems described above, influenza outbreaks include a number of cases in which elderly and other high-risk individuals develop influenza and subsequently experience a gradual deterioration of underlying cardiovascular, pulmonary, or renal function—changes that occasionally are irreversible and lead to death. These fatalities contribute to the overall excess mortality associated with influenza A outbreaks.

LABORATORY FINDINGS AND DIAGNOSIS Laboratory diagnosis is accomplished during acute influenza by isolation of the virus from throat swabs, nasopharyngeal washes, or sputum. Virus is usually detected in tissue culture or less commonly is found in the amniotic cavity of chick embryos within 48 to 72 h after inoculation. The rapid viral diagnostic tests now available detect viral nucleoprotein or neuraminidase with high specificity and sensitivities of 57 to 81% compared with tissue culture. Viral nucleic acids have been detected in clinical samples by reverse transcriptase polymerase chain reaction. The type of influenza virus (A or B) may be determined by either immunofluorescence or HI techniques, and the hemagglutinin subtype of influenza A virus (H1, H2, or H3) may be identified by HI with use of subtype-specific antisera. Serologic methods for diagnosis require comparison of antibody titers in sera obtained during the acute illness with those in sera obtained 10 to 14 days after the onset of illness and are useful primarily in retrospect. Fourfold or greater titer rises as detected by HI or CF or significant rises as measured by ELISA are diagnostic of acute infection. CF tests are generally less sensitive than other serologic techniques, but, as they detect type-specific antigens, they may be particularly useful when subtype-specific reagents are not available.

Other laboratory tests are generally not helpful in making a specific diagnosis of influenza virus infection. Leukocyte counts are variable, frequently being low early in illness and normal or slightly elevated later. Severe leukopenia has been described in overwhelming viral or bacterial infection, while leukocytosis with more than 15,000 cells/μL raises the suspicion of secondary bacterial infection.

DIFFERENTIAL DIAGNOSIS On clinical grounds alone, an individual case of influenza may be difficult to differentiate from an acute respiratory illness caused by any of a variety of respiratory viruses or by *Mycoplasma pneumoniae*. Severe streptococcal pharyngitis or early bacterial pneumonia may mimic acute influenza, although bacterial pneumonias generally do not run a self-limited course. Purulent sputum in which a bacterial pathogen can be detected by Gram's staining is an important diagnostic feature in bacterial pneumonia. The fact that influenza occurs in characteristic outbreaks during the winter months may facilitate a clinical diagnosis. When local health authorities indicate that influenza is present in the community, an acute febrile respiratory illness can be attributed to influenza with a high degree of certainty, particularly if the typical features of abrupt onset and systemic symptoms are present.

℞ **TREATMENT** In uncomplicated cases of influenza, symptom-based therapy with acetaminophen for the relief of headache, myalgia, and fever may be considered, but the use of salicylates should be avoided in children below 18 years of age because of the possible association of salicylates with Reye's syndrome. Since cough is ordinarily self-limited, treatment with cough suppressants generally is not indicated, although codeine-containing compounds may be employed if the cough is particularly troublesome. Patients should be advised to rest and maintain hydration during acute illness and should return to full activity only gradually after the illness has resolved, especially if the illness has been severe.

Specific antiviral therapy is available for influenza: amantadine and rimantadine for influenza A and the neuraminidase inhibitors zanamivir and oseltamivir for both influenza A and influenza B. If begun within 48 h of the onset of illness, treatment with amantadine or rimantadine has reduced the duration of systemic and respiratory symptoms of influenza by ~50%. From 5 to 10% of individuals who receive amantadine experience mild CNS side effects, primarily jitteriness, anxiety, insomnia, or difficulty in concentrating. These side effects disappear promptly upon cessation of the drug. Rimantadine appears to be equally efficacious and is associated with less frequent CNS side effects than is amantadine. In adults, the usual dose of amantadine or rimantadine is 200 mg/d for 3 to 7 days. Since both drugs are excreted via the kidney, the dose should be reduced to ≤100 mg/d in elderly patients and patients with renal insufficiency. Zanamivir, inhaled orally at a dose of 10 mg twice a day for 5 days, or oseltamivir, ingested orally at a dose of 75 mg twice a day for 5 days, has reduced the duration of signs and symptoms of influenza by 1 to 1.5 days if treatment is started within 2 days of the onset of illness. Zanamivir may exacerbate bronchospasm in asthmatic patients, and oseltamivir has been associated with nausea and vomiting, whose frequency can be reduced by drug administration with food. Currently, only amantadine and zanamivir are approved in the United States for treatment of children (the latter for use in children ≥7 years old). Ribavirin, a nucleoside analogue with activity against a variety of viral agents, has been reported to be effective against both influenza A and influenza B virus infections when administered as an aerosol, although it is relatively ineffective when administered orally.

Studies demonstrating the therapeutic efficacy of antiviral compounds in influenza have primarily involved young adults with uncomplicated disease; it is not known whether such compounds are effective in the treatment of complications such as influenza pneumonia. Therapy for primary influenza pneumonia is directed at maintaining oxygenation and is most appropriately undertaken in an intensive care unit, with aggressive respiratory and hemodynamic support as needed. Bypass membrane oxygenators have been employed in this setting with variable results. When an acute respiratory distress syndrome develops, fluids must be administered cautiously, with close monitoring of blood gases and hemodynamic function.

Antibacterial drugs should be reserved for the therapy of bacterial complications of acute influenza, such as secondary bacterial pneumonia. The choice of antibiotics should be guided by Gram's staining and culture of appropriate specimens of respiratory secretions, such as sputum or transtracheal aspirates. If the etiology of a case of bacterial pneumonia is unclear from an examination of respiratory secretions, empirical antibiotics effective against the most common bacterial pathogens in this setting (*S. pneumoniae*, *S. aureus*, and *H. influenzae*) should be selected (Chaps. 138, 139, and 149).

PROPHYLAXIS The major public health measure for prevention of influenza has been the use of inactivated influenza vaccines derived from influenza A and B viruses that circulated during the previous influenza season. If the vaccine virus and the currently circulating viruses are closely related, 50 to 80% protection against influenza would be expected. Presently available vaccines have been highly purified and are associated with few reactions. Up to 5% of individuals experience low-grade fever and mild systemic symptoms 8 to 24 h after vaccination, and up to one-third develop mild redness or tenderness at the vaccination site. Since the vaccine is produced in eggs, individuals with true hypersensitivity to egg products either should be desensitized or should not be vaccinated. Although the 1976 swine influenza vaccine appears to have been associated with an increased frequency of Guillain-Barré syndrome, influenza vaccines administered since 1976 generally have not been. Possible exceptions were noted during the 1992–1993 and 1993–1994 influenza seasons, when there may have been an excess risk of Guillain-Barré syndrome of slightly more than one case per million among vaccine recipients. However, the overall health risk following influenza outweighs the potential risk associated with vaccination. Investigational live attenuated ("cold-adapted") influenza A and B vaccines also have been developed and have been highly effective in preventing influenza in studies in adults and children. Such vaccines are administered intranasally and stimulate local antibody production more efficiently than conventional inactivated vaccines.

The U.S. Public Health Service recommends influenza vaccination for any individual >6 months of age who is at an increased risk for complications of influenza. Included are individuals with chronic cardiovascular or pulmonary disorders (including asthma) and residents of nursing homes and other chronic-care facilities. Other populations for whom the vaccine is recommended include healthy individuals >65 years of age and individuals who have required regular medical attention for diabetes mellitus, renal disease, hemoglobinopathies, or immunosuppression. Individuals who provide care for high-risk patients or who come into frequent contact with such patients, including household members, should also receive vaccine to reduce the likelihood of transmission of infection. Vaccination is recommended for women who will be in the second or third trimester of pregnancy during the influenza season and for individuals 6 months to 18 years of age who are receiving long-term aspirin therapy and may be at risk for Reye's syndrome. Since commercially available vaccines are inactivated ("killed"), they may be administered safely to immunocompromised patients. Influenza vaccination is not associated with exacerbations of chronic nervous-system diseases such as multiple sclerosis. Vaccine should be administered early in the autumn before influenza outbreaks occur and should be repeated annually to maintain immunity against the most current influenza virus strains.

Of the vaccines currently available (inactivated whole-virus vaccine, subvirion vaccine, and purified surface-antigen vaccine), only the "split-virus" preparations (i.e., the subvirion and purified surface-antigen vaccines) should be given to children <13 years old, since the whole-virus preparations have been associated with higher rates of adverse reactions in this age group.

Studies have shown amantadine and rimantadine to be 70 to 100% effective in the prophylaxis of illness associated with influenza A virus infection. Such prophylaxis is most likely to be used for high-risk individuals who have not received influenza vaccine or in a situation where the vaccines previously administered are relatively ineffective because of antigenic changes in the circulating virus. During an outbreak, amantadine or rimantadine can be administered simultaneously with inactivated vaccine, since neither drug interferes with an immune response to the vaccine. In fact, there is evidence that the protective effects of amantadine and vaccine may be additive. Amantadine has also been employed to control nosocomial outbreaks of influenza A. For prophylaxis, administration of amantadine or rimantadine should be instituted promptly when influenza A activity is detected and must be continued daily for the duration of the outbreak. The dosage most frequently employed has been 200 mg/d for adults, but the dose should be reduced for patients with renal insufficiency and for the elderly. Viruses resistant to both amantadine and rimantadine can emerge quickly after therapy with these drugs, and the possible transmission of these resistant viruses has been reported. The neuraminidase inhibitors zanamivir and oseltamivir have also been reported to be highly effective in the prophylaxis of influenza A and offer the advantage of efficacy against influenza B as well. They are currently under review for use as prophylaxis. As with amantadine and rimantadine, the neuraminidase inhibitors must be administered daily to maintain prophylaxis.

BIBLIOGRAPHY

BELSHE RB et al: The efficacy of live attenuated, cold adapted trivalent, intranasal influenza vaccine in children. N Engl J Med 38:1405, 1998

CENTERS FOR DISEASE CONTROL AND PREVENTION: Prevention and control of influenza. MMWR 47(RR–6):1, 1998

DOLIN R et al: A controlled trial of amantadine and rimantadine in the prophylaxis of influenza A infection. N Engl J Med 307:580, 1982

GLEZEN WP: Serious morbidity and mortality associated with influenza epidemics. Epidemiol Rev 4:25, 1982

GROSS PA et al: Association of influenza immunization with reduction in mortality in an elderly population: A prospective study. Arch Intern Med 148:562, 1988

HAYDEN FG et al: Use of the selective oral neuraminidase inhibitor oseltamivir to prevent influenza. N Engl J Med 341:1336, 1999

——— et al: Use of the oral neuraminidase inhibitor oseltamivir in experimental human influenza: Randomized controlled trials for prevention and treatment. JAMA 282:1240, 1999

MIST (MANAGEMENT OF INFLUENZA IN THE SOUTHERN HEMISPHERE TRIALISTS) STUDY GROUP: Randomized trial of efficacy and safety of inhaled zanamivir in treatment of influenza A and B infections. Lancet 352:1871, 1998

MURPHY BR, WEBSTER RG: Orthomyxoviruses, in Virology, 3d ed, BN Fields (ed). New York, Raven Press, 1995, pp 1091-1152

SIMONSEN L et al: Pandemic vs epidemic mortality: A pattern of changing age distribution. J Infect Dis 178:53, 1998

191
Anthony S. Fauci, Dan L. Longo

THE HUMAN RETROVIRUSES

The retroviruses, which make up a large family (Retroviridae), infect mainly vertebrates. They have a unique replication cycle whereby their genetic information is encoded by RNA rather than DNA. Retroviruses contain an RNA-dependent DNA polymerase (a reverse transcriptase) that directs the synthesis of a DNA form of the viral genome after infection of a host cell. The designation *retrovirus* denotes that information in the form of RNA is transcribed into DNA in the host cell—a sequence that overturned a central dogma of molecular biology: that information passes unidirectionally from DNA to RNA to protein. The observation that RNA was the source of genetic information in the causative agents of certain animal tumors led to a number of paradigm-shifting biologic insights regarding not only the direction of genetic-information passage but also the viral etiology of certain cancers and the concept of oncogenes as normal host genes scavenged and altered by a viral vector.

The family Retroviridae includes three subfamilies (Table 191-1): Oncovirinae, of which human T-cell lymphotropic virus (HTLV) type I is the most important in humans; Lentivirinae, of which HIV is the most important in humans; and Spumavirinae, the "foamy" viruses, named for the pathologic appearance of infected cells. A number of spumaviruses have been isolated from humans; however, they are not associated with any known disease and therefore are not discussed further in this chapter.

The wide variety of interactions of a retrovirus with its host range from completely benign events (e.g., silent carriage of endogenous retroviral sequences in the germ-line genome of many animal species) to rapidly fatal infections (e.g., exogenous infection with an oncogenic virus such as Rous sarcoma virus in chickens). The ability of retroviruses to acquire and alter the structure and function of host cell sequences has revolutionized our understanding of molecular carcinogenesis. The viruses can insert into the germ-line genome of the host cell and behave as a transposable or movable genetic element. They can activate or inactivate genes near the site of integration into the genome. They can rapidly alter their own genome by recombination and mutation under selective environmental stimuli.

Most human viral diseases occur as a consequence of either tissue destruction by the virus itself or the host's response to the virus. Although these mechanisms are operative in retroviral infections, retroviruses have additional mechanisms of inducing disease, including the malignant transformation of an infected cell and the induction of an immunodeficiency state that leads to opportunistic diseases (infections and neoplasms; Chap. 309).

STRUCTURE AND LIFE CYCLE
Despite the wide range of biologic consequences of retroviral infection, all retroviruses are similar in structure, genome organization, and mode of replication. Retroviruses are 70 to 130 nm in diameter and have a lipid-containing envelope surrounding an icosahedral capsid with a dense inner core. The core contains two identical copies of the single-stranded RNA genome. The RNA molecules are 8 to 10 kb

long and are complexed with reverse transcriptase and tRNA. Other viral proteins, such as integrase, are also components of the virion particle. The RNA has features usually found in mRNA: a cap site at the 5' end of the molecule, which is important in the initiation of mRNA translation, and a polyadenylation site at the 3' end, which influences mRNA turnover (i.e., messages with shorter polyA tails turn over faster than messages with longer polyA tails). However, the retroviral RNA is not translated; instead it is transcribed into DNA. The DNA form of the retroviral genome is called a *provirus*.

The replication cycle of retroviruses proceeds in two phases (Fig. 191-1). In the first phase, the virus enters the cytoplasm after binding to a specific cell-surface receptor (with HIV, a cell-surface coreceptor is also utilized for binding and entry); the viral RNA and reverse transcriptase synthesize a double-stranded DNA version of the RNA template; and the provirus moves into the nucleus and integrates into the host cell genome. This proviral integration is permanent. Although some animal retroviruses integrate into a single specific site of the host genome in every infected cell, the four known pathogenic human retroviruses (HTLV-I, HTLV-II, HIV-1, and HIV-2) integrate randomly. This first phase of replication depends entirely on gene products in the virus. The second phase includes the synthesis and processing of viral genomes, mRNAs, and proteins using host cell machinery, often under the influence of viral gene products. Virions are assembled and released from the cell by budding from the membrane; host cell membrane proteins are frequently incorporated into the envelope of the virus. Proviral integration occurs during the S phase of the cell cycle; thus, in general, nondividing cells are resistant to retroviral infection. Only the lentiviruses are able to infect nondividing cells. Once a host is infected, it is infected for life.

Retroviral genomes include both coding and noncoding sequences (Fig. 191-2). In general, noncoding sequences are important recognition signals for DNA or RNA synthesis or processing events and are located in the 5' and 3' terminal regions of the genome. All retroviral genomes are terminally redundant, containing identical sequences called *long terminal repeats* (LTRs). The ends of the retroviral RNA genome differ slightly in sequence from the integrated retroviral DNA. In the latter, the LTR sequences are repeated in both the 5' and the 3' terminus of the virus. The LTRs contain sequences involved in initiating the expression of the viral proteins, the integration of the provirus, and the polyadenylation of viral RNAs. The primer binding site, which is critical for the initiation of reverse transcription, and the viral

Table 191-1   Classification of Retroviruses: The Family Retroviridae

Subfamily, Group[a]	Example	Feature
Oncovirinae (oncogenic viruses)		
Avian leukosis	Rous sarcoma virus	Contains *src* oncogene
Mammalian C-type	Abelson leukemia virus	Contains *abl* oncogene
B-type	Murine mammary tumor virus	Can be endogenous or exogenous
D-type	Mason-Pfizer monkey virus	—
HTLV-BLV	HTLV-I	Causes T-cell lymphoma and neurologic disease
Lentivirinae (slow viruses)	HIV-1, HIV-2	Causes AIDS
	Visna virus	Causes lung and brain diseases in sheep
	Feline immunodeficiency virus	Causes immunodeficiency in cats
Spumavirinae (foamy viruses)	Simian foamy virus, human foamy virus	Causes no known disease

[a] The Oncovirinae were originally grouped into types A–D on the basis of morphologic features (size, core location, budding) under electron microscopy; however, this system has been replaced by groupings based on relationships of genome structure and sequence.

NOTE: HTLV, human T-lymphotropic virus; BLV, bovine leukemia virus.

FIGURE 191-1 The life cycle of retroviruses. *A.* Overview of virus replication. The retrovirus enters a target cell by binding to a specific cell-surface receptor; once the virus is internalized, its RNA is released from the nucleocapsid and is reverse-transcribed into proviral DNA. The provirus is inserted into the genome and then transcribed into RNA; the RNA is translated; and virions assemble and are extruded from the cell membrane by budding. *B.* Overview of retroviral gene expression. The provirus is transcribed, capped, and polyadenylated. Viral RNA molecules then have one of three fates: They are exported to the cytoplasm, where they are packaged as the viral RNA in infectious viral particles; they are spliced to form the message for the envelope polyprotein; or they are translated into Gag and Pol proteins. Most of the messages for the Pol protein fail to initiate Pol translation because of a stop codon before its initiation; however, in a fraction of the messages, the stop codon is missed and the Pol proteins are translated. *(Modified from JM Coffin, in BN Fields, DM Knipe (eds): Fields Virology. New York, Raven, 1990.)*

packaging sequences are located outside the LTR sequences. The coding regions include the *gag* (group-specific antigen, core protein), *pol* (RNA-dependent DNA polymerase), and *env* (envelope) genes. The *gag* gene encodes a precursor polyprotein that is cleaved to form three to five capsid proteins; a fraction of the Gag precursor proteins also contain a protease responsible for cleaving the Gag and Pol polyproteins. A Gag-Pol polyprotein gives rise to the protease that is responsible for cleaving the Gag-Pol polyprotein. The *pol* gene encodes three proteins: the reverse transcriptase, the integrase, and the protease. The reverse transcriptase functions to copy the viral RNA into the double-stranded DNA provirus, which can attach to the host cell DNA via the action of integrase. The protease functions to cleave the Gag-Pol polyprotein into smaller protein products. The *env* gene encodes the envelope glycoproteins: one protein that binds to specific surface receptors and determines what cell types can be infected and a smaller

transmembrane protein that anchors the complex to the envelope. The cartoon in Fig. 191-3 shows how the retroviral gene products make up the virus structure.

HTLVs have a region between *env* and the 3′ LTR that encodes at least two proteins in overlapping reading frames; Tax, a 40-kD protein that does not bind to DNA but induces the expression of host cell transcription factors that alter host cell gene expression; and Rex, a 27-kD protein that regulates the expression of viral mRNAs. These two proteins are produced from messages that are similar but that are spliced differently from overlapping but distinct exons.

The lentiviruses in general, and HIV-1 and -2 in particular, contain a larger genome than other pathogenic retroviruses. They contain an untranslated region between *pol* and *env* that encodes portions of several proteins, varying with the reading frame into which the mRNA is spliced. Tat is a 14-kD protein that augments the expression of virus from the LTR. The Rev protein of HIV-1, similar to the Rex protein of HTLV, regulates RNA splicing and/or RNA transport. The Nef protein downregulates CD4, the cellular receptor for HIV; alters host T cell activation pathways; and enhances viral infectivity. The Vif protein is necessary for the proper assembly of the HIV nucleoprotein core in many types of cells; without Vif, proviral DNA is not efficiently produced in these infected cells. Vpr, Vpu (HIV-1 only), and Vpx (HIV-2 only) are viral proteins encoded by translation of the same message in different reading frames. As noted above, oncogenic retroviruses depend on cell proliferation for their replication; lentiviruses can infect nondividing cells, largely owing to effects mediated by Vpr. Vpr facilitates transport of the provirus into the nucleus and can induce other cellular changes, such as G2 growth arrest and differentiation of some target cells. Vpx is structurally related to Vpr, but its functions are not fully defined. Vpu promotes the degradation of CD4 in the endoplasmic reticulum and stimulates the release of virions from infected cells.

Retroviruses can be either exogenously acquired by infection with a virion capable of replication or transmitted in the germ line as endogenous virus. Endogenous retroviruses are often replication-defective. The human genome contains endogenous retroviral sequences, but there are no known replication-competent endogenous retroviruses in humans.

In general, viruses that contain only the *gag*, *pol*, and *env* genes either are not pathogenic or take a long time to induce disease because the pathogenesis of neoplastic transformation relies on the chance integration of the provirus at a spot in the genome that will result in the expression of a cellular gene (proto-oncogene) that becomes transforming by virtue of its unregulated expression. For example, avian leukosis virus causes B cell leukemia by inducing the expression of *myc*. Some retroviruses possess captured and altered cellular genes near their integration site, and these viral oncogenes are capable of transforming the infected host cell. Viruses that have oncogenes often have lost a portion of their genome that is required for replication. Such viruses need helper viruses to reproduce, a feature that may explain why these acute transforming retroviruses are rare in nature. All human retroviruses identified to date are exogenous and are not acutely transforming (that is, they lack a transforming oncogene).

These remarkable properties of retroviruses have led to experimental efforts to use them as vectors to insert specific genes into particular cell types, a process known as *gene therapy* or *gene transfer*. The process could be used to repair a genetic defect or to introduce a new property that could be used therapeutically; for example, a gene (e.g., thymidine kinase) that would make a tumor cell susceptible to killing by a drug (e.g., ganciclovir) could be inserted. One source of concern about the use of retroviral vectors in humans is that replication-competent viruses might rescue endogenous retroviral replication, with unpredictable results. This concern is not merely hypothetical: The detection of proteins encoded by endogenous retroviral sequences on the surface of cancer cells implies that the genetic events leading to the cancer were able to activate the synthesis of these usually silent genes.

HUMAN T-CELL LYMPHOTROPIC VIRUS

HTLV-I was isolated in 1980 from a T-cell lymphoma cell line from a patient originally thought to have cutaneous T cell lymphoma. Later it became clear that the patient had a distinct form of lymphoma (originally reported in Japan) called *adult T cell leukemia/lymphoma* (ATL). Serologic data have determined that HTLV-I is the cause of at least two important diseases: ATL and tropical spastic paraparesis, also called *HTLV-I–associated myelopathy* (HAM). HTLV-I may also play a role in infective dermatitis and uveitis syndromes.

Two years after the isolation of HTLV-I, HTLV-II was isolated from a patient with an unusual form of hairy cell leukemia that affected T cells. Although early epidemiologic studies of HTLV-II failed to reveal a consistent disease association, more recent studies suggest an association of HTLV-II with human disease (see "Associated Diseases" under "Features of HTLV-II Infection," below), particularly among injection drug users.

FIGURE 191-2 Genomic structure of retroviruses. The murine leukemia virus MuLV has the typical three structural genes: *gag*, *pol*, and *env*. The *gag* region gives rise to three proteins: matrix (MA), capsid (CA), and nucleic acid–binding (NC) proteins. The *pol* region encodes both a protease (PR) responsible for cleaving the viral polyproteins and a reverse transcriptase (RT). In addition, HIV *pol* encodes an integrase (IN). The *env* region encodes a surface protein (SU) and a small transmembrane protein (TM). The human retroviruses have additional gene products translated in each of the three possible reading frames. HTLV-I and HTLV-II have *tax* and *rex* genes with exons on either side of the *env* gene. HIV-1 and HIV-2 have six accessory gene products: *tat*, *rev*, *vif*, *nef*, *vpr*, and either *vpu* (in HIV-1) or *vpx* (in HIV-2). The genes for these proteins are located mainly between the *pol* and *env* genes.

BIOLOGY AND MOLECULAR BIOLOGY

Because the biology of HTLV-I and that of HTLV-II are similar, the following discussion will focus on HTLV-I.

The cellular receptor for HTLV-I has not yet been identified, but it maps to chromosome 17. Generally, only T cells are productively infected, but infection of B cells and other cell types is occasionally detected. The most common outcome of HTLV-I infection is latent carriage of randomly integrated provirus in CD4+ T cells. HTLV-I does not contain an oncogene and does not insert into a unique site in the genome. Indeed, most infected cells express no viral gene products. The only viral gene product that is routinely expressed in tumor cells transformed by HTLV-I in vivo is *tax*, and even *tax* is not expressed in the tumor cells of many ATL patients. Cells transformed in vitro, by contrast, actively transcribe HTLV-I RNA and produce infectious virions. Most HTLV-I–transformed cell lines are the result of the infection of a normal host T cell in vitro. It is difficult to establish cell lines derived from authentic ATL cells.

Although *tax* does not itself bind to DNA, it does induce the expression of a wide range of host-cell gene products, including transcription factors (especially *c-rel*, *ets*-1 and -2, and members of the *fos/jun* family), cytokines [e.g., interleukin (IL) 2, granulocyte-macrophage colony-stimulating factor, and tumor necrosis factor (TNF)], and membrane proteins and receptors [major histocompatibility (MHC) molecules and IL-2 receptor α]. The genes activated by *tax* are generally controlled by transcription factors of the *c-rel* and cyclic AMP response element binding (CREB) protein families. It is unclear how this induction of host gene expression leads to neoplastic transformation. Induction of a cytokine-autocrine loop has been proposed; however, IL-2 is not the crucial cytokine. The involvement of IL-4, IL-7, and IL-15 has been proposed.

In light of the irregular expression of *tax* in ATL cells, it has been suggested that *tax* is important in the early phases of transformation but is not essential for the maintenance of the transformed state. As is clear from the epidemiology of HTLV-I infection, transformation of an infected cell is a rare event and may depend on heterogeneous second, third, or fourth genetic hits. No consistent chromosomal abnormalities have been described in ATL; however, individual cases with *p53* mutations and translocations involving the T cell receptor genes on chromosome 14 have been reported. *Tax* may repress certain DNA repair enzymes, permitting the accumulation of genetic damage that would normally be repaired. However, the molecular pathogenesis of HTLV-I–induced neoplasia is not fully understood.

FEATURES OF HTLV-I INFECTION   Epidemiology

HTLV-I infection is transmitted in at least three ways: from mother to child, especially in breast milk; through sexual activity, more com-

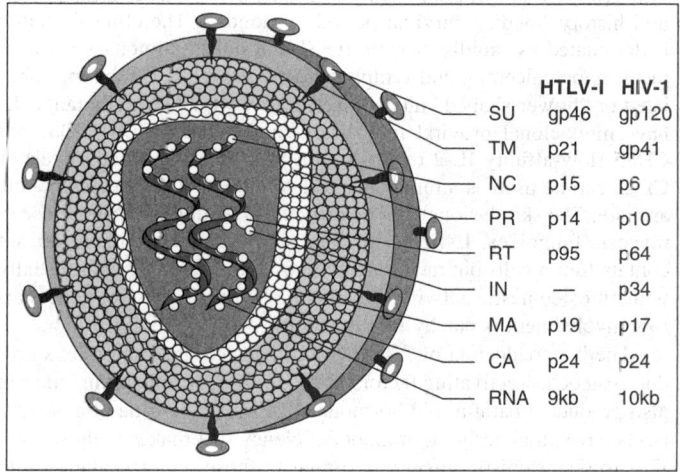

	HTLV-I	HIV-1
SU	gp46	gp120
TM	p21	gp41
NC	p15	p6
PR	p14	p10
RT	p95	p64
IN	—	p34
MA	p19	p17
CA	p24	p24
RNA	9kb	10kb

FIGURE 191-3 Schematic structure of human retroviruses. The surface glycoprotein (SU) is responsible for binding to receptors of host cells. The transmembrane protein (TM) anchors SU to the virus. NC is a nucleic acid–binding protein found in association with the viral RNA. A protease (PR) cleaves the polyproteins encoded by the *gag*, *pol*, and *env* genes into their functional components. RT is reverse transcriptase, and IN is an integrase present in some retroviruses (e.g., HIV-1) that facilitates insertion of the provirus into the host genome. MA is a Gag protein closely associated with the lipid of the envelope. The capsid protein (CA) forms the major internal structure of the virus, the core shell.

monly from men to women; and through the blood—via contaminated transfusions or contaminated needles. The virus is most commonly transmitted perinatally. Compared with HIV, which can be transmitted in cell-free form, HTLV-I is less infectious, and its transmission usually requires cell-to-cell contact.

HTLV-I is endemic in southwestern Japan and Okinawa, where more than 1 million persons are infected. Antibodies to HTLV-I are present in the serum of up to 35% of Okinawans, 10% of residents of the Japanese island of Kyushu, and <1% of persons in nonendemic regions of Japan. Despite this high prevalence of infection, only about 500 cases of ATL are diagnosed in this area each year. Clusters of infection have been noted in other areas of the Orient, such as Taiwan; in the Caribbean basin, including northeastern South America; in central Africa; in Italy; in Israel; in the Arctic; and in the southeastern part of the United States.

A progressive spastic or ataxic myelopathy that develops in an individual who is HTLV-I positive (i.e., who has serum antibodies to HTLV-I) is likely to be due to direct nervous system infection with the virus; a similar disorder may result from infection with HIV or HTLV-II. In rare instances, patients with HAM are seronegative but have detectable antibody to HTLV-I in the cerebrospinal fluid (CSF).

The cumulative lifetime risk of developing ATL is 2% among HTLV-I–infected patients; a similar risk is projected for HAM. The distribution of the two diseases overlaps the distribution of HTLV-I, with >95% of affected patients showing serologic evidence of HTLV-I infection. The latent period between infection and the emergence of disease is 20 to 30 years for ATL. For HAM, the median latency period is about 3.3 years (range, 4 months to 30 years). The development of ATL is rare among persons infected by blood products; however, ~20% of patients with HAM acquire HTLV-I from contaminated blood.

Associated Diseases • *ATL*   Four clinical types of HTLV-I–induced neoplasia have been described: acute, lymphomatous, chronic, and smoldering. All of these tumors are monoclonal proliferations of CD4+ post-thymic T cells with clonal proviral integrations and clonal T-cell receptor gene rearrangements.

About 60% of patients who develop malignancy have classic *acute* ATL, which is characterized by a short clinical prodrome (~2 weeks between the first symptoms and the diagnosis) and an aggressive natural history (median survival period, 6 months). The clinical picture is dominated by rapidly progressive skin lesions, pulmonary involvement, hypercalcemia, and lymphocytosis with cells containing lobulated or "flower-shaped" nuclei (**see Plate V-40**). The malignant cells have monoclonal proviral integrations and express CD4, CD3, and CD25 (low-affinity IL-2 receptors) on their surface. Serum levels of CD25 can be used as a tumor marker. Anemia and thrombocytopenia are rare. The skin lesions may be difficult to distinguish from those in mycosis fungoides. Lytic bone lesions, which are common, do not contain tumor cells but rather are composed of osteolytic cells, usually without osteoblastic activity. Despite the leukemic picture, bone marrow involvement is patchy in most cases.

The hypercalcemia of ATL is multifactorial; the tumor cells produce osteoclast-activating factors (TNF-α, IL-1, lymphotoxin) and can also produce a parathyroid hormone–like molecule. The affected patients have an underlying immunodeficiency that makes them susceptible to opportunistic infections similar to those seen in patients with AIDS (Chap. 309). The pathogenesis of the immunodeficiency is unclear. Pulmonary infiltrates in ATL patients reflect leukemic infiltration half the time and opportunistic infections with organisms such as *Pneumocystis carinii* and other fungi the other half. Gastrointestinal symptoms are nearly always related to opportunistic infection. Serum concentrations of lactate dehydrogenase (LDH) and alkaline phosphatase are often elevated. About 10% of patients have leptomeningeal involvement leading to weakness, altered mental status, paresthesia, and/or headache. Unlike other forms of central nervous system (CNS) lymphoma, ATL may be accompanied by normal CSF protein levels. The diagnosis depends on finding ATL cells in the CSF (Chap. 112).

The *lymphomatous* type of ATL occurs in ~20% of patients and is similar to the acute form in its natural history and clinical course, except that circulating abnormal cells are rare and lymphadenopathy is evident. The histology of the lymphoma is variable but does not influence the natural history. In general, the diagnosis is suspected on the basis of the patient's birthplace and the presence of skin lesions and hypercalcemia. The diagnosis is confirmed by the detection of antibodies to HTLV-I in serum.

Patients with the *chronic* form of ATL generally have normal serum levels of calcium and LDH and no involvement of the CNS, bone, or gastrointestinal tract. The median duration of survival for these patients is 2 years. In some cases, chronic ATL progresses to the acute form of the disease.

Fewer than 5% of patients have the *smoldering* form of ATL. In this form, the malignant cells have monoclonal proviral integration; <5% of peripheral-blood cells exhibit typical morphologic abnormalities; hypercalcemia, adenopathy, and hepatosplenomegaly do not develop; the CNS, the bones, and the gastrointestinal tract are not involved; and skin and pulmonary lesions may be present. The median survival period of this small subset of patients appears to be ≥5 years.

HAM (tropical spastic paraparesis)   In contrast to ATL, in which there is a slight predominance of male patients, HAM affects females disproportionately. HAM resembles multiple sclerosis in certain ways (Chap. 371). The onset is insidious. Symptoms include weakness or stiffness in one or both legs, back pain, and urinary incontinence. Sensory changes are usually mild, but peripheral neuropathy may develop. The disease generally takes the form of slowly progressive and unremitting thoracic myelopathy; one-third of patients are bedridden within 10 years of diagnosis, and one-half are unable to walk unassisted by this point. Patients display spastic paraparesis or paraplegia with hyperreflexia, ankle clonus, and extensor plantar responses. Cognitive function is usually spared; cranial nerve abnormalities are unusual.

Magnetic resonance imaging (MRI) reveals lesions in both the white matter and the paraventricular regions of the brain as well as in the spinal cord. Pathologic examination of the spinal cord shows symmetric degeneration of the lateral columns, including the corticospinal tracts; some cases involve the posterior columns as well. The spinal meninges and cord parenchyma contain an inflammatory infiltrate with myelin destruction.

HTLV-I is not usually found in cells of the CNS but may be detected in a small population of lymphocytes present in the CSF. In general, HTLV-I replication is greater in HAM than in ATL, and patients with HAM have a stronger immune response to the virus. Antibodies to HTLV-I are present in the serum and appear to be produced in the CSF of HAM patients, where titers are often higher than in the serum. The pathophysiology of HAM may involve the induction of autoimmune destruction of neural cells by T cells with specificity for viral components such as Tax or Env proteins. One theory is that susceptibility to HAM may be related to the presence of human leukocyte antigen (HLA) alleles capable of presenting viral antigens in a fashion that leads to autoimmunity. Insufficient data are available to confirm an HLA association.

Other putative HTLV-I–related diseases   In areas where HTLV-I is endemic, diverse inflammatory and autoimmune diseases have been attributed to the virus, including uveitis, dermatitis, pneumonitis, rheumatoid arthritis, and polymyositis. However, a causal relationship between HTLV-I and these illnesses has not been rigorously established.

Prevention   Women in endemic areas should not breast-feed their children, and blood donors should be screened for serum antibodies to HTLV-I. As in the prevention of HIV infection, the practice of safe sex and the avoidance of needle sharing are important.

℞   **TREATMENT**   For the small number of patients who develop HTLV-I–related disease, therapies are not curative. In patients with the acute and lymphomatous types of ATL, the disease progresses rapidly. Hypercalcemia is generally controlled by glucocorticoid administration and cytotoxic therapy directed against the neoplasm. The tumor is highly responsive to combination chemotherapy that is employed against other forms of lymphoma; however, patients are susceptible to overwhelming bacterial and opportunistic infections, and ATL relapses within 4 to 10 months after remission in most patients. The combination of interferon α and zidovudine may extend survival. Because viral replication is not clearly associated with ATL progression, zidovudine is probably effective through its cytotoxic effects (as a chain-terminating thymidine analogue) rather than its antiviral effects. An experimental approach using an yttrium 90–labeled antibody to the IL-2 receptor appears promising but is not widely available. Patients with the chronic or smoldering form of ATL may be managed with an expectant approach: Treat any infections, and watch and wait for signs of progression to acute disease.

Patients with HAM may obtain some benefit from the use of glucocorticoids to reduce inflammation. Antiretroviral regimens have not been effective. In one study, danazol (200 mg tid) produced significant neurologic improvement in five of six treated patients, with resolution of urinary incontinence in two cases, decreased spasticity in three, and the restoration of the ability to walk after confinement to a wheelchair in two. Physical therapy and rehabilitation are important components of management.

FEATURES OF HTLV-II INFECTION   Epidemiology
HTLV-II is endemic in certain Native American tribes. It is generally considered to be a New World virus that was brought from Asia to the Americas 10,000 to 40,000 years ago during the migration of infected populations across the Bering land bridge.

The mode of transmission of HTLV-II is probably the same as that of HTLV-I (see above). HTLV-II may be less readily transmitted sexually than HTLV-I.

Studies of large cohorts of injection drug users with serologic assays that reliably distinguish HTLV-I from HTLV-II indicate that the vast majority of HTLV-positive subjects are infected with HTLV-II. The seroprevalence of HTLV in a cohort of 7841 injection drug users from drug treatment centers in Baltimore, Chicago, Los Angeles, New Jersey (Asbury Park and Trenton), New York City (Brooklyn and Harlem), Philadelphia, and San Antonio was 20.9%, with >97% of cases due to HTLV-II. The seroprevalence of HTLV-II was higher in the Southwest and the Midwest than in the Northeast. In contrast, the seroprevalence of HIV-1 was higher in the Northeast than in the Southwest or the Midwest. Approximately 3% of the cohort members were infected with both HTLV-II and HIV-1. The seroprevalence of HTLV-II increased linearly with age. Women were significantly more likely to be infected with HTLV-II than were men; the virus is thought to be more efficiently transmitted from male to female than from female to male.

Associated Diseases   Although HTLV-II was isolated from a patient with a T cell variant of hairy cell leukemia, this virus has not been consistently associated with a particular disease and in fact has been thought of as "a virus searching for a disease." However, evidence is accumulating that HTLV-II may play a role in certain neurologic, hematologic, and dermatologic diseases. These data require confirmation, particularly in light of the previous confusion regarding the relative prevalences of HTLV-I and HTLV-II among injection drug users.

Prevention   Avoidance of needle sharing, safe-sex practices, screening of blood (by assays for HTLV-I, which also detect HTLV-II), and avoidance of breast-feeding by infected women are important principles in the prevention of spread of HTLV-II.

HUMAN IMMUNODEFICIENCY VIRUS

HIV-1 and HIV-2 are members of the lentivirus subfamily of Retroviridae and are the only lentiviruses known to infect humans. The lentiviruses are slow-acting by comparison with viruses that cause acute infection (e.g., influenza virus) but not by comparison with other retroviruses. The features of acute primary infection with HIV resemble those of more classic acute infections. The characteristic chronicity

of HIV disease is consistent with the designation *lentivirus*. →*For a detailed discussion of HIV, see Chap. 309.*

BIBLIOGRAPHY

BLATTNER WA: Human retroviruses: Their role in cancer. Proc Assoc Am Physicians 111:563, 1999

DECOCK KM et al: Prevention of mother-to-child HIV transmission in resource-poor countries: Translating research into policy and practice. JAMA 283:1175, 2000

FAUCI AS: The AIDS epidemic—considerations for the 21st century. N Engl J Med 341: 1046, 1999

HARRINGTON WJ JR et al: Tropical spastic paraparesis/HTLV-I-associated myelopathy (TSP/HAM): Treatment with an anabolic steroid danazol. AIDS Res Hum Retroviruses 7:1031, 1991

HOLLSBERG P, HAFLER DA: Pathogenesis of diseases induced by human lymphotropic virus type I infection. N Engl J Med 328:1173, 1993

MURPHY RL (Chairman): Critical issues surrounding treatment in the era of active antiretroviral therapeutics: Proceedings of a Northwestern University Medical School Conference. Clin Infect Dis 30(Suppl 2):S95–197, 2000

NEUVEUT C, JEANG KT: HTLV-I Tax and cell cycle progression. Prog Cell Cycle Res 4:157, 2000

POIESZ BJ et al: Detection and isolation of type C retrovirus particles from fresh and cultured lymphocytes of a patient with cutaneous T-cell lymphoma. Proc Natl Acad Sci USA 77:7415, 1980

TOBINAI K: Adult T-cell leukemia, in *Clinical Oncology*, 2d ed, MD Abeloff et al (eds). New York, Churchill-Livingstone, 2000, p 2748

TRONO D: HIV accessory proteins: Leading roles for the supporting cast. Cell 82:189, 1995

YAO J, WIGDAHL B: Human T-cell lymphotropic virus type I genomic expression and impact on intracellular signaling pathways during neurodegenerative disease and leukemia. Front Biosci 5:D138, 2000

192   Harry B. Greenberg

VIRAL GASTROENTERITIS

In less developed countries, acute infectious diarrheal disease is a leading cause of morbidity in all age groups and of mortality in infants and young children. In developed countries, acute diarrheal illness remains an important cause of morbidity among both children and adults. Two distinct groups of viruses—the rotaviruses and the enteric caliciviruses, such as Norwalk virus—as well as a variety of bacterial pathogens (Chap. 131) have emerged as important etiologic agents of gastroenteritis. The rotaviruses are primarily pathogens of young children. The Norwalk and related enteric caliciviruses affect adults as well as children. Several important gastrointestinal viruses are characterized in Table 192-1 and depicted in Fig. 192-1.

ROTAVIRUS   Classification and Characterization   Rotaviruses are members of the Reoviridae family. The rotavirus virion consists of a 100-nm triple-shelled icosahedral capsid surrounding a genome composed of 11 segments of double-stranded RNA. Several genetically distinct groups of rotaviruses (groups A, B, C, etc.) have been identified, but group A strains account for the great majority of illnesses in humans. With only one exception, the rotavirus gene segments are monocistronic. The virus has two surface proteins (VP4 and VP7), both of which are involved in viral neutralization. The major internal capsid protein (VP6) is the target of cross-reactive antibody to different virus strains. This protein also appears to induce protective immunity, although the mechanism is not clear. Because rotaviruses have a segmented genome, they are capable of undergoing gene reassortment at high frequency. The role of gene reassortment in generating rotavirus antigenic diversity is not known. In immunocompetent humans and animals, rotavirus infection is characterized by replication that is localized almost exclusively in the epithelial cells of the small intestine.

Epidemiology   Rotavirus infection occurs worldwide. By the age of 3 years, virtually every individual has been infected by rotaviruses

Table 192-1 Characteristics of Several Gastrointestinal Viruses

Virus Type	Genome Structure	Major Risk Groups	Seasonality	Diagnostic Tests[a]	Treatment
Rotavirus (group A)	Double-stranded segmented RNA	Children <3 years	Winter	ELISA	1. Oral rehydration 2. Vaccination
Adenovirus (types 40, 41)	Double-stranded DNA	Children <3 years	Year-round	ELISA	Oral rehydration
Caliciviruses (genogroup III, SLVs)	Plus-sense single-stranded RNA	Young children	Unknown	Experimental and EM	Oral rehydration
Astrovirus	Plus-sense single-stranded RNA	Young children ?Immunocompromised individuals	Winter	Experimental and EM	Oral rehydration
Norwalk-like viruses (genogroups I, II)	Plus-sense single-stranded RNA	Children and adults, epidemics	Winter	Experimental and EM	Oral rehydration
Parvovirus[b]	Single-stranded DNA	No enteric disease	Year-round	EM	None needed
Picornavirus[c] (enterovirus)	Plus-sense single-stranded RNA	Usually no enteric disease	Depends on strain	Culture and EM	None needed
Coronavirus	Plus-sense single-stranded RNA, enveloped	Unknown, no well-characterized enteric disease	Unknown	EM	None

[a] ELISA, enzyme-linked immunosorbent assay; EM, electron microscopy.
[b] See also Chap. 187.
[c] See also Chap. 193.

at least once. Most rotavirus infections are subclinical or cause mild gastrointestinal illnesses that do not require hospitalization. The first infection is the most likely to be symptomatic; subsequent infections are often mild or asymptomatic. In areas with a temperate climate, rotavirus infection is seasonal, occurring in the colder winter months. In the United States, the annual seasonal rotavirus epidemic tends to spread from west to east, starting in California and ending in New England. In tropical areas, rotavirus infection tends to occur throughout the year, with some increase in incidence during the cooler rainy season.

Rotaviruses are the single most important cause of severe dehydrating diarrhea in infants and children <3 years old in both developed and less developed countries; they account for 25 to 50% of all cases of diarrhea requiring hospitalization or intensive rehydration therapy. During a rotavirus outbreak in a temperate climate, this percentage can be as high as 80%. In the United States, between 5 and 10% of all diarrheal episodes among children under the age of 5 years are caused by rotavirus. Infection due to rotavirus accounts for ~500,000 physician visits per year in the United States. Although severe rotavirus infections are confined primarily to infants and young children, these agents are frequently associated with mild diarrhea in adults, particularly family members of affected infants, geriatric patients, and immunocompromised hosts. They are responsible for up to 10% of cases of traveler's diarrhea (Chap. 131). Rotaviruses also may cause occasional cases of acute and chronic diarrhea in patients with AIDS.

Rotavirus serotypes have been defined by the antigenicity of both VP4 (P serotype) and VP7 (G serotype). At least 14 distinct G serotypes of rotavirus have been described, but only four types are commonly encountered in the United States. At least 20 P serotypes have been identified to date, of which only two are common among children in this country. The relationship of the frequency of infection with these multiple serotypes to host immune status is unclear. It does appear, however, that infection with one or two serotypes induces some degree of heterotypic immunity to severe disease.

A large variety of mammalian and avian species can be infected by rotavirus, but these animal rotavirus strains do not frequently cause disease in humans. Rotaviruses are shed in very large numbers in the stool (up to 10^{10} particles per gram of feces). Although transmission presumably takes place via the fecal-oral route, rotavirus infection spreads with great efficacy in developed as well as less developed countries.

Pathophysiology Rotavirus infects and kills the mature villus tip cells of the small intestine. The mature epithelial cells are replaced by immature absorptive cells that cannot absorb carbohydrates or other nutrients efficiently. Rotavirus infection thus leads to osmotic diarrhea due to nutrient malabsorption. Changes in intracellular cyclic adenosine monophosphate or guanosine monophosphate are not involved in the etiology of rotavirus diarrhea. Rotavirus also encodes a nonstructural protein (NSP4) that appears to function as an enterotoxin during infection. It is not known whether immunity to NSP4 plays a role in protection or disease resolution.

Manifestations The manifestations of rotavirus infection range from subclinical infection through mild diarrhea to severe, occasionally fatal dehydrating illness. Most information concerning the signs and symptoms of rotavirus infection has been derived from studies of hospitalized young children. The onset of illness is usually abrupt. More than 80% of affected children develop vomiting followed by diarrhea. About one-third of hospitalized children have a temperature of >39°C (>102.2°F). Mucus is commonly found in the stool, but white and red blood cells are present in the stool in fewer than 15% of cases.

Rotavirus infection frequently occurs in conjunction with respiratory tract symptoms, but there is little evidence to indicate that rotavirus replicates in the respiratory tract. Rotavirus infection has been observed in association with a wide variety of other clinical syndromes, including sudden infant death syndrome, Reye's syndrome, encephalitis, aseptic meningitis, pneumonia, exanthema subitum, Kawasaki's syndrome, necrotizing enterocolitis, intussusception, Schönlein-Henoch purpura, hemolytic-uremic syndrome, disseminated intravascular coagulation, and Crohn's disease. The etiologic relationship between these clinical syndromes and rotavirus infection is probably coincidental rather than causal. Rotavirus infection may be especially severe or even fatal in immunocompromised children.

Clinical Immunity Relative immunity to rotavirus illness is acquired early in childhood, after one or two natural infections. Subclinical infections in neonates have been shown to protect these children against severe rotavirus gastroenteritis for up to 3 years. Immunity is not complete, and adults with low levels of antibody can be symptomatically infected. Local humoral immunity appears to be the critical determinant in protection, and cellular immune mechanisms seem to be involved as well.

Diagnosis Because rotavirus is shed in large amounts in the stool, detection is relatively easy. Various specific and highly sensitive commercial immunoassays are available to detect rotavirus antigen in fecal specimens. DNA probe diagnosis appears to be sensitive and specific, as do polymerase chain reaction (PCR)–based assays, but these detection methods have been used primarily for research purposes. No particular signs or symptoms are pathognomonic for rotavirus infection, but this infection is more frequently associated with severe dehydration than are infections caused by other enteric bacterial or viral pathogens.

℞ **TREATMENT** Although rotavirus diarrhea appears to be caused primarily by intestinal epithelial-cell lysis and death, it can be adequately managed with standard oral rehydration therapy. Only rarely is intravenous rehydration required. Since rotavirus infections have persisted in developed countries with advanced sanitation facilities and widely available clean water, it is unlikely that these infections will prove to be preventable by hygienic measures alone. Progress with a number of candidate live attenuated vaccines suggests that prevention through vaccination may be feasible. In 1998, a multivalent rotavirus vaccine was licensed for use in children under the age of 6 months in the United States. The vaccine virus was a live attenuated animal rotavirus containing genes encoding the four human G serotypes most common in the United States. The licensed vaccine was administered orally as three doses and was highly effective in preventing severe rotavirus illness. Reports of intussusception associated with the administration of rotavirus vaccine have been published; further studies are required to define the relative risk. However, because of the apparent association with intussusception, this first rotavirus vaccine has been withdrawn from use.

NORWALK AND RELATED ENTERIC CALICIVIRUSES Classification and Characterization Various round 27- to 32-nm particles, some with clearly defined ultrastructure, have been identified in the stools of individuals with acute nonbacterial gastroenteritis. In the past, these agents have been difficult to classify because they are shed in the stool in small amounts for only a few days and have not been adapted to cell culture or to animal models. The Norwalk virus is the most extensively studied and best-characterized member of this group of enteric caliciviruses, which also in-

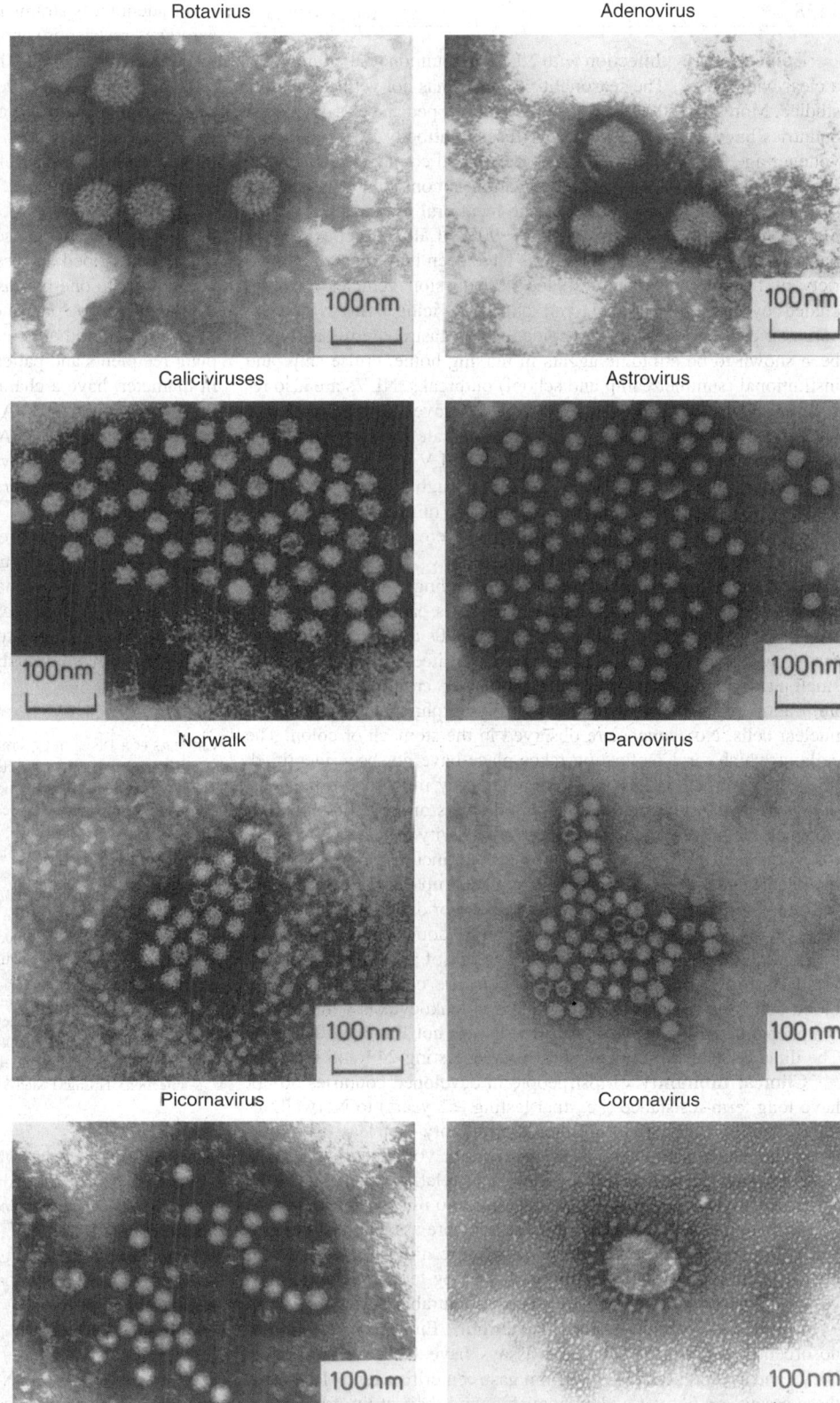

FIGURE 192-1 Electron micrographs of selected viruses found in the intestine. *(From S Monroe et al: J Med Virol 33:193, 1991, with permission.)*

cludes such serologically or genetically distinct viruses as Hawaii virus, Snow Mountain virus, Southampton virus, Lordsdale virus, Mexico virus, Sapporo virus, and a number of agents described as calicivirus-like. Molecular biologic studies have shown that all these viruses have a protein structure similar to that of typical caliciviruses, with a single structural protein of ~60 kDa. The genomes of Norwalk virus and numerous related viruses have been cloned and sequenced.

The genomes are plus-stranded RNA molecules of ~7.5 kb. On the basis of these molecular biologic studies, the human enteric caliciviruses can be divided into two groups: the Norwalk-like viruses (NLVs) and the Sapporo-like viruses (SLVs). The SLVs have a more typical calicivirus-like ultrastructure and cause diarrhea in young children. Unlike the NLVs, the SLVs may not cause frequent epidemics in adults.

Epidemiology Infection with NLVs is common year-round, with a clear winter peak. The seasonality of SLVs has not yet been widely studied. More than 80% of adults in both developed and less developed countries have antibodies to these viruses. Antibody is acquired at a younger age among children in less developed countries than among those in developed areas; this observation is consistent with the assumption that NLVs are spread by the fecal-oral route. In the United States, the NLVs are responsible for ~90% of all epidemics of non-bacterial gastroenteritis. These agents have been incriminated in a variety of food-borne epidemics, and transmission vehicles have included oysters, green salad, and chocolate icing. The NLVs are common causes of waterborne epidemics of gastroenteritis and have been shown to be etiologic agents in nursing home, cruise ship, and institutional (summer camp and school) outbreaks. NLVs are also responsible for a small proportion of cases of traveler's diarrhea. NLV infection is a common cause of mild to moderate childhood diarrhea.

In less developed countries, the role of NLV infection in the etiology of diarrhea in adults has not been thoroughly investigated. Preliminary studies indicate that NLVs can cause mild diarrhea in young children, but they do not appear to cause severe illness in infants in either developed or less developed countries.

Pathophysiology Information concerning the pathologic changes induced by the enteric caliciviruses is based almost entirely on a few studies of volunteers during the 1970s and 1980s. After infection with Norwalk or Hawaii virus, the architecture of the proximal small intestine is altered, with villus shortening, crypt hyperplasia, and infiltration of the lamina propria by polymorphonuclear and mononuclear cells. No changes are observed in the stomach or colon. The cells in which viral replication takes place have not been identified. The histologic alterations are accompanied by mild steatorrhea, carbohydrate malabsorption, and decreased levels of some brush border enzymes. No changes in adenylate cyclase activity have been observed.

Manifestations Norwalk illness has an incubation period of 18 to 72 h. The disease is characterized by the abrupt onset of nausea and abdominal cramps followed by vomiting and/or diarrhea. Vomiting is reported more frequently for children than for adults. Low-grade fever [>37.5° C (>99.5° F)] develops in about half of affected individuals. Headache, myalgias, and abdominal pain are common. The white blood cell count is normal; rarely, there is leukocytosis with relative lymphopenia. Red and white blood cells are not found in the stool. The illness is usually mild and self-limited, lasting 24 to 48 h.

Clinical Immunity Most people in developed countries do not have long-term resistance (i.e., that lasting ≥2 years) to Norwalk reinfection. Short-term (several-month) immunity—at least to homotypic challenge—does appear to develop. In volunteers challenged with Norwalk agent, there is a paradoxical relationship between the level of antibody to NLVs and susceptibility to illness: Low levels of Norwalk antibody in the serum and intestine are associated with clinical resistance to illness. It appears, therefore, that immune mechanisms are not the primary determinants of long-term protection from NLVs. Immunity to the SLVs may be more durable.

Diagnosis, Treatment, and Prevention Enzyme-linked immunosorbent assays and PCR-based assays have been developed for NLVs and several other 27- to 32-nm gastroenteritis agents. However, these assays are not yet widely available, and their utility for general diagnosis has not been tested. Because Norwalk illness is acute and self-limited, treatment is not usually required. In the rare case of severe vomiting or diarrhea, oral or intravenous rehydration is indicated. Because long-term immunity to the NLVs does not usually follow natural infection, the role of vaccination may be limited to specific settings (e.g., the military). Recombinant NLV particles have been produced and are capable of inducing an immune response when administered orally to volunteers.

MISCELLANEOUS ENTERIC VIRAL PATHOGENS
Enteric adenoviruses are a minor cause of diarrheal illness in infants and children, accounting for 10% of cases. These viruses differ from other adenovirus strains in a variety of ways, including neutralization serotype, restriction endonuclease digestion pattern, and ability to grow in tissue culture. The role of enteric adenovirus illness in adults or in persons in less developed countries is not known.

Several strains of antigenically distinct rotaviruses, presently called *atypical rotaviruses* or *groups B and C rotaviruses*, have been identified as the cause of occasional episodes of diarrhea in humans and animals.

Preliminary epidemiologic studies have indicated that *astroviruses* are a fairly frequent cause of mild to moderate diarrhea in young children in developed and less developed countries, accounting for about one-quarter to one-half as much illness as group A rotaviruses. Moreover, preliminary data indicate that astroviruses are a common cause of diarrhea in immunocompromised hosts, such as bone marrow transplant recipients and patients with AIDS. Astroviruses are 27 to 32 nm in diameter, have a characteristic icosahedral ultrastructure, and contain a plus-stranded RNA genome with a size of ~7.0 kb and a unique genomic organization. At least seven distinct serotypes have been identified. The current availability of sensitive and specific diagnostic assays should allow more complete assessment of the importance of these agents.

Coronaviruses are frequent causes of diarrheal disease in a variety of animals. Using electron microscopy, several investigators have identified putative coronavirus-like particles in the stools of patients with diarrhea. In most cases, however, these particles do not have the typical morphologic features of coronaviruses and may represent bacterial breakdown products or cellular fragments.

BIBLIOGRAPHY

CENTERS FOR DISEASE CONTROL AND PREVENTION: Intussusception among recipients of rotavirus vaccine—United States, 1998–1999. MMWR 48:577, 1999

JIANG X et al: Sequence and genomic organization of Norwalk virus. Virology 195:51, 1993

JOENSUU J et al: Prolonged efficacy of rhesus-human reassortant rotavirus vaccine. Pediatr Infect Dis J 17:427, 1998

NOEL JS et al: Identification of a distinct common strain of "Norwalk-like viruses" having a global distribution. J Infect Dis 179:1334, 1999

PANG XL et al: Human calicivirus-associated sporadic gastroenteritis in Finnish children less than two years of age followed prospectively during a rotavirus vaccine trial. Pediatr Infect Dis J 18:420, 1999

PARASHAR UD et al: Hospitalizations associated with rotavirus diarrhea in the United States, 1993 through 1995: Surveillance based on the new ICD-9-CM rotavirus specific diagnostic code. J Infect Dis 177:13, 1998

PÉREZ-SCHAEL I et al: Efficacy of the rhesus rotavirus-based quadrivalent vaccine in infants and young children in Venezuela. N Engl J Med 337:1181, 1997

VELAZQUEZ FR et al: Rotavirus infection in infants as protection against subsequent infections. N Engl J Med 335:1022, 1996

193 *Jeffrey I. Cohen*

ENTEROVIRUSES AND REOVIRUSES

ENTEROVIRUSES

CLASSIFICATION AND CHARACTERIZATION Enteroviruses are so named because of their ability to multiply in the gastrointestinal tract. Despite their name, these viruses are not a prominent cause of gastroenteritis. Enteroviruses encompass 64 human serotypes: 3 serotypes of poliovirus, 23 serotypes of coxsackievirus A, 6 serotypes of coxsackievirus B, 28 serotypes of echovirus, and enteroviruses 68 through 71.

Human enteroviruses contain a single-stranded RNA genome surrounded by an icosahedral capsid comprising four viral proteins. These viruses have no lipid envelope and are stable in acidic environments, including the stomach. They are resistant to inactivation by standard disinfectants (e.g., alcohol, detergents) and can persist for days at room temperature.

Much of what is known about the pathogenesis of enteroviruses has been derived from studies of poliovirus infection. After ingestion, poliovirus is thought to infect epithelial cells in the mucosa of the gastrointestinal tract and then to spread to and replicate in the submucosal lymphoid tissue of the tonsils and Peyer's patches. The virus next spreads to the regional lymph nodes, a viremic phase ensues, and the virus replicates in organs of the reticuloendothelial system. In some cases, a second viremia occurs and the virus replicates further in various tissues, sometimes causing symptomatic disease.

It is uncertain whether poliovirus reaches the central nervous system (CNS) during viremia or whether it also spreads via peripheral nerves. Since viremia precedes the onset of neurologic disease in humans and in experimentally infected chimpanzees, it has been assumed that the virus enters the CNS via the bloodstream. The poliovirus receptor is a member of the immunoglobulin superfamily. Poliovirus infection is limited to primates, largely because of the ability of their cells to express the viral receptor. Studies demonstrating the poliovirus receptor in the end-plate region of muscle at the neuromuscular junction suggest that if the virus enters the muscle during viremia, it could travel across the neuromuscular junction up the axon to the anterior horn cells. Studies of monkeys or transgenic mice expressing the poliovirus receptor show that, after intramuscular injection, poliovirus does not reach the spinal cord if the sciatic nerve is cut. Taken together, these findings suggest that poliovirus can spread directly from muscle to the CNS by neural pathways. The receptor for echovirus types 1 and 8 is VLA-2 integrin, that for echovirus 7 is CD55, and that for coxsackievirus B is CAR (also used by adenovirus).

Poliovirus can usually be cultured from the blood 3 to 5 days after infection, before the development of neutralizing antibodies. While viral replication at secondary sites begins to slow 1 week after infection, it continues in the gastrointestinal tract. Poliovirus is shed from the oropharynx for up to 3 weeks after infection and from the gastrointestinal tract for as long as 12 weeks; immunodeficient patients can shed poliovirus for more than 1 year. During replication in the gastrointestinal tract, attenuated oral poliovirus can mutate, reverting to a more neurovirulent phenotype within a few days. The clinical significance of this increased neurovirulence is unknown.

Humoral and secretory immunity in the gastrointestinal tract is important for the control of enterovirus infections. Enteroviruses induce specific IgM, which usually persists for < 6 months, and specific IgG, which persists for life. Capsid protein VP1 is the predominant target of neutralizing antibody, which generally confers lifelong protection against subsequent disease caused by the same serotype but does not prevent infection or virus shedding. Enteroviruses also induce cellular immunity, but the importance of this mechanism in limiting infection is uncertain. Patients with impaired cellular immunity are not known to develop unusually severe disease when infected with enteroviruses. In contrast, the severe infections in patients with agammaglobulinemia emphasize the importance of humoral immunity in controlling enterovirus infections. IgA antibodies are important in reducing poliovirus replication in and shedding from the gastrointestinal tract. Breast milk contains IgA specific for enteroviruses and can protect humans from infection.

EPIDEMIOLOGY Enteroviruses have a worldwide distribution. More than 50% of nonpoliovirus enterovirus infections and more than 90% of poliovirus infections are subclinical. When symptoms do develop, they are usually nonspecific and occur in conjunction with fever; only a minority of infections are associated with specific clinical syndromes. The incubation period for most enterovirus infections ranges from 2 to 14 days but usually is less than a week.

Enterovirus infection is more common in socioeconomically disadvantaged areas, especially in those where conditions are crowded and in tropical areas where hygiene is poor. Infection is most common among infants and young children; serious illness develops most often during the first few days of life and in older children and adults. In developing countries, where children are infected at an early age, poliovirus infection has less often been associated with paralysis; in

countries with better hygiene, older children and adults are more likely to be seronegative, become infected, and develop paralysis. Passively acquired maternal antibody reduces the risk of symptomatic infection in neonates. Young children are the most frequent shedders of enteroviruses and are usually the index cases in family outbreaks. In temperate climates, enterovirus infections occur most often in the summer and fall; no seasonal pattern is apparent in the tropics.

Most enteroviruses are transmitted primarily by the fecal-oral route from fecally contaminated fingers or inanimate objects. Patients are most infectious shortly before and after the onset of symptomatic disease, when virus is present in the stool and throat. The ingestion of virus-contaminated food or water can also cause disease. Certain enteroviruses (such as enterovirus 70, which causes acute hemorrhagic conjunctivitis) can be transmitted by direct inoculation from the fingers to the eye. Airborne transmission is important for some viruses that cause respiratory tract disease, such as coxsackievirus A21. Enteroviruses can be transmitted across the placenta from mother to fetus, causing severe disease in the newborn. The transmission of enteroviruses through blood transfusions or insect bites has not been documented. Nosocomial spread of coxsackievirus and echovirus has taken place in hospital nurseries.

DIAGNOSIS Isolation of enterovirus in cell culture is the most common procedure for the diagnosis of infection. While cultures of stool, nasopharyngeal, or throat samples from patients with enterovirus diseases are often positive, isolation of the virus from these sites does not prove that it is directly associated with disease because these sites are frequently colonized for weeks in patients with subclinical infections. Isolation of virus from the throat is more likely to be associated with disease than isolation from the stool since virus is shed for shorter periods from the throat. Cultures of cerebrospinal fluid (CSF), serum, fluid from body cavities, or tissues are positive less frequently, but a positive result is indicative of disease caused by enterovirus. In some cases the virus can be isolated only from the blood or only from the CSF; therefore, it is important to culture multiple sites. Cultures are more likely to be positive earlier than later in the course of infection. Most human enteroviruses can be detected within a week after inoculation of cell cultures. Cultures may be negative because of the presence of neutralizing antibody, lack of susceptibility of the cells used, or inappropriate handling of the specimen. Coxsackievirus A may require inoculation into special cell-culture lines or into suckling mice.

Identification of the serotype of an enterovirus is useful primarily for epidemiologic studies and, with a few exceptions, has little clinical utility. It is important to identify serious infections with enterovirus during epidemics and to distinguish the vaccine strain of poliovirus from the other enteroviruses in the throat or in the feces. Stool and throat samples for culture as well as acute- and convalescent-phase serum specimens should be obtained from all patients with suspected poliomyelitis. In the absence of a positive CSF culture, a positive culture of stool obtained within the first 2 weeks after the onset of symptoms is most often used to confirm the diagnosis of poliomyelitis. If poliovirus is isolated, it should be sent to the Centers for Disease Control and Prevention (CDC) in Atlanta for identification as either a wild-type or a vaccine virus.

The polymerase chain reaction (PCR) has been used to amplify viral nucleic acid from CSF, serum, urine, throat swabs, and tissues. A single pair of PCR primers can detect more than 92% of the serotypes that infect humans. With the proper controls, PCR of the CSF is highly sensitive ($\geq$95%) and specific (>80%) and is more rapid than culture. PCR of serum is also highly sensitive and specific in the diagnosis of disseminated disease. PCR may be particularly helpful for the diagnosis and follow-up of enterovirus disease in immunodeficient patients receiving immunoglobulin therapy, whose viral cultures may be negative. Antigen detection and hybridization of enterovirus sequences in human tissues with a specific probe are additional options, but these techniques are generally less sensitive than PCR.

Serologic diagnosis of enterovirus infection is limited by the large number of serotypes and the lack of a common antigen. Demonstration of seroconversion may be useful in rare cases for confirmation of culture results, but serologic testing is usually limited to epidemiologic studies. Serum should be collected and frozen soon after the onset of disease and again about 4 weeks later. Measurement of neutralizing titers is the most accurate method for antibody determination; measurement of complement-fixation titers is usually less sensitive. Titers of virus-specific IgM are elevated in both acute and chronic infection.

℞ TREATMENT Most enterovirus infections are mild and resolve spontaneously; however, intensive supportive care may be needed for cardiac, hepatic, or CNS disease. Intravenous, intrathecal, or intraventricular immunoglobulin has been used with apparent success for the treatment of chronic enterovirus meningoencephalitis and dermatomyositis in patients with hypo- or agammaglobulinemia. The disease may stabilize or resolve during therapy; however, some patients decline inexorably despite therapy. Intravenous administration of immunoglobulin with high titers of antibody to the infecting virus has been successful in the treatment of some cases of life-threatening infection in neonates, who may not have maternally acquired antibody. In one trial involving neonates with enterovirus infections, immunoglobulin containing very high titers of antibody to the infecting virus reduced rates of viremia; however, the study was too small to show a substantial clinical benefit. Oral pleconaril, a capsid-binding antiviral agent, reduced symptoms in a placebo-controlled trial of enteroviral aseptic meningitis and in a challenge study with coxsackievirus. This drug is available for compassionate use in patients with certain severe enterovirus infections. Glucocorticoids are contraindicated.

Good hand-washing practices and the use of gowns and gloves are important in limiting nosocomial transmission of enteroviruses during epidemics. Enteric precautions are indicated for 7 days after the onset of enterovirus infections.

POLIOVIRUS Manifestations Most infections with poliovirus are asymptomatic. After an incubation period of 3 to 6 days, about 5% of patients present with a minor illness (abortive poliomyelitis) manifested by fever, malaise, sore throat, anorexia, myalgias, and headache. This condition usually resolves in 3 days. About 1% of patients present with aseptic meningitis (nonparalytic poliomyelitis). Examination of CSF reveals lymphocytic pleocytosis, a normal glucose level, and a normal or slightly elevated protein level; CSF polymorphonuclear leukocytes may be present early. In some patients, especially children, malaise and fever precede the onset of aseptic meningitis.

The least common presentation is that of paralytic disease. After one or several days, signs of aseptic meningitis are followed by severe back, neck, and muscle pain and by the rapid or gradual development of motor weakness. In some cases the disease appears to be biphasic, with aseptic meningitis followed first by apparent recovery but then (1 or 2 days later) by the return of fever and the development of paralysis; this form is more common among children than among adults. Weakness is generally asymmetric, is proximal more than distal, and may involve the legs (most commonly); the arms; or the abdominal, thoracic, or bulbar muscles. Paralysis develops during the febrile phase of the illness and usually does not progress after defervescence. Urinary retention may also occur. Examination reveals weakness, fasciculations, decreased muscle tone, and reduced or absent reflexes in affected areas. Transient hyperreflexia sometimes precedes the loss of reflexes. Patients frequently report sensory symptoms, but objective sensory testing usually yields normal results. Bulbar paralysis may lead to dysphagia, difficulty in handling secretions, or dysphonia. Respiratory insufficiency due to aspiration, involvement of the respiratory center in the medulla, or paralysis of the phrenic or intercostal nerves may develop, and severe medullary involvement may lead to circulatory collapse. Most patients with paralysis recover some function weeks to months after infection. About two-thirds of patients have residual neurologic sequelae.

Paralytic disease is more common among older individuals, pregnant women, and persons exercising strenuously or undergoing trauma at the time of CNS symptoms. Tonsillectomy predisposes to bulbar poliomyelitis, and intramuscular injections increase the risk of paralysis in the involved limb(s).

At present, the only cases of poliomyelitis in the United States are due to live poliovirus vaccine; of the four cases reported in the United States in 1997 and 1998, three occurred in recipients of the first or second dose of oral poliovirus vaccine (OPV), and one occurred in an adult contact of a recipient of OPV. The median interval from vaccination to the onset of symptoms is usually 3 weeks. About 5% of the cases of poliomyelitis associated with vaccine occur in members of the community who have had no known direct contact with vaccinees. About 15% of all cases of vaccine-associated poliomyelitis involve immunodeficient children or adults, most of whom have hypo- or agammaglobulinemia. In these patients the median interval between vaccination and the onset of symptoms is 6 weeks, but disease can develop up to 6 months after vaccination. The risk of developing poliomyelitis after oral vaccination is estimated at 1 case per 2.5 million doses administered. The risk of developing paralytic disease after oral vaccination is about 2000 times higher among immunodeficient patients than among immunocompetent children.

The *postpolio syndrome* presents as a new onset of weakness, fatigue, fasciculations, and pain with additional atrophy of the muscle group involved during the initial paralytic disease 20 to 40 years earlier. The syndrome is more common among women and with increasing time after acute disease. The onset is insidious, and weakness occasionally extends to muscles that were not involved during the initial illness. The prognosis is generally good; progression to further weakness is usually slow, with plateau periods that range from 1 to 10 years. The postpolio syndrome is thought to be due to progressive dysfunction and loss of motor neurons that compensated for the neurons lost during the original infection and not to persistent or reactivated poliovirus infection.

Prevention and Eradication (See also Chap. 122) After a peak of 57,879 cases of poliomyelitis in the United States in 1952, the introduction of inactivated vaccine in 1955 and of oral vaccine in 1961 ultimately eradicated disease due to wild-type poliovirus in the western hemisphere. Such disease has not been documented in the United States since 1979, when cases occurred among religious groups who had declined immunization. In the western hemisphere, paralysis due to wild-type poliovirus was last documented in 1991.

In 1988, the World Health Organization adopted a resolution to eradicate poliomyelitis by the year 2000. From 1988 to 1997, the number of cases worldwide decreased by 89%, with about 6227 cases reported from 46 countries in 1998. More than 80% of the world's cases of confirmed polio in 1998 occurred in India, Pakistan, Bangladesh, and Nigeria. Polio is a source of concern for unimmunized or partially immunized travelers to these regions. Outbreaks of polio in Europe and North America have been traced to cases imported from the Indian subcontinent. Clearly, global eradication of polio is necessary to eliminate the risk of importation of wild-type virus. Outbreaks are thought to have been facilitated by suboptimal rates of vaccination, isolated pockets of unvaccinated children, poor sanitation and crowding, improper vaccine-storage conditions, and a reduced level of response to one of the serotypes in the vaccine.

For the development of live OPV containing all three poliovirus serotypes, wild-type virus was attenuated by passage in monkey kidney cell cultures. OPV strains differ from the wild-type strains in a limited number of nucleotide changes (i.e., fewer than 60). Multiple doses are required to ensure infection and development of immunity to all three serotypes. While intramuscular injections of other vaccines (live or attenuated) can be given concurrently with OPV, unnecessary intramuscular injections should be avoided during the first month after vaccination because they increase the risk of vaccine-associated paralysis. Inactivated poliovirus vaccine is generated by formalin inac-

Table 193-1 Recommendations for Poliovirus Vaccination of Adults

1. Routine primary poliovirus vaccination is not indicated for unvaccinated adults residing in the United States, except for:
   a. travelers to areas where poliovirus is or may be epidemic or endemic;
   b. members of communities or population groups with disease caused by wild-type polioviruses;
   c. laboratory workers handling specimens that may contain wild-type polioviruses;
   d. health care workers in close contact with patients who may be excreting wild-type polioviruses;
   e. persons whose children will be receiving OPV.
2. Three doses of IPV are recommended for adults who need to be immunized.

ABBREVIATIONS: IPV, inactivated poliovirus vaccine; OPV, oral poliovirus vaccine.
SOURCE: Modified from 1997 Redbook, Report of the Committee on Infectious Diseases.

tivation of the three serotypes of live poliovirus. Since 1988 an enhanced-potency inactivated poliovirus vaccine (IPV) has been available in the United States.

OPV and IPV induce antibodies that persist for at least 5 years. Both vaccines induce IgG and IgA antibodies. Compared with recipients of IPV, recipients of OPV shed less virus and less frequently develop reinfection with wild-type virus after exposure to poliovirus. Although IPV is safe and efficacious, OPV offers the advantages of ease of administration, lower cost, and induction of intestinal immunity resulting in a reduction in the risk of community transmission of wild-type virus. Because of progress toward global eradication of polio (with a reduced risk of imported cases) and the continued occurrence of cases of vaccine-associated polio, the CDC recommended in 1997 that children receive a sequential schedule of two doses of IPV followed by two doses of OPV or a four-dose schedule of IPV alone. To further reduce the risk of vaccine-associated polio, the Advisory Committee for Immunization Practices recommended (in June 1999) an all-IPV regimen for childhood poliovirus vaccination. Beginning in January 2000, children should receive IPV at 2, 4, and 6 to 18 months and 4 to 6 years of age. OPV will be used only in special circumstances: (1) for mass immunization campaigns to control outbreaks of polio; (2) for vaccination of unimmunized children who will be traveling to a polio-endemic area within 4 weeks; and (3) for children whose parents do not accept an all-IPV regimen. The latter children should receive at least two doses of IPV before receiving OPV. The risk of vaccine-associated polio should be discussed before administering OPV. Recommendations for vaccination of adults are listed in Table 193-1.

COXSACKIEVIRUS, ECHOVIRUS, AND OTHER ENTEROVIRUSES An estimated 5 to 10 million cases of symptomatic enterovirus disease occur in the United States each year. Enteroviruses are the most common cause of aseptic meningitis and nonspecific febrile illnesses of neonates. Certain clinical syndromes are more likely to be caused by certain serotypes (Table 193-2), but there is much overlap. From 1970 to 1983, 70% of enterovirus infections were caused by only 10 of the 64 human serotypes. Echoviruses 9 and 11 alone accounted for 24% of recognized enterovirus infections; echoviruses 4, 6, and 30 and coxsackieviruses A9 and B2 through B5 accounted for 46%.

Nonspecific Febrile Illness (Summer Grippe) The most common clinical manifestation of enterovirus infection is a nonspecific febrile illness. After an incubation period of 3 to 6 days, patients present with an acute onset of fever, malaise, and headache. Occasional cases are associated with upper respiratory symptoms, and some cases include nausea and vomiting. Symptoms often last for 3 to 4 days, and most cases resolve in a week. While infections with other respiratory viruses occur more often from late fall to early spring, enterovirus febrile illness frequently occurs in the summer and early fall.

Generalized Disease of the Newborn Most serious enterovirus infections in infants develop during the first week of life, although severe disease can occur up to 3 months of age. Neonates often present with an illness resembling bacterial sepsis, with fever, irritability, and lethargy. Laboratory abnormalities include leukocytosis with a left shift, thrombocytopenia, elevated values in liver function tests, and CSF pleocytosis. The illness can be complicated by myocarditis and hypotension, fulminant hepatitis and disseminated intravascular coagulation, meningitis or meningoencephalitis, or pneumonia. It may be difficult to distinguish enterovirus infection from bacterial sepsis, although a history of a recent virus-like illness in the mother provides a clue.

Aseptic Meningitis and Encephalitis Enteroviruses are the cause of up to 90% of cases of aseptic meningitis in children and young adults in which an etiologic agent can be identified. Patients with aseptic meningitis typically present with an acute onset of fever, chills, headache, photophobia, and pain on eye movement. Nausea and vomiting are also common. Examination reveals meningismus without localizing neurologic signs; drowsiness or irritability may also be apparent. In some cases, a febrile illness may be reported that remits but returns several days later in conjunction with signs of meningitis. Other systemic manifestations may provide clues to an enteroviral cause, including diarrhea, myalgias, rash, pleurodynia, myocarditis, and herpangina. Examination of the CSF invariably reveals pleocytosis; early in the course, polymorphonuclear leukocytes may be present or even predominant, raising the possibility of bacterial or other nonviral causes of meningitis. Partially treated bacterial meningitis may be particularly difficult to exclude in some instances. A useful rule is that the CSF cell count in enteroviral meningitis shows a shift to lymphocytic predominance within 24 h of presentation, and the total count generally does not exceed 1000 cells/μL. Additional CSF findings consist of a normal glucose content and a normal or only slightly elevated (by ≤ 100 mg/mL) level of protein. Enteroviruses and mumps virus may produce a similar picture of meningitis; a low CSF glucose level suggests mumps, whereas a normal CSF glucose level and transient CSF polymorphonuclear pleocytosis suggest enterovirus infection. Symptoms ordinarily resolve within a week, although CSF abnormalities can persist for several weeks. Enteroviral meningitis is often more severe in adults than in children. Neurologic sequelae are rare, and most patients have an excellent prognosis.

Enteroviral encephalitis is much less common than enteroviral aseptic meningitis. Occasional highly inflammatory cases of enteroviral meningitis may be complicated by a mild form of encephalitis that is recognized on the basis of progressive lethargy, disorientation, and sometimes seizures. Less commonly, severe primary encephalitis may develop. It is estimated that 10 to 20% of cases of viral encephalitis are due to enteroviruses. Immunocompetent patients generally have a good prognosis.

Table 193-2 Manifestations Commonly Associated with Enterovirus Serotypes

Manifestation	Serotype(s) of Indicated Virus	
	Coxsackievirus	Echovirus (E) and Enterovirus (Ent)
Aseptic meningitis	A2, 4, 7, 9, 10; B1-5	E4, 6, 7, 9, 11, 16, 18, 19, 30, 33; Ent70, 71
Exanthem	A4, 5, 9, 10, 16; B1, 3-5	E4-7, 9, 11, 16-19, 25, 30; Ent71
Generalized disease of the newborn	B2-5	E4-6, 9, 11, 14, 16, 19
Hand-foot-and-mouth disease	A5, 7, 9, 10, 16; B2, 5	Ent71
Herpangina	A1-10, 16, 22; B1-5	E6, 9, 11, 16, 17, 25; Ent71
Myocarditis, pericarditis	A4, 9, 16; B1-5	E6, 9, 11
Paralysis	A4, 7, 9; B1-5	E2, 4, 6, 9, 11, 30; Ent70, 71
Pleurodynia	A1, 2, 4, 6, 9, 10, 16; B1-6	E1-3, 6, 7, 9, 11, 12, 14, 16, 19, 24, 25, 30
Pneumonia	A9, 16; B1-5	E6, 7, 9, 11, 12, 19, 20, 30; Ent68, 71

Patients with hypo- or agammaglobulinemia or severe combined immunodeficiency may develop chronic meningitis or encephalitis; about half of these patients have a dermatomyositis-like syndrome, with peripheral edema, rash, and myositis. They may also have chronic hepatitis. Patients may develop neurologic disease while receiving gamma globulin replacement therapy. Echoviruses (especially echovirus 11) are the most common pathogens in this situation.

Paralytic disease due to enteroviruses other than poliovirus occurs sporadically and is usually less severe than poliomyelitis. Most cases are due to enterovirus 70 or 71 or to coxsackievirus A7 or A9. Guillain-Barré syndrome is also associated with enterovirus infection. While some studies have suggested a link between enteroviruses and the chronic fatigue syndrome, most recent studies have not demonstrated such an association.

Pleurodynia (Bornholm Disease) Patients with pleurodynia present with an acute onset of fever and spasms of pleuritic chest or upper abdominal pain. Chest pain is more frequent in adults, and abdominal pain is more common in children. Paroxysms of severe, knifelike pain usually last 15 to 30 min and are associated with diaphoresis and tachypnea. Fever peaks within an hour after the onset of paroxysms and subsides when pain resolves. The involved muscles are tender to palpation, and a pleural rub may be detected. The white blood cell count and chest x-ray are usually normal. Most cases are due to coxsackievirus B and occur during epidemics. Symptoms resolve in a few days, and recurrences are rare. Treatment includes the administration of nonsteroidal anti-inflammatory agents or the application of heat to the affected muscles.

Myocarditis and Pericarditis Enteroviruses are estimated to cause up to one-third of cases of acute myocarditis. Coxsackievirus B and its RNA have been detected in pericardial fluid and myocardial tissue in some cases of acute myocarditis and pericarditis. Most cases of enteroviral myocarditis or pericarditis occur in newborns, adolescents, or young adults. More than two-thirds of patients are male. Patients often present with an upper respiratory tract infection that is followed by fever, chest pain, dyspnea, arrhythmias, and occasionally heart failure. A pericardial friction rub is documented in half of cases, and the electrocardiogram shows ST segment elevations or ST- and T-wave abnormalities. Serum levels of myocardial enzymes are often elevated. Neonates commonly have severe disease, while most older children and adults recover completely. Up to 10% of cases progress to chronic dilated cardiomyopathy. Chronic constrictive pericarditis may also be a sequela.

Exanthems Enterovirus infection is the leading cause of exanthems in children in the summer and fall. While exanthems are associated with many enteroviruses, certain types have been linked to specific syndromes. Echoviruses 9 and 16 have frequently been associated with exanthem and fever. Rashes may be discrete (rubelliform) or confluent (morbilliform), beginning on the face and spreading to the trunk and extremities. Echovirus 9 is the most common cause of rubelliform rash. Unlike the rash of rubella, the enteroviral rash occurs in the summer and is not associated with lymphadenopathy. Roseola-like rashes develop after defervescence, with macules and papules on the face and trunk. The Boston exanthem, caused by echovirus 16, is a roseola-like rash that often affects multiple members of a family. A variety of other rashes have been associated with enteroviruses, including erythema multiforme and vesicular, urticarial, petechial, or purpuric lesions. Enanthems also occur, including lesions that resemble the Koplik's spots seen with measles.

Hand-Foot-and-Mouth Disease After an incubation period of 4 to 6 days, patients with hand-foot-and-mouth disease present with fever, anorexia, and malaise; these manifestations are followed by the development of sore throat and vesicles (**Plate IID-39**) on the buccal mucosa and often on the tongue and then by the appearance of tender vesicular lesions on the dorsum of the hands, sometimes with involvement of the palms. The vesicles may form bullae and quickly ulcerate. About one-third of patients also have lesions on the palate, uvula, or tonsillar pillars, and one-third have a rash on the feet (including the soles) or on the buttocks. The disease is highly infectious, with attack rates of close to 100% among young children. The lesions usually resolve in 1 week. Most cases are due to coxsackievirus A16 or enterovirus 71.

An epidemic of enterovirus 71 infection in Taiwan in 1998 resulted in thousands of cases of hand-foot-and-mouth disease or herpangina. Severe complications included CNS disease, myocarditis, and pulmonary hemorrhage. About 90% of those who died were children ≤5 years old, and these deaths were associated with pulmonary edema or pulmonary hemorrhage. CNS disease included aseptic meningitis, flaccid paralysis (similar to poliomyelitis), or rhombencephalitis with myoclonus and tremor or ataxia. The mean age of patients with CNS complications was 2.5 years, and magnetic resonance imaging in cases with encephalitis usually showed brain-stem lesions.

Herpangina Herpangina is usually caused by coxsackievirus A and presents as acute-onset fever, sore throat, dysphagia, and grayish-white papulovesicular lesions on an erythematous base that ulcerate. The lesions can persist for weeks; are present on the soft palate, anterior pillars of the tonsils, and uvula; and are concentrated in the posterior portion of the mouth. In contrast to herpes stomatitis, enteroviral herpangina is not associated with gingivitis. Acute lymphonodular pharyngitis associated with coxsackievirus A10 presents as white or yellow nodules surrounded by erythema in the posterior oropharynx. The lesions do not ulcerate.

Acute Hemorrhagic Conjunctivitis Patients with acute hemorrhagic conjunctivitis present with an acute onset of severe eye pain, blurred vision, photophobia, and watery discharge from the eye. Examination reveals edema, chemosis, and subconjunctival hemorrhage and often shows punctate keratitis and conjunctival follicles as well. Preauricular adenopathy is often found. Epidemics and nosocomial spread have been associated with enterovirus 70 and coxsackievirus A24. Systemic symptoms, including headache and fever, develop in 20% of cases, and recovery is usually complete in 10 days. The sudden onset and short duration of the illness help to distinguish acute hemorrhagic conjunctivitis from other ocular infections such as those due to adenovirus and *Chlamydia*. Paralysis has been associated with some cases of acute hemorrhagic conjunctivitis due to enterovirus 70 during epidemics.

Other Manifestations Enteroviruses are an infrequent cause of childhood pneumonia and the common cold. Coxsackievirus B has been isolated at autopsy from the pancreas of a few children presenting with insulin-dependent diabetes mellitus; however, most attempts to isolate the virus have been unsuccessful. Other diseases that have been associated with enterovirus infection include bronchitis, bronchiolitis, croup, infectious lymphocytosis, polymyositis, acute arthritis, and acute nephritis.

REOVIRUSES

Reoviruses are double-stranded RNA viruses encompassing three serotypes. Serologic studies indicate that most humans are infected with reoviruses during childhood; however, it has been difficult to establish a definite link of reovirus infection with a particular disease. It is likely that most infections either are asymptomatic or cause very mild disease. One outbreak of reovirus infection in children resulted in minor upper respiratory tract symptoms. Reovirus is considered a rare cause of mild gastroenteritis in infants and children. Speculation regarding an association of reovirus type 3 with idiopathic neonatal hepatitis and extrahepatic biliary atresia is based on an elevated prevalence of antibody to reovirus among some of these patients, detection of viral RNA by PCR in hepatobiliary tissues in some studies, and detection of virus in the porta hepatis in one case.

BIBLIOGRAPHY

ABZUG MJ et al: Neonatal enterovirus infection: Virology, serology, and effects of intravenous immune globulin. Clin Infect Dis 20:1201, 1995

AHMED A et al: Clinical utility of the polymerase chain reaction for diagnosis of enteroviral meningitis in infancy. J Pediatr 131:393, 1997

CHEN RT et al: Seroprevalence of antibody against poliovirus in inner-city preschool children: Implications for vaccination policy in the United States. JAMA 275:1639, 1996

COCHI SL et al (eds): *Global Poliomyelitis Eradication Initiative: Status Report.* J Infect Dis 175(Suppl 1):S1–S292, 1997

DALAKAS MC et al: The postpolio syndrome: Advances in the pathogenesis and treatment. Ann NY Acad Sci 753:1, 1995

HO M et al: An epidemic of enterovirus 71 infection in Taiwan. N Engl J Med 341:929, 1999

HUANG C-C et al: Neurologic complications in children with enterovirus 71 infection. N Engl J Med 341:936, 1999

MCKINNEY R et al: Chronic enteroviral meningoencephalitis in agammaglobulinemic patients. Rev Infect Dis 9:334, 1987

PREVOTS DR et al: Poliomyelitis prevention in the United States: New recommendations for routine childhood vaccination place greater reliance on inactivated poliovirus vaccine. Pediatr Ann 26:378, 1997

ROTBART HA (ed): *Human Enterovirus Infections.* Washington, DC, ASM Press, 1995

ROTBART HA et al: Treatment of human enterovirus infections. Antiviral Res 38:1, 1998

STREBEL PM et al: Intramuscular injections within 30 days of immunization with oral poliovirus vaccine—a risk factor for vaccine-associated paralytic poliomyelitis. N Engl J Med 332:500, 1995

194   *Anne Gershon*

MEASLES (RUBEOLA)

DEFINITION   Measles (rubeola) is a highly contagious, acute, exanthematous respiratory disease with a characteristic clinical picture and pathognomonic enanthem. A successful live attenuated measles vaccine became available in 1963 in the United States and elsewhere, and measles is now an unusual disease in most developed countries where this vaccine is widely used. However, measles continues to occur sporadically in mini-epidemics in the United States, and major epidemics in developing nations make this disease a persistent cause of childhood morbidity and mortality.

ETIOLOGIC AGENT   Measles virus is a member of the genus *Morbillivirus* and the family Paramyxoviridae. It is closely related to the viruses causing canine and porcine distemper, rinderpest of cattle, and *peste des petits ruminants* of goats and sheep. There is only one antigenic type. Measles virions are pleomorphic spherical structures having a diameter of 100 to 250 nm and consisting of six proteins. The inner capsid is composed of a coiled helix of RNA and three proteins, and the outer envelope consists of a matrix protein bearing two types of short surface-glycoprotein projections or peplomers. One peplomer is a conical hemagglutinin (H) and the other a dumbbell-shaped fusion (F) protein. The genome has been sequenced, and it is thereby possible to distinguish vaccine-type measles virus from the wild type. In addition, genetic variability of wild-type measles virus occurs; eight genotypes have been identified.

EPIDEMIOLOGY   Measles has a worldwide distribution; humans are the only natural hosts, although other primates can be experimentally infected. During the prevaccination era in the United States, measles epidemics occurred every 2 to 5 years in the winter and spring. In an epidemic year, roughly half a million measles cases were reported; 99% of adults had serologic evidence of previous measles infection. After the live attenuated vaccine became available, the number of cases reported to the Centers for Disease Control and Prevention (CDC) fell, with a nadir of 1497 cases in 1983. After an upsurge to more than 27,000 cases (with 89 deaths) in 1990, the disease was once more brought under control (with only 312 cases reported to the CDC in 1993), in part through the routine administration of two doses of vaccine. The foremost reason for the resurgence of measles was failure to immunize infants and young children, especially in inner-city areas. Primary vaccine failure (documented in about 5% of individuals) and secondary vaccine failure or waning immunity accounted for some cases.

In recent years the majority of cases of measles have involved preschool children. Between 1993 and 1996, fewer than 1000 cases were reported annually in the United States; in 1995 there were 309 reported cases, and in 1996 there were 508. Molecular studies indicated interruption of transmission of indigenous measles in 1993. Most cases have since resulted from international importations of the virus. Mortality is highest among children under 2 years of age and among adults. Patients with impaired cell-mediated immunity are at especially high risk for severe or even fatal measles. The measles-associated mortality rate in the United States is about 0.3%; in developing countries, mortality frequently exceeds 1% and sometimes approaches 10%.

Measles virus is transmitted by respiratory secretions, predominantly through exposure to aerosols but also through direct contact with larger droplets. Patients are contagious from 1 or 2 days before the onset of symptoms until 4 days after the appearance of the rash. Infectivity peaks during the prodromal phase. The mean intervals from infection to onset of symptoms and to appearance of rash are 10 and 14 days, respectively.

PATHOGENESIS AND PATHOLOGY   Measles virus invades the respiratory epithelium and spreads via the bloodstream to the reticuloendothelial system, from which it infects all types of white blood cells, thereby establishing infection of the skin, respiratory tract, and other organs. Both viremia and viruria develop. Multinucleated giant cells with inclusion bodies in the nucleus and cytoplasm (Warthin-Finkeldey cells) are found in respiratory and lymphoid tissues and are pathognomonic for measles. Direct invasion of T lymphocytes and increased levels of suppressive cytokines, such as interleukin 4, may play a role in the temporary depression of cellular immunity that accompanies and transiently follows measles. The major infected cell in the blood is the monocyte. Infection of the entire respiratory tract accounts for the characteristic cough and coryza of measles and for the less frequent manifestations of croup, bronchiolitis, and pneumonia. Generalized damage to the respiratory tract, with resultant loss of cilia, predisposes to secondary bacterial infections such as pneumonia and otitis media.

Specific antibodies are not detectable before the onset of rash. Cellular immunity (consisting of cytotoxic T cells and possibly natural killer cells) plays a prominent role in host defense, and patients who are deficient in cellular immunity are at high risk for severe measles. Children with isolated agammaglobulinemia are not at increased risk. Immune reactions to the virus in the endothelial cells of dermal capillaries play a substantial role in the development of Koplik's spots (the pathognomonic enanthem) as well as in that of rash; in immunodeficient hosts, measles may be severe despite the absence of these manifestations. Measles antigens have been demonstrated in involved skin during early stages of the illness.

Pathologic changes in measles encephalitis include focal hemorrhage, congestion, and perivascular demyelination. Measles virus is rarely isolated from cerebrospinal fluid (CSF) in cases of encephalitis, which are thought to be due to the interaction of virus-infected cells with local cellular immune factors.

CLINICAL MANIFESTATIONS   Measles begins with a 2- to 4-day respiratory prodrome of malaise, cough, coryza, conjunctivitis with lacrimation, nasal discharge, and increasing fever [with temperatures as high as 40.6°C (105°F), probably reflecting secondary viremia]. At this stage of the illness, in which the rash has not yet developed, influenza may be suspected. Just before the onset of the rash, Koplik's spots appear as 1- to 2-mm blue-white spots on a bright red background. Without adequate illumination for examination, they may be overlooked. Koplik's spots are typically located on the buccal mucosa alongside the second molars and may be extensive; they are not associated with any other infectious disease. The spots wane after the onset of rash and soon disappear. The entire buccal and inner labial mucosa may be inflamed, and the lips may be reddened.

The characteristic erythematous, nonpruritic, maculopapular rash of measles begins at the hairline and behind the ears, spreads down the trunk and limbs to include the palms and soles, and often becomes confluent. At this time, the patient is at the most severe point of the illness. By the fourth day, the rash begins to fade in the order in which it appeared. Brownish discoloration of the skin and desquamation may occur later. Fever usually resolves by the fourth or fifth day after the onset of rash; prolonged fever suggests a complication of measles. Lymphadenopathy, diarrhea, vomiting, and splenomegaly are common features. The chest x-ray may be abnormal, even in uncomplicated measles, because of the propensity of this virus to invade the respiratory tract. The entire illness usually lasts about 10 days. The disease tends to be more severe in adults than in children, with higher fever, more prominent rash, and a higher incidence of complications.

Milder forms of the illness with less intense symptoms and a milder rash, termed *modified measles*, may occur in individuals with preexisting partial immunity induced by active or passive vaccination. These patients include infants under 1 year of age who retain some proportion of passively acquired maternal antibodies. On occasion, individuals with a history of immunization may develop modified measles.

COMPLICATIONS   The complications of measles can conveniently be divided into three groups, according to the site involved: the respiratory tract, the central nervous system (CNS), and the gastrointestinal tract. Respiratory tract involvement, manifested as laryngitis, croup, or bronchitis, occurs in the majority of cases of uncomplicated measles. In young children, otitis media is the most common complication. Pneumonia is a frequent reason for hospitalization, especially of adults. The pneumonia is of viral origin in the majority of cases, but secondary bacterial infection (most commonly caused by streptococci, pneumococci, or staphylococci) also takes place with some frequency. Primary giant cell (Hecht's) pneumonia is most often documented in immunocompromised and/or malnourished patients.

Encephalographic abnormalities in the absence of symptoms of CNS disease are extremely frequent in measles. Symptomatic CNS disease, with fever, headache, drowsiness, coma, and/or seizures, occurs in about 1 case in 1000. Symptoms usually begin within days after the onset of rash but occasionally appear for the first time several weeks later. About 10% of patients do not survive acute measles encephalitis; a significant percentage of surviving patients develop permanent sequelae, such as mental retardation or epilepsy. Most cases appear to result from an immune-mediated response to myelin proteins (postinfectious encephalomyelitis) and not directly from viral infection of the CNS (Chap. 371). Rarely, transverse myelitis follows measles. Immunocompromised patients are at risk for progressive fatal encephalitis 1 to 6 months after measles; in some cases, even though prior measles has not been recognized, the virus is identified at autopsy. Subacute sclerosing panencephalitis (SSPE)—a protracted, chronic, extremely rare form of measles encephalitis—sometimes follows measles and is particularly common among children who have measles before the age of 2 years (Chap. 373). SSPE has virtually disappeared in the United States as a result of widespread vaccination. Typically, progressive dementia evolves over several months. SSPE is thought to be due to a complex interaction of the host with defective measles virus. It is associated with extremely high levels of antibodies to measles virus in the blood and CSF.

Gastrointestinal complications of measles include gastroenteritis, hepatitis, appendicitis, ileocolitis, and mesenteric adenitis. It is not uncommon to detect high levels of alanine and aspartate aminotransferases in the absence of gastrointestinal signs such as jaundice.

Other, rare complications include myocarditis, glomerulonephritis, and postinfectious thrombocytopenic purpura. Measles can exacerbate preexisting tuberculosis, presumably through depression of cellular immunity induced by the virus. Natural measles and immunization against measles can result in tuberculin skin-test anergy lasting for about 1 month.

ATYPICAL MEASLES   An atypical form of measles has been reported in individuals who received formalin-inactivated measles vac-
cine (used in the United States from 1963 through 1967 and in Canada until 1970) and subsequently were exposed to measles virus. After a several-day prodrome of fever, myalgia, and headache, the rash appears. Unlike the rash of typical measles, that of atypical measles begins peripherally and moves centrally; it can be urticarial, maculopapular, hemorrhagic, and/or vesicular. Fever is usually high and is accompanied by edema of the extremities, interstitial pulmonary infiltrates, hepatitis, and (on occasion) pleural effusion. The differential diagnosis often includes Rocky Mountain spotted fever, Henoch-Schönlein purpura, meningococcemia, drug allergy, toxic shock syndrome, and varicella. Despite the severity of atypical measles, patients invariably recover after a convalescence that may be prolonged. Measles virus is not isolated from these patients, and they do not spread the virus to others. This disease is believed to be due to hypersensitivity to measles virus induced by the inactivated vaccine. Formalin inactivation destroys the antigenicity of the F protein, antibodies to which are important in preventing spread of the virus from one cell to another. The role of cellular immunity in this process is unknown. Extremely high convalescent titers of antibody to measles virus (e.g., 1:1,000,000) are diagnostic of atypical measles. To prevent this syndrome, adults who received formalin-inactivated measles vaccine should be reimmunized with at least one dose of live attenuated measles vaccine. Since inactivated measles vaccine has not been available for more than 25 years, atypical measles has now virtually disappeared.

MEASLES IN THE IMMUNOCOMPROMISED HOST   Patients with defects in cell-mediated immunity are at risk for severe protracted and fatal measles. Included in this category are patients with congenital cellular immune defects or malignancy, recipients of immunosuppressive therapy, or persons infected with HIV. In these patients, measles may not be accompanied by a rash. Complications are primary measles (giant cell) pneumonia, progressive encephalitis beginning weeks to months after initial infection, and (in HIV-infected patients) progression to AIDS.

MEASLES IN ADULTS   Measles is naturally a disease of childhood and, like many other viral infections, is more severe in adults than in children. About 3% of young adults with measles develop primary viral pneumonia and require hospitalization. Hepatitis and bronchospasm are more common among adults with measles than among children, and the rash is more severe and more confluent in adults. Bacterial superinfection is more common among adults, more than one-third of whom develop respiratory complications such as otitis media, sinusitis, and pneumonia. Adults may develop measles because they were never immunized or (more rarely) because their vaccine-induced immunity has waned. Very low titers of antibody to measles virus have been associated with lack of protection.

LABORATORY FINDINGS   Lymphopenia and neutropenia are common in measles and may be due to invasion of leukocytes by the virus, with subsequent cell death. Leukocytosis may herald a bacterial superinfection. Patients with measles encephalitis usually have an elevated protein concentration in CSF as well as lymphocytosis. A specific diagnosis of measles can be made quickly by immunofluorescent staining of a smear of respiratory secretions for measles antigen; monoclonal antibodies conjugated to fluorescein are commercially available for this purpose. Secretions can also be examined microscopically for multinucleated giant cells. Measles virus can be isolated from respiratory secretions or urine and rapidly identified in tissue culture with fluorescein-labeled monoclonal antibodies. Measles virus RNA has been demonstrated by diagnostic reverse-transcription polymerase chain reaction. A number of serologic tests are available for the diagnosis of measles; however, a serologic diagnosis cannot necessarily be made quickly since both acute- and convalescent-phase sera are usually tested, ideally at the same time. The older hemagglutination inhibition test has been replaced by enzyme immunoassay (EIA), which is more sensitive and simpler to perform. EIA can be used to measure specific IgM and thus to diagnose measles on the basis of an acute-phase serum sample alone. Specific IgM antibodies are detectable within 1 to 2 days after the appearance of rash, and the IgG titer rises significantly after 10 days. As already mentioned, atypical measles and SSPE are associated with extremely high titers of antibody.

DIFFERENTIAL DIAGNOSIS Classic measles—with Koplik's spots, cough, coryza, conjunctivitis, and a rash beginning on the head—is easily diagnosed on clinical grounds. Modified measles is more difficult to diagnose clinically since one or more characteristic signs may be lacking. The differential diagnosis of measles includes Kawasaki's syndrome, scarlet fever, infectious mononucleosis, toxoplasmosis, drug eruption, and *Mycoplasma pneumoniae* infection. Most of these conditions can be identified by either culture or serologic assay. In the differential diagnosis of measles, attention should be paid to the current epidemiology of the disease in the community and to the patient's history of measles vaccination and foreign travel.

PREVENTION The development of live attenuated measles vaccine by Enders and his colleagues was a milestone in American medicine. This vaccine, used in the United States for the routine immunization of children since 1963, induces seroconversion in about 95% of recipients and probably confers lifelong protection. Waning immunity to measles after immunization has been documented only on rare occasions. For the past 25 years, measles vaccine has been available as the combination vaccine measles-mumps-rubella (MMR); MMR vaccine should be administered to children between the ages of 12 and 15 months. (Vaccination at 12 months is preferred for infants whose mothers were immunized against measles in childhood. These mothers have lower antibody titers than women who have had natural measles, and their infants correspondingly have transplacental antibodies of lower titer and shorter duration.) A second dose of MMR vaccine is recommended for school-aged children at 4 to 12 years of age. This two-dose policy was developed in the late 1980s in response to measles outbreaks in the United States. Since the institution of the two-dose regimen and the increased effort to immunize all children, measles has again become an unusual disease in the United States. Regional guidelines that reflect the current local epidemiology of measles should be followed.

Older susceptible persons should also be immunized. Individuals should be considered susceptible to measles unless they have documentation of physician-diagnosed measles or of the receipt of two doses of vaccine, have laboratory evidence of measles immunity, or were born before 1957. Rarely, individuals born before 1957 develop measles, and those who are at risk of exposure to measles (e.g., health workers, teachers, and international travelers) should be tested for measles antibody and immunized if necessary. Approximately 10% of healthy vaccinees develop a fever, with temperatures up to 39.4°C (103°F), 5 to 7 days after vaccination; this fever lasts 1 to 5 days and is accompanied by a transient rash. Individuals previously immunized only with killed vaccine are considered susceptible and should receive at least one dose—and preferably two doses—of MMR vaccine. Transient adverse reactions in these individuals include fever, malaise, and redness and swelling at the injection site.

Because of the severity of measles in this group and the lack of reported problems following vaccination, children with asymptomatic HIV infection should receive MMR vaccine; those with severe immunosuppression (<15% CD4 lymphocytes) should not. A case of fatal measles due to vaccine-type virus was reported in a college student with AIDS. Measles vaccine is contraindicated for persons with impaired cell-mediated immunity, for pregnant women, and for persons with a history of anaphylaxis due to egg protein or neomycin. Minor illnesses, with or without fever and a history of convulsions, are not contraindications to vaccination. Vaccination should be deferred for 6 to 11 months after the receipt of immune globulin or of blood products containing antibodies and for at least 3 months after the discontinuation of immunosuppressive treatment. Vaccine failures have been ascribed to faulty storage of the preparation used, immunization of infants with preexisting (maternally derived) antibodies, and simultaneous administration of measles vaccine and immune globulin.

Children and adults who are susceptible to measles and are exposed to the disease should receive postexposure prophylaxis. Standard immune globulin, given intramuscularly within 6 days of expo-

sure, can exert a protective or modifying effect; the earlier it is given, the better the outcome. The dose is 0.25 mL/kg for healthy persons and 0.5 mL/kg for immunocompromised persons, with a maximum dose of 15 mL. Immune globulin is particularly strongly indicated for susceptible household contacts, especially those less than 1 year of age, and for immunocompromised persons. HIV-infected persons, particularly those with severe immunosuppression, should be given immune globulin after exposure, regardless of their measles immune status and whether or not they are receiving intravenous immunoglobulin. Vaccination within 72 h of exposure may also provide protection against clinical measles, but this strategy is contraindicated as postexposure prophylaxis for immunocompromised individuals. Vaccine and immune globulin should not be given concurrently.

℞ TREATMENT Therapy for measles is largely supportive and symptom-based. Patients with otitis media and pneumonia should be given standard antibiotics. Patients with encephalitis need supportive care, including observation for increased intracranial pressure. Controlled trials suggest clinical benefit from high doses of vitamin A in severe or potentially severe measles, especially in children under the age of 2 years. A dose of 50,000 IU is used for infants age 1 to 6 months, 100,000 IU for infants age 7 to 12 months, and 200,000 IU for children over 1 year. A single dose is administered on two consecutive days. Transient vomiting and headache may be associated with the administration of vitamin A. Ribavirin is effective against measles virus in vitro and may be considered for use in immunocompromised individuals.

BIBLIOGRAPHY

CENTERS FOR DISEASE CONTROL AND PREVENTION: Measles, mumps, and rubella—vaccine use and strategies for elimination of measles, rubella, and congenital rubella syndrome and control of mumps. MMWR 47:1, 1998

EBERHART-PHILLIPS JE et al: Measles in pregnancy: A descriptive study of 58 cases. Obstet Gynecol 82:797, 1993

FORNI AL et al: Severe measles pneumonitis in adults: Evaluation of clinical characteristics and therapy with intravenous ribavirin. Clin Infect Dis 19:454, 1994

GREMILLION DH et al: Measles pneumonia in young adults. An analysis of 106 cases. Am J Med 71:539, 1981

HUSSEY GD et al: A randomized, controlled trial of vitamin A in children with severe measles. N Engl J Med 323:160, 1990

KAPLAN LJ et al: Severe measles in immunocompromised patients. JAMA 267:1237, 1992

LA BOCCETTA AC et al: Measles encephalitis. Report of 61 cases. Am J Dis Child 107:247, 1964

MARKOWITZ LE et al: Duration of live measles vaccine–induced immunity. Pediatr Infect Dis J 9:101, 1990

PELTOLA H et al: The elimination of indigenous measles, mumps, and rubella from Finland by a 12-year, two-dose vaccination program. N Engl J Med 331:1397, 1994

SMARON MF et al: Diagnosis of measles by fluorescent antibody and culture of nasopharyngeal secretions. J Virol Methods 33:223, 1991

TAKAHASHI H et al: Detection and comparison of viral antigens in measles and rubella rashes. Clin Infect Dis 22:36, 1996

195 *Anne Gershon*

RUBELLA (GERMAN MEASLES)

DEFINITION Rubella is an acute viral infection of children and adults that characteristically includes rash, fever, and lymphadenopathy and has a broad spectrum of other possible manifestations. However, a high percentage of rubella infections in both children and adults are subclinical. In addition, the illness can resemble a mild attack of measles (rubeola) and can cause arthritis, especially in adults. Rubella during pregnancy can lead to fetal infection, with the production of a significant constellation of malformations (*congenital rubella syndrome*) in a high proportion of infected fetuses.

ETIOLOGIC AGENT Rubella virus, a togavirus, is the only member of the *Rubivirus* genus and is closely related to the alphaviruses. Unlike these agents, however, it does not require a vector for transmission. Moreover, there is no RNA sequence homology between rubella virus and the alphaviruses.

The rubella virion is composed of an inner icosahedral capsid of RNA and protein that is surrounded by a lipid-containing envelope with a diameter of about 60 nm. The structural proteins associated with rubella virus are E1 and E2 (transmembrane envelope glycoproteins) and C (the capsid protein that surrounds the viral RNA). Only one serotype has been identified.

EPIDEMIOLOGY In the United States during the prevaccine era, rubella was most common in the spring and most often affected school-age children; only 80 to 90% of adults were immune; and major epidemics occurred every 6 to 9 years. The most recent epidemic in the United States occurred in 1964 to 1965, when there were more than 12 million reported cases of postnatal rubella and more than 20,000 cases of the congenital rubella syndrome. Since the introduction of live attenuated rubella vaccine in 1969, there have been no epidemics; limited outbreaks have been reported in settings where susceptible individuals come into close contact with one another (e.g., schools and workplaces). In 1996, only 213 cases of postnatally acquired rubella—most of them in young adults—and 2 confirmed cases of congenital rubella syndrome were reported to the Centers for Disease Control and Prevention (CDC).

Whether symptomatic or subclinical, rubella is contagious, albeit less so than measles. Its incubation period is 18 days on average, with a range of 12 to 23 days. The virus, which is spread in droplets shed in respiratory secretions, infects the respiratory tract and then the bloodstream. In postnatally acquired infections, rubella virus is shed during the prodromal phase of the illness, and shedding from the pharynx can continue for about a week after onset. Despite high titers of specific neutralizing antibodies, infants with congenital rubella may excrete rubella virus from the respiratory tract and in the urine until the age of 2 years. This excretion raises important issues related to infection control in hospital and day-care settings. Persons recently immunized with live attenuated rubella vaccine do not transmit the vaccine virus to others, although low titers of rubella virus may be detected transiently in the pharynx.

After an attack of rubella, specific antibodies and cell-mediated immunity develop and probably play a significant role in protection against future disease. Asymptomatic reinfection at the level of the respiratory tract is common upon reexposure to the virus but is rarely if ever associated with viremia.

Rubella virus has been cultured from respiratory secretions during reinfection. Fetal infection may occur during maternal reinfection but is acknowledged to be extremely rare because of the absence of maternal viremia under these circumstances. Viremia following reinfection of individuals immunized against rubella is also rare. Thus the current level of congenital rubella in the United States is exceedingly low.

PATHOGENESIS AND PATHOLOGY Little is known about the microscopic pathology of postnatally acquired rubella since the disease is invariably self-limited. Like that of measles, the rash of rubella is immunologically mediated; its onset coincides with the development of specific antibodies. Viremia can be demonstrated for about a week before and ends within a few days after the onset of rash.

The cause of the damage to cells and organs in congenital rubella is not well understood. Proposed mechanisms of fetal damage include mitotic arrest of cells, tissue necrosis without inflammation, and chromosomal damage. The growth of the fetus may be retarded. Other findings may include decreased numbers of megakaryocytes in the bone marrow, extramedullary hematopoiesis, and interstitial pneumonia.

CLINICAL MANIFESTATIONS **Postnatally Acquired Rubella** Infection acquired after birth usually results in an extremely mild or subclinical illness. A prodromal phase is uncommon in children; adults may have more severe disease, with a brief prodrome of malaise, fever, and anorexia. The foremost symptoms of postnatally acquired rubella include posterior auricular, cervical, and suboccipital lymphadenopathy; fever; and rash. The rash often begins on the face and spreads down the body. It is maculopapular but not confluent, is sometimes accompanied by mild coryza and conjunctivitis, and generally lasts for 3 to 5 days. A petechial enanthem on the soft palate, designated *Forschheimer spots*, may occur but is not specific for rubella. Fever may be absent entirely or may be present for only several days in the early phase of the illness.

Complications of postnatally acquired rubella are uncommon; bacterial superinfection is rare. One particularly troublesome complication is seen almost exclusively in women: arthritis, most frequently involving the fingers, wrists, and/or knees, develops as the rash is appearing and may take several weeks to resolve. Chronic arthritis resulting from rubella is extremely rare. Rubella virus has been isolated from joint fluid during acute rubella arthritis and from peripheral blood in chronic rubella arthritis.

Another complication of postnatally acquired rubella is hemorrhage due to both thrombocytopenia and vascular damage, which occurs in 1 of every 3000 patients. Thrombocytopenia may last for weeks or months; it can have long-term consequences if there is bleeding into organs such as the eye or the brain.

Both children and adults may develop encephalitis after rubella; the incidence is about five times lower than that of encephalitis following measles. Adults are more likely than children to develop encephalitis; the mortality rate from this complication is 20 to 50%. Mild hepatitis is an unusual complication. Immunosuppressed patients are not at increased risk for rubella as they are for measles.

Congenital Rubella Maternal infection in early pregnancy can lead to fetal infection, with resultant congenital rubella. The classic signs of congenital rubella are cataract, heart disease, and deafness, but a myriad of other defects have been reported. These abnormalities include signs and symptoms that are transient, such as low birth weight, thrombocytopenia, hepatosplenomegaly, jaundice, and pneumonia; those that are permanent, such as deafness, pulmonic stenosis, patent ductus arteriosus, glaucoma, and cataract; and those that are developmental, such as mental retardation, diabetes mellitus, and behavioral disorders.

The most important factor in the pathogenicity of rubella virus for the fetus is gestational age at the time of infection. Maternal infection during the first trimester leads to fetal infection in about 50% of cases; maternal infection early in the second trimester leads to fetal infection in about one-third of cases. Fetal malformations not only are more common after maternal infection in the first trimester but also tend to be more severe and to involve more organ systems. While a fetus infected in the fourth week of gestation may develop many problems, one infected later (e.g., in the 20th week) may have isolated deafness as the only symptom.

DIAGNOSIS Since postnatally acquired rubella is such a mild disease and since many cases are subclinical, diagnosis on clinical grounds can be difficult. Other diseases that may mimic rubella include toxoplasmosis, scarlet fever, modified measles, roseola, fifth disease (erythema infectiosum due to parvovirus B19), and enteroviral infection. Routine laboratory tests usually reveal leukopenia and atypical lymphocytes.

The isolation of rubella virus in cell cultures of throat samples, urine, or other secretions is difficult and expensive but is sometimes undertaken. This technique is most useful when congenital rubella is suspected. A laboratory diagnosis is more often made serologically. The most commonly used test is an enzyme-linked immunosorbent assay (ELISA) for IgG and IgM antibodies. Acute rubella is diagnosed by the documentation of a fourfold or greater rise in the titer of IgG antibodies in paired acute- and convalescent-phase serum specimens or by the detection of rubella-specific IgM antibodies in one serum specimen. However, false-negative and -positive IgM reactions are sometimes obtained. Moreover, true-positive IgM reactions can be obtained in both primary infection and reinfection. Congenital rubella is diagnosed by the isolation of rubella virus, the detection of IgM antibodies in a single serum sample, and/or the documentation of either the persistence of rubella antibodies in serum beyond 1 year of age or a rising antibody titer anytime during infancy in an unvaccinated child. Biopsied tissues and/or blood and cerebrospinal fluid have also been used for the demonstration of rubella antigens with monoclonal antibodies and for the detection of rubella RNA by in situ hybridization and polymerase chain reaction.

PREVENTION   Live attenuated rubella vaccine was licensed in 1969, 7 years after the virus was first isolated in culture. This vaccine was developed as a strategy to prevent congenital rubella by ensuring that very few pregnant women would be susceptible and that there would be little circulating wild-type virus. Rubella vaccine induces seroconversion in more than 95% of recipients. Since its licensure, there have been no major epidemics in the United States, and the number of cases has declined by 98%. The vaccine currently licensed in the United States, RA 27/3, is propagated in human diploid cells and is more immunogenic (particularly with regard to the stimulation of secretory immunity) than previously licensed vaccines. The present vaccination strategy, developed in part when measles was not being adequately controlled, is to immunize all infants at 12 to 15 months of age with measles-mumps-rubella (MMR) vaccine and to administer a second dose at 4 to 12 years of age. Rubella vaccine may also be administered to anyone who is thought to be susceptible to the infection and is not pregnant; it is particularly important that hospital workers of either sex be immune to rubella so that nosocomial transmission is avoided. While there has been little change in the prevalence of immunity to rubella among women of childbearing age (about 80%), the incidence of congenital rubella is extremely low—about 10 cases annually. It is likely that, although antibody may be undetectable years after immunization, protection against infection—possibly due to cell-mediated immunity—is the rule. At present, there is little if any evidence of significant waning of clinically important immunity to rubella with time.

On occasion, rubella vaccine may cause arthralgia or arthritis, especially in young women. Very rarely, rubella vaccination results in chronic arthritis; however, even cases of frank arthritis in vaccinees are self-limited, lasting only about 1 week.

After investigation of a series of more than 400 women who were inadvertently immunized during pregnancy and who carried their infants to term, the CDC has concluded that vaccine-type rubella virus either does not cause the congenital rubella syndrome at all or does so at an incidence too low to be detected. Nonetheless, rubella vaccine is contraindicated for use in pregnant women, and it is recommended that pregnancy be avoided for at least 3 months after rubella vaccination. It is acceptable for rubella-susceptible children whose mothers are also susceptible to be immunized, since vaccinated individuals do not shed rubella virus or transmit it to susceptible individuals. Although it is recommended that rubella vaccine not be given to immunosuppressed persons, the vaccine is given to children infected with HIV. No adverse effects of rubella vaccine have been reported in immunocompromised patients.

℞ **TREATMENT**   There is no specific therapy for rubella. At one time, immune globulin was used in an effort to prevent congenital rubella when pregnant women became infected. However, since administration of immune globulin did not prevent maternal viremia, this approach was discarded. Treatment is given for symptoms such as fever, arthralgia, and arthritis.

BIBLIOGRAPHY

BOSMA TJ et al: Use of PCR for prenatal and postnatal diagnosis of congenital rubella. J Clin Microbiol 33:2881, 1995

CENTERS FOR DISEASE CONTROL AND PREVENTION: Measles, mumps, and rubella—vaccine use and strategies for elimination of measles, rubella, and congenital rubella syndrome and control of mumps. MMWR 47:1, 1998

CHANTLER JK et al: Persistent rubella virus infection associated with chronic arthritis in children. N Engl J Med 313:1117, 1985

CUSI MG et al: Serological evidence of reinfection among vaccinees during rubella outbreak. Lancet 336:1071, 1991

FREY TK et al: Molecular analysis of rubella virus epidemiology across three continents, North America, Europe, and Asia. J Infect Dis 178:642, 1998

GREGG NM: Congenital cataract following German measles in the mother. Trans Ophthalmol Soc Aust 3:35, 1941

HERRMANN KL: Available rubella serologic tests. Rev Infect Dis 7:S108, 1985

HORSTMANN D et al: Persistence of vaccine-induced immune responses to rubella. Rev Infect Dis 7:S80, 1985

MELLINGER AK et al: High incidence of congenital rubella syndrome after a rubella outbreak. Pediatr Infect Dis J 14:573, 1995

TOWNSEND JJ et al: Progressive rubella panencephalitis: Late onset after congenital rubella. N Engl J Med 292:990, 1975

WEIBEL RE, BENOR DE: Chronic arthropathy and musculoskeletal symptoms associated with rubella vaccines: A review of 124 claims submitted to the National Vaccine Injury Compensation Program. Arthritis Rheum 39:1529, 1996

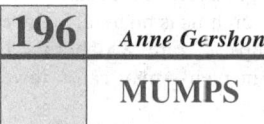

196   *Anne Gershon*

MUMPS

DEFINITION   Mumps is an acute, systemic, communicable viral infection whose most distinctive feature is swelling of one or both parotid glands. Involvement of other salivary glands, the meninges, the pancreas, and the gonads is also common.

ETIOLOGIC AGENT   Mumps virus, a paramyxovirus, is pleomorphic and has a diameter ranging from 100 to 600 nm. The virion is composed of RNA and five proteins. The RNA is surrounded by an envelope with glycoprotein projections. There are two envelope glycoproteins—a hemagglutinin-neuraminidase (HN) and a hemolysis cell fusion antigen (F)—as well as a matrix envelope protein (M). There are two internal components: a nucleocapsid protein (NP) and an RNA polymerase protein. There is only one antigenic type of mumps virus.

EPIDEMIOLOGY   After the introduction of mumps vaccine in 1967, the incidence of clinical mumps declined significantly in the United States. In 1968 (before widespread immunization), 185,691 cases of mumps were reported in this country. The 906 cases reported in 1995 represent a reduction in the number of cases by >99% from prevaccine levels; this is the lowest number of cases ever reported in a year. Before widespread vaccination, the incidence of mumps was highest in the winter and spring, with epidemics every 2 to 5 years. At that time, mumps was principally a disease of childhood, although today more than 50% of cases occur in young adults. Epidemics tended to occur in confined populations, such as those in schools and the military services.

The incubation period of mumps generally ranges from 14 to 18 days, with extremes of 7 and 23 days. However, because a contact may be shedding virus before the onset of clinical disease or (like one-third of patients) may have subclinical infection, the incubation period in individual cases is often uncertain. One attack of mumps usually confers lifelong immunity. Long-term immunity is also associated with immunization.

PATHOGENESIS   Mumps virus is transmitted by droplet nuclei, saliva, and fomites. Replication of the virus in the epithelium of the upper respiratory tract leads to viremia, which is followed by infection of glandular tissues and/or the central nervous system (CNS).

Little is known of the pathology of mumps since the disease is rarely fatal. The affected glands contain perivascular and interstitial mononuclear cell infiltrates with prominent edema. Necrosis of acinar and epithelial duct cells is evident in the salivary glands and in the germinal epithelium of the seminiferous tubules.

CLINICAL MANIFESTATIONS   The prodrome of mumps consists of fever, malaise, myalgia, and anorexia. Parotitis, if it develops, usually does so within the next 24 h but may be delayed for as long as a week; it is generally bilateral, although the onset on the two sides may not be synchronous and at times only one side is affected. The submaxillary and sublingual glands are involved less often than the parotid and are almost never involved alone. Swelling of the parotid is accompanied by tenderness and obliteration of the space between the ear lobe and the angle of the mandible. The patient frequently reports an earache and finds it difficult to eat, swallow, or talk. Glandular swelling increases for a few days and then gradually subsides, disappearing within a week. The orifice of Stensen's duct is commonly red and swollen. Presternal pitting edema has been described in about 5% of mumps cases, often in association with submandibular adenitis.

Other than parotitis, orchitis is the most common manifestation of mumps among postpubertal males, developing in about 20% of cases. The testis is painful and tender and is enlarged to several times its normal size; accompanying fever is common. Later, testicular atrophy develops in half of the affected men. Since orchitis is bilateral in fewer than 15% of cases, sterility after mumps is rare. Oophoritis in women—far less common than orchitis in men—may cause lower abdominal pain but does not lead to sterility.

Aseptic meningitis, which may develop before, during, after, or in the absence of parotitis, is a common manifestation of mumps in both children and adults. Symptoms include stiff neck, headache, and drowsiness. Pleocytosis of the cerebrospinal fluid (CSF), with up to 1000 cells/μL, may develop in up to 50% of cases of clinical mumps, but clinical signs of meningeal irritation are documented in only 5 to 25% of cases. Within the first 24 h, polymorphonuclear leukocytes may predominate in CSF, but by the second day nearly all the cells are lymphocytes. The glucose level in CSF may be abnormally low, and this finding may arouse suspicion of bacterial meningitis. Aseptic meningitis due to mumps without parotitis is indistinguishable clinically from that caused by other viruses. Mumps meningitis is almost invariably self-limited, although cranial nerve palsies have occasionally led to permanent sequelae, particularly deafness. More rarely, mumps virus may cause encephalitis, which presents as high fever with marked changes in the level of consciousness and frequently results in permanent sequelae in survivors. Other CNS problems occasionally associated with mumps include cerebellar ataxia, facial palsy, transverse myelitis, Guillain-Barré syndrome, and aqueductal stenosis leading to hydrocephalus.

Mumps pancreatitis, which may present as abdominal pain, is difficult to diagnose because an elevated serum amylase level can be associated with either parotitis or pancreatitis. Other unusual complications of mumps include myocarditis, mastitis, thyroiditis, nephritis, arthritis, and thrombocytopenic purpura. An excessive number of spontaneous abortions are associated with gestational mumps when the disease occurs during the first trimester. Mumps in pregnancy does not lead to premature birth or fetal malformations.

DIFFERENTIAL DIAGNOSIS The diagnosis of mumps is made easily in patients with acute bilateral parotitis and a history of recent exposure. When parotitis is unilateral or absent or when sites other than the parotid gland are involved, laboratory diagnosis is required (see below).

The myriad causes of bilateral parotid swelling other than mumps virus include infection with other viruses, such as parainfluenza virus type 3, coxsackieviruses, and influenza A virus; metabolic diseases, such as diabetes mellitus and uremia; and drugs, such as phenylbutazone and thiouracil. Unilateral parotid swelling can result from a tumor, a cyst, or a ductal obstruction due to stones or strictures. Other conditions associated with chronic parotid swelling include sarcoidosis, Sjögren's syndrome, and infection with HIV. Suppurative parotitis, usually caused by *Staphylococcus aureus*, is most often unilateral.

Other entities should be considered when manifestations consistent with mumps appear in organs other than the parotid. Testicular torsion may produce a painful scrotal mass resembling that seen in mumps orchitis. Other viruses (e.g., enteroviruses) may cause aseptic

meningitis that is clinically indistinguishable from that due to mumps virus.

LABORATORY DIAGNOSIS Mumps virus is readily isolated after inoculation of appropriate clinical specimens into a variety of host systems, such as rhesus monkey kidney cells and human embryonic lung fibroblasts. The virus can be rapidly identified by the use of cells grown in shell vials and of fluorescein-labeled monoclonal antibodies. Mumps virus may be recovered from saliva, throat, and urine during the first few days of illness and from the CSF of patients with mumps meningitis. Shedding of virus in the urine may persist for as long as 2 weeks. No particular peripheral blood cell count is characteristic of mumps.

Highly sensitive enzyme-linked immunosorbent assays are useful for diagnosis of mumps and for determination of susceptibility to the disease. Acute mumps can be diagnosed either by the examination of acute- and convalescent-phase sera for a significant increase in IgG antibody titer or by the demonstration of specific IgM in one serum specimen. Use of a skin-test antigen to assess immunity to mumps has been replaced by serologic testing.

PREVENTION Live attenuated mumps vaccine (Jeryl Lynn strain) induces antibodies that protect against infection in more than 95% of cases. The subcutaneously administered vaccine may be given to children older than 1 year but is not recommended for younger infants because of the potential for interference by passive maternal antibodies. Mumps vaccine is usually administered as part of the measles-mumps-rubella (MMR) vaccine at the age of 12 to 15 months and again at 4 to 12 years of age. This MMR vaccine is also recommended for susceptible older children, adolescents, and adults, particularly adolescent males who have not had mumps. For these patients, either MMR or monovalent mumps vaccine may be given; two doses are preferred. Inadvertent immunization of individuals who are already immune is not associated with significant adverse reactions. Mumps vaccine is not recommended for pregnant women, for patients receiving glucocorticoids, or for other immunocompromised hosts. However, children with HIV infection who are not severely immunocompromised can safely be immunized against mumps; MMR vaccine is usually used for this purpose (Chap. 194).

R̲x̲ **TREATMENT** Therapy for parotitis and other manifestations of mumps is symptom-based. The administration of analgesics and the application of warm or cold compresses to the parotid area may be helpful. Mumps immune globulin is of no value in the prophylaxis or treatment of established disease. Testicular pain may be minimized by the local application of cold compresses and gentle support for the scrotum. Anesthetic blocks may also be used. Neither the administration of glucocorticoids nor incision of the tunica albuginea is of proven value for the treatment of severe orchitis. Anecdotal information on a small number of patients with orchitis suggests that administration of interferon α may be helpful.

BIBLIOGRAPHY

BROWN E et al: The Urabe AM9 mumps vaccine is a mixture of viruses differing at amino acid 335 of the hemagglutinin-neuraminidase gene with one form associated with disease. J Infect Dis 174:619, 1996

CENTERS FOR DISEASE CONTROL AND PREVENTION: Update on adult immunization: Recommendations of the Immunization Practices Advisory Committee (ACIP). MMWR 40:22, 1991

———: Measles, mumps, and rubella—vaccine use and strategies for elimination of measles, rubella, and congenital rubella syndrome and control of mumps. MMWR 47:1, 1998

CHAUDARY S et al: Fulminant mumps myocarditis. Ann Intern Med 110:569, 1989

GUT JP et al: Symptomatic mumps reinfections. J Med Virol 45:17, 1995

HAREL L et al: Mumps arthritis in children. Pediatr Infect Dis J 9:928, 1990

HERSH BS et al: Mumps outbreak in a highly vaccinated population. J Pediatr 119:187, 1991

LYON RP et al: Mumps epididymo-orchitis: Treatment by anesthetic block of the spermatic cord. JAMA 196:736, 1966

MCDONALD JC et al: Clinical and epidemiologic features of mumps encephalitis and possible causes of vaccine-related disease. Pediatr Infect Dis J 8:751, 1989

RUTHER U et al: Successful interferon-alpha 2 therapy for a patient with acute mumps orchitis. Eur Urol 27:174, 1995

RABIES VIRUS AND OTHER RHABDOVIRUSES

RABIES VIRUS

DEFINITION Rabies is an acute viral disease of the central nervous system (CNS) that affects all mammals and that is transmitted by infected secretions, usually saliva. Most exposures to rabies are through the bite of an infected animal, but on occasion contact with a virus-containing aerosol or the ingestion or transplantation of infected tissues may initiate the disease process.

ETIOLOGY The rabies virus is a bullet-shaped, enveloped, single-stranded RNA virus that is 75 to 80 nm in diameter and belongs to the genus *Lyssavirus* within the rhabdovirus family. The envelope glycoproteins of rabies viruses are arranged in knoblike structures that cover the surface of the virion. Genetic and phenotypic analyses of the envelope have been used to detail the molecular epidemiology and spread of unique variants within animal species. The viral glycoproteins bind to acetylcholine receptors, contribute to the neurovirulence of rabies virus, elicit neutralizing and hemagglutination-inhibiting antibodies, and stimulate cytotoxic T cell immunity. The nucleocapsid antigen induces a complement-fixing antibody as well as T helper cell reactivity. Neutralizing antibodies to the surface glycoproteins appear to be protective and are directed at conformational epitopes of the viral envelope glycoprotein. The antibodies to rabies virus used in diagnostic immunofluorescence assays are generally directed against the nucleocapsid antigens. Isolates of rabies virus from different animal species and locales differ in their antigenic and biologic properties. These variations may account for differences in virulence between isolates. Interferon is induced by rabies virus, particularly in those tissues with high virus concentrations, and may play some role in retarding progressive infection.

EPIDEMIOLOGY Rabies is found in animals in all regions of the world except Australasia and Antarctica. Rabies exists in two epidemiologic forms: *urban rabies*, propagated chiefly by unimmunized domestic dogs and cats, and *sylvatic rabies*, propagated by skunks, foxes, raccoons, mongooses, wolves, and bats. Infection in domestic animals usually represents a "spillover" from sylvatic reservoirs of infection. Human infection occurs through contact with unimmunized domestic animals or from exposure to wild animals in locales where rabies is enzootic or epizootic. The worldwide incidence of rabies is estimated at more than 30,000 cases per year. Southeast Asia, the Philippines, Africa, the Indian subcontinent, and tropical South America are areas where the disease is especially common. In some endemic areas, 1 to 2% of autopsies yield evidence of rabies. Increased spread of terrestrial rabies (i.e., rabies in animals that walk on the ground rather than rabies in animals that fly) and increased travel to countries where urban rabies exists have made the recognition of clinical rabies and its prevention of increasing importance. While focal epidemics of terrestrial rabies have occurred in the United States and Europe, human rabies is uncommon, largely because of successful domestic-animal vaccination programs. Since 1980, 36 human cases of rabies have been diagnosed in the United States; 58% of these cases were associated with exposure to bats, while one-third were acquired through dog bites sustained outside the United States. Most persons with proven clinical rabies in this country report no history of an animal bite. More than one-third of recent cases have been diagnosed post-mortem.

In most areas of the world, the dog is the most important vector of rabies virus for humans. However, the wolf (in eastern Europe and Arctic regions), the mongoose (in South Africa and the Caribbean), the fox (in western Europe), and the vampire bat (in Latin America) may also be prominent vectors. Although rabies in wildlife is common throughout both the developed and the undeveloped world, most cases of postexposure prophylaxis are associated with domesticated animals such as dogs and cats. In the United States, local governments are charged with initiating and maintaining programs for rabies vaccination of all dogs, cats, and ferrets. Rodents and lagomorphs are rarely infected with rabies virus. Several cases of human-to-human transmission of rabies through corneal transplantation have also been documented. Bite and nonbite exposures to infected humans could theoretically transmit rabies. Because of delayed diagnosis, postexposure prophylaxis of health care workers and close contacts of cases is common.

PATHOGENESIS The first event in rabies is the introduction of live virus through the epidermis or onto a mucous membrane. Initial viral replication appears to occur within striated muscle cells at the site of inoculation. The peripheral nervous system is exposed at the neuromuscular and/or neurotendinous spindles of unmyelinated sensory nerve cell endings. The virus then spreads centripetally up the nerve to the CNS, probably via peripheral nerve axoplasm, at a rate of ~3 mm/h. Viremia has been documented in experimental conditions but is thought not to play a role in naturally acquired disease. Once the virus reaches the CNS, it replicates almost exclusively within the gray matter and then passes centrifugally along autonomic nerves to other tissues—the salivary glands, adrenal medulla, kidneys, lungs, liver, skeletal muscles, skin, and heart. Passage of the virus into the salivary glands and viral replication in mucinogenic acinar cells facilitate further transmission via infected saliva. The incubation period of rabies is exceedingly variable, ranging from 7 days to >1 year (mean, 1 to 2 months) and apparently depending on the amount of virus introduced, the amount of tissue involved, host defense mechanisms, and the actual distance that the virus has to travel from the site of inoculation to the CNS. Rates of infection and mortality are highest from bites on the face, intermediate from bites on the hands and arms, and lowest from bites on the legs. Cases of human rabies with an extended incubation period (2 to 7 years) have been reported, but they are rare. Host immune responses and viral strains also influence disease expression.

The neuropathology of rabies resembles that of other viral diseases of the CNS: hyperemia, varying degrees of chromatolysis, nuclear pyknosis, and neuronophagia of the nerve cells; infiltration by lymphocytes and plasma cells of the Virchow-Robin space; microglial infiltration; and parenchymal areas of nerve cell destruction. In experimental animal models, adenohypophyseal infection with rabies virus, with reduction in growth hormone and vasopressin release, is common. The most characteristic pathologic finding of rabies in the CNS is the formation of cytoplasmic inclusions called *Negri bodies* within neurons. Each eosinophilic mass measures ~10 nm and is made up of a finely fibrillar matrix and rabies virus particles. Negri bodies are distributed throughout the brain, particularly in Ammon's horn, the cerebral cortex, the brainstem, the hypothalamus, the Purkinje cells of the cerebellum, and the dorsal spinal ganglia. Negri bodies are not demonstrated in at least 20% of cases of rabies, and their absence from brain material does not rule out the diagnosis.

CLINICAL MANIFESTATIONS The clinical manifestations of rabies can be divided into four stages: (1) a nonspecific prodrome, (2) an acute encephalitis similar to other viral encephalitides, (3) a profound dysfunction of brainstem centers that produces the classic features of rabies encephalitis, and (4) death or, in rare cases, recovery.

The prodromal period usually lasts 1 to 4 days and is marked by fever, headache, malaise, myalgias, increased fatigability, anorexia, nausea and vomiting, sore throat, and a nonproductive cough. The prodromal symptom suggestive of rabies is the complaint of paresthesia and/or fasciculations at or around the site of inoculation of virus. These sensations, which may be related to the multiplication of virus in the dorsal root ganglion of the sensory nerve supplying the area of the bite, are reported by 50 to 80% of patients.

The encephalitic phase is usually ushered in by periods of excessive motor activity, excitation, and agitation. Confusion, hallucinations, combativeness, bizarre aberrations of thought, muscle spasms, meningismus, opisthotonic posturing, seizures, and focal paralysis soon appear. Characteristically, the periods of mental aberration are interspersed with completely lucid periods, but as the disease progresses the lucid periods get shorter until the patient lapses into coma. Hyperesthesia, with excessive sensitivity to bright light, loud noise, touch, and even gentle breezes, is very common. On physical examination, the temperature may be found to be as high as 40.6°C (105°F). Abnormalities of the autonomic nervous system include dilated irregular pupils; increased lacrimation, salivation, and perspiration; and postural hypotension. Evidence of upper motor neuron paralysis, with weakness, increased deep tendon reflexes, and extensor plantar responses, is the rule. Paralysis of the vocal cords is common. Unfortunately, the presenting signs and symptoms of rabies are indistinguishable from those of other viral and neurologic diseases. Thus delays in diagnosis are frequent. The presence of hydrophobia or aerophobia (seen in about two-thirds of recent cases) increases the likelihood of antemortem diagnosis.

The manifestations of brainstem dysfunction begin shortly after the onset of the encephalitic phase. Cranial nerve involvement causes diplopia, facial palsies, optic neuritis, and the characteristic difficulty with deglutition. The combination of excessive salivation and difficulty in swallowing produces the traditional picture of "foaming at the mouth." Hydrophobia, the painful, violent, involuntary contraction of the diaphragmatic, accessory respiratory, pharyngeal, and laryngeal muscles initiated by swallowing liquids, is seen in ~50% of cases. Involvement of the amygdaloid nucleus may result in priapism and spontaneous ejaculation. The patient lapses into coma, and involvement of the respiratory center produces an apneic death. The prominence of early brainstem dysfunction distinguishes rabies from other viral encephalitides and accounts for the rapid downhill course. The median period of survival after the onset of symptoms is 4 days, with a maximum of 20 days, unless artificial supportive measures are instituted.

If intensive respiratory support is used, a number of late complications may appear. These include inappropriate secretion of antidiuretic hormone, diabetes insipidus, cardiac arrhythmias, vascular instability, adult respiratory distress syndrome, gastrointestinal bleeding, thrombocytopenia, and paralytic ileus. Recovery is very rare and, when it occurs, gradual.

Rabies may also present as an ascending paralysis resembling the Landry/Guillain-Barré syndrome (dumb rabies, *rage tranquille*). Initially, this clinical pattern was reported most frequently among persons given postexposure rabies prophylaxis after being bitten by vampire bats. Paralytic rabies also occurs in Southeast Asia among persons with canine exposures.

The difficulty of diagnosing rabies associated with ascending paralysis is illustrated by cases of person-to-person transmission of the virus by tissue transplantation. Corneal transplants from donors who died of presumed Landry/Guillain-Barré syndrome produced clinical rabies in and caused the deaths of the recipients. Retrospective pathologic examinations of the brains of recipients demonstrated Negri bodies, and rabies virus was subsequently isolated from each donor's frozen eye.

LABORATORY FINDINGS Early in the disease, hemoglobin values and routine blood chemistry results are normal; abnormalities develop as hypothalamic dysfunction, gastrointestinal bleeding, and other complications ensue. The peripheral white blood cell count is usually slightly elevated (12,000 to 17,000/μL) but may be normal or as high as 30,000/μL.

The specific diagnosis of rabies depends on (1) the isolation of virus from infected secretions [saliva or, rarely, cerebrospinal fluid (CSF)] or tissue (brain), (2) the serologic demonstration of acute infection, (3) the detection of viral antigen in infected tissue (e.g., corneal impression smears, skin biopsies, or brain), or (4) the detection of viral nucleic acid (RNA) by polymerase chain reaction (PCR). A reference laboratory evaluating antemortem samples can confirm rabies with high sensitivity and specificity. Isolation of virus from saliva,

demonstration of viral nucleic acid in saliva, or detection of viral antigen in a nuchal skin biopsy specimen is most sensitive. Examination of corneal epithelium specimens appears less sensitive. In the unvaccinated person, demonstration of rabies antibodies in serum or CSF may be useful, although such antibodies may not appear until late in the course of disease. Samples of brain obtained at postmortem examination or brain biopsy should be subjected to (1) mouse inoculation studies for virus isolation, (2) fluorescent antibody (FA) staining for viral antigen, and (3) histologic and/or electron microscopic examination for Negri bodies or reverse transcription PCR for rabies virus RNA.

Postexposure rabies prophylaxis rarely elicits CSF neutralizing antibody to rabies virus. If present after prophylaxis, such antibody is usually found at a low titer (<1:64), whereas CSF titers in human rabies may vary from 1:200 to 1:160,000.

DIFFERENTIAL DIAGNOSIS There is little to distinguish rabies from other viral encephalitides. The most helpful clue to the diagnosis is a history of a bite or other salivary exposure to a potentially infected animal. As bite exposures are infrequent among U.S. cases, a history of relatively recent travel to a rabies-endemic area should be sought. Other problems to be considered in the differential diagnosis include hysterical reactions to animal bites (pseudohydrophobia), Landry/Guillain-Barré syndrome, poliomyelitis, and allergic encephalomyelitis developing in response to rabies vaccine; this last problem is usually associated with receipt of nerve tissue–derived vaccine and usually begins 1 to 4 weeks after vaccination.

℞ **TREATMENT Postexposure Prophylaxis** (See Fig. 197-1) Although rabies among humans is rare in the United States, each year ~35,000 persons receive postexposure prophylaxis. The decision to initiate postexposure prophylaxis should include the following considerations: (1) whether the individual came into physical contact with saliva or another substance likely to contain rabies virus, (2) whether rabies is known or suspected in the species and area associated with

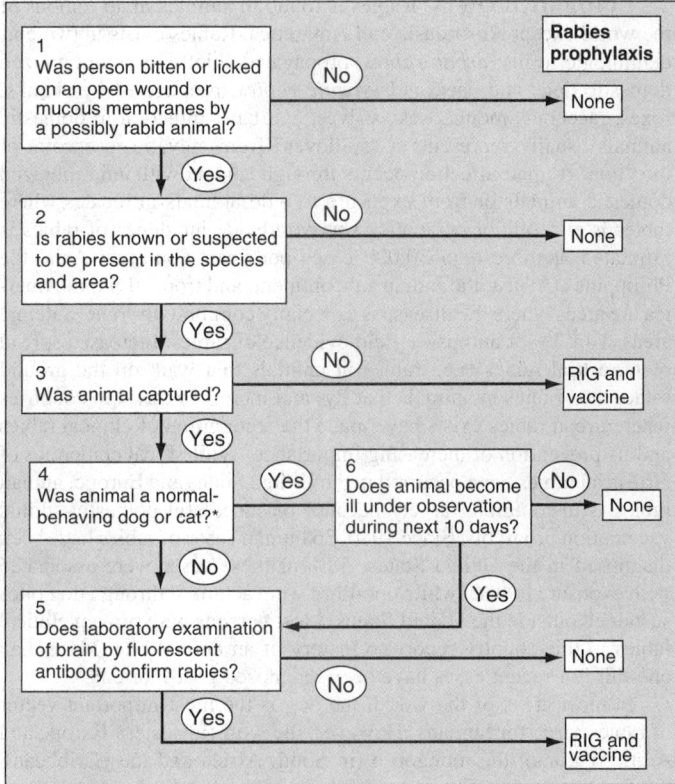

FIGURE 197-1 Postexposure rabies prophylaxis algorithm. *Instances of exposure to livestock or to normal-behaving, unvaccinated dogs or cats should be considered individually, and local and state public health officials should be consulted.

the exposure (e.g., all persons within the continental United States bitten by a bat that escapes should receive postexposure prophylaxis), and (3) the circumstances surrounding the exposure (e.g., whether the bite was provoked or unprovoked). Bites associated with the feeding of an animal are considered to have been provoked.

If rabies is known or suspected to be present in the animal species involved in a human exposure, the implicated animal should be captured if possible. Any wild animal involved in a rabies exposure; any ill, unvaccinated, or stray domestic animal involved in a rabies exposure; and any animal inflicting an unprovoked bite, exhibiting abnormal behavior, or suspected of being rabid should be humanely killed. The animal's head should be sent immediately to an appropriate laboratory for rabies FA examination. If examination of the brain by the FA technique gives negative results, it can be assumed that the saliva contains no virus, and the exposed person need not be treated. Persons exposed to wild animals that subsequently escape, that are capable of carrying rabies (bats, skunks, coyotes, foxes, raccoons, etc.), and that inhabit an area where rabies is known or suspected to be present should undergo both passive and active immunization against rabies (see below) as soon as possible after exposure.

In an area in which feline or canine rabies is not prevalent, a healthy biting dog, cat, or ferret can be confined and observed for 10 days. Persons in such an area should not begin a course of prophylaxis unless the animal develops clinical signs of rabies. If the animal becomes ill or behaves abnormally during the observation period, it should be killed for FA examination. Experimental and epidemiologic evidence suggests that animals that remain healthy for 10 days after a bite will not have transmitted rabies virus at the time of the bite. In areas of high endemicity for canine rabies, immediate examination of the animal's brain, especially in the case of a severe bite, may be warranted. Bites of rodents, rabbits, and hares almost never require antirabies postexposure prophylaxis. Unless the exposed person can rule out a bite, scratch, or mucous membrane exposure, postexposure prophylaxis should be considered after direct contact between a human and a bat.

Postexposure prophylaxis of rabies includes rigorous cleansing and treatment of the wound and the administration of rabies vaccine together with antirabies immunoglobulin. Postexposure prophylaxis should be initiated as soon as possible after exposure. As the incubation period of rabies is quite variable, postexposure prophylaxis should be begun as long as clinical signs of rabies are not present.

1. *Wound cleansing and treatment.* Thorough cleansing and treatment of the bite wound constitute an important component of rabies prevention. The wound should be scrubbed with soap and then flushed with water. Both mechanical cleansing and chemical cleansing are important. Quaternary ammonium compounds such as 1 to 4% benzalkonium chloride, 1% cetrimonium bromide, or povidone-iodine solutions should be utilized. Tetanus toxoid and antibiotic prophylaxis should be administered as needed.

2. *Passive immunization with antirabies antiserum of either equine or human origin.* Postexposure antirabies vaccination should include the administration of both passive antibody and vaccine, except when the individual has previously received preexposure prophylaxis. Human rabies immune globulin (RIG) is preferred because equine antiserum may cause serum sickness. RIG is administered only once, at the beginning of the postexposure prophylaxis regimen. The recommended dose of RIG is 20 IU/kg. The dose of equine antiserum is 40 units/kg. The full dose should be thoroughly infiltrated into the area around the wound and into the wound itself. Any remaining portion of the dose is injected intramuscularly at a site distant from the vaccine.

3. *Active immunization with antirabies vaccine.* Three rabies vaccines are available in the United States: (1) human diploid cell vaccine (HDCV), which can be given either intramuscularly or intradermally; (2) rabies vaccine absorbed (RVA); and (3) purified chick embryo cell vaccine. The latter two vaccines are administered intramuscularly. Each vaccine is derived from a different strain of rabies virus and prepared in a slightly different formulation. The three vac-

cines are considered equally efficacious and safe, and any of the three can be administered in conjunction with RIG. Five 1-mL doses of HDCV are given intramuscularly, preferably in the deltoid or anterolateral thigh area: the gluteal area should not be utilized. The five doses of HDCV should be administered within 28 days on the following schedule: days 0, 3, 7, 14, and 28. The World Health Organization also recommends 21- and 90-day injections. Severe reactions to these vaccines are uncommon. Immediate hypersensitivity responses, such as urticaria, have been reported in ~1 of every 650 recipients. Systemic reactions, such as fever, headache, and nausea, are generally mild and are reported in 1 to 4% of recipients. Local reactions, such as swelling, erythema, and induration at the injection site, occur in 15 to 20% of vaccinees. Guillain-Barré syndrome has been reported but appears to be quite rare.

In the developing world, several other effective rabies vaccines have been licensed and used extensively. They include vaccines made in chick embryonic cells, primary hamster cells, Vero cells, and duck embryonic cells. As some of these preparations are somewhat less immunogenic than the vaccines approved by the U.S. Food and Drug Administration (FDA), evaluation of serum antibodies after immunization is suggested by some authorities.

The combination of RIG and HDCV elicits high titers of neutralizing antibodies in almost all recipients. Only rarely has this regimen proved unsuccessful in preventing the development of rabies. None of the patients in whom rabies was diagnosed in the United States between 1980 and 1996 had received postexposure prophylaxis. Administration of vaccine alone appears to be associated with a higher failure rate than use of the combination, especially in severe bite exposures. Because of cost, postexposure prophylaxis consisting of intradermal injections of rabies vaccine is being used increasingly in the developing world. The combination of RIG plus 0.1-mL intradermal doses of HDCV at eight sites on day 0, four sites on day 7, and one site on days 28 and 91 produces good antibody responses and has had excellent clinical results. Alternatively, the World Health Organization has approved a regimen of two 0.1-mL doses at two intradermal sites on days 0, 3, and 7 and a 0.1-mL intradermal injection at a single site on days 21 and 90. The FDA has not approved the intradermal route for postexposure prophylaxis.

Preexposure Prophylaxis   Individuals at high risk of contact with rabies virus, including veterinarians, cave explorers, laboratory workers, and animal handlers, should receive preexposure prophylaxis with rabies vaccine. Three 1-mL intramuscular or three 0.1-mL intradermal injections of HDCV on days 0, 7, and 21 or 28 should be administered. Concomitant chloroquine administration interferes with the antibody response to rabies vaccine. Depending on the level of risk, serologic testing should be done at 6-month to 2-year intervals.

An immune complex reaction consisting of urticaria, arthralgia, arthritis, angioedema, and systemic symptoms has been reported in up to 6% of persons receiving intramuscular booster doses of HDCV. This reaction is self-limited and appears to be associated with the presence of β-propiolactone-altered human serum albumin in the vaccine and the development of IgE antibodies to this antigen.

Persons who work in high-risk areas should undergo periodic measurement of antibodies. When neutralizing titers fall below 1:5, booster doses should be given. Booster doses may be administered as a single 1-mL intramuscular or 0.1-mL intradermal injection. Postexposure prophylaxis in individuals previously given preexposure prophylaxis consists of two intramuscular doses of HDCV on days 0 and 3. RIG is not given in these situations.

MOKOLA VIRUS

Mokola virus was first isolated from wild shrews captured in Nigeria and was shown to be related morphologically and serologically to rabies virus. The subsequent isolation of the virus from cats in South Africa suggested a wider prevalence of the agent than had previously

NOAH DL et al: Epidemiology of human rabies in the United States, 1980 to 1996. Ann Intern Med 128:922, 1998

PAPE WS et al: Risk for rabies transmission from encounters with bats, Colorado 1977–1996. Emerg Infect Dis 5:433, 1999

SMITH JS: New aspects of rabies with emphasis on epidemiology, diagnosis, and prevention of the disease in the United States. Clin Microbiol Rev 9:166, 1996

STRADY A et al: Antibody persistence following preexposure regimens of cell-culture rabies vaccines: 10-year follow-up and proposal for a new booster policy. J Infect Dis 177:1290, 1998

TANTAWICHIEN T et al: Antibody response after a far site intradermal booster vaccination with cell culture rabies vaccine. Clin Infect Dis 28:1100, 1999

been expected. Only two cases of clinical infection have been reported; both were in children. One patient had a nonfatal illness characterized by fever, pharyngitis, and convulsions; Mokola virus was recovered from CSF. In the second patient, fever with cough and vomiting was followed within several days by drowsiness, confusion, and generalized flaccid weakness. The CSF was normal. The patient progressed to deep coma and died within 10 days of onset. Mokola virus was isolated from the brain, and examination of histopathologic sections revealed finely granular cytoplasmic inclusions that were distinguishable from Negri bodies in many neurons.

VESICULAR STOMATITIS VIRUS

Vesicular stomatitis is a viral illness of animals that occasionally affects humans. It presents as an acute, self-limited, influenza-like disease. The disease in animals is found in the United States and South America and affects chiefly domestic cattle, horses, swine, wild deer, raccoons, skunks, and bobcats.

In animals, vesicular stomatitis is characterized by the development of vesicles on the oral mucosa, particularly the tongue; the udders; and the heels. The mode of spread is probably by direct contact; however, epidemics tend to occur in warm weather, and isolation of the virus from *Phlebotomus* sandflies in Panama and *Aedes* species in New Mexico suggests that these insects may be vectors. Two distinct serotypes, New Jersey and Indiana, have been recognized, and most outbreaks in North America have been attributed to the New Jersey strain.

In humans, vesicular stomatitis is most common among laboratory workers. In one report, three-fourths of laboratory personnel handling experimentally infected animals or manipulating the virus developed neutralizing antibodies. The disease is also transmissible, however, under natural conditions among workers having direct contact with infected animals, especially cattle. An incubation period ranging from 1 to 6 days is followed by the sudden onset of fever [with temperatures of up to 40°C (104°F)], chills, profuse sweating, myalgias, malaise, headache, and pain on ocular movement. One-third to one-half of patients have a sore throat and cervical and/or submandibular adenopathy. Small raised vesicular lesions may appear on the buccal mucosa. Conjunctivitis and coryza are evident in ~20% of cases. Occasionally, small subcorneal, intraepithelial vesicles appear on the fingers, usually in association with direct inoculation of the virus. Symptoms generally last 3 to 4 days, but occasionally the course is diphasic. Inapparent infection is common: among laboratory workers with serologic evidence of infection, only about one-half report symptoms. In some areas of Panama, 17 to 35% of the population have neutralizing antibodies to vesicular stomatitis virus.

The differential diagnosis includes hand-foot-and-mouth disease, herpangina, primary herpetic pharyngitis and other mucocutaneous syndromes, and influenza. The virus is not commonly isolated from patients. However, a rise in titer of complement-fixation and/or neutralizing antibody to vesicular stomatitis virus between acute- and convalescent-phase sera helps to confirm the diagnosis. Treatment is nonspecific.

BIBLIOGRAPHY

ADVISORY COMMITTEE ON IMMUNIZATION PRACTICES (ACIP): Human rabies prevention—United States, 1999. MMWR 48:RR-1,1999

Case records of the MGH 21-1998: A 32-year-old woman with pharyngeal spasms and paresthesia after a dog bite. N Engl J Med 339:105, 1998

Compendium of animal rabies control 1999. MMWR 48:RR-31-9, 1999

DIETZSCHOLD B et al: Human diploid cell culture rabies vaccine (HDCV) and purified chick embryo cell culture (PCEC) both confer protective immunity against infection with the silver fixed rabies virus strain (SH BRV). Vaccine 16:1656, 1998

FISHBEIN DB, ROBINSON LE: Current concepts. Rabies. N Engl J Med 329:1632, 1993

JAVADI MA et al: Transmission of rabies by corneal graft. Cornea 15:431, 1996

| **198** | *C. J. Peters* |

INFECTIONS CAUSED BY ARTHROPOD- AND RODENT-BORNE VIRUSES

Most viral infections that come to medical attention in office or hospital practice in the developed countries are caused by viruses that can be latent in the human host, such as the herpesviruses, or by viruses that are continuously transmitted among humans, such as measles virus, influenza virus, and HIV. However, some other viruses are transmitted in nature without regard to humans and only incidentally infect and produce disease in humans; in addition, a few agents are regularly spread among humans by arthropods. Most of these viruses either are maintained by arthropods or chronically infect rodents. Obviously, the mode of transmission is not a rational basis for taxonomic classification. Indeed, zoonotic viruses from at least seven virus families act as significant human pathogens (Table 198-1). The virus families differ fundamentally from one another in terms of morphology, replication mechanisms, and genetics. Information on a virus's membership in a family or genus is enlightening with regard to maintenance strategies, sensitivity to antivirals, and some aspects of pathogenesis but does not necessarily predict which clinical syndromes—if any—the virus will cause in humans.

FAMILIES OF ARTHROPOD- AND RODENT-BORNE VIRUSES The Arenaviridae The Arenaviridae are spherical, 110- to 130-nm particles that bud from the cell's plasma membrane and utilize ambisense RNA genomes with two segments for replication. There are two main phylogenetic branches of Arenaviridae: the Old World viruses, such as Lassa fever and lymphocytic choriomeningitis (LCM) viruses, and the New World viruses, including those causing the South American hemorrhagic fevers (HFs). Arenaviruses persist in nature by chronically infecting rodents with a striking one-virus–one-rodent species relationship. These rodent infections result in long-term virus excretion and perhaps in lifelong viremia; vertical infection is common with some arenaviruses. Humans become infected through the inhalation of aerosols containing arenaviruses, which are then deposited in the terminal air passages, and probably also through close contact with rodents and their excreta, which results in the contamination of mucous membranes or breaks in the skin.

The Bunyaviridae The family Bunyaviridae includes four medically significant genera. All of these spherical viruses have three negative-sense RNA segments maturing into 90- to 120-nm particles in the Golgi complex and exiting the cell by exocytosis. Viruses of the genus *Bunyavirus* are largely mosquito-borne and have a viremic vertebrate intermediate host; many are also transovarially transmitted in their specific mosquito host. One serologic group also uses biting midges as vectors. Sandflies or mosquitoes are the vectors for the genus *Phlebovirus* (named after phlebotomus fever or sandfly fever, the best-known disease associated with the genus), while ticks serve as vectors for the genus *Nairovirus*. Viruses of both of these genera are also associated with vertical transmission in the arthropod host and with horizontal spread through viremic vertebrate hosts. The genus

Table 198-1 Major Zoonotic Virus Families and Some Characteristics of Typical Members

Family	Genus or Group	Syndrome(s): Typical Viruses	Maintenance Strategy
Arenaviridae	Old World complex	FM, E: Lymphocytic choriomeningitis virus HF: Lassa fever virus	Chronic infection of rodents, often with persistent viremia; vertical transmission common
	New World or Tacaribe complex	HF: South American HF viruses (Machupo, Junin, Guanarito, Sabia)	Chronic infection of rodents, sometimes with persistent viremia; vertical infection may occur
Bunyaviridae	*Bunyavirus*	E: California serogroup viruses (La Crosse, Jamestown Canyon, California encephalitis)	Mosquito-vertebrate cycle; transovarial transmission in mosquito common
		FM: Bunyamwera, group C, Tahyna viruses	
		FM: Oropouche virus	Transmitted by *Culicoides*
	Phlebovirus	FM: Sandfly fever, Toscana viruses	Sandfly transmission between vertebrates, with prominent transovarial component in sandfly
		FM: Punta Toro virus	
		HF, FM, E: Rift Valley fever virus	Mosquito-vertebrate transmission, with transovarial component in mosquito
	Nairovirus	HF: Crimean Congo HF virus	Tick-vertebrate, with transovarial transmission in tick
	Hantavirus	HF: Hantaan, Dobrava, Puumala viruses	Rodent reservoir; chronic virus shedding, but chronic viremia unknown
		HF: Sin Nombre and related hantaviruses	Sigmodontine rodent reservoir
Filoviridae*a*		HF: Marburg viruses, Ebola viruses (4 subtypes)	Unknown
Flaviviridae	*Flavivirus* (mosquito-borne)	HF: Yellow fever virus	Mosquito-vertebrate; transovarial rare
		FM, HF: Dengue viruses (4 subtypes)	
		E: St. Louis, Japanese, West Nile, and Murray Valley encephalitis viruses; Rocio viruses	
	Flavivirus (tick-borne)	E: Central European tick-borne encephalitis, Russian spring-summer encephalitis, Powassan viruses	Tick-vertebrate
		HF: Omsk HF, Kyasanur Forest disease viruses	
Reoviridae	*Coltivirus*	FM, E: Colorado tick fever virus	Tick-vertebrate
	Orbivirus	FM, E: Orungo, Kemerova viruses	Arthropod-vertebrate
Rhabdoviridae*b*	*Vesiculovirus*	FM: Vesicular stomatitis virus (Indiana, New Jersey); Chandipura, Piry viruses	Sandfly-vertebrate, with prominent transovarial component in sandfly
Togaviridae	*Alphavirus*	AR: Sindbis, chikungunya, Mayaro, Ross River, Barmah Forest viruses	Mosquito-vertebrate
		E: Eastern, western, and Venezuelan equine encephalitis viruses	

a The Filoviridae are discussed in Chap. 199.
b The Rhabdoviridae are discussed in Chap. 197.

NOTE: Abbreviations refer to the disease syndrome most commonly associated with the virus: FM, fever, myalgia; AR, arthritis, rash; E, encephalitis; HF, hemorrhagic fever.

Hantavirus is unique among the Bunyaviridae in that it is not transmitted by arthropods but is maintained in nature by rodent hosts that chronically shed virus. Like the arenaviruses, the hantaviruses usually display striking virus-rodent species specificity. Hantaviruses do not cause chronic viremia in their rodent host and are transmitted only horizontally from rodent to rodent.

Other Families The Flaviviridae are positive-sense, single-stranded RNA viruses that form particles of 40 to 50 nm in the endoplasmic reticulum. The flaviviruses discussed here are from the genus *Flavivirus* and make up two phylogenetically and antigenically distinct divisions transmitted among vertebrates by mosquitoes and ticks, respectively. The mosquito-borne viruses fall into phylogenetic groups that include yellow fever virus, the four dengue viruses, and encephalitis viruses, while the tick-borne group encompasses a geographically varied spectrum of species, some of which are responsible for encephalitis or for hemorrhagic disease with encephalitis. The Reoviridae are double-stranded RNA viruses with multisegmented genomes. These 80-nm particles are the only viruses discussed in this chapter that do not have a lipid envelope and thus are insensitive to detergents. The Togaviridae have a single positive strand RNA genome and bud particles of ~60 to 70 nm from the plasma membrane. The togaviruses discussed here are all members of the genus *Alphavirus* and are transmitted among vertebrates by mosquitoes in their natural cycle.→*The Filoviridae and the Rhabdoviridae are discussed in Chaps. 199 and 197, respectively.*

PROMINENT FEATURES OF ARTHROPOD- AND RODENT-BORNE VIRUSES Although this chapter discusses the major features of selected arthropod- and rodent-borne viruses, it does not deal with more than 500 other distinct recognized zoonotic viruses, about one-fourth of which infect humans. Zoonotic viruses are undergoing genetic evolution, "new" zoonotic viruses are being discovered, and the epidemiology of zoonotic viruses is continuing to evolve

through environmental changes affecting vectors, reservoirs, and humans. These zoonotic viruses are most numerous in the tropics but are also found in temperate and frigid climates. Their distribution and seasonal activity may be variable and often depend largely on ecologic conditions such as rainfall and temperature, which in turn affect the density of vectors and reservoirs and the development of infection therein.

Maintenance and Transmission Arthropod-borne viruses infect their vectors after the ingestion of a blood meal from a viremic vertebrate. The vectors then develop chronic, systemic infection as the viruses penetrate the gut and spread throughout the body. The viruses eventually reach the salivary glands during a period that is referred to as *extrinsic incubation* and that typically lasts 1 to 3 weeks in mosquitoes. At this point an arthropod is competent to continue the chain of transmission by infecting another vertebrate when a subsequent blood meal is taken. The arthropod generally is unharmed by the infection, and the natural vertebrate partner usually has only transient viremia with no overt disease. An alternative mechanism for virus maintenance in its arthropod host is transovarial transmission, which is common among members of the family Bunyaviridae.

Rodent-borne viruses such as the hantaviruses and arenaviruses are maintained in nature by chronic infection transmitted between rodents. As in arthropod-borne virus cycles, there is usually a high degree of rodent-virus specificity, and there is no overt disease in the reservoir/vector.

Epidemiology The distribution of arthropod- and rodent-borne viruses is restricted by the areas inhabited by their reservoir/vectors and provides an important clue in the differential diagnosis. Table 198-2 shows the approximate geographic distribution of the most important of these viruses. Members of each family, each genus, and even each serologically related group usually occur in each area but may not be pathogenic in all areas or may not be a commonly rec-

Table 198-2 Geographic Distribution of Some Important and Commonly Encountered Human Zoonotic Viral Diseases

Area	Arenaviridae	Bunyaviridae	Flaviviridae	Rhabdoviridae	Togaviridae
North America	Lymphocytic chorio-meningitis	La Crosse, Jamestown Canyon, California encephalitis; hantavirus pulmonary syndrome	St. Louis, Powassan encephalitis; dengue	Vesicular stomatitis	Eastern, western equine encephalitis
South America	Bolivian, Argentine, Venezuelan, and Brazilian HF; lymphocytic choriomeningitis	Oropouche, group C, Punta Toro infection; hantavirus pulmonary syndrome	Yellow fever, dengue, Rocio virus infection	Vesicular stomatitis, Piry virus infection	Mayaro virus infection, Venezuelan equine encephalitis
Europe	Lymphocytic chorio-meningitis	Tahyna, Toscana, sandfly fever, HF with renal syndrome	West Nile, Central European tick-borne, Russian spring-summer encephalitis	—	Sindbis virus infection
Middle East	—	Sandfly fever, Crimean Congo HF	West Nile encephalitis, dengue	—	—
Eastern Asia	—	Sandfly fever; Hantaan, Seoul virus infection	Dengue; Japanese, Russian spring-summer encephalitis; Omsk HF	Chandipura virus infection	—
Southwestern Asia	—	Sandfly fever, Crimean Congo HF	West Nile, Japanese encephalitis; dengue; Kyasanur Forest disease	—	Chikungunya
Southeast Asia	—	Seoul virus infection	Japanese encephalitis, dengue	—	Chikungunya
Africa	Lassa fever	Bunyamwera virus infection, Rift Valley fever	Yellow fever, dengue	—	Sindbis virus infection, chikungunya
Australia	—	—	Murray Valley encephalitis, dengue	—	Ross River, Barmah Forest virus infection

NOTE: HF, hemorrhagic fever.

ognized cause of disease in all areas and so may not be included in the table. Although there is generally no overt disease in the vertebrate reservoirs, disease in nonhuman target species may be a useful diagnostic clue, and serologic testing of selected animals may be a useful way to monitor virus circulation.

Most of these diseases are acquired in a rural setting; a few have urban vectors. Seoul, sandfly fever, and Oropouche viruses are examples of urban viruses, but the most notable are yellow fever, dengue, and chikungunya viruses, which are transmitted between humans with the mosquito *Aedes aegypti* as a principal or alternate vector. A history of mosquito bite has little diagnostic significance in the individual; a history of tick bite is more diagnostically specific. Rodent exposure is often reported by persons infected with an arenavirus or a hantavirus but again has little specificity. Indeed, aerosols may infect persons who have no recollection of having even seen rodents.

Syndromes Human disease caused by arthropod- and rodent-borne viruses is often subclinical. The spectrum of possible responses to infection is wide, and our knowledge of the outcome of most of these infections is limited. The usual disease syndromes associated with these viruses have been grouped into four categories: fever and myalgia, arthritis and rash, encephalitis, and hemorrhagic fever. Although for the purposes of this discussion most viruses have been placed in a single group, the categories often overlap. For example, West Nile and Venezuelan equine encephalitis viruses are discussed as encephalitis viruses, but during epidemics they may cause many cases of milder febrile syndromes and relatively uncommon cases of encephalitis. Similarly, Rift Valley fever virus is best known as a cause of HF, but the attack rates for febrile disease are far higher, and encephalitis is occasionally seen as well. LCM virus is classified as a cause of fever and myalgia because this syndrome is its most common disease manifestation and, even when central nervous system (CNS) disease occurs, it is usually mild and is preceded by fever and myalgia. Dengue virus infection is considered as a cause of fever and myalgia (dengue fever) because this is by far the most common manifestation worldwide and is the syndrome most likely to be seen in the United

States; however, dengue HF is also discussed in the HF section because of its complicated pathogenesis and importance in pediatric practice in certain areas of the world.

Diagnosis Laboratory diagnosis is required in any given case, although epidemics occasionally provide clinical and epidemiologic clues on which an educated guess as to etiology can be based. For most arthropod- and rodent-borne viruses, acute-phase serum samples (collected within 3 or 4 days of onset) have yielded isolates, and paired sera have been used to demonstrate rising antibody titers by a variety of tests. Intensive efforts to develop rapid tests for HF have resulted in an antigen-detection enzyme-linked immunosorbent assay (ELISA) and an IgM-capture ELISA that can provide a diagnosis based on a single serum sample within a few hours and are particularly useful in severe cases. More sensitive reverse transcription polymerase chain reaction (RT-PCR) tests may yield diagnoses based on samples without detectable antigen and may also provide useful genetic information about the virus. Preliminary data suggest that similar tests applied to some fever-myalgia syndromes would give positive results if developed further. Hantavirus infections differ from others discussed here in that severe acute disease is immunopathologic; patients present with serum IgM that serves as the basis for a sensitive and specific test. Every ELISA must include a control incorporating a negative antigen with each serum sample tested; the frequent failure to include such a control has resulted in numerous false-positive results in diagnostic tests.

At the time of diagnosis, patients with encephalitis are generally no longer viremic or antigenemic and usually do not have virus in cerebrospinal fluid (CSF). In this situation, the value of serologic methods and RT-PCR is being validated. IgM capture is increasingly being used for the simultaneous testing of serum and CSF. IgG ELISA or classic serology is useful in the evaluation of past exposure to the viruses, many of which circulate in areas with a minimal medical infrastructure and sometimes cause mild or subclinical infection.

The remainder of this chapter offers general descriptions of the broad syndromes caused by arthropod- and rodent-borne viruses and then addresses specific differences between diseases. It is important to remember that most of the diseases under consideration have not been studied in detail with modern medical approaches and thus available data may be incomplete or biased.

FEVER AND MYALGIA

Fever and myalgia constitute the syndrome most commonly associated with zoonotic virus infection. Many of the numerous viruses belonging to the families listed in Table 198-1 probably cause this syndrome, but several viruses have been selected for inclusion in the table because of their prominent associations with the syndrome and their biomedical importance.

The syndrome typically begins with the abrupt onset of fever, chills, intense myalgia, and malaise. Patients may also report joint pains, but no true arthritis is detectable. Anorexia is characteristic and may be accompanied by nausea or even vomiting. Headache is common and may be severe, with photophobia and retroorbital pain. Physical findings are minimal and are usually confined to conjunctival injection with pain on palpation of muscles or the epigastrium. The duration of symptoms is quite variable but generally is 2 to 5 days, with a biphasic course in some instances. The spectrum of disease varies from subclinical to temporarily incapacitating.

Less constant findings include a maculopapular rash. Epistaxis may occur but does not necessarily indicate a bleeding diathesis. A minority of the cases caused by some viruses are known or suspected to include aseptic meningitis, but this diagnosis is difficult in remote areas, given the patients' photophobia and myalgia as well as the lack of opportunity to examine the CSF. Although pharyngitis may be noted or radiographic evidence of pulmonary infiltrates found in some cases, these viruses are not primary respiratory pathogens. The differential diagnosis includes anicteric leptospirosis, rickettsial diseases, and the early stages of other syndromes discussed in this chapter. These diseases are often described as "flulike," but the usual absence of cough and coryza makes influenza an unlikely confounder except at the earliest stages.

Complete recovery is generally the outcome in this syndrome, although prolonged asthenia and nonspecific symptoms have been described in some cases, particularly after infection with LCM or dengue virus. Treatment is supportive, with aspirin avoided because of the potential for exacerbated bleeding and Reye's syndrome. Efforts at prevention are best based on vector control, which, however, may be expensive or impossible. For mosquito control, destruction of breeding sites is generally the most economically and environmentally sound approach; spraying to kill adult mosquitoes and thus to reduce their numbers transiently may have a preventive role in selected settings but has not been notably effective in the past. Measures taken by the individual to avoid the vector can be valuable. Avoiding the vector's habitat and times of peak activity, preventing the vector from entering dwellings by using screens or other barriers, judiciously applying arthropod repellents such as diethyltoluamide (DEET) to the skin, and wearing permethrin-impregnated clothing are all possible approaches, depending on the vector and its habits.

LYMPHOCYTIC CHORIOMENINGITIS LCM is transmitted from the common house mouse (*Mus musculus*) to humans by aerosols of excreta and secreta. LCM virus, an arenavirus, is maintained in the mouse mainly by vertical transmission from infected dams. The vertically infected mouse remains viremic for life, with high concentrations of virus in all tissues. Infected colonies of pet hamsters have also served as a link to humans. LCM virus is widely used in immunology laboratories as a model of T cell function and can silently infect cell cultures and passaged tumor lines, resulting in infections among scientists and animal caretakers. Patients with LCM may have a history of residence in rodent-infested housing or other exposure to rodents. An antibody prevalence of ~5 to 10% has been reported in adults from the United States, Argentina, and endemic areas of Germany.

LCM differs from the general syndrome of fever and myalgia in that its onset is gradual. Among the conditions occasionally associated with LCM are orchitis, transient alopecia, arthritis, pharyngitis, cough, and maculopapular rash. An estimated one-fourth of patients or fewer suffer a febrile phase of 3 to 6 days and then, after a brief remission, develop renewed fever accompanied by severe headache, nausea and vomiting, and meningeal signs lasting for about a week. These patients virtually always recover fully, as do the uncommon patients with clear-cut signs of encephalitis. Recovery may be delayed by transient hydrocephalus.

During the initial febrile phase, leukopenia and thrombocytopenia are common and virus can usually be isolated from blood. During the CNS phase of the illness, virus may be found in the CSF, but antibodies are present in blood. The pathogenesis of LCM is thought to resemble that following direct intracranial inoculation of the virus into adult mice; the onset of the immune response leads to T cell–mediated immunopathologic meningitis. During the meningeal phase, CSF mononuclear-cell counts range from the hundreds to the low thousands per microliter, and hypoglycorrhachia is found in one-third of cases. The IgM-capture ELISA of serum and CSF is usually positive; RT-PCR assays have been developed for application to CSF.

Infection with LCM virus should be suspected in acutely ill febrile patients with marked leukopenia and thrombocytopenia. In cases of aseptic meningitis, any of the following should suggest LCM: well-marked febrile prodrome, adult age, autumn seasonality, low CSF glucose levels, or CSF mononuclear cell counts >1000/μL.

In pregnant women, LCM virus infection may lead to fetal invasion with consequent congenital hydrocephalus and chorioretinitis. Since the maternal infection may be mild, consisting of only a short febrile illness, antibodies to the virus should be sought in both the mother and the fetus in suspicious circumstances, particularly TORCH-negative neonatal hydrocephalus. [TORCH is a battery of tests encompassing *t*oxoplasmosis, *o*ther conditions (congenital syphilis and viruses), *r*ubella, *c*ytomegalovirus, and *h*erpes simplex virus.]

BUNYAMWERA VIRUS INFECTION The mosquito-transmitted Bunyamwera serogroup viruses are found on every continent except Australia and Antarctica. Bunyamwera virus and its close relative Ilesha virus commonly cause febrile disease in Africa. Other related viruses are implicated in such disease in Southeast Asia (Batai virus), Europe (Calovo virus), and South America (Wyeomyia virus). In North America, Cache Valley virus has been implicated in febrile human disease and in rare instances of more serious systemic illness; the presence of serum antibodies to this virus may be associated with congenital malformations. In Central America, the closely related Fort Sherman virus causes the fever-myalgia syndrome.

GROUP C VIRUS INFECTION The group C viruses include at least 11 agents transmitted by mosquitoes in neotropical forests. These agents are among the most common causes of arboviral infection in humans entering American jungles and cause acute febrile disease.

TAHYNA VIRUS INFECTION This California serogroup virus (see discussion of California encephalitis, below) occurs in central and western Europe, and related viruses are emerging in Russia. The significance of Tahyna virus in human health has been studied only in the Czech and Slovak Republics; there, the virus was found to be a prominent cause of febrile disease, in some cases causing pharyngitis, pulmonary syndromes, and aseptic meningitis. The potential for arboviruses to be unexpectedly involved in such cases in areas of high mosquito prevalence needs to be kept in mind.

OROPOUCHE FEVER Oropouche virus is transmitted in Central and South America by a biting midge, *Culicoides paraensis*, which often breeds to high density in cacao husks and other vegetable detritus found in towns and cities. Explosive epidemics involving thousands of cases have been reported from several towns in Brazil and Peru. Rash and aseptic meningitis have been detected in a number of cases.

SANDFLY FEVER The sandfly *Phlebotomus papatasi* transmits sandfly fever. Female sandflies may be infected by the oral route as they take a blood meal and may transmit the virus to offspring when they lay their eggs after a second blood meal. This prominent transovarial pattern was the first to be recognized among dipterans and complicates virus control. A previous designation for sandfly fever, "3-day fever," instructively describes the brief, debilitating course associated with this essentially benign infection. There is neither a rash nor CNS involvement, and complete recovery is the rule.

Sandfly fever is found in the circum-Mediterranean area, extending to the east through the Balkans into China as well as into the Middle East and southwestern Asia. The vector is found in both rural and urban settings and is known for its small size, which enables it to penetrate standard mosquito screens and netting, and for its short flight range. Epidemics have been described in the wake of natural disasters and wars. In parts of Europe, sandfly populations and virus transmission were greatly reduced by the extensive residual spraying conducted after World War II to control malaria, and the incidence continues to be low. A common pattern of disease in endemic areas consists of high attack rates among travelers and military personnel with little or no disease in the local population, who are protected after childhood infection. In addition to the two well-characterized, non-cross-protective Sicilian and Naples virus species, more than 30 related phleboviruses are transmitted by sandflies and mosquitoes, but most are of unknown significance in terms of human health.

TOSCANA VIRUS DISEASE Toscana virus is a *Phlebovirus* (family Bunyaviridae) transmitted primarily by the circum-Mediterranean sandfly *P. perniciosus*. The vertebrate amplifying host, if one exists, is unknown. Toscana virus infection is common during the summer among rural residents and vacationers; a number of cases have been identified in travelers returning to Germany and Scandinavia. The disease may manifest as an uncomplicated febrile illness but is often associated with aseptic meningitis, with virus isolated from the CSF.

PUNTA TORO VIRUS DISEASE Of the several phleboviruses that are associated with New World sandflies and infect humans, Punta Toro virus is the best known. The disease caused by this virus is clinically similar to but epidemiologically different from that caused by the Naples or Sicilian sandfly fever viruses. Punta Toro virus infections are sporadic and are acquired in the tropical forest, where the vectors rest on tree buttresses. Epidemics have not been reported, but antibody prevalences among inhabitants of villages in the endemic areas indicate a cumulative lifetime exposure rate of >50%.

DENGUE FEVER All four distinct dengue viruses (dengue 1–4) have *A. aegypti* as their principal vector, and all cause a similar clinical syndrome. In rare cases, second infection with a serotype of dengue virus different from that involved in the primary infection leads to dengue HF with severe shock (see below). Sporadic cases are seen in the settings of endemic transmission and epidemic disease. Year-round transmission between latitudes 25°N and 25°S has been established, and seasonal forays of the viruses to points as far north as Philadelphia are thought to have taken place in the United States. With increasing spread of the vector mosquito throughout the tropics and subtropics, large areas of the world have become vulnerable to the introduction of dengue viruses, particularly through air travel by infected humans, and both dengue fever and the related dengue HF are becoming increasingly common. Conditions favorable to dengue transmission exist in the southern United States, and bursts of dengue fever activity are to be expected in this region, particularly along the Mexican border, where water may be stored in containers and *A. aegypti* numbers may therefore be greatest: this mosquito, which is also an efficient vector of the yellow fever and chikungunya viruses, typically breeds near human habitation, using relatively fresh water from sources such as water jars, vases, discarded containers, coconut husks, and old tires. *A. aegypti* usually inhabits dwellings and bites during the day.

After an incubation period of 2 to 7 days, the typical patient experiences the sudden onset of fever, headache, retroorbital pain, and back pain along with the severe myalgia that gave rise to the colloquial designation "break-bone fever." There is often a macular rash on the first day as well as adenopathy, palatal vesicles, and scleral injection. The illness may last a week, with additional symptoms usually including anorexia, nausea or vomiting, marked cutaneous hypersensitivity, and—near the time of defervescence—a maculopapular rash beginning on the trunk and spreading to the extremities and the face. Epistaxis and scattered petechiae are often noted in uncomplicated dengue, and preexisting gastrointestinal lesions may bleed during the acute illness.

Laboratory findings include leukopenia, thrombocytopenia, and, in many cases, serum aminotransferase elevations. The diagnosis is made by IgM ELISA or paired serology during recovery or by antigen-detection ELISA or RT-PCR during the acute phase. Virus is readily isolated from blood in the acute phase if mosquito inoculation or mosquito cell culture is used.

COLORADO TICK FEVER Several hundred cases of Colorado tick fever are reported annually in the United States. The infection is acquired between March and November through the bite of an infected *Dermacentor andersoni* tick in mountainous western regions at altitudes of 1200 to 3000 m (4000 to 10,000 ft). Small mammals serve as the amplifying host. The most common presentation consists of fever and myalgia; meningoencephalitis is not uncommon, and hemorrhagic disease, pericarditis, myocarditis, orchitis, and pulmonary presentations are also reported. Rash develops in a substantial minority of cases. The disease usually lasts 7 to 10 days and is often biphasic. The most important differential diagnostic considerations since the beginning of the twentieth century have been Rocky Mountain spotted fever and tularemia.

Infection of erythroblasts and other marrow cells by Colorado tick fever virus results in the appearance and persistence (for several weeks) of erythrocytes containing the virus. This feature, detected in smears stained by immunofluorescence, can be diagnostically helpful. The clinical laboratory detects leukopenia and thrombocytopenia.

ORBIVIRUS INFECTION The orbiviruses encompass many human and veterinary pathogens. For example, Orungo virus is widely transmitted by mosquitoes in tropical Africa and causes febrile disease in humans. The Kemerova complex includes the Kemerova, Lipovnik, and Tribec viruses of Russia and central Europe; these viruses are transmitted by ticks and are associated with febrile and neurologic disease.

VESICULAR STOMATITIS See Chap. 197.

ENCEPHALITIS

Arboviral encephalitis is a seasonal disease, commonly occurring in the warmer months. Its incidence varies markedly with time and place, depending on ecologic factors. The causative viruses differ substantially in terms of case-infection ratio (i.e., the ratio of clinical to subclinical infection), mortality, and residua (Table 198-3). Humans are not an important amplifier of these viruses.

All the viral encephalitides discussed in this section have a similar pathogenesis as far as is known. An infected arthropod ingests a blood meal from a human and infects the host. The initial period of viremia is thought to originate most commonly from the lymphoid system. Viremia leads to CNS invasion, presumably through infection of olfactory neuroepithelium with passage through the cribiform plate or through infection of brain capillaries and multifocal entry into the CNS. During the viremic phase, there may be little or no recognized disease except in the case of tick-borne flaviviral encephalitis, in which there may be a clearly delineated phase of fever and systemic illness. The disease process in the CNS arises partly from direct neuronal infection and subsequent damage and partly from edema, inflammation, and other indirect effects. The usual pathologic picture is one of focal necrosis of neurons, inflammatory glial nodules, and perivascular lymphoid cuffing; the severity and distribution of these abnormalities

Table 198-3 Prominent Features of Arboviral Encephalitis

Virus	Natural Cycle	Incubation Period, Days	Annual No. of Cases	Case-to-Infection Ratio	Age of Cases	Case-Fatality Rate, %	Residua
La Crosse	*Aedes triseriatus*–chipmunk (transovarial component in mosquito also important)	~3–7	70 (U.S.)	<1:1000	<15 years	<0.5	Recurrent seizures in ~10%; severe deficits in rare cases; decreased school performance and behavioral change suspected in small proportion
St. Louis	*Culex tarsalis, C. pipiens, C. quinquefasciatus*–birds	4–21	85, with hundreds to thousands in epidemic years (U.S.)	<1:200	Milder cases in the young; more severe cases in adults >40 years old, particularly the elderly	7	Common in the elderly
Japanese	*Culex tritaeniorhyncus*–birds	5–15	>25,000	1:200–300	All ages; children in highly endemic areas	20–50	Common (approximately half of cases); may be severe
West Nile	*Culex* mosquitoes–birds	3–6	?	Very low	Mainly the elderly and children	—	Uncommon
Central European	*Ixodes ricinus*–rodents, insectivores	7–14	Thousands	1:12	All ages; milder in children	1–5	20%
Russian spring-summer	*I. persulcatus*–rodents, insectivores	7–14	Hundreds	—	All ages; milder in children	20	Approximately half of cases; often severe; limb-girdle paralysis
Powassan	*I. cookei*–wild mammals	~10	~1 (U.S.)	—	All ages; some predilection for children	~10	Common (approximately half of cases)
Eastern equine	*Culiseta melanura*–birds	~5–10	5 (U.S.)	1:40 adult 1:17 child	All ages; predilection for children	50–75	Common
Western equine	*Culex tarsalis*–birds	~5–10	~20 (U.S.)	1:1000 adult 1:50 child 1:1 infant	All ages; predilection for children <2 years old (increased mortality in elderly)	3–7	Common only among infants < 1 year old
Venezuelan equine (epidemic)	Unknown (multiple mosquito species and horses in epidemics)	1–5	?	1:250 adult 1:25 child (approximate)	All ages; predilection for children	~10	—

vary with the infecting virus. Involved areas display the "luxury perfusion" phenomenon, with normal or increased total blood flow and low oxygen extraction.

The typical patient presents with a prodrome of nonspecific constitutional symptoms, including fever, abdominal pain, vertigo, sore throat, and respiratory symptoms. Headache, meningeal signs, photophobia, and vomiting follow quickly. Involvement of deeper structures may be signaled by lethargy, somnolence, and intellectual deficit (as disclosed by the mental status examination or failure at serial 7 subtraction); more severely affected patients will be obviously disoriented and may be comatose. Tremors, loss of abdominal reflexes, cranial nerve palsies, hemiparesis, monoparesis, difficulty in swallowing, and frontal lobe signs are all common. Convulsions and focal signs may be evident early or may appear during the course of the disease. Some patients present with an abrupt onset of fever, convulsions, and other signs of CNS involvement. The results of human infection range from no significant symptoms through febrile headache to aseptic meningitis and finally to full-blown encephalitis; the proportions and severity of these manifestations vary with the infecting virus.

The acute encephalitis usually lasts from a few days to as long as 2 to 3 weeks, but recovery may be slow, with weeks or months required for the return of maximal recoupable function. Common complaints during recovery include difficulty concentrating, fatigability, tremors, and personality changes. The acute illness requires management of a comatose patient who may have intracranial pressure elevations, inappropriate secretion of antidiuretic hormone, respiratory failure, and convulsions. There is no specific therapy for these viral encephalitides. The only practical preventive measures are vector management and personal protection against the arthropod transmitting the virus; for Japanese encephalitis or tick-borne encephalitis, vaccination should be considered in certain circumstances (see relevant sections below).

The diagnosis of arboviral encephalitis depends on the careful evaluation of a febrile patient with CNS disease, with rapid identification of treatable herpes simplex encephalitis, ruling out of brain abscess, exclusion of bacterial meningitis by serial CSF examination, and performance of laboratory studies to define the viral etiology. Leptospirosis, neurosyphilis, Lyme disease, cat-scratch fever, and newer viral encephalitides such as Nipah virus infection from Malaysia should be considered. The CSF examination usually shows a modest cell count—in the tens or hundreds or perhaps a few thousand. Early in the process, a significant proportion of these cells may be polymorphonuclear leukocytes, but usually there is a mononuclear cell predominance. CSF glucose levels are usually normal. There are exceptions to this pattern of findings. In eastern equine encephalitis, for example, polymorphonuclear leukocytes may predominate during the first 72 h of disease and hypoglycorrhachia may be detected. In LCM, lymphocyte counts may be in the thousands, and the glucose concentration may be diminished. Experience with imaging studies is still evolving; clearly however, both computed tomography (CT) and magnetic resonance imaging (MRI) may be normal except for evidence of preexisting conditions or sometimes may suggest diffuse edema. Several patients with eastern equine encephalitis have had focal abnormalities, and individuals with severe Japanese encephalitis have presented with bilateral thalamic lesions that have often been hemorrhagic. Electroencephalography usually shows diffuse abnormalities and is not directly helpful.

A humoral immune response is usually detectable at or near the onset of disease. Both serum and CSF should be examined for IgM antibodies. Virus generally cannot be isolated from blood or CSF, although Japanese encephalitis virus has been recovered from CSF in severe cases. Virus can be obtained from and viral antigen is present in brain tissue, although its distribution may be focal.

CALIFORNIA, LA CROSSE, AND JAMESTOWN CANYON VIRUS ENCEPHALITIS The isolation of California encephalitis virus established the California serogroup of viruses as a cause of encephalitis, and its use as a diagnostic antigen led to the description of many cases of "California encephalitis." In fact, however, this virus has been implicated in only a few cases of encephalitis, and the serologically related La Crosse virus is the major cause of encephalitis among viruses in the California serogroup. "California encephalitis" due to La Crosse virus infection is most commonly reported from the upper Midwest but is also found in other areas of the central and eastern United States, most often in West Virginia, Tennessee, North Carolina, and Georgia. The serogroup includes 13 other viruses, some of which may also be involved in human disease that is misattributed because of the complexity of the group's serology; these viruses include the Jamestown Canyon, snowshoe hare, Inkoo, and Trivittatus viruses, all of which have *Aedes* mosquitoes as their vector and all of which have a strong element of transovarial transmission in their natural cycles.

The mosquito vector of La Crosse virus is *A. triseriatus*. In addition to a prominent transovarial component of transmission, a mosquito can also become infected through feeding on viremic chipmunks and other mammals as well as through venereal transmission from another mosquito. The mosquito breeds in sites such as tree holes and abandoned tires and bites during daylight hours; these findings correlate with the risk factors for cases: recreation in forested areas, residence at the forest's edge, and the presence of abandoned tires around the home. Intensive environmental modification based on these findings has reduced the incidence of disease in a highly endemic area in the Midwest. Most cases occur from July through September. The Asian tiger mosquito, *A. albopictus*, efficiently transmits the virus to mice and also transmits the agent transovarially in the laboratory; this aggressive anthropophilic mosquito has the capacity to urbanize, and its possible impact on transmission to humans is of concern.

An antibody prevalence of ≥20% in endemic areas indicates that infection is common, but CNS disease has been recognized primarily in children <15 years of age. The illness varies from a picture of aseptic meningitis accompanied by confusion to severe and occasionally fatal encephalitis. Although there may be prodromal symptoms, the onset of CNS disease is sudden, with fever, headache, and lethargy often joined by nausea and vomiting, convulsions (in one-half of patients), and coma (in one-third of patients). Focal seizures, hemiparesis, tremor, aphasia, chorea, Babinski's sign, and other evidence of significant neurologic dysfunction are common, but residua are not. Perhaps 10% of patients have recurrent seizures in the succeeding months. Other serious sequelae are rare, although a decrease in scholastic standing has been reported and mild personality change has occasionally been suggested. Treatment is supportive over a 1- to 2-week acute phase during which status epilepticus, cerebral edema, and inappropriate secretion of antidiuretic hormone are important concerns. Ribavirin has been used in severe cases, and a clinical trial of this drug is under way.

The blood leukocyte count is commonly elevated, sometimes reaching levels of 20,000/μL, and there is usually a left shift. CSF cell counts are typically 30 to 500/μL with a mononuclear cell predominance (although 25 to 90% of cells are polymorphonuclear in some cases). The protein level is normal or slightly increased, and the glucose level is normal. Specific virologic diagnosis based on IgM-capture assays of serum and CSF is efficient. The only human anatomic site from which virus has been isolated is the brain.

Jamestown Canyon virus has been implicated in several cases of encephalitis in adults; in these cases the disease was usually associated with a significant respiratory illness at onset. Human infection with this virus has been documented in New York, Wisconsin, Ohio, Michigan, Ontario, and other areas of North America where the vector mosquito, *A. stimulans*, feeds on its main host, the white-tailed deer.

ST. LOUIS ENCEPHALITIS St. Louis encephalitis virus is transmitted between *Culex* mosquitoes and birds. This virus causes low-level endemic infection among rural residents of the western and central United States, where *C. tarsalis* is the vector (see "Western Equine Encephalitis," below), but the more urbanized mosquito species *C. pipiens* and *C. quinquefasciatus* have been responsible for epidemics resulting in hundreds or even thousands of cases in cities of the central and eastern United States. Most cases occur in June through October. The urban mosquitoes breed in accumulations of stagnant water and sewage with high organic content and readily bite humans in and around houses at dusk. The elimination of open sewers and trash-filled drainage systems is expensive and may not be possible, but screening of houses and implementation of personal protective measures may be an effective approach for individuals. The rural vector is most active at dusk and outdoors; its bites can be avoided by modification of activities and use of repellents.

Disease severity increases with age: infections that result in aseptic meningitis or mild encephalitis are concentrated in children and young adults, while severe and fatal cases primarily affect the elderly. Infection rates are similar in all age groups; thus the greater susceptibility of older persons to disease is a biologic consequence of aging. The disease has an abrupt onset, sometimes following a prodrome, and begins with fever, lethargy, confusion, and headache. In addition, nuchal rigidity, hypotonia, hyperreflexia, myoclonus, and tremor are common. Severe cases can include cranial nerve palsies, hemiparesis, and convulsions. Patients often complain of dysuria and may have viral antigen in urine as well as pyuria. The overall mortality is generally ~7% but may reach 20% among patients over the age of 60. Recovery is slow. Emotional lability, difficulties in concentration and memory, asthenia, and tremor are commonly prolonged in older patients.

The CSF of patients with St. Louis encephalitis usually contains tens to hundreds of cells, with a lymphocytic predominance and a normal glucose level. Leukocytosis with a left shift is often documented.

JAPANESE ENCEPHALITIS Japanese encephalitis virus is found throughout Asia, including far eastern Russia, Japan, China, India, Pakistan, and Southeast Asia, and causes occasional epidemics on western Pacific islands. The virus has been detected in the Torres Strait islands, and a human encephalitis case has been identified on the nearby Australian mainland. This flavivirus is particularly common in areas where irrigated rice fields attract the natural avian vertebrate hosts and provide abundant breeding sites for mosquitoes such as *C. tritaeniorhyncus*, which transmit the virus to humans. Additional amplification by pigs, which suffer abortion, and horses, which develop encephalitis, may be significant as well. Vaccination of these additional amplifying hosts may reduce the transmission of the virus. An effective, formalin-inactivated vaccine purified from mouse brain is produced in Japan and licensed for human use in the United States. It is given on days 0, 7, and 30 or—with some sacrifice in serum neutralizing titer—on days 0, 7, and 14. Vaccination is indicated for summer travelers to rural Asia, where the risk of clinical disease may be 0.05 to 2.1/10,000 per week. The severe and often fatal disease reported in expatriates must be balanced against the 0.1 to 1% chance of a late systemic or cutaneous allergic reaction. These reactions are rarely fatal but may be severe and have been known to begin 1 to 9 days after vaccination, with associated pruritus, urticaria, and angioedema. Live attenuated vaccines are being used in China but are not recommended in the United States at this time.

WEST NILE VIRUS INFECTION West Nile virus is transmitted among wild birds by *Culex* mosquitoes in Africa, the Middle East, southern Europe, and Asia. It is a frequent cause of febrile disease without CNS involvement, but it occasionally causes aseptic meningitis and severe encephalitis; these serious infections are particularly common among children and the elderly. The febrile-myalgic syndrome caused by West Nile virus differs from many others by the frequent appearance of a maculopapular rash concentrated on the trunk and lymphadenopathy. Headache, ocular pain, sore throat, nausea and vomiting, and arthralgia (but not arthritis) are common accompaniments. In addition, the virus has been implicated in severe and fatal hepatic necrosis in Africa.

In 1996 West Nile virus caused more than 300 cases of CNS disease, with 10% mortality, in the Danube flood plain, including Bucharest. In 1999 the virus appeared in New York City and other areas of the northeastern United States, causing more than 60 cases of aseptic meningitis or encephalitis among humans as well as die-offs among crows, exotic zoo birds, and other avians. The encephalitis was most severe among the elderly and was often associated with notable muscle weakness and even with flaccid paralysis. The virus, thought to have been transmitted in New York City by the ubiquitous *C. pipiens* mosquito, returned to larger areas of the northeastern United States in the summer of 2000 and threatens to spread farther in the Americas via bird migration.

West Nile virus falls into the same phylogenetic group of flaviviruses as St. Louis and Japanese encephalitis viruses, as do Murray Valley and Rocio viruses. The latter two viruses are both maintained in mosquitoes and birds and produce a clinical picture resembling that of Japanese encephalitis. Murray Valley virus has caused occasional epidemics and sporadic cases in Australia. Rocio virus caused recurrent epidemics in a focal area of Brazil in 1975 to 1977 and then virtually disappeared.

CENTRAL EUROPEAN TICK-BORNE ENCEPHALITIS AND RUSSIAN SPRING-SUMMER ENCEPHALITIS A spectrum of tick-borne flaviviruses has been identified across the Eurasian land mass. Many are known mainly as agricultural pathogens (e.g., louping ill virus in the United Kingdom). From Scandinavia to the Urals, central European tick-borne encephalitis is transmitted by *Ixodes ricinus*. Human cases occur between April and October, with a peak in June and July. A related and more virulent virus is that of Russian spring-summer encephalitis, which is associated with *I. persulcatus* and is distributed from Europe across the Urals to the Pacific Ocean. The ticks transmit the disease primarily in the spring and early summer, with a lower rate of transmission later in summer. Small mammals are the vertebrate amplifiers for both viruses. The risk varies by geographic area and can be highly localized within a given area; human cases usually follow outdoor activities or consumption of raw milk from infected goats or other infected animals.

After an incubation period of 7 to 14 days or perhaps longer, the central European viruses classically result in a febrile-myalgic phase that lasts for 2 to 4 days and is thought to correlate with viremia. A subsequent remission for several days is followed by the recurrence of fever and the onset of meningeal signs. The CNS phase varies from mild aseptic meningitis, which is more common among younger patients, to severe encephalitis with coma, convulsions, tremors, and motor signs lasting for 7 to 10 days before improvement begins. Spinal and medullary involvement can lead to typical limb-girdle paralysis and to respiratory paralysis. Most patients recover, only a minority with significant deficits. Infections with the far eastern viruses generally run a more abrupt course. The encephalitic syndrome caused by these viruses sometimes begins without a remission and has more severe manifestations than the European syndrome. Mortality is high, and major sequelae—most notably, lower motor neuron paralyses of the proximal muscles of the extremities, trunk, and neck—are common.

In the early stage of the illness, virus may be isolated from the blood. In the CNS phase, IgM antibodies are detectable in serum and/or CSF. Thrombocytopenia sometimes develops during the initial febrile illness, which resembles the early hemorrhagic phase of some other tick-borne flaviviral infections, such as Kyasanur Forest disease. Other tick-borne flaviviruses are less common causes of encephalitis, including louping ill virus in the United Kingdom and Powassan virus.

There is no specific therapy for infection with these viruses. However, effective alum-adjuvanted, formalin-inactivated vaccines are produced in Austria, Germany, and Russia. Two doses of the Austrian vaccine separated by an interval of 1 to 3 months appear to be effective in the field, and antibody responses are similar when vaccine is given

on days 0 and 14. Other vaccines have elicited similar neutralizing antibody titers. Since rare cases of postvaccination Guillain-Barré syndrome have been reported, vaccination should be reserved for persons likely to experience rural exposure in an endemic area during the season of transmission. Cross-neutralization for the central European and far eastern strains has been established, but there are no published field studies on cross-protection of formalin-inactivated vaccines. Because 0.2 to 4% of ticks in endemic areas may be infected, tick bites raise the issue of immunoglobulin prophylaxis. Prompt administration of high-titered specific preparations should probably be undertaken, although no controlled data are available to prove the efficacy of this measure. Immunoglobulin should not be administered late because of the risk of antibody-mediated enhancement.

POWASSAN ENCEPHALITIS Powassan virus is a member of the tick-borne encephalitis virus complex and is transmitted by *I. cookei* among small mammals in eastern Canada and the United States, where it has been responsible for 20 recognized cases of human disease. Other ticks may transmit the virus in a wider geographic area, and there is some concern that *I. scapularis* (also called *I. dammini*), a competent vector in the laboratory, may become involved as it becomes more prominent in the United States. Patients with Powassan encephalitis—often children—present in May through December after outdoor exposure and an incubation period thought to be about 1 week. Powassan encephalitis is severe, and sequelae are common.

EASTERN EQUINE ENCEPHALITIS Eastern equine encephalitis is found primarily within endemic swampy foci along the eastern coast of the United States, with a few inland foci as far removed as Michigan. Human cases present from June through October, when the bird–*Culiseta* mosquito cycle spills over into other mosquito species such as *A. sollicitans* or *A. vexans*, which are more likely to bite mammals. There is concern over the potential role of the introduced anthropophilic mosquito species *A. albopictus*, which has been found to be naturally infected and is an effective vector in the laboratory. Horses are a common target for the virus; if not vaccinated, they serve as a harbinger of human disease but probably do not play a significant role in amplification of the virus.

Eastern equine encephalitis is one of the most destructive of the arboviral conditions, with a brusque onset, rapid progression, high mortality, and frequent residua. This severity is reflected in the extensive necrotic lesions and polymorphonuclear infiltrates found at postmortem examination of the brain and the acute polymorphonuclear CSF pleocytosis often occurring during the first 1 to 3 days of disease. In addition, leukocytosis with a left shift is a common feature. A formalin-inactivated vaccine has been used to protect laboratory workers but is not generally available or applicable.

WESTERN EQUINE ENCEPHALITIS The primary maintenance cycle for western equine encephalitis virus in the United States is between *C. tarsalis* and birds, principally sparrows and finches. Equines and humans become infected, and both species suffer encephalitis without amplifying the virus in nature. St. Louis encephalitis is transmitted in a similar cycle in the same region but causes human disease about a month earlier than the period (July through October) in which western equine encephalitis virus is active. Large epidemics of western equine encephalitis took place in the western and central United States and Canada during the 1930s to 1950s, but in recent years the disease has been uncommon. There were 41 reported cases in the United States in 1987 but only 4 reported cases from 1988 to 1995. This decline in incidence may reflect in part the integrated approach to mosquito management that has been employed in irrigation projects and the increasing use of agricultural pesticides; it almost certainly reflects the increased tendency for humans to be indoors behind closed windows at dusk, the peak period of biting by the major vector.

Western equine encephalitis virus causes a typical diffuse viral encephalitis with an increased attack rate and increased morbidity in the young, particularly children <2 years old. In addition, mortality is high among the young and the very elderly. One-third of individuals who have convulsions during the acute illness have subsequent seizure activity. Infants <1 year old—particularly those in the first months of life—are at serious risk of motor and intellectual damage. Twice as many males as females develop clinical encephalitis after 5 to 9 years of age; this difference may be related to greater outdoor exposure of boys to the vector but is also likely due in part to biologic differences. A formalin-inactivated vaccine has been used to protect laboratory workers but is not generally available or applicable.

VENEZUELAN EQUINE ENCEPHALITIS There are six known types of virus in the Venezuelan equine encephalitis complex. An important distinction is between the "epizootic" viruses (subtypes IAB and IC) and the "enzootic" viruses (subtypes ID to IF and types II to VI). The epizootic viruses have an unknown natural cycle but periodically cause extensive epidemics in equines and humans in the Americas. These epidemics rely on the high-level viremia in horses and mules that results in the infection of several species of mosquitoes, which in turn infect humans and perpetuate virus transmission. Humans also have high-level viremia but probably are not important in virus transmission. Enzootic viruses are found primarily in humid tropical forest habitats and are maintained between *Culex* mosquitoes and rodents; these viruses cause human disease but are not pathogenic for horses and do not cause epizootics.

Epizootics of Venezuelan equine encephalitis occurred repeatedly in Venezuela, Colombia, Ecuador, Peru, and other South American countries at intervals of ≤10 years from the 1930s until 1969, when a massive epizootic spread throughout Central America and Mexico, reaching southern Texas in 1972. Genetic sequencing of the virus from the 1969 to 1972 outbreak suggested that it originated from residual "un-inactivated" virus in veterinary vaccines. The outbreak was terminated in Texas with the use of a live attenuated vaccine (TC-83) originally developed for human use by the U.S. Army; this virus was then used for further production of inactivated veterinary vaccines. No further epizootic disease was identified until 1995 and subsequently, when additional epizootics took place in Colombia, Venezuela, and Mexico. The viruses involved in these epizootics as well as previously epizootic subtype IC viruses have been shown to be close phylogenetic relatives of known enzootic subtype ID viruses. This finding suggests that active evolution and selection of epizootic viruses are under way in northern South America.

During epizootics, extensive human infection is the rule, with clinical disease in 10 to 60% of infected individuals. Most infections result in notable acute febrile disease, while relatively few result in encephalitis. A low rate of CNS invasion is supported by the absence of encephalitis among the many infections resulting from exposure to aerosols in the laboratory or from vaccine accidents. The most recent large epizootic of Venezuelan equine encephalitis occurred in Colombia and Venezuela in 1995; of the more than 85,000 clinical cases, 4% (with a higher proportion among children than adults) included neurologic symptoms and 300 ended in death.

Enzootic strains of Venezuelan equine encephalitis virus are common causes of acute febrile disease, particularly in areas such as the Florida Everglades and the humid Atlantic coast of Central America. Encephalitis has been documented only in the Florida infections; the three cases were caused by type II enzootic virus, also called *Everglades virus*. All three patients had preexisting cerebral disease. Extrapolation from the rate of genetic change suggests that Everglades virus may have been introduced into Florida <200 years ago and that it is most closely related to the ID subtypes that appear to have given evolutionary rise to the epizootic strains active in South America.

The prevention of epizootic Venezuelan equine encephalitis depends on vaccination of horses with the attenuated TC-83 vaccine or with an inactivated vaccine prepared from that strain. Humans can be protected with similar vaccines, but the use of such products is restricted to laboratory personnel because of reactogenicity and limited availability. In addition, wild-type virus and perhaps TC-83 vaccine

may have some degree of fetal pathogenicity. Enzootic viruses are genetically and antigenically different from epizootic viruses, and protection against the former with vaccines prepared from the latter is relatively ineffective.

ARTHRITIS AND RASH

True arthritis is a common accompaniment of several viral diseases, such as rubella (caused by a non-alphavirus togavirus), parvovirus B19 infection, and hepatitis B; it is an occasional accompaniment of infection due to mumps virus, enteroviruses, herpesviruses, and adenoviruses. It is not generally appreciated that the alphaviruses are also common causes of arthritis. In fact, the alphaviruses discussed below all cause acute febrile diseases accompanied by the development of true arthritis and a maculopapular rash. Rheumatic involvement includes arthralgia alone, periarticular swelling, and (less commonly) joint effusions. Most of these diseases are less severe and have fewer articular manifestations in children than in adults. In temperate climates, these are summer diseases. No specific therapy or licensed vaccines exist.

SINDBIS VIRUS INFECTION Sindbis virus is transmitted among birds by mosquitoes. Infections with the northern European strains of this virus (which cause, for example, Pogosta disease in Finland, Karelian fever in the independent states of the former Soviet Union, and Okelbo disease in Sweden) and with the genetically related southern African strains are particularly likely to result in the arthritis-rash syndrome. Exposure to a rural environment is commonly associated with this infection, which has an incubation period of <1 week.

The disease begins with rash and arthralgia. Constitutional symptoms are not marked, and fever is modest or lacking altogether. The rash, which lasts about a week, begins on the trunk, spreads to the extremities, and evolves from macules to papules that often vesiculate. The arthritis of this condition is multiarticular, migratory, and incapacitating, with resolution of the acute phase in a few days. Wrists, ankles, phalangeal joints, knees, elbows, and—to a much lesser extent—proximal and axial joints are involved. Persistence of joint pains and occasionally of arthritis is a major problem and may go on for months or even years despite a lack of deformity.

CHIKUNGUNYA VIRUS INFECTION It is likely that chikungunya virus ("that which bends up") is of African origin and is maintained among nonhuman primates on that continent by *Aedes* mosquitoes of the subgenus *Stegomyia* in a fashion similar to yellow fever virus. Like yellow fever virus, chikungunya virus is readily transmitted among humans in urban areas by *A. aegypti*. The *A. aegypti*–chikungunya virus transmission cycle has also been introduced into Asia, where it poses a prominent health problem. The disease is endemic in rural areas of Africa, and intermittent epidemics take place in towns and cities of Africa and Asia. Chikungunya is one more reason (in addition to dengue and yellow fever) that *A. aegypti* must be controlled.

Full-blown disease is most common among adults, in whom the clinical picture may be dramatic. The brusque onset follows an incubation period of 2 to 3 days. Fever and severe arthralgia are accompanied by chills and constitutional symptoms such as headache, photophobia, conjunctival injection, anorexia, nausea, and abdominal pain. Migratory polyarthritis mainly affects the small joints of the hands, wrists, ankles, and feet, with lesser involvement of the larger joints. Rash may appear at the outset or several days into the illness; its development often coincides with defervescence, which takes place around day 2 or day 3 of disease. The rash is most intense on the trunk and limbs and may desquamate. Petechiae are occasionally seen, and epistaxis is not uncommon, but this virus is not a regular cause of the HF syndrome, even in children. A few patients develop leukopenia. Elevated levels of aspartate aminotransferase (AST) and C-reactive protein have been described, as have mildly decreased platelet counts. Recovery may require weeks. Some older patients continue to suffer from stiffness, joint pain, and recurrent effusions for several years; this persistence may be especially common in HLA-B27 patients. An investigational live attenuated vaccine has been developed but requires further testing.

A related virus, O'nyong-nyong, caused a major epidemic of arthritis and rash involving at least 2 million people as it moved across eastern and central Africa in the 1960s. After its mysterious emergence, the virus virtually disappeared, leaving only occasional evidence of its persistence in Kenya until a transient resurgence of epidemic activity in 1997.

MAYARO FEVER Mayaro virus is maintained in the forests of the Americas by *Haemagogus* mosquitoes and nonhuman primates. It causes a frequently endemic and sometimes epidemic infection of humans and appears to produce a syndrome resembling chikungunya.

EPIDEMIC POLYARTHRITIS (ROSS RIVER VIRUS INFECTION) Ross River virus has caused epidemics of distinctive clinical disease in Australia since the beginning of the twentieth century and continues to be responsible for thousands of cases in rural and suburban areas annually. The virus is transmitted by *A. vigilax* and other mosquitoes, and its persistence is thought to involve transovarial transmission. No definitive vertebrate host has been identified, but several mammalian species, including wallabies, have been suggested. Endemic transmission has also been documented in New Guinea, and in 1979 the virus swept through the eastern Pacific Islands, causing hundreds of thousands of illnesses. The virus was carried from island to island by infected humans and was believed to have been transmitted among humans by *A. polynesiensis* and *A. aegypti*.

The incubation period is 7 to 11 days long, and the onset of illness is sudden, with joint pain usually ushering in the disease. The rash generally develops coincidentally or follows shortly but in some cases precedes joint pains by several days. Constitutional symptoms such as low-grade fever, asthenia, myalgia, headache, and nausea are not prominent and indeed are absent in many cases. Most patients are incapacitated for considerable periods by joint involvement, which interferes with sleeping, walking, and grasping. Wrist, ankle, metacarpophalangeal, interphalangeal, and knee joints are the most commonly involved, although toes, shoulders, and elbows may be affected with some frequency. Periarticular swelling and tenosynovitis are common, and one-third of patients have true arthritis. Only half of all arthritis patients can resume normal activities within 4 weeks, and 10% still must limit their activity at 3 months. Occasional patients are symptomatic for 1 to 3 years but without progressive arthropathy. Aspirin and nonsteroidal anti-inflammatory drugs are effective for the treatment of symptoms.

Clinical laboratory values are normal or variable in Ross River virus infection. Tests for rheumatoid factor and antinuclear antibodies are negative, and the erythrocyte sedimentation rate is acutely elevated. Joint fluid contains 1000 to 60,000 mononuclear cells per microliter, and Ross River virus antigen is demonstrable in macrophages. IgM antibodies are valuable in the diagnosis of this infection, although they occasionally persist for years. The isolation of the virus from blood by mosquito inoculation or mosquito cell culture is possible early in the illness. Because of the great economic impact of annual epidemics in Australia, an inactivated vaccine is being developed and has been found to be protective in mice.

Perhaps because of the local interest in arboviruses in general and in Ross River virus in particular, other arthritogenic arboviruses have been identified in Australia, including Gan Gan virus, a member of the family Bunyaviridae; Kokobera virus, a flavivirus; and Barmah Forest virus, an alphavirus. The last virus is a common cause of infection and must be differentiated from Ross River virus by specific testing.

HEMORRHAGIC FEVERS

The viral HF syndrome is a constellation of findings based on vascular instability and decreased vascular integrity. An assault, direct or indirect, on the microvasculature leads to increased permeability and (particularly when platelet function is decreased) to actual disruption and local hemorrhage. Blood pressure is decreased, and in severe cases

shock supervenes. Cutaneous flushing and conjunctival suffusion are examples of common, observable abnormalities in the control of local circulation. The hemorrhage is inconstant and is in most cases an indication of widespread vascular damage rather than a life-threatening loss of blood volume. Disseminated intravascular coagulation is occasionally found in any severely ill patient with HF but is thought to occur regularly only in the early phases of HF with renal syndrome, Crimean Congo HF, and perhaps some cases of filovirus HF. In some viral HF syndromes, specific organs may be particularly impaired, such as the kidney in HF with renal syndrome, the lung in hantavirus pulmonary syndrome, or the liver in yellow fever, but in all these diseases the generalized circulatory disturbance is critically important.

The pathogenesis of HF is poorly understood and varies among the viruses regularly implicated in the syndrome, which number more than a dozen. In some cases direct damage to the vascular system or even to parenchymal cells of target organs is important, whereas in others soluble mediators are thought to play the major role. The acute phase in most cases of HF is associated with ongoing virus replication and viremia. Exceptions are the hantavirus diseases and dengue HF/dengue shock syndrome (DHF/DSS), in which the immune response plays a major pathogenic role.

The HF syndromes all begin with fever and myalgia, usually of abrupt onset. Within a few days the patient presents for medical attention because of increasing prostration that is often accompanied by severe headache, dizziness, photophobia, hyperesthesia, abdominal or chest pain, anorexia, nausea or vomiting, and other gastrointestinal disturbances. Initial examination often reveals only an acutely ill patient with conjunctival suffusion, tenderness to palpation of muscles or abdomen, and borderline hypotension or postural hypotension, perhaps with tachycardia. Petechiae (often best visualized in the axillae), flushing of the head and thorax, periorbital edema, and proteinuria are common. Levels of AST are usually elevated at presentation or within a day or two thereafter. Hemoconcentration from vascular leakage, which is usually evident, is most marked in hantavirus diseases and in DHF/DSS. The seriously ill patient progresses to more severe symptoms and develops shock and other findings typical of the causative virus. Shock, multifocal bleeding, and CNS involvement (encephalopathy, coma, convulsions) are all poor prognostic signs.

One of the major diagnostic clues is travel to an endemic area within the incubation period for a given syndrome (Table 198-4). Except for Seoul, dengue, and yellow fever virus infections, which have urban vectors, travel to a rural setting is especially suggestive of a diagnosis of HF.

Early recognition is important because of the need for virus-specific therapy and supportive measures, including prompt, atraumatic hospitalization; judicious fluid therapy that takes into account the patient's increased capillary permeability; administration of cardiotonic drugs; use of pressors to maintain blood pressure at levels that will support renal perfusion; treatment of the relatively common secondary bacterial infections; replacement of clotting factors and platelets as indicated; and the usual precautionary measures used in the treatment of patients with hemorrhagic diatheses. Disseminated intravascular coagulation should be treated only if clear laboratory evidence of its existence is found and if laboratory monitoring of therapy is feasible; there is no proven benefit of such therapy. The available evidence suggests that HF patients have a decreased cardiac output and will respond poorly to fluid loading as it is often practiced in the treatment of shock associated with bacterial sepsis. Specific therapy is available for several of the HF syndromes. In addition, several diseases considered in the differential diagnosis—malaria, shigellosis, typhoid, leptospirosis, relapsing fever, and rickettsial disease—are treatable and potentially lethal. Strict barrier nursing and other precautions against infection of medical staff and visitors are indicated in HF except that due to hantaviruses, yellow fever, Rift Valley fever, and dengue.

LASSA FEVER Lassa virus is known to cause endemic and epidemic disease in Nigeria, Sierra Leone, Guinea, and Liberia, al-

Table 198-4 Viral Hemorrhagic Fever (HF) Syndromes and Their Distribution

Disease	Incubation Period, Days	Case-Infection Ratio	Case-Fatality Rate, %	Geographic Range	Target Population
Lassa fever	5–16	Mild infections probably common	15	West Africa	All ages, both sexes
South American HF	7–14	Most infections (more than half) result in disease	15–30	Selected rural areas of Bolivia, Argentina, Venezuela, and Brazil	Bolivia: Men in countryside; all ages, both sexes in villages Argentina: All ages, both sexes; excess exposure and disease in men Venezuela: All ages, both sexes
Rift Valley fever	2–5	~1:100 (most infections result in fever and myalgia)	~50	Sub-Saharan Africa, Madagascar, Egypt	All ages, both sexes; more often diagnosed in men; preexisting liver disease may predispose
Crimean Congo HF	3–12	≥1:5 or higher	15–30	Africa, Middle East, Balkans, southern region of former Soviet Union, western China	All ages, both sexes; men more exposed in some settings
HF with renal syndrome	9–35	Hantaan, >1:1.25; Puumala, 1:20	5–15, Hantaan; <1, Puumala	Worldwide, depending on rodent reservoir	Excess of male patients (partly due to greater exposure); mainly adults
Hantavirus pulmonary syndrome	~7–28	Very high	40–50	Americas	Excess of male patients due to some occupational exposure; mainly adults
Marburg or Ebola HF	3–16	High	25–90	Sub-Saharan Africa	All ages, both sexes; children less exposed
Yellow fever	3–6	1:2–1:20	20	Africa, South America	All ages, both sexes; adults more exposed in jungle setting; preexisting flavivirus immunity may cross-protect
Dengue HF/dengue shock syndrome	2–7	1:10,000, nonimmune; 1:100, heterologous immune	<1 with supportive treatment	Tropics and subtropics worldwide	Predominantly children; previous heterologous dengue infection predisposes to HF
Kyasanur Forest/ Omsk HF	3–8	Variable	0.5–10	Mysore State, India/ western Siberia	Variable

though it is probably more widely distributed in West Africa. This virus and its relatives exist elsewhere in Africa, but their health significance is unknown. Like other arenaviruses, Lassa virus is spread to humans by small-particle aerosols from chronically infected rodents and may also be acquired during the capture or eating of these animals. It can be transmitted by close person-to-person contact. The virus is often present in urine during convalescence and is suspected to be present in seminal fluid early in recovery. Nosocomial spread has occurred but is uncommon if proper sterile parenteral techniques are used. People of all ages and both sexes are affected; the incidence of disease is highest in the dry season, but transmission takes place year-round. In countries where Lassa virus is endemic, Lassa fever can be a prominent cause of febrile disease. For example, in one hospital in Sierra Leone, laboratory-confirmed Lassa fever is consistently responsible for one-fifth of admissions to the medical wards. There are probably tens of thousands of Lassa fever cases annually in West Africa alone.

The average case has a gradual onset (among the HF agents, only the arenaviruses are typically associated with a gradual onset) that gives way to more severe constitutional symptoms and prostration. Bleeding is seen in only ~15 to 30% of cases. A maculopapular rash is often noted in light-skinned Lassa patients. Effusions are common, and male-dominant pericarditis may develop late. The fetal death rate is 92% in the last trimester, when maternal mortality is also increased from the usual 15% to 30%; these figures suggest that interruption of the pregnancy of infected women should be considered. White blood cell counts are normal or slightly elevated, and platelet counts are normal or somewhat low. Deafness coincides with clinical improvement in ~20% of cases and is permanent and bilateral in some. Reinfection may occur but has not been associated with severe disease.

High-level viremia or a high serum concentration of AST statistically predicts a fatal outcome. Thus patients with an AST level of >150 IU/mL should be treated with intravenous ribavirin. This antiviral nucleoside analogue appears to be effective in reducing mortality from rates among retrospective controls, and its only major side effect is reversible anemia that usually does not require transfusion. The drug should be given by slow intravenous infusion in a dose of 32 mg/kg; this dose should be followed by 16 mg/kg q6h for 4 days and then by 8 mg/kg q8h for 6 days.

SOUTH AMERICAN HF SYNDROMES (ARGENTINE, BOLIVIAN, VENEZUELAN, AND BRAZILIAN) These diseases are similar to one another clinically, but their epidemiology differs with the habits of their rodent reservoirs and the interactions of these animals with humans (Table 198-4). Person-to-person or nosocomial transmission is rare but has occurred.

The basic disease resembles Lassa fever with two marked differences. First, thrombocytopenia—often marked—is the rule, and bleeding is quite common. Second, CNS dysfunction is much more common than in Lassa fever and is often manifest by marked confusion, tremors of the upper extremities and tongue, and cerebellar signs. Some cases follow a predominantly neurologic course, with a poor prognosis. The clinical laboratory is helpful in diagnosis since thrombocytopenia, leukopenia, and proteinuria are typical findings.

Argentine HF is readily treated with convalescent-phase plasma given within the first 8 days of illness. In the absence of passive antibody therapy, intravenous ribavirin in the dose recommended for Lassa fever is likely to be effective in all the South American HF syndromes. The transmission of the disease from men convalescing from Argentine HF to their wives suggests the need for counseling of arenavirus HF patients concerning the avoidance of intimate contacts for several weeks after recovery. A safe, effective, live attenuated vaccine exists for Argentine HF. In experimental animals, this vaccine is cross-protective against the Bolivian HF virus.

RIFT VALLEY FEVER This mosquito-borne virus is also a pathogen of domestic animals such as sheep, cattle, and goats. It is maintained in nature by transovarial transmission in floodwater *Aedes* mosquitoes and presumably also has a vertebrate amplifier. Epizootics and epidemics occur when sheep or cattle become infected during particularly heavy rains; developing high-level viremia, these animals infect many different species of mosquitoes. Remote sensing via satellite can detect the ecologic changes associated with high rainfall that predict the likelihood of Rift Valley fever transmission; it can also detect the special depressions from which the floodwater *Aedes* mosquito vectors emerge. In addition, the virus is infectious when transmitted by contact with blood or aerosols from domestic animals or their abortuses. The slaughtered meat is not infectious; anaerobic glycolysis in postmortem tissues results in an acidic environment that rapidly inactivates Bunyaviridae such as Rift Valley fever virus and Crimean-Congo HF virus. The natural range of Rift Valley fever virus is confined to sub-Saharan Africa, where its circulation is markedly enhanced by substantial rainfall such as that which occurred during the El Niño phenomenon of 1997. The virus has also been found in Madagascar and has been introduced into Egypt, where it caused major epidemics in 1977 to 1979, 1993, and subsequently. Neither person-to-person nor nosocomial transmission has been documented.

Rift Valley fever virus is unusual in that it causes at least four different clinical syndromes. Most infections are manifested as the febrile-myalgic syndrome. A small proportion result in HF with especially prominent liver involvement. Perhaps 10% of otherwise mild infections lead to retinal vasculitis; funduscopic examination reveals edema, hemorrhages, and infarction, and some patients have permanently impaired vision. A small proportion of cases (<1 in 200) are followed by typical viral encephalitis. One of the complicated syndromes does not appear to predispose to another.

There is no proven therapy for any of the syndromes described above. The sensitivity of animal models of Rift Valley fever to antibody or ribavirin therapy suggests that either could be given intravenously to persons with HF. Both retinal disease and encephalitis occur after the acute febrile syndrome has ended and serum neutralizing antibody has developed—events suggesting that only supportive care need be given. Epidemic disease is best prevented by vaccination of livestock. The established ability of this virus to propagate after an introduction into Egypt suggests that other potentially receptive areas, including the United States, should have a response ready for such an eventuality. It seems likely that this disease, like Venezuelan equine encephalitis, can be controlled only with adequate stocks of an effective live attenuated vaccine, and there are no such global stocks. A formalin-inactivated vaccine confers immunity to humans, but quantities are limited and three injections are required; this vaccine is recommended for exposed laboratory workers and for veterinarians working in sub-Saharan Africa.

CRIMEAN CONGO HF This severe HF syndrome has a wide geographic distribution, potentially being found wherever ticks of the genus *Hyalomma* occur (Table 198-4). The propensity of these ticks to feed on domestic livestock and certain wild mammals means that veterinary serosurveys are the most effective mechanism for the surveillance of virus circulation in a region. Human infection is acquired via a tick bite or during the crushing of infected ticks. Domestic animals do not become ill but do develop viremia; thus there is danger

of infection at the time of slaughter and for a brief interval thereafter (through contact with hides or carcasses). Cases have followed sheep shearing. An epidemic in South Africa was associated with slaughter of tick-infested ostriches. Nosocomial epidemics are common and are usually related to extensive blood exposure or needle sticks.

Although generally similar to other HF syndromes, Crimean Congo HF causes extensive liver damage, resulting in jaundice in some cases. Clinical laboratory values indicate disseminated intravascular coagulation and show elevations in AST, creatine phosphokinase, and bilirubin. Patients with fatal cases generally have more marked changes, even in the early days of illness, and also develop leukocytosis rather than leukopenia. Thrombocytopenia is also more marked and develops earlier in cases with a fatal outcome.

No controlled trials have been performed with intravenous ribavirin, but clinical experience and retrospective comparison of patients with ominous clinical laboratory values suggest that ribavirin is efficacious and should be given. No human or veterinary vaccines are recommended.

HF WITH RENAL SYNDROME This disease, the first to be identified as an HF, is widely distributed over Europe and Asia; the major causative viruses and their rodent reservoirs on these two continents are Puumala virus (bank vole, *Clethrionomys glareolus*) and Hantaan virus (striped field mouse, *Apodemus agrarius*), respectively. Other potential causative viruses exist, including Dobrava virus (yellow-necked field mouse, *A. flavicollus*), which causes severe HF with renal syndrome in the Balkans. Seoul virus is associated with the Norway or sewer rat, *Rattus norvegicus*, and has a worldwide distribution through the migration of the rodent; it is associated with mild or moderate HF with renal syndrome in Asia, but in many areas of the world the human disease has been difficult to identify. Most cases occur in rural residents or vacationers; the exception is Seoul virus disease, which may be acquired in an urban or rural setting or from contaminated laboratory rat colonies. Classic Hantaan disease in Korea (Korean HF) and in rural China (epidemic HF) is most common in spring and fall and is related to rodent density and agricultural practices. Human infection is acquired primarily through aerosols of rodent urine, although virus is also present in saliva and feces. Patients with hantavirus diseases are not infectious. HF with renal syndrome is the most important form of HF today, with more than 100,000 cases of severe disease in Asia annually and milder Puumala infections numbering in the thousands as well.

Severe cases of HF with renal syndrome caused by Hantaan virus evolve in identifiable stages: the febrile stage with myalgia, lasting 3 to 4 days; the hypotensive stage, often associated with shock and lasting from a few hours to 48 h; the oliguric stage with renal failure, lasting 3 to 10 days; and the polyuric stage with diuresis and hyposthenuria.

The *febrile period* is initiated by the abrupt onset of fever, headache, severe myalgia, thirst, anorexia, and often nausea and vomiting. Photophobia, retroorbital pain, and pain on ocular movement are common, and the vision may become blurred with ciliary body inflammation. Flushing over the face, the V area of the neck, and the back are characteristic, as are pharyngeal injection, periorbital edema, and conjunctival suffusion. Petechiae often develop in areas of pressure, the conjunctivae, and the axillae. Back pain and tenderness to percussion at the costovertebral angle reflect massive retroperitoneal edema. Laboratory evidence of mild to moderate disseminated intravascular coagulation is present. Other laboratory findings include proteinuria and an active urinary sediment.

The *hypotensive phase* is ushered in by falling blood pressure and sometimes by shock. The relative bradycardia typical of the febrile phase is replaced by tachycardia. Kinin activation is marked. The rising hematocrit reflects increasing vascular leakage. Leukocytosis with a left shift develops, and thrombocytopenia continues. Atypical lymphocytes—which in fact are activated CD8+ and to a lesser extent CD4+ T cells—circulate. Proteinuria is marked, and the urine's specific gravity falls to 1.010. The renal circulation is congested and compromised from local and systemic circulatory changes resulting in necrosis of tubules, particularly at the corticomedullary junction, and oliguria.

During the *oliguric phase*, hemorrhagic tendencies continue, probably in large part because of uremic bleeding defects. The oliguria persists for 3 to 10 days before renal function returns and marks the onset of the *polyuric stage*, which carries the danger of dehydration and electrolyte abnormalities.

Mild cases of HF with renal syndrome may be much less stereotypical. The presentation may include only fever, gastrointestinal abnormalities, and transient oliguria followed by hyposthenuria.

HF with renal syndrome should be suspected in patients with rural exposure in an endemic area. Prompt recognition of the disease will permit rapid hospitalization and expectant management of shock and renal failure. Useful clinical laboratory parameters include leukocytosis, which may be leukemoid and is associated with a left shift; thrombocytopenia; and proteinuria. Mainstays of therapy are the management of shock, reliance on pressors, modest crystalloid infusion, intravenous use of human serum albumin, and treatment of renal failure with prompt dialysis for the usual indications. Hydration may result in pulmonary edema, and hypertension should be avoided because of the possibility of intracranial hemorrhage. Use of intravenous ribavirin has reduced mortality and morbidity in severe cases provided treatment is begun within the first 4 days of illness. The case-fatality ratio may be as high as 15% but with proper therapy should be <5%. Sequelae have not been definitely established, but there is a correlation in the United States between chronic hypertensive renal failure and the presence of antibodies to Seoul virus.

Infections with Puumala virus, the most common cause of HF with renal syndrome in Europe, result in a much attenuated picture but the same general presentation. The syndrome may be referred to by its former name, *nephropathia epidemica*. Bleeding manifestations are found in only 10% of cases, hypotension rather than shock is usually seen, and oliguria is present in only about half of patients. The dominant features may be fever, abdominal pain, proteinuria, mild oliguria, and sometimes blurred vision or glaucoma followed by polyuria and hyposthenuria in recovery. Mortality is <1%.

The diagnosis is readily made by IgM-capture ELISA, which should be positive at admission or within 24 to 48 h thereafter. The isolation of virus is difficult, but RT-PCR of a blood clot collected early in the clinical course or of tissues obtained postmortem will give positive results. Such testing is usually undertaken only if definitive identification of the infecting viral species is required or if molecular epidemiologic questions exist.

HANTAVIRUS PULMONARY SYNDROME Hantavirus pulmonary syndrome was discovered in 1993, but retrospective identification of cases by immunohistochemistry (1978) and serology (1959) support the idea that it is a recently discovered rather than a truly new disease. The causative viruses are hantaviruses of a distinct phylogenetic lineage that is associated with the rodent subfamily Sigmodontinae. Sin Nombre virus chronically infects the deer mouse (*Peromyscus maniculatus*) and is the most important virus causing hantavirus pulmonary syndrome in the United States. The disease is also caused by a Sin Nombre virus variant from the white-footed mouse (*P. leucopus*), by Black Creek Canal virus (*Sigmodon hispidus*, the cotton rat), and by Bayou virus (*Oryzomys palustris*, the rice rat). Several other related viruses cause the disease in South America, but Andes virus is unusual in that it, alone among hantaviruses, has been implicated in human-to-human transmission. The disease is linked to rodent exposure and particularly affects rural residents living in dwellings permeable to rodent entry or working at occupations that pose a risk of rodent exposure. Each rodent species has its own particular habits; in the case of the deer mouse, these behaviors include living in and around human habitation.

The disease begins with a prodrome of about 3 to 4 days (range,

1 to 11 days) comprising fever, myalgia, malaise, and often gastrointestinal disturbances such as nausea, vomiting, and abdominal pain. Dizziness is common and vertigo occasional. Severe prodromal symptoms bring some individuals to medical attention, but patients are usually recognized as the cardiopulmonary phase begins. Typically, there is slightly lowered blood pressure, tachycardia, tachypnea, mild hypoxemia, and early radiographic signs of pulmonary edema. Physical findings in the chest are often surprisingly scant. The conjunctival and cutaneous signs of vascular involvement seen in other types of HF are absent. During the next few hours, decompensation may progress rapidly to severe hypoxemia and respiratory failure. Most patients surviving the first 48 h of hospitalization are extubated and discharged within a few days, with no apparent residua.

Management during the first few hours after presentation is critical. The goal is to prevent severe hypoxemia by oxygen therapy and, if needed, intubation and intensive respiratory management. During this period, hypotension and shock with increasing hematocrit invite aggressive fluid administration, but this intervention should be undertaken with great caution. Because of low cardiac output with myocardial depression and increased pulmonary vascular permeability, shock should be managed expectantly with pressors and modest infusion of fluid guided by the pulmonary capillary wedge pressure. Mild cases can be managed by frequent monitoring and oxygen administration without intubation. Many patients require intubation to manage hypoxemia and also develop shock. Mortality remains at ~30 to 40% with good management. The antiviral drug ribavirin inhibits the virus in vitro but did not have a marked effect on patients treated in an open-label study.

During the prodrome, the differential diagnosis of hantavirus pulmonary syndrome is difficult, but by the time of presentation or within 24 h thereafter, a number of diagnostically helpful clinical features become apparent. Cough is not usually present at the outset but may develop later. Interstitial edema is evident on the chest x-ray. Later, bilateral alveolar edema with a central distribution develops in the setting of a normal-sized heart; occasionally, the edema is initially unilateral. Pleural effusions are often visualized. Thrombocytopenia, circulating atypical lymphocytes, and a left shift (often with leukocytosis) are almost always evident; thrombocytopenia has been a particularly important early clue. Hemoconcentration, proteinuria, and hypoalbuminemia should also be sought. Although thrombocytopenia virtually always develops and prolongation of the partial thromboplastin time is the rule, clinical evidence for coagulopathy or laboratory indications of disseminated intravascular coagulation are found in only a minority of cases, usually in severely ill patients. Severely ill patients also have acidosis and elevated serum levels of lactate. Mildly increased values in renal function tests are common, but patients with severe cases often have markedly elevated concentrations of serum creatinine; some of the viruses other than Sin Nombre virus have been associated with more kidney involvement, but few such cases have been studied. The differential diagnosis includes abdominal surgical conditions and pyelonephritis as well as rickettsial disease, sepsis, meningococcemia, plague, tularemia, influenza, and relapsing fever.

A specific diagnosis is best made by IgM testing of acute-phase serum, which has yielded positive results even in the prodrome. Tests using a Sin Nombre virus antigen detect the related hantaviruses causing the pulmonary syndrome in the Americas. Occasionally, heterologous viruses will react only in the IgG ELISA, but this finding is highly suspicious given the very low seroprevalence of these viruses in normal populations. RT-PCR is usually positive when used to test blood clots obtained in the first 7 to 9 days of illness as well as tissues; this test is useful in identifying the infecting virus in areas outside the home range of the deer mouse and in atypical cases.

YELLOW FEVER Yellow fever virus caused major epidemics in the Americas, Africa, and Europe before the discovery of mosquito transmission in 1900 led to its control through attacks on its urban vector, *A. aegypti*. Only then was it found that a jungle cycle also existed in Africa, involving other *Aedes* mosquitoes and monkeys, and that colonization of the New World with *A. aegypti*, originally an African species, had established urban yellow fever as well as an independent sylvatic yellow fever cycle in American jungles involving *Haemagogus* mosquitoes and New World monkeys. Today, urban yellow fever transmission occurs only in some African cities, but the threat exists in the great cities of South America, where reinfestation by *A. aegypti* has taken place and dengue transmission by the same mosquito is common. As late as 1905, New Orleans suffered more than 3000 cases with 452 deaths from "yellow jack." Despite the existence of a highly effective and safe vaccine, several hundred jungle yellow fever cases occur annually in South America, and thousands of jungle and urban cases occur each year in Africa.

Yellow fever is a typical HF accompanied by prominent hepatic necrosis. A period of viremia, typically lasting 3 or 4 days, is followed by a period of "intoxication." During the latter phase in severe cases, the characteristic jaundice, hemorrhages, black vomit, anuria, and terminal delirium occur, perhaps related in part to extensive hepatic involvement. Blood leukocyte counts may be normal or reduced and are often high in terminal stages. Albuminuria is usually noted and may be marked; as renal function fails in terminal or severe cases, the level of blood urea nitrogen rises proportionally. Abnormalities detected in liver function tests range from modest elevations of AST levels in mild cases to severe derangement.

Urban yellow fever can be prevented by the control of *A. aegypti*. The continuing sylvatic cycle requires vaccination of all visitors to areas of potential transmission. With few exceptions (in the very young and the elderly), reactions to vaccine are minimal; immunity is provided within 10 days and lasts for at least 10 years. An egg allergy dictates caution in vaccine administration. Although there are no documented harmful effects of the vaccine on the fetus, pregnant women should be immunized only if they are definitely at risk of yellow fever exposure. Since vaccination has been associated with several cases of encephalitis in children under 6 months of age, it should be delayed until after 12 months of age unless the risk of exposure is very high. Timely information on changes in yellow fever distribution and yellow fever vaccine requirements can be obtained from Health Information for Travelers, Centers for Disease Control and Prevention, Atlanta, GA 30333; by fax request (404-332-4565; document number 220022#); by phone (404-332-4559); or on the World-Wide Web at www.cdc.gov.

DENGUE HEMORRHAGIC FEVER/DENGUE SHOCK SYNDROME A syndrome of HF noted in the 1950s among children in the Philippines and Southeast Asia was soon associated with dengue virus infections, particularly those occurring against a background of previous exposure to another serotype. The transient heterotypic protection after dengue virus infection is replaced within several weeks by the potential for heterotypic infection resulting in typical dengue fever (see above) or—uncommonly—for enhanced disease (secondary DHF/DSS). In rare instances, primary dengue infections lead to an HF syndrome, but much less is known about pathogenesis in this situation. In the past 20 years, *A. aegypti* has progressively reinvaded Latin America and other areas, and frequent travel by infected individuals has introduced multiple strains of dengue virus from many geographic areas. Thus the pattern of hyperendemic transmission of multiple dengue serotypes has now been established in the Americas and the Caribbean and has led to the emergence of DHF/DSS as a major problem there as well. Millions of dengue infections, including many thousands of cases of DHF/DSS, occur annually. The severe syndrome is unlikely to be seen in U.S. citizens since few children have the dengue antibodies that can trigger the pathogenetic cascade when a second infection is acquired.

Macrophage/monocyte infection is central to the pathogenesis of dengue fever and to the origin of DHF/DSS. Previous infection with a heterologous dengue-virus serotype may result in the production of nonprotective antiviral antibodies that nevertheless bind to the virion's surface and through interaction with the Fc receptor focus secondary dengue viruses on the target cell, the result being enhanced infection. The host is also primed for a secondary antibody response when viral

antigens are released and immune complexes lead to activation of the classic complement pathway, with consequent phlogistic effects. Cross-reactivity at the T cell level results in the release of physiologically active cytokines, including interferon γ and tumor necrosis factor α. The induction of vascular permeability and shock depends on multiple factors, including the following:

1. *Presence of enhancing and nonneutralizing antibodies*—Transplacental maternal antibody may be present in infants <9 months old, or antibody elicited by previous heterologous dengue infection may be present in older individuals. T cell reactivity is also intimately involved.
2. *Age*—Susceptibility to DHF/DSS drops considerably after 12 years of age.
3. *Sex*—Females are more often affected than males.
4. *Race*—Caucasians are more often affected than blacks.
5. *Nutritional status*—Malnutrition is protective.
6. *Sequence of infection*—For example, serotype 1 followed by serotype 2 seems to be more dangerous than serotype 4 followed by serotype 2.
7. *Infecting serotype*—Type 2 is apparently more dangerous than other serotypes.

In addition, there is considerable variation among strains of a given serotype, with Southeast Asian serotype 2 strains having more potential to cause DHF/DSS than others.

Dengue HF is identified by the detection of bleeding tendencies (tourniquet test, petechiae) or overt bleeding in the absence of underlying causes such as preexisting gastrointestinal lesions. Dengue shock syndrome, usually accompanied by hemorrhagic signs, is much more serious and results from increased vascular permeability leading to shock. In mild DHF/DSS, restlessness, lethargy, thrombocytopenia (<100,000/μL), and hemoconcentration are detected 2 to 5 days after the onset of typical dengue fever, usually at the time of defervescence. The maculopapular rash that often develops in dengue fever may also appear in DHF/DSS. In more severe cases, frank shock is apparent, with low pulse pressure, cyanosis, hepatomegaly, pleural effusions, ascites, and in some cases severe ecchymoses and gastrointestinal bleeding. The period of shock lasts only 1 or 2 days, and most patients respond promptly to close monitoring, oxygen administration, and infusion of crystalloid or—in severe cases—colloid. The case-fatality rates reported vary greatly with case ascertainment and the quality of treatment; however, most DHF/DSS patients respond well to supportive therapy, and overall mortality in an experienced center in the tropics is probably as low as 1%.

A virologic diagnosis can be made by the usual means, although multiple flavivirus infections lead to a broad immune response to several members of the group, and this situation may result in a lack of virus specificity of the IgM and IgG immune responses. A secondary antibody response can be sought with tests against several flavivirus antigens to demonstrate the characteristic wide spectrum of reactivity.

The key to control of both dengue fever and DHF/DSS is the control of *A. aegypti*, which also reduces the risk of urban yellow fever and chikungunya virus circulation. Control efforts have been handicapped by the presence of nondegradable tires and long-lived plastic containers in trash repositories, insecticide resistance, urban poverty, and an inability of the public health community to mobilize the populace to respond to the need to eliminate mosquito breeding sites. Live attenuated dengue vaccines are in the late stages of development and have produced promising results in early tests. Whether vaccines can provide safe, durable immunity to an immunopathologic disease such as DHF/DSS in endemic areas is an issue that will have to be tested, but it is hoped that vaccination will reduce transmission to negligible levels.

KYASANUR FOREST DISEASE AND OMSK HEMORRHAGIC FEVER Kyasanur Forest virus and Omsk HF virus are geographically restricted, tick-borne flaviviruses that cause a syndrome of viral HF during a wave of viremia and that may also enter the CNS to cause subsequent viral encephalitis (see discussion of tick-borne encephalitis above). There is no therapy for these infections, but an inactivated vaccine has been used in India against Kyasanur Forest disease. A new and related virus isolate has been obtained from butchers with HF in the Middle East; the implication is that there are more agents in this group.

FILOVIRUS HEMORRHAGIC FEVER　　See Chap. 199.

BIBLIOGRAPHY

ZOONOTIC VIRUSES

CALISHER CH: Medically important arboviruses of the United States and Canada. Clin Microbiol Rev 7:89, 1994

TSAI TF: Arboviral infections in the US. Infect Dis Clin North Am 5:73, 1991

HEMORRHAGIC FEVERS

CENTERS FOR DISEASE CONTROL AND PREVENTION: Management of patients with suspected viral hemorrhagic fever. MMWR 37(S-3):1, 1988

———: Update: Management of patients with suspected viral hemorrhagic fever—United States. MMWR 44:475, 1995

PETERS CJ et al: Management of patients infected with high-hazard viruses. Arch Virol 11(Suppl):141, 1996

——— et al: Pathogenesis of viral hemorrhagic fevers, in *Viral Pathogenesis*, N Nathanson et al (eds). Philadelphia, Lippincott-Raven, 1996

ARENAVIRUSES

BARRY M et al: Treatment of a laboratory-acquired Sabiá virus infection. N Engl J Med 333:294, 1995

ENRIA D, MAIZTEGUI JI: Antiviral treatment of Argentine hemorrhagic fever. Antiviral Res 23:23, 1994

——— et al: Arenaviruses, in *Tropical Infectious Diseases: Principles, Pathogens, & Practice*, RL Guerrant et al (eds). New York, Saunders, 1999, pp 1189–1212

JOHNSON KM et al: Clinical virology of Lassa fever in hospitalized patients. J Infect Dis 155:456, 1987

McCORMICK JB et al: A case-control study of the clinical diagnosis and course of Lassa fever. J Infect Dis 155:445, 1987

SALAS R et al: Venezuelan hemorrhagic fever. Lancet 338:1033, 1991

BUNYAVIRIDAE

ANTONIADIS A et al: Direct genetic detection of Dobrava virus in Greek and Albanian haemorrhagic fever with renal syndrome (HFRS) patients. J Infect Dis 174:407, 1996

BRUNO P et al: The protean manifestations of hemorrhagic fever with renal syndrome. A retrospective review of 26 cases from Korea. Ann Intern Med 113:385, 1990

DUCHIN JS et al: Hantavirus pulmonary syndrome: A clinical description of 17 patients with a newly recognized disease. N Engl J Med 330:949, 1994

HUGGINS JW et al: Prospective, double-blind, concurrent, placebo controlled clinical trial of intravenous ribavirin therapy of hemorrhagic fever with renal syndrome. J Infect Dis 164:1119, 1991

KETAI LH et al: Hantavirus pulmonary syndrome (HPS): Radiographic findings in 16 patients. Radiology 191:665, 1994

LAUGHLIN LW et al: Epidemic Rift Valley fever in Egypt: Observations of the spectrum of human illness. Trans R Soc Trop Med Hyg 73:630, 1979

PETERS CJ: Hantavirus pulmonary syndrome in the Americas, in *Emerging Infections II*, WM Scheld et al (eds). Washington, DC, ASM Press, 1998, pp 17–64

———, LEDUC JW: Bunyaviridae: Bunyaviruses, phleboviruses, and related viruses, in *Textbook of Human Virology*, 2d ed, R Belshe (ed). St Louis, Mosby Year Book, 1991, pp 571–614

SEXTON DJ et al: Life-threatening Cache Valley virus infection. N Engl J Med 336:547, 1997

SWANEPOEL R et al: Epidemiologic and clinical features of Crimean-Congo hemorrhagic fever in South Africa. Am J Trop Med Hyg 6:120, 1987

——— et al: The clinical pathology of Crimean-Congo hemorrhagic fever. Rev Infect Dis 11(Suppl 4):S794, 1989

ZAKI SR: Hantavirus-associated diseases, in *The Pathology of Infectious Diseases*, DH Connor et al (eds). Stamford, CT, Appleton & Lange, 1997

FLAVIVIRUSES

BARROS MLB, BOECKEN G: Jungle yellow fever in the central Amazon. Lancet 348:969, 1996

HALSTEAD SB: Antibody, macrophages, dengue virus infection, shock, and hemorrhage: A pathogenic cascade. Rev Infect Dis 11(Suppl 4):S830, 1989

KURANE I et al: Immunopathologic mechanisms of dengue hemorrhagic fever and dengue shock syndrome. Arch Virol 9:59, 1994

LUBY JP: St. Louis encephalitis, Rocio encephalitis, and West Nile fever, in *Kass Hand-*

book of Infectious Diseases. Exotic Viral Infections, JS Porterfield (ed). New York, Chapman and Hall, 1995, pp 183–202

MONATH TP, HEINZ FX: Flaviviruses, in *Fields Virology*, 3d ed, BN Fields et al (eds). Philadelphia, Lippincott-Raven, 1996, pp 961–1034

TSAI T, YU XX: Japanese encephalitis vaccines, in *Vaccines*, 2d ed, SW Plotkin and E Mortimer (eds). Philadelphia, WB Saunders, 1994, pp 671–713

——— et al: West Nile encephalitis epidemic in southeastern Romania. Lancet 352:767, 1998

WALDVOGEL K et al: Severe tick-borne encephalitis following passive immunization. Eur J Pediatr 155:775, 1996

REOVIRUSES

EMMONS RW: Colorado tick fever, in *Handbook Series of Zoonoses, Section B: Viral Zoonoses, vol 1*, GW Beran (ed). Boca Raton, FL, CRC Press, 1981, pp 113–124

MONATH TP, GUIRAKHOO F: Orbiviruses and coltiviruses, in *Fields Virology*, 3d ed, BN Fields et al (eds). Philadelphia, Lippincott-Raven, 1996, pp 1735–1766

TOGAVIRUSES

FRASER JRE: Epidemic polyarthritis and Ross River virus disease. Clin Rheum Dis 12:369, 1986

JOHNSTON RE, PETERS CJ: Alphaviruses, in *Fields Virology*, 3d ed, BN Fields et al (eds). Philadelphia, Lippincott-Raven, 1996, pp 843–898

MACKENZIE JS: Mosquito-borne viruses and epidemic polyarthritis. Med J Aust 164:90, 1996

PHILLIPS DA et al: Clinical and subclinical Barmah Forest virus infection in Queensland. Med J Aust 152:463, 1990

RIVAS F et al: Epidemic Venezuelan equine encephalitis in La Guajira, Colombia, 1995. J Infect Dis 175:828, 1997

 199　　*C. J. Peters*

FILOVIRIDAE (MARBURG AND EBOLA VIRUSES)

DEFINITION　　Both Marburg virus and Ebola virus cause an acute febrile illness associated with high mortality. This illness is characterized by multisystem involvement that begins with the abrupt onset of headache, myalgias, and fever and proceeds to prostration, rash, shock, and often bleeding manifestations. Epidemics usually begin with a single case acquired from an unknown reservoir in nature and spread mainly through close contact with sick persons or their body fluids, either in the home or at the hospital.

ETIOLOGY　　The family Filoviridae comprises two antigenically and genetically distinct viruses: Marburg virus and Ebola virus. Ebola virus has four readily distinguishable subtypes named for their original site of recognition (Zaire, Sudan, Cote d'Ivoire, and Reston). Except for Ebola virus subtype Reston, all the Filoviridae are African viruses that cause severe and often fatal disease in humans. The Reston virus, which has been exported from the Philippines on several occasions, has caused fatal infections in monkeys but only subclinical infections in humans. Different isolates of the four Ebola subtypes made over time and space exhibit remarkable sequence conservation, indicating marked genetic stability in their selective niche. Typical filovirus particles contain a single linear, negative-sense, single-stranded RNA arranged in a helical nucleocapsid. The virions are 790 to 970 nm in length; they may also appear in elongated, contorted forms. The lipid envelope confers sensitivity to lipid solvents and common detergents. The viruses are largely destroyed by heat (60°C, 30 min) and by acidity but may persist for weeks in blood at room temperature. The surface glycoprotein self-associates to form the virion surface spikes, which presumably mediate attachment to cells and fusion. The glycoprotein's high sugar content may contribute to its low capacity to elicit neutralizing antibodies. A smaller form of the glycoprotein, bearing many of its antigenic determinants, is produced by in vitro–infected cells and is found in the circulation in human disease; it has been speculated that this circulating soluble protein may suppress the immune response to the virion surface protein or block antiviral effector mechanisms. Both Marburg virus and Ebola virus are biosafety level 4 pathogens because of their high associated mortality rate and aerosol infectivity.

EPIDEMIOLOGY Marburg virus was first identified in Germany in 1967, when infected African green monkeys (*Cercopithecus aethiops*) imported from Uganda transmitted the agent to vaccine-laboratory workers. Of the 25 human cases acquired from monkeys, 7 ended in death. The six secondary cases were associated with close contact or parenteral exposure. Secondary spread to the wife of one patient was documented, and virus was isolated from the husband's semen despite the presence of circulating antibodies. Subsequently, isolated cases of Marburg virus infection have been reported from eastern and southern Africa, with limited spread.

In 1999, repeated transmission of Marburg virus to workers in a gold mine in eastern Democratic Republic of Congo was documented. The secondary spread of the virus among patients' families was more extensive than previously noted, resembling that of Ebola virus and emphasizing the importance of hygiene and proper barrier nursing in the epidemiology of these viruses in Africa.

In 1976, epidemics of severe hemorrhagic fever (550 human cases) occurred simultaneously in Zaire and Sudan, and Ebola virus was found to be the etiologic agent. Later, it was shown that different subtypes of virus—associated with 90% and 50% mortality, respectively—caused the two epidemics. Both epidemics were associated with interhuman spread (particularly in the hospital setting) and the use of unsterilized needles and syringes, a common practice in developing-country hospitals. The epidemics dwindled as the clinics were closed and people in the endemic area increasingly shunned affected persons and avoided traditional burial practices.

The Zaire subtype of Ebola virus recurred in a major epidemic (317 cases, 88% mortality) in Democratic Republic of Congo in 1995 and in smaller epidemics in Gabon in 1994–1996. Mortality was high, transmission to caregivers and others who had direct contact with body fluids was common, and poor hygiene in hospitals exacerbated spread. In the Congo epidemic, an index case was infected in Kikwit in January 1995. The epidemic smoldered until April, when intense nosocomial transmission forced closure of the hospitals; samples were finally sent to the laboratory for Ebola testing, which yielded positive results within a few hours. International assistance, with barrier nursing instruction and materials, was provided; nosocomial transmission ceased, hospitals reopened, and patients were segregated to prevent intrafamilial spread. The last case was reported in June 1995.

Three separate emergences of Ebola virus (subtype Zaire) were detected in Gabon from 1994 through 1996, all associated with deep forest exposure and subsequent familial and nosocomial transmission. In the 1996 episode, a physician exposed to Ebola-infected patients traveled to South Africa with a fever; a nurse who assisted in a cutdown on the physician developed Ebola hemorrhagic fever and died in spite of intensive care. The index patient was identified retrospectively on the basis of serum antibodies and virus isolation from semen. Thus, distant transport of Ebola virus is an established risk, and limited nosocomial spread is possible even under hygienic conditions.

The Reston subtype of Ebola virus was first seen in the United States in 1989, when it caused a fatal, highly transmissible disease among cynomolgus macaques imported from the Philippines and quarantined in Reston, VA, pending distribution to biomedical researchers. This and other appearances of the Reston virus have been traced to a single export facility in the Philippines, but no source in nature has been established.

Epidemiologic studies (including a specific search in the Kikwit epidemic) have failed to yield evidence for an important role of airborne particles in human disease. This lack of epidemiologic evidence is surprising and seems to conflict with the viruses' classification as biosafety level 4 pathogens based in part on their aerosol infectivity and with formal laboratory assessments showing a high degree of aerosol infectivity for monkeys. Sick humans apparently do not usually generate sufficient amounts of infectious aerosols to pose a significant hazard to those around them.

Available evidence points to a nonprimate reservoir for these viruses, but an intensive search has failed to elucidate what this reservoir might be. Speculation has centered on a possible role for bats, but that hypothesis has arisen in part merely because of the ubiquity of bats when sought in affected areas and the frustration of researchers in identifying a source of virus.

PATHOLOGY AND PATHOGENESIS In humans and in animal models, Ebola and Marburg viruses replicate well in virtually all cell types, including endothelial cells, macrophages, and parenchymal cells of multiple organs. Viral replication is associated with cellular necrosis both in vivo and in vitro. Significant findings at the light-microscopic level include liver necrosis with Councilman bodies (intracellular inclusions that correlate with extensive collections of viral nucleocapsids), interstitial pneumonitis, cerebral glial nodules, and small infarcts. Antigen and virions are abundant in fibroblasts, interstitium, and (to a lesser extent) the appendages of the subcutaneous tissues in fatal cases; escape through small breaks in the skin or possibly through sweat glands may occur and, if so, may be correlated with the established epidemiologic risk of close contact with patients and the touching of the deceased. Inflammatory cells are not prominent, even in necrotic areas.

In addition to sustaining direct damage from viral infection, patients infected with Ebola virus (Zaire subtype) have high circulating levels of proinflammatory cytokines, which presumably contribute to the severity of the illness. In fact, the virus interacts intimately with the cellular cytokine system. It is resistant to the antiviral effects of interferon α, although this mediator is amply induced. Viral infection of endothelial cells selectively inhibits the expression of MHC class I molecules and blocks the induction of several genes by the interferons. In addition, glycoprotein expression inhibits αV integrin expression, an effect that has been shown in vitro to lead to detachment and subsequent death of endothelial cells.

Acute infection is associated with high levels of circulating virus and viral antigen. Clinical improvement takes place when viral titers decrease concomitantly with the onset of a virus-specific immune response, as detected by enzyme-linked immunosorbent assay (ELISA) or fluorescent antibody test. In fatal cases, there is usually little evidence of an antibody response and there is extensive depletion of spleen and lymph nodes. Recovery is apparently mediated by the cellular immune response: convalescent-phase plasma has little in vitro virus-neutralizing capacity and is not protective in passive transfer experiments in monkey and guinea pig models.

CLINICAL MANIFESTATIONS After an incubation period of ~7 to 10 days (range, 3 to 16 days), the patient abruptly develops fever, severe headache, malaise, myalgia, nausea, and vomiting. Continued fever is joined by diarrhea (often severe), chest pain (accompanied by cough), prostration, and depressed mentation. In light-skinned patients (and less often in blacks), a maculopapular rash appears around day 5 to 7 and is followed by desquamation. Bleeding may begin about this time and is apparent from any mucosal site and into the skin. In some epidemics, fewer than half of patients have had overt bleeding, and this manifestation has been absent even in some fatal cases. Additional findings include edema of the face, neck, and/or scrotum; hepatomegaly; flushing; conjunctival injection; and pharyngitis. Around 10 to 12 days after the onset of disease, the sustained fever may break, with improvement and eventual recovery of the patient. Recrudescence of fever may be associated with secondary bacterial infections or possibly with localized virus persistence. Late hepatitis, uveitis, and orchitis have been reported, with isolation of virus from semen or detection of polymerase chain reaction (PCR) products in vaginal secretions for several weeks.

LABORATORY FINDINGS Leukopenia is common early on; neutrophilia has its onset later. Platelet counts fall below (sometimes much below) 50,000/μL. Laboratory evidence of disseminated intravascular coagulation may be found, but its clinical significance and the need for therapy are controversial. Serum levels of alanine and aspartate aminotransferases (particularly the latter) rise progressively, and jaundice develops in some cases. The serum amylase level may be elevated, and this elevation may be associated with abdominal pain suggesting pancreatitis. Proteinuria is usual; decreased kidney function is proportional to shock.

DIAGNOSIS Most patients acutely ill with Ebola or Marburg viruses have high concentrations of virus in blood. Antigen-detection ELISA is a sensitive, robust diagnostic modality. Virus isolation and reverse transcriptase PCR are also effective and provide additional sensitivity in some cases. Patients who are recovering develop IgM and IgG antibodies that are best detected by ELISA but are also reactive in the less specific fluorescent antibody test. Skin biopsies are an extremely useful adjunct in postmortem diagnosis of Ebola and, to a lesser extent, Marburg virus infections because of the presence of large amounts of viral antigen, the relative safety of obtaining the sample, and the freedom from cold-chain requirements for formalin-fixed tissues.

℞ **TREATMENT** No virus-specific therapy is available, and, given the extensive viral involvement in fatal cases, supportive treatment may not be as useful as was once hoped. Vigorous treatment of shock should take into account the likelihood of vascular leak in the pulmonary and systemic circulation and of myocardial functional compromise. The membrane fusion mechanism of Ebola resembles that of retroviruses, and the identification of "fusogenic" sequences

suggests that inhibitors of cell entry may be developed. Despite the poor neutralizing capacity of polyclonal convalescent-phase sera, phage display of immunoglobulin mRNA from convalescent bone marrow has produced monoclonal antibodies that have in vitro neutralizing capacity and mediate protection in guinea pig models.

PREVENTION No vaccine is available, but barrier nursing precautions in African hospitals can greatly decrease the spread of the virus beyond the index case and thus prevent epidemics of filoviruses and other agents as well.

BIBLIOGRAPHY

HARCOURT BH et al: Ebola virus selectively inhibits responses to interferons, but not to IL-1beta in endothelial cells. J Virol 73:3491, 1999

KLENK HD (ed): Marburg and Ebola viruses. Curr Top Microbiol Immunol 235:1, 1999

MALASHKEVICH VN et al: Core structure of the envelope glycoprotein GP2 from Ebola virus at 1.9-Å resolution. Proc Natl Acad Sci USA 96:2662, 1999

MARTINI GA, SIEGERT R (eds): *Marburg Virus Disease.* Berlin, Springer-Verlag, 1971, pp 1–230

PATTYN SR (ed): *Ebola Virus Haemorrhagic Fever.* Amsterdam, Elsevier/North-Holland, 1978, pp 1–436 (Also available at www.itg.be/ebola)

PETERS CJ, LEDUC JW: An introduction to Ebola: The virus and the disease. J Infect Dis 179(Suppl 1): Six, 1999 (Also available at www.journals.uchicago.edu/JID/)

WORLD HEALTH ORGANIZATION: Ebola haemorrhagic fever in Zaire, 1976. Report of an international commission. Bull World Health Organ 56:271, 1978

———: Ebola haemorrhagic fever in Sudan, 1976. Report of a World Health Organization International Study Team. Bull World Health Organ 56:247, 1978

Section 15
FUNGAL AND ALGAL INFECTIONS

---

200 *John E. Bennett*

DIAGNOSIS AND TREATMENT OF FUNGAL INFECTIONS

MYCOLOGY FUNDAMENTALS

Fungi can appear microscopically as either rounded, budding forms (yeastlike organisms) or hyphae (molds). Yeastlike colonies are smooth, while mold colonies are fuzzy; fungi that grow as yeasts include species of *Candida* and *Cryptococcus*, while fungi that grow as molds include species of *Aspergillus, Rhizopus,* and dermatophytes (ringworm fungi). The fungi that cause histoplasmosis, blastomycosis, sporotrichosis, coccidioidomycosis, and paracoccidioidomycosis are called *dimorphic* ("having two forms") because they are spherical in tissue but grow like molds when cultured at room temperature. *Candida* species other than *Candida glabrata* appear in tissue as both budding yeasts and tubular elements called *pseudohyphae. Pneumocystis carinii* is closer to fungi than to parasites by ribosomal sequences (Chap. 209). Because the drugs used to treat *Pneumocystis* pneumonia are also used to treat parasitic or bacterial infections, those drugs will not be discussed in this chapter.

Many fungi can form two different types of spores and are given different names, depending on the spore-bearing structures. When the spores are produced by mitosis, the fungus is said to be an *anamorph,* or to be in the imperfect state. Many fungi can have different sporulating structures in which genetic recombination occurs, often as a result of coculture with a strain of the opposite mating type. A fungus producing those distinctive spores is said to be a *teleomorph,* or to be in the perfect state. Diagnostic laboratories usually use the name of

the anamorph because they do not use culture conditions that would produce the teleomorph. One exception is *Scedosporium apiospermum,* which is often observed as a teleomorph in the diagnostic laboratory and identified as *Pseudallescheria boydii.*

Most fungi that are pathogenic for humans are saprophytes in nature; they cause infection when airborne spores reach the lung or paranasal sinus or when hyphae or spores are accidentally inoculated into the skin or cornea. Acquisition of infection from another person or an animal has been reported in the case of ringworm but is very rare in other mycoses. Thus, hospitalized patients with fungal infections do not require special isolation. Most fungi infect hosts preferentially by one route and only infrequently by other routes. For example, the agents of ringworm, pityriasis versicolor, and piedra infect the epidermis and its appendages. Sporotrichosis and mycetoma usually arise from subcutaneous inoculation. Inhalation is the route of inoculation for the agents of most deep mycoses. Ingestion of fungi rarely causes infection; *Candida albicans,* a normal commensal in the mouth and intestine, reaches deeper tissues only when mucosal or cutaneous barriers are breached by disease, surgery, trauma, or catheterization. Histoplasmosis, blastomycosis, coccidioidomycosis, and paracoccidioidomycosis have been called "endemic" mycoses to emphasize their restricted geographic distribution. Some fungi, such as *Aspergillus,* are said to be opportunists in that they usually infect hosts with compromised immunity. This distinction is relative, not absolute.

Immunity after exposure to fungi may confer partial protection against reinfection. Residents of areas in which mycoses are endemic are less subject to infection than are newcomers. Predisposing factors are helpful in defining host defense. Immunoglobulin deficiencies do not appear to predispose to any mycosis, whereas neutropenia is common among patients who develop invasive aspergillosis or deep candidiasis. Cell-mediated immunity appears to be of paramount importance in most other deep mycoses.

COLOR ATLASES

I. Atlas of Cardiology

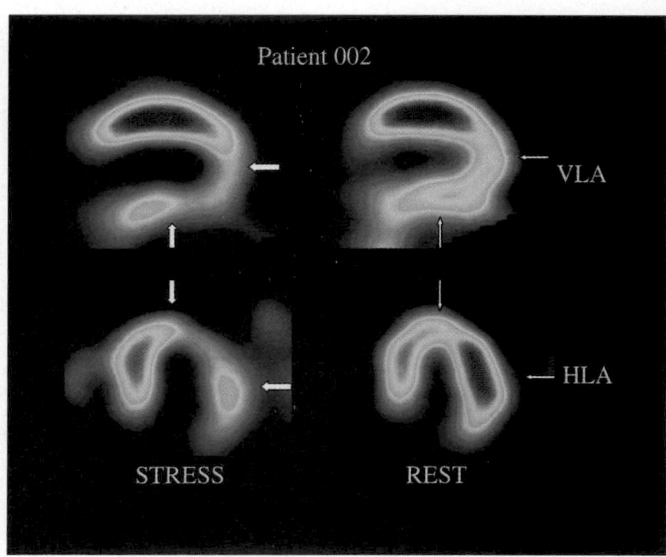

I-1A **Exercise sestamibi study** on a 71-year-old, white female with atypical angina. *Left:* stress images; *right:* rest images. The images are normal. There is even sestamibi update throughout the myocardium at rest and during stress. SA, short axis. Mid, middle of the left ventricle. VLA, vertical long axis. HLA, horizontal long axis.

I-1B **Exercise sestamibi study** on a 75-year-old male with a history of typical angina. *Left:* stress images; *right:* rest images. The stress images show a large defect involving the apex, lateral, and inferior walls (*thick arrows*), which improves at rest (*thin arrows*). Subsequent coronary angiography demonstrates severe three-vessel coronary artery disease.

I-2 **Transesophageal echocardiographic view** of a patient with severe mitral regurgitation due to a flail posterior leaflet. The *arrow* points to the portion of the posterior leaflet that is unsupported and moves into the left atrium during systole. *Right:* color flow imaging demonstrating a large mosaic jet of mitral regurgitation during systole. LA, left atrium; LV, left ventricle; AV, aortic valve.

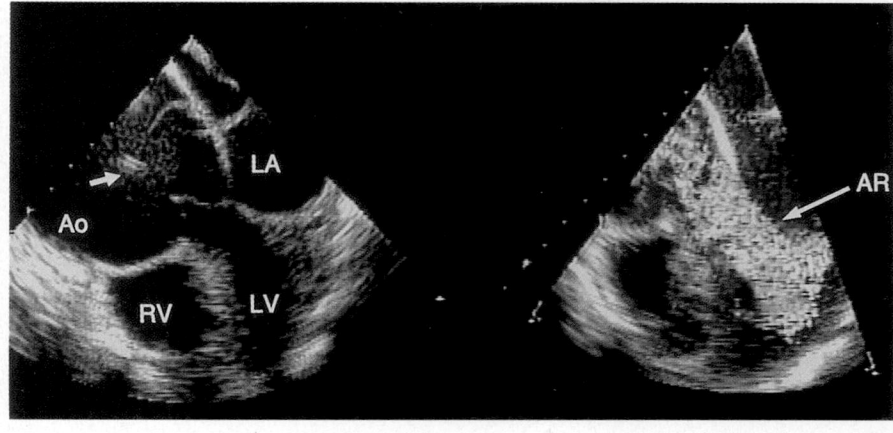

I-3 **Transesophageal echocardiographic view** of a patient with a dilated aorta, aortic dissection, and severe aortic regurgitation. The *arrow* points to the intimal flap that is seen in the dilated ascending aorta. *Left:* the long axis apex down view of the black and white two-dimensional image in diastole. *Right:* color flow imaging that demonstrates a large mosaic jet of aortic regurgitation. AO, aorta; RV, right ventricle; AR, aortic regurgitation.

II. Atlas of Dermatology

Stephen F. Templeton / Thomas J. Lawley

A. Common Skin Diseases and Lesions

IIA-1 **Acne vulgaris** with inflammatory papules, pustules, and comedones

IIA-2 **Acne rosacea** with prominent facial erythema, telangiectasias, scattered papules, and small pustules.

IIA-3 **Psoriasis** is characterized by small and large erythematous plaques with adherent silvery scale.

IIA-4 **Atopic dermatitis** with hyperpigmentation, lichenification, and scaling in the antecubital fossae.

IIA-5 **Dyshidrotic eczema,** characterized by deep-seated vesicles and scaling on palms and lateral fingers, is often associated with an atopic diathesis.

IIA-6 **Seborrheic dermatitis** showing central facial erythema with overlying greasy, yellowish scale.

IIA-7 **Stasis dermatitis** showing erythematous, scaly, and oozing patches over the lower leg. Several stasis ulcers are also seen in this patient.

IIA-8A **Allergic contact dermatitis,** acute phase, with sharply demarcated, weeping, eczematous plaques in a perioral distribution.

IIA-8B **Allergic contact dermatitis** to nickel, chronic phase demonstrating an erythematous, lichenified, weeping plaque on skin chronically exposed to a metal snap.

IIA-9 **Lichen planus** showing multiple flat-topped, violaceous papules and plaques. Nail dystrophy as seen in this patient's thumbnail may also be a feature.

IIA-10 **Seborrheic keratoses** are seen as "stuck on," waxy, verrucous papules and plaques with a variety of colors ranging from light tan to black.

IIA-11 **Vitiligo** in a typical acral distribution demonstrating striking cutaneous depigmentation, as a result of loss of melanocytes.

IIA-12 **Alopecia areata** characterized by a sharply demarcated circular patch of scalp completely devoid of hairs. Follicular orifices are preserved, indicating a nonscarring alopecia.

IIA-13 **Pityriasis rosea** Multiple round to oval erythematous patches with fine central scale are distributed along the skin tension lines on the trunk.

IIA-14A **Urticaria** showing characteristic discrete and confluent, edematous, erythematous papules and plaques.

IIA-14B **Dermatographism** Erythema and whealing that developed after firm stroking of the skin.

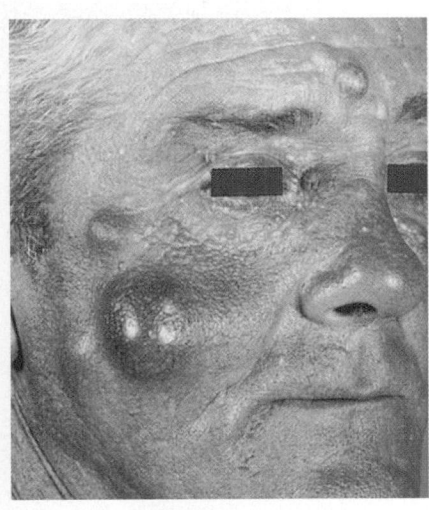

IIA-15 **Epidermoid cysts** Several inflamed and noninflamed firm, cystic nodules are seen in this patient. Often a patulous follicular punctum is observed on the overlying epidermal surface.

IIA-16 **Keloids** resulting from ear piercing, with firm exophytic flesh-colored to erythematous nodules of scar tissue.

IIA-17 **Cherry hemangiomas** are very common and arise in middle-aged to older adults. They are characterized by multiple erythematous to dark purple papules usually located on the trunk.

IIA-18 **Frostbite** with vesiculation, surrounded by edema and erythema.

IIA-19 **Frostbite** with vesiculation, surrounded by edema and erythema.

B. Cutaneous Neoplasms

IIB-20 **Kaposi's sarcoma** in a patient with AIDS demonstrating patch, plaque, and tumor stages.

IIB-21 **Non-Hodgkin's lymphoma** involving the skin with typical violaceous, "plum-colored" nodules.

IIB-22 **Basal cell carcinoma** showing central ulceration and a pearly, rolled, telangiectatic tumor border.

IIB-23 **Mycosis fungoides** is a cutaneous T cell lymphoma, and plaque stage lesions are seen in this patient.

IIB-24 **Metastatic carcinoma** to the skin is characterized by inflammatory, often ulcerated dermal nodules.

IIB-25 **Keratoacanthoma** is a low-grade squamous cell carcinoma that presents as an exophytic nodule with central keratinous debris.

IIB-26 **Squamous cell carcinoma** seen here as a hyperkeratotic crusted and somewhat eroded plaque on the lower lip. Sun-exposed skin such as the head, neck, hands, and arms are other typical sites of involvement.

IIB-27 **Actinic keratoses** consists of hyperkeratotic erythematous papules and patches on sun-exposed skin. They arise in middle-aged to older adults and have some potential for malignant transformation.

IIC-28 **Nevus** Nevi are benign proliferations of nevomelanocytes characterized by regularly shaped hyperpigmented macules or papules of a uniform color.

IIC-29 **Dysplastic nevi** are irregularly pigmented and shaped nevomelanocytic lesions which may be associated with familial melanoma.

IIC-30 **Superficial spreading melanoma** is the most common type of malignant melanoma and demonstrates color variegation (black, blue, brown, pink, and white) and irregular borders.

IIC-31 **Lentigo maligna melanoma** occurs on sun-exposed skin as a large, hyperpigmented macule or plaque with irregular borders and variable pigmentation.

IIC-32 **Nodular melanoma** most commonly manifests itself as a rapidly growing, often ulcerated or crusted black nodule.

IIC-33 **Acral lentiginous melanoma** is more common in blacks, Asians, and Hispanics and occurs as an enlarging hyperpigmented macule or plaque on the palms and soles. Lateral pigment diffusion is present.

D. Infectious Disease and the Skin

IID-34 **Erysipelas** is a streptococcal infection of the superficial dermis and consists of well-demarcated, erythematous, edematous, warm plaques.

IID-35 **Spread of herpes zoster with chemotherapy** The patient reported external ear pain. A vesticular rash on the concha and antihelix suggested Ramsay Hunt syndrome.

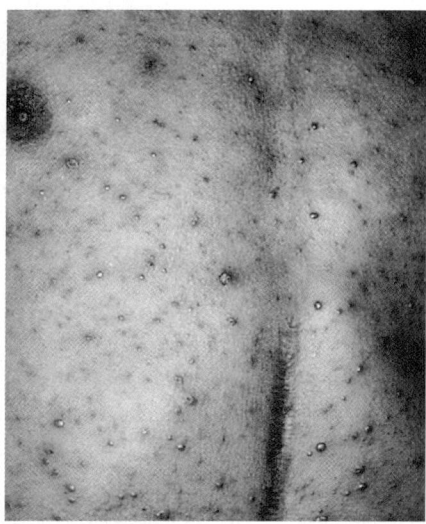

IID-36 **Varicella** showing numerous lesions in various stages of evolution: vesicles on an erythematous base, umbilicated vesicles, and crusts.

IID-37 **Herpes zoster** is seen in this HIV-infected patient as hemorrhagic vesicles and pustules on an erythematous base grouped in a dermatomal distribution.

IID-38 **Impetigo contagiosa** is a superficial streptococcal or *Staphylococcus aureus* infection consisting of honey-colored crusts and erythematous weeping erosions. Occasionally, bullous lesions may be seen.

IID-39 **Tender vesicles and erosions** in the mouth of a patient with hand-foot-and-mouth disease.

IID-40 **Lacy reticular rash of erythema infectiosum** (fifth disease).

IID-41 **Molluscum contagiosum** is a cutaneous poxvirus infection characterized by multiple umbilicated flesh-colored or hypopigmented papules.

IID-42 **Oral hairy leukoplakia** often presents as white plaques on the lateral tongue and is associated with Epstein-Barr virus infection.

IID-43 **Pseudomembranous oral candidiasis** Adherent white, mucoid plaques with an erythematous halo seen here on the palate often indicate an immunocompromised state.

IID-44 **Fulminant meningococcemia** with extensive angular purpuric patches.

IID-45 **Rocky Mountain spotted fever** demonstrating pinpoint petechial lesions on the palm and volar aspect of the wrist.

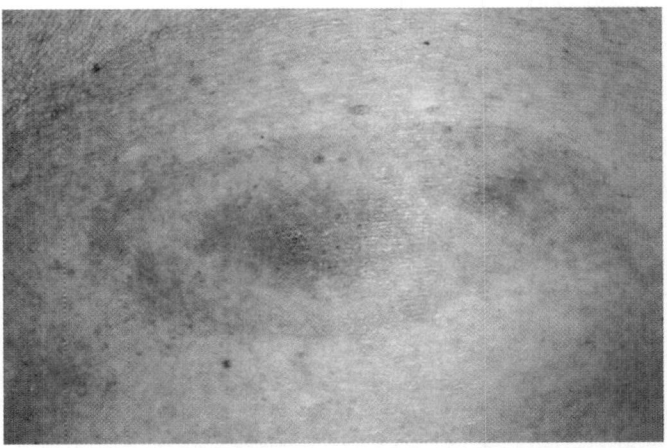

IID-46 **Erythema chronicum migrans** is the early cutaneous manifestation of Lyme disease and is characterized by erythematous annular patches, often with a central erythematous papule at the tick bite site.

IID-47 **Primary syphilis** with a firm, nontender chancre.

IID-48 **Secondary syphilis** commonly affects the palms and soles with scaling, firm, red-brown papules.

IID-49 **Condylomata lata** are moist, somewhat verrucous intertriginous plaques seen in secondary syphilis.

IID-50 **Secondary syphilis** demonstrating the papulosquamous truncal eruption.

IID-51 **Tinea corporis** is a superficial fungal infection, seen here as an erythematous annular scaly plaque with central clearing.

IID-52 **Scabies** showing typical scaling erythematous papules and few linear burrows.

IID-53 **Skin lesions** caused by *Chironex fleckeri* sting.

IID-54 **Chancroid** with characteristic penile ulcers and associated left inguinal adenitis (bubo).

IID-55 **Condylomata acuminata** are lesions induced by human papillomavirus and in this patient are seen as multiple verrucous papules coalescing into plaques.

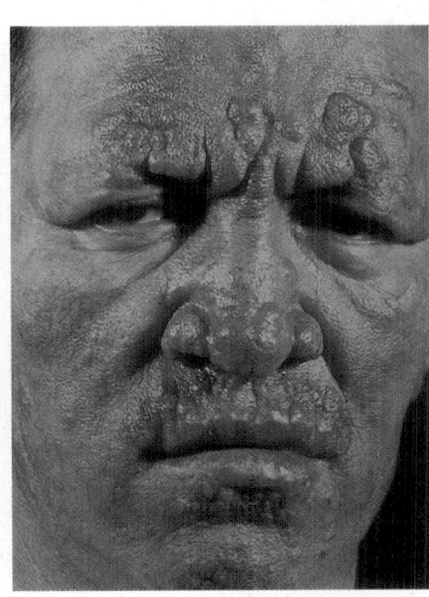

IID-56 **A patient with features of polar lepromatous leprosy;** multiple nodular skin lesions, particularly of the forehead, and loss of eyebrows.

A

B

C

D

IID-57 **Skin lesions of neutropenic patients** *A.* Papules related to *Escherichia coli* bacteremia in a neutropenic patient with acute lymphocytic leukemia. *B.* The same lesion the following day. *C.* Ecthyma gangrenosum in a neutropenic patient with *Pseudomonas aeruginosa* bacteremia. *D.* Papule in a neutropenic patient with *Candida tropicalis* fungemia.

IID-58 **Septic emboli** with hemorrhage and infarction due to acute *Staphylococcus aureus* endocarditis.

IID-59 Vegetations (*arrows*) due to viridans streptococcal endocarditis involving the mitral valve.

IID-60 **Disseminated gonococcemia** in the skin is seen as hemorrhagic papules and pustules with purpuric centers in an acral distribution.

E. Immunologically Mediated Skin Disease

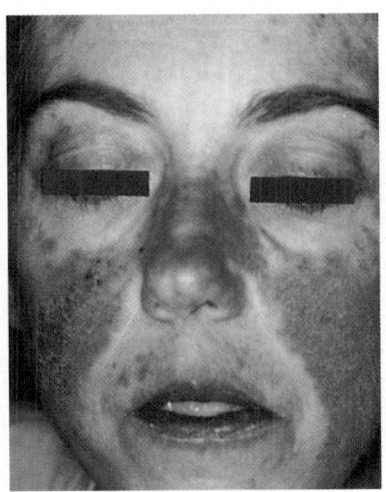

IIE-61A **Systemic lupus erythematosus** showing prominent, scaly, malar erythema. Involvement of other sun-exposed sites is also common.

IIE-61B **Acute LE** on the upper chest demonstrating brightly erythematous and slightly edematous coalescence papules and plaques.

IIE-62 **Discoid lupus erythematosus** Violaceous, hyperpigmented, atrophic plaques, often with evidence of follicular plugging, which may result in scarring, are characteristic of this cutaneous form of lupus.

IIE-63 **Dermatomyositis** Periorbital violaceous erythema characterizes the classic heliotrope rash.

IIE-64 **Scleroderma** characterized by typical expressionless, mask-like facies.

IIE-65 **Dermatomyositis** often involves the hands as erythematous flat-topped papules over the knuckles (Gottron's sign) and periungal telangiectasias.

IIE-66 **Scleroderma** showing acral sclerosis and focal digital ulcers.

IIE-67 **Erythema multiforme** is characterized by multiple erythematous plaques with a target or iris morphology and usually represents a hypersensitivity reaction to drugs or infections (especially herpes simplex virus).

IIE-68 **Dermatitis herpetiformis** manifested by pruritic, grouped vesicles in a typical location. The vesicles are often excoriated and may occur on knees, buttocks, and posterior scalp.

IIE-69A **Pemphigus vulgaris** demonstrating flaccid bullae that are easily ruptured, resulting in multiple erosions and crusted plaques.

IIE-69B **Pemphigus vulgaris** almost invariably involves the oral mucosa and may present with erosions involving the gingiva, buccal mucosa, palate, posterior pharynx, or the tongue.

IIE-70 **Erythema nodosum** is a panniculitis characterized by tender deep-seated nodules and plaques usually located on the lower extremities.

IIE-71 **Vasculitis** Palpable purpuric papules on the lower legs are seen in this patient with cutaneous small vessel vasculitis.

IIE-72 **Bullous pemphigoid** with tense vesicles and bullae on an erythematous, urticarial base.

F. Skin Manifestations of Internal Disease

IIF-73 **Acanthosis nigricans** demonstrating typical hyperpigmented axillary plaques with a velvet-like, verrucous surface.

IIF-74 **Pretibial myxedema** manifesting as waxy, infiltrated plaques in a patient with Graves' disease.

IIF-75 **Plaque of Sweet's syndrome** demonstrating an erythematous indurated plaque with a pseudo-vesicular border.

IIF-76 **Bilateral rheumatoid nodules** of the upper extremities.

IIF-77 **Neurofibromatosis** demonstrating numerous flesh-colored cutaneous neurofibromas.

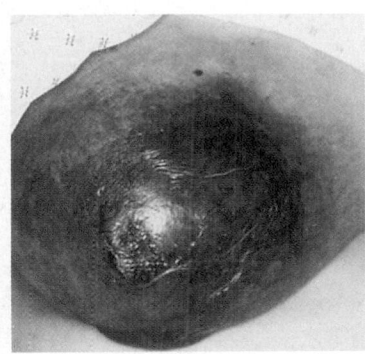

IIF-78 **Coumarin** necrosis showing cutaneous and subcutaneous necrosis of a breast. Other fatty areas such as buttocks and thighs are also common sites of involvement.

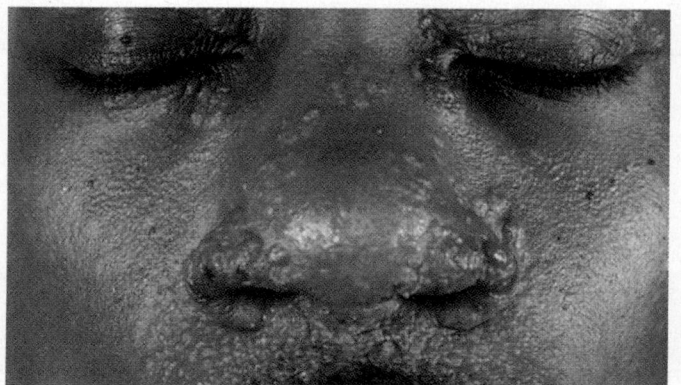

IIF-79A **Sarcoid** Infiltrated papules and plaques of variable color are seen in a typical paranasal and periorbital location.

IIF-79B **Sarcoid** Infiltrated, hyperpigmented, and slightly erythematous coalescent papules and plaques on the upper arm.

IIF-80 **Pyoderma gangrenosum** on the posterior-lateral aspect of the lower leg demonstrating multiple purulent draining ulcers on an infiltrated erythematous plaque.

III. Atlas of Endoscopic Findings

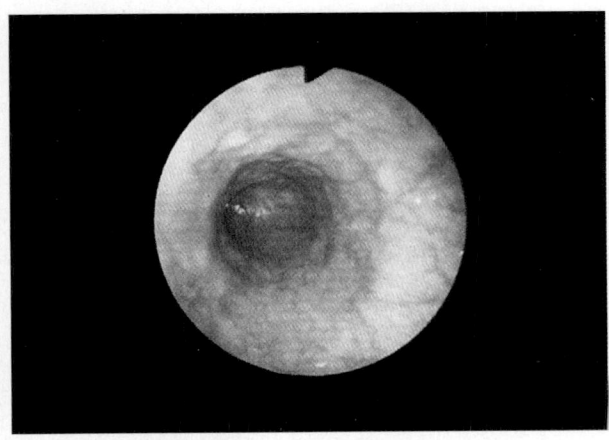

III-1 **Normal esophagus** Fine vasculature can be seen.

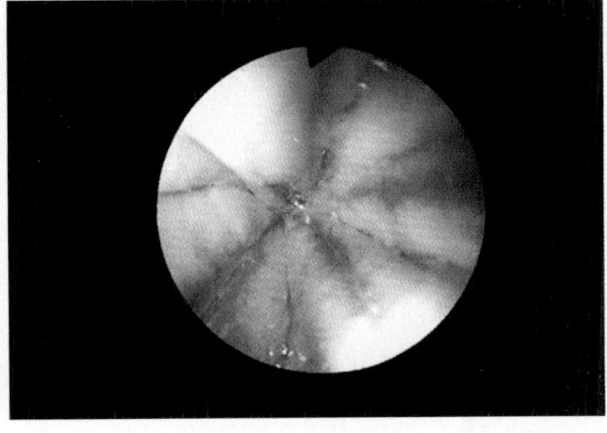

III-2 **Peptic regurgitant esophagitis** Linear red streaks with a central white streak extend up the esophagus.

III-3 **Ulcerated squamous cell carcinoma,** with a depressed center, involving one wall of the esophagus.

III-4 **Moniliasis of the esophagus** A white exudate is seen with underlying erythematous mucosa.

III-5 **Barrett's metaplasia of the esophagus with an adenocarcinoma** The squamocolumnar junction is noted in the proximal esophagus. A mucosal irregularity in the center of the photograph was an adenocarcinoma.

III-6 **Normal body of the stomach with rugal folds**

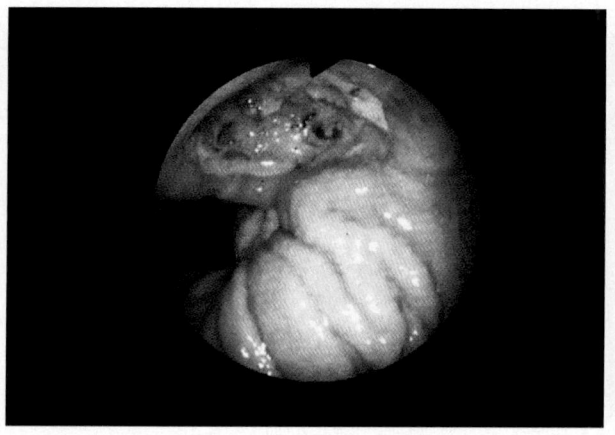

III-7 **Large, benign, lesser curve gastric ulcer**   The folds end at the ulcer margin.

III-8 **Gastric polyp**   The histologic type must be determined by excision and pathologic examination.

III-9 **Arteriovenus malformation of the gastric mucosa**

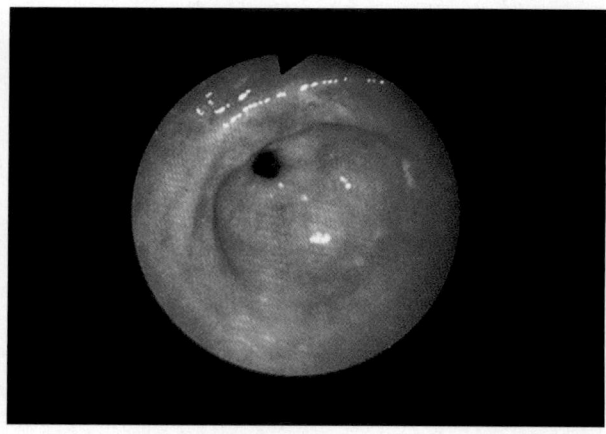

III-10 **Normal pylorus**   Note the absence of gastric rugal folds in the antrum proximal to the pylorus.

III-11 **Normal duodenal bulb**

III-12 **Duodenal ulcer**   A typical ulcer with a clean base is seen on the anterior surface of the duodenal bulb.

III-13 **Normal papilla of Vater** The fold pattern surrounding the papilla is normal; bile is seen adjacent to the papilla.

III-14 **Periampullary carcinoma** The mass at the papilla of Vater has been catheterized during ERCP.

III-15 **Endoscopic papillotomy** A papillotome has been passed into the papilla, the wire bowed, and an incision made, with electrosurgical current, in the superior aspect of the papilla.

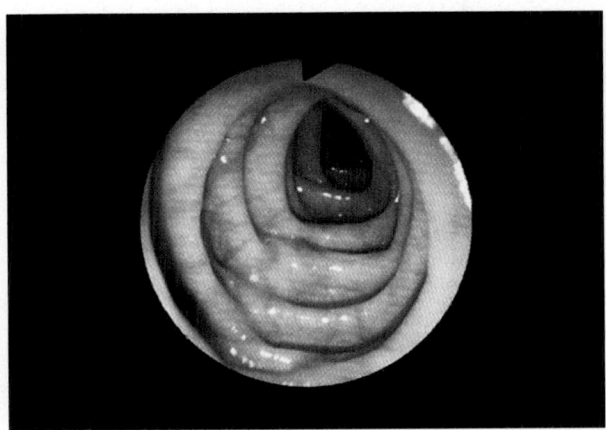

III-16 **Normal colon** Typical folds and vascular pattern can be seen.

III-17 **Colonic adenomatous polyp** The polyp is erythematous; a stalk is seen covered with normal mucosa.

III-18 **Multiple, small, colonic adenomatous polyps in a case of familial polyposis coli** This colon must be removed to prevent the development of cancer.

III-19 **Colon adenocarcinoma** The cancer is multilobed and growing into the lumen.

III-20 **Crohn's colitis** with linear, serpiginous, white-based ulcers surrounded by colonic mucosa which is relatively normal.

III-21 **Severe ulcerative colitis** with diffuse ulceration, bleeding, and exudation.

III-22 **Kaposi's sarcoma involving the colon in a patient with AIDS** The erythematous lesions involve most of the colonic mucosa in the photograph.

III-23 **Colonic varices** Multiple, serpiginous, subephithelial structures impinge on the colonic lumen.

III-24 **Ileal pouch** The mucosa appears normal in this pouch reconstructed from ileum to provide a reservoir after total proctocolectomy and ileoanal anastomosis.

IV. Atlas of Funduscopic Findings

IV-1 **Retinal vasculitis, uveitis, and hemorrhage** in a 32-year-old woman with Crohn's disease. Note that the veins are frosted with a white exudate. Visual acuity improved from 20/400 to 20/20 following treatment with intravenous methylprednisolone.

IV-2 **Cytomegalovirus** in a patient with AIDS appears as an arcuate zone of retinitis with hemorrhages and optic disc swelling. Often CMV is confined to the retinal periphery, beyond view of the direct ophthalmoscope.

IV-3 **Hollenhorst plaque** lodged at the bifurcation of a retinal arteriole proves that a patient is shedding emboli from either the carotid artery, great vessels, or heart.

IV-4 **Central retinal artery occlusion** combined with ischemic optic neuropathy in a 19-year-old woman with an elevated titer of anticardiolipin antibodies. Note the orange dot (rather than cherry red) corresponding to the fovea and the spared patch of retina just temporal to the optic disc.

IV-5 **Hypertensive retinopathy** with scattered flame (splinter) hemorrhages and cotton wool spots (nerve fiber layer infarcts) in a patient with headache and a blood pressure of 234/120.

IV-6 **Central retinal vein occlusion** can produce massive retinal hemorrhage ("blood and thunder"), ischemia, and vision loss.

IV-7 **Anterior ischemic optic neuropathy** from temporal arteritis in a 78-year old woman with pallid disc swelling, hemorrhage, visual loss, myalgia, and an erythrocyte sedimentation rate of 86 mm/h..

IV-8 **Retrobulbar optic neuritis** is characterized by a normal fundus examination initially, hence the rubric, "the doctor sees nothing, and the patient sees nothing." Optic atrophy develops after severe or repeated attacks.

IV-9 **Optic atrophy** is not a specific diagnosis, but refers to the combination of optic disc pallor, arteriolar narrowing, and nerve fiber layer destruction produced by a host of eye diseases, especially optic neuropathies.

IV-10 **Papilledema** means optic disc edema from raised intracranial pressure. This obese young woman with pseudotumor cerebri was misdiagnosed as a migraineur until fundus examination was performed, showing optic disc elevation, hemorrhages, and cotton wool spots.

IV-11 **Optic disc drusen** are calcified deposits of unknown etiology within the optic disc. They are sometimes confused with papilledema.

IV-12 **Retinal detachment** appears as an elevated sheet of retinal tissue with folds. In this patient the fovea was spared, so acuity was normal, but a superior detachment produced an inferior scotoma.

IV-13 **Glaucoma** results in "cupping" as the neural rim is destroyed and the central cup becomes enlarged and excavated. The cup-to-disc ratio is about 0.7/1.0 in this patient.

IV-14 **Age-related macular degeneration** begins with the accumulation of drusen within the macula. They appear as scattered yellow subretinal deposits.

IV-15 **Diabetic retinopathy** results in scattered hemorrhages and yellow exudates. This patient has neovascular vessels proliferating from the optic disc, requiring urgent pan retinal laser photocoagulation.

IV-16 **Retinitis pigmentosa** with black clumps of pigment in the retinal periphery known as "bone spicules." There is also atrophy of the retinal pigment epithelium, making the vasculature of the choroid easily visible.

IV-17 **Melanoma of the choroid,** appearing as an elevated dark mass in the inferior temporal fundus, just encroaching upon the fovea.

IV-18 **Kayser-Fleischer ring** develops in Wilson's disease from copper deposition in Descemet's membrane, producing brownish discoloration of the peripheral cornea. It should not be confused with the yellow-white lipid ring of arcus senilis, which is common in the elderly and occasionally signifies hyperlipidemia, especially when it appears at a young age.

V. Atlas of Hematology

V-1 **Normal blood smear** Normal red blood cells are round, possess an area of central pallor, appear slightly smaller than the nucleus of a mature lymphocyte, and vary little in size (anisocytosis) or in shape (poikilocytosis).

V-2 **β-Thalassemia intermedia** Microcytic and hypochromic red blood cells are seen that resemble the red blood cells of severe iron deficiency anemia shown in Fig. IV-4. Many elliptical and teardrop-shaped red blood cells are noted.

V-3 **Uremia** The red blood cells in uremia may acquire numerous, regularly spaced, small spiny projections. Such cells, called burr cells or echinocytes, are readily distinguishable from irregularly spiculated acanthocytes shown in Fig. V-27.

V-4 **Burkitt's lymphoma** The neoplastic cells are homogenous, medium-sized B cells with frequent mitotic figures, a morphologic correlate of high growth fraction. Reactive macrophages are scattered through the tumor and their pale cytoplasm in a background of blue-staining tumor cells gives the tumor a so-called "starry sky" appearance.

V-5 **Marrow iron stores** This marrow section is stained with Prussian blue. Iron takes up the stain and is concentrated in reticuloendothelial cells. This picture shows normal iron stores. In iron deficiency states, no stainable iron is detectable. In the anemia of chronic disease, iron is present but cytokines prevent its mobilization and utilization in heme synthesis.

V-6 **Multiple myeloma (marrow)** The cells bear characteristic morphologic features of plasma cells, round or oval cells with an eccentric nucleus composed of coarsely clumped chromatin, a densely basophilic cytoplasm, and a perinuclear clear zone (hof) containing the Golgi apparatus. Binucleate and multinucleate malignant plasma cells also can be seen.

V-7 **Reactive lymphocytes (infectious mononucleosis)** Reactive lymphocytes are usually large and contain abundant cytoplasm. The nucleus may be eccentrically placed and may have irregular borders and indentations (not seen on this plate). The cytoplasm contains areas that stain a darker blue due to their increased content of RNA. The cytoplasm may be indented where it abuts against a red blood cell.

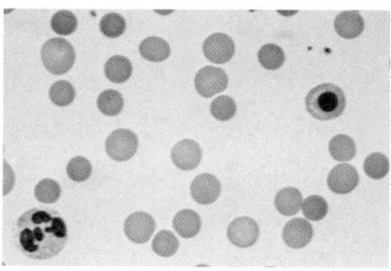

V-8 **Immunohemolytic anemia** Microspherocytes are seen on this blood smear along with several macrocytes with a slight purple tinge (polychromasia). The latter represent new red blood cells released early from the bone marrow. The microspherocytes seen in immunohemolytic anemia may be indistinguishable from the microspherocytes seen in hereditary spherocytosis (Fig. V-26).

V-9 **Leukoerythroblastic smear** Teardrop-shaped red blood cells indicative of membrane damage from collagen fibers, a nucleated red blood cell indicative of premature release of erythroid precursors, and immature myeloid cells indicative of extramedullary hematopoiesis are noted. This peripheral blood smear is related to marrow fibrosis, either primary myelofibrosis or secondary myelophthisis.

A B

V-10 A. **Normal granulocyte** The normal granulocyte has a segmented nucleus with heavy, clumped chromatin; fine neutrophilic granules are dispersed throughout its cytoplasm. *B.* **Normal monocyte and lymphocyte** The normal monocyte is a large cell with an indented or folded nucleus containing loose, strand-like chromatin; the cytoplasm is a blue-gray color and usually contains fine azurophilic granules. The normal lymphocyte is a smaller cell. Its nucleus is usually round but may be indented, as in the cell shown in this plate. The nuclear chromatin has a smudgy appearance; the cytoplasm is blue.

V-11 **Normal granulocyte precursors in marrow** The earliest granulocytic precursor (myeloblast) possesses a round nucleus with fine, punctate chromatin and one or more nucleoli; the cytoplasm is blue. As nuclear differentiation proceeds, the nucleoli disappear, the chromatin coarsens, and the nucleus becomes increasingly indented and finally segmented. As cytoplasmic differentiation proceeds, azurophilic granules appear and cytoplasm changes color from blue to the yellow-pink-gray hue of the mature granulocyte, and as this occurs the azurophilic granules become obscured by fine neutrophilic granules.

V-12 **Leukemic cell in acute promyelocytic leukemia** Note multiple Auer rods.

V-13 **Aplastic anemia** This marrow section shows only fat with nearly complete absence of hematopoietic tissue.

V-14 **Normal bone marrow biopsy** This a low power view of an H&E-stained section of normal marrow. Note that the nucleated cellular elements account for about 40 to 50 percent and the fat *(clear areas)* accounts for about 50 to 60 percent of the area.

V-15 **Erythroid hyperplasia** This marrow section shows an increase in the fraction of cells in the erythroid lineage as might be seen in a healthy marrow compensating for acute blood loss or hemolysis. The E/G ratio is greater than 1/1.

V-16 **Iron-deficiency anemia** In severe iron deficiency, the red blood cells are smaller than normal (microcytosis), and their central area of pallor is expanded (hypochromia) so that the cells appear to have only a thin rim of hemoglobin.

V-17 **Chronic lymphocytic leukemia** The peripheral WBC count is high due to increased numbers of small, well-differentiated lymphocytes. However, the leukemic lymphocytes are fragile, and substantial numbers of broken, smudged cells are usually also present on the blood smear.

V-18 **Hodgkin's disease, mixed cellularity** A Reed-Sternberg cell is present near the center of the field; a large cell with a bilobed nucleus and prominent nucleoli. The majority of the cells are normal lymphocytes, neutrophils, and eosinophils that form a pleiomorphic cellular infiltrate.

V-19 **Marrow fibrosis** This marrow section shows the marrow cavity replaced by fibrous tissue composed of reticulin fibers and collagen. When this fibrosis is due to a primary hematologic process, it is called *myelofibrosis*. When the fibrosis is secondary to a tumor or a granulomatous process, it is called *myelophthisis*.

V-20 **Acute myelocytic leukemia** This marrow section shows sheets of primitive myeloblasts with numerous large nucleoli.

V-21 **Liver disease** Round macrocytes of rather uniform size are seen. Many of the macrocytes are also target cells.

V-22 **Diffuse large B cell lymphoma** The neoplastic cells are large with vesicular nuclear chromatin and prominent nucleoli.

V-23 **Neutrophils with toxic granulation** In infection and other toxic states, azurophilic granules may become visible in mature granulocytes as coarse, dark-staining cytoplasmic granules.

V-24 **Megaloblastic anemia** Oval macrocytes, well filled with hemoglobin, are admixed with lesser numbers of small teardrop-shaped red blood cells. Note also hypersegmented granulocyte.

V-25 **Leukemic cells in acute lymphoblastic leukemia** characterized by round or convoluted nuclei, high nuclear/cytoplasmic ratio and absence of cytoplasmic granules.

V-26 **Hereditary spherocytosis** Small, densely staining red blood cells are seen that have lost their central area of pallor (microspherocytes). Microspherocytes may also be found in other hemolytic disorders (Fig. V-8).

V-27 **Spur cell anemia** Spur cells are recognized as distorted red blood cells containing several irregularly distributed thornlike projections. Cells with this morphologic abnormality are also called acanthocytes.

V-28 **Traumatic hemolysis** The helmet-shaped red blood cell and the small triangular-shaped red blood cells seen on this smear represent morphologic evidence of mechanical damage to red blood cells within the blood vessels.

V-29 **Granulocytic hyperplasia** This marrow section shows an increase in the fraction of cells in the myeloid or granulocytic lineage as might be seen in a healthy marrow responding to infection. The E/G ratio is less than 1/3.

V-30 **Follicular lymphoma** The normal nodal architecture is effaced by nodular expansions of tumor cells. Nodules vary in size and mimic normal lymphoid follicles.

V-31 **Auer rod** This peripheral blood smear shows a myeloblast with a single Auer rod in the cytoplasm. Auer rods, when present, are usually seen in acute myelocytic leukemia.

A *B*

V-32 A. **Normal eosinophil** The eosinophil contains large, bright-orange granules; the nucleus is bilobed. *B.* **Basophil** The basophil contains large, purple-black granules that fill the cell and obscure the nucleus.

V-33 **Megaloblastic erythropoiesis** This marrow section demonstrates so-called nuclear-cytoplasmic dissociation; the cytoplasm of erythroblasts is filled with hemoglobin demonstrating nearly complete maturation while the nuclei have loose chromatin characteristic of more immature erythroid cells. The slow nuclear maturation is related to a decrease in DNA synthesis related to an insufficient supply of reduced folate to synthesize thymidylate. DNA synthesis inhibitors can produce this picture, as can folate and B_{12} deficiency.

A *B*

V-34 A. **Chédiak-Higashi anomaly** In this ultimately fatal disorder, the granulocytes contain huge cytoplasmic granules, formed from aggregation and fusion of azurophilic and specific granules. Large abnormal granules are found in other granule-containing cells throughout the body. *B.* **Pelger-Hüet anomaly** In this benign disorder, the majority of granulocytes are bilobed. The nucleus frequently has a spectacle-like or "pince-nez" configuration.

V-35 **Band with Döhle body** (center) Döhle bodies are discrete, blue-staining non-granular areas found in the periphery of the cytoplasm of the neutrophil in infections and other toxic states. They represent aggregates of rough endoplasmic reticulum.

V-36 **Chronic granulocytic leukemia** The peripheral WBC count is high due to increased numbers of granulocytes and their precursors. The majority of the WBCs are segmented granulocytes or band forms, but myelocytes (as seen on this plate) and promyeloblasts (not seen on this plate) may also be found on review of the blood smear.

V-37 **Ringed sideroblast** Refractory anemia with ringed sideroblasts (RARS) is in the spectrum of myelodysplastic syndromes. This marrow Prussian blue stain shows an orthochromatic normoblast with a collar of blue granules surrounding the nucleus. The blue granules represent iron-laden mitochondria.

V-38 **Hypersegmentation** Frequent five-lobed granulocytes on a blood smear or granulocytes with more than five lobes are evidence of hypersegmentation, an important clue to the diagnosis of megaloblastic anemia.

V-39 **Sickle cell anemia** The elongated and crescent-shaped red blood cells seen on this smear represent circulating irreversibly sickled cells. Target cells and a nucleated red blood cell are also seen.

V-40 **Adult T cell leukemia/lymphoma** This peripheral blood smear reveals leukemia cells with the typical "flower-shaped" nucleus.

VI. Atlas of Diagnostic Microbiology

VI-1 **Gram-stained sputum** from a patient with acute purulent tracheobronchitis. Many polymorphonuclear neutrophils and a few macrophages are seen along with many gram-negative cocci, (*Moraxella catarrhalis*), a few of which appear as pairs. Nearly all organisms are cell associated and probably have been taken up by phagocytes, consistent with the notion that *Moraxella* is a lower-grade pathogen than organisms such as *Streptococcus pneumoniae*.

VI-2 The microbiologist can easily identify *Streptococcus pneumoniae* as the etiologic agent of pneumonia when microscopic examination of Gram-stained sputum specimen reveals this kind of picture.

Plates VI-3 through VI-33 are photomicrographs reproduced from "Benchaids for the Diagnosis of Malaria Infections," 2d ed, with the permission of the World Health Organization.

P. falciparum—thin film

VI-3 Trophozoites–young

VI-4 Trophozoites–old

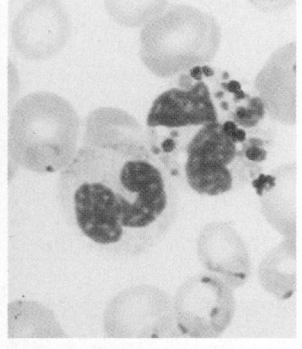

VI-5 Pigment in polymorphonuclear cell and trophozoites

VI-6 Schizonts–mature

VI-7 Gametocytes–female

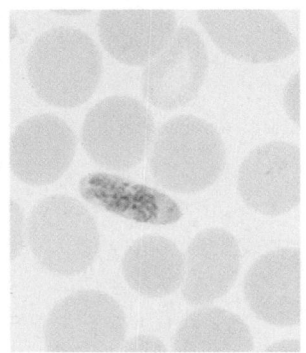

VI-8 Gametocytes–male

P. vivax—thin film

VI-9 Trophozoites–young

VI-10 Trophozoites–old

VI-11 Schizonts–mature

VI-12 Gametocytes–female

VI-13 Gametocytes–male

P. ovale—thin film

VI-14 Trophozoites–old

VI-15 Schizonts–mature

VI-16 Gametocytes–male

VI-17 Gametocytes–female

VI-18   Trophozoites–old

VI-19   Schizonts–mature

VI-20   Gametocytes–male

VI-21   Gametocytes–female

Babesia—thin film

VI-22   Trophozoites

P. vivax—thick film

VI-25   Trophozoites

P. ovale—thick film

VI-28   Trophozoites

P. malariae—thick film

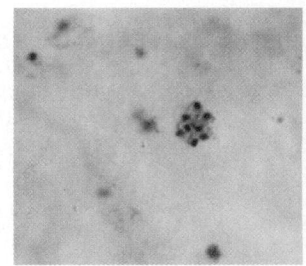

VI-31   Trophozoites

P. falciparum—thick film

VI-23   Trophozoites

VI-26   Schizonts

VI-29   Schizonts

VI-32   Schizonts

VI-24   Gametocytes

VI-27   Gametocytes

VI-30   Gametocytes

VI-33   Gametocytes

SOURCES OF PHOTOGRAPHS

I. CARDIOLOGY

R. Gibbons, MD I-1A, I-1B Exercise sestamibi study

II. DERMATOLOGY

L. Baden, MD IID-58 Septic emboli
Jean Bolognia, MD IIA-6 Seborrheic dermatitis; IIB-21 Non-Hodgkin's lymphoma
S. Wright Caughman, MD IIC-32 Nodular melanoma; IID-55 Condylomata acuminatum
Gregory Cox, MD IID-47 Primary syphilis
Daniel F. Danzl, MD IIA-18, IIA-19 Frostbite
Robert Gelber, MD IID-56 Polar lepromatous leprosy
Stephen E. Gellis, MD IID-39 Hand foot-and-mouth disease; IID-44 Fulminant meningococcemia
John Greenspan, PhD IID-42 Oral hairy leukoplakia; IID-43 Pseudomembranous oral candidiasis
Robert Hartman, MD IID-36 Varicella
A.W. Kerchner, MD IID-59 Veridans streptococcal endocarditis
James Krell, MD IIE-63 Dermatomyositis
Marilynne McKay, MD IIE-62 Discoid lupus erythematosus
V. Pranava Murthy, MD IID-53 Skin lesions
Daniel M. Musher, MD IID-60 Disseminated gonococcemia
Alvin Solomon, MD IIC-31 Lentigo maligna melanoma; IID-48 Secondary syphilis of the palms
Mary Spraker, MD IID-38 Impetigo contagiosa
Robert Swerlick, MD IIA-2 Acne rosacea; IIA-4 Atopic dermatitis; IIA-8*B* Allergic contact dermatitis; IIA-9 Lichen planus; IIA-12 Alopecia areata; IIA-14*B* Dermatographism; IIB-27 Actinic keratoses; IID-37 Disseminated herpes zoster; IID-45 Rocky Mountain spotted fever; IIE-61*B* Acute lupus erythematosus; IIE-63 Dermatomyositis; IIE-69*B* Pemphigus vulgaris; IIE-70 Erythema nodosum; IIE-71 Vasculitis; IIF-75 Sweet's syndrome; IIF-76 Rheumatoid nodules; IIF-79B Sarcoid; IIF-80 Pyoderma gangrenosum
Kalman Watsky, MD IIA-1 Acne vulgaris
Yale Resident's Slide Collection IID-41 Molluscum contagiosum; IID-46 Erythema chronicum migrans; IID-49 Condylomata lata; IIE-67 Erythema multiforme; IIE-72 Bullous pemphigoid
Kim Yancey, MD IIF-78 Coumarin necrosis

III. ENDOSCOPIC FINDINGS

FE Silverstein and **GN Tytgat** *Atlas of Gastrointestinal Endoscopy,* New York, Gower Medical Publishing, 1987. All photographs except III-12, III-23, III-24
GN Tytgat III-12; III-23; III-24

IV FUNDUSCOPIC FINDINGS

Jonathan C. Horton, MD, PhD IV-1 to IV-18

V. HEMATOLOGY

Robert S. Hillman, MD, and **Kenneth A. Ault, MD** *Hematology in General Practice,* New York, McGraw-Hill, 1995. Courtesy of the American Society of Hematology Slide Bank. V-30 to V-39
Elaine Jaffe, MD V-25 to V-29

VI. DIAGNOSTIC MICROBIOLOGY

Elil Renganathan, MD, WHO, Geneva VI-3 to VI-33

Many fungi can be identified to the genus or even the species level by microscopic examination of smears or biopsy specimens. Calcofluor white staining with fluorescence microscopy is a sensitive technique for smears of sputum, bronchoalveolar lavage fluid, or pus. India ink smear remains the method of choice for detecting cryptococci in cerebrospinal fluid (CSF). *Candida* yeast cells and pseudohyphae are the only fungi that are usually gram-positive on smears. For other fungi, Gram's staining is distinctly suboptimal. For histopathology slides, Gomori methenamine silver and a neutral counterstain are preferred.

The method used has a marked effect on the rapidity and sensitivity of blood cultures for fungi except in the case of *Candida* species, which are relatively easy to grow. For most other fungi, concentration of the blood by lysis centrifugation and culture on solid medium constitute the optimal technique. Commercially available nucleic acid hybridization techniques can speed the identification of slow-growing molds, such as *Histoplasma capsulatum* and *Coccidioides immitis*. Serology has limited value, but testing of serum or CSF for cryptococcal antigen or antibody to *C. immitis* can be diagnostic. Detection of *Histoplasma* antigen in urine or serum is helpful in diagnosis and in following the results of treatment for disseminated histoplasmosis. Skin testing with fungal antigens is not useful in detecting active infection.

ANTIFUNGAL THERAPY

TOPICAL AGENTS   Imidazoles and Triazoles (See also "Systemic Antifungals," below)   These synthetic compounds act by inhibiting ergosterol synthesis in the fungal cell wall and, when given topically, may cause direct damage to the fungal cytoplasmic membrane. The imidazoles available for cutaneous application include clotrimazole, econazole, ketoconazole, sulconazole, oxiconazole, and miconazole. Vaginal formulations include four imidazoles (miconazole, clotrimazole, tioconazole, and butoconazole) and one triazole (terconazole). As yet, no substantial differences in the efficacy of or local intolerance to the various topical azoles have become apparent. All are effective in the treatment of cutaneous candidiasis, tinea (pityriasis) versicolor, and mild to moderately severe ringworm of the glabrous skin. Vaginal formulations are effective for vulvovaginal candidiasis. Clotrimazole is poorly absorbed from the gastrointestinal tract, but the oral troche is useful as a topical treatment for oral and esophageal candidiasis.

Polyene Macrolide Antibiotics   These broad-spectrum antifungal agents combine with sterol in the fungal cytoplasmic membrane, increasing membrane permeability. Topically, they are not active against ringworm but are effective against candidiasis of the skin and mucous membranes. Nystatin and amphotericin B suspensions are effective in oral thrush, and vaginal troches are effective in vulvovaginal candidiasis. Both nystatin and amphotericin B are available in topical preparations for cutaneous candidiasis.

Other Topical Antifungals   Ciclopirox olamine, haloprogin, terbinafine, and naftifine have the same clinical spectrum among the cutaneous mycoses as the imidazoles. Tolnaftate and undecylenic acid are effective against ringworm but not candidiasis. Keratolytic agents, such as salicylic acid, are helpful as accessory drugs for some hyperkeratotic skin lesions.

SYSTEMIC ANTIFUNGALS   Griseofulvin   Griseofulvin is a useful drug in the treatment of certain kinds of ringworm; however, it is ineffective in the treatment of candidiasis. The microcrystalline and ultramicrocrystalline preparations differ in dose but not in efficacy. Absorption of both is enhanced when the drug is ingested with fat-containing foods. Griseofulvin interacts with phenobarbital and coumarin-type anticoagulants.

Terbinafine   Oral terbinafine (250 mg once daily) is at least as effective as itraconazole and more effective than griseofulvin in onychomycosis and ringworm. Treatment duration ranges from 3 months for fingernails to 6 months for toenails. Gastrointestinal distress is the most common side effect. Rash, hepatitis, and pancytopenia have oc-

curred, but serious adverse effects have been uncommon. Terbinafine decreases cyclosporine levels. Cimetidine increases and rifampin decreases terbinafine levels in blood.

Imidazoles and Triazoles • *General features*   The azole antifungals include imidazoles and triazoles. Fluconazole, itraconazole, and investigational azoles are all triazoles, so named because they have three nitrogens in the ring structure. This class has less impact on human hormonal synthesis and less hepatotoxicity than the only widely used systemic imidazole, ketoconazole. Itraconazole has many structural features in common with ketoconazole; however, it has a broader spectrum of activity and has largely replaced ketoconazole.

Reported interactions of itraconazole and fluconazole with other drugs are listed in Table 200-1. Ketoconazole interactions (not listed) appear to be the same as those listed for itraconazole. Azole interactions with any one class of drugs, such as benzodiazepines, HMG-CoA reductase inhibitors, or drugs that decrease gastric acidity, should be considered to apply to all drugs of that class until proven otherwise. Fluconazole differs substantially from itraconazole: unlike that of itraconazole, the absorption of fluconazole is independent of food or gastric acid, and fluconazole has much less effect on the hepatic metabolism of other drugs than does itraconazole. High fluconazole blood levels engendered by azotemia or by dosages above those used in pharmacologic studies may lead to new and profound drug interactions.

All azoles have the potential for embryotoxicity and teratogenicity. In fact, it seems likely that azoles should not be given during pregnancy without a discussion of the serious risks and possible benefits with the mother. Four infants born to mothers taking at least 400 mg of fluconazole daily for coccidioidal meningitis have had severe bone, craniofacial, or cardiac abnormalities. Similarity of these abnormalities to those in pregnant animals given fluconazole suggests that fluconazole caused the defects.

Table 200-1   Interactions of Itraconazole and Fluconazole with Other Drugs

Interaction, Drug(s)	Intraconazole	Fluconazole
Azole increases blood level of other drug		
Antihistamines (nonsedating astemizole, terfenadine)	+	0
Antimetabolites (busulfan, vincristine, vinblastine)	+	0
Benzodiazepines (midazolam, triazolam)	+	0
Calcium channel inhibitors (felodipine)	+	0
Cisapride	+	0
Cyclosporine	+	+
Digoxin	+	0
HMG-CoA reductase inhibitors (lovastatin, simvastatin)	+	?
Phenytoin	+	+
Prednisolone	±[a]	0
Protease inhibitors (indinavir, ritonavir)	+	0
Quinidine	+	?
Sulfonylureas (glipizide, glyburide, tolbutamide)	+	+
Tacrolimus	+	?
Warfarin	±	±
Other drug decreases azole blood level		
Antacids (simultaneous administration)	+	0
Carbamazepine	+	0
H$_2$ receptor antagonists (cimetidine, ranitidine, famotidine, nizatidine)	+	0
Isoniazid	+	0
Phenobarbital	+	0
Phenytoin	+	0
Proton pump inhibitors (omeprazole, lansoprazole)	+	0
Rifampin, rifabutin	+	±

[a] The symbol "±" indicates that interaction is variable but is more likely with a high azole blood concentration.

Itraconazole Itraconazole is useful in the treatment of blastomycosis, histoplasmosis, candidiasis, coccidioidomycosis, sporotrichosis, pseudallescheriasis, onychomycosis, ringworm, tinea versicolor, and some cases of aspergillosis. Its efficacy in mycoses of the central nervous system has been modest at best. Almost no bioactive drug appears in urine. Itraconazole is metabolized in the liver, with the hydroxy metabolite accounting for at least half of the antifungal activity in serum. Food increases absorption of itraconazole capsules by about threefold but substantially reduces absorption of the cyclodextrin suspension. Ability of the suspension to exert a topical as well as a systemic effect probably accounts for its improved efficacy in oropharyngeal candidiasis. The usual dosage of either oral itraconazole formulation is 100 to 200 mg once daily for oropharyngeal and esophageal candidiasis. For deep infections, itraconazole capsules are given at an initial dosage of 600 to 800 mg daily for 3 days and a subsequent dosage of 200 to 400 mg once daily continued for 6 to 12 months. Itraconazole blood levels are helpful in documenting absorption of oral itraconazole when the drug is used for the treatment of deep mycoses. An intravenous formulation is commercially available and should be considered for initial therapy in hospitalized patients in whom itraconazole absorption may be suboptimal. Immunosuppressed patients with rapidly progressing pseudallescheriasis, an infection that does not respond to amphotericin B, are candidates for intravenous itraconazole treatment.

Fluconazole This triazole can be administered in tablet form, as a suspension, or as an intravenous infusion. With a half-life of about 31 h, fluconazole can be given once a day. Approximately 80% of the drug is excreted unchanged in the urine. Patients with creatinine clearance rates of 21 to 50 mL/min and 11 to 20 mL/min should have their fluconazole doses reduced by 50 and 75%, respectively. The drug penetrates the CSF and other body fluids very well.

Nausea and abdominal distress are the most common forms of dose-limiting fluconazole toxicity. An allergic rash may develop and is particularly common among patients infected with HIV. Fatal cases of Stevens-Johnson syndrome have been described in the HIV-infected population. Alopecia commonly follows prolonged administration of ≥400 mg daily but resolves when therapy is discontinued. Rare cases of anaphylaxis, hepatic necrosis, and neutropenia have been described.

Fluconazole is useful in the treatment of oropharyngeal and esophageal candidiasis in adults. A single 150-mg tablet is effective in vulvovaginal candidiasis. Catheter-acquired candidemia in the immunocompetent host responds to 400 mg of fluconazole daily in conjunction with the removal of the infected catheter. Treatment should be continued for 10 to 14 days after the patient has become afebrile. Fluconazole is also effective in initial and maintenance therapy for cryptococcal meningitis in patients with AIDS, although most of these patients should initially receive a 2-week course of intravenous amphotericin B. Patients with coccidioidal meningitis can often be given fluconazole rather than intrathecal amphotericin B as maintenance therapy.

The incidence of deep candidiasis among recipients of allogeneic bone marrow transplants can be reduced by the administration of fluconazole (400 mg daily) for 75 days after initiation of the transplantation-preparative regimen. Prophylaxis in other neutropenic patients has not appeared useful. Fluconazole (200 mg daily) reduced the incidence of cryptococcosis and mucosal candidiasis among AIDS patients whose CD4+ cell counts were <200/μL and was particularly effective among those with counts of <50/μL. However, this regimen is not recommended because it does not reduce mortality, is expensive, and can lead to drug resistance.

Fluconazole is less effective than itraconazole in blastomycosis, histoplasmosis, and sporotrichosis. The drug is not active in aspergillosis or mucormycosis.

Amphotericin B A colloidal deoxycholate complex of the polyene drug amphotericin B is available for intravenous or intrathecal administration. In-line filters with a 0.22-μm pore diameter may trap some of the colloid. The catabolism of amphotericin B is extremely slow and is not influenced by renal failure, hepatic failure, or hemodialysis. The drug's penetration into CSF and vitreous humor is poor; however, the concentrations in pleural, peritoneal, and articular exudates are adequate for many mycoses. Histoplasmosis, blastomycosis, paracoccidioidomycosis, candidiasis, and cryptococcosis are the most responsive mycoses; coccidioidomycosis, extraarticular sporotrichosis, aspergillosis, and mucormycosis are less responsive; and chromoblastomycosis, mycetoma, and pseudallescheriasis respond little, if at all. The usual course is 0.5 to 0.7 mg/kg daily for 8 to 10 weeks. Infusions are generally given in 5% dextrose over 2 to 4 h.

Initial doses of amphotericin B occasionally cause marked febrile reactions that may be poorly tolerated by adult patients with limited cardiac or pulmonary function. It may be prudent to give such patients an initial 1-mg test dose followed by rapidly escalating doses, depending on tolerance. Premedication with aspirin or acetaminophen or the addition of hydrocortisone (25 mg) to the infusion decreases chills and fever. Azotemia during treatment is usual, the extent depending on the daily dose. Saline infusions have been advocated to reduce azotemia. Permanent loss of renal function is related to the total dose of amphotericin B; this condition is generally noted in adults who have received >3 g. Other side effects include anemia, hypokalemia, renal tubular acidosis, nausea, anorexia, weight loss, phlebitis, and occasionally hypomagnesemia. Intrathecal amphotericin B has been used in coccidioidal meningitis and refractory cryptococcal meningitis, although this therapy is associated with considerable toxicity.

Three lipid formulations of amphotericin B are commercially available in the United States: amphotericin B lipid complex (ABLC), amphotericin B colloidal dispersion (ABCD), and liposomal amphotericin B (L-AB). All cause less nephrotoxicity than the older amphotericin B deoxycholate complex (ABD). Acute, febrile infusion-related reactions occur with all three lipid formulations but are most severe with ABCD. The recommended duration for initial infusions of ABCD is 1 mg/kg per hour, somewhat slower than the 2-h duration of ABLC or L-AB infusions, with the intent of decreasing febrile reactions. Premedication with acetaminophen is also an option. Use of these remarkably expensive formulations should be confined to patients who cannot tolerate the nephrotoxicity of ABD. Although the lipid formulations are also approved for patients failing to respond to ABD, there is no indication that these formulations are more effective than ABD for any mycosis.

Flucytosine Flucytosine (5-fluorocytosine) is a synthetic oral drug useful in cryptococcosis, candidiasis, and chromoblastomycosis. Within the fungal cell, flucytosine is converted to the antimetabolite 5-fluorouracil. Drug resistance appears rather rapidly when flucytosine is used alone. For this reason, the drug is generally used in combination with amphotericin B. The usual dose of flucytosine is 25 to 37.5 mg/kg every 6 h. Flucytosine is well absorbed from the gastrointestinal tract. The drug penetrates well into the CSF and is excreted unchanged in the urine. Even modest reductions in renal function may elevate flucytosine blood levels into the toxic range (≥100 to 125 μg/mL). Elevated levels are associated with a significant incidence of neutropenia and thrombocytopenia and also seem to predispose to colitis, the other major toxic effect of this drug. Hepatotoxicity is idiosyncratic and uncommon. An allergic rash may develop.

BIBLIOGRAPHY

BOWDEN RA et al: Phase 1 study of amphotericin B colloidal dispersion for the treatment of invasive fungal infections after bone marrow transplant. J Infect Dis 173:1208, 1996

DISMUKES WE: Introduction to antifungal drugs. Clin Infect Dis 30:653, 2000

KWON-CHUNG KJ, BENNETT JE: *Medical Mycology*. Philadelphia, Lea & Febiger, 1992

MANGINO JE, PAPPAS PG: Itraconazole for the treatment of histoplasmosis and blastomycosis. Int J Antimicrob Agents 5:219, 1995

PAPPAS PG et al: Alopecia associated with fluconazole therapy. Ann Intern Med 123:354, 1995

POWDERLY WG et al: A randomized trial comparing fluconazole with clotrimazole troches for the prevention of fungal infections in patients with advanced human immunodeficiency virus infection. N Engl J Med 332:700, 1995

REX J et al: A randomized trial comparing fluconazole with amphotericin B for the treatment of candidemia in patients with neutropenia. N Engl J Med 331:1325, 1994

SLAVIN MA et al: Efficacy and safety of fluconazole prophylaxis for fungal infections after marrow transplantation—a prospective, randomized, double-blind trial. J Infect Dis 171:1545, 1995

SOBEL JD: Practice guidelines for the treatment of fungal infections. Clin Infect Dis 30: 652, 2000

VAN DER HORST CM et al: Treatment of cryptococcal meningitis associated with the acquired immunodeficiency syndrome. N Engl J Med 337:15, 1997

WHITE MH et al: Randomized, double-blind clinical trial of amphotericin B colloidal dispersion vs amphotericin B in the empirical treatment of fever and neutropenia. Clin Infect Dis 27:296, 1998

WONG-BERINGER A et al: Lipid formulations of amphotericin B: Clinical efficacy and toxicities. Clin Infect Dis 27:603, 1998

201

John E. Bennett

HISTOPLASMOSIS

ETIOLOGIC AGENT *Histoplasma capsulatum* is a dimorphic fungus that grows as a mold in nature or on Sabouraud's agar at room temperature. Hyphae bear both large and small spores, which are used for identification. Nucleic acid hybridization can also be used to identify the organism in culture. *H. capsulatum* grows as a small budding yeast in host tissue and on enriched agar, such as blood cysteine glucose, at 37°C. Despite its name, the fungus is unencapsulated. Coculture of isolates with opposite mating types can produce different sporulating structures in which genetic recombination occurs. When these structures, referred to as a *teleomorph* or the *perfect state*, are seen in culture, the name *Ajellomyces capsulatus* is used.

EPIDEMIOLOGY Infection with *H. capsulatum* has been encountered in many areas of the world but is much more frequent in certain areas. Within the United States, infection is most common in the southeastern, mid-Atlantic, and central states. Endemicity is probably contingent on the availability of proper conditions in nature for growth of the fungus. *H. capsulatum* prefers moist surface soil, particularly soil enriched by droppings of certain birds and bats. The fungus has been isolated repeatedly from such sites, and many case clusters have occurred 5 to 18 days after the exposure of groups of people to dust while (for example) cleaning dirt-floored chicken coops; raking soil beneath bird-roosting sites; exploring caves; and cleaning, remodeling, or demolishing old buildings. Skin-test reactivity in many endemic areas indicates that ≥80% of residents over age 16 have been exposed.

PATHOGENESIS AND PATHOLOGY Microconidia, or small spores, of *H. capsulatum* are small enough to reach the alveoli on inhalation and are transformed there to budding forms. With time, an intense granulomatous reaction occurs. Caseation necrosis or calcification may mimic tuberculosis. In children, the primary infection usually heals completely but may leave spotty calcification in the hilar nodes or lung. Transient dissemination may leave calcified granulomas in the spleen. In adults, a rounded mass of scar tissue, with or without central calcification, may remain in the lung. This mass has been called a *histoplasmoma*. Previous exposure is thought to confer some protection against reinfection, but infection in persons with prior positive skin tests clearly has occurred.

In a small proportion of patients, histoplasmosis becomes a progressive, potentially fatal infection. The disease occurs either as chronic fibrocavitary pneumonia or, less commonly, as disseminated infection. Patients with either form lack a history of acute primary pulmonary histoplasmosis. Chronic pulmonary infection favors otherwise healthy males over the age of 40. A history of cigarette use or the presence of emphysema is elicited from nearly all patients with chronic progressive pulmonary histoplasmosis. An acute, rapidly fatal disseminated infection is most likely to be encountered among young children and immunosuppressed patients, including those with AIDS. A more chronic but equally lethal disseminated infection is more common among previously healthy adults.

CLINICAL MANIFESTATIONS The vast majority of infections are either asymptomatic or mild, and the diagnosis is elusive. Cough, fever, malaise, and chest x-ray findings of hilar adenopathy with or without one or more areas of pneumonitis are typical features. Erythema nodosum and erythema multiforme have been reported in a few outbreaks. Hilar adenopathy may cause temporary compression of the right-middle-lobe bronchus in children and young adults. Subacute pericarditis may develop, probably by extension from contiguous lymph nodes. Rarely, hilar nodes undergo a caseous, granulomatous reaction with perinodal fibrosis. Mediastinal structures become encased by progressive fibrosis, and compression of the pulmonary veins, superior vena cava, pulmonary arteries, and esophagus may take place over many years. Late in mediastinal disease, only rare nonviable *Histoplasma* cells can be found in caseous residua of lymph nodes.

Chronic pulmonary histoplasmosis is characterized by a gradual onset (over weeks or months) of increasing productive cough, weight loss, and sometimes night sweats. Chest x-ray reveals uni- or bilateral fibronodular apical infiltrates. Approximately one-third of cases stabilize or improve spontaneously early in the course. The remainder progress insidiously. Retraction and cavitation of the upper lobes occur, with spread to the apex of the lower lobes and other areas of the lung. Emphysema and bulla formation further compromise pulmonary function. Death from cor pulmonale, bacterial pneumonia, or histoplasmosis occurs after months or years.

Acute disseminated histoplasmosis may be mistaken for miliary tuberculosis (Chap. 169). Common findings include fever, emaciation, hepatosplenomegaly, lymphadenopathy, jaundice, anemia, leukopenia, and thrombocytopenia. A high index of suspicion is necessary in patients with AIDS, in whose cases there may be other explanations for the abnormalities caused by disseminated histoplasmosis. All these features may be noted in chronic dissemination as well, but chronic disease tends to be more localized. Indurated ulcers of the mouth, tongue, nose, or larynx are reported in about one-fourth of cases. Other focal findings include granulomatous hepatitis, Addison's disease, gastrointestinal ulceration, endocarditis, and chronic meningitis. Chest x-ray abnormalities are evident in half of cases and characteristically consist of discrete nodules or a miliary pattern.

Infection with *H. capsulatum* var. *duboisii* is rare outside of Africa. The yeast form is larger in tissue than that of *H. capsulatum* var. *capsulatum*. Clinical manifestations resemble those of blastomycosis more than those of histoplasmosis in that skin and bone lesions are very common.

DIAGNOSIS Culture of the etiologic organism is the preferred method for diagnosis of histoplasmosis but is often difficult. Blood cultures are best done by the lysis-centrifugation technique, with plates held at 30°C for at least 2 weeks. Approximately 15 mL of blood should be cultured from adults. Routine blood cultures in broth are generally unsuitable. Cultures of bone marrow, mucosal lesions, liver, and bronchoalveolar lavage fluid are diagnostically useful in disseminated histoplasmosis. Sputum culture is the preferred method for the diagnosis of chronic pulmonary histoplasmosis. However, growth may require 2 to 4 weeks to become visible, and other organisms may overgrow the plate. Diagnosis based on Giemsa-stained smears of blood or bronchoalveolar lavage fluid or on methenamine silver staining of infected lung, bone marrow, lymph node, or mucosal lesions requires considerable expertise, although these techniques yield results rapidly and provide specimens that can easily be sent to a referral laboratory. Organisms may be very scanty in lesions with marked caseous necrosis. An assay for *Histoplasma* antigen in blood or urine is commercially available and is useful both for diagnosis and for monitoring of the response to therapy in patients with AIDS who have disseminated infection. Diagnosis by antigen detection requires confirmation by culture or histopathology because false-positive results have occasionally been obtained. Tests for antibody to *H. capsulatum* have been of limited value in diagnosis. Histoplasmin skin testing has proven useful in epidemiologic studies but not in clinical diagnosis. Neither skin testing nor serology has been predictive of histoplasmosis in patients infected with HIV.

℞ **TREATMENT**   Acute pulmonary histoplasmosis requires no therapy. Oral itraconazole (200 mg/d) can be given to shorten the course of illness, although this effect has not been proven. Patients with mediastinal fibrosis may benefit from surgery, but their ultimate prognosis is poor. All patients with disseminated or chronic fibronodular pulmonary histoplasmosis should receive chemotherapy. Intravenous amphotericin B (0.6 mg/kg daily) is the drug of choice for the initial treatment of patients with disseminated histoplasmosis who are severely ill or immunosuppressed or whose infection involves the central nervous system; the regimen can be changed to itraconazole (200 mg twice daily) once clinical improvement is evident in these patients. Measuring itraconazole trough blood levels should be considered in those patients (e.g., patients with AIDS) who may not be absorbing the drug well (Chap. 200). Itraconazole suspension, taken fasting, is better absorbed than the capsule formulation. Fluconazole is reliably absorbed, even in patients taking drugs to block gastric acid secretion, but at doses up to 400 mg/d has been less effective in treatment of chronic pulmonary or disseminated histoplasmosis. Patients with AIDS whose disseminated histoplasmosis has responded to 10 weeks of therapy should receive itraconazole (200 mg/d) for life to prevent relapse. It remains unknown whether patients with a sustained response to highly active antiretroviral therapy can discontinue maintenance therapy with itraconazole.

Immunocompetent patients can initially be given itraconazole (200 mg twice daily) and are generally treated for 6 to 12 months. Ketoconazole (400 to 800 mg once daily) can be used instead of itraconazole for the treatment of immunocompetent patients without central nervous system disease when the lower cost is more important than the higher incidence of side effects. Alternatively, immunocompetent patients can be given a 10-week course of amphotericin B (0.5 mg/kg daily).

Long-term maintenance therapy with an azole is not recommended for patients other than those with AIDS. However, relapse of chronic pulmonary and disseminated histoplasmosis is not rare and warrants careful follow-up for 1 year after therapy.

BIBLIOGRAPHY

GOODWIN RA et al: Histoplasmosis in normal hosts. Medicine 60:231, 1981

HECHT FM et al: Itraconazole maintenance treatment for histoplasmosis in AIDS: A prospective, multicenter trial. J Acquir Immune Defic Syndr 16:100, 1997

PEDDI VR et al: Disseminated histoplasmosis in renal allograft recipients. Clin Transplant 10:160, 1996

RAYMOND LW et al: Scars without wounds: Spectrum of delayed manifestations of histoplasmosis outside of the endemic area. Crit Rev Diagn Imaging 14:37, 1980

WHEAT J: Histoplasmosis. Experience during outbreaks in Indianapolis and review of the literature. Medicine (Baltimore) 76:339, 1997

——— et al: Disseminated histoplasmosis in the acquired immune deficiency syndrome: Clinical findings, diagnosis and treatment, and review of the literature. Medicine 69: 361, 1990

——— et al: Prevention of relapse of histoplasmosis with itraconazole in patients with the acquired immunodeficiency syndrome. Ann Intern Med 118:610, 1993

——— et al: Endemic mycoses in AIDS: A clinical review. Clin Microbiol Rev 8:146, 1995

——— et al: Itraconazole treatment of disseminated histoplasmosis in patients with the acquired immunodeficiency syndrome. Am J Med 98:336, 1995

——— et al: Practice guidelines for the management of patients with histoplasmosis. Clin Infect Dis 30:688, 2000

202   *John E. Bennett*

COCCIDIOIDOMYCOSIS

ETIOLOGIC AGENT   *Coccidioides immitis* has two forms, growing as a white fluffy mold on most culture media but as a nonbudding spherical form (a spherule) in host tissue or under special conditions. The organism reproduces in host tissue by forming small endospores within mature spherules. After rupture of the spherule, the released endospores enlarge, become spherules, and repeat the cycle. The fungus is identified by its appearance and by the formation of thick-walled, barrel-shaped spores, called *arthrospores*, in the hyphae of the mold form.

EPIDEMIOLOGY, PATHOGENESIS, AND PATHOLOGY
C. immitis is a soil saprophyte found in certain arid regions of the United States, Mexico, Central America, and South America. Within the United States, most cases of infection with *C. immitis* are acquired in California, Arizona, and western Texas. A few cases are acquired by exposure to fomites from endemic areas (e.g., in cotton bales).

Infection in humans and animals results from inhalation of windborne arthrospores from soil sites. This primary pulmonary infection is symptomatic in only 40% of cases, with symptoms ranging from a mild influenza-like illness to severe pneumonia. Mild self-limited infections may come to medical attention because of case clusters or hypersensitivity reactions: erythema nodosum, erythema multiforme, toxic erythema, arthralgia, arthritis, conjunctivitis, or episcleritis. Case clusters occur 10 to 14 days after a group of susceptible individuals is exposed to dust in an endemic area through such activities as archaeologic excavation, rock hunting, military maneuvers, or construction work. Windstorms can carry spores to adjacent nonendemic areas and cause case clusters. The usual course of primary pneumonia is complete healing, although an area of pneumonitis (detected on radiographs) may heal by the formation of a coinlike lesion called a *coccidioidoma*. Less commonly, a single thin-walled cavity remains as a chronic sequela in the area of consolidation. Alternatively, an area of consolidation may persist as chronic pneumonia or progress to fibronodular cavitary disease.

Pleural effusion may be the only manifestation of primary infection. Spontaneous healing of this form is common.

An uncommon but dreaded complication of coccidioidomycosis is dissemination beyond the lung and hilar lymph nodes. Dissemination is especially frequent among blacks, Filipinos, Native Americans, Mexican-Americans, pregnant women, and immunosuppressed patients, including those with AIDS.

C. immitis incites a chronic granulomatous reaction in host tissue, often with caseation necrosis. Lung and hilar node lesions may show calcification. Both IgM and IgG antibodies to *C. immitis* are induced by infection, but neither type of antibody appears to be protective. The amount of specific IgG antibody is a rough measure of the antigenic mass (i.e., of the intensity of infection), and a high titer is a poor prognostic sign. Appearance of delayed hypersensitivity to antigens of *C. immitis* is most common in clinical forms of disease with a good prognosis, such as self-limited primary pulmonary disease. In skin tests for *Coccidioides* antigens, about half of patients with disseminated disease have negative results that portend a poor outcome.

CLINICAL MANIFESTATIONS   Symptomatic primary pulmonary infection is manifested by fever, cough, chest pain, malaise, and sometimes the hypersensitivity reactions listed above. Chest radiographs may show an infiltrate, hilar adenopathy, or pleural effusion. Mild peripheral-blood eosinophilia may be found. Spontaneous improvement begins after several days to 2 weeks of illness and usually culminates in complete recovery.

The symptoms of a chronic thin-walled cavity include cough or hemoptysis in half of cases; the other half are asymptomatic. Chronic progressive pulmonary coccidioidomycosis causes cough, sputum production, variable degrees of fever, and weight loss. The first indications of dissemination usually appear during primary infection. Reactivation with dissemination in later years occurs occasionally, especially if Hodgkin's disease, non-Hodgkin's lymphoma, renal transplantation, AIDS, or immunosuppression of some other etiology has supervened. Dissemination should be suspected when fever, malaise, hilar or paratracheal lymphadenopathy, elevated sedimentation rate, and high complement fixation titers signal abnormal persistence in patients with primary pulmonary coccidioidomycosis. With time, lesions appear in the bone, skin, subcutaneous tissue, meninges, joints, and other sites. Chronic meningitis presents as headache of indolent onset, with or without other signs of disseminated coccidioidomycosis. Cultures and smears of cerebrospinal fluid (CSF) are most often negative, but antibody is usually detectable in CSF by complement fixation. Skin lesions are indolent and maculopapular; soft tissue and bony lesions contain pus and may present as a draining sinus. Without treatment, disseminated coccidioidomycosis progresses to death over weeks to years.

Disseminated coccidioidomycosis can progress rapidly in patients with advanced HIV infection. Fever with skin or bone lesions may be the first sign. Those who present with diffuse pulmonary infiltrates have a poor prognosis. Blood cultures are positive late in the disease, if at all.

DIAGNOSIS When coccidioidomycosis is suspected, sputum, urine, and pus should be examined for *C. immitis* by wet smear and culture. *The laboratory request should indicate clearly that coccidioidomycosis is suspected, because the mold form must be handled with extreme care to prevent infection of laboratory personnel.* On biopsy, smaller spherules must be distinguished from nonbudding forms of *Blastomyces* and *Cryptococcus*, but the appearance of the mature spherule is diagnostic.

Serologic tests are very helpful in the diagnosis of coccidioidomycosis. Latex agglutination and agar gel diffusion tests are useful in screening sera for antibody to *Coccidioides*. The complement fixation test is used for CSF determinations and for the confirmation and quantitation of serum antibody detected by screening tests. The number of cases with a positive complement fixation test depends on the severity of disease and on the laboratory performing the test. Positive tests are least common among patients with solitary pulmonary cavities or primary pulmonary infection, while sera from patients with disseminated disease in multiple organs are nearly all positive. Seroconversion is helpful in primary pulmonary coccidioidomycosis but may not occur for up to 8 weeks after onset. A positive complement fixation test of unconcentrated CSF is diagnostic of meningitis. Rarely, a parameningeal focus causes a positive complement fixation test of CSF.

Conversion of the skin test from negative to positive ($\geq$5 mm of induration at 24 or 48 h) with spherulin may take place between days 3 and 21 of symptoms in primary pulmonary coccidioidomycosis. Skin testing can be helpful in epidemiologic studies, such as investigations of case clusters or the definition of endemic areas. The utility of skin testing as a diagnostic tool is limited by the persistence of positive tests resulting from remote exposures to *Coccidioides* and by the frequency of negative skin tests among patients with either thin-walled cavities or disseminated coccidioidomycosis. A positive skin test has not predicted dissemination in HIV-infected patients. The presence of complement-fixing antibody to *C. immitis* in AIDS patients should prompt a search for active infection.

TREATMENT Primary pulmonary coccidioidomycosis usually resolves spontaneously. Some physicians give a few weeks of treatment with intravenous amphotericin B or itraconazole to patients with unusually severe or protracted primary infection in the hope of aborting disseminated or chronic pulmonary disease.

Patients with severe or rapidly progressing disseminated coccidioidomycosis are first given intravenous amphotericin B at a dose of 0.5 to 0.7 mg/kg daily. Patients whose condition improves after 2 to 3 months of treatment with amphotericin B or who have more indolent

disseminated infection are given itraconazole (200 mg twice daily) or fluconazole (400 to 600 mg/d). These oral agents are useful for long-term suppression of infection, and treatment should be continued for years. Patients with coccidioidal meningitis usually are initially given fluconazole (400 to 800 mg/d) but may require intrathecal amphotericin B. Hydrocephalus is a frequent complication of uncontrolled meningitis. Surgical debridement of bone lesions or drainage of abscesses can be helpful. The prognosis for ultimate cure of disseminated coccidioidomycosis is guarded.

Resection of chronic progressive pulmonary lesions is a helpful adjunct to chemotherapy when infection is confined to the lung and to one lobe. A single thin-walled cavity tends to close spontaneously and ordinarily is not resected. Such a cavity responds poorly to chemotherapy.

BIBLIOGRAPHY

CATANZARO A et al: Fluconazole in the treatment of chronic pulmonary and nonmeningeal disseminated coccidioidomycosis. Am J Med 98:249, 1995

FISH DG et al: Coccidioidomycosis during human immunodeficiency virus infection. A review of 77 patients. Medicine 69:384, 1990

GALGIANI JN: Coccidioidomycosis: A regional disease of national importance. Rethinking approaches for control. Ann Intern Med 130:293, 1999

——— et al: Practice guidelines for the treatment of coccidioidomycosis. Clin Infect Dis 30:658, 2000

KIM K et al: Chronic pulmonary coccidioidomycosis: Computed tomographic and pathologic findings in 18 patients. Can Assoc Rad J 49:401, 1998

KIRKLAND TN, FIERER J: Coccidioidomycosis: A reemerging infectious disease. Emerg Infect Dis 2:192, 1996

SCHNEIDER E et al: A coccidioidomycosis outbreak following the Northridge, California, earthquake. JAMA 277:904, 1997

---

203 John E. Bennett

BLASTOMYCOSIS

ETIOLOGIC AGENT *Blastomyces dermatitidis* is a dimorphic fungus that grows at room temperature as a white or tan mold but grows within the host or at 37°C as budding, round yeastlike cells. The fungus can be identified on the basis of its appearance, its dimorphism, the small spores borne on hyphae of the mold form, or the results of nucleic acid hybridization. When isolates of the two opposite mating types are grown close together on special culture medium, such as yeast extract or soil extract agar, sporulating structures that characterize the perfect state (teleomorph), called *Ajellomyces dermatitidis*, appear.

EPIDEMIOLOGY The infection is restricted by geography and age. Blastomycosis is uncommon in any locality, but most cases occur in the southeastern, central, and mid-Atlantic areas of the United States, with occasional cases in other localities in the United States and Canada. Cases have also been encountered in Africa, Mexico, Central America, and (rarely) South America. Most patients are between 20 and 69 years old. The male-to-female ratio is about 10:1. There is no occupational predisposition to the development of blastomycosis.

PATHOGENESIS AND PATHOLOGY Infection with *B. dermatitidis* appears to be acquired by inhalation of the fungus from soil, decomposed vegetation, or rotting wood. Several case clusters have resulted from participation in recreational activities in wooded areas along waterways. Infection is not transmissible from person to person. The initial pulmonary infection may either heal spontaneously or become chronic. Spread to other portions of the lung, cavitation, or endobronchial lesions may be found in patients with chronic disease.

Whether or not the lung lesion resolves spontaneously, infection commonly spreads hematogenously to the skin, subcutaneous tissue, bone, prostate, epididymis, or mucosa of the nose, mouth, or larynx. Less commonly, infection spreads to the brain, meninges, liver, lymph nodes, or spleen. Dissemination may not be evident for weeks or years after the appearance of the lung lesion. Progressive infection is only rarely attributable to an underlying disease, to HIV infection, or to immunosuppressive treatment. The inflammatory response includes lymphocytes, giant cells, and neutrophils. Pseudoepitheliomatous hyperplasia may be striking and may lead to a mistaken diagnosis of squamous cell carcinoma.

CLINICAL MANIFESTATIONS   A few patients have acute, self-limited pneumonia. Fever, productive cough, myalgia, and malaise usually resolve within a month. Pulmonary infiltrates clear slowly as *B. dermatitidis* disappears from the sputum.

In the vast majority of patients, blastomycosis has an indolent onset and a chronically progressive course. Fever, cough, weight loss, lassitude, skin lesions, and chest ache are common. Skin lesions favor exposed areas and enlarge over many weeks from pimples to well-circumscribed, verrucous, crusted, or ulcerated lesions. Pain and regional lymphadenopathy are minimal. Large chronic lesions may undergo central healing with scarring and contracture. Mucous membrane lesions resemble squamous cell carcinoma. Chest x-ray findings are abnormal in two-thirds of patients, with one or more pneumonic or nodular infiltrates. Calcification, hilar adenopathy, and large pleural effusions are rare. Osteolytic lesions may be found in nearly any bone and present as a cold abscess or a draining sinus. Extension to a contiguous joint may cause indolent swelling, pain, and restricted motion. Prostatic and epididymal lesions clinically resemble those of tuberculosis.

DIAGNOSIS   The diagnosis of blastomycosis is made by demonstration of the fungus in a culture of sputum, pus, or urine. An expert can diagnose blastomycosis on the basis of the appearance of the organism in wet smear or histopathologic section. The fungus may be visible in a sputum cytology smear but is easily overlooked.

℞ **TREATMENT**   A few patients have developed only transitory lung lesions, but no guidelines are known to distinguish these patients from those whose disease will progress locally or disseminate. Therefore, every patient should receive treatment. Intravenous amphotericin B is the drug of choice for patients with rapidly progressive infections, severe illness, or central nervous system lesions. Skin and noncavitary lung lesions should be treated for about 8 to 10 weeks. The recommended total dose for an adult is about 2 g. Cavitary lung disease or infection extending beyond the lung and skin should be treated for about 10 to 12 weeks with ≥2.5 g.

Oral itraconazole (200 mg twice daily with food) is the drug of choice for the treatment of patients who have indolent nonmeningeal blastomycosis of mild to moderate severity and who take the drug reliably. Therapy with itraconazole is continued for 6 to 12 months.

The mortality rate in appropriately treated cases is ≤15%.

BIBLIOGRAPHY

BAUMGARDNER DJ et al: Epidemiology of blastomycosis in a region of high endemicity in north-central Wisconsin. Clin Infect Dis 15:629, 1992

BRADSHER RW: Blastomycosis: Fungal infections of the lung. Update 1989. Semin Respir Infect 5:105, 1990

CHAPMAN SW et al: Endemic blastomycosis in Mississippi: Epidemiological and clinical studies. Semin Respir Infect 12:219, 1997

———— et al: Practice guidelines for the management of patients with blastomycosis. Clin Infect Dis 30:679, 2000

MANGINO JE, PAPPAS PG: Itraconazole for the treatment of histoplasmosis and blastomycosis. Int J Antimicrob Agents 5:219, 1995

PAPPAS PG et al: Blastomycosis in immunocompromised patients. Medicine 72:311, 1993

SACCENTE M et al: Vertebral blastomycosis with paravertebral abscess: Report of eight cases and review of the literature. Clin Infect Dis 26:413, 1998

204   *John E. Bennett*

CRYPTOCOCCOSIS

ETIOLOGIC AGENT   Cryptococcosis is an infection caused by the yeastlike fungus *Cryptococcus neoformans*. This fungus reproduces by budding and forms round, yeastlike cells. Within the host and on certain culture media, a large polysaccharide capsule surrounds each yeast cell. The fungus grows well in smooth, creamy-white colonies on Sabouraud's or other simple media at 20 to 37°C. Identification of the organism is based on gross and microscopic appearance, biochemical test results, and growth at 37°C. The results of nucleic acid hybridization or the formation of brown pigment on Niger seed agar can also be used for identification.

The fungus has four capsular serotypes, designated A, B, C, and D. There are also two mating types. Coculture of opposite mating types creates a transient diploid state called *Filobasidiella neoformans* var. *neoformans* for serotypes A and D and *F. neoformans* var. *bacillispora* for serotypes B and C. Organisms not cultured under mating conditions are designated *C. neoformans* var. *neoformans* for serotypes A and D and *C. neoformans* var. *gattii* for serotypes B and C; a simple color medium distinguishes the two varieties.

EPIDEMIOLOGY   Weathered pigeon droppings commonly contain serotype A or D (*C. neoformans* var. *neoformans*). *C. neoformans* var. *gattii* has been isolated from the litter around trees of the species *Eucalyptus camaldulensis* and *E. tereticornis*. Eucalyptus isolates have so far typed as serotype B. The distribution of these eucalyptus species in Australia corresponds to the distribution of infections due to *C. neoformans* var. *gattii* in that country. The high prevalence of these trees in other subtropical climates has been postulated to explain the relative restriction of such infections to warm climates.

Cryptococcosis due to *C. neoformans* var. *neoformans* is a common complication of late infection with HIV. The incidence appears to be declining in some areas of the United States, probably as a result of highly active antiretroviral therapy and use of fluconazole for oropharyngeal candidiasis. Patients who have undergone solid-organ transplantation or glucocorticoid therapy and those with sarcoidosis are also at increased risk for infections with *C. neoformans* var. *neoformans*. Almost all such infections are caused by serotype A, although serotype D occurs in up to 20% of cases in Western Europe. Infections with var. *gattii* have been rare among AIDS patients and other immunocompromised patients, even in subtropical climates, where var. *gattii* infection occurs in previously healthy individuals.

Animals, particularly cats, can acquire cryptococcosis but have not transmitted the infection to other animals or to humans. The source from which humans acquire the infection is unknown, with the rare exception of cases acquired through a transplanted cornea, kidney, or other solid organ. Cryptococcosis is rare before puberty.

PATHOGENESIS AND PATHOLOGY   Infection is thought to be acquired by inhalation of fungus into the lungs. Pulmonary infection has a tendency toward spontaneous resolution and is frequently asymptomatic. Silent hematogenous spread to the brain leads to clusters of cryptococci in the perivascular areas of cortical gray matter, in the basal ganglia, and, to a lesser extent, in other areas of the central nervous system. The inflammatory response around these foci is usually scant. In the more chronic cases, a dense basilar arachnoiditis is typical. Lung lesions are characterized by intense granulomatous inflammation. Cryptococci are best seen in tissue by staining with methenamine silver or periodic acid–Schiff. Although a strongly positive result on mucicarmine staining of tissue is diagnostic, staining varies from intense to absent.

CLINICAL MANIFESTATIONS   Most patients have *meningoencephalitis* at the time of diagnosis. This form of the infection is invariably fatal without appropriate therapy; death occurs any time from 2 weeks to several years after the onset of symptoms. Early manifestations include headache, nausea, staggering gait, dementia, irritability, confusion, and blurred vision. Both fever and nuchal rigidity are often mild or lacking. Papilledema is evident in one-third of cases at the time of diagnosis. Cranial nerve palsies, typically asymmetric, occur in about one-fourth of cases. Other lateralized signs are rare. With progression of the infection, deepening coma and signs of brainstem compression appear. Autopsy often reveals cerebral edema in more acute cases and hydrocephalus in more chronic cases.

Pulmonary cryptococcosis causes chest pain in about 40% of patients and cough in 20%. The chest x-ray shows one or more dense infiltrates, which are often well circumscribed. Cavitation, pleural effusions, and hilar adenopathy are infrequent. Calcification is not evident, and fibrotic stranding is rarely noticeable.

Ten percent of patients with cryptococcosis have skin lesions, and the vast majority of patients with skin lesions have disseminated infection. One or a few asymptomatic tiny papular lesions appear and slowly enlarge; they display a tendency toward central softening leading to ulceration. Osteolytic lesions occur in 4% of cases and usually present as a cold abscess. Rare manifestations of cryptococcosis include prostatitis, endophthalmitis, hepatitis, pericarditis, endocarditis, and renal abscess.

DIAGNOSIS Fever and headache in a patient with AIDS or with risk factors for HIV infection suggest the possibility of cryptococcosis, toxoplasmosis, or central nervous system lymphoma. Evidence of a focal lesion on magnetic resonance imaging is unusual in cryptococcosis. Most cryptococcal cerebral mass lesions occur in patients infected with *C. neoformans* var. *gattii* who also have meningitis. In patients without AIDS, meningitis due to *C. neoformans* resembles that due to *Mycobacterium tuberculosis*, *Histoplasma capsulatum*, *Coccidioides immitis*, or metastatic cancer. Lumbar puncture is the single most useful diagnostic test. An india ink smear of centrifuged cerebrospinal fluid (CSF) sediment reveals encapsulated yeast in more than half of cases, although artifacts can cause confusion. In patients without AIDS, levels of glucose in CSF are reduced in half of all cases; protein levels are usually increased; and lymphocytic pleocytosis is usually found. CSF abnormalities are less pronounced in patients with AIDS, although india ink smear is more often positive.

Approximately 90% of patients with cryptococcal meningoencephalitis, including all those with a positive CSF smear, have capsular antigen detectable in CSF or serum by latex agglutination. An enzyme immunoassay for cryptococcal antigen is also available. Occasional false-positive results in the above tests make culture the definitive diagnostic test and have prevented serum antigen from being a useful screening test in asymptomatic patients with AIDS. *C. neoformans* is often present in urine from patients with meningoencephalitis. Fungemia occurs in 10 to 30% of patients and is particularly common among patients with AIDS.

Pulmonary cryptococcosis mimics malignancy with regard to radiographic findings and symptoms. Sputum culture is positive in only 10% of cases, and serum antigen tests are positive in only one-third. Occasionally, *C. neoformans* appears in one or more sputum specimens as an endobronchial saprophyte. Biopsy is usually required for diagnosis.

Cutaneous cryptococcosis may be mistaken for a comedo, basal cell carcinoma, or sarcoidosis. In patients with AIDS, skin lesions may be numerous and are sometimes mistaken for molluscum contagiosum. Biopsy reveals myriad cryptococci. Osseous cryptococcosis resembles tuberculosis.

℞ **TREATMENT** Patients with AIDS and cryptococcosis are treated initially with intravenous amphotericin B (0.7 mg/kg daily) for at least 2 weeks and until their clinical condition is stable; thereafter, they receive fluconazole. The addition of flucytosine (25 mg/kg every 6 h) to amphotericin B for 2 weeks has minimal impact on morbidity and mortality. After treatment with amphotericin B, fluconazole (400 mg) is given once daily. Daily doses of 800 mg have

been used with marginal changes in toxicity or efficacy. The addition of flucytosine to fluconazole increases gastrointestinal intolerance. After infection is controlled, treatment with a smaller dose of fluconazole (200 mg/d) is continued indefinitely. Itraconazole is less effective than fluconazole for maintenance therapy. It is not yet known whether patients whose CD4+ T lymphocyte counts have exhibited a sustained rise in response to antiretroviral therapy can safely discontinue fluconazole maintenance therapy.

In patients without AIDS, the therapeutic goal is to cure the infection, not merely to control its symptoms. A single intensive course is given until cultures from all previously positive sites (particularly CSF) become convincingly negative. Normalization of the glucose level in lumbar CSF is desirable, but complete clearing of CSF or serum antigen during therapy is not essential. Amphotericin B (0.6 to 0.7 mg/kg daily for $\geq$10 weeks) is the best-studied regimen. Flucytosine has been added to amphotericin B to accelerate the culture response, but grave toxicity can result unless flucytosine blood levels are kept below 100 μg/mL. Case reports have described patients without HIV infection who have responded to fluconazole or liposomal amphotericin B, but the dose and duration of treatment required to cure cryptococcal meningitis are undefined. Amphotericin B lipid complex and amphotericin B colloidal dispersion are not recommended pending further study.

Hydrocephalus may be the presenting manifestation or a later complication of cryptococcosis. Blindness, dementia, and personality change are among the other sequelae. Daily lumbar puncture or CSF shunting has been advocated—in the hope of averting permanent blindness—for patients with marked cerebral edema who have incipient blurred vision.

Patients with extraneural cryptococcosis most often require treatment with intravenous amphotericin B, with or without flucytosine. Observation or excision of lesions may suffice for some patients who have previously been healthy; who have a single focus in lung, skin, or bone; and who have no cryptococci in CSF, urine, or blood.

PREVENTION Fluconazole (200 mg/d) has been shown to decrease the incidence of cryptococcosis in HIV-infected patients with CD4+ cell counts of <200/μL and particularly in those with counts of <50/μL. Weekly fluconazole has not provided this protection. Daily fluconazole has not conferred a survival advantage; in light of its cost and the currently low incidence of cryptococcosis in patients with AIDS in the United States, prophylaxis is strongly discouraged.

BIBLIOGRAPHY

MEYOHAS M-C et al: Pulmonary cryptococcosis: Localized and disseminated infections in 27 patients with AIDS. Clin Infect Dis 21:628, 1995

MURAKAWA GJ et al: Cutaneous *Cryptococcus* infection and AIDS: Report of 12 cases and review of the literature. Arch Dermatol 132:545, 1996

POWDERLY WG et al: Measurement of cryptococcal antigen in serum and cerebrospinal fluid: Value in the management of AIDS-associated cryptococcal meningitis. Clin Infect Dis 18:789, 1994

——— et al: A randomized trial comparing fluconazole with clotrimazole troches for the prevention of fungal infections in patients with advanced human immunodeficiency virus infection. NIAID AIDS Clinical Trials Group. N Engl J Med 332:700, 1995

REX JR et al: Catastrophic visual loss due to *Cryptococcus neoformans* meningitis. Medicine 72:207, 1993

SAAG MS et al: A comparison of itraconazole versus fluconazole as maintenance therapy for AIDS-associated cryptococcal meningitis. Clin Infect Dis 28:291, 1999

——— et al: Practice guidelines for the management of cryptococcal disease. Clin Infect Dis 30:710, 2000

SPEED B, DUNT D: Clinical and host differences between infections with the two varieties of *Cryptococcus neoformans*. Clin Infect Dis 21:28, 1995

VAN DER HORST CM et al: Treatment of cryptococcal meningitis associated with the acquired immunodeficiency syndrome. NIAID Mycoses Study Group and AIDS Clinical Trials Group. N Engl J Med 337:15, 1997

205

John E. Bennett

CANDIDIASIS

ETIOLOGIC AGENTS *Candida albicans* is the most common cause of mucosal candidiasis and is responsible for about half of all cases of candidemia in hospitalized patients. A small proportion of *C. albicans* isolates have been transferred to a new species, *C. dubliniensis*. *C. tropicalis*, *C. parapsilosis*, *C. guilliermondii*, *C. glabrata* (formerly *Torulopsis glabrata*), *C. krusei*, and a few other *Candida* species also cause potentially fatal bloodstream infection. Many of these non-*albicans* species can enter the bloodstream through an intravascular catheter. *Candida* species, taken together, are the fifth most common cause of nosocomial bloodstream infections in the United States.

All *Candida* species pathogenic for humans are also encountered as commensals of humans, particularly in the mouth, stool, and vagina. These species grow rapidly at 25° to 37°C on simple media as oval, budding cells. In special culture media and in tissue, hyphae or elongated branching structures called *pseudohyphae* are formed. *C. glabrata* differs from other members of the genus in that it forms no true hyphae or pseudohyphae in vitro or in infected tissue. *C. albicans* and *C. dubliniensis* can be identified presumptively by their ability to form germ tubes in serum or by the formation of thick-walled large spores called *chlamydospores*. Final identification of all *Candida* species requires biochemical tests.

PATHOGENESIS Candidiasis is often preceded by increased colonization of the mouth, vagina, and stool with *Candida* due to broad-spectrum antibiotic therapy. Additional local and systemic factors favor infection. Oropharyngeal thrush is particularly likely to occur in neonates and in patients with diabetes mellitus, HIV infection, or dentures. Vulvovaginal candidiasis (Chap. 132) is especially common in the third trimester of pregnancy. *Candida* from the perineum can enter the urinary tract via an indwelling bladder catheter. Cutaneous candidiasis most often involves macerated skin, such as that in the diapered area of infants, under pendulous breasts, or on hands constantly in water or covered by occlusive gloves. *Candida* can pass from the colonized surface into deep tissue when the integrity of the mucosa or skin is violated, as, for example, by perforation of the gastrointestinal tract through trauma, surgery, or peptic ulceration or by mucosal damage due to cytotoxic agents used for cancer chemotherapy. Although *Candida* is not normally a resident of the skin, secretions from the mouth, rectum, or vagina as well as drainage from surgical wounds or tracheostomy sites can contaminate the hub or skin site of a catheter in an umbilical or central vein. Intravenous drug abuse or third-degree burns can also provide a skin portal for *Candida* that can lead to deep candidiasis. Once *Candida* has passed the integumentary barrier, very low birth weight (in neonates) and neutropenia or glucocorticoid therapy (in any patient) markedly compromise host defense. Hematogenous seeding is particularly evident in the retina, kidney, spleen, and liver.

CLINICAL MANIFESTATIONS *Oral thrush* presents as discrete and confluent adherent white plaques on the oral and pharyngeal mucosa, particularly in the mouth and on the tongue. These lesions are usually painless, but fissuring at the corners of the mouth can be painful. Unexplained oropharyngeal thrush raises the possibility of HIV infection. Oral thrush is common in acute HIV infection and becomes increasingly common as the CD4+ cell count falls. At CD4+ counts <50/μL, esophageal thrush also becomes common. HIV infection appears not to be an independent risk factor for vulvovaginal thrush.

Cutaneous candidiasis presents as red macerated intertriginous areas, paronychia, balanitis, or pruritus ani. Candidiasis of the perineal and scrotal skin may be accompanied by discrete pustular lesions on the inner aspects of the thighs. *Chronic mucocutaneous candidiasis* or *candidal granuloma* typically presents as circumscribed hyperkeratotic skin lesions, crumbling dystrophic nails, partial alopecia in areas of scalp lesions, and both oral and vaginal thrush. Systemic infection is very rare, but disfigurement of the face and hands can be severe. Other findings may include chronic epidermophytosis, dental dysplasia, and hypofunction of the parathyroid, adrenal, or thyroid gland. A variety of defects in T cell function have been described in these patients. Vulvovaginal thrush (Chap. 132) causes pruritus, discharge, and sometimes pain on intercourse or urination. Speculum examination reveals an inflamed mucosa and a thin exudate, often with white curds.

Esophageal candidiasis is often asymptomatic but can cause substernal pain or a sense of obstruction on swallowing. Most lesions are in the distal third of the esophagus and appear on endoscopy as areas of redness and edema, focal white patches, or ulcers. Biopsy or brushing is required for diagnosis and for detection of concomitant infections, particularly herpes simplex in patients with hematologic malignancies and cytomegalovirus infection in AIDS patients. Esophagography (barium swallow) is diagnostically insensitive but may reveal spasm or mucosal irregularities. *Candida* esophagitis can cause bleeding and impaired alimentation. Hematogenous dissemination from the esophagus probably occurs in some neutropenic patients but is rarely reported in HIV-infected patients.

Candida can cause cystitis, pyelitis, or renal papillary necrosis in an obstructed urinary tract. When a colonized urinary tract is operated on or instrumented, candidemia may result. However, most patients with *Candida* cultured from the urine simply have bladder colonization from a Foley catheter or a sizable volume of residual urine. Contamination of a voided midstream specimen by vaginal *Candida* is also common.

Candidemia originating from an intravascular catheter may clear in the immunocompetent patient when the catheter is removed. Focal seeding of the retina can take place even if candidemia clears and the patient becomes afebrile. Unilateral or bilateral small white retinal exudates appear within 2 weeks of the onset of candidemia. Lesions may regress spontaneously or enlarge slowly. The vitreous humor becomes cloudy, and the patient notices blurring, ocular pain, or a scotoma. Retinal detachment, vitreous abscess, and extension to the anterior chamber can occur over the ensuing weeks. These retinal lesions, present in ~10% of nonneutropenic patients with candidemia, are the principal reason that systemic antifungal therapy is recommended for all patients with candidemia. Funduscopy should be performed to be certain that retinal lesions, if present, resolve completely. Most cases with ocular involvement have occurred in nonneutropenic patients. In contrast, so-called hepatosplenic candidiasis is usually recognized in patients with acute leukemia who are recovering from profound neutropenia. This entity, better called *chronic disseminated candidiasis*, originates from intestinal seeding of the portal and venous circulation. Fever, modestly elevated serum concentrations of alkaline phosphatase, and multiple small abscesses evident on ultrasonography, magnetic resonance imaging, or computed tomography of the liver, spleen, or kidney suggest the diagnosis. During acute candidemia in neutropenic patients, small erythematous papules may appear anywhere on the skin (**Plate IID-57D**). If the patient does not expire promptly from disseminated candidiasis, the lesions will develop a necrotic center. Painful muscle lesions may also be found. Punch biopsy of a skin lesion helps distinguish this extremely grave condition from *Malassezia* folliculitis, a similar-appearing but benign condition that can involve the cape area of the chest or the extremities of a sweaty febrile patient.

Hematogenous seeding in the neutropenic patient is occasionally visible radiologically as tiny pulmonary nodules. *Candida* pneumonia, apart from hematogenous candidiasis, is very rare. Organisms seeding a native or prosthetic cardiac valve originate principally from central venous catheters; occasionally, valvular seeding is encountered in intravenous drug abusers. Emboli to large arteries, such as the iliac or femoral artery, are characteristic. Intravenous injection of impure brown heroin has caused a clinical syndrome consisting of *Candida* endophthalmitis and purulent folliculitis, sometimes accompanied by vertebral osteomyelitis. This diffuse folliculitis favors hairy areas, including the scalp and bearded facial skin.

Candida can cause indolent arthritis, most commonly of the knee, in patients who have received glucocorticoid injections into the joint, in patients who are immunosuppressed, and in low-birth-weight neonates. Prosthetic joints may become infected during implantation. Scanty growth of *Candida* from joint fluid can cause the laboratory to incorrectly dismiss the organism as a contaminant.

Hematogenous dissemination can lead to brain abscess or chronic meningitis. Diagnosis of infections of ventriculoperitoneal shunts is difficult because symptoms are indolent and cultures of lumbar fluid are usually sterile.

DIAGNOSIS Demonstration of pseudohyphae on wet smear with confirmation by culture is the procedure of choice for diagnosing superficial candidiasis. Scrapings for the smear may be obtained from skin, nails, and oral and vaginal mucosa. Culture alone is not diagnostic; however, recovery of *Candida* species from multiple superficial sites in immunosuppressed patients may portend visceral invasion.

Deeper lesions due to *Candida* may be diagnosed by histologic section of biopsy specimens or by culture of cerebrospinal fluid, blood, joint fluid, or surgical specimens. Blood cultures are useful in the diagnosis of *Candida* endocarditis and intravenous catheter–induced sepsis but are positive less often in other forms of disseminated disease. Serologic tests for antibody or antigen are not useful.

TREATMENT Cutaneous candidiasis of macerated areas responds to measures that reduce moisture and chafing plus topical application of an antifungal agent in a nonocclusive base. Nystatin powder or a cream containing ciclopirox or an azole is useful. Clotrimazole, miconazole, econazole, ketoconazole, sulconazole, and oxiconazole are available as creams or lotions. *Candida* vulvovaginitis responds better to an azole than to nystatin suppositories. There is little difference in efficacy among miconazole, clotrimazole, tioconazole, butoconazole, and terconazole vaginal formulations. Systemic treatment of *Candida* vulvovaginitis with a single 150-mg capsule of fluconazole is more convenient than topical treatment but also poses a higher risk of adverse effects. Clotrimazole troches, used five times a day, are more effective in oral and esophageal candidiasis than nystatin suspension. Oral fluconazole (100 to 200 mg once daily) is more convenient and more effective in esophagitis than clotrimazole troches. Esophagitis not responding to fluconazole may warrant repeat endoscopy to exclude other conditions. Itraconazole suspension (100 to 200 mg/d) alleviates *Candida* esophagitis in some patients in whom fluconazole treatment fails. Amphotericin B suspension has limited use but can be tried in patients whose oropharyngeal candidiasis does not respond to azoles.

Management of recurrent oropharyngeal candidiasis in the HIV-infected patient presents special problems. Patients with CD4+ cell counts <100/μL who have received prolonged fluconazole therapy are at risk of developing azole resistance, requiring an increased dose to mount a response, relapsing early, and eventually failing to respond well to any dose of fluconazole. The increasing azole resistance in this population suggests that HIV-infected patients with oropharyngeal candidiasis should be treated for each individual episode and that only when episodes become intolerably frequent should weekly or daily preventive therapy be given and even then at the lowest dose required to maintain remission. In contrast, AIDS patients with *Candida* esophagitis are so prone to relapse that preventive therapy with fluconazole is recommended for all proven cases. Most HIV-infected patients with azole-resistant oropharyngeal candidiasis also have esophagitis. Nearly all patients with azole-resistant oropharyngeal or esophageal candidiasis respond to intravenous amphotericin B (0.3 to 0.5 mg/kg daily) but relapse promptly after the completion of therapy.

Bladder thrush responds to bladder irrigations with amphotericin B (50 μg/mL for 5 days). If no bladder catheter is in place, oral flu-conazole can be used to control candiduria. In all forms of superficial candidiasis, relapse after successful treatment is common unless the underlying factor can be eliminated.

Intravenous amphotericin B is the drug of choice in disseminated candidiasis. The deoxycholate formulation is usually given at a dosage of 0.5 to 0.7 mg/kg daily. Open, noncomparative studies of the lipid formulations of amphotericin B have suggested that they may be useful in disseminated candidiasis, but the optimal dose and formulation remain unknown. Fluconazole in an adult dose of 100 mg/d is probably the drug of choice for chronic mucocutaneous candidiasis.

In immunocompetent patients with intravenous catheter–acquired *C. albicans* fungemia, the catheter should be removed in conjunction with the administration of either fluconazole (400 mg/d) or amphotericin B (0.5 mg/kg daily). Patients with suppurative phlebitis of a peripheral vein should have the infected portion of the vein excised. Therapy for candidemia is continued for 2 weeks after the patient becomes afebrile. The *Candida* species involved should be considered in choosing between fluconazole and amphotericin B. *C. krusei* and *C. inconspicua* are rare causes of candidemia but are resistant to fluconazole in vitro. *C. glabrata* exhibits intermediate susceptibility to fluconazole, but too few cases have been studied to determine whether candidemia involving that species will respond as well to fluconazole as to amphotericin B. Strains of *C. lusitaniae* resistant to amphotericin B but susceptible to azoles have been encountered. Intravenous amphotericin B, with or without flucytosine, is the preferred treatment for *Candida* endophthalmitis, although cures have been reported with fluconazole. Pars plana vitrectomy may facilitate diagnosis and cure when a *Candida* vitreous abscess is present. Injection of amphotericin B into the vitreous humor can also be helpful.

Injection of amphotericin B into an infected joint, pleural cavity, or peritoneum is rarely indicated. Removal of prostheses, including prosthetic joints, cardiac valves, peritoneal dialysis catheters, and central venous catheters, is usually essential. Collections of pus, such as those in the postoperative abdomen, need to be drained surgically or by percutaneous, computed tomography–guided catheterization; an exception relates to the numerous small abscesses in liver, spleen, or kidney in chronic disseminated candidiasis, which cannot be drained effectively and require prolonged antifungal therapy. In general, treatment should continue until the patient with chronic disseminated candidiasis has been afebrile and nonneutropenic for at least 2 weeks. Defects may persist on imaging studies long after cure. Relapse during another episode of neutropenia is common unless the patient is receiving amphotericin B. Repeat cytotoxic therapy or even bone marrow transplantation can be undertaken in patients with prior chronic disseminated candidiasis, but amphotericin B should be given prophylactically during neutropenia.

Fluconazole can decrease the incidence of deep candidiasis in recipients of allogeneic bone marrow transplants when 400 mg is given daily until engraftment. Although the incidence of superficial candidiasis is also decreased by fluconazole prophylaxis, superficial infection can be readily detected and treated. Aspergillosis is not prevented by prophylactic fluconazole. Studies of leukemic and other neutropenic patients have found no beneficial effect of prophylactic fluconazole.

BIBLIOGRAPHY

BENOIT D et al: Management of candidal thrombophlebitis of the central veins: Case report and review. Clin Infect Dis 26:393, 1998

CASADO JL et al: Candidal meningitis in HIV-infected patients: Analysis of 14 cases. Clin Infect Dis 25:673, 1997

DONAHUE SP et al: Intraocular candidiasis in patients with candidemia. Clinical implications derived from a prospective multicenter study. Ophthalmology 101:1302, 1994

EDWARDS JE et al: International Conference for the Development of a Consensus on the Management and Prevention of Severe Candidal Infections. Clin Infect Dis 25:43, 1997

MELGAR GR et al: Fungal prosthetic valve endocarditis in 16 patients. An 11-year experience in a tertiary care hospital. Medicine 76:94, 1997

NGUYEN MH et al: *Candida* prosthetic valve endocarditis: Prospective study of six cases and review of the literature. Clin Infect Dis 22:262, 1996

ODDS FC: *Candida and Candidosis*. Philadelphia, Saunders, 1988

PFALLER MA et al: National surveillance of nosocomial bloodstream infection due to *Candida albicans*: Frequency of occurrence and antifungal susceptibility in the SCOPE Program. Diagn Microbiol Infect Dis 31:327, 1998

REX JH et al: A randomized trial comparing fluconazole with amphotericin B for the treatment of candidemia in patients without neutropenia. N Engl J Med 331:1325, 1994

——— et al: Practice guidelines for the treatment of candidiasis. Clin Infect Dis 30:662, 2000

SLAVIN MA et al: Efficacy and safety of fluconazole prophylaxis for fungal infections after marrow transplantation—a prospective, randomized, double-blind study. J Infect Dis 171:1545, 1995

SOBEL JD et al: Vulvovaginal candidiasis: Epidemiologic, diagnostic, and therapeutic considerations. Am J Obstet Gynecol 178:203, 1998

THALER M et al: Hepatic candidiasis in cancer patients: The evolving picture of the syndrome. Ann Intern Med 198:88, 1988

WILCOX CM et al: A randomized, double-blind comparison of itraconazole oral solution and fluconazole tablets in the treatment of esophageal candidiasis. J Infect Dis 176:227, 1997

206   *John E. Bennett*

ASPERGILLOSIS

ETIOLOGIC AGENTS *Aspergillus fumigatus* is the most common cause of aspergillosis, but *A. flavus*, *A. niger*, and several other species can also cause disease. *Aspergillus* is a mold with septate hyphae about 2 to 4 μm in diameter. The fungus is identified by its gross and microscopic appearance in culture.

PATHOGENESIS AND PATHOLOGY All the common species of *Aspergillus* that cause disease in humans are ubiquitous in the environment, growing on dead leaves, stored grain, compost piles, hay, and other decaying vegetation. Inhalation of *Aspergillus* spores must be extremely common, but disease is rare. Invasion of lung tissue is confined almost entirely to immunosuppressed patients, in roughly 90% of whom two of the following three conditions will be operative: a granulocyte count in peripheral blood of <500/μL, treatment with supraphysiologic doses of adrenal glucocorticoids, and a history of treatment with cytotoxic drugs such as cyclosporine. Invasive aspergillosis is an occasional complication of AIDS. *Aspergillus* infection is characterized by hyphal invasion of blood vessels, thrombosis, necrosis, and hemorrhagic infarction. Chronic granulomatous disease of childhood also predisposes to invasive pulmonary aspergillosis, but in that situation the inflammatory response is a pyogranuloma and blood vessel invasion is rare.

Massive inhalation of *Aspergillus* spores by healthy persons can lead to acute, diffuse, self-limited pneumonitis. Epithelioid granulomas with giant cells and central pyogenic areas containing hyphae are detected in these cases. Spontaneous recovery taking several weeks is the usual course.

Aspergillus can colonize the damaged bronchial tree, pulmonary cysts, or cavities of patients with underlying lung disease. Balls of hyphae within cysts or cavities (aspergillomas), usually in the upper lobe, may reach several centimeters in diameter and may be visible on chest x-ray. Tissue invasion does not occur. The term *allergic bronchopulmonary aspergillosis* denotes the condition of patients with pre-existing asthma who have eosinophilia, IgE antibody to *Aspergillus*, and fleeting pulmonary infiltrates from bronchial plugging.

CLINICAL MANIFESTATIONS *Endobronchial saprophytic pulmonary aspergillosis* presents as chronic productive cough, often with hemoptysis, in a patient with prior chronic lung disease, such as tuberculosis, sarcoidosis, bronchiectasis, or histoplasmosis. *Aspergillus* may be spread from its endocavitary or endobronchial site to the pleura during the course of bacterial lung abscess or surgery. Patients reported to have chronic necrotizing *Aspergillus* pneumonia appear in most instances to have had saprophytic endobronchial colonization and a pulmonary process attributable to another disease, with or without superimposed bacterial infections. Patients with chronic pneumonia and *Aspergillus* in the sputum should be assumed to have either pneumonia of a different etiology (e.g., histoplasmosis) or *Aspergillus* pneumonia with underlying immunosuppression (e.g., chronic granulomatous disease or infection with HIV).

Invasive aspergillosis in the immunocompromised host presents as an acute, rapidly progressive, densely consolidated pulmonary infiltrate and is most common among patients with acute leukemia and recipients of tissue transplants. Infection progresses by direct extension across tissue planes and by hematogenous dissemination to lung, brain, and other organs. Computed tomography (CT) has been particularly valuable in suggesting the diagnosis of invasive pulmonary aspergillosis in patients with neutropenia. The earliest CT finding is one or more small pulmonary nodules. As a nodule enlarges, the dense central core of infarcted tissue becomes surrounded by edema or hemorrhage, forming a hazy rim called the *halo sign*. This rim disappears in a few days as the dense core enlarges. When bone marrow function recovers, the infarcted central core cavitates, creating the *crescent sign*. *Aspergillus* may invade immunosuppressed patients through the skin at a site of minor trauma or through the upper airway mucosa. Early lesions in the nose should be sought in patients with neutropenia who have fever and minimal epistaxis. Scarlet-red patches of the mucosa rapidly become necrotic and white, then black. Rapid extension into the adjacent paranasal sinus, orbit, or face is usual, with or without the appearance of lung lesions.

Aspergillus sinusitis in immunocompetent patients may take three forms. A ball of hyphae may form in a chronically obstructed paranasal sinus, without tissue invasion. Much less commonly, a chronic, fibrosing granulomatous inflammation associated with *Aspergillus* hyphae within tissue may begin in the sinus and spread slowly to the orbit and the brain. *Aspergillus* is also a cause of allergic fungal sinusitis, but dark-walled fungi (e.g., *Cladosporium*, *Alternaria*) are more common in this setting. Patients usually have a history of chronic allergic rhinitis, sometimes with nasal polyps, but are otherwise healthy, presenting with painless proptosis, nasal obstruction, or dull aching pain. On CT or magnetic resonance imaging, a solid soft tissue mass pushing out the lateral wall of the ethmoid sinus or the medial wall of the maxillary sinus may be detected. On sinus exploration, the mucosa is found to be thickened and inflamed but intact. Within the sinus cavity, sticky mucopus with strands of neutrophils, eosinophils, Charcot-Leyden crystals, and occasional hyphae can be found.

Aspergillosis in HIV-infected patients most commonly involves the lung, presenting as fever, cough, and dyspnea. Typically, the CD4 cell count is below 50/μL. Roughly half of these patients have neutropenia or have recently been treated with glucocorticoids. Bilateral diffuse or focal pulmonary infiltrates with a tendency to cavitate constitute the most common radiologic manifestation. Well-localized, white, necrotic pseudomembranes full of hyphae or ulcers may develop in the trachea or the major bronchi. Progression of bronchitis to pneumonia is usual, but hematogenous dissemination is uncommon. Either allergic or invasive *Aspergillus* sinusitis can occur in HIV-infected patients; the allergic form can develop even at CD4 cell counts above 50/μL.

The growth of *Aspergillus* on cerumen and detritus within the external auditory canal is termed *otomycosis*. Trauma to the cornea may cause *Aspergillus* keratitis. Endophthalmitis follows the introduction of *Aspergillus* into the globe by trauma or surgery. *Aspergillus* may infect intracardiac or intravascular prostheses.

DIAGNOSIS The repeated isolation of *Aspergillus* from sputum or the demonstration of hyphae in sputum or bronchoalveolar lavage fluid suggests endobronchial colonization or infection. Even a single isolation of *Aspergillus* from the sputum of a neutropenic patient with pneumonia, particularly a child or a nonsmoker, suggests the diagnosis of invasive aspergillosis. In patients with advanced AIDS, fever, and cough, the isolation of *Aspergillus* from respiratory secretions raises the possibility of aspergillosis and thus should prompt bronchoscopy. Fungus ball of the lung is usually detectable by chest x-ray. IgG antibody to *Aspergillus* antigens is demonstrable in the serum of many colonized patients and of virtually all patients with fungus ball.

Biopsy is usually required for the diagnosis of invasive aspergillosis of the lung, nose, paranasal sinus, bronchi, or sites of dissemination. Blood cultures are rarely positive, even in patients with infected cardiac valves (native or prosthetic). Detection of galactomannan antigen in serum suggests the diagnosis, but false-positives are frequent, particularly in children. *Aspergillus* hyphae can be identified presumptively by histology, but culture is required for confirmation and for determination of the species. Only culture can reliably distinguish aspergillosis from pseudallescheriasis; drug therapy for these two diseases differs.

℞ TREATMENT Patients with severe hemoptysis due to fungus ball of the lung may benefit from lobectomy. Poor pulmonary function in residual lung and dense pleural adhesions around the lesion can complicate the resection. Systemic chemotherapy is of no value in endobronchial or endocavitary aspergillosis.

Treatment with intravenous amphotericin B (1.0 to 1.5 mg/kg daily) has resulted in the arrest or cure of invasive aspergillosis when immunosuppression is not severe. Liposomal amphotericin B at daily doses of 1 to 4 mg/kg has given results that seem roughly comparable to those obtained with amphotericin B deoxycholate. Itraconazole (200 mg twice daily) is useful in some less immunosuppressed patients with indolent or slowly progressive invasive aspergillosis. Surgery is the only treatment needed for fungus ball of the sinus and for allergic fungal sinusitis. Antifungal therapy has little effect on either entity if used alone, but chronic suppressive therapy has been begun postoperatively for relapse of allergic fungal sinusitis. The prognosis for cure of invasive aspergillosis in the paranasal sinus is very poor when the patient has profound and unremitting neutropenia. The prognosis is better in less immunosuppressed patients.

BIBLIOGRAPHY

DENNING DW: Invasive aspergillosis. Clin Infect Dis 26:781, 1998

LOGAN PM et al: Invasive aspergillosis of the airways: Radiographic, CT and pathologic findings. Radiology 193:383, 1994

LOTHLOLARY O et al: Invasive aspergillosis in patients with acquired immunodeficiency syndrome: Report of 33 cases. Am J Med 95:177, 1993

SHIRAKUSA T et al: Surgical treatment of pulmonary aspergilloma and *Aspergillus* empyema. Ann Thorac Surg 48:779, 1989

STEVENS DA et al: Practice guidelines for diseases caused by *Aspergillus*. Clin Infect Dis 30:696, 2000

TALBOT GH et al: Invasive *Aspergillus* rhinosinusitis in patients with acute leukemia. Rev Infect Dis 13:219, 1991

WALD A et al: Epidemiology of *Aspergillus* infections in a large cohort of patients undergoing bone marrow transplantation. J Infect Dis 175:1459, 1997

207 *John E. Bennett*

MUCORMYCOSIS

ETIOLOGIC AGENTS Species of *Rhizopus*, *Rhizomucor*, and *Cunninghamella* are the most common causes of mucormycosis, but species of *Apophysomyces*, *Saksenaea*, *Mucor*, and *Absidia* also are occasionally responsible for this infection. The organism in tissue is composed of broad, rarely septate hyphae of uneven diameter (6 to 50 μm). The organisms are inexplicably difficult to grow from infected tissue. When growth does take place, it is rapid and profuse on most media at room temperature. Identification is based on the gross and microscopic appearance of the mold.

Zygomycosis is a term that includes mucormycosis and entomophthoramycosis. The latter is a tropical infection of the subcuta-

neous tissue or paranasal sinuses caused by species of *Basidiobolus* and *Conidiobolus*, respectively.

EPIDEMIOLOGY AND PATHOLOGY *Rhizopus* and *Rhizomucor* species are ubiquitous, appearing on decaying vegetation, dung, and foods of high sugar content. Mucormycosis is uncommon and is largely confined to patients with serious preexisting diseases. Mucormycosis originating in the paranasal sinuses and nose predominantly affects patients with poorly controlled diabetes mellitus. Patients who have undergone organ transplantation, who have a hematologic malignancy, or who are receiving long-term deferoxamine therapy are predisposed to mucormycosis of either sinus or lung. Gastrointestinal mucormycosis occurs in a variety of conditions, including uremia, severe malnutrition, and diarrheal diseases. The infection is acquired from nature, with no person-to-person spread. In all forms of mucormycosis, vascular invasion by hyphae is a prominent feature. Ischemic or hemorrhagic necrosis is the foremost histologic finding.

CLINICAL MANIFESTATIONS Mucormycosis originating in the nose and paranasal sinuses produces a characteristic clinical picture. Low-grade fever, dull sinus pain, and sometimes nasal congestion or a thin, bloody nasal discharge are followed in a few days by double vision, increasing fever, and obtundation. Examination reveals a unilateral generalized reduction of ocular motion, chemosis, and proptosis. The nasal turbinates on the involved side may be dusky red or necrotic. A sharply delineated area of necrosis, strictly respecting the midline, may appear in the hard palate. The skin of the cheek may become inflamed. Fungal invasion of the globe or ophthalmic artery leads to blindness. Opacification of one or more sinuses is detected by computed tomography (CT) or by magnetic resonance imaging (MRI). Carotid arteriography may show invasion or obstruction of the carotid siphon. Coma is due to direct invasion of the frontal lobe. Early symptoms mimic those of bacterial sinusitis. Clouding of the sensorium may be attributed to diabetic acidosis. Cavernous sinus thrombosis may be considered when orbital invasion occurs. Without treatment, the patient may die after an interval ranging from a few days to a few weeks.

Pulmonary mucormycosis manifests as progressive severe pneumonia accompanied by high fever and toxicity. The necrotic center of large infiltrates may cavitate. Hematogenous spread to other areas of the lung, as well as to the brain and other organs, is common. Survival beyond 2 weeks is unusual. Gastrointestinal invasion presents as one or more ulcers that tend to perforate. Hematogenous dissemination can originate from the gastrointestinal tract, lung, or paranasal sinuses. Sometimes no portal of entry can be found.

DIAGNOSIS CT or MRI is very helpful in assessing the extent of sinusitis before surgery and in evaluating the patient afterward. CT is better for detecting bony erosion; MRI better visualizes extension into the frontal lobe or carotid artery in the siphon. Lesions of the lung and craniofacial structures are best diagnosed by biopsy and histologic section. Cultural confirmation should be attempted. Wet smear of crushed tissue can provide a rapid diagnosis. Cultures of blood and cerebrospinal fluid are negative. Smear and culture of sputum may be positive during cavitation of a lung lesion.

℞ TREATMENT Regulation of diabetes mellitus and a decrease in the dose of immunosuppressive drugs facilitate the treatment of mucormycosis. Extensive debridement of craniofacial lesions appears to be very important. Orbital exenteration may be required. Intravenous amphotericin B is clearly of value in craniofacial mucormycosis and should be employed in the other forms of mucormycosis as well. The maximal tolerated doses are given until progression is halted. With the deoxycholate formulation, 1 to 1.5 mg/kg daily is indicated. Therapy is continued for a total of 10 to 12 weeks. Azoles are of no value. Appropriate management results in cure of about half of craniofacial infections. The survival of patients with pulmonary, gastrointestinal, or disseminated mucormycosis is rare.

BIBLIOGRAPHY

GALETTA SL et al: Rhinocerebral mucormycosis: Management and survival after carotid occlusion. Ann Neurol 28:103, 1990

HOLLAND J: Emerging zygomycoses of humans: *Saksenaea vasiformis* and *Apophysomyces elegans*. Curr Top Med Mycol 8:27, 1997

MCADAMS HP et al: Pulmonary mucormycosis: Radiologic findings in 32 cases. Am J Radiol 168:1541, 1997

PETERSON KL et al: Rhinocerebral mucormycosis: Evolution of the disease and treatment options. Laryngoscope 107:855, 1997

SINGH N et al: Invasive gastrointestinal zygomycosis in a liver transplant recipient: Case report and review of zygomycosis in solid-organ transplant recipients. Clin Infect Dis 20:617, 1995

TEDDER M et al: Pulmonary mucormycosis: Results of medical and surgical therapy. Ann Thorac Surg 57:1044, 1994

208   *John E. Bennett*

MISCELLANEOUS MYCOSES AND ALGAL INFECTIONS

CHROMOBLASTOMYCOSIS This chronic subcutaneous mycosis, rarely seen in the United States, presents as a verrucoid, ulcerated, or crusted skin lesion. The disease follows the introduction of any of several fungi into subcutaneous tissue by thorns or bits of vegetation. The infection spreads over ensuing months and years to contiguous tissue, causing few symptoms. The appearance of thick-walled, dark-colored, rounded forms ("copper pennies") in histopathologic section is diagnostic. Surgical excision is the treatment of choice. Itraconazole has ameliorated some relatively small and incompletely excised lesions.

DERMATOPHYTOSIS **Definition** Dermatophytosis, also known as ringworm or tinea, is a chronic fungal infection of the skin, hair, or nails.

Etiology Species of *Trichophyton*, *Microsporum*, and *Epidermophyton* are called *dermatophytes*. These organisms grow in and remain confined to the keratinous structures of the body. Other mycoses, such as candidiasis, pityriasis versicolor, and tinea nigra, sometimes include fungal invasion of keratinous structures but traditionally are not called dermatophytoses.

Pathology and Pathogenesis Dermatophyte species are referred to as *anthropophilic*, *zoophilic*, or *geophilic*, depending on whether their usual reservoir in nature appears to be humans, animals, or soil, respectively. The infectivity of organisms from all these sources is low, and outbreaks are largely confined to occasional clusters of cases of scalp infection in children. Acquisition of a dermatophytosis appears to be favored by minor trauma, maceration, and poor hygiene of the skin. Infection does not seem to confer solid immunity: Repeated infection with the same species is common, particularly with anthropophilic species. The infrequency of scalp infection among adults has been attributed to local factors rather than immunity.

Invasion of the stratum corneum by dermatophytes may cause inflammation that is either mild or (particularly with zoophilic fungi) intense. Shedding of the stratum corneum is increased by inflammation. To the extent that fungal growth cannot keep up with shedding, inflammation may help terminate infection. Conversely, infection is probably favored when shedding is reduced by treatment with glucocorticoids and cytotoxic drugs. Antifungal drugs interfere with the ability of fungal growth to keep up with shedding.

Clinical Manifestations The disease varies with the site of infection and the fungal species involved. Foot infection (athlete's foot, tinea pedis) may present as fissuring of the toe webs, scaling of the plantar surfaces, or vesicles around the toe webs and soles. Interdigital lesions may be pruritic or, when bacterial superinfection occurs, may be painful. Hand infection is less common but resembles foot infection.

Scalp dermatophytosis (tinea capitis) is characterized by areas of alopecia and scaling. In so-called endothrix infection, the hair shaft breaks off at the skin surface, leaving the hairs visible as black dots in the scalp. Some forms of scalp infection include an area of intense boggy suppuration called a *kerion*.

Dermatophytosis of the glabrous skin (tinea corporis, **Plate IID-51**) presents as circumscribed lesions with a wide variety of appearances, including scales, vesicles, and pustules. Inflammation may be minimal or intense. Central healing of less inflamed lesions may take place. The serpiginous border of inflammation is the source of the name *ringworm*.

Dermatophytosis of the bearded area (tinea barbae) appears as a pustular folliculitis. Onychomycosis (tinea unguium) presents as a white discoloration of the nails or as thickening, chalkiness, and crumbling of the nails. Peeling and fissuring of paronychial nail folds or keratotic debris under the nail edge also may be evident.

Diagnosis Discolored hairs, scales, and keratotic debris under infected nails should be collected for KOH smear and culture. In the scraping of skin lesions, a drop of water on the skin site may keep the removed scales from flying off and thus may aid in their collection. Culture is important in distinguishing dermatophytes from *Candida* and fungal saprophytes growing in keratinaceous debris.

℞ **TREATMENT** Noninflammatory lesions of the trunk, groin, hands, and feet usually respond to twice-daily applications of clotrimazole, miconazole, ketoconazole, econazole, naftifine, terbinafine, or ciclopirox olamine cream. Hyperkeratotic lesions of the palms and soles respond slowly to these agents and may benefit from Whitfield's ointment initially to thin the keratin. Ointment should not be used between the toes, in the groin, or in the gluteal crease because maceration promotes bacterial infection.

Ringworm that is moderately severe, that is unresponsive to topical therapy, or that involves the scalp, nails, or bearded area should be treated systemically. Once-daily therapy with itraconazole (200 mg), terbinafine (250 mg), microcrystalline griseofulvin (500 mg), or ultramicrocrystalline griseofulvin (375 mg) is effective. Treatment must be continued until all infected keratin is gone. Cutting off infected hair and cleansing interdigital webs can expedite cure. Secondary bacterial infection of the foot may require soaks or antibacterial agents. The likelihood of relapse of dermatophyte foot infections may be decreased by keeping the feet clean and dry. For nail infections, itraconazole or terbinafine is preferred. In distal subungual onychomycosis, a single course of either drug results in initial improvement in half of patients, of whom half relapse. Results are better with fingernails than with toenails and for more distal rather than lateral nail involvement. To save money, itraconazole can be given as a double dose (400 mg) for 1 week each month with only marginal loss of efficacy. The duration of therapy is 2 to 3 months for fingernails and 4 to 6 months for toenails.

PROTOTHECOSIS *Prototheca* species are ubiquitous achlorophyllic algae that enter the skin through contaminated wounds and cause localized infections in the olecranon bursa, skin, subcutaneous tissue, tendon sheaths, or deeper tissue. Diagnosis is based on culture or histopathologic demonstration of sporangia with endospores in tissue. Surgical debridement and treatment with intravenous amphotericin B are useful.

FUSARIOSIS *Fusarium* species can cause localized or hematogenously disseminated infection. Localized infection results from contaminated wounds. Almost all patients with hematogenously disseminated infection are severely immunosuppressed and profoundly neutropenic. Skin lesions occur in two-thirds of patients. Several painful red indurated lesions appear on the extremities or sometimes the trunk. These lesions often develop an ecchymotic center that ulcerates. A portal of infection is not usually apparent. Blood cultures have been positive in 59% of cases. Amphotericin B is probably the drug of choice for the treatment of fusariosis, but recovery depends on the diminution of neutropenia.

MALASSEZIA INFECTION (PITYRIASIS) *Malassezia furfur* is part of the normal flora of the human skin but can cause tinea (pityriasis) versicolor or catheter-acquired sepsis. Tinea versicolor appears as asymptomatic, well-delineated, hyperpigmented or hypopigmented macules centered on the upper trunk and upper arms. Confluent lesions may cover large areas, making the border difficult to find. A fine "branny" scale or folliculitis is sometimes visible. When examined microscopically by KOH mount, skin sections are seen to contain characteristic round and elongated cells. On inspection with Wood's light, lesions either do not fluoresce or appear yellow-green. *Erythrasma* resembles tinea versicolor but is characterized by gram-positive bacilli on smear and coral-red fluorescence. Azole creams are effective for the treatment of small areas of tinea versicolor; however, the application of selenium sulfide shampoo (Selsun) for 10 min daily, followed by showering to remove the shampoo, is more practical for large areas. Itraconazole is also effective. Catheter-acquired sepsis due to *M. furfur* develops in patients (particularly neonates) receiving intravenous lipid. The organism requires special culture conditions for growth, and the infection is cured by catheter removal.

MYCETOMA Etiology *Actinomycetoma* refers to infection by actinomycetes of the genera *Nocardia*, *Nocardiopsis*, *Streptomyces*, and *Actinomadura*. *Eumycetoma* is caused by true fungi of many different genera. The predominant agent varies with the locality.

Pathogenesis and Pathology The pathogens live in the soil and enter the skin through minor trauma. The most common site of infection is the foot. The infection runs a relentless course over many years, with destruction of contiguous bone and fascia. Grains are found in purulent foci surrounded by fibrosis and a mononuclear cell inflammatory response.

Clinical Manifestations Mycetoma is a chronic suppurative infection originating in subcutaneous tissue and characterized by the presence of grains, which are tightly clumped colonies of the causative agent. The infected site is characterized by painless swelling, woody induration, and sinus tracts that discharge pus intermittently. Systemic symptoms do not develop, and spread to distant sites in the body does not take place.

Diagnosis Although the clinical picture is characteristic, mycetoma is sometimes confused with chronic osteomyelitis or botryomycosis. The diagnosis requires demonstration of grains in pus from the draining sinus or in biopsy sections. Many histologic sections may need to be examined to locate a grain.

R_x **TREATMENT** Actinomycetoma may respond to prolonged combination chemotherapy—e.g., with streptomycin and either dapsone or trimethoprim-sulfamethoxazole. Eumycetoma rarely responds to chemotherapy; some cases caused by *Madurella mycetomatis* have appeared to respond to ketoconazole or itraconazole.

PARACOCCIDIOIDOMYCOSIS Etiology Formerly called *South American blastomycosis*, this mycosis is caused by *Paracoccidioides brasiliensis*. A dimorphic fungus, *P. brasiliensis* grows as a budding yeast in tissue but may be grown as either a yeast or a mold on culture medium. The organism is identified by its gross and microscopic appearance.

Pathogenesis and Pathology Infection is thought to be acquired by inhalation of spores from environmental sources, possibly soil. Pulmonary infection produces few symptoms initially. Hematogenous spread to the mucous membranes of the mouth and nose, the lymph nodes, and other sites causes patients to seek medical attention. In fatal cases, the infection spreads to the adrenals, the gastrointestinal tract, and many other viscera.

Clinical Manifestations Common signs include indurated ulcers of the mouth, oropharynx, larynx, and nose; enlarged and draining lymph nodes; lesions of the skin and genitalia; and productive cough, weight loss, dyspnea, and sometimes fever. Paracoccidioidomycosis is acquired only in South America, Central America, and Mexico, but its extreme indolence may delay its recognition until many years after the patient has left the endemic area. Chest radiography most often shows bilateral patchy pneumonia.

Diagnosis Cultures of sputum, pus, and mucosal lesions are often diagnostic. The diagnosis can be made by smear or histologic section, although confirmation by culture is preferable. Serologic tests are useful in suggesting the diagnosis and monitoring the response to therapy.

R_x **TREATMENT** Relatively mild cases of paracoccidioidomycosis may be cured by 1 year of treatment with oral ketoconazole or itraconazole (200 to 400 mg daily). More advanced cases are treated with intravenous amphotericin B followed by itraconazole.

PHAEOHYPHOMYCOSIS This is the name given to infections caused by fungi with dark-walled hyphae, excluding those given conventional names like chromoblastomycosis. Although an extraordinary variety of fungi and clinical syndromes are encompassed by this definition, most patients have brain abscess, subcutaneous abscess, or allergic fungal sinusitis. Most of the brain abscesses are due to *Cladophialophora bantiana*, *Ochroconis gallopavum*, *Exophiala dermatitidis*, *Bipolaris* species, and *Ramichloridium mackenziei*. Patients are previously healthy. Subcutaneous abscesses are usually single, arise at the site of minor trauma, and occur in both immunosuppressed and immunocompetent individuals. A large number of dematiaceous (dark-walled) mold species cause subcutaneous phaeohyphomycosis as well as allergic fungal sinusitis. The latter entity develops in patients with allergic rhinitis and presents as an expanding mucoid mass in one or more paranasal sinuses. The tenacious mucus contains eosinophils, Charcot-Leyden crystals, and occasional hyphae. Surgical excision of phaeohyphomycotic lesions is important. Antifungal therapy may retard recurrences but is of little value unless surgical excision has been performed.

PSEUDALLESCHERIASIS Etiology Also called *Petriellidium boydii*, *Pseudallescheria boydii* is a mold frequently found in soil. When the fungus is isolated in the imperfect state, it is called *Scedosporium apiospermum*.

Pathogenesis and Pathology Wind-borne spores of *P. boydii*, arising from the soil, are the presumed source of infection. The fungus grows as a mold within tissue, causing necrosis and abscess formation.

Clinical Manifestations *P. boydii* resembles *Aspergillus* in its ability to colonize the endobronchial tree, to form fungus balls in the lungs or paranasal sinuses, and to invade the cornea or globe of the eye, the soft tissues, the joints, or the bones after trauma or surgery and in its propensity to invade the lungs and paranasal sinuses of immunosuppressed hosts, including patients with AIDS. Hyphae of *P. boydii* in tissue may be difficult to distinguish from those of *Aspergillus*. Infection with *P. boydii* is much less common than that with *Aspergillus*. Intravascular hyphae, a hallmark of invasive aspergillosis, are also found in pseudallescheriasis. Near-drowning in polluted water has led to severe *P. boydii* pneumonia, often with dissemination and fatal brain abscesses.

Diagnosis Demonstration of hyphae in tissue and culture confirmation are required for diagnosis.

R_x **TREATMENT** Itraconazole at the maximal tolerated doses is the regimen of choice. Surgical drainage or debridement can be helpful. The prognosis is poor.

Scedosporium prolificans, a fungus closely related to *P. boydii*, has caused infections in bones, joints, or soft tissue, usually after trauma. These infections have responded to surgical debridement. Disseminated infection with *S. prolificans* in immunosuppressed patients has been fatal. The response to treatment with all antifungal agents has been poor.

SPOROTRICHOSIS Etiology *Sporothrix schenckii* lives as a saprophyte on plants in many areas of the world. In nature and on culture at room temperature, the fungus grows as a mold; within host tissue or at 37°C on enriched media, it grows as a budding yeast. It is identified by its appearance in mold and yeast forms.

Pathogenesis and Pathology   Infection results from the inoculation of *S. schenckii* into subcutaneous tissue through minor trauma. Nursery workers, florists, and gardeners acquire the illness from roses, sphagnum moss, and other plants. Infection may be limited to the site of inoculation (plaque sporotrichosis) or extend along proximal lymphatic channels (lymphangitic sporotrichosis). Spread beyond an extremity—the usual site of infection—is rare, and hematogenous dissemination from the skin remains unproven. The portal for osteoarticular, pulmonary, and other extracutaneous forms of sporotrichosis is unknown but is likely the lung.

Untreated sporotrichosis persists for months. The inflammatory response includes both the clustering of neutrophils and a marked granulomatous response with epithelioid cells and giant cells.

Clinical Manifestations   In lymphangitic sporotrichosis, which is by far the most common manifestation, a nearly painless red papule forms at the site of inoculation. Over the next several weeks, similar nodules form along proximal lymphatic channels. The nodules intermittently discharge small amounts of pus. Ulceration may occur. The proximal extension of these lesions, often with skip areas, is quite distinctive but may be mimicked by lesions of *Nocardia brasiliensis*, *Mycobacterium marinum*, or (in rare cases) *Leishmania brasiliensis* or *Mycobacterium kansasii*.

Plaque sporotrichosis manifests as a nontender red maculopapular granuloma confined to the site of inoculation. Osteoarticular sporotrichosis presents as mono- or polyarticular arthritis of indolent onset and progression over months or years, involving the elbows, knees, wrists, ankles, and (rarely) smaller joints of the extremities. Periarticular bone develops areas of demineralization detectable on x-ray, and draining sinuses may appear over joints and bursae. Hematogenous spread to the skin may take place during polyarticular disease, but none of the skin lesions shows lymphangitic spread. Immunosuppression, including that due to advanced infection with HIV, predisposes to hematogenous spread. Pulmonary sporotrichosis usually presents as a single chronic cavitary upper-lobe lung lesion. Chronic meningitis can develop in the absence of skin or lung lesions. *S. schenckii* is difficult to recover from cerebrospinal fluid.

Diagnosis   Culture of pus, joint fluid, sputum, or a skin biopsy specimen is the preferred method of diagnosis. The appearance of *S. schenckii* in tissue is quite variable. In skin lesions, the organisms are hard to find.

℞ **TREATMENT**   Cutaneous sporotrichosis can be cured with a saturated solution of potassium iodide given orally in increasing divided doses of up to 4.5 to 9 mL/d for adults, as tolerated. Gastrointestinal disturbance or acneiform rash over the cape area and face is common, but therapy should be continued for 1 month after the resolution of all lesions. Itraconazole (100 to 200 mg daily) is an effective and better-tolerated alternative. Extracutaneous sporotrichosis rarely responds to iodides, but more than half of cases have been cured by prolonged courses of intravenous amphotericin B. Itraconazole (200 mg once or twice daily) is effective in some cases of extracutaneous sporotrichosis.

TRICHOSPORONOSIS   A recent change in taxonomy of the genus *Trichosporon* has moved most of the agents causing deep infections from *T. beigelii* into the species *T. asahii*, with a few categorized as *T. mucoides*. White piedra of the scalp is caused by *T. ovoides* and that of the pubic hair by *T. inkin*. *T cutaneum* and *T. asteroides* cause superficial infections. Most of what is currently known about *Trichosporon* infections is not species specific, so the following description refers to *T. beigelii*. *T. capitatum*, which causes disseminated infection in patients with neutropenia, was previously reclassified as *Blastoschizomyces capitatus* and will not be covered here.

T. beigelii can colonize the human gastrointestinal tract and skin and can enter the bloodstream of patients with severe neutropenia through an inapparent source. Hematogenously disseminated infection is manifested by fever and often by the development of several erythematous or purpuric tender papules anywhere on the body. Lesions can form large, tense hemorrhagic bullae. In some patients, native or prosthetic cardiac valves become infected. In tissue, hyphae and yeastlike cells are seen. Amphotericin B is probably the drug of choice for treatment, but recovery is dependent on the return of bone marrow function.

BIBLIOGRAPHY

BARBER GR et al: Catheter-related *Malassezia furfur* fungemia in immunocompromised patients. Am J Med 95:365, 1993

BOUTATI EI, ANAISSIE EJ: *Fusarium*, a significant emerging pathogen in patients with hematologic malignancy: Ten years' experience at a cancer center and implications for management. Blood 90:999, 1997

CAREY WP et al: Cutaneous protothecosis in a patient with AIDS and severe functional defect: Successful therapy with amphotericin B. Clin Infect Dis 25:1265, 1997

DUONG TA: Infection due to *Penicillium marneffei*, an emerging pathogen: Review of 155 reported cases. Clin Infect Dis 23:125, 1996

ENGLAND DM, HOCHHOLZER L: Adiaspiromycosis: An unusual fungal infection of the lung. Am J Surg Pathol 17:876, 1993

HAY RJ et al: Mycetoma. J Med Vet Mycol 30(Suppl 1):41, 1992

KAUFFMAN CA et al: Practice guidelines for the management of patients with sporotrichosis. Clin Infect Dis 30:684, 2000

MARCON MJ, POWELL DA: Human infections due to *Malassezia* spp. Clin Microbiol Rev 5:101, 1992

MEYER RD et al: Fungal sinusitis in patients with AIDS: Report of 4 cases and review of the literature. Medicine 73:69, 1994

NARANJO MS et al: Treatment of paracoccidioidomycosis with itraconazole. J Med Vet Mycol 28:67, 1990

REIDY JJ et al: Infection of the conjunctiva by *Rhinosporidium seeberi*. Surv Ophthalmol 41:409, 1997

RESTREPO A: Treatment of tropical mycoses. J Am Acad Dermatol 31:S91, 1994

RINALDI MG: Phaeohyphomycosis. Dermatol Clin 14:147, 1996

RUXIN TA et al: *Pseudallescheria boydii* in an immunocompromised host: Successful treatment with debridement and itraconazole. Arch Dermatol 132:382, 1996

SUGITA T et al: Taxonomic position of deep-seated, mucosa associated, and superficial isolates of *Trichosporon cutaneum* from trichosporonosis patients. J Clin Microbiol 33:1368, 1995

SUPPARATPINYO K et al: A controlled trial of itraconazole to prevent relapse of *Penicillium marneffei* infection in patients infected with the human immunodeficiency virus. N Engl J Med 339:1739, 1998

SUTTON DA et al: U.S. case report of cerebral phaeohyphomycosis caused by *Ramichloridium obovoideum* (*R. mackenziei*): Criteria for identification, therapy, and review of other known dematiaceous neurotropic taxa. J Clin Microbiol 36:708, 1998

VARTIVARIAN SE et al: Emerging fungal pathogens in immunocompromised patients: Classification, diagnosis, and management. Clin Infect Dis 17(Suppl 2):487, 1993

WINN RE et al: Systemic sporotrichosis treated with itraconazole. Clin Infect Dis 17:210, 1993

209   *Peter D. Walzer*

PNEUMOCYSTIS CARINII INFECTION

DEFINITION AND DESCRIPTION   *Pneumocystis carinii* is an opportunistic pathogen whose natural habitat is the lung. The organism is an important cause of pneumonia in the compromised host.

Although the taxonomic status of *P. carinii* has long been controversial, molecular studies during the past decade have clearly placed the organism among the fungi. This classification is based on analysis of gene sequences for ribosomal RNA, mitochondrial proteins, and major enzymes. The cell wall of *P. carinii* contains β-1,3-glucan; drugs that inhibit β-glucan synthesis in fungi are highly active against *P. carinii* in animal models. However, in contrast to most fungi, *P. carinii* lacks ergosterol and is not susceptible to antifungal drugs that inhibit ergosterol synthesis.

Study of the basic biology of *P. carinii* has been severely hampered by the lack of a reliable in vitro cultivation system. Major developmental stages of the organism include the small (1- to 4-μm) pleomorphic trophozoite or trophic form; the 5- to 8-μm cyst, which has a thick cell wall and contains up to eight intracystic bodies; and the precyst, an intermediate stage. The life cycle of *P. carinii* probably involves asexual replication by the trophic form and sexual reproduction by the cyst, which ends in release of the intracystic bodies; an intracellular stage has not been identified. Ultrastructurally, *P. carinii* has a primitive organelle system, but little is known about its metabolism.

P. carinii contains two prominent antigen groups. The 95- to 140-kDa major surface glycoprotein (MSG) complex represents a family of proteins encoded by multiple genes. The MSG complex is highly immunogenic, contains shared and species-specific antigenic determinants, and exhibits protective B and T cell epitopes in animal models. The MSG complex plays a pivotal role in the host-parasite relationship in *P. carinii* infection. It facilitates adherence to host proteins via extracellular matrix proteins, surfactant proteins, and the mannose receptor; and its ability to undergo antigenic variation may represent a mechanism by which *P. carinii* evades the host immune response. The other antigen, which migrates as a band of 35 to 55 kDa, is the most common antigen recognized by the host and thus may serve as a marker of infection.

EPIDEMIOLOGY *P. carinii* has a worldwide distribution among humans and has been detected in a variety of animals. The organisms found in these hosts are morphologically identical, but recent studies have revealed a high degree of genetic diversity and host specificity. Serologic surveys indicate that most healthy children have been exposed to the organism by 3 to 4 years of age. Animal model experiments have demonstrated that *P. carinii* is transmitted by the airborne route. Person-to-person transmission has been suggested by the occurrence of outbreaks of pneumocystosis among institutionalized debilitated infants and in hospitals caring for immunosuppressed patients. On the basis of animal studies, the incubation period is thought to be 4 to 8 weeks.

PATHOGENESIS AND PATHOLOGY The host factors that predispose to the development of pneumocystosis involve defects in cellular and humoral immunity. People at risk for the disease include patients infected with HIV; persons receiving immunosuppressive therapy (particularly glucocorticoids) for cancer, organ transplantation, and other disorders; children with primary immunodeficiency diseases; and premature malnourished infants. The central role of CD4+ cells in host resistance to *P. carinii* has been shown by research in experimental animals and by studies that have correlated the risk of pneumocystosis in HIV-infected patients with CD4+ cell counts. Evidence supporting the importance of impaired humoral immunity consists of the occurrence of pneumocytosis in patients and animals with B cell defects and the beneficial effect of passively administered antibodies.

The principal host effector cells against *P. carinii* are alveolar macrophages, which ingest and kill the organism, releasing a variety of inflammatory mediators. Tumor necrosis factor α and interleukin (IL) 1 are important in the early host defenses against *P. carinii*, but the role of other cytokines is less clear. Recent evidence suggests that HIV alters the mannose receptor–mediated binding and phagocytosis of *P. carinii*.

After being inhaled, *P. carinii* takes up residence in the alveoli, where it attaches tightly to type I cells but maintains an extracellular existence. In some cases, the organism remains in the host for long periods, and pneumonia develops by reactivation of latent infection; in other cases, pneumonia arises from a new bout of infection. As the immune system of the host becomes compromised, *P. carinii* organisms propagate and gradually fill the alveoli. This scenario is accompanied by a complex series of events that result in increased alveolar-capillary permeability and damage to type I cells. Surfactant abnormalities include a fall in bronchoalveolar lavage (BAL) fluid phospholipids and an increase in surfactant proteins A and D. Contri-

butions of the host inflammatory response to lung injury are suggested by the correlation of increased IL-8 levels and neutrophil counts in BAL fluid from patients with relatively severe disease.

On lung sections stained with hematoxylin and eosin, the alveoli are filled with a typical foamy, vacuolated exudate. Severe disease may include interstitial edema, fibrosis, and hyaline membrane formation. The host inflammatory changes usually consist of hypertrophy of alveolar type II cells, a typical reparative response, and a mild mononuclear cell interstitial infiltrate. Malnourished infants display an intense plasma cell infiltrate that gave the disease its early name: interstitial plasma cell pneumonia.

CLINICAL FEATURES Patients with *P. carinii* pneumonia develop dyspnea, fever, and nonproductive cough. Symptoms in non-HIV-infected patients often begin after the glucocorticoid dose has been tapered and typically last 1 to 2 weeks. HIV-infected patients are usually ill for several weeks or longer and have relatively subtle manifestations. However, the clinical picture in individual patients is quite variable, and a high index of suspicion and elicitation of a careful history are key factors in early detection.

Physical findings include tachypnea, tachycardia, and cyanosis, but lung auscultation reveals few abnormalities. The white blood cell count is variable and is usually governed by the patient's underlying disease. Assessment of arterial blood gases demonstrates hypoxia, an increased alveolar-arterial oxygen gradient ($PA_{O_2} - Pa_{O_2}$), and respiratory alkalosis. There also may be changes in pulmonary function test values (diffusing capacity) and increased uptake with nuclear imaging techniques (gallium scan). Elevated serum concentrations of lactate dehydrogenase (LDH) have been reported; they probably reflect lung parenchymal damage but are not specific to *P. carinii* infection. In general, laboratory abnormalities are less severe in HIV-infected patients than in non-HIV-infected patients.

The classic findings on chest radiography consist of bilateral diffuse infiltrates beginning in the perihilar regions (Fig. 209-1), but various atypical manifestations (nodular densities, cavitary lesions) have also been reported. Patients who receive aerosolized pentamidine have an increased frequency of upper-lobe infiltrates and pneumothorax. Early in the course of pneumocystosis, the chest radiograph may be normal.

Although *P. carinii* usually remains confined to the lungs, cases of disseminated infection have occurred in both HIV-infected and non-HIV-infected patients. One risk factor for extrapulmonary spread in patients with HIV is the administration of aerosolized pentamidine. The most common sites of extrapulmonary involvement are the lymph

FIGURE 209-1 Chest radiograph depicting diffuse infiltrates in an HIV-infected patient with pneumocystosis.

nodes, spleen, liver, and bone marrow. Clinical manifestations range from incidental findings at autopsy to specific organ involvement. Histopathologic examination reveals the presence of *P. carinii* and the characteristic associated foamy material. Treatment for the extrapulmonary forms of pneumocystosis is the same as that for pneumonia.

DIAGNOSIS   Because the clinical picture of *P. carinii* infection can be produced by many other infectious and noninfectious agents, the diagnosis must be based on specific identification of the organism. A definitive diagnosis is made by histopathologic staining. Traditional stains have included reagents such as methenamine silver, toluidine blue, and cresyl echt violet, which selectively stain the wall of *P. carinii* cysts, and reagents such as Wright-Giemsa, which stain the nuclei of all developmental stages. Other reagents include nonspecific fluorochrome stains (calcofluor white) and Papanicolaou's stain. Immunofluorescence with monoclonal antibodies is more sensitive than histologic staining but is also more expensive. DNA amplification by the polymerase chain reaction offers the greatest sensitivity and may find a place in the routine diagnosis of *P. carinii* when commercial kits become available.

The successful diagnosis of pneumocystosis depends upon the collection of proper specimens. In general, the yield from different diagnostic procedures is higher in HIV-infected patients than in non-HIV-infected patients because of the higher organism burden in the former group. Sputum induction has gained popularity as a simple, noninvasive technique; this procedure requires trained and dedicated personnel, and its success has varied at different institutions. Fiberoptic bronchoscopy with BAL, which is more sensitive than sputum induction, remains the mainstay of *P. carinii* diagnosis. This procedure also provides information about the organism burden, the host inflammatory response, and the presence of other opportunistic infections. Transbronchial biopsy and open lung biopsy, which are the most invasive procedures, are reserved for situations in which a diagnosis cannot be made by BAL.

COURSE AND PROGNOSIS   In the typical case of untreated *P. carinii* pneumonia, progressive respiratory embarrassment leads to death. Therapy is most effective when instituted early in the course of the disease, before there is extensive alveolar damage. If induced sputum is nondiagnostic and BAL cannot be performed in a timely manner, it is reasonable to begin empiric therapy with drugs active against *P. carinii*. However, this practice does not obviate the need for a specific etiologic diagnosis. With improvements in management, the case-fatality rate has been lowered to about 15% in HIV-infected patients but remains high (40%) in non-HIV-infected patients. The most widely used prognostic indicators have been the arterial oxygen pressure and the alveolar-arterial oxygen gradient. Other factors that may influence survival include neutrophil counts and IL-8 levels in BAL fluid, chest radiographic abnormalities, serum LDH and albumin levels, and the expertise of the hospital in caring for patients with HIV infection. Concurrent pulmonary infections complicate management, but the presence of cytomegalovirus usually does not affect the outcome of pneumocystosis.

℞ **TREATMENT**   Trimethoprim-sulfamethoxazole (TMP-SMZ), which acts by inhibiting folic acid synthesis, is considered the drug of choice for all forms of pneumocystosis. The daily dosage, administered orally or intravenously in three or four divided doses, is 15 to 20 mg TMP/kg and 75 to 100 mg SMZ/kg. Therapy is continued for 14 days in non-HIV-infected patients and for 21 days in persons infected with HIV. Since HIV-infected patients respond more slowly than non-HIV-infected patients, it is prudent to wait at least 7 days after the initiation of treatment before concluding that therapy has failed. The addition of drugs to an existing regimen is no more effective than switching regimens and may increase the risk of toxicity. TMP-SMZ is well tolerated by non-HIV-infected patients, but more than half of HIV-infected patients experience serious adverse reactions, including fever, rash, neutropenia, thrombocytopenia, hepatitis, and hyperkalemia.

Several alternative regimens are available for the treatment of mild to moderate cases of *P. carinii* pneumonia: TMP (15 mg/kg per day orally) plus dapsone (100 mg/d orally), clindamycin (600 mg every 6 h intravenously or 300 to 450 mg every 6 h orally) plus primaquine (15 to 30 mg of base per day orally), or atovaquone alone (750 mg twice daily orally). Dapsone and primaquine should be used with caution in patients with glucose-6-phosphate dehydrogenase deficiency.

Two alternative drugs are available for the treatment of moderate to severe forms of pneumocystosis. Pentamidine, which has been used against *P. carinii* for many years, is administered as a single daily dose of 4 mg/kg by slow intravenous infusion. Pentamidine is highly toxic; its major side effects are hypotension, cardiac arrhythmias, dysglycemias, azotemia, electrolyte changes, and neutropenia. Trimetrexate is administered intravenously as a single daily dose of 45 mg/m^2; in conjunction with trimetrexate therapy, folinic acid is given orally or intravenously at a dose of 20 mg/m^2 every 6 h to prevent bone marrow suppression.

Patients with HIV frequently experience deterioration in respiratory function shortly after receiving anti–*P. carinii* drugs. Several studies have shown that the administration of glucocorticoids to patients with HIV and moderate to severe pneumocystosis (a P_{O_2} of ≤ 70 mmHg or a $PA_{O_2} - Pa_{O_2}$ of ≥ 35 mmHg) can prevent this problem and improve the rate of survival. The administration of steroids should be started early in the course of the illness (usually when antimicrobial drugs are begun) for maximal benefit; the recommended regimen is 40 mg of prednisone orally twice daily on days 1 to 5, 40 mg/d on days 6 to 10, and 20 mg/d on days 11 to 20. This regimen has generally proven to be safe despite concern about its effects on other opportunistic infections. The use of steroids as adjunctive therapy in HIV-infected patients with mild pneumocystosis or in non-HIV-infected patients remains to be evaluated.

PREVENTION   Primary prophylaxis is indicated for HIV-infected patients at high risk of developing pneumocystosis—that is, those who have CD4+ cell counts of $<200/\mu L$, unexplained fever [$>37.8°C$ ($100°$ F)] for ≥ 2 weeks, or a history of oropharyngeal candidiasis. Guidelines for the administration of primary prophylaxis to other immunocompromised hosts are less clear. Secondary prophylaxis is indicated for all patients who have recovered from *P. carinii* pneumonia. Among HIV-infected patients, the risk of recurrent episodes of pneumocystosis is high and lifelong; among non-HIV-infected patients, the risk is lower and exists for as long as the immunosuppressive condition persists.

Several antimicrobial drugs are effective in preventing pneumocystosis, although some concern has been raised about possible resistance. One double-strength tablet of TMP-SMZ (160 mg TMP, 800 mg SMZ) per day is the prophylactic regimen of choice. The major limitation of TMP-SMZ treatment is the high frequency of adverse reactions among HIV-infected patients. Recommended alternative regimens include TMP-SMZ at a reduced dose (80 mg TMP, 400 mg SMZ) or frequency (3 times per week), dapsone alone at a daily oral dose of 100 mg, dapsone at a dose of 50 mg/d combined with weekly oral doses of pyrimethamine (50 mg) and folinic acid (25 mg), pentamidine at a monthly dose of 300 mg administered by Respigard nebulizer, and atovaquone at an oral dose of 1500 mg/d.

Although there are no specific recommendations for preventing the spread of *P. carinii* in health care facilities, it seems prudent to prevent direct contact between patients with pneumocystosis and other susceptible hosts.

BIBLIOGRAPHY

BENEFIELD TL et al: Prognostic value of interleukin-8 in AIDS-associated *Pneumocystis carinii* pneumonia. Am J Respir Crit Care Med 151:1058, 1995

HORNER RD et al: Relationship between procedures and health insurance for critically ill patients with *Pneumocystis carinii* pneumonia. Am J Respir Crit Care Med 152:1435, 1995

KAZANJIAN P et al: *Pneumocystis carinii* mutations associated with sulfa and sulfone prophylaxis failures in AIDS patients. AIDS 12:873, 1998

KOZIEL H et al: Reduced binding and phagocytosis of *Pneumocystis carinii* by alveolar macrophages from persons infected with HIV-1 correlates with mannose receptor down regulation. J Clin Invest 102:1322, 1998

LIMPER AH et al: Interactions of parasite and host epithelial cell cycle regulation during *Pneumocystis carinii* pneumonia. J Lab Clin Med 130:132, 1997

SAFRIN S et al: Comparison of three regimens for treatment of mild to moderate *Pneumocystis carinii* pneumonia in patients with AIDS. Ann Intern Med 124:792, 1996

STRINGER JR, WALZER PD: Molecular biology and epidemiology of *Pneumocystis carinii* infection in AIDS. AIDS 10:561, 1996

THEUS SA et al: Adoptive transfer of lymphocytes sensitized to the major surface glycoprotein of *Pneumocystis carinii* confers protection in the rat. J Clin Invest 95:2587, 1995

US PUBLIC HEALTH SERVICE/INFECTIOUS DISEASES SOCIETY OF AMERICA: Guidelines for the prevention of opportunistic infections in persons infected with human immunodeficiency virus: A summary. MMWR 46(RR-12):1, 1997

WALZER PD: Immunological features of *Pneumocystis carinii* infection in humans. Clin Diagn Lab Immunol 6:149, 1999

Section 16
PROTOZOAL AND HELMINTHIC INFECTIONS: GENERAL CONSIDERATIONS

210

Peter F. Weller

APPROACH TO THE PATIENT WITH PARASITIC INFECTION

Because diverse parasitic organisms may infect humans, a range of factors are germane to an assessment of the possible parasitic etiology of a patient's disease. These factors include issues related to the patient's history, immune status, and presenting clinical and laboratory characteristics, especially eosinophilia. Complementing historical information, a full clinical evaluation and laboratory testing provide additional data to direct the assessment for parasitic infection. The specific tests required, ranging from standard blood biochemical assays to imaging of selected organs, are dictated by the nature of the patient's illness. Additional diagnostic testing for parasitic infections (Chap. 211) completes the evaluation.

HISTORY   Geographic History   The history can provide valuable information about potential exposures to parasitic infections. A history of travel to, residence or work in, or immigration from areas of the world in which various parasites not endemic in the United States are encountered offers a clue to possible parasitic or other infectious etiologies of a patient's disease (Chap. 123). Some parasitic infections may become manifest early after a traveler's return home; paramount among these in terms of preventable mortality is malaria. If a patient has been in a region of the world where malaria is endemic (even only briefly, as in an airport layover), fever mandates a consideration of malaria, whether or not malaria chemoprophylaxis has been used. Falciparum malaria, which in a nonimmune patient may progress rapidly to serious and even life-threatening consequences (Chap. 214), is a potential medical emergency and must be considered at the initial evaluation, even if symptoms and fever patterns are suggestive of less specific flulike or gastrointestinal illness. Rarely, malaria transmission has been reported within the United States.

For patients with a history of recent travel, the onset of gastrointestinal symptoms only after return suggests protozoal diseases characterized by a 1- to 2-week delay between acquisition and appearance of symptoms—notably, giardiasis, cyclosporiasis, and cryptosporidiosis (Chap. 218). Gastrointestinal symptoms lasting longer than a week also suggest protozoan etiologies, including giardiasis, amebiasis, and cyclosporiasis. For patients who have traveled less recently, information on the specific countries and the types of regions (urban or rural) visited and on the nature and duration of the visit, whether for general tourism or for activities related to specific occupations, is helpful in concert with presenting clinical features and hematologic and other laboratory findings. Diseases that may become manifest only some years after an individual leaves an endemic region include schistosomiasis, some forms of filariasis, strongyloidiasis, echinococcosis, and cysticercosis.

For the illnesses of patients who have never left the United States, various parasitic etiologies should be considered, depending on the presenting disease. Trichomoniasis, trichinellosis, strongyloidiasis, giardiasis, cryptosporidiosis, cyclosporiasis, echinococcosis, and pinworm are among the parasitic infections endemic in settings within the United States. Diseases that are more frequent where there is fecal contamination of soil or other environmental sites include hookworm, ascariasis, trichuriasis, amebiasis, and strongyloidiasis; dermal exposure, as by walking barefoot on soil contaminated with parasitic larvae, predisposes residents of such an area as well as travelers to the acquisition of cutaneous larva migrans, hookworm, and strongyloidiasis.

Dietary History   If more than one patient develops similar symptoms in a given situation, common-source water- or foodborne diseases (giardiasis, cryptosporidiosis, cyclosporiasis) should be considered. Waterborne infections are more likely to be acquired from surface water supplies, ranging from mountain streams to municipal reservoirs. Likewise, attention to dietary history may be helpful. Trichinellosis should be considered when the patient may have consumed contaminated pork, bear, walrus, or other meat from carnivores. Ingestion of undercooked fish predisposes to anisakiasis and to infection with other fish-dwelling nematodes, tapeworms (*Diphyllobothrium latum*), or flukes (*Nanophyetus salmincola*). Ingestion of snails or of produce contaminated with land snails can lead to infection with *Angiostrongylus cantonensis* (eosinophilic meningitis; Chap. 219). Ingestion of more exotic animal foodstuffs, including snakes, can result in the transmission of gnathostomiasis (Chap. 219). For children with a propensity for pica, ingestion of soil containing *Toxocara* eggs may lead to visceral larva migrans. Consumption of ground-grown vegetables, including those shipped in from distant fields contaminated with human feces, provides an opportunity for the ingestion of nematode eggs of *Ascaris lumbricoides* or *Trichuris trichiura*.

Other Exposure Histories   An antecedent blood transfusion raises the possibility of malaria (especially that due to *Plasmodium malariae* or *P. falciparum*), babesiosis, or Chagas' disease. A history of wading or swimming in fresh water is germane to the acquisition of schistosomiasis or avian schistosome dermatitis. Fresh water may be a source of infection with free-living amebae, and these protozoa may cause meningoencephalitis or ocular infections. Arthropod vector–borne parasitic infections include malaria and lymphatic filariasis (carried by mosquitoes) and babesiosis (carried by ticks); the latter is transmitted in some regions of the United States.

Residence in an institutional setting where fecal-oral hygiene may be imperfect raises the possibility of giardiasis, cryptosporidiosis, or strongyloidiasis. Child-care centers provide opportunities for young children and their family members to acquire giardiasis, cryptosporidiosis, and pinworm infections. Trichomoniasis is transmitted sexually;

giardiasis, cryptosporidiosis, amebiasis, and strongyloidiasis can be transmitted during anal intercourse or oral-anal contact.

IMMUNE STATUS   The patient's immune status is relevant in determining which parasitic infections need to be considered. In patients infected with HIV-1, especially those with depressed CD4+ lymphocyte counts, specific protozoan diseases may develop opportunistically. These infections include toxoplasmosis, isosporiasis, cyclosporiasis, cryptosporidiosis, visceral leishmaniasis, American trypanosomiasis, microsporidiosis, and infections with free-living amebae (*Acanthamoeba* and related genera). In individuals infected with human T-lymphotropic virus type 1, strongyloidiasis is a prominent consideration. Patients who are asplenic are at risk not only for overwhelming infections due to encapsulated bacteria but also for fulminant infections caused by intraerythrocytic protozoa, including malaria and babesiosis. Patients with hypogammaglobulinemia or cystic fibrosis may develop refractory giardiasis. In patients developing symptoms of enterocolitis while receiving glucocorticoids, the possibility of an exacerbation of unsuspected strongyloidiasis or amebic colitis should be considered.

EOSINOPHILIA   Eosinophilia may offer a hematologic clue to the presence of some parasites. Only two protozoan parasites have been associated with eosinophilia: *Isospora belli* and, on occasion, *Dientamoeba fragilis*. The detection of eosinophilia generally mandates a consideration of the multicellular helminthic parasites that characteristically elicit interleukin 5–mediated eosinophilia. (Helminth-elicited eosinophilia, however, may be suppressed by glucocorticoid therapy or by intercurrent bacterial or viral infections.) The magnitude of eosinophilia tends to correlate with the extent of tissue invasion by helminths. Marked blood eosinophilia (more than 3000 eosinophils per microliter) develops during the early transpulmonary migration of intestinal nematodes, including *Ascaris* and hookworms, at a time when eggs (whose presence confirms the diagnosis) have not yet been produced in the intestinal tract.

Eosinophilia is also marked in the early stages of fluke infections, including schistosomiasis (Katayama fever), paragonimiasis, clonorchiasis, and fascioliasis; during the stage of muscle invasion in trichinellosis; during tissue migration of adult worms in loiasis and gnathostomiasis; and with heavy infections in visceral larva migrans. Eosinophilia persisting for more than a year may be indicative of hookworm infection, strongyloidiasis, visceral larva migrans (especially in children), filarial infection (including onchocerciasis, loiasis, and tropical pulmonary eosinophilia), fluke infections (including schistosomiasis, fascioliasis, clonorchiasis, and paragonimiasis), and cysticercosis. Leakage of fluids from echinococcal cysts can cause intermittent increases in eosinophilia.

Eosinophilia sometimes provides the only clue to the presence of helminthic infection and should prompt an evaluation for such infection. Serologic testing for schistosomiasis, filariasis, visceral larva migrans, and strongyloidiasis will be helpful in an assessment for some of the diseases most likely to elicit eosinophilia. Serologic evaluation for strongyloidiasis is especially important since autoinfection may permit persistence of the organisms for decades and put the patient at risk for disseminated disease if immunosuppressive glucocorticoids are later administered for any reason.

BIBLIOGRAPHY

GYORKOS TW et al: Intestinal parasite infection in the Kampuchean refugee population 6 years after resettlement in Canada. J Infect Dis 166:413, 1992

JONES JL et al: Surveillance for AIDS-defining opportunistic illnesses, 1992–1997. MMWR Surveill Summ 48(SS-2):1, 1999

KAPPUS KD et al: Intestinal parasitism in the United States: Update on a continuing problem. Am J Trop Med Hyg 50:705, 1994

KARP CL, NEVA FA: The human immunodeficiency virus and tropical infectious disease coinfection, in *Tropical Infectious Diseases: Principles, Pathogens and Practice,* RL Guerrant et al (eds). Philadelphia, Churchill Livingstone, 1999, pp 1586–1630

LEVY DA et al: Surveillance for waterborne-disease outbreaks—United States, 1995–1996. MMWR Surveill Summ 47(SS-5):1, 1998

LIBMAN MD et al: Screening for schistosomiasis, filariasis, and strongyloidiasis among expatriates returning from the tropics. Clin Infect Dis 17:353, 1993

SVENSON JE et al: Imported malaria. Clinical presentation and examination of symptomatic travelers. Arch Intern Med 155:861, 1995

WILSON ME, WELLER PF: Eosinophilia, in *Tropical Infectious Diseases: Principles, Pathogens and Practice,* RL Guerrant et al (eds). Philadelphia, Churchill Livingstone, 1999, pp 1400–1419

211	*Charles E. Davis*

LABORATORY DIAGNOSIS OF PARASITIC INFECTIONS

The cornerstone for the diagnosis of parasitic infections is a thorough history of the patient's illness. Epidemiologic aspects of the illness are especially important because the risks of acquiring many parasites are closely related to occupation, recreation, or travel to areas of high endemicity. Without a basic knowledge of the epidemiology and life cycles of the major parasites, it is difficult to approach the diagnosis of parasitic infections systematically. Accordingly, the medical classification of important human parasites in this chapter emphasizes their geographic distribution, their transmission, and the anatomic location and stages of their life cycle in humans. The text and tables are intended to serve as a guide to the correct diagnostic procedures for the major parasitic infections and to direct the reader to other chapters that contain more comprehensive information about each infection. Tables 211-1, 211-2, and 211-3 summarize the geographic distributions, the anatomic locations, and the laboratory methods employed for the diagnosis of flatworm, roundworm, and protozoal infections, respectively.

In addition to selecting the correct diagnostic procedures, physicians must counsel their patients to ensure that specimens are collected properly and arrive at the laboratory promptly. For example, the diagnosis of bancroftian filariasis is unlikely to be confirmed by the laboratory unless blood is drawn near midnight, when the nocturnal microfilariae are active. Laboratory personnel and surgical pathologists should be notified in advance when a parasitic infection is suspected. Continuing interaction with the laboratory staff and the surgical pathologists increases the likelihood that parasites in body fluids or biopsy specimens will be examined carefully by the most capable individuals.

INTESTINAL PARASITES   Most helminths and protozoa exit the body in the fecal stream. The patient or the patient's attendant should be instructed to collect feces in a clean cardboard container and to record the time of collection on the container. Contamination with water, which could contain free-living protozoa, or with urine should be avoided. Fecal samples should be collected before ingestion of barium or other contrast agents for radiologic procedures and before treatment with antidiarrheal agents and antacids, because these substances change the consistency of the feces and interfere with microscopic detection of parasites. Because of the cyclic shedding of most parasites in the feces, a minimum of three samples collected on alternate days should be examined. When delays in transport to the laboratory are unavoidable or specimens must be shipped by mail, fecal samples should be kept in polyvinyl alcohol to preserve protozoal trophozoites. Refrigeration will also preserve trophozoites for a few hours and protozoal cysts and helminthic ova for several days.

Analysis of fecal samples consists of both a macroscopic and a microscopic examination. Watery or loose stools are more likely to contain protozoal trophozoites, but protozoal cysts and all stages of helminths may be found in formed feces. If adult worms or tapeworm segments are observed, they should be transported promptly to the laboratory or washed and preserved in fixative for later examination. The only tapeworm with motile segments is *Taenia saginata*, the beef tapeworm, which patients sometimes bring to the physician. Motility is an important distinguishing characteristic, because the ova of *T.*

Table 211-1 Flatworm Infections

| Parasite | Geographic Distribution | Life-Cycle Hosts | | Diagnosis | | | |
		Intermediate (Transmission)	Definitive	Parasite Stage	Body Fluid or Tissue	Serologic Tests	Other
TAPEWORMS (CESTODES)							
Intestinal tapeworms							
Taenia saginata (beef tapeworm)	Worldwide	Beef	Humans	Ova, segments	Feces	—	Motile segments
Hymenolepis nana (dwarf tapeworm)	Worldwide	Grain beetles	Humans, mice[a]	Ova	Feces	—	—
Diphyllobothrium latum (fish tapeworm)	Worldwide	Copepods–fish[c]	Humans, other mammals	Ova, segments	Feces	—	Megaloblastic anemia in 1%
T. solium[b] (pork tapeworm)	Worldwide	Swine	Humans	Ova, segments	Feces	WB	Especially Mexico, Central and South America, Africa
Somatic tapeworms							
Echinococcus granulosus (hydatid disease)	Sheep-raising and hunting areas	Sheep, camels, humans, others	Dogs	Hydatid	Lung, liver	WB, EIA	Chest radiography, CT, MRI
E. multilocularis (hydatid disease)	Subarctic areas	Rodents, humans	Foxes, dogs, cats	Hydatid	Liver	—	May resemble cholangiocellular carcinoma
T. solium[b] (pork tapeworm)	Worldwide	Swine, humans	Humans	Cysticercus	Muscles, CNS	WB	CT, MRI, radiography
FLUKES (TREMATODES)							
Intestinal flukes							
Fasciolopsis buski	China, India	Snails–water chestnuts	Humans	Ova	Feces	—	—
Heterophyes heterophyes	Far East, India	Snails–fish	Humans	Ova	Feces	—	—
Metagonimus yokogawai	Focal in Europe and North Africa	Snails–fish	Humans	Ova	Feces	—	—
Liver flukes							
Clonorchis sinensis	China, Southeast Asia	Snails–fish	Humans	Ova	Feces, bile	—	Recurrent bacterial cholangitis
Fasciola hepatica	Sheep-raising areas	Snails–watercress	Humans, sheep	Ova	Feces,[d] bile	—	Cirrhosis, portal hypertension
Lung flukes							
Paragonimus spp.	Orient, Africa, South America	Snails–crabs/crayfish	Humans, other mammals	Adults, ova	Lung, sputum, feces	WB	Chest radiography, CT, MRI
Blood flukes							
Schistosoma mansoni	Africa, Central and South America, West Indies	Snails	Humans	Ova, adults	Feces	EIA, WB	Rectal snips, liver biopsy
S. haematobium	Africa	Snails	Humans	Ova, adults	Urine	WB	Liver, urine, or bladder biopsy
S. japonicum	Far East	Snails	Humans	Ova, adults	Feces	WB	Liver biopsy

[a] Larvae also can mature in intestinal villi of humans and mice.
[b] *T. solium* can cause either intestinal infections or cysticercosis. Its ova are identical to those of *T. saginata*; scolices and segments of the two species differ.
[c] When there are two intermediate hosts, the first is separated from the second by a dash. Definitive hosts are infected by the second intermediate host.

[d] Ova seldom reach the fecal stream during acute disease.
NOTE: WB, western blot; CT, computed tomography; MRI, magnetic resonance imaging; CNS, central nervous system; EIA, enzyme immunoassay. Serologic tests listed in Tables 211-1, 211-2, and 211-3 are available from the Centers for Disease Control and Prevention, Atlanta, GA.

saginata and *T. solium*, the cause of cysticercosis, are morphologically indistinguishable.

Microscopic examination of feces (Table 211-4) is not complete until direct wet mounts have been evaluated and concentration techniques as well as permanent stains have been applied. Before accepting a report of negativity for ova and parasites as final, the physician should insist that the laboratory undertake each of these procedures. Some intestinal parasites are more readily detected in material other than feces. For example, use of the string test (or one of its commercial substitutes) to sample duodenal contents is sometimes necessary to detect *Giardia lamblia*, *Cryptosporidium*, and *Strongyloides* larvae. Use of the "Scotch tape" technique to detect pinworm ova on the perianal skin sometimes also reveals ova of *T. saginata*

deposited perianally when the motile segments disintegrate (Table 211-4).

Two routine solutions are used to make wet mounts for the identification of the various life stages of helminths and protozoa: physiologic saline for trophozoites, cysts, ova, and larvae and dilute iodine solution for protozoal cysts and ova. Iodine solution must never be used to examine specimens for trophozoites because it kills the parasites and thus eliminates their characteristic motility.

The two most common concentration procedures for detecting small numbers of cysts and ova are formalin-ether sedimentation and zinc sulfate flotation. The formalin-ether technique is preferable, because all parasites sediment but not all float. Slides permanently stained for trophozoites should be prepared before concentration. Ad-

Table 211-2   Roundworm Infections

Parasite	Geographic Distribution	Life-Cycle Hosts Intermediate (Transmission)	Definitive	Parasite Stage	Body Fluid or Tissue	Serologic Tests	Other
INTESTINAL ROUNDWORMS							
Enterobius vermicularis (pinworm)	Temperate and tropical zones	Fecal-oral	Humans	Ova	Perianal skin	—	"Scotch tape" test
Trichuris trichiura (whip-worm)	Temperate and tropical zones	Soil, fecal-oral	Humans	Ova	Feces	—	Rectal prolapse
Ascaris lumbricoides (roundworm of humans)	Temperate and tropical zones	Soil, fecal-oral	Humans	Ova	Feces	—	Sx of pulmonary migration
Ancylostoma duodenale (Old World hookworm)	Eurasia, Africa, Pacific	Soil→skin	Humans	Ova/larvae	Feces	—	Sx of pulmonary migration, anemia
Necator americanus (New World hookworm)	U.S., Africa, worldwide	Soil→skin	Humans	Ova/larvae	Feces	—	Sx of pulmonary migration, anemia
Strongyloides stercoralis (strongyloidiasis)	Moist tropics and subtropics	Soil→skin	Humans	Larvae	Feces, sputum, duodenal fluid	EIA	Dissemination in immunodeficiency
TISSUE ROUNDWORMS							
Trichinella spiralis (trichinosis)	Worldwide	Swine/humans	Swine/humans	Larvae	Muscle	BF, EIA	Muscle biopsy
Wuchereria bancrofti (filariasis)	Coastal areas in tropics and subtropics	Mosquitoes	Humans	Microfilariae	Blood, lymph nodes	—	Nocturnal periodicity[a]
Brugia malayi (filariasis)	Asia, Indian subcontinent	Mosquitoes	Humans	Microfilariae	Blood	—	Nocturnal
Loa loa (African eye worm)	West and Central Africa	Mango flies (*Chrysops*)	Humans	Microfilariae	Blood	—	May be visible in eye, diurnal
Onchocerca volvulus (river blindness)	Africa, Mexico, Central and South America	Blackflies	Humans	Adults/larvae	Skin/eye	—	Examine nodules or skin snips
Dracunculus medinensis (guinea worm)	Africa	*Cyclops*	Humans	Adults/larvae	Skin	—	May be visible in lesion
LARVA MIGRANS SYNDROMES							
Ancylostoma braziliense (creeping eruption)	Tropical and temperate zones	Soil→skin	Dogs/cats, humans	Larvae	Skin	—	Dog and cat hookworm
Toxocara canis and *cati* (visceral larva migrans)	Tropical and temperate zones	Soil, fecal-oral	Dogs/cats, humans	Larvae	Viscera, CNS, eye	EIA[b]	Also caused by roundworms of other species

[a] Blood should be drawn at midnight, except for infection acquired in the South Pacific.
[b] The presence of hemagglutinins is a useful clue.

NOTE: BF, bentonite flocculation; Sx, signs/symptoms; EIA, enzyme immunoassay; CNS, central nervous system.

ditional slides stained for cysts and ova may be made from the concentrate.

In many instances, especially in the differentiation of *Entamoeba histolytica* from other amebas, identification of parasites from wet mounts or concentrates must be considered tentative. Permanently stained smears allow study of the cellular detail necessary for definitive identification. The iron-hematoxylin stain is excellent for critical work, but trichrome staining, which can be completed in 1 h, is a satisfactory alternative that also reveals parasites in specimens preserved in polyvinyl alcohol fixative.

BLOOD AND TISSUE PARASITES   Invasion of tissue by protozoa and helminths renders the choice of diagnostic techniques more difficult. For example, physicians must understand that aspiration of an amebic liver abscess rarely reveals *E. histolytica* because the trophozoites are located primarily in the abscess wall. They must remember that the urine sediment offers the best opportunity to detect *Schistosoma haematobium* in the Ethiopian youngster or the American traveler who returns from Africa with hematuria (Table 211-5). Tables 211-1, 211-2, and 211-3, which offer a quick guide to the geographic distribution and anatomic locations of the major tissue parasites,

should help the physician to select the appropriate body fluid or biopsy site for microscopic examination. Tables 211-5, 211-6, and 211-7 provide additional information about the identification of parasites in samples from specific anatomic locations. The laboratory procedures for detection of parasites in other body fluids are similar to those used in the examination of feces. The physician should insist on wet mounts, concentration techniques, and permanent stains for all body fluids. The trichrome or iron-hematoxylin stain is satisfactory for all tissue helminths in body fluids other than blood, but microfilarial worms and blood protozoa are more easily visualized when stained with Giemsa or Wright's stain.

The most common parasites detected in Giemsa-stained blood smears are the plasmodia, microfilariae, and African trypanosomes (Table 211-5). Most patients with Chagas' disease present in the chronic phase, when *Trypanosoma cruzi* is no longer microscopically detectable in blood smears. Wet mounts are sometimes more sensitive than stained smears for the detection of microfilariae and African trypanosomes because these active parasites cause noticeable movement of the erythrocytes in the microscopic field. Nuclepore filtration of blood facilitates the detection of microfilariae. The intracellular amas-

Table 211-3 Protozoal Infections

Parasite	Geographic Distribution	Life-Cycle Hosts — Intermediate (Transmission)	Life-Cycle Hosts — Definitive	Diagnosis — Parasite Stage	Diagnosis — Body Fluid or Tissue	Diagnosis — Serologic Tests	Diagnosis — Other
INTESTINAL PROTOZOANS							
Entamoeba histolytica (amebiasis)	Worldwide, especially tropics	Fecal-oral	Humans	Troph, cyst	Feces, liver	EIA, ID, antigen detection	Ultrasound, liver CT, PCR
Giardia lamblia (giardiasis)	Worldwide	Fecal-oral	Humans	Troph, cyst	Feces	Antigen detection	String test
Isospora belli	Worldwide	Fecal-oral	Humans	Oocyst	Feces	—	Acid-fast
Cryptosporidium	Worldwide	Fecal-oral	Humans, other animals	Oocyst	Feces	Antigen detection	Acid-fast, biopsy, PCR
Cyclospora cayetanensis	Worldwide?	Fecal-oral	Humans, other animals?	Oocyst	Feces	—	Modified safranin, epifluorescence, PCR
Enterocytozoon bieneusi (microsporidiosis)	Worldwide?	?	Animals, humans	Spore	Feces	—	Modified trichrome, biopsy, PCR
FREE-LIVING AMEBAS							
Naegleria	Worldwide	Warm water	Humans	Troph, cyst	CNS, nares	—	Biopsy, nasal swab
Acanthamoeba	Worldwide	Soil, water	Humans	Troph, cyst	CNS, skin, cornea	—	Biopsy, scrapings
BLOOD AND TISSUE PROTOZOANS							
Plasmodium spp. (malaria)	Subtropics and tropics	Mosquitoes	Humans	Asexual	Blood	Limited use	PCR
Babesia microti (babesiosis)	U.S., especially New England	Ticks	Rodents, humans	Asexual	Blood	IIF	Animal spp. in asplenia, PCR
Trypanosoma rhodesiense (African sleeping sickness)	Sub-Saharan East Africa	Tsetse flies	Humans, herbivores	Tryp	Blood, CSF	Card agglutination, IIF[a]	Also chancre, lymph nodes
T. gambiense (African sleeping sickness)	Sub-Saharan West Africa	Tsetse flies	Humans, swine	Tryp	Blood, CSF	Card agglutination, IIF[a]	Also chancre, lymph nodes
T. cruzi (Chagas' disease)	Mexico→South America	Reduviid bugs (triatomes)	Humans, dogs, wild animals	Amastigote, tryp	Multiple organs/blood	IIF	Reactivation in immunosuppression
Leishmania tropica, etc.	Widespread in tropics and subtropics	Sandflies (*Phlebotomus*)	Humans, dogs, rodents	Amastigote	Skin	IFA[b]	Biopsy, scraping, culture
L. braziliensis (mucocutaneous)	Mexico→South America	Sandflies (*Lutzomyia*)	Humans, dogs, rodents	Amastigote	Skin, mucous membranes	IFA[b]	Biopsy, scraping, culture
L. donovani (kala-azar)	Widespread in tropics and subtropics	Sandflies (*Phlebotomus*)	Humans, dogs, wild animals	Amastigote	RE system	IFA[b]	Biopsy, culture
Toxoplasma gondii (toxoplasmosis)	Worldwide	Humans, other mammals	Cats	Cyst, troph	CNS, eye, muscles, other	EIA, IIF	Reactivation in immunosuppression

[a] Card agglutination provided to endemic countries by the World Health Organization; contact the CDC.

[b] Limited specificity. Most sensitive for *L. donovani* (kala-azar).

NOTE: ID, immunodiffusion by commercial kit (not available from the CDC); CT, computed tomography; troph, trophozoite; tryp, trypomastigote form; IIF, indirect immunofluorescence; RE, reticuloendothelial; PCR, polymerase chain reaction; EIA, enzyme immunoassay; CNS, central nervous system; IFA, indirect fluorescent antibody.

tigote forms of *Leishmania* spp. and *T. cruzi* can sometimes be visualized in stained smears of peripheral blood, but aspirates of the bone marrow, liver, and spleen are the best sources for microscopic detection and culture of *Leishmania* in kala-azar and of *T. cruzi* in chronic Chagas' disease.

The diagnosis of malaria and the critical distinction among the various *Plasmodium* spp. are made by microscopic examination of stained thick and thin blood films (Table 211-6; **Plates VI-3 through VI-33**). Most malariologists prefer Giemsa stain because of its overall high quality, suitability for staining of both thick and thin smears, and stability in tropical climates. Wright's stain can produce high-quality thin smears and is widely used in the Americas, but it deteriorates rapidly in the tropics because its methanol base is highly hygroscopic. Specimens of capillary or venous blood should be obtained every 4 to 12 h until a diagnosis is established. The thin smear is made on clean slides exactly like a blood film for a white blood cell differential. The thick film is made by placing one drop of blood on the slide and stirring it in a circular motion to a diameter of about 2 cm. The erythrocytes in the thick film are lysed with water, but the thin film is fixed in methanol to preserve erythrocyte morphology.

Although most tissue parasites stain with the traditional hematoxylin and eosin, surgical biopsy specimens should also be stained with appropriate special stains. The surgical pathologist who is accustomed to applying silver stains for *Pneumocystis carinii* to induced sputum and transbronchial biopsies may have to be reminded to examine wet mounts and iron-hematoxylin–stained preparations of pulmonary specimens for helminthic ova and *E. histolytica*. The clinician should also be able to advise the surgeon and pathologist about optimal techniques for the identification of parasites in specimens obtained by certain specialized minor procedures (Table 211-7). For example, the excision of skin snips for the diagnosis of onchocerciasis, the collection of rectal snips for the diagnosis of schistosomiasis, and punch biopsy of skin lesions for the identification and culture of cutaneous and mucocutaneous species of *Leishmania* are simple procedures, but the diagnosis can be missed if the specimens are improperly obtained or processed.

NONSPECIFIC TESTS Eosinophilia is a common accompaniment of infections with most of the tissue helminths; absolute numbers of eosinophils may be high in trichinosis and the migratory phases of filariasis (Table 211-8). Intestinal helminths provoke eosinophilia

Table 211-4   Laboratory Diagnosis of Parasites Found in Feces[a]

Parasites and Fecal Stages	Alternative Diagnostic Procedures
TAPEWORMS (CESTODES)	
Taenia saginata ova and segments	Perianal "Scotch tape" test for ova
Hymenolepis nana ova	None
Diphyllobothrium ova and segments	None
T. solium ova and segments	Serology; brain biopsy for neurocysticercosis
FLUKES (TREMATODES)	
Fasciolopsis buski ova	None
Heterophyes heterophyes ova	None
Metagonimus yokogawai ova	None
Clonorchis (Opisthorchis) sinensis ova	Examination of bile for ova and adults in cholangitis
Fasciola hepatica ova	Examination of bile for ova and adults in cholangitis
Paragonimus spp. ova	Serology; sputum; biopsy of lung or brain for ova
Schistosoma ova	Serology for all; rectal snips (especially for *S. mansoni*), urine (*S. haematobium*), liver biopsy and liver ultrasound
ROUNDWORMS	
Enterobius vermicularis ova and adults	Perianal "Scotch tape" test for ova and adults
Trichuris trichiura ova	None
Ascaris lumbricoides ova and adults	Examination of sputum for larvae in lung disease
Hookworm ova and occasional larvae	Examination of sputum for larvae in lung disease
Strongyloides larvae	Duodenal aspirate or jejunal biopsy; serology; sputum or lung biopsy for filariform larvae in disseminated disease
Capillaria philippinensis ova[b]	None
PROTOZOANS	
Entamoeba histolytica trophozoites and cysts	Serology; liver biopsy for trophozoites
Giardia lamblia trophozoites and cysts	Duodenal aspirate or jejunal biopsy[c]
Isospora belli oocysts	Duodenal aspirate or jejunal biopsy[c]
Cryptosporidium oocysts	Duodenal aspirate or jejunal biopsy[c]
Enterocytozoon bieneusi spores	Duodenal aspirate or jejunal biopsy[c]

[a] Stains and concentration techniques are discussed in the text.
[b] Can be confused with *T. trichiura*.
[c] Commercial string test or Crosby capsule is satisfactory; *Isospora* and *Cryptosporidium* are acid-fast.

only during pulmonary migration of the larval stages. Eosinophilia is not a manifestation of protozoal infections, with the possible exceptions of those due to *Isospora* and *Dientamoeba fragilis*.

Like the hypochromic, microcytic anemia of heavy hookworm infections, other nonspecific laboratory abnormalities may suggest parasitic infection in patients with appropriate geographic and/or environmental exposures. Biochemical evidence of cirrhosis or an abnormal urine sediment in an African immigrant certainly raises the possibility of schistosomiasis, and anemia and thrombocytopenia in a febrile traveler or immigrant are among the hallmarks of malaria. Computed tomography and magnetic resonance imaging also contribute to the diagnosis of infections with many tissue parasites and have become invaluable adjuncts in the diagnosis of neurocysticercosis and cerebral toxoplasmosis.

ANTIBODY AND ANTIGEN DETECTION Useful antibody assays for many of the important tissue parasites are available; those listed in Table 211-9 can be obtained from the Centers for Disease Control and Prevention (CDC) in Atlanta. The results of most

serologic tests not listed in the tables and not offered by the CDC should be interpreted with caution.

The value of antibody assays is limited in the case of the filarial worms and plasmodia. The detection of antibody to plasmodia is of limited use for establishing the diagnosis of malaria in individual patients because diagnostic titers develop slowly and the tests must be sent to the CDC. Filarial antigens cross-react with those from other nematodes, and antibody assays do not distinguish between past and current infection. In contrast, a negative result in an American or European traveler virtually rules out the diagnosis of bancroftian or brugian filariasis. Promising new assays for filarial antigens and antibodies in lymphatic filariasis are not yet available in commercial kits or from the CDC.

Despite these specific limitations, the restricted geographic distribution of many tropical parasites increases the diagnostic usefulness of antibody detection in travelers from industrialized countries. On the other hand, a large proportion of the world has been exposed to *Toxoplasma gondii*, and the presence of IgG antibody does not constitute proof of active disease.

Fewer antibody assays are available for the diagnosis of infection with intestinal parasites. Cross-reactivity and lack of efficient cultivation techniques, along with the ability to establish diagnoses without invasive procedures, have discouraged intensive investigation of these methods. *E. histolytica* is the major exception. Sensitive, specific serologic tests are invaluable in the diagnosis of amebiasis. Commercial kits for the detection of antigen by enzyme-linked immunosorbent assay or of whole organisms by fluorescent antibody assay are now available for several protozoan parasites (Table 211-9).

Table 211-5   Identification of Parasites in Blood and Other Body Fluids

Body Fluid, Parasite	Enrichment/Stain	Culture Technique
BLOOD		
Plasmodium spp.	Thick and thin smears/Giemsa or Wright's	Not useful for diagnosis
Leishmania spp.	Buffy coat/Giemsa	Media available from CDC
African trypanosomes[a]	Buffy coat, anion column/wet mount and Giemsa	Mouse or rat inoculation[b]
Trypanosoma cruzi[c]	As for African species	As above and xenodiagnosis
Toxoplasma gondii	Buffy coat/Giemsa	Fibroblast cell lines
Microfilariae[d]	Nuclepore filtration/wet mount and Giemsa	None
URINE[e]		
Schistosoma haematobium	Centrifugation/wet mount	None
Microfilariae (in chyluria)	As for blood	None
SPINAL FLUID		
African trypanosomes	Centrifugation, anion column/wet mount and Giemsa	As for blood
Naegleria fowleri	Centrifugation/wet mount and Giemsa or trichrome	Nonnutrient agar overlaid with *Escherichia coli*

[a] *Trypanosoma rhodesiense* and *T. gambiense*.
[b] Inject mice intraperitoneally with 0.2 mL of whole heparinized blood (0.5 mL for rats). After 5 days, tail blood should be checked daily for trypanosomes as described above.
[c] Detectable in blood by conventional techniques only during acute disease. Xenodiagnosis is successful in about 50% of patients with chronic Chagas' disease.
[d] Day (1000–1400 h) and night (2200–0200 h) blood should be drawn to maximize the chance of detecting *Wuchereria* (nocturnal except for Pacific strains), *Brugia* (nocturnal), and *Loa loa* (diurnal).
[e] *Trichomonas vaginalis* is often detectable in urine, but examination of vaginal secretions is probably the preferable technique.

Table 211-6 Differential Diagnosis of *Plasmodium* Spp. in Blood Smears[a]

Feature	*P. falciparum*	*P. vivax*	*P. malariae*	*P. ovale*
FEATURE OF RED CELLS				
Size	All sizes	Large (young)	Small (old)	Large (young)
Shape	Round; may be crenated	Round or oval	Round	Round or pear-shaped, fimbriated
Stippling	Maurer's clefts: large, red (up to 20)	Schüffner's dots: numerous, small, red	None	Schüffner's dots
FEATURE OF PARASITE				
Ring trophozoites	Threadlike, multiple infections, double chromatin dots, accolé forms[b]	Thicker	Compact	Compact
Mature trophozoites	Absent	Ameboid, may fill cell	More regular, smaller band forms[c]	Less ameboid and smaller than those of *P. vivax*
Schizonts	Absent	12 to 24 merozoites	8 to 12 merozoites, often rosetted around pigment	8 to 12 merozoites
Gametocytes	Banana-shaped, central chromatin (female) or diffuse (male)	Round, fills cell, pigment often central	Round, large, coarse pigment	Smaller and oval, but similar to those of *P. vivax*
DIAGNOSTIC KEYS				
	Gametocyte, multiple rings, double chromatin dots, accolé forms, heavy infections	Schizont, large RBCs, ameboid forms	Schizont, small RBCs, band forms	Schizont and large RBCs, pear-shaped, fimbriated RBCs

[a] See Plates VI-3 through VI-33.
[b] At periphery of RBCs; may be flattened into rod shape.
[c] Stretch across RBCs, but not banana-shaped.
NOTE: RBCs, red blood cells.

MOLECULAR TECHNIQUES DNA hybridization with probes that are repeated many times in the genome of a specific parasite and amplification of a specific DNA fragment by the polymerase chain reaction (PCR) are promising techniques for the diagnosis of parasitic infections. Although molecular techniques for the detection of many parasites are already being used in insect vectors, animal models, and human trials, few are available for routine use in patients at this time. The only available commercial kit is that for the identi-

Table 211-7 Minor Procedures for Diagnosis of Parasitic Infections

Procedure	Parasite(s) and Stage
Skin snips: Lift skin with a needle and excise about 1 mg to a depth of 0.5 mm from several sites. Weigh each sample, place it in 0.5 mL of saline for 4 h, and examine wet mounts and Giemsa stains of the saline either directly or after filtration. Count microfilariae.[a]	*Onchocerca volvulus* and *Mansonella streptocerca* microfilariae
Biopsies of subcutaneous nodules: Stain routine histopathologic sections and impression smears with Giemsa.	*Loa loa* adults and *O. volvulus* adults and microfilariae
Muscle biopsies: Excise about 1.0 g of deltoid or gastrocnemius muscle and squash between two glass slides for direct microscopic examination.	*Trichinella spiralis* larvae (and perhaps *Taenia solium* cysticerci)
Rectal snips: From four areas of mucosa take 2-mg snips, tease onto a glass slide, and flatten with a second slide before examining directly at 10×. Preparations may be fixed in alcohol or stained.	*Schistosoma* ova of all species, but especially *S. mansoni*
Aspirate of chancre or lymph node[b]: Aspirate center with 18-gauge needle, place a drop on a slide, and examine for motile forms. An otherwise insufficient volume of material may be stained with Giemsa.	*Trypanosoma gambiense* and *T. rhodesiense* trypomastigotes
Corneal scrapings: Obtain sample from ophthalmologist for immediate Giemsa staining and culture on nutrient agar overlaid with *Escherichia coli*.	*Acanthamoeba* spp. trophozoites or cysts
Swabs, aspirates, or punch biopsies of skin lesions: Obtain specimen from margin of lesion for Giemsa staining of impression smears, and section and culture on special media from CDC.	Cutaneous and mucocutaneous *Leishmania* spp.

[a] Counts of >100/mg are associated with significant risk of complications.
[b] Lymph node aspiration is contraindicated in some infections and should be used judiciously.

Table 211-8 Parasites Frequently Associated with Eosinophilia[a]

Parasite	Comment
TAPEWORMS (CESTODES)	
Echinococcus granulosus	When hydatid cyst leaks
Taenia solium	During muscle encystation and in CSF with neurocysticercosis
FLUKES (TREMATODES)	
Paragonimus spp.	Uniformly high in acute stage
Fasciola hepatica	May be high in acute stage
Clonorchis (Opisthorchis) sinensis	Variable
Schistosoma mansoni	50% of infected travelers
S. haematobium	25% of infected travelers
S. japonicum	Up to 6000/μL in acute infection
ROUNDWORMS	
Ascaris lumbricoides	During larval migration
Hookworm species	During larval migration
Strongyloides stercoralis	Profound during migration and early years of infection
Trichinella spiralis	Up to 7000/μL
Filarial species[b]	Varies but can reach 5000 to 8000/μL
Toxocara spp.	>3000/μL
Ancylostoma braziliense	With extensive cutaneous eruption
Gnathostoma spinigerum	In visceral larva migrans and eosinophilic meningitis
Angiostrongylus cantonensis	In eosinophilic meningitis
A. costaricensis	During larval migration in mesenteric vessels
POSSIBLE PROTOZOAL CAUSES	
Isospora belli	A few reports of profound eosinophilia
Dientamoeba fragilis	Possible pathogenicity and eosinophilia

[a] Virtually every helminth has been associated with eosinophilia. This table includes both common and uncommon parasites that frequently elicit eosinophilia during infection.
[b] *Wuchereria bancrofti*, *Brugia* spp., *Loa loa*, and *Onchocerca volvulus*.

Table 211-9 Serologic and Molecular Tests for Parasitic Infections

Parasite, Infection	Antibody	Antigen or DNA/RNA
TAPEWORMS		
Echinococcosis	WB, EIA	
Cysticercosis	WB	
FLUKES		
Paragonimiasis	WB	
Schistosomiasis	EIA, WB	
ROUNDWORMS		
Strongyloidiasis	EIA	
Trichinellosis	BF, EIA	
Toxocariasis	EIA	
PROTOZOANS		
Amebiasis	EIA	EIA, PCR
Giardiasis		EIA, IIF, DFA
Cryptosporidiosis		IIF, EIA, DFA, PCR
Malaria (all species)	IIF[a]	PCR
Babesiosis	IIF	PCR
Chagas' disease	IIF	
Leishmaniasis	IIF	
Toxoplasmosis	IIF, EIA (IgM)	
Microsporidiosis		PCR
Cyclosporiasis		PCR

[a] Of limited use for management of acute disease.

NOTE: BF, bentonite flocculation; EIA, enzyme immunoassay; WB, western blot; IIF, indirect immunofluorescence; DFA, direct fluorescent antibody; PCR, polymerase chain reaction. All antibody tests listed are available from the CDC. Antigen and parasite detection kits are available commercially. The PCRs listed are those currently available from the CDC.

fication of *Trichomonas vaginalis* by hybridization of secretions from vaginal swabs with synthetic oligonucleotide probes. The CDC will perform PCR for microsporidia, cryptosporidia, *Cyclospora*, and *E. histolytica* on stools (frozen or fixed in either potassium dichromate or ethanol) and on biopsy and bronchoalveolar lavage samples (fixed in methanol or ethanol). For *Plasmodium* and *Babesia*, PCR is performed on blood treated with EDTA or collected in IsoCode Stix (Schleicher and Schuell).

BIBLIOGRAPHY

EBERHARD M et al: Laboratory diagnosis of *Cyclospora* infections. Acta Pathol Lab Med 121:792, 1997

FLECK SL, MOODY AH: *Diagnostic Techniques in Medical Parasitology*. London, Wright, 1988

GARCIA LS et al: Diagnosis of parasitic infections: Collection, processing, and examination of specimens, in *Manual of Clinical Microbiology*, 6th ed, PR Murray et al (eds). Washington, DC, ASM Press, 1995, pp 1145–1158

HAQUE R et al: Comparison of PCR, isoenzyme analysis, and antigen detection for diagnosis of *Entamoeba histolytica* infection. J Clin Microbiol 36:449, 1998

MOLYNEUX DH: Vector-borne parasitic diseases—an overview of recent changes. Int J Parasitol 28:927, 1998

TOMECKI JK (ed): *Dermatologic Clinics, Systemic Mycoses and Parasitic Diseases*. Philadelphia, Saunders, 1989, vol 7

WEBER R et al: Improved light-microscopical detection of microsporidia spores in stool and duodenal aspirates. N Engl J Med 326:161, 1992

WELLER PF: Eosinophilia in travelers. Med Clin North Am 76:1413, 1992

WILSON M et al: Evaluation of six commercial kits for detection of human immunoglobulin M antibodies to *Toxoplasma gondii*. J Clin Microbiol 35:3112, 1997

——— et al: Clinical immunoparasitology, in *Manual of Clinical Laboratory Immunology*, 5th ed, NR Rose et al (eds). Washington, DC, ASM Press, 1997, pp 575–584

212 *Thomas A. Moore*

THERAPY FOR PARASITIC INFECTIONS

Over the last few decades, the reach of some parasitic diseases such as malaria has extended because of factors such as deforestation, population shifts, global warming, and other climatic events (e.g., "El Niño"). Efforts to combat this trend are complicated by the development and spread of drug resistance among parasites and the limited introduction of new antiparasitic agents. However, significant advances toward the reduction of the burden of parasitic disease have been made. The generous donation of ivermectin and albendazole for global eradication programs has improved the health of countless individuals and offers the promise of disease eradication. The expanded use of traditionally nonparasitic agents, such as amphotericin B for visceral leishmaniasis, has offered hope against the specter of drug resistance. The introduction of newer agents, such as triclabendazole, also appears promising.

Currently recommended treatment options for most parasitic diseases of humans are listed in Table 212-1. A brief summary of some of the agents can be found below; each agent is listed by its generic name. Many of the agents are approved by the Food and Drug Administration (FDA) but are considered investigational for the treatment of certain infections; these drugs are marked accordingly in Table 212-1. Drugs marked in the text with an asterisk (*) are available only through the Centers for Disease Control and Prevention (CDC) Drug Service (telephone: 404-639-3670). Other drugs, marked with a dagger (†), are available only through the manufacturer; contact information for these manufacturers may be available from the CDC. Information on dosing in children and pregnant women can be obtained in the references at the end of the chapter.

Albendazole This benzimidazole derivative has recently become generally available and is active against a broad range of helminths and protozoa. All benzimidazoles act by binding to free β-tubulin, inhibiting the polymerization of tubulin and the microtubule-dependent uptake of glucose. In helminths, the result is the depletion of glycogen stores, but this fundamental disruption of cellular metabolism also offers treatment for a wide range of parasitic diseases. Like all benzimidazoles, albendazole is poorly absorbed from the gastrointestinal tract. However, since the active metabolite attains higher serum and cyst concentrations than mebendazole, it is more effective against echinococcal disease. Significant adverse reactions are usually limited to prolonged use and include abdominal pain and reversible hepatic dysfunction. Rarely, leukopenia and reversible alopecia occur. Albendazole is contraindicated in early pregnancy.

Artesunate and Artemether Artesunate, artemether, and the parent compound artemisinin are sesquiterpene lactones derived from the wormwood plant *Artemisia annua*. These agents have become first-line treatments for severe falciparum malaria in some areas of the world where drug resistance is a major problem. They are rapidly effective against the asexual blood forms of *Plasmodium* spp., including multidrug-resistant *P. falciparum*, but they are not active against intrahepatic forms. Their mechanism of action is not completely understood, but they are believed to act by converting to free radicals and other intermediates in the presence of intraparasitic iron; the result is alkylation of parasite proteins or membrane damage. Artemisinin derivatives presently show no cross-resistance with known antimalarials and thus are important for treating severe malaria in areas of multidrug resistance. However, long treatment courses are required and, when these agents are used alone, recrudescence may occur. Artemisinin and its derivatives are cleared rapidly from the circulation, and their short half-lives limit their use for prophylaxis. Adverse events are usually infrequent and mild and include drug fever and contact dermatitis. Animal data suggest that neurotoxicity can develop if the compounds are administered chronically, and cerebellar dysfunction

Infection: Organism (See Also Chapter[a])	Treatment of Choice	Alternative Treatment
Amebiasis: *Entamoeba histolytica* (213)		
Asymptomatic infection	Paromomycin 500 mg PO tid for 10 days	Iodoquinol 650 mg PO tid for 20 days
Intestinal disease	Metronidazole 750 mg PO or IV tid for 5–10 days *plus* luminal agent as for asymptomatic infection	Tinidazole 2 g PO once *plus* luminal agent as for asymptomatic infection
Hepatic abscess	Metronidazole 750 mg PO or IV tid for 5–10 days *plus* luminal agent as for asymptomatic infection	Tinidazole 2 g PO once (repeat as needed) *plus* luminal agent as for asymptomatic infection
Amebic Meningoencephalitis: *Naegleria fowleri* (213)	Amphotericin B[b] 1 mg/kg per day IV; duration of treatment uncertain; benefit of adding rifampin 600 mg PO bid uncertain	—
Angiostrongyliasis (219)		
Angiostrongylus cantonensis	Supportive therapy with serial lumbar punctures and glucocorticoids as needed; benefit of medical therapy unclear	—
A. costaricensis	Thiabendazole[b] 25 mg/kg PO tid for 3 days (max 3 g/d); repeat 3 times within 3 weeks	—
Anisakiasis: *Anisakis, Pseudoterranova* spp. (220)	Surgical or endoscopic removal, if possible	—
Ascariasis: *Ascaris lumbricoides* (220)	Albendazole[b] 400 mg PO once	Mebendazole 100 mg PO bid for 3 days or 500 mg once, *or* pyrantel pamoate 11 mg/kg PO once (max 1 g)
Babesiosis: *Babesia* spp. (214)	Clindamycin[b] 1.2 g IV bid or 600 mg PO tid for 7–10 days *plus* quinine 650 mg PO tid for 7–10 days; consider exchange transfusion for critically ill patients	Atovaquone[b] 750 mg PO bid for 7–10 days *plus* azithromycin[b] 0.5–1 g/d PO for 7–10 days, *or* quinine 650 mg PO tid for 7–10 days *plus* azithromycin[b] 0.5–1 g/d PO for 7–10 days
Balantidiasis: *Balantidium coli* (218)	Tetracycline[b] 500 mg PO qid for 10 days, *or* doxycycline[b] 100 mg PO bid for 10 days	Metronidazole[b] 750 mg PO tid for 5 days, *or* iodoquinol[b] 650 mg PO tid for 20 days
Capillariasis: *Capillaria philippinensis* (220)	Albendazole[b] 400 mg/d PO for 10 days	Mebendazole[b] 200 mg PO bid for 20 days
Cestode Infections (223)		
Intestinal stage (adults)		
Diphyllobothrium latum, Dipylidium caninum, Taenia saginata, T. solium	Praziquantel[b] 5–10 mg/kg PO once	—
Hymenolepis nana	Praziquantel 25 mg/kg PO once	—
Tissue stage (larvae)		
Cysticercosis: *T. solium*[c]	Praziquantel 50–60 mg/kg per day PO in 3 divided doses for 15 days, with glucocorticoids and cimetidine for CNS lesions; *or* praziquantel 25 mg/kg PO q2h for 3 doses followed by dexamethasone 10 mg IM 4 h later and 10 mg/d IM for the next 2 days	Albendazole 7.5 mg/kg PO q12h for 8 days, with dexamethasone 10 mg/d IM for the first 4 days for CNS lesions
Echinococcosis		
Echinococcus granulosus	PAIR[d] or surgical excision *plus* albendazole 15 mg/kg per day for at least 4 days before procedure and continued for at least 4 weeks afterward; for uncomplicated lesions, albendazole 400 mg PO bid for 12 weeks (repeat as needed)	Mebendazole 40–50 mg/d PO for 3–6 months, repeat as needed
E. multilocularis	Surgical resection *plus* albendazole 400 mg PO bid for up to 2 years	—
Cryptosporidiosis: *Cryptosporidium parvum* (218)	Supportive care in normal hosts; paromomycin[b] 500–750 mg PO qid may be effective in HIV-infected patients	Nitazoxanide[b] 500 mg PO bid for 7 days
Cutaneous Larva Migrans: *Ancylostoma* spp. (219)	Ivermectin[b] 150–200 μg/kg PO once, *or* thiabendazole 25 mg/kg PO bid or 10% suspension topically for 2–5 days	Albendazole[b] 200 mg PO bid for 2–7 days
Cyclosporiasis: *Cyclospora cayetanensis* (218)	Trimethoprim-sulfamethoxazole[b] 160/800 mg PO bid for 7 days	—
Dientamebiasis: *Dientamoeba fragilis* (218)	Paromomycin[b] 10 mg/kg PO tid for 7 days	Iodoquinol 650 mg PO tid for 20 days, *or* tetracycline[b] 500 mg PO qid for 10 days
Dracunculiasis: *Dracunculus medinensis* (221)	Worm removal *plus* metronidazole[b] 250 mg PO tid for 10 days	Worm removal *plus* thiabendazole 25 mg/kg PO bid/tid for 3 days
Enterobiasis: *Enterobius vermicularis* (220)	Mebendazole 100 mg PO once, repeat in 2 weeks	Albendazole[b] 400 mg PO once, repeat in 2 weeks; *or* pyrantel pamoate 11 mg/kg once (max 1 g), repeat in 2 weeks
Filariasis (221)		
Lymphatic filariasis: *Wuchereria bancrofti, Brugia* spp.[e]	DEC[f] 2 mg/kg PO tid for 12 days[g]	Albendazole[b] 400 mg PO bid for 21 days (macrofilaricidal only)
Tropical pulmonary eosinophilia: *W. bancrofti, Brugia* spp.	DEC 2 mg/kg PO tid for 14 days	—
Loiasis: *Loa loa*		
Microfilariae present in concentrated blood[e]	Prednisone 40–60 mg/d followed by DEC 0.5 mg/kg per day; if well tolerated, taper prednisone and gradually increase DEC dose to 8–10 mg/kg per day for 21 days	—

(continued)

Infection: Organism (See Also Chapter[a])	Treatment of Choice	Alternative Treatment
Microfilariae absent in concentrated blood[h]	DEC 8–10 mg/kg per day (divided into 3 doses) PO for 21 days	—
Mansonellosis		
Mansonella ozzardi	Ivermectin 6 mg PO once	—
M. perstans	DEC as for loiasis; no treatment has been proven completely effective	Mebendazole 100 mg PO bid for 30 days, *or* albendazole 400 mg PO bid for 10 days
M. streptocerca	Ivermectin[b] 150 μg/kg PO once	DEC 2 mg/kg PO tid for 14–21 days
Onchocerciasis: *Onchocerca volvulus*	Ivermectin 150 μg/kg once, repeat every 6–12 months; onchocercal nodules on head should be surgically excised	—
Flukes (222)		
Biliary duct-dwelling flukes: *Clonorchis sinensis, Opisthorchis* spp.	Praziquantel 25 mg/kg PO tid for 1 day	Albendazole[b] 400 mg PO bid for 7 days
Liver-dwelling flukes		
Fasciola hepatica	Triclabendazole 10 mg/kg PO once	Bithionol 30–50 mg/kg PO qod for 10–15 doses
Metorchis conjunctus	Praziquantel[b] 25 mg/kg PO tid for 1 day	—
Intestine-dwelling flukes		
Fasciolopsis buski, Heterophyes heterophyes, Metagonimus yokogawai, Echinostoma spp.	Praziquantel[b] 25 mg/kg PO tid for 1 day	—
Nanophyetus salmincola	Praziquantel[b] 20 mg/kg PO tid for 1 day	—
Lung-dwelling flukes: *Paragonimus* spp.	Praziquantel[b] 25 mg/kg PO tid for 2 days	Triclabendazole 10 mg/kg PO bid for 1 day
Giardiasis: *Giardia lamblia* (218)	Metronidazole[b] 250 mg PO tid for 5 days	Tinidazole 2 g PO once, *or* furazolidone 100 mg PO qid for 7–10 days, *or* paromomycin[b] 10 mg/kg PO tid for 7 days, *or* albendazole 400 mg/d PO for 5 days, *or* quinacrine 100 mg PO tid for 5 days
Gnathostomiasis: *Gnathostoma spinigerum* (219)	Albendazole[b] 400–800 mg/d PO for 21 days	Surgical removal if possible
Hookworm: *Ancylostoma duodenale, Necator americanus* (220)	Mebendazole 100 mg PO bid for 3 days or 500 mg PO once	Albendazole[b] 400 mg PO once
Isosporiasis: *Isospora belli* (218)	Trimethoprim-sulfamethoxazole[b] 160/800 mg PO qid for 10 days, then bid for 3 weeks	Pyrimethamine 50–75 mg/d PO for 3 weeks
Leishmaniasis: *Leishmania donovani, L. major, L. infantum, L chagasi, L mexicana, L. tropica, Viannia* spp. (215)		
Cutaneous leishmaniasis	Sodium stibogluconate *or* meglumine antimonate 20 mg Sb/kg per day IV or IM for 20 days	Pentamidine 3 mg/kg IV or IM qod for 4 doses or 2 mg/kg qod for 7 doses, *or* amphotericin B[b] 0.5–1 mg/kg IV qod or qd to a total dose of 20 mg/kg
Mucosal leishmaniasis	Sodium stibogluconate *or* meglumine antimonate 20 mg Sb/kg per day IV or IM for 28 days	Amphotericin B[b] 1 mg/kg IV qod or qd to a total dose of 20–40 mg/kg, *or* pentamidine 2–4 mg/kg IV or IM qod or 3 times weekly for ≥15 doses
Visceral leishmaniasis	Sodium stibogluconate *or* meglumine antimonate 20 mg Sb/kg per day IV or IM for 28 days, *or* lipid-complexed amphotericin B 2–5 mg/kg per day (total dose 15–40 mg/kg)[i]	Amphotericin B[b] deoxycholate 0.5–1 mg/kg IV qod or qd to a total dose of 15–20 mg/kg, *or* pentamidine 4 mg/kg qod or 3 times weekly for 15–30 doses
Malaria: *Plasmodium vivax, P. falciparum, P. ovale, P. malariae* (214)		
Severe malaria (parenteral therapy)	Quinidine gluconate 10 mg base/kg (max 600 mg) by continuous infusion over 1–2 h followed by 0.02 mg/kg per min, until patient can take oral therapy; consider exchange transfusion in critically ill patients	Artesunate 2.4 mg/kg IV or IM followed by 1.2 mg/kg at 12 and 24 h, then daily; *or* artemether 3.2 mg/kg IM, then 1.6 mg/kg per day
Uncomplicated malaria (oral therapy)		
All *except* chloroquine-resistant *Plasmodium* spp.	Chloroquine phosphate 10 mg base/kg followed by 10 mg/kg at 24 h and 5 mg/kg at 48 h or by 5 mg/kg at 12, 24, and 36 h (total dose, 25 mg/kg); treatment of infections due to *P. vivax* or *P. ovale* should be followed by radical cure	—
Chloroquine-resistant *P. falciparum*	Quinine sulfate 10 mg salt/kg tid for 7 days *plus* tetracycline[b] 4 mg/kg qid or doxycycline[b] 3 mg/kg per day for 7 days	Mefloquine 15 mg base/kg PO once for semi-immunes or followed 8–12 h later by second dose of 10 mg/kg for nonimmunes or in areas with mefloquine resistance; *or* atovaquone 1 g/d for 3 days *plus* either proguanil 400 mg/d for 3 days or doxycycline[b] 100 mg bid for 3 days; *or* artesunate 4 mg/kg per day for 3 days *plus* mefloquine 1.25 g once; *or* halofantrine 500 mg qid for 3 doses, repeat in 1 week

(*continued*)

Table 212-1—(continued)

Infection: Organism (See Also Chapter[a])	Treatment of Choice	Alternative Treatment
Chloroquine-resistant *P. vivax*	Quinine sulfate 650 mg PO q8h for 3–7 days *plus* either doxycycline[b] 100 mg PO bid for 7 days or pyrimethamine/sulfadoxine 3 tablets once on last day of quinine; treatment should be followed by radical cure	Mefloquine 1.25 g PO once
Radical cure (*P. vivax* and *P. ovale* only)	Primaquine phosphate 26.3 mg (15 mg base)/d for 14 days, or 79 mg (45 mg base)/week for 8 weeks	—
Microsporidiosis (218)		
Ocular: *Encephalitozoon hellem, E. cuniculi, Vittaforma corneae*	Albendazole[b] 400 mg PO bid for 4 weeks, repeat as needed	—
Intestinal: *Enterocytozoon bieneusi, Encephalitozoon intestinalis*	Albendazole[b] 400 mg PO bid for 3 weeks, repeat as needed	—
Disseminated: *E. hellem, E. cuniculi, E. intestinalis, Pleistophora* spp.	Albendazole[b] 400 mg PO bid; duration of therapy uncertain	—
Schistosomiasis (222)		
Schistosoma haematobium	Praziquantel 20 mg/kg PO bid for 1 day	Metrifonate 7.5–10 mg/kg PO once every other week for 3 doses
S. japonicum, S. mekongi	Praziquantel 20 mg/kg PO tid for 1 day	
S. mansoni	Praziquantel 20 mg/kg PO bid for 1 day	Oxamniquine 15 mg/kg PO once for disease acquired in the western hemisphere; 15 mg/kg PO bid for 2 days for disease acquired in Africa or the Middle East
Strongyloidiasis: *Strongyloides stercoralis* (220)	Ivermectin 200 μg/kg per day PO for 1–2 days; in hyperinfection syndrome, continue treatment until parasites are eradicated	Albendazole 400 mg/d PO for 3 days, *or* thiabendazole 25 mg/kg PO bid (max 3 g/d) for 2 days
Toxoplasmosis: *Toxoplasma gondii* (217)		
Acute infection or relapse	Pyrimethamine 200 mg PO once, then 50–75 mg/d PO *plus* sulfadiazine 4–6 g/d in 4 divided doses *plus* folinic acid 10 mg/d PO for 6 weeks; adjunctive therapy with prednisone 80–120 mg/d PO is indicated in ocular disease	Pyrimethamine 200 mg PO once, then 50–75 mg/d PO *plus* folinic acid 10 mg/d PO *plus* either clindamycin 1.2–4.8 g/d IV or atovaquone 750 mg PO qid for 6 weeks
Infection in pregnancy	Spiramycin 10–15 mg/kg IV tid until delivery; if fetal infection is suspected or confirmed, treat after first trimester for immunocompetent patients	—
Trichinellosis: *Trichinella* spp. (219)	Glucocorticoids (for severe symptoms) *plus* albendazole[b] 400 mg PO bid for 8 days	Mebendazole[b] 200–300 mg PO tid for 3 days, then 400–500 mg PO tid for 10 days; *or* thiabendazole[b] 25 mg/kg PO bid (max 3 g) for 7 days
Trichomoniasis: *Trichomonas vaginalis* (218)	Metronidazole 2 g PO once or 250 mg PO tid for 7 days	Tinidazole 2 g PO once
Trichostrongyliasis: *Trichostrongylus* spp. (220)	Albendazole[b] 400 mg PO once	Mebendazole[b] 100 mg PO bid for 3 days
Trichuriasis: *Trichuris trichiura* (220)	Albendazole[b] 400 mg PO once	Mebendazole 100 mg PO bid for 3 days or 500 mg PO once
Trypanosomiasis (216)		
Chagas' disease: *Trypanosoma cruzi*	Nifurtimox 2–2.5 mg/kg PO qid for 90–120 days	Benznidazole 5 mg/kg per day PO for 60–90 days
Sleeping sickness		
West African trypanosomiasis: *T. brucei gambiense*		
Stage 1	Suramin 1 g IV on days 1, 3, 7, 14, and 21	Eflornithine 100 mg IV qid for 2 weeks, then 300 mg/kg per day PO for 3–4 weeks; *or* pentamidine[b] 4 mg/kg per day IV or IM for 10 days
Stage 2	Eflornithine 100 mg IV qid for 2 weeks, then 300 mg/kg/d PO for 3–4 weeks	—
East African trypanosomiasis: *T. brucei rhodesiense*		
Stage 1	Suramin 1 g IV on days 1, 3, 7, 14, and 21	Pentamidine[b] 4 mg/kg per day IV or IM for 10 days, *or* melarsoprol 2–3.6 mg/kg per day IV in 3 divided doses for 3 days
Stage 2	Melarsoprol 2–3.6 mg/kg per day IV in 3 divided doses for 3 days	Tryparsamide 30 mg/kg (max 2 g) *plus* suramin 10 mg/kg IV every 5 days, to a total of 12 doses of each drug
Visceral Larva Migrans: *Toxocara* spp. (219)	Supportive therapy; glucocorticoids as needed	DEC 2 mg/kg PO tid for 7–10 days, *or* albendazole[b] 400 mg PO bid for 3–5 days, *or* mebendazole[b] 100–200 mg PO bid for 5 days

[a] See also the indicated chapters on specific parasitic diseases, which present more detailed information on topics such as alternative regimens, contraindications, and adverse reactions.

[b] Not specifically approved by the U.S. Food and Drug Administration (FDA) for use in this infection.

[c] Surgery indicated for ocular and spinal lesions.

[d] Percutaneous aspiration, infusion of scolicidal agents, and reaspiration.

[e] Apheresis before treatment may be beneficial to heavily infected individuals.

[f] Diethylcarbamazine.

[g] Coinfection with *Onchocerca volvulus* or *Loa loa* must be ruled out before initiation of therapy because of potentially fatal adverse effects.

[h] When microfilariae are absent from concentrated blood, coinfection with *O. volvulus* must be ruled out before initiation of therapy because of potentially adverse effects (Mazzotti reaction).

[i] See Table 215-2 for detailed information on regimens approved by the FDA.

has been reported in persons treated with artesunate. These drugs are not available in the United States.

Amphotericin B   Amphotericin exerts its effect by inserting itself into the cytoplasmic membrane of the organism and binding sterols, causing membrane permeability. Amphotericin B deoxycholate, a lipophilic polyene drug, is an effective agent for the treatment of leishmaniasis and amebic meningoencephalitis due to *Naegleria* spp., but its use is associated with significant nephrotoxicity and occasional allergic reactions. Three lipid-complexed formulations of amphotericin B have been released: amphotericin B colloidal dispersion (ABCD), amphotericin B lipid complex (ABLC), and liposomal amphotericin B. These agents are effective against antimony-resistant visceral leishmaniasis and offer the benefits of shorter courses and less toxicity.

Atovaquone   Atovaquone is a hydroxynaphthoquinone that exerts its broad-spectrum antiprotozoal activity via inhibition of parasite mitochondrial electron transport. Although it has relatively poor bioavailability, atovaquone exhibits potent activity against toxoplasmosis when used with pyrimethamine. When combined with proguanil or doxycycline, it is effective for both treatment and prophylaxis of malaria. Side effects are rare but can include nausea and a maculopapular rash.

Azithromycin   An azalide antibiotic, azithromycin has been used to treat a number of protozoal infections such as babesiosis, malaria, toxoplasmosis, and cryptosporidiosis. Azithromycin acts by inhibiting protein synthesis; in apicomplexan parasites, this inhibition occurs in the plastid. Most adverse reactions are gastrointestinal (diarrhea, nausea, abdominal pain) and uncommon and rarely require discontinuation of the drug.

Benznidazole   This oral nitroimidazole derivative is used to treat acute Chagas' disease, and cure rates of 80 to 90% have been recorded. Benznidazole acts by generating oxygen radicals to which the parasite is more sensitive than mammalian cells because of a relative deficiency in antioxidant enzymes. Adverse effects are frequent and include rashes, nausea, paresthesias, and leukopenia. The safety of benznidazole in early pregnancy has not been established, but the drug should be used immediately after the first trimester to prevent congenital transmission. Benznidazole is currently unavailable in the United States.

Bithionol*   Bithionol is a phenolic substance structurally related to hexachlorophene. Its antihelminthic activity is poorly understood, but the agent is believed to inhibit oxidative phosphorylation. Bithionol is no longer manufactured. A dwindling supply is available from the CDC for treatment of fascioliasis and paragonimiasis. The drug's distribution is limited to physicians treating patients with one of these diseases who are unable to use praziquantel because of previous idiosyncratic or allergic reactions or in whom a course of praziquantel has failed to eradicate infection. Significant side effects are common and include abdominal pain, diarrhea, and urticaria.

Chloroquine   The best-known of the 4-aminoquinolines, chloroquine has marked, rapid schizonticidal and gametocidal activity against blood forms of *P. ovale* and *P. malariae* and against susceptible strains of *P. vivax* and *P. falciparum*. It is not active against intrahepatic forms (*P. vivax* and *P. ovale*). Chloroquine is concentrated in the acidic food vacuoles of intraerythrocytic parasites, where it reaches levels 600-fold higher than plasma levels. The drug inhibits a parasite heme polymerase that protects the parasite from the membrane-damaging byproducts of hemoglobin degradation; as a result of this inhibition, the parasite is effectively killed with its own metabolic waste. Chloroquine resistance appears to arise as a result of a decreased level of chloroquine uptake. This drug is safe for use in pregnancy. Adverse reactions include pruritus, transient headaches, and nausea.

Clindamycin   This macrolide is an effective adjunct for the treatment of several protozoal infections, including toxoplasmosis, malaria,

and babesiosis. The most significant potential adverse reaction is the development of *Clostridium difficile*–associated diarrhea. When administered with quinine, clindamycin is active against drug-resistant falciparum malaria; this combination is the therapy of choice for babesiosis.

Diethylcarbamazine*   A piperazine derivative with a long history of successful use, this drug remains the treatment of choice for lymphatic filariasis and loiasis and has also been used for visceral larva migrans. Diethylcarbamazine exerts effects on helminths, including immobilization due to a decrease in muscle activity, disruption of microtubule formation, and alteration of helminthic surface membranes resulting in enhanced killing by the host's immune system. In addition, this agent enhances adherence properties of eosinophils. It is safe for use in pregnancy and well tolerated. Significant adverse events associated with the drug, including encephalopathy and death, are attributable to the parasite burden, which is best assessed by the degree of microfilaremia. Use in patients with onchocerciasis can precipitate a Mazzotti reaction with pruritus, fever, and arthralgias. Untoward effects produced directly by diethylcarbamazine usually involve the gastrointestinal tract and are dose-related.

Eflornithine (Difluoromethylornithine, DFMO)†   This ornithine derivative has specific activity against all stages of infection with *Trypanosoma brucei gambiense* and acts by irreversibly inhibiting ornithine decarboxylase—an enzyme critical to the formation of polyamines, which are essential to trypanosomatids. Eflornithine readily crosses the blood-brain barrier and is excreted mainly by the kidneys. Its use is contraindicated in pregnancy. Adverse reactions, which are usually mild and reversible, include pancytopenia, diarrhea, and transient hearing loss.

Furazolidone   This nitrofuran derivative, which is an effective alternative agent for the treatment of giardiasis, acts by damaging parasite DNA. Since it is the only agent active against *Giardia* that is available in liquid form, it is often used to treat young children. Side effects include allergic reactions, nausea, vomiting, and disulfiram-like reactions when ingested with alcohol. Because hemolytic anemia due to glutathione instability can occur, furazolidone treatment is contraindicated in mothers who are breast-feeding and in neonates.

Halofantrine   An oral alternative drug for treatment of malaria due to chloroquine-resistant *P. falciparum*, this 9-phenanthrenemethanol is one of three classes of arylaminoalcohols first identified as potential antimalarial agents by the World War II Malaria Chemotherapy Program. Its activity is believed to be similar to that of chloroquine. Halofantrine is generally well tolerated; the most commonly reported adverse effects are abdominal pain and diarrhea. The incidence of pruritus is lower than that with chloroquine. Halofantrine causes dose-related prolongation of the PR and QT intervals, and its use is contraindicated in persons who have cardiac disease or who have taken mefloquine in the preceding 3 weeks. Halofantrine treatment is also contraindicated in pregnant and lactating women. The drug is currently unavailable in the United States.

Iodoquinol   This hydroxyquinoline is an effective luminal agent for the treatment of amebiasis, balantidiasis, and infection with *Dientamoeba fragilis*. Its mechanism of action is unknown. Adverse effects include headache, diarrhea, nausea, vomiting, abdominal pain, pruritus, fever, seizures, and encephalopathy. Most serious are the reactions related to prolonged high-dose therapy, which should not occur if the dosage regimens recommended in Table 212-1 are followed. Because the drug contains iodine, it should be used with caution in patients with thyroid disease.

Ivermectin   This derivative of avermectin is used to treat infections caused by a wide range of helminths. It is the drug of choice for the treatment of onchocerciasis, strongyloidiasis, and cutaneous larva migrans. While active against the intestinal helminths *Ascaris lumbricoides* and *Enterobius vermicularis*, it is variably effective in trichuriasis and ineffective against hookworms. Recent data suggest that ivermectin acts by opening neuromuscular membrane-associated glutamate-dependent chloride channels (unique to nematodes and arthropods)—an event resulting in an influx of chloride ions, worm paralysis, and subsequent death by immune or other mechanisms. Ivermectin is generally safe, easy to administer, and well tolerated, but encephalopathy and occasional deaths have been reported when the drug is given to persons with high burdens of *Loa loa* microfilaremia. Ivermectin is not approved for use during pregnancy.

Mebendazole   This benzimidazole derivative is widely used for treatment of intestinal helminths and exhibits activity against *Echinococcus granulosus*. Benzimidazoles block parasite microtubule assembly and glucose uptake. Because mebendazole is poorly absorbed, its incidence of side effects is low, but its usefulness in treating tissue helminths is limited. Transient abdominal pain and diarrhea sometimes occur, usually in persons with massive parasite burdens. The use of mebendazole is contraindicated in pregnancy.

Mefloquine   Like quinine and chloroquine, this quinoline is active only against the asexual erythrocytic stages of malarial parasites. The mode of action of mefloquine is similar to that of chloroquine, but mefloquine is not concentrated so extensively in the food vacuole and may act on alternative targets in the parasite. Taken as a single dose, it is the preferred drug for prophylaxis of chloroquine-resistant malaria; high doses can be used for treatment. The development of drug-resistant strains of *P. falciparum* in parts of Africa and Southeast Asia is ominous, but mefloquine is still an effective drug in most of the world. It is well tolerated by most persons, but its safety in pregnancy is unknown. Adverse effects are usually dose-related and include nausea and dizziness. Psychosis and seizures occur rarely, but treatment of patients with neuropsychiatric conditions warrants caution. Concomitant use of quinine, quinidine, or drugs causing β-adrenergic blockade may produce electrocardiographic disturbances or cardiac arrest.

Melarsoprol*   This trivalent arsenical is used for the treatment of late-stage East African trypanosomiasis and is not uniformly effective. The drug enters the parasite via an adenosine transporter; resistant strains lack this transport system. Arsenicals react avidly with sulfhydryl groups on proteins and inhibit their function. This is the likely mechanism of action and the cause of the severe adverse effects commonly seen. Encephalopathy is the most serious side effect, usually occurring within 4 days of the initiation of therapy and resulting in death in 6% of recipients.

Metrifonate   This organophosphorus compound has selective activity against *Schistosoma haematobium*. It is partially metabolized to 2,2-dimethyldichlorovinyl phosphate (DDVP), a highly active chemical that irreversibly inhibits the acetylcholinesterase enzyme. Schistosomal cholinesterase is more susceptible to this metabolite than is the corresponding human enzyme. Metrifonate's exact mechanism of action is uncertain, but it is believed to inhibit tegumental acetylcholine receptors that mediate glucose transport. Although the drug is well tolerated, recipients experience a transient decrease in plasma cholinesterase activity and should not be exposed to neuromuscular blocking agents or organophosphate insecticides for at least 48 h after treatment. Metrifonate's safety in pregnancy is not established. The drug is currently unavailable in the United States.

Metronidazole   Of the nitroimidazoles, only metronidazole has been licensed in the United States. This drug has FDA approval only for the treatment of amebiasis and trichomoniasis, although it is currently the drug of choice for giardiasis and trichomoniasis and is an alternative agent for balantidiasis. Metronidazole is reduced by anaerobic metabolism, and the metabolite acts as an electron sink, depriving anaerobes of reducing equivalents. Covalent binding or other interactions of intermediate metabolites of metronidazole with parasite macromolecules may partly explain the efficacy of this agent. Its benefit in dracunculiasis appears to be due to a reduction in inflammation rather than to any specific antihelminthic effect. Metronidazole is generally well tolerated despite common side effects such as nausea, headache, and a metabolic aftertaste. Alcohol should be avoided due to disulfiram-like effects. Although metronidazole has not been approved

or recommended for use during pregnancy, it has not been associated with birth defects.

Nifurtimox*   This nitrofuran compound is an effective oral agent for the treatment of acute Chagas' disease. Intracellular reduction followed by auto-oxidation yielding oxygen radicals has been suggested as the mode of action of nifurtimox on *Trypanosoma cruzi* and as the basis of its toxicity in humans. Prolonged use is required, but the course may have to be interrupted due to drug toxicity, which develops in 40 to 70% of recipients. Adverse reactions are common, dose related, and reversible. They include nausea, vomiting, abdominal pain, insomnia, seizures, and polyneuritis. Nifurtimox should be avoided in early pregnancy.

Nitazoxanide†   This 5-nitrothiazole compound appears to be a safe and effective alternative agent for the treatment of cryptosporidiosis. Its mechanism of action is unknown. It is currently available only from Romark Laboratories in the United States.

Oxamniquine   This tetrahydroquinoline derivative is an effective alternative agent for the treatment of schistosomiasis, although susceptibility to this drug exhibits regional variation. In treated adult schistosomes, oxamniquine produces marked tegumental alterations similar to those seen with praziquantel but less rapid (evident 4 to 8 days after treatment). Patients should be warned that their urine may have an intense orange-red color. Side effects are uncommon and usually mild, although hallucinations and seizures have been reported. Oxamniquine has not been shown to be teratogenic or embryotoxic, but its use in pregnancy has not been approved.

Paromomycin   This aminoglycoside is an effective oral agent for the treatment of infections due to intestinal protozoa. Like other aminoglycosides, it is poorly absorbed after oral administration and binds to the 30S ribosomal RNA in the aminoacyl-tRNA site, resulting in inhibition of protein synthesis. Paromomycin is well tolerated and safe for use in pregnancy.

Pentamidine Isethionate   This diamine is an effective alternative agent for some forms of leishmaniasis and trypanosomiasis. While its mechanism of action remains undefined, it is known to exert a wide range of effects, including interaction with trypanosomal kinetoplast DNA, interference with polyamine synthesis through a decrease in the activity of ornithine decarboxylase, and inhibition of RNA polymerase, ribosomal function, and the synthesis of nucleic acids and proteins. Adverse reactions are common and include hypotension, pancreatitis, hypoglycemia, arrhythmias, and reversible renal failure.

Praziquantel   This heterocyclic prazino-isoquinoline derivative is highly active against a broad spectrum of trematodes and cestodes. It disrupts the parasite tegument, resulting in contracture with loss of adherence to host tissues and ultimately disintegration or expulsion. Drug levels are reduced by concomitantly administered glucocorticoids, but cimetidine can be used to offset this problem. Praziquantel is generally well tolerated, but seizures may result in persons with neurocysticercosis. Patients with schistosomiasis who have heavy parasite burdens may develop abdominal discomfort, nausea, headache, dizziness, and drowsiness. Although praziquantel has not been shown to be mutagenic, teratogenic, or embryotoxic, it is preferable to delay treatment until after delivery unless immediate intervention is essential. Because praziquantel is excreted in breast milk, it is recommended that women not nurse on the day(s) of drug administration or for 72 h thereafter.

Primaquine Phosphate   This drug is the only agent available for eradication of the hepatic stage of malarial parasites. In order to be effective, it must be metabolized by the host. Although their parasiticidal activity remains unclear, the metabolites are believed to affect both pyrimidine synthesis and the mitochondrial electron transport chain. The major adverse effect of this drug is acute hemolysis in patients with glucose-6-phosphate dehydrogenase (G6PD) deficiency. Primaquine phosphate is otherwise well tolerated. Its use in pregnancy is contraindicated.

Proguanil (Chloroguanide) This agent, which inhibits plasmodial dihydrofolate reductase, is used with atovaquone for oral treatment of uncomplicated malaria or with chloroquine for prophylaxis in parts of Africa without widespread chloroquine-resistant *P. falciparum*. Proguanil is quite well tolerated at the usually prescribed doses, but higher doses can produce nausea, vomiting, abdominal pain, and diarrhea. It is not available in the United States.

Pyrantel Pamoate This safe, well-tolerated, and inexpensive pyrimidine derivative depolarizes the neuromuscular junctions of most intestinal nematodes, resulting in irreversible paralysis and allowing natural expulsion of the worms with the host's feces. The drug is poorly absorbed from the gastrointestinal tract and is usually effective in a single dose. It has minimal toxicity at the oral doses used to treat intestinal helminthic infection.

Pyrimethamine When combined with short-acting sulfonamides, this diaminopyrimidine is effective in malaria, toxoplasmosis, and isosporiasis. Unlike mammalian cells, the parasites that cause these infections cannot utilize preformed pyrimidines obtained through salvage pathways but rather rely completely on de novo synthesis of pyrimidines, for which folate derivatives are essential cofactors.

Pyrimethamine-sulfadoxine is an effective adjunctive agent for the oral treatment of uncomplicated malaria due to chloroquine-resistant organisms. However, its usefulness as a first-line agent is limited by the development of resistant strains of *P. falciparum* and *P. vivax*.

When combined with sulfadiazine, pyrimethamine is the treatment of choice for toxoplasmosis, but the duration of the required course of therapy often results in the development of folate deficiency requiring folinic acid supplementation. Sulfadiazine crystals can cause hematuria, and allergic drug reactions due to sulfadiazine often require a switch to clindamycin.

Quinacrine* Quinacrine is the only drug approved by the FDA for the treatment of giardiasis. It is not commercially available but can be obtained from alternative sources through the CDC Drug Service. Quinacrine intercalates into parasite DNA and inhibits nucleic acid synthesis. Side effects are common and include nausea and vomiting, headache, and skin discoloration. Alcohol is best avoided due to a disulfiram-like effect.

Quinine and Quinidine When combined with another agent, the cinchona alkaloid quinine is effective for the oral treatment of both uncomplicated malaria due to chloroquine-resistant strains and babesiosis. Quinine acts rapidly against the asexual blood stages of all forms of human malaria. For severe malaria, only quinidine (the dextroisomer of quinine) is available in the United States. Its use requires cardiac monitoring, and dose reduction is necessary in persons with severe renal impairment. Both quinine and quinidine can produce hypoglycemia. Symptoms of cinchonism (tinnitus, headache, nausea, and visual disturbances) are dose-related and reversible.

Spiramycin† This macrolide antibiotic is used to treat acute toxoplasmosis in pregnancy and congenital toxoplasmosis. Although not yet licensed in the United States, it is available through the FDA. Complications of treatment are rare but can include life-threatening ventricular arrhythmias in neonates.

Sodium Stibogluconate* and Meglumine Antimonate These pentavalent antimony compounds are first-line agents for the treatment of all forms of leishmaniasis. Despite their use in leishmaniasis for almost 100 years, their mechanism of action against *Leishmania* spp. remains unknown. Presumably, the compounds interfere with parasite metabolism. The drugs are taken up by the reticuloendothelial system, and their activity against *Leishmania* spp. may be enhanced by this localization. Resistance is a major problem in some areas of the world. Side effects are common and generally reversible but require temporary interruption of therapy in many cases. Chemical pancreatitis is almost universal, although it is often asymptomatic. In rare instances, pentavalent antimony compounds produce prolongation of the QT interval, and sudden death due to arrhythmia or cardiac failure has been reported. Arthralgias, myalgias, and headaches occur frequently. Since the drugs' safety in pregnancy has not been established, their use should be avoided if possible in pregnant women. These agents may be used in children >18 months of age.

Suramin* This derivative of urea is the drug of choice for the early stage of African trypanosomiasis. The drug acts by forming stable complexes with proteins, inhibiting multiple enzymes. Suramin has a variety of potentially severe side effects, including anaphylaxis, exfoliative dermatitis, paresthesias, photophobia, and renal dysfunction.

Tetracycline and Doxycycline These antibiotics are useful in the treatment of balantidiasis and *D. fragilis* infection as well as in the oral treatment of uncomplicated malaria due to chloroquine-resistant strains. The tetracyclines inhibit protein synthesis in prokaryotic ribosomes, and they probably have the same activity in parasites. Potential side effects in adults include nausea, vomiting, and photosensitivity dermatitis. Because they can impair normal development of bones and teeth, tetracyclines are contraindicated in pregnant women and children <8 years of age.

Thiabendazole This benzimidazole derivative is a potent antihelminthic agent, but its use in strongyloidiasis and other infections is limited by frequent, severe side effects. Patients most often report dizziness, headache, nausea, and vomiting. Less commonly, hepatitis and severe hypersensitivity reactions develop. The drug's mechanism of action is similar to that of other benzimidazoles. Treatment with thiabendazole is contraindicated in pregnancy.

Tinidazole This nitroimidazole is effective for the treatment of amebiasis, giardiasis, and trichomoniasis. Its mechanism of action and side effects are similar to those seen with metronidazole, but adverse events appear to be less frequent and severe with tinidazole. In addition, tinidazole is potentially curative in a single dose. This agent is currently unavailable in the United States.

Triclabendazole This benzimidazole is effective against paragonimiasis and all stages of *Fasciola hepatica*, a trematode with inherent resistance to praziquantel. The sulfoxide metabolite, which is believed to be responsible for the drug's activity, binds to fluke tubulin and disrupts microtubule-based processes. Triclabendazole is safe and well tolerated and offers single-dose cure. It is currently unavailable in the United States.

Trimethoprim-Sulfamethoxazole This synergistic antifolate compound is active against cyclosporiasis, isosporiasis, and encephalitis due to *Toxoplasma gondii*. Trimethoprim is a dihydrofolate reductase inhibitor whose effect is enhanced by sulfamethoxazole. Adverse effects, which can be severe, are usually attributable to the sulfonamide component and involve allergic skin reactions, bone marrow suppression, and hemolysis.

BIBLIOGRAPHY

ABRAMOWICZ M (ed): Drugs for parasitic infections. Med Lett Drugs Ther 40:1, 2000

LIU LX, WELLER PF: Antiparasitic drugs. N Engl J Med 334:1178, 1996

MOORE TA, NASH TE: Tissue Nematodes, in *Current Therapy of Infectious Disease*, 2d ed, D Schlossberg (ed). St. Louis, Mosby, 2000, pp 660–665

ROSENBLATT JE: Antiparasitic agents. Mayo Clin Proc 74:1161, 1999

WORLD HEALTH ORGANIZATION: *Model Prescribing Information: Drugs Used in Parasitic Diseases*, 2d ed. Geneva, WHO, 1995

213 | *Sharon L. Reed*

AMEBIASIS AND INFECTION WITH FREE-LIVING AMEBAS

AMEBIASIS

DEFINITION   Amebiasis is an infection with the intestinal protozoan *Entamoeba histolytica*. About 90% of infections are asymptomatic, and the remaining 10% produce a spectrum of clinical syndromes ranging from dysentery to abscesses of the liver or other organs.

LIFE CYCLE AND TRANSMISSION   *E. histolytica* is acquired by ingestion of viable cysts from fecally contaminated water, food, or hands. Food-borne exposure is most prevalent and is particularly likely when food handlers are shedding cysts or food is being grown with feces-contaminated soil, fertilizer, or water. Less common means of transmission include contaminated water, oral and anal sexual practices, and—in rare instances—direct rectal inoculation through colonic irrigation devices. Motile trophozoites are released from cysts in the small intestine and, in most patients, remain as harmless commensals in the large bowel. After encystation, infectious cysts are shed in the stool and can survive for several weeks in a moist environment. In some patients, the trophozoites invade either the bowel mucosa, causing symptomatic colitis, or the bloodstream, causing distant abscesses of the liver, lungs, or brain. The trophozoites may not encyst in patients with active dysentery, and motile hematophagous trophozoites are frequently present in fresh stools. Trophozoites are rapidly killed by exposure to air or stomach acid, however, and therefore cannot cause infection.

EPIDEMIOLOGY   About 10% of the world's population is infected with *Entamoeba*, the majority with noninvasive *Entamoeba dispar*. Amebiasis results from infection with *E. histolytica* and is the third most common cause of death from parasitic disease (after schistosomiasis and malaria). Areas of highest incidence (due to inadequate sanitation and crowding) include most developing countries in the tropics, particularly Mexico, India, and nations of Central and South America, tropical Asia, and Africa. The main groups at risk in developed countries are travelers, recent immigrants, homosexual men, and inmates of institutions.

The wide spectrum of clinical disease is caused in part by infection with the two different species of *Entamoeba*. Isolates of *E. histolytica* from patients with invasive amebiasis have unique isoenzymes, surface antigens, DNA markers, and virulence properties and now are recognized as a distinct species from the noninvasive *E. dispar*.

Most asymptomatic carriers, including homosexual men and AIDS patients, harbor *E. dispar* and have self-limited infections. These observations suggest that *E. dispar* is incapable of causing invasive disease, since *Cryptosporidium* and *Isospora belli*, which also cause only self-limited illnesses in immunocompetent people, cause devastating diarrhea in patients with AIDS. However, host factors play a role as well. In one study, 10% of asymptomatic patients who were colonized with *E. histolytica* went on to develop amebic colitis, while the rest remained asymptomatic and cleared the infection within 1 year.

PATHOGENESIS AND PATHOLOGY   Both trophozoites (Fig. 213-1) and cysts (Fig. 213-2) are found in the intestinal lumen, but only trophozoites of *E. histolytica* invade tissue. The trophozoite is 20 to 60 μm in diameter and contains vacuoles and a nucleus with a characteristic central karyosome. In animals, depletion of intestinal mucus, diffuse inflammation, and disruption of the epithelial barrier occur before trophozoites actually come into contact with the colonic mucosa. Trophozoites attach to colonic mucus and epithelial cells by a galactose-inhibitable lectin. The earliest intestinal lesions are mi-

FIGURE 213-1   Trophozoite of *E. histolytica* demonstrating a single nucleus with a central, dotlike karyosome (trichrome stain).

croulcerations of the mucosa of the cecum, sigmoid colon, or rectum that release erythrocytes, inflammatory cells, and epithelial cells. Proctoscopy reveals small ulcers with heaped up margins and normal intervening mucosa. Submucosal extension of ulcerations under viable-appearing surface mucosa causes the classic "flask-shaped" ulcer containing trophozoites at the margins of dead and viable tissues. Although neutrophilic infiltrates may accompany the early lesions in animals, human intestinal infection is marked by a paucity of inflammatory cells, probably in part because of the killing of neutrophils by trophozoites. Treated ulcers characteristically heal with little or no scarring. Occasionally, however, full-thickness necrosis and perforation occur.

Rarely, intestinal infection results in the formation of a mass lesion, or *ameboma*, in the bowel lumen. The overlying mucosa is usually thin and ulcerated, while other layers of the wall are thickened, edematous, and hemorrhagic; this condition results in exuberant formation of granulation tissue with little fibrous-tissue response.

A number of virulence factors have been linked to the ability of *E. histolytica* to invade through the interglandular epithelium. One is an extracellular cysteine proteinase that degrades collagen, elastin, secretory IgA, and the anaphylatoxins C3a and C5a. Other enzymes may

FIGURE 213-2   Cyst of *E. histolytica* showing three of the four nuclei (trichrome stain).

disrupt glycoprotein bonds between mucosal epithelial cells in the gut. Amebas can lyse neutrophils, monocytes, lymphocytes, and cells of colonic and hepatic cell lines. The cytolytic effect of amebas appears to require direct contact with target cells and may be linked to the release of phospholipase A and pore-forming peptides.

Liver abscesses are always preceded by intestinal colonization, which may be asymptomatic. Blood vessels may be compromised early by lysis of the wall and thrombus formation. Trophozoites invade veins to reach the liver through the portal venous system. *E. histolytica* is resistant to complement-mediated lysis, a property critical to survival in the bloodstream. In contrast, *E. dispar* is rapidly lysed by complement and is thus restricted to the bowel lumen. Inoculation of amebas into the portal system of hamsters results in an acute cellular infiltrate consisting predominantly of neutrophils. Later, the neutrophils are lysed by contact with amebas, and the release of neutrophil toxins may contribute to necrosis of hepatocytes. The liver parenchyma is replaced by necrotic material that is surrounded by a thin rim of congested liver tissue. The necrotic contents of a liver abscess are classically described as "anchovy paste," although the fluid is variable in color and is composed of bacteriologically sterile granular debris with few or no cells. Amebas, if seen, tend to be found near the capsule of the abscess.

Clinical infection does not induce immunity to recurrent colonization with *E. histolytica*, but repeated episodes of colitis or liver abscess are unusual. Antibody is not protective; titers correlate with the length of illness rather than with the severity of disease. Studies of animals suggest that cell-mediated immunity may be important for protection, although patients with AIDS appear not to be predisposed to more severe disease.

CLINICAL SYNDROMES **Intestinal Amebiasis** The most common type of amebic infection is asymptomatic cyst passage. Even in highly endemic areas, most patients harbor *E. dispar*.

Symptomatic amebic colitis develops 2 to 6 weeks after the ingestion of infectious cysts. Lower abdominal pain and mild diarrhea develop gradually and are followed by malaise, weight loss, and diffuse lower abdominal or back pain. Cecal involvement may mimic acute appendicitis. Patients with full-blown dysentery may pass 10 to 12 stools per day. The stools contain little fecal material and consist mainly of blood and mucus. In contrast to those with bacterial diarrhea, fewer than 40% of patients with amebic dysentery are febrile. Virtually all patients have heme-positive stools.

More fulminant intestinal infection, with severe abdominal pain, high fever, and profuse diarrhea, is rare and occurs predominantly in children. Patients may develop toxic megacolon, in which there is severe bowel dilation with intramural air. Patients receiving glucocorticoids are at risk for severe amebiasis. Uncommonly, patients develop a chronic form of amebic colitis, which can be confused with inflammatory bowel disease. The association between severe amebiasis complications and glucocorticoid therapy emphasizes the importance of excluding amebiasis when inflammatory bowel disease is suspected. An occasional patient presents with only an asymptomatic or tender abdominal mass caused by an ameboma, which is easily confused with cancer on barium studies. A positive serologic test or biopsy can prevent unnecessary surgery in this setting. The syndrome of postamebic colitis—persistent diarrhea following documented cure of amebic colitis—is controversial; no evidence of recurrent amebic infection can be found, and re-treatment usually has no effect.

Amebic Liver Abscess Extraintestinal infection by *E. histolytica* most often involves the liver. Of travelers who develop an amebic liver abscess after leaving an endemic area, 95% do so within 5 months. Young patients with an amebic liver abscess are more likely than older patients to present in the acute phase with prominent symptoms of <10 days duration. Most patients are febrile and have right-upper-quadrant pain, which may be dull or pleuritic in nature and radiate to the shoulder. Point tenderness over the liver and right-sided pleural effusion are common. Jaundice is rare. Although the initial site

of infection is the colon, fewer than one-third of patients with an amebic abscess have active diarrhea. Older patients from endemic areas are more likely to have a subacute course lasting 6 months, with weight loss and hepatomegaly. About one-third of patients with chronic presentations are febrile. Thus, the clinical diagnosis of an amebic liver abscess may be difficult to establish because the symptoms and signs are often nonspecific. Since 10 to 15% of patients present only with fever, amebic liver abscess must be considered in the differential diagnosis of fever of unknown origin (Chap. 125).

Complications of Amebic Liver Abscess Pleuropulmonary involvement, which is reported in 20 to 30% of patients, is the most frequent complication of amebic liver abscess. Manifestations include sterile effusions, contiguous spread from the liver, and rupture into the pleural space. Sterile effusions and contiguous spread usually resolve with medical therapy, but frank rupture into the pleural space requires drainage. A hepatobronchial fistula may cause cough productive of large amounts of necrotic material that may contain amebas. This dramatic complication carries a good prognosis. Abscesses that rupture into the peritoneum may present as an indolent leak or an acute abdomen and require both percutaneous catheter drainage and medical therapy. Rupture into the pericardium, usually from abscesses of the left lobe of the liver, carries the gravest prognosis; it can occur during medical therapy and requires surgical drainage.

Other Extraintestinal Sites The genitourinary tract may become involved by direct extension of amebiasis from the colon or by hematogenous spread of the infection. Painful genital ulcers, characterized by a punched-out appearance and profuse discharge, may develop secondary to extension from either the intestine or the liver. Both these conditions respond well to medical therapy. Cerebral involvement has been reported in fewer than 0.1% of patients in large clinical series. Symptoms and prognosis depend on the size and location of the lesion.

DIAGNOSTIC TESTS **Laboratory Diagnosis** Stool examinations, serologic tests, and noninvasive imaging of the liver are the most important procedures in the diagnosis of amebiasis. Fecal findings suggestive of amebic colitis include a positive test for heme, a paucity of neutrophils, and the presence of Charcot-Leyden crystal protein (double pyramid-shaped crystals normally found in the cytoplasm of eosinophils). The definitive diagnosis of amebic colitis is made by the demonstration of hematophagous trophozoites of *E. histolytica* (Fig. 213-1). Because trophozoites are killed rapidly by water, drying, or barium, it is important to examine at least three fresh stool specimens. Examination of a combination of wet mounts, iodine-stained concentrates, and trichrome-stained preparations of fresh stool and concentrates for cysts (Fig. 213-2) or trophozoites (Fig. 213-1) confirms the diagnosis in 75 to 95% of cases. Cultures of amebas are more sensitive but are not routinely available. If stool examinations are negative, sigmoidoscopy with biopsy of the edge of ulcers may increase the yield, but this procedure is dangerous during fulminant colitis because of the risk of perforation. Trophozoites in a biopsy specimen from a colonic mass confirm the diagnosis of ameboma, but trophozoites are rare in liver aspirates. Accurate diagnosis requires experience, since the trophozoites may be confused with neutrophils and the cysts must be differentiated morphologically from *Entamoeba hartmanni*, *Entamoeba coli*, and *Endolimax nana*, which do not cause clinical disease and do not warrant therapy. Unfortunately, the cysts of *E. histolytica* cannot be distinguished microscopically from those of *E. dispar*. Therefore, the microscopic diagnosis of *E. histolytica* can be made only by the detection of *Entamoeba* trophozoites that have ingested erythrocytes (Fig. 213-1). Diagnostic tests based on the detection of the galactose-inhibitable lectin of *E. histolytica* are now available and compare favorably with the polymerase chain reaction and with isolation in culture followed by isoenzyme analysis in terms of sensitivity.

Serology is an important addition to the methods used for the parasitologic diagnosis of invasive amebiasis. Kits for the performance of agar gel diffusion assays and ELISAs are commercially available, and the results of these tests are positive in more than 90% of patients with colitis, amebomas, or liver abscess. Positive results in conjunction with the appropriate clinical syndrome suggest active disease because serologic findings usually revert to negative within 6 to 12 months. Even in highly endemic areas such as South Africa, fewer than 10% of asymptomatic individuals have a positive amebic serology. The interpretation of the indirect hemagglutination test is more difficult because titers may remain positive for as long as 10 years.

Up to 10% of patients with acute amebic liver abscess may have negative serologic findings; in suspected cases with an initially negative result, testing should be repeated in a week. In contrast to carriers of *E. dispar*, most asymptomatic carriers of *E. histolytica* develop antibodies. Thus, serologic tests are helpful in assessing the risk of invasive amebiasis in asymptomatic, cyst-passing individuals in nonendemic areas. Serologic tests also should be performed in patients with ulcerative colitis before the institution of glucocorticoid therapy to prevent the development of severe colitis or toxic megacolon owing to unsuspected amebiasis.

Routine hematology and chemistry tests are usually not very helpful in the diagnosis of invasive amebiasis. About three-fourths of patients with an amebic liver abscess have leukocytosis (>10,000 cells/μL); this condition is particularly likely if symptoms are acute or complications have developed. Invasive amebiasis does not elicit eosinophilia. Anemia, if present, is usually multifactorial. Even with large liver abscesses, liver enzyme levels are normal or minimally elevated. The alkaline phosphatase level is most often elevated and may remain so for months. Aminotransferase elevations suggest acute disease or a complication.

Radiographic Studies Radiographic barium studies are potentially dangerous in acute amebic colitis. Amebomas are usually identified first by a barium enema, but biopsy is necessary for differentiation from carcinoma.

Radiographic techniques such as ultrasonography, computed tomography (Fig. 213-3), and magnetic resonance imaging are all useful for detection of the round or oval hypoechoic cyst. More than 80% of patients who have had symptoms for >10 days have a single abscess of the right lobe of the liver. Approximately 50% of patients who have had symptoms for <10 days have multiple abscesses. Findings associated with complications include large abscesses (>10 cm) in the superior part of the right lobe, which may rupture into the pleural space; multiple lesions, which must be differentiated from pyogenic abscesses; and lesions of the left lobe, which may rupture into the pericardium. Because abscesses resolve slowly and may increase in size in patients who are responding clinically to therapy, frequent follow-up ultrasonography may prove confusing. Complete resolution of a liver abscess within 6 months can be anticipated in two-thirds of patients, but 10% may have persistent abnormalities for a year.

DIFFERENTIAL DIAGNOSIS The differential diagnosis of intestinal amebiasis includes bacterial diarrheas caused by *Campylobacter*; enteroinvasive *Escherichia coli*; and *Shigella*, *Salmonella*, and *Vibrio* species. Although the typical patient with amebic colitis has less prominent fever than in these other conditions as well as heme-positive stools with few neutrophils, correct diagnosis requires bacterial cultures, microscopic examination of stools, and amebic serologic testing. As has already been mentioned, amebiasis must be ruled out in any patient thought to have inflammatory bowel disease.

Because of the variety of presenting signs and symptoms, amebic liver abscess can easily be confused with pulmonary or gallbladder disease or with any febrile illness with few localizing signs, such as malaria or typhoid fever. The diagnosis should be considered in members of high-risk groups who have recently traveled outside the United States and in inmates of institutions. Once radiographic studies have identified an abscess in the liver, the most important differential diagnosis is between amebic and pyogenic abscess. Patients with pyogenic abscess typically are older and have a history of underlying bowel disease or recent surgery. Amebic serology is helpful, but aspiration of the abscess, with Gram's staining and culture of the material, may be required for differentiation of the two diseases.

℞ TREATMENT Intestinal Disease The drugs used to treat amebiasis can be classified according to their primary site of action. Luminal amebicides are poorly absorbed and reach high concentrations in the bowel, but their activity is limited to cysts and trophozoites close to the mucosa. Only two luminal drugs are available in the United States: iodoquinol and paromomycin (Table 213-1). Indications for the use of luminal agents include eradication of cysts in patients with colitis or a liver abscess and treatment of asymptomatic carriers. The majority of asymptomatic individuals who pass cysts are colonized with *E. dispar*, which does not warrant specific therapy. However, unless the presence of *E. dispar* can be proven by specific antigen detection tests and the lack of an antibody response, it may be prudent to treat asymptomatic individuals who pass cysts.

Tissue amebicides reach high concentrations in the blood and tissue after oral or parenteral administration. The development of nitroimidazole compounds, especially metronidazole, was a major advance in the treatment of invasive amebiasis. Patients with amebic colitis should be treated with intravenous or oral metronidazole (750 mg three times daily for 5 to 10 days). Side effects include nausea, vomiting, abdominal discomfort, and a disulfiram-like reaction. Other imidazole compounds, such as tinidazole and ornidazole, are as effective but are

FIGURE 213-3 Abdominal computed tomography scan of a large amebic abscess of the right lobe of the liver. (*Courtesy of the Department of Radiology, UCSD Medical Center, San Diego.*)

Table 213-1 Drug Therapy for Amebiasis

Drug	Dosage
ASYMPTOMATIC CARRIER (LUMINAL AGENTS)	
Iodoquinol (650-mg tablets)	650 mg tid for 20 days
Paromomycin (250-mg tablets)	500 mg tid for 10 days
ACUTE COLITIS	
Metronidazole (250- or 500-mg tablets) plus	750 mg PO or IV tid for 5 to 10 days
Luminal agent as above	
AMEBIC LIVER ABSCESS	
Metronidazole	750 mg PO or IV tid for 5 to 10 days
Tinidazole[a]	2 g PO
Ornidazole[a] plus	2 g PO
Luminal agent as above	

[a] Not available in the United States.

not available in the United States. All patients should also receive a full course of therapy with a luminal agent, since metronidazole does not eradicate cysts. Resistance to metronidazole has not been identified. Relapses are not uncommon and probably represent reinfection or failure to eradicate amebas from the bowel because of an inadequate dosage or duration of therapy.

Amebic Liver Abscess Metronidazole is the drug of choice for amebic liver abscess. The usefulness of nitroimidazoles in single-dose or abbreviated regimens is important in endemic areas where access to hospitalization is limited. With early diagnosis and therapy, mortality from uncomplicated amebic liver abscess is <1%. The second-line therapeutic agents emetine and chloroquine should be avoided if possible because of the potential cardiovascular and gastrointestinal side effects of the former and the higher relapse rates with the latter. There is no evidence that combined therapy with two drugs is more effective than the single-drug regimen. Studies of South Africans with liver abscesses demonstrated that 72% of patients without intestinal symptoms had bowel infection with *E. histolytica*; thus, all treatment regimens should include a luminal agent to eradicate cysts and prevent further transmission. Amebic liver abscess recurs rarely.

Aspiration of Liver Abscesses More than 90% of patients respond dramatically to metronidazole therapy with decreases in both pain and fever within 72 h. Indications for aspiration of liver abscesses are (1) the need to rule out a pyogenic abscess, particularly in patients with multiple lesions; (2) the failure to respond clinically in 3 to 5 days; (3) the threat of imminent rupture; and (4) the prevention of rupture of left-lobe abscesses into the pericardium. There is no evidence that aspiration, even of large abscesses (up to 10 cm), accelerates healing. Percutaneous drainage may be successful even if the liver abscess has already ruptured. Surgery should be reserved for instances of bowel perforation and rupture into the pericardium.

PREVENTION Amebic infection is spread by ingestion of food or water contaminated with cysts. Since an asymptomatic carrier may excrete up to 15 million cysts per day, prevention of infection requires adequate sanitation and eradication of cyst carriage. In high-risk areas, infection can be minimized by the avoidance of unpeeled fruits and vegetables and the use of bottled water. Because cysts are resistant to readily attainable levels of chlorine, disinfection by iodination (tetraglycine hydroperiodide) is recommended. There is no effective prophylaxis.

INFECTION WITH FREE-LIVING AMEBAS

EPIDEMIOLOGY Free-living amebas of the genera *Acanthamoeba*, *Naegleria*, and *Balamuthia* are distributed throughout the world and have been isolated from a wide variety of fresh and brackish water, including that from lakes, taps, hot springs, swimming pools, and heating and air-conditioning units, and even from the nasal passages of healthy children. Encystation may protect the protozoa from desiccation and food deprivation. The persistence of *Legionella pneumophila* in water supplies may be attributable in part to chronic infection of free-living amebas, particularly *Naegleria*.

NAEGLERIA INFECTIONS Primary amebic meningoencephalitis caused by *Naegleria fowleri* follows the aspiration of water contaminated with trophozoites or cysts or the inhalation of contaminated dust, leading to invasion of the olfactory neuroepithelium. After an incubation period of 2 to 15 days, severe headache, high fever, nausea, vomiting, and meningismus develop. Photophobia and palsies of the third, fourth, and sixth cranial nerves are common. Rapid progression to seizures and coma may follow, and most patients die within a week. Infection is most common in otherwise healthy children or young adults, who often report recent swimming in lakes or heated swimming pools.

Diagnosis depends on the detection of motile trophozoites in wet mounts of fresh spinal fluid. Other laboratory findings resemble those for fulminant bacterial meningitis, with elevated intracranial pressure, high white blood cell counts (up to 20,000 cells/μL), and elevated protein concentrations and low glucose levels in cerebrospinal fluid. The diagnosis should be considered in any patient who has purulent meningitis without evidence of bacteria on Gram's staining, antigen detection assay, and culture. The prognosis is uniformly poor. Only four survivors, treated with high-dose amphotericin B and rifampin, have been reported. Antibodies to *Naegleria* spp. have been detected in normal adults; serologic testing is not useful in the diagnosis of acute infection.

ACANTHAMOEBA INFECTIONS **Granulomatous Amebic Encephalitis** Infection with *Acanthamoeba* species follows a more indolent course and occurs typically in chronically ill or debilitated patients. Risk factors include lymphoproliferative disorders, chemotherapy, glucocorticoid therapy, lupus erythematosus, and AIDS. Infection usually reaches the central nervous system hematogenously from a primary focus in the sinuses, skin, or lungs. In the central nervous system, the onset is insidious, and the syndrome often mimics a space-occupying lesion. Altered mental status, headache, and stiff neck may be accompanied by focal findings such as cranial nerve palsies, ataxia, and hemiparesis. In the United States, cutaneous ulcers or hard nodules containing amebas were detected in 8 of 13 AIDS patients with disseminated *Acanthamoeba* infection.

Examination of the cerebrospinal fluid for trophozoites may be diagnostically helpful, but lumbar puncture may be contraindicated because of increased intracerebral pressure. Computed tomography frequently reveals cortical and subcortical lesions of decreased density consistent with embolic infarcts. In other patients, multiple enhancing lesions with edema may mimic the computed tomographic appearance of toxoplasmosis. Demonstration of the trophozoites and cysts of *Acanthamoeba* on wet mounts or in biopsy specimens establishes the diagnosis. Culture on nonnutrient agar plates seeded with *Escherichia coli* may also be helpful. Fluorescein-labeled antiserum is available from the Centers for Disease Control and Prevention (CDC) for the detection of protozoa in biopsy specimens. At least nine cases of granulomatous amebic encephalitis have been reported in patients with AIDS, in whom the disease may have an accelerated course (with survival for only 3 to 40 days) because of their difficulty in forming granulomas. Although studies in animals suggest that rifampin may be useful, the infection is almost uniformly fatal.

Keratitis The incidence of keratitis caused by *Acanthamoeba* has increased in the past 20 years, in part as a result of improved diagnosis. The first of these infections to be recognized were associated with trauma to the eye and exposure to contaminated water. At present, most infections are linked to extended-wear contact lenses. Risk factors include the use of homemade saline, the wearing of lenses while swimming, and inadequate disinfection. Since contact lenses presumably cause microscopic trauma, the early corneal findings may be nonspecific. The first symptoms usually include tearing and the painful sensation of a foreign body. Once infection is established, progression is rapid; the characteristic clinical sign is an annular, paracentral corneal ring representing a corneal abscess. Deeper corneal invasion and loss of vision may follow.

The differential diagnosis includes bacterial, mycobacterial, and herpetic infection. The irregular polygonal cysts of *Acanthamoeba* (Fig. 213-4) may be identified in corneal scrapings or biopsy material, and trophozoites can be grown on special media. Cysts are resistant to available drugs, and the results of medical therapy have been disappointing. Some reports have suggested partial responses to propamidine isethionate eyedrops. Severe infections usually require keratoplasty.

BALAMUTHIA INFECTIONS *Balamuthia mandrillaris*, a free-living ameba previously referred to as a leptomyxid ameba, is an important etiologic agent of amebic meningoencephalitis in immunocompetent hosts. The course is typically subacute, with focal neurologic signs, fever, seizures, and headaches leading to death within 1 week to several months after onset. Examination of cerebrospinal fluid reveals mononuclear pleocytosis, elevated protein levels, and normal to low glucose concentrations. Multiple hypodense lesions are usually

FIGURE 213-4 Double-walled cyst of *Acanthamoeba castellani*, as seen by phase-contrast microscopy. *[From DJ Krogstad et al, in A Balows et al (eds): Manual of Clinical Microbiology, 5th ed. Washington, DC, American Society for Microbiology, 1991.]*

detected with imaging studies. The diagnosis is almost always made post-mortem, and specific identification may require immunofluorescence with antibodies from the CDC to differentiate the trophozoites from *Acanthamoeba*.

BIBLIOGRAPHY

AMEBIASIS

HAQUE R et al: Comparison of PCR, isoenzyme analysis, and antigen detection for diagnosis of *Entamoeba histolytica* infection. J Clin Microbiol 36:449, 1998

IRUSEN EM et al: Asymptomatic intestinal colonization by pathogenic *Entamoeba histolytica* in amebic liver abscess: Prevalence, response to therapy, and pathogenic potential. Clin Infect Dis 14:889, 1992

PETRI WA: Amebiasis and the *Entamoeba histolytica* Gal/GalNAc lectin: From bench to bedside. J Invest Med 44:24, 1996

————, SINGH U: Diagnosis and management of amebiasis. Clin Infect Dis 29:1117, 1999

QUE X, REED SL: The role of extracellular cysteine proteinases in pathogenesis of *Entamoeba histolytica* invasion. Parasitol Today 13:190, 1997

REED SL et al: *Entamoeba histolytica* infection and AIDS. Am J Med 90:269, 1991

STANLEY SL: Progress toward development of a vaccine for amebiasis. Clin Microbiol Rev 10:637, 1997

THOMPSON JE et al: Amebic liver abscess: A therapeutic approach. Rev Infect Dis 7:171, 1985

ACANTHAMOEBA, *NAEGLERIA*, AND *BALAMUTHIA*

DENNEY CF et al: Amebic meningoencephalitis caused by *Balamuthia mandrillaris*: Case report and review. Clin Infect Dis 25:1354, 1997

LARKIN DFP : *Acanthamoeba* keratitis. Int Ophthalmol Clin 31:163, 1991

MARTINEZ AJ, VISVESVARA GS: Free-living, amphizoic and opportunistic amebas. Brain Pathol 7:583, 1997

SISON JP et al: Disseminated *Acanthamoeba* infection in patients with AIDS: Case reports and review. Clin Infect Dis 20:1207, 1995

214

Nicholas J. White, Joel G. Breman

MALARIA AND BABESIOSIS: DISEASES CAUSED BY RED BLOOD CELL PARASITES

"Humanity has but three great enemies: Fever, famine and war; of these by far the greatest, by far the most terrible, is fever."

William Osler

MALARIA

Malaria is a protozoan disease transmitted by the bite of infected *Anopheles* mosquitoes. It is the most important of the parasitic diseases of humans, with transmission in 103 countries affecting more than 1 billion people and causing between 1 and 3 million deaths each year. Malaria has now been eradicated from North America, Europe, and Russia but, despite enormous control efforts, has resurged in many parts of the tropics. Added to this resurgence are the increasing problems of drug resistance of the parasite and insecticide resistance of the vectors. Occasional local transmission following importation of malaria has occurred recently in several southern and eastern areas of the United States and in Europe, indicating the continual danger to nonmalarious countries. Malaria remains today, as it has been for centuries, a heavy burden on tropical communities, a threat to nonendemic countries, and a danger to travelers.

ETIOLOGY AND PATHOGENESIS Four species of the genus *Plasmodium* cause nearly all malarial infections in humans (although rare infections involve species normally affecting other primates). These are *P. falciparum*, *P. vivax*, *P. ovale*, and *P. malariae* (Table 214-1). Almost all deaths are caused by falciparum malaria. Human infection begins when a female anopheline mosquito inoculates plasmodial sporozoites from its salivary gland during a blood meal (Fig. 214-1). These microscopic motile forms of the malarial parasite are carried rapidly via the bloodstream to the liver, where they invade hepatic parenchymal cells and begin a period of asexual reproduction. By this amplification process (known as intrahepatic or preerythrocytic schizogony or merogony), a single sporozoite eventually may produce 10,000 to more than 30,000 daughter merozoites. The swollen liver cell eventually bursts, discharging motile merozoites into the bloodstream; at this point the symptomatic stage of the infection begins. In *P. vivax* and *P. ovale* infections, a proportion of the intrahepatic forms do not divide immediately but remain dormant for months to years before reproduction begins. These dormant forms, or hypnozoites, are the cause of the relapses that characterize infection with these two species.

After entry into the bloodstream, merozoites rapidly invade erythrocytes and become trophozoites. Attachment is mediated via a specific erythrocyte surface receptor. In the case of *P. vivax*, this receptor is related to the Duffy blood-group antigen Fy^a or Fy^b. Most West Africans and people with origins in that region carry the Duffy-negative FyFy phenotype and are therefore resistant to *P. vivax* malaria. During the early stage of intraerythrocytic development, the small "ring forms" of the four parasitic species appear similar under light microscopy. As the trophozoites enlarge, species-specific characteristics become evident, pigment becomes visible, and the parasite assumes an irregular or ameboid shape. By the end of the 48-h intraerythrocytic life cycle (72 h for *P. malariae*), the parasite has consumed nearly all the hemoglobin and grown to occupy most of the red cell. Multiple nuclear divisions take place (merogony), and the red cell ruptures to release 6 to 30 daughter merozoites, each capable of invading a new red cell and repeating the cycle. The disease in human beings is caused by the direct effects of red cell invasion and destruction by the asexual parasite and the host's reaction. After a series of asexual cycles (*P. falciparum*) or immediately (*P. vivax*, *P. ovale*, *P. malariae*), some of the parasites develop into morphologically distinct long-lived sexual forms (gametocytes) that can transmit malaria.

After being ingested in the blood meal of a biting female anopheline mosquito, the male and female gametocytes form a zygote in the insect's midgut. This zygote matures into an ookinete, which penetrates and encysts in the mosquito's gut wall. The resulting oocyst expands by asexual division until it bursts to liberate myriad motile sporozoites, which then migrate in the hemolymph to the salivary gland of the mosquito to await inoculation into another human at the next feeding.

EPIDEMIOLOGY Malaria occurs throughout most of the tropical regions of the world (Fig. 214-2). *P. falciparum* predominates in Africa, New Guinea, and Haiti; *P. vivax* is more common in Central America and the Indian subcontinent. The prevalence of these two

Table 214-1 Characteristics of *Plasmodium* Species Infecting Humans

Characteristic	Finding for Indicated Species			
	P. falciparum	*P. vivax*	*P. ovale*	*P. malariae*
Duration of intrahepatic phase (days)	5.5	8	9	15
Number of merozoites released per infected hepatocyte	30,000	10,000	15,000	15,000
Duration of erythrocytic cycle (hours)	48	48	50	72
Red cell preference	Younger cells (but can invade cells of all ages)	Reticulocytes	Reticulocytes	Older cells
Morphology	Usually only ring forms[a]; banana-shaped gametocytes	Irregularly shaped large rings and trophozoites; enlarged erythrocytes; Schüffner's dots	Infected erythrocytes, enlarged and oval; Schüffner's dots	Band or rectangular forms of trophozoites common
Pigment color	Black	Yellow-brown	Dark brown	Brown-black
Ability to cause relapses	No	Yes	Yes	No

[a] Parasitemia sometimes exceeds 2% with multiple infections of a single erythrocyte.

species is approximately equal in South America, eastern Asia, and Oceania. *P. malariae* is found in most endemic areas, especially throughout sub-Saharan Africa, but is much less common than the other species mentioned. *P. ovale* is relatively unusual outside of Africa and, where it is found, comprises <1% of isolates.

The epidemiology of malaria is complex and may vary considerably even within relatively small geographic areas. Endemicity traditionally has been defined in terms of parasitemia rates or palpable-spleen rates in children 2 to 9 years of age as hypoendemic (<10%), mesoendemic (11 to 50%), hyperendemic (51 to 75%), and holoendemic (>75%). In holo- and hyperendemic areas—e.g., certain regions of tropical Africa or coastal New Guinea, where there is intense *P. falciparum* transmission and there can be more than one human bite per infected mosquito per day—people are infected repeatedly throughout their lives. Here, morbidity and mortality during childhood are considerable. Immunity against disease is hard won in these areas, and the young-childhood burden of disease is high; by adulthood, however, most malarial infections are asymptomatic. This situation, with frequent year-round infection, is termed *stable transmission* and generally occurs where there is holo- and hyperendemicity. In areas where transmission is low, erratic, or focal, full protective immunity is not acquired, and symptomatic disease may occur at all ages. This situation usually exists in hypoendemic areas and is termed *unstable transmission*. Even in areas with stable transmission, there is often an increased incidence coinciding with increased mosquito breeding during the rainy season. Malaria behaves like an epidemic disease in some areas, particularly those with unstable malaria, such as northern India, Sri Lanka, Southeast Asia, Ethiopia, southern Africa, and Madagascar. An epidemic can develop when there are changes in environmental, economic, or social conditions, such as heavy rains following drought or migrations (usually of refugees or workers) from a nonmalarious region to an area of high transmission; a breakdown in malaria control and prevention services can intensify epidemic conditions. This situation usually results in considerable mortality among all age groups.

The principal determinants of the epidemiology of malaria are the number (density), the human-biting habits, and the longevity of the anopheline mosquito vectors. Not all anophelines can transmit malaria, and those that do vary considerably in their efficiency as malaria vectors. More specifically, the transmission of malaria is directly proportional to the density of the vector, the square of the number of human bites per day per mosquito, and the tenth power of the probability of the mosquito's surviving for 1 day. Mosquito longevity is particularly important, because the portion of the parasite's life cycle that takes place within the mosquito—from gametocyte ingestion to subsequent inoculation (sporogony)—lasts for 8 to 30 days, depending on ambient temperature; thus, to transmit malaria, the mosquito must survive for longer than 7 days. In general, at temperatures below 16 to 18°C, sporogony is not completed and transmission does not occur. Therefore, the most effective mosquito vectors of malaria are those such as *A. gambiae*, which are long-lived, occur in high densities in tropical climates, breed readily, and bite humans in preference to other animals. The entomologic inoculation rate—the number of sporozoite-positive mosquito bites per year—is the most common measure of malarial transmission and varies from <1 in some parts of Latin America and Southeast Asia to >300 in parts of tropical Africa.

ERYTHROCYTE CHANGES IN MALARIA After invading an erythrocyte, the growing parasite progressively consumes and degrades intracellular proteins, principally hemoglobin. The potentially toxic heme is polymerized to biologically inert hemozoin, or malaria pigment. The parasite also alters the red cell membrane by changing its transport properties, exposing cryptic surface antigens, and inserting new parasite-derived proteins. The red cell becomes more irregular in shape, more antigenic, and less deformable.

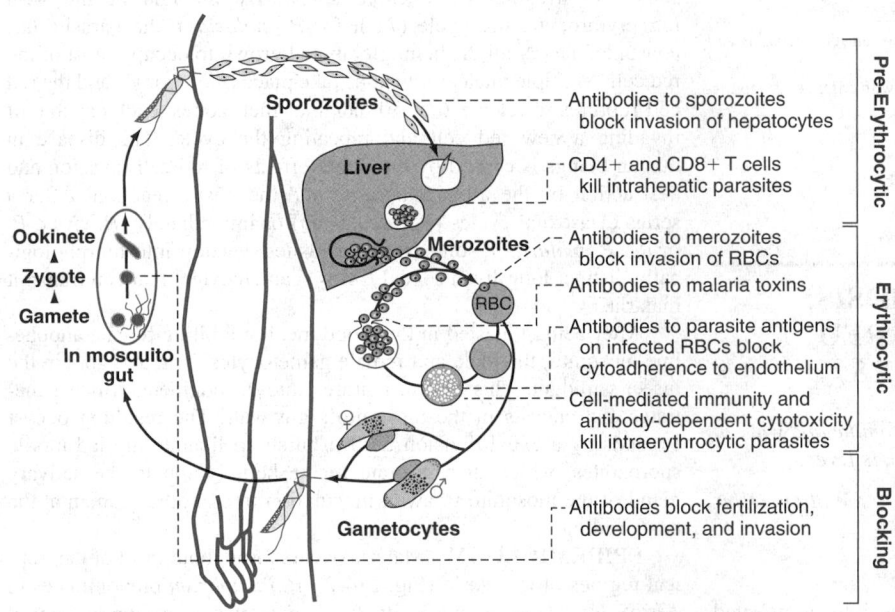

FIGURE 214-1 The malaria transmission cycle.

In *P. falciparum* infections, membrane protuberances appear on the erythrocyte's surface in the second 24 h of the asexual cycle. These "knobs" extrude a high-molecular-weight, antigenically variant, strain-specific, adhesive protein (PfEMP1) that mediates attachment to receptors on venular and capillary endothelium—an event termed *cytoadherence*. Several receptors have been identified, of which intercellular adhesion molecule 1 is probably the most important in the brain, chondroitin sulfate B in the placenta, and CD36 in most other organs. Thus the infected erythrocytes stick inside the small blood vessels. At the same stage, these *P. falciparum*–infected red cells may also adhere to uninfected red cells to form rosettes. The processes of cytoadherence and rosetting are central to the pathogenesis of falciparum malaria. They result in the sequestration of red cells containing mature forms of the parasite in vital organs (particularly the brain), where they interfere with microcirculatory flow and metabolism. Sequestered parasites continue to develop out of reach of the principal host defense mechanism: splenic processing and filtration. As a consequence, only the younger ring forms of the asexual parasites are seen in the peripheral blood in falciparum malaria, and the level of peripheral parasitemia underestimates the true number of parasites within the body. Severe malaria is also associated with reduced deformability of the uninfected erythrocytes, which compromises their passage through the partially obstructed capillaries and venules and shortens red cell survival.

In the other three "benign" malarias, sequestration does not occur, and all stages of the parasite's development are evident on peripheral blood smears. Whereas *P. vivax*, *P. ovale*, and *P. malariae* show a marked predilection for either old red cells or reticulocytes and produce a level of parasitemia seldom exceeding 2%, *P. falciparum* can invade erythrocytes of all ages and may be associated with very high levels of parasitemia.

HOST RESPONSE Initially, the host responds to plasmodial infection by activating nonspecific defense mechanisms. Splenic immunologic and filtrative clearance functions are augmented in malaria, and the removal of both parasitized and uninfected erythrocytes is accelerated. The parasitized cells escaping splenic removal are destroyed when the schizont ruptures. The material released induces the activation of macrophages and the release of proinflammatory mononuclear cell–derived cytokines, which cause fever and exert other pathologic effects. Temperatures of ≥40°C damage mature parasites; in untreated infections, the effect of such temperatures is to synchronize further the parasitic cycle with eventual production of the regular fever spikes and rigors that originally served to characterize the different malarias. These regular fever patterns (tertian, every 2 days; quartan, every 3 days) are seldom seen in patients who receive prompt and effective antimalarial treatment.

The geographic distributions of sickle cell disease, thalassemia, and glucose-6-phosphate dehydrogenase (G6PD) deficiency closely resemble that of malaria before the introduction of control measures. This observation suggests that these genetic disorders confer protection against death from falciparum malaria. For example, HbA/S heterozygotes (sickle cell trait) have a sixfold reduction in the risk of dying from severe falciparum malaria. This decrease in risk appears to be related to impaired parasite growth at low oxygen tensions. In Melanesia, children with α-thalessemia appear to have more frequent malaria (both vivax and falciparum) in the early years of life, and this pattern of infection appears to protect against severe disease. In Mel-

anesian ovalocytosis, rigid erythrocytes resist merozoite invasion and the intraerythrocytic milieu is hostile.

The specific immune response to malaria eventually controls the infection and, with exposure to sufficient strains, confers protection from high-level parasitemia and disease but not from infection. As a result of this state of infection without illness (premunition), asymptomatic parasitemia is common among adults and older children living in regions with stable and intense transmission (i.e., holo- or hyperendemic areas). Immunity is specific for both the species and the strain of infecting malarial parasite. Both humoral immunity and cellular immunity are necessary for protection, but the mechanisms of each are incompletely understood (Fig. 214-1). Immune individuals have a polyclonal increase in serum levels of IgM, IgG, and IgA, although much of this antibody is unrelated to protection. Antibodies to a variety of parasitic antigens presumably act in concert to limit in vivo replication of the parasite. In the case of falciparum malaria, the most important of these is the antigenically variant protein PfEMP1 mentioned above. Passively transferred IgG from immune adults has been shown to reduce levels of parasitemia in children, and passive transfer of maternal antibody contributes to the relative protection of infants from severe malaria in the first months of life. This complex immunity to disease is lost when a person lives outside an endemic area for several months or longer.

Several factors retard the development of cellular immunity to malaria. These factors include the absence of major histocompatibility antigens on the surface of infected red cells, which precludes direct T cell recognition; malaria antigen–specific immune unresponsiveness; and the enormous strain diversity of malarial parasites along with the ability of the parasites to express immunodominant variant antigens on the erythrocyte surface that change during the period of infection. Strain diversity also has an impact on the heterogeneity of the humoral antibody response. Immunity to all strains is never achieved. Parasites may persist in the blood for months (or, in the case of *P. malariae*, for many years) if treatment is not given. The complexity of the immune response in malaria, the sophistication of the parasites' evasion mechanisms, and the lack of a good in vitro correlate with clinical immunity have all slowed progress toward an effective vaccine.

CLINICAL FEATURES The first symptoms of malaria are nonspecific; the lack of a sense of well-being, headache, fatigue, abdominal discomfort, and muscle aches followed by fever are all similar to the symptoms of a minor viral illness. In some instances, a prominence of headache, chest pain, abdominal pain, arthralgia, myalgia, or diarrhea may suggest another diagnosis. Although headache may be severe in malaria, there is no neck stiffness or photophobia resembling that in meningitis. While myalgia may be prominent, it is not usually

FIGURE 214-2 Worldwide distribution of malaria and drug-resistant *Plasmodium falciparum*, 1999.

||||| Chloroquine-resistant malaria ● Chloroquine-sensitive malaria ○ Multiple drug-resistant malaria

as severe as in dengue fever, and the muscles are not tender as in leptospirosis or typhus. Nausea, vomiting, and orthostatic hypotension are common. The classic malarial paroxysms, in which fever spikes, chills, and rigors occur at regular intervals, suggest infection with *P. vivax* or *P. ovale*. The fever is irregular at first (that of falciparum malaria may never become regular); the temperature of nonimmune individuals and children often rises above 40°C in conjunction with tachycardia and sometimes delirium. Although childhood febrile convulsions may occur with any of the malarias, generalized seizures are specifically associated with falciparum malaria and may herald the development of cerebral disease. Many clinical abnormalities have been described in acute malaria, but most patients with uncomplicated infections have few abnormal physical findings other than fever, malaise, mild anemia, and (in some cases) a palpable spleen. Anemia may be quite common among young children living in areas with stable transmission, particularly where there is parasite resistance to chloroquine or other drugs. Splenic enlargement is very common among otherwise-healthy individuals in malaria-endemic areas and reflects repeated infections; however, in nonimmune individuals with malaria, the spleen takes several days to become palpable. Slight enlargement of the liver is also common, particularly in young children. Mild jaundice is common in adults; it may develop in patients with otherwise uncomplicated falciparum malaria and usually resolves over 1 to 3 weeks. Malaria is not associated with a rash like those seen in meningococcal septicemia, typhus, enteric fever, viral exanthems, and drug reactions. Petechial hemorrhages in the skin or mucous membranes—features of viral hemorrhagic fevers and leptospirosis—develop only rarely in severe falciparum malaria.

Severe Falciparum Malaria Appropriately treated, uncomplicated falciparum malaria carries a mortality rate of ~0.1%. However, once vital organ dysfunction occurs or the proportion of erythrocytes infected increases to >3%, mortality rises steeply. The major manifestations of severe falciparum malaria are shown in Table 214-2.

Cerebral malaria Coma is a characteristic and ominous feature of falciparum malaria and, despite treatment, is associated with death rates of ~20% among adults and 15% among children. Lesser degrees of obtundation, delirium, and abnormal behavior should also be taken very seriously. The onset may be gradual or sudden following a convulsion.

Cerebral malaria manifests as diffuse symmetric encephalopathy; focal neurologic signs are unusual. Although some passive resistance to head flexion may be detected, signs of meningeal irritation are lacking. The eyes may be divergent and a pout reflex is common, but other primitive reflexes are usually absent. The corneal reflexes are preserved except in deep coma. Muscle tone may be either increased or decreased. The tendon reflexes are variable, and the plantar reflexes may be flexor or extensor; the abdominal and cremasteric reflexes are absent. Flexor or extensor posturing may be documented. Approximately 15% of patients have retinal hemorrhages; with pupillary dilatation and indirect ophthalmoscopy, this figure increases to 30 to 40%. Other abnormalities include discrete spots of retinal opacification (30 to 60%), papilledema (8% of children, rare in adults), cotton wool spots (<5%), and decolorization of a retinal vessel or segment of vessel (occasional cases). Convulsions, usually generalized and often repeated, occur in up to 50% of children with cerebral malaria. More covert seizure activity is common, particularly in children, and may manifest as repetitive tonic-clonic eye movements. Whereas adults rarely suffer neurologic sequelae, ~10% of children surviving cerebral malaria—especially those with hypoglycemia, severe anemia, repeated seizures, and deep coma—have some residual neurologic deficit when they regain consciousness; hemiplegia, cerebral palsy, cortical blindness, deafness, and impaired cognition and learning—all of varying duration—have been reported.

Hypoglycemia An important and common complication of severe malaria, hypoglycemia is associated with a poor prognosis and is particularly problematic in children and pregnant women. Hypogly-

cemia in malaria results from a failure of hepatic gluconeogenesis and an increase in the consumption of glucose by both host and parasite. To compound the situation, quinine and quinidine—drugs used commonly for the treatment of severe chloroquine-resistant malaria—are powerful stimulants of pancreatic insulin secretion. Hyperinsulinemic hypoglycemia is especially troublesome in pregnant women receiving quinine treatment. In severe disease, the clinical diagnosis of hypoglycemia is difficult: the usual physical signs (sweating, gooseflesh, tachycardia) are absent, and the neurologic impairment caused by hypoglycemia cannot be distinguished from that caused by malaria.

Lactic acidosis Lactic acidosis commonly coexists with hypoglycemia in patients with malaria and is an important contributor to death from severe malaria. In adults, coexisting renal impairment often compounds the acidosis. Acidotic breathing, sometimes called respiratory distress, is a sign of poor prognosis. It is often followed by circulatory failure refractory to volume expansion or inotropic drugs or by respiratory arrest. The plasma concentrations of bicarbonate or lactate are the best biochemical prognosticators in severe malaria. Lactic acidosis is caused by the combination of anaerobic glycolysis in tissues where sequestered parasites interfere with microcirculatory flow, lactate production by the parasites, and a failure of hepatic and renal lactate clearance. The prognosis of lactic acidosis is poor.

Noncardiogenic pulmonary edema Adults with severe falciparum malaria may develop noncardiogenic pulmonary edema even after several days of antimalarial therapy. This manifestation may also develop in otherwise-uncomplicated vivax malaria, where recovery is usual. The pathogenesis of this variant of the adult respiratory distress

Table 214-2 Manifestations of Severe Falciparum Malaria

Signs	Manifestations
Major	
Unarousable coma/ cerebral malaria	Failure to localize or respond appropriately to noxious stimuli; coma persisting for >30 min after generalized convulsion
Acidemia/acidosis	Arterial pH <7.25 or plasma bicarbonate level of <15 mmol/L; venous lactate level of >15 mmol/L manifests as labored deep breathing, often termed "respiratory distress"
Severe normo- chromic, normo- cytic anemia	Hematocrit of <15% or hemoglobin level of <50 g/L (<5 g/dL) with parasitemia level of >100,000/μL
Renal failure	Urine output (24 h) of <400 mL in adults or <12 mL/kg in children; no improvement with rehydration; serum creatinine level of >265 μmol/L (>3.0 mg/dL)
Pulmonary edema/ adult respiratory distress syndrome	Noncardiogenic pulmonary edema, often aggravated by overhydration
Hypoglycemia	Plasma glucose level of <2.2 mmol/L (<40 mg/dL)
Hypotension/shock	Systolic blood pressure of <50 mmHg in children 1–5 years or <80 mmHg in adults; core/ skin temperature difference of >10°C
Bleeding/dissemi- nated intravascular coagulation	Significant bleeding and hemorrhage from the gums, nose, and gastrointestinal tract and/or evidence of disseminated intravascular coagulation
Convulsions	More than two generalized seizures in 24 h
Hemoglobinuria[a]	Macroscopic black, brown, or red urine; not associated with effects of oxidant drugs and red blood cell enzyme defects (such as G6PD deficiency)
Other	
Impaired conscious- ness	Obtunded but arousable
Extreme weakness	Prostration
Hyperparasitemia	Parasitemia level of >5% in nonimmune patients
Jaundice	Serum bilirubin level of >50 mmol/L (>3.0 mg/dL)

[a] Hemoglobinuria may occur in uncomplicated malaria.
NOTE: G6PD, glucose-6-phosphate dehydrogenase.

Renal impairment Renal impairment is common among adults with severe falciparum malaria but rare among children. The pathogenesis of renal failure is unclear but may be related to erythrocyte sequestration interfering with renal microcirculatory flow and metabolism. Clinically and pathologically, this syndrome manifests as acute tubular necrosis; renal cortical necrosis never develops. Mortality in the initial phase of hypercatabolic acute renal failure is high; in survivors, urine flow resumes in a median of 4 days, and serum creatinine levels return to normal in a mean of 17 days (Chap. 269). Dialysis or hemofiltration considerably enhances the likelihood of a patient's survival.

Hematologic abnormalities Anemia results from accelerated red cell destruction and removal by the spleen in conjunction with ineffective erythropoiesis. In severe malaria, both infected and uninfected red cells show reduced deformability, which correlates with prognosis and development of anemia. Splenic clearance of cells is also increased. In nonimmune individuals and in areas with unstable transmission, anemia can develop rapidly and transfusion is often required. In many areas of Africa, children may develop severe anemia as a result of repeated malarial infections. Anemia is a common consequence of antimalarial drug resistance, which results in repeated or continued infection.

Slight coagulation abnormalities are common in falciparum malaria, and mild thrombocytopenia is usual. As mentioned above, fewer than 5% of patients with severe malaria have significant bleeding with evidence of disseminated intravascular coagulation. Hematemesis, presumably from stress ulceration or acute gastric erosions, may also occur.

Liver dysfunction Mild hemolytic jaundice is common in malaria. Severe jaundice is associated with *P. falciparum* infections, is more common among adults than among children, and results from hemolysis, hepatocyte injury, and cholestasis. When accompanied by other vital organ dysfunction (often renal impairment), liver dysfunction carries a poor prognosis. Hepatic dysfunction contributes to hypoglycemia, lactic acidosis, and impaired drug metabolism.

Other complications Aspiration pneumonia following convulsions is an important cause of death in cerebral malaria. Chest infections and catheter-induced urinary tract infections are common among patients who are unconscious for >3 days. Septicemia may complicate severe malaria; in endemic areas *Salmonella* bacteremia has been associated specifically with *P. falciparum* infections.

Malaria in Pregnancy In hyper- and holoendemic areas, falciparum malaria in primi- and secundigravid women is associated with low birth weight (average reduction, ~170 g) and consequently increased infant and childhood mortality. In general, infected mothers in areas of stable transmission remain asymptomatic despite intense parasitization of the placenta due to sequestration of parasitized erythrocytes in the placental microcirculation. Maternal HIV infection predisposes pregnant women to a higher prevalence of malaria and parasite density and predisposes their newborns to congenital malaria infection and low birth weight.

In areas with unstable transmission of malaria, pregnant women are prone to severe infections and are particularly vulnerable to high-level parasitemia with anemia, hypoglycemia, and acute pulmonary edema. Fetal distress, premature labor, and stillbirth or low birth weight are common results. Congenital malaria occurs in fewer than 5% of newborns whose mothers are infected and is related directly to the parasite density in maternal blood and in the placenta. *P. vivax* malaria in pregnancy is also associated with a reduction in birth weight (average, 100 g), but, in contrast with the situation in falciparum malaria, this effect is greater in multigravid than in primigravid women.

Malaria in Children Most of the estimated 1 to 3 million persons who die of falciparum malaria each year are young African children. Convulsions, coma, hypoglycemia, metabolic acidosis, and severe anemia are relatively common among children with severe malaria, whereas deep jaundice, acute renal failure, and acute pul-

monary edema are unusual. Severely anemic children may present with labored deep breathing, which in the past has been attributed incorrectly to "anemic congestive cardiac failure" but is in fact usually caused by metabolic acidosis, often compounded by hypovolemia. In general, children tolerate antimalarial drugs well and respond rapidly to treatment.

Transfusion Malaria Malaria can be transmitted by blood transfusion, needle-stick injury, sharing of needles by infected drug addicts, or organ transplantation. The incubation period in these settings is often short because there is no preerythrocytic stage of development. The clinical features and management of these cases are the same as for naturally acquired infections, although falciparum malaria tends to be especially severe in drug addicts. Radical chemotherapy with primaquine is unnecessary for *P. vivax* and *P. ovale* infections.

CHRONIC COMPLICATIONS OF MALARIA **Tropical Splenomegaly (Hyperreactive Malarial Splenomegaly)** Chronic or repeated malarial infections produce hypergammaglobulinemia; normochromic, normocytic anemia; and, in certain situations, splenomegaly. Some residents of malaria-endemic areas in tropical Africa and Asia exhibit an abnormal immunologic response to repeated infections that is characterized by massive splenomegaly, hepatomegaly, marked elevations in serum titers of IgM and malarial antibody, hepatic sinusoidal lymphocytosis, and (in Africa) peripheral B cell lymphocytosis. This syndrome has been associated with the production of cytotoxic IgM antibodies to suppressor (CD8+) lymphocytes, antibodies to CD5+ T cells, and an increase in the ratio of CD4+ T cells to CD8+ T cells. It is believed that these events lead to uninhibited B cell production of IgM and the formation of cryoglobulins (IgM aggregates and immune complexes). This immunologic process stimulates reticuloendothelial hyperplasia and clearance activity and eventually produces splenomegaly. Patients with hyperreactive malarial splenomegaly (HMS) present with an abdominal mass or a dragging sensation in the abdomen and occasional sharp abdominal pains suggesting perisplenitis. Anemia and some degree of pancytopenia are usually evident, but in many cases malarial parasites cannot be found in peripheral blood smears. Vulnerability to respiratory and skin infections is increased; many patients die of overwhelming sepsis. Persons with HMS who are living in endemic areas should receive antimalarial chemoprophylaxis: the results are usually good. In nonendemic areas, treatment is advised. In some cases refractory to therapy, clonal lymphoproliferation may develop and then evolve into a malignant lymphoproliferative disorder.

Quartan Malarial Nephropathy Chronic or repeated infections with *P. malariae*, and possibly other malarial species, may cause soluble immune-complex injury to the renal glomeruli, resulting in the nephrotic syndrome. Other, unidentified factors must contribute to this process since only a very small proportion of infected patients develop renal disease. The histologic appearance is that of focal or segmental glomerulonephritis with splitting of the capillary basement membrane. Subendothelial dense deposits are seen on electron microscopy, and immunofluorescence reveals deposits of complement and immunoglobulins; in samples of renal tissue from children, *P. malariae* antigens are often visible. A coarse-granular pattern of basement membrane immunofluorescent deposits (predominantly IgG3) with selective proteinuria carries a better prognosis than a fine-granular, predominantly IgG2 pattern with nonselective proteinuria. Quartan nephropathy usually responds poorly to treatment with either antimalarial agents or glucocorticoids and cytotoxic drugs.

Burkitt's Lymphoma and Epstein-Barr Virus Infection It is possible that malaria-related immunosuppression provokes infection with lymphoma viruses. Burkitt's lymphoma is strongly associated with Epstein-Barr virus. The prevalence of this childhood tumor is high in malarious areas of Africa.

DIAGNOSIS **Demonstration of the Parasite** The diagnosis of malaria rests on the demonstration of asexual forms of the parasite in peripheral blood smears subjected to Romanovsky staining. Following a negative blood smear, repeat smears should be made if there is a high degree of suspicion. Giemsa at pH 7.2 is preferred; Wright's, Field's, or Leishman's stain can also be used. Both thin and thick blood smears should be examined (**See Plates VI-3 through VI-21 and VI-23 through VI-33**).

The thin blood smear should be rapidly air-dried, fixed in anhydrous methanol, and stained, and the red cells in the tail of the film should then be examined under oil immersion. The level of parasitemia is expressed as the number of parasitized erythrocytes among 1000 cells, and this figure is converted to the number of parasitized erythrocytes per microliter. Simple, sensitive, and specific antibody–based diagnostic stick or card tests that detect *P. falciparum*–specific, histidine-rich protein (HRP) 2 or lactate dehydrogenase antigens in fingerprick blood samples have been introduced. Some of these tests carry a second antibody, which allows falciparum malaria to be distinguished from the less dangerous malarias. The relationship between parasitemia and prognosis is complex; in general, patients with $>10^5$ parasites per microliter are at increased risk of dying, but nonimmune patients may die with much lower counts and semi-immune persons may tolerate parasitemia levels many times higher with only minor symptoms. In severe malaria, a poor prognosis is indicated by a predominance of more mature *P. falciparum* parasites (i.e., >20% of parasites with visible pigment), by the presence of circulating schizonts in the peripheral blood film, or by the presence of phagocytosed malarial pigment in >5% of neutrophils. Gametocytes may remain evident for several days after treatment has begun; unless trophozoites are also visible on the blood film, their presence does not constitute evidence of drug resistance.

The thick blood film should be of uneven thickness. The smear should be dried thoroughly and stained without fixing. As many layers of erythrocytes overlie one another and are lysed during the staining procedure, the thick film has the advantage of concentrating the parasites (by 20- to 40-fold compared with a thin blood film) and thus increasing diagnostic sensitivity. Both parasites and white cells are counted, and the number of parasites per unit volume is calculated from the total leukocyte count. Alternatively, a white count of 8000/ μL is assumed. A minimum of 200 white cells should be counted. Interpretation of thick films requires some experience because artifacts are common. Before a thick smear is judged to be negative, 100 to 200 fields should be examined under oil immersion. Phagocytosed malarial pigment is sometimes seen inside peripheral blood monocytes or polymorphonuclear leukocytes and may provide a clue to recent infection if malarial parasites are not detectable. After the clearance of the parasites, malarial pigment is often evident for several days in peripheral blood phagocytes, bone marrow aspirates, or smears of fluid expressed after intradermal puncture. Staining of parasites with the fluorescent dye acridine orange allows more rapid diagnosis of cases in which the level of parasitemia is low.

Laboratory Findings Normochromic, normocytic anemia is usually documented. The leukocyte count is generally low to normal, although it may be raised in very severe infections. The erythrocyte sedimentation rate, degree of plasma viscosity, and level of C-reactive protein are high. The platelet count is usually reduced to $\sim10^5/\mu$L. Severe infections may be accompanied by prolonged prothrombin and partial thromboplastin times and by severe thrombocytopenia. Levels of antithrombin III are reduced even in mild infection. In uncomplicated malaria, plasma concentrations of electrolytes, blood urea nitrogen, and creatinine are usually normal. Findings in severe malaria may include metabolic acidosis, with low plasma concentrations of glucose, sodium, bicarbonate, calcium, phosphate, and albumin together with elevations in lactate, blood urea nitrogen, creatinine, urate, muscle and liver enzymes, and conjugated and unconjugated bilirubin. Hypergammaglobulinemia is usual in immune and semi-immune subjects, and urinalysis generally gives normal results. In adults and children with cerebral malaria, the mean opening pressure at lumbar puncture is $\sim$160 mm of cerebrospinal fluid (CSF); the CSF is usually normal or

has a slightly elevated total protein level [<1.0 g/L (100 mg/dL)] and cell count (<20/μL).

PREVENTION In most of the tropics, the eradication of malaria is not yet feasible because of the widespread distribution of *Anopheles* breeding sites; the great number of infected persons; and inadequacies in resources, infrastructure, and control programs. Where possible, the disease is contained by judicious use of insecticides to kill the mosquito vector, rapid diagnosis and appropriate patient management, and administration of chemoprophylaxis to high-risk groups. Malaria researchers are intensifying their efforts to better understand parasite-human-mosquito-environmental interactions and develop more effective control and prevention interventions. Despite the enormous investment in efforts to develop a malaria vaccine, no safe, effective, long-lasting vaccine is likely to be available for general use in the near future (Chap. 122). While there is promise for one or more malaria vaccines on the more distant horizon, prevention and control measures continue to rely on antivector and drug use strategies.

Personal Protection Against Malaria Simple measures to reduce the frequency of mosquito bites in malarious areas are very important. These measures include the avoidance of exposure to mosquitoes at their peak feeding times (usually dusk and dawn, but also throughout the night) and the use of insect repellents, suitable clothing, and insecticide-impregnated bed nets. Widespread use of bed nets, particularly those treated with residual pyrethroids, reduces the incidence of malaria and has been shown to reduce mortality in western and eastern Africa.

Chemoprophylaxis (Table 214-3) Few areas of therapeutics are as controversial as antimalarial drug prophylaxis. Recommendations for prophylaxis depend on knowledge of local patterns of plasmodial drug sensitivity and the likelihood of acquiring malarial infection. Chemoprophylaxis is never entirely reliable, and malaria should always be considered in the differential diagnosis of fever in patients who have traveled to endemic areas, even if they are taking prophylactic antimalarial drugs.

Pregnant women traveling to malarious areas should be warned about the potential risks. All pregnant women at risk in endemic areas should be encouraged to attend regular antenatal clinics and should receive either prophylaxis with chloroquine or proguanil (chloroguanide) or intermittent treatment with pyrimethamine-sulfadoxine, provided there is not high-level resistance to these drugs. In addition, antimalarial prophylaxis should be considered for children between the ages of 3 months and 4 years in areas where malaria causes high childhood mortality; such prophylaxis may not be logistically or economically feasible in many countries. Children born to nonimmune mothers in endemic areas (usually expatriates moving to these areas) should receive prophylaxis from birth.

Travelers should start taking antimalarial drugs at least 1 week before departure so that any untoward reactions can be detected and therapeutic antimalarial blood concentrations will be present when needed. Antimalarial prophylaxis should continue for 4 weeks after the traveler has left the endemic area.

Mefloquine has become the antimalarial prophylactic agent of choice for much of the tropics because it is usually effective against multidrug-resistant falciparum malaria and is reasonably well tolerated. Mild nausea, dizziness, fuzzy thinking, disturbed sleep patterns, and malaise are relatively common. Approximately 1 in every 10,000 recipients develops an acute reversible neuropsychiatric reaction manifested by confusion, psychosis, convulsions, or encephalopathy. The role of mefloquine prophylaxis in pregnancy remains uncertain; in studies in Africa, mefloquine prophylaxis was found to be effective and safe during pregnancy. However, in one study from Thailand, treatment of malaria with mefloquine was associated with an increased risk of stillbirth.

Daily administration of doxycycline is an effective alternative to mefloquine that also exhibits some causal (preerythrocytic) prophylactic activity. Doxycycline is generally well tolerated but may cause vulvovaginal thrush, diarrhea, and photosensitivity and cannot be used by children <8 years old or by pregnant women. The combination drug atovaquone-proguanil hydrochloride (3.75/1.5 mg/kg, or 250/100 mg daily, adult dose) has recently been shown to be a very effective alternate to mefloquine chemoprophylaxis in drug-resistant areas. This drug must be taken with food or a milky drink because it is highly lipophilic: it is well-tolerated by adults and children.

Chloroquine remains the drug of choice for the prevention of infection with drug-sensitive *P. falciparum* and with the other human malarial species (although chloroquine-resistant *P. vivax* has been reported from parts of eastern Asia, Oceania, and South America). Unfortunately, there are few areas of the world with chloroquine-sensitive *P. falciparum*. Chloroquine is generally well tolerated, although some patients are unable to take the drug because of malaise, headache, or (in dark-skinned patients) pruritus. A concomitant filarial infection may provoke or aggravate chloroquine-induced pruritus. Chloroquine is considered safe in pregnancy. With chronic administration for >5 years, a characteristic dose-related retinopathy may develop, but this condition is rare at the doses used for antimalarial prophylaxis. Idiosyncratic or allergic reactions are also rare. Skeletal and cardiac myopathy are potential problems with protracted prophylactic use; they occur most often at the high doses used in the treatment of rheumatoid arthritis. Neuropsychiatric reactions and skin rashes are unusual. Amodiaquine, a related aminoquinoline, is associated with a high risk of agranulocytosis (~1 person in 2000 with continuous use) and should not be used for prophylaxis.

Table 214-3 Prophylaxis and Self-Treatment for Malaria

Drug	Usage	Adult Dosage	Child Dosage
Prophylaxis			
Mefloquine	Used in areas where chloroquine-resistant malaria has been reported	228 mg of base (250 mg of salt) orally, once/week[a]	<15 kg: 4.6 mg of base/kg (5 mg of salt/kg) 15–19 kg: ¼ tablet/week 20–30 kg: ½ tablet/week 31–45 kg: ¾ tablet/week >45 kg: 1 tablet/week
Doxycycline[b]	Used as alternative to mefloquine	100 mg orally, once/day	>8 years of age: 2 mg/kg per day orally; maximum dose, 100 mg/d
Chloroquine	Used in areas where chloroquine-resistant malaria has *not* been reported	300 mg of base (500 mg of salt) orally, once/week	5 mg of base/kg (8.3 mg of salt/kg) orally, once/week; maximum dose, 300 mg of base
Proguanil (not available in U.S.)	Used simultaneously *with* chloroquine as alternative to mefloquine or doxycycline	200 mg orally, once/day, in combination with weekly chloroquine	<2 years: 50 mg/d 2–6 years: 100 mg/d 7–10 years: 150 mg/d >10 years: 200 mg/d
Primaquine[c]	Used for travelers only after testing for G6PD deficiency; postexposure prevention for relapsing malaria or prophylaxis	Postexposure: 15 mg of base (26.3 mg of salt) orally, once/day for 14 days Prophylaxis: 30 mg of base daily	0.3 mg of base/kg (0.5 mg of salt/kg) orally, once/day for 14 days
Atovaquone-proguanil[c]	Used as alternative to mefloquine	250/100 mg orally once/day	11–20 kg 62.5 mg/100 mg 21–30 kg 125 mg/50 mg 31–40 kg 187.5 mg/75 mg >40 kg 250 mg/100 mg
Self-treatment			
Pyrimethamine-sulfadoxine[d]	In areas with chloroquine-resistant malaria, should be carried during travel by persons taking mefloquine or doxycycline	3 tablets (75 mg of pyrimethamine and 1500 mg of sulfadoxine) orally, as a single dose	5–10 kg: ½ tablet 11–20 kg: 1 tablet 21–30 kg: 1½ tablets 31–45 kg: 2 tablets >45 kg: 3 tablets

[a] Tablets manufactured outside the United States contain 250 mg of base.
[b] Not in pregnant women or children <8 years old.
[c] Primaquine and atovaquone-proguanil have both proved safe and effective for antimalarial chemoprophylaxis in areas with chloroquine-resistant falciparum malaria, but more data are needed, particularly in children. These drugs should not be used in pregnancy.
[d] Regimen is used for treatment only, *not* prophylaxis.

In the past, the dihydrofolate reductase inhibitors pyrimethamine and proguanil (chloroguanide) have been administered widely, but resistant strains of both *P. falciparum* and *P. vivax* have limited their use. Whereas antimalarial quinolines such as chloroquine act on the erythrocyte stage of parasitic development, the dihydrofolate reductase inhibitors also inhibit preerythrocytic growth in the liver (causal prophylaxis) and development in the mosquito (sporonticidal activity). Proguanil is safe and well tolerated, although mouth ulceration occurs in ~8% of persons using this drug; it is considered safe for antimalarial prophylaxis in pregnancy. The prophylactic use of the combination of pyrimethamine and sulfadoxine is not recommended because of an unacceptable incidence of severe toxicity, principally exfoliative dermatitis and other skin rashes, agranulocytosis, hepatitis, and pulmonary eosinophilia. The combination of pyrimethamine with dapsone (0.2/1.5 mg/kg weekly; 25/200 mg maximum) is a second-line alternative available in some countries and can be used in areas with chloroquine-resistant *P. falciparum*. This combination is generally well tolerated; however, resistance is increasing, and dapsone may cause methemoglobinemia and allergic reactions and (at higher doses) may pose a significant risk of agranulocytosis. Primaquine (0.5 mg/kg, or 30 mg daily) has also proved safe and effective in clinical trials in drug-resistant areas and can be considered when all other options are containdicated. Proguanil and the pyrimethamine-dapsone combination are not available in the United States.

Because of the increasing spread and intensity of plasmodial resistance to chloroquine in Africa and other areas of the world (Fig. 214-2), the Centers for Disease Control and Prevention (CDC; www.cdc.gov/travel/index.htm), which recommends a weekly dose of mefloquine for all travelers, maintains an updated 24-h travel and malaria information audiotape that can be accessed by touch-tone telephone (888-232-3228). Regional and disease-specific documents may be requested from the CDC Fax Information Service (888-232-3299). Consultation for the evaluation of prophylaxis failures or treatment of malaria can be obtained from state and local health departments and the CDC (770-488-7788).

℞ **TREATMENT** When a patient in or from a malarious area presents with fever, thick and thin blood smears should be prepared and examined immediately to confirm the diagnosis and identify the species of infecting parasite. Repeat blood smears should be performed at least every 12 h for 2 days if the first smears are negative. Patients with severe malaria or those unable to take oral drugs should receive parenteral antimalarial therapy. If there is any doubt about the resistance status of the infecting organism, then quinine or quinidine should be given. Several drugs are available for oral treatment, and the choice of drug depends on the likely sensitivity of the infecting parasites. Despite recent evidence of chloroquine resistance in *P. vivax* (from parts of Indonesia, Oceania, and Brazil), chloroquine remains the treatment of choice for the "benign" human malarias (*P. vivax*, *P. ovale*, *P. malariae*). Characteristics of various antimalarial agents are shown in Table 214-4, and drug regimens approved by the U.S. Food and Drug Administration are detailed in Table 214-5. The avail-

Table 214-4 Properties of Antimalarial Drugs

Drug(s)	Pharmacokinetic Properties	Antimalarial Activity	Minor Toxicity	Major Toxicity
Quinine, quinidine	Good oral and IM absorption (quinine); Cl and V_d reduced, but plasma protein binding (principally to $\propto1$ acid glycoprotein) increased (90%) in malaria; quinine $t_{1/2}$: 16 h in malaria, 11 h in healthy persons; quinidine $t_{1/2}$: 13 h in malaria, 8 h in healthy persons	Acts mainly on trophozoite blood stage; kills gametocytes of *P. vivax, P. ovale*, and *P. malariae*; no action on liver stages	*Common:* "Cinchonism": tinnitus, high-tone hearing loss, nausea, vomiting, dysphoria, postural hypotension; ECG QT_c interval prolongation (quinine usually by <10% but quinidine by up to 25%) *Rare:* Diarrhea, visual disturbance, rashes *Note:* Very bitter taste	*Common:* Hypoglycemia *Rare:* Hypotension, blindness, deafness, cardiac arrhythmias, thrombocytopenia, hemolysis, hemolytic-uremic syndrome, vasculitis, cholestatic hepatitis, neuromuscular paralysis *Note:* Quinidine more cardiotoxic
Chloroquine	Good oral absorption, very rapid IM and SC absorption; complex pharmacokinetics; enormous Cl and V_d (unaffected by malaria); blood concentration profile determined by distribution processes in malaria; $t_{1/2}$: 1–2 months	As for quinine but acts slightly earlier in asexual cycle	*Common:* Nausea, dysphoria, pruritus in dark-skinned patients, postural hypotension *Rare:* Accommodation difficulties, rash *Note:* Bitter taste, well tolerated	*Acute:* Hypotensive shock (parenteral), cardiac arrhythmias, neuropsychiatric reactions *Chronic:* Retinopathy (cumulative dose, >100 g), skeletal and cardiac myopathy
Mefloquine	Adequate oral absorption; no parenteral preparation; $t_{1/2}$: 14–20 days (shorter in malaria)	As for quinine	Nausea, giddiness, dysphoria, fuzzy thinking, sleeplessness, nightmares, sense of dissociation	Neuropsychiatric reactions, convulsions, encephalopathy
Tetracycline, doxycycline[a]	Excellent absorption; $t_{1/2}$: 8 h for tetracycline, 18 h for doxycycline	Weak antimalarial activity; should not be used alone for treatment	Gastrointestinal intolerance, deposition in growing bones and teeth, photosensitivity, moniliasis, benign intracranial hypertension	Renal failure in patients with impaired renal function (tetracycline)
Halofantrine[b]	Highly variable absorption related to fat intake; $t_{1/2}$: 1–3 days (active desbutyl metabolite $t_{1/2}$: 3–7 days)	As for quinine	Diarrhea	Cardiac conduction disturbances; atrioventricular block; ECG QT_c interval prolongation; potentially lethal ventricular tachyarrhythmias
Artemisinin and derivatives (artemether, artesunate)	Good oral absorption, variable absorption of IM artemether; artesunate and artemether biotransformed to active metabolite dihydroartemisinin; all drugs eliminated rapidly; $t_{1/2}$: <1 h	Broader stage specificity and more rapid than other drugs; no action on liver stages	Reduction in reticulocyte count; fever; allergy	Neurotoxicity of oil-based IM preparations reported in animals, but no evidence in humans
Pyrimethamine	Good oral absorption, variable IM absorption; $t_{1/2}$: 4 days	For blood stages, acts mainly on mature forms; causal prophylactic	Well tolerated	Megaloblastic anemia, pancytopenia, pulmonary infiltration
Proguanil (chloroguanide)	Good oral absorption; biotransformed to active metabolite cycloguanil; $t_{1/2}$: 16 h	Causal prophylactic; not used alone for treatment	Well tolerated; mouth ulcers and rare alopecia	Megaloblastic anemia in renal failure
Primaquine	Complete oral absorption; active compound not known; $t_{1/2}$: 7 h	Radical cure; eradicates hepatic forms of *P. vivax* and *P. ovale*; kills gametocytes of *P. falciparum*	Nausea, vomiting, diarrhea, abdominal pain, hemolysis, methemoglobinemia	Massive hemolysis in subjects with severe G6PD deficiency
Atovaquone	Highly variable absorption related to fat intake; $t_{1/2}$: 30–70 h	Acts mainly on trophozoite blood stage	None identified	—
Lumefantrine	Highly variable absorption related to fat intake; $t_{1/2}$: 3–4 days	As for quinine	None identified	—

[a] Tetracycline and doxycycline should not be given to pregnant women or to children <8 years of age.
[b] Halofantrine should not be used by patients with long ECG QT_c intervals or known conduction disturbances or by those taking drugs that may affect ventricular repolarization, e.g., quinidine, quinine, mefloquine, chloroquine, neuroleptics, antiarrhythmics, tricyclic antidepressants, terfenadine, or astemizole.

ABBREVIATIONS: Cl, systemic clearance; V_d, total apparent volume of distribution; IM, intramuscular; SC, subcutaneous; ECG, electrocardiogram; G6PD, glucose-6-phosphate dehydrogenase.

ability of antimalarial drugs varies considerably between countries. Many of the drugs used to treat malaria in endemic areas are not available in temperate countries such as the United States.

Severe Malaria Because of resistance, chloroquine can no longer be relied upon in most countries for the treatment of severe malaria. The antiarrhythmic quinidine gluconate is as effective as quinine and, as it is more readily available, has replaced quinine for the treatment of malaria in the United States. The administration of quinidine must be closely monitored if dysrrhythmias and hypotension are to be avoided. Total plasma levels in excess of 8 μg/mL, a QT_c interval of >0.6 s, or QRS widening beyond 25% of baseline are indications for slowing infusion rates. If arrhythmia or saline-unresponsive hypotension develops, treatment with this drug should be discontinued. Quinine is safer than quinidine; cardiovascular monitoring is not required except when the recipient has cardiac disease. In some areas of Asia, the Chinese drugs derived from artemisinin (artemether and artesunate) have become first-line treatments for severe malaria. These agents are rapidly effective against multidrug-resistant falciparum malaria and are at least as effective as and safer than quinine or quinidine. They are not available in the United States.

Severe falciparum malaria constitutes a medical emergency requiring intensive nursing care and careful management. The patient should be weighed and, if comatose, placed on his or her side. Frequent evaluation of the patient's condition is essential. Ancillary drugs such as high-dose glucocorticoids, urea, heparin, and dextran are of no value.

Parenteral antimalarial treatment should be started as soon as possible. An initial loading dose should be given so that therapeutic concentrations are reached as soon as possible. Both quinine and quinidine will cause dangerous hypotension if injected rapidly; when given intravenously, they must be administered carefully by rate-controlled infusion only. The optimal therapeutic range for quinine and quinidine in severe malaria is not known with certainty, but total plasma concentrations of 8 to 15 mg/mL for quinine and 3.5 to 8.0 mg/mL for quinidine are effective and do not cause serious toxicity. The systemic clearance and apparent volume of distribution of these alkaloids are markedly reduced and plasma protein binding is increased in severe malaria, so that the blood concentrations attained with a given dose are higher. If the patient remains seriously ill or in acute renal failure for >2 days, the maintenance doses of quinine or quinidine should be reduced by 30 to 50% to prevent toxic accumulation of the drugs. The initial doses should never be reduced. If one of the artemisinin derivatives or chloroquine is given, dose reductions are unnecessary, even in renal failure. Exchange transfusion should be considered for severely ill patients, although the precise indications for this procedure have not been agreed upon. It has been recommended that—if safe and feasible—exchange should be considered for parasitemia levels of 5 to 15% and is indicated for parasitemia levels of $>15\%$. The role of prophylactic intramuscular phenobarbital in preventing convulsions in cerebral malaria also remains uncertain.

Table 214-5 Recommended Therapeutic Doses of Antimalarial Drugs

Drug	Uncomplicated Malaria (Oral)	Severe Malaria[a] (Parenteral)
Chloroquine	10 mg of base/kg followed by 10 mg/kg at 24 h and 5 mg/kg at 48 h *or* by 5 mg/kg at 12, 24, and 36 h (total dose, 25 mg/kg); for *P. vivax* or *P. ovale*, primaquine (0.25 mg of base/kg per day for 14 days[c]) added for radical cure	10 mg of base/kg by constant-rate infusion over 8 h followed by 15 mg/kg over 24 h *or* by 3.5 mg of base/kg by IM or SC injection every 6 h (total dose, 25 mg/kg)[b]
Sulfadoxine/ pyrimethamine	25/1.25 mg/kg, single oral dose (3 tablets for adults)	—
Mefloquine	15 mg/kg followed 8–12 h later by second dose of 10 mg/kg	—
Quinine	10 mg of salt/kg q8h for 7 days combined with tetracycline[d] (4 mg/kg qid) or doxycycline (3 mg/kg once daily) or clindamycin (10 mg/kg bid) for 7 days	20 mg of salt/kg by IV infusion over 4 h[e] followed by 10 mg/kg infused over 2–8 h every 8 h
Quinidine gluconate	—	10 mg of base/kg by constant-rate infusion over 1–2 h followed by 0.02 mg/kg per min, with ECG monitoring[f]
Artesunate	In combination with 25 mg of mefloquine/kg, 12 mg/kg given in divided doses over 3–5 days (e.g., 4 mg/kg for 3 days or 4 mg/kg followed by 2 mg/kg per day for 4 days); if used alone, give for 7 days (usually 4 mg/kg initially followed by 2 mg/kg daily)	2.4 mg/kg IV or IM stat followed by 1.2 mg/kg at 12 and 24 h and then daily
Artemether	Same regimen as for artesunate	3.2 mg/kg IM stat followed by 1.6 mg/kg per day
Atovaquone-proguanil	For adults >40 kg, each dose comprises 4 tablets (each containing atovaquone 250 mg and proguanil 100 mg) taken once daily for 3 days with food	—
Artemether-lumefantrine	For adults ≥35 kg, each dose comprises 4 tablets (each containing artemether 20 mg and lumefantrine 120 mg) at 0, 8, 24, and 48 h (semi-immunes) or at 0, 8, 24, 36, 48, and 60 h (nonimmunes) taken after food	—

[a] Oral treatment should be substituted for parenteral therapy as soon as the patient can take tablets by mouth.
[b] Chloroquine-resistant *P. falciparum* is now very widespread.
[c] In Oceania and Southeast Asia, the dose should be 0.33 to 0.5 mg of base/kg. This regimen should not be used in patients with severe variants of G6PD deficiency.
[d] Neither tetracycline nor doxycycline should be given to pregnant women or to children <8 years old.
[e] Alternatively, infusion of 7 mg of salt/kg over 30 min can be followed by 10 mg of salt/kg over 4 h.
[f] Some authorities recommend a lower dose of intravenous quinidine: 6.2 mg of base/kg over 1–2 h followed by 0.0125 mg/kg per min.
NOTE: In severe malaria, quinine or quinidine should be used if there is any doubt about the infecting strain's sensitivity to chloroquine.
ABBREVIATIONS: IM, intramuscular; SC, subcutaneous; IV, intravenous; ECG, electrocardiogram; G6PD, glucose-6-phosphate dehydrogenase.

When the patient is unconscious, the blood glucose level should be measured every 4 to 6 h, and values below 2.2 mmol/L (40 mg/dL) should prompt treatment with intravenous dextrose. All patients treated with intravenous quinine or quinidine should receive a continuous infusion of 5 to 10% dextrose. The parasite count and hematocrit level should be measured every 6 to 12 h. Anemia develops rapidly; if the hematocrit falls below 20%, then whole blood (preferably fresh) or packed cells should be transfused slowly, with careful attention to circulatory status. Renal function should be checked daily. Judicious use of small doses of a diuretic to prevent fluid overload may be needed, particularly in the elderly. Children presenting with severe anemia and acidotic breathing are often hypovolemic; in this situation, resuscitation with crystalloids or blood is indicated. Accurate assessment is vital. Management of fluid balance is difficult in severe malaria, particularly in adults, because of the thin dividing line between overhydration (leading to pulmonary edema) and underhydration (contributing to renal impairment). If necessary, pulmonary artery occlusion pressures should be measured and maintained in the low-normal range. As soon as the patient can take fluids, oral therapy should be substituted for parenteral treatment.

Uncomplicated Malaria Infections due to *P. vivax*, *P. malariae*, *P. ovale*, and known sensitive strains of *P. falciparum* should be treated with oral chloroquine (total dose, 25 mg of base/kg). In Africa,

1211

chloroquine-resistant strains are usually sensitive to sulfadoxine/pyrimethamine. Where there is resistance to the latter combination, either (1) quinine plus tetracycline or doxycycline (or clindamycin) or (2) mefloquine should be used; tetracycline and doxycycline cannot be given to pregnant women or to children <8 years of age. Oral quinine is extremely bitter and regularly produces cinchonism comprising tinnitus, high-tone deafness, nausea, vomiting, and dysphoria. Compliance is poor with the required 5- to 7-day regimens of this drug. Mefloquine should be given at a total dosage of 25 mg/kg (15 mg/kg followed 8 to 12 h later by 10 mg/kg) and, where available and approved for use, combined with artesunate or artemether (4 mg/kg per day for 3 days). Although significant resistance to mefloquine has been documented in Thailand, Burma, Vietnam, and Cambodia, this agent is usually effective against multidrug-resistant strains of *P. falciparum* outside these areas. Artemether-lumefantrine and atovaquone-proguanil are recently introduced, well-tolerated antimalarial drugs used in 3-day regimens. They are both effective against multidrug-resistant falciparum malaria.

Patients should be monitored for vomiting for 1 h after the administration of any oral antimalarial drug. Symptom-based treatment, with tepid sponging and acetaminophen administration, lowers fever and thereby reduces the patient's propensity to vomit these drugs. Minor central nervous system reactions (nausea, dizziness, sleep disturbances) are common. The incidence of serious adverse neuropsychiatric reactions to mefloquine treatment is ~1 in 1000 in Asia but may be as high as 1 in 200 among Africans and Caucasians. All the antimalarial quinolines (chloroquine, mefloquine, and quinine) exacerbate the orthostatic hypotension associated with malaria, and all are tolerated better by children than by adults. Pregnant women, young children, patients unable to tolerate oral therapy, and nonimmune subjects (e.g., travelers) with suspected malaria should be evaluated carefully and hospitalization considered. If there is any doubt as to the identity of the infecting malarial species, treatment for falciparum malaria should be given. A negative blood smear does not rule out malaria; thick blood films should be checked 1 and 2 days later to exclude the diagnosis. Nonimmune subjects receiving treatment for malaria should have daily parasite counts performed until negative thick films indicate clearance of the parasite. If the level of parasitemia does not fall below 25% of the admission value in 48 h or if parasitemia has not cleared by 7 days (and compliance is assured), drug resistance is likely and the regimen should be changed. Quinine (or quinidine) and tetracycline should be reserved for multidrug-resistant infections, but if falciparum malaria has been contracted in an area of known drug sensitivity, then treatment with chloroquine, sulfadoxine/pyrimethamine, or mefloquine is preferable because these agents are better tolerated and simpler to administer.

Primaquine (0.3 mg of base/kg; 15 mg of base, adult dose) should be given daily for 14 days to patients with *P. vivax* or *P. ovale* infections after laboratory tests for G6PD deficiency have proved negative. A dose of 22.5 to 30 mg for an adult is recommended for infections acquired in Southeast Asia and Oceania. If the patient has a mild variant of G6PD deficiency, primaquine can be given in a dose of 0.6 mg of base/kg (45 mg maximum) once weekly for 8 weeks.

PREVENTING DRUG RESISTANCE In much of the tropics, drug-resistant *P. falciparum* is increasing in distribution, frequency, and intensity. There is a growing belief among malariologists that, to prevent resistance, falciparum malaria should no longer be treated with single drugs in endemic areas; the same rationale has been applied in the treatment of tuberculosis and HIV/AIDS. This strategy is based upon simultaneous use of two or more drugs with different modes of action: one, an artemisinin derivative (artesunate, artemether, or dihydroartemisinin), given for 3 days; and the other, a slower-acting antimalarial. In areas where *P. falciparum* is still sensitive, chloroquine is used as the second drug; where there is low-grade chloroquine resistance (e.g., many areas of Africa), either amodiaquine or sulfadox-

ine/pyrimethamine can be used in combination with the artemisinin derivative. Where there is also resistance to sulfadoxine/pyrimethamine, the combinations artesunate plus mefloquine, artemether plus lumefantrine, or quinine plus tetracycline or clindamycin can be considered (although tetracycline cannot be given to pregnant women or to children <8 years of age). Atovaquone/proguanil, which is also effective against drug-resistant malaria, can also be combined with artesunate to prevent the emergence of resistance. While significant resistance to mefloquine occurs in Thailand, Burma, and Cambodia, the mefloquine/artesunate combinations are still reliably effective in these areas. The artemisinin derivatives and lumefantrine (all unlicensed in the United States) and atovaquone-proguanil are tolerated well with no significant adverse effects.

COMPLICATIONS **Acute Renal Failure** If the level of blood urea nitrogen or creatinine rises despite adequate rehydration, fluid administration should be restricted to prevent volume overload. The indications for dialysis are the same as those in other forms of hypercatabolic acute renal failure (Chap. 269). Even with adequate peritoneal dialysis, secondary bacterial infections are common in the tropics, and hemodialysis or hemofiltration is preferable. Some patients pass small volumes of urine sufficient to allow control of fluid balance; these cases can be managed conservatively if other indications for dialysis do not arise. Renal function usually improves within days, but full recovery may take weeks.

Acute Pulmonary Edema Patients should be positioned at 45° and given oxygen and intravenous diuretics. Pulmonary artery occlusion pressures may be normal, indicating increased pulmonary capillary permeability. Positive pressure ventilation should be started early if the immediate measures fail (Chap. 233).

Hypoglycemia An initial slow injection of 50% dextrose (0.5 g/kg) should be followed by an infusion of 10% dextrose (0.10 g/kg per hour). The blood glucose level should be checked regularly thereafter, as recurrent hypoglycemia is common, particularly in patients receiving quinine or quinidine. In severely ill patients, hypoglycemia commonly occurs together with metabolic (lactic) acidosis and carries a poor prognosis.

Other Complications Patients who develop spontaneous bleeding should be given fresh blood and intravenous vitamin K. Convulsions should be treated with intravenous or rectal benzodiazepines and, if necessary, respiratory support. Aspiration pneumonia should be suspected in any unconscious patient with convulsions, particularly with persistent hyperventilation; intravenous antimicrobial agents and oxygen should be administered, and pulmonary toilet should be undertaken. Treatment for systemic *Salmonella* and other infections common in African children with falciparum malaria should be considered. Hypoglycemia or gram-negative septicemia should be suspected when the condition of any patient suddenly deteriorates for no obvious reason during antimalarial treatment.

BABESIOSIS

Babesiosis is a protozoan disease of animals that is transmitted by ticks; humans are infected incidentally and initially develop a nonspecific febrile illness. *Babesia* organisms enter red blood cells and resemble malarial parasites morphologically, thus posing a diagnostic problem.

ETIOLOGY AND NATURAL CYCLE Of the more than 100 species of *Babesia*, *B. microti* and *B. divergens* are the two that cause most human infections. Ixodid (hard-bodied) ticks, in particular *Ixodes scapularis* (*I. dammini*) and *I. ricinus*, are the vectors of the parasite. Ticks ingest *Babesia* while feeding, and the parasite multiplies within the tick's gut wall. The organisms then spread to the salivary glands; their inoculation into a vertebrate host by a tick larva, nymph, or adult completes the cycle of transmission. Asexual reproduction of *Babesia* within red blood cells produces two or four parasites.

EPIDEMIOLOGY While *Babesia* infections in wild and domestic animals are distributed globally, almost all *B. microti* infections in the United States occur along the northeastern coast, including Nantucket Island, Martha's Vineyard, and Cape Cod in Massachusetts; Block Island in Rhode Island; Long Island, Shelter Island, and Fire Island in New York; and the nearby mainland, including Connecticut. Cases also have been reported from Wisconsin, Minnesota, Virginia, Maryland, Georgia, and Mexico. *Babesia* isolates from patients in Washington and California have been characterized as WA-1-type parasites, a category that is genetically and antigenically distinct from *B. microti*. A strain isolated in Missouri differs from these isolates, suggesting that babesiosis may be an "emerging infection." The deer tick, *I. scapularis*, is the vector associated with *B. microti*. In Europe, *B. divergens* has been responsible for the majority of the 22 reported cases of babesiosis; Yugoslavia, Russia, France, the United Kingdom, and Ireland have accounted for most of these infections.

Transfusions are another source of babesiosis. In the more than 20 transfusion-associated cases reported, parasites were uncommonly detected in blood donors, but serologic testing of their blood for *Babesia* gave positive results.

Infections with *B. divergens* have occurred sporadically in previously splenectomized patients in several countries in Europe. *I. ricinus* is probably the vector in these cases, as it is for the transmission of this organism among cattle. The infected persons were predisposed to illness by their asplenic status.

I. scapularis feeds on rodents as a larva and a nymph and on deer as an adult; nymphs are abundant during the spring and summer and feed on humans readily. In some endemic areas, the seroprevalence in the human population may be >2%. This figure indicates that asymptomatic infection is more frequent than is generally thought.

CLINICAL PRESENTATION The incubation period for *B. microti* infection is about 1 to 4 weeks. Immunosuppressed patients, splenectomized individuals, and the elderly have the most severe illness. The clinical presentation varies widely; symptoms and signs include a gradual onset of irregular fever, chills, sweating, muscle pain, and fatigue. Mild hepatosplenomegaly and mild hemolytic anemia may develop. The level of parasitemia may exceed 10%. The illness may continue for weeks or months.

Patients infected with *B. divergens* have a more severe illness, with a rapid onset of chills, fever, nausea, vomiting, and hemolytic anemia progressing to jaundice, hemoglobinemia, and renal failure. *B. divergens* infections are often fatal.

DIAGNOSIS Whether or not they have a history of exposure to ticks or tick bites, febrile persons living in endemic areas should have Giemsa-stained thick and thin blood films **(see Plate VI-22)** examined for small intraerythrocytic parasites. *B. microti* appears as a small ring form resembling *P. falciparum*. Unlike infection with *Plasmodium*, however, that with *Babesia* does not cause the production of pigment in parasites, nor are schizonts or gametocytes formed. Dividing within red blood cells, *B. microti* can form four daughter parasites attached by strands of cytoplasm; these "tetrad" forms are seen infrequently in human blood films but are a distinguishing feature. An indirect immunofluorescence antibody test is useful for the diagnosis of infection with *B. microti* but does not replace the blood smear. The serum antibody titer rises 2 to 4 weeks after the onset of illness and then wanes over 6 to 12 months; cross-reactions can occur with other species of *Babesia* and with *Plasmodium*.

About 50% of patients infected with *B. microti* have antibody to *Borrelia burgdorferi*, the agent of Lyme disease (Chap. 176); this figure varies with the geographic area. The occurrence of mixed infections is not surprising since both organisms are transmitted by *I. scapularis*. This tick species is also a potential vector of human granulocytic ehrlichiosis; the same tick may carry more than one tickborne disease. Intraperitoneal inoculation of blood from patients with babesiosis into hamsters or gerbils results in detectable parasitemia within 2 to 4 weeks.

℞ TREATMENT *B. microti* infections in patients with intact spleens are often self-limiting without treatment, although symptoms may persist for months with or without treatment. Because silent parasitemia may have prolonged symptoms and signs, treatment is advised for all patients infected with *Babesia*. Treatment with the combination of quinine sulfate (650 mg of salt orally tid) plus clindamycin (600 mg orally tid or 1.2 g parenterally bid) for 7 to 10 days is usually effective but may not always eliminate parasites. The pediatric dose is 20 to 40 mg/kg per day for quinine sulfate and 25 mg/kg per day for clindamycin, both given in three divided doses over 7 to 10 days. Atovaquone suspension (750 mg bid) plus azithromycin (500 to 1000 mg/d) may be effective when quinine and clindamycin fail. Especially severe infections with high-level *B. microti* parasitemia in asplenic patients have been successfully treated with exchange transfusions in addition to quinine and clindamycin.

BIBLIOGRAPHY

BAIRD JK et al: Primaquine for prophylaxis against malaria among nonimmune transmigrants in Irian Jaya, Indonesia. Am J Trop Med Hyg 52:479, 1995

CENTERS FOR DISEASE CONTROL AND PREVENTION: *Health Information for International Travel, 1999–2000*. Atlanta, Department of Health and Human Services, 1999

GARNHAM PCC: Malaria parasites of man: Life cycles and morphology (excluding ultrastructure) in malaria, in *Principles and Practice of Malariology*, WH Wernsdorfer, I McGregor (eds). Edinburgh, Churchill Livingstone, 1988, pp 61–96

GELFAND JA, CALLAHAN MV: Babesiosis. Curr Clin Top Infect Dis 18:201, 1998

HERWALDT BL et al: Babesiosis in Wisconsin: A potentially fatal disease. Am J Trop Med Hyg 53:146, 1995

HOFFMAN SL, MILLER LH: Perspectives on malaria vaccine development, in *Malaria Vaccine Development*, SL Hoffman (ed). Washington, DC, ASM Press, 1996, pp 1–13

KRAUSE PJ et al: Persistent parasitemia after acute babesiosis. N Engl J Med 339:160, 1998

NEWTON P, WHITE N: Malaria: New developments in treatment and prevention. Annu Rev Med 50:179, 1999

PASLOSKE BL, HOWARD RJ: Malaria, the red cell and the endothelium. Annu Rev Med 45:283, 1994

SHANKS GD: Malaria prevention and prophylaxis, in *Bailliere's Clinical Infectious Diseases*, vol 2-2, G Pasvol (ed). London, Bailliere Tindall, 1995, pp 331–349

SNOW RW: Estimating mortality, morbidity and disability due to malaria among Africa's non-pregnant population. Bull World Health Org 77:624, 1999

STEKETEE RW et al: Impairment of a pregnant woman's acquired ability to limit *Plasmodium falciparum* by infection with human immunodeficiency virus type-1. Am J Trop Med Hyg 55(Suppl):43, 1996

WHITE NJ: The treatment of malaria. N Engl J Med 335:800, 1996

———: Malaria pathophysiology, in *Malaria: Parasite Biology, Pathogenesis, Protection*, I. Sherman (ed). Washington, DC, ASM Press, 1998, pp 371–385

WORLD HEALTH ORGANIZATION: Control of tropical diseases. Severe and complicated malaria. Trans R Soc Trop Med Hyg 84(Suppl 2):1, 1990

215 *Barbara L. Herwaldt*

LEISHMANIASIS

OVERVIEW

DEFINITION The term *leishmaniases* refers collectively to various clinical syndromes caused by obligate intracellular protozoa of the genus *Leishmania* (order Kinetoplastida). Leishmaniasis is endemic in diverse ecologic settings in the tropics, the subtropics, and southern Europe that range from deserts to rain forests and from rural to periurban areas. It typically is a vector-borne zoonosis, with rodents and canids as common reservoir hosts and humans as incidental hosts. In humans, visceral, cutaneous, and mucosal leishmaniasis result from infection of macrophages throughout the mononuclear-phagocyte system, in the skin, and in the naso-oropharyngeal mucosa, respectively. Current challenges include the emergence of leishmaniasis in new geographic areas and host populations (e.g., visceral leishmaniasis in persons infected with HIV) as well as the need for field-applicable, rapid diagnostic tests and for effective, safe, and affordable oral therapies, control measures, and immunoprophylactic agents.

Table 215-1 Major *Leishmania* Species That Cause Disease in Humans

Species[a]	Clinical Syndrome[b]	Geographic Distribution
SUBGENUS *LEISHMANIA*		
L. donovani complex		
L. donovani	VL (PKDL, OWCL)	China, Indian subcontinent, southwestern Asia, Ethiopia, Kenya, Sudan; possibly sporadic in sub-Saharan Africa
L. infantum	VL (OWCL)	China, central and southwestern Asia, Middle East, southern Europe, North Africa, Ethiopia, Sudan; sporadic in sub-Saharan Africa
L. chagasi	VL (NWCL)	Central and South America
L. mexicana complex		
L. mexicana	NWCL (DCL)	Texas, Mexico, Central and South America
L. amazonensis	NWCL (ML, DCL, VL)	Panama and South America
L. tropica	OWCL (VL)[c]	Central Asia, India, southwestern Asia, Middle East, Turkey, Greece, North Africa, Ethiopia, Kenya, Namibia
L. major	OWCL[d]	Central Asia, India, southwestern Asia, Middle East, Turkey, North Africa, Sahel region of north-central Africa, Ethiopia, Sudan, Kenya
L. aethiopica	OWCL (DCL)	Ethiopia, Kenya
SUBGENUS *VIANNIA*		
L. (V.) braziliensis	NWCL (ML)	Central and South America
L. (V.) guyanensis	NWCL (ML)	South America
L. (V.) panamensis	NWCL (ML)	Central America, Venezuela, Colombia, Ecuador, Peru
L. (V.) peruviana	NWCL[e]	Peru (western slopes of Andes)

[a] Species other than those listed here have been reported to infect humans.
[b] Abbreviations: VL, visceral leishmaniasis; PKDL, post–kala-azar dermal leishmaniasis; OWCL, Old World cutaneous leishmaniasis; NWCL, New World (American) cutaneous leishmaniasis; DCL, diffuse cutaneous leishmaniasis; ML, mucosal leishmaniasis. Clinical syndromes less frequently associated with the various species are shown in parentheses.
[c] *L. tropica* also causes leishmaniasis recidivans and viscerotropic leishmaniasis.
[d] *L. major*–like organisms also cause New World cutaneous leishmaniasis.
[e] The cutaneous leishmaniasis syndrome caused by this species is called *uta*.

ETIOLOGY The organisms that cause the various forms of leishmaniasis in humans are listed in Table 215-1. Visceral leishmaniasis is typically but not exclusively caused by organisms of the *Leishmania donovani* complex; Old World cutaneous leishmaniasis by *L. tropica*, *L. major*, and *L. aethiopica*; New World (or American) cutaneous leishmaniasis by organisms of the *L. mexicana* complex and the *Viannia* subgenus; and mucosal leishmaniasis by some organisms in the *Viannia* subgenus.

LIFE CYCLE *Leishmania* parasites are transmitted by the bite of female phlebotomine sandflies [genus *Phlebotomus* (Old World) or *Lutzomyia* (New World)]. As the flies attempt to feed, they regurgitate the parasite's flagellated promastigote stage into the skin of mammalian hosts. Promastigotes attach to receptors on macrophages, are phagocytized, and transform within phagolysosomes into the nonflagellated amastigote stage, which multiplies by binary fission. After rupture of infected macrophages, amastigotes are phagocytized by other macrophages. If ingested by feeding sandflies, amastigotes transform back into promastigotes, which require at least 7 days to become infective.

IMMUNOLOGY Advances in the understanding of the immunology of leishmaniasis have made this parasitic disease the paradigm for studies of the T cell subsets and cytokines that govern resistance and susceptibility to intracellular pathogens. The paradigm is best demonstrated in murine *L. major* infection. In inbred mice, production of interferon γ (IFN-γ) by T_H1 and natural killer cells confers resistance. Interleukin (IL)12 induces naive T cells to differentiate into T_H1 cells and induces T cells and natural killer cells to produce IFN-γ. In contrast, expansion of IL-4-producing T_H2 cells mediates susceptibility.

Not all aspects of leishmaniasis in mice, whose susceptibility to leishmanial infection is genetically determined, apply to human infection, for which the genetic determinants are being investigated. However, a consistent principle is that healing and resistance to reinfection are associated with expanding numbers of *Leishmania*-specific T_H1 cells, production of IFN-γ, and activation of macrophages to kill intracellular amastigotes. In human visceral leishmaniasis, IL-10 appears to be associated with pathology; in addition, IL-4 may contribute to progression of disease.

GENERAL DIAGNOSTIC PRINCIPLES Definitive diagnosis of leishmaniasis requires demonstration of the parasite. To identify amastigotes by light-microscopic examination, the specimen obtained from an infected site (e.g., thin smear, histologic section) should be stained with Giemsa or another Romanovsky stain and presumptive amastigotes (2 to 4 μm in diameter) examined under oil immersion for the presence of a nucleus and a rod-shaped kinetoplast (Fig. 215-1); the latter is a specialized mitochondrial structure that contains extranuclear DNA. Other means of parasitologic confirmation include in vitro culture (e.g., on Novy-MacNeal-Nicolle medium), animal inoculation, and use of molecular techniques that are under investigation (e.g., polymerase chain reaction).

The *Leishmania* species that infect humans are morphologically similar. They can be distinguished by isoenzyme analysis of cultured promastigotes, determination of monoclonal antibody specificity, or various molecular methods.

Indirect immunologic methods for diagnosis include serologic assays and tests for *Leishmania*-specific cell-mediated immunity (e.g., skin testing for delayed-type hypersensitivity reactions). The usefulness of such methods depends in part on the clinical syndrome (see below). Traditional serologic assays (e.g., indirect immunofluorescent antibody testing) do not reliably distinguish past from current infec-

FIGURE 215-1 Amastigotes (the tissue form of the *Leishmania* parasite) in a bone marrow specimen from a patient with visceral leishmaniasis. Each amastigote has a nucleus and kinetoplast. The extracellular amastigotes probably were released from mononuclear phagocytes during specimen manipulation.

tion, and no leishmanin skin-test preparation has been approved for use in the United States. Advances in molecular methods (e.g., production of recombinant/synthetic antigens) may lead to the development of better diagnostic techniques.

GENERAL THERAPEUTIC PRINCIPLES For a given case of leishmaniasis, it is important to consider whether the patient's illness could result in substantial morbidity or in death and therefore requires expeditious treatment with a regimen that generally is highly effective. For decades, the pentavalent antimonial (Sb^V) compounds sodium stibogluconate and meglumine antimonate have been the mainstays of antileishmanial therapy (Table 215-2). Toxicity (with such manifestations as myalgia, arthralgia, fatigue, elevated amino-

Table 215-2 Drug Regimens for Treatment of Leishmaniasis[a]

Clinical Syndrome, Drug	Route of Administration	Regimen
VISCERAL LEISHMANIASIS		
First-line		
Pentavalent antimony[b]	IV, IM	20 mg Sb^V/kg qd for 28 days
Amphotericin B, lipid formulation[c]	IV	2–5 mg/kg qd (total: usually ~15–21 mg/kg)
Alternatives		
Amphotericin B (deoxycholate)	IV	0.5–1 mg/kg qod or qd (total: usually ~15–20 mg/kg)
Paromomycin sulfate[d]	IV, IM	15–20 mg/kg qd for ~21 days
Pentamidine isethionate	IV, IM	4 mg/kg qod or thrice weekly for ~15–30 doses
CUTANEOUS LEISHMANIASIS		
First-line		
Pentavalent antimony[b]	IV, IM	20 mg Sb^V/kg qd for 20 days
Parenteral alternatives		
Pentamidine isethionate	IV, IM	3 mg/kg qod for 4 doses or 2 mg/kg qod for 7 doses
Amphotericin B (deoxycholate)	IV	0.5–1 mg/kg qod or qd (total: up to ~20 mg/kg)
Oral alternatives		
Ketoconazole	PO	600 mg/d for 28 days[e]
Itraconazole	PO	200 mg bid for 28 days[e]
Dapsone	PO	100 mg bid for 6 weeks[e]
MUCOSAL LEISHMANIASIS		
First-line		
Pentavalent antimony[b]	IV, IM	20 mg Sb^V/kg qd for 28 days
Alternatives		
Amphotericin B (deoxycholate)	IV	1 mg/kg qod or qd (total: usually ~20–40 mg/kg)
Pentamidine isethionate	IV, IM	2–4 mg/kg qod or thrice weekly for ≥15 doses

[a] See text for additional details. To maximize effectiveness and minimize toxicity, the listed regimens should be individualized according to the particularities of the case.

[b] The Centers for Disease Control and Prevention (CDC) provides the pentavalent antimonial (Sb^V) compound sodium stibogluconate (Pentostam; Glaxo Wellcome, PLC, United Kingdom; 100 mg Sb^V/mL) to U.S.-licensed physicians through the CDC Drug Service (404-639-3670). The other widely used pentavalent antimonial compound, meglumine antimonate (Glucantime; Rhône Poulenc, France; 85 mg Sb^V/mL), is available primarily in Spanish- and French-speaking areas of the world.

[c] The lipid formulations of amphotericin B include liposomal amphotericin B, amphotericin B lipid complex, and amphotericin B cholesteryl sulfate. The U.S. Food and Drug Administration recently approved the following regimen of liposomal amphotericin B for immunocompetent patients: 3 mg/kg qd on days 1–5, 14, and 21, for a total of 21 mg/kg; for immunosuppressed patients, the approved regimen is 4 mg/kg qd on days 1–5, 10, 17, 24, 31, and 38, for a total of 40 mg/kg. Alternative regimens that have been proposed for immunocompetent patients include treatment on days 1–5 and 10 with 3–4 mg/kg qd for cases from Europe or Brazil, with 3 mg/kg qd for cases from Africa, and with 2–3 mg/kg qd for cases from India.

[d] Not commercially available as of this writing.

[e] Adult dosage.

transferase levels, chemical pancreatitis, and electrocardiographic abnormalities) becomes increasingly common as the course of treatment progresses but usually does not limit therapy and is reversible.

The traditional parenteral alternatives to Sb^V—amphotericin B and pentamidine isethionate—are generally considered more apt to induce serious or irreversible toxicity (e.g., nephrotoxicity). However, these agents are being advocated for use in some situations (see below; Table 215-2), in part because of the benefits of new formulations (e.g., lipid formulations of amphotericin B) or dosage regimens of these drugs and the decreasing effectiveness of Sb^V in some settings. Many other agents have been touted as alternatives or adjuncts to Sb^V, often on the basis of suboptimal data. Some of these agents may be useful in certain situations, with one caveat: even the results of well-conducted clinical trials are not always generalizable to the treatment of patients in other settings. Most of the nonparenteral agents evaluated to date have at best modest activity against some of the *Leishmania* species.

PREVENTION AND CONTROL The transmission of *Leishmania* species typically is focal, with local "hot spots," in part because of the limited flight range of sandflies; these insects have a short, hopping flight style and usually remain within a few hundred meters of their breeding site. They rest in dark, moist places in habitats ranging from deserts to rain forests; peridomestic sandflies rest in debris or rubble near buildings.

Personal protective measures include the avoidance of outdoor activities when sandflies are most active (dusk to dawn); the use of mechanical barriers such as screens and bed-nets that keep out sandflies, which are about one-third the size of mosquitoes; the wearing of protective clothing; and the application of insect repellent to exposed skin. Impregnation of clothing, bed-nets, and screens with permethrin may also be useful, as may spraying of dwellings with residual-action insecticide. Vaccine strategies are being investigated. Treatment of human cases is an effective control measure only where humans are the primary reservoirs of infection. Vector control and elimination of reservoir hosts may be useful in select settings—for example, where transmission is intra- or peridomiciliary.

VISCERAL LEISHMANIASIS

More than 90% of the world's cases of visceral leishmaniasis occur in Bangladesh, northeastern India (particularly Bihar State), Nepal, Sudan, and northeastern Brazil. The causative species typically are those of the *L. donovani* complex (Table 215-1). The organisms can be transmitted not only by sandflies but also congenitally and parenterally (e.g., through blood transfusions or sharing of needles). Infection begins in macrophages at the inoculation site (e.g., in dermal macrophages at the site of a sandfly bite) and disseminates throughout the mononuclear-phagocyte system in the context of both specific (i.e., to leishmanial antigens) and nonspecific (e.g., to tuberculin) anergy.

CLINICAL MANIFESTATIONS Visceral infection can remain subclinical or become symptomatic, with an acute, subacute, or chronic course. In some settings, inapparent infections far outnumber clinically apparent ones; malnutrition is among the risk factors for the development of disease. The incubation period usually ranges from weeks to months but can be as long as years. Whereas the general term *visceral leishmaniasis* covers a broad spectrum of severity and manifestations, the term *kala-azar* (Hindi for "black fever," indicating that the skin of some patients turns gray) generally conjures up the classic image of profoundly cachectic, febrile patients who are heavily infected with parasites and have life-threatening disease. Splenomegaly (with the spleen most often soft and nontender) typically is more impressive than hepatomegaly, and the spleen can in fact be massive; both splenomegaly and hepatomegaly result from reticuloendothelial cell hyperplasia. Peripheral lymphadenopathy is common in some settings, including Sudan.

The abnormal laboratory findings associated with advanced disease include pancytopenia—anemia, leukopenia (neutropenia, marked eosinopenia, relative lymphocytosis and monocytosis), and thrombocytopenia—as well as hypergammaglobulinemia (chiefly involving IgG, from polyclonal B cell activation) and hypoalbuminemia. Causes of anemia can include bone-marrow infiltration, hypersplenism, autoimmune hemolysis, and bleeding.

Some patients develop post–kala-azar dermal leishmaniasis. This syndrome is manifested by skin lesions (including macules, papules, nodules, and patches) that typically are most prominent on the face. These lesions can develop during therapy or within a few months thereafter (e.g., in East Africa) or can develop years later (e.g., in India); relapse of visceral infection can occur. Persons with persistent skin lesions can serve as reservoir hosts of infection.

Viscerotropic leishmaniasis caused by *L. tropica*, which typically is dermotropic, was recognized among U.S. soldiers who participated in Operation Desert Storm in the Persian Gulf. The affected persons had light parasite burdens and nonspecific manifestations of visceral infection (e.g., fatigue, fever, and gastrointestinal symptoms).

DIAGNOSIS   Although molecular techniques are under investigation, parasitologic diagnosis of visceral leishmaniasis has traditionally been accomplished by demonstration of the parasite on stained slides or in cultures of a tissue aspirate or a biopsy specimen (e.g., of spleen, liver, bone marrow, or lymph node). The diagnostic yield is highest for splenic aspiration (specifically, as high as 98% vs. <90% for other specimens), but this procedure can cause hemorrhage.

Patients with florid kala-azar commonly have relatively heavy parasite burdens, develop high titers of antibody to *Leishmania* (diagnostically useful but not protective), and have undetectable *Leishmania*-specific cell-mediated immunity (with leishmanin skin-test reactivity as well as lymphocyte proliferation and IFN-γ responses to leishmanial antigens typically noted only after recovery). In contrast, viscerotropic leishmaniasis can be difficult to diagnose because of a light parasite burden and a minimal antibody response. A promising noninvasive serologic method for diagnosing kala-azar uses nitrocellulose paper strips impregnated with K39, a recombinant leishmanial polypeptide; this technique is being field-tested.

The differential diagnosis of visceral leishmaniasis includes other tropical infectious diseases that cause fever or organomegaly (e.g., typhoid fever, miliary tuberculosis, brucellosis, malaria, tropical splenomegaly syndrome, and schistosomiasis) as well as diseases such as leukemia and lymphoma. Post–kala-azar dermal leishmaniasis should be differentiated from syphilis, yaws, and leprosy.

℞ TREATMENT   Because persons who have kala-azar generally die if not appropriately treated, highly effective therapy is essential, as is close monitoring for bleeding and intercurrent infectious conditions such as pneumonia and diarrhea. Outside of India, treatment with a pentavalent antimonial compound still is common (Table 215-2). The use of an alternative parenteral agent (Table 215-2) should be considered even for first-line therapy if unresponsiveness to Sb^V therapy is prevalent, as it is in India, or if nonantimonial therapy would be advantageous for other reasons (e.g., toxicity profile or duration of therapy).

A major advance has been the advent of lipid formulations of amphotericin B, in which various lipids have replaced deoxycholate. These formulations, which passively target amphotericin to macrophage-rich organs, are more costly than conventional amphotericin B but are associated with less nephrotoxicity and can be given in shorter courses. Other parenteral alternatives that have merit in some settings include the aminoglycoside paromomycin (the chemical equivalent of aminosidine; not commercially available as of this writing), which has been used as monotherapy (in India) or as an adjunct to Sb^V, and pentamidine. The oral agent miltefosine is being evaluated in clinical trials and preliminarily appears to be highly effective and acceptably tolerated.

Typically, patients feel better and become afebrile during the first week of treatment. Abnormal laboratory findings and splenomegaly may take weeks or months to resolve. The best indicator of permanent cure is freedom from clinical relapse during at least 6 months of follow-up. Repeat tissue sampling is indicated if the patient's status is in question. The persistence of some parasites is not necessarily a poor prognostic indicator, whereas the apparent absence of parasites does not ensure that the patient will not have a relapse.

VISCERAL LEISHMANIASIS IN PERSONS INFECTED WITH HIV   Visceral leishmaniasis has become an important opportunistic infection among persons infected with HIV-1 in geographic areas in which both infections are endemic. To date, most dual infections have been reported from southern Europe, where *L. infantum* (of the *L. donovani* complex) is endemic. In patients infected with HIV, even relatively avirulent *Leishmania* strains can disseminate to the viscera. Clinical leishmaniasis in coinfected patients can represent newly acquired or reactivated infection; most coinfected patients with clinically evident leishmaniasis have fewer than 200 CD4+ lymphocytes per microliter. Recent data suggest that leishmaniasis is a cofactor in the pathogenesis of HIV infection; the lipophosphoglycan (a major surface molecule) of *L. donovani* induces transcription of HIV in CD4+ cells.

A diagnosis of visceral leishmaniasis should be considered for patients infected with HIV who have ever been in leishmaniasis-endemic areas and who have manifestations such as unexplained fever, organomegaly, anemia, or pancytopenia. Coinfected patients can develop unusual manifestations of visceral leishmaniasis, in part because of atypical localization of the parasite (e.g., in the gastrointestinal tract).

The diagnostic sensitivity of classic serologic methods is lower in coinfected than in immunocompetent patients (~50% vs. >90%). However, parasitologic diagnosis by noninvasive means is easier in coinfected patients. Parasites are more commonly found in the circulating blood monocytes of these patients; the sensitivities are ~50% for a Giemsa-stained peripheral-blood smear and ~70% for culture of a buffy-coat preparation. Invasive methods of parasitologic diagnosis (e.g., microscopic examination or culture of a bone marrow aspirate) typically are highly sensitive, especially for previously untreated patients, who commonly have heavy parasite burdens.

Coinfected patients may initially respond well to standard antileishmanial therapy, albeit with more drug toxicity than is experienced by most immunocompetent persons. However, coinfected patients commonly have a chronic or relapsing course, seemingly irrespective of the drug regimens used for induction and suppression therapy.

CUTANEOUS LEISHMANIASIS

Cutaneous leishmaniasis has traditionally been classified as New World (American) or Old World disease. Local names for New World disease include *chiclero ulcer, pian bois* (bush yaws), and *uta*; those for Old World disease include *oriental sore, bouton d'orient, Aleppo evil,* and *Baghdad boil*. More than 90% of the world's cases of cutaneous leishmaniasis occur in Afghanistan, Algeria, Iran, Iraq, Saudi Arabia, Syria, Brazil, and Peru. In the Americas, the leishmaniasis-endemic area extends from southern Texas to northern Argentina; the etiologic agents typically are those of the *L. mexicana* complex and the *Viannia* subgenus (Table 215-1) but also include *L. major*–like organisms and *L. chagasi*. Old World cutaneous leishmaniasis is caused by *L. tropica, L. major,* and *L. aethiopica* as well as by *L. infantum* and *L. donovani*.

CLINICAL MANIFESTATIONS   The incubation period for clinically evident disease typically ranges from weeks to months. The first manifestation is usually a papule at the site of the sandfly bite but can be regional lymphadenopathy (sometimes bubonic) in *L. (V.) braziliensis* infection. Most skin lesions evolve from papular to nodular to ulcerative, with a central depression (which can be several centimeters in diameter) surrounded by a raised indurated border (Fig. 215-2). Some lesions persist as nodules or plaques. Multiple primary lesions, satellite lesions, regional adenopathy, sporotrichoid subcuta-

FIGURE 215-2 Ulcerative skin lesions with raised outer borders on the arm of a patient with New World (American) cutaneous leishmaniasis acquired in Costa Rica. (*Photograph courtesy of Dr. A. Wright.*)

neous nodules, lesion pain or pruritus, and secondary bacterial infection are variably present. The infecting species, the location of the lesion, and the host's immune response are among the determinants of the clinical manifestations and chronicity of untreated lesions. For example, in the New World, lesions caused by *L. mexicana* tend to be smaller and less chronic than those caused by *L. (V.) braziliensis*; in the Old World, *L. major* tends to cause "wet" exudative lesions that are less chronic than the "dry" lesions with central crusting that are caused by *L. tropica*. The spontaneous resolution of lesions does not preclude reactivation or reinfection.

The polyparasitic and oligoparasitic ends of the spectrum of cutaneous leishmaniasis are respectively represented by the rare syndromes of diffuse cutaneous leishmaniasis (DCL) and leishmaniasis recidivans, both of which are notoriously difficult to treat. DCL caused by *L. aethiopica* (Old World) or by the *L. mexicana* complex (New World), develops in the context of *Leishmania*-specific anergy and is manifested by chronic, disseminated, nonulcerative skin lesions: on histopathologic examination of specimens from these lesions, abundant parasites but few lymphocytes are noted. Leishmaniasis recidivans, a hyperergic variant with scarce parasites, is usually caused by *L. tropica* and manifested by a chronic solitary lesion on the cheek that expands slowly despite central healing.

DIAGNOSIS Dermal scrapings of debrided ulcerative lesions are useful for histologic examination, aspirates of skin lesions and lymph nodes for in vitro culture, and biopsy specimens for both examination and culture. Although examination of histologic sections of biopsy specimens can help exclude other diagnoses, amastigotes appear larger and are more easily recognizable on Giemsa-stained thin smears (e.g., smears of dermal scrapings, touch preparations of biopsy specimens). As lesions age, amastigotes become scarcer, and parasitologic confirmation becomes more difficult.

Serologic testing is an insensitive means for diagnosing cutaneous leishmaniasis; antibody titers usually are at most minimally elevated except in patients who have DCL. In contrast, leishmanin skin-test reactivity usually develops during active infection in persons who have simple cutaneous or recidivans leishmaniasis but not in those who have DCL.

Cutaneous leishmaniasis is frequently confused with tropical, traumatic, and venous-stasis ulcers; foreign-body reactions; superinfected insect bites; myiasis; impetigo; fungal infections (e.g., sporotrichosis); mycobacterial infections; and other diseases (e.g., sarcoidosis, neoplasms). DCL and leishmaniasis recidivans should be differentiated from lepromatous leprosy and lupus vulgaris, respectively.

℞ **TREATMENT** Decisions about whether and how to treat cutaneous leishmaniasis should take into account whether mucosal dissemination is possible (as it is in the Americas with some organisms in the *Viannia* subgenus; Table 215-1) as well as the location (e.g., on the face), number, size, evolution, and chronicity of the cutaneous lesions. When optimal effectiveness is important, intravenous or intramuscular Sb^V therapy is recommended (Table 215-2). In studies in Colombia (predominantly with the *Viannia* subgenus), relatively short

courses of treatment with pentamidine (Table 215-2) were effective (cure rate, 96%) and quite well tolerated. Thus pentamidine may be a good parenteral alternative to Sb^V. The clinical response to antileishmanial therapy begins with lessening induration; healing often continues after the end of therapy. Relapse typically is manifested by clinical reactivation at the margin of the lesion.

Although many oral agents have been touted for treatment of leishmaniasis, even those that are the most effective typically are moderately active at best and are effective only against some *Leishmania* species or strains. The oral agent miltefosine is being evaluated. In the New World, ketoconazole has some activity against *L. mexicana* and *L. (V.) panamensis* and may be more active than itraconazole (at least against the *Viannia* subgenus), which is better tolerated (Table 215-2). Dapsone has looked promising in India but not in Colombia. Adjunctive immunotherapy remains highly experimental but may be useful in DCL. Local or topical therapy can be considered for some cases of infection in which there is no risk of mucosal dissemination (e.g., for relatively benign lesions caused by *L. mexicana* or *L. major*). Examples of local approaches include the application of an ointment containing paromomycin and methylbenzethonium chloride (not licensed in the United States), the intralesional administration of Sb^V, heat therapy, and cryotherapy.

MUCOSAL LEISHMANIASIS

Leishmanial infection of the naso-oropharyngeal mucosa is a relatively rare but potentially disfiguring metastatic complication of cutaneous leishmaniasis. Mucosal disease develops despite antileishmanial cell-mediated immunity and most commonly is caused by organisms of the *Viannia* subgenus, typically *L. (V.) braziliensis* but also *L. (V.) panamensis* and *L. (V.) guyanensis*. Although mucosal disease usually becomes clinically evident within several years after the healing of the original cutaneous lesions, cutaneous and mucosal lesions can coexist or appear decades apart. Typically, the original cutaneous lesions of patients who develop mucosal disease were not treated or were suboptimally treated.

Mucosal involvement generally is manifested first by persistent unusual nasal symptoms (e.g., epistaxis), with erythema and edema of the nasal mucosa, and then by progressive, ulcerative, naso-oropharyngeal destruction. Supportive laboratory data (e.g., a positive serologic test) are useful, but the scarcity of amastigotes makes parasitologic confirmation difficult. The differential diagnosis includes sarcoidosis, neoplasms, midline granuloma, rhinoscleroma, paracoccidioidomycosis, histoplasmosis, leprosy, syphilis, and tertiary yaws.

Treatment with a pentavalent antimonial compound is moderately effective for mild mucosal disease, whereas advanced disease may not respond to such treatment or may relapse repeatedly (Table 215-2). Amphotericin B (deoxycholate) is the best alternative drug currently available. Patients who develop signs of respiratory compromise during therapy may benefit from the concomitant administration of glucocorticoids.

BIBLIOGRAPHY

ALVAR J et al: *Leishmania* and human immunodeficiency virus coinfection: The first 10 years. Clin Microbiol Rev 10:298, 1997

BERMAN JD: Human leishmaniasis: Clinical, diagnostic, and chemotherapeutic developments in the last 10 years. Clin Infect Dis 24:684, 1997

———: Editorial response: U.S. Food and Drug Administration approval of AmBisome (liposomal amphotericin B) for treatment of visceral leishmaniasis. Clin Infect Dis 28:49, 1999

BERNIER R et al: The lipophosphoglycan of *Leishmania donovani* up-regulates HIV-1 transcription in T cells through the nuclear factor-κB elements. J Immunol 160:2881, 1998

HERWALDT BL: Leishmaniasis. Lancet 354:1191, 1999

———, BERMAN JD: Recommendations for treating leishmaniasis with sodium stibogluconate (Pentostam) and review of pertinent clinical studies. Am J Trop Med Hyg 46:296, 1992

JHA TK et al: Miltefosine, an oral agent, for the treatment of Indian visceral leishmaniasis. N Engl J Med 341:1795, 1999

KENNEY RT et al: Splenic cytokine responses in Indian kala-azar before and after treatment. J Infect Dis 177:815, 1998

LAGUNA F et al: Treatment of visceral leishmaniasis in HIV-infected patients: A randomized trial comparing meglumine antimonate with amphotericin B. AIDS 13:1063, 1999

MAGILL AJ et al: Visceral infection caused by *Leishmania tropica* in veterans of Operation Desert Storm. N Engl J Med 328:1383, 1993

MEYERHOFF A: U.S. Food and Drug Administration approval of AmBisome (liposomal amphotericin B) for treatment of visceral leishmaniasis. Clin Infect Dis 28:42, 1999

REED SG: Diagnosis of leishmaniasis. Clin Dermatol 14:471, 1996

SUNDAR S et al: Rapid accurate field diagnosis of Indian visceral leishmaniasis. Lancet 351:563, 1998

WEIGLE K, SARAVIA NG: Natural history, clinical evolution, and the host-parasite interaction in New World cutaneous leishmaniasis. Clin Dermatol 14:433, 1996

WORLD HEALTH ORGANIZATION: Control of the leishmaniases. Technical Report Series 793. Geneva, World Health Organization, 1990

216   *Louis V. Kirchhoff*

TRYPANOSOMIASIS

CHAGAS' DISEASE

DEFINITION Chagas' disease, or American trypanosomiasis, is a zoonosis caused by the protozoan parasite *Trypanosoma cruzi*. Acute Chagas' disease is usually a mild febrile illness that results from initial infection with the organism. After spontaneous resolution of the acute illness, most infected persons remain for life in the indeterminate phase of chronic Chagas' disease, which is characterized by subpatent parasitemia, easily detectable antibodies to *T. cruzi*, and an absence of symptoms. In a minority of chronically infected patients, cardiac and gastrointestinal lesions develop that can result in serious morbidity and even death.

LIFE CYCLE AND TRANSMISSION *T. cruzi* is transmitted among its mammalian hosts by hematophagous triatomine insects, often called reduviid bugs. The insects become infected by sucking blood from animals or humans who have circulating parasites. Ingested organisms multiply in the gut of the triatomines, and infective forms are discharged with the feces at the time of subsequent blood meals. Transmission to a second vertebrate host occurs when breaks in the skin, mucous membranes, or conjunctivae become contaminated with bug feces that contain infective parasites. *T. cruzi* also can be transmitted by the transfusion of blood donated by infected persons, from mother to fetus, and in laboratory accidents.

PATHOLOGY An indurated inflammatory lesion called a *chagoma* often appears at the site of the parasite's entry. Local histologic changes include the presence of parasites within leukocytes and cells of subcutaneous tissues and the development of interstitial edema, lymphocytic infiltration, and reactive hyperplasia of adjacent lymph nodes. After dissemination of the organisms through the lymphatics and the bloodstream, muscles (including the myocardium) may become heavily parasitized. The characteristic pseudocysts present in sections of infected tissues are intracellular aggregates of multiplying parasites.

The pathogenesis of chronic Chagas' disease is poorly understood. The heart is the organ most commonly affected, and changes include biventricular enlargement, thinning of the ventricular walls, apical aneurysms, and mural thrombi. Widespread lymphocytic infiltration, diffuse interstitial fibrosis, and atrophy of myocardial cells are often demonstrated, but parasites are rarely seen in myocardial tissue. Conduction-system involvement often affects the right branch and the left anterior branch of the bundle of His. In chronic Chagas' disease of the gastrointestinal tract (megadisease), the esophagus and colon may exhibit varying degrees of dilatation. On microscopic examination, focal inflammatory lesions with lymphocytic infiltration are seen, and the number of neurons in the myenteric plexus may be markedly reduced.

EPIDEMIOLOGY *T. cruzi* is found only in the Americas. Wild and domestic mammals harboring *T. cruzi* and infected triatomines are found in spotty distributions from the southern United States to southern Argentina. Humans become involved in the cycle of transmission when infected vectors take up residence in the primitive wood, adobe, and stone houses common in much of Latin America. Thus, human *T. cruzi* infection is a health problem primarily among the poor in rural areas of Central and South America. Most new *T. cruzi* infections in rural settings occur in children, but the incidence is unknown because most cases go undiagnosed. Thousands of individuals also become infected every year through blood transfusions in urban areas. Several dozen patients with HIV and chronic *T. cruzi* infections who underwent acute recrudescence of the latter have been described. These patients generally presented with *T. cruzi* brain abscesses, a manifestation of the illness that does not occur in immunocompetent persons. Currently, it is estimated that 16 to 18 million people, more than a third of whom live in Brazil, are chronically infected with *T. cruzi*. Chronic Chagas' disease is a major cause of morbidity and mortality in many Latin American countries, including Mexico, since many chronically infected persons eventually develop symptomatic cardiac lesions or gastrointestinal disease.

In recent years, the rate of *T. cruzi* transmission has been decreasing in several endemic countries as a result of successful vector and blood-bank control programs. A major program in the "southern cone" nations of South America (Uruguay, Paraguay, Bolivia, Brazil, Chile, and Argentina), begun in 1991, has provided the framework for much of the progress achieved. If current trends continue, transmission will be essentially eliminated in much of the endemic range by the year 2003.

Acute Chagas' disease is rare in the United States. Five cases of autochthonous transmission and four instances of transmission by blood transfusion have been reported. Moreover, in the last 26 years, seven laboratory-acquired infections and nine imported cases of acute Chagas' disease were reported to the Centers for Disease Control and Prevention (CDC). In contrast, the prevalence of chronic *T. cruzi* infections in the United States has increased considerably in recent years. Since the mid-1970s, enormous numbers of Latin Americans have emigrated to the United States. In one study conducted in Washington, D.C., 5% of Salvadoran and Nicaraguan immigrants were found to have chronic *T. cruzi* infections. Estimates based on the latter study and on studies done in several United States blood banks put the total number of infected immigrants now living in the United States at more than 50,000. The presence of these carriers of *T. cruzi* creates a substantial risk of transmission by blood transfusion, as is evidenced by the four transfusion-associated cases just cited.

CLINICAL COURSE The first signs of acute Chagas' disease develop at least 1 week after invasion by the parasites. When the organisms enter through a break in the skin, an indurated area of erythema and swelling (the chagoma), accompanied by local lymphadenopathy, may appear. Romaña's sign—the classic finding in acute Chagas' disease, which consists of unilateral painless edema of the palpebrae and periocular tissues—can result when the conjunctiva is the portal of entry. These initial local signs are followed by malaise, fever, anorexia, and edema of the face and lower extremities. A morbilliform rash may also appear. Generalized lymphadenopathy and hepatosplenomegaly may develop. Severe myocarditis develops rarely; most deaths in acute Chagas' disease are due to heart failure. Neurologic signs are not common, but meningoencephalitis has been reported. The acute symptoms resolve spontaneously in virtually all patients, who then enter the asymptomatic or indeterminate phase of chronic *T. cruzi* infection.

Symptomatic chronic Chagas' disease becomes apparent years or even decades after the initial infection. The heart is commonly involved, and symptoms are caused by rhythm disturbances, cardiomyopathy, and thromboembolism. Right bundle-branch block is the most common electrocardiographic abnormality, but other types of atrioventricular block, premature ventricular contractions, and tachy-

and bradyarrhythmias occur frequently. Cardiomyopathy often results in right-sided or biventricular heart failure. Embolization of mural thrombi to the brain or other areas may take place. Patients with mega-esophagus suffer from dysphagia, odynophagia, chest pain, and re-gurgitation. Aspiration can occur, especially during sleep, and repeated episodes of aspiration pneumonitis are common. Weight loss, ca-chexia, and pulmonary infection can result in death. Patients with megacolon are plagued by abdominal pain and chronic constipation, and advanced megacolon can cause obstruction, volvulus, septicemia, and death.

DIAGNOSIS The diagnosis of acute Chagas' disease requires the detection of parasites. Microscopic examination of fresh anticoag-ulated blood or of the buffy coat is the simplest way to see the motile organisms. Parasites also can be seen in Giemsa-stained thin and thick blood smears. When repeated attempts to visualize the organisms are unsuccessful, mouse inoculation, culture of blood in specialized me-dia, or xenodiagnosis can be performed. In the last technique, unin-fected triatomine insects are allowed to feed on the patient's blood. When done properly, all of these methods yield positive results in a high proportion of patients with acute Chagas' disease and in at least half of those with chronic infections. Since early treatment of acute Chagas' disease is extremely important, however, the decision to ini-tiate therapy for *T. cruzi* infection despite negative wet preparations and smears must be made on clinical and epidemiologic grounds be-fore the results of these indirect methods become available. Serologic testing is of limited usefulness in diagnosing acute Chagas' disease.

The diagnosis of chronic Chagas' disease is made by the detection of antibodies that bind to *T. cruzi* antigens. Demonstration of the para-site is not of primary importance. Several highly sensitive serologic tests for antibodies to *T. cruzi* are used widely in Latin America, in-cluding complement-fixation and immunofluorescence tests and en-zyme-linked immunosorbent assays (ELISAs). However, a persistent problem with these conventional assays is the occurrence of false-positive reactions, typically with sera from patients who have other parasitic infections or autoimmune diseases. For this reason, it is gen-erally recommended that positivity in one assay be confirmed by two other tests and that well-characterized positive and negative compar-ison sera be included in each run. A highly sensitive and specific method for detecting antibodies to *T. cruzi* [approved by the Clinical Laboratory Improvement Amendment (CLIA) and available in the au-thor's laboratory] employs immunoprecipitation of radiolabeled *T. cruzi* antigens and electrophoresis. Serodiagnostic assays that employ recombinant *T. cruzi* proteins as target antigens are being developed, as are tests based on the amplification of *T. cruzi* DNA sequences by polymerase chain reaction. However, these tests are not yet available for general use.

℞ **TREATMENT** Therapy for Chagas' disease is unsatisfactory. Nifurtimox is the only drug active against *T. cruzi* that is available in the United States. In acute Chagas' disease, nifurtimox markedly reduces the duration of symptoms and parasitemia and decreases the mortality rate. Nevertheless, its efficacy at eradicating parasites is low. Limited studies have shown that only ~70% of acute infections are cured parasitologically by a full course of treatment. Despite its lim-itations, nifurtimox treatment should be initiated as early as possible in acute Chagas' disease. Moreover, when laboratory accidents occur in which it appears likely that *T. cruzi* infection could become estab-lished, nifurtimox therapy should be initiated without waiting for clin-ical or parasitologic indications of infection.

Common adverse effects of nifurtimox include abdominal pain, anorexia, nausea, vomiting, and weight loss. Neurologic reactions to the drug may include restlessness, disorientation, insomnia, twitching, paresthesia, polyneuritis, and seizures. These symptoms usually dis-appear when the dosage is reduced or treatment is discontinued. The recommended daily dosage is 8 to 10 mg/kg for adults, 12.5 to 15 mg/kg for adolescents, and 15 to 20 mg/kg for children 1 to 10 years of age. The drug should be given orally in four divided doses each day, and therapy should be continued for 90 to 120 days. Nifurtimox is

available from the Drug Service of the CDC in Atlanta, Georgia (tele-phone number, 770-639-3670).

Benznidazole is a second agent used to treat Chagas' disease. Its efficacy is similar to that of nifurtimox, and its adverse effects include peripheral neuropathy, rash, and granulocytopenia. The recommended oral dosage is 5 mg/kg per day for 60 days. Benznidazole is used widely in Latin America.

The question of whether patients in the indeterminate or chronic symptomatic phases of Chagas' disease should be treated with nifur-timox or benznidazole has been debated for years. Studies of *T. cruzi*–infected laboratory animals and humans suggest that elimination of the parasites reduces the appearance or progression of cardiac pathol-ogy. In view of these findings, an international panel of experts has recommended that all patients infected with *T. cruzi* be treated with one drug or the other, regardless of their clinical status or the duration of infection.

The usefulness of allopurinol, fluconazole, and itraconazole for the treatment of acute Chagas' disease has been studied extensively in laboratory animals and to a lesser extent in humans. None of these drugs has exhibited a level of anti–*T. cruzi* activity that warrants its use in patients. Studies in mice have shown that recombinant interferon γ decreases the duration and severity of acute *T. cruzi* infection; how-ever, its usefulness in persons with acute Chagas' disease has not been evaluated systematically.

Patients who develop cardiac and/or gastrointestinal disease in as-sociation with *T. cruzi* infection should be referred to appropriate sub-specialists for further evaluation and treatment. Cardiac transplantation is an option for patients with end-stage chagasic cardiopathies. Post-operative prophylaxis with nifurtimox or benznidazole should be con-sidered because without it the immunosuppression required after sur-gery has been shown to result in reactivation of *T. cruzi* infection, often with serious consequences or even death.

PREVENTION Since drug therapy is unsatisfactory and vac-cines are not available, the control of *T. cruzi* transmission in endemic countries must depend on reduction of domiciliary vector populations by spraying of insecticides, improvement of housing, and education. In addition, in endemic areas, programs for the screening of donated blood for *T. cruzi* need to be expanded and improved to reduce rates of transmission by transfusion. Tourists traveling in endemic areas should avoid sleeping in dilapidated houses outside urban areas. Mos-quito nets and insect repellent provide additional protection.

In the United States, the question of how best to avoid transmission of *T. cruzi* by blood transfusion is not easily resolved. Since no assay for *T. cruzi* infection has received clearance from the Food and Drug Administration (FDA) for use in blood banks, serologic screening is not yet an option. The FDA currently mandates the use of a question-naire for identifying and deferring donors at high risk for *T. cruzi* infection. This approach may be effective and not reduce the blood supply intolerably, but it is important to bear in mind that approaches based solely on questionnaires have not been entirely successful at eliminating transfusion-associated transmission of other infectious agents.

In view of the possibly serious consequences of chronic *T. cruzi* infection, it would be prudent for all immigrants from endemic regions to be tested for evidence of infection. Identification of infected persons is also important because the implantation of pacemakers benefits some patients who develop ominous rhythm disturbances. The possi-bility of congenital transmission is yet another justification for screening.

Laboratory personnel should wear gloves and eye protection when working with *T. cruzi* and infected vectors.

SLEEPING SICKNESS

DEFINITION Sleeping sickness, or human African trypanoso-miasis (HAT), is caused by flagellated protozoan parasites that belong to the *T. brucei* complex and are transmitted to humans by tsetse flies. In untreated patients, the trypanosomes first cause a febrile illness that is followed months or years later by progressive neurologic impairment and death.

THE PARASITES AND THEIR TRANSMISSION The East African (*rhodesiense*) and the West African (*gambiense*) forms of sleeping sickness are caused, respectively, by two trypanosome subspecies: *T. brucei rhodesiense* and *T. brucei gambiense*. These subspecies are morphologically indistinguishable but cause illnesses that are epidemiologically and clinically distinct. The parasites are transmitted by blood-sucking tsetse flies of the genus *Glossina*. The insects acquire the infection when they ingest blood from infected mammalian hosts. After many cycles of multiplication in the midgut of the vector, the parasites migrate to the salivary glands. Their transmission takes place when they are inoculated during a subsequent blood meal. The injected trypanosomes multiply in the blood and other extracellular spaces and evade immune destruction in mammalian hosts for long periods by undergoing antigenic variation, in which the antigenic structure of their surface coat of glycoproteins changes periodically.

PATHOGENESIS AND PATHOLOGY A self-limited inflammatory lesion (trypanosomal chancre) may appear a week or so after the bite of an infected tsetse fly. A systemic febrile illness then evolves as the parasites are disseminated through the lymphatics and bloodstream. Systemic HAT without central nervous system (CNS) involvement is generally referred to as *stage I disease*. In this stage, widespread lymphadenopathy and splenomegaly reflect marked lymphocytic and histiocytic proliferation and invasion of morular cells, which are plasmacytes that may be involved in the production of IgM. Endarteritis, with perivascular infiltration of both parasites and lymphocytes, may develop in lymph nodes and spleen. Myocarditis develops frequently in patients with stage I disease and is especially common in *T. b. rhodesiense* infections.

Hematologic manifestations that accompany stage I HAT include moderate leukocytosis, thrombocytopenia, and anemia. High levels of immunoglobulins, consisting primarily of polyclonal IgM, are a constant feature, and heterophile antibodies, antibodies to DNA, and rheumatoid factor are often detected. High levels of antigen-antibody complexes may play a role in the tissue damage and increased vascular permeability that facilitate dissemination of the parasites.

Stage II disease involves invasion of the CNS. The presence of trypanosomes in perivascular areas is accompanied by intense infiltration of mononuclear cells. Abnormalities in cerebrospinal fluid (CSF) include increased pressure, elevated total protein concentration, and pleocytosis. In addition, trypanosomes are frequently found in CSF.

EPIDEMIOLOGY The trypanosomes that cause sleeping sickness are found only in Africa. Approximately 50 million persons are at risk of acquiring HAT, and tens of thousands of new cases occur every year. Precise data are not available because health statistics are often incomplete in the developing countries where HAT is endemic. Sleeping sickness has undergone a resurgence in recent years, with major epidemics in the Sudan, Ivory Coast, Chad, the Central African Republic, and several other endemic countries.

Humans are the only reservoir of *T. b. gambiense*, which occurs in widely distributed foci in tropical rain forests of Central and West Africa. Gambiense trypanosomiasis is primarily a problem in rural populations; tourists rarely become infected. Trypanotolerant antelope species in savanna and woodland areas of Central and East Africa are the principal reservoir of *T. b. rhodesiense*. Cattle also can become infected but generally succumb to the parasite. Since risk results for the most part from contact with tsetse flies that feed on wild animals, humans acquire *T. b. rhodesiense* infection only incidentally, usually while working in areas where infected game and vectors are present. In addition, occasional cases occur among visitors to game parks in East Africa. During the past 22 years, 21 cases of imported HAT have

been reported to the CDC, most of which were caused by *T. b. rhodesiense*.

CLINICAL COURSE A painful trypanosomal chancre appears in some patients at the site of inoculation of the parasite. Hematogenous and lymphatic dissemination (stage I disease) is marked by the onset of fever. Typically, bouts of high temperatures lasting several days are separated by afebrile periods. Lymphadenopathy is prominent in *T. b. gambiense* trypanosomiasis. The nodes are discrete, movable, rubbery, and nontender. Cervical nodes are often visible, and enlargement of the nodes of the posterior cervical triangle, or Winterbottom's sign, is a classic finding. Pruritus and maculopapular rashes are common. Inconstant findings include malaise, headache, arthralgias, weight loss, edema, hepatosplenomegaly, and tachycardia.

CNS invasion (stage II disease) is characterized by the insidious development of protean neurologic manifestations that are accompanied by progressive abnormalities in the CSF. A picture of progressive indifference and daytime somnolence develops (hence the designation "sleeping sickness"), sometimes alternating with restlessness and insomnia at night. A listless gaze accompanies a loss of spontaneity, and speech may become halting and indistinct. Extrapyramidal signs may include choreiform movements, tremors, and fasciculations. Ataxia is frequent, and the patient may appear to have Parkinson's disease, with a shuffling gait, hypertonia, and tremors. In the final phase, progressive neurologic impairment ends in coma and death.

The most striking difference between the West African and East African trypanosomiases is that the latter illness tends to follow a more acute course. Typically, in tourists, systemic signs of infection, such as fever, malaise, and headache, appear before the end of the trip or shortly after the return home. Persistent tachycardia unrelated to fever is common early in the course of *T. b. rhodesiense* trypanosomiasis, and death may result from arrhythmias and congestive heart failure before CNS disease develops. In general, untreated *T. b. rhodesiense* trypanosomiasis leads to death in a matter of weeks to months, often without a clear distinction between the hemolymphatic and CNS stages.

DIAGNOSIS A definitive diagnosis of HAT requires detection of the parasite. If a chancre is present, fluid should be expressed and examined directly by light microscopy for the highly motile trypanosomes. The fluid also should be fixed and stained with Giemsa. Material obtained by needle aspiration of lymph nodes early in the course of the illness should be examined similarly. Examination of wet preparations and Giemsa-stained thin and thick films of serial blood samples is also useful. If parasites are not seen in blood, efforts should be made to concentrate the organisms; the simplest method involves the use of quantitative buffy coat analysis tubes (QBC, Becton-Dickinson, Franklin Lakes, NJ). In these tubes, which are coated with acridine orange, the parasites are separated from blood cells by centrifugation and are easily seen under light microscopy because of the stain. The buffy coat from 10 to 15 mL of anticoagulated blood or the pellet obtained by centrifugation of the eluate from 25 to 50 mL of blood passed through a DEAE-cellulose column also can be examined. Trypanosomes may be seen in material aspirated from the bone marrow; the aspirate can be inoculated into liquid culture medium, as can blood, buffy coat, lymph node aspirates, and CSF. Finally, *T. b. rhodesiense* infection can be detected by inoculation of these specimens into mice or rats, which results in patent parasitemias in a week or two. Although this method is highly sensitive for the detection of *T. b. rhodesiense*, it does not detect *T. b. gambiense* because of host specificity.

It is essential to examine CSF from all patients in whom HAT is suspected. An increase in the CSF cell count is the first abnormality to be detected; increases in opening pressure and in levels of total protein and IgM develop later. Trypanosomes may be seen in the sediment of centrifuged CSF. Any CSF abnormality in a patient in whom trypanosomes have been found at other sites must be viewed as pathognomonic for CNS involvement and thus must prompt specific treatment for CNS disease.

A number of serologic assays are available to aid in the diagnosis of HAT, but their variable sensitivity and specificity mandate that decisions about treatment be based on demonstration of the parasite. These tests are of value for epidemiologic surveys.

℞ **TREATMENT** The drugs traditionally used for treatment of HAT are suramin, pentamidine, and organic arsenicals. An addition to this list is eflornithine (difluoromethylornithine), which was approved by the FDA in November 1990 for the treatment of West African trypanosomiasis. In the United States these drugs can be obtained from the CDC. Therapy for HAT must be individualized on the basis of the infecting organism (*T. b. gambiense* or *T. b. rhodesiense*), the presence or absence of CNS disease, adverse reactions, and (occasionally) drug resistance. The choices of drugs for the treatment of HAT are summarized in Table 216-1.

Suramin is highly effective against stage I disease. However, it can cause serious adverse effects and must be administered under the close supervision of a physician. A 100- to 200-mg intravenous test dose should be administered to detect hypersensitivity. The dosage for adults is 1 g intravenously on days 1, 3, 7, 14, and 21. The regimen for children is 20 mg/kg (maximum, 1 g) intravenously on days 1, 3, 7, 14, and 21. The drug is given by slow intravenous infusion of a freshly prepared 10% aqueous solution. Approximately 1 patient in 20,000 has an immediate, severe, and potentially fatal reaction to the drug, developing nausea, vomiting, shock, and seizures. Less severe reactions include fever, photophobia, pruritus, arthralgias, and skin eruptions. Renal damage is the most common important adverse effect of suramin. Transient proteinuria often appears during treatment. A urinalysis should be done before each dose, and treatment should be discontinued if proteinuria increases or if casts and red cells appear in the sediment. Suramin should not be given to patients with renal insufficiency.

Eflornithine is highly effective for treatment of both stages of West African trypanosomiasis. In the trials on which the FDA based its approval, this agent cured more than 90% of 600 patients with stage II disease. The recommended treatment schedule is 400 mg/kg per day intravenously in four divided doses for 2 weeks. Adverse reactions include diarrhea, anemia, thrombocytopenia, seizures, and hearing loss. The high dosage and duration of therapy required are disadvantages that make widespread use of eflornithine difficult.

Pentamidine is the alternative drug for patients with stage I HAT, although some *T. b. rhodesiense* infections are unresponsive to this agent. The dose for both adults and children is 4 mg/kg per day intramuscularly or intravenously for 10 days. Frequent, immediate adverse reactions include nausea, vomiting, tachycardia, and hypotension. These reactions are usually transient and do not warrant cessation of therapy. Other adverse reactions include nephrotoxicity, abnormal liver function tests, neutropenia, rashes, hypoglycemia, and sterile abscesses.

The arsenical melarsoprol is the drug of choice for the treatment of East African trypanosomiasis with CNS involvement. Melarsoprol cures both stages of the disease and therefore is also indicated for the treatment of stage I disease in patients who fail to respond to or cannot tolerate suramin and/or pentamidine. However, because of its relatively high toxicity, melarsoprol is never the first choice for the treatment of stage I disease. The drug should be given to adults in three courses of 3 days each. The dosage is 2 to 3.6 mg/kg per day intravenously in three divided doses for 3 days followed 1 week later by 3.6 mg/kg per day, also in three divided doses and for 3 days. The latter course is repeated 10 to 21 days later. In debilitated patients, suramin is administered for 2 to 4 days before therapy with melarsoprol is initiated. An 18-mg initial dose of the latter drug, followed by progressive increases to the standard dose, has been recommended. For children, a total of 18 to 25 mg/kg should be given over 1 month. A starting dose of 0.36 mg/kg intravenously should be increased gradually to a maximum of 3.6 mg/kg at 1- to 5-day intervals, for a total of 9 or 10 doses.

Melarsoprol is highly toxic and should be administered with great care. The incidence of reactive encephalopathy has been reported to be as high as 18% in some series. Clinical manifestations of reactive encephalopathy include high fever, headache, tremor, impaired speech, seizures, and even coma and death. Treatment with melarsoprol should be discontinued at the first sign of encephalopathy but may be restarted cautiously at lower doses a few days after signs have resolved. Extravasation of the drug results in intense local reactions. Vomiting, abdominal pain, nephrotoxicity, and myocardial damage can occur.

The treatment of patients with stage II East African disease who cannot tolerate melarsoprol is problematic. The combination of the arsenical tryparsamide and suramin is one possible approach, but its efficacy is limited because suramin does not penetrate the CNS well and tryparsamide is much less effective against *T. b. rhodesiense* than it is against *T. b. gambiense*. The schedule for tryparsamide therapy is 30 mg/kg (maximum, 2 g) in a single intravenous dose every 5 days for a total of 12 doses; that for suramin treatment is 10 mg/kg intravenously every 5 days, also for a total of 12 injections. Tryparsamide can cause encephalopathy, fever, vomiting, abdominal pain, rash, tinnitus, and a variety of ocular symptoms. Alternatively, eflornithine can be administered as outlined above to patients who cannot tolerate melarsoprol, but, as noted, its effectiveness against *T. b. rhodesiense* is variable.

PREVENTION HAT poses complex public-health and epizootic problems in Africa. Considerable progress has been made in some areas through control programs that focus on eradication of vectors and drug treatment of infected humans; however, there is no consensus on the best approach to solving the overall problem, and major epidemics continue to occur. Individuals can reduce their risk of acquiring trypanosomiasis by avoiding areas known to harbor infected insects, by wearing protective clothing, and by using insect repellent. Chemoprophylaxis is not recommended, and no vaccine is available to prevent transmission of the parasites.

BIBLIOGRAPHY

CHAGAS' DISEASE

BOCCHI EA et al: Higher incidence of malignant neoplasms after heart transplantation for treatment of chronic Chagas' heart disease. J Heart Lung Transplant 17:399, 1998

GOMES ML et al: Chagas' disease diagnosis: Comparative analysis of parasitologic, molecular, and serologic methods. Am J Trop Med Hyg 60:205, 1999

GUZMAN BRACHO C et al: Risk of transmission of *Trypanosoma cruzi* by blood transfusion in Mexico [Spanish]. Pan Am J Public Health 4:94, 1998

KIRCHHOFF LV: American trypanosomiasis (Chagas' disease): A persistent problem in Latin America now affects the United States. N Engl J Med 329:639, 1993

———: American trypanosomiasis (Chagas' disease). Gastroenterol Clin North Am 25:517, 1996

——— et al: Increased specificity of serodiagnosis of Chagas' disease by detection of antibody to the 72- and 90-kilodalton glycoproteins of *Trypanosoma cruzi*. J Infect Dis 155:561, 1987

LEIBY DA et al: Seroepidemiology of *Trypanosoma cruzi*, etiologic agent of Chagas' disease, in U.S. blood donors. J Infect Dis 176:1047, 1997

OCHS DE et al: Postmortem diagnosis of autochthonous acute chagasic myocarditis by PCR amplification of a species-specific DNA sequence of *Trypanosoma cruzi*. Am J Trop Med Hyg 54:526, 1996

PARADA H et al: Cardiac involvement is a constant finding in acute Chagas' disease: A clinical, parasitological and histopathological study. Int J Cardiol 60:49, 1997

Table 216-1 Treatment of Human African Trypanosomiases[a]

Causative Organism	Clinical Stage	
	I (Normal CSF)	II (Abnormal CSF)
T. brucei gambiense (West African)	Suramin or eflornithine Alternative: Pentamidine	Eflornithine Alternative: Tryparsamide plus suramin
T. brucei rhodesiense (East African)	Suramin Alternative: Pentamidine	Melarsoprol

[a] For doses and duration, see text.

SARTORI AM et al: Follow-up of 18 patients with human immunodeficiency virus infection and chronic Chagas' disease, with reactivation of Chagas' disease causing cardiac disease in three patients. Clin Infect Dis 26:177, 1998

SCHMUNIS GA et al: Interruption of Chagas' disease transmission through vector elimination. Lancet 348:1171, 1996

SLEEPING SICKNESS

DONELSON JE et al: Multiple mechanisms of immune evasion by African trypanosomes. Mol Biochem Parasitol 91:51, 1998

Drugs for parasitic infections. Med Lett Drugs Ther 40:1, 1998

EKWANZALA M et al: In the heart of darkness: Sleeping sickness in Zaire. Lancet 348: 1427, 1996

HUNTER CA, KENNEDY PGE: Immunopathology in central nervous system human African trypanosomiasis. J Neuroimmunol 36:91, 1992

JORDAN AM: *Trypanosomiasis Control and African Rural Development*. London, Longman, 1986

PEPIN J, MILORD F: The treatment of African trypanosomiasis. Adv Parasitol 33:1, 1994

STERNBERG JM: Immunobiology of African trypanosomiasis. Chem Immunol 70:186, 1998

TRUC P et al: Parasitological diagnosis of human African trypanosomiasis: A comparison of the QBC® and miniature anion-exchange centrifugation techniques. Trans R Soc Trop Med Hyg 92:288, 1998

217   *Lloyd H. Kasper*

TOXOPLASMA INFECTION

DEFINITION   Toxoplasmosis is the disease caused by infection with the obligate intracellular parasite *Toxoplasma gondii*. Acute infection acquired after birth may be asymptomatic but frequently results in the chronic persistence of cysts within the tissues of the host. Both acute and chronic toxoplasmosis are conditions in which the parasite is responsible for the development of clinically evident disease, including lymphadenopathy, encephalitis, myocarditis, and pneumonitis. Congenital toxoplasmosis is an infection of newborns that results from the transplacental passage of parasites from an infected mother to the fetus. These infants usually are asymptomatic at birth but later manifest a wide range of signs and symptoms, including chorioretinitis, strabismus, epilepsy, and psychomotor retardation.

ETIOLOGY   *T. gondii* is an intracellular coccidian that infects both birds and mammals. There are two distinct stages in the life cycle of *T. gondii*: the nonfeline and feline stages. In the nonfeline stage, tissue cysts that contain bradyzoites or sporulated oocysts are ingested by an intermediate host (e.g., a human, mouse, sheep, or pig). The cyst is rapidly digested by the acidic-pH gastric secretions. Bradyzoites or sporozoites are released, enter the small-intestinal epithelium, and transform into rapidly dividing tachyzoites. The tachyzoites can infect and replicate in all mammalian cells except red blood cells. Once attached to the host cell, the parasite penetrates the cell and forms a parasitophorous vacuole within which it divides. Parasite replication continues until the number of parasites within the cell approaches a critical mass and the cell ruptures, releasing parasites that infect adjoining cells.

As a result of this process, an infected organ soon shows evidence of cytopathology. Most tachyzoites are eliminated by means of the host's humoral and cell-mediated immune responses. Tissue cysts containing many bradyzoites develop 7 to 10 days after the systemic tachyzoite infection. These tissue cysts occur in a variety of host organs but persist principally within the central nervous system (CNS) and muscle. The development of this chronic stage completes the nonfeline portion of the life cycle. Active infection in the immunocompromised host is most likely due to the spontaneous release of encysted parasites that undergo rapid transformation into tachyzoites within the CNS.

The principal stage in the life cycle of the parasite takes place in the cat (the definitive host) and its prey. The parasite's sexual phase is defined by the formation of oocysts within the feline host. This enteroepithelial cycle begins with the ingestion of the bradyzoite tissue cysts and culminates after several intermediate stages in the production of gametes. Gamete fusion produces a zygote, which envelops itself in a rigid wall and is secreted in the feces as an unsporulated oocyst. After 2 to 3 days of exposure to air at ambient temperature, the noninfectious oocyst sporulates to produce eight sporozoite progeny. The sporulated oocyst can be ingested by an intermediate host, such as a person emptying a cat's litter box, a pig rummaging in a barnyard, or perhaps a mouse. It is in the intermediate host that the parasite completes its life cycle.

EPIDEMIOLOGY   *T. gondii* infects a wide range of mammals and birds. Its seroprevalence depends on the locale and the age of the population. Generally, hot arid climatic conditions are associated with a low prevalence of infection. In the United States and most European countries, the prevalence of seroconversion increases with age and exposure. For example, in the United States, 5 to 30% of individuals 10 to 19 years old and 10 to 67% of those over the age of 50 years show serologic evidence of exposure; seroprevalence increases by approximately 1% per year. In Central America, France, Turkey, and Brazil, the seroprevalence is higher.

TRANSMISSION   Oral Transmission   The principal source of human *Toxoplasma* infection remains uncertain. Transmission usually takes place by the oral route and can be attributable to ingestion of either sporulated oocysts from contaminated soil or bradyzoites from undercooked meat. During acute feline infection, a cat may excrete as many as 100 million parasites per day. These very stable sporozoite-containing oocysts are highly infectious and may remain viable for many years in the soil. Humans infected during a well-documented outbreak of oocyst-transmitted infection develop stage-specific antibodies to the oocyst/sporozoite.

Children and adults also can acquire infection from tissue cysts containing bradyzoites. The ingestion of a single cyst is all that is required for human infection. Undercooking or insufficient freezing of meat is an important source of infection in the developed world. In the United States, 10 to 20% of lamb products and 25 to 35% of pork products show evidence of cysts that contain bradyzoites. The incidence in beef is much lower—perhaps as low as 1%. Direct ingestion of bradyzoite cysts in these various meat products leads to acute infection.

Transmission via Blood or Organs   In addition to oral transmission, direct transmission of the parasite by blood or organ products during transplantation takes place at a low rate. Viable parasites can be cultured from refrigerated anticoagulated blood, which may be a source of infection in individuals receiving blood transfusions. *T. gondii* infection also has been reported in kidney and heart transplant recipients who were uninfected before transplantation.

Transplacental Transmission   About one-third of all women who acquire infection with *T. gondii* during pregnancy transmit the parasite to the fetus; the remainder give birth to normal, uninfected babies. Of the various factors that influence fetal outcome, gestational age at the time of infection is the most critical (see below). Few data support a role for recrudescent maternal infection as the source of congenital disease. Thus, women who are seropositive before pregnancy usually are protected against acute infection and do not give birth to congenitally infected neonates.

The following general guidelines can be used to evaluate congenital infection. There is essentially no risk if the mother becomes infected ≥6 months before conception. If infection is acquired <6 months before conception, the likelihood of transplacental infection increases as the interval between infection and conception decreases. In pregnancy, if the mother becomes infected during the first trimester, the incidence of transplacental infection is lowest (about 15%), but the disease in the neonate is most severe. If maternal infection occurs during the third trimester, the incidence of transplacental infection is greatest (65%), but the infant is usually asymptomatic at birth. Infected infants who are normal at birth may have a higher incidence of learning disabilities and chronic neurologic sequelae than uninfected children.

Only a small proportion (20%) of women infected with *T. gondii* develop clinical signs of infection. Often the diagnosis is first appreciated when routine postconception serologic tests show evidence of specific antibody.

PATHOGENESIS Upon the host's ingestion of either tissue cysts containing bradyzoites or oocysts containing sporozoites, the parasites are released from the cysts by a digestive process. Bradyzoites are resistant to the effect of pepsin and invade the host's gastrointestinal tract. Within enterocytes, the parasites undergo morphologic transformation, giving rise to invasive tachyzoites. These tachyzoites induce a parasite-specific secretory IgA response. From the gastrointestinal tract, parasites are disseminated to a variety of organs, particularly lymphatic tissue, skeletal muscle, myocardium, retina, placenta, and the CNS. At these sites, the parasite infects host cells, replicates, and invades the adjoining cells. In this fashion, the hallmarks of the infection develop: cell death and focal necrosis surrounded by an acute inflammatory response.

In the normal immune host, both the humoral and the cellular immune responses control infection; parasite virulence and tissue tropism may be strain specific. Tachyzoites are sequestered by a variety of immune mechanisms, including induction of parasiticidal antibody, activation of macrophages with radical intermediates, production of interferon γ (IFN-γ), and stimulation of cytotoxic T lymphocytes of the CD8+ phenotype. These antigen-specific lymphocytes are capable of killing both extracellular parasites and target cells infected with parasites. As tachyzoites are cleared from the acutely infected host, tissue cysts containing bradyzoites begin to appear, usually within the CNS and the retina. In the immunocompromised or fetal host, the immune factors necessary to control the spread of tachyzoite infection are lacking. This altered immune state allows the persistence of tachyzoites and gives rise to the progressive focal destruction that results in organ failure (i.e., necrotizing encephalitis, pneumonia, and myocarditis).

Persistence of infection with cysts containing bradyzoites is common in the immunocompetent host. This lifelong infection usually remains subclinical. Although bradyzoites are in a slow metabolic phase, cysts do degenerate and rupture within the CNS. This degenerative process, with the development of new bradyzoite-containing cysts, is the most probable source of recrudescent infection in immunocompromised individuals and the most likely stimulus for the persistence of antibody titers in the immunocompetent host.

PATHOLOGY Cell death and focal necrosis due to replicating tachyzoites induce an intense mononuclear inflammatory response in any tissue or cell type infected. Tachyzoites rarely can be visualized by routine histopathologic staining of these inflammatory lesions. However, immunofluorescence staining with parasitic antigen-specific antibodies can reveal either the organism itself or evidence of antigen. In contrast to this inflammatory process caused by tachyzoites, bradyzoite-containing cysts cause inflammation only at the early stages of development, and even this inflammation may be a response to the presence of tachyzoite antigens. Once the cysts reach maturity, the inflammatory process can no longer be detected, and the cysts remain immunologically quiescent within the brain matrix until they rupture.

Lymph Nodes During acute infection, lymph node biopsy demonstrates characteristic findings, including follicular hyperplasia and irregular clusters of tissue macrophages with eosinophilic cytoplasm. Granulomas rarely are evident in these specimens. Although tachyzoites are not usually visible, they can be sought either by subinoculation of infected tissue into mice, with resultant disease, or by the polymerase chain reaction (PCR). PCR amplification of DNA fragments representing either p30 (SAG-1) or p22 (SAG-2) surface antigen or B1 antigen is an effective and sensitive assay for establishing infection of lymph node tissue by tachyzoites.

Eyes In the eye, infiltrates of monocytes, lymphocytes, and plasma cells may produce uni- or multifocal lesions. Granulomatous lesions and chorioretinitis can be observed in the posterior chamber following acute necrotizing retinitis. Other ocular complications of infection include iridocyclitis, cataracts, and glaucoma.

Central Nervous System During CNS involvement, both focal and diffuse meningoencephalitis can be documented, with evidence of necrosis and microglial nodules. Necrotizing encephalitis in patients without AIDS is characterized by small diffuse lesions with perivascular cuffing in contiguous areas. In the AIDS population, polymorphonuclear leukocytes may be present in addition to monocytes, lymphocytes, and plasma cells. Cysts containing bradyzoites frequently are found contiguous with the necrotic tissue border.

Lungs Among patients with AIDS who die of toxoplasmosis, 40 to 70% have involvement of the heart and lung. Interstitial pneumonitis can develop in the neonate and the immunocompromised patient. Thickened and edematous alveolar septa infiltrated with mononuclear and plasma cells are apparent. This inflammation may extend to the endothelial walls. Tachyzoites and bradyzoite-containing cysts have been observed within the alveolar membrane. Superimposed bronchopneumonia can be caused by other microbial agents.

Heart Cysts and aggregates of parasites in cardiac muscle tissue are evident in patients with AIDS who die of toxoplasmosis. Focal necrosis surrounded by inflammatory cells is associated with hyaline necrosis and disrupted myocardial cells. Pericarditis is associated with toxoplasmosis in some patients.

Other Sites Pathologic changes during disseminated infection are similar to those described for the lymph nodes, eyes, and CNS. In patients with AIDS, the skeletal muscle, pancreas, stomach, and kidneys can be involved, with necrosis, invasion by inflammatory cells, and (rarely) the presence of tachyzoites detectable by routine staining. Large necrotic lesions may cause direct tissue destruction. In addition, secondary effects from acute infection of these various organs, including pancreatitis, myositis, and glomerulonephritis, have been reported.

HOST IMMUNE RESPONSE Acute *Toxoplasma* infection evokes a cascade of protective immune responses in the normal host. *Toxoplasma* enters the host at the gut mucosal level and evokes a mucosal immune response that includes the production of antigen-specific secretory IgA. Titers of serum IgA antibody directed at p30 (SAG-1) have been shown to be a useful marker of congenital and acute toxoplasmosis. Milk-whey IgA from acutely infected mothers contains a high titer of antibody to *T. gondii* and can block infection of enterocytes in vitro. In mice, IgA intestinal secretions directed at the parasite are abundant and are associated with the induction of mucosal T cells.

Within the host, *T. gondii* rapidly induces detectable levels of both IgM and IgG serum antibodies. Monoclonal gammopathy of the IgG class can occur in congenitally infected infants. IgM levels may be increased in newborns with congenital infection. The polyclonal IgG antibodies evoked by infection are parasiticidal in vitro in the presence of serum complement and are the basis for the Sabin-Feldman dye test. However, cell-mediated immunity is the major protective response evoked by the parasite during host infection. Macrophages are activated following phagocytosis of antibody-opsonized parasites. This activation can lead to death of the parasite by either an oxygen-dependent or an oxygen-independent process. If the parasite is not phagocytosed and enters the macrophage by active penetration, it continues to replicate, and this replication may represent the mechanism for transport and dissemination to distant organs. *Toxoplasma* stimulates a robust interleukin (IL) 12 response by human dendritic cells. The CD4+ and CD8+ T cell responses are antigen-specific and further stimulate the production of a variety of important lymphokines that expand the T cell and natural killer cell repertoire. *T. gondii* is a potent inducer of a T_H1 phenotype, with IL-12 and IFN-γ playing an essential role in the control of the parasites' growth in the host. Regulation of the inflammatory response is at least partially under the control of a T_H2 response that includes the production of IL-4 and IL-10 in seropositive individuals. Both asymptomatic patients and those with active infection may show a depression in the ratio of CD4+ to CD8+ lymphocytes. This shift may be correlated with a disease syndrome but is not necessarily correlated with disease outcome. Human T cell clones of both the CD4+ and the CD8+ phenotypes are cytolytic against parasite-infected macrophages. These T cell clones produce cytokines that are "microbistatic." IL-18, IL-7, and IL-15 upregulate the production of IFN-γ and may be important during acute and chronic infection. The effect of IFN-γ may be paradoxical, with stimulation of a host downregulatory response as well.

Although in patients with AIDS *T. gondii* infection is believed to be recrudescent, determination of antibody titers is not helpful in establishing reactivation. Because of the severe depletion in CD4+ T cells, quite frequently there is no observed increase in antibody titer during exacerbation of infection. T cells from AIDS patients with reactivation of toxoplasmosis fail to secrete both IFN-γ and IL-2. This alteration in the production of these critical immune cytokines contributes to the persistence of infection. *Toxoplasma* infection frequently develops late in the course of AIDS, when the loss of T cell–dependent protective mechanisms, particularly CD8+ T cells, becomes most pronounced.

CLINICAL MANIFESTATIONS In persons whose immune systems are intact, acute toxoplasmosis is usually asymptomatic and self-limited. This condition can go unrecognized in 80 to 90% of adults and children with acquired infection. The asymptomatic nature of this infection makes diagnosis difficult in mothers infected during pregnancy. In contrast, the wide range of clinical manifestations in congenitally infected children includes severe neurologic complications such as hydrocephalus, microcephaly, mental retardation, and chorioretinitis. If prenatal infection is severe, multiorgan failure and subsequent intrauterine fetal death can occur. In children and adults, chronic infection can persist throughout life, with little consequence to the immunocompetent host.

Toxoplasmosis in the Immunocompetent Person The most common manifestation of acute toxoplasmosis is cervical lymphadenopathy. The nodes may be single or multiple, are usually nontender, are discrete, and vary in firmness. Lymphadenopathy also may be found in suboccipital, supraclavicular, inguinal, and mediastinal areas. Generalized lymphadenopathy occurs in 20 to 30% of symptomatic patients. Between 20 and 40% of patients with lymphadenopathy also have headache, malaise, fatigue, and fever [usually with a temperature of <40°C (<104°F)]. A smaller proportion of symptomatic individuals have myalgia, sore throat, abdominal pain, maculopapular rash, meningoencephalitis, and confusion. Rare complications associated with infection in the normal immune host include pneumonia, myocarditis, encephalopathy, pericarditis, and polymyositis. Symptoms associated with acute infection usually resolve within several weeks, although the lymphadenopathy may persist for some months. In a recent epidemic, toxoplasmosis was diagnosed correctly in only 3 of the 25 patients who consulted physicians. If toxoplasmosis is considered in the differential diagnosis, routine laboratory and serologic screening should be performed before node biopsy.

The results of routine laboratory studies are usually unremarkable except for minimal lymphocytosis, an elevated sedimentation rate, and a nominal increase in liver aminotransferases. Evaluation of cerebrospinal fluid (CSF) in cases with evidence of encephalopathy or meningoencephalitis shows an elevation of intracranial pressure, mononuclear pleocytosis (10 to 50 cells/mL), a slight increase in protein concentration, and (occasionally) an increase in the gamma globulin level. PCR amplification of the *Toxoplasma* DNA target sequence in the CSF may be beneficial. The CSF of chronically infected individuals is normal.

Ocular Infection Infection with *T. gondii* is estimated to cause 35% of all cases of chorioretinitis in the United States and Europe. Most ocular involvement is believed to be due to congenital infection, with a very low incidence following acquired infection. Between 1 and 3% of all patients with AIDS develop debilitating chorioretinitis due to *T. gondii*. A variety of ocular manifestations are documented, including blurred vision, scotoma, photophobia, and eye pain. Macular

involvement occurs with loss of central vision, and nystagmus is secondary to poor fixation. Involvement of the extraocular muscles may lead to disorders of convergence and to strabismus. Ophthalmologic examination should be undertaken in newborns with suspected congenital infection. As the inflammation resolves, vision improves, but episodic flare-ups of chorioretinitis, which progressively destroy retinal tissue and lead to glaucoma, are common.

The ophthalmologic examination reveals yellow-white, cotton-like patches with indistinct margins of hyperemia. As the lesions age, white plaques with distinct borders and black spots within the retinal pigment become more apparent. Lesions usually are located near the posterior pole of the retina; they may be single but are more commonly multiple. Congenital lesions may be unilateral or bilateral and show evidence of massive chorioretinal degeneration with extensive fibrosis. Surrounding these areas of involvement are a normal retina and vasculature. In patients with AIDS, retinal lesions are often large, with diffuse retinal necrosis, and include both free tachyzoites and cysts containing bradyzoites. Toxoplasmic chorioretinitis may be a prodrome to the development of encephalitis.

Infection of the Immunocompromised Person Patients with AIDS and those receiving immunosuppressive therapy for lymphoproliferative disorders are at greatest risk for developing acute toxoplasmosis. This predilection may be due either to reactivation of latent infection or to acquisition of parasites from exogenous sources such as blood or transplanted organs. In individuals with AIDS, more than 95% of cases of *Toxoplasma* encephalitis are believed to be due to recrudescent infection. In most of these cases, encephalitis develops when the CD4+ cell count falls below $100/\mu L$. In the immunocompromised individual, the disease may be rapidly fatal if untreated. Thus accurate diagnosis and initiation of appropriate therapy are necessary to prevent fulminant infection.

Toxoplasmosis is a principal opportunistic infection of the CNS in persons with AIDS. Although geographic origin may be related to frequency of infection, it has no correlation with the severity of disease in the immunocompromised host. Individuals with AIDS who are seropositive for *T. gondii* are at a very high risk for developing encephalitis. In the United States, about one-third of the 15 to 40% of adult patients with AIDS who are latently infected with the parasite develop *Toxoplasma* encephalitis.

The signs and symptoms of acute toxoplasmosis in the immunocompromised patient are principally within the CNS. More than 50% of patients with clinical manifestations have intracerebral involvement. Clinical findings at the time of presentation range from nonfocal to focal dysfunction. These findings include encephalopathy, meningoencephalitis, and mass lesions. Patients may present with altered mental status (75%), fever (10 to 72%), seizures (33%), headaches (56%), and focal neurologic findings (60%), including motor deficits, cranial nerve palsies, movement disorders, dysmetria, visual-field loss, and aphasia. Patients who present with evidence of diffuse cortical dysfunction develop evidence of focal neurologic disease as the infection progresses. This altered condition is due not only to the necrotizing encephalitis caused by direct invasion of the parasite but also to secondary effects, including vasculitis, edema, and hemorrhage. The onset of infection can range from an insidious process over several weeks to an acute confusional state with fulminant focal deficits, including hemiparesis, hemiplegia, visual-field defects, localized headache, and focal seizures.

Although lesions can occur anywhere within the CNS, the areas most involved appear to be the brainstem, basal ganglia, pituitary gland, and corticomedullary junction. Brainstem involvement gives rise to a variety of neurologic dysfunctions, including cranial nerve palsy, dysmetria, and ataxia. With basal ganglionic infection, patients may develop hydrocephalus, choreiform movements, and choreoathetosis. Because *Toxoplasma* usually causes encephalitis, meningeal involvement is uncommon, and thus CSF findings may be unremarkable or may include a modest increase in cell count and in protein—but not glucose—concentration.

Cerebral toxoplasmosis needs to be differentiated from other opportunistic infections or tumors within the CNS of those afflicted with AIDS. The differential diagnosis includes herpes simplex encephalitis, cryptococcal meningitis, progressive multifocal leukoencephalopathy, and primary CNS lymphoma. Involvement of the pituitary gland can give rise to panhypopituitarism and hyponatremia from inappropriate secretion of vasopressin (antidiuretic hormone). AIDS-dementia complex may present as cognitive impairment, attention loss, and altered memory. Brain biopsy in those patients who have been treated for *Toxoplasma* encephalitis but who continue to exhibit neurologic dysfunction often fails to identify organisms.

Autopsies of patients infected with *Toxoplasma* have demonstrated the involvement of multiple organs, including the lungs, gastrointestinal tract, pancreas, skin, eyes, heart, and liver. *Toxoplasma* pneumonia can occur and can be confused with *Pneumocystis carinii* infection. Respiratory involvement usually presents as dyspnea, fever, and a nonproductive cough and may rapidly progress to acute respiratory failure with hemoptysis, metabolic acidosis, hypotension, and (occasionally) disseminated intravascular coagulation. Histopathologic studies demonstrate necrosis and a mixed cellular infiltrate. The presence of organisms is a helpful diagnostic indicator, but organisms can also be found in healthy tissue. Infection of the heart is usually asymptomatic but can be associated with cardiac tamponade or biventricular failure. Infections of the gastrointestinal tract and the liver have been documented.

A presumptive clinical diagnosis of toxoplasmic encephalitis in patients with AIDS is based on clinical presentation, history of exposure as evidenced by positive serology, and radiologic evaluation. When these criteria are used, the predictive value is as high as 80%. More than 97% of patients with AIDS and toxoplasmosis have IgG antibody to the parasite in their sera. IgM serum antibody is usually not demonstrable. Intrathecal antibody to *T. gondii* may be present. Neuroradiologic evaluation should include double-dose contrast computed tomography (CT) of the head. By this test, single and frequently multiple contrast-enhancing lesions (<2 cm) may be identified. Magnetic resonance imaging (MRI) usually demonstrates multiple lesions and provides a more sensitive evaluation of the efficacy of therapy than does CT. Patients with primary CNS lymphoma are four times more likely than patients with *Toxoplasma* encephalitis to have solitary lesions on an MRI scan. A therapeutic trial of anti-*Toxoplasma* medications is frequently used to assess the diagnosis. Treatment of presumptive *Toxoplasma* encephalitis with pyrimethamine/clindamycin results in quantifiable clinical improvement in more than 50% of patients by day 3. By day 7, more than 90% of treated patients show evidence of improvement. In contrast, if patients fail to respond or have lymphoma, clinical signs and symptoms worsen by day 7. Patients in this category require brain biopsy with or without a change in therapy. This procedure can now be performed by a stereotactic CT-guided method that reduces the potential for complications. Brain biopsy for *T. gondii* identifies organisms in 50 to 75% of cases. Some studies indicate that PCR amplification of target genes significantly increases the sensitivity of detection of parasites.

Congenital Toxoplasmosis Between 400 and 4000 infants born each year in the United States are affected by congenital toxoplasmosis. Infection of the placenta leads to hematogenous infection of the fetus. As has already been stated, the proportion of fetuses that become infected increases but the clinical severity of the infection declines as gestation proceeds. Persistence of the parasite can ultimately result in reactivation and further damage decades later. Factors associated with relatively severe disabilities include delayed diagnosis and initiation of therapy, neonatal hypoxia and hypoglycemia, profound visual impairment, uncorrected hydrocephalus, and increased intracranial pressure. If treated appropriately, upwards of 70% of children have normal developmental, neurologic, and ophthalmologic findings at follow-up evaluations. Treatment for 1 year with pyrimethamine and sulfonamide is tolerated with minimal toxicity (see below).

DIAGNOSIS Tissue and Body Fluids The diagnosis of acute toxoplasmosis can be made by isolation of the parasite from blood or other body fluids after subinoculation of the sample into the peritoneal cavity of mice. Mice should be tested for organisms in the peritoneal fluid 6 to 10 days after inoculation. If no parasites are found in the mouse's peritoneal fluid, its anti-*Toxoplasma* serum titer can be evaluated 4 to 6 weeks after inoculation. Isolation of *T. gondii* from the patient's body fluids reflects acute infection, whereas isolation from biopsied tissue is an indication only of the presence of tissue cysts and should not be misinterpreted as acute toxoplasmosis. Persistent parasitemia in patients with latent, asymptomatic infection is rare. Histologic examination of lymph nodes may suggest the characteristic changes described above. Demonstration of tachyzoites in lymph nodes establishes the diagnosis of acute toxoplasmosis. Like subinoculation into mice, histologic demonstration of cysts containing bradyzoites confirms prior infection with *T. gondii* but is nondiagnostic for acute infection.

Serology The procedures just described have great diagnostic value but are limited by difficulties encountered either in the growth of parasites in vivo or in the identification of tachyzoites by histochemical methods. Serologic testing has become the routine method of diagnosis. A wide range of serologic tests that can be used to measure antibody to *T. gondii* are available commercially.

Diagnosis of acute infection with *T. gondii* can be established by detection of the simultaneous presence of IgG and IgM antibody to *Toxoplasma* in serum. The presence of circulating IgA favors the diagnosis of an acute infection. The Sabin-Feldman dye test, the indirect fluorescent antibody test, and the enzyme-linked immunosorbent assay (ELISA) all satisfactorily measure circulating IgG antibody to *Toxoplasma*. Positive IgG titers (>1:10) can be detected as early as 2 to 3 weeks after infection. These titers usually peak at 6 to 8 weeks and decline slowly to a new baseline level that persists for life. It is necessary to measure the serum IgM titer in concert with the IgG titer to better establish the time of infection. The methods currently available for this determination are the double-sandwich IgM-ELISA and the IgM-immunosorbent assay (IgM-ISAGA). Both of these assays are specific and sensitive, and their use precludes the false-positive results associated with rheumatoid factor and antinuclear antibody. The double-sandwich IgA-ELISA is more sensitive than the IgM-ELISA for detecting congenital infection in the fetus and newborn.

The Immunocompetent Adult or Child For the patient who presents with lymphadenopathy only, a positive IgM titer is an indication of acute infection—and an indication for therapy, if that is clinically warranted (see "Treatment" below). The serum IgM titer should be determined again in 3 weeks. An elevation in the IgG titer without an increase in the IgM titer suggests that infection is present but that it is not acute. If there is a borderline increase in either IgG or IgM, the titers should be assessed again in 3 to 4 weeks.

Ocular Toxoplasmosis Because of the congenital nature of ocular toxoplasmosis, the serum antibody titer may not correlate with the presence of active lesions in the fundus. In general, a positive IgG titer (measured in undiluted serum if necessary) in conjunction with typical lesions establishes the diagnosis. If lesions are atypical and the titer is in the low-positive range, the diagnosis is presumptive. The parasitic antigen-specific polyclonal IgG assay as well as the parasitic antigen-specific PCR may facilitate the diagnosis.

The Immunocompromised Host As discussed above, in patients with AIDS, the presence of IgG and radiologic findings consistent with toxoplasmosis are grounds for a presumptive diagnosis. Attempts to evaluate rising IgG titers or to determine whether IgM is present are not productive. Serologic evidence of infection virtually always precedes the development of *Toxoplasma* encephalitis. It is therefore important to determine the *Toxoplasma* antibody status of all patients infected with HIV. Antibody titers may range from negative to 1:1024 in patients with AIDS and *Toxoplasma* encephalitis. Fewer than 3% of patients have no demonstrable antibody to *Toxoplasma* at the time of diagnosis. Determination of the intrathecal antibody titer may be useful in identifying prior infection. PCR amplification of genetic material of the parasite found in the CSF may prove diagnostically beneficial in the future.

Patients with toxoplasmic encephalitis have focal or multifocal abnormalities demonstrable by CT or MRI. These findings are not pathognomonic of *Toxoplasma* infection since 40% of CNS lymphomas are multifocal and 50% are ring-enhancing. Lesions on MRI scan are multiple and are located in both hemispheres, with the basal ganglia and corticomedullary junction most commonly involved. For both MRI and CT scans, the rate of false-negative results is approximately 10%. The finding of a single lesion on an MRI scan increases the suspicion of primary lymphoma and strengthens the argument for the performance of a brain biopsy.

Now used in some centers, SPECT (single-photon emission CT) has been touted as a definitive means of detecting or ruling out *Toxoplasma* infection when a CNS lesion is suspected. In the future, SPECT may well be widely used for this purpose.

As in other conditions, the radiologic response may lag behind the clinical response. Resolution of lesions may take from 3 weeks to 6 months. Some patients show clinical improvement despite worsening radiographic findings.

A presumptive diagnosis of *Toxoplasma* encephalitis should prompt the immediate initiation of therapy. After 3 weeks, repeat radiologic studies should detect improvement. If glucocorticoids have been administered, radiologic studies should be repeated at the time of discontinuation to determine whether an exacerbation of disease has occurred. If the patient's clinical condition becomes worse, performance of a biopsy must be strongly considered.

Congenital Infection   The issue of concern when a pregnant woman has evidence of recent *T. gondii* infection is obviously whether the fetus is infected. PCR of the amniotic fluid to detect the B1 gene of the parasite has replaced fetal blood sampling. Serologic diagnosis is based on the persistence of IgG antibody or a positive IgM titer after the first week of life (a time frame that excludes placental leak). The IgG determination should be repeated every 2 months. An increase in IgM beyond the first week of life is indicative of acute infection. However, up to 25% of infected newborns may be seronegative and have normal routine physical examinations. Thus assessment of the eye and the brain, with ophthalmologic testing, CSF evaluation, and radiologic studies, is important in establishing the diagnosis.

TREATMENT   Current therapeutic protocols are directed at folate metabolism, protein synthesis, or nucleic acid synthesis of the parasite. Pyrimethamine and trimethoprim inhibit the enzyme dihydrofolate reductase. Inhibitors of protein synthesis, including clindamycin, chlortetracycline, and azithromycin, affect growth of the parasite. Inhibitors of purine synthesis, such as arprinocid, may prove to be important. Atovaquone, which blocks pyrimidine salvage, has demonstrated activity against both *T. gondii* and *P. carinii*.

Immunologically competent adults and older children who have only lymphadenopathy do not require specific therapy unless they have persistent and severe symptoms. Patients with ocular toxoplasmosis should be treated for 1 month with pyrimethamine plus either sulfadiazine or clindamycin. Prenatal antibiotic therapy can reduce the number of infants severely affected by *Toxoplasma* infection.

Congenital Infection   Congenitally infected neonates are treated with daily oral pyrimethamine (0.5 to 1 mg/kg) and sulfadiazine (100 mg/kg) for 1 year. In addition, therapy with spiramycin (100 mg/kg per day) plus prednisone (1 mg/kg per day) has been shown to be efficacious for congenital infection.

Infection in Immunocompromised Patients   Patients with AIDS should be treated for acute toxoplasmosis; in the immunocompromised patient, toxoplasmosis is rapidly fatal if untreated. The main-

stay of treatment for *Toxoplasma* encephalitis in immunocompromised patients is a combination regimen. Administered together for 4 to 6 weeks or until radiologic improvement is documented, pyrimethamine (a 200-mg loading dose followed by 50 to 75 mg/d) and sulfadiazine (4 to 6 g/d in four divided doses) block folic acid metabolism and reduce the parasite burden. Leucovorin (calcium folinate, 10 to 15 mg/d) is given as an adjunct to prevent the bone marrow toxicity associated with pyrimethamine. Both pyrimethamine and sulfadiazine cross the blood-brain barrier. A prominent consequence of dual therapy is the high incidence of associated toxicity (40%). Rash may develop during the first 3 weeks in up to 20% of patients but does not preclude the use of this combination. Other complications include hematologic effects, crystalluria, hematuria, radiolucent renal stones, and nephrotoxicity. During therapy, serum levels of these drugs may be erratic, but such fluctuations have not been correlated with these complications.

Pyrimethamine and sulfadiazine are active only against the tachyzoite stage of the parasite. Thus, after immunocompromised patients complete the initial 4- to 6-week course, they must receive lifelong suppressive therapy with pyrimethamine (25 to 50 mg/d) and sulfadiazine (2 to 4 g/d). If sulfadiazine cannot be tolerated, a combination of pyrimethamine (75 mg/d) plus clindamycin (450 mg tid) can be used. It is possible that pyrimethamine (50 to 75 mg/d) is sufficient for chronic suppressive therapy.

Alternative Regimens   Alternative therapies have been established because of the toxicity associated with the long-term antimicrobial therapy necessary for many individuals infected with *T. gondii*. Dapsone (diaminodiphenyl sulfone), with its longer serum half-life and decreased toxicity, is an effective alternative to sulfadiazine. Spiramycin, which has been used in Europe to treat pregnant women, reduces transplacental transmission. However, spiramycin has been ineffective as primary prophylaxis in patients with AIDS. Clindamycin is well absorbed from the gastrointestinal tract, and serum levels peak 1 to 2 h after administration. The combination of oral pyrimethamine (25 to 75 mg/d) plus intravenous clindamycin (1200 to 4800 mg/d) is effective for patients with AIDS who have *Toxoplasma* encephalitis. Toxic effects of clindamycin include nausea, vomiting, neutropenia, rash, and pseudomembranous colitis. Other macrolides that have been evaluated include roxithromycin, clarithromycin, and azithromycin. Evidence suggests that the macrolides are not beneficial by themselves, but a combination of pyrimethamine and clarithromycin appears to be effective. Atovaquone (750 mg tid or qid) is an optional agent for the treatment of individuals who are intolerant of other agents. Glucocorticoids can be used to treat intracerebral edema, but their benefit has not yet been established. It is difficult to assess the benefit of glucocorticoids when they are administered in conjunction with anti-*Toxoplasma* medication. Anticonvulsants are sometimes necessary for the treatment of seizures, but attention should be given to the potential interaction between sulfadiazine and phenytoin. A regimen of trimethoprim-sulfamethoxazole or dapsone plus pyrimethamine with leucovorin may prevent the development of *Toxoplasma* encephalitis in individuals infected with HIV who are seropositive for *T. gondii* after their CD4+ T lymphocyte count falls to 100/μL.

PREVENTION   The chances of primary infection with *Toxoplasma* can be reduced by not eating undercooked meat and by avoiding oocyst-contaminated material (i.e., a cat's litter box). Meat should be heated to 60°C or frozen to kill cysts. Hands should be washed thoroughly after work in the garden, and all fruits and vegetables should be washed. Blood intended for transfusion into *Toxoplasma*-seronegative immunocompromised individuals should be screened for antibody to *T. gondii*. Although such serologic screening is not routinely performed, seronegative women should be screened for evidence of infection several times during pregnancy if they are exposed to environmental conditions that put them at risk for infection with *T. gondii*. HIV-positive individuals should adhere closely to these preventive measures.

FICHERA ME, ROOS DS: A plastid organelle as a drug target in apicomplexa parasites. Nature 390:407, 1997

FOULON W et al: Treatment of toxoplasmosis during pregnancy. Am J Obstet Gynecol 180:410, 1999

HOWE D, SIBLEY LD: *T. gondii* comprises three clonal lineages: Correlation of genotype with human disease. J Infect Dis 172:1561, 1995

MCLEOD R et al: Immunogenetics in pathogenesis of and protection against toxoplasmosis. Curr Top Microbiol Immunol 219:95, 1996

METS MB et al: Eye manifestations of congenital toxoplasmosis. Am J Ophthalmol 123: 1, 1997

PODZAMCZER D et al: Intermittent trimethoprim-sulfamethoxazole compared with dapsone-pyrimethamine for the simultaneous primary prophylaxis of *Pneumocystis* pneumonia and toxoplasmosis in patients infected with HIV. Ann Intern Med 122:755, 1995

REMINGTON JS et al: Toxoplasmosis, in *Infectious Diseases of the Fetus and Newborn Infant*, 4th ed, JS Remington, JO Klein (eds). Philadelphia, Saunders, 1994

ROBERTS F et al: Evidence for the shikimato pathway in apicomplexa parasites. Nature 393:801, 1998

SEGUIN R, KASPER LH: Sensitized lymphocytes and CD40 ligation augment IL-12 production by human dendritic cells in response to *T. gondii*. J Infect Dis 179:467, 1999

VILLENA I et al: Pyrimethamine-sulfadoxine treatment of congenital toxoplasmosis. Scand J Infect Dis 30:295, 1998

---

218 *Peter F. Weller*

PROTOZOAL INTESTINAL INFECTIONS AND TRICHOMONIASIS

PROTOZOAL INFECTIONS

GIARDIASIS *Giardia lamblia* is a cosmopolitan protozoal parasite that inhabits the small intestines of humans and other mammals. Giardiasis is one of the most common parasitic diseases worldwide and causes both endemic and epidemic intestinal disease and diarrhea.

Life Cycle and Epidemiology Infection follows the ingestion of the environmentally hardy cysts, which excyst in the small intestine, releasing trophozoites that multiply by binary fission, occasionally to enormous numbers. *Giardia* remains a pathogen of the proximal small bowel and does not disseminate hematogenously. Trophozoites remain free in the lumen or attach to the mucosal epithelium by means of a ventral sucking disk. As a trophozoite encounters altered conditions, it forms a morphologically distinct cyst, which is the stage of the parasite usually found in the feces. Trophozoites may be present and even predominate in loose or watery stools, but it is the resistant cyst that survives outside the body and is responsible for transmission. Cysts do not tolerate heating, desiccation, or continued exposure to feces but do remain viable for months in cold fresh water. The number of cysts excreted varies widely but can approach 10^7 per gram of stool.

Giardia infections are common in both developed and developing countries. Ingestion of as few as 10 cysts is sufficient to cause infection in humans. Because cysts are infectious when excreted or shortly thereafter, person-to-person transmission occurs where fecal hygiene is poor. Giardiasis, as a symptomatic or an asymptomatic infection, is especially prevalent in day-care centers; person-to-person spread also takes place in other institutional settings with poor fecal hygiene and during homosexual contact. If food is contaminated with *Giardia* cysts after cooking or preparation, food-borne transmission can occur. Waterborne transmission accounts for episodic infections (e.g., in campers and other travelers) and for massive epidemics in metropolitan areas. Surface water, ranging from mountain streams to large municipal res-

ervoirs, can become contaminated with fecally derived *Giardia* cysts; outmoded water systems are subject to cross-contamination from leaking sewer lines. The efficacy of water as a means of transmission is enhanced by the small infectious inoculum of *Giardia*, the prolonged survival of cysts in cold water, and the resistance of cysts to killing by routine chlorination methods that are adequate for controlling bacteria. Viable cysts can be eradicated from water by either boiling or filtration. In the United States, *Giardia* is a common agent identified in waterborne epidemics of gastroenteritis; it is also common in developing countries.

The importance of animal reservoirs as sources of infection for humans is unclear. *Giardia* parasites morphologically similar to those in humans are found in a large number of mammals, including beavers from reservoirs implicated in epidemics, dogs, cats, and ruminants. Although the high degree of isolate heterogeneity noted in humans is consistent with infections originating from different animal sources, animals have not been directly established as sources of human infection.

Giardiasis, like cryptosporidiosis, creates a significant economic burden because of the costs incurred in the installation of water filtration systems required to prevent waterborne epidemics, in the management of epidemics that involve large communities, and in the evaluation and treatment of endemic infections.

Pathophysiology The reasons that some, but not all, infected patients develop clinical manifestations and the mechanisms by which *Giardia* causes alterations in small-bowel function are largely unknown. Although trophozoites adhere to the epithelium, they do not cause invasive or locally destructive alterations. The lactose intolerance and significant malabsorption that develop in a minority of infected adults and children are clinical signs of the loss of brush border enzyme activities. In most infections the morphology of the bowel is unaltered, but in a few cases—usually in chronically infected, symptomatic patients—the histopathologic findings (including flattened villi) and the clinical manifestations resemble those of tropical sprue and gluten-sensitive enteropathy. The pathogenesis of diarrhea in giardiasis is not known.

The natural history of *Giardia* infection varies markedly. Infections may be aborted, transient, recurrent, or chronic. Parasite as well as host factors may be important in determining the course of infection and disease. Both cellular and humoral responses develop in human infections, but their precise roles in the control of infection and/or disease are unknown. Because patients with hypogammaglobulinemia commonly suffer from prolonged, severe infections that are poorly responsive to treatment, humoral immune responses appear to be important. The greater susceptibility of the young than of the old and of newly exposed persons than of chronically exposed populations also suggests that at least partial protective immunity may develop. Although no strains of the parasite that are clearly nonpathogenic have been identified, *Giardia* isolates vary biochemically and biologically. The marked biochemical differences among some isolates may help account for the different courses of infection in experimentally infected humans and animals. The surface of trophozoites is covered by a family of related cysteine-rich proteins that undergo surface antigenic variation and may contribute to prolonged and/or repeated infections.

Clinical Manifestations Disease manifestations of giardiasis range from asymptomatic carriage to fulminant diarrhea and malabsorption. Most infected persons are asymptomatic, but in epidemics the proportion of symptomatic cases may be higher. Symptoms may develop suddenly or gradually. In persons with acute giardiasis, symptoms develop after an incubation period that lasts at least 5 to 6 days and usually 1 to 3 weeks. Prominent early symptoms include diarrhea, abdominal pain, bloating, belching, flatus, nausea, and vomiting. Although diarrhea is common, upper intestinal manifestations such as nausea, vomiting, bloating, and abdominal pain may predominate. The duration of acute giardiasis is usually in excess of 1 week, although diarrhea often subsides. Individuals with chronic giardiasis may present with or without having experienced an antecedent acute symptomatic episode. Diarrhea is not necessarily prominent, but increased flatus, loose stools, sulfurous burping, and (in some instances) weight loss occur. Symptoms may be continual or episodic and can persist for years. Some persons who have relatively mild symptoms for long periods recognize the extent of their discomfort only in retrospect. Fever, the presence of blood and/or mucus in the stools, and other signs and symptoms of colitis are uncommon and suggest a different diagnosis or a concomitant illness. Symptoms tend to be intermittent yet recurring and gradually debilitating, in contrast with the acute disabling symptoms associated with many enteric bacterial infections. Because of the less severe illness and the propensity for chronic infections, patients may seek medical advice late in the course of the illness; however, disease can be severe, resulting in malabsorption, weight loss, growth retardation, dehydration, and (in rare cases) death. A number of extraintestinal manifestations have been described, such as urticaria, anterior uveitis, and arthritis; whether these are caused by giardiasis or concomitant processes is unclear.

Giardiasis can be life-threatening in patients with hypogammaglobulinemia and is typically difficult to treat and eradicate. *Giardia* infections can complicate other preexisting intestinal diseases, such as cystic fibrosis. Although *Giardia* can cause enteric illness in patients with AIDS, neither the course of infection nor the response to treatment differs for patients with and without AIDS.

Diagnosis Giardiasis is diagnosed by the detection of parasite antigen in the feces or by the identification of cysts in the feces or of trophozoites in the feces or small intestines. Cysts are oval, measure 8 to 12 μm $\times$ 7 to 10 μm, and characteristically contain four nuclei. Trophozoites are pear-shaped, dorsally convex, flattened parasites with two nuclei and four pairs of flagella. The diagnosis is sometimes difficult to establish. Direct examination of fresh or properly preserved stools as well as concentration methods should be used. Because cyst excretion is variable and may be undetectable at times, repeated examination of stool, sampling of duodenal fluid, and biopsy of the small intestine may be required to detect the parasite. Tests for parasitic antigen in stool are at least as sensitive and specific as good microscopic examinations and are easier to perform. All of these methods occasionally yield false-negative results.

TREATMENT Cure rates with metronidazole (250 mg tid for 5 days) are usually >80%; those with furazolidone (100 mg qid for 7 to 10 days) are somewhat lower. The latter agent is frequently used to treat children because it is available as a palatable elixir that is not bitter. Quinacrine, the first effective drug for the treatment of giardiasis, is available from a limited number of pharmacies. Albendazole (400 mg/d for 5 days) may be effective.

Patients in whom initial treatment fails can be re-treated with a longer course. Almost all patients respond to therapy and are cured, although some with chronic giardiasis experience delayed resolution of symptoms after eradication of *Giardia*. Those who remain infected after repeated treatments should be evaluated for reinfection through family members, close personal contacts, and environmental sources as well as for hypogammaglobulinemia. In cases refractory to multiple treatment courses, prolonged therapy with metronidazole (750 mg tid for 21 days) has been successful. Tinidazole, not available in the United States, is considered more effective than metronidazole or quinacrine. When children attending day-care centers infect an entire family, treatment of all infected family members, including asymptomatic carriers, may be required to prevent reinfection. Paromomycin, an oral aminoglycoside that is not well absorbed, can be given to symptomatic pregnant women, although the experience accumulated thus far is not a sufficient basis on which to judge how often this agent either eradicates infection or ameliorates symptoms.

Prevention Although *Giardia* is extremely infectious, disease can be prevented by the exclusive consumption of noncontaminated food and water. Cooking food adequately and boiling or filtering potentially contaminated water prevent infection.

CRYPTOSPORIDIOSIS The coccidian parasite *Cryptosporidium* is now known to cause diarrheal disease in immunocompetent human hosts and to be especially common among persons with AIDS or other forms of immunodeficiency.

Life Cycle and Epidemiology Cryptosporidiosis is acquired by the consumption of oocysts (50% infectious dose: ~132 oocysts in nonimmune individuals), which excyst to liberate sporozoites that in turn enter and infect intestinal epithelial cells. The parasite's further development involves both asexual and sexual cycles, which produce forms capable of infecting other epithelial cells and of generating oocysts that are passed in the feces. *Cryptosporidium* spp. infect a number of animals and can spread from infected animals to humans. Since oocysts are immediately infectious when passed in feces, person-to-person transmission takes place in day-care centers and among household contacts and medical providers. Waterborne transmission accounts for infections in travelers and for common-source epidemics. Oocysts are quite hardy and resist killing by routine chlorination. Both drinking water and recreational water (e.g., pools, waterslides) have been increasingly recognized as sources of infection.

Pathophysiology Although intestinal epithelial cells harbor the parasite in an intracellular vacuole, the means by which secretory diarrhea is elicited remain uncertain. No characteristic pathologic changes are found by biopsy. The distribution of infection can be spotty within the principal site of infection, the small bowel. Cryptosporidia are found in some patients in the pharynx, stomach, and large bowel and at times in the respiratory tract. Especially in patients with AIDS, involvement of the biliary tract can cause papillary stenosis, sclerosing cholangitis, or cholecystitis.

Clinical Manifestations Asymptomatic infections can occur in both immunocompetent and immunocompromised hosts. In immunocompetent persons, symptoms develop after an incubation period of about a week and consist principally of watery nonbloody diarrhea, at times in conjunction with abdominal pain, nausea, anorexia, fever, and/or weight loss. In these hosts, the illness usually subsides after 1 to 2 weeks, whereas in immunocompromised hosts, especially those with AIDS, diarrhea can be chronic, persistent, and remarkably profuse, causing clinically significant fluid and electrolyte depletion. Stool volumes may range from 1 to 25 L/d. Weight loss, wasting, and abdominal pain may be severe. Biliary tract involvement can manifest as midepigastric or right upper quadrant pain.

Diagnosis Evaluation usually starts with fecal examination for small oocysts, which are 4 to 5 μm in diameter and are smaller than the fecal stages of most other parasites. Detection is enhanced by evaluation of stools (obtained on multiple days) by several techniques, including modified acid-fast and direct immunofluorescent stains and enzyme immunoassays. Cryptosporidia also can be identified by light and electron microscopy at the apical surfaces of intestinal epithelium from biopsy specimens of the small bowel and, less frequently, the large bowel.

TREATMENT To date, no chemotherapeutic agents effective against *Cryptosporidium* have been identified, although paromomycin (500 to 750 mg qid) may be partially effective for some patients infected with HIV. Improvement in immune status with antiretroviral therapy can lead to amelioration of cryptosporidiosis. Otherwise, treatment includes supportive care with replacement of fluids and electrolytes and administration of antidiarrheal agents. Biliary tract obstruction may require papillotomy or T-tube placement. Prevention requires minimizing exposure to infectious oocysts in human or animal feces. Use of submicron water filters may minimize acquisition of infection from drinking water.

ISOSPORIASIS The coccidian parasite *Isospora belli* causes human intestinal disease. Infection is acquired by the consumption of oocysts, after which the parasite invades intestinal epithelial cells and undergoes both sexual and asexual cycles of development. Oocysts excreted in stool are not immediately infectious but must undergo further maturation. Although *I. belli* infects many animals, little is known about the epidemiology or prevalence of this parasite in humans. It appears to be most common in tropical and subtropical countries. Acute infections can begin abruptly with fever, abdominal pain, and watery nonbloody diarrhea and can last for weeks or months. In patients who have AIDS or are immunocompromised for other reasons, infections often are not self-limited but rather resemble cryptosporidiosis, with chronic, profuse watery diarrhea. Eosinophilia, which is not found in other enteric protozoan infections, may be detectable. The diagnosis is usually made by detection of the large (~25-μm) oocysts in stool by modified acid-fast staining. Oocyst excretion may be low-level and intermittent; if repeated stool examinations are unrevealing, sampling of duodenal contents by aspiration or small-bowel biopsy (often with electron-microscopic examination) may be necessary.

In contrast to cryptosporidiosis, isosporiasis responds to chemotherapy. Trimethoprim-sulfamethoxazole (160/800 mg qid for 10 days and then bid for 3 weeks) has been effective; for patients intolerant of sulfonamides, pyrimethamine (50 to 75 mg/d) can be used. Relapses can occur in persons with AIDS and necessitate maintenance therapy with trimethoprim-sulfamethoxazole (160/800 mg three times a week) or combined sulfadoxine (500 mg) and pyrimethamine (25 mg) once weekly.

CYCLOSPORIASIS Coccidian parasites of the genus *Cyclospora* have been identified as the causative organisms in diarrheal illness formerly ascribed to blue-green algal or *Cyanobacteria*-like forms. This parasite is globally distributed: illness due to *Cyclospora cayetanensis* has been reported in the United States, Asia, Africa, Latin America, and Europe. The epidemiology of this parasite has not yet been fully defined, but waterborne transmission and especially transmission in imported raspberries have been recognized. The full spectrum of illness attributable to *Cyclospora* has not been delineated. Some patients may harbor the infection without symptoms, but many with cyclosporiasis have diarrhea, flulike symptoms, and flatulence and burping. The illness can be self-limited, can wax and wane, or (in many cases) can involve prolonged diarrhea, anorexia, and upper gastrointestinal symptoms, with sustained fatigue and weight loss in some instances. Diarrheal illness may persist for longer than a month. *Cyclospora* can cause enteric illness in patients infected with HIV, albeit at an unknown frequency.

The parasite is detectable in epithelial cells of small-bowel biopsy samples and elicits secretory diarrhea by an unknown means. The absence of fecal blood and leukocytes indicates that disease due to *Cyclospora* is not caused by destruction of the small-bowel mucosa. The diagnosis can be made by detection of spherical 8- to 10-μm oocysts in the stool, although routine stool O and P examinations are not sufficient. Specific fecal examinations must be requested to detect the oocysts, which are variably acid-fast and are fluorescent when viewed with ultraviolet light microscopy. Cyclosporiasis should be considered in the differential diagnosis of prolonged diarrhea, with or without a history of travel by the patient to other countries.

Cyclosporiasis is effectively treated with trimethoprim-sulfamethoxazole (160/800 mg bid for 7 days). Patients infected with HIV, however, may experience relapses after such treatment and thus may require longer-term suppressive maintenance therapy.

MICROSPORIDIOSIS Microsporidia are obligate intracellular spore-forming protozoa that infect many animals and cause disease in humans, especially as opportunistic pathogens in AIDS. Microsporidia are members of a distinct phylum, Microspora, which contains dozens of genera and hundreds of species. The various microsporidia are differentiated by their developmental life cycles, by ultrastructural features, and by molecular taxonomy based on ribosomal RNA. The com-

plex life cycles of the organisms result in the production of infectious spores. Currently, six genera of microsporidia—*Encephalitozoon*, *Pleistophora*, *Nosema*, *Vittaforma*, *Trachipleistophora*, and *Enterocytozoon*—are recognized as causes of human disease; a seventh genus—*Microsporidium*, which includes organisms of uncertain taxonomic status—also causes disease in humans. Though some microsporidia are probably prevalent causes of self-limited or asymptomatic infections in immunocompetent patients, little is known of how microsporidiosis is acquired.

Microsporidiosis is most common among patients with AIDS, less common among patients with other types of immunocompromise, and rare among immunocompetent hosts. In patients with AIDS, intestinal infections with *Enterocytozoon bieneusi* and *Encephalitozoon* (formerly *Septata*) *intestinalis* are increasingly recognized to contribute to chronic diarrhea and wasting; these infections are found in 10 to 40% of patients with chronic diarrhea. Both organisms have been found in the biliary tracts of patients with cholecystitis. *E. intestinalis* may also disseminate to cause fever, diarrhea, sinusitis, cholangitis, and bronchiolitis. In patients with AIDS, *E. hellem* has caused superficial keratoconjunctivitis as well as sinusitis, respiratory tract disease, and disseminated infection. Myositis due to *Pleistophora* has been documented. *Nosema*, *Vittaforma*, and *Microsporidium* have caused stromal keratitis associated with trauma in immunocompetent patients.

Microsporidia are small gram-positive organisms with mature spores measuring 0.5 to 2 μm × 1 to 4 μm. Diagnosis of microsporidial infections in tissue often requires electron microscopy, although intracellular spores can be visualized by light microscopy with hematoxylin and eosin, Giemsa, or tissue Gram's stains. For the diagnosis of intestinal microsporidiosis, modified trichrome or chromotrope 2R-based staining and Uvitex 2B or calcofluor fluorescent staining reveal spores in smears of feces or duodenal aspirates. Definitive therapies for microsporidial infections remain to be established. For superficial keratoconjunctivitis due to *E. hellem*, topical therapy with fumagillin suspension has shown promise (Chap. 211). For enteric infections with *E. bieneusi* and *E. intestinalis* in HIV-infected patients, therapy with albendazole may be efficacious (Chap. 211).

OTHER INTESTINAL PROTOZOA **Balantidiasis** *Balantidium coli* is a large ciliated protozoal parasite that can produce a spectrum of large-intestinal disease analogous to amebiasis. The parasite is widely distributed in the world. Since it infects pigs, cases in humans are more common where pigs are raised; in Muslim countries, rodents may be important carriers. Infective cysts can be transmitted from person to person and through water, but many cases are due to the ingestion of cysts derived from porcine feces in association with slaughtering, with use of pig feces for fertilizer, or with contamination of water supplies by pig feces.

Ingested cysts liberate trophozoites, which reside and replicate in the large bowel. Many patients remain asymptomatic, but some have persisting intermittent diarrhea, and a few develop more fulminant dysentery. In symptomatic individuals, the pathology in the bowel—both gross and microscopic—is similar to that seen in amebiasis, with varying degrees of mucosal invasion, focal necrosis, and ulceration. Balantidiasis, unlike amebiasis, does not spread hematogenously to other organs. The diagnosis is usually made by detection of the trophozoite stage in stool or sampled colonic tissue. Tetracycline (500 mg qid for 10 days) is an effective therapeutic agent.

***Blastocystis hominis* Infection** *B. hominis*, long considered a nonpathogenic yeast, is believed by some to be a protozoan capable of causing intestinal disease, although its taxonomy and inherent pathogenicity remain uncertain. Some patients who pass *B. hominis* in their stools are asymptomatic, whereas others have diarrhea and associated intestinal symptoms. Diligent evaluation reveals other potential bacterial, viral, or protozoal causes of diarrhea in some but not all patients with symptoms. Because the pathogenicity of *B. hominis* is uncertain and because therapy for *Blastocystis* infection is neither specific nor uniformly effective, patients with prominent intestinal symptoms should be fully evaluated for other infectious causes of diarrhea. If diarrheal symptoms associated with *Blastocystis* are prominent, either metronidazole (750 mg tid for 10 days) or iodoquinol (650 mg tid for 20 days) can be used.

Dientamoeba fragilis Infection   *D. fragilis* is unique among intestinal protozoa in that it has a trophozoite stage but not a cyst stage. How trophozoites survive to transmit infection is not known, but the unusually high prevalence of *D. fragilis* infection among persons with pinworm infection raises the possibility that eggs or larvae of *Enterobius* facilitate the transmission of *D. fragilis*. When symptoms develop in patients with *D. fragilis* infection, they are generally mild and include intermittent diarrhea, abdominal pain, and anorexia. The diagnosis is made by the detection of trophozoites in stool; the lability of these forms accounts for the greater yield when fecal samples are preserved immediately after collection. Since fecal excretion rates vary, examination of several samples obtained on alternate days increases the rate of detection. Iodoquinol (650 mg tid for 20 days), paromomycin (25 to 30 mg/kg per day in three doses for 7 days), or tetracycline (500 mg qid for 10 days) is appropriate for treatment.

Sarcosporidiosis   Various *Sarcocystis* spp. of coccidian parasites are widely distributed agents of infection in numerous animals. These parasites have an obligatory cycle of development involving two hosts. Sexual reproduction occurs in the intestine, with sporocysts passed in the feces; asexual multiplication leads to the development of muscle cysts. Humans can develop intestinal infections—albeit apparently infrequently—by ingesting muscle-stage cysts in undercooked pork or beef. While the full spectrum of the intestinal disease is not defined, a diarrheal illness can ensue, and sporocysts are found in the stool. Alternatively, ingestion of fecally derived sporocysts can lead to the development of cysts in striated or cardiac muscle. Some patients experience muscle pain and swelling, but the frequency and nature of symptoms elicited by muscle involvement are not clear, and these cysts, measuring 100 to 325 μm, also have been found incidentally in muscle specimens. Muscle-stage infections are not followed by further spread in humans. No specific therapy exists for either intestinal or muscle-stage *Sarcocystis* infections in humans.

TRICHOMONIASIS

Various species of trichomonads can be found in the mouth (in association with periodontitis) and occasionally in the gastrointestinal tract. *Trichomonas vaginalis*—one of the most prevalent protozoal parasites in the United States—is a pathogen of the genitourinary tract and a major cause of symptomatic vaginitis.

Life Cycle and Epidemiology   *T. vaginalis* is a pear-shaped, actively motile organism that measures about 10 by 7 μm, replicates by binary fission, and inhabits the lower genital tract of females and the urethra and prostate of males. In the United States, it accounts for about 3 million infections per year in women. While the organism can survive for a few hours in moist environments and could be acquired by direct contact, person-to-person venereal transmission accounts for virtually all cases of trichomoniasis. Its prevalence is greatest among persons with multiple sexual partners and among those with other sexually transmitted diseases.

Clinical Manifestations   Most men infected with *T. vaginalis* are asymptomatic, although some develop urethritis and a few have epididymitis or prostatitis. In contrast, infection in women, which has an incubation period of 5 to 28 days, is usually symptomatic and manifests with malodorous vaginal discharge (often yellow), vulvar erythema and itching, dysuria or urinary frequency (in 30 to 50% of pa-

tients), and dyspareunia. These manifestations, however, do not clearly distinguish trichomoniasis from other types of infectious vaginitis.

Diagnosis   Detection of motile trichomonads by microscopy of wet mounts of vaginal or prostatic secretions has been the conventional means of diagnosis. Although such microscopy provides an immediate diagnosis, its sensitivity for the detection of *T. vaginalis* is only ~50 to 60% in routine evaluations of vaginal secretions. Direct immunofluorescent antibody staining is more sensitive (70 to 90%) than wet-mount examinations. *T. vaginalis* can be recovered from the urethra of both males and females and is detectable in males after prostatic massage. Culture of the parasite is the most sensitive means of detection; however, the facilities for culture are not generally available, and detection of the organism takes 3 to 7 days.

R̲x̲ TREATMENT   Metronidazole is the mainstay of treatment and may be given either as a single 2-g dose or as 250 mg tid for 7 days. All sexual partners must be treated concurrently to prevent reinfection, especially from asymptomatic males. Alternatives to metronidazole for treatment during pregnancy are not readily available, although use of 100-mg clotrimazole vaginal suppositories nightly for 2 weeks may cure some infections in pregnant women. Reinfection often accounts for apparent treatment failures, but strains of *T. vaginalis* exhibiting high-level resistance to metronidazole have been encountered. Treatment of these resistant infections with higher oral doses, parenteral doses, or concurrent oral and vaginal doses of metronidazole has been successful.

BIBLIOGRAPHY

CHAPPELL CL et al: Infectivity of *Cryptosporidium parvum* in heathy adults with pre-existing anti–*C. parvum* serum immunoglobulin G. Am J Trop Med Hyg 60:157, 1999

EBERHARD ML et al: Laboratory diagnosis of *Cyclospora* infections. Arch Pathol Lab Med 121:792, 1997

EBRAHIMZADEH A, BOTTONE EJ: Persistent diarrhea caused by *Isospora belli*: Therapeutic response to pyrimethamine and sulfadiazine. Diagn Microbiol Infect Dis 26:87, 1996

FLEMING CA et al: A foodborne outbreak of *Cyclospora cayetanensis* at a wedding: Clinical features and risk factors for illness. Arch Intern Med 158:1121, 1998

GRIFFITHS JK: Human cryptosporidiosis: Epidemiology, transmission, clinical disease, treatment, and diagnosis. Adv Parasitol 40:37, 1998

HERWALDT BL, BEACH MJ: The return of *Cyclospora* in 1997: Another outbreak of cyclosporiasis in North America associated with imported raspberries. Cyclospora Working Group. Ann Intern Med 130:210, 1999

HORIKI N et al: Epidemiologic survey of *Blastocystis hominis* infection in Japan. Am J Trop Med Hyg 56:370, 1997

HOXIE NJ et al: Cryptosporidiosis-associated mortality following a massive waterborne outbreak in Milwaukee, Wisconsin. Am J Public Health 87:2032, 1997

KOTLER DP, ORENSTEIN JM: Clinical syndromes associated with microsporidiosis. Adv Parasitol 40:321, 1998

KRAMER MH et al: First reported outbreak in the United States of cryptosporidiosis associated with a recreational lake. Clin Infect Dis 26:27, 1998

LENGERICH EJ et al: Severe giardiasis in the United States. Clin Infect Dis 18:760, 1994

MANABE YC et al: Cryptosporidiosis in patients with AIDS: Correlates of disease and survival. Clin Infect Dis 27:536, 1998

MANK TG et al: Sensitivity of microscopy versus enzyme immunoassay in the laboratory diagnosis of giardiasis. Eur J Clin Microbiol Infect Dis 16:615, 1997

MOLINA JM et al: Albendazole for treatment and prophylaxis of microsporidiosis due to *Encephalitozoon intestinalis* in patients with AIDS: A randomized double-blind controlled trial. J Infect Dis 177:1373, 1998

OBERHUBER G et al: Giardiasis: A histologic analysis of 567 cases. Scand J Gastroenterol 32:48, 1997

ORTEGA YR et al: *Cyclospora cayetanensis*. Adv Parasitol 40:399, 1998

PETRIN D et al: Clinical and microbiological aspects of *Trichomonas vaginalis*. Clin Microbiol Rev 11:300, 1998

STEINER TS et al: Protozoal agents: What are the dangers for the public water supply? Annu Rev Med 48:329, 1997

219

Leo X. Liu, Peter F. Weller

TRICHINELLA AND OTHER TISSUE NEMATODES

Nematodes are elongated, symmetric roundworms. Parasitic nematodes of medical significance may be broadly classified as intestinal or tissue nematodes, but such a classification system is imprecise. This chapter covers trichinellosis, visceral and ocular larva migrans, cutaneous larva migrans, cerebral angiostrongyliasis, and gnathostomiasis. All are zoonotic infections caused by incidental exposure to infectious nematodes. The clinical symptoms of these infections are due largely to invasive larval stages that (except in the case of *Trichinella*) do not reach maturity in humans.

TRICHINELLOSIS   Trichinellosis develops after the ingestion of meat containing cysts of *Trichinella*—for example, pork or other meat from a carnivore. While most infections are mild and asymptomatic, heavy infections can cause severe enteritis, periorbital edema, myositis, and (infrequently) death.

Life Cycle and Epidemiology   Five species of *Trichinella* are now recognized as causes of infection in humans. Two species are distributed worldwide: *T. spiralis*, which is found in a great variety of carnivorous and omnivorous animals, and *T. pseudospiralis*, which is found in mammals and birds. *T. nativa* is present in Arctic regions and infects bears; *T. nelsoni* is found in equatorial Africa, where it is common among felid predators and scavengers such as hyenas and bush pigs; and *T. bitovi* is found in temperate areas of Europe and western Asia among carnivores but not among domestic swine.

After the consumption of trichinous meat by the host, encysted larvae are liberated by digestive acid and pepsin (Fig. 219-1). The larvae invade the small-bowel mucosa and mature rapidly into adult worms. After about 1 week, female worms release newborn larvae that migrate via the circulation to striated muscle. The larvae of all species except *T. pseudospiralis* then encyst by inducing a radical transformation in the muscle cell architecture. Although host immune responses may help to expel adult worms, they have little effect on muscle-dwelling larvae.

Human trichinellosis is most often caused by the ingestion of infected pork products and thus can occur in almost any location where the meat of domestic or wild swine is eaten. Human trichinellosis also may be acquired from the meat of other animals, including dogs (in parts of Asia and Africa), horses (in Italy and France), and bears and walruses (in northern regions). Although cattle (being herbivores) are not natural hosts of *Trichinella*, beef has been implicated in outbreaks when contaminated or adulterated with trichinous pork. Laws that prohibit the feeding of uncooked garbage to pigs have greatly reduced the transmission of trichinellosis in the United States. About 40 cases of trichinellosis are reported annually in this country, but most mild cases probably remain undiagnosed. Recent U.S. outbreaks have been attributable to undercooked ethnic pork dishes, homemade and commercial sausage, wild boar meat, and walrus meat.

Pathogenesis and Clinical Features   Clinical symptoms of trichinellosis arise from the successive phases of parasite enteric invasion, larval migration, and muscle encystment (Fig. 219-1). Most light infections (those with <10 larvae per gram of muscle) are asymptomatic, whereas heavy infections (which can involve >50 larvae per gram of muscle) can be life-threatening. Invasion of the gut by large numbers of parasites occasionally provokes diarrhea during the first week after infection. Abdominal pain, constipation, nausea, or vomiting also may be prominent. The prolonged and fulminant diarrhea

noted with Arctic trichinellosis probably reflects a response to repeated infection.

Symptoms due to larval migration and muscle invasion begin to appear in the second week after infection. The migrating *Trichinella* larvae provoke a marked local and systemic hypersensitivity reaction, with fever and hypereosinophilia. Periorbital and facial edema is common, as are hemorrhages in the subconjunctivae, retina, and nail beds ("splinter" hemorrhages). A maculopapular rash, headache, cough, dyspnea, or dysphagia sometimes develops. Myocarditis with tachyarrhythmias or heart failure—and, less commonly, encephalitis or pneumonitis—may develop and accounts for most deaths of patients with trichinellosis.

Upon onset of larval encystment in muscle 2 to 3 weeks after infection, symptoms of myositis with myalgias, muscle edema, and weakness develop, usually overlapping with the inflammatory reactions to migrating larvae. The most commonly involved muscle groups include the extraocular muscles; the biceps; and the muscles of the jaw, neck, lower back, and diaphragm. Peaking about 3 weeks after infection, symptoms subside only gradually during a prolonged convalescence.

Laboratory Findings and Diagnosis   Blood eosinophilia develops in >90% of patients with symptomatic trichinellosis and may peak at a level of >50% between 2 and 4 weeks after infection. Serum levels of IgE and muscle enzymes, including creatine phosphokinase, lactate dehydrogenase, and aspartate aminotransferase, are elevated in most symptomatic patients. Patients should be questioned thoroughly

Larvae migrate to penetrate striated muscle, reside in "nurse cells," and encyst, causing: **Muscle pain, fever, periorbital edema, eosinophilia, occasional CNS or cardiac damage**

Larvae are released in the stomach and mature into adult worms over 1–2 wks in small bowel, causing: **Irritation and mild abdominal cramping or even diarrhea**

Encysted larvae are ingested in undercooked pork, boar, horse, or bear

Similar cycle (as in humans) in swine or other carnivores (rats, bears, foxes, dogs, cats, or horses)

FIGURE 219-1   Life cycle of *Trichinella*. (*From Bruschi and Murrell, with permission.*)

about their consumption of pork or wild-animal meat and about illness in other individuals who ate the same meat. A presumptive clinical diagnosis can be based on fevers, eosinophilia, periorbital edema, and myalgias after a suspect meal. A rise in the titer of parasite-specific antibody, which usually does not occur until after the third week of infection, confirms the diagnosis. Alternatively, a definitive diagnosis requires surgical biopsy of at least 1 g of involved muscle; the yields are highest near tendon insertions. The fresh muscle tissue should be compressed between glass slides and examined microscopically, because larvae may be overlooked by examination of routine histopathologic sections alone.

℞ **TREATMENT** Current anthelmintic drugs are ineffective against *Trichinella* larvae in muscle. Fortunately, most lightly infected patients recover uneventfully with bed rest, antipyretics, and analgesics. Glucocorticoids like prednisone (1 mg/kg daily for 5 days) are beneficial for severe myositis and myocarditis. Mebendazole and albendazole, like thiabendazole, appear to be active against enteric stages of the parasite, but their efficacy against encysted larvae has not been conclusively demonstrated.

Prevention Larvae may be killed by cooking pork until it is no longer pink or by freezing it at −15°C for 3 weeks. However, Arctic *T. nativa* larvae in walrus or bear meat are relatively resistant and may remain viable despite freezing.

VISCERAL AND OCULAR LARVA MIGRANS Visceral larva migrans is a syndrome caused by nematodes that are normally parasitic for nonhuman host species. In humans, the nematode larvae do not typically develop into adult worms but instead migrate through host tissues and elicit eosinophilic inflammation. The most common form of visceral larva migrans is toxocariasis due to larvae of the canine ascarid *Toxocara canis* or, less commonly, the feline ascarid *T. cati*. Rare cases with eosinophilic meningoencephalitis have been caused by the raccoon ascarid *Baylisascaris procyonis*.

Life Cycle and Epidemiology The canine roundworm *T. canis* is distributed among dogs worldwide. Ingestion of infective eggs by dogs is followed by liberation of *Toxocara* larvae, which penetrate the gut wall and migrate intravascularly into the canine liver, muscle, and other tissues, where most remain in a developmentally arrested state. During pregnancy, some larvae resume migration in bitches and infect puppies prenatally (through transplacental transmission) or after birth (through suckling). Thus, in lactating bitches and puppies, larvae return to the intestinal tract and develop into adult worms, which produce eggs that are released in the feces. Humans acquire toxocariasis mainly by eating soil contaminated by puppy feces containing infective *T. canis* eggs. Visceral larva migrans is most common among children who habitually eat dirt, but most toxocaral infections are subclinical. Reported rates of *Toxocara* seropositivity range from 2% in an unselected American population to >20% among kindergarten children in the United States and England.

Pathogenesis and Clinical Features Clinical disease most commonly afflicts preschool children. After humans ingest *Toxocara* eggs, the larvae hatch and penetrate the intestinal mucosa, from which they are carried by the circulation to a wide variety of organs and tissues. The larvae invade the liver, lungs, central nervous system, and other sites, releasing toxic products and provoking intense local eosinophilic granulomatous responses. The degree of clinical illness depends on larval number and tissue distribution, reinfection, and host immune responses. Most light infections are asymptomatic and may be manifest only by blood eosinophilia. Characteristic symptoms of visceral larva migrans include fever, malaise, anorexia and weight loss, cough, wheezing, and rashes. Hepatosplenomegaly is common. These features are often accompanied by extraordinary peripheral eosinophilia, which may approach 90%. Uncommonly, seizures or behavioral disorders develop. The rare deaths in this disease are due to severe neurologic, pneumonic, or myocardial involvement.

Diagnosis In addition to prominent eosinophilia, leukocytosis and hypergammaglobulinemia are usually evident. Transient pulmonary infiltrates are apparent on chest x-rays of about half of patients with symptoms of pneumonitis. The clinical diagnosis can be confirmed by an enzyme-linked immunosorbent assay for toxocaral antibodies. Stool examination, while important in the evaluation of unexplained eosinophilia, is worthless for toxocariasis, since the larvae do not develop into egg-producing adults in humans.

The ocular form of the larva migrans syndrome occurs when *Toxocara* larvae invade the eye. An eosinophilic granulomatous mass, most commonly in the posterior pole of the retina, develops around the entrapped larva. The retinal lesion can mimic retinoblastoma in appearance, and mistaken diagnosis of the latter condition can lead to unnecessary enucleation. The spectrum of eye involvement also includes endophthalmitis, uveitis, and chorioretinitis. Unilateral visual disturbances, strabismus, and eye pain are the most common presenting symptoms. In contrast to visceral larva migrans, ocular toxocariasis usually develops in older children or young adults with no history of pica; these patients seldom have eosinophilia or visceral manifestations.

℞ **TREATMENT** The vast majority of *Toxocara* infections are self-limited and resolve without specific therapy. In patients with severe myocardial, central nervous system, or pulmonary involvement, glucocorticoids may be employed to reduce inflammatory complications. Available anthelmintic drugs, including diethylcarbamazine, mebendazole, and albendazole, have not been shown conclusively to alter the course of larva migrans. Control measures include prohibiting dog excreta in public parks and playgrounds, deworming dogs, and preventing pica in children. Treatment of ocular disease is unsatisfactory, and the role of glucocorticoids or anthelmintic drugs in management is controversial.

CUTANEOUS LARVA MIGRANS Cutaneous larva migrans ("creeping eruption") is a serpiginous skin eruption caused by burrowing larvae of animal hookworms, usually the dog and cat hookworm *Ancylostoma braziliense*. The larvae hatch from eggs passed in dog and cat feces and mature in the soil. Humans become infected after skin contact with soil in areas frequented by dogs and cats, such as areas underneath house porches or scrub vegetation. Cutaneous larva migrans is especially prevalent among children and in regions with warm humid climates, including the southeastern United States.

After larvae penetrate the skin, erythematous lesions form along the tortuous tracts of their migration through the dermal-epidermal junction; the larvae advance several centimeters in a day. The intensely pruritic lesions may occur anywhere on the body and can be numerous if the patient has lain on the ground. Vesicles and bullae may form later. The animal hookworm larvae do not mature in humans and, without treatment, will die out after several weeks, with resolution of skin lesions. The diagnosis is made readily on clinical grounds, and a skin biopsy only rarely yields diagnostic parasite material. Symptoms can be alleviated by thiabendazole administered orally (25 mg/kg bid) or topically (10% aqueous or petroleum jelly suspension) for 2 to 5 days, by ivermectin (a single dose of 150 to 200 μg/kg), or by albendazole (200 mg bid for 2 days).

***ANGIOSTRONGYLUS CANTONENSIS* INFECTION** *A. cantonensis*, the rat lungworm, is the most common cause of human eosinophilic meningitis.

Life Cycle and Epidemiology This infection occurs principally in Southeast Asia and the Pacific Basin. *A. cantonensis* larvae produced by adult worms in the rat lung migrate to the gastrointestinal tract and are expelled with the feces. They develop into infective larvae in land snails and slugs. Humans acquire the infection by ingesting raw infected mollusks; vegetables contaminated by mollusk slime; or crabs, freshwater shrimp, and certain marine fish that have themselves eaten infected mollusks. The larvae then migrate to the brain.

Pathogenesis and Clinical Features The parasites eventually die in the central nervous system, but not before initiating pathologic consequences that, in heavy infections, can result in permanent neurologic sequelae or death. Migrating larvae cause proteolytic damage and marked local eosinophilic inflammation and hemorrhage, with subsequent necrosis and granuloma formation around dying worms. Clinical symptoms develop between 2 and 35 days after the ingestion of larvae. Patients usually present with an insidious or abrupt excruciating frontal, occipital, or bitemporal headache. Neck stiffness, nausea and vomiting, and paresthesias are also common. Fever, cranial and extraocular nerve palsies, seizures, paralysis, and lethargy are uncommon.

Laboratory Findings Examination of the cerebrospinal fluid is mandatory in suspected cases and usually reveals an elevated opening pressure, a white blood cell count of 150 to 2000/μL, and an eosinophilic pleocytosis of >20%. The protein concentration is usually elevated and the glucose level normal. The motile larvae of *A. cantonensis* are only rarely seen in the cerebrospinal fluid. Peripheral-blood eosinophilia may be mild. The diagnosis is generally based on the clinical presentation of eosinophilic meningitis together with a compatible epidemiologic history.

R_X **TREATMENT** Specific chemotherapy is not of benefit in angiostrongyliasis; larvicidal agents may actually exacerbate inflammatory brain lesions. Management consists of supportive measures, including the administration of analgesics, sedatives, and—in severe cases—glucocorticoids. In most patients, cerebral angiostrongyliasis has a self-limited course, and recovery is complete. The infection may be prevented by adequately cooking snails, crabs, and prawns and inspecting vegetables for mollusk infestation. Other parasitic causes of eosinophilic meningitis in endemic areas may include gnathostomiasis, paragonimiasis, schistosomiasis, and neurocysticercosis.

GNATHOSTOMIASIS Infection of human tissues with larvae of *Gnathostoma spinigerum* can cause eosinophilic meningoencephalitis, migratory cutaneous swellings, or invasive masses of the eye and visceral organs.

Life Cycle and Epidemiology Human gnathostomiasis occurs in many countries and is notably endemic in Southeast Asia and parts of China and Japan. In nature, the mature adult worms parasitize the gastrointestinal tract of dogs and cats. First-stage larvae hatch from eggs passed into water and are ingested by *Cyclops* species (water fleas). Infective third-stage larvae develop in the flesh of many animal species (including fish, frogs, eels, snakes, chickens, and ducks) that have eaten either infected *Cyclops* or another infected second intermediate host. Humans typically acquire the infection by eating raw or undercooked fish or poultry. The raw fish dishes of *somfak* in Thailand and *sashimi* in Japan account for most cases of human gnathostomiasis. Some cases in Thailand result from the local practice of applying frog or snake flesh as a poultice.

Pathogenesis and Clinical Features Clinical symptoms are due to the aberrant migration of a single larva into cutaneous, visceral, neural, or ocular tissues. After invasion, larval migration may cause local inflammation, with pain, cough, or hematuria accompanied by fever and eosinophilia. Painful, itchy, migratory swellings may develop in the skin, particularly in the distal extremities or periorbital area. Cutaneous swellings usually last about a week but often recur intermittently over many years. Larval invasion of the eye can provoke a sight-threatening inflammatory response. Finally, invasion of the central nervous system results in eosinophilic meningitis with myeloencephalitis, a serious complication due to ascending larval migration along a large nerve track. Patients characteristically present with agonizing radicular pain and paresthesias in the trunk or a limb, which are followed shortly by paraplegia. Cerebral involvement, with focal hemorrhages and tissue destruction, is often fatal.

Diagnosis and Treatment Cutaneous migratory swellings with marked peripheral eosinophilia, supported by an appropriate geographic and dietary history, generally constitute an adequate basis for a clinical diagnosis of gnathostomiasis. However, patients may present with ocular or cerebrospinal involvement without antecedent cutane

ous swellings. In the latter case, eosinophilic pleocytosis is demonstrable (usually along with hemorrhagic or xanthochromic cerebrospinal fluid), but worms are almost never recovered from the cerebrospinal fluid. Surgical removal of the parasite from subcutaneous or ocular tissue, though rarely feasible, is both diagnostic and therapeutic. Albendazole (400 to 800 mg daily for 21 days) may be helpful. At present, cerebrospinal involvement is managed with supportive measures and generally with a course of glucocorticoids. Gnathostomiasis can be prevented by adequate cooking of fish and poultry in endemic areas.

BIBLIOGRAPHY

BALDISSEROTTO M et al: Ultrasound findings in children with toxocariasis: Report on 18 cases. Pediatr Radiol 29:316, 1999
BRUSCHI F, MURRELL KD: Trichinellosis, in *Tropical Infectious Diseases: Principles, Pathogens and Practice,* RL Guerrant et al (eds). Philadelphia, Churchill Livingstone, 1999, pp 917–926
DIAZ CAMACHO SP et al: Clinical manifestations and immunodiagnosis of gnathostomiasis in Culiacan, Mexico. Am J Trop Med Hyg 59:908, 1998
HOTEZ PJ: Visceral and ocular larva migrans. Semin Neurol 13:175, 1993
JELINEK T et al: Cutaneous larva migrans in travelers: Synopsis of histories, symptoms, and treatment of 98 patients. Clin Infect Dis 19:1062, 1994
JONGWUTIWES S et al: First outbreak of human trichinellosis caused by *Trichinella pseudospiralis.* Clin Infect Dis 26:111, 1998
KAPEL CM et al: Freeze tolerance, morphology, and RAPD-PCR identification of *Trichinella nativa* in naturally infected Arctic foxes. J Parasitol 85:144, 1999
LUCCHINA LC et al: Dermatology and the recently returned traveler: Infectious diseases with dermatologic manifestations. Int J Dermatol 36:167, 1997
MOORHEAD A et al: Trichinellosis in the United States, 1991–1996: Declining but not gone. Am J Trop Med Hyg 60:66, 1999
WELLER PF, LIU LX: Eosinophilic meningitis. Semin Neurol 13:161, 1993

220 *Peter F. Weller, Thomas B. Nutman*

INTESTINAL NEMATODES

More than a billion people worldwide are infected with one or more species of intestinal nematodes. Table 220-1 summarizes biologic and clinical features of infections due to the major intestinal parasitic nematodes. These parasites are most common in regions with poor fecal sanitation, particularly in developing countries in the tropics and subtropics but also in the United States. Although nematode infections are not usually fatal, they contribute to malnutrition and diminished work capacity. Humans may on occasion be infected with nematode parasites that ordinarily infect animals; these zoonotic infections include trichostrongyliasis, anisakiasis, capillariasis, and abdominal angiostrongyliasis.

Intestinal nematodes are roundworms; they range in length from 1 mm to many centimeters when mature (Table 220-1). Their life cycles are complex and highly varied; some species, including *Strongyloides stercoralis* and *Enterobius vermicularis,* can be transmitted directly from person to person, while others, such as *Ascaris lumbricoides, Necator americanus,* and *Ancylostoma duodenale,* require a soil phase for development. Because most helminth parasites do not self-replicate, the acquisition of a heavy burden of adult worms requires repeated exposure to the parasite in its infectious stage, whether larva or egg. Hence, clinical disease, as opposed to asymptomatic infection, generally develops only with prolonged residence in an endemic area. In persons with marginal nutrition, intestinal helminth infections may impair growth and development. Eosinophilia and elevated serum IgE levels are features of many helminthic infections and, when unexplained, should always prompt a search for occult helminthiasis. Significant protective immunity to intestinal nematodes appears not to develop in humans, although mechanisms of parasite im

Table 220-1 Major Human Intestinal Parasitic Nematodes

Feature	Ascaris lumbricoides (Roundworm)	Necator americanus, Ancylostoma duodenale (Hookworm)	Strongyloides stercoralis	Trichuris trichiura (Whipworm)	Enterobius vermicularis (Pinworm)
Global prevalence in humans (millions)	1273	1277	50	902	300
Endemic areas	Worldwide	Hot, humid regions	Hot, humid regions	Worldwide	Worldwide
Infective stage	Egg	Filariform larva	Filariform larva	Egg	Egg
Route of infection	Oral	Percutaneous	Percutaneous or auto-infection	Oral	Oral
Gastrointestinal location of worms	Jejunal lumen	Jejunal mucosa	Small-bowel mucosa	Cecum, colonic mucosa	Cecum, appendix
Adult worm size	15–40 cm	7–12 mm	2 mm	30–50 mm	8–13 mm (female)
Pulmonary passage of larvae	Yes	Yes	Yes	No	No
Incubation period[a] (days)	60–75	40–100	17–28	70–90	35–45
Longevity	1 y	N. americanus: 2–5 y A. duodenale: 6–8 y	Decades (owing to autoinfection)	5 y	2 months
Fecundity (eggs/day/worm)	240,000	N. americanus: 4000–10,000 A. duodenale: 10,000–25,000	5000–10,000	3000–7000	2000
Principal symptoms	Rarely gastrointestinal or biliary obstruction	Iron-deficiency anemia in heavy infection	Gastrointestinal symptoms; malabsorption or sepsis in hyperinfection	Gastrointestinal symptoms, anemia	Perianal pruritus
Diagnostic stage	Eggs in stool	Eggs in fresh stool, larvae in old stool	Larvae in stool or duodenal aspirate; sputum in hyperinfection	Eggs in stool	Eggs from perianal skin on cellulose acetate tape
Treatment	Mebendazole Albendazole Pyrantel pamoate Piperazine citrate	Mebendazole Pyrantel pamoate Albendazole	1. Ivermectin 2. Albendazole 3. Thiabendazole	Mebendazole Albendazole	Mebendazole Pyrantel pamoate Albendazole

> Parasitic Nematode (spanning header over the five nematode columns)

[a] Time from infection to egg production by mature female worm.

mune evasion and host immune responses to these infections have not been elucidated in detail.

ASCARIASIS *A. lumbricoides* is the largest intestinal nematode parasite of humans, reaching up to 40 cm in length. Most infected individuals have low worm burdens and are asymptomatic. Clinical disease arises from larval migration in the lungs or effects of the adult worms in the intestines.

Life Cycle Adult worms live in the lumen of the small intestine. Mature female *Ascaris* worms are extraordinarily fecund, each producing up to 240,000 eggs a day, which pass with the feces. Ascarid eggs, which are remarkably resistant to environmental stresses, become infective after several weeks of maturation in the soil and can remain infective for years. After infective eggs are swallowed, larvae hatched in the intestine invade the mucosa, migrate through the circulation to the lungs, break into the alveoli, ascend the bronchial tree, and return via swallowing to the small intestine, where they develop into adult worms. Between 2 and 3 months elapse between initial infection and egg production. The adult worms live for ~1 to 2 years.

Epidemiology *Ascaris* is widely distributed in tropical and subtropical regions as well as in other humid areas, including the rural southeastern United States. Transmission typically occurs through fecally contaminated soil and is due either to a lack of sanitary facilities or to the use of human manure ("night soil") as fertilizer. With their propensity for hand-to-mouth fecal carriage, younger children in impoverished rural areas are most affected. Infection outside endemic areas, though uncommon, can occur from eggs borne on transported vegetables.

Clinical Features During the lung phase of larval migration, about 9 to 12 days after egg ingestion, patients may develop an irritating nonproductive cough and burning substernal discomfort that is aggravated by coughing or deep inspiration. Dyspnea and blood-tinged sputum are less common. Fever is usually reported, with temperatures sometimes exceeding 38.5°C (101.3°F). Eosinophilia develops during this symptomatic phase and subsides slowly over weeks. Chest x-rays may reveal evidence of eosinophilic pneumonitis (Löffler's syndrome), with round or oval infiltrates a few millimeters to several centimeters in size. These infiltrates may be transient and intermittent, clearing after several weeks. Where there is seasonal transmission of the parasite, seasonal pneumonitis with eosinophilia may develop in previously infected and sensitized hosts.

In established infections, adult worms in the small intestine usually cause no symptoms. In heavy infections, particularly in children, a large bolus of entangled worms can cause pain and small-bowel obstruction, sometimes complicated by perforation, intussusception, or volvulus. Single worms may cause disease when they migrate into aberrant sites. A large worm can enter and occlude the biliary tree, causing biliary colic, cholecystitis, cholangitis, pancreatitis, or (rarely) intrahepatic abscesses. Migration of an adult worm up the esophagus can provoke coughing and oral expulsion of the worm. In highly endemic areas, intestinal and biliary ascariasis can rival acute appendicitis and gallstones as causes of surgical acute abdomen.

Laboratory Findings Most cases of ascariasis can be diagnosed by the microscopic detection of characteristic mamillated *Ascaris* eggs (65 by 45 μm) in fecal samples. Occasionally, patients present after passing an adult worm—identifiable by its large size and smooth cream-colored surface—in the stool or through the mouth or nose. During the early transpulmonary migratory phase, when eosinophilic pneumonitis occurs, larvae can be found in sputum or gastric aspirates before diagnostic eggs appear in the stool. The eosinophilia that is prominent during this early stage usually decreases to minimal levels in established infection. The large adult worms may be visualized, occasionally serendipitously, on contrast studies of the gastrointestinal tract. A plain abdominal film may reveal masses of worms in gas-filled loops of bowel in patients with intestinal obstruction. Pancreatico-biliary worms can be detected by ultrasound and endoscopic retrograde cholangiopancreatography; the latter method also has been used to extract biliary *Ascaris* worms.

Rx **TREATMENT** Ascariasis should always be treated to prevent potentially serious complications. Mebendazole or albendazole (which is considered an investigational drug by the Food and Drug Administration for this indication) is effective. These benzimidazoles are contraindicated in pregnancy and in heavy infections, in which they may provoke ectopic migration. Pyrantel pamoate and piperazine citrate are safe in pregnancy. Mild diarrhea and abdominal pain are uncommon side effects of these agents. Partial intestinal obstruction should be managed with nasogastric suction, intravenous fluid administration, and instillation of piperazine through the nasogastric tube, but complete obstruction and its severe complications require immediate surgical intervention.

HOOKWORM One-fourth of the world's population is infected with one of the two hookworm species (*A. duodenale* and *N. americanus*). Most infected individuals are asymptomatic. Hookworm disease develops from a combination of factors—a heavy worm burden, a prolonged duration of infection, and an inadequate iron intake—and results in iron-deficiency anemia and, on occasion, hypoproteinemia.

Life Cycle Adult hookworms, which are about 1 cm long, use buccal teeth (*Ancylostoma*) or cutting plates (*Necator*) to attach to the small-bowel mucosa and suck blood (0.2 mL/d per *Ancylostoma* adult) and interstitial fluid. The adult hookworms produce thousands of eggs daily. The eggs are deposited with feces in soil, where rhabditiform larvae hatch and develop over a 1-week period into infectious filariform larvae. Infective larvae penetrate the skin and reach the lungs by way of the bloodstream. There they invade alveoli and ascend the airways before being swallowed and reaching the small intestine. The prepatent period from skin invasion to appearance of eggs in the feces is about 6 to 8 weeks, but it may be longer with *A. duodenale*. Larvae of *A. duodenale*, if swallowed, can survive and develop directly in the intestinal mucosa. Adult hookworms may survive over a decade but usually live about 6 to 8 years for *A. duodenale* and 2 to 5 years for *N. americanus*.

Epidemiology *A. duodenale* is prevalent in southern Europe, North Africa, and northern Asia, and *N. americanus* is the predominant species in the western hemisphere and equatorial Africa. The two species overlap in many tropical regions, particularly Southeast Asia. In most areas, older children have the greatest incidence and intensity of hookworm infection. In rural areas where fields are fertilized with night soil, older working adults also may be heavily affected.

Clinical Features Most hookworm infections are asymptomatic. Infective larvae may provoke pruritic maculopapular dermatitis ("ground itch") at the site of skin penetration as well as serpiginous tracts of subcutaneous migration (similar to cutaneous larva migrans) in previously sensitized hosts. Larvae migrating through the lungs occasionally cause mild transient pneumonitis, but this condition develops less frequently in hookworm infection than in ascariasis. In the early intestinal phase, infected persons may develop epigastric pain (often with postprandial accentuation), inflammatory diarrhea, or other abdominal symptoms accompanied by eosinophilia. The major consequence of chronic hookworm infection is iron deficiency. Symptoms are minimal if iron intake is adequate, but marginally nourished individuals develop symptoms of progressive iron-deficiency anemia and hypoproteinemia, including weakness, shortness of breath, and skin depigmentation.

Laboratory Findings The diagnosis is established by the finding of characteristic 40- by 60-μm oval hookworm eggs in the feces. Stool-concentration procedures may be required to detect light infections. Eggs of the two species are indistinguishable. In a stool sample that is not fresh, the eggs may have hatched to release rhabditiform larvae, which need to be differentiated from those of *S. stercoralis*.

Hypochromic microcytic anemia, occasionally with eosinophilia or hypoalbuminemia, is characteristic of hookworm disease.

Rx **TREATMENT** Hookworm infection can be eradicated with several safe and highly effective anthelmintic drugs, including mebendazole, albendazole, and pyrantel pamoate (Chap. 212). Mild iron-deficiency anemia often can be treated with oral iron alone. Severe hookworm disease with protein loss and malabsorption necessitates nutritional support and oral iron replacement along with deworming.

Ancylostoma caninum This parasite, the canine hookworm, has been identified as a cause of human eosinophilic enteritis, especially in northeastern Australia. In this zoonotic infection, adult hookworms attach to the small intestine (where they may be visualized by endoscopy) and elicit abdominal pain and intense local eosinophilia. Treatment with mebendazole (100 mg twice daily for 3 days) is effective.

STRONGYLOIDIASIS *S. stercoralis* is distinguished by its ability, unusual among helminths, to replicate in the human host. This capacity permits ongoing cycles of autoinfection as infective larvae are internally produced. Strongyloidiasis can thus persist for decades without further exposure of the host to exogenous infective larvae. In immunocompromised hosts, large numbers of invasive *Strongyloides* larvae can disseminate widely and can be fatal.

Life Cycle In addition to a parasitic cycle of development, *Strongyloides* can undergo a free-living cycle of development in the soil. This adaptability facilitates the parasite's survival in the absence of mammalian hosts. Rhabditiform larvae passed in feces can transform into infectious filariform larvae either directly or after a free-living phase of development. Humans acquire strongyloidiasis when filariform larvae in fecally contaminated soil penetrate the skin or mucous membranes. The larvae then travel through the bloodstream to the lungs, where they break into the alveolar spaces, ascend the bronchial tree, are swallowed, and thereby reach the small intestine. There the larvae mature into adult worms that penetrate the mucosa of the proximal small bowel. The minute (2-mm-long) parasitic adult female worms reproduce by parthenogenesis; parasitic adult males do not exist. Eggs hatch locally in the intestinal mucosa, releasing rhabditiform larvae that migrate to the lumen and pass with the feces into soil. Alternatively, rhabditiform larvae in the bowel can develop directly into filariform larvae that penetrate the colonic wall or perianal skin and enter the circulation to repeat the migration that establishes ongoing internal reinfection. This autoinfection cycle allows strongyloidiasis to persist for decades after the host has left an endemic area.

Epidemiology *S. stercoralis* is spottily distributed in tropical areas and other hot, humid regions and is particularly common in Southeast Asia, sub-Saharan Africa, and Brazil. In the United States, the parasite is endemic in parts of the South and is found in residents of mental institutions who practice poor hygiene and in immigrants and military veterans who have lived in endemic areas abroad.

Clinical Features In uncomplicated strongyloidiasis, many patients are asymptomatic or have mild cutaneous and/or abdominal symptoms. Recurrent urticaria, often involving the buttocks and wrists, is the most common cutaneous manifestation. Migrating larvae can elicit a pathognomonic serpiginous eruption, *larva currens* ("running larva")—a pruritic, raised, erythematous lesion that advances as rapidly as 10 cm/h along the course of larval migration. Adult parasites burrow into the duodenojejunal mucosa and can cause abdominal (usually midepigastric) pain, which resembles peptic ulcer pain except that it is aggravated by food ingestion. Nausea, diarrhea, gastrointestinal bleeding, mild chronic colitis, and weight loss can occur. Small-bowel obstruction may develop with early, heavy infection. Pulmonary symptoms are rare in uncomplicated strongyloidiasis. Eosinophilia is common, with levels fluctuating over time.

The ongoing autoinfection cycle of strongyloidiasis is normally contained by unknown factors of the host's immune system. Abrogation of host immunity, especially with glucocorticoid therapy and much less commonly with other immunosuppressive medications, leads to hyperinfection, with the generation of large numbers of filariform larvae. Colitis, enteritis, or malabsorption may develop. In disseminated strongyloidiasis, larvae may invade not only gastrointestinal tissues and the lungs but also the central nervous system, peritoneum, liver, and kidney. Moreover, bacteremia may develop because of the entry of enteric flora through disrupted mucosal barriers. Gram-negative sepsis, pneumonia, or meningitis may complicate or dominate the clinical course. Eosinophilia is often absent in severely infected patients. Disseminated strongyloidiasis, particularly in patients with unsuspected infection who are given glucocorticoids, can be fatal. Strongyloidiasis is a frequent complication of infection with human T cell lymphotropic virus type I, but disseminated strongyloidiasis is not common among patients infected with HIV.

Diagnosis   In uncomplicated strongyloidiasis, the finding of rhabditiform larvae in feces is diagnostic. The eggs are almost never detectable because they hatch in the intestine. Rhabditiform larvae are 200 to 250 μm long, with a short buccal cavity that distinguishes them from hookworm rhabditiform larvae. Single stool examinations detect only about one-third of uncomplicated infections, in which few larvae are passed. Serial examinations and the use of the agar plate detection method improve the sensitivity of stool diagnosis. In uncomplicated—but not hyperinfection—strongyloidiasis, stool examinations may be repeatedly negative. If stool examinations are negative, *Strongyloides* can be assayed by sampling of the duodenojejunal contents by aspiration or biopsy. An enzyme-linked immunosorbent assay for antibodies to excretory-secretory or somatic antigens of *Strongyloides* is a sensitive method of diagnosing uncomplicated infections. In disseminated strongyloidiasis, filariform larvae (550 μm long) should be sought in stool as well as in samples obtained from sites of potential larval migration, including sputum, bronchoalveolar lavage fluid, or surgical drainage fluid.

TREATMENT   Even in the asymptomatic state, strongyloidiasis must be treated because of the potential for fatal hyperinfection. Ivermectin (200 μg/kg daily for 1 or 2 days) is more effective and better tolerated than thiabendazole (25 mg/kg bid for 2 days), whose common adverse effects include nausea, vomiting, diarrhea, dizziness, and neuropsychiatric disturbances. Because thiabendazole is not uniformly effective, stool examinations, eosinophil counts, and monitoring of clinical symptoms should be continued after treatment. For disseminated strongyloidiasis, treatment should be extended for at least 5 to 7 days or until the parasites are eradicated.

Strongyloides fülleborni   This unusual species, which has been encountered in Africa and Papua New Guinea, is thought to be transmitted from person to person and through maternal milk. *S. fülleborni* releases membranous sacs filled with eggs into the stool. Most commonly affected are infants and young children, who present with abdominal distention, respiratory distress, vomiting, or diarrhea.

TRICHURIASIS   Most infections with the whipworm *Trichuris trichiura* are asymptomatic, but heavy infections may cause gastrointestinal symptoms. Like the other soil-transmitted helminths, whipworm is distributed globally in the tropics and subtropics and is most common among poor children.

Life Cycle   A broad posterior section and a thin anterior portion give *Trichuris* its characteristic whiplike shape. The adult worms reside in the colon and cecum, the anterior portions threaded into the superficial mucosa. Thousands of eggs laid daily by adult female worms pass with the feces and mature in the soil. After ingestion, infective eggs hatch in the duodenum, releasing larvae that mature before migrating to the large bowel. The entire cycle takes about 3 months, and adult worms may live for several years.

Clinical Features   Tissue reactions to whipworms are mild. Most infected individuals have no symptoms or eosinophilia. Heavy infections may result in abdominal pain, anorexia, and bloody or mucoid diarrhea resembling inflammatory bowel disease. Rectal prolapse can result from massive infections in children, who often suffer from malnourishment and other diarrheal illnesses. Moderately heavy whipworm burdens also contribute to growth retardation.

Diagnosis and Treatment   The characteristic 50- by 20-μm lemon-shaped whipworm eggs are readily detected on stool examination. Adult worms, which are 3 to 5 cm long, occasionally can be seen on proctoscopy. Mebendazole or albendazole is safe and effective for treatment (Chap. 212).

ENTEROBIASIS (PINWORM)   *E. vermicularis* is more common in temperate countries than in the tropics. More than 40 million Americans, particularly schoolchildren, are estimated to be infected with pinworms.

Life Cycle and Epidemiology   *Enterobius* adult worms are about 1 cm long and dwell in the bowel lumen. The gravid female worm migrates nocturnally out into the perianal region and releases up to 10,000 immature eggs. The eggs become infective within hours and are transmitted by hand-to-mouth passage. The larvae hatch and mature entirely within the intestine. This life cycle takes about 1 month, and adult worms survive for about 2 months. Self-infection results from perianal scratching and transport of infective eggs on the hands or under the nails to the mouth. Owing to the ease of person-to-person spread, pinworm infections are common among family members and institutionalized populations.

Clinical Features   Most pinworm infections are asymptomatic. Perianal pruritus is the cardinal symptom. The itching is often worse at night owing to the nocturnal migration of the female worms, and it may lead to excoriation and bacterial superinfection. Heavy infections have been claimed to cause abdominal pain and weight loss. On rare occasions, pinworms invade the female genital tract, causing vulvovaginitis and pelvic or peritoneal granulomas. Eosinophilia or elevated levels of serum IgE are rare.

Diagnosis   Since pinworm eggs are not usually released in the bowel, the diagnosis cannot be made by looking for eggs in the feces. Instead, eggs deposited in the perianal region are detected by the application of clear cellulose acetate tape to the perianal region in the morning. After the tape is transferred to a microscope slide, low-power examination will reveal the characteristic pinworm eggs, which are oval, measure 55 by 25 μm, and are flattened along one side.

TREATMENT   All affected individuals should be given a dose of mebendazole or pyrantel pamoate, with treatment repeated after 10 to 14 days (Chap. 212). Treatment of household members is also advocated to eliminate asymptomatic reservoirs of potential reinfection.

TRICHOSTRONGYLIASIS   *Trichostrongylus* species that are normally parasites of herbivorous animals occasionally infect humans, particularly in Asia and Africa. This parasite has been termed *pseudo hookworm* because of similarities to the hookworms in life cycle and egg morphology. Humans acquire the infection by accidentally ingesting *Trichostrongylus* larvae on contaminated leafy vegetables. The larvae do not migrate in humans but mature directly into adult worms in the small bowel. These worms ingest far less blood than hookworms; most infected people are asymptomatic, but heavy infections may give rise to mild anemia and eosinophilia. *Trichostrongylus* eggs encountered on stool examination resemble those of hookworms but are larger (85 by 115 μm). Appropriate treatment consists of mebendazole or albendazole (Chap. 212).

ANISAKIASIS   Anisakiasis is a gastrointestinal infection caused by the accidental ingestion in uncooked saltwater fish of nematode larvae belonging to the family Anisakidae. The incidence of anisakiasis in the United States has increased as a result of the growing popularity of raw fish dishes. Most cases occur in Japan, the Netherlands, and Chile, where raw fish—sushi, pickled green herring, and seviche, respectively—are national culinary staples. Anisakid nematodes parasitize large sea mammals such as whales, dolphins, and seals. As part of a complex parasitic life cycle involving marine food chains, infectious larvae migrate to the musculature of a variety of fish. Both *Anisakis simplex* and *Pseudoterranova decipiens* have been implicated in human anisakiasis, but an identical gastric syndrome may be caused by the red larvae of eustrongylid parasites of fish-eating birds.

When humans consume infected raw fish, live larvae may be coughed up within 48 h. Alternatively, larvae may immediately penetrate the mucosa of the stomach. Within hours, violent upper abdominal pain accompanied by nausea and occasionally vomiting ensues, mimicking an acute abdomen. The diagnosis can be established by direct visualization on upper endoscopy, outlining of the worm by contrast radiographic studies, or histopathologic examination of extracted tissue. In experienced hands, the first technique is preferable because extraction of the burrowing larvae by endoscopic technique is curative. In addition, larvae may pass to the small bowel, where they penetrate the mucosa and provoke a vigorous eosinophilic granulomatous response. Symptoms may appear 1 or 2 weeks after the infective meal, with intermittent abdominal pain, diarrhea, nausea, and fever resembling the manifestations of Crohn's disease. The diagnosis may be suggested by barium studies and confirmed by curative surgical resection of a granuloma in which the worm is embedded. Anisakid eggs are not found in the stool, since the larvae do not mature in humans. Anisakid larvae in saltwater fish are killed by cooking to 60°C, freezing at −20°C for 3 days, or commercial blast freezing, but not usually by salting, marinating, or cold smoking. No medical treatment is available; if possible, surgical or endoscopic removal should be undertaken.

CAPILLARIASIS Intestinal capillariasis is caused by ingestion of raw fish infected with *Capillaria philippinensis*. Subsequent autoinfection can lead to a severe wasting syndrome. The disease occurs in the Philippines and Thailand and, on occasion, elsewhere in Asia. The natural cycle of *C. philippinensis* involves fish from fresh and brackish water. When humans eat infected raw fish, the larvae mature in the intestine into adult worms, which produce invasive larvae that cause intestinal inflammation and villus loss. Capillariasis has an insidious onset with nonspecific abdominal pain and watery diarrhea. If untreated, progressive autoinfection can lead to protein-losing enteropathy and severe malabsorption and ultimately to death from cachexia, cardiac failure, or superinfection. The diagnosis is established by identification of the characteristic peanut-shaped (20- by 40-μm) eggs on stool examination. Severely ill patients require hospitalization and supportive therapy in addition to prolonged anthelmintic treatment with mebendazole or albendazole (Chap. 212).

ABDOMINAL ANGIOSTRONGYLIASIS Abdominal angiostrongyliasis is found in Latin America and Africa. The zoonotic parasite *Angiostrongylus costaricensis* causes eosinophilic ileocolitis after the ingestion of contaminated vegetation. *A. costaricensis* normally parasitizes the cotton rat and other rodents, with slugs and snails serving as intermediate hosts. Humans become infected by accidentally ingesting infective larvae in mollusk slime deposited on fruits and vegetables; children are at highest risk. The larvae penetrate the gut wall and migrate to the mesenteric artery, where they develop into adult worms. Eggs deposited in the gut wall provoke an intense eosinophilic granulomatous reaction, and adult worms may cause mesenteric arteritis, thrombosis, or frank bowel infarction. Symptoms may mimic those of appendicitis, including abdominal pain and tenderness, fever, vomiting, and a palpable mass in the right iliac fossa. Leukocytosis and eosinophilia are prominent. A barium enema may reveal ileocecal filling defects, but a definitive diagnosis is usually made surgically with partial bowel resection. Pathologic study reveals a thickened bowel wall with eosinophilic granulomas surrounding the *Angiostrongylus* eggs. In nonsurgical cases, the diagnosis rests solely on clinical grounds because larvae and eggs cannot be detected in the stool. Medical therapy for abdominal angiostrongyliasis (thiabendazole; Chap. 212) is of uncertain efficacy. Careful observation and surgical resection for severe symptoms are the mainstays of treatment.

BIBLIOGRAPHY

BECKINGHAM IJ et al: Management of hepatobiliary and pancreatic *Ascaris* infestation in adults after failed medical treatment. Br J Surg 85:907, 1998

CHAN M-S:The global burden of intestinal nematode infections—fifty years on. Parasitol Today 13:438, 1997

CROESE J et al: Human enteric infection with canine hookworms. Ann Intern Med 120: 369, 1994

CROSS JH: Intestinal capillariasis. Clin Microbiol Rev 5:120, 1992

DUARTE Z et al: Abdominal angiostrongyliasis in Nicaragua: A clinico-pathological study on a series of 12 case reports. Ann Parasitol Hum Comp 66:259, 1991

GENTA RM et al: Strongyloidiasis in US veterans of the Vietnam and other wars. JAMA 258:49, 1987

GOTUZZO E et al: *Strongyloides stercoralis* hyperinfection associated with human T cell lymphotropic virus type-1 infection in Peru. Am J Trop Med Hyg 60:146, 1999

GYORKOS TW et al: Intestinal parasite infection in the Kampuchean refugee population 6 years after resettlement in Canada. J Infect Dis 166:413, 1992

HAQUE AK et al: Pathogenesis of human strongyloidiasis: Autopsy and quantitative parasitological analysis. Mod Pathol 7:276, 1994

HOTEZ PJ, PRITCHARD DI: Hookworm infection. Sci Am 272:68, 1995

OCHOA B: Surgical complications of ascariasis. World J Surg 15:222, 1991

REEDER MM: The radiological and ultrasound evaluation of ascariasis of the gastrointestinal, biliary, and respiratory tracts. Semin Roentgenol 33:57, 1998

SCHANTZ PM: The dangers of eating raw fish (editorial). N Engl J Med 320:1143, 1989

TAKABE K et al: Anisakidosis: A cause of intestinal obstruction from eating sushi. Am J Gastroenterol 93:1172, 1998

UPARANUKRAW P et al: Fluctuations of larval excretion in *Strongyloides stercoralis* infection. Am J Trop Med Hyg 60:967, 1999

221 *Thomas B. Nutman, Peter F. Weller*

FILARIASIS AND RELATED INFECTIONS (LOIASIS, ONCHOCERCIASIS, AND DRACUNCULIASIS)

Filarial worms are nematodes that dwell in the subcutaneous tissues and the lymphatics. Eight filarial species infect humans (Table 221-1); of these, four—*Wuchereria bancrofti*, *Brugia malayi*, *Onchocerca volvulus*, and *Loa loa*—are responsible for most serious filarial infections. Filarial parasites, which infect an estimated 170 million persons worldwide, are transmitted by specific species of mosquitoes or other arthropods and have a complex life cycle including infective larval stages carried by insects and adult worms that reside in either lymphatic or subcutaneous tissues of humans. The offspring of adults are microfilariae, which, depending on their species, are 200 to 250 μm long and 5 to 7 μm wide, may or may not be enveloped in a loose sheath, and either circulate in the blood or migrate through the skin (Table 221-1). To complete the life cycle, microfilariae are ingested by the arthropod vector and develop over 1 to 2 weeks into new infective larvae. Adult worms live for many years, whereas microfilariae survive from 3 to 36 months.

Usually, infection is established only with repeated and prolonged exposures to infective larvae. Since the clinical manifestations of filarial diseases develop relatively slowly, these infections should be considered chronic diseases with possible long-term debilitating effects. In terms of the nature, severity, and timing of clinical manifestations, patients with filariasis who are native to endemic areas and undergo lifelong exposure may differ significantly from those who are travelers or who have recently moved to these areas. Characteristically, the disease is more acute and intense in newly exposed individuals than in natives of endemic areas.

LYMPHATIC FILARIASIS

Lymphatic filariasis is caused by *W. bancrofti*, *B. malayi*, or *B. timori*. The threadlike adult parasites reside in lymphatic channels or

Table 221-1   Characteristics of the Filariae

Organism	Periodicity	Distribution	Vector	Location of Adult	Microfilarial Location	Sheath
Wuchereria bancrofti	Nocturnal	Cosmopolitan areas worldwide, including South America and Africa	*Culex* (mosquitoes)	Lymphatic tissue	Blood	+
		Mainly India China, Indonesia	*Anopheles* (mosquitoes) *Aedes* (mosquitoes)			
	Subperiodic	Eastern Pacific	*Aedes* (mosquitoes)	Lymphatic tissue	Blood	+
Brugia malayi	Nocturnal	Southeast Asia, Indonesia, India	*Mansonia, Anopheles* (mosquitoes)	Lymphatic tissue	Blood	+
	Subperiodic	Indonesia, Southeast Asia	*Coquillettidia, Mansonia* (mosquitoes)	Lymphatic tissue	Blood	+
B. timori	Nocturnal	Indonesia	*Anopheles* (mosquitoes)	Lymphatic tissue	Blood	+
Loa loa	Diurnal	West and Central Africa	*Chrysops* (deerflies)	Subcutaneous tissue	Blood	+
Onchocerca volvulus	None	South and Central America, Africa	*Simulium* (blackflies)	Subcutaneous tissue	Skin, eye	−
Mansonella ozzardi	None	South and Central America Caribbean	*Culicoides* (midges) *Simulium* (blackflies)	Undetermined site	Blood	−
M. perstans	None	South and Central America, Africa	*Culicoides* (midges)	Body cavities, mesentery, perirenal tissue	Blood	−
M. streptocerca	None	West and Central Africa	*Culicoides* (midges)	Subcutaneous tissue	Skin	−

lymph nodes, where they may remain viable for more than two decades.

EPIDEMIOLOGY   *W. bancrofti*, the most widely distributed human filarial parasite, affects an estimated 115 million people and is found throughout the tropics and subtropics, including Asia and the Pacific Islands, Africa, areas of South America, and the Caribbean basin. Humans are the only definitive host for the parasite. Generally, the subperiodic form is found only in the Pacific Islands; elsewhere, *W. bancrofti* is nocturnally periodic. (Nocturnally periodic forms of microfilariae are scarce in peripheral blood by day and increase at night, whereas subperiodic forms are present in peripheral blood at all times and reach maximal levels in the afternoon.) Natural vectors for *W. bancrofti* are *Culex fatigans* mosquitoes in urban settings and anopheline or aedean mosquitoes in rural areas.

Brugian filariasis due to *B. malayi* occurs primarily in China, India, Indonesia, Korea, Japan, Malaysia, and the Philippines. *B. malayi* also has two forms distinguished by the periodicity of microfilaremia. The more common nocturnal form is transmitted in areas of coastal rice fields, while the subperiodic form is found in forests. *B. malayi* naturally infects cats as well as humans. *B. timori* exists only on islands of the Indonesian archipelago.

PATHOLOGY   The principal pathologic changes result from inflammatory damage to the lymphatics, which is caused by adult worms and not by microfilariae. Adult worms live in afferent lymphatics or sinuses of lymph nodes and cause lymphatic dilatation and thickening of the vessel walls. The infiltration of plasma cells, eosinophils, and macrophages in and around the infected vessels, along with endothelial and connective tissue proliferation, leads to tortuosity of the lymphatics and damaged or incompetent lymph valves. Lymphedema and chronic-stasis changes with hard or brawny edema develop in the overlying skin. These consequences of filariasis are due both to direct effects of the worms and to the immune response of the host to the parasite. These immune responses are believed to cause the granulomatous and proliferative processes that precede total lymphatic obstruction. It is thought that the vessel remains patent as long as the worm remains viable and that death of the worm leads to enhanced granulomatous reaction and fibrosis. Lymphatic obstruction results, and, despite collateralization of the lymphatics, lymphatic function is compromised.

CLINICAL FEATURES   The most common presentations of the lymphatic filariases are asymptomatic (or subclinical) microfilaremia, hydrocele, acute adenolymphangitis (ADL), and chronic lymphatic disease. In areas where *W. bancrofti* or *B. malayi* is endemic,

the overwhelming majority of infected individuals have few overt clinical manifestations of filarial infection despite large numbers of circulating microfilariae in the peripheral blood. Although they may be clinically asymptomatic, virtually all persons with *W. bancrofti* or *B. malayi* microfilaremia have some degree of subclinical disease that includes microscopic hematuria and/or proteinuria, dilated (and tortuous) lymphatics (visualized by imaging), and—in men—scrotal lymphangiectasia (detectable by ultrasound). Despite these findings, the majority of individuals appear to remain clinically asymptomatic for years; relatively few progress to the acute and chronic stages of infection.

ADL is characterized by high fever, lymphatic inflammation (lymphangitis and lymphadenitis), and transient local edema. The lymphangitis is retrograde, extending peripherally from the lymph node draining the area where the adult parasites reside. Regional lymph nodes are often enlarged, and the entire lymphatic channel can become indurated and inflamed. Concomitant local thrombophlebitis can occur as well. In brugian filariasis, a single local abscess may form along the involved lymphatic tract and subsequently rupture to the surface. The lymphadenitis and lymphangitis involve both the upper and lower extremities in both bancroftian and brugian filariasis, but involvement of the genital lymphatics occurs almost exclusively with *W. bancrofti* infection. This genital involvement can be manifested by funiculitis, epididymitis, scrotal pain, and tenderness. In endemic areas, another type of acute disease—dermatolymphangioadenitis (DLA)—is recognized as a syndrome that includes high fever, chills, myalgias, and headache. Edematous inflammatory plaques clearly demarcated from normal skin are seen. Vesicles, ulcers, and hyperpigmentation may also be noted. There is often a history of trauma, burns, radiation, insect bites, punctiform lesions, or chemical injury. Entry lesions, especially in the interdigital area, are common. DLA is often diagnosed as cellulitis.

If lymphatic damage progresses, transient lymphedema can develop into *lymphatic obstruction* and the permanent changes associated with elephantiasis. Brawny edema follows early pitting edema, and thickening of the subcutaneous tissues and hyperkeratosis occur. Fissuring of the skin develops, as do hyperplastic changes. Superinfection of these poorly vascularized tissues becomes a problem. In bancroftian filariasis, in which genital involvement is common, hydroceles may develop; in advanced stages, this condition may evolve into scrotal lymphedema and scrotal elephantiasis. Furthermore, if there is obstruction of the retroperitoneal lymphatics, the increased renal lymphatic pressure leads to rupture of the renal lymphatics and the development of chyluria, which is usually intermittent and most prominent in the morning.

The clinical manifestations of filarial infections in travelers or transmigrants who have recently entered an endemic region are distinctive. Given a sufficient number of bites by infected vectors, usually over a 3- to 6-month period, recently exposed patients can develop acute lymphatic or scrotal inflammation with or without urticaria and localized angioedema. Lymphadenitis of epitrochlear, axillary, femoral, or inguinal lymph nodes is often followed by retrogradely evolving lymphangitis. Acute attacks are short-lived and, in contrast to filarial fevers in patients native to endemic areas, are usually not accompanied by fever. With prolonged exposure to infected mosquitoes, these attacks, if untreated, become more severe and lead to permanent lymphatic inflammation and obstruction.

DIAGNOSIS A definitive diagnosis can be made only by detection of the parasites and hence can be difficult. Adult worms localized in lymphatic vessels or nodes are largely inaccessible. Microfilariae can be found in blood, in hydrocele fluid, or (occasionally) in other body fluids. Such fluids can be examined microscopically, either directly or—for greater sensitivity—after concentration of the parasites by the passage of fluid through a polycarbonate cylindrical pore filter (pore size, 3 μm) or by the centrifugation of fluid fixed in 2% formalin (Knott's concentration technique). The timing of blood collection is critical and should be based on the periodicity of the microfilariae in the endemic region involved. Many infected individuals do not have microfilaremia, and definitive diagnosis in such cases can be difficult. Assays for circulating antigens of *W. bancrofti* permit the diagnosis of microfilaremic and cryptic (amicrofilaremic) infection. Two tests are commercially available: one is an enzyme-linked immunosorbent assay (ELISA) and the other a rapid-format immunochromatographic card test. Both assays have sensitivities that range from 96 to 100% and specificities that approach 100%. There are currently no tests for circulating antigens in brugian filariasis.

Polymerase chain reaction (PCR)–based assays for DNA of *W. bancrofti* and *B. malayi* in blood have been developed. A number of studies indicate that this diagnostic method is of equivalent or greater sensitivity compared with parasitologic methods, detecting patent infection in almost all infected subjects.

In cases of suspected lymphatic filariasis, examination of the scrotum or the female breast using high-frequency ultrasound in conjunction with Doppler techniques may result in the identification of motile adult worms within dilated lymphatics. Worms may be visualized in the lymphatics of the spermatic cord in up to 80% of infected men. Live adult worms have a distinctive pattern of movement within the lymphatic vessels (termed the *filaria dance sign*).

Radionuclide lymphoscintigraphic imaging of the limbs reliably demonstrates widespread lymphatic abnormalities in both asymptomatic microfilaremic persons and those with clinical manifestations of lymphatic pathology. While of potential utility in the delineation of anatomic changes associated with infection, lymphoscintigraphy is unlikely to assume primacy in the diagnostic evaluation of individuals with suspected infection; it is principally a research tool, and the radionuclide-protein conjugates are not commercially available or approved by the U.S. Food and Drug Administration (FDA).

Eosinophilia and elevated serum concentrations of IgE and antifilarial antibody support the diagnosis of lymphatic filariasis. There is, however, extensive cross-reactivity between filarial antigens and antigens of other helminths, including the common intestinal roundworms; thus, interpretations of serologic findings can be difficult. In addition, residents of endemic areas can become sensitized to filarial antigens through exposure to infected mosquitoes without having patent filarial infections.

In acute episodes, lymphatic filariasis must be distinguished from thrombophlebitis, infection, and trauma. Retrogradely evolving lymphangitis is a characteristic feature that helps distinguish filarial lymphangitis from typically ascending bacterial lymphangitis. Chronic filarial lymphedema must be distinguished from the lymphedema of

malignancy, postoperative scarring, trauma, chronic edematous states, and congenital lymphatic system abnormalities.

℞ **TREATMENT** With new definitions of clinical syndromes in lymphatic filariasis and new tools to assess clinical status (e.g., ultrasound, lymphoscintigraphy, circulating filarial antigen assays), approaches to treatment based on infection status can be considered. Diethylcarbamazine (DEC, 6 mg/kg daily for 12 days), which has both macro- and microfilaricidal properties, remains the treatment of choice for the individual with active lymphatic filariasis (microfilaremia, antigen positivity, or adult worms on ultrasound), although albendazole (400 mg twice daily for 21 days) has demonstrated macrofilaricidal efficacy.

As has already been mentioned, a growing body of evidence indicates that, although they may be asymptomatic, virtually all persons with *W. bancrofti* or *B. malayi* microfilaremia have some degree of subclinical disease (hematuria, proteinuria, abnormalities on lymphoscintigraphy). Thus, early treatment of asymptomatic persons is recommended to prevent further lymphatic damage. For ADL, supportive treatment (including the administration of antipyretics and analgesics) is recommended, as is antibiotic therapy if secondary bacterial infection is likely. Similarly, because lymphatic disease is associated with the presence of adult worms, treatment with DEC is recommended for microfilaria-negative adult-worm carriers.

In persons with chronic manifestations of lymphatic filariasis, treatment regimens that emphasize hygiene, prevention of secondary bacterial infections, and physiotherapy have gained wide acceptance for morbidity control. These regimens are similar to those recommended for lymphedema of most nonfilarial causes and known by a variety of names, including *complex decongestive physiotherapy* and *complex lymphedema therapy*. Hydroceles can be drained repeatedly or managed surgically. In patients with chronic manifestations of lymphatic filariasis, drug treatment should be reserved for cases with evidence of active infection.

The recommended course of DEC treatment (12 days; total dose, 72 mg/kg) has remained standard for many years; however, data indicate that single-dose DEC treatment with 6 mg/kg may be equally efficacious. The 12-day course provides more rapid short-term microfilarial suppression. Regimens that utilize single-dose DEC or ivermectin or combinations of single doses of albendazole and either DEC or ivermectin have all been demonstrated to have a sustained microfilaricidal effect.

Side effects of DEC treatment include fever, chills, arthralgias, headaches, nausea, and vomiting. Both the development and the severity of these reactions are directly related to the number of microfilariae circulating in the bloodstream and may represent an acute hypersensitivity reaction to the antigens being released by dead and dying parasites.

PREVENTION AND CONTROL Avoidance of mosquito bites is usually not feasible for residents of endemic areas, but visitors should make use of insect repellent and mosquito nets. DEC can kill developing forms of filarial parasites and has been shown to be useful as a prophylactic agent in humans.

Community-based intervention is the current approach to elimination of lymphatic filariasis as a public health problem. The underlying tenet of this approach is that mass annual distribution of antimicrofilarial chemotherapy (albendazole with either DEC or ivermectin) will profoundly suppress microfilaremia. If the suppression is sustained, then transmission can be interrupted. As an added benefit, these combinations have secondary effects on gastrointestinal helminths. An alternative approach to the control of lymphatic filariasis is the use of salt fortified with DEC. Community use of DEC-fortified salt dramatically reduces microfilarial density with no apparent adverse reactions. Community education and clinical care for persons already suffering from the chronic sequelae of lymphatic filariasis are important components of filariasis control and elimination programs.

TROPICAL PULMONARY EOSINOPHILIA

Tropical pulmonary eosinophilia (TPE) is a distinct syndrome that develops in some individuals infected with lymphatic filarial species. This syndrome affects males and females at a ratio of 4:1, often during the third decade of life. The majority of cases have been reported from India, Pakistan, Sri Lanka, Brazil, and Southeast Asia.

CLINICAL FEATURES The main features include a history of residence in filarial endemic regions, paroxysmal cough and wheezing that are usually nocturnal (and probably related to the nocturnal periodicity of microfilariae), weight loss, low-grade fever, adenopathy, and pronounced blood eosinophilia (>3000 eosinophils/μL). Chest x-rays may be normal but generally show increased bronchovascular markings; diffuse miliary lesions or mottled opacities may be present in the middle and lower lung fields. Tests of pulmonary function show restrictive abnormalities in most cases and obstructive defects in half. Total serum IgE levels (10,000 to 100,000 ng/mL) and antifilarial antibody titers are characteristically elevated.

PATHOLOGY In TPE there is rapid clearance of microfilariae and parasite antigens from the bloodstream by the lungs, and the clinical symptoms result from allergic and inflammatory reactions elicited by the cleared parasites. In some subjects, trapping of microfilariae in other reticuloendothelial organs can cause hepatomegaly, splenomegaly, or lymphadenopathy. A prominent, eosinophil-enriched, intra-alveolar infiltrate is often reported. In the absence of successful treatment, interstitial fibrosis can lead to progressive pulmonary damage.

DIFFERENTIAL DIAGNOSIS TPE must be distinguished from asthma, Löffler's syndrome, allergic bronchopulmonary aspergillosis, allergic granulomatosis with angiitis (Churg-Strauss syndrome), the systemic vasculitides (most notably periarteritis nodosa and Wegener's granulomatosis), chronic eosinophilic pneumonia, and the idiopathic hypereosinophilic syndrome. In addition to a geographic history of filarial exposure, useful features for distinguishing TPE include wheezing that is solely nocturnal, very high levels of antifilarial antibodies, and a rapid initial response to treatment with DEC.

℞ TREATMENT DEC is used at a dosage of 4 to 6 mg/kg of body weight per day for 14 days. Symptoms usually resolve within 3 to 7 days after the initiation of therapy. Relapse, which occurs in ~12 to 25% of cases (sometimes after an interval of years), requires re-treatment.

ONCHOCERCIASIS

Onchocerciasis ("river blindness") is caused by the filarial nematode *O. volvulus*, which infects an estimated 13 million individuals. The majority of individuals infected with *O. volvulus* live in the equatorial region of Africa extending from the Atlantic coast to the Red Sea. About 70,000 persons are infected in Guatemala and Mexico, with smaller foci in Venezuela, Colombia, Brazil, Ecuador, Yemen, and Saudi Arabia. Onchocerciasis is the second leading cause of infectious blindness worldwide.

ETIOLOGY AND EPIDEMIOLOGY Infection in humans begins with the deposition of infective larvae on the skin by the bite of an infected blackfly. The larvae develop into adults, which are typically found in subcutaneous nodules. About 7 months to 3 years after infection, the gravid female releases microfilariae that migrate out of the nodule and throughout the tissues, concentrating in the dermis. Infection is transmitted to other persons when a female fly ingests microfilariae from the host's skin and these microfilariae then develop into infective larvae. Adult *O. volvulus* females and males are about 40 to 60 cm and 3 to 6 cm in length, respectively. The life span of

adults can be as long as 18 years, with an average of ~9 years. Because the blackfly vector breeds along free-flowing rivers and streams (particularly in rapids) and generally restricts its flight to an area within several kilometers of these breeding sites, both biting and disease transmission are most intense in these locations.

PATHOLOGY Onchocerciasis affects primarily the skin, eyes, and lymph nodes. In contrast to that in lymphatic filariasis, the damage in onchocerciasis is elicited by microfilariae and not by adults. In the skin, there are mild but chronic inflammatory changes that can result in loss of elastic fibers, atrophy, and fibrosis. The subcutaneous nodules, or onchocercomata, consist primarily of fibrous tissues surrounding the adult worm, often with a peripheral ring of inflammatory cells. In the eye, neovascularization and corneal scarring lead to corneal opacities and blindness. Inflammation in the anterior and posterior chambers frequently results in anterior uveitis, chorioretinitis, and optic atrophy. Although punctate opacities are due to an inflammatory reaction surrounding dead or dying microfilariae, the pathogenesis of most manifestations of onchocerciasis is still unclear.

CLINICAL FEATURES **Skin** Pruritus and rash are the most frequent manifestations of onchocerciasis. The pruritus can be incapacitating; the rash is typically a papular eruption that is generalized rather than localized to a particular region of the body. Long-term infection results in exaggerated and premature wrinkling of the skin, loss of elastic fibers, and epidermal atrophy that can lead to loose, redundant skin and hypo- or hyperpigmentation. Localized eczematoid dermatitis can cause hyperkeratosis, scaling, and pigmentary changes. Such lesions are often seen in the lower extremities but can be distributed more extensively.

Onchocercomata These subcutaneous nodules, which can be palpable and/or visible, contain the adult worm. In African patients, they are common over the coccyx and sacrum, the trochanter of the femur, the lateral anterior crest, and other bony prominences; in Latin American patients, they tend to develop preferentially in the upper part of the body, particularly on the head, neck, and shoulders. Nodules vary in size and characteristically are firm and not tender. It has been estimated that, for every palpable nodule, there are four deeper nonpalpable ones.

Ocular Tissue Visual impairment is the most serious complication of onchocerciasis and usually affects only those persons with moderate or heavy infections. Lesions may develop in all parts of the eye. The most common early finding is conjunctivitis with photophobia. In the cornea, punctate keratitis—consisting of acute inflammatory reactions surrounding dying microfilariae manifested as "snowflake" opacities—is frequent in younger patients and resolves without apparent complications. Sclerosing keratitis occurs in 1 to 5% of infected persons and is the leading cause of onchocercal blindness in Africa. Anterior uveitis and iridocyclitis develop in ~5% of infected persons in Africa. In Latin America, complications of the anterior uveal tract (pupillary deformity) may cause secondary glaucoma. Characteristic chorioretinal lesions develop as a result of atrophy and hyperpigmentation of the retinal pigment epithelium. Constriction of the visual field and frank optic atrophy may occur.

Lymph Nodes Mild to moderate lymphadenopathy is frequent, particularly in the inguinal and femoral areas, where the enlarged nodes may hang down in response to gravity ("hanging groin"), sometimes predisposing to inguinal and femoral hernias.

Systemic Manifestations Some heavily infected individuals develop cachexia with loss of adipose tissue and muscle mass. Among adults who become blind, there is a three- to fourfold increase in the mortality rate.

DIAGNOSIS Definitive diagnosis depends on the detection of an adult worm in an excised nodule or, more commonly, of microfilariae in a skin snip. Skin snips are obtained with a corneal-scleral punch, which collects a blood-free skin biopsy sample extending to just below the epidermis, or by lifting of the skin with the tip of a needle and excision of a small (1- to 3-mm) piece with a sterile scalpel blade. The biopsy tissue is incubated in tissue culture medium or in saline on a glass slide or flat-bottomed microtiter plate. After incubation for 2 to 4 h (or occasionally overnight in light infections), microfilariae emergent from the skin can be visualized by low-power microscopy.

Eosinophilia and elevated serum IgE levels are common but, because they occur in many parasitic infections, are not diagnostic in themselves. Assays to detect specific antibodies to *Onchocerca* and PCR to detect onchocercal DNA in skin snips are now in use in specialized laboratories and are highly sensitive and specific.

The *Mazzotti test* is a provocative technique that can be used in cases where the diagnosis of onchocerciasis is still in doubt (i.e., when skin snips and ocular examination reveal no microfilariae). A small dose of DEC (0.5 to 1.0 mg/kg) is given orally; the development or exacerbation of pruritus or rash within hours is highly suggestive of onchocerciasis.

℞ **TREATMENT** The main goals of therapy are to prevent the development of irreversible lesions and to alleviate symptoms. Surgical excision is recommended when nodules are located on the head (because of the proximity of microfilaria-producing adult worms to the eye), but chemotherapy is the mainstay of management. Ivermectin, a semisynthetic macrocyclic lactone active against microfilariae, is the first-line agent for the treatment of onchocerciasis. It is given orally in a single dose of 150 μg/kg, either yearly or semiannually. After treatment, most individuals have few or no reactions. Pruritus, cutaneous edema, and/or maculopapular rash occurs in ~1 to 10% of treated individuals. In areas of Africa coendemic for *O. volvulus* and *L. loa*, however, ivermectin is contraindicated (as it is for pregnant or breastfeeding women) because of severe posttreatment encephalopathy seen in patients, especially children, who are heavily microfilaremic for *L. loa* (>2000 to 5000 microfilariae per milliliter). Although ivermectin treatment results in a marked drop in microfilarial density, its effect can be short-lived (<6 months in some cases). Thus, it is occasionally necessary to give ivermectin more frequently for persistent symptoms. No currently available agent kills adult *O. volvulus*.

PREVENTION Vector control has been beneficial in highly endemic areas in which breeding sites are vulnerable to insecticide spraying, but most areas endemic for onchocerciasis are not suited to this type of control. Community-based administration of ivermectin every 6 to 12 months is now being used to interrupt transmission in endemic areas. This measure, in conjunction with vector control, has already helped reduce the prevalence of disease in endemic foci in Africa and Latin America. No drug has proven useful for prophylaxis of *O. volvulus* infection.

LOIASIS

ETIOLOGY AND EPIDEMIOLOGY Loiasis is caused by *L. loa* (the African eye worm), which is present in the rain forests of West and Central Africa. Adult parasites (females, 50 to 70 mm long and 0.5 mm wide; males, 25 to 35 mm long and 0.25 mm wide) live in subcutaneous tissues; microfilariae circulate in the blood with a diurnal periodicity that peaks between 12:00 noon and 2:00 P.M.

CLINICAL FEATURES Manifestations of loiasis in natives of endemic areas may differ from those in temporary residents or visitors. Among the indigenous population, loiasis is often an asymptomatic infection with microfilaremia. Infection may be recognized only after subconjunctival migration of an adult worm or may be manifested by episodic Calabar swellings, evanescent localized areas of angioedema and erythema developing on the extremities and less frequently at other sites. Nephropathy, encephalopathy, and cardiomyopathy are rare. In patients who are not residents of endemic areas, allergic symptoms predominate, episodes of Calabar swelling tend to be more frequent and debilitating, microfilaremia is rare, and eosinophilia and increased levels of antifilarial antibodies are characteristic.

PATHOLOGY The pathogenesis of the manifestations of loiasis is poorly understood. Calabar swellings are thought to result from a hypersensitivity reaction to the adult worm.

DIAGNOSIS Definitive diagnosis of loiasis requires the detection of microfilariae in the peripheral blood or the isolation of the adult worm from the eye or from a subcutaneous biopsy specimen from a site of swelling developing after treatment. PCR-based assays for the detection of *L. loa* DNA in blood are now available in specialized laboratories and are highly sensitive and specific. In practice, the diagnosis must often be based on a characteristic history and clinical presentation, blood eosinophilia, and elevated levels of antifilarial antibodies, particularly in travelers to an endemic region, who are usually amicrofilaremic. Other clinical findings in the latter individuals include hypergammaglobulinemia, elevated levels of serum IgE, and elevated leukocyte and eosinophil counts.

℞ **TREATMENT** DEC (8 to 10 mg/kg per day for 21 days) is effective against both the adult and the microfilarial forms of *L. loa*, but multiple courses are frequently necessary before the disease resolves completely. In cases of heavy microfilaremia, allergic or other inflammatory reactions can take place during treatment, including central nervous system involvement with coma and encephalitis. Heavy infections can be treated initially with apheresis to remove the microfilariae and with glucocorticoids (40 to 60 mg of prednisone per day) followed by doses of DEC (0.5 mg/kg per day). If antifilarial treatment has no adverse effects, the prednisone dose can be rapidly tapered and the dose of DEC gradually increased to 8 to 10 mg/kg per day.

Albendazole and ivermectin (although not approved by the FDA) have been shown to be effective in reducing microfilarial loads. DEC (300 mg weekly) is an effective prophylactic regimen for loiasis.

STREPTOCERCIASIS

Mansonella streptocerca, found mainly in the tropical forest belt of Africa from Ghana to Zaire, is transmitted by biting midges. The major clinical manifestations involve the skin and include pruritus, papular rashes, and pigmentation changes. Many infected individuals have inguinal adenopathy, although most are asymptomatic. The diagnosis is made by detection of the characteristic microfilariae in skin snips. DEC (6 mg/kg per day in divided doses for 14 to 21 days) is effective in killing both microfilariae and adult worms. As in onchocerciasis, treatment is sometimes accompanied by urticaria, arthralgias, myalgias, headaches, and abdominal discomfort. Ivermectin at a single dose of 150 μg/kg leads to sustained suppression of microfilariae in the skin and is likely to assume primacy in the treatment of streptocerciasis.

MANSONELLA PERSTANS INFECTION

Mansonella perstans, distributed across the center of Africa and in northeastern South America, is transmitted by midges. Adult worms reside in serous cavities—pericardial, pleural, and peritoneal—as well as in the mesentery and the perirenal and retroperitoneal tissues. Microfilariae circulate in the blood without periodicity. The clinical and pathologic features of the infection are poorly defined. Most patients appear to be asymptomatic, but manifestations may include transient angioedema and pruritus of the arms, face, or other parts of the body (analogous to the Calabar swellings of loiasis); fever; headache; arthralgias; and right upper quadrant pain. Occasionally, pericarditis and hepatitis occur. The diagnosis is based on the demonstration of microfilariae in blood or serosal effusions. Perstans filariasis is often associated with peripheral blood eosinophilia and antifilarial antibody elevations. Although DEC (8 to 10 mg/kg per day for 21 days) is the standard therapeutic agent, there is little evidence that it is effective. Cure is indicated by the disappearance of symptoms and eosinophilia; multiple courses of therapy are usually required. Both mebendazole (100 mg twice daily for 30 days) and albendazole (400 mg twice daily for 10 days) have been reported to be effective.

MANSONELLA OZZARDI INFECTION

The distribution of *Mansonella ozzardi* is restricted to Central and South America and certain Caribbean islands. Adult worms are rarely recovered from humans. Microfilariae circulate in the blood without periodicity. Although this organism has often been considered nonpathogenic, headache, articular pain, fever, pulmonary symptoms, adenopathy, hepatomegaly, pruritus, and eosinophilia have been ascribed to *M. ozzardi* infection. Diagnosis is made by the detection of microfilariae in peripheral blood. Ivermectin (a single dose of 6 mg) has been shown to be effective in treating this infection.

DRACUNCULIASIS (GUINEA WORM INFECTION)

ETIOLOGY AND EPIDEMIOLOGY   Dracunculiasis, caused by *Dracunculus medinensis*, is a parasitic infection whose incidence has declined dramatically because of global eradication efforts. Current estimates suggest that there are only 78,000 cases worldwide, the majority in Sudan. Humans acquire this infection when they ingest water containing infective larvae derived from *Cyclops*, a crustacean that is the intermediate host. Larvae penetrate the stomach or intestinal wall, mate, and mature. The adult male probably dies; the female *Dracunculus* develops over a year and migrates to subcutaneous tissues, usually in the lower extremity. As the thin female *Dracunculus*, ranging in length from 300 cm to 1 m, approaches the skin, a blister forms that, over days, breaks down and forms an ulcer. When the blister opens, large numbers of motile, rhabditiform larvae can be released into stagnant water; ingestion by *Cyclops* completes the life cycle.

CLINICAL FEATURES   Few or no clinical manifestations of dracunculiasis are evident until just before the blister forms, when there is an onset of fever and generalized allergic symptoms, including periorbital edema, wheezing, and urticaria. The emergence of the worm is associated with local pain and swelling. When the blister ruptures (usually as a result of immersion in water), the adult worm releases larva-rich fluid, and this release is associated with a relief of symptoms. The shallow ulcer surrounding the emerging adult worm heals over weeks to months. Such ulcers, however, can become secondarily infected, the result being cellulitis, local inflammation, abscess formation, or (uncommonly) tetanus. Occasionally, the adult worm does not emerge but becomes encapsulated and calcified.

DIAGNOSIS   The diagnosis is based on the findings developing with the emergence of the adult worm, as described above.

℞ **TREATMENT**   Gradual extraction of the worm by winding of a few centimeters on a stick each day remains the common and effective practice. Worms may be excised surgically. The administration of thiabendazole (25 mg/kg twice daily for 3 days) or metronidazole (250 mg three times daily for 10 days) may relieve symptoms but has no proven activity against the worm.

PREVENTION   Prevention, which remains the only real control measure, depends on the provision of safe drinking water.

ZOONOTIC FILARIAL INFECTIONS

Dirofilariae that affect primarily dogs, cats, and raccoons and *Brugia* parasites that affect small mammals occasionally infect humans incidentally. Because humans are an abnormal host, the parasites never develop fully. Pulmonary dirofilarial infection caused by the canine heartworm *Dirofilaria immitis* generally presents in humans as a solitary pulmonary nodule. Chest pain, hemoptysis, and cough are uncommon. Infections with *D. repens* (from dogs) or *D. tenuis* (from raccoons) can cause local subcutaneous nodules in humans. Zoonotic *Brugia* infection can produce isolated lymph node enlargement. Eosinophilia levels and antifilarial antibody titers are not commonly elevated. Excisional biopsy is both diagnostic and curative; these infections usually do not respond to chemotherapy.

BIBLIOGRAPHY

ADDISS DA, DREYER G: Treatment of lymphatic filariasis, in *Lymphatic Filariasis*, TB Nutman (ed). London, Imperial College Press, 1999, pp 151–199

BURNHAM GJ: Onchocerciasis. Lancet 351:1341, 1998

DREYER G et al: Acute attacks in the extremities of persons living in an area endemic for bancroftian filariasis: Differentiation of two syndromes. Trans R Soc Trop Med Hyg 93:413, 1999

FREEDMAN DO et al: Lymphoscintigraphic analysis of lymphatic abnormalities in symptomatic and asymptomatic human filariasis. J Infect Dis 170:927, 1994

GARDON J et al: Serious reactions after mass treatment of onchocerciasis with ivermectin in an area endemic for *Loa loa* infection. Lancet 350:18, 1997

HOPKINS DR: Perspectives from the dracunculiasis eradication programme. Bull World Health Organ 76(Suppl 2):38, 1998

KLION AD et al: Loiasis in endemic and non-endemic populations: Immunologically mediated differences in clinical presentation. J Infect Dis 163:1318, 1991

MCCARTHY JS: Diagnosis of lymphatic filarial infections, in *Lymphatic Filariasis*, TB Nutman (ed). London, Imperial College Press, 1999, pp 127–149

NOROES J et al: Occurrence of living adult *Wuchereria bancrofti* in the scrotal area of men with microfilaraemia. Trans R Soc Trop Med Hyg 90:55, 1996

ORIHEL TC, EBERHARD ML: Zoonotic filariasis. Clin Microbiol Rev 11:366, 1998

OTTESEN EA et al: The role of albendazole in programmes to eliminate lymphatic filariasis. Parasitol Today 15:382, 1999

WHO EXPERT COMMITTEE ON ONCHOCERCIASIS: Onchocerciasis and its control: Fourth report. Technical Report Series No. 852, Geneva, WHO, 1995

222   Adel A.F. Mahmoud

SCHISTOSOMIASIS AND OTHER TREMATODE INFECTIONS

Trematodes, or flatworms, are a group of morphologically and biologically heterogeneous parasitic helminths that belong to the phylum Platyhelminthes. Human infection with trematodes occurs in many geographic areas and can cause considerable morbidity and mortality. For clinical purposes, the significant trematode infections of humans may be divided according to the tissues invaded by adult flukes: blood, biliary tree, intestines, and lungs (Table 222-1).

Trematodes share some common morphologic features, including macroscopic size (from 1 cm to several cm); dorsoventral, flattened, bilaterally symmetric bodies (adult worms); and the prominence of two suckers. Except for the schistosomes, all trematodes that parasitize humans are hermaphroditic. The life cycle of trematodes involves a definitive host (mammalian/human), in which adult worms initiate sexual reproduction, and an intermediate host (snails, fish, etc.), in which asexual multiplication of the larval forms occurs. More than one intermediate host may be necessary for some species of trematodes. Human infection is initiated either by direct penetration of intact skin or by ingestion. Upon maturation within the human host, adult flukes initiate sexual reproduction that results in egg production. Helminth ova leave the definitive host in excreta or sputum and, upon reaching suitable environmental conditions, they hatch, releasing free-living miracidia that must find a specific snail intermediate host. After asexual reproduction, cercariae are released from infected snails; these organisms either infect humans (schistosomes) or must find another intermediate host to allow encystment into metacercariae.

The host-parasite relationship in trematode infections is a product of the biologic features of these organisms: they are multicellular, undergo several developmental changes within the host, and usually result in chronic infections. In general, the distribution of worm infections in human populations is overdispersed; i.e., it follows a negative binomial mathematical relationship in which most infected individuals harbor low worm burdens while a small percentage are heavily infected. It is the heavily infected minority who are particularly prone to disease sequelae and who represent an epidemiologically significant

Table 222-1 Major Human Trematode Infections

Trematode	Transmission	Endemic Area(s)
BLOOD FLUKES		
Shistosoma mansoni	Skin penetration by cercariae	Africa, South America, Middle East
S. japonicum	Skin penetration by cercariae	China, Philippines, Indonesia
S. intercalatum	Skin penetration by cercariae	West Africa
S. mekongi	Skin penetration by cercariae	Southeast Asia
S. haematobium	Skin penetration by cercariae	Africa, Middle East
BILIARY (HEPATIC) FLUKES		
Clonorchis sinensis	Ingestion of metacercariae in freshwater fish	Far East
Opisthorchis viverrini	Ingestion of metacercariae in freshwater fish	Far East, Thailand
O. felineus	Ingestion of metacercariae in freshwater fish	Far East, Europe
Fasciola hepatica	Ingestion of metacercariae on aquatic plants or in water	Worldwide
F. gigantica	Ingestion of metacercariae on aquatic plants or in water	Sporadic, Africa
INTESTINAL FLUKES		
Fasciolopsis buski	Ingestion of metacercariae on aquatic plants	Southeast Asia
Heterophyes heterophyes	Ingestion of metacercariae in freshwater or brackish-water fish	Far East, North Africa
LUNG FLUKES		
Paragonimus westermani	Ingestion of metacercariae in crayfish or crabs	Global except North America and Europe

reservoir of infection in endemic areas. It is important to appreciate that worms do not multiply within the definitive host and that they have a relatively long life span, ranging from a few months to a few years. Morbidity and mortality due to trematode infections reflect a multifactorial process that results from the tipping of a delicate balance based on the intensity of infection and the host reactions that initiate and modulate pathologic outcome. The genetics of the parasite and the human host contribute to the outcome of infection and disease. Furthermore, infections with trematodes that migrate through or reside in host tissues are associated with a moderate to high degree of peripheral blood eosinophilia; this association is of significance in protective and immunopathologic sequelae and is a useful clinical indicator of infection.

Approach to the Patient

The approach to individuals with suspected trematode infection begins with the question: Where have you been? Details of geographic history, exposure to freshwater bodies, and indulgence in local eating habits without ensuring safety of food and drink are all essential elements in the history. The workup plan must include a detailed physical examination and tests appropriate for the suspected infection. Diagnosis is based either on detection of the relevant stage of the parasite in excreta, sputum, or (rarely) tissue samples or on sensitive and specific serologic tests. Consultation with physicians familiar with these infections or with the U.S. Centers for Disease Control and Prevention (CDC) is helpful in guiding diagnosis and selecting therapy.

BLOOD FLUKES: SCHISTOSOMIASIS

Human schistosomiasis is caused by five species of this parasitic trematode belonging to the subclass Digenea: the intestinal species *Schistosoma mansoni*, *S. japonicum*, *S. mekongi*, and *S. intercalatum* and the urinary species *S. haematobium*. Infection may cause considerable morbidity in the intestines, liver, and urinary tract, and a proportion of affected individuals die. Other schistosome species (e.g., avian species) may invade human skin but then die in subcutaneous tissue, producing only self-limiting cutaneous manifestations.

Information on the prevalence and geographic distribution of human schistosomiasis is inexact. The five species are estimated to infect 200 to 300 million people in South America, the Caribbean, Africa, the Middle East, and Southeast Asia. The total population living under conditions favoring transmission approximates double or triple that number—a fact reflecting the public health significance of schistosomiasis.

ETIOLOGY Human infection is initiated by penetration of intact skin with infective cercariae. These organisms are released from infected snails in freshwater bodies; they measure ~2 mm in length and possess an anterior and a ventral sucker that attaches to the skin surface and facilitates penetration. Once in the subcutaneous tissue, the organism transforms into the next stage: the schistosomula. This transformation involves morphologic, membrane, and immunologic changes, prominent among which is the transformation of the cercarial outer membrane from a trilaminar to a heptalaminar structure that is then maintained throughout the life span of the worms in humans. The transformation to a heptalaminar structure is thought to be the schistosome's main adaptive mechanism for survival in humans. Schistosomula begin their migration within 2 to 4 days via venous or lymphatic vessels, reaching the lungs and finally the liver parenchyma. Sexually mature worms descend in pairs into the venous system at specific anatomic locations: intestinal veins (*S. mansoni*, *S. japonicum*, *S. mekongi*, and *S. intercalatum*) and vesical veins (*S. haematobium*). Adult gravid females then travel against venous blood flow to small tributaries, where they deposit their ova intravascularly. Schistosome ova have specific morphologic features that can be used to differentiate species. Aided by enzymatic secretions through minipores in eggshells, ova move through the venous wall, traversing host tissues to reach the lumen of the intestinal or urinary tract, and are voided with stools or urine. Approximately 50% of ova, however, fail in their attempt to be transported to the outside environment and are either retained in host tissues locally (intestines or urinary tract) or carried by venous blood flow to the liver and other organs. Schistosome ova that reach freshwater bodies hatch, releasing free-living miracidia that seek the snail intermediate host to undergo several asexual multiplication cycles. Finally, infective cercariae are shed from snails.

Adult schistosome worms measure ~1 to 2 cm in length. The male is slightly shorter, with a flattened body; its edges curve anteriorly to form the gynecophoral canal, in which mature adult females are usually held. The females are longer, slender, and rounded in cross-section. The precise nature of biochemical and reproductive exchanges between the two sexes is unknown, as are the regulatory mechanisms for pairing. Adult schistosomes parasitize specific sites in the host venous system. What guides adult intestinal schistosomes to branches of the superior or inferior mesenteric veins or adult *S. haematobium* worms to the vesical plexus is unknown. In addition, the evasion mechanisms by which adult worms inhibit the coagulation cascade and the effector arms of the host immune responses are not fully understood.

A systematic examination of schistosomal molecular phylogeny as well as gene structure and organization has begun. Analysis of the sequence of nuclear ribosome and internal transcribed spacer 2 and mitochondrial 16 sRNA indicates that human schistosomes may be divided into three monophyletic groups: the *S. haematobium* group, including *S. haematobium* and *S. intercalatum*; the *S. mansoni* group, including *S. mansoni* and *S. rodhaini*; and a group containing the two Asian schistosomes, *S. japonicum* and *S. mekongi*. These molecular groupings coincide with results of previous attempts to use morphologic or nucleic acid data to produce a taxonomic framework. In other studies, the schistosome genome was determined to be made up of 16 chromosomes; sexual differentiation is related to the presence of ZW chromosomes in females and ZZ chromosomes in males.

EPIDEMIOLOGY The distribution of schistosome infection and related disease syndromes in human populations is dependent on both parasite and host factors. In endemic areas, the rate of yearly onset of new infection, or incidence, is low. Prevalence, on the other hand, starts to be appreciable by the age of 3 to 4 years and builds to a maximum that varies by endemic region (up to 100%) in the 15- to 20-year age group. Prevalence then stabilizes or decreases slightly in older age groups (>40 years). Intensity of infection (as measured by fecal or urinary egg counts, which correlate with adult worm burdens in most circumstances) follows the increase in prevalence up to the age of 15 to 20 years and then declines markedly in older age groups. This decline may reflect acquisition of resistance, or it may be due to changes in water contact patterns, since older people are exposed less. Furthermore, the unique distribution of schistosomes in human populations, which fits a negative binomial pattern (see above), may be due to heterogeneity of worm populations, with some more invasive than others; alternatively, it may be due to differences in the genetic susceptibility of host populations.

Disease due to schistosomiasis is the outcome of parasitologic, host, and additional infectious, nutritional, and environmental factors. Most of the disease syndromes relate to the presence of one or more of the parasite stages in the human host. The distribution of disease manifestations in the populations of endemic areas correlates with the intensity and duration of infection as well as with the age and genetic susceptibility of the host. Overall, disease manifestations are clinically relevant in only a small proportion of persons infected with any of the intestinal schistosomes. In contrast, urinary schistosomiasis manifests clinically in most infected individuals.

Patients with both HIV infection and schistosomiasis have been found to excrete far fewer eggs in their stools than those infected with *S. mansoni* alone. The two groups have responded equally to treatment with praziquantel.

PATHOGENESIS AND IMMUNITY During the invasive stage, cercaria-associated dermatitis reflects dermal and subdermal inflammatory responses—both humoral and cell-mediated. As the parasites approach sexual maturity and the commencement of oviposition, acute schistosomiasis or Katayama fever (a serum sickness–like illness; see "Clinical Features," below) may occur. The associated antigen excess results in the formation of soluble immune complexes, which may be deposited in several tissues, initiating the sequence of pathologic events. In chronic schistosomiasis, most disease manifestations are due to eggs retained in host tissue. The granulomatous response around these ova is cell-mediated and is regulated both positively and negatively by a cascade of cytokine, cellular, and humoral responses. Granuloma formation begins with recruitment of a host of inflammatory cells in response to antigens secreted by the living organism within the ova. Cells recruited initially include phagocytes, antigen-specific T cells, and eosinophils. Fibroblasts, giant cells, and B lymphocytes predominate later. Once activated, T cells produce cytokines [such as tumor necrosis factor α (TNF-α), interleukin (IL) 2, IL-4, and IL-5, which in turn activate endothelial cells] and produce specific chemokines such as monocyte chemotactic protein 1 (MCP-1). The result is recruitment of the cellular elements that organize in the form of granulomas around parasite eggs. These lesions reach a size many times that of the eggs, thus inducing organomegaly and obstruction. Immunomodulation or downregulation of host responses to schistosome eggs plays a significant role in limiting the extent of the granulomatous lesions—and consequently disease—in chronically infected experimental animals or humans. The underlying mechanisms involve another cascade of regulatory cytokines (IL-10, IL-12) and idiotypic antibodies. Subsequent to the granulomatous response, fibrosis sets in, resulting in more permanent disease sequelae. Because schistosomiasis is a chronic infection, the accumulation of antigen-antibody complexes results in deposits in renal glomeruli and may cause significant kidney disease.

The better-studied pathologic sequelae in schistosomiasis are those observed in liver disease. Ova that are carried by portal blood embolize to the liver. Because of their size (~150 × 60 μm in the case of *S. mansoni*), they lodge at presinusoidal sites, where granulomas are formed. The granulomas contribute to the liver enlargement observed in infected individuals. Schistosomal hepatomegaly is also associated with certain class I and class II HLA markers; its genetic basis appears to be multigenic. Presinusoidal portal blockage causes several hemodynamic changes, including portal hypertension and associated development of portosystemic collaterals at the esophagogastric junction and other sites. Esophageal varices are most likely to break and cause repeated episodes of hematemesis. Because changes in liver hemodynamics in schistosomiasis are slow, compensatory arterialization of blood flow through the liver is established. While this compensatory mechanism may be associated with certain metabolic side effects, the retention of hepatocyte perfusion may permit the maintenance of normal liver function for several years.

After granuloma formation, the second most significant pathologic change in the liver relates to the onset of fibrosis. It is characteristically periportal (Symmers' clay-pipe stem fibrosis) but may be diffuse. Fibrosis, when diffuse, may be seen in areas of egg deposition and granuloma formation, but it is also seen in distant locations such as portal tracts. Schistosomiasis alone results in pure fibrotic lesions in the liver; cirrhosis occurs when other nutritional or infectious agents (e.g., hepatitis B or C virus) are involved. In recent years, it has been recognized that deposition of fibrotic tissue in the extracellular matrix results from the interaction of T lymphocytes with cells of the fibroblast series; several cytokines, such as IL-2, IL-4, IL-1, and transforming growth factor β (TGF-β), are known to stimulate fibrogenesis. The process may be dependent on the genetic constitution of the host. Furthermore, regulatory cytokines that can suppress fibrogenesis, such as interferon γ (IFN-γ) or IL-12, may play a role in modulating the response.

While the above description focuses on granuloma formation and fibrosis of the liver, similar processes occur in urinary schistosomiasis. Granuloma formation at the lower end of the ureters obstructs urinary flow, with subsequent development of hydroureter and hydronephrosis. Similar lesions in the urinary bladder cause the protrusion of papillomatous structures into its cavity; these may ulcerate and/or bleed. The chronic stage of infection is associated with scarring and deposition of calcium in the bladder wall.

Immunomodulation is an essential mechanism in shaping the clinical and pathologic outcome of schistosomiasis. While most detailed immunologic analyses have been performed in experimental animals, enough evidence exists from studies in humans to delineate the suppression of T cell responses in association with active infections and a regulatory role for IL-10.

Studies on immunity to schistosomiasis, whether innate or acquired, have expanded our knowledge of the components of these responses and the target antigens. The concept of innate immunity is illustrated by the inability of avian schistosomes, which cause swimmers' itch, to reach maturity in humans. The critical question, however, is whether humans acquire immunity to schistosomes. Epidemiologic evidence suggests the onset of acquired immunity during the course of infection in young adults. Curative treatment of infection divides populations in endemic areas into those who acquire reinfection rapidly (susceptible) and those who follow a protracted course (resistant). This difference may be explained by differences in transmission, immunologic response, or genetic susceptibility. The mechanism of acquired immunity involves antibodies, complement, and several effector cells, particularly eosinophils. Furthermore, the intensity of schistosome infection has been correlated with a region in chromosome 5. In other studies, several protective schistosome antigens have been identified as vaccine candidates.

CLINICAL FEATURES In general, disease manifestations of schistosomiasis occur in three stages, which vary not only by species but also by intensity of infection and other host factors, such as age and genetics. During the phase of cercarial invasion, a form of dermatitis may be observed. This so-called swimmers' itch occurs most often with *S. mansoni* and *S. japonicum* infections, manifesting 2 or

3 days after invasion as an itchy maculopapular rash on the affected areas of the skin. The condition is particularly severe when humans are exposed to avian schistosomes. This form of cercarial dermatitis is seen around the freshwater lakes in the northern United States, particularly in the spring. Cercarial dermatitis is a self-limiting clinical entity. During worm maturation and at the beginning of oviposition (i.e., 4 to 8 weeks after skin invasion), acute schistosomiasis or Katayama fever—a serum sickness–like syndrome with fever, generalized lymphadenopathy, and hepatosplenomegaly—may develop. Individuals suffering from acute schistosomiasis show a high degree of peripheral blood eosinophilia. Parasite-specific antibodies may be detected before schistosome eggs are identified in excreta. Acute schistosomiasis has become an important clinical entity worldwide because of increased travel to endemic areas. Travelers are exposed to the parasite while swimming or wading in freshwater bodies and upon their return present with the acute manifestations of the disease. The course of acute schistosomiasis is generally benign, but deaths are occasionally reported in association with heavy exposure to schistosomes.

The main clinical manifestations of chronic schistosomiasis are species-dependent. Intestinal species (*S. mansoni*, *S. japonicum*, *S. mekongi*, and *S. intercalatum*) cause intestinal and hepatosplenic disease as well as several manifestations associated with portal hypertension. During the intestinal phase, which may begin a few months after infection and may last for years, symptomatic patients characteristically have colicky abdominal pain and bloody diarrhea. Patients may also report fatigue and an inability to perform daily routine functions and may show evidence of growth retardation. The severity of intestinal schistosomiasis is often related to the intensity of the worm burden. The disease runs a chronic course but rarely progresses to a functional level (e.g., malabsorption) or to anatomic lesions of the gut. The exception is colonic polyposis, which has been seen in some endemic areas, such as Egypt.

The hepatosplenic phase of disease manifests early (during the first year of infection, particularly in children) with enlargement of the liver due to parasite-induced granulomatous lesions. Hepatomegaly is seen in ~15 to 20% of infected individuals when whole communities in endemic areas are studied. It correlates roughly with the intensity of infection, occurs more often in children than in adults, and may be related to specific HLA haplotypes. In subsequent phases of infection, presinusoidal blockage of blood flow leads to portal hypertension and splenomegaly. Moreover, portal hypertension may lead to varices at the lower end of the esophagus and at other sites. Patients with schistosomal liver disease may have right-upper-quadrant "dragging" pain during the hepatomegaly phase, and this pain may move to the left upper quadrant as splenomegaly progresses. Bleeding from esophageal varices may, however, be the first clinical manifestation of this phase. Patients may experience repeated bleeding but seem to tolerate its impact, since an adequate total hepatic blood flow permits normal liver function for a considerable period in schistosomal hepatomegaly. In late-stage disease, typical fibrotic changes occur along with liver function deterioration and the onset of ascites, hypoalbuminemia, and defects in coagulation. Intercurrent viral infections of the liver or nutritional deficiencies may well accelerate or exacerbate the deterioration of hepatic function.

The extent and severity of intestinal and hepatic disease in schistosomiasis mansoni and japonica have been well described. While it was originally thought that *S. japonicum* might induce more severe disease manifestations because the adult worms can produce ten times more eggs than *S. mansoni*, subsequent field studies have not supported this claim. Clinical observations of individuals infected with *S. mekongi* or *S. intercalatum* have been less detailed, partly because of the far more limited geographic distribution of these organisms.

The clinical manifestations of *S. haematobium* infection occur relatively early and involve a relatively high percentage of individuals. Up to 80% of children infected with *S. haematobium* have dysuria, frequency, and hematuria, which may be terminal. Urine examination reveals blood and albumin as well as an unusually high frequency of bacterial urinary tract infection. These manifestations correlate with intense infection, the presence of urinary bladder granulomas, and subsequent ulceration. Along with the local effects of granuloma formation in the urinary bladder, obstruction of the lower end of the ureters results in hydroureter and hydronephrosis, which can be seen in 25 to 50% of infected children. As infection progresses, bladder granulomas undergo fibrosis; the result is the presence of typical sandy patches visible on cystoscopy. In many endemic areas, an association between squamous cell carcinoma of the bladder and *S. haematobium* infection has been observed. Such malignancy is detected in a younger age group than transitional cell carcinoma. In fact, *S. haematobium* has now been classified as a human carcinogen.

Significant disease may occur in other organs during chronic schistosomiasis. Most important is disease in the lungs and central nervous system; other locations, such as the skin and the genital organs, are far less frequently affected. In pulmonary schistosomiasis, embolized eggs lodge in small arterioles, producing acute necrotizing arteriolitis and granuloma formation. During *S. mansoni* and *S. japonicum* infection, schistosome eggs reach the lungs after the development of portosystemic collateral circulation; in *S. haematobium* infection, ova may reach the lungs directly via connections between the vesical and systemic circulation. After the development of arteriolitis and granuloma formation, fibrous tissue deposition is detected and leads to endarteritis obliterans, pulmonary hypertension, and cor pulmonale. This clinical entity is an uncommon presentation during chronic schistosomiasis. The most frequent symptoms are cough, fever, and dyspnea; ascites and hemoptysis are less frequently encountered. Cor pulmonale may be diagnosed radiologically on the basis of prominent right side of the heart and dilation of the pulmonary artery. Frank evidence of right-sided heart failure may be seen in late cases.

Central nervous system schistosomiasis is important but less frequent than pulmonary schistosomiasis. It characteristically occurs as cerebral disease due to *S. japonicum* infection. Migratory worms deposit eggs in the brain and induce a granulomatous response. The frequency of this manifestation among infected individuals in some endemic areas (e.g., the Philippines) is calculated at 2 to 4%. Jacksonian epilepsy due to *S. japonicum* infection is the second most common cause of epilepsy in these areas. *S. mansoni* and *S. haematobium* infections have been associated with transverse myelitis. This syndrome is thought to be due to eggs traveling to the venous plexus around the spinal cord. In schistosomiasis mansoni, transverse myelitis is usually seen in the chronic stage after the development of portal hypertension and portosystemic shunts, which allow ova to travel to the spinal cord veins. This proposed sequence of events has been challenged because of a few reports of transverse myelitis occurring early in the course of *S. mansoni* infection. More information is needed to confirm these observations. During schistosomiasis haematobia, ova may travel through communication between vesical and systemic veins, resulting in spinal cord disease that may be detected at any stage of infection. Pathologic study of lesions in schistosomal transverse myelitis may reveal eggs along with necrotic or granulomatous lesions. Patients usually present with acute or rapidly progressing lower-leg weakness accompanied by sphincter dysfunction.

DIAGNOSIS Physicians in areas not endemic for schistosomiasis face considerable diagnostic challenges. In the most common clinical presentation, a returning traveler exhibits symptoms and signs of any of the acute syndromes of schistosomiasis—namely, cercarial dermatitis or Katayama fever. Central to correct diagnosis is a thorough inquiry into travel history and exposure to freshwater bodies, whether slow or fast running. Differential diagnosis of fever in returned travelers includes a spectrum of infections whose etiologies are viral (e.g., Dengue fever), bacterial (e.g., enteric fever, leptospirosis), rickettsial, or protozoal (e.g., malaria). In cases of Katayama fever, prompt diagnosis is essential and is based on clinical presentation, high-level peripheral blood eosinophilia, and a positive serologic assay for schistosomal antibodies. Two tests are available at the CDC: the Falcon assay screening test/enzyme-linked immunosorbent assay (FAST-

ELISA) and the confirmatory enzyme-linked immunoelectrotransfer blot (EITB). Both tests are highly sensitive and ~96% specific. In some instances, examination of stool or urine for ova may yield positive results.

Individuals with established infection are diagnosed by a combination of geographic history, characteristic clinical presentation, and presence of schistosome ova in excreta. The diagnosis may also be established with the serologic assays mentioned above or with those that detect circulating schistosome antigens. These assays can be applied either to blood or to other body fluids (e.g., cerebrospinal fluid). For stool examination, the Kato thick smear or any other concentration method generally identifies all but the most lightly infected individuals. Urine may be examined by microscopy of sediment or by filtration of a known volume through Nuclepore filters. Kato thick smear and Nuclepore filtration provide quantitative data on the intensity of infection, which is of value in assessing the degree of tissue damage and in monitoring the effect of chemotherapy. Finally, schistosome infection may be diagnosed by examination of tissue samples, typically rectal biopsies; other biopsy procedures (e.g., liver biopsy) are not needed, except in special circumstances.

Differential diagnosis of schistosomal hepatomegaly must include viral hepatitis of all etiologies, miliary tuberculosis, malaria, visceral leishmaniasis, ethanol abuse, and causes of hepatic and portal vein obstruction. Of patients with these conditions, only a few may present with organomegaly and relatively intact liver function. The differential diagnosis of hematuria in *S. haematobium* infection includes bacterial cystitis, tuberculosis, urinary stones, and malignancy.

℞ **TREATMENT**   Treatment of schistosomiasis depends on the stage of infection and the clinical presentation. Other than topical dermatologic applications for relief of itching, no specific treatment is indicated for cercarial dermatitis caused by avian schistosomes. Therapy for acute schistosomiasis or Katayama fever needs to be adjusted appropriately for each case. While antischistosomal chemotherapy is indicated, it does not address immediate pathologic changes. In severe acute schistosomiasis, management in an acute-care setting is necessary, with supportive measures and consideration of glucocorticoid treatment. Once the acute critical phase is over, specific chemotherapy is indicated. For all individuals with infection established by either the demonstration of schistosome eggs or positive serology, treatment to eradicate the parasite should be administered. The drug of choice is praziquantel, which—depending on the infecting species (Table 222-2)—is administered orally as 40 or 60 mg/kg in two or three doses over a single day. Praziquantel treatment results in parasitologic cure in ~85% of cases and reduces egg counts by >90%. Few side effects

Table 222-2   Drug Therapy for Human Trematode Infections

Infection	Drug of Choice	Adult Dose and Duration
BLOOD FLUKES		
S. mansoni, S. intercalatum, S. haematobium	Praziquantel	20 mg/kg, 2 doses in 1 day
S. japonicum, S. mekongi	Praziquantel	20 mg/kg, 3 doses in 1 day
BILIARY FLUKES		
C. sinensis, O. viverrini, O. felineus	Praziquantel	25 mg/kg, 3 doses in 1 day
F. hepatica, F. gigantica	Triclabendazole	10 mg/kg once
INTESTINAL FLUKES		
F. buski, H. heterophyes	Praziquantel	25 mg/kg, 3 doses in 1 day
LUNG FLUKES		
P. westermani	Praziquantel	25 mg/kg, 3 doses per day for 2 days

have been encountered, and those that do develop usually do not interfere with completion of treatment. Other antischistosomal chemotherapeutic agents are currently considered only as alternatives when praziquantel is unavailable. The effect of antischistosomal treatment on disease manifestations varies by stage. Early hepatomegaly and bladder lesions are known to resolve following chemotherapy, but the late established manifestations, such as fibrosis, do not change. Additional management modalities are needed for individuals with other manifestations, such as hepatocellular failure or recurrent hematemesis. The use of these interventions is guided by general medical and surgical principles.

PREVENTION AND CONTROL   Since transmission of schistosomiasis is dependent on human behavior, it is theoretically possible to devise an effective preventive strategy. The geographic distribution of infections in endemic regions of the world is not clearly demarcated. It is therefore prudent for travelers to avoid contact with all freshwater bodies, irrespective of the speed of water flow or unsubstantiated claims of safety. Some topical agents, when applied to the skin, may conceivably inhibit cercarial penetration, but none of these agents is currently available. If exposure occurs, a follow-up visit with a health care provider is strongly recommended. Prevention of infection in inhabitants of endemic areas is a significant challenge. People of these regions use freshwater bodies for sanitary, domestic, recreational, and agricultural purposes. In the absence of adequate alternatives, several control measures have been used, including application of molluscicides, provision of sanitary water and means for sewage disposal, chemotherapy, and health education. Current recommendations to countries endemic for schistosomiasis emphasize the use of multiple approaches. Particularly with the advent of a single-oral-dose, safe, and effective antischistosomal agent, chemotherapy has been most successful in reducing the intensity of infection and reversing disease. The duration of this positive impact depends on transmission dynamics in a specific endemic region. The ultimate goal of research on prevention and control is the development of a vaccine. Although there are a few promising leads, this goal is probably not within reach during the next decade or so.

LIVER (BILIARY) FLUKES

Several species of biliary fluke infecting humans are particularly common in Southeast Asia and Russia. Other species are transmitted in Europe, Africa, and the Americas. On the basis of their migratory pathway in humans, these infections may be divided into the *Clonorchis* and *Fasciola* groups.

CLONORCHIASIS AND OPISTHORCHIASIS   Infection with *C. sinensis*, the Chinese or oriental fluke, is endemic among fish-eating mammals in Southeast Asia. Humans are an incidental host; the prevalence of human infection is highest in China, Vietnam, and Korea. Infection with *Opisthorchis viverrini* and *O. felineus* is zoonotic in cats and dogs. Transmission to humans occurs occasionally, particularly in Thailand (*O. viverrini*) and in Southeast Asia and eastern Europe (*O. felineus*). Data on the exact geographic distribution of these infectious agents in human populations are rudimentary.

Infection with any of these three species is established by ingestion of raw or inadequately cooked freshwater fish harboring metacercariae. These organisms excyst in the duodenum, releasing larvae that travel through the ampulla of Vater and mature into adult worms in the bile canaliculi. Mature flukes are flat and elongated, measuring 1 to 2 cm in length. The hermaphroditic worms reproduce by releasing small operculated eggs, which pass with bile into the intestines and are voided with stools. The life cycle is completed in the environment in specific freshwater snails (the first intermediate host) and encystment of metacercariae in freshwater fish.

Except for late sequelae, the exact clinical syndromes caused by clonorchiasis and opisthorchiasis are not well defined. Since most infected individuals harbor a low worm burden, many are asymptomatic. Moderate to heavy infection may be associated with vague right-upper-quadrant pain. In contrast, chronic or repeated infection is associated with manifestations such as cholangitis, cholangiohepatitis, and biliary obstruction. Cholangiocarcinoma is epidemiologically related to *C. sinensis* infection in China and to *O. viverrini* infection in northeastern Thailand. This association has resulted in the classification of these infectious agents as human carcinogens.

FASCIOLIASIS   Infections with *F. hepatica* and *F. gigantica* are worldwide zoonoses that are particularly endemic in sheep-raising countries. Human cases have been reported in South America, Europe, Africa, Australia, and the Far East. Recent estimates indicate a worldwide prevalence of 17 million cases. High endemicity has been reported in certain areas of Peru and Bolivia. In most endemic areas the predominant species is *F. hepatica*, but in Asia and Africa a varying degree of overlap with *F. gigantica* has been observed.

Humans acquire fascioliasis by ingestion of metacercariae attached to certain aquatic plants, such as watercress. Infection may also be acquired by consumption of contaminated water or ingestion of food items washed with such water. Acquisition of human infection through consumption of freshly prepared raw liver containing immature flukes has been reported. Infection is initiated when metacercariae excyst, penetrate the gut wall, and travel through the peritoneal cavity to invade the liver capsule. Adult worms finally reach the bile ducts, where they produce large operculated eggs, which are voided in the bile and through the gastrointestinal tract to the outside environment. The flukes' life cycle is completed in specific snails (the first intermediate host) and encystment on aquatic plants.

The clinical features of fascioliasis relate to the intensity of infection, but even more to the stage of infection. Acute disease develops during the parasites' migration (1 to 2 weeks after infection) and includes fever, right-upper-quadrant pain, hepatomegaly, and eosinophilia. Computed tomography of the liver may show migratory tracks. Symptoms and signs usually subside as the parasites reach their final habitat. In individuals with chronic infection, bile duct obstruction and biliary cirrhosis are infrequently demonstrated. No relation to hepatic malignancy has been ascribed to fascioliasis.

DIAGNOSIS   The diagnosis of infection with any of the biliary flukes depends on a high degree of suspicion, the elicitation of an appropriate geographic history, and stool examination for the characteristically shaped parasite ova. Additional evidence may be obtained by documenting peripheral blood eosinophilia or imaging the liver. Serologic testing is helpful, particularly in lightly infected individuals.

℞ **TREATMENT**   Drug therapy (praziquantel or triclabendazole) is summarized in Table 222-2. Patients with anatomic lesions in the biliary tract or malignancy are managed according to general medical guidelines.

INTESTINAL FLUKES

Two species of intestinal flukes cause human infection in defined geographic areas worldwide. The large *Fasciolopsis buski* (adults measure 2 by 7 cm) is endemic in Southeast Asia, while the smaller *Heterophyes heterophyes* is found in the Nile Delta of Egypt and in the Far East. Infection is initiated by ingestion of metacercariae attached to aquatic plants (*F. buski*) or encysted in freshwater or brackish-water fish (*H. heterophyes*). Flukes mature in human intestines, and eggs are passed with stools. Most individuals infected with intestinal flukes are asymptomatic. In heavy *F. buski* infection, diarrhea, abdominal pain, and malabsorption may be encountered. Heavy infection with *H. heterophyes* may be associated with abdominal pain and mucous diarrhea. The diagnosis is established by detection of the characteristically shaped ova in stool samples. The drug of choice for treatment is praziquantel (Table 222-2).

LUNG FLUKES

Infection with the lung fluke *Paragonimus westermani* and related species (e.g., *P. africanus*) is endemic in many parts of the world, excluding North America and Europe. Endemicity is particularly noticeable in West Africa, Central and South America, and Asia. In nature, the reservoir hosts of *P. westermani* are wild and domestic felines. In Africa, *P. africanus* has been found in other species, such as dogs. Adult lung flukes, which are 7 to 12 mm in length, are found encapsulated in the lungs of infected persons. In rare circumstances, flukes are found encysted in the central nervous system (cerebral paragonimiasis) or abdominal cavity. Humans acquire lung fluke infection by ingesting infective metacercariae encysted in the muscles and viscera of crayfish and freshwater crabs. In endemic areas, these crustaceans are consumed either raw or pickled. Once the organisms reach the duodenum, they excyst, penetrate the gut wall, and travel through the peritoneal cavity, diaphragm, and pleural space to reach the lungs. Mature flukes are found in the bronchioles surrounded by cystic lesions. Parasite eggs are either expectorated with sputum or swallowed and passed to the outside environment with feces. The life cycle is completed in snails and freshwater crustacea.

When maturing flukes lodge in lung tissues, they cause hemorrhage and necrosis, resulting in cyst formation. The adjacent lung parenchyma shows evidence of inflammatory infiltration, predominantly by eosinophils. Cysts usually measure 1 to 2 cm in diameter and may contain 1 or 2 worms each. With the onset of oviposition, cysts usually rupture in adjacent bronchioles—an event allowing ova to exit from the human host. Older cysts develop thickened walls, which may undergo calcification. During the active phase of paragonimiasis, lung tissues surrounding parasite cysts may contain evidence of pneumonia, bronchitis, bronchiectasis, and fibrosis.

Pulmonary paragonimiasis is particularly symptomatic in persons with moderate to heavy infection. Productive cough with brownish sputum or frank hemoptysis associated with peripheral blood eosinophilia is usually the presenting feature. Chest examination may reveal signs of pleurisy. In chronic cases, bronchitis or bronchiectasis may predominate, but these conditions rarely proceed to lung abscess. Imaging of the lungs demonstrates characteristic features, including patchy densities, cavities, pleural effusion, and ring shadows. Cerebral paragonimiasis presents as either space-occupying lesions or epilepsy. Pulmonary paragonimiasis is diagnosed by the detection of parasite ova in sputum and/or stools. Serology is of considerable help in egg-negative cases and in cerebral paragonimiasis. The drug of choice for treatment is praziquantel (Table 222-2). Other medical or surgical management may be needed for pulmonary or cerebral lesions.

CONTROL AND PREVENTION OF TISSUE FLUKES

For residents of nonendemic areas who are visiting an endemic region, the only effective preventive measure is to avoid ingestion of local plants, fish, or crustaceans; if their ingestion is necessary, they should be washed or cooked thoroughly. Instruction on water and food preparation and consumption should be included in physicians' advice to travelers (Chap. 123). Interruption of transmission among residents of endemic areas depends on avoiding ingestion of the infective stage of the helminths and appropriate disposal of feces and sputum to prevent the hatching of eggs in the environment. These two approaches rely greatly on socioeconomic development and health education. In countries where economic progress has resulted in financial and social improvements, transmission has decreased. The third approach to control in endemic communities entails selective use of chemotherapy for individuals posing the highest risk of transmission—i.e., those with heavy infections. The availability of praziquantel—a broad-spectrum, safe, and effective antihelminthic agent—provides a means for reducing the reservoirs of infection in human populations. However, the existence of most of these helminths as zoonoses in several animal species complicates control efforts.

BIBLIOGRAPHY

Drugs for parasitic infections. Med Lett Drugs Ther 40:1, 1998

GUYATT H et al: Assessing the public health importance of *Schistosoma mansoni* in different endemic areas: Attributable fraction estimates as an approach. Am J Trop Med Hyg 53:660, 1995

LIU LX, HARINASUTA KT: Liver and intestinal flukes. Gastroenterol Clin North Am 25: 627, 1996

MAHMOUD AAFM (ed): Parasitic lung diseases, in *Lung Biology in Health and Disease*, vol 101, C Lenfaut (ex ed). New York, Marcel Dekker, 1997, pp 1–235

———: Schistosomiasis from the bench to the field, in *Tropical Medicine: Science and Practice*, G Pasvol and S Hoffman (eds). London, Imperial College Press, 2000

MAS-COMA MS et al: Epidemiology of human fascioliasis: A review and proposed new classification. Bull World Health Organ 77:340, 1999

MONTENEGRO SML et al: Cytokine production in acute versus chronic human schistosomiasis: The cross-regulatory role of interferon γ and interleukin-10 in the responses of peripheral blood mononuclear cells and splenocytes to parasite antigens. J Infect Dis 179:1502, 1999

SUBRAMANIAN AK et al: Long-term suppression of adult bladder morbidity and severe hydronephrosis following selective population chemotherapy for *Schistosoma haematobium*. Am J Trop Med Hyg 61:476, 1999

TSANG VCW, WILKINS PP: Immunodiagnosis of schistosomiasis. Immunol Invest 26: 175, 1997

VISSER LG et al: Outbreak of acute schistosomiasis among travelers returning from Mali, West Africa. Clin Infect Dis 20:280, 1995

223 A. Clinton White, Jr., Peter F. Weller

CESTODES

Cestodes, or tapeworms, are segmented worms. The adults reside in the gastrointestinal tract, but the larvae can be found in almost any organ. Human tapeworm infections can be divided into two major clinical groups. In one group, humans are the definitive hosts, and the adult tapeworms live in the gastrointestinal tract (*Taenia saginata, Diphyllobothrium, Hymenolepis,* and *Dipylidium caninum*). In the other, humans are intermediate hosts, and larval-stage parasites are present in the tissues. Diseases in this category include echinococcosis, sparganosis, and coenurosis. For *T. solium,* the human may be either the definitive or the intermediate host.

The ribbon-shaped tapeworm attaches to the intestinal mucosa by means of sucking cups or grooves located on the head (scolex). Behind the scolex is a short, narrow neck from which proglottids (segments) form. As each proglottid matures, it is displaced further back from the neck by the formation of new, less mature segments. The progressively elongating chain of attached proglottids, called the *strobila,* constitutes the bulk of the tapeworm. The length varies among species. In some, the tapeworm may consist of more than 1000 proglottids and may be several meters long. As each proglottid becomes gravid, eggs are released. Since eggs of the different *Taenia* species are morphologically identical, differences in the morphology of the scolex or proglottids provide the basis for diagnostic identification to the species level. Most human tapeworms require at least one intermediate host for complete larval development. After ingestion by an intermediate host, an egg releases the larval oncosphere, which penetrates the intestinal mucosa. The oncosphere migrates to tissues and develops into an encysted form known as a *cysticercus* (single scolex), a *coenurus* (multiple scolices), or a *hydatid* (cyst with daughter cysts, each containing several protoscolices). Ingestion by the definitive host of tissues containing a cyst enables a scolex to develop into a tapeworm.

TAENIASIS SAGINATA The beef tapeworm *T. saginata* occurs in all countries where raw or undercooked beef is eaten. It is most prevalent in sub-Saharan African and Middle Eastern countries.

Etiology and Pathogenesis Humans are the only definitive host for the adult stage of *T. saginata.* This tapeworm, which can reach 8 m in length, inhabits the upper jejunum and has a scolex with four prominent suckers and 1000 to 2000 proglottids. Each gravid segment has 15 to 30 uterine branches (in contrast to 8 to 12 for *T. solium*). The eggs are indistinguishable from those of *T. solium*; each measures 30 to 40 μm and has a thick brown striated shell containing the embryo. Eggs deposited on vegetation can live for months to years until they are ingested by cattle or other herbivores. The embryo released after ingestion invades the intestinal wall and is carried to striated muscle, where it transforms into a cysticercus. When ingested in raw or undercooked beef, this form can infect humans. After the cysticercus is ingested, it takes about 2 months for an adult worm to develop.

Clinical Manifestations Patients become aware of the infection most commonly by noting passage of proglottids in their feces. The proglottids are often motile, and patients may experience perianal discomfort when proglottids are discharged. Mild abdominal pain or discomfort, nausea, change in appetite, weakness, and weight loss can occur with *T. saginata* infection.

Diagnosis The diagnosis is made by the detection of eggs or proglottids in the stool. Eggs may also be present in the perianal area; thus, if proglottids or eggs are not found in the stool, the perianal region should be examined with use of a cellophane-tape swab (as in pinworm infection). Distinguishing *T. saginata* from *T. solium* requires examination of mature proglottids or the scolex. Serologic tests are not helpful diagnostically. Eosinophilia and elevated levels of serum IgE may be detected.

℞ TREATMENT A single dose of praziquantel (5 to 10 mg/kg) is highly effective.

Prevention The major method of preventing infection is the adequate cooking of beef; exposure to temperatures as low as 56°C for 5 min will destroy cysticerci. Refrigeration or salting for long periods or freezing at −10°C for 9 days also kills cysticerci in beef. General preventive measures include inspection of beef and proper disposal of human feces.

TAENIASIS SOLIUM AND CYSTICERCOSIS The pork tapeworm *T. solium* can cause two distinct forms of infection. The form that develops depends on whether humans are infected with adult tapeworms in the intestine or with larval forms in the tissues (cysticercosis). Humans are the only definitive hosts for *T. solium*; pigs are the usual intermediate hosts, although dogs, cats, and sheep may harbor the larval forms. *T. solium* exists worldwide but is most prevalent in Latin America, Africa, South and Southeast Asia, and eastern Europe. Cysticercosis occurs in industrialized nations largely as a result of the immigration of infected persons from endemic areas.

Etiology and Pathogenesis The adult tapeworm generally resides in the upper jejunum. Its globular scolex attaches by both sucking disks and two rows of hooklets. Often only one adult worm is present, but that worm may live for years. The tapeworm, usually about 3 m in length, may have as many as 1000 proglottids, each of which produces up to 50,000 eggs. Groups of three to five proglottids are generally released and excreted into the feces, and the eggs in these proglottids are infective for both humans and animals. The eggs may survive in the environment for several months. After ingestion by the intermediate host, eggs embryonate, penetrate the intestinal wall, and are carried to many tissues, with a predilection for striated muscle of the neck, tongue, and trunk. Within 60 to 90 days, the encysted larval stage develops. These cysticerci can survive for long periods. Humans acquire infections that lead to intestinal tapeworms by ingesting undercooked pork containing cysticerci. Infections that cause human cysticercosis follow the ingestion of *T. solium* eggs, usually from fecally contaminated food. Autoinfection may occur if an individual with an egg-producing tapeworm ingests eggs derived from his or her own feces.

Clinical Manifestations Intestinal infections with *T. solium* may be asymptomatic. Epigastric discomfort, nausea, a sensation of hunger, weight loss, and diarrhea are infrequent. Fecal passage of proglottids may be noted by patients.

In cysticercosis, the clinical manifestations are entirely different.

Cysticerci can be found anywhere in the body, most commonly in the brain and the skeletal muscle. The clinical presentation of cysticercosis depends on the number and location of cysticerci as well as the extent of associated inflammatory responses or scarring. Neurologic manifestations are the most common. When inflammation surrounds cysticerci in the brain parenchyma, seizures are frequent. These seizures may be generalized, focal, or Jacksonian. Hydrocephalus results from obstruction of cerebrospinal fluid (CSF) flow by cysticerci and accompanying inflammation or by CSF outflow obstruction from arachnoiditis. Signs of increased intracranial pressure, including headache, nausea, vomiting, changes in vision, dizziness, ataxia, or confusion, are often evident. Patients with hydrocephalus may develop papilledema or display altered mental status. When cysticerci develop at the base of the brain or in the subarachnoid space, they cause chronic meningitis or arachnoiditis, communicating hydrocephalus, or strokes.

Diagnosis The diagnosis of intestinal *T. solium* infection is made by the detection of eggs or proglottids, as described for *T. saginata*. In cysticercosis, diagnosis can be difficult. A consensus conference has proposed absolute, major, minor, and epidemiologic criteria for diagnosis (Table 223-1). Diagnostic certainty is possible only with definite demonstration of the parasite (absolute criteria). This task can be accomplished by histologic observation of the parasite in excised tissue, by funduscopic visualization of the parasite in the eye (in the anterior chamber, vitreous, or subretinal spaces), or by neuroimaging studies demonstrating cystic lesions containing a scolex. In most cases, diagnostic certainty is not possible. Instead, a clinical diagnosis is made on the basis of a combination of clinical presentation, radiographic studies, serologic tests, and exposure history.

Neuroimaging findings suggestive of neurocysticercosis constitute the primary major diagnostic criterion. These findings include cystic lesions with or without enhancement (e.g., ring enhancement), one or more calcifications (which may also have associated enhancement), or focal enhancing lesions. Cysticerci in the brain parenchyma are usually 5 to 10 mm in diameter and rounded. Cystic lesions in the subarachnoid space or fissures may enlarge up to 5 cm in diameter and may be lobulated. For cysticerci within the subarachnoid space or ventricles, the walls may be very thin and the cyst fluid is often isodense with CSF. Thus, obstructive hydrocephalus or enhancement of the basilar meninges may be the only finding on computed tomography (CT) in neurocysticercosis. Cysticerci in the ventricles or subarachnoid space are usually visible to an experienced neuroradiologist on magnetic resonance imaging (MRI) or with intraventricular contrast injection. CT is more sensitive than MRI in identifying calcified lesions, whereas MRI is better for identifying cystic lesions and enhancement. Typical

Table 223-1 Proposed Diagnostic Criteria for Human Cysticercosis, 1996

1. Absolute criteria
   a. Demonstration of cysticerci by histologic or microscopic examination of biopsy material
   b. Visualization of the parasite in the eye by funduscopy
   c. Neuroradiologic demonstration of cystic lesions containing a scolex
2. Major criteria
   a. Neuroradiologic lesions suggestive of neurocysticercosis
   b. Demonstration of antibodies to cysticerci in serum by immunoblot or in cerebrospinal fluid by immunoblot or ELISA
   c. Identification of characteristic "cigar-shaped" calcifications on soft tissue x-rays
3. Minor criteria
   a. Presence of subcutaneous nodules suggestive of cysticerci
   b. Punctate calcifications on radiographic studies
   c. Clinical manifestations suggestive of neurocysticercosis
   d. Disappearance of intracranial lesions during treatment with anticysticercal drugs
4. Epidemiologic criteria
   a. Residence in a cysticercosis-endemic area
   b. Frequent travel to a cysticercosis-endemic area
   c. Household contact with an individual infected with *Taenia solium*

NOTE: ELISA, enzyme-linked immunosorbent assay.
SOURCE: Modified from Del Brutto et al.

cigar-shaped calcifications in muscle are a second major diagnostic criterion.

The third major diagnostic criterion is detection of specific antibodies to cysticerci. While most tests employing unfractionated antigen have high rates of false-positive and -negative results, this problem can be overcome by using the more specific immunoblot assay. An immunoblot assay using lentil-lectin purified glycoproteins has >99% specificity and is highly sensitive. However, patients with single intracranial lesions or with calcifications may be seronegative. With this assay, serum samples provide greater diagnostic sensitivity than CSF. However, CSF may be useful when only unfractionated antigens are used.

Minor diagnostic criteria include the presence of subcutaneous nodules, punctate soft tissue or intracranial calcifications, clinical manifestations suggestive of neurocysticercosis (such as seizures, hydrocephalus, or altered mental status), or disappearance of lesions in conjunction with anticysticercal drug therapy. Epidemiologic criteria include current or prior residence in an endemic area, frequent travel to an endemic area, or exposure to a tapeworm carrier or household member infected with *T. solium*. Diagnosis is confirmed in patients with a combination of either two major criteria or one major criterion with two minor criteria and one epidemiologic criterion. The fulfillment of one major criterion and two other criteria or of three minor criteria with epidemiologic exposure supports a probable diagnosis. While the CSF is usually abnormal in neurocysticercosis, CSF abnormalities are not pathognomonic. Patients may have CSF pleocytosis with a predominance of lymphocytes, neutrophils, or eosinophils. The protein level in CSF may be elevated; the glucose concentration is usually normal but may be depressed.

TREATMENT Intestinal *T. solium* infection is treated with a single dose of praziquantel (5 to 10 mg/kg). However, praziquantel can evoke an inflammatory response in the central nervous system if concomitant cryptic cysticercosis is present.

The management of neurocysticercosis focuses primarily on symptomatic treatment of seizures or hydrocephalus. Seizures can usually be controlled with anticonvulsants. If parenchymal lesions resolve without development of calcifications and patients remain free of seizures, anticonvulsant therapy can usually be discontinued after 2 years. Four placebo-controlled trials failed to identify any clinical advantage of antiparasitic drugs for parenchymal neurocysticercosis. However, trends toward faster resolution of neuroradiologic abnormalities were observed. Thus, some authorities favor use of antiparasitic drugs, including praziquantel (50 to 60 mg/kg daily in three divided doses for 15 days or 100 mg/kg in three doses given over a single day) or albendazole (15 mg/kg per day for 8 to 28 days). Both agents may exacerbate the inflammatory response around the dying parasite, exacerbating seizures or hydrocephalus. Thus, patients receiving these drugs should be carefully monitored. High-dose glucocorticoids can be used during treatment or if symptoms worsen. Since glucocorticoids induce first-pass metabolism of praziquantel and may decrease its antiparasitic effect, cimetidine should be coadministered to inhibit praziquantel metabolism.

For patients with hydrocephalus, the emergent reduction of intracranial pressure is the mainstay of therapy. In the case of obstructive hydrocephalus, this task requires either a diverting procedure, such as ventriculoperitoneal shunting, or removal of the cysticerci by craniotomy or via ventriculoscopy. Historically, shunts have usually failed. However, low failure rates have been attained with treatment with antiparasitic drugs or chronic glucocorticoids or with use of flow-sensitive shunts. In patients with subarachnoid cysts, glucocorticoids are needed to reduce arachnoiditis and accompanying vasculitis. Patients may benefit from prolonged courses of antiparasitic drugs and shunting for hydrocephalus. In patients with elevated intracranial pressure due to multiple inflamed lesions, glucocorticoids are the mainstay of therapy, and antiparasitic drugs should be avoided until the elevated pressure resolves. For ocular and spinal medullary lesions, drug-induced inflammation may cause irreversible damage. Most patients should be managed surgically, although case reports have described cures with medical therapy.

Prevention Measures for the prevention of intestinal *T. solium* infection consist of the application to pork of precautions similar to those described above for beef with regard to *T. saginata* infection. The prevention of cysticercosis involves minimizing the opportunities for ingestion of fecally derived eggs by means of good personal hygiene, effective fecal disposal, and treatment and prevention of human intestinal infections.

ECHINOCOCCOSIS Echinococcosis is an infection of humans caused by the larval stage of *Echinococcus granulosus, E. multilocularis,* or *E. vogeli. E. granulosus,* which produces unilocular cystic lesions, is prevalent in areas where livestock is raised in association with dogs. This tapeworm species is found in Australia, Argentina, Chile, Africa, eastern Europe, the Middle East, New Zealand, and the Mediterranean region, particularly Lebanon and Greece. *E. multilocularis,* which causes multilocular alveolar lesions that are locally invasive, is found in Alpine, sub-Arctic, or Arctic regions, including Canada, the United States, and central and northern Europe and Asia. *E. vogeli* causes polycystic hydatid disease and is found only in Central and South America. Like other cestodes, echinococcal species have both intermediate and definitive hosts. The definitive hosts are dogs that pass eggs in their feces. Cysts develop in the intermediate hosts—sheep, cattle, humans, goats, camels, and horses for *E. granulosus* and mice and other rodents for *E. multilocularis*—after the ingestion of eggs. When a dog ingests beef or lamb containing cysts, the life cycle is completed.

Etiology The small (5 mm long) adult *E. granulosus* worm, which lives for 5 to 20 months in the jejunum of dogs, has only three proglottids—one immature, one mature, and one gravid. The gravid segment splits to release eggs that are morphologically similar to *Taenia* eggs and are extremely hardy. After humans ingest the eggs, embryos escape from the eggs, penetrate the intestinal mucosa, enter the portal circulation, and are carried to various organs, most commonly the liver and lungs. Larvae develop into fluid-filled unilocular hydatid cysts that consist of an external membrane and an inner germinal layer. Daughter cysts develop from the inner aspect of the germinal layer, as do germinating cystic structures called *brood capsules.* New larvae, called *protoscolices,* develop in large numbers within the brood capsule. The cysts expand slowly over a period of years.

The life cycle of *E. multilocularis* is similar except that small rodents serve as the intermediate hosts. The cyst of *E. multilocularis,* however, is quite different in that the larval form remains in the proliferative phase, the hydatid cyst is always multilocular, and vesicles progressively invade the host tissue by peripheral extension of processes from the germinal layer.

Clinical Manifestations Slowly enlarging echinococcal cysts generally remain asymptomatic until their expanding size or their space-occupying effect in an involved organ elicits symptoms. The liver and the lungs are the most common sites of these cysts. Since a period of years elapses before cysts enlarge sufficiently to cause symptoms, they may be discovered incidentally on a routine x-ray or ultrasound study.

Patients with hepatic echinococcosis who are symptomatic most often present with abdominal pain or a palpable mass in the right upper quadrant. Compression of a bile duct or leakage of cyst fluid into the biliary tree may mimic recurrent cholelithiasis, and biliary obstruction can result in jaundice. Rupture of or episodic leakage from a hydatid cyst may produce fever, pruritus, urticaria, eosinophilia, or anaphylaxis. Pulmonary hydatid cysts may rupture into the bronchial tree or peritoneal cavity and produce cough, chest pain, or hemoptysis. Rupture of hydatid cysts may lead to multifocal dissemination of protoscolices, which can form additional cysts. Rupture can occur spontaneously or at surgery. Other presentations are due to the involvement

of bone (invasion of the medullary cavity with slow bone erosion producing pathologic fractures), the central nervous system (space-occupying lesions), and the heart (conduction defects, pericarditis).

The cysts of *E. multilocularis* characteristically present as a slowly growing hepatic tumor, with progressive destruction of the liver and extension into vital structures. Patients commonly complain of upper quadrant and epigastric pain, and obstructive jaundice may be apparent. A minority of patients experience the metastasis of lesions to the lung and brain.

Diagnosis Radiographic and related imaging studies are important in detecting and evaluating echinococcal cysts. Plain films will define pulmonary cysts—usually as rounded irregular masses of uniform density—but may miss cysts in other organs unless there is cyst wall calcification (as occurs in the liver). MRI, CT, and ultrasound reveal well-defined cysts with thick or thin walls. When older cysts contain a layer of hydatid sand that is rich in accumulated scolices, these imaging methods may detect this fluid layer of different density. However, the most pathognomonic finding, if demonstrable, is that of daughter cysts within the larger cyst. This finding, like eggshell or mural calcification on CT, is indicative of *E. granulosus* infection and helps to distinguish the cyst from carcinomas, bacterial or amebic liver abscesses, or hemangiomas. CT of alveolar hydatid cysts reveals indistinct solid masses with central necrosis and plaquelike calcifications.

A specific diagnosis can be made by the examination of aspirated fluids for scoliceal hooklets, but diagnostic aspiration is not usually recommended because of the risk of fluid leakage resulting in either dissemination of infection or anaphylactic reactions. Serodiagnostic assays can be useful, although a negative test does not exclude the diagnosis of echinococcosis. Cysts in the liver elicit positive antibody responses in ~90% of cases, whereas up to 50% of individuals with cysts in the lungs are seronegative. Detection of antibody to specific echinococcal antigens by immunoblotting has the highest degree of specificity.

℞ TREATMENT Therapy for echinococcosis is based on considerations of the size, location, and manifestations of cysts and the overall health of the patient. Surgery has traditionally been the principal definitive method of treatment; *E. granulosus* cysts are excised, or tissue containing *E. multilocularis* cysts is resected. Risks at surgery from leakage of fluid include anaphylaxis and dissemination of infectious scolices. The latter complication has been minimized by the instillation of scolicidal solutions such as hypertonic saline or ethanol, which may cause hypernatremia, intoxication, or sclerosing cholangitis. Albendazole, which is active against *Echinococcus,* should be administered adjunctively, beginning before resection and continuing for several weeks for *E. granulosus* and for up to 2 years for *E. multilocularis.* Percutaneous *aspiration, infusion* of scolicidal agents, and *reaspiration* (PAIR) can be used instead of surgery in many cases of cystic echinococcosis. PAIR is contraindicated for superficially located cysts (because of the risk of rupture), for cysts with multiple thick internal septal divisions (honeycombing pattern), and for cysts communicating with the biliary tree. Therapy with albendazole (15 mg/kg daily in two divided doses) should be initiated at least 4 days before the procedure and continued for at least 4 weeks afterward. Ultrasound- or CT-guided aspiration allows confirmation of the diagnosis by demonstration of protoscolices in the aspirate. Either alcohol or hypertonic saline should then be infused. Daughter cysts within the primary cyst may need to be punctured separately. In experienced hands, this approach yields rates of cure and relapse equivalent to those following surgery, with less perioperative morbidity and shorter hospitalization. Medical therapy with albendazole alone for 12 weeks to 6 months results in cure in ~30% of cases and improvement in another 50%. Many of the failures are subsequently treated successfully with PAIR or additional courses of medical therapy. Response to treatment is best assessed by serial imaging studies with attention to cyst size and consistency.

Prevention In endemic areas, echinococcosis can be prevented by administering praziquantel to infected dogs, by denying dogs access to infected animals, or by vaccinating sheep. Limitation of the number of stray dogs is helpful in reducing the prevalence of infection among humans.

HYMENOLEPIASIS NANA Infection with *Hymenolepis nana*, the dwarf tapeworm, is the most common of all the cestode infections. *H. nana* is endemic in both temperate and tropical regions of the world. Infection is spread by fecal/oral contamination and is common among institutionalized children.

Etiology and Pathogenesis *H. nana* is the only cestode of humans that does not require an intermediate host. Both the larval and adult phases take place in the human. The adult, the smallest tapeworm parasitizing humans, is about 2 cm long and dwells in the proximal ileum. Proglottids, which are quite small and are rarely seen in the stool, release spherical eggs 30 to 44 μm in diameter, each of which contains an oncosphere with six hooklets. The eggs are immediately infective and are unable to survive in the external environment for more than 10 days. *H. nana* can also be acquired by the ingestion of infected insects (especially larval meal-worms and larval fleas). When the egg is ingested by a new host, the oncosphere is freed and penetrates the intestinal villi, becoming a cysticercoid larva. Larvae migrate back into the intestinal lumen, attach to the mucosa, and mature over 10 to 12 days into adult worms. Eggs may also hatch before passing into the stool, causing internal autoinfection with increasing numbers of intestinal worms. Although the life span of adult *H. nana* is only about 4 to 10 weeks, the autoinfection cycle perpetuates the infection.

Clinical Manifestations *H. nana* infection, even with many intestinal worms, is usually asymptomatic. When infection is intense, anorexia, abdominal pain, and diarrhea develop.

Diagnosis Infection is diagnosed by the finding of eggs in the stool.

℞ **TREATMENT** Praziquantel (25 mg/kg once) is the treatment of choice, since it acts against both the adult worms and the cysticercoids in the intestinal villi.

Prevention Good personal hygiene and improved sanitation can eradicate the disease. Epidemics have been controlled by mass chemotherapy coupled with improved hygiene.

HYMENOLEPIASIS DIMINUTA *Hymenolepis diminuta*, a cestode of rodents, occasionally infects small children, who ingest the adult worm in uncooked cereal foods contaminated by fleas and other insects in which larvae develop. Infection is usually asymptomatic and is diagnosed by the detection of eggs in the stool. Treatment with praziquantel results in cure in most cases.

DIPHYLLOBOTHRIASIS *Diphyllobothrium latum* and other *Diphyllobothrium* species are found in the lakes, rivers, and deltas of the northern hemisphere, Central Africa, and Chile.

Etiology and Pathogenesis The adult worm, the longest tapeworm (up to 25 m), attaches to the ileal and occasionally to the jejunal mucosa by its suckers, which are located on its elongated scolex. The adult worm has 3000 to 4000 proglottids, which release approximately 1 million eggs daily into the feces. If an egg reaches water, it hatches and releases a free-swimming embryo that can be eaten by small freshwater crustaceans (*Cyclops* or *Diaptomus* species). After an infected crustacean containing a developed procercoid is swallowed by a fish, the larva migrates into the fish's flesh and grows into a plerocercoid, or sparganum larva. Humans acquire the infection by ingesting infected raw fish. Within 3 to 5 weeks, the tapeworm matures into an adult in the human intestine.

Clinical Manifestations Most *D. latum* infections are asymptomatic, although manifestations may include transient abdominal discomfort, diarrhea, vomiting, weakness, and weight loss. Occasionally, infection can cause acute abdominal pain and intestinal obstruction; in rare cases cholangitis or cholecystitis may be produced by migrating proglottids. Because the tapeworm absorbs large quantities of vitamin B_{12} and interferes with ileal B_{12} absorption, vitamin B_{12} deficiency can develop. Up to 2% of infected patients, especially the elderly, have megaloblastic anemia resembling pernicious anemia and may exhibit neurologic sequelae of B_{12} deficiency.

Diagnosis The diagnosis is made readily by the detection of the characteristic eggs in the stool. The eggs possess a single shell with an operculum at one end and a knob at the other. Mild to moderate eosinophilia may be detected.

℞ **TREATMENT** Praziquantel (5 to 10 mg/kg once) is highly effective. Parenteral vitamin B_{12} should be given if B_{12} deficiency is manifest.

Prevention Infection can be prevented by heating fish to 54°C for 5 min or by freezing it at -18°C for 24 h. Placing fish in brine with a high salt concentration for long periods kills the eggs.

DIPYLIDIASIS *Dipylidium caninum*, a common tapeworm of dogs and cats, may accidentally infect humans. Dogs, cats, and occasionally humans become infected by ingesting fleas harboring cysticercoids. Children are more likely to become infected than adults. Most infections are asymptomatic, but abdominal pain, diarrhea, anal pruritus, urticaria, eosinophilia, or passage of segments in the stool may occur. The diagnosis is made by the detection of proglottids in the stool. As in *D. latum* infection, therapy consists of praziquantel. Prevention requires anthelmintic treatment and flea control for pet dogs or cats.

SPARGANOSIS Humans can be infected by the sparganum, or plerocercoid larva, of a diphyllobothrid tapeworm of the genus *Spirometra*. Infection can be acquired by the consumption of water containing infected *Cyclops*; by the ingestion of infected snakes, birds, or mammals; or by the application of infected flesh as poultices. The worm migrates slowly in tissues, and infection commonly presents as a subcutaneous swelling. Periorbital tissues can be involved, and ocular sparganosis may destroy the eye. Surgical excision is used to treat localized sparganosis.

COENUROSIS This rare infection of humans by the larval stage (coenurus) of the dog tapeworm *Taenia multiceps* or *T. serialis* results in a space-occupying cystic lesion. As in cysticercosis, involvement of the central nervous system and subcutaneous tissue is most common. Both definitive diagnosis and treatment require surgical excision of the lesion. Chemotherapeutic agents generally are not effective.

BIBLIOGRAPHY

AMMANN RW, ECKERT J: Cestodes: *Echinococcus*. Gastroenterol Clin North Am 25:655, 1996

BOTERO D et al: Taeniasis and cysticercosis. Infect Dis Clin North Am 7:683, 1993

DEL BRUTTO OH et al: Proposal for diagnostic criteria for human cysticercosis and neurocysticercosis. J Neurol Sci 142:1, 1996

FLISSER A: Taeniasis and cysticercosis due to *Taenia solium*. Prog Clin Parasitol 4:77, 1994

FRANCHI C et al: Long-term evaluation of patients with hydatidosis treated with benzimidazole carbamates. Clin Infect Dis 29:304, 1999

GIL-GRANDE LA et al: Randomised controlled trial of efficacy of albendazole in intra-abdominal hydatid disease. Lancet 342:1269, 1993

KAMMERER WS, SCHANTZ PM: Echinococcal disease. Infect Dis Clin North Am 7:605, 1993

KHUROO MS et al: Percutaneous drainage compared with surgery for hepatic hydatid cysts. N Engl J Med 337:881, 1997

PAWLOWSKI Z, SCHANTZ P (eds): Advances in clinical management of cystic echinococcosis. Acta Trop 64:1; 67:1, 1997

SALINAS R, PRASAD K: Drugs in neurocysticercosis (tapeworm infection of the brain), in *The Cochrane Library*, issue 4. Oxford, Update Software, 1998

SCHAEFER JW, KHAN MY: Echinococcosis (hydatid disease): Lessons from experience with 59 patients. Rev Infect Dis 13:243, 1991

SCHANTZ PM, KRAMER HJ: Larval cestode infections: Cysticercosis and echinococcosis. Curr Opin Infect Dis 8:342, 1995

SCHARF D: Neurocysticercosis: Two hundred thirty eight cases from a California hospital. Arch Neurol 46:77, 1989

WHITE AC JR: Neurocysticercosis: A major cause of neurologic disease worldwide. Clin Infect Dis 24:101, 1997

———: Neurocysticercosis: Updates on epidemiology, pathogenesis, diagnosis and management. Annu Rev Med 51:187, 2000

——— et al: *Taenia solium* cysticercosis: Host-parasite interactions and the immune response. Chem Immunol 66:209, 1997

WORLD HEALTH ORGANIZATION INFORMAL WORKING GROUP ON ECHINOCOCCOSIS: Guidelines for treatment of cystic and alveolar echinococcosis in humans. Bull World Health Organ 74:231, 1996

NOBEL PRIZE IN PHYSIOLOGY OR MEDICINE, 1945

Alexander Fleming was born on August 6, 1881, the youngest child of Hugh and Grace Fleming in Lochfield, Scotland. After attending local schools, he moved to London to join his two brothers, Tom and John, and attended Regent Street Polytechnic for two years. At age 16 he became a shipping clerk, but with the good fortune of a legacy of 250 British pounds from an uncle, he decided to enroll in medical school at St. Mary's in London. Fleming was a brilliant student, capturing virtually every academic prize. More important, when he graduated in 1906 he joined the laboratory of Almroth Wright, his future mentor. During World War I, Fleming and Wright moved to Boulogne, France, where they tended the wounds of injured soldiers. At the end of the war, Fleming returned to St. Mary's to become assistant director of the Inoculation Department. Although Fleming was a skilled laboratory worker, his laboratory was not very neat, as he stacked old culture plates on his bench until there was no more room. In 1928 he was growing various strains of staphylococcus and prepared some culture plates just before leaving for 2 weeks of vacation. On his return he saw one plate that was contaminated with a mold and observed that no bacteria were growing around the mold. In 1929 he published a paper entitled "On the Antibacterial Actions of Cultures of a Penicillium."

In the 1930s, Fleming used penicillin primarily to prepare pure strains of bacteria for vaccines. He no doubt felt that enhanced natural immunity with vaccines, rather than chemotherapy, would be the future treatment of bacterial infections in humans. Moreover, he observed that staphylococci developed rapid immunity to penicillin in culture and that penicillin was unstable; in the impure state, large quantities would be necessary to treat humans. In fact, had it not been for the work of Florey and Chain on penicillin at Oxford, the drug might have remained of interest only to bacteriologists and not to physicians caring for patients.

Howard Florey was born in Adelaide, Australia, on September 24, 1898, the only son of Joseph and Bertha Florey. He attended Saint Peter's Collegiate School in Adelaide and then attended medical school at the University of Adelaide. After graduation, Florey studied at Oxford University in England on a Rhodes scholarship. He spent a year abroad in the United States as a Rockefeller Fellow and then completed his Ph.D. at Cambridge in 1927 under the direction of the internationally renowned biochemist, Frederick G. Hopkins. In 1932 Florey was appointed Chair in Pathology at the University of Sheffield; and then in 1936 he became director of Oxford's Sir William Dunn School of Pathology. It was there that Florey began his long association with Ernst Chain. With a mutual interest in antibacterial chemicals produced by microbes, Florey and Chain began to study the crude form of penicillin, which could be obtained from the culture medium in which the mold, *Penicillium notatum*, had been grown. In 1940 Florey and his co-workers published a paper, "Penicillin as a Chemotherapeutic Agent," which showed that mice infected with fatal doses of staphylococci or clostridia (gangrene) uniformly survived when treated with penicillin. Moreover, in contrast to earlier attempts to develop chemotherapeutic agents, penicillin demonstrated no evidence of toxicity.

The initial stumbling block for its use in humans was that it took hundreds of gallons of culture media to yield enough penicillin to treat a single individual. This problem was overcome in Florey's laboratory, and in 1941 infections in 10 humans were treated with penicillin and the results reported in a paper entitled "Further Observations of Penicillin." Great Britain was in the throes of World War II and could not provide adequate funding to produce enough penicillin for widespread use. Florey went to the United States and convinced the American Office of Scientific Research, along with industry, to fund the effort. This led to the widespread use of penicillin to treat the casualties during the Normandy invasion.

Ernst Chain was born in Berlin, Germany, on June 19, 1906, the son of Michael, an immigrant from White Russia, and Margarete, his German wife. Both Russian and German were spoken at home, where music was important and Ernst became an accomplished pianist. He attended the Luisen *Gymnasium* (German high school) and then the Friedrich Wilhelm University. Ernst earned his degree in 1930 in chemistry and physiology. After graduation he worked first at the Kaiser-Wilhelm Institute and then the Charité Hospital in Berlin in biochemical research. With the rise of Nazism and being a Jew, Chain left Germany and worked with Sir Frederick G. Hopkins at Cambridge from 1933 to 1935. He then went as a lecturer in clinical pathology to Sir William Dunn School of Pathology at Oxford where he met Howard Florey. In 1939 they began to work on penicillin together with some funding from the Rockefeller Institute. Chain focused on the fundamental chemical properties and structure of penicillin. Eventually penicillin was identified by x-ray analysis of the crystals as a beta-lactam in 1945. In 1948 he moved to Rome and with Beecham researchers, Chain discovered a process for producing 6-aminopenicillanic acid from which all known penicillins could be produced by a simple reaction. This observation led to the production of an oral penicillin. In 1961 he returned to Britain to Imperial College, University of London, as Chair of Biochemistry where he facilitated the movement of discoveries from the laboratory to pilot studies and then to production.

REFERENCES

1. Aaseng N: *The Disease Fighters*. Minneapolis, Lerner Publications, 1987
2. Magill FN (ed): *Nobel Prize Winners: Physiology or Medicine*, vol 2. Pasadena, Salem Press, 1993
3. Schrier RW: *A Salute to Nobel Laureates in Physiology and Medicine*, Proceedings of the Association of American Physicians 108(1): Jan 1996
4. Sourkes TL: *Nobel Prize Winners in Medicine and Physiology 1901–1965*. London, Abelard-Schuman, 1967

Robert W. Schrier, MD

Section 1
DIAGNOSIS

224

Eugene Braunwald

APPROACH TO THE PATIENT WITH HEART DISEASE

The symptoms caused by heart disease result most commonly from myocardial ischemia, from disturbance of the contraction and/or relaxation of the myocardium, from obstruction to blood flow, or from an abnormal cardiac rhythm or rate. Ischemia is manifest most frequently as chest discomfort, while reduction of the pumping ability of the heart commonly leads to weakness and fatigability or, when severe, produces cyanosis, hypotension, syncope, and elevated intravascular pressure behind a failing ventricle. The latter results in abnormal fluid accumulation, which in turn leads to dyspnea, orthopnea, and systemic or pulmonary edema. Obstruction to blood flow, as in valvular stenosis, can cause symptoms resembling those resulting from congestive heart failure. Cardiac arrhythmias often develop suddenly, and the resulting signs and symptoms—palpitation, dyspnea, hypotension, presyncope and syncope—generally occur abruptly and may disappear as rapidly as they develop. Ischemic heart disease, by far the most common form of heart disease in adults, may present with chest discomfort but also as heart failure, tachyarrhythmia, and sudden cardiac death.

Myocardial or coronary function that may be adequate at rest may be inadequate during exertion. Thus a history of chest discomfort and/or dyspnea that appears only during activity is characteristic of heart disease, while the opposite pattern, i.e., the appearance of these symptoms at rest and their remission during exertion, is rarely observed in patients with organic heart disease.

Many patients with cardiocirculatory disease also may be asymptomatic, both at rest and during exertion, but may present an abnormal physical finding, such as a heart murmur, elevated arterial pressure, or an abnormality of the electrocardiogram (ECG) or of the cardiac silhouette on the chest roentgenogram. Patients may exhibit asymptomatic ischemia on an exercise stress test. In some asymptomatic patients the first clinical event may be catastrophic—sudden cardiac death, acute myocardial infarction, or stroke.

Diseases of the heart and circulation are so common and the laity is so well acquainted with the major symptoms resulting from these disorders that patients, and occasionally physicians, erroneously attribute many noncardiac complaints to cardiovascular disease. The combination of the widespread fear of heart disease with the deep-seated emotional connotations concerning this organ's function results in the frequent development of symptoms that mimic those of organic disease in persons with normal cardiovascular systems. The unraveling of symptoms and signs due to organic heart disease from those not directly related is an important and challenging task in such patients.

Patients in whom heart disease has been confirmed, especially those who have experienced a major cardiovascular event such as a myocardial infarction or a serious arrhythmia, are often frightened and anxious about hospital discharge and resuming normal activity, including sexual relations. Attention to these matters is vital in the care of cardiac patients.

Dyspnea, one of the cardinal manifestations of heart failure, is not limited to patients with heart disease but is also observed in conditions as diverse as pulmonary disease, marked obesity, and anxiety (Chap. 32). Similarly, chest discomfort may result from a variety of causes other than myocardial ischemia (Chap. 13). Whether heart disease is responsible for these symptoms can frequently be determined by carrying out a careful clinical examination. Noninvasive testing using electrocardiography at rest and during exercise (Chap. 226), echocardiography (Chap. 227), roentgenography, and myocardial imaging usually provides important additional information to permit the correct interpretation of symptoms; more specialized invasive examinations (catheterization and angiography; Chap. 228) are occasionally necessary.

DIAGNOSIS As outlined by the New York Heart Association, the elements of a complete cardiac diagnosis include consideration of the following:

1. *The underlying etiology.* Is the disease congenital, infectious, hypertensive, or ischemic in origin?
2. *The anatomic abnormalities.* Which chambers are involved? Are they hypertrophied, dilated, or both? Which valves are affected? Are they regurgitant and/or stenotic? Is there pericardial involvement? Has there been a myocardial infarction?
3. *The physiologic disturbances.* Is an arrhythmia present? Is there evidence of congestive heart failure or of myocardial ischemia?

One example may serve to illustrate the importance of establishing a complete diagnosis. The identification of myocardial ischemia as the etiology of a patient's exertional chest discomfort is of great clinical importance. However, the simple recognition of ischemia is insufficient to formulate a therapeutic strategy or prognosis until the underlying anatomic abnormalities responsible for the myocardial ischemia, e.g., coronary atherosclerosis or aortic stenosis, are identified and a judgment made as to whether other physiologic disturbances that cause an imbalance between myocardial oxygen supply and demand, such as severe anemia, thyrotoxicosis, or supraventricular tachycardia, play a contributory role.

The fourth element of the diagnosis involves an assessment of *functional disability.* How strenuous is the physical activity required to elicit symptoms? The functional classification provided by the New York Heart Association has been found to be useful (Table 224-1).

The establishment of a correct and complete cardiac diagnosis often commences with the history and physical examination (Chap. 225). Indeed the clinical examination remains the basis for the diagnosis of a wide variety of disorders (Table 224-2). The clinical examination may then be supplemented by four types of laboratory tests: (1) ECG (Chap. 226); (2) chest roentgenogram; (3) noninvasive graphic examinations [echocardiogram, radionuclide and imaging techniques] (Chap. 227); and occasionally (4) specialized invasive examinations, i.e., cardiac catheterization, angiocardiography, and coronary angiography (Chap. 228).

In the diagnostic process, the results obtained from each of these several modalities should be analyzed independently of one another as well as together. Only in this way can one avoid overlooking a subtle, though important, finding. For example, an ECG should be obtained in every patient suspected of heart disease. It may provide the critical clue in establishing the correct diagnosis, e.g., the finding of a mild atrioventricular conduction disturbance in a patient with unexplained syncope, even when all other methods of examination reveal no abnormal findings, can be the clue that advanced heart block and asystole might be the cause and can dictate electrophysiologic

Table 224-1 New York Heart Association Functional Classification

Class I	Class III
No limitation of physical activity	Marked limitation of physical activity
No symptoms with ordinary exertion	Less than ordinary activity causes symptoms
Class II	Asymptomatic at rest
Slight limitation of physical activity	Class IV
Ordinary activity causes symptoms	Inability to carry out any physical activity without discomfort
	Symptoms at rest

SOURCE: Modified from The Criteria Committee of the New York Heart Association.

testing. On the other hand, when combined intelligently with the results of other methods of examination, the ECG may provide essential confirmatory data. Thus, the knowledge that a patient has an apical diastolic rumbling murmur may direct particular attention to the P waves, and the recognition of electrocardiographic left atrial enlargement supports the suggestion that the murmur is caused by mitral stenosis. The diagnosis can then be confirmed by echocardiography, a technique that can also determine the severity of the obstruction and its effects on pulmonary artery pressure and on right and left ventricular function.

Family History In eliciting the history of a patient with known or suspected cardiovascular disease, particular attention should be directed to the family history. Familial clustering is common in many forms of heart disease. Mendelian transmission of single-gene defects may occur, as in hypertrophic cardiomyopathy (Chap. 238), the Marfan syndrome (Chap. 351), and sudden death associated with a prolonged QT syndrome (Chap. 230). Essential hypertension or coronary atherosclerosis are often polygenic disorders. While familial transmission may be less obvious than in the single-gene disorders, it is also helpful in assessing risk and prognosis. Familial clustering of cardiovascular diseases may occur not only on a genetic basis but also may be related to familial dietary or behavior patterns, such as excessive ingestion of salt or calories or cigarette smoking.

Assessment of Functional Impairment When an attempt is made to determine the severity of functional impairment in a patient with heart disease, it is helpful to ascertain with as much precision as possible the level of activity and the rate at which it is performed before symptoms develop. Thus, breathlessness that occurs after running up two long flights of stairs denotes far less functional impairment than similar symptoms occurring after taking a few steps on the level. Also, the degree of customary physical activity at work and during recreation should be considered. The development of two-flight dyspnea in a marathon runner may be far more significant than the development of one-flight dyspnea in a previously sedentary person. Similarly, the history must include a detailed consideration of the patient's therapeutic regimen. For example, the persistence or development of edema, breathlessness, and other manifestations of heart failure in a patient whose diet is rigidly restricted in sodium content and who is receiving optimal doses of diuretics is far more grave than are similar manifestations in the absence of these measures. In an effort to determine the rate of progression of symptoms, and thereby of the severity

Table 224-2 Conditions in Which Clinical Examination Is an Important Determinant of Diagnosis: Confirmation by Echocardiography Is Often Useful

Mitral valve prolapse	Tricuspid regurgitation
Congestive heart failure	Aortic stenosis
Cardiac tamponade	Acute pulmonary hypertension
Hypertension	Chronic pulmonary hypertension
Mitral stenosis	High-output states
Chronic mitral regurgitation	Atrial septal defect
Chronic aortic regurgitation	Anginal syndrome

of the underlying illness, it may be useful to ascertain what, if any, specific tasks the patient could carry out 1 year earlier that he or she cannot carry out at present.

Electrocardiogram (See also Chap. 226) Although an ECG should be recorded in every patient with known or suspected heart disease, with the exception of the identification of arrhythmias and of acute myocardial infarction, it rarely permits establishment of a specific diagnosis. In the absence of other abnormal findings, electrocardiographic changes must not be overinterpreted. The range of normal electrocardiographic findings is wide, and the tracing can be affected significantly by many noncardiac factors, such as age, body habitus, and serum electrolyte concentrations.

Natural History The natural history of cardiovascular disease must be appreciated. Cardiovascular disorders often present acutely, as in a previously asymptomatic patient with extensive coronary atherosclerosis who develops an acute myocardial infarction or the previously asymptomatic patient with hypertrophic cardiomyopathy whose first clinical manifestation is syncope or even sudden death. However, in both instances, the alert physician may recognize the patient at risk of these complications long before they occur and can often take measures to prevent their occurrence. For example, the patient with acute myocardial infarction may well have had risk factors for atherosclerosis for many years. Had these been recognized, their elimination or reduction might have delayed or even prevented the infarction. Similarly, the patient with hypertrophic cardiomyopathy may have had a heart murmur for years, and a positive family history might have led to an echocardiographic examination and the recognition of the condition and appropriate therapy long before the acute manifestations.

PITFALLS IN CARDIOVASCULAR MEDICINE Increasing subspecialization in internal medicine and the perfection of advanced diagnostic techniques in cardiology can lead to several undesirable consequences. Examples include:

1. Failure by the *noncardiologist* to recognize important cardiac manifestations of systemic illnesses. Examples of the latter are (a) stroke (atrial fibrillation, mitral stenosis); (b) skeletal muscular dystrophies (associated with cardiomyopathy); (c) hemochromatosis (associated with myocardial infiltration and restrictive cardiomyopathy); (d) congenital deafness (associated with prolonged QT interval and serious cardiac arrhythmias); (e) Raynaud's disease (associated with primary pulmonary hypertension and coronary vasospasm); (f) connective tissue disorders, e.g., the Marfan syndrome, (aortic dilatation and aneurysm, prolapsed mitral valve); (g) hyperthyroidism (heart failure, atrial fibrillation); (h) hypothyroidism (pericardial effusion, coronary artery disease); (i) rheumatoid arthritis (pericarditis, aortic valve disease); (j) scleroderma (cor pulmonale, myocardial fibrosis, pericarditis); (k) systemic lupus erythematosus (valvulitis, myocarditis, pericarditis); and (l) sarcoidosis (arrhythmias, cardiomyopathy). In patients with these and other systemic disorders a cardiovascular examination should be carried out to identify and estimate the severity of cardiovascular involvement.

2. Failure by the cardiologist to recognize underlying systemic disorders, such as those listed above, in patients with a cardiac disorder. Patients with heart disease should be assessed for the frequent *noncardiac* manifestations of systemic disorders with cardiovascular manifestations. For example, Lyme disease should be considered in patients with unexplained fluctuating atrioventricular block. A cardiovascular abnormality may provide the clue critical to the recognition of some systemic disorders. For instance, unexplained atrial fibrillation may provide the first clue to the diagnosis of thyrotoxicosis.

3. Overreliance on and overutilization of laboratory tests, particularly invasive techniques for the examination of the cardiovascular system. Cardiac catheterization and coronary arteriography (Chap. 228) provide precise diagnostic information under many circumstances. For example, they aid in establishing a specific anatomic diagnosis, which, in turn, may be critical to developing a therapeutic plan in patients with known or suspected ischemic heart disease. Although a great deal of attention has been lavished on these expensive

examinations, it should be recognized that they serve to *supplement*, not *supplant*, a careful examination carried out by clinical and non-invasive techniques. A coronary arteriogram should not be carried out in lieu of a careful history in patients with chest pain suspected of having ischemic heart disease. Although coronary arteriography may establish whether the coronary arteries are obstructed, the results often do not provide a definite answer to the question of whether a patient's complaint of chest pain is attributable to coronary arteriosclerosis. Catheterization of the left side of the heart is all too frequently employed to assess patients with valvular heart disease when echocardiographic examination would actually provide more useful information.

Despite the enormous value of these invasive tests in certain circumstances, they entail some small risk to the patient, involve discomfort and substantial cost, and place a strain on existing medical facilities. Therefore, they should be carried out only if, after clinical examination and assessment by noninvasive tests, the results of the invasive examination can be expected to modify the patient's management.

℞ **TREATMENT** After a complete diagnosis has been established, a number of therapeutic options are usually available. Several examples may be used to demonstrate some of the principles of cardiovascular therapeutics:

1. In the absence of evidence of heart disease, a clear, definitive statement to that effect should be made and the patient should *not* be asked to return at intervals for repeated examinations. If there is no evidence for disease, such continued attention may lead to the patient developing inappropriate anxiety and fixation on the heart.
2. If there is no evidence of cardiovascular disease but the patient has one or more risk factors for the development of ischemic heart disease (Chap. 242), a plan for their reduction should be developed and the patient should be retested at intervals to assess that he or she is complying and that these risk factors are in fact being reduced.
3. Asymptomatic or mildly symptomatic patients with valvular heart disease that is anatomically severe should be evaluated periodically, every 6 to 12 months, by clinical and noninvasive examinations. Early signs of deterioration of ventricular function can be detected in this manner and in appropriate patients may signify the need for surgical treatment before the development of disabling symptoms, irreversible myocardial damage, and excessive risk of surgical treatment (Chap. 236).
4. It is critical to establish clear criteria for deciding on the form of treatment (medical, percutaneous coronary intervention, or surgical revascularization) in patients with ischemic heart disease (Chap. 244). Mechanical revascularization, i.e., the latter two modalities, represents a major therapeutic advance in the treatment of this most common form of heart disease in developed nations, but these techniques are probably being employed too frequently in the United States; the mere presence of angina pectoris and/or the demonstration of critical coronary arterial narrowing at angiography should not reflexly evoke a decision to treat the patient surgically or by percutaneous coronary intervention. Instead, coronary revascularization should be limited to those patients with ischemic heart disease who have not responded adequately to medical treatment (e.g., intractable angina) or in whom the procedure has been shown to improve the natural history (e.g., three-vessel coronary artery disease with left ventricular dysfunction.)

BIBLIOGRAPHY

BRAUNWALD E, ZIPES D, LIBBY P (eds): *Heart Disease*, 6th ed. Philadelphia, Saunders, 2001
CONSTANT J: *Bedside Cardiology*, 4th ed. Boston, Little, Brown, 1993
THE CRITERIA COMMITTEE OF THE NEW YORK HEART ASSOCIATION: *Nomenclature and Criteria for Diagnosis*, 9th ed. Boston, Little, Brown, 1994
HURST JW: *Cardiovascular Diagnosis: The Initial Examination*. St. Louis, Mosby, 1993

MARRIOTT HJL: *Bedside Cardiac Diagnosis*. Philadelphia, Lippincott, 1993
O'ROURKE RA et al: The history, physical examination, and cardiac auscultation, in *Hurst's The Heart*, 9th ed, RW Alexander et al (eds). New York, McGraw-Hill, 1998, pp 229–342
VANDEN BELT J: The history, in *Classic Teachings in Clinical Cardiology: A Tribute to W. Proctor Harvey*, M Chizner (ed). Cedar Grove, NJ, Laennec, 1996, pp 41–54

225   *Robert A. O'Rourke, Eugene Braunwald*

PHYSICAL EXAMINATION OF THE CARDIOVASCULAR SYSTEM

A meticulous physical examination is an often inadequately utilized low-cost method for assessing the cardiovascular system and frequently provides important information for the appropriate selection of additional tests. First, the general physical appearance should be evaluated. The patient may appear tired because of a chronic low cardiac output; the respiratory rate may be rapid in cases of pulmonary venous congestion. Central cyanosis, often associated with clubbing of the fingers and toes, indicates right-to-left cardiac or extracardiac shunting or inadequate oxygenation of blood by the lungs. Cyanosis in the distal extremities, cool skin, and increased sweating result from vasoconstriction in patients with severe heart failure (Chap. 36). Non-cardiovascular details can be equally important. For example, infective endocarditis is the likely diagnosis in patients with petechiae, Osler's nodes, and Janeway lesions (Chap. 126).

The blood pressure should be taken in both arms and with the patient supine and upright; the heart rate should be timed for 30 s. Orthostatic hypotension and tachycardia may indicate a reduced blood volume, while resting tachycardia may be due to heart failure.

Careful examination of the optic fundi is essential (Chap. 246), and the retinal vessels may show evidence of systemic hypertension, arteriosclerosis, or embolism. The latter may result from atherosclerosis in larger arteries (e.g., the carotid) or may represent a complication of valvular heart disease (e.g., endocarditis).

Palpation of the peripheral arterial pulses in the upper and lower extremities is necessary to define the adequacy of systemic blood flow and to detect the presence of occlusive arterial lesions. It is also important to examine both legs for evidence of edema, varicose veins, or thrombophlebitis (Chap. 248). The cardiovascular examination includes careful evaluation of both the carotid arterial and the jugular venous pulses, as well as deliberate precordial palpation and attentive cardiac auscultation.

ARTERIAL PRESSURE PULSE The normal central aortic pulse wave is characterized by a fairly rapid rise to a somewhat rounded peak (Fig. 225-1). The anacrotic shoulder, present on the ascending limb, occurs at the time of peak rate of aortic flow just before maximum pressure is reached. The less steep descending limb is interrupted by a sharp downward deflection, coincident with aortic valve closure, called the *incisura*. As the pulse wave is transmitted peripherally, the initial upstroke becomes steeper, the anacrotic shoulder becomes less apparent, and the incisura is replaced by the smoother dicrotic notch. Accordingly, palpation of a peripheral arterial pulse (e.g., the radial pulse) frequently gives less information than examination of a more central pulse (e.g., the carotid pulse) regarding alterations in left ventricular ejection or aortic valve function. However, certain findings, such as the bisferiens pulse of aortic regurgitation or pulsus alternans, are more evident in peripheral arteries (Fig. 225-2). The carotid pulse is best examined with the sternocleidomastoid muscle relaxed and with the head rotated slightly toward the examiner. In palpating the brachial arterial pulse, the examiner can support the subject's relaxed elbow with the right arm while compressing the brachial pulse with the thumb. The usual technique is to compress the artery

FIGURE 225-1 *A.* Schematic representation of electrocardiogram, aortic pressure pulse (AOP), phonocardiogram recorded at the apex, and apex cardiogram (ACG). On the phonocardiogram, S_1, S_2, S_3, and S_4 represent the first through fourth heart sounds; OS represents the opening snap of the mitral valve, which occurs coincident with the O point of the apex cardiogram. S_3 occurs coincident with the termination of the rapid-filling wave (RFW) of the ACG, while S_4 occurs coincident with the *a* wave of the ACG. *B.* Simultaneous recording of electrocardiogram, indirect carotid pulse (CP), phonocardiogram along the left sternal border (LSB), and indirect jugular venous pulse (JVP). ES, ejection sound; SC, systolic click.

with the thumb or forefinger until the maximum pulse is sensed. Varying degrees of pressure should then be applied while concentrating on the separate phases of the pulse wave. This method, known as *trisection*, is useful for assessing the sharpness of the upstroke, systolic peak, and diastolic slope of the arterial pulse. In most normal persons, a dicrotic wave is not palpable.

A small weak pulse, *pulsus parvus*, is common in conditions with a diminished left ventricular stroke volume, a narrow pulse pressure, and increased peripheral vascular resistance (Fig. 225-2). A *hypokinetic* pulse may be due to hypovolemia, to left ventricular failure, to restrictive pericardial disease, or to mitral valve stenosis. In aortic valve stenosis, the delayed systolic peak, *pulsus tardus*, results from obstruction to left ventricular ejection. In contrast, a large, bounding (*hyperkinetic*) pulse is usually associated with an increased left ventricular stroke volume, a wide pulse pressure, and a decrease in peripheral vascular resistance. This pattern occurs characteristically in

FIGURE 225-2 Schematic representation of arterial pulse waveforms that occur with alterations in cardiac hemodynamics, which may result from normal physiologic responses or may be due to cardiac disease. S, systole; D, diastole. *[Modified from RA O'Rourke, in Hurst's The Heart, 9th ed, RW Alexander et al (eds). New York, McGraw-Hill, 1990, with permission.]*

patients with an elevated stroke volume, as in complete heart block; with hyperkinetic circulation due to anxiety, anemia, exercise, or fever; or with a rapid runoff of blood from the arterial system (as caused by a patent ductus arteriosus or peripheral arteriovenous fistula). Patients with mitral regurgitation or a ventricular septal defect may also have a bounding pulse, since vigorous left ventricular ejection produces a rapid upstroke in the arterial pulse, even though the duration of systole and the forward stroke volume may be reduced. In aortic regurgitation, the rapidly rising, bounding arterial pulse results from an increased left ventricular stroke volume and an increased rate of ventricular ejection.

The *bisferiens pulse*, which has two systolic peaks, is characteristic of aortic regurgitation (with or without accompanying stenosis) and of hypertrophic cardiomyopathy (Chap. 238). In the latter condition, the pulse wave upstroke rises rapidly and forcefully, producing the first systolic peak ("percussion wave"). A brief decline in pressure follows because of the sudden midsystolic decrease in the rate of left ventricular ejection, when severe obstruction often develops. This pressure trough is followed by a smaller and more slowly rising positive pulse wave ("tidal wave") produced by continued ventricular ejection and by reflected waves from the periphery. The *dicrotic pulse* has two palpable waves, one in systole and one in diastole. It usually denotes a very low stroke volume, particularly in patients with dilated cardiomyopathy.

Pulsus alternans is a pattern in which there is regular alteration of the pressure pulse amplitude, despite a regular rhythm (Fig. 225-2). It is due to alternating left ventricular contractile force, usually indicates severe impairment of left ventricular function, and commonly occurs in patients who also have a loud third heart sound. Pulsus alternans may also occur during or following paroxysmal tachycardia or for several beats following a premature beat in patients without heart disease. In *pulsus bigeminus*, there is also a regular alteration of pressure pulse amplitude, but it is caused by a premature ventricular contraction that follows each regular beat. In *pulsus paradoxus*, the decrease in systolic arterial pressure that normally accompanies the reduction in arterial pulse amplitude during inspiration is accentuated. In patients with pericardial tamponade (Chap. 239), airway obstruction, or superior vena cava obstruction, the decrease in systolic arterial pressure frequently exceeds the normal decrease of 10 mmHg and the peripheral pulse may disappear completely during inspiration.

Simultaneous palpation of the radial and femoral arterial pulses, which normally are virtually coincident, is important to rule out aortic coarctation, in which the latter pulse is weakened and delayed (Chap. 234).

JUGULAR VENOUS PULSE (JVP) The two main objectives of the examination of the neck veins are inspection of their waveform and estimation of the central venous pressure (CVP). In most patients, the right internal jugular vein is best for both purposes. Usually, the pulsation of the internal jugular vein is greatest when the trunk is inclined by less than 30°. In patients with elevated venous pressure, it may be necessary to elevate the trunk further, sometimes to as much as 90°. When the neck muscles are relaxed, shining a beam of light tangentially across the skin overlying the vein exposes the pulsations of the internal jugular vein. Simultaneous palpation of the left carotid artery aids the examiner in deciding which pulsations are venous and in relating the venous pulsations to their timing in the cardiac cycle.

The normal JVP reflects phasic pressure changes in the right atrium and consists of two or sometimes three positive waves and two negative troughs (Fig. 225-1). The positive presystolic *a* wave is produced by venous distention due to right atrial contraction and is the dominant wave in the JVP, particularly during inspiration. Large *a* waves indicate that the right atrium is contracting against an increased resistance (Fig. 225-3), such as occurs with tricuspid stenosis or more commonly with increased resistance to right ventricular filling (pulmonary hypertension or pulmonic stenosis). Large *a* waves also occur during arrhythmias whenever the right atrium contracts while the tricuspid valve is closed by right ventricular systole. Such "cannon" *a* waves may occur regularly (as during junctional rhythm) or irregularly (as in

FIGURE 225-3 Abnormal jugular venous pulse waveforms commonly present in patients with cardiac disease and/or arrhythmias. See text. [*Modified from RA O'Rourke, in Hurst's The Heart, 9th ed, RW Alexander et al (eds). New York, McGraw-Hill, 1990, with permission.*]

atrioventricular dissociation with ventricular tachycardia or complete heart block). The *a* wave is absent in patients with atrial fibrillation, and there is an increased delay between the *a* wave and the carotid arterial pulse in patients with first-degree atrioventricular block.

The *c* wave, often observed in the JVP, is a positive wave produced by the bulging of the tricuspid valve into the right atrium during right ventricular isovolumetric systole and by the impact of the carotid artery adjacent to the jugular vein. The *x* descent is due both to atrial relaxation and to the downward displacement of the tricuspid valve during ventricular systole. The *x* descent wave during systole is often accentuated in patients with constrictive pericarditis (Fig. 225-3), but the nadir of this wave is reduced with right ventricular dilation and is often reversed in tricuspid regurgitation. The positive, late systolic *v* wave results from the increasing volume of blood in the right atrium during ventricular systole when the tricuspid valve is closed. Tricuspid regurgitation causes the *v* wave to be more prominent; when tricuspid regurgitation becomes severe, the combination of a prominent *v* wave and obliteration of the *x* descent results in a single large positive systolic wave. After the *v* wave peaks, the right atrial pressure falls because of the decreased bulging of the tricuspid valve into the right atrium as right ventricular pressure declines and the tricuspid valve opens (Fig. 225-3).

This negative descending limb—the *y* descent of the JVP—is produced mainly by the opening of the tricuspid valve and the subsequent rapid inflow of blood into the right ventricle. A rapid, deep *y* descent in early diastole occurs with severe tricuspid regurgitation. A venous pulse characterized by a sharp *y* descent, a deep *y* trough, and a rapid ascent to the baseline is seen in patients with constrictive pericarditis or with severe right-sided heart failure and a high venous pressure. A slow *y* descent in the JVP suggests an obstruction to right ventricular filling, as occurs with tricuspid stenosis or right atrial myxoma.

The right internal jugular is the best vein to use for accurate estimation of the CVP. The sternal angle is used as the reference point, because the center of the right atrium lies approximately 5 cm below the sternal angle in the average patient, regardless of body position. The patient is examined at the optimal degree of trunk elevation for visualization of venous pulsations. The vertical distance between the top of the oscillating venous column and the level of the sternal angle is determined; generally it is less than 3 cm (3 cm + 5 cm = 8 cm blood). The most common cause of a high venous pressure is an elevated right ventricular diastolic pressure. In patients suspected of having right ventricular failure who have a normal CVP at rest, the abdominojugular reflux test may be helpful. The palm of the examiner's hand is placed over the abdomen, and firm pressure is applied for 10 s or more. In normal persons, this maneuver does not alter the jugular venous pressure significantly, but when right heart function is impaired, the upper level of venous pulsation usually increases. A positive abdominojugular test is best defined as an increase in JVP during 10 s of firm midabdominal compression followed by a rapid

drop in pressure of 4 cm blood on release of the compression. The most common cause of a positive test is right-sided heart failure secondary to elevated left heart filling pressures. Also, abdominal compression may elicit the JVP pattern typical of tricuspid regurgitation when the resting pulse wave is normal. *Kussmaul's sign*—an increase rather than the normal decrease in the CVP during inspiration—is most often caused by severe right-sided heart failure; it is a frequent finding in patients with constrictive pericarditis or right ventricular infarction.

PRECORDIAL PALPATION The location, amplitude, duration, and direction of the cardiac impulse usually can be best appreciated with the fingertips. The normal left ventricular apex impulse is located at or medial to the left midclavicular line in the fourth or fifth intercostal space and is a tapping, early systolic outward thrust localized to a point usually less than 2.5 cm in diameter. It is due primarily to recoil of the heart as blood is ejected and should be evaluated with the patient supine and in the left lateral position. Left ventricular hypertrophy results in exaggeration of the amplitude, duration, and often size of the normal left ventricular thrust. The impulse may be displaced laterally and downward into the sixth or seventh interspace, particularly in patients with a left ventricular volume load such as occurs in cases of aortic regurgitation or dilated cardiomyopathy.

Additional abnormal features that are detectable at the left ventricular apex include marked presystolic distention of the left ventricle, which is often accompanied by a fourth heart sound in patients with an excessive left ventricular pressure load or myocardial ischemia/infarction, and a prominent early diastolic rapid-filling wave, which is often accompanied by a third heart sound in patients with left ventricular failure or mitral valve regurgitation (Fig. 225-1). A double systolic apical impulse is often palpable in patients with hypertrophic cardiomyopathy.

Right ventricular hypertrophy often results in a sustained systolic lift at the lower left parasternal area, which starts in early systole and is synchronous with the left ventricular apical impulse.

Abnormal precordial pulsations occur during systole in patients with left ventricular dyssynergy due to ischemic heart disease or to diffuse myocardial disease from some other cause. These pulsations often occur in patients with a recent myocardial infarction and may be present in some patients only during episodes of angina. They are most commonly felt in the left midprecordium one or two interspaces above and/or 1 to 2 cm medial to the left ventricular apex. A systolic bulge occurring in the region of the apex is difficult to distinguish from the impulse of left ventricular hypertrophy.

A left parasternal lift is frequently present in patients with severe mitral regurgitation. This pulsation occurs distinctly later than the left ventricular apical impulse, is synchronous with the *v* wave in the left atrial pressure curve, and is due to anterior displacement of the right ventricle by an enlarged, expanding left atrium. A similar impulse occurs to the right of the sternum in some patients with severe tricuspid regurgitation and a giant right atrium. Pulsation of the right sternoclavicular joint may indicate a right-sided aortic arch or aneurysmal dilation of the ascending aorta. Pulmonary artery pulsation is often visible and palpable in the second left intercostal space. While it may be normal in children or thin young adults, this pulsation usually denotes pulmonary hypertension, increased pulmonary blood flow, or poststenotic pulmonary artery dilation.

Thrills are palpable, low-frequency vibrations associated with heart murmurs. The systolic murmur of mitral regurgitation may be palpated at the cardiac apex. When the palm of the hand is placed over the precordium, the thrill of aortic stenosis crosses the palm toward the right side of the neck, while the thrill of pulmonic stenosis radiates more often to the left side of the neck. The thrill due to a ventricular septal defect is usually located in the third and fourth intercostal spaces near the left sternal border.

Percussion should be performed in each patient to identify normal or abnormal position of the heart, stomach, and liver. However, in patients with a normal cardiac situs, percussion adds little to careful inspection and palpation in the recognition of cardiac enlargement.

CARDIAC AUSCULTATION

To obtain the most information from cardiac auscultation, the observer should keep in mind several principles: (1) Auscultation should be performed in a quiet room to avoid the distracting noises of normal activity. (2) For optimal auscultation, attention must be focused on the phase of the cardiac cycle during which the auscultatory event is expected to occur. (3) The timing of a heart sound or murmur can be determined accurately from its relation to other observable events in the cardiac cycle—the carotid arterial pulse, the apical impulse, or the JVP. (4) To define the significance of a cardiac sound or murmur, it is often necessary to observe alterations in its timing or intensity during various physiologic and/or pharmacologic interventions (Table 225-1).

HEART SOUNDS   The major components of heart sounds are vibrations associated with the abrupt acceleration or deceleration of blood in the cardiovascular system. Studies using simultaneous echocardiographic-phonocardiographic recordings indicate that the first and second heart sounds are produced primarily by the closure of the atrioventricular (AV) and semilunar valves and the events that accompany these closures. The intensity of the *first heart sound* (S_1) is influenced by (1) the position of the mitral leaflets at the onset of ventricular systole; (2) the rate of rise of the left ventricular pressure pulse; (3) the presence or absence of structural disease of the mitral valve; and (4) the amount of tissue, air, or fluid between the heart and the stethoscope. S_1 is louder if diastole is shortened because of tachycar-

Table 225-1   Effects of Physiologic and Pharmacologic Interventions on the Intensity of Heart Murmurs and Sounds

Respiration   Systolic murmurs due to TR or pulmonic blood flow through a normal or stenotic valve and diastolic murmurs of TS or PR generally increase with inspiration, as do right-sided S_3 and S_4. Left-sided murmurs and sounds usually are louder during expiration.

Valsalva maneuver   Most murmurs decrease in length and intensity. Two exceptions are the systolic murmur of HCM, which usually becomes much louder, and that of MVP, which becomes longer and often louder. Following release of the Valsalva maneuver, right-sided murmurs tend to return to control intensity earlier than left-sided murmurs.

After VPB or AF   Murmurs originating at normal or stenotic semilunar valves increase in the cardiac cycle following a VPB or in the cycle after a long cycle length in AF. By contrast, systolic murmurs due to AV valve regurgitation either do not change, diminish (papillary muscle dysfunction), or become shorter (MVP).

Positional changes   With *standing*, most murmurs diminish, two exceptions being the murmur of HCM, which becomes louder, and that of MVP, which lengthens and often is intensified. With *squatting*, most murmurs become louder, but those of HCM and MVP usually soften and may disappear. Passive leg raising usually produces the same results.

Exercise   Murmurs due to blood flow across normal or obstructed valves (e.g., PS, MS) become louder with both isotonic and submaximal isometric (handgrip) exercise. Murmurs of MR, VSD, and AR also increase with handgrip exercise. However, the murmur of HCM often decreases with near maximum handgrip exercise. Left-sided S_4 and S_3 are often accentuated by exercise, particularly when due to ischemic heart disease.

Pharmacologic interventions   During the initial relative hypotension following amyl nitrite inhalation, murmurs of MR, VSD, and AR decrease, while murmurs of aortic stenosis or sclerosis increase. During the later tachycardia phase, murmurs of MS and right-sided lesions also increase. The response in MVP often is biphasic (first softer and then louder than control). The arterial constrictor phenylephrine tends to produce the opposite effects.

Transient arterial occlusion   Transient external compression of both arms by bilateral cuff inflation to 20 mmHg over peak systolic pressure augments the murmurs of MR, VSD, and AR, but not murmurs due to other causes.

NOTE: TR, tricuspid regurgitation; TS, tricuspid stenosis; PR, pulmonic regurgitation; HCM, hypertrophic cardiomyopathy; MVP, mitral valve prolapse; PS, pulmonic stenosis; MS, mitral stenosis; MR, mitral regurgitation; VSD, ventricular septal defect; AR, aortic regurgitation; VPB, ventricular premature beat; and AF, atrial fibrillation.

dia, if atrioventricular flow is increased because of high cardiac output or prolonged because of mitral stenosis, or if atrial contraction precedes ventricular contraction by an unusually short interval, reflected in a short PR interval. The loud S_1 in mitral stenosis usually signifies that the valve is pliable and that it remains open at the onset of isovolumetric contraction because of the elevated left atrial pressure. A soft S_1 may be due to poor conduction of sound through the chest wall, a slow rise of the left ventricular pressure pulse, a long PR interval, or imperfect closure due to reduced valve substance, as in mitral regurgitation. S_1 is also soft when the anterior mitral leaflet is immobile because of rigidity and calcification, even in the presence of predominant mitral stenosis.

Splitting of the two high-pitched components of S_1 by 10 to 30 ms is a normal phenomenon (Fig. 225-1). The first component of S_1 is attributed to mitral valve closure, and the second to tricuspid valve closure. Widening of the S_1 is due most often to complete right bundle branch block and the resulting delay in onset of the right ventricular pressure pulse. Reversed splitting of the S_1, in which the mitral component follows the tricuspid component, may be present in patients with severe mitral stenosis, left atrial myxoma, and left bundle branch block.

Splitting of the *second heart sound* (S_2) into audibly distinct aortic (A_2) and pulmonic (P_2) components normally occurs during inspiration, when the augmented inflow into the right ventricle increases its stroke volume and ejection period and thus delays closure of the pulmonic valve. P_2 is coincident with the incisura of the pulmonary artery pressure curve, which is separated from the right ventricular pressure tracing by an interval termed the "hangout time." The absolute value of this interval reflects the resistance to pulmonary blood flow and the impedance characteristics of the pulmonary vascular bed. This interval is prolonged, and physiologic splitting of S_2 is accentuated, in conditions associated with right ventricular volume overload and a distensible pulmonary vascular bed. However, in patients with an increase in pulmonary vascular resistance, the hangout time is markedly reduced, and narrow splitting of S_2 is present. Splitting that persists with expiration (heard best at the pulmonic area or left sternal border) is usually abnormal when the patient is in the upright position. Such splitting may be due to many causes: delayed activation of the right ventricle (right bundle branch block); left ventricular ectopic beats; a left ventricular pacemaker; prolongation of right ventricular contraction with an increased right ventricular pressure load (pulmonary embolism or pulmonic stenosis); or delayed pulmonic valve closure because of right ventricular volume overload associated with right ventricular failure or diminished impedance of the pulmonary vascular bed and a prolonged hangout time (atrial septal defect).

In pulmonary hypertension, P_2 is loud, and splitting of the second heart sound may be diminished, normal, or accentuated, depending on the cause of the pulmonary hypertension, the pulmonary vascular resistance, and the presence or absence of right ventricular decompensation. Early aortic valve closure, occurring with mitral regurgitation or a ventricular septal defect, may also produce splitting that persists during expiration. It may also occur with constrictive pericarditis. In patients with an atrial septal defect, the proportion of right atrial filling contributed by the left atrium and the venae cavae varies reciprocally during the respiratory cycle, so that right atrial inflow remains relatively constant. Therefore, the volume and duration of right ventricular ejection are not significantly increased by inspiration, and there is little inspiratory exaggeration of the splitting of S_2. This phenomenon, termed *fixed splitting* of the second heart sound, is of considerable diagnostic value.

A delay in aortic valve closure causing P_2 to precede A_2 results in so-called reversed (paradoxic) splitting of S_2. Splitting is then maximal in expiration and decreases during inspiration with the normal delay of pulmonic valve closure. The most common causes of reversed splitting of S_2 are left bundle branch block and delayed excitation of the left ventricle from a right ventricular ectopic beat. Mechanical prolongation of left ventricular systole, resulting in reversed splitting of S_2, may also be caused by severe aortic outflow obstruction, a large aorta-to-pulmonary artery shunt, systolic hypertension, and ischemic heart disease or cardiomyopathy with left ventricular failure. P_2 is normally softer than A_2 in the second left intercostal space; a P_2 that is greater than A_2 in this area suggests pulmonary hypertension, except in patients with atrial septal defect.

The *third heart sound* (S_3) is a low-pitched sound produced in the ventricle 0.14 to 0.16 s after A_2, at the termination of rapid filling. This sound is frequent in normal children and in patients with high cardiac output. However, in patients over 40 years old, an S_3 usually indicates impairment of ventricular function, AV valve regurgitation, or other conditions that increase the rate or volume of ventricular filling. The left-sided S_3 is best heard with the bell piece of the stethoscope at the left ventricular apex during expiration and with the patient in the left lateral position. The right-sided S_3 is best heard at the left sternal border or just beneath the xiphoid and is usually louder with inspiration. Often it is accompanied by the systolic murmur of functional tricuspid regurgitation. Third heart sounds often disappear with treatment of heart failure.

An S_3 that is earlier (0.10 to 0.12 s after A_2) and higher-pitched than normal (a pericardial knock) often occurs in patients with constrictive pericarditis (Chap. 239); its presence depends on the restrictive effect of the adherent pericardium, which halts diastolic filling abruptly.

The *opening snap* (OS) is a brief, high-pitched, early diastolic sound, which is usually due to stenosis of an AV valve, most often the mitral valve. It is generally heard best at the lower left sternal border and radiates well to the base of the heart. The A_2-OS interval is inversely related to the height of the mean left atrial pressure and ranges from 0.04 to 0.12 s. In the second intercostal space, an OS is often confused with P_2. However, careful auscultation will reveal both components of S_2, followed by the OS. The OS of tricuspid stenosis occurs later in diastole than the mitral OS and is often overlooked in patients with more prominent mitral valve disease.

The *fourth heart sound* (S_4) is a low-pitched, presystolic sound produced in the ventricle during ventricular filling; it is associated with an effective atrial contraction and is best heard with the bell piece of the stethoscope. The sound is absent in patients with atrial fibrillation. The S_4 occurs when diminished ventricular compliance increases the resistance to ventricular filling, and it is frequently present in patients with systemic hypertension, aortic stenosis, hypertrophic cardiomyopathy, ischemic heart disease, and acute mitral regurgitation. Most patients with an acute myocardial infarction and sinus rhythm have an audible S_4. The fourth heart sound is frequently accompanied by visible and palpable presystolic distention of the left ventricle. It is loudest at the left ventricular apex when the patient is in the left lateral position and is accentuated by mild isotonic or isometric exercise in the supine position. The right-sided S_4 is present in patients with right ventricular hypertrophy secondary to either pulmonic stenosis or pulmonary hypertension and frequently accompanies a prominent presystolic *a* wave in the JVP.

An S_4 frequently accompanies delayed AV conduction even in the absence of clinically detectable heart disease. The incidence of an audible S_4 increases with increasing age. Whether an audible S_4 in adults without other evidence of cardiac disease is abnormal remains controversial.

The *ejection sound* is a sharp, high-pitched event occurring in early systole and closely following the first heart sound. Ejection sounds occur in the presence of semilunar valve stenosis and in conditions associated with dilation of the aorta or pulmonary artery. The aortic ejection sound is usually heard best at the left ventricular apex and the second right intercostal space; the pulmonary ejection sound is loudest at the upper left sternal border. The latter, unlike most other right-sided acoustical events, is heard better during expiration.

Nonejection or *midsystolic clicks*, occurring with or without a late systolic murmur, often denote prolapse of one or both leaflets of the mitral valve (Chap. 236). They also may be caused by tricuspid valve prolapse. They probably result from chordae tendineae that are functionally unequal in length on either or both AV valves and are heard

best along the lower left sternal border and at the left ventricular apex. Systolic clicks may be single or multiple, and they may occur at any time in systole but are usually later than the systolic ejection sound.

HEART MURMURS (See also Chap. 34) Cardiac murmurs result from vibrations set up in the bloodstream and the surrounding heart and great vessels as a result of turbulent blood flow, the formation of eddies, and cavitation (bubble formation as a result of sudden decrease in pressure).

The intensity (loudness) of murmurs may be graded from I to VI. A grade I murmur is so faint that it can be heard only with special effort; a grade IV murmur is commonly accompanied by a thrill; and a grade VI murmur is audible with the stethoscope removed from contact with the chest. The configuration of a murmur may be crescendo, decrescendo, crescendo-decrescendo (diamond-shaped), or plateau. The precise time of onset and time of cessation of a murmur depend on the instant in the cardiac cycle at which an adequate pressure difference between two chambers arises and disappears (Fig. 225-4).

The location on the chest wall where the murmur is best heard and the areas to which it radiates can aid in identifying the cardiac structure from which the murmur originates. For example, the murmur of aortic valve stenosis is usually loudest in the second right intercostal space and radiates to the carotid arteries. By contrast, the murmur of mitral regurgitation is most often loudest at the cardiac apex. It may radiate to the left sternal border and base of the heart when the posterior mitral leaflet is predominantly involved or to the axilla and back when the anterior leaflet is more severely affected. In the latter case, the regurgitant blood is directed toward the posterior left atrial wall.

It is often difficult to classify a cardiac murmur with certainty on the basis of its timing, configuration, location, radiation, pitch, or intensity. However, by noting changes in the characteristics of the murmur during maneuvers that alter cardiac hemodynamics, the auscultator can often identify its correct origin and significance (Table 225-1).

FIGURE 225-4 *A.* Schematic representation of ECG, aortic pressure (AOP), left ventricular pressure (LVP), and left atrial pressure (LAP). The shaded areas indicate a transvalvular pressure difference during systole. HSM, holosystolic murmur; MSM, midsystolic murmur. *B.* Graphic representation of ECG, aortic pressure (AOP), left ventricular pressure (LVP) and left atrial pressure (LAP) with shaded areas indicating transvalvular diastolic pressure difference. EDM, early diastolic murmur; PSM, presystolic murmur; MDM, middiastolic murmur.

Accentuation of a murmur during inspiration (a maneuver that augments systemic venous return) implies that it originates on the right side of the circulation; expiratory exaggeration has less significance. Prolonged expiratory pressure against a closed glottis (i.e., the Valsalva maneuver) reduces the intensity of most murmurs by diminishing both right and left ventricular filling (i.e., ventricular preload). The systolic murmur associated with *hypertrophic cardiomyopathy* and the late systolic murmur due to *mitral valve prolapse* are exceptions and may be paradoxically accentuated during the Valsalva maneuver. Murmurs due to flow across a normal or obstructed semilunar valve increase in intensity in the cycle following a premature ventricular beat or a long RR interval in atrial fibrillation. In contrast, murmurs due to AV valve regurgitation or a ventricular septal defect do not change appreciably during the beat following a prolonged diastole. Standing, which decreases left ventricular volume, accentuates the murmur of hypertrophic cardiomyopathy and occasionally the murmur due to mitral valve prolapse. Squatting, which increases both venous return and systemic arterial resistance and thus ventricular afterload, increases most murmurs, except those due to hypertrophic cardiomyopathy and mitral regurgitation due to a prolapsed mitral valve, which often decrease. Sustained handgrip exercise, which increases systemic arterial pressure and heart rate, often accentuates the murmurs of mitral regurgitation, aortic regurgitation, and mitral stenosis but usually diminishes those due to aortic stenosis or hypertrophic cardiomyopathy. Pharmacologic interventions include inhalation of amyl nitrite, which reduces systemic arterial pressure and increases blood flow, thereby increasing the intensity of murmurs due to valvular stenosis while diminishing those due to aortic or mitral regurgitation (Table 225-1). Transient external arterial occlusion by the inflation of bilateral arm cuffs to 20 mmHg (2.66 kPa) above systolic blood pressure for 5 s usually intensifies murmurs due to left-sided regurgitant lesions; this method is applicable to almost all patients and does not require administration of any drug.

Systolic Murmurs   *Holosystolic (pansystolic) murmurs* are generated when there is flow between two chambers that have widely different pressures throughout systole, such as the left ventricle and either the left atrium or the right ventricle (Fig. 225-4). The pressure gradient occurs early in contraction and lasts until relaxation is almost complete. Therefore, holosystolic murmurs begin before aortic ejection, and at the area of maximal intensity they begin with S_1 and end after S_2. Holosystolic murmurs accompany mitral or tricuspid regurgitation, ventricular septal defect, and, under certain circumstances, aortopulmonary shunts. Although the typical high-pitched murmur of mitral regurgitation usually continues throughout systole, the shape of the murmur may vary considerably. The holosystolic murmurs of mi-

tral regurgitation and ventricular septal defect are augmented by transient exercise and are diminished by lowering the left ventricular systolic pressure by inhalation of amyl nitrite. The murmur of tricuspid regurgitation associated with pulmonary hypertension is holosystolic and frequently increases during inspiration. Not all patients with mitral or tricuspid regurgitation or ventricular septal defect have holosystolic murmurs (Chap. 236). Often, a mild valvular regurgitant jet, detected by color flow Doppler techniques, is not associated with an audible murmur despite optimal auscultation. Such regurgitant jets usually do not indicate clinical heart disease. Trivial mitral regurgitation can be detected by Doppler in up to 45% of normal individuals; tricuspid regurgitation in up to 70%; and pulmonic regurgitation in up to 88%. Normal aortic regurgitation is encountered much less frequently, and its incidence increases with advancing age (Fig. 225-5).

Midsystolic murmurs, also called *systolic ejection murmurs*, which are often crescendo-decrescendo in shape, occur when blood is ejected across the aortic or pulmonic outflow tracts (Fig. 225-4). The murmur starts shortly after S_1, when the ventricular pressure becomes high enough to open the semilunar valve. As the velocity of ejection increases, the murmur gets louder; as ejection declines, it diminishes. The murmur ends before the ventricular pressure falls enough to permit closure of the aortic or pulmonic leaflets. When the semilunar valves are normal, an increased flow rate (as occurs in states of elevated cardiac output), ejection into a dilated vessel beyond the valve, or increased transmission of sound through a thin chest wall may be responsible for this murmur. Most benign, functional murmurs are midsystolic and originate from the pulmonary outflow tract. Valvular or subvalvular obstruction of either ventricle may also cause such a midsystolic murmur, the intensity being related to the flow rate.

The murmur of aortic stenosis is the prototype of the left-sided midsystolic murmur. The location and radiation of this murmur are influenced by the direction of the high-velocity jet within the aortic root. In *valvular aortic stenosis*, the murmur is usually maximal in the second right intercostal space, with radiation into the neck. In *supravalvular aortic stenosis*, the murmur is occasionally loudest even higher, with disproportionate radiation into the right carotid artery. In hypertrophic cardiomyopathy, the midsystolic murmur originates in the left ventricular cavity and is usually maximal at the lower left sternal edge and apex, with relatively little radiation to the carotids. When the aortic valve is immobile (calcified), the aortic closure sound (A_2) may be soft and inaudible so that the length and configuration of the murmur are difficult to determine. Midsystolic murmurs also occur in patients with mitral regurgitation or, less frequently, tricuspid regurgitation resulting from papillary muscle dysfunction. Such murmurs due to mitral regurgitation are often confused with those originating in the aorta, particularly in elderly patients.

The patient's age and the area of maximal intensity aid in determining the significance of midsystolic murmurs. Thus, in a young adult with a thin chest and a high velocity of blood flow, a faint or moderate midsystolic murmur heard only in the pulmonic area is usually without clinical significance, while a somewhat louder murmur in the aortic area may indicate congenital aortic stenosis. In elderly patients, pulmonic flow murmurs are rare, while aortic systolic murmurs are common and may be due to aortic dilation, to a significant degree of valvular aortic stenosis, or to nonstenotic thickening of the aortic valve leaflets. Midsystolic aortic and pulmonic murmurs are intensified after amyl nitrite inhalation and during the cardiac cycle following a premature ventricular beat, while those due to mitral regurgitation are unchanged or softer. Aortic systolic murmurs are diminished by interventions that increase aortic impedance, such as transient arterial occlu-

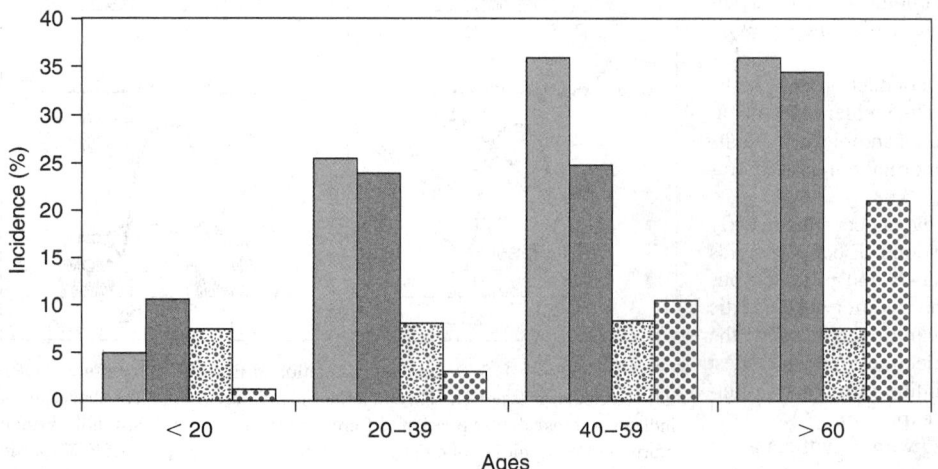

FIGURE 225-5   Percent incidence of mitral (shaded blue), tricuspid (shaded gray), pulmonic (stippled blue), and aortic (blue dots) regurgitation by Doppler echocardiography in clinically normal subjects at various ages. (*Modified from Choong et al.*)

sion. Echocardiography or cardiac catheterization may be necessary to separate a prominent and exaggerated functional murmur from one due to congenital or acquired semilunar valve stenosis.

Early systolic murmurs begin with the first heart sound and end in midsystole. In *large ventricular septal defects with pulmonary hypertension*, the shunting at the end of systole may be small or absent, resulting in an early systolic murmur. A similar murmur may occur with very *small muscular ventricular septal defects*, the shunt being interrupted in late systole. An early systolic murmur is a feature of *tricuspid regurgitation occurring in the absence of pulmonary hypertension*. This lesion is common in narcotics abusers with infective endocarditis, in whom a tall regurgitant right atrial *v* wave reaches the level of the normal right ventricular pressure in late systole, confining the murmur to early systole. Patients with acute mitral regurgitation into a noncompliant left atrium and a large *v* wave often have a loud early systolic murmur that diminishes as the pressure gradient between the left ventricle and left atrium decreases in late systole (Chap. 236).

Late systolic murmurs are faint or moderately loud, high-pitched apical murmurs that start well after ejection and do not mask either heart sound. They are probably related to papillary muscle dysfunction caused by infarction or ischemia of these muscles or to their distortion by left ventricular dilation. They may appear only during angina but are common in patients with myocardial infarction or diffuse myocardial disease. Late systolic murmurs following midsystolic clicks are due to late systolic mitral regurgitation caused by prolapse of the mitral valve into the left atrium (Chap. 236).

Diastolic Murmurs *Early diastolic murmurs* (Fig. 225-4) begin with or shortly after S_2, as soon as the corresponding ventricular pressure falls enough below that in the aorta or pulmonary artery. The high-pitched murmurs of aortic regurgitation or of pulmonic regurgitation due to pulmonary hypertension are generally decrescendo, since there is a progressive decline in the volume or rate of regurgitation during diastole. Faint, high-pitched murmurs of aortic regurgitation are difficult to hear unless they are specifically sought by applying firm pressure with the diaphragm over the left midsternal border while the patient sits leaning forward and holds a breath in full expiration. The diastolic murmur of aortic regurgitation is enhanced by an acute elevation of the arterial pressure, such as occurs with handgrip exercise; it diminishes with a decrease in arterial pressure, as with amyl nitrite inhalation. The diastolic murmur of congenital pulmonic regurgitation without pulmonary hypertension is low- to medium-pitched. The onset of this murmur is delayed because the regurgitant flow is minimal at the onset of pulmonic valve closure when the reverse pressure gradient responsible for the regurgitation is negligible.

Middiastolic murmurs usually arise from the mitral or tricuspid valves (Fig. 225-4), occur during early ventricular filling, and are due to disproportion between valve orifice size and flow rate. Such murmurs may be quite loud (grade III), despite only slight AV valve stenosis, when there is normal or increased blood flow. Conversely, the murmurs may be soft or even absent despite severe obstruction if the cardiac output is markedly reduced. When stenosis is marked, the diastolic murmur is prolonged, and the duration of the murmur is more reliable than its intensity as an index of the severity of valve obstruction.

The low-pitched, middiastolic murmur of mitral stenosis characteristically follows the OS. It should be specifically sought by placing the bell of the stethoscope at the site of the left ventricular impulse, which is best localized with the patient on the left side. Frequently, the murmur of mitral stenosis is present only at the left ventricular apex, and it may be increased in intensity by mild supine exercise or by inhalation of amyl nitrite. In tricuspid stenosis, the middiastolic murmur is localized to a relatively limited area along the left sternal edge and may be louder during inspiration.

Middiastolic murmurs may be generated across the mitral valve in cases of mitral regurgitation, patent ductus arteriosus, or ventricular septal defect, and across the tricuspid valve in cases of tricuspid regurgitation or atrial septal defect. These murmurs are related to the torrential flow across an AV valve, usually follow an S_3, and tend to

occur with large left-to-right shunts or severe AV valve regurgitation. A soft middiastolic murmur may sometimes be heard in patients with acute rheumatic fever (Carey-Coombs murmur). It has been attributed to inflammation of the mitral valve cusps or excessive left atrial blood flow as a consequence of mitral regurgitation.

In acute, severe aortic regurgitation, the left ventricular diastolic pressure may exceed the left atrial pressure, resulting in a middiastolic murmur due to "diastolic mitral regurgitation." In severe, chronic aortic regurgitation, a murmur is frequently present that may be either middiastolic or presystolic (Austin-Flint murmur). This murmur appears to originate at the anterior mitral valve leaflet when blood enters the left ventricle simultaneously from both the aortic root and the left atrium.

Presystolic murmurs begin during the period of ventricular filling that follows atrial contraction and therefore occur in sinus rhythm. They are usually due to AV valve stenosis and have the same quality as the middiastolic filling rumble, but they are usually crescendo, reaching peak intensity at the time of a loud S_1. The presystolic murmur corresponds to the AV valve gradient, which may be minimal until the moment of right or left atrial contraction. It is the presystolic murmur that is most characteristic of tricuspid stenosis and sinus rhythm. A right or left *atrial myxoma* may occasionally cause either middiastolic or presystolic murmurs that resemble the murmurs of mitral or tricuspid stenosis.

Continuous Murmurs These begin in systole, peak near S_2, and continue into all or part of diastole. These murmurs result from continuous flow due to a communication between high- and low-pressure areas that persists through the end of systole and the beginning of diastole. A *patent ductus arteriosus* causes a continuous murmur as long as the pressure in the pulmonary artery is much below that in the aorta. The murmur is intensified by elevation of the systemic arterial pressure and is reduced by amyl nitrite inhalation. When pulmonary hypertension is present, the diastolic portion may disappear, leaving the murmur confined to systole. A continuous murmur is uncommon in cases of aortopulmonary septal defect, which usually is associated with severe pulmonary hypertension. Surgically produced connections and the subclavian–pulmonary artery anastomosis result in murmurs similar to that of a patent ductus.

Continuous murmurs may result from congenital or acquired *systemic arteriovenous fistula, coronary arteriovenous fistula*, anomalous origin of the left coronary artery from the pulmonary artery, and communications between the *sinus of Valsalva and the right side of the heart*. Continuous murmurs may also occur in patients with a small atrial septal defect with a high left atrial pressure. Murmurs associated with *pulmonary arteriovenous fistulas* may be continuous but are usually only systolic. Continuous murmurs may also be due to disturbances of flow pattern in constricted systemic (e.g., renal) or pulmonary arteries when marked pressure differences between the two sides of the narrow segment persist; a continuous murmur in the back may be present in *coarctation of the aorta; pulmonary embolism* may cause continuous murmurs in partially occluded vessels.

In nonconstricted arteries, continuous murmurs may be due to rapid flow through a tortuous bed. Such murmurs typically occur within the bronchial arterial collateral circulation in cyanotic patients with severe pulmonary outflow obstruction. The "mammary souffle," an innocent murmur heard over the breasts during late pregnancy and in the early postpartum period, may be systolic or continuous. The innocent cervical venous hum is a continuous murmur usually audible over the medial aspect of the right supraclavicular fossa with the patient upright. The hum is usually louder during diastole and can be abolished instantaneously by digital compression of the ipsilateral internal jugular vein. Transmission of a loud venous hum to the area below the clavicles may result in a mistaken diagnosis of patent ductus arteriosus.

Pericardial Friction Rub These adventitious sounds may have presystolic, systolic, and early diastolic scratchy components, may be confused with a murmur or extracardiac sound when heard only in systole. It is best appreciated with the patient upright and leaning forward and may be accentuated during inspiration.

The evaluation of the patient with a heart murmur may vary greatly depending on many of the considerations discussed above. These include the intensity of the cardiac murmur, its timing in the cardiac cycle, its location and radiation, and its response to various physiologic maneuvers. Also of importance are the presence or absence of cardiac and noncardiac symptoms and whether other cardiac or noncardiac physical findings suggest that the cardiac murmur is clinically significant. The skill and confidence of the cardiac auscultator, the relative costs of various diagnostic approaches, and the accuracy and reliability of additional tests in the laboratory where they are performed are also important factors. One systematic approach to the patient with a heart murmur is depicted in Fig. 34-3. This algorithm is particularly applicable to children and adults under age 40.

BIBLIOGRAPHY

BRAUNWALD E: The clinical examination, in *Primary Cardiology*, L Goldman, E Braunwald (eds). Philadelphia, Saunders, 1998, pp 27–43

————: Physical examination of the heart and circulation, in *Heart Disease*, 6th ed, E Braunwald et al (eds). Philadelphia, Saunders, 2001

CHOONG CY et al: Prevalence of valvular regurgitation by Doppler echocardiography in patients with structurally normal hearts by 2-dimensional echocardiography. Am Heart J 117:636, 1989

CLEMENT DL, COHN JN: Salvaging the history, physical examination and doctor-patient relationship in a technological cardiology environment. J Am Coll Cardiol 33:892, 1999

CRAWFORD MH: *Examination of the Heart*, Part 2: *Inspection and Palpation of Venous and Arterial Pulses.* Chicago, American Heart Association, 1990

EILEN SD et al: Accuracy of precordial palpation for detecting increased left ventricular volume. Ann Intern Med 99:628, 1983

EWY GA: The abdominojugular test: Technique and hemodynamic correlates. Ann Intern Med 109:456, 1988

LEMBO NJ et al: Bedside diagnosis of systolic murmurs. N Engl J Med 318:1572, 1988

O'ROURKE RA: Approach to a patient with a heart murmur, in *Primary Cardiology*, L Goldman, E Braunwald (eds). Philadelphia, Saunders, 1998, pp 155–173

PERLOFF JK (ed): *Physical Examination of the Heart and Circulation*, 2d ed. Philadelphia, Saunders, 1990

SHAVER JA: Cardiac auscultation: A cost-effective diagnostic skill. Curr Probl Cardiol 20(7):441, 1995

YOSHIDA K et al: Color Doppler evaluation of valvular regurgitation in normals. Circulation 78:840, 1988

---

226   *Ary L. Goldberger*

ELECTROCARDIOGRAPHY

The electrocardiogram (ECG or EKG) is a graphic recording of electric potentials generated by the heart. The signals are detected by means of metal electrodes attached to the extremities and chest wall and are then amplified and recorded by the electrocardiograph. ECG *leads* actually display the instantaneous *differences* in potential between these electrodes.

The clinical utility of the ECG derives from its immediate availability as a noninvasive, inexpensive, and highly versatile test. In addition to its use in detecting arrhythmias, conduction disturbances, and myocardial ischemia, electrocardiography may reveal other findings related to life-threatening metabolic disturbances (e.g., hyperkalemia) or increased susceptibility to sudden cardiac death (e.g., QT prolongation syndromes). The advent of coronary thrombolysis or angioplasty in the early therapy of acute myocardial infarction (Chap. 243) has refocused particular attention on the sensitivity and specificity of ECG signs of myocardial ischemia.

ELECTROPHYSIOLOGY   (See also Chaps. 229 and 230)

Depolarization of the heart is the initiating event for cardiac contraction. The electric currents that spread through the heart are produced by three components: cardiac pacemaker cells, specialized conduction tissue, and the heart muscle itself. The ECG, however, records only the depolarization (stimulation) and repolarization (recovery) potentials generated by the atrial and ventricular myocardium. Under resting conditions, myocardial cells are *polarized*; that is, they carry an electric charge on their surface due to transmembrane ion concentration differences. The charge measured across atrial and ventricular cell membranes is about 90 mV, with the inside negative relative to the outside. When these cells are stimulated above a critical threshold potential, they rapidly depolarize and transiently reverse their membrane polarity. This depolarization process spreads in a wavelike manner through the atria and ventricles. The return of myocardial fibers to their original resting state occurs during repolarization.

The depolarization stimulus for the normal heartbeat originates in the sinoatrial (SA) *node* (Fig. 226-1) or *sinus node*, a collection of *pacemaker* cells. These cells fire spontaneously; that is, they exhibit *automaticity*. The first phase of cardiac electrical activation is the spread of the depolarization wave through the right and left atria, followed by atrial contraction. Next, the impulse stimulates pacemaker and specialized conduction tissues in the atrioventricular (AV) nodal and His-bundle areas; together, these two regions constitute the AV junction. The bundle of His bifurcates into two main branches, the right and left bundles, which rapidly transmit depolarization wavefronts to the right and left ventricular myocardium by way of Purkinje fibers. The main left bundle bifurcates into two primary subdivisions, a left anterior fascicle and a left posterior fascicle. The depolarization wavefronts then spread through the ventricular wall, from endocardium to epicardium, triggering ventricular contraction.

Since the cardiac depolarization and repolarization waves have direction and magnitude, they can be represented by vectors. *Vectorcardiograms* that measure and display these instantaneous potentials are no longer used much in clinical practice. However, the general principles of vector analysis remain fundamental to understanding the genesis of normal and pathologic ECG waveforms. Vector analysis illustrates a central concept of electrocardiography—that the ECG records the complex spatial and temporal summation of electrical potentials from multiple myocardial fibers conducted to the surface of the body. This principle accounts for inherent limitations in both ECG *sensitivity* (activity from certain cardiac regions may be canceled out or may be too weak to be recorded) and *specificity* (the same vectorial sum can result from either a selective gain or a loss of forces in opposite directions).

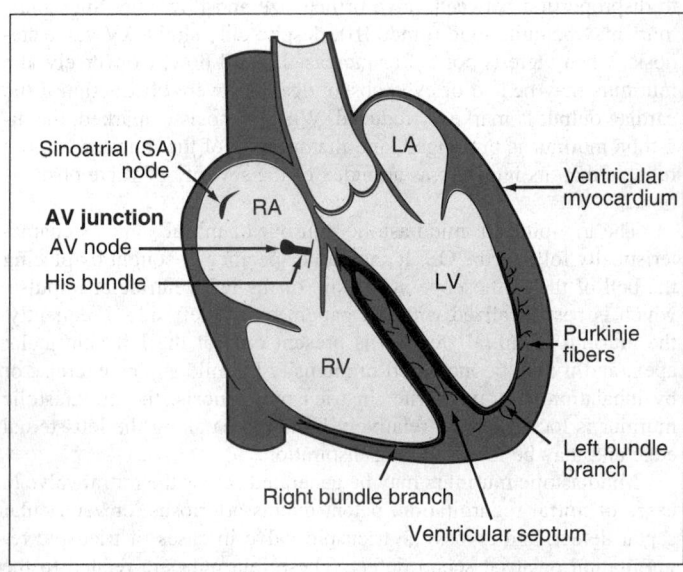

FIGURE 226-1 Schematic of the cardiac conduction system.

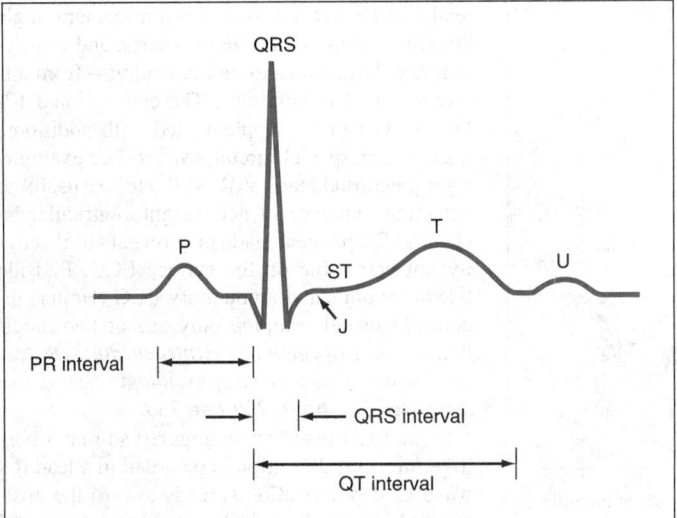

FIGURE 226-2 Basic ECG waveforms and intervals. Not shown is the R-R interval, the time between consecutive QRS complexes.

FIGURE 226-3 The QRS-T cycle corresponds to different phases of the ventricular action potential as described in Chap. 229.

ECG WAVEFORMS AND INTERVALS The ECG waveforms are labeled alphabetically, beginning with the P wave, which represents atrial depolarization (Fig. 226-2). The QRS complex represents ventricular depolarization, and the ST-T-U complex (ST segment, T wave, and U wave) represents ventricular repolarization. The J point is the junction between the end of the QRS complex and the beginning of the ST segment. Atrial repolarization is usually too low in amplitude to be detected, but it may become apparent in such conditions as acute pericarditis or atrial infarction.

The QRS-T waveforms of the surface (extracellular) ECG correspond in a general way with the different phases of simultaneously obtained ventricular *action potentials*, the intracellular recordings from single myocardial fibers (Fig. 226-3) (Chap. 229). The rapid upstroke (phase 0) of the action potential corresponds to the onset of QRS. The plateau (phase 2) corresponds to the

isoelectric ST segment, and active repolarization (phase 3) to the inscription of the T wave. Factors that decrease the slope of phase 0 by impairing the influx of Na^+ (e.g., drugs such as quinidine or procainamide, or hyperkalemia) tend to increase QRS duration. Conditions that prolong phase 2 (amiodarone, hypocalcemia) increase the QT interval. In contrast, shortening of ventricular repolarization (phase 2), as by digitalis or hypercalcemia, abbreviates the ST segment.

The electrocardiogram is ordinarily recorded on special graph paper which is divided into 1-mm² gridlike boxes (Fig. 226-4). Since the ECG paper speed is generally 25 mm/s, the smallest (1 mm) horizontal divisions correspond to 0.04 s (40 ms), with heavier lines at intervals of 0.20 s (200 ms). Vertically, the ECG graph measures the amplitude of a given wave or deflection (1 mV = 10 mm with standard calibration; the voltage criteria for hypertrophy mentioned below are given in millimeters). There are four major ECG intervals: R-R, PR, QRS, and QT (Fig. 226-2). The heart rate (beats per minute) can be readily computed from the interbeat (R-R) interval by dividing the number of large (0.20 s) time units between consecutive R waves into 300 or the number of small (0.04 s) units into 1500. The PR interval measures the time (normally 120 to 200 ms) between atrial and ventricular depolarization, which includes the physiologic delay imposed by stimulation of cells in the AV junction area. The QRS interval (normally 100 ms or less) reflects the duration of ventricular depolarization. The QT interval includes both ventricular depolarization and repolarization times and varies inversely with the heart rate. A rate-related ("corrected") QT interval, QT_c, can be calculated as $QT/\sqrt{R\text{-}R}$ and normally is ≤ 0.44 s.

The QRS complex is subdivided into specific deflections or waves. If the initial QRS deflection in a given lead is negative, it is termed a *Q wave*; the first positive deflection is termed an *R wave*. A negative deflection after an R wave is an *S wave*. Subsequent positive or negative waves are labeled R′ and S′, respectively. Lowercase letters (qrs) are used for waves of relatively small amplitude. An entirely negative QRS complex is termed a *QS wave*.

ECG LEADS The 12 conventional ECG leads record the difference in potential between electrodes placed on the surface of the body. These leads are divided into two groups: six extremity (limb) leads and six chest (precordial) leads. The extremity leads record potentials transmitted onto the *frontal plane* (Fig. 226-5A), and the chest leads record potentials transmitted onto the *horizontal plane* (Fig. 226-5B). The six extremity leads are further subdivided into three *bipolar* leads (I, II, and III) and three *unipolar* leads (aVR, aVL, and aVF). Each bipolar lead measures the difference in potential between electrodes at two extremities: lead I = left arm–right arm voltages, lead II = left leg–right arm, and lead III = left leg–left arm. The unipolar

FIGURE 226-4 The ECG graph paper records the time (interval) between cardiac electrical events along the horizontal axis and their amplitude (voltage) along the vertical axis.

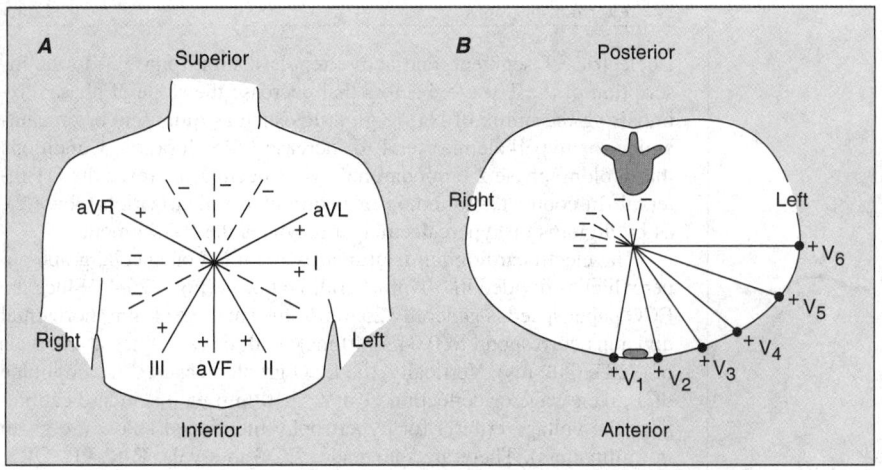

FIGURE 226-5 The six frontal plane (*A*) and six horizontal plane (*B*) leads provide a three-dimensional representation of cardiac electrical activity.

leads measure the voltage (V) at one locus relative to an electrode (called the *central terminal* or *indifferent electrode*) that has approximately zero potential. Thus, aVR = right arm, aVL = left arm, and aVF = left leg (foot). The lowercase *a* indicates that these unipolar potentials are electrically augmented by 50 percent. The right leg electrode functions as a ground. The spatial orientation and polarity of the six frontal plane leads is represented on the hexaxial diagram (Fig. 226-6).

The six chest leads (Fig. 226-7) are unipolar recordings obtained by electrodes in the following positions: lead V_1, fourth intercostal space, just to the right of the sternum; lead V_2, fourth intercostal space, just to the left of the sternum; lead V_3, midway between V_2 and V_4; lead V_4, midclavicular line, fifth intercostal space; lead V_5, anterior axillary line, same level as V_4; and lead V_6, midaxillary line, same level as V_4 and V_5.

Together, the frontal and horizontal plane electrodes provide a three-dimensional representation of cardiac electrical activity. Each

lead can be likened to a different camera angle "looking" at the same events—atrial and ventricular depolarization and repolarization—from different spatial orientations. The conventional 12-lead ECG can be supplemented with additional leads under special circumstances. For example, right precordial leads V_3R, V_4R, etc. are useful in detecting evidence of acute right ventricular ischemia. Esophageal leads may reveal atrial activity not detectable on the surface ECG. Bedside telemetry units and ambulatory ECG (Holter) recordings usually employ only one or two modified leads, respectively. →*Intracardiac electrocardiography and electrophysiologic testing are discussed in Chaps. 229 and 230.*

The ECG leads are configured so that a positive (upright) deflection is recorded in a lead if a wave of depolarization spreads toward the positive pole of that lead, and a negative deflection if the wave spreads toward the negative pole. If the mean orientation of the depolarization vector is at right angles to a given lead axis, a biphasic (equally positive and negative) deflection will be recorded.

GENESIS OF THE NORMAL ECG

P WAVE The normal atrial depolarization vector is oriented downward and toward the subject's left, reflecting the spread of depolarization from the sinus node to the right and then the left atrial myocardium. Since this vector points toward the positive pole of lead II and toward the negative pole of lead aVR, the normal P wave will be positive in lead II and negative in lead aVR. By contrast, activation of the atria from an ectopic pacemaker in the lower part of either atrium or in the AV junction region may produce retrograde P waves (negative in lead II, positive in lead aVR).

QRS COMPLEX Normal ventricular depolarization proceeds as a rapid, continuous spread of activation wavefronts. This complex process can be divided into two major, sequential phases, and each phase can be represented by a mean vector (Fig. 226-8). The first phase is depolarization of the interventricular septum from the left to the right (vector 1). The second results from the simultaneous depolarization of the main mass of the right and left ventricles; it is normally dominated by the more massive left ventricle, so that vector 2 points leftward and posteriorly. Therefore, a right precordial lead (V_1) will record this biphasic depolarization process with a small positive deflection (septal r wave) followed by a larger negative deflection (S

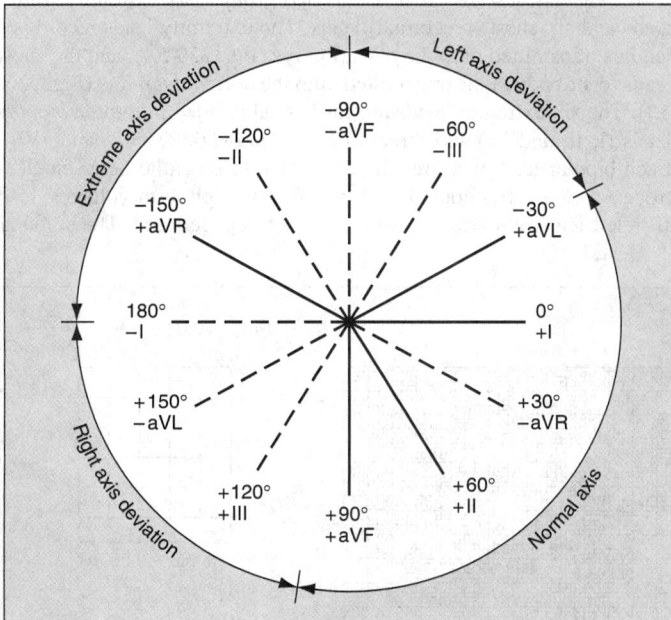

FIGURE 226-6 The frontal plane (extremity or limb) leads are represented on a hexaxial diagram. Each ECG lead has a specific spatial orientation and polarity. The positive pole of each lead axis (*solid line*) and negative pole (*hatched line*) are designated by their angular position relative to the positive pole of lead I (0°). The mean electrical axis of the QRS complex is measured with respect to this display.

FIGURE 226-7 The horizontal plane (chest or precordial) leads are obtained with electrodes in the locations shown.

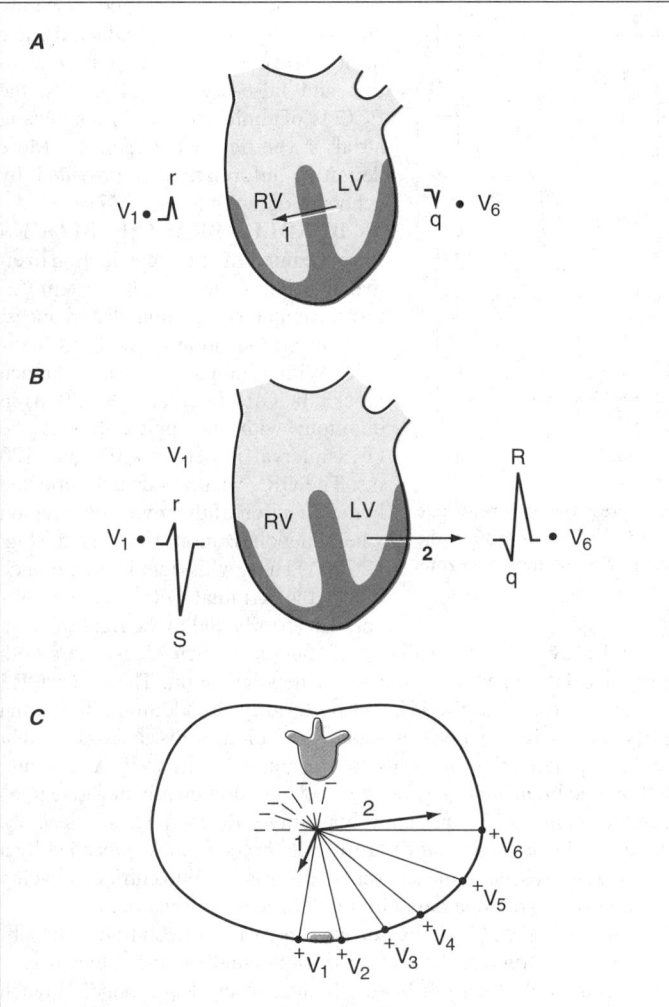

FIGURE 226-8 Ventricular depolarization can be divided into two major phases, each represented by a vector. *A*. The first phase (*arrow 1*) denotes depolarization of the ventricular septum, beginning on the left side and spreading to the right. This process is represented by a small "septal" r wave in lead V_1 and a small septal q wave in lead V_6. *B*. Simultaneous depolarization of the left and right ventricles (LV and RV) constitutes the second phase. Vector 2 is oriented to the left and posteriorly, reflecting the electrical predominance of the LV. *C*. Vectors (*arrows*) representing these two phases are shown in reference to the horizontal plane leads. (*After Goldberger, 1999.*)

wave). A left precordial lead, e.g., V_6, will record the same sequence with a small negative deflection (septal q wave) followed by a relatively tall positive deflection (R wave). Intermediate leads show a relative increase in R-wave amplitude (normal R-wave progression) and a decrease in S-wave amplitude progressing across the chest from the right to left. The precordial lead where the R and S waves are of approximately equal amplitude is referred to as the *transition zone* (usually V_3 or V_4) (Fig. 226-9).

The QRS pattern in the extremity leads may vary considerably from one normal subject to another depending on the *electrical axis* of the QRS, which describes the mean orientation of the QRS vector with reference to the six frontal plane leads. Normally, the QRS axis ranges from $-30°$ to $+100°$ (Fig. 226-6). An axis more negative than $-30°$ is referred to as *left axis deviation*, while an axis more positive than $+100°$ is referred to as *right axis deviation*. Left axis deviation may occur as a normal variant but is more commonly associated with left ventricular hypertrophy, a block in the anterior fascicle of the left bundle system (left anterior fascicular block or hemiblock), or inferior myocardial infarction. Right axis deviation also may occur as a normal variant (particularly in children and young adults), as a spurious find-

ing due to reversal of the left and right arm electrodes, or in conditions such as right ventricular overload (acute or chronic), infarction of the lateral wall of the left ventricle, dextrocardia, left pneumothorax, or left posterior fascicular block.

T WAVE AND U WAVE   Normally, the mean T-wave vector is oriented roughly concordant with the mean QRS vector. Since depolarization and repolarization are electrically opposite processes, this normal QRS–T-wave vector concordance indicates that repolarization must normally proceed in the reverse direction from depolarization (i.e., from ventricular epicardium to endocardium). The normal U wave is a small, rounded deflection (≤ 1 mm) that follows the T wave and usually has the same polarity as the T wave. An abnormal increase in U-wave amplitude is most commonly due to drugs (e.g., quinidine, procainamide, disopyramide) or hypokalemia. Very prominent U waves are a marker of increased susceptibility to the *torsades de pointes* type of ventricular tachycardia (Chap. 230). Inversion of the U wave in the precordial leads is abnormal and may be a subtle sign of ischemia.

MAJOR ECG ABNORMALITIES

CARDIAC ENLARGEMENT AND HYPERTROPHY
Right atrial overload (acute or chronic) may lead to an increase in P-wave amplitude (≥ 2.5 mm) (Fig. 226-10). Left atrial overload typically produces a biphasic P wave in V_1 with a broad negative component or a broad (≥ 120 ms), often notched P wave in one or more limb leads (Fig. 226-10). This pattern also may occur with left atrial conduction delays in the absence of actual atrial enlargement, leading to the more general designation of *left atrial abnormality*.

Right ventricular hypertrophy due to a pressure load (as from pulmonic valve stenosis or pulmonary artery hypertension) is characterized by a relatively tall R wave in lead V_1 (R $\geq$ S wave), usually with right axis deviation (Fig. 226-11); alternatively, there may be a qR pattern in V_1 or V_3R. ST depression and T-wave inversion in the right to midprecordial leads are also often present. This so-called ventricular strain pattern is attributed to repolarization abnormalities in hypertrophied muscle. Right ventricular hypertrophy due to ostium secundum–type atrial septal defects, with the accompanying right ventricular volume overload, is commonly associated with an incomplete or complete right bundle branch block pattern with a rightward QRS axis.

Acute cor pulmonale due to pulmonary embolism (Chap. 261) for example, may be associated with a normal ECG or a variety of abnormalities. Sinus tachycardia is the most common arrhythmia, although other tachyarrhythmias, such as atrial fibrillation or flutter, may occur. The QRS axis may shift to the right, sometimes in concert with the so-called $S_1Q_3T_3$ pattern (prominence of the S wave in lead I, Q wave in lead III, with T-wave inversion in lead III). Acute right ventricular dilation also may be associated with poor R-wave progression and T-wave inversions in V_1 to V_4 (right ventricular "strain") simulating acute anterior infarction. A right ventricular conduction disturbance may appear.

Chronic cor pulmonale due to obstructive lung disease (Chap. 237) usually does not produce the classic ECG patterns of right ventricular hypertrophy noted above. Instead of tall right precordial R waves, chronic lung disease more typically is associated with small R waves in right to midprecordial leads (poor R-wave progression) due in part to downward displacement of the diaphragm and the heart. Low-voltage complexes are commonly present, owing to hyperaeration of the lungs.

A number of different voltage criteria for *left ventricular hypertrophy* (Fig. 226-11) have been proposed on the basis of the presence of tall left precordial R waves and deep right precordial S waves [e.g., $SV_1 + (RV_5 \text{ or } RV_6) \geq 35$ mm; or $(RV_5 \text{ or } RV_6) \geq 25$ mm]. Repolarization abnormalities (ST depression with T-wave inversions) also may appear (left ventricular "strain" pattern) in leads with prominent

FIGURE 226-9 Normal electrocardiogram from a healthy subject. Sinus rhythm is present with a heart rate of 75 beats per minute. PR interval is 0.16 s; QRS interval (duration) is 0.08 s; QT interval is 0.36 s; the mean QRS axis is about +70°. The precordial leads show normal R-wave progression with the transition zone (R wave = S wave) in lead V_3.

R waves. However, prominent precordial voltages may occur as a normal variant, especially in athletic or thin-chested individuals. Left ventricular hypertrophy may increase limb lead voltage (e.g., RaVL ≥ 11 to 13 mm, RaVF ≥ 20 mm; $R_1 + S_{III} \geq 25$ mm) with or without increased precordial voltage. The presence of left atrial abnormality increases the likelihood of underlying left ventricular hypertrophy in cases with borderline voltage criteria. Left ventricular hypertrophy often progresses to incomplete or complete left bundle branch block. The sensitivity of conventional voltage criteria for left ventricular hypertrophy is decreased in obese persons and in women. ECG evidence for left ventricular hypertrophy is a major noninvasive marker of in-

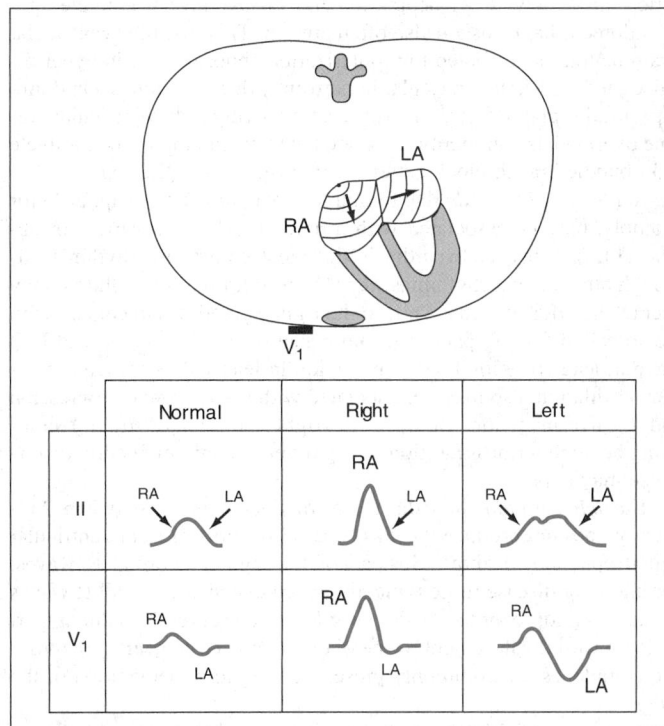

FIGURE 226-10 Right atrial (RA) overload may cause tall, peaked P waves in the limb or precordial leads. Left atrial (LA) abnormality may cause broad, often notched P waves in the limb leads and a biphasic P wave in lead V_1 with a prominent negative component representing delayed depolarization of the LA. *(After MK Park, WG Guntheroth: How to Read Pediatric ECGs, 2d ed. St. Louis, Mosby–Year Book, 1987.)*

creased risk of cardiovascular morbidity and mortality, including sudden cardiac death. However, because of false-positive and false-negative diagnoses, the ECG is of limited utility in diagnosing atrial or ventricular enlargement. More definitive information is provided by echocardiography (Chap. 227).

BUNDLE BRANCH BLOCKS
Intrinsic impairment of conduction in either the right or left bundle system (intraventricular conduction disturbances) leads to prolongation of the QRS interval. With complete bundle branch blocks the QRS interval is ≥ 120 ms in duration; with incomplete blocks the QRS interval is between 100 and 120 ms. The QRS vector is usually oriented in the direction of the myocardial region where depolarization is delayed (Fig. 226-12). Thus, with right bundle branch block, the terminal QRS vector is oriented anteriorly and to the right (rSR′ in V_1 and qRS in V_6, typically). Left bundle branch block alters both early and later phases of ventricular depolarization. The major QRS vector is directed to the left and posteriorly. In addition, the normal early left-to-right pattern of septal activation is disrupted such that septal depolarization proceeds from right to left as well. As a result, left bundle branch block generates wide, predominantly negative (QS) complexes in lead V_1 and entirely positive (R) complexes in lead V_6. A pattern identical to that of left bundle branch block, preceded by a sharp spike, is seen in most cases of electronic right ventricular pacing because of the relative delay in left ventricular activation.

Bundle branch block may occur in a variety of conditions. In subjects without structural heart disease, right bundle branch block is seen more commonly than left bundle branch block. Right bundle branch block also occurs with heart disease, both congenital (e.g., atrial septal defect) and acquired (e.g., valvular, ischemic). Left bundle branch block is often a marker of one of four underlying conditions: ischemic heart disease, long-standing hypertension, severe aortic valve disease, and cardiomyopathy. Bundle branch blocks may be chronic or intermittent. A bundle branch block may be rate-related; for example, often it occurs when the heart rate exceeds some critical value.

Bundle branch blocks and depolarization abnormalities secondary to artificial pacemakers not only affect ventricular depolarization (QRS) but are also characteristically associated with *secondary repolarization* (ST-T) abnormalities. With bundle branch blocks, the T-wave is typically opposite in polarity to the last deflection of the QRS (Fig. 226-12). This discordance of the QRS–T-wave vectors is caused by the altered sequence of repolarization that occurs secondary to altered depolarization. In contrast, *primary repolarization* abnormalities are independent of QRS changes and are related instead to actual alterations in the electrical properties of the myocardial fibers themselves (for example, in the resting membrane potential or action potential duration), not just to changes in the sequence of repolarization. Ischemia, electrolyte imbalance, and drugs such as digitalis all cause such primary ST–T-wave changes. Primary and secondary T-wave changes may coexist. For example, T-wave inversions in the right precordial leads with left bundle branch block or in the left precordial leads with right bundle branch block may be important markers of underlying ischemia or other abnormalities.

Partial blocks ("hemiblocks") in the left bundle system (left anterior or posterior fascicular blocks) generally do not prolong the QRS duration substantially but instead are associated with shifts in the frontal plane QRS axis (leftward or rightward, respectively). More complex combinations of fascicular and bundle branch blocks may occur involving the left and right bundle system. Examples of *bifascicular block* include right bundle branch block and left posterior fascicular block, right bundle branch block with left anterior fascicular block, and complete left bundle branch block. Chronic bifascicular block in an asymptomatic individual is associated with a relatively low risk of progression to high-degree AV heart block. In contrast, new bifascicular block with acute anterior myocardial infarction carries a much greater risk of complete heart block. Alternation of right and left bundle branch block is a sign of *trifascicular disease*. However, the presence of a prolonged PR interval and bifascicular block does not necessarily indicate trifascicular involvement, since this combination may arise with AV node disease and bifascicular block. Intraventricular conduction delays also can be caused by extrinsic (toxic) factors that slow ventricular conduction, particularly hyperkalemia or drugs (type 1 antiarrhythmic agents, tricyclic antidepressants, phenothiazines).

Prolongation of QRS duration does not necessarily indicate a conduction delay but may be due to *preexcitation* of the ventricles via a bypass tract, as in the Wolff-Parkinson-White (WPW) syndrome (Chap. 230) and related variants. The diagnostic triad of WPW consists of a wide QRS complex associated with a relatively short PR interval and slurring of the initial part of the QRS (delta wave), the latter effect due to aberrant activation of ventricular myocardium. The presence of a bypass tract predisposes to reentrant supraventricular tachyarrhythmias (Chap. 230).

MYOCARDIAL ISCHEMIA AND INFARCTION (See also Chap. 243) The ECG is a cornerstone in the diagnosis of acute and chronic ischemic heart disease. The findings depend on several key factors: the nature of the process [reversible (i.e., ischemia) versus irreversible (i.e., infarction)], the duration (acute versus chronic), extent (transmural versus subendocardial), and localization (anterior versus inferoposterior), as well as the presence of other underlying abnormalities (ventricular hypertrophy, conduction defects).

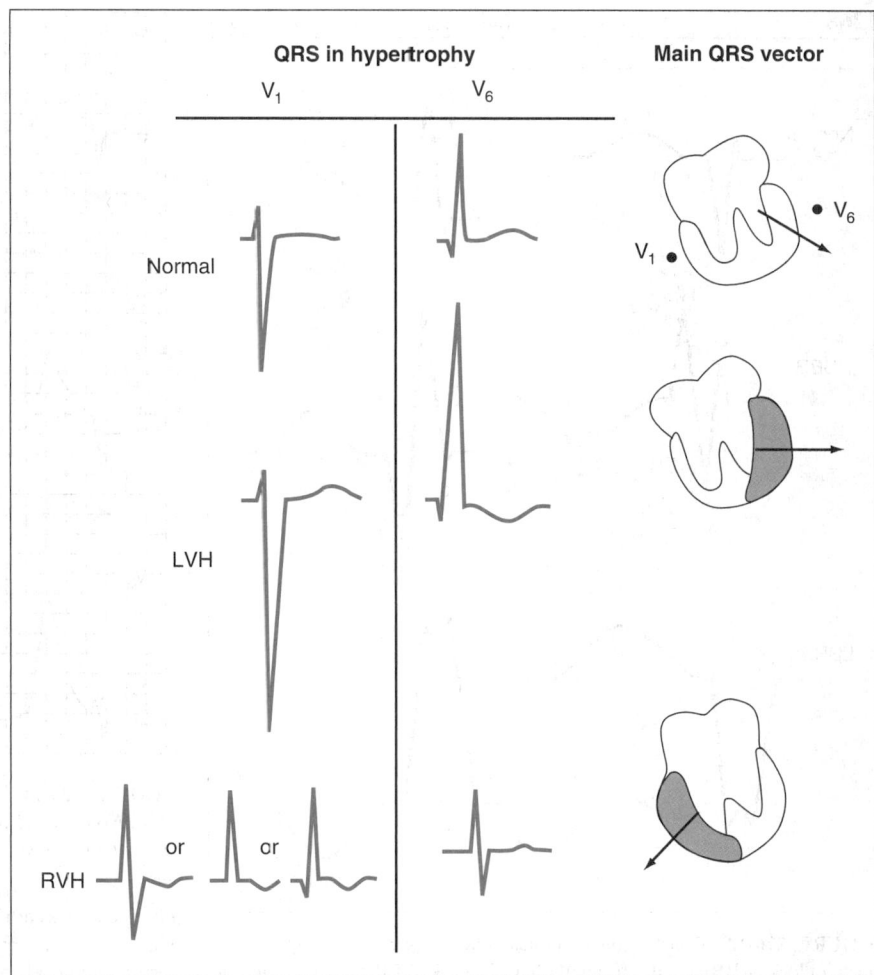

FIGURE 226-11 Left ventricular hypertrophy (LVH) increases the amplitude of electrical forces directed to the left and posteriorly. In addition, repolarization abnormalities may cause ST-segment depression and T-wave inversion in leads with a prominent R wave ("strain" pattern). Right ventricular hypertrophy (RVH) may shift the QRS vector to the right; this effect usually is associated with an R, RS, or qR complex in lead V_1. T-wave inversions may be present in right precordial leads ("strain" pattern).

Ischemia exerts complex time-dependent effects on the electrical properties of myocardial cells. Severe, acute ischemia lowers the resting membrane potential and shortens the duration of the action potential. Such changes cause a voltage gradient between normal and ischemic zones. As a consequence, current flows between these regions. These so-called currents of injury are represented on the surface ECG by deviation of the ST segment (Fig. 226-13). When the acute ischemia is *transmural*, the ST vector is usually shifted in the direction of the outer (epicardial) layers, producing ST elevations and sometimes, in the earliest stages of ischemia, tall, positive so-called hyperacute T waves over the ischemic zone. With ischemia confined primarily to the *subendocardium*, the ST vector typically shifts toward the subendocardium and ventricular cavity, so that overlying (e.g., anterior precordial) leads show ST-segment depression (with ST elevation in lead aVR). Multiple factors affect the amplitude of acute ischemic ST deviations. Profound ST elevation or depression in multiple leads usually indicates very severe ischemia. From a clinical viewpoint, the division of acute myocardial infarction into ST segment elevation and non-ST elevation (NSTEMI) types is useful since the efficacy of acute reperfusion therapy is limited to the former group (Chap. 243).

The ECG leads are more helpful in localizing regions of ST elevation than non-ST elevation ischemia. For example, acute transmural anterior wall ischemia is reflected by ST elevations or increased T-wave positivity (Fig. 226-14) in one or more of the precordial leads (V_1 to V_6) and leads I and aVL. Anteroseptal ischemia produces these changes in leads V_1 to V_3, apical or lateral ischemia in leads V_4 to V_6. Transmural inferior wall ischemia produces changes in leads II, III, and aVF. Posterior wall ischemia may be indirectly recognized by *reciprocal* ST depressions in leads V_1 to V_3. Prominent reciprocal ST depressions in these leads also occur with certain inferior wall infarcts, particularly those with posterior or lateral wall extension. Right ventricular ischemia usually produces ST elevations in right-sided chest leads (Fig. 226-7). When ischemic ST elevations occur as the earliest sign of acute infarction, they are typically followed within a period ranging from hours to days by evolving T-wave inversions and often by Q waves occurring in the same lead distribution. (T-wave inversions due to evolving or chronic ischemia correlate with prolongation of repolarization and are often associated with QT lengthening.) Reversible transmural ischemia, for example, due to coronary vasospasm (Prinzmetal's variant angina), may cause transient ST-segment elevations without development of Q waves. Depending on the severity and duration of such ischemia, the ST elevations may either resolve completely in minutes or be followed by T-wave inversions that persist for hours or even days. Patients with ischemic chest pain who present with deep T-wave inversions in multiple precordial leads (e.g., V_1 to V_4) with or without cardiac enzyme elevations typically have severe obstruction in the left anterior descending coronary artery system (Fig. 226-15). In contrast, patients whose baseline ECG already shows abnormal T-wave inversions may develop T-wave normalization (pseudonormalization) during episodes of acute transmural ischemia.

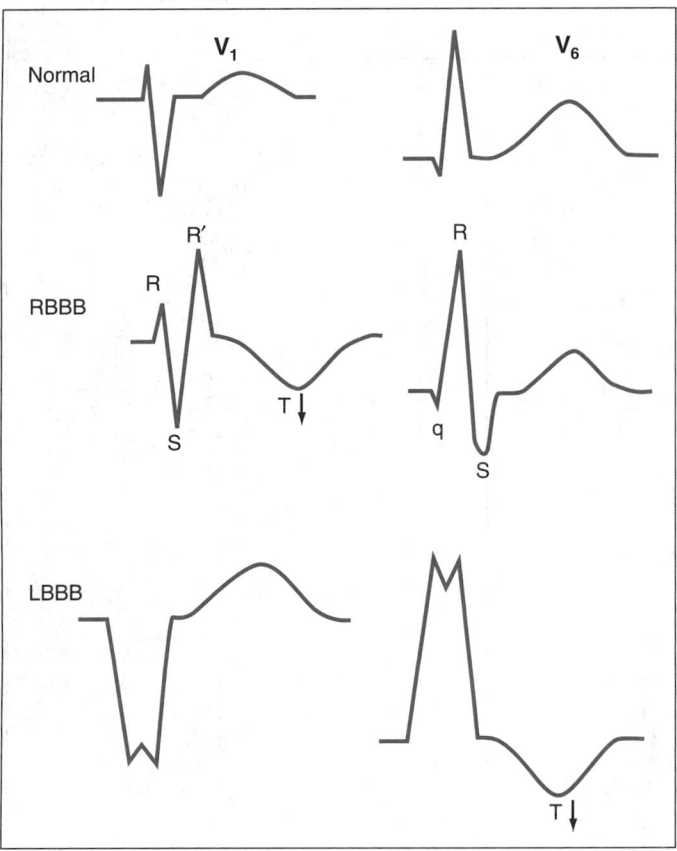

FIGURE 226-12   Comparison of typical QRS-T patterns in right bundle branch block (RBBB) and left bundle branch block (LBBB) with the normal pattern in leads V_1 and V_6. Note the secondary T-wave inversions (*arrows*) in leads with an rSR' complex with RBBB and in leads with a wide R wave with LBBB.

FIGURE 226-14   Hyperacute phase of anteroseptal myocardial infarction (MI). Note the tall positive T waves (V_2 to V_3) along with ST-segment elevations and Q waves (V_1 to V_3).

With infarction, depolarization (QRS) changes often accompany repolarization (ST-T) abnormalities. Necrosis of sufficient myocardial tissue may lead to decreased R-wave amplitude or frank abnormal Q waves in the anterior or inferior leads (Fig. 226-16). Previously, abnormal Q waves were considered to be markers of transmural myocardial infarction, while subendocardial infarcts were thought not to produce Q waves. However, careful ECG-pathology correlative studies have indicated that transmural infarcts may occur without Q waves and that subendocardial (nontransmural) infarcts may sometimes be associated with Q waves. Therefore, infarcts are more appropriately classified as "Q-wave" or "non-Q-wave." The major acute ECG changes in syndromes of ischemic heart disease are schematically summarized in Fig. 226-17. Loss of depolarization forces due to posterior or lateral infarction may cause reciprocal increases in R-wave amplitude in leads V_1 and V_2 without diagnostic Q waves in any of the conventional leads. Atrial infarction may be associated with PR-segment deviations due to an atrial current of injury, changes in P-wave morphology, or atrial arrhythmias. In the weeks and months following infarction, these ECG changes may persist or begin to resolve. Complete normalization of the ECG following Q-wave infarction is uncommon but may occur, particularly with smaller infarcts. In contrast, ST-segment elevations that persist for several weeks or more after a Q-wave infarct usually correlate with a severe underlying wall motion disorder (akinetic or dyskinetic zone), although not necessarily a frank ventricular aneurysm.

ECG changes due to ischemia may occur spontaneously or may be provoked by various exercise protocols (stress electrocardiography) (Chap. 244). In patients with severe ischemic heart disease, exercise testing is most likely to elicit signs of subendocardial ischemia (horizontal or downsloping ST depression in multiple leads). ST-segment elevation during exercise is most often observed after a Q-wave infarct. This repolarization change does not necessarily indicate active ischemia but correlates strongly with the presence of an underlying ventricular wall motion abnormality. However, in patients *without* prior infarction, transient ST-segment elevation with exercise is a reliable sign of transmural ischemia.

The ECG has important limitations in both sensitivity and specificity in the diagnosis of ischemic heart disease. Although a single normal ECG does not exclude ischemia or even acute infarc-

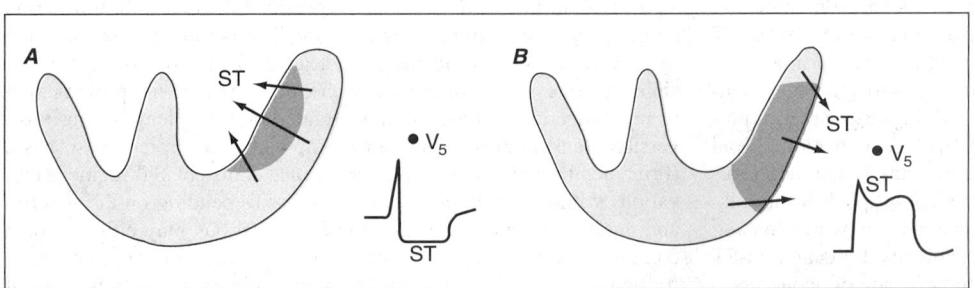

FIGURE 226-13   Acute ischemia causes a current of injury. With predominant subendocardial ischemia (*A*), the resultant ST vector will be directed toward the inner layer of the affected ventricle and the ventricular cavity. Overlying leads therefore will record ST depression. With ischemia involving the outer ventricular layer (*B*) (transmural or epicardial injury), the ST vector will be directed outward. Overlying leads will record ST elevation.

tion, a normal ECG *throughout* the course of an acute infarct is distinctly uncommon. Prolonged chest pain without diagnostic ECG changes, therefore, should always prompt a careful search for other noncoronary causes of chest pain (Chap. 13). Furthermore, the diagnostic changes of acute or evolving ischemia are often masked by the presence of left bundle branch block, electronic ventricular pacemaker patterns, and WPW preexcitation. On the other hand, clinicians may overdiagnose ischemia or infarction based on the presence of ST-segment elevations or depressions, T-wave inversions, tall positive T waves, or Q waves *not* related to ischemic heart disease (pseudoinfarct patterns). For example, ST-segment elevations simulating ischemia may occur with acute pericarditis (Fig. 226-18) or myocarditis, or as a normal variant ("early repolarization" pattern). Similarly, tall, positive T waves do not invariably represent hyperacute ischemic changes but also may be caused by normal variants, hyperkalemia, cerebrovascular injury, and left ventricular volume overload due to mitral or aortic regurgitation, among other causes. ST-segment elevations and tall, positive T waves are common findings in leads V_1 and V_2 in left bundle branch block or left ventricular hypertrophy in the absence of ischemia. The differential diagnosis of Q waves (Table 226-1) includes physiologic or positional variants, ventricular hypertrophy, acute or chronic noncoronary myocardial injury, hypertrophic cardiomyopathy, and ventricular conduction disorders. Digitalis, ventricular hypertrophy, hypokalemia, and a variety of other factors may cause ST-segment depression mimicking subendocardial ischemia. Prominent T-wave inversion may occur with ventricular hypertrophy, cardiomyopathy, myocarditis, and cerebrovascular injury (particularly intracranial bleeds; Fig. 226-19), among many other conditions.

METABOLIC FACTORS AND DRUG EFFECTS A variety of metabolic and pharmacologic agents alter the ECG and, in particular, cause changes in repolarization (ST-T-U) and sometimes QRS prolongation. Certain life-threatening electrolyte disturbances may be diagnosed initially and monitored from the ECG. *Hyperkalemia* produces a sequence of changes usually beginning with narrowing and peaking (tenting) of the T waves. Further elevation of extracellular K^+ leads to AV conduction disturbances, diminution in P-wave amplitude, and widening of the QRS interval. Severe hyperkalemia eventually causes cardiac arrest with a slow sinusoidal type of mechanism ("sine-wave" pattern) followed by asystole. *Hypokalemia* (Fig. 226-19) prolongs ventricular repolarization, often with prominent U waves. Prolongation of the QT interval (Fig. 226-19) is also seen with drugs that increase the duration of the ventricular action potential—type 1A antiarrhythmic agents and related drugs (e.g., quinidine, disopyramide, procainamide, tricyclic antidepressants, phenothiazines) and type III agents (amiodarone, sotalol). Marked QT prolongation, sometimes with deep, wide T-wave inversions, may occur with intracranial bleeds, particularly subarachnoid hemorrhage ("CVA T-wave" pattern) (Fig. 226-19). Systemic *hypothermia* (Fig. 226-19) also prolongs repolarization, usually with a distinctive convex elevation of the J point (Osborn wave). *Hypocalcemia* typically prolongs the QT interval (ST portion), while *hypercalcemia* shortens it (Fig. 226-20). Digitalis glycosides also shorten the QT interval, often with a characteristic "scooping" of the ST–T-wave complex (*digitalis effect*).

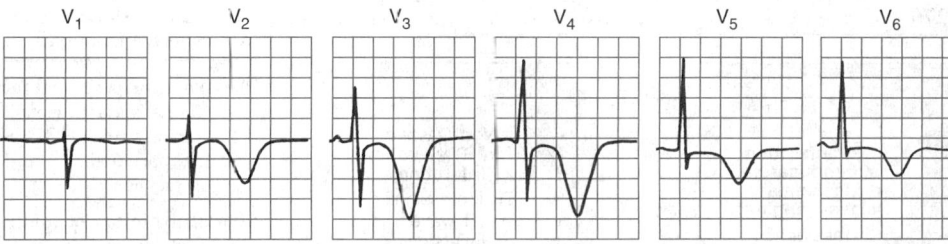

FIGURE 226-15 Severe anterior wall ischemia (with or without infarction) may cause prominent T-wave inversions in the precordial leads. This pattern is usually associated with a high-grade stenosis of the left anterior descending coronary artery.

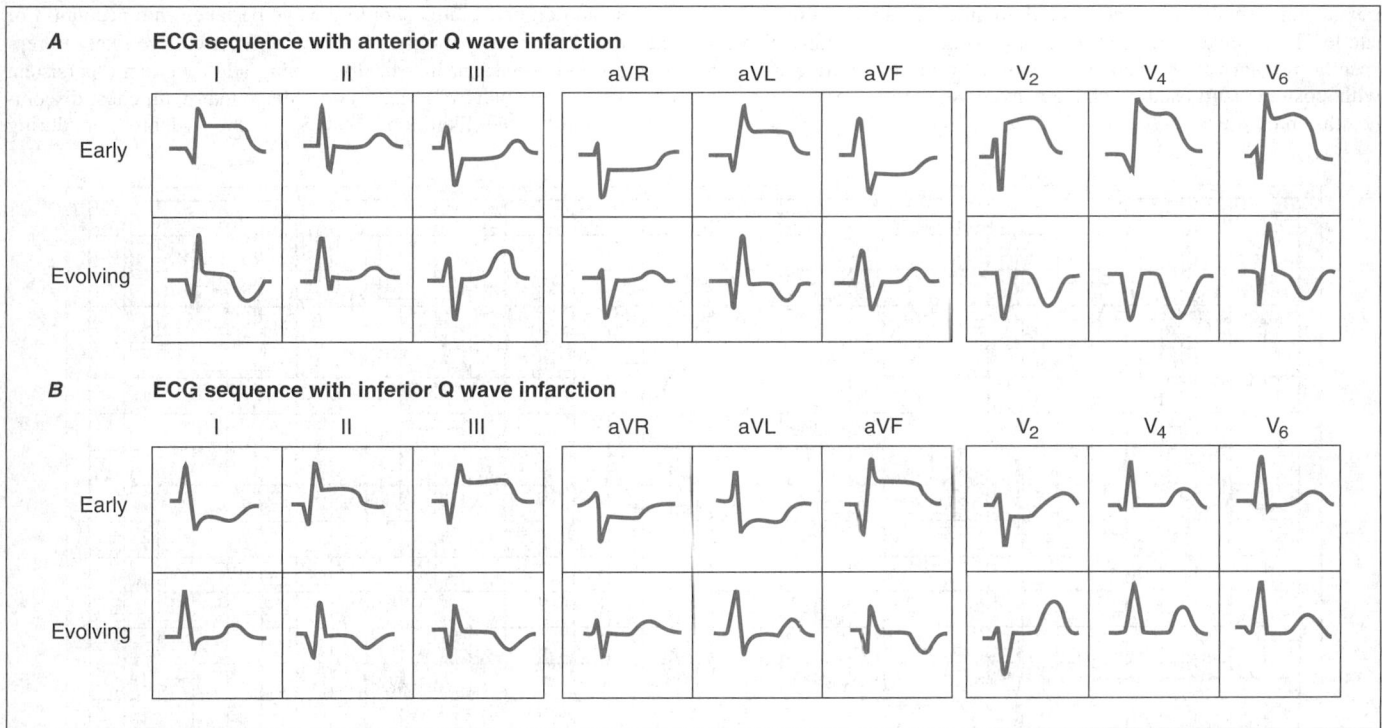

FIGURE 226-16 Sequence of depolarization and repolarization changes with (*A*) acute anterior and (*B*) acute inferior wall Q-wave infarctions. With anterior infarcts, ST elevation in leads I, aVL, and the precordial leads may be accompanied by reciprocal ST depressions in leads II, III, and aVF. Conversely, acute inferior (or posterior) infarcts may be associated with reciprocal ST depressions in leads V_1 to V_3. (*After Goldberger, 1999.*)

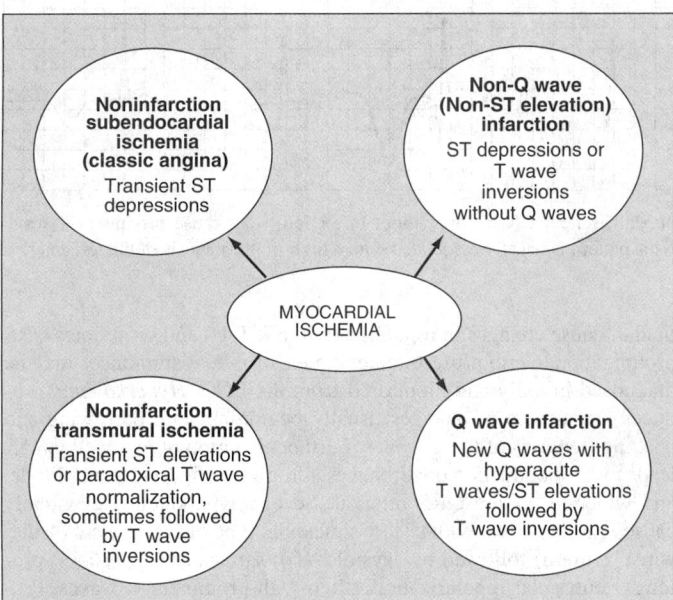

FIGURE 226-17   Variability of ECG patterns with acute myocardial ische-mia. The ECG also may be normal or nonspecifically abnormal. Furthermore, these categorizations are not mutually exclusive. For example, a non-ST ele-vation infarct may evolve into a Q-wave infarct; ST elevations may be followed by a non-Q-wave infarct; or ST depressions and T-wave inversions may be followed by a Q-wave infarct. *(After Goldberger, 1991.)*

Many other factors are associated with ECG changes, particularly alterations in ventricular repolarization. T-wave flattening, minimal T-wave inversions or slight ST-segment depression ("nonspecific ST–T-wave changes") may occur with a variety of electrolyte and acid-base disturbances, a variety of infectious processes, central nervous system disorders, endocrine abnormalities, many drugs, ischemia, hy-poxia, and virtually any type of cardiopulmonary abnormality. While subtle ST–T-wave changes may be markers of ischemia, transient non-specific repolarization changes also may occur following a meal or with postural (orthostatic) change, hyperventilation, or exercise in healthy individuals.

Table 226-1   Differential Diagnosis of Q Waves (with Selected Examples)

Physiologic or positional factors
1. Normal variant "septal" q waves
2. Normal variant Q waves in V_1 to V_2, aVL, III, and aVF
3. Left pneumothorax or dextrocardia: loss of lateral R-wave progression

Myocardial injury or infiltration
1. Acute processes: myocardial ischemia or infarction, myocarditis, hyper-kalemia
2. Chronic processes: myocardial infarction, idiopathic cardiomyopathy, myocarditis, amyloid, tumor, sarcoid, scleroderma, Chagas' disease, echinococcus cyst

Ventricular hypertrophy/enlargement
1. Left ventricular (poor R-wave progression[a])
2. Right ventricular (reversed R-wave progression[b] or poor R-wave pro-gression, particularly with chronic obstructive lung disease)
3. Hypertrophic cardiomyopathy (may simulate anterior, inferior, posterior, or lateral infarcts)

Conduction abnormalities
1. Left bundle branch block (poor R-wave progression[b])
2. Wolff-Parkinson-White patterns

---

[a] Small or absent R waves in the right to midprecordial leads.
[b] Progressive decrease in R-wave amplitude from V_1 to the mid- or lateral precordial leads.
SOURCE: After Goldberger, 1991.

ELECTRICAL ALTERNANS   Electrical alternans—a beat-to-beat alternation in one or more components of the ECG signal—is a common type of nonlinear cardiovascular response to a variety of perturbations. For example, total electrical alternans (P-QRS-T) with sinus tachycardia is a relatively specific sign of pericardial effusion, often with cardiac tamponade. The mechanism relates to a periodic swinging motion of the heart in the effusion at a frequency exactly one-half the heart rate. ST-T alternans is a sign of electrical instability and may precede ventricular fibrillation.

CLINICAL INTERPRETATION OF THE ECG   Accurate analysis of ECGs requires thoroughness and care. The patient's age, gender, and clinical status should always be taken into account. For example, T-wave inversions in leads V_1 to V_3 are more likely to rep-resent a normal variant in a healthy young adult woman ("persistent juvenile T-wave pattern") than in an elderly man with chest discom-fort. Similarly, the likelihood that ST-segment depression during

FIGURE 226-18   Acute pericarditis often produces diffuse ST-segment ele-vations (in this case in leads I, II, aVF, and V_2 to V_6) due to a ventricular current of injury. Note also the characteristic PR-segment deviation (opposite in polarity to the ST segment) due to a concomitant atrial injury current.

exercise testing represents ischemia depends partly on the prior probability of coronary artery disease.

Many mistakes in ECG interpretation are errors of omission. Therefore, a systematic approach is desirable. The following 14 points should be analyzed carefully in every ECG: (1) standardization (calibration) and technical features (including lead placement and artifacts); (2) heart rate; (3) rhythm; (4) PR interval; (5) QRS interval; (6) QT interval; (7) P waves; (8) QRS voltages; (9) mean QRS electrical axis; (10) precordial R-wave progression; (11) abnormal Q waves; (12) ST segments; (13) T waves; (14) U waves.

Only after analyzing all these points should the interpretation be formulated. Where appropriate, important clinical correlates or inferences should be mentioned. For example, prolonged ventricular repolarization with prominent U waves should suggest hypokalemia or drug toxicity (e.g., due to quinidine or procainamide) (Fig. 226-19). The combination of left atrial abnormality (enlargement) and signs of right ventricular hypertrophy suggests mitral stenosis. Low voltage with sinus tachycardia raises the possibility of pericardial tamponade or chronic obstructive lung disease. Sinus tachycardia with QRS and QT (U) prolongation suggests tricyclic antidepressant overdose (Fig. 226-19). Comparison with previous ECGs is essential. →*The diagnosis and management of specific cardiac arrhythmias and conduction disturbances are discussed in Chaps. 229 and 230.*

COMPUTERIZED ELECTROCARDIOGRAPHY Computerized ECG systems are increasingly used. Digital systems provide for convenient storage and immediate retrieval of thousands of ECG records. In recent years, computer programs for ECG analysis have become more reliable. However, despite these advances, computer interpretation of ECGs has important limitations. Incomplete or inaccurate readings are most likely with arrhythmias and complex abnormalities. Therefore, computerized interpretation (including measurements of basic ECG intervals) should not be accepted without careful physician review.

FIGURE 226-19 A variety of metabolic derangements, drug effects, and other factors may prolong ventricular repolarization with QT prolongation or prominent U waves. Repolarization prolongation, particularly if due to hypokalemia or pharmacologic agents, indicates increased susceptibility to torsades de pointes type ventricular tachycardia. Hypothermia is associated with a distinctive convex "hump" at the J point (Osborn wave, *arrow*). Note QRS and QT prolongation along with sinus tachycardia in the case of tricyclic antidepressant overdose.

BIBLIOGRAPHY

BRADY WJ et al: Electrocardiographic manifestations: Patterns that confound the EKG diagnosis of acute myocardial infarction—left bundle branch block, ventricular paced rhythm, and left ventricular hypertrophy. J Emerg Med 18:71, 2000

GOLDBERGER AL: *Myocardial Infarction: Electrocardiographic Differential Diagnosis,* 4th ed. St. Louis, Mosby–Year Book, 1991

GOLDBERGER AL: *Clinical Electrocardiography: A Simplified Approach,* 6th ed. St. Louis, Mosby, 1999

MIRVIS DM: *Electrocardiography: A Physiologic Approach.* St. Louis, Mosby–Year Book, 1993

MIRVIS DM, GOLDBERGER AL: Electrocardiography, in *Heart Disease: A Textbook of Cardiovascular Medicine,* 6th ed, E Braunwald, DP Zipes, P Libby (eds). Philadelphia, Saunders, 2001

227 *Rick A. Nishimura, Raymond J. Gibbons, A. Jamil Tajik*

NONINVASIVE CARDIAC IMAGING: ECHOCARDIOGRAPHY AND NUCLEAR CARDIOLOGY

Cardiovascular imaging has significantly enhanced the practice of cardiology over the past few decades. Two-dimensional echocardiography is able to visualize the heart directly in real time using ultrasound, providing instantaneous assessment of the myocardium, valves, pericardium, and great vessels. Doppler echocardiography measures the velocity of moving red blood cells and has become a noninvasive alternative to cardiac catheterization for assessment of hemodynamics. Transesophageal echocardiography has provided a new window for high-resolution imaging of posterior structures of the heart, particularly the left atrium, mitral valve, and aorta. Nuclear cardiology uses isotopes to assess myocardial perfusion and function and has contributed greatly to the evaluation of patients with ischemic heart disease. This chapter provides an overview of the basic concepts of both echocardiography and nuclear cardiology and the clinical indications for each procedure.

ECHOCARDIOGRAPHY

TWO-DIMENSIONAL ECHOCARDIOGRAPHY **Basic Principles** Two-dimensional echocardiography uses the principle of

FIGURE 226-20 Prolongation of the Q-T interval (ST-segment portion) is typical of hypocalcemia. Hypercalcemia may cause abbreviation of the ST segment and shortening of the QT interval.

ultrasound reflection off cardiac structures to produce images of the heart (Table 227-1). The imaging is performed from multiple acoustic windows with different transducer rotations so that the entire heart and great vessels can be displayed in real time and in various two-dimensional planes. Most information from a study is obtained from a visual analysis of the two-dimensional images. Some laboratories use a concomitant M-mode study (one-dimensional echocardiogram) derived from the two-dimensional image for objective measurements of chamber size and function. For a transthoracic echocardiogram, the imaging is performed with a hand-held transducer placed directly on the chest wall. In selected patients, a transesophageal echocardiogram may be performed, in which an ultrasound transducer is mounted on the tip of an endoscope placed in the esophagus and directed towards the cardiac structures, so that high-resolution images of the posterior structures are obtained.

The frequency of the ultrasound used in clinical practice is usually between 2.5 and 5.0 MHz. The images produced depend on the acoustic reflection of the ultrasound off the various structures. Ultrasound passes readily through liquid, such as blood or pericardial fluid, and these are displayed as black on the two-dimensional image. When ultrasound is reflected off more solid structures, such as the myocardium and valves, there is a gray scale display. Structures such as calcium produce intense acoustic reflection and are displayed as bright white on the two-dimensional image. In a standard echocardiographic examination, the images are obtained from parasternal, apical, subcostal, and suprasternal windows. Multiple transducer rotations and angulations from each window are used to ensure that all parts of the cardiac structures are imaged. Most echocardiographic studies are recorded on videotape for off-line analysis, but direct digital acquisition units are enhancing the ability for storage and retrieval of images.

Current echocardiographic machines are portable, which allows them to be wheeled directly to the patient's bedside. Thus, a major advantage of echocardiography over other imaging modalities is the ability to obtain instantaneous images of the cardiac structures for immediate interpretation, even in emergency or trauma units or in critical care settings.

A limitation of a two-dimensional echocardiogram performed via a transthoracic approach is the inability to obtain high-quality images in all patients, especially those with a thick chest wall or severe lung disease. Ultrasound waves are poorly transmitted through lung parenchyma. In patients with inadequate transthoracic echocardiographic images, transesophageal echocardiography can be performed.

Table 227-1 Clinical Uses of Echocardiography

Two-Dimensional Echocardiography	**Stress Echocardiography**
Cardiac chambers	Two-dimensional
Chamber size	Myocardial ischemia
Left ventricular	Viable myocardium
Hypertrophy	Doppler
Regional wall motion abnormalities	Valve disease
Valve	**Transesophageal**
Morphology and motion	**Echocardiography**
Pericardium	Inadequate transthoracic images
Effusion	Aortic disease
Tamponade	Infective endocarditis
Masses	Source of embolism
Great vessels	Valve prosthesis
Doppler Echocardiography	Intraoperative
Valve stenosis	
Gradient	
Valve area	
Valve regurgitation	
Semiquantitation	
Intracardiac pressures	
Volumetric flow	
Diastolic filling	
Intracardiac shunts	

The diagnostic accuracy of an echocardiogram is highly dependent upon both the operator of the echocardiographic equipment and the interpreter of the study. There are many important technical aspects to obtaining and interpreting the two-dimensional images, requiring training, experience, and expertise.

Chamber Size and Function   Two-dimensional echocardiography is an ideal imaging modality for assessing left ventricular size and function (Fig. 227-1). A qualitative assessment of the cavity size of the ventricle and systolic function can be made directly from the two-dimensional image by experienced observers (Fig. 227-2). Quantitative assessment of left ventricular size and function can be made by M-mode echocardiography (measuring systolic and diastolic dimensions of the short axis of the left ventricle) or quantitative two-dimensional echocardiography. With quantitative two-dimensional echocardiography, endocardial outlines of the left ventricular cavity are traced in systole and diastole and the left ventricular cavity areas are then fitted to computer models of the left ventricle to obtain systolic and diastolic volumes, making it more cumbersome and less reproducible than the M-mode method. However, the M-mode method can be used only in patients with symmetrically contracting ventricles, as the M-mode samples only the septum and free wall at the mid-ventricle level. The presence or absence of regional wall motion abnormalities can be visually assessed by examining endocardial motion as well as wall thickening. M-mode and two-dimensional echocardiography are useful in the diagnosis of left ventricular hypertrophy, seen as an increase in wall thickness. Other chamber sizes are assessed by visual analysis, including the left atrium and right-sided chambers. There is no method for quantitative analysis of right ventricular size and function by two-dimensional echocardiography, due to the complex geometry of the right ventricle.

Valve Abnormalities (See also Chap. 236)   Valve morphology and motion can be visualized by two-dimensional echocardiography (Figs. 227-1 and 227-2). Leaflet thickness and mobility, valve calcification, and the appearance of subvalvular and supravalvular struc-

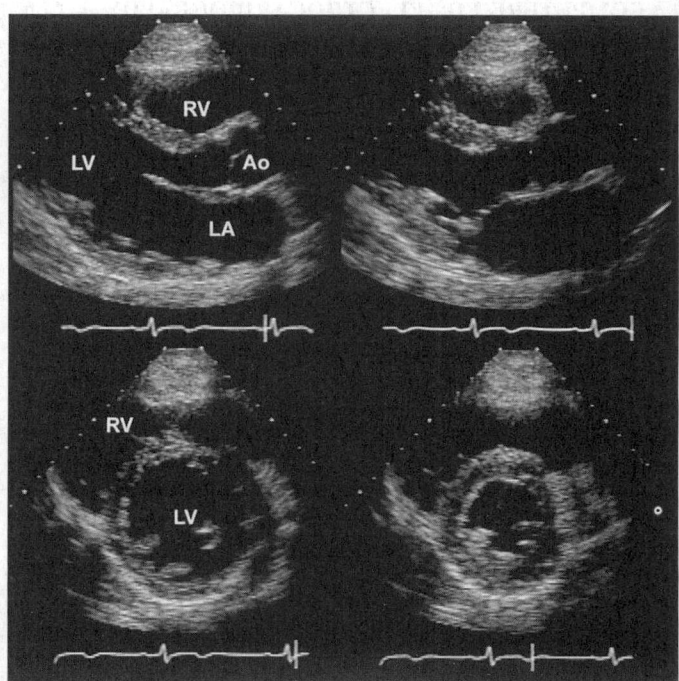

FIGURE 227-1   Two-dimensional echocardiographic still frame images from a normal patient with a normal heart. *Upper*: Parasternal long axis view during systole and diastole (*left*) and systole (*right*). During systole, there is thickening of the myocardium and reduction in the size of the left ventricle (LV). The valve leaflets are thin and open widely. *Lower*: Parasternal short axis view during diastole (*left*) and systole (*right*) demonstrating a decrease in the left ventricular cavity size during systole as well as an increase in wall thickening. LA, left atrium; RV, right ventricle; Ao, aorta.

FIGURE 227-2 Apical four-chamber view from a patient with a dilated cardiomyopathy. The left ventricle (LV) is dilated, and there is little change in the LV cavity size from diastole (*left*) to systole (*right*). RV, right ventricle; LA, left atrium.

tures can be assessed. Valve stenosis is reliably diagnosed by the thickening and decreased mobility of the valve. Two-dimensional echocardiography is the "gold standard" for the diagnosis of mitral stenosis, which produces typical tethering and diastolic doming. The severity of the stenosis can be obtained from a direct planimeter measurement of the mitral valve orifice from the short axis view. The presence and etiology of stenosis of the semilunar valves can be made by two-dimensional echocardiography (**Plate I-1**). Estimating the severity of the stenosis by two-dimensional echocardiography alone is less reliable and requires Doppler echocardiography. The diagnosis of valvular regurgitation must be made by Doppler echocardiography, but two-dimensional echocardiography is valuable for determining the etiology of the regurgitation. Annular dilatation, prolapse, flail leaflets, vegetation, and rheumatic involvement can be diagnosed and the left ventricular response to volume overload can be assessed by two-dimensional echocardiography.

Pericardial Disease (See also Chap. 239) Two-dimensional echocardiography is the imaging modality of choice for the detection of pericardial effusion, which is easily visualized as a black echolucent ovoid structure surrounding the heart. In the hemodynamically unstable patient with pericardial tamponade, typical echo findings of right ventricular collapse, right atrial collapse, and a dilated inferior vena cava are seen (see Fig. 239-1). In patients with subclinical tamponade, these two-dimensional echocardiographic features may not be present, but the diagnosis of elevated pericardial pressure can be made by Doppler findings of variations of inflow velocities with respiration (see Figs. 239-2 and 239-4). Echocardiographically guided pericardiocentesis has now become a standard of care. A two-dimensional echocardiogram can directly visualize the location of the pericardial fluid in relationship to the entry point, and this technique has led to a low complication rate. Increased thickness of the pericardium is difficult to assess by two-dimensional echocardiography. Subtle clues to pericardial constriction can be seen on two-dimensional echocardiography from enhanced ventricular interaction, but Doppler imaging is required for confirmation of this diagnosis.

Intracardiac Masses (See also Chap. 240) Intracardiac masses can be visualized on two-dimensional echocardiography, provided that image quality is adequate. Solid masses appear as echo-dense structures, which can be located inside the cardiac chambers or infiltrating into the myocardium or pericardium (see Fig. 240-1). Although an echocardiographic examination cannot provide pathologic confirmation of the etiology of a mass, there are several instances in which the diagnosis of the mass can be suspected from its appearance, mobility, and the concomitant abnormalities seen. *Left ventricular thrombus* appears as an echo-dense structure, usually in the apical region associated

with regional wall motion abnormalities. The appearance and mobility of the thrombus are predictive of embolic events. *Atrial myxoma* can be diagnosed by the appearance of a well-circumscribed mobile mass with attachments to the atrial septum. Prominent benign structures, such as *lipomatous infiltration of the atrial septum* and a *calcified mitral annulus*, may appear as cardiac masses. The high-resolution images provided by transesophageal echocardiography may be required for further delineation of myocardial masses.

Aortic Disease (See also Chap. 247) Two-dimensional echocardiography can provide information on diseases of the aorta. The proximal ascending aorta, the arch, and the distal descending aorta can usually be visualized via the transthoracic approach. For patients in whom a dilated aorta is well visualized, two-dimensional echocardiography can be used for serial follow-up. Aortic dissection can be diagnosed when an intimal flap is visualized on a transthoracic echocardiogram. However, the definitive diagnosis of an aortic dissection usually requires a transesophageal echocardiogram (**Plate I-2**).

DOPPLER ECHOCARDIOGRAPHY **Basic Principles** Doppler echocardiography uses ultrasound reflecting off moving red blood cells to measure the velocity of blood flow across valves, within cardiac chambers, and through the great vessels. Normal and abnormal blood flow patterns can be assessed noninvasively. Color flow Doppler imaging (**Plates I-1 and I-2**) displays the blood velocities in real time superimposed upon a two-dimensional echocardiographic image. The different colors indicate the direction of blood flow (blue towards and red away from the transducer), with green color superimposed when there is turbulent flow. Thus regurgitant lesions and shunts may be assessed by color flow Doppler. Pulsed-wave Doppler measures the blood flow velocity in a specific location on the two-dimensional echocardiographic image and displays the velocities in a spectral pattern using time as the *x*-axis. Continuous-wave Doppler echocardiography can measure high velocities of blood flow directed along the line of the Doppler beam, such as occur in the presence of valve stenosis, valve regurgitation, or intracardiac shunts. These high velocities can be used to determine intracardiac pressure gradients by a modified Bernoulli equation:

$$\text{Pressure change} = 4 \times (\text{velocity})^2$$

In this equation, the contribution from viscous friction and flow acceleration to the change in pressure is assumed to be negligible. The derived pressure gradient can be used to determine intracardiac pressures and stenosis severity.

Valve Gradients (See also Chap. 236) In the presence of valvular stenosis, there is an increase in the velocity of blood flow across the stenotic valve. A continuous-wave Doppler beam can be placed into this jet of blood, and the measured velocity used to determine an instantaneous gradient across the valve by applying the modified Bernoulli equation. Integration of this velocity over time provides an accurate measurement of the mean gradient across the valve. If the Doppler beam is directed parallel to the jet, the Doppler-derived valve gradient is accurate and reproducible and correlates with that obtained from cardiac catheterization. Since the valve gradient is dependent upon transvalvular flow, a valve area should be derived noninvasively. An accurate assessment of the mean gradient and valve area can be obtained in most patients, provided that the Doppler beam is parallel to the stenotic jet. The Doppler examination is highly operator-dependent, especially in patients with aortic stenosis. If the Doppler beam is not parallel to the stenotic jet, there may be a significant underestimation of the valve gradient. In patients with mitral stenosis, it is technically easier to align the Doppler beam with the stenotic jet; thus the mean transmitral gradient is usually accurate and reproducible. A Doppler-derived transmitral gradient may be more reliable than that obtained by conventional cardiac catheterization, given the inherent errors that may occur with a pulmonary artery wedge pressure measurement.

Valvular Regurgitation (See also Chap. 236) Valvular regurgitation is diagnosed by Doppler echocardiography when there is an abnormal retrograde flow across the valve. Color flow imaging is the Doppler method used most frequently to detect valve regurgitation by visualization of a high-velocity turbulent jet in the chamber proximal to the regurgitant valve. The sensitivity of Doppler echocardiography for the detection of regurgitant lesions is high, and even trivial or mild regurgitation in the absence of clinical auscultatory evidence of a regurgitant murmur may be detected. The size and extent of the color flow jet into the receiving cardiac chamber provide a qualitative estimate of the severity of regurgitation, but there are many limitations to using color jet size alone. Indirect clues for the severity of valvular regurgitation are available from other Doppler interrogation sites (e.g., intensity of a continuous-wave signal, volume of forward flow across a regurgitant valve). Methods for quantitation of regurgitation severity are now available, such as the measurement of the proximal isovelocity surface area, and these may be employed for determining effective orifice area and regurgitant volumes. As with other quantitative Doppler measurements, these methods are operator-dependent, and reliable data require an experienced high-volume laboratory.

Intracardiac Pressures These can be calculated from the peak continuous-wave Doppler signal of a regurgitant lesion. The Bernoulli equation is applied to the peak velocity to obtain the pressure gradient between two cardiac chambers. This is commonly applied to a tricuspid regurgitant jet, from which the systolic pressure gradient between the right atrium and right ventricle can be calculated. Adding an assumed right atrial pressure to this gradient will give a derived right ventricular systolic pressure. Change in pressure over time during isovolumic contraction can be derived from a mitral regurgitation signal. This measurement provides an index of systolic contractility.

Cardiac Output Volume flow rates can be reliably measured noninvasively from Doppler echocardiography. Using the hydrodynamic principle of flow through a rigid tube, the volume of flow can be calculated from the area of an orifice through which blood flows multiplied by the time of the velocity. The most accurate site for this measurement is through the left ventricular outflow tract. The product of the outflow area and velocity provides a beat-to-beat measurement of stroke volume, which, when multiplied by heart rate, provides a measurement of cardiac output.

Diastolic filling (See also Chap. 231) Doppler echocardiography allows noninvasive evaluation of ventricular diastolic filling. The transmitral velocity curves reflect the relative pressure gradients between the left atrium and left ventricle throughout the diastolic filling period. They are influenced by the rate of ventricular relaxation, the driving force across the valve, and the compliance of the left ventricle. There is a progression of diastolic dysfunction in disease states, which can be assessed by Doppler flow velocity curves (Fig. 227-3). In the early phase of diastolic dysfunction there is primarily an abnormality of relaxation, with decreased early transmitral flow and a compensatory increase in flow during atrial contraction. As disease progresses, there is a higher left atrial pressure and reduced compliance of the left ventricle, resulting in a higher early transmitral velocity and shortening of the deceleration of flow in early diastole, termed *restriction to filling*. These transmitral flow curves can be used to estimate ventricular filling pressures and to determine prognosis in certain disease entities. The addition of Doppler interrogation of pulmonary venous flow as well as right-sided chamber flow provides further information concerning the diastolic properties.

Congenital Heart Disease (See also Chap. 234) Doppler echocardiography has been useful in the evaluation of patients with congenital heart disease. Congenital stenotic or regurgitant valve lesions can be assessed. The detection and semiquantitation of intracardiac shunts is possible by Doppler echocardiography. Patency of surgical shunts and conduits can be determined.

STRESS ECHOCARDIOGRAPHY (See also Chap. 244) Two-dimensional and Doppler echocardiography are usually per-

Abnormal Relaxation   **Restriction**

LVEDP 6 mmHg   LVEDP 34 mmHg

FIGURE 227-3 High-fidelity left ventricular pressure curve superimposed upon a mitral inflow velocity curve obtained by Doppler echocardiography. The ratio of early and late diastolic flows is termed an *E:A ratio*. *Left*: In early stages of diastolic dysfunction, there is an abnormality of relaxation. There is a decrease in the early diastolic filling and an increase with filling at atrial contraction, resulting in a low E:A ratio of 0.5, with deceleration time (DT) of 280 ms. In this instance, the left ventricular end-diastolic pressure (LVEDP) is low at 6 mmHg. *Right*: As diastolic dysfunction progresses, there is a restriction to filling, in which there is a high early diastolic velocity and low velocity at atrial contraction resulting in a high E:A ratio of 3.0, with DT of 120 ms. In this instance, the LVEDP is markedly elevated to 34 mmHg. The DT reflects the rate of decline of the early velocity and is a measure of the effective operative compliance of the left ventricle. (See text for explanation.)

formed in the resting state. Further information can be obtained by reimaging during either exercise or pharmacologic stress. The primary indications for stress echocardiography are to confirm the suspicion of coronary artery disease and estimate its severity. Doppler stress testing provides additional information for the patient with valvular heart disease.

The response of the myocardium to ischemia consists of a cascade of events. A decrease in systolic contraction of the ischemic area, termed a *regional wall motion abnormality*, occurs before symptoms or electrocardiographic changes. During a stress echocardiogram, two-dimensional echocardiographic images at rest and during stress are digitized and displayed in a side-by-side format so that induced regional wall motion abnormalities may be detected. Changes in overall systolic function as well as end-systolic volume are also assessed. New regional wall motion abnormalities, a decline in ejection fraction, and an increase in end-systolic volume with stress are all indicators of myocardial ischemia (Fig. 227-4).

Stress testing is usually done with exercise protocols using either upright treadmill or bicycle exercise. The echocardiographic imaging is done at baseline and then immediately after exercise. In patients who are not able to exercise, pharmacologic testing can be performed by infusing dobutamine, which increases myocardial oxygen demand. Dobutamine echocardiography has also been used to assess myocardial viability in patients with poor systolic function and concomitant coronary artery disease. In this type of study, dobutamine is given at a low dose of 5 to 10 μg/kg per minute. In the presence of viable myocardium, an increase in the systolic contraction of the myocardium is evident.

There are limitations to stress echocardiography. It is important that the images be obtained as soon as possible after exercise is stopped since regional wall motion abnormalities may dissipate rapidly with time. Optimal image quality is essential for proper interpretation, and this depends on not only patient habitus but also the ability of the sonographer to obtain the image. Interpretation of the images is highly operator-dependent, and thus this technique requires an experienced echocardiographer.

FIGURE 227-4 Stress echocardiographic images in a patient with known coronary artery disease. *Left*: The systolic views from a patient in the resting state is shown. The upper frame is taken from a four-chamber view and the lower frame is taken from a two-chamber view. *Right*: The systolic views are shown immediately after exercise. The arrows point to the appearance of a regional wall motion abnormality in the anterior and apical segments. LV, left ventricle; RV, right ventricle. *(From Oh JK et al, with permission.)*

Doppler echocardiography can be used at rest and during exercise in patients with valvular heart disease to determine the hemodynamic response to stress. Gradients across stenotic valves can be measured at rest and immediately after exercise, which provides information previously obtained by right heart catheterization during exercise. Pulmonary pressures can be obtained from the tricuspid regurgitation velocities at rest and during exercise.

TRANSESOPHAGEAL ECHOCARDIOGRAPHY This technique has provided a new window on the heart. Because of the close proximity of the esophagus to the heart, high-resolution images of posterior structures are consistently obtained. Transesophageal echocardiography should be performed when further information is required after comprehensive two-dimensional and Doppler transthoracic echocardiograms. Diseases of the aorta, such as aortic dissection, can be readily diagnosed and quantitated by transesophageal echocardiography (**Plate I-2**; Chap. 247). Defining the source of embolism is a common indication for transesophageal echocardiography, as abnormalities such as atrial thrombi, patent foramen ovale, and aortic debris can be detected. Other masses, particularly those in the atria, can be visualized. The presence of vegetations for the diagnosis of infective endocarditis and its complications can be assessed by transesophageal echocardiography (Chap. 126). The evaluation of suspected abnormalities of a mitral prosthesis is an indication for transesophageal echocardiography, as the posterior imaging window will avoid the problems of acoustic reflection caused by the prosthetic valve seen with transthoracic echocardiography. Transesophageal echocardiography can be used during cardiac surgery to guide various operations, such as mitral valve repair and septal myectomy. When limited information is obtained from a transthoracic echocardiogram due to poor imaging windows, transesophageal echocardiography can be useful.

ADVANCES IN ECHOCARDIOGRAPHY There are several areas of technological advances in the field of echocardiography. Digital conversion of images allows zoom functions and endless loop playback and facilitates storage and retrieval. Harmonic imaging is a technologic advance that may significantly improve image quality, particularly in patients with poor acoustic windows. Echo contrast agents containing microbubbles cause reflection of ultrasound waves and produce bright echo-dense images. Newer contrast agents have been developed that traverse the pulmonary circulation, entering the

left-sided chambers from an intravenous injection. Two-dimensional echocardiographic imaging during the appearance of echo contrast in the left ventricle enhances definition of the endocardial border. The appearance of contrast directly in the myocardium may be useful for examining myocardial blood flow. Three-dimensional reconstruction of ultrasound images is an exciting new area of investigation that will add further to the utility of echocardiography.

NUCLEAR CARDIOLOGY

BASIC PRINCIPLES OF NUCLEAR CARDIOLOGY
All nuclear cardiology studies depend upon the injection into the patient of an isotope that emits photons, generally gamma rays generated during radioactive decay when the nucleus of an isotope changes from one energy level to a lower one. Radionuclide imaging uses a special camera that images these photons. A common problem with all nuclear studies is that photons are emitted in all directions from the point of origin, and scattering, attenuation, and absorption of the photons can occur. The higher the energy of the isotope, the less chance for scatter or absorption.

The two most commonly used isotopes are technetium 99m (^{99m}Tc) and thallium 201 (^{201}Tl). Technetium is used in both myocardial perfusion studies and radionuclide angiography and is formed on site from molybdenum 99 (^{99}Mo). The parent compound has a half-life of 66 h and thus is easily transported. ^{99m}Tc, which is a metastable compound, is constantly formed from ^{99}Mo in the on-site generator. During the decay of ^{99m}Tc to ^{99}Tc, photons are emitted with a characteristic 140-keV photopeak and a half-life of 6 h. ^{201}Tl, on the other hand, needs to be generated in a cyclotron facility and transported as a finished product, with a half-life of 73 h. The thallium isotope decay process is more complex than that of technetium, with most photons in the 80-keV range. Due to its higher energy and shorter half-life, technetium is a more desirable imaging agent.

ASSESSMENT OF VENTRICULAR FUNCTION Equilibrium radionuclide angiography, also known as *multiple-gated blood pool imaging*, is useful for the noninvasive assessment of ventricular function. It involves the imaging of ^{99m}Tc-labeled albumin or red cells that are uniformly distributed throughout the blood volume. Resting images of the blood pool of isotopes within the cardiac chambers are obtained by electrocardiographic gating through multiple cycles, so that sufficient counts can be detected to obtain an image. This requires that the heart rate be reasonably constant without significant arrhythmia. Resting images are usually obtained in the anterior, lateral, and left anterior oblique views. Each image lasts approximately 2 to 4 min.

Ejection fraction is determined by a count-based program from equilibrium radionuclide angiography; this does not require any assumptions regarding the geometry of the ventricle. It provides an accurate, reproducible method for assessment of left ventricular function. Regional wall motion analysis can be done by visual qualitative assessment, although there are programs for quantitative analysis. Left ventricular volume can also be assessed by a count-based method, using a regression equation. Other clinical variables that can be obtained include size and function of the right ventricle, size of atrial chambers and great vessels, and diastolic filling parameters. The severity of valvular regurgitant lesions can be assessed by measurement of a regurgitant fraction, which compares right ventricular stroke volume with left ventricular stroke volume.

First-pass radionuclide angiography is an alternative method for the noninvasive assessment of ventricular function. In contrast to equilibrium radionuclide angiography, first-pass radionuclide angiography involves the recording of the movement of a bolus of radionuclide during its "first pass" through the central circulation. This does not require labeling of red blood cells. ^{99m}Tc is utilized because of its low cost and short half-life. During this testing, the passage of the radioisotope through the right atrium, right ventricle, pulmonary circulation, left atrium, left ventricle, and aorta is recorded with a high count (usually multicrystal) camera. The high count rates allow temporal definition of the passage of the bolus. The change in counts of a sample placed over a ventricle reflects its function. One major advantage of first-pass angiography is the short acquisition time required, as an injected bolus will complete its passage within 30 s. In contrast to equilibrium radionuclide angiography, the right and left sides of the heart can be scanned separately. The disadvantage of first-pass radionuclide angiography compared to equilibrium testing is its poorer resolution of ventricular wall motion. It is also inaccurate in instances where the injected bolus becomes delayed in its transit, such as with severe tricuspid regurgitation or pulmonary hypertension.

Ejection fraction and regional wall motion may also be assessed using gating of single-photon emission computed tomographic (SPECT) myocardial perfusion images using technetium-labeled perfusion agents (see below).

ASSESSMENT OF MYOCARDIAL PERFUSION   Myocardial perfusion imaging by nuclear techniques is now widely applied for the evaluation of ischemic heart disease. Injection of radioisotopes at rest and during stress is performed to produce images of myocardial regional uptake proportional to regional blood flow. With maximal exercise, myocardial blood flow is increased up to fivefold above the resting condition. In the presence of a fixed coronary stenosis, there is an inability to increase myocardial perfusion in the territory supplied by the stenosis, creating a flow differential and inhomogeneous distribution of the isotope (see Fig. 244-2). In patients who are unable to exercise, pharmacologic agents are used to increase blood flow and create similar inhomogeneities. The preferred pharmacologic agents are adenosine or dipyridamole, which increase blood flow to a similar degree as exercise. In patients with bronchospastic lung disease, which is a contraindication to the use of adenosine or dipyridamole, dobutamine may be used as an alternative, although it does not increase blood flow to the same extent.

^{201}Tl is a potassium analogue and is avidly taken up by viable myocardial cells. The degree of uptake is related directly to the coronary blood flow. An initial injection is usually performed at peak exercise, and hypoperfused myocardium will have less thallium uptake than a region of normal perfusion (see Fig. 244-2). Over the next several hours, a complex process occurs that is known as "redistribution." There is a continuous input of thallium into the myocardium from a large reservoir of thallium in the blood pool. At the same time, thallium continuously washes out of portions of the myocardium at a rate that is dependent on local myocardial perfusion. The final result is that a region of ischemia that initially appears as an area of reduced uptake becomes apparently normal over time; this redistribution is seen on delayed imaging. In regions of fibrosis (infarction), there will be no redistribution on delayed imaging. A "reinjection" of an additional small amount of thallium before acquisition of the delayed images enhances the detection of ischemia. The presence of redistribution in areas of hypokinesia has been associated with recovery of left ventricular function after revascularization.

Other findings on thallium imaging may be of considerable clinical importance. Increased lung uptake of thallium may be seen immediately after stress and assessed either quantitatively or qualitatively. This finding reflects increased pulmonary capillary wedge pressure during stress. It occurs in the presence of severe coronary artery disease and/or left ventricular dysfunction. It provides important adverse prognostic information that is incremental to other clinical, stress, and coronary angiographic variables. Thallium images may also show evidence of transient poststress left ventricular dilatation. This finding is also associated with severe coronary artery disease and/or left ventricular dysfunction as well as with an adverse prognosis.

^{99m}Tc-labeled compounds have a higher photon energy and shorter half-life than ^{201}Tl, permitting the injection of larger doses. As a result, these compounds generally provide higher quality scans with fewer artifacts. Three technetium-labeled agents have been approved for general use: teboroxime, tetrofosmin, and sestamibi. The latter is the best

studied of these agents and is currently used most frequently. Like thallium, sestamibi distributes to the myocardium in relation to blood flow, and its uptake requires a viable myocardial cell and an intact cell membrane. It is transported through the cytoplasm and bound to the mitochondria in a nearly irreversible fashion. Compared to thallium, there is far less redistribution. As a result, the agent must generally be injected twice—once at rest and once during stress.

Myocardial Perfusion Imaging Protocols (Plate I-1)   The use of ^{201}Tl usually involves one of three protocols. The first protocol (stress-redistribution-delayed imaging) involves stress imaging, followed by redistribution imaging 3 or 4 h later (see Fig. 244-2). If fixed defects are present, delayed imaging is performed at a later time (usually 24 h) to detect additional redistribution. The second protocol (stress-redistribution-reinjection) also involves stress images and redistribution images 3 or 4 h later. In those patients with fixed defects on redistribution imaging, reinjection of a small amount of thallium is then performed. Repeat imaging is performed approximately 30 min later to identify a difference in myocardial uptake consistent with ischemia. In the third protocol (stress-reinjection-delayed imaging) patients are reinjected with a small amount of thallium before performing delayed imaging at 3 or 4 h. In those patients who have fixed defects on these reinjection images, more delayed imaging is then performed (usually at 24 h) in order to detect redistribution of both the initial stress dose as well as the reinjection dose. All three protocols therefore involve the use of stress images and delayed images in all patients, with a third set of images in a small subset of patients in order to improve the detection of thallium redistribution.

Stress imaging with sestamibi may utilize a 2-day protocol with different days for the injections of sestamibi at rest and during stress. Either the stress image or the rest image may be performed first. The protocol may also be carried out in one day. When the rest study is performed first a low dose is used, followed by a stress study using a larger injected dose. Alternatively, the order of these two studies may be reversed.

COMPARISON   OF   THALLIUM   AND   SESTAMIBI Both ^{201}Tl and ^{99m}Tc sestamibi provide clinically useful myocardial perfusion images in the majority of patients. The choice between the two is often dictated by local experience and economics. However, in selected patients, there may be factors that suggest a clear advantage for one or the other. The relative advantages of both agents are listed in Table 227-2.

NUCLEAR   CARDIOLOGY   IN   CLINICAL   DECISION MAKING   Stress-myocardial-perfusion imaging with either ^{201}Tl or ^{99m}Tc sestamibi plays a pivotal role in both the diagnosis and risk stratification of patients with established or suspected coronary artery disease.

For the diagnosis of coronary artery disease, stress-myocardial-perfusion imaging is an appropriate initial test (as opposed to a treadmill exercise electrocardiogram) in patients with left bundle branch

Table 227-2   Relative Advantages of Thallium-201 and Technetium-99m Sestamibi

Thallium
  Lower radiopharmaceutical cost
  Greater experience, including long-term prognostic value
  Measurement of increased pulmonary uptake
  Detection of resting ischemia (hibernating myocardium)
Sestamibi
  Better image quality (particularly in obese patients or female patients with
    breast attenuation)
  Ventricular function assessment (first-pass or gated SPECT)
  Shorter imaging times (lower cost)
  Shorter imaging protocols (patient/scheduling convenience)
  Acute imaging in myocardial infarction (myocardium at risk) and unstable
    angina (chest pain triage)
  Superior quantification, particularly of resting perfusion defect (infarct
    size)

NOTE: SPECT, single-positron emission computed tomography.

block, an electronically paced ventricular rhythm, >1 mm of ST segment depression at rest, or prior coronary artery revascularization, or in patients who are unable to exercise to a level high enough to give meaningful results. Stress-myocardial-perfusion imaging is also performed as a second test to clarify the significance of an equivocal treadmill exercise electrocardiogram.

For risk stratification, stress perfusion imaging can identify the extent, severity, and location of ischemia. These findings are often pivotal in defining the need for coronary angiography and coronary revascularization. Normal stress-myocardial-perfusion scans are highly predictive of both the absence of significant coronary artery disease and a low risk of cardiac death (less than 1% per year); coronary angiography is usually not required. Patients with markedly abnormal myocardial perfusion scans (large stress-induced defects, multiple stress-induced defects of moderate size, large fixed defect with left ventricular dilatation or increased ^{201}Tl lung uptake) are at high risk (>3 percent annual mortality rate). In such patients, coronary angiography and possible revascularization are appropriate.

POSITRON EMISSION TOMOGRAPHY (PET) The underlying physics of PET scanning is quite different from that involved in the standard radionuclide techniques described above. The annihilation of the positron leads to the simultaneous emission of two very high energy (511 keV) photons in opposite directions. These can then be imaged by a series of detectors placed in a ring around the patient. The very high energy of the photons results in far less scatter and attenuation than with conventional nuclear cardiology techniques. The sophistication of the required equipment and the associated expense have generally limited the availability of this technique. PET cameras are considerably more expensive than conventional nuclear cardiology cameras. The radiopharmaceuticals involved require a cyclotron for production and generally have half-lives that are so short that transportation beyond the immediate local region is not feasible.

Positron emitters can be employed to study both myocardial blood flow and myocardial metabolism. Nitrogen-13 ammonia, oxygen-15 water, and rubidium-82 have all been employed to assess myocardial blood flow. They permit measurement of absolute regional blood flows, in contrast to the relative blood flows that are assessed with ^{201}Tl or ^{99m}Tc sestamibi. This advantage has been utilized for research purposes but has not yet been exploited clinically. Myocardial metabolism is most often assessed using fluorine-18 deoxyglucose. This agent permits the detection and quantification of exogenous glucose utilization in areas of hypoperfused myocardium.

The clinical application of PET scanning that has been most well studied is the assessment of myocardial viability. The pattern of enhanced fluorodeoxyglucose uptake in regions of decreased perfusion (termed *glucose/blood flow "mismatch"*) indicates the presence of ischemic myocardium that has preferentially shifted its metabolic substrate towards glucose rather than fatty acid or lactate. This pattern identifies regions of ischemic or hibernating myocardium that are likely to improve in function after revascularization (Chap. 244).

Careful studies have consistently shown the ability of PET to identify ischemic or hibernating myocardium in 10 to 20% of regions that would be classified as fibrotic (infarcted) by ^{201}Tl or ^{99m}Tc sestamibi. For that reason, this technique is generally regarded as the "gold standard" for the assessment of myocardial viability. However, because of its greater cost, national clinical practice guidelines have suggested that its usage be restricted to the specific situations where it is most beneficial.

Within the past few years, specially modified conventional gamma cameras have been employed to image fluorodeoxyglucose in an attempt to avoid the expense related to cameras dedicated to PET. The limited evidence available suggests that this approach is inferior to standard PET.

BIBLIOGRAPHY

BELLER GA: Perfusion imaging: 50th Anniversary Historical Article. J Am Coll Cardiol 34:49, 1999

FLEISCHMANN KE et al: Exercise echocardiography or exercise SPECT imaging? A meta-analysis of diagnostic test performance. JAMA 180(10):913, 1998

GIBBONS RJ: Role of nuclear cardiology for determining management of patients with stable coronary artery disease. J Nucl Cardiol 1 (Suppl):S118–130, 1994

—— et al: Long-term outcome of patients with intermediate-risk exercise electrocardiograms who do not have myocardial perfusion defects on radionuclide imaging. Circulation (in press)

—— et al: Infarct size measured by SPECT imaging with technetium-99m sestamibi—a measure of the efficacy of therapy in acute myocardial infarction. Circulation (in press).

NISHIMURA RA, TAJIK AJ: Evaluation of diastolic filling of the left ventricle in health and disease: Doppler echocardiography is the clinicians' Rosetta stone. J Am Coll Cardiol 30(1):8, 1997

OH JK et al: *The Echo Manual*, 2d ed. Lippincott-Williams & Wilkins, Philadelphia 1999

RITCHIE JL et al: ACC/AHA guidelines for clinical use of radionuclide imaging: A report of the ACC/AHA task force on practice guidelines. J Am Coll Cardiol 25:521, 1995

228   *Donald S. Baim, William Grossman*

DIAGNOSTIC CARDIAC CATHETERIZATION AND ANGIOGRAPHY

Despite progressive improvements in noninvasive techniques, cardiac catheterization remains a key clinical tool for assessing the anatomy and physiology of the heart and its associated vasculature. It involves the insertion of small (diameter, 2 to 3 mm), hollow plastic tubes or catheters into a peripheral artery or vein under local anesthesia, and passage of their tips into the heart for pressure measurement or for the injection of a liquid radiographic contrast agent. The findings characterize the extent and severity of cardiac disease and thereby help in deciding on the most appropriate plan for medical, surgical, or catheter-based treatment. While most patients with coronary artery disease (CAD) or valvular disease can be managed using only clinical and noninvasive test data, more than 1.5 million cardiac catheterization and angiographic procedures are performed each year for diagnostic or interventional purposes, or both. This chapter focuses on the uses of cardiac catheterization as a diagnostic tool. →*For further discussion of catheter-based interventions, see Chap. 245.*

INDICATIONS, CONTRAINDICATIONS, AND COMPLICATIONS   Indications Given the expense and small, but real, risks of cardiac catheterization, it is not performed routinely whenever cardiac disease is diagnosed or suspected. Instead, cardiac catheterization is recommended only when there is a need to confirm the presence of a clinically suspected condition, define its anatomic and physiologic severity, and determine whether important associated conditions are present. This need most commonly arises when a patient is experiencing limiting or escalating symptoms of cardiac dysfunction (Chap. 232) or myocardial ischemia (Chap. 244) or when objective measures (such as exercise testing or echocardiography) suggest that the patient has a high risk of progressing to rapid functional deterioration, myocardial infarction, or other adverse events. Under these circumstances, catheterization is often a prelude to treatment by cardiac surgery or a catheter-based intervention. In the past, cardiac catheterization was considered mandatory in *all* patients being considered for cardiac surgery. Today, many patients with congenital or valvular heart disease can undergo surgical correction based solely on clinical and noninvasive test data; however, cardiac catheterization and coronary arteriography remain the only techniques that can define coronary anatomy with sufficient precision to support decisions regarding coronary surgery or catheter-based interventions in patients with CAD. In patients with other forms of heart disease (e.g., dilated cardiomyopathy, valvular heart disease), cardiac catheterization can provide hemody-

Table 228-1   Relative Contraindications to Cardiac Catheterization and Angiography

Uncontrolled ventricular irritability: increased risk of ventricular tachycardia and fibrillation during catheterization if ventricular irritability is uncontrolled

Uncorrected hypokalemia or digitalis toxicity

Uncorrected hypertension: predisposes to myocardial ischemia and/or heart failure during angiography

Intercurrent febrile illness

Decompensated heart failure: especially acute pulmonary edema, unless catheterization can be done with patient sitting up

Anticoagulated state: prothrombin time >18 s

Severe allergy to radiographic contrast agent

Severe renal insufficiency and/or anuria: unless dialysis is planned to remove fluid and radiographic contrast load

namic characterization essential for the design of an appropriate medical regimen as well as for an assessment of prognosis.

Contraindications   When there is a clinical "need to know," there are very few absolute contraindications in a patient who understands and accepts the associated risks. Some relative contraindications to cardiac catheterization, however, are listed in Table 228-1. Most center on factors that increase the risk of the procedure above the baseline mortality risk of roughly 1 in 1000 for clinically stable patients. This risk is increased more than tenfold in patients with severe symptoms, certain types of coronary anatomy, valve disease, left ventricular dysfunction, or severe noncardiac disease, as outlined in Table 228-2.

Complications   Beyond the mortality risk, cardiac catheterization carries a 1 in 1000 risk of stroke or myocardial infarction. Other problems, such as transient tachy- or bradyarrhythmias or bruising or bleeding at the catheter insertion site, occur in fewer than 1% of patients and respond to drug therapy, countershock, or vascular surgical repair, without long-term sequelae. Although serious, problems such as cardiac perforation or arterial dissection are very rare in the modern era of cardiac catheterization.

Some patients, however, are intolerant of the iodinated contrast agents used for angiography, which may produce transient deterioration in renal function (particularly in patients with baseline renal dysfunction or proteinuria who are not adequately prehydrated) or *allergic reactions* ranging from urticaria to frank anaphylaxis in sensitive patients. These allergic reactions can be suppressed by pretreatment with glucocorticoids (prednisone, 20 to 40 mg every 6 h), conventional antihistamines (e.g., diphenhydramine, 25 mg every 6 h), and H$_2$ antagonists (cimetidine, 300 mg every 6 h), starting 18 to 24 h prior to

Table 228-2   Patient Characteristics Associated with Increased Mortality from Cardiac Catheterization

Age: Infants (<1 month old) and the elderly (>80 years old) are at increased risk of death during cardiac catheterization. Elderly women appear to be at higher risk than elderly men.

Functional class: Mortality in class IV patients is more than 10 times greater than in class I–II patients.

Severity of coronary obstruction: Mortality for patients with left main coronary artery disease is more than 10 times greater than in patients with one- or two-vessel disease.

Valvular heart disease: Especially when severe and combined with coronary disease, is associated with a higher risk of death at cardiac catheterization than coronary artery disease alone.

Left ventricular dysfunction: Mortality in patients with a left ventricular ejection fraction <30% is more than 10 times greater than in patients with an ejection fraction ≥50%.

Severe noncardiac disease: Patients with renal insufficiency, insulin-requiring diabetes, advanced cerebrovascular and/or peripheral vascular disease, or severe pulmonary insufficiency have an increased incidence of death and other major complications from cardiac catheterization.

the procedure. Despite these precautions, occasional individuals still develop anaphylactic reactions during radiographic contrast angiography, and intravenous epinephrine must be at hand to treat such instances. Alternatively, one of the newer nonionic contrast agents may be used with less risk of a severe allergic reaction. Unlike the original high-osmolar agents, the newer low-osmolar contrast agents (including true nonionic contrast agents and the ionic dimer ioxaglate) have a lesser myocardial depressant effect and produce fewer side effects (hypotension, nausea, bradycardia, or a sensation of marked warmth following injection) than earlier high-osmolar agents. They are, however, somewhat more expensive than traditional high-osmolar ionic agents, so that many catheterization laboratories reserve their use for patients who are at higher risk for contrast-related problems.

TECHNIQUES

Cardiac catheterization is performed with the patient in the fasting state and awake but sedated. Although cardiac catheterization used to be performed exclusively as an inpatient procedure, current practice is to perform most elective procedures on an outpatient basis, with the patient discharged 4 to 6 h after the procedure is completed. Typical preprocedure sedatives include diazepam (Valium, 5 to 10 mg orally) or midazolam (Versed, 1 mg intravenously). It is also customary to give the antihistamine diphenhydramine (Benadryl, 25 to 50 mg orally) before the procedure in the hope of suppressing minor allergic reactions to iodinated contrast. Since cardiac catheterization is a sterile procedure, prophylactic antibiotics are not necessary. To minimize the risks of bleeding at the local catheter insertion site, patients who have been anticoagulated chronically with warfarin should have this agent discontinued at least 48 h prior to the procedure, so that the INR falls below 2.

Most (>95%) cardiac catheterizations are performed by the percutaneous femoral technique, in which a needle puncture is performed in the femoral artery (for left heart catheterization) and the femoral vein (for right heart catheterization). A flexible guidewire is inserted through this needle, allowing placement of a vascular access sheath through which the desired catheters can be advanced. This percutaneous technique has been modified for other sites, including the brachial and even the radial artery. The brachial or radial approach has an advantage in the patient with peripheral vascular disease involving the abdominal aorta and iliac or femoral arteries or in whom immediate postprocedure ambulation is desired, but it involves some limitations in the range of devices that can be used if the diagnostic procedure evolves into a catheter-based intervention. With these alternatives, the original cut-down, or Sones, technique of cardiac catheterization by direct exposure of the brachial artery and vein in the antecubital fossa is rarely used.

Cardiac catheterization may include a variety of different measurements of pressure and flow (hemodynamics) as well as a variety of different contrast injections recorded as x-ray movies (angiography). The exact types of testing performed in any given procedure depend on the nature of the clinical problem being evaluated. In patients with CAD, the procedure may include only left ventriculography and coronary angiography, while in patients with valvular heart disease, full left and right heart hemodynamic studies may be performed.

RIGHT HEART CATHETERIZATION   Measurement of the pressures in the right side of the heart was once a routine part of each cardiac catheterization, but it is now used in fewer than 25% of procedures because it adds little to the evaluation of the patient with CAD. It is still useful, however, when significant left and/or right ventricular dysfunction, valve disease, myopericardial disease, or intracardiac shunting is suspected. The right heart catheterization procedure is similar to the placement of a Swan-Ganz catheter at the bedside in the intensive care unit, except that it is performed under fluoroscopic guidance. A balloon flotation catheter is advanced from a suitable vein (femoral, brachial, subclavian, or internal jugular) into the superior vena cava, where blood is sampled for oximetry. The

Table 228-3   Normal Values for Hemodynamic Parameters

Pressures (mmHg)

Systemic arterial	
Peak systolic/end-diastolic	100–140/60–90
Mean	70–105
Left ventricle	
Peak systolic/end-diastolic	100–140/3–12
Left atrium (or pulmonary capillary wedge)	
Mean	2–10
a wave	3–15
v wave	3–15
Pulmonary artery	
Peak systolic/end-diastolic	15–30/4–12
Mean	9–18
Right ventricle	
Peak systolic/end-diastolic	15–30/2–8
Right atrium	
Mean	2–8
a wave	2–10
v wave	2–10
Resistances [(dyn·s)/cm^5]	
Systemic vascular resistance	700–1600
Pulmonary vascular resistance	20–130
Cardiac index [(L/min)/m^2]	2.6–4.2
Oxygen consumption index [(L/min)/m^2]	110–150
Arteriovenous oxygen difference (mL/L)	30–50

catheter is then positioned in the right atrium, where pressure is measured. The balloon is inflated with air (or carbon dioxide, if intracardiac shunting is supected) and advanced sequentially into the right ventricle, pulmonary artery, and pulmonary artery wedge position. Pressure is recorded at each of these locations, with normal values for pressures measured during cardiac catheterization summarized in Table 228-3. After the pulmonary wedge pressure (which approximates left atrial pressure) is recorded, the balloon is deflated so that pulmonary artery pressure can be monitored and blood samples obtained for oximetry. Comparison of oxygen saturations in the superior and inferior vena cava, the chambers of the right heart, and pulmonary artery permits assessment of the presence of a left-to-right shunt at the atrial, ventricular, or pulmonary artery level, which will be manifested as an increase ("step-up") in oxygen saturation of blood as it traverses these vessels and chambers.

Measurement of Cardiac Output   Measurements of the pulmonary artery and aortic oxygen content and oxygen consumption allow calculation of the cardiac output by the Fick principle, which states that

$$Q \; (\text{L/min}) = \frac{O_2 \; \text{consumption (mL/min)}}{\text{arteriovenous } O_2 \; \text{difference (mL/L)}}$$

In order to compare individuals of different body weights and sizes, O_2 consumption and cardiac output (Q) are commonly divided by body surface area. Normal values for O_2 consumption and cardiac output are given in Table 228-3. What is calculated by dividing O_2 consumption by the arteriovenous O_2 difference across the lungs (estimated pulmonary venous − pulmonary arterial O_2 content) is actually the pulmonary blood flow (Q_p). In patients with left-to-right shunt at the atrial, ventricular, or pulmonary artery levels, pulmonary blood flow will exceed systemic blood flow. In such cases, systemic blood flow (Q_s) is calculated by dividing O_2 consumption by the systemic arteriovenous O_2 difference. The latter is calculated as the systemic arterial blood O_2 content minus the mixed venous blood O_2 content as estimated using blood from the chamber immediately proximal to the level of the shunt. The Fick method is most dependable when the cardiac output is low and the arteriovenous oxygen difference is large.

Another approach to the measurement of cardiac output during right heart catheterization is the thermodilution technique, in which a thermistor is mounted on the tip of a balloon flotation catheter and positioned in the pulmonary artery. Cold dextrose solution or saline is injected via a proximal port on the catheter into the vena cava or right atrium, and the change in temperature monitored at the thermistor is integrated electronically. This integral is inversely proportional to the volume flow rate past the thermistor, and if the temperatures of the injectate and pulmonary artery blood are measured, cardiac output (actually, pulmonary blood flow) can be calculated. In contrast to the Fick method, the indicator-dilution method is least reliable when the cardiac output is low.

LEFT HEART CATHETERIZATION   Whether performed using the femoral, brachial, or radial approach, the left heart catheter is advanced under fluoroscopic guidance into the central aorta, where pressure is measured and recorded. Next, the catheter is advanced in retrograde fashion across the aortic valve into the left ventricle, where pressure is measured. If a right heart catheter is in place, this is an appropriate time for simultaneous measurement and recording of left heart, right heart, and peripheral arterial pressures together with a determination of cardiac output by either thermodilution or the Fick principle. These measures allow assessment of possible pressure gradients across the mitral and aortic valves, and catheter pullback on the right side permits assessment of possible gradients across the pulmonic and tricuspid valves. Simultaneous measurement of pressures and cardiac output provides the data for calculation of systemic and pulmonary vascular resistances. The resistance to blood flow through the systemic vascular bed is

$$SVR = 80(MAP - RA)/SBF$$

where *SVR* is systemic vascular resistance [(dyn·s)/cm^5], *MAP* and *RA* are mean aortic and right atrial pressures (mmHg), 80 is a constant for converting to metric units, and *SBF* is systemic blood flow (L/min). Resistance to blood flow through the pulmonary vascular bed is

$$PVR = 80(PA - PCW \text{ or } LA)/PBF$$

where *PVR* is pulmonary vascular resistance [(dyn·s)/cm^5]; *PA*, *PCW*, and *LA* are pulmonary artery, pulmonary capillary wedge, and left atrial mean pressures, respectively (mmHg); and *PBF* is pulmonary blood flow (L/min). Normal values for pulmonary and systemic vascular resistances are given in Table 228-3.

When valvular stenosis is present, the measurements of the upstream and downstream pressures and flow allow calculation of the valve orifice using the Gorlin formula.

$$A = flow/K\sqrt{\Delta P}$$

where *A* is the valve orifice area (cm^2), *flow* is the blood flow (mL/s) across the stenotic valve; Δ*P* is the mean pressure gradient (mmHg) during the period of blood flow; and *K* is a constant (44.3 for the aortic valve and 37.7 for the mitral valve).

As seen in Fig. 228-1, normal left ventricular and aortic pressures are essentially equal during systole, while normal left atrial (pulmonary capillary wedge) and left ventricular pressures are equal during diastole in the normal heart. The presence of a systolic pressure gradient between the left ventricle and aorta indicates obstruction at the level of the aortic valve (e.g., calcific *aortic stenosis*) or at subaortic level (e.g., *hypertrophic obstructive cardiomyopathy*). Similarly, the presence of a diastolic pressure gradient between the left atrium (or pulmonary capillary wedge pressure) and the left ventricle generally indicates *mitral stenosis*, although it may also be seen in rare conditions such as cor triatriatum and left atrial myoxoma. An example of a large diastolic pressure gradient in a patient with mitral stenosis is seen in Fig. 228-2. As seen in Fig. 228-3, patients with significant mitral regurgitation may have a prominent *v* wave in the pulmonary capillary wedge pressure, which often increases substantially during modest exercise. Severe *aortic regurgitation* produces a widening of

FIGURE 228-1 Left ventricular (LV), radial artery, and pulmonary capillary wedge (PCW) pressures in a patient with normal cardiovascular function. Note the absence of a pressure gradient between the LV and radial artery in systole and between the LV and PCW in diastole.

the aortic pulse pressure, with equilibration of aortic and left ventricular pressures in diastole (Fig. 228-4). Right-sided pressures exhibit a characteristic deformity in the presence of valvular heart disease affecting the tricuspid or pulmonic valves. In patients with severe *tricuspid regurgitation*, the right atrial pressure resembles the right ventricular pressure closely in appearance. Mean right atrial pressure and right ventricular end-diastolic pressure are both elevated in tricuspid regurgitation. In *tricuspid stenosis*, there is a pressure gradient between the right atrium and ventricle during diastole.

Abnormalities in pressure waveforms may also be suggestive of conditions such as *cardiac tamponade* or *pericardial constriction* (Chap. 239). In both conditions there is equalization of left and right ventricular diastolic pressures. However, in constrictive pericarditis, nearly all ventricular filling occurs shortly after mitral and tricuspid valve opening; after this period of rapid filling, ventricular volumes cannot increase further owing to the constricting pericardium. This abnormality produces an abrupt early ventricular diastolic pressure rise with a mid- and late-ventricular pressure plateau, giving the so-called square root sign (Fig. 228-5). In contrast, in tamponade there is equalization of diastolic pressures with a gradual increase throughout diastole.

Congestive heart failure due to myocardial contractile dysfunction is associated with characteristic alterations in the ventricular pressure waveforms seen at cardiac catheterization. Neither the rise nor the decline in isovolumic pressure is as steep as in the normal heart. The reduced slopes of pressure rise and decline are associated with an

FIGURE 228-2 Pulmonary capillary wedge (PCW) and left ventricular (LV) pressure tracings in a 40-year-old woman with mitral stenosis. This patient also had systemic hypertension and significant elevation of her LV diastolic pressure. *[From BA Carabello, W Grossman, in Grossman's Cardiac Catheterization, Angiography, and Intervention, 6th ed, DS Baim, W Grossman (eds). Baltimore, Lippincott Williams & Wilkins, 2000.]*

abbreviated ejection period, giving the left ventricular pressure tracing a triangular appearance (Fig. 228-6). Also, the pressure decline does not continue to zero, so the minimal left ventricular pressure may be elevated. This hemodynamic finding correlates with an increased ventricular end-systolic volume, which is a sign of depressed contractile function of the left ventricular myocardium.

CARDIAC ANGIOGRAPHY

LEFT VENTRICULOGRAPHY   Following the measurement of cardiac pressures, the angiographic portion of the cardiac catheterization usually begins with left ventriculography—the injection of radiographic contrast material directly into the left ventricular cavity. A power injector is used to inject 30 to 45 mL of radiographic contrast material into the left ventricular chamber at a rate of 10 to 12 mL/s. The resulting radiographic images are recorded, and the left ventricular silhouette is defined at end-diastole and end-systole. This permits calculation of the left ventricular chamber volumes and ejection fraction, as well as qualitative assessment of regional wall motion abnormalities. The normal left ventricle ejects 50 to 80% of its end-diastolic volume with each beat; i.e., its *ejection fraction* is 0.50 to 0.80. In adults, normal values for left ventricular volumes are, for end-diastolic volume, 72 ± 15 mL/m^2 (mean $\pm$ standard deviation) and, for end-systolic volume, 20 ± 8 mL/m^2. Regional abnormalities of wall motion are illustrated in Fig. 228-7 and include diminished inward motion of a myocardial segment (*hypokinesis*), absence of inward movement of a myocardial segment (*akinesis*), and paradoxical systolic expansion of a regional myocardial segment (*dyskinesis*).

Left ventriculography is usually performed in the right anterior oblique projection, which allows assessment of the mitral and aortic valves. Mitral regurgitation is easily visualized as the leakage of radiographic contrast material back into the left atrium during left ventricular systole. Its severity can be estimated qualitatively using a grading system of 1+ (mild; radiographic contrast material clears with each beat and never opacifies the entire left atrium) to 4+ (severe; opacification of the entire left atrium occurs within one beat, and contrast material can be seen refluxing into the pulmonary veins).

Left ventriculography performed in the *left* anterior oblique projection permits detection of abnormal communications, such as a ventricular septal defect (Chap. 234). In the most common form of hypertrophic cardiomyopathy (idiopathic hypertrophic subaortic stenosis; Chap. 238), left ventriculography in this projection shows anterior motion of the anterior leaflet of the mitral valve during systole and bulging of the interventricular septum into the left ventricular cavity, especially in the subaortic region. Mural thrombi within the left ventricular chamber may be well visualized during left ventriculography; they occur most commonly in the left ventricular apex.

AORTOGRAPHY Rapid injection of radiographic contrast material into the ascending aorta allows detection of abnormalities that involve the aorta and aortic valve. When suspected clinically, aortography permits detection and qualitative assessment of the severity of abnormalities such as aortic regurgitation, which is graded using a 1+ to 4+ scale, as for mitral regurgitation. Abnormal communications between the aorta and right side of the heart, such as a patent ductus arteriosus or ruptured aneurysm of a sinus of Valsalva, may be visualized. Aortography can permit identification of aortic aneurysm and of aortic dissection (Chap. 247) by visualizing an intimal flap within the aortic lumen.

CORONARY ANGIOGRAPHY This common procedure involves the selective injection of a radiographic contrast agent into the coronary arteries. Placement of the catheter tip into the right and left coronary arteries is carried out under fluoroscopic guidance, and contrast agent is injected by hand during recording of the radiographic image. Each coronary artery is usually viewed in several projections to permit assessment of the severity of stenosis and to minimize the overlap of adjacent vessels. In addition to the detection of coronary artery stenoses, coronary angiography is useful for the detection of congenital abnormalities of the coronary circulation, coronary arteriovenous fistulas, and patency of coronary artery bypass grafts. Examples of normal and abnormal coronary anatomy are shown in Figs. 228-8 and 228-9. The location, severity, and morphology of the stenotic lesions can be analyzed in great detail, and the resulting information is essential to planning either bypass surgery or catheter-based intervention (Fig. 228-10). This is usually done by visual estimation of percent diameter stenosis of each lesion relative to the "uninvolved" adjacent reference segment, with stenosis > 50% taken as being hemodynamically significant (interfering with maximal increases in perfusion of the subserved myocardial territory during stress).

POSTPROCEDURE CARE The average cardiac catheterization procedure takes between 30 and 45 min. Intravenous heparin (2000 to 3000 IU) may or may not be given at the time of catheter insertion. At the completion of the procedure, heparin may be reversed

FIGURE 228-3 Hemodynamic findings at rest and during exercise in a patient with mitral regurgitation. Left ventricular (LV), pulmonary capillary wedge (PCW), and radial artery pressure tracings are shown before (*left*) and during (*right*) the sixth minute of supine bicycle exercise. PCW mean pressure and v wave increase substantially with exercise. [*From BH Lorell, W Grossman, in Grossman's Cardiac Catheterization, Angiography, and Intervention, 6th ed, DS Baim, W Grossman (eds). Baltimore, Lippincott Williams & Wilkins, 2000.*]

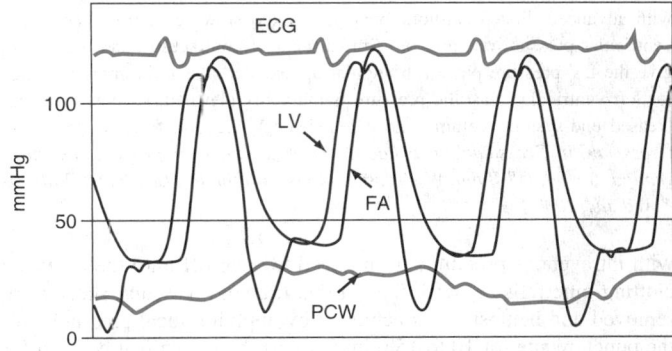

FIGURE 228-4 Severe aortic regurgitation. There is equilibration between the left ventricular (LV) and aortic or femoral artery (FA) pressures in diastole. Also, LV diastolic pressure exceeds pulmonary capillary wedge (PCW) pressure early in diastole, indicating premature closure of the mitral valve (a characteristic feature of severe aortic regurgitation). [*From W Grossman, in Grossman's Cardiac Catheterization, Angiography, and Intervention, 6th ed, DS Baim, W Grossman (eds). Baltimore, Lippincott Williams & Wilkins, 2000.*]

FIGURE 228-5 Left ventricular (LV), right ventricular (RV), and pulmonary capillary wedge (PCW) pressure tracings in a patient with severe constrictive pericarditis. Note the diastolic dip and plateau ("square root sign") pattern for left and right ventricular diastolic pressures (*left*). The wedge pressure (*right*) shows early systolic and early diastolic dips.

FIGURE 228-6 Left ventricular (LV) and aortic (Ao) pressures in a patient with advanced dilated cardiomyopathy. Marked slowing of the rates of left ventricular pressure rise and fall (impairment of contractility and relaxation) give the LV pressure pulse a triangular appearance. Also, the minimal value for left ventricular diastolic pressure is markedly elevated, suggesting an increased end-systolic volume and a reduced LV ejection fraction. *[From W Grossman, in Grossman's Cardiac Catheterization, Angiography, and Intervention, 6th ed, DS Baim, W Grossman (eds). Baltimore, Lippincott Williams & Wilkins, 2000.]*

with intravenous protamine or allowed to wear off until the activated clotting time falls below 160 s. At that time, the vascular sheaths are removed and hemostasis is achieved by applying local pressure over the puncture site for 10 to 15 min. Patients then remain at bed rest for

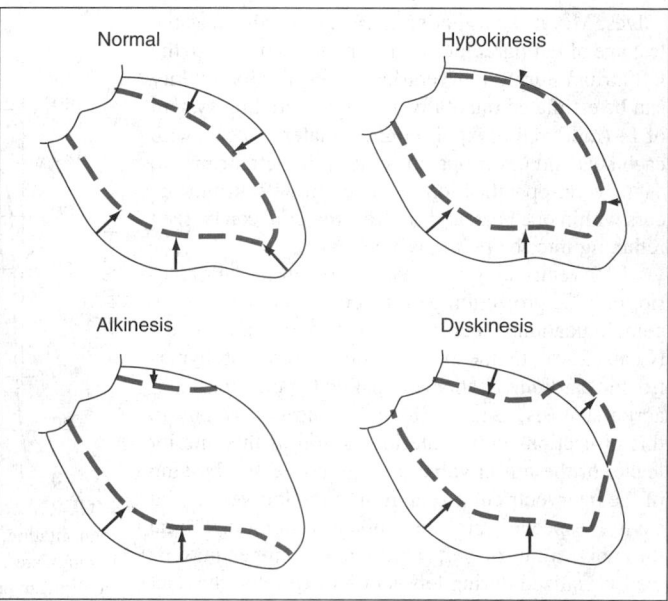

FIGURE 228-7 Diagrammatic representation of end-diastolic (*solid line*) and end-systolic (*dashed line*) silhouettes of left ventricular cineangiograms in various forms of localized wall motion disorder in patients with coronary heart disease. Normal wall motion is symmetric; a patient with *hypokinesis* exhibits reduced contraction, seen here over the anterior and apical surfaces; a patient with *akinesis* exhibits absent wall motion, seen here over the anteroapical surface; a patient with *dyskinesis* exhibits paradoxic bulging of a small portion of the anterior wall with systole.

4 to 6 h before ambulating and being discharged to home. A variety of devices for sealing the arterial puncture site can allow a shorter period of bed rest and earlier ambulation. Patients with suitable anatomy may return at a later date for either catheter-based intervention or bypass surgery, although it is now common practice to perform a catheter-based intervention during the same procedure as the diagnostic cardiac catheterization, if appropriate.

FIGURE 228-8 Representation of coronary anatomy relative to the interventricular and atrioventricular valve planes. Coronary branches are indicated as L Main (left main), LAD (left anterior descending), D (diagonal), S (septal), CX (circumflex), OM (obtuse marginal), RCA (right coronary artery), CB (conus branch), SN (sinus node), AcM (acute marginal), PD (posterior descend- ing), PL (posterolateral left ventricular). RAO, right anterior oblique, LAO, left anterior oblique. *[From DS Baim, W Grossman, in Grossman's Cardiac Catheterization, Angiography, and Intervention, 6th ed, DS Baim, W Grossman (eds). Baltimore, Lippincott Williams & Wilkins, 2000.]*

FIGURE 228-9 Coronary angiogram showing a right coronary artery (RCA) with a severe (95%) stenosis at its midpoint (*arrow*).

BIBLIOGRAPHY

BAIM DS, GROSSMAN W (eds): *Grossman's Cardiac Catheterization, Angiography, and Intervention*, 6th ed. Baltimore, Lippincott Williams & Wilkins, 2000

DAVIDSON CJ et al: Cardiac catheterization, in *Heart Disease*, 6th ed, E Braunwald (ed). Philadelphia, Saunders, 2001

JOHNSON LW, KRONE R: Cardiac catheterization 1991: A report of the Registry of the Society for Cardiac Angiography and Interventions (SCA&I). Cathet Cardiovasc Diagn 28:219, 1993

KERN MJ et al: Interpretation of cardiac pathophysiology from pressure waveform anal-

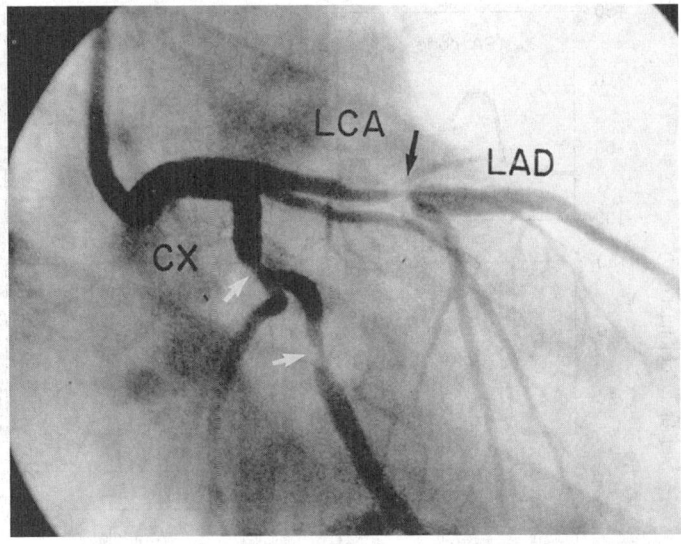

FIGURE 228-10 Coronary angiogram of a left coronary artery (LCA) with a tight stenosis in the proximal left anterior descending (LAD) artery (*black arrow*) immediately prior to the origin of a large septal branch. The circumflex artery (CX) has two moderately severe stenoses (*white arrows*).

ysis: Simultaneous left and right ventricular pressure measurements. Cathet Cardiovasc Diagn 28:51, 1993

SCANLON PJ et al: AHA/ACC guidelines or coronary angiography—executive summary and recommendations. Circulation 99:2345, 1999

Section 2
DISORDERS OF RHYTHM

229

Mark E. Josephson, Peter Zimetbaum

THE BRADYARRHYTHMIAS: DISORDERS OF SINUS NODE FUNCTION AND AV CONDUCTION DISTURBANCES

ANATOMY OF THE CONDUCTING SYSTEM Under normal conditions, the pacemaker function of the heart resides in the sinoatrial (SA) node, which lies at the junction of the right atrium and superior vena cava. The SA node is approximately 1.5 cm long and 2 to 3 mm wide and is supplied by the sinus node artery, which arises from either the right coronary artery (60%) or the left circumflex coronary artery (40%). Once the impulse exits the sinus node and perinodal tissue, it traverses the atrium until it reaches the atrioventricular (AV) node. The blood supply of the AV node is derived from the posterior descending coronary artery (90%). The AV node lies at the base of the interatrial septum just above the tricuspid annulus and anterior to the coronary sinus. The electrophysiologic properties of the AV node result in slow conduction, which is responsible for the normal delay in AV conduction, i.e., the PR interval.

The bundle of His emerges from the AV node, enters the fibrous skeleton of the heart, and courses anteriorly across the membranous interventricular septum. It has a dual blood supply from the AV nodal artery and a branch of the anterior descending coronary artery. The branching (distal) portion of the bundle of His gives rise to a broad sheet of fibers that course over the left side of the interventricular septum to form the left bundle branch and a narrow cable-like structure on the right side that forms the right bundle branch. The arborization of both the right and left bundle branches gives rise to the distal His-Purkinje system, which ultimately extends throughout the endocardium of the right and left ventricles.

The SA node, atrium, and AV node are significantly influenced by autonomic tone. Vagal influences depress automaticity of the SA node, depress conduction, and prolong refractoriness in the tissue surrounding the SA node; inhomogeneously decrease atrial refractoriness and slow atrial conduction; and prolong AV nodal conduction and refractoriness. Sympathetic influences exert the opposite effect.

ELECTROPHYSIOLOGIC PRINCIPLES

In the resting state, the interior of most cardiac cells, with the exception of the SA and AV nodes, is approximately −80 to −90 mV, negative with respect to a reference extracellular electrode. The resting membrane potential is determined primarily by the concentration gradient of potassium across the cell membrane. Activation of cardiac cells results from movement of ions across the cell membrane, causing a transient depolarization known as the *action potential*. The ionic species responsible for the action potential varies among the cardiac tissues, and the configuration of the action potential is therefore unique to each tissue (Fig. 229-1).

The action potential of the His-Purkinje system and ventricular myocardium has five phases (Fig. 229-2). The rapid depolarizing current (phase 0) is mainly determined by an influx of sodium into my-

FIGURE 229-1 Action potential configurations in different regions of the mammalian heart. *(From AM Katz, Physiology of the Heart, 2e, New York, Raven, 1992, with permission.)*

ocardial cells followed by a secondary (slower) influx of calcium, which produces a slow inward current. The repolarization phases of the action potential (phases 1 to 3) are primarily related to outward flux of potassium. The resting membrane potential is phase 4.

The bradyarrhythmias result from abnormalities either of impulse formation, i.e., automaticity, or of conduction. *Automaticity,* which is normally observed in the sinus node, the specialized fibers of the His-

FIGURE 229-2 Schematic representation of the action potential in normal ventricle depicting the direction, strength, and period of flow of the ionic currents underlying the action potential. The arrow's direction and size indicate whether current is inward- or outward-directed and the approximate current strength of the ion identified at the arrow's base. The horizontal position of the arrow corresponds to the same moment in the time course of action potential (see text). The five phases of the action potential are indicated by the numerals placed along the waveform. *(From Ten Eick et al, Prog Cardiovasc Dis 24(2): 157, 1981, with permission.)*

Purkinje system, and some specialized atrial fibers, is the property of a cardiac cell that causes it to depolarize spontaneously during phase 4 of the action potential, leading to the generation of an impulse. To exhibit automaticity, the resting membrane potential must decrease spontaneously until threshold potential is reached and an all-or-none regenerative response occurs. The ionic currents producing spontaneous diastolic depolarization appear to involve the inward current of either sodium or calcium and a decreasing outward potassium current. The velocity of *conduction,* i.e., impulse propagation through cardiac tissues, depends on the magnitude of inward current, which is directly related to the rate of rise and amplitude of phase 0 of the action potential. The more positive the threshold potential and the slower the rate of depolarization toward threshold, the slower is the rate of rise of phase 0 of the action potential and the slower is the conduction velocity. Disease states or drugs may result in lower rates of rise of phase 0 at any given membrane potential. Passive membrane properties (e.g., intracellular resistance and intercellular coupling) can also affect impulse propagation. Propagation is more rapid parallel to fiber orientation than transverse to it, a property termed *anisotropic conduction.*

Refractoriness is a property of cardiac cells that defines the period of recovery that cells require after being discharged before they can be reexcited by a stimulus. The *absolute refractory period* is defined by that portion of the action potential during which no stimulus, regardless of its strength, can evoke another response. The *effective refractory period* is that part of the action potential during which a stimulus can evoke only a local, nonpropagated response. The *relative refractory period* extends from the end of the effective refractory period to the time that the tissue is fully recovered. During this time, a stimulus of greater than threshold strength is required to evoke a response, which is propagated more slowly than normal. In the normal His-Purkinje system or ventricular myocytes, excitability is recovered following completion of the action potential, and evoked responses have characteristics similar to the spontaneous normal response. In the AV node, recovery of excitability occurs well after completion of the action potential.

INTRACARDIAC RECORDINGS OF THE SPECIALIZED CONDUCTING SYSTEM Electrode catheters allow the recording of activation of portions of the specialized conducting system, including the bundle of His. To obtain a recording from the bundle of His, the electrode catheter is positioned across the tricuspid valve (Fig. 229-3). The interval from local atrial depolarization in the His bundle recording to the onset of depolarization of the His bundle deflection is called the *AH interval* (normal = 60 to 125 ms) and represents an indirect method of assessing AV nodal conduction time. The interval from the beginning of the His bundle deflection to the earliest onset of ventricular activation, as measured from any of multiple-surface electrocardiogram (ECG) leads or the intracardiac ventricular electrogram, is called the *HV interval* (normal = 35 to 55 ms) and represents conduction time through the His-Purkinje system. Electrode catheters can be positioned in the area of the sinus node to record high right atrial activity. Left atrial activity may be recorded directly via a catheter placed across a patent foramen ovale or indirectly using a catheter inserted into the coronary sinus. The atrial activation sequence may be "mapped," and sites of intra- and interatrial conduction abnormalities may be ascertained.

SINUS NODE DYSFUNCTION

The SA node is normally the dominant cardiac pacemaker because its intrinsic discharge rate is the highest of all potential cardiac pacemakers. Its responsiveness to alterations in autonomic nervous system tone is responsible for the normal acceleration of heart rate during exercise and the slowing that occurs during rest and sleep. Increases in sinus rate normally result from an increase in sympathetic tone acting via β-adrenergic receptors and/or a decrease in parasympathetic tone acting via muscarinic receptors. Slowing of the heart rate is normally due to opposite alterations. In adults, the normal sinus rate under basal conditions is 60 to 100 beats per minute. *Sinus bradycardia* is said to exist when the sinus rate is less than 60 beats per minute, and *sinus*

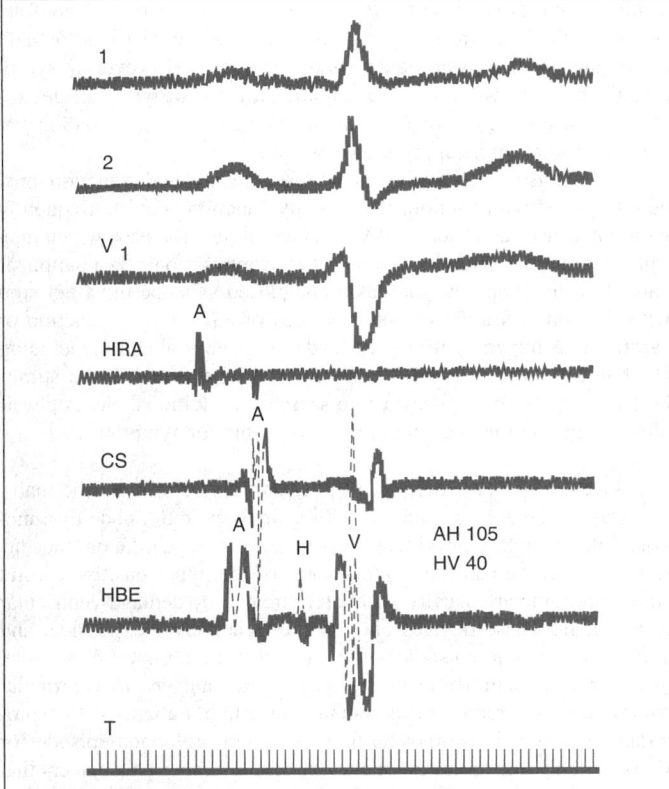

FIGURE 229-3 Normal intracardiac recording. Surface ECG leads I, II, and V$_1$ are displayed with intracardiac ECGs from the high right atrium (HRA), left atrium from the coronary sinus (CS), and AV junction to obtain a His bundle electrogram (HBE). T, time lines; A, atrial activation; H, His bundle activation; V, ventricular activation. Atrial activation begins in the HRA and spreads inferiorly to the low atrial septum, as recorded in the HBE, and the left atrium, as recorded in the CS. The AH and HV intervals represent AV nodal and His-Purkinje conduction times, respectively. Vertical lines = 0.10 s. *(From ME Josephson, SF Seides, Clinical Cardiac Electrophysiology: Techniques and Interpretations. Philadelphia, Lea & Febiger, 1979, with permission.)*

tachycardia when it exceeds 100 beats per minute. However, there is wide variation among individuals, and rates less than 60 beats per minute do not necessarily indicate pathologic states. For example, trained athletes often exhibit resting rates under 50 beats per minute due to increases in vagal tone. Normal elderly individuals may also show marked sinus bradycardia at rest.

ETIOLOGY SA node dysfunction is most often found in the elderly as an isolated phenomenon. Although interruption of the blood supply to the SA node may produce dysfunction, the correlation between obstruction of the sinus node artery and clinical evidence of SA node dysfunction is poor. Specific disease states associated with SA node dysfunction include senile amyloidosis and other conditions associated with infiltration of the atrial myocardium. Sinus bradycardia is associated with hypothyroidism, advanced liver disease, hypothermia, typhoid fever, and brucellosis; it occurs during episodes of hypervagotonia (vasovagal syncope), severe hypoxia, hypercapnia, acidemia, and acute hypertension. However, most cases of SA node dysfunction are due to idiopathic degeneration or are secondary to pharmacologic agents.

MANIFESTATIONS Although marked (≤50 beats per minute) sinus bradycardia may cause fatigue and other symptoms due to inadequate cardiac output, more commonly sinus node dysfunction is manifest as paroxysmal dizziness, presyncope, or syncope.

These symptoms usually result from abrupt, prolonged sinus pauses caused by failure of sinus impulse formation (sinus arrest) or block of conduction of sinus impulses to the surrounding atrial tissue (sinus exit block). In either case, the ECG manifestation is a prolonged period (>3 s) of atrial asystole. In some patients, SA node dysfunction is accompanied by abnormalities in AV conduction. In addition to the absence of atrial activity, lower pacemakers fail to emerge during the sinus pauses, resulting in periods of ventricular asystole and syncope. Occasionally, SA node dysfunction is manifested by an inadequate acceleration in sinus rate in response to a stress such as exercise or fever. In some patients, SA node dysfunction may become manifest only in the presence of certain cardioactive drugs: cardiac glycosides, β-adrenergic blocking drugs, calcium channel blockers, amiodarone, and other antiarrhythmic agents. These agents, which do not usually cause sinus node dysfunction in normal people, may unmask evidence of sinus node dysfunction in susceptible individuals.

The *sick sinus syndrome* refers to a combination of symptoms (dizziness, confusion, fatigue, syncope, and congestive heart failure) caused by SA node dysfunction and manifested by marked sinus bradycardia, sinoatrial block, or sinus arrest. Because these symptoms are nonspecific, and because ECG manifestations of sinus node dysfunction are often intermittent, it may be difficult to prove that such symptoms are actually caused by SA node dysfunction.

Atrial tachyarrhythmias such as atrial fibrillation, atrial flutter, or atrial tachycardia may be accompanied by SA node dysfunction. The *bradycardia-tachycardia syndrome* refers to paroxysmal atrial arrhythmia that upon termination is followed by prolonged sinus pauses (Fig. 229-4) or in which there are alternating periods of tachyarrhythmia and bradyarrhythmia. Syncope or presyncope may result from failure of the sinus node to recover function following suppression of automaticity by atrial tachyarrhythmia.

DIAGNOSIS *First-degree sinoatrial exit block* denotes a prolonged conduction time from the SA node to the surrounding atrial tissue. It cannot be recognized on a standard (surface) ECG but requires invasive intracardiac recordings, which can detect this condition indirectly, by measuring the sinus response to atrial premature beats, or directly, by recording SA node electrograms. *Second-degree sinoatrial exit block* denotes the intermittent failure of conduction of sinus impulses to the surrounding atrial tissue; it is manifested as the intermittent absence of P waves (Fig. 229-5). *Third-degree*, or *complete, sinoatrial block* is characterized by a lack of atrial activity or by the presence of an ectopic subsidiary atrial pacemaker. On the standard ECG it cannot be distinguished from sinus arrest, but direct intracardiac recordings of SA node activity permit this distinction. The *bradycardia-tachycardia syndrome* is manifested on the standard ECG as tachyarrhythmias (Fig. 229-4). Most often these are atrial flutter or fibrillation, although any tachycardia during which the atria are activated may cause overdrive suppression of the sinus node resulting in clinical appearance of this syndrome.

The most important step in the diagnosis is to correlate symptoms with ECG evidence of SA node dysfunction. While ambulatory ECG (Holter) monitoring remains a mainstay in evaluating sinus node function, most episodes of syncope are paroxysmal and unpredictable. Sin-

FIGURE 229-4 Tachycardia-bradycardia syndrome. Rhythm strip of ECG lead II showing spontaneous cessation of supraventricular tachycardia followed by a 6-s pause prior to resumption of sinus activity. The patient was asymptomatic during supraventricular tachycardia, but the sinus pause caused severe light-headedness.

FIGURE 229-5   Second-degree sinoatrial exit block. Surface ECG denoting abrupt absence of P wave during sinus rhythm. Prior to the pause, the sinus rate is regular. The interval of the pause is exactly twice the basal sinus cycle length. The arrow marks the appropriate location for the absent P wave. SA exit block can be 2:1 as above or longer, as shown in Fig. 229-6.

gle and even multiple 24-h Holter monitor recordings may fail to include a symptomatic episode.

Caution must be taken in interpreting the Holter monitor results. For instance, a pause during sleep is often a normal finding associated with heightened vagal tone. This should not be interpreted as sinus node dysfunction requiring pacemaker implantation.

Continuous-loop event records represent a more specific diagnostic tool. These devices may be worn for prolonged periods of time and allow close correlation between electrocardiographic findings and symptoms. They do require the patient's ability to activate the monitor at the time of symptoms. More recently, an implantable event recorder, which can be interrogated like a pacemaker, has been developed for patients with rare events.

The response to carotid sinus pressure and pharmacologic autonomic "denervation" of the heart may be helpful. Carotid sinus pressure can be particularly useful in patients in whom paroxysmal dizziness or syncope is compatible with the hypersensitive carotid sinus syndrome (Chap. 21). In such patients, the response can be dramatic, and sinus pauses in excess of 5 s may occur. Although pauses in excess of 3 s are considered abnormal, in elderly patients such pauses are common and do not necessarily signify a diagnostic response. This is a major limitation of the use of carotid sinus pressure as a diagnostic test in the elderly. The other noninvasive test of SA node function involves the use of pharmacologic agents to manipulate the autonomic nervous system and assess the balance of parasympathetic and sympathetic activity on the sinus node. Physiologic or pharmacologic maneuvers that are vagomimetic (Valsalva maneuver or phenylephrine-induced hypertension), vagolytic (atropine), sympathomimetic (isoproterenol or hypotension by nitroprusside), or sympatholytic (β-adrenergic blocking agents) can be utilized, singly and in combination. These studies are designed to test the response of the sinus node to autonomic stimulation and inhibition and thereby characterize the status of autonomic regulation of the sinus node. Abnormalities of the autonomic control of sinus function are particularly common in patients in whom asymptomatic sinus bradycardia is documented.

Intrinsic Heart Rate   This is a manifestation of the primary activity of the SA node, and its determination requires chemical autonomic blockade of the heart with a combination of atropine and a beta blocker. Normal values of intrinsic heart rate (in beats per minute) are calculated by the formula $118.1 - (0.57 \times \text{age})$. The use of autonomic blockade can separate patients with asymptomatic sinus bradycardia into a group with primary sinus node dysfunction (slow intrinsic heart rate) and a group with autonomic imbalance (normal intrinsic heart rate). Autonomic blockade is particularly useful when combined with invasive assessment of sinus node function. Autonomic blockade may depress conduction in patients with intrinsic disease of the conduction system and should be carried out only in a setting where arrhythmias can be monitored and treated rapidly.

EVALUATION   The invasive electrophysiologic investigation of SA node dysfunction should be undertaken in patients who have had symptoms compatible with SA node dysfunction and in whom no documentation of the arrhythmia responsible for these symptoms has been obtained by prolonged Holter monitoring. Asymptomatic patients with sinus bradycardia need *not* be tested, since no therapy is indicated.

Similarly, symptomatic patients with ECG documentation of asystole, sinoatrial block or arrest, or the bradycardia-tachycardia syndrome do not require electrophysiologic tests for diagnosis. However, in symptomatic patients without documentation of an arrhythmia, electrophysiologic assessment of SA node function can yield information that may be used to guide appropriate therapy.

The results of electrophysiologic tests of sinus node function must be interpreted with caution. SA node dysfunction coexists frequently with other disorders such as AV conduction disturbances, which may cause symptoms such as syncope. Electrophysiologic evaluation of patients with symptoms such as undiagnosed syncope must not stop with the demonstration of abnormalities of SA node dysfunction or carotid sinus hypersensitivity. Instead, complete evaluation, including His bundle recordings and programmed atrial and ventricular stimulation (Chap. 230), is necessary to search for additional electrophysiologic abnormalities that could be responsible for symptoms.

℞ TREATMENT   Permanent pacemakers (p. 1290) are the mainstay of therapy for patients with symptomatic SA node dysfunction. Patients with intermittent paroxysms of bradycardia or sinus arrest and with the cardioinhibitory form of the hypersensitive carotid sinus syndrome are usually adequately treated by demand ventricular pacemakers. These devices are reliable, relatively inexpensive, and suffice to prevent episodic symptoms due to abrupt bradycardia. Whether dual-chamber pacing offers any advantages to ventricular pacing in such circumstances remains uncertain. Patients with symptomatic chronic sinus bradycardia or frequent prolonged episodes of sinus node dysfunction do better with dual-chamber pacemakers that preserve the normal AV activation sequence. Although theoretically an atrial demand pacemaker should be adequate for patients with SA node dysfunction, the frequent accompaniment of dysfunction in other portions of the cardiac conduction system usually mandates placement of a pacemaker capable of ventricular pacing. Recent studies suggest that AV sequential pacing may also be useful in preventing atrial fibrillation, an important component of the bradycardia-tachycardia syndrome.

AV CONDUCTION DISTURBANCES

The specialized cardiac conducting system normally ensures synchronous conduction of each sinus impulse from the atria to the ventricles. Abnormalities of conduction of the sinus impulse to the ventricles may portend the development of heart block, which can ultimately lead to syncope or cardiac arrest. In order to evaluate the clinical significance of conduction abnormalities, the physician must assess (1) the site of conduction disturbance, (2) the risk of progression to complete block, and (3) the probability that a subsidiary escape rhythm arising distal to the site of block will be electrophysiologically and hemodynamically stable. This latter point is perhaps the most important, since the rate and stability of the escape pacemaker determine what symptoms result from heart block. The escape pacemaker following AV nodal block is usually in the His bundle, which generally has a stable rate of 40 to 60 beats per minute and is associated with a QRS complex of normal duration (in the absence of a preexisting intraventricular conduction defect). This contrasts with escape rhythms arising in the distal His-Purkinje system, which have lower intrinsic rates (25 to 45 beats per minute), manifest wide QRS complexes with prolonged duration, and are unstable. Thus, the most important issue is to assess the risk of infra- or intra-His block (which always mandates a pacemaker) or AV nodal block in which the frequency of the escape pacemaker is not sufficient to meet hemodynamic requirements (Table 229-1). Although prolonged QRS complexes are invariable when the distal His-Purkinje pacemakers form the escape mechanism, wide QRS complexes can also coexist with AV nodal block and a His bundle rhythm. Therefore, QRS morphology alone may not be adequate to identify the site of block.

ETIOLOGY   The AV node is supplied by the parasympathetic and sympathetic nervous systems and is sensitive to variations in au-

1. Atrial activation times: Measurement of intraatrial conduction times. Prolonged activation times may be associated with atrial flutter or fibrillation.
2. Measurement of AH and HV intervals: Prolongation of AH interval (>125 ms) or prolongation of the HV interval (>55 ms) may help localize the site of delay.
3. Incremental atrial pacing: To determine the cycle length at which block occurs in the AV node and/or His-Purkinje system. Block below the His bundle at rates of <150 beats per minute portends the development of infra-His block.

tonomic tone. Chronic slowing of AV nodal conduction may be seen in highly trained athletes who have hypervagotonia at rest. A variety of diseases and drugs can also influence AV nodal conduction. These include acute processes such as myocardial infarction (particularly inferior), coronary spasm (usually of the right coronary artery), digitalis intoxication, excesses of beta and/or calcium blockers, acute infections such as viral myocarditis, acute rheumatic fever, infectious mononucleosis, and miscellaneous disorders such as Lyme disease, sarcoidosis, amyloidosis, and neoplasms, particularly cardiac mesotheliomas. AV nodal block may also be congenital.

Two degenerative diseases are commonly responsible for damage to the specialized conducting system and produce AV block usually associated with bundle branch block (Chap. 226). In *Lev's disease*, there is calcification and sclerosis of the fibrous cardiac skeleton, which frequently involves the aortic and mitral valves, the central fibrous body, and the summit of the ventricular septum. *Lenegre's disease* appears to be a primary sclerodegenerative disease within the conducting system itself with no involvement of the myocardium or the fibrous skeleton of the heart. These two diseases are probably the most common causes of isolated chronic heart block in adults. Hypertension and aortic and/or mitral stenosis are specific disorders that either accelerate the degeneration of the conducting system or have a direct effect by calcification and fibrosis involving the conducting system.

First-degree AV block, more properly termed *prolonged AV conduction*, is classically characterized by a PR interval >0.20 s, but use of this value may be misleading in terms of clinical significance. Since the PR interval is determined by atrial, AV nodal, and His-Purkinje activation, delay in any one or more of these structures can contribute to a prolonged PR interval. In the presence of a QRS complex of normal duration, a PR interval >0.24 s almost invariably is due to a delay within the AV node. If the QRS is prolonged, delays may be present at any of the levels mentioned above. Delay within the His-Purkinje system is always accompanied by a prolonged QRS duration but can occur with a relatively normal PR interval (Fig. 229-6). However, as indicated below, it is only with intracardiac recordings that the exact site of delay can be determined.

Second-degree heart block (intermittent AV block) is present when some atrial impulses fail to conduct to the ventricles. Mobitz type I second-degree AV block (AV Wenckebach block) is characterized by progressive PR interval prolongation prior to block of an atrial impulse (Fig. 229-7A). The pause that follows is less than fully compensatory (i.e., is less than two normal sinus intervals), and the PR interval of the first conducted impulse is shorter than the last conducted atrial impulse prior to the blocked P wave. Usually the difference between the longest and shortest PR intervals exceeds 100 ms. This type of block is almost always localized to the AV node and associated with a normal QRS duration, although bundle branch block may be present. It is seen most often as a transient abnormality with inferior wall infarction or with drug intoxication, particularly digitalis, beta blockers, and occasionally calcium channel antagonists. This type of block can also be observed in normal individuals with heightened vagal tone. Although Mobitz type I block can progress to complete heart block, this is uncommon, except in the setting of acute inferior wall myocardial infarction. Even when it does, however, the heart block is usually well tolerated because the escape pacemaker usually arises in the

proximal His bundle and provides a stable rhythm. As a result, the presence of Mobitz type I second-degree AV block rarely mandates aggressive therapy. Therapeutic decisions depend on the ventricular response and the symptoms of the patient. If the ventricular rate is adequate and the patient is asymptomatic, observation is sufficient.

In Mobitz type II second-degree AV block, conduction fails suddenly and unexpectedly without a preceding change in PR intervals (Fig. 229-7B). It is generally due to disease of the His-Purkinje system and is most often associated with a prolonged QRS duration. When Mobitz type II block occurs with a normal QRS duration, an intra-His site of block should be expected (Fig. 229-7C). It is important to recognize this type of block because it has a high incidence of progression to complete heart block with an unstable, slow, lower escape pacemaker. Therefore, pacemaker implantation is necessary in this condition. Mobitz type II block may occur in the setting of anteroseptal infarction or in the primary or secondary sclerodegenerative or calcific disorders of the fibrous skeleton of the heart. In so-called high-degree AV block there are periods of two or more consecutively blocked P waves, but intermittent conduction can be demonstrated. Block is usually in the His-Purkinje system, but simultaneous block in the AV node may also be present. Regardless of the site of origin of the escape rhythm, if it is slow and the patient is symptomatic, a cardiac pacemaker is mandatory.

Third-degree AV block is present when no atrial impulse propagates to the ventricles. If the QRS complex of the escape rhythm is of normal duration, occurs at a rate of 40 to 55 beats per minute, and increases with atropine or exercise, AV nodal block is probable. Congenital complete AV block is usually localized to the AV node. If the block is within the His bundle, the escape pacemaker is usually less responsive to these perturbations. If the escape rhythm of the QRS is wide and associated with rates ≤40 beats per minute, block is usually localized in, or distal to, the His bundle and mandates a pacemaker, since the escape rhythm in this setting is unreliable (Fig. 229-8). Some patients with infra-His bundle block are capable of retrograde conduction. In such patients, a "pacemaker syndrome" (see below) may develop if a simple ventricular pacemaker is used. Dual-chamber pacemakers eliminate this potential problem.

FIGURE 229-6 Example of marked His-Purkinje system disease with a relatively normal PR interval. Surface leads I, aVF, and V₁ are shown with electrograms from the high right atrium (HRA), His bundle electrogram (HBE), and time lines (T). The QRS shows right bundle branch block and left anterior hemiblock; the PR interval is minimally elevated at 205 ms, but the HV interval exceeds 100 ms. Such a prolonged HV interval mandates a pacemaker.

FIGURE 229-7 *A.* Mobitz type I second-degree AV block. Intracardiac recordings demonstrate that the PR prolongation (320, 615 ms) is localized to the AV node (AH 240, 535 ms, respectively). HBE, His bundle electrogram; A, atrium; H, His; V, ventricle. Time lines (T) = 100 ms. *B.* Mobitz type II second-degree AV block. Intracardiac recordings document block below the His bundle. *(A and B from ME Josephson, SF Seides, Clinical Cardiac Electrophysiology: Techniques and Interpretations. Philadelphia, Lea & Febiger, 1979.) C.* 2:1 heart block. Surface leads 1, aVF, V₁, demonstrate 2:1 heart block. The intracardiac leads, high right atrium (HRA), coronary sinus (CS), and HBE, demonstrate a diseased His bundle with marked intra-His conduction delay (split-His = HH′) during conducted beats and block in the His bundle every other beat (i.e., between H and H′). *(From ME Josephson, Clinical Cardiac Electrophysiology: Techniques and Interpretations. Philadelphia, Williams & Wilkins, 1993, with permission.)*

AV DISSOCIATION AV dissociation exists whenever the atria and ventricles are under the control of two separate pacemakers and, while present in complete AV block, can occur in the absence of a primary conduction disturbance. AV dissociation unrelated to heart block may occur under two circumstances: First, it may develop with an AV junctional rhythm in response to severe sinus bradycardia. When the sinus rate and the escape rate are similar and the P waves occur just before, in, or following the QRS complex, *isorhythmic AV dissociation* is said to be present. Treatment usually consists of removal of the offending cause of sinus bradycardia (i.e., discontinuation of digitalis, beta blockers, or calcium antagonists), accelerating the sinus node by vagolytic agents, or insertion of a pacemaker if the

escape rhythm is slow and results in symptoms. Second, AV dissociation can be caused by an enhanced lower (junctional or ventricular) pacemaker that competes with normal sinus rhythm and frequently exceeds it. This has been called *interference AV dissociation* because the rapid lower pacemaker results in bombardment of the AV node in a retrograde fashion, rendering it refractory to the normal sinus impulses. Thus failure of antegrade conduction is a physiologic response in this circumstance. Interference dissociation commonly occurs during ventricular tachycardia, accelerated junctional or ventricular rhythms seen with digitalis intoxication, myocardial ischemia and/or infarction, or local irritation following cardiac surgery. The accelerated rhythm should be treated with either antiarrhythmic drugs (Chap. 230), removal of an offending drug, or correction of the metabolic abnormality or ischemia.

INTRACARDIAC ELECTROCARDIOGRAPHIC RECORDINGS IN DIAGNOSIS AND MANAGEMENT The main therapeutic decision in patients with AV conduction disturbance is whether or not a permanent pacemaker is required, and a number of circumstances exist in which His bundle electrocardiography can be a useful diagnostic tool upon which to base this decision. It is unquestionable that patients with *symptomatic* second- or third-degree AV block should be paced, and therefore, these patients do not require electrophysiologic study. However, intracardiac ECG recordings can be useful in at least the following four groups of patients:

1. *Patients with syncope and bundle branch or bifascicular block without documentation of AV block.* In such patients, the demonstration of marked infra-His bundle conduction disturbances, i.e., a prolonged HV interval (>100 ms), may usually be taken as an indication of the need for the insertion of the permanent pacemaker. Complete electrophysiologic evaluation, including atrial and ventricular programmed stimulation, is indicated to help identify other possible cardiac etiologies for the syncope. Since the incidence of significant advanced AV block is low in *asymptomatic* patients who have bifascicular block, electrophysiologic evaluation or permanent pacemakers are not cost-effective. In this group, observation appears most reasonable.

2. *Patients with 2:1 AV conduction.* Intracardiac recordings are necessary to ascertain the site of the conduction disturbance because the typical ECG features of Mobitz type I or Mobitz type II block cannot be discerned during a 2:1 pattern of AV conduction on the surface ECG. Intracardiac recordings may demonstrate that AV nodal block, intra-His bundle block, infra-His bundle block, or combinations of block may be responsible (Figs. 229-7 and 229-8). A surface ECG finding that suggests an infra-His bundle lesion is the presence of alternating bundle branch block associated with changing PR intervals. Intracardiac recordings in such patients confirm that the block is almost always in the His-Purkinje system. Increasing block with exercise or following atropine suggests intra- or infra-His block (Table 229-2). The finding of infra- or intra-His bundle block in patients with asymptomatic second-degree AV block mandates pacemaker therapy because of the high likelihood of the development of symptomatic high-grade AV block and syncope.

3. *Patients with Wenckebach block in the presence of bundle branch block.* This situation, particularly when the maximal change in PR interval is ≤ 50 ms, can suggest intra- or infra-His Wenckebach

block, in which case a pacemaker is mandated. Intracardiac recordings are necessary to make this diagnosis.

4. *Asymptomatic patients with third-degree AV block.* In such patients, electrophysiologic studies may be useful in assessing the stability of the junctional pacemaker. Pacing is indicated when the His bundle escape pacemaker is shown to be unstable by an inadequate response to exercise, atropine, or isoproterenol or by a prolonged junctional recovery time following ventricular pacing.

GENETIC CONSIDERATIONS

A number of congenital and familial syndromes involving the cardiac conduction system have been described. An example of a congenital condition that is transmitted but not genetic is congenital complete heart block associated with material systemic lupus erythematosus. This disorder is associated

FIGURE 229-8   Third-degree AV block. The figure shows surface leads 1, aVF, V$_1$, and an intracardiac His bundle recording (HBE). Complete heart block is evident on the surface leads. The intracardiac recording demonstrates an absence of QRS deflection (V) after a His bundle (H) spike. This indicates block below the His bundle. Note that following the second QRS complex (V), there is an atrial (A) deflection indicating retrograde conduction. Retrograde conduction is often present when block is in the His-Purkinje system but is virtually never present when block is in the AV node. *(From ME Josephson, Clinical Cardiac Electrophysiology: Techniques and interpretations, Philadelphia. Williams & Wilkins, 1993.)*

with maternal IgG autoantibodies to several ribonucleoproteins that are transplacentally transmitted to the fetus and damage the fetal AV node. The fetal conduction disease is generally clinically evident by the second trimester and is associated with significant fetal mortality and neonatal requirement of cardiac pacing.

The embryonic development of the cardiac septa and conduction system occur together, and clinical disorders have been described, including the Holt-Oram syndrome, an autosomal dominant disorder including upper limb dysplasia and atrial septal defect, often with conduction disturbances in the AV node. Studies of families with a high incidence of congenital heart disease, including ostium secundum atrial septal defect and conduction disorders in the AV node, have identified the gene NKX2-5 on chromosome 5q35 as important in the regulation of septation and in the development and function of the AV node. A familial syndrome of progressive complete heart block has also long been recognized. The gene for this disorder has been mapped to a region on chromosome 19q13. Familial disorders of SA node function have also been described, but specific details of abnormal genetic sites are not available. ■

TREATMENT   **Pharmacologic Therapy**   Pharmacologic therapy is usually reserved for acute situations. Atropine (0.5 to 2.0 mg intravenously) and isoproterenol (1 to 4 μg/min intravenously) are useful in increasing heart rate and decreasing symptoms in patients with sinus bradycardia or AV block localized to the AV node. They

have an insignificant effect on lower pacemakers. In patients with neurovascular syncope, beta blockers and disopyramide have been suggested as methods to depress left ventricular function and decrease mechanoreceptor-related reflexes. Mineralocorticoids, ephedrine, and theophylline have also been reported to be of benefit to occasional patients. Unfortunately, no controlled study has shown that any of these pharmacologic modalities works in a predictable fashion in all patients. Further work on delineating different mechanisms in different patient groups may allow us to apply pharmacologic agents more appropriately. Long-term therapy of bradyarrhythmias is best accomplished by pacemakers.

Pacemakers   External energy sources can be used to stimulate the heart when disorders in impulse formation and/or transmission lead to symptomatic bradyarrhythmias. Pacer stimuli can be applied to the atria and/or ventricles. Indications for pacemaker insertion are listed in the guidelines summarized on p. 1290.

Temporary pacing   This is usually instituted to provide immediate stabilization prior to permanent pacemaker placement or to provide pacemaker support when a bradycardia is precipitated by what is presumed to be a transient event such as ischemia or drug toxicity. Temporary pacing is usually achieved by the transvenous insertion of an electrode catheter with the catheter positioned in the right ventricular apex and attached to an external generator. This procedure is associated with a small risk of cardiac perforation, infection at the insertion site, and thromboembolism; the risk of the latter two complications increases markedly if the pacing wire is left in place for more than 48 h. The development of an entirely external transthoracic cardiac pacing system may preclude the need for transvenous pacing in selected patients. However, occasional failure of ventricular capture and significant discomfort related to the large current required for effective transthoracic ventricular stimulation preclude the uniform use of this approach.

Permanent pacing   This mode of pacing is instituted for persistent or intermittent symptomatic bradycardia not related to a self-limiting precipitating factor or for documented infranodal second- or third-degree AV block. Permanent pacing leads are usually inserted transvenously through the subclavian or cephalic vein with the leads positioned in the right atrial appendage for atrial pacing and the right ventricular apex for ventricular pacing. The leads are then attached to the pulse generator, which is inserted into a subcutaneous pocket below the clavicle. Epicardial lead placement is used when (1) transvenous access cannot be obtained; (2) the chest is already open, i.e., in the course of a cardiac operation; and (3) adequate endocardial lead placement cannot be achieved. Most pacemaker generators are pow-

Table 229-2   Site of 2:1 Atrioventricular Block

Characteristic	Observation—Site of Block
1. QRS width	BBB—anywhere
	Normal QRS—in AV node or His bundle
2. PR interval of conducted P wave	>0.30 s—in AV node
	≤0.16 s—in HPS or His bundle[a]
3. Atropine or exercise	Improve conduction—in AV node
	Worsen conduction—in HPS or His bundle[a]
4. CSP	Worsen conduction—in AV node
	Improve conduction—in HPS or His bundle[a]
5. Retrograde conduction	Present—in HPS or His bundle[a]
	Absent—may be anywhere

[a] Use of a pacemaker is indicated.

NOTE: BBB, bundle branch block; HPS, His-Purkinje system; CSP, carotid sinus pressure.

ered by lithium batteries. The life expectancy of the generator is related to (1) voltage output required for capture, (2) requirement for incessant or intermittent pacing, and (3) number of cardiac chambers paced. Life expectancy of the simple ventricular demand pacemaker can exceed 10 years.

Pacing code A code consisting of three to five letters has been developed for describing pacemaker type and function (Table 229-3). The first letter indicates the chamber(s) paced and is designated *V* for ventricular pacing, *A* for atrial pacing, or *D* for dual-chamber (both atrial and ventricular) pacing. The second letter indicates the chamber in which electrical activity is sensed and is also indicated by *A*, *V*, or *D*. An additional designation, *O*, has been used when pacemaker discharge is not dependent on a sensed electrical activity. The third letter refers to the response to a sensed electric signal. The letter *O* represents no response to an underlying electric signal, usually related to the absence of associated sensing function; *I* represents inhibition of pacing function; *T* represents triggering of pacing function; and *D* indicates a dual response, i.e., spontaneous atrial and ventricular activity inhibiting atrial and ventricular pacing and atrial activity triggering a ventricular response. Additional fourth and fifth letters of the pacing code have been recommended to indicate whether the pacemaker is programmable and has rate modulation (fourth) and whether special

---

Guidelines for Permanent Pacing*

Acquired AV Block in Adults

Class I

1. Complete heart block, permanent or intermittent, at any anatomic level, associated with any anatomic level, associated with any one of the following complications:
   a. Symptomatic bradycardia. In the presence of complete heart block, symptoms must be presumed to be due to the heart block unless proved to be otherwise.
   b. Congestive heart failure.
   c. Ectopic rhythms and other medical conditions that require drugs that suppress the automaticity of escape pacemakers and result in symptomatic bradycardia.
   d. Documented periods of asystole $\geq$ 3.0 s or any escape rate < 40 beats per minute in symptom-free patients.
   e. Confusional states that clear with temporary pacing.
   f. Post-AV junction ablation, myotonic dystrophy.
2. Second-degree AV block, permanent or intermittent, regardless of the type or the site of block, with symptomatic bradycardia.
3. Atrial fibrillation, atrial flutter, or rare cases of supraventricular tachycardia with complete heart block or advanced AV block, bradycardia, and any of the conditions described under a. The bradycardia must be related to digitalis or drugs known to impair AV conduction.

Class II

1. Asymptomatic complete heart block, permanent or intermittent, at any anatomic site, with ventricular rates of 40 beats per minute or faster.
2. Asymptomatic type II second-degree AV block, permanent or intermittent.
3. Asymptomatic type I second-degree AV block at infra-His or intra-His levels.

Class III

1. First-degree AV block.
2. Asymptomatic type I second-degree AV block at the supra-His (AV node) level.

After Myocardial Infarction

Class I

1. Persistent advanced second-degree AV block or complete heart block after acute myocardial infarction with block in the His-Purkinje system (bilateral bundle branch block).
2. Transient advanced AV block and associated bundle branch block.

Class II

1. Persistent advanced block at the AV node.

Class III

1. Transient AV conduction disturbances in the absence of intraventricular conduction defects.
2. Transient AV block in the presence of isolated left anterior hemiblock.
3. Acquired left anterior hemiblock in the absence of AV block.
4. Persistent first-degree AV block in the presence of bundle branch block not demonstrated previously.

Bifascicular and Trifascicular Block

Class I

1. Bifascicular block with intermittent complete heart block associated with symptomatic bradycardia.

2. Bifascicular or trifascicular block with intermittent type II second-degree AV block without symptoms attributable to the heart block.

Class II

1. Bifascicular or trifascicular block with syncope that is not proved to be due to complete heart block, but other possible causes for syncope are not identifiable.
2. Markedly prolonged HV (>100 ms).
3. Pacing-induced infra-His block.

Class III

1. Fascicular block without AV block or symptoms.
2. Fascicular block with first-degree AV block without symptoms.

Sinus Node Dysfunction

Class I

1. Sinus node dysfunction with documented symptomatic bradycardia. In some patients this will occur as a consequence of long-term (essential) drug therapy of a type and dose for which there are no acceptable alternatives.

Class II

1. Sinus node dysfunction, occurring spontaneously or as a result of necessary drug therapy, with heart rates < 40 beats per minute when a clear association between significant symptoms consistent with bradycardia and the actual presence of bradycardia has not been documented.

Class III

1. Sinus node dysfunction in asymptomatic patients, including those in whom substantial sinus bradycardia (heart rate < 40 beats per minute) is a consequence of long-term drug treatment.
2. Sinus node dysfunction in patients in whom symptoms suggestive of bradycardia are clearly documented not to be associated with a slow heart rate.

Hypersensitive Carotid Sinus and Neurovascular Syndromes

Class I

1. Recurrent syncope associated with clear, spontaneous events provoked by carotid sinus stimulation; minimal carotid sinus pressure induces asystole of >3 s duration in the absence of any medication that depresses the sinus node or AV conduction.

Class II

1. Recurrent syncope without clear, provocative events and with a hypersensitive cardioinhibitory response.
2. Syncope with associated bradycardia reproduced by a head-up tilt with or without isoproterenol or other forms of provocative maneuvers and in which a temporary pacemaker and a second provocative test can establish the likely benefits of a permanent pacemaker.

Class III

1. A hyperactive cardioinhibitory response to carotid sinus stimulation in the absence of symptoms.
2. Vague symptoms, such as dizziness, light-headedness, or both, with a hyperactive cardioinhibitory response to carotid sinus stimulation.
3. Recurrent syncope, light-headedness, or dizziness in the absence of a cardioinhibitory response.

---

* Class I: agreement that permanent pacemaker should be implanted. Class II: divergence of opinion regarding need for implantation. Class III: agreement that pacemaker is unnecessary.

SOURCE: Guidelines for The Implantation of Cardiac Pacemakers and Antiarrhythmic Devices. Am Coll Cardiol/Am Heart Assoc.

antitachycardia functions are available (i.e., antitachycardia pacing, *T*, and delivery of high- or low-energy shocks). In the fourth category, *M* represents multiprogrammability and *R* represents rate response ("physiologic") pacing. It follows from the described code that the standard VVIR (ventricular demand pacemaker) paces the ventricle, senses the ventricle, is inhibited by sensed spontaneous ventricular activity, and has rate modulation, while the DDDR pulse generator is capable of sensing and pacing both the atria and ventricles and has a dual response to the sensed atrial and ventricular activity as described above (Fig. 229-9). Both pacemakers have rate modulation (*R*). "Physiologic" pacemakers use sensors (muscular activity, respiratory rate, temperature, O_2 saturation, QT interval, etc.) as methods to allow the pacemaker to increase the heart rate in response to physiologic demands, i.e., exercise. These pacemakers are essential when chronotropic incompetence is present and an increase in heart rate is required to enhance physiologic performance. Studies have shown that such "physiologic" pacemakers improve exercise tolerance and relieve symptoms to a greater degree than fixed-rate pacemakers.

Selection of the appropriate pacemaker and pacing mode depends on the clinical condition and the type of bradyarrhythmia being treated. The two most common pacing mode selections are DDD and VVI. DDD provides AV sequential pacing, which is ideally suited for the relatively young and active patient who has intact sinus node function or intermittent dysfunction and high-grade persistent or intermittent AV block. The DDD mode will allow for physiologic atrial sensed and ventricular paced rates and improve exercise tolerance. AV synchrony and dual-chamber pacing may also be desirable in patients with borderline hemodynamic reserve who are dependent on atrial contribution to cardiac output and in those patients who develop the pacemaker syndrome (see below) in response to ventricular demand pacing.

Rate-responsive DDD (i.e., DDDR) pacing is indicated when chronotropic incompetence is present in a patient who requires AV synchrony. The DDD pacing mode is contraindicated in chronic atrial fibrillation or flutter, because rapid and irregular ventricular pacing will occur to the upper rate limit. In some cases this will produce a more rapid ventricular rate than the patient's own rate in the absence of a pacemaker. DDD pacemakers must either automatically switch (i.e., mode-switching function) or be reprogrammed to the VVI mode. Almost all such pacemakers are now combined with some form of rate responsiveness so that when the device functions in the VVI mode, it also will respond to physiologic demands (VVIR).

Chronotropic insufficiency (i.e., the inability of the sinus rate to accelerate) is a contraindication for a DDD pacemaker, since such a pacemaker will act as a "fixed-rate" pacemaker at the programmed lower rate. In these situations, a rate-adaptive or "physiologic" pacemaker is indicated (VVIR or DDDR). In patients with impaired sinus node function or chronic atrial fibrillation, a sensor-driven, rate-adaptive pacemaker must be implanted. As mentioned earlier, these pacemakers automatically adjust ventricular pacing rates to a sensed indicator of exertion. The DDD pacing mode may also be contraindicated in patients with intermittent or persistent ventriculoatrial conduction, who may develop pacemaker-mediated tachycardia (see below).

Programmability of pacemakers This allows for modification of

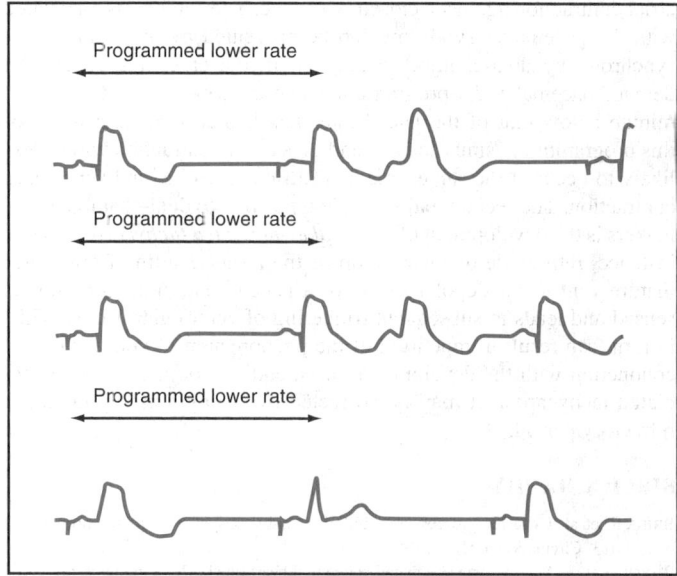

FIGURE 229-9 Normally functioning DDD pacemaker. All three panels show a lead II rhythm strip at 50 mm/s. The programmed lower rate is approximately 55 beats per minute. (*Top*) AV sequential pacing with a paced AV interval of 160 ms is shown for the first two complexes. A VPC occurs and is sensed, resetting the cycle. (*Middle*) The first beat is AV paced, but spontaneous sinus P waves and APC trigger a ventricular paced complex with a sensed P to QRS of 120 ms. (*Bottom*) After the first AV paced complex, a paced atrial complex conducts to the ventricle with a PR of 120 ms, inhibiting the ventricular pacemaker.

pacing function after implantation and for adaptation to changes in clinical needs. Pacemaker programming is accomplished by activation of the programming head positioned over the implanted pulse generator after making the desired changes in programmable parameters (Table 229-3). A radio frequency system is routinely used to communicate the program to the pacemaker. A high degree of sophistication is required to recognize the presence and causes of pacemaker malfunction and their treatment.

Complications Adverse effects of permanent pacing are usually associated with failure or malfunction of the pacing system. These problems are usually secondary to over- or undersensing, output failure, and/or lead fracture or displacement. Two other problems may occur. The *pacemaker syndrome* consists of fatigue, dizziness, syncope, and distressing pulsations in the neck and chest and can be associated with adverse hemodynamic effects. The pathophysiologic contributors to the pacemaker syndrome include (1) loss of atrial contribution to ventricular systole; (2) vasodepressor reflex initiated by cannon *a* waves, which are caused by atrial contractions against a closed tricuspid valve and observed in the jugular venous pulse (Chap. 225); and (3) systemic and pulmonary venous regurgitation due to

Table 229-3 The NASPE/BPEG Generic Pacemaker Code

Position Category	I Chamber(s) Paced	II Chamber(s) Sensed	III Response to Sensing	IV Programmability, Rate Modulation	V Antitachyarrhythmia Function(s)
	O, None	O, None	O, None	O, None	O, None
	A, Atrium	A, Atrium	T, Triggered	P, Simple programmable	P, pacing (antitachyarrhythmia)
	V, Ventricle	V, Ventricle	I, Inhibited	M, Multiprogrammable	S, Shock
	D, Dual (A + V)	D, Dual (A + V)	D, Dual (T + I)	C, Communicating	D, Dual (P + S)
				R, Rate modulation	
Manufacturer's designation	S, single (A or V)	S, (A or V)			

SOURCE: From DP Zipes, in E Braunwald (ed): *Heart Disease: A Textbook of Cardiovascular Medicine*, 5th ed. Philadelphia, Saunders, 1997.

atrial contraction against a closed AV valve. The symptoms associated with the pacemaker syndrome can be prevented by maintaining AV synchrony by dual-chamber pacing or, in the case of a ventricular demand pacemaker, by programming an escape rate 15 to 20 beats per minute below that of the paced rate (i.e., hysteresis). As a result of this programming, sinus activity and thus atrial contraction will be less likely to occur at the same time as ventricular pacing and ventricular contraction. The second major problem peculiar to dual-chamber pacemakers is the development of *pacemaker-mediated tachycardia*. In this instance, retrograde depolarization of the atria, resulting from a premature ventricular depolarization or a paced ventricular complex, is sensed and leads to subsequent triggering of ventricular pacing. This, in turn, can result in repetition of the phenomenon of ventriculoatrial conduction with the development of an endless-loop, pacemaker-mediated tachycardia. It may be corrected by reprogramming the atrial refractory period.

BIBLIOGRAPHY

BRINK P et al: Gene for progressive familial heart block type 1 maps to chromosome 19q13. Circulation 91:1633, 1995

BUYON J et al: Autoimmune associated congenital heart block: Demographics, mortality, morbidity and recurrence rates obtained from a national neonatal lupus registry. J Am Coll Cardiol 31:1685, 1998

DREIFUS LS et al: Guidelines for implantation of cardiac pacemakers and antiarrhythmic devices: A report of the American College of Cardiology/American Heart Association Task Force on Assessment of Diagnostic and Therapeutic Cardiovascular Procedures (Committee on Pacemaker Implantation). J Am Coll Cardiol 18:1, 1991

ELLENBOGEN KA et al: New insights into pacemaker syndrome gained from hemodynamic, humoral and vascular responses during ventriculo-atrial pacing. Am J Cardiol 65(1):53, 1990

GROH SS, ZIPES DP: Cardiac pacemakers, in *Heart Disease: A Textbook of Cardiovascular Medicine*, 6th ed, E Braunwald et al (eds). Philadelphia, Saunders, 2001

HUANG SK et al: Carotid sinus hypersensitivity in patients with unexplained syncope: Clinical, electrophysiologic and long-term follow-up observations. Am Heart J 116: 989, 1988

JOSEPHSON ME: *Clinical Electrophysiology*, 2d ed. Philadelphia, Lea and Febiger, 1993, chaps 4, 5, 6, 13

MENDES LA, DAVIDOFF R: Cardiogenic seizure with bradyarrhythmia: Documentation of the mechanism during asystole. Am Heart J 125:1786, 1993

MICHAËLSON M, JANZON A: Isolated congenital complete atrioventricular block in adult life. A prospective study. Circulation 92:442, 1995

SCHOTT J et al: Congenital heart disease caused by mutations in the transcription factor NKX2-5. Science, in press

SRA JS et al: Comparison of cardiac pacing with drug therapy in the treatment of neurocardiogenic (vasovagal) syncope with bradycardia or asytole. N Engl J Med 328: 1085, 1993

WALLER BF et al: Anatomy, histology and pathology of the cardiac conduction system: Part II. Clin Cardiol 16:347, 1993

230

Mark E. Josephson, Peter Zimetbaum

THE TACHYARRHYTHMIAS

AF	atrial fibrillation	PSVT	paroxysmal supraventricular tachycardias
APCs	atrial premature complexes		
AV	atrioventricular	SVT	supraventricular tachycardia
CAST	cardiac arrhythmia suppression trial	VA	ventriculoatrial
		VF	ventricular fibrillation
ECG	electrocardiogram	VPCs	ventricular premature complexes
ICD	implantable cardioverter/defibrillator		
		VT	ventricular tachycardia
LQTS	long QT syndrome	WPW	Wolff-Parkinson-White
MAT	multifocal atrial tachycardia		

MECHANISMS OF TACHYARRHYTHMIAS

Tachyarrhythmias may be divided into disorders of impulse propagation and disorders of impulse formation.

REENTRY   Disorders of impulse propagation (reentry) are generally considered to be the most common mechanism of sustained paroxysmal tachyarrhythmia. The requirements for initiating reentry include (1) electrophysiologic inhomogeneity (i.e., differences in conduction and/or refractoriness) in two or more regions of the heart connected with each other to form a potentially closed loop; (2) unidirectional block in one pathway; (3) slow conduction over an alternative pathway, allowing time for the initially blocked pathway to recover excitability; and (4) reexcitation of the initially blocked pathway to complete a loop of activation (Fig. 230-1). Repetitive circulation of the impulse over this loop can produce a sustained tachyarrhythmia. While anatomic obstacles may underlie reentry and provide an inexcitable center around which the impulse can circulate, they are not essential. Reentrant arrhythmias can be reproducibly initiated and terminated by premature complexes and rapid stimulation. The response of these arrhythmias to stimulation can help distinguish them from arrhythmias caused by triggered activity.

ENHANCED AUTOMATICITY   Disorders of impulse formation can be subdivided into tachyarrhythmias caused by enhanced automaticity and those caused by triggered activity. In addition to the sinus node, automatic pacemaker activity can be observed in specialized atrial fibers, fibers of the atrioventricular (AV) junction, and Purkinje fibers (Chap. 229). Myocardial cells do not normally possess pacemaker activity. Enhancement of normal automaticity in latent pacemaker fibers or the development of abnormal automaticity due to partial depolarization of the resting membrane occurs as a consequence of a variety of pathophysiologic states, which include (1) increased endogenous or exogenous catecholamines, (2) electrolyte disturbances (e.g., hyperkalemia), (3) hypoxia or ischemia, (4) mechanical effects (e.g., stretch), and (5) drugs (e.g., digitalis). Tachycardia caused by automaticity cannot be started or stopped by pacing.

TRIGGERED ACTIVITY   Rhythms due to triggered activity are events that do not occur spontaneously but require a change in cardiac electrical frequency as a trigger. Triggered activity may be caused by early afterdepolarizations, which occur during phases 2 and 3 of the action potential, or delayed afterdepolarizations, which occur following completion of phase 3 of the action potential (Fig. 229-2). Triggered activity has been observed in atrial, ventricular, and His-Purkinje tissue under conditions such as increased local catecholamine concentration, hyperkalemia, hypercalcemia, and digitalis intoxication (delayed afterdepolarizations) or during bradycardia, hypokalemia, or

FIGURE 230-1   Schema of reentry. Y branching of the Purkinje system to ventricular muscle is shown in panels *A* through *C*. The right limb (*gray area*) of the Purkinje system has a longer refractory period than the left. *A*. During a slow stimulated rate (S_1), conduction proceeds normally over both Purkinje fibers, resulting in collision in the ventricular muscle. *B*. An early premature stimulus (S_2) results in block in the Purkinje fiber on the right and slow conduction down the left. The impulse conducts through the ventricle and attempts to reenter the initial site of block but fails because this site has not fully recovered excitability. *C*. An earlier stimulus (S_3) again results in block on the left. The resulting slower propagation down the left fiber provides enough time for the initial site of block to recur and allows the impulse to conduct through it to produce a reentrant circuit.

other situations prolonging action potential duration (early afterdepolarizations). All of these conditions produce an accumulation of intracellular calcium. With increasing amplitude of the afterdepolarizations, threshold can be reached and repetitive activity produced. The exact role of triggered activity in spontaneous clinical arrhythmias is unknown, but tachyarrhythmias associated with digitalis intoxication, accelerated idioventricular rhythm in acute infarction and/or reperfusion, and exercise-induced ventricular tachycardia (VT) are believed to be caused by triggered activity due to delayed afterdepolarizations. *Torsade de pointes* ("twisting of the points"; polymorphic VT associated with long QT intervals) may be caused by triggered activity due to early afterdepolarizations, although reentry may also be operative.

FIGURE 230-2 ECG lead II. Sinus rhythm with one atrial premature complex (*arrow*). Note the difference in P-wave configuration between sinus and the premature atrial complexes. In addition, note that the PR interval of the premature complex is prolonged, due to slowed conduction of the premature impulse through the AV conduction system.

The use of electrophysiologic studies, i.e., intracardiac recordings and programmed stimulation, has greatly expanded the understanding of the mechanisms of tachyarrhythmias. In addition to helping diagnose arrhythmias, these techniques may be of value in determining the most appropriate types of therapy because they allow the physician to observe the hemodynamic and symptomatic consequences of the arrhythmia in the presence or absence of therapy. Electrophysiologic studies of tachycardias require the positioning of multiple electrode catheters at critical areas within the heart. These electrodes must be capable of both stimulating and recording from multiple sites in the atria and/or ventricles.

PREMATURE COMPLEXES

ATRIAL PREMATURE COMPLEXES (APC) APCs can be found on 24-h Holter monitoring in over 60% of normal adults. APCs are usually asymptomatic and benign, although at times they may be associated with palpitations. In susceptible patients, they can initiate paroxysmal supraventricular tachycardias. APCs may originate from any location in either atrium, and they are recognized on the electrocardiogram (ECG) as early P waves with a morphology that differs from the sinus P wave (Fig. 230-2). While APCs usually conduct to the ventricles when they occur late in the cardiac cycle, early APCs may reach the AV conduction system while it is still in its relative refractory period, resulting in a conduction delay manifested by prolonged PR interval following the premature P wave (Fig. 230-2). Very early APCs may even block in the AV node if this structure is encountered during its effective refractory period. APCs, whether conducted or not, are usually followed by a pause before a return to sinus activity. Most commonly, an APC enters and resets the sinus node, so the sum of the pre- and postextrasystolic PP intervals is less than the sum of two sinus PP intervals (Fig. 230-2). In this case, the pause is said to be less than fully compensatory. The QRS complex following most APCs is normal, although early APCs may be followed by aberrantly conducted QRS complexes due to the premature complex falling within the relative refractory period of the His-Purkinje system.

Since most APCs are asymptomatic, treatment is not required. When they cause palpitations or trigger paroxysmal supraventricular tachycardias (see below), treatment may be useful. Factors that precipitate APCs, such as alcohol, tobacco, or adrenergic stimulants, should be identified and eliminated; in their absence, mild sedation or the use of a beta blocker may be tried.

AV JUNCTIONAL COMPLEXES The site of origin of these complexes is thought to be in the bundle of His, since the normal AV node in vivo possesses no automaticity. AV junctional complexes are less common than either atrial or ventricular premature complexes and are more often associated with cardiac disease or digitalis intoxication. Junctional premature impulses can conduct both antegradely to the ventricles and retrogradely to the atrium and, on rare occasions, may fail to conduct in either direction. Premature AV junctional complexes can be recognized by normal-appearing QRS complexes that are not preceded by a P wave. Retrograde P waves (inverted in leads II, III, and aVF) may be observed after the QRS complex.

While often asymptomatic, junctional premature complexes may be associated with palpitations and cause cannon *a* waves, which may result in distressing pulsations in the neck. When symptomatic, they should be treated like APCs.

VENTRICULAR PREMATURE COMPLEXES (VPCs) These are among the most common arrhythmias and occur in patients with and without heart disease. Of adult males, ≥60% will exhibit VPCs during a 24-h Holter monitoring. In patients without heart disease, VPCs have not been shown to be associated with any increased incidence in mortality or morbidity. VPCs may occur in up to 80% of patients with previous myocardial infarction, and in this setting, if frequent (>10 per hour) and/or complex (occurring in couplets), they have been associated with increased mortality. However, cardiac mortality in such patients usually occurs in association with significantly impaired ventricular function. While frequent and complex ventricular ectopy is an independent risk factor, it is not as strong a risk factor as is impaired ventricular function. Moreover, even though ventricular tachycardia and/or fibrillation may be the basis for the sudden death in these patients, this does not a priori establish a cause-and-effect relation between spontaneous ectopy and life-threatening ventricular tachycardia or fibrillation. Very early cycle (R-on-T) VPCs have been stated by some to increase the risk of sudden death. Although this has been observed during acute ischemia and in the setting of QT prolongation, frequently, VT or fibrillation is precipitated by VPCs that occur after the T wave of the prior beat.

VPCs are recognized by wide (usually >0.14 s), bizarre QRS complexes that are not preceded by P waves (Fig. 230-3*A*). They may bear a relatively fixed relationship to the preceding sinus complex (i.e., fixed coupled VPCs). When fixed coupling is not present and the interval between VPCs has a common denominator, *ventricular parasystole* is said to be present (Fig. 230-4). Under these circumstances, the VPCs are a manifestation of abnormal automaticity of a protected ventricular focus. Because this focus is not penetrated by sinus impulses, it is not reset by them, and the interectopic intervals remain relatively fixed (≤120 ms variation of mean RR cycle length).

VPCs may occur singly; in patterns of bigeminy, in which every sinus beat is followed by a VPC; in trigeminy, in which two sinus beats are followed by a VPC; in quadrigeminy, etc. Two successive VPCs are termed *pairs* or *couplets*, while three or more consecutive VPCs are termed *ventricular tachycardia* when the rate exceeds 100 beats per minute (Fig. 230-3*B*). VPCs may have similar morphologies (monomorphic, or uniform) or different morphologies (polymorphic, or multiformed).

Most commonly, VPCs are not conducted retrogradely to the atrium to reset the sinoatrial node. Thus they produce a fully compensatory pause; i.e., the interval between conducted sinus beats that

A

B

FIGURE 230-3 *A.* Single ventricular ectopy. During sinus rhythm, five premature ventricular complexes (filled circles) occur. Note that the QRS configuration is bizarre and different from that during sinus rhythm. The premature ventricular complexes are not preceded by P waves. The QRS widths of the premature complexes are 120–160 ms and multiple morphologies are present. The pause following the premature complexes is fully compensatory, the sinus beat after the premature complex occurring on time. *B.* Nonsustained ventricular tachycardia (VT). Following two sinus beats, an atrial premature contraction with long PR interval initiates an 8-beat run of wide complex tachycardia. Atrial activity can be seen following the fourth and seventh beats. The greater number of QRS complexes compared with P waves confirms the diagnosis of VT.

bracket the VPC equals two basic RR intervals. Ventricular impulses may also manifest retrograde conduction to the atrium and cause inverted P waves in leads II, III, and aVF. This retrograde atrial activation can reset the sinus node, and the pause that results may therefore be less than compensatory. In many instances, the VPC will not be associated with retrograde ventriculoatrial (VA) conduction but may block retrogradely in the AV node. This renders the AV node refractory to the subsequent sinus beat and causes slowed conduction (i.e., prolonged PR interval) or block of the next sinus P wave. This prolonged PR interval is said to be a manifestation of concealed retrograde conduction of the ventricular impulse into the AV node. A VPC that does not produce any manifestation of retrograde concealed conduction and fails to influence the oncoming sinus impulse is termed an *interpolated VPC.*

VPCs can cause palpitations or neck pulsations secondary to either the occurrence of cannon *a* waves or the increased force of contraction due to postextrasystolic potentiation of ventricular contractility. Pa-

FIGURE 230-4 Ventricular parasystole. At varying sinus cycle lengths during exercise, interectopic intervals remain constant at 1620 to 1640 ms. However, the coupling intervals between sinus and ectopic complexes vary between 510 and 310 ms.

tients with frequent VPCs or bigeminy may rarely develop syncope or lightheadedness because the VPCs do not result in an adequate stroke volume and the cardiac output is reduced by the "halving" of the heart rate.

TREATMENT In the absence of cardiac disease, isolated asymptomatic VPCs, regardless of configuration and frequency, need no treatment. When arrhythmias are symptomatic, the symptoms should first be addressed by either allaying the patient's anxiety or, if this is not successful, reducing the frequency of the VPCs with antiarrhythmic agents. β-Adrenergic blockers may be successful in managing VPCs that occur primarily in the daytime or under stressful situations and in specific settings such as mitral valve prolapse and thyrotoxicosis. While other antiarrhythmic agents may be tried should this be unsuccessful, their risk may outweigh any benefits. In patients with cardiac disease, frequent VPCs are associated with an increased risk of sudden and nonsudden cardiac death, and many physicians have attempted to eliminate or reduce the frequency of these VPCs in an attempt to reduce this risk. However, the cause-and-effect relationship of the VPCs to fatal events has never been established. The ability of pharmacologic antiarrhythmic therapy guided by continuous ECG monitoring to reduce the risk of sudden death in postmyocardial infarction patients with frequent (≥6 per minute) VPCs was tested by the Cardiac Arrhythmia Suppression Trial (CAST). This study compared mortality in patients whose ectopy was suppressed by one of three agents (encainide, flecainide, or moricizine) and then randomized to treat with either the "effective" drug or placebo. After a mean follow-up of 2 years, the study was discontinued because both the sudden death and overall mortality rate were significantly increased in patients receiving antiarrhythmic agents. This study has shown that in patients having the characteristics of the study population, abolition of ventricular ectopy by pharmacologic therapy cannot be used as a marker to define reduction of the risk of sudden death after myocardial infarction and, in fact, may increase mortality. Recent studies have evaluated the use of electrophysiologic testing and implantable cardioverter/defibrillator (ICD) placement in the management of patients at high risk for sudden death (i.e., those with left ventricular ejection fractions <40% and nonsustained VT). These studies have found that induction of a sustained ventricular arrhythmia through programmed electrical stimulation selects a group of these patients whose prognosis is improved with implantation of a defibrillator. These studies have found no correlation between the rate, morphology, or duration of nonsustained episodes of VT and the likelihood of having a sustained ventricular arrhythmia.

Antiarrhythmic agents can also produce the lethal arrhythmias that they are given to prevent (proarrhythmic effects). Thus therapy directed toward VPCs in the setting of chronic cardiac disease may result in an inappropriate and costly use of agents without proven efficacy and with potential side effects in many patients. The high incidence of side effects and the frequent exacerbation of arrhythmias caused by all antiarrhythmic drugs make it mandatory to monitor patients being treated with such agents.

In acute myocardial infarction, the greatest incidence of primary ventricular fibrillation occurs within the first 24 h (Chap. 243). Temporary prophylactic antiarrhythmic therapy with lidocaine or procainamide was formerly recommended for all patients with acute infarction, regardless of the presence or degree of spontaneous ectopy.

However, failure to improve overall survival and drug toxicity have led most physicians to recommend prophylactic antiarrhythmic therapy only to young patients with complicated infarctions, where a favorable risk-benefit ratio may be obtained. Other studies have shown that intravenous beta blockers may also reduce the incidence of primary ventricular fibrillation.

TACHYCARDIAS

Tachycardias refer to arrhythmias with three or more complexes at rates exceeding 100 beats per minute; they occur more often in structurally diseased than in normal hearts. Those paroxysmal tachycardias that are initiated by APCs or VPCs are considered to be due to reentry, except some of the digitalis-induced tachyarrhythmias, which are probably due to triggered activity (see below).

If the patient is hemodynamically stable, an attempt should be made to determine the mechanism and origin of the tachycardia, since this will usually lead to an appropriate therapeutic decision. Information to be obtained from the ECG includes (1) the presence, frequency, morphology, and regularity of P waves and QRS complexes; (2) the relationship between atrial and ventricular activity; (3) a comparison of the QRS morphology during sinus rhythm and during the tachycardia; and (4) the response to carotid sinus massage or other vagal maneuvers. It is useful first to compare a 12-lead ECG during the tachycardia with one recorded during sinus rhythm. One can also utilize the electrodes situated at the end of a flexible pacing catheter inserted into the esophagus behind the left atrium to record atrial activity.

Observation of the jugular venous pulse can provide clues to the presence of atrial activity and its relationship to ventricular ectopy. Intermittent cannon *a* waves suggest AV dissociation, while persistent cannon a waves suggest 1:1 VA conduction. Flutter waves may be seen or no atrial activity may be apparent, as in the presence of atrial flutter and fibrillation, respectively. The arterial pulse may also manifest AV dissociation or atrial fibrillation by demonstrating variations in amplitude. A first heart sound of variable intensity during a regular rhythm also suggests AV dissociation or atrial fibrillation (AF).

Carotid sinus pressure should only be applied while the patient is electrocardiographically monitored with resuscitative equipment available to manage the rare episode of asystole and/or ventricular fibrillation associated with this procedure. Carotid sinus massage should not be performed in patients with carotid arterial bruits. The patient should be positioned flat with the neck extended. Massage of one carotid bulb at a time should be performed by applying firm pressure just underneath the angle of the jaw for up to 5 s. Alternative vagomimetic maneuvers include the Valsalva maneuver, immersion of the face in cold water, and administration of 5 to 10 mg edrophonium.

SINUS TACHYCARDIA   In the adult, sinus tachycardia is said to be present when the heart rate exceeds 100 beats per minute (bpm): sinus tachycardia rarely exceeds 200 bpm and is not a primary arrhythmia; instead, it represents a physiologic response to a variety of stresses, such as fever, volume depletion, anxiety, exercise, thyrotoxicosis, hypoxemia, hypotension, or congestive heart failure. Sinus tachycardia has a gradual onset and offset. The ECG demonstrates P waves with sinus contour preceding each QRS complex. Carotid sinus pressure usually produces modest slowing with a gradual return to the previous rate upon cessation. This contrasts with the response of paroxysmal supraventricular tachycardias, which may slow slightly and terminate abruptly.

℞ **TREATMENT**   Sinus tachycardia should not be treated as a primary arrhythmia, since it is almost always a physiologic response to a demand placed on the heart. As such, the therapy should be directed to the primary disorder. This may involve institution of digitalis and/or diuretics for heart failure and oxygen for hypoxemia, treatment of thyrotoxicosis, volume repletion, aspirin for fever, or tranquilizers for emotional upset.

ATRIAL FIBRILLATION   AF is a common arrhythmia that may occur in paroxysmal and persistent forms. It may be seen in normal subjects, particularly during emotional stress or following surgery, exercise, acute alcoholic intoxication, or a prominent surge of vagal tone (i.e., vasovagal response). It may also occur in patients with heart or lung disease who develop acute hypoxia, hypercapnia, or metabolic or hemodynamic derangements. Persistent AF usually occurs in patients with cardiovascular disease, most commonly rheumatic heart disease, nonrheumatic mitral valve disease, hypertensive cardiovascular disease, chronic lung disease, atrial septal defect, and a variety of miscellaneous cardiac abnormalities. AF may be the presenting finding in thyrotoxicosis. So-called lone AF, which occurs in patients without underlying heart disease, often represents the tachycardia phase of the tachycardia-bradycardia syndrome.

The morbidity associated with AF is related to (1) excessive ventricular rate, which in turn may lead to hypotension, pulmonary congestion, or angina pectoris in susceptible individuals; (2) the pause following cessation of AF, which can cause syncope; (3) systemic embolization, which occurs most commonly in patients with rheumatic heart disease (Table 230-1); (4) loss of the contribution of atrial contraction to cardiac output, which may cause fatigue; and (5) anxiety secondary to palpitations. In patients with severe cardiac dysfunction, particularly those with hypertrophied, noncompliant ventricles, the combination of the loss of the atrial contribution to ventricular filling and the abbreviated filling period due to the rapid ventricular rate in AF can produce marked hemodynamic instability, resulting in hypotension, syncope, or heart failure. In patients with mitral stenosis, in whom ventricular filling time is critical, development of AF with a rapid ventricular rate may precipitate pulmonary edema (Chap. 236). AF may also cause a cardiomyopathy related to persistent rapid rates (so-called tachycardia-induced cardiomyopathy).

AF is characterized by disorganized atrial activity without discrete P waves on the surface ECG (Fig. 230-5A). Atrial activation is manifested by an undulating baseline or by more sharply inscribed atrial deflections of varying amplitude and frequency ranging from 350 to 600 beats per minute. The ventricular response is irregularly irregular. This results from the large number of atrial impulses that penetrate the AV node, making it partially refractory to subsequent impulses. This effect of nonconducted atrial impulses to influence the response to subsequent atrial impulses is termed *concealed conduction*. As a result, the ventricular response is relatively slow, considering the actual atrial rate. AF may convert to atrial flutter, especially in response to antiarrhythmic drugs like quinidine or flecainide. If AF converts to atrial flutter, which has a slower atrial rate, the effect of concealed conduction may be diminished, and a paradoxic increase in the ventricular response may occur. The main factor determining the rate of the ventricular response is the functional refractory period of the AV node or the most rapid paced rate at which 1:1 conduction through the AV node can be observed.

If, in the presence of AF, the ventricular rhythm becomes regular and slow (e.g., 30 to 60 bpm), complete heart block is suggested, and if the ventricular rhythm is regular and rapid (e.g., ≥100 bpm), a tachycardia arising in the AV junction or ventricle should be suspected. Digitalis intoxication is a common cause of both phenomena.

Table 230-1   Factors Associated with High Risk of Stroke in Patients with Atrial Fibrillation

1. Age >65
2. Hypertension
3. Rheumatic heart disease
4. Prior stroke or TIA
5. Diabetes mellitus
6. Congestive heart failure
7. Left atrial dimension >5 cm

NOTE: TIA, transient ischemic attack.

V₁

A

II

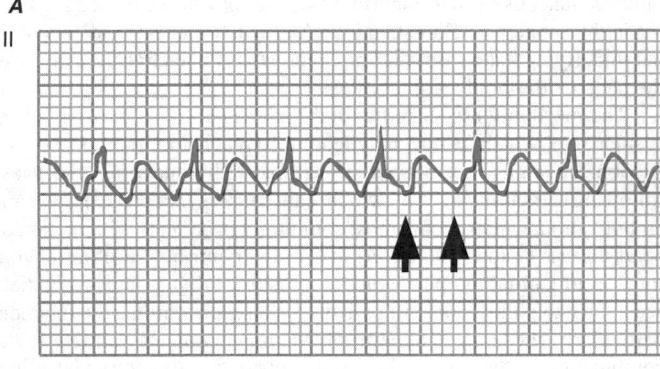

B

FIGURE 230-5 Atrial fibrillation and atrial flutter. *A*. Lead V₁ demonstrating an irregular ventricular rhythm associated with poorly defined irregular atrial activity consistent with atrial fibrillation. *B*. Lead II demonstrates atrial flutter, identified by the regular "sawtooth-like" activity (*arrows*) at an atrial rate of 300 bpm with 2:1 ventricular response.

Patients with AF exhibit a loss of *a* waves in the jugular venous pulse and variable pulse pressures in the carotid arterial pulse. The first heart sound usually varies in intensity. On echocardiography, the left atrium is frequently enlarged, and in patients in whom the left atrial diameter exceeds 4.5 cm, it may be difficult to convert AF to sinus rhythm and/or maintain the latter, despite therapy.

℞ **TREATMENT** In acute AF, a precipitating factor such as fever, pneumonia, alcoholic intoxication, thyrotoxicosis, pulmonary emboli, congestive heart failure, or pericarditis should be sought. When such a factor is present, therapy should be directed toward the primary abnormality. If the patient's clinical status is severely compromised, electrical cardioversion is the treatment of choice. In the absence of severe cardiovascular compromise, slowing of ventricular rate becomes the initial therapeutic goal. This may be most rapidly accomplished with β-adrenergic blockers and/or calcium channel antagonists. Both prolong the refractory period of the AV node and slow conduction within it. When catecholamine levels or sympathetic nervous system tone is likely to be elevated, beta blockers may be favored. Digitalis preparations are less effective, take longer to act, and are associated with more toxicity. Conversion to sinus rhythm may then be attempted. Prior to cardioversion, precautions must be taken to reduce the risk of systemic embolization. Patients should be anticoagulated to an INR of at least 1.8 for the prior 3 consecutive weeks or have had AF for <48 h. Alternatively, for those patients with AF for >48 h who are not anticoagulated, a transesophageal echocardiogram can exclude the presence of left atrial thrombus and allow safe cardioversion. Following cardioversion, anticoagulation must be maintained for at least 4 weeks until atrial mechanical function returns to normal.

Antiarrhythmic medications in either oral or intravenous form may be employed but are only modestly effective in restoring sinus rhythm. When antiarrhythmic agents such as the quinidine-like drugs (type 1A) or the flecainide-like agents (type 1C) are used (Table 230-2), it is important to increase AV node refractoriness prior to administering such drugs because their vagolytic effect and/or their ability to convert

Table 230-2 Classification of Antiarrhythmic Drugs

Class I	Drugs that reduce maximal velocity of phase of depolarization (V_max) due to block of inward Na⁺ current in tissue with fast response action potentials
	A ↓ V_max at all heart rates and ↑ action potential duration, e.g., quinidine, procainamide, disopyramide
	B Little effect at slow rates on V_max in normal tissue; ↓ V_max in partially depolarized cells with fast response action potentials
	Effects increased at faster rates
	No change or ↓ in action potential duration, e.g., lidocaine, phenytoin, tocainide, mexiletine
	C ↓ V_max at normal rates in normal tissue
	Minimal effect on action potential duration, e.g., flecainide, propafenone, moricizine
Class II	Antisympathetic agents, e.g., propranolol and other β-adrenergic blockers: ↓ SA nodal automaticity, ↑ AV nodal refractoriness, and ↓ AV nodal conduction velocity
Class III	Agents that prolong action potential duration in tissue with fast-response action potentials, e.g., bretylium, amiodarone, sotalol
Class IV	Calcium (slow) channel blocking agents: ↓ conduction velocity and ↑ refractoriness in tissue with slow-response action potentials, e.g., verapamil, diltiazem

Drugs that cannot be classified by this schema:
  Digitalis
  Adenosine

NOTE: SA, sinoatrial; AV, atrioventricular.

AF to atrial flutter may reduce the concealed conduction in the AV node and lead to an excessively rapid ventricular response. β-Adrenergic blockers are especially useful in this regard.

Direct-current electrical cardioversion is a highly effective method to restore sinus rhythm, either as a primary method of therapy or following the failure of antiarrhythmic medications. Electrical cardioversion is accomplished through the delivery of at least 200 W · s of energy between electrodes placed to the right of the sternum and the cardiac apex or to the left of the scapula. If external cardioversion is unsuccessful, internal cardioversion with energy delivered between two catheters inside the heart or one inside and a patch outside the heart may prove effective.

It is unlikely that patients with chronic AF will convert to and remain in sinus rhythm in the presence of long-standing rheumatic heart disease and/or when the atria are markedly enlarged. It is also unlikely for patients with recurrent, paroxysmal lone AF to be converted to and maintained in sinus rhythm.

The goal of therapy in patients in whom AF cannot be converted to sinus rhythm is control of the ventricular response. This can usually be accomplished by digitalis, beta blockers, or calcium channel blockers singly or in combination. In occasional patients, the ventricular response cannot be controlled by pharmacologic therapy alone. In such patients, the creation of complete heart block by radiofrequency catheter ablation of the AV junction followed by permanent pacemaker implantation is appropriate. Surgical or direct-current catheter ablation of the AV junction is rarely required to achieve AV block.

If sinus rhythm is restored electrically or pharmacologically, quinidine or related agents as well as the class IC agents (e.g., flecainide), sotalol, or amiodarone may be used to prevent recurrence. In patients in whom cardioversion is unsuccessful or in whom AF has recurred or is likely to recur despite antiarrhythmic therapy, it is probably wisest to allow the patient to remain in AF and to control the ventricular response with calcium antagonists, β-adrenergic blockers, or digitalis glycosides. Since such patients are always at risk of systemic embolization, particularly in the presence of organic heart disease, chronic anticoagulation must be considered (Table 230-3). Chronic anticoagulation is particularly important in the elderly, where the attributable

Table 230-3 Recommendations for Long-Term Anticoagulation in Patients with Chronic Atrial Fibrillation

Age, years	Risk Factors[a]	Recommendations
<65	Absent	Aspirin
	Present	Warfarin [target INR 2.5 (range 2.0–3.0)]
65–75	Absent	Aspirin or warfarin
	Present	Warfarin [target INR 2.5 (range 2.0–3.0)]
>75	All patients	Warfarin [target INR 2.5 (range 2.0–3.0)]

[a] Risk factors are prior transient ischemic attack, systemic embolus or stroke, hypertension, poor left ventricular function, rheumatic mitral valve disease, prosthetic heart valve.
SOURCE: From A Laupacis et al: Chest 114:579S, 1998.

risk of AF for stroke approaches 30%. Several studies have now demonstrated conclusively that the incidence of embolization in patients with AF not associated with valvular heart disease is reduced by chronic anticoagulation with warfarin-like agents. Aspirin also may be effective for this purpose in patients who are not at high risk for stroke. Although anticoagulation may be associated with hemorrhagic complications, the risk is largely associated with INRs above the recommended range of 1.8 to 3.0. Recommendations for the selection of antiarrhythmic medications to prevent the recurrence of AF are shown in Fig. 230-6.

Ablation therapy for cure of AF is an active area of investigation. This therapy is particularly attractive for the small subset of patients who have a focal atrial tachycardia that degenerates into AF. These automatic foci are often located in the pulmonary veins, and a targeted ablation in these areas may be curative. While ablation of these foci is possible, the procedure can result in pulmonary vein stenosis, pulmonary hypertension, and stroke. Further technologic advances are necessary before this procedure can be more widely and safely performed. A more morbid approach involves making multiple lesions in the right and left atria (MAZE procedure) to compartmentalize the electrical conductance of these chambers and disallow the propagation of fibrillatory waves. The morbidity, mortality, and success rate of such catheter-based procedures renders them experimental at this time.

ATRIAL FLUTTER This arrhythmia occurs most often in patients with organic heart disease. Flutter may be paroxysmal, in which

FIGURE 230-6 Recommendations for the selection of antiarrhythmic medications to prevent the recurrence of atrial fibrillation. See Tables 230-2 and 230-4 for definition of types IA and IC drugs. An atrioventricular nodal blocking agent (i.e., beta blocker, calcium channel blocker, or digoxin) should be added to all type IC and IA agents as well as to dofetilide. LVEF, left ventricular ejection fraction; CHF, congestive heart failure; CAD, coronary artery disease; EF, ejection fraction.

case there is usually a precipitating factor, such as pericarditis or acute respiratory failure, or it may be persistent. Atrial flutter (as well as AF) is very common during the first week following open-heart surgery. Atrial flutter is usually less long-lived than is AF, although on occasion it may persist for months to years. Most commonly, if it lasts for more than a week, atrial flutter will convert to AF. Systemic embolization is less common in atrial flutter than in AF.

Atrial flutter is characterized by an atrial rate between 250 and 350 bpm. Typically, the ventricular rate is half the atrial rate, i.e., approximately 150 bpm. If the atrial rate is slowed to <220 beats per minute by antiarrhythmic agents such as quinidine, which also possess vagolytic properties, the ventricular rate may rise suddenly because of the development of 1:1 AV conduction. Classically, flutter waves are seen as regular sawtooth-like atrial activity, most prominent in the inferior leads (Fig. 230-5B). When the ventricular response is regular and not a simple fraction of the atrial rate, complete AV block is present, which may be a manifestation of digitalis toxicity. Activation mapping suggests that atrial flutter is a form of atrial reentry localized to the right atrium.

TREATMENT The most effective treatment of atrial flutter is direct-current cardioversion, which can be accomplished at low energy (25 to 50 W · s) under mild sedation. Higher energies (100 to 200 W · s) are often used because they are less likely to cause AF, which not infrequently occurs following lower energy delivery. Although atrial flutter is associated with a slightly lower risk of embolization than AF, the same precautions should be followed in regard to anticoagulation as are used with AF. In patients who develop atrial flutter following open-heart surgery or recurrent flutter in the setting of acute myocardial infarction, particularly if they are being treated with digitalis, atrial pacing (using temporary pacing wires implanted at the time of operation or a pacing lead inserted into the atrium pervenously) at rates of 115 to 130% of the atrial flutter rate can usually convert the atrial flutter to sinus rhythm. Atrial pacing may also result in the conversion of atrial flutter to AF, which allows for easier control of the ventricular response. If immediate conversion of atrial flutter is not mandated by the patient's clinical status, the ventricular response should first be slowed by blocking the AV node with a beta blocker, calcium antagonist, or digitalis. Digitalis is the least effective and occasionally converts atrial flutter into AF. Once AV nodal conduction is slowed with any of these drugs, an attempt to convert flutter to sinus rhythm using a class I (A or C) agent or amiodarone should be made. Increasing doses of the drug selected are administered until the rhythm converts or side effects occur. Ibutilide is a new antiarrhythmic agent that is administered intravenously and appears to be particularly effective for conversion of atrial flutter to sinus rhythm.

Quinidine, other Class IA drugs, flecainide, propafenone, sotalol, and amiodarone (Table 230-4) may be useful in preventing recurrences of atrial flutter. Radiofrequency ablation is a highly effective treatment for patients with the most typical forms of atrial flutter, which are due to reentry around the tricuspid valve in a counterclockwise or clockwise fashion. The coronary sinus and inferior vena cava cause the wavefront of activation to pass between them and the tricuspid valve. Ablation of the narrowed isthmus using radiofrequency energy can cure flutter in >85% of cases.

PAROXYSMAL SUPRAVENTRICULAR TACHYCARDIAS (PSVT) In most cases, functional differences in conduction and refractoriness in the AV node or the presence of an AV bypass tract provide the substrate for the development of PSVT (previously termed *paroxysmal atrial tachycardia*). Electrophysiologic studies have demonstrated that reentry is responsible for the vast majority of cases of PSVT (Fig. 230-7). Reentry has been localized to the sinus node, atrium, AV node, or a macroreentrant circuit involving conduction in the antegrade direction through the AV node and retrograde through an AV bypass tract. Such a bypass tract may also conduct

Table 230-4 Drugs Used to Treat Cardiac Tachyarrhythmias

Drug	Mode of Administration	$t_{1/2}$ (oral), h	Route of Metabolism	Clinical Effects and/or Indications for Use
Digoxin	IV, 0.25–1.5 mg Oral, 0.75–1.5 mg loading dose over 12–24 h Maintenance, 0.23–0.50 mg/kg	36	Renal	Slowing of ventricular rate during AF, flutter, and other atrial tachycardias in the absence of preexcitation; slowing, termination, and/or prevention of SVT due to AV nodal reentry and AV reentry utilizing bypass tracts; may terminate or prevent intra-atrial reentrant tachycardias; ineffective in prevention of automatic atrial tachycardias
Adenosine	IV bolus, 6–12 mg	<10s		Acute termination of regular reentrant SVT involving the AV node
Quinidine (class IA)	Oral, 200–400 mg q6h	8–9	Hepatic, 80% Renal, 20%	Atrial and ventricular tachyarrhythmias; all types of SVT; control of ventricular rate in patients with preexcitation and AF and flutter
Procainamide (class IA)	IV, 40–50 mg/min to total of 10–20 mg/kg. Oral, 500–1000 mg q6h (sustained-release forms)	3–5	Hepatic, 50% Renal, 50%	Same as quinidine
Disopyramide (class IA)	Oral, 100–300 mg q6h	8–9	Hepatic, 50% Renal, 50%	Same as quinidine
Lidocaine (class IB)	IV, 20–50 mg/min to total of 5 mg/kg loading dose, followed by 1–4 mg/kg	1–2	Hepatic	VT and VF, especially during acute ischemia and myocardial infarction
Phenytoin (class IB)	IV, 20 mg/kg to total dose of 1000 mg Oral, 1000-mg loading dose over 24 h Maintenance, 100–400 mg/d	18–36	Hepatic	Tachyarrhythmias induced by digitalis; occasionally effective for ventricular tachyarrhythmias not induced by digitalis alone or in combination with other antiarrhythmic agents; polymorphic VT associated with increased QT interval
Mexiletine (class IB)	Oral, 100–300 mg q6–8h	9–12	Hepatic	Ventricular tachyarrhythmias; secondary agent in combination with other class 1 medication
Flecainide (class IC)	Oral, begin at 50–100 mg bid, increase by ≤50 mg in 4-day intervals to a maximum of mg daily	7–23	Hepatic, 75% Renal, 25%	Supraventricular tachyarrhythmias including atrial fibrillation and flutter; also ventricular arrhythmias refractory to other medications or radiofrequency ablation
Propafenone (class IC)	Oral, 150–300 mg q8h	5–8	Hepatic	Same as flecainide
Moricizine (class IC)	Oral, 200–400 mg q8h	2–6	Hepatic	Same as flecainide
Beta blockers (class II) e.g., metoprolol	IV, load with 5–10 mg q5min for 3 doses, then 3 mg q6h Oral, 25–100 mg bid	3–4	Hepatic	Slowing of ventricular rate during AF, atrial flutter, and other atrial tachyarrhythmias in the absence of preexcitation; SVT due to AV nodal reentry; reentry utilizing bypass tracts; arrhythmias (e.g., VT) induced by exercise or occurring in the presence of hyperthyroidism; polymorphic VT associated with congenital long QT syndrome
Bretylium (class III)	IV, 1–2 mg/kg per min to total load, 5–10 mg/kg Maintenance, 0.5–2 mg/kg	8–14	Renal	Refractory VT and VF, especially due to acute ischemia
Amiodarone (class III)	IV, 5–10 mg/kg load over 20 min, then 1 g/24 h		Hepatic	Sustained VT and VF
	Oral, load 800–1600 mg/d for 1 week, then 400–600 mg/d for 3 weeks, then 200–400 mg/d thereafter	13–103		AF and atrial flutter, other types of SVT, VT, VF
Sotalol (class III)	Oral, 80–320 mg q12h	10–20	Renal, 90% Hepatic, 10%	Atrial and ventricular tachyarrhythmias
Ibutilide (class III)	IV, <60 kg: 0.01 mg/kg over 10 min IV, ≥60 kg: 1 mg over 10 min, repeat after 10 min if no effect	2–6	Hepatic	AF, atrial flutter, and other SVTs including preexcitation tachycardias
Dofetilide	125–250 mg PO bid	8–12	Renal	AF, atrial flutter, and other SVTs
Calcium channel blockers (class IV) e.g., verapamil	IV, 2.5–10 mg over 1–2 min to total of 0.15 mg/kg Oral, 240–480 qd	6–24	Hepatic	Slowing of ventricular rate during AF and flutter, and other SVTs in the absence of preexcitation; idiopathic VT
Diltiazem	IV, load with 0.25 mg/kg over 2 min; if needed, repeat after 15 min with 0.35 mg over 2 min Maintenance, 10–15 mg/h		Hepatic	Same as verapamil

NOTE: AF, atrial fibrillation; AV, atrioventricular; SVT, supraventricular tachycardia; VF, ventricular fibrillation; VT, ventricular tachycardia.

antegradely, in which case the Wolff-Parkinson-White (WPW) syndrome is said to be present. When the bypass tract manifests only retrograde conduction, it is termed a *concealed bypass tract* (Fig. 230-7B). In these cases, the QRS complex during sinus rhythm is normal. In the absence of the WPW syndrome, reentry through the AV node or through a concealed bypass tract makes up more than 90% of all PSVTs.

AV NODAL REENTRANT TACHYCARDIA There is no age or disease predisposition for the development of AV nodal reentrant tachycardia, the most common cause of supraventricular tachy-

A

B

C

FIGURE 230-7 Examples of reentrant supraventricular tachycardia (SVT). *A.* AV nodal reentry. No P waves are visible. *B.* AV reentry using a concealed bypass tract. Inverted retrograde P waves are superimposed on the T wave. *C.* Intraatrial reentry. Inverted P waves follow the T waves and precede the QRS complex.

Clinical Features AV nodal reentry may produce palpitations, syncope, and heart failure depending on the rate and duration of the arrhythmia and the presence and severity of any underlying heart disease. Hypotension and syncope may occur because of the sudden loss of the atrial contribution to ventricular filling; this can also lead to a marked increase in atrial pressure, acute pulmonary edema, and a reduction in ventricular filling. Simultaneous atrial and ventricular contraction produces cannon *a* waves with each heartbeat.

TREATMENT In patients without hypotension, vagal maneuvers, particularly carotid sinus massage, can terminate the arrhythmia in 80% of cases. If hypotension is present, raising the blood pressure by the cautious use of intravenous phenylephrine in 0.1-mg increments may terminate the arrhythmia alone or in combination with carotid sinus pressure. If these maneuvers are unsuccessful, verapamil (2.5 to 10 mg intravenously) or adenosine (6 to 12 mg intravenously) is the agent of choice. We prefer to use adenosine because of its extremely short half-life, lessening the consequences of any side effects. Beta blockers may also be used to slow or terminate the tachycardia but are agents of second choice. Digitalis glycosides have a slower onset of action and should *not* be used for acute therapy. When these drugs fail to terminate the tachycardia, or when the tachycardia is recurrent, atrial or ventricular pacing via a temporary pacemaker inserted pervenously may be used to terminate the arrhythmia. However, if severe ischemia and/or hypotension is caused by the tachycardia, dc cardioversion should be considered.

AV nodal reentry can usually be prevented by the use of drugs that act primarily on the antegrade slow pathway (such as digitalis, beta blockers, or calcium channel antagonists) or on the fast pathway (class IA or IC; Table 230-4). We favor initial therapy with beta blockers, calcium channel antagonists, or digoxin because the risk-benefit ratio associated with treatment with these agents is more favorable than that of IA or IC agents. Drugs most likely to avert recurrences prevent induction of the arrhythmias by programmed stimulation. This technique utilizes temporary pacemaker catheters connected to a physiologic stimulator capable of variable rate pacing and stimulation with one or more precisely timed premature impulses. In symptomatic patients who require chronic therapy, radiofrequency catheter modification of the AV node should be considered. This technique can cure AV nodal reentry in >90% of cases and has been proven to be safe, although a 1 to 2% risk of AV block requiring a permanent pacemaker exists.

AV REENTRANT TACHYCARDIA PSVT due to AV reentry incorporates a concealed AV bypass tract as part of the tachycardia circuit. Thus the impulse passes antegradely from the atria through the AV node and His-Purkinje system to the ventricles and then retrogradely through the (concealed) bypass tract back to the atrium. Patients with this disorder manifest the same type of PSVT as do patients with the WPW syndrome (see below), but the bypass tract cannot conduct in an antegrade direction during sinus rhythm or other atrial tachyarrhythmias.

AV reentrant tachycardia can be initiated and terminated by either APCs or VPCs. Initiation of PSVT by a VPC is virtually diagnostic of AV reentry. Alternation of the QRS complexes occurs in approximately one-third of such tachycardias. Since atrial activation must follow ventricular activation during AV reentry, the P wave usually occurs after the QRS complex (Fig. 230-7*B*).

Atrial activation mapping is of major value in evaluating the origin of these tachycardias. Most concealed bypass tracts are left-sided. Thus, during PSVT or during ventricular pacing, the earliest activation sequence is recorded in the left atrium, usually via a catheter in the coronary sinus. This eccentric atrial activation is quite distinct from the normal retrograde activation sequence in which the earliest activation of the atria is in the area of the AV junction. The ability of a ventricular stimulus to conduct to the atrium at a time when the bundle

cardia. It is, however, more commonly observed in women. It usually presents as a regular narrow QRS complex tachycardia at rates of 120 to 250 bpm. APCs that initiate the arrhythmia are almost always associated with a prolonged PR interval. Retrograde P waves may be absent, buried in the QRS complex, or appear as distortions at the terminal parts of the QRS complex (Fig. 230-7*A*).

AV nodal reentrant PSVT (Fig. 230-8) can be reproducibly initiated and terminated by appropriately timed atrial premature stimuli. The onset of the tachycardia is almost always associated with prolongation of the PR interval due to marked AV nodal conduction delay (prolonged AH interval) following the APC that is critical for the genesis of the arrhythmia. The sudden prolongation of the AH interval is consistent with the concept of dual AV nodal pathways: a *fast pathway*, which exhibits rapid conduction and a long refractory period, and a *slow pathway*, which has a short refractory period but conducts slowly. During sinus rhythm, only conduction over the fast pathway is manifest, resulting in a normal PR interval (Fig. 230-8). Atrial extrastimuli at a critical coupling interval are blocked in the fast pathway because of its longer refractory period and are conducted slowly through the slow pathway. If conduction down the slow pathway is slow enough to allow the previously refractory fast pathway time to recover excitability, a single atrial (echo) reentrant beat or sustained tachycardia ensues. A critical balance between conduction velocity and refractoriness within the node is required to sustain AV nodal reentry. Retrograde atrial and antegrade ventricular activation occur simultaneously, explaining why P waves may not be apparent on the surface ECG.

FIGURE 230-8 Mechanism of AV nodal reentry: The atrium, AV node (AVN), and His bundle are shown schematically. The AV node is longitudinally dissociated into two pathways, slow and fast, with different functional properties (see text). In each panel of this diagram, blue lines denote excitation in the AV node, which is manifest on the surface electrocardiogram, while black lines denote conduction, which is concealed and not apparent on the surface electrocardiogram. *A.* During sinus rhythm (NSR) the impulse from the atrium conducts down both pathways. However, only conduction over the fast pathway is manifest on the surface ECG, producing a normal PR interval of 0.16 s. *B.* An atrial premature depolarization (APD) blocks in the fast pathway. The impulse conducts over the slow pathway to the His bundle and ventricles,

producing a PR interval of 0.24 s. Because the impulse is premature, conduction over the slow pathway occurs more slowly than it would during sinus rhythm. *C.* A more premature atrial impulse blocks in the fast pathway, conducting with increased delay in the slow pathway, producing a PR interval of 0.28 s. The impulse conducts retrogradely up the fast pathway producing a single atrial echo. Sustained reentry is prevented by subsequent block in the slow pathway. *D.* A still more premature atrial impulse blocks initially in the fast pathway, conducting over the slow pathway with increasing delay producing a PR interval of 0.36 s. Retrograde conduction occurs over the fast pathway and reentry occurs, producing a sustained tachycardia (SVT). *(After ME Josephson: Clinical Cardiac Electrophysiology, 2d ed. Phildelphia, Lea & Febiger, 1993.)*

of His is refractory and the termination of the tachycardia by a ventricular stimulus that does not reach the atrium are diagnostic of retrograde conduction over a concealed bypass tract.

℞ **TREATMENT** This is similar to the treatment for AV nodal reentry tachycardia. Although pharmacologic agents may be used, patients who require chronic therapy should be considered candidates for radiofrequency catheter ablation of the bypass tract. This requires detailed electrophysiologic study to exclude other arrhythmias that may be responsible for patients' symptoms and to determine the location of the bypass tract(s). The efficacy of this procedure exceeds 90%, with minimal risks. In the remaining small number of patients failing catheter ablation, surgical ablation or pharmacologic therapy can be used.

SINUS NODE REENTRY AND OTHER ATRIAL TACHYCARDIAS Reentry in the region of the sinus node or within the atria is invariably initiated by APCs. These arrhythmias are less common than AV nodal or AV reentry and are more often associated with underlying cardiac disease. During sinus node reentry, the P-wave morphology is identical to that occurring in sinus rhythm, but the PR interval is prolonged. This is in contrast to sinus tachycardia,

in which the PR interval tends to shorten. With intraatrial reentry, the P-wave configuration differs from that during sinus rhythm, and the PR interval is prolonged (Fig. 230-7*C*).

℞ **TREATMENT** Sinus node and atrial reentrant arrhythmias are managed like other reentrant PSVTs, except that catheter ablation is less successful because multiple foci may be present.

NONREENTRANT ATRIAL TACHYCARDIAS These may be a manifestation of digitalis intoxication or may be associated with severe pulmonary or cardiac disease, with hypokalemia, or with the administration of theophylline or adrenergic drugs. Multifocal atrial tachycardia (MAT) (Fig. 230-9) is particularly common following theophylline administration. By definition, MAT requires three or more consecutive P waves of different morphologies at rates greater than 100 beats per minute. MAT usually has an irregular ventricular rate because of varying AV conduction. There is a high incidence of atrial fibrillation (50 to 70%) in patients with MAT. Treatment should be directed at the underlying disorder. The digitalis-induced arrhythmias are caused by triggered activity. In such atrial tachycardias with AV block secondary to digitalis intoxication, the atrial rate rarely exceeds 180 bpm, and typically 2:1 block is present. Atrial arrhythmias

FIGURE 230-9 Multifocal atrial tachycardia. A lead I rhythm strip demonstrates a multifocal atrial tachycardia defined by ≥3 consecutive P waves of variable morphology and rate >100 bpm (*arrows*).

precipitated by digitalis can usually be treated by withdrawal of the drug.

Automatic atrial tachycardias not caused by digitalis are difficult to terminate, and in such cases the main goal of therapy should be to control the ventricular response, either by drugs that affect the AV node, such as digitalis, beta blockers, or calcium channel antagonists, or by ablation techniques. Catheter ablation and surgery have been employed to eradicate the arrhythmia's focus or create heart block for rate control.

PREEXCITATION (WPW) SYNDROME The most frequently encountered type of ventricular preexcitation is that associated with AV bypass tracts. These connections are composed of strands of atrial-like muscle which may occur almost anywhere around the AV rings. The term *Wolff-Parkinson-White syndrome* is applied to patients with both preexcitation on the ECG and paroxysmal tachycardias. AV bypass tracts can be associated with certain congenital abnormalities, the most important of which is Ebstein's anomaly.

AV bypass tracts that conduct in an antegrade direction produce a typical ECG pattern of a short PR interval (<0.12 s), a slurred upstroke of the QRS complex (delta wave), and a wide QRS complex. This pattern results from a fusion of activation of the ventricles over both the bypass tract and the AV nodal His-Purkinje system (Fig. 230-10). The relative contribution of activation over each system determines the amount of preexcitation.

During PSVT in WPW, the impulse is usually conducted antegradely over the normal AV system and retrogradely through the bypass tract. The characteristics are identical to those described on p. 1299. Rarely (approximately 5%), tachycardias occurring in patients with WPW will exhibit a reverse pattern with antegrade conduction through the bypass tract and retrograde conduction through the normal AV system. This produces a tachycardia with a wide QRS complex in which the ventricles are totally activated by the bypass tract. Atrial flutter and AF also occur commonly in patients with WPW syndrome. Since the bypass tract does not have the same decremental conducting properties as the AV node, the ventricular responses during atrial flutter or fibrillation may be unusually rapid and may cause ventricular fibrillation (VF).

The goals of electrophysiologic evaluation in patients suspected of having the WPW syndrome are (1) to confirm the diagnosis, (2) to localize the bypass tract and determine how many bypass tracts are present, (3) to demonstrate the role of the bypass tract in the genesis of the arrhythmias, (4) to determine the potential for the development of possibly life-threatening rates during atrial flutter or fibrillation, and (5) to evaluate therapeutic options.

Rx **TREATMENT** Pharmacologic therapy is aimed at altering the electrophysiologic properties (i.e., refractoriness or conduction velocity) of one or more components of the reentrant circuit. This is most often accomplished by agents such as beta blockers or calcium channel blockers that slow conduction and increase refractoriness of the AV node or by agents such as quinidine or flecainide that slow conduction and increase refractoriness primarily in the bypass tract. Some drugs may affect multiple sites (Fig. 230-11).

Acute management of episodes of PSVT in patients with WPW syndrome is similar to that of PSVT in patients with concealed bypass tracts.

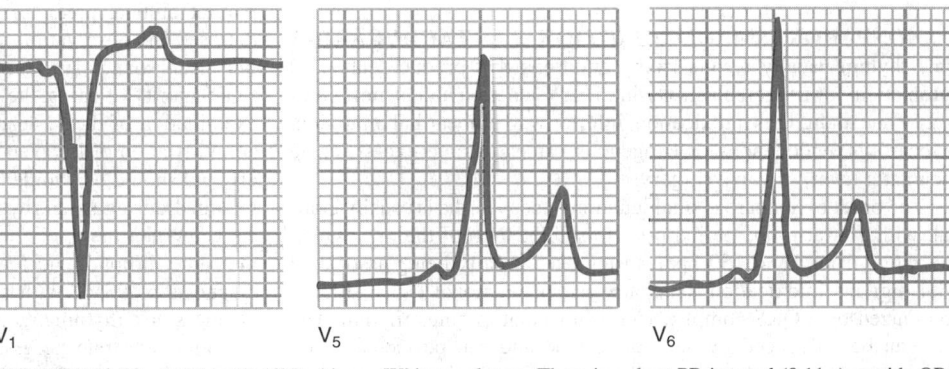

FIGURE 230-10 ECG in Wolff-Parkinson-White syndrome. There is a short PR interval (0.11 s), a wide QRS complex (0.12 s), and slurring on the upstroke of the QRS produced by early ventricular activation over the bypass tract (delta wave, d in lead I). The negative delta waves in V_1 are diagnostic of a right-sided bypass tract. Note the Q wave (negative delta wave) in lead III, mimicking myocardial infarction.

In patients with the WPW syndrome and AF, dc cardioversion should be carried out if there is a life-threatening, rapid ventricular response. In non-life–threatening situations, lidocaine (3 to 5 mg/kg) or procainamide (15 mg/kg) administered intravenously over 15 to 20 min will usually slow the ventricular response. More recently, ibutilide has become available as an alternative therapy for preexcitation tachycardia. Caution should be employed when using digitalis or intravenous verapamil in patients with the WPW syndrome and AF, since these drugs can shorten the refractory period of the accessory pathway and can increase the ventricular rate, thereby placing the patient at increased risk for VF. Chronic oral therapy with verapamil is not associated with this risk. In addition to these drugs, beta-blocking agents are of no utility in controlling the ventricular response during AF when conduction proceeds over the bypass tract. Although atrial or ventric-

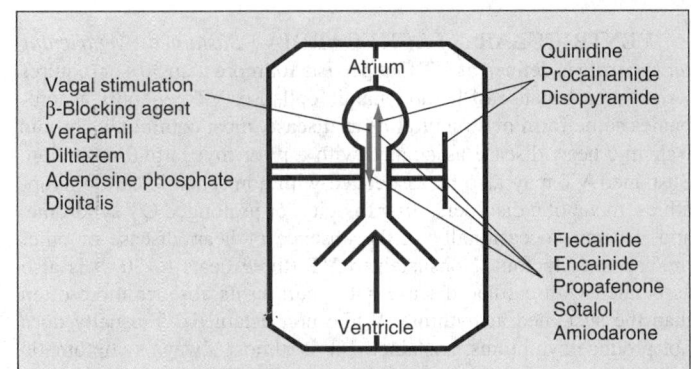

FIGURE 230-11 Site of action of antiarrhythmic agents in the Wolff-Parkinson-White syndrome. The atrium, ventricle, antegrade conduction through the AV node (↓), retrograde conduction through the AV node (↑), and the bypass tract are shown. Drugs on the left affect antegrade AV nodal conduction. Type IA drugs on the upper right affect retrograde conduction over the node and antegrade conduction over the bypass tract. Drugs on the lower right affect conduction in both directions in the AV node and the bypass tract.

ular pacing can almost always terminate PSVT in patients with the WPW syndrome, they can induce AF. As such, chronic pacemaker therapy is to be discouraged.

While surgical ablation of bypass tracts offers a permanent cure of supraventricular tachycardia (SVT) and most AFs associated with SVT, the advent of radiofrequency catheter ablation has virtually eliminated the need for surgery. Catheter ablation of bypass tracts is possible in >90% of patients and is the treatment of choice in patients with symptomatic arrhythmias. It is safer, more cost-effective, and just as successful as surgery. Nevertheless, surgical ablation may be required in the occasional patient in whom catheter ablation fails.

NONPAROXYSMAL JUNCTIONAL TACHYCARDIA

This rhythm usually results from conditions that produce enhanced automaticity or triggered activity in the AV junction and is most commonly due to digitalis intoxication, inferior wall myocardial infarction, myocarditis, endogenous or exogenous catecholamine excess, acute rheumatic fever, or valve surgery.

The onset of nonparoxysmal junctional tachycardia is usually gradual, with a "warm-up" period prior to stabilization of the rate, which can range from 70 to 150 bpm, faster rates usually being associated with digitalis intoxication. Nonparoxysmal junctional tachycardia is recognized by a QRS complex identical to that of sinus rhythm. The rate can be influenced by autonomic tone and can be increased by catecholamines, vagolytic agents, or exercise and slowed somewhat by carotid sinus pressure. When this rhythm is due to digitalis intoxication, it usually is associated with AV block and/or dissociation. Soon after cardiac surgery, retrograde conduction is more likely to be present because of the heightened sympathetic state.

℞ **TREATMENT** This is directed toward elimination of the underlying etiologic factors. Since digitalis is the most common cause of this rhythm, discontinuation of this drug is indicated. If the rhythm is associated with other serious manifestations of digitalis intoxication, such as ventricular or atrial irritability, active intervention with lidocaine or a beta blocker may be useful, and in some instances, use of digitalis antibodies (Fab fragments) should be considered. Cardioversion of this rhythm should not be attempted, particularly in the setting of digitalis intoxication. When AV conduction is intact, atrial pacing can capture and override the junctional focus and provide the AV synchrony necessary to maximize cardiac output. Nonparoxysmal junctional tachycardia is usually not a chronic, recurrent problem, and attention to the acute precipitating events can often resolve the tachycardia.

VENTRICULAR TACHYCARDIA *Sustained ventricular tachycardia* is defined as VT that persists for more than 30 s or requires termination because of hemodynamic collapse. VT generally accompanies some form of structural heart disease, most commonly chronic ischemic heart disease associated with a prior myocardial infarction. Sustained VT may also be associated with nonischemic cardiomyopathies, metabolic disorders, drug toxicity, or prolonged QT syndrome, and it occurs occasionally in the absence of heart disease or other predisposing factors. Nonsustained VT (three beats to 30 s) is also associated with cardiac disease but occurs in its absence more often than the sustained arrhythmia. While nonsustained VT usually does not produce symptoms, sustained VT is almost always symptomatic and is often associated with marked hemodynamic compromise and/or the development of myocardial ischemia. A fixed anatomic substrate, not acute ischemia, is responsible for most recurrent episodes of sustained uniform VT. Acute ischemia appears to have little role in the genesis of sustained uniform VT associated with chronic infarction but may play a role in the degeneration of stable VT into VF or initiation of polymorphic VT. Most episodes of VF begin with VT.

The ECG diagnosis of VT is suggested by a wide-complex QRS tachycardia at a rate exceeding 100 bpm. The QRS configuration dur-

ing any episode of VT may be uniform (monomorphic), or it may vary from beat to beat (polymorphic). *Bidirectional tachycardia* refers to VT that shows an alternation in QRS amplitude and axis. Typically this appears as a QRS with a right bundle branch block pattern with alternating superior (leftward) and inferior axes (rightward). While the rhythm is usually quite regular, slight irregularity may exist. Atrial activity may be dissociated from ventricular activity, or the atria may be depolarized retrogradely. The onset of the tachycardia is generally abrupt, but in nonparoxysmal tachycardias it can be gradual. Paroxysmal VT is usually initiated by a VPC.

It is important to distinguish SVT with aberration of intraventricular conduction from VT because the clinical implications and management of these two arrhythmias are totally different. The most important clinical predictor of VT is the presence of structural heart disease. The observation of intermittent cannon *a* waves and varying first heart sounds suggests AV dissociation and is diagnostic of VT. In a majority of cases, the diagnosis can and should be made by close examination of the 12-lead ECG. Pharmacologic maneuvers, such as administration of intravenous verapamil or adenosine, can be hazardous and should be avoided. It is always useful to have a 12-lead ECG recorded during sinus rhythm for comparison with that during tachycardia. When the tracing obtained during sinus rhythm demonstrates the same morphologic features as those during the tachycardia, the diagnosis of PSVT with aberration is favored. An infarction pattern on the sinus rhythm tracing suggests the potential presence of the anatomic substrate necessary for VT. Characteristics of the 12-lead ECG during the tachycardia that suggest a ventricular origin for the arrhythmia are (1) a QRS complex >0.14 s in the absence of antiarrhythmic therapy, (2) AV dissociation (with or without fusion or captured beats) or variable retrograde conduction (Fig. 230-12), (3) a superior QRS axis in the presence of a right bundle branch block pattern, (4) concordance of the QRS pattern in all precordial leads (i.e., all positive or all negative deflections), and (5) other QRS patterns (morphology) with prolonged duration that are inconsistent with typical right or left bundle branch block patterns. (See Table 230-5 for a detailed synopsis of ECG criteria that favor the diagnosis of VT over SVT for wide complex tachycardia.) A wide, complex, bizarre tachycardia that is very irregular suggests AF with conduction over an AV bypass tract. Similarly, a QRS complex in excess of 0.20 s is uncommon during VT in the absence of drug therapy and is more common with preexcitation. Intravenous verapamil will stop most recalcitrant SVTs involving the AV junction, but it is rarely effective for VT. Because of this property, verapamil has been utilized to attempt to differentiate SVT with aberrant conduction from VT. However, this is extremely hazardous, since intravenous verapamil can precipitate cardiac arrest in patients with VT.

It has been possible to replicate sustained uniform VT in more than 95% of patients with this arrhythmia using programmed electrical stimulation. In most patients the tachycardia is initiated with ventricular premature stimuli. A sustained monomorphic VT with a morphology identical to that of the spontaneous arrhythmia is the rule. The clinical significance of polymorphic VT initiated by programmed stimulation is not clear, since more aggressive stimulation (i.e., the use of three or four extrastimuli) can induce polymorphic VT and even VF in some normal subjects and in patients who have never had a clinical arrhythmia.

Sustained uniform VT can be terminated by programmed stimulation or rapid pacing in at least 75% of patients; the remainder require cardioversion. The ability to reproducibly initiate and terminate a sustained, uniform VT permits assessment of pharmacologic and electrical therapy of these arrhythmias.

The reproducible termination of VT by programmed stimulation permits evaluation of the effectiveness of antitachycardia pacemakers for long-term therapy of paroxysmal episodes of arrhythmia. Unfortunately, rapid pacing, the most effective form of therapy, can accelerate the tachycardia and/or produce VF. Therefore, antitachycardia pacing is a viable form of therapy only when the pacing device includes backup defibrillation capabilities.

Clinical Features Symptoms resulting from VT depend on the ventricular rate, duration of the tachycardia, and presence and extent of underlying cardiac disease. When the tachycardia is rapid and associated with severe myocardial dysfunction and cerebrovascular disease, hypotension and syncope are common. However, the presence of hemodynamic stability does not preclude a diagnosis of VT. The rate, loss of the atrial contribution to ventricular filling, and abnormal sequence of ventricular activation are important factors producing a decreased cardiac output during VT.

The *prognosis* of VT depends on the underlying disease state. If sustained VT develops within the first 6 weeks following acute myocardial infarction, the prognosis is poor, with a 75% mortality rate at 1 year. Patients with nonsustained VT following myocardial infarction have a threefold greater risk of death than a comparable group of patients without this arrhythmia. However, a cause-and-effect relationship between the nonsustained tachycardia and subsequent sudden death has not been established. Patients without heart disease who have uniform VT have a good prognosis and an extremely low risk of sudden death.

FIGURE 230-12 Ventricular tachycardia with AV dissociation. P waves are dissociated from the underlying wide complex rhythm (best seen on lead V_1).

![Rx] **TREATMENT** The risk-benefit ratio of treating each specific type of VT should be considered before beginning therapy. This is important because antiarrhythmic agents can produce or exacerbate the very arrhythmias that they are given to prevent. In general, patients with VT but without organic heart disease have a benign course; such patients with asymptomatic, nonsustained VT need not be treated because their prognosis will not be affected. An exception is the patient with congenital long QT syndrome. Such patients have recurrent polymorphic VT and a high mortality from sudden death if untreated. Patients with sustained VT in the absence of heart disease usually require therapy because the arrhythmia causes symptoms. These tachycardias may respond to beta blockers; verapamil; class IA, IC, or III agents; or amiodarone. In patients with VT and organic heart disease, if marked hemodynamic compromise is present or if there is evidence of ischemia, congestive heart failure, or central nervous system hypoperfusion, the rhythm should be promptly terminated by dc cardioversion (see below). If the patient with organic heart disease tolerates the VT well, pharmacologic therapy may be tried. Procainamide is probably the most effective agent for acute therapy. It may or may not terminate the tachycardia but almost always slows the rate. In stable patients in whom these drugs do not terminate the arrhythmia, a pacing catheter can be inserted pervenously into the right ventricular apex, and the tachycardia can be terminated by overdrive pacing.

Programmed stimulation is probably the most effective way to select the appropriate antiarrhythmic agent to prevent recurrent, sustained VT. After demonstrating that the tachycardia can be initiated reproducibly in the absence of antiarrhythmic agents, drugs can be studied serially, and the drug that prevents initiation of the tachycardia can be selected; long-term (>2 years) successful prevention of the arrhythmia can then be expected in 80% of patients if a complete stimulation protocol is used following drug administration. Failure to perform a complete protocol will lead to recurrences, which are often blamed on the lack of utility of programmed stimulation as a method of evaluating drug efficacy. Drug levels demonstrated to be successful in the laboratory need to be maintained chronically. Unfortunately, prevention of inducible VT is expected in only 50% of cases. Use of Holter monitor for guided therapy, although advocated by some, is of less value.

Antitachycardia pacing has been used as a means to terminate tachycardias that have been reproducibly terminated by pacing in the electrophysiology laboratory. Automatic antitachycardia pacing devices are not used alone because pacing during VT may accelerate tachycardia, converting a stable arrhythmia into an unstable one and resulting in severe hemodynamic compromise. However, devices combining antitachycardia pacing with an ICD (see below) afford a "backup" means of terminating unstable arrhythmias.

The advent of endocardial catheter and intraoperative mapping led to the development of surgical techniques for the management of VT. Activation mapping permits localization of the site of origin of the

Table 230-5   Wide Complex Tachycardia

ECG CRITERIA THAT FAVOR VENTRICULAR TACHYCARDIA

1. AV dissociation
2. QRS width: >0.14 s with RBBB configuration
   >0.16 s with LBBB configuration
3. QRS axis: Left axis deviation with RBBB morphology
   Extreme left axis deviation (northwest axis) with LBBB morphology
4. Concordance of QRS in precordial leads
5. Morphologic patterns of the QRS complex
   RBBB: Mono- or biphasic complex in V_1
   RS (*only with left axis deviation*) or QS in V_6

LBBB: Broad R wave in V_1 or V_2 ≥0.04 s
   Onset of QRS to nadir of S wave in V_1 or V_2 of ≥0.07 s
   Notched downslope of S wave in V_1 or V_2
   Q wave in V_6

NOTE: AV, atrioventricular; BBB, bundle branch block.

arrhythmia. In centers in which expertise in mapping is available, operation has been successfully employed to cure tachycardias in the majority of patients in whom it has been undertaken. Even though most patients with VT and ischemic heart disease have markedly impaired left ventricular function and multivessel coronary artery disease, the operative mortality rate has ranged between 8 and 15%. Following operation, >90% of survivors are controlled either off (two-thirds of patients) or on (one-third) antiarrhythmic agents that were previously ineffective in controlling these rhythms. With the development of radiofrequency ablation and refinement of mapping criteria to locate critical sites of the VT circuit, precisely, catheter ablation can be performed as a curative procedure in selected patients. In experienced centers cure of VT in these *selected* patients approaches 75%.

Specific Types of VT   *Torsade de pointes* (Fig. 230-13) refers to VT characterized by polymorphic QRS complexes that change in amplitude and cycle length, giving the appearance of oscillations around the baseline. This rhythm is, by definition, associated with QT prolongation. The latter may result from electrolyte disturbances (particularly hypokalemia and hypomagnesemia), use of a variety of antiarrhythmic drugs (especially quinidine), phenothiazines and tricyclic antidepressants, liquid protein diets, intracranial events, and bradyarrhythmias, particularly third-degree AV block. It also may occur as a congenital anomaly that most often presents with torsade de pointes (syncope or sudden death) at a young age.

The electrocardiographic hallmark is polymorphic VT preceded by marked QT prolongation, often in excess of 0.60 s. These patients often have multiple episodes of nonsustained polymorphic VT associated with recurrent syncope, but they also may develop VF and sudden cardiac death.

Therapy should be directed at removing the precipitating factors, i.e., correcting metabolic abnormalities and removing drugs that have induced the prolonged QT interval. In the setting of drug-induced torsade de pointes, atrial or ventricular overdrive pacing and the administration of magnesium have also been useful in terminating and preventing the arrhythmia. For patients with the congenital prolonged QT interval syndrome, β-adrenergic blocking agents have been the mainstay of therapy; agents that shorten the QT interval may also be useful (e.g., phenytoin). Cervicothoracic sympathectomy has been proposed as a form of therapy for congenital prolonged QT syndrome, but it is not often effective as the sole therapy. Pacing in combination with beta blockers and sympathectomy has been used by some investigators when beta blockers fail, but it is not uniformly successful and results

in a Horner's syndrome. More recently, ICDs with dual chambered pacing capability and beta blockers have become the treatment of choice for patients with recurrent episodes despite beta blockers.

Polymorphic tachycardias associated with normal QT intervals in patients with ischemic heart disease that are initiated by "R-on-T" VPCs are probably caused by reentry, and their treatment is totally different. This is not true torsade de pointes. In such cases, class I or III agents may be the most effective form of therapy and should be administered in full antiarrhythmic doses. However, these arrhythmias may also result from acute, severe ischemia and will only respond to abolition of the ischemia, usually by revascularization.

Accelerated idioventricular rhythm, also termed *slow VT*, with a rate that ranges from 60 to 120 bpm, usually occurs in acute myocardial infarction, often during reperfusion. It may also be seen following cardiac operations; in patients with cardiomyopathy, rheumatic fever, or digitalis intoxication; and in patients with no evidence of heart disease. The rhythm is usually transient and rarely causes significant hemodynamic compromise or symptoms.

Treatment is rarely necessary and should usually be considered only if symptoms arise due to impaired hemodynamics, most commonly due to AV dissociation. In most cases, atropine can accelerate the sinus rate to overdrive the ventricular rhythm.

VENTRICULAR FLUTTER AND VENTRICULAR FIBRILLATION (Fig. 230-14; See also Chap. 39)   These arrhythmias occur most often in patients with ischemic heart disease. They also occur following administration of antiarrhythmic drugs, particularly those that induce prolonged QT intervals and torsade de pointes (see above), in patients with severe hypoxia or ischemia, and in those with WPW who develop AF with an extremely rapid ventricular response (p. 1299). Electrical accidents frequently cause cardiac arrest due to the development of VF. The onset of these arrhythmias is rapidly followed by loss of consciousness and, if untreated, death. Episodes of cardiac arrest recorded during Holter monitoring reveal that approximately three-fourths of the sudden deaths are due to VT or VF.

In patients with nonischemic VF, the onset usually begins with a short run of rapid VT, which is initiated by a relatively late coupled VPC. In patients with acute myocardial infarction or ischemia, however, VF is usually precipitated by a single early ventricular complex beat falling on the T wave (the vulnerable period), which produces a rapid VT that degenerates into VF (Fig. 230-14).

The clinical setting in which VF occurs is important. Most patients who have primary VF within the first 48 h of the onset of acute infarction have a good long-term prognosis, with a very low rate of recurrence or sudden cardiac death. Their short-term mortality may, however, be slightly increased. In contrast, patients who experience VF unassociated with the development of acute myocardial infarction

FIGURE 230-13 Rhythm strips of patients with drug (disopyramide)-induced torsade de pointes. The polymorphic ventricular tachycardia is associated with very long QT intervals.

FIGURE 230-14 Ventricular fibrillation. In a patient with coronary disease, ventricular fibrillation is initiated by an early ventricular premature complex that produces a rapid polymorphic ventricular tachycardia which rapidly de- generates to ventricular fibrillation (note the undulating baseline with indistinguishable systole and diastole).

have a recurrence rate of 20 to 30% in the year following the event (Chap. 39).

Ventricular flutter usually appears as a sine wave with a rate between 150 and 300 bpm. These oscillations make it impossible to assign a specific morphology to the arrhythmia and in some cases to distinguish it from rapid VT. VF is recognized by grossly irregular undulations of varying amplitudes, contours, and rates (Fig. 230-14). Electrophysiologic studies have demonstrated that regardless of the apparent gross irregularity on the surface ECG, VF usually starts out with a rapid repetitive sequence of VT that ultimately breaks down into multiple wavelets of reentry.

Electrophysiologic studies have been useful in patients who have been resuscitated from cardiac arrest. In approximately 70% of patients with prior infarction, programmed stimulation can reproducibly initiate a sustained VT. Ablation may be possible in some of these patients, particularly if the VT can be slowed so that it can be mapped. Several recent secondary prevention trials have demonstrated superior survival (3 years) in patients treated with ICDs versus amiodarone (Table 230-6). However, in patients with ejection fractions >35% or <20%, survival was comparable. Further subgroup analysis is necessary to identify those patients most likely to be benefited by ICDs.

⟨ **GENETIC CONSIDERATIONS** Many advances have been ⟩ made in the identification of genes responsible for syndromes associated with ventricular tachycardias and sudden cardiac death. Four specific examples include the congenital long QT syndrome (LQTS), hypertrophic obstructive cardiomyopathy (Chap. 238), arrhythmogenic right ventricular dysplasia, and the Brugada syndrome. The latter is a recently described disorder characterized by the electrocardiographic profile of a pseudo bundle branch block pattern with ST elevation and terminal T-wave inversion in leads V_1-V_3 (Fig. 230-15). The clinical presentation is VF in patients with structurally normal hearts. A mutation in the cardiac sodium channel, SCN 5A, is believed to be responsible. While the same gene is responsible for the LQTS, the mutation is different in the two syndromes. ∎

℞ **TREATMENT**

Pharmacologic Antiarrhythmic Therapy Prior to initiation of pharmacologic antiarrhythmic therapy, potential aggravating factors such as transient metabolic abnormalities, congestive heart failure, or acute ischemia must be corrected; in some cases this may suffice to control arrhythmias. In addition, the potential role of drugs as a cause or exacerbating factor in the development of the arrhythmia must be

Table 230-6   Trials of ICD Therapy vs. Antiarrythmic Drugs (AAD): VT/VF Patients

	AVID			CIDS	CASH
Protocol	ICD vs. empiric amiodarone or sotolol (mainly amiodarone)			ICD vs. empiric amiodarone	ICD vs. empiric amiodarone, metoprolol, and propafenone[a]
Sample size	n = 1016 AAD = 509 ICD = 507			n = 659 Amiodarone = 331 ICD = 328	n = 346 Amiodarone = 92 Metoprolol = 97 Propafenone* = 58 ICD = 99
Patient inclusion criteria	Survivors of VF VT with syncope VT with EF ≤ 40%			Survivors of VF VT with syncope VT with EF ≤ 35% and cycle length ≤ 400 ms	Survivors of VF (no EF requirement)
Mortality in "drug" or "control" arm	17.7% 1 year	25.3% 2 years	35.9% 3 years	30% 3 years	19.6% 2 years
Mortality in ICD arm	10.7% 1 year	18.4% 2 years	24.6% 3 years	25% 3 years	12.1% 2 years
Reduction in mortality with ICD	39% 1 year	27% 2 years	31% 3 years	20% 3 years	37% 2 years

[a] Following an interim analysis in March, 1992, enrollment in propafenone arm was discontinued because mortality was increased significantly over mortality in the ICD arm.
NOTE: EF, ejection fraction; ICD, implanted cardioverter/defibrillator; VF, ventricular fibrillation; VT, ventricular tachycardia.
SOURCES: AVID Investigators: N Engl J Med 337(22):1576, 1997; K Kuck, S Connolly: ACC NewsOnline, 1998.

V1

V2

V3

FIGURE 230-15 Brugada syndrome. Note ST elevation with terminal T wave inversion in leads V_1-V_2 mimicking right bundle branch block.

considered. It must be recognized that we do not have a good understanding of the effects of antiarrhythmic agents on the spontaneous onset of tachyarrhythmias. In some cases, they may facilitate the onset.

Antiarrhythmic drugs are used in three principal situations: (1) to

Table 230-7 Toxicity of Most Frequently Used Antiarrhythmic Agents

Drug	Nonarrhythmic Toxicity	Proarrhythmic Toxicity			
		TDP[a]	A Flutter 1:1	VT/VF	Bradycardia
Digoxin	Anorexia, nausea, vomiting, visual changes	Atrial tachycardia, VT, AV nodal block, accelerated junctional rhythms, atrial and ventricular premature depolarizations; acceleration of ventricular rate during atrial fibrillation or flutter in the presence of preexcitation			
Quinidine[b]	Anorexia, nausea, vomiting, diarrhea, cinchonism, tinnitus, hearing and visual changes, thrombocytopenia, hemolytic anemia, rash, potentiation of digoxin levels	2%	++	++	+
Procainamide[b]	Lupus erythematosus–like syndrome, anorexia, nausea	2%	+	++	+
Disopyramide[b]	Anticholinergic actions: dry mouth, urinary retention, visual disturbances (avoid in narrow-angle glaucoma) constipation, congestive heart failure	2%	+	++	+
Lidocaine	Dizziness, confusion, delirium, seizures, coma; side effects potentiated by liver and heart failure	—	—	—	+[b]
Mexiletine	Ataxia, tremor, gait disturbances, rash, vomiting	—	—	—	—
Flecainide	Dizziness, nausea	Rare	+++	++	++
Propafenone[c]	Taste disturbance, bronchospasm	Rare	+++	++	++
Amiodarone	Pulmonary infiltrates and fibrosis, hepatitis, hypo- and hyperthyroidism, photosensitivity, peripheral neuropathy, tremor	Rare	+++	+++	+++
Sotalol	Bronchospasm	+++	+	+	+++

[a] TDP (torsade de pointes) occurs most often in the setting of slow heart rates, QT prolongation, and hypokalemia or hypomagnesemia and at the time of conversion from atrial fibrillation to sinus rhythm. QT prolongation and torsade de pointes are not dose-related phemonema. QRS prolongation is a dose-related phenomena and will occur at toxic concentrations. QT and WRS intervals should be monitored and dose reductions made for interval prolongations.

[b] May suppress sinus node function in patients with underlying sinus node dysfunction. May suppress escape foci in patients with complete heart block.

[c] Avoid in patients with prior myocardial infarction and depressed left ventricular function. Use in combination with AV nodal blocking agent to limit risk of atrial flutter with 1:1 conduction.

NOTE: A flutter 1:1, atrial flutter with 1:1 atrioventricular (AV) conduction; VT/VF, ventricular tachycardia/ventricular fibrillation.

terminate an acute arrhythmia; (2) to prevent recurrence of an arrhythmia; and (3) to prevent a life-threatening arrhythmia for which the patient is perceived to be at risk but which has never occurred.

Most currently available antiarrhythmic agents (Table 230-4) have a relatively low toxic/therapeutic ratio; all can exert proarrhythmic effects (Table 230-7), and therefore they may exacerbate underlying arrhythmias. Serum levels can be determined for most currently available antiarrhythmic agents. Standards for therapeutic and toxic levels can serve only as a rough guide for selecting the appropriate dose in any individual patient. In the final analysis, the therapeutic level in a given patient is the concentration that achieves the desired antiarrhythmic effect, and the toxic level for each patient is the concentration at which undesirable side effects occur. Since many adverse effects are directly related to drug concentrations, the lowest serum level that achieves an effective antiarrhythmic response should be chosen.

In order to determine the therapeutic level for a patient, one must have a standard to judge drug efficacy. For a patient with an incessant arrhythmia, antiarrhythmic drugs may be administered empirically until the arrhythmia is suppressed. If a reproducible precipitating factor such as exercise can be identified, serial drug testing during such a provocative maneuver may be performed. Unfortunately, most arrhythmias are sporadic and occur unpredictably without identifiable precipitating factors. In these cases, if one waits to observe spontaneous recurrences on each antiarrhythmic drug, assessment of drug efficacy may require months. This type of assessment of efficacy may be adequate for arrhythmias that are not life-threatening. However, this mode of assessment is inadequate for arrhythmias that compromise hemodynamic stability, result in syncope, or cause cardiac arrest. In such cases, two methods for determination of arrhythmic drug efficacy have been utilized. The first, which consists of continuous ECG monitoring in the control state and then in the presence of antiarrhythmic drugs, has been used in order to determine the effect that each drug has on spontaneous atrial or ventricular ectopy. This method presupposes that the mechanism responsible for sustained arrhythmias is the same as that causing isolated premature depolarizations (which may or may not be true) and that therefore eradication of isolated ectopy will correlate with prevention of sustained arrhythmias. This method has a number of limitations. First, patients frequently show marked degrees of spontaneous variation in frequency of ectopy, which may mimic antiarrhythmic drug effects. Second, 25 to 30% of patients with sustained ventricular arrhythmias such as VT or VF demonstrate only rare spontaneous ectopy. Finally, many patients demonstrate a dissociation between the effects of antiarrhythmic agents on spontaneous ectopy and the effects of the same agent on sustained arrhythmias.

An alternative method to assess drug efficacy is programmed stimulation. Numerous studies have demonstrated that most clinically occurring supraventricular and ventricular tachyarrhythmias may be reproducibly initiated and terminated safely using this technique. Studies are performed initially in a baseline state in the absence of antiarrhythmic drugs. If the patient's clinical arrhythmia can be reproducibly initiated, then the ability of individual antiarrhythmic drugs to prevent reinduction of the arrhythmia can be assessed either after the drug is administered intravenously or after several days of oral loading in order to achieve a steady-state serum concentration. Use of this method assumes that (1) the induced and spontaneous arrhythmias are identical, and (2) prevention of induction of arrhythmias will correlate with prevention of recurrent spontaneous tachycardias on the same drug regimen. This technique has been validated in patients with a variety of reentrant PSVTs, VT, and VF. The technique is safe when carefully performed, the potential complications being those of any intravascular catheterization. Appropriate interpretation of the results of programmed stimulation is critically dependent on correlating the patient's spontaneous arrhythmias with those induced in the laboratory, with regard to rate and morphology, in order to be certain that the arrhythmia induced in the laboratory represents the same arrhythmia that occurred spontaneously and caused symptoms.

Classification of Antiarrhythmic Drugs A number of classifications of antiarrhythmic drugs have been proposed; the most frequently used is a modification of one proposed by Vaughan-Williams (Table 230-2). This classification is based in part on the ability of antiarrhythmic drugs to modify the cardiac cellular (1) excitatory currents (Na$^+$ or Ca^{2+}), (2) action potential duration, and (3) automaticity (phase 4 depolarization). These effects of the drugs on isolated cardiac cells are thought to account for some of the antiarrhythmic properties of the drugs. Thus depression of excitatory currents by class I and class IV antiarrhythmics results in slowing of conduction velocity and may interrupt arrhythmias by blocking conduction in areas of marginal excitability, where conduction velocity is already slow. Class III antiarrhythmics allegedly exert their action by increasing refractoriness through prolongation of the action potential duration. However, this classification has a number of limitations. The electrophysiologic effects of these drugs in vivo may differ from their effects on isolated cells. Also, the effects of heart rate and fiber geometry are not considered. Not all drugs (e.g., adenosine) fit into the classifications. Finally, some drugs (e.g., amiodarone) exhibit properties consistent with multiple classes. The uses, actions, and toxic actions of currently available antiarrhythmic drugs are summarized in Tables 230-4 and 230-7.

Electrical Therapy of Tachyarrhythmias • *Pacemakers*
Cardiac pacing can be used to terminate and in selected cases prevent recurrent supraventricular and ventricular arrhythmias. Because many tachyarrhythmias appear to be due to a reentrant mechanism with the impulse traveling in a circuit, a properly timed paced impulse can penetrate and prematurely depolarize part of the circuit, rendering it refractory to the next circulating wavefront and thereby interrupting the circus movement. Pacing therapy for arrhythmias is generally reserved for patients whose arrhythmias are refractory to drug therapy and who remain hemodynamically stable during the tachycardia. All forms of pacing therapy require repeated demonstration of their effectiveness and reliability in terminating the arrhythmias during electrophysiologic testing prior to implantation of the pacing device.

The type of pacing device and modality selected for arrhythmia termination depends on (1) the rate of the tachycardia (rates >160 bpm are rarely terminated by a single premature stimulus), (2) the type of arrhythmia (atrial flutter and VT are rarely terminated by single extrastimuli), and (3) concomitant drug therapy.

Because many tachycardias cannot be terminated by single premature stimuli, pacemakers have been developed that allow for multiple extrastimuli (burst pacing) to be introduced. In the current era, antitachycardia pacing is almost exclusively for ventricular arrhythmias because of the success of radiofrequency ablative therapy for supraventricular arrhythmias.

Cardiac pacing has also been used to prevent ventricular tachyarrhythmias. Polymorphic VT associated with a long QT interval and bradycardia (torsade de pointes, p. 1304) is most likely to respond. Pacing the atrium and/or ventricle at rates between 90 and 120 bpm appears to increase the homogeneity of electrical recovery and markedly reduces the propensity for a recurrence of arrhythmias.

Pacemakers may be self-contained or energized by an external radiofrequency source. The self-contained pacemaker may function automatically [i.e., it incorporates an arrhythmia recognition program (circuit)], or it may be activated by an external magnet. The major advantage of a fully automatic system is that there is no need for the patient to recognize the arrhythmia in order for termination to occur. The advantages of the externally activated system (rarely used today) include (1) the decreased risk of unnecessary treatment because of faulty sensing, and (2) the opportunity to initiate monitoring at the time of attempted termination of arrhythmia. This type of monitoring is frequently helpful if pacing techniques are employed to terminate VT, given the risk of acceleration of the arrhythmia by pacing.

The limitations of pacing therapy are primarily related to (1) the changes in the characteristics of the arrhythmia over time such that programmed pacing parameters no longer terminate the tachycardia, (2) the risk of acceleration of the tachycardia with the development of AF when stimulating the atrium and the development of rapid VT and VF when stimulating the ventricles, and (3) inappropriate recognition of supraventricular tachyarrhythmias as ventricular tachycardias, leading to delivery of therapy unnecessarily, which can initiate VT or VF. Future pacing generators that can perform cardioversion and defibril-

lation will increase the applicability of pacing therapy for the treatment of arrhythmias (see below).

Cardioversion and defibrillation Electrical cardioversion and defibrillation remain the most reliable methods for terminating arrhythmias. By depolarizing all or at least a large portion of excitable myocardium in a near homogeneous fashion, the electrical shock can interrupt reentrant arrhythmias. External cardioversion is routinely performed by placing two paddles 12 cm in diameter in firm contact with the chest wall, with one paddle usually located to the right of the sternum at the level of the second rib and the other in the left anterior axillary line in the fifth intercostal space. If the patient is conscious, a short-acting barbiturate to act as an anesthetic or an amnesic drug such as diazepam or medazolam should be administered to prevent patient discomfort. A person skilled in maintaining an airway should be present.

Energy is delivered synchronously with the QRS complex for all arrhythmias except ventricular flutter and VF, since asynchronous shocks can produce VF. The amount of energy used will vary with the type of tachycardia being treated. With the exception of AF, SVTs can frequently be terminated with energy levels in the range of 25 to 50 W · s, while AF usually requires ≥100 W · s for termination. For terminating VT, energy levels ≥100 W · s should probably be employed. While energies as low as 25 W · s may be used successfully, they also have a higher incidence of producing VF or AF. At least 200 W · s of energy should be used for initial attempts at terminating VF. If the initial shock fails, all repeated attempts at defibrillation should be with the maximum energy that the defibrillator is capable of delivering (320 to 400 W · s).

Indications for cardioversion depend on the clinical setting and the patient's general condition. Any tachycardia (except sinus tachycardia) that produces hypotension, myocardial ischemia, or heart failure warrants consideration of prompt termination using external cardioversion. Arrhythmias that fail to terminate with pharmacologic therapy may also be terminated by electrical cardioversion. Transient bradycardias and supraventricular and ventricular irritability following cardioversion are common and usually do not warrant antiarrhythmic intervention.

Implanted cardioverter/defibrillator ICD devices have been developed that will promptly recognize and terminate life-threatening ventricular arrhythmias. These devices can deliver <1 to 40 W · s, the amount of which can be programmed. Current devices have antitachycardia pacing capabilities such that VT can be sensed and terminated without resorting to a painful shock. In such devices, high-energy shocks are reserved for hypotensive VT, acceleration of VT, or failure to terminate VT after a programmed duration (Fig. 230-16). ICDs now can be implanted transvenously, and some are small enough to be implanted in a manner similar to pacemakers. Clinical trials testing the function of these devices in patients with drug-refractory ventricular arrhythmias have demonstrated survival from sudden death at 1 year ranging between 92 and 100%. Currently, ICDs should be considered for patients with VT that is not hemodynamically tolerated. As mentioned earlier, recent randomized trials suggest that ICDs confer improved mortality over amiodarone in patients with hemodynamically untolerated VT and a cardiac arrest not due to reversible causes (Table 230-6). Finally, they are indicated for patients with depressed left ventricular function, prior myocardial infarction, nonsustained and sustained VT at electrophysiologic study (Table 230-8). Guidelines for their use are given in Table 230-9.

The most frequent problem with the ICD has been its inappropriate discharge in the absence of sustained ventricular arrhythmias. Additional potential problems include an increase in defibrillation threshold and decrease in tachycardia rates below the rate cut-off of the device in response to many antiarrhythmic drugs. Permanently implanted ventricular pacemakers may interfere with the device's ability to sense VF. This can be avoided by using committed bipolar pacing systems that are better able to sense local ventricular activity. Diagnostic fea-

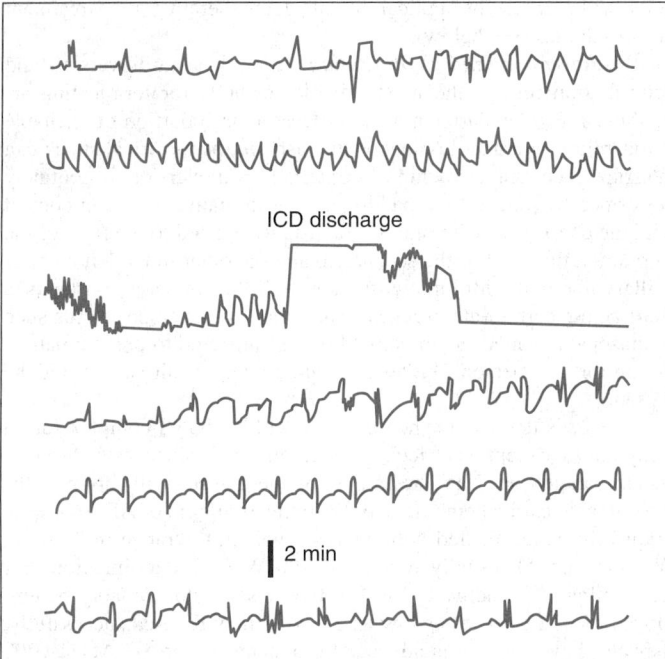

FIGURE 230-16 Normally functioning implantable defibrillators. A continuous Holter monitoring tracing is shown. On the top strip, a rapid polymorphic tachycardia is initiated which beats more uniformly. The automatic implantable cardioverter/defibrillator (ICD) senses the rhythm and delivers a shock which restores sinus rhythm.

tures of newer, all-in-one devices are able to identify the probable cause of an ICD discharge (e.g., AF, SVT, fractured lead) and to adjust pharmacologic therapy or reprogram the device to avoid such inappropriate shocks. These newer devices have the capability to take a "second look" prior to shock delivery and thus may abort delivery for self-terminating arrhythmias. In addition, the range of candidates suitable for implantation will be expanded because the newer devices have the capability of shock therapy for patients whose arrhythmias do not cause loss of consciousness.

Table 230-9   ACC/AHA Guidelines for ICD Implantation

CLASS 1[a]

1. Cardiac arrest due to VF or VT not due to a transient or reversible cause.
2. Spontaneous sustained VT.
3. Syncope of undetermined origin with clinically relevant, hemodynamically significant sustained VT or VF induced at EP study when drug therapy is ineffective, not tolerated, or not preferred.
4. Nonsustained VT with coronary disease, prior MI, LV dysfunction, and inducible VF or sustained VT at EP study that is not suppressible by a class I antiarrhythmic drug.

CLASS 2[b]

1. Cardiac arrest presumed to be due to VF when EP testing is precluded by other medical conditions.
2. Severe symptoms attributable to sustained ventricular tachyarrhythmias while awaiting cardiac transplantation.
3. Familial or inherited conditions with a high risk for life-threatening ventricular tachyarrhythmias such as long QT syndrome or hypertrophic cardiomyopathy.
4. Nonsustained VT with coronary artery disease, prior MI, and LV dysfunction, and inducible sustained VT or VF at EP study.
5. Recurrent syncope of undetermined etiology in the presence of ventricular dysfunction and inducible ventricular arrhythmias at EP study, when other causes of syncope have been excluded.

CLASS 3[c]

1. Syncope of undetermined cause in a patient without inducible ventricular tachyarrhythmias
2. Incessant VT or VF
3. VF or VT resulting from arrhythmias amenable to surgical or catheter ablation; for example, atrial arrhythmias associated with the Wolff-Parkinson-White syndrome, right ventricular outflow tract VT, idiopathic LV tachycardia, or fascicular VT.
4. Ventricular tachyarrhythmias due to a transient or reversible disorder.

[a] Evidence and/or agreement that procedure is indicated.
[b] Divergence in evidence opinion that procedure is indicated.
[c] Evidence/agreement that procedure is not indicated or is harmful.
NOTE: EP, electrophysiology; LV, left ventricular; MI, myocardial infarction; VF, ventricular fibrillation; VT, ventricular tachycardia.
SOURCE: Adapted from American College of Cardiology/American Heart Association: J Am Coll Cardiol 31:1175, 1998.

Newer generations of ICDs are smaller and frequently allow placement of a second lead in the right atria. This lead senses atrial activity and provides enhanced discrimination of atrial from ventricular electrical activity. This enhanced discrimination of SVT from VT prevents inappropriate shocks for SVT that may be misinterpreted as VT and allows the device to switch from a dual-chamber to a single-chamber device should an SVT-like AF develop. These dual-chamber devices also allow AV sequential pacing. Finally, ICDs are now available that have defibrillation coils in the right atrium as well as right ventricle. These devices are suited for patients with infrequent but highly symptomatic atrial fibrillation. Patients with these atrial defibrillators can activate the device themselves and terminate their atrial fibrillation without going to the hospital.

Ablative Therapy for Arrhythmias Catheter-based mapping techniques have provided a nonoperative approach to the identification and cure of a variety of arrhythmias. In fact, catheter ablation techniques are now the procedures of choice for symptomatic patients with (1) concealed or manifest (WPW) bypass tracts, (2) AV nodal reentrant SVT, (3) typical atrial flutter, and (4) poorly controlled ventricular responses to atrial arrhythmias, most commonly AF. Successful ablation of bypass tracts and modifications of the AV node by radiofrequency energy are extremely successful and

Table 230-8   ICD Therapy for Primary Prevention of Sudden Cardiac Death

	MADIT	MUSTT
Protocol	ICD vs. conventional (AAD, primarily empiric amiodarone)	EP-guided Rx (AAD or ICD) vs. control

Sample size	n = 196
	    Conventional = 101
	    ICD = 95
		n = 704
		    EP-guided Rx = 351
		    Control = 353

Patient inclusion	S/P MI, EF ≤ 35% NSVT, inducible sustained VT not suppressible by procainamide	CAD, EF ≤ 40%, NSVT, inducible sustained VT
Total mortality	Conventional = 39% ICD = 16% (27 months)	Control = 48% EP-guided Rx = 42% AAD = 55% ICD = 24% (60 months)
Reduction in mortality by ICD	54%	55% (vs. control or AAD)
SCD or cardiac arrest	Conventional = 13% ICD = 3.2%	Control = 32% EP-guided Rx = 25% AAD = 37% ICD = 9%
Reduction in SCD or cardiac arrest by ICD	62.5%	75% (vs. control or AAD)

NOTE: AAD, antiarrhythmic drug; CAD, coronary artery disease; EF, ejection fraction; EP, electrophysiology; ICD, implantable cardioverter/defibrillator; MADIT, multicenter automatic defibrillator trial; MUSTT, multicenter unsustained tachycardia trial; NSVT, nonsustained ventricular tachycardia; RX, therapy; SCD, sudden cardiac death; S/P MI, status post-myocardial infarction; VT, ventricular tachycardia.
SOURCE: From Buxton; Moss.

FIGURE 230-17 Radiofrequency ablation of idiopathic ventricular tachycardia in a patient with prior infarction. Leads I, II, and III are shown. Ventricular tachycardia with a right bundle branch block and left axis deviation is shown in a patient with a prior inferior wall infarction. Radiofrequency applied to the site of origin terminates the tachycardia.

cost-effective and are the procedure of choice for patients with recurrent episodes. The creation of AV block with implantation of a pacemaker is the method of choice in managing patients with AF and poorly controlled ventricular response. Idiopathic VTs (Fig. 230-17) and some VTs that are associated with coronary artery disease are also amenable to ablation, but the result is less successful than for ablation of SVTs.

Surgical therapy is now relegated to cases of sustained VT associated with coronary artery disease when operative intervention is needed for coronary bypass surgery and/or aneurysmectomy or VT associated with specific structural abnormalities (e.g., idiopathic left ventricle aneurysm, s/p surgery for tetralogy of Fallot). It also may be undertaken for the unusual instances of failed catheter ablation for SVTs associated with bypass tracts.

BIBLIOGRAPHY

BRUGADA R et al: Identification of a genetic locus for familial atrial fibrillation. N Engl J Med 336:905, 1997

BUXTON AE et al: A randomized study of the prevention of sudden death in patients with coronary artery disease. N Engl J Med 341:1882, 1999

GILLIS AM: Pacing to prevent atrial fibrillation. Cardiol Clin 18:25, 2000

GREGORATAS G: ACC/AHA Guidelines for Implantation of Cardiac Pacemakers and Antiarrhythmia Devices: A report of the American College of Cardiology/American Heart Association Task Force on Practice Guidelines (Committee on Pacemaker Implantation). J Am Coll Cardiol 31:1175, 1998

HOLMES DR JR et al: The effect of medical and surgical treatment on subsequent sudden cardiac death in patients with coronary artery disease. A report from the Coronary Artery Surgery Study. Circulation 73:1254, 1986

HUANG DT et al: Hybrid pharmacologic and ablative therapy: A novel and effective approach for the management of atrial fibrillation. J Cardiovasc Electrophysiol 9:462, 1998

KIRCHOFF CJHJ, JOSEPHSON ME: In Role of Anisotopy in Clinical Arrhythmias, PM Spooner, RW Joyner, J Jalife (eds): New York, Futura, 1998, pp 135–157

LEVY S: Classification system of atrial fibrillation. Curr Opin Cardiol 15:54, 2000

MOSS AJ et al: Improved survival with an implanted defibrillator in patients with coronary disease at high risk for ventricular arrhythmia. N Engl J Med 335:1933, 1996

OLGIN JE, MILES W: Ablation of atrial tachycardia, in I Singer, S Barold, AJ Camm (eds): Pharmacologic Therapy in the 21st Century. New York, Futura, 1998, pp 197–217

PRIORI SG: Genetic and molecular basis of cardiac arrhythmias: Impact on clinical management. Circulation 99:518, 1995

ROY D et al: Amiodarone to prevent recurrence of atrial fibrillation. Canadian trial of Atrial Fibrillation Investigators. N Engl J Med 342:913, 2000

WYSE DG: Pharmacologic therapy in patients with ventricular tachyarrhythmias. Cardiol Clin 11:65, 1993

ZIPES DP: Specific arrhythmias: Diagnosis and treatment, in Heart Disease: A Textbook of Cardiovascular Medicine, 6th ed, E Braunwald (ed). Philadelphia, Saunders, 2001

Section 3
DISORDERS OF THE HEART

231

Eugene Braunwald

NORMAL AND ABNORMAL MYOCARDIAL FUNCTION

CELLULAR BASIS OF CARDIAC CONTRACTION

THE CARDIAC ULTRASTRUCTURE About three-fourths of the ventricular *myocardium* is composed of individual striated muscle cells (myocytes), normally 17 to 25 μm in diameter and 60 to 140 μm in length (Fig. 231-1A). Each fiber contains multiple, rodlike crossbanded strands (myofibrils) that run the length of the fiber and are, in turn, composed of serially repeating structures, the sarcomeres. The cytoplasm between the myofibrils contains other cell constituents (Fig. 231-1B), such as the single centrally located nucleus, numerous mitochondria, and intracellular membrane system, the sarcoplasmic reticulum.

The *sarcomere*, the structural and functional unit of contraction, is delimited by two adjacent dark lines, the Z lines (Fig. 231-1C). The distance between Z lines varies with the degree of contraction or stretch of the muscle and ranges between 1.6 and 2.2 μm. Within the confines of the sarcomere are alternating light and dark bands, giving the myocardial fibers their striated appearance under the light microscope. At the center of the sarcomere is a dark band of constant length (1.5 μm), the A band, which is flanked by two lighter bands, the I bands, which are of variable length. The sarcomere of heart muscle, like that of skeletal muscle, is made up of two sets of interdigitating myofilaments (Fig. 232-1D). Thicker filaments, composed principally of the protein myosin, traverse the A band. They are about 10 nm (100 Å) in diameter, with tapered ends, and measure 1.5 to 1.6 μm in length. Thinner filaments, composed primarily of actin, course from the Z line through the I band into the A band. They are approximately 5 nm (50 Å) in diameter and 1.0 μm in length. Thus there is overlapping of thick and thin filaments only within the A band, while the I band contains only thin filaments (Fig. 232-1C). On electron-micro-

FIGURE 231-1 *A.* Microscopic evidence of heart muscle. *B.* Cardiac contraction and relaxation result from changing concentrations of Ca²⁺ ions in the myocardial cytosol. Ca²⁺ ions are shown schematically as entering via the calcium channel, which opens in response to the wave of depolarization that travels along the sarcolemma. These Ca²⁺ ions "trigger" the release of more calcium from the sarcoplasmic reticulum (SR) and thereby initiate a contraction-relaxation cycle. Eventually, the small amount of calcium that has entered the cell leaves, predominantly by a Na⁺-Ca²⁺ exchanger with a lesser role for the sarcolemmal calcium pump. *C.* The varying actin-myosin overlap is shown for systole and diastole. *D.* The myosin heads, attached to the thick filaments, interact with the thin actin filaments. *(Reprinted with permission. Copyright 1997 LH Opie.)*

In forming the thick myofilament, which is composed of ~300 longitudinally stacked myosin molecules, the rodlike segments of the myosin molecules are laid down in an orderly, polarized manner, leaving the globular portions projecting outward so that they can interact with actin to generate force and shortening (Fig. 231-2). *Actin* has a molecular weight of about 47,000. The thin filament is composed of a double helix of two chains of actin molecules wound about each other on a larger molecule, tropomyosin, which serves as a "backbone" to the thin filament. A group of these regulatory proteins, troponins C, I, and T, are spaced at regular intervals on this filament (Fig. 231-3). In contrast to myosin, actin has no intrinsic enzymatic activity, but it has the ability to combine reversibly with myosin in the presence of ATP and Ca²⁺. The latter activates the myosin ATPase, which in turn breaks down ATP, the energy source for contraction. In relaxed muscle this interaction is inhibited by tropomyosin. *Titin* (Fig. 231-1D) is a large, flexible, myofibrillar protein that connects myosin to the Z line. Its stretching is believed to contribute to the elasticity of the heart.

During activation of the myocyte, Ca²⁺ becomes attached to troponin C, which results in a conformational change in the regulatory protein tropomyosin, which in turn exposes the actin cross-bridge interaction sites. Repetitive interaction between myosin heads and actin filaments is termed *cross-bridge cycling*, which results in sliding of the actin along the myosin filaments, ultimately causing muscle shortening and/or the development of tension. The splitting of ATP, which is synthesized in the mitochondria, then dissociates the myosin cross-bridge from the actin. In the presence of ATP (Fig. 231-2), linkages between actin and myosin filaments are made and broken cyclically as long as sufficient Ca²⁺ is present; these linkages cease when [Ca²⁺] falls below a critical level, and the troponin-tropomyosin complex once more prevents interactions between the myosin cross-bridges and the actin filaments. Intracytoplasmic Ca²⁺ is a principal mediator of the inotropic state of the heart; the fundamental action of most positive inotropic drugs, including the digitalis glycosides, β-adrenergic agonists, and phosphodiesterase inhibitors, is to raise the [Ca²⁺] in the vicinity of the myofilaments. Cyclic AMP enhances the phosphorylation of troponin I, a protein that accelerates cardiac relaxation.

The *sarcoplasmic reticulum* (SR) (Fig. 231-1B) is a complex network of anastomosing intracellular channels that invests the myofibrils. It is less profuse in cardiac than in skeletal muscle. Its longitudinally disposed membrane-lined tubules are closely applied to the surfaces of individual sarcomeres but have no direct continuity with the outside of the cell. However, closely related to the SR, both structurally and functionally, are the transverse tubules, or T system, formed by tubelike invaginations of the sarcolemma that extend into the myocardial fiber along the Z lines, i.e., the ends of the sarcomeres.

CARDIAC ACTIVATION At rest, the cardiac cell is polarized, i.e., the interior has a negative charge relative to the outside of the cell, with a transmembrane potential of −80 to −100 mV (Chap. 229). The sarcolemma, which in the resting state is largely impermeable to Na⁺, has a Na⁺- and K⁺-stimulating pump energized by ATP

scopic examination, bridges may be seen to extend between the thick and thin filaments within the A band.

THE CONTRACTILE PROCESS The sliding model for muscle rests on the fundamental observation that the thick and thin filaments are constant in overall length during both contraction and relaxation. With activation, the actin filaments are propelled further into the A band. In the process, the A band remains constant in length, whereas the I band shortens and the Z lines move toward one another.

The *myosin* molecule is a complex, asymmetric fibrous protein with a molecular weight of about 500,000; it has a rodlike portion that is about 150 nm (1500 Å) in length with a globular portion at its end (Fig. 231-1D). This globular portion of the myosin is the site of ATPase activity and also forms the bridges between the myosin and actin.

that extrudes Na+ from the cell; the pump plays a critical role in establishing this resting potential. Thus, on the inside of the cell [K+] is relatively high and [Na+] is far lower, while in the extracellular milieu [Na+] is high and [K+] is low. At the same time, in the resting state, the extracellular [Ca2+] greatly exceeds the free intracellular [Ca2+].

During the plateau of the action potential (phase 2) there is a slow inward current through L-type Ca2+ channels in the sarcolemma (Fig. 231-4). The absolute quantity of Ca2+ that crosses the surface membrane is relatively small and itself appears to be incapable of bringing about full activation of the contractile apparatus. The depolarizing current not only extends across the surface of the cell but penetrates deeply into the cell by way of the ramifying T system; this Ca2+ current triggers the release of much larger quantities of Ca2+ from the SR, a process termed *Ca2+-induced Ca2+ release*.

The Ca2+ released from the SR then diffuses toward the sarcomere and, as already described, combines with troponin C. By repressing this inhibitor of contraction, Ca2+ activates the myofilaments to shorten. During repolarization the activity of the Ca2+ pump in the SR reaccumulates Ca2+ against a concentration gradient, and the Ca2+ is stored by its attachment to a protein *calsequestrin*. This is an energy-requiring process that lowers the [Ca2+] in the vicinity of the myofibrils to a level that inhibits the actin-myosin interaction responsible for contraction and in this manner leads to relaxation. Also, there is an exchange of Ca2+ for Na+ at the sarcolemma, reducing the cytoplasmic [Ca2+]. Thus, the combination of the cell membrane, transverse tubules, and SR, with their ability to transmit the action potential, to release, and then to reaccumulate Ca2+, appears to play a fundamental role in the rhythmic contraction and relaxation of heart muscle.

The ATP formed from substrate oxidation is the principal source of energy for almost all of the mechanical work of contraction performed by the myocardial cell. The high-energy phosphate stores in ATP are in equilibrium with those in the form of creatine phosphate. The activity of myosin ATPase determines the rate of forming and breaking of the actin-myosin cross-bridges and ultimately the velocity of muscle contraction.

THE ROLE OF MUSCLE LENGTH In all striated muscle, including cardiac muscle, the force of contraction depends on initial muscle length. The sarcomere length associated with the most forceful contraction is approximately 2.2 μm. At this length the two sets of myofilaments of the sarcomere are configured so as to provide the greatest area for their interaction. The length of the sarcomere also regulates the extent of activation of the contractile system, i.e., its sensitivity to Ca2+. According to this concept, termed *length-dependent activation*, at the optimal sarcomere length of 2.2 μm, the myofilament sensitivity to Ca2+ is maximal.

The relation between the initial length of the muscle fibers and the developed force is of prime importance for the function of heart muscle. This forms the basis of the Frank-Starling relation (Starling's law of the heart), which states that, within limits, the force of ventricular contraction is a function of the end-diastolic length of the cardiac muscle, which in turn is closely related to the ventricular end-diastolic volume.

FIGURE 231-2 Reaction mechanism of actomyosin ATPase, simplified to show four steps. In relaxed muscle (*upper left*), ATP bound to the myosin cross-bridge dissociates the thick and thin filaments. *Step 1:* Hydrolysis of myosin-bound ATP by the ATPase site on the myosin head transfers the chemical energy of the nucleotide to the activated cross-bridge (*upper right*). When cytosolic Ca2+ concentration is low, as in relaxed muscle, the reaction cannot proceed because tropomyosin and the troponin complex on the thin filament do not allow the active sites on actin to interact with the cross-bridges. Therefore, even though the cross-bridges are energized, they cannot interact with actin. *Step 2:* When Ca2+ binding to troponin C has exposed active sites on the thin filament, actin interacts with the myosin cross-bridges to form an active complex (lower right) in which the energy derived from ATP is retained in the actin-bound cross-bridge, whose orientation has not yet shifted. *Step 3:* The muscle contracts when ADP dissociates from the cross-bridge; this step leads to the formation of the low-energy rigor complex (lower left), in which the chemical energy derived from ATP hydrolysis has been expended to perform mechanical work (the "rowing" motion of the cross-bridge). *Step 4:* The muscle returns to its resting state, and the cycle ends when a new molecule of ATP binds to the rigor complex and dissociates the cross-bridge from the thin filament. This cycle continues until calcium is dissociated from troponin C in the thin filament, which causes the contractile proteins to return to the resting state with the cross-bridge in the energized state. [*From AM Katz, in WS Colucci (ed): Heart Failure: Cardiac Function and Dysfunction, in Atlas of Heart Diseases, 2d ed, E Braunwald (series ed). Philadelphia, Current Medicine, 1999.*]

MYOCARDIAL MECHANICS

THE FORCE-VELOCITY CURVE The mechanical activity of striated muscle, skeletal and cardiac, may be expressed externally in two ways: by shortening and by the development of tension. In both forms of striated muscle the velocity of shortening is inversely related to the tension development, an expression of the so-called force-velocity relation (Fig. 231-5). Expressed simply, the greater the load the muscle is called upon to lift, the lower the velocity (and extent) of shortening, and vice versa. Skeletal muscle fibers have a single, essentially fixed, force-velocity curve; i.e., at any given muscle length, the inverse relation between force and velocity is fixed. The contractile activity of skeletal muscle is controlled by varying the frequency of nerve impulses stimulating the muscle, and thereby the number of contractions of each fiber per unit of time, as well as by the number of muscle fibers, i.e., motor units, that contact, while the contractile properties of each individual fiber remain constant. Although the muscle's resting length also influences the characteristics of contraction, this variable remains essentially fixed in vivo because of the muscles' skeletal attachments. In contrast to skeletal muscle, the number of myocardial cells and within them the myofibrils and sarcomeres that become activated during each contraction is constant. However, the contractile activity of the myocardium is readily altered under physiologic conditions by changes in resting fiber length and by changes

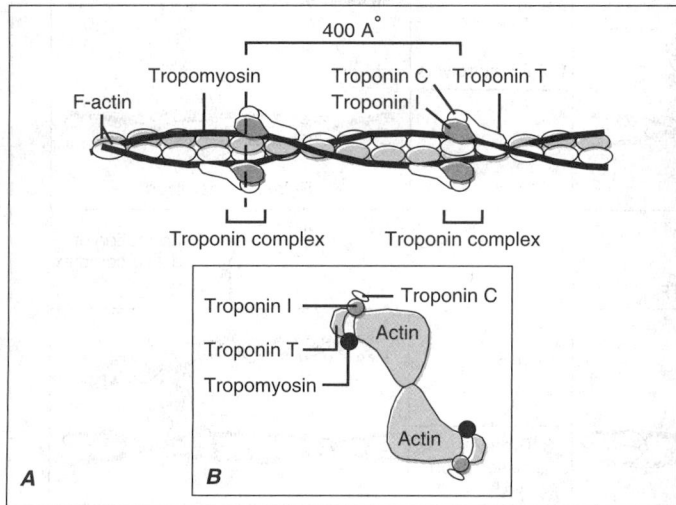

FIGURE 231-3 Structure of the thin filament. *A.* The "backbone" of the thin filament, seen in a longitudinal view, is F-actin, which contains two strands of actin monomers (light blue and white). Troponin complexes, made up of one molecule each of troponin C, troponin I, and troponin T, are distributed at approximately 40-nm (400-Å) intervals along the thin filament. Elongated tropomyosin molecules (solid line in the grooves between the two actin strands). *B.* A cross-section of the thin filament at the level where the troponin complexes are located shows probable relationships between actin, tropomyosin, and the three components of the troponin complex. The strength of the bond linking troponin I and actin varies, depending on whether Ca²⁺ is bound to troponin C. *[Adapted from AM Katz, in WS Colucci (ed): Heart Failure: Cardiac Function and Dysfunction, in Atlas of Heart Diseases, 2d ed, E Braunwald (series ed). Philadelphia, Current Medicine, 1999, with permission of the publisher.]*

in the inotropic state, i.e., the contractility, both of which shift the myocardial force-velocity curve. Many neurohumoral influences affect contractility, but the most important influence is the adrenergic nervous system operating via its neurotransmitter, norepinephrine.

VENTRICULAR EJECTION AND FILLING

Analysis of the heart as a pump has classically centered on the relation between the end-diastolic volume of the ventricle (which is related to the length of the muscle fibers) and its stroke volume (the Frank-Starling relation). The end-diastolic or "filling" pressure of the ventricle is sometimes used as a surrogate for the end-diastolic volume. In the heart-lung preparation the stroke volume varies directly with the diastolic fiber length (preload) and inversely with the arterial resistance (afterload), and as the heart fails it delivers a progressively smaller stroke volume from a normal or even elevated end-diastolic volume. The relation between the ventricular end-diastolic pressure and the stroke work of the ventricle (the ventricular function curve) provides a useful definition of the level of *myocardial contractility* (also termed the contractile, or inotropic, state of the ventricle). An increase in ventricular contractility is accompanied by a shift of the ventricular function curve upward and to the left [greater stroke work at any level of ventricular end-diastolic pressure (or volume), or lower end-diastolic pressure at any level of stroke work], while depression of contractility is characterized by a shift downward and to the right (Fig. 231-6).

During the adrenergic stimulation of the myocardium that accompanies exercise, relatively little change in ventricular end-diastolic volume occurs, while cardiac output, aortic flow velocity, stroke work, and the rate of ventricular pressure development are all augmented, reflecting an increase in myocardial contractility.

The important influence of the adrenergic neurotransmitter, norepinephrine (Chap. 72), on the mechanical properties of the myocar-

dium has long been recognized. Direct stimulation of the cardiac adrenergic nerves augments ventricular function as a consequence of the release of norepinephrine from adrenergic nerve endings in the heart. Norepinephrine activates myocardial β receptors and through a series of G (guanine nucleotide binding) protein mediated changes activates the enzyme adenylate cyclase, which leads to the formation of cyclic AMP from ATP (Fig. 231-7). The latter, in turn, activates protein kinase, which causes a more rapid, forceful contraction by phosphorylating the Ca²⁺ channel in the myocardial sarcolemma, thereby enhancing the influx of Ca²⁺ into the myocyte. Ca²⁺ acts on the contractile apparatus, as described on p. 1311. Cyclic AMP also phosphorylates the SR protein phospholamban, which increases the uptake of Ca²⁺ by the SR, thereby enhancing the rate of relaxation. Adrenergic activation is evidenced by tachycardia, a reduction in cardiac dimensions, and increased rates of ejection and filling.

FIGURE 231-4 The Ca²⁺ fluxes and key structures involved in cardiac excitation-contraction coupling. The *arrows* denote the direction of Ca²⁺ fluxes. The thickness of each arrow indicates the magnitude of the calcium flux. Two Ca²⁺ cycles regulate excitation-contraction coupling and relaxation. The larger cycle is entirely intracellular and involves Ca²⁺ fluxes into and out of the sarcoplasmic reticulum, and Ca²⁺ binding to and release from troponin C. The smaller extracellular Ca²⁺ cycle occurs when this cation moves into and out of the cell. The action potential opens plasma membrane Ca²⁺ channels to allow passive entry of Ca²⁺ into the cell from the extracellular fluid (*arrow A*). Only a small portion of the Ca²⁺ that enters the cell directly activates the contractile proteins (*arrow A₁*). The extracellular cycle is completed when Ca²⁺ is actively transported back out to the extracellular fluid by way of two plasma membrane fluxes mediated by the sodium-calcium exchanger (*arrow B₁*) and the plasma membrane calcium pump (*arrow B₂*). In the intracellular Ca²⁺ cycle, passive Ca²⁺ release occurs through channels in the cisternae (*arrow C*) and initiates contraction, and active Ca²⁺ uptake by the Ca²⁺ pump of the sarcotubular network (*arrow D*) relaxes the heart. Diffusion of Ca²⁺ within the sarcoplasmic reticulum (*arrow G*) returns this activator cation to the cisternae, where it is stored in a complex with calsequestrin and other calcium-binding proteins. Ca²⁺ released from the sarcoplasmic reticulum initiates systole when it binds to troponin C (*arrow E*). Lowering of cytosolic [Ca²⁺] by the SR cause this ion to dissociate from troponin (*arrow F*) and relaxes the heart. Ca²⁺ may also move between mitochondria and cytoplasm (H). *(Adapted from Katz, with permission.)*

FIGURE 231-5 Effects of the addition of norepinephrine (NE) and the development of heart failure on the force-velocity relation of the cat papillary muscle. NE induces an increase in the velocity of shortening at any load, in the maximum force and isometric contraction (Po), and in the maximum velocity of zero load shortening (V_{max}). Heart failure has the opposite effect. *Key:* o, control; -x-x, failure. *(Modified from E Braunwald in Heart Disease, 4th ed. Philadelphia, Saunders, 1992.)*

ASSESSMENT OF CARDIAC FUNCTION

Several techniques are available for defining impaired cardiac function in patients. With the patient at rest, and at a normal or elevated ventricular end-diastolic pressure, the cardiac output and stroke volume may be depressed in the presence of heart failure, but not uncommonly these variables are within normal limits. A more sensitive index is the ejection fraction, i.e., the ratio of stroke volume to end-diastolic volume (normal value 67 ± 8%), which may be estimated by radiocontrast or radionuclide angiography or echocardiography, and it is frequently depressed in systolic heart failure even when the stroke volume itself is normal. Alternatively, the detection of abnormally elevated ventricular end-diastolic volumes (normal value 70 ± 20 mL/m²) in the presence of a normal stroke volume signifies impairment of left ventricular systolic function. A limitation of cardiac output, ejection fraction, and ventricular volume in the assessment of cardiac function is that these variables are influenced strongly by ventricular loading conditions. Thus, a depressed ejection fraction and lowered cardiac output may be observed in patients with normal ventricular function but reduced preload, as occurs in hypovolemia, or with increased afterload, as occurs in acutely elevated arterial pressure.

The end-systolic left ventricular pressure-volume relationship is a particularly useful index of ventricular performance since it is independent of both preload and afterload (Fig. 231-8). At any level of myocardial contractility, left ventricular end-systolic volume varies inversely with end-systolic pressure; as contractility declines, end-systolic volume (at any level of end-systolic pressure) rises. Noninvasive techniques, particularly echocardiography and radionuclide angiography (Chap. 227), are of great value in the clinical assessment of myocardial function. They provide measurements of end-systolic volume (or end-systolic dimension) that can be related to systolic arterial pressure. In addition, they provide convenient measurements of ejection fraction and systolic shortening rate and allow measurement of ventricular filling (see below).

Exercise A useful technique for evaluating ventricular performance involves the measurement of the circulatory changes occurring during exercise. Thus, left ventricular performance may be estimated

accurately by measuring the left ventricular end-diastolic pressure, cardiac output, and total-body O_2 consumption at rest and during exercise. In persons with normal cardiac function, the cardiac output rises by more than 500 mL/min for each 100-mL increase in O_2 consumption per minute. The left ventricular end-diastolic pressure at rest is less than 12 mmHg and changes little during exercise, while cardiac output, and to a lesser extent stroke volume, rise, the latter especially when exercise is carried out in the upright position. The failing left ventricle, on the other hand, is characterized by an elevation of end-diastolic pressure during exercise to above 12 mmHg, accompanied by either no change or a fall in stroke volume and a subnormal increase in cardiac output related to the increase in minute O_2 consumption. The overall performance of the cardiopulmonary system in delivering oxygen to the metabolizing tissue can also be estimated by measuring the maximal O_2 consumption achieved during escalating treadmill exercise ($\dot{V}_{max_{O_2}}$). Normal values exceed 20 mL/min per kilogram, while values under 10 mL/min per kilogram represent severe impairment of function, usually seen in patients with severe heart failure and a poor prognosis.

The potential value of stressing the left ventricle in assessing its performance is emphasized by the fact that the normal range of left ventricular end-diastolic pressure, cardiac index, and ventricular stroke work in the resting state are wide, with values that frequently overlap those seen in patients with ventricular dysfunction.

DIASTOLIC FUNCTION (Fig. 231-9) This important variable is best assessed by continuously measuring the flow velocity across the mitral valve using Doppler echocardiography. Normally, the velocity of inflow is more rapid in early diastole than during atrial systole; with impaired relaxation the rate of early diastolic filling declines, while the rate of presystolic filling rises. With severe impairment of filling the pattern is "pseudo-normalized" and early ventricular filling becomes more rapid as left atrial pressure upstream to the stiff left ventricle rises.

FIGURE 231-6 Diagram showing the interrelations among influences on ventricular end-diastolic volume (EDV) through stretching of the myocardium and the contractile state of the myocardium. Levels of ventricular EDV associated with filling pressures that result in dyspnea and pulmonary edema are shown on the abscissa. Levels of ventricular performance required when the subject is at rest, while walking, and during maximal activity are designated on the ordinate. The broken lines are the descending limbs of the ventricular-performance curves, which are rarely seen during life but which show the level of ventricular performance if end-diastolic volume could be elevated to very high levels. For further explanation see text. *(Modified from E Braunwald et al: Mechanisms of Contraction of the Normal and Failing Heart. Boston, Little, Brown, 1976.)*

β - ADRENERGIC AGONIST

Ca²⁺

SL

β receptor

GTP

αs

β

γ

Adenyl cyclase

P

cAMP

Via protein kinase A

Ca²⁺

⊕

Ca²⁺

⊕

SR

⊕

P

Metabolism
• glycolysis
• lipolysis
• citrate cycle

Ca²⁺

ADP + Pᵢ

ATP ⊕

Myosin ATPase

ADP + Pᵢ ⊕

troponin C

⊕

②

①

cAMP via TnI

cAMP via PL

⊕

INCREASED

β ⎰ 1. rate of contraction
   ⎱ 2. peak force
     3. rate of relaxation

③

⊕

Control

Pattern of contraction

FIGURE 231-7 Signal systems involved in positive intropic and lusitropic (enhanced relaxation) effects of β-adrenergic stimulation. When the β-adrenergic agonist interacts with the β receptor, a series of G protein-mediated changes leads to activation of adenylate cyclase and formation of cyclic AMP (cAMP). The latter acts via protein kinase A to stimulate metabolism (left) and to phosphorylate the Ca²⁺ channel protein. The result is an enhanced opening probability of the Ca²⁺ channel, thereby increasing the inward movement of Ca²⁺ ions through the sarcolemma (SL) of the T tubule. These Ca²⁺ ions release more calcium from the sarcoplasmic reticulum (SR) to increase cytosolic Ca²⁺ and to activate troponin C. Ca²⁺ ions also increase the rate of breakdown of ATP to ADP and inorganic phosphate (Pᵢ). Enhanced myosin ATPase activity explains the increased rate of contraction, with increased activation of troponin C explaining increased peak force development. An increased rate of relaxation is explained because cyclic AMP also activates the protein phospholamban, situated on the membrane of the SR, that controls the rate of uptake of calcium into the SR. The latter effect explains enhanced relaxation (lusitropic effect). P, phosphorylation; PL, phospholamban; SL, sarcolemma; SR, sarcoplasmic reticulum; TnI, troponin I. *(Reprinted with permission. Copyright 1997 L Opie.)*

CONTROL OF CARDIAC PERFORMANCE AND OUTPUT

The extent of shortening of heart muscle and, therefore, the stroke volume of the intact ventricle are determined by three influences: (1) the length of the muscle at the onset of contraction, i.e., the preload; (2) the inotropic state of the muscle, i.e., the position of its force-velocity-length relation and its end-diastolic–shortening–relation; and (3) the tension that the muscle is called upon to develop during contraction, i.e., the afterload. Within wide limits, heart rate determines the cardiac output at any stroke volume as long as the other three influences remain constant. Ventricular filling is influenced by the extent and speed of myocardial relaxation, which in turn is determined by the rate of uptake of Ca²⁺ by the SR; the latter may be reduced by

ischemia. Filling may be also impeded by the stiffness of the ventricular wall, which may be increased by ventricular hypertrophy and conditions that infiltrate the ventricle, such as amyloid, or by an extrinsic constraint (e.g., pericardial compression).

VENTRICULAR END-DIASTOLIC VOLUME (PRELOAD) At any level of inotropic state and afterload, the performance of the myocardium is influenced profoundly by ventricular end-diastolic fiber length and therefore by diastolic ventricular volume, i.e., by operation of the Frank-Starling mechanism (Fig. 231-6). The following are the major determinants of ventricular preload in the intact organism:

Total Blood Volume When blood volume is depleted, as in hemorrhage or dehydration, venous return to the heart declines (Chap. 38) and ventricular end-diastolic volume (preload) falls, as does ventricular performance, as reflected in stroke volume and ventricular work.

Distribution of Blood Volume The ventricular end-diastolic volume is influenced by the distribution of blood volume between the intra- and extrathoracic compartments. This distribution in turn is influenced by the following:

1. *Body position.* Gravitational forces pool blood in dependent portions of the body; upright posture augments extrathoracic at the expense of intrathoracic blood volume and reduces ventricular work.

2. *Intrathoracic pressure.* Normally, mean intrathoracic pressure is negative, which increases thoracic blood volume and ventricular end-diastolic volume and enhances the return of blood to the heart, particularly during inspiration, when this pressure becomes more negative. Elevation of intrathoracic pressure, as occurs during the Valsalva maneuver or prolonged bouts of coughing or with positive-pressure ventilation, has the opposite effect. It impedes venous return, diminishes intrathoracic blood volume, and reduces stroke volume and ventricular work.

3. *Intrapericardial pressure.* When this pressure is elevated, as in pericardial tamponade (Chap. 239), there is interference with cardiac filling, and the resultant reduction in ventricular diastolic volume reduces stroke volume and ventricular work.

4. *Venous tone.* The venous system is not a simple system of passive conduits between the systemic capillary bed and the right atrium. Instead, the smooth muscle in the walls of the venules and veins responds to a variety of neural and humoral stimuli. Venoconstriction occurs during muscular exercise, deep respiration, fright, or marked hypovolemic shock, reducing extrathoracic and augmenting intrathoracic and intraventricular blood volumes and ventricular performance.

5. *The pumping action of skeletal muscle.* During muscular exercise the contracting skeletal muscles squeeze blood out of the venous bed and, with the aid of the venous valves, displace it centrally, thereby increasing intrathoracic blood volume, ventricular end-diastolic volume, and ventricular work.

Atrial Contraction Vigorous, appropriately timed atrial contraction augments ventricular filling and end-diastolic volume. The atrial contribution to ventricular filling, the so-called atrial kick, is of particular importance in patients with concentric ventricular hypertrophy. In such patients, the loss of atrial systole (as occurs with the development of atrial fibrillation) reduces ventricular end-diastolic pressure and volume, ultimately lowering myocardial performance. The atrial contribution to ventricular filling may also be reduced by atrioventricular dissociation, prolongation or abbreviation of the P-R interval, and depression of atrial contractility.

INOTROPIC STATE (MYOCARDIAL CONTRACTILITY) A number of factors determine the level of ventricular performance at any given ventricular end-diastolic volume, i.e., the position of the ventricular function curve (Fig. 231-6) as well as the position of the left ventricular pressure-volume plane (Fig. 231-8). These influences may be considered to operate by modifying myocardial force-velocity relations. In the final analysis, most of these influences act by altering the $[Ca^{2+}]$ in the vicinity of the myofilaments, which in turn trigger cross-bridge cycling (p. 1293).

Adrenergic Nerve Activity (See also Chap. 72) The quantity of norepinephrine released by adrenergic nerve endings in the heart is determined by the adrenergic nerve impulse traffic; alterations in the frequency of these nerve impulses modify the quantity of norepinephrine released and acting on the β-adrenergic receptors in the myocardium. This mechanism is the most important one that acutely modifies myocardial contractility under physiologic conditions.

Circulating Catecholamines (See also Chap. 72) When it is stimulated by adrenergic nerve impulse, the adrenal medulla releases catecholamines, which, when they reach the heart, augment both heart rate and myocardial contractility.

FIGURE 231-8 The responses of the left ventricle to increased afterload, increased preload, and increased and reduced contractility are shown in the pressure-volume plane. ESPVR, end-systolic pressure-volume relation; E_{ES}, the slope of the end-systolic pressure-volume relation. *Left*. Effects of increases in preload and afterload on the pressure-volume loop. Since there has been no change in contractility, ESPVR is unchanged. With an increase in afterload, stroke volume falls ($1 \rightarrow 2$); with an increase in preload, stroke volume rises ($1 \rightarrow 3$). *Right*. With increased myocardial contractility, the normal ESPVR moves to the left of the normal line (lower end-systolic volume at any end-systolic pressure) and stroke volume rises ($1 \rightarrow 3$). With reduced myocardial contractility, the ESPVR moves to the right; end-systolic volume is increased and stroke volume falls ($1 \rightarrow 2$).

The Force-Frequency Relation The position of the myocardial force-velocity curve is also influenced by the rate and rhythm of cardiac contraction; e.g., ventricular extrasystoles result in postextrasystolic potentiation, presumably by increasing the quantity of Ca^{2+} that enters the cardiac cell. The contractility of the normal (but not of the failing) heart is augmented by an increase in frequency of contraction.

Exogenously Administered Inotropic Agents Isoproterenol, dopamine, dobutamine, and other sympathomimetic agents, cardiac glycosides, Ca^{2+}, amrinone, milrinone, and other phosphodiesterase inhibitors all improve the myocardial force-velocity relation and therefore may be used to stimulate ventricular performance.

Physiologic Depressants Included among these are severe myocardial hypoxia, ischemia, and acidosis. Acting either singly or in combination, these influences depress the myocardial force-velocity curve and left ventricular work at any given ventricular end-diastolic volume.

Pharmacologic Depressants These include many antiarrhythmic drugs such as procainamide and disopyramide; calcium antagonists such as verapamil; beta blockers; and large doses of barbiturates, alcohol, and general anesthetics as well as many other drugs.

Loss of Myocytes When a sufficiently large portion of ventricular myocardium becomes nonfunctional or necrotic, as occurs transiently during ischemia (Chap. 244) and permanently in myocardial infarction (Chap. 243), total ventricular performance at any given level of end-diastolic volume becomes depressed. Programmed cell death (apoptosis) can also cause loss of myocytes and, when sufficiently widespread, can impair ventricular function and cause heart failure.

Intrinsic Myocardial Depression Although the fundamental mechanisms responsible for depression of myocardial contractility in most cases of chronic congestive heart failure secondary to prolonged ventricular overload or cardiomyopathy remain to be elucidated (p. 1316), it is now apparent that in this condition the inotropic state of individual surviving myocytes is depressed, and as a consequence the ventricular performance at any ventricular preload and afterload is lowered.

VENTRICULAR AFTERLOAD The stroke volume is ultimately a function of the extent of ventricular fiber shortening. In the intact heart, as in isolated cardiac muscle, the velocity and extent of shortening of ventricular muscle fibers at any level of preload and myocardial contractility are inversely related to the afterload, i.e., the load that opposes shortening. In the intact heart the afterload may be defined as the tension or stress developed in the ventricular wall during ejection. Therefore, the afterload is determined by the aortic pressure as well as the volume and thickness of the ventricular cavity. Laplace's law indicates that the tension of the myocardial fiber is a function of the product of the intracavitary ventricular pressure and ventricular radius divided by the wall thickness. Therefore, at any given level of aortic pressure, the afterload faced by a dilated left ventricle of normal thickness is higher than that encountered by a normal-sized ventricle. Conversely, at the same aortic pressure and ventricular diastolic volume, the afterload of a thick-walled ventricle is lower than of a thin-walled chamber. The aortic pressure, in turn, is determined by the peripheral vascular resistance, the physical characteristics of the arterial tree, and the volume of blood it contains at the onset of ejection.

The critical role played by the ventricular afterload in cardiovascular regulation is shown in Fig. 231-10. As already noted, increases in both preload and contractility increase myocardial fiber shortening, while increases in afterload reduce it. The extent of myocardial fiber shortening and left ventricular size are the determinants of stroke volume. Arterial pressure, in turn, is related to the product of cardiac output and systemic vascular resistance, while afterload is a function of left ventricular volume, wall thickness, and arterial pressure. An increase in arterial pressure induced by vasoconstriction, for example, augments afterload, which opposes myocardial fiber shortening, reducing stroke volume. This in turn tends to limit the increase in pressure.

When myocardial contractility becomes impaired and the ventricle dilates, afterload rises and becomes increasingly important in determining cardiac output. Increases in afterload may result from neural and humoral stimuli that occur in response to a fall in cardiac output. This increased afterload may reduce cardiac output further while myocardial oxygen requirements are increased. This can cause a vicious cycle. Treatment with vasodilators has the opposite effect; by reducing afterload, cardiac output rises (Chap. 232).

Under normal circumstances, the various influences acting on cardiac performance enumerated above interact in a complex fashion to maintain cardiac output at a level appropriate to the requirements of the metabolizing tissues, and interference with any one of these mechanisms may not influence the cardiac output. For example, a moderate reduction of blood volume *or* the loss of the atrial contribution to

1315

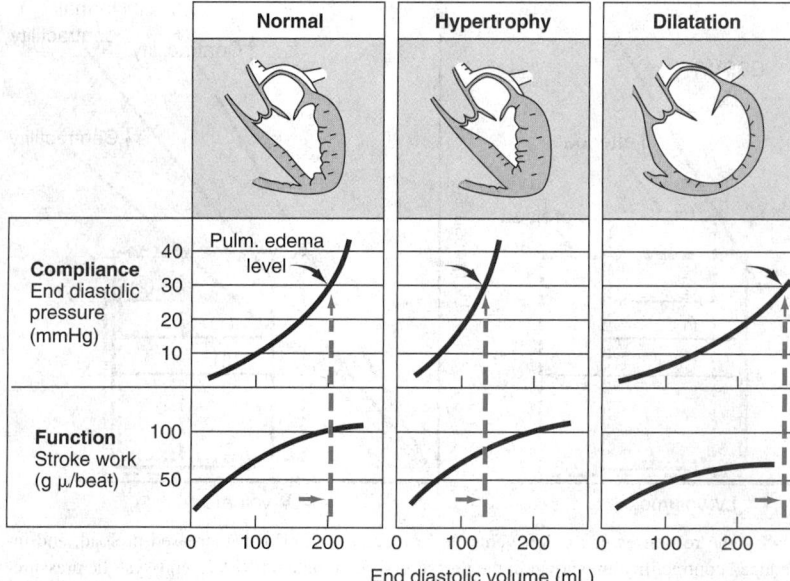

FIGURE 231-9 Relationship between left ventricular end-diastolic volume and (1) end-diastolic pressure (*top*), describing the *compliance* of the left ventricle, i.e., its *diastolic* properties; and (2) left ventricular stroke work (*bottom*), describing the ventricle's *systolic* function curve. The normal left ventricle (*left*) reaches an end-diastolic pressure of 30 mmHg (pulmonary edema level) when its end-diastolic volume is elevated to 200 mL. The concentrically hypertrophied left ventricle (*center*) exhibits normal systolic function since the relation between left ventricular end-diastolic volume and stroke work is unchanged, but there is "diastolic failure" in that end-diastolic pressure reaches pulmonary edema level (i.e., 30 mmHg) at a lower level than normal (i.e., 130 mL). The dilated ventricle (*right*) exhibits "systolic failure" in that the maximal stroke work and the stroke volume at any level of end-diastolic volume are depressed. The left ventricle displays increased diastolic compliance, i.e., distensibility, with a higher than normal end-diastolic volume (280 mL) required to reach the pulmonary edema level. (*Reprinted with permission from R Gorlin, Prim Cardiol 6:84, 1980.*)

ventricular contraction can ordinarily be sustained without a reduction in the cardiac output at rest. Other factors, such as increases in the frequency of adrenergic nerve impulses to the heart and in heart rate, will, in a normal individual, serve as compensatory mechanisms, augment contractility, and sustain cardiac output.

EXERCISE The hemodynamic changes that occur normally during exercise in the upright position are complex (Fig. 231-6). Hyperventilation, the pumping action of the exercising muscles, and the venoconstriction during exercise all augment venous return and hence ventricular filling and preload. Simultaneously, the increase in the adrenergic nerve impulse traffic to the myocardium, the increased concentration of circulating catecholamines, and the tachycardia that occur during exercise combine to augment the contractile state of the myocardium (Fig. 231-6, curves 1 and 2) and lead to an elevation of stroke

work and stroke volume, without change or even a reduction of end-diastolic pressure and volume (Fig. 231-6, points A and B). Vasodilatation occurs in the exercising muscles, thus tending to limit the increase in arterial pressure that would otherwise occur as cardiac output rises to levels as high as five times basal during maximal exercise. This vasodilatation ultimately allows the achievement of a greatly elevated cardiac output during exercise, at an arterial pressure only moderately higher than in the resting state.

THE FAILING HEART

Although heart failure may be readily described as a clinical syndrome, characterized by well-known symptoms and physical signs (Chap. 232), a precise physiologic or biochemical definition is far more difficult. However, from the clinical point of view, heart failure may be considered to be the condition in which *an abnormality of cardiac function is responsible for the inability of the heart to pump blood at a rate commensurate with the requirements of the metabolizing tissues and/or allows it to do so only from an abnormally elevated ventricular diastolic volume.* Abnormalities during systole and/or diastole may be present in heart failure (Fig. 231-9). In so-called *systolic heart failure* (p. 1320), an impairment of myocardial contractility causes weakened systolic contraction, which leads, ultimately, to a reduction in stroke volume and cardiac output, inadequate ventricular emptying, cardiac dilatation, and often elevation of ventricular diastolic pressure. Idiopathic dilated cardiomyopathy (Chap. 238) is the prototype of systolic heart failure. In *diastolic heart failure* (p. 1320), the principal abnormality is impaired relaxation and filling of the ventricle, which leads to an elevation of ventricular diastolic pressure at any given diastolic volume (Fig. 231-9). Failure of relaxation can be functional and transient, as during ischemia, which reduced the ATP required for the SR pump to lower cytoplasmic Ca^{2+}. Chronically impaired ventricular filling can be caused by a stiffened, thickened ventricle. Typical conditions in which diastolic failure occurs are restrictive cardiomyopathy secondary to infiltrative conditions, such as amyloidosis or hemochromatosis, as well as hypertrophic cardiomyopathy (Chap. 238). The concentric hypertrophy associated with chronic hypertension can also impair ventricular filling but rarely causes overt heart failure. In many patients with cardiac hypertrophy and dilatation, systolic and diastolic failure coexist; the left ventricle both empties and fills abnormally. There may be cardiac dilatation, but the ventricle's pressure-volume relation is shifted, raising the ventricular diastolic pressure at any given volume.

Although a defect in myocardial contraction is characteristic of systolic heart failure, many conditions may cause such a defect. These include a primary abnormality in the heart muscle, as occurs in cardiomyopathy, or an abnormality secondary to a chronic excessive work load as in hypertension or valvular heart disease. In ischemic heart disease, systolic heart failure results from a loss in the quantity of normally contracting cells (secondary to myocardial necrosis and apoptosis) and/or from transient loss of function in reversibly ischemic (hibernating) myocardium (Chap. 244).

Heart failure should be distinguished from conditions that resemble it, such as (1) states of circulatory insufficiency in which myocardial function is not primarily impaired, such as cardiac tamponade or hemorrhagic shock; (2) conditions in which there is circulatory congestion because of abnormal salt and water retention but in which there is no serious disturbance of the heart's function, such as acute glomerulonephritis; and

FIGURE 231-10 Scheme of interactions among various components that regulate cardiac activity. Solid lines indicate an augmenting effect; broken line represents an inhibiting effect. (*From E Braunwald, N Engl J Med 290:1124–1129, 1420–1425, 1974.*)

(3) conditions in which a normal myocardium is suddenly presented with a load that exceeds its capacity, such as accelerated hypertension or rupture of a valve cusp secondary to infective endocarditis.

ADAPTIVE MECHANISMS A number of mechanisms aid the heart faced with an increased hemodynamic burden (such as pressure or volume overload) or that has sustained loss of myocardium or contractility. These mechanisms include the following:

1. The *Frank-Starling mechanism* operating through an increase in preload (p. 1314). As outlined above, an increase in the end-diastolic volume of the ventricle is associated with stretching of the sarcomeres, which increases the interaction between actin and myosin filaments and their sensitivity to Ca^{2+}. Ventricular dilatation may become maladaptive when it becomes excessive, as may occur in severe aortic or mitral regurgitation; this increases wall stress through the operation of LaPlace's law and reduces shortening.

2. *Increased afterload*, as occurs in aortic stenosis and hypertension, also augments wall tension, leading to concentric hypertrophy, which in turn restores elevated ventricular wall stress to normal. However, ventricular hypertrophy impairs ventricular filling, and if the hypertrophy is insufficient to restore wall stress to normal, the ventricle dilates and this increases wall stress further, leading to a vicious circle.

3. *Redistribution of a subnormal cardiac output* away from the skin, skeletal muscle, and kidneys with maintenance of blood flow to the brain and the heart.

4. *Neurohumoral adjustments*, which tend to maintain arterial pressure and are discussed in Chap. 72. Like the other adaptive mechanisms, when neurohumoral adjustments are severe and chronic they impair cardiac function (see below).

BIOCHEMICAL ABNORMALITIES IN HEART FAILURE There is no unifying theory providing a biochemical basis for heart failure. However, a number of abnormalities have been described.

Reduction in Cardiac Efficiency The common forms of low-output systolic heart failure, secondary to coronary atherosclerosis, hypertension, cardiomyopathy, and certain valvular and congenital lesions, are characterized by an absolute or a relative reduction in the external work delivered by the heart, while myocardial oxygen consumption remains normal or nearly so. Therefore, the external efficiency, i.e., the ratio of external work performed to energy consumed, is often depressed.

Alterations in Energy Metabolism When heart failure occurs in the presence of acute or chronic ischemia, it can be attributed to reduced myocardial energy supplies. Severe ventricular hypertrophy and/or dilatation of any etiology can also cause relative ischemia, especially in the subendocardium, and this can impair both ventricular contraction and filling. In some forms of experimental and clinical heart failure without ischemia, myocardial energy stores in the form of creatine phosphate are decreased, as is the activity of the enzyme creatin kinase required for the shuttling of high-energy phosphate between creatine phosphate and adenosine diphosphate, suggesting that reductions in myocardial energy reserves may play a role.

Alterations in Regulatory Proteins Changes in the cardiac regulatory proteins frequently occur in chronic heart failure. These include a reduction of myosin ATPase activity, which may be caused by an alteration in the expression of troponin T and/or of myosin light chain kinase 2, alterations that could be responsible for lowering the rate of interaction between myosin and actin myofilaments, leading to systolic heart failure.

Abnormalities of Excitation-Contraction Coupling Substantial evidence supports the view that in many forms of heart failure the delivery of Ca^{2+} to the contractile sites is reduced, thereby impairing cardiac performance (Table 231-1). However, the molecular basis of this abnormality—indeed of the subcellular structures involved, i.e., the sarcolemma, T tubules, and/or SR—has yet to be defined. There is, however, evidence for a reduction in the activity of the Ca^{2+} release channel in the SR and of messenger RNAs of the proteins regulating Ca^{2+} movements. These include the sarcolemmal Ca^{2+} channels, the Ca^{2+} release channels, and the Ca^{2+} uptake pump, which play critical roles in the movement of Ca^{2+} between the SR and the cytoplasm.

Table 231-1 Calcium Homeostasis in Failing Human Myocardium

Intracellular Calcium Concentration	Calcium-Handling Proteins (mRNA Levels)
Basal (diastolic) ↑	Voltage-dependent Ca^{2+} channels ↓
Peak (systolic) ↓	Na^+/Ca^{2+} exchanger ↑
Rate of fall ↓	SR Ca^{2+}-ATPase ↓
	Phospholamban ↓
	Phospholamban/SR Ca^{2+} ATPase ↑
	Ca^{2+} release channel ↓
	Calsequestrin ↔

SOURCE: From DB Sawyer, WS Colucci, in WS Colucci (ed): *Heart Failure: Cardiac Function and Dysfunction*, in *Atlas of Heart Diseases*, 2d ed, E Braunwald (series ed). Philadelphia, Current Medicine, 1999.

Impaired expression of the genes encoding these proteins can impair both myocardial contraction and relaxation and thereby contribute to the development of heart failure.

NEUROHUMORAL AND CYTOKINE ADJUSTMENTS A reduction in cardiac performance evokes a series of neurohumoral adjustments, which, at different times, may be adaptive and maladaptive. Although they are useful because they maintain arterial perfusion pressure in the face of a sudden reduction of cardiac output, these neurohumoral adjustments increase the hemodynamic burden and oxygen requirements of the failing ventricle (Fig. 231-11).

The Adrenergic Nervous System In patients with heart failure the levels of circulating norepinephrine may be markedly elevated, reflecting the increased activity of the adrenergic nervous system; indeed the prognosis in patients with heart failure varies inversely with the concentration of plasma norepinephrine. This increased activity of the adrenergic neurons supports ventricular contractility in *acute* heart failure. Heart failure is intensified when large doses of β-adrenergic blocking agents are administered acutely, providing evidence for the protective action of adrenergic nervous activation. However, the *chronic* adrenergic stimulation that occurs in heart failure may increase afterload by raising vascular resistance, cause cardiac arrhythmias, and may damage myocytes further, perhaps by causing Ca^{2+} overload.

The density of adrenergic receptors, their coupling to G proteins,

FIGURE 231-11 Interplay between cardiac function and neurohumoral and cytokine systems. Myocardial injury, of many etiologies, can depress cardiac function, which in turn causes activation of the sympathoadrenal system (SAS) and the renin-angiotensin-aldosterone system (RAAS) and the elaboration of endothelin, arginine vasopressin (AVP), and cytokines such as tumor necrosis factor (TNF) α. In acute heart failure (*left*), these are adaptive and tend to maintain arterial pressure and cardiac function. In chronic heart failure (*right*), they cause maladaptive hypertrophic remodeling and apoptosis, which cause further myocardial injury and impairment of cardiac function. The horizontal line on the right (*) shows that chronic maladaptive influences can be inhibited by angiotensin converting enzyme inhibitors, β-adrenergic blockers, angiotensin type I receptor blockers, aldosterone antagonists, and endothelin type A blockers.

and the concentration of cardiac norepinephrine stores are all reduced in chronic, severe heart failure. These changes are accompanied by a reduction in the activity of adenylate cyclase, which may lower the intracellular concentration of cyclic AMP. The latter in turn reduces the activation of protein kinase, the phosphorylation of Ca^{2+} channels, transarcolemmal Ca^{2+} entry, as well as the phosphorylation of phospholamban, a protein in the SR, which reduces the reuptake of Ca^{2+} by the latter (Fig. 231-7). Changes in the G proteins, which couple the β receptor to the catalytic adenylate cyclase (which is responsible for the production of cyclic AMP), may also occur in heart failure, with increased activity of the inhibitory subunit.

The Renin-Angiotensin-Aldosterone System   When cardiac output declines, the renin-angiotensin-aldosterone system (Chap. 331) is activated. Concentrations of both circulating angiotensin II and aldosterone are increased, the former contributing to excess vasoconstriction and the latter to the retention of salt and water and perhaps to cardiac fibrosis. The local (tissue) renin-angiotensin system is also activated in heart failure. Patients with heart failure are usually improved by blocking this system with angiotensin-converting enzyme inhibitors, angiotensin II receptor blockers, and aldosterone antagonists (Chap. 232).

Endothelin   The concentration of circulatory endothelin, a polypeptide that is a very powerful vasoconstrictor, is increased in heart failure. A number of studies have shown that blockade of endothelin receptors improves left ventricular function in patients and experimental animals with heart failure.

Tumor Necrosis Factor α The overexpression of a number of cytokines also appears to play a prominent role in the pathogenesis of heart failure. It has now been well established that patients exhibit elevated levels of tumor necrosis factor (TNF) α, both in the circulation and in cardiac muscle; the pathophysiologic significance of this finding is just unfolding. Transgenic mice with overexpressed cardiac TNF-α have systolic dysfunction, myocarditis, ventricular dilatation, heart failure, and shortened survival. The infusion of TNF-α impairs ventricular function, and this can be reversed with a TNF-α antagonist.

Vasodilator Peptides   A number of vasodilator peptides are released by the dilated heart. Best known are the natriuretic peptides atrial natriuretic peptide (ANP) and brain natriuretic peptide (BNP). When stretch receptors in the atria (ANP and BNP) and ventricles (BNP) are activated, these hormones (or their prohormones) are released and act on specific natriuretic peptide receptors, which increase the concentrations of cyclic GMP in the kidney, adrenal glomerulose, vascular smooth muscle, and platelets. Urine volume and sodium excretion are augmented, vascular resistance is reduced, and the release of renin and the secretion of aldosterone are reduced. These effects, while beneficial, are not sufficiently powerful to oppose the sodium-retaining and vasoconstrictor influences of the other neurohumoral systems activated in heart failure. Elevated circulating concentrations of ANP and particularly BNP correlate with a poor prognosis in heart failure. Drugs that augment the concentrations of these compounds are under development.

Figure 231-11 illustrates current concepts of neurohumoral-cytokine activation in heart failure. The activation of the adrenergic nervous system and the renin-angiotensin-aldosterone system and the enhanced elaboration of endothelin and arginine vasopressin appear to be adaptive in *acute*, severe heart failure. However, they all appear to exert a maladaptive response in chronic heart failure. Inflammatory cytokines and oxidative stress are emerging as potent noxious stimuli as well. Together they result in a vicious circle, causing myocyte hypertrophy, remodeling, and cell death, the latter often due to myocardial apoptosis, all resulting in further impairment of cardiac function and myocardial injury. Effective agents that interfere with the adverse effects of these stimuli on cardiac function, such as endothelin receptor blockers and TNF-α antagonists, are becoming available, and these neurohumoral and cytokine blockers appear capable of interrupting the vicious circle.

HEART FAILURE—A DISTURBANCE OF THE MYOCARDIAL PUMP   In the final analysis, in systolic heart failure the basic problem is depression of the myocardial force-velocity relationship and of the length–active tension curve, reflecting reductions in the contractile state of the myocardium (Fig. 231-6, curves 1 to 3, Fig. 231-8, right). In diastolic failure there is upward displacement of the diastolic pressure–volume relation (Fig. 231-9). In many instances, cardiac output and external ventricular performance at rest are within normal limits but are maintained at these levels only by an increased end-diastolic fiber length and an elevated ventricular end-diastolic volume, i.e., through the operation of the Frank-Starling mechanism (Fig. 231-6, points A to D). The elevation of left ventricular preload is associated with increases in the pulmonary capillary pressure, contributing to the dyspnea experienced by patients with heart failure, while elevation of right ventricular preload raises systemic venous pressure and contributes to the development of edema. The improvement of contractility that normally accompanies augmented adrenergic activity during exercise is attenuated or even prevented by norepinephrine depletion and downregulation of myocardial β receptors, which occur in severe heart failure (Fig. 231-6, curves 3 and 3′).

The factors that augment ventricular filling during exercise in the normal individual push the failing myocardium along its flattened length–active tension curve, and although the left ventricle may perform somewhat better at this higher diastolic volume, this occurs only as a consequence of an inordinate elevation of ventricular end-diastolic volume and pressure and, therefore, of the pulmonary capillary pressure. The latter intensifies dyspnea and therefore plays an important role in limiting the intensity of exercise that the patient can perform. Left ventricular failure becomes fatal when the myocardial length–active tension curve is depressed (Fig. 231-6, curve 4) to the point at which cardiac performance fails to satisfy the requirements of the peripheral tissues even at rest, and/or the left ventricular end-diastolic and pulmonary capillary pressures are elevated to levels that result in pulmonary edema (Fig. 231-6, point E).

BIBLIOGRAPHY

ANVERSA P et al: Myocyte death in heart failure. Curr Opin Cardiol 11:245, 1996

ARAI M et al: Sarcoplasmic reticulum gene expression in cardiac hypertrophy and heart failure. Circ Res 74:555, 1994

COLUCCI WS (ed): *Heart Failure: Cardiac Function and Dysfunction*, in *Atlas of Heart Diseases*, 2d ed, E Braunwald (series ed). Philadelphia, Current Medicine, 1999

———, BRAUNWALD E: Pathophysiology of heart failure, in *Heart Disease*, 6th ed, E Braunwald (ed). Philadelphia, Saunders, 2001

HEIN S et al: Altered expression of titin and contractile proteins in failing human myocardium. J Mol Cell Biol 26:1291, 1994

KATZ AM: *Heart Failure*, New York, Raven, 2000, pp 381

LITTLE WC, BRAUNWALD E: Assessment of cardiac function, in *Heart Disease*, 6th ed, E Braunwald (ed). Philadelphia, Saunders, 2001

OPIE LH: Mechanisms of cardiac contraction and relaxation, in *Heart Disease*, 6th ed, E Braunwald (ed). Philadelphia, Saunders, 2001

SCHWARTZ K, MERCADIER J-J: Molecular and cellular biology of heart failure. Curr Opin Cardiol 11:227, 1996

SOLARO RJ et al: Regulatory proteins and diastolic relaxation, in *Diastolic Relaxation of the Heart*, BH Lorell, W Grossman (eds). Boston, Kluwer Academic, 1994, pp 43–53

WOLFF MR et al: Rate of tension development in cardiac muscle varies with level of activator calcium. Circ Res 76:154, 1995

232   *Eugene Braunwald*

HEART FAILURE

Heart failure (HF) is the pathophysiologic state in which an abnormality of *cardiac* function is responsible for the failure of the heart to pump blood at a rate commensurate with the requirements of the metabolizing tissues *and/or* allows it to do so only from an abnormally elevated diastolic volume. HF is frequently, but not always, caused by a defect in myocardial contraction, and then the term *myocardial failure* is appropriate. The latter may result from a primary abnormality in heart muscle, as occurs in the cardiomyopathies, in viral myocarditis (Chap. 238), and with excessive programmed cell death (apoptosis). HF also results commonly from coronary atherosclerosis, which interferes with cardiac contraction by causing myocardial infarction and ischemia. HF may also occur in valvular and/or congenital heart disease in which the heart muscle is damaged by the long-standing excessive hemodynamic burden imposed by the valvular abnormality or cardiac malformation.

In other patients with HF, however, a similar clinical syndrome is present but without any detectable abnormality of *myocardial* function. In some of these patients the normal heart is suddenly presented with a mechanical load that exceeds its capacity, such as an acute hypertensive crisis, rupture of an aortic valve cusp, or massive pulmonary embolism. HF in the presence of normal myocardial function also occurs in chronic conditions in which there is impaired filling of the ventricles due to a mechanical abnormality such as tricuspid and/or mitral stenosis, constrictive pericarditis without myocardial involvement, endocardial fibrosis, and some forms of hypertrophic cardiomyopathy. In many patients with HF, particularly those with valvular or congenital heart disease, there is a combination of impaired myocardial function and hemodynamic overload.

Heart failure should be distinguished from (1) conditions in which there is circulatory congestion secondary to abnormal salt and water retention but in which there is no disturbance of cardiac function per se, as occurs in renal failure; and (2) noncardiac causes of inadequate cardiac output, such as hypovolemic shock (Chap. 38).

The ventricles respond to a chronically increased hemodynamic burden with the development of hypertrophy (Fig. 232-1). When the ventricle is called on to deliver an elevated cardiac output for prolonged periods, as in valvular regurgitation, it develops *eccentric hypertrophy*, i.e., cavity dilatation, with an increase in muscle mass so that the ratio between wall thickness and ventricular cavity size remains relatively constant early in the process. With chronic pressure overload, as in valvular aortic stenosis or untreated hypertension, *concentric ventricular hypertrophy* develops; in this condition the ratio between wall thickness and ventricular cavity size increases. In both eccentric and concentric hypertrophy, a stable hyperfunctioning state may exist for many years, but myocardial function may ultimately deteriorate, leading to HF. Often at this time, the ventricle dilates and the ratio between wall thickness and cavity size declines, leading to increased stress on each unit of myocardium, further dilatation, and a vicious circle.

Heart failure represents a major public health problem in industrialized nations. It appears to be the only common cardiovascular condition that is increasing in prevalence and incidence. In the United States, HF is responsible for almost 1 million hospital admissions and 40,000 deaths annually. Since HF is more common in the elderly, its prevalence is likely to continue to increase as the population ages.

CAUSES OF HEART FAILURE

In evaluating patients with HF, it is important to identify not only the *underlying* but also the *precipitating cause*. The cardiac abnormality produced by a congenital or acquired lesion such as valvular aortic stenosis may exist for many years and cause no clinical disability. Frequently, however, clinical manifestations of HF are precipitated for the first time in the course of some acute disturbance that places an additional load on a myocardium that is chronically excessively burdened (see below). Such a heart may be compensated but have little additional reserve, and the additional load imposed by a precipitating cause results in further deterioration of cardiac function. Identification of such precipitating causes is of critical importance because their

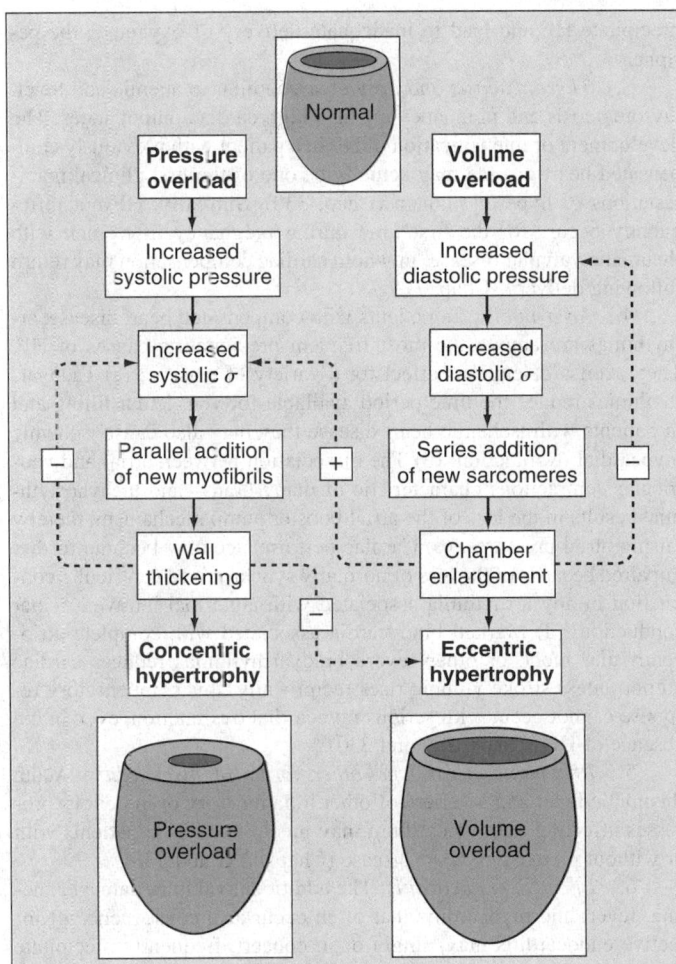

FIGURE 232-1 Patterns of ventricular hypertrophy. Specific patterns of ventricular remodeling occur in response to the imposed augmentation in work load. A pattern of hypertrophic growth characterized as concentric, in which increased mass is out of proportion to chamber volume, is particularly effective in reducing systolic wall stress (σ) under conditions of heightened pressure load. In contrast, in volume overload conditions, in which the major stimulus is diastolic loading, a predominant finding is a great increase in the cavity size or volume. Although there can be extensive increases in mass, the relationship between mass and volume is either preserved or, in severe cases, reduced. The fundamental response is generated by cellular hypertrophy. However, the configuration of the new contractile tissue is specific and offsets the mechanical stimulus. [*Modified from W Grossman et al in NR Alpert (ed): Perspectives in Cardiovascular Research. Myocardial Hypertrophy and Failure, vol 7. New York, Raven Press, 1993, with permission.*]

prompt alleviation may be lifesaving. In the absence of underlying heart disease, these acute disturbances do not by themselves lead to HF.

PRECIPITATING CAUSES

1. *Infection.* Patients with pulmonary vascular congestion due to left ventricular failure are more susceptible to pulmonary infection than are normal persons; any infection may precipitate HF. The resulting fever, tachycardia, and hypoxemia and the increased metabolic demands may place a further burden on an overloaded, but compensated, myocardium of a patient with chronic heart disease.

2. *Anemia.* In the presence of anemia, the oxygen needs of the metabolizing tissues can be met only by an increase in the cardiac output (Chap. 61). Although such an increase in cardiac output can be sustained by a normal heart, a diseased, overloaded, but otherwise compensated heart may be unable to augment sufficiently the volume of blood that it delivers to the periphery. In this manner, the combination of anemia and previously compensated heart disease can

precipitate HF and lead to inadequate delivery of oxygen to the periphery.

3. *Thyrotoxicosis and pregnancy.* Similar to anemia and fever, thyrotoxicosis and pregnancy are also high cardiac output states. The development or intensification of HF in a patient with previously compensated heart disease may actually be one of the first clinical manifestations of hyperthyroidism (Chap. 330). Similarly, HF not infrequently occurs for the first time during pregnancy in women with rheumatic valvular disease, in whom cardiac compensation may return following delivery (Chap. 7).

4. *Arrhythmias.* In patients with compensated heart disease, arrhythmias are among the most frequent precipitating causes of HF. They exert a deleterious effect for a variety of reasons: (a) Tachyarrhythmias reduce the time period available for ventricular filling and in patients with ischemic heart disease they may also cause ischemic myocardial dysfunction. (b) The dissociation between atrial and ventricular contractions characteristic of many brady- and tachyarrhythmias results in the loss of the atrial booster pump mechanism, thereby raising atrial pressures. (c) Cardiac performance may become further impaired because of the loss of normally synchronized ventricular contraction in any arrhythmia associated with abnormal intraventricular conduction. (d) Marked bradycardia associated with complete atrioventricular block or other severe bradyarrhythmias reduces cardiac output unless stroke volume rises reciprocally; this compensatory response cannot occur with serious myocardial dysfunction, even in the absence of HF (Chaps. 229 and 230).

5. *Rheumatic, viral, and other forms of myocarditis.* Acute rheumatic fever and a variety of other inflammatory or infectious processes affecting the myocardium may precipitate HF in patients with or without preexisting heart disease (Chaps. 235 and 238).

6. *Infective endocarditis.* The additional valvular damage, anemia, fever, and myocarditis that often occur as a consequence of infective endocarditis may, singly or in concert, frequently precipitate HF (Chap. 126).

7. *Physical, dietary, fluid, environmental, and emotional excesses.* The sudden augmentation of sodium intake as with a large meal, the inappropriate discontinuation of pharmaceuticals to treat HF, blood transfusions, physical overexertion, excessive environmental heat or humidity, and emotional crises all may precipitate HF in patients with heart disease who were previously compensated.

8. *Systemic hypertension.* Rapid elevation of arterial pressure, as may occur in some instances of hypertension of renal origin or upon discontinuation of antihypertensive medication in patients with essential hypertension, may result in cardiac decompensation (Chap. 246).

9. *Myocardial infarction.* In patients with chronic but compensated ischemic heart disease, a fresh infarct, sometimes otherwise silent clinically, may further impair ventricular function and precipitate HF (Chap. 243).

10. *Pulmonary embolism.* Physically inactive patients with low cardiac output are at increased risk of developing thrombi in the veins of the lower extremities or the pelvis. Pulmonary emboli may result in further elevation of pulmonary arterial pressure, which in turn may produce or intensify ventricular failure. In the presence of pulmonary vascular congestion, such emboli also may cause pulmonary infarction (Chap. 261).

A systematic search for these precipitating causes should be made in every patient with the new development or recent intensification of HF. If properly recognized, the precipitating cause of HF usually can be treated more effectively than the underlying cause. Therefore, the prognosis in patients with HF in whom a precipitating cause can be identified, treated, and eliminated is more favorable than in patients in whom the underlying disease process has progressed to the point of producing HF without a precipitating cause.

HF may be described as *systolic* or *diastolic*, *high-output* or *low-output*, *acute* or *chronic*, *right-sided* or *left-sided*, and *forward* or *backward*. These descriptors are often useful in a clinical setting, particularly early in the patient's course, but late in the course of chronic HF the differences between them often become blurred.

SYSTOLIC VERSUS DIASTOLIC FAILURE   The distinction between these two forms of HF, described in Fig. 231-9, relates to whether the principal abnormality is the inability of the ventricle to contract normally and expel sufficient blood (systolic failure) or to relax and/or fill normally (diastolic failure). The major clinical manifestations of systolic failure relate to an inadequate cardiac output with weakness, fatigue, reduced exercise tolerance, and other symptoms of hypoperfusion, while in diastolic HF the manifestations relate principally to the elevation of filling pressures. Many patients, particularly those who have both ventricular hypertrophy *and* dilatation, exhibit abnormalities both of contraction and relaxation coexist.

Diastolic HF may be caused by increased resistance to ventricular inflow and reduced ventricular diastolic capacity (constrictive pericarditis and restrictive, hypertensive, and hypertrophic cardiomyopathy), impaired ventricular relaxation (acute myocardial ischemia), and myocardial fibrosis and infiltration (restrictive cardiomyopathy).

HIGH-OUTPUT VERSUS LOW-OUTPUT HEART FAILURE   It is useful to classify patients with HF into those with a low cardiac output, i.e., *low-output HF*, and those with an elevated cardiac output, i.e., *high-output HF*. The former occurs secondary to ischemic heart disease, hypertension, dilated cardiomyopathy, and valvular and pericardial disease, while the latter is seen in patients with HF and hyperthyroidism, anemia, pregnancy, arteriovenous fistulas, beriberi, and Paget's disease. In clinical practice, however, low-output and high-output HF cannot always be readily distinguished. The normal range of cardiac output is wide [2.2 to 3.5 (L/min)/m^2]; in many patients with so-called low-output HF, the cardiac output may actually be just within the normal range at rest (although lower than it had been previously), but it fails to rise normally during exertion. On the other hand, in patients with so-called high-output HF, the output may not exceed the upper limits of normal (although it would have been elevated had it been measured before HF supervened); rather, it may have fallen to within normal limits. Regardless of the *absolute* level of the cardiac output, however, cardiac failure may be said to be present when the characteristic clinical manifestations described below are accompanied by a depression of the curve relating ventricular end-diastolic volume to cardiac performance (see Fig. 231-6).

An integral physiologic component of *systolic* HF is the delivery of an inadequate quantity of oxygen required by the metabolizing tissues. In the absence of peripheral shunting of blood, this is reflected in an abnormal widening of the normal arterial–mixed venous oxygen difference (35 to 50 mL/L in the basal state). In mild cases, such an abnormality may not be present at rest but becomes evident only during exertion or other hypermetabolic states. In patients with high cardiac output states, such as those associated with arteriovenous fistula or thyrotoxicosis, the arterial–mixed venous oxygen difference is normal or low. The mixed venous oxygen saturation is raised by the admixture of blood that has been diverted away from the metabolizing tissues, and it may be presumed that even in these patients the delivery of oxygen to the latter is reduced despite the normal or even elevated mixed venous oxygen saturation. When HF occurs in such patients, the arterial–mixed venous oxygen difference, regardless of the absolute value, still exceeds the level that existed prior to the development of HF. Therefore, the cardiac output, though normal or even elevated, is lower than before HF supervened.

In most forms of high-output HF, the heart is called on to pump abnormally large quantities of blood in order to deliver the oxygen required by the metabolizing tissues. The hemodynamic burden placed on the myocardium by the increased flow load resembles that produced by chronic aortic regurgitation. In addition, thyrotoxicosis and beriberi may also impair myocardial metabolism directly, while very severe anemia may interfere with myocardial function by producing myocardial anoxia, especially in the subendocardium and in the presence of underlying obstructive coronary artery disease.

ACUTE VERSUS CHRONIC HEART FAILURE The prototype of *acute HF* is the sudden development of a large myocardial infarction or rupture of a cardiac valve in a patient who previously was entirely well. *Chronic HF* is typically observed in patients with dilated cardiomyopathy or multivalvular heart disease that develops or progresses slowly. Acute HF is usually predominantly systolic, and the sudden reduction in cardiac output often results in systemic hypotension without peripheral edema. In contrast, in chronic HF, arterial pressure is ordinarily well maintained until very late in the course, but there is often accumulation of edema.

RIGHT-SIDED VERSUS LEFT-SIDED HEART FAILURE Many of the clinical manifestations of HF result from the accumulation of excess fluid behind either one or both ventricles (Chaps. 32 and 37). This fluid usually localizes upstream to (behind) the ventricle that is initially affected. For example, patients in whom the left ventricle is hemodynamically overloaded (e.g., aortic stenosis) or weakened (e.g., postmyocardial infarction) develop dyspnea and orthopnea as a result of pulmonary congestion, a condition referred to as *left-sided HF*. In contrast, when the underlying abnormality affects the right ventricle primarily (e.g., congenital valvular pulmonic stenosis or pulmonary hypertension secondary to pulmonary thromboembolism), symptoms resulting from pulmonary congestion are uncommon, and edema, congestive hepatomegaly, and systemic venous distention, i.e., clinical manifestations of *right-sided HF*, are more prominent. When HF has existed for months or years, such localization of excess fluid behind the failing ventricle may no longer exist. For example, patients with long-standing aortic valve disease or systemic hypertension may develop ankle edema, congestive hepatomegaly, and systemic venous distention late in the course of their disease, even though the abnormal hemodynamic burden initially was placed on the left ventricle. This occurs in part because of the secondary pulmonary hypertension and resultant right-sided HF but also because of the retention of salt and water characteristic of HF (Chap. 37). The muscle bundles composing both ventricles are continuous, and both ventricles share a common wall, the interventricular septum. Also, biochemical changes that occur in HF and that may be involved in the impairment of myocardial function (Chap. 231), such as norepinephrine depletion and alterations in the activity of myosin ATPase, occur in the myocardium of *both* ventricles, regardless of the specific chamber on which the abnormal hemodynamic burden is placed initially.

BACKWARD VERSUS FORWARD HEART FAILURE For many years a controversy has revolved around the question of the mechanism of the clinical manifestations resulting from HF. The concept of *backward HF* contends that in HF, one or the other ventricle fails to discharge its contents or fails to fill normally. As a consequence, the pressures in the atrium and venous system behind the failing ventricle rise, and retention of sodium and water occurs as a consequence of the elevation of systemic venous and capillary pressures and the resultant transudation of fluid into the interstitial space (Chap. 37). In contrast, the proponents of the *forward HF* hypothesis maintain that the clinical manifestations of HF result directly from an inadequate discharge of blood into the arterial system. According to this concept, salt and water retention is a consequence of diminished renal perfusion and excessive proximal tubular sodium reabsorption and of excessive distal tubular reabsorption through activation of the renin-angiotensin-aldosterone (RAA) system.

A rigid distinction between *backward* and *forward* HF (like a rigid distinction between right and left HF) is artificial, since both mechanisms appear to operate to varying extents in most patients with HF. However, the rate of onset of HF often influences the clinical manifestations. For example, when a large portion of the left ventricle is suddenly destroyed, as in myocardial infarction, although stroke vol-

ume and blood pressure are suddenly reduced (both manifestations of forward failure), the patient may succumb to acute pulmonary edema, a manifestation of backward failure. If the patient survives the acute insult, clinical manifestations resulting from a chronically depressed cardiac output, including the abnormal retention of fluid within the systemic vascular bed, may develop. Similarly, in the case of massive pulmonary embolism, the right ventricle may dilate and the systemic venous pressure may rise to high levels (backward failure), or the patient may develop shock secondary to low cardiac output (forward failure), but this low-output state may have to be maintained for some days before sodium and water retention sufficient to produce peripheral edema occurs.

REDISTRIBUTION OF CARDIAC OUTPUT In HF, systemic blood flow is redistributed so that the delivery of oxygen to vital organs, such as the brain and myocardium, is maintained at normal or near-normal levels, while flow to less critical areas, such as the cutaneous and muscular beds and the viscera, is reduced. This redistribution serves as an important compensatory mechanism when cardiac output is reduced. It is most marked when a patient with HF exercises, but as HF advances, redistribution occurs even in the basal state. Vasoconstriction mediated by the adrenergic nervous system is largely responsible for redistribution, which in turn may be responsible for many of the clinical manifestations of HF, such as fluid accumulation (reduction of renal blood flow), low-grade fever (reduction of cutaneous flow), and fatigue (reduction of muscle flow).

SALT AND WATER RETENTION (See also Chap. 37) When the volume of blood pumped by the left ventricle into the systemic vascular bed is reduced, a complex sequence of adjustments occurs that ultimately results in the abnormal accumulation of fluid. On the one hand, many of the troubling clinical manifestations of HF are secondary to this excessive retention of fluid; on the other, this abnormal fluid accumulation and the expansion of blood volume that accompanies it also constitute an important compensatory mechanism that tends to maintain cardiac output and therefore perfusion of the vital organs. Except in the terminal stages of HF, the ventricle operates on an ascending, albeit depressed and flattened, function curve (Fig. 231-6, p. 1313), and the augmented ventricular end-diastolic volume and pressure characteristic of HF must be regarded as helping to maintain the reduced cardiac output, despite causing pulmonary and/or systemic venous congestion.

Congestive HF is also characterized by a complex series of neurohumoral adjustments. The activation of the adrenergic nervous system is discussed on p. 1315; there is also activation of the RAA system and increased release of antidiuretic hormone and endothelin. These influences elevate systemic vascular resistance and enhance sodium and water retention and potassium excretion. These actions are, to a minor extent, opposed by the release of atrial and brain natriuretic peptide, which also occurs in congestive HF. Patients with severe HF may exhibit a reduced capacity to excrete a water load, which may result in dilutional hyponatremia. In the presence of HF, effective filling of the systemic arterial bed is reduced, a condition that initiates the renal and hormonal changes mentioned above (Fig. 37-2).

The elevation of systemic venous pressure and the alterations of renal and adrenal function characteristic of HF vary in their relative importance in the production of edema in different patients. The RAA axis is activated most intensely by acute HF, and its activity tends to decline as HF becomes chronic. In patients with tricuspid valve disease or constrictive pericarditis, the elevated venous pressure and the transudation of fluid from systemic capillaries appear to play the dominant role in edema formation. On the other hand, severe edema may be present in patients with ischemic or hypertensive heart disease, in whom systemic venous pressure is within normal limits or is only minimally elevated. In such patients, the retention of salt and water is probably due primarily to a redistribution of cardiac output and a concomitant reduction in renal perfusion, as well as activation of the RAA axis. Regardless of the mechanisms involved in fluid retention, untreated patients with chronic congestive HF have elevations of total blood volume, interstitial fluid volume, and body sodium. These abnormalities diminish after clinical compensation has been achieved by effective treatment, especially with diuretics.

CLINICAL MANIFESTATIONS OF HEART FAILURE

DYSPNEA Respiratory distress that occurs as the result of increased effort in breathing is the most common symptom of HF (Chap. 32). In early HF, dyspnea is observed only during activity, when it may simply represent an aggravation of the breathlessness that occurs normally under these circumstances. As HF advances, however, dyspnea appears with progressively less strenuous activity and ultimately is present even when the patient is at rest. The principal difference between exertional dyspnea in normal persons and in patients with HF is the degree of activity necessary to induce this symptom. Cardiac dyspnea is observed most frequently in patients with elevations of pulmonary venous and capillary pressures. Such patients usually have engorged pulmonary vessels and interstitial pulmonary edema, which may be evident on radiologic examination. This interstitial pulmonary edema reduces the compliance of the lungs and thereby increases the work of the respiratory muscles required to inflate the lungs. The activation of receptors in the lungs results in the rapid, shallow breathing characteristic of cardiac dyspnea. The oxygen cost of breathing is increased by the excessive work of the respiratory muscles. This is coupled with the diminished delivery of oxygen to these muscles, which occurs as a consequence of the reduced cardiac output and which may contribute to fatigue of the respiratory muscles and the sensation of shortness of breath.

Orthopnea Dyspnea in the recumbent position is usually a later manifestation of HF than exertional dyspnea. Orthopnea occurs because of the redistribution of fluid from the abdomen and lower extremities into the chest during recumbency causing an increase in the pulmonary capillary hydrostatic pressure, as well as elevation of the diaphragm accompanying supine posture. Patients with orthopnea must elevate their heads on several pillows at night and frequently awaken short of breath or coughing (the so-called nocturnal cough) if their heads slip off the pillows. The sensation of breathlessness is usually relieved by sitting upright, since this position reduces venous return and pulmonary capillary pressure, and many patients report that they find relief from sitting in front of an open window. In advanced HF, orthopnea may become so severe that patients cannot lie down at all and must spend the entire night in a sitting position. On the other hand, in other patients with long-standing, severe left ventricular failure, symptoms of pulmonary congestion may actually diminish with time as the function of the right ventricle becomes impaired.

Paroxysmal (Nocturnal) Dyspnea This term refers to attacks of severe shortness of breath and coughing that generally occur at night, usually awaken the patient from sleep, and may be quite frightening. Though simple orthopnea may be relieved by sitting upright at the side of the bed with legs dependent, in the patient with paroxysmal nocturnal dyspnea, coughing and wheezing often persist even in this position. Paradoxical nocturnal dyspnea may be caused in part by the depression of the respiratory center during sleep, which may reduce ventilation sufficiently to lower arterial oxygen tension, particularly in patients with interstitial lung edema and reduced pulmonary compliance. Also, ventricular function may be further impaired at night because of reduced adrenergic stimulation of myocardial function. *Cardiac asthma* is closely related to paroxysmal nocturnal dyspnea and nocturnal cough and is characterized by wheezing secondary to bronchospasm—most prominent at night. *Acute pulmonary edema* (Chap. 32) is a severe form of cardiac asthma due to marked elevation of

pulmonary capillary pressure leading to alveolar edema, associated with extreme shortness of breath, rales over the lung fields, and the transudation and expectoration of blood-tinged fluid. If not treated promptly, acute pulmonary edema may be fatal.

CHEYNE-STOKES RESPIRATION Also known as *periodic respiration* or *cyclic respiration*, Cheyne-Stokes respiration is characterized by diminished sensitivity of the respiratory center to arterial P_{CO_2}. There is an apneic phase, during which the arterial P_{O_2} falls and the arterial P_{CO_2} rises. These changes in the arterial blood stimulate the depressed respiratory center, resulting in hyperventilation and hypocapnia, followed in turn by recurrence of apnea. Cheyne-Stokes respiration occurs most often in patients with cerebral atherosclerosis and other cerebral lesions, but the prolongation of the circulation time from the lung to the brain that occurs in HF, particularly in patients with hypertension and coronary artery disease and associated cerebral vascular disease, also appears to precipitate this form of breathing.

FATIGUE AND WEAKNESS These nonspecific but common symptoms of HF are related to the reduction of perfusion of skeletal muscle. Exercise capacity is reduced by the limited ability of the failing heart to increase its output and deliver oxygen to the exercising muscle.

ABDOMINAL SYMPTOMS Anorexia and nausea associated with abdominal pain and fullness are frequent complaints and may be related to the congested liver and portal venous system.

CEREBRAL SYMPTOMS In severe HF, particularly in elderly patients with accompanying cerebral arteriosclerosis, reduced cerebral perfusion, and arterial hypoxemia, there may be alterations in the mental state characterized by confusion, difficulty in concentration, impairment of memory, headache, insomnia, and anxiety. *Nocturia* is common in HF and may contribute to insomnia.

PHYSICAL FINDINGS (See Chap. 225) In moderate HF, the patient is in no distress at rest except that he or she may be uncomfortable when lying flat for more than a few minutes. In more severe HF, the pulse pressure may be diminished, reflecting a reduction in stroke volume, and the diastolic arterial pressure may be elevated as a consequence of generalized vasoconstriction. In acute HF, severe hypotension may be present. There may be cyanosis of the lips and nail beds (Chap. 36) and sinus tachycardia, and the patient may insist on sitting upright. *Systemic venous pressure* is often abnormally elevated in HF, and this may be reflected in distention of the jugular veins. In the early stages of HF, the venous pressure may be normal at rest but may become abnormally elevated during and immediately after exertion as well as with sustained pressure on the abdomen (positive abdominojugular reflux).

Third and fourth heart sounds are often audible but are not specific for HF, and *pulsus alternans*, i.e., a regular rhythm in which there is alternation of strong and weak cardiac contractions and therefore alternation in the strength of the peripheral pulses, may be present. Pulsus alternans, a sign of severe HF, may be detected by sphygmomanometry and in more severe instances by palpation; it frequently follows an extrasystole and is observed most commonly in patients with cardiomyopathy or hypertensive or ischemic heart disease.

Pulmonary Rales Moist, inspiratory, crepitant rales and dullness to percussion over the lung bases are common in patients with HF and elevated pulmonary venous and capillary pressures. In patients with pulmonary edema, rales may be heard widely over both lung fields; they are frequently coarse and sibilant and may be accompanied by expiratory wheezing. Rales may, however, be caused by many conditions other than left ventricular failure. Some patients with long-standing HF have no rales because of increased lymphatic drainage of alveolar fluid.

Cardiac Edema (See Chap. 37) This is usually symmetric and dependent, occurring in the legs, particularly in the pretibial region and ankles in ambulatory patients, in whom it is most prominent in the evening. Cardiac edema occurs in the sacral region of patients who are bed-ridden. Pitting edema of the arms and face occurs rarely and then only late in the course of HF.

Hydrothorax and Ascites Pleural effusion in congestive HF results from the elevation of pleural capillary pressure and transudation of fluid into the pleural cavities. Since the pleural veins drain into *both* the systemic and pulmonary veins, hydrothorax occurs most commonly with marked elevation of pressure in both venous systems but also may be seen with marked elevation of pressure in either venous bed. It is more frequent in the right pleural cavity than in the left. *Ascites* also occurs as a consequence of transudation and results from increased pressure in the hepatic veins and the veins draining the peritoneum (Chap. 46). Marked ascites occurs most frequently in patients with tricuspid valve disease and constrictive pericarditis.

Congestive Hepatomegaly An enlarged, tender, pulsating liver also accompanies systemic venous hypertension and is observed not only in the same conditions in which ascites occurs but also in milder forms of HF from any cause. With prolonged, severe hepatomegaly, as in patients with tricuspid valve disease or chronic constrictive pericarditis, enlargement of the spleen, i.e., congestive splenomegaly, may also occur.

Jaundice This is a late finding in HF and is associated with elevations of both the direct- and indirect-reacting bilirubin; it results from impairment of hepatic function secondary to hepatic congestion and the hepatocellular hypoxia associated with central lobular atrophy. Hepatic enzymes are frequently elevated. If hepatic congestion occurs acutely, the jaundice may be severe and the enzymes strikingly elevated.

Cardiac Cachexia With severe chronic HF there may be serious weight loss and cachexia because of (1) elevation of circulating concentrations of tumor necrosis factor; (2) elevation of the metabolic rate, which results in part from the extra work performed by the respiratory muscles, the increased oxygen needs of the hypertrophied heart, and/or the discomfort associated with severe HF; (3) anorexia, nausea, and vomiting due to central causes, to digitalis intoxication, or to congestive hepatomegaly and abdominal fullness; (4) impairment of intestinal absorption due to congestion of the intestinal veins; and (5) rarely, due to protein-losing enteropathy in patients with particularly severe failure of the right side of the heart.

Other Manifestations With reduction of blood flow, the extremities may be cold, pale, and diaphoretic. Urine flow is depressed, and the urine contains albumin and has a high specific gravity and a low concentration of sodium. In addition, prerenal azotemia may be present. In patients with long-standing severe HF, impotence and depression are common.

ROENTGENOGRAPHIC AND ECHOCARDIOGRAPHIC FINDINGS In addition to the enlargement of the particular chambers characteristic of the lesion responsible for HF, distention of pulmonary veins and redistribution to the apices is common in patients with HF and elevated pulmonary vascular pressures. Also, pleural effusions may be evident and associated with interlobar effusions.

DIFFERENTIAL DIAGNOSIS The diagnosis of congestive HF may be established by observing some combination of the clinical manifestations of HF described above, together with the findings characteristic of one of the etiologic forms of heart disease. Table 232-1 shows the Framingham criteria, which are useful in the diagnosis of HF. Since chronic HF is often associated with cardiac enlargement, the diagnosis should be questioned, but is by no means excluded, when all chambers are normal in size. Two-dimensional echocardiography (Chap. 227) is particularly useful in assessing the dimensions of each cardiac chamber. HF is sometimes difficult to distinguish from pulmonary disease, and the differential diagnosis is discussed in Chap. 32. Pulmonary embolism also presents many of the manifestations of HF, but hemoptysis, pleuritic chest pain, a right ventricular lift, and the characteristic mismatch between ventilation and perfusion on lung scan should point to this diagnosis (Chap. 261).

Ankle edema may be due to varicose veins, cyclic edema, or grav-

Table 232-1 Framingham Criteria for Diagnosis of Congestive Heart Failure[a]

MAJOR CRITERIA

Paroxysmal nocturnal dyspnea
Neck vein distention
Rales
Cardiomegaly
Acute pulmonary edema
S_3 gallop
Increased venous pressure (>16 cmH$_2$O)
Positive hepatojugular reflux

MINOR CRITERIA

Extremity edema
Night cough
Dyspnea on exertion
Hepatomegaly
Pleural effusion
Vital capacity reduced by one-third from normal
Tachycardia (≥120 bpm)

MAJOR OR MINOR

Weight loss ≥4.5 kg over 5 days' treatment

[a] To establish a clinical diagnosis of congestive heart failure by these criteria, at least one major and two minor criteria are required.
SOURCE: KKL Ho et al, Circulation 88:107, 1993.

itational effects (Chap. 37), but in these patients there is no jugular venous hypertension at rest or with pressure over the abdomen. Edema secondary to renal disease can usually be recognized by appropriate renal function tests and urinalysis and is rarely associated with elevation of venous pressure. Enlargement of the liver and ascites occur in patients with hepatic cirrhosis and also may be distinguished from HF by normal jugular venous pressure and absence of a positive abdominojugular reflux.

TREATMENT (See Practice Guidelines) The treatment of HF may be divided into four components: (1) removal of the precipitating cause, (2) correction of the underlying cause, (3) prevention of deterioration of cardiac function, and (4) control of the congestive HF state. The first two components are discussed in other chapters together with each specific disease entity or complication. Examples of removal of precipitating causes are the treatment of pneumococcal pneumonia or the restoration of sinus rhythm in a patient with atrial fibrillation. In many instances, surgical treatment will correct or at least alleviate the underlying cause of HF. The third component of the treatment of HF, i.e., the prevention of deterioration of cardiac function, involves the administration of angiotensin-converting enzyme (ACE) inhibitors and β-adrenergic blockers as well as reduction of cardiac work load. Control of the congestive heart failure state requires reduction of the excessive retention of salt and water as well as enhancement of myocardial contractility. The vigor with which each of these measures is pursued in any individual patient should depend on the severity of HF and the tempo of the disease. Following effective treatment, recurrence of the clinical manifestations of HF can often be prevented by continuing those measures that were originally effective.

While a simple rule for the treatment of all patients with HF cannot be formulated because of its varied etiologies, hemodynamic features, clinical manifestations, and severity of HF, insofar as the treatment of chronic congestive failure is concerned, the administration of an ACE inhibitor retards the development of HF and should be begun early in patients with left ventricular systolic dysfunction (ejection fraction < 0.40), even if they are asymptomatic. Then, as symptoms develop, simple measures such as moderate restriction of activity and sodium intake and oral diuretics should be tried. β-adrenergic receptor blockers and digitalis glycosides are given for patients with systolic HF. If

I. Evaluation
  A. Assess functional status by NY Heart Association classification
  B. Assess fluid status to determine need for diuretics
  C. Assess left ventricular (LV) ejection fraction to distinguish between systolic, diastolic, or combined HF (echocardiography or radionuclide angiography)
  D. Assess invasive hemodynamics in patients unresponsive to treatment and/or transplant candidates

II. Prevention
  A. Control coronary risk factors (Chap. 241)
  B. Institute reperfusion strategies in acute myocardial infarction (Chap. 242)
  C. Prescribe ACE inhibition and/or beta blockade in patients with LV dysfunction without HF

III. General therapeutic measures
  A. Restrict salt intake to <3 g qd
  B. Recommend regular, moderate exercise
  C. Avoid antiarrhythmic agents for asymptomatic arrhythmias
  D. Avoid nonsteroidal anti-inflammatory agents
  E. Provide influenzal and pneumococcal immunization

IV. Diuretics
  A. Administer diuretics for all pts with HF with fluid accumulation to achieve normal jugular venous pressure and relief of edema
  B. Weigh daily to select/adjust dose
  C. Treat diuretic resistance
    1. IV administration
    2. Use ≥2 diuretics in combination (e.g. furosemide and metolazone)
  D. Administer short-term dopamine to enhance renal blood flow

V. ACE inhibitors
  A. Administer to all patients with LV systolic failure and LV dysfunction without heart failure
  B. Contraindications:
    1. High-output angioedema or anuric renal failure
    2. Pregnancy
    3. Hypotension
    4. Creatinine > 265 μmol/L (3 mg/dL)
    5. Serum K > 5.5 mmol/L
    6. Bilateral renal artery stenosis.

VI. β-Adrenergic blockers
  A. Administer to all NYHA class II or III pts with systolic HF, often together with ACE inhibitors and diuretics
  B. Contraindications
    1. Bronchospastic disease
    2. Symptomatic bradycardia or advanced heart block
    3. Instability

VII. Digitalis
  A. Use in pts with LV systolic HF along with diuretics, ACE inhibitors, beta blocker; especially useful in pts with atrial fibrillation

VIII. Other measures
  A. Consider hydralazine-iosorbide combination in patients intolerant of ACE inhibition
  B. Use angiotensin-receptor blocker in pts who develop angioedema or cough with ACE inhibitor
  C. Consider spironolactone in patients with class IV symptoms
  D. Do *not* use calcium antagonists for treatment of heart failure and avoid them for treatment of angina or hypertension in pts with heart failure

IX. Antiarrhythmic therapy
  A. Antiarrhythmic drugs (Chap. 230) are not recommended for pts with asymptomatic or nonsustained ventricular arrhythmias
  B. Class I antiarrhythmics should be avoided except in acute life-threatening arrhythmias
  C. Class III antiarrhythmics, especially amiodarone, may be used to treat atrial arrhythmias but not for the prevention of sudden death.

SOURCE: Modified from Packer and Cohn.

these measures are insufficient, the next step is more rigorous restriction of salt intake and higher doses and multiple diuretics. If HF persists, hospitalization with rigid salt restriction, bed rest, intravenous vasodilators, and positive inotropic agents are tried. Assisted circulation and cardiac transplantation (Chap. 233) are considered for patients with severe, intractable HF and a poor prognosis.

Prevention of Deterioration of Myocardial Infarction Chronic activation of the RAA axis and of the sympathetic nervous systems in HF result in a maladaptive response and cause further deterioration of cardiac function and/or potentially fatal arrhythmias (Chap. 231). Drugs that block these two systems have been found to be useful in the management of HF (Tables 232-2 and 232-3).

Angiotensin-converting enzyme inhibitors In many patients with HF, the left ventricular afterload is increased as a consequence of the several neural and humoral influences that act to constrict the peripheral vascular bed. In addition to the vasoconstriction, the ventricular end-diastolic and -systolic volumes rise in systolic HF. As a consequence of the operation of Laplace's law, which relates myocardial wall tension to the product of intraventricular pressure and radius (both of which may become elevated in HF), the aortic impedance, i.e., the force that opposes left ventricular ejection, or the ventricular afterload, rises, which reduces stroke volume (Fig. 231-10, p. 1316). In many patients with systolic HF, a modest reduction of systemic vascular resistance and afterload elevates the stroke volume and reduces the elevated ventricular filling pressure of the failing ventricle.

The pharmacologic reduction of impedance to left ventricular ejection with an ACE inhibitor represents an important component of the management of HF. This approach may be particularly helpful in (but is by no means limited to) patients with systolic HF due to myocardial infarction (Chap. 243), and in patients with valvular regurgitation (Chap. 236). ACE inhibition should not be used in hypotensive patients. In patients with both acute and chronic systolic HF who are treated with ACE inhibitors, cardiac output rises, the pulmonary wedge pressure falls, the signs and symptoms of HF are relieved, and a new steady state is achieved in which cardiac output is higher and afterload lower with no or only mild reduction of arterial pressure. The administration of ACE inhibitors has been shown to prevent or retard the development of HF in patients with left ventricular dysfunction without HF, to reduce symptoms, enhance exercise performance, and to reduce long-term mortality when they are begun in such patients shortly after acute myocardial infarction. These beneficial effects are related only in part to the salutary hemodynamic effects, i.e., the reduction of preload and afterload. Their major effect appears to be on inhibition of local (tissue) renin-angiotensin systems.

Lisinopril in doses of 20 mg qd or enalapril 10 mg bid have been shown to be useful in the management of heart failure.

Angiotensin Receptor Blockers In patients who cannot tolerate ACE inhibitors (because of cough, angioneurotic edema, leukopenia),

Table 232-2   Overview of Angiotensin-Converting Enzyme Inhibitors in Heart Failure

	Odds Ratio	95% Confidence Interval
Total mortality	0.77	0.67–0.88
Mortality or hospitalization	0.65	0.57–0.74
Progressive heart failure	0.69	0.58–0.83
Sudden death	0.91	0.73–1.12
Fatal myocardial infarction	0.82	0.60–1.11
Total mortality		
Class 1	0.75	0.46–1.23
Class 2	0.83	0.68–1.01
Class 3	0.76	0.60–0.96
Class 4	0.55	0.36–0.84
EF >0.25	0.98	0.78–1.23
EF ≤0.25	0.69	0.57–0.85

NOTE: EF, ejection fraction
SOURCE: From Garg and Yusuf. Copyright 1995, American Medical Association.

	Beta Blockade		Aldosterone Antagonist
Trial name	CIBIS II	MERIT-HF	RALES
Drug	Bisoprolol (B1 selective)	Metoprolol (B1 selective)	Spironolactone
Age (avg, years)	61	64	65
CAD%	50	65	54
Male %	80	77	73
NYHA II %		41	
III %	83	55	71
IV	17	4	29
ACE I %	90	90	95
LVEF %	28	28	<35%
Placebo Annual mortality, %	13	10	22
Mortality reduction			
All cause	34	34	30
Sudden death	42	41	29
Pump failure death	26	49	36
Hospital admissions for HF	32		35

an angiotensin II receptor blocker (type AT1) antagonist (e.g., losartan 50 mg qid) may be used instead.

Aldosterone Antagonist The activation of the RAA axis in HF increases not only circulating and tissue angiotensin II but also aldosterone. The latter, in addition to causing sodium retention and worsening edema (Chaps. 331 and 37), causes sympathetic activation, myocardial, vascular, and perivascular fibrosis and reduces arterial compliance. In one large multicenter trial in patients with advanced heart failure and reduced ejection fraction (RALES), spironolactone, 25 mg/d reduced total mortality, as well as sudden death and death from pump failure (Table 232-3). Since spironolactone is also a useful diuretic (see below), its widespread use in systolic heart failure should be considered.

β-adrenoceptor blockers While the abrupt administration of large doses of β-adrenergic receptor blockers can intensify HF, the administration of gradually escalating doses of metoprolol, carvedilol, and bisoprolol have been reported to improve the symptoms of HF, and to reduce all-cause death, cardiovascular death, sudden death, and pump failure death (Table 232-3). In patients with moderately severe HF (classes II and III), the administration of 12.5 mg metoprolol CR/XL qd, increasing over 4 weeks to a target dose of 200 mg qid, has been shown to be beneficial. β-Adrenoceptor blockers are not indicated in HF patients who are unstable, in New York Heart Association Class IV, in HF patients shortly after acute myocardial infarction, or in those with HF and normal ejection fraction, i.e., with diastolic HF.

Reduction of Cardiac Work Load This consists of reducing physical activity, instituting emotional rest, and reducing afterload (see above). Modest restriction of physical activity in mild cases and rest in bed or in a chair in severe failure are useful. In acute, severe failure, meals should be small in quantity, but more frequent, and every effort should be made to diminish the patient's anxiety; sometimes drugs such as diazepam (2 to 5 mg tid) for several days are useful. Physical and emotional rest tends to lower arterial pressure and reduce the load on the myocardium by diminishing the requirements for cardiac output.

Reduced physical exertion should be continued for several days after the patient's condition has stabilized. The hazards of phlebothrombosis and pulmonary embolism which occur with bed rest may be reduced with anticoagulants, leg exercises, and elastic stockings. *Absolute* bed rest is rarely required or advisable, and the patient should ordinarily be encouraged to sit in a chair. Heavy sedation should be avoided. In ambulatory patients with chronic, moderately severe HF, additional periods of rest on weekends frequently allow continuation of gainful employment. Following recovery from HF, the patient's activities should be assessed, and often, professional, community, and/or family responsibilities should be curtailed. Intermittent rest during the day (e.g., a scheduled 1-h nap or rest following lunch) and the avoidance of strenuous exertion are often helpful. Regular, nonexhausting exercise such as walking or riding a stationary-bicycle ergometer as tolerated should be employed once the patient has become compensated. Weight reduction by restriction of caloric intake in obese patients with HF also diminishes cardiac work load and is an essential component of the therapeutic program.

Control of Excessive Fluid Many of the clinical manifestations of HF result from expansion of the extracellular fluid volume. A negative sodium balance can be achieved by reducing the dietary intake and increasing the urinary excretion of this ion with the aid of diuretics. Rarely, in severe HF, mechanical removal of extracellular fluid by means of thoracentesis and paracentesis may be necessary.

Diet In patients with mild HF, symptomatic improvement may result simply from reducing the sodium intake, particularly if accompanied by periods of physical rest. The normal diet contains approximately 6 to 10 g sodium chloride; this intake can be reduced by half simply by excluding salt-rich foods and salt added at the table. Reduction of the ordinary dietary intake to approximately one-fourth of normal may be achieved if, in addition, all salt is omitted from cooking. In patients with severe HF who have fluid accumulation despite diuretic therapy (see below), the dietary intake of sodium chloride should be reduced to between 500 and 1000 mg, and in order to achieve this, milk, cheese, bread, cereals, canned vegetables and soups, some salted cuts of meat, and some fresh vegetables (including spinach, celery, and beets) must be eliminated. A variety of fresh fruit, green vegetables, specially processed breads and milk, and salt substitutes are permissible. Late in the course of HF, dilutional hyponatremia may develop in patients who are unable to excrete a water load, sometimes because of excessive secretion of antidiuretic hormone. In such cases, water intake as well as sodium intake must be restricted.

Calories should be restricted in obese patients with HF. In patients with severe HF and cardiac cachexia, on the other hand, an attempt must be made to maintain nutritional intake and to avoid caloric and vitamin deficiencies; nutritional supplements may be in order.

Diuretics Diuretics should be given to relieve fluid accumulation and thus reduce or prevent edema and jugular venous distention. A variety of diuretic agents are available (Table 246-6, p. 1422), and almost all are effective in patients with mild HF. However, in the more severe forms of HF, the selection of diuretics is more difficult, and abnormalities in serum electrolytes must be taken into account. Overtreatment must be avoided, since the resultant hypovolemia may reduce cardiac output, interfere with renal function, and produce profound weakness and lethargy.

THIAZIDE DIURETICS These agents are used widely and are useful by themselves in patients with mild HF and in combination with other diuretics in those with severe HF. In patients with chronic mild or moderate HF, the continued administration of a thiazide diuretic abolishes or diminishes the need for rigid dietary sodium restriction, although salty foods and table salt still should be avoided. Thiazide diuretics reduce the reabsorption of sodium and chloride in the first half of the distal convoluted tubule and a portion of the cortical ascending limb of the loop of Henle, and water follows the unreabsorbed salt. Thiazides fail to increase free water clearance and in some instances reduce it. This may result in the excretion of a hypertonic urine and may contribute to dilutional hyponatremia. As a consequence of increased delivery of sodium to the distal nephron, sodium-potassium ion exchange is enhanced, and kaliuresis results. In contrast to the loop diuretics, which enhance calcium excretion, the thiazides have the opposite effect.

Thiazide diuretics are effective and useful in the treatment of HF as long as the glomerular filtration rate exceeds approximately 50% of normal. Chlorothiazide is administered in doses of up to 500 mg every 6 h. Many derivatives of this compound are available but differ principally in dosage and duration of action. Chlorthalidone (25 to 50 mg/d) is especially useful since it may be administered once daily.

Potassium depletion and metabolic alkalosis (the latter due to increased H⁺ secretion as a substitute for the depleted intracellular stores of potassium) are the chief adverse metabolic effects following prolonged administration of the thiazides, of metolazone, and of the loop diuretics. Hypokalemia may seriously enhance the dangers of digitalis intoxication (see below), and induce fatigue and lethargy; these may be prevented by oral supplementation with potassium chloride or preferably by the addition of a potassium-retaining diuretic, such as a spironolactone or triamterene. Other side effects of thiazides include reduction of the excretion of uric acid, which may lead to hyperuricemia, and impaired glucose tolerance, which rarely may precipitate hyperosmolar coma in poorly regulated diabetic patients. Skin rashes, thrombocytopenia, and granulocytopenia have also been reported.

METOLAZONE   This quinethazone derivative has a site of action and potency similar to those of the thiazides but has been reported to be effective in the presence of moderate renal failure. The usual dose is 5 to 10 mg/d. Metolazone may be added to thiazide and loop diuretics in severe HF.

FUROSEMIDE, BUMETANIDE, ETHACRYNIC ACID, PIRETANIDE, AND TORSEMIDE   These "loop" diuretics are similar physiologically but differ chemically from one another. These drugs reversibly inhibit the reabsorption of sodium, potassium, and chloride in the thick ascending limb of Henle's loop, apparently by blocking a cotransport system in the luminal membrane. They may induce renal cortical vasodilatation and can produce rates of urine formation that may be as high as one-fourth of the glomerular filtration rate. Metabolic alkalosis may be caused by a large increase in the urinary excretion of chloride, hydrogen, and potassium ions. Hypokalemia, hyperuricemia, and hyperglycemia are observed occasionally, as with thiazide diuretics. The reabsorption of free water is decreased. All five of these drugs are readily absorbed orally, are excreted in the bile and urine, and are usually effective both intravenously and by mouth. Weakness, nausea, and dizziness may complicate the administration of all loop diuretics; ethacrynic acid has been associated with transient or even permanent deafness as well as with skin rash and granulocytopenia.

These powerful diuretics are useful in all forms of HF, particularly in patients with otherwise refractory HF and pulmonary edema. They have been shown to be effective in patients with hypoalbuminemia, hyponatremia, hypochloremia, hypokalemia, and with reductions in the glomerular filtration rate and to produce a diuresis in patients in whom thiazide diuretics and aldosterone antagonists, alone and in combination, are ineffective. In patients with refractory HF, the action of loop diuretics may be potentiated by intravenous administration and by the addition of other diuretics, i.e., thiazides, metozalone, osmotic diuretics, and the potassium-sparing diuretics—spironolactone, triamterene, and amiloride.

ALDOSTERONE ANTAGONISTS   These agents act on the cortical collecting ducts, are relatively weak, and therefore are rarely indicated as sole agents. However, their potassium-sparing properties make them particularly useful in conjunction with the more potent kaliuretic agents, i.e., the loop diuretics, thiazides, and metozalone. The potassium-sparing agents fall into two classes.

The spironolactones resemble aldosterone structurally and act by competitive inhibition of aldosterone, thereby blocking the exchange between sodium and both potassium and hydrogen in the distal tubules and collecting ducts. These agents produce a sodium diuresis, and in contrast to the thiazides, ethacrynic acid, and furosemide, they result in potassium retention. Although secondary hyperaldosteronism exists in some patients with congestive HF, the spironolactones are effective even in patients in whom the serum aldosterone concentration is within normal limits.

Spironolactone may be administered in doses of 25 mg daily to 50 mg three to four times daily by mouth. The maximal effect of this regimen is not observed for approximately 4 days. Spironolactones are most effective when administered in combination with loop and/or thiazide diuretics. The opposing action of these drugs on urine and serum potassium makes possible a sodium diuresis without either hyper- or hypokalemia when spironolactone and one of these other agents are administered in combination. Also, since spironolactone, triamterene, and amiloride act on the distal tubule, they are particularly effective when used in combination with one of these other diuretics that act more proximally. Spironolactone, triamterene, and amiloride should not be administered alone to patients with hyperkalemia, renal failure, or hyponatremia. Reported complications of Aldactone A include nausea, epigastric distress, mental confusion, drowsiness, gynecomastia, and erythematous eruptions.

As mentioned above, a lower dose of spironolactone (25 mg/d), which exerts little if any diuretic effect, has been shown to prolong life in patients with advanced HF (Table 232-3).

Triamterene and *amiloride* exert renal effects similar to those of the spironolactones; i.e., they block sodium reabsorption and secondarily inhibit potassium secretion in the distal tubules. However, their action does not depend on the presence of aldosterone. The effective dose of triamterene is 100 mg once or twice daily, and that of amiloride is 5 mg daily. Side effects include nausea, vomiting, diarrhea, headache, granulocytopenia, eosinophilia, and skin rash. Both triamterene and the chemically unrelated diuretic amiloride resemble Aldactone A in that their diuretic potency is not great, but they are effective in preventing the hypokalemia characteristic of loop diuretics and thiazides. A number of diuretic preparations contain a combination of a thiazide and either triamterene or amiloride in a single capsule. They may be useful in patients who develop hypokalemia with a thiazide but should not be used in patients with impaired renal function and/or hyperkalemia.

When *choosing a diuretic*, orally administered loop diuretics or thiazides are the agents of choice in the treatment of chronic cardiac edema of mild to moderate degree in patients without hyperglycemia, hyperuricemia, or hypokalemia. Spironolactones, triamterene, and amiloride are not potent diuretics when used alone, but they potentiate the thiazide and loop diuretics. Loop diuretics, given alone or with spironolactone or triamterene, are the agents of choice in patients with severe HF refractory to other diuretics. In very severe HF, the combination of a loop diuretic, a thiazide, and a potassium-sparing diuretic is required.

Vasodilators   Direct vasodilators may be useful in patients with severe, acute HF who demonstrate systemic vasoconstriction despite ACE inhibitor therapy. The ideal vasodilator for the treatment of *acute* HF should have a rapid onset and brief duration of action when administered by intravenous infusion; sodium nitroprusside (0.1 to 3.0 μg/kg per minute) qualifies as such a drug, but its use requires careful monitoring of the arterial pressure and, if possible, of the pulmonary artery wedge pressure. The combination of hydralazine (up to 300 mg qd orally) and isosorbide diuretics (up to 160 mg qd orally) may be useful for chronic oral administration.

Enhancement of Myocardial Contractility • *Digitalis*   The improvement of myocardial contractility by means of cardiac glycosides is useful in the control of HF. *Digoxin*, which has a half-life of 1.6 days, is filtered in the glomeruli and secreted by the renal tubules. Significant reductions of the glomerular filtration rate reduce the elimination of digoxin and, therefore, may prolong digoxin's effect, allowing it to accumulate to toxic levels. In patients with normal renal function, a plateau concentration in the blood and tissue is reached after 5 days of daily maintenance treatment without a loading dose (see Fig. 70-2).

MECHANISM OF ACTION   The most important effect of digitalis on cardiac muscle is to shift its force-velocity relation upward (Fig. 231-5, p. 1313). Cardiac glycosides inhibit the monovalent cation transport enzyme–coupled Na⁺,K⁺-ATPase and increase intracellular sodium content; this, in turn, increases intracellular Ca^{2+} through a

Na^+-Ca^{2+} exchange carrier mechanism. The increased myocardial uptake of Ca^{2+} augments Ca^{2+} released to the myofilaments during excitation and, therefore, invokes a positive inotropic response.

Cardiac glycosides also produce alterations in the electrical properties of both the contractile cells and the specialized automatic cells, leading to increased automaticity and ectopic impulse activity. They also prolong the effective *refractory period* of the atrioventricular node and thereby slow ventricular rate in atrial flutter and fibrillation.

USE IN HEART FAILURE Digitalis is particularly effective in patients with systolic HF complicated by atrial flutter and fibrillation and a rapid ventricular rate, who benefit from both slowing of the ventricular rate and the positive inotropic effect. Although digitalis does not improve survival in patients with systolic HF and sinus rhythm, it reduces the need for hospitalization. By stimulating myocardial contractility moderately, digitalis improves ventricular emptying; i.e., it increases cardiac output, augments the ejection fraction, promotes diuresis, and reduces the elevated diastolic pressure and volume and the end-systolic volume of the failing ventricle. This action reduces symptoms resulting from pulmonary vascular congestion and elevated systemic venous pressure. Digitalis is of little or no value in patients with HF, sinus rhythm, and the following conditions: hypertrophic cardiomyopathy, myocarditis, mitral stenosis, chronic constrictive pericarditis, and any form of diastolic HF.

The maintenance dose of digoxin is 0.25 mg qd for most adults; in the elderly and others with mild impairment of renal function, it is 0.125 mg qd. Loading doses, four times the maintenance dose, may be administered in acute systolic failure.

DIGITALIS INTOXICATION This is a serious and potentially fatal complication. Advanced age, acute myocardial infarction or ischemia, hypoxemia, magnesium depletion, renal insufficiency, hypercalcemia, electrical cardioversion, and hypothyroidism all may reduce tolerance to digitalis. The most common precipitating cause of digitalis intoxication, however, is depletion of potassium stores, which often occurs in patients with HF as a result of diuretic therapy and secondary hyperaldosteronism.

Anorexia, nausea, and vomiting are among the earliest signs of digitalis intoxication. The most frequent disturbances of cardiac rhythm are ventricular premature beats, bigeminy, ventricular tachycardia, and, rarely, ventricular fibrillation. Atrioventricular block of varying degrees of severity may occur. Nonparoxysmal atrial tachycardia with variable atrioventricular block is characteristic of digitalis intoxication. Chronic digitalis intoxication may be insidious in onset and characterized by exacerbations of HF, weight loss, cachexia, neuralgias, gynecomastia, yellow vision, and delirium.

The administration of quinidine, verapamil, amiodarone, and propafenone to patients receiving digoxin raises the serum concentration of the latter by reducing both the renal and nonrenal elimination of digoxin and by reducing its volume of distribution. These drugs increase the propensity to digitalis intoxication, and the dose of digitalis should be reduced by half in patients receiving these drugs.

TREATMENT OF DIGITALIS INTOXICATION When tachyarrhythmias result from digitalis intoxication, withdrawal of the drug and treatment with β-adrenoceptor blocker or lidocaine are indicated. If hypokalemia is present, potassium should be administered cautiously and by the oral route. Fab fragments of purified, intact digitalis antibodies are a potentially lifesaving approach to the treatment of severe intoxication.

Sympathomimetic amines (See also Chap. 72) Two sympathomimetic amines that act largely on β-adrenergic receptors—dopamine and dobutamine—improve myocardial contractility (Table 72-1) and are effective in the management of HF; they must be administered by constant intravenous infusion for up to 1 week and are useful in patients with intractable, severe HF, particularly those with a reversible component, such as exists in patients who have undergone cardiac surgery, in patients with acute myocardial infarction and shock or pulmonary edema, and in patients with refractory HF as a "bridge" to transplantation. While these sympathomimetic amines improve the hemodynamics and symptoms in these conditions, it is not clear that they

improve survival. Their administration should be accompanied by careful and continuous monitoring of the electrocardiogram, arterial pressure, and, if possible, pulmonary artery wedge pressure.

Dopamine is a naturally occurring immediate precursor of norepinephrine and has a combination of actions that makes it particularly useful in the treatment of a variety of hypotensive states of HF. At very low doses, i.e., 1 to 2 (μg/kg)/min, it dilates renal and mesenteric blood vessels through stimulation of specific dopaminergic receptors, thereby augmenting renal and mesenteric blood flow and sodium excretion. In the range of 2 to 10 (μg/kg)/min, dopamine stimulates myocardial β_1 receptors but induces relatively little tachycardia, while at higher doses it also stimulates α-adrenergic receptors and elevates arterial pressure.

Dobutamine is a synthetic catecholamine that acts on β_1, β_2, and α receptors. It exerts a potent inotropic action, has only a modest cardioaccelerating effect, and lowers peripheral vascular resistance, but since it simultaneously raises cardiac output, it may not lower systemic arterial pressure in patients with severe HF. Dobutamine, given in continuous infusions of 2.5 to 10 (μg/kg)/min, is useful in the treatment of acute HF without hypotension.

A major problem with sympathomimetics is the loss of responsiveness, apparently due to "downregulation" of adrenergic receptors, which becomes evident within 8 h of continuous administration. This problem may be managed by intermittent therapy.

Phosphodiesterase inhibitors These bipyridines, amrinone and milrinone, are noncatecholamine, nonglycoside agents that exert both positive inotropic and vasodilator actions by inhibiting a specific phosphodiesterase. They are suitable for intravenous use only; by simultaneously stimulating cardiac contractility and dilating the systemic vascular bed they reverse the major hemodynamic abnormalities associated with intractable HF. Amrinone and milrinone may be administered for the same conditions in which sympathomimetics are useful and may be employed together with dopamine or dobutamine.

Other Measures • *Anticoagulants* Patients with severe HF are at increased risk of pulmonary emboli secondary to venous thrombosis and of systemic emboli secondary to intracardiac thrombi and should be treated with warfarin. Patients with HF and atrial fibrillation, previous venous thrombosis, and pulmonary or systemic emboli are at especially high risk and should receive heparin followed by warfarin.

Diastolic heart failure The major goal in the treatment of this condition is to eliminate or reduce the causes of diastolic dysfunction, such as ventricular hypertrophy, fibrosis, or ischemia. The second is to reduce pulmonary and/or systemic venous congestion, a major consequence of diastolic dysfunction.

Management of arrhythmias (See also Chap. 230) Premature ventricular contractions and episodes of asymptomatic ventricular tachycardia are common in advanced HF. Sudden death, presumably due to ventricular fibrillation, is responsible for about one-half of all deaths in this condition. (The remainder are due to failure of the cardiac pump.) The management of arrhythmias should commence with correction of electrolyte and acid-base disturbances (Chaps. 49 and 50), especially diuretic-induced hypokalemia, as well as digitalis intoxication (see above). Treatment with class I antiarrhythmics such as quinidine, procainamide, or flecainide (Chap. 230) is fraught with danger because these drugs are proarrhythmic in patients with HF. Amiodarone, a class III antiarrhythmic, on the other hand, is well tolerated and is the drug of choice for patients with heart failure and atrial fibrillation. Patients who have been resuscitated from sudden death, those with syncope or presyncope due to ventricular arrhythmias, and those with asymptomatic ventricular tachyarrhythmias in whom ventricular tachycardia can be induced during electrophysiologic testing should be considered for the implantable automatic defibrillator. This may prevent recurrence of the arrhythmia and sudden death; back-up pacing may prevent sudden death due to bradyarrhythmias.

Refractory heart failure When the response to ordinary treatment is inadequate, HF is considered to be refractory. Before assuming that this condition simply reflects advanced, terminal, myocardial depression, careful consideration must be given to several possibilities: (1) an underlying and overlooked cause of the heart disease that may be amenable to specific surgical or medical therapy, such as infective endocarditis, hypertension, thyrotoxicosis, or silent aortic or mitral stenosis; (2) one or a combination of the precipitating causes of HF, such as pulmonary or urinary tract infection, recurrent pulmonary emboli, arterial hypoxemia, anemia, or arrhythmia; and (3) complications of overly vigorous therapy, such as digitalis intoxication, hypovolemia, or electrolyte imbalance. Recognition and proper treatment of the aforementioned complications are likely to restore responsiveness to therapy.

Hyponatremia is a manifestation of advanced refractory HF. It may be a complication of overaggressive diuresis leading to reduced glomerular filtration rate and decreased delivery of NaCl to the diluting sites in the distal tubule. Hyponatremia may also result from nonosmotic stimuli for the continued secretion of antidiuretic hormone. Therapy involves improvement of the cardiovascular status, if possible (sometimes requiring the administration of a sympathomimetic amine), as well as temporary cessation of diuretic therapy and restriction of oral water intake. Hypertonic saline is very rarely indicated because total-body sodium is usually elevated, not depressed, in HF.

The combination of the intravenously administered vasodilator sodium nitroprusside, a phosphodiesterase inhibitor (amrinone or milrinone), together with a sympathomimetic amine (dopamine or dobutamine) often results in additive effects, raising cardiac output and lowering filling pressure.

In hospitalized patients with refractory HF, therapy guided by hemodynamic measurements provided by a balloon flotation (Swan-Ganz) catheter may be helpful. The goal of manipulating diuretics, vasodilators, and inotropic agents is to achieve a pulmonary capillary wedge pressure of 15 to 18 mmHg, a right atrial pressure of 5 to 8 mmHg, a cardiac index > 2.2 (L/min)/m^2, and a systemic vascular resistance of 800 to 1200 dyne $\cdot$ s/cm^5. Once these values are achieved, an attempt should be made to convert the patient from intravenous to oral vasodilator therapy.

Assisted circulation/cardiac transplantation When patients with HF become unresponsive to a combination of all the aforementioned therapeutic measures, are in New York Heart Association class IV, and are deemed unlikely to survive 1 year, they should be considered for temporary assisted circulation and/or cardiac transplantation (see Chap. 233).

Treatment of Acute Pulmonary Edema Pulmonary edema secondary to left ventricular failure or mitral stenosis is described in Chap. 32. It is life-threatening and must be considered a medical emergency. As is the case for the more chronic forms of HF, in the treatment of pulmonary edema, attention must be directed to identifying and removing any precipitating causes of decompensation, such as an arrhythmia or infection. However, because of the acute nature of the problem, a number of additional nonspecific measures are necessary. If it does not delay treatment unduly, recording pulmonary vascular pressures through a Swan-Ganz catheter and intraarterial pressure directly is advisable. The first six measures listed below are ordinarily applied simultaneously or nearly so.

1. Morphine is administered intravenously repetitively, as needed, in doses from 2 to 5 mg. This drug reduces anxiety, reduces adrenergic vasoconstrictor stimuli to the arteriolar and venous beds, and thereby helps to break a vicious cycle. Naloxone should be available in case respiratory depression occurs.
2. Because the alveolar edema interferes with O$_2$ diffusion resulting in arterial hypoxemia, 100% O$_2$ should be administered, preferably under positive pressure. The latter increases intraalveolar pressure, reduces transudation of fluid from the alveolar capillaries, and impedes venous return to the thorax, reducing pulmonary capillary pressure.

3. The patient should be maintained in the sitting position, with the legs dangling along the side of the bed, if possible, which tends to reduce venous return.
4. Intravenous loop diuretics, such as furosemide or ethacrynic acid (40 to 100 mg) or bumetanide (1 mg), will, by rapidly establishing a diuresis, reduce circulating blood volume and thereby hasten the relief of pulmonary edema. In addition, when given intravenously, furosemide also exerts a venodilator action, reduces venous return, and thereby improves pulmonary edema even before the diuresis commences.
5. Afterload reduction is achieved with intravenous sodium nitroprusside at 20 to 30 μg/min in patients whose systolic arterial pressures exceed 100 mmHg.
6. Inotropic support should be provided by dopamine or dobutamine as described on p. 1327. Patients with systolic HF who are not receiving digitalis should receive 0.75 to 1.0 mg digoxin intravenously over 15 min.
7. Sometimes, aminophylline (theophylline ethylenediamine), 240 to 480 mg intravenously, is effective in diminishing bronchoconstriction, increasing renal blood flow and sodium excretion, and augmenting myocardial contractility.
8. If the above-mentioned measures are not sufficient, rotating tourniquets should be applied to the extremities.

After these emergency measures have been instituted and the precipitating factors treated, the diagnosis of the underlying cardiac disorder responsible for the pulmonary edema must be established, if it is not already known. After stabilization of the patient's condition, a long-range strategy for prevention of future episodes of pulmonary edema must be established, and this may require surgical treatment.

PROGNOSIS

The prognosis in patients with HF depends primarily on the nature of the underlying heart disease and on the presence or absence of a precipitating factor that can be treated. When one of the latter can be identified and removed, the outlook for immediate survival is far better than if HF occurs without any obvious precipitating cause. In the latter situation, survival usually ranges between 6 months and 4 years depending on the severity (Fig. 232-2). The long-term prognosis is more favorable when the underlying forms of heart disease, e.g., valvular heart disease, can be treated effectively. The prognosis can be estimated by observing the response to treatment. When clinical improvement occurs with only modest dietary sodium restriction and small doses of diuretics, the outlook is far better than if, in addition to these measures, intensive diuretic therapy and vasodilators are necessary. Other factors that have been shown to be associated with a poor prog-

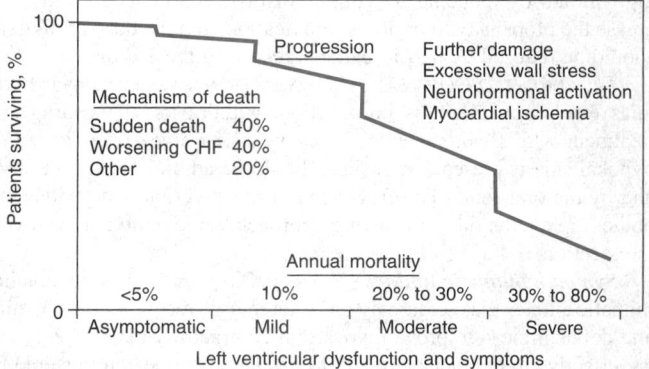

FIGURE 232-2 The natural history of congestive heart failure (CHF). Once left ventricular systolic dysfunction is present, it usually progresses, albeit not predictably. As left ventricular dysfunction progresses and symptoms increase, mortality rate increases and the process becomes inexorable. Myocyte loss and fibrosis become irreversible. An effective preventive measure must be introduced before onset or early in the course of progressive left ventricular dysfunction. *(From Massie and Shah, with permission.)*

nosis include a severely depressed ejection fraction ($<25\%$), a reduced maximal O_2 uptake [<10 (mL/kg)/min], the inability to walk on the level and at a normal pace for more than 3 min, reduced (<133 mEq/L) serum sodium concentration, reduced (<3 mEq/L) serum potassium concentration, elevated circulating atrial and brain natriuretic peptide and norepinephrine concentrations, as well as frequent ventricular extrasystoles. A large fraction of patients with HF die suddenly, presumably of ventricular fibrillation. Unfortunately, there is no evidence that this complication can be prevented by the administration of antiarrhythmic agents. See guideline material.

BIBLIOGRAPHY

BRISTOW M et al: Clinical management of heart failure, in *Heart Disease*, 6th ed, E Braunwald (ed). Philadelphia, Saunders, 2001

BRISTOW MR: Beta adrenergic receptor blockade in chronic heart failure. Circulation 101: 558, 2000

CIBIS II INVESTIGATORS AND COMMITTEES: The Cardiac Insufficiency Bisoprolol Study II (CIBIS II): A randomised trial. Lancet 353:9–13, 1999

COLUCCI WS, BRAUNWALD E (eds): *Heart Failure: Cardiac Function and Dysfunction*, in *Atlas of Heart Diseases*, 2d ed, E Braunwald (series ed). Philadelphia, Current Medicine, 1999

COLUCCI WS et al: Clinical aspects of heart failure, in *Heart Disease*, 6th ed, E Braunwald (ed). Philadelphia, Saunders, 2001

FRANCIS GS et al: Neurohumoral activation in preclinical heart failure. Remodeling and the potential for intervention. Circulation 87 (Suppl 5):IV90, 1993

GARG R, YUSUF S: Overview of randomized trials of angiotensin-converting enzyme inhibitors on mortality and morbidity in patients with heart failure. Collaborative Group on ACE Inhibitor Trials. JAMA 274:462, 1995

GHEORGHIADE M et al: Current medical therapy for advanced heart failure. Heart Lung 29:16, 2000

KUBO SH, COHN JN: Long-term treatment of the ambulatory patient with heart failure, in *Cardiovascular Therapeutics*, TW Smith (ed). Philadelphia, Saunders, 1996, pp 210–231

MASSIE BM, SHAH NH: The heart failure epidemic: Magnitude of the problem and potential mitigating approaches. Curr Opin Cardiol 11:221, 1996

MERIT-HF STUDY GROUP: Effect of metoprolol CR/XL in chronic heart failure: Metoprolol CR/XL Randomised Intervention Trial in Congestive Heart Failure (MERIT-HF). Lancet 353:2001, 1999

PACKER M, COHN JN (eds): Consensus recommendations for the management of chronic heart failure. Am J Cardiol 83:1a-38a, 1999

PITT B et al: The effect of spironolactone on morbidity and mortality in patients with severe heart failure. N Engl J Med 341:709, 1999

WILCOX CS: Diuretics, in *The Kidney*, 6th ed, BM Brenner (ed). Philadelphia, Saunders, 2000, pp 2219–2252

233

John S. Schroeder

CARDIAC TRANSPLANTATION

Orthotopic allograft cadaver cardiac transplantation as a treatment for end-stage cardiac disease achieved its thirty-third anniversary on December 7, 2000. On that day in 1967 Dr. Christiaan Barnard accomplished the first successful cardiac transplant in a human, quickly followed by Dr. Norman Shumway and Dr. Richard Lower at Stanford University. After an initial early wave of enthusiasm, the problems of immunosuppression slowed application of the procedure until the introduction of cyclosporine in 1980. A subsequent worldwide expansion of cardiac transplantation has resulted in approximately 2500 cardiac transplants per year, with further increases limited only by the donor supply. Current 1- and 5-year survival rates of 85 and 70% indicate that cardiac transplantation is the therapy of choice in patients with end-stage heart disease who are unlikely to survive the next 6 to 12 months.

INDICATIONS AND SELECTION OF CANDIDATES

The limited donor supply and relatively high cost of cardiac transplantation have restricted it to patients most likely to survive and re-

sume a functional life after transplantation. It is estimated that only 2000 potential donors in the United States, for a pool of at least 20,000 candidates based on current guidelines, become available yearly. Attempts to increase donor awareness in both physicians and the public are being made. Optimal candidates for this procedure are those who would be expected to return to a functional life if their hearts were replaced (Table 233-1). This requires a mentally vigorous, medically compliant person who has not suffered extensive other end-stage organ damage from cardiac failure, does not have other systemic disease such as severe diabetes mellitus or collagen vascular disease, or is not positive for HIV. Long-standing pulmonary hypertension or recurrent pulmonary emboli and infarction may result in irreversible pulmonary hypertension leading to intraoperative death. Several heart transplant centers have initiated cardiac transplantation for newborns with left ventricular hypoplasia, but long-term survival experience is still very limited.

Timing of the recommendation to undergo cardiac transplantation can be difficult and requires assessment of the patient's current disability, stability of course, and likelihood of surviving the next 6 to 12 months. Generally, left ventricular ejection fractions under 15 to 20% and presence of serious ventricular arrhythmias indicate a 1-year survival rate of 50% or less. Estimating prognosis remains very challenging. A maximal oxygen uptake during exercise (maximal $\dot{V}_{O_2}$) of <10 mL O_2 per kilogram per minute usually indicates poor likelihood of survival for 1 year and has been a criterion for transplant candidacy in some programs. Maximal $\dot{V}_{O_2}$ values between 10 and 14 mL O_2 per kilogram per minute are in a borderline range, with values >14 usually predicting good 1- to 2-year survival. The increasing acceptance of cardiac transplantation as a treatment modality for heart failure without a corresponding increase in donor availability has led to prolonged waiting times of as much as 2 years or more. This longer waiting time has led to more rigorous medical care of the patient awaiting transplant with meticulous monitoring of electrolytes, fluid status, and overall well-being. Aggressive therapy for congestive heart failure with high-dose angiotensin-converting enzyme inhibitors and beta blockers and meticulous monitoring of serum electrolytes and renal function have led to stabilization and many times some improvement in the functional status of patients awaiting a donor. This has led to as many as 30 to 40% of listed patients being placed "on hold" based on their improved status. Whether these patients can maintain their improved

---

Table 233-1   Indications and Contraindications for Cardiac Transplantation

Indications
1. End-stage heart disease that limits prognosis for survival over 2 years or severely limits daily quality of life despite optimal medical and other surgical therapy
2. No secondary exclusion criteria
3. Suitable psychosocial profile and social support system
4. Suitable physiologic/chronologic age

Exclusion Criteria
1. Active infectious process
2. Recent pulmonary infarction
3. Insulin-requiring diabetes with evidence of end-organ damage
4. Irreversible pulmonary hypertension [pulmonary vascular resistance (PVR) poorly responsive to nitroprusside with PVR > 2 or pulmonary systolic pressure > 50 mmHg at peak dose or at mean arterial pressure of 65–70 mmHg]
5. Presence of circulating cytotoxic antibodies
6. Presence of active peptic ulcer disease
7. Active or recent malignancy
8. Presence of severe chronic obstructive pulmonary disease or chronic bronchitis
9. Substance or alcohol abuse
10. Presence of peripheral or cerebrovascular disease
11. Other systemic diseases that would jeopardize rehabilitation post-transplant

state or will subsequently deteriorate remains to be seen. Recurrent hospitalizations may be required. Patients may become dopamine/dobutamine-dependent to maintain adequate cardiac output. This dependency on an inotropic agent plus the need for a balloon flotation catheter for hemodynamic monitoring moves the patient to the highest priority (1a) for a donor heart.

In addition to these pharmacologic bridges to transplantation, mechanical bridges are occasionally used where pharmacologic therapy is no longer effective. Three approaches are currently used. The first is intraaortic balloon pumping, which can increase cardiac output by 15 to 20%. The second is a left ventricular assist device (LVAD), which empties blood via a tube placed in the apex of the left ventricle and pumps it with an electrically driven "bellows-type" mechanism into the abdominal aorta. This approach is highly effective and has been used for several months with successful subsequent transplantation. Limitations include right ventricular failure and/or high pulmonary vascular resistance, since the LVAD does not "unload" the right ventricle. Blood clotting in the device remains a problem, in addition to the obvious problems of infection. Finally, total mechanical heart replacement is also applied in some transplant centers. This complete replacement circumvents the problem of right ventricular failure but is limited by the greater complexity of the device, which can lead to clotting and systemic emboli. Patients who underwent mechanical assistance *and* received a donor heart have 1-year survival statistics similar to those who went directly to transplantation.

Tissue cross-matching between donor and recipient has generally not been done because of difficulty in obtaining good matches and lack of correlation between match and outcome. Size, ABO matching, negative lymphocyte cross-match, and avoidance of a transplantation from a cytomegalovirus (CMV)-positive donor to a CMV-negative recipient are more important.

OPERATIVE PROCEDURE   The surgeon removes the diseased heart but leaves the posterior wall of the right atrium in place and the superior and inferior venae cavae intact. The posterior wall of the left atrium is also left in situ with pulmonary veins intact. The donor heart is then removed in toto with the posterior wall of the right and left atria incised, which allows suturing of left atrial donor rim to recipient rim and right atrial donor rim to recipient rim, with anastomosis of the aorta and pulmonary artery.

IMMUNOSUPPRESSION AND REJECTION   Controlling rejection while avoiding the adverse side effects of immunosuppressive agents is pivotal to successful transplantation. Rejection is characterized by perivascular infiltration of killer T lymphocytes, which migrate into the myocardium and cause cellular necrosis if not checked. Since early rejection can be silent, it is important to detect it before necrosis occurs. Immunologic monitoring of activated T lymphocytes in peripheral blood offers clues to the timing of a rejection process but has not been sufficiently reliable to dictate antirejection therapy. Therefore, repeated percutaneous transvenous right ventricular endomyocardial biopsies via the right internal jugular vein are required for histologic determination of the state of immunosuppression and rejection.

One widely used scheme for grading the stages of rejection is as follows: cannot rule out rejection, mild early rejection, moderate rejection, and severe rejection. Serial biopsies are taken every 1 to 2 weeks early after transplantation, with gradually widening intervals depending on the patient's course and rejection history. Prolongation of isovolumic relaxation time measured by echocardiography may also provide early clues to rejection.

Immunosuppressive therapy regimens vary but usually include triple therapy with cyclosporine, azathioprine, and prednisone. The immunosuppressive agent tacrolimus, as either "rescue therapy" for graft rejection unresponsive to cyclosporine or as initial immunosuppressive therapy, is increasingly popular. Another immunosuppressive agent, mycophenolate mofetil, has been introduced initially as a substitute for azathioprine, and in one trial appeared to be superior in reducing transplant coronary atherosclerosis and mortality. Prophylactic courses of monoclonal antibody OKT3 or antithymocyte globulin may also be given early after transplantation. Careful monitoring of the adverse side effects of these agents is extremely important because they include nephrotoxicity, bone marrow suppression, and opportunistic infections. For discussion of immunosuppressive drugs, see Chap. 272.

EARLY COURSE AND COMPLICATIONS   It is rare for a cardiac transplant patient to have a completely uncomplicated postoperative course. In the immediate postoperative period, right-sided heart failure due to pulmonary vascular disease is most life-threatening. During the 2 to 3 weeks after transplantation, the patient is hospitalized with meticulous monitoring for evidence of rejection and infections, repeated percutaneous transvenous endomyocardial biopsies, and adjustment of immunosuppressive drugs. During the ensuing 4 to 6 weeks, infectious complications, including bacterial, viral, and protozoan infections, are common. A successful transplant program requires a highly aggressive and sophisticated approach to diagnosis and therapy of infections in the immunocompromised host. CMV infection involving multiple organs is common and accelerates graft rejection as well. Prophylaxis with ganciclovir can dramatically reduce severe CMV infections and graft rejection, leading to less morbidity and improved survival. Depending on the degree of cardiac cachexia preoperatively, the patient is usually functional at 1 week and discharged from the hospital at 2 to 3 weeks if no major complication occurs.

The average first-year cost ranges from $100,000 to $150,000, depending on the need for repeated hospitalization and cardiac biopsies, and is occasionally much higher. Yearly costs for immunosuppressive agents range from $10,000 to $30,000, in addition to the expense of medical surveillance for rejection or complications.

PHYSIOLOGY AND FUNCTION   Since the allografted heart remains denervated, cardiac function differs from that of the innervated heart during both rest and exercise. The electrocardiogram of a recipient shows two P waves; the P wave of the recipient's heart reflects the residual sinus node and posterior walls of the remaining native atria but is dissociated from the QRS, since the depolarization impulse does not cross the suture line. Although it does not control donor heart rate, the recipient's sinus node remains innervated and under the influence of the autonomic nervous system. The donor sinus node controls the rate of the transplanted heart. The donor heart's P wave has a regular PR interval, reflecting conduction to the ventricles. Since the controlling sinus node is denervated, it maintains a heart rate of 100 to 110 beats per minute, and rate increase depends on alterations in chronotropic agents perfusing the sinus node. Partial reinnervation may occur in some patients late after transplantation. This is manifested primarily by the occurrence of angina-like symptoms in patients who have developed accelerated graft atherosclerosis (see below).

Ventricular function in response to isometric and isotonic exercise has been studied extensively. The early response to exercise is more dependent on the Frank-Starling mechanism and change in ventricular volume and filling pressure. As exercise proceeds and catecholamines are released with their positive inotropic and chronotropic effects, cardiac output begins to rise. The cardiac transplant recipient can achieve approximately 70% of the maximal cardiac output expected for his or her age, easily sufficient for the stresses of everyday life.

LATE COURSE AND COMPLICATIONS   Although the rejection process partially subsides, lifelong administration of immunosuppressive drugs, albeit at lower doses, is still required and remains a hazard. Infectious complications and unsuspected rejection continue to occur, requiring ongoing surveillance and monitoring. Routine cardiac biopsies are performed at 3-month intervals to monitor for unsuspected early rejection. Acute rejection or infection predominates in the first year after transplantation. Chronic rejection (i.e., accelerated coronary vascular disease) becomes the most important cause of death after the first year. The process is a fibrointimal hyperplasia that can go undetected by coronary arteriography at first and then cause diffuse atherosclerotic changes. Risk factors for its development may include repeated rejection episodes and elevated lipid levels. CMV infections have also been associated with higher frequency of this disease. Immunocytochemistry on endomyocardial biopsies in cardiac transplant recipients has shown a high incidence of arterial endothelial cell activation, as reflected by the presence of intercellular adhesion molecule 1 and histocompatibility antigen HLA-DR during the first 3 months after transplantation. The presence of these markers has been associated with a high risk of the subsequent development of graft coronary artery atherosclerosis, with death or the need for a second transplant. Thus, activation of the arterial/arteriolar endothelium predicts development of coronary artery disease in and the subsequent failure of the transplanted heart.

Angina is rare, and patients may present with sudden death or silent myocardial infarction. This diffuse accelerated vascular process affects both proximal and distal coronary vessels so that standard approaches, such as angioplasty or coronary artery bypass grafting, are not generally useful but occasionally are successful.

Uncontrolled trials with anticoagulation, aspirin, and improved immunosuppression with cyclosporine have done little to lower this frequency; 40 to 50% of patients show arteriographic evidence of coronary vascular disease 5 years after transplantation. Retransplantation has been employed for some patients with severe graft atherosclerosis, but it is limited by the scarcity of donors and poorer survival expectations after the second transplant. Diltiazem has been reported to reduce the severity and occurrence of this accelerated vascular process when started at the time of transplantation. Calcium channel blockers are the agents of choice for cyclosporine-induced hypertension, a common complication in the posttransplant patient. Pravastatin and simvastatin have been reported not only to lower lipid levels but also to reduce graft vessel coronary artery disease and improve survival. Administration of one of these drugs is advisable for all heart transplant recipients. A comparative trial of azathioprine versus mycophenolate mofetil reported less graft disease and cardiovascular mortality in the latter group.

In addition to the well-known hazards of long-term glucocorticoid usage, the immunosuppressed patient is at increased risk for neoplasia. An unusual form of lymphoma can occur frequently in extranodal locations, which is linked to prior Epstein-Barr viral infection. This lymphoma can be polyclonal or monoclonal, is associated with excessive immunosuppression, and may respond to simply lowering doses of cyclosporine and administration of acyclovir rather than requiring more aggressive chemo- or radiotherapy. Many cases regress fully and do not recur.

HEART-LUNG TRANSPLANTATION

Patients with congenital heart disease with Eisenmenger's complex (Chap. 234) or primary pulmonary hypertension (Chap. 260) are now considered for heart-lung transplantation. The surgical technique is similar to that for heart transplantation, except that the pulmonary venous attachments to the left atrium are left intact, and a tracheal anastomosis is required. The postoperative period is more complex, since the lungs may be rejected separately from the heart, requiring repeated endobronchoscopic biopsies when rejection is suspected. The immunosuppressive regimen is similar to that for heart transplants, except that glucocorticoids are avoided in the first 1 to 2 weeks to allow healing of the tracheal anastamosis. Long-term survival has in the past been limited by obliterative bronchiolitis due to chronic unrecognized rejection; survival rates have been approximately 60% at 1 year and 50% at 2 years but appear to be improving. Heart-lung transplants have also been applied to primary pulmonary hypertension, but more recent experience with single-lung transplants for these patients has been satisfactory, thus utilizing scarce donors more effectively. Single-lung transplants are also being applied increasingly for patients with advanced emphysema. Double-lung transplants for pa-

tients with cystic fibrosis have also become the operation of choice for this group. →*For further discussion, see Chap. 267.*

BIBLIOGRAPHY

BENIAMINOVITZ A et al: Prevention of rejection in cardiac transplantation by blockade of the interleukin-2 receptor with a monoclonal antibody. N Engl J Med 342:613, 2000

HOSENPUD JD et al: The Registry of the International Society for Heart and Lung Transplantation: Fifteenth official Report—1998. Transplantation 17:656, 1999

HUNT SA: Current status of cardiac transplantation. JAMA 280:1692, 1998

KAPADIA SR et al: Intravascular ultrasound imaging after cardiac transplantation: Advantage of multi-vessel imaging. J Heart Lung Trans 19:167, 2000

KOBASHIGAWA JA: Mycophenolate mofetil in cardiac transplantation. Curr Opin Cardiol 13:117, 1998

LABARRERE CA et al: Endothelial activation and development of coronary artery disease in transplanted human hearts. JAMA 278:1169, 1997

ROBBINS R, REITZ B: Therapy of heart failure: Heart-lung transplantation, in E Braunwald, D Zipes, P Libby (eds): *Heart Disease*, 6th ed. Philadelphia, Saunders, 2001

WENKE K et al: Simvastatin reduces graft vessel disease and mortality after heart transplantation: A four year randomized trial. Circulation 96:1398, 1997

234 *William F. Friedman, John S. Child*

CONGENITAL HEART DISEASE IN THE ADULT

Congenital heart disease complicates approximately 1% of all live births. It occurs in about 4% of offspring of women with congenital heart disease. Substantial numbers of affected infants reach adulthood because of successful medical and/or surgical management, or because the alteration caused in cardiovascular physiology is well tolerated.

ETIOLOGY AND PREVENTION Congenital cardiovascular malformations are generally the result of aberrant embryonic development of a normal structure, or failure of such a structure to progress beyond an early stage of embryonic or fetal development. Malformations are due to complex multifactorial genetic and environmental causes. Recognized chromosomal aberrations and mutations of single genes account for <10% of all cardiac malformations (Table 234-1).

The presence of a cardiac malformation as one component of the multiple system involvement in Down's, Turner's, and the trisomy 13-15(D1) and 17-18 (E) syndromes may be anticipated in occasional pregnancies by detection of abnormal chromosomes in fetal cells obtained from amniotic fluid or chorionic villus biopsy. Identification in such cells of the enzyme disorders characteristic of Hurler's syndrome, homocystinuria, or type II glycogen storage disease may also allow one to predict cardiac disease.

PATHOPHYSIOLOGY The anatomic and physiologic changes in the heart and circulation due to any specific congenital cardiocirculatory lesion are not static but rather progress from prenatal life to adulthood. Thus, malformations that are benign or escape detection in childhood may become clinically significant in the adult. For example, the functionally normal, congenitally bicuspid aortic valve may thicken and calcify with time, resulting in significant aortic stenosis; or the well-tolerated left-to-right shunt of an atrial septal defect may not result in cardiac decompensation, with or without pulmonary hypertension, until the fourth or fifth decade.

Pulmonary Hypertension This is a common companion of many congenital cardiac lesions, and the status of the pulmonary vascular bed is often the principal determinant of the clinical manifestations, the course, and the feasibility of surgical repair. Increases in pulmonary arterial pressure result from elevation of pulmonary blood flow and/or resistance, the latter due sometimes to an increase in vascular tone but usually the result of obstructive, obliterative structural

Table 234-1　Syndromes with Associated Cardiovascular Involvement

Syndrome (Genetic Locus)	Major Cardiovascular Manifestations	Major Noncardiac Abnormalities
HERITABLE AND POSSIBLY HERITABLE		
Ellis–van Creveld	Single atrium or atrial septal defect	Chondrodystrophic dwarfism, nail dysplasia, polydactyly
TAR (thrombocytopenia-absent radius)	Atrial septal defect, tetralogy of Fallot	Radial aplasia or hypoplasia, thrombocytopenia
Holt-Oram (12q21–q3)	Atrial septal defect (other defects common)	Skeletal upper limb defect, hypoplasia of clavicles
Kartagener	Dextrocardia	Situs inversus, sinusitis, bronchiectasis
Laurence-Moon-Biedl-Bardet	Variable defects	Retinal pigmentation, obesity, polydactyly
Noonan (12q24)	Pulmonic valve dysplasia, cardiomyopathy (usually hypertrophic)	Webbed neck, pectus excavatum, cryptorchidism
Tuberous sclerosis (type 1—4q; type 2—16p)	Rhabdomyoma, cardiomyopathy	Phakomatosis, bone lesions, hamartomatous skin lesions
Multiple lentigines (LEOPARD) syndrome	Pulmonic stenosis	Basal cell nevi, broad facies, rib anomalies, deafness
Rubenstein-Taybi (16p13.3)	Patent ductus arteriosus (others)	Broad thumbs and toes, hypoplastic maxilla, slanted palpebral fissures
Familial deafness	Arrhythmias, sudden death	Sensorineural deafness
Weber-Osler-Rendu (9q33)	Arteriovenous fistulas (lung, liver, mucous membranes)	Multiple telangiectasias
Apert (10q26)	Ventricular septal defect	Craniosynostosis, midfacial hypoplasia, syndactyly
Crouzon (10q26, 4p16.3)	Patent ductus arteriosus, aortic coarctation	Ptosis with shallow orbits, craniosynostosis, maxillary hypoplasia
Hypertrophic cardiomyopathy (locus heterogeneity, 14q11.2–12, 1q32, 15q22, 11p11.2, etc.)	Asymmetric septal hypertrophy	Family history of sudden death
Incontinentia pigmenti	Patent ductus arteriosus	Irregular pigmented skin lesions, patchy alopecia, hypodontia
Alagille (arteriohepatic dysplasia) (20p12)	Peripheral pulmonic stenosis, pulmonic stenosis	Biliary hypoplasia, vertebral anomalies, prominent forehead, deep-set eyes
Catch-22 (DiGeorge) (22q11)	Interrupted aortic arch, tetralogy of Fallot, truncus arteriosus	Thymic hypoplasia or aplasia, parathyroid aplasia or hypoplasia, abnormal facies
Shprintzen (velocardiofacial) (22q11.2)	Ventricular septal defect, tetralogy of Fallot, right aortic arch	Cleft palate, prominent nose, slender hands, learning disability
Williams (7q11.23)	Supravalvular aortic stenosis, peripheral pulmonic stenosis	Mental deficiency, elfin facies, loquacious personality, hoarse voice
Long QT (Jervell and Lange-Nielsen, Romano-Ward) (11p15.5, 7q35, 3p21, 21q22)	Long QT interval, ventricular arrhythmias	Family history of sudden death, congenital deafness (not in Romano-Ward)
Friedreich's ataxia (9q)	Cardiomyopathy and conduction defects	Ataxia, speech defect, degeneration of spinal cord dorsal columns
Muscular dystrophy	Cardiomyopathy	Pseudohypertrophy of calf muscles, weakness of trunk and proximal limb muscles
Cystic fibrosis (7q)	Cor pulmonale	Pancreatic insufficiency, malabsorption, chronic lung disease
Sickle cell anemia	Cardiomyopathy, mitral regurgitation	Hemoglobin SS
Conradi-Hunermann	Ventricular septal defect, patent ductus arteriosus	Asymmetrical limb shortness, early punctate mineralization, large skin pores
Cockayne	Accelerated atherosclerosis	Cachectic dwarfism, retinal pigment abnormalities, photosensitivity dermatitis
Progeria	Accelerated atherosclerosis	Premature aging, alopecia, atrophy of subcutaneous fat, skeletal hypoplasia
CONNECTIVE TISSUE DISORDERS		
Cutis laxa	Peripheral pulmonic stenosis	Generalized disruption of elastic fibers, diminished skin resilience, hernias
Ehlers-Danlos (2q31)	Arterial dilatation and rupture, mitral regurgitation	Hyperextensible joints, hyperelastic and friable
Marfan (15q21.1)	Aortic dilatation, aortic and mitral incompetence	Gracile habitus, arachnodactyly with hyperextensibility, lens subluxation
Osteogenesis imperfecta (4.17)	Aortic incompetence	Fragile bones, blue sclerae
Pseudoxanthoma elasticum	Peripheral and coronary arterial disease	Degeneration of elastic fibers in skin, retinal angioid streaks
INBORN ERRORS OF METABOLISM		
Pompe disease	Glycogen storage disease of heart	Acid maltase deficiency, muscular weakness
Homocystinuria	Aortic and pulmonary arterial dilatation, intravascular thrombosis	Cystathionine synthetase deficiency, lens subluxation, osteoporosis
Mucopolysaccharidoses: Hurler; Hunter	Multivalvular and coronary and great artery disease, cardiomyopathy	Hurler: Deficiency of α-L-iduronidase, corneal clouding, coarse features, growth and mental retardation
		Hunter: Deficiency of L-iduranosulfate sulfatase, coarse facies, clear cornea, growth and mental retardation

(continued)

Table 234-1—(continued)

Syndrome (Genetic Locus)	Major Cardiovascular Manifestations	Major Noncardiac Abnormalities
Morquio; Scheie; Maroteaux-Lamy	Aortic regurgitation	Morquio: Deficiency of *N*-acetylhexosamine sulfate sulfatase, cloudy cornea, severe bone changes involving vertebrae and epiphyses Scheie: Deficiency of α-L-iduronidase, cloudy cornea, normal intelligence, peculiar facies Maroteaux-Lamy: Deficiency of arylsulfatase B, cloudy cornea, osseous changes
CHROMOSOMAL ABNORMALITIES		
Trisomy 21 (Down syndrome)	Endocardial cushion defect, atrial or ventricular septal defect, tetralogy of Fallot	Hypotonia, hyperextensible joints, mongoloid facies, mental retardation
Trisomy 13 (D)	Ventricular septal defect, RV patent ductus arteriosus, double-outlet RV	Single midline intracerebral ventricle with midfacial defects, polydactyly, nail changes, mental retardation
Trisomy 18 (E)	Congenital polyvalvular dysplasia, ventricular septal defect, patent ductus	Clenched hand, short sternum, low arch dermal ridge pattern on fingertips, mental retardation
Cri du chat (short-arm deletion-5)	Ventricular septal defect	Cat cry, microcephaly, antimongoloid slant of palpebral fissures, mental retardation
XO (Turner)	Coarctation of aorta, bicuspid aortic valve, aortic dilatation	Short female, broad chest, lymphedema, webbed neck
XXXY and XXXXX	Patent ductus arteriosus	XXXY: Hypogenitalism, mental retardation, radial-ulnar synostosis XXXXX: Small hands, incurving of fifth fingers, mental retardation
SPORADIC DISORDERS		
VATER association	Ventricular septal defect	Vertebral anomalies, anal atresia, tracheo-esophageal fistula, radial and renal anomalies
CHARGE association	Tetralogy of Fallot (other defects common)	Colobomas, choanal atresia, mental and growth deficiency, genital and ear anomalies
Cornelia de Lange	Ventricular septal defect	Micromelia, synophrys, mental and growth deficiency
TERATOGENIC DISORDERS		
Rubella	Patent ductus arteriosus, pulmonic valvular and/or arterial stenosis, atrial septal defect	Cataracts, deafness, microcephaly
Alcohol	Ventricular septal defect (other defects)	Microcephaly, growth and mental deficiency, short palpebral fissures, smooth philtrum, thin upper lip
Dilantin	Pulmonic stenosis, aortic stenosis, coarctation, patent ductus arteriosus	Hypertelorism, growth and mental deficiency, short phalanges, bowed upper lip
Thalidomide	Variable	Phocomelia
Lithium	Ebstein's anomaly, tricuspid atresia	None

SOURCE: Modified from WF Friedman.

changes within the pulmonary vascular bed. Because pulmonary vascular obstructive disease can be the determining factor in assessing the advisability of operation, it is important to quantitate and compare pulmonary to systemic flows and resistances in patients with severe pulmonary hypertension. The causes of pulmonary vascular obstructive disease are unknown, although increased pulmonary blood flow, increased pulmonary arterial blood pressure, elevated pulmonary venous pressure, erythrocytosis, systemic hypoxemia, acidosis, and the bronchial circulation have been implicated. The designation *Eisenmenger syndrome* is applied to patients with a large communication between the two circulations at the aortopulmonary, ventricular, or atrial levels and bidirectional or predominantly right-to-left shunts because of high-resistance and obstructive pulmonary hypertension. No specific treatment has proved beneficial for obstructive pulmonary vascular disease, although both single lung transplantation with intracardiac defect repair, and total heart-lung transplantation show promise (Chaps. 233 and 267).

Erythrocytosis The chronic hypoxemia in cyanotic congenital heart disease results in *erythrocytosis* due to increased erythropoietin production (Chap. 36). The commonly used term *polycythemia* is a misnomer because white cell counts are normal and platelet counts are normal to decreased. Cyanotic patients with erythrocytosis may have compensated or decompensated hematocrits. Compensated erythrocytosis with iron-replete equilibrium hematocrits rarely results in symptoms of hyperviscosity at hematocrits <65% and occasionally not even with hematocrits ≥70%. Therapeutic phlebotomy is rarely required in compensated erythrocytosis. In contrast, patients with decompensated erythrocytosis fail to establish equilibrium with unstable, rising hematocrits and recurrent hyperviscosity symptoms. Therapeutic phlebotomy, a two-edged sword, allows temporary relief of symptoms but begets instability of the hematocrit and compounds the problem by iron depletion. Iron-deficiency symptoms are usually indistinguishable from those of hyperviscosity; progressive symptoms after recurrent phlebotomy are usually due to iron depletion with hypochromic microcytosis. Iron depletion results in a larger number of smaller (microcytic) hypochromic red cells that are less capable of carrying oxygen and less deformable in the microcirculation. Because these microcytes are less deformable in the microcirculation and there are more of them relative to the plasma volume, the viscosity is greater than for an equivalent hematocrit with fewer, larger, iron-replete, deformable cells. As such, iron-depleted erythrocytosis results in increasing symptoms due to decreased oxygen delivery to the tissues.

Hemostasis is abnormal in cyanotic congenital heart disease, due in part to the increased blood volume and engorged capillaries, abnormalities in platelet function and sensitivity to aspirin or nonsteroidal anti-inflammatory agents, and abnormalities of the extrinsic and intrinsic coagulation system. Oral contraceptives are contraindicated for cyanotic women because of the enhanced risk of vascular thrombosis.

The risk of stroke is greatest in children younger than 4 years with cyanotic heart disease and iron deficiency, often with dehydration as an aggravating cause. In contrast, adults with cyanotic congenital heart disease do not appear to be at increased risk for stroke, unless there are excessive injudicious phlebotomies, inappropriate use of aspirin or anticoagulants, or the presence of atrial arrhythmias or infective endocarditis.

Symptoms of hyperviscosity can be produced in any cyanotic patient with erythrocytosis if dehydration causes a reduction of plasma volume. Phlebotomy, when required for symptoms of hyperviscosity not due to dehydration or iron deficiency, is a simple outpatient removal of 500 mL of blood over 45 min with isovolumetric replacement with isotonic saline (5% dextrose if congestive heart failure exists). Acute phlebotomy without volume replacement is contraindicated. Iron repletion in decompensated iron-depleted erythrocytosis ameliorates iron-deficiency symptoms but must be done gradually to avoid a sudden excessive rise in hematocrit and resultant hyperviscosity.

Pregnancy The physiologic alterations during normal gestation (Chap. 7) can create symptoms and physical findings that may be attributed erroneously to heart disease. Dyspnea due to the hormonal influence of progesterone and elevation of the diaphragm in association with peripheral edema and fatigability may be attributed inappropriately to heart failure. The jugular venous pulsations normally become more apparent after the twentieth week. Elevation of the diaphragm can cause basal rales (which disappear with deep breathing). Both ventricles are more easily palpated due to the normal increase in ventricular volumes and elevation of the diaphragm. Third heart sounds, already relatively frequent in normal nongravid young women, increase in frequency and intensity with pregnancy because of increased heart rate and volume of flow across the mitral and tricuspid valves. Midsystolic murmurs across the pulmonary outflow tract and supraclavicular systolic murmurs are caused by increased cardiac output. Venous hums and mammary souffles are usual during pregnancy.

These normal circulatory changes may impinge upon the woman's cardiac reserve. The mother is most at risk if she has a cardiovascular lesion associated with pulmonary vascular disease and pulmonary hypertension (e.g., Eisenmenger's physiology or mitral stenosis) or left ventricular (LV) outflow tract obstruction (e.g., aortic stenosis) but also risks death with any malformation that may cause heart failure or a hemodynamically important arrhythmia (Table 234-2). The fetus is most at risk in the presence of maternal cyanosis, heart failure, or pulmonary hypertension. Women with aortic coarctation or Marfan's syndrome are at risk for aortic dissection. Patients with cyanotic heart disease, pulmonary hypertension, or Marfan's syndrome should not become pregnant; those with correctable lesions should be counseled about the risks of pregnancy with an uncorrected malformation versus repair and later pregnancy. The effect of pregnancy in postoperative patients depends on the outcome of the repair including the presence and severity of residua, sequelae, or complications. Contraception is an important topic with such patients. Tubal ligation should be considered in those in whom pregnancy is strictly contraindicated.

INFECTIVE ENDOCARDITIS (See also Chap. 126) Routine antimicrobial prophylaxis is recommended for most patients with congenital heart disease whether operated on or not. Antibiotic prophylaxis is not uniformly effective. Nonetheless, it is recommended for all dental procedures, gastrointestinal and genitourinary surgery, and diagnostic procedures such as proctosigmoidoscopy and cystoscopy. The clinical and bacteriologic profile of infective endocarditis in patients with congenital heart disease has changed with the advent of intracardiac surgery and of prosthetic devices. Two major predisposing causes of infective endocarditis are a susceptible cardiovascular substrate and a source of bacteremia. Prophylaxis includes both chemotherapeutic (antimicrobial) and nonchemotherapeutic (hygienic) measures. Meticulous dental and skin care is required.

EXERCISE Advice on athletics and exercise is governed by the nature of the exercise and by the type and severity of the congenital cardiovascular lesion. Patients with lesions characterized by LV outflow tract obstruction, if more than mild to moderate, or pulmonary vascular disease, risk syncope or even sudden death. In Fallot's tetralogy, isotonic exercise–induced decrease in systemic vascular resistance relative to the right ventricular (RV) outflow obstruction augments the right-to-left shunt, increases hypoxemia, and causes an increase in subjective breathlessness due to the response of the respiratory center to the changes in blood gases and pH.

INSURABILITY AND EMPLOYABILITY Most patients with congenital heart disease must pay significantly more than standard life insurance rates, assuming their anomaly places them in a category that companies have determined is eligible for insurance. A paucity of actuarial survival data beyond adolescence for persons with most congenital cardiac lesions that have undergone operative repair has made it difficult to convince insurance companies to offer reasonable cost insurance even to individual patients whose long-term prognosis is quite good.

Employment is affected by the patient's physical capacity relative to the type of job sought. Job discrimination exists, often because the employer is reluctant to accept health insurance responsibilities. Eligibility for some occupations is governed by public safety regulations, e.g., airline pilots, bus drivers.

SPECIFIC CARDIAC DEFECTS

Table 234-3 provides a classification of cardiac anomalies that recognizes the general categories of clinical presentation, functional consequences, and site of origin of congenital defects.

Categorizing the defect(s) in an individual patient requires an answer to a number of basic questions. Is the patient acyanotic or cyanotic? Is pulmonary arterial blood flow increased or not? Does the malformation originate in the left or right side of the heart? Which is the dominant ventricle? Is pulmonary hypertension present or not? With the above information as a foundation, the use of more refined diagnostic techniques such as transthoracic (precordial) and transesophageal echocardiography and Doppler imaging, magnetic resonance imaging, and/or hemodynamic study and angiocardiography leads to a precise anatomic and functional assessment.

ACYANOTIC CONGENITAL HEART DISEASE WITH A LEFT-TO-RIGHT SHUNT

ATRIAL SEPTAL DEFECT This common cardiac anomaly in adults occurs more frequently in females. The *sinus venosus* type occurs high in the atrial septum near the entry of the superior vena cava and is associated frequently with anomalous connection of pul-

Table 234-2 Tolerance of Pregnancy by Patients with Various Congenital Cardiac Malformations

Well Tolerated	Intermediate Effect	Poorly Tolerated
NYHA class I	NYHA class II–III	NYHA class IV
Left-right shunts without PHTN	Repaired transposition of the great arteries	Right-left shunt, unrepaired cyanotic heart disease
Aortic or mitral valvular regurgitation (mild-moderate)	Fontan repairs	PHTN and/or pulmonary vascular disease (e.g., Eisenmenger's, "primary PHTN")
Pulmonic or tricuspid regurgitation (if low pressure, even severe)	Aortic or mitral stenosis (moderate)	Aortic or mitral stenosis (severe)
Pulmonic stenosis (mild-moderate)	Ebstein's anomaly	Pulmonic stenosis (severe)
Well-repaired tetralogy of Fallot		Marfan's or aortic coarctation

NOTE: NYHA, New York Heart Association; PHTN, pulmonary hypertension.

monary veins from the right lung to the junction of the superior vena cava and right atrium (RA). *Ostium primum* anomalies are a form of atrioventricular septal defect that lie immediately adjacent to the atrioventricular valves, either of which may be deformed and incompetent. Ostium primum defects occur commonly in patients with Down's syndrome, although the more complex atrioventricular septal defects with a common atrioventricular valve and a posterior defect of the basal portion of the interventricular septum are more characteristic of this chromosomal defect. The most common atrial septal defect involves the fossa ovalis, is midseptal in location, and is of the *ostium secundum* type. This type of defect should not be confused with a *patent foramen ovale*. Anatomic obliteration of the foramen ovale ordinarily follows its functional closure soon after birth, but residual "probe patency" is a normal variant; atrial septal defect denotes a true deficiency of the atrial septum and implies functional and anatomic patency.

The magnitude of the left-to-right shunt through an atrial septal defect depends on the defect size, the diastolic properties of both ventricles, and the relative impedance in the pulmonary and systemic circulations. The left-to-right shunt causes diastolic overloading of the RV and increased pulmonary blood flow.

Patients with atrial septal defect are usually asymptomatic in early life, although there may be some physical underdevelopment and an increased tendency for respiratory infections; cardiorespiratory symptoms occur in many older patients. Beyond the fourth decade, a significant number of patients develop atrial arrhythmias, pulmonary arterial hypertension, bidirectional and then right-to-left shunting of blood,

Table 234-3 Classification of Congenital Heart Disease

ACYANOTIC WITH LEFT-TO-RIGHT SHUNT

I. Atrial level shunt
  A. Atrial septal defect
    1. Ostium primum
    2. Ostium secundum
    3. Sinus venosus
  B. Atrial septal defect with mitral stenosis (Lutembacher's syndrome)
  C. Partial anomalous pulmonary venous connection
II. Ventricular level shunt
  A. Ventricular septal defect
    1. Inlet septum
    2. Muscular septum
    3. Perimembranous septum
    4. Infundibular septum
  B. Ventricular septal defect with aortic regurgitation
  C. Ventricular septal defect with left ventricular to right atrial shunt

III. Aortic root to right heart shunt
  A. Ruptured sinus of Valsalva aneurysm
  B. Coronary arteriovenous fistula
  C. Anomalous origin of the left coronary artery from the pulmonary trunk
IV. Aortopulmonary level shunt
  A. Aortopulmonary window
  B. Patent ductus arteriosus
V. Multiple level shunts
  A. Complete common atrioventricular canal
  B. Ventricular septal defect with atrial septal defect
  C. Ventricular septal defect with patent ductus arteriosus

ACYANOTIC WITHOUT A SHUNT

I. Left heart malformations
  A. Congenital obstruction to left atrial inflow
    1. Pulmonary vein stenosis
    2. Mitral stenosis
    3. Cor triatriatum
  B. Mitral regurgitation
    1. Atrioventricular septal (endocardial cushion)
    2. Congenitally corrected transposition of the great arteries
    3. Anomalous origin of the left coronary artery from the pulmonary trunk
    4. Miscellaneous (double-orifice mitral valve, congenital perforations, accessory commissures with anomalous chordal insertion, congenitally short or absent chordae, cleft posterior leaflet, parachute mitral valve, etc.)
  C. Primary dilated endocardial fibroelastosis

  D. Aortic stenosis
    1. Discrete subvalvular
    2. Valvular
    3. Supravalvular
  E. Aortic valve regurgitation
  F. Coarctation of the aorta
II. Right heart malformations
  A. Acyanotic Ebstein's anomaly of the tricuspid valve
  B. Pulmonic stenosis
    1. Subinfundibular
    2. Infundibular
    3. Valvular
    4. Supravalvular (stenosis of pulmonary artery and its branches)
  C. Congenital pulmonary valve regurgitation
  D. Idiopathic dilatation of the pulmonary trunk

CYANOTIC

I. Increased pulmonary blood flow
  A. Complete transposition of the great arteries
  B. Double-outlet right ventricle of the Taussig-Bing type
  C. Truncus arteriosus
  D. Total anomalous pulmonary venous connection
  E. Single ventricle without pulmonic stenosis
  F. Common atrium
  G. Tetralogy of Fallot with pulmonary atresia and increased collateral arterial flow
  H. Tricuspid atresia with large ventricular septal defect and no pulmonic stenosis
  I. Hypoplastic left heart (aortic atresia, mitral atresia)

II. Normal or decreased pulmonary blood flow
  A. Tricuspid atresia
  B. Ebstein's anomaly with right-to-left atrial shunt
  C. Pulmonary atresia with intact ventricular septum
  D. Pulmonic stenosis or atresia with ventricular septal defect (tetralogy of Fallot)
  E. Pulmonic stenosis with right-to-left atrial shunt
  F. Complete transposition of the great arteries with pulmonic stenosis
  G. Double-outlet right ventricle with pulmonic stenosis
  H. Single ventricle with pulmonic stenosis
  I. Pulmonary arteriovenous fistula
  J. Vena caval to left atrial communication

OTHER

I. Congenitally corrected transposition of the great arteries

II. The cardiac malpositions
III. Congenital complete heart block

SOURCE: Modified from JK Perloff, *The Clinical Recognition of Congenital Heart Disease,* Philadelphia, Saunders, 1991.

and cardiac failure. Patients exposed to the chronic environmental hypoxia of high altitude tend to develop pulmonary hypertension at younger ages. In some older patients, left-to-right shunting across the defect increases as progressive systemic hypertension and/or coronary artery disease result in reduced compliance of the LV.

Physical Examination Examination usually reveals a prominent RV cardiac impulse and palpable pulmonary artery pulsation. The first heart sound is normal or split, with accentuation of the tricuspid valve closure sound. Increased flow across the pulmonic valve is responsible for a midsystolic pulmonary ejection murmur. The second heart sound is widely split and is relatively fixed in relation to respiration. A mid-diastolic rumbling murmur, loudest at the fourth intercostal space and along the left sternal border, reflects increased flow across the tricuspid valve. In patients with ostium primum defects, an apical thrill and holosystolic murmur indicate associated mitral or tricuspid incompetence or a ventricular septal defect.

The physical findings are altered when an increase in the pulmonary vascular resistance results in diminution of the left-to-right shunt. Both the pulmonary and tricuspid murmurs decrease in intensity, the pulmonic component of the second heart sound and a systolic ejection sound are accentuated, the two components of the second heart sound may fuse, and a diastolic murmur of pulmonic regurgitation appears. Cyanosis and clubbing accompany the development of a right-to-left shunt.

In adults with an atrial septal defect and atrial fibrillation, the physical findings may be confused with the findings of mitral stenosis with pulmonary hypertension because the tricuspid flow murmur and widely split second heart sound may be mistakenly thought to represent the diastolic murmur of mitral stenosis and the mitral "opening snap," respectively.

Electrocardiogram In patients with an ostium secundum defect, the electrocardiogram (ECG) usually shows right axis deviation and an rSr′ pattern in the right precordial leads representing delayed posterobasal activation of the ventricular septum and enlargement of the RV outflow tract. An ectopic atrial pacemaker or first-degree heart block occurs occasionally in patients with defects of the sinus venosus type. In patients with an ostium primum defect, the RV conduction defect is characteristically accompanied by left axis deviation and by superior orientation and counterclockwise rotation of the QRS loop in the frontal plane. Varying degrees of RV and RA hypertrophy may occur with each type of defect, depending on the height of the pulmonary artery pressure. *Chest roentgenograms* reveal enlargement of the RA and RV, dilatation of the pulmonary artery and its branches, and increased pulmonary vascular marking.

Echocardiogram This test shows pulmonary arterial and RV dilatation, and anterior systolic (paradoxical) or flat interventricular septal motion if a significant RV volume overload is present. The defect may be visualized directly from subcostal, right parasternal, or apical echocardiographic windows. In most institutions, two-dimensional echocardiography, supplemented by conventional or color Doppler flow examination, has supplanted cardiac catheterization as the confirmatory test for atrial septal defect. Transesophageal echocardiography is indicated if the transthoracic echocardiogram is ambiguous, which is often the case with sinus venosus defects. Cardiac catheterization is then performed if inconsistencies exist in the clinical data, if significant pulmonary hypertension or associated malformations are suspected, or if coronary artery disease is a possibility.

℞ **TREATMENT** Operative repair, ideally in children age 3 to 6 years, should be advised for all patients with uncomplicated atrial septal defects in whom there is significant left-to-right shunting, i.e., with pulmonary-to-systemic flow ratios exceeding ~2.0:1.0. Excellent results may be anticipated, at low risk, even in patients older than 40 years in the absence of pulmonary hypertension. The defect is closed, usually with a patch of pericardium or of prosthetic material, with the patient on cardiopulmonary bypass. In patients with ostium primum defects, cleft, deformed, and incompetent valves often require repair. Intraoperative transesophageal echocardiography is used to monitor the surgical results of mitral valve repair. Operation should not be carried out in patients with small defects and trivial left-to-right shunts, or in those with severe pulmonary vascular disease without a significant left-to-right shunt.

Patients with atrial septal defect of the sinus venosus or ostium secundum types rarely die before the fifth decade. During the fifth and sixth decades the incidence of progressive symptoms, often leading to severe disability, increases substantially. Medical management should include prompt treatment of respiratory tract infections, antiarrhythmic medications for atrial fibrillation or supraventricular tachycardia, and the usual measures for hypertension, coronary disease, or heart failure (Chap. 232), if these complications occur. The risk of infective endocarditis is quite low unless the defect is complicated by valvular regurgitation or has recently been repaired with a patch (Chap. 126).

VENTRICULAR SEPTAL DEFECT Defects of the ventricular septum are common as isolated defects and as one component of a combination of anomalies. The opening is usually single and situated in the membranous portion of the septum. The functional disturbance is dependent primarily on its size and on the status of the pulmonary vascular bed, rather than on the location of the defect. Only small or moderate-size defects are usually seen initially in adulthood as most

patients with isolated large defects come to medical and, often, surgical attention very early in life.

A wide spectrum exists in the natural history of ventricular septal defect, ranging from spontaneous closure to congestive cardiac failure and death in early infancy. Within this spectrum is the possible development of pulmonary vascular obstruction, RV outflow tract obstruction, aortic regurgitation, and infective endocarditis. Spontaneous closure is more common in patients born with a small ventricular septal defect and occurs in early childhood in most patients.

Patients with large ventricular septal defects and pulmonary hypertension are those at greatest risk for developing pulmonary vascular obstruction. Thus, large defects should be corrected surgically early in life when pulmonary vascular disease is still reversible or not yet developed. In patients with severe pulmonary vascular obstruction (Eisenmenger syndrome), symptoms in adult life consist of exertional dyspnea, chest pain, syncope, and hemoptysis. The right-to-left shunt leads to cyanosis, clubbing, and erythrocytosis. In all patients, the degree to which pulmonary vascular resistance is elevated before operation is a critical factor determining prognosis. If the pulmonary vascular resistance is one-third or less of the systemic value, progression of pulmonary vascular disease after operation is unusual. However, if a moderate to severe increase in pulmonary vascular resistance exists preoperatively, either no change or a progression of pulmonary vascular disease is common postoperatively.

RV outflow tract obstruction develops in ~5 to 10% of patients who present in infancy with a moderate to large left-to-right shunt. With time, as subvalvular RV outflow tract obstruction progresses, the findings in these patients begin to resemble more closely those of the cyanotic tetralogy of Fallot.

In ~5% of patients, incompetence of the aortic valve results from insufficient cusp tissue or prolapse of the cusp through the interventricular defect; the aortic regurgitation then complicates and usually dominates the clinical course.

Two-dimensional *echocardiography* with conventional or color Doppler examination can usually define the number and location of defects in the ventricular septum and detect associated anomalies. Hemodynamic and angiographic study may be employed to assess the status of the pulmonary vascular bed and clarify details of the altered anatomy.

℞ **TREATMENT** Surgery is not recommended for patients with normal pulmonary arterial pressures with small shunts (pulmonary-to-systemic flow ratios of less than 1.5 to 2.0:1.0). Operative correction is indicated when there is a moderate to large left-to-right shunt with a pulmonary-to-systemic flow ratio >1.5:1.0 or 2.0:1.0, in the absence of prohibitively high levels of pulmonary vascular resistance.

PATENT DUCTUS ARTERIOSUS The ductus arteriosus is a vessel leading from the bifurcation of the pulmonary artery to the aorta just distal to the left subclavian artery. Normally, the vascular channel is open in the fetus but closes immediately after birth. The flow across the ductus is determined by the pressure and resistance relationships between the systemic and pulmonary circulations and by the cross-sectional area and length of the ductus. In most adults with this anomaly, pulmonary pressures are normal and a gradient and shunt from aorta to pulmonary artery persist throughout the cardiac cycle, resulting in a characteristic thrill and a continuous "machinery" murmur with a late systolic accentuation at the upper left sternal edge. In adults who were born with a large left-to-right shunt through the ductus arteriosus, pulmonary vascular obstruction (Eisenmenger syndrome) with pulmonary hypertension, right-to-left shunting, and cyanosis have usually developed. Severe pulmonary vascular disease results in reversal of flow through the ductus, unoxygenated blood is shunted to the descending aorta, and the toes, but not the fingers, become cyanotic and clubbed, a finding termed *differential cyanosis*. The leading causes of death in adults with patent ductus are cardiac failure and infective endocarditis; occasionally severe pulmonary vascular obstruction may cause aneurysmal dilatation, calcification, and rupture of the ductus.

234 Congenital Heart Disease: Adult   **1337**

Rx **TREATMENT** In the absence of severe pulmonary vascular disease and predominant left-to-right shunting of blood, the patent ductus should be surgically ligated or divided. Transcatheter closure is experimental, using coils, buttons, plugs, and umbrellas. Thoracoscopic surgical approaches are considered experimental. Operation should be deferred for several months in patients treated successfully for infective endocarditis, because the ductus may remain somewhat edematous and friable.

AORTIC ROOT TO RIGHT HEART SHUNTS The three most common causes of aortic root to right heart shunts are congenital aneurysm of an aortic sinus of Valsalva with fistula, coronary arteriovenous fistula, and anomalous origin of the left coronary artery from the pulmonary trunk. *Aneurysm of an aortic sinus of Valsalva* consists of a separation or lack of fusion between the media of the aorta and the annulus fibrosis of the aortic valve. Rupture usually occurs in the third or fourth decade of life; most often the aorticocardiac fistula is between the right coronary cusp and the RV, but occasionally, when the noncoronary cusp is involved, the fistula drains into the RA. Abrupt rupture causes chest pain, bounding pulses, a continuous murmur accentuated in diastole, and volume overload of the heart. Diagnosis is confirmed by two-dimensional and Doppler echocardiographic studies; cardiac catheterization quantitates the left-to-right shunt, and thoracic aortography visualizes the fistula. Medical management is directed at cardiac failure, arrhythmias, or endocarditis. At operation, the aneurysm is closed and amputated, and the aortic wall is reunited with the heart, either by direct suture or with a prosthesis.

Coronary arteriovenous fistula, an unusual anomaly, consists of a communication between a coronary artery and another cardiac chamber, usually the coronary sinus, RA, or RV. The shunt is usually of small magnitude, and myocardial blood flow is not usually compromised. Potential complications include infective endocarditis, thrombus formation with occlusion or distal embolization, rupture of an aneurysmal fistula, and rarely, pulmonary hypertension and congestive failure. A loud, superficial, continuous murmur at the lower or midsternal border usually prompts a further evaluation of asymptomatic patients. Doppler echocardiography demonstrates the site of drainage; if the site of origin is proximal, it may be detectable by two-dimensional echocardiography. Retrograde thoracic aortography or coronary arteriography permits identification of the size and anatomic features of the fistulous tract, which may be closed by suture or transcatheter obliteration.

The third anomaly causing a shunt from the aortic root to the right heart is *anomalous origin of the left coronary artery from the pulmonary artery*. Myocardial infarction and fibrosis commonly lead to death within the first year, though up to 20% of patients survive to adolescence and beyond without surgical correction. The diagnosis is supported by the ECG findings of an anterolateral myocardial infarction. Operative management of adults consists of coronary artery bypass with an internal mammary artery graft or saphenous vein–coronary artery graft.

ACYANOTIC CONGENITAL HEART DISEASE WITHOUT A SHUNT

CONGENITAL AORTIC STENOSIS Malformations that cause obstruction to LV outflow include congenital valvular aortic stenosis, discrete subaortic stenosis, supravalvular aortic stenosis, and hypertrophic obstructive cardiomyopathy (Chap. 238).

Valvular Aortic Stenosis This malformation occurs three to four times more often in males than in females. The congenital bicuspid aortic valve, which is not necessarily stenotic, is one of the most common congenital malformations of the heart, although it may go undetected in early life. Because bicuspid valves may become stenotic with time or be the site of infective endocarditis, the lesion may be difficult to distinguish in adults from acquired rheumatic or degenerative calcific aortic stenosis.

The dynamics of blood flow associated with a congenitally deformed, rigid aortic valve commonly lead to thickening of the cusps and, in later life, to calcification. Hemodynamically significant obstruction causes concentric hypertrophy of the LV wall and dilatation of the ascending aorta.→*The clinical manifestations and hemodynamic abnormalities are discussed in Chap. 236.*

Rx **TREATMENT** The medical management of congenital valvular aortic stenosis includes prophylaxis against infective endocarditis and, in patients with diminished cardiac reserve, the administration of digitalis and diuretics and sodium restriction while awaiting operation. If severe aortic stenosis is present, strenuous physical activity should be avoided even when the patient is asymptomatic, and participation in competitive sports should probably be restricted in patients with milder degrees of obstruction. Aortic valve replacement is indicated in adults with critical obstruction, i.e., with an aortic valve area <0.5 cm^2/m^2, with symptoms secondary to LV dysfunction or myocardial ischemia, or with hemodynamic evidence of LV dysfunction. In asymptomatic children or adolescents or young adults with critical aortic stenosis without valvular calcification or these features, aortic balloon valvuloplasty is often useful (Chap. 245). If surgery is contraindicated in older patients because of a complicating medical problem such as malignancy or renal or hepatic failure, balloon valvuloplasty may provide short-term improvement. It may serve as a bridge to aortic valve replacement in patients with severe heart failure.

Subaortic Stenosis The most common form of subaortic stenosis is the *idiopathic hypertrophic* variety, also termed *hypertrophic cardiomyopathy*, which is present at birth in about one-third of the patients and is discussed in Chap. 238. In contrast, both clinically and physiologically, the *discrete* form of subaortic stenosis resembles valvular aortic stenosis. The lesion usually consists of a membranous diaphragm or fibrous ring encircling the LV outflow tract just beneath the base of the aortic valve. Echocardiography demonstrates the subaortic obstruction; Doppler studies show turbulence proximal to the aortic valve and also detect and quantitate the pressure gradient and severity of aortic regurgitation. Treatment consists of excision of the membrane or fibrous ridge.

Supravalvular Aortic Stenosis This anomaly consists of a localized or diffuse narrowing of the ascending aorta originating just above the level of the coronary arteries at the superior margin of the sinuses of Valsalva. In contrast to other forms of aortic stenosis, the coronary arteries are subjected to elevated systolic pressures from the LV, are often dilated and tortuous, and are susceptible to premature atherosclerosis. New information indicates that a genetic defect for the anomaly is located in the same chromosomal subunit as elastin on chromosome 7.

COARCTATION OF THE AORTA Narrowing or constriction of the lumen of the aorta may occur anywhere along its length but is most common distal to the origin of the left subclavian artery near the insertion of the ligamentum arteriosum. Coarctation occurs in ~7% of patients with congenital heart disease, is twice as common in males as in females, and is most frequent in patients with gonadal dysgenesis. Clinical manifestations depend on the site and extent of obstruction and the presence of associated cardiac anomalies, most commonly a bicuspid aortic valve. Aneurysmal arterial dilatation of the circle of Willis produces a high risk of sudden rupture and death.

Most children and young adults with isolated, discrete coarctation are asymptomatic. Headache, epistaxis, cold extremities, and claudication with exercise may occur, and attention is usually directed to the cardiovascular system when a heart murmur or hypertension in the upper extremities and absence, marked diminution, or delayed pulsations in the femoral arteries are detected on physical examination.

Enlarged and pulsatile collateral vessels may be palpated in the intercostal spaces anteriorly, in the axillae, or posteriorly in the interscapular area. The upper extremities and thorax may be more developed than the lower extremities. A midsystolic murmur over the anterior part of the chest, back, and spinous processes may become continuous if the lumen is narrowed sufficiently to result in a high-velocity jet across the lesion throughout the cardiac cycle. Additional systolic and continuous murmurs over the lateral thoracic wall may reflect increased flow through dilated and tortuous collateral vessels. The ECG usually reveals LV hypertrophy. Roentgenograms may show a dilated left subclavian artery high on the left mediastinal border and a dilated ascending aorta. Indentation of the aorta at the site of coarctation and pre- and poststenotic dilatation (the "3" sign) along the left paramediastinal shadow are almost pathognomonic. Notching of the ribs, an important radiographic sign, is due to erosion by dilated collateral vessels. Two-dimensional echocardiography from para- or suprasternal windows identifies the site and length of coarctation, while Doppler studies record and quantitate the pressure gradient. Transesophageal echocardiography and magnetic resonance imaging or digital angiography allow visualization of the length and severity of the obstruction and the associated collateral arteries. In adults, cardiac catheterization is indicated primarily to evaluate the coronary arteries.

The chief hazards result from severe hypertension and include the development of cerebral aneurysms and hemorrhage, rupture of the aorta, premature coronary arteriosclerosis, LV failure, and infective endocarditis.

℞ **TREATMENT**   Treatment is usually surgical; resection and end-to-end anastomosis or subclavian flap angioplasty are used commonly, although it may be necessary to use a tubular graft, patch, or bypass conduit if the narrowed segment is long. Systemic hypertension postoperatively, in the absence of residual coarctation, appears to be related to the duration of preoperative hypertension. Percutaneous balloon dilatation is controversial in native unoperated aortic coarctation but commonly successful for postsurgical recoarctation, often with deployment of a stent.

PULMONARY STENOSIS WITH INTACT VENTRICULAR SEPTUM   Obstruction to RV outflow may be localized to the supravalvular, valvular, or subvalvular levels or occur at a combination of these sites. Multiple sites of narrowing of the peripheral pulmonary arteries are a feature of *rubella embryopathy* and may occur with both the familial and sporadic forms of supravalvular aortic stenosis. Valvular pulmonic stenosis is the most common form of isolated RV obstruction.

The severity of the obstructing lesion, rather than the site of narrowing, is the most important determinant of the clinical course. In the presence of a normal cardiac output, a peak systolic transvalvular pressure gradient between 50 and 80 mmHg is considered to be moderate stenosis; levels below and above that range are classified as mild and severe, respectively. Patients with mild pulmonic stenosis are generally asymptomatic and demonstrate little or no progression in the severity of obstruction with age. In patients with more significant stenosis, the severity may increase with time. Symptoms vary with the degree of obstruction. Fatigue, dyspnea, RV failure, and syncope may limit the activity of older patients, in whom moderate or severe obstruction may prevent an augmentation of cardiac output with exercise. In patients with severe obstruction, the systolic pressure in the RV may exceed that in the LV, since the ventricular septum is intact. RV ejection is prolonged with moderate or severe stenosis, and the sound of pulmonary valve closure is delayed and soft. RV hypertrophy reduces the compliance of that chamber, and a forceful RA contraction is necessary to augment RV filling. A fourth heart sound, prominent *a* waves in the jugular venous pulse, and, occasionally, presystolic pulsations of the liver reflect vigorous atrial contraction. The clinical diagnosis is supported by a right parasternal lift and harsh systolic

ejection murmur and thrill at the upper left sternal border, typically preceded by a systolic ejection sound, if the obstruction is valvular. The holosystolic decrescendo murmur of tricuspid regurgitation may accompany severe pulmonic stenosis, especially in the presence of congestive heart failure. Cyanosis usually reflects right-to-left shunting through a patent foramen ovale or atrial septal defect. In patients with supravalvular or peripheral pulmonary arterial stenosis, the murmur is systolic or continuous and is best heard over the area of narrowing, with radiation to the peripheral lung fields.

The ECG may be helpful in assessing the degree of RV obstruction. In mild cases, the ECG is often normal, whereas moderate and severe stenoses are associated with right axis deviation and RV hypertrophy. A ventricular strain pattern, as well as high-amplitude P waves in leads II and V_1, indicating RA enlargement, is associated with severe stenosis. The chest roentgenogram with mild or moderate pulmonic stenosis often shows a heart of normal size and normal vascularity of the lungs. In the presence of valvular stenosis, poststenotic dilatation of the main and left pulmonary arteries may be evident. With severe obstruction and resultant RV failure, RA and RV enlargement are generally evident. The pulmonary vascularity may be reduced with severe stenosis, RV failure, and/or a right-to-left shunt at the atrial level. Two-dimensional echocardiography visualizes pulmonary valve morphology; the outflow tract pressure gradient can be estimated by Doppler ultrasonography.

℞ **TREATMENT**   The cardiac catheter technique of balloon valvuloplasty (Chap. 228) is usually effective. Direct surgical relief of moderate and severe obstruction may be accomplished at a low risk. Multiple stenoses of the peripheral pulmonary arteries are usually inoperable, but narrowing of a single branch or at the bifurcation of the main pulmonary trunk may be corrected.

CYANOTIC CONGENITAL HEART DISEASE WITH INCREASED PULMONARY BLOOD FLOW

COMPLETE TRANSPOSITION OF THE GREAT ARTERIES   In this condition the aorta arises from the RV to the right of and anterior to the pulmonary artery, which emerges from the LV (Fig. 234-1, *left panel*). This results in two separate and parallel circulations, and some communication between them must exist after birth to sustain life. Most patients have an interatrial communication, two-thirds have a patent ductus arteriosus, and about one-third have

FIGURE 234-1   Complete transposition of the great arteries is depicted in the left panel. The aorta arises from the RV and the pulmonary artery from the LV. The only mixing between the two circulations occurs across a patent foramen ovale. In the right panel, the tetralogy of Fallot cartoon illustrates the two most important anatomic findings, a large ventricular septal defect and RV outflow tract obstruction. A right-to-left shunt is shown across the ventricular septum.

an associated ventricular septal defect. Transposition is more common in males and accounts for ~10% of cyanotic heart disease.

The course is determined by the degree of tissue hypoxia, the ability of each ventricle to sustain an increased work load in the presence of reduced coronary arterial oxygenation, the nature of the associated cardiovascular anomalies, and the status of the pulmonary vascular bed. Pulmonary vascular obstruction develops by 1 to 2 years of age in patients with an associated large ventricular septal defect or large patent ductus arteriosus in the absence of obstruction to LV outflow.

℞ **TREATMENT** The balloon or blade catheter or surgical creation or enlargement of an interatrial communication in the neonate is the simplest procedure for providing increased intracardiac mixing of systemic and pulmonary venous blood. Systemic–pulmonary artery anastomosis may be indicated in the patient with severe obstruction to LV outflow and diminished pulmonary blood flow. Intracardiac repair may be accomplished by rearranging the venous returns (intraatrial switch, i.e., Mustard or Senning operation) so that the systemic venous blood is directed to the mitral valve and thence to the LV and pulmonary artery, while the pulmonary venous blood is diverted through the tricuspid valve and RV to the aorta. The late survival after these repairs is good, but late sudden death is the most worrisome feature. Preferably, this malformation is corrected in infancy by transposing both coronary arteries to the posterior artery and transecting, contraposing, and anastomosing the aorta and pulmonary arteries (arterial switch operation). For those patients with a ventricular septal defect in whom it is necessary to bypass a severely obstructed LV outflow tract, corrective operation employs an intracardiac ventricular baffle and extracardiac prosthetic conduit to replace the pulmonary artery (Rastelli procedure).

SINGLE VENTRICLE This is a family of complex lesions with both atrioventricular valves or a common atrioventricular valve opening to a single ventricular chamber. Associated anomalies include abnormal great artery positional relationships, pulmonic valvular or subvalvular stenosis, and subaortic stenosis.

Survival to adulthood depends on a relatively normal pulmonary blood flow and good ventricular function. Modifications of the Fontan approach are generally applied to these patients with creation of a pathway(s) from the systemic veins to the pulmonary arteries.

CYANOTIC CONGENITAL HEART DISEASE WITH DECREASED PULMONARY BLOOD FLOW

TRICUSPID ATRESIA This malformation is characterized by atresia of the tricuspid valve, an interatrial communication, and, frequently, hypoplasia of the RV and pulmonary artery. The clinical picture is usually dominated by severe cyanosis due to obligatory admixture of systemic and pulmonary venous blood in the LV. The ECG characteristically shows RA enlargement, left axis deviation, and LV hypertrophy.

Atrial septostomy and palliative operations to increase pulmonary blood flow, often by anastomosis of a systemic artery or vein to a pulmonary artery, may allow survival to the second or third decade. A Fontan atriopulmonary connection may then allow functional correction in those patients with normal or low pulmonary arterial resistance pressure and good LV function.

EBSTEIN'S ANOMALY Characterized by a downward displacement of the tricuspid valve into the RV, due to anomalous attachment of the tricuspid leaflets, the Ebstein tricuspid valve tissue is dysplastic and results in tricuspid regurgitation. The abnormally situated tricuspid orifice produces an "atrialized" portion of the RV lying between the atrioventricular ring and the origin of the valve, which is continuous with the RA chamber. Often the RV is hypoplastic. Although the clinical manifestations are variable, some patients come to initial attention because of progressive cyanosis from right-to-left atrial shunting, or symptoms due to tricuspid regurgitation and RV

dysfunction, or paroxysmal atrial tachyarrhythmias. Diagnostic findings by two-dimensional echocardiography include the abnormal positional relation between the tricuspid and mitral valves with apical displacement of the septal tricuspid leaflet. Tricuspid regurgitation is quantitated by Doppler examination. Surgical approaches include prosthetic replacement of the tricuspid valve when the leaflets are tethered or repair of the native valve.

TETRALOGY OF FALLOT The four components of the tetralogy of Fallot are ventricular septal defect, obstruction to RV outflow, aortic override (straddle) of the ventricular septal defect, and RV hypertrophy (Fig. 234-1, right panel).

The severity of RV outflow obstruction determines the clinical presentation. The severity of hypoplasia of the RV outflow tract varies from mild to complete (pulmonary atresia). Pulmonary valve stenosis and supravalvular and peripheral pulmonary arterial obstruction may coexist; rarely there is unilateral absence of a pulmonary artery (usually the left). A right-sided aortic arch and descending aorta occur in ~25% of patients with tetralogy.

The relationship between the resistance to blood flow from the ventricles into the aorta and into the pulmonary vessels plays a major role in determining the hemodynamic and clinical picture. Thus, the severity of obstruction to RV outflow is of fundamental significance. When the obstruction is severe, the pulmonary blood flow is reduced markedly, and a large volume of desaturated systemic venous blood is shunted from right to left across the ventricular septal defect. Severe cyanosis and erythrocytosis occur, and symptoms and sequelae of systemic hypoxemia are prominent. In many infants and children the obstruction is mild but progressive.

The ECG ordinarily shows RV and, less often, RA hypertrophy. Radiologic examination characteristically reveals a normal-sized, boot-shaped heart (*coeur en sabot*) with prominence of the RV and a concavity in the region of the pulmonary conus. The pulmonary vascular markings are typically diminished, and the aortic arch and knob may be on the right side. Two-dimensional echocardiography from the parasternal or subcostal windows demonstrates the malalignment of the ventricular septal defect and the subpulmonary stenosis. Selective angiocardiography with RV injection provides architectural details of the RV outflow tract, pulmonary valve and annulus, and caliber of the main branches of the pulmonary artery; coronary arteriography identifies the anatomy and course of the coronary arteries.

℞ **TREATMENT** Factors that may complicate the treatment of patients with tetralogy of Fallot include infective endocarditis, paradoxic embolism, excessive erythrocytosis, coagulation defects, and cerebral infarction or abscess. Corrective operation is advisable at some point for almost all patients with this anomaly. Successful correction avoids progressive infundibular obstruction, delayed growth, and complications due to hypoxemia and excessive erythrocytosis. The size of the pulmonary arteries rather than the age or size of the infant or child is the most important determinant in establishing candidacy for primary repair. Pronounced hypoplasia of the pulmonary arteries is a relative contraindication for an early corrective surgical procedure. When this problem is present, a palliative operation, such as creation of a systemic arterial–pulmonary arterial shunt, is carried out and is usually followed by complete correction, which can be carried out at a lower risk later in childhood.

OTHER FORMS OF CONGENITAL HEART DISEASES

CONGENITALLY CORRECTED TRANSPOSITION The two fundamental anatomic abnormalities in this malformation are transposition of the ascending aorta and pulmonary trunk and inversion of the ventricles. This arrangement results in desaturated systemic venous blood passing from the RA through the mitral valve to the LV and into the pulmonary trunk, whereas arterialized pulmonary venous blood flows from the left atrium (LA) through the tricuspid valve to the RV and into the aorta. Thus, the circulation is corrected functionally. The clinical presentation, course, and prognosis of patients with congenitally corrected transposition vary depending on the nature and severity of any complicating intracardiac anomalies. Ebstein-type anomalies of the left-side tricuspid atrioventricular valve, ventricular septal defect, obstruction to outflow from the venous ventricle, and congenital heart block are often associated with corrected transposition. The diagnosis of the malformation and associated lesions can often be established by two-dimensional echocardiography and Doppler examination.

MALPOSITIONS OF THE HEART Positional anomalies refer to conditions in which the cardiac apex is in the right side of the chest (dextrocardia), or at the midline (mesocardia), or in which there is a normal location of the heart in the left side of the chest but abnormal position of the viscera (isolated levocardia). Knowledge of the position of the abdominal organs and of the branching pattern of the main stem bronchi is important in categorizing these malpositions. When dextrocardia occurs without situs inversus, when the visceral situs is indeterminate, or if isolated levocardia is present, associated, often complex, multiple cardiac anomalies are usually present. In contrast, mirror-image dextrocardia is usually observed with complete situs inversus, which occurs most frequently in individuals whose hearts are otherwise normal.

SURGICALLY MODIFIED CONGENITAL HEART DISEASE

Because of the enormous strides in cardiovascular surgical techniques that have occurred in the past 20 years, a large number of long-term survivors of corrective operations in infancy and childhood have reached adulthood. These patients are often challenging because of the diversity of anatomic, hemodynamic, and electrophysiologic residua and sequelae of cardiac operations.

The proper care of the survivor of operation for congenital heart disease requires that the clinician understand the details of the malformation before operation; pay meticulous attention to the details of the operative procedure; and recognize the postoperative residua (conditions left totally or partially uncorrected), the sequelae (conditions caused by surgery), and the complications that may have resulted from the operation. With the exception of ligation and division of an uncomplicated patent ductus arteriosus, almost every other surgical repair of an anomaly leaves behind or causes some abnormality of the heart and circulation that may range from trivial to serious. Intraoperative transesophageal echocardiography assists in detecting unsuspected lesions, in monitoring the repair, and in verifying a satisfactory result or directing further repair. Thus, even with results that are considered clinically to be good to excellent, continued long-term postoperative follow-up is advisable.

Table 234-4 lists the categories of common late postoperative problems. Cardiac operations importantly involving the atria, such as closure of atrial septal defect, repair of total or partial anomalous pulmonary venous return, or venous switch corrections of complete transposition of the great arteries (the Mustard or Senning operations), may be followed years later by sinus node or atrioventricular node dysfunction or by atrial arrhythmias. Intraventricular surgery may also result in electrophysiologic consequences, including complete heart block necessitating pacemaker insertion to avoid sudden death. In ad-

Table 234-4 Potential Late Postoperative Problems

Residual shunts	Arrhythmias and conduction defects
Residual ventricular outflow obstruction	Myocardial dysfunction
	Prosthetic valve malfunction
Residual valvular anomalies	Prosthetic conduit obstruction
Systemic arterial hypertension	Infective endocarditis
Pulmonary vascular obstruction	

dition, valvular problems may arise late after initial cardiac operation. An example is the progressive stenosis of an initially nonobstructive bicuspid aortic valve in the patient who underwent aortic coarctation repair. Such aortic valves may also be the site of infective endocarditis. After repair of the ostium primum atrial septal defect, the cleft mitral valve may become progressively incompetent. Tricuspid regurgitation may also be progressive in the postoperative patient with tetralogy of Fallot if RV outflow tract obstruction was not relieved adequately at initial surgery. In many patients with surgically modified congenital heart disease, inadequate relief of an obstructive lesion, or a residual regurgitant lesion, or a residual shunt will cause or hasten the onset of clinical signs and symptoms of myocardial dysfunction. Despite a good hemodynamic repair, many patients with a subaortic RV develop RV decompensation and signs of "left heart failure." In many patients, particularly those who were cyanotic for many years before operation, a preexisting compromise in ventricular performance is due to the original underlying malformation.

A final category of postoperative problems involves the use of prosthetic valves, patches, or conduits in the operative repair. The special risks include infective endocarditis, thrombus formation, and premature degeneration and calcification of the prosthetic materials. There are many patients in whom extracardiac conduits are required to correct the circulation functionally and often to carry blood to the lungs from the RA or RV. These conduits may develop intraluminal obstruction, and, if they include a prosthetic valve, it may show progressive calcification and thickening.

BIBLIOGRAPHY

BRICKNER ME et al: Congenital heart disease in adults. N Engl J Med 342:256, 334, 2000

BURN J et al: Recurrence risks in offspring of adults with major heart defects: Results from first cohort of British collaborative study. Lancet 351:311, 1998

CHILD JS (section editor): Congenital heart disease. Curr Treatment Options Cardiovasc Med 1:301-379, 1999

CONNELLY MS et al: Canadian consensus conference on adult congenital heart disease 1996. Can J Cardiol 14:395, 1998

FRIEDMAN WF: Congenital heart disease in infancy and childhood, in *Heart Disease*, 6th ed, E Braunwald et al (eds). Philadelphia, Saunders, 2001

GATZOULIS MA et al: Atrial arrhythmia after surgical closure of atrial septal defects in adults. N Engl J Med 340:839, 1999

LIP GYH et al: Percutaneous balloon valvuloplasty for congenital pulmonary valve stenosis in adults. Clin Cardiol 22:733, 1999

MORRIS CD et al: Thirty-year incidence of infective endocarditis after surgery for congenital heart defect. JAMA 279:599, 1998

NIWA K et al: Eisenmenger syndrome in adults: Ventricular septal defect, truncus arteriosus, univentricular heart. J Am Coll Cardiol 34:223, 1999

SAIDI AS et al: Outcome of pregnancy following intervention for coarctation of the aorta. Am J Cardiol 82:786, 1998

235 *Edward L. Kaplan*

RHEUMATIC FEVER

In many parts of the world, especially in industrialized countries, acute rheumatic fever is less common than it was during the early and midyears of the twentieth century. In the late 1940s, patients with rheumatic fever and rheumatic heart disease accounted for more than half of schoolchildren recognized to have cardiovascular problems in the United States. During the Second World War, there were more than 20,000 cases of acute rheumatic fever in U.S. Navy personnel alone. The incidence of rheumatic fever has declined remarkably in the industrialized countries of the world, where the disease has become rare. However, in many developing countries, which account for almost two-thirds of the world's population, streptococcal infections, rheumatic fever, and rheumatic heart disease remain a very significant public health problem. The magnitude of the problem in these countries today is similar to that in North America 50 years ago.

The decreased incidence of acute rheumatic fever and the low prevalence of rheumatic heart disease in industrialized countries have led many physicians and public health authorities to the incorrect conclusion that these conditions are no longer a problem. However, starting in the 1980s, unexpected scattered outbreaks of acute rheumatic fever among both adults and children in North America have confirmed the capacity for this potentially serious illness to reappear and pose significant public health problems. Neither antimicrobial agents nor other public health measures have been totally effective in the control of rheumatic fever in the industrialized or industrializing world.

EPIDEMIOLOGY The epidemiology of acute rheumatic fever is identical to that of group A streptococcal upper respiratory tract infections (Chap. 140). As is the case for streptococcal sore throat, acute rheumatic fever most often occurs in children; the peak age-related incidence is between 5 and 15 years. Most initial attacks in adults take place at the end of the second and beginning of the third decades of life. Rarely, initial attacks occur as late as the fourth decade and recurrent attacks have been documented as late as the fifth decade.

Epidemiologic risk factors classically associated with individual attacks and especially with outbreaks of acute rheumatic fever include lower standards of living, especially crowding; the disease has been more common among socially and economically disadvantaged populations. However, the outbreaks in the United States in the late 1980s and early 1990s cannot be explained entirely by these factors. The large Utah outbreak of more than 500 cases during 13 years has affected primarily middle class patients with ready access to medical care. Therefore, one can conclude that the organism itself as well as the degree of host/herd immunity to the prevalent serotypes in an affected community are equally important risk factors.

Studies have shown that approximately 3% of individuals with untreated group A streptococcal pharyngitis will develop rheumatic fever. The epidemiology of rheumatic fever is also influenced by the serotypes of group A streptococci present in a population. The concept of "rheumatogenecity" of specific strains is largely based upon epidemiologic evidence associating certain serotypes with rheumatic fever (e.g., serotypes 1, 3, 5, 6, 18, etc.). Mucoid isolates are frequently associated with virulence and with rheumatic fever.

PATHOGENESIS More than half a century ago the pioneering studies of Lancefield differentiated beta-hemolytic streptococci into serologic groups. This ultimately led to the association of infection by the group A organism of the pharynx and tonsils (not of the skin) and the subsequent development of acute rheumatic fever. However, the mechanism(s) responsible for the development of rheumatic fever after an infection remains incompletely defined. Historically, approaches to understanding the pathogenesis of rheumatic fever have been grouped into three major categories: (1) direct infection by the group A streptococcus; (2) a toxic effect of streptococcal extracellular products on the host tissues; and (3) an abnormal or dysfunctional immune response to one or more as yet unidentified somatic or extracellular antigens produced by all (or perhaps only by some) group A streptococci.

There is insufficient evidence to support direct infection of the heart as the inciting event. Additionally, while toxins such as streptolysin O and others have been postulated to have a pathogenetic role, there is relatively little convincing evidence of this at the present time. Major efforts have focused on an abnormal immune response by the human host to one or more group A streptococcal antigens.

The hypothesis of "antigenic mimicry" between human and group A streptococcal antigens has been studied extensively and has concentrated on two interactions. The first is the similarity between the group-specific carbohydrate of the group A streptococcus and the glycoprotein of heart valves; the second involves the molecular similarity among the streptococcal cell membrane, streptococcal M protein sarcolemma, and other moieties of the human myocardial cell.

The possibility of a predisposing genetic influence in some individuals is one of the most tantalizing of the incompletely understood factors that might contribute to susceptibility to rheumatic fever. The precise genetic factors influencing the attack rate have never been adequately defined. Observations have been described that support the concept that this nonsuppurative sequel to a group A streptococcal upper respiratory tract infection results from an abnormal immune response by the human host. Thus, differences in immune responses to streptococcal antigens have been reported. Further, new data suggest that a unique surface marker on non-T lymphocytes in patients with rheumatic fever and rheumatic heart disease may prove helpful in defining which individuals are susceptible to developing rheumatic fever after a streptococcal infection because of abnormal immune responses.

DIAGNOSIS There is no specific laboratory test that can establish a diagnosis of rheumatic fever. The diagnosis, therefore, is a clinical one but requires supporting evidence from the clinical microbiology and clinical immunology laboratories. Because of the variety of signs and symptoms associated with the rheumatic fever syndrome, in 1944 Jones first proposed criteria to assist the clinician in standardizing the diagnosis of rheumatic fever. The most recent modification of the *Jones criteria* (Updated Jones Criteria) was published in 1992 by a Special Writing Group of the American Heart Association (Table 235-1).

There are five criteria termed *major* because they are most commonly found in patients with rheumatic fever: carditis, migratory polyarthritis, Sydenham's chorea, subcutaneous nodules, and erythema marginatum.

The *carditis* of acute rheumatic fever is a pancarditis involving the pericardium, myocardium, and endocardium. In most published series, between 40 and 60% of patients with acute rheumatic fever have evidence of carditis, which is characterized by one or more of the following: sinus tachycardia, the murmur of mitral regurgitation, an S_3 gallop, a pericardial friction rub, and cardiomegaly. The introduction of echocardiography has assisted in the identification of subtle abnormalities of the mitral valve, and these may be present in an additional 20% of patients who do not have an audible heart murmur. A prolonged PR interval and evidence of heart failure may be present as well, but these are nonspecific and may be found in a number of other diseases.

Healing of the rheumatic valvulitis may cause fibrous thickening and adhesion, resulting in the most serious complication of rheumatic fever, i.e., valvular stenosis and/or regurgitation (Chap. 236). The mitral valve is involved most frequently, followed by the aortic valve. However, isolated aortic valve disease as a consequence of acute rheumatic fever is quite rare. In patients with aortic valve disease due to rheumatic fever, the mitral valve is almost always simultaneously affected. Even minor degrees of rheumatic valvular involvement can lead to susceptibilities to infective endocarditis (Chap. 126). Although rheumatic pericarditis can cause a serous effusion, fibrin deposits, and even pericardial calcification, it does not lead to constrictive pericarditis.

A *migratory polyarthritis* is present in as many as 75% of cases, most often affecting the ankles, wrists, knees, and elbows over a period of days. It usually does not affect the small joints of the hands or feet

Table 235-1 The Jones Criteria for Rheumatic Fever, Updated 1992

Major Criteria	Minor Criteria
Carditis	Clinical
Migratory polyarthritis	Fever
Sydenham's chorea	Arthralgia
Subcutaneous nodules	Laboratory
Erythema marginatum	Elevated acute phase reactants
	Prolonged PR interval

plus
Supporting evidence of a recent group A streptococcal infection
(e.g., positive throat culture or rapid antigen detection test; and/
or elevated or increasing streptococcal antibody test)

SOURCE: Modified from the Special Writing Group of the American Heart Association.

and seldom involves the hip joints. Since salicylates and other anti-inflammatory drugs usually cause prompt resolution of joint symptoms, it is important that the clinician *not* prescribe these medications until it is determined whether the arthritis is migratory. The arthritis of acute rheumatic fever is extremely painful. Pain can be controlled with codeine or similar analgesics until the diagnosis is established. The difference between arthralgia (subjective joint pain) and arthritis (joint pain and swelling) must be understood. Too often, arthralgia is used (incorrectly) as a major criterion.

Sydenham's chorea occurs in fewer than 10% of patients with rheumatic fever. The latent period between the onset of the initiating streptococcal infection and the onset of Sydenham's chorea may be as long as several months. While differing from the other manifestations, this central nervous system disorder is a part of the rheumatic fever complex and should be managed as such. Many patients who appear to have only chorea may present several decades later with evidence of typical rheumatic valvular disease. There is no definitive laboratory test for establishing a diagnosis of Sydenham's chorea, and the diagnosis is one of exclusion. Patients with Sydenham's chorea should be given secondary prophylaxis for prevention of recurrent attacks, even if they do not appear to have rheumatic heart disease.

Subcutaneous nodules and *erythema marginatum* are rare major manifestations, usually present in fewer than 10% of cases. Subcutaneous nodules are found over extensor surfaces of joints, are seen most often in patients with long-standing rheumatic heart disease, and are extremely rare in patients experiencing an initial attack. Erythema marginatum is an uncommon manifestation. It is an evanescent macular eruption with rounded borders—usually concentrated on the trunk.

The *minor criteria* (Table 235-1) are nonspecific and may be present in many clinical conditions.

To fulfill the Jones criteria, either two major criteria, or one major criterion and two minor criteria, *plus* evidence of an antecedent streptococcal infection are required. The latter may be provided by recovery of the organism on culture or by evidence of an immune response to one of the commonly measured group A streptococcal antibodies (e.g., anti-streptolysin O, anti-deoxyribonuclease B, anti-hyaluronidase). Since the accurate diagnosis of rheumatic fever has future medical and financial implications, the clinician is obligated to evaluate any patient completely until the suspected diagnosis is either established or excluded.

Both the clinical microbiology and the clinical immunology laboratories have important roles in confirming the diagnosis of rheumatic fever. An attempt should be made to recover the organism from a throat culture, although group A streptococci can be recovered from the upper respiratory tract of only 25 to 40% of patients at the time the diagnosis is made. If a rapid antigen detection test is used but is negative, a confirmatory throat culture must be performed. It is helpful to obtain two or three cultures from the throat at the time the diagnosis is suspected but before initiating antibiotic therapy in order to confirm the presence of the organism.

At least 80% of patients with acute rheumatic fever have an elevated anti-streptolysin O titer at presentation. If one employs two additional streptococcal antibody tests such as the anti-DNAse B or anti-hyaluronidase test, the percentage of patients who show evidence of a preceding group A streptococcal infection will rise to more than 95%. While an initially elevated titer is convincing, being able to demonstrate a rise in titer from the acute to the convalescent phase is a more reliable means of documenting the recent infection. If three antibody tests are done and there is no evidence of a preceding infection, the diagnosis must be seriously reconsidered.

℞ **TREATMENT**   There are two necessary therapeutic approaches to patients with acute rheumatic fever: anti-streptococcal antibiotic therapy and therapy for the clinical manifestations of the disease. At the time of diagnosis, *all* patients with acute rheumatic fever should be treated as if they have a group A streptococcal infection, whether or not the organism is recovered by culture. In addition to the relatively large percentage of such patients who may have a negative throat culture at the time of diagnosis, others may have only a few organisms present in the throat. Conventional antibiotic treatment should be started immediately: a complete 10-day course in adults of either oral penicillin V (500 mg twice daily), or erythromycin (250 mg four times daily) for those with penicillin allergy. Many choose intramuscular benzathine penicillin G (a single intramuscular injection of 1.2 million units) for the treatment of the presumed streptococcal infection; this will also serve as the first dose of secondary prophylaxis for the prevention of recolonization of the upper respiratory tract in the future. Intramuscular benzathine penicillin G has been reported to result in a transient elevation of the erythrocyte sedimentation rate, which can prove confusing in the acute phase of the disease.

Following the initial anti-streptococcal therapy, secondary prophylaxis should be initiated to prevent subsequent colonization of the upper respiratory tract with group A streptococci. Recommendations of the American Heart Association and of the World Health Organization are for intramuscular injection of 1.2 million units of benzathine penicillin G every 4 weeks or for oral penicillin V (250 mg twice daily) or oral sulfadiazine (1.0 g daily). Recent studies have shown that in those individuals who are at high risk for recurrence of rheumatic fever, intramuscular benzathine penicillin G given every 3 weeks is more effective in reducing the risk of recurrence. Since it is known that the risk of recurrence of rheumatic fever is highest during the first 5 years after the attack, secondary prophylaxis is always given for at least this period. After that the decision to continue or discontinue secondary prophylaxis is dependent upon whether the patient has documented rheumatic heart disease and whether the patient is at high risk of exposure to streptococci (e.g., students, school teachers, medical and military personnel, etc.). Many believe that those with documented recurrences and/or documented rheumatic valvular heart disease should receive secondary prophylaxis for life. The duration of prophylaxis is often individualized for specific patients.

Medical therapy for the manifestations of rheumatic fever depends on the clinical status of the patient. For adult patients with the arthritis of rheumatic fever, salicylates in doses escalating to 2 g four times daily are very effective and will result in marked clinical improvement, often within 12 h. When this prompt relief does not occur, one should reexamine the original diagnosis. Salicylates may be given for 4 to 6 weeks and gradually tapered so as to prevent a rebound. The erythrocyte sedimentation rate is one method for determining the rate of taper for salicylates. Usually this requires at least 2 weeks. There are no conclusive data to support using nonsteroidal anti-inflammatory drugs for acute rheumatic fever. There is no indication for the use of steroids (usually prednisone) solely for the treatment of the arthritis of rheumatic fever.

Most experienced physicians believe that there is a role for steroids in patients with severe carditis accompanied by congestive heart failure. However, neither salicylates nor glucocorticoids influence the future development of valvular heart disease. In adults, prednisone can be started in doses as high as 30 mg four times daily in especially severe cases, and, as the patient improves, salicylates can be added during the tapering of the steroid dose; this may require 4 to 6 weeks.

In the presence of congestive heart failure, conventional medical measures (Chap. 232) are indicated. In the past, patients with acute rheumatic fever were kept at complete bed rest for months. This is inappropriate unless there is a specific reason such as persistent active carditis or severe heart failure. Patients with arthritis will begin to feel better very soon after anti-inflammatory therapy with salicylates is begun. They may be released from bed rest but should not resume full activity until signs of inflammatory process have abated and the acute-phase reactants have returned to normal.

BIBLIOGRAPHY

COMMITTEE ON RHEUMATIC FEVER, ENDOCARDITIS AND KAWASAKI DISEASE OF THE COUNCIL ON CARDIOVASCULAR DISEASE IN THE YOUNG OF THE AMERICAN HEART ASSOCIATION: Treatment of acute streptococcal pharyngitis and prevention of rheumatic fever: A statement for health professionals. Pediatrics 96:758, 1995

DAJANI A: Rheumatic fever, in *Heart Disease*, 6th ed, E Braunwald et al (eds). Philadelphia, Saunders, 2001

KAPLAN EL: Global assessment of rheumatic fever and rheumatic heart disease at the close of the century. The influences and dynamics of population and pathogens: A failure to realize prevention? (The T. Duckett Jones Memorial Lecture.) Circulation 88:1964, 1993

KAPLAN EL: The group A streptococcal upper respiratory tract carrier state: An enigma. J Pediatr 97:337, 1980

KIM EJ: Index of suspicion. Diagnosis: acute rheumatic fever (ARF). Pediatr Rev 21:21, 26, 2000

NARULA J et al (eds): Rheumatic fever, in *American Registry of Pathology*. Washington, DC, 1999

SPECIAL WRITING GROUP OF THE COMMITTEE ON RHEUMATIC FEVER, ENDOCARDITIS AND KAWASAKI DISEASE OF THE COUNCIL ON CARDIOVASCULAR DISEASE IN THE YOUNG OF THE AMERICAN HEART ASSOCIATION: Guidelines for the diagnosis of rheumatic fever. Jones criteria, 1992 Update. JAMA 268:2069, 1992

STEVENS DL, KAPLAN EL (eds): *Streptococcal Infections: Clinical Aspects, Microbiology, and Molecular Pathogenesis*. New York, Oxford Univ Press, 2000

VEASY GL et al: Persistence of acute rheumatic fever in the intermountain area of the United States. J Pediatr 24:9, 1994

236

Eugene Braunwald

VALVULAR HEART DISEASE

AF	atrial fibrillation	MVP	mitral valve prolapse
AR	aortic regurgitation	MVR	mitral valve replacement
AS	aortic stenosis	OS	opening snap
AVR	aortic valve replacement	PA	pulmonary arterial
CO	cardiac output	PAP	pulmonary arterial pressure
EF	ejection fraction	PR	pulmonary regurgitation
LA	left atrium	RA	right atrial
LV	left ventricle	RV	right ventricle
MR	mitral regurgitation	TR	tricuspid regurgitation
MS	mitral stenosis	TS	tricuspid stenosis

The role of physical examination in the evaluation of patients with valvular disease is also considered in Chap. 225; of electrocardiography in Chap. 226; of echocardiography in Chap. 227; and of cardiac catheterization and angiography in Chap. 228.

MITRAL STENOSIS

ETIOLOGY AND PATHOLOGY   Two-thirds of all patients with mitral stenosis (MS) are female. MS is generally rheumatic in origin; very rarely, it is congenital. Pure or predominant MS occurs in approximately 40% of all patients with rheumatic heart disease. In others, lesser degrees of MS may accompany mitral regurgitation (MR) and aortic valve lesions. With reductions in the incidence of acute rheumatic fever, particularly in temperate climates and developed nations, the incidence of MS is declining. In rheumatic stenosis the valve leaflets are diffusely thickened by fibrous tissue and/or calcific deposits. The mitral commissures fuse, the chordae tendineae fuse and shorten, the valvular cusps become rigid, and these changes, in turn, lead to narrowing at the apex of the funnel-shaped (fish-mouth) valve. Although the initial insult to the mitral valve is rheumatic, the later changes may be a nonspecific process resulting from trauma to the valve caused by altered flow patterns due to the initial deformity. Calcification of the stenotic mitral valve immobilizes the leaflets and narrows the orifice further. Thrombus formation and arterial embolization may arise from the calcific valve itself, but more frequently arise from the dilated left atrium (LA) in patients with atrial fibrillation (AF).

PATHOPHYSIOLOGY   In normal adults the mitral valve orifice is 4 to 6 cm². In the presence of significant obstruction, i.e., when the orifice is less than approximately 2 cm², blood can flow from the LA to the left ventricle (LV) only if propelled by an abnormally elevated left atrioventricular pressure gradient (see Fig. 228-2), the hemodynamic hallmark of MS. When the mitral valve opening is reduced to 1 cm², a LA pressure of approximately 25 mmHg is required to maintain a normal cardiac output (CO). The elevated pulmonary venous and pulmonary arterial (PA) wedge pressures reduce pulmonary compliance, contributing to exertional dyspnea. The first bouts of dyspnea are usually precipitated by clinical events that increase the rate of blood flow across the mitral orifice, resulting in further elevation of the LA pressure (see below). To assess the severity of obstruction, both the transvalvular pressure gradient and the flow rate must be measured (Chap. 228). The latter depends not only on the CO but on the heart rate as well. An increase in heart rate shortens diastole proportionately more than systole and diminishes the time available for flow across the mitral valve. Therefore, at any given level of CO, tachycardia augments the transvalvular gradient and elevates further the LA pressure. (Similar considerations apply to the tricuspid valve.)

The LV diastolic pressure is normal in isolated MS; coexisting aortic valve disease, systemic hypertension, MR, ischemic heart disease, and perhaps the residua of damage produced by rheumatic myocarditis are sometimes responsible for elevations that reflect impaired LV function and/or reduced LV compliance. LV dysfunction, as reflected in reduced LV ejection fraction (EF), occurs in about one-fourth of patients with severe, chronic MS and may be a consequence of prolonged reduction of preload and/or extension of scarring from the valve into the adjacent myocardium. In pure MS and sinus rhythm, the elevated LA and PA wedge pressures exhibit a prominent atrial contraction (*a* wave) and a gradual pressure decline after mitral valve opening (*y* descent) (see Fig. 228-4). In severe MS and whenever the pulmonary vascular resistance is significantly increased, the pulmonary arterial pressure (PAP) is elevated even when the patient is at rest, and in extreme cases it may approach the systemic arterial pressure. Further elevations of LA, PA wedge, and PAP occur during exercise. When the PA systolic pressure exceeds approximately 50 mmHg in patients with MS, or for that matter with any lesion affecting the left side of the heart, the increased right ventricle (RV) afterload impedes the emptying of this chamber, and the RV end-diastolic pressure and volume usually rise.

Cardiac Output   The hemodynamic response to mitral obstruction ranges from a normal CO and a high left atrioventricular pressure gradient to a markedly reduced CO and low transvalvular pressure gradient. In most patients with moderate MS, the CO is normal or almost so at rest but rises subnormally during exertion. In patients with severe MS, particularly those in whom the pulmonary vascular resistance is strikingly elevated, the CO is subnormal at rest and may fail to rise or may even decline during activity.

Pulmonary Hypertension   The clinical and hemodynamic features of MS are influenced importantly by the level of the PAP. Pulmonary hypertension results from (1) passive backward transmission of the elevated LA pressure; (2) pulmonary arteriolar constriction, which presumably is triggered by LA and pulmonary venous hypertension (reactive pulmonary hypertension); (3) interstitial edema in the walls of the small pulmonary vessels; and (4) organic obliterative changes in the pulmonary vascular bed. Severe pulmonary hypertension results in tricuspid regurgitation (TR) and pulmonary incompetence as well as right-sided heart failure. The changes in the pulmonary vascular bed also may be considered to exert a protective effect; the elevated precapillary resistance reduces the likelihood of symptoms of pulmonary congestion by reducing the surge of blood into the pulmonary capillary bed during activity. However, this protection occurs at the expense of a reduced, fixed CO.

SYMPTOMS   In temperate climates the latent period between the initial attack of rheumatic carditis (in the increasingly rare circumstances in which a history of one can be elicited) and the development of symptoms due to MS is generally about two decades; most patients begin to experience disability in the fourth decade. Studies carried out before the development of mitral valvotomy revealed that once a patient with MS became seriously symptomatic, the disease progressed continuously to death within 2 to 5 years. In economically deprived areas, in tropical and subtropical climates, particularly on the Indian subcontinent, in Central America, and in the Middle East, MS tends to progress more rapidly and frequently causes serious symptoms in patients less than the age of 20 years. In contrast, slowly progressive MS in the elderly is being recognized with increasing frequency in the United States and western Europe.

When valvular obstruction is mild, the physical signs of MS may be present without symptoms. However, even in patients whose mitral orifices are large enough to accommodate a normal blood flow with only mild elevations of LA pressure, marked elevations of this pressure leading to dyspnea and cough may be precipitated by severe exertion, excitement, fever, severe anemia, paroxysmal tachycardia, sexual intercourse, pregnancy, and thyrotoxicosis. As MS progresses, lesser stresses precipitate dyspnea, and the patient becomes limited in daily activities. The redistribution of blood from the dependent portions of the body to the lungs, which occurs when the recumbent position is assumed, leads to orthopnea and paroxysmal nocturnal dyspnea. *Pulmonary edema* develops when there is a sudden surge in flow across a markedly narrowed mitral orifice. When moderately severe MS has existed for several years, *atrial arrhythmias*—premature contractions, paroxysmal tachycardia, flutter, and AF—occur with increasing frequency. The rapid ventricular rate associated with untreated or inadequately treated AF is frequently responsible for acute exacerbations of dyspnea. The development of permanent AF often marks a turning point in the patient's course and is generally associated with acceleration of the rate at which symptoms progress.

Hemoptysis (Chap. 33) results from rupture of pulmonary-bronchial venous connections secondary to pulmonary venous hypertension. It occurs most frequently in patients who have elevated LA pressures without markedly elevated pulmonary vascular resistances and is almost never fatal.

As the severity of MS progresses and the pulmonary vascular resistance rises or when tricuspid stenosis (TS) or TR develop, symptoms secondary to pulmonary congestion sometimes diminish, and the episodes of acute pulmonary edema and hemoptysis may become reduced in frequency and severity. The elevation of pulmonary vascular resistance further increases RV systolic pressure, leading to RV failure, fatigue, abdominal discomfort due to hepatic congestion, and edema.

Recurrent pulmonary emboli (Chap. 261), sometimes with infarction, are an important cause of morbidity and mortality late in the course of MS. *Pulmonary infections*, i.e., bronchitis, bronchopneumonia, and lobar pneumonia, commonly complicate untreated MS. *Infective endocarditis* (Chap. 126) is rare in pure MS but is not uncommon in patients with combined MS and MR. *Chest pain* occurs in about 10% of patients with severe MS; it may be due to pulmonary hypertension or myocardial ischemia secondary to accompanying coronary atherosclerosis.

Pulmonary Changes   In addition to the aforementioned changes in the pulmonary vascular bed, fibrous thickening of the walls of the alveoli and pulmonary capillaries occurs commonly in MS. The vital capacity, total lung capacity, maximal breathing capacity, and oxygen uptake per unit of ventilation are reduced (Chap. 250), and the latter fails to rise normally during exertion. Pulmonary compliance falls further as pulmonary capillary pressure rises during exercise. In some patients, airway resistance is abnormally increased. These alterations in pulmonary mechanics contribute to an increase in the work of breathing and dyspnea. The diffusing capacity may be reduced, particularly during exertion, as a result of structural changes in the diffusing surface and reduction of the pulmonary capillary blood volume. These changes in the lungs are due, in part, to increased transudation of fluid from the pulmonary capillaries into the interstitial and alveolar spaces. However, the increased capacity of the pulmonary lymphatic system to drain excess fluid retards the development of alveolar edema.

Thrombi and Emboli   *Thrombi* may form in the left atria, particularly in the enlarged atrial appendages of patients with MS. If they *embolize*, they do so most commonly to the brain, kidneys, spleen, and extremities. Embolization occurs much more frequently in patients with AF or other unstable atrial arrhythmias, in older patients, and in those with a reduced cardiac output. However, systemic embolization may be the presenting complaint in otherwise asymptomatic patients with mild MS. At operation, thrombi are not found more frequently in the LA of patients with a past history of embolization than in those without this complication, indicating that usually the freshly formed clots are the ones that dislodge. Patients who have had one or more systemic emboli have an increased predilection for further embolic episodes. Rarely, a large pedunculated thrombus or a free-floating clot may suddenly obstruct the stenotic mitral orifice. Such "ball valve" thrombi produce syncope, angina, and changing auscultatory signs with alterations in position, findings that resemble those produced by an LA myxoma (Chap. 240).

PHYSICAL FINDINGS   (See also Chap. 225)   **Inspection and Palpation**   In patients with severe MS, there may be a malar flush with pinched and blue facies. In patients with sinus rhythm and severe pulmonary hypertension or associated TS, the jugular venous pulse reveals prominent *a* waves due to vigorous right atrial systole. In patients with AF, the jugular pulse reveals only a single expansion during systole (*c-v* wave). The systemic arterial pressure is usually normal or slightly low. A RV tap along the left sternal border signifies an enlarged RV. A diastolic thrill is frequently present at the cardiac apex, particularly with the patient in the left lateral recumbent position.

Auscultation   The first heart sound (S_1) is generally accentuated and snapping, and since the mitral valve does not close until the LV pressure reaches the level of the elevated LA pressure, this sound is often slightly delayed, causing a prolonged Q-S_1 interval on the phonocardiogram. The pulmonary component of the second heart sound (P_2) is often accentuated, and the two components of the second heart sound (S_2) are closely split. A pulmonary systolic ejection click may be heard in patients with severe pulmonary hypertension. The opening snap (OS) of the mitral valve is most readily audible in expiration at, or just medial to, the cardiac apex but also may be easily heard along the left sternal edge or at the base of the heart. This sound generally follows the sound of aortic valve closure (A_2) by 0.05 to 0.12 s; that is, it follows P_2. Since the OS occurs when the LV pressure falls below the LA pressure, the time interval between A_2 and OS varies inversely with the severity of the MS. The intensities of the OS and S_1 correlate with the mobility of the anterior mitral leaflet.

The OS is followed by a low-pitched, rumbling, diastolic murmur, heard best at the apex with the patient in the left lateral recumbent position (see Fig. 225-4). It is accentuated by mild exercise (e.g., a few rapid sit-ups) carried out just before auscultation. In general, the duration of this murmur correlates with the severity of the stenosis. In patients with sinus rhythm, the murmur often reappears or becomes reaccentuated during atrial systole, as atrial contraction reelevates the rate of blood flow across the narrowed orifice. Soft (grade I or II/VI) systolic murmurs are commonly heard at the apex or along the left sternal border in patients with pure MS and do not necessarily signify the presence of MR. Hepatomegaly, ankle edema, ascites, and pleural effusion, particularly in the right pleural cavity, may occur in patients with MS and RV failure.

Associated Lesions   With severe pulmonary hypertension, a pansystolic murmur produced by functional TR may be audible along the left sternal border. Characteristically, this murmur is accentuated by inspiration and diminishes during forced expiration (Carvallo's sign) or during performance of the Valsalva maneuver; it should not be confused with the apical pansystolic murmur of MR.

The recognition of associated MR is of considerable clinical importance in patients with MS. A presystolic murmur and an accentuated S_1 speak against the presence of serious associated MR, but when the S_1 and/or the OS are soft or absent in a patient with mitral valve disease who also has an apical systolic murmur, it is likely that significant MR and/or serious calcification of the deformed mitral valve leaflets are present. A third heart sound (S_3) at the apex often signifies that the MR is serious; this sound is generally duller, is lower pitched, and follows the OS. Occasionally, in patients with pure MS, physical signs may falsely suggest MR. A RV S_3 and an enlarged RV that forms the cardiac apex may give the erroneous impression of LV enlargement. The rumbling diastolic murmur of MS become less prominent or may even disappear and be replaced by the systolic murmur of functional TR, which is mistaken for MR. When CO is markedly reduced in a patient with MS, the typical auscultatory findings, including the diastolic rumbling murmur, may not be detectable (silent MS), but they may reappear as compensation is restored. Associated TS also tends to obscure many of the physical signs of MS.

The Graham Steell murmur of pulmonary regurgitation (PR), a high-pitched, diastolic, decrescendo blowing murmur along the left sternal border, results from dilatation of the pulmonary valve ring and occurs in patients with mitral valve disease and severe pulmonary hypertension. This murmur may be indistinguishable from the more common murmur produced by aortic regurgitation (AR), except that it is rarely audible at the second right intercostal space and may disappear after successful surgical treatment of the MS.

LABORATORY EXAMINATION **Electrocardiogram** In MS and sinus rhythm, the P wave usually suggests LA enlargement (see Fig. 226-10). It may become tall and peaked in lead II and upright in lead V_1 when severe pulmonary hypertension or TS complicates MS and right atrial (RA) enlargement occurs. The QRS complex is usually normal. However, with severe pulmonary hypertension, right axis deviation and RV hypertrophy are often present.

Roentgenogram The earliest changes are straightening of the left border of the cardiac silhouette, prominence of the main pulmonary arteries, dilatation of the upper lobe pulmonary veins, and backward displacement of the esophagus by an enlarged LA. In severe MS, however, all chambers and vessels upstream to the narrowed valve are prominent, including both atria, pulmonary arteries and veins, RV, and superior vena cava. Kerley B lines are fine, dense, opaque, horizontal lines that are most prominent in the lower and midlung fields and that result from distention of interlobular septa and lymphatics with edema when the resting mean LA pressure exceeds approximately 20 mmHg.

Echocardiogram (See also Chap. 227) This is the most sensitive and specific noninvasive method for diagnosing MS. Transthoracic two-dimensional color flow Doppler echocardiographic imaging and Doppler ultrasound provide critical information, including an estimate of the transvalvular gradient and of mitral orifice size, the presence and severity of accompanying MR, the extent of restriction of valve leaflets, their thickness, and the degree of distortion of the subvalvular apparatus, and the anatomic suitability for balloon mitral valvotomy. In addition, echocardiography provides an assessment of the size of the cardiac chambers, an estimation of the PAP, and an indication of the presence and severity of associated TR and PR. Transesophageal echocardiography provides superior images and should be employed when transthoracic imaging is inadequate for guiding therapy.

DIFFERENTIAL DIAGNOSIS Significant MR may also be associated with a prominent diastolic murmur at the apex, but this murmur commences slightly later in patients with MR than in patients with MS, and there is often clear-cut evidence of LV enlargement. An apical pansystolic murmur of at least grade III/VI intensity as well as an S_3 should arouse the suspicion of significant associated MR. Similarly, the apical middiastolic murmur associated with AR (Austin Flint murmur) may be mistaken for MS. TS, which occurs rarely in the absence of MS, may mask many of the clinical features of MS. Echocardiography is particularly useful in detecting MS in patients who have or are suspected of having other valve lesions and in defining the severity of the various lesions.

Primary pulmonary hypertension (Chap. 260) results in a number of the clinical and laboratory features of MS. It occurs most frequently in young women. However, the OS and diastolic rumbling murmur are absent, and the pulmonary artery wedge and LA pressures are normal, as is the size of the LA on echocardiography. *Atrial septal defect* (Chap. 234) also may be mistaken for MS; in both conditions

there is often clinical, electrocardiographic, and roentgenographic evidence of RV enlargement and accentuation of the pulmonary vascularity. The widely split S_2 of atrial septal defect may be confused with the mitral OS, and the diastolic flow murmur across the tricuspid valve may be mistaken for the mitral diastolic murmur. However, the absence of LA enlargement and of Kerley B lines and the demonstration of fixed splitting of S_2 favor atrial septal defect over MS.

Left atrial myxoma (Chap. 240) may obstruct LA emptying, causing dyspnea, a diastolic murmur, and hemodynamic changes resembling those of MS. However, patients with an LA myxoma often have features suggestive of a systemic disease, such as weight loss, fever, anemia, systemic emboli, and elevated erythrocyte sedimentation rate and serum IgG concentration. Usually an OS is not audible, and the auscultatory findings may change markedly with body position. The diagnosis can be established by the demonstration of a characteristic echo-producing mass in the LA with two-dimensional echocardiography.

CARDIAC CATHETERIZATION AND ANGIOCARDIOGRAPHY Left heart catheterization is useful for clarifying the picture when there is a discrepancy between clinical and echocardiographic findings (see Fig. 228-2). It is helpful in assessing associated lesions such as aortic stenosis (AS) and AR. Catheterization and coronary arteriography are not usually necessary to aid in the decision about surgery in younger patients with typical findings of severe obstruction on clinical examination and echocardiography. In males over 45 years of age, females over 55 years of age, and younger patients with coronary risk factors, especially those with positive noninvasive stress tests for myocardial ischemia, coronary angiography is usually advisable preoperatively to detect patients with critical coronary obstructions that should be bypassed at the time of operation. Catheterization and LV angiography are also indicated in most patients who have undergone balloon mitral valvotomy or previous mitral valve operations and who have redeveloped serious symptoms.

℞ TREATMENT In the asymptomatic adolescent with mitral valve disease, penicillin prophylaxis of β-hemolytic streptococcal infections (Chap. 235) and prophylaxis for infective endocarditis (Chap. 126) are important. In symptomatic patients, some improvement usually occurs with restriction of sodium intake and maintenance doses of oral diuretics. Digitalis glycosides do not alter the hemodynamics and usually do not benefit patients with pure MS and sinus rhythm but are necessary for slowing the ventricular rate of patients with AF. Small doses of beta blockers (e.g., atenolol 25 to 50 mg/d) may be added when cardiac glycosides fail to control ventricular rate in such patients. Anticoagulants should be administered for at least 1 year to patients with MS who have suffered systemic and/or pulmonary embolization and permanently to those with AF.

If AF is of relatively recent origin in a patient whose MS is not severe enough to warrant balloon mitral valvotomy or surgical valvotomy, reversion to sinus rhythm pharmacologically or by means of electrical countershock is indicated. Usually this reversion should be undertaken after the patient has had 3 weeks of anticoagulant treatment. Conversion to sinus rhythm is rarely helpful in patients with severe MS, particularly those in whom the LA is especially enlarged or in whom AF has been present for more than 1 year, since sinus rhythm is rarely sustained.

Mitral valvotomy Unless there is a specific contraindication, mitral valvotomy is indicated in the symptomatic patient with isolated MS whose effective orifice is less than approximately 1.0 cm²/m² body surface area, or <1.6 cm² in normal-sized adults. Mitral valvotomy can be carried out by two techniques: percutaneous balloon mitral valvotomy and surgical valvotomy. In balloon mitral valvotomy (Figs. 236-1 and 236-2), a catheter is directed into the LA after transseptal puncture and a balloon (Inoue balloon) is directed across the valve and inflated in the valvular orifice. This has become the procedure of choice for patients with uncomplicated MS.

FIGURE 236-1 Technique of double balloon mitral valvuloplasty. *A.* The position of the guidewire in the left atrium after left atrial puncture using the Brockenbrough needle. *B.* The position of the guidewire as it is advanced into the left ventricle across the stenotic mitral valve. C. Partial inflation of a balloon catheter across the stenotic mitral valve. *[From JP Srebro, TA Ports, Catheter-balloon valvuloplasty, in K Chatterjee et al (eds): Cardiology: An Illustrated Text. Philadelphia, Lippincott, 1991.]*

An "open" valvotomy with cardiopulmonary bypass is usually preferable to closed valvotomy. In addition to opening the valve commissures, it is important to loosen any subvalvular fusion of papillary muscles and chordae tendineae and to remove large deposits of calcium, thereby improving valvular function, as well as to remove atrial thrombi.

Valvotomy, whichever technique is used, usually results in striking symptomatic and hemodynamic improvement and prolongs survival. In uncomplicated cases, the mortality rate is <2%. However, there is no evidence that the procedure improves the prognosis of patients with slight or no functional impairment unless they develop severe pulmonary hypertension on exertion. Therefore, unless recurrent systemic embolization has occurred, valvotomy is *not* recommended for patients who are entirely asymptomatic, regardless of hemodynamic findings. When there is little symptomatic improvement after valvotomy, it is likely that the procedure was ineffective, that it induced MR, or that associated valvular or myocardial disease was present. The recurrence of symptoms several years after what appeared to be a satisfactory initial result is usually due to an inadequate valvotomy, but progression of other valvular lesions, mitral restenosis, or some combination of these conditions also may be responsible. About half of all patients undergoing mitral valvotomy require reoperation by 10 years. In the pregnant patient with MS, valvotomy should be carried out if pulmonary congestion occurs despite intensive medical treatment.

FIGURE 236-2 Simultaneous left atrial (LA) and left ventricular (LV) pressure before and after balloon mitral valvuloplasty in a patient with severe mitral stenosis. *[From Braunwald (Courtesy of Raymond G. McKay, MD).]*

PREDILATATION

ECG

40

Pressure (mmHg)

20

0

Mean mitral gradient 15 mmHg
Cardiac output 3.0 L/min
Mitral valve area 0.6 cm²

POSTDILATATION

ECG

40

20

0

Mean mitral gradient 3 mmHg
Cardiac output 3.8 L/min
Mitral valve area 1.8 cm²

Table 236-1 Mortality Rates After Valve Replacement and Repair

Operative Category	Number	Operative Mortality (%)
AVR (isolated)	26,317	4.3
MVR (isolated)	13,936	6.4
Multiple valve replacement	3,840	9.6
AVR + CAB	22,713	8.0
MVR + CAB	8,788	15.3
Multiple valve replacement + CAB	1,424	18.8
AVR + any valve repair	938	7.4
MVR + any valve repair	1,266	12.5
Aortic valve repair	597	5.9
Mitral valve repair	4,167	3.0
Tricuspid valve repair	144	13.9

NOTE: AVR, aortic valve replacement; CAB, coronary artery bypass; MVR, mitral valve replacement.
SOURCE: Modified from WRE Jamieson et al.

In patients with MS and significant associated MR, those in whom the valve has been severely distorted by previous transcatheter or operative manipulation, or those in whom the surgeon does not find it possible to improve valve function significantly, mitral valve replacement (MVR) may have to be carried out. Since the operative mortality rate of isolated MVR is still approximately 6% (Table 236-1), and since there are long-term complications of valve replacement, patients in whom preoperative evaluation suggests the possibility that MVR may be required should be operated on only if they have critical MS, i.e., an orifice <0.6 cm²/m² body surface area and are in New York Heart Association class III, i.e., symptomatic with ordinary activity, despite optimal medical therapy. The overall 10-year survival of surgical survivors is approximately 70%. Long-term prognosis is worse in older patients and those with marked disability and striking depression of the cardiac index preoperatively.

MITRAL REGURGITATION

ETIOLOGY Chronic rheumatic heart disease is the cause of severe MR in about one-third of cases. In contrast to MS, rheumatic MR occurs more frequently in males. The rheumatic process produces rigidity, deformity, and retraction of the valve cusps and commissural fusion, as well as shortening, contraction, and fusion of the chordae tendineae. Mitral valve prolapse (MVP), an important cause of MR, is considered in the next section. MR also may occur as a congenital anomaly (Chap. 234), most commonly as a defect of the endocardial cushions (atrioventricular cushion defects). MR may occur with fibrosis of a papillary muscle in patients with healed myocardial infarction as well as in patients with infarction involving the base of a papillary muscle. Transient MR also may occur during periods of ischemia involving a papillary muscle or the adjacent myocardium and may accompany bouts of angina pectoris. MR may occur with marked LV enlargement of any cause in which dilatation of the mitral annulus and lateral displacement of the papillary muscles interfere with coaptation of the valve leaflets. In hypertrophic cardiomyopathy, the anterior leaflet of the mitral valve is displaced anteriorly during systole, leading to regurgitation (Chap. 238). Calcification of the mitral annulus of unknown cause, presumably degenerative, which occurs most commonly in elderly women, also can be responsible for significant MR. Acute MR may occur secondary to infective endocarditis involving the valve or chordae tendineae, in acute myocardial infarction with rupture of a papillary muscle or one of its heads, as a consequence of trauma, or after chordal rupture.

Regardless of cause, severe MR is often progressive, since enlargement of the LA places tension on the posterior mitral leaflet, pulling it away from the mitral orifice and thereby aggravating the valvular dysfunction. Similarly, the dilatation of the LV increases the regurgitation, which in turn enlarges the LA and LV further, causing chordal rupture and resulting in a vicious circle; hence the aphorism, "mitral regurgitation begets mitral regurgitation."

PATHOPHYSIOLOGY The resistance to LV emptying is reduced in patients with MR. As a consequence, the LV is decompressed into the LA during ejection, and with the reduction in LV size there is a rapid decline in LV tension. The initial compensation to acute MR is more complete LV emptying. However, LV volume increases progressively as the severity of the regurgitation increases and as LV function deteriorates. This increase in LV volume is often accompanied by a depressed forward CO. The regurgitant volume varies directly with the LV systolic pressure and the size of the regurgitant orifice; the latter, in turn, is influenced profoundly by the extent of LV dilatation.

The v wave in the LA pressure pulse is usually prominent (see Fig. 228-3). During early diastole, as the distended LA empties, there is a particularly rapid y descent (as long as there is no associated MS). In chronic MR, there is often an increase in LV compliance, so that LV volume rises with little elevation in LV diastolic pressure. The effective (forward) CO is usually reduced in seriously symptomatic patients. A brief, early diastolic atrioventricular pressure gradient may occur in patients with pure MR as a result of the very rapid flow of blood across a normal-sized mitral orifice.

The prompt appearance of contrast material in the LA after its injection into the LV signifies the presence of MR. The regurgitant volume can be measured by determining the difference between the total LV stroke volume, estimated angiocardiographically, and the effective forward stroke volume determined by the Fick method (Chap. 228). In severe cases, as much as 50% of the total LV stroke volume regurgitates with each beat. Qualitative, but clinically useful, estimates of the severity of regurgitation may be made by observation on cineangiograms of the degree of LA opacification after the injection of contrast material into the LV. Color flow Doppler imaging is most commonly used for this purpose (see below).

The compliance, i.e., the pressure-volume relationship, of the LA and pulmonary venous bed affects the clinical picture. Patients with acute MR usually have *normal or reduced compliance*, little enlargement of the LA, but marked elevation of the LA pressure, particularly of the v wave. Pulmonary edema is common. Patients with a *marked increase in LA compliance* are at the opposite end of the spectrum, having long-standing, severe MR, marked enlargement of the LA, and normal or only slightly elevated LA and PA pressures. These patients usually complain of severe fatigue and exhaustion secondary to a low CO, while symptoms resulting from pulmonary congestion are less prominent; AF is almost invariably present. Most common are patients whose clinical and hemodynamic features are between those in the two aforementioned groups, with variable degrees of enlargement of the LA and with significant elevation of the LA pressure. Symptoms are secondary to a combination of reduced forward CO and pulmonary congestion.

SYMPTOMS Fatigue, exertional dyspnea, and orthopnea are the most prominent complaints in patients with chronic, severe MR. Systemic embolism occurs less frequently than in MS. Right-sided heart failure, with painful hepatic congestion, ankle edema, distended neck veins, ascites, and TR, occurs in patients with MR who have associated pulmonary vascular disease and marked pulmonary hypertension. In patients with acute, severe MR, LV failure with acute pulmonary edema is common.

PHYSICAL FINDINGS The arterial pressure is usually normal, and in patients with severe MR the arterial pulse may show a sharp upstroke. The jugular venous pulse shows abnormally prominent *a* waves in patients with sinus rhythm and marked pulmonary hypertension and prominent *v* waves in those with accompanying severe TR. A systolic thrill is often palpable at the cardiac apex, the LV is hyperdynamic with a brisk systolic impulse and a palpable rapid-filling wave, and the apex beat is often displaced laterally. An RV tap and the shock of pulmonary valve closure may be palpable in patients with marked pulmonary hypertension.

Auscultation The S_1 is generally absent, soft, or buried in the systolic murmur; indeed, an accentuated mitral closure sound is useful in excluding severe MR. In patients with severe MR, the aortic valve may close prematurely, resulting in wide splitting of the S_2. An OS indicates associated MS but does not exclude predominant regurgitation. A low-pitched S_3 occurring 0.12 to 0.17 s after the aortic valve closure sound, i.e., at the completion of the rapid-filling phase of the LV, is believed to be caused by the sudden tensing of the papillary muscles, chordae tendineae, and valve leaflets and is an important auscultatory feature of severe MR. The absence of an S_3 indicates that if MR exists, it may not be severe. The S_3 may be followed by a short, rumbling, diastolic murmur, even in the absence of MS. A fourth heart sound (S_4) is often audible in patients with acute, severe MR of recent onset who are in sinus rhythm. A presystolic murmur is not ordinarily heard with isolated MR but is present in patients with sinus rhythm and associated MS.

A systolic murmur of at least grade III/VI intensity, is the most characteristic auscultatory finding in severe MR. It is usually holosystolic (see Fig. 225-4), but it may be decrescendo and cease in late systole in patients with acute, severe MR when the tall v wave in the LA pressure pulse reduces the late systolic LV-LA (reverse) pressure gradient. In MR due to papillary muscle dysfunction or MVP, the systolic murmur commences in midsystole (see below). The systolic murmur is usually most prominent at the apex and radiates into the axilla. However, in patients with ruptured chordae tendineae or primary involvement of the posterior mitral leaflet, the regurgitant jet strikes the LA wall adjacent to the aortic root. In this situation, the systolic murmur is transmitted to the base of the heart and therefore may be confused with the murmur of AS. In patients with ruptured chordae tendineae the systolic murmur may have a cooing or "sea gull" quality, while a flail leaflet may cause a murmur with a musical quality. The systolic murmur of MR is intensified by isometric strain but is reduced during the Valsalva maneuver.

LABORATORY EXAMINATION **Electrocardiogram** In patients with sinus rhythm there is evidence of LA enlargement, but RA enlargement also may be present when pulmonary hypertension is severe. Chronic, severe MR is generally associated with AF. In many patients there is no clear-cut electrocardiographic evidence of enlargement of either ventricle. In others the signs of LV hypertrophy are present.

Roentgenogram The LA and LV are the dominant chambers; in chronic cases, the former may be massively enlarged and forms the right border of the cardiac silhouette. Pulmonary venous congestion, interstitial edema, and Kerley B lines are sometimes noted. Marked calcification of the mitral leaflets occurs commonly in patients with long-standing combined MR and MS. Calcification of the mitral annulus may be visualized.

Echocardiogram Color flow Doppler imaging is the most accurate noninvasive technique for the detection and estimation of MR. Two-dimensional echocardiography is useful for assessing LV function from end systolic and end-diastolic volumes and EF. The LA is usually enlarged and/or exhibits increased pulsations; the LV may be hyperdynamic. Findings that help to determine the etiology of MR can often be identified by two-dimensional echocardiography. Transesophageal imaging provides greater detail than transthoracic imaging. With ruptured chordae tendineae or a flail leaflet, coarse, errative motion of the involved leaflets may be noted. Vegetations associated with infective endocarditis, incomplete coaptation of the anterior and posterior mitral leaflets, and annular calcification, as well as MR secondary to LV dilatation, aneurysm, or dyskinesis may be recognized. The echocardiogram in patients with MVP is described in the next section.

R_x **TREATMENT** **Medical** The nonsurgical management of patients with severe MR begins with restricting those physical activities that regularly produce dyspnea and excessive fatigue, reducing sodium intake, and enhancing sodium excretion with the appropriate use of diuretics (Chap. 232). Vasodilators and digitalis glycosides increase the forward output of the failing LV. Intravenous nitroprusside or nitroglycerin to reduce afterload and thereby the volume of regurgitant flow are useful in stabilizing patients with acute and/or severe MR. Angiotensin-converting enzyme inhibitors are useful in the treatment of chronic MR. The same considerations as in patients with MS apply to the reversion of AF to sinus rhythm. In the late stages of heart failure anticoagulants and leg binders are used to diminish the likelihood of venous thrombi and pulmonary emboli.

Surgical In the selection of patients with severe MR for surgical treatment, the chronic, often slowly progressive nature of the condition must be balanced against the immediate and long-term risks associated with valve reconstruction or replacement. Patients with MR who are asymptomatic or who are limited only during strenuous exertion are not considered to be candidates for surgical treatment, since their condition may remain stable for many years. By contrast, unless there are contraindications, surgical treatment should be offered to patients with severe MR whose limitations do not allow full time employment or the performance of normal household activities despite optimal medical management. Surgical treatment of severe MR is indicated even for asymptomatic patients or those with mild symptoms when LV dysfunction is progressive, with LV ejection fraction declining below 60% and/or end-systolic cavity dimension on echocardiography rising above 50 mm. In patients with impaired LV function, the risk of surgery rises sharply, the recovery of LV performance is incomplete, and the long-term survival is reduced (Fig. 236-3). However, conservative management has little to offer these patients, so operative treatment may be indicated even at an advanced stage of the disease; and occasionally, the clinical and hemodynamic improvement that follows surgical treatment of patients with advanced disease is dramatic. Though most patients who survive surgery appear to be greatly improved, some degree of myocardial dysfunction may persist.

When surgical treatment is contemplated, left-sided heart catheterization and angiocardiography may be helpful in confirming the presence of severe MR in patients in whom there is a discrepancy between the clinical picture and the echocardiographic findings; these procedures may also aid in detecting and assessing the severity of associated valve lesions. Importantly, coronary arteriography identifies patients who require concomitant coronary revascularization.

Surgical treatment of MR, especially that caused by valves that are markedly deformed, with shrunken, calcified leaflets secondary to rheumatic fever, requires MVR with a prosthesis. However, in an increasing fraction of patients, particularly those with severe annular dilatation, flail leaflets, MVP, ruptured chordae, or infective endocarditis, reconstruction of the mitral valve apparatus (mitral valvuloplasty) and/or mitral annuloplasty with an annuloplasty ring may be successful. Valve reconstruction should be carried out whenever feasible since the operative risk is about half (~3%) of that associated with MVR (Table 236-1). Also, reconstruction spares the patient the long-term adverse consequences of valve replacement (i.e., thromboembolic and hemorrhagic complications in the case of mechanical

prostheses and late valve failure necessitating repeat valve replacement in the case of bioprostheses). In addition, by preserving the integrity of the papillary muscles and subvalvular apparatus, mitral valvuloplasty maintains LV function.

MITRAL VALVE PROLAPSE

MVP, also variously termed the *systolic click-murmur syndrome, Barlow's syndrome, floppy-valve syndrome,* and *billowing mitral leaflet syndrome,* is a relatively common, but highly variable, clinical syndrome resulting from diverse pathogenic mechanisms of the mitral valve apparatus. Among these are excessive or redundant mitral leaflet tissue, which is commonly involved with myxomatous degeneration and greatly increased concentration of acid mucopolysaccharide. It is a frequent finding in patients with heritable disorders of connective tissue, including the Marfan syndrome (Chap. 351), osteogenesis imperfecta, and the Ehler-Danlos syndrome. In most patients with MVP, however, myxomatous degeneration is confined to the mitral (or less commonly the tricuspid or aortic) valves without other clinical or pathologic manifestations of disease; the posterior leaflet is usually more affected than the anterior, and the mitral valve annulus is often greatly dilated. In many patients, elongated redundant chordae tendineae cause or contribute to the regurgitation.

In most patients with MVP, the cause is unknown, but in some it appears to be a genetically determined collagen tissue disorder. A reduction in the production of type III collagen has been incriminated, and electron microscopy has revealed fragmentation of collagen fibrils. MVP may be associated with thoracic skeletal deformities similar to but not as severe as those in the Marfan syndrome, including a high arched palate and alterations of the chest and thoracic spine, including the so-called straight back syndrome. MVP also may occur as a sequel of acute rheumatic fever, in ischemic heart disease, and in cardiomyopathies, as well as in 20% of patients with ostium secundum atrial septal defect.

MVP may lead to excessive stress on the papillary muscles, which in turn leads to dysfunction and ischemia of the papillary muscles and subjacent ventricular myocardium; rupture of chordae tendineae and progressive annular dilatation and calcification also contribute to valvular regurgitation, which then places more stress on the diseased mitral valve apparatus, thereby creating a vicious cycle. The electrocardiographic changes (see below) and ventricular arrhythmias appear to result from regional ventricular dysfunction related to increased stress placed on the papillary muscles.

CLINICAL FEATURES MVP is more common in females. It affects individuals in a wide age range but most commonly between the ages of 14 and 30 years. The clinical course is often benign. MVP may also be observed in older (>50 years) patients, often males, and in them MR is more often severe and requires surgical treatment. There is an increased familial incidence for some patients, suggesting an autosomal dominant form of inheritance. MVP encompasses a broad spectrum of severities in patients, ranging from only a systolic click and murmur and mild prolapse of the posterior leaflet of the mitral valve to severe MR due to chordal rupture and massive prolapse of both leaflets. In many patients, this condition progresses over years or decades.

Most patients are asymptomatic and remain so for their entire lives. However, MVP is now the most common cause of isolated severe MR requiring surgical treatment in North America. Arrhythmias, most commonly ventricular premature contractions and paroxysmal supraventricular and ventricular tachycardia, have been reported and may cause palpitations, light-headedness, and syncope. Sudden death has been noted but is a very rare complication. Many patients have chest pain that is difficult to evaluate. It is often substernal, prolonged, poorly related to exertion, and rarely resembles typical angina pectoris. Transient cerebral ischemic attacks secondary to emboli from the mitral valve due to endothelial disruption have been reported. Infective endocarditis may occur in patients with MR associated with MVP.

FIGURE 236-3 Late survival rates of patients surviving surgical correction of MR according to preoperative echocardiographic ejection fraction (EF). *(From M Enriquez-Sarano et al: Echocardiographic prediction of survival after surgical correction of organic mitral regurgitation. Circulation 90:833, 1994, with permission.)*

Auscultation The most important finding is the mid- or late (nonejection) systolic click, which occurs 0.14 s or more after the S_1 and is thought to be generated by the sudden tensing of slack, elongated chordae tendineae or by the prolapsing mitral leaflet when it reaches its maximum excursion. Systolic clicks may be multiple and may be followed by a high-pitched, late systolic crescendo-decrescendo murmur, which occasionally is "whooping" or "honking," and is heard best at the apex. The click and murmur occur earlier with standing, during the strain of the Valsalva maneuver, and any intervention that decreases LV volume, exaggerating the propensity of mitral leaflet prolapse. Conversely, squatting and isometric exercise, which increase LV volume, diminish mitral prolapse, and the click-murmur complex is delayed and may even disappear. Some patients have a midsystolic click without the murmur; others have the murmur without a click. Still others have both sounds at different times.

LABORATORY EXAMINATION The *electrocardiogram* most commonly is normal but may show biphasic or inverted T waves in leads II, III, and aVF, and occasionally supraventricular or ventricular premature contractions. *Two-dimensional echocardiography* is particularly effective in identifying the abnormal position and prolapse of the mitral valve leaflets; a useful echocardiographic definition of MVP is systolic displacement (in the parasternal view) of the mitral valve leaflets by at least 2 mm into the LA superior to the plane of the mitral annulus. Thickening of the mitral valve leaflets identifies a subgroup of patients at higher risk of infective endocarditis and the development of severe MR. Prolapse of the tricuspid and/or aortic valve may be found. *Color-imaging* and *Doppler studies* are helpful in revealing and evaluating accompanying MR. *Angiocardiography* generally shows prolapse of the posterior and sometimes of both mitral valve leaflets.

℞ **TREATMENT** The management of patients with MVP consists of reassurance of the asymptomatic patient without severe MR or arrhythmias and the prevention of infective endocarditis with antibiotic prophylaxis in patients with a systolic murmur and/or thickening of mitral valve leaflets on endocardiography. Beta blockers have been found to relieve chest pain. If symptomatic tachyarrhythmias have occurred, antiarrhythmic agents as dictated by electrophysiologic studies should be administered. If the patient is symptomatic from severe MR, mitral valve repair (or rarely, replacement) is indicated. Antiplatelet aggregation agents such as aspirin should be given to patients with transient ischemic attacks, and if these are not effective, anticoagulants should be used.

AORTIC STENOSIS

AS occurs in about one-fourth of all patients with chronic valvular heart disease; approximately 80% of adult patients with symptomatic valvular AS are male.

ETIOLOGY AS in adults may be congenital in origin, it may be secondary to rheumatic inflammation of the aortic valve, or it may be due to degenerative calcification of the aortic cusps of unknown cause. The *congenitally affected valve* may already be stenotic at birth (Chap. 234) and may become progressively more fibrotic, calcified, and stenotic. In other cases the valve may be congenitally deformed, usually bicuspid, without serious narrowing of the aortic orifice during childhood; its abnormal architecture makes its leaflets susceptible to otherwise ordinary hemodynamic stresses, which ultimately lead to valvular thickening, calcification, increased rigidity, and narrowing of the aortic orifice.

Rheumatic endocarditis of the aortic leaflets produces commissural fusion, sometimes resulting in a bicuspid valve. This condition in turn, makes the leaflets more susceptible to trauma and ultimately leads to fibrosis, calcification, and further narrowing. By the time the obstruction to LV outflow causes serious clinical disability, the valve is usually a rigid calcified mass, and careful examination may make it difficult or even impossible to determine the etiology of the underlying process. Rheumatic AS is almost always associated with rheumatic

involvement of the mitral valve. A rheumatic etiology is favored by a history of active rheumatic fever and by associated severe AR.

Age-related degenerative calcific AS (also known as senile or sclerocalcific AS) is now the most common cause of AS in adults in North America and Western Europe. About 30% of persons >65 years exhibit aortic valve sclerosis, many of whom have a systolic murmur of AS but without obstruction, while an additional 2% exhibit frank stenosis.

OTHER FORMS OF OBSTRUCTION TO LEFT VENTRICULAR OUTFLOW Besides valvular AS, three other lesions may be responsible for obstruction to LV outflow.

1. *Hypertrophic cardiomyopathy* (Chap. 238). This condition is characterized by marked hypertrophy of the LV and involves in particular the interventricular septum; it may cause subaortic obstruction.
2. *Discrete congenital subvalvular AS* (Chap. 234). This congenital anomaly is produced by either a membranous diaphragm or a fibrous ridge just below the aortic valve.
3. *Supravalvular AS* (Chap. 234). This uncommon congenital anomaly is produced by narrowing of the ascending aorta or by a fibrous diaphragm with a small opening just above the aortic valve.

PATHOPHYSIOLOGY The obstruction to LV outflow produces a systolic pressure gradient between the LV and aorta. When severe obstruction is suddenly produced experimentally, the LV responds by dilatation and reduction of stroke volume. However, in patients the obstruction may be present at birth and/or increases gradually over the course of many years, and LV output is maintained by the presence of concentric LV hypertrophy. This serves as a useful compensatory mechanism because it reduces toward normal the systolic stress developed by the myocardium. A large transaortic valvular pressure gradient may exist for many years without a reduction of CO or LV dilatation; ultimately, however, these changes occur.

A peak systolic pressure gradient >50 mmHg in the face of a normal cardiac output or an effective aortic orifice less than approximately 0.5 cm²/m² body surface area, i.e., less than approximately one-third of the normal orifice, is generally considered to represent critical obstruction to LV outflow. The elevated LV end-diastolic pressure observed in many patients with severe AS signifies the presence of LV dilatation and/or diminished compliance of the hypertrophied LV wall. A large *a* wave in the LA pressure pulse is usually present. Loss of an appropriately timed, vigorous atrial contraction, as occurs in AF or atrioventricular dissociation, may result in a rapid aggravation of symptoms. Although the CO at rest is within normal limits in most patients with severe AS, it usually fails to rise normally during exercise. Late in the course the CO and LV–aortic pressure gradient decline, and the mean LA, PA, and RV pressures rise.

The hypertrophied LV muscle mass elevates myocardial oxygen requirements. In addition, even in the absence of obstructive coronary artery disease, there may be interference with coronary blood flow, because the pressure compressing the coronary arteries exceeds the coronary perfusion pressure, often causing ischemia, especially in the subendocardium and during tachycardia both in the presence and in the absence of coronary arterial narrowing.

A significant fraction of patients with rheumatic AS has associated mitral valve disease. AS intensifies the severity of accompanying MR by increasing the pressure driving blood from the LV to the LA.

SYMPTOMS AS is rarely of hemodynamic or clinical importance until the valve orifice has narrowed to approximately 0.5 cm²/m² body surface area in adults. Even critical AS may exist for many years without producing any symptoms because of the ability of the hypertrophied LV to generate the elevated intraventricular pressures required for a normal stroke volume.

Most patients with pure or predominant AS have gradually increasing obstruction for years but do not become symptomatic until the sixth to eighth decades. Exertional dyspnea, angina pectoris, and syncope are the three cardinal symptoms. Often there is a history of insidious progression of fatigue and dyspnea associated with gradual curtailment of activities. *Dyspnea* results primarily from elevation of the pulmonary capillary pressure caused by elevations of LA and LV diastolic pressures secondary to reduced compliance and/or LV dilatation. *Angina pectoris* usually develops somewhat later and reflects an imbalance between the augmented myocardial oxygen requirements and reduced oxygen availability; the former results from the increased myocardial mass and intraventricular pressure, while the latter may result from accompanying coronary artery disease, which is not uncommon in patients with AS, as well as from compression of the coronary vessels by the hypertrophied myocardium. Therefore, angina may occur in severe AS even without obstructive epicardial coronary artery disease. *Exertional syncope* may result from a decline in arterial pressure caused by vasodilatation in the exercising muscles and inadequate vasoconstriction in nonexercising muscles in the face of a fixed CO or from a sudden fall in CO produced by an arrhythmia.

Since the CO at rest is usually well maintained until late in the course, marked fatigability, weakness, peripheral cyanosis, and other clinical manifestations of a low CO are usually not prominent until this stage is reached. Orthopnea, paroxysmal nocturnal dyspnea, and pulmonary edema, i.e., symptoms of LV failure, also occur only in the advanced stages of the disease. Severe pulmonary hypertension leading to RV failure and systemic venous hypertension, hepatomegaly, AF, and TR are usually late findings in patients with isolated, severe AS.

When AS and MS coexist, the reduction of cardiac output induced by MS lowers the pressure gradient across the aortic valve and thereby masks many of the clinical findings produced by AS. Left heart catheterization is helpful in defining the relative importance of each valvular abnormality.

PHYSICAL FINDINGS   The rhythm is generally regular until very late in the course; at other times, AF should suggest the possibility of associated mitral valve disease. The systemic arterial pressure is usually within normal limits. In the late stages, however, when stroke volume declines, the systolic pressure may fall and the pulse pressure narrow. Systemic hypertension is unusual in patients with marked AS, and a basal systolic arterial pressure >200 mmHg essentially excludes severe narrowing of this valve. The peripheral arterial pulse, as palpated in the carotid or brachial arteries, rises slowly to a delayed sustained peak (pulsus parvus et tardus) (see Fig. 225-2*B*). In the elderly, the stiffening of the arterial wall may mask this important physical sign. A palpable double systolic arterial pulse, the so-called bisferiens pulse, excludes pure or predominant AS and signifies dominant AR. In the late stages of AS, when the pulse pressure is reduced, the pulse amplitude may be so small that the anacrotic nature of the pulse and the delay in its upstroke may become difficult to appreciate. In many patients the *a* wave in the jugular venous pulse is accentuated. This results from the diminished distensibility of the RV cavity caused by the bulging, hypertrophied interventricular septum.

The LV impulse is usually active and displaced laterally, reflecting the presence of LV hypertrophy. A double apical impulse may be recognized, particularly with the patient in the left lateral recumbent position. A systolic thrill is generally present at the base of the heart, in the jugular notch, and along the carotid arteries. In patients who do not have marked pulmonary emphysema, a thick chest wall, thoracic deformity, or heart failure, the absence of a systolic thrill suggests that the AS is relatively mild.

Auscultation   An early systolic ejection sound, actually the OS of the aortic valve, is frequently audible in children and adolescents with congenital noncalcific valvular AS. This sound usually disappears when the valve becomes calcified and rigid. As AS increases in severity, LV systole may become prolonged so that the aortic valve closure sound no longer precedes the pulmonic valve closure sound, and the two components may become synchronous, or aortic valve closure may even follow pulmonic valve closure, causing paradoxic

splitting of the S_2 (Chap. 225). The sound of aortic valve closure can be heard most frequently in patients with AS who have pliable valves, and calcification diminishes the intensity of this sound. Frequently, an S_4 is audible at the apex and reflects the presence of LV hypertrophy and an elevated LV end-diastolic pressure; an S_3 generally occurs when the LV dilates.

The murmur of AS is characteristically an ejection (mid) systolic murmur that commences shortly after the S_1, increases in intensity to reach a peak toward the middle of ejection, and ends just before aortic valve closure (see Fig. 225-4). It is characteristically low-pitched, rough, and rasping in character, loudest at the base of the heart, most commonly in the second right intercostal space. It is transmitted upward along the carotid arteries. Occasionally, it is transmitted downward and to the apex where it may be confused with the systolic murmur of MR; the latter, however, is usually holosystolic. In almost all patients with severe obstruction, the murmur is at least grade III/VI. In patients with mild degrees of obstruction or in those with severe stenosis with heart failure in whom the stroke volume and therefore the transvalvular flow rate are reduced, the murmur may be relatively soft and brief.

LABORATORY EXAMINATION   **Electrocardiogram**   The main finding in most patients with severe AS is LV hypertrophy (see Fig. 226-10). In advanced cases, ST-segment depression and T-wave inversion (LV "strain") in standard leads I and aVL and in the left precordial leads are evident. However, there is no close correlation between the electrocardiogram and the hemodynamic severity of obstruction, and the absence of electrocardiographic signs of LV hypertrophy does not exclude severe obstruction. The presence of LA enlargement should suggest the possibility of associated mitral valve disease.

Roentgenogram   The chest roentgenogram may show no or little overall cardiac enlargement for many years, since the development of concentric LV hypertrophy is the initial response to obstruction to LV outflow. Hypertrophy without dilatation may produce some rounding of the cardiac apex in the frontal projection and slight backward displacement in the lateral view; critical AS is often associated with poststenotic dilatation of the ascending aorta. Aortic calcification is usually readily apparent on fluoroscopic examination or by echocardiography; *the absence of valvular calcification in an adult suggests that severe valvular AS is not present.* In later stages of the disease as the LV dilates, there is increasing roentgenographic evidence of LV enlargement; pulmonary congestion; and enlargement of the LA, PA, and right side of the heart.

Echocardiogram   The key findings are LV hypertrophy and, in patients with valvular calcification (i.e., most adult patients with symptomatic AS), multiple, bright, thick, echoes from within the aortic root. Eccentricity of the aortic valve cusps is characteristic of congenitally bicuspid valves (**Plate I-3**). Transesophageal imaging displays the obstructed orifice extremely well. LV dilatation and reduced systolic shortening reflect impairment of LV function. The transaortic valvular gradient can be estimated by Doppler echocardiography. Echocardiography is particularly useful for identifying valvular abnormalities such as MS and AR, which sometimes accompany AS, and for differentiating valvular AS from obstructive hypertrophic cardiomyopathy.

Catheterization   Catheterization of the left side of the heart and coronary arteriography should generally be carried out in patients suspected of having severe AS who are being considered for operative treatment. These investigations are especially indicated in the following:

1.   Patients with clinical signs of AS and symptoms of myocardial ischemia, in whom associated coronary artery disease is suspected. An effort should be made to determine whether AS or coronary atherosclerosis is primarily responsible for the symptoms, and coronary arteriography should be carried out in an effort to identify patients who require coronary bypass grafting at the time of aortic valve surgery.

2.   Patients with multivalvular disease, in whom the role played by each valvular deformity should be defined to aid in the planning of definitive operative treatment.

3. Young, asymptomatic patients with noncalcific congenital AS, to define the severity of obstruction to LV outflow, since operation [which does not usually require aortic valve replacement (AVR)] or balloon valvotomy may be indicated for them if severe AS is present, even in the absence of symptoms. Balloon valvotomy may follow left heart catheterization immediately.

4. Patients in whom it is suspected that the obstruction to LV outflow may not be at the aortic valve but rather in the sub- or supra-valvular regions.

NATURAL HISTORY Death in patients with severe AS occurs most commonly in the seventh and eighth decades. Based on data obtained at postmortem examination in patients not treated surgically, the average time to death after the onset of various symptoms was as follows: angina pectoris, 3 years; syncope, 3 years; dyspnea, 2 years; and congestive heart failure, 1.5 to 2 years. Moreover, in >80% of patients who died with AS, symptoms had existed for <4 years. Congestive heart failure was considered to be the cause of death in one-half to two-thirds of patients. Among adults dying with valvular AS, sudden death, which presumably results from an arrhythmia, occurred in 10 to 20% and at an average age of 60 years. However, most sudden deaths occur in patients who had previously been symptomatic.

TREATMENT All patients with moderate or severe AS require careful periodic follow-up. In patients with severe AS, strenuous physical activity should be avoided even in the asymptomatic stage. Digitalis glycosides, sodium restriction, and the cautious administration of diuretics are indicated in the treatment of congestive heart failure, but care must be taken to avoid volume depletion since this may cause a marked reduction of CO. While nitroglycerin is helpful in relieving angina pectoris, vasodilator therapy for heart failure is usually of little value and may, in fact, be harmful.

Surgical Treatment The most critical decision in the management of AS concerns the advisability of surgical treatment which, in most adults with calcific AS and critical obstruction (aortic orifice <0.5 cm²/m² body surface area), consists of AVR. In most instances, it is prudent to postpone operation in patients with severe calcific AS who are asymptomatic (unless they exhibit LV dysfunction), since their future course is difficult to predict and they may continue to do well for many years. However, they should be followed carefully by clinical examination for the development of symptoms and by serial echocardiograms for evidence of deteriorating LV function. Operation is generally indicated in patients with severe AS who are asymptomatic, irrespective of their LV function, as well as those who exhibit LV dysfunction, even if they are asymptomatic. In patients without heart failure, the operative risk of AVR is approximately 4% (Table 236-1).

When angina pectoris, syncope, or LV decompensation develops in adults with severe valvular AS, the outlook, despite medical treatment, is very poor and can be improved significantly by AVR. The operative risk is considerably lower than the risk of nonoperative treatment; moreover, the symptomatic improvement in some survivors of operation has been remarkable. Regression of LV hypertrophy may occur after relief of obstruction.

Operation should, if possible, be carried out before frank LV failure develops; at this late stage, the operative risk is high (15 to 20%), and evidence of myocardial disease may persist even when the operation is technically successful. Furthermore, long-term postoperative survival also correlates inversely with preoperative LV dysfunction. Nonetheless, in view of the very poor prognosis of such patients when they are treated medically, there is usually little choice but to advise surgical treatment. In patients in whom severe AS and coronary artery disease coexist, relief of the AS and revascularization of the myocardium by means of aortocoronary bypass grafting may result in striking clinical and hemodynamic improvement.

Because many patients with calcific AS are elderly, particular attention must be directed to the adequacy of hepatic, renal, and pulmonary function before AVR is recommended. The mortality rate depends to a substantial extent on the patient's preoperative clinical and

hemodynamic state. The 10-year survival rate of patients with AVR is approximately 60%. Approximately 30% of bioprosthetic valves evidence primary valve failure in 10 years, requiring re-replacement, and an approximately equal percentage of patients with mechanical prostheses develop significant hemorrhagic complications as a consequence of treatment with anticoagulants.

Percutaneous Balloon Aortic Valvuloplasty This procedure is preferable to operation in children and young adults with congenital, noncalcific AS. It is not commonly used in elderly patients with severe calcific AS because of a high restenosis rate. Nonetheless, this procedure has been used successfully in patients who are too ill or frail to undergo operation, in patients with life-threatening AS and advanced extracardiac disease, and as a "bridge to operation" in patients with severe LV dysfunction.

AORTIC REGURGITATION

ETIOLOGY AR may be caused by primary valve disease or by primary aortic root disease.

Primary Valve Disease Approximately three-fourths of patients with pure or predominant valvular AR are males; females predominate among patients with AR who have associated mitral valve disease. In approximately two-thirds of patients with AR the disease is rheumatic in origin, resulting in thickening, deformity, and shortening of the individual aortic valve cusps, changes that prevent their proper opening during systole and closure during diastole. A rheumatic origin is less common in patients with isolated AR. Acute AR may result from infective endocarditis, which can develop on a valve previously affected by rheumatic disease, a congenitally deformed valve, or, rarely, a normal aortic valve, and perforate or erode one or more of the leaflets. Patients with congenital membranous subaortic stenosis often develop thickening of the aortic valve leaflets, which makes the valves particularly susceptible to endocarditis. AR also may occur in patients with congenital bicuspid aortic valves. Prolapse of an aortic cusp, resulting in progressive chronic AR, occurs in approximately 15% of patients with ventricular septal defect (Chap. 234). Congenital fenestrations of the aortic valve occasionally produce mild AR. Although traumatic rupture of the aortic valve is an uncommon cause of acute AR, it does represent the most frequent serious lesion in patients surviving nonpenetrating cardiac injuries. The coexistence of hemodynamically significant AS with AR usually excludes all the rarer forms of AR because it occurs almost exclusively in patients whose AR is rheumatic or congenital in origin. In patients with AR due to primary valvular disease, dilatation of the aortic annulus may occur secondarily and intensify the regurgitation.

Primary Aortic Root Disease AR, both acute and chronic, also may be due entirely to marked aortic dilatation, i.e., aortic root disease, without primary involvement of the valve leaflets; widening of the aortic annulus and separation of the aortic leaflets are responsible for the AR (Chap. 247). Cystic medial necrosis of the ascending aorta, which may or may not be associated with other manifestations of the Marfan syndrome, idiopathic dilatation of the aorta, osteogenesis imperfecta, and severe hypertension all may widen the aortic annulus and lead to progressive AR. Occasionally, AR is caused by retrograde dissection of the aorta involving the aortic annulus. Syphilis and ankylosing rheumatoid spondylitis may be associated with cellular infiltration and scarring of the media of the thoracic aorta, leading to aortic dilatation, aneurysm formation, and severe regurgitation. In syphilis of the aorta, the involvement of the intima may narrow the coronary ostia, which in turn may be responsible for myocardial ischemia.

PATHOPHYSIOLOGY The total stroke volume ejected by the LV (i.e., the sum of the effective forward stroke volume and the volume of blood that regurgitates back into the LV) is increased in patients with AR. In patients with wide-open (free) AR, the volume of regurgitant flow may equal the effective forward stroke volume. In contrast to MR, in which a fraction of the LV stroke volume is delivered into the low-pressure LA, in AR the entire LV stroke volume is ejected into a high-pressure zone, the aorta. An increase in the LV end-diastolic volume (increased preload) constitutes the major hemodynamic compensation for AR. The dilatation of the LV allows this chamber to eject a larger stroke volume without requiring any increase in the relative shortening of each myofibril. Therefore, severe AR may occur with a normal effective forward stroke volume and a normal left ventricular/ejection fraction (EF) [total (forward plus regurgitant) stroke volume/end-diastolic volume], together with an elevated LV end-diastolic pressure and volume. However, through the operation of Laplace's law (which holds that myocardial wall tension is the product of intracavitary pressure and LV radius), LV dilatation increases the LV systolic tension required to develop any given level of systolic pressure. As LV function deteriorates, the end-diastolic volume rises and the forward stroke volume and EF decline. Deterioration of LV function often precedes the development of symptoms. Considerable thickening of the LV wall also occurs with chronic AR, and at autopsy the hearts of these patients may be among the largest encountered, sometimes weighing >1000 g.

The reverse pressure gradient from aorta to LV, which is responsible for the AR flow, falls progressively during diastole (see Fig. 228-4), accounting for the decrescendo nature of the diastolic murmur. Equilibration between aortic and LV pressures may occur toward the end of diastole in patients with severe AR, particularly when the heart rate is slow, and the LV end-diastolic pressure may be elevated, occasionally to extremely high levels (>40 mmHg). Rarely, in acute, severe AR, the LV pressure exceeds the LA pressure toward the end of diastole, and this reversed pressure gradient closes the mitral valve prematurely or causes diastolic MR.

In patients with severe AR, the effective forward CO usually is normal or only slightly reduced at rest, but often it fails to rise normally during exertion. Early signs of LV dysfunction include reduction in the EF, determined by echocardiography or radionuclide angiography. In advanced stages there may be considerable elevation of the LA, PA wedge, PA, and RV pressures and lowering of the forward CO at rest.

Myocardial ischemia may occur in patients with AR because myocardial oxygen requirements are elevated by both LV dilatation and elevated LV systolic tension. However, the major portion of coronary blood flow occurs during diastole, when arterial pressure is subnormal, thereby reducing coronary perfusion pressure. This combination of increased oxygen demand and reduced supply may cause myocardial ischemia, particularly of the subendocardium.

HISTORY A family history may frequently be elicited from patients with AR associated with the Marfan syndrome. A history compatible with infective endocarditis may sometimes be elicited from patients with rheumatic or congenital involvement of the aortic valve, and the infection often precipitates or seriously aggravates preexisting symptoms. Ankylosing spondylitis is usually self-evident.

Chronic, severe AR may have a long latent period, and patients may remain relatively asymptomatic for as long as 10 to 15 years. However, uncomfortable awareness of the heartbeat, especially on lying down, may be an early complaint. Sinus tachycardia during exertion or with emotion or premature ventricular contractions may produce particularly uncomfortable palpitations, as well as head pounding. These complaints may persist for many years before the development of exertional dyspnea, usually the first symptom of diminished cardiac reserve. The dyspnea is followed by orthopnea, paroxysmal nocturnal dyspnea, and excessive diaphoresis. Chest pain occurs frequently, even in younger patients, and it is not necessary to invoke the presence of coronary artery disease to explain this symptom in patients with severe AR. Anginal pain may develop at rest as well as during exertion. Nocturnal angina may be a particularly troublesome symptom, and it may be accompanied by marked diaphoresis. The anginal episodes can be prolonged and often do not respond satisfac-

torily to sublingual nitroglycerin. Systemic fluid accumulation, including congestive hepatomegaly and ankle edema may develop late in the course of the disease.

In patients with acute, severe AR, as may occur in infective endocarditis or trauma, the LV cannot dilate sufficiently to maintain stroke volume, and LV diastolic pressure rises rapidly with associated elevations of LA and PA wedge pressures. Pulmonary edema and/or cardiogenic shock may develop rapidly.

PHYSICAL FINDINGS In severe AR, the jarring of the entire body and the bobbing motion of the head with each systole can be appreciated, and the abrupt distention and collapse of the larger arteries are easily visible. The examination should be directed toward the detection of conditions predisposing to AR, such as the Marfan syndrome, rheumatoid spondylitis, and ventricular septal defect.

Arterial Pulse A rapidly rising "water-hammer" pulse, which collapses suddenly as arterial pressure falls rapidly during late systole and diastole (Corrigan's pulse), and capillary pulsations, an alternate flushing and paling of the skin at the root of the nail while pressure is applied to the tip of the nail (Quincke's pulse), are characteristic of free AR. A booming, "pistol-shot" sound can be heard over the femoral arteries (Traube's sign), and a to-and-fro murmur (Duroziez's sign) is audible if the femoral artery is lightly compressed with a stethoscope.

The arterial pulse pressure is widened, with an elevation of the systolic pressure, sometimes to as high as 300 mmHg, and a depression of the diastolic pressure. The measurement of arterial diastolic pressure with a sphygmomanometer may be complicated by the fact that systolic sounds are frequently heard with the cuff completely deflated. However, the level of cuff pressure at the time of muffling of the Korotkoff sounds generally corresponds fairly closely to the true intraarterial diastolic pressure. The severity of AR does not always correlate directly with the arterial pulse pressure, and severe regurgitation may exist in patients with arterial pressures in the range of 140/60 mmHg. As the disease progresses and the LV end-diastolic pressure rises markedly, the arterial diastolic pressure may actually rise also, since the aortic diastolic pressure cannot fall below the LV end-diastolic pressure.

Palpation The LV impulse is heaving and displaced laterally and inferiorly. The systolic expansion and diastolic retraction of the apex are prominent and contrast with the sustained systolic thrust characteristic of severe AS. A diastolic thrill is often palpable along the left sternal border, and a prominent systolic thrill may be palpable in the jugular notch and transmitted upward along the carotid arteries. This thrill and the accompanying systolic murmur are due to the markedly increased blood flow across the aortic orifice and do not necessarily signify the coexistence of AS. In many patients with pure AR or with combined AS and AR, the carotid arterial pulse is bisferiens, i.e., with two systolic waves separated by a trough.

Auscultation In patients with severe AR, the aortic valve closure sound is usually absent. An S_3 and systolic ejection sound are frequently audible, and occasionally, an S_4 also may be heard. The murmur of AR is typically a high-pitched, blowing, decrescendo diastolic murmur, heard best in the third intercostal space along the left sternal border (see Fig. 225-4). In patients with mild AR, this murmur is brief, but as the severity increases, generally becomes louder and longer, indeed holodiastolic. When the murmur is soft, it can be heard best with the diaphragm of the stethoscope and with the patient sitting up, leaning forward, and with the breath held in forced expiration. In patients in whom the AR is caused by primary valvular disease, the diastolic murmur is usually louder along the left than the right sternal border. However, when the murmur is heard best along the right sternal border, it suggests that the AR is caused by aneurysmal dilatation of the aortic root. "Cooing" or musical diastolic murmurs suggest eversion of an aortic cusp vibrating in the regurgitant stream. Unless it is trivial in magnitude, the AR is usually accompanied by peripheral signs such as a widened pulse pressure or a collapsing pulse. By contrast, with the Graham Steell murmur of pulmonary regurgitation, which may be confused with the diastolic murmur of AR, there usually is clinical evidence of severe pulmonary hypertension, including a loud and palpable pulmonary component of the S_2.

A midsystolic ejection murmur is frequently audible in AR. It is generally heard best at the base of the heart and is transmitted along the carotid vessels. This murmur may be quite loud without signifying aortic obstruction; it is often higher pitched, shorter, and less rasping in quality than the ejection systolic murmur heard in patients with predominant AS. A third murmur frequently heard in patients with severe AR is the Austin Flint murmur, a soft, low-pitched, rumbling middiastolic bruit. It is probably produced by the displacement of the anterior leaflet of the mitral valve by the AR stream but does not appear to be associated with hemodynamically significant mitral obstruction. Both the Austin Flint murmur and the rumbling diastolic murmur of MS are loudest at the apex, but the murmur of MS is usually accompanied by a loud S_1 and immediately follows the OS of the mitral valve, whereas the Austin Flint murmur is often shorter in duration than the murmur of MS; in patients with sinus rhythm the latter exhibits presystolic accentuation. The auscultatory features of AR are intensified by isometric exercise such as strenuous handgrip, which augments systemic resistance, and reduced by inhalation of amyl nitrite. A blowing holosystolic murmur at the apex, which is transmitted to the axilla, also may be heard in patients with AR who have marked LV dilatation and functional MR.

In acute, severe AR, the elevation of LV end-diastolic pressure may lead to early closure of the mitral valve, an associated middiastolic sound, a soft or absent S_1, a pulse pressure that is not particularly wide, and a soft, short diastolic murmur.

LABORATORY EXAMINATION Electrocardiogram In patients with mild AR, there may be no electrocardiographic abnormalities, but with severe, chronic AR, the electrocardiographic signs of LV hypertrophy become manifest (Chap. 226). In addition, these patients frequently exhibit ST-segment depression and T-wave inversion in leads I, aVL, V_5, and V_6 ("LV strain"). Left axis deviation and/or QRS prolongation denote diffuse myocardial disease, generally associated with patchy fibrosis, and usually signify a poor prognosis.

Roentgenogram In severe chronic AR, the apex is displaced downward and to the left in the frontal projection, and frequently the cardiac shadow extends below the left diaphragm. LV enlargement also may be apparent in the left anterior oblique and lateral projections, in which the LV is displaced posteriorly and encroaches on the spine. In patients in whom primary valvular disease is responsible for the AR, the ascending aorta and aortic knob may be moderately dilated. When AR is caused by primary disease of the aortic wall, aneurysmal dilatation of the aorta may be noted, and the aorta may fill the retrosternal space in the lateral view.

Echocardiogram Increased systolic excursion of the posterior left ventricular wall is evident; the extent and velocity of wall motion are normal or even supernormal, until myocardial contractility declines. A rapid, high-frequency fluttering of the anterior mitral leaflet produced by the impact of the regurgitant jet is a characteristic finding. The echocardiogram is also useful in determining the cause of AR, by detecting dilatation of the aortic annulus (**Plate I-3**). Thickening and failure of coaptation of the leaflets also may be noted. Color flow Doppler echocardiographic imaging is very sensitive in the detection of AR, and Doppler echocardiography is helpful in assessing its severity. Serial two-dimensional echocardiography is valuable in evaluating LV performance and in detecting progressive myocardial dysfunction.

Cardiac Catheterization and Angiography In addition to providing an accurate confirmation of the magnitude of regurgitation and the status of LV function, the condition of the coronary arterial bed may be evaluated preoperatively.

TREATMENT Although operation constitutes the principal treatment of AR and should be carried out before the development of heart failure, the latter usually responds briefly to treatment with digitalis glycosides, salt restriction, diuretics, and vasodilators, especially ACE inhibitors. Digitalis also may be indicated in patients with severe regurgitation and dilated left ventricles without frank LV failure. Cardiac arrhythmias and infections are poorly tolerated in patients with free AR and must be treated promptly and vigorously. Although nitroglycerin and long-acting nitrates are not as helpful in relieving anginal pain as in patients with ischemic heart disease, they are worth a trial. Long-acting nifedipine has been found to delay the need for operation. Patients with syphilitic aortitis should receive a full course of penicillin therapy (Chap. 172).

Surgical Treatment In deciding on the advisability and proper timing of surgical treatment, two points should be kept in mind: (1) patients with chronic AR usually do not become symptomatic until after the development of myocardial dysfunction, and (2) surgical treatment often does not restore normal LV function. Therefore, in patients with severe AR, careful clinical follow-up and noninvasive testing with echocardiography at approximately 6-month intervals are necessary if operation is to be undertaken at the optimal time, i.e., *after* the onset of LV dysfunction but *prior* to the development of severe symptoms. Operation can be deferred as long as the patient both remains asymptomatic and retains normal LV function. In general, operation should be carried out even in asymptomatic patients with progressive LV dysfunction and an LVEF $<55\%$ or a LV end-systolic volume >55 mL/m^2. (The latter has been referred to as the "55/55 rule.")

AVR with a suitable mechanical or tissue prosthesis is generally necessary in patients with rheumatic AR and in many patients with other forms of regurgitation. Rarely, when a leaflet has been perforated during an episode of infective endocarditis or torn from its attachments to the aortic annulus, surgical repair may be possible. When AR is due to aneurysmal dilatation of the annulus and ascending aorta rather than to primary valvular involvement, it may be possible to reduce the regurgitation by narrowing the annulus or by excising a portion of the aortic root without replacing the valve. More frequently, however, regurgitation can be eliminated only by replacing the aortic valve, excising the dilated or aneurysmal ascending aorta responsible for the regurgitation, and replacing the latter with a graft. This formidable procedure entails a higher risk than isolated AVR.

As in patients with other valvular abnormalities, both the operative risk and the late mortality are largely dependent on the stage of the disease and on myocardial function at the time of operation. The overall operative mortality for isolated AVR is 4.3% (Table 236-1). However, patients with marked cardiac enlargement and prolonged LV dysfunction experience an operative mortality rate of approximately 10% and a late mortality rate of approximately 5% per year due to LV failure despite a technically satisfactory operation. Nonetheless, because of the very poor prognosis with medical management, even patients with LV failure should be considered for operation.

ACUTE AORTIC REGURGITATION Infective endocarditis, aortic dissection, and trauma are the most common causes of severe, acute AR. Since the LV has not had time to dilate in this condition, stroke volume declines and ventricular diastolic pressure rises markedly; the arterial pulse pressure is often not markedly widened, and the physical signs characteristic of severe chronic AR may be absent. Premature closure of the mitral valve is common and can be recognized by echocardiography. The S_1 is soft or absent; the aortic diastolic murmur is characteristically brief. Patients present with pulmonary congestion and edema, as well as hypotension secondary to a low cardiac output. Acute, severe AR requires prompt surgical treatment, which may be lifesaving.

TRICUSPID STENOSIS

TS, a relatively uncommon valvular lesion in North America and western Europe, is more common in tropical and subtropical climates, especially on the Indian subcontinent, and in Latin America. It is generally rheumatic in origin and is more common in women than in men. It does not occur as an isolated lesion but is usually associated with MS. Hemodynamically significant TS occurs in 5 to 10% of patients with severe MS; rheumatic TS is commonly associated with some degree of TR.

PATHOPHYSIOLOGY   A diastolic pressure gradient between the RA and RV can be recorded with a double-lumen cardiac catheter. It is augmented when the transvalvular blood flow increases during inspiration and declines during expiration. A mean diastolic pressure gradient >4 mmHg is usually sufficient to elevate the mean RA pressure to levels that result in systemic venous congestion and, unless sodium intake has been restricted and diuretics administered, it is associated with ascites and edema, sometimes severe. In patients with sinus rhythm, the RA *a* wave may be extremely tall and may even approach the level of the RV systolic pressure. The resting CO is usually depressed and fails to rise during exercise. The low CO is responsible for the normal or only slightly elevated LA, PA, and RV systolic pressures despite the presence of MS.

SYMPTOMS   Since the development of MS generally precedes that of TS, many patients initially have symptoms of pulmonary congestion. Amelioration of these symptoms should raise the possibility that TS may be developing. Characteristically, patients complain of relatively little dyspnea for the degree of hepatomegaly, ascites, and edema that they have. Fatigue secondary to a low cardiac output and discomfort due to refractory edema, ascites, and marked hepatomegaly are common in patients with TS and/or TR. In some patients, TS may be suspected for the first time when symptoms of RV failure persist after an adequate mitral valvulotomy.

PHYSICAL FINDINGS   Since TS usually occurs in the presence of other obvious valvular disease, the diagnosis may be missed unless it is specifically considered and searched for. Severe TS is associated with marked hepatic congestion, often resulting in cirrhosis, jaundice, serious malnutrition, anasarca, and ascites. Congestive hepatomegaly and, in cases of severe tricuspid valve disease, splenomegaly are present. The jugular veins are distended, and in patients with sinus rhythm there may be giant *a* waves. The *v* waves are less conspicuous, and since tricuspid obstruction impedes RA emptying during diastole, there is a slow *y* descent. In patients with sinus rhythm there may be prominent presystolic pulsations of the enlarged liver as well.

On auscultation, the pulmonic valve closure sound is not accentuated, and occasionally, an OS of the tricuspid valve may be heard approximately 0.06 s after pulmonic valve closure. The diastolic murmur of TS has many of the qualities of the diastolic murmur of MS, and since TS almost always occurs in the presence of MS, the less common valvular lesion may be missed. However, the tricuspid murmur is generally heard best along the left lower sternal margin and over the xiphoid process and is most prominent during presystole in patients with sinus rhythm. The diastolic murmur is reduced in amplitude as the stethoscope is inched laterally, only to intensify or reappear as the mitral murmur at the apex. The murmur of TS is augmented during inspiration, and it is reduced during expiration and particularly during the strain of Valsalva maneuver, when tricuspid blood flow is reduced. This finding is often most easily elicited when the patient is in the erect position.

LABORATORY EXAMINATION   The electrocardiographic features of RA enlargement (Chap. 226) include tall, peaked P waves in lead II, as well as prominent, upright P waves in lead V_1. The *absence* of electrocardiographic evidence of renovascular hypertension (RVH) in a patient with right-sided heart failure who is believed to have MS should suggest associated tricuspid valve disease. The chest roentgenogram in patients with combined TS and MS show particular prominence of the RA and superior vena cava without much enlargement of the PA and with less evidence of pulmonary vascular congestion than occurs in patients with isolated MS. On echocardiographic

examination, the tricuspid valve is usually thickened; the transvalvular gradient can be estimated by Doppler echocardiography.

℞ **TREATMENT**   Patients with TS generally exhibit marked systemic venous congestion; intensive salt restriction and diuretic therapy are required during the preoperative period. Such a preparatory period may diminish hepatic congestion and thereby improve hepatic function sufficiently so that the risks of operation are diminished. Surgical relief of the TS should be carried out, preferably at the time of mitral valvotomy, in patients with moderate or severe TS who have mean diastolic pressure gradients exceeding approximately 4 mmHg and tricuspid orifices less than 1.5 to 2.0 cm². TS is almost always accompanied by significant TR. Open-heart repair may permit substantial improvement of tricuspid valve function. If this cannot be accomplished, the tricuspid valve may have to be replaced with a prosthesis, preferably a large bioprosthetic valve.

TRICUSPID REGURGITATION

Most commonly, TR is functional and secondary to marked dilatation of the RV and the tricuspid annulus. Functional TR may complicate RV enlargement of any cause, including inferior wall infarcts that involve the RV, and it is commonly seen in the late stages of heart failure due to rheumatic or congenital heart disease with severe pulmonary hypertension, as well as in ischemic heart disease, cardiomyopathy, and cor pulmonale. It is in part reversible if pulmonary hypertension is relieved. Rheumatic fever may produce organic TR, often associated with TS. Infarction of RV papillary muscles, tricuspid valve prolapse, carcinoid heart disease, endomyocardial fibrosis, infective endocarditis, and trauma all may produce TR. Less commonly, TR results from congenitally deformed tricuspid valves, and it occurs with defects of the atrioventricular canal as well as with Ebstein's malformation of the tricuspid valve (Chap. 234).

As is the case for TS, the clinical features of TR result primarily from systemic venous congestion and reduction of CO. With the onset of TR in patients with pulmonary hypertension, symptoms of pulmonary congestion diminish, but the clinical manifestations of right-sided heart failure become intensified. The neck veins are distended with prominent *v* waves; and marked hepatomegaly, ascites, pleural effusions, edema, systolic pulsations of the liver, and positive hepatojugular reflux are common. A prominent RV pulsation along the left parasternal region and a blowing holosystolic murmur along the lower left sternal margin, which may be intensified during inspiration and reduced during expiration or the strain of the Valsalva maneuver, are characteristic findings; AF is usually present.

The electrocardiogram usually shows changes characteristic of the lesion responsible for the enlargement of the RV that leads to TR. Roentgenographic examination usually reveals enlargement of both the RA and RV. Echocardiography may be helpful by demonstrating RV dilatation and prolapsing or flail tricuspid leaflets; the diagnosis of TR can be made by color flow Doppler echocardiography, and the severity estimated by Doppler examination. The latter is also useful in estimating PA pressure.

In patients with severe TR, the CO is usually markedly reduced, and the RA pressure pulse may exhibit no *x* descent during early systole but a prominent *c-v* wave with a rapid *y* descent. The mean RA and the RV end-diastolic pressures are often elevated.

℞ **TREATMENT**   Isolated TR, in the absence of pulmonary hypertension, such as that occurring as a consequence of infective endocarditis or trauma, is usually well tolerated and does not require operation. Indeed, even total excision of an infected tricuspid valve is often well tolerated if the PA pressure is normal. Treatment of the underlying cause of heart failure usually reduces the severity of functional TR. In patients with mitral valve disease and TR secondary to pulmonary hypertension and massive RV enlargement, effective surgical correction of the mitral valvular abnormality results in lowering of the PA pressures and gradual reduction or disappearance of the TR without direct treatment of the tricuspid valve. However, recovery may be much more rapid in patients with severe secondary TR if, at the time of mitral valve surgery, tricuspid annuloplasty (generally with the insertion of a plastic ring), open tricuspid valve repair, or, in the rare instance of severe organic tricuspid valve disease, tricuspid valve replacement is performed. Surgical treatment of the TR also should be carried out in patients with severe regurgitation secondary to deformity of the tricuspid valve due to rheumatic fever, particularly those *without* severe pulmonary hypertension.

PULMONIC VALVE DISEASE

The pulmonic valve is affected by rheumatic fever far less frequently than are the other valves, and it is uncommonly the seat of infective endocarditis. The most common *acquired* abnormality affecting the pulmonic valve is regurgitation secondary to dilatation of the pulmonic valve ring as a consequence of severe pulmonary hypertension. This produces the Graham Steell murmur, a high-pitched, decrescendo, diastolic blowing murmur along the left sternal border, which is difficult to differentiate from the far more common murmur produced by AR. It is usually of little hemodynamic significance; indeed, surgical removal or destruction of the pulmonic valve by infective endocarditis does not produce heart failure unless serious pulmonary hypertension is also present. The *carcinoid syndrome* may cause pulmonic stenosis and/or regurgitation. →*Congenital pulmonic stenosis is discussed in Chap. 234.*

VALVE REPLACEMENT

The results of replacement of any valve are dependent primarily on (1) the patient's myocardial function and general medical condition at the time of operation, (2) the technical abilities of the operative team and the quality of the postoperative care, and (3) the durability, hemodynamic characteristics, and thrombogenicity of the prosthesis. Increased operative mortality is associated with the higher levels of preoperative functional disability and pulmonary hypertension. Late complications of replacement of any valve, which are declining in incidence, include paravalvular leakage, thromboemboli, bleeding due to anticoagulants, mechanical dysfunction of the prosthesis, and infective endocarditis.

The considerations involved in the choice between a bioprosthetic (tissue) and artificial mechanical valve are similar in the mitral and aortic positions and in the treatment of stenotic, regurgitant, or mixed lesions. All patients who have undergone replacement of any valve with a mechanical prosthesis must be maintained permanently on anticoagulants, but this treatment imposes a hazard of hemorrhage. The primary advantage of bioprostheses over mechanical prostheses is the reduction of thromboembolic complications; and except for patients with chronic AF, few such instances have been associated with their use. The major disadvantage of bioprosthetic valves is their mechanical deterioration, the incidence of which is inversely proportional with age. This results in the need to replace the prosthesis in 30% of patients by 10 years and in 50% by 15 years. Bioprostheses are ordinarily not used in younger patients (<35 years) because of accelerated deterioration but are particularly useful in the elderly (>70 years), in whom there is more concern about chronic anticoagulation than about long-term (>15 years) valve durability. These valves are also indicated in women who expect to become pregnant, as well as others in whom anticoagulation may be contraindicated. Alternative bioprostheses are homograft (allograft) aortic valves obtained from cadavers and cryopreserved, pericardial autografts as well as pulmonary autograft transplanted into the aortic position. In patients without contraindications to anticoagulants, particularly those under 65 years, a mechanical prosthesis may be preferable. Many surgeons now select the St. Jude prosthesis, a double-disk tilting prosthesis, for replacement of both aortic and mitral valves because of somewhat more favorable hemodynamic characteristics and a suggestion of lower thrombogenicity.

BIBLIOGRAPHY

BONOW RO et al: ACC/AHA Guidelines for the management of patients with valvular heart disease. J Am Coll Cardiol 32:1486, 1998

BRAUNWALD E: Valvular heart disease, in *Heart Disease*, 6th ed, E Braunwald, D Zipes, P Libby (eds). Philadelphia, Saunders, 2001

BYRNE JG et al: Repair versus replacement of mitral valve for treating severe ischemic mitral regurgitation. Coron Artery Dis 11:31, 2000

CANNEGIETER SC et al: Oral anticoagulant treatment in patients with mechanical heart valves: How to reduce the risk of thromboembolic and bleeding complications. J Intern Med 245:369, 1999

CARABELLO BA, CRAWFORD FA: Valvular heart disease. N Engl J Med 337:32, 1997

HA JW et al: Tricuspid stenosis and regurgitation: Doppler and color flow echocardiography and cardiac catheterization findings. Clin Cardiol 23:51, 2000

JAMIESON WRE et al: Risk stratification for cardiac valve replacement. National Cardiac Surgery Database. Ann Thorac Surg 67:943, 1999

KIRKLIN JW, BARRATT-BOYES BG: Part III. Acquired valvular heart disease, in *Cardiac Surgery*, 2d ed, JW Kirklin, BG Barratt-Boyes (eds). New York, Wiley, 1993, p 425

KVIDAL P et al: Observed and relative survival after aortic valve replacement. J Am Coll Cardiol 35:747, 2000

OTTO CM (ed): *Valvular Heart Disease*. Philadelphia, Saunders, 1999, 468 pp

RAHIMTOOLA S (ed): *Valvular Heart Disease*, in *Atlas of Heart Diseases*, vol 11, E Braunwald (series ed). Philadelphia, Current Medicine, 1996

SENTHILNATHAN V et al: Heart valves: Which is the best choice? Cardiovasc Surg 7:393, 1999

VON SEGESSER LK et al: Less invasive aortic valve surgery: Rationale and technique. Eur J Cardiothorac Surg 15:781, 1999

237 *Eugene Braunwald*

COR PULMONALE

DEFINITIONS *Cor pulmonale* is defined as enlargement of the right ventricle (RV) secondary to abnormalities of the lungs, thorax, pulmonary ventilation, or circulation. It sometimes leads to RV failure, with an elevation of transmural RV end-diastolic pressure. Cor pulmonale and RV failure may be acute, as in pulmonary thromboembolism; or chronic, as in stable, severe chronic obstructive lung disease (COLD); or "acute on chronic," as in COLD with a superimposed infection and intensification of hypoxia. Approximately 20% of hospital admissions for heart failure are caused by RV failure associated with cor pulmonale. More than half of the patients with COLD have cor pulmonale, and this condition constitutes between 5 and 10% of all adult heart diseases in the United States. Cor pulmonale constitutes a higher percentage of all forms of heart disease in countries where the incidence of COLD is higher, such as the United Kingdom, and in areas such as Mexico City where air pollution is severe.

NORMAL FUNCTION OF THE PULMONARY CIRCULATION

The pulmonary circulation is interposed between the right and left ventricles for the purpose of gas exchange, the filtering out of particles, and the chemical modification of the blood, such as the conversion of angiotensin I to angiotensin II. Normally, flow through the pulmonary vascular bed depends not only on the pumping action of the RV but also on respiratory movements and on the filling and contraction of the left ventricle. Respiratory motion facilitates pulmonary blood flow by enhancing venous return into the thorax on inhalation; the positive pressure of exhalation then aids in propelling blood into the systemic vascular bed.

The stroke volume of the RV, as of the left, is regulated by its preload, contractility, and afterload (Chap. 231). Since the RV is a

Table 237-1   Cor Pulmonale

Mechanisms	Responses	Characteristics
PULMONARY VASCULAR DISEASES		
Emboli, large or multiple	Fall in cardiac output due to acute obstruction	Acute cor pulmonale Right ventricular distention Shock
Emboli, small; vasculitis; widespread lung damage (ARDS)	Pulmonary hypertension due to widespread hypoxia and microvascular obstruction	Subacute cor pulmonale Right ventricular distention Breathlessness and fever
Emboli, medium and recurrent; primary pulmonary hypertension; diet or drug vasopathy	Pulmonary hypertension due to vascular obstruction Low or normal cardiac output	Chronic cor pulmonale Right heart hypertrophy Breathlessness
RESPIRATORY DISEASES		
Obstructive Chronic bronchitis and emphysema; chronic asthma	Pulmonary hypertension due to hypoxia, vascular stretching, and loss of vessels Heart beat impeded externally by lung hyperinflation Normal or high output	Chronic cor pulmonale "Blue bloater" or "Pink puffer" (see Chap. 258)
Restrictive 1. Intrinsic: interstitial fibrosis, lung resection	Hypertension due to hypoxia, vascular distortion and loss Normal or low output	Chronic cor pulmonale Breathlessness Hyperventilation
2. Extrinsic: obesity, myxedema, muscle weakness, kyphoscoliosis, upper airway obstruction, diminished respiratory drive, high altitude	Hypertension due to alveolar hypoxia Normal or high output	Chronic cor pulmonale Peripheral edema Hypoventilation

NOTE: ARDS, acute respiratory distress syndrome.

relatively thin, compliant reservoir, acute changes in venous return (e.g., an increase with inhalation and decline with exhalation) can occur with little change in transmural RV pressure. However, the ability of the RV to increase its systolic pressure is limited. Normally, the RV afterload, which is closely related to the pulmonary artery pressure, is low. The pulmonary artery pressure normally rises slightly when blood is displaced into the chest at the start of exercise; on assuming recumbency; or with cold, anxiety, or pain. A driving pressure of only about 5 cmH$_2$O between the pulmonary artery (15 cmH$_2$O) and the left atrium (10 cmH$_2$O) normally propels the entire cardiac output of approximately 5 L/min at rest through the lungs, and only a modest increase in pressure is necessary to drive a flow of up to 25 L/min through the pulmonary capillary bed during maximal exercise.

The resistance of the pulmonary circulation (R), i.e., the pulmonary vascular resistance (Chap. 228), is calculated as the intravascular driving pressure (DP), i.e., pulmonary artery pressure minus pulmonary venous or left atrial pressure, divided by the pulmonary blood flow rate ($\dot{Q}$). The caliber of a distensible vessel depends on its transmural pressure. Calculated R increases when vessels collapse, narrow, or lengthen, or when the viscosity of the blood increases.

$$R = \frac{Kl\mu}{r^4}$$

where K = constant; l = length; r = radius; and μ = viscosity. Calculated R decreases with increasing pulmonary blood flow because pulmonary vessels are distended and collapsed vessels are recruited.

PATHOPHYSIOLOGY   The severity of RV enlargement in cor pulmonale is a function of the increase in afterload. When the pulmonary vascular resistance is elevated and relatively fixed, as in pulmonary vascular or severe parenchymal lung disease, an elevation in cardiac output as occurs with physical exertion can elevate pulmonary artery pressure markedly. RV afterload may be augmented when the lungs are hyperinflated, as in COLD, due to the compression of the alveolar capillaries and the lengthening of the pulmonary vessels. RV afterload can also increase when lung volume is reduced following extensive pulmonary resection, as well as in restrictive lung diseases in which pulmonary vessels are compressed and distorted. RV afterload rises with hypoxic pulmonary vasoconstriction caused by hypoxia or acidosis, which are important causes of pulmonary hypertension. Hypoxic vasoconstriction in regions of the lung affected by disease distributes blood flow to normally ventilated regions. Hypoxic vasoconstriction results from alveolar, rather than intravascular, hypoxia and is exaggerated by hypercapnia, probably because of the associated acidosis. When the hematocrit becomes markedly elevated with chronic hypoxemia (secondary polycythemia), the increase in blood viscosity can also aggravate the pulmonary hypertension. Chronic hypoxic pulmonary vasoconstriction may cause pulmonary vascular disease with endothelial swelling and medial hypertrophy (see below).

The elevation of RV afterload responsible for cor pulmonale is caused principally by pulmonary vascular or parenchymal disease. The principal syndromes and their pathophysiologic mechanisms are summarized in Table 237-1.

PULMONARY VASCULAR DISEASES

In these conditions the RV afterload is elevated as a consequence of restriction to pulmonary blood flow. In cor pulmonale secondary to pulmonary vascular disease, pulmonary hypertension is usually more severe than in pulmonary parenchymal disease. Chronic cor pulmonale secondary to pulmonary vascular disease may result from repeated pulmonary emboli, pulmonary vasculitis, pulmonary vasoconstriction secondary to high altitude, congenital heart disease with left-to-right shunting (e.g., atrial or ventricular septal defect, patent ductus arteriosus; Chap. 234), as well as pulmonary venoocclusive disease. When the cause of elevated pulmonary vascular resistance responsible for cor pulmonale cannot be defined, the condition is referred to as *primary pulmonary hypertension* (Chap. 260).

COR PULMONALE DUE TO PULMONARY EMBOLI
This condition is associated with two distinct syndromes.

Acute Cor Pulmonale   It has been estimated that in the United States about 50,000 people die each year from pulmonary thromboembolism (Chap. 261). Probably half die within the first hour from acute right heart failure due to massive or multiple emboli. A sudden, large embolic burden causes a low-output state resulting from the RV's inability to generate the pressure necessary to drive blood through the acutely compromised pulmonary vascular bed. Depression of cardiac output can also occur with a moderate-sized embolism if the pulmonary circulation has been critically compromised by previous pulmonary vascular or parenchymal disease. The RV begins to fail when systolic pressure is forced to double acutely, i.e., to exceed approximately 50 mmHg. Acute RV failure secondary to pulmonary embolism is suggested by the history of the sudden onset of severe dyspnea and cardiovascular collapse in a patient with, or predisposed to, venous thrombosis.

Clinical manifestations   Acute RV failure causes pallor, sweating, hypotension, and a rapid pulse of small amplitude. The neck veins are distended and often exhibit prominent *v* waves secondary to tricuspid regurgitation. The liver may be pulsatile, distended, and tender. A systolic murmur of tricuspid regurgitation along the left sternal border may be accompanied by a presystolic (S_4) gallop sound. Arterial blood gas frequently shows reduced Pa_{O_2} due to ventilation/perfusion mismatching and a low Pa_{CO_2} due to hyperventilation.

℞ **TREATMENT** If the cardiac output remains adequate to sustain the patient during the critical first 2 or 3 h, endogenous thrombolysis usually results in fragmentation of the clot and the pulmonary artery pressure returns to normal rapidly. Although it has been shown that treatment with thrombolytic agents lyses clots more rapidly than does heparin (Chap. 261), this therapy is probably indicated only when cardiac output is critically reduced and the RV fails. In acute cor pulmonale [and in RV failure due to acute RV infarction (Chap. 243)], an increase in RV preload can be achieved by a cautious expansion of blood volume, which helps to maintain cardiac output. When hypoxic pulmonary vasoconstriction contributes to pulmonary hypertension, inhalation of 100% O_2 reduces RV afterload.

Chronic Cor Pulmonale Secondary to Pulmonary Vascular Disease In contrast to acute, massive thromboembolism, when the elevation in pulmonary vascular resistance and the RV hypertrophy develop gradually, higher pulmonary vascular pressures, sometimes even approaching systemic arterial levels, may be generated. Chronic cor pulmonale can be caused by recurrent, medium-sized emboli that fail to lyse, but organize, resulting in chronic thromboembolic pulmonary hypertension. Particles from intravenous drug abuse, parasites, or tumor tissue that embolizes into the pulmonary vascular bed may also cause persistent pulmonary hypertension. Chronic cor pulmonale can also be caused by *primary pulmonary hypertension* (Chap. 260) or any chronic widespread vasculitis, such as occurs in association with collagen vascular disorders and that may affect the pulmonary vascular bed, particularly the CREST syndrome (Chap. 313).

Clinical Manifestations Dyspnea and tachypnea are characteristic features of pulmonary hypertension secondary to pulmonary vascular disease. They may be distressing during mild exertion or even at rest and are *not* relieved by sitting upright. An unproductive cough is another frequent complaint. Anterior chest pain, due to acute dilation of the root of the pulmonary artery or RV ischemia, can occur. The elevation in systemic venous pressure can cause hepatomegaly and ankle edema.

Occasionally there is cyanosis due to arterial hypoxemia and low cardiac output. A RV heave may be palpable along the left sternal border or in the epigastrium, and a high-pitched pulmonary ejection click may be audible to the left of the upper sternum. The second (pulmonary) component of the second heart sound is intensified and may be palpable; fixed narrow splitting of the second heart sound and a right ventricular protodiastolic gallop (S_3) that may increase during inspiration can be present. A systolic murmur of tricuspid regurgitation, which is augmented by inspiration, is often audible; occasionally, a diastolic murmur of pulmonary regurgitation is also heard. Prominent *a* (and sometimes also *v*) waves in the jugular venous pulse are evident. The onset of RV failure is reflected by an increase of venous pressure, the development of larger *v* waves associated with increasing tricuspid regurgitation, a positive hepatojugular reflux, and a gallop rhythm with both third and fourth heart sounds. These physical findings of RV failure can disappear rapidly when pulmonary artery pressure is reduced by relief of hypoxemia.

Hypocapnia due to alveolar hyperventilation is an important feature of chronic pulmonary hypertension secondary to pulmonary vascular disease. Usually there are no abnormalities on spirometry, but the ratio of dead space to tidal volume may be high, particularly when large-vessel obstruction is present. The diffusing capacity of the lung is reduced when the pulmonary vascular disease is associated with a capillary vasculitis and/or loss of capillary blood volume. Typically,

exertion causes a marked fall in Pa_{O_2}. The assessment of exercise capacity may be a useful way of following changes in the severity of pulmonary vascular disease in patients with chronic cor pulmonale, because exercise ability is limited by cardiac output and the latter, in turn, by the severity of the pulmonary vascular obstruction.

Laboratory Examination On *radiologic examination* the pulmonary trunk and hilar vessels are enlarged, as is the descending right pulmonary artery. Ventilation and perfusion lung scans and systemic venography showing deep vein thrombosis in the lower extremities are helpful in confirming the diagnosis of embolic pulmonary vascular disease. In the presence of severe pulmonary hypertension, the *electrocardiogram* (ECG) shows P pulmonale, right axis deviation, and RV hypertrophy (Chap. 226).

Echocardiography allows measurement of the thickness of the RV wall and may show enlargement of the RV cavity in relation to the left. The interventricular septum may be displaced leftward and may move paradoxically during the cardiac cycle. Pulmonary artery and RV systolic pressure can be estimated from measurement of the peak tricuspid regurgitant flow and pulmonic regurgitant flow with Doppler echocardiography.

Magnetic resonance imaging is useful for measuring RV mass, wall thickness, cavity volume, and ejection fraction.

Failure of the RV ejection fraction (measured by radionuclide ventriculography) to increase on exercise is a good indicator of pulmonary hypertension and/or intrinsic RV dysfunction. *Myocardial perfusion scintigraphy* with thallium 201 or sestamibi is also useful in diagnosing cor pulmonale, since the hypertrophied RV is visualized by these radionuclides. (Normally the RV is not imaged by these radionuclides because of the much greater uptake by the left ventricle.)

Cardiac catheterization provides precise measurement of pulmonary vascular pressures, calculation of pulmonary vascular resistance, and their responses to oxygen and vasodilators. Catheterization is sometimes helpful in patients with cor pulmonale to exclude congenital and left heart diseases, and it allows pulmonary angiography to be carried out to confirm the nature of the pulmonary vascular obstruction. Measurements of pulmonary vascular pressure and flow during exercise may reveal abnormal pressure increments of pulmonary artery systolic and diastolic and RV diastolic pressures and an inadequate responses of cardiac output.

Lung biopsy can be useful in demonstrating vasculitis in some types of pulmonary vascular disease such as the collagen vascular diseases, rheumatoid arthritis, and Wegener's granulomatosis.

PARENCHYMAL PULMONARY DISEASES

The pathogenesis of cor pulmonale in patients with chronic parenchymal pulmonary disease is shown in Fig. 237-1. Cor pulmonale may be caused by both obstructive and restrictive lung diseases, more frequently the former. In these conditions there are usually only modest elevations of pulmonary artery pressure. The development of cor pulmonale confers a poor prognosis on patients with respiratory disease, not because RV failure cannot be treated, but because it reflects the seriousness of the underlying pulmonary disease.

CHRONIC OBSTRUCTIVE LUNG DISEASE (See also Chap. 258) This is the most common cause of chronic cor pulmonale. The enlargement of the RV is attributed to the mild-to-moderate pulmonary hypertension that is common in severe obstructive bronchitis and emphysema. Pulmonary artery systolic pressure is typically in the range of 50 to 60 mmHg, far below the systemic levels that may occur in patients with congenital heart disease and in those with primary pulmonary hypertension. Patients with cor pulmonale due to COLD usually have an advanced form of the disease with $FEV_1 <$ 1.0 L and $Pa_{O_2} < 60$ mmHg (Chap. 250). RV failure secondary to COLD often occurs when there is "acute-on-chronic" respiratory failure with intensification of hypoxemia.

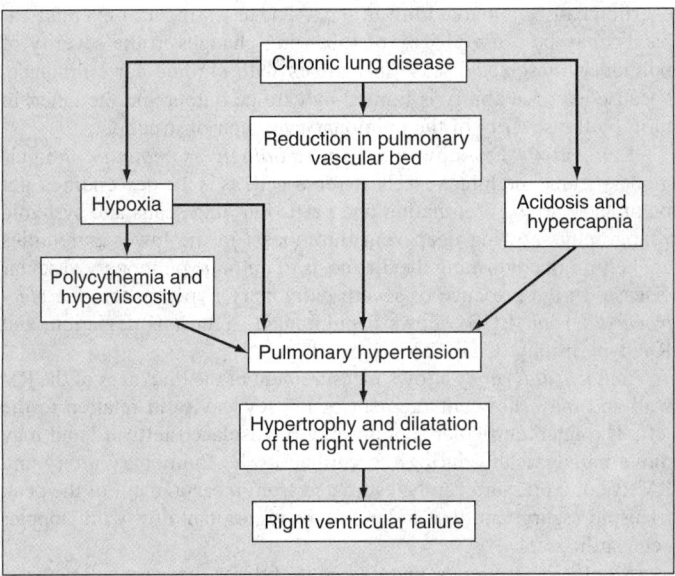

FIGURE 237-1   Pathogenesis of cor pulmonale. *[Reproduced with permission from WR Summer, in LJ Rubin (ed): Pulmonary Heart Disease. Boston, Martinus Nijhoff, 1984, p 285.]*

Pulmonary hypertension in COLD is caused by one or more of the following:

1. Pulmonary vasoconstriction secondary to alveolar hypoxia, acidemia, and hypercapnia. When these vasoconstrictor stimuli persist, medial thickening of the smaller muscular arteries develops by the mechanical effects of the high lung volume on the pulmonary vessels.
2. The loss of small vessels in the vascular bed in regions of emphysema and lung destruction.
3. The increased cardiac output and blood viscosity caused by polycythemia secondary to hypoxia.

Of these causes, hypoxia is the most important. Pulmonary artery pressure rises further on exercise and often falls acutely on inspiration of 100% O_2. Cardiac output tends to be high in the absence of heart failure if hypoxia and hypercapnia are present. Because of the importance of hypoxic pulmonary vasoconstriction in causing pulmonary hypertension, the hypoventilating "blue bloater" with alveolar hypoxia and hypercapnia more frequently suffers from pulmonary hypertension and consequent cor pulmonale than does the emphysematous "pink puffer" without alveolar hypoxia. Ischemic left ventricular dysfunction is a frequent accompaniment since patients with cor pulmonale secondary to COLD usually have a history of heavy cigarette smoking, a major risk factor for ischemic heart disease. The elevation of pulmonary artery pressure may be secondary, in part, to the increase in left atrial pressure resulting from left heart dysfunction. Almost half of all patients who die with cor pulmonale due to COLD also have left ventricular hypertrophy on postmortem examination.

Right ventricular failure often complicates cor pulmonale when patients with COLD develop ventilatory failure and/or a superimposed acute respiratory infection with hypoxia and hypercapnia, and worsening of pulmonary hypertension. Both supraventricular and ventricular arrhythmias may occur. The liver is engorged, tender, and displaced downward by the low diaphragm; a hepatojugular reflux may be present.

An exacerbation of airway obstruction elevates intrathoracic pressure, which impedes venous return, raises jugular venous pressure, and may cause peripheral edema. The venous hypertension due to airflow obstruction declines, sometimes very rapidly, with relief of the obstruction.

Pathology   The RV hypertrophies progressively in COLD. The main pulmonary arteries are enlarged, and the muscular pulmonary arteries show prominent longitudinal muscle, fibrosis, and elastic changes that continue into the arterioles, where the media becomes muscularized. The small vessels and capillaries are distorted or disappear in regions of lung hyperinflation.

Clinical Manifestations   A history of a productive cough and dyspnea, perhaps with wheezing, is frequently elicited. Breathlessness limits the patient's ability in the minor stresses of daily living. Frequently there is a history of emergency hospital admissions because of respiratory infection, sometimes necessitating mechanical ventilation. In breathing oxygen, there may be increasing somnolence or other symptoms of hypercapnia such as recurring headaches, confusion, and even vomiting which, when combined with blurred optic discs (also due to cerebral vasodilation), constitutes the "pseudo tumor cerebri" syndrome. Hypoxia due to hypoventilation is usually worse at night.

Physical findings   Often there is nicotine staining of the fingers, a tell-tale sign reflecting many years of heavy cigarette smoking. The skin may be warm and the arterial pulse bounding in the high cardiac output state induced by hypoxia and hypercapnia. The distention of the chest due to the airflow obstruction and the presence of rhonchi and wheezes secondary to chronic bronchitis usually make cardiac auscultation difficult. A right-sided protodiastolic gallop sound (S_3) and a systolic murmur of tricuspid regurgitant may be audible. Signs of right heart failure are, as discussed above, difficult to separate from those due to severe airflow obstruction. Peripheral edema may worsen with elevation of systemic venous pressure when atrial fibrillation occurs or when pulmonary infection supervenes. A positive hepatojugular reflux suports the diagnosis of RV failure.

Laboratory Examination   *Pulmonary function studies* show marked airflow obstruction with hypoxemia and hypercapnia. Exercise is limited by ventilatory rather than cardiac dysfunction until RV failure develops. The *chest roentgenogram* reveals hyperinflation, which makes the degree of right heart enlargement difficult to assess. The central pulmonary arteries are large, but at the periphery the vessels are narrowed and disappear, particularly in regions of the lungs that are markedly emphysematous. The ECG is relatively insensitive in demonstrating right heart enlargement because the enlarged lungs are poor electrical conductors and the inspiratory position of the chest is associated with a vertically positioned heart. Arrhythmias, particularly atrial fibrillation and multifocal atrial tachycardia, are common.

Echocardiographic imaging is often difficult because of the air in the distended lungs but usually reveals an increased cross-section of the right ventricular cavity, abnormal thickening of the RV wall, and pulmonary hypertension. Myocardial perfusion scintigraphy shows an abnormally high ratio of right-to-left ventricular uptake.

Right heart catheterization can be carried out at the bedside with a balloon-tipped, flow-directed, multilumen catheter fitted with thermocouples for measuring cardiac output by thermodilution (Chap. 228). The pulmonary artery wedge pressure is usually normal at rest in patients with uncomplicated cor pulmonale. Cardiac catheterization may be useful in assessing the severity of the pulmonary hypertension and its response to respiring oxygen.

℞ TREATMENT   First, medical management of the acute and/or chronic lung disease must be optimal (Chaps. 258 and 265). Acute respiratory infection, often the precipitant of RV failure, must be treated promptly and vigorously. Alveolar hypoxia at rest and during exertion and sleep should be corrected by improving alveolar ventilation through relieving the airflow obstruction and by judiciously increasing the inspired O_2 concentration. Long-term O_2 therapy is helpful in patients with severe COLD and reduces pulmonary artery pressure and pulmonary vascular resistance. When the lung disease improves and pulmonary vasoconstriction secondary to the alveolar hypoxia and hypercapnia are corrected, tachypnea and the signs attributed to right heart failure are relieved. Bronchodilators and antibiotics lessen airflow obstruction, and diuretics relieve the edema. Loop diuretics must be used with care since they may cause a metabolic alkalosis and thereby blunt the respiratory drive. Digitalis should be used cautiously in the presence of overt RV failure, and small phlebotomies should be considered when the hematocrit exceeds 55 to 60%. Inhalation of nitric oxide and infusion of prostacyclin are undergoing evaluation as agents to reduce pulmonary hypertension.

The prognosis in cor pulmonale depends on that of the underlying pulmonary disease.

RESTRICTIVE LUNG DISEASES (See also Chap. 259) Cor pulmonale in a variety of restrictive disorders of the lung is often associated with obliteration of the pulmonary vascular bed by lung destruction and fibrosis. Treatment of the underlying disorder and management of RV failure, as described above, are indicated.

DISORDERS OF VENTILATION A variety of disorders of the neuromuscular apparatus, diaphragm, and chest wall cause pulmonary hypertension and cor pulmonale secondary to chronic hypoxia and/or compression of pulmonary vessels. Disorders of ventilatory control, including the sleep apnea syndrome, and upper airways obstruction may be responsible for chronic hypoxia, secondary pulmonary hypertension, cor pulmonale, and eventual RV failure. Management consists of treating the underlying disorder, as discussed in Chaps. 263 and 264; the inhalation of oxygen; and the management of RV failure with diuretics and digoxin.

CHRONIC MOUNTAIN SICKNESS (MONGE'S DISEASE) Residents at high altitudes with chronic hypoxia and secondary polycythemia may develop pulmonary hypertension and cor pulmonale. Psychiatric symptoms—confusion and loss of mental acuity—are common features. Descent to a lower altitude and/or cautious phlebotomy result in lowering of pulmonary artery pressure and relief of symptoms.

BIBLIOGRAPHY

HARALDSSON A et al: Comparison of inhaled nitric oxide and inhaled aerosolized prostacyclin in the evaluation of heart transplant candidates with elevated pulmonary vascular resistance. Chest 114:780, 1998

INCALZI RA et al: Electrocardiographic signs of cor pulmonale: A negative prognostic finding in chronic obstructive pulmonary disease. Circulation 99:1600, 1999

JAIN D, ZARET BJ: Assessment of right ventricular function. Role of nuclear imaging techniques. Cardiol Clin 10:23, 1992

LOH E: Cor pulmonale, in *Cardiopulmonary Diseases and Cardiac Tumors*, S Goldhaber (ed), in *Atlas of Heart Diseases*, vol 3, E Braunwald (series ed). Philadelphia, Current Medicine, 1995, pp 1.1–1.24

MACNEE W: Pathophysiology of cor pulmonale in chronic obstructive pulmonary disease. Am J Respir Crit Care Med 150:833, 1994

RAPAPORT E: Cor pulmonale, in *Textbooks of Respiratory Medicine*, JF Murray, JA Nadel (eds). Philadelphia, Saunders, 2000

RICH S: Cor pulmonale, in *Heart Disease*, 6th ed, E Braunwald (ed). Philadelphia, Saunders, 2001

TUTAR E et al: Echocardiographic evaluation of left ventricular diastolic function in chronic cor pulmonale. Am J Cardiol 83:1414, 1999

VIZZA CD et al: Right and left ventricular dysfunction in patients with severe pulmonary disease. Chest 113:576, 1998

WEITZENBLUM E et al: Benefit from long-term O₂ therapy in chronic obstructive pulmonary disease patients. Respiration 59(Suppl I):14, 1992

——— et al: Pulmonary hemodynamics in patients with chronic obstructive pulmonary disease before and during an episode of peripheral edema. Chest 105:1377, 1994

238 *Joshua Wynne, Eugene Braunwald*

THE CARDIOMYOPATHIES AND MYOCARDITIDES

The cardiomyopathies are diseases that involve the myocardium directly and are not the result of hypertension or congenital, valvular, coronary, arterial, or pericardial abnormalities.* When the cardiomyopathies are classified on an etiologic basis, two fundamental forms are recognized: (1) a primary type, consisting of heart muscle disease of unknown cause; and (2) a secondary type, consisting of myocardial disease of known cause or associated with a disease involving other organ systems (Table 238-1). (In the World Health Organization classification, *specific cardiomyopathy* is used to describe heart muscle diseases associated with certain systemic or cardiac disorders; examples include hypertensive and metabolic cardiomyopathy.) In many cases, however, it is not possible to arrive at a specific etiologic diagnosis, and thus it is often more desirable to classify the cardiomyopathies on the basis of differences in their pathophysiology and clinical presentation (Tables 238-2 and 238-3).

DILATED CARDIOMYOPATHY

Left and/or right ventricular systolic pump function is impaired, leading to progressive cardiac enlargement, a process called *remodeling*, and often, but not invariably, producing symptoms of congestive heart failure. There is, however, no close correlation between the degree of contractile dysfunction and the severity of symptoms. Mural thrombi may be present, particularly in the left ventricular apex. Histologic examination reveals extensive areas of interstitial and perivascular fibrosis. Myocyte necrosis and cellular infiltration may be present but are not prominent.

Although no cause is apparent in many cases, dilated cardiomyopathy is probably the end result of myocardial damage produced by a variety of toxic, metabolic, or infectious agents. Dilated cardiomyopathy may be the late sequel of acute viral myocarditis, possibly mediated through an immunologic mechanism. Most commonly a disease of middle-aged men and more common in African Americans than in whites, it may occur in any patient population. The prevalence of this condition appears to be increasing. A reversible form of dilated cardiomyopathy may be found with alcohol abuse, pregnancy, selenium deficiency, hypophosphatemia, hypocalcemia, thyroid disease, cocaine use, and chronic uncontrolled tachycardia. Approximately 20% of patients have familial forms of the disease, with mutations of genes encoding myocardial structure proteins as well as transcription factors that control the expression of other myocyte genes. The disease is genetically heterogeneous; autosomal dominant, autosomal recessive, and X-linked transmission have been documented.

Right ventricular dysplasia is a unique cardiomyopathy marked by progressive replacement of the right ventricular wall with adipose tissue. Often associated with ventricular arrhythmias, the clinical course is variable, but sudden death is a constant threat. Catheter ablation of putative arrhythmia sites and insertion of an implantable cardioverter-defibrillator are often employed.

CLINICAL MANIFESTATIONS Symptoms of left- and right-sided congestive failure (Chap. 232), manifested by exertional

---

*Diffuse myocardial fibrosis secondary to multiple myocardial scars produced by extensive coronary arterial narrowing and occlusion can impair left ventricular function and is frequently referred to as *ischemic cardiomyopathy*. This is a colloquial use of the term, however, and should be avoided; the term *cardiomyopathy* should be restricted to a condition *primarily* involving heart muscle. In so-called ischemic cardiomyopathy the *primary* involvement is of the coronary vessels.

Table 238-1   Etiologic Classification of Cardiomyopathies

PRIMARY MYOCARDIAL INVOLVEMENT

Idiopathic (D,R,H)
Familial (D,R,H)
Eosinophilic endomyocardial disease (R)
Endomyocardial fibrosis (R)

SECONDARY MYOCARDIAL INVOLVEMENT

Infective (D)	Connective tissue disorders (D)
Viral myocarditis	Systemic lupus erythematosus
Bacterial myocarditis	Polyarteritis nodosa
Fungal myocarditis	Rheumatoid arthritis
Protozoal myocarditis	Progressive systemic sclerosis
Metazoal myocarditis	Dermatomyositis
Spirochetal	Infiltrations and granulomas (R,D)
Rickettsial	Amyloidosis
Metabolic (D)	Sarcoidosis
Familial storage disease (D,R)	Malignancy
Glycogen storage disease	Neuromuscular (D)
Mucopolysaccharidoses	Muscular dystrophy
Hemochromatosis	Myotonic dystrophy
Fabry's disease	Friedreich's ataxia (H,D)
Deficiency (D)	Sensitivity and toxic reactions (D)
Electrolytes	Alcohol
Nutritional	Radiation
	Drugs
	Peripartum heart disease (D)

NOTE: The principal clinical manifestation(s) of each etiologic grouping is denoted by D (dilated), R (restrictive), or H (hypertrophic) cardiomyopathy.
SOURCE: Adapted from the WHO/ISFC task force report on the definition and classification of cardiomyopathies, 1980.

dyspnea, fatigue, orthopnea, paroxysmal nocturnal dyspnea, peripheral edema, and palpitations, develop gradually in most patients. Some patients have left ventricular dilatation for months or even years before becoming symptomatic. Others develop symptoms after recovery from a viral infection. Although vague chest pain may be present, typical angina pectoris is unusual and suggests the presence of concomitant ischemic heart disease. Systemic embolism, stroke, and syncope may occur.

PHYSICAL EXAMINATION   Variable degrees of cardiac enlargement and findings of congestive heart failure are noted. In patients with advanced disease, the pulse pressure is narrow and the jugular venous pressure is elevated. Third and fourth heart sounds are common, and mitral or tricuspid regurgitation may occur.

LABORATORY EXAMINATIONS   The chest roentgenogram demonstrates enlargement of the cardiac silhouette due to left ventricular enlargement, although generalized cardiomegaly is often seen. The lung fields may demonstrate evidence of pulmonary venous hypertension and interstitial or alveolar edema. The electrocardiogram often shows sinus tachycardia or atrial fibrillation, ventricular arrhythmias, left atrial abnormality, diffuse nonspecific ST-T wave abnormalities, and sometimes intraventricular conduction defects and low voltage. Echocardiography and radionuclide ventriculography show left ventricular dilatation, with normal or minimally thickened or thinned walls, and systolic dysfunction (reduced ejection fraction).

Cardiac catheterization and coronary angiography are usually performed to exclude ischemic heart disease, although hemodynamic monitoring may occasionally be helpful in the management of the

Table 238-2   Clinical Classification of Cardiomyopathies

1. Dilated: Left and/or right ventricular enlargement, impaired systolic function, congestive heart failure, arrhythmias, emboli
2. Restrictive: Endomyocardial scarring or myocardial infiltration resulting in restriction to left and/or right ventricular filling
3. Hypertrophic: Disproportionate left ventricular hypertrophy, typically involving septum more than free wall, with or without an intraventricular systolic pressure gradient; usually of a nondilated left ventricular cavity

acutely decompensated patient. The left ventricular end-diastolic, left atrial, and pulmonary capillary wedge pressures are usually elevated; when failure of the right side of the heart supervenes, the right ventricular end-diastolic, right atrial, and central venous pressures also rise. Angiography reveals a dilated, diffusely hypokinetic left ventricle, often with some degree of mitral regurgitation; the coronary arteries are normal, thereby excluding so-called ischemic cardiomyopathy. Transvenous endomyocardial biopsy is usually not necessary in idiopathic or familial dilated cardiomyopathy, in which it reveals nonspecific findings of myocyte hypertrophy and fibrosis. However, it may be helpful in the recognition of secondary cardiomyopathies such as myocardial infiltration with amyloid and of acute myocarditis.

℞ TREATMENT   Most patients pursue an inexorably downhill course, and the majority, particularly those over 55 years of age, die within 3 years of the onset of symptoms. African Americans are more likely to suffer progressive heart failure and death than Caucasians. Spontaneous improvement or stabilization occurs in about a quarter of patients. Death is due to either congestive heart failure or ventricular tachy- or bradyarrhythmia; sudden death is a constant threat. Systemic embolization is a concern, and patients with heart failure secondary to cardiomyopathy should be considered for chronic anticoagulation. Standard therapy of heart failure with salt restriction, angiotensin-converting enzyme (ACE) inhibitors, diuretics, and digitalis produces symptomatic improvement (Chap. 232). An angiotensin II receptor blocker may be substituted in ACE-intolerant patients. Most ambulatory patients profit as well from the addition of a β-adrenergic blocker. Some patients with dilated cardiomyopathy who have biopsy evidence of myocardial inflammation have been treated with immunosuppressive therapy, but long-term evidence of efficacy is lacking. Alcohol should be avoided because of its cardiac toxic effects. Antiarrhythmic agents are best avoided for fear of proarrhythmic and other side effects, unless they are needed to treat symptomatic or serious arrhythmias. Insertion of an implantable cardioverter-defibrillator is useful in patients with malignant arrhythmias. In patients with advanced disease who are refractory to medical therapy, cardiac transplantation should be considered (Chap. 233).

ALCOHOLIC CARDIOMYOPATHY   Individuals who consume large quantities of alcohol over many years may develop a clinical picture identical to idiopathic dilated cardiomyopathy; indeed, alcoholic cardiomyopathy is the major form of secondary dilated cardiomyopathy in the western world. Ceasing alcohol consumption before severe heart failure has developed may halt the progression or even reverse the course of this disease, unlike the idiopathic variety, which is marked by progressive deterioration. Alcoholic patients with advanced heart failure have a poor prognosis, particularly if they continue to drink; fewer than one-quarter survive 3 years. The key to the treatment of alcoholic cardiomyopathy is total and permanent abstinence.

A second presentation of alcoholic cardiotoxicity may be found in individuals without overt heart failure and consists of recurrent supraventricular or ventricular tachyarrhythmias. Termed the *holiday heart syndrome*, it typically appears after a drinking binge; atrial fibrillation is seen most frequently, followed by atrial flutter and ventricular premature depolarizations. Other patients develop left ventricular hypertrophy, perhaps related to concomitant systemic hypertension; they may present with symptoms of pulmonary congestion due to abnormal diastolic stiffness (diminished compliance) of the left ventricle (Chap. 231).

PERIPARTUM CARDIOMYOPATHY   (See Chap. 7)   Cardiac dilatation and congestive heart failure of unexplained cause may develop during the last trimester of pregnancy or within 6 months after delivery; most women develop symptoms in the month before or immediately after delivery. The cause of this disorder is unknown, but in some patients endomyocardial biopsy has shown evidence of a myocarditis. Necropsy shows cardiac enlargement, often with mural thrombi, along with histologic evidence of myocardial degeneration and fibrosis. The patient who develops peripartum cardiomyopathy typically is multiparous, African American, and over the age of 30, although the disease may be found in a wide spectrum of patients. The symptoms, signs, and treatment are similar to those in patients with idiopathic dilated cardiomyopathy. The mortality rate is quite variable but may be as high as 25 to 50%. The prognosis in these patients appears to be closely related to whether the heart size returns to normal after the first episode of congestive heart failure. If it does, subsequent pregnancies may sometimes be well tolerated; if the heart remains enlarged, however, further pregnancies frequently produce increasing myocardial damage, ultimately leading to refractory congestive heart failure and death. Those who recover should be encouraged to avoid further pregnancies, particularly if cardiomegaly persists.

NEUROMUSCULAR DISEASE

(See also Chap. 381) Cardiac involvement is common in many of the muscular dystrophies. In *Duchenne's progressive muscular dystrophy*, mutations in a gene that encodes a cardiac structural protein called *dystrophin* lead to myocyte death. Myocardial involvement is most frequently indicated by a distinctive and unique electrocardiographic pattern consisting of tall R waves in right precordial leads with an R/S ratio greater than 1.0, often associated with deep Q waves in the limb and lateral precordial leads. These electrocardiographic abnormalities appear to result from selective transmural necrosis of the posterobasal left ventricle and associated papillary muscle. A variety of supraventricular and ventricular arrhythmias are frequently found. Rapidly progressive congestive heart failure may develop despite extended periods of apparent circulatory stability during which the only detectable abnormalities are in the electrocardiogram. *Myotonic dystrophy* is characterized by a variety of electrocardiographic abnormalities, especially disorders of impulse formation and conduction, but other overt clinical evidence of heart disease is uncommon. Because of these abnormalities, syncope and sudden death are major hazards; in appropriate patients, insertion of a permanent pacemaker may be effective. In *limb-girdle dystrophy* and *fascioscapulohumeral dystrophy*, cardiac involvement is uncommon and seldom severe, although arrhythmias and conduction disturbances may be seen on occasion. Involvement of the heart is very common in *Friedreich's ataxia* (manifested by abnormal electrocardiographic or echocardiographic findings), with as many as half the patients developing cardiac symptoms. The electrocardiogram most commonly demonstrates ST-segment and T-wave abnormalities. The echocardiogram may demonstrate left ventricular hypertrophy, with either symmetric or asymmetric hypertrophy of the left ventricular septum compared with the free wall. Although morphologically similar to some cases of hypertrophic cardiomyopathy, cellular disarray is lacking.

DRUGS

A variety of pharmacologic agents may damage the myocardium acutely, producing a pattern of inflammation (myocarditis), or they may lead to chronic damage of the type seen with idiopathic dilated cardiomyopathy (Chap. 71). Certain drugs produce only electrocardiographic abnormalities, while others may precipitate fulminant congestive heart failure and death.

The anthracycline derivatives, particularly *doxorubicin* (Adriamycin), are powerful antineoplastic agents that, when given in high doses (more than 550 mg/m² for doxorubicin), may produce fatal heart failure. The incidence of heart failure is related not only to the dose of the drug but also to the presence or absence of several risk factors

(cardiac irradiation, age >70 years, underlying heart disease, hypertension, treatment with cyclophosphamide); at any dose, patients with these risk factors have an eight- to tenfold greater frequency of developing heart failure than do patients lacking them. Radionuclide ventriculography and echocardiography, usually combined with exercise stress, may document preclinical deterioration of left ventricular function and allow appropriate dose adjustments; by so monitoring left ventricular function, it is often possible to continue doxorubicin even in patients at high risk for developing heart failure. Efforts to modify the dose schedule by giving the drug more slowly, along with the selective use of potentially cardioprotective agents such as the iron-chelator dexrazoxone, have further reduced the risk of cardiotoxicity. Some patients with congestive heart failure, even those with severe depression of left ventricular function, have demonstrated recovery of cardiac function with aggressive management with ACE inhibitors and diuretics. In others, late asymptomatic contractile dysfunction is common, even in those without initial cardiotoxicity. Children may demonstrate reduced myocardial hypertrophy and mass over time, presumably due to doxorubicin's inhibition of myocardial cell growth.

High-dose *cyclophosphamide* may produce congestive heart failure acutely or within 2 weeks of administration; a characteristic histopathologic feature is myocardial edema and hemorrhagic necrosis. Rarely, patients treated with *5-fluorouracil* will develop chest pain and electrocardiographic changes of myocardial ischemia or infarction. Electrocardiographic changes and arrhythmias may result from treatment with tricyclic antidepressants, the phenothiazines, emetine, lithium, and various aerosol propellants. *Cocaine abuse* is associated with a variety of life-threatening cardiac complications, including sudden death, myocarditis, dilated cardiomyopathy, and acute myocardial infarction (resulting from coronary spasm and/or thrombosis with or without underlying coronary artery stenosis). Nitrates and calcium channel blockers have been used to treat cocaine-induced cardiotoxicities; β-adrenergic blockers should be avoided.

HYPERTROPHIC CARDIOMYOPATHY

Hypertrophic cardiomyopathy (HCM) is characterized by left ventricular hypertrophy, typically of a nondilated chamber, without obvious cause such as hypertension or aortic stenosis. It is found in about 1 in 500 of the general population. Two features of HCM have attracted

Table 238-3 Laboratory Evaluation of the Cardiomyopathies

	Dilated	Restrictive	Hypertrophic
Chest roentgenogram	Moderate to marked cardiac silhouette enlargement Pulmonary venous hypertension	Mild cardiac silhouette enlargement	Mild to moderate cardiac silhouette enlargement
Electrocardiogram	ST-segment and T-wave abnormalities	Low voltage, conduction defects	ST-segment and T-wave abnormalities Left ventricular hypertrophy Abnormal Q waves
Echocardiogram	Left ventricular dilatation and dysfunction	Increased left ventricular wall thickness Normal or mildly reduced systolic function	Asymmetric septal hypertrophy (ASH) Systolic anterior motion (SAM) of the mitral valve
Radionuclide studies	Left ventricular dilatation and dysfunction (RVG)	Normal or mildly reduced systolic function (RVG)	Vigorous systolic function (RVG) Perfusion defect (²⁰¹Tl)
Cardiac catheterization	Left ventricular dilatation and dysfunction Elevated left- and often right-sided filling pressures Diminished cardiac output	Normal or mildly reduced systolic function Elevated left- and right-sided filling pressures	Vigorous systolic function Dynamic left ventricular outflow obstruction Elevated left- and right-sided filling pressures

NOTE: RVG, radionuclide ventriculogram; ²⁰¹Tl, thallium 201.

the greatest attention: (1) heterogeneous left ventricular hypertrophy, often with preferential hypertrophy of the interventricular septum resulting in asymmetric septal hypertrophy; and (2) a dynamic left ventricular outflow tract pressure gradient, related to a narrowing of the subaortic area as a consequence of the midsystolic apposition of the anterior mitral valve leaflet against the hypertrophied septum, i.e., systolic anterior motion (SAM) of the mitral valve. Initial studies of this disease emphasized the dynamic "obstructive" features, and it has been termed *idiopathic hypertrophic subaortic stenosis* and *hypertrophic obstructive cardiomyopathy*. It has become clear, however, that only about one-quarter of patients with HCM demonstrate an outflow tract pressure gradient. The ubiquitous pathophysiologic abnormality is not systolic but rather *diastolic* dysfunction (Chap. 231), characterized by increased stiffness of the hypertrophied muscle. This results in elevated diastolic filling pressures and is present despite a hyperdynamic left ventricle.

The pattern of hypertrophy is distinctive in HCM and differs from that seen in secondary hypertrophy (as in hypertension). Most patients have striking regional variations in the extent of hypertrophy in different portions of the left ventricle, and the majority demonstrate a ventricular septum whose thickness is disproportionately increased when compared with the free wall. Other patients may demonstrate disproportionate involvement of the apex or left ventricular free wall; 10% or more of patients have concentric involvement of the ventricle. A bizarre and disorganized arrangement of cardiac muscle cells in the septum occurs, with disorganization of the myofibrillar architecture, along with a variable degree of myocardial fibrosis and thickening of the small intramural coronary arteries. In some children, systolic compression of an intramyocardial segment of a coronary artery may lead to ischemia and death.

§ **GENETIC CONSIDERATIONS** About half of all patients with HCM have a positive family history compatible with autosomal-dominant transmission, and more than 100 different mutations have been identified. About 40% of these are associated with mutations of the cardiac β-myosin heavy chain gene on chromosome 14, with certain mutations associated with more malignant prognoses. About 15% have a mutation of the cardiac troponin T gene on chromosome 1, 20% a mutation of myosin-binding protein C (chromosome 11), and about 5% a mutation of the α-tropomyosin gene. The remainder of familial cases are due to mutations of other genes such as the gene for troponin I. Echocardiographic studies have confirmed that about one-third of the first-degree relatives of patients with familial HCM have evidence of the disease, although in many of these patients the extent of hypertrophy is mild, no outflow tract pressure gradient is present, and symptoms are not prominent. Since the hypertrophic characteristics may not be apparent in childhood and often appear first in adolescence, a single normal echocardiogram in a child does not exclude the presence of the disease. Many sporadic cases of HCM probably represent spontaneous mutations. ■

HEMODYNAMICS In contrast to the obstruction produced by a fixed narrowed orifice, such as valvular aortic stenosis, the pressure gradient in HCM, when present, is dynamic and may change between examinations and even from beat to beat. Obstruction appears to result from further narrowing of an already small left ventricular outflow tract by SAM of the mitral valve against the hypertrophied septum. While SAM is occasionally found in a variety of conditions besides HCM, it is *always* found when obstruction is present in HCM. Three basic mechanisms are involved in the production and intensification of the dynamic pressure gradient: (1) increased left ventricular contractility, (2) decreased ventricular volume (preload), and (3) decreased aortic impedance and pressure (afterload). Interventions that increase myocardial contractility, such as exercise, sympathomimetic amines, and digitalis glycosides, and those that reduce ventricular volume, such as the Valsalva maneuver, sudden standing, nitroglycerin, amyl nitrite, or tachycardia, may all cause an increase in the gradient and the mur-

mur. Conversely, elevation of arterial pressure by phenylephrine, squatting, sustained handgrip, augmentation of venous return by passive leg raising, and expansion of the blood volume all increase ventricular volume and ameliorate the gradient and murmur.

CLINICAL FEATURES The clinical course of HCM is highly variable. Many patients are asymptomatic or mildly symptomatic and may be relatives of patients with known disease. Unfortunately, the first clinical manifestation of the disease may be sudden death, frequently occurring in children and young adults, often during or after physical exertion. In symptomatic patients, the most common complaint is dyspnea, largely due to increased stiffness of the left ventricular walls, which impairs ventricular filling and leads to elevated left ventricular diastolic and left atrial pressures. Other symptoms include angina pectoris, fatigue, syncope, and near-syncope ("graying-out spells"). Symptoms are not closely related to the presence or severity of an outflow pressure gradient. Most patients with gradients demonstrate a double or triple apical precordial impulse, a rapidly rising carotid arterial pulse, and a fourth heart sound. The hallmark of obstructive HCM is a systolic murmur, which is typically harsh, diamond-shaped, and usually begins well after the first heart sound, since ejection is unimpeded early in systole. The murmur is best heard at the lower left sternal border as well as at the apex, where it is often more holosystolic and blowing in quality, no doubt due to the mitral regurgitation that usually accompanies obstructive HCM.

LABORATORY EVALUATION The *electrocardiogram* commonly shows left ventricular hypertrophy and widespread, deep, broad Q waves that suggest an old myocardial infarction. Many patients demonstrate arrhythmias, both atrial (supraventricular tachycardia or atrial fibrillation) and ventricular (ventricular tachycardia), during ambulatory (Holter) monitoring. *Chest roentgenography* may be normal, although a mild to moderate increase in the cardiac silhouette is common. The mainstay of the diagnosis of HCM is the *echocardiogram*, which demonstrates left ventricular hypertrophy, often with the septum 1.3 or more times the thickness of the high posterior left ventricular free wall. The septum may demonstrate an unusual "ground-glass" appearance, probably related to its abnormal cellular architecture and myocardial fibrosis. SAM of the mitral valve is found in patients with pressure gradients. The left ventricular cavity typically is small in HCM, with vigorous posterior wall motion but reduced septal excursion. A rare form of HCM, characterized by apical hypertrophy, is often associated with giant negative T waves on the electrocardiogram and a "spade-shaped" left ventricular cavity on angiography; it usually has a benign clinical course. *Radionuclide scintigraphy* with thallium 201 frequently reveals evidence of myocardial perfusion defects even in asymptomatic patients.

Although cardiac catheterization is not required to diagnose HCM, the two typical *hemodynamic* features are an elevated left ventricular diastolic pressure due to diminished left ventricular compliance and, when obstruction is present, a systolic pressure gradient between the body of the left ventricle and the subaortic region. When a gradient is not present, it can be induced in some patients by provocative maneuvers such as infusion of isoproterenol, inhalation of amyl nitrite, or the Valsalva maneuver.

℞ **TREATMENT** Since sudden death often occurs during or just after physical exertion, competitive sports and probably strenuous activity should be proscribed. Dehydration should be avoided, and diuretics should be used with caution. β-Adrenergic blockers are often used and ameliorate angina pectoris and syncope in one-third to one-half of patients. Resting intraventricular pressure gradients are usually unchanged, although these drugs may limit the increase in the gradient that occurs during exercise. It is not known whether β-adrenergic blockers offer any protection against sudden death. Amiodarone appears to be effective in reducing the frequency of supraventricular as well as life-threatening ventricular arrhythmias, and anecdotal data suggest that it may reduce the risk of sudden death. Verapamil and diltiazem may reduce the stiffness of the ventricle, reduce the elevated diastolic pressures, increase exercise tolerance, and, in some instances, reduce the severity of outflow tract pressure gradients, although adverse side effects occur in about one-quarter of patients. Nifedipine should be avoided. The combination of beta blockers and calcium antagonists should be used with caution. Disopyramide has been used in some patients to reduce left ventricular contractility and the outflow pressure gradient.

If atrial fibrillation occurs, a strenuous effort should be made to restore and then maintain sinus rhythm. Dual-chamber permanent pacing with a short PR interval has been reported to improve symptoms and reduce the outflow gradient in some patients with severe symptoms, presumably by altering the pattern of ventricular depolarization and contraction. Infarction of the interventricular septum induced by ethanol injections into the septal artery has also been reported to reduce obstruction. The insertion of an implantable cardioverter defibrillator should be considered in patients surviving cardiac arrest and those with high-risk ventricular tachyarrhythmias (Chap. 230). A surgical myotomy/myectomy of the hypertrophied septum may result in lasting symptomatic improvement in about three-quarters of severely symptomatic patients with large pressure gradients who are unresponsive to medical management. The effect of any of these therapies on the natural history is not clear. Digitalis, diuretics, nitrates, vasodilators, and β-adrenergic agonists are best avoided if possible, particularly in patients with known left ventricular outflow tract pressure gradients. Even social alcohol ingestion may produce sufficient vasodilatation to exacerbate an outflow pressure gradient.

First-degree relatives of patients with HCM should be screened by echocardiography.

PROGNOSIS The natural history of HCM is variable, although many patients never exhibit any clinical manifestations. Others demonstrate an improvement of symptoms with time. Atrial fibrillation is common late in the course of the disease; its onset may lead to an increase in symptoms, due to loss of the atrial contribution to filling of the thickened ventricle. Infective endocarditis occurs in fewer than 10% of patients, and endocarditis prophylaxis is indicated, particularly in patients with resting obstruction and mitral regurgitation. Progression of HCM to left ventricular dilatation and dysfunction without an outflow pressure gradient has been reported but is unusual; in about 5 to 10% of patients, however, some degree of left ventricular systolic impairment, wall thinning, and chamber enlargement occurs over time. The major cause of mortality in HCM is sudden death, which may occur in asymptomatic patients or interrupt an otherwise stable course in symptomatic ones. Predictors of sudden death include age less than 30 years, ventricular tachycardia on ambulatory monitoring, marked ventricular hypertrophy, syncope (especially in children), genetic mutations associated with an increased risk, and a family history of sudden death. There is no correlation between the risk of sudden death and the severity of symptoms or the presence or severity of an outflow tract pressure gradient.

RESTRICTIVE CARDIOMYOPATHY

The hallmark of the restrictive cardiomyopathies is abnormal diastolic function (Chap. 231); the ventricular walls are excessively rigid and impede ventricular filling. Myocardial fibrosis, hypertrophy, or infiltration due to a variety of causes is usually responsible. The infiltrative diseases, which represent important causes for secondary restrictive cardiomyopathy, may also show some impairment of systolic function. Myocardial involvement with *amyloid* is a common cause of secondary restrictive cardiomyopathy, although restriction is also seen in hemochromatosis, glycogen deposition, endomyocardial fibrosis, sarcoidosis, Fabry's disease, the eosinophilias, and scleroderma; in the transplanted heart and following mediastinal radiation; and in neoplastic infiltration and myocardial fibrosis of diverse causes. In many of these conditions, particularly those with substantial concomitant endocardial involvement, partial obliteration of the ventricular cavity by fibrous tissue and thrombus contributes to the abnormally increased

resistance to ventricular filling. Thromboembolic complications ensue in about a third of patients.

The inability of the ventricle to fill limits cardiac output and raises filling pressure. Therefore, exercise intolerance and dyspnea are usually the most prominent symptoms. As a result of persistently elevated venous pressure, these patients commonly have dependent edema, ascites, and an enlarged, tender, and often pulsatile liver. The jugular venous pressure is elevated and does not fall normally, or it may rise with inspiration (Kussmaul's sign). The heart sounds may be distant, and third and fourth heart sounds are common. In contrast to constrictive pericarditis, which the restrictive cardiomyopathies resemble in many respects, the apex impulse is usually easily palpable, and mitral regurgitation is more common. The electrocardiogram often shows low-voltage, nonspecific ST-T-wave changes and various arrhythmias. Pericardial calcification on x-ray, which would suggest constrictive pericarditis, is absent. Echocardiography typically reveals symmetrically thickened left ventricular walls and normal or slightly reduced ventricular volumes and systolic function. Doppler recordings demonstrate accentuated early diastolic filling. Cardiac catheterization shows a decreased cardiac output, elevation of the right and left ventricular end-diastolic pressures, and a dip-and-plateau configuration of the diastolic portion of the ventricular pressure pulse resembling that seen in constrictive pericarditis.

Differentiation from constrictive pericarditis may be challenging (Chap. 239). This distinction is of importance because the latter condition is potentially curable by operation. Helpful in the differentiation of these two diseases are right ventricular transvenous endomyocardial biopsy (by revealing myocardial infiltration or fibrosis in restrictive cardiomyopathy) and computed tomography or magnetic resonance imaging (by demonstrating a thickened pericardium in constrictive pericarditis). Treatment is usually disappointing, except for hemochromatosis (where desferoxamine has been helpful in reducing myocardial iron content). Chronic anticoagulation is often recommended to reduce the risk of embolization from the heart.

ENDOMYOCARDIAL FIBROSIS This is a progressive disease of unknown cause that occurs most commonly in children and young adults residing in tropical and subtropical Africa, particularly Uganda and Nigeria. Endomyocardial fibrosis is a frequent cause of heart failure in Africa, accounting for up to one-quarter of deaths due to heart disease. The condition is characterized by fibrous endocardial lesions of the inflow portion of the right or left ventricle (or both) and often involves the atrioventricular valves, producing valvular regurgitation. The apex of the ventricles may be obliterated by a mass of thrombus and fibrous tissue. In some ways this disease resembles eosinophilic endomyocardial disease (see below), although they occur in quite different geographic areas and age groups and generally are felt to be different diseases.

The clinical picture depends on which ventricle and atrioventricular valve show predominant involvement; left-sided involvement results in symptoms of pulmonary congestion, while predominant right-sided disease presents features of a restrictive cardiomyopathy. Medical treatment is often disappointing, and surgical excision of the fibrotic endocardium and replacement of the involved atrioventricular valve have led to substantial symptomatic improvement in some patients.

EOSINOPHILIC ENDOMYOCARDIAL DISEASE Also called *Loeffler's endocarditis* and *fibroplastic endocarditis*, this disease appears to be a subcategory of the hypereosinophilic syndrome in which the heart is predominantly involved, with cardiac damage the apparent result of the toxic effects of eosinophilic proteins. Typically, the endocardium of either or both ventricles thickens markedly, with involvement of the underlying myocardium. Large mural thrombi may develop in either ventricle, thereby compromising the size of the ventricular cavity and serving as a source of pulmonary and systemic emboli. Hepatosplenomegaly and localized eosinophilic infiltration of other organs are usually present. Management usually includes diuretics, afterload-reducing agents, and anticoagulation. The use of glucocorticoids and cytotoxic drugs (hydroxyurea in particular) appears to have improved survival substantially. Surgical treatment, as for endomyocardial fibrosis, may be helpful in selected patients.

DIFFERENTIAL DIAGNOSIS Involvement of the heart is the most frequent cause of death in *primary amyloidosis* (Chap. 319), while clinically significant cardiac involvement is uncommon in the secondary form. Focal deposits of amyloid in elderly patients (*senile cardiac amyloidosis*) are common and usually clinically insignificant. Aspiration of abdominal fat or biopsy of the rectal mucosa, gingiva, liver, kidney, or myocardium permits the diagnosis to be made before death in over three-quarters of cases. The heart is firm, rubbery, and noncompliant, and four clinical presentations (alone or in combination) are seen: (1) diastolic dysfunction (restrictive cardiomyopathy), (2) systolic dysfunction, (3) arrhythmias and conduction disturbances, and (4) orthostatic hypotension. The two-dimensional echocardiogram may be helpful in making the diagnosis of amyloidosis and may show a thickened myocardial wall with a distinctive "speckled" appearance. Chemotherapy, often with alkylating agents, appears to have improved survival in specific cases, but the overall prognosis is poor.

Hemochromatosis (Chap. 345) is often the result of multiple transfusions or a hemoglobinopathy; the familial (autosomal recessive) form should be suspected if cardiomyopathy occurs in the setting of diabetes mellitus, hepatic cirrhosis, and increased skin pigmentation. The diagnosis may be confirmed by endomyocardial biopsy. Phlebotomy may be of some benefit if employed early in the course of the disease. Continuous subcutaneous administration of deferoxamine may reduce body iron stores and result in clinical improvement.

Myocardial *sarcoidosis* (Chap. 318) is generally associated with other manifestations of systemic disease and may cause restrictive as well as congestive features, since cardiac infiltration by sarcoid granulomas results not only in increased stiffness of the myocardium but also in diminished systolic contractile function. A variety of arrhythmias, including high-grade atrioventricular block, have been noted. A common cardiac manifestation of systemic sarcoidosis is right heart overload due to pulmonary artery hypertension as a result of parenchymal pulmonary involvement. The *carcinoid syndrome* results in endocardial fibrosis and stenosis and/or regurgitation of the tricuspid and/or pulmonary valve (Chap. 236); morphologically similar lesions have been seen with the use of the anorexic agents fenfluramine and phentermine.

MYOCARDITIDES

Myocarditis, i.e., cardiac inflammation, is most commonly the result of an infectious process. Myocarditis may also result from a hypersensitivity to drugs or may be caused by radiation, chemicals, or physical agents. In an unknown number of cases, acute myocarditis progresses to chronic dilated cardiomyopathy. While almost every infectious agent is capable of producing myocarditis (Table 238-1), clinically significant acute myocarditis in the United States is caused most commonly by viruses, especially coxsackievirus B. The clinical manifestations range from an asymptomatic state, with the presence of myocarditis inferred only by the finding of transient electrocardiographic ST-T-wave abnormalities, to a fulminant condition with arrhythmias, heart failure, and death. In some patients, myocarditis simulates acute myocardial infarction, with chest pain, electrocardiographic changes, and elevated serum levels of myocardial enzymes.

The physical examination is often normal, although more severe cases may show a muffled first heart sound, along with a third heart sound and a murmur of mitral regurgitation. A pericardial friction rub may be audible in patients with associated pericarditis.

Though viral myocarditis is most often self-limited and without sequelae, severe involvement may recur, and it is likely that acute viral myocarditis occasionally progresses to a chronic form and to dilated cardiomyopathy. Patients with viral myocarditis often give a history of a preceding upper respiratory febrile illness or a flulike syndrome, and viral nasopharyngitis or tonsillitis may be evident clinically. The isolation of virus from the stool, pharyngeal washings, or other body fluids and changes in specific antibody titers are helpful clinically. Endomyocardial biopsy, carried out early in the illness, may show round-cell infiltration and necrosis of adjacent myocytes.

Experimental studies suggest that exercise may be deleterious in patients with viral myocarditis, and strenuous activity should be proscribed until the electrocardiogram has returned to normal. Patients who develop congestive heart failure respond to the usual measures (ACE inhibitors, diuretics, and salt restriction), but they appear to be unusually sensitive to digitalis. Arrhythmias are common and are occasionally difficult to manage. Deaths attributed to heart failure, tachyarrhythmias, and heart block have been reported, and it seems prudent to monitor the electrocardiogram of patients with arrhythmias, especially during the acute illness.

HIV MYOCARDITIS (See also Chap. 309) Many HIV-infected patients have subclinical cardiac involvement, including pericardial effusion, right-sided chamber enlargement, and neoplastic involvement. Overt clinical involvement is seen in 10% of HIV patients, and the most common finding is left ventricular dysfunction that in some cases appears to be due to infiltration of the myocardium by the virus itself. In other patients, the heart is affected by any of the various opportunistic infections common in AIDS, such as toxoplasmosis, as well as by cardiac metastases in Kaposi's sarcoma. The clinical manifestations of cardiac involvement may be incorrectly attributed to concurrent noncardiac problems such as pneumonia. This is unfortunate, since the dilated cardiomyopathy of HIV infection may respond at least transiently to standard therapy with digitalis, diuretics, and ACE inhibitors.

BACTERIAL MYOCARDITIS Bacterial involvement of the heart is uncommon, but when it does occur, it is usually as a complication of bacterial endocarditis (typically due to *Staphylococcus aureus* and enterococci). Myocardial abscess formation may involve the valve rings and interventricular septum. *Diphtheritic myocarditis* develops in over one-quarter of the patients with diphtheria, is one of the most serious complications, and is the most common cause of death (Chap. 141). Cardiac damage is due to the liberation of a toxin that inhibits protein synthesis and leads to a dilated, flabby, hypocontractile heart; the conducting system is frequently involved as well. Cardiomegaly and severe congestive heart failure typically appear after the first week of illness. Prompt therapy with antitoxin is crucial; antibiotic therapy is also indicated but is of less urgency.

CHAGAS' DISEASE Chagas' disease, caused by the protozoan *Trypanosoma cruzi* and transmitted by an insect vector (Chap. 216), produces an extensive myocarditis that typically becomes evident years after the initial infection. It is one of the most common causes of heart disease encountered in Central and South America; in rural endemic areas 20 to 75% of the population may be affected. An increasing number of cases are found in the United States as patients migrate from endemic areas. Although only about 1% of infected individuals have an acute illness, which may include acute myocarditis, upwards of one-third develop chronic myocardial damage many years later. The chronic form is characterized by dilatation of several cardiac chambers, fibrosis and thinning of the ventricular wall, aneurysm formation (especially at the left ventricular apex), and mural thrombi. Chronic progressive heart failure is the rule and is associated with poor survival. The electrocardiogram is abnormal in most patients with cardiac involvement and typically shows right bundle branch block and left anterior hemiblock, which may progress to complete atrioventricular block. The *echocardiogram* may reveal a unique pattern of hypokinesis of the posterior left ventricular wall and relatively preserved septal motion. Ventricular arrhythmias are common and are seen especially during and after exertion; oral amiodarone appears to be particularly effective in treating ventricular tachyarrhythmias. The cause of death is either intractable congestive heart failure or an arrhythmia, with a minority of patients dying from embolic phenomena.

℞ TREATMENT Therapy is directed toward amelioration of the congestive heart failure and arrhythmias; progressive conduction system disease and heart block may require implantation of a pacemaker. Anticoagulation (if feasible) may reduce the risk of thromboembolism. Medical therapy is often unsatisfactory or unavailable (especially in poor rural areas), however, and a more promising tactic in endemic areas has been the institution of public health measures, particularly the use of insecticides to eliminate the vector.

GIANT CELL MYOCARDITIS This rare myocarditis of unknown cause is characterized by the presence of multinucleated giant cells in the myocardium. It usually causes rapidly fatal congestive heart failure and arrhythmia in young to middle-aged adults. At necropsy, the distinctive features include cardiac enlargement, ventricular thrombi, grossly visible serpiginous areas of myocardial necrosis in both ventricles, and microscopic evidence of giant cells within an extensive inflammatory infiltrate. The cause of giant cell myocarditis remains obscure, although it occurs in association with thymoma, systemic lupus erythematosus, and thyrotoxicosis. While treatment with immunosuppressive therapy may help in some patients, cardiac transplantation is the treatment of choice.

LYME CARDITIS (See also Chap. 176) Lyme disease is caused by a tick-borne spirochete and is most common in the Northeast, upper Midwest, and Pacific Coastal regions of the United States during the summer months. About 10% of patients develop symptomatic cardiac involvement during the acute phase of the disease. Atrioventricular nodal conduction abnormalities are the most common manifestations of involvement, and may lead to syncope. Concomitant myopericarditis is not uncommon, and mild asymptomatic left ventricular dysfunction may occur. Intravenous ceftriaxone or penicillin is used in all but the mildest forms of Lyme carditis, in which case oral amoxicillin or doxycycline is employed. Hospitalization with electrocardiographic monitoring is indicated in patients with second- or third-degree atrioventricular block. A temporary pacemaker may be needed for symptomatic heart block; the utility of glucocorticoids in reversing heart block is uncertain, but they are usually employed. Long-term cardiac manifestations of Lyme disease are uncommon.

BIBLIOGRAPHY

BORGGREFE M, BREITHARDT G: Is the implantable defribrillator indicated in patients with hypertrophic cardiomyopathy and aborted sudden death? J Am Coll Cardiol 31: 1086, 1998

BRODSKY GL et al: Lamin A/C gene mutation associated with dilated cardiomyopathy with variable skeletal muscle involvement. Circulation 101:473, 2000

BROWN CS, BERTOLET BD: Peripartum cardiomyopathy: A comprehensive review. Am J Obstet Gynecol 178:409, 1998

DEC GW, FUSTER V: Medical progress: Idiopathic dilated cardiomyopathy. N Engl J Med 331:1564, 1994

DOEVENDANS PA: Hypertrophic cardiomyopathy: Do we have the algorithm for life and death? Circulation 10:1224, 2000

FAUCHIER L et al: Comparison of long-term outcome of alcoholic and idiopathic dilated cardiomyopathy. Eur Heart J 21:306, 2000

FRUSTACI A et al: Giant cell myocarditis responding to immunosuppressive therapy. Chest 117:905, 2000

GARG A et al: The ineffectiveness of immunosuppressive therapy in lymphocytic myocarditis: An overview. Ann Intern Med 129:317, 1998

HAGAR JM, RAHIMTOOLA SH: Chagas' heart disease. Curr Probl Cardiol 20:827, 1995

KUSHWAHA SS et al: Restrictive cardiomyopathy. N Engl J Med 336:267, 1997

KYLE RA: Amyloidosis. Circulation 91:1269, 1995

LEIDEN JM: The genetics of dilated cardiomyopathy—emerging clues to the puzzle. N Engl J Med 337:1080, 1997

MACHADO CR et al: Cardiac autonomic denervation in congestive heart failure: Comparison of Chagas' heart disease with other dilated cardiomyopathy. Hum Pathol 31:3, 2000

MARON BJ et al: Impact of laboratory molecular diagnosis on contemporary diagnostic criteria for genetically transmitted cardiovascular diseases: Hypertrophic cardiomyopathy, long-QT syndrome, and Marfan syndrome. Circulation 98:1460, 1998

MASON JW et al: A clinical trial of immunosuppressive therapy for myocarditis. N Engl J Med 333:269, 1995

NIIMURA H et al: Mutations in the gene for cardiac myosin-binding protein C and late-onset familial hypertrophic cardiomyopathy. N Engl J Med 338:1248, 1998

RICHARDSON P et al: Report of the 1995 World Health Organization/International Society and Federation of Cardiology Task Force on the Definition and Classification of Cardiomyopathies. Circulation 93:841, 1996

ROBIOLIO PA et al: Carcinoid heart disease. Correlation of high serotonin levels with valvular abnormalities detected by cardiac catheterization and echocardiography. Circulation 92:790, 1995

SANGHA O et al: Lack of cardiac manifestations among patients with previously treated Lyme disease. Ann Intern Med 128:346, 1998

SINGAL PK, ILISKOVIC N: Doxorubicin-induced cardiomyopathy. N Engl J Med 339:900, 1998

SORAJJA P et al: Pacing in hypertrophic cardiomyopathy. Cardiol Clin 18:67, 2000

THANIGARAJ S, PEREZ JE: Apical hypertrophic cardiomyopathy: Echocardiographic diagnosis with the use of intravenous contrast image enhancement. J Am Soc Echocardiogr 13:146, 2000

WYNNE J, BRAUNWALD E: The cardiomyopathies and myocarditides, in Heart Disease, 6th ed, E. Braunwald (ed). Philadelphia, Saunders, 2001

239 *Eugene Braunwald*

PERICARDIAL DISEASE

NORMAL FUNCTIONS OF THE PERICARDIUM The visceral pericardium is a serous membrane that is separated by a small quantity (15 to 50 mL) of fluid, an ultrafiltrate of plasma, from a fibrous sac, the parietal pericardium. The pericardium normally prevents sudden dilatation of the cardiac chambers during exercise and with hypervolemia. As the result of the development of a negative intrapericardial pressure during ejection, the pericardial sac facilitates atrial filling during ventricular systole. The pericardium also restricts the anatomic position of the heart, minimizes friction between the heart and surrounding structures, prevents displacement of the heart and kinking of the great vessels, and probably retards the spread of infections from the lungs and pleural cavities to the heart. Notwithstanding the foregoing, total absence of the pericardium does not produce obvious clinical disease. In partial left pericardial defects the main pulmonary artery and left atrium may bulge through the defect; very rarely, herniation and subsequent strangulation of the left atrium may cause sudden death.

ACUTE PERICARDITIS

Acute pericarditis, by far the most common pathologic process involving the pericardium, may be classified both clinically and etiologically (Table 239-1). Pain, a pericardial friction rub, electrocardiographic changes, and pericardial effusion with cardiac tamponade and paradoxic pulse are cardinal manifestations of many forms of acute pericarditis and will be considered prior to a discussion of the most common forms of the disorder.

Chest pain is an important but not invariable symptom in various forms of acute pericarditis (Chap. 13); it is usually present in the acute infectious types and in many of the forms presumed to be related to hypersensitivity or autoimmunity. Pain is often absent in a slowly developing tuberculous, postirradiation, neoplastic, or uremic pericarditis. The pain of pericarditis is often severe. It is characteristically retrosternal and left precordial, referred to the back and the left trapezius ridge. Often the pain is pleuritic consequent to accompanying pleural inflammation, i.e., sharp and aggravated by inspiration, coughing, and changes in body position, but sometimes it is a steady, constricting pain that radiates into either arm or both arms and resembles that of myocardial ischemia; therefore, confusion with myocardial infarction is common. Characteristically, however, pericardial pain may be relieved by sitting up and leaning forward and is intensified by lying supine. The differentiation of acute myocardial infarction from acute pericarditis becomes perplexing when, with acute pericarditis, the serum creatine kinase level rises, presumably because of concomitant involvement of the epicardium. However, these enzyme

Table 239-1 Classification of Pericarditis

CLINICAL CLASSIFICATION

I. Acute pericarditis (<6 weeks)
  A. Fibrinous
  B. Effusive (serous or sanguineous)
II. Subacute pericarditis (6 weeks to 6 months)
  A. Effusive-constrictive
  B. Constrictive
III. Chronic pericarditis (<6 months)
  A. Constrictive
  B. Effusive
  C. Adhesive (nonconstrictive)

ETIOLOGIC CLASSIFICATION

I. Infectious pericarditis
  A. Viral (coxsackievirus A and B, echovirus, mumps, adenovirus, hepatitis, HIV)
  B. Pyogenic (pneumococcus, streptococcus, staphylococcus, *Neisseria, Legionella*)
  C. Tuberculous
  D. Fungal (histoplasmosis, coccidioidomycosis, *Candida*, blastomycosis)
  E. Other infections (syphilitic, protozoal, parasitic)
II. Noninfectious pericarditis
  A. Acute myocardial infarction
  B. Uremia
  C. Neoplasia
    1. Primary tumors (benign or malignant, mesothelioma)
    2. Tumors metastatic to pericardium (lung and breast cancer, lymphoma, leukemia)
  D. Myxedema
  E. Cholesterol
  F. Chylopericardium
  G. Trauma
    1. Penetrating chest wall
    2. Nonpenetrating
  H. Aortic dissection (with leakage into pericardial sac)
  I. Postirradiation
  J. Familial Mediterranean fever
  K. Familial pericarditis
    1. Mulibrey nanism*a*
  L. Acute idiopathic
  M. Whipple's Disease
  N. Sarcoidosis
III. Pericarditis presumably related to hypersensitivity or autoimmunity
  A. Rheumatic fever
  B. Collagen vascular disease (SLE, rheumatoid arthritis, ankylosing spondylitis, scleroderma, acute rheumatic fever, Wegener's granulomatosis)
  C. Drug-induced (e.g., procainamide, hydralazine, phenytoin, isoniazide, minoxidil, anticoagulants, methysergide)
  D. Postcardiac injury
    1. Postmyocardial infarction (Dressler's syndrome)
    2. Postpericardiotomy
    3. Posttraumatic

a An autosomal recessive syndrome, characterized by growth failure, muscle hypotonia, hepatomegaly, ocular changes, enlarged cerebral ventricles, mental retardation, and chronic constrictive pericarditis.

elevations, if they occur, are quite modest, given the extensive electrocardiographic ST-segment elevation in pericarditis.

The *pericardial friction rub* is the most important physical sign of acute pericarditis; it may have up to three components per cardiac cycle and is high-pitched, scratching, and grating, as described in Chap. 225; it can sometimes be elicited only when firm pressure with the diaphragm of the stethoscope is applied to the chest wall at the left lower sternal border. It is heard most frequently during expiration with the patient in the sitting position. The rub is often inconstant and the loud to-and-fro leathery sound may disappear within a few hours, possibly to reappear the following day.

The *electrocardiogram* (ECG) in acute pericarditis without massive effusion usually displays changes secondary to acute subepicar-

dial inflammation (see Fig. 226-18, p. 1270). There is widespread elevation of the ST segments, often with upward concavity, involving two or three standard limb leads and V_2 to V_6, with reciprocal depressions only in aVR and sometimes V_1. Usually there are no significant changes in QRS complexes, except for some reduction in voltage in patients with large pericardial effusions. After several days, the ST segments return to normal, and only then do the T waves become inverted. In contrast, in acute myocardial infarction, reciprocal depression of ST segments is usually more prominent; QRS changes occur, particularly the development of Q waves, as well as notching and loss of R-wave amplitude; and T-wave inversions usually occur within hours *before* the ST segments have become isoelectric. Sequential ECGs are useful in distinguishing acute pericarditis from acute myocardial infarction. In the latter, elevated ST segments return to normal within hours. Early repolarization is a normal variant and may also cause widespread ST-segment elevation, most prominent in left precordial leads. However, in this condition the T waves are usually tall and the ST/T ratio is under 0.25, but this ratio is higher in acute pericarditis. Depression of the PR segment (below the TP segment) is also common and reflects atrial involvement. With large pericardial effusions, the QRS voltage is reduced; atrial premature beats and atrial fibrillation are sometimes noted.

PERICARDIAL EFFUSION In acute pericarditis, pericardial effusion is usually associated with pain and/or the above-mentioned ECG changes characteristic of pericarditis and an enlargement of the cardiac silhouette. Pericardial effusion is especially important clinically when it develops within a relatively short time, since it may lead to cardiac tamponade (see below). Differentiation from cardiac enlargement may be difficult on physical examination, but heart sounds tend to become faint with pericardial effusion; the friction rub may disappear, and the apex impulse may vanish, but sometimes it remains palpable, albeit medial to the left border of cardiac dullness. The base of the left lung may be compressed by pericardial fluid, producing Ewart's sign, a patch of dullness beneath the angle of the left scapula. The chest roentgenogram may show a "water bottle" configuration of the cardiac silhouette but may also be normal or almost so. Lucent pericardial fat lines may be seen deep within the cardiopericardial silhouette. Fluoroscopic examination may show the ventricular pulsations to be diminished. Pericardial effusion is common after cardiac surgery and myocardial infarction.

Diagnosis *Echocardiography* is the most effective diagnostic laboratory technique available, since it is sensitive, specific, simple, noninvasive, may be performed at the bedside, and can identify accompanying cardiac tamponade (see below). The presence of pericardial fluid is recorded by two-dimensional transthoracic echocardiography as a relatively echo-free space between the posterior pericardium and left ventricular epicardium in patients with small effusions and as a space between the anterior right ventricle and the parietal pericardium just beneath the anterior chest wall in those with larger effusions. In the latter the heart may swing freely within the pericardial sac; when severe, the extent of this motion alternates and may be associated with electrical alternans. Echocardiography allows localization and estimation of the quantity of pericardial fluid. The diagnosis of pericardial fluid or thickening may be confirmed by computed tomography (CT) or magnetic resonance imaging (MRI); these techniques may be superior to echocardiography in detecting loculated pericardial effusions and pericardial thickening.

Pericardiocentesis When pericardial fluid is removed for diagnostic and/or therapeutic purposes, a needle attached to a properly grounded ECG lead is inserted into the pericardial space, usually through a subxiphoid approach, and, if possible, using echocardiographic control. Intrapericardial pressure should be measured before fluid is withdrawn. Pericardial effusion nearly always has the physical characteristics of an exudate. Bloody fluid is commonly due to tuberculosis or tumor but may also be found in the effusion of rheumatic fever, post-cardiac injury, and post-myocardial infarction (especially following the administration of anticoagulant), and in uremic pericarditis. Transudative pericardial effusions may occur in heart failure.

CARDIAC TAMPONADE The accumulation of fluid in the pericardium in an amount sufficient to cause serious obstruction to the inflow of blood to the ventricles results in cardiac tamponade. This complication may be fatal if it is not recognized and treated promptly. The three most common causes of tamponade are neoplastic disease, idiopathic pericarditis, and uremia. Tamponade may also result from bleeding into the pericardial space either following cardiac operations and trauma (including cardiac perforation during diagnostic procedures) or from tuberculosis and hemopericardium. The latter may occur when a patient with any form of acute pericarditis is treated with anticoagulants.

The three principal features of tamponade are elevation of intracardiac pressures, limitation of ventricular filling, and reduction of cardiac output. The quantity of fluid necessary to produce this critical state may be as small as 200 mL when the fluid develops rapidly or more than 2000 mL in slowly developing effusions when the pericardium has had the opportunity to stretch and adapt to an increasing volume. The volume of fluid required to produce tamponade also varies directly with the thickness of the ventricular myocardium and inversely with the thickness of the parietal pericardium.

Table 239-2 lists the features that distinguish cardiac tamponade from constrictive pericarditis. The classic findings of falling arterial pressure, rising venous pressure, and faint heart sounds usually occur only with severe, acute tamponade, as occurs with cardiac trauma or rupture. Tamponade may also develop more slowly, and under these circumstances the clinical manifestations may resemble those of heart failure, including dyspnea, orthopnea, hepatic engorgement, and jugular venous hypertension. A high index of suspicion for cardiac tamponade is required, since, in many instances, no obvious cause for pericardial disease is apparent. Tamponade should be considered in any patient with hypotension and elevation of jugular venous pressure with a prominent *x* descent; in contrast to constrictive pericarditis, in which the *y* descent is prominent (Chap. 225), in cardiac tamponade it is diminutive or absent. A positive Kussmaul sign (see below) is rare in cardiac tamponade, as is a pericardial knock. Their presence suggests that an organizing process and epicardial constriction are present in addition to effusion. A widening of the area of flatness to percussion across the anterior aspect of the chest wall, a paradoxical pulse (see below), hypotension, relatively clear lung fields, diminished pulsations of the cardiac silhouette on fluoroscopy, enlargement of the cardiac silhouette (especially in subacute or chronic tamponade), reduction in amplitude of the QRS complexes, and *electrical alternans* of the P, QRS, and T waves should raise the suspicion of cardiac tamponade.

Paradoxical Pulse This important clue to the presence of cardiac tamponade consists of *a greater than normal (10 mmHg) inspiratory decline in systolic arterial pressure*. When severe, it may be detected by palpating weakness or disappearance of the arterial pulse during inspiration, but usually sphygmomanometric measurement of systolic pressure during slow respiration is required.

Table 239-2 Features That Distinguish Cardiac Tamponade from Constrictive Pericarditis and Similar Clinical Disorders

Characteristic	Tamponade	Constrictive Pericarditis	Restrictive Cardiomyopathy	RVMI[a]
Clinical				
Pulsus paradoxus	Common	Usually absent	Rare	Rare
Jugular veins				
Prominent *y* descent	Absent	Usually present	Rare	Rare
Prominent *x* descent	Present	Usually present	Present	Rare
Kussmaul's sign	Absent	Present	Absent	Absent
Third heart sound	Absent	Absent	Rare	May be present
Pericardial knock	Absent	Often present	Absent	Absent
Electrocardiogram				
Low ECG voltage	May be present	May be present	May be present	Absent
Electrical alternans	May be present	Absent	Absent	Absent
Echocardiography				
Thickened pericardium	Absent	Present	Absent	Absent
Pericardial calcification	Absent	Often present	Absent	Absent
Pericardial effusion	Present	Absent	Absent	Absent
RV size	Usually small	Usually normal	Usually normal	Enlarged
Myocardial thickness	Normal	Normal	Usually increased	Normal
Right atrial collapse and RVDC	Present	Absent	Absent	Absent
Increased early filling, ↑ mitral flow velocity	Absent	Present	Present	May be present
Exaggerated respiratory variation in flow velocity	Present	Present	Absent	Absent
CT/MRI				
Thickened/calcific pericardium	Absent	Present	Absent	Absent
Cardiac catheterization				
Equalization of diastolic procedures	Usually present	Usually present	Usually absent	Absent or present
Cardiac biopsy helpful?	No	No	Sometimes	No

[a] RV, right ventricle; RVMI, right ventricular myocardial infarction; RVDC, right ventricular diastolic collapse; ECG, electrocardiograph.
SOURCE: From GM Brockington et al, Cardiol Clin 8:645, 1990.

Since both ventricles share a tight incompressible covering, i.e., the pericardial sac, the inspiratory enlargement of the right ventricle in cardiac tamponade compresses and reduces left ventricular volume; leftward bulging of the interventricular septum further reduces the left ventricular cavity as the right ventricle enlarges during inspiration. Thus in cardiac tamponade the normal inspiratory augmentation of right ventricular volume causes an exaggerated reciprocal reduction in left ventricular volume. Also, respiratory distress increases the fluctuations in intrathoracic pressure, which exaggerates the mechanism just described. Right ventricular infarction (Chap. 243) may resemble cardiac tamponade with hypotension, elevated jugular venous pressure, an absent *y* descent in the jugular venous pulse, and occasionally pulsus paradoxus. The differences between these two conditions are shown in Table 239-2

Paradoxical pulse occurs not only in cardiac tamponade but also in approximately one-third of patients with constrictive pericarditis. Paradoxical pulse is not pathognomonic of pericardial disease because it may be observed in some cases of hypovolemic shock, acute and chronic obstructive airways disease, and pulmonary embolus.

Low-pressure tamponade refers to mild tamponade in which the intrapericardial pressure is increased from its slightly subatmospheric levels to +5 to +10 mmHg; in some instances hypovolemia coexists. As a consequence, the central venous pressure is normal or only slightly elevated, while arterial pressure is unaffected and there is no paradoxical pulse. The patients are asymptomatic or complain of mild weakness and dyspnea The diagnosis is aided by echocardiography, and both hemodynamic and clinical manifestations improve following pericardiocentesis.

FIGURE 239-1 Parasternal long-axis (*A*) and apical four-chamber (*B*) images from a patient with cardiac tamponade, demonstrating the presence of right ventricular diastolic collapse and right atrial collapse. In this patient, even the left atrium is seen to collapse because of tamponade. LV, left ventricle; LA, left atrium; Ao, aorta; PE, pericardial effusion; RVDC, right ventricular diastolic collapse; RAC, right atrial collapse; LAC, left atrial collapse. *(From Cujer et al.)*

sion is carried out, an attempt should be made to remove as much fluid as possible. Surgical drainage through a limited thoracotomy may be required in recurrent tamponade and/or when it is necessary to obtain tissue for diagnosis.

VIRAL OR IDIOPATHIC FORM OF ACUTE PERICARDITIS

In some cases of this common disorder, an A or B coxsackievirus or the virus of influenza, echovirus, mumps, herpes simplex, chickenpox, adenovirus, or Epstein-Barr has been isolated from pericardial fluid and/or appropriate elevations in viral antibody titers have been noted. In many instances, acute pericarditis occurs in association with illnesses of known viral origin and, presumably, are caused by the same agent. Commonly, there is an antecedent infection of the respiratory tract, but in many patients such an association is not evident and viral isolation and serologic studies are negative. Most frequently, a viral causation cannot be established; the term *acute idiopathic pericarditis* is then appropriate. Acute pericarditis is a common complication in patients infected with AIDS (Chap. 309). It may be caused by HIV itself; by opportunistic infections, such as cytomegalovirus and tuberculosis; or by associated neoplasms, such as lymphoma or Kaposi's sarcoma.

Acute pericarditis occurs at all ages

Diagnosis Since immediate treatment of cardiac tamponade may be lifesaving, prompt measures to establish the diagnosis by echocardiography should be undertaken (Fig 239-1). When pericardial effusion causes tamponade, during inspiration right ventricular diameter increases while left ventricular diameter and mitral valve opening decrease. Often the right ventricular cavity is reduced in diameter, and there is late diastolic inward motion (collapse) of the right ventricular free wall and of the right atrium. Doppler ultrasound shows exaggerated pulmonic (and tricuspid) flow during inspiration, with reciprocal changes in aortic (and mitral) flow (Fig 239-2).

If measured, the pericardial pressure is elevated and equal to the right atrial pressure. There is "equalization" of pressures, i.e., the pulmonary artery wedge is equal, or close, to right atrial, right ventricular, and pulmonary artery diastolic pressures. The "square root" sign in the ventricular pressure pulses and the prominent *y* descent in atrial and jugular venous pressure are characteristic of constrictive pericarditis (see below) and are rarely present in tamponade.

℞ **TREATMENT** Patients with acute pericarditis should be observed frequently for the development of an effusion; if a large effusion is present, the patient should be hospitalized and watched closely for signs of tamponade. In the presence of an effusion, arterial and venous pressures and heart rate should be monitored or followed carefully and serial echocardiograms obtained. If manifestations of tamponade appear, pericardiocentesis must be carried out at once, since relief of the intrapericardial pressure may be lifesaving. It is helpful, though not essential, to carry this out in the catheterization laboratory with hemodynamic and fluoroscopic monitoring. A small catheter advanced over the needle inserted into the pericardial cavity may be left in place to allow draining of the pericardial space if fluid reaccumulates. When a *diagnostic* pericardiocentesis of a large effu-

FIGURE 239-2 Pulmonary artery and aortic blood flow velocity recordings in cardiac tamponade. There is a marked increase in the pulmonary flow velocity during inspiration. Simultaneously, there is a marked decrease in aortic flow velocity. In, inspiration; Ex, expiration. *(From Cujer et al.)*

but is more frequent in young adults. Regardless of the specific cause, the clinical manifestations are similar. Acute pericarditis is often associated with pleural effusions and pneumonitis. The almost simultaneous development of fever and precordial pain, often 10 to 12 days after a presumed viral illness, constitutes an important feature in the differentiation of acute pericarditis from myocardial infarction, in which pain precedes fever. The constitutional symptoms are usually mild to moderate, but occasionally the initial symptoms are stormy, the temperature rising to 40°C. A pericardial friction rub is often audible. The disease ordinarily runs its course in a few days to 4 weeks, but one or more recurrences occur in about one-fourth of patients. Although accumulation of some pericardial fluid is common, tamponade is unusual, and constrictive pericarditis is a possible complication. The ST-segment alterations in the ECG usually disappear after 1 or more weeks, but the abnormal T waves may persist for several years and be a source of confusion in persons without a clear history of pericarditis. Pleuritis and pneumonitis frequently accompany pericarditis. Granulocytosis followed by lymphocytosis is common.

℞ TREATMENT There is no specific therapy, but bed rest and anti-inflammatory treatment with aspirin, if necessary up to 900 mg qid, may be given. If this is ineffective, one of the nonsteroidal anti-inflammatory agents, such as indomethacin (25 to 75 mg qid) or a glucocorticoid (e.g., prednisone, 40 to 80 mg daily) usually suppresses the clinical manifestations of the acute illness and may be useful in patients in whom the purulent and tuberculous forms of pericarditis have been excluded. Anticoagulants should be avoided. After the patient has been asymptomatic and afebrile for about a week, the dose of the anti-inflammatory agent is gradually tapered. When recurrences are multiple, frequent, disabling, and continue beyond 2 years, pericardiectomy may be effective in terminating the illness.

POST-CARDIAC INJURY SYNDROME Acute pericarditis may appear under a variety of circumstances that have one common feature: previous injury to the myocardium, with blood in the pericardial cavity. The syndrome may develop after a cardiac operation (postpericardiotomy syndrome); after cardiac trauma (Chap. 240), e.g., a stab wound, contusions after a nonpenetrating blow to the chest; or after perforation of the heart with a catheter. Rarely, it follows myocardial infarction.

The clinical picture of the post-cardiac injury syndrome mimics acute viral or acute idiopathic pericarditis. The principal symptom is the pain of acute pericarditis, which usually develops 1 to 4 weeks following the cardiac injury but sometimes appears only after an interval of months. Recurrences of pericarditis are common and may occur up to 2 years or more after the injury. Fever with temperature up to 40°C, pericarditis, pleuritis, and pneumonitis are the outstanding features, and the bout of illness usually subsides in 1 or 2 weeks. The pericarditis may be of the fibrinous variety, or it may be a pericardial effusion, which is often serosanguineous, and may be accompanied by arthralgias, but rarely causes tamponade. Leukocytosis, an increased sedimentation rate, and electrocardiographic changes typical of acute pericarditis also may occur.

The mechanisms responsible for this syndrome have not been identified, but they are probably the result of a hypersensitivity reaction in which the antigen originates from injured myocardial tissue and/or pericardium; the suggested designation of *post-cardiac injury syndrome* for this group of disorders implies that they may have a common pathogenetic mechanism. Circulating autoantibodies to myocardium occur frequently, but their precise role has not been defined. Viral infection may also play an etiologic role, since antiviral antibodies are often elevated in patients who develop this syndrome following cardiac surgery.

Often no treatment is necessary aside from aspirin and analgesics. The management of pericardial effusion and tamponade has already been discussed. When the illness is followed by a series of disabling recurrences, therapy with a nonsteroidal anti-inflammatory agent or a glucocorticoid is usually effective.

Differential Diagnosis Since there is no specific test for *acute idiopathic pericarditis*, the diagnosis is one of exclusion. Consequently, all other disorders that may be associated with acute fibrinous pericarditis must be considered. A common diagnostic error is mistaking acute viral or idiopathic pericarditis for acute myocardial infarction and vice versa. When it is associated with *acute myocardial infarction*, acute fibrinous pericarditis may be confused with acute viral or idiopathic pericarditis; this complication of infarction, described in Chap. 243, is characterized by fever, pain, and a friction rub in the first 4 days following the development of the infarct (to be distinguished from the pericarditis in Dressler's syndrome, which is a form of post-cardiac injury pericarditis and which occurs a week or two following myocardial infarction). ECG abnormalities (such as the appearance of Q waves, brief ST-segment elevations with reciprocal changes, and earlier T-wave changes in myocardial infarction) and the extent of the elevations of myocardial enzymes are helpful in differentiating pericarditis from acute myocardial infarction.

Pericarditis secondary to post-cardiac injury is differentiated from acute idiopathic pericarditis chiefly by timing. If it occurs within a few weeks of a myocardial infarction or a chest blow, it may be justified to conclude that the two are probably related. If the infarct has been silent or the chest blow forgotten, the relationship to the pericarditis may not be recognized.

It is important to distinguish *pericarditis due to collagen vascular disease* from acute idiopathic pericarditis. Most important in the differential diagnosis is the pericarditis due to systemic lupus erythematosus (SLE; Chap. 311) or drug-induced (procainamide or hydralazine) lupus. In these conditions, pain is often present; sometimes in SLE the pericarditis appears as an asymptomatic effusion, and rarely, tamponade develops. When pericarditis occurs in the absence of any obvious underlying disorder, the diagnosis may be made on discovery of lupus erythematosus cells or a rise in the titer of antinuclear antibodies. Acute pericarditis may complicate the viral, pyogenic, mycobacterial, and fungal infections that occur in AIDS. Acute pericarditis is an occasional complication of *rheumatoid arthritis*, *scleroderma*, and *polyarteritis nodosa*, and other evidence of these diseases is usually obvious. Asymptomatic pericardial effusion is also frequent in these disorders. It is important to question every patient with acute pericarditis about the ingestion of procainamide, hydralazine, isoniazid, cromolyn, and minoxidil, since these drugs can cause this syndrome.

The pericarditis of *acute rheumatic fever* is generally associated with evidence of severe pancarditis and with cardiac murmurs (Chap. 235). *Pyogenic (purulent) pericarditis* is usually secondary to cardiothoracic operations, immunosuppressive therapy, rupture of the esophagus into the pericardial sac, or rupture of a ring abscess in a patient with infective endocarditis and with septicemia complicating aseptic pericarditis. It is accompanied by fever, chills, septicemia, and evidence of infection elsewhere. *Tuberculous pericarditis* (Chap. 169) may present as an acute pericarditis associated with fever, weight loss, and other clinical manifestations of active systemic tuberculosis; the diagnosis may be aided by a positive tuberculin test and evidence of pulmonary or mediastinal tuberculosis. Tubercle bacilli can be cultured from the pericardial space only infrequently, and a biopsy of the pericardium with bacteriologic and histologic examination may be required. Alternatively, tuberculous pericarditis may present as a chronic asymptomatic effusion, as subacute effusive-constrictive pericarditis, or as frank chronic constrictive pericarditis (see below).

Uremic pericarditis (Chap. 270) occurs in up to one-third of patients with chronic uremia and is seen most frequently in patients undergoing chronic hemodialysis. It may be fibrinous and is generally associated with an effusion that may be sanguineous. A friction rub is common, but pain is usually absent. Treatment with an anti-inflammatory agent and intensification of hemodialysis is usually adequate. Occasionally, tamponade occurs and pericardiocentesis is required. When uremic pericarditis is recurrent, persistent, or very troubling, pericardiectomy may be necessary. Pericarditis due to *neoplastic diseases* results from extension or invasion of metastatic tumors (most commonly carcinoma of the lung and breast, malignant melanoma, lymphoma, and leukemia) to the pericardium; pain, atrial arrhythmias, and tamponade are complications that occur occasionally. *Mediastinal irradiation* for neoplasm may cause acute pericarditis and/or chronic constrictive pericarditis after eradication of the tumor. Unusual causes of acute pericarditis include syphilis, fungal infection (histoplasmosis, blastomycosis, aspergillosis, and candidiasis), and parasitic infestation (amebiasis, toxoplasmosis, echinococcosis, trichinosis).

CHRONIC PERICARDIAL EFFUSIONS   Chronic pericardial effusions are sometimes encountered in patients without an antecedent history of acute pericarditis. They may cause few symptoms per se, and their presence may be detected by finding an enlarged cardiac silhouette on chest roentgenogram.

Tuberculosis   This is a common cause of chronic pericardial effusion, although less so in the United States than in other parts of the world (Chap. 169). The clinical picture is that of a chronic, systemic illness in a patient with pericardial effusion. It is important to consider this condition in a middle-aged or elderly person with fever and enlargement of the cardiac silhouette of undetermined origin, with or without elevation of venous pressure. Weight loss, fever, and fatigability are sometimes observed. Inasmuch as treatment is quite effective, overlooking a tuberculous pericardial effusion may have serious consequences. A chest roentgenogram for pulmonary tuberculosis should be obtained, and a search for tuberculosis in other organs carried out; tuberculin skin tests should be performed and repeated after several weeks. If the etiology of chronic pericardial effusion remains obscure, a pericardial biopsy, preferably by a limited thoracotomy, should be performed. If definitive evidence is then still lacking but the specimen shows caseation necrosis, antituberculous chemotherapy is indicated. If the biopsy specimen shows a thickened pericardium, pericardiectomy should be carried out in order to prevent the development of constriction.

Other Causes of Chronic Pericardial Effusion   *Myxedema* may be responsible for a pericardial effusion that is sometimes massive but rarely, if ever, causes cardiac tamponade. The cardiac silhouette is markedly enlarged, and an echocardiogram is necessary to distinguish cardiomegaly from pericardial effusion. The diagnosis of myxedema is frequently overlooked. It is important, therefore, to carry out appropriate tests for thyroid function (Chap. 330) as well as echocardiography in patients with an enlarged cardiac outline of undetermined origin. *Cholesterol pericardial disease* is sometimes associated with myxedema. It is characterized by large pericardial effusions with a high cholesterol content, which may induce an inflammatory response and constrictive pericarditis.

Neoplasms, SLE, rheumatoid arthritis, mycotic infections, radiation therapy, pyogenic infections, severe chronic anemia, and chylopericardium may also cause chronic pericardial effusion and should be considered and specifically looked for in such patients.

Aspiration and analysis of the pericardial fluid are often helpful in diagnosis. In infections the organism can often be identified by smear or culture. Grossly sanguineous pericardial fluid results most commonly from a neoplasm, tuberculosis, uremia, or slow leakage from an aortic aneurysm.

CHRONIC CONSTRICTIVE PERICARDITIS

This disorder results when the healing of an acute fibrinous or serofibrinous pericarditis or a chronic pericardial effusion is followed by obliteration of the pericardial cavity with the formation of granulation tissue. The latter gradually contracts and forms a firm scar, encasing the heart and interfering with filling of the ventricles. In some reports, a high percentage of cases has been of tuberculous origin. In North America, tuberculosis is now an infrequent cause. Chronic constrictive pericarditis may also follow purulent infection, trauma, cardiac oper-

ation of any type, mediastinal irradiation, histoplasmosis, neoplastic disease (especially breast cancer, lung cancer, and lymphoma), acute viral or idiopathic pericarditis, rheumatoid arthritis, SLE, and chronic renal failure with uremia treated by chronic dialysis. In many patients the cause of the pericardial disease is undetermined, and in them an asymptomatic or forgotten bout of viral pericarditis, acute or idiopathic, may have been the inciting event. The heart may also be constricted and compressed by malignant tumors or organized blood clot in the pericardial cavity.

The basic physiologic abnormality in symptomatic patients with chronic constrictive pericarditis, as in those with cardiac tamponade, is the inability of the ventricles to fill because of the limitations imposed by the rigid, thickened pericardium or the tense pericardial fluid. In constrictive pericarditis, ventricular filling is unimpeded during early diastole but is reduced abruptly when the elastic limit of the pericardium is reached, while in cardiac tamponade, ventricular filling is impeded throughout diastole. In chronic constrictive pericarditis, ventricular end-diastolic and stroke volumes are reduced and the end-diastolic pressures in both ventricles and the mean pressures in the atria, pulmonic veins, and systemic veins are all elevated to similar levels, i.e., within 5 mmHg. The fibrotic process may extend into the myocardium and cause myocardial scarring, and venous congestion may then be due to the combined effects of the myocardial and pericardial lesions. Despite these hemodynamic changes, myocardial function may be normal or only slightly impaired.

In constrictive pericarditis, the central venous and right and left atrial pressure pulses display an M-shaped contour, with prominent *x* and *y* descents; the *y* descent, which is absent or diminished in cardiac tamponade, is the most prominent deflection in constrictive pericarditis and is interrupted by a rapid rise in pressure during early diastole, when ventricular filling is impeded by the constricting pericardium. These characteristic changes are transmitted to the jugular veins, where they may be recognized by inspection. In constrictive pericarditis, the ventricular pressure pulses in both ventricles exhibit characteristic "square root" signs during diastole (Fig. 239-3). These hemodynamic changes, although characteristic, are not pathognomonic of constrictive pericarditis but may also be observed in cardiomyopathies characterized by restriction of ventricular filling (Chap. 238).

CLINICAL AND LABORATORY FINDINGS (Table 239-2) Weakness, fatigue, weight gain, increased abdominal girth, abdominal discomfort, and edema are common. The patient often appears to be

FIGURE 239-3 Left (LV) and right ventricular (RV) pressure recording from a patient with constrictive pericarditis showing the characteristic dip and plateau ("square root" sign) in both ventricular pressure pulses. End-diastolic pressures are equal in the two ventricles. *[Modified from BH Lorell, W Grossman, in W Grossman (ed): Cardiac Catheterization and Angiography. Philadelphia, Lea & Febiger, 1986, p 430.]*

chronically ill with decreased skeletal muscle mass and a protuberant abdomen. Exertional dyspnea is common, and orthopnea may occur, although it is usually not severe. Acute left ventricular failure (acute pulmonary edema) is very uncommon. The cervical veins are distended and may remain so even after intensive diuretic treatment, and venous pressure may fail to decline during inspiration (Kussmaul's sign). The latter is frequent in chronic pericarditis but may also occur in tricuspid stenosis, right ventricular infarction, and restrictive cardiomyopathy. The pulse pressure is normal or reduced. In about one-third of the cases a paradoxical pulse can be detected. Congestive hepatomegaly is pronounced and may impair hepatic function; ascites is common and is usually more prominent than dependent edema. In about half of patients the heart is normal in size; if it is enlarged, the enlargement is rarely extreme. The apical pulse is reduced in intensity, retracts in systole, and moves outward in diastole. The heart sounds may be distant; an early third heart sound, i.e., a pericardial knock, occurring 0.09 to 0.12 s after aortic valve closure that coincides with a sudden deceleration in ventricular filling, is often conspicuous, and murmurs are usually absent. Because of the high sustained venous pressure, congestive splenomegaly may make the spleen palpable. In the absence of infective endocarditis or tricuspid valve disease, splenomegaly in a patient with congestive heart failure should arouse suspicion of constrictive pericarditis. Protein-losing gastroenteropathy, due to impaired lymphatic drainage from the small intestine, and marked proteinuria or hypoalbuminemia may complicate chronic constrictive pericarditis.

The *ECG* frequently displays low voltage of the QRS complex and diffuse flattening or inversion of the T waves. P mitrale may be present in patients with sinus rhythm; atrial fibrillation is present in about one-third of patients. The *chest roentgenogram* shows a normal or slightly enlarged heart, sometimes with pericardial calcification.

Inasmuch as the usual physical signs of cardiac disease (murmurs, cardiac enlargement) may be inconspicuous or absent in chronic constrictive pericarditis, hepatic enlargement and dysfunction associated with intractable ascites may lead to a mistaken diagnosis of cirrhosis of the liver. This error can be avoided if the neck veins are inspected carefully in patients with ascites and hepatomegaly. *Given a clinical picture resembling hepatic cirrhosis, but with the added feature of distended neck veins, careful search for calcification of the pericardium by chest roentgenography and CT or MRI should be carried out and may disclose this curable or remediable form of heart disease.*

The echocardiogram typically shows pericardial thickening, atrial enlargement, dilatation of the inferior vena cava and hepatic veins, and a sharp halt in ventricular filling in early diastole, with normal ventricular systolic function; there is a distinctive pattern of transvalvular flow velocity on Doppler echocardiography. There is an exaggerated reduction in blood flow velocity in the pulmonary veins and across the mitral valve during inspiration, with the opposite occurring during expiration. Diastolic flow velocity in the vena cavae into the right atrium and across the tricuspid valve increases in an exaggerated manner during inspiration and declines during expiration (Fig. 239-4). However, echocardiography cannot definitively exclude the diagnosis. MRI and CT scanning, especially the latter (Fig. 239-5), are more accurate than echocardiography in establishing or excluding the presence of a thickened pericardium. Pericardial thickening and even pericardial calcification, however, are not synonymous with constrictive pericarditis since they may occur without seriously impairing ventricular filling.

DIFFERENTIAL DIAGNOSIS Like cor pulmonale (Chap. 237), chronic constrictive pericarditis may be associated with severe systemic venous hypertension but little pulmonary congestion; the heart usually is not enlarged, and a paradoxical pulse may be present. However, in cor pulmonale advanced parenchymal pulmonary disease is usually obvious and venous pressure *falls* during inspiration, i.e., Kussmaul's sign is negative. *Tricuspid stenosis* (Chap. 236) may also simulate chronic constrictive pericarditis; congestive hepatomegaly, splenomegaly, ascites, and venous distention may be equally prominent, and the manifestations of left-sided heart failure may be incon-

Inspiration   Expiration

FIGURE 239-4 Schematic of respiratory variation in transvalvular and central venous flow velocities in constrictive pericarditis. With inspiration, the driving pressure gradient from the pulmonary capillaries to the left cardiac chambers decreases, resulting in a decrease in mitral and diastolic pulmonary venous (PV) flow velocity. The decreased left ventricular filling results in ventricular septal shift to the left (small arrow), allowing augmented flow to the right-sided chambers, shown as increased tricuspid inflow and diastolic hepatic venous (HV) flow velocity (downward deflection = increased flow to the right atrium) because the cardiac volume is relatively fixed as a result of the thickened shell of pericardium. The opposite changes occur during expiration. D, diastole; LA, left atrium; LV, left ventricle; RA, right atrium; RV, right ventricle; S, systole. *(From Oh et al.)*

spicuous. However, in tricuspid stenosis, a characteristic murmur as well as mitral stenosis are usually present. In tricuspid stenosis, a paradoxical pulse and a steep, deep *y* descent in the jugular venous pulse do not occur, serving to differentiate it from chronic constrictive pericarditis.

Because constrictive pericarditis can be corrected surgically, it is important, though often difficult, to distinguish chronic constrictive pericarditis from restrictive cardiomyopathy (Chap. 238), which has a

FIGURE 239-5 Computed tomographic scan showing thickened pericardium encases the right (arrowhead) and left ventricles (arrow), producing constriction. The cause of the constriction was thought to be an inflammatory process. *[From W Stanford, in LP Elliott (ed): The Fundamentals of Cardiac Imaging in Infants, Children and Adults. Philadelphia, Lippincott, 1991, p 418, with permission.]*

similar physiologic abnormality, i.e., restriction of ventricular filling. In many of these patients the ventricular wall is thickened on echocardiographic examination (Table 239-2). The features favoring the diagnosis of restrictive cardiomyopathy over chronic constrictive pericarditis include a well-defined apex beat, cardiac enlargement, and pronounced orthopnea with attacks of acute left ventricular failure, left ventricular hypertrophy, gallop sounds (in place of a pericardial knock), bundle branch block, and in some cases abnormal Q waves on the ECG. The echocardiogram in chronic constrictive pericarditis characteristically shows pericardial thickening, i.e., a distinct echo posterior to the left ventricular wall, and paradoxical septal motion. The left ventricular wall moves sharply outward in early diastole and then remains flat. Marked respiratory variations in atrioventricular flow velocities on Doppler echocardiography are characteristic of constrictive pericarditis but not restrictive cardiomyopathy (Fig. 239-4). The definitive diagnosis of restrictive cardiomyopathy, when it is due to an infiltrative disease such as amyloidosis, can often be established by endomyocardial biopsy. CT scanning and MRI are very useful in distinguishing between restrictive cardiomyopathy and chronic constrictive pericarditis. In the former, the ventricular walls are hypertrophied, while in the latter the pericardium is thickened and sometimes calcified.

When a patient has progressive, disabling, and unresponsive congestive failure and displays any of the features of constrictive heart disease, the most careful and detailed clinical and laboratory studies must be carried out in order to detect or exclude constrictive pericarditis, since the latter is usually curable.

Occult Constrictive Disease Patients with this condition may have unexplained fatigue, dyspnea, and chest pain. No overt manifestations of pericardial disease are present, but following the rapid intravenous infusion of 1 L of saline solution, diastolic equilibration of intracardiac atrial and ventricular pressures found in overt constrictive pericarditis occur. Although symptomatic improvement may follow pericardiectomy, this procedure should not be carried out in asymptomatic persons.

TREATMENT Pericardial resection is the only definitive treatment of constrictive pericarditis, but dietary sodium restriction and diuretics are useful during preoperative preparation. The benefits derived from cardiac decortication are often striking, and the improvement, though slight at first, usually is progressive over a period of months. The risk of this operation depends on the extent of penetration of the myocardium by the calcific process, by the severity of myocardial atrophy, by the extent of secondary impairment of hepatic and/or renal function, and by the patient's general condition. Operative mortality is in the range of 3 to 10%; the patients with the most severe and/or advanced disease are at highest risk. Therefore, surgical treatment should be carried out relatively early in the course.

Many cases of constrictive pericarditis are of tuberculous origin. Antituberculous therapy during the phase of effusion may prevent the development of constriction, and such therapy should be carried out before and after operation if a tuberculous origin can be diagnosed, is suspected, or cannot be excluded in a patient with chronic constrictive pericarditis (Chap. 169).

Subacute Effusive-Constrictive Pericarditis This form of pericardial disease is characterized by the combination of a tense effusion in the pericardial space and constriction of the heart by thickened pericardium. It shares a number of features both with chronic pericardial effusion (p. 1366) producing cardiac compression and with pericardial constriction. It may be caused by tuberculosis, multiple attacks of acute idiopathic pericarditis, radiation, traumatic pericarditis, uremia, and scleroderma. The heart is generally enlarged, and a paradoxical pulse and a prominent x descent (without a prominent y descent) are present in the atrial and jugular venous pressure pulses. Following pericardiocentesis, the physiologic findings may change from those of cardiac

tamponade to those of pericardial constriction, with a "square root" sign in the ventricular pressure pulse and a prominent y descent in the atrial and jugular venous pressure pulses. Furthermore, the intrapericardial pressure and the central venous pressure may decline, but not to normal. In many patients the condition progresses to the chronic constrictive form of the disease. Wide excision of both the visceral and parietal pericardium is usually effective.

OTHER DISORDERS OF THE PERICARDIUM

Pericardial cysts appear as rounded or lobulated deformities of the cardiac silhouette, most commonly at the right cardiophrenic angle. They do not cause symptoms, and their major clinical significance lies in the possibility of confusion with a tumor, ventricular aneurysm, or massive cardiomegaly. *Tumors* involving the pericardium are most commonly secondary to malignant neoplasms originating in or invading the mediastinum, including carcinoma of the bronchus and breast, lymphoma, and melanoma. The most common *primary* malignant tumor is the mesothelioma. The usual clinical picture of malignant pericardial tumor is an insidiously developing, often bloody, pericardial effusion. Surgical exploration is required to establish a definitive diagnosis and to carry out definitive or, more commonly, palliative treatment.

BIBLIOGRAPHY

CUJER B et al: Echocardiography in pericardial diseases, in *Marcus' Cardiac Imaging: A Companion to Braunwald's Heart Disease*, 2d ed, DJ Skorton et al (eds). Philadelphia, Saunders, 1996, pp 404–419

FOWLER NO: Constrictive pericarditis: Its history and current status. Clin Cardiol 18:341, 1995

HEIDENREICH PA et al: Pericardial effusions in AIDS: Incidence and survival. Circulation 92:3229, 1995

HOIT BD, SHAW D: The paradoxical pulse in tamponade, mechanisms and echocardiographic correlates. Echocardiography 11:477, 1994

KHAN AH: The postcardiac injury syndromes. Clin Cardiol 15:67, 1992

LING LH et al: Calcific constrictive pericarditis: Is it still with us? Ann Intern Med 132:444, 2000

OH JK et al: Diagnostic role of Doppler echocardiography in constrictive pericarditis. J Am Coll Cardiol 23:154, 1994

SAGRISTA SAULEDA J et al: Purulent pericarditis: Review of a 20-year experience in a general hospital. J Am Coll Cardiol 22:1661, 1993

SHABETAI R: Treatment of pericardial disease, in *Cardiovascular Therapeutics: A Companion to Braunwald's Heart Disease*, TW Smith (ed). Philadelphia, Saunders, 1996, pp 742–750

SPODICK D: Pericardial diseases, in *Heart Disease*, 6th ed, E Braunwald, D Zipes, P Libby (eds): Philadelphia, Saunders, 2001

TSANG TS et al: Outcomes of primary and secondary treatment of pericardial effusion in patients with malignancy. Mayo Clin Proc 75:248, 2000

VAITKUS PT, KUSSMAUL WG: Treatment of malignant pericardial effusion. JAMA 272:59, 1994

ZAYAS R et al: Incidence of specific etiology and role of methods for specific etiologic diagnosis of primary acute pericarditis. Am J Cardiol 75:378, 1995

240 *Wilson S. Colucci, Daniel T. Price*

CARDIAC TUMORS, CARDIAC MANIFESTATIONS OF SYSTEMIC DISEASES, AND TRAUMATIC CARDIAC INJURY

TUMORS OF THE HEART

PRIMARY TUMORS Primary tumors of the heart are rare. Approximately three-quarters are histologically benign, and the remainder, which in almost all cases are sarcomas, are malignant (Table 240-1). Because all cardiac tumors have the potential for causing life-

Type	Number	Percent
Benign	199	58.0
Myxoma	114	33.2
Rhabdomyoma	20	5.8
Fibroma	20	5.8
Hemangioma	17	5.0
Atrioventricular nodal	10	2.9
Granular cell	4	1.2
Lipoma	2	0.6
Paraganglioma	2	0.6
Myocytic hamartoma	2	0.6
Histiocytoid cardiomyopathy	2	0.6
Inflammatory psuedotumor	2	0.6
Other benign tumors	4	1.2
Malignant	144	42.0
Sarcoma	137	39.9
Lymphoma	7	2.1

SOURCE: Modified from A Burke; R Virmani: *Atlas of Tumor Pathology. Tumors of the Heart and Great Vessels.* Washington, DC, Armed Forces Institute of Pathology 1996, p 231.

threatening complications, and many are now curable by surgery, it is important that the diagnosis be made whenever possible.

Clinical Presentation Cardiac tumors may present with a wide array of cardiac and noncardiac manifestations. The location and the size of the tumor are the major determinants of the specific signs and symptoms, many of which are present in more common forms of heart disease, such as chest pain, syncope, heart failure, murmurs, arrhythmias, conduction disturbances, and pericardial effusion with or without tamponade.

Myxoma Myxomas are the most common type of primary cardiac tumor in all age groups, accounting for one-third to one-half of all cases at postmortem and for about three-quarters of the tumors treated surgically. They occur at all ages, most commonly in the third through sixth decades. There is a female predilection. Although most myxomas are sporadic, some are familial with autosomal dominant transmission or are part of a syndrome that involves a complex of abnormalities including lentigines or pigmented nevi, primary nodular adrenal cortical disease with or without Cushing's syndrome, myxomatous mammary fibroadenomas, testicular tumors, and/or pituitary adenomas with gigantism or acromegaly. Certain constellations of findings have been referred to as the *NAME* syndrome (nevi, atrial myxoma, myxoid neurofibroma, and ephelides) or the *LAMB* syndrome (lentigines, atrial myxoma, and blue nevi). Approximately 7% of cardiac myxomas are familial or part of the syndrome myxoma with the complex of abnormalities described above.

Pathologically, myxomas are gelatinous structures consisting of myxoma cells imbedded in a stroma rich in glycosaminoglycans. Most are pedunculated on a fibrovascular stalk and average 4 to 8 cm in diameter. The majority are solitary and located in the atria, particularly the left, where they arise from the interatrial septum in the vicinity of the fossa ovalis. In contrast to sporadic tumors, familial or syndrome myxoma tumors tend to occur in younger individuals, be multiple or ventricular in location, and have more postoperative recurrences, probably reflecting their multicentric nature.

Myxomas commonly present with obstructive, embolic, or constitutional signs and symptoms. The most common clinical presentation mimics that of mitral valve disease, either stenosis due to tumor prolapse into the mitral orifice or regurgitation due to tumor-induced valvular trauma. Ventricular myxomas may cause outflow obstruction similar to that caused by subaortic or subpulmonic stenosis. The symptoms and signs of myxoma may be of sudden onset or positional in nature, reflecting changes in tumor position due to gravity. An auscultatory finding, termed a "tumor plop," is a characteristic low-pitched sound that may be audible during early or

middiastole and is thought to result from the tumor abruptly stopping as it strikes the ventricular wall. Myxomas may also present with peripheral or pulmonary emboli, or constitutional signs and symptoms including fever, weight loss, cachexia, malaise, arthralgia, rash, clubbing, Raynaud's phenomenon, hypergammaglobulinemia, anemia, polycythemia, leukocytosis, elevated erythrocyte sedimentation rate, thrombocytopenia, or thrombocytosis. Not surprisingly, myxomas are frequently misdiagnosed as endocarditis, collagen vascular disease, or noncardiac tumor.

Two-dimensional transthoracic or transesophageal echocardiography is useful in the diagnosis of cardiac myxoma and allows determination of the site of tumor attachment and tumor size, which are important considerations in the planning of surgical excision (Fig. 240-1). Computed tomography and particularly magnetic resonance imaging may provide important information regarding size, shape, composition, and surface characteristics of the tumor. Because myxomas may be familial, echocardiographic screening of first-degree relatives is appropriate, particularly if the patient is young and has multiple tumors or evidence of syndrome myxoma. Although cardiac catheterization and angiography have previously been performed routinely before surgery, catheterization of the chamber from which the tumor arises is attended by the risk of tumor emboli. Catheterization is no longer considered mandatory when adequate noninvasive information is available and other cardiac diseases (e.g., coronary artery disease) are not considered likely.

TREATMENT Surgical excision utilizing cardiopulmonary bypass is indicated and is generally curative. Myxomas recur in approximately 12 to 22% of familial cases and in about 1 to 2% of sporadic cases. Tumor recurrence is most likely due to multifocal lesions in the former and inadequate resection in the latter.

Other Benign Tumors Cardiac *lipomas*, although relatively common, are usually incidental findings at postmortem examination. However, they may grow as large as 15 cm and may present with symptoms due to mechanical interference with cardiac function, arrhythmias, or conduction disturbances, or as an abnormality of the cardiac silhouette on chest x-ray. *Papillary fibroelastomas*, similarly, are relatively common findings on cardiac valves or the adjacent endothelium at postmortem, but seldom result in clinical symptoms. Occasionally, these growths may cause mechanical interference with valve function. *Rhabdomyomas* and *fibromas*, the most frequent tu-

FIGURE 240-1 Transthoracic echocardiogram during diastole demonstrating a large myocardial mass, which is an atrial myxoma (Myx) that prolapses into the left ventricle (LV). RA, right atrium; RV, right ventricle. *(Courtesy of Dr. Rick Nishimura.)*

mors in infants and children, most commonly occur in the ventricles and therefore produce signs and symptoms by mechanical obstruction that may mimic valvular stenosis, congestive heart failure, restrictive or hypertrophic cardiomyopathy, and pericardial constriction. Rhabdomyomas are probably hamartomatous growths; are multiple in 90% of cases; and may be associated with tuberous sclerosis, adenoma sebaceum, and benign kidney tumors in approximately 30% of patients. Calcification of a cardiac tumor strongly suggests that it is a fibroma, although myxomas and sarcomas also may be calcified. *Hemangiomas* and *mesotheliomas* are generally small tumors, most often intramyocardial in location, and may cause atrioventricular conduction disturbances and even sudden death as a result of their propensity for location in the region of the AV node. Other benign tumors arising from the heart include *teratoma, chemodectoma, neurilemoma, granular cell myoblastoma,* and *bronchogenic cysts.*

Sarcoma   Almost all primary cardiac malignancies are sarcomas, which may be of several histologic types. In general, these tumors are characterized by a rapidly downhill course leading to the patient's death in weeks to months from the time of presentation as a result of hemodynamic compromise, local invasion, or distant metastases. Sarcomas commonly involve the right side of the heart, and because of their rapid growth, invasion of the pericardial space and obstruction of the cardiac chambers or venae cavae are common. Sarcomas can also occur on the left side of the heart and may be mistaken for myxomas.

℞ TREATMENT   At the time of presentation these tumors have often spread too extensively for surgical excision. Although scattered reports exist of palliation with surgery, radiotherapy, and/or chemotherapy, the overall experience with cardiac sarcomas is poor. The one exception appears to be cardiac lymphosarcomas, which may respond to a combination of chemo- and radiotherapy.

TUMORS METASTATIC TO THE HEART   Tumors metastatic to the heart are many times more common than primary tumors; and as the life expectancy of patients with various forms of malignant neoplasms is extended by more effective therapy, the frequency of cardiac metastases will also increase. Although cardiac metastases occur in 1 to 20% of all tumor types, the relative incidence is especially high in malignant melanoma and, to a somewhat lesser extent, in leukemia and lymphoma. In absolute numbers, the most common primary originating sites of cardiac metastases are carcinoma of the breast and lung, reflecting the high incidence of these cancers. Cardiac metastases almost always occur in the setting of widespread primary disease, and most often either primary or metastatic disease exists elsewhere in the thoracic cavity. Nevertheless, a cardiac metastasis may occasionally be the initial presentation of a tumor elsewhere in the body.

Cardiac metastases reach the heart from the blood stream, the lymphatics, or by direct invasion. They generally are small, firm nodules. Diffuse infiltration may also occur, especially with sarcomas or hematologic neoplasms. The pericardium is most often involved, followed by myocardial involvement of any chamber, and, rarely, by involvement of the endocardium or cardiac valves.

Cardiac metastases result in clinical manifestations only about 10% of the time and rarely are the cause of death. In most instances the metastases are not the cause of the presenting clinical features but occur in the setting of a previously recognized malignant neoplasm. Although cardiac metastases may present with a large number of nonspecific signs and symptoms, the most common are dyspnea, signs of acute pericarditis, cardiac tamponade, a rapid increase in the cardiac silhouette on chest x-ray, new onset of ectopic tachyarrhythmia or AV block, and congestive heart failure. As with primary cardiac tumors, the clinical presentation is more closely related to the location and size of the tumor rather than histologic type. Many of these signs and

symptoms also occur with myocarditis, pericarditis, or cardiomyopathy resulting from radiotherapy or chemotherapy.

Electrocardiographic findings are nonspecific. On chest roentgenography the cardiac silhouette is most often normal but may reveal a pericardial effusion or bizarre contour. Echocardiography is useful for the diagnosis of pericardial effusion and the visualization of larger metastases. Computed tomography, magnetic resonance imaging, and radionuclide imaging with gallium or thallium may provide useful anatomic information. Angiography may delineate discrete lesions, and pericardiocentesis can allow a specific cytologic diagnosis.

℞ TREATMENT   Because most patients with cardiac metastases have widespread disease, therapy generally consists of treatment of the primary tumor. Symptomatic malignant effusions are treated by removal of fluid by pericardiocentesis, with or without concomitant instillation of a sclerosing agent (e.g., tetracycline), or placement of a pericardial window for drainage to the pleural space to palliate symptoms and delay or prevent reaccumulation of the effusion.

CARDIAC EFFECTS OF CANCER THERAPY   →*See Chap. 238.*

CARDIOVASCULAR MANIFESTATIONS OF SYSTEMIC DISEASES

DIABETES MELLITUS (See also Chap. 333)   There is an increased incidence of large vessel atherosclerosis and myocardial infarction in patients with both insulin- and non-insulin-dependent diabetes mellitus. Coronary artery disease is the most common cause of death in adults with diabetes mellitus. Diabetes mellitus is an independent risk factor for coronary artery disease (Chap. 241), and the incidence of coronary artery disease is related to the duration of diabetes. In patients with diabetes mellitus, myocardial infarctions are not only more frequent but also tend to be larger in size and more likely to result in complications such as heart failure, shock, and death. Patients with diabetes mellitus are more likely to have an abnormal or absent pain response to myocardial ischemia, probably as a result of generalized autonomic nervous system dysfunction. Ambulatory electrocardiographic monitoring has shown that up to 90% of episodes of ischemia are silent in diabetic patients with coronary artery disease; the presentation of ischemia may be exertional or episodic dyspnea, flash pulmonary edema, arrhythmias, heart block, or syncope. Since coronary artery disease is more common in in patients with diabetes mellitus and often is not associated with typical anginal symptoms, the threshold for the diagnosis should be low, particularly when the duration of disease is long and concomitant risk factors for coronary artery disease (e.g., hypertension, smoking, hyperlipidemia) are present.

Patients with diabetes mellitus may also have myocardial dysfunction characteristic of a restrictive cardiomyopathy in the absence of large-vessel (epicardial) coronary artery disease, with abnormal relaxation of the myocardium, and evidenced clinically by elevated left ventricular filling pressures. Histologically, these patients have interstitial fibrosis with increased amounts of collagen, glycoprotein, triglycerides, and cholesterol in the myocardial interstitium; and in some cases intimal thickening, hyaline deposition, and inflammatory changes have been observed in small intramural arteries. Patients with diabetes mellitus have an increased risk of developing clinical heart failure, even after correction for the presence of coronary artery disease, hypertension, and obesity, and it is likely that diabetic cardiomyopathy contributes to excessive cardiovascular morbidity and mortality in these patients. There is some evidence that insulin therapy results in an amelioration of the myocardial dysfunction.

MALNUTRITION AND VITAMIN DEFICIENCY MALNUTRITION (See also Chap. 74)   In patients whose intake of protein, calories, or both is severely deficient, the heart may become thin, pale, and flabby with myofibrillar atrophy and interstitial edema. The systolic pressure and cardiac output are low, and the pulse pressure is narrow. Generalized edema is common and is due to a combination of factors, including reduced serum oncotic pressure and myocardial dysfunction. Such profound states of malnutrition, termed *marasmus* in the case of caloric deficiency and *kwashiorkor* in the case of relative protein deficiency, are most common in underdeveloped countries. However, significant nutritional heart disease may also occur in developed nations, particularly in patients with chronic diseases such as AIDS, in patients with anorexia nervosa, and in patients with severe cardiac failure in whom gastrointestinal hypoperfusion and venous congestion may lead to anorexia and malabsorption. Open-heart surgery poses increased risk in malnourished patients, and they may benefit from preoperative hyperalimentation.

Thiamine Deficiency (Beriberi) (See also Chap. 75) In many cases, malnutrition is accompanied by thiamine deficiency, although this hypovitaminosis may also occur in the presence of an adequate protein and caloric intake, particularly in the Far East, where polished rice deficient in thiamine may be a major dietary component. In western nations, the widespread use of thiamine-enriched flour limits the presence of deficiency primarily to alcoholics and food faddists. The measurement of the thiamine-pyrophosphate effect (TPPE) can biochemically quantitate thiamine stores. An elevated TPPE, indicative of thiamine deficiency, has been found in 20 to 90% of patients with chronic heart failure. The deficiency appears to result from both reduced dietary intake and a diuretic-induced increase in the urinary excretion of thiamine. The acute administration of thiamine to these patients increases the left ventricular ejection fraction and the excretion of salt and water.

Clinically, there is usually evidence of generalized malnutrition, peripheral neuropathy, glossitis, and anemia. The characteristic cardiovascular syndrome is heart failure with increased cardiac output, tachycardia, and often elevated filling pressures in the left and right sides of the heart. The major cause of the high-output state is vasomotor depression, the precise mechanism of which is not understood but which leads to a reduced systemic vascular resistance. The cardiac examination reveals a wide pulse pressure, tachycardia, a third heart sound, and, frequently, an apical systolic murmur. The electrocardiogram may show decreased voltage, a prolonged QT interval, and T-wave abnormalities. The chest x-ray generally shows a large heart with signs of congestive heart failure. The response to thiamine is often dramatic, with an increase in systemic vascular resistance, decrease in cardiac output, clearing of pulmonary congestion, and a reduction in heart size often occurring in 12 to 48 h. Although the response to digitalis and diuretics may be poor before thiamine therapy, these agents may be important *after* thiamine is given, since the left ventricle may not be capable of dealing with the increased workload presented by the return of vascular tone.

Vitamin B₆, B₁₂, and Folate Deficiency (See also Chap. 241) These vitamin cofactors in the metabolism of homocysteine probably contribute to the majority of cases of hyperhomocysteinemia in the general population. Hyperhomocysteinemia is associated with increased risk of atherosclerosis. Supplementation of these vitamins has reduced the incidence of hyperhomocysteinemia in the United States. The clinical benefit of normalizing elevated homocysteine levels, however, remains unproven.

OBESITY (See also Chap. 77) Severe obesity, particularly when it occurs in an upper-body distribution, is associated with an increase in cardiovascular morbidity and mortality. Although obesity itself is not considered a disease, there is clearly an increased prevalence of hypertension, glucose intolerance, and atherosclerotic coronary artery disease in obese patients. In addition, these patients have a distinct abnormality of the cardiovascular system characterized by increases in total and central blood volumes, cardiac output, and left ventricular filling pressure. The elevated cardiac output appears to be required to support the metabolic needs of the excessive adipose tissue. Left ventricular filling pressure is often at the upper limits of normal and rises excessively with exercise. As a result of chronic volume overload, eccentric cardiac hypertrophy with cardiac dilatation and abnormal ventricular function may develop. Pathologically, there are

left and, in some cases, right ventricular hypertrophy and generalized cardiac dilatation, which is not due simply to fatty infiltration of the myocardium. Although these patients may develop pulmonary congestion, peripheral edema, and exercise intolerance, the recognition of these findings may be difficult in massively obese patients.

Weight reduction is the most effective therapy and results in reduction in blood volume and in the return of cardiac output toward normal. However, rapid weight reduction may be dangerous, as cardiac arrhythmias and sudden death due to electrolyte imbalance have been described. Digitalis, sodium restriction, and diuretics may also be useful. This form of heart disease should be distinguished from the Pickwickian syndrome (Chap. 263), which may share several of the cardiovascular features of heart disease secondary to severe obesity but, in addition, frequently has components of central apnea, hypoxemia, pulmonary hypertension, and cor pulmonale.

THYROID DISEASE (See also Chap. 330) Thyroid hormone exerts a major influence on the cardiovascular system by a number of direct and indirect mechanisms, and not surprisingly, cardiovascular effects are prominent in both hypo- and hyperthyroidism. Thyroid hormone causes increases in total-body metabolism and oxygen consumption that indirectly place an increased workload on the heart. In addition, although the exact mechanism has not been defined, thyroid hormone exerts direct inotropic, chronotropic, and dromotropic effects that are similar to those seen with adrenergic stimulation (e.g., tachycardia, increased cardiac output). Thyroid hormone increases the synthesis of myosin and of Na^+,K^+-ATPase, as well as the density of myocardial beta-adrenergic receptors.

Hyperthyroidism Cardiovascular presentations of hyperthyroidism include palpitations, systolic hypertension, fatigue, or, in patients with underlying heart disease, angina or heart failure. Sinus tachycardia is found in about 40% of patients and atrial fibrillation in about 15%. Other findings include a hyperdynamic precordium, a widened pulse pressure, an increase in the intensity of the first heart sound and the pulmonic component of the second heart sound, and a third heart sound. An increased incidence of mitral valve prolapse has been associated with hyperthyroidism, and in some cases there may be a midsystolic murmur heard best at the left sternal border with or without a systolic ejection click. A *Means-Lerman scratch* is a systolic scratchy sound, heard at the left second intercostal space during expiration; it is thought to result from the rubbing of the hyperdynamic pericardium against the pleura. Elderly patients with hyperthyroidism, so-called apathetic hyperthyroidism, may present with only the cardiovascular manifestations of thyrotoxicosis, such as atrial fibrillation, which may be resistant to therapy until the hyperthyroidism is controlled. Angina pectoris and congestive heart failure are unusual unless there is coexistent underlying heart disease, and in many cases symptoms resolve with treatment of the hyperthyroidism.

Hypothyroidism Cardiac manifestations of hypothyroidism include a reduction in cardiac output, stroke volume, heart rate, blood pressure, and pulse pressure. In about one-third of patients there is a pericardial effusion which only rarely results in tamponade. Increased capillary permeability results in pleural and pericardial effusions. Other clinical signs include cardiomegaly, bradycardia, weak arterial pulses, and distant heart sounds. Although the signs and symptoms of myxedema may suggest the diagnosis of congestive heart failure, in the absence of other cardiac disease, myocardial failure is uncommon. The electrocardiogram generally shows sinus bradycardia and low voltage and may show prolongation of the QT interval, decreased P-wave voltage, prolonged AV conduction time, intraventricular conduction disturbances, and nonspecific ST-T wave abnormalities. Chest x-ray may show cardiomegaly, often with a "water bottle" configuration, pleural effusions, and, in some cases, evidence of congestive heart failure. Pathologically, the heart is pale, dilated, and flabby, often with myofibrillar swelling, loss of striations, and interstitial fibrosis.

Patients with hypothyroidism frequently have elevations of cholesterol and triglycerides and severe atherosclerotic coronary artery disease. Before treatment with thyroid hormone, patients with hypothyroidism frequently do not have angina pectoris, presumably because of the low metabolic demands made by their condition. However, angina and myocardial infarction may be precipitated during initiation of thyroid hormone replacement, especially in elderly patients with underlying heart disease. Therefore, replacement should be done with care, starting with low doses that are increased gradually.

MALIGNANT CARCINOID (See also Chap. 93)   These tumors elaborate a variety of vasoactive amines (e.g., serotonin), kinins, indoles, and other substances believed to be responsible for the diarrhea, flushing, and labile blood pressure in these patients. The cardiac lesions due to gastrointestinal carcinoids are almost exclusively in the right side of the heart and occur only when there are hepatic metastases, suggesting that the substance responsible for the cardiac lesions is inactivated by passage through the liver and lungs. Similar lesions occur in the left side of the heart when there exists a right-to-left shunt or the tumor is located in the lungs. These lesions are fibrous plaques on the endothelium of the cardiac chambers, valves, and great vessels. These plaques, which result in distortion of the cardiac valves, consist of smooth-muscle cells embedded in a stroma of acid mucopolysaccharide and collagen and presumably result from healing of endothelial injury. The clinical syndrome is most often that of tricuspid regurgitation, pulmonic stenosis, or both. In some cases a high-output state may occur, presumably as a result of a decrease in systemic vascular resistance due to a vasoactive substance released by the tumor. Progression of the cardiac lesions does not appear to be affected by treatment with serotonin antagonists, and in some severely symptomatic patients valve replacement is indicated. Coronary artery spasm, presumably due to a circulating vasoactive substance, may occur in patients with carcinoid syndrome.

PHEOCHROMOCYTOMA (See also Chap. 332)   In addition to causing labile or sustained hypertension, the high circulating levels of catecholamines may also cause direct myocardial injury. Focal myocardial necrosis and inflammatory cell infiltration are present in about 50% of patients who die with pheochromocytoma and may contribute to clinically significant left ventricular failure and pulmonary edema. Left ventricular function and congestive heart failure may resolve after removal of the tumor. In addition, hypertension results in left ventricular hypertrophy.

RHEUMATOID ARTHRITIS AND THE COLLAGEN VASCULAR DISEASES Rheumatoid Arthritis   (See also Chap. 312)   There may be inflammation of any or all parts of the heart in patients with rheumatoid arthritis. Pericarditis is the most common cause of clinically apparent disease and may be found by echocardiography in 10 to 50% of all patients with rheumatoid arthritis, particularly those with subcutaneous nodules. However, only a small fraction of these patients have clinical evidence of pericarditis, which usually follows a benign course but occasionally may progress to cardiac tamponade or constrictive pericarditis. The pericardial fluid is generally an exudate, with decreased concentrations of complement and glucose and elevated cholesterol. Coronary arteritis with intimal inflammation and edema is present in about 20% of cases but only rarely results in angina pectoris or myocardial infarction. The cardiac valves, most often the mitral and aortic, may be involved by inflammation and granuloma formation that in some cases may cause clinically significant regurgitation due to valve deformity. Myocarditis rarely results in cardiac dysfunction.

Treatment is directed at the underlying rheumatoid arthritis and may include glucocorticoids. Pericardiectomy is usually required in cases of tamponade or persistent effusion.

Seronegative Arthropathies   The seronegative arthropathies (Chaps. 315 and 324), ankylosing spondylitis, Reiter's syndrome, psoriatic arthritis, and the arthritides associated with ulcerative colitis and regional enteritis may be accompanied by a pancarditis and proximal aortitis; the latter may result in aortic regurgitation and may extend into the anterior mitral valve ring and/or AV node. Conduction disturbances are common, occurring in up to one-third of patients; they are more common in patients with aortic valve disease and appear to be associated with the presence of the HLA-B27 antigen. Both aortic regurgitation and AV block are more common in patients with peripheral joint involvement and long-standing disease; treatment with aortic valve replacement and permanent pacemaker placement may be required. Up to one-fifth of patients with peripheral joint involvement and disease for more than 30 years have significant aortic regurgitation. Occasionally, aortic regurgitation precedes the onset of arthritis, and, therefore, the diagnosis of a seronegative arthritis should be considered in young males with isolated aortic regurgitation.

Systemic Lupus Erythematosus (SLE) (See also Chap. 311)   Pericarditis is common, occurring in about two-thirds of patients, and generally pursues a benign course, although rarely tamponade or constriction may result. The characteristic *endocardial lesions* of SLE, described by Libman and Sacks, consist of wartlike lesions most often located at the angles of the AV valves or on the ventricular surface of the mitral valve. Hemodynamically important valvular regurgitation is rare. Patients with the antiphospholipid syndrome have a higher incidence of cardiovascular abnormalities, including valvular disease (particularly regurgitant lesions), a variety of thrombotic disorders (venous and arterial thrombosis, thrombocytopenia, premature stroke), myocardial infarction, pulmonary hypertension, and cardiomyopathy. Myocarditis generally parallels the activity of the disease, and although common histologically, seldom results in clinical heart failure unless associated with hypertension. Although arteritis of large coronary arteries may rarely result in myocardial ischemia, there is also an increased frequency of coronary atherosclerosis that may be related to hypertension or glucocorticoid therapy.

TRAUMATIC HEART DISEASE

Cardiac damage may be due to either penetrating or nonpenetrating injuries. The most frequent cause of a *nonpenetrating injury* is the impact of the chest against the steering wheel of an automobile. The absence of external signs of thoracic trauma does not exclude serious injury of the heart. Although the commonest injury is myocardial contusion, any structure of the heart may be affected by the trauma.

Myocardial contusions are often not immediately recognized in trauma patients due to focus on more obvious injuries. Myocardial contusion may cause arrhythmias, bundle branch block, or electrocardiographic abnormalities resembling those of infarction or pericarditis, and so it is important to bear trauma in mind as a cause of otherwise unexplained electrocardiographic changes. Serum creatine kinase (CK) MB isoenzyme levels are increased in about 20% of patients, but false-positive elevations of MB may occur in the presence of massive injuries associated with large increases in total CK. Cardiac troponin levels may have a greater diagnostic value than CK-MB. Echocardiography can detect abnormal wall motion and the presence of pericardial effusion, in addition to aiding in diagnosis of other forms of cardiac trauma. Myocardial contusion may produce positive radionuclide scans and regional impairment of ventricular function, as occurs in myocardial infarction (Chap. 243). Pericardial effusion may occur weeks or even months after the accident. In these cases, the pericardial effusion is a manifestation of the postcardiac injury syndrome, which resembles the postpericardiotomy syndrome (Chap. 239).

Rupture of the heart valves or the supporting structures leads to acute valvular incompetence. The presence of a loud heart murmur followed by the development of rapidly progressive heart failure after trauma heralds this diagnosis, which can be made by either transthoracic or transesophageal echocardiography.

The most serious consequence of nonpenetrating injury is myocardial rupture, leading to tamponade or intracardiac shunting. Although it is generally immediately fatal, up to 40 percent of patients with cardiac rupture have been reported to survive long enough to reach a specialized trauma center. Hemopericardium may also follow tearing of a pericardial vessel or coronary artery.

Rupture of the aorta is a common consequence of nonpenetrating chest trauma. Indeed, rupture of the aorta at the isthmus or just above the aortic valve is the most common vascular deceleration injury. The clinical presentation is similar to that in aortic dissection (Chap. 247). The arterial pressure and pulse amplitude may be increased in the upper extremities and decreased in the lower extremities, and on chest roentgenogram there may be widening of the mediastinum. Occasionally, aortic rupture is limited by the aortic adventitia and results in a silent false aneurysm that may be discovered months or years after the injury.

Penetrating injuries of the heart, produced by bullets or stab wounds, usually result in immediate or very rapid death because of hemopericardium or massive hemorrhage. However, up to half of such patients may survive if they are resuscitated and/or survive long enough to reach a specialized trauma center. Perforation complicating the placement of an intravenous intracardiac catheter or pacemaker lead is another common cause of penetrating injuries to the heart and great vessels.

When great vessel rupture is due to a penetrating injury, there is usually a hemothorax and, less often, a hemopericardium. Hematoma formation may compress major vessels, and arteriovenous fistulae may form, sometimes resulting in high-output congestive heart failure.

Patients who suffer penetrating injuries of the heart should be carefully examined several weeks after the event to rule out a ventricular septal defect or mitral regurgitation that may have gone undetected at the time of emergency surgery. Sometimes the patient survives the acute incident and presents with a cardiac murmur and congestive heart failure. A left-to-right shunt due to traumatic ventricular septal defect, aortopulmonary artery fistula, or coronary arteriovenous fistula may be suspected and confirmed by cardiac catheterization and angiocardiography.

Rx **TREATMENT** The treatment of an uncomplicated myocardial contusion, with or without myocardial infarction, is similar to that for a myocardial infarction, except that anticoagulation is contraindicated, and should include monitoring for the development of complications such as arrhythmia and cardiac rupture (Chap. 243). Acute myocardial failure resulting from the rupture of a valve usually requires operative correction. Immediate thoracotomy should be carried out for most cases of penetrating injury or if there is evidence of cardiac tamponade and/or shock regardless of the type of trauma. Pericardiocentesis may be helpful in patients with tamponade, but usually only as holding maneuver on the way to the operating room. Pericardial hemorrhage often leads to constriction, which must be treated by decortication.

BIBLIOGRAPHY

COLUCCI WS et al: Primary tumors of the heart, in *Heart Disease*, 6th ed, E Braunwald et al (eds). Philadelphia, Saunders, 2001

DUFLOU J et al: Sudden cardiac death as a result of heart disease in morbid obesity. Am Heart J 130:306, 1996

HOFFMAN : Rheumatic diseases and the heart, in *Heart Disease*, 6th ed, E Braunwald et al (eds). Philadelphia, Saunders, 2001

KLEIN I: Thyroid hormone and the cardiovascular system. Am J Med 88:631, 1990

KLUKE MH, MAYER RJ: Carcinoid tumors. N Engl J Med 340:858, 1999

MATTOX : Traumatic heart disease, in *Heart Disease*, 6th ed, E Braunwald et al (eds). Philadelphia, Saunders, 2001

MCALLISTER HA Jr et al: Tumors of the heart and pericardium. Curr Probl Cardiol 24: 57, 1999

NATAN DM: Long-term complications of diabetes mellitus. N Engl J Med 328:1676, 1993

O'NEILL TW et al: The heart in ankylosing spondylitis. Ann Rheum Dis 51:705, 1992

PRETRE R, CHILCOTT M: Blunt trauma to the heart and great vessels. N Engl J Med. 336: 626, 1997

REYMON K: Cardiac myxomas. N Engl J Med 333:1610, 1995

RHEE PM et al: Penetrating cardiac injuries: a population-based study. J Trauma 45:366, 1998

ROBERTS WC: A unique heart disease associated with a unique cancer: carcinoid heart disease. Am J Cardiol 80:251, 1997

———, HIGH ST: The heart in systemic lupus erythematosus. Curr Probl Cardiol 24:1, 1999

SHIMON I et al: Improved left ventricular function after thiamine supplementation in patients with congestive heart failure receiving long-term furosemide therapy. Am J Med 98:485, 1995

SOWERS JR: Diabetes mellitus and cardiovascular disease in women. Arch Intern Med 158:617, 1998

WELCH GN, LOSCALZO J: Homocysteine and atherothrombosis. N Engl J Med 338:1042, 1998

Section 4
VASCULAR DISEASE

---

241 *Peter Libby*

THE PATHOGENESIS OF ATHEROSCLEROSIS

HDL	high-density lipoproteins	PAI	plasminogen-activator inhibitor
ICAM	intercellular adhesion	PDGF	platelet-derived growth factors
	molecule	TGF	transforming growth
IFN	interferon		factor
IL	interleukin	TNF	tumor necrosis factor
LDL	low-density lipoprotein	VCAM	vascular cell adhesion
Lp(a)	lipoprotein		molecule

Atherosclerosis is the leading cause of death and disability in the developed world. Despite our familiarity with this disease, some of its fundamental characteristics remain poorly recognized and understood. Although many generalized or systemic risk factors predispose to its development, atherosclerosis affects various regions of the circulation preferentially and yields distinct clinical manifestations depending on the particular circulatory bed affected. Atherosclerosis of the coronary arteries commonly causes myocardial infarction (Chap. 243) and angina pectoris (Chap. 244). Atherosclerosis of the arteries supplying the central nervous system frequently provokes strokes and transient cerebral ischemia (Chap. 361). In the peripheral circulation, atherosclerosis causes intermittent claudication and gangrene and can jeopardize limb viability (Chap. 248). Involvement of the splanchnic circulation can cause mesenteric ischemia. Atherosclerosis can affect the kidneys either directly (e.g., renal artery stenosis) or as a frequent site of atheroembolic disease (Chap. 278).

Even within a given arterial bed, atherosclerosis tends to occur focally, typically in certain predisposed regions. In the coronary circulation, for example, the proximal left anterior descending coronary artery exhibits a particular predilection for developing atherosclerotic occlusive disease. Likewise, atherosclerosis preferentially affects the proximal portions of the renal arteries and, in the extracranial circulation to the brain, the carotid bifurcation. Indeed, atherosclerotic lesions often form at branching points of arteries, regions of disturbed blood flow. Not all manifestations of atherosclerosis result from stenotic, occlusive disease. Ectasia and development of aneurysmal disease, for example, frequently occur in the aorta (Chap. 247). The mechanisms that underlie this discontinuous anatomic distribution of atherosclerosis remain uncertain.

Legend:
- Endothelial cells
- Smooth muscle cells
- Proteoglycan
- Lipoprotein particles
- Leukocytes adhesion molecules
- Monocytes
- T-lymphocyte

FIGURE 241-1 *A.* The normal artery. The normal artery consists of three layers. The intima, lined by a monolayer of endothelial cells in contact with the blood, contains resident smooth-muscle cells embedded in extracellular matrix. The internal elastic lamina forms the border of the intima with the underlying tunica media. The media contains layers of smooth-muscle cells

Atherosclerosis manifests itself focally not only in space, as just described, but in time as well. Atherogenesis in humans typically occurs over a period of many years, usually many decades. Growth of atherosclerotic plaques probably does not occur in a smooth linear fashion, but rather discontinuously, with periods of relative quiescence punctuated by periods of rapid evolution. After a generally prolonged "silent" period, atherosclerosis may become clinically manifest. The clinical expressions of atherosclerosis may be chronic, as in the development of stable, effort-induced angina pectoris or of predictable and reproducible intermittent claudication. Alternatively, a much more dramatic acute clinical event, such as myocardial infarction, a cerebrovascular accident, or sudden cardiac death, may first herald the presence of atherosclerosis. Other individuals may never experience clinical manifestations of arterial disease despite the presence of widespread atherosclerosis demonstrated post mortem.

INITIATION OF ATHEROSCLEROSIS   Lipoprotein Accumulation and Modification • *Fatty streak formation* An integrated view of experimental results in animals and study of human atherosclerosis suggests that the "fatty streak" represents the initial lesion of atherosclerosis (Fig. 241-1). The formation of these early lesions of atherosclerosis most often seems to arise from focal increases in the content of lipoproteins within regions of the intima (Fig. 241-1*B*). This accumulation of lipoprotein particles may not result simply from an increased permeability, or "leakiness," of the overlying endothelium. Rather, these lipoproteins may collect in the intima of arteries because they bind to constituents of the extracellular matrix, increasing the residence time of the lipid-rich particles within the arterial wall. Lipoproteins that accumulate in the extracellular space of the intima of arteries often associate with proteoglycan molecules of

FIGURE 241-1—*(continued)*

invested with a collagen- and elastin-rich extracellular matrix. Elastic arteries such as the aorta contain concentric lamellae of smooth-muscle cells sandwiched between dense bands of elastin. Muscular arteries have a looser organization of smooth-muscle cells dispersed within the matrix. The external elastic lamina forms the border of the media with the adventitia. The adventitia contains nerves and some mast cells and is the origin of the vasa vasorum, which supply blood to the outer two-thirds of the tunica media.

B. Accumulation of lipoprotein particles. Lipoprotein particles can accumulate in the intima of arteries, particularly when the ambient concentration is increased by hypercholesterolemic states. The lipoprotein particles often associate with constituents of the extracellular matrix, notably proteoglycans. Sequestration within the intima separates lipoproteins from some plasma antioxidants and can favor oxidative modification. Such modified lipoprotein particles may trigger a local inflammatory response responsible for signaling subsequent steps in lesion formation.

C. Adhesion of leukocytes. In hypercholesterolemia, adhesion of mononuclear leukocytes to the luminal endothelial occurs early. The augmented expression of various adhesion molecules for leukocytes probably triggers this first step in the recruitment of white blood cells to the site of a nascent arterial lesion.

D. Penetration of leukocytes. Once adherent, some white blood cells will migrate into the intima. The directed migration of leukocytes probably depends on chemoattractant factors including modified lipoprotein particles themselves and chemoattractant cytokines such as the chemokine macrophage chemoattractant protein 1 produced by vascular wall cells in response to modified lipoproteins.

E. Accumulation of leukocytes. Leukocytes resident in the evolving fatty streak can divide and exhibit augmented expression of receptors for modified lipoproteins (scavenger receptors). These mononuclear phagocytes imbibe lipids and transform into foam cells whose cytoplasm is filled with lipid droplets.

F. Formation of the fibrous cap and lipid core. As the fatty streak evolves into a more complicated atherosclerotic lesion, smooth-muscle cells accumulate within the expanding intima and the amount of extracellular matrix increases. The fibrous cap, formed of extracellular matrix elaborated by the smooth-muscle cells in the intima, characteristically overlies a lipid core filled with macrophages. In addition to dividing, these cells in the lipid core can die, releasing their lipid contents into the extracellular space.

the arterial extracellular matrix. At sites of lesion formation, the balance of different matrix constituents may vary in important ways. Of the three major classes of proteoglycans, for example, a relative excess of heparan sulfate molecules in relation to keratan sulfate or chondritin sulfate may promote the retention of lipoprotein particles by binding them and slowing their egress from nascent lesions.

Lipoprotein particles in the extracellular space of the intima, particularly those bound to matrix macromolecules, may undergo chemical modifications. Accumulating evidence supports a pathogenic role for such modifications of lipoproteins in atherogenesis. Two types of such alterations in lipoproteins bear particular interest in the context of understanding how risk factors actually promote atherogenesis: oxidation and nonenzymatic glycation.

Lipoprotein oxidation Lipoproteins sequestered from plasma antioxidants in the extracellular space of the intima may be particularly susceptible to oxidative modification. Oxidatively modified low-density lipoprotein (LDL), rather than being a defined homogenous entity, actually comprises a variable and incompletely defined mixture. Both the lipid and protein moieties of these particles can participate in oxidative modification. Modifications of the lipids may include formation of hydroperoxides, lysophospholipids, oxysterols, and aldehydic breakdown products of fatty acids. Recently recognized phospholipid oxidation products include palmitoyl-oxovaleroyl-glycero-phosphoryl choline (POVPC), palmitoyl-glutarolyl-glycero-phosphoryl choline (PGPC), and epoxyisoprostane E$_2$-glycero-phosphocholine (PEIPC). Modifications of the apoprotein moieties may include breaks in the peptide backbone as well as derivatization of certain amino acid residues. The side chain amino group of lysine may condense with components of the oxidized lipids (4-hydroxynonenol, or malondialdehyde). A more recently recognized modification may result from local hypochlorous acid production by inflammatory cells within the plaque, giving rise to chlorinated species such as chlorotyrosyl moieties. Ongoing work is characterizing specific chemical constituents of oxidized lipoproteins responsible for various biologic effects. Examples include oxovaleryl-phosphoryl choline. Considerable evidence supports the presence of such chemical entities in atherosclerotic lesions.

Nonenzymatic glycation In diabetic patients with sustained hyperglycemia, nonenzymatic glycation of apolipoproteins and other arterial proteins likely occurs that may likewise alter their function and propensity to accelerate atherogenesis. A good deal of experimental work suggests that both oxidatively modified and glycated lipoproteins or their constituents can contribute to many of the subsequent cellular events of lesion development.

Leukocyte Recruitment After the accumulation of extracellular lipid, recruitment of leukocytes occurs as a second step in formation of the fatty streak (Fig. 241-1C). The white blood cell types typically found in the evolving atheroma include primarily cells of the mononuclear lineage: monocytes and lymphocytes. A number of adhesion molecules or receptors for leukocytes expressed on the surface of the arterial endothelial cell likely participate in the recruitment of leukocytes to the nascent fatty streak. Adhesion molecules of particular interest include vascular cell adhesion molecule (VCAM) 1 and intercellular adhesion molecule (ICAM) 1 (members of the immunoglobulin gene superfamily) and P-selectin (a member of a distinct family of leukocyte receptors known as selectins). Lysophosphatidylcholine, a constituent of oxidatively modified LDL, can augment expression of VCAM-1. This example illustrates how the accumulation of lipoproteins in the arterial intima may link mechanistically with leukocyte recruitment and subsequent events in lesion formation.

Laminar shear forces, such as those encountered in most regions of normal arteries, can also suppress the expression of leukocyte adhesion molecules such as VCAM-1. Sites of predilection for forming atherosclerotic lesions (e.g., branch points) often have disturbed laminar flow. Ordered laminar shear of normal blood flow augments the production of nitric oxide by endothelial cells. This molecule, in addition to its vasodilator properties, can act at the low levels constitutively produced by arterial endothelium as a local anti-inflammatory autacoid, for example, limiting local VCAM-1 expression. These examples indicate how hemodynamic forces may influence the cellular events that underlie atherosclerotic lesion initiation and illustrate a potential explanation for the focal distribution of atherosclerotic lesions at certain sites predetermined by altered flow patterns.

Once adherent to the surface of the arterial endothelial cell via interaction with a receptor such as VCAM-1, the monocytes and lymphocytes penetrate the endothelial layer and take up residence in the intima (Fig. 241-1D). In addition to products of modified lipoproteins, cytokines (a class of protein mediators of inflammation) can regulate the expression of adhesion molecules involved in leukocyte recruitment. For example, the cytokines interleukin (IL) 1 or tumor necrosis factor (TNF) α induce or augment the expression of VCAM-1 and ICAM-1 on endothelial cells. Because modified lipoproteins can induce cytokine release from vascular wall cells, this pathway may provide an additional link between accumulation and modification of lipoproteins and leukocyte recruitment. The directed migration of leukocytes into the arterial wall may also result from the actions of modified lipoprotein. For example, oxidized LDL may promote the chemotaxis of leukocytes. Also, oxidatively modified lipoproteins can elicit the production by vascular wall cells of chemoattractant cytokines such as monocyte chemoattractant protein 1.

Foam-cell formation Once resident within the intima, the mononuclear phagocytes differentiate into macrophages and transform into lipid-laden foam cells. Transformation of mononuclear phagocytes into foam cells requires the uptake of lipoprotein particles by receptor-mediated endocytosis. One might suppose that the well-known recognized receptor for LDL mediates this lipid uptake. Patients or animals lacking effective LDL receptors due to genetic alterations (e.g., familial hypercholesterolemia), however, have abundant arterial le-

sions and extraarterial xanthomata rich in macrophage-derived foam-cells. Also, the exogenous cholesterol suppresses expression of the LDL receptor, such that under hypercholesterolemic conditions the level of this cell-surface receptor for LDL decreases. Candidates for alternative receptors that can mediate lipid-loading of foam cells include a growing number of macrophage "scavenger" receptors, which preferentially endocytose modified lipoproteins, and other receptors for oxidized LDL or β-VLDL (very low density lipoprotein), a type of lipoprotein commonly encountered in certain hypercholesterolemic states (Chap. 344). By imbibing lipids from the extracellular space, the mononuclear phagocytes bearing such scavenger receptors may remove lipoproteins from the developing lesion. Some lipid-loaded macrophages may leave the artery wall, functioning to clear lipid from the artery. Lipid accumulation, and hence propensity to form atheroma, ensues if the amount of lipid entering the artery wall exceeds that exported by mononuclear phagocytes or other pathways. Macrophages may thus play a vital role in the dynamic economy of lipid accumulation in the arterial wall during atherogenesis. Some lipid-laden foam cells within the expanding intimal lesion perish. Some of the death of foam cells may result from a program of cell death known as *apoptosis*. This death of mononuclear phagocytes results in formation of the lipid-rich center of more complicated atherosclerotic plaques, often called the *necrotic core* of the lesion.

Macrophages taking up modified lipoproteins, much like intrinsic vascular wall cells, may elaborate cytokines and growth factors that can further signal some of the cellular events in lesion complication. A number of growth factors or cytokines elaborated by mononuclear phagocytes can stimulate smooth-muscle cell proliferation and production of extracellular matrix, which accumulates in atherosclerotic plaques. IL-1 and TNF-α are examples of cytokines that can induce local production of growth factors such as forms of platelet-derived growth factor, fibroblast growth factor, and others that may play a role in plaque evolution and complication. Other cytokines, notably interferon (IFN) γ derived from activated T cells within lesions, can inhibit smooth-muscle proliferation and synthesis of interstitial forms of collagen. These examples illustrate how atherogenesis likely depends on a complex balance between mediators that can promote lesion formation and other pathways that can mitigate the atherogenic process.

Factors That Modulate Inhibition of Atheroma Elaboration of small molecules by activated mononuclear phagocytes and vascular wall cells in the evolving lesion may also modulate atherogenesis. Notably, reactive oxygen species can modulate growth of smooth-muscle cells, activate inflammatory gene expression via the nuclear factor kappa B (NFκB) transcriptional control system, and annihilate NO radicals, decreasing the effect of this endogenous vasodilator. However, the macrophage in the lesion may be activated to express the inducible form of the enzyme that can synthesize NO, known as inducible NO synthase. This high-capacity form of the enzyme can produce relatively large, potentially cytotoxic amounts of NO radicals. While at low concentrations of ·NO produced by the constitutive NO synthase in endothelial cells, this radical may produce beneficial effects; when overproduced by activated phagocytes, it may prove deleterious.

Export by phagocytes may constitute one response to local lipid overload in the evolving lesion. Another mechanism, reverse cholesterol transport mediated by high-density lipoproteins (HDL), may provide an independent pathway for lipid removal from atheroma. Multiple observational studies have established a tight inverse relationship between the level of HDL cholesterol and the risk for coronary events. Increased HDL may explain why premenopausal women have less atherosclerosis than age-matched men. In various in vitro models, HDL can mediate net cholesterol removal from lipid-laden macrophages. This process likely involves a family of scavenger receptors (the "B" family), highly expressed by steroidogenic tissues and by cells within atheroma as well. Such "reverse cholesterol transport" may also pertain during human atherogenesis and help to explain HDL's protective effect on lesion formation.

Although clear evidence supports lipoprotein disorders as predisposing factors for atheroma formation, other etiologies may contribute to or modulate atherogenesis (Table 242-1). For example, hypertension constitutes an independent risk factor for coronary events. Male gender and the postmenopausal state also augment the risk of developing coronary artery disease. Premenopausal women have increased HDL levels compared to age-matched men. However, a favorable lipoprotein pattern only partially accounts for the protection against atherosclerosis conferred by the premenopausal state. Thus, as yet poorly understood direct effects of estrogens on the arterial wall may account for some of this benefit. Studies in progress are investigating possible mechanisms of estrogen's possible "vasculoprotective" effect and the role of estrogen replacement therapy as an antiatherogenic strategy in postmenopausal women.

Diabetes mellitus accelerates atherogenesis. In addition to the well-known microvascular complications of diabetes (Chap. 333), macrovascular disease such as atherosclerosis causes a great deal of excess mortality in the diabetic populations. Diabetes-associated dyslipidemias strongly promote atherogenesis. In particular, the constellation of insulin resistance, high triglycerides, and low HDL, often in association with central adiposity and hypertension frequent in type 2 diabetic patients, seems to accelerate atherogenesis potently. As noted above, hyperglycemia may promote the nonenzymatic glycation of LDL. LDL modified in this manner, like oxidatively modified LDL, may signal many of the initial events in atherogenesis. Other lipoproteins such as triglyceride-rich particles or lipoprotein (a) [Lp(a)] may also prove particularly atherogenic.

Lp(a) (often pronounced "lipoprotein little a" to distinguish it from apolipoprotein AI and others found in HDL) provides a potential link between hemostasis and blood lipids. The Lp(a) particle consists of an apoprotein (a) molecule bound by a sulfhydryl link to the apolipoprotein B moiety of a LDL particle. Apoprotein (a) has homology with plasminogen and may inhibit fibrinolysis by competing with plasminogen. Other risk factors for atherosclerosis related to blood clotting include elevated levels of fibrinogen or of the inhibitor of fibrinolysis, plasminogen-activator inhibitor (PAI) 1. Another nonlipid risk factor for coronary events, elevated levels of *homocysteine*, may act by promoting thrombosis, although the pathophysiology of this association is uncertain at present.

The relationship between *tobacco use* and atherosclerosis also remains poorly understood (Chap. 390). The rapid reduction in risk for cardiac events after cessation of cigarette smoking implies that tobacco may promote thrombosis or some other determinant of plaque stability as well as evolution of the atherosclerotic lesion itself. For example, tobacco smokers have elevated fibrinogen levels, a variable associated with increased atherosclerosis and acute cardiovascular events.

In other situations, antecedent inflammatory states may predispose towards atherosclerosis. For example, *Kawasaki disease* in childhood may promote development of vascular lesions in the arteries of adults (Chap. 317). Infectious agents continue to be proposed as instigators or potentiators of atherogenesis. Both viral and microbial pathogens have been invoked in this context (e.g., Herpesviridae, including cytomegalovirus, or *Chlamydia*). In some patients, immune or autoimmune reactions may contribute to atherogenesis. In the particular example of the accelerated form of coronary arteriopathy that plagues heart transplant recipients, immunologic factors may contribute importantly to the pathogenesis. The roles of the immune response and of infectious diseases in usual atherosclerosis remain speculative.

Known genetic defects in lipoprotein metabolism account for only a fraction of the familial risk for coronary artery disease. Thus, other as yet undefined genetic factors must contribute to coronary risk. Mechanisms of disease susceptibility involving the arterial wall might account for some of the genetic predisposition to atherosclerosis unexplained by lipoprotein disorders. Application of molecular genetic techniques should help identify new polymorphisms linked to coronary risk and may eventually shed light on new pathophysiologic mechanisms. For example, some data suggest a link between certain alleles of the genes encoding angiotensin-converting enzyme or PAI-1 with increased risk of myocardial infarction. Large studies currently in progress should clarify these and other potential markers of genetic susceptibility to atherosclerosis.

ATHEROMA EVOLUTION AND COMPLICATION Involvement of Arterial Smooth-Muscle Cells Although the fatty streak commonly precedes the development of a more advanced atherosclerotic plaque, not all fatty streaks progress to yield atheroma. Fatty streaks occur in populations not prone to develop late lesions (e.g., indigenous Africans). These findings raise several questions. Why do some fatty streaks progress to fibrous lesions but not others? By what mechanisms do fatty streaks evolve into more complex lesions? While accumulation of lipid-laden macrophages is the hallmark of the fatty streaks, accumulation of fibrous tissue typifies the more advanced atherosclerotic lesion. The smooth-muscle cell synthesizes the bulk of the extracellular matrix of the complex atherosclerotic lesion. Hence, arrival of smooth-muscle cells and their elaboration of extracellular matrix probably provides a critical transition, yielding a fibrofatty lesion in place of a simple accumulation of macrophage-derived foam cells.

Recent research has provided insight into the mechanisms that may trigger migration and proliferation of smooth-muscle cells into and within the evolving intimal lesion and signal the accumulation of extracellular matrix. Cytokines and growth factors elicited by modified lipoproteins or other agents from both vascular wall cells and infiltrating leukocytes can modulate functions of the smooth-muscle cell. For example, platelet-derived growth factors (PDGF) elaborated by activated endothelial cells can stimulate the migration of smooth-muscle cells. In this manner, smooth-muscle cells resident in the tunica media may migrate into the intima. Various growth factors produced locally can stimulate the proliferation of both resident smooth-muscle cells in the intima and those that have migrated from the media. Transforming growth factor (TGF) β, among other mediators, potently stimulates interstitial collagen production by smooth-muscle cells. These mediators may arise not only from neighboring vascular cells or leukocytes (a "paracrine" pathway) but in some instances from the same cell that responds to the factor (an "autocrine" pathway). Together, these alterations in smooth-muscle cells, signaled by these mediators acting at short distances, can hasten transformation of the fatty streak into a more fibrous smooth-muscle cell and extracellular matrix–rich lesion.

In addition to locally produced mediators, atherogenic risk factor signals related to blood coagulation and thrombosis likely contribute to atheroma evolution and complication. Current evidence suggests that fatty streak formation begins without frank denuding endothelial injury or desquamation. In advanced fatty streaks, however, microscopic breaches in endothelial integrity may occur. Microthrombi rich in platelets can form at such sites of limited endothelial denudation, due to exposure of the highly thrombogenic extracellular matrix of underlying basement membrane. Activated platelets release numerous factors that can promote the fibrotic response. In addition to PDGF and TGF-β, low-molecular-weight mediators such as serotonin can also alter smooth-muscle function. Most of these microthrombi probably resolve without clinical manifestation by a process of local fibrinolysis, resorption, and endothelial repair.

As atherosclerotic lesions advance, abundant plexi of microvessels develop in connection with the artery's vasa vasorum. These newly developing microvascular networks may contribute to lesion complication in several ways. These blood vessels provide an abundant surface area for leukocyte trafficking and may serve as the portal of entry and exit of white blood cells from the established atheroma. The plaques' microvessels may also furnish foci for intraplaque hemorrhage. Like the neovessels in the diabetic retina, microvessels of the plaque may be friable and prone to rupture and produce focal hemorrhage. Such a vascular leak leads to thrombosis in situ and thrombin

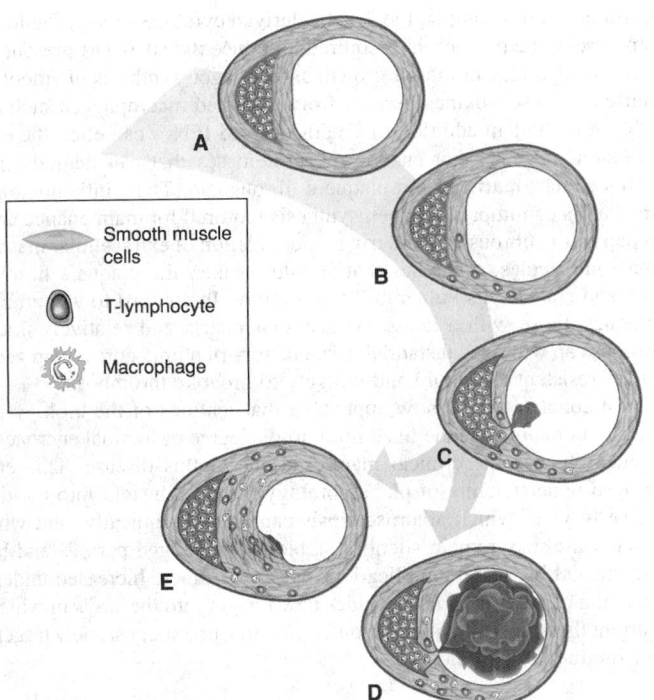

FIGURE 241-2 Plaque rupture, thrombosis, and healing. *A.* Arterial remodeling during atherogenesis. During the initial part of the life history of an atheroma, growth is often outward, preserving the caliber of lumen. This phenomenon of "compensatory enlargement" accounts in part for the tendency of coronary arteriography to underestimate the degree of atherosclerosis.

B. Focal inflammation characterizes unstable atherosclerotic plaques. Foci of inflammation often occur in atheroma. Analysis of lesions that have ruptured and caused fatal myocardial infarction characteristically show a prominent infiltration of macrophages and T lymphocytes. Both the leukocytes and the intrinsic vascular cells around points of plaque rupture show markers of inflammatory activation.

C. Rupture of the plaque's fibrous cap causes thrombosis. Physical disruption of the atherosclerotic plaque commonly causes arterial thrombosis by allowing blood coagulant factors to contact thrombogenic collagen found in the

generation from prothrombin. In addition to its role in blood coagulation, thrombin can modulate many aspects of vascular cell function including stimulation of proliferation and cytokine release from smooth-muscle cells and production of growth factors such as PDGF from endothelial cells. Atherosclerotic plaques often contain fibrin and hemosiderin, indicating episodes of intraplaque hemorrhage as an element in plaque complication.

As they advance, atherosclerotic plaques also accumulate calcium. Proteins specialized in binding of calcium usually associated with bone also occur in atherosclerotic lesions. For example, osteocalcin, osteopontin, and bone morphogenetic proteins localize in atherosclerotic plaques. In fact, complication of the atherosclerotic plaque recapitulates many aspects of bone formation.

Traditionally, atherosclerosis research has focused much attention on proliferation of smooth-muscle cells, yet these cells actually replicate rather slowly in complicated atherosclerotic lesions. Estimates of the rate of smooth-muscle cell division at a given time point in such lesions show replicative rate below 1%. Such observations do not exclude bursts of proliferative activity at certain junctures in the history of an atheroma, perhaps in association with local thrombin generation due to microvascular hemorrhage or formation of a microthrombus at a site of localized endothelial denudation, as discussed above. On the other hand, cell death has been recognized as a component of atherogenesis since the time of Virchow in the mid-nineteenth century. Indeed, complex atheroma often have a primarily fibrous character lacking the hypercellular appearance of less advanced lesions and actually exhibiting a paucity of smooth-muscle cells. This relative lack

FIGURE 241-2—(*continued*)

arterial extracellular matrix and tissue factor produced by macrophage-derived foam cells in the lipid core of lesions. In this manner, sites of plaque rupture form the nidus for thrombi. The normal artery wall possesses several fibrinolytic or antithrombotic mechanisms that tend to resist thrombosis and lyse clots that begin to form in situ. Such antithrombotic or thrombolytic molecules include thrombomodulin tissue and urokinase-type plasminogen activators, heparan sulfate proteoglycans, prostacyclin, and nitric oxide. When the clot overwhelms the endogenous fibrinolytic mechanisms, it may propagate and lead to arterial occlusion (*E*). In some cases, the thrombus may lyse or organize into a mural thrombus without occluding the vessel. Such instances may be clinically silent. The subsequent thrombin-induced fibrosis and healing causes a fibroproliferative response that can lead to a more fibrous lesion, one that can produce an eccentric plaque that causes a hemodynamically significant stenosis (*D*).

D. Healing of a mural thrombus leads to lesion fibrosis and progression and luminal narrowing. Local thrombin activation can stimulate smooth-muscle proliferation. Proteins released from platelets including platelet-derived growth factors and transforming growth factor β may also augment collagen production by smooth-muscle cells and modulate their growth. In this way, a nonocclusive mural thrombus, even if clinically silent or causing unstable angina rather than infarction, can provoke a healing response that can promote lesion fibrosis and luminal encroachment. Such a sequence of events may convert a "vulnerable" atheroma with a thin fibrous cap prone to rupture into a more "stable" fibrous plaque with a reinforced cap. Angioplasty of unstable coronary lesions may "stabilize" the lesions by a similar mechanism, producing a wound followed by healing.

E. Plaque rupture with a propagated, occlusive thrombus can cause acute myocardial infarction. When a stable, occlusive thrombus forms in a coronary artery, the consequences depend on the degree of existing collateral vessels. In a patient with chronic multivessel, occlusive coronary artery disease, collateral channels have usually formed. In such circumstances, even a total arterial occlusion may not lead to myocardial infarction, or may produce an unexpectedly modest or a non-Q-wave infarct because of collateral flow. In the patient with less advanced disease and without substantial stenotic lesions to provide a stimulus to collateral vessel formation, sudden plaque rupture and arterial occlusion commonly produce Q wave infarction. These are the types of patients who may present with myocardial infarction or sudden death as a first manifestation of coronary atherosclerosis.

of smooth-muscle cells in advanced atheroma may result from the ultimate predominance of cytostatic mediators such as TGF-β or IFN-γ, which can inhibit smooth-muscle cell proliferation. Also, smooth-muscle cells as well as macrophages in advanced atherosclerotic lesions can undergo programmed cell death, or apoptosis. Some of the same cytokines that activate atherogenic functions of vascular wall cells can also trigger the program of apoptosis in these cells.

Thus, during the evolution of the atherosclerotic plaque, a complex balance between entry and egress of lipoproteins and leukocytes, cell proliferation and cell death, extracellular matrix production and remodeling, as well as calcification and neovascularization contribute to lesion formation. Multiple and often competing signals trigger these various cellular events. Increasingly, we appreciate links between atherogenic risk factors and the altered behavior of intrinsic vascular wall cells and infiltrating leukocytes that underlie the complex pathogenesis of these lesions.

CLINICAL SYNDROMES OF ATHEROSCLEROSIS

Atherosclerotic lesions occur ubiquitously in western societies. Most atheroma produce no symptoms, and many never cause clinical manifestations. Numerous patients with diffuse atherosclerosis may succumb to unrelated illnesses without ever having experienced a clinically significant manifestation of atherosclerosis. What accounts for this variability in the clinical expression of atherosclerotic disease?

Arterial remodeling during atheroma formation (Fig. 241-2*A*) represents a frequently overlooked but clinically important feature of lesion evolution. During the initial phases of atheroma development, the plaque usually grows outward, in an abluminal direction. Vessels affected by atherogenesis tend to increase in diameter, a phenomenon known as *compensatory enlargement*, a type of vascular remodeling. The growing atheroma does not encroach upon the arterial lumen until the burden of atherosclerotic plaque exceeds approximately 40% of the area encompassed by the internal elastic lamina. Thus, during much of its life history, an atheroma will not cause stenosis that can limit blood flow.

Flow-limiting stenoses commonly form later in the history of the plaque. Many such plaques manifest themselves by stable syndromes such as demand-induced angina pectoris or intermittent claudication in the extremities. In the coronary and other circulations, even occlusion due to atheroma does not invariably lead to infarction. The hypoxic stimulus of repeated bouts of ischemia characteristically induces formation of collateral vessels in the myocardium, mitigating the consequences of an acute occlusion of an epicardial coronary artery. On the other hand, we now appreciate that many lesions that cause acute or unstable atherosclerotic syndromes, particularly in the coronary circulation, may arise from atherosclerotic plaques that do not produce a flow-limiting stenosis. Such lesions may produce only minimal luminal irregularities on traditional angiograms and often do not meet the traditional criteria for "significance" by arteriography. Instability of such nonocclusive stenoses may explain the frequency of myocardial infarction as an initial manifestation of coronary artery disease (in about a third of cases) in patients who report no prior history of angina pectoris, a syndrome usually caused by flow-limiting stenoses.

Pathologic studies afford considerable insight into the microanatomic substrate underlying "instability" of plaques that are not critically stenotic. A superficial erosion of the endothelium or a frank plaque rupture or fissure usually produces the thrombus that causes episodes of unstable angina pectoris or the occlusive and relatively persistent thrombus that causes acute myocardial infarction (Fig. 241-2C). In the case of carotid atheroma, a deeper ulceration that provides a nidus for formation of platelet thrombi may underlie the unstable syndromes that cause transient ischemic attacks.

Rupture of the plaque's fibrous cap (Fig. 241-2C) permits contact of coagulation factors in the blood with highly thrombogenic tissue factor expressed by macrophage foam cells in the plaque's lipid-rich core. If the ensuing thrombus is nonocclusive or transient, the episode of plaque disruption may not cause symptoms or may result in ischemic symptoms such as rest angina. Occlusive thrombi that endure will often cause acute myocardial infarction, particularly in the absence of a well-developed collateral circulation supplying the affected territory. Repetitive episodes of plaque disruption and healing provide one likely mechanism of transition of the fatty streak to a more complex fibrous lesion (Fig. 241-2D). The healing process in arteries, as in skin wounds, involves the laying down of new extracellular matrix and fibrosis.

Not all atheroma exhibit the same propensity to rupture. Studies of the pathology of culprit lesions that have caused acute myocardial infarction reveal several characteristic features. Plaques that have proven vulnerable tend to have thin fibrous caps, relatively large lipid cores, and a high content of macrophages. Morphometric studies of such culprit lesions show that macrophages and T lymphocytes predominate at the site of plaque rupture. On the other hand, sites of plaque rupture contain relatively few smooth-muscle cells. The cells that concentrate at sites of plaque rupture bear markers of inflammatory activation. The presence of the transplantation, or histocompatibility, antigen HLA-DR provides one convenient gauge of the degree of inflammation in cells in atheroma. Resting cells in normal arteries seldom express this transplantation antigen. However, macrophages and smooth-muscle cells at sites of human coronary artery plaque disruption do bear this inducible cell-surface marker. Therefore, the presence of HLA-DR-positive macrophages and T cells indicates an ongoing inflammatory response at sites of plaque rupture.

Inflammatory mediators may actually regulate processes that govern the integrity of the plaque's fibrous cap and hence its propensity

to rupture. For example, the T cell–derived cytokine IFN-γ, found in atherosclerotic plaques and required to induce the HLA-DR present at sites of rupture, can inhibit growth and collagen synthesis of smooth-muscle cells. Cytokines derived from activated macrophages such as TNF-α or IL-1 in addition to T cell–derived IFN-γ can elicit the expression of genes that encode the proteinases that can degrade the extracellular matrix of the plaque's fibrous cap. Thus, inflammatory mediators can impair collagen synthesis required for maintenance and repair of the fibrous cap and trigger degradation of extracellular matrix macromolecules, processes that should weaken the plaque's fibrous cap and enhance its vulnerability to rupture. In contrast to vulnerable plaques, those with a dense extracellular matrix and relatively thick fibrous cap without substantial tissue factor–rich lipid cores seem generally resistant to rupture and unlikely to provoke thrombosis.

In conclusion, we now appreciate that features of the biology of the atheromatous plaque in addition to its degree of luminal encroachment influence the clinical manifestations of this disease. This enhanced understanding of plaque biology provides insight into the diverse ways in which atherosclerosis can present clinically, and why the disease may remain silent or stable for prolonged periods and be punctuated by acute complications at certain times. Increased understanding of atherogenesis provides new insight into the ways in which current therapies may improve outcomes and also suggests new targets for future intervention.

BIBLIOGRAPHY

DAVIES MJ: The composition of coronary-artery plaques. N Engl J Med 336:1312, 1997

FUSTER V et al: Pathogenesis of coronary disease: The biologic role of risk factors. J Am Coll Cardiol 27:964, 1996

LIBBY P: The molecular bases of the acute coronary syndromes. Circulation 91:2844, 1995

LIBBY P: The vascular biology of atherosclerosis, in *Heart Disease*, 6th ed., E Braunwald, D Zipes, P Libby (eds). Philadelphia, Saunders, 2001

ROSS R: Atherosclerosis—an inflammatory disease. N Engl J Med 340:115, 1999

WITZUM JL, BERLINER JA: Oxidized phospholipids and isoprostanes in atherosclerosis. Curr Opin Lipidol 9:441, 1998

---

242   *Peter Libby*

PREVENTION AND TREATMENT OF ATHEROSCLEROSIS

Atherosclerosis remains the major cause of death and premature disability in developed societies. Moreover, current predictions estimate that by the year 2020 cardiovascular diseases, notably atherosclerosis, will become the leading global cause of total disease burden, defined as the years subtracted from healthy life by disability or premature death. Substantial success has been achieved in recent years in reducing morbidity and mortality due to acute coronary events. However, the opportunity for treating the underlying disease process, atherosclerosis, and preventing its acute complications presents an enormous challenge and opportunity at the same time.

THE CONCEPT OF ATHEROSCLEROTIC RISK FACTORS

During the first half of the twentieth century, animal experiments and clinical observation linked certain variables, such as hypercholesterolemia, to the risk of atherosclerotic events. The systematic study of risk factors in humans, however, began approximately mid-century. The prospective, community-based Framingham Heart Study provided rigorous support for the concept that hypercholesterolemia, hypertension, and other factors correlated with cardiovascular risk. Similar observational studies performed in the United States and abroad provided independent support for the concept of "risk factors" for cardiovascular disease. Numerous studies, including the Seven Countries Study per-

Modifiable risk factors	Unmodifiable risk factors
By life-style	Age
Smoking	Male gender
Obesity	Genetics
Physical inactivity	
By pharmacotherapy and or life-style	
Lipid disorders	
Hypertension	
Insulin resistance	

formed by Keys and colleagues, suggested a link between dietary habits and cardiovascular risk based upon population studies.

From a practical viewpoint, it is useful to group the cardiovascular risk factors that have emerged from such studies into two categories: (1) those modifiable by lifestyle and/or pharmacotherapy, and (2) those that are essentially unmodifiable (Table 242-1). The weight of evidence supporting various risk factor differs. For example, hypercholesterolemia and hypertension indubitably predict coronary risk, but other so-called nontraditional risk factors, such as levels of homocysteine, lipoprotein (a) [Lp(a)], or infection, remain controversial. It is worth distinguishing further between factors that actually participate in the pathogenesis of atherosclerosis and those that may merely serve as markers of risk without themselves playing a primary role in pathogenesis. The sections below will consider some of these risk factors and approaches to their modification.

LIPID DISORDERS (See also Chap. 344) Abnormalities in plasma lipoproteins and derangements in lipid metabolism rank as the most firmly established and best understood risk factors for atherosclerosis. Descriptions of the lipoprotein classes, and a detailed explication of lipoprotein metabolism are given in Chap. 344. The mechanisms by which lipoproteins may influence atherogenesis are considered in Chap. 241. Therefore this section will focus on preventive aspects of treatment of lipid disorders.

Current national guidelines recommend cholesterol screening in all adults. The screen should include a fasting lipid profile [total cholesterol, triglycerides, low-density lipoprotein (LDL) cholesterol and high-density lipoprotein (HDL) cholesterol]. Dietary measures, including specific consultation by practitioners with training in nutrition, should be offered to all patients with hyperlipidemia as defined by the National Cholesterol Education Project Adult Treatment Panel II (Table 242-2). A "normal" total cholesterol level should not falsely reassure individuals with additional risk factors for coronary heart disease or when the HDL level is below 1 mmol/L (40 mg/dL). Many patients with established atherosclerosis fall into this category. Such individuals should receive particular encouragement to adopt life-style measures such as diet and exercise aimed at increasing their HDL levels.

The addition of drug therapy to dietary and other nonpharmacologic measures to reduce the risk of atherosclerotic events in asymptomatic patients without manifest vascular disease remains unsettled. In asymptomatic patients with heterozygous familial hypercholesterolemia, LDL lowering by pharmacologic measures reduces atherosclerosis in both men and women. The West of Scotland Study established that lipid lowering with the HMG-CoA inhibitor pravastatin can effectively reduce cardiac events and total mortality in a cohort of patients with hypercholesterolemia but without prior myocardial infarction (Table 242-3). The recent AFCAPS/TexCAPS Study showed that treatment with lovastatin similarly reduced coronary events in patients without previous myocardial infarction but with "average" total and LDL cholesterol levels and somewhat decreased HDL levels.

Although the role of drug therapy in primary prevention of the manifestations of atherosclerosis remains incompletely defined, abundant evidence establishes the benefit of drug therapy in patients with hypercholesterolemia and established coronary artery disease (Table 242-3). A number of well-designed and -executed large-scale clinical trials have now shown that treatment with statins reduces recurrent myocardial infarction, reduces strokes, and lessens the need for revascularization or hospitalization for unstable angina pectoris. These studies have enrolled patients in numerous countries on at least three continents and encompass individuals with clearly elevated levels of cholesterol and those with "average" total and LDL cholesterol levels.

Lipid-lowering therapies do not appear to exert their beneficial effect on cardiovascular events by causing a marked "regression" of obstructive coronary lesions. Angiographically monitored studies of lipid lowering have shown at best a modest reduction in coronary artery stenoses over the duration of study. Yet these same studies consistently show substantial decreases in coronary events. These results suggest that the mechanism of benefit of lipid lowering does not require a substantial reduction in the fixed stenoses. Rather, the benefit may derive from "stabilization" of atherosclerotic lesions without decreased stenosis. Such stabilization of atherosclerotic lesions and the attendant decrease in coronary events may result from the egress of lipids or by favorably influencing aspects of the biology of atherogenesis discussed in Chap. 241. In addition, as sizeable lesions may protrude abluminally rather than into the lumen, shrinkage of such plaques might not be apparent on angiograms.

The benefit of LDL lowering by HMG-CoA reductase inhibitor (statin) therapy on cardiovascular events seems to require 6 to 24 months of treatment. Improvement of vasomotor responses to endothelial-dependent vasodilators occurs much more rapidly, requiring 6 months or less. Thus, HMG-CoA reductase inhibitors may act by two or more mechanisms on the arteries of hypercholesterolemic individuals. The relatively rapid improvement in endothelial-dependent vasomotion may reflect enhanced production or reduced destruction of the endogenous vasodilator nitric oxide at the level of the arterial endothelium. Reduction in the thrombotic complications of atherosclerosis, such as myocardial infarction or unstable angina, probably requires more prolonged treatment to effect removal of lipid from deeper within the atheroma, yielding improvements in the biology underlying plaque destabilization described in Chap. 241.

Our current understanding of the mechanism by which elevated LDL levels promote atherogenesis relates to oxidative modification of these particles within the artery wall, promoting formation of macrophage-derived foam cells and providing a stimulus for inflammation (Chap. 241). These concepts have given rise to considerable interest in the possibility that antioxidants, either dietary or pharmacologic, might reduce atherogenesis. Considerable experimental evidence supports this notion. In addition, many observational studies show a correlation of antioxidant consumption and reduced cardiovascular risk. Rigorous, controlled clinical trial evidence, however, has not yet proven the effectiveness of antioxidant therapy, whether dietary or with supplements of vitamins or drugs, for prevention or treatment of

Table 242-2 Treatment Decisions Based on LDL Cholesterol Level

Patient Category	Initiation Level, mmol/L (mg/dL)		LDL Goal, mmol/L (mg/dL)	
	Dietary Therapy	Drug Treatment	Dietary Therapy	Drug Treatment
Without CHD and with fewer than two risk factors	≥4.1(160)	≥4.9(190)	<4.1(160)	<4.1(160)
Without CHD and with two or more risk factors	≥3.4(130)	≥4.1(160)	<3.4(130)	<3.4(130)
With CHD	>2.6(100)	≥3.4(130)	≤2.6(100)	≤2.6(100)

NOTE: LDL, low-density lipoprotein; CHD, coronary heart disease.
SOURCE: From the guidelines issued by the National Cholesterol Education Project Adult Treatment Panel II: JAMA 269:3025, 1993.

Table 242-3 Selected Clinical Trials of Statin Therapy for Prevention of Coronary or CHD Events

Trial	Previous MI	Lipids	Before lipid lowering, mmol/L (mg/dL)	Decrease in cholesterol, mmol/L(mg/dL)	CHD event reduction, %
WOSCOPS	−	Total cholesterol	7.0(272)	0.52(20)	31
		LDL	5.0(192)	0.67(26)	
AFCAPS/TexCAPS	−	Total cholesterol	5.7(220)	0.47(18)	36
		LDL	4.0(156)	0.65(25)	
4S	+	Total cholesterol	6.7(261)	0.65(25)	34
		LDL	4.9(188)	0.91(35)	
CARE	+	Total cholesterol	5.4(209)	0.52(20)	24
		LDL	3.6(139)	0.72(28)	
LIPID	+	Total cholesterol	5.7(219)	0.47(18)	24
		LDL	3.9(150)	0.65(25)	

NOTE: MI, myocardial infarction; CHD, coronary heart disease; LDL, low-density lipoprotein.
SOURCES: WOSCOPS: J Shepherd et al: West of Scotland Coronary Prevention Study Group. N Engl J Med 333:1301, 1995. AFCAPS/TexCAPS: JR Downs et al: Air Force/Texas Coronary Atherosclerosis Prevention Study. JAMA 279:1615, 1998. 4S: Anonymous: The Scandinavian Simvastin Survival Study. Lancet 344:1383, 1994. CARE: FM Sacks et al: Cholesterol and Recurrent Events Trial (CARE) Investigators. N Engl J Med 335:1001, 1996. LIPID: Anonymous: The Long-Term Intervention with Pravastatin in Ischemic Disease (LIPID) Study Group. N Engl J Med 339:1349, 1998.

atherosclerosis. Indeed, controlled trials with β-carotene have demonstrated no reduction in cardiovascular events. For these reasons, as its efficacy remains speculative, it is premature to consider antioxidant administration as a replacement for established therapies. Furthermore, general use of such treatments, particularly in lower risk individuals, should await the results of rigorous prospective studies designed to define the doses, appropriate patient groups, and evaluate the possibility of adverse or unwanted effects of antioxidants.

HYPERTENSION (See also Chap. 246) The preponderance of epidemiologic data supports a relationship between hypertension and atherosclerotic risk. Clinical trial evidence available since the 1970s established that pharmacologic treatment of hypertension can reduce the risk of stroke and heart failure. However, clinical trial evidence demonstrating reduced risk of coronary events due to antihypertensive therapy has lagged. At present, the combined weight of the evidence supports a reduction in coronary risk by antihypertensive therapy. Some of the difficulty in demonstrating this benefit may derive from the potentially adverse effects of certain classes of antihypertensive drugs on the lipid profile, notably, thiazide diuretics and beta-blocking agents. Indeed, studies of patients with previous myocardial infarction or reduced left ventricular function have shown that treatment with angiotensin-converting enzyme (ACE) inhibitors can reduce the risk of coronary events, an unanticipated outcome. Therefore "lipid-neutral" antihypertensive agents such as ACE inhibitors or α_1-adrenergic blocking agents merit consideration in patients with other risk factors for coronary artery disease or with established atherosclerosis.

DIABETES MELLITUS AND INSULIN RESISTANCE (See also Chap. 333) Most patients with diabetes mellitus die of atherosclerosis and its complications. Secular trends towards aging of the population and increased girth will make type 2 (noninsulin-dependent) diabetes mellitus an increasing public health problem in the coming years. The criteria for diagnosis of diabetes have recently undergone revision. Currently, a fasting plasma glucose level of 6.9 mmol/L (125 mg/dL) establishes the diagnosis of diabetes. In the intermediate range, plasma glucose levels between 6.1 and 6.9 mmol/L (110 and 125 mg/dL) indicate impaired fasting glucose. Thus, fasting glucose >6.1 mmol/L (110 mg/dL) indicates abnormal glucose tolerance. These definitions based on fasting plasma glucose alone obviate the need for performing glucose tolerance tests.

A major feature of elevated cardiovascular risk in patients with type 2 diabetes probably relates to the abnormal lipoprotein profile associated with insulin resistance known as *diabetic dyslipidemia*. While diabetic patients may often have LDL cholesterol levels near average, the LDL particles tend to be smaller and denser and thus more atherogenic (Chap. 344). Other features of diabetic dyslipidemia include low HDL and elevated triglycerides. Establishing that strict glycemic control reduces the risk of macrovascular complications of di-

abetes has proven much more elusive than the established beneficial effects on microvascular complications such as retinopathy or renal disease. In the absence of clear-cut evidence that tight glycemic control reduces coronary risk in diabetic patients, attention to other aspects of risk in this patient population assumes even greater importance. In this regard, recent clinical trials have demonstrated unequivocal benefit of HMG-CoA reductase inhibitor therapy in diabetic patients, including those with "average" LDL cholesterol levels. Having diabetes places patients in the same risk category as those with established atherosclerotic disease. Therefore, recent guidelines promulgated by the American Diabetes Association recommend an aggressive approach to lipid lowering in the diabetic population, as supported by recent clinical trials. These guidelines establish a target LDL cholesterol level of 2.6 mmol/L (100 mg/dL) for the patient with diabetes.

MALE GENDER/POSTMENOPAUSAL STATE Decades of observational studies have verified excess coronary risk in males compared with premenopausal females. After menopause, however, coronary risk accelerates in women. At least part of the apparent protection against coronary heart disease in premenopausal women derives from their relatively higher HDL levels compared with those of men. After menopause, HDL values fall in concert with increased coronary risk. Estrogen therapy lowers LDL cholesterol and raises HDL cholesterol, changes that should decrease coronary risk. A multitude of observational studies has suggested that estrogen-replacement therapy (ERT) reduces coronary risk. Substantial experimental data support the biologic plausibility of a beneficial effect of estrogen in reducing atherosclerotic events, but a number of potential confounding factors render clinical trials necessary to establish the cardiovascular benefits of ERT. In men, high-dose estrogen treatment caused excess mortality, probably due to increased thromboembolic complications.

The recently reported Heart and Estrogen/Progestin Replacement Study (HERS) has highlighted the need for clinical trial evidence to substantiate the observational and experimental data regarding estrogen's beneficial effects on the vasculature and lipid profile. In this trial, postmenopausal female survivors of acute myocardial infarction were randomized to an estrogen/progestin combination or to placebo. This study showed no overall reduction in recurrent coronary events in the active treatment arm. Indeed, early in the 5-year course of this trial, there was a trend toward an actual increase in vascular events in the treated women. As in the previous Coronary Drug Project trial, the excess events may have resulted from an increase in thromboembolism. HERS does not definitively exclude a potential benefit of other combinations of estrogens with progestins or a benefit of estrogens alone in patients lacking a uterus. A more prolonged follow-up might have disclosed an accrual of benefit in the treatment group, as the excess events appeared in the first years of the trial in the treated group. Moreover, drugs of the selective estrogen receptor modulator class might dissociate the increased risk of breast and/or uterine cancer from cardiovascular benefit. This possibility will likewise require randomized clinical trial evidence evaluating coronary events to validate widespread application. The current quandary surrounding ERT as a means of reducing cardiovascular risk highlights the need for redoubled attention to known modifiable risk factors in women. In the recent clinical trials with HMG-CoA reductase inhibitors, women, when included, have derived benefits at least commensurate with those seen in men. Data from HERS itself showed that application of lipid-lowering therapy to female survivors of myocardial infarction lagged far behind guidelines. Choices regarding ERT in postmenopausal women remain complex. Physicians should work together with women to provide information and help weigh the risks and benefits of ERT, taking personal preferences into account.

242 Prevention, Treatment of Atherosclerosis   **1385**

DYSREGULATED COAGULATION OR FIBRINOLYSIS

Thrombosis ultimately causes the gravest complications of atherosclerosis. The propensity to form thrombi and/or to lyse clots once they form could clearly influence the manifestations of atherosclerosis. Thrombosis provoked by atheroma rupture and subsequent healing may promote plaque growth, as described in Chap. 241. Certain individual characteristics can influence thrombosis or fibrinolysis and have received attention as potential coronary risk factors. For example, fibrinogen levels correlate with coronary risk and provide information regarding coronary risk independent of the lipoprotein profile. Elevated fibrinogen levels might promote a thrombotic diathesis. Alternatively, fibrinogen, an acute-phase reactant, may serve as a marker of inflammation rather than directly participating in the pathogenesis of coronary events.

The stability of an arterial thrombus depends on the balance between fibrinolytic factors, such as plasmin, and inhibitors of the fibrinolytic system, such as plasminogen activator inhibitor (PAI) 1. Certain genotypes of the PAI-1 gene appear to correlate with increased coronary risk. Yet, overall, the levels of tissue plasminogen activator and PAI-1 in plasma have not proven to add information beyond the lipid profile to assessment of cardiovascular risk. Likewise, the role of Lp(a) (Chap. 344) as a modulator of fibrinolysis remains controversial. Apo Lp(a) has high homology to plasminogen but lacks the enzymatic activity of this fibrinolytic molecule. Thus, Lp(a) might antagonize fibrinolysis, serving as a type of "dominant negative" competitor of plasminogen. However, in vivo evidence for this mechanism, and, indeed, the independent contribution of Lp(a), is clouded by difficulties in standardizing the assays and the highly polymorphic nature of this protein in humans.

HOMOCYSTEINE

A large body of literature suggests a relationship between hyperhomocysteinemia and coronary events. Several mutations in the enzymes involved in homocysteine accumulation correlate with thrombosis and, in some studies, coronary risk. Although thrombosis and atherosclerosis seem intimately linked, direct evidence of an atherogenic effect of hyperhomocysteinemia in humans remains weak. The role of hyperhomocysteinemia in atherosclerotic complications, however, has important practical implications. The plasma level of homocysteine can vary with diet. Nutritional supplementation with folic acid can lower homocysteine levels in many individuals. A substantial portion of the elderly population in the United States has only a marginal sufficiency of folate intake. A fortification of the American diet with folic acid, aimed at reduction of neural tube defects, is lowering homocysteine levels in the population at large. Recommending a diet rich in folate or consumption of multivitamin supplements containing folic acid should be considered in individuals with atherosclerosis out of proportion to traditional or established risk factors and with elevated levels of homocysteine. The possibility that folate treatment might mask pernicious anemia should be considered when advising such supplementation. No clinical trial evidence currently establishes a reduction in coronary events in patients with hyperhomocysteinemia treated with folate.

INFECTION/INFLAMMATION

Recent years have witnessed a resurgence of interest in the possibility that infections may cause or contribute to atherosclerosis. A spate of recent publications has furnished evidence in support for a role of *Chlamydia pneumoniae*, cytomegalovirus, or other infectious agents in atherosclerosis and restenosis following coronary intervention. Some microorganisms exist in human atherosclerotic plaques. However, seroepidemiologic evidence for an association between infection with various agents and atherosclerosis remains inconclusive. Several ongoing large trials of antibiotic treatment in survivors of myocardial infarction may provide support for an etiologic or contributory role of microbial infection in recurrent coronary events. Even if positive, however, such clinical trials would neither inculpate any particular microorganisms nor even prove that a benefit derived from the antimicrobial action of the agent employed.

Although direct infection may not cause atherosclerosis, the infectious agents and the host defenses against these invaders might potentiate atherogenesis, acting as inflammatory stimuli. Just as inflammation may mediate some of the altered arterial biology in response to hyperlipoproteinemia, so might infectious agents incite an inflammatory response that could promote atherosclerosis and its complications. Thus, microbial pathogens might act in concert with traditional risk factors to accelerate atherogenesis or cause complication or aggravation of existing atheroma.

In this regard, evidence is accumulating that markers of inflammation correlate with coronary risk. For example, elevated plasma levels of C-reactive protein (CRP) can prospectively predict risk of myocardial infarction and correlate with outcome of patients with acute coronary syndromes. As in the case of fibrinogen, elevated levels of the acute-phase reactant CRP may merely reflect ongoing inflammation rather than a direct etiologic role for CRP in coronary artery disease. It remains uncertain whether elevations in acute-phase reactants such as fibrinogen or CRP serve as a marker for the overall atherosclerotic burden, and hence of coronary events. Alternatively, the elevation in acute-phase reactants could reflect extravascular inflammation that could potentiate atherosclerosis or its complications. In all likelihood, both factors contribute to elevation of inflammatory markers in patients at risk for coronary events. These observations raise the possibility that anti-inflammatory therapies might reduce atherosclerotic events. Indeed, lipid-lowering therapy may reduce coronary events in part by reducing the inflammatory aspects of the pathogenesis of atherosclerosis.

LIFE-STYLE MODIFICATION

The prevention of atherosclerosis presents a long-term challenge to all health care professionals and for public health policy. Both individual practitioners and organizations providing health care should strive to help patients optimize their risk factor profile long before atherosclerotic disease might become manifest. The care plan for all patients seen by internists should include measures to assess and minimize cardiovascular risk. Physicians must counsel patients regarding the health risks of tobacco use and provide guidance regarding smoking cessation. Likewise, physicians should advise all patients about prudent dietary and exercise habits for maintaining ideal body weight. The recent National Institutes of Health Consensus Panel on Physical Activity and Cardiovascular Health established a goal of accumulating at least 30 min of moderate-intensity physical activity on a daily basis. Obesity, particularly the male pattern of centripetal or visceral fat accumulation, can promote an atherogenic dyslipidemia characterized by elevated triglycerides, a low HDL level, and glucose intolerance. Physicians should encourage their patients to take responsibility for behavior related to modifiable risk factors for development of premature atherosclerotic disease. Conscientious counseling and patient education may forestall the need for pharmacologic measures intended to reduce coronary risk.

ISSUES IN RISK ASSESSMENT

A growing panel of markers of coronary risk presents a perplexing array to the practitioner. Such markers include size fractionation of LDL particles, measurement of concentrations of homocysteine, Lp(a), fibrinogen, CRP, and PAI-1, among others. In general, such specialized tests add little to the information available from a careful history and physical examination and measurement of a plasma lipoprotein profile and fasting blood sugar. Evaluation of such specialized markers might be considered in individuals without evident risk factors other than premature vascular disease or a worrisome family history. A similar confusion surrounds the use of specialized radiographic estimations of coronary artery calcification. Information is accumulating that the amount of calcium determined by such techniques as electron beam computed tomography correlates with coronary risk. However, the utility of using such estimates of coronary artery calcium content as a guide to therapy remains unproven, particularly in asymptomatic individuals. Inappropriate use of such imaging modalities might promote excessive inva-

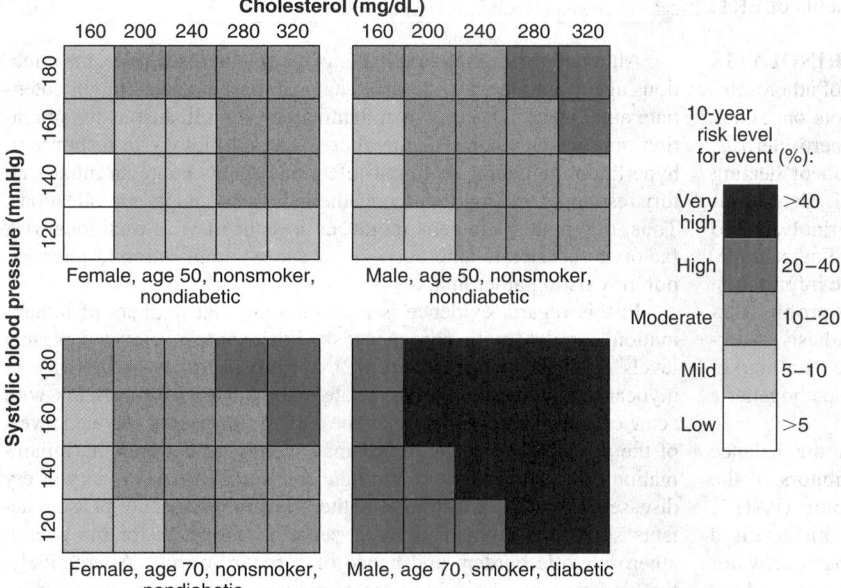

Cholesterol (mg/dL)

Systolic blood pressure (mmHg)

Female, age 50, nonsmoker, nondiabetic

Male, age 50, nonsmoker, nondiabetic

Female, age 70, nonsmoker, nondiabetic

Male, age 70, smoker, diabetic

10-year risk level for event (%):

Very high		>40
High		20–40
Moderate		10–20
Mild		5–10
Low		>5

FIGURE 242-1 *The multi-factorial nature of coronary risk*: examples from the European Treatment Guidelines. Shown are four matrices derived from the guidelines currently used in Europe to stratify individuals for treatment. Each matrix shows differing levels of systolic blood pressure (columns) and increasing levels of serum cholesterol (rows). The 10-year risk levels for a coronary heart disease event are plotted according to the scale shown on the far right. The darkness of the color indicates higher risk. These examples illustrate the differences between a female (top left matrix) versus a male (top right matrix), both age 50 and nonsmokers. The bottom pair of matrices illustrate the risk ascribed to individuals both age 70, one with three additional risk factors (male gender, tobacco use, and diabetes mellitus, lower right) versus a nonsmoking, nondiabetic female (lower left). *(From D Wood et al: Prevention of coronary heart disease in clinical practice. Summary of recommendations of the Second Joint Task Force of European and other Societies on Coronary Prevention. Hypertension 16:1407, 1998.)*

sive diagnostic and therapeutic procedures. Widespread application of such modalities for screening should await proof that clinical benefit derives from their application.

THE CONCEPT OF GLOBAL RISK

Adoption of hygienic life-style changes to ameliorate coronary risk entails little expense or possibility of adverse effects. In contrast, pharmacotherapy can prove costly. Although lipid-lowering drugs such as the HMG-CoA reductase inhibitors have proven exceedingly well tolerated in clinical trials, the use of these or other lipid-lowering agents could produce adverse reactions in some individuals. The decision to initiate drug treatment for reduction of risk of atherosclerotic events requires careful consideration, particularly in the setting of "primary prevention" or in patients without known atherosclerotic disease. In this regard, it is prudent to consider not only the LDL cholesterol but also the individual patient's global cardiovascular risk. For example, an individual with an average LDL but a low HDL, hypertension, and a family history of premature coronary artery disease might warrant initiation of drug therapy more than an individual with the same LDL level in the absence of the other risk factors. Rather than considering plasma lipoprotein values in insolation, current European guidelines reserve drug treatment for individuals with a calculated absolute coronary heart disease risk of greater than 20% over 10 years. The calculation of coronary risk includes taking gender, smoking history, and systolic blood pressure into account, in addition to plasma cholesterol levels. This policy illustrates how estimations of global risk may be applied to optimize decisions regarding initiation of drug therapy to prevent atherosclerotic events (Fig. 242-1).

THE CHALLENGE OF IMPLEMENTATION: CHANGING PHYSICIAN AND PATIENT BEHAVIOR Enormous strides have been made in the prevention and treatment of atherosclerosis. Despite declining age-adjusted rates of coronary death, cardio-

vascular mortality is on the rise due to the aging of the population overall. There is a powerful global trend toward increased atherosclerotic disease. Enormous challenges remain regarding translation of the current evidence base into practice. The obstacles to implementation of current evidence-based prevention and treatment of atherosclerosis include economics, education, physician awareness, and patient adherence to recommended regimens. Future goals in the field of treatment of atherosclerosis should include application of the current knowledge regarding risk factor management and, when appropriate, drug therapy.

BIBLIOGRAPHY

ANONYMOUS: Management of dyslipidemia in adults with diabetes. Diabetes Care 22 (Suppl 1):S56, 1999

BROWN BG et al: Lipid lowering and plaque regression: New insights into prevention of plaque disruption and clinical events in coronary disease. Circulation 87:1781, 1993

GAZIANO JM, MANSON JE, RIDKER PM: Primary and secondary prevention of coronary heart disease, in *Heart Disease*, 6th ed., E Braunwald, D Zipes, P Libby (eds). Philadelphia, Saunders, 2001

GOTTO AM Jr.: Lipid-lowering therapy for the primary prevention of coronary heart disease. J Am Coll Cardiol 33:2078, 1999

LIBBY P et al: Roles of infectious agents in atherosclerosis and restenosis: An assessment of the evidence and need for future research. Circulation 96:4095, 1997

MURRAY CH, LOPEZ AD: Alternative projections of mortality and disability by cause 1990–2020: Global Burden of Disease Study. Lancet 349:1498, 1997

PETITTI DB: Hormone replacement therapy and heart disease prevention: Experimentation trumps observation. JAMA 280:650, 1998

RIDKER P, LIBBY P: Nontraditional coronary risk factors and vascular biology: The frontiers of preventive cardiology. J Invest Med 46:338, 1998

243

Elliott M. Antman, Eugene Braunwald

ACUTE MYOCARDIAL INFARCTION

ACE	angiotensin-converting enzyme
AIVR	accelerated idioventricular rhythm
AMI	acute myocardial infarction
APSAC	anisoylated plasminogen streptokinase activator complex
AV	atrioventricular
CHF	congestive heart failure
CK	creatine phosphokinase
cTnI	cardiac-specific troponin I
cTnT	cardiac-specific troponin T
ECG	electrocardiogram
LMWHs	low-molecular-weight heparin preparations
LV	left ventricular
MI	myocardial infarction
MR	mitral regurgitation
NSTEMI	non-ST elevation MI
PCI	percutaneous coronary intervention
rPA	reteplase
RV	right ventricular
tPA	tissue plasminogen activator
UFH	unfractionated heparin

Acute myocardial infarction (AMI) is one of the most common diagnoses in hospitalized patients in industrialized countries. In the United States, approximately 1.1 million AMIs occur each year. The mortality rate with AMI is approximately 30%, with more than half of these deaths occurring before the stricken individual reaches the hospital. Although the mortality rate after admission for AMI has declined by about 30% over the last two decades, approximately 1 of every 25 patients who survives the initial hospitalization dies in the first year after AMI. Survival is markedly reduced in elderly patients (over age 75), whose mortality rate is 20% at 1 month and 30% at 1 year after AMI.

AMI generally occurs when coronary blood flow decreases abruptly after a thrombotic occlusion of a coronary artery previously narrowed by atherosclerosis. Slowly developing, high-grade coronary artery stenoses usually do not precipitate AMI because of the development of a rich collateral network over time. Instead, AMI occurs when a coronary artery thrombus develops rapidly at a site of vascular injury. This injury is produced or facilitated by factors such as cigarette smoking, hypertension, and lipid accumulation. In most cases, infarction occurs when an atherosclerotic plaque fissures, ruptures, or ulcerates and when conditions (local or systemic) favor thrombogenesis, so that a mural thrombus forms at the site of rupture and leads to coronary artery occlusion. Histologic studies indicate that the coronary plaques prone to rupture are those with a rich lipid core and a thin fibrous cap (Chap. 241). After an initial platelet monolayer forms at the site of the ruptured plaque, various agonists (collagen, ADP, epinephrine, serotonin) promote platelet activation. After agonist stimulation of platelets, there is production and release of thromboxane A_2 (a potent local vasoconstrictor), further platelet activation, and potential resistance to thrombolysis.

In addition to the generation of thromboxane A_2, activation of platelets by agonists promotes a conformational change in the glycoprotein IIb/IIIa receptor (Chap. 116). Once converted to its functional state, this receptor develops a high affinity for amino acid sequences on soluble adhesive proteins (i.e., integrins) such as von Willebrand factor (vWF) and fibrinogen. Since vWF and fibrinogen are multivalent molecules, they can bind to two different platelets simultaneously, resulting in platelet cross-linking and aggregation.

The coagulation cascade is activated on exposure of tissue factor in damaged endothelial cells at the site of the ruptured plaque. Factors VII and X are activated, ultimately leading to the conversion of prothrombin to thrombin, which then converts fibrinogen to fibrin (Chap. 117). Fluid-phase and clot-bound thrombin participate in an autoamplification reaction that leads to further activation of the coagulation cascade. The culprit coronary artery eventually becomes occluded by a thrombus containing platelet aggregates and fibrin strands.

In rare cases, AMI may be due to coronary artery occlusion caused by coronary emboli, congenital abnormalities, coronary spasm, and a wide variety of systemic—particularly inflammatory—diseases. The amount of myocardial damage caused by coronary occlusion depends on (1) the territory supplied by the affected vessel, (2) whether or not the vessel becomes totally occluded, (3) the duration of coronary occlusion, (4) the quantity of blood supplied by collateral vessels to the affected tissue, (5) the demand for oxygen of the myocardium whose blood supply has been suddenly limited, (6) native factors that can produce early spontaneous lysis of the occlusive thrombus, and (7) the adequacy of myocardial perfusion in the infarct zone when flow is restored in the occluded epicardial coronary artery.

Patients at increased risk of developing AMI include those with multiple coronary risk factors (Chap. 241) and those with unstable angina or Prinzmetal's variant angina (Chap. 244). Less common underlying medical conditions predisposing patients to AMI include hypercoagulability, collagen vascular disease, cocaine abuse, and intracardiac thrombi or masses that can produce coronary emboli.

CLINICAL PRESENTATION

In up to one-half of cases, a precipitating factor appears to be present before AMI, such as vigorous physical exercise, emotional stress, or a medical or surgical illness. Although AMI may commence at any time of the day or night, circadian variations have been reported such that clusters are seen in the morning within a few hours of awakening. The increased frequency early in the day may be due to a combination of an increase in sympathetic tone and an increased tendency to thrombosis between 6:00 A.M. and 12 noon.

Pain is the most common presenting complaint in patients with AMI. In some instances, it may be severe enough to be described as the worst pain the patient has ever felt. The pain is deep and visceral; adjectives commonly used to describe it are *heavy*, *squeezing*, and *crushing*, although occasionally it is described as stabbing or burning (Chap. 13). It is similar in character to the discomfort of angina pectoris but usually is more severe and lasts longer. Typically the pain involves the central portion of the chest and/or the epigastrium, and on occasion it radiates to the arms. Less common sites of radiation include the abdomen, back, lower jaw, and neck. The frequent location of the pain beneath the xiphoid and patients' denial that they may be suffering a heart attack are chiefly responsible for the common mistaken impression of indigestion. The pain of AMI may radiate as high as the occipital area but not below the umbilicus. It is often accompanied by weakness, sweating, nausea, vomiting, anxiety, and a sense of impending doom. The pain may commence when the patient is at rest. When the pain begins during a period of exertion, it does not usually subside with cessation of activity, in contrast to angina pectoris.

Although pain is the most common presenting complaint, it is by no means always present. The proportion of painless AMIs is greater in patients with diabetes mellitus, and it increases with age. In the elderly, AMI may present as sudden-onset breathlessness, which may progress to pulmonary edema. Other less common presentations, with or without pain, include sudden loss of consciousness, a confusional state, a sensation of profound weakness, the appearance of an arrhythmia, evidence of peripheral embolism, or merely an unexplained drop in arterial pressure. The pain of AMI can simulate pain from acute pericarditis (Chap. 239), pulmonary embolism (Chap. 261), acute aortic dissection (Chap. 247), costochondritis, and gastrointestinal disorders. These conditions should therefore be considered in the differential diagnosis.

PHYSICAL FINDINGS Most patients are anxious and restless, attempting unsuccessfully to relieve the pain by moving about in bed, altering their position, and stretching. Pallor associated with perspiration and coolness of the extremities occurs commonly. The combination of substernal chest pain persisting for >30 min and diaphoresis strongly suggests AMI. Although many patients have a normal pulse rate and blood pressure within the first hour of AMI, about one-fourth of patients with anterior infarction have manifestations of sympathetic nervous system hyperactivity (tachycardia and/or hypertension), and up to one-half with inferior infarction show evidence of parasympathetic hyperactivity (bradycardia and/or hypotension).

The precordium is usually quiet, and the apical impulse may be difficult to palpate. In patients with anterior wall infarction, an abnormal systolic pulsation caused by dyskinetic bulging of infarcted myocardium may develop in the periapical area within the first days of the illness and then may resolve. Other physical signs of ventricular dysfunction that may be present include, in order of decreasing incidence, fourth (S_4) and third (S_3) heart sounds, decreased intensity of heart sounds, and, in more severe cases, paradoxical splitting of the second heart sound (Chap. 225). A transient apical systolic murmur due to dysfunction of the mitral valve apparatus may be midsystolic or late systolic in timing. A pericardial friction rub is heard in many patients with transmural AMI at some time in the course of the disease, if they are examined frequently. The carotid pulse is often decreased in volume, reflecting reduced stroke volume. Jugular venous distention with clear lung fields should raise suspicion of right ventricular infarction. Temperature elevations up to 38°C may be observed during the first week after AMI; however, a temperature exceeding 38°C should prompt a search for other causes. The arterial pressure is variable; in most patients with transmural infarction, systolic pressure declines by approximately 10 to 15 mmHg from the preinfarction state.

LABORATORY FINDINGS

Myocardial infarction (MI) progresses through the following temporal stages: (1) acute (first few hours to 7 days), (2) healing (7 to 28 days), and (3) healed (29 days and beyond). When evaluating the results of diagnostic tests for AMI, the temporal phase of the infarction process must be considered. The laboratory tests of value in confirming the diagnosis may be divided into 4 groups: (1) electrocardiogram (ECG), (2) serum cardiac markers, (3) cardiac imaging, and (4) nonspecific indexes of tissue necrosis and inflammation.

ELECTROCARDIOGRAM   The electrocardiographic manifestations of AMI are described in Chap. 226. During the initial stage of the acute phase of MI, total occlusion of the infarct artery produces ST-segment elevation. Most patients initially presenting with ST-segment elevation evolve Q waves on the ECG and are ultimately diagnosed as having sustained a Q-wave MI. A small proportion may sustain only a non-Q-wave MI. When the obstructing thrombus is not totally occlusive, obstruction is transient, or if a rich collateral network is present, no ST-segment elevation is seen. Such patients are initially considered to be experiencing either unstable anigna or a non-ST-segment elevation MI (NSTEMI). Among patients presenting without ST-segment elevation, if a serum cardiac marker is detected and no Q wave develops, the diagnosis of non-Q-wave MI is ultimately made. A minority of patients who present initially without ST-segment elevation may develop a Q-wave MI. Previously it was believed that transmural MI is present if the ECG demonstrates Q waves or loss of R waves, and nontransmural MI may be present if the ECG shows only transient ST-segment and T-wave changes. However, electrocardiographic-pathologic correlations are far from perfect; and therefore a more rational nomenclature for designating electrocardiographic infarction is now commonly in use, with the terms Q-wave and non-Q-wave MI replacing the terms transmural and nontransmural MI, respectively.

The presentations that comprise the spectrum ranging from unstable angina through non-Q-wave MI to Q-wave MI are called the *acute coronary syndromes* (Fig. 243-1). This classification scheme provides a conceptual framework for interpreting the diagnostic and prognostic information gleaned from serum cardiac marker measurements as well as for planning antithrombotic therapy.

SERUM CARDIAC MARKERS   Certain proteins, called *serum cardiac markers*, are released into the blood in large quantities

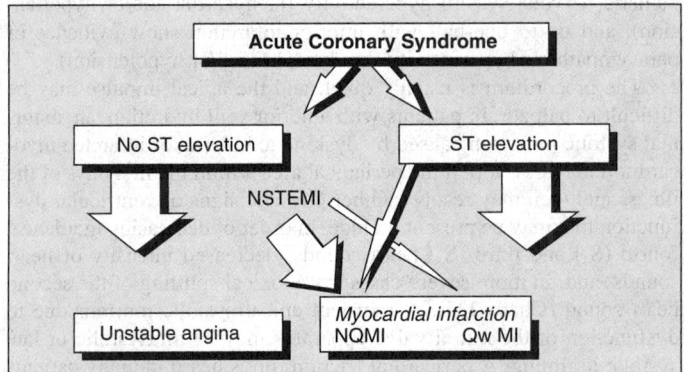

FIGURE 243-1   Acute coronary syndromes. Patients with ischemic discomfort may present with or without ST-segment elevation on the ECG. Of patients with ST-segment elevation, most (*large arrow*) ultimately develop a Q-wave AMI (QwMI), while a few (*small arrow*) develop a non-Q-wave AMI (NQMI). Patients who do not present without ST-segment elevation are suffering from either unstable angina or a non-ST segment elevation MI (NSTEMI) (*large arrows*), a distinction that is ultimately made on the presence or absence of a serum cardiac marker such as CKMB or a cardiac troponin detected in the blood. Most patients presenting with NSTEMI ultimately develop a NQMI on the ECG; a few may develop a QwMI. The spectrum of clinical presentations ranging from unstable angina through NQMI and QwMI are referred to as the actue coronary syndromes. [*Adapted from EM Antman, E Braunwald: Acute myocardial infarction, in Heart Disease, A Textbook of Cardiovascular Medicine, 5th ed, E Braunwald (ed). Philadelphia, Saunders, 1997.*]

from necrotic heart muscle after AMI. The rate of liberation of specific proteins differs depending on their intracellular location and molecular weight, and the local blood and lymphatic flow. The temporal pattern of protein release is of diagnostic importance, but contemporary urgent reperfusion strategies necessitate making a decision (based largely on a combination of clinical and ECG findings) before the results of blood tests have returned from the central laboratory. Rapid whole-blood bedside assays for serum cardiac markers are now available and may facilitate management decisions, particularly in patients with nondiagnostic ECGs.

Creatine phosphokinase (CK) rises within 4 to 8 h and generally returns to normal by 48 to 72 h. An important drawback of total CK measurement is its lack of specificity for AMI, as CK may be elevated with skeletal muscle trauma. A two- to threefold elevation of total CK may follow an intramuscular injection, for example. This ambiguity may lead to the erroneous diagnosis of AMI in a patient who has been given an intramuscular injection of a narcotic for chest pain of noncardiac origin. Other potential sources of total CK elevation are (1) skeletal muscular diseases, including muscular dystrophy, myopathies, and polymyositis; (2) electrical cardioversion; (3) hypothyroidism; (4) stroke; (5) surgery; and (6) skeletal muscle damage secondary to trauma, convulsions, and prolonged immobilization.

The MB isoenzyme of CK has the advantage over total CK that it is not present in significant concentrations in extracardiac tissue and therefore is considerably more specific. However, cardiac surgery, myocarditis, and electrical cardioversion often result in elevated serum levels of the MB isoenzyme. A ratio (relative index) of CKMB mass: CK activity ≥ 2.5 suggests but is not diagnostic of a myocardial rather than a skeletal muscle source for the CKMB elevation. This ratio is less useful when levels of total CK are high owing to skeletal muscle injury or when the total CK level is within the normal range but CKMB is elevated.

Rather than attempting to make the diagnosis of AMI on the basis of a single measurement of CK and CKMB, clinicians should evaluate a series of measurements obtained over the first 24 h. Skeletal muscle release of CKMB typically produces a "plateau" pattern, whereas AMI produces a CKMB elevation that peaks approximately 20 h after the onset of coronary occlusion. When released into the circulation, the myocardial form of CKMB (CKMB2) is acted on by the enzyme carboxypeptidase, which cleaves a lysine residue from the carboxyl terminus to produce an isoform (CKMB1) with a different electrophoretic mobility. A CKMB2:CKMB1 ratio of >1.5 is highly sensitive for the diagnosis of AMI, particularly 4 to 6 h after the onset of coronary occlusion.

Cardiac-specific troponin T (cTnT) and *cardiac-specific troponin I (cTnI)* have amino acid sequences different from those of the skeletal muscle forms of these proteins. These differences have permitted the development of quantitative assays for cTnT and cTnI with highly specific monoclonal antibodies. Since cTnT and cTnI are not normally detectable in the blood of healthy individuals but may increase after AMI to levels over 20 times higher than the cutoff value (usually set only slightly above the noise level of the assay), the measurement of cTnT or cTnI is of considerable diagnostic usefulness, and they are now the preferred biochemical markers for MI. The cardiac troponins are particularly valuable when there is clinical suspicion of either skeletal muscle injury or a small MI that may be below the detection limit for CK and CKMB measurements. Levels of cTnI may remain elevated for 7 to 10 days after AMI, and cTnT levels may remain elevated for up to 10 to 14 days. Thus, measurement of cTnT or cTnI has replaced measurement of lactate dehydrogenase (LDH) and its isoenzymes in patients with suspected MI who come to medical attention more than 24 to 48 h after the onset of symptoms.

Myoglobin is released into the blood within only a few hours of the onset of AMI. Although myoglobin is one of the first serum cardiac markers that rises above the normal range after AMI, it lacks cardiac specificity, and it is rapidly excreted in the urine, so that blood levels return to the normal range within 24 h of the onset of infarction.

Many hospitals are using cTnT or cTnI rather than CKMB as the routine serum cardiac marker for diagnosis of AMI, although any of these analytes remains clinically acceptable. It is not cost-effective to measure both a cardiac-specific troponin and CKMB at all time points in every patient. However, in view of the prolonged elevation of cardiac-specific troponins (>1 week), episodes of recurrent ischemic discomfort and suspected recurrent MI are more readily diagnosed with a serum cardiac marker that remains elevated in the blood more briefly, such as CKMB or myoglobin.

While it has long been recognized that the total quantity of protein released correlates with the size of the infarct, the peak protein concentration correlates only weakly with infarct size. Recanalization of a coronary artery occlusion (either spontaneously or by mechanical or pharmacologic means) in the early hours of AMI causes earlier and higher peaking (at about 8 to 12 h after reperfusion) of serum cardiac markers.

Characteristic rises occur in serum cardiac markers in virtually all patients with clinically proven MI. CK and CKMB levels generally do not rise in unstable angina. However, approximately one-third of patients who are considered to have unstable angina on the basis of a lack of CK or CKMB elevation have elevations of cTnT or cTnI, probably indicating the presence of microinfarction. The finding of an elevated cardiac-specific troponin level, even in the presence of normal CK and CKMB values, is indicative of an adverse prognosis, and such patients should be considered to have sustained MI and managed as described below.

For the purposes of confirming the diagnosis of MI, serum cardiac markers should be measured on admission, 6 to 9 h after admission, and 12 to 24 h after admission if the diagnosis remains uncertain.

The *nonspecific reaction* to myocardial injury is associated with polymorphonuclear leukocytosis, which appears within a few hours after the onset of pain, persists for 3 to 7 days, and often reaches levels of 12,000 to 15,000 leukocytes per microliter. The erythrocyte sedimentation rate rises more slowly than the white blood cell count, peaking during the first week and sometimes remaining elevated for 1 or 2 weeks.

CARDIAC IMAGING *Two-dimensional echocardiography* (Chap. 227) is the most frequently employed imaging modality in patients with AMI. Abnormalities of wall motion are almost universally present. Even when no ST-segment elevation is seen, echocardiographically detectable wall motion abnormalities may be observed. Although AMI cannot be distinguished from an old myocardial scar or from acute severe ischemia by echocardiography, the ease and safety of the procedure make its use appealing as a screening tool. In the emergency department setting, early detection of the presence or absence of wall motion abnormalities by echocardiography can aid in management decisions, such as whether the patient should receive reperfusion therapy [e.g., thrombolysis or a percutaneous coronary intervention (PCI)]. Echocardiographic estimation of left ventricular (LV) function is useful prognostically; detection of reduced function serves as an indication for therapy with an angiotensin-converting enzyme inhibitor (see "Angiotensin-Converting Enzyme Inhibitors," below). Echocardiography may also identify the presence of right ventricular (RV) infarction, ventricular aneurysm, pericardial effusion, and LV thrombus. In addition, Doppler echocardiography is useful in the detection and quantitation of a ventricular septal defect and mitral regurgitation, two serious complications of AMI (see below).

Several radionuclide imaging techniques are available for evaluating patients with suspected AMI. However, these imaging modalities are used less often than echocardiography because they are more cumbersome and they lack sensitivity and specificity in many clinical circumstances. Myocardial perfusion imaging with ^{201}Tl or ^{99m}Tc-sestamibi, which are distributed in proportion to myocardial blood flow and concentrated by viable myocardium (Chap. 244) reveal a defect ("cold spot") in most patients during the first few hours after development of a transmural infarct. However, although perfusion scanning is extremely sensitive, it cannot distinguish acute infarcts from chronic scars and thus is not specific for the diagnosis of *acute* MI. Radionuclide ventriculography, carried out with ^{99m}Tc-labeled red blood cells, frequently demonstrates wall motion disorders and reduction in the ventricular ejection fraction in patients with AMI. While of value in assessing the hemodynamic consequences of infarction and in aiding in the diagnosis of RV infarction when the RV ejection fraction is depressed, this technique is also quite nonspecific, as many cardiac abnormalities other than MI alter the radionuclide ventriculogram.

MANAGEMENT

PREHOSPITAL CARE The prognosis in AMI is largely related to the occurrence of two general classes of complications: (1) electrical complications (arrhythmias) and (2) mechanical problems ("pump failure"). Most out-of-hospital deaths from AMI are due to the sudden development of ventricular fibrillation. The vast majority of deaths due to ventricular fibrillation occur within the first 24 h of the onset of symptoms, and, of these, over half occur in the first hour. Therefore, the major elements of prehospital care of patients with suspected AMI include (1) recognition of symptoms by the patient and prompt seeking of medical attention; (2) rapid deployment of an emergency medical team capable of performing resuscitative maneuvers, including defibrillation; and (3) expeditious transportation of the patient to a hospital facility that is continuously staffed by physicians and nurses skilled in managing arrhythmias, providing advanced cardiac life support, and (4) expeditious implementation of reperfusion therapy. The biggest delay usually occurs not during transportation to the hospital but rather between the onset of pain and the patient's decision to call for help. This delay can best be reduced by education of the public by health care professionals concerning the significance of chest pain and the importance of seeking early medical attention. Increasingly, monitoring and treatment are carried out by trained personnel in the ambulance, further shortening the time between the onset of the infarction and appropriate treatment.

INITIAL MANAGEMENT IN THE EMERGENCY DEPARTMENT In the emergency department, the goals for the management of patients with suspected AMI include control of cardiac pain, rapid identification of patients who are candidates for urgent reperfusion therapy, triage of lower-risk patients to the appropriate location in the hospital, and avoidance of inappropriate discharge of patients with AMI. Many aspects of the treatment of AMI are initiated in the emergency department and then continued during the in-hospital phase of management.

Aspirin is now considered an essential element in the management of patients with suspected AMI and is effective across the entire spectrum of acute coronary syndromes (Fig. 243-2 and 243-3). Rapid inhibition of cyclooxygenase in platelets followed by a reduction of thromboxane A_2 levels is achieved by buccal absorption of a chewed 160 to 325 mg tablet in the emergency department. This measure should be followed by daily oral administration of aspirin in a dose of 160 to 325 mg.

Since patients with AMI may develop hypoxemia secondary to ventilation-perfusion abnormalities from LV failure and intrinsic pulmonary disease, it has been a common practice to routinely administer *supplemental oxygen*. In patients whose arterial oxygen saturation is normal as estimated by pulse oximetry or measured by an arterial blood gas specimen, supplemental oxygen is of limited if any clinical benefit and therefore is not cost effective. However, when hypoxemia is present, oxygen should be administered by nasal prongs or face mask (2 to 4 L/min) for the first 6 to 12 h after infarction; the patient should then be reassessed to determine if there is a continued need for such treatment.

CONTROL OF PAIN *Morphine* is a very effective analgesic for the pain associated with AMI. However, it may reduce sympathetically mediated arteriolar and venous constriction, and the resulting venous pooling may reduce cardiac output and arterial pressure. This complication does not contraindicate the use of morphine. Hypotension associated with venous pooling usually responds promptly to elevation of the legs, but in some patients volume expansion with intra-

FIGURE 243-2 Management strategy for patients suspected of having an ST-segment elevation. AMI patients should receive aspirin (ASA), beta blockers (in the absence of contraindications), and an antithrombin (particularly if a relatively fibrin-specific thrombolytic agent is used). Adjunctive antithrombin therapy is probably not required for patients receiving streptokinase. Patients treated within 12 h who are eligible for thrombolytic therapy should expeditiously receive such treatment or be considered for primary percutaneous transluminal coronary angioplasty (PCI). Immediate, primary PCI is also to be considered when lytic therapy is contraindicated. An intravenous glycoprotein IIb/IIIa (GPIIb/IIIa) inhibitor may be helpful for reducing thrombotic complications during primary PCI. *[Modified from EM Antman: Overview of medical therapy, in RM Califf (ed): Acute Myocardial Infarction and Other Acute Ischemic Syndromes, in E Braunwald (Series ed): Atlas of Heart Diseases, vol. 8. Philadelphia, Current Medicine 1996.]*

venous saline is required. The patient may experience diaphoresis and nausea, but these events usually pass and are replaced by a feeling of well-being associated with the relief of pain. Morphine also has a vagotonic effect and may cause bradycardia or advanced degrees of heart block, particularly in patients with posteroinferior infarction. These side effects usually respond to atropine (0.5 mg intravenously). Morphine is routinely administered by repetitive (every 5 min) intravenous injection of small doses (2 to 4 mg) rather than by the subcutaneous administration of a larger quantity, because absorption may be unpredictable by the latter route.

Before morphine is administered, sublingual *nitroglycerin* can be given safely to most patients with AMI. Up to three 0.4-mg doses should be administered at about 5-min intervals. In addition to diminishing or abolishing chest discomfort, nitroglycerin, once considered contraindicated in the setting of AMI, may be capable of both decreasing myocardial oxygen demand (by lowering preload) and increasing myocardial oxygen supply (by dilating infarct-related coronary vessels or collateral vessels). In patients whose initially favorable response to sublingual nitroglycerin is followed by the return of chest pain, particularly if accompanied by other evidence of ongoing ischemia such as further ST-segment or T-wave shifts, the use of intravenous nitroglycerin should be considered. Therapy with nitrates should be avoided in patients who present with low systolic arterial pressure (<100 mmHg) or in whom there is clinical suspicion of right ventricular infarction (inferior infarction on electrocardiogram, elevated jugular venous pressure, clear lungs, and hypotension). Nitrates should not be administered to patients who have taken the phosphodiasterase 5 inhibitor sildenafil for erectile dysfunction within the preceding 24 h

since it may potentiate the hypotensive effects of nitrates. An idiosyncratic reaction to nitrates, consisting of sudden marked hypotension, sometimes occurs but can usually be reversed promptly by the rapid administration of intravenous atropine.

Intravenous *beta blockers* are also useful in the control of the pain of AMI. These drugs control pain effectively in some patients, presumably by diminishing myocardial oxygen demand and hence ischemia. More important, there is evidence that intravenous beta blockers reduce in-hospital mortality, particularly in high-risk patients (see "β-Adrenoceptor Blockers," below). A commonly employed regimen is metoprolol, 5 mg every 2 to 5 min for a total of three doses, provided the patient has a heart rate >60 beats per minute (bpm), systolic pressure >100 mmHg, a PR interval <0.24 s, and rales that are no higher than 10 cm up from the diaphragm. Fifteen minutes after the last intravenous dose, an oral regimen is initiated of 50 mg every 6 h for 48 h followed by 100 mg every 12 h.

FIGURE 243-3 Management strategy for patients with unstable angina and AMI without ST-segment elevation. These patients should be treated with an antithrombin and aspirin. Nitrates should be administered for recurrent episodes of angina. The risk of death and cardiac ischemic events may be reduced in high risk patients if an intravenous GPIIb/IIIa inhibitor is administered. Adequate beta blockade should be established; when that is not possible or contraindications exist, a calcium antagonist can be considered. Patients at high risk should be triaged to cardiac catheterization with plans for revascularization if clinically suitable, while patients who are clinically stable can be treated more conservatively with continued observation in the hospital and consideration of a stress test to screen for any provocable myocardial ischemia. CABG, coronary artery bypass grafting; LV, left ventricular. *[Modified from EM Antman: Overview of medical therapy, in RM Califf (ed): Acute Myocardial Infarction and Other Acute Ischemic Syndromes, in E Braunwald (Series ed): Atlas of Heart Diseases, vol. 8. Philadelphia, Current Medicine 1996.]*

Unlike beta blockers, calcium antagonists are of little value in the acute setting, and there is evidence that short-acting dihydropyridines may be associated with an increased mortality risk.

MANAGEMENT STRATEGIES (Figs. 243-2 and 243-3) The primary tool for screening patients and making triage decisions is the initial 12-lead ECG. When ST-segment elevation in at least two contiguous leads of at least 2 mm in V1-V3 and 1 mm in other leads is present, a patient should be considered a candidate for *reperfusion therapy* (Fig. 243-2). If no contraindications are present (see "Contra-indications and Complications," under "Thombolysis," below), thrombolytic therapy should ideally be initiated within 30 min. The process of selecting patients for thrombolysis versus primary PCI (angioplasty, or stenting) (Chap. 245) is discussed below. In the absence of ST-segment elevation, thrombolysis is not helpful, and evidence exists suggesting that it may be harmful. Pharmacotherapy for patients presenting without ST-segment elevation (Fig. 243-3) typically includes measures to control cardiac pain (as discussed above), aspirin, anti-thrombin therapy (preferably with low-molecular-weight heparin), and infusion of nitroglycerin as needed to control recurrent ischemia. For high-risk patients an intravenous infusion of a glycoprotein IIb/IIIa inhibitor should be considered. Further management recommendations for patients without ST-segment elevation are outlined in Fig. 243-3.

LIMITATION OF INFARCT SIZE The quantity of myocardium that becomes necrotic as a consequence of a coronary artery occlusion is determined by factors other than just the site of occlusion. While the central zone of the infarct contains necrotic tissue that is irretrievably lost, the fate of the surrounding ischemic myocardium may be improved by timely restoration of coronary perfusion, reduction of myocardial oxygen demands, prevention of the accumulation of noxious metabolites, and blunting of the impact of mediators of reperfusion injury (e.g., calcium overload and oxygen-derived free radicals). Up to one-third of patients with AMI may achieve *spontaneous* reperfusion of the infarct-related coronary artery within 24 h and experience improved healing of infarcted tissue. Reperfusion either pharmacologically (by thrombolysis) or mechanically (by angioplasty and/or stenting) accelerates the process of opening the occluded infarct-related artery in those patients in whom spontaneous thrombolysis ultimately would have occurred and also greatly increases the number of patients in whom restoration of flow in the infarct-related artery is accomplished. Timely restoration of flow in the epicardial infarct-related artery combined with improved perfusion of the downstream zone of infarcted myocardium results in a limitation of infarct size. Protection of the ischemic myocardium by the maintenance of an optimal balance between myocardial oxygen supply and demand through pain control, treatment of congestive heart failure, and minimization of tachycardia and hypertension extends the "window" of time for the salvage of myocardium by reperfusion strategies.

Glucocorticoids and nonsteroidal anti-inflammatory agents, with the exception of aspirin, should be avoided in the setting of AMI. They can impair infarct healing and increase the risk of myocardial rupture, and their use may result in a larger infarct scar. In addition, they can increase coronary vascular resistance, thereby potentially reducing flow to ischemic myocardium.

THROMBOLYSIS The thrombolytic agents tissue plasminogen activator (tPA), streptokinase, anisoylated plasminogen streptokinase activator complex (APSAC) and reteplase (rPA) have been approved by the Food and Drug Administration for intravenous use in the setting of AMI. These drugs all act by promoting the conversion of plasminogen to plasmin, which subsequently lyses fibrin thrombi. Although considerable emphasis was first placed on a distinction between more fibrin-specific agents, such as tPA, and non-fibrin-specific agents, such as streptokinase, it is now recognized that these differences are only relative, as some degree of systemic fibrinolysis occurs with tPA. The principal goal of thrombolysis is prompt restoration of coronary arterial patency.

When assessed angiographically, flow in the culprit coronary artery is described by a simple qualitative scale called the TIMI grading

system: grade 0 indicates complete occlusion of the infarct-related artery; grade 1 indicates some penetration of the contrast material beyond the point of obstruction but without perfusion of the distal coronary bed; grade 2 indicates perfusion of the entire infarct vessel into the distal bed but with flow that is delayed compared with that of a normal artery; and grade 3 indicates full perfusion of the infarct vessel with normal flow. Early reports frequently lumped TIMI grades 2 and 3 under the general category of *patency*, but it is now recognized that grade 3 flow is the goal of reperfusion therapy, because full perfusion of the infarct-related coronary artery yields far better results in terms of infarct size, maintenance of LV function, and reduction of both short- and long-term mortality rates. Relatively new methods of angiographic assessment of the efficacy of thrombolysis include counting the number of frames required on the cine film for dye to flow from the origin of the infarct-related artery to a landmark in the distal vascular bed (TIMI frame count) and determining the rate of entry and exit of contrast dye from the microvasculature in the myocardial infarct zone (TIMI Myocardial Perfusion Grade).

Thrombolytic therapy can reduce the relative risk of in-hospital death by up to 50% when administered within the first hour of the onset of symptoms of AMI, and much of this benefit is maintained for at least 10 years. Appropriately used thrombolytic therapy appears to reduce infarct size, limit LV dysfunction, and reduce the incidence of serious complications such as septal rupture, cardiogenic shock, and malignant ventricular arrhythmias. Since myocardium can be salvaged only before it has been irreversibly injured, the timing of reperfusion therapy, by thrombolysis or a catheter-based approach, is of extreme importance in achieving maximum benefit. While the upper time limit depends on specific factors in individual patients, it is clear that "every minute counts" and that patients treated within 1 to 3 h of the onset of symptoms generally benefit most. Although reduction of the mortality rate is more modest, the therapy remains of benefit for many patients seen 3 to 6 h after the onset of infarction, and some benefit appears to be possible up to 12 h, especially if chest discomfort is still present and ST segments remain elevated in ECG leads that do not yet demonstrate new Q waves. In addition to the possibility of early treatment, clinical factors that favor proceeding with thrombolytic therapy include anterior wall injury, hemodynamically complicated infarction, and widespread ECG evidence of myocardial jeopardy. Although patients (younger than 65 years) achieve a greater relative reduction in the mortality rate than elderly patients, the higher *absolute* mortality rate (15 to 25%) in elderly patients results in similar absolute reductions in the mortality rates for both age groups.

Intriguing data are accumulating to indicate that improved ventricular function and reduced mortality may also be achieved by *late coronary reperfusion*. The benefits of late reperfusion cannot be attributed to a reduction of infarct size but appear to result from improvement of tissue healing in the infarct zone with prevention of infarct expansion, enhancement of collateral flow, improvement of myocardial contractile performance, and reduction in the tendency to electrical instability. In addition, *hibernating myocardium* (i.e., poorly contractile myocardium in a zone that is supplied by a stenotic infarct-related coronary artery with slow antegrade perfusion, Chap. 244) may show improved contraction after angioplasty to increase coronary blood flow.

tPA is more effective than streptokinase at restoring full perfusion—i.e., TIMI grade 3 coronary flow—and has a small edge in improving survival as well. The current recommended regimen of tPA consists of a 15-mg bolus followed by 50 mg intravenously over the first 30 min, followed by 35 mg over the next 60 min. Streptokinase is administered as 1.5 million units (MU) intravenously over 1 h. Reteplase is administered in a double bolus regimen consisting of a 10-MU bolus given over 2 to 3 min followed by a second 10-MU bolus 30 min later.

Promising new pharmacologic regimens for reperfusion combine an intravenous glycoprotein IIb/IIIa inhibitor with a reduced dose of a thrombolytic agent. Such combination reperfusion regimens appear to facilitate the rate and extent of thrombolysis by inhibiting platelet aggregation, weakening the clot structure, and allowing penetration of the thrombolytic agent deeper into the clot.

Contraindications and Complications   Clear contraindications to the use of thrombolytic agents include a history of cerebrovascular hemorrhage at any time, a nonhemorrhagic stroke or other cerebrovascular event within the past year, marked hypertension (a reliably determined systolic arterial pressure >180 mmHg and/or a diastolic pressure >110 mmHg) at any time during the acute presentation, suspicion of aortic dissection, and active internal bleeding (excluding menses). While advanced age is associated with an increase in hemorrhagic complications, the benefit of thrombolytic therapy in the elderly appears to justify its use if no other contraindications are present and the amount of myocardium in jeopardy appears to be substantial.

Relative contraindications to thrombolytic therapy, which require careful assessment of the risk:benefit ratio, include current use of anticoagulants (international normalized ratio ≥2), a recent (<2 weeks) invasive or surgical procedure or prolonged (>10 min) cardiopulmonary resuscitation, known bleeding diasthesis, pregnancy, a hemorrhagic ophthalmic condition (e.g., hemorrhagic diabetic retinopathy), active peptic ulcer disease, and a history of severe hypertension that is currently adequately controlled. Because of the risk of an allergic reaction, patients should not receive streptokinase if that agent had been received within the preceding 5 days to 2 years.

Allergic reactions to streptokinase occur in approximately 2% of patients who receive it. While a minor degree of hypotension occurs in 4 to 10% of patients given this agent, marked hypotension occurs, although rarely, in association with severe allergic reactions.

Hemorrhage is the most frequent and potentially the most serious complication. Because bleeding episodes that require transfusion are more common when patients require invasive procedures, unnecessary venous or arterial interventions should be avoided in patients receiving thrombolytic agents. Hemorrhagic stroke is the most serious complication and occurs in approximately 0.5 to 0.9% of patients being treated with these agents. This rate increases with advancing age, with patients older than 70 years experiencing roughly twice the rate of intracranial hemorrhage as those younger than 65 years. Large-scale intervention trials have suggested that the rate of intracranial hemorrhage with tPA or rPA is slightly higher than that with streptokinase.

Routine angiography after thrombolysis with the intent of performing a PCI on underlying coronary artery stenoses in the culprit vessel is not recommended. Higher rates of abrupt closure of the infarct-related coronary artery with a need for urgent coronary artery bypass surgery as well as a trend toward an increase in mortality rate have been noted with this approach. Instead, after thrombolytic therapy, cardiac catheterization and coronary angiography should be carried out if there is evidence of either (1) failure of reperfusion (persistent chest pain and ST-segment elevation beyond 90 min) in which case a *rescue PCI* should be considered, or (2) coronary artery reocclusion (reelevation of ST segments and/or recurrent chest pain) or the development of recurrent ischemia (such as recurrent angina in the early hospital course or a positive exercise stress test before discharge), in which case an *elective PCI* should be considered. Coronary artery bypass surgery should be reserved for patients whose coronary anatomy is unsuited to angioplasty but in whom revascularization appears to be advisable because of extensive jeopardized myocardium or recurrent ischemia.

Primary Percutaneous Coronary Intervention (See also Chap. 245)   PCI, usually angioplasty and/or stenting without preceding thrombolysis, is also effective in restoring perfusion in AMI when carried out on an emergency basis in the first few hours of MI. It has the advantage of being applicable to patients who have contraindications to thrombolytic therapy but otherwise are considered appropriate candidates for reperfusion. It appears to be more effective than thrombolysis in opening occluded coronary arteries and, *when performed by*

experienced operators in dedicated medical centers, is associated with better short-term and long-term clinical outcomes. It remains to be determined whether the advantages of primary PCI reported from organized research efforts can be replicated in routine clinical practice. However, PCI is expensive in terms of personnel and facilities, and its applicability is seriously limited by its availability, around the clock, in only a minority of hospitals.

HOSPITAL PHASE MANAGEMENT

CORONARY CARE UNITS   These units are routinely equipped with a system that permits continuous monitoring of the cardiac rhythm of each patient and hemodynamic monitoring in selected patients. Defibrillators, respirators, noninvasive transthoracic pacemakers, and facilities for introducing pacing catheters and flow-directed balloon-tipped catheters are also usually available. Equally important is the organization of a highly trained team of nurses who can recognize arrhythmias; adjust the dosage of antiarrhythmic, vasoactive, and anticoagulant drugs; and perform cardiac resuscitation, including electroshock, when necessary.

Patients should be admitted to a coronary care unit early in their illness when it is expected that they will derive benefit from the sophisticated and expensive care provided. The availability of electrocardiographic monitoring and trained personnel outside the coronary care unit has made it possible to admit lower-risk patients (e.g., those not hemodynamically compromised and without active arrhythmias) to "intermediate care units."

The duration of stay in the coronary care unit is dictated by the ongoing need for intensive care. If AMI has been ruled out (ideally within 8 to 12 h) and symptoms are controlled with oral therapy, patients may be transferred out of the coronary care unit. Also, patients who have a confirmed AMI but who are considered to be at low risk (no prior infarction and no persistent chest discomfort, congestive heart failure, hypotension, or cardiac arrhythmias) may be safely transferred out of the coronary care unit in 24 to 36 h.

Activity   Factors that increase the work of the heart during the initial hours of infarction may increase the size of the infarct. Therefore, patients with AMI should be kept at bed rest for the first 12 h. However, in the absence of complications, patients should be encouraged, under supervision, to resume an upright posture by dangling their feet over the side of the bed and sitting in a chair within the first 24 h. This practice is both psychologically beneficial and usually results in a reduction in the pulmonary capillary wedge pressure. In the absence of hypotension and other complications, by the second or third day patients typically are ambulating in their room with increasing duration and frequency, and they may shower or stand at the sink to bathe. By day 3 or 4 after infarction, patients should be increasing their ambulation progressively to a goal of 600 ft at least three times a day.

Diet   Because of the risk of emesis and aspiration soon after MI, patients should receive either nothing or only clear liquids by mouth for the first 4 to 12 h. The typical coronary care unit diet should provide ≤30% of total calories as fat and have a cholesterol content of ≤300 mg/d. Complex carbohydrates should make up 50 to 55% of total calories. Portions should not be unusually large, and the menu should be enriched with foods that are high in potassium, magnesium, and fiber but low in sodium. Diabetes mellitus and hypertriglyceridemia are managed by restriction of concentrated sweets in the diet.

Bowels   Bed rest and the effect of the narcotics used for the relief of pain often lead to constipation. A bedside commode rather than a bedpan, a diet rich in bulk, and the routine use of a stool softener such as dioctyl sodium sulfosuccinate (200 mg/d) are recommended. If the patient remains constipated despite these measures, a laxative can be prescribed. Contrary to prior belief, it is safe to perform a gentle rectal examination on patients with AMI.

Sedation   Many patients require sedation during hospitalization to withstand the period of enforced inactivity with tranquillity. Diazepam (5 mg), oxazepam (15 to 30 mg), or lorazepam (0.5 to 2 mg), given three or four times daily, is usually effective. An additional dose of any of the above medications may be given at night to ensure adequate sleep. Attention to this problem is especially important during the first few days in the coronary care unit, where the atmosphere of 24-h vigilance may interfere with the patient's sleep. However, sedation is no substitute for reassuring, quiet surroundings. Many drugs used in the coronary care unit, such as atropine, H_2 blockers, and narcotics, can produce delirium, particularly in the elderly. This effect should not be confused with agitation, and it is wise to conduct a thorough review of the patient's medications before arbitrarily prescribing additional doses of anxiolytics.

PHARMACOTHERAPY

ANTITHROMBOTIC AGENTS The use of antiplatelet and antithrombin therapy during the initial phase of AMI is based on extensive laboratory and clinical evidence that thrombosis plays an important role in the pathogenesis of this condition. The primary goal of treatment with antiplatelet and antithrombin agents is to establish and maintain patency of the infarct-related artery. A secondary goal is to reduce the patient's tendency to thrombosis and thus the likelihood of mural thrombus formation or deep venous thrombosis, either of which could result in pulmonary embolization. The degree to which antiplatelet and antithrombin therapy achieves these goals partly determines how effectively it reduces the risk of mortality from AMI.

As noted previously (see "Initial Management in the Emergency Department," above), aspirin is the standard antiplatelet agent for patients with AMI. The most compelling evidence for the benefits of antiplatelet therapy (mainly with aspirin) in AMI is found in the comprehensive overview by the Antiplatelet Trialists' Collaboration. Data from nearly 20,000 patients with AMI enrolled in nine randomized trials were pooled and revealed a reduction in the mortality rate from 11.7% in control patients to 9.3% in patients receiving antiplatelet agents. This difference corresponds to the prevention of 24 deaths for every 1000 patients treated. Similarly, 2 strokes and 12 recurrent infarctions are prevented for every 1000 patients treated with antiplatelet therapy.

The glycoprotein IIb/IIIa receptor is the focus of intense investigation by basic and clinical scientists (Chap. 116). Because platelet-rich thrombi are more resistant to thrombolytic agents than platelet-poor thrombi and because platelet aggregates appear to play a role in reocclusion after initially successful thrombolysis, glycoprotein IIb/IIIa inhibition may facilitate thrombolysis and reduce the rate of reocclusion of reperfused vessels. Compounds have been developed that block the glycoprotein IIb/IIIa receptor. These drugs appear useful for preventing thrombotic complications in patients with AMI undergoing PCI and reduce the rate of the composite endpoint of death and recurrent AMI in the medical management of patients without ST-segment elevation at presentation.

The standard antithrombin agent used in clinical practice is unfractionated heparin (UFH). Despite numerous clinical trials, the precise role of heparin in patients treated with thrombolytic agents remains uncertain. The available data fail to show any convincing benefit of UFH with respect to either coronary arterial patency or mortality rate when UFH is added to a regimen of aspirin and a non-fibrin-specific thrombolytic agent such as streptokinase. Although not conclusively proven, it appears that the immediate administration of intravenous UFH, in addition to a regimen of aspirin and tPA, helps to facilitate thrombolysis and to establish and maintain patency of the infarct-related artery. This effect is achieved at the cost of a small increased risk of bleeding. Most clinicians who use tPA also administer a bolus and infusion of UFH, which should be administered as a bolus of 60 U/kg followed by a maintenance infusion of 12 U/kg per hour. The activated partial thromboplastin time during maintenance therapy should be 1.5 to 2 times the control value.

An alternative to UFH for anticoagulation of patients with AMI that is being used with increased frequency are the low-molecular-weight heparin preparations (LMWHs), which are formed by enzymatic or chemical depolymerization to produce saccharide chains of

varying length but with a mean molecular weight of about 5000 Da. The LMWHs have several advantages over UFH including an increased anti-factor Xa:IIa ratio, decreased sensitivity to platelet factor IV, a more stable reliable anticoagulant effect, and enhanced bioavailability, thereby permitting administration via the subcutaneous route. Because of the stable anticoagulant effect when LMWHs are used, routine monitoring of hematologic tests such as the activated partial thromboplastin time (aPTT) is not required. Although the LMWHs share many pharmacologic similarities, they also vary in a number of important features; and therefore these agents should be considered individually rather than as members of an interchangeable class of compounds. Of the LMWHs, nadroparin and dalteparin have been found to be similar to UFH in therapeutic effectiveness, while enoxaparin (1 mg/kg subcutaneously every 12 h) appears to be superior to UFH for reducing the mortality rate and cardiac ischemic events in patients with AMI who do not present with ST-segment elevation. Direct comparisons among the LMWHs have not been carried out.

Patients with an anterior location of the infarction, severe LV dysfunction, congestive heart failure, a history of embolism, two-dimensional echocardiographic evidence of mural thorombus, or atrial fibrillation are at increased risk of systemic or pulmonary thromboembolism. Such individuals should receive full therapeutic levels of antithrombin therapy (UFH or LMWHs) while hospitalized, followed by at least 3 months of warfarin therapy.

BETA-ADRENOCEPTOR BLOCKERS The benefits of beta blockers in patients with AMI can be divided into those that occur immediately when the drug is given acutely and those that accrue over the long term when the drug is given for secondary prevention after an index infarction. Acute intravenous beta blockade improves the myocardial oxygen supply-demand relationship, decreases pain, reduces infarct size, and decreases the incidence of serious ventricular arrhythmias. An overview of the data from 27,000 patients enrolled in nine randomized trials in the prethrombolytic era indicates that intravenous followed by oral beta blockade is associated with a 15% relative reduction in mortality, nonfatal reinfarction, and nonfatal cardiac arrest. In patients who undergo thrombolysis soon after the onset of chest pain, no incremental reduction in mortality rate is seen with beta blockers, but recurrent ischemia and reinfarction are reduced.

Beta blocker therapy after AMI thus is useful for most patients except those in whom it is specifically contraindicated (patients with heart failure or severely compromised LV function, heart block, orthostatic hypotension, or a history of asthma) and perhaps those whose excellent long-term prognosis (defined as an expected mortality rate of <1% per year) markedly diminishes any potential benefit (patients younger than 55 years with normal ventricular function, no complex ventricular ectopy, and no angina).

Although the data supporting the use of beta blockers in patients with AMI who do not present with ST-segment elevation are limited, the available evidence suggests that even among such patients, the use of beta blockers decreases the rates of cardiovascular mortality and reinfarction, and increases the probability of long-term survival.

ANGIOTENSIN CONVERTING ENZYME INHIBITORS Angiotensin-converting enzyme (ACE) inhibitors reduce the mortality rate after AMI, and the mortality benefits are additive to those achieved with aspirin and beta blockers. The maximum benefit is seen in high-risk patients (those who are elderly or have an anterior infarction, a prior infarction, and/or globally depressed LV function), but evidence suggests that a short-term benefit occurs when ACE inhibitors are prescribed unselectively to all hemodynamically stable patients with AMI (i.e., those with a systolic pressure >100 mmHg). The mechanism involves a reduction in ventricular remodeling after infarction (see "Ventricular Dysfunction," below) with a subsequent reduction in the risk of congestive heart failure (CHF). The rate of recurrent infarction also may be lower in patients treated chronically with ACE inhibitors after infarction.

ACE inhibitors should be prescribed within 24 h to all patients with AMI and overt CHF as well as to hemodynamically stable patients with ST-segment elevation or left bundle branch block. There is little evidence to support the immediate use of ACE inhibitors in patients with AMI who present without ST-segment changes or only with ST-segment depression without CHF. Before hospital discharge, LV function should be assessed with an imaging study. ACE inhibitors should be continued indefinitely in patients who have clinically evident CHF, in patients whom an imaging study shows a reduction in global LV function or a large regional wall motion abnormality, or in those who are hypertensive.

OTHER AGENTS   Although the actual impact on the mortality rate is slight (three to four lives saved per 1000 patients treated), *nitrates* (intravenous or oral) may be useful in the relief of pain associated with AMI. Favorable effects on the ischemic process and ventricular remodeling (see below) have led many physicians to routinely use intravenous nitroglycerin (5 to 10 μg/min initial dose and up to 200 μg/min as long as hemodynamic stability is maintained) for the first 24 to 48 h after the onset of infarction.

Results of multiple trials of different calcium antagonists have failed to establish a role for these agents in the treatment of most patients with AMI, in contrast to the more consistent data that exist for other drugs (e.g., beta blockers, aspirin, thrombolytic agents). The routine use of calcium antagonists cannot be recommended.

A metabolic supportive measure that has shown promise in several small-scale trials of patients with AMI is the administration of a solution of glucose-insulin-potassium (GIK). A GIK infusion lowers the concentration of plasma free fatty acids and improves ventricular performance. Strict control of blood glucose in diabetic patients with AMI has been shown to reduce the mortality rate. It remains to be determined whether infusions of GIK should be administered to all patients with AMI.

Intracellular *magnesium* levels are frequently reduced in patients with AMI, but this deficit is not adequately reflected in serum measurements, as magnesium is predominantly an intracellular ion and <1% of its total body stores is intravascular. Whether giving routine empirical supplemental infusions of magnesium to high-risk patients with AMI is beneficial remains an open question. At present, serum magnesium should be measured in all patients on admission, and any demonstrated deficits should be corrected to minimize the risk of arrhythmias. There does not appear to be any benefit in the routine use of magnesium when it is administered relatively late (after more than 6 h) or to patients with an uncomplicated AMI who have a low mortality risk. Its role in high-risk patients is under investigation.

COMPLICATIONS AND THEIR TREATMENT

VENTRICULAR DYSFUNCTION   After AMI, the LV undergoes a series of changes in shape, size, and thickness in both the infarcted and noninfarcted segments. This process is referred to as *ventricular remodeling* and generally precedes the development of clinically evident CHF in the months to years after infarction. Soon after AMI, the LV begins to dilate. Acutely, this results from expansion of the infarct (i.e., slippage of muscle bundles, disruption of normal myocardial cells, and tissue loss within the necrotic zone, resulting in disproportionate thinning and elongation of the infarct zone). Later, lengthening of the noninfarcted segments occurs as well. The overall chamber enlargement that occurs is related to the size and location of the infarct, with greater dilation following infarction of the apex of the LV and causing more marked hemodynamic impairment, more frequent heart failure, and a poorer prognosis. Progressive dilation and its clinical consequences may be ameliorated by therapy with ACE inhibitors and other vasodilators (e.g., nitrates). Thus, in patients with an ejection fraction <40%, regardless of whether or not heart failure is present, ACE inhibitors should be prescribed.

HEMODYNAMIC ASSESSMENT   Pump failure is now the primary cause of in-hospital death from AMI. The extent of ischemic

necrosis correlates well with the degree of pump failure and with mortality, both early (within 10 days of infarction) and later. The most common clinical signs are pulmonary rales and S_3 and S_4 gallop rhythms. Pulmonary congestion is also frequently seen on the chest roentgenogram. Elevated LV filling pressure and elevated pulmonary artery pressure are the characteristic hemodynamic findings, but these findings may result from a reduction of ventricular compliance (diastolic failure) and/or a reduction of stroke volume with secondary cardiac dilation (systolic failure) (Chap. 231).

A classification originally proposed by Killip divides patients into four groups: class I, no signs of pulmonary or venous congestion; class II, moderate heart failure as evidenced by rales at the lung bases, S_3 gallop, tachypnea, or signs of failure of the right side of the heart, including venous and hepatic congestion; class III, severe heart failure, pulmonary edema; and class IV, shock with systolic pressure <90 mmHg and evidence of peripheral vasoconstriction, peripheral cyanosis, mental confusion, and oliguria. When this classification was established in 1967, the expected hospital mortality rate of patients in these classes was as follows: class I, 0 to 5%; class II, 10 to 20%; class III, 35 to 45%; and class IV, 85 to 95%. With advances in management, the mortality rate in each class has fallen, perhaps by as much as one-third to one-half.

Hemodynamic evidence of abnormal LV function appears when contraction is seriously impaired in 20 to 25% of the LV. Infarction of $\geq$40% of the LV usually results in cardiogenic shock (see below). Positioning of a balloon flotation catheter in the pulmonary artery permits monitoring of LV filling pressure; this technique is useful in patients who exhibit hypotension and/or clinical evidence of CHF. Cardiac output can also be determined with a pulmonary artery catheter. With the addition of intraarterial pressure monitoring, systemic vascular resistance can be calculated as a guide to adjusting vasopressor and vasodilator therapy. Some patients with AMI have markedly elevated LV filling pressures (>22 mmHg) and normal cardiac indexes [>2.6 and >3.6 L/(min/m²)], while others have relatively low LV filling pressures (<15 mmHg) and reduced cardiac indexes. The former patients usually benefit from diuresis, while the latter may respond to volume expansion by means of intravenous administration of colloid-containing solutions.

Hypovolemia   Hypovolemia is an easily corrected condition that may contribute to the hypotension and vascular collapse associated with AMI in some patients. It may be secondary to previous diuretic use, to reduced fluid intake during the early stages of the illness, and/or to vomiting associated with pain or medications. Consequently, hypovolemia should be identified and corrected in patients with AMI and hypotension before more vigorous forms of therapy are begun. Central venous pressure reflects RV rather than LV filling pressure and is an inadequate guide for adjustment of blood volume, since LV function is almost always affected much more adversely than RV function in patients with AMI. The optimal LV filling or pulmonary artery wedge pressure may vary considerably among patients. Each patient's ideal level (generally ~20 mmHg) is reached by cautious fluid administration during careful monitoring of oxygenation and cardiac output. Eventually, the cardiac output level plateaus, and further increases in LV filling pressure only increase congestive symptoms and decrease systemic oxygenation without raising arterial pressure.

℞ **TREATMENT**   The management of CHF in association with AMI is similar to that of acute heart failure secondary to other forms of heart disease (avoidance of hypoxemia, diuresis, afterload reduction, inotropic support) (Chap. 232), except that the benefits of digitalis administration to patients with AMI are unimpressive. By contrast, diuretic agents are extremely effective, as they diminish pulmonary congestion in the presence of systolic and/or diastolic heart failure. Left ventricular filling pressure falls and orthopnea and dyspnea improve after the intravenous administration of furosemide or other loop diuretics. These drugs should be used with caution, however, as they can result in a massive diuresis with associated decreases in plasma volume, cardiac output, systemic blood pressure, and hence coronary perfusion. Nitrates in various forms may be used to decrease preload and congestive symptoms. Oral isosorbide dinitrate, topical nitroglycerin ointment, or intravenous nitroglycerin all have the advantage over a diuretic of lowering preload through venodilation without decreasing the total plasma volume. In addition, nitrates may improve ventricular compliance if ischemia is present, as ischemia causes an elevation of LV filling pressure. The patient with pulmonary edema is treated as described in Chap. 232, but vasodilators must be used with caution to prevent serious hypotension. As noted earlier, ACE inhibitors are an ideal class of drugs for management of ventricular dysfunction after AMI, especially for the long term.

CARDIOGENIC SHOCK   In recent years, efforts to reduce infarct size and prompt treatment of ongoing ischemia and other complications of MI appear to have reduced the incidence of cardiogenic shock from 20% to about 7%. Only 10% of patients with this condition present with it on admission, while 90% develop it during hospitalization. Typically, patients who develop cardiogenic shock have severe multivessel coronary artery disease with evidence of "piecemeal" necrosis extending outward from the original infarct zone (Fig. 243-4).

Cardiogenic shock should be considered to be a form of severe LV failure. This syndrome is characterized by marked hypotension with systolic arterial pressure of <80 mmHg and a markedly reduced cardiac index [<1.8 L/(min/m²)] in the face of an elevated LV filling (pulmonary capillary wedge) pressure (>18 mmHg). Hypotension alone is not a basis for the diagnosis of cardiogenic shock, because many patients who make an uneventful recovery have serious hypotension (systolic pressure of <80 mmHg) for several hours. Such patients often have low LV filling pressures, and their hypotension usually resolves with the administration of intravenous fluids. In contrast to hypovolemic hypotension, cardiogenic shock is generally associated

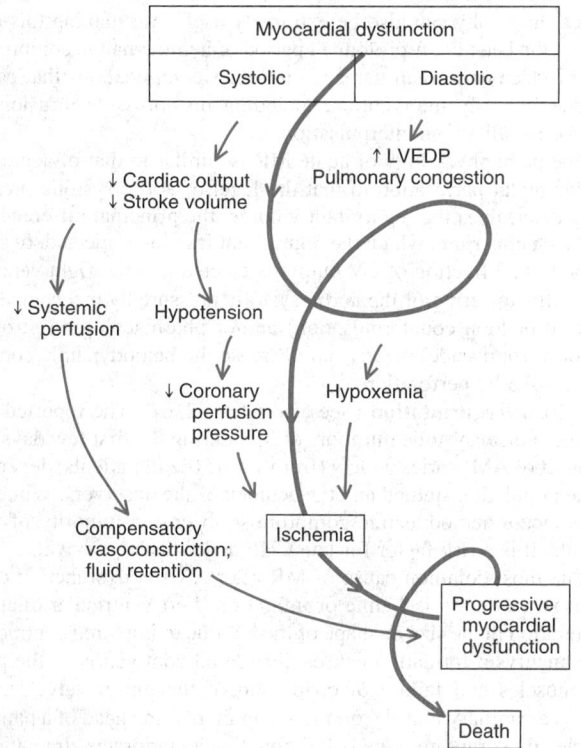

FIGURE 243-4 Pathophysiology of cardiogenic shock: Systolic and diastolic myocardial dysfunction occurs after MI, resulting in pulmonary congestion and a reduction in cardiac output. Systemic and coronary hypoperfusion occur, resulting in progressive ischemia. Although a number of compensatory mechanisms are activated in an attempt to support the circulation, these compensatory mechanisms may become maladaptive and produce a worsening of hemodynamics. A vicious circle of progressive myocardial dysfunction occurs that ultimately results in death if it is not interrupted. LVEDP, left ventricular end-diastolic pressure. (*From Hollenberg et al.*)

with a mortality rate of >70%; however, recent efforts to restore perfusion by coronary angioplasty or surgical revascularization suggest that this high mortality rate can be lowered by as much as one-half.

Risk factors for the in-hospital development of shock include advanced age, a depressed LV ejection fraction on admission, a large infarct, previous MI, and a history of diabetes mellitus. Patients with several of these risk factors should be considered for cardiac catheterization and mechanical reperfusion (by PCI or surgery) before the development of shock.

Pathophysiology of Severe Power Failure   A marked reduction in the quantity of contracting myocardium is the cause of cardiogenic shock in AMI. The initial insult reduces arterial pressure, and the reduction in coronary perfusion pressure and myocardial blood flow initiates a vicious cycle that impairs myocardial function further and may increase the size of the infarct (Fig. 243-4). Arrhythmias and metabolic acidosis also contribute to this deterioration, because they are the result of inadequate perfusion. This positive feedback loop accounts for the high mortality rate associated with the shock syndrome.

TREATMENT   The physiology and ominous prognosis of cardiogenic shock dictate that all patients with this condition should, if possible, have continuous monitoring of arterial pressure and of LV filling pressure (as reflected in the pulmonary capillary wedge pressure measured with a pulmonary artery balloon catheter) as well as frequent determinations of cardiac output. When pulmonary edema coexists, endotracheal intubation may be necessary to ensure oxygenation. The relief of pain is important, as some vasodepressor reflex activity may be a response to severe pain. However, narcotics should be used cautiously, in view of their propensity to lower arterial pressure. The primary objective of treatment is to maintain coronary perfusion by raising the arterial blood pressure with vasopressors (see below), intraaortic balloon counterpulsation, and manipulation of blood volume to a level that ensures an optimum LV filling pressure (~20 mmHg). The latter may require either infusion of crystalloid or diuresis.

Vasopressors   Various intravenous drugs may be used to augment arterial pressure and cardiac output in patients with cardiogenic shock. All have important disadvantages or problems, and none has been shown to change the outcome in patients with established shock. *Isoproterenol* is a sympathomimetic amine that is now rarely used in the treatment of shock due to MI. Although this agent increases contractility, it also produces peripheral vasodilation and increases the heart rate. The resulting increase in myocardial oxygen consumption and reduction of coronary perfusion pressure may extend the area of ischemic injury. *Norepinephrine* (Chap. 72) is a potent α-adrenergic agonist with powerful vasoconstrictor properties that also possesses β-adrenergic activity and therefore enhances contractility. Because the increase in afterload and contractility associated with its use causes a marked increase in myocardial oxygen consumption, norepinephrine should be reserved for patients in desperate situations or for those with cardiogenic shock and reduced systemic vascular resistance. It should be started at a dosage of 2 to 4 μg/min. If pressure cannot be maintained with a dosage of 15 μg/min, it is unlikely that a further increase will be beneficial.

Dopamine (Chap. 72) is useful in many patients with severe power failure. At low doses (2 to 10 μg/kg per min), the drug has positive chronotropic and inotropic effects as a consequence of β receptor stimulation. At higher doses, a vasoconstrictor effect results from α receptor stimulation. At lower doses (≤2 μg/kg per min), dopamine also has the unique effect of dilating the renal and splanchnic vascular beds, and it apparently has little effect on myocardial oxygen consumption. Intravenous dopamine is started at an infusion rate of 2 to 5 μg/kg per min, and the dosage is increased every 2 to 5 min up to a maximum of 20 to 50 μg/kg per min. Systolic arterial blood pressure should be maintained at ~90 mmHg. *Dobutamine* is a synthetic sympathomimetic amine with positive inotropic action and minimal positive chronotropic or peripheral vasoconstrictive activity in the usual dosage range of 2.5 to 10 μg/kg per min. It should not be used when a vasoconstrictor effect is required. However, in patients with less profound degrees of hypotension, dobutamine may be an extremely useful agent, particularly if positive chronotropy is to be avoided.

Amrinone and *milrinone* are positive inotropic agents without catecholamine structure or activity that inhibit phosphodiesterase. These drugs resemble dobutamine in pharmacologic activity, although they have a more potent vasodilating action. For amrinone, an initial loading dose of 0.75 mg/kg is given over 2 to 3 min. If effective, it is followed by an infusion of 5 to 10 μg/kg per min. If necessary, the dose may then be increased up to 15 μg/kg per min for short periods. Milrinone is given as a loading dose of 50 μg/kg over 10 min followed by a maintenance infusion of 0.375 to 0.75 μg/kg per min.

Aortic Counterpulsation In cardiogenic shock, mechanical assistance with an intraaortic balloon pumping (IABP) system capable of augmenting both diastolic pressure and cardiac output may be helpful. A sausage-shaped balloon at the end of a catheter is introduced percutaneously into the aorta via the femoral artery, and the balloon is automatically inflated during early diastole, thereby augmenting coronary blood flow. The balloon collapses in early systole, thereby reducing the afterload against which LV ejection takes place. Improvement in hemodynamic status has been achieved with balloon pumping in a large number of patients. In the absence of early revascularization, however, long-term survival after this mode of therapy in patients with cardiogenic shock is still disappointing. Intraaortic balloon pumping may best be reserved for patients whose condition merits mechanical (surgical or angioplastic) intervention (e.g., patients with continuing ischemia, ventricular septal rupture, or mitral regurgitation) and in whom a successful result is likely to reverse the cardiogenic shock. This technique is contraindicated if aortic regurgitation is present or aortic dissection is suspected.

Therapy for the shock syndrome secondary to MI, while improving gradually as a result of meticulous attention to the details outlined above, continues to be disappointing overall because a large fraction of patients with the syndrome have large areas of infarcted myocardium with severe, diffuse coronary atherosclerosis. The SHOCK trial was a randomized study comparing emergency revascularization (PCI or coronary artery bypass grafting) with initial medical stabilization and delayed revascularization as clinically indicated for patients with cardiogenic shock. Although the 30-day mortality rates in the two groups did not differ significantly, the 6-month and 1-year mortality rates in the emergency revascularization group were significantly lower than the corresponding rates in the stabilization and delayed revascularization group. Patients younger than 75 years showed particular benefit from emergency revascularization. However, few patients developing cardiogenic shock have prompt access to these expensive techniques. It is hoped that the widespread and early application of thrombolytic therapy will reduce the amount of myocardium that becomes necrotic and thereby reduce the incidence of this syndrome.

RIGHT VENTRICULAR INFARCTION Approximately one-third of patients with inferoposterior infarction demonstrate at least a minor degree of RV necrosis. An occasional patient with inferoposterior LV infarction also has extensive RV infarction, and rare patients present with infarction limited primarily to the RV. Clinically significant RV infarction causes signs of severe RV failure [jugular venous distention, Kussmaul's sign (Chap. 225), hepatomegaly] with or without hypotension. ST-segment elevations of right-sided precordial ECG leads, particularly lead V_4R, are frequently present in the first 24 h in patients with RV infarction. Two-dimensional echocardiography is helpful in determining the degree of RV dysfunction. Catheterization of the right side of the heart often reveals a distinctive hemodynamic pattern resembling cardiac tamponade or constrictive pericarditis (steep right atrial "y" descent and an early diastolic dip and plateau in

right ventricular waveforms) (Chap. 239). Therapy consists of volume expansion to maintain adequate RV preload and efforts to improve LV performance with attendant reduction in pulmonary capillary wedge and pulmonary arterial pressures.

MECHANICAL CAUSES OF HEART FAILURE Free Wall Rupture Myocardial rupture is a dramatic complication of AMI that is most likely to occur during the first week after the onset of symptoms; its frequency increases with the age of the patient. First infarction, a history of hypertension, no history of angina pectoris, and a relatively large Q-wave infarct are associated with a higher incidence of cardiac rupture. The clinical presentation typically is a sudden loss of pulse, blood pressure and consciousness while the ECG continues to show sinus rhythm (apparent electromechanical dissociation or pulseless electrical activity). The myocardium continues to contract, but forward flow is not maintained as blood escapes into the pericardium. Cardiac tamponade (Chap. 239) ensues, and closed-chest massage is ineffective. This condition is almost universally fatal, although dramatic cases of urgent pericardiotensis followed by successful surgical repair have been reported.

Ventricular Septal Defect The pathogenesis of perforation of the ventricular septum is similar to that of free wall rupture, but the chance of successful therapy is greater. Patients with ventricular septal rupture present with sudden, severe LV failure in association with the appearance of a pansystolic murmur, often accompanied by a parasternal thrill. It is often impossible to differentiate this condition from rupture of a papillary muscle with resulting mitral regurgitation (MR), and the presence in both conditions of a tall "v" wave in the pulmonary capillary wedge pressure further complicates the differentiation. The diagnosis of ventricular septal defect can be established by the demonstration of a left-to-right shunt (i.e., an oxygen step-up at the level of the RV) by means of limited cardiac catheterization performed at the bedside with a flow-directed balloon catheter. Color flow Doppler echocardiography can also be extremely useful for making this diagnosis at the bedside. A prolonged period of hemodynamic compromise may produce end-organ damage and other complications that can be avoided by early intervention, including nitroprusside infusion and intraaortic balloon counterpulsation.

The pathophysiology of acute MR is similar to that of acute ventricular septal perforation in that the level of aortic systolic pressure partly determines the regurgitant volume, the principal difference being the chamber into which the regurgitant fraction is ejected. In septal perforation, a fraction of LV output is ejected into the right ventricle. As in MR, lowering of the aortic systolic pressure by mechanical (intraaortic balloon counterpulsation) and/or pharmacologic (nitroglycerin or nitroprusside) means can decrease the hemodynamic compromise caused by perforation.

Mitral Regurgitation (See also Chap. 236) The reported incidence of apical systolic murmurs of MR during the first few days after the onset of AMI varies widely (from 10 to 50% of patients) depending on the population studied and the acumen of the observers. While MR causes acute hemodynamic compromise in only a minority of these patients, it is a risk factor for late CHF and reduced survival.

The most common cause of MR after AMI is dysfunction of the mitral valve due to ischemia or infarction. Left ventricular dilatation or alteration in the size or shape of the LV due to impaired contractility or to aneurysm formation causes disordered contraction of the papillary muscles and failure of coaptation of the mitral valve leaflets. Rarely, a papillary muscle, or, more commonly, the head of a papillary muscle, may rupture. Then, LV function deteriorates dramatically, with superimposition of severe MR. The major element in the differential diagnosis is perforation of the ventricular septum as discussed above. Surgical repair or replacement of the mitral valve may lead to dramatic improvement in patients in whom acute heart failure results primarily from severe MR due to papillary muscle rupture or dysfunction and in whom global ventricular function is relatively good.

If aortic systolic pressure is lowered in patients with MR, a greater fraction of the LV output will be ejected antegrade, thus lessening the regurgitant fraction. To this end, both intraaortic balloon counterpulsation (IABC), which lowers the aortic systolic pressure mechanically, and the infusion of nitroglycerin or sodium nitroprusside, which reduce systemic vascular resistance, have been used with success in the interim management of patients with severe MR in the presence of AMI. Ideally, definitive operative treatment should be postponed until pulmonary congestion has cleared and the infarct has had time to heal. However, if the patient's hemodynamic and/or clinical condition does not improve or stabilize, surgical treatment should be undertaken, even in the acute stage.

ARRHYTHMIAS (See also Chaps. 229 and 230) The incidence of arrhythmias after AMI is higher in patients seen early after the onset of symptoms. The mechanisms responsible for infarction-related arrhythmias include autonomic nervous system imbalance, electrolyte disturbances, ischemia, and slowed conduction in zones of ischemic myocardium. An arrhythmia can usually be managed successfully if trained personnel and appropriate equipment are available when it develops. Since most deaths from arrhythmia occur during the first few hours after infarction, the effectiveness of treatment relates directly to the speed with which patients come under medical observation. The prompt management of arrhythmias constitutes a significant advance in the treatment of myocardial infarction.

Ventricular Premature Beats Infrequent, sporadic ventricular premature depolarizations occur in almost all patients with AMI and do not require therapy. Whereas in the past, frequent, multifocal, or early diastolic ventricular extrasystoles (so-called warning arrhythmias) were routinely treated with antiarrhythmic drugs to reduce the risk of development of ventricular tachycardia and ventricular fibrillation, pharmacologic therapy is now reserved for patients with sustained ventricular arrhythmias. Prophylactic antiarrhythmic therapy (either intravenous lidocaine early or oral agents later) is contraindicated for ventricular premature beats in the absence of clinically important ventricular tachyarrhythmias, as such therapy may actually increase the mortality rate. β-Adrenoceptor blocking agents are effective in abolishing ventricular ectopic activity in patients with AMI and in the prevention of ventricular fibrillation. As described above (see "β-Adrenoceptor Blockers"), they should be used routinely in patients without contraindications. In addition, hypokalemia and hypomagnesemia are risk factors for ventricular fibrillation in patients with AMI; the serum potassium concentration should be adjusted to approximately 4.5 mmol/L and magnesium to about 2.0 mmol/L.

Ventricular Tachycardia and Fibrillation Within the first 24 h of AMI, ventricular tachycardia and fibrillation can occur without prior warning arrhythmias. The occurrence of ventricular fibrillation can be reduced by prophylactic administration of intravenous lidocaine. However, prophylactic use of lidocaine has not been shown to reduce overall mortality from AMI. In fact, in addition to causing possible noncardiac complications, lidocaine may predispose to an excess risk of bradycardia and asystole. For these reasons, and with earlier treatment of active ischemia, more frequent use of beta-blocking agents, and the nearly universal success of electrical cardioversion or defibrillation, routine prophylactic antiarrhythmic drug therapy is no longer recommended. It should be reserved for patients who cannot reach a hospital or for those treated in hospitals that lack the constant presence in the coronary care unit of a physician or nurse trained in the recognition and treatment of ventricular fibrillation.

Sustained ventricular tachycardia that is well tolerated hemodynamically should be treated with an intravenous regimen of lidocaine (bolus of 1.0 to 1.5 mg/kg; infusion of 20 to 50 μg/kg per min), procainamide (bolus of 15 mg/kg over 20 to 30 min; infusion of 1 to 4 mg/min), or amiodarone (bolus of 75 to 150 mg over 10 to 15 min followed by infusion of 1.0 mg/min for 6 h and then 0.5 mg/min); if it does not stop promptly, electroversion should be used (Chap. 230). An unsynchronized discharge of 200 to 300 J (defibrillation) is used immediately in patients with ventricular fibrillation or when ventricular tachycardia causes hemodynamic deterioration. Ventricular tachycardia or fibrillation that is refractory to electroshock may be more responsive after the patient is treated with epinephrine (1 mg intravenously or 10 mL of a 1:10,000 solution via the intracardiac route), bretylium (a 5 mg/kg bolus), or amiodarone (a 75 to 150 mg bolus).

Ventricular arrhythmias, including the unusual form of ventricular tachycardia known as *torsade de pointes* (Chap. 230), may occur in patients with AMI as a consequence of other concurrent problems (such as hypoxia, hypokalemia, or other electrolyte disturbances) or of the toxic effects of an agent being administered to the patient (such as digoxin or quinidine). A search for such secondary causes should always be undertaken.

Although the in-hospital mortality rate is increased, the long-term survival is good in patients who survive to hospital discharge after *primary* ventricular fibrillation, i.e., ventricular fibrillation that is a primary response to acute ischemia and is not associated with predisposing factors such as CHF, shock, bundle branch block, or ventricular aneurysm. This result is in sharp contrast to the poor prognosis for patients who develop ventricular fibrillation *secondary* to severe pump failure. For patients who develop ventricular tachycardia or ventricular fibrillation late in their hospital course (i.e., after the first 48 h), the mortality rate is increased both in-hospital and during long-term follow-up. Such patients should be considered for electrophysiologic study (Chap. 230).

Accelerated Idioventricular Rhythm Accelerated idioventricular rhythm (AIVR, "slow ventricular tachycardia"), a ventricular rhythm with a rate of 60 to 100 beats per minute, occurs in 25% of patients with AMI. It often occurs transiently during thrombolytic therapy at the time of reperfusion. The rate of AIVR is usually similar to that of the sinus rhythm that precedes and follows it, and this similarity of rate plus the relatively minor hemodynamic effects make this rhythm more difficult to detect except by electrocardiographic monitoring. For the most part, AIVR is benign and does not presage the development of classic ventricular tachycardia. Most episodes of AIVR do not require treatment if the patient is monitored carefully, as degeneration into a more serious arrhythmia is rare, and, if it occurs, AIVR can generally be readily treated with a drug that increases the sinus rate (atropine).

Supraventricular Arrhythmias Sinus tachycardia is the most common supraventricular arrhythmia. If it occurs secondary to another cause (such as anemia, fever, heart failure, or a metabolic derangement), the primary problem should be treated first. However, if it appears to be due to sympathetic overstimulation, for example, as part of a hyperdynamic state, then treatment with a beta blocker is indicated. Other common arrhythmias in this group are atrial flutter and atrial fibrillation, which are often secondary to LV failure. Digoxin is usually the treatment of choice for supraventricular arrhythmias if heart failure is present. If heart failure is absent, beta blockers, verapamil, or diltiazem are suitable alternatives for controlling the ventricular rate, as they may also help to control ischemia. If the abnormal rhythm persists for >2 h with a ventricular rate in excess of 120 beats per minute, or if tachycardia induces heart failure, shock, or ischemia (as manifested by recurrent pain or ECG changes), a synchronized electroshock (100 to 200 J) should be used.

Accelerated junctional rhythms have diverse causes but may occur in patients with inferoposterior infarction. Digitalis excess must be ruled out. In some patients with severely compromised LV function, the loss of appropriately timed atrial systole results in a marked decrease in cardiac output. Right atrial or coronary sinus pacing is indicated in such instances.

Sinus Bradycardia Treatment of sinus bradycardia is indicated if hemodynamic compromise results from the slow heart rate. Atropine is the most useful drug for increasing heart rate and should be given intravenously in doses of 0.5 mg initially. If the rate remains below 50 to 60 bpm, additional doses of 0.2 mg, up to a total of 2.0 mg, may be given. Persistent bradycardia (<40 bpm) despite atropine may be treated with electrical pacing. Isoproterenol should be avoided.

Atrioventricular and Intraventricular Conduction Disturbances (See also Chap. 229) Both the in-hospital mortality rate and the post-discharge mortality rate of patients who have complete atrioventricular (AV) block in association with anterior infarction are markedly higher than those of patients who develop AV block with inferior infarction. This difference is related to the fact that heart block in inferior infarction is commonly a result of increased vagal tone and/or the release of adenosine and therefore is transient. In anterior wall infarction, heart block is usually related to ischemic malfunction of the conduction system, which commonly is associated with extensive myocardial necrosis.

Temporary electrical pacing provides an effective means of increasing the heart rate of patients with bradycardia due to AV block. However, acceleration of the heart rate may have only a limited impact on prognosis in patients with anterior wall infarction and complete heart block in whom the large size of the infarct is the major factor determining outcome. It should be carried out if it improves hemodynamics, however. Pacing does appear to be beneficial in patients with inferoposterior infarction who have complete heart block associated with heart failure, hypotension, marked bradycardia, or significant ventricular ectopic activity. A subgroup of these patients, those with RV infarction, often respond poorly to ventricular pacing because of the loss of the atrial contribution to ventricular filling. In such patients, dual-chamber AV sequential pacing may be required.

External noninvasive pacing electrodes should be positioned in a "demand" mode for patients with sinus bradycardia (rate <50 bpm) that is unresponsive to drug therapy, Mobitz II second-degree AV block, third-degree heart block, or bilateral bundle branch block (e.g., right bundle branch block plus left anterior fascicular block). Retrospective studies suggest that permanent pacing may reduce the long-term risk of sudden death due to bradyarrhythmias in the rare patient who develops combined persistent bifascicular and transient third-degree heart block during the acute phase of MI.

OTHER COMPLICATIONS   Recurrent Chest Discomfort
Recurrent angina develops in ~25% of patients hospitalized for AMI. This percentage is even higher in patients who undergo successful thrombolysis. Since recurrent or persistent ischemia often heralds extension of the original infarct or reinfarction in a new myocardial zone and is associated with a doubling of risk after AMI, patients with these symptoms should be considered for repeat thrombolysis or referred for prompt coronary arteriography and mechanical revascularization. Repeat administration of a thrombolytic agent is an alternative to early mechanical revascularization.

Pericarditis (See also Chap. 239)   Pericardial friction rubs and/or pericardial pain are frequently encountered in patients with transmural AMI. This complication can usually be managed with aspirin (650 mg qid). It is important to diagnose the chest pain of pericarditis accurately, since failure to recognize it may lead to the erroneous diagnosis of recurrent ischemic pain and/or infarct extension, with resulting inappropriate use of anticoagulants, nitrates, beta blockers, or coronary arteriography. When it occurs, complaints of pain radiating to either trapezius muscle is helpful since such a pattern of discomfort is typical of pericarditis but rarely occurs with ischemic discomfort. Anticoagulants potentially could cause tamponade in the presence of acute pericarditis (as manifested by either pain or persistent rub) and therefore should not be used unless there is a compelling indication.

Thromboembolism Clinically apparent thromboembolism complicates AMI in ~10% of cases, but embolic lesions are found in 20% of patients in necropsy series, suggesting that thromboembolism is often clinically silent. Thromboembolism is considered to be at least an important contributing cause of death in 25% of patients with AMI who die after admission to the hospital. Arterial emboli originate from LV mural thrombi, while most pulmonary emboli arise in the leg veins.

Thromboembolism typically occurs in association with large infarcts (especially anterior), CHF, and a LV thrombus detected by echocardiography. The incidence of arterial embolism from a clot originating in the ventricle at the site of an infarction is small but real. Two-dimensional echocardiography reveals LV thrombi in about one-third of patients with anterior wall infarction but in few patients with inferior or posterior infarction. Arterial embolism often presents as a major complication, such as hemiparesis when the cerebral circulation is involved or hypertension if the renal circulation is compromised. When a thrombus has been clearly demonstrated by echocardiographic or other techniques or when a large area of regional wall motion abnormality is seen even in the absence of a detectable mural thrombus, systemic anticoagulation should be undertaken (in the absence of contraindications), as the incidence of embolic complications appears to be markedly lowered by such therapy. The appropriate duration of therapy is unknown, but 3 to 6 months is probably prudent.

Left Ventricular Aneurysm   The term *ventricular aneurysm* is usually used to describe *dyskinesis* or local expansile paradoxical wall motion. Normally functioning myocardial fibers must shorten more if stroke volume and cardiac output are to be maintained in patients with ventricular aneurysm; if they cannot, overall ventricular function is impaired. True aneurysms are composed of scar tissue and neither predispose to nor are associated with cardiac rupture.

The complications of LV aneurysm do not usually occur for weeks to months after AMI; they include CHF, arterial embolism, and ventricular arrhythmias. Apical aneurysms are the most common and the most easily detected by clinical examination. The physical finding of greatest value is a double, diffuse, or displaced apical impulse. Ventricular aneurysms are readily detected by two-dimensional echocardiography, which may also reveal a mural thrombus in an aneurysm.

Rarely, myocardial rupture may be contained by a local area of pericardium, along with organizing thrombus and hematoma. Over time, this *pseudoaneurysm* enlarges, maintaining communication with the LV cavity through a narrow neck. Because a pseudoaneurysm often ruptures spontaneously, it should be surgically repaired if recognized.

POSTINFARCTION RISK STRATIFICATION AND MANAGEMENT

Many clinical factors have been identified that are associated with an increase in cardiovascular risk after initial recovery from AMI. Some of the most important factors include persistent ischemia (spontaneous or provoked), depressed LV ejection fraction (<40%), rales above the lung bases on physical examination or congestion on chest radiograph, and symptomatic ventricular arrhythmias. Other features associated with increased risk include a history of previous myocardial infarction, age over 70 years, diabetes, prolonged sinus tachycardia, hypotension, ST-segment changes at rest without angina ("silent ischemia"), an abnormal signal-averaged ECG, nonpatency of the infarct-related coronary artery (if angiography is undertaken), and persistent advanced heart block or a new intraventricular conduction abnormality on the ECG. Therapy must be individualized on the basis of the relative importance of the risk(s) present.

The goal of preventing reinfarction and death after recovery from AMI has led to strategies to evaluate risk after infarction. Early after AMI, this evaluation generally involves the use of noninvasive testing. In stable patients, submaximal exercise stress testing may be carried out before hospital discharge to detect residual ischemia and ventricular ectopy and to provide the patient with a guideline for exercise in the early recovery period. Alternatively, or in addition, a maximal (symptom-limited) exercise stress test may be carried out 4 to 6 weeks after infarction. Evaluation of LV function at rest and during exercise is usually warranted as well. Recognition of a depressed LV ejection fraction by echocardiography or radionuclide ventriculography identifies patients who should receive ACE inhibitors (see "Angiotensin-Converting Enzyme Inhibitors," above). Patients in whom angina is induced at relatively low workloads, those who have a large reversible defect on perfusion imaging or a depressed ejection fraction, those with demonstrable ischemia, and those in whom exercise provokes symptomatic ventricular arrhythmias should be considered at high risk for recurrent MI or death from arrhythmia; and cardiac catheterization with coronary angiography and/or invasive electrophysiologic evaluation is advised.

Exercise tests also aid in formulating an individualized exercise prescription, which can be much more vigorous in patients who tolerate exercise without any of the above-mentioned adverse signs. Additionally, predischarge stress testing may provide an important psychological benefit, building the patient's confidence by demonstrating a reasonable exercise tolerance. Furthermore, particularly when no arrhythmias or signs of ischemia are identified, the patient benefits by the physician's reassurance that objective evidence suggests no immediate jeopardy.

In many hospitals a cardiac rehabilitation program with progressive exercise is initiated in the hospital and continued after discharge. Ideally, such programs should include an educational component that informs patients about their disease and its risk factors.

The usual duration of hospitalization for an uncomplicated AMI is about 5 days. The remainder of the convalescent phase may be accomplished at home. During the first 2 weeks, the patient should be encouraged to increase activity by walking about the house and outdoors in good weather. Normal sexual activity may be resumed during this period. After 2 weeks, the physician must regulate the patient's activity on the basis of exercise tolerance. Most patients will be able to return to work within 2 to 4 weeks.

SECONDARY PREVENTION OF INFARCTION

Various secondary preventive measures are at least partly responsible for the improvement in the long-term mortality and morbidity rates after AMI. Long-term treatment with an antiplatelet agent (usually aspirin) after AMI is associated with a 25% reduction in the risk of recurrent infarction, stroke, or cardiovascular mortality (36 fewer events for every 1000 patients treated). In addition, in patients taking aspirin chronically, AMIs tend to be smaller and are more likely to be non-Q-wave in nature. An alternative antiplatelet agent that may be used for secondary prevention in patients intolerant of aspirin is the ADP receptor antagonist clopidogrel (75 mg orally daily). ACE inhibitors should be used indefinitely by patients with clinically evident heart failure, a moderate decrease in global ejection fraction, or a large regional wall motion abnormality to prevent late ventricular remodeling and recurrent ischemic events.

The chronic routine use of oral β-adrenoceptor blockers for at least 2 years after AMI is supported by well-conducted, placebo-controlled trials that have convincingly demonstrated reductions in the rates of total mortality, sudden death, and, in some instances, reinfarction. In contrast, calcium antagonists are not recommended for routine secondary prevention.

Evidence suggests that warfarin lowers the risk of late mortality and the incidence of reinfarction after AMI. Since studies comparing aspirin and warfarin therapy separately or in combination have not yet been completed, most physicians prescribe aspirin routinely for all patients without contraindications and add warfarin for patients at increased risk of embolism (see "Thromboembolism," above).

Finally, risk factors for *atherosclerosis* (Chap. 241) should be discussed with the patient, and, when possible, favorably modified. In particular, efforts should be made to ensure the cessation of smoking and the control of hypertension and hyperlipidemia (the target low-density lipoprotein level is <100 mg/dL). In addition, regular physical exercise and reduction of emotional stress should be encouraged. The benefits of hormone replacement therapy in postmenopausal women recovering from MI remain controversial. The initiation of a combination of estrogen plus progestin is associated with an increased risk of cardiovascular events within the first year but may reduce events in later years (HERS Trial). Thus, hormone replacement therapy prevention of coronary events should not be given *de novo* to postmenopausal women after AMI. Postmenopausal women already taking estrogen plus progestin at the time of AMI may continue that therapy.

BIBLIOGRAPHY

AMERICAN HEART ASSOCIATION: *Heart and Stroke Facts: 2000 Statistical Supplement.* Dallas, American Heart Association, 2000

ANTMAN EM, BRAUNWALD E: Acute myocardial infarction, in *Heart Disease*, 6th ed, E Braunwald, Zipes DP, Libby P (eds). Philadelphia, Saunders, 2001

—— et al: Abciximab facilitates the rate and extent of thrombolysis: Results of the Thrombolysis in Myocardial Infarction (TIMI) 14 trial. Circulation 99:2720, 1999

—— et al: Assessment of the treatment effect of enoxaparin for unstable angina/non-Q-wave myocardial infarction: TIMI 11B-ESSENCE meta-analysis. Circulation 100: 1602, 1999

BARRON HV et al: Use of reperfusion therapy for acute myocardial infarction in the United States: Data from the National Registry of Myocardial Infarction 2. Circulation 97: 1150, 1998

CAIRNS JA et al: Antithrombotic agents in coronary artery disease. Chest 114:611S, 1998

FALK E et al: Coronary plaque disruption. Circulation 92:657, 1995

FIBRINOLYTIC THERAPY TRIALISTS (FTT) COLLABORATIVE GROUP: Indications for fibrinolytic therapy in suspected acute myocardial infarction: Collaborative overview of early mortality and major morbidity results from all randomised trials of more than 1000 patients. Lancet 343:311, 1994

FUTTERMAN LG, LEMBERG L: Update on management of acute myocardial infarction: Facilitated percutaneous coronary intervention. Am J Crit Care 9:70, 2000

GOLDMAN LE, EISENBERG MJ: Identification and management of patients with failed thrombolysis after acute myocardial infarction. Ann Intern Med 132:556, 2000

GOTTLIEB SS et al: Effect of beta-blockade on mortality among high-risk and low-risk patients after myocardial infarction. N Engl J Med 339:489, 1998

HOCHMAN JS et al: Early revascularization in acute myocardial infarction complicated by cardiogenic shock. N Engl J Med 341:625, 1999

HOLLENBERG SM et al: Cardiogenic shock. Ann Intern Med 131:47, 1999

KINCH JW, RYAN TJ: Right ventricular infarction. N Engl J Med 330:1211, 1994

MICHAELS AD, GOLDSCHLAGER N: Risk stratification after acute myocardial infarction in the reperfusion era. Prog Cardiovasc Dis 42:273, 2000

NATIONAL HEART ATTACK ALERT PROGRAM COORDINATING COMMITTEE—60 MINUTES TO TREATMENT WORKING GROUP: Emergency department: Rapid identification and treatment of patients with acute myocardial infarction. Ann Emerg Med 23:311, 1994

PFEFFER JM et al: Angiotensin-converting enzyme inhibition and ventricular remodeling after myocardial infarction. Annu Rev Physiol 57:805, 1995

RYAN TJ et al: 1999 Update: ACC/AHA guidelines for the management of patients with acute myocardial infarction. A report of the American College of Cardiology/American Heart Association Task Force on Practice Guidelines (Committee on Management of Acute Myocardial Infarction). J Am Coll Cardiol 34:890, 1999

SCARBOROUGH RM et al: Platelet glycoprotein IIb/IIIa antagonists: What are the relevant issues concerning their pharmacology and clinical use? Circulation 100:437, 1999

THE GUSTO INVESTIGATORS: An international randomized trial comparing four thrombolytic strategies for acute myocardial infarction. N Engl J Med 329:673, 1993

TIEFEBRUNN AJ et al: Clinical experience with primary percutaneous transluminal coronary angioplasty compared with alteplase (recombinant tissue-type plasminogen activator) in patients with acute myocardial infarction: A report from the Second National Registry of Myocardial Infarction (NRMI-2). J Am Coll Cardiol 31:1240, 1998

TOPOL EJ: Acute myocardial infarction: Thrombolysis. Heart 83:122, 2000

YUSUF S et al: Beta blockade during and after myocardial infarction: An overview of the randomized trials. Prog Cardiovasc Dis 27:335, 1985

ZIMMERMAN J et al: Diagnostic marker cooperative study for the diagnosis of myocardial infarction. Circulation 99:1671, 1999

244

Andrew P. Selwyn, Eugene Braunwald

ISCHEMIC HEART DISEASE

ETIOLOGY AND PATHOPHYSIOLOGY

Ischemia refers to a lack of oxygen due to inadequate perfusion, which results from an imbalance between oxygen supply and demand. The most common cause of myocardial ischemia is atherosclerotic disease of epicardial coronary arteries. Ischemic heart disease (IHD) is the most common, serious, chronic, life-threatening illness in the United States, where more than 11 million persons have IHD. This condition causes more deaths and disability and incurs greater economic costs than any other illness in the developed world.

By reducing the lumen of the coronary arteries, atherosclerosis reduces myocardial perfusion in the basal state or limits appropriate increases in perfusion when the demand for flow is augmented, as occurs during exertion or excitement. Coronary blood flow can also be limited by spasm, arterial thrombi, and, rarely, coronary emboli as well as by ostial narrowing due to luetic aortitis. Congenital abnormalities, such as anomalous origin of the left anterior descending coronary artery from the pulmonary artery, may cause myocardial ischemia and infarction in infancy, but this cause is very rare in adults. Myocardial ischemia can also occur if myocardial oxygen demands are markedly increased, as in severe ventricular hypertrophy due to aortic stenosis. The latter can present with angina that is indistinguishable from that caused by coronary atherosclerosis. A reduction in the oxygen-carrying capacity of the blood, as in extremely severe anemia or in the presence of carboxyhemoglobin, is a rare cause of myocardial ischemia. Not infrequently, two or more causes of ischemia will coexist, such as an increase in oxygen demand due to left ventricular hypertrophy and a reduction in oxygen supply secondary to coronary atherosclerosis and anemia. Often such a combination leads to clinical manifestations of ischemia.

Although the large epicardial coronary arteries are capable of constriction and relaxation, in healthy persons they serve largely as conduits and are referred to as *conductance vessels*, while the intramyocardial arterioles normally exhibit striking changes in tone and are therefore referred to as *resistance vessels*. Abnormal constriction or failure of normal dilation of the coronary resistance vessels can also cause ischemia. When it causes angina this condition is referred to as *microvascular angina*.

The normal coronary circulation is dominated and controlled by the heart's requirements for oxygen. This need is met by the ability of the coronary vascular bed to vary its resistance (and therefore blood flow) considerably while the myocardium extracts a high and relatively fixed percentage of oxygen. Normally, intramyocardial resistance vessels demonstrate an immense capacity for dilation. For example, the changing oxygen needs with exercise and emotional stress affect coronary vascular resistance and in this manner regulate the supply of oxygen and substrate to the myocardium (*metabolic regulation*). The coronary resistance vessels also adapt to physiologic alterations in blood pressure in order to maintain coronary blood flow at levels appropriate to myocardial needs (*autoregulation*).

CORONARY ATHEROSCLEROSIS (See also Chap. 241) Epicardial coronary arteries are a major site of atherosclerotic disease. The major risk factors for atherosclerosis [high plasma low-density lipoprotein (LDL), low plasma high-density lipoprotein (HDL), cigarette smoking, hypertension, and diabetes mellitus] are thought to disturb the normal functions of the vascular endothelium. These functions include local control of vascular tone, maintenance of an anticoagulant surface, and defense against inflammatory cells. The loss of these defenses leads to inappropriate constriction, luminal clot formation, and abnormal interactions with blood monocytes and platelets. The latter leads to subintimal collections of fat, cells, and debris (i.e., atherosclerotic plaques), which develop at irregular rates in different segments of the epicardial coronary tree and lead eventually to segmental reductions in cross-sectional area (stenosis). The relationship between pulsatile flow and luminal stenosis is complex, but experiments have shown that when a stenosis reduces the cross-sectional area by approximately 75%, a full range of increases in flow to meet increased myocardial demand is not possible. When the luminal area is reduced by more than approximately 80%, blood flow at rest may be reduced, and further minor decreases in the stenotic orifice can reduce coronary flow dramatically and cause myocardial ischemia.

Segmental atherosclerotic narrowing of epicardial coronary arteries is caused most commonly by the formation of a plaque, which is subject to fissuring, hemorrhage, and thrombosis. Any of these events can temporarily worsen the obstruction, reduce coronary blood flow, and cause clinical manifestations of myocardial ischemia, as described below. The location of the obstruction will influence the quantity of myocardium rendered ischemic and thus determine the severity of the clinical manifestations. Severe coronary narrowing and myocardial ischemia are frequently accompanied by the development of collateral vessels, especially when the narrowing develops gradually. When well developed, such vessels can, by themselves, provide sufficient blood flow to sustain the viability of the myocardium at rest but not during conditions of increased demand.

Once stenosis of a proximal epicardial artery has reduced the cross-sectional area by more than approximately 70%, the distal resistance vessels (when they function normally) dilate to reduce vascular resistance and maintain coronary blood flow. A pressure gradient develops across the proximal stenosis, and poststenotic pressure falls. When the resistance vessels are maximally dilated, myocardial blood flow becomes dependent on the pressure in the coronary artery distal to the obstruction. In these circumstances ischemia in the region perfused by the stenotic artery can be precipitated by increases in myocardial oxygen demands caused by physical activity, emotional stress, and/or tachycardia. Changes in the caliber of the stenosed coronary artery due to physiologic vasomotion, loss of endothelial control of dilation, pathologic spasm, or small platelet plugs can all upset the critical balance between oxygen supply and demand and thus precipitate myocardial ischemia.

EFFECTS OF ISCHEMIA The inadequate perfusion induced by coronary atherosclerosis may cause transient disturbances of the mechanical, biochemical, and electrical functions of the myocardium. The abrupt development of severe ischemia, as occurs with total or subtotal occlusion, is associated with almost instantaneous failure of normal muscle contraction and relaxation. The relatively poor perfusion of the subendocardium causes more intense ischemia of this portion of the wall. Ischemia of large portions of the ventricle will cause transient left ventricular failure, and if the papillary muscles are involved, mitral regurgitation can complicate this event. When ischemia is transient, it may be associated with angina pectoris; when it is prolonged, it can lead to myocardial necrosis and scarring with or without the clinical picture of acute myocardial infarction (Chap. 243). Coronary atherosclerosis is a focal process that usually causes nonuniform ischemia. Regional disturbances of ventricular contractility cause segmental akinesis or, in severe cases, bulging (dyskinesia), which can greatly reduce myocardial pump function.

Underlying these mechanical disturbances are a wide range of abnormalities in cell metabolism, function, and structure. When oxygenated, the normal myocardium metabolizes fatty acids and glucose to carbon dioxide and water. With severe oxygen deprivation, fatty acids cannot be oxidized, and glucose is broken down to lactate; intracellular pH is reduced, as are the myocardial stores of high-energy phosphates, ATP, and creatine phosphate. Impaired cell membrane function leads to potassium leakage and the uptake of sodium by myocytes. The severity and duration of the imbalance between myocardial oxygen supply and demand will determine whether the damage is reversible (0 to 20 min for total occlusion) or whether it is permanent, with subsequent myocardial necrosis (>20 min).

Ischemia also causes characteristic changes in the electrocardiogram (ECG) such as repolarization abnormalities, as evidenced by inversion of the T wave and, when more severe, by displacement of the ST segment (Chap. 226). Transient ST-segment depression often reflects subendocardial ischemia, while transient ST-segment elevation is thought to be caused by more severe transmural ischemia. Another important consequence of myocardial ischemia is electrical instability, which may lead to ventricular tachycardia or ventricular fibrillation (Chap. 230). Most patients who die suddenly from IHD do so as a result of ischemia-induced malignant ventricular tachyarrhythmias (Chap. 39).

ASYMPTOMATIC VERSUS SYMPTOMATIC ISCHEMIC HEART DISEASE (IHD) Postmortem studies on accident victims and military casualties in western countries have shown that coronary atherosclerosis often begins to develop prior to age 20 and is widespread even among adults who were asymptomatic during life.

When all age groups are considered, IHD is the most common cause of death not only in men but also in women (Chap. 6). Exercise stress tests in asymptomatic persons may show evidence of silent myocardial ischemia, i.e., exercise-induced ECG changes not accompanied by angina; coronary angiographic studies of such persons may reveal obstructive [coronary artery disease (CAD) (Chap. 228)]. Postmortem examination of patients with obstructive CAD without a history of any clinical manifestations of myocardial ischemia often shows macroscopic scars secondary to myocardial infarction in regions supplied by diseased coronary arteries. According to population studies, approximately 25% of patients who survive acute myocardial infarction may not reach medical attention, and these patients carry the same adverse prognosis as those who present with the classic clinical syndrome (Chap. 243). Sudden death may be unheralded and is a common presenting manifestation of IHD (Chap. 39). Patients can also present with cardiomegaly and heart failure secondary to ischemic damage of the left ventricular myocardium that may have caused no symptoms prior to the development of heart failure; this condition is referred to as *ischemic cardiomyopathy*. In contrast to the asymptomatic phase of IHD, the symptomatic phase is characterized by chest discomfort due to either angina pectoris or acute myocardial infarction (Chap. 243). Having entered the symptomatic phase, the patient may exhibit a stable or progressive course, revert to the asymptomatic stage, or suddenly die.

STABLE ANGINA PECTORIS

This episodic clinical syndrome is due to transient myocardial ischemia. Various diseases that cause myocardial ischemia as well as the numerous forms of discomfort with which it may be confused are discussed in Chap. 13. Males constitute approximately 70% of all patients with angina pectoris and an even greater fraction of those younger than 50 years of age.

HISTORY The typical patient with angina is a 50- to 60-year-old man or 65- to 75-year-old woman who seeks medical help for chest discomfort, usually described as heaviness, pressure, squeezing, smothering, or choking and only rarely as frank pain. When the patient is asked to localize the sensation, he or she will typically press on the sternum, sometimes with a clenched fist, to indicate a squeezing, central, substernal discomfort. This symptom is usually crescendo-decrescendo in nature and lasts 1 to 5 min. Angina can radiate to the left shoulder and to both arms and especially to the ulnar surfaces of the forearm and hand. It can also arise in or radiate to the back, neck, jaw, teeth, and epigastrium.

Although episodes of angina are typically caused by exertion (e.g., exercise, hurrying, or sexual activity) or emotion (e.g., stress, anger, fright, or frustration) and are relieved by rest, they may also occur at rest (see "Unstable Angina Pectoris," p. 1408) and at night while the patient is recumbent (angina decubitus). The patient may be awakened at night distressed by typical chest discomfort and dyspnea. Nocturnal angina may be due to episodic tachycardia or activities such as micturition. It can also be due to the expansion of the intrathoracic blood volume that occurs with recumbency, which causes an increase in cardiac size and myocardial oxygen demand that lead to ischemia and transient left ventricular failure.

The threshold for the development of angina pectoris varies from person to person and may vary by time of day and emotional state. Many patients report a fixed threshold for angina, which occurs predictably at a certain level of activity. In these patients coronary stenosis and myocardial oxygen supply are fixed and ischemia is precipitated by an increase in myocardial oxygen demand. In other patients the threshold for angina may vary considerably within any given day and from day to day. In such patients variations in oxygen supply, most likely due to changes in coronary vascular tone, may play an important role. A patient may report symptoms upon minor exertion in the morning (a short walk or shaving) yet by midday may be capable of much greater effort without symptoms. Angina may also be precipitated by unfamiliar tasks, a heavy meal, or exposure to cold.

Sharp, fleeting chest pain or prolonged, dull aches localized to the left submammary area are rarely due to myocardial ischemia. However, angina pectoris may be atypical in location and may not be strictly related to provoking factors. In addition, this symptom may exacerbate and remit over days, weeks, or months. Its occurrence can be seasonal, being more frequent in the winter in temperate climates. Anginal "equivalents" are symptoms of myocardial ischemia other than angina. These include dyspnea, fatigue, and faintness and are more common in the elderly.

Systematic questioning of the patient with suspected IHD is important to uncover a positive family history of premature IHD (under the age of 45 years in first-degree male relatives and under 55 in female relatives), diabetes, hyperlipidemia, hypertension, cigarette smoking, and other risk factors for coronary atherosclerosis. The history of typical angina pectoris establishes the diagnosis of IHD until proven otherwise. In patients with atypical angina (Chap. 13), coexistence of advanced age, male sex, the postmenopausal state, and risk factors for atherosclerosis (Chap. 241) increase the likelihood of important coronary disease.

PHYSICAL EXAMINATION The physical examination is often normal in the patient with stable angina. Rarely, the general examination reveals signs of risk factors associated with coronary atherosclerosis such as xanthelasma, xanthomas (Chap. 241), or diabetic skin lesions. There may also be signs of anemia, thyroid disease, and nicotine stains on the fingertips from cigarette smoking. Palpation can reveal thickened or absent peripheral arteries, signs of cardiac enlargement, and abnormal contraction of the cardiac impulse (left ventricular akinesia or dyskinesia). Examination of the fundi may reveal increased light reflexes and arteriovenous nicking as evidence of hypertension (Table 35-2), while auscultation can uncover arterial bruits, a third and/or fourth heart sound, and, if acute ischemia or previous infarction has impaired papillary muscle function, an apical systolic murmur due to mitral regurgitation. These auscultatory signs are best appreciated with the patient in the left decubitus position. Aortic stenosis, aortic regurgitation (Chap. 236), pulmonary hypertension (Chap. 260), and hypertrophic cardiomyopathy (Chap. 238) must be excluded, since these disorders may cause angina in the absence of coronary atherosclerosis. Examination during an anginal attack is useful, since ischemia can cause transient left ventricular failure with the appearance of a third and/or fourth heart sound, a dyskinetic cardiac apex, mitral regurgitation, and even pulmonary edema.

LABORATORY EXAMINATION Although the diagnosis of IHD can be made with confidence from the clinical examination, a number of simple laboratory tests can be helpful. The urine should be examined for evidence of diabetes mellitus and renal disease, since both of these conditions accelerate atherosclerosis. Similarly, examination of the blood should include measurements of lipids (cholesterol—total, low density, high density—and triglycerides), glucose, creatinine, hematocrit, and, if indicated based on the physical examination, thyroid function. A chest x-ray is important, since it may show the consequences of IHD, i.e., cardiac enlargement, ventricular aneurysm, or signs of heart failure. These signs can support the diagnosis of IHD and are important in assessing the degree of cardiac damage and the effects of treatment for heart failure.

Electrocardiogram A 12-lead ECG recorded at rest is normal in about half the patients with typical angina pectoris, but there may be signs of an old myocardial infarction (Chap. 226). Although repolarization abnormalities, i.e., T-wave and ST-segment changes and intraventricular conduction disturbances at rest, are suggestive of IHD, they are nonspecific, since they can also occur in pericardial, myocardial, and valvular heart disease or transiently with anxiety, changes in posture, drugs, or esophageal disease. Typical ST-segment and T-wave changes that accompany episodes of angina pectoris and disappear thereafter are more specific. The most characteristic changes include displacement of the ST segment that is similar in every way to that induced during a stress test (see below). The ST segment is usually depressed during angina but may be elevated—sometimes strikingly so—in Prinzmetal's angina.

Stress Testing   The most widely used test both for the diagnosis of IHD and establishing the prognosis involves recording the 12-lead ECG before, during, and after exercise on a treadmill or using a bicycle ergometer. The test consists of a standardized incremental increase in external workload while the patient's ECG, symptoms, and arm blood pressure are monitored. Performance is usually symptom-limited, and the test is discontinued upon evidence of chest discomfort, severe shortness of breath, dizziness, fatigue, ST-segment depression of >0.2 mV (2 mm), a fall in systolic blood pressure exceeding 10 mmHg, or the development of a ventricular tachyarrhythmia. This test seeks to discover any limitation in exercise performance and establish the relationship between chest discomfort and the typical ECG signs of myocardial ischemia. The ischemic ST-segment response is generally defined as flat depression of the ST segment of more than 0.1 mV below the baseline (i.e., the PR segment) and lasting longer than 0.08 s (Fig. 244-1). Upsloping or junctional ST-segment changes are not considered characteristic of ischemia and do not constitute a positive test. Although T-wave abnormalities, conduction disturbances, and ventricular arrhythmias that develop during exercise should be noted, they are also not diagnostic. Negative exercise tests in which the target heart rate (85% of maximal heart rate for age and sex) is not achieved are considered to be nondiagnostic. When applying and interpreting ECG stress testing, one must first consider the probability that CAD exists in the patient or population under study (i.e., pretest probability). Overall, false-positive or -negative results can occur in one-third of cases. However, a positive result on exercise indicates that the likelihood of CAD is 98% in males over 50 years of age with a history of typical angina pectoris who develop chest discomfort during the test. The likelihood decreases progressively and significantly if the patient has atypical or no chest pain by history and/or during the test. The incidence of false-positive tests is significantly increased in asymptomatic men under the age of 40 or in premenopausal women with no risk factors for premature atherosclerosis. It is also increased in patients taking cardioactive drugs, such as digitalis and quinidine, or in those with intraventricular conduction disturbances, resting abnormalities of the ST segment and T wave, myocardial hypertrophy, or abnormal serum potassium levels. Obstructive disease limited to the circumflex coronary artery may result in a false-negative stress test since the posterior portion of the heart which this vessel supplies is not well represented on the surface 12-lead ECG. Since the overall

sensitivity of exercise stress electrocardiography is only about 75%, a negative result does not exclude CAD, although it makes the likelihood of three-vessel or left main CAD extremely unlikely.

The physician should be present throughout the exercise test, and it is important to measure total duration of exercise, the times to the onset of ischemic ST-segment change and chest discomfort, the external work performed (generally expressed as a stage of exercise), and the internal cardiac work performed; the last is represented by the heart rate–blood pressure product. The depth of the ST-segment depression and the time needed for recovery of these ECG changes are also important. Because the risks of exercise testing are small but real—estimated at one fatality and two nonfatal complications per 10,000 tests—equipment for resuscitation should be available. Modified (heart rate–limited rather than symptom-limited) exercise tests can be performed safely in patients as early as 6 days after myocardial infarction. Contraindications to exercise stress testing include acute myocardial infarction (<4–5 days), rest angina <48 h, unstable rhythm, severe aortic stenosis, acute myocarditis, uncontrolled heart failure, and active infective endocarditis.

The normal response to graded exercise includes a progressive increase in heart rate and blood pressure. Failure of the blood pressure to increase or an actual decrease in blood pressure with signs of ischemia during the test is an important adverse prognostic sign, since it may reflect ischemia-induced global left ventricular dysfunction. The development of angina and/or severe (>0.2 mV) ST-segment depression at a low workload, i.e., before completion of stage II of the Bruce protocol, and ST-segment depression that persists for more than 5 min after the termination of exercise increases the specificity of the test and suggests severe ischemic heart disease and a high risk of future adverse events.

When the resting ECG is abnormal (e.g., Wolff-Parkinson-White syndrome, >1 mm of resting ST-segment depression, left bundle branch block, paced ventricular rhythm), information gained from an exercise test can be enhanced by stress myocardial perfusion imaging after the intravenous administration of a radioisotope such as thallium 201 or technetium 99m sestamibi during exercise (or a pharmacologic stress) (Chap. 227); the imaging is carried out both immediately after cessation of exercise to detect reversible ischemia and 4 h later to confirm reversible ischemia and regions of infarction (Fig. 244-2).

An important fraction of patients who need noninvasive stress testing to identify myocardial ischemia and increased risk of coronary events cannot exercise because of peripheral vascular or musculoskeletal disease, exertional dyspnea, or deconditioning. In these circumstances intravenous dipyridamole or adenosine can be used in place of exercise. The development of a transient perfusion defect with a tracer such as radioactive thallium or technetium 99m sestamibi is used to detect myocardial ischemia. Ambulatory monitoring of the ECG can assess myocardial ischemia as episodes of ST-segment depression. These techniques are sensitive and capable of identifying patients with ischemia who are at increased risk of coronary events.

Two-dimensional echocardiography of the left ventricle can assess both global and regional wall motion abnormalities due to myocardial infarction or persistent ischemia (Chap. 227). Stress (exercise or dobutamine) echocardiography may cause the emergence of regions of akinesis or dyskinesis not present at rest. Stress echocardiography, like stress myocardial perfusion imaging, is more sensitive than exercise electrocardiography in the diagnosis of IHD. The relative advantages of stress echocardiography and stress radionuclide perfusion imaging in the diagnosis of IHD are shown in Table 244-1.

Echocardiography or radionuclide angiography should be carried out to assess left ventricular function in patients with chronic stable angina and in patients with a history of a prior myocardial infarction, pathologic Q waves, or clinical evidence of heart failure.

Coronary Arteriography   (See also Chap. 228)   This diagnostic method outlines the coronary anatomy and can be used to detect important evidence of coronary atherosclerosis or to exclude this condition. By this means, one can assess the severity of obstructive lesions and, when coronary arteriography is combined with left ventricular

FIGURE 244-1   Lead V₄ at rest (*top*) and after 4½ min of exercise (*bottom*). There is 3 mm (0.3 mV) of horizontal ST-segment depression, indicating a positive test for ischemia. [*Modified from BR Chaitman, in E Braunwald et al (eds): Heart Disease, 6th ed, Philadelphia, Saunders, 2001.*]

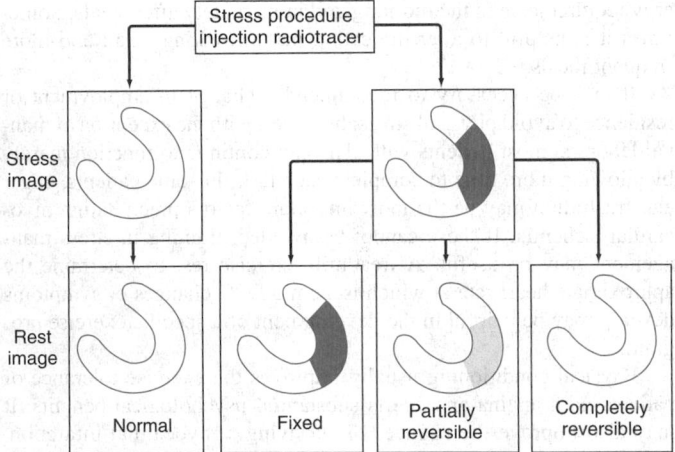

FIGURE 244-2 Interpretation of stress (exercise) and rest myocardial perfusion images. A normal image will show homogeneous accumulation of radiotracer on the exercise and rest (or delayed) image. An area with decreased uptake of the radiotracer (which appears as a darker area on a perfusion image) is referred to as a *defect*. A patient with a fixed perfusion defect will have an abnormal exercise image and an identical rest or delayed redistribution image (scarring). A partially reversible perfusion defect appears as an abnormal exercise image and an improved but still abnormal rest image (ischemia and scarring). A reversible perfusion defect appears as an abnormal exercise image and a normal rest or delayed image (ischemia). *[From FJ Wackers, in GA Beller (ed), Chronic Ischemic Heart Disease, in E Braunwald (series ed), Atlas of Heart Diseases, Philadelphia, Current Medicine, 1994.]*

angiocardiography, can evaluate both global and regional function of the left ventricle.

Indications Coronary arteriography is indicated in (1) patients with chronic stable angina pectoris who are severely symptomatic despite medical therapy and who are being considered for revascularization, i.e., a percutaneous coronary intervention (PCI) or coronary artery bypass grafting (CABG); (2) patients with troublesome symptoms that present diagnostic difficulties in whom there is need to confirm or rule out the diagnosis of IHD; (3) patients with known or possible angina pectoris who have survived sudden cardiac death; and (4) patients judged to be at high risk of sustaining coronary events based on signs of severe ischemia on noninvasive testing, regardless of the presence or severity of symptoms (see below).

Examples of other clinical situations include:

1. Patients with chest discomfort suggestive of angina pectoris but a negative or nondiagnostic stress test who require a definitive diagnosis for guiding medical management, alleviating psychological stress, career or family planning, or insurance purposes.
2. Patients who have been admitted repeatedly to the hospital for suspected acute myocardial infarction but in whom this diagnosis has not been established and in whom the presence or absence of CAD should be determined.
3. Patients with careers that involve the safety of others (e.g., airline pilots) who have questionable symptoms, suspicious or positive noninvasive tests, and in whom there are reasonable doubts about the state of the coronary arteries.
4. Patients with aortic stenosis or hypertrophic cardiomyopathy and angina in whom the chest pain could be due to IHD.
5. Male patients aged 45 and females aged 55 years of age or older who are to undergo a cardiac operation, such as valve replacement or repair and who may or may not have clinical evidence of myocardial ischemia.
6. Patients who are at high risk after myocardial infarction because of the recurrence of angina or the presence of heart failure, frequent ventricular premature contractions, or signs of ischemia in the stress test.
7. Patients with angina pectoris, regardless of severity, in whom noninvasive testing indicates a high risk of coronary events.

8. Patients in whom coronary spasm or another nonatherosclerotic cause of myocardial ischemia (e.g., coronary artery anomaly, Kawasaki's disease) is suspected.

PROGNOSIS

The principal prognostic indicators in patients with IHD are the functional state of the left ventricle, the location and severity of coronary artery narrowing, and the severity or activity of myocardial ischemia. Angina pectoris of recent onset, unstable angina, angina that is unresponsive or poorly responsive to medical therapy or is accompanied by symptoms of congestive heart failure all indicate an increased risk for adverse coronary events. The same is true for the physical signs of heart failure, episodes of pulmonary edema, transient third heart sounds, or mitral regurgitation or for echocardiographic (or roentgenographic) evidence of cardiac enlargement. An abnormal resting ECG or positive evidence of myocardial ischemia during a stress test also indicates increased risk. Most importantly, the following signs during noninvasive testing indicate a high risk for coronary events: a strongly positive exercise test showing onset of myocardial ischemia at low workloads [≥0.1 mV ST-segment depression before completion of stage II (Bruce protocol) of the exercise test; ≥0.2 mV ST depression in any stage; ST depression for >5 min following the cessation of exercise; a decline in systolic pressure >10 mmHg during exercise; the development of ventricular tachyarrhythmias during exercise]; the development of large or multiple perfusion defects or increased lung uptake during stress radioisotope perfusion imaging; and a decrease in left ventricular ejection fraction during exercise on radionuclide ventriculography or during stress echocardiography. Conversely, patients who can complete stage III of the Bruce exercise protocol and have a normal stress perfusion scan or negative stress echocardiographic evaluation are at very low risk of future coronary events.

On cardiac catheterization, elevations in left ventricular end-diastolic pressure and ventricular volume and a reduced ejection fraction are the most important signs of left ventricular dysfunction and are associated with a poor prognosis. Patients with chest discomfort but normal left ventricular function and normal coronary arteries have an excellent prognosis. In patients with normal left ventricular function and mild angina but with critical stenoses (≥70% luminal diameter) of one, two, or three epicardial coronary arteries, the 5-year mortality rates are approximately 2, 8, and 11 percent, respectively. Obstructive lesions of the left anterior descending coronary artery proximal to the origin of the first septal artery are associated with a greater risk than are lesions of the right or left circumflex coronary artery, since the former vessel usually perfuses a greater quantity of myocardium. Stenosis (>50% luminal diameter) of the left main coronary artery is

Table 244-1 Comparative Advantages of Stress Echocardiography and Stress Radionuclide Perfusion Imaging in Diagnosis of CAD

Advantages of stress echocardiography
1. Higher specificity
2. Versatility—more extensive evaluation of cardiac anatomy and function
3. Greater convenience/efficacy/availability
4. Lower cost

Advantages of stress perfusion imaging
1. Higher technical success rate
2. Higher sensitivity—especially for single vessel coronary disease involving the left circumflex
3. Better accuracy in evaluating possible ischemia when multiple resting LV wall motion abnormalities are present
4. More extensive published data base—especially in evaluation of prognosis

SOURCE: ACC/AHA/ACP-ASIM Guidelines for the Management of Patients with Chronic Stable Angina: A report of the American College of Cardiology/American Heart Association Task Force on Practice Guidelines (Committee on Management of Patients with Chronic Stable Angina). J Am Coll Cardiol 33:2092, 1999.

associated with a mortality rate of about 15% per year. The segmental atherosclerotic plaques in epicardial arteries go through phases of inflammatory cellular activity, degeneration, endothelial instability, abnormal vasomotion, platelet aggregation, and fissuring or hemorrhage. These factors can temporarily worsen the stenosis and cause abnormal reactivity of the vessel wall, thus exacerbating the manifestations of ischemia. The recent onset of symptoms, the appearance of severe ischemia during stress testing, and unstable angina pectoris (p. 1508) all reflect episodes of rapid progression in coronary lesions.

With any degree of obstructive CAD, mortality is greatly increased when left ventricular function is impaired; conversely, at any level of left ventricular function, the prognosis is influenced importantly by the quantity of myocardium perfused by the critically obstructed vessels. Therefore, it is useful to collect all the evidence substantiating past myocardial damage (ECG and ventriculographic evidence of myocardial infarction), residual left ventricular function (ejection fraction and wall motion), and risk of future damage from coronary events (extent of coronary disease and severity of ischemia defined by noninvasive stress testing). The larger the amount of established myocardial necrosis, the less the heart is able to withstand additional damage and the poorer the prognosis. All the above signs of past damage plus the risk of future damage should be considered indicators of risk.

℞ **TREATMENT** Each patient must be evaluated individually with respect to his or her expectations and goals, control of symptoms, and prevention of adverse clinical outcomes such as myocardial infarction and premature death. The degree of disability as well as the physical and emotional stress that precipitate angina must be carefully recorded in order to set treatment goals. Each management plan should consist of the following: (1) explanation and reassurance, (2) identification and treatment of aggravating conditions, (3) adaptation of activity, (4) treatment of risk factors that will decrease the occurrence of adverse coronary outcomes, (5) drug therapy for angina, and (6) consideration of mechanical revascularization.

Explanation and Reassurance Patients with IHD need to understand their condition as best they can and to realize that a long and useful life is possible even though they suffer from angina pectoris or have experienced and recovered from an acute myocardial infarction. Offering case histories of persons in public life who have lived with coronary disease as well as results of national studies showing improved outcomes can be of great value when encouraging patients to resume or maintain activity and return to their occupation. A planned program of rehabilitation can encourage patients to lose weight, improve exercise tolerance, and control risk factors with more confidence.

Identification and Treatment of Aggravating Conditions A number of conditions may either increase oxygen demand or decrease oxygen supply to the myocardium and may precipitate or exacerbate angina. Aortic valve disease and hypertrophic cardiomyopathy may cause angina and should be excluded or treated. Obesity, hypertension, and hyperthyroidism may be managed successfully in order to reduce the frequency of anginal attacks. Decreased myocardial oxygen supply may be due to reduced oxygenation of the blood (e.g., in pulmonary disease or, when carboxyhemoglobin is present, due to cigarette or cigar smoking) or decreased oxygen-carrying capacity (e.g., in anemia). Correction of these abnormalities, if present, may reduce or even eliminate angina pectoris.

Adaptation of Activity Therapy of angina due to episodes of myocardial ischemia consists of eliminating the discrepancy between the demand of the heart muscle for oxygen and the ability of the coronary circulation to meet this demand. Most patients can be made to understand this fundamental concept and utilize it in the rational programming of activity. Many tasks that ordinarily evoke angina may be accomplished without symptoms simply by reducing the speed at which they are performed. Patients must appreciate the diurnal variation in their tolerance of certain activities and should reduce their energy requirements in the morning and immediately after meals. Sometimes it is helpful to alter the eating pattern, taking small and more frequent meals.

It may be necessary to recommend a change in employment or residence to avoid physical stress; however, with the exception of manual laborers, most patients with IHD can continue to function merely by allowing more time to complete each task. In some patients, anger and frustration may be the most important factors precipitating myocardial ischemia. If these cannot be avoided, training in stress management may be useful. A treadmill exercise test to determine the approximate heart rate at which ischemic ECG changes or symptoms develop may be helpful in the development of a specific exercise program.

Physical conditioning usually improves the exercise tolerance of patients with angina and exerts substantial psychological benefits. It may also improve the chances of surviving a myocardial infarction. An exercise program within the limits of each patient's threshold for the development of angina pectoris should be encouraged.

Treatment of Risk Factors Although the treatment of risk factors was developed for the primary prevention of coronary atherosclerosis, there is growing evidence that it can reduce the occurrence of angina, myocardial infarction, and death both in subjects without proven IHD as well as in those with a history of chronic angina or an acute coronary syndrome. A *family history* of premature IHD is an important indicator of increased risk and should trigger a search for treatable risk factors such as hyperlipidemia, hypertension, and diabetes. *Obesity* impairs the treatment of other risk factors and increases the risk of adverse coronary events. In addition, obesity is often accompanied by two other risk factors—hypertension and hyperlipidemia. The treatment of obesity and these accompanying risk factors is an important component of any management plan.

Cigarette smoking accelerates coronary atherosclerosis in both sexes and at all ages and increases the risk of myocardial infarction and death. By increasing myocardial oxygen needs and reducing oxygen supply it aggravates angina. Smoking cessation studies have demonstrated important benefits with a significant decline in the occurrence of these adverse outcomes. The physician's message must be clear and strong and supported by programs that achieve and monitor abstinence (Chap. 390). *Hypertension* (Chaps. 35 and 246) is associated with increased risk of adverse clinical events from coronary atherosclerosis as well as stroke. In addition, the left ventricular hypertrophy that results from sustained hypertension aggravates ischemia. There is evidence that long-term, effective treatment of hypertension can decrease the occurrence of adverse coronary events. *Diabetes mellitus* (Chap. 333) accelerates coronary and peripheral atherosclerosis and is frequently associated with dyslipidemias and increases in the risk of angina, myocardial infarction, and sudden coronary death. Strict control of the dyslipidemia that is frequently found in diabetic patients is essential, as described below.

Treatment of dyslipidemia The adverse interactions between the atherogenic lipids (LDL, triglycerides, and lipid remnants) play a critical role in the development of atherosclerosis and the ischemic syndromes. The treatment of dyslipidemia is central when aiming for long-term relief from angina, reduced need for revascularization, and reduction in myocardial infarction and death. Epidemiology, angiographic trials, and controlled trails have shown that (1) men over 45 years and women over 55 years with two risk factors (family history of premature IHD, cigarette smoking, hypertension, diabetes mellitus) or evidence of atherosclerotic disease should have a total cholesterol ≤ 5.17 mmol/L (≤ 200 mg/dL), LDL ≤ 2.58 mmol/L (≤ 100 mg/dL), and HDL ≥ 1.03 mmol/L (≤ 40 mg/dL); and (2) diabetic patients any age need to achieve the same goals as the likelihood of adverse coronary events is so high. The controlled trials have shown equal benefit for women, the elderly, and even smokers. The control of lipids can be achieved by the combination of a diet low in saturated fatty acids, exercise, and weight loss. Frequently, HMG CoA reductase inhibitors (statins) are required and can lower LDL cholesterol (25 to 60%), raise HDL cholesterol (5 to 9%), and lower triglycerides (5 to 45%). Niacin and fibrates can be used to raise HDL cholesterol and lower triglycerides (Chaps. 242 and 341).

Risk reduction in women with IHD The incidence of clinical IHD in premenopausal women is very low. However, following the menopause, the atherogenic risk factors increase (e.g., increased LDL, reduced HDL) and the rate of clinical coronary events accelerates to the levels observed in men. Women have not given up cigarette smoking as effectively as have men. Diabetes mellitus, which is more common in women, greatly increases the occurrence of clinical IHD and amplifies the deleterious effects of hypertension, hyperlipidemia, and smoking. Cardiac catheterization and coronary revascularization are often applied more sparingly in women and at a later, and more severe, stage of the disease than in men. These factors likely explain the modest increase in complications. Although many of the clinical trials to date have not represented women adequately, the evidence is that when cholesterol lowering, beta blockers after myocardial infarction, and CABG are applied in the appropriate patient groups, women enjoy the same benefits of improved outcome as do men.

Drug Therapy The commonly used drugs for angina pectoris are summarized in Table 244-2.

Nitrates This valuable class of drugs in the management of angina pectoris acts by causing systemic venodilation, thereby reducing myocardial wall tension and oxygen requirements, as well as by dilating the epicardial coronary vessels and increasing blood flow in collateral vessels. The absorption of these agents is most rapid and complete through the mucous membranes. For this reason, nitroglycerin is administered sublingually in tablets of 0.4 or 0.6 mg. Patients with angina should be instructed to take the medication both to relieve angina and also in anticipation of stress (exercise or emotional) that is likely to induce an episode. The value of this prophylactic use of the drug cannot be overemphasized.

Headache and a pulsating feeling in the head are the most common side effects of nitroglycerin and fortunately only rarely become disturbing at the doses usually required to relieve or prevent angina. Nitroglycerin deteriorates with exposure to air, moisture, and sunlight, so that if the drug neither relieves discomfort or headache nor produces a slight sensation of burning at the sublingual site of absorption, the preparation may be inactive and a fresh supply should be obtained. If relief is not achieved after the first dose of nitroglycerin, a second or third dose may be given at 5-min intervals. If discomfort continues despite treatment, the patient should consult a physician or report promptly to a hospital emergency room for evaluation of possible unstable angina or acute myocardial infarction (Chap. 243).

A diary of angina and nitroglycerin use may be valuable for detecting changes in the frequency or severity of discomfort that may signify the development of unstable angina pectoris and/or herald an impending myocardial infarction.

None of the long-acting nitrates is as effective as sublingual nitroglycerin for the acute relief of angina. These preparations can be swallowed, chewed, or administered as a patch or paste by the transdermal route. They provide effective plasma levels for up to 24 h, but the therapeutic response is highly variable. Different preparations and/or administration during the daytime should be tried only to prevent discomfort in the individual patient while avoiding side effects such as

Table 244-2 Drugs Commonly Used for Angina Pectoris

Drug	Usual Dose	Side Effects	Contraindications
NITRATES			
Sublingual NTG	0.3–0.6 mg	Flushing, headache	Intolerance of side effects
Isosorbide dinitrate SR			
Oral	10–60 mg q8h	Flushing, headache, tolerance after 24 h	As above, worsening ischemia on withdrawal
Sublingual	2.5–10 mg q4–6h		
Transdermal NTG patch	0.4–1.2 mg/h for 12–14 h	Flushing, headache, tolerance after 24 h	As above, worsening ischemia on withdrawal
Isosorbide-5-monitrate			
Oral	20–30 mg bid	Flushing, headache, tolerance after 24 h	As above, worsening ischemia on withdrawal
Oral SR	60–240 mg once daily		
BETA BLOCKERS			
Propranolol	20–80 mg qid	Depression, constipation, impotence, bronchospasm, heart failure, bradycardia	Asthma, AV conduction block, heart failure
Metoprolol	25–200 mg bid	As above	As above
Atenolol	50–150 mg once daily	As above	As above
CALCIUM CHANNEL BLOCKING DRUGS			
Nifedipine XL	30–90 mg daily	Hypotension, flushing, edema, worsening angina	Hypotension, intolerance of side effects
Diltiazem SR	60–120 mg bid	Constipation, AV conduction block, worsening heart failure	AV conduction block, impaired LV function, bradycardia
Verapamil SR	180–240 mg daily	Constipation, AV conduction block, worsening heart failure	AV conduction delay, impaired LV function, bradycardia
Amlodipine	5–10 mg daily	Edema	Intolerance of side effects

NOTE: NTG, nitroglycerin; SR, slow release; XL, slow release preparation.

headache and dizziness. Individual dose titration is important in order to prevent side effects. Useful preparations include isosorbide dinitrate (10 to 60 mg PO bid or tid), nitroglycerin ointment (0.5 to 2.0 in. qid), or sustained-release transdermal patches (5 to 25 mg/d). The nitrates likely bind to guanylate cyclase in vascular smooth muscle cells, oxidize sulfhydryl groups, and are converted to *S*-nitrosothiols. This leads to an increase in cyclic guanosine monophosphate which causes relaxation of vascular smooth muscle. Tolerance with loss of efficacy develops with 12 to 24 h of continuous exposure to all of the long-acting nitrates due to depletion of sulfhydryl groups and to counterregulatory alterations in intravascular fluid balance with fluid retention. In order to minimize the effects of tolerance, the minimum effective dose should be used and a minimum of 8 h each day kept free of the drug so as to restore any useful response(s).

Beta blockers (See also Chap. 72) These drugs represent an important component of the pharmacologic treatment of angina pectoris. They reduce myocardial oxygen demand by inhibiting the increases in heart rate and myocardial contractility caused by adrenergic activation. Beta blockade reduces these variables most strikingly during exercise while causing only small reductions in heart rate, cardiac output, and arterial pressure at rest. Long-acting beta-blocking drugs (atenolol, 50 to 100 mg/d, and nadolol, 40 to 80 mg/d) offer the advantage of once-a-day dosage (Tables 72-1 and 244-2). The therapeutic aims include relief of angina and ischemia. These drugs can also reduce mortality and reinfarction when given to patients after myocardial infarction. Relative contraindications to the use of beta blockers include asthma and reversible airway obstruction in patients with chronic lung disease, atrioventricular conduction disturbances, severe bradycardia, Raynaud's phenomenon, and a history of depression. Side effects include fatigue, impotence, cold extremities, intermittent claudication, bradycardia (sometimes severe), impaired atrioventricular conduction, left ventricular failure, bronchial asthma, and intensification of the hypoglycemia produced by oral hypoglycemic agents and insulin. Reducing the dose or even discontinuation of the drug may be necessary if these side effects develop and persist.

Calcium antagonists Slow-release nifedipine (30 to 90 mg once daily), verapamil (80 to 120 mg tid), diltiazem (30 to 90 mg qid), amlodipine (2.5 to 10 mg daily), and other calcium antagonists are coronary vasodilators that produce variable and dose-dependent reductions in myocardial oxygen demand, contractility, and arterial pressure. These combined pharmacologic effects are advantageous and make these agents effective in the treatment of angina pectoris. They are indicated when beta blockers are contraindicated, poorly tolerated, or ineffective. Verapamil and diltiazem may produce symptomatic disturbances in cardiac conduction and bradyarrhythmias, exert negative inotropic actions, and are more likely to worsen left ventricular failure, particularly when used in patients with left ventricular dysfunction. Although useful effects are usually achieved when calcium antagonists are combined with beta blockers and nitrates, careful individual titration of dose is essential with these potent combinations. Variant (Prinzmetal's) angina responds particularly well to calcium antagonists, supplemented when necessary by nitrates. Nifedipine as well as other calcium antagonists are now formulated as long-acting preparations including diltiazem (60 to 120 mg twice daily) and verapamil (180 to 240 mg once daily).

Verapamil should not ordinarily be combined with beta blockers because of the combined effects on heart rate and contractility. Diltiazem can be combined with beta blockers with caution and only in patients with normal ventricular function and no conduction disturbances. Nifedipine or amlodipine and the beta blockers have complementary actions on coronary blood supply and myocardial oxygen demands. While the former decreases blood pressure and dilates coronary arteries, the latter slows heart rate and decreases contractility. Nifedipine and the other second-generation dihydropyridine calcium antagonists (nicardipine, isradipine, amlodipine, and felodipine) are potent vasodilators and useful in the simultaneous treatment of angina and hypertension. Short-acting dihydropyridines should be avoided because of the risk of precipitating infarction, particularly in the absence of beta blockers.

Choice between beta blockers and calcium antagonists for initial therapy Since beta blockers have been shown to improve life expectancy following myocardial infarction (p. 1393), they may be preferable in patients with chronic IHD. However, calcium antagonists are indicated in patients with the following: (1) angina and a history of asthma or chronic obstructive pulmonary disease; (2) sick-sinus syndrome or significant atrioventricular conduction disturbances; (3) Prinzmetal's angina; (4) symptomatic peripheral vascular disease; and (5) adverse reactions to beta blockers—depression, sexual disturbances, fatigue. Many patients with angina do well with a combination of a beta blocker and dihydropyridine calcium antagonist.

Antiplatelet drugs Aspirin is an irreversible inhibitor of platelet cyclooxygenase activity and thereby interferes with platelet activation. Chronic administration of 100 to 325 mg orally per day has been shown to reduce coronary events in asymptomatic adult men, patients with asymptomatic ischemia after myocardial infarction, patients with chronic stable angina, and patients with or who have survived unstable angina and myocardial infarction. Administration of this drug should be considered in all patients with IHD in the absence of side effects such as gastrointestinal bleeding, allergy, or dyspepsia. Clopidogrel is an oral agent that blocks ADP receptor–mediated platelet aggregation. It provides the same benefits as aspirin, if not better, particularly if aspirin causes the side effects listed above.

In summary, a regimen of exercise, smoking cessation, treatment of hypertension and dyslipidemia, aspirin, and beta blockers after infarction are medical interventions that reduce angina, the need for revascularization, myocardial infarction and coronary death.

Treatment of angina and heart failure Transient left ventricular failure with angina can be controlled by the use of nitrates. For patients with established congestive heart failure the increased left ventricular wall tension raises myocardial oxygen demand. Treatment of congestive heart failure with angiotensin-converting enzyme inhibitors, diuretics, and digitalis (Chap. 232) will decrease heart size, wall tension, and myocardial oxygen demands, which, in turn, will help to control angina and ischemia. Nocturnal angina can often be relieved by the treatment of heart failure; however, there is no proven benefit when these drugs are used in patients with angina, a normal heart size, and no evidence of heart failure. Nitrates are particularly useful and can simultaneously improve the disturbed hemodynamics of congestive heart failure by vasodilatation, thereby reducing preload, and relieve angina by preventing or reversing myocardial ischemia. There is some evidence that amlodipine is a calcium antagonist that is well tolerated by patients with left ventricular dysfunction and a valuable agent in the treatment of angina in patients with heart failure. The combination of congestive heart failure and angina in patients with IHD usually indicates a poor prognosis and warrants serious consideration of cardiac catheterization and mechanical revascularization.

CORONARY REVASCULARIZATION

While the basic management of patients with CAD, which is a lifelong condition, is medical, as described above, many patients are improved by coronary revascularization procedures, as described below. These interventions should be employed in conjunction with but do not replace the continuing need to modify risk factors.

PERCUTANEOUS CORONARY INTERVENTION (See also Chap. 245) PCI, most commonly percutaneous transluminal coronary angioplasty (PTCA) or stenting, is a widely used method to achieve revascularization of the myocardium in patients with symptomatic IHD and suitable stenoses of epicardial coronary arteries. Whereas patients with stenosis of the left main coronary artery and those with three-vessel CAD (especially with associated impaired left ventricular function) who require revascularization are best treated with CABG, PCI is widely employed in patients with symptoms and evidence of ischemia due to stenoses of one or two vessels, and even selected patients with three-vessel disease, and may offer many advantages over surgery.

Indications and Patient Selection The most common clinical indication for PCI is angina pectoris, stable or unstable, accompanied by evidence of ischemia in an exercise test. PCI is more effective than medical therapy for the relief of angina. The value of this procedure in reducing the occurrence of coronary death and myocardial infarction has not been established, and therefore it is not generally indicated in asymptomatic or mildly symptomatic patients. PCI can be used to treat stenoses in native coronary arteries as well as in bypass grafts in patients who have recurrent angina following coronary artery surgery. This is an important indication when the technical difficulties and the increased mortality that accompanies reoperation are considered. PCI has also been carried out in patients with recent total occlusion (within 3 months) of a coronary artery and severe angina; in this group the primary success rate is slightly decreased.

Risks When coronary stenoses are discrete and symmetric, two and three vessels can be dilated in sequence. However, case selection is essential in order to avoid a prohibitive risk of complications. Advanced age, stenoses with thrombus, left ventricular dysfunction, stenosis of an artery perfusing a large segment of myocardium without collaterals, long eccentric or irregular stenoses, and calcified plaques all increase the likelihood of complications but are not absolute contraindications, while left main coronary artery stenosis *is* generally regarded as an absolute contraindication. The major complications are usually due to dissection or thrombosis with vessel occlusion, uncontrolled ischemia, and ventricular failure. Oral aspirin and intravenous heparin are always given to reduce coronary thrombus formation. In unstable angina and when intracoronary thrombus is seen, the use of specific platelet glycoprotein receptor antagonists further reduce thrombotic complications and increase success. In experienced hands, the overall mortality rate should be less than 0.5%, the need for emergency coronary surgery less than 1%, and the occurrence of clinical myocardial infarction less than 2%. Minor complications occur in 5 to 10% of patients and include occlusion of a branch of a coronary artery, myocardial infarction with release of CK-MB into the circulation, and complications of arterial catheterization.

Efficacy Primary success, i.e., adequate dilation (an increase in luminal diameter to a residual diameter obstruction <50%) with relief of angina, is achieved in approximately 95% of cases. Recurrent stenosis of the dilated vessels occurs in 30 to 45% of cases within 6 months of PTCA, and angina will recur within 6 to 12 months in 25% of cases. This recurrence of symptoms and restenosis is more common in patients with diabetes mellitus, unstable angina, incomplete dilation of the stenosis, dilation of the left anterior descending coronary artery, and stenoses containing thrombi. Dilation of arteries that are totally occluded and of stenotic or occluded vein grafts also exhibits a high incidence of restenosis. It is usual clinical practice to administer aspirin for months after the procedure. Although aspirin and the antiplatelet drug Clopidogrel may help prevent acute coronary thrombosis during and shortly following PCI, there are no controlled clinical trials that have demonstrated that these medications or any other can clearly reduce the incidence of restenosis. Successful deployment of a metal stent lowers the restenosis rate to 10 to 30% at 6 months but initially requires vigorous antiplatelet therapy (aspirin and Clopidogrel). There is early evidence that local radiation can further reduce restenosis.

If patients do not develop restenosis or angina within the first year after angioplasty, the prognosis for maintaining improvement over the subsequent 4 years is excellent. If restenosis occurs, PTCA can be repeated with the same success and risk, but the likelihood of restenosis increases with the third or subsequent attempt.

Successful PCI produces effective relief of angina in over 95% of cases and has been shown to be more effective than medical therapy for up to 2 years. Between 30 and 50% of patients with symptomatic IHD who require revascularization can be treated by PCI and need not undergo CABG. Successful PCI is less invasive and expensive than CABG, usually requires only 1 to 2 days in the hospital, and permits considerable savings in the initial cost of care. Successful PCI also allows earlier return to work and the resumption of an active life. However, this economic benefit is reduced over time because of the greater need for follow-up and for repeat procedures.

CORONARY ARTERY BYPASS GRAFTING In CABG, a section of a vein (usually the saphenous) is used to form a connection between the aorta and the coronary artery distal to the obstructive lesion. Alternatively, anastomosis of one or both of the internal mammary arteries or a radial artery to the coronary artery distal to the obstructive lesion may be employed and is now preferred whenever possible.

Although some indications for coronary artery bypass surgery are controversial, certain areas of agreement exist:

1. The operation is relatively safe, with mortality rates less than 1% in patients without serious comorbid disease and normal left ventricular function, when the procedure is performed by an experienced surgical team.
2. Intraoperative and postoperative mortality increase with the degree of ventricular dysfunction, comorbidities, age above 80 years, and surgical inexperience. The effectiveness and risk of CABG vary widely depending on case selection and the skill and experience of the surgical team.
3. Occlusion of vein grafts is observed in 10 to 20% during the first postoperative year and in approximately 2% per year during 5- to 7-year follow-up and 4% per year thereafter. Long-term patency rates are considerably higher for internal mammary and radial artery implantations; in patients with left anterior descending coronary artery obstruction, survival is better when coronary bypass involves the internal mammary artery rather than a saphenous vein. Graft patency and outcomes are improved by meticulous treatment of risk factors, particularly dyslipidemia.
4. Angina is abolished or greatly reduced in approximately 90% of

patients following complete revascularization. Although this is usually associated with graft patency and restoration of blood flow, the pain may also have been alleviated as a result of infarction of the ischemic segment or a placebo effect. Within 3 years, angina recurs in about one-fourth of patients but is rarely severe.

5. CABG does not appear to reduce the incidence of myocardial infarction in patients with chronic IHD; perioperative myocardial infarction occurs in 5 to 10% of cases, but in most instances these infarcts are small and have little effect on left ventricular function.
6. Mortality is reduced by operation in patients with stenosis of the left main coronary artery as well as in patients with three- or two-vessel disease with significant obstruction of the proximal left anterior descending coronary artery. The survival benefit is greater in patients with abnormal left ventricular function (ejection fraction <50%). Mortality *may* also be reduced in the following patients: (1) with one- or two-vessel CAD without significant proximal left anterior descending artery CAD but with high-risk criteria on noninvasive testing; (2) with obstructive CAD who have survived sudden cardiac death or sustained ventricular tachycardia; (3) who have undergone previous CABG and who have multiple saphenous vein graft stenoses, especially of a graft supplying the left anterior descending coronary artery; and (4) with prior PCI recurrent stenosis, and high-risk criteria on noninvasive testing.

Indications for CABG are usually based on the severity of symptoms, coronary anatomy, and ventricular function. The ideal candidate is male, less than 75 years of age, has no other complicating disease, has troublesome or disabling symptoms that are not adequately controlled by medical therapy or does not tolerate medical therapy and wishes to lead a more active life, and has severe stenoses of several epicardial coronary arteries with objective evidence of myocardial ischemia as a cause of the chest discomfort. Great symptomatic benefit can be anticipated in such patients.

Congestive heart failure and/or left ventricular dysfunction (ejection fraction <40%), advanced age (>75 years), reoperation, urgent need for surgery, and the presence of diabetes are all associated with higher perioperative mortality.

Left ventricular dysfunction can be due to noncontractile segments that are viable (hibernating myocardium). These can be detected by using radionuclide scans of myocardial perfusion and metabolism, positron emission tomography, or delayed scanning with thallium-201 or by return of contractile function provoked by low-dose dobutamine. Revascularization can return function and improve survival.

The Choice Between PCI and CABG (See Table 244-3) A number of randomized trials have compared PTCA and CABG in patients with multivessel CAD who were suitable technically for both procedures. The redevelopment of angina requiring repeat coronary angiography and repeat revascularization due to restenosis was higher in the PTCA group. However, the occurrence of death or myocardial infarction has been found to be similar between both groups for up to 5 years. In patients with diabetes plus disease of two or more coronary arteries, bypass surgery results in significantly better outcomes and survival and should be the technique of choice. In addition, the recurrence of angina and stenosis and the need for additional revascularization was much higher in the angioplasty group (about 50%) than in the surgery group (about 10%). Based on these trials and observational studies, we now recommend that patients with an unacceptable level of angina despite optimal medical management should be considered for revascularization. Patients with single- or two-vessel disease with normal or slightly depressed global left ventricular function and anatomically suitable lesions are ordinarily advised initially to undergo PCI (Chap. 245). Patients with two- or three-vessel disease and impaired global left ventricular function (left ventricular ejection fraction <45%) or diabetes mellitus or those with left main disease or other

Table 244-3 Comparison of Revascularization Procedures in Multivessel Disease

Procedure	Advantages	Disadvantages
Percutaneous coronary intervention (PCI)	Less invasive Shorter hospital stay Lower initial cost Easily repeated Effective in relieving symptoms	Restenosis High incidence of incomplete revascularization Unknown effect on outcomes in patients with severe left ventricular dysfunction Limited to specific anatomic subsets Poor outcome in diabetics with 2 or 3 vessel coronary disease
Coronary artery bypass grafting (CABG)	Effective in relieving symptoms Improved survival in certain subsets Ability to achieve complete revascularization	Cost Increased risk of a repeat procedure due to late graft closure Morbidity and mortality of major surgery

SOURCE: Modified from DP Faxon, in GA Beller (ed), *Chronic Ischemic Heart Disease*, in E Braunwald (series ed), *Atlas of Heart Diseases*, Philadelphia, Current Medicine, 1994.

lesions unsuitable for catheter-based procedures should be considered for CABG as the initial method of revascularization (Table 244-3).

UNSTABLE ANGINA PECTORIS

The following three patient groups may be said to have unstable angina pectoris: (1) patients with new onset (<2 months) angina that is severe and/or frequent (≥3 episodes per day); (2) patients with accelerating angina, i.e., those with chronic stable angina who develop angina that is distinctly more frequent, severe, prolonged, or precipitated by less exertion than previously; (3) those with angina at rest. Five mechanisms for unstable angina have been described: (1) a nonocclusive thrombus—often a platelet plug—overlying a fissured atherosclerotic plaque; (2) dynamic obstruction—either spasm of an epicardial coronary artery, as in Prinzmetal's variant angina (see below), or abnormal vasoconstriction of the coronary microcirculation, as in microvascular angina; (3) severe, organic luminal narrowing, as in restenosis following a PCI; (4) arterial inflammation leading to thrombosis; and (5) increase in myocardial oxygen demands caused by conditions such as tachycardia, fever, and thyrotoxicosis in the presence of fixed, severe coronary obstruction. More than one of these may be operative.

When unstable angina is accompanied by objective ECG evidence of transient myocardial ischemia (ST-segment changes and/or T-wave inversions during episodes of chest pain), it is associated with critical stenoses in one or more major epicardial coronary arteries in about 85% of cases.

℞ **TREATMENT** The management of unstable angina is outlined in Fig. 244-3. The patient is admitted to the hospital, placed at rest, sedated, and reassured. In all instances, concomitant conditions that can intensify ischemia, such as tachycardia, hypertension, diabetes mellitus, cardiomegaly, heart failure, arrhythmias, thyrotoxicosis, and any acute febrile illness, should be sought and vigorously treated. Acute myocardial infarction should be ruled out by means of serial ECGs and measurements of plasma cardiac enzyme activity.

Continuous ECG monitoring should be carried out. Since thrombus formation frequently complicates this condition, intravenous heparin should be given for 3 to 5 days to maintain the partial thrombo-plastin time at 2 to 2.5 times control, together with or followed by oral aspirin at a dose of 325 mg/d. Alternatively, low-molecular-weight heparin (e.g., enoxaparin, 1 mg/kg subcutaneously b.i.d.) may be used. High-risk unstable angina patients, i.e., those with rest pain, and ST-segment deviations and/or release of a marker of myocardial injury (such as troponin I or T) should also receive an intravenous infusion of a platelet GpIIb/IIIa inhibitor. A beta blocker should be administered and a calcium antagonist added if ischemia persists despite the aforementioned therapy, but with caution and an awareness of the possible side effects discussed above. Dosages of these agents should be raised rapidly, but the patient must be observed carefully to avoid bradycardia, heart failure, and hypotension. Nitroglycerin should be given by the sublingual route as needed for symptoms. Intravenous nitroglycerin is quite effective, especially in patients with episodes of ischemia that are particularly severe or prolonged. It is begun at a dosage of 10 μg/min and is raised in 5 μg/min increments to a level at which chest pain is abolished but systolic arterial pressure is maintained or reduced only slightly and other side effects are avoided. After initial stabilization, either an early invasive strategy (coronary angiography and revascularization) or early conservative strategy (continued medical therapy) can be pursued (Fig. 244-3).

The majority of patients (approximately 80%) improve with rest and medical treatment over a 48-h period. If angina at rest and/or ECG evidence of ischemia persist despite 24 to 48 h of the comprehensive treatment described above, then cardiac catheterization and coronary arteriography should be performed in patients with no obvious contraindications for revascularization. If the anatomy is suitable, PCI can be performed. If the coronary anatomy is not suitable for PCI, CABG should be considered to relieve symptoms and myocardial ischemia and as a means of preventing myocardial damage. The factors that influence the choice between catheter-based and surgical revascularization are similar to those in chronic stable angina.

In the early conservative strategy, if the patient's symptoms and signs are controlled on medical therapy, a diagnostic exercise ECG or perfusion scan or, if exercise is not possible, a pharmacologic stress test (p. 1402) should be carried out near the time of hospital discharge. If there is evidence of severe myocardial ischemia and/or evidence of a high risk of coronary events (p. 1402), consideration should be given to catheterization and, depending on the findings, revascularization. Following discharge, patients with unstable angina should be managed similar to chronic angina patients (p. 1404). Severe obstructive CAD is often present in patients with unstable angina who respond to medical therapy. Many patients in whom the unstable state is controlled are left with severe chronic stable angina and ultimately require mechanical revascularization.

PRINZMETAL'S VARIANT ANGINA This relatively uncommon form of unstable angina is characterized by recurrent, prolonged attacks of severe ischemia, caused by episodic focal spasm of an epicardial coronary artery. Approximately three-fourths of patients with Prinzmetal's angina exhibit a mild or moderately severe fixed obstruction (with a luminal diameter 50 to 70% of normal) within 1 cm of the site of spasm. Patients with this condition are often smokers and are younger than patients with unstable angina secondary to coronary atherosclerosis. Ischemic pain usually occurs at rest, sometimes awakens the patient from sleep, and is characterized by multilead ST-segment elevation. The diagnosis may be confirmed by detecting transient spasm occurring spontaneously or following a provocative stimulus (intracoronary acetylcholine, hyperventilation) on coronary arteriography. While long-term survival is excellent, complications include episodes of disabling pain, myocardial infarction, serious ventricular arrhythmias, atrioventricular block, and, rarely, sudden death.

℞ **TREATMENT** Management of the acute attack consists of multiple doses of sublingual nitroglycerin, an intravenous infusion of nitroglycerin, and short-acting nifedipine (10 to 30 mg); hypotension should be avoided. In chronic management, long-acting nitrates and calcium antagonists are useful. Beta blockers are of little value, while prazosin, a selective alpha-adrenoceptor blocker, may be useful. Occasionally, mechanical revascularization is helpful in patients with accompanying severe discrete obstructive lesions.

ASYMPTOMATIC (SILENT) ISCHEMIA

Obstructive CAD, acute myocardial infarction, and transient myocardial ischemia are frequently asymptomatic. During continuous ambulatory ECG monitoring, the majority of ambulatory patients with typical chronic stable angina are found to have objective evidence of myocardial ischemia (ST-segment depression) during episodes of chest discomfort while they are active outside the hospital, but many of these patients also appear to have more frequent episodes of asymptomatic ischemia. In addition, there is a large (but as yet unknown) number of totally asymptomatic people with severe coronary atherosclerosis who exhibit ST-segment changes during activity. Some of these patients exhibit higher thresholds to electrically induced pain, others show higher endorphin levels, and still others may be diabetic patients with autonomic dysfunction.

Evidence of frequent episodes of ischemia (symptomatic and asymptomatic) during daily life appears to indicate an increased likelihood of adverse coronary events such as death and myocardial infarction. The widespread use of exercise ECG during routine examinations has also defined some of these heretofore unrecognized patients with asymptomatic CAD. Longitudinal studies have demonstrated an increased incidence of coronary events (sudden death, myocardial infarction, and angina) in asymptomatic patients with positive exercise tests. In addition, patients with asymptomatic ischemia after suffering a myocardial infarction are at greater risk for a second coronary event.

Rx **TREATMENT** The management of patients with asymptomatic ischemia must be individualized. Thus, the physician should consider the following: (1) the degree of positivity of the stress test, particularly the stage of exercise at which ECG signs of ischemia appear, the magnitude and number of the perfusion defect(s) on thallium scintigraphy, and the change in left ventricular ejection fraction which occurs on radionuclide ventriculography or echocardiography during ischemia and/or during exercise; (2) the ECG leads showing a positive response, with changes in the anterior precordial leads indicating a less favorable prognosis than changes in the inferior leads; and (3) the patient's age, occupation, and general medical condition. Most would agree that an asymptomatic 45-year-old commercial airline pilot with 0.4-mV ST-segment depression in leads V_1 to V_4 during mild exercise should undergo coronary arteriography, whereas the asymptomatic, sedentary 75-year-old retiree with 0.1-mV ST-segment depression in leads II and III during maximal activity need not. However, there is no consensus about the appropriate procedure in the large majority of patients for whom the situation is less extreme. Patients with evidence of severe ischemia on noninvasive testing (as outlined

FIGURE 244-3 Management algorithm for unstable angina. CCSC, Canadian Cardiovascular Society classification; CCU, coronary care unit; CABG, coronary artery bypass grafting; PCI, percutaneous coronary intervention. (*Modified from Braunwald et al.*)

earlier) should undergo coronary arteriography. Asymptomatic patients with silent ischemia, three-vessel CAD, and impaired left ventricular function may be considered appropriate candidates for CABG.

The treatment of risk factors, particularly lipid lowering as described above, as well as the use of aspirin and beta blockers have been shown to reduce events and improve outcomes in asymptomatic as well as symptomatic patients with ischemia and proven CAD. While the incidence of asymptomatic ischemia can be reduced by treatment with beta blockers, calcium channel antagonists, and long-acting nitrates, it is not clear whether this is necessary or desirable in patients who have not suffered a myocardial infarction. However, there is evidence that beta-adrenoceptor blockade begun 7 to 35 days after acute myocardial infarction improves survival (Chap. 243).

BIBLIOGRAPHY

BRAUNWALD E et al: Diagnosing and managing unstable angina. Circulation 90:613, 1994

CAIRNS JA et al: Antithrombotic agents in coronary artery disease. Chest 114:61S, 1998

CREAGER MA et al: Results of the CAPTURE trial. Clopidogrel versus aspirin in patients at risk of ischemic events. Vasc Med 3:257, 1998

FARMER JA et al: Aggressive lipid therapy in the statin era. Prog Cardiovasc Dis 41:71, 1998

FAVOLARO RG et al: Landmarks in the development of coronary artery bypass surgery. Circulation 98:466, 1998

GERSH BJ et al: Chronic ischemic heart disease, in *Heart Disease*, 6th ed, E Braunwald et al (eds). Philadelphia, Saunders, 2001

GOTTO AM Jr et al: Risk factor modification: Rationale for management of dyslipidemia. Am J Med 104:6S, 1998

——— et al: Preventing coronary disease in women: Brief observations from the clinical data. J Women's Health 7:195, 1998

HENDERSON RA et al: Long-term results of RITA-1 trial, clinical and cost comparisons of coronary angioplasty and coronary artery bypass grafting. Randomized intervention treatment of angina. Lancet 352:1419, 1998

HE ZX et al: Severity of coronary artery calcification by electron beam computed tomography predicts silent myocardial ischemia. Circulation 101:244, 2000

HEUSCH G et al: Alpha-adrenergic coronary vasoconstriction and myocardial ischemia in humans. Circulation 101:689, 2000

KING SB et al: Balloon angioplasty versus new device intervention: Clinical outcomes. A comparison of the NHLBI PTCA and NACI registries. J Am Coll Cardiol 31:558, 1998

MAYER S et al: Prinzmetal's variant angina. Clin Cardiol 21:243, 1998

NAKAO S et al: Hyperventilation as a specific test for diagnosis of coronary artery spasm. Am J Cardiol 80:545, 1997

SOLOMON AJ et al: Management of chronic stable angina: Medical therapy, percutaneous transluminal coronary angioplasty, and coronary artery bypass graft surgery. Lessons from the randomized trials. Ann Intern Med 128:216, 1998

FIGURE 245-1   Focal discrete stenosis of the mid-right coronary angioplasty in a patient with unstable angina, shown before (*left panel*) and after (*right panel*) inflation of the PTCA balloon catheter. The lesion is typical of the straightforward lesion anatomy treated by early (pre-1985) coronary angioplasty.

245   *Donald S. Baim*

PERCUTANEOUS CORONARY REVASCULARIZATION

Before 1977, bypass surgery was the only form of revascularization available to treat coronary artery disease. In that year, Andreas Gruntzig performed the first catheter-based coronary revascularization, which he named percutaneous transluminal coronary angioplasty (PTCA). With crude early equipment and limited anatomic capability, fewer than 1000 such procedures were performed worldwide annually until 1981. Through the 1980s and early 1990s, however, progressive improvements in the balloon angioplasty equipment led to improved results, expanded indications for use, and explosive growth in PTCA to the point that in the United States, the annual number of procedures (~300,000) roughly matched the number of surgical bypass operations. This growth has been sustained during the late 1990s with the introduction of a number of newer devices (including stents and atherectomy devices) that further improved the acute success and safety as well as the long-term durability of what is now known more broadly as percutaneous coronary revascularization (PCR) or intervention (PCI). The current annual number of PCRs (~600,000) is thus now greater than the number of coronary bypass operations (~400,000). The dominant role that catheter-based intervention has assumed in the treatment of coronary artery disease has led to definition of the field known as *interventional cardiology*, which now has its own fellowship requirements and Board certification of additional qualifications based on training (a specialized interventional cardiology fellowship beyond basic cardiology training), ongoing experience (75 procedures per year), and a written examination.

All catheter-based coronary interventions are derivatives of diagnostic cardiac catheterization (Chap. 228), in which catheters are introduced into the arterial circulation by needle puncture, advanced into the heart under fluoroscopic guidance, and used for pressure measurements or injections of radio-opaque liquid contrast agents. Interventional procedures differ in that the catheter placed into the ostium of the narrowed coronary artery has a slightly larger diameter, and its lumen is used to convey a flexible, steerable guidewire (diameter <0.5 mm) down the coronary artery lumen, through the narrowing, and into the vessel beyond. This guidewire then serves as the rail over which angioplasty balloons or other therapeutic devices are run to enlarge the narrowed segment of coronary artery (Fig. 245-1). Because PCR is performed with local anesthesia and requires only a short (1- to 2-day) hospitalization, its use in suitable patients can greatly decrease expense and recovery time compared to those associated with coronary bypass surgery. Not all types of coronary narrowing are well

suited to catheter-based intervention, but such intervention is the treatment of choice for roughly 70% of patients with symptomatic single vessel disease and roughly 20% of patients with symptomatic three-vessel disease. Given these anatomic restrictions and the small but definite risk of catheter-based intervention (elective mortality rate 0.4 to 1.0%, compared to a rate of 1 to 3% for elective surgical bypass), PCR should still be viewed as an invasive procedure whose risks and benefits for each individual patient need to be weighed before use. Beyond the decision of which patients should undergo revascularization (versus continued medical management), the selection of which patients should undergo catheter-based rather than surgical revascularization requires detailed understanding of both clinical and coronary angiographic factors, as well as the applicability of various interventional techniques.

INDICATIONS   The main indication for PCR remains the presence of one or more coronary stenoses that are approachable by catheter-based techniques and are thought to be responsible for a clinical syndrome that warrants revascularization. Moreover, the risks and benefits of revascularization by PCR should compare favorably with those of surgery. In patients with significant narrowing of a single coronary artery, the main benefit of revascularization lies in relief of anginal symptoms rather than in increasing their already good prognosis with medical therapy. By contrast, for the patient with significant left main stenosis or multivessel disease, revascularization may both relieve angina *and* improve long-term survival. Most patients with multivessel coronary disease, however, currently undergo surgical rather than catheter-based revascularization, particularly when one or more vessels supplying significant areas of viable myocardium are not well-suited to PCR (owing to chronic total occlusion or other unfavorable anatomic features). In patients for whom either PCR or bypass surgery is a possible treatment for multivessel coronary artery disease, a number of randomized trials have suggested that the two procedures have equivalent in-hospital and 3- to 5-year mortality rates, but that more patients undergoing PCR (40 to 50% versus 7 to 10% surgical patients) will require a second revascularization procedure (generally a repeat PCR to treat restenosis) by 5 years to maintain an equivalent level of symptom relief. One exception may be diabetic patients with multivessel coronary artery disease, for whom some studies have suggested better survival with surgical treatment than with PCR.

The clinical indications for PCR cover the spectrum from patients with unstable angina or acute infarction to patients with silent ischemia, as summarized in the 1999 guidelines. For most patients, PCR is used to treat anatomically approachable lesions that are responsible for the clinical syndrome of *moderately severe, chronic, stable angina*, which persists despite medical antianginal therapy (Chap. 244). Approximately 15% of current patients undergoing PCR, however, have only mild anginal symptoms despite suitable coronary anatomy but have objective evidence of ischemia on noninvasive testing (i.e., an abnormal exercise test). At the other extreme, many patients have more pressing indications for revascularization, including unstable angina or even acute myocardial infarction (with or without prior thrombolytic therapy). An aggressive approach to the treatment of unstable angina involving initial stabilization with beta blockers, nitrates, heparin, and antiplatelet agents (aspirin and frequently a platelet glycoprotein IIb/IIIa receptor blocker), followed by diagnostic catheterization, and same-procedure PCR of the underlying blockage, offers the patient a more rapid return to work, fewer readmissions and late revascularizations, and potentially a reduction in late events compared to prolonged initial trials of medical therapy before proceeding with invasive evaluation and treatment.

In the early 1980s the introduction of intravenous fibrinolytic agents to reopen the occluded infarct-related vessel was a major advance in the treatment of acute myocardial infarction (Chap. 243). It seemed reasonable that

FIGURE 245-2 Left coronary angiogram in a patient with acute anterior myocardial infarction and cardiogenic shock shows occlusion of the proximal left anterior descending coronary artery (*top panel, arrow*) with only faint filling beyond the obstructing thrombus. After initial PTCA (*lower left panel*), there is restored antegrade flow with residual stenosis. After stent placement (*lower right panel*), there is no residual stenosis and brisk flow. This improvement was associated with reversal of shock hemodynamics, including normalization of severe lactic acidosis.

PCR might further improve the results of thrombolytic therapy by treating the underlying atherosclerotic stenosis, opening those arteries that failed to reperfuse with a thrombolytic alone and preventing the 10 to 20% incidence of in-hospital reocclusion that occurs after even successful thrombolysis. Randomized trials, however, showed that none of the routine PCR strategies tested after thrombolytic administration improved the outcome more than a "watchful waiting" strategy in which PCR was reserved for patients with spontaneous or exercise-induced ischemia. In contrast, there is evidence that *primary* or direct angioplasty (used instead of thrombolytic therapy) can reduce the in-hospital mortality rate (from roughly 7 to 4%) when performed promptly by a skilled operator (Fig. 245-2). Another advantage of PCR is that it can be performed even in the approximately 30% of patients with acute myocardial infarction with contraindications to thrombolytic therapy.

As the clinical indications for PCR have broadened, so have its anatomic capabilities. PCR thus is no longer restricted to proximal, discrete, subtotal, concentric, noncalcified lesions, as was the case initially. Calcified, complex, or diffuse disease lesions respond well to coronary stent placement, sometimes after pretreatment with rotational atherectomy. Even totally occluded coronary arteries (particularly ones that have been occluded for less than 6 months) can be crossed and dilated effectively, although the success rate remains somewhat lower than for subtotal lesions (60% versus 90% for subtotal stenotic lesions). In addition to lesions in the native coronary tree, obstructions in saphenous vein (Fig. 245-3) or internal mammary artery bypass grafts also can be dilated successfully to treat postbypass angina. If multiple lesions are responsible for the clinical syndrome, they generally can be dilated during a single procedure.

RESULTS The success rate for PCR exceeds 95% for dilating a target lesion so that its residual diameter stenosis is <50% (<30% when a stent has been used), without producing an associated complication. About half of the failures result from inability to cross the target lesion with the guidewire or balloon catheter, particularly when that target lesion is a chronic total occlusion. With balloon dilatation alone, some local dissection is present in virtually all successful procedures. Before the introduction of stent technology (see below), more extensive dissection (particularly in association with local thrombus formation or vasospasm) led to abrupt closure of the dilated segment soon after withdrawal of the balloon catheter, and necessitated emergency bypass surgery in approximately 3% of angioplasty attempts. However, such dissections are now routinely treated by stent placement, reducing the incidence of emergency bypass surgery to <1%. Other than dissection, the main hazards of PCR concern spasm, thrombosis, and perforation.

Coronary spasm is controlled by the routine use of vasodilators (nitrates and calcium channel antagonists), whereas thrombosis is con-

FIGURE 245-3 Stent placement in a diseased saphenous vein graft. *Left*: Severe eccentric stenosis in an 8-year-old saphenous vein graft to the left anterior descending coronary artery. *Middle*: After balloon angioplasty, the lumen remains stenotic due to elastic recoil of the vessel wall and disruption (dissection) of the plaque. *Right*: After placement of a coronary stent, both recoil and dissection have been overcome, providing a large smooth lumen.

trolled by systemic anticoagulation (heparin, 7000 to 10,000 units during the procedure to maintain an activated clotting time of 250 to 300 s), and antiplatelet therapy (aspirin, 325 mg/d starting at least 24 h before PCR and continued for at least 3 to 6 months after the procedure). If a coronary stent has been placed, aspirin is supplemented by a blocker of the platelet ADP receptor (ticlopidine or clopidogrel) to reduce the likelihood of stent thrombosis (see below). Newer potent intravenous antiplatelet agents (blockers of the platelet glycoprotein IIb/IIIa receptors) may reduce further the incidence of ischemic complications within 72 h of PCR, and are used prophylactically in what are perceived to be high-risk interventions or provisionally in interventions that have left behind an imperfect mechanical result (e.g., an unstented distal dissection).

Perforation of a coronary artery was an extremely rare complication of conventional balloon angioplasty but may occur in up to 1% of patients undergoing more aggressive atherectomy procedures (see below). Even small perforations of the distal vessel by the angioplasty guidewire may lead to significant hemopericardium requiring urgent pericardiocentesis in the setting of intense anticoagulant and antiplatelet therapy. Finally, catheter-based interventions are subject to all of the complications of diagnostic catheterization, including adverse reactions to iodinated contrast agents and groin hematoma. By and large, however, catheter-based coronary revascularization has reached the point of being a safe and effective alternative to surgical revascularization.

FOLLOW-UP   After successful PCR of all "culprit" lesions, marked improvement or complete resolution of the presenting ischemic syndrome should be evident. In approximately 20% of patients, however, evidence of recurrent ischemia develops within 6 months, due to restenosis of the dilated segment. This restenosis appears to result from excessive local fibrointimal proliferation and vessel constriction, occurring in response to the local injury that is part of enlarging the stenotic lumen. When recurrent ischemia develops more than 6 months after PCR, it usually reflects progression of disease at another site, rather than restenosis. Whether due to restenosis or disease progression, most post-PCR problems can be treated by repeat PCR, so that only about 10% of patients require bypass surgery during the 5 years after a successful procedure. When a patient has provided evidence of severe obstructive coronary atherosclerosis requiring revascularization, either by bypass surgery or PCR, the opportunity to implement an aggressive program to reduce atherosclerotic risk factors and thereby slow the pace of development of new lesions should not be overlooked (Chap. 244).

NONBALLOON TECHNIQUES   Conventional balloon angioplasty (PTCA) was the only catheter-based coronary revascularization technique that was widely available before 1990. Although it offered anatomic versatility and acceptable short- and long-term results, the difficulty of using this technique for certain anatomic lesion types (e.g., calcified eccentric, ostial, thrombus-containing, or bifurcation lesions) and the persistence of problems such as abrupt closure and restenosis fostered the development of a number of newer, nonballoon techniques that include stent placement and atherectomy. These treatments moved from clinical investigation to routine clinical practice during the early 1990s and now account for 70 to 80% of percutaneous coronary interventions. Used appropriately, these new techniques have improved the success, safety, and long-term results (restenosis rate) in most lesion types. Most of these procedures cost more than PTCA, but much of this cost can be recouped by the reduction in long-term expenses for the treatment of restenosis. Given these developments, stand-alone balloon angioplasty is now used in a minority of procedures (20% of all PCRs), although adjunctive balloon angioplasty is still routinely used to pre- or postdilate, before or after a newer interventional device.

STENTS   Stents are metallic scaffolds that are inserted into a diseased vessel segment in their collapsed form and are then expanded (by balloon expansion, or by self-expansion after removal of a con-

straining membrane) to establish a normal-appearing vessel lumen. Stents overcome two of the principal limitations of balloon dilatation—the tendency for elastic recoil of the vessel wall and local dissection of the plaque. As such, stents provide a larger acute lumen than does conventional balloon angioplasty, which allows them to reduce the incidence of subsequent restenosis by roughly one-third (e.g., angiographic restenosis rates of 20% versus 33%, and clinical restenosis rates of 10% versus 16 to 20%). When in-stent restenosis does occur, it is almost never the result of stent crush but rather the consequence of excessive neointimal hyperplasia within the stent (Fig. 245-4). In-stent restenosis can be treated by atherectomy to remove the excess tissue (see below), balloon dilatation, and then local delivery of β or γ radiation to suppress neointimal regrowth.

Two balloon-expandable stent designs were approved by the Food and Drug Administration (FDA) in the early 1990s—a wire coil design for use in stabilizing actual or threatened abrupt closure and a slotted tube design for elective treatment of native coronary lesions. After their release, the efficacy of the slotted tube design was demonstrated in a variety of other circumstances, including restenotic lesions and saphenous vein grafts (Fig. 245-3). In the late 1990s, a number of second generation stent designs were developed that offer easier delivery to tortuous or distal lesions as well as a wider variety of sizes and lengths. The approval of these devices has allowed them to completely replace the first generation devices in clinical practice (Fig. 245-5). Still further refinements in stent coverings (to seal aneurysms or perforations) and coatings (to suppress stent thrombosis and in-stent proliferation) are in progress.

Early experience suggested that metallic stents were prone to thrombotic occlusion, either acute (<24 h) or subacute (1 to 14 days with a peak at 6 days), and that an aggressive anticoagulation regimen (aspirin, dipyridamole, and warfarin) was needed to prevent such thrombosis. This aggressive anticoagulant regimen reduced the incidence of stent thrombosis to ~3% but led to longer hospitalization and an increased incidence of local vascular complications at the femoral arterial entry site. Subsequent data suggested that many of these thrombotic complications were the result of incomplete stent expansion and that more attention to full initial deployment would allow the same stents to be used with only antiplatelet drugs (aspirin plus the platelet ADP-receptor blockers, ticlopidine or clopidogrel) with more

FIGURE 245-4   Short- and long-term results in a long lesion in the right coronary artery. *Left*: A long (~50 mm) area of disease (*arrows*) is present in the right coronary artery. *Right center*: Contrast injection after placement of two long second generation stents (25 and 35 mm long) shows excellent patency throughout the proximal- and mid-portions of the vessel. *Right*: Follow-up angiogram 6 months after stent placement shows mild lumen reduction throughout the stented segment due to neointimal hyperplasia within the stent (note the separation between the stent shadows and the contrast-filled lumen. Mild degrees of proliferative narrowing are benign and common within stents (particularly long stents such as this one). Had the degree of lumen reduction been greater and associated with recurrent symptoms or an abnormal exercise test, however, re-intervention would have been performed with a debulking technique (e.g., rotational atherectomy) followed by balloon angioplasty, and possibly local radiation delivery (brachytherapy) to inhibit excessive tissue regrowth.

acceptable thrombosis and vascular complication rates (each <1%). This rapid evolution in devices, concomitant medications, and indications has led to the dominance of stent placement in catheter-based coronary revascularization, with placement of one or more stents in 70 to 80% of all procedures.

Atherectomy Whereas both balloon angioplasty and stent placement enlarge the coronary lumen by displacing plaque, atherectomy catheters enlarge the lumen by removing plaque mass from the treated lesion. Directional atherectomy achieves this result by use of a special catheter with a windowed steel cylinder at its tip. Inflation of a low-pressure positioning balloon on the back of the cylinder presses plaque into the window, where it is cut and trapped by a spinning cup-shaped cutter. This device was the first (1990) approved nonballoon technology to reach clinical practice, and it is still the treatment of choice for noncalcified lesions at the origin of the left anterior descending artery or at major coronary bifurcations (Fig. 245-6). Although its efficacy over conventional balloon angioplasty has been demonstrated, the ease and result of stent placement are much greater for most other lesion types. Rotational atherectomy uses burrs of various sizes (diameter 1.25 to 2.50 mm) that are coated on their leading half with small diamond chips. The burr is spun at 140,000 to 160,000 rpm as it is advanced through a coronary lesion over a leading guidewire. As the burr is advanced, the diamond chips grind through the obstructing plaque, and pulverize it into small (5 to 25 μm) particles, which pass through the distal coronary microcirculation. This device has emerged as an effective treatment for long (>20 mm), calcified, ostial lesions or in-stent restenotic lesions, frequently followed by balloon dilation or stent placement. *Extraction* atherectomy uses a combination of distal cutting blades rotating at low speed and continuous vacuum aspiration to remove coronary obstructions. The device has limited cutting efficiency, and its use is now confined to softer lesions (e.g., atherosclerotic saphenous vein grafts) or thrombotic lesions. Newer aspiration devices based on the Bernoulli principle appear better able to remove clot and cause less vessel disruption.

Although it is not mechanical, laser light [at wavelengths from the ultraviolet (308 mm) to the midinfrared (2000 μm)] can be delivered to obstructing coronary plaques through bundles of small optical fibers housed in flexible catheters whose outer diameter is between 1.2 and 2.0 mm. When these catheters are pulsed with laser energy as they are advanced through a coronary obstruction over a guidewire, they can ablate noncalcified coronary plaque by a combination of photoacoustic (blast), thermal, and photochemical effects. Although lasers have been used to treat ostial as well as diffuse coronary lesions, acceptance of the technique has been limited by the expense of the device and the fact that these lesions can be treated by other techniques, such as rotational atherectomy.

SUMMARY With the development of new techniques such as stent placement and atherectomy, new drug regimens, and a preponderance of "evidence-based" practices, over the last 20 years catheter-based revascularization (PCR) has developed from a procedural curiosity to one of the mainstays of coronary revascularization. As short- and long-term results have improved and the number of procedures

FIGURE 245-5 Second generation stent. *Left*: The flexibility typical of second generation stents is shown in bending the collapsed stent on its delivery balloon. *Right*: The same stent design is shown in its balloon-expanded configuration, in some of the available lengths [32 mm (top), 16 mm, and 9 mm]. The availability of a variety of second generation stents since 1997 has helped make stent placement a part of more than 70% of all PCRs.

FIGURE 245-6 Treatment of a bifurcation lesion in the circumflex coronary artery. *Upper left*: Stenosis (*arrow*) involves both the main circumflex and a large marginal branch. *Upper right*: Directional atherectomy as performed in the main circumflex. *Middle left*: Interim result after atherectomy in the main circumflex shows resolution of stenosis in that vessel (*curved arrow*) but persistent stenosis in the marginal branch (*small arrow*). *Lower right*: Additional atherectomy cuts are made in the marginal branch. *Lower left*: The final result (*arrow*) shows no residual stenosis in either the main circumflex or the marginal branch.

has continued to grow, the pace of development, if anything, has intensified.

BIBLIOGRAPHY

BAIM DS: Coronary angioplasty, in *Cardiac Catheterization, Angiography and Intervention*, 6th ed, D Baim, W Grossman (eds). Baltimore, Lippincott, Williams & Wilkins, 2000

CARROZZA JP et al: Coronary intervention: Angioplasty, stents, and atherectomy, in *Evidence Based Cardiology*, S Yusuf et al (eds). London, BMJ Books, 1998

DETRE KM et al: Coronary revascularization in diabetic patients—a comparison of the randomized and observational components of the Bypass Angioplasty Revascularization Investigation (BARI). Circulation 99:633, 1999

FISCHMAN DL et al: A randomized comparison of coronary stent placement and balloon angioplasty in the treatment of coronary artery disease. N Engl J Med 331:496, 1994

GIBBONS RJ et al: ACC/AHA/ACP-ASIM guidelines for the management of patients with chronic stable angina—executive summary and recommendations. Circulation 99: 2829, 1999

HIRSHFELD JW et al: Recommendations for the assessment and maintenance of proficiency in coronary interventional procedures. J Am Coll Cardiol 31:722, 1998

KONG DF et al: Outcomes of therapeutic agents that block the platelet glycoprotein IIb/IIIa integrin in ischemic heart disease. Circulation 98:2829, 1998

KUNTZ RE, BAIM DS: Defining coronary restenosis: Newer clinical and angiographic paradigms. Circulation 88:1310, 1993

LEON MB et al: A randomized trial comparing three anti-thrombotic drug regimens following coronary-artery stenting. N Engl J Med 339:1665, 1998

POPMA J: Interventional cardiology, in *Heart Disease*, 6th ed, E Braunwald, D Zipes, P Libby (eds). Philadelphia, Saunders, 2001

WEAVER WD et al: Comparison of primary coronary angioplasty and intravenous thrombolytic therapy for acute myocardial infarction—a quantitative review. JAMA 278: 2093, 1997

246   *Gordon H. Williams*

HYPERTENSIVE VASCULAR DISEASE

An elevated arterial pressure is probably the most important public health problem in developed countries. It is common, asymptomatic, readily detectable, usually easily treatable, and often leads to lethal complications if left untreated (Chap. 35). As a result of extensive educational programs in the late 1960s and 1970s by both private and government agencies, the number of undiagnosed and/or untreated patients was reduced significantly by the late 1980s to a level of about 25%, with a concomitant decline in cardiovascular mortality. Unfortunately, by the mid-1990s, this beneficial trend began to wane. The number of undiagnosed patients with hypertension increased to nearly 33%, the decline in cardiovascular mortality flattened, and the number of individuals with chronic diseases with untreated or poorly treated hypertension increased. For example, the prevalence of end-stage renal disease per million population increased from <100 in 1982 to >250 in 1995, and the prevalence of congestive heart failure from ages 55 to 75 more than doubled between 1976 to 1980 and 1988 to 1991. Thus, although our understanding of the pathophysiology of elevated arterial pressure has increased, in 90 to 95% of cases the etiology (and thus potentially the means of prevention or cure) is still largely unknown. As a consequence, in most cases the hypertension is treated nonspecifically, resulting in a large number of minor side effects and a relatively high (50 to 60%) noncompliance rate.

PREVALENCE   The prevalence of hypertension depends on both the racial composition of the population studied and the criteria used to define the condition. In a white suburban population like that in the Framingham Study, nearly one-fifth of individuals have blood pressures >160/95, while almost one-half have pressures >140/90. An even higher prevalence has been documented in the nonwhite population. In females the prevalence is closely related to age, with a substantial increase occurring after age 50. This increase is presumably related to the hormonal changes of menopause, although the mechanism is unclear. Thus, the ratio of hypertension frequency in women versus men increases from 0.6 to 0.7 at age 30 to 1.1 to 1.2 at age 65.

The prevalence of various forms of secondary hypertension depends on the nature of the population studied and on how extensive the evaluation is. There are no available data to define the frequency of secondary hypertension in the general population, although in middle-aged males it has been reported to be 6%. On the other hand, in referral centers where patients undergo an extensive evaluation, it has been reported to be as high as 35%. The various forms of hypertension are outlined in Table 246-1, and their relative frequencies are given in Table 246-2.

ESSENTIAL HYPERTENSION

Patients with arterial pressure and no definable cause are said to have *primary*, *essential*, or *idiopathic hypertension*. Undoubtedly, the primary difficulty in uncovering the mechanism(s) responsible for the hypertension in these patients is attributable to the variety of systems

Table 246-1   Classification of Arterial Hypertension

SYSTOLIC HYPERTENSION WITH WIDE PULSE PRESSURE

I. Decreased compliance of aorta (arteriosclerosis)
II. Increased stroke volume
   A. Aortic regurgitation
   B. Thyrotoxicosis
   C. Hyperkinetic heart syndrome
   D. Fever
   E. Arteriovenous fistula
   F. Patent ductus arteriosus

SYSTOLIC AND DIASTOLIC HYPERTENSION (INCREASED PERIPHERAL VASCULAR RESISTANCE)

I. Renal
   A. Chronic pyelonephritis
   B. Acute and chronic glomerulonephritis
   C. Polycystic renal disease
   D. Renovascular stenosis or renal infarction
   E. Most other severe renal diseases (arteriolar nephrosclerosis, diabetic nephropathy, etc.)
   F. Renin-producing tumors
II. Endocrine
   A. Oral contraceptives
   B. Adrenocortical hyperfunction
      1. Cushing's disease and syndrome
      2. Primary hyperaldosteronism
      3. Congenital or hereditary adrenogenital syndromes (17α-hydroxylase and 11β-hydroxylase defects)
   C. Pheochromocytoma
   D. Myxedema
   E. Acromegaly
III. Neurogenic
   A. Psychogenic
   B. Diencephalic syndrome
   C. Familial dysautonomia (Riley-Day)
   D. Polyneuritis (acute porphyria, lead poisoning)
   E. Increased intracranial pressure (acute)
   F. Spinal cord section (acute)
IV. Miscellaneous
   A. Coarctation of aorta
   B. Increased intravascular volume (excessive transfusion, polycythemia vera)
   C. Polyarteritis nodosa
   D. Hypercalcemia
   E. Medications, e.g., glucocorticoids, cyclosporine
V. Unknown etiology
   A. Essential hypertension (>90% of all cases of hypertension)
   B. Toxemia of pregnancy
   C. Acute intermittent porphyria

Table 246-2   Prevalence of Various Forms of Hypertension in the General Population and in Specialized Referral Clinics[a]

Diagnosis	General Population, %	Specialty Clinic, %
Essential hypertension	92–94	65–85
Renal hypertension:		
Parenchymal	2–3	4–5
Renovascular	1–2	4–16
Endocrine hypertension:		
Primary aldosteronism	0.3	0.5–12
Cushing's syndrome	<0.1	0.2
Pheochromocytoma	<0.1	0.2
Oral contraceptive–induced	0.5–1	1–2
Miscellaneous	0.2	1

[a] Estimates based on a number of reports in the literature.

that are involved in the regulation of arterial pressure—peripheral and/or central adrenergic, renal, hormonal, and vascular—and to the complexity of the interrelations of these systems. Several abnormalities have been described in patients with essential hypertension, often with a claim that one or more of them are primarily responsible for the hypertension. While it is still uncertain whether these individual abnormalities are primary or secondary, varying expressions of a single disease process or reflective of separate disease entities, the accumulating data increasingly support the latter hypothesis. Therefore, just as pneumonia is caused by a variety of infectious agents, even though the clinical picture observed may be similar, so essential hypertension likely has a number of distinct causes. Thus, the distinction between primary and secondary hypertension has become blurred, and the approach to both the diagnosis and therapy of hypertensive patients has been modified. For example, when a group of patients with essential hypertension is separated into a distinct subset (e.g., low-renin essential hypertension), the patients have not been reclassified as having a form of secondary hypertension but rather remain in the essential hypertensive group. In this chapter, individuals in whom a specific structural organ or gene defect is responsible for hypertension are defined as having a *secondary* form of hypertension. In contrast, individuals in whom generalized or functional abnormalities may be the cause of hypertension, even if the abnormalities are discrete, are defined as having *essential* hypertension.

GENETIC CONSIDERATIONS   Genetic factors have long been assumed to be important in the genesis of hypertension. Data supporting this view can be found in animal studies as well as in population studies in humans. One approach has been to assess the correlation of blood pressure in families (familial aggregation). From these studies, the minimum size of the genetic factor can be expressed by a correlation coefficient of approximately 0.2. However, the variation in the size of the genetic factor in different studies reemphasizes the probably heterogeneous nature of the essential hypertensive population. In addition, most studies support the concept that the inheritance is probably multifactorial or that a number of different genetic defects each have an elevated blood pressure as one of their phenotypic expressions. Finally, both monogenic defects (e.g., glucocorticoid-remediable aldosteronism and Liddle's syndrome) and susceptibility genes (e.g., the angiotensinogen and α adducin genes) have now been reported which have as one of their consequences an increased arterial pressure (see below and Chap. 331). Yet, as can be seen in Table 246-3, most studies of likely genes have failed to document linkage

Table 246-3   Genesis Hypothesized to be Involved in Essential Hypertension

Gene	Intermediate Phenotype Used	Statistical Approach	
		Association	Linkage
11β Hydroxylase/aldosterone synthase	Urine 18 OH cortisol	Not done	Positive
β Subunit epithelial sodium channel	None	Not done	Positive
Angiotensinogen	Severe, early-onset hypertension	Positive	Positive
Angiotensin-converting enzyme	None	Negative[a]	Negative
Renin	None	Negative	Negative
Angiotensin II AT1 receptor	None	Negative	Negative
Glucocorticoid receptor	Increased plasma cortisol	Positive	Not done
Renal kallikrein	None	Negative	Not done
Endothelin 1	None	Negative	Not done
Insulin receptor	None	Positive	Not done
Human SA locus	None	Positive	Negative
α Adducin	None	Positive	Not done
Endothelial cell adducin	None	Positive	Not done
Endothelial cell NO synthase	None	Positive	Not done
Apoliproprotein C III	None	Positive	Not done
Lipoprotein lipase	None	Positive	Not done

[a] One positive study.
NOTE: OH, hydroxy; NO, nitric oxide.
SOURCE: From GH Williams, NDL Fisher, in E Braunwald (ed): *The Genetics of Human Hypertension in Heart Disease, Update 5.* Philadelphia, Saunders, 1995.

or consistent association with hypertension. However, uncertainty exists as to the validity of these negative conclusions. A positive relationship between hypertension and a gene could be obscured by the high probability of a false-negative result because of the heterogeneity of the hypertensive population. Thus, intermediate phenotypes in the hypertensive population need to be identified to differentiate patients into more homogeneous subgroups; the role of a specific candidate gene can then be more readily assessed. Such an approach is illustrated in Table 246-4. ■

ENVIRONMENT   A number of environmental factors have been implicated in the development of hypertension, including salt intake, obesity, occupation, alcohol intake, family size, and crowding. These factors have all been assumed to be important in the increase in blood pressure with age in more affluent societies, in contrast to the decline in blood pressure with age in less affluent groups.

SALT SENSITIVITY   The environmental factor that has received the greatest attention is salt intake. Even this factor illustrates the heterogeneous nature of the essential hypertensive population, in that the blood pressure in only approximately 60% of hypertensives is particularly responsive to the level of sodium intake. The cause of this special sensitivity to salt varies, with primary aldosteronism, bilateral renal artery stenosis, renal parenchymal disease, and low-renin essential hypertension accounting for about half the patients. In the remainder, the pathophysiology is still uncertain, but postulated contributing factors include chloride intake, calcium intake, a generalized cellular membrane defect, insulin resistance, and "nonmodulation" (see below).

ROLE OF RENIN   Renin is an enzyme secreted by the juxtaglomerular cell of the kidney and linked with aldosterone in a negative feedback loop (Chap. 331). While a variety of factors can modify its rate of secretion, the primary determinant is the volume status of the individual, particularly as related to changes in dietary sodium intake. The end product of the action of renin on its substrate is the generation of the peptide angiotensin II. The response of target tissues to this peptide is uniquely determined by the prior dietary electrolyte intake. For example, sodium intake normally modulates adrenal and renal vascular responses to angiotensin II. With sodium restriction, adrenal responses are enhanced and the renal vascular responses reduced. Sodium loading has the opposite effect. The range of plasma renin activities observed in hypertensive subjects is broader than in normotensive individuals. In consequence, some hypertensive patients have been defined as having *low-renin* and others as having *high-renin* essential hypertension.

Low-Renin Essential Hypertension   Approximately 20% of patients who by all other criteria have essential hypertension have suppressed plasma renin activity. This situation is more common in individuals of African descent than in white patients. Though these patients are not hypokalemic, they have been reported to have expanded extracellular fluid volumes, and it has been suggested but not proved that they have sodium retention and renin suppression due to excessive production of an unidentified mineralocorticoid. On the other hand, some, but not all, studies have suggested that the adrenal cortex of some of these patients has an increased sensitivity to angi-

Table 246-4   Role of Intermediate Phenotypes in Genetic Analysis

Gene	Phenotype	
	Intermediate	Distant
Converting enzyme	Angiotensin II effect on kidney	Increases BP
Angiotensinogen		Increases BP
Aldo synthase	Increases 18 OH cortisol	Increases BP
Kallikrein	Decreases urine kallikrein	Increases BP
Na+/H+ exchanger	Increases Na/Li CTT	Increases BP

NOTE: BP, blood pressure; OH, hydroxy; CTT, countertransport.
SOURCE: From GH Williams, NDL Fisher, in E Braunwald (ed): *The Genetics of Human Hypertension in Heart Disease, Update 5.* Philadelphia, Saunders, 1995.

otensin II as the underlying mechanism. Not only does this hypothesis potentially explain their low plasma renin activity, it also suggests the cause of their hypertension. On a diet with a normal or high sodium content, aldosterone production will not be suppressed normally, leading to a mild degree of hyperaldosteronism with its resulting increased sodium retention, volume expansion, and increase in blood pressure. Since this altered sensitivity has been reported even in patients with normal-renin hypertension, it is likely that patients with low-renin hypertension are not a distinct subset but rather form part of a continuum of patients with essential hypertension.

Nonmodulating Essential Hypertension   Another subset of hypertensive patients has an adrenal defect opposite to that observed in some low-renin patients—a reduced adrenal response to sodium restriction. In these individuals, sodium intake does not modulate either adrenal or renal vascular responses to angiotensin II. Hypertensives in this subset have been termed *nonmodulators* because of the absence of the sodium-mediated modulation of target tissue responses to angiotensin II. These individuals make up 25 to 30% of the hypertensive population, have plasma renin activity levels that are normal to high if measured when the patient is on a low-salt diet, and have hypertension that is salt-sensitive because of a defect in the kidney's ability to excrete sodium appropriately. They also are more insulin-resistant than ohter hypertensive patients, and the pathophysiologic characteristics can be corrected by the administration of a converting-enzyme inhibitor. Furthermore, the nonmodulation characteristic appears to be genetically determined (associated with a certain allele of the angiotensinogen gene). Thus, nonmodulators are probably the most completely characterized intermediate phenotype in the hypertensive population.

High-Renin Essential Hypertension   Approximately 15% of patients with essential hypertension have plasma renin activity levels above the normal range. It has been suggested that plasma renin plays an important role in the pathogenesis of the elevated arterial pressure in these patients. However, most studies have found that saralasin (a substance that, like losartan, acts as a competitive antagonist of angiotensin II) significantly reduces blood pressure in fewer than half of these patients. This finding has led some investigators to postulate that the elevated renin levels and blood pressure may both be secondary to an increase in adrenergic system activity. It has been proposed that, in patients with angiotensin-dependent high-renin hypertension whose arterial pressures are lowered by an angiotensin II antagonist, the mechanism responsible for the increase in renin and, therefore, for the hypertension is the nonmodulating defect.

SODIUM ION VERSUS CHLORIDE OR CALCIUM Most studies assessing the role of salt in the hypertensive process have assumed that it is the sodium ion that is important. However, some investigators have suggested that the chloride ion may be equally important. This suggestion is based on the observation that feeding chloride-free sodium salts to salt-sensitive hypertensive animals fails to increase arterial pressure. Calcium has also been implicated in the pathogenesis of some forms of essential hypertension. A low-calcium intake has been associated with an increase in blood pressure in epidemiologic studies; an increase in leukocyte cytosolic calcium levels has been reported in some hypertensives. Finally, calcium entry blockers are effective antihypertensive agents. Several studies have reported a potential link between the salt-sensitive forms of hypertension and calcium. It has been postulated that salt loading in combination with a defect in the kidney's ability to excrete salt may lead to a secondary increase in circulating natriuretic factors. One of these factors, the so-called digitalis-like natriuretic factor, inhibits ouabain-sensitive Na^+, K^+-ATPase and thereby leads to intracellular calcium accumulation and a hyperreactive vascular smooth muscle.

CELL MEMBRANE DEFECT   Another postulated explanation for salt-sensitive hypertension is a generalized cell membrane defect. This hypothesis derives most of its data from studies on circulating blood elements, particularly red blood cells, in which abnormalities in the transport of sodium across the cell membrane have

been documented. Since both increases and decreases in the activity of different transport systems have been reported, it is likely that some abnormalities are primary and some are secondary. It has been assumed that this abnormality in sodium transport reflects an undefined alteration in the cell membrane and that this defect occurs in many, perhaps all, cells of the body, particularly the vascular smooth-muscle cells. The defect leads to an abnormal accumulation of calcium in vascular smooth muscle, resulting in a heightened vascular responsiveness to vasoconstrictor agents. This defect has been proposed to be present in 35 to 50% of essential hypertensive persons on the basis of studies using red cells. Other studies suggest that the abnormality in red cell sodium transport is not fixed but can be modified by environmental factors.

The common final pathway in all these hypotheses is an increase in cytosolic calcium resulting in increased vascular reactivity. However, as described above, several mechanisms might produce this calcium accumulation.

INSULIN RESISTANCE   Insulin resistance and/or hyperinsulinemia have been suggested as being responsible for the increased arterial pressure in some patients with hypertension. While it is clear that a substantial fraction of the hypertensive population has insulin resistance and hyperinsulinemia, it is less certain that this is more than an association. Insulin resistance is common in patients with non-insulin-dependent diabetes mellitus (NIDDM) or obesity. Both obesity and NIDDM are more common in hypertensive than in normotensive subjects. However, several studies have found that hyperinsulinemia and insulin resistance are present even in lean hypertensive patients without NIDDM, suggesting that this relationship is more than a coincidence. As noted earlier, these individuals seem to be concentrated in the nonmodulation phenotype.

Hyperinsulinemia can increase arterial pressure by one or more of four mechanisms. An underlying assumption in each case is that some, but not all, of the target tissues of insulin are resistant to its effects. Specifically, tissues involved in glucose homeostasis are resistant (thereby producing the hyperinsulinemia), while tissues involved in the hypertensive process are not. First, hyperinsulinemia produces renal sodium retention (at least acutely) and increases sympathetic activity. Either or both of these effects could lead to an increase in arterial pressure. Another mechanism is vascular smooth-muscle hypertrophy secondary to the mitogenic action of insulin. Third, insulin also modifies ion transport across the cell membrane, thereby potentially increasing the cytosolic calcium levels of insulin-sensitive vascular or renal tissues. This mechanism would increase arterial pressure for reasons similar to those described above for the membrane-defect hypothesis. Finally, insulin resistance may be a marker for another pathologic process, e.g., nonmodulation, which could be the primary mechanism increasing blood pressure. It is important to point out, however, that the role of insulin in controlling arterial pressure is only vaguely understood, and, therefore, its potential as a pathogenic factor in hypertension remains unclear.

Few of the features of hypertension discussed above remain constant in a given patient. Some may be a reflection of the current metabolic and hormonal status of the patient rather than a permanent feature of the disease process. For example, at one point a patient might have insulin resistance secondary to obesity, which could lead to sodium retention, intravascular volume expansion, and renin suppression. This patient would be labeled as having "low-renin essential hypertension." If the patient lost weight, however, the salt-retaining tendency would be reversed. If the blood pressure did not normalize, the patient might then have "normal or high-renin essential hypertension." Thus, the features reviewed above should not be considered mutually exclusive or permanent characteristics in a given patient with hypertension.

FACTORS THAT MODIFY THE COURSE OF ESSENTIAL HYPERTENSION   Age, race, sex, smoking, alcohol intake, serum cholesterol, glucose intolerance, and weight may all alter the prognosis of this disease. The younger the patient when hypertension is first noted, the greater is the reduction in life expectancy if the hypertension is left untreated. In the United States, urban blacks have

Black race
Youth
Male sex
Persistent diastolic pressure >115 mmHg
Smoking
Diabetes mellitus
Hypercholesterolemia
Obesity
Excess alcohol intake
Evidence of end organ damage
  1. Cardiac
    a. Cardiac enlargement
    b. Electrocardiographic signs of ischemia or left ventricular strain
    c. Myocardial infarction
    d. Congestive heart failure
  2. Eyes
    a. Retinal exudates and hemorrhages
    b. Papilledema
  3. Renal: impaired renal function
  4. Nervous system: cerebrovascular accident

about twice the prevalence of hypertension as whites and more than four times the hypertension-induced morbidity rate. At all ages and in both white and nonwhite populations, females with hypertension fare better than males up to the age of 65, and the prevalence of hypertension in premenopausal females is substantially less than that in age-matched males or postmenopausal women. Yet, compared with their normotensive counterparts, females with hypertension run the same relative risk of a morbid cardiovascular event as males do. Accelerated atherosclerosis is an invariable companion of hypertension. Thus, it is not surprising that independent risk factors associated with the development of atherosclerosis, such as an elevated serum cholesterol, glucose intolerance, and/or cigarette smoking, significantly enhance the effect of hypertension on mortality rate regardless of age, sex, or race (Chap. 241). There also is no question that a positive correlation exists between obesity and arterial pressure. A gain in weight is associated with an increased frequency of hypertension in persons with normal blood pressure, and weight loss in obese persons with hypertension lowers their arterial pressure and, if they are being treated for hypertension, the intensity of therapy required to keep them normotensive. Whether these changes are mediated by changes in insulin resistance is unknown.

NATURAL HISTORY Because essential hypertension is a heterogeneous disorder, variables other than the arterial pressure modify its course. Thus, the probability of developing a morbid cardiovascular event with a given arterial pressure may vary as much as 20-fold depending on whether associated risk factors are present (Table 246-5). Although exceptions have been reported, most untreated adults with hypertension will develop further increases in arterial pressure with time. Furthermore, it has been demonstrated from both actuarial data and experience in the era prior to effective therapy that untreated hypertension is associated with a shortening of life by 10 to 20 years, usually related to an acceleration of the atherosclerotic process, with the rate of acceleration in part related to the severity of the hypertension. Even individuals who have relatively mild disease—i.e., without evidence of end organ damage—that is left untreated for 7 to 10 years have a high risk of developing significant complications. Nearly 30% will exhibit atherosclerotic complications, and more than 50% will have end organ damage related to the hypertension itself, such as cardiomegaly, congestive heart failure, retinopathy, a cerebrovascular accident, and/or renal insufficiency. Thus, even in its mild forms, hypertension is a progressive and lethal disease if left untreated.

SECONDARY HYPERTENSION

As noted earlier, in only a small minority of patients with elevated arterial pressure can a specific cause be identified. Yet these patients should not be ignored for at least two reasons: (1) correction of the cause may cure their hypertension, and (2) these secondary forms of the disease may provide insight into the etiology of essential hypertension. Nearly all the secondary forms of hypertension are related to an alteration in hormone secretion and/or renal function and are discussed in detail in other chapters.

RENAL HYPERTENSION (See also Chap. 278) Hypertension produced by renal disease is the result of either (1) a derangement in the renal handling of sodium and fluids leading to volume expansion or (2) an alteration in renal secretion of vasoactive materials resulting in a systemic or local change in arteriolar tone. The main subdivisions of renal hypertension are renovascular hypertension, including preeclampsia and eclampsia, and renal parenchymal hypertension. A simple explanation for *renal vascular hypertension* is that decreased perfusion of renal tissue due to stenosis of a main or branch renal artery activates the renin-angiotensin system, described in Chap. 331. Circulating angiotensin II elevates arterial pressure by directly causing vasoconstriction, by stimulating aldosterone secretion with resulting sodium retention, and/or by stimulating the adrenergic nervous system. In practice, only about one-half of patients with renovascular hypertension have an absolute elevation in renin activity in peripheral plasma, although when renin measurements are referenced against an index of sodium balance, a much higher fraction have inappropriately high values.

Activation of the renin-angiotensin system has also been offered as an explanation for the hypertension in both acute and chronic *renal parenchymal disease*. In this formulation, the only difference between renovascular and renal parenchymal hypertension is that the decreased perfusion of renal tissue in the latter case results from inflammatory and fibrotic changes involving multiple small intrarenal vessels. There are enough differences between the two conditions, however, to suggest that other mechanisms are active in renal parenchymal disease. Specifically, (1) peripheral plasma renin activity is elevated far less frequently in renal parenchymal than in renovascular hypertension; (2) cardiac output is said to be normal in renal parenchymal hypertension (unless uremia and anemia are present) but slightly elevated in renovascular hypertension; (3) circulatory responses to tilting and to the Valsalva maneuver are exaggerated in the latter condition; and (4) blood volume tends to be high in patients with severe renal parenchymal disease and low in patients with severe unilateral renovascular hypertension. Alternative explanations for the hypertension in renal parenchymal disease include the possibilities that the damaged kidneys (1) produce an unidentified vasopressor substance other than renin, (2) fail to produce a necessary humoral vasodilator substance (perhaps prostaglandin or bradykinin), (3) fail to inactivate circulating vasopressor substances, and/or (4) are ineffective in disposing of sodium. In the last case, the retained sodium would be responsible for the hypertension as outlined earlier. Although all these explanations, including participation of the renin-angiotensin system, probably have some validity in individual patients, the hypothesis involving sodium retention is particularly attractive. It is supported by the observation that those patients with chronic pyelonephritis or polycystic renal disease who are salt wasters do not develop hypertension and by the observation that removal of salt and water by dialysis or diuretics is effective in controlling arterial pressure in most patients with renal parenchymal disease.

A rare form of renal hypertension results from the excess secretion of renin by juxtaglomerular cell tumors or nephroblastomas. The initial presentation is similar to that of hyperaldosteronism, with hypertension, hypokalemia, and overproduction of aldosterone. However, in contrast to primary aldosteronism, peripheral renin activity is *elevated instead of subnormal*. This disease can be distinguished from other forms of secondary aldosteronism by the presence of normal renal function and unilateral increases in renal vein renin concentration without a renal artery lesion.

ENDOCRINE HYPERTENSION **Adrenal Hypertension** Hypertension is a feature of a variety of adrenal cortical abnormalities. In *primary aldosteronism* (Chap. 331), there is a clear relationship between the aldosterone-induced sodium retention and the hypertension. Normal individuals given aldosterone develop hypertension only if they also ingest sodium. Since aldosterone causes sodium retention by stimulating renal tubular exchange of sodium for potassium, hypokalemia is a prominent feature in most patients with primary aldosteronism, and, therefore, the measurement of serum potassium provides a simple screening test. The effect of sodium retention and volume expansion in chronically suppressing plasma renin activity is critical for the definitive diagnosis. In most clinical situations, plasma renin activity and plasma or urinary aldosterone levels parallel each other, but in patients with primary aldosteronism, aldosterone levels are high and relatively fixed because of autonomous aldosterone secretion, whereas plasma renin activity levels are suppressed and respond sluggishly to sodium depletion. Primary aldosteronism may be secondary to either a tumor or bilateral adrenal hyperplasia. It is important to distinguish between these two conditions preoperatively, since the hypertension in the latter case is usually not modified by operation.

The sodium-retaining effect of large amounts of glucocorticoids (perhaps resulting in part from saturation of the 11β-hydroxysteroid hydrogenase enzyme system in the kidney by the increased concentration of cortisol) also offers an explanation for the hypertension in severe cases of Cushing's syndrome (Chap. 331). Moreover, increased production of mineralocorticoids has also been documented in some patients with Cushing's syndrome. However, the hypertension in many cases of Cushing's syndrome does not seem volume-dependent, leading investigators to speculate that it may be secondary to glucocorticoid-induced production of renin substrate (angiotensin-mediated hypertension). In the forms of the adrenogenital syndrome due to C-11 or C-17 hydroxylase deficiency (Chap. 331), deoxycorticosterone accounts for the sodium retention and the resulting hypertension, which is accompanied by suppression of plasma renin activity.

In patients with pheochromocytoma (Chap. 332), increased secretion of epinephrine and norepinephrine by a tumor (most often located in the adrenal medulla) causes excessive stimulation of adrenergic receptors, which results in peripheral vasoconstriction and cardiac stimulation. This diagnosis is confirmed by demonstrating increased urinary excretion of epinephrine and norepinephrine and/or their metabolites.

Acromegaly (See also Chap. 328) Hypertension, coronary atherosclerosis, and cardiac hypertrophy are frequent complications of this condition.

Hypercalcemia (See also Chap. 340) The hypertension that occurs in up to one-third of patients with hyperparathyroidism ordinarily can be attributed to renal parenchymal damage due to nephrolithiasis and nephrocalcinosis. However, increased calcium levels can also have a direct vasoconstrictive effect. In some cases, the hypertension disappears when the hypercalcemia is corrected. Thus, paradoxically, the increased serum calcium level in hyperparathyroidism raises blood pressure, while epidemiologic studies suggest that a high calcium intake lowers blood pressure. To further confuse the issue, calcium entry–blocking agents are effective antihypertensive agents. Additional studies are needed to resolve these seemingly conflicting observations.

Oral Contraceptives Several years ago, a common cause of endocrine hypertension was the use of estrogen-containing oral contraceptives. However, several studies have since suggested that this is no longer true, probably owing to the lower estrogen content of modern oral contraceptives. In patients receiving these agents who do become hypertensive, the mechanism is likely to be activation of the renin-angiotensin-aldosterone system. Thus, both volume (aldosterone) and vasoconstrictor (angiotensin II) factors are important. The estrogen component of oral contraceptive agents stimulates the hepatic synthesis of the renin substrate angiotensinogen, which in turn favors the increased production of angiotensin II and secondary aldosteronism. Some women taking oral contraceptives have increased plasma concentrations of angiotensin II and aldosterone with some increase in

arterial pressure. However, only a small number actually have an increase in arterial pressure to a level >140/90, and, in about half of these, the hypertension will remit within 6 months of stopping the drug.

Why some women taking oral contraceptives develop hypertension and others do not is unclear but may be related to (1) increased vascular sensitivity to angiotensin II, (2) the presence of mild renal disease, (3) familial factors (over one-half have a positive family history for hypertension), (4) age (hypertension is significantly more prevalent in women over age 35), (5) the estrogen content of the contraceptive, and/or (6) obesity. Indeed some investigators have suggested that the oral contraceptives are simply unmasking women with essential hypertension.

COARCTATION OF THE AORTA (See also Chap. 234) The hypertension associated with coarctation may be caused by the constriction itself or perhaps by the changes in the renal circulation, which result in an unusual form of renal arterial hypertension. The diagnosis of coarctation is usually evident from physical examination and routine x-ray findings.

EFFECTS OF HYPERTENSION

Patients with hypertension die prematurely; the most common cause of death is heart disease, with stroke and renal failure also frequent, particularly in patients with significant retinopathy.

EFFECTS ON THE HEART Cardiac compensation for the excessive workload imposed by increased systemic pressure is at first sustained by concentric left ventricular hypertrophy, characterized by an increase in wall thickness. Ultimately, the function of this chamber deteriorates, the cavity dilates, and the symptoms and signs of heart failure appear (Chap. 231). Angina pectoris may also occur because of the combination of accelerated coronary arterial disease and increased myocardial oxygen requirements as a consequence of the increased myocardial mass (Chap. 244). On physical examination, the heart is enlarged and has a prominent left ventricular impulse. The sound of aortic closure is accentuated, and there may be a faint murmur of aortic regurgitation. Presystolic (atrial, fourth) heart sounds appear frequently in hypertensive heart disease, and a protodiastolic (ventricular, third) heart sound or summation gallop rhythm may be present. Electrocardiographic changes of left ventricular hypertrophy (Chap. 226) may occur, but the electrocardiogram substantially underestimates the frequency of cardiac hypertrophy compared with that observed with the echocardiogram. Evidence of ischemia or infarction may be observed late in the disease. Most deaths due to hypertension result from myocardial infarction or congestive heart failure. Recent data suggest that some of the myocardial damage may be mediated by aldosterone in the presence of a normal/high salt intake rather than just the increased blood pressure or an increase in angiotensin II levels per se.

NEUROLOGIC EFFECTS The neurologic effects of longstanding hypertension may be divided into retinal and central nervous system changes. Because the retina is the only tissue in which the arteries and arterioles can be examined directly, repeated ophthalmoscopic examination provides the opportunity to observe the progress of the vascular effects of hypertension (Table 35-2). The Keith-Wagener-Barker classification of the *retinal changes* in hypertension has provided a simple and excellent means for serial evaluation of hypertensive patients. Increasing severity of hypertension is associated with focal spasm and progressive general narrowing of the arterioles, as well as the appearance of hemorrhages, exudates, and papilledema. These retinal lesions often produce scotomata, blurred vision, and even blindness, especially when there is papilledema or hemorrhages of the macular area. Hypertensive lesions may develop acutely and, if therapy results in significant reduction of blood pressure, may show rapid resolution. Rarely, these lesions resolve without therapy. In contrast, retinal arteriolosclerosis results from endothelial and muscular proliferation, and it accurately reflects similar changes in other organs. Sclerotic changes do not develop as rapidly as hypertensive lesions, nor do they regress appreciably with therapy. As a consequence of increased wall thickness and rigidity, sclerotic arterioles distort and compress the veins where the two vessel types cross in their common fibrous sheath, and the reflected light streak from the arterioles is changed by the increased opacity of the vessel wall.

Central nervous system dysfunction also occurs frequently in patients with hypertension. Occipital headaches, most often occurring in the morning, are among the most prominent early symptoms of hypertension. Dizziness, light-headedness, vertigo, tinnitus, and dimmed vision or syncope may also be observed, but the more serious manifestations are due to vascular occlusion, hemorrhage, or encephalopathy (Chap. 361). The pathogeneses of the former two disorders are quite different. *Cerebral infarction* is secondary to the increased atherosclerosis observed in hypertensive patients, whereas *cerebral hemorrhage* is the result of both the elevated arterial pressure and the development of cerebral vascular microaneurysms (Charcot-Bouchard aneurysms). Only age and arterial pressure are known to influence the development of the microaneurysms. Thus, it is not surprising that arterial pressure shows a better association with cerebral hemorrhage than with either cerebral or myocardial infarction.

Hypertensive encephalopathy consists of the following symptom complex: severe hypertension, disordered consciousness, increased intracranial pressure, retinopathy with papilledema, and seizures. The pathogenesis is uncertain but is probably not related to arteriolar spasm or cerebral edema. Focal neurologic signs are infrequent and, if present, suggest that infarction, hemorrhage, or transient ischemic attacks are more likely diagnoses. Although some investigators have suggested that prompt lowering of arterial pressure in these patients may adversely affect cerebral blood flow, most studies indicate that this is not the case.

EFFECTS ON THE KIDNEY (See also Chap. 278)   Arteriosclerotic lesions of the afferent and efferent arterioles and the glomerular capillary tufts are the most common renal vascular lesions in hypertension and result in a decreased glomerular filtration rate and tubular dysfunction. Proteinuria and microscopic hematuria occur because of glomerular lesions, and approximately 10% of the deaths caused by hypertension result from renal failure. Blood loss in hypertension occurs not only from renal lesions; epistaxis, hemoptysis, and metrorrhagia also occur frequently in these patients.

Approach to the Patient

The detailed initial evaluation of the hypertensive patient is outlined in Chap. 35. It includes the critical elements of the history, physical examination, and basic laboratory investigation that aid in arriving at appropriate diagnostic and therapeutic decisions (Table 35-2).

DIAGNOSIS OF SECONDARY HYPERTENSION   Certain clues from the history, physical examination, and basic laboratory studies may suggest an unusual cause for the hypertension and dictate the need for special studies. For example, the abrupt onset of severe hypertension and/or the onset of hypertension of any severity in a patient under the age of 25 or over the age of 50 should lead to laboratory tests to exclude renovascular hypertension and pheochromocytoma. A history of headaches, palpitations, anxiety attacks, unusual sweating, hyperglycemia, and weight loss should also lead to tests to exclude pheochromocytoma. The presence of an abdominal bruit should lead to a workup for renovascular hypertension, and the finding on physical examination of bilateral upper abdominal masses consistent with polycystic renal disease should lead to the performance of an abdominal ultrasound examination or intravenous pyelogram (IVP). An elevated creatinine or blood urea nitrogen level, associated with proteinuria and hematuria, should prompt a detailed workup for renal insufficiency (Chap. 268). Special studies for secondary hypertension are also indicated if there is therapeutic failure with the initial drug program. The specific diagnostic measures depend on the most likely causes of secondary hypertension.

Pheochromocytoma (See also Chap. 332)   The easiest and best screening procedure for pheochromocytoma is the measurement of catecholamines and their metabolites in a 24-h urine sample collected while the patient is hypertensive. Measurement of plasma catecholamine levels may also be useful. These tests may be indicated even in patients who do not have episodic hypertension, since over half the patients with pheochromocytoma have fixed hypertension. Provocative tests are seldom, if ever, indicated, although occasionally a suppressive test may be useful.

Cushing's Syndrome (See also Chap. 331)   A 24-h urine test for cortisol and creatinine or the administration of 1 mg of dexamethasone at bedtime, followed by the measurement of plasma cortisol at 7 to 10 A.M., is the best test to screen for the presence of Cushing's syndrome. A urine cortisol level of <2750 nmol (100 μg) or suppression of the plasma cortisol level to <140 nmol/L (5 μg/dL) effectively rules out Cushing's syndrome.

Renovascular Hypertension (See also Chap. 278)   Over the past decades the standard approach to screen for renovascular hypertension has progressed from the rapid-sequence IVP to one of three noninvasive techniques: the captopril-enhanced radionuclide renal scan (the preferred choice), a duplex Doppler flow study, or magnetic resonance (MRI) angiography. However, perhaps the most sensitive and specific screening test, the spiral computed tomography (CT) scan, which gives a three-dimensional view, unfortunately also requires giving an intravenous contrast agent.

The definitive test for surgically correctable renal disease is the combination of a renal angiogram and renal vein renin determinations. The renal arteriogram both establishes the presence of a renal arterial lesion and aids in the determination of whether the lesion is due to atherosclerosis or to one of the fibrous or fibromuscular dysplasias. It does not, however, prove that the lesion is responsible for the hypertension, nor does it permit prediction of the chances of surgical cure. It must be noted that (1) renal artery stenosis is a frequent finding by angiography and at postmortem in normotensive individuals, and (2) essential hypertension is a common condition and may occur in combination with renal arterial stenosis that is not responsible for the hypertension. Bilateral renal vein catheterization for measurement of plasma renin activity is therefore used to assess the functional significance of any lesion noted on arteriography. When one kidney is ischemic and the other is normal, all the renin released comes from the involved kidney. In the most straightforward situation, the ischemic kidney has a significantly higher venous plasma renin activity than the normal kidney, by a factor of 1.5 or more. Moreover, the renal venous blood draining the uninvolved kidney exhibits levels similar to those in the inferior vena cava below the entrance of the renal veins.

Significant benefit from operative correction may be anticipated in at least 80% of patients with the findings described above if care is taken to prepare the patient properly before renal vein blood sampling, i.e., by discontinuing renin-suppressing drugs, such as beta blockers, for at least 10 days; restricting the patient to a low-sodium intake for 4 days; and/or giving a converting-enzyme inhibitor for 24 h. When obstructing lesions in the *branches* of the renal arteries are demonstrated by arteriography, an attempt to obtain blood samples from the main *branches* of the renal vein should be made in an effort to identify a localized intrarenal arterial lesion responsible for the hypertension.

Primary Aldosteronism (See also Chap. 331)   These patients usually exhibit hypokalemia. Diuretic therapy often complicates the picture when the hypokalemia is first observed and needs to be assessed. Given the presence of hypokalemia, the relation between plasma renin activity and the aldosterone level becomes the key to the diagnosis of primary aldosteronism. The aldosterone concentration or excretion rate is high and plasma renin activity is low in primary aldosteronism, and these levels are relatively unaffected by changes in sodium balance. Thus, the aldosterone:renin ratio is high. A critical part of the evaluation after primary aldosteronism has been established is to determine whether disease is unilateral or bilateral, because surgical removal of the lesion usually reduces arterial pressure only in patients with unilateral disease.

Plasma Renin Activity Measurements   Some studies have suggested that the plasma renin level should be measured in most hypertensive patients and related to a 24-h urine sodium excretion rate to assess whether high, low, or normal renin levels are present. It has been proposed that this information may be important for both therapeutic and prognostic reasons. However, as noted earlier, it is unclear, on the basis of the available data and treatment programs, that these random measurements are really useful except in patients with findings suggestive of renal vascular disease or mineralocorticoid excess in whom lateralizing renal vein renin levels or suppressed peripheral renin levels may be of diagnostic and/or therapeutic significance.

℞ **TREATMENT   Indications for Therapy**   Virtually every patient with a diastolic arterial pressure that persistently exceeds 90 mmHg, or any patient over 65 years of age with a systolic arterial pressure >160 mmHg, is a candidate for diagnostic studies and for subsequent treatment. Furthermore, at any given level of blood pressure elevation, the ultimate risk of developing hypertensive vascular complications is greater in men than in women, in younger than in older persons, and in diabetic than nondiabetic patients. It may be argued, then, that it is hard to justify producing the uncomfortable side effects of therapy in, for example, an asymptomatic woman over 70 years of age with a diastolic pressure of 90 mmHg. On the other hand, it is easy to justify side effects in a man of 30 with a diastolic pressure exceeding 110 mmHg because such a person may be expected to receive the greatest benefit from therapy. Fortunately, the choice of treatment is such that a satisfactory program to control arterial pressure with minimal side effects can be developed for most patients, particularly as more studies assessing the impact of specific therapeutic agents on the patient's quality of life are reported.

A reasonable guideline would be that all patients with a diastolic pressure repeatedly >90 mmHg or systolic pressure >140 mmHg should be treated unless specific contraindications exist. Patients with isolated *systolic* hypertension (levels >160 mmHg with diastolic pressure <89 mmHg) should also be treated if they are over age 65. It is uncertain that individuals under age 65 who have isolated systolic hypertension will benefit from therapy until the results of a well-controlled, prospective study are completed. Patients with labile hypertension or isolated systolic hypertension who are not treated should have regular follow-up examinations at 6-month intervals because of the frequent development of progressive and/or sustained hypertension. Finally, if coronary artery disease or associated cardiovascular risks are present, then treatment of a patient with a lower blood pressure may be warranted. For example, patients with angina pectoris or diabetes mellitus with diastolic blood pressures between 85 and 90 mmHg may be candidates for antihypertensive therapy.

What should the blood pressure goal be? Previously it was assumed that 140/90 mmHg was the desired level. This still seems reasonable for nondiabetic patients since the Hypertension Optimal Treatment (HOT) study did not detect a significant difference in cardiovascular risk between patients with treatment goal diastolic blood pressures of 90 and 80 mmHg. However, in patients with diabetes this is not the case. In the UK Prospective Diabetes Study (UKPDS), individuals with a blood pressure of 144/82 mmHg had a substantially lower risk compared to those with a blood pressure of 154/87 mmHg. The HOT study investigators documented a similar finding in their diabetic subset. Thus, it seems reasonable to target a blood pressure in the normal range for diabetic patients, i.e., 130/85 mmHg. While not definitively proven, it seems prudent to use the same goal in all young and middle-aged patients depending on what other cardiovascular risk factors are present. For elderly individuals, a goal of 140/90 mmHg is appropriate, although definitive data for lowering systolic blood pressure below 160 mmHg is still lacking. Importantly, how aggressive one should be in achieving these blood pressure goals depends on the number and severity of other risk factors present.

The identification of an operable form of secondary hypertension does not automatically mean that surgical treatment is indicated. The decision depends on the age and general health of the patient, the natural history of the lesion, and the response of the arterial pressure to drug therapy. In patients with renovascular hypertension, the feasibility of renal angioplasty, the advantages of surgical repair versus nephrectomy, and the degree of overall renal functional impairment must be considered. Age and general health are important in patients with renovascular hypertension due to arteriosclerosis, because there is no evidence that repair of the stenosis increases life expectancy in the elderly patient with other evidence of vascular disease. Knowledge of the natural history of the disease is especially important when making a decision in the case of a young patient with renal artery stenosis due to fibrous dysplasia. If the arteriographic appearance suggests that the stenosis is due to intimal or subadventitial fibroplasia, the lesion may be expected to progress, and operation or angioplasty is required. Medial fibroplasia, on the other hand, often remains stable, and operation or angioplasty may not be necessary if pressure can be controlled by drug therapy.

The decision regarding operation should also be considered carefully in patients with primary aldosteronism when neither abdominal CT nor bilateral adrenal venous sampling for aldosterone demonstrates a tumor, because such patients may prove to have multinodular hyperplasia. In that case, bilateral adrenalectomy would be required to eliminate the aldosterone excess, and, even then, hypertension would usually persist. If hypokalemia can be controlled by an aldosterone receptor antagonist, e.g., spironolactone, or other drug therapy and arterial pressure lowered with antihypertensive agents, then it is reasonable to withhold operative treatment.

GENERAL MEASURES   Nondrug therapeutic intervention is probably indicated in all patients with sustained hypertension and probably in most with labile hypertension. The general measures employed include (1) relief of stress, (2) dietary management, (3) regular aerobic exercise, (4) weight reduction (if needed), and (5) control of other risk factors contributing to the development of arteriosclerosis. Relief of emotional and environmental stress is one of the reasons for the improvement in hypertension that occurs when a patient is hospitalized. Though it is usually impossible to extricate the hypertensive patient from all internal and external stresses, he or she should be advised to avoid unnecessary tensions. In rare instances, it may be appropriate to recommend a change of job or of life-style. It has been suggested that relaxation techniques may also lower arterial pressure. However, it is uncertain that these techniques alone have much long-term effect.

Dietary management has three aspects:

1.   Because of the documented efficacy of sodium restriction and volume contraction in lowering blood pressure, patients previously were instructed to curtail sodium intake drastically. Some investigators have suggested that this is not necessary. They base their conclusion on two observations: (1) In many patients the blood pressure is not sensitive to the level of sodium intake, and (2) diuretics provide another method of decreasing body sodium stores in individuals whose blood pressure is sodium-sensitive. However, meta-analyses of previous diet studies have documented a 5-mmHg reduction in systolic pressure and a 2.6-mmHg reduction in diastolic pressure when sodium intake is reduced by approximately 75 meq/d. In addition, several reports have documented that, while mild sodium restriction has little if any direct action on blood pressure, it significantly potentiates the efficacy of nearly all antihypertensive agents. Thus, by making it possible to control blood pressure with lower doses of drugs, sodium restriction leads to a reduction in side effects. In addition, it is quite clear that in some hypertensive patients, as noted above, the level of sodium intake does influence the blood pressure. Thus, since there is no apparent risk to mild sodium restriction, the most practical approach now is to advise mild dietary sodium restriction (up to 5 g NaCl per

day), which can be achieved by eliminating all additions of salt to food that is prepared normally. Some studies have also reported a lowering of arterial pressure related to an *increase* in potassium and/or calcium intake. For example, in one meta-analysis, dietary potassium supplements of 50 to 120 meq/d reduced blood pressure by about the same amount as salt restriction (by 6 mmHg systolic and 3.4 mmHg diastolic). While the advisability of these forms of dietary alteration is still controversial, the fact that a moderately high calcium intake (1.5 g elemental calcium daily) probably also reduces the extent of age-related osteoporosis, combined with the results of the potassium supplementation studies, indicate that they are probably useful adjuncts. A particularly useful approach is the DASH (Dietary Approaches to Stop Hypertension) diet, which uses natural foods that are high in potassium and low in saturated and total fat. This diet significantly lowered blood pressure in borderline and stage 1 hypertensive subjects (see Table 35-1 for definitions).

2. Caloric restriction should be urged for patients who are overweight. Some obese patients will show a significant reduction in blood pressure simply as a consequence of weight loss. In the Trial of Antihypertensive Interventions and Management (TAIM) study, weight reduction (average 4.4 kg over 6 months) lowered blood pressure by 2.5 mmHg.

3. A restriction in the intake of cholesterol and saturated fats is recommended, as this diet modification may diminish the incidence of arteriosclerotic complications. Reducing alcohol intake to <15 mL daily is also beneficial. Regular exercise is indicated within the limits of the patient's cardiovascular status. Not only is exercise helpful in controlling weight, but there is also evidence that physical conditioning itself may lower arterial pressure. Isotonic exercises (jogging, swimming) are better than isometric exercises (weight lifting) since the latter, if anything, raises arterial pressure. The dietary management outlined above is aimed at the control of other risk factors. Probably the most significant additional step that could be taken in this area would be to convince the smoker to give up cigarettes.

DRUG THERAPY FOR HYPERTENSION
(Table 246-6)

To make rational use of antihypertensive drugs, the sites and mechanisms of their action must be understood. In general, there are six classes of drugs: diuretics, antiadrenergic agents, vasodilators, calcium entry blockers, angiotensin-converting enzyme (ACE) inhibitors, and angiotensin receptor antagonists.

DIURETICS (See also Chap. 232) The thiazides are the most frequently used and most extensively investigated members of this group, and their early effect is certainly related to sodium diuresis and volume depletion. A reduction in peripheral vascular resistance has also been reported by some workers to be important in the long term. Traditionally, thiazide diuretics have formed the cornerstone of most therapeutic programs designed to lower arterial pressure, and they are usually effective within 3 to 4 days. Furthermore, they have been shown to reduce mortality and morbidity in long-term trials. However, in recent years there has been increasing resistance to their routine use, primarily because of their adverse metabolic effects, which include hypokalemia due to renal potassium loss, hyperuricemia due to uric acid retention, carbohydrate intolerance, and hyperlipidemia. These effects are minimized if the dose is kept below the equivalent of 25 mg/d of hydrochlorothiazide. The more potent loop-acting diuretics furosemide and bumetanide have also been shown to be antihypertensive but have been used less extensively for this indication, primarily because of their shorter duration of action. Spironolactone causes renal sodium loss by blocking the effect of mineralocorticoids, and, therefore, it may be more effective in patients whose mineralocorticoid levels are excessive, such as patients with primary or secondary aldosteronism. However, a clinical trial in heart failure using low doses of spironolactone achieved a 30% reduction in mortality, suggesting that an aldosterone receptor antagonist may be beneficial even when aldosterone levels are relatively normal. Although they do not compete directly with aldosterone, triamterene and amiloride act at the same site as spironolactone to impede sodium reabsorption. They are effective in the same situations as an aldosterone receptor antagonist, except that triamterene has little intrinsic antihypertensive effect. Their major disadvantage is that they can produce hyperkalemia, particularly in patients with impaired renal function. Any of these three potassium-sparing diuretics can also be given along with thiazide diuretics to minimize renal potassium loss.

ANTIADRENERGIC AGENTS (See also Chap. 72) These drugs act at one or more sites—centrally on the vasomotor center, in peripheral neurons, where they modify catecholamine release, or in target tissues, where they block adrenergic receptor sites. Drugs that appear to have predominant *central actions* are *clonidine, methyldopa, guanabenz,* and *guanfacine*. These drugs and their metabolites are predominantly α-receptor agonists. Stimulation of α_2 receptors in the vasomotor centers of the brain *reduces* sympathetic outflow, thereby reducing arterial pressure. Usually a fall in cardiac output and heart rate also occurs, more commonly with clonidine and guanabenz, but the baroreceptor reflex is intact. Thus, postural symptoms are absent. However, rebound hypertension may occur rarely when these drugs, particularly clonidine and guanabenz, are stopped. This effect is probably secondary to an increase in norepinephrine release, which is inhibited by these agents owing their agonist effect on presynaptic α receptors. They are usually not used as first-line therapy.

Another class of antiadrenergic agents consists of the *ganglionic blocking drugs,* which are used infrequently now. Because of their side effects, ganglionic blocking agents are now usually reserved for the rapid lowering of arterial pressure by parenteral administration of the short-acting agent *trimethaphan* in patients with severe hypertension.

Various drugs act at *postganglionic adrenergic nerve endings,* but they are rarely used now because of their side effects. *Guanethidine* and its shorter-acting analogue guanadrel block the release of norepinephrine from adrenergic nerve endings. They usually reduce cardiac output and lower systolic more than diastolic blood pressure. They also produce a greater postural effect than the other drugs that act at the nerve endings, and orthostatic hypotension is a frequent side effect.

The last group of drugs affecting the adrenergic system are those that block the *peripheral adrenergic receptors,* α, β, or both (Chap. 72).

α-Adrenergic Receptor Blockers These agents also usually are not used as first-line therapy. *Phentolamine* and *phenoxybenzamine* block the action of norepinephrine at α-adrenergic receptor sites. These two compounds block both presynaptic (α_2) and postsynaptic (α_1) α receptors, and the former action accounts for the tolerance that develops. *Prazosin* is more effective because it selectively blocks only *postsynaptic* α receptors, i.e., α_1 receptors. Thus, presynaptic α activity remains, suppressing norepinephrine release, and tolerance occurs only infrequently. Accordingly, prazosin produces less tachycardia but more postural hypotension than direct-acting vasodilators, such as hydralazine, and rarely can produce substantial hypotension following the first dose. Its use has decreased with a report of its association with an increase in cardiovascular events.

β-Adrenergic Receptor Blockers (See also Chap. 244) A number of effective *β-adrenergic receptor blocking agents* are available that block sympathetic effects on the heart and should be most effective in reducing cardiac output and in lowering arterial pressure when there is increased cardiac sympathetic nerve activity. These agents *are* often used as first-line therapy. In addition, they block the adrenergic nerve–mediated release of renin from the renal juxtaglomerular cells. This action may be an important component of their blood pressure–lowering action. β-Adrenergic blockers are particularly useful when employed in conjunction with vascular smooth-muscle relaxants, which tend to evoke a reflex increase in heart rate, and with diuretics, the administration of which often results in an elevation of circulating renin activity. In practice, beta blockers appear to be effective even when there is no evidence of increased sympathetic tone, with about

Table 246-6   Drugs Used in Treatment of Hypertension—Listed According to Site of Action

Site of Action	Drug	Dosage	Indications	Contraindications/Cautions	Frequent or Peculiar Side Effects
DIURETICS					
Renal tubule	Thiazides: e.g., hydro-chlorothiazide	Depends on specific drug Oral: 12.5–25 mg daily	Mild hypertension; as adjunct in treatment of moderate to severe hypertension	Diabetes mellitus, hyperuricemia, primary aldosteronism	Potassium depletion, hyperglycemia, hyperuricemia, hypercholesterolemia, dermatitis, purpura, depression, hypercalcemia
	Loop-acting: e.g., furosemide	Oral: 20–80 mg 2 or 3 times a day	Mild hypertension; as adjunct in severe or malignant hypertension, particularly with renal failure	Hyperuricemia, primary aldosteronism	Potassium depletion, hyperuricemia, hyperglycemia, hypocalcemia, blood dyscrasias, rash, nausea, vomiting, diarrhea
	Potassium-sparing: Spironolactone	Oral: 25 mg 2 to 4 times daily	Hypertension due to hypermineralocorticoidism; as adjunct to thiazide therapy	Renal failure	Hyperkalemia, diarrhea, gynecomastia menstrual irregularities
	Triamterene	Oral: 25–100 mg daily			Hyperkalemia, nausea, vomiting, leg cramps, nephrolithiasis, GI disturbances
	Amiloride	Oral: 5–10 mg daily			
ANTIADRENERGIC AGENTS					
Central	Clonidine	Oral: 0.05–0.6 mg twice daily	Mild to moderate hypertension, renal disease with hypertension		Postural hypotension, drowsiness, dry mouth, rebound hypertension after abrupt withdrawal, insomnia
	Guanabenz	Oral: 4–16 mg twice daily			
	Guanfacine	Oral: 1–3 mg daily			
	Methyldopa (also acts by blocking sympathetic nerves)	Oral: 250–1000 mg twice daily IV: 250–1000 mg every 4–6 h (tolerance may develop)	Mild to moderate hypertension (oral), malignant hypertension (IV)	Pheochromocytoma, active hepatic disease (IV), during MAO inhibitor administration	Postural hypotension, sedation, fatigue, diarrhea, impaired ejaculation, fever, gynecomastia, lactation, positive Coombs' tests (occasionally associated with hemolysis), chronic hepatitis, acute ulcerative colitis, lupus-like syndrome
Autonomic ganglia	Trimethaphan	IV: 1–6 mg/min	Severe or malignant hypertension	Severe coronary artery disease, cerebrovascular insufficiency, diabetes mellitus (on hypoglycemic therapy), glaucoma, prostatism	Postural hypotension, visual symptoms, dry mouth, constipation, urinary retention, impotence
Nerve endings	Guanethidine	Oral: 10–150 mg daily	Moderate to severe hypertension	Pheochromocytoma, severe coronary artery disease, cerebrovascular insufficiency, during MAO inhibitor administration	Postural hypotension, bradycardia, dry mouth, diarrhea, impaired ejaculation, fluid retention, asthma
	Guanadrel	Oral: 5–50 mg twice daily			
α Receptors	Phentolamine	IV: 1–5 mg bolus	Suspected or proved pheochromocytoma	Severe coronary artery disease	Tachycardia, weakness, dizziness, flushing
	Phenoxybenzamine	Oral: 10–50 mg once or twice daily (tolerance may develop)	Proved pheochromocytoma		Postural hypotension, tachycardia, miosis, nasal congestion, dry mouth
	Prazosin	Oral: 1–10 mg twice daily	Mild to moderate hypertension	Use with caution in the elderly	Sudden syncope, headache, sedation, dizziness, tachycardia, anticholinergic effect, fluid retention
	Terazosin	Oral: 1–20 mg daily			
	Doxazosin	Oral: 1–16 mg daily			
β Receptors	Propranolol	Oral: 10–120 mg 2 to 4 times daily	Mild to moderate hypertension (especially with evidence of hyperdynamic circulation); as adjunct to hydralazine therapy	Congestive heart failure, asthma, diabetes mellitus (on hypoglycemic therapy), during MAO inhibitor administration, COPD, sick sinus syndrome, 2d or 3d degree heart block	Dizziness, depression, bronchospasm, nausea, vomiting, diarrhea, constipation, heart failure, fatigue, Raynaud's phenomenon, hallucinations, hypertriglyceridemia, hypercholesterolemia, psoriasis; sudden withdrawal may precipitate angina or myocardial injury in patients with heart disease
	Metoprolol	Oral: 25–150 mg twice daily			
	Nadolol	Oral: 20–120 mg daily			
	Atenolol	Oral: 25–100 mg daily			
	Timolol	Oral: 5–15 mg twice daily			
	Betaxolol	Oral: 10–20 mg daily			

(continued)

Table 246-6—(continued)

Site of Action	Drug	Dosage	Indications	Contraindications/Cautions	Frequent or Peculiar Side Effects
	Carteolol	Oral: 2.5–10 mg daily			
	Pindolol	Oral: 5–30 mg twice daily			Less resting bradycardia than other beta blockers
	Acebutolol	Oral: 200–600 mg twice daily			
α/β Receptors	Labetalol	Oral: 100–600 mg twice daily IV: 2 mg/min			Similar to beta blockers with more postural effects
	Carvediol	Oral: 12.5–50 mg daily or in divided doses			

VASODILATORS

Vascular smooth muscle	Hydralazine	Oral: 10–75 mg 4 times daily IV or IM: 10–50 mg every 6 h (tolerance may develop)	As adjunct in treatment of moderate to severe hypertension (oral), malignant hypertension (IV or IM), renal disease with hypertension	Lupus erythematosus, severe coronary artery disease	Headache, tachycardia, angina pectoris, anorexia, nausea, vomiting, diarrhea, lupuslike syndrome, rash, fluid retention
	Minoxidil	Oral: 2.5–40 mg twice daily	Severe hypertension	Severe coronary artery disease	Tachycardia, aggravates angina, marked fluid retention, hair growth on face and body, coarsening of facial features, possible pericardial effusions
	Diazoxide	IV: 1–3 mg/kg up to 150 mg rapidly	Severe or malignant hypertension	Diabetes mellitus, hyperuricemia, congestive heart failure	Hyperglycemia, hyperuricemia, sodium retention
	Nitroprusside	IV: 0.5–8 (μg/kg)/min	Malignant hypertension		Apprehension, weakness, diaphoresis, nausea, vomiting, muscle twitching, cyanide toxicity

ANGIOTENSIN-CONVERTING ENZYME INHIBITORS

Converting enzyme	Captopril	Oral: 12.5–75 mg twice daily	Mild to severe hypertension, renal artery stenosis	Renal failure (reduction of dose), bilateral renal artery stenosis, pregnancy	Leukopenia, pancytopenia, hypotension, cough, angioedema, urticarial rash, fever, loss of taste, acute renal failure in bilateral renal artery stenosis, hyperkalemia
	Benazepril	Oral: 5–40 mg daily			Same as captopril, but little evidence for leukopenia, but perhaps increased frequency of cough and angioedema. All can be given once daily, but side effects are reduced if one-half dose is given twice daily. Fosinopril is excreted more in bile than the others.
	Enalapril	Oral: 2.5–40 mg daily			
	Enalaprilat	IV: 0.625–1.25 mg over 5 min every 6–8 h			
	Fosinopril	Oral: 10–40 mg daily			
	Lisinopril	Oral: 5–40 mg daily			
	Quinapril	Oral: 5–80 mg daily			
	Ramipril	Oral: 1.25–20 mg daily			
	Trandolapril	Oral: 1–4 mg daily			

ANGIOTENSIN RECEPTOR ANTAGONISTS

	Losartan	Oral: 25–50 mg once or twice daily	Mild to severe hypertension, renal artery stenosis	Pregnancy, bilateral renal artery stenosis	Hypotension, acute renal failure in bilateral renal artery stenosis, hyperkalemia
	Valsartan	Oral: 80–320 mg			
	Irbesartan	Oral: 150–300 mg daily			

(continued)

Site of Action	Drug	Dosage	Indications	Contraindications/Cautions	Frequent or Peculiar Side Effects
CALCIUM CHANNEL ANTAGONISTS					
Vascular smooth muscle	Dihydropyridines:				
	Nifedipine XL	Oral: 30–90 mg daily	Mild to moderate hypertension	Heart failure, 2d or 3d degree heart block	Tachycardia, flushing, gastrointestinal disturbances, hyperkalemia, edema, headache
	Amlodipine	Oral: 2.5–10 mg daily			
	Felodipine XL	Oral: 5–10 mg daily			
	Isradipine	Oral: 2.5–10 mg daily			
	Nicardipine	Oral: 20–40 mg 3 times daily			
	Benzothiazepines:				
	Diltiazem	Oral: 30–90 mg 4 times daily or as CD form 180–300 mg daily	Mild to moderate hypertension	Heart failure, 2d or 3d degree heart block	Same as amlodipine, except no tachycardia or edema, but can cause heart block, constipation, and liver dysfunction
	Phenylalkylamine:				
	Verapamil	Oral: 30–120 mg 4 times daily or as SR form 120–480 mg daily	Mild to moderate hypertension	Heart failure, 2d or 3d degree heart block	

NOTE: MAO, monoamine oxidase; COPD, chronic obstructive pulmonary disease; XL, CD, SR are long-acting or sustained-release formulations.

one-half or more of all hypertensive patients showing a fall in pressure. Furthermore, like diuretics, they have been shown to reduce morbidity and mortality in long-term clinical trials. However, these agents can precipitate congestive heart failure and asthma in susceptible individuals, and they must be used with caution in diabetic patients receiving hypoglycemic therapy because they inhibit the usual sympathetic responses to hypoglycemia. Cardioselective beta-blocking agents (so-called beta$_1$ blockers, e.g., metoprolol, atenolol) have been developed and may be superior to nonselective beta blockers such as propranolol and timolol in patients with bronchospasm. Nadolol, a nonselective beta blocker, unlike other drugs of this class, is excreted unchanged in the urine and has a half-life of 14 to 20 h; only one dose a day is required. Atenolol also usually needs to be given only once a day. Pindolol and acebutolol are nonselective beta blockers that have partial agonist activity and, therefore, produce less bradycardia. Labetalol exerts both α- and β-adrenergic blocking actions. It is usually not used as first-line therapy as there is no mortality study in which it has been tested. Thus, it lowers arterial pressure not only by the same complex actions as do beta blockers but also directly by reducing systemic vascular resistance. Usually it has a more rapid onset of action but produces more postural symptoms and chronic sexual dysfunction than the other beta blockers.

VASODILATORS   These agents are usually not used for initial therapy. *Hydralazine* is the most versatile of the drugs that cause direct relaxation of vascular smooth muscle; it is effective both orally and parenterally and acts mainly on arterial resistance rather than on venous capacitance vessels, as evidenced by lack of postural effects. Unfortunately, the effect of hydralazine on peripheral resistance is partly negated by a reflex increase in sympathetic discharge that raises heart rate and cardiac output. This response limits the usefulness of hydralazine, especially in patients with severe coronary artery disease. However, the efficacy of hydralazine can be increased if it is given in conjunction with a beta blocker or a drug such as methyldopa or clonidine, all of which block reflex sympathetic stimulation of the heart. A serious side effect of doses of hydralazine exceeding 300 mg/d has been the production of a lupus erythematosus–like syndrome.

Minoxidil is even more potent than hydralazine but unfortunately produces significant hypertrichosis and fluid retention and, therefore, is mainly limited to patients with severe hypertension and renal insufficiency.

Diazoxide, a thiazide derivative, is restricted in its application to acute situations. It is not a diuretic; in fact, it causes sodium retention. However, like other thiazides, it reduces carbohydrate tolerance. It must be given rapidly intravenously to guarantee an effect. It begins to act immediately to lower blood pressure, and its effects may last for several hours. *Nitroprusside* given intravenously also acts as a direct vasodilator, with onset and offset of actions that are almost immediate. *Nitroglycerin* is a third direct-acting vasodilator useful as an intravenous agent. These latter three drugs are useful only for the treatment of hypertensive emergencies (Table 246-7).

Table 246-7   Therapeutic Agents Used to Treat Malignant Hypertension

Drug	Route	Starting Dose	Time Course of Action			Oral Preparation Available
			Onset	Peak	Duration	
IMMEDIATE ONSET						
Nitroprusside	Continuous IV	0.25 μg/kg/min	<1 min	1–2 min	2–5 min	No
Nitroglycerin	Continuous IV	5 μg/min	1–5 min	2–6 min	3–10 min	No
Diazoxide	IV bolus	50 mg q 5–10 min up to 600 mg	1–5 min	2–4 min	4–12 h	No
Fenoldopan	Continuous IV	0.1–0.3 μg/kg per min	<5 min	5–10 min	30 min	No
Esmolol	Continuous IV	250–500 μg/min × 1 min; then 50–100 μg/kg per min × 4 min	1–2 min	2–3 min	10–20 min	No
DELAYED ONSET						
Enalaprilat	IV	1.25 mg q 6 h	10–15 min	3–4 h	6–24 h	Yes
Hydralazine	IV, IM	5–10 mg q 20 min × 3	10–20 min	20–40 min	4–12 h	Yes
Labetalol	IV	20–80 mg q 10 min up to 300 mg	5 min	20–30 min	3–6 h	Yes
Nicardipine	IV	5–15 mg/h	5–10 min	20–40 min	1–4 h	Yes

ACE INHIBITORS Drugs from several of the categories discussed above have been shown to possess an additional action resulting in inhibition of renin secretion. These include clonidine, reserpine, methyldopa, and beta blockers. A second group of drugs inhibit the enzyme converting angiotensin I into angiotensin II—ACE. These agents are an increasingly popular choice for initial therapy. They are useful because they not only inhibit the generation of a potent vasoconstrictor (angiotensin II) but also may retard the degradation of a potent vasodilator (bradykinin), alter prostaglandin production (an effect most notable with captopril), and can modify the activity of the adrenergic nervous system. They are especially useful in renal or renovascular hypertension and in diabetic patients, as well as in accelerated and malignant hypertension. However, in patients with bilateral renal artery stenosis, rapid deterioration of renal function may occur. They are also as effective in mild, uncomplicated hypertension as beta blockers and thiazides—and have fewer side effects, particularly ones that adversely affect the patient's quality of life.

These drugs should be used with caution when the renin system is activated (e.g., by severe heart failure, prior diuretic therapy, or substantial salt restriction) to avoid profound hypotension. Usually, diuretics are stopped 2 to 3 days before administration of an ACE inhibitor is begun and are added back later if needed.

ANGIOTENSIN RECEPTOR ANTAGONISTS These drugs have effects similar to those of ACE inhibitors. However, instead of blocking the production of angiotensin II, they competitively inhibit its binding to the angiotensin II AT_1 receptor subtype. Their utility and tolerability are similar to those of the ACE inhibitors, but they do not cause cough or angioedema.

CALCIUM CHANNEL ANTAGONISTS There are three subclasses of calcium channel antagonists: the phenylalkylamine derivatives (e.g., verapamil), the benzothiazepines (e.g., diltiazem), and the dihydropyridines (e.g., amlodipine). To date, there is only one therapeutic agent in each of the first two classes but a number of agents in the third class. All three subclasses modify calcium entry into cells by interacting with specific binding sites on the α_1 subunit of the L-type voltage-dependent calcium channel. Thus, since there are other calcium channels (e.g., the T and N types), the actions of these drugs only partially modify total calcium transport into cells. The relative specificity of each agent stems from the fact that each class has a unique binding site on the α_1 subunit, and these sites are variably expressed in different tissues. Thus, while agents from all three subclasses cause vasodilation, usually only dihydropyridines produce reflex tachycardia. Diltiazem and verapamil can both slow atrioventricular conduction—a feature not observed with the dihydropyridines. While calcium channel antagonists are also useful in angina pectoris (Chap. 244), because of their negative inotropic actions, they should be used with caution in hypertensive patients with heart failure. Considerable controversy has surrounded the use of calcium channel antagonists in the treatment of hypertension. In part the controversy was secondary to the inadequacy of the data and the confusion between the use of short-acting agents (e.g., nifedipine) and long-acting agents. Several facts have helped partially to resolve this controversy. First has been the general recognition that despite its previously frequent use as an antihypertensive agent, short-acting nifedipine rarely, if ever, should be used to treat hypertension, since it has been reported to increase the incidence of acute coronary events. Second, the results of the SYST-EUR (Systolic Hypertension in Europe) trial documented that a long-acting calcium channel antagonist reduced mortality to an extent equivalent to that previously reported for diuretics and beta blockers. Thus, long-acting calcium channel antagonists are often used as first-line therapy.

APPROACH TO DRUG THERAPY The aim of drug therapy is to use the agents just described, alone or in combination, to return arterial pressure to normal levels with minimal side effects. Ideally, one would choose a therapeutic program that specifically corrects the underlying defect resulting in the elevated blood pressure—for example, treatment with spironolactone for patients with primary aldosteronism. As our knowledge of the mechanisms underlying the

hypertension in individual patients increases, more specific drug programs will become available. Such programs presumably will result in normalization of blood pressure with fewer side effects. In the absence of this information, an empirical approach is used, which takes into consideration efficacy, safety, impact on the quality of life, compliance, ease of administration, and cost. When used in combination, drugs are chosen for their different sites of action. However, except for those patients with severe hypertension (average diastolic blood pressure >130 mmHg), in whom intensive therapy with several agents simultaneously is usually required, most patients are treated *initially* with a single agent.

Since many effective antihypertensive agents are available, a number of useful therapeutic regimens have been developed. There are two major authoritative groups who have treatment guidelines when the patient's condition does not require a specific approach: World Health Organization–International Society of Hypertension (WHO-ISH) (Figs. 246-1 and 246-2) and the Sixth U.S. Joint National Committee (JNC) on Prevention, Detection, Evaluation, and Treatment of High Blood Pressure (JNC VI). In the absence of specific therapy, their approaches are similar in most respects, relying heavily on the results of randomized clinical trials (Table 246-8), except for which drugs should be used to initiate therapy. JNC VI recommends starting with diuretics and/or beta blockers because they are the ones where mortality trials have demonstrated a positive effect of treatment. The WHO-ISH guidelines recommends initiating therapy with any of six classes of agents (Table 246-9). The different recommendations, in part, reflect the fact that the WHO-ISH committee reviewed more recent data from mortality clinical trials that, in one case, documented a reduction in morbidity and mortality with a long-acting calcium

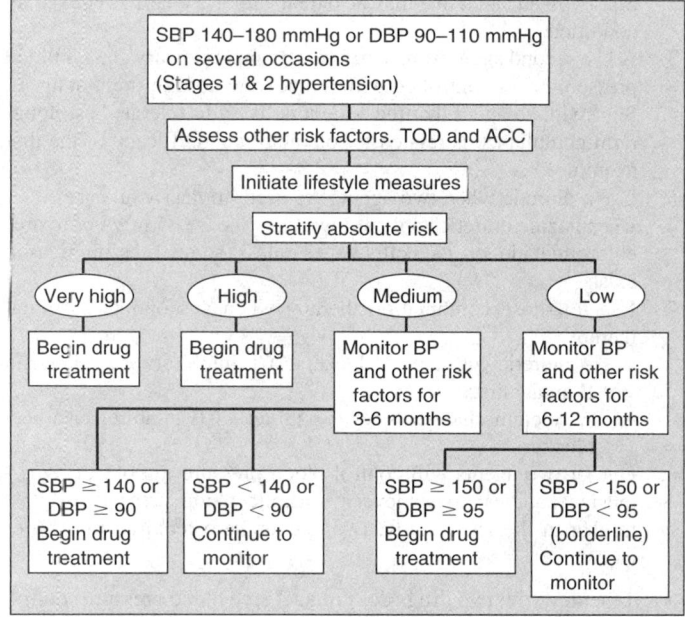

FIGURE 246-1 Initiation of treatment in patients with hypertension. See Table 246-9 for listing of classes of agents to use initially. In the initial evaluation the patients are stratified for cardiovascular risk using three categories: level of blood pressure (stages 1 to 3 varying from low to high risk); the presence of risk factors—smoking, obesity, male gender, etc.—which vary from 0 factors (low risk) to three or more factors (high risk equivalent to having diabetes mellitus), target organ damage (TOD), or diabetes (both high risk if present regardless of other risk factors); and clinical cardiovascular or renal disease (very high risk if present regardless of other risk factors). SBP, systolic blood pressure; DBP, diastolic blood pressure; TOD, target organ damage (previous WHO stage 2 hypertension); ACC, associated clinical conditions including clinical cardiovascular disease and renal disease (previous WHO stage 3 hypertension). (*Adapted with permission from 1999 WHO.*)

FIGURE 246-2 Approach to the hypertensive patient after initiating antihypertensive drug treatment. See Fig. 246-1 for initial steps and definition of risk and Table 246-9 for initial choice of agents. *(Adapted with permission from 1999 WHO.)*

channel antagonist versus placebo that was similar to previous reports for diuretics and beta blockers and, in another case, reported that ACE inhibitors were as effective as beta blockers and diuretics in reducing mortality (Table 246-8).

There are several critical caveats common to both approaches:

1. Start with a low dose of an agent and, if blood pressure is not controlled, increase only moderately.
2. Start with an agent that may also treat and/or not harm a coexisting condition.
3. Add a second agent from a different, complementary class if blood pressure is not controlled with a moderate dose of the first agent.
4. Start with an agent that the patient is likely to tolerate best; long-term compliance is related to tolerability and efficacy of the first agent used.
5. Use a diuretic when two agents are used, in nearly all cases.
6. Use thiazide diuretics only at low doses, i.e., ≤25 mg/d of hydrochlorothiazide or its equivalent, unless some pressing reason exists.
7. Use low-dose combination therapy when appropriate as initial therapy:
   a. A diuretic with a beta blocker, ACE inhibitor, or angiotensin II antagonist;
   b. A calcium channel blocker with an ACE inhibitor or a beta blocker
8. One or two agents will control blood pressure in 90% of hypertensive patients; to achieve a diastolic blood pressure of <90 mmHg in the HOT study, two agents were required in 70% of cases.

If therapy with two drugs does not achieve blood pressure control, the primary agent should be increased to full dose, e.g., 100 mg of captopril or atenolol, 20 mg of enalapril, or 360 mg of diltiazem. If the blood pressure is still not controlled, then a detailed search for a secondary cause of hypertension, as outlined above, is indicated. If none is found, then a dietary assessment will often reveal a high sodium intake. With reduction in salt intake to 5 g/d or less, blood pressure is often controlled. If the blood pressure is still not controlled, then the primary agent should be switched, maintaining the thiazide. Caution should be used if an ACE inhibitor was not the original agent, as administration of such an agent to a patient who is already taking a diuretic occasionally may lead to profound hypotension. If none of these changes produces better control of arterial pressure, then the combination of a calcium channel antagonist and an ACE inhibitor, or

triple therapy, usually with a diuretic, ACE inhibitor, and hydralazine, may be effective.

If the blood pressure is controlled, then a stepwise reduction in the dose and/or withdrawal of some of the agents should be carried out to determine the minimal therapeutic program that will maintain the blood pressure at 140/90 mmHg or less. Whether triple or quadruple drug therapy is warranted to lower blood pressure further is uncertain.

Fewer than 5% of patients will still be hypertensive at this point. For these, one first should consider the reasons for therapeutic failure, as shown in Table 246-10. If none can be identified, then one of the other agents, such as one of the vasodilators listed in Table 246-6 (e.g., hydralazine) or an antiadrenergic agent (e.g., prazosin or clonidine), should be added. If blood pressure is controlled, previous drugs are withdrawn sequentially to determine the minimal therapeutic program that will maintain a normal blood pressure.

While the recommendations outlined above are satisfactory for a large majority of patients, it is important to use a flexible approach, because individual patients may respond differently to individual drugs and drug combinations. For those patients requiring multiple drugs, once the appropriate combination has been found, the use of a single formulation with the appropriate combination of drugs may simplify the regimen and thereby increase compliance. Every effort should be made to reduce the number of times each day the patients must interrupt their schedules for the medication. Pharmacologic treatment of essential hypertension is usually lifelong, and since most patients are asymptomatic, compliance with a complex regimen may be a serious problem, particularly if the therapeutic regimen has a negative impact on the quality of the patient's life. Finally, it is uncertain what level of arterial pressure should be accepted as representing adequate control. It is clear that reducing diastolic blood pressure to <90 mmHg is appropriate and reduces morbidity and/or mortality.

Five groups of patients with hypertension require special consideration because of associated conditions. These groups are considered in the following sections.

RENAL DISEASE Reduction of arterial pressure in hypertensive patients with impaired renal function is often accompanied initially by an increase in serum creatinine. This change does not represent further structural renal damage and should not deter the physician from continuing the therapy, since achievement of blood pressure control may eventually reduce the value toward normal. However, if serum creatinine increases in a patient treated with a converting-enzyme inhibitor, care needs to be exercised, because these patients may have bilateral renal artery disease. Their renal function will continue to de-

Table 246-8   Randomized Clinical Trials in Hypertension

Trial Reference	Patient Number and Characteristics	Trial Arms	Endpoints	Results	Conclusion
SYST-EUR, Staessen et al, 1997	4695, >60 years old 2 years' follow-up	Nitrendipine/enalapril or HTZ Placebo	Primary: Death, all cardiovascular events, strokes	Active treatment reduced total stroke rate 42% ($p = .003$); nonfatal stroke decreased 44% ($p = .007$). All fatal and nonfatal cardiac endpoints declined 26% ($p = .03$). Cardiovascular mortality decreased 27% ($p = .07$).	Among elderly patients with isolated systolic hypertension, nitrendipine reduced cardiovascular complications; treatment of 1000 patients for 5 years with this regimen may prevent 29 strokes and/or 53 major cardiovascular endpoints
SYST-EUR, Tuomilehto et al, 1999	4695 (diabetic = 492) >60 years old 2 years' follow-up	Nitrendipine/enalapril or HTZ Placebo	Primary: Death, all cardiovascular events, strokes	In diabetics total mortality reduced 55%; mortality from cardiovascular disease by 76%; all cardiovascular events combined by 69%; nonfatal stroke by 73% Reductions in mortality and all cardiovascular events were significantly larger among diabetic than nondiabetic patients ($p = .04$ to $.01$).	Calcium channel antagonist significantly reduces cardiovascular morbidity and mortality in elder hypertensive patients; the effect is greater in diabetic than nondiabetic subjects
CAPPP Trial, Hansson et al, 1999	10,985, age 25–66, diastolic BP ≥ 100 mmHg 2–3 years' follow-up	Captopril Diuretics/beta blocker	Primary: Composite of fatal and nonfatal myocardial infarction, stroke, and other cardiovascular deaths	Primary endpoint relative risk 1.05, $p = .52$; Cardiovascular mortality was lower with captopril, relative risk 0.77, $p = .092$ Fatal and nonfatal stroke was more common with captopril, relative risk 1.25, $p = .044$	Captopril and conventional treatment did not differ in preventing cardiovascular morbidity and mortality
HOT Study, Hansson et al, 1998	18,790, 50–80 years with diastolic BP 100–115 mmHg 3–4 years' follow-up	Felodipine plus four other agents to reduce diastolic BP to 90 mmHg or 85 mmHg or 80 mmHg	Major cardiovascular events	Lowest cardiovascular mortality occurred at 86.5 mmHg; further reduction below these BPs was safe but no further reduction in risk; in patients with diabetes, a 51% reduction in cardiovascular events in target group = 80 mmHg compared with target group = 90 mmHg (p for trend = $.006$)	Intensive lowering of BP was associated with a low rate of cardiovascular events down to a diastolic BP of 82.6 mmHg
DASH Trial, Appel et al, 1997	459 with diastolic blood pressure 80–95 mmHg; 8 wks. Sodium intake and body weight were maintained constant.	Diet rich in fruits and vegetables Diet rich in fruits, vegetables, and low-fat dairy products Control (average U.S. diet)	Blood pressure.	Combination diet reduced systolic and diastolic BP by 5.5 and 3.0 mmHg more than the control diet ($p < .001$); the fruit and vegetable diet had an intermediate effect	A diet rich in fruits, vegetables, and low-fat dairy food can substantially lower BP
Messerli et al, 1998	Meta-analysis of efficacy of beta blockers vs. Diuretics as first-line therapy for elderly patients (60 years) with hypertension Approximate mean of 5 years' follow-up	Diuretics, 8 trials Beta blockers, 2 trials	Cerebrovascular events, coronary heart disease, stroke mortality, cardiovascular mortality, all-cause mortality	Diuretics significantly reduced cerebrovascular events odds ratio (0.61), coronary heart disease odds ratio (0.74), stroke mortality odds ratio (0.67), cardiovascular mortality odds ratio (0.75), and all-cause mortality odds ratio (0.86); beta blockers significantly reduced only cerebrovascular events odds ratio (0.74)	In elderly patients with hypertension, first-line diuretics reduced morbidity and mortality better than beta blockers

NOTE: HTZ, hydrochlorothiazine; BP, blood pressure.

Table 246-9 Guidelines for Selecting Drug Treatment of Hypertension

Class of Drug	Compelling Indications	Possible Indications	Compelling Contraindications	Possible Contraindications
Diuretics	Heart failure Elderly patients Systolic hypertension	Diabetes	Gout	Dyslipidemia Sexually active males
β-Blockers	Angina After myocardial infarct Tachyarrhythmias	Heart failure Pregnancy Diabetes	Asthma and COPD Heart block[a]	Dyslipidemia Athletes and physically active patients Peripheral vascular disease
ACE inhibitors	Heart failure Left ventricular dysfunction After myocardial infarct Diabetic nephropathy		Pregnancy Hyperkalaemia Bilateral renal artery stenosis	
Calcium antagonists	Angina Elderly patients Systolic hypertension	Peripheral vascular disease	Heart block[b]	Congestive heart failure[c]
α-Blockers	Prostatic hypertrophy	Glucose intolerance Dyslipidaemia		Orthostatic hypotension
Angiotensin II antagonists	ACE inhibitor cough	Heart failure	Pregnancy Bilateral renal artery stenosis Hyperkalaemia	

[a] Grade 2 or 3 atrioventricular block.
[b] Grade 2 or 3 atrioventricular block with verapamil or diltiazem.
[c] Verapamil or diltiazem.

NOTE: COPD, chronic obstructive pulmonary disease; ACE, angiotensin-converting enzyme.
SOURCE: Adapted with permission from 1999 WHO.

teriorate as long as the converting-enzyme inhibitor is given. Thus, converting-enzyme inhibitors should be used cautiously in patients with impaired renal function, and renal function should be assessed frequently (every 4 to 5 days) for the first 3 weeks. While converting-enzyme inhibitors are contraindicated in patients with bilateral renal artery stenosis, these are the drugs of choice in patients with unilateral renal artery stenosis and a normally functioning contralateral kidney and probably also in patients with chronic renal failure with or without diabetes mellitus.

CORONARY ARTERY DISEASE In these patients, who also may be taking cardiac glycosides, thiazides should be used judiciously, and a reduction in serum potassium levels should be watched for and, if found, should be corrected rapidly. Beta blockers should be withdrawn carefully, if at all, in these patients. Finally, calcium channel antagonists and converting-enzyme inhibitors may be useful in these patients because they minimize a number of potential adverse reactions that accompany the use of other therapeutic agents, particularly nonspecific vasodilators.

DIABETES MELLITUS The diabetic patient with hypertension is particularly challenging to treat because many of the agents used to lower blood pressure can affect glucose metabolism adversely. Converting-enzyme inhibitors may be particularly useful in these individuals. They have no known adverse effects on glucose or lipid metabolism and minimize the development of diabetic nephropathy by reducing renal vascular resistance and renal perfusion pressure—the primary factor underlying renal deterioration in these patients.

PREGNANCY The patient who is pregnant and hypertensive or who develops hypertension during pregnancy (pregnancy-induced hy-

Table 246-10 Reasons for Poor Therapeutic Response in Patients with Hypertension

Inadequate patient compliance
Volume expansion
  Caused by excessive sodium intake
  Caused by nondiuretic antihypertensive agent
  Caused by renal damage
Excessive weight gain
Inadequate doses
Drug antagonism
Cold remedies
Sympathomimetics
Oral contraceptives (estrogens)
Adrenal steroids
Secondary forms of hypertension

pertension, preeclampsia, eclampsia) is particularly difficult to treat. Because it is uncertain whether autoregulation of uterine blood flow occurs, lowering blood pressure in the pregnant hypertensive patient may result in reduced placental and fetal perfusion. Thus, a conservative approach to lowering blood pressure is usually indicated. In the second and third trimesters, antihypertensive agents are often not indicated unless the diastolic pressure exceeds 95 mmHg. In general, severe salt restriction and/or diuretics are not used because of the associated increase in fetal wastage. Beta blockers need to be used cautiously for similar reasons. Methyldopa and hydralazine, and to a lesser extent calcium channel antagonists, are the antihypertensive agents used most often, because they have no known adverse effects on the fetus. Little is known about the safety of other antihypertensive agents in pregnancy, except that nitroprusside and converting-enzyme inhibitors may cause adverse effects on the fetus and are contraindicated.

ELDERLY PATIENTS Hypertensive patients who are over age 65, and particularly those over age 75, offer substantial challenges to the physician. Several studies have reported that healthy elderly patients, whether male or female, who are treated with relatively modest doses of antihypertensive agents show a substantial reduction in strokes and stroke-related deaths. This is true whether the patient has systolic and diastolic hypertension or isolated systolic hypertension. What is not clear from these studies is how broadly the results can be extrapolated, since the studies were performed in healthy elderly patients, while many such patients have other diseases. Thus, in the elderly hypertensive patient, individualization of therapy still seems warranted.

Probably fewer than one-third of hypertensive patients in the United States are being treated effectively. Only a small number of these failures are related to drug unresponsiveness. Most are related to (1) failure to detect hypertension, (2) failure to institute effective treatment of an asymptomatic hypertensive patient, and (3) failure of the asymptomatic hypertensive patient to adhere to therapy. To help with the latter problem, patients must be educated to continue treatment once an effective regimen has been identified. Side effects and inconveniences of treatment must be minimized or counteracted in order to obtain the patient's continued cooperation.

MALIGNANT HYPERTENSION

In addition to marked blood pressure elevation in association with papilledema and retinal hemorrhages and exudates, the full-blown picture of malignant hypertension may include manifestations of hypertensive encephalopathy, such as severe headache, vomiting, visual disturbances (including transient blindness), transient paralyses, convulsions, stupor, and coma. These manifestations have been attributed to spasm of cerebral vessels and to cerebral edema. In some patients who have died, multiple small thrombi have been found in the cerebral vessels. Cardiac decompensation and rapidly declining renal function are other critical features of malignant hypertension. Oliguria may, in fact, be the presenting feature. The vascular lesion characteristic of malignant hypertension is fibrinoid necrosis of the walls of small arteries and arterioles, and this development can be reversed by effective antihypertensive therapy.

The pathogenesis of malignant hypertension is unknown. However, at least two independent processes—dilation of cerebral arteries and generalized arteriolar fibrinoid necrosis—contribute to the associated signs and symptoms. The cerebral arteries dilate because the normal autoregulation of cerebral blood flow decompensates as a result of the markedly elevated arterial pressure. Cerebral blood flow therefore is excessive, producing the encephalopathy associated with malignant hypertension. Many patients also show evidence of a microangiopathic hemolytic anemia; this secondary phenomenon could contribute to the deterioration of renal function. Most patients also have elevated levels of peripheral plasma renin activity and increased aldosterone production, and these effects may be involved in causing vascular damage.

Perhaps fewer than 1% of hypertensive patients develop the malignant phase, which can occur in the course of both essential and secondary hypertension. Rarely, it is the first recognized manifestation of the blood pressure problem, and it is unusual for it to occur in patients under treatment. The average age at diagnosis is 40, and men are affected more often than women. Prior to the availability of effective therapy, the life expectancy after diagnosis of malignant hypertension was less than 2 years, with most deaths being due to renal failure, cerebral hemorrhage, or congestive heart failure. With the advent of effective antihypertensive therapy, at least half the patients survive for more than 5 years.

℞ **TREATMENT** Malignant hypertension is a medical emergency that requires immediate therapy. However, it needs to be distinguished from severe hypertension, since overly aggressive therapy in malignant hypertension could result in a potentially hazardous reduction in myocardial and cerebral perfusion. The initial aims of therapy should be (1) correction of medical complications and (2) reduction of diastolic pressure by one-third, but not to a level <95 mmHg. The drugs available for treatment of malignant hypertension can be divided into two groups on the basis of time of onset of action (Table 246-7). Those in the first group act within a few minutes but are not satisfactory for long-term management. If the patient is having convulsions, and if arterial pressure must be reduced rapidly, then one from the immediate-acting group should be used.

The first three agents in this group require continuous infusion and close monitoring. *Nitroprusside* is given by continuous intravenous infusion at a dose of 0.25 to 8.0 μg/kg per min. It is probably the agent of choice in this condition, since it dilates both arterioles and veins. It has the advantage over the ganglionic blockers of not being associated with the development of tachyphylaxis and can be used for days with few side effects. The dosage must be controlled with an infusion pump. *Nitroglycerin* affects veins more than arterioles and is given by continuous infusion at a rate of 5 to 100 μg/min. It is particularly useful in the treatment of hypertension following coronary bypass surgery, myocardial infarction, left ventricular failure, or unstable angina pectoris. *Diazoxide* is the easiest agent to administer, for no individual titration of dosage is required. However, it is probably less effective than the other agents. It primarily affects arteriolar and not venous tone. A dose of 50 to 100 mg is given rapidly intravenously, and the antihypertensive effect appears in 1 to 5 min. The same dose can be repeated in 5 to 10 min, if necessary, or when the pressure begins to rise, usually after several hours. The total dose should not exceed 600 mg/d. In an occasional patient, pressure may drop below normal levels after diazoxide administration. This drug should not be

used in patients in whom aortic dissection or myocardial infarction is suspected. Because it can increase the force of myocardial contraction, often a beta blocker is given concomitantly. *Enalaprilat*, an intravenous form of the ACE inhibitor *enalapril*, has also proven effective, particularly in individuals with left heart failure. Finally, intravenous *labetalol* may be particularly useful in patients with a myocardial infarct or angina because it prevents an increase in heart rate. However, it may be ineffective in patients previously treated with beta blockers and is contraindicated in patients with heart failure, asthma, bradycardia, or heart block. It may also serve as an alternative therapy in patients with eclampsia who are unresponsive to hydralazine.

Patients given any of these agents also should receive other medications effective for long-term control. Those in the second group in Table 246-7 require 30 min or more to produce their full effect, but they have the advantage of being satisfactory for subsequent oral administration and for long-term management of the patient's hypertension. If such a delay in the achievement of the full effect is acceptable, intravenous *hydralazine* is effective in many patients within 10 min; an effective protocol involves giving 10-mg doses intravenously every 10 to 15 min until the desired effect has been obtained or until a total of 50 mg has been administered. The total amount required for response may then be repeated intramuscularly or intravenously every 6 h. Hydralazine should be used with caution in patients with significant coronary artery disease and should be avoided in patients manifesting myocardial ischemia or aortic dissection. It is effective in preeclampsia. *Esmolol*, a beta blocker with an onset of action of 1 to 2 min, is particularly useful in aortic dissection and for perioperative hypertensive crisis. Its major disadvantage is that it can have a negative inotropic effect. Its use in individuals with congestive heart failure, obstructive lung disease, or asthma is problematic.

Furosemide is an important adjunct to the therapy just discussed. Given either orally or intravenously, it serves to maintain sodium diuresis in the face of a falling arterial pressure and thus will speed recovery from encephalopathy and congestive heart failure as well as maintain the sensitivity to the primary antihypertensive drug. Digitalis (Chap. 232) may also be indicated if there is evidence of cardiac decompensation.

In patients with malignant hypertension in whom the existence of pheochromocytoma is suspected, urine should be collected for measurement of the products of catecholamine metabolism, and drugs that might release additional catecholamines, such as methyldopa, reserpine, and guanethidine, must be avoided. The parenteral drug of choice in these patients is phentolamine, administered with care to avoid a precipitous reduction in arterial pressure.

There is hope even for patients who fail to respond sufficiently to any of the forms of therapy and who show progressive deterioration in renal function. In some, a period of peritoneal dialysis or hemodialysis to deplete extracellular fluid has resulted in better blood pressure control and eventual improvement in renal function. In those patients with refractory hypertension and renal failure who do not respond to volume depletion or hypotensive therapy, including minoxidil administration—particularly those with marked elevation of plasma renin activity—bilateral nephrectomy has resulted in amelioration of hypertension; subsequently, these patients have been maintained on chronic dialysis or have received renal homografts. However, bilateral nephrectomy should be avoided where possible because (1) the loss of renal erythropoietin will contribute to the associated anemia, (2) vitamin D metabolism may be adversely affected, and (3) all residual renal function will be lost.

BIBLIOGRAPHY

APPEL LJ et al: A clinical trial of the effects of dietary patterns on blood pressure. DASH Collaborative Research Group N Engl J Med 336:1117, 1997
CONLIN PH, WILLIAMS GH: Use of calcium blockers in hypertension. Adv Intern Med, 43:533, 1998

DAHLOF B et al: Morbidity and mortality in the Swedish Trial in Old Patients with Hypertension (STOP-Hypertension). Lancet 338:1281, 1991

DE WARDENER HE: Salt reduction and cardiovascular risk: The anatomy of a myth. J Hum Hypertens 13:1, 1999

DOMINICZAK AF et al: Genes and hypertension: From gene mapping in experimental models to vascular gene transfer strategies. Hypertension 35:164, 2000

GRIFFITH LE et al: The influence of dietary and nondietary calcium supplementation on blood pressure. Am J Hypertens 12:84, 1999

HANSSON L et al: Effects of intensive blood-pressure lowering and low-dose aspirin in patients with hypertension: Principal results of the Hypertension Optimal Treatment (HOT) randomized trial. Lancet 351:1755, 1998

——— et al: Effect of angiotensin-converting-enzyme inhibition compared with conventional therapy of cardiovascular morbidity and mortality in hypertension: The Captopril Prevention Project (CAPPP) randomized trial. Lancet 353:611, 1999

HIRSCHL MM: Guidelines for the drug treatment of hypertensive crises. Drugs 50:991, 1995

JAFFE LS, SEELY EW: The heterogeneity of the blood pressure response to hormonal contraceptives. Curr Opin Endo Diab 2:257, 1995

JULIUS S et al: Overweight and hypertension: A 2-way street? Hypertension 35:807, 2000

KAPLAN N: Systemic hypertension: Mechanisms and diagnosis, in *Heart Disease*, 6th ed, E Braunwald et al (eds). Philadelphia, WB Saunders, 2001

LAKSHMAN MR et al: Diuretics and beta-blockers do not have adverse effects at 1 year on plasma lipid and lipoprotein profiles in men with hypertension. Arch Intern Med 159:551, 1999

MESSERLI FG, GRODZICKI T: Antihypertensive therapy in the elderly: Evidence-based guidelines and reality. Arch Intern Med 159:1621, 1999

——— et al: Are beta-blockers efficacious as first line therapy for hypertension in the elderly? A systematic review. JAMA 279:1903, 1998

MORTENSEN RM, WILLIAMS GH: Aldosterone action (physiology), in *Endocrinology*, 4th ed, LJ DeGroot et al (eds). Philadelphia, Saunders, 2000

PRISANT LM, MOSER M: Hypertension in the elderly: Can we improve results of therapy? Arch Intern Med 160:283, 2000

PUSCHETT JB: Diuretics and the therapy of hypertension. Am J Med Sci 319:1, 2000

Sixth Report of the Joint National Committee on Prevention, Detection, Evaluation, and Treatment of High Blood Pressure. Arch Intern Med 157:2413, 1997

STAESSEN JA et al: Randomized double-blind comparison of placebo and active treatment for older patients with isolated systolic hypertension. The Systolic Hypertension in Europe (SYST-EUR) trial investigators. Lancet 350:757, 1997

WARNOCK DG: Low renin hypertension in the next milennium. Semin Nephrol 20:40, 2000

WILLIAMS GH: Quality of life considerations in therapeutic decision-making: Antihypertensive therapy as a model, in *Aging, Health and Healing*, M Bergener et al (eds). New York, Springer, 1995, p 257

1999 World Health Organization–International Society of Hypertension Guidelines for the Management of Hypertension. J Hypertens 17:151, 1999

247   *Victor J. Dzau, Mark A. Creager*

DISEASES OF THE AORTA

The aorta is the conduit through which the blood ejected from the left ventricle is delivered to the systemic arterial bed. In adults, its diameter is approximately 3 cm at the origin, 2.5 cm in the descending portion in the thorax, and 1.8 to 2 cm in the abdomen. The aortic wall consists of a thin intima composed of endothelium, subendothelial connective tissue, and an internal elastic lamina; a thick tunica media composed of smooth-muscle cells and extracellular matrix; and an adventitia composed primarily of connective tissue enclosing the vasa vasorum and nervi vascularis. In addition to its conduit function, the viscoelastic and compliant properties of the aorta also subserve a buffering function. The aorta is distended during systole to enable a portion of the stroke volume to be stored, and it recoils during diastole so that blood continues to flow to the periphery. Because of its continuous exposure to high pulsatile pressure and shear stress, the aorta is particularly prone to injury and disease resulting from mechanical trauma (Table 247-1). The aorta is also more prone to rupture than any other vessel, especially with the development of aneurysmal dilatation, since its

Table 247-1   Diseases of the Aorta: Etiology and Associated Factors

Aortic aneurysm	Aortic occlusion
Atherosclerosis	Atherosclerosis
Cystic medial necrosis	Thromboembolism
Tuberculosis	**Aortitis**
Syphilitic infection	Syphilitic aortitis
Mycotic infection	Rheumatic aortitis
Rheumatic aortitis	Takayasu's arteritis
Trauma	Giant cell arteritis
Aortic dissection	
Cystic medial necrosis	
Systemic hypertension	
Atherosclerosis	
Takayasu's arteritis	
Giant cell arteritis	

wall tension, as governed by Laplace's law (i.e., proportional to the product of pressure and radius), would be increased.

AORTIC ANEURYSM

An *aneurysm* is defined as a pathologic dilatation of a segment of a blood vessel. A *true aneurysm* involves all three layers of the vessel wall and is distinguished from a *pseudoaneurysm*, in which the intimal and medial layers are disrupted and the dilatation is lined by adventitia only and sometimes by perivascular clot. Aneurysms also may be classified accordingly to their gross appearance. A *fusiform aneurysm* affects the entire circumference of a segment of the vessel, resulting in a diffusely dilated lesion. In contrast, a *saccular aneurysm* involves only a portion of the circumference, resulting in an outpouching of the vessel wall. Aortic aneurysms are also classified according to location, i.e., abdominal versus thoracic. Aneurysms of the descending thoracic aorta are usually contiguous with infradiaphragmatic aneurysms and are referred to as *thoracoabdominal aortic aneurysms*.

ETIOLOGY   The most common pathologic condition associated with aortic aneurysm is *atherosclerosis*. It is controversial whether atherosclerosis itself actually causes aortic aneurysms or whether atherosclerosis develops as a secondary event in the dilated aorta. Causality is implied by studies that have shown that many patients with aortic aneurysms have coexisting risk factors for atherosclerosis (Chap. 241), particularly cigarette smoking, as well as atherosclerosis in other blood vessels. Seventy-five percent of atherosclerotic aneurysms are located in the distal abdominal aorta, below the renal arteries.

Cystic medial necrosis is the term used to describe the degeneration of collagen and elastic fibers in the tunica media of the aorta, as well as the loss of medial cells that are replaced by multiple clefts of mucoid material. Cystic medial necrosis characteristically affects the proximal aorta, results in circumferential weakness and dilatation, and leads to development of fusiform aneurysms involving the ascending aorta and the sinuses of Valsalva. This condition is particularly prevalent in patients with Marfan syndrome and Ehrlers-Danlos syndrome type IV (Chap. 351) but also occurs in pregnant women, in patients with hypertension, and in those with valvular heart disease. Sometimes it appears as an isolated condition in patients without any other apparent disease. Familial clusterings of aortic aneurysms occur in 20% of patients, suggesting a hereditary basis of the disease. A mutation of the gene encoding type III procollagen has been implicated. *Syphilis* (Chap. 172) is a relatively uncommon cause of aortic aneurysm. Syphilitic periaortitis and mesoaortitis damage elastic fibers, resulting in thickening and weakening of the aortic wall. Approximately 90% of syphilitic aneurysms are located in the ascending aorta or aortic arch. *Tuberculous aneurysms* (Chap. 169) typically affect the thoracic aorta and result from direct extension of infection from hilar lymph nodes or contiguous abscesses or from bacterial seeding. Loss of aortic wall elasticity results from granulomatous destruction of the medial layer. A *mycotic aneurysm* is a rare condition that develops as a result of staphylococcal, streptococcal, or salmonella infections of the aorta, usually at an atherosclerotic plaque. These aneurysms are usually saccular. Blood cultures are often positive and reveal the nature of the infecting agent.

Vasculitides associated with aortic aneurysm include Takayasu's arteritis and giant cell arteritis, which may cause aneurysms of the aortic arch and descending thoracic aorta. Spondyloarthropathies such as ankylosing spondylitis, rheumatoid arthritis, psoriatic arthritis, relapsing polychondritis, Behçet's syndrome, and Reiter's syndrome are associated with dilatation of the ascending aorta. *Traumatic aneurysms* may develop after penetrating or non-penetrating chest trauma and most commonly affect the descending thoracic aorta just beyond the site of insertion of the ligamentum arteriosum. *Congenital aortic aneurysms* may be primary or associated with anomalies such as a bicuspid aortic valve or aortic coarctation.

THORACIC AORTIC ANEURYSMS The clinical manifestations and natural history of thoracic aortic aneurysms depend on their location. Cystic medial necrosis is the most common cause of ascending aortic aneurysms, whereas atherosclerosis is the condition most frequently associated with aneurysms of the aortic arch and descending thoracic aorta. The average growth rate of thoracic aneurysms is 0.1 to 0.4 cm per year. The risk of rupture is related to the size of the aneurysm and the presence of symptoms; it increases substantially for ascending aortic aneurysms >6 cm and descending thoracic aneurysms >7 cm. Most thoracic aortic aneurysms are asymptomatic. However, compression or erosion of adjacent tissue by aneurysms may cause symptoms such as chest pain, shortness of breath, cough, hoarseness, or dysphagia. Aneurysmal dilatation of the ascending aorta may cause congestive heart failure as a consequence of aortic regurgitation; and compression of the superior vena cava may produce congestion of the head, neck, and upper extremities.

A chest x-ray may be the first test to suggest the diagnosis of a thoracic aortic aneurysm. Findings include widening of the mediastinal shadow and displacement or compression of the trachea or left mainstem bronchus. Two-dimensional echocardiography, and particularly transesophageal echocardiography, can be used to assess the proximal ascending aorta and descending thoracic aorta. Both contrast-enhanced computed tomography (CT) and magnetic resonance imaging (MRI) are sensitive and specific tests for assessment of aneurysms of the thoracic aorta. In asymptomatic patients whose aneurysms are too small to justify surgery, noninvasive testing with either contrast-enhanced CT or MRI should be performed at least every 6 to 12 months to monitor expansion. Contrast aortography is frequently required preoperatively to assess the length of the aneurysm and involvement of branch vessels.

Patients with thoracic aortic aneurysms, and particularly patients with Marfan syndrome who have evidence of aortic root dilatation, should receive long-term beta-blocker therapy. Additional medical therapy should be given, as necessary, to control hypertension. Operative repair with placement of a prosthetic graft is indicated in patients with symptomatic thoracic aortic aneurysms and in those in whom the aortic diameter is >6 cm. In patients with Marfan syndrome, thoracic aortic aneurysms >5 cm should be considered for surgery.

ABDOMINAL AORTIC ANEURYSMS Abdominal aortic aneurysms occur more frequently in males than in females, and the incidence increases with age. Abdominal aortic aneurysms may affect 1 to 2% of men older than 50 years. At least 90% of all abdominal aortic aneurysms are affected by atherosclerosis, and most of these aneurysms are below the level of the renal arteries. Prognosis is related to both the size of the aneurysm and the severity of coexisting coronary artery and cerebrovascular disease. The risk of rupture increases with the size of the aneurysm. The 5-year risk of rupture for aneurysms <5 cm is 1 to 2%, whereas it is 20 to 40% for aneurysms >5 cm in diameter. The formation of mural thrombi within the aneurysm may predispose to peripheral embolization.

An abdominal aortic aneurysm commonly produces no symptoms. It is usually detected on routine examination as a palpable, pulsatile, and nontender mass, or it is an incidental finding during an abdominal x-ray or ultrasound performed for other reasons. However, as abdom-

inal aortic aneurysms expand, they may become painful. Some patients complain of strong pulsations in the abdomen; others experience pain in the chest, lower back, or scrotum. Aneurysmal pain is usually a harbinger of rupture and represents a medical emergency. More often, acute rupture occurs without any prior warning, and this complication is always life-threatening. Rarely, there is leakage of the aneurysm with severe pain and tenderness. Acute pain and hypotension occur with rupture of the aneurysm, which requires emergency operation.

Abdominal radiography may demonstrate the calcified outline of the aneurysm. However, about 25% of aneurysms are not calcified and cannot be visualized by plain x-ray. An abdominal ultrasound can delineate the transverse and longitudinal dimensions of an abdominal aortic aneurysm and may detect mural thrombus. Abdominal ultrasound in useful for serial documentation of aneurysm size and can be used to screen patients at risk for developing aortic aneurysm, such as those with affected siblings, peripheral atherosclerosis, or peripheral artery aneurysms. CT with contrast and MRI are accurate, noninvasive tests to determine the location and size of abdominal aortic aneurysms. Contrast aortography is used commonly for the evaluation of patients with aneurysms before surgery; but the procedure carries a small risk of complications, such as bleeding, allergic reactions, and atheroembolism. This technique is useful in documenting the length of the aneurysm, especially its upper and lower limits, and the extent of associated atherosclerotic vascular disease. However, since the presence of mural clots may reduce the luminal size, aortography may underestimate the diameter of an aneurysm.

TREATMENT Operative repair of the aneurysm and insertion of a prosthetic graft is indicated for abdominal aortic aneurysms of any size that are expanding rapidly or are associated with symptoms. For asymptomatic aneurysms, operation is indicated if the diameter is >5 cm. Operation may be recommended in patients with aneurysm diameters of 4 to 5 cm, except for patients with exceptionally high operative risk. However, in a recent randomized trial of patients with abdominal aortic aneurysms <5.5 cm, there was no difference in the 6-year mortality rate between those followed with ultrasound surveillance and those undergoing elective aneurysm repair. Thus, serial noninvasive follow-up of smaller aneurysms (<5 cm) is an alternative to immediate surgery. Percutaneous placement of endovascular stent grafts (Fig. 247-1) for treatment of infrarenal abdominal aortic aneurysms is currently available for selected patients, and initial reports have been favorable.

In surgical candidates, careful preoperative cardiac and general medical evaluations (followed by appropriate therapy of complicating conditions) are essential. Preexisting coronary artery disease, congestive heart failure, pulmonary disease, diabetes, and advanced age add to the risk of surgery. Perioperative management should include the placement of a Swan-Ganz catheter and arterial line to monitor and optimize left ventricular filling pressure, cardiac output, and arterial pressure, especially during clamping and unclamping of the aorta, as well as during the immediate postoperative period. With careful preoperative cardiac evaluation and postoperative care the operative mortality rate approximates 1 to 2%. After acute rupture, the mortality rate of emergent operation generally exceeds 50%.

AORTIC DISSECTION

Aortic dissection is caused by a circumferential or, less frequently, transverse tear of the intima. It often occurs along the right lateral wall of the ascending aorta where the hydraulic shear stress is high. Another common site is the descending thoracic aorta just below the ligamentum arteriosum. The initiating event is either a primary intimal tear with secondary dissection into the media or a medial hemorrhage that dissects into and disrupts the intima. The pulsatile aortic flow then dissects along the elastic lamellar plates of the aorta and creates a false lumen. The dissection usually propagates distally down the descending

FIGURE 247-1 Example of stent grafts used for the endoluminal treatment of infrarenal aortic aneurysms. The left panel shows a straight stent graft that is inserted into the abdominal aorta. The right panel shows a bifurcated graft with two components that are inserted separately and then joined. *(From Blum et al., with permission.)*

FIGURE 247-2 Classification of aortic dissections. Stanford classification: Type A dissections (*top panels*) involve the ascending aorta independent of site of tear and distal extension; type B dissections (*bottom panels*) involve transverse and/or descending aorta without involvement of the ascending aorta. DeBakey classification: Type I dissection involves ascending to descending aorta (*top left*); type II dissection is limited to ascending or transverse aorta, without descending aorta (*top center + top right*); type III dissection involves descending aorta only (*bottom left*). [*From DC Miller, in RM Doroghazi, EE Slater (eds): Aortic Dissection. New York, McGraw-Hill, 1983, with permission.*]

aorta and into its major branches, but it also may propagate proximally. In some cases, a secondary distal intimal disruption occurs, resulting in the reentry of blood from the false to the true lumen.

There are at least two important pathologic and radiologic variants: intramural hematoma without an intimal flap and penetrating ulcer. The clinical picture and therapeutic management of intramural hematoma are similar to those for classic aortic dissection. By contrast, penetrating ulcers are usually localized and are not associated with extensive propagation. They are primarily found in the distal portion of the descending thoracic aorta and are associated with extensive atherosclerotic disease. The ulcer can erode beyond the intimal border, leading to medial hematoma, and may progress to false aneurysm formation or rupture.

DeBakey and coworkers initially classified aortic dissections as type I, in which an intimal tear occurs in the ascending aorta but which involves the descending aorta as well; type II, in which the dissection is limited to the ascending aorta; and type III, in which the intimal tear is located in the descending area with distal propagation of the dissection (Fig. 247-2). Another classification (Stanford) is that of type A, in which the dissection involves the ascending aorta (proximal dissection), and type B, in which it is limited to the descending aorta (distal dissection). From a management standpoint, classification into type A or B is more practical and useful, since DeBakey types I and II are managed in a similar manner.

The factors that predispose to aortic dissection include systemic hypertension, a coexisting condition in 70% of patients, and cystic medial necrosis. Aortic dissection is the major cause of morbidity and mortality in patients with Marfan syndrome (Chap. 351) and similarly may affect patients with Ehlers-Danlos syndrome. The incidence is

also increased in patients with inflammatory aortitis (i.e., Takayasu's arteritis, giant cell arteritis), congenital aortic valve anomalies (e.g., bicuspid valve), in those with coarctation of the aorta, and in otherwise normal women during the third trimester of pregnancy.

CLINICAL MANIFESTATIONS The peak incidence is in the sixth and seventh decades. Men are more affected than women by a ratio of 2:1. The presentations of aortic dissection and its variants are the consequences of intimal tear, dissecting hematoma, occlusion of involved arteries, and compression of adjacent tissues. Acute aortic dissection presents with the sudden onset of pain (Chap. 13), which is often described as very severe and tearing and is associated with diaphoresis. The pain may be localized to the front or back of the chest, often the interscapular region, and typically migrates with propagation of the dissection. Other symptoms include syncope, dyspnea, and weakness. Physical findings may include hypertension or hypotension, loss of pulses, aortic regurgitation, pulmonary edema, and neurologic findings due to carotid artery obstruction (hemiplegia, hemianesthesia) or spinal cord ischemia (paraplegia). Bowel ischemia, hematuria, and myocardial ischemia have all been observed. These clinical manifestations reflect complications resulting from the dissection occluding the major arteries. Furthermore, clinical manifestations may result from the compression of adjacent structures (e.g., superior cervical ganglia, superior vena cava, bronchus, esophagus) by the expanding dissection causing aneursymal dilatation, and include Horner's syndrome, superior vena caval syndrome, hoarseness, dysphagia, and airway compromise. Hemopericardium and cardiac tamponade may complicate a type A lesion with retrograde dissection. Acute aortic regurgitation is an important and common (>50%) complication of proximal dissection. It is the outcome of either a circumferential tear that widens the aortic root or a disruption of the annulus by dissecting hematoma that tears a leaflet(s) or displaces it below the line of closure. Signs of aortic regurgitation include bounding pulses, a wide pulse pressure, a diastolic murmur often radiating along the right sternal border, and evidence of congestive heart failure. The clinical manifestation depends on the severity of the regurgitation.

In dissections involving the ascending aorta, the chest x-ray often reveals a widened superior mediastinum. A pleural effusion (usually left-sided) also may be present. This effusion is typically serosanguinous and not indicative of rupture unless accompanied by hypotension and falling hematocrit. In dissections of the descending thoracic aorta, a widened mediastinum also may be observed on chest x-ray. In addition, the descending aorta may appear to be wider than the ascending portion. An electrocardiogram that shows no evidence of ischemia is helpful in distinguishing aortic dissection from myocardial infarction. Rarely, the dissection involves the right or left coronary ostium and causes acute myocardial infarction. The diagnosis of aortic dissection can be established by aortography or by the use of noninvasive techniques such as echocardiography, CT, or MRI. Aortography may be used to document the diagnosis; identify the entry point, the intimal flap, and the false and true lumina; and to establish the extent of dissection into the major arteries. Coronary angiography may be performed concomitantly in high-risk patients in the evaluation and preparation for surgery. The sensitivity of aortography is 70% for visualizing an intimal flap, 56% for the site of intimal tear, and 87% for false lumen. It is unable to recognize intramural hemorrhage. Transthoracic echocardiography can be performed simply and rapidly and has an overall sensitivity of 60 to 85%. For diagnosing proximal ascending aortic dissections, its sensitivity exceeds 80%; it is less useful for detecting dissection of the arch and descending thoracic aorta. Transesophageal echocardiography (Fig. 247-3) requires greater skill and patient cooperation but is very accurate in identifying dissections of the ascending and descending thoracic aorta, but not the arch, achieving 98% sensitivity and approximately 90% specificity. CT and MRI are both highly accurate in identifying the intimal flap and the extent of the dissection; each has a sensitivity and specificity exceeding 90%. They are useful in recognizing intramural hemorrhage and penetrating ulcers. MRI also can detect blood flow, which may be useful in characterizing antegrade versus retrograde dissection. These noninvasive tests are now becoming the diagnostic procedures of choice. Their relative utility depends on the availability and expertise in individual institutions as well as on the hemodynamic stability of the patient, with CT and MRI obviously less suitable for more unstable patients.

FIGURE 247-3 Aortic dissection. *Left*. Transesophageal echocardiogram of the ascending aorta demonstrating a freely mobile flap within the lumen of the vessel. Ao, aorta; La, left atrium; Fl, flap. *Right*. When color Doppler was superimposed on the image, the true lumen (*open arrow*) was easily separated from the false lumen (*solid arrow*).

℞ **TREATMENT** Medical therapy should be initiated as soon as the diagnosis is considered. The patient should be admitted to an intensive care unit for monitoring hemodynamics and urine output. Unless hypotension is present, therapy should be aimed at reducing cardiac contractility and systemic arterial pressure, and thereby shear stress. For acute dissection, unless contraindicated, β-adrenergic blockers should be administered parenterally, using intravenous propranolol, metoprolol, or the short-acting esmolol to achieve a heart rate of approximately 60 beats per minute. This should be accompanied by sodium nitroprusside infusion to lower systolic blood pressure to 120 mmHg or less. Labetalol (Chap. 246), a drug with both β- and α-adrenergic blocking properties, also has been used as a parenteral agent in the acute therapy of dissection.

The calcium channel antagonists, verapamil and diltiazem, may be used intravenously if nitroprusside or labetalol cannot be employed. Experience with calcium antagonists is limited. Direct vasodilators, such as diazoxide and hydralazine, are contraindicated because these agents can increase hydraulic shear and may propagate dissection.

Emergent or urgent surgical correction is the preferred treatment for ascending aortic dissections (type A) and complicated type B dissections including those characterized by propagation, compromise of major aortic branches, impending rupture, or continued pain. Surgery involves excision of the intimal flap, obliteration of the false lumen,

and placement of an interposition graft. A composite valve-graft conduit is used if the aortic valve is disrupted. The overall in-hospital mortality rate after surgical treatment of patients with aortic dissection is reported to be 15 to 20%. The major causes of perioperative mortality and morbidity include myocardial infarction, paraplegia, renal failure, tamponade, hemorrhage, and sepsis. Recent reports of the use of endoluminal stent grafts in selected patients with type B dissection have been encouraging. Other transcatheter techniques, such as fenestration of the intimal flaps and stenting of narrowed branch vessels to increase flow to compromised organs, are also under investigation. For uncomplicated and stable distal dissection (type B), medical therapy is the preferred treatment. The in-hospital mortality rate of medically treated patients with type B dissection is 15 to 20%. Long-term therapy for patients with aortic dissection (with or without surgery) consists of the control of hypertension and reduction of cardiac contractility with the use of beta blockers plus other antihypertensive agents such as angiotensin-converting enzyme inhibitor or calcium antagonist. Patients with chronic type B dissection should be followed on an outpatient basis every 6 to 12 months by contrast-enhanced CT or MRI to detect propagation. Patients with Marfan syndrome are at high risk for postdissection complications. The long-term prognosis for patients with treated dissections is generally good with careful follow-up; the 10-year survival rate is approximately 60%.

AORTIC OCCLUSION

CHRONIC ATHEROSCLEROTIC OCCLUSIVE DISEASE

Atherosclerosis may affect the thoracic and abdominal aorta, but occlusive aortic disease caused by atherosclerosis usually is confined to the distal abdominal aorta below the renal arteries. Frequently the disease extends to the iliac arteries (Chap. 248). Claudication characteristically involves the lower back, buttocks, and thighs and may be associated with impotence in males (Leriche syndrome). The severity of the symptoms depends on the adequacy of collaterals. With sufficient collateral blood flow, a complete occlusion of the abdominal aorta may occur without the development of ischemic symptoms. The physical findings include absence of femoral and other distal pulses bilaterally and the detection of an audible bruit over the abdomen (usually at or below the umbilicus) and the common femoral arteries. Atrophic skin, loss of hair, and coolness of the lower extremities are usually observed. In advanced ischemia, rubor on dependency and pallor on elevation can be seen.

The diagnosis is usually established by the physical examination and noninvasive testing, including leg pressure measurements, Doppler velocity analysis, and pulse volume recordings. The anatomy may be defined by abdominal aortography before revascularization. Operative treatment is indicated in patients with debilitating symptoms and/or with the development of leg ischemia.

ACUTE OCCLUSION   Acute occlusion in the distal abdominal aorta represents a medical emergency because it threatens the viability of the lower extremities. It usually results from an occlusive embolus that almost always originates from the heart. Rarely, acute occlusion may occur as the result of in situ thrombosis in a preexisting severely narrowed segment of the aorta or plaque rupture and hemorrhage into such an area.

The clinical picture is one of acute ischemia of the lower extremities. Severe rest pain, coolness, and pallor of the lower extremities and the absence of distal pulses bilaterally are the usual manifestations. Diagnosis should be established rapidly by aortography. Emergency thrombectomy or revascularization is indicated.

AORTITIS

Aortitis frequently affects the ascending aorta and may result in aneurysmal dilatation and aortic regurgitation; it occasionally obstructs branch vessels of the aorta.

SYPHILITIC AORTITIS   This late manifestation of luetic infection (Chap. 172) usually affects the proximal ascending aorta, particularly the aortic root, resulting in aortic dilatation and aneurysm formation. Syphilitic aortitis may occasionally involve the aortic arch or the descending aorta. The aneurysms may be saccular or fusiform and are usually asymptomatic, but compression of and erosion into adjacent structures may result in symptoms; rupture also may occur.

The initial lesion is an obliterative endarteritis of the vasa vasorum, especially in the adventitia. This is an inflammatory response to the invasion of the adventitia by the spirochetes. Destruction of the aortic media occurs as the spirochetes spread into this layer, usually via the lymphatics accompanying the vasa vasorum. Destruction of collagen and elastic tissues leads to dilation of the aorta, scar formation, and calcification. These changes account for the characteristic radiographic appearance of a calcified ascending aortic aneurysm.

The disease typically presents as an incidental radiographic finding 15 to 30 years after initial infection. Symptoms may result from aortic regurgitation, narrowing of coronary ostia due to syphilitic aortitis, compression of adjacent structures (e.g., esophagus), or rupture. Diagnosis is established by a positive serologic test, i.e., rapid plasmin reagin (RPR) or fluorescent treponemal antibody. Treatment includes penicillin and surgical excision and repair.

RHEUMATIC AORTITIS   Rheumatoid arthritis (Chap. 312), ankylosing spondylitis (Chap. 315), psoriatic arthritis (Chap. 324), Reiter's syndrome (Chap. 315), Behçet's syndrome (Chap. 316), relapsing polychondritis, and inflammatory bowel disorders may all be associated with aortitis involving the ascending aorta. The inflammatory lesions usually involve the ascending aorta and may extend to the sinuses of Valsalva, the mitral valve leaflets, and adjacent myocardium. The clinical manifestations are aneurysm, aortic regurgitation, and involvement of the cardiac conduction system.

TAKAYASU'S ARTERITIS   Inflammatory diseases of the aortic arch resulting in obstruction of the aorta and its major arteries characterize this major group of diseases. Takayasu's arteritis is also termed *pulseless disease* because of the frequent occlusion of the large arteries originating from the aorta. It also may involve the descending thoracic and abdominal aorta and occlude large branches such as the renal arteries. Aortic aneurysms may also occur. The pathology is a panarteritis, characterized by mononuclear cells and occasionally giant cells, with marked intimal hyperplasia, medial and adventitial thickening, and, in chronic form, fibrotic occlusion. The disease is most prevalent in young females of Asian descent. During the acute stage, fever, malaise, weight loss, and other systemic symptoms may be evident. An elevation of the erythrocyte sedimentation rate is common. The chronic stages of the disease present with symptoms related to large artery occlusion, such as upper extremity claudication, cerebral ischemia, and syncope. The chronic disease is intermittently active. Since the process is progressive and there is no definitive therapy, the prognosis is usually poor. Glucocorticoids and immunosuppressive agents have been reported to be effective in some patients during the acute phase. Occasionally, anticoagulation prevents thrombosis and complete occlusion of a large artery. Surgical bypass of a critically stenotic artery may be necessary.

GIANT CELL ARTERITIS   (See also Chap. 317)   This vasculitis occurs in older individuals and affects women more often than men. Primarily large and medium-sized arteries are affected. The pathology is that of focal granulomatous lesions involving the entire arterial wall. It may be associated with polymyalgia rheumatica. Obstruction of medium-sized arteries (e.g., temporal and ophthalmic arteries) and of major branches of the aorta and the development of aortitis and aortic regurgitation are some of the complications of the disease. High-dose glucocorticoid therapy may be effective when given early.

BIBLIOGRAPHY

BLANCHARD JF et al: Risk factors for abdominal aortic aneurysm: results of a case-control study. Am J Epidem 151:575, 2000

BLUM U et al: Endoluminal stent-grafts for infrarenal abdominal aortic aneurysms. N Engl J Med 336:13, 1997

CREAGER MA et al: Aneurysmal disease of the aorta and its branches, in *Vascular Medicine*, J Loscalzo et al (eds). Boston, Little, Brown, 1996, pp 907–925

DAKE MD et al: Endovascular stent-graft placement for the treatment of acute aortic dissection. N Engl J Med 340:1546, 1999

HAGAN PG et al: The International Registry of Acute Aortic Dissection (IRAD): New insights into an old disease. JAMA 283:897, 2000

HASHIMOTO H: Takayasu's arteritis and giant cell (temporal or cranial) arteritis. Intern Med 39:4, 2000

ISSELBACHER EM et al: Diseases of the aorta, in *Heart Disease*, 6th ed, E Braunwald (ed). Philadelphia, Saunders, 2001

NIENABER CA et al: Nonsurgical reconstruction of thoracic aortic dissection by stent-graft placement. N Engl J Med 340:1539, 1999

O'GARA PT, DESANCTIS RN: Aortic dissection in vascular medicine. J Loscalzo et al (eds). Boston, Little, Brown, 1996, pp 927–950

PALOMBI M et al: Endovascular treatment of a ruptured thoracic aortic aneurysm. Eur J Vasc Endovasc Surg 19:101, 2000

THE UK SMALL ANEURYSM TRIAL PARTICIPANTS: Mortality results from randomised controlled trial of early elective surgery or ultrasonographic surveillance for small abdominal aortic aneurysms. Lancet 352:1649, 1998

| **248** | *Mark A. Creager, Victor J. Dzau* |

VASCULAR DISEASES OF THE EXTREMITIES

ARTERIAL DISORDERS

PERIPHERAL ARTERIAL DISEASE   Atherosclerosis (arteriosclerosis obliterans) is the leading cause of occlusive arterial disease of the extremities in patients over 40 years old; the highest incidence occurs in the sixth and seventh decades of life. As in patients with atherosclerosis of the coronary and cerebral vasculature, there is an increased prevalence of peripheral atherosclerotic disease in individuals with diabetes mellitus, hypercholesterolemia, hypertension, or hyperhomocysteinemia and in cigarette smokers.

Pathology   (See also Chap. 241)   Segmental lesions causing stenosis or occlusion are usually localized in large and medium-sized vessels. The pathology of the lesions includes atherosclerotic plaques with calcium deposition, thinning of the media, patchy destruction of muscle and elastic fibers, fragmentation of the internal elastic lamina, and thrombi composed of platelets and fibrin. The primary sites of involvement are the abdominal aorta and iliac arteries (30% of symptomatic patients), the femoral and popliteal arteries (80 to 90% of patients), and the more distal vessels, including the tibial and peroneal arteries (40 to 50% of patients). Atherosclerotic lesions occur preferentially at arterial branch points, sites of increased turbulence, altered shear stress, and intimal injury. Involvement of the distal vasculature is most common in elderly individuals and patients with diabetes mellitus.

Clinical Evaluation The most common *symptom* is intermittent claudication, which is defined as a pain, ache, cramp, numbness, or a sense of fatigue in the muscles; it occurs during exercise and is relieved by rest. The site of claudication is distal to the location of the occlusive lesion. For example, buttock, hip, and thigh discomfort occurs in patients with aortoiliac disease (Leriche syndrome), whereas calf claudication develops in patients with femoral-popliteal disease. Symptoms are far more common in the lower than in the upper extremities because of the higher incidence of obstructive lesions in the former region. In patients with severe arterial occlusive disease, critical limb ischemia may develop. Patients will complain of rest pain or a feeling of cold or numbness in the foot and toes. Frequently, these symptoms occur at night when the legs are horizontal and improve when the legs are in a dependent position. With severe ischemia, rest pain may be persistent.

Important *physical findings* of peripheral arterial disease include decreased or absent pulses distal to the obstruction, the presence of bruits over the narrowed artery, and muscle atrophy. With more severe disease, hair loss, thickened nails, smooth and shiny skin, reduced skin temperature, and pallor or cyanosis are frequent physical signs. In addition, ulcers or gangrene may occur. Elevation of the legs and repeated flexing of the calf muscles produce pallor of the soles of the feet, whereas rubor, secondary to reactive hyperemia, may develop when the legs are dependent. The time required for rubor to develop or for the veins in the foot to fill when the patient's legs are transferred from an elevated to a dependent position is related to the severity of the ischemia and the presence of collateral vessels. Patients with severe ischemia may develop peripheral edema because they keep their legs in a dependent position much of the time. Ischemic neuritis can result in numbness and hyporeflexia.

Noninvasive Testing The history and physical examination are usually sufficient to establish the diagnosis of peripheral arterial disease. An objective assessment of the severity of disease is obtained by noninvasive techniques. These include digital pulse volume recordings, Doppler flow velocity waveform analysis, duplex ultrasonography (which combines B-mode imaging and pulse-wave Doppler examination), segmental pressure measurements, transcutaneous oximetry, stress testing (usually using a treadmill), and tests of reactive hyperemia. In the presence of significant peripheral arterial disease, the volume displacement in the leg is decreased with each pulse, and the Doppler velocity contour becomes progressively flatter. Duplex ultrasonography is often useful in detecting stenotic lesions in native arteries and bypass grafts.

Arterial pressure can be recorded noninvasively along the legs by serial placement of sphygmomanometric cuffs and use of a Doppler device to auscultate or record blood flow. Normally, systolic blood pressure in the legs and arms is similar. Indeed, ankle pressure may be slightly higher than arm pressure due to pulse-wave reflection. In the presence of hemodynamically significant stenoses, the systolic blood pressure in the leg is decreased. Thus, if one were to obtain a ratio of the ankle and brachial artery pressures, it would be ≥ 1.0 in normal individuals and <1.0 in patients with peripheral arterial disease. A ratio of <0.5 is consistent with severe ischemia.

Treadmill testing allows the physician to assess functional limitations objectively. Decline of the ankle-brachial systolic pressure ratio immediately after exercise may provide further support for the diagnosis of peripheral arterial disease in patients with equivocal symptoms and findings on examination. Exercise testing also allows simultaneous evaluation for the presence of coronary artery disease.

Contrast angiography should not be used for routine diagnostic testing but is performed prior to potential revascularization. It is useful in defining the anatomy to assist operative planning and is also indicated if nonsurgical interventions are being considered, such as percutaneous transluminal angioplasty (PTA) or thrombolysis. Recent studies have suggested that magnetic resonance angiography has diagnostic accuracy comparable to that of contrast angiography.

Prognosis The natural history of patients with peripheral arterial disease is influenced primarily by the extent of coexisting coronary artery and cerebral vascular disease. Studies using coronary angiography have estimated that approximately one-half of patients with symptomatic peripheral arterial disease also have significant coronary artery disease. Life-table analysis has indicated that patients with claudication have a 70% 5-year and a 50% 10-year survival rate. Most deaths are either sudden or secondary to myocardial infarction. The likelihood of symptomatic progression of peripheral arterial disease appears less than the chance of succumbing to coronary artery disease. Approximately 75% of nondiabetic patients who present with mild to moderate claudication remain symptomatically stable or improve. Deterioration is likely to occur in the remainder, with approximately 5% of the group ultimately undergoing amputation. The prognosis is worse in patients who continue to smoke cigarettes or who have diabetes mellitus.

TREATMENT Therapeutic options include supportive measures, pharmacologic treatment, nonoperative interventions, and surgery. Supportive measures include meticulous care of the feet, which should be kept clean and protected against excessive drying with moisturizing creams. Well-fitting and protective shoes are advised to reduce trauma. Sandals and shoes made of synthetic materials that do not "breathe" should be avoided. Elastic support hose should be avoided, as they reduce blood flow to the skin. In patients with ischemia at rest, shock blocks under the head of the bed together with a canopy over the feet may improve perfusion pressure and ameliorate some of the rest pain.

Treatment of associated factors that contribute to the development of atherosclerosis should be initiated. The importance of discontinuing cigarette smoking cannot be overemphasized. The physician must assume a major role in this life-style modification. It is important to control blood pressure in hypertensive patients but to avoid hypotensive levels. Treatment of hypercholesterolemia is advocated, although reduction in cholesterol levels has not been shown unequivocally to reverse peripheral atherosclerotic lesions. However, it has been shown to prevent or to slow progression of the disease and to improve survival in patients with coronary atherosclerosis. Patients with claudication should also be encouraged to exercise regularly and at progressively more strenuous levels. Supervised exercise training programs may improve muscle efficiency and prolong walking distance. Patients also should be advised to walk for 30 to 45 min daily, stopping at the onset of claudication and resting until the symptoms resolve before resuming ambulation.

Pharmacologic Management This form of treatment of patients with peripheral arterial disease has not been as successful as the medical treatment of coronary artery disease (Chap. 244). In particular, vasodilators as a class have not proved to be beneficial. During exercise, peripheral vasodilation occurs distal to sites of significant arterial stenoses. As a result, perfusion pressure falls, often to levels less than that generated in the interstitial tissue by the exercising muscle. Drugs such as α-adrenergic blocking agents, calcium channel antagonists, papaverine, and other vasodilators have not been shown to be effective in patients with peripheral arterial disease. Pentoxifylline, a substituted xanthine derivative, has been reported to decrease blood viscosity and to increase red cell flexibility, thereby increasing blood flow to the microcirculation and enhancing tissue oxygenation. Several placebo-controlled studies have reported that pentoxifylline increased the duration of exercise in patients with claudication, but its efficacy has not been confirmed in all clinical trials. Cilostazol, a phosphodiesterase inhibitor with vasodilator and antiplatelet properties, has been reported to increase claudication distance and recently received an indication for treatment of peripheral arterial disease by the U.S. Food and Drug Administration. Other drugs are being studied that potentially may improve claudication, such as L-arginine, which is the precursor of the endothelium-dependent vasodilator, nitric oxide, and vasodilator prostaglandins. Several studies have suggested that long-term parenteral administration of vasodilator prostaglandins decreases pain and facilitates healing of ulcers in patients with severe limb ischemia. Clinical trials with angiogenic growth factors such as vascular endothelial growth factor (VEGF) and basic fibroblast growth factor (bFGF) are proceeding. A preliminary report suggested that intramuscular gene transfer of DNA encoding VEGF may promote collateral blood vessel growth in patients with critical limb ischemia.

Platelet inhibitors, particularly aspirin, reduce the risk of adverse cardiovascular events in patients with peripheral atherosclerosis. Clopidogril, a drug that inhibits platelet aggregation via its effect on ADP-dependent platelet-fibrinogen binding, appears to be more effective than aspirin in reducing cardiovascular morbidity and mortality in patients with peripheral arterial disease. The anticoagulants heparin and warfarin have not been shown to be effective in patients with chronic peripheral arterial disease but may be useful in acute arterial obstruction secondary to thrombosis or systemic embolism. Similarly, thrombolytic intervention using drugs such as streptokinase, urokinase, or recombinant tissue plasminogen activator (tPA) may have a role in the treatment of acute thrombotic arterial occlusion but is not effective in patients with chronic arterial occlusion secondary to atherosclerosis.

Revascularization   Revascularization procedures, including nonoperative as well as operative interventions, are usually reserved for patients with progressive, severe, or disabling symptoms and ischemia at rest, as well as for individuals who must be symptom-free because of their occupation. Angiography should be performed mainly in patients who are being considered for a revascularization procedure. Nonoperative interventions include PTA, stent placement, and atherectomy (Chap. 245). PTA of the iliac artery is associated with a higher success rate than PTA of the femoral and popliteal arteries. Approximately 90 to 95% of iliac PTAs are initially successful, and the 3-year patency rate is in excess of 75%. Patency rates may be higher if a stent is placed in the iliac artery. The initial success rate for femoral-popliteal PTA is approximately 80%, with a 60% 3-year patency rate. Patency rates are influenced by the severity of pretreatment stenoses; the prognosis of total occlusive lesions is worse than that of nonocclusive stenotic lesions.

Several operative procedures are available for treating patients with aortoiliac and femoral-popliteal artery disease. The preferred operative procedure depends on the location and extent of the obstruction(s) and general medical condition of the patient. Operative procedures for aortoiliac disease include aortobifemoral bypass, axillofemoral bypass, femoral-femoral bypass, and aortoiliac endarterectomy. The most frequently used procedure is the aortobifemoral bypass using knitted Dacron grafts. Immediate graft patency approaches 99%, and 5- and 10-year graft patency in survivors is in excess of 90 and 80%, respectively. Operative complications include myocardial infarction and stroke, infection of the graft, peripheral embolization, and sexual dysfunction from interruption of autonomic nerves in the pelvis. Operative mortality ranges from 1 to 3%, mostly due to ischemic heart disease.

Operative therapy for femoral-popliteal artery disease includes in situ and reverse autogenous saphenous vein bypass grafts, placement of polytetrafluoroethylene (PTFE) or other synthetic grafts, and thromboendarterectomy. Operative mortality ranges from 1 to 3%. The long-term patency rate depends on the type of graft used, the location of the distal anastomosis, and the patency of runoff vessels beyond the anastomosis. Patency rates of femoral-popliteal saphenous vein bypass grafts at 1 year approach 90% and at 5 years, 70 to 80%. Five-year patency rates of infrapopliteal saphenous vein bypass grafts are 60 to 70%. In contrast, 5-year patency rates of infrapopliteal PTFE grafts are less than 30%. Lumbar sympathectomy alone or as an adjunct to aortofemoral reconstruction has fallen into disfavor.

Preoperative cardiac risk assessment may identify individuals especially likely to experience an adverse cardiac event during the perioperative period. Patients with angina, prior myocardial infarction, ventricular ectopy, heart failure, or diabetes are among those at increased risk. Noninvasive tests, such as treadmill testing (if feasible), dipyridamole thallium or sestamibi scintigraphy, dobutamine echocardiography, and ambulatory ischemia monitoring permit further stratification of patient risk (Chap. 245). Patients with abnormal test results require close supervision and adjunctive management with antianginal medications. It is not known whether coronary angiography and coronary arterial revascularization reduce overall perioperative mortality in high-risk patients undergoing peripheral vascular surgery, but cardiac catheterization should be considered in patients suspected of having left main or three-vessel coronary artery disease.

FIBROMUSCULAR DYSPLASIA   This is a hyperplastic disorder affecting medium-sized and small arteries. It occurs predominantly in females and usually involves renal and carotid arteries but can affect extremity vessels such as the iliac and subclavian arteries. The histologic classification includes intimal, medial, and periadventitial dysplasia. Medial dysplasia is the most common type and is characterized by hyperplasia of the media with or without fibrosis of the elastic membrane. It is identified angiographically by a "string of beads" appearance caused by thickened fibromuscular ridges contiguous with thin, less involved portions of the arterial wall. When limb vessels are involved, clinical manifestations are similar to those for atherosclerosis, including claudication and rest pain. PTA and surgical reconstruction have been beneficial in patients with debilitating symptoms or threatened limbs.

THROMBOANGIITIS OBLITERANS   Thromboangiitis obliterans (Buerger's disease) is an inflammatory occlusive vascular disorder involving small and medium-sized arteries and veins in the distal upper and lower extremities. Cerebral, visceral, and coronary vessels may also be affected. This disorder develops most frequently in men under age 40. The prevalence is higher in Asians and individuals of eastern European descent. While the cause of thromboangiitis obliterans is not known, there is a definite relationship to cigarette smoking in patients with this disorder.

In the initial stages of thromboangiitis obliterans, polymorphonuclear leukocytes infiltrate the walls of the small and medium-sized arteries and veins. The internal elastic lamina is preserved, and thrombus may develop in the vascular lumen. As the disease progresses, mononuclear cells, fibroblasts, and giant cells replace the neutrophils. Later stages are characterized by perivascular fibrosis and recanalization.

The clinical features of thromboangiitis obliterans often include a triad of claudication of the affected extremity, Raynaud's phenomenon (p. 1438), and migratory superficial vein thrombophlebitis. Claudication is usually confined to the calves and feet or the forearms and hands, because this disorder primarily affects distal vessels. In the presence of severe digital ischemia, trophic nail changes, painful ulcerations, and gangrene may develop at the tips of the fingers. The physical examination shows normal brachial and popliteal pulses but reduced or absent radial, ulnar, and/or tibial pulses. Arteriography is helpful in making the diagnosis. Smooth, tapering segmental lesions in the distal vessels are characteristic, as are collateral vessels at sites of vascular occlusion. Proximal atherosclerotic disease is usually absent. The diagnosis can be confirmed by excisional biopsy and pathologic examination of an involved vessel.

There is no specific treatment except abstention from tobacco. The prognosis is worse in individuals who continue to smoke, but results are discouraging even in those who do stop smoking. Arterial bypass of the larger vessels may be used in selected instances, as well as local debridement, depending on the symptoms and severity of ischemia. Antibiotics may be useful; anticoagulants and glucocorticoids are not helpful. If these measures fail, amputation may be required.

VASCULITIS   Other vasculitides may affect the arteries supplying the upper and lower extremities. →*Takayasu's arteritis and giant cell (temporal) arteritis are discussed in Chap. 317.*

ACUTE ARTERIAL OCCLUSION   This results in the sudden cessation of blood flow to an extremity. The severity of ischemia and the viability of the extremity depend on the location and extent of the occlusion and the presence and subsequent development of collateral blood vessels. There are two principal causes of acute arterial occlusion: embolism and thrombus in situ.

The most common sources of arterial emboli are the heart, aorta, and large arteries. Cardiac disorders that cause thromboembolism include atrial fibrillation, both chronic and paroxysmal; acute myocardial infarction; ventricular aneurysm; cardiomyopathy; infectious and marantic endocarditis; prosthetic heart valves; and atrial myxoma. Emboli to the distal vessels may also originate from proximal sites of atherosclerosis and aneurysms of the aorta and large vessels. Less frequently, an arterial occlusion results paradoxically from a venous thrombus that has entered the systemic circulation via a patent foramen ovale or other septal defect. Arterial emboli tend to lodge at vessel bifurcations because the vessel caliber decreases at these sites; in the lower extremities, emboli lodge most frequently in the femoral artery, followed by the iliac artery, aorta, and popliteal and tibioperoneal arteries.

Acute arterial thrombosis in situ occurs most frequently in atherosclerotic vessels at the site of a stenosis or aneurysm and in arterial bypass grafts. Trauma to an artery may also result in the formation of an acute arterial thrombus. Arterial occlusion may complicate arterial punctures and placement of catheters. Less frequent causes include the thoracic outlet compression syndrome, which causes subclavian artery occlusion, and entrapment of the popliteal artery by abnormal placement of the medial head of the gastrocnemius muscle. Polycythemia and hypercoagulable disorders (Chaps. 110 and 118) are also associated with acute arterial thrombosis.

Clinical Features The symptoms of an acute arterial occlusion depend on the location, duration, and severity of the obstruction. Often, severe pain, paresthesia, numbness, and coldness develop in the involved extremity within 1 h. Paralysis may occur with severe and persistent ischemia. Physical findings include loss of pulses distal to the occlusion, cyanosis or pallor, mottling, decreased skin temperature, muscle stiffening, loss of sensation, weakness, and/or absent deep tendon reflexes. If acute arterial occlusion occurs in the presence of an adequate collateral circulation, as is often the case in acute graft occlusion, the symptoms and findings may be less impressive. In this situation, the patient complains about an abrupt decrease in the distance walked before claudication occurs or of modest pain and paresthesia. Pallor and coolness are evident, but sensory and motor functions are generally preserved. The diagnosis of acute arterial occlusion is usually apparent from the clinical presentation. Arteriography is useful for confirming the diagnosis and demonstrating the location and extent of occlusion.

℞ **TREATMENT** Once the diagnosis is made, the patient should be anticoagulated with intravenous heparin to prevent propagation of the clot. In cases of severe ischemia of recent onset, and particularly when limb viability is jeopardized, immediate intervention to ensure reperfusion is indicated. Surgical thromboembolectomy or arterial bypass procedures are used to restore blood flow to the ischemic extremity promptly, particularly when a large proximal vessel is occluded.

Intraarterial thrombolytic therapy is effective when acute arterial occlusion is caused by a thrombus in an atherosclerotic vessel or arterial bypass graft. Thrombolytic therapy may also be indicated when the patient's overall condition contraindicates surgical intervention or when smaller distal vessels are occluded, thus preventing surgical access. One approach for administering intraarterial urokinase is to give 240,000 IU/h for 4 h, followed by 120,000 IU/h for a maximum of 48 h. Intraarterial recombinant tPA may be administered at infusion rates of 1 mg/h or 0.05 mg/kg per hour. Meticulous observation for hemorrhagic complications is required during intraarterial thrombolytic therapy.

If the limb is not in jeopardy, a more conservative approach that includes observation and administration of anticoagulants may be taken. Anticoagulation prevents recurrent embolism and reduces the likelihood of thrombus propagation. It can be initiated with intrave-

nous heparin and followed by oral warfarin. Recommended dosages are the same as those used for deep vein thrombosis (see below). Emboli resulting from infectious endocarditis, the presence of prosthetic heart valves, or atrial myxoma often require surgical intervention to remove the cause.

ATHEROEMBOLISM Atheroembolism constitutes a subset of acute arterial occlusion. In this condition, multiple small deposits of fibrin, platelet, and cholesterol debris embolize from proximal atherosclerotic lesions or aneurysmal sites. Atheroembolism may occur after intraarterial procedures. Since the emboli tend to lodge in the small vessels of the muscle and skin and may not occlude the large vessels, distal pulses usually remain palpable. Patients complain of acute pain and tenderness at the site of embolization. Digital vascular occlusion may result in ischemia and the "blue toe" syndrome; digital necrosis and gangrene may develop. Localized areas of tenderness, pallor, and livedo reticularis (see below) occur at sites of emboli. Skin or muscle biopsy may demonstrate cholesterol crystals.

Ischemia resulting from atheroemboli is notoriously difficult to treat. Usually neither surgical revascularization procedures nor thrombolytic therapy is helpful because of the multiplicity, composition, and distal location of the emboli. Some evidence suggests that platelet inhibitors prevent atheroembolism. Surgical intervention to remove or bypass the atherosclerotic vessel or aneurysm that causes the recurrent atheroemboli may be necessary.

THORACIC OUTLET COMPRESSION SYNDROME This is a symptom complex resulting from compression of the neurovascular bundle (artery, vein, or nerves) at the thoracic outlet as it courses through the neck and shoulder. Cervical ribs, abnormalities of the scalenus anticus muscle, proximity of the clavicle to the first rib, or abnormal insertion of the pectoralis minor muscle may compress the subclavian artery and brachial plexus as these structures pass from the thorax to the arm. Patients may develop shoulder and arm pain, weakness, paresthesia, claudication, Raynaud's phenomenon, and even ischemic tissue loss and gangrene. Examination is often normal unless provocative maneuvers are performed. Occasionally, distal pulses are decreased or absent and digital cyanosis and ischemia may be evident. Tenderness may be present in the supraclavicular fossa. Abducting the affected arm by 90° and externally rotating the shoulder may precipitate symptoms. Several additional maneuvers are used to confirm the diagnosis of vascular compression and to suggest the location of the abnormality. These include the scalene maneuver (extension of the neck and rotation of the head to the side of the symptoms), the costoclavicular maneuver (posterior rotation of shoulders), and the hyperabduction maneuver (raising the arm 180°), which may cause subclavian bruits and loss of pulses in the arm. A chest x-ray will indicate the presence of cervical ribs. The electromyogram will be abnormal if the brachial plexus is involved.

℞ **TREATMENT** Most patients can be managed conservatively. They should be advised to avoid the positions that cause symptoms. Many patients benefit from shoulder girdle exercises. Surgical procedures such as removal of the first rib or resection of the scalenus anticus muscle are necessary occasionally for relief of symptoms or treatment of ischemia.

ARTERIOVENOUS FISTULA Abnormal communications between an artery and a vein, bypassing the capillary bed, may be congenital or acquired. Congenital arteriovenous fistulas are the result of persistent embryonic vessels that fail to differentiate into arteries and veins; they may be associated with birthmarks, can be located in almost any organ of the body, and frequently occur in the extremities. Acquired arteriovenous fistulas are either created to provide vascular access for hemodialysis or occur as a result of a penetrating injury such as a gunshot or knife wound or as complications of arterial catheterization or surgical dissection. An infrequent cause of arteriovenous fistula is rupture of an arterial aneurysm into a vein.

The clinical features depend on the location and size of the fistula. Frequently, a pulsatile mass is palpable, and a thrill and bruit lasting throughout systole and diastole are present over the fistula. With long-standing fistulas, clinical manifestations of chronic venous insufficiency, including peripheral edema, large, tortuous varicose veins, and stasis pigmentation become apparent because of the high venous pressure. Evidence of ischemia may occur in the distal portion of the extremity. Skin temperature is higher over the arteriovenous fistula. Large arteriovenous fistulas may result in an increased cardiac output with consequent cardiomegaly and high-output heart failure (Chap. 232).

Diagnosis   The diagnosis is often evident from the physical examination. Compression of a large arteriovenous fistula may cause reflex slowing of the heart rate (Nicoladoni-Branham sign). Arteriography can confirm the diagnosis and is useful in demonstrating the site and size of the arteriovenous fistula.

℞ **TREATMENT**   Management of arteriovenous fistulas may involve surgery, radiotherapy, or embolization. Congenital arteriovenous fistulas are often difficult to treat because the communications may be numerous and extensive, and new ones frequently develop after ligation of the most obvious ones. Many of these lesions are best treated conservatively using elastic support hose to reduce the consequences of venous hypertension. Occasionally, embolization with autologous material, such as fat or muscle, or with hemostatic agents, such as gelatin sponges or silicon spheres, is used to obliterate the fistula. Acquired arteriovenous fistulas are usually amenable to surgical treatment that involves division or excision of the fistula. Occasionally, autogenous or synthetic grafting is necessary to reestablish continuity of the artery and vein.

RAYNAUD'S PHENOMENON   Raynaud's phenomenon is characterized by episodic digital ischemia, manifested clinically by the sequential development of digital blanching, cyanosis, and rubor of the fingers or toes following cold exposure and subsequent rewarming. Emotional stress may also precipitate Raynaud's phenomenon. The color changes are usually well demarcated and are confined to the fingers or toes. Typically, one or more digits will appear white when the patient is exposed to a cold environment or touches a cold object. The blanching, or pallor, represents the ischemic phase of the phenomenon and results from vasospasm of digital arteries. During the ischemic phase, capillaries and venules dilate, and cyanosis results from the deoxygenated blood that is present in these vessels. A sensation of cold or numbness or paresthesia of the digits often accompanies the phases of pallor and cyanosis.

With rewarming, the digital vasospasm resolves, and blood flow into the dilated arterioles and capillaries increases dramatically. This "reactive hyperemia" imparts a bright red color to the digits. In addition to rubor and warmth, patients often experience a throbbing, painful sensation during the hyperemic phase. Although the triphasic color response is typical of Raynaud's phenomenon, some patients may develop only pallor and cyanosis; others may experience only cyanosis.

Pathophysiology   Raynaud originally proposed that cold-induced episodic digital ischemia was secondary to exaggerated reflex sympathetic vasoconstriction. This theory is supported by the fact that α-adrenergic blocking drugs as well as sympathectomy decrease the frequency and severity of Raynaud's phenomenon in some patients. An alternative hypothesis is that the digital vascular responsiveness to cold or to normal sympathetic stimuli is enhanced. It is also possible that normal reflex sympathetic vasoconstriction is superimposed on local digital vascular disease or that there is enhanced adrenergic neuroeffector activity.

Raynaud's phenomenon is broadly separated into two categories: the idiopathic variety, termed *Raynaud's disease*, and the secondary variety, which is associated with other disease states or known causes of vasospasm (Table 248-1).

Table 248-1   Classification of Raynaud's Phenomenon

Primary or idiopathic Raynaud's phenomenon: Raynaud's disease
Secondary Raynaud's phenomenon
  Collagen vascular diseases: scleroderma, systemic lupus erythematosus, rheumatoid arthritis, dermatomyositis, polymyositis
  Arterial occlusive diseases: atherosclerosis of the extremities, thromboangiitis obliterans, acute arterial occlusion, thoracic outlet syndrome
Pulmonary hypertension
  Neurologic disorders: intervertebral disk disease, syringomyelia, spinal cord tumors, stroke, poliomyelitis, carpal tunnel syndrome
  Blood dyscrasias: cold agglutinins, cryoglobulinemia, cryofibrinogenemia, myeloproliferative disorders, Waldenström's macroglobulinemia
  Trauma: vibration injury, hammer hand syndrome, electric shock, cold injury, typing, piano playing
  Drugs: ergot derivatives, methysergide, β-adrenergic receptor blockers, bleomycin, vinblastine, cisplatin

Raynaud's Disease   This appellation is applied when the secondary causes of Raynaud's phenomenon have been excluded. Over 50% of patients with Raynaud's phenomenon have Raynaud's disease. Women are affected about five times more often than men, and the age of presentation is usually between 20 and 40 years. The fingers are involved more frequently than the toes. Initial episodes may involve only one or two fingertips, but subsequent attacks may involve the entire finger and may include all the fingers. The toes are affected in 40% of patients. Although vasospasm of the toes usually occurs in patients with symptoms in the fingers, it may happen alone. Rarely, the earlobes and the tip of the nose are involved. Raynaud's phenomenon occurs frequently in patients who also have migraine headaches or variant angina. These associations suggest that there may be a common predisposing cause for the vasospasm.

Results of physical examination often are entirely normal; the radial, ulnar, and pedal pulses are normal. The fingers and toes may be cool between attacks and may perspire excessively. Thickening and tightening of the digital subcutaneous tissue (*sclerodactyly*) develop in 10% of patients. Angiography of the digits for diagnostic purposes is not indicated.

In general, patients with Raynaud's disease appear to have the milder forms of Raynaud's phenomenon. Fewer than 1% of these patients lose a part of a digit. After the diagnosis is made, the disease improves spontaneously in approximately 15% of patients and progresses in about 30%.

Secondary Causes of Raynaud's Phenomenon   Raynaud's phenomenon occurs in 80 to 90% of patients with systemic sclerosis (scleroderma) and is the presenting symptom in 30% (Chap. 313). It may be the only symptom of scleroderma for many years. Abnormalities of the digital vessels may contribute to the development of Raynaud's phenomenon in this disorder. Ischemic fingertip ulcers may develop and progress to gangrene and autoamputation. About 20% of patients with systemic lupus erythematosus (SLE) have Raynaud's phenomenon (Chap. 311). Occasionally, persistent digital ischemia develops and may result in ulcers or gangrene. In most severe cases, the small vessels are occluded by a proliferative endarteritis. Raynaud's phenomenon occurs in about 30% of patients with dermatomyositis or polymyositis (Chap. 382). It frequently develops in patients with rheumatoid arthritis and may be related to the intimal proliferation that occurs in the digital arteries.

Atherosclerosis of the extremities is a frequent cause of Raynaud's phenomenon in men over age 50. Thromboangiitis obliterans is an uncommon cause of Raynaud's phenomenon but should be considered in young men, particularly in those who are cigarette smokers. The development of cold-induced pallor in these disorders may be confined to one or two digits of the involved extremity. Occasionally, Raynaud's phenomenon may follow acute occlusion of large and medium-sized arteries by a thrombus or embolus. Embolization of atheroembolic debris may cause digital ischemia. The latter situation often involves one or two digits and should not be confused with Raynaud's phenomenon. In patients with the thoracic outlet syndrome, Raynaud's phenomenon may result from diminished intravascular pressure, stim-

Raynaud's phenomenon occurs in patients with primary pulmonary hypertension (Chap. 260); this is more than coincidental and may reflect a neurohumoral abnormality that affects both the pulmonary and digital circulations.

A variety of blood dyscrasias may be associated with Raynaud's phenomenon. Cold-induced precipitation of plasma proteins, hyperviscosity, and aggregation of red cells and platelets may occur in patients with cold agglutinins, cryoglobulinemia, or cryofibrinogenemia. Hyperviscosity syndromes that accompany myeloproliferative disorders and Waldenström's macroglobulinemia should also be considered in the initial evaluation of patients with Raynaud's phenomenon.

Raynaud's phenomenon occurs often in patients whose vocations require the use of vibrating hand tools, such as chain saws or jackhammers. The frequency of Raynaud's phenomenon also seems to be increased in pianists and typists. Electric shock injury to the hands or frostbite may lead to the later development of Raynaud's phenomenon.

Several drugs have been causally implicated in Raynaud's phenomenon. These include ergot preparations, methysergide, β-adrenergic receptor antagonists, and the chemotherapeutic agents bleomycin, vinblastine, and cisplatin.

℞ **TREATMENT** Most patients with Raynaud's phenomenon experience only mild and infrequent episodes. These patients need reassurance and should be instructed to dress warmly and avoid unnecessary cold exposure. In addition to gloves and mittens, patients should protect the trunk, head, and feet with warm clothing to prevent cold-induced reflex vasoconstriction. Tobacco use is contraindicated.

Drug treatment should be reserved for the severe cases. The calcium channel antagonists, especially nifedipine and diltiazem, decrease the frequency and severity of Raynaud's phenomenon. Adrenergic blocking agents, such as reserpine, have been shown to increase nutritional blood flow to the fingers. Some, but not all, patients achieve satisfactory results with long-term reserpine therapy. Moreover, systemic use of this drug is limited by side effects of hypotension, nasal stuffiness, lethargy, and depression. The postsynaptic α_1-adrenergic antagonist prazosin has been used with favorable responses. Doxazosin and terazosin may also be effective. Other sympatholytic agents, such as methyldopa, guanethidine, and phenoxybenzamine, may be useful in some patients. Surgical sympathectomy is helpful in some patients who are unresponsive to medical therapy, but benefit is often transient.

ACROCYANOSIS In this condition, there is arterial vasoconstriction and secondary dilation of the capillaries and venules with resulting persistent cyanosis of the hands and, less frequently, the feet. Cyanosis may be intensified by exposure to a cold environment. Women are affected much more frequently than men, and the age of onset is usually less than 30 years. Generally, patients are asymptomatic but seek medical attention because of the discoloration. Examination reveals normal pulses, peripheral cyanosis, and moist palms. Trophic skin changes and ulcerations do *not* occur. The disorder can be distinguished from Raynaud's phenomenon because it is persistent and not episodic, the discoloration extends proximally from the digits, and blanching does not occur. Ischemia secondary to arterial occlusive disease can usually be excluded by the presence of normal pulses. Central cyanosis and decreased arterial oxygen saturation are not present. Patients should be reassured and advised to dress warmly and avoid cold exposure. Pharmacologic intervention is not indicated.

LIVEDO RETICULARIS In this condition, localized areas of the extremities develop a mottled or netlike appearance of reddish to blue discoloration. The mottled appearance may be more prominent following cold exposure. The idiopathic form of this disorder occurs equally in men and women, and the most common age of onset is in the third decade. Patients with the idiopathic form are usually asymptomatic and seek attention for cosmetic reasons. Livedo reticularis can also occur following atheroembolism (see above). Rarely, skin ulcerations develop. Patients should be reassured and advised to avoid cold environments. No drug treatment is indicated.

PERNIO (CHILBLAINS) This is a vasculitic disorder associated with exposure to cold; acute forms have been described. Raised erythematous lesions develop on the lower part of the legs and feet in cold weather. These are associated with pruritus and a burning sensation, and they may blister and ulcerate. Pathologic examination demonstrates angiitis characterized by intimal proliferation and perivascular infiltration of mononuclear and polymorphonuclear leukocytes. Giant cells may be present in the subcutaneous tissue. Patients should avoid exposure to cold, and ulcers should be kept clean and protected with sterile dressings. Sympatholytic drugs may be effective in some patients.

ERYTHROMELALGIA (ERYTHERMALGIA) This disorder is characterized by burning pain and erythema of the extremities. The feet are involved more frequently than the hands, and males are affected more frequently than females. Erythromelalgia may occur at any age but is most common in middle age. It may be primary or secondary to myeloproliferative disorders such as polycythemia vera and essential thrombocytosis, or it may occur as an adverse effect of drugs such as nifedipine or bromocriptine. Patients complain of burning in the extremities that is precipitated by exposure to a warm environment and aggravated by a dependent position. The symptoms are relieved by exposing the affected area to cool air or water or by elevation. Erythromelalgia can be distinguished from ischemia secondary to peripheral arterial disorders and peripheral neuropathy because the peripheral pulses are present and the neurologic examination is normal. There is no specific treatment; aspirin may produce relief in patients with erythromelalgia secondary to myeloproliferative disease. Treatment of associated disorders in secondary erythromelalgia may be helpful.

FROSTBITE In this condition, tissue damage results from severe environmental cold exposure or from direct contact with a very cold object. Tissue injury results from both freezing and vasoconstriction. Frostbite usually affects the distal aspects of the extremities or exposed parts of the face, such as the ears, nose, chin, and cheeks. Superficial frostbite involves the skin and subcutaneous tissue. Patients experience pain or paresthesia, and the skin appears white and waxy. After rewarming, there is cyanosis and erythema, wheal- and-flare formation, edema, and superficial blisters. Deep frostbite involves muscle, nerves, and deeper blood vessels. It may result in edema of the hand or foot, vesicles and bullae, tissue necrosis, and gangrene.

Initial treatment is rewarming, performed in an environment where reexposure to freezing conditions will not occur. Rewarming is accomplished by immersion of the affected part in a water bath at temperatures of 40 to 44°C (104 to 111°F). Massage, application of ice water, and extreme heat are contraindicated. The injured area should be cleansed with soap or antiseptic and sterile dressings applied. Analgesics are often required during rewarming. Antibiotics are used if there is evidence of infection. The efficacy of sympathetic blocking drugs is not established. Following recovery, the affected extremity may exhibit increased sensitivity to cold.

VENOUS DISORDERS

Veins in the extremities can be broadly classified as either superficial or deep. In the lower extremity, the superficial venous system includes the greater and lesser saphenous veins and their tributaries. The deep veins of the leg accompany the major arteries. Perforating veins connect the superficial and deep systems at multiple locations. Bicuspid valves are present throughout the venous system to direct the flow of venous blood centrally.

VENOUS THROMBOSIS The presence of thrombus within a superficial or deep vein and the accompanying inflammatory response in the vessel wall is termed *venous thrombosis* or *thrombophlebitis*. Initially, the thrombus is composed principally of platelets and fibrin. Red cells become interspersed with fibrin, and the thrombus tends to propagate in the direction of blood flow. The inflammatory response in the vessel wall may be minimal or characterized by granulocyte infiltration, loss of endothelium, and edema.

The factors that predispose to venous thrombosis were initially described by Virchow in 1856 and include stasis, vascular damage, and hypercoagulability. Accordingly, a variety of clinical situations are associated with increased risk of venous thrombosis (Table 248-2). Venous thrombosis may occur in more than 50% of patients having orthopedic surgical procedures, particularly those involving the hip or knee, and in 10 to 40% of patients who undergo abdominal or thoracic operations. The prevalence of venous thrombosis is particularly high in patients with cancer of the pancreas, lungs, genitourinary tract, stomach, and breast. Approximately 10 to 20% of patients with idiopathic deep vein thrombosis have or develop clinically overt cancer; there is no consensus on whether these individuals should be subjected to intensive diagnostic workup to search for occult malignancy. Risk of thrombosis is increased following trauma, such as fractures of the spine, pelvis, femur, and tibia. Immobilization, regardless of the underlying disease, is a major predisposing cause of venous thrombosis. This fact may account for the relatively high incidence in patients with acute myocardial infarction or congestive heart failure. The incidence of venous thrombosis is increased during pregnancy, particularly in the third trimester and in the first month postpartum, and in individuals who use oral contraceptives or receive postmenopausal hormone replacement therapy. A variety of clinical disorders that produce systemic hypercoagulability, including resistance to activated protein C (factor V Leiden); antithrombin III, protein C, and protein S deficiencies; antiphospholipid syndrome; SLE; myeloproliferative diseases; dysfibrinogenemia; and disseminated intravascular coagulation, are associated with venous thrombosis. Venulitis occurring in thromboangiitis obliterans, Behçet's disease, and homocysteinuria may also cause venous thrombosis.

DEEP VENOUS THROMBOSIS   The most important consequences of this disorder are pulmonary embolism (Chap. 261) and the syndrome of chronic venous insufficiency. Deep venous thrombosis of the iliac, femoral, or popliteal veins is suggested by unilateral leg swelling, warmth, and erythema. Tenderness may be present along the course of the involved veins, and a cord may be palpable. There may be increased tissue turgor, distention of superficial veins, and the appearance of prominent venous collaterals. In some patients, deoxygenated hemoglobin in stagnant veins imparts a cyanotic hue to the limb, a condition called *phlegmasia cerulea dolens*. In markedly edematous legs, the interstitial tissue pressure may exceed the capillary perfusion pressure, causing pallor, a condition designated *phlegmasia alba dolens*.

The diagnosis of deep venous thrombosis of the calf is often difficult to make at the bedside. This is so because only one of multiple veins may be involved, allowing adequate venous return through the remaining patent vessels. The most common complaint is calf pain.

Examination may reveal posterior calf tenderness, warmth, increased tissue turgor or modest swelling, and, rarely, a cord. Increased resistance or pain during dorsiflexion of the foot (Homans' sign) is an unreliable diagnostic sign.

Deep venous thrombosis occurs less frequently in the upper extremity than in the lower extremity, but the incidence is increasing because of greater utilization of indwelling central venous catheters. The clinical features and complications are similar to those described for the leg.

Diagnosis   The noninvasive test used most often to diagnose deep venous thrombosis is duplex venous ultrasonography (B-mode, i.e., two-dimensional, imaging, and pulse-wave Doppler interrogation). By imaging the deep veins, thrombus can be detected either by direct visualization or by inference when the vein does not collapse on compressive maneuvers. The Doppler ultrasound measures the velocity of blood flow in veins. This velocity is normally affected by respiration and by manual compression of the foot or calf. Flow abnormalities occur when deep venous obstruction is present. The positive predictive value of duplex venous ultrasonography approaches 95% for proximal deep vein thrombosis. In the calf, because calf veins are more difficult to visualize than proximal veins, the sensitivity of this technique is only 50 to 75%, although its specificity is 95%.

Impedance plethysmography measures changes in venous capacitance during physiologic maneuvers. Venous obstruction blunts the normal changes in venous capacitance that occur following inflation and deflation of a thigh cuff. The predictive value of this test for detecting occlusive thrombi in proximal veins is approximately 90%. However, it is much less sensitive for diagnosing deep venous thrombosis of the calves.

Magnetic resonance imaging (MRI) is another noninvasive means to detect deep vein thrombosis. Its diagnostic accuracy for assessing proximal deep vein thrombosis is similar to that of duplex ultrasonography. It is useful in patients with suspected thrombosis of the superior and inferior venae cavae or pelvic veins.

Deep venous thrombosis can also be diagnosed by venography. Contrast medium is injected into a superficial vein of the foot and directed to the deep system by the application of tourniquets. The presence of a filling defect or absence of filling of the deep veins is required to make the diagnosis.

Deep vein thrombosis must be differentiated from a variety of disorders that cause unilateral leg pain or swelling, including muscle rupture, trauma, or hemorrhage; a ruptured popliteal cyst; and lymphedema. It may be difficult to distinguish swelling caused by the postphlebitic syndrome from that due to acute recurrent deep venous thrombosis. Leg pain may also result from nerve compression, arthritis, tendinitis, fractures, and arterial occlusive disorders. A careful history and physical examination can usually determine the cause of these symptoms.

Table 248-2   Conditions Associated with an Increased Risk for Development of Venous Thrombosis

Surgery
  Orthopedic, thoracic, abdominal, and genitourinary procedures
Neoplasms
  Pancreas, lung, ovary, testes, urinary tract, breast, stomach
Trauma
  Fractures of spine, pelvis, femur, or tibia; spinal cord injuries
Immobilization
  Acute myocardial infarction, congestive heart failure, stroke, postoperative
    convalescence
Pregnancy
Estrogen use (for replacement or contraception)
Hypercoagulable states
  Resistance to activated protein C; deficiencies of antithrombin III, protein
    C, or protein S; antiphospholipid antibodies; myeloproliferative diseases;
    dysfibrinogenemia; disseminated intravascular coagulation
Venulitis
  Thromboangiitis obliterans, Behçet's disease, homocysteinuria
Previous deep vein thrombosis

℞   **TREATMENT   Anticoagulants** (See also Chap. 261)   Prevention of pulmonary embolism is the most important reason for treating patients with deep vein thrombosis, since in the early stages the thrombus may be loose and poorly adherent to the vessel wall. Patients should be placed in bed, and the affected extremity should be elevated above the level of the heart until the edema and tenderness subside. Anticoagulants prevent thrombus propagation and allow the endogenous lytic system to operate. Initial therapy should include either unfractionated heparin or low-molecular-weight heparin. Unfractionated heparin should be administered intravenously as an initial bolus of 7500 to 10,000 IU, followed by a continuous infusion of 1000 to 1500 IU/h. The rate of the heparin infusion should be adjusted so that the activated partial thromboplastin time (aPTT) is approximately twice the control value. Subcutaneous injection of heparin has been used as an alternative form of therapy. In fewer than 5% of patients, heparin therapy may cause thrombocytopenia. Infrequently, these patients develop arterial thrombosis and ischemia. Low-molecular-weight (4000 to 6000 Da) heparins are reported to be as effective as or better than conventional, unfractionated heparin in preventing extension or recurrence of venous thrombosis. Depending on the specific preparation, low-molecular-weight heparin is administered subcutaneously, in fixed doses, once or twice daily; for example, the dose of enoxaparin is 1 mg/kg subcutaneously bid. The incidence of thrombocytopenia is less with low-molecular-weight heparin than with conventional preparations. Hirudin, a direct thrombin inhibitor, may be used as initial anticoagulant therapy for patients in whom heparin is contraindicated because of heparin-induced thrombocytopenia. Warfarin is administered during the first week of treatment with heparin and may be started as early as the first day of heparin treatment if the aPTT is therapeutic. It is important to overlap heparin treatment with oral anticoagulant therapy for at least 4 to 5 days because the full anticoagulant effect of warfarin is delayed. The dose of warfarin should be adjusted to maintain the prothrombin time at an international normalized ratio (INR) of 2.0 to 3.0.

Anticoagulant treatment is indicated for patients with proximal deep vein thrombosis, since pulmonary embolism may occur in approximately 50% of untreated individuals. The use of anticoagulants for isolated deep vein thrombosis of the calf is controversial. However, approximately 20 to 30% of calf thrombi propagate to the thigh, thereby increasing the risk of pulmonary embolism. The overall incidence of pulmonary embolism in patients presenting initially with deep calf vein thrombosis is 5 to 20%. Also, isolated calf vein thrombosis has been identified as a cause of embolic stroke via a patent foramen ovale. Therefore, patients with calf vein thrombosis should either receive anticoagulants or be followed with serial noninvasive tests to determine whether proximal propagation has occurred. Anticoagulant treatment should be continued for at least 3 to 6 months for patients with acute idiopathic deep vein thrombosis and for those with a temporary risk factor for venous thrombosis to decrease the chance of recurrence. The duration of treatment is indefinite for patients with recurrent deep vein thrombosis and for those in whom associated causes, such as malignancy or hypercoagulability, have not been eliminated. If treatment with anticoagulants is contraindicated because of a bleeding diathesis or risk of hemorrhage, protection from pulmonary embolism can be achieved by mechanically interrupting the flow of blood through the inferior vena cava. Inferior vena cava plication generally has been replaced by percutaneous insertion of a filter.

Thrombolytics Thrombolytic drugs such as streptokinase, urokinase, and tPA may also be used, but there is no evidence that thrombolytic therapy is more effective than anticoagulants in preventing pulmonary embolism. However, early administration of thrombolytic drugs may accelerate clot lysis, preserve venous valves, and decrease the potential for developing postphlebitic syndrome.

Prophylaxis Prophylaxis should be considered in clinical situations where the risk of deep vein thrombosis is high. Low-dose unfractionated heparin (5000 units 2 h prior to surgery and then 5000 units every 8 to 12 h postoperatively), warfarin, and external pneumatic compression are all useful. Low-dose heparin reduces the risk of deep vein thrombosis associated with thoracic and abdominal surgery and with prolonged bed rest. Low-molecular-weight heparins have been shown to prevent deep vein thrombosis in patients undergoing general or orthopedic surgery and in acutely ill medical patients. They are said to be more effective than conventional heparin and to cause an equal or lower incidence of bleeding. Danaparoid, a low-molecular-weight heparinoid, may be used for prophylaxis in patients undergoing hip surgery. Warfarin in a dose that yields a prothrombin time equivalent to an INR of 2.0 to 3.0 is effective in preventing deep vein thrombosis associated with bone fractures and orthopedic surgery. Warfarin is started the night before surgery and continued throughout the convalescent period. External pneumatic compression devices applied to the legs are used to prevent deep vein thrombosis when even low doses of heparin or warfarin might cause serious bleeding, as during neurosurgery or transurethral resection of the prostate.

SUPERFICIAL VEIN THROMBOSIS Thrombosis of the greater or lesser saphenous veins or their tributaries—i.e., superficial vein thrombosis—does not result in pulmonary embolism. It is asso-

ciated with intravenous catheters and infusions, occurs in varicose veins, and may develop in association with deep vein thrombosis. Migrating superficial vein thrombosis is often a marker for a carcinoma and may also occur in patients with vasculitides, such as thromboangiitis obliterans. The clinical features of superficial vein thrombosis are easily distinguished from those of deep vein thrombosis. Patients complain of pain localized to the site of the thrombus. Examination reveals a reddened, warm, and tender cord extending along a superficial vein. The surrounding area may be red and edematous.

℞ TREATMENT Treatment is primarily supportive. Initially, patients can be placed at bed rest with leg elevation and application of warm compresses. Nonsteroidal antiinflammatory drugs may provide analgesia but may also obscure clinical evidence of thrombus propagation. If a thrombosis of the greater saphenous vein develops in the thigh and extends toward the saphenofemoral vein junction, it is reasonable to consider anticoagulant therapy to prevent extension of the thrombus into the deep system and a possible pulmonary embolism.

VARICOSE VEINS Varicose veins are dilated, tortuous superficial veins that result from defective structure and function of the valves of the saphenous veins, from intrinsic weakness of the vein wall, from high intraluminal pressure, or, rarely, from arteriovenous fistulas. Varicose veins can be categorized as primary or secondary. Primary varicose veins originate in the superficial system and occur two to three times as frequently in women as in men. Approximately half of patients have a family history of varicose veins. Secondary varicose veins result from deep venous insufficiency and incompetent perforating veins or from deep venous occlusion causing enlargement of superficial veins that are serving as collaterals.

Patients with venous varicosities are often concerned about the cosmetic appearance of their legs. Symptoms consist of a dull ache or pressure sensation in the legs after prolonged standing; it is relieved with leg elevation. The legs feel heavy, and mild ankle edema develops occasionally. Extensive venous varicosities may cause skin ulcerations near the ankle. Superficial venous thrombosis may be a recurring problem, and, rarely, a varicosity ruptures and bleeds. Visual inspection of the legs in the dependent position usually confirms the presence of varicose veins.

Varicose veins can usually be treated with conservative measures. Symptoms often decrease when the legs are elevated periodically, when prolonged standing is avoided, and when elastic support hose are worn. External compression stockings provide a counterbalance to the hydrostatic pressure in the veins. Small symptomatic varicose veins can be treated with sclerotherapy, in which a sclerosing solution is injected into the involved varicose vein and a compression bandage is applied. Surgical therapy usually involves extensive ligation and stripping of the greater and lesser saphenous veins and should be reserved for patients who are very symptomatic, suffer recurrent superficial vein thrombosis, and/or develop skin ulceration. Surgical therapy may also be indicated for cosmetic reasons.

CHRONIC VENOUS INSUFFICIENCY Chronic venous insufficiency may result from deep vein thrombosis and/or valvular incompetence. Following deep vein thrombosis, the delicate valve leaflets become thickened and contracted so that they cannot prevent retrograde flow of blood; the vein becomes rigid and thick-walled. Although most veins recanalize after an episode of thrombosis, the large proximal veins may remain occluded. Secondary incompetence develops in distal valves because high pressures distend the vein and separate the leaflets. Primary deep venous valvular dysfunction may also occur without previous thrombosis. Patients with venous insufficiency often complain of a dull ache in the leg that worsens with prolonged standing and resolves with leg elevation. Examination demonstrates increased leg circumference, edema, and superficial varicose veins. Erythema, dermatitis, and hyperpigmentation develop along the distal aspect of the leg, and skin ulceration may occur near the medial and lateral malleoli. Cellulitis may be a recurring problem. Patients should be advised to avoid prolonged standing or sitting; frequent leg elevation is helpful. Graduated compression stockings should be worn during the day. These efforts should be intensified if skin ulcers develop. Ulcers should be treated with applications of wet to dry dressings and, occasionally, dilute topical antibiotic solutions. Commercially available dressings comprising antiseptic solutions and compressive bandages may be applied and should be changed weekly until healing occurs. Recurrent ulceration and severe edema may be treated by surgical interruption of incompetent communicating veins. Rarely, surgical valvuloplasty and bypass of venous occlusions are employed.

LYMPHATIC DISORDERS

Lymphatic capillaries are blind-ended tubes formed by a single layer of endothelial cells. The absent or widely fenestrated basement membrane of lymphatic capillaries allows access to interstitial proteins and particles. Lymphatic capillaries merge to form larger vessels which contain smooth muscle and are capable of vasomotion. Small and medium-sized lymphatic vessels empty into progressively larger channels, most of which drain into the thoracic duct. The lymphatic circulation is involved in the absorption of interstitial fluid and in the response to infection.

LYMPHEDEMA   Lymphedema may be categorized as primary or secondary (Table 248-3). The prevalence of primary lymphedema is approximately 1 per 10,000 individuals. Primary lymphedema may be secondary to agenesis, hypoplasia, or obstruction of the lymphatic vessels. It may be associated with Turner syndrome, Klinefelter syndrome, Noonan syndrome, the yellow nail syndrome, the intestinal lymphangiectasia syndrome, and lymphangiomyomatosis. Women are affected more frequently than men. There are three clinical subtypes: congenital lymphedema, which appears shortly after birth; lymphedema praecox, which has its onset at the time of puberty; and lymphedema tarda, which usually begins after age 35. Familial forms of congenital lymphedema (Milroy's disease) and lymphedema praecox (Meige's disease) may be inherited in an autosomal dominant manner with variable penetrance; autosomal or sex-linked recessive forms are less common.

Secondary lymphedema is an acquired condition resulting from damage to or obstruction of previously normal lymphatic channels (Table 248-3). Recurrent episodes of bacterial lymphangitis, usually caused by streptococci, are a very common cause of lymphedema. The most common cause of secondary lymphedema worldwide is filariasis (Chap. 221). Tumors, such as prostate cancer and lymphoma, can also obstruct lymphatic vessels. Both surgery and radiation therapy for breast carcinoma may cause lymphedema of the upper extremity. Less common causes include tuberculosis, contact dermatitis, lymphogranuloma venereum, rheumatoid arthritis, pregnancy, and self-induced or factitious lymphedema following application of tourniquets.

Lymphedema is generally a painless condition, but patients may

Table 248-3   Causes of Lymphedema

Primary
   Congenital (includes Milroy's disease)
   Lymphedema praecox (includes Meige's disease)
   Lymphedema tarda
Secondary
   Recurrent lymphangitis
   Filariasis
   Tuberculosis
   Neoplasm
   Surgery
   Radiation therapy

experience a chronic dull, heavy sensation in the leg, and most often they are concerned about the appearance of the leg. Lymphedema of the lower extremity, initially involving the foot, gradually progresses up the leg so that the entire limb becomes edematous. In the early stages, the edema is soft and pits easily with pressure. In the chronic stages, the limb has a woody texture, and the tissues become indurated and fibrotic. At this point the edema may no longer be pitting. The limb loses its normal contour, and the toes appear square. Lymphedema should be distinguished from other disorders that cause unilateral leg swelling, such as deep vein thrombosis and chronic venous insufficiency. In the latter condition, the edema is softer, and there is often evidence of a stasis dermatitis, hyperpigmentation, and superficial venous varicosities.

The evaluation of patients with lymphedema should include diagnostic studies to clarify the cause. Abdominal and pelvic ultrasound and computed tomography can be used to detect obstructing lesions such as neoplasms. MRI may reveal edema in the epifascial compartment and identify lymph nodes and enlarged lymphatic channels. Lymphoscintigraphy and lymphangiography are rarely indicated, but either can be used to confirm the diagnosis or to differentiate primary from secondary lymphedema. Lymphoscintigraphy involves the injection of radioactively labeled technetium-containing colloid into the distal subcutaneous tissue of the affected extremity. In lymphangiography, contrast material is injected into a distal lymphatic vessel that has been isolated and cannulated. In primary lymphedema, lymphatic channels are absent, hypoplastic, or ectatic. In secondary lymphedema, lymphatic channels are usually dilated, and it may be possible to determine the level of obstruction.

℞ **TREATMENT**   Patients with lymphedema of the lower extremities must be instructed to take meticulous care of their feet to prevent recurrent lymphangitis. Skin hygiene is important, and emollients can be used to prevent drying. Prophylactic antibiotics are often helpful, and fungal infection should be treated aggressively. Patients should be encouraged to participate in physical activity; frequent leg elevation can reduce the amount of edema. Physical therapy, including massage to facilitate lymphatic drainage, may be helpful. Patients can be fitted with graduated compression hose to reduce the amount of lymphedema that develops with upright posture. Occasionally, intermittent pneumatic compression devices can be applied at home to facilitate reduction of the edema. Diuretics are contraindicated and may cause depletion of intravascular volume and metabolic abnormalities. Recently, microsurgical lymphatico-venous anastomotic procedures have been performed to rechannel lymph flow from obstructed lymphatic vessels into the venous system.

BIBLIOGRAPHY

AQEL MB, OLIN JW: Thromboangiitis obliterans (Buerger's disease). Vasc Med 2:61, 1997

BAUMGARTNER I et al: Constitutive expression of VEGF165 after intramuscular gene transfer promotes collateral vessel development in patients with critical limb ischemia. Circulation 97:1114, 1998

DAWSON DL et al: Cilostazol has beneficial effects in treatment of intermittent claudication. Circulation 98:678, 1998

DORMANDY JA, RUTHERFORD RB: Management of peripheral arterial disease (PAD). J Vasc Surg 31:51, 2000

DE CATERINA R: Endothelial dysfunctions: Common denominators in vascular disease. Curr Opin Lipid 11:9, 2000

GOULD MK et al: Low-molecular-weight heparins compared with unfractionated heparin for treatment of acute venous thrombosis. Ann Intern Med 130:789, 1999

KEARON C et al: A comparison of three months of anticoagulation with extended anticoagulation for a first episode of idiopathic venous thromobembolism. N Engl J Med 340:901, 1999

LOSCALZO J et al:*Vascular Medicine*, 2d ed. Boston, Little, Brown, 1996

SZUBA A, ROCKSON SG: Lymphedema: Classification, diagnosis and therapy. Vasc Med 3:145, 1998

THE COLUMBUS INVESTIGATORS: Low-molecular-weight heparin in the treatment of patients with venous thromboembolism. N Engl J Med 337:657, 1997

WORKING PARTY ON THROMBOLYSIS IN THE MANAGEMENT OF LIMB ISCHEMIA: Thrombolysis in the management of lower limb peripheral arterial occlusion—a consensus document. Am J Cardiol 81:207, 1998

Section 1
DIAGNOSIS

249

Jeffrey M. Drazen, Steven E. Weinberger

APPROACH TO THE PATIENT WITH DISEASE OF THE RESPIRATORY SYSTEM

Patients with disease of the respiratory system generally present because of symptoms, an abnormality on a chest radiograph, or both. A set of diagnostic possibilities is often suggested by the initial problems at presentation, including the particular symptom(s) and the appearance of any radiographic abnormalities. The differential diagnosis is then refined on the basis of additional information gleaned from physical examination, pulmonary function testing, additional imaging studies, and bronchoscopic examination. This chapter will consider the approach to the patient based on the major patterns of presentation, focusing on the history, the physical examination, and the chest radiograph. →*For further discussion of pulmonary function testing, see Chap. 250, and of other diagnostic studies, see Chap. 251.*

CLINICAL PRESENTATION

HISTORY Dyspnea (shortness of breath) and cough are the primary presenting symptoms for patients with respiratory system disease. Less common symptoms include hemoptysis (the coughing up of blood) and chest pain, often with a pleuritic quality.

Dyspnea (See also Chap. 32) When evaluating a patient with shortness of breath, one should first determine the time course over which the symptom has become manifest. Patients who were well previously and developed *acute* shortness of breath (over a period of hours to days) can have acute disease affecting the airways (an acute attack of asthma), the pulmonary parenchyma (acute pulmonary edema or an acute infectious process such as a bacterial pneumonia), the pleural space (a pneumothorax), or the pulmonary vasculature (a pulmonary embolus). A *subacute* presentation (over days to weeks) can suggest an exacerbation of preexisting airways disease (asthma or chronic bronchitis), a parenchymal infection or a noninfectious inflammatory process that proceeds at a relatively slow pace (*Pneumocystis carinii* pneumonia in a patient with AIDS, mycobacterial or fungal pneumonia, Wegener's granulomatosis, eosinophilic pneumonia, bronchiolitis obliterans with organizing pneumonia, and many others), neuromuscular disease (Guillain-Barré syndrome, myasthenia gravis), pleural disease (pleural effusion from a variety of possible causes), or chronic cardiac disease (congestive heart failure). A *chronic* presentation (over months to years) often indicates chronic obstructive lung disease, chronic interstitial lung disease, or chronic cardiac disease. Chronic diseases of airways (not only chronic obstructive lung disease but also asthma) are characterized by exacerbations and remissions. Patients often have periods when they are severely limited by shortness of breath, but these may be interspersed with periods in which symptoms are minimal or absent. In contrast, many of the diseases of pulmonary parenchyma are characterized by a slow but inexorable progression.

Other Respiratory Symptoms *Cough* (Chap. 33) may indicate the presence of lung disease, but cough per se is not useful for the differential diagnosis. The presence of sputum accompanying the cough often suggests airway disease and may be seen in asthma, chronic bronchitis, or bronchiectasis.

Hemoptysis (Chap. 33) can originate from disease of the airways, the pulmonary parenchyma, or the vasculature. Diseases of the airways can be inflammatory (acute or chronic bronchitis, bronchiectasis, or cystic fibrosis) or neoplastic (bronchogenic carcinoma or bronchial carcinoid tumors). Parenchymal diseases causing hemoptysis may be either localized (pneumonia, lung abscess, tuberculosis, or infection with *Aspergillus*) or diffuse (Goodpasture's syndrome, idiopathic pulmonary hemosiderosis). Vascular diseases potentially associated with hemoptysis include pulmonary thromboembolic disease and pulmonary arteriovenous malformations.

Chest pain (Chap. 13) caused by diseases of the respiratory system usually originates from involvement of the parietal pleura. As a result, the pain is accentuated by respiratory motion and is often referred to as *pleuritic*. Common examples include primary pleural disorders, such as neoplasm or inflammatory disorders involving the pleura, or pulmonary parenchymal disorders that extend to the pleural surface, such as pneumonia or pulmonary infarction.

Additional Historic Information Information about risk factors for lung disease should be explicitly explored to assure a complete basis of historic data. A history of current and past smoking, especially of cigarettes, should be sought from all patients. The smoking history should include the number of years of smoking, the intensity (i.e., number of packs per day), and, if the patient no longer smokes, the interval since smoking cessation. The risk of lung cancer falls progressively with the interval following discontinuation of smoking, and loss of lung function above the expected age-related decline ceases with the discontinuation of smoking. Even though chronic obstructive lung disease and neoplasia are the two most important respiratory complications of smoking, other respiratory disorders (e.g., spontaneous pneumothorax, respiratory bronchiolitis–interstitial lung disease, eosinophilic granuloma of the lung, and pulmonary hemorrhage with Goodpasture's syndrome) are also associated with smoking. A history of significant secondhand (passive) exposure to smoke, whether in the home or at the workplace, should also be sought as it may be a risk factor for neoplasia or an exacerbating factor for airways disease.

The patient may have been exposed to other inhaled agents associated with lung disease, which act either via direct toxicity or through immune mechanisms (Chaps. 253 and 254). Such exposures can be either occupational or avocational, indicating the importance of detailed occupational and personal histories, the latter stressing exposures related to hobbies or the home environment. Important agents include the inorganic dusts associated with pneumoconiosis (especially asbestos and silica dusts) and organic antigens associated with hypersensitivity pneumonitis (especially antigens from molds and animal proteins). Asthma, which is more common in women than men, is often exacerbated by exposure to environmental allergens (dust mites, pet dander, or cockroach allergens in the home or allergens in the outdoor environment such as pollen and ragweed) or may be caused by occupational exposures (diisocyanates). Exposure to particular infectious agents can be suggested by contacts with individuals with known respiratory infections (especially tuberculosis) or by residence in an area with endemic pathogens (histoplasmosis, coccidioidomycosis, blastomycosis).

A history of coexisting nonrespiratory disease or of risk factors for or previous treatment of such diseases should be sought, as they may

Table 249-1 Typical Chest Examination Findings in Selected Clinical Conditions

Condition	Percussion	Fremitus	Breath Sounds	Voice Transmission	Adventitious Sounds
Normal	Resonant	Normal	Vesicular (at lung bases)	Normal	Absent
Consolidation or atelectasis (with patent airway)	Dull	Increased	Bronchial	Bronchophony, whispered pectoriloquy, egophony	Crackles
Consolidation or atelectasis (with blocked airway)	Dull	Decreased	Decreased	Decreased	Absent
Asthma	Resonant	Normal	Vesicular	Normal	Wheezing
Interstitial lung disease	Resonant	Normal	Vesicular	Normal	Crackles
Emphysema	Hyperresonant	Decreased	Decreased	Decreased	Absent or wheezing
Pneumothorax	Hyperresonant	Decreased	Decreased	Decreased	Absent
Pleural effusion	Dull	Decreased	Decreased[a]	Decreased[a]	Absent or pleural friction rub

[a] May be altered by collapse of underlying lung, which will increase transmission of sound.
SOURCE: Adapted from Weinberger.

predispose a patient to both infectious and noninfectious respiratory system complications. Common examples include systemic rheumatic diseases that are associated with pleural or parenchymal lung disease (Chap. 312), metastatic neoplastic disease in the lung, or impaired host defense mechanisms and secondary infection, which occur in the case of hematologic and lymph node malignancies. Risk factors for AIDS should be sought, as the lungs are not only the most common site of AIDS-defining infection but also can be involved by nonfectious complications of AIDS (Chap. 309). Treatment of nonrespiratory disease can be associated with respiratory complications, either because of effects on host defense mechanisms (immunosuppressive agents, cancer chemotherapy) with resulting infection or because of direct effects on the pulmonary parenchyma (cancer chemotherapy, radiation therapy, or treatment with other agents, such as amiodarone) or on the airways (beta-blocking agents causing airflow obstruction, angiotensin-converting enzyme inhibitors causing cough) (Chap. 253).

Family history is important for evaluating diseases that have a genetic component. These include disorders such as cystic fibrosis, α_1-antitrypsin deficiency, and asthma.

PHYSICAL EXAMINATION The general principles of inspection, palpation, percussion, and auscultation apply to the examination of the respiratory system. However, the physical examination should be directed not only toward ascertaining abnormalities of the lungs and thorax but also toward recognizing other findings that may reflect underlying lung disease.

On *inspection*, the rate and pattern of breathing as well as the depth and symmetry of lung expansion are observed. Breathing that is unusually rapid, labored, or associated with the use of accessory muscles of respiration generally indicates either augmented respiratory demands or an increased work of breathing. Asymmetric expansion of the chest is usually due to an asymmetric process affecting the lungs, such as endobronchial obstruction of a large airway, unilateral parenchymal or pleural disease, or unilateral phrenic nerve paralysis. Visible abnormalities of the thoracic cage include kyphoscoliosis and ankylosing spondylitis, either of which can alter compliance of the thorax, increase the work of breathing, and cause dyspnea.

On *palpation*, the symmetry of lung expansion can be assessed, generally confirming the findings observed by inspection. Vibration produced by spoken sounds is transmitted to the chest wall and is assessed by the presence or absence and symmetry of tactile fremitus. Transmission of vibration is decreased or absent if pleural liquid is interposed between the lung and the chest wall or if an endobronchial obstruction alters sound transmission. In contrast, transmitted vibration may increase over an area of underlying pulmonary consolidation.

The relative resonance or dullness of the tissue underlying the chest wall is assessed by *percussion*. The normal sound of underlying air-containing lung is resonant. In contrast, consolidated lung or a pleural effusion sounds dull, while emphysema or air in the pleural space results in a hyperresonant percussion note.

On *auscultation* of the lungs, the examiner listens for both the quality and intensity of the breath sounds and for the presence of extra, or adventitious, sounds. Normal breath sounds heard through the stethoscope at the periphery of the lung are described as *vesicular breath sounds*, in which inspiration is louder and longer than expiration. If sound transmission is impaired by endobronchial obstruction or by air or liquid in the pleural space, breath sounds are diminished in intensity or absent. When sound transmission is improved through consolidated lung, the resulting *bronchial breath sounds* have a more tubular quality and a more pronounced expiratory phase. Sound transmission can also be assessed by listening to spoken or whispered sounds; when these are transmitted through consolidated lung, *bronchophony* and *whispered pectoriloquy*, respectively, are present. The sound of a spoken E becomes more like an A, though with a nasal or bleating quality, a finding that is termed *egophony*.

The primary adventitious (abnormal) sounds that can be heard include crackles (rales), wheezes, and rhonchi. *Crackles* represent the typically inspiratory sound created when alveoli and small airways open and close with respiration, and they are often associated with interstitial lung disease, microatelectasis, or filling of alveoli by liquid. *Wheezes*, which are generally more prominent during expiration than inspiration, reflect the oscillation of airway walls that occurs when there is airflow limitation, as may be produced by bronchospasm, airway edema or collapse, or intraluminal obstruction by neoplasm or secretions. *Rhonchi* is the term applied to the sounds created when there is free liquid in the airway lumen; the viscous interaction between the free liquid and the moving air creates a low-pitched vibratory sound. Other adventitious sounds include pleural friction rubs and stridor. The gritty sound of a *pleural friction rub* indicates inflamed pleural surfaces rubbing against each other, often during both inspiratory and expiratory phases of the respiratory cycle. *Stridor*, which occurs primarily during inspiration, represents flow through a narrowed upper airway, as occurs in an infant with croup.

A summary of the patterns of physical findings on pulmonary examination in common types of respiratory system disease is shown in Table 249-1.

A meticulous *general physical examination* is mandatory in patients with disorders of the respiratory system. Enlarged lymph nodes in the cervical and supraclavicular regions should be sought. Disturbances of mentation or even coma can occur in patients with acute carbon dioxide retention and hypoxemia. Telltale stains on the fingers point to heavy cigarette smoking; infected teeth and gums may occur in patients with aspiration pneumonitis and lung abscess.

Clubbing of the digits can be found in lung cancer, interstitial lung disease, and chronic infections in the thorax, such as bronchiectasis, lung abscess, and empyema. Clubbing can also be seen with congenital heart disease associated with right-to-left shunting and with a variety of chronic inflammatory or infectious diseases, such as inflammatory bowel disease and endocarditis. A number of systemic diseases, such as systemic lupus erythematosus, scleroderma, and rheumatoid arthritis, may be associated with pulmonary complications, even though their primary clinical manifestations and physical findings are not primarily related to the lungs. Conversely, other diseases that most commonly affect the respiratory system, such as sarcoidosis, can have findings on physical examination not related to the respiratory system, including ocular findings (uveitis, conjunctival granulomas) and skin findings (erythema nodosum, cutaneous granulomas).

CHEST RADIOGRAPHY

Chest radiography is often the initial diagnostic study performed to evaluate patients with respiratory symptoms, but it can also provide the initial evidence of disease in patients who are free of symptoms. Perhaps the most common example of the latter situation is the finding of one or more nodules or masses when the radiograph is performed for a reason other than evaluation of respiratory symptoms.

A number of diagnostic possibilities are often suggested by the radiographic pattern (Figs. 249-1 and 249-2). A localized region of opacification involving the pulmonary parenchyma can be described as a nodule (usually <6 cm in diameter), a mass (usually ≥ 6 cm in diameter), or an infiltrate. Diffuse disease with increased opacification is usually characterized as having an alveolar, an interstitial, or a nodular pattern. In contrast, increased radiolucency can be localized, as seen with a cyst or bulla, or generalized, as occurs with emphysema. The chest radiograph is also particularly useful for the detection of pleural disease, especially if manifested by the presence of air or liquid in the pleural space. An abnormal appearance of the hila and/or the mediastinum can suggest a mass or enlargement of lymph nodes.

A summary of representative diagnoses suggested by these common radiographic patterns is presented in Table 249-2.

Additional Diagnostic Evaluation Further information for clarification of radiographic abnormalities is frequently obtained with computed tomographic scanning of the chest (Chap. 251; see Fig. 265-2). This technique is more sensitive than plain radiography in detecting subtle abnormalities and can suggest specific diagnoses based on the pattern of abnormality. →*For further discussion of the use of other imaging studies, including magnetic resonance imaging, scintigraphic studies, ultrasound, and angiography, see Chap. 251.*

Alteration in the function of the lungs as a result of respiratory system disease is assessed objectively by pulmonary function tests, and effects on gas exchange are evaluated by measurement of arterial blood gases or by oximetry (Chap. 250). As part of pulmonary function testing, quantitation of forced expiratory flow assesses the presence of obstructive physiology, which is consistent with diseases affecting the

FIGURE 249-2 Anteroposterior (AP) chest radiograph demonstrating a diffuse alveolar filling pattern due to the acute respiratory distress syndrome (ARDS).

structure or function of the airways, such as asthma and chronic obstructive lung disease. Measurement of lung volumes assesses the presence of restrictive disorders, seen with diseases of the pulmonary parenchyma or respiratory pump and with space-occupying processes within the pleura.

Bronchoscopy is useful in some settings for visualizing abnor-

Table 249-2 Major Respiratory Diagnoses with Common Chest Radiographic Patterns

Solitary circumscribed density—nodule (<6 cm) or mass (≥6 cm)
  Primary or metastatic neoplasm
  Localized infection (bacterial abscess, mycobacterial or fungal infection)
  Wegener's granulomatosis (one or several nodules)
  Rheumatoid nodule (one or several nodules)
  Vascular malformation
  Bronchogenic cyst

Localized opacification (infiltrate)
  Pneumonia (bacterial, atypical, mycobacterial, or fungal infection)
  Neoplasm
  Radiation pneumonitis
  Bronchiolitis obliterans with organizing pneumonia
  Bronchocentric granulomatosis
  Pulmonary infarction

Diffuse interstitial disease
  Idiopathic pulmonary fibrosis
  Pulmonary fibrosis with systemic rheumatic disease
  Sarcoidosis
  Drug-induced lung disease
  Pneumoconiosis
  Hypersensitivity pneumonitis
  Infection (*Pneumocystis*, viral pneumonia)
  Eosinophilic granuloma

Diffuse alveolar disease
  Cardiogenic pulmonary edema
  Acute respiratory distress syndrome
  Diffuse alveolar hemorrhage
  Infection (*Pneumocystis*, viral or bacterial pneumonia)
  Sarcoidosis

Diffuse nodular disease
  Metastatic neoplasm
  Hematogenous spread of infection (bacterial, mycobacterial, fungal)
  Pneumoconiosis
  Eosinophilic granuloma

FIGURE 249-1 Posteroanterior (PA) chest radiograph of a patient with diffuse interstitial lung disease due to idiopathic pulmonary fibrosis. (*From Weinberger, Principles of Pulmonary Medicine, 3d ed. Philadelphia, Saunders, 1998, with permission*).

malities of the airways and for obtaining a variety of samples from either the airway or the pulmonary parenchyma (Chap. 251).

INTEGRATION OF THE PRESENTING CLINICAL PATTERN AND DIAGNOSTIC STUDIES

Patients with respiratory symptoms but a normal chest radiograph most commonly have diseases affecting the airways, such as asthma or chronic obstructive pulmonary disease. However, the latter diagnosis is also commonly associated with radiographic abnormalities, such as diaphragmatic flattening and attenuation of vascular markings. Other disorders of the respiratory system for which the chest radiograph is normal include disorders of the respiratory pump (either the chest wall or the neuromuscular apparatus controlling the chest wall) or pulmonary circulation and occasionally interstitial lung disease. Chest examination and pulmonary function tests are generally helpful in sorting out these diagnostic possibilities. Obstructive diseases associated with a normal or relatively normal chest radiograph are often characterized by findings on physical examination and pulmonary function testing that are typical for these conditions. Similarly, diseases of the respiratory pump or interstitial diseases may also be suggested by findings on physical examination or by particular patterns of restrictive disease seen on pulmonary function testing.

When respiratory symptoms are accompanied by radiographic abnormalities, diseases of the pulmonary parenchyma or the pleura are usually present. Either diffuse or localized parenchymal lung disease is generally visualized well on the radiograph, and both air and liquid in the pleural space (pneumothorax and pleural effusion, respectively) are usually readily detected by radiography.

Radiographic findings in the absence of respiratory symptoms often indicate localized disease affecting the airways or the pulmonary parenchyma. One or more nodules or masses can suggest intrathoracic malignancy, but they also can be the manifestation of a current or previous infectious process. Patients with diffuse parenchymal lung disease on radiographic examination may be free of symptoms, as is sometimes the case with pulmonary sarcoidosis.

In approaching the patient with pulmonary disease, consideration must be given to the observation that substantial changes in the relative incidence of diseases affecting the respiratory system have taken place in the United States during the past four decades. The prevalence of chronic infectious disorders such as lung abscess and bronchiectasis has decreased. Tuberculosis declined only to undergo resurgence when two susceptible populations, patients with AIDS and immigrants from Southeast Asia, increased in number. Patients with chronic bronchitis and with emphysema now survive longer and form an increasing fraction of patients with chronic respiratory disease, as do patients with environmental lung disease and with drug-induced pulmonary disease. Modern intercontinental travel has increased the appearance in the western world of parasitic infestations of the lung. Also, the reduction of immune competence that occurs in patients with AIDS and in those with diabetes as well as in patients being treated for a variety of malignancies and those receiving immunosuppressive drugs has led to an increasing incidence of opportunistic infections of the lungs with a variety of microorganisms that were rarely pathogenic in the past.

BIBLIOGRAPHY

ALBERT RK et al (eds): *Comprehensive Respiratory Medicine*. St. Louis, Mosby, 1999

DeGOWIN R et al: *DeGowin & DeGowin's Diagnostic Examination*, 7th ed. New York, McGraw-Hill, 2000

EBI-KRYSTON KL: Respiratory symptoms and pulmonary function as predictors of 10-year mortality from respiratory disease, cardiovascular disease, and all causes in the Whitehall Study. J Clin Epidemiol 41:251, 1988

IRWIN RS, MADISON JM: Anatomical diagnostic protocol in evaluating chronic cough with specific reference to gastroesophageal reflux disease. Am J Med 108:1265, 2000

JUNIPER EF: Impact of upper respiratory allergic diseases on quality of life. J Allergy Clin Immunol 101:5386, 1998

MARTINEZ FD et al: Asthma and wheezing in the first six years of life. N Engl J Med 332:133, 1995

WEINBERGER SE: *Principles of Pulmonary Medicine*, 3d ed. Philadelphia, Saunders, 1998

WELTY C et al: The relationship of airways responsiveness to cold air, cigarette smoking, and atopy to respiratory symptoms and pulmonary function in adults. Am Rev Respir Dis 130:198, 1984

250　Steven E. Weinberger, Jeffrey M. Drazen

DISTURBANCES OF RESPIRATORY FUNCTION

CNS	central nervous system	MIP	maximal inspiratory pressure
ERV	expiratory reserve volume	MMFR	maximal midexpiratory flow rate
FEF	forced expiratory flow		
FEV	forced expiratory volume	PAP	pulmonary arterial pressure
FRC	functional residual capacity	PVR	pulmonary vascular resistance
FVC	forced vital capacity	RV	residual volume
IC	inspiratory capacity	TLC	total lung capacity
MEP	maximal expiratory pressure	VC	vital capacity

The respiratory system includes the lungs, the central nervous system (CNS), the chest wall (with the diaphragm and intercostal muscles), and the pulmonary circulation. The CNS controls the activity of the muscles of the chest wall, which constitute the pump of the respiratory system. Because these components of the respiratory system act in concert to achieve gas exchange, malfunction of an individual component or alteration of the relationships among components can lead to disturbances in function. In this chapter we consider three major aspects of disturbed respiratory function: (1) disturbances in ventilatory function, (2) disturbances in the pulmonary circulation, and (3) disturbances in gas exchange. →*For further discussion of disorders relating to CNS control of ventilation, see Chap. 263.*

DISTURBANCES IN VENTILATORY FUNCTION

Ventilation is the process whereby the lungs replenish the gas in the alveoli. Measurements of ventilatory function in common diagnostic use consist of quantification of the gas volume contained in the lungs under certain circumstances and the rate at which gas can be expelled from the lungs. Two measurements of lung volume commonly used for respiratory diagnosis are total lung capacity (TLC) and residual volume (RV). The former is the volume of gas contained in the lungs after a maximal inspiration, whereas the latter is the volume of gas remaining in the lungs at the end of a maximal expiration. The volume of gas that is exhaled from the lungs in going from TLC to RV is called the *vital capacity* (VC) (Fig. 250-1).

Common clinical measurements of airflow are obtained from maneuvers in which the subject inspires to TLC and then forcibly exhales to RV. Three measurements are commonly made from a recording of exhaled volume versus time—i.e., a spirogram—obtained during such a forced expiratory maneuver: (1) the volume of gas exhaled during the first second of expiration [forced expiratory volume (FEV) in 1 s, or FEV_1], (2) the total volume exhaled [forced vital capacity (FVC)], and (3) the average expiratory flow rate during the middle 50% of the VC [forced expiratory flow (FEF) between 25 and 75% of the VC, or $FEF_{25-75\%}$, also called the maximal midexpiratory flow rate (MMFR)] (Fig. 250-2).

PHYSIOLOGIC FEATURES　The lungs are elastic structures, containing collagen and elastic fibers that resist expansion. For normal lungs to contain air, they must be distended either by a positive internal pressure—i.e., by a pressure in the airways and alveolar spaces—or by a negative external pressure—i.e., by a pressure outside the lung. The relationship between the volume of gas contained in the lungs and the distending pressure (the *transpulmonary pressure*, or P_{TP}, defined

FIGURE 250-1 Lung volumes, shown by block diagrams *(left)* and by a spirographic tracing *(right)*. TLC, total lung capacity; VC, vital capacity; RV, residual volume; IC, inspiratory capacity; ERV, expiratory reserve volume; FRC, functional residual capacity; V_T, tidal volume. *(From Weinberger, with permission.)*

as internal pressure minus external pressure) is described by the pressure-volume curve of the lungs (Fig. 250-3*A*).

The chest wall is also an elastic structure, with properties similar to those of an expandable and compressible spring. The relationship between the volume enclosed by the chest wall and the distending pressure for the chest wall is described by the pressure-volume curve of the chest wall (Fig. 250-3*B*). For the chest wall to assume a volume different from its resting volume, the internal or external pressures acting on it must be altered.

At functional residual capacity (FRC), defined as the volume of gas in the lungs at the end of a normal exhalation, the lungs are partially inflated, so their elastic recoil exerts a force tending to empty the lungs. At the same time, chest wall volume is such that its elastic recoil promotes outward expansion. FRC occurs at the lung volume at which the tendency of the lungs to contract is opposed by the equal and opposite tendency of the chest wall to expand (Fig. 250-3*C*).

For the lungs and the chest wall to achieve a volume other than the resting volume (FRC), either the pressures acting on them must be changed passively—e.g., by a mechanical ventilator that delivers positive pressure to the airways and alveoli—or the respiratory muscles must actively oppose the tendency of the lungs and the chest wall to return to FRC. During inhalation to volumes above FRC, the inspiratory muscles actively overcome the tendency of the respiratory sys-

FIGURE 250-3 *A.* Pressure-volume curve of the lungs. *B.* Pressure-volume curve of the chest wall. *C.* Pressure-volume curve of the respiratory system, showing the superimposed component curves of the lungs and the chest wall. RV, residual volume; FRC, functional residual capacity; TLC, total lung capacity. *(From Weinberger, with permission.)*

tem to decrease volume back to FRC. During active exhalation to volumes below FRC, expiratory muscle activity must overcome the tendency of the respiratory system to increase volume back to FRC.

At TLC, the maximal force applied by the inspiratory muscles to expand the lungs is opposed mainly by the inward recoil of the lungs. As a consequence, the major determinants of TLC are the stiffness of the lungs and inspiratory muscle strength. If the lungs become stiffer—i.e., less compliant—TLC is decreased. If the lungs become less stiff (more compliant), TLC is increased. If the inspiratory muscles are significantly weakened, they are less able to overcome the inward elastic recoil of the lungs, and TLC is lowered.

At RV, the force exerted by the expiratory muscles to decrease lung volume further is balanced by the outward recoil of the chest wall, which becomes extremely stiff at low lung volumes. Two factors influence the volume of gas contained in the lungs at RV. The first is the ability of the subject to exert a prolonged expiratory effort, which is related to muscle strength and the ability to overcome sensory stimuli from the chest wall. The second is the ability of the lungs to empty to a small volume. In normal lungs, as P_{TP} is lowered, lung volume decreases. In lungs with diseased airways, as P_{TP} is lowered, flow limitation or airway closure may limit the amount of gas that can be expired. Consequently, either weak expiratory muscles or intrinsic airways disease can result in an elevation in measured RV.

Dynamic measurements of ventilatory function are made by having the subject inhale to TLC and then perform a forced expiration to RV. If a subject performs a series of such expiratory maneuvers using increasing muscular intensity, expiratory flow rates will increase until a certain level of effort is reached. Beyond this level, additional effort at any given lung volume will not increase the forced expiratory flow rate; this phenomenon is known as the *effort independence* of forced expiratory flow. The physiologic mechanisms determining the flow rates during this effort-independent phase of FEF have been shown to

FIGURE 250-2 Spirographic tracings of forced expiration, comparing a normal tracing *(A)* and tracings in obstructive *(B)* and parenchymal restrictive *(C)* disease. Calculations of FVC, FEV$_1$, and FEF$_{25-75\%}$ are shown only for the normal tracing. Since there is no measure of absolute starting volume with spirometry, the curves are artificially positioned to show the relative starting lung volumes in the different conditions.

be the elastic recoil of the lung, the airflow resistance of the airways between the alveolar zone and the physical site of flow limitation, and the airway wall compliance at the site of flow limitation. Physical processes that decrease elastic recoil, increase airflow resistance, or increase airway wall compliance decrease the flow rate that can be achieved at any given lung volume. Conversely, processes that increase elastic recoil, decrease resistance, or stiffen airway walls increase the flow rate that can be achieved at any given lung volume.

MEASUREMENT OF VENTILATORY FUNCTION

Ventilatory function is measured under static conditions for determination of lung volumes and under dynamic conditions for determination of forced expiratory flow rates. VC, expiratory reserve volume (ERV), and inspiratory capacity (IC) (Fig. 250-1) are measured by having the patient breathe into and out of a spirometer, a device capable of measuring expired or inspired gas volume while plotting volume as a function of time. Other volumes—specifically, RV, FRC, and TLC —cannot be measured in this way because they include the volume of gas present in the lungs even after a maximal expiration. Two techniques are commonly used to measure these volumes: helium dilution and body plethysmography. In the helium dilution method, the subject repeatedly breathes in and out from a reservoir with a known volume of gas containing a trace amount of helium. The helium is diluted by the gas previously present in the lungs and very little is absorbed into the pulmonary circulation. From knowledge of the reservoir volume and the initial and final helium concentrations, the volume of gas present in the lungs can be calculated. The helium dilution method may underestimate the volume of gas in the lungs if there are slowly communicating airspaces, such as bullae. In this situation, lung volumes can be measured more accurately with a body plethysmograph, a sealed box in which the patient sits while panting against a closed mouthpiece. Because there is no airflow into or out of the plethysmograph, the pressure changes in the thorax during panting cause compression and rarefaction of gas in the lungs and simultaneous rarefaction and compression of gas in the plethysmograph. By measuring the pressure changes in the plethysmograph and at the mouthpiece, the volume of gas in the thorax can be calculated using Boyle's law.

Lung volumes and measurements made during forced expiration are interpreted by comparing the values measured with the values expected given the age, height, sex, and race of the patient (Appendix A). Regression curves have been constructed on the basis of data obtained from large numbers of normal, nonsmoking individuals without evidence of lung disease. Predicted values for a given patient can then be obtained by using the patient's age and height in the appropriate regression equation; different equations are used depending on the patient's race and gender. Because there is some variability among normal individuals, values between 80 and 120% of the predicted value have traditionally been considered normal. Increasingly, calculated percentiles are used in determining normality. Specifically, values of individual measurements falling below the fifth percentile are considered to be below normal.

The normal value for the ratio FEV_1/FVC is approximately 0.75 to 0.80, although this value does fall somewhat with advancing age. The $FEF_{25-75\%}$ is often considered a more sensitive measurement of early airflow obstruction, particularly in small airways. However, this measurement must be interpreted cautiously in patients with abnormally small lungs (low TLC and VC). These patients exhale less air during forced expiration, and the $FEF_{25-75\%}$ may appear abnormal relative to the usual predicted value, even though it is normal relative to the size of the patient's lungs.

It is also a common practice to plot expiratory flow rates against lung volume (rather than against time); the close linkage of flow rates to lung volumes produces a typical *flow-volume curve* (Fig. 250-4). In addition, the spirometric values mentioned above can be calculated from the flow-volume curve. Commonly, flow rates during a maximal inspiratory effort performed as rapidly as possible are plotted as well, making the flow-volume curve into a *flow-volume loop*. At TLC, be-

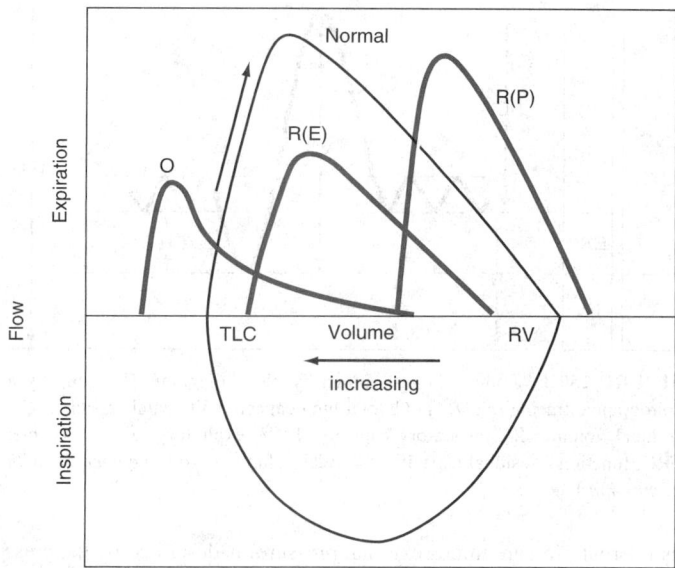

FIGURE 250-4 Flow-volume curves in different conditions: O, obstructive disease; R(P), parenchymal restrictive disease; R(E), extraparenchymal restrictive disease with limitation in inspiration and expiration. Forced expiration is plotted in all conditions; forced inspiration is shown only for the normal curve. TLC, total lung capacity; RV, residual volume. By convention, lung volume increases to the left on the abscissa. The arrow alongside the normal curve indicates the direction of expiration from TLC to RV.

fore expiratory flow starts, the flow rate is zero; once forced expiration has begun, a high peak flow rate is rapidly achieved. As expiration continues and lung volume approaches RV, the flow rate falls progressively, in a nearly linear fashion as a function of lung volume for a person with normal lung function. During maximal inspiration from RV to TLC, inspiratory flow is most rapid at the midpoint of inspiration, so the inspiratory portion of the loop is U-shaped or saddle-shaped. The flow rates achieved during maximal expiration can be analyzed quantitatively by comparing the flow rates at specified lung volumes with the predicted values or qualitatively by analyzing the shape of the descending limb of the expiratory curve.

Assessing the strength of respiratory muscles is an additional part of the overall evaluation of some patients with respiratory dysfunction. When a patient exhales completely to RV and then tries to inspire maximally against an occluded airway, the pressure that can be generated is called the *maximal inspiratory pressure* (MIP). On the other hand, when a patient inhales to TLC and then tries to expire maximally against an occluded airway, the pressure generated is called the *maximal expiratory pressure* (MEP). In the proper clinical setting, these studies may provide useful information regarding the cause of abnormal lung volumes and the possibility that respiratory muscle weakness may be causally related to the lung volume abnormalities.

PATTERNS OF ABNORMAL FUNCTION The two major patterns of abnormal ventilatory function, as measured by static lung volumes and spirometry, are restrictive and obstructive patterns. In the *obstructive pattern*, the hallmark is a decrease in expiratory flow rates. With fully established disease, the ratio FEV_1/FVC is decreased, as is the $FEF_{25-75\%}$ (Fig. 250-2, line *B*). The expiratory portion of the flow-volume loop demonstrates decreased flow rates for any given lung volume. Nonuniform emptying of airways is reflected by a coved (concave upward) configuration of the curve (Fig. 250-4). With early obstructive disease, which originates in the small airways, FEV_1/FVC may be normal; the only abnormalities noted on routine testing of pulmonary function may be a depression in $FEF_{25-75\%}$ and an abnormal, i.e., coved, configuration in the terminal portion of the forced expiratory flow-volume curve.

In *obstructive* disease, the TLC is normal or increased. When helium equilibration tests are used to measure lung volumes, the measured volume may be less than the actual volume if helium was not well distributed to all regions of the lung. Residual volume is elevated as a result of airway closure during expiration, and the ratio RV/TLC is increased. VC is frequently decreased in obstructive disease because of the striking elevations in RV with only minor changes in TLC.

A *restrictive pattern* can be broadly divided into two subgroups, depending on the location of the pathology: pulmonary parenchymal and extraparenchymal. For extraparenchymal disease, dysfunction can be predominantly in inspiration or in both inspiration and expiration (Table 250-1). The hallmark of a restrictive pattern, found in all these subcategories, is a decrease in lung volumes, primarily TLC and VC. In pulmonary parenchymal disease, RV is also generally decreased, and forced expiratory flow rates are preserved. In fact, when FEV$_1$ is considered as a percentage of the FVC, the flow rates are often supranormal, i.e., disproportionately high relative to the size of the lungs (Fig. 250-2, line *C*). The flow-volume curve may graphically demonstrate this disproportionate relationship between flow rates and lung volumes, since the expiratory portion of the curve appears relatively tall (preserved flow rates) but narrow (decreased lung volumes), as shown in Fig. 250-4.

In the extraparenchymal pattern characterized by *inspiratory dysfunction*, caused by either inspiratory muscle weakness or a stiff chest wall, inadequate distending forces are exerted on an otherwise normal lung. As a result, TLC values are less than predicted, RV is often not significantly affected, and expiratory flow rates are preserved. If inspiratory muscle weakness is the cause of this pattern, then MIP is decreased. In the extraparenchymal pattern characterized by *inspiratory and expiratory dysfunction*, the ability to expire to a normal RV is also limited, because of either expiratory muscle weakness or a deformed chest wall that is abnormally rigid at volumes below FRC. Consequently, RV is often elevated, unlike the pattern observed in the other restrictive subcategories. The ratio FEV$_1$/FVC is variable and depends on expiratory muscle strength. If expiratory muscle strength is significantly decreased, then MEP is decreased, the ability to expire rapidly is impaired, and FEV$_1$/FVC may be decreased even though there is no airflow obstruction. If expiratory muscle strength is normal but the chest wall is abnormally stiff below FRC, then FEV$_1$/FVC is normal or increased.

CLINICAL CORRELATIONS Table 250-1 summarizes the expected alterations in ventilatory function as indicated by pulmonary function testing. One reason to establish a ventilatory diagnosis is to categorize the functional disorder. This information can be useful in diagnosis, as outlined in Table 250-2. Note that lung disease such as pulmonary vascular disease or lung nodules can be present without abnormal ventilatory function, but the presence of specific diagnostic findings is an aid in differential diagnosis.

DISTURBANCES IN THE PULMONARY CIRCULATION

PHYSIOLOGIC FEATURES The pulmonary vasculature must handle the entire output of the right ventricle, approximately 5 L/min in a normal adult at rest. The comparatively thin-walled vessels of the pulmonary arterial system provide relatively little resistance to flow and are capable of handling this large volume of blood at perfusion pressures that are low compared with those of the systemic circulation. The normal mean pulmonary artery pressure is 15 mmHg, as compared to approximately 95 mmHg for the normal mean aortic pressure. Regional blood flow in the lung is dependent on hydrostatic forces. In an upright person, pulmonary arterial pressure (PAP) is lowest at the apex of the lung and highest at the lung base. As a result, in the upright position, perfusion is least at the apex and greatest at the base. When cardiac output increases, as occurs during exercise, the

Table 250-1 Alterations in Ventilatory Function

	TLC	RV	VC	FEV$_1$/FVC	MIP	MEP
Obstructive	N to ↑	↑	↓	↓ [a]	N	N
Restrictive						
Pulmonary parenchymal	↓	↓	↓	N to ↑	N	N
Extraparenchymal—inspiratory	↓	N to ↓	↓	N	↓/N[b]	N
Extraparenchymal—inspiratory + expiratory	↓	↑	↓	Variable	↓/N[b]	↓/N[b]

[a] Mild obstructive (small airways) disease may have decreased FEF$_{25-75\%}$ with normal FEV$_1$/FVC.
[b] Reduced if due to respiratory muscle weakness; normal if due to chest wall stiffness.
NOTE: N, normal; for other abbreviations, see text.

pulmonary vasculature is capable of recruiting previously unperfused vessels and distending underperfused vessels, thus responding to the increase in flow with a decrease in pulmonary vascular resistance. In consequence, the increase in mean PAP, even with a three- to fourfold increase in cardiac output, is small.

METHODS OF MEASUREMENT Assessment of circulatory function in the pulmonary vasculature depends on measuring pulmonary vascular pressures and cardiac output. Clinically, these measurements are commonly made in intensive care units capable of invasive monitoring and in cardiac catheterization laboratories. With a flow-directed pulmonary arterial (Swan-Ganz) catheter, PAP and pulmonary capillary wedge pressure can be measured directly, and cardiac output can be obtained by the thermodilution method. Pulmonary vascular resistance (PVR) can then be calculated according to the equation

$$PVR = 80(PAP - PCW)/CO$$

where PVR = pulmonary vascular resistance (dyn·s/cm^5); PAP = mean pulmonary arterial pressure (mmHg); PCW = pulmonary capillary wedge pressure (mmHg); and CO = cardiac output (L/min).

The normal value for pulmonary vascular resistance is approximately 50 to 150 dyn·s/cm^5.

MECHANISMS OF ABNORMAL FUNCTION (See also Chap. 260) PVR may increase by a variety of mechanisms. Pulmonary arterial and arteriolar vasoconstriction is a prominent response to alveolar hypoxia. PVR also increases if intraluminal thrombi or proliferation of smooth muscle in vessel walls diminishes the luminal cross-sectional area. If small pulmonary vessels are destroyed, either

Table 250-2 Common Respiratory Diseases by Diagnostic Categories

OBSTRUCTIVE

Asthma
Chronic obstructive lung disease (chronic bronchitis, emphysema)
Bronchiectasis
Cystic fibrosis
Bronchiolitis

RESTRICTIVE—PARENCHYMAL

Sarcoidosis
Idiopathic pulmonary fibrosis
Pneumoconiosis
Drug- or radiation-induced interstitial lung disease

RESTRICTIVE—EXTRAPARENCHYMAL

Neuromuscular
  Diaphragmatic weakness/paralysis
  Myasthenia gravis[a]
  Guillain-Barré syndrome[a]
  Muscular dystrophies[a]
  Cervical spine injury[a]
Chest wall
  Kyphoscoliosis
  Obesity
  Ankylosing spondylitis[a]

[a] Can have inspiratory and expiratory limitation (see text).

by scarring or by loss of alveolar walls, the total cross-sectional area of the pulmonary vascular bed diminishes, and PVR increases. When PVR is elevated, either PAP rises to maintain normal cardiac output or cardiac output falls if PAP does not increase.

CLINICAL CORRELATIONS   Disturbances in the function of the pulmonary vasculature as a result of primary cardiac disease, either congenital heart disease or conditions that elevate left atrial pressure, such as mitral stenosis, are beyond the scope of this chapter and are discussed in Chaps. 234 and 236, respectively. Instead, the focus will be on the pulmonary vasculature as its function is affected by diseases primarily involving the respiratory system, including the pulmonary vessels themselves.

All diseases of the respiratory system causing hypoxemia are potentially capable of increasing PVR, since alveolar hypoxia is a very potent stimulus for pulmonary vasoconstriction. The more prolonged and intense the hypoxic stimulus, the more likely it is that a significant increase in PVR producing pulmonary hypertension will result. In practice, patients with hypoxemia caused by chronic obstructive lung disease, interstitial lung disease, chest wall disease, and the obesity hypoventilation–sleep apnea syndrome are particularly prone to developing pulmonary hypertension. If there are additional structural changes in the pulmonary vasculature secondary to the underlying process, these will increase the likelihood of developing pulmonary hypertension.

With diseases directly affecting the pulmonary vessels, a decrease in the cross-sectional area of the pulmonary vascular bed is primarily responsible for increased PVR, while hypoxemia generally plays a lesser role. In the case of recurrent pulmonary emboli, parts of the pulmonary arterial system are occluded by intraluminal thrombi originating in the systemic venous system. With primary pulmonary hypertension (Chap. 260) or with pulmonary vascular disease secondary to scleroderma, the small pulmonary arteries and arterioles are affected by a generalized obliterative process that narrows and occludes these vessels. PVR increases, and significant pulmonary hypertension often results.

DISTURBANCES IN GAS EXCHANGE

PHYSIOLOGIC FEATURES   The primary functions of the respiratory system are to remove the appropriate amount of CO_2 from blood entering the pulmonary circulation and to provide adequate O_2 to blood leaving the pulmonary circulation. For these functions to be carried out properly, there must be adequate provision of fresh air to the alveoli for delivery of O_2 and removal of CO_2 (ventilation), adequate circulation of blood through the pulmonary vasculature (perfusion), adequate movement of gas between alveoli and pulmonary capillaries (diffusion), and appropriate contact between alveolar gas and pulmonary capillary blood (ventilation-perfusion matching).

A normal individual at rest inspires approximately 12 to 16 times per minute, each breath having a tidal volume of approximately 500 mL. A portion (approximately 30%) of the fresh air inspired with each breath does not reach the alveoli but remains in the conducting airways of the lung. This component of each breath, which is not generally available for gas exchange, is called the *anatomic dead space component*. The remaining 70% reaches the alveolar zone, mixes rapidly with the gas already there, and can participate in gas exchange. In this example, the total ventilation each minute is approximately 7 L, composed of 2 L/min of dead space ventilation and 5 L/min of alveolar ventilation. In certain diseases, some alveoli are ventilated but not perfused, so that some ventilation in addition to the anatomic dead space component is wasted. If total dead space ventilation is increased but total minute ventilation is unchanged, then alveolar ventilation must fall correspondingly.

Gas exchange is dependent on alveolar ventilation rather than total minute ventilation, as outlined below. The partial pressure of CO_2 in arterial blood (Pa_{CO_2}) is directly proportional to the amount of CO_2

produced per minute ($\dot{V}_{CO_2}$) and inversely proportional to alveolar ventilation ($\dot{V}A$), according to the relationship

$$Pa_{CO_2} = 0.863 \times \dot{V}_{CO_2}/\dot{V}A$$

where $\dot{V}_{CO_2}$ is expressed in mL/min, $\dot{V}A$ in L/min, and Pa_{CO_2} in mmHg. At fixed $\dot{V}_{CO_2}$, when alveolar ventilation increases, Pa_{CO_2} falls, and when alveolar ventilation decreases, Pa_{CO_2} rises. Maintaining a normal level of O_2 in the alveoli (and consequently in arterial blood) also depends on provision of adequate alveolar ventilation to replenish alveolar O_2. This principle will become more apparent from consideration of the alveolar gas equation below.

Diffusion of O_2 and CO_2   Both O_2 and CO_2 diffuse readily down their respective concentration gradients through the alveolar wall and pulmonary capillary endothelium. Under normal circumstances, this process is rapid, and equilibration of both gases is complete within one-third of the transit time of erythrocytes through the pulmonary capillary bed. Even in disease states in which diffusion of gases is impaired, the impairment is unlikely to be severe enough to prevent equilibration of CO_2 and O_2. Consequently, a diffusion abnormality rarely results in arterial hypoxemia at rest. If erythrocyte transit time in the pulmonary circulation is shortened, as occurs with exercise, and diffusion is impaired, then diffusion limitation may contribute to hypoxemia. Exercise testing can often demonstrate such physiologically significant abnormalities due to impaired diffusion. Even though diffusion limitation rarely makes a clinically significant contribution to resting hypoxemia, clinical measurements of what is known as *diffusing capacity* (see below) can be a useful measure of the integrity of the alveolar-capillary membrane.

Ventilation-Perfusion Matching   In addition to the absolute levels of alveolar ventilation and perfusion, gas exchange depends critically on the proper matching of ventilation and perfusion. The spectrum of possible ventilation-perfusion ($\dot{V}/\dot{Q}$) ratios in an alveolar-capillary unit ranges from zero, in which ventilation is totally absent and the unit behaves as a shunt, to infinity, in which perfusion is totally absent and the unit behaves as dead space. The P_{O_2} and P_{CO_2} of blood leaving each alveolar-capillary unit depend on the gas tension (of blood and air) entering that unit and on the particular $\dot{V}/\dot{Q}$ ratio of the unit. At one extreme, when an alveolar-capillary unit has a $\dot{V}/\dot{Q}$ ratio of 0 and behaves as a shunt, blood leaving the unit has the composition of mixed venous blood entering the pulmonary capillaries, i.e., $P\bar{v}_{O_2} \approx 40$ mmHg and $P\bar{v}_{CO_2} \approx 46$ mmHg. At the other extreme, when an alveolar-capillary unit has a high $\dot{V}/\dot{Q}$ ratio, it behaves almost like dead space, and the small amount of blood leaving the unit has partial pressures of O_2 and CO_2 ($P_{O_2} \approx 150$ mmHg, $P_{CO_2} \approx 0$ mmHg while breathing room air) approaching the composition of inspired gas.

In the ideal situation, all alveolar-capillary units have equal matching of ventilation and perfusion, i.e., a ratio of approximately 1 when each is expressed in L/min. However, even in the normal individual, some $\dot{V}/\dot{Q}$ mismatching is present, since there is normally a gradient of blood flow from the apices to the bases of the lungs. There is a similar gradient of ventilation from the apices to the bases, but it is less marked than the perfusion gradient. As a result, ventilation-perfusion ratios are higher at the lung apices than at the lung bases. Therefore, blood coming from the apices has a higher P_{O_2} and lower P_{CO_2} than blood coming from the bases. The net P_{O_2} and P_{CO_2} of the blood mixture coming from all areas of the lung is a flow-weighted average of the individual components, which reflects both the relative amount of blood from each unit and the O_2 and CO_2 *content* of the blood coming from each unit. Because of the sigmoid shape of the oxyhemoglobin dissociation curve (see Fig. 106-2), it is important to distinguish between the partial pressure and the content of O_2 in blood. Hemoglobin is almost fully (~90%) saturated at a P_{O_2} of 60 mmHg, and little additional O_2 is carried by hemoglobin even with a substantial elevation of P_{O_2} above 60 mmHg. On the other hand, significant O_2 desaturation of hemoglobin occurs once P_{O_2} falls below 60 mmHg and onto the steep descending limb of the curve. As a result, blood

P_{O_2} has only a small elevation in O_2 content and cannot compensate for blood coming from regions with a low $\dot{V}/\dot{Q}$ ratio and a low P_{O_2}, which has a significantly decreased O_2 content. Although $\dot{V}/\dot{Q}$ mismatching can influence P_{CO_2}, this effect is less marked and is often overcome by an increase in overall minute ventilation.

MEASUREMENT OF GAS EXCHANGE **Arterial Blood Gases** The most commonly used measures of gas exchange are the partial pressures of O_2 and CO_2 in arterial blood, i.e., Pa_{O_2} and Pa_{CO_2}, respectively. These partial pressures do not measure directly the quantity of O_2 and CO_2 in blood but rather the driving pressure for the gas in blood. The actual quantity or content of a gas in blood also depends on the solubility of the gas in plasma and the ability of any component of blood to react with or bind the gas of interest. Since hemoglobin is capable of binding large amounts of O_2, oxygenated hemoglobin is the primary form in which O_2 is transported in blood. The actual content of O_2 in blood therefore depends both on the hemoglobin concentration and on the Pa_{O_2}. The Pa_{O_2} determines what percentage of hemoglobin is saturated with O_2, based on the position on the oxyhemoglobin dissociation curve. Oxygen content in normal blood (at 37°C, pH 7.4) can be determined by adding the amount of O_2 dissolved in plasma to the amount bound to hemoglobin, according to the equation

$$O_2 \text{ content} = 1.34 \times [\text{hemoglobin}] \times \text{saturation} + 0.0031 \times P_{O_2}$$

since each gram of hemoglobin is capable of carrying 1.34 mL O_2 when fully saturated, and the amount of O_2 that can be dissolved in plasma is proportional to the P_{O_2}, with 0.0031 mL O_2 dissolved per deciliter of blood per mmHg P_{O_2}. In arterial blood, the amount of O_2 transported dissolved in plasma (approximately 0.3 mL O_2 per deciliter of blood) is trivial compared with the amount bound to hemoglobin (approximately 20 mL O_2 per deciliter of blood).

Most commonly, P_{O_2} is the measurement used to assess the effect of respiratory disease on the oxygenation of arterial blood. Direct measurement of O_2 saturation in arterial blood by oximetry is also important in selected clinical conditions. For example, in patients with carbon monoxide intoxication, carbon monoxide preferentially displaces O_2 from hemoglobin, essentially making a portion of hemoglobin unavailable for binding to O_2. In this circumstance, carbon monoxide saturation is high and O_2 saturation is low, even though the driving pressure for O_2 to bind to hemoglobin, reflected by P_{O_2}, is normal. Measurement of O_2 saturation is also important for the determination of O_2 content when mixed venous blood is sampled from a pulmonary arterial catheter to calculate cardiac output by the Fick technique. In mixed venous blood, the P_{O_2} is normally about 40 mmHg, but small changes in P_{O_2} may reflect relatively large changes in O_2 saturation.

A useful calculation in the assessment of oxygenation is the alveolar-arterial O_2 difference ($PA_{O_2} - Pa_{O_2}$), commonly called the *alveolar-arterial O_2 gradient* (or A − a gradient). This calculation takes into account the fact that alveolar and, hence, arterial P_{O_2} can be expected to change depending on the level of alveolar ventilation, reflected by the arterial P_{CO_2}. When a patient hyperventilates and has a low P_{CO_2} in arterial blood and alveolar gas, alveolar and arterial P_{O_2} will rise; conversely, hypoventilation and a high P_{CO_2} are accompanied by a decrease in alveolar and arterial P_{O_2}. These changes in arterial P_{O_2} are independent of abnormalities in O_2 transfer at the alveolar-capillary level and reflect only the dependence of alveolar P_{O_2} on the level of alveolar ventilation.

In order to determine the alveolar-arterial O_2 difference, the alveolar P_{O_2} (PA_{O_2}) must first be calculated. The equation most commonly used for this purpose, a simplified form of the alveolar gas equation, is

$$PA_{O_2} = FI_{O_2} \times (P_B - P_{H_2O}) - Pa_{CO_2}/R$$

where FI_{O_2} = fractional concentration of inspired O_2 (≈ 0.21 when breathing room air); P_B = barometric pressure (approximately 760

mmHg at sea level); P_{H_2O} = water vapor pressure (47 mmHg when air is fully saturated at 37°C); and R = respiratory quotient (the ratio of CO_2 production to O_2 consumption, usually assumed to be 0.8). If the preceding values are substituted into the equation for the patient breathing air at sea level, the equation becomes

$$PA_{O_2} = 150 - 1.25 \times Pa_{CO_2}$$

The alveolar-arterial O_2 difference can then be calculated by subtracting measured Pa_{O_2} from calculated PA_{O_2}. In a healthy young person breathing room air, the $PA_{O_2} - Pa_{O_2}$ is normally less than 15 mmHg; this value increases with age and may be as high as 30 mmHg in elderly patients.

The adequacy of CO_2 elimination is measured by the partial pressure of CO_2 in arterial blood, i.e., Pa_{CO_2}. A more complete understanding of the mechanisms and chronicity of abnormal levels of P_{CO_2} also requires measurement of pH and/or bicarbonate (HCO_3^-), since P_{CO_2} and the patient's acid-base status are so closely intertwined (Chap. 50).

Pulse Oximetry Because measurement of Pa_{O_2} requires arterial puncture, it is not ideal either for office use or for routine or frequent measurement in the inpatient setting. Additionally, because it provides intermittent rather than continuous data about the patient's oxygenation, it is not ideal for close monitoring of unstable patients. Pulse oximetry, an alternative method for assessing oxygenation, is readily available in many clinical settings. Using a probe usually clipped over a patient's finger, the pulse oximeter calculates oxygen saturation (rather than Pa_{O_2}) based on measurements of absorption of two wavelengths of light by hemoglobin in pulsatile, cutaneous arterial blood. Because of differential absorption of the two wavelengths of light by oxygenated and nonoxygenated hemoglobin, the percentage of hemoglobin that is saturated with oxygen, i.e., the Sa_{O_2}, can be calculated and displayed instantaneously.

Although the pulse oximeter has been a major advance in the noninvasive, continuous monitoring of oxygenation, there are several issues and potential problems concerning its use. First, the clinician must be aware of the relationship between oxygen saturation and tension as shown by the oxyhemoglobin dissociation curve (Fig. 106-2). Because the curve becomes relatively flat above an arterial P_{O_2} of 60 mmHg (corresponding to Sa_{O_2} = 90%), the oximeter is relatively insensitive to changes in Pa_{O_2} above this level. In addition, the position of the curve and therefore the specific relationship between Pa_{O_2} and Sa_{O_2} may change depending on factors such as temperature, pH, and the erythrocyte concentration of 2,3-diphosphoglycerate. Second, when cutaneous perfusion is decreased, e.g., owing to low cardiac output or the use of vasoconstrictors, the signal from the oximeter may be less reliable or even unobtainable. Third, other forms of hemoglobin, such as carboxyhemoglobin and methemoglobin, are not distinguishable from oxyhemoglobin when only two wavelengths of light are used. The Sa_{O_2} values reported by the pulse oximeter are not reliable in the presence of significant amounts of either of these forms of hemoglobin. In contrast, the device used to measure oxygen saturation in samples of arterial blood, called the CO-oximeter, uses at least four wavelengths of light and is capable of distinguishing oxyhemoglobin, deoxygenated hemoglobin, carboxyhemoglobin, and methemoglobin. Finally, the clinician must remember that the often-used goal of $Sa_{O_2} \geq$ 90% does not indicate anything about CO_2 elimination and therefore does not ensure a clinically acceptable P_{CO_2}.

Diffusing Capacity The ability of gas to diffuse across the alveolar-capillary membrane is ordinarily assessed by the diffusing capacity of the lung for carbon monoxide (DL_{CO}). In this test, a small concentration of carbon monoxide (0.3%) is inhaled, usually in a single breath that is held for approximately 10 s. The carbon monoxide is diluted by the gas already present in the alveoli and is also taken up by hemoglobin as the erythrocytes course through the pulmonary capillary system. The concentration of carbon monoxide in exhaled gas is measured, and DL_{CO} is calculated as the quantity of carbon monoxide absorbed per minute per mmHg pressure gradient from the alveoli to the pulmonary capillaries. The value obtained for DL_{CO} depends on the alveolar-capillary surface area available for gas exchange and on the pulmonary capillary blood volume. In addition, the thickness of the alveolar-capillary membrane, the degree of $\dot{V}/\dot{Q}$ mismatching, and the patient's hemoglobin level will affect the measurement. Because of this effect of hemoglobin levels on DL_{CO}, the measured DL_{CO} is frequently corrected to take the patient's hemoglobin level into account. The value for DL_{CO}, ideally corrected for hemoglobin, can then be compared with a predicted value, based either on age, height, and gender or on the alveolar volume (V_A) at which the value was obtained. Alternatively, the DL_{CO} can be divided by V_A and the resulting value for DL_{CO}/V_A compared with a predicted value.

Approach to the Patient

Arterial Blood Gases   Hypoxemia is a common manifestation of a variety of diseases affecting the lungs or other parts of the respiratory system. The broad clinical problem of hypoxemia is often best characterized according to the underlying mechanism. The four basic, and not mutually exclusive, mechanisms of hypoxemia are (1) a decrease in inspired P_{O_2}, (2) hypoventilation, (3) shunting, and (4) $\dot{V}/\dot{Q}$ mismatching. Hypoxemia due to decreased diffusion occurs only under selected clinical circumstances and is not usually included among the general categories of hypoxemia. Determining the underlying mechanism for hypoxemia depends on measurement of the Pa_{CO_2}, calculation of $PA_{O_2} - Pa_{O_2}$, and knowledge of the response to supplemental O_2. A flowchart summarizing the approach to the hypoxemic patient is given in Fig. 250-5.

A decrease in the inspired P_{O_2} and hypoventilation both cause hypoxemia by lowering PA_{O_2} and therefore Pa_{O_2}. In each case, gas exchange at the alveolar-capillary level occurs normally, and $PA_{O_2} - Pa_{O_2}$ is not elevated. Hypoxemia due to decreased inspired P_{O_2} can be diagnosed from knowledge of the clinical situation. Inspired P_{O_2} is lowered either because the patient is at a high altitude, where barometric pressure is low, or, much less commonly, because the patient is breathing a gas mixture containing less than 21% O_2. The hallmark

of hypoventilation as a cause of hypoxemia is an elevation in Pa_{CO_2}. This is associated with an increase in PA_{CO_2} and a fall in PA_{O_2}. When hypoxemia is due purely to a low inspired P_{O_2} or to alveolar hypoventilation, $PA_{O_2} - Pa_{O_2}$ is normal. If $PA_{O_2} - Pa_{O_2}$ and Pa_{CO_2} are both elevated, then an additional mechanism, such as $\dot{V}/\dot{Q}$ mismatching or shunting, is contributing to hypoxemia.

Shunting is a cause of hypoxemia when desaturated blood effectively bypasses oxygenation at the alveolar-capillary level. This situation occurs either because a structural problem allows desaturated blood to bypass the normal site of gas exchange or because perfused alveoli are not ventilated. Shunting is associated with an elevation in the $PA_{O_2} - Pa_{O_2}$ value. When shunting is an important contributing factor to hypoxemia, the lowered Pa_{O_2} is relatively refractory to improvement by supplemental O_2.

Finally, the largest clinical category of hypoxemia is $\dot{V}/\dot{Q}$ mismatching. With $\dot{V}/\dot{Q}$ mismatching, regions with low $\dot{V}/\dot{Q}$ ratios contribute blood with a low P_{O_2} and a low O_2 content. Corresponding regions with high $\dot{V}/\dot{Q}$ ratios contribute blood with a high P_{O_2}. However, because blood is already almost fully saturated at a normal P_{O_2}, elevation of the P_{O_2} to a high value does not significantly increase O_2 saturation or content and therefore cannot compensate for the reduction of O_2 saturation and content in blood coming from regions with a low $\dot{V}/\dot{Q}$ ratio. When $\dot{V}/\dot{Q}$ mismatch is the primary cause of hypoxemia, $PA_{O_2} - Pa_{O_2}$ is elevated, and P_{CO_2} generally is normal. Supplemental O_2 corrects the hypoxemia by raising the P_{O_2} in blood coming from regions with a low $\dot{V}/\dot{Q}$ ratio; this response distinguishes hypoxemia due to $\dot{V}/\dot{Q}$ mismatching from that due to true shunt.

The essential mechanism underlying all cases of hypercapnia is alveolar ventilation that is inadequate for the amount of CO_2 produced. It is conceptually useful to characterize CO_2 retention further, based on a more detailed examination of the potential contributing factors. These include (1) increased CO_2 production; (2) decreased ventilatory drive ("won't breathe"); (3) malfunction of the respiratory pump or increased airways resistance, which makes it more difficult to sustain adequate ventilation ("can't breathe"); and (4) inefficiency of gas exchange (increased dead space or $\dot{V}/\dot{Q}$ mismatch) necessitating a compensatory increase in overall minute ventilation. In practice, more than one of these mechanisms is commonly responsible for hypercapnia, since increased minute ventilation is capable of compensating for increased CO_2 production and for inefficiencies of gas exchange.

FIGURE 250-5   Flow diagram outlining the diagnostic approach to the patient with hypoxemia ($Pa_{O_2} < 80$ mmHg). $PA_{O_2} - Pa_{O_2}$ is usually < 15 mmHg for subjects ≤ 30 years old and increases by ~ 3 mmHg per decade after age 30.

Diffusing Capacity Although abnormalities in diffusion are rarely responsible for hypoxemia, clinical measurement of diffusing capacity is frequently used to assess the functional integrity of the alveolar-capillary membrane, which includes the pulmonary capillary bed. Diseases that affect solely the airways generally do not lower DL_{CO}, whereas diseases that affect the alveolar walls or the pulmonary capillary bed will have an effect on DL_{CO}. Even though DL_{CO} is a useful marker for assessing whether disease affecting the alveolar-capillary bed is present, an abnormal DL_{CO} does not necessarily imply that diffusion limitation is responsible for hypoxemia in a particular patient.

CLINICAL CORRELATIONS Useful clinical correlations can be made with the mechanisms underlying hypoxemia (Fig. 250-5). A lowered inspired P_{O_2} contributes to hypoxemia if either the patient is at high altitude or if the concentration of inspired O_2 is less than 21%. The latter problem occurs if a patient receiving anesthesia or ventilatory support is inadvertently given a gas mixture to breathe containing less than 21% O_2 or if O_2 is consumed from the ambient gas, as can occur during smoke inhalation from a fire. The primary feature of hypoventilation as a cause of hypoxemia is an elevation in arterial P_{CO_2}. →*For further discussion of the clinical correlations with hypoventilation, see Chap. 263.*

Shunting as a cause of hypoxemia can reflect transfer of blood from the right to the left side of the heart without passage through the pulmonary circulation, as occurs with an intracardiac shunt. This problem is most common in the setting of cyanotic congenital heart disease, when an interatrial or interventricular septal defect is associated with pulmonary hypertension so that shunting is in the right-to-left rather than the left-to-right direction. Shunting of blood through the pulmonary parenchyma is most frequently due to disease causing absence of ventilation to perfused alveoli. This can occur if the alveoli are atelectatic or if they are filled with fluid, as in pulmonary edema (both cardiogenic and noncardiogenic), or with extensive intraalveolar exudation of fluid due to pneumonia. Less commonly, vascular anomalies with arteriovenous shunting in the lung can cause hypoxemia. These anomalies can be hereditary, as found with hereditary hemorrhagic telangiectasia (Osler-Rendu-Weber syndrome), or acquired, as in pulmonary vascular malformations secondary to hepatic cirrhosis, which are similar to the commonly recognized cutaneous vascular malformations ("spider hemangiomas").

Ventilation-perfusion mismatch is the most common cause of hypoxemia clinically. Most of the processes affecting either the airways or the pulmonary parenchyma are distributed unevenly throughout the lungs and do not necessarily affect ventilation and perfusion equally. Some areas of lung may have good perfusion and poor ventilation, whereas others may have poor perfusion and relatively good ventilation. Important examples of airways diseases in which $\dot{V}/\dot{Q}$ mismatch causes hypoxemia are asthma and chronic obstructive lung disease. Parenchymal lung diseases causing $\dot{V}/\dot{Q}$ mismatch and hypoxemia include interstitial lung disease and pneumonia.

Clinically important alterations in CO_2 elimination range from excessive ventilation and hypocapnia to inadequate CO_2 elimination and hypercapnia. →*For further discussion of these clinical problems, see Chap. 263.*

Diffusing Capacity Measurement of DL_{CO} may be useful for assessing disease affecting the alveolar-capillary bed or the pulmonary vasculature. In practice, three main categories of disease are associated with lowered DL_{CO}: interstitial lung disease, emphysema, and pulmonary vascular disease. With interstitial lung disease, scarring of alveolar-capillary units diminishes the area of the alveolar-capillary bed as well as pulmonary blood volume. With emphysema, alveolar walls are destroyed, so the surface area of the alveolar-capillary bed is again diminished. In patients with disease causing a decrease in the cross-sectional area and volume of the pulmonary vascular bed, such as recurrent pulmonary emboli or primary pulmonary hypertension, DL_{CO} is commonly diminished.

Diffusing capacity may be elevated if pulmonary blood volume is increased, as may be seen in congestive heart failure. However, once interstitial and alveolar edema ensue, the net DL_{CO} depends on the opposing influences of increased pulmonary capillary blood volume elevating DL_{CO} and pulmonary edema decreasing it. Finding an elevated DL_{CO} may be useful in the diagnosis of alveolar hemorrhage, as in Goodpasture's syndrome. Hemoglobin contained in erythrocytes in the alveolar lumen is capable of binding carbon monoxide, so the exhaled carbon monoxide concentration is diminished and the measured DL_{CO} is increased.

BIBLIOGRAPHY

AMERICAN THORACIC SOCIETY: Lung function testing: Selection of reference values and interpretive strategies. Am Rev Respir Dis 144:1202, 1991

CELLI BR: The importance of spirometry in COPD and asthma: effect on approach to management. Chest 117:15S, 2000

CRAPO RO: Pulmonary-function testing. N Engl J Med 331:25, 1994

———, FORSTER RE II: Carbon monoxide diffusing capacity. Clin Chest Med 10:187, 1989

LEVITZKY MG: Pulmonary Physiology, 5th ed. New York, McGraw-Hill, 1999

QUANJER PH et al: Lung volumes and forced ventilatory flows. Report Working Party Standardization of Lung Function Tests, European Community for Steel and Coal. Official Statement of the European Respiratory Society. Eur Respir J [Suppl] 16:5, 1993

SHAPIRO BA et al: *Clinical Application of Blood Gases*, 5th ed. St. Louis, Mosby, 1994

SOCIETY OF CRITICAL CARE MEDICINE: A model for technology assessment applied to pulse oximetry. Crit Care Med 21:615, 1993

WEINBERGER SE: *Principles of Pulmonary Medicine*, 3d ed. Philadelphia, Saunders, 1998

WEST JB, WAGNER PD: Pulmonary gas exchange. Am J Respir Crit Care Med 157 (Pt 2): S82, 1998

---

251   *Steven E. Weinberger, Jeffrey M. Drazen*

DIAGNOSTIC PROCEDURES IN RESPIRATORY DISEASE

The diagnostic modalities available for assessing the patient with suspected or known respiratory system disease include imaging studies and techniques for acquiring biologic specimens, some of which involve direct visualization of part of the respiratory system. →*Methods used to characterize the functional changes developing as a result of disease, including pulmonary function tests and measurements of gas exchange, are discussed in Chap. 250.*

IMAGING STUDIES

ROUTINE RADIOGRAPHY Routine chest radiography, which generally includes both posteroanterior and lateral views, is an integral part of the diagnostic evaluation of diseases involving the pulmonary parenchyma, the pleura, and, to a lesser extent, the airways and the mediastinum (see Figs. 249-1 and 249-2). Lateral decubitus views are often useful for determining whether pleural abnormalities represent freely flowing fluid, whereas apical lordotic views can often visualize disease at the lung apices better than the standard posteroanterior view. Portable equipment, which is often used for acutely ill patients who either cannot be transported to a radiology suite or cannot stand up for posteroanterior and lateral views, generally yields just a single radiograph taken in the anteroposterior direction. →*Common radiographic patterns and their clinical correlates are reviewed in Chap. 249.*

COMPUTED TOMOGRAPHY Computed tomography (CT) offers several advantages over routine chest radiography. First, the use of cross-sectional images often makes it possible to distinguish between densities that would be superimposed on plain radiographs. Second, CT is far better than routine radiographic studies at characterizing tissue density, distinguishing subtle differences in density between adjacent structures, and providing accurate size assessment of lesions. As a result, CT is particularly valuable in assessing hilar and mediastinal disease (which is often poorly characterized by plain radiography), in identifying and characterizing disease adjacent to the chest wall or spine (including pleural disease), and in identifying areas of fat density or calcification in pulmonary nodules (Fig. 251-1). Its utility in the assessment of mediastinal disease has made CT an important tool in the staging of lung cancer (Chap. 88), as an assessment of tumor involvement of mediastinal lymph nodes is critical to proper staging. With the additional use of contrast material, CT also makes it possible to distinguish vascular from nonvascular structures, which is particularly important in distinguishing lymph nodes and masses from vascular structures.

Helical CT scanning allows the collection of continuous data over a larger volume of lung during a single breath-holding maneuver than is possible with conventional CT. With CT angiography, in which intravenous contrast is administered and images are acquired rapidly by helical scanning, pulmonary emboli can be detected in segmental and larger pulmonary arteries. With high-resolution CT (HRCT), the thickness of individual cross-sectional images is approximately 1 to 2 mm, rather than the usual 10 mm, and the images are reconstructed with high-spatial-resolution algorithms. The detail that can be seen on HRCT scans allows better recognition of subtle parenchymal and airway disease, such as bronchiectasis, emphysema, and diffuse parenchymal disease (Fig. 251-2). Certain nearly pathognomonic patterns have now been recognized for many of the interstitial lung diseases, such as lymphangitic carcinoma, idiopathic pulmonary fibrosis, sarcoidosis, and eosinophilic granuloma; at present it is not yet clear in what settings these patterns will obviate the need for obtaining lung tissue.

MAGNETIC RESONANCE IMAGING   The role of magnetic resonance imaging (MRI) in the evaluation of respiratory system disease is less well defined than that of CT. Because MRI generally provides a less detailed view of the pulmonary parenchyma as well as poorer spatial resolution, its usefulness in the evaluation of parenchymal lung disease is limited at present. However, MRI has advantages over CT in certain clinical settings. Because its images can be reconstructed in sagittal and coronal as well as transverse planes, MRI may be better for imaging abnormalities near the lung apex, the spine, and the thoracoabdominal junction. In addition, vascular structures can be distinguished from nonvascular structures without the need for contrast. Flowing blood does not produce a signal on MRI, so

FIGURE 251-1   CT scan demonstrating a mediastinal mass of heterogeneous density. CT is superior to plain radiography for the detection of abnormal mediastinal densities and the distinction of masses from adjacent vascular structures.

FIGURE 251-2   High-resolution CT scan demonstrating pulmonary parenchyma with a heterogeneous appearance. Most of the parenchyma has a subtle "ground-glass" pattern of increased density, best recognized by comparison with the intervening areas of normal lung, which have irregular but well-defined borders. The ground-glass pattern in this patient was due to hypersensitivity pneumonitis. *(From Weinberger, with permission.)*

vessels appear as hollow tubular structures. This feature can be useful in determining whether abnormal hilar or mediastinal densities are vascular in origin and in defining aortic lesions such as aneurysms or dissection.

SCINTIGRAPHIC IMAGING   Radioactive isotopes, administered by either intravenous or inhaled routes, allow the lungs to be imaged with a gamma camera. The most common use of such imaging is ventilation-perfusion lung scanning performed for evaluation of pulmonary embolism. When injected intravenously, albumin macroaggregates labeled with technetium 99m become lodged in pulmonary capillaries; therefore, the distribution of the trapped radioisotope follows the distribution of blood flow. When inhaled, radiolabeled xenon gas can be used to demonstrate the distribution of ventilation. For example, pulmonary thromboembolism usually produces one or more regions of ventilation-perfusion mismatch—that is, regions in which there is a defect in perfusion that follows the distribution of a vessel and that is not accompanied by a corresponding defect in ventilation (Chap. 261). Another common use of such radioisotope scans is in a patient with impaired lung function who is being considered for lung resection. The distribution of the isotope(s) can be used to assess the regional distribution of blood flow and ventilation, allowing the physician to estimate the level of postoperative lung function.

Another scintigraphic imaging technique, gallium imaging, has been of diagnostic value in patients with *Pneumocystis carinii* pneumonia and other opportunistic infections. Use of gallium imaging may provide clues to sort out the differential diagnosis of pulmonary infiltrates in immunosuppressed patients, especially patients with AIDS.

PULMONARY ANGIOGRAPHY   The pulmonary arterial system can be visualized by pulmonary angiography, in which radiopaque contrast medium is injected through a catheter previously threaded into the pulmonary artery. When performed in cases of pulmonary embolism, pulmonary angiography demonstrates the consequences of an intravascular clot—either a defect in the lumen of a vessel (a "filling defect") or an abrupt termination ("cutoff") of the vessel. Other, less common indications for pulmonary angiography include visualization of a suspected pulmonary arteriovenous malformation and assessment of pulmonary arterial invasion by a neoplasm.

ULTRASOUND   Because ultrasound energy is rapidly dissipated in air, ultrasound imaging is not useful for evaluation of the pulmonary parenchyma. However, it is helpful in the detection and localization of pleural abnormalities and is often used as a guide to placement of a needle for sampling of pleural liquid (i.e., for thoracentesis).

COLLECTION OF SPUTUM Sputum can be collected either by spontaneous expectoration or after inhalation of an irritating aerosol, such as hypertonic saline. The latter method, called *sputum induction*, is commonly used to obtain sputum for diagnostic studies, either because sputum is not spontaneously being produced or because of an expected higher yield of certain types of findings. Knowledge of the appearance and quality of the sputum specimen obtained is especially important when one is interested in Gram's staining and culture. Because sputum consists mainly of secretions from the tracheobronchial tree rather than the upper airway, the finding of alveolar macrophages and other inflammatory cells is consistent with a lower respiratory tract origin of the sample, whereas the presence of squamous epithelial cells in a "sputum" sample indicates contamination by secretions from the upper airways.

Besides processing for routine bacterial pathogens by Gram's staining and culture, sputum can be processed for a variety of other pathogens, including staining and culture for mycobacteria or fungi, culture for viruses, and staining for *P. carinii*. In the specific case of sputum obtained for evaluation of *P. carinii* pneumonia in a patient infected with HIV, for example, sputum should be collected by induction, rather than spontaneous expectoration, and an immunofluorescent stain should be used to detect the organisms. Cytologic staining of sputum for malignant cells, using the traditional Papanicolaou method, allows noninvasive evaluation for suspected lung cancer. Traditional stains and cultures are now also being supplemented in some cases by immunologic techniques and by molecular biologic methods, including the use of polymerase chain reaction amplification and DNA probes.

PERCUTANEOUS NEEDLE ASPIRATION A needle can be inserted through the chest wall into a pulmonary lesion for the purpose of aspirating material for analysis by cytologic or microbiologic techniques. The procedure is usually carried out under CT guidance, which assists in the positioning of the needle and assures that it is localized in the lesion. Although the potential risks of this procedure include intrapulmonary bleeding and creation of a pneumothorax with collapse of the underlying lung, the low risk of complication in experienced hands is usually worth the information obtained. However, a limitation of the technique is sampling error due to the small amount of material obtained. Thus, findings other than a specific cytologic or microbiologic diagnosis are of limited clinical value.

THORACENTESIS Sampling of pleural liquid by thoracentesis is commonly performed for diagnostic purposes or, in the case of a large effusion, for palliation of dyspnea. Diagnostic sampling, either by blind needle aspiration or after localization by ultrasound, allows the collection of liquid for microbiologic and cytologic studies. Analysis of the fluid obtained for its cellular composition and chemical constituents, including glucose, protein, and lactate dehydrogenase, allows the effusion to be classified as either exudative or transudative (Chap. 262). In some cases, particularly in the setting of possible tuberculous involvement of the pleura (tuberculous pleuritis), closed biopsy of the parietal pleura is also performed, using a cutting needle (either an Abrams or a Cope biopsy needle) to sample tissue for histopathologic examination and culture.

BRONCHOSCOPY Bronchoscopy is the process of direct visualization of the tracheobronchial tree. Bronchoscopy with a rigid bronchoscope is generally performed in an operating room on a patient under general anesthesia. The development of a flexible fiberoptic bronchoscope has revolutionized the diagnostic use of bronchoscopy. Although bronchoscopy is now performed almost exclusively with fiberoptic instruments, rigid bronchoscopes still have a role in selected circumstances, primarily because of their larger suction channel and the fact that the patient can be ventilated through the bronchoscope channel. These situations include the retrieval of a foreign body and the suctioning of a massive hemorrhage, for which the small suction channel of the bronchoscope may be insufficient.

Flexible Fiberoptic Bronchoscopy This is an outpatient procedure that is usually performed in an awake but sedated patient. The bronchoscope is passed through either the mouth or the nose, between the vocal cords, and into the trachea. The ability to flex the scope makes it possible to visualize virtually all airways to the level of subsegmental bronchi. The bronchoscopist is able to identify endobronchial pathology, including tumors, granulomas, bronchitis, foreign bodies, and sites of bleeding. Samples from airway lesions can be taken by several methods, including washing, brushing, and biopsy. Washing involves instillation of sterile saline through a channel of the bronchoscope and onto the surface of a lesion. A portion of the liquid is collected by suctioning through the bronchoscope, and the recovered material can be analyzed for cells (cytology) or organisms (by standard stains and cultures). Brushing or biopsy of the surface of the lesion, using a small brush or biopsy forceps at the end of a long cable inserted through a channel of the bronchoscope, allows recovery of cellular material or tissue for analysis by standard cytologic and histopathologic methods.

The bronchoscope can be used to sample material not only from the regions that can be directly visualized (i.e., the airways) but also from the more distal pulmonary parenchyma. With the bronchoscope wedged into a subsegmental airway, aliquots of sterile saline can be instilled through the scope, allowing sampling of cells and organisms even from alveolar spaces. This procedure, called *bronchoalveolar lavage*, has been particularly useful for the recovery of organisms such as *P. carinii* in patients with HIV infection.

Brushing and biopsy of the distal lung parenchyma can also be performed with the same instruments that are used for endobronchial sampling. These instruments can be passed through the scope into small airways, where they penetrate the airway wall, allowing biopsy of peribronchial alveolar tissue. This procedure, called *transbronchial biopsy*, is used when there is either relatively diffuse disease or a localized lesion of adequate size. With the aid of fluoroscopic imaging, the bronchoscopist is able to determine not only whether and when the instrument is in the area of abnormality, but also the proximity of the instrument to the pleural surface. If the forceps are too close to the pleural surface, there is a risk of violating the visceral pleura and creating a pneumothorax; the other potential complication of transbronchial biopsy is pulmonary hemorrhage. The incidence of these complications is less than several percent.

Another procedure involves use of a hollow-bore needle passed through the bronchoscope for sampling of tissue adjacent to the trachea or a large bronchus. The needle is passed through the airway wall, and cellular material can be aspirated from mass lesions or enlarged lymph nodes, generally in a search for malignant cells. This procedure can facilitate the staging of lung cancer by identifying mediastinal lymph node involvement and in some cases obviates the need for a more invasive procedure.

The bronchoscope may provide the opportunity for treatment as well as diagnosis. For example, an aspirated foreign body may be retrieved with an instrument passed through the scope, and bleeding may be controlled with a balloon catheter similarly introduced. Newer interventional techniques performed through a bronchoscope include methods for achieving and maintaining patency of airways that are partially or completely occluded, especially by tumors. These techniques include laser therapy, cryotherapy, electrocautery, and stent placement.

VIDEO-ASSISTED THORACIC SURGERY Recent advances in video technology have allowed the development of thoracoscopy, or video-assisted thoracic surgery (VATS), for the diagnosis and management of pleural as well as parenchymal lung disease. This procedure, done under general anesthesia, involves the passage of a rigid scope with a distal lens through a trocar inserted into the pleura. A high-quality image is shown on a monitor screen, allowing the operator to manipulate instruments passed into the pleural space through separate small intercostal incisions. With these instruments, the operator can biopsy lesions of the pleura under direct vision, which provides an obvious advantage over closed pleural biopsy. In addition, this procedure is now used commonly to biopsy peripheral lung tissue or to remove peripheral nodules, for both diagnostic and therapeutic purposes. Because this procedure is much less invasive than the traditional thoracotomy performed for lung biopsy, it has largely supplanted "open lung biopsy."

THORACOTOMY Although frequently replaced by VATS, thoracotomy remains an option for the diagnostic sampling of lung tissue. It provides the largest amount of material, and it can be used to biopsy and/or excise lesions that are too deep or too close to vital structures for removal by VATS. The choice between VATS and thoracotomy needs to be made on a case-by-case basis, and the relative indications for each are still evolving as more experience is being gained with VATS.

MEDIASTINOSCOPY AND MEDIASTINOTOMY Tissue biopsy is often critical for the diagnosis of mediastinal masses or enlarged mediastinal lymph nodes. Although CT is useful for determining the size of mediastinal lymph nodes as part of the staging of lung cancer, confirmation that enlarged lymph nodes are actually involved with tumor generally requires biopsy and histopathologic examination. The two major procedures used to obtain specimens from masses or nodes in the mediastinum are mediastinoscopy (via a suprasternal ap-

proach) and mediastinotomy (via a parasternal approach). Both procedures are performed under general anesthesia by a qualified surgeon. In the case of suprasternal mediastinoscopy, a rigid mediastinoscope is inserted at the suprasternal notch and passed into the mediastinum along a pathway just anterior to the trachea. Tissue can be obtained with biopsy forceps passed through the scope, sampling masses or nodes that are in a paratracheal or pretracheal position. Left paratracheal and aortopulmonary lymph nodes are not accessible by this route and thus are commonly sampled by parasternal mediastinotomy (the Chamberlain procedure). This approach involves either a right or left parasternal incision and dissection directly down to a mass or node that requires biopsy.

BIBLIOGRAPHY

ALBERT RK et al (eds): *Comprehensive Respiratory Medicine.* Philadelphia, Mosby, 1999

DICHTER JR et al: Approach to the immunocompromised host with pulmonary symptoms. Hematol Oncol Clin North Am 7:887, 1993

ETTINGER NA: Invasive diagnostic approaches to pulmonary infiltrates. Semin Respir Infect 8:168, 1993

HARRIS RJ et al: The diagnostic and therapeutic utility of thoracoscopy. A review. Chest 108:828, 1995

MCELVEIN RB: Procedures in the evaluation of chest disease. Clin Chest Med 13:1, 1992

WANG K-P, MEHTA AC: *Flexible Bronchoscopy,* Cambridge, MA, Blackwell, 1995

WEBB WR et al: *High-Resolution CT of the Lung,* 2d ed. Philadelphia, Lippincott-Raven, 1996

WEINBERGER SE: *Principles of Pulmonary Medicine,* 3d ed. Philadelphia, Saunders, 1998

Section 2
DISEASES OF THE RESPIRATORY SYSTEM

252   *E. R. McFadden, Jr.*

ASTHMA

DEFINITION Asthma is defined as a chronic inflammatory disease of airways that is characterized by increased responsiveness of the tracheobronchial tree to a multiplicity of stimuli. It is manifested physiologically by a widespread narrowing of the air passages, which may be relieved spontaneously or as a result of therapy, and clinically by paroxysms of dyspnea, cough, and wheezing. Asthma is an episodic disease, with acute exacerbations interspersed with symptom-free periods. Typically, most attacks are short-lived, lasting minutes to hours, and clinically the patient seems to recover completely after an attack. However, there can be a phase in which the patient experiences some degree of airway obstruction daily. This phase can be mild, with or without superimposed severe episodes, or much more serious, with severe obstruction persisting for days or weeks; the latter condition is known as *status asthmaticus*. In unusual circumstances, acute episodes can cause death.

PREVALENCE AND ETIOLOGY Asthma is very common; it is estimated that 4 to 5% of the population of the United States is affected. Similar figures have been reported from other countries. Bronchial asthma occurs at all ages but predominantly in early life. About one-half of cases develop before age 10, and another third occur before age 40. In childhood, there is a 2:1 male/female preponderance, but the sex ratio equalizes by age 30.

From an etiologic standpoint, asthma is a heterogeneous disease. It is useful for epidemiologic and clinical purposes to classify asthma by the principal stimuli that incite or are associated with acute episodes. However, it is important to emphasize that this distinction may

often be artificial, and the response of a given subclassification usually can be initiated by more than one type of stimulus. Furthermore, the application of molecular and cell biologic techniques to asthma pathogenesis is also beginning to blur this type of classification. With these reservations in mind, one can describe two broad types of asthma: allergic and idiosyncratic.

Atopy is the single largest risk factor for the development of asthma. *Allergic asthma* is often associated with a personal and/or family history of allergic diseases such as rhinitis, urticaria, and eczema, with positive wheal-and-flare skin reactions to intradermal injection of extracts of airborne antigens, with increased levels of IgE in the serum, and/or with a positive response to provocation tests involving the inhalation of specific antigen.

A significant fraction of patients with asthma present with no personal or family history of allergy, with negative skin tests, and with normal serum levels of IgE, and therefore have disease that cannot be classified on the basis of defined immunologic mechanisms. These patients are said to have *idiosyncratic asthma*. Many develop a typical symptom complex on contracting an upper respiratory illness. The initial insult may be little more than a common cold, but after several days the patient begins to develop paroxysms of wheezing and dyspnea that can last for days to months. These individuals should not be confused with persons in whom the symptoms of bronchospasm are superimposed on chronic bronchitis or bronchiectasis (Chaps. 256 and 258).

Many patients have disease that does not fit clearly into either of the preceding categories but instead falls into a mixed group with features of each. In general, asthma that has its onset in early life tends to have a strong allergic component, whereas asthma that develops late tends to be nonallergic or to have a mixed etiology.

PATHOGENESIS OF ASTHMA The common denominator underlying the asthmatic diathesis is a nonspecific hyperirritability of the tracheobronchial tree. When airway reactivity is high, symptoms are more severe and persistent, and the amount of therapy required to control the patient's complaints is greater. In addition, the magnitude of diurnal fluctuations in lung function is greater, and the patient tends to awaken at night or in the early morning with breathlessness.

In both normal and asthmatic individuals, airway reactivity rises after viral infections of the respiratory tract and exposure to oxidant air pollutants such as ozone and nitrogen dioxide (but not sulfur dioxide). Viral infections have more profound consequences, and airway responsiveness may remain elevated for many weeks after a seemingly trivial upper respiratory tract infection. In contrast, airway reactivity remains high for only a few days after exposure to ozone. Allergens can cause airway responsiveness to rise within minutes and to remain elevated for weeks. If the dose of antigen is high enough, acute episodes of obstruction may occur daily for a prolonged period after a single exposure.

The most popular hypothesis at present for the pathogenesis of asthma is that it derives from a state of persistent subacute inflammation of the airways. An active inflammatory process is frequently observed in endobronchial biopsy specimens even from asymptomatic patients. The airways can be edematous and infiltrated with eosinophils, neutrophils, and lymphocytes, with or without an increase in the collagen content of the epithelial basement membrane. There may also be glandular hypertrophy. The most ubiquitous finding is a generalized increase in cellularity associated with an elevated capillary density. Occasionally, denudation of the epithelium may also be observed.

Although the translation of these histologic observations into a disease process is still incomplete, it is widely believed that the physiologic and clinical features of asthma derive from an interaction among the resident and infiltrating inflammatory cells in the airway surface epithelium, inflammatory mediators, and cytokines. The cells thought to play important parts in the inflammatory response are mast cells, eosinophils, lymphocytes, and epithelial cells. The roles of neutrophils and macrophages are less well defined. Each of these cell types can contribute mediators and cytokines to initiate and amplify both acute inflammation and the long-term pathologic changes described above. The mediators released—histamine; bradykinin; the leukotrienes C, D, and E; platelet-activating factor; and prostaglandins (PGs) E_2, $F_2\alpha$, and D_2—produce an intense, immediate inflammatory reaction involving bronchoconstriction, vascular congestion, and edema formation. In addition to their ability to evoke prolonged contraction of airway smooth muscle and mucosal edema, the leukotrienes may also account for some of the other pathophysiologic features of asthma, such as increased mucus production and impaired mucociliary transport. This intense local event can then be followed by a more chronic one. The chemotactic factors elaborated (eosinophil and neutrophil chemotactic factors of anaphylaxis and leukotriene B_4) bring eosinophils, platelets, and polymorphonuclear leukocytes to the site of the reaction. These infiltrating cells as well as resident macrophages and the airway epithelium itself potentially are an additional source of mediators to enhance both the immediate and the cellular phase. The airway epithelium is both the target of, and a contributor to, the inflammatory cascade. These cells amplify bronchoconstriction by elaborating endothelin-1 and promoting vasodilatation through the release of nitric oxide, PGE_2 and the 15-hydroxyeicosatetraenoic acid (15-HETE) products of arachidonic acid metabolism. They also generate cytokines such as granulocyte-macrophage colony stimulating factor (GM-CSF), interleukin (IL)8, Rantes, and eotaxin.

Like the mast cell in the early reaction, the eosinophil appears to play an important part in the infiltrative component. The granular proteins in this cell (major basic protein and eosinophilic cationic protein) and oxygen-derived free radical are capable of destroying the airway epithelium, which then is sloughed into the bronchial lumen in the form of Creola bodies. Besides resulting in a loss of barrier and secretory function, such damage elicits the production of chemotactic cytokines, leading to further inflammation. In theory, it also can expose sensory nerve endings, thus initiating neurogenic inflammatory pathways. That, in turn, could convert a primary local event into a generalized reaction via a reflex mechanism.

T lymphocytes also appear to be important in the inflammatory response. These cells are present in increased numbers in asthmatic airways and produce cytokines that activate cell-mediated immunity, as well as humoral (IgE) immune responses. Activated T cells recovered from the lungs of persons with asthma express messenger RNA for the cytokines known to play a part in the recruitment and activation of mast cells and eosinophils. Furthermore, the T_H1 and T_H2 lymphocyte subtypes have functions that may influence the asthmatic response. The T_H1 cytokines IL-2 and interferon (IFN) γ can promote the growth and differentiation of B cells and the activation of macrophages, respectively. The T_H2 cytokines IL-4 and IL-5 stimulate B-cell growth and immunoglobulin secretion, and IL-5 promotes eosinophil proliferation, differentiation, and activation. It can also facilitate granule release from basophils.

Cytokine production is another central component of the inflammation of asthma. Cytokines are synthesized and released from many of the inflammatory cells mentioned above, as well as from epithelial cells, fibroblasts, endothelial cells, and airway smooth muscle. Cytokines activate specific cell-surface receptors that are coupled to signal transduction pathways, which often result in alterations of gene regulation and enzyme production. The cytokines that are particularly relevant to asthma are secreted by T lymphocytes and include IL-3 enhanced (mast cell survival), IL-4 and IL-13 (switching of B lymphocytes to IgE production and expression of adhesion molecules), and IL-5 (differentiation and enhanced survival of eosinophils). Other cytokines, such as IL-1B, IL-6, IL-11, tumor necrosis factor α (TNF-α) and GM-CSF, are proinflammatory and may amplify the inflammatory response.

The relative roles of each of the above elements in the production of heightened airway reactivity and clinical asthma have yet to be determined. Although inflammation is clearly important, recent evidence indicates that the intensity of the cellular infiltrate in the airways is not related either to the severity of the disease state or to the level of airway reactivity. Furthermore, it is unlikely that any one cell type or mediator accounts for every feature. For example, mast cell–derived mediators cannot explain the whole picture, for they have been found in the blood of individuals with mast cell–related diseases such as cold-induced and cholinergic-induced urticaria and in the airways of atopic individuals without asthma. Since these individuals had no lower respiratory illness or complaints, these alleged mediators of asthma would appear to need a unique background from which to exhibit their effects. Similarly, the inflammatory cells believed to be relevant to asthma are also found in the airways of atopic individuals without asthma, raising the possibility that they are merely nonspecific markers of atopy rather than specific indexes of asthma. Finally, the therapeutic administration of IL-2 and GM-CSF to patients with cancer results in eosinophilia with cell activation but not in asthma.

GENETIC CONSIDERATIONS   Although there is little doubt that asthma has a strong familial component, the identification of the genetic mechanisms underlying the illness has proven difficult for multiple reasons, including such fundamental issues as a lack of uniform agreement on the definition of the disease, the inability to define a single phenotype, non-Mendelian modes of inheritance, and an incomplete understanding of how environmental factors modify genetic expression. Screening families for candidate genes has identified multiple chromosomal regions that relate to atopy, elevated IgE levels, and airway hyperresponsiveness. Evidence for genetic linkage of high total serum IgE levels and atopy has been observed on chromosomes 5q, 11q, and 12q in a number of populations scattered throughout the world. Regions of the genome demonstrating evidence for linkage to bronchial hyperreactivity also typically show evidence for linkage to elevated total serum IgE levels. Excellent candidate genes exist for specific abnormalities in asthma within the regions that were identified in the linkage studies. For example, chromosome 5q contains cytokine clusters including IL-4, IL-5, IL-9, and IL-13. Other regions on chromosome 5q also contain the beta-adrenergic receptors and the glucocorticoid receptors. Chromosome 6p contains regions that are important in antigen presentation and mediation of the inflammatory response. Chromosome 12q contains two genes that could influence atopy and airway hyperresponsiveness, including nitric oxide synthase. ■

The stimuli that interact with airway responsiveness and incite acute episodes of asthma can be grouped into seven major categories: allergenic, pharmacologic, environmental, occupational, infectious, exercise-related, and emotional.

Allergens   Allergic asthma is dependent on an IgE response controlled by T and B lymphocytes and activated by the interaction of antigen with mast cell–bound IgE molecules. The airway epithelium and submucosa contain dendritic cells that capture and process antigen. After taking up an immunogen, these cells migrate to the local lymph nodes where they present the material to T cell receptors. In the appropriate genetic setting, the interaction of antigen with a naïve T cell T_H0 in the presence of IL-4 leads to the differentiation of the cell to a T_H2 subset. This process not only helps facilitate the inflammation of asthma but also causes B lymphocytes to switch their antibody production from IgG and IgM to IgE. Most of the allergens that provoke asthma are airborne, and to induce a state of sensitivity they must be reasonably abundant for considerable periods of time. Once sensitization has occurred, however, the patient can exhibit exquisite responsivity, so that minute amounts of the offending agent can produce significant exacerbations of the disease. Immune mechanisms appear to be causally related to the development of asthma in 25 to 35% of all cases and to be contributory in perhaps another third. Higher prevalences have been suggested, but it is difficult to know how to interpret the data because of confounding factors. Allergic asthma is frequently seasonal, and it is most often observed in children and young adults. A nonseasonal form may result from allergy to feathers, animal danders, dust mites, molds, and other antigens that are present continuously in the environment. Exposure to antigen typically produces an immediate response in which airway obstruction develops in minutes and then resolves. In 30 to 50% of patients, a second wave of bronchoconstriction, the so-called late reaction, develops 6 to 10 h later. In a minority, only a late reaction occurs. It was formerly thought that the late reaction was essential to the development of the increase in airway reactivity that follows antigen exposure. Recent data show that not to be the case.

The mechanism by which an inhaled allergen provokes an acute episode of asthma depends in part on antigen-antibody interactions on the surface of pulmonary mast cells, with the subsequent generation and release of the mediators of immediate hypersensitivity. Current hypotheses hold that very small antigenic particles penetrate the lung's defenses and come in contact with mast cells that interdigitate with the epithelium at the luminal surface of the central airways. The subsequent elaboration of mediators and cytokines then produces the sequence outlined above.

Pharmacologic Stimuli   The drugs most commonly associated with the induction of acute episodes of asthma are aspirin, coloring agents such as tartrazine, β-adrenergic antagonists, and sulfiting agents. It is important to recognize drug-induced bronchial narrowing because its presence is often associated with great morbidity. Furthermore, death sometimes has followed the ingestion of aspirin (or other nonsteroidal anti-inflammatory agents) or β-adrenergic antagonists. The typical aspirin-sensitive respiratory syndrome primarily affects adults, although the condition may occur in childhood. This problem usually begins with perennial vasomotor rhinitis that is followed by a hyperplastic rhinosinusitis with nasal polyps. Progressive asthma then appears. On exposure to even very small quantities of aspirin, affected individuals typically develop ocular and nasal congestion and acute, often severe episodes of airways obstruction. The prevalence of aspirin sensitivity in patients with asthma varies from study to study, but many

authorities feel that 10% is a reasonable figure. There is a great deal of cross reactivity between aspirin and other nonsteroidal anti-inflammatory compounds that inhibit prostaglandin G/H synthase 1 (cyclooxygenase type 1). Indomethacin, fenoprofen, naproxen, zomepirac sodium, ibuprofen, mefenamic acid, and phenylbutazone are particularly important in this regard. However, acetaminophen, sodium salicylate, choline salicylate, salicylamide, and propoxyphene are well tolerated. The exact frequency of cross reactivity to tartrazine and other dyes in aspirin-sensitive individuals with asthma is also controversial; again, 10% is the commonly accepted figure. This peculiar complication of aspirin-sensitive asthma is particularly insidious, however, in that tartrazine and other potentially troublesome dyes are widely present in the environment and may be unknowingly ingested by sensitive patients.

Patients with aspirin sensitivity can be desensitized by daily administration of the drug. After this form of therapy, cross tolerance also develops to other nonsteroidal anti-inflammatory agents. The mechanism by which aspirin and other such drugs produce bronchospasm appears to be a chronic overexcretion of cysteinyl leukotrienes, which activate mast cells. The adverse reaction to aspirin can be inhibited with the use of leukotriene synthesis blockers or receptor antagonists.

Beta-adrenergic antagonists regularly obstruct the airways in individuals with asthma as well as in others with heightened airway reactivity and should be avoided by such individuals. Even the selective $beta_1$ agents have this propensity, particularly at higher doses. In fact, the local use of $beta_1$ blockers in the eye for the treatment of glaucoma has been associated with worsening asthma.

Sulfiting agents, such as potassium metabisulfite, potassium and sodium bisulfite, sodium sulfite, and sulfur dioxide, which are widely used in the food and pharmaceutical industries as sanitizing and preserving agents, also can produce acute airway obstruction in sensitive individuals. Exposure usually follows ingestion of food or beverages containing these compounds, e.g., salads, fresh fruit, potatoes, shellfish, and wine. Exacerbation of asthma has been reported after the use of sulfite-containing topical ophthalmic solutions, intravenous glucocorticoids, and some inhalational bronchodilator solutions. The incidence and mechanism of action of this phenomenon are unknown. When suspected, the diagnosis can be confirmed by either oral or inhalational provocations.

Environment and Air Pollution   (See also Chap. 254)   Environmental causes of asthma are usually related to climatic conditions that promote the concentration of atmospheric pollutants and antigens. These conditions tend to develop in heavily industrial or densely populated urban areas and are frequently associated with thermal inversions or other situations creating stagnant air masses. In these circumstances, although the general population can develop respiratory symptoms, patients with asthma and other respiratory diseases tend to be more severely affected. The air pollutants known to have this effect are ozone, nitrogen dioxide, and sulfur dioxide. Sulfur dioxide needs to be present in high concentrations and produces its greatest effects during periods of high ventilation. In some regions of North America, seasonal concentrations of airborne antigens such as pollen can rise high enough to result in epidemics of asthma admissions to hospitals and an increase in the death rate. These events may be ameliorated by treating patients prophylactically with anti-inflammatory drugs before the allergy season begins.

Occupational Factors   (See also Chap. 254)   Occupation-related asthma is a significant health problem, and acute and chronic airway obstruction has been reported to follow exposure to a large number of compounds used in many types of industrial processes. Bronchoconstriction can result from working with or being exposed to *metal salts* (e.g., platinum, chrome, and nickel), *wood and vegetable dusts* (e.g., those of oak, western red cedar, grain, flour, castor bean, green coffee bean, mako, gum acacia, karay gum, and tragacanth), *pharmaceutical agents* (e.g., antibiotics, piperazine, and cimetidine), *industrial chemicals and plastics* (e.g., toluene diisocyanate, phthalic acid anhydride, trimellitic anhydride, persulfates, ethylenediamine, *p*-phenylenediamine, and various dyes), *biologic enzymes* (e.g., laundry detergents and pancreatic enzymes), and *animal and insect dusts, serums, and secretions*. It is important to recognize that exposure to sensitizing chemicals, particularly those used in paints, solvents, and plastics, also can occur during leisure or non-work-related activities.

There seem to be three underlying mechanisms for this airway obstruction: (1) In some cases, the offending agent results in the formation of a specific IgE, and the cause seems immunologic (the immunologic reaction can be immediate, late, or dual); (2) in other cases, the substance causes a direct liberation of bronchoconstrictor substances; and (3) in other instances, the substance causes direct or reflex stimulation of the airways of individuals with either latent or frank asthma. If the occupational agent causes an immediate or dual immunologic reaction, the history is similar to that which occurs with exposure to other antigens. Often, however, patients will give a characteristic cyclic history. They are well when they arrive at work, and symptoms develop toward the end of the shift, progress after the work site is left, and then regress. Absence from work during weekends or vacations brings about remission. Frequently, there are similar symptoms in fellow employees.

Infections Respiratory infections are the most common of the stimuli that evoke acute exacerbations of asthma. Well-controlled investigations have demonstrated that respiratory viruses and not bacteria or allergy to microorganisms are the major etiologic factors. In young children, the most important infectious agents are respiratory syncytial virus and parainfluenza virus. In older children and adults, rhinovirus and influenza virus predominate as pathogens. Simple colonization of the tracheobronchial tree is insufficient to evoke acute episodes of bronchospasm, and attacks of asthma occur only when symptoms of an ongoing respiratory tract infection are, or have been, present. Viral infections can actively and chronically destabilize asthma, and they are perhaps the only stimuli that can produce constant symptoms for weeks. The mechanism by which viruses induce exacerbations of asthma may be related to the production of T cell–derived cytokines that potentiate the infiltration of inflammatory cells into already susceptible airways.

Exercise Exercise is a very common precipitant of acute episodes of asthma. This stimulus differs from other naturally occurring provocations, such as antigens, viral infections, and air pollutants, in that it does not evoke any long-term sequelae, nor does it increase airway reactivity. Exercise can be made to provoke bronchospasm in every patient with asthma, and in some it is the only trigger that produces symptoms. When such patients are followed for sufficient periods, however, they often develop recurring episodes of airway obstruction independent of exercise; thus, the onset of this problem frequently is the first manifestation of the full-blown asthmatic syndrome. The critical variables that determine the severity of the postexertional airway obstruction are the levels of ventilation achieved and the temperature and humidity of the inspired air. The higher the ventilation and the lower the heat content of the air, the greater the response. For the same inspired air conditions, running produces a more severe attack of asthma than walking. Conversely, for a given task, the inhalation of cold air markedly enhances the response, while warm, humid air blunts or abolishes it. Consequently, activities such as ice hockey, cross-country skiing, and ice skating are more provocative than is swimming in an indoor, heated pool. The mechanism by which exercise produces obstruction may be related to a thermally produced hyperemia and engorgement of the microvasculature of the bronchial wall and does not appear to involve smooth-muscle contraction.

Emotional Stress Abundant objective data demonstrate that psychological factors can interact with the asthmatic diathesis to worsen or ameliorate the disease process. The pathways and nature of the interactions are complex but are operational to some extent in almost half the patients studied. Changes in airway caliber seem to be mediated through modification of vagal efferent activity, but endorphins also may play a role. The most frequently studied variable has been that of suggestion, and the weight of current evidence indicates

that it can be quite important in selected individuals with asthma. When psychically responsive individuals are given the appropriate suggestion, they can actually decrease or increase the pharmacologic effects of adrenergic and cholinergic stimuli on their airways. The extent to which psychological factors participate in the induction and/or continuation of any given acute exacerbation is not established but probably varies from patient to patient and in the same patient from episode to episode.

PATHOLOGY In a patient who has died of acute asthma, the most striking feature of the lungs at necropsy is their gross overdistention and failure to collapse when the pleural cavities are opened. When the lungs are cut, numerous gelatinous plugs of exudate are found in most of the bronchial branches down to the terminal bronchioles. Histologic examination shows hypertrophy of the bronchial smooth muscle, hyperplasia of mucosal and submucosal vessels, mucosal edema, denudation of the surface epithelium, pronounced thickening of the basement membrane, and eosinophilic infiltrates in the bronchial wall. There is an absence of any of the well-recognized forms of destructive emphysema.

PATHOPHYSIOLOGY The pathophysiologic hallmark of asthma is a reduction in airway diameter brought about by contraction of smooth muscle, vascular congestion, edema of the bronchial wall, and thick, tenacious secretions. The net result is an increase in airway resistance, a decrease in forced expiratory volumes and flow rates, hyperinflation of the lungs and thorax, increased work of breathing, alterations in respiratory muscle function, changes in elastic recoil, abnormal distribution of both ventilation and pulmonary blood flow with mismatched ratios, and altered arterial blood gas concentrations. Thus, although asthma is considered to be primarily a disease of airways, virtually all aspects of pulmonary function are compromised during an acute attack. In addition, in very symptomatic patients there frequently is electrocardiographic evidence of right ventricular hypertrophy and pulmonary hypertension. When a patient presents for therapy, his or her forced vital capacity tends to be $\leq 50\%$ of normal. The 1-s forced expiratory volume (FEV_1) averages 30% or less of predicted, while the maximum and minimum midexpiratory flow rates are reduced to 20% or less of expected. In keeping with the alterations in mechanics, the associated air trapping is substantial. In acutely ill patients, residual volume (RV) frequently approaches 400% of normal, while functional residual capacity doubles. The patient tends to report that the attack has ended clinically when the RV has fallen to 200% of its predicted value and the FEV_1 reaches 50% of the predicted level.

Hypoxia is a universal finding during acute exacerbations, but frank ventilatory failure is relatively uncommon, being observed in 10 to 15% of patients presenting for therapy. Most individuals with asthma have hypocapnia and a respiratory alkalosis. In acutely ill patients, the finding of a normal arterial carbon dioxide tension tends to be associated with quite severe levels of obstruction. Consequently, when found in a symptomatic individual, it should be viewed as representing impending respiratory failure, and the patient should be treated accordingly. Equally, the presence of metabolic acidosis in the setting of acute asthma signifies severe obstruction. Usually, there are no clinical counterparts to the derangements in blood gases. Cyanosis is a very late sign. Hence, a dangerous level of hypoxia can go undetected. Likewise, signs attributable to carbon dioxide retention, such as sweating, tachycardia, and wide pulse pressure, or to acidosis, such as tachypnea, tend not to be of great value in predicting the presence of hypercapnia or hydrogen ion excess in individual patients, because they are too frequently seen in anxious patients with more moderate disease. Trying to judge the state of an acutely ill patient's ventilatory status on clinical grounds alone can be extremely hazardous, and clinical indicators should not be relied on with any confidence. Therefore, in patients with suspected alveolar hypoventilation, arterial blood gas tensions must be measured.

CLINICAL FEATURES The symptoms of asthma consist of a triad of dyspnea, cough, and wheezing, the last often being regarded as the *sine qua non*. In its most typical form, asthma is an episodic disease, and all three symptoms coexist. At the onset of an attack, patients experience a sense of constriction in the chest, often with a nonproductive cough. Respiration becomes audibly harsh, wheezing in both phases of respiration becomes prominent, expiration becomes prolonged, and patients frequently have tachypnea, tachycardia, and mild systolic hypertension. The lungs rapidly become overinflated, and the anteroposterior diameter of the thorax increases. If the attack is severe or prolonged, there may be a loss of adventitial breath sounds, and wheezing becomes very high pitched. Furthermore, the accessory muscles become visibly active, and a paradoxical pulse often develops. These two signs are extremely valuable in indicating the severity of the obstruction. In the presence of either, pulmonary function tends to be significantly more impaired than in their absence. It is important to note that the development of a paradoxical pulse depends on the generation of large negative intrathoracic pressures. Thus, if the patient's breathing is shallow, this sign and/or the use of accessory muscles could be absent even though obstruction is quite severe. The other signs and symptoms of asthma only imperfectly reflect the physiologic alterations that are present. Indeed, if the disappearance of subjective complaints or even of wheezing is used as the end point at which therapy for an acute attack is terminated, an enormous reservoir of residual disease will be missed.

The end of an episode is frequently marked by a cough that produces thick, stringy mucus, which often takes the form of casts of the distal airways (Curschmann's spirals) and, when examined microscopically, often shows eosinophils and Charcot-Leyden crystals. In extreme situations, wheezing may lessen markedly or even disappear, cough may become extremely ineffective, and the patient may begin a gasping type of respiratory pattern. These findings imply extensive mucus plugging and impending suffocation. Ventilatory assistance by mechanical means may be required. Atelectasis due to inspissated secretions occasionally occurs with asthmatic attacks. Spontaneous pneumothorax and/or pneumomediastinum occur but are rare.

Less typically, a patient with asthma may complain of intermittent episodes of nonproductive cough or exertional dyspnea. Unlike other individuals with asthma, when these patients are examined during symptomatic periods, they tend to have normal breath sounds but may wheeze after repeated forced exhalations and/or may show ventilatory impairments when tested in the laboratory. In the absence of both these signs, a bronchoprovocation test may be required to make the diagnosis.

DIFFERENTIAL DIAGNOSIS   The differentiation of asthma from other diseases associated with dyspnea and wheezing is usually not difficult, particularly if the patient is seen during an acute episode. The physical findings and symptoms listed above and the history of periodic attacks are quite characteristic. A personal or family history of allergic diseases such as eczema, rhinitis, or urticaria is valuable contributory evidence. An extremely common feature of asthma is nocturnal awakening with dyspnea and/or wheezing. In fact, this phenomenon is so prevalent that its absence raises doubt about the diagnosis. *Upper airway obstruction by tumor* or *laryngeal edema* can occasionally be confused with asthma. Typically, a patient with such a condition will present with stridor, and the harsh respiratory sounds can be localized to the area of the trachea. Diffuse wheezing throughout both lung fields is usually absent. However, differentiation can sometimes be difficult, and indirect laryngoscopy or bronchoscopy may be required. Asthma-like symptoms have been described in patients with glottic dysfunction. These individuals narrow their glottis during inspiration and expiration, producing episodic attacks of severe airway obstruction. Occasionally, carbon dioxide retention develops. However, unlike asthma, the arterial oxygen tension is well preserved, and the alveolar-arterial gradient for oxygen narrows during the episode, instead of widening as with lower airway obstruction. To establish the diagnosis of glottic dysfunction, the glottis should be examined when the patient is symptomatic. Normal findings at such a time exclude the diagnosis; normal findings during asymptomatic periods do not.

Persistent wheezing localized to one area of the chest in association with paroxysms of coughing indicates *endobronchial disease* such as foreign-body aspiration, a neoplasm, or bronchial stenosis.

The signs and symptoms of *acute left ventricular failure* occasionally mimic asthma, but the findings of moist basilar rales, gallop rhythms, blood-tinged sputum, and other signs of heart failure (Chap. 232) allow the appropriate diagnosis to be reached.

Recurrent episodes of bronchospasm can occur with *carcinoid tumors* (Chap. 93), *recurrent pulmonary emboli* (Chap. 261), and *chronic bronchitis* (Chap. 258). In chronic bronchitis there are no true symptom-free periods, and one can usually obtain a history of chronic cough and sputum production as a background on which acute attacks of wheezing are superimposed. Recurrent emboli can be very difficult to separate from asthma. Frequently, patients with this condition present with episodes of breathlessness, particularly on exertion, and they sometimes wheeze. Pulmonary function studies may show evidence of peripheral airway obstruction (Chap. 250); when these changes are present, lung scans also may be abnormal. The therapeutic response to bronchodilators and to the institution of anticoagulant therapy may be helpful, but pulmonary angiography may be necessary to establish the correct diagnosis.

Eosinophilic pneumonias (Chap. 253) are often associated with asthmatic symptoms, as are various chemical pneumonias and exposures to insecticides and cholinergic drugs. Bronchospasm occasionally is a manifestation of *systemic vasculitis* with pulmonary involvement.

DIAGNOSIS   The diagnosis of asthma is established by demonstrating reversible airway obstruction. *Reversibility* is traditionally defined as a 15% or greater increase in FEV_1 after two puffs of a β-adrenergic agonist. When the spirometry results are normal at presentation, the diagnosis can be made by showing heightened airway responsiveness to challenges with histamine, methacholine, or isocapnic hyperventilation of cold air. Once the diagnosis is confirmed, the course of the illness and the effectiveness of therapy can be followed by measuring peak expiratory flow rates (PEFRs) at home and/or the FEV_1 in the laboratory. Positive wheal-and-flare reactions to skin tests can be demonstrated to various allergens, but such findings do not necessarily correlate with the intrapulmonary events. Sputum and blood eosinophilia and measurement of serum IgE levels are also helpful but are not specific for asthma. Chest roentgenograms showing hyperinflation are also nondiagnostic.

℞ **TREATMENT**   Elimination of the causative agent(s) from the environment of an allergic individual with asthma is the most successful means available for treating this condition (for details on avoidance, see Chap. 310). Desensitization or immunotherapy with extracts of the suspected allergens has enjoyed widespread favor, but controlled studies are limited and have not proved it to be highly effective.

Drug Treatment   The available agents for treating asthma can be divided into two general categories: drugs that inhibit smooth muscle contraction, i.e., the so-called "quick relief medications" (beta-adrenergic agonists, methylxanthines, and anticholinergics) and agents that prevent and/or reverse inflammation, i.e., the "long-term control medications" (glucocorticoids, leukotriene inhibitors and receptor antagonists, and mast cell–stabilizing agents).

Adrenergic stimulants   The drugs in this category consist of the catecholamines, resorcinols, and saligenins. These agents are analogues and produce airway dilation through stimulation of beta-adrenergic receptors and activation of G proteins with the resultant formation of cyclic adenosine monophosphate (AMP). They also decrease release of mediators and improve mucociliary transport. The catecholamines available for clinical use are epinephrine, isoproterenol, and isoetharine. As a group, these compounds are short-acting (30 to 90 min) and are effective only when administered by inhalational or parenteral routes. Epinephrine and isoproterenol are not β_2-selective and have considerable chronotropic and inotropic cardiac effects. Epinephrine also has substantial alpha-stimulating effects. The usual dose is 0.3 to 0.5 mL of a 1:1000 solution administered subcutaneously. Isoproterenol is devoid of alpha activity and is the most potent agent of this group. It is usually administered in a 1:200 solution by inhalation. Isoetharine is the most β_2-selective compound of this class, but it is a relatively weak bronchodilator. It is employed as an aerosol and supplied as a 1% solution. The use of these agents in treating asthma has been superceded by longer acting selective β_2 agonists.

The commonly used resorcinols are metaproterenol, terbutaline, and fenoterol, and the most widely known saligenin is albuterol (salbutamol). With the exception of metaproterenol, these drugs are highly selective for the respiratory tract and virtually devoid of significant cardiac effects except at high doses. Their major side effect is tremor. They are active by all routes of administration, and because their chemical structures allow them to bypass the metabolic processes used to degrade the catecholamines, their effects are relatively long-lasting (4 to 6 h). Differences in potency and duration among agents can be eliminated by adjusting doses and/or administration schedules.

Inhalation is the preferred route of administration because it allows maximal bronchodilation with fewer side effects. In the past it was fashionable to treat episodes of severe asthma with intravenous sympathomimetics such as isoproterenol. This approach no longer appears justifiable. Isoproterenol infusions clearly can induce myocardial damage, and even for the β_2-selective agents such as terbutaline and albuterol, intravenous administration offers no advantages over the inhaled route.

Salmeterol is a very long-lasting (9 to 12 h) congener of albuterol. When given every 12 h, it is effective in providing sustained symptomatic relief. It is particularly helpful for conditions such as nocturnal and exercise-induced asthma. It is not recommended for the treatment of acute episodes because of its relatively slow onset of action (approximately 30 min), nor is it intended as a rescue drug for breakthrough symptoms. In addition, its long half-life means that administration of extra doses can cause cumulative side effects.

Methylxanthines Theophylline and its various salts are medium-potency bronchodilators that work by increasing cyclic AMP by the inhibition of phosphodiesterase. The therapeutic plasma concentrations of theophylline traditionally have been thought to lie between 10 and 20 μg/mL. Some sources, however, recommend a lower target range between 5 and 15 μg/mL to avoid toxicity. The dose required to achieve the desired level varies widely from patient to patient owing to differences in the metabolism of the drug. Theophylline clearance, and thus the dosage requirement, is decreased substantially in neonates and the elderly and those with acute and chronic hepatic dysfunction, cardiac decompensation, and cor pulmonale. Clearance is also decreased during febrile illnesses. Clearance is increased in children. In addition, a number of important drug interactions can alter theophylline metabolism. Clearance falls with the concurrent use of erythromycin and other macrolide antibiotics, the quinolone antibiotics, and troleandomycin, allopurinol, cimetidine, and propranolol. It rises with use of cigarettes, marijuana, phenobarbital, phenytoin, or any other drug that is capable of inducing hepatic microsomal enzymes.

For maintenance therapy, long-acting theophylline compounds are available and are usually given once or twice daily. The dose is adjusted on the basis of the clinical response with the aid of serum theophylline measurements. Single-dose administration in the evening reduces nocturnal symptoms and helps keep the patient complaint-free during the day. Aminophylline and theophylline are available for intravenous use. The recommendations for intravenous therapy in children aged 9 to 16 and in young adult smokers not currently receiving theophylline products are a loading dose of 6 mg/kg followed by an infusion of 1 mg/kg per hour for the next 12 h and then 0.8 mg/kg per hour thereafter. In nonsmoking adults, older patients, and those with cor pulmonale, congestive heart failure, and liver disease, the loading dose remains the same, but the maintenance dose is reduced to between 0.1 and 0.5 mg/kg per hour. In patients already receiving theophylline, the loading dose is frequently withheld or, in extreme situations, reduced to 0.5 mg/kg.

The most common side effects of theophylline are nervousness, nausea, vomiting, anorexia, and headache. At plasma levels greater than 30 μg/mL there is a risk of seizures and cardiac arrhythmias.

Anticholinergics Anticholinergic drugs such as atropine sulfate produce bronchodilation in patients with asthma, but their use is limited by systemic side effects. Nonabsorbable quaternary ammonium congeners (atropine methylnitrate and ipratropium bromide) have been found to be both effective and free of untoward effects. They may be of particular benefit for patients with coexistent heart disease, in whom the use of methylxanthines and β-adrenergic stimulants may be dangerous. The major disadvantages of the anticholinergics are that they are slow to act (60 to 90 min may be required before peak bronchodilation is achieved) and they are only of modest potency.

Glucocorticoids Glucocorticoids are the most potent and most effective anti-inflammatory medications available. Systemic or oral steroids are most beneficial in acute illness when severe airway obstruction is not resolving or is worsening despite intense optimal bronchodilator therapy, and in chronic disease when there has been failure of a previously optimal regimen with frequent recurrences of symptoms of increasing severity. Inhaled glucocorticoids are used in the long-term control of asthma.

Glucocorticoids are not bronchodilators and the correct dose to use in acute situations is a matter of debate. The available data indicate that very high doses do not offer any advantage over more conventional amounts. In the United States, a usual starting dose is 40 to 60 mg of methylprednisolone intravenously every 6 h. Since intravenous and oral administration produce the same effects, prednisone, 60 mg every 6 h, can be substituted. Clinical impressions suggest that smaller quantities may work as effectively, but there are no confirmatory data. In the United Kingdom and elsewhere, acute asthma both in and out of hospital is frequently treated with doses of prednisolone ranging from 30 to 40 mg given once daily. It should be emphasized that the effects of steroids in acute asthma are not immediate and may not be seen for 6 h or more after the initial administration. Consequently, it is mandatory to continue vigorous bronchodilator therapy during this interval. Irrespective of the regimen chosen, it is important to appreciate that rapid tapering of glucocorticoids frequently results in recurrent obstruction. Most authorities recommend reducing the dose by one-half every third to fifth day after an acute episode. In situations in which it appears that continued steroid therapy will be needed, an alternate-day schedule should be instituted to minimize side effects. This is particularly important in children, since continuous glucocorticoid administration interrupts growth. Long-acting preparations such as dexamethasone should not be used in this approach, for they defeat the purpose of alternate-day schedules by causing prolonged suppression of the pituitary-adrenal axis. The availability of inhaled agents has all but eliminated the need for this form of therapy.

INHALED GLUCOCORTICOIDS These drugs are indicated in patients with persistent symptoms. The agents currently available in the United States are beclomethasone, budesonide, flunisolide, fluticasone propionate, and triamcinolone acetonide. Each has relative advantages and disadvantages, and they are not absolutely interchangeable on either a microgram or a per puff basis. However, all of these drugs share the ability to control inflammation, facilitate the long-term prevention of symptoms, and reduce the need for oral glucocorticoids.

There is no fixed dose of inhaled steroid that works for all patients. Requirements are dictated by the response of the individual and wax and wane in concert with progression of the disease. Generally, the worse the patient's condition, the more inhaled steroid is needed to gain control. Once achieved, however, remission can often be maintained with quantities as low as one or two puffs/day. Inhaled steroids can take up to a week or more to produce improvements; consequently, in rapidly deteriorating situations, it is best to prescribe oral preparations and initiate inhaled drugs as the dose of the former is reduced. In less emergent circumstances, the quantity of inhaled drug can be increased up to 2 to 2.5 times the recommended starting doses. It is critical to remember that the side effects increase in proportion to the dose-time product. In addition to thrush and dysphonia, the increased systemic absorption that accompanies larger doses of inhaled steroids has been reported to produce adrenal suppression, cataract formation, decreased growth in children, interference with bone metabolism, and purpura. As is the case with oral agents, suppression of inflammation, per se, cannot be relied upon to provide optimal results. It is essential to continue adrenergic or methylxanthine bronchodilators if the patient's disease is unstable.

Mast cell–stabilizing agents   Cromolyn sodium and nedocromil sodium do not influence airway tone. Their major therapeutic effect is to inhibit the degranulation of mast cells, thereby preventing the release of the chemical mediators of anaphylaxis.

Cromolyn sodium and nedocromil, like the inhaled steroids, improve lung function, reduce symptoms, and lower airway reactivity in persons with asthma. They are most effective in atopic patients who have either seasonal disease or perennial airway stimulation. A therapeutic trial of two puffs four times daily for 4 to 6 weeks frequently is necessary before the beneficial effects of the drug appear. Unlike steroids, nedocromil and cromolyn sodium, when given prophylactically, block the acute obstructive effects of exposure to antigen, industrial chemicals, exercise, or cold air. With antigen, the late response is also abolished. Therefore, a patient who has intermittent exposure to either antigenic or nonantigenic stimuli that provoke acute episodes of asthma need not use these drugs continuously but instead can obtain protection by taking the drug only 15 to 20 min before contact with the precipitant.

Leukotriene modifiers   As mentioned earlier, the cysteinyl leukotrienes (LTC_4, LTD_4, and LTE_4) produce many of the critical elements of asthma, and drugs have been developed to either reduce the synthesis of all of the leukotrienes by inhibiting 5-lipoxygenase (5-LO), the enzyme involved in their production, or competitively antagonizing the principal moiety (LTD_4). Zileuton is the only 5-lipoxygenase synthesis inhibitor that is available in the United States. It is a modest bronchodilator that reduces asthma morbidity, provides protection against exercise-induced asthma, and diminishes nocturnal symptoms, but it has limited effectiveness against allergens. Hepatic enzyme levels can be elevated after its use, and there are significant interactions with other drugs metabolized in the liver. The LTD_4 receptor antagonists (zafirlukast and montelukast) have therapeutic and toxicologic profiles similar to that of zileuton but are long acting and permit twice to single daily dose schedules.

This class of drugs does not appear to be uniformly effective in all patients with asthma. Although precise figures are lacking, most authorities put the number of positive responders at less than 50%. As yet, there is no way of determining prospectively who will benefit, so clinical trials are required. Typically, if there is no improvement after one month, treatment can be discontinued.

Miscellaneous agents   It has been suggested that steroid-dependent patients might benefit from the use of immunosuppressant agents such as methotrexate or gold salts. The effects of these agents on steroid dosage and disease activity are minor, and side effects can be considerable. Consequently, this form of treatment can be viewed only as experimental. Opiates, sedatives, and tranquilizers should be absolutely avoided in the acutely ill patient with asthma because the risk of depressing alveolar ventilation is great, and respiratory arrest has been reported to occur shortly after their use. Admittedly, most individuals are anxious and frightened, but experience has shown that they can be calmed equally well by the physician's presence and reassurances. β-Adrenergic blockers and parasympathetic agonists are contraindicated because they can cause marked deterioration in lung function.

Expectorants and mucolytic agents have enjoyed great vogue in the past, but they do not add significantly to the treatment of the acute or chronic phases of this disease. Mucolytic agents such as acetylcysteine may actually produce bronchospasm when administered to susceptible patients with asthma. This effect can be overcome by aerosolizing them in solution with a β-adrenergic agent. The use of intravenous fluids in the treatment of acute asthma also has been advocated. There is little evidence that this adjunct hastens recovery. Nonstandard bronchodilators, such as intravenous magnesium sulfate, for the treatment of acute asthma attacks are not yet warranted in clinical practice because of the controversy surrounding their efficacy.

Special instructions   The treatment of patients with asthma who have coexisting conditions such as heart disease or pregnancy does not differ materially from that outlined above. Therapy with inhaled β_2-selective and anti-inflammatory agents is the mainstay. The lowest doses of adrenergics that produce the desired effects should be used.

FRAMEWORK FOR MANAGEMENT   Emergency Situations   The most effective treatment for acute episodes of asthma requires a systematic approach based on the aggressive use of sympathomimetic agents and serial monitoring of key indices of improvement. Reliance on empirism and subjective assessment is no longer acceptable. Multiple inhalations of a short-acting sympathomimetic, such as albuterol, are the cornerstone of most regimens. These drugs provide three to four times more relief than does intravenous aminophylline. Anticholinergic drugs are not first-line therapy because of their long lag time to onset ($\sim$ 30 to 40 min) and their relatively modest bronchodilator properties. In emergency situations, β_2 agonists can be given every 20 min by handheld nebulizer for 2 to 3 doses. The optimum cumulative dose of albuterol appears to lie between 5 and 10 mg. It does not matter how the adrenergic agonists are inhaled. Treatment with albuterol administered by jet nebulizer, metered dose inhaler, or dry powder inhaler all provide equal resolution in acute situations. Aminophylline or ipratropium can be added to the regimen after the first hour in an attempt to speed resolution. Recent studies in a large series of patients demonstrate that β_2 agonists alone terminate attacks in approximately two-thirds of patients, and that another 5 to 10% benefit from a methylxanthine or ipratropium in combination with a sympathomimetic. The remainder have a poor acute response to all forms of therapy.

Acute episodes of bronchial asthma are one of the most common respiratory emergencies seen in the practice of medicine, and it is essential that the physician recognize which episodes of airway obstruction are life-threatening and which patients demand what level of care. These distinctions can be made readily by assessing selected clinical parameters in combination with measures of expiratory flow and gas exchange. The presence of a paradoxical pulse, use of accessory muscles, and marked hyperinflation of the thorax signify severe airways obstruction, and failure of these signs to remit promptly after aggressive therapy mandates objective monitoring of the patient with measurements of arterial blood gases and the peak expiratory flow rate (PEFR) or FEV_1.

In general, there is a correlation between the severity of the obstruction with which the patient presents and the time it takes to resolve it. Those individuals with the most impairment typically require the most extensive therapy for resolution. If the PEFR or FEV_1 is equal to or less than 20% of predicted on presentation and does not double within an hour of receiving the preceding therapy, the patient is likely to require extensive treatment including glucocorticoids before the obstruction dissipates. This group represents approximately 20% of all the patients who present for acute care. They generally require 3 to 4 days of inpatient treatment before becoming asymptomatic. In such individuals, if the clinical signs of a paradoxical pulse and accessory muscle use are diminishing, and/or if PEFR is increasing, there is no need to change medications or doses; the patient need only be followed. However, if the PEFR falls by more than 20% of its previous value or if the magnitude of the pulsus paradoxicus is increasing, serial measures of arterial blood gases are required, as well as a reconsideration of the therapeutic modalities being employed. If the patient has hypocarbia, one can afford to continue the current approaches a while longer. On the other hand, if the Pa_{CO_2} is within the normal range or is elevated, the patient should be monitored in an intensive care setting, and therapy should be intensified to reverse or arrest the patient's respiratory failure.

Chronic Treatment The goal of chronic therapy is to achieve a stable, asymptomatic state with the best pulmonary function possible using the least amount of medication. The first step is to educate patients to function as partners in their management. The severity of the illness needs to be assessed and monitored with objective measures of lung function. Asthma triggers should be avoided or controlled, and plans should be made for both chronic management and treatment of exacerbations. Regular follow-up care is mandatory. With respect to pharmacologic interventions, in general, the simplest approach works best. Infrequent symptoms require only the use of an inhaled sympathomimetic on an "as needed" basis. When the disease worsens, as manifested by nocturnal awakenings and daytime symptoms, inhaled steroids and/or mast cell–stabilizing agents should be added. If symptoms do not abate, the dose of inhaled steroids can be increased. An upper limit has not yet been established, but side effects of glucocorticoid excess begin to appear more frequently when the dose exceeds 2.0 mg/d. Persistent asthma complaints can be treated with long-acting inhaled β_2 agonists, sustained-release theophylline, and/or parasympatholytics. In patients with recurrent or perennial symptoms and unstable lung function, oral steroids in a single daily dose are added to the regimen. Once control is reached and sustained for several weeks, a step-down reduction in therapy should be undertaken, beginning with the most toxic drug, to find the minimum amount of medication required to keep the patient well. During this process, the PEFR should be monitored and medication adjustments should be based on objective changes in lung function as well as on the patient's symptoms.

PROGNOSIS AND CLINICAL COURSE The mortality rate from asthma is small. The most recent figures indicate fewer than 5000 deaths per year out of a population of approximately 10 million patients at risk. Death rates, however, appear to be rising in inner-city areas where there is limited availability of health care.

Information on the clinical course of asthma suggests a good prognosis particularly for those whose disease is mild and develops in childhood. The number of children who still have asthma 7 to 10 years after the initial diagnosis varies from 26 to 78%, averaging 46%; however, the percentage who continue to have severe disease is relatively low (6 to 19%).

Although there are reports of patients with asthma developing irreversible changes in lung function, these individuals frequently have comorbid stimuli such as cigarette smoking that could account for these findings. Even when untreated, individuals with asthma do not continuously move from mild to severe disease with time. Rather, their clinical course is characterized by exacerbations and remissions. Some studies suggest that spontaneous remissions occur in approximately 20% of those who develop the disease as adults and that 40% or so can be expected to experience improvement, with less frequent and severe attacks, as they grow older.

BIBLIOGRAPHY

AMERICAN THORACIC SOCIETY: Guidelines for the evaluation of impairment/disability in patients with asthma. Am Rev Respir Dis 147:1056, 1993

———: Progress of the interface of inflammation and asthma. Am J Respir Crit Care Med 152:385, 1995

BARNES PJ, ADCOCK IM: Transcription factors and asthma. Eur Respir J 12:221, 1998

BURR ML: Epidemiology of asthma. Monogr Allergy 31:80, 1993

HOLGATE ST: The cellular and mediator basis of asthma in relation to natural history. Lancet 350 (Suppl 2):5, 1997

MCFADDEN ER JR: Evolving concepts in the pathogenesis and management of asthma. Adv Intern Med 39:357, 1994

———, GILBERT IA: Exercise-induced asthma. N Engl J Med 330:1362, 1994

——— et al: Protocol therapy for acute asthma: Therapeutic benefits and cost savings. Am J Med 99:651, 1995

——— et al: Comparison of two dose regimens of albuterol in acute asthma. Am J Med 105:12, 1998

SANDFORD A et al: The genetics of asthma. Am J Respir Crit Care Med 153:1749, 1996

SHEFFER AL, TAGGART VS: The National Asthma Education Program. Expert panel report guidelines for the diagnosis and management of asthma. Med Care 31:MS20, 1993

WARDLAW AJ: The role of air pollution in asthma. Clin Exp Allergy 23:81, 1993

253

Joel N. Kline, Gary W. Hunninghake

HYPERSENSITIVITY PNEUMONITIS AND PULMONARY INFILTRATES WITH EOSINOPHILIA

HYPERSENSITIVITY PNEUMONITIS

Hypersensitivity pneumonitis (HP), or extrinsic allergic alveolitis, is an immunologically induced inflammatory disorder of the lung parenchyma, involving alveolar walls and terminal airways, secondary to repeated inhalation of a variety of organic agents by a susceptible host. Causes of HP are typically designated with colorful names denoting the occupational or avocational risk associated with the disease; "farmer's lung" is the term most commonly used for HP due to inhalation of antigens present in moldy hay, such as thermophilic actinomyces, *Micropolyspora faeni*, and *Aspergillus* species. The prevalence of HP is unknown but varies with the environmental exposure and the specific antigen involved. The prevalence of farmer's lung among Wisconsin dairy farmers has been reported as 4.2 per 1000. The diagnosis of HP requires a constellation of clinical, radiographic, physiologic, pathologic, and immunologic criteria, each of which is rarely pathognomonic alone; and the preferred treatment is avoidance of the causative antigen when practical.

ETIOLOGY Agents implicated as causes of HP include those listed in Table 253-1. Many cases of HP occurring in various occupations involve exposure to similar agents, particularly the thermophilic actinomycetes. In the United States, the most common types of HP are farmer's lung, bird fancier's lung, and chemical worker's lung. In *farmer's lung*, inhalation of proteins such as thermophilic bacteria and fungal spores that are present in moldy bedding and feed are most commonly responsible for the development of HP. These antigens are probably also responsible for the etiology of *mushroom worker's disease* (moldy composted growth medium is the source of the proteins) and *bagassosis* (moldy sugar cane is the source). *Bird fancier's lung* (and the related disorders of duck fever, turkey handler's lung, and dove pillow's lung) is a response to inhalation of bird proteins from feathers and droppings. *Chemical worker's lung* is an example of how simple chemicals, such as isocyanates, may also cause immune-mediated diseases. In this case, antihapten antibodies may be responsible for the development of HP.

PATHOGENESIS The finding that precipitating antibodies against extracts of moldy hay were demonstrable in most patients with farmer's lung led to the early conclusion that HP was an immune-complex–mediated reaction. Subsequent investigations of HP in humans and animal models provided evidence for the importance of cell-mediated hypersensitivity. The very early (acute) reaction is characterized by an increase in polymorphonuclear leukocytes in the alveoli and small airways. This early lesion is followed by an influx of mononuclear cells into the lung and the formation of granulomas that appear to be the result of a classic delayed (T cell mediated) hypersensitivity reaction to repeated inhalation of antigen and adjuvant-active materials. Recent studies in animal models suggest that the disease is mediated as a classic T_H1 cell-mediated immune response to antigen.

Bronchoalveolar lavage in patients with HP consistently demonstrates an increase in the number of T lymphocytes in lavage fluid (a finding that is also observed in patients with other granulomatous lung disorders). Patients with recent or continual exposure to antigen may have an increase in the number of polymorphonuclear leukocytes in lavage fluid. Increased numbers of mast cells have also been reported. In most patients examined during recovery from acute disease, the T lymphocytes in lavage fluid are predominantly the CD8+ T cell subset.

Table 253-1   Selected Examples of Hypersensitivity Pneumonitis (HP)

Disease	Antigen	Source of Antigen
Bagassosis	Thermophilic actinomycetes[a]	"Moldy" bagasse (sugar cane)
Bird fancier's, breeder's, or han-dler's lung[b]	Parakeet, pigeon, chicken, turkey proteins	Avian droppings or feathers
Cephalosporium HP	Contaminated basement (sewage)	Cephalosporium
Cheese washer's lung	Penicillium casei	Moldy cheese
Chemical worker's lung[b]	Isocyanates	Polyurethane foam, varnishes, lac-quer
Coffee worker's lung	Coffee bean dust	Coffee beans
Compost lung	Aspergillus	Compost
Detergent worker's disease	Bacillus subtilis enzymes	Detergent
Familial HP	B. subtilis	Contaminated wood dust in walls
Farmer's lung[b]	Thermophilic actinomycetes[a]	"Moldy" hay, grain, silage
Fish meal worker's lung	Fish meal dust	Fish meal
Furrier's lung	Animal fur dust	Animal pelts
Hot tub lung	Cladosporium sp.	Mold on ceiling
Humidifier or air-conditioner lung (ventilation pneumonitis)	Aureobasidium pullulans or other microorganisms	Contaminated water in humidifica-tion or forced-air air-conditioning systems
Japanese summer house HP	Trichosporon cutaneum	House dust? Bird droppings
Laboratory worker's HP	Male rat urine	Laboratory rat
Lycoperdonosis	Lycoperdon puffballs	Puffball spores
Malt worker's lung	A. fumigatus or A. clavatus	Moldy barley
Maple bark disease	Cryptostroma corticale	Maple bark
Miller's lung	Sitophilus granarius (wheat wee-vil)	Infested wheat flour
Mushroom worker's lung	Thermophilic actinomycetes,[a] other	Mushroom compost
Paulis HP	Paulis reagent	Laboratory reagent
Pituitary snuff taker's lung	Animal proteins	Heterologous pituitary snuff
Potato riddler's lung	Thermophilic actinomycetes,[a] Aspergillus	"Moldy" hay around potatoes
Sauna taker's lung	Aureobasidium sp., other	Contaminated sauna water
Sequoiosis	Aureobasidium, Graphium sp.	Redwood sawdust
Streptomyces albus HP	Streptomyces albus	Contaminated fertilizer
Suberosis	Cork dust mold	Cork dust
Tap water lung	Unknown	Contaminated tap water
Thatched roof disease	Saccharomonospora viridis	Dried grasses and leaves
Tobacco worker's disease	Aspergillus sp.	Mold on tobacco
Winegrower's lung	Botrytis cinerea	Mold on grapes
Wood trimmer's disease	Rhizopus sp., Mucor sp.	Contaminated wood trimmings
Woodman's disease	Penicillium sp.	Oak and maple trees
Woodworker's lung	Wood dust, Alternaria	Oak, cedar, pine, and mahogany dusts

[a] Thermophilic actinomycetes species include Micropolyspora faeni, Thermoactinomyces vulgaris, T. saccharrii, T. viridis, and T. candidus.

[b] Most common causes of hypersensitivity pneumonitis in the United States.

In patients with very recent exposure to antigen, however, the numbers of CD4+ T cells may increase in lavage fluid. Similar findings may be present in similarly exposed, asymptomatic individuals. These observations and others in animal models suggest that there is an active modulation of granuloma formation in the lung by immunoregulatory T cells and associated cytokines in this disorder.

CLINICAL PRESENTATION   The clinical picture is that of an interstitial pneumonitis, although it varies from patient to patient and seems related to the frequency and intensity of exposure to the causative antigen and perhaps other host factors. The presentation can be *acute, subacute,* or *chronic.* In the *acute form,* symptoms such as cough, fever, chills, malaise, and dyspnea may occur 6 to 8 h after exposure to the antigen and usually clear within a few days if there is no further exposure to antigen. The *subacute form* often appears insidiously over a period of weeks marked by cough and dyspnea and may progress to cyanosis and severe dyspnea requiring hospitalization. In some patients, a subacute form of the disease may persist after an acute presentation of the disorder, especially if there is continued exposure to antigen. In most patients with the acute or subacute form of HP, the symptoms, signs, and other manifestations of HP disappear within days, weeks, or months if the causative agent is no longer inhaled. Transformation to a chronic form of the disease may occur in patients with continued antigen exposure, but the frequency of such

progression is uncertain. The *chronic form* of HP may be clinically indistinguishable from pulmonary fibrosis due to a wide variety of causes. Physical examination may reveal clubbing. This stage may progressively worsen, resulting in dependence on supplemental O_2, pulmonary hypertension, and death from respiratory failure. An indolent gradually progressive form of the disease can be associated with cough and exertional dyspnea without a prior history consistent with acute or subacute manifestations. Such a gradual onset frequently occurs with low-dose exposure to the antigen.

Because strict definitions of acute, subacute, and chronic stages of HP have not been generally agreed on, interpretation of epidemiologic and clinical studies can be difficult. Therefore, it has been proposed that HP be described as recently diagnosed, recurrent or progressive, or residual disease. For these categories, required diagnostic criteria include the presence of an appropriate exposure; exertional dyspnea; inspiratory crackles; and, if performed, lymphocytic alveolitis on bronchoalveolar lavage. Supportive criteria include recurrent febrile episodes, radiographic infiltrates, diminished pulmonary diffusing capacity, precipitating antibodies to appropriate antigens, histopathologic demonstration of granulomas, and improvement in symptoms with avoidance of exposure.

DIAGNOSIS   After acute exposure to antigen, neutrophilia and lymphopenia are frequently present. Eosinophilia is not a feature. All forms of the disease may be associated with elevations in erythrocyte sedimentation rate, C-reactive protein, rheumatoid factor, and serum immunoglobulins. Antinuclear antibodies are rarely present and appear to have no pathogenic role. Examination for *serum precipitins* against suspected antigens, such as those listed in Table 253-1, is an important part of the diagnostic workup and should be performed on any patient with interstitial lung disease, especially if a suggestive exposure history is elicited. If found, precipitins indicate sufficient exposure to the causative agent for generation of an immunologic response. The diagnosis of HP is not established solely by the presence of precipitins, however, as precipitins are found in sera of many individuals exposed to appropriate antigens who demonstrate no other evidence of HP. False-negative results may occur because of poor-quality antigens or an inappropriate choice of antigens. Extraction of antigens from the suspected source may at times be helpful.

No specific or distinctive *chest roentgenogram* occurs in HP. It can be normal even in symptomatic patients. The acute or subacute phase may be associated with poorly defined, patchy, or diffuse infiltrates or with discrete, nodular infiltrates (Fig. 253-1). In the chronic phase, the chest x-ray usually shows a diffuse reticulonodular infiltrate. Honeycombing may eventually develop as the condition progresses. Apical sparing is common, suggesting that disease severity correlates with inhaled antigen load, but no particular distribution or pattern is classic for HP. Abnormalities rarely seen in HP include pleural effusion or thickening, and hilar adenopathy. High-resolution chest computed tomography (CT) has been reported to show a characteristic constellation of abnormalities, including (1) global lung involvement with increased lung density, (2) prominence of medium-sized bronchial walls, (3) patchy air space opacification with reticular and nodular patterns and midzone prominence, and (4) absence of hilar lymph node enlargement. No pathognomonic CT features of HP have been described (Fig. 253-2).

Pulmonary function studies in all forms of HP may show a restrictive or obstructive pattern with loss of lung volumes, impaired diffusion capacity, decreased compliance, and an exercise-induced hypoxemia. Resting hypoxemia may also be found. Bronchospasm and bronchial hyperreactivity are sometimes found in acute HP. With antigen avoidance, the pulmonary function abnormalities are usually reversible, but they may gradually increase in severity or may occur rapidly after acute or subacute exposure to antigen.

Bronchoalveolar lavage is used in some centers to aid in diagnostic evaluation. A marked lymphocytic alveolitis on bronchoalveolar lavage is almost universal, although not pathognomonic. Lymphocytes typically have a decreased helper/suppressor ratio and are activated. Alveolar neutrophilia is also prominent acutely but tends to fade in the absence of recurrent exposure. Bronchoalveolar mastocytosis may correlate with disease activity. *Lung biopsy*, obtained through flexible bronchoscopy, open-lung procedures, or thoracoscopy, may be diagnostic. Although the histopathology is distinctive, it may not be pathognomonic of HP. When the biopsy is taken during the active phase of disease, typical findings include an interstitial alveolar infiltrate consisting of plasma cells, lymphocytes, and occasional eosinophils and neutrophils, usually with accompanying granulomas. Interstitial fibrosis may be present but most often is mild in earlier stages of the disease. Some degree of bronchiolitis is found in about half the cases, whereas vasculitis is not a feature of the disorder. The triad of mononuclear bronchiolitis; interstitial infiltrates of lymphocytes and plasma cells; and single, nonnecrotizing, and randomly scattered parenchymal granulomas without mural vascular involvement is consistent with but not specific for HP.

Inhalation challenge studies have been described as useful to differentiate between HP and other interstitial lung diseases. These tests should be performed in a center that specializes in provocation testing for reasons of both safety and accuracy. Moveover, because the antigens used for provocation testing are not standardized, interpretation of these tests is difficult. In general, these tests may be used to support a diagnosis of HP, but they are not sufficiently accepted to either confirm or deny the diagnosis. The lack of standardized, nonirritating antigens and of proven controlled protocols makes *skin testing* useful only for research purposes. Similarly, in vitro tests of cell-mediated (delayed) hypersensitivity have not consistently been shown to correlate with clinical HP and have no place in the routine diagnostic workup.

In summary, the diagnosis in most cases is established by (1) consistent history, physical findings, pulmonary function tests, and chest x-ray; (2) exposure to a recognized antigen; and (3) finding an antibody to that antigen. In a few circumstances, bronchoalveolar lavage and/ or lung biopsy may be needed. Provocation tests may be useful but are not essential for the diagnosis.

DIFFERENTIAL DIAGNOSIS Chronic HP may often be difficult to distinguish from a number of other interstitial lung disorders such as idiopathic pulmonary fibrosis, sarcoidosis, interstitial lung disease associated with a collagen vascular disorder, and drug-induced lung diseases. A negative history for use of relevant drugs and no evidence of a systemic disorder usually exclude the presence of drug-induced lung disease or a collagen vascular disorder. Bronchoalveolar lavage often shows predominance of neutrophils in idiopathic pulmonary fibrosis and a predominance of CD4+ lymphocytes in sarcoidosis. Hilar/paratracheal lymphadenopathy or evidence of multisystem involvement also favors the diagnosis of sarcoidosis. In some patients, a lung biopsy may be required to differentiate chronic HP from other interstitial diseases. The lung disease associated with acute or subacute HP may clinically resemble other disorders that present

FIGURE 253-1 Chest X-ray of acute HP demonstrating interstitial infiltrates most prominently in the lower lung fields bilaterally. *(Courtesy of JS Wilson.)*

with systemic symptoms and recurrent pulmonary infiltrates, including the allergic bronchopulmonary mycoses and other eosinophilic pneumonias.

Eosinophilic pneumonia is often associated with asthma and is typified by peripheral eosinophilia; neither of these is a feature of HP. Allergic bronchopulmonary aspergillosis (ABPA) is the most common example of the allergic bronchopulmonary mycoses and is sometimes confused with HP because of the presence of precipitating antibodies to *A. fumigatus*. ABPA is associated with allergic (atopic) asthma. Acute HP may be confused with *organic dust toxic syndrome* (ODTS), a condition that is more common than HP. ODTS follows heavy exposure to organic dusts and is characterized by transient fever and muscle aches, with or without dyspnea and cough. Serum precipitins are absent, and the chest x-ray is usually normal. Studies have shown no immunologic basis for ODTS, and endotoxin is suspected to be involved in its pathogenesis. This distinction is important, as ODTS is a self-limited disorder without significant long-term sequellae, whereas continued antigen exposure in HP can result in permanent disability. Massive exposure to moldy silage may result in a syndrome

FIGURE 253-2 Chest CT scan of a case of acute hypersensitivity pneumonitis in which scattered regions of ground glass and nodular infiltrates are seen bilaterally. *(Courtesy of JS Wilson.)*

termed *pulmonary mycotoxicosis*, or *atypical farmer's lung*, with fever, chills, and cough and the presence of pulmonary infiltrates within a few hours of exposure. No previous sensitization is required, and precipitins are absent to *Aspergillus*, the suspected causative agent.

℞ **TREATMENT**   Because effective treatment depends largely on avoiding the antigen, identification of the causative agent and its source is essential. This identification is usually possible if the physician takes a careful environmental and occupational history or, if necessary, visits the patient's environment. The simplest way to avoid the incriminated agent is to remove the patient from the environment or the source of the agent from the patient's environment. This recommendation cannot be taken lightly when it completely changes the life-style or livelihood of the patient. In many cases, however, the source of exposure (birds, humidifiers) can easily be removed. If occupational exposure is involved, an initial attempt can be made at antigen avoidance maneuvers that are least disruptive to the patient's livelihood, which usually means avoiding areas associated with heavy exposure and wearing an appropriate mask. This will not protect against small-molecular-weight agents such as isocyanates, which require more elaborate respiratory systems. Pollen masks, personal dust respirators, airstream helmets, and ventilated helmets with a supply of fresh air are increasingly efficient means of purifying inhaled air. If symptoms recur or physiologic abnormalities progress in spite of these measures, then more effective measures to avoid antigen exposure must be pursued. Compromises with environmental control pertain primarily to the acute, recurrent, transient clinical form of HP and must be accompanied by careful follow-up. Subacute forms are ordinarily the result of a heavy, sustained exposure. The chronic form typically results from low-grade or recurrent exposure over many months or years, and the lung disease may already be partially irreversible. These patients are usually advised to avoid completely all possible contact with the offending agent, although follow-up studies of individuals with farmer's lung and bird fancier's lung have found resolution of the disease despite continued exposure in some patients.

Patients with the *acute*, recurrent form of HP usually recover without need for glucocorticoids. *Subacute* HP may be associated with severe symptoms and marked physiologic impairment and may continue to progress for several days despite hospitalization. Urgent establishment of the diagnosis and prompt institution of glucocorticoid treatment are indicated in such patients. Such therapy may also hasten recovery in patients with lesser involvement. Prednisone at a dosage of 1 mg/kg per day or its equivalent is continued for 7 to 14 days and then tapered over the ensuing 2 to 6 weeks at a rate that depends on the patient's clinical status. Patients with *chronic* HP may gradually recover without therapy after the institution of environmental control. In many patients, however, a trial of prednisone may be useful to obtain maximal reversibility of the lung disease. After initial prednisone therapy (1 mg/kg per day for 2 to 4 weeks), the drug is tapered to the lowest dosage that will maintain the functional status of the patient. Many patients will not require or benefit from long-term therapy if there is no further exposure to antigen. Available studies report no effect of glucocorticoid therapy on long-term prognosis of farmer's lung.

PULMONARY INFILTRATES WITH EOSINOPHILIA

Pulmonary infiltrates with eosinophilia (PIE, eosinophilic pneumonias) include distinct individual syndromes characterized by eosinophilic pulmonary infiltrates and, commonly, peripheral blood eosinophilia. Since Loeffler's initial description of a transient, benign syndrome of migratory pulmonary infiltrates and peripheral blood eosinophilia of unknown cause, this group of disorders has been enlarged to include several diseases of both known and unknown etiology (Table 253-2). These diseases may be considered as putative hypersen-

Table 253-2   Pulmonary Infiltrates with Eosinophilia

ETIOLOGY KNOWN

Allergic bronchopulmonary mycoses
Parasitic infestations
Drug reactions
Eosinophilia-myalgia syndrome

IDIOPATHIC

Loeffler's syndrome
Acute eosinophilic pneumonia
Chronic eosinophilic pneumonia
Allergic granulomatosis of Churg and Strauss
Hypereosinophilic syndrome

sitivity lung diseases but are not to be confused with HP (extrinsic allergic alveolitis), in which eosinophilia is not a feature. When an eosinophilic pneumonia is associated with bronchial asthma, it is important to determine if the patient has atopic asthma and has wheal-and-flare skin reactivity to *Aspergillus* or other relevant fungal antigens. If so, other criteria should be sought for diagnosis of ABPA (Table 253-3) or other, rarer examples of allergic bronchopulmonary mycosis such as those caused by *Penicillium*, *Candida*, *Curvularia*, or *Helminthosporium* spp. *A. fumigatus* is the most common cause of ABPA, although other *Aspergillus* species have also been implicated. ABPA has been reported to complicate cystic fibrosis. The chest roentgenogram in ABPA may show transient, recurrent infiltrates or may suggest the presence of proximal bronchiectasis. High-resolution chest CT is a sensitive, noninvasive technique for the recognition of proximal bronchiectasis. The bronchial asthma of ABPA likely involves an IgE-mediated hypersensitivity, whereas the bronchiectasis associated with this disorder is thought to result from a deposition of immune complexes in proximal airways. Treatment usually requires the long-term use of systemic glucocorticoids.

Tropical eosinophilia is usually caused by filarial infection; however, eosinophilic pneumonias also occur with other parasites such as *Ascaris*, *Ancyclostoma* sp., *Toxocara* sp., and *Strongyloides stercoralis*. Tropical eosinophilia due to *Wuchereria bancrofti* or *W. malayi* occurs most commonly in southern Asia, Africa, and South America, and is treated successfully with diethylcarbamazine.

Drug-induced eosinophilic pneumonias are exemplified by acute reactions to nitrofurantoin, which may begin 2 h to 10 days after nitrofurantoin is started, with symptoms of dry cough, fever, chills, and dyspnea; an eosinophilic pleural effusion accompanying patchy or diffuse pulmonary infiltrates may also occur. Other drugs associated with eosinophilic pneumonias include sulfonamides, penicillin, chlorpropamide, thiazides, tricyclic antidepressants, hydralazine, mephenesin, mecamylamine, nickel carbonyl vapor, gold salts, isoniazid, para-aminosalicylic acid, and others. Treatment consists of withdrawal of the incriminated drugs and the use of glucocorticoids, if necessary. The eosinophilia-myalgia syndrome, caused by dietary supplements of L-tryptophan, is occasionally associated with pulmonary infiltrates.

Table 253-3   Diagnostic Features of Allergic Bronchopulmonary Aspergillosis (ABPA)

MAIN DIAGNOSTIC CRITERIA

Bronchial asthma
Pulmonary infiltrates
Peripheral eosinophilia ($>1000/\mu L$)
Immediate wheal-and-flare response to *A. fumigatus*
Serum precipitins to *A. fumigatus*
Elevated serum IgE
Central bronchiectasis

OTHER DIAGNOSTIC FEATURES

History of brownish plugs in sputum
Culture of *A. fumigatus* from sputum
Elevated IgE (and IgG) class antibodies specific for *A. fumigatus*

The group of idiopathic eosinophilic pneumonias consists of diseases of varying severity. *Loeffler's syndrome* was originally reported as a benign, acute eosinophilic pneumonia of unknown cause characterized by migrating pulmonary infiltrates and minimal clinical manifestations. In some patients, these clinical characteristics may prove to be secondary to parasites or drugs. *Acute eosinophilic pneumonia* has been described recently as an idiopathic acute febrile illness lasting less than 7 days with severe hypoxemia, pulmonary infiltrates, and no history of asthma. *Chronic eosinophilic pneumonia* presents with significant systemic symptoms including fever, chills, night sweats, cough, anorexia, and weight loss lasting for several weeks to months. The chest x-ray classically shows peripheral infiltrates resembling a photographic negative of pulmonary edema. Some patients also have bronchial asthma of the intrinsic or nonallergic type. Dramatic clearing of symptoms and chest x-rays is often noted within 48 h after initiation of glucocorticoid therapy.

Allergic angiitis and granulomatosis of Churg and Strauss is a multisystem vasculitic disorder that frequently involves the skin, kidney, and nervous system in addition to the lung. The disorder may occur at any age and favors persons with a history of bronchial asthma. The asthma often is progressive until the onset of fever and exaggerated eosinophilia, at which time the symptoms of asthma may ease. The illness may be fulminating and the prognosis grave unless treated aggressively with glucocorticoids and, at times, immunosuppressive therapy. The recent introduction of leukotriene-modifying agents (zafirlukast, zyleuton, and montelukast) has unmasked a number of cases of unrecognized Churg-Strauss syndrome when individuals with asthma have been weaned from glucocorticoids with the use of these antigens.

The *hypereosinophilic syndrome* is characterized by the presence of more than 1500 eosinophils per microliter of peripheral blood for 6 months or longer; lack of evidence for parasitic, allergic, or other known causes of eosinophilia; and signs or symptoms of multisystem organ dysfunction. Consistent features are blood and bone marrow eosinophilia with tissue infiltration by relatively mature eosinophils. The heart may be involved with tricuspid valve abnormalities or endomyocardial fibrosis and a restrictive, biventricular cardiomyopathy. Other organs affected typically include the lungs, liver, spleen, skin, and nervous system. Treatment consists of glucocorticoids and/or hydroxyurea, plus treatment as needed for cardiac dysfunction, which is frequently responsible for much of the morbidity and mortality in this syndrome.

BIBLIOGRAPHY

HYPERSENSITIVITY PNEUMONITIS

DENIS M: Proinflammatory cytokines in hypersensitivity pneumonitis. Am J Respir Crit Care Med 151:164, 1995

GUDMUNDSSON G et al: IL-12 modulates expression of hypersensitivity pneumonitis. J Immunol 161:991, 1998

GURNEY JW et al: Agricultural disorders of the lung. Radiographics 11:625, 1991

KOKKARINEN JI et al: Recovery of pulmonary function in farmer's lung. A five-year followup study. Am Rev Respir Dis 147:793, 1993

MARX JJ et al: Cohort studies of immunologic lung disease among Wisconsin dairy farmers. Am J Int Med 18:263, 1990

RAMIREZ-VENEGAS A et al: Utility of a provocation test for diagnosis of chronic pigeon breeder's disease. Am J Respir Crit Care Med 158:862, 1998

RICHERSON HB et al: Guidelines for the clinical evaluation of hypersensitivity pneumonitis. J Allergy Clin Immunol 84:839, 1989

ROSE CS: Hypersensitivity pneumonitis, in *Textbook of Respiratory Medicine*, Murray JF, Nadel JA (eds). Philadelphia, Saunders, 2000, pp 1867–1884

ROSE C, KING TE: Controversies in hypersensitivity pneumonitis. Am Rev Respir Dis 145:1, 1992

EOSINOPHILIC PNEUMONIA

MROUEH S, SPOCK A: Allergic bronchopulmonary aspergillosis in patients with cystic fibrosis. Chest 105:32, 1994

PATTERSON R, GREENBERGER PA, ROBERTS ML (eds): *Allergic Bronchopulmonary Aspergillosis.* Providence, RI, OceanSide Pub, 1995

ROSENOW EC III et al: Drug-induced pulmonary disease: An update. Chest 102:239, 1992

SHINTANI H et al: Acute eosinophilic pneumonia caused by cigarrette smoking. Intern Med 39:66, 2000

254 *Frank E. Speizer*

ENVIRONMENTAL LUNG DISEASES

This chapter provides perspectives on ways to assess pulmonary diseases for which environmental causes are suspected. This assessment is important because removal of the patient from a harmful environment is often the only intervention that might prevent further significant deterioration or lead to improvement in a patient's condition. Furthermore, the identification of an environment-associated disease in a single patient may lead to primary preventive strategies affecting other similarly exposed people who have not yet developed disease.

The exact magnitude of the problem is unknown, but there is no question that large numbers of people are at risk for developing serious respiratory disease as a result of occupational or environmental exposures. For example, recent estimates suggest that approximately 2.4 million workers in the United States have been exposed to crystalline silica or asbestos dust in mining and nonmining industries. Even if only 5% of these workers (a conservative estimate) are to suffer from respiratory disease as a result of their exposure, this figure represents more than 100,000 individuals.

Although industries are required to spend substantial amounts of capital in efforts to protect their workers, occupationally related respiratory diseases continue to occur. These diseases are often attributed to exposures in the past, at a time when we were not aware of the risk incurred and the need for worker protection to the degree that we are today.

HISTORY AND PHYSICAL EXAMINATION The patient's history is of paramount importance in assessing any potential occupational or environmental exposure, and the physician must ask the patient to describe a suspected environmental exposure in detail.

Inquiry into specific work practices should include questions about specific contaminants involved, the availability and use of personal respiratory protection devices, the size and ventilation of workspaces, and whether coworkers have similar complaints. In addition, the patient must be questioned about alternative sources for potentially toxic exposures, including hobbies or other environmental exposures at home. Short-term exposures to potential toxic agents in the distant past must also be considered (Chap. 391).

Many people are aware of the potential hazards in their workplaces, and many states require that employees be informed about potentially hazardous exposures. These requirements include the provision of specific educational materials (including Material Safety Data Sheets), personal protective equipment and instructions in its use, and information on environmental control procedures. Reminders posted in the workplace may warn workers about hazardous substances. Protective clothing, lockers, and shower facilities may be considered necessary parts of the job. However, even in these more progressive industries, the introduction of new processes, particularly when related to the use of new chemical compounds, may change exposure significantly, and often only the employee on the production line is aware of the change. For the physician who regularly sees patients from a particular industry, a visit to the work site can be very instructive. Alternatively, physicians can request inspections by appropriate federal and/or state authorities.

The physical examination of patients with environment-related lung diseases may help to determine the nature and severity of the pulmonary condition. Unfortunately, the pulmonary response to most injurious agents is the development of a limited number of nonspecific physical signs. These findings do not point to the specific causative agent, and other types of information must be used to arrive at an etiologic diagnosis.

PULMONARY FUNCTION TESTS AND CHEST RADIOGRAPHY   Many mineral dusts produce characteristic alterations in the mechanics of breathing and lung volumes that clearly indicate a restrictive pattern (Chaps. 250 and 259). Exposures to a number of organic dusts or chemical agents capable of producing occupational asthma result in pronounced obstructive patterns of pulmonary dysfunction that may be reversible (Chap. 252). Measurement of change in forced expiratory volume (FEV_1) before and after a working shift can be used to detect an acute inflammatory or bronchoconstrictive response. An acute decrement of FEV_1 over the first work shift of the week is a characteristic feature of cotton textile workers with byssinosis.

The chest radiograph is useful in detecting and monitoring the pulmonary response to mineral dusts. The International Labour Organization (ILO) International Classification of Radiographs of Pneumoconioses classifies chest radiographs according to the nature and size of opacities seen and the extent of involvement of the parenchyma. In general, opacities may be round or irregular, small (<10 mm in diameter) or large. They may be few in number, with visible normal lung markings, partially obscure normal markings, or totally obscure normal markings. Although useful for screening large numbers of workers, the ILO system lacks specificity and may over- or underestimate the functional impact of pneumoconiosis. With dusts causing rounded, regular opacities like those evident in coal worker's pneumoconiosis, the degree of involvement on the chest radiograph may be extensive, while pulmonary function may be only minimally impaired.

In contrast, in pneumoconiosis causing linear, irregular opacities like those seen in asbestosis, the radiograph may lead to underestimation of the severity of the impairment. It is possible for a patient to have a history of exposure, a moderately reduced forced vital capacity (FVC), and a reduced diffusion capacity in asbestosis with a relatively normal chest radiograph. The radiographic findings of irregular or linear opacities are simply more difficult to separate from normal markings until relatively late in the disease. When shadows become large, as shown in Fig. 254-1, the condition is termed *complicated pneumoconiosis*, sometimes called progressive massive fibrosis (PMF). For the individual patient with a history of exposure, conventional computed tomography (CT) and high-resolution computed tomography

FIGURE 254-1   Progressive Massive Fibrosis ILO Classification C. Lesions are bilateral relatively homogeneous, symmetric and stable over at least one year. *(With permission of the ILO International Classification of Radiographs of Pneumoconiosis–revised 1980.)*

(HRCT) have improved the sensitivity of identifying diffuse parenchymal abnormalities of the lung. The procedures have been shown to provide earlier detection of silicosis and asbestosis.

Other diagnostic procedures of use in identifying environment-induced lung disease include evaluation of heavy metal concentrations in urine (arsenic in smelter workers, cadmium in battery plant workers); bacteriologic studies (tuberculosis in medical care personnel, anthrax in wool sorters); fungal studies (coccidioidomycosis in southwestern farm workers, histoplasmosis in poultry or pigeon handlers); and serologic studies (psittacosis in pet shop workers or owners of sick birds, Q fever in tanners or slaughterhouse workers). Ultimately, a lung biopsy may be required both for morphologic diagnosis of the underlying pulmonary disease and for attempted identification of the specific etiologic agent.

MEASUREMENT OF EXPOSURE   If reliable environmental sampling data are available, this information should be used in assessing a patient's exposure. Since many of the chronic diseases result from exposure over many years, current environmental measurements should be combined with work histories to arrive at estimates of past exposure. Even in acute conditions, when monitoring of exposure may be possible, little may be known about the actual dose received by the lung. Most of the research on health effects of air pollutants (discussed later in this chapter) has relied on fixed-station monitoring of outdoor air, often at locations somewhat distant from the residences of the people being studied. In addition, most people spend less than 20% of their time outdoors. Therefore, outdoor measurements can be used only in a relative sense, and they cannot be relied on to estimate actual dose.

In situations where individual exposure to specific agents—either in a work setting or via ambient air pollutants—has been determined, transport of these agents through the airways may be an important factor affecting dose. Highly soluble gases such as sulfur dioxide are absorbed in the upper airway and presumably produce their effects by reflex response of sensitive neural fibrils in the trachea or larger airways. In contrast, nitrogen dioxide, which is less soluble, may reach the bronchioles and alveoli in sufficient quantities to result in an acute life-threatening disease in farmers exposed even briefly to the gas evolved from moldy hay in silos (silo-filler's disease).

Particle size and chemistry of air contaminants also must be considered. Particles above 10 to 15 μm in diameter, because of their settling velocities in air, do not penetrate beyond the upper airways. These larger particles are often referred to as "fugitive dusts" and include pollens, other windblown dusts, and dusts resulting from mechanical industrial processes. They have little or no role in chronic respiratory disease except perhaps as related to cancer (see below).

Particles below 10 μm in size are created by the burning of fossil fuels or high-temperature industrial processes resulting in condensation products from gases, fumes, or vapors. These particles are divided into two size fractions on the basis of their chemical characteristics. Particles of approximately 2.5 to 10 μm (coarse-mode fraction) contain crustal elements, such as silica, aluminum, and iron. These particles mostly deposit relatively high in the tracheobronchial tree. Although the total mass of an ambient sample is dominated by these larger respirable particles, the number of particles, and therefore the surface area on which potential toxic agents can deposit and be carried to the lower airways, is dominated by particles smaller than 2.5 μm (fine-mode fraction or accumulation mode). The smallest particles, those less than 0.1 μm in size, remain in the airstream and deposit in the lung only on a random basis as they come into contact with the alveolar walls.

Besides the size characteristics of particles and the solubility of gases, the actual chemical composition, mechanical properties, and immunogenicity or infectivity of inhaled material determine in large part the nature of the diseases found among exposed persons. Few studies to date have directly measured those characteristics. However, they are of increasing concern as management strategies for environmental and occupational exposures are developed.

ASBESTOSIS Except in localized regions with single industrial exposures, such as coal-mining or granite-quarrying regions, the most frequent inorganic dust-related chronic pulmonary diseases are associated with industries using *asbestiform fibers*. *Asbestos* is a generic term for several different mineral silicates, including chrysolite, amosite, anthophyllite, and crocidolite. Besides workers involved in the mining, milling, and manufacturing of asbestos products, workers in the building trades, including pipe fitters and boilermakers, were exposed to asbestos, which was widely used in construction because of its exceptional thermal and electric insulation properties. In addition, asbestos was used in the manufacture of fire-smothering blankets and safety garments, as filler for plastic materials, in cement and floor tiles, and in friction materials, such as brake and clutch linings.

Exposure to asbestos is not limited to persons who directly handle the material. Cases of asbestos-related diseases have been encountered in individuals with only moderate exposure, such as the painter or electrician who works alongside the insulation worker in a shipyard or the housewife who does no more than shake out and wash her husband's work clothes. Community exposure has probably resulted from the use of asbestos-containing material sprayed on steel girders in many large buildings as a safety feature to prevent buckling in case of fire.

Asbestos was first used extensively in the 1940s. Starting in 1975 it was mostly replaced with synthetic mineral fibers, such as fiberglass or slag wool. However, asbestos is still used in the manufacture of brake linings and remains as pipe and boiler insulation in hundreds of thousands of workplaces and homes. Despite current regulations mandating adequate training for any worker potentially exposed to asbestos, exposure probably continues among inexperienced demolition workers. The major health effects from exposure to asbestos are pulmonary fibrosis (asbestosis) and cancers of the respiratory tract, the pleura, and (in rare cases) the peritoneum.

Asbestosis is a diffuse interstitial fibrosing disease of the lung that is directly related to the intensity and duration of exposure. Except for its association with a history of exposure to asbestos (generally in a work setting), asbestosis resembles the other forms of diffuse interstitial fibrosis (Chap. 259). Usually, moderate to severe exposure has taken place for at least 10 years before the disease becomes manifest.

Physiologic studies reveal a restrictive pattern with a decrease in lung volumes. Flow rates are commonly reduced less than would be predicted on the basis of the volume reduction. An early sign of severe disease may be a reduction in diffusing capacity.

Pulmonary fibrosis may occur following sufficient exposure to any of the asbestiform fiber types. The fibrotic lesions do not appear to relate to either shape or chemical composition of any fiber type. During phagocytosis of the asbestos fiber, the membrane of the macrophage is damaged and this damage results in the release of lysosomes containing enzymes that may act to damage the lung parenchyma. The clinical manifestations are typical of those physical findings in any patient with pulmonary fibrosis (Chap. 259).

Diagnosis The chest radiograph can be used to detect a number of manifestations of asbestos exposure as well as to identify specific lesions. Past exposure is specifically indicated by pleural plaques, which are characterized by either thickening or calcification along the parietal pleura, particularly along the lower lung fields, the diaphragm, and the cardiac border. Without additional manifestations, pleural plaques imply only exposure, not pulmonary impairment. Benign pleural effusions may occur, particularly in patients with asbestosis, but are not necessarily restricted to those with overt disease. The fluid is sterile but may be a serous or blood-stained exudate and may occur bilaterally. The effusion may be slowly progressive or may resolve spontaneously.

The radiographic diagnosis of asbestosis depends on the presence of irregular or linear opacities, usually first noted in the lower lung fields and spreading into the middle and upper lung fields as the disease progresses. An indistinct heart border or a "ground glass" appearance in the lung fields is seen in some cases. As the fibrotic changes in the parenchyma begin to coalesce, the patient develops obliteration of entire acinar units, with eventual formation of the classical honeycombed lung, which appears on chest radiographs as coarse infiltrates with small (about 7- to 10-μm) air spaces. In cases in which the x-ray changes are less obvious, HRCT may show distinct changes of subpleural curvilinear lines 5 to 10 cm in length that appear to be parallel to the pleural surface; these alterations increase the positive predictive value of radiographic evidence from approximately 85% to about 100%.

In general, newly diagnosed cases will have resulted from exposure levels that were present many years before and, in spite of the patients' having left the industry, are attributable to that former exposure. Since the patient may be eligible for compensation within a specific time frame after the diagnosis of an asbestos-related disease is made, the physician making the diagnosis should be certain to inform the patient promptly. On occasion, the physician may have reason to suspect ongoing exposure from a patient's current job description or actual monitoring data. In such cases, federal or state health authorities may need to be notified. Present-day occupational safety and health regulations, if followed properly, protect workers from exposure.

Casual, nonoccupational exposure to undisturbed sources of asbestos-containing materials—e.g., in walls of schools or other buildings—represents little if any hazard to people who inhabit or work in such buildings. Because the association of smoking and asbestos exposure increases the risk of developing lung cancer (see below), it is extremely important to advise patients with a history of exposure to asbestos to stop smoking. No specific therapy is available in the management of patients with asbestosis. The supportive care is the same as that given to any patient with diffuse interstitial fibrosis from any cause.

Lung cancer (Chap. 88), either squamous cell carcinoma or adenocarcinoma, is the most frequent cancer associated with asbestos exposure. The excess frequency of lung cancer in asbestos workers is associated with a minimum lapse of 15 to 19 years between first exposure and development of the disease. Persons with more exposure are at greater risk of disease. In addition, there appears to be a significant multiplicative effect that leads to a far greater risk of lung cancer in persons who are cigarette smokers and have asbestos exposure than would be expected from the additive risk of each factor. To date, efforts to consider these high-risk individuals for special surveillance studies, including sputum cytologic examinations and repeated chest x-rays as frequently as every 4 to 6 months, have resulted in neither significant early detection nor prolonged survival once the lung cancer is found.

Mesotheliomas (Chap. 262), both pleural and peritoneal, are also associated with asbestos exposure. In contrast to lung cancers, these tumors do not appear to be associated with smoking. Relatively short-term asbestos exposures of 1 to 2 years or less occurring some 20 to 25 years in the past have been associated with the development of mesotheliomas (an observation that emphasizes the importance of obtaining a complete environmental exposure history). The risk for this type of tumor peaks 30 to 35 years after initial exposure. Since maximum exposure took place in the United States between 1930 and 1960, peak incidence of disease in men occurred in 1997, with a total of 2300 cases. Incidence is expected to decline over the next 30+ years to about 500 cases per year.

Although approximately 50% of mesotheliomas metastasize, the tumor generally is locally invasive, and death usually results from local extension. Most patients present with effusions that may obscure the underlying pleural tumor. In contrast to the findings in effusion due to other causes, because of the restriction placed on the chest wall, no shift of mediastinal structures toward the opposite side of the chest will be seen. The major diagnostic problem is differentiation from peripherally spreading pulmonary adenocarcinoma or from adenocarcinoma metastasized to pleura from an extrathoracic primary site. Although a needle biopsy may be diagnostic, an open biopsy is often necessary, and even the latter procedure may not provide a definitive diagnosis of the origin of the tumor.

Since epidemiologic studies have shown that more than 80% of mesotheliomas may be associated with asbestos exposure, documented mesothelioma in a worker with occupational exposure to asbestos may be compensable in many parts of the United States.

SILICOSIS   In spite of the technical adequacy of existing protective equipment, *free silica* (SiO_2), or crystalline quartz, is still a major occupational hazard. In the United States, estimates of potential numbers of exposed workers range between 1.2 and 3 million people. The major occupational exposures include: mining; stonecutting; employment in abrasive industries, such as stone, clay, glass, and cement manufacturing; foundry work; packing of silica flour; and quarrying, particularly of granite. Most often, progressive pulmonary fibrosis (silicosis) occurs in a dose-response fashion after many years of exposure.

Workers exposed through sandblasting in confined spaces, tunneling through rock with high quartz content (15 to 25%), or the manufacture of abrasive soaps may develop acute silicosis with as little as 10 months' exposure. The disease may be rapidly fatal in less than 2 years, despite the discontinuation of exposure. A radiographic picture of profuse miliary infiltration or consolidation is characteristic of acute silicosis.

In long-term, less intense exposure, small rounded opacities in the upper lobes, with retraction and hilar adenopathy, classically appear on the radiograph after 15 to 20 years. Calcification of hilar nodes may occur in as many as 20% of cases and produces the characteristic "eggshell" pattern. These changes may be preceded by or associated with a reticular pattern of irregular densities that are uniformly present throughout the upper lung zones.

The nodular fibrosis may be progressive in the absence of further exposure, with coalescence and formation of nonsegmental conglomerates of irregular masses in excess of 1 cm in diameter. These masses become quite large and are characteristic of PMF (Figure 254-1). Significant functional impairment with both restrictive and obstructive components may be associated with this form of silicosis. In the late stages of the disease, ventilatory failure may develop. In more subtle cases, CT may be helpful both in identifying nodules, which are preferentially located in the posterior aspect of the upper lobes, as well as in identifying larger opacities and more coalescence than might be noted on regular chest x-rays. Patients with silicosis are at greater risk of acquiring *Mycobacterium tuberculosis* infections (silicotuberculosis) and atypical mycobacterial infections. Because the frequency with which tuberculosis has been found at autopsy in patients with PMF exceeds considerably the frequency of premorbid diagnosis, treatment for tuberculosis is indicated in any patient with silicosis and a positive tuberculin test.

Other less hazardous silicates include Fuller's earth, kaolin, mica, diatomaceous earths, silica gel, soapstone, carbonate dusts, and cement dusts. The production of fibrosis in workers exposed to these agents is believed to be related either to the free silica content of these dusts or, for substances that contain no free silica, to the potentially large dust loads to which these workers may be exposed.

Other silicates, including *talc dusts*, may be contaminated with asbestos and/or free silica. Accidental exposure to significant quantities of talc may result in an acute syndrome with cough, cyanosis, and labored breathing (acute talcosis). Severe progressive fibrosis with respiratory failure may ensue within a few years. Far more common is the fibrosis and/or pleural or lung cancer associated with chronic exposure in rubber workers who use commercial talc as a lubricant in tire molds. Pure talc does not produce fibrosis; thus, it is difficult to sort out whether the effects are due to the contamination of commercial talc by asbestos or by free silica.

COAL WORKER'S PNEUMOCONIOSIS (CWP) *Coal dust* is associated with CWP, which has enormous social, economic, and medical significance in every nation in which coal mining is an important industry. Simple radiographically identified CWP is seen in 12% of all miners and in as many as 50% of anthracite miners with more than 20 years' work on the coal face. The prevalence of disease is lower in workers in bituminous coal mines. Since much western U.S. coal is bituminous, CWP is less prevalent in that region.

Much of the symptomatology associated with simple CWP appears to be similar and additive to the effects of cigarette smoking on the development of chronic bronchitis and obstructive lung disease (Chap. 258). In the early stages of simple CWP, radiographic abnormalities consist of small, irregular opacities (reticular pattern). With prolonged exposure, one sees small, rounded, regular opacities, 1 to 5 mm in diameter (nodular pattern). Calcification is generally not seen, although approximately 10% of older anthracite miners have calcified nodules.

Complicated CWP is manifested by the appearance on the chest radiograph of nodules ranging from 1 cm in diameter to the size of an entire lobe, generally confined to the upper half of the lungs. This condition, considered a form of PMF, is accompanied by a significant reduction in diffusing capacity and is associated with premature mortality. In contrast to patients with silicosis, underground miners with simple CWP develop PMF at a rate of only 5 to 15%, depending on the type of coal.

The mechanism whereby PMF occurs in CWP is not fully understood. Several hypotheses have been proposed, including: (1) sufficient free silica is present in the dust; (2) normal clearance mechanisms are unable to clear the excessive dust loads; and (3) atypical reactions to *M. tuberculosis* occur. As previously described, PMF in silicosis is associated with prolonged duration and high intensity of exposure to free silica. Heavy exposure to carbon particles free of silica occurs in carbon black, graphite, and charcoal workers. The prolonged exposure of these workers may result in sufficient accumulation of carbon in the lung to produce PMF. The mechanism appears to relate to a breakdown of the clearance capacity of the airways.

Caplan's syndrome (Chap. 312), first described in coal miners but subsequently found in patients with a variety of pneumoconioses, includes seropositive rheumatoid arthritis with characteristic PMF. The syndrome suggests an immunopathologic mechanism. Over the last decade, the mechanisms by which the chronic inhalation of mineral dusts produce an increase in inflammatory cells (including macrophages and neutrophils), which in turn causes PMF, have been explored. Coal dust can: (1) be a source of reactive oxygen species causing lung injury; (2) result in stimulation of macrophages to produce cytokines and enhance production of (anti)fibrogenic factors such as TNF-α; (3) increase protease activity; and (4) increase inactivation of α_1-antitrypsin and leukocyte elastase activity. The final pathologic pathway may be fibrosis resulting from the interactions of a variety of these mechanisms.

BERYLLIOSIS   Beryllium may produce an acute pneumonitis or, far more commonly, a chronic interstitial pneumonitis. Unless one inquires specifically about occupational exposures to beryllium in the manufacture of alloys, ceramics, high-technology electronics, and (before the 1950s) the production of fluorescent lights, one may miss entirely the etiologic relationship to an occupational exposure. Nonspecific pulmonary function tests may be normal or may indicate evidence of restrictive disease. Between 2 and 15 years of exposure, depending on its intensity, are required for the disease to become manifest. On open lung biopsy, granulomatous formation similar to that seen in sarcoidosis (Chap. 318) may make differentiation impossible unless tissue levels of beryllium are measured.

Other hard metals, including aluminum powders, chromium, cobalt, titanium dioxide, and tungsten, may produce an interstitial pneumonitis, but this is rare.

OTHER INORGANIC DUSTS   Other dusts are considered *nuisance dusts* because their major environmental and health effects seem to be reduction in visibility and irritation of eyes, ears, nasal passages, and other mucous membranes, respectively. If they penetrate to the lower airways, these dusts do not affect the architecture of the terminal bronchioles or acinar spaces nor do they destroy collagen. Generally, clinical effects are reversible. Pulmonary function tests are usually normal unless another disease process coexists. If the dusts are radiodense, macular collections may produce striking radiographic pictures that are so characteristic that patients with a history of significant exposure are easily diagnosed as having the condition that bears the name reflecting the nature of the dust. Examples of radiodense dusts include iron and iron oxides from welding or silver finishing (*siderosis*); tin oxide used in metallurgy, color stabilization, printing, and the manufacture of porcelain, glass, and fabric (*stannosis*); and barium sulfate used as a catalyst for organic reactions, drilling mud components, and electroplating (*baritosis*). Other metal dusts producing similar radiodense pictures include *cerium dioxide* and *antimony salts*.

Most of the inorganic dusts discussed thus far are associated with the production of either dust macules or interstitial fibrotic changes in the lung. Another set of dusts (Table 254-1), along with some of the dusts previously discussed, is associated with chronic mucous hypersecretion (chronic bronchitis), with or without reduction of expiratory flow rates. These conditions are caused by cigarette smoking, and any effort to attribute some component of the disease to occupational and environmental exposures must take cigarette smoking into account. Most studies suggest an additive effect of dust exposure and smoking. The pattern of the effect is similar to that of cigarette smoking, suggesting that small airway inflammation may be the initial site of pathologic response in those cases associated with the development of obstructive lung disease. Cigarette smoke is usually the more noxious agent, and dust effects may be discernible only in nonsmokers.

ORGANIC DUSTS Some of the specific diseases associated with organic dusts are discussed in detail in the chapters on asthma (Chap. 252) and hypersensitivity pneumonitis (Chap. 253). Many of these diseases are named for the specific setting in which they are found, e.g., farmer's lung, malt worker's disease, or mushroom worker's disease. Occupational and other environmental exposures must be sought when these conditions are suspected. Often the temporal relation of symptoms to exposure furnishes the best evidence for the diagnosis. Three occupational groups are singled out for discussion because they represent the largest proportion of people affected by the diseases resulting from organic dusts.

Cotton Dust (Byssinosis) Estimates of the number of exposed persons in the United States vary, but probably over 800,000 persons are exposed occupationally to cotton, flax, or hemp in the production of yarns for cotton, linen, and rope making. Although this discussion focuses on cotton, the same syndrome—albeit somewhat less severe—has been reported in association with exposure to flax, hemp, and jute.

Exposure occurs throughout the manufacturing process but is most pronounced in those portions of the factory involved with the treatment of the cotton prior to spinning—i.e., blowing, mixing, and carding (straightening of fibers). Attempts to control dust levels by use of exhaust hoods, general increases in ventilation, and wetting procedures in some settings have been highly successful. However, respiratory protective equipment appears to be required during certain operations to prevent workers from being exposed to levels of dust that exceed the current U.S. cotton dust standard.

Byssinosis is characterized clinically as occasional (early stage) and then regular (late stage) chest tightness toward the end of the first day of the workweek ("Monday chest tightness"). In epidemiologic studies, depending on the level of exposure via the carding room air, up to 80% of employees may show a significant drop in their FEV_1 over the course of a Monday shift.

Initially the symptoms do not recur on subsequent days of the week. However, in 10 to 25% of workers, the disease may be progressive, with chest tightness recurring or persisting throughout the

Table 254-1 Selected Occupational Dusts Believed to Be Associated with Mucous Hypersecretion and/or Obstructive Airway Disease and Other Respiratory Diseases[a]

Agent (Exposure)	Mucous Hypersecretion	Obstruction	Other Conditions[b]
INORGANIC DUSTS			
Antimony (storage batteries, solder, ceramics, glass, plastics)	X		P
Arsenic (manufacture of pesticides, pigments, glass, alloys)	X		C
Barium and compounds including BaO, $BaSO_4$, $BaCO_3$ (catalysts, drilling mud, electroplating)	X		P
Cadmium dust (electroplating, battery manufacture, welding, smelting, aluminum soldering)	X	X	P
Cement dust (construction trades, manufacture of cement blocks)	X	X	
Chromium and CrO_3, CrF_2 (corrosion inhibitor pigment, metallurgy, electroplating)	X		C
Coal dust (mining)	X		P
Coke oven emissions (retort house, coke ovens)	X	X	P, C
Graphite (steelmaking, lubricants, pencils, paints, stove polish)	X	X	P
Iron dust (steel and nonferrous foundry workers, welding)	X		P
Mica (insulation, roofing shingles, oil refining, rubber manufacturing)	X		P
Phosphorus, elemental chlorides, sulfides (manufacture of fireworks, agricultural chemicals, insecticides, pesticides)	X	X	
Rock dusts (miners, tunnelers, quarry workers)	X		P
Vanadium pentoxide (welding electrodes, additive to steel, by-product in ash from oil burning)	X	X	
ORGANIC DUSTS (see Chap. 253)			
Cotton dust, flax, hemp (manufacture of yarns for linen, rope, cotton; ginning, cottonseed crushing; waste fiber processing)	X	X	
Grain dusts (farmers, workers in grain elevators, barge and grain ship crew members)	X	X	
Moldy hay (farmers, other animal attendants)	X		HP

[a] The table excludes agents associated with asthma as the primary disease (see Chap. 252).
[b] Other conditions include hypersensitivity pneumonitis (HP), pneumoconiosis (P), and cancers (C).
NOTE: X indicates that mucous hypersecretion or obstruction is associated with exposure.

workweek. After more than 10 years of exposure, workers with recurrent symptoms are more likely to have an obstructive pattern on pulmonary function testing. These higher grades of impairment are seen in workers exposed both to high levels of dust and for greater durations. There is an additive effect of cotton dust exposure plus cigarette smoking. The highest grades of impairment are generally seen in smokers.

Treatment in the early stages of the disease is directed toward reversing the bronchospasm with bronchodilators; however, the chest tightness appears to relate, at least in part, to histamine release, and antihistamines have been shown to lessen the anticipated fall in FEV_1 the first day of the week. Clearly, reduction of dust exposure is of primary importance. All workers with persistent symptoms or significantly reduced levels of pulmonary function should be moved to areas of lower risk of exposure. Regular surveillance of pulmonary function in the industry has made it easier to identify affected persons. Persons with reduced pulmonary function, a personal history of respiratory allergy, and a history of continued cigarette smoking should be considered at increased risk of developing byssinosis in association with work in the cotton industry.

Grain Dust   Although the exact number of workers at risk in the United States is not known, at least 500,000 people work in grain elevators, and over 2 million farmers are potentially exposed to grain dust. The presentation of disease in grain elevator employees or in workers in flour or feed mills is virtually identical to the characteristic findings in cigarette smokers, i.e., persistent cough, mucous hypersecretion, wheeze and dyspnea on exertion, and reduced FEV_1 and FEV_1/FVC ratio (Chap. 250).

Dust concentrations in grain elevators vary greatly but appear to be in excess of 10,000 $\mu g/m^3$; approximately one-third of the particles, by weight, are in the respirable range. The effect of grain dust exposure is additive to that of cigarette smoking, with approximately 50% of workers who smoke having symptoms. Among nonsmoking grain elevator operators, approximately one-quarter have mucous hypersecretion, about five times the number that would be expected in unexposed nonsmokers. However, evidence of obstruction on pulmonary function studies is observed only in workers who smoke. It is not clear whether the reason is an enhancement of the cigarette smoking effect in exposed workers or a greater susceptibility of smokers to the effects of grain dust.

Farmer's Lung   This condition results from exposure to moldy hay containing spores of thermophilic actinomycetes that produce a hypersensitivity pneumonitis (Chap. 253). There are few good population-based estimates of the frequency of occurrence of this condition in the United States. However, among farmers in Great Britain, the rate of disease ranges from approximately 10 to 50 per 1000. The prevalence of disease varies in association with rainfall, which determines the amount of fungal growth, and with differences in agricultural practices related to turning and stacking hay.

The patient with acute farmer's lung presents 4 to 8 h after exposure with fever, chills, malaise, cough, and dyspnea without wheezing. The history of exposure is obviously essential to distinguish this disease from influenza or pneumonia with similar symptoms. In the chronic form of the disease, the history of repeated attacks after similar exposure is important in differentiating this syndrome from other causes of patchy fibrosis (e.g., sarcoidosis).

A wide variety of other organic dusts are associated with the occurrence of hypersensitivity pneumonitis (Chap. 253). For those patients who present with hypersensitivity pneumonitis, specific and careful inquiry about occupations, hobbies, or other home environmental exposures will, in most cases, reveal the source of the etiologic agent.

ASSESSMENT OF DISABILITY   Significant reduction of dust levels in coal mines has resulted from federal legislation, enacted in the United States in 1969, that requires that respirable dust levels in underground mines be reduced to less than 2000 $\mu g/m^3$. This same legislation authorizes payment to coal miners (or their survivors) totally disabled by CWP. The criteria for disability from CWP remain unclear and arbitrary. It is critical that physicians involved in occupational lung disease claim cases be aware of detailed exposure histories of their patients, in terms of both occupational exposures and other environmental exposures (cigarette smoking). To assess disability properly may require input not only from physicians but also from experts in ergonomics and vocational rehabilitation, lawyers, and employer and employee representatives.

Most commonly, the patient presents with asthma, and it is the physician's task to decide whether the asthma is occupation-induced or work-aggravated asthma. The distinction is important not only because of the implications for disability compensation but also because the longer one is exposed to an inciting agent, the worse the prognosis for recovery from occupation-induced asthma. The clinical evaluation of such a patient requires adherence to a prescribed protocol that may include not only the components of the evaluation previously described but also rechallenge of the patient in a controlled setting or under a carefully monitored program in a work setting.

TOXIC CHEMICALS   Exposure to toxic chemicals affecting the lung generally involves gases and vapors. A common accident is one in which the victim is trapped in a confined space where the chemicals have accumulated to toxic levels. In addition to the specific toxic effects of the chemical, the victim will often sustain considerable anoxia, which can play a dominant role in determining whether the individual survives.

Table 254-2 lists a variety of toxic agents that can produce acute and sometimes life-threatening reactions in the lung. All these agents in sufficient concentrations have been demonstrated, at least in animal studies, to affect the lower airways and disrupt alveolar architecture, either acutely or as a result of chronic exposure. Some of these agents may be generated acutely in the environment. For example, when plastics burn, a number of compounds, including hydrogen cyanide and hydrochloric acid, may be formed and released. →*The effects and treatment of exposure to these toxic gases are discussed in Chap. 391.*

Firefighters and fire victims are at risk of *smoke inhalation*, a numerically important cause of acute cardiorespiratory failure. Smoke inhalation kills more fire victims than does thermal injury. Carbon monoxide poisoning with resulting significant hypoxemia can be life-threatening (Chap. 396). Firefighters may inappropriately use the "blackness" of the smoke to indicate the degree of incomplete combustion and thus of carbon monoxide elevation. The use of synthetic materials (plastic, polyurethanes), which, when burned, may release a variety of other toxic agents, must be considered when evaluating smoke inhalation victims. Exposed victims may suffer some degree of lower respiratory tract inflammation, similar to that seen with exposure to other irritant gases (e.g., chlorine). Severe cases may include pulmonary edema.

Firefighters and victims also may be exposed to large quantities of particulate smoke. Significant long-term effects are not clearly associated with this particulate exposure except as related to the production of irritating effects on the upper airways; however, increased airway responsiveness in firefighters with repeated episodes of smoke inhalation has been demonstrated.

Some agents used in the manufacture of synthetic materials such as plastics, polyurethanes, and other polymers have resulted in some workers' being sensitized to extremely low levels of *isocyanates, aromatic amines,* or *aldehydes*. Repeated exposure to these agents causes some workers to develop chronic cough and sputum production, asthma, or episodes of low-grade fever and malaise.

Exposure occurs by an unusual route in *polymer fume fever*. Polymers, notably fluorocarbons, which at normal temperatures produce no reaction, may be transmitted from a worker's hands to his or her cigarettes. As the cigarette burns, the polymer is volatilized, and the inhaled agent causes a characteristic syndrome of fever, chills, malaise, and occasionally mild wheezing. The same scenario applies when workers are exposed to heated polymers without cigarette use—*meat wrappers' asthma*. A similar self-limited, influenza-like syndrome—*metal fume fever*—results from acute exposure to fumes or smoke of zinc, copper, magnesium, and other volatilized metals. The syndrome may begin several hours after work and resolves within 24 h, only to

Table 254-2 Selected Common Toxic Chemical Agents Affecting the Lung

Agent(s)	Selected Exposures	Acute Effects from High or Accidental Exposure	Chronic Effects from Relatively Low Exposure
Acid fumes; H_2SO_4, HNO_3	Manufacture of fertilizers, chlorinated organic compounds, dyes, explosives, rubber products, metal etching, plastics	Mucous membrane irritation, followed by chemical pneumonitis 2–3 days later	Bronchitis and suggestion of mildly reduced pulmonary function in children with life-long residential exposure to high levels; clinical significance unknown
Ammonia	Refrigeration; petroleum refining; manufacture of fertilizers, explosives, plastics, and other chemicals	Same as for acid fumes	Chronic bronchitis
Cyanides	Electroplating; extraction of gold or silver; manufacture of mirrors, fumigants, photo supplies	Increase in respiratory rate followed by respiratory arrest, lactic acidosis, pulmonary edema, death	No data
Diazomethane	Methylating agent for acid compounds; laboratory workers	Violent coughing, dyspnea, wheezing, pulmonary edema	No data
Formaldehyde	Manufacture of resins, leathers, rubber, metals, and woods; laboratory workers, embalmers; emission from urethane foam insulation	Same as for acid fumes	Cancers in one species; no data on humans
Halides (Cl, Br, F)	Bleaching in pulp, paper, textile industry; manufacture of chemical compounds; synthetic rubber, plastics, disinfectant, rocket fuel, gasoline	Mucous membrane irritation, pulmonary edema; possible reduced FVC 1–2 yrs after exposure	Dryness of mucous membrane, epistaxis, dental fluorosis, tracheobronchitis
Hydrogen sulfide	By-product of many industrial processes, oil, other petroleum processes and storage	Respiratory paralysis similar to cyanides	Conjunctival irritation, chronic bronchitis, recurrent pneumonitis
Isocyanates (TDI, HDI, MDI)	Production of polyurethane foams, plastics, adhesives, surface coatings	Mucous membrane irritation, dyspnea, cough, wheeze, pulmonary edema	Upper respiratory tract irritation, cough, asthma, allergic alveolitis
Nitrogen dioxide	Silage, metal etching, explosives, rocket fuels, welding, by-product of burning fossil fuels	Cough, dyspnea, pulmonary edema may be delayed 4–12 h; possible result from acute exposure: bronchiolitis obliterans in 2–6 wks	Emphysema in animals, ?chronic bronchitis, associated with reduced lung function in children with lifelong residential exposure, clinical significance unknown
Ozone	Arc welding, flour bleaching, deodorizing, emissions from copying equipment, photochemical air pollutant	Mucous membrane irritant, pulmonary hemorrhage and edema, reduced pulmonary function transiently in children and adults exposed to summer haze	Chronic eye irritation
Phosgene	Organic compound, metallurgy, volatilization of chlorine-containing compounds	Delayed onset of bronchiolitis and pulmonary edema	Chronic bronchitis
Phthalic anhydride	Manufacture of resin esters, polyester resins, thermoactivated adhesives	Nasal irritation, cough	Asthma, chronic bronchitis
Sulfur dioxide	Manufacture of sulfuric acid, bleaches, coating of nonferrous metals, food processing, refrigerant, burning of fossil fuels, wood pulp industry	Mucous membrane irritant, epistaxis	?Chronic bronchitis

return on repeated exposure. A proper occupational history should make the diagnosis evident.

ENVIRONMENTAL RESPIRATORY CARCINOGENS
Historically, it has been the astute clinician who has recognized a higher incidence of malignant tumors associated with certain environmental exposures. When these observations are linked to an occupational setting, they must be pursued by epidemiologic studies of relatively large groups of both current and former workers. Often the concentration and/or exact nature of the substances involved in the putative exposures cannot be determined. Rarely, the possibility that a substance can play an etiologic role in cancer is supported by observing that a few cases of a very rare tumor in a particular group represent "an epidemic." Examples are nasal sinus and lung cancer in nickel workers, angiosarcomas of the liver in vinyl chloride workers, and adenocarcinomas of the nose in woodworkers.

Only in those few cases in which animal studies have been carried out can one confirm that a given suspected agent is really a carcinogen. For example, bis(chloromethyl)ether (BCME) has been shown to produce tumors in animals and oat cell cancer of the lung in humans. In this particular case, BCME, used as a chemical intermediary in the manufacture of a number of organic compounds, was found to produce tumors in animals at about the same time as the substance was introduced into industry.

In addition to asbestos exposures, other occupational exposures associated with either proven or suspected respiratory carcinogens include those to acrylonitrile, arsenic compounds, beryllium (animal studies only), BCME, chromium, polycyclic hydrocarbons (through coke oven emissions), iron oxide, isopropyl oil (nasal sinuses), mustard gas, the various ores used to produce pure nickel, talc (possible asbestos contamination in both mining and milling), vinyl chloride, welding materials, wood used in woodworking (nasal cancer only), and uranium. The occurrence of excess cancers in uranium miners raises the possibility that a large number of workers are at risk by virtue of exposure to similar radiation hazards. This number includes not only workers involved in processing uranium but also workers exposed in underground mining operations where radon daughters may be emitted from rock formations.

GENERAL ENVIRONMENTAL EXPOSURES

AIR POLLUTION Dramatic and disastrous episodes of air pollution inversion have been documented in many industrialized centers in the world. Each of these episodes has been associated with excess acute mortality in the very old, the very young, and those with chronic cardiopulmonary diseases. The most dramatic event was the London fog of 1952, in which approximately 4000 excess deaths occurred over a 2-week period following 5 days of severe cold and dense fog. Similar episodes in the United States, although less dramatic in terms of total deaths, occurred in Donora, Pennsylvania, in 1948 and in New York City in the 1960s. In these episodes, which were generally associated with cold temperature and air stagnation, patients with underlying cardiopulmonary disease were most severely affected.

In addition to significant excess mortality during these episodes, a large number of people required medical care for cardiorespiratory complaints. Subsequent follow-up studies failed to implicate these episodic disasters in the etiology of chronic respiratory disease in adults. On the other hand, many epidemiologic studies of both international and regional differences in the prevalences of chronic respiratory disease suggest that long-term exposures in polluted areas in the early to middle part of the twentieth century were associated with excess chronic respiratory disease.

In 1970, the U.S. government established air quality standards for several pollutants believed to be responsible for excess cardiorespiratory diseases. Primary standards regulated by the Environmental Protection Agency (EPA) designed to protect the public health with an adequate margin of safety exist for sulfur dioxide, particulates <10 μm in size, nitrogen dioxide, ozone, lead, and carbon monoxide. Standards for each of these pollutants are updated regularly through an extensive review process conducted by the EPA. In 1997, a new standard was added for particles less than 2.5 μm; however, the standard does not become effective until year 2002.

Pollutants are generated from both stationary sources (power plants and industrial complexes) and mobile sources (automobiles), and none of the pollutants occurs in isolation. Thus, except for the change in carboxyhemoglobin from carbon monoxide exposure, it becomes extremely difficult to relate any specific health effect to any single pollutant. Furthermore, pollutants may be changed by chemical reactions after being emitted. For example, reducing agents, such as sulfur dioxide and particulate matter from a power plant stack, may react in air to produce acid sulfates and aerosols, the precursors of acid rain, which can be transported long distances in the atmosphere. Oxidizing substances, such as oxides of nitrogen and oxidants from automobile exhaust, may react with sunlight to produce ozone. Although originally a problem confined to the southwestern part of the United States, in recent years, at least during the summertime, elevated ozone and acid aerosol levels have been documented throughout the United States. Both acute and chronic effects of these exposures are currently under investigation.

The symptoms and diseases associated with air pollution are the same as the nononcogenic conditions commonly associated with cigarette smoking. In addition, respiratory illness in early childhood has been associated with chronic exposure to only modestly elevated levels of SO_2 and respirable particles. Recent population-based studies comparing cities that have relatively high levels of particulate exposures with less polluted communities suggest excess morbidity and mortality from cardiorespiratory conditions in long-term residents of the former communities. This finding, in part, has led to greater emphasis on publicizing pollution alert levels. One can only advise individuals with significant cardiopulmonary impairment to stay indoors during periods when pollution exceeds current standards.

INDOOR EXPOSURE   Because of increased concern about energy costs, efforts to become energy efficient have led to reduced air-exchange rates in indoor environments. The unintentional effect of these efforts has been to increase exposures to a variety of air contaminants heretofore not considered important.

Until relatively recently, little attention was given to the effects of *passive cigarette smoking* (Chap. 390). Several studies have shown that the respirable particulate load in any household is directly proportional to the number of cigarette smokers living in the home. Increases in prevalence of respiratory illnesses and reduced levels of pulmonary function measured with simple spirometry have been found in children of smoking parents in a number of studies.

Evidence from numerous case-control and cohort studies shows modest excess disease associations for cardiopulmonary diseases and lung cancer. Because most of these excess relative risks appear to be below 50%, it is virtually impossible for any one of the studies to be considered definitive. Thus, the techniques of meta-analysis have been used effectively to combine data from the best of these studies. The most recent meta-analyses for lung cancer, cardiac disease, and respiratory disease in terms of excess mortality suggest an approximately 25% increase for each condition, even after adjustment for major potential confounders. According to measures of plasma cotinine, a metabolite of nicotine, a nonsmoker living with a smoker is exposed to approximately 1% of the level of tobacco smoke to which a smoker of 20 cigarettes a day is exposed. In spite of some prominent detractors, these combined relative risks appear to be consistent with the estimated exposure levels and suggest a consensus that the associations are causal.

Radon gas is believed to be a risk factor for lung cancer. The main radon product (radon 222) is a gas that results from the decay series of uranium 238, with the immediate precursor being radium 226. The amount of radium in earth materials determines how much radon gas will be emitted. Outdoors, the concentrations are trivial. Indoors, levels are dependent on the ventilation rate and the size of the space into which the gas is emitted. Levels associated with excess lung cancer risk may be present in as many as 10% of the houses in the United States. When smokers reside in the household, the problem is potentially greater, since the molecular size of radon particles allows them to readily attach to smoke particles that are inhaled. Fortunately, technology is available for assessing and reducing the level of exposure.

Other indoor exposures associated with an increased risk of atopy and asthma include those to such specific recognized putative biologic agents as cockroach antigen, dust mites, and pet danders. Other indoor chemical agents include formaldehyde, perfumes, and latex particles. Of recent interest are the nonspecific responses associated with "tight-building syndrome," in which no particular agent has been implicated; the affected individuals suffer from a wide variety of complaints, including respiratory symptoms, that are relieved only by avoiding exposure in the building in question. The degree to which "smells" or other sensory stimuli are involved in the triggering of potentially incapacitating psychological or physical responses has yet to be determined, and the long-term consequences of such environmental exposures are as yet unknown.

PORTAL OF ENTRY   The lung is a primary point of entry into the body for a number of toxic agents that affect other organ systems. For example, the lung is a route of entry for benzene (bone marrow), carbon disulfide (cardiovascular and nervous systems), cadmium (kidney), and metallic mercury (kidney, central nervous system). Thus, in any disease state of obscure origin, it is important to consider the possibility of inhaled environmental agents. Such consideration can sometimes furnish the clue needed to identify a specific external cause for a disorder that might otherwise be labeled "idiopathic."

BIBLIOGRAPHY

BALAAN MR et al: Clinical aspects of coal workers' pneumoconiosis and silicosis. Occup Med 8:19, 1993

BECKLAKE MR et al: The relationship between acute and chronic airway responses to occupational exposures. Curr Pulmonol 9:25, 1988

BLANC PD: Acute pulmonary responses to toxic exposures. In *Textbook of Respiratory Medicine*, 3d ed. Murray JF, Nadel JA (eds). Philadelphia, WB Saunders, 2000, pp 1903–1914

CHAN-YEUNG M, MALO J-L: Occupational asthma. N Engl J Med 333: 107, 1995

CHECKOWAY H, FRANZBLAU A: Is silicosis required for silica-associated lung cancer? Am J Indust Med 37:252, 2000

COCHRANE AL, MOORE FA: A 20-year follow-up of men aged 55–64 including coal miners and foundry workers in Staveley. Br J Ind Med 37:226, 1980

Guidelines for the Use of International Labour Office Classification of Radiographs of Pneumoconiosis. Occupational Safety and Health Sciences 22 (Revised 1980). Geneva, ILO, 1980

HACKSHAW AK et al: The accumulated evidence on lung cancer and environmental tobacco smoke. Br Med J 315:980, 1997

HE J et al: Passive smoking and the risk of coronary heart disease—a meta-analysis of epidemiologic studies. New Engl J Med 340:920, 1999

LEONARD JF, TEMPLETON PA: Pulmonary imaging techniques in the diagnosis of occupational interstitial lung disease, in *Occupational Medicine: State of the Art Reviews*, vol 7, no 2, WS Beckett, R Bascon (eds). Philadelphia, Hanley and Belfus,
1992, pp 241–260

MULLOY KB et al: Use of chest radiographs in epidemiological investigations of pneumoconioses. Br J Ind Med 50:273, 1993

PARKES WR: *Occupational Lung Disorders*, 3d ed. Oxford, Butterworth-Heinemann, 1994

PRICE B: Analysis of current trends in United States mesothelioma incidence. Am J Epidemiol 145:211, 1997

ROSENMAN KD et al: Silicosis in the 1990s. Chest 111:779, 1997

SAMET JM, SPENGLER JD: *Indoor Air Pollution: A Health Perspective*, Baltimore, The
Johns Hopkins University, 1991, Chaps. 2 and 15

SCHENKER MB: Regulatory and policy issues, in *Occupational and Environmental Respiratory Disease*, P Harber et al: (eds). St Louis, Mosby Year Books, 1996

SCHINS RP, BORM PJ: Mechanisms and mediators in coal dust induced toxicity: A review.
Ann Occup Hyg 43:7, 1999

Table 255-1 Microbial Pathogens That Cause Pneumonia

Community-Acquired	Hospital-Acquired	HIV Infection–Associated
Mycoplasma pneumoniae	Enteric aerobic gram-negative bacilli	*Pneumocystis carinii*
Streptococcus pneumoniae	*Pseudomonas aeruginosa*	*M. tuberculosis*
Haemophilus influenzae	*S. aureus*	*S. pneumoniae*
Chlamydia pneumoniae	Oral anaerobes	*H. influenzae*
Legionella pneumophila		
Oral anaerobes		
Moraxella catarrhalis		
Staphylococcus aureus		
Nocardia spp.		
Viruses[a]		
Fungi[b]		
Mycobacterium tuberculosis		
Chlamydia psittaci		

[a] Influenza virus, cytomegalovirus, respiratory syncytial virus, measles virus, varicella-
zoster virus, and hantavirus.

[b] *Histoplasma*, *Coccidioides*, and *Blastomyces* spp.

255 Matthew E. Levison

PNEUMONIA, INCLUDING NECROTIZING PULMONARY INFECTIONS (LUNG ABSCESS)

BAL	bronchoalveolar lavage	PCP	*P. carinii* pneumonia
CFU	colony-forming units	PORT	Pneumonia Patient Outcomes
HPS	hantavirus pulmonary syndrome		Research Team
ICU	intensive care unit	PSB	protected double-sheathed brush
IDSA	Infectious Diseases Society of	TMP-SMZ	trimethoprim-
	America		sulfamethoxazole
MIC	minimal inhibitory	TTA	transtracheal aspiration
	concentration		

Pneumonia is an infection of the pulmonary parenchyma that can be
caused by various bacterial species, including mycoplasmas, chlamydiae, and rickettsiae; viruses; fungi; and parasites (Table 255-1). Thus
pneumonia is not a single disease but a group of specific infections,
each with a different epidemiology, pathogenesis, clinical presentation, and clinical course. Identification of the etiologic microorganism
is of primary importance, since this is the key to appropriate antimicrobial therapy. However, because of the serious nature of the infection, antimicrobial therapy generally needs to be started immediately,
often before laboratory confirmation of the causative agent. The specific microbial etiology remains elusive in more than one-third of
cases—e.g., when no sputum is available for examination, blood cultures are sterile, and there is no pleural fluid. Serologic confirmation
requires weeks because of the late formation of specific antibody.

Thus initial antimicrobial therapy is often empirical and is based
on the setting in which the infection was acquired, the clinical presentation, patterns of abnormality on chest radiography, results of staining
of sputum or other infected body fluids, and current patterns of susceptibility of the suspected pathogens to antimicrobial agents. After
the etiologic agent is identified, specific antimicrobial therapy can be
chosen.

DEFENSE MECHANISMS The lung is a complex structure
composed of aggregates of units that are formed by the progressive
branching of the airways. Approximately 80% of the cells lining the
central airways are ciliated, pseudostratified, columnar epithelial cells;
the percentage decreases in the peripheral airways. Each ciliated cell
contains about 200 cilia that beat in coordinated waves ~1000 times
per minute, with a fast forward stroke and a slower backward recovery.
Ciliary motion is also coordinated between adjacent cells so that each
wave is propagated toward the oropharynx. The cilia are covered by
a liquid film that is ~5 to 10 μm thick and is composed of two layers.
The outer, or gel, layer is viscous and traps deposited particles. The
cilia beat in the less viscous inner, or sol, layer. During the forward
stroke, the tips of the cilia just touch the viscous gel and propel it
toward the oropharynx. During recovery, the cilia move entirely within

the low-resistance sol layer. Ciliated cells are interspersed with mucus-
secreting cells in the trachea and bronchi but not in the bronchioles.

The alveolar walls, from blood to air, consist of the endothelium
that lines the network of anastomotic capillaries, the capillary basement membrane, the interstitial tissue, the alveolar basement membrane, the alveolar lining epithelial cells (which are either flattened
type I pneumocytes that cover 95% of the alveolar surface or rounded,
granular, surfactant-producing type II pneumocytes), and epithelial lining fluid. The epithelial lining fluid contains surfactant, fibronectin,
and immunoglobulin, which may opsonize or—in the presence of
complement—lyse microbial pathogens deposited on the alveolar surface. Loosely attached to the lining cells or lying free within the lumen
are the alveolar macrophages, lymphocytes, and a few polymorphonuclear leukocytes.

The lower respiratory tract is normally sterile, despite being adjacent to enormous numbers of microorganisms that reside in the oropharynx and being exposed to environmental microorganisms in inhaled air. This sterility is the result of efficient filtering and clearance
mechanisms.

Infectious particles deposited on the squamous epithelium of distal
nasal surfaces normally are removed by sneezing, while those deposited on the more proximal ciliated surfaces are swept posteriorly in
the mucus lining into the nasopharynx, where they are swallowed or
expectorated. Reflex closure of the glottis and cough protect the lower
respiratory tract. Those particles deposited on the tracheobronchial surface are swept by ciliary motion toward the oropharynx. Infectious
particles that bypass defenses in the airways and are deposited on the
alveolar surface are cleared by phagocytic cells and humoral factors.
Alveolar macrophages are the major phagocytes in the lower respiratory tract. Some phagocytosed microorganisms are killed by the phagocyte's oxygen-dependent systems, lysosomal enzymes, and cationic
proteins. Other microorganisms can evade microbicidal mechanisms
and persist within the macrophage. For example, *Mycobacterium tuberculosis* persists within the lysosome, while *Legionella* resides
within intracellular inclusions that fail to fuse with lysosomes. Intracellular pathogens can then be transported to the ciliated surfaces and
into the oropharynx or via the lymphatics to regional lymph nodes.
The alveolar macrophages process and present microbial antigens to
the lymphocyte and also secrete cytokines (e.g., tumor necrosis factor
and interleukin 1) that modulate the immune process in T and B lymphocytes. Cytokines facilitate the generation of an inflammatory response, activate alveolar macrophages, and recruit additional phagocytes and other immunologic factors from plasma. The inflammatory
exudate is responsible for many of the local signs of pulmonary consolidation and for the systemic manifestations of pneumonia, such as
fever, chills, myalgias, and malaise.

TRANSMISSION   Microbial pathogens may enter the lung by one of several routes.

Aspiration of Organisms That Colonize the Oropharynx Most pulmonary pathogens originate in the oropharyngeal flora. Aspiration of these pathogens is the most common mechanism for the production of pneumonia. At various times during the year, healthy individuals transiently carry common pulmonary pathogens in the nasopharynx; these pathogens include *Streptococcus pneumoniae*, *S. pyogenes*, *Mycoplasma pneumoniae*, *Haemophilus influenzae*, and *Moraxella catarrhalis*. The sources of anaerobic pulmonary pathogens, such as *Porphyromonas gingivalis*, *Prevotella melaninogenica*, *Fusobacterium nucleatum*, *Actinomyces* spp., spirochetes, and anaerobic streptococci, are the gingival crevice and dental plaque, which contain more than 10^{11} colony-forming units (CFU) of microorganisms per gram. The frequency of aerobic gram-negative bacillary colonization of the oropharyngeal mucosa, which is unusual in healthy persons (<2%), increases with hospitalization, worsening debility, severe underlying illness, alcoholism, diabetes, and advanced age. This change may be a consequence of increased salivary proteolytic activity, which destroys fibronectin, a glycoprotein coating the surface of the mucosa. Fibronectin is the receptor for the normal gram-positive flora of the oropharynx. Loss of fibronectin exposes the receptors for aerobic gram-negative bacilli on the epithelial cell surface. The source of aerobic gram-negative bacilli may be the patient's own stomach (which can become colonized with these organisms as the result of an increase in gastric pH with atrophic gastritis or after the use of H_2-blocking agents or antacids), contaminated respiratory equipment, hands of health care workers, or contaminated food and water. Nasogastric tubes can facilitate the transfer of gastric bacteria to the pharynx.

About 50% of healthy adults aspirate oropharyngeal secretions into the lower respiratory tract during sleep. Aspiration occurs more frequently and may be more pronounced in individuals with an impaired level of consciousness (e.g., alcoholics; drug abusers; and patients who have seizures, strokes, or general anesthesia), neurologic dysfunction of the oropharynx, and swallowing disorders or mechanical impediments (e.g., nasogastric or endotracheal tubes). Pneumonia due to anaerobes is an especially likely outcome if the aspirated material is large in volume or contains virulent components of the anaerobic microbial flora or foreign bodies, such as aspirated food or necrotic tissue. Impairment of the cough reflex increases the risk of pneumonia, as does mucociliary or alveolar macrophage dysfunction.

Inhalation of Infectious Aerosols   Deposition of inhaled particles within the respiratory tract is determined primarily by particle size. Particles >10 μm in diameter are deposited mostly in the nose and upper airways. Particles <5 μm in diameter (also called *airborne droplet nuclei*) and containing one or perhaps two microorganisms fail to settle out by gravity but rather remain suspended in the atmosphere for long periods unless removed by ventilation or by filtration in the lungs of the individual breathing the contaminated air. Transmission of an infectious agent in the form of an aerosol is particularly efficient. These infectious aerosols are small enough to bypass host defenses in the upper respiratory tract and airways. A greater percentage of particles are deposited in small bronchioles and alveoli as particle size decreases below 5 μm. One inhaled particle of appropriate size may be sufficient to reach the alveolus and initiate infection. The etiologies of pneumonia typically acquired by inhalation of infectious aerosols include tuberculosis, influenza, legionellosis, psittacosis, histoplasmosis, Q fever, and hantavirus pulmonary syndrome (HPS).

Hematogenous Dissemination from an Extrapulmonary Site Infection, usually with *Staphylococcus aureus*, disseminates hematogenously to the lungs in patients (such as intravenous drug users) who have either right- or left-sided bacterial endocarditis and in patients with intravenous catheter infections. *Fusobacterium* infections of the retropharyngeal tissues (Lemierre's syndrome—i.e., retropharyngeal abscess and jugular venous thrombophlebitis) also disseminate hematogenously to the lungs.

Direct Inoculation and Contiguous Spread   Two additional routes of transmission of bacteria to the lungs are direct inoculation (as a result of either tracheal intubation or stab wounds to the chest) and contiguous spread from an adjacent site of infection.

PATHOLOGY   The pneumonic process may involve primarily the interstitium or the alveoli. Involvement of an entire lobe is called *lobar pneumonia*. When the process is restricted to alveoli contiguous to bronchi, it is called *bronchopneumonia*. Confluent bronchopneumonia may be indistinguishable from lobar pneumonia. Cavities develop when necrotic lung tissue is discharged into communicating airways, resulting in either necrotizing pneumonia (multiple small cavities, each <2 cm in diameter, in one or more bronchopulmonary segments or lobes) or lung abscess (one or more cavities >2 cm in diameter). The classification of pneumonia is best based upon the causative microorganism rather than upon these anatomic characteristics (the criteria used in the past).

EPIDEMIOLOGY   The patient's living circumstances, occupation, travel history, pet or animal exposure history, and contacts with other ill individuals as well as the physician's knowledge of the epidemic curve of community outbreaks provide clues to the microbial etiology of a given case of pneumonia (Table 255-1). The relative frequency of various pulmonary pathogens varies with the setting in which the infection was acquired—e.g., community, nursing home, or hospital. In patients hospitalized with community-acquired pneumonia, the most frequent pathogens are *S. pneumoniae*, *H. influenzae*, *Chlamydia pneumoniae*, and *Legionella pneumophila*. *C. pneumoniae* is often found in association with other pathogens, including *S. pneumoniae*, and the associated pathogen appears to influence the course of the pneumonia. *M. pneumoniae*, which usually causes mild illness, is common among outpatients with community-acquired pneumonia, but may also be an underappreciated cause in all age groups of severe pneumonia that requires hospitalization. In contrast, enteric aerobic gram-negative bacilli and *Pseudomonas aeruginosa*, uncommon causes of community-acquired pneumonia, are estimated to account for >50% of cases of hospital-acquired pneumonia, while *S. aureus* is responsible for >10%. The relative frequencies of pathogens in pneumonia acquired in nursing homes fall somewhere between those of community- and hospital-acquired pneumonia. Enteric aerobic gram-negative bacilli and *P. aeruginosa* are more common among nursing home residents than among patients who acquire pneumonia in noninstitutional settings.

The season of the year and the geographic location are other predictors of etiology. The frequency of influenza virus as a cause of both community-acquired and institutionally acquired pneumonia increases during the winter months. Moreover, influenza virus infection causes an increase in the frequency of secondary bacterial pneumonia due to *S. pneumoniae*, *S. aureus*, and *H. influenzae*. Outbreaks of influenza in a community tend to be explosive and widespread, with many secondary cases resulting from the short incubation period of several days and the high degree of communicability. *Legionella* colonizes hot-water storage systems that provide favorable conditions for its proliferation, such as warm temperature, stagnation, and sediment accumulation. Acquisition of *Legionella* pneumonia requires exposure to aerosols generated from these contaminated water supplies—e.g., during an overnight stay in a hotel with a faulty air-handling system or after repair of domestic plumbing in buildings with contaminated water supplies. Legionellosis also occurs in explosive outbreaks when large numbers of susceptible people are exposed to an infectious aerosol; however, no secondary cases occur because of the low level of communicability of *L. pneumophila*. *Mycoplasma* causes outbreaks, usually in relatively closed populations such as those at military bases, at colleges, or in households; however, because of its long incubation period (2 to 3 weeks) and its relatively low degree of communicability, *Mycoplasma* infection moves through the community slowly, affecting another person as the first is recovering. In communities where infection with HIV type 1 is endemic, *Pneumocystis carinii* and *M. tuberculosis* are more prominent causes of community-acquired pneumonia. *Chlamydia psittaci* produces illness in bird handlers. Histoplasmosis, blastomycosis, and coccidioidomycosis are causes of pneumonia that have specific geographic distributions.

255 Pneumonia, Including Necrotizing Pulmonary Infections **1477**

HPS is a newly described, frequently fatal disease caused by one of several hantaviruses. Most cases in the United States have been reported from the Four Corners area (New Mexico, Arizona, Utah, and Colorado), where the pathogen is the Sin Nombre virus. The primary hosts are rodents, which apparently remain healthy but excrete the virus in urine, feces, and saliva. Hantavirus infection is acquired by inhalation of infectious aerosols when rodent nests are disturbed by human domestic, occupational, or recreational activities. The appearance of HPS in the southwestern United States is thought to have occurred because of increased rainfall in the region, which increased the rodent food supply and thus the rodent population. No person-to-person transmission of HPS is thought to have taken place, except perhaps in an outbreak in southern Argentina in 1996.

AGE AND COMORBIDITY Age is an important predictor of the infecting agent in pneumonia. *Chlamydia trachomatis* and respiratory syncytial virus are common among infants < 6 months of age; *H. influenzae* among children 6 months to 5 years of age; *M. pneumoniae, C. pneumoniae,* and hantavirus among young adults; *H. influenzae* and *M. catarrhalis* among elderly individuals with chronic lung disease; and *L. pneumophila* among elderly persons, smokers, and persons with compromised cell-mediated immunity (e.g., transplant recipients), renal or hepatic failure, diabetes, or systemic malignancy.

Oral anaerobes, frequently in combination with aerobic bacterial components of the human flora (e.g., viridans streptococci), are causes of community-acquired pneumonia and anaerobic lung abscess in patients who are prone to aspiration. Edentulous persons, who have lower numbers of oral anaerobes, are less likely to develop pneumonia due to anaerobes. When the etiology of community-acquired pneumonia in unselected hospitalized patients has been studied by methods that entail strict anaerobic bacteriology and that avoid contamination of lower respiratory tract secretions by the oral flora, anaerobic bacteria have been found to account for as many as 20 to 30% of cases. In hospital-acquired pneumonia, anaerobes are the pathogens—with or without aerobic copathogens—in about one-third of cases. However, the aerobic copathogens in hospital-acquired pneumonia are frequently virulent microorganisms in their own right (e.g., enteric aerobic gram-negative bacilli, *P. aeruginosa,* and *S. aureus*).

The patient's underlying disease may be characterized by specific immunologic or inflammatory defects that predispose to pneumonia due to specific pathogens (Table 255-2). For example, immunoglobulin deficiencies—especially those involving IgG subtypes 2 and 4, which are important in the immune response to encapsulated organisms (e.g., *S. pneumoniae* and *H. influenzae*)—may be associated with recurrent sinopulmonary infections. Immunoglobulin deficiencies may be inherited, or they may be acquired (i.e., as a result of either decreased production, as in lymphoproliferative malignancies, or excessive protein loss, as in nephrosis or protein-losing enteropathy). Inherited immunoglobulin deficiencies may be global or selective. Patients with recurrent sinopulmonary infections and a selective deficiency of IgG2 and/or IgG4 may have a total plasma IgG level within the normal range, as these particular IgG subtypes constitute only 25% of total IgG. HIV-infected patients may also exhibit ineffective antibody formation, which predisposes to infection with these encapsulated bacteria. Severe neutropenia (<500 neutrophils/μL) increases the risk of infections due to *P. aeruginosa,* Enterobacteriaceae, *S. aureus,* and (if neutropenia is prolonged) *Aspergillus.* The risk is unusually high for infections due to *M. tuberculosis* among HIV-infected patients with circulating CD4− lymphocyte counts of <500/μL; for infections due to *P. carinii, Histoplasma capsulatum,* and *Cryptococcus neoformans* among those with CD4+ counts of <200/μL; and for infections due to *M. avium-intracellulare* and cytomegalovirus among those with counts of <50/μL. Long-term glucocorticoid therapy increases the risk of tuberculosis and nocardiosis.

CLINICAL MANIFESTATIONS **Community-Acquired Pneumonia** Community-acquired pneumonia has traditionally been thought to present as either of two syndromes: the typical presentation or the atypical presentation. Although current data suggest that these two syndromes may be less distinct than was once thought, the characteristics of the clinical presentation may nevertheless have some diagnostic value.

The "typical" pneumonia syndrome is characterized by the sudden onset of fever, cough productive of purulent sputum, shortness of breath, and (in some cases) pleuritic chest pain; signs of pulmonary consolidation (dullness, increased fremitus, egophony, bronchial breath sounds, and rales) may be found on physical examination in areas of radiographic abnormality. The typical pneumonia syndrome is usually caused by the most common bacterial pathogen in community-acquired pneumonia, *S. pneumoniae,* but can also be due to other bacterial pathogens, such as *H. influenzae* and mixed anaerobic and aerobic components of the oral flora.

The "atypical" pneumonia syndrome is characterized by a more gradual onset, a dry cough, shortness of breath, a prominence of extrapulmonary symptoms (such as headache, myalgias, fatigue, sore throat, nausea, vomiting, and diarrhea), and abnormalities on chest radiographs despite minimal signs of pulmonary involvement (other than rales) on physical examination. Atypical pneumonia is classically produced by *M. pneumoniae* but can also be caused by *L. pneumophila, C. pneumoniae,* oral anaerobes, and *P. carinii* as well as by *S. pneumoniae* and the less frequently encountered pathogens *C. psittaci, Coxiella burnetii, Francisella tularensis, H. capsulatum,* and *Coccidioides immitis.* *Mycoplasma* pneumonia (Chap. 178) may be complicated by erythema multiforme, hemolytic anemia, bullous myringitis, encephalitis, and transverse myelitis. *Legionella* pneumonia (Chap. 151) is frequently associated with deterioration in mental status, renal and hepatic abnormalities, and marked hyponatremia; pneumonia due to *H. capsulatum* (Chap. 201) or *C. immitis* (Chap. 202) is often accompanied by erythema nodosum. In *C. pneumoniae* pneumonia (Chap. 179), sore throat, hoarseness, and wheezing are relatively common. The atypical pneumonia syndrome in patients whose behavioral history places them at risk of HIV infection suggests *Pneumocystis* infection. These patients may have concurrent infections caused by other opportunistic pathogens, such as pulmonary (and frequently extrapulmonary) tuberculosis, oral thrush due to *Candida albicans,* or extensive perineal ulcers due to herpes simplex virus.

Certain viruses also produce pneumonia that is usually characterized by an atypical presentation—i.e., chills, fever, shortness of breath, dry nonproductive cough, and predominance of extrapulmonary symptoms. Primary viral pneumonia can be caused by influenza virus (usually as part of a community outbreak in winter), by respiratory syncytial virus (in children and immunosuppressed individuals), by measles or varicella-zoster virus (accompanied by the characteristic rash), and by cytomegalovirus (in patients immunocompromised by HIV infection or by therapy given in association with organ trans-

Table 255-2 Pulmonary Pathogens Associated with Specific Defects in Host Defenses

Defect	Pathogens
Severe hypogammaglobulinemia	Encapsulated bacteria: *Streptococcus pneumoniae, Haemophilus influenzae*
Severe neutropenia	*Pseudomonas aeruginosa,* Enterobacteriaceae, *Staphylococcus aureus, Aspergillus*
Defective cell-mediated immunity CD4+ lymphocyte count	
<500/μL	*Mycobacterium tuberculosis*
<200/μL	*Pneumocystis carinii, Histoplasma capsulatum, Cryptococcus neoformans*
<50/μL	*Mycobacterium avium-intracellulare,* cytomegalovirus
Long-term glucocorticoid therapy	*M. tuberculosis, Nocardia*

plantation). Hantavirus causes an initial nonspecific febrile prodrome, after which the patient develops rapidly progressive respiratory failure and diffuse pulmonary infiltrates on chest radiographs as a result of exudation into the pulmonary interstitium and alveoli, with thrombocytopenia, neutrophilic leukocytosis, circulating immunoblasts, and laboratory evidence of hemoconcentration. In addition, influenza and measles can predispose to secondary bacterial pneumonia as a result of the destruction of the mucociliary barrier of the airways. Secondary bacterial infection may either follow the viral infection without interruption or be separated from the viral infection by several days of transient relief of symptoms. Bacterial infection may be heralded by sudden worsening of the patient's clinical condition, with persisting or renewed chills, fever, and cough productive of purulent sputum, possibly accompanied by pleuritic chest pain.

Patients with hematogenous *S. aureus* pneumonia may present with fever and dyspnea only. In these cases the inflammatory response is initially confined to the pulmonary interstitium. Cough, sputum production, and signs of pulmonary consolidation develop only after the infection extends into the bronchi. These patients are usually gravely ill, with intravascular infection as well as pneumonia, and may have signs of endocarditis (Chap. 126).

Nocardiosis (Chap. 165) is frequently complicated by metastasis of lesions to the skin and central nervous system. Signs of pulmonary consolidation, cough, and sputum production may be lacking in patients who are unable to mount an inflammatory response, such as those with agranulocytosis. The major manifestations in these patients may be limited to fever, tachypnea, agitation, and altered mental status. Elderly or severely ill patients may fail to develop fever.

Tuberculosis also produces an atypical presentation that is characterized by fever, night sweats, cough, and shortness of breath and sometimes by pleuritic chest pain and blood-streaked sputum. Several weeks usually elapse before the patient seeks medical attention because of the gradual worsening of these symptoms, by which time he or she will have lost considerable weight.

Nosocomial Pneumonia   Patients with nosocomial pneumonia often pose a diagnostic challenge. The differential diagnosis of acute respiratory disease in critically ill, hospitalized patients is diverse and includes noninfectious entities, such as congestive heart failure, acute respiratory distress syndrome, preexisting lung disease, atelectasis, and oxygen- or drug-related toxicities, that may be difficult to distinguish clinically or radiologically from pneumonia. The usual criteria for nosocomial pneumonia, which include new or progressive pulmonary infiltrates, purulent tracheobronchial secretions, fever, and leukocytosis, are frequently unreliable in these patients, who often have preexisting pulmonary disease, endotracheal tubes that irritate the tracheal mucosa and may elicit an inflammatory exudate in respiratory secretions, or multiple other problems likely to produce fever and leukocytosis. Patients with nosocomial pneumonia complicating an underlying illness associated with significant neutropenia often have no purulent respiratory tract secretions or pulmonary infiltrates, and patients with nosocomial pneumonia complicating uremia or cirrhosis often remain afebrile. In addition, the patients at greatest risk for nosocomial pneumonia are most likely to be heavily colonized with potential pulmonary pathogens in the oropharyngeal or tracheobronchial mucosa; thus the presence of these organisms in gram-stained preparations or cultures of respiratory tract secretions does not necessarily confirm the diagnosis of pneumonia.

Aspiration Pneumonia and Anaerobic Lung Abscess   Aspiration of a sufficient volume of gastric acid produces a chemical pneumonitis characterized by acute dyspnea and wheezing with hypoxemia and infiltrates on chest radiographs in one or both lower lobes. Clinical findings following aspiration of particulate matter depend on the extent of endobronchial obstruction and range from acute apnea to persistent cough with or without recurrent infection. Although the aspiration of oral anaerobes can initially lead to an infiltrative process, it ultimately results in putrid sputum, tissue necrosis, and pulmonary cavities. In

about three-quarters of cases, the clinical course of an abscess of anaerobic polymicrobial etiology is indolent and mimics that of pulmonary tuberculosis, with cough, shortness of breath, chills, fever, night sweats, weight loss, pleuritic chest pain, and blood-streaked sputum lasting for several weeks or more. In other patients the disease may present more acutely. Patients with anaerobic abscesses are usually prone to aspiration of oropharyngeal contents and have periodontal disease. One genus of oral anaerobes, *Actinomyces*, produces a chronic fibrotic necrotizing process that crosses tissue planes and may involve the pleural space, ribs, vertebrae, and subcutaneous tissue, with eventual discharge of sulfur granules (macroscopic bacterial masses) through the skin (empyema necessitatis).

DIAGNOSIS   Radiography   Chest radiography is more sensitive than physical examination for detection of pulmonary infiltrates. Indeed, *P. carinii* pneumonia (PCP) is the only relatively common form of pneumonia associated with false-negative chest radiographs; up to 30% of patients with PCP have false-negative results. Chest radiographs can confirm the presence and location of the pulmonary infiltrate; assess the extent of the pulmonary infection; detect pleural involvement, pulmonary cavitation, or hilar lymphadenopathy; and gauge the response to antimicrobial therapy. However, chest radiographs may be normal when the patient is unable to mount an inflammatory response (e.g., in agranulocytosis) or is in the early stage of an infiltrative process (e.g., in hematogenous *S. aureus* pneumonia or PCP associated with AIDS). High-resolution computed tomography of the lungs can improve the accuracy of diagnosis of pneumonia, especially when the process involves lung obscured by the diaphragm, liver, ribs and clavicles, or heart.

The anatomic localization of the inflammatory process, as visualized in chest radiographs, occasionally has diagnostic implications. Most pulmonary pathogens produce focal lesions. A multicentric distribution suggests hematogenous infection, in which case the remote location of the primary infection (e.g., endocarditis or thrombophlebitis) should be sought. Hematogenous pneumonia, which results from septic embolization in patients with thrombophlebitis or right-sided endocarditis and from bacteremia in patients with left-sided endocarditis, appears on the chest radiograph as multiple areas of pulmonary infiltration that subsequently may cavitate. A diffuse distribution suggests the involvement of *P. carinii*, cytomegalovirus, hantavirus, measles virus, or herpes zoster virus (with pneumonia due to the last two pathogens diagnosed by the characteristic accompanying rash). Pleurisy and hilar nodal enlargement are unusual with PCP and cytomegalovirus pneumonia; their presence suggests another etiology. Diffuse lesions in immunocompromised patients also suggest legionellosis, tuberculosis, histoplasmosis, *Mycoplasma* infection, or disseminated strongyloidiasis.

Oral anaerobes, *S. aureus, S. pneumoniae* serotype III, aerobic gram-negative bacilli, *M. tuberculosis*, and fungi as well as certain noninfectious conditions can produce tissue necrosis and pulmonary cavities (Table 255-3). In contrast, *H. influenzae, M. pneumoniae*, viruses, and most other serotypes of *S. pneumoniae* almost never cause cavities. Apical disease, with or without cavities, suggests reactivation tuberculosis. Anaerobic abscesses are located in dependent, poorly ventilated, and poorly draining bronchopulmonary segments and characteristically have air-fluid levels, unlike the well-ventilated, well-

Table 255-3   Causes of Pulmonary Cavities

INFECTIOUS

Bacteria: Oral anaerobes (*Bacteroides* spp., fusobacteria, *Actinomyces* spp., anaerobic and microaerophilic cocci), enteric aerobic gram-negative bacilli, *Pseudomonas aeruginosa*, *Legionella* spp., *Staphylococcus aureus*, *Streptococcus pneumoniae* serotype III, *Mycobacterium tuberculosis*, *Nocardia* spp.

Fungi: *Histoplasma capsulatum*, *Coccidioides immitis*, *Blastomyces* spp.

NONINFECTIOUS

Neoplasms, Wegener's granulomatosis, infarction, infected bullae and cysts drained upper-lobe cavities caused by *M. tuberculosis*, an obligate aerobe. Air-fluid levels may also be present in cavities due to pulmonary necrosis of other infectious etiologies, such as *S. aureus* and aerobic gram-negative bacilli. *Mucor* and *Aspergillus* invade blood vessels and cause pleural-based, wedge-shaped areas of pulmonary infarction; these infarcts may subsequently cavitate.

In the patient with an uncomplicated course, chest radiographs need not be repeated before discharge, since the resolution of infiltrates may take up to 6 weeks after initial presentation. However, patients who do not respond clinically, who have a pleural effusion on admission, who may have postobstructive pneumonia, or who are infected with certain pathogens (e.g., *S. aureus*, aerobic gram-negative bacilli, or oral anaerobes) need more intensive surveillance. At times, computed tomography may be especially helpful in distinguishing different processes—e.g., pleural effusion versus underlying pulmonary consolidation, hilar adenopathy versus pulmonary mass, and pulmonary abscess versus empyema with an air-fluid level.

Sputum Examination   Examination of the sputum remains the mainstay of the evaluation of a patient with acute bacterial pneumonia. Unfortunately, expectorated material is frequently contaminated by potentially pathogenic bacteria that colonize the upper respiratory tract (and sometimes the lower respiratory tract) without actually causing disease. This contamination reduces the diagnostic specificity of any lower respiratory tract specimen. In addition, it has been estimated that the usual laboratory processing methods detect the pulmonary pathogen in fewer than 50% of expectorated sputum samples from patients with bacteremic *S. pneumoniae* pneumonia. This low sensitivity may be due to misidentification of the α-hemolytic colonies of *S. pneumoniae* as nonpathogenic α-hemolytic streptococci ("normal flora"), overgrowth of the cultures by hardier colonizing organisms, or loss of more fastidious organisms due to slow transport or improper processing. In addition, certain common pulmonary pathogens, such as anaerobes, mycoplasmas, chlamydiae, *Pneumocystis*, mycobacteria, fungi, and legionellae, cannot be cultured by routine methods.

Since expectorated material is routinely contaminated by oral anaerobes, the diagnosis of anaerobic pulmonary infection is frequently inferred. Confirmation of such a diagnosis requires the culture of anaerobes from pulmonary secretions that are uncontaminated by oropharyngeal secretions, which in turn requires the collection of pulmonary secretions by special techniques, such as transtracheal aspiration (TTA), transthoracic lung puncture, and protected brush via bronchoscopy. These procedures are invasive and are usually not used unless the patient fails to respond to empirical therapy.

Gram's staining of sputum specimens, screened initially under low-power magnification ($10\times$ objective and $10\times$ eyepiece) to determine the degree of contamination with squamous epithelial cells, is of utmost diagnostic importance. In patients with the typical pneumonia syndrome who produce purulent sputum, the sensitivity and specificity of Gram's staining of sputum minimally contaminated by upper respiratory tract secretions (>25 polymorphonuclear leukocytes and <10 epithelial cells per low-power field) in identifying the pathogen as *S. pneumoniae* are 62 and 85%, respectively. Gram's staining in this case is more specific and probably more sensitive than the accompanying sputum culture. The finding of mixed flora on Gram's staining of an uncontaminated sputum specimen suggests an anaerobic infection. Acid-fast staining of sputum should be undertaken when mycobacterial infection is suspected. Examination by an experienced pathologist of Giemsa-stained expectorated respiratory secretions from patients with AIDS has given satisfactory results in the diagnosis of PCP. The sensitivity of sputum examination is enhanced by the use of monoclonal antibodies to *Pneumocystis* and is diminished by prior prophylactic use of inhaled pentamidine. Blastomycosis can be diagnosed by the examination of wet preparations of sputum. Sputum stained directly with fluorescent antibody can be examined for *Legionella*, but this test yields false-negative results relatively often. Thus sputum should also be cultured for *Legionella* on special media.

Expectorated sputum usually is easily collected from patients with a vigorous cough but may be scant in patients with an atypical syndrome, in the elderly, and in persons with altered mental status. If the patient is not producing sputum and can cooperate, respiratory secretions should be induced with ultrasonic nebulization of 3% saline. An attempt to obtain lower respiratory secretions by passage of a catheter through the nose or mouth rarely achieves the desired results in an alert patient and is discouraged; usually the catheter can be found coiled in the oropharynx.

In some cases that do not require the patient's hospitalization (see "Decision to Hospitalize," below), an accurate microbial diagnosis may not be crucial, and empirical therapy can be started on the basis of clinical and epidemiologic evidence alone. This approach may also be appropriate for hospitalized patients who are not severely ill and who are unable to produce an induced sputum specimen. Use of invasive procedures to establish a microbial diagnosis carries risks that must be weighed against potential benefits. However, the decision to initiate empirical therapy without an evaluation of induced sputum should be undertaken with caution and, in the case of hospitalized patients, should always be accompanied by the culture of several blood samples. The ability to understand the cause of a poor response to empirical antimicrobial therapy (Table 255-4) may be compromised by the lack of initial sputum and blood cultures. Establishing a specific microbial etiology in the individual patient is important, for it allows institution of specific pathogen–directed antimicrobial therapy and reduces the use of broad-spectrum combination regimens to cover multiple possible pathogens. Use of a single narrow-spectrum antimicrobial agent exposes the patient to fewer potential adverse drug reactions and reduces the pressure for selection of antimicrobial resistance. Emergence of antimicrobial resistance is a type of adverse drug reaction unlike others, because it is "contagious." In addition, establishing a microbial diagnosis can help define local community outbreaks and antimicrobial resistance patterns.

Invasive Procedures   The sensitivities and specificities of the invasive procedures described below for obtaining pulmonary material vary with the type of immunocompromised patient, the type of pulmonary lesion, and the degree of prior exposure to therapeutic or prophylactic antimicrobial agents.

Transtracheal aspiration   Popular several decades ago, TTA is rarely performed today. Although the sensitivity of the procedure is high (approaching 90%), the specificity is low. The material obtained by TTA (from a catheter inserted through the cricothyroid cartilage and advanced toward the carina) is not contaminated by upper respiratory tract secretions but can contain organisms that colonize the tracheobronchial tree without necessarily causing pneumonia. Significant morbidity and even death have attended the use of TTA. Contraindicated in patients with a bleeding diathesis, TTA may cause infection at the puncture site and may lead to severe subcutaneous and mediastinal emphysema in patients who are coughing vigorously.

Percutaneous transthoracic lung puncture   This procedure employs a skinny (small-gauge) needle that is advanced into the area of pulmonary consolidation with computed tomographic guidance. It requires that the patient cooperate, have good hemostasis, and be able to tolerate a possible associated pulmonary hemorrhage or pneumothorax. Patients on mechanical ventilation cannot undergo lung puncture because of the high incidence of complicating pneumothorax.

Table 255-4   Factors Involved in Poor Response to Empirical Antimicrobial Therapy

Incorrect microbiologic diagnosis
Inappropriate antimicrobial agent or dosing regimen
Drug hypersensitivity or other adverse effect (e.g., *Clostridium difficile* colitis)
Infectious complication: empyema, metastatic spread, superinfection
Atelectasis, parapneumonic effusion, phlebitis
Poor host defenses (e.g., endobronchial obstruction, life-threatening comorbidity)

Step 1	Step 2

Step 1

Patients with community-acquired pneumonia

↓

Is the patient more than 50 years of age? — **Yes** →

↓ No

Does the patient have a history of any of the following coexisting conditions?
Neoplastic disease
Congestive heart failure
Cerebrovascular disease
Renal disease
Liver disease — **Yes** →

↓ No

Does the patient have any of the following abnormalities on physical examination?
Altered mental status
Pulse ≥125/minute
Respiratory rate ≥30/minute
Systolic blood pressure <90 mmHg
Temperature <35°C or ≥40°C — **Yes** →

↓ No

Assign patient to risk class I

(center box) → Assign patient to risk class II–V according to step 2 of the prediction rule

Step 2

Characteristic	Points Assigned*
Demographic factor	
Age	
Men	Age (yr)
Women	Age (yr) − 10
Nursing home resident	+10
Coexisting illnesses	
Neoplastic disease	+30
Liver disease	+20
Congestive heart failure	+10
Cerebrovascular disease	+10
Renal disease	+10
Physical examination findings	
Altered mental status	+20
Respiratory rate ≥30/min	+20
Systolic blood pressure <90 mmHg	+20
Temperature <35°C or ≥40°C	+15
Pulse ≥125/min	+10
Laboratory and radiographic findings	
Arterial pH <7.35	+30
Blood urea nitrogen >30 mg/dL (11 mmol/L)	+20
Sodium <130 mmol/L	+20
Glucose >250 mg/dL (14 mmol/L)	+10
Hematocrit <30%	+10
Partial pressure of arterial oxygen <60 mmHg or O$_2$ saturation <90%	+10
Pleural effusion	+10

Risk class	No. of points	Recommendations for site of care
I	No predictors	Outpatient
II	≤70	Outpatient
III	71–90	Inpatient (briefly)
IV	91–130	Inpatient
V	>130	Inpatient

FIGURE 255-1 Criteria for hospitalization of patients with pneumonia: the PORT score. *A risk score (total point score) for a given patient is obtained by summing the patient's age in years (age minus 10 for females) and the points for each applicable patient characteristic. †Oxygen saturation of <90% is also considered abnormal. (*Adapted from Fine et al. and Bartlett et al.*)

Fiberoptic bronchoscopy Fiberoptic bronchoscopy is safe and relatively well tolerated and has become the standard invasive procedure used to obtain lower respiratory tract secretions from seriously ill or immunocompromised patients with complex or progressive pneumonia. This technique provides a direct view of the lower airways. Specimens obtained by bronchoscopy should be subjected to Gram's, acid-fast, *Legionella* direct fluorescent antibody, and Gomori's methenamine silver staining and should be cultured for routine aerobic and anaerobic bacteria, legionellae, mycobacteria, and fungi. Samples are collected with a protected double-sheathed brush (PSB), by bronchoalveolar lavage (BAL), or by transbronchial biopsy (TBB) at the site of pulmonary consolidation. The PSB sample is usually contaminated by oropharyngeal flora; quantitative cultures of the 1 mL of sterile culture medium into which the brush is placed after withdrawal from the inner catheter must be performed to differentiate contamination (<1000 CFU/mL) from infection (≥1000 CFU/mL). The results of PSB are highly specific and highly sensitive, especially when the patient has not received antibiotics before culture. BAL is usually performed with 150 to 200 mL of sterile, nonbacteriostatic saline. When used to facilitate endoscopy, local anesthetic agents with antibacterial activity can lower the sensitivity of culture results. Quantitative bacteriologic evaluation of BAL fluid has given results similar to those obtained with the PSB technique. Gram's staining of the cytocentrifuged BAL fluid specimen can serve as an immediate guide in the selection of antimicrobial therapy to be administered while culture results are awaited.

Open-lung biopsy This procedure is most commonly needed when specimens obtained bronchoscopically from an immunocompromised patient with progressive pneumonia have been unrevealing. Limitations on the performance of an open-lung biopsy include hypoxemia and a bleeding diathesis, which may supervene while the physician is deciding whether to undertake this procedure. Results of an open-lung biopsy are considered diagnostic because of the large size of the tissue sample. The diagnostic yield of this procedure is greatest in focal lesions, whereas bronchoscopic evaluation is most useful in diffuse lesions.

Other Diagnostic Tests In the initial evaluation of a patient with pneumonia, at least two blood samples for culture should be obtained from different venipuncture sites; if empyema is a clinical consideration, diagnostic thoracentesis is indicated. Positive blood or pleural fluid culture is generally considered diagnostic of the etiology of pneumonia. However, bacteremia and empyema each occur in fewer than 10 to 30% of patients with pneumonia.

Serologic studies are sometimes helpful in defining the etiology of certain types of pneumonia, although serologic diagnosis—because it is often delayed by the need to demonstrate at least a fourfold rise in convalescent-phase antibody titer—is usually retrospective. A single IgM antibody titer of >1:16, a single IgG antibody titer of >1:128, or a fourfold or greater rise in the IgG titer obtained by indirect immunofluorescence is diagnostic of *M. pneumoniae* infection. A single IgM antibody titer of ≥1:20, a single IgG antibody titer of ≥1:128, or a fourfold or greater rise in the IgG titer obtained by micro-indirect immunofluorescence is diagnostic of *C. pneumoniae* infection. A single *Legionella* antibody titer of ≥1:256 or a fourfold rise to a titer of ≥1:128 suggests acute legionellosis. A highly sensitive and specific urinary antigen test is available to detect *L. pneumophila* serogroup 1 in patients with pneumonia; this organism accounts for ~70% of *L. pneumophila* infections. The diagnosis of hantavirus infection is confirmed by detection of IgM serum antibodies, a rising titer of IgG serum antibodies, hantavirus-specific RNA by polymerase chain reaction in clinical specimens, and hantavirus-specific antigen by immunohistochemistry.

DECISION TO HOSPITALIZE Approximately 20% of patients with community-acquired pneumonia are hospitalized, some perhaps unnecessarily. Use of inpatient hospital services is costly and at times poses risks to the patient (e.g., the risk of nosocomial infections). Thus hospitalization must be justified by anticipation of a poor outcome if the case is managed in an outpatient setting.

The Pneumonia Patient Outcomes Research Team (PORT) has attempted to quantify the risk of death and other adverse outcomes of community-acquired pneumonia by assignment of points to 19 variables (Fig. 255-1), with stratification of patients into five classes based on cumulative point score. This prediction rule was derived and validated in a large number of patients. On the basis of their observations, the PORT investigators suggest that outpatient management is appropriate for many patients in classes I and II, in whom the risks of subsequent hospitalization (≤8.2%) and of death (<0.6%) are low. They suggest outpatient management after a short hospital stay for patients in class III, whose risk of subsequent hospitalization if initially treated at home is 16.7% but whose risk of admission to the intensive care unit (ICU) is 5.9%—similar to that for patients in classes I and II. The PORT investigators further suggest that patients in classes IV and V (risk of death, 8.2 and 29.2%, respectively; risk of ICU admission, 11.4 and 17.3%, respectively) should receive traditional inpatient care. An expert panel from the Infectious Diseases Society of America (IDSA) endorses the PORT recommendations.

Other characteristics that favor a decision to hospitalize the patient include the known presence of certain etiologic microorganisms (e.g., *S. aureus*) that are associated with a poor prognosis, multilobe pulmonary involvement, suppurative complications (e.g., empyema or septic arthritis), evidence of poor functional status (e.g., hypotension or hypoxemia on presentation in patients otherwise in classes I, II, and III), evidence of a patient's inability to comply with treatment recommendations, anticipated difficulty in assessing the response to outpatient treatment, and an inadequate home support system that may compromise outpatient care. Discharge from the hospital should be guided by similar considerations.

TREATMENT Community-Acquired Pneumonia: Outpatient Management Most cases of community-acquired pneumonia in otherwise-healthy adults do not require hospitalization. Although desirable, it is often impractical in the outpatient setting to obtain a chest radiograph and sputum Gram's stain and culture in order to confirm the clinical diagnosis of pneumonia and its microbial etiology before starting antimicrobial therapy. Consequently, the oral antimicrobial treatment administered in the outpatient setting is frequently empirical (Table 255-5). The pathogen in such a situation is likely to be *M. pneumoniae*, *S. pneumoniae*, or *C. pneumoniae*. In older patients with underlying chronic respiratory disease, *L. pneumophila*, *H. influenzae*, or *M. catarrhalis* should also be considered. In patients at risk of aspiration, oral anaerobes may be involved. Few oral antimicrobial drugs have a reliable spectrum encompassing all of these pathogens (Table 255-5). Whatever regimen is chosen, its antimicrobial activity should encompass *S. pneumoniae*, the most common cause of pneumonia. Increasing resistance among pneumococci to all the available oral antimicrobial agents precludes the designation of any one agent as the clear drug of choice.

Strains of *S. pneumoniae* for which the minimal inhibitory concentration (MIC) of penicillin (as determined by the broth dilution method) is 0.1 to 1.0 μg/mL are considered to have intermediate-level resistance, while strains whose MIC is >1.0 μg/mL are considered to have high-level resistance. The current, less time-consuming method to screen for penicillin resistance is the use of a 1-μg oxacillin disk in a disk diffusion assay. Penicillin resistance (i.e., an MIC $\geq$0.1 μg/mL) is indicated by a zone of growth inhibition of $\leq$19 mm. Antimicrobial gradient paper strips (the E-test), which yield the exact MIC, are as accurate as the broth dilution technique, can be performed as rapidly as the oxacillin disk diffusion assay, and have replaced the oxacillin disk test in many institutions.

The resistance of *S. pneumoniae* to penicillin varies greatly with the source of the clinical sample tested (e.g., strains isolated from middle-ear fluid are most often resistant), the age of the patient (e.g., resistance is more frequent among children than among adults), the setting (e.g., resistance is more common in day-care centers), the patient's socioeconomic status (the frequency of resistance is highest in samples from suburban and white patients), and the geographic region in which the specimen was collected. Caution must be exercised in the interpretation of surveys of antimicrobial resistance among pneumococci in the United States, which can be strongly affected by these types of sampling bias. In a national survey of clinical isolates from normally sterile body sites that was conducted in 1997 in various surveillance areas throughout the United States by the Centers for Disease Control and Prevention (CDC), 11% (range, 6 to 19%) of 3110 isolates of *S. pneumoniae* exhibited intermediate-level resistance to penicillin, and 14% (range, 8 to 26%) displayed high-level resistance. However, in another national survey of the antimicrobial susceptibility of clinical isolates obtained from respiratory tract sites between February and June 1997 at 27 U.S. medical centers (SENTRY surveillance program), 28% of 845 isolates (with a range of 11 to 52% at the various medical centers) displayed intermediate-level penicillin resistance, and an additional 16% (with a range of 0 to 33%) displayed high-level penicillin resistance.

As a consequence of the production of altered penicillin-binding proteins with decreased β-lactam affinity, penicillin-resistant *S. pneumoniae* exhibits at least some degree of cross-resistance to all β-lactams, including the extended-spectrum third- and fourth-generation cephalosporins. Since the mechanism of penicillin resistance does not involve β-lactamase production, β-lactam/β-lactamase inhibitor combinations (e.g., amoxicillin/clavulanate) offer no advantage. Indeed, the MICs of penicillin and amoxicillin are nearly identical, but the serum levels after equivalent doses are much higher for amoxicillin than for penicillin, a difference that may reflect a therapeutic advantage of amoxicillin. Among the oral cephalosporins, cefaclor, cefadroxil, and cephalexin have variable activity against penicillin-sensitive strains; cefuroxime and cefpodoxime have activity against penicillin-susceptible strains but variable activity against penicillin-intermediate strains and no activity against highly penicillin-resistant strains.

Table 255-5 Empirical Oral Antimicrobial Therapy for Outpatient Management of Community-Acquired Pneumonia

Pathogen	Value of Indicated Antimicrobial[a]							
	Penicillin G	Amoxicillin/ Clavulanate	Cefuroxime	Trimethoprim-Sulfamethoxazole	Doxycycline	Erythromycin	Ciprofloxacin	Newer Fluoroquinolones[b]
Streptococcus pneumoniae	±[c]	±[c]	±[c]	±[c]	+[c]	±[c]	±	+[c]
Haemophilus influenzae	−	+	+	+	+	−[d]	+	+
Moraxella catarrhalis	−	+	+	+	+	+	+	+
Anaerobes	±	+	±	−	−	−	−	±
Mycoplasma pneumoniae	−	−	−	−	+	+	+	+
Chlamydia pneumoniae	−	−	−	−	+	+	+	+
Legionella pneumophila	−	−	−	±	±	+	+	+

[a] +, effective; −, ineffective; ±, sometimes effective.
[b] Levofloxacin, gatifloxacin, moxifloxacin, and sparfloxacin.
[c] In the United States, about 42% of strains are currently resistant to penicillin (15% with high-level penicillin resistance), 20% to amoxicillin and cefuroxime, 20–30% to trimethoprim-sulfamethoxazole, 7–10% to doxycycline (tetracycline), 14% to erythromycin, and <4% to the newer fluoroquinolones.
[d] The new macrolides azithromycin and clarithromycin are more active against *H. influenzae* than erythromycin and are equally or more active against other respiratory pathogens.

Resistance to other antimicrobial agents, such as the macrolides (erythromycin, clarithromycin, and azithromycin), clindamycin, tetracycline and doxycycline, and trimethoprim-sulfamethoxazole (TMP-SMZ), is also more common among penicillin-intermediate strains than among penicillin-susceptible strains, and it is most common among highly penicillin-resistant strains. Overall rates of resistance among *S. pneumoniae* strains are ~14% for the macrolides, 4% for clindamycin, up to 10% for tetracyclines, and 20 to 30% for TMP-SMZ. Rates of resistance to the newer fluoroquinolones levofloxacin, gatifloxacin, moxifloxacin, and sparfloxacin are <4%, regardless of penicillin susceptibility. At best, the older fluoroquinolones (e.g., ciprofloxacin) have borderline activity, as judged by serum levels in relation to MICs of these drugs against the pneumococcus.

Optimally, the choice of antimicrobial drugs for empirical therapy should be guided by local resistance patterns, if known. Options for empirical antimicrobial therapy should be modified in light of continually evolving antimicrobial resistance patterns resulting from the introduction of new resistant clones into the community from other regions or the emergence of resistant mutants under the selective pressure of local patterns of antimicrobial use. The IDSA has published guidelines for the treatment of community-acquired pneumonia. These guidelines emphasize the need for a chest radiograph when pneumonia is suspected and for the establishment of a microbial diagnosis (e.g., by sputum Gram's stain with or without culture) whenever possible. Doxycycline and the newer fluoroquinolones are recommended alternatives for initial empirical oral therapy, especially when penicillin-resistant pneumococci are suspected. The utility of the macrolides and amoxicillin depends on susceptibility of pneumococci in the local community.

The regimen should be modified for patients with particular epidemiologic factors or comorbidities related to specific pathogens—e.g., structural lung disease or suspected aspiration. Aspiration pneumonia can be treated with amoxicillin/clavulanate, clindamycin, or amoxicillin plus metronidazole because these regimens are active against oral anaerobes. Metronidazole alone has inadequate activity against microaerophilic gram-positive cocci and must be supplemented with a β-lactam agent that compensates for this defect in spectrum. If macrolides are used and *H. influenzae* is suspected, azithro-mycin or clarithromycin is preferred because of erythromycin's poor activity against this organism. Alternative agents for *H. influenzae* include amoxicillin/clavulanate, doxycycline, or a fluoroquinolone. The β-lactams are not active against pathogens causing atypical pneumonia (e.g., *Mycoplasma*, *C. pneumoniae*, or *Legionella*), in which case doxycycline, a macrolide, or a fluoroquinolone is preferred.

The IDSA guidelines recommend that pneumococcal pneumonia be treated for 7 to 10 days or until the patient has been afebrile for 72 h. Pneumonia caused by *Legionella*, *C. pneumoniae*, or *Mycoplasma* should be treated for 2 to 3 weeks unless azithromycin is used, in which case a 5-day course is acceptable because of the drug's prolonged half-life in tissues.

Community-Acquired Pneumonia: Inpatient Management
Patients who have community-acquired pneumonia and are ill enough to be hospitalized (Fig. 255-1) must have a chest radiograph to establish the diagnosis of pneumonia, must undergo prompt microbiologic evaluation (including Gram's staining and culture of sputum and culture of two blood samples drawn by separate venipuncture), and must receive empirical antimicrobial therapy based on Gram's staining of sputum and knowledge of the current antimicrobial sensitivities of the pulmonary pathogens in the local geographic area (Tables 255-6 and 255-7). Antimicrobial therapy should be initiated promptly (e.g., within 8 h of admission). Parenteral antimicrobial therapy in the hospitalized patient is usually mandatory. A lack of sputum production, an atypical clinical presentation, the presence of diffuse radiographic infiltrates, a rapidly progressive downhill course, and a poor response to prior empirical therapy are among the indications for the use of invasive procedures to detect the pulmonary pathogen, especially in the immunocompromised patient. Although broad-spectrum antibacterial therapy should be started during a full evaluation in severely ill patients with rapidly progressing illness, these empirical regimens cannot encompass all the possible pathogens without producing unnecessary toxicity and expense. Indeed, in immunocompromised patients (including those with neutropenia or HIV infection), the number of microbial and noninfectious causes of pulmonary disease is large and increasing. Since failure to provide specific treatment can prove rapidly fatal, a diagnosis should be sought aggressively so that optimal therapy can be started promptly.

Penicillin or ampicillin remains the drug of choice for infection due to penicillin-susceptible pneumococci. Studies suggest that high-

Table 255-6   Empirical Antimicrobial Therapy for the Management of Hospitalized Patients with Community-Acquired Pneumonia

Pathogen	Penicillin G	Second-Generation Cephalosporins	Third- and Fourth-Generation Cephalosporins[b]	Metronidazole	Trimethoprim-Sulfamethoxazole	Erythromycin	Ampicillin/Sulbactam	Newer Fluoro-quinolones[c]
Streptococcus pneumoniae	±[d]	±[d]	+[d]	−	±[d]	±[d]	±[d]	+[d]
Staphylococcus aureus	−	+	+	−	+	+	+	+
Haemophilus influenzae	−	+	+	−	+	−	+	+
Moraxella catarrhalis	−	+	+	−	+	+	+	+
Anaerobic gram-positive cocci	+	+	+	±	−	±	+	±
Anaerobic gram-negative bacilli	−	−	−	+	−	−	+	±
Chlamydia pneumoniae	−	−	−	−	−	+	−	+
Legionella pneumophila	−	−	−	−	±	+	−	+
Mycoplasma pneumoniae	−	−	−	−	−	+	−	+

Value of Indicated Antimicrobial[a]

[a] +, effective; −, ineffective; ±, sometimes effective.
[b] Ceftriaxone, cefotaxime, and cefepime.
[c] Levofloxacin, gatifloxacin, moxifloxacin, and sparfloxacin.
[d] In the United States, about 42% of strains are currently resistant to penicillin (15% with high-level penicillin resistance; ampicillin slightly less active than penicillin), 20% are resistant to cefuroxime (similar activity displayed by the first-generation cephalosporin cephalothin), 4–5% are highly resistant to third- or fourth-generation cephalosporins, 20–30% are resistant to trimethoprim-sulfamethoxazole, 7–10% are resistant to doxycycline (tetracycline), 14% are resistant to erythromycin, and <4% are resistant to the newer fluoroquinolones.

Drug	Dosage
Ampicillin/sulbactam	3 g IV q6h
Aztreonam	2 g IV q8h
Cefazolin	1–2 g IV q8h
Cefepime	2 g IV q8h
Cefotaxime, ceftizoxime	1–2 g IV q8–12h
Ceftazidime	2 g IV q8h
Ceftriaxone	1–2 g IV q12h
Cefuroxime	750 mg IV q8h
Ciprofloxacin	400 mg IV or 750 mg PO q12h
Clindamycin	600–900 mg IV q8h
Erythromycin	0.5–1.0 g IV q6h
Gentamicin (or tobramycin)	5 mg/kg/d in 3 equally divided doses IV q8h
Imipenem	500 mg IV q6h
Levofloxacin	500 mg IV or PO q24h
Metronidazole	500 mg IV or PO q6h
Nafcillin	2 g IV q4h
Penicillin G	3 million units IV q4–6h
Piperacillin/tazobactam	4.5 g IV q6h
Ticarcillin/clavulanate	3.1 g IV q4h
Vancomycin	1 g (15 mg/kg) IV q12h

[a] Dosage must be modified for patients with renal failure. Guidelines on the duration of therapy for each pathogen are given in the text of this chapter and of chapters on specific infecting agents.

dose intravenous penicillin G (e.g., 10 to 20 million units daily), ampicillin (2 g every 6 h), ceftriaxone (1 or 2 g every 24 h), or cefotaxime (1 to 2 g every 6 h) constitutes adequate therapy for pneumonia due to strains exhibiting intermediate resistance to penicillin (MIC, 0.1 to 1 μg/mL). The effectiveness of high-dose intravenous penicillin against pneumonia due to highly resistant pneumococcal strains is unknown, but MICs of cefotaxime and ceftriaxone for these strains are usually lower than those of penicillin or ampicillin and most other β-lactam antibiotics. Ceftriaxone or cefotaxime may be effective when the MIC of penicillin is ≥ 1 μg/mL and those of ceftriaxone and cefotaxime are ≤ 2 μg/mL. However, highly cephalosporin-resistant strains have become a problem in certain geographic areas. Since all penicillin-resistant strains are sensitive to vancomycin, initial empirical therapy should include this antibiotic (1 g intravenously every 12 h) when the patient with pneumococcal pneumonia is severely ill, has significant comorbidity, and lives in a region where highly penicillin- or cephalosporin-resistant strains have become common.

If the result of Gram's staining of sputum is not interpretable or not available, then the IDSA guidelines recommend empirical therapy for patients hospitalized on a general medical unit with a β-lactam (e.g., ceftriaxone, cefotaxime) or a β-lactam/β-lactamase inhibitor combination, with or without a macrolide, or with one of the fluoroquinolones alone. Seriously ill patients who are hospitalized in the ICU should always receive a macrolide or a newer fluoroquinolone in addition to the β-lactam to cover Legionella. The therapeutic regimens should be modified further in the following situations: structural disease of the lung (e.g., bronchiectasis) requires treatment with an anti-Pseudomonas β-lactam plus a macrolide or with a newer fluoroquinolone plus an aminoglycoside; penicillin allergy requires treatment with a newer fluoroquinolone, with or without clindamycin; and suspected aspiration requires treatment with a newer fluoroquinolone plus either clindamycin or metronidazole or with a β-lactam/β-lactamase inhibitor combination alone. A recent study of almost 13,000 elderly hospitalized patients with pneumonia, which controlled for severity of illness, baseline differences in patient characteristics, and processes of care, documented 30-day mortality that was 26 to 36% lower among those treated initially with a fluoroquinolone alone or a macrolide combined with a second- or nonpseudomonal third-generation cephalosporin than among those initially given a nonpseudomonal third-generation cephalosporin alone. This result may reflect the importance of pathogens such as Mycoplasma, Legionella, and C. pneumoniae in these patients.

Therapy can be switched from intravenous to oral agents within 3 days to complete a 7- to 10-day course if the patient's clinical condition improves rapidly and if antimicrobial agents that are readily absorbed after oral administration and that reach tissue levels above the MIC are available. The presence of S. aureus or aerobic gram-negative bacilli or the development of suppurative complications requires a more prolonged course of therapy. Pneumonia caused by Legionella, C. pneumoniae, or Mycoplasma should be treated for 2 to 3 weeks unless azithromycin is used. Anaerobic lung abscess should be treated with the regimens suggested for aspiration pneumonia until a chest radiograph (with radiography performed at 2-week intervals) is clear or shows only a small stable scar. Therapy is prolonged for ≥ 6 weeks to prevent relapse, although shorter courses are probably sufficient for many patients. Surgery is rarely required for lung abscess; indications for surgery include massive hemoptysis and suspected neoplasm. Supportive measures include the administration of supplemental oxygen and intravenous fluids, assistance in clearing secretions, fiberoptic bronchoscopy, and (if necessary) ventilatory support. Caution should be exercised in bronchoscopic drainage of large, fluid-filled lung abscesses because of the potential for sudden massive spillage of large collections of pus into the airways.

Patients with risk factors for HIV infection and an atypical pneumonia syndrome should be evaluated for PCP because of its frequency as an index diagnosis in HIV infection and its potential severity. Tuberculosis and other causes of atypical pneumonia must be excluded as part of the evaluation of these patients. Empirical therapy can consist of either TMP-SMZ (15 to 20 mg of trimethoprim per kg, given daily in four divided doses intravenously or by mouth) or pentamidine (3 to 4 mg/kg daily, given intravenously), and therapy is continued for 3 weeks in confirmed cases of PCP. Although some data suggest that TMP-SMZ is more effective than pentamidine, further studies directly comparing the two agents are needed. The frequency and severity of the adverse effects of the two drugs are generally thought to be equivalent. The addition of glucocorticoids (prednisone, 40 mg twice daily, with subsequent tapering of the dose) early in the course of PCP in patients with an arterial P_{O_2} of <70 mmHg decreases the need for mechanical ventilation and improves the patient's chances of survival and functional status. Prophylaxis for recurrent PCP must be started at the end of therapy.

Institutionally Acquired Pneumonia Pneumonia acquired in institutions such as nursing homes or hospitals is frequently caused by enteric aerobic gram-negative bacilli, P. aeruginosa, or S. aureus, with or without oral anaerobes. Again, the selection of empirical antimicrobial therapy should be guided by Gram's staining of sputum (Tables 255-7 and 255-8) and knowledge of the prevalent nosocomial pathogens and their current in vitro antimicrobial sensitivity patterns in the institution involved. An aggressive diagnostic approach is needed in some circumstances, especially for the immunocompromised patient (as outlined above).

S. aureus acquired in some institutions is frequently methicillin resistant. Such strains are resistant to all β-lactam antibiotics and may also be resistant to clindamycin, erythromycin, and the fluoroquinolones. Only vancomycin is predictably active against these organisms, and this drug should be added to the empirical regimen when methicillin-resistant organisms may be involved in pneumonia.

When multiantibiotic resistance is a problem, pneumonia due to gram-negative bacilli in the institutionalized patient can be treated initially with a β-lactam active against P. aeruginosa (ceftazidime, cefepime, piperacillin/tazobactam, ticarcillin/clavulanate, aztreonam, or imipenem) or with a parenterally administered fluoroquinolone (ciprofloxacin, ofloxacin, gatifloxacin, or levofloxacin). Among the fluoroquinolones, ciprofloxacin remains the most potent antipseudomonal agent. Ticarcillin/clavulanate and piperacillin/tazobactam are preferred over other penicillins with activity against P. aeruginosa (e.g., ticarcillin or piperacillin alone), which are not sufficiently active against Klebsiella pneumoniae, a relatively common pathogen. However, for

Table 255-8 Empirical Antimicrobial Therapy, Based on Gram's Staining of Sputum, for Institutionally Acquired Pneumonia

Etiology	Regimen
Presumptive *Staphylococcus aureus*	Nafcillin or vancomycin[a]
Presumptive enteric aerobic gram-negative bacilli or *Pseudomonas aeruginosa*	1. Ceftazidime or cefepime ± aminoglycoside 2. Ticarcillin/clavulanate or piperacillin/tazobactam ± aminoglycoside 3. Aztreonam ± aminoglycoside 4. Imipenem[b,c] ± aminoglycoside 5. Fluoroquinolone[c] ± aminoglycoside or β-lactam
Mixed flora	1. Ceftazidime or cefepime + clindamycin (or metronidazole) ± aminoglycoside[e] 2. Ticarcillin/clavulanate or piperacillin/tazobactam ± aminoglycoside[e] 3. Aztreonam + clindamycin (or metronidazole[d]) ± aminoglycoside[e] 4. Imipenem[b,c] ± aminoglycoside[e] 5. Fluoroquinolone[c] + clindamycin (or metronidazole[d,e]) ± aminoglycoside or β-lactam

[a] If methicillin-resistant *S. aureus* is known to exist in the institution, use vancomycin; otherwise, use an antistaphylococcal β-lactam such as nafcillin or cefazolin.
[b] Use when extended-spectrum β-lactamase producers are endemic in the institution.
[c] Use when chromosomally encoded, inducible β-lactamase producers are endemic in the institution.
[d] Metronidazole must be combined with vancomycin or another antimicrobial that covers microaerophilic and anaerobic gram-positive cocci.
[e] Add vancomycin if methicillin-resistant *S. aureus* is present in the institution.

infection suspected to be due to *P. aeruginosa*, the higher dose recommended by the package insert is required; a lower dose contains less piperacillin or ticarcillin than is needed to be effective against this organism. Ampicillin/sulbactam, the other parenterally administered β-lactam/β-lactamase inhibitor combination, is not active against many nosocomial pathogens, such as *P. aeruginosa*, *Enterobacter* spp., and *Serratia* spp., and therefore is inappropriate as empirical therapy for nosocomial pneumonia.

In seriously ill patients, especially those infected with organisms in which resistance frequently emerges during therapy (e.g., *P. aeruginosa*), use of a β-lactam/aminoglycoside or β-lactam/fluoroquinolone combination is prudent. Combinations of a β-lactam plus an aminoglycoside are used for bactericidal synergy. Combinations of a β-lactam or an aminoglycoside with a fluoroquinolone are not expected to enhance the already-rapid bactericidal activity of the fluoroquinolone alone. However, such combinations are also used to broaden the spectrum of antibacterial activity, to cover the possibility of infection with resistant pathogens, to treat polymicrobial infection, and to prevent the emergence of antimicrobial resistance.

Pneumonia due to possible coinfection with aerobic gram-negative bacilli and anaerobes, as reflected by a polymicrobial flora on Gram's staining of sputum, can usually be treated with any of the following regimens: (1) cefepime or ceftazidime plus metronidazole or clindamycin, (2) aztreonam or a fluoroquinolone plus clindamycin, or (3) imipenem, piperacillin/tazobactam, or ticarcillin/clavulanate. The regimens should include double coverage for *P. aeruginosa* when this organism is suspected (Table 255-8).

The production of chromosomally encoded, inducible β-lactamases by some aerobic gram-negative bacilli, including *Serratia marcescens*, *Enterobacter cloacae*, *Citrobacter freundii*, *Morganella morganii*, *P. aeruginosa*, and *Acinetobacter calcoaceticus*, has important implications for the treatment of nosocomial pneumonia in institutions where these organisms are common nosocomial pathogens. Antibiotic resistance in these pathogens has been attributed to two related mechanisms: inducible production of chromosomally encoded β-lactamases

and selection of mutants that have lost the genes that control expression of β-lactamase production. The control genes repress β-lactamase production in the absence of a β-lactam agent and allow β-lactamase production in the presence of a β-lactam agent. This group of organisms has a relatively high mutation rate for loss of these control genes, and their loss results in continuous production of large amounts of β-lactamase (*stable derepression*). The derepressed mutants are resistant to third-generation cephalosporins, aztreonam, and broad-spectrum penicillins. These chromosomally encoded, inducible β-lactamases are not inhibited by clavulanic acid, tazobactam, or sulbactam.

Selection by the β-lactam antibiotic of the derepressed mutants present in the dense bacterial populations of infected pulmonary tissue at the initiation of antibiotic therapy apparently accounts for the emergence of resistance during therapy, which is especially problematic in severely compromised patients whose defective host defenses are unable to control the growth of a few resistant mutants. The only β-lactam agents that maintain activity against the derepressed mutants are the fourth-generation cephalosporin cefepime and the carbapenem imipenem. The fluoroquinolones and aminoglycosides may also retain activity against these mutants. TMP-SMZ may remain active against all of these gram-negative bacilli except *P. aeruginosa*, which is inherently resistant to this agent. Some clinicians have questioned the efficacy of aminoglycosides alone for the treatment of gram-negative bacillary pneumonia. The poor clinical efficacy of aminoglycosides has been attributed to the low drug levels attained in bronchial secretions and to a loss of antimicrobial activity due to the relative acidity of purulent secretions, the anaerobic conditions in infected lung, and (in the case of *P. aeruginosa*) the divalent cations calcium and magnesium. The nephrotoxicity and ototoxicity of aminoglycosides frequently lead to underdosing with these agents. These problems are compounded by unpredictable pharmacokinetics that necessitate measurement of serum levels of aminoglycosides. If multiantibiotic-resistant nosocomial organisms are likely to be the pathogens infecting severely compromised patients, reliable empirical agents may be fluoroquinolones, cefepime, and imipenem—unless resistance to these drugs is also endemic in the institution. Some strains of *K. pneumoniae* and *Escherichia coli* have acquired a plasmid encoding the production of an extended-spectrum β-lactamase that can be detected as in vitro resistance to ceftazidime or aztreonam. The presence of an extended-spectrum β-lactamase confers resistance to all third-generation cephalosporins and aztreonam. Some of these strains may also be resistant to piperacillin/tazobactam and cefepime, and many are also resistant to the fluoroquinolones. The only reliable agents are the carbapenems, such as imipenem. Up-to-date knowledge of the antimicrobial sensitivities of an institution's nosocomial pathogens and use of various preventive practices are mandatory.

Amantadine (200 mg/d for most adults and 100 mg/d for persons >65 years of age) is effective for the prevention of influenza A virus infection in the unimmunized patient during an influenza A outbreak and for the treatment (for 5 to 7 days) of early influenza A virus infection. Ribavirin is effective for respiratory syncytial virus infection. Intravenous acyclovir (5 to 10 mg/kg every 8 h for 7 to 14 days) is appropriate for varicella pneumonia. Treatment of cytomegalovirus pneumonia has yielded unsatisfactory results, but intravenous immunoglobulin combined with ganciclovir may be effective in some instances. Therapy for hantavirus pulmonary syndrome is supportive, and overall mortality has been 55%.

PREVENTION The prevention of pneumonia involves either (1) decreasing the likelihood of encountering the pathogen or (2) strengthening the host's response once the pathogen is encountered. The first approach can include measures such as hand washing and glove use by persons who care for patients infected with contact-transmitted pathogens (e.g., aerobic gram-negative bacilli); use of face masks or negative-pressure isolation rooms for patients with pneumonia due to pathogens spread by the aerosol route (e.g., *M. tuberculosis*); prompt institution of effective chemotherapy for patients with contagious illnesses; and correction of conditions that facilitate aspiration. The second approach includes the use of chemoprophylaxis or immunization for patients at risk. Chemoprophylaxis may be administered to patients who have encountered or are likely to encounter the pathogen before they become symptomatic (e.g., amantadine during a community outbreak of influenza A, as mentioned above; isoniazid for tuberculosis; or TMP-SMZ for pneumocystosis) or to patients who are likely to have a recurrence following recovery from a symptomatic episode (e.g., TMP-SMZ for pneumocystosis in patients with HIV infection). The prevention of nosocomial pneumonia requires good infection control practices, judicious use of broad-spectrum antimicrobial agents, and maintenance of patients' gastric acidity—a major factor that prevents colonization of the gastrointestinal tract by nosocomial gram-negative bacillary pathogens. To prevent stress ulceration, it is preferable to use sucralfate, which maintains gastric acidity, rather than H_2-blocking agents. To prevent ventilator-associated nosocomial pneumonia, the following strategies have been proposed: use of the semirecumbent position, of endotracheal tubes that allow continuous aspiration of secretions accumulating above the cuff, and of heat and moisture exchangers that reduce the formation of condensate within the tubing circuitry. Vaccines (Chaps. 122, 138, 149, 190, and 194) are available for immunization against *S. pneumoniae*, *H. influenzae* type b, influenza viruses A and B, and measles virus. Influenza and pneumococcal vaccines are strongly recommended for individuals >65 years of age and for persons of any age who are at risk of adverse consequences of influenza or pneumonia because of underlying conditions. Pneumococcal, *Haemophilus*, and influenza vaccines are recommended for HIV-infected patients who are still capable of responding to a vaccine challenge. The currently available 23-valent pneumococcal vaccine covers 88% of the serotypes causing systemic disease as well as 8% of related serotypes. The increasing prevalence of multiantibiotic resistance among pneumococci makes pneumococcal immunization of high-risk individuals of utmost importance. Immune serum globulin is available for intravenous replacement therapy in those patients with congenital or acquired hypogammaglobulinemia. Some patients who have selective IgG2 subtype deficiency and recurrent sinopulmonary infections and who are immunologically unresponsive to capsular polysaccharide vaccines may nevertheless have an antibody response to the capsular polysaccharide that is covalently linked to a protein, as it is in the conjugate *H. influenzae* type b vaccine and a similar experimental conjugate pneumococcal vaccine.

BIBLIOGRAPHY

BARTLETT JG et al: Community-acquired pneumonia in adults: Guidelines for management. Clin Infect Dis 26:811, 1998

BOWTON DL: Nosocomial pneumonia in the ICU—year 2000 and beyond. Chest 115:28S, 1999

DOERN GV et al: Prevalence of antimicrobial resistance among respiratory tract isolates of *Streptococcus pneumoniae* in North America: 1997 results from the SENTRY Antimicrobial Surveillance Program. Clin Infect Dis 27:764, 1998

FINE MJ et al: A prediction rule to identify low risk patients with community-acquired pneumonia. N Engl J Med 236:243, 1987

GLEASON PP et al: Associations between initial antimicrobial therapy and the medical outcomes for hospitalized elderly patients with pneumonia. Arch Intern Med 159:2562, 1999

HAHN DL et al: Association of *Chlamydia pneumoniae* (strain TWAR) infection with wheezing, asthmatic bronchitis and adult-onset asthma. JAMA 266:225, 1991

JACOBS MR: Treatment and diagnosis of infections caused by drug-resistant *Streptococcus pneumoniae*. Clin Infect Dis 15:119, 1992

LEVISON ME, BUSH L: Pharmacodynamics of antimicrobial agents. Bactericidal and postantibiotic effects. Infect Dis Clin North Am 3:415, 1989

——— et al: Clindamycin compared with penicillin for the treatment of anaerobic lung abscess. Ann Intern Med 98:466, 1983

MEEHAN TP et al: Quality of care, process and outcome in elderly patients with pneumonia. JAMA 278:2080, 1997

PALLARES R et al: Resistance to penicillin and cephalosporin and mortality from severe pneumococcal pneumonia in Barcelona, Spain. N Engl J Med 333:474, 1995

RAMIREZ JA et al: Early switch from intravenous to oral cephalosporins in the treatment of hospitalized patients with community-acquired pneumonia. Arch Intern Med 155:1273, 1995

SANDERS CC, SANDERS WE JR: Clinical significance of inducible β-lactamase in gram-negative bacteria. Eur J Clin Microbiol 6:435, 1987

SHELHAMER JH et al: NIH Conference: Respiratory disease in the immunosuppressed patient. Ann Intern Med 117:415, 1992

STEINHOFF D et al: *Chlamydia pneumoniae* as a cause of community-acquired pneumonia in hospitalized patients in Berlin. Clin Infect Dis 22:958, 1996

WOODHEAD MA et al: Prospective study of the aetiology and outcome of pneumonia in the community. Lancet 1:671, 1987

---

256   *Steven E. Weinberger*

BRONCHIECTASIS

DEFINITION Bronchiectasis is an abnormal and permanent dilatation of bronchi. It may be either focal, involving airways supplying a limited region of pulmonary parenchyma, or diffuse, involving airways in a more widespread distribution. Although this definition is based on pathologic changes in the bronchi, diagnosis is often suggested by the clinical consequences of chronic or recurrent infection in the dilated airways and the associated secretions that pool within these airways.

PATHOLOGY The bronchial dilatation of bronchiectasis is associated with destructive and inflammatory changes in the walls of medium-sized airways, often at the level of segmental or subsegmental bronchi. The normal structural components of the wall, including cartilage, muscle, and elastic tissue, are destroyed and may be replaced by fibrous tissue. The dilated airways frequently contain pools of thick, purulent material, while more peripheral airways are often occluded by secretions or obliterated and replaced by fibrous tissue. Additional microscopic features include bronchial and peribronchial inflammation and fibrosis, ulceration of the bronchial wall, squamous metaplasia, and mucous gland hyperplasia. The parenchyma normally supplied by the affected airways is abnormal, containing varying combinations of fibrosis, emphysema, bronchopneumonia, and atelectasis. As a result of the inflammation, vascularity of the bronchial wall increases, with associated enlargement of the bronchial arteries and anastomoses between the bronchial and pulmonary arterial circulations.

Three different patterns of bronchiectasis were described by Reid in 1950. In *cylindrical bronchiectasis* the bronchi appear as uniformly dilated tubes that end abruptly at the point that smaller airways are obstructed by secretions. In *varicose bronchiectasis* the affected bronchi have an irregular or beaded pattern of dilatation resembling varicose veins. In *saccular (cystic) bronchiectasis* the bronchi have a ballooned appearance at the periphery, ending in blind sacs without recognizable bronchial structures distal to the sacs.

ETIOLOGY AND PATHOGENESIS Bronchiectasis is a consequence of inflammation and destruction of the structural components of the bronchial wall. Infection is the usual cause of the inflammation; microorganisms such as *Pseudomonas aeruginosa* and *Haemophilus influenzae* produce pigments, proteases, and other toxins that injure the respiratory epithelium and impair mucociliary clearance. The host inflammatory response induces epithelial injury, largely as a result of mediators released from neutrophils. As protection against infection is compromised, the dilated airways become more susceptible to colonization and growth of bacteria. Thus, a reinforcing cycle can result, with inflammation producing airway damage, impaired clearance of microorganisms, and further infection, which then completes the cycle by inciting more inflammation.

Infectious Causes Adenovirus and influenza virus are the main viruses that cause bronchiectasis in association with lower respiratory tract involvement. Virulent bacterial infections, especially with potentially necrotizing organisms such as *Staphylococcus aureus*, *Kleb-*

siella, and anaerobes, remain important causes of bronchiectasis when antibiotic treatment of a pneumonia is not given or is significantly delayed. Bronchiectasis has been reported in patients with HIV infection, perhaps at least partly due to recurrent bacterial infection. Tuberculosis can produce bronchiectasis by a necrotizing effect on pulmonary parenchyma and airways and indirectly as a consequence of airway obstruction from bronchostenosis or extrinsic compression by lymph nodes. Nontuberculous mycobacteria are frequently cultured from patients with bronchiectasis, often as secondary infections or colonizing organisms. However, it has now also been recognized that these organisms, especially those of the *Mycobacterium avium* complex, can serve as primary pathogens associated with the development and/or progression of bronchiectasis. Mycoplasmal and necrotizing fungal infections are rare causes of bronchiectasis.

Impaired host defense mechanisms are often involved in the predisposition to recurrent infections. The major cause of localized impairment of host defenses is endobronchial obstruction. Bacteria and secretions cannot be cleared adequately from the obstructed airway, which develops recurrent or chronic infection. Slowly growing endobronchial neoplasms such as carcinoid tumors may be associated with bronchiectasis. Foreign-body aspiration is another important cause of endobronchial obstruction, particularly in children. Airway obstruction can also result from bronchostenosis, from impacted secretions, or from extrinsic compression by enlarged lymph nodes.

Generalized impairment of pulmonary defense mechanisms occurs with immunoglobulin deficiency, primary ciliary disorders, or cystic fibrosis. Infections and bronchiectasis are therefore often more diffuse. With panhypogammaglobulinemia, the best described of the immunoglobulin disorders associated with recurrent infection and bronchiectasis, patients often also have a history of sinus or skin infections. Selective deficiency of an IgG subclass, especially IgG2, has also been described in a small number of patients with bronchiectasis.

The primary disorders associated with ciliary dysfunction, termed *primary ciliary dyskinesia*, are responsible for 5 to 10% of cases of bronchiectasis. Numerous defects are encompassed under this category, including structural abnormalities of the dynein arms, radial spokes, and microtubules. The cilia become dyskinetic; their coordinated, propulsive action is diminished, and bacterial clearance is impaired. The clinical effects include recurrent upper and lower respiratory tract infections, such as sinusitis, otitis media, and bronchiectasis. Because normal sperm motility also depends on proper ciliary function, males are generally infertile (Chap. 335). Approximately half of patients with primary ciliary dyskinesia fall into the subgroup of *Kartagener's syndrome*, in which situs inversus accompanies bronchiectasis and sinusitis.

In cystic fibrosis (Chap. 257), the tenacious secretions in the bronchi are associated with impaired bacterial clearance, resulting in colonization and recurrent infection with a variety of organisms, particularly mucoid strains of *P. aeruginosa* but also *S. aureus*, *H. influenzae*, *Escherichia coli*, and *Burkholderia cepacia*.

Noninfectious Causes   Some cases of bronchiectasis are associated with exposure to a toxic substance that incites a severe inflammatory response. Examples include inhalation of a toxic gas such as ammonia or aspiration of acidic gastric contents, though the latter problem is often also complicated by aspiration of bacteria. An immune response in the airway may also trigger inflammation, destructive changes, and bronchial dilatation. This mechanism is presumably responsible at least in part for bronchiectasis with allergic bronchopulmonary aspergillosis (ABPA), which is due to an immune response to *Aspergillus* organisms that have colonized the airway (Chap. 253). Bronchiectasis accompanying ABPA often involves proximal airways and is associated with mucoid impaction. Bronchiectasis also occurs rarely in ulcerative colitis, rheumatoid arthritis, and Sjögren's syndrome, but it is not known whether an immune response triggers airway inflammation in these patients.

In α_1-antitrypsin deficiency, the usual respiratory complication is the early development of panacinar emphysema, but affected individuals may occasionally have bronchiectasis. In the *yellow nail syndrome*, which is due to hypoplastic lymphatics, the triad of lymphedema, pleural effusion, and yellow discoloration of the nails is accompanied by bronchiectasis in approximately 40% of patients.

CLINICAL MANIFESTATIONS   Patients typically present with persistent or recurrent cough and purulent sputum production. Hemoptysis occurs in 50 to 70% of cases and can be due to bleeding from friable, inflamed airway mucosa. More significant, even massive bleeding is often a consequence of bleeding from hypertrophied bronchial arteries.

When a specific infectious episode initiates bronchiectasis, patients may describe a severe pneumonia followed by chronic cough and sputum production. Alternatively, patients without a dramatic initiating event often describe the insidious onset of symptoms. In some cases, patients are either asymptomatic or have a nonproductive cough, often associated with "dry" bronchiectasis in an upper lobe. Dyspnea or wheezing generally reflects either widespread bronchiectasis or underlying chronic obstructive pulmonary disease. With exacerbations of infection, the amount of sputum increases, it becomes more purulent and often more bloody, and patients may become febrile. Such episodes may be due solely to exacerbations of the airway infection, but associated parenchymal infiltrates sometimes reflect an adjacent pneumonia.

Physical examination of the chest overlying an area of bronchiectasis is quite variable. Any combination of crackles, rhonchi, and wheezes may be heard, all of which reflect the damaged airways containing significant secretions. As with other types of chronic intrathoracic infection, clubbing may be present. Patients with severe, diffuse disease, particularly those with chronic hypoxemia, may have associated cor pulmonale and right ventricular failure. Amyloidosis can result from chronic infection and inflammation but is now seldom seen.

RADIOGRAPHIC AND LABORATORY FINDINGS
Though the chest radiograph is important in the evaluation of suspected bronchiectasis, the findings are often nonspecific. At one extreme, the radiograph may be normal with mild disease. Alternatively, patients with saccular bronchiectasis may have prominent cystic spaces, either with or without air-liquid levels, corresponding to the dilated airways. These may be difficult to distinguish from enlarged airspaces due to bullous emphysema or from regions of honeycombing in patients with severe interstitial lung disease. Other findings are due to dilated airways with thickened walls, which result from peribronchial inflammation. Because of decreased aeration and atelectasis of the associated pulmonary parenchyma, these dilated airways are often crowded together in parallel. When seen longitudinally, the airways appear as "tram tracks"; when seen in cross-section, they produce "ring shadows." Because the dilated airways may be filled with secretions, the lumen may appear dense rather than radiolucent, producing an opaque tubular or branched tubular structure.

Bronchography, which involves coating the airways with a radiopaque, iodinated lipid dye instilled through a catheter or bronchoscope, can provide excellent visualization of bronchiectatic airways. However, this technique has now been replaced by computed tomography (CT), which also provides an excellent view of dilated airways as seen in cross-sectional images (Fig. 256-1). With the advent of high-resolution CT scanning, in which the images are 1.0 to 1.5 mm thick, the sensitivity for detecting bronchiectasis has improved even further. Other features on high-resolution CT scanning can suggest a specific etiology of the bronchiectasis. For example, bronchiectasis of relatively proximal airways suggests ABPA, whereas the presence of multiple small pulmonary nodules (nodular bronchiectasis) suggests infection with *M. avium* complex.

Examination of sputum often reveals an abundance of neutrophils and colonization or infection with a variety of possible organisms. Appropriate staining and culturing of sputum often provide a guide to antibiotic therapy.

Additional evaluation is aimed at diagnosing the cause for the bronchiectasis. When bronchiectasis is focal, fiberoptic bronchoscopy

FIGURE 256-1 High-resolution CT scan of bronchiectasis showing dilated airways in both lower lobes and in the lingula. When seen in cross section, the dilated airways have a ringlike appearance. *(From Weinberger, with permission).*

may reveal an underlying endobronchial obstruction. In other cases, upper lobe involvement may be suggestive of either tuberculosis or ABPA. With more widespread disease, measurement of sweat chloride levels for cystic fibrosis, structural or functional assessment of nasal or bronchial cilia or sperm for primary ciliary dyskinesia, and quantitative assessment of immunoglobulins may explain recurrent airway infection. In an asthmatic person with proximal bronchiectasis or other historical features to suggest ABPA, skin testing, serology, and sputum culture for *Aspergillus* are helpful in confirming the diagnosis.

Pulmonary function tests may demonstrate airflow obstruction as a consequence of diffuse bronchiectasis or associated chronic obstructive lung disease. Bronchial hyperreactivity, e.g., to methacholine challenge, and some reversibility of the airflow obstruction with inhaled bronchodilators are relatively common.

℞ **TREATMENT** Therapy has four major goals: (1) elimination of an identifiable underlying problem; (2) improved clearance of tracheobronchial secretions; (3) control of infection, particularly during acute exacerbations; and (4) reversal of airflow obstruction. Appropriate treatment should be instituted when a treatable cause is found, for example, treatment of hypogammaglobulinemia with immunoglobulin replacement, tuberculosis with antituberculous agents, and ABPA with glucocorticoids.

Secretions are typically copious and thick and contribute to the symptoms. Chest physical therapy with vibration, percussion, and postural drainage frequently helps patients with copious secretions. Mucolytic agents to thin secretions and allow better clearance are controversial. Aerosolized recombinant DNase, which decreases viscosity of sputum by breaking down DNA released from neutrophils, has been shown to improve pulmonary function in cystic fibrosis, but similar benefits have not been found with bronchiectasis due to other etiologies.

Antibiotics have an important role in management. For patients with infrequent exacerbations characterized by an increase in quantity and purulence of the sputum, antibiotics are commonly used only during acute episodes. Although choice of an antibiotic may be guided by Gram's stain and culture of sputum, empiric coverage (e.g., with ampicillin, amoxicillin, trimethoprim-sulfamethoxazole, or cefaclor) is often given initially. When *P. aeruginosa* is present, oral therapy with a quinolone or parenteral therapy with an aminoglycoside or third-generation cephalosporin may be appropriate. In patients with chronic purulent sputum despite short courses of antibiotics, more prolonged courses, e.g., with oral amoxicillin or inhaled aminoglycosides, or intermittent but regular courses of single or rotating antibiotics have been used.

Bronchodilators to improve obstruction and aid clearance of secretions are particularly useful in patients with airway hyperreactivity

and reversible airflow obstruction. Although surgical therapy was common in the past, more effective antibiotic and supportive therapy has largely replaced surgery. However, when bronchiectasis is localized and the morbidity is substantial despite adequate medical therapy, surgical resection of the involved region of lung should be considered.

When massive hemoptysis, often originating from the hypertrophied bronchial circulation, does not resolve with conservative therapy, including rest and antibiotics, therapeutic options are either surgical resection or bronchial arterial embolization (Chap. 33). Although resection may be successful if disease is localized, embolization is preferable with widespread disease. In patients with extensive disease, chronic hypoxemia and cor pulmonale may indicate the need for long-term supplemental oxygen. For selected patients who are disabled despite maximal therapy, lung transplantation is a therapeutic option.

BIBLIOGRAPHY

AFZELIUS BA: Immotile cilia syndrome: Past, present, and prospects for the future. Thorax 53:894, 1998

JONES A, ROWE BH: Bronchopulmonary hygiene physical therapy in bronchiectasis and chronic obstructive pulmonary disease: a systemic review. Heart & Lung 29:125, 2000

KANG EY et al: Bronchiectasis: Comparison of preoperative thin-section CT and pathologic findings in resected specimens. Radiology 195:649, 1995

KING MA et al: Bronchial dilatation in patients with HIV infection: CT assessment and correlation with pulmonary function tests and findings at bronchoalveolar lavage. AJR Am J Roentgenol 168:1535, 1997

LUCE JM: Bronchiectasis, in *Textbook of Respiratory Medicine*, 3d ed, JF Murray, JA Nadel (eds). Philadelphia, Saunders, 2000, pp 1325–1342

NICOTRA MB et al: Clinical, pathophysiologic, and microbiologic characterization of bronchiectasis in an aging cohort. Chest 108:955, 1995

WALLACE RJ JR et al: Polyclonal *Mycobacterium avium* complex infections in patients with nodular bronchiectasis. Am J Respir Crit Care Med 158:1235, 1998

WEINBERGER SE: *Principles of Pulmonary Medicine*, 3d ed. Philadelphia, Saunders, 1998

257   *Richard C. Boucher*

CYSTIC FIBROSIS

Cystic fibrosis (CF) is a monogenetic disorder that presents as a multisystem disease. The first signs and symptoms typically occur in childhood, but about 7% of patients in the United States are diagnosed as adults. Due to improvements in therapy, more than 36% of patients are now adults ≥ 18 years of age and 12% are past the age of 30. The median survival is over 32 years for males and 29 years for females with CF. Thus, CF is no longer only a pediatric disease, and internists must be prepared to recognize and treat its many complications. This disease is characterized by chronic airways infection that ultimately leads to bronchiectasis and bronchiolectasis, exocrine pancreatic insufficiency and intestinal dysfunction, abnormal sweat gland function, and urogenital dysfunction.

PATHOGENESIS

GENETIC CONSIDERATIONS CF is an autosomal recessive disease resulting from mutations in a gene located on chromosome 7. The prevalence of CF varies with the ethnic origin of a population. CF is detected in approximately 1 in 3000 live births in the Caucasian population of North America and northern Europe, 1 in 17,000 live births of African-Americans, and 1 in 90,000 live births of the Asian population of Hawaii. The most common mutation in the CF gene (~70% of CF chromosomes) is a 3-bp deletion that results in an absence of phenylalanine at amino acid position 508 (ΔF_{508}) of the CF gene protein product, known as the CF transmembrane regulator (CFTR). The large number (>800) of relatively uncommon (<2%) mutations identified in the CF gene makes it difficult to use DNA diagnostic technologies for identifying heterozygotes in populations at large, and no simple physiologic measurements allow heterozygote detection. ■

CFTR PROTEIN The CFTR protein is a single polypeptide chain containing 1480 amino acids that appears to function both as a cyclic AMP–regulated Cl⁻ channel and, as its name implies, a regulator of other ion channels. The fully processed form of CFTR is found in the plasma membrane in normal epithelia (Fig. 257-1). Biochemical studies indicate that the ΔF_{508} mutation leads to improper processing and intracellular degradation of the CFTR protein. Thus, absence of CFTR at appropriate cellular sites is often part of the pathophysiology of CF. However, other mutations in the CF gene produce CFTR proteins that are fully processed but are nonfunctional or only partially functional at the appropriate cellular sites.

EPITHELIAL DYSFUNCTION The epithelia affected by CF exhibit different functions in their native state; i.e., some are volume-absorbing (airways and distal intestinal epithelia), some are salt-absorbing but not volume absorbing (sweat duct), and others are volume-secretory (proximal intestine and pancreas). Given this diverse array of native activities, it should not be surprising that CF produces very different effects on patterns of electrolyte and water transport. However, the unifying concept is that all affected tissues express abnormal ion transport function.

ORGAN-SPECIFIC PATHOPHYSIOLOGY   Lung The diagnostic biophysical hallmark of CF is the raised transepithelial electric potential difference (PD) detected in airway epithelia. The transepithelial PD reflects components of both the rate of active ion transport and the resistance to ion flow of the superficial epithelium. CF airway epithelia exhibit both raised transport rates (Na⁺) and decreased Cl⁻ permeability (Fig. 257-2). The Cl⁻ permeability defect reflects at least in part the absence of cyclic AMP–dependent kinase and protein kinase C–regulated Cl⁻ transport that is mediated by the Cl⁻ channel functions of CFTR. An important observation is that there is an alternative Cl⁻ channel expressed in airway epithelia. This "alternative" Cl⁻ channel (Cl_a^-) is different from CFTR and is regulated by intracellular Ca^{2+} levels. This channel can substitute for CFTR with regard to net Cl⁻ transport and may be a potential therapeutic target.

Raised Na⁺ absorption is a routine feature of CF airway epithelia. Na⁺ transport abnormalities in CF are not a widespread feature of the CF epithelial phenotype and appear confined to volume-absorbing epi-

FIGURE 257-2 Comparison of ion transport properties of normal (*top*) and CF (*bottom*) airway epithelia. The vectors describe routes and magnitudes of Na⁺ and Cl⁻ transport. The normal basal pattern for ion transport is absorption of Na⁺ from the lumen via an amiloride-sensitive Na⁺ channel. This process is accelerated in CF. The capacity to initiate cyclic AMP–mediated Cl⁻ secretion is diminished in CF airway epithelia due to absence/dysfunction of the CFTR Cl⁻ channel. The accelerated Na⁺ absorption in CF reflects the absence of CFTR inhibitory effects on Na⁺ channels. Cl_a^-, alternative Cl⁻ channel; PD, potential difference; CFTR, cystic fibrosis transmembrane regulator.

thelia. Recent studies demonstrate that the increased Na⁺ transport reflects the absence of CFTR's tonic inhibitory regulatory function on Na⁺ channel activity. It appears that CFTR inhibits Na⁺ channel activity as a part of its general function to act as a "switch" that coordinates the balance between Na⁺ absorption and Cl⁻ secretion.

The central hypothesis of CF airways pathophysiology has been that an abnormally high rate of Na⁺ absorption and low rate of Cl⁻ secretion reduce the salt and water content of mucus and deplete the volume of the perciliary liquid (PCL). Both the thickening of mucins and the depletion of the PCL lead to a failure to clear mucus normally from the airways by either ciliary or airflow-dependent (cough) mechanisms. An alternative hypothesis suggests that the central defect in CF airways is raised salt concentration in secretions that inhibits the function of antimicrobial substances. Direct measurements of salt concentration *in vivo* have, however, provided no evidence that there are differences in salt concentration in CF versus normal airway secretions.

The unique predisposition of CF airways to chronic infection by *Staphylococcus aureus* and *Pseudomonas aeruginosa* raises the issue that other as yet undefined abnormalities in airway surface liquids also may contribute to the failure of lung defense. However, it may be that *Pseudomonas* is selected by its propensity to grow in biofilm

FIGURE 257-1 Cellular metabolism of the CFTR protein. In a normal cell (*left*), CFTR is synthesized in the rough endoplasmic reticulum (RER), is glycosylated in the Golgi apparatus, and functions as a Cl⁻ channel and regulator of other ion channels when located in the plasma membrane. Two possible outcomes of mutations in the CF gene are shown (*right*). (1) If a mutation disturbs protein folding, e.g., the ΔF_{508} mutation, CFTR is degraded intracellularly so that no protein is transported to the plasma membrane. (2) With other mutations, the abnormal protein is processed and traffics to the plasma membrane but functions abnormally at that site.

colonies on the surfaces of thickened, retained mucus plaques in CF airways.

257 Cystic Fibrosis **1489**

Gastrointestinal Tract The gastrointestinal effects of CF are diverse. In the exocrine pancreas, the absence of the CFTR Cl^- channel in the apical membrane of pancreatic ductal epithelia limits the function of an apical membrane Cl^--HCO_3^- exchanger to secrete HCO_3^- and Na^+ (by a passive process) into the duct. The failure to secrete Na^+-HCO_3^- and water leads to retention of enzymes in the pancreas and ultimately destruction of virtually all pancreatic tissue. The CF intestinal epithelium, because of the lack of Cl^- and water secretion, fails to flush the secreted mucins and other macromolecules from intestinal crypts. The diminished CFTR-mediated secretion of liquid may be exacerbated by excessive absorption of liquid in the distal intestine, reflecting abnormalities of CFTR-mediated regulation of Na^+ absorption (both mediated by Na^+ channels and possibly other Na^+ transporters, e.g., Na^+-H^+ exchangers). Both dysfunctions lead to desiccated intraluminal contents and obstruction of both the small and large intestines. In the hepatobiliary system, defective hepatic ductal Cl^- and water secretion causes retention of biliary secretions and focal biliary cirrhosis and bile duct proliferation in approximately 25 to 30% of patients with CF. The inability of the CF gallbladder epithelium to secrete salt and water can lead to both chronic cholecystitis and cholelithiasis.

Sweat Gland Patients with CF secrete nearly normal volumes of sweat in the sweat acinus. However, they are not able to absorb NaCl from sweat as it moves through the sweat duct due to the inability to absorb Cl^- across the ductal epithelial cells.

CLINICAL FEATURES

Most patients with CF present with signs and symptoms of the disease in childhood. Approximately 15% of patients present within the first 24 h of life with gastrointestinal obstruction, termed *meconium ileus.* Other common presentations within the first year or two of life include respiratory tract symptoms, most prominently cough and/or recurrent pulmonary infiltrates, and failure to thrive. A significant proportion of patients (~7%), however, are diagnosed after age 18.

RESPIRATORY TRACT Upper respiratory tract disease is almost universal in patients with CF. Chronic sinusitis is common in childhood and leads to nasal obstruction and rhinorrhea. The occurrence of nasal polyps approaches 25% and often requires surgery.

In the lower respiratory tract, the first symptom of CF is cough. With time, the cough becomes persistent and produces viscous, purulent, often greenish colored sputum. Inevitably, periods of clinical stability are interrupted by "exacerbations," defined by increased cough, weight loss, increased sputum volume, and decrements in pulmonary function. These exacerbations require aggressive therapy, including frequent postural drainage and oral antibiotics, and often intravenous antibiotics (see below), with the goal being recovery of lung function. Over the course of years, the exacerbations become more frequent and the recovery of lost lung function incomplete, leading to respiratory failure.

Patients with CF exhibit a characteristic sputum microbiology. *Haemophilus influenzae* and *S. aureus* are often the first organisms recovered from samples of lung secretions in newly diagnosed patients with CF. *P. aeruginosa* is typically cultured from lower respiratory tract secretions thereafter. After repetitive antibiotic exposure, *P. aeruginosa*, often in a mucoid form, is usually the predominant organism recovered from sputum and may be present as several strains with different antibiotic sensitivities. *Burkholderia* (formerly *Pseudomonas*) *cepacia* has been recovered from CF sputum and is pathogenic. Patient-to-patient spread of certain strains of this organism indicates that infection control in the hospital should be practiced. Other gram-negative rods recovered from CF sputum include *Xanthomonas zylosoxida* and *P. gladioli*, and occasionally, mucoid forms of *Proteus*, *Escherichia coli*, and *Klebsiella*. Up to 50% of patients with CF have *Aspergillus fumigatus* in their sputum, and up to 10% of these patients exhibit the syndrome of allergic bronchopulmonary aspergillosis. *My-cobacterium tuberculosis* is rare in patients with CF. However, 10 to 20% of adult patients with CF have sputum cultures positive for nontuberculous mycobacteria, and in some patients these microorganisms are associated with disease.

The first lung function abnormalities observed in children with CF, increased ratios of residual volume to total lung capacity, suggest that small airways disease is the first functional lung abnormality in CF. As the disease progresses, both reversible and irreversible changes in forced vital capacity and forced expiratory volume in 1 s are noted. The reversible component reflects the accumulation of intraluminal secretions and/or airway reactivity, which occurs in 40 to 60% of patients with CF. The irreversible component reflects chronic destruction of the airway wall and bronchiolitis.

The earliest chest x-ray change in CF lungs is hyperinflation, reflecting small airways obstruction. Later, signs of luminal mucus impaction, bronchial cuffing, and finally, bronchiectasis, e.g., ring shadows, are noted. For reasons that are still unknown, the right upper lobe displays the earliest and most severe changes. Neither CT nor MRI scanning is routinely performed on patients with CF.

CF pulmonary disease is associated with many intermittent complications. Pneumothorax is common (>10% of patients). The production of small amounts of blood in sputum is common in CF patients with advanced pulmonary disease and appears to be associated with lung infection. Massive hemoptysis is life-threatening and difficult to localize bronchoscopically. With advanced lung disease, digital clubbing becomes evident in virtually all patients with CF. As late events, respiratory failure and cor pulmonale are prominent features of CF.

GASTROINTESTINAL TRACT The syndrome of meconium ileus in infants presents with abdominal distention, failure to pass stool, and emesis. The abdominal flat plate can be diagnostic with small intestinal air fluid levels, a granular appearance representing meconium, and a small colon. In children and young adults, a syndrome termed *meconium ileus equivalent* or distal intestinal obstruction occurs. The syndrome presents with right lower quadrant pain, loss of appetite, occasional emesis, and often a palpable mass. The syndrome can be confused with appendicitis, which occurs frequently in patients with CF. The characteristic intestinal abnormalities are complicated by exocrine pancreatic insufficiency in more than 90% of patients with CF. Insufficient pancreatic enzyme release yields the typical pattern of protein and fat malabsorption, with frequent, bulky, foul-smelling stools. Signs and symptoms of malabsorption of fat-soluble vitamins, including vitamins E and K, are also noted. Pancreatic beta cells are typically spared, but function decreases with age, causing hyperglycemia and increasing requirements for insulin in older patients with CF.

GENITOURINARY SYSTEM Late onset of puberty is common in both males and females with CF. The delayed maturational pattern is likely secondary to the effects of chronic lung disease and inadequate nutrition on reproductive endocrine function. More than 95% of male patients with CF are azoospermic, reflecting obliteration of the vas deferens that probably reflects defective liquid secretion. Twenty percent of women with CF are infertile due to effects of chronic lung disease on the menstrual cycle; thick, tenacious cervical mucus that blocks sperm migration; and possibly fallopian tube/uterine wall abnormalities in liquid transport. More than 90% of completed pregnancies produce viable infants, and women with CF are generally able to breast-feed infants normally.

DIAGNOSIS

Because of the large number of CF mutations, DNA analysis is not used for primary diagnosis. The primary diagnosis of CF rests on a combination of clinical criteria and analyses of sweat Cl^- values. The values for the Na^+ and Cl^- concentration in sweat vary with age, but typically in adults a Cl^- concentration of >70 mEq/L discriminates between patients with CF and patients with other lung diseases.

DNA analyses are being performed increasingly in patients with CF. Comprehensive genotype-phenotype relationships have not yet been established sufficiently for prognosis. A relationship between ΔF_{508} homozygosity and pancreatic insufficiency has been established, but no predictive relationship holds for ΔF_{508} homozygosity and lung disease.

Between 1 and 2% of patients with the clinical syndrome of CF have normal sweat Cl^- values. In most of these patients, the nasal transepithelial PD is raised into the diagnostic range for CF, and sweat acini do not secrete in response to injected beta-adrenergic agonists. A single mutation of the CFTR gene, 3849 + 10 kb C → T, is associated with approximately 50% of CF patients with normal sweat Cl^- values.

℞ **TREATMENT** The major objectives of therapy for CF are to promote clearance of secretions and control infection in the lung, provide adequate nutrition, and prevent intestinal obstruction. Ultimately, gene therapy may become the treatment of choice.

Lung Disease The principal techniques for clearing pulmonary secretions are breathing exercises, flutter valves, and chest percussion. Regular use of these maneuvers is effective in preserving lung function. There is increasing interest in the use of hypertonic saline (3 to 7%) aerosols to augment the clearance of secretions.

More than 95% of patients with CF die of complications resulting from lung infection. Antibiotics are the principal agents available for treating lung infection, and their use should be guided by sputum culture results. Early intervention with antibiotics is useful, and long courses of treatment are the rule. Because of increased total-body clearance and volume of distribution of antibiotics in patients with CF, the required doses are higher for patients with CF than for patients with similar chest infections who do not have CF.

Increased cough and mucus production are treated with antibiotics given orally. Typical oral agents used to treat *Staphylococcus* include a semisynthetic penicillin or a cephalosporin. Oral ciprofloxacin may reduce pseudomonal bacterial counts and control symptoms. However, its clinical usefulness may be limited by rapid emergence of resistant organisms, and accordingly, courses should be intermittent (2 to 3 weeks) and not chronic. More severe exacerbations, or exacerbations associated with bacteria resistant to oral antibiotics, require intravenous antibiotics. Traditionally, intravenous therapy has been given in the hospital, but outpatient intravenous antibiotic administration has gained widespread acceptance. Usually, two drugs, often one of them an aminoglycoside, are used to treat *P. aeruginosa* to hinder emergence of resistant organisms. Drug dosage should be monitored so that levels for gentamicin or tobramycin peak at ranges of ~10 $\mu g/mL$ and exhibit troughs of <2 $\mu g/mL$. Usually, a cephalosporin, e.g., ceftazadime, and/or a penicillin derivative is used as the second drug. Antibiotics directed at *Staphylococcus* and/or *H. influenzae* are added depending on the results of the culture. Aerosolization of antibiotics also may have an important role in treating CF lung infection. Large doses of aminoglycosides, e.g., 600 mg tobramycin twice daily, via aerosol may be effective at delaying exacerbations. Aerosol administration also permits the use of other drugs, e.g., colistin, that are relatively ineffective by the intravenous route.

A number of pharmacologic agents for promoting mucus clearance are in use. *N*-acetyl-cysteine, which solubilizes mucus glycoproteins, has not been shown to have clinically significant effects on mucus clearance and/or lung function. Recombinant human DNAse, however, degrades the concentrated DNA in CF sputum, decreases sputum viscosity, and increases airflow during short-term administration. Long-term (6 months) DNAse treatment increases the time between pulmonary exacerbations. Most patients receive a therapeutic trial of DNAse to test for efficacy, and a sizeable minority appear to demonstrate persistent objective benefits. Clinical trials of experimental drugs aimed at restoring salt and water content of secretions are underway.

The most promising may be long-acting nucleotide (UTP)-based compounds that appear active in inducing liquid secretion in CF airways.

Inhaled β-adrenergic agonists can be useful to control airways constriction. They achieve a short-term increase in airflow, but long-term benefit has not been shown. Inhaled anticholinergics provide an alternative. Oral steroids are not first-line agents for controlling airways constriction and are of no use in improving the nonreversible component of lung function. Steroids may be useful for treating allergic bronchopulmonary aspergillosis.

The chronic damage to airway walls reflects to some extent the destructive activities of inflammatory enzymes generated in part by inflammatory cells. To date, specific therapies with antiproteases have not been successfully developed. However, a subset of adolescents with CF appears to benefit from long-term, high-dose non-steroidal (ibuprofen) therapy.

A number of pulmonary complications require acute interventions. Atelectasis is best treated with chest physiotherapy and antibiotic therapy. Pneumothoraces involving 10% or less of the lung can be observed without intervention. The use of chest tubes to expand collapsed, diseased lung often requires long periods of time, and sclerosing agents should be used with caution because of possible limitations for subsequent lung transplantation. Small-volume hemoptysis requires no specific therapy other than treatment of lung infection and assessment of coagulation and vitamin K status. If massive hemoptysis occurs, bronchial artery embolization can be successful. The most ominous complications of CF are respiratory failure and cor pulmonale. The most effective conventional therapy for these conditions is vigorous medical management of the lung disease and O_2 supplementation. Noninvasive positive pressure ventilation through a face mask may be an effective adjunctive therapy. Ultimately, the only effective treatment for respiratory failure in CF is lung transplantation (Chap. 267). The 2-year survival for lung transplantation exceeds 60%, and deaths in transplant patients result principally from graft rejection, often involving obliterative bronchiolitis. The transplanted lungs do not develop a CF-specific phenotype.

Gastrointestinal Disease Maintenance of adequate nutrition is critical for the health of the patient with CF. Most (>90%) of patients with CF benefit from pancreatic enzyme replacement. Capsules generally contain between 4000 and 29,000 units of lipase. The dose of enzymes (typically no more than 20,000 units/kg per meal) should be adjusted on the basis of weight gain, abdominal symptomatology, and character of stools. Replacement of fat-soluble vitamins, particularly vitamins E and K, is usually required. Hyperglycemia most often becomes manifest in the adult and typically requires insulin treatment.

For treatment of acute obstruction due to meconium ileus equivalent, megalodiatrizoate or other hypertonic radiocontrast materials delivered by enema to the terminal ileum are utilized. For control of symptoms, adjustment of pancreatic enzymes and the supplementation of intake by salt solutions containing osmotically active agents, e.g., propyleneglycol or lactulose, are utilized. Persistent symptoms may indicate a diagnosis of gastrointestinal malignancy, which is increased in incidence in patients with CF. Hepatic and gallbladder complications are treated as for patients without CF. End-stage liver disease can be treated by transplantation, which has a 2-year survival rate exceeding 50%.

Psychosocial Factors CF imposes a tremendous burden on patients. Health insurance, career options, family planning, and life expectancy become major issues. Thus, assisting patients with the psychosocial adjustments required by CF is critical.

BIBLIOGRAPHY

BEAR CE et al: Purification and functional reconstitution of the cystic fibrosis transmembrane conductance regulator (CFTR). Cell 68:809, 1992
BOUCHER RC et al: Cystic fibrosis, in *Textbook of Respiratory Medicine*, 3d ed, JF Murray, JA Nadel (eds). Philadelphia, Saunders, 2000, pp 1291–1324
CHENG SH et al: Defective intracellular transport and processing of CFTR is the molecular basis of most cystic fibrosis. Cell 63:827, 1990

DINWIDDIE R: Pathogenesis of lung disease in cystic fibrosis. Respiration 67:3, 2000

DRUMM M: What happens to DeltaF508 *in vivo*? J Clin Invest 103:1369, 1999

FITZSIMMONS SC: *CFF Patient Registry. 1997 Annual Report.* Bethesda, MD, Cystic Fibrosis Foundation, 1998

HIGHSMITH WE et al: A novel mutation in the cystic fibrosis gene in patients with pulmonary disease but normal sweat chloride concentrations. N Engl J Med 331:974, 1994

HULL J et al: Elemental content of airway surface liquid from infants with cystic fibrosis. Am J Respir Crit Care Med 157:10, 1998

KNOWLES MR et al: Ion compositon of airway surface liquid of patients with cystic fibrosis as compared to normal and disease-control subjects. J Clin Invest 100:2588, 1997

KONSTAN MW, BERGER M: Current understanding of the inflammatory process in cystic fibrosis: Onset and etiology. Pediatr Pulmonol 24:137, 1997

———— et al: Effect of high-dose ibuprofen in patients with cystic fibrosis. N Engl J Med 332:848, 1995

MATSUI H et al: Evidence for perciliary liquid layer depletion, not abnormal ion composition, in the pathogenesis of cystic fibrosis airways disease. Cell 95:1005, 1998

O'LOUGHLIN EV et al: Abnormal epithelial transport in cystic fibrosis jejunum. Am J Physiol 260:G758, 1991

RAMSEY BW et al: Efficacy of aerosolized tobramycin in patients with cystic fibrosis. N Engl J Med 328:1740, 1993

SMITH JJ et al: Cystic fibrosis airway epithelia fail to kill bacteria because of abnormal airway surface fluid. Cell 85:229, 1996

ZIELENSKI J, TSUI LC: Cystic fibrosis: Genotypic and phenotypic variations. Annu Rev Genet 29:777, 1995

258

Eric G. Honig, Roland H. Ingram, Jr.

CHRONIC BRONCHITIS, EMPHYSEMA, AND AIRWAYS OBSTRUCTION

DEFINITION Chronic obstructive pulmonary disease (COPD) is the name of a group of chronic and slowly progressive respiratory disorders characterized by reduced maximal expiratory flow during forced exhalation. Most of the airflow obstruction is fixed, but a variable degree of reversibility and bronchial hyperreactivity may be seen. COPD may coexist with asthma and, when abnormal airway reactivity is present, differentiation between these disorders can be challenging. COPD comprises emphysema and chronic bronchitis, two distinct processes, although most often present in combination. The definition excludes other causes of chronic airflow obstruction such as cystic fibrosis (Chap. 257), bronchiolitis obliterans (Chap. 259), and bronchiectasis (Chap. 256).

Emphysema is defined anatomically as a permanent and destructive enlargement of airspaces distal to the terminal bronchioles without obvious fibrosis and with loss of normal architecture. *Chronic bronchitis* is defined clinically as the presence of a cough productive of sputum not attributable to other causes on most days for at least 3 months over 2 consecutive years. Chronic bronchitis may be present in the absence of airflow limitation, but COPD always involves clinically significant airflow limitation.

EPIDEMIOLOGY COPD is a common medical problem affecting an estimated 16 million Americans. Males are more frequently affected than females, and Caucasians more frequently than African Americans. There is a higher prevalence of COPD among persons with a lower socioeconomic status and in those with a history of low birth weight. COPD is the fourth leading cause of death in the United States and is the only one of the 10 leading causes of death for which mortality rates are still rising. Prevalence peaks in the seventh and eighth decades, then levels off, largely due to mortality.

DISEASE MECHANISMS

PATHOGENESIS COPD evolves from an inflammatory process involving the airways and distal airspaces. Increased activity of oxidants combined with decreased activity of antioxidants, termed *oxidative stress*, have been implicated in the development of inflammation and COPD. Cigarette smoke produces high concentrations of oxygen free radicals including superoxide, hydrogen peroxide, and hypochlorous acid. Cigarette smoke is an independent source of Fe^{2+}, releases Fe^{2+} from ferritin, and catalyzes the formation of the highly active hydroxyl radical from O_2^- and H_2O_2 by eosinophils, neutrophils, and alveolar macrophages. Cigarette tar contains nitric oxide and induces nitric oxide synthase. In the presence of oxidants, NO is metabolized to cytotoxic peroxynitrates. In order for elastase to degrade elastin, α_1 antitrypsin (α_1AT) must be inactivated. Cigarette smoke, oxidants, activated neutrophils, and type II alveolar pneumocytes are all capable of inactivating α_1AT as well as matrix metalloproteinase inhibitors. Oxidant stress is also capable of inducing mucus hypersecretion. Cigarette smoke also acts as a chemoattractant and upregulates adhesion molecules. Smoke increases neutrophil transit time through the pulmonary circulation, increases adhesion, and decreases deformability. Smoke and elastase both increase the expression of the proinflammatory nuclear transcription factor κB (NfκB) as well as interleukin 8, a chemokine found to be elevated in COPD patients, that recruits neutrophils, basophils, eosinophils, and T lymphocytes.

The submucosa of the small airway in patients with COPD has increased numbers of CD8 lymphocytes and eosinophils, macrophages, and mast cells. Neutrophils are increased in smokers, but their numbers do not correlate with the presence of airflow obstruction. Patients with chronic airflow obstruction show higher levels of myeloperoxidase and eosinophilic cationic protein than do patients with normal airflow. Macrophages and mast cells produce transforming growth factor β (TGF-β), a peptide related to fibrogenesis. Patients with chronic airflow obstruction show a twofold elevation of TGF-β in lavage liquid; the amount of TGF-β shows a significant negative correlation with FEV_1 (the forced expiratory volume in 1 s). Smoke also leads to lipid peroxidation and to DNA damage. Widespread point mutations of the p53 gene locus have been identified in patients with lung cancer and precancerous dysplasia. These may predispose to the development of lung cancer.

RISK FACTORS COPD is characterized by a reduced FEV_1 and an accelerated rate of decline of FEV_1. The reduction in FEV_1 can occur by any of three pathways: (1) impaired childhood growth and development, with a lower peak in early adulthood and a normal rate of decline with aging (e.g., early childhood infection and passive smoke exposure); (2) normal growth and development with a premature peak but normal subsequent decline (e.g., asthma and passive smoking); and (3) normal growth and development and peak with accelerated decline (e.g., active smoking and, to a lesser degree, environmental exposures).

Smoking Cigarette smoking is the most commonly identified correlate with both chronic bronchitis during life and extent of emphysema at postmortem. The prevalence of COPD shows a dose-response relationship with the number of pack-years of tobacco consumed. Some 90% of all COPD patients are current or former tobacco smokers. Experimental studies have shown that prolonged cigarette smoking impairs respiratory epithelial ciliary movement, inhibits function of alveolar macrophages, and leads to hypertrophy and hyperplasia of mucus-secreting glands; massive exposure in dogs can produce emphysematous changes. Cigarette smoke also inhibits antiproteases and causes polymorphonuclear leukocytes to release proteolytic enzymes acutely. Cigarette smoke can produce an acute increase in airways resistance due to vagally mediated smooth-muscle constriction by stimulating submucosal irritant receptors. Increased airways responsiveness is associated with more rapid progression in patients with chronic airways obstruction. Obstruction of small airways is the earliest demonstrable mechanical defect in young cigarette smokers and may disappear completely after cessation of smoking.

Although smoking cessation does not result in complete reversal of more pronounced obstruction, there is a significant slowing of the decline in lung function in all smokers who give up cigarettes. Passive exposure to tobacco smoke correlates with respiratory symptoms such as cough, wheeze, and sputum production. Not only is cigarette smoking the most common single factor leading to chronic airways obstruction, it also adds to the effects of every other contributory factor to be discussed below.

Air Pollution   The incidence and mortality rates of both chronic bronchitis and emphysema may be higher in heavily industrialized urban areas. Exacerbations of bronchitis are clearly related to periods of heavy pollution with sulfur dioxide (SO_2) and particulate matter. While nitrogen dioxide (NO_2) can produce small-airways obstruction (bronchiolitis) in experimental animals exposed to high concentrations, there are no data convincingly implicating NO_2, at even the highest pollutant levels, in the pathogenesis or worsening of airways obstruction in humans (Chap. 254).

Occupation   Chronic bronchitis is more prevalent in workers who engage in occupations exposing them to either inorganic or organic dusts or to noxious gases. Epidemiologic surveys have succeeded in demonstrating an accelerated decline in lung function in many such workers—e.g., workers in plastics plants exposed to toluene diisocyanate, and carding room workers in cotton mills (Chap. 254)—suggesting that their occupational exposure contributes to their future disability.

Infection   Morbidity, mortality, and frequency of acute respiratory illnesses are higher in patients with chronic bronchitis. Many attempts have been made to relate these illnesses to infection with viruses, mycoplasmas, and bacteria. However, only the rhinovirus is found more often during exacerbations; that is to say, pathogenic bacteria, mycoplasmas, and viruses other than rhinovirus are found just as often between as during exacerbations. Epidemiologic studies, however, implicate acute respiratory illness as one of the major factors associated with the etiology as well as the progression of chronic airways obstruction. Cigarette smokers may either transitorily develop or worsen small-airways obstruction in association with even mild viral respiratory infections. There is also some evidence that severe viral pneumonia early in life may lead to chronic obstruction, predominantly in small airways.

GENETIC CONSIDERATIONS   Despite the strong etiologic association between smoking and COPD, only 15 to 20% of smokers lose FEV_1 at a rate fast enough to manifest COPD. Epidemiologic evidence of familial clustering of COPD cases is strong and repeated, suggesting that susceptibility to the effects of tobacco smoke has genetic determinants. Twin studies show that even after controlling for active and passive smoking, FEV_1 correlated more closely in monozygotic than dizygotic twins and more than in other family members with a lesser percentage of shared genotype. In first-degree relatives of a cohort of COPD patients with normal α_1AT levels, FEV_1 was reduced compared to controls but only among current or ex-smokers. Smoking and nonsmoking relatives of control subjects both had normal FEV_1. These data suggest genetic risk factors that are expressed in response to smoking.

α_1 Antitrypsin Deficiency   Thus far, deficiency of α_1AT is the only genetic abnormality that has been specifically linked to COPD. α_1AT is a 394–amino acid serine proteinase inhibitor whose synthesis is governed by a 12.2-kB 7-exon gene located at 14q32.1. α_1AT synthesis is expressed primarily in the liver and to a lesser degree in neutrophils and monocytes. Hepatic α_1AT escapes into the general circulation, where it counteracts neutrophil elastase. Normal levels of α_1AT are 20 to 48 μmol/L; levels above 11 μmol/L (35% of normal) are considered protective. There are 75 known alleles of α_1AT, which are inherited in an autosomal codominant manner and are generally classified as normal (MM), deficient, null, or dysfunctional. The most common deficient allele, termed ZZ (or Pi^{ZZ} phenotype), results from a single amino acid substitution $^{342}Glu \rightarrow Lys$, which causes sponta-

neous polymerization of the polypeptide, markedly impeding its release into the circulation from the liver. What does escape is vulnerable to oxidation and spontaneous polymerization, further impeding its function. The retained material is associated with hepatic cirrhosis (Chap. 299), while diminished circulating levels (2.5 to 7 μmol/L, averaging 16% of normal) lead to antiprotease deficiency. Pi^{ZZ}, the most common disease-related α_1AT abnormality, occurs in 1:2000 to 1:7000 persons of European descent and is rare in those of Oriental and African lineage. Pi^{SS} phenotypes are associated with α_1AT levels of 15 to 33 μmol (mean 52% of normal). Pi^{null} have no detectable antiprotease levels. Heterozygotes have intermediate levels of antiprotease.

Clinically significant deficiency of α_1AT, with levels below 11 μmol/L, has been associated with homozygous Pi^{ZZ}, $Pi^{nullnull}$, or Pi^{nullZ} and the premature development of severe emphysema, chronic bronchitis, or bronchiectasis. α_1AT deficiency accounts for 2% of observed cases of emphysema. Rare below age 25, the disease usually presents as dyspnea and cough in patients in their fourth decade. Although not a true population-based study, a large national registry of 1129 severe α_1AT-deficiency cases indicated that the typical patient was in the mid-forties, with an FEV_1 and a pulmonary diffusing capacity at or below 50% of the predicted levels. Most had exertional dyspnea and wheezing, but fewer than half reported a chronic cough. Nearly 80% had a positive family history of lung disease, and 25% reported a positive family history for liver disease. The average rate of decline of FEV_1 is reported to be 100 to 130 mL per year for smokers and 50 to 80 mL per year for ex-smokers or lifetime nonsmokers with α_1AT deficiency.

Pathologically, panacinar emphysema predominates, and radiographically, changes are more marked in the lower lobes. It is becoming increasingly apparent that tobacco smoking is an extremely important cofactor for the development of disease in α_1AT-deficient individuals. Only a few lifetime nonsmokers with Pi^{ZZ} develop emphysema. Most never have symptoms, have a normal rate of decline of FEV_1, and live a normal life span. Many cases are discovered only as a consequence of family screening of emphysema patients. Because the total number of Pi^{ZZ} individuals is unknown, the risk of disease for smokers is difficult to ascertain accurately. The risk of disease is lower still for heterozygotes with one M or S allele. Smoking is again an important cofactor. ■

PATHOLOGY   The pathologic changes of COPD involve large and small airways and the terminal respiratory unit. Airway narrowing is seen in large and small airways and is caused by changes in their normal constituents in response to persistent inflammation.

The airway epithelium is characterized by squamous metaplasia, atrophy of ciliated cells, and hypertrophy of mucus glands. The remodeled epithelium actively produces cytokines that amplify and sustain the inflammatory process. The small airways are the major site of airflow limitation. Small airways show a variety of lesions narrowing their lumina, including goblet cell hyperplasia, mucosal and submucosal inflammatory cells, edema, peribronchial fibrosis, intraluminal mucus plugs, and increased smooth muscle. CD8+ T lymphocytes and B lymphocytes characterize the inflammatory infiltrate. The marked thickening of the subepithelial lamina reticularis, characteristic of asthma, is absent in COPD.

In the central airways, subepithelial inflammation is present with increased numbers of eosinophils and CD8+ T lymphocytes. Unlike asthma, the eosinophils are not activated and do not degranulate. Neutrophils are present in the epithelium but not in the subepithelial layers. In larger cartilaginous airways, chronic bronchitis is associated with hypertrophy of submucosal mucus-producing glands. Quantitation of this anatomic change, known as the *Reid index*, is based on the ratio of the thickness of the submucosal glands to that of the bronchial wall. In persons without a history of chronic bronchitis, the mean ratio is 0.44 ± 0.09, whereas in those with such a history, the mean ratio is 0.52 ± 0.08. Although a low index is rarely associated with symptoms and a high index is commonly associated with symptoms during life, there is a great deal of overlap. Therefore, many persons will have morphologic changes in large airways without having had chronic bronchitis.

Emphysema begins as an increase in the number and size of alveolar fenestrae and results in the eventual destruction of alveolar septae and their attachments to terminal and respiratory bronchioles. Emphysema is classified according to the pattern of involvement of the gas-exchanging units (acini) of the lung distal to the terminal bronchiole. With *centriacinar emphysema*, the distention and destruction are mainly limited to the respiratory bronchioles with relatively less change peripherally in the acinus. Because of the large functional reserve in the lung, many units must be involved in order for overall dysfunction to be detectable. The centrally destroyed regions of the acinus have a high ventilation/perfusion ratio because the capillaries are missing, yet ventilation continues. This results in a deficit of perfusion relative to ventilation, while the peripheral portions of the acinus have crowded and small alveoli with intact, perfused capillaries giving a low ventilation/perfusion ratio. This results in a deficit of ventilation relative to blood flow, giving a high alveolar-arterial P_{O_2} difference ($PA_{O_2} - Pa_{O_2}$) (Chap. 250).

During normal aging, airspaces enlarge and alveolar ducts increase in diameter. These changes are extremely common in lungs from persons over age 50 and may be misidentified as emphysema.

Panacinar emphysema involves both the central and peripheral portions of the acinus, which results, if the process is extensive, in a reduction of the alveolar-capillary gas exchange surface and loss of elastic recoil properties. When emphysema is severe, it may be difficult to distinguish between the two types, which most often coexist in the same lung.

PATHOPHYSIOLOGY **Airflow Limitation** Although both chronic bronchitis and emphysema can exist without evidence of obstruction, by the time a patient begins to experience dyspnea as a result of these processes, obstruction is always demonstrable. Airflow limitation and increased airways resistance may be caused by loss of elastic recoil driving passive exhalation due to emphysema, by increased collapsibility of small airways through loss of radial traction on airways, or to increased resistance due to intrinsic narrowing of small airways.

In addition to providing radial support to airways during quiet breathing, the elastic recoil properties of the lung serve as a major determinant of maximal expiratory flow rates. The static recoil pressure of the lung is the difference between alveolar and intrapleural pressure. During forced exhalations, when alveolar and intrapleural pressures are high, there are points in the airway at which bronchial pressure equals pleural pressure. Flow does not increase with higher pleural pressure after these points become fixed, so that the effective driving pressure between alveoli and such points is the elastic recoil pressure of the lung (Fig. 258-1). Hence maximal expiratory flow rates represent a complex and dynamic interplay among airways caliber, elastic recoil pressures, and collapsibility of airways. Correlative studies of structure and function suggest that small-airway narrowing is the most important correlate of airflow obstruction, followed by loss of elastic recoil. Collapsibility is probably a less important factor. As a direct consequence of the altered pressure-airflow relationships, the work of breathing is increased in bronchitis and emphysema. Since flow-resistive work is flow rate-dependent, there is a disproportionate increase in the work of breathing when ventilation must be increased, as in exercise.

Hyperinflation The designated subdivisions of the lung volume outlined in Chap. 250 are abnormal to varying degrees in both bronchitis and emphysema. The residual volume and functional residual capacity (FRC) are almost always higher than normal. Since the normal FRC is the volume at which the inward recoil of the lung is balanced by the outward recoil of the chest wall, loss of elastic recoil of the lung results in a higher FRC. In addition, prolongation of expiration in association with obstruction would lead to a dynamic increase in FRC (dynamic hyperinflation) if inspiration is initiated before the respiratory system reaches its static balance point. Dynamic hyperinflation contributes additionally to the discomfort associated with airflow obstruction by flattening the diaphragm and placing it at a me-

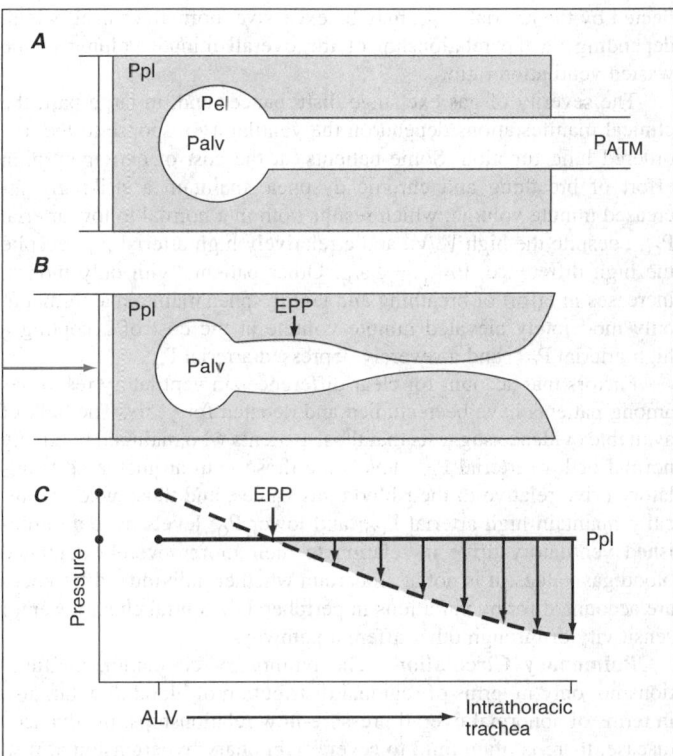

FIGURE 258-1 *A.* A schematic diagram of the lung and intrathoracic airways with no airflow. The alveolar pressure (Palv) is greater than pleural pressure (Ppl) by an amount equal to the elastic recoil pressure of the lung (Pel)—i.e., Palv is the algebraic sum of Ppl + Pel. With no airflow Palv equals atmospheric pressure (P_{ATM}), and for all of the intrathoracic airways, pressure outside is less than the pressure inside due to the Pel. *B.* The same schematic lung during forced exhalation when pleural pressure becomes quite positive (*arrow*). Palv is still greater than Ppl by an amount equal to Pel. However, there is a pressure drop along the airway associated with flow, and at some point Ppl equals local bronchial pressure (so-called equal pressure point, EPP). Mouthward from this point, Ppl exceeds local bronchial pressure and hence acts to compress the airways. *C.* Pressure within the airways from alveoli to the intrathoracic trachea is shown as a dashed line (---) and Ppl is shown as a constant (—). Therefore, the driving pressure from alveoli to EPP is equal to Pel, and a decrease in Pel (i.e., loss of elastic recoil) would mean a smaller driving pressure and smaller flow rates.

chanical disadvantage due to shortened diaphragmatic fiber length and a perpendicular insertion with the lower ribs. The exertional increase in end-expiratory lung volume and consequent decrease in inspiratory capacity have been strongly associated with the degree of dyspnea. Elevations of total lung capacity (TLC) are frequent. The exact cause is uncertain, but increases in total lung capacity are often found in association with decreases in the elastic recoil of the lung. Although the vital capacity is frequently reduced, significant airways obstruction can be present with a normal to near-normal vital capacity.

Impaired Gas Exchange Maldistribution of inspired gas and blood flow is always present to some extent. When the mismatching is severe, impairment of gas exchange is reflected in abnormalities of arterial blood gases. Small-airway narrowing causes a decrease in ventilation of their distal alveolar acini. When alveolar capillaries remain intact, this results in mismatching of ventilation and blood flow, reduced ventilation-perfusion ratios, and mild to moderate hypoxemia. With emphysema, destruction of alveolar walls may decrease alveolar capillary perfusion as well, better preserving ventilation-perfusion matching, and Pa_{O_2}. Shunt hypoxemia is unusual. There are regions of the lung with a deficit of perfusion in relation to ventilation that increase the wasted ventilation ratio (i.e., V_d/V_t; Chap. 250). At a normal resting CO_2 production, the net effective alveolar ventilation, as reflected by the arterial P_{CO_2}, may be excessive, normal, or insufficient, depending on the relationship of the overall minute volume to the wasted ventilation ratio.

The severity of gas exchange disturbances and, in large part, the clinical manifestations depend on the ventilatory response to the disordered lung function. Some patients, at the cost of extremely high effort of breathing and chronic dyspnea, maintain a strikingly increased minute volume, which results both in a normal to low arterial P_{CO_2}, despite the high V_d/V_t, and a relatively high arterial P_{O_2}, despite the high difference, $PA_{O_2} - Pa_{O_2}$. Other patients with only modest increases in effort of breathing and less dyspnea maintain a normal to only moderately elevated minute volume at the cost of accepting a high arterial P_{CO_2} and a severely depressed arterial P_{O_2}.

Factors that account for clear differences in ventilatory responses among patients have been studied and debated for years. The bulk of available evidence suggests that those patients who maintain relatively normal or low arterial P_{CO_2} levels are those with an increased ventilatory drive relative to their blood gas values, and those who chronically maintain high arterial P_{CO_2} and lower P_{O_2} levels have a diminished ventilatory drive in relation to their more severely deranged blood gas values. It is not at all certain whether individual differences are accounted for by variations in peripheral or central chemoreceptor sensitivity or through other afferent pathways.

Pulmonary Circulation   The pulmonary circulation malfunctions not only in terms of regional distribution of blood flow but also in terms of abnormal overall pressure-flow relationships. In advanced disease, there is often mild to severe pulmonary hypertension at rest, with further increases disproportionate to cardiac output elevations during exercise. A reduction in the total cross-sectional area of the pulmonary vascular bed can be attributed to thickening of medium and large muscular pulmonary arteries, to enhanced contraction of vascular smooth muscle in pulmonary arteries and arterioles, as well as to destruction of alveolar septa with loss of capillaries. Rarely does loss of capillaries alone lead to severe pulmonary hypertension with cor pulmonale, except as a near-terminal event (Chap. 237). Of more importance is the constriction of pulmonary vessels in response to alveolar hypoxia. The pulmonary arteries of patients with severe hypoxemia COPD have been shown to exhibit increased contractility and impaired relaxation in response to pharmacologic stimuli in vitro. These differences between the pulmonary arteries of COPD patients and normal individuals are abolished by inhibition of NO synthase, suggesting that patients develop an endothelial defect in NO synthesis. The constriction is somewhat reversible by an increase in alveolar P_{O_2} with therapy.

There is a synergism between hypoxia and acidosis that assumes importance during episodes of acute or chronic respiratory insufficiency. Chronic hypoxia, especially in concert with carboxyhemoglobinemia, often seen with heavy cigarette smoking, leads not only to pulmonary vascular constriction but also to secondary erythrocytosis. The latter, although not proved to be a significant contributor to pulmonary hypertension, could add to pulmonary vascular resistance. As discussed in Chap. 237, chronic afterload on the right ventricle leads to hypertrophy and, in association with disordered blood gases, ultimately to failure. Hypoventilation may occur during rapid eye movement sleep and lead to desaturation, which may be severe. Repeated desaturation may cause pulmonary hypertension.

Renal and Hormonal Dysfunction   Chronic hypoxemia and hypercapnia have been shown to cause increased circulating levels of norepinephrine, renin, and aldosterone and decreased levels of antidiuretic hormone. Renal arterial endothelium in COPD patients exhibits defects similar to those seen in the pulmonary arteries, shifting renal blood flow from the cortex to the medulla and impairing renal functional reserve. The combination of hemodynamic and hormonal disturbances leads to defective excretion of salt and water loads and, together with right ventricular dysfunction, to the plethoric and cyanotic manifestations of some patients with COPD.

Cachexia   Weight loss sometimes occurs in patients with advanced COPD. A body-mass index (BMI) < 25 kg/m^2 is associated with increased frequency of exacerbations and with significantly reduced survival. Cachexia has been attributed to caloric intake failing to keep pace with energy expenditures associated with increased work of breathing, but more recent evidence suggests that a biochemical basis is more likely. Hypoxemia leads to increased circulating levels of tumor necrosis factor α (TNF-α), and weight loss has now been correlated with levels of the latter.

Peripheral Muscle Dysfunction   Protein and muscle are lost as part of wasting in advanced COPD. Skeletal muscle bulk is lost with proportional reductions in strength. Proximal limb girdle muscles of the upper and lower extremities are particularly affected, contributing to dyspnea with activities of daily living. Fiber composition in skeletal muscle changes, favoring endurance over strength. These changes occur in parallel with FEV_1 and independently of glucocorticoid use, which can also cause myopathy and muscle weakness.

Osteoporosis   Loss of bone density is common in advanced disease. Over half of COPD patients lose more than 1 SD of bony density, and more than one-third have values more than 2 SDs below normal. Vertebral fractures are especially common. These changes are even more severe in patients receiving chronic glucocorticoid therapy.

NATURAL HISTORY   COPD is identified by the presence of an abnormal FEV_1 in middle age, usually early in the fifth decade, and is characterized by an accelerated decline of FEV_1 with aging. In normal individuals, FEV_1 normally reaches a lifetime peak at age 25 and undergoes a linear decline of about 35 mL per year thereafter. Annual loss of FEV_1 among susceptible individuals who develop COPD is between 50 and 100 mL per year. Greater rates of decline have been associated with mucus hypersecretion, especially in men, and with bronchial hyperreactivity. Acute exacerbations do not alter the rate of decline. Dyspnea and impairment of physical work capacity are characteristic only of moderately severe to severe airways obstruction. There is considerable variation among individual patients. The majority of patients usually experience exertional dyspnea when FEV_1 falls below 40% of predicted and have dyspnea at rest when the FEV_1 <25% of predicted. In addition to dyspnea at rest, CO_2 retention and cor pulmonale frequently occur when the FEV_1 falls to 25% of predicted. With a respiratory infection, small changes in the degree of obstruction can make a large difference in symptoms and gas exchange. Thus small therapeutic gains may have rewarding results.

Exacerbation   The clinical course of COPD can be characterized as one of slow progression and relative stability punctuated by episodic exacerbations occurring, on average, a little more than once per year. Exacerbations are generally described as a worsening of previously stable disease characterized by increased dyspnea, wheeze, and cough and sputum volume, tenacity, and purulence, with variable degrees of water retention and with worsening gas exchange and ventilation-perfusion relationships. Hyperinflation and work of breathing are increased. To the extent that diaphragmatic function and neuromuscular drive can compensate for the increased work, Pa_{CO_2} will not rise, but when work demands exceed respiratory pump capacity, hypercapnia and respiratory acidemia ensue. Cardiac output often does not increase sufficiently to compensate for the increased oxygen consumption from respiratory muscles, thereby compounding the hypoxemia due to $\dot{V}/\dot{Q}$ mismatching and hypercapnia.

Most COPD exacerbations are thought to be a consequence of acute tracheobronchitis, usually infectious. Most infections are primarily bacterial or the consequence of bacterial superinfection of a primary viral process. Exacerbations may also be triggered by, and must be distinguished from, left ventricular failure, cardiac arrhythmias, pneumothorax, pneumonia, and pulmonary thromboembolism. Upper airway obstruction, aspiration, rhinitis or sinusitis, asthma, or gastroesophageal reflux should be excluded. Although COPD exacerbations are individually serious and potentially life-threatening, they do not cause accelerated declines of FEV_1 over time.

HISTORY Patients with COPD are most often tobacco smokers with a history of at least one pack per day for at least 20 years. The disease is only rarely seen in nonsmokers. Onset is typically in the fifth decade and often comes to attention as a productive cough or acute chest illness. Exertional dyspnea is usually not encountered until the sixth or seventh decade. The patient's perception of dyspnea correlates poorly with physiologic measurements, especially among older patients. A morning "smoker's cough" is frequent, usually mucoid in character but becoming purulent during exacerbations, which in early disease are intermittent and infrequent. Volume is generally small. Production of more than 60 mL/d should prompt investigation for bronchiectasis. The frequency and severity of cough generally do not correlate with the degree of functional impairment. Wheezing may be present but does not indicate severity of illness. As COPD progresses, exacerbations become more severe and more frequent. Gas exchange disturbances, worsen and dyspnea becomes progressive. Exercise tolerance becomes progressively limited. With worsening hypoxemia, erythrocytosis and cyanosis may occur. The development of morning headache may indicate the onset of significant CO_2 retention. In advanced disease, weight loss is frequent and correlates with an adverse prognosis. When blood gas derangements are severe, cor pulmonale may manifest itself by peripheral edema and water retention. Anxiety, depression, and sleep disturbances are not infrequent.

PHYSICAL FINDINGS The physical examination has poor sensitivity and variable reproducibility in COPD. Findings may be minimal or even normal in mild disease, requiring objective laboratory data for confirmation. In early disease, the only abnormal findings may be wheezes on forced expiration and a forced expiratory time prolonged beyond 6 s. With progressive disease, findings of hyperinflation become more apparent. These include an increased anteroposterior diameter of the chest, inspiratory retraction of the lower rib margins (Hoover's sign), decreased cardiac dullness, and distant heart and breath sounds. Coarse inspiratory crackles and rhonchi may be heard, especially at the bases. To gain better mechanical advantage for their compromised respiratory muscles, patients with severe airflow obstruction may adopt a characteristic tripod sitting posture with the neck angled forward and the upper torso supported on the elbows and arms. Breathing through pursed lips prolongs expiratory time and may help reduce dynamic hyperinflation.

Cor pulmonale and right heart failure may be evidenced by dependent edema and an enlarged, tender liver (Chap. 237). With pulmonary hypertension, a loud pulmonic component of the second heart sound may be audible, along with a right ventricular heave and a murmur of tricuspid regurgitation; these findings may be obscured by hyperinflation. If right-sided pressures are sufficiently high, neck veins may elevate instead of collapse with inspiration (Kussmaul's sign). Cyanosis is a somewhat unreliable manifestation of severe hypoxemia and is seen when severe hypoxemia and erythrocytosis are present.

Radiographic Findings A posteroanterior and lateral chest film should be obtained primarily to exclude competing diagnoses. They may be entirely normal in mild disease. As COPD progresses, abnormalities reflect emphysema, hyperinflation, and pulmonary hypertension. Emphysema is manifested by an increased lucency of the lungs. In smokers, these changes are more prominent in the upper lobes, while in α_1AT deficiency, they are more likely in basal zones. Local radiolucencies >1 cm in diameter and surrounded by hairline arcuate shadows indicate the presence of bullae and are highly specific for emphysema. With hyperinflation, the chest becomes vertically elongated with low flattened diaphragms. The heart shadow is also vertical and narrow. The retrosternal airspace is increased on the lateral view, and the sternal-diaphragmatic angle exceeds 90°. In the presence of pulmonary hypertension, the pulmonary arteries become enlarged and taper rapidly. The right heart border may become prominent and impinge on the retrosternal airspace. The presence of "dirty lung fields" may reflect the presence of bronchiolitis.

Computed tomography has greater sensitivity and specificity for emphysema than the plain film but is rarely necessary except for the diagnosis of bronchiectasis and evaluation of bullous disease. Nonhomogeneous distribution of emphysema is thought by some to be an indicator of suitability for lung volume reduction surgery (LVRS).

PULMONARY FUNCTION TESTING (See also Chap. 250) Because of the imprecision of clinical findings, objective evaluation of the presence, severity, and reversibility of airflow obstruction is essential in the diagnostic evaluation of COPD. A normal FEV_1 essentially excludes the diagnosis. The spirogram in COPD shows decreased volume changes with time and a failure to reach a plateau after 3 to 5 s. Continued airflow may be evident for 10 s or more on forced exhalation. The flow-volume curve shows diminished expiratory flow at all lung volumes. Expiratory flow is concave to the volume axis. When flow is plotted against absolute lung volume, the entire curve is shifted to higher volumes, reflecting hyperinflation. Serial spirometry is important in assessing the rate of decline of FEV_1.

Reversibility is assessed by spirometry before and after administration of an inhaled bronchodilator, most often a short-acting β_2-adrenergic agonist. Testing should be performed when the patient is clinically stable. Short-acting bronchodilators should be withheld for 6 h, long-acting dilators for 12 h, and theophylline for 24 h prior to testing. A significant response is an increase of at least 12% and 200 mL in either FEV_1 or forced vital capacity (FVC). Postbronchodilator FEV_1 is useful for prognostication. Although only one-third of COPD patients show a significant response to an inhaled bronchodilator in the pulmonary function laboratory on any one day, two-thirds will show a significant response when tested with different bronchodilators on several different occasions. The degree of bronchodilator response at any one testing session does not predict the degree of clinical benefit to the patient. Therefore, bronchodilators are given irrespective of the acute response obtained in the pulmonary function laboratory. The American Thoracic Society recommends staging COPD by FEV_1. Stage I, mild disease, is defined as $FEV_1 \geq 50\%$ predicted; stage II, moderate disease, 35 to 49% predicted; and stage III, severe disease, <35% predicted.

Lung volumes are useful for the assessment of hyperinflation. Transfer factor for carbon monoxide (DL_{CO}) correlates negatively with the degree of emphysema but is not specific and may miss mild disease. Neither test is indicated routinely, but DL_{CO} may help distinguish chronic asthma from emphysema.

Measurements for arterial blood gas are not needed for mild disease, but they should be assessed routinely for stage II or stage III COPD. Patients with pulmonary hypertension or cor pulmonale with normal daytime blood gases should be evaluated for nocturnal desaturation by overnight oximetry. Polysomnography to exclude concurrent sleep apnea should be obtained for patients who also complain of excessive daytime somnolence or who have a history of snoring.

α_1AT levels are not needed routinely but should be obtained for chronic airflow obstruction or chronic bronchitis in nonsmokers, as well as in COPD patients with bronchiectasis, cirrhosis without apparent risks, premature emphysema, or basilar emphysema; in patients under age 50 with unremitting asthma; and in individuals with a family history of α_1AT deficiency.

℞ TREATMENT Treatment of COPD is based on the principles of prevention of further evolution of disease, preservation of airflow, preservation and enhancement of functional capacity, management of physiologic complications, and avoidance of exacerbations.

Smoking Cessation (See also Chap. 390) The Lung Health Study has demonstrated that elimination of tobacco smoking confers significant survival benefit to patients with COPD. Prolonged survival is associated with reduced rates of malignancy and cardiovascular disease as well as with a significant increment in FEV_1 in the first year after smoking cessation. The rate of decline of FEV_1 reverts back to that of a nonsmoker. Although bronchodilator therapy produces similar first-year gains in FEV_1, pharmacotherapy alone does not modify the decline of airflow over time. Even unsuccessful quitters show significant benefits when compared to continuing smokers.

Despite the demonstrated benefits of smoking cessation, sustained quitting is difficult to achieve. Overall, only 6% of smokers succeed in quitting long term, and 70 to 80% of short-term quitters start smoking again. Successful quitting requires concerted active and continuing intervention by the physician. The physician should address the issue in regular patient visits, assess the patient's readiness to quit, advise the patient as to the best methods for smoking cessation, provide emotional and pharmacologic support, and arrange close follow-up of the patient's efforts. The concept of "lung age" may be helpful in promoting smoking cessation by determining the age at which the observed FEV_1 would be a normal finding. Lungs of 50- to 60-year-old smokers may be "normal" for a 70- to 80-year-old individual. Nicotine patches and nicotine polacrilex gum improve quit rates, especially among nicotine-dependent smokers. The addition of oral bupropion at 150 mg twice daily produces significant additional benefit, with a 1-year sustained abstinence rate of 22.5% compared to 6% for placebo. Smoking cessation is typically associated with weight gain of 3 to 4 kg. To minimize weight gain, reluctance to quit, and relapse, prospective quitters should be counseled to reduce caloric intake and to increase physical activity.

Bronchodilators These drugs improve dyspnea and exercise tolerance by improving airflow and by reducing end-expiratory lung volume and air-trapping. Although airflow limitation is relatively fixed, some degree of response to bronchodilator medication is usually present. Bronchodilator medication is available in metered-dose inhaler (and some dry-powder inhalers) and in nebulizable and oral forms. Inhalers deliver medications directly to the airways and have limited systemic absorption and side effects. Proper use requires timing and coordination of inspiration and inhaler actuation and presents frequent difficulties for chronic lung patients. These problems can usually be overcome with education and with the use of holding chambers. Aerosol nebulizers have no pharmacologic advantage over metered-dose inhalers. Their use should be limited to patients who remain unable to master metered dose inhalers adequately. Oral medication is associated with higher rates of adherence than inhalers but shows higher rates of systemic side effects without superior bronchodilation.

Three major classes of bronchodilators are commonly employed in the treatment of patients with COPD: short- and long-acting β_2-adrenergic agonists, anticholinergics, and theophylline derivatives. Short-acting β_2-agonists (albuterol, pirbuterol, terbutaline, metaproterenol) are relatively bronchoselective with minimal effects on heart rate and blood pressure. They produce significant bronchodilation at 5 to 15 min and remain effective for 4 to 6 h. Long-acting β_2-agonists (oral sustained-release albuterol and inhaled salmeterol) have an onset of action of 15 to 30 min and a 12-h duration of action. Anticholinergic agents (ipratropium bromide) have a 30- to 60-min onset of action and a 4- to 6-h duration. Theophyllines are generally administered orally in 12- or 24-h preparations. Recommended bronchodilator regimens are shown in Table 258-1.

Regular use of ipratropium may lead to improvements in baseline

FEV_1 when compared with short-acting β_2-agonists. When used together, ipratropium and short-acting β_2-agents show greater clinical efficacy than either agent alone, without an increase in side effects. Salmeterol as a single agent produces longer lasting bronchodilation than ipratropium, improves baseline FEV_1 over time, and is not associated with loss of efficacy over a period of several months. Salmeterol, however, has not yet been evaluated as a component of combination therapy.

Theophylline is a weak bronchodilator with a narrow therapeutic window. Much of its clinical benefit derives from effects other than bronchodilation; therapeutic doses of theophylline increase ventilatory drive, enhance diaphragmatic contractility, and increase cardiac output. About 20% of COPD patients respond to theophylline with improved airflow, exercise tolerance, and quality of life. Theophylline produces additional benefits in exercise capacity and quality of life when used in combination with short-acting β_2-adrenergic agonists. The therapeutic range for theophylline is commonly given as 10 to 20 μg/mL, with greater efficacy but greater toxicity seen at higher serum levels. The risk of toxicity is greater in older patients and in those with heart and kidney disease. Optimal dosing must balance the competing considerations of risk and benefit for each individual patient.

Glucocorticoids Because COPD, like asthma, is a disease associated with airway inflammation, glucocorticoids are an intuitively attractive therapeutic modality. Nevertheless, results of clinical trials of glucocorticoid therapy in COPD patients have shown less impressive benefits when compared to patients with asthma. The degree of response to glucocorticoids appears to correlate with the presence of asthmatic features, but data supporting their use is limited. Only 10% more patients show subjective benefit and increase their FEV_1 or forced vital capacity by at least 20% when compared to those on placebo. Responders cannot be reliably identified on clinical grounds, although response to an inhaled β_2-agonist is commonly used as a predictor. The benefits of a 10- to 14-day trial of 30 to 40 mg/d of prednisone for patients with stage III disease who have not responded adequately to mixed bronchodilator therapy remain to be proven. Long-term systemic glucocorticoid use is associated with multiple side effects. In particular, they have been associated with worsened osteoporosis and increased risk of vertebral fracture. If systemic steroids are used, the lowest effective dose should be employed and alternate-day dosing used whenever possible. The use of inhaled glucocorticoids ameliorates systemic side effects. Three large clinical trials have shown that inhaled glucocorticoids do not alter the rate of decline of FEV_1. While an inhaled glucocorticoid does not decrease the number or frequency of COPD exacerbations, it may decrease their severity and reduce the need for hospitalization. Symptoms and exercise tolerance improve on inhaled glucocorticoids.

Management of α_1AT Deficiency Given the central role of smoking in the pathogenesis of disease, smoking cessation is an important cornerstone in the management of α_1AT deficiency. Exogenous α_1AT derived from pooled human plasma administered intravenously in a weekly dose of 60 mg/kg has been shown to induce protective levels of α_1AT in deficient individuals. Because of the expense and inconvenience of the treatment, replacement of α_1AT is used only for patients over age 18 with α_1AT levels below 11 μmol/L who have stopped smoking and who have airflow obstruction. A recently published large nonrandomized trial showed that augmentation therapy significantly decreased 5-year mortality (RR 0.64) for patients receiving replacement. The rate of decline of FEV_1 also decreased with augmentation therapy. In both instances, benefit was largely restricted to those patients with FEV_1 35 to 49% of predicted. These findings require confirmation in randomized controlled trials.

Oxygen Severe and progressive hypoxemia is often seen in advanced COPD and may result in cellular hypoxia with deleterious physiologic consequences. The establishment of adequate systemic oxygen transport is essential to the prevention of tissue hypoxia and requires attention to cardiac output and hemoglobin concentration as well as to arterial O_2 saturation (Sa_{O_2}). Long-term O_2 therapy has been shown to reverse secondary polycythemia; improve body weight; ame-

Table 258-1 Recommended Bronchodilator Therapy for Chronic Obstructive Pulmonary Disease

Stage	FEV_1, % predicted	Treatment
I	> 50	β_2-agonist prn
II	35–49	Combined anticholinergic and β_2-agonist
III	<35	Above plus long-acting β_2-agonist and/or sustained release theophylline
		Consider oral glucocorticoid trial

SOURCE: Celli et al, 1995, and Pearson et al, 1997.

liorate cor pulmonale; and enhance neuropsychiatric function, exercise tolerance, and activities of daily living. Two major studies, one in the United States and one in the United Kingdom, established a survival benefit for long-term O_2 therapy that increased with the number of hours per day that O_2 was used. The mechanism for this benefit has not been conclusively elucidated, but it appears to be related to the stabilization of pulmonary hemodynamics.

The need for long-term O_2 therapy should be documented with measurement of arterial blood gases obtained at rest and confirmed by a separate determination of resting arterial blood gases during a period of medical stability after 30 to 90 days of optimum medical therapy. Once the need for O_2 has been demonstrated in a stable patient, the requirement is generally for the duration of the patient's life. Patients with a $Pa_{O_2} \leq 55$ mmHg or $Sa_{O_2} \leq 88\%$ should be provided with oxygen titrated to raise Sa_{O_2} to $\geq 90\%$. Oxygen is likewise indicated for patients who have a PaO_2 of 56 to 59 mmHg with $Sa_{O_2} \geq 89\%$ when hematocrit is 55% or when cor pulmonale or other objective evidence of pulmonary hypertension is present. Oxygen may be appropriate for patients whose resting awake $Pa_{O_2} \geq 60$ mmHg with $Sa_{O_2} \geq 90\%$ if they become hypoxic during exercise or sleep. Once oxygen is prescribed, the dose should be titrated to maintain $Sa_{O_2} \geq 90\%$ during sleep and normal walking, as well as at rest, and it should be used for a minimum of 15 h a day to realize a survival benefit.

Oxygen is most frequently delivered through a nasal cannula at rates of 2 to 5 L/min. Oxygen-sparing cannulae are available. Transtracheal administration provides further O_2-sparing benefits but requires scrupulous attention to catheter maintenance and hygiene and is not suitable for all patients. Oxygen is packaged as compressed gas or compressed liquid or can be delivered from an O_2 concentrator, a molecular sieve that enriches O_2 by removing nitrogen from ambient air. O_2 should be prescribed from sources that are appropriate to the individual patient's life-style and needs. It is customary to provide a stationary O_2 source, either an O_2 concentrator, which is dependent on a reliable source of electricity, or 100-kg (200-lb) H cylinders of compressed O_2. Flow resistance imposes a 15-m (50-ft) practical limit to the length of tubing connecting the O_2 source to the patient's cannula. For patients whose activities of daily living require ambulation beyond this limit, ambulatory or portable systems should be provided. Ambulatory O_2 needs may be met with rolling 10-kg (22-lb) E cylinders of compressed O_2, or with portable 2-kg (4.5-lb) aluminum cylinders or 3-kg (6.6-lb) liquid oxygen packs. The duration of O_2 availability from an O_2 concentrator is unlimited. For compressed gas and liquid sources, the amount of available oxygen is determined by the size of the system and the patient's liter flow needs. Portable systems generally provide 4 to 5 h of O_2 flow.

Oxygen therapy is generally safe. Cylinders should be secured to prevent tipping over or potentially explosive disconnection of the regulator valve. Oxygen should be stored away from open flames or other source of heat, and patients and family members should be educated to be especially scrupulous about avoiding smoking in the presence of flowing O_2.

Prophylaxis No evidence supports the prophylactic use of antibiotics in stable COPD. Yearly influenza vaccination is recommended for all patients with chronic cardiopulmonary disease, although objective benefit has not been conclusively demonstrated. Pneumococcal vaccination with 23-valent polysaccharide is also recommended. Amantadine should be used for unvaccinated patients who are placed at risk by an outbreak of influenza A.

Rehabilitation Airflow limitation, dyspnea, and muscle loss and deconditioning all compromise cardiopulmonary fitness and contribute to a progressively constrained daily life and unsatisfactory quality of life. Pulmonary rehabilitation is a multidisciplinary program of care for patients with chronic respiratory impairments that is individually tailored and designed to optimize physical and social performance. A pulmonary rehabilitation program consists of exercise training, patient education, psychosocial and behavioral intervention, and regular assessment of outcomes and is designed to minimize the disability and handicap imposed by the physiologic impairments consequent to

COPD. Rehabilitation in COPD should be considered for patients with persistent symptoms and disability despite optimal medical management. Spirometric criteria should not be the primary basis for referral into rehabilitation programs. Exercise consists of 20 to 30 min of upper and lower extremity exercise at 60 to 75% maximum $\dot{V}_{O_2}$ or heart rate two to five times a week. Both strength and endurance exercises are provided. Education covers pursed lip and other breathing strategies to minimize dyspnea, energy-conservation skills, principles of medications and proper use of metered-dose inhalers, nutrition, and end-of-life decision-making. Behavioral interventions focus on dyspnea, depression, and self-sufficiency and on issues of control, coping, and role function. Dyspnea, exercise tolerance, activity level, and quality of life are followed at regular intervals. Pulmonary rehabilitation programs have been shown to improve endurance time for submaximal exercise by 38 to 80% and 6-min walking distance by 80 to 113 m. Clinically meaningful reduction in dyspnea and improvement of quality of life have been reported. No clinical trials have been adequately designed to address the issue of survival benefit. Reductions in costs of care and resource consumption have not reached statistical significance.

Despite maximal medical therapy, when COPD progresses to stage III and is complicated by hypercapnia or pulmonary hypertension, surgical approaches to treatment may be considered.

Transplantation (See also Chap. 267) Owing to its frequency in the general population, emphysema is the most common indication for lung transplantation. Transplantation should be actively considered for end-stage COPD patients when the prognosis from the disease is worse than the survival statistics for the surgery. Lung transplantation should be considered for COPD patients who, despite maximal medical therapy, have an $FEV_1 < 25\%$ predicted and with pulmonary hypertension or cor pulmonale. Precedence is given to those patients with a Pa_{CO_2} of 55 mmHg and progressive deterioration. Asthma and other reversible airflow limitation must be excluded. Rehabilitation and long-term O_2 therapy, where appropriate, should be provided prior to transplant evaluation.

Lung Volume Reduction Surgery LVRS, or pneumectomy, is designed to relieve dyspnea and improve exercise function in severely disabled patients with stage III emphysema. At operation, severely emphysematous lung tissue is resected, leading to improvement in elastic recoil in the remaining pulmonary parenchyma. This decreases hyperinflation and enhances diaphragmatic function, with consequent 25 to 50% improvement of airflow and exercise capacity. In early uncontrolled studies, hospital mortality for LVRS ranged from 5 to 18% and hospital stays averaged 9 to 18 days, with frequent significant air leaks. Cost of LVRS was $33,000 to $70,000 per case. Because of the large number of potential candidates, the high cost involved, and unanswered questions about the benefits of the operation, use of LVRS in the United States has been restricted to a multicenter randomized controlled trial, the National Emphysema Treatment Trial (NETT), comparing LVRS with best medical therapy. Stage III emphysema patients accepted for evaluation into NETT are under age 75, are severely hyperinflated, and have severe dyspnea despite optimal medical therapy. Contraindications to LVRS are similar to those for lung transplantation, including active smoking, marked obesity or cachexia, and inability to undertake pulmonary rehabilitation successfully. There has been little consensus regarding features identifying ideal and suboptimal candidates for the surgery. Radiographic heterogeneity of disease and the absence of significant intrinsic airway disease have been suggested characteristics of patients likely to benefit. Results from the NETT suggest that physiologic benefits from LVRS may begin to be lost as early as 1 year after surgery. Accelerated declines of FEV_1 have been reported, averaging 100 mL per year and particularly marked in those patients with the greatest postoperative gains in airflow. Improvements in dyspnea and exercise tolerance may be sustained for as long as 3 years but may decline thereafter. Until these issues are satisfactorily resolved, LVRS will remain an experimental procedure.

Treatment of Exacerbations • *Triage* The initial decision in the management of an exacerbation of COPD is whether hospitalization is necessary. Rapidity of evolution of symptoms and response to initial therapy, level of consciousness, presence or absence of respiratory distress, severity of gas exchange disturbance, and arterial blood gas deviation from the patient's stable baseline should influence the decision to hospitalize. The patient's ability to manage at home and the resources available for home care should weigh heavily in the decision-making process.

Home therapy For patients with mild exacerbations for whom outpatient therapy is appropriate, a combination of anticholinergic and short-acting β_2-adrenergic agonist bronchodilators should be prescribed. Although β_2-agonists may be given as frequently as once an hour, there is no advantage to administering anticholinergic bronchodilators more frequently than every 4 to 6 h. Metered-dose inhalers should be used with spacers. There is no evidence that the use of nebulizers provides any improvement in outcome.

The presence of increased sputum volume or purulence suggest an infectious cause of an exacerbation. With either of these features is present in conjunction with increased breathlessness or when both are present, antibiotics should be prescribed. The organisms most frequently associated with mild COPD exacerbations include *Streptococcus pneumoniae*, *Haemophilus influenzae*, and *Moraxella catarrhalis*. Trimethoprim/sulfamethoxazole, doxycycline, or amoxicillin is an appropriate management option, although choices may be modified by local antibiotic sensitivity data.

There is a need for well-controlled studies on the utility of glucocorticoids in the outpatient management of COPD exacerbations. Oral glucocorticoids may be continued in patients already receiving such treatment or given to patients who do not show a satisfactory response to bronchodilator therapy. The usual dose is 20 to 40 mg daily for 7 to 10 days. Short-term glucocorticoid therapy lasting less than 3 weeks may be discontinued without the use of a tapering dose.

Hospital management For patients with exacerbations of sufficient severity to warrant hospitalization, improvement of airflow, gas exchange, and acid-base status are of central importance. Hospitalized patients should receive bronchodilators, antibiotics, oral glucocorticoids, and sufficient O_2 to keep the $Sa_{O_2} \geq 90\%$. β_2-agonists and anticholinergic agents should be given together every 4 to 6 h. The frequency of sympathomimetic bronchodilator administration may be increased as needed to as often as every 20 min. Because high doses of β_2-agonists may cause hypokalemia, serum potassium levels and heart rate should be monitored closely for patients receiving frequent doses of these agents. Data are contradictory regarding the addition of theophylline to the bronchodilator regiment of patients showing an inadequate initial response, yet the current American and British Thoracic Societies' guidelines recommend consideration of its use to produce plasma theophylline levels between 10 and 20 μg/mL. Oral glucocorticoids have been shown to produce modest improvements in FEV_1 and in the duration of hospitalization for COPD exacerbations. Recent data indicate that more severe COPD exacerbations are associated with the recovery of enterobacteriaciae in respiratory secretions. For this reason, a second- or third-generation cephalosporin, a fluoroquinolone, a second-generation macrolide, or an extended-spectrum penicillin is now recommended as initial therapy. Attempts to obtain diagnostically adequate sputum should be made, and, when available, sputum results should be used to individualize therapy in the light of local microbial sensitivity spectra. Oxygen therapy is an important component of the management of a severe exacerbation of COPD. It is important to maintain the $Sa_{O_2} > 90\%$ and Pa_{O_2} between 60 and 65 mmHg for most patients. In many cases, administration of O_2 will result in worsening hypercapnia, although rarely to a clinically significant degree if the O_2 is used only in amounts to achieve the minimal goals. The elevation of Pa_{CO_2} is multifactorial, resulting from increased dead space due to reduced tidal volume as well as from the Haldane effect, i.e., a right wave shift of the CO_2 dissociation curve in the presence of increased saturated hemoglobin. The lower the initial Pa_{O_2} and the greater the increase, the larger the increase in Pa_{CO_2} observed. Patients whose pH on presentation is below 7.25 and with $Pa_{O_2} < 50$ mmHg are at particular risk and should be observed closely.

For patients at increased risk of hypercapnia, administration of controlled concentrations of O_2 through a Venturi mask is reasonable. Inspired O_2 concentrations (FI_{O_2}) of 0.24 to 0.28 are usually sufficient to keep $Sa_{O_2} \geq 90\%$.

MECHANICAL VENTILATION (See also Chap. 266) Patients with impaired consciousness, respiratory distress evidenced by tachypnea with a respiratory rate greater than 35 breaths per minute and/or abdominal paradox, severe hypoxemia, or significant respiratory acidosis with pH < 7.25 and who deteriorate despite treatment are candidates for immediate ventilatory support using either noninvasive (mask) or invasive (intubation) approaches. The goals are to buy time for medical treatments to take effect, to rest the respiratory muscles, and to improve gas exchange abnormalities while avoiding the major complications of mechanical ventilatory support.

Noninvasive positive-pressure ventilation (NIPPV) delivered by nasal mask should be considered in units that have experience with the technique for patients who remain alert and cooperative, who are not heavily sedated, who are hemodynamically stable, and who are able to clear their airways by coughing up secretions. In these circumstances, NIPPV has been shown to be successful in avoiding the need for endotracheal intubation in up to 70% of cases. Success, as evidenced by improved Pa_{CO_2} and pH, should be evident within the first 60 min. Part-time NIPPV for 6 to 8 h per day may afford sufficient respiratory muscle rest to avert the need for invasive conventional ventilation. Failed attempts at NIPPV can be followed by intubation and conventional ventilation and do not appear to carry a worse prognosis. Successful application of NIPPV has been associated with a decrease in intensive care and hospital stays, incidence of nosocomial pneumonia, and costs.

Before committing to endotracheal intubation and conventional ventilatory support, the patient's wishes for such support, the patient's quality of life, and the benefits and costs of care should be thoroughly reviewed. Where the patient's wishes cannot be clearly ascertained or there is uncertainty about the appropriateness of the intervention, intubation and ventilation should proceed. If mechanical ventilatory support is subsequently determined to be inappropriate, support may then be withdrawn.

Once intubation is accomplished, the patient can be ventilated in the controlled ventilation, assist-control, intermittent mandatory ventilation, or pressure support modes. FI_{O_2} should be sufficient to obtain $Sa_{O_2} \geq 90\%$ and Pa_{O_2} of 60 to 65 mmHg. An FI_{O_2} of 0.24 to 0.40 is usually adequate for the purpose. Minute volume should be adequate to keep pH ≥ 7.25, but one should not strive to achieve a "normal" Pa_{CO_2}. It is important to try to avoid overventilation and hyperinflation in ventilated COPD patients. Because the time constant for exhalation is abnormally prolonged, it is essential to allow adequate expiratory time to permit as complete emptying of each breath as possible, preferably at least 3 to 4 s. This is best accomplished by minimizing tidal volume and respiratory rate. Lesser gains in expiratory (E) time can be obtained by high inspiratory (I) flow rates and I:E ratios of 1:2 or higher. Inadequate expiratory time leads to dynamic hyperinflation and in turn to the development of intrinsic positive end-expiratory pressure (PEEPi). PEEPi is just as capable of producing hypotension as extrinsically applied PEEP. When a mechanically ventilated patient with obstructive lung disease abruptly develops hypotension, PEEPi should be excluded, either by direct measurement or by disconnecting the patient from the ventilator for 30 to 60 s. PEEPi and dynamic hyperinflation increase the work of breathing, place the diaphragm at mechanical disadvantage, and contribute significantly to difficulties in weaning from ventilatory support. Over a period of days, as the underlying precipitants of the exacerbation are controlled, airway obstruction gradually remits and gas exchange improves and it becomes appropriate to consider removal from mechanical ventilatory support.

The principles of weaning from mechanical ventilation are discussed in detail in Chap. 266.

Prognosis after exacerbation The hospital mortality rate for an episode of respiratory failure in COPD ranges from 11 to 25% and depends on the severity of the episode, the patient's chronic health and nutritional status, and the presence of cor pulmonale or congestive heart failure. Data regarding subsequent course may be helpful in educating COPD patients and in guiding their subsequent management decisions. Among survivors of mechanical ventilation, the 6-month mortality rate is approximately 40%. Two-thirds of survivors have frequent recurrences of exacerbations, and functional status thereafter is often poor.

BIBLIOGRAPHY

BERNARD S et al: Peripheral muscle weakness in patients with chronic obstructive pulmonary disease. Am J Respir Crit Care Med 158:629, 1998

BROCHARD L et al: Noninvasive ventilation for acute exacerbations of chronic obstructive pulmonary disease. N Engl J Med 333:817, 1995

CELLI B et al: Standards for the diagnosis and care of patients with chronic obstructive pulmonary disease. Am J Respir Crit Care Med 152:S77, 1995

CONNORS AF et al: Outcomes following acute exacerbation of severe chronic obstructive lung disease. The SUPPORT investigators (Study to Understand Prognoses and Preferences for Outcomes and Risks of Treatments). Am J Respir Crit Care Med 154: 959, 1996

FEIN A: Lung volume reduction surgery: Answering the crucial questions. Chest 113: 277S, 1998.

HOGG JC: Chronic bronchitis: The role of viruses. Semin Respir Infect 15:32, 2000

LAREAU SC et al: Pulmonary rehabilitation 1999. Am J Respir Crit Care Med 159:1666, 1999

MADISON J, IRWIN R: Chronic obstructive pulmonary disease. Lancet 352:467, 1998

NIEWOEHNER DE et al: Effect of systemic glucocorticoids on exacerbations of chronic obstructive pulmonary disease. N Engl J Med 340:1941, 1999

O'BYRNE PM, POSTMA DS: The many faces of airway inflammation. Asthma and chronic obstructive pulmonary disease. Am J Respir Crit Care Med 159:S1, 1999

PEARSON M et al: BTS Guidelines for the management of chronic obstructive pulmonary disease. Thorax 52(Suppl 5):S1, 1997

PIQUETTE CA et al: Chronic bronchitis and emphysema, in *Textbook of Respiratory Medicine*, 3d ed, JF Murray, JA Nadel (eds). Philadelphia, Saunders, 2000, pp 1187–1246

SCHOLS AM: Nutrition in chronic obstructive pulmonary disease. Curr Opin Pulm Med 6:110, 2000

SETHI JM, ROCHESTER CL: Smoking and chronic obstructive pulmonary disease. Clin Chest Med 21:67, 2000

259   *Talmadge E. King, Jr.*

INTERSTITIAL LUNG DISEASES

AIP	acute interstitial pneumonia	FEV$_1$	forced expiratory volume in one second
ARDS	acute respiratory distress syndrome	FVC	forced vital capacity
BAL	bronchoalveolar lavage	GM-CSF	granulocyte-macrophage colony stimulating factor
BG	bronchocentric granulomatosis	HRCT	high-resolution computed tomography
BOOP	bronchiolitis obliterans with organizing pneumonia	ILDs	interstitial lung diseases
COP	cryptogenic organizing pneumonia	IPF	idiopathic pulmonary fibrosis
CTDs	connective tissue diseases	LAM	lymphangioleiomyomatosis
DAHs	diffuse alveolar hemorrhage syndromes	NSIP	nonspecific interstitial pneumonia
DIP	desquamative interstitial pneumonitis	PAP	pulmonary alveolar proteinosis
D$_{LCO}$	diffusing capacity of the lung for carbon monoxide	PLCH	pulmonary Langerhans cell histiocytosis
DTPA	diethylenetriamene pentaacetate	SLE	systemic lupus erythematosus
		TLC	total lung capacity
		UIP	usual interstitial pneumonia

The interstitial lung diseases (ILDs) represent a large number of conditions that involve the parenchyma of the lung—the alveoli, the alveolar epithelium, the capillary endothelium, and the spaces between these structures, as well as the perivascular and lymphatic tissues. This heterogeneous group of disorders is classified together because of similar clinical, roentgenographic, physiologic, or pathologic manifestations. These disorders are often associated with considerable morbidity and mortality, and there is little consensus regarding the best management of most of them.

ILDs have been difficult to classify because more than 200 known individual diseases are characterized by diffuse parenchymal lung involvement, either as the primary condition or as a significant part of a multiorgan process, as may occur in the connective tissue diseases (CTDs). One useful approach to classification is to separate the ILDs into two groups, those of known and those of unknown causes (Table 259-1). Each of these groups can be subdivided into subgroups according to the presence or absence of histologic evidence of granulomas in interstitial or vascular areas. For each ILD there may be an acute phase, and there is usually a chronic one as well. Rarely, some are recurrent, with intervals of subclinical disease.

Sarcoidosis (Chap. 318), idiopathic pulmonary fibrosis (IPF), and pulmonary fibrosis associated with CTDs (Chaps. 311 to 317) are the

Table 259-1   Major Categories of Alveolar and Interstitial Inflammatory Lung Disease

Lung Response: Alveolitis, Interstitial Inflammation, and Fibrosis

KNOWN CAUSE

Asbestos	Radiation
Fumes, gases	Aspiration pneumonia
Drugs (antibiotics, amiodarone, gold) and chemotherapy drugs	Residual of adult respiratory distress syndrome

UNKNOWN CAUSE

Idiopathic interstitial pneumonias	Pulmonary alveolar proteinosis
Idiopathic pulmonary fibrosis (usual interstitial pneumonia)	Lymphocytic infiltrative disorders (lymphocytic interstitial pneumonias associated with connective tissue disease)
Desquamative interstitial pneumonia	
Respiratory bronchiolitis-associated interstitial lung disease	Eosinophilic pneumonias
Acute interstitial pneumonia (diffuse alveolar damage)	Lymphangioleiomyomatosis
	Amyloidosis
Cryptogenic organizing pneumonia (bronchiolitis obliterans with organizing pneumonia)	Inherited diseases
	Tuberous sclerosis, neurofibromatosis, Niemann-Pick disease, Gaucher's disease, Hermansky-Pudlak syndrome
Nonspecific interstitial pneumonia	
Connective tissue diseases	
Systemic lupus erythematosus, rheumatoid arthritis, ankylosing spondylitis, systemic sclerosis, Sjögren's syndrome, polymyositis-dermatomyositis	Gastrointestinal or liver diseases (Crohn's disease, primary biliary cirrhosis, chronic active hepatitis, ulcerative colitis)
	Graft-vs.-host disease (bone marrow transplantation; solid organ transplantation)
Pulmonary hemorrhage syndromes	
Goodpasture's syndrome, idiopathic pulmonary hemosiderosis, isolated pulmonary capillaritis	

Lung Response: Granulomatous

KNOWN CAUSE

Hypersensitivity pneumonitis (organic dusts)	Inorganic dusts: beryllium silica

UNKNOWN CAUSE

Sarcoidosis	Bronchocentric granulomatosis
Langerhans cell granulomatosis (eosinophilic granuloma of the lung)	Lymphomatoid granulomatosis
Granulomatous vasculitides	
Wegener's granulomatosis, allergic granulomatosis of Churg-Strauss	

most common ILDs of unknown etiology. Among the ILDs of known cause, the largest group comprises occupational and environmental exposures, especially the inhalation of inorganic dusts, organic dusts, and various fumes or gases (Chaps. 253 and 254). A clinical diagnosis is possible for many forms of ILD, especially if an occupational and environmental history is aggressively pursued. For other forms, tissue examination, usually obtained by thoracoscopic or open lung biopsy is critical to confirmation of the diagnosis. High-resolution computed tomography (HRCT) scanning promises to improve diagnostic accuracy further as histologic-image correlation is perfected.

PATHOGENESIS

The ILDs are nonmalignant disorders and are not caused by identified infectious agents. The precise pathway(s) leading from injury to fibrosis is not known. Although there are multiple initiating agent(s) of injury, the immunopathogenic responses of lung tissue are limited, and the mechanisms of repair have common features. Two major histopathologic patterns are found in patients with ILD: a granulomatous pattern (Fig. 259-1) and a pattern in which inflammation and fibrosis predominate.

GRANULOMATOUS LUNG DISEASE   This process is characterized by an accumulation of T lymphocytes, macrophages, and epithelioid cells organized into discrete structures (granulomas) in the lung parenchyma. The granulomatous lesions can progress to fibrosis. Many patients with granulomatous lung disease remain free of severe impairment of lung function, or, when symptomatic, they improve after treatment. The main differential diagnosis is between sarcoidosis (Chap. 318) and hypersensitivity pneumonitis (Chap. 253).

INFLAMMATION AND FIBROSIS   The initial insult is an injury to the epithelial surface causing inflammation in the air spaces and alveolar walls. If the disease becomes chronic, inflammation spreads to adjacent portions of the interstitium and vasculature and eventually causes interstitial fibrosis. Other important histopathologic patterns in ILDs include diffuse alveolar damage (acute or organizing), desquamative interstitial pneumonia, respiratory bronchiolitis, lymphocytic interstitial pneumonia, and an organizing pneumonia [bronchiolitis obliterans with organizing pneumonia (BOOP) pattern]. The development of irreversible scarring (fibrosis) of alveolar walls, airways, or vasculature is the most feared outcome in all of these conditions because it is often progressive and leads to significant derangement of ventilatory function and gas exchange.

FIGURE 259-1 Hypersensitivity pneumonitis. Granulomatous inflammation with scattered, small, ill-formed granulomas, which in this case manifest primarily as clusters of giant cells.

INITIAL EVALUATION

Patients with ILDs come to medical attention mainly because of the onset of progressive exertional dyspnea or a persistent, nonproductive cough. Hemoptysis, wheezing, and chest pain may be present. Often, the identification of interstitial opacities on chest x-ray focuses the diagnostic approach toward one of the ILDs.

HISTORY   Duration of Illness   *Acute presentation* (days to weeks), while unusual, occurs with allergy (drugs, fungi, helminths), acute idiopathic interstitial pneumonia, eosinophilic pneumonia, and hypersensitivity pneumonitis. These conditions may be confused with atypical pneumonias because of diffuse alveolar opacities on chest x-ray. *Subacute presentation* (weeks to months) may occur in all ILDs but is seen especially in sarcoidosis, drug-induced ILDs, the alveolar hemorrhage syndromes, cryptogenic organizing pneumonia (COP), and the acute immunologic pneumonia that complicates systemic lupus erythematosus (SLE) or polymyositis. In most ILDs the symptoms and signs are *chronic* (months to years). Examples include IPF, sarcoidosis, pulmonary Langerhans cell histiocytosis (PLCH) (also known as Langerhans cell granulomatosis, eosinophilic granuloma, and histiocytosis X), pneumoconioses, and CTDs. *Episodic presentations* are unusual and include eosinophilic pneumonia, hypersensitivity pneumonitis, cryptogenic organizing pneumonia, vasculitides, pulmonary hemorrhage, and Churg-Strauss syndrome.

Age   Most patients with sarcoidosis, ILD associated with CTD, lymphangioleiomyomatosis (LAM), PLCH, inherited forms of ILD (familial IPF, Gaucher's disease, Hermansky-Pudlak syndrome) present between the ages of 20 and 40 years. Most patients with IPF are older than 50 years.

Gender   LAM and pulmonary involvement in tuberous sclerosis occur exclusively in premenopausal women. Also, ILD in Hermansky-Pudlak syndrome and in the CTDs is more common in women; an exception is ILD in rheumatoid arthritis, which is more common in men. Because of occupational exposures, pneumoconioses also occur more frequently in men.

Family History   Family history is occasionally helpful because familial associations (with an autosomal dominant pattern) have been identified in tuberous sclerosis and neurofibromatosis. An autosomal recessive pattern of inheritance occurs in Niemann-Pick disease, Gaucher's disease, and the Hermansky-Pudlak syndrome. Familial clustering has been increasingly identified in sarcoidosis and familial pulmonary fibrosis, a process similar to IPF.

Smoking History   Patients with PLCH, desquamative interstitial pneumonia (DIP), Goodpasture's syndrome, and respiratory bronchiolitis are almost always current or former smokers. Two-thirds to 75% of patients with IPF have a history of smoking.

Occupation and Environmental History   A strict chronological listing of the patient's lifelong employment must be sought, including specific duties and known exposures. In hypersensitivity pneumonitis (Fig. 259-1), respiratory symptoms, fever, chills, and an abnormal chest roentgenogram are often temporally related to a hobby (pigeon breeder's disease) or to the workplace (Farmer's lung) (Chap. 253). Symptoms may diminish or disappear after the patient leaves the site of exposure for several days; similarly, symptoms may reappear on returning to the exposure site.

Other Important Past History   Parasitic infections may cause pulmonary eosinophilia, and therefore a travel history should be taken in patients with known or suspected ILD. History of risk factors for HIV infection should be elicited from all patients with ILD because several processes may occur at the time of initial presentation or during the clinical course, e.g., HIV infection, BOOP, acute interstitial pneumonia, lymphocytic interstitial pneumonitis, or diffuse alveolar hemorrhage.

RESPIRATORY SYMPTOMS AND SIGNS   Dyspnea is a common and prominent complaint in patients with ILD, especially the idiopathic interstitial pneumonias, hypersensitivity pneumonitis, COP, sarcoidosis, eosinophilic pneumonias, and PLCH. Some patients, especially patients with sarcoidosis, silicosis, PLCH, hypersensitivity pneumonitis, lipoid pneumonia, or lymphangitis carcinomatosis may have extensive parenchymal lung disease on chest x-ray without significant dyspnea, especially early in the course of the illness. Wheezing is an uncommon manifestation of ILD but has been described in patients with chronic eosinophilic pneumonia, Churg-Strauss syndrome, respiratory bronchiolitis, and sarcoidosis. Clinically significant chest pain is uncommon in most ILDs. However, substernal discomfort is common in sarcoidosis. Sudden worsening of dyspnea, especially if associated with acute chest pain, may indicate a spontaneous pneumothorax, which occurs in PLCH, tuberous sclerosis, LAM, and neurofibromatosis. Frank hemoptysis and blood-streaked sputum are rarely presenting manifestations of ILD but can be seen in the diffuse alveolar hemorrhage syndromes (DAHs), LAM, tuberous sclerosis, and the granulomatous vasculitides. Fatigue and weight loss are common in all ILDs.

PHYSICAL EXAMINATION The findings are usually not specific. Most commonly, physical examination reveals tachypnea, and bibasilar end-inspiratory dry crackles, which are common in most forms of ILD associated with inflammation but are less likely to be heard in the granulomatous lung diseases. Crackles may be present in the absence of radiographic abnormalities on the chest radiograph. Scattered late inspiratory high-pitched rhonchi—so-called inspiratory squeaks—are heard in patients with bronchiolitis. The cardiac examination is usually normal except in the mid or late stages of the disease when findings of pulmonary hypertension and cor pulmonale may become evident (Chap. 237). Cyanosis and clubbing of the digits occurs in some patients with advanced disease.

LABORATORY Antinuclear antibodies, anti-immunoglobulin antibodies (rheumatoid factors), and circulating immune complexes are identified in some patients, even in the absence of a defined CTD. A raised LDH is a nonspecific finding common to ILDs. Elevation of the serum angiotensin-converting enzyme level is common in sarcoidosis. Serum precipitins confirm exposure when hypersensitivity pneumonitis is suspected, although they are not diagnostic of the process. Antineutrophil cytoplasmic or anti-basement membrane antibodies are useful if vasculitis is suspected. The electrocardiogram is usually normal unless pulmonary hypertension is present; then it demonstrates right-axis deviation or right ventricular hypertrophy. Echocardiography also reveals right ventricular dilatation and/or hypertrophy in the presence of pulmonary hypertension.

CHEST IMAGING STUDIES **Chest X-ray** ILD may be first suspected on the basis of an abnormal chest radiograph, which most commonly reveals a bibasilar reticular pattern. A nodular or mixed pattern of alveolar filling and increased reticular markings may also be present (see Fig. 249-1). A subgroup of ILDs exhibit nodular opacities with a predilection for the upper lung zones [sarcoidosis, PLCH, chronic hypersensitivity pneumonitis, silicosis, berylliosis, rheumatoid arthritis (necrobiotic nodular form), ankylosing spondylitis]. The chest x-ray correlates poorly with the clinical or histopathologic stage of the disease. The radiographic finding of honeycombing correlates with pathologic findings of small cystic spaces and progressive fibrosis; when present, it portends a poor prognosis. In most cases, the chest radiograph is nonspecific and usually does not allow a specific diagnosis.

Computed Tomography HRCT is superior to the plain chest x-ray for early detection and confirmation of suspected ILD. Also, HRCT allows better assessment of the extent and distribution of disease, and it is especially useful in the investigation of patients with a normal chest radiograph. Coexisting disease is often best recognized on HRCT scanning, e.g., mediastinal adenopathy, carcinoma, or emphysema. In the appropriate clinical setting HRCT may be sufficiently characteristic to preclude the need for lung biopsy in IPF, sarcoidosis, hypersensitivity pneumonitis, asbestosis, lymphangitic carcinoma, and PLCH. When a lung biopsy is required, HRCT scanning is useful for determining the most appropriate area from which biopsy samples should be taken.

Radionuclide Scanning Gallium-67 lung scanning is of limited value in evaluating the inflammatory component of ILD. An accelerated clearance from the lung of soluble aerosolized hydrophilic radionuclides such as ^{99m}Tc-diethylenetriamene pentaacetate (DTPA) is an index of pulmonary epithelial permeability that results from inflammation. This test may provide a means of assessing the activity of ILD. Normal ^{99m}Tc-DTPA clearance in IPF predicts stable disease, while rapid clearance identifies patients at risk for deterioration.

PULMONARY FUNCTION TESTING **Spirometry and Lung Volumes** Measurement of lung function is important in assessing the extent of pulmonary involvement in patients with ILD. Most forms of ILD produce a restrictive defect with reduced total lung capacity (TLC), functional residual capacity, and residual volume (Chap. 250). Forced expiratory volume in one second (FEV_1) and forced vital capacity (FVC) are reduced, but these changes are related to the decreased TLC. The FEV_1/FVC ratio is usually normal or increased. Reductions in lung volumes increase as lung stiffness worsens with disease progression. A few disorders (uncommon in sarcoidosis and hypersensitivity pneumonitis, while common in tuberous sclerosis and LAM) produce interstitial opacities on chest x-ray and obstructive airflow limitation on lung function testing.

Diffusing Capacity A reduction in the diffusing capacity of the lung for carbon monoxide D_{LCO} is a common but nonspecific finding in most ILDs. This decrease is due, in part, to effacement of the alveolar capillary units but, more importantly, to mismatching of ventilation and perfusion ($\dot{V}/\dot{Q}$). Lung regions with reduced compliance due to either fibrosis or cellular infiltration may be poorly ventilated but may still maintain adequate blood flow and $\dot{V}/\dot{Q}$ in these regions act like true venous admixture. The severity of the reduction in D_{LCO} does not correlate with disease stage.

Arterial Blood Gas The resting arterial blood gas may be normal or reveal hypoxemia (secondary to a mismatching of ventilation to perfusion) and respiratory alkalosis. A normal arterial O_2 tension (or saturation by oximetry) at rest does not rule out significant hypoxemia during exercise or sleep. CO_2 retention is rare and is usually a manifestation of end-stage disease.

Cardiopulmonary Exercise Testing Because hypoxemia at rest is not always present and because severe exercise-induced hypoxemia may go undetected, it is useful to perform exercise testing with measurement of arterial blood gases to detect abnormalities of gas exchange. Arterial oxygen desaturation, a failure to decrease dead space appropriately with exercise [i.e., a high V_D/V_T ratio (Chap. 250)], and an excessive increase in respiratory rate with a lower-than-expected recruitment of tidal volume provide useful information about physiologic abnormalities and extent of disease. Serial assessment of resting and exercise gas exchange is an excellent method for following disease activity and responsiveness to treatment, especially in patients with IPF.

FIBEROPTIC BRONCHOSCOPY AND BRONCHOALVEOLAR LAVAGE (BAL) In selected diseases (e.g., sarcoidosis, hypersensitivity pneumonitis, DAHs, cancer, pulmonary alveolar proteinosis), cellular analysis of BAL fluid may be useful in narrowing the differential diagnostic possibilities among various types of ILD. The role for BAL in defining the stage of disease and assessment of disease progression or response to therapy remains poorly understood, and the usefulness of BAL in the clinical assessment and management remains to be established.

TISSUE AND CELLULAR EXAMINATION Lung biopsy is the most effective method for confirming the diagnosis and assessing disease activity. The findings may identify a more treatable process than originally suspected, particularly chronic hypersensitivity pneumonitis, COP, respiratory bronchiolitis-associated ILD, or sarcoidosis. Biopsy should be obtained before initiation of treatment. A definitive diagnosis avoids confusion and anxiety later in the clinical course if the patient does not respond to therapy or suffers serious side effects from it.

Fiberoptic bronchoscopy with multiple transbronchial lung biopsies (4 to 8 biopsy samples) is often the initial procedure of choice, especially when sarcoidosis, lymphangitic carcinomatosis, eosinophilic pneumonia, Goodpasture's syndrome, or infection are suspected. If a specific diagnosis is not made by transbronchial biopsy, then surgical lung biopsy by video-assisted thoracic surgery or open thoracotomy is indicated. Adequate-sized biopsies from multiple sites, usually from two lobes, should be obtained. Relative contraindications to lung biopsy include serious cardiovascular disease, "honeycombing" and other roentgenographic evidence of diffuse end-stage disease, severe pulmonary dysfunction, or other major operative risks, especially in the elderly.

℞ **TREATMENT**   Although the course of ILD is variable, progression is common and often insidious. All treatable possibilities should be carefully considered. Since therapy does not reverse fibrosis, the major goals of treatment are permanent removal of the offending agent when known and early identification and aggressive suppression of the acute and chronic inflammatory process, thereby reducing further lung damage.

Hypoxemia (PaO_2 <55 mmHg) at rest and/or with exercise should be managed by supplemental oxygen. If cor pulmonale develops, diuretic therapy and phlebotomy may occasionally be required (Chap. 237).

Drug Therapy   Glucocorticoids are the mainstay of therapy for suppression of the alveolitis present in ILD, but the success rate is low. There have been no placebo-controlled trials of glucocorticoids in ILD, so there is no direct evidence that steroids improve survival in many of the diseases for which they are commonly used. Glucocorticoid therapy is recommended for symptomatic ILD patients with idiopathic interstitial pneumonias, eosinophilic pneumonias, COP, CTD, sarcoidosis, acute inorganic dust exposures, acute radiation pneumonitis, DAH, and drug-induced ILD. In organic dust disease, glucocorticoids are recommended for both the acute and chronic stages.

The optimal dose and proper length of therapy with glucocorticoids in the treatment of most ILDs is not known. A common starting dose is prednisone, 0.5 to 1 mg/kg in a once-daily oral dose (based on the patient's lean body weight). This dose is continued for 4 to 12 weeks, at which time the patient is reevaluated. If the patient is stable or improved, the dose is tapered to 0.25 to 0.5 mg/kg and is maintained at this level for an additional 4 to 12 weeks depending on the course. Rapid tapering or a shortened course of glucocorticoid treatment can result in recurrence. If the patient's condition continues to decline while on glucocorticoids, a second agent (see below) is often added and the prednisone dose is lowered to or maintained at 0.25 mg/kg per day.

Cyclophosphamide and azathioprine (1 to 2 mg/kg lean body weight per day) with or without glucocorticoids, have been tried with variable success in IPF, vasculitis, and other ILDs. An objective response usually requires at least 8 to 12 weeks to occur. In situations in which these drugs have failed or could not be tolerated, other agents, including methotrexate, colchicine, penicillamine, and cyclosporine, have been tried. However, their role in the treatment of ILDs remains to be determined.

Many cases of ILD are chronic and irreversible despite the therapy discussed above, and lung transplantation may then be considered (Chap. 267).

INDIVIDUAL FORMS OF ILD

IDIOPATHIC PULMONARY FIBROSIS   Several risk factors appear to be associated with the development of IPF, a common ILD of unknown etiology. These include cigarette smoking; exposure to antidepressants; a history of chronic aspiration secondary to gastroesophageal reflux; and exposures to metal dust, wood dust, and solvents. Numerous viruses have been implicated in the pathogenesis of

IPF, but no clear evidence for a viral etiology has been confirmed. The most compelling evidence for participation of genetic factors is the description fo familial cases of pulmonary fibrosis, which is transmitted as an autosomal dominant trait with variable penetrance. An association has been reported between IPF and α, antitrypsin inhibition (Pi) alleles on chromosome 14.

Clinical Manifestations   Exertional dyspnea, a nonproductive cough, and inspiratory crackles with or without digital clubbing may be present on physical examination. The chest roentgenogram and HRCT typically show patchy, predominantly peripheral, subpleural, reticular opacities in the lower lung zones. There may also be a ground-glass opacity usually associated with traction bronchiectasis and bronchiolectasis or subpleural honeycombing. Pulmonary function tests often reveal a restrictive pattern, a reduced D_{LCO}, and arterial hypoxemia that is exaggerated or elicited by exercise.

Histologic Findings   Confirmation of the presence of the usual interstitial pneumonia (UIP) pattern on histologic examination is essential to confirm this diagnosis (Fig. 259-2). Transbronchial biopsies are not helpful in making the diagnosis of UIP, and surgical biopsy is usually required. The histologic hallmark and chief diagnostic criterion of UIP is a heterogeneous appearance at low magnification with alternating areas of normal lung, interstitial inflammation, fibrosis, and honeycomb changes. The latter are composed of cystic fibrotic air spaces that are frequently lined by bronchiolar epithelium and filled with mucin. Smooth muscle hyperplasia is commonly present in areas of fibrosis and honeycomb change. Biopsies taken from patients during an accelerated phase of their illness may show a combination of UIP and diffuse alveolar damage. These histologic abnormalities affect the peripheral, subpleural parenchyma most severely. The interstitial inflammation is usually patchy and consists of a lymphoplasmacytic infiltrate in the alveolar septa, associated with hyperplasia of type 2 pneumocytes. The fibrotic zones are composed mainly of dense collagen, although scattered foci of proliferating fibroblasts are a consistent finding. The extent of fibroblastic proliferation is predictive of disease progression. A UIP-like pattern can also be seen with CTDs, pneumoconioses (e.g., asbestosis), radiation injury, certain drug-induced lung diseases (e.g., nitrofurantoin), and chronic aspiration. Also, a fibrotic pattern may be found in the chronic stage of several specific disorders such as sarcoidosis, chronic hypersensitivity pneumonitis, organized chronic eosinophilic pneumonia, and PLCH. Since other histopathologic features are frequently present in these syndromes, the term UIP is used for those patients in whom the lesion is idiopathic and not associated with another condition.

℞ **TREATMENT**   The clinical course is variable with a 5-year survival rate of 30 to 50% after diagnosis. Treatment options in-

FIGURE 259-2   Usual interstitial pneumonia (UIP). Interstitial fibrous thickening emanates from peribronchiolar regions. Microhoneycombing is present. Few discernable normal alveolar walls are present. The bronchiole and vessel are unaffected.

clude glucocorticoids, cytotoxic agents (e.g., azathioprine, cyclophosphamide), and antifibrotic agents (e.g., colchicine, perfenidone, or interferon gamma-1b), alone or in combination with glucocorticoids. However, there is no firm evidence that any of these treatment approaches improves survival or the quality of life. Because of the poor prognosis in untreated patients, a therapeutic trial may be tried. If therapy is recommended, it should be started at the first identification of clinical or physiologic evidence of impairment of lung function. Lung transplantation should be considered for those patients who experience progressive deterioration despite optimal medical management and who meet the established criteria (Chap. 267).

DESQUAMATIVE INTERSTITIAL PNEUMONIA DIP is a rare but distinct clinical and pathologic entity found exclusively in cigarette smokers. The histologic hallmark is the extensive accumulation of macrophages in intraalveolar spaces with minimal interstitial fibrosis. The peak incidence is in the fourth and fifth decades. Most patients present with dyspnea. Lung function testing shows a restrictive pattern with reduced DL_{CO} and arterial hypoxemia. The chest x-ray usually shows diffuse hazy opacities. Clinical recognition of DIP is important because the process is associated with a better prognosis (10-year survival rate is ~70%) and a better response to smoking cessation and systemic glucocorticoids than the more common IPF. Respiratory bronchiolitis-associated ILD is considered to be a subset of DIP and is characterized by the accumulation of macrophages in peribronchical alveoli.

ACUTE INTERSTITIAL PNEUMONIA (AIP) (HAMMAN-RICH SYNDROME) This is a rare, fulminant form of lung injury characterized by diffuse alveolar damage on lung biopsy. Most patients are older than 40 years. AIP is similar in presentation to the acute respiratory distress syndrome (ARDS) (Chap. 265) and probably corresponds to the subset of cases of idiopathic ARDS. The onset is usually abrupt in a previously healthy individual. A prodromal illness, usually lasting 7 to 14 days before presentation, is common. Fever, cough, and dyspnea are frequent manifestations at presentation. Diffuse, bilateral, air-space opacification is present on chest radiograph. HRCT scans show bilateral, patchy, symmetric areas of ground-glass attenuation. Bilateral areas of air-space consolidation may also be present. A predominantly subpleural distribution may be seen. The diagnosis of AIP requires the presence of a clinical syndrome of idiopathic ARDS and pathologic confirmation of organizing diffuse alveolar damage. Therefore, lung biopsy is required to confirm the diagnosis. Most patients have moderate to severe hypoxemia and develop respiratory failure. Mechanical ventilation is often required. The mortality rate is high (>60%), with most patients dying within 6 months of presentation. Recurrences have been reported. However, those who recover often have substantial improvement in lung function. The main treatment is supportive. It is not clear that glucocorticoid therapy is effective.

NONSPECIFIC INTERSTITIAL PNEUMONIA (NSIP) This condition defines a subgroup of the idiopathic interstitial pneumonias that can be distinguished clinically and pathologically from UIP, DIP, AIP, and idiopathic BOOP. Lung biopsy shows varying proportions of chronic interstitial inflammation and fibrosis. NSIP is a subacute restrictive process that usually occurs at a younger age than UIP. It is often associated with a febrile illness, relative lack of clubbing, and HRCT findings that show ground-glass opacities and areas of consolidation. Unlike patients with IPF, most patients with NSIP have a good prognosis, and most show improvement after treatment with glucocorticoids.

ILD ASSOCIATED WITH CONNECTIVE TISSUE DISORDERS Clinical findings suggestive of a CTD (musculoskeletal pain, weakness, fatigue, fever, joint pains or swelling, photosensitivity, Raynaud's phenomenon, pleuritis, dry eyes, dry mouth) should be sought in any patient with ILD. The CTDs may be difficult to rule out since the pulmonary manifestations occasionally precede the more typical systemic manifestations by months or years. The most common form of pulmonary involvement is a chronic interstitial pattern similar to that in patients with IPF. However, determining the precise nature of lung involvement in most of the CTDs is difficult due to the high incidence of lung involvement caused by disease-associated complications of esophageal dysfunction (predisposing to aspiration and secondary infections), respiratory muscle weakness (atelectasis and secondary infections), complications of therapy (opportunistic infections), and associated malignancies.

Progressive Systemic Sclerosis (PSS) (See also Chap. 313) Clinical evidence of ILD is present in about one-half of patients with progressive systemic sclerosis, and pathologic evidence in three-quarters. Pulmonary function tests show a restrictive pattern and impaired diffusing capacity, often before any clinical or radiographic evidence of lung disease appears. Pulmonary vascular disease alone or in association with pulmonary fibrosis, pleuritis, or recurrent aspiration pneumonitis is strikingly resistant to current modes of therapy.

Rheumatoid Arthritis (RA) (See also Chap. 312) ILD associated with rheumatoid arthritis is more common in men. Pulmonary manifestations of rheumatoid arthritis include pleurisy with or without effusion, ILD in up to 20% of cases, necrobiotic nodules (nonpneumoconiotic intrapulmonary rheumatoid nodules) with or without cavities, Caplan's syndrome (rheumatoid pneumoconiosis), pulmonary hypertension secondary to rheumatoid pulmonary vasculitis, BOOP, and upper airway obstruction due to arytenoid arthritis.

Systemic Lupus Erythematosus (See also Chap. 311) Lung disease is a common complication in SLE. Pleuritis with or without effusion is the most common pulmonary manifestation. Other lung manifestations include the following: atelectasis, diaphragmatic dysfunction with loss of lung volumes, pulmonary vascular disease, pulmonary hemorrhage, uremic pulmonary edema, infectious pneumonia, and BOOP. Acute lupus pneumonitis characterized by pulmonary capillaritis leading to alveolar hemorrhage is common. Chronic, progressive ILD is uncommon. It is important to exclude pulmonary infection. Although pleuropulmonary involvement may not be evident clinically, pulmonary function testing, particularly D_{LCO} reveals abnormalities in many patients with SLE.

Polymyositis and Dermatomyositis (PM/DM) (See also Chap. 382) ILD occurs in ~10% of patients with polymyositis and dermatomyositis, and the clinical features are similar to those of IPF. Diffuse reticular or nodular opacities with or without an alveolar component occur radiographically, with a predilection for the lung bases. ILD occurs more commonly in the subgroup of patients with an anti-Jo-1 antibody that is directed to histidyl tRNA synthetase. Weakness of respiratory muscles contributing to aspiration pneumonia may be present. A rapidly progressive illness characterized by diffuse alveolar damage may cause respiratory failure.

Sjögren's Syndrome (See also Chap. 314) General dryness and lack of airways secretion cause the major problems of hoarseness, cough, and bronchitis. Lymphocytic interstitial pneumonitis, lymphoma, pseudolymphoma, bronchiolitis, and bronchiolitis obliterans are associated with this condition. Lung biopsy is frequently required to establish a precise pulmonary diagnosis. Glucocorticoids have been used in the management of ILD associated with Sjögren's syndrome with some degree of clinical success.

DRUG-INDUCED ILD (See also Chap. 71) Many classes of drugs have the potential to induce diffuse ILD, which is manifest most commonly as exertional dyspnea and nonproductive cough. A detailed history of the medications taken by the patient is needed to identify drug-induced disease, including over-the-counter medications, oily nose drops, or petroleum products (mineral oil). In most cases, the pathogenesis is unknown, although a combination of direct toxic effects of the drug (or its metabolite) and indirect inflammatory and immunologic events is likely. The onset of the illness may be abrupt and fulminant, or it may be insidious, extending over weeks to months. The drug may have been taken for several years before a reaction develops (e.g., amiodarone), or the lung disease may occur weeks to years after the drug has been discontinued (e.g., carmustine). The extent and severity of disease are usually dose related. Treatment consists of discontinuation of any possible offending drug and supportive care.

CRYPTOGENIC ORGANIZING PNEUMONIA (COP) Also known as idiopathic BOOP, COP is a clinicopathologic syndrome of unknown etiology. The onset is usually in the fifth and sixth decades. The presentation may be of a flu-like illness with cough, fever, malaise, fatigue, and weight loss. Inspiratory crackles are frequently present on examination. Pulmonary function is usually impaired, with a restrictive defect and arterial hypoxemia being most common. The roentgenographic manifestations are distinctive, revealing bilateral, patchy, or diffuse alveolar opacities in the presence of normal lung volume. Recurrent and migratory pulmonary opacities are common. HRCT shows areas of air-space consolidation, ground-glass opacities, small nodular opacities and bronchial wall thickening and dilation. These changes occur more frequently in the periphery of the lung and in the lower lung zone. Lung biopsy shows granulation tissue within small airways, alveolar ducts, and airspaces, with chronic inflammation in the surrounding alveoli. Glucocorticoid therapy induces clinical recovery in two-thirds of patients. A few patients have rapidly progressive courses with fatal outcomes despite glucocorticoids.

Foci of organizing pneumonia (i.e., a "BOOP pattern") is a nonspecific reaction to lung injury found adjacent to other pathologic processes or as a component of other primary pulmonary disorders (e.g., cryptococcosis, Wegener's granulomatosis, lymphoma, hypersensitivity pneumonitis, and eosinophilic pneumonia). Consequently, the clinician must carefully reevaluate any patient found to have this histopathologic lesion to rule out these possibilities.

EOSINOPHILIC PNEUMONIA See Chap. 253

PULMONARY ALVEOLAR PROTEINOSIS Although not strictly an ILD, pulmonary alveolar proteinosis (PAP) resembles and is therefore considered with these conditions. It has been proposed that a defect in macrophage function, more specifically an impaired ability to process surfactant, may play a role in the pathogenesis of PAP. This diffuse disease is characterized by the accumulation of an amorphous, periodic acid-Schiff–positive lipoproteinaceous material in the distal air spaces. There is little or no lung inflammation, and the underlying lung architecture is preserved. Mutant mice lacking the gene for granulocyte-macrophage colony stimulating factor (GM-CSF) have a similar accumulation of surfactant and surfactant apoprotein in the alveolar spaces. Moreover, reconstitution of the respiratory epithelium of GM-CSF knockout mice with the GM-CSF gene completely corrects the alveolar proteinosis. Data from BAL studies in patients suggest that PAP is an autoimmune disease with neutralizing antibody of immunoglobulin G isotype against GM-CSF. These findings suggest that neutralization of GM-CSF bioactivity by the antibody causes dysfunction of alveolar macrophages, which results in reduced surfactant clearance.

The typical age of presentation is 30 to 50 years, and males predominate. The clinical presentation is usually insidious and manifested by progressive exertional dyspnea, fatigue, weight loss, and low-grade fever. A nonproductive cough is common, but occasionally expectoration of "chunky" gelatinous material may occur. Polycythemia, hypergammaglobulinemia, and increased LDH levels are frequent. Markedly elevated serum levels of lung surfactant proteins A and D have been found in PAP. Radiographically, bilateral symmetrical alveolar opacities located centrally in mid and lower lung zones result in a "bat-wing" distribution. HRCT shows a ground-glass opacification and thickened intralobular structures and interlobular septa. Whole lung lavage(s) through a double-lumen endotracheal tube provides relief to many patients with dyspnea or progressive hypoxemia and also may provide long-term benefit.

PULMONARY LYMPHANGIOLEIOMYOMATOSIS Pulmonary LAM is a rare condition that afflicts premenopausal women and should be suspected in young women with emphysema, recurrent pneumothorax, or chylous pleural effusion. It is often misdiagnosed as asthma or chronic obstructive pulmonary disease. Pathologically,

LAM is characterized by the proliferation of atypical pulmonary interstitial smooth muscle and cyst formation. The immature-appearing smooth-muscle cells react with monoclonal antibody HMB45, which recognizes a 100-kDa glycoprotein (gp100) originally found in human melanoma cells. Caucasians are affected much more commonly than members of other racial groups. The disease accelerates during pregnancy and abates after oopherectomy. Common complaints at presentation are dyspnea, cough, and chest pain. Hemoptysis may be life threatening. Spontaneous pneumothorax occurs in 50% of patients; it may be bilateral and necessitate pleurodesis. Chylothorax, chyloperitonium (chylous ascites), chyluria, and chylopericardium are other complications. Pulmonary function testing usually reveals an obstructive or mixed obstructive-restrictive pattern, and gas exchange is often abnormal. HRCT shows thin-walled cysts surrounded by normal lung without zonal predominance. Progression is common, with a median survival of 8 to 10 years from diagnosis. Oophorectomy, progesterone (10 mg/d), and, more recently, tamoxifen and luteinizing hormone-releasing hormone analogs have been used. Lung transplantation offers the only hope for cure despite reports of recurrent disease in the transplanted lung.

SYNDROMES OF ILD WITH DIFFUSE ALVEOLAR HEMORRHAGE Injury to arterioles, venules, and the alveolar septal (alveolar wall or interstitial) capillaries can result in hemoptysis secondary to disruption of the alveolar-capillary basement membrane. This results in bleeding into the alveolar spaces, which characterizes DAH. Pulmonary capillaritis, characterized by a neutrophilic infiltration of the alveolar septae, may lead to necrosis of these structures, loss of capillary structural integrity, and the pouring of red blood cells into the alveolar space. Fibrinoid necrosis of the interstitium and red blood cells within the interstitial space are sometimes seen. Bland pulmonary hemorrhage (i.e., DAH without inflammation of the alveolar structures) may also occur.

The clinical onset is often abrupt, with cough, fever, and dyspnea. Severe respiratory distress requiring ventilatory support may be evident at initial presentation. Although hemoptysis is expected, it can be absent at the time of presentation in one-third of the cases. For patients without hemoptysis, new alveolar opacities, a falling hemoglobin level, and hemorrhagic BAL fluid point to the diagnosis. The chest radiograph is nonspecific and most commonly shows new patchy or diffuse alveolar opacities. Recurrent episodes of DAH may lead to pulmonary fibrosis, resulting in interstitial opacities on the chest radiograph. An elevated white blood cell count and falling hematocrit are frequent. Evidence for impaired renal function caused by focal segmental necrotizing glomerulonephritis, usually with crescent formation, may also be present.

Varying degrees of hypoxemia may occur and often are severe enough to require ventilatory support. The D_{LCO} may be increased, resulting from the increased hemoglobin within the alveoli compartment. Evaluation of either lung or renal tissue by immunofluorescent techniques indicates an absence of immune complexes (pauci-immune) in Wegener's granulomatosis, microscopic polyangiitis pauci-immune glomerulonephritis, and isolated pulmonary capillaritis. A granular pattern is found in the CTDs, particularly SLE, and a characteristic linear deposition is found in Goodpasture's syndrome. Granular deposition of IgA-containing immune complexes are present in Henoch-Schönlein purpura.

The mainstay of therapy for the DAH associated with systemic vasculitis, CTD, Goodpasture's syndrome, and isolated pulmonary capillaritis is intravenous methylprenisolone, 0.5 to 2.0 g daily in divided doses for up to 5 days, followed by a gradual tapering, and then maintenance on an oral preparation. Prompt initiation of therapy is important, particularly in the face of renal insufficiency, since early initiation of therapy has the best chance of preserving renal function. The decision to start other immunosuppressive therapy (cyclophosphamide or azathioprine) acutely depends on the severity of illness.

Goodpasture's Syndrome Pulmonary hemorrhage and glomerulonephritis are features in most patients with this disease (Chap. 275). Autoantibodies to renal glomerular and lung alveolar basement membranes are present. This syndrome can present and recur as DAH without an associated glomerulonephritis. In such case, circulating antibasement membrane antibody is often absent, and the only way to establish the diagnosis is by demonstrating linear immunofluorescence in lung tissue. The underlying histology may be bland hemorrhage or DAH associated with capillaritis. Plasmapheresis has been recommended as adjunctive treatment.

Idiopathic Pulmonary Hemosiderosis This condition is a diagnosis of exclusion. Only 20% of reported cases occur in adults. In children, the condition is associated with celiac disease, and elevated IgA levels are found in 50% of patients. These associations are lacking in most adults. A lung biopsy is usually necessary to document the lack of inflammatory injury in the lung tissues and to exclude other diseases with confidence.

INHERITED DISORDERS ASSOCIATED WITH ILD Pulmonary opacities and respiratory symptoms typical of ILD can develop in related family members and in several inherited diseases. These include the phakomatoses, tuberous sclerosis and neurofibromatosis (Chap. 370), and the lysosomal storage diseases, Niemann-Pick disease and Gaucher's disease (Chap. 349). The Hermansky-Pudlak syndrome (Chap. 116) is an autosomal recessive disorder in which granulomatous colitis and ILD may occur. It is characterized by oculocutaneous albinism, bleeding diathesis secondary to platelet dysfunction, and the accumulation of a chromolipid, lipofuscin material in cells of the reticuloendothelial system. The pulmonary fibrosis is similar to IPF, but the alveolar macrophages may contain cytoplasmic ceroid-like inclusions.

ILD WITH A GRANULOMATOUS RESPONSE IN LUNG TISSUE OR VASCULAR STRUCTURES Inhalation of organic dusts, which cause hypersensitivity pneumonitis, or of inorganic dust, such as silica, which elicits a granulomatous inflammatory reaction leading to ILD, produces diseases of known etiology (Table 259-1) that are discussed in Chaps. 253 and 254. Sarcoidosis (Chap. 318) is prominent among granulomatous diseases of unknown cause in which ILD is an important feature.

Pulmonary Langerhans Cell Histiocytosis (PLCH, Pulmonary Histiocytosis X, Langerhans Cell Granulomatosis, or Eosinophilic Granuloma PLCH is a rare, smoking-related, diffuse lung disease that primarily affects men between the ages of 20 and 40 years. The clinical presentation varies from an asymptomatic state to a rapidly progressive condition. The most common clinical manifestations at presentation are cough, dyspnea, chest pain, weight loss, and fever. Pneumothorax occurs in about 25% of patients. Hemoptysis and diabetes insipidus are rare manifestations. The radiographic features vary with the stage of the disease. The combination of ill-defined or stellate nodules (2 to 10 mm in diameter), reticular or nodular opacities, bizarre-shaped upper zone cysts, preservation of lung volume, and sparing of the costophrenic angles are characteristics of PLCH. HRCT that reveals a combination of nodules and thin-walled cysts is virtually diagnostic of PLCH. The most frequent pulmonary function abnormality is a markedly reduced D_{LCO}, although varying degrees of restrictive disease, airflow limitation, and diminished exercise capacity may occur. Discontinuance of smoking is the key treatment, resulting in clinical improvement in one-third of patients. Most patients with PLCH suffer persistent or progressive disease. Death due to respiratory failure occurs in ~10% of patients.

Granulomatous Vasculitides (See also Chap. 317) The granulomatous vasculitides are characterized by pulmonary angiitis (i.e., inflammation and necrosis of blood vessels) with associated granuloma formation (i.e., infiltrates of lymphocytes, plasma cells, epithelioid cells, or histiocytes, with or without the presence of multinucleated giant cells, sometimes with tissue necrosis). The lungs are almost always involved, although any organ system may be affected. Wegener's granulomatosis and allergic angiitis and granulomatosis (Churg-Strauss syndrome) primarily affect the lung but are associated with a systemic vasculitis as well. The granulomatous vasculitides generally limited to the lung include necrotizing sarcoid granulomatosis and benign lymphocytic angiitis and granulomatosis. Granulomatous infection and pulmonary angiitis due to irritating embolic material (e.g., talc) are important known causes of pulmonary vasculitis.

LYMPHOCYTIC INFILTRATIVE DISORDERS This group of disorders features lymphocyte and plasma cell infiltration of the lung parenchyma. The disorders either are benign or can behave as low-grade lymphomas. Included are angioimmunoblastic lymphadenopathy with dysproteinemia, a rare lymphoproliferative disorder characterized by diffuse lymphadenopathy, fever, hepatosplenomegaly, and hemolytic anemia, with ILD in some cases.

Lymphocytic Interstitial Pneumonitis This rare form of ILD occurs in adults, some of whom have an autoimmune disease or dysproteinemia. It has been reported in patients with Sjögren's syndrome and HIV infection.

Lymphomatoid Granulomatosis This multisystem disorder of unknown etiology is an angiocentric malignant (T cell) lymphoma characterized by a polymorphic lymphoid infiltrate, an angiitis, and granulomatosis. Although it may affect virtually any organ, it is most frequently characterized by pulmonary, skin, and central nervous system involvement.

BRONCHOCENTRIC GRANULOMATOSIS Rather than a specific clinical entity, bronchocentric granulomatosis (BG) is a descriptive histologic term that describes an uncommon and nonspecific pathologic response to a variety of airway injuries. There is evidence that BG is caused by a hypersensitivity reaction to *Aspergillus* or other fungi in patients with asthma. About half of the patients described have chronic asthma with severe wheezing and peripheral blood eosinophilia. In patients with asthma, BG probably represents one pathologic manifestation of allergic bronchopulmonary aspergillosis, or another allergic mycosis. In patients without asthma, BG has been associated with rheumatoid arthritis and a variety of infections, including tuberculosis, echinococcosis, histoplasmosis, coccidiodomycosis, and nocardiosis. The chest roentgenogram reveals irregularly shaped nodular or mass lesions with ill-defined margins, which are usually unilateral and solitary, with an upper-lobe predominance. Glucocorticoids are the treatment of choice, often with excellent outcome, although recurrences may occur as therapy is tapered or stopped.

BIBLIOGRAPHY

AMERICAN THORACIC SOCIETY: Idiopathic pulmonary fibrosis: Diagnosis and treatment. International Consensus Statement. Am J Resp Crit Care Med 161:646, 2000

BJORAKER JA et al: Prognostic significance of histiopathologic subsets in idiopathic pulmonary fibrosis. Am J Respir Crit Care Med 157:199, 1998

BRITISH THORACIC SOCIETY: The Diagnosis, Assessment and Treatment of Diffuse Parenchymal Lung Disease in Adults. Thorax 54 (Suppl 1):S1-S28, 1999

GOLDSTEIN LS et al: Pulmonary alveolar proteinosis: Clinical features and outcomes. Chest 114:1357, 1998

JENNINGS CA et al: Pauci-immune pulmonary capillaritis and diffuse alveolar hemorrhage: A vasculitic process limited to the lungs. Am J Respir Crit Care Med 155:1101, 1997

KALASSIAN KG, RAFFIN TA: Lymphangioleiomyomatosis, in *Textbook of Respiratory Medicine*, 3d ed, JF Murray, JA Nadel (eds). Philadelphia, Saunders, 2000, pp 1775–1788

KATZENSTEIN ALA, MYERS JL: Idiopathic pulmonary fibrosis. Clinical relevance of pathologic classification. Am J Respir Crit Care Med 157:1310, 1998

KING TE Jr: Connective tissue disease, *Interstitial Lung Diseases*, 3d ed, MI Schwarz, TE King, Jr. (eds). Hamilton, BC Decker, 1998, 451-505

LIMPER AH, ROSENOW III EC: Drug-induced interstitial lung disease. Curr Opin Pulm Med 2:396, 1996

NAGAI S et al: Idiopathic nonspecific interstitial pneumonia/fibrosis: Comparison with idiopathic pulmonary fibrosis and BOOP. Europ Respir J 12:1010, 1998

TAZI A et al: Adult pulmonary Langerhans' cell histiocytosis. Thorax 55:405, 2000

260   *Stuart Rich*

PRIMARY PULMONARY HYPERTENSION

Primary pulmonary hypertension is an uncommon disease characterized by increased pulmonary artery pressure and pulmonary vascular resistance. The incidence has been estimated at approximately 2 cases per million. There is a female-to-male preponderance (1.7:1), with patients most commonly presenting in the third and fourth decades, although the age range is from infancy to greater than 60 years. Because the predominant symptom of primary pulmonary hypertension is dyspnea, which can have an insidious onset in an otherwise healthy person, the disease is typically diagnosed late in its course. By that time, the clinical and laboratory findings of severe pulmonary hypertension are usually present.

PATHOLOGY   The histopathology of primary pulmonary hypertension is not pathognomonic for the disease but represents a pulmonary arteriopathy that is observed in pulmonary hypertension from a variety of causes. A wide spectrum of vascular abnormalities involving the endothelium, smooth muscle cells, and extracellular matrix is present. Heterogeneity with respect to these abnormalities is often seen from patient to patient, and within patients. The most common features noted are medial hypertrophy, concentric and eccentric intimal fibrosis, recanalized thrombi appearing as fibrous webs, and plexiform lesions. In most patients, varying degrees of these abnormalities can be found. Rare variant forms of primary pulmonary hypertension also exist.

Pulmonary venoocclusive disease is a rare and distinct pathologic entity, found in fewer than 10% of patients with primary pulmonary hypertension. Histologically, it is manifest by widespread intimal proliferation and fibrosis of the intrapulmonary veins and venules, occasionally extending to the arteriolar bed. The pulmonary venous obstruction explains the increased pulmonary capillary wedge pressure observed in patients with advanced disease. These patients may develop orthopnea that can mimic left ventricular failure.

Pulmonary capillary hemangiomatosis is also a very rare form of primary pulmonary hypertension. Histologically, it is characterized by infiltrating thin-walled blood vessels that are widespread throughout the pulmonary interstitium and walls of the pulmonary arteries and veins. These patients often have hemoptysis as a clinical feature.

ETIOLOGY   It is likely that there are several pathobiologic processes that result in pulmonary hypertension as a final common pathway. These include inhibition of the voltage-regulated (Kv) potassium channel producing vasoconstriction secondary to contraction of the pulmonary artery smooth muscle cells, an imbalance in vasocontricting and vasodilating mediators that are involved in the control of pulmonary vascular tone (including prostacyclin and thromboxane), reduced expression of nitric oxide synthase in the endothelium of the pulmonary arterial bed, inflammation, thrombosis in situ of the pulmonary vascular bed from a procoagulant state, and persistent matrix protein synthesis in the pulmonary arteries. The types of abnormalities that occur are likely influenced by the patient's genotype and exposure to risk factors that serve to trigger these processes. Risk factors that have been linked to the development of pulmonary hypertension include anorexigens, collagen vascular diseases, congenital systemic to pulmonary shunts, portal hypertension, and HIV infection.

Recently, a marked increase in the incidence of primary pulmonary hypertension occurred in Europe and the United States as a result of the widespread use of the fenfluramine appetite suppressants. The clinical and pathologic features of these cases were identical to patients with primary pulmonary hypertension who were unexposed. Atlhough very limited exposure to the fenfluramines can cause primary pulmonary hypertension, the risk increased dramatically with prolonged use. Like the experience with aminorex, an anorexigen that produced a similar epidemic in the 1960s, the incidence of primary pulmonary hypertension fell when the drugs were withdrawn from the market. The mechanism by which these agents produce pulmonary hypertension is unknown.

GENETIC CONSIDERATIONS   The locus of a gene linked to familial primary pulmonary hypertension has been identified on chromosome 2q31-32. Familial primary pulmonary hypertension occurs in approximately 6 to 12% of cases and is characterized by autosomal dominant inheritance, variable age of onset, and incomplete penetrance. The clinical and pathologic features of familial and sporadic primary pulmonary hypertension are virtually identical. Genetic anticipation, which relates to offspring of subsequent generations manifesting the disease at younger ages or with greater severity, is also a feature. Trinucleotide repeat expansion, originally described in several neurologic disorders, remains the only biologic explanation for genetic anticipation and raises the possibility that the pathogenesis of familial primary pulmonary hypertension may have a neurologic basis. Patients who present with sporadic disease probably possess a genetic predisposition that becomes expressed following exposure to an external trigger or risk factor. ∎

PATHOPHYSIOLOGY   The underlying hemodynamic derangement in primary pulmonary hypertension is an increased resistance to pulmonary blood flow. Early in the disease there is a marked elevation in pulmonary artery pressure with relatively normal cardiac function. Over time the cardiac output becomes progressively reduced rather than the pulmonary artery pressure becoming progressively increased. Initially, the pulmonary arteries may respond to vasodilators, but as the disease progresses, the elevated pulmonary vascular resistance becomes fixed. The pulmonary capillary wedge pressure remains normal until the late stages, when it tends to rise in response to impaired diastolic filling of the left ventricle due to the altered configuration of the intraventricular septum. Eventually, as the right ventricle fails, the right atrial and right ventricular end-diastolic pressures rise in an attempt to compensate for the myocardial depression that has developed in response to chronic severe right ventricular pressure overload.

Pulmonary function is usually normal in primary pulmonary hypertension, although a mild restrictive pattern (Chap. 250) is sometimes seen. Hypoxemia is common and is believed to be due to a mismatch between pulmonary ventilation and perfusion, magnified by a low cardiac output. Occasional patients with a patent foramen ovale may develop right-to-left shunting, which can also contribute to systemic arterial desaturation.

DIAGNOSIS   Primary pulmonary hypertension refers to pulmonary arterial hypertension wihtout an identifiable risk factor. Clinically, primary pulmonary arterial hypertension should be distinguished from pulmonary venous hypertension, pulmonary hypertension associated with disorders of the respiratory system and/or hypoxema, and pulmonary hypertension due to chronic thrombotic and/or embolic disease (Chap. 261).

A thorough diagnostic evaluation to look for all potential causes should be undertaken (Fig. 260-1). The history usually reveals the gradual onset of shortness of breath with effort, progressing until the patient is dyspneic with minimal activity. The average duration from symptom onset until diagnosis is 2.5 years. Other common symptoms are fatigue, angina pectoris that likely represents right ventricular ischemia, syncope, near syncope, and peripheral edema.

The physical examination is characteristic. Increased jugular venous pressure, a reduced carotid pulse, and an easily palpable right ventricular lift are typical. Most patients have an increased pulmonic component of the second heart sound and right-sided third and fourth heart sounds. Tricuspid regurgitation is a clinical feature of right ventricular failure. Peripheral cyanosis and/or edema tend to occur in later stages of the disease. Clubbing is not a feature.

The chest x-ray generally shows enlarged central pulmonary arteries and clear lung fields. The electrocardiogram usually reveals right axis deviation and right ventricular hypertrophy. The echocardiogram

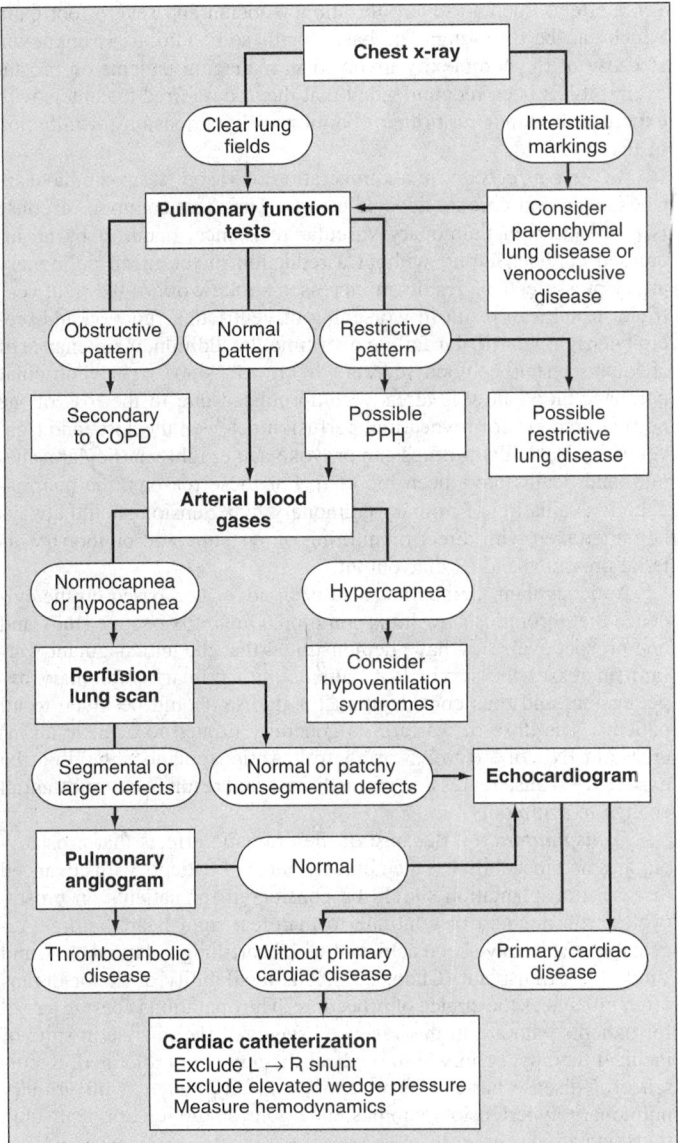

FIGURE 260-1 An algorithm for the workup of a patient with unexplained pulmonary hypertension.

demonstrates right ventricular enlargement, a reduction in left ventricular cavity size, and abnormal septal configuration consistent with right ventricular pressure overload. Doppler studies have revealed a marked dependence on atrial systole for ventricular filling. Hypoxemia, hypocapnia, and an abnormal diffusing capacity for carbon monoxide are almost invariable findings. A mild restrictive pattern on pulmonary function is sometimes observed, but evidence of airways obstruction suggests a secondary etiology for the pulmonary hypertension. The presence of significant restrictive changes on pulmonary function testing (Chap. 250) should prompt a high-resolution computed tomographic scan to look for interstitial lung disease, which may otherwise not be obvious. A perfusion lung scan may be normal or abnormal with multiple diffuse patchy filling defects of a nonsegmental nature and not suggestive of pulmonary thromboembolism. If the lung scan reveals perfusion defects of a segmental or subsegmental nature, a pulmonary angiogram must be done. Severe pulmonary hypertension in a patient with a high-probability lung scan should suggest a chronic process and *not* acute pulmonary embolism, since the non-conditioned right ventricle is unable to generate high systolic pressures acutely in the face of pulmonary thromboembolism. Chronic thromboembolic obstruction of the large pulmonary arteries (Chap. 261) can mimic primary pulmonary hypertension but can be amenable to treatment with surgical thromboendarterectomy.

There is risk in performing pulmonary angiography in patients with primary pulmonary hypertension, and it is recommended that selective or subselective injections with small amounts of low-osmolar, nonionic contrast material be made following the pretreatment with 1 mg atropine to prevent vagally mediated bradycardia.

Cardiac catheterization is mandatory to characterize the disease and exclude an underlying cardiac shunt as the cause. The use of balloon-flotation catheters, especially those with removable guidewires, can facilitate right heart catheterization. A right-to-left shunt might be attributable to a patent foramen ovale, but any left-to-right shunting implies the presence of a congenital defect. Although it may be difficult to obtain, the pulmonary capillary wedge pressure is normal. If it is increased, left heart catheterization should also be performed to exclude mitral stenosis or increased left ventricular end-diastolic pressures as the cause of the pulmonary hypertension. Although the diagnostic evaluation of these patients can be hazardous, experience from a national multicenter study revealed no mortality or serious morbidity in more than 300 patients whose evaluation included pulmonary angiography and cardiac catheterization. It is not necessary to perform an open lung biopsy in these patients to make an accurate diagnosis. Laboratory tests should also be performed, including antinuclear antibody and HIV testing.

On occasion, a patient may have marked elevations in pulmonary artery pressure in association with mild obstructive or interstitial lung disease, essential hypertension, ischemic heart disease, or valvular heart disease. Although it may appear that the pulmonary hypertension is out of proportion to the underlying associated condition, it likely represents a pulmonary vasoconstrictive response to the associated condition, which is serving as a trigger of pulmonary arterial hypertension. Thus severe pulmonary hypertension can coexist with mild chronic obstructive pulmonary disease, small intracardiac shunts, mild mitral stenosis, and even ischemic heart disease. The distinction is important because the treatment of pulmonary hypertension should always include treating the underlying associated cause.

NATURAL HISTORY The natural history of primary pulmonary hypertension is unknown because initially the disease is largely asymptomatic. Several older series have reported a mean survival of 2 to 3 years for patients from the time of diagnosis. Functional class is a strong predictor of survival, since patients who are New York Heart Association functional classes II and III have a mean survival of 3.5 years compared with those who are functional class IV, in whom the mean survival is 6 months. The cause of death is usually right ventricular failure or sudden death; sudden death appears to be a late feature of the disease. Increased right atrial pressure above 15 mmHg and reduced cardiac index below 2 (L/min)/m² are hemodynamic predictors of a poor prognosis.

TREATMENT Because the pulmonary vascular resistance increases dramatically with exercise, patients should be cautioned against participating in activities that demand increased physical stress. Digoxin may increase cardiac output and lower circulating levels of norepinephrine. Diuretic therapy relieves dyspnea and peripheral edema and may be useful in reducing right ventricular volume overload in the presence of tricuspid regurgitation.

It is recommended that all patients in whom primary pulmonary hypertension is confirmed undergo acute drug testing with short-acting pulmonary vasodilators to determine the extent of pulmonary vasodilator reserve or reactivity (Fig. 260-2). Intravenous adenosine, inhaled nitric oxide, and intravenous prostacyclin all appear to have similar effects in reducing pulmonary vascular resistance acutely with little effect on the systemic vascular bed. Adenosine is given as a constant infusion in doses of 50 (μg/kg)/min and increased every 2 min until side effects develop. Similarly, prostacyclin is given in doses of 2 (ng/kg)/min and increased every 30 min until side effects develop. Maximal physiologic effectiveness of the therapy is determined at the highest tolerated dose. Nitric oxide is generally administered via in-

FIGURE 260-2 An algorithm for the evaluation and drug treatment of a patient with primary pulmonary hypertension.

halation in 5 to 10 parts per million and increased every few minutes until no further effectiveness is obtained.

Calcium channel antagonists Patients who have substantial reductions in pulmonary vascular resistance from the short-acting vasodilators may be candidates to receive oral calcium channel blockers. These drugs should be administered under direct hemodynamic guidance in order to determine effectiveness and safety. Typically, patients will require high doses (e.g., nifedipine, 120 to 240 mg/d, or diltiazem, 540 to 900 mg/d*). Patients who manifest significant reductions in mean pulmonary artery pressure and pulmonary vascular resistance should demonstrate improved symptoms, regression of right ventricular hypertrophy, and improved survival with chronic therapy. However, fewer than half the patients who are responsive to the short-acting vasodilators will respond to this regimen. It is unknown whether the response to calcium blockers depends on the histologic subtype, but the therapy appears to be more successful in patients who are diagnosed early and have less advanced disease.

Prostacyclin This agent has been approved as a treatment of primary pulmonary hypertension for patients who are functional class III or IV and unresponsive to conventional therapy. Clinical trials have demonstrated that patients realize an improvement in symptoms and exercise tolerance and reduction in mortality, even if no acute hemodynamic response to drug challenge occurs. The drug can only be administered intravenously and requires placement of a permanent central venous catheter and continuous dose titration, as tolerance develops in all patients over a short period of time. The optimal dose has not been determined. Patients may deteriorate clinically from too much or too little drug. The side effects of prostacyclin, which include flushing, jaw pain, and diarrhea, are generally tolerated by most patients. The major problems with this therapy have been infections related to the venous catheter, which requires close monitoring and diligence on behalf of the patient. Recent data suggest that prostacyclin, in addition to its vasodilator and antithrombotic properties, may lead to reversal of the vascular remodeling that occurs in primary pulmonary hypertension. Long-term use of prostacyclin has been associated with ad-

---

*These agents have not been approved for the treatment of primary pulmonary hypertension by the U.S. Food and Drug Administration.

verse effects such as severe thrombocytopenia and severe foot pain, which can be disabling. The basis for these conditions is unknown. Because of the complexity involved in managing patients on prostacyclin, it has been recommended that they be referred to centers with expertise in managing primary pulmonary hypertension for initiation of therapy.

Adverse effects The administration of vasodilators can have serious acute and chronic adverse effects. The most common response is a reduction in pulmonary vascular resistance, manifest by an increased cardiac output, without a reduction in the mean pulmonary artery pressure. This results in increased stroke work of the right ventricle, which can result in worsening of ventricular function and precipitate right ventricular failure over time. In addition, maintenance of adequate systemic blood pressure is crucial, since right ventricular coronary blood flow is already compromised due to the loss of the normal gradient for myocardial perfusion between the aorta and right ventricle. Vasodilator drugs can provoke acute right ventricular ischemia, and deaths have been reported. For these reasons, the pharmacologic evaluation of primary pulmonary hypertension should always be undertaken with direct monitoring of systemic and pulmonary arterial pressures and cardiac output.

Anticoagulant therapy has also been advocated based on the evidence that thrombosis in situ is common. One retrospective study and one prospective study have demonstrated that the anticoagulant warfarin increases the survival of patients with primary pulmonary hypertension, and thus consideration for its use should be given to all patients. The dose of warfarin is generally titrated to achieve an increase in INR of 2.0 to 2.5 of control. Anticoagulants should not be expected to cause regression of the disease and result in any substantial change in symptoms.

Transplantation Because of the dramatic effects that prostacyclin has had in stabilizing the clinical course of patients with advanced disease, transplantation should be considered for patients on prostacyclin who develop or continue to manifest right heart failure. Acceptable results have been achieved with heart-lung, bilateral lung, and single lung transplant (Chap. 267). The availability of donor organs often influences the choice of procedure. The operation is best reserved for patients who are in the advanced stages of the disease in spite of medical therapy, or in whom medical therapy is not tolerated. Recurrence of disease has not been reported in any patient with primary pulmonary hypertension who has undergone single lung or heart-lung transplantation.

BIBLIOGRAPHY

ARROLIGA AC et al: Primary pulmonary hypertension: Update on pathogenesis and novel therapies. Cleve Clin J Med 67:175, 181, 189, 2000
MCLAUGHLIN VV et al: Reduction in pulmonary vascular resistance with long-term prostacyclin therapy in primary pulmonary hypertension. N Engl J Med 338:273, 1998
RICH S, BRAUNWALD E: Pulmonary hypertension, in *Heart Disease*, 6th ed, E Braunwald (ed). Philadelphia, Saunders, 2001, Chap. 53
RICH S (ed): Primary Pulmonary Hypertension: Executive Summary from the World Symposium—Primary Pulmonary Hypertension 1998. Available from the World Health Organization via the Internet (www.who.int/ncd/cvd/pph.html)
RUBIN LJ et al: Pulmonary vasculitis and primary pulmonary hypertension, in *Textbook of Respiratory Medicine*, 3d ed, JF Murray, JA Nadel (eds). Philadelphia, Saunders, 2000, pp 1533–1556

261   *Samuel Z. Goldhaber*

PULMONARY THROMBOEMBOLISM

GENETIC CONSIDERATIONS Rudolf Virchow postulated more than a century ago that three potentially overlapping factors predisposed to venous thrombosis: (1) local trauma to the vessel wall; (2) hypercoagulability; and (3) stasis. We now believe that many patients who suffer pulmonary thromboembolism (PTE) have an under-

Table 261-1   Stressors That May Precipitate Pulmonary Thromboembolism

Table 261-1   Stressors That May Precipitate Pulmonary
Thromboembolism

Surgery, trauma
Obesity
Oral contraceptives, pregnancy, postpartum, postmenopausal hormone replacement
Cancer (sometimes occult) or cancer chemotherapy
Immobilization (stroke or intensive care unit patients)
Indwelling central venous catheter

lying inherited predisposition that remains clinically silent until an acquired stressor occurs such as surgery, obesity, or pregnancy (Table 261-1). When PTE is identified, a detailed family history for venous thromboembolism should be obtained.

Factor V Leiden   The most frequent inherited predisposition to hypercoagulability is resistance to the endogenous anticoagulant protein, activated protein C. The phenotype of activated protein C resistance is associated with a single point mutation, designated *factor V Leiden*, in the factor V gene. This missense mutation—a single nucleotide substitution of adenine for guanine 1691—causes an amino acid substitution of glutamine for arginine at position 506.

The prevalence of the heterozygous state was about 6% in healthy American male physicians participating in the Physicians' Health Study and was three times higher among those physicians who subsequently developed venous thrombosis. Furthermore, after anticoagulation (for at least 3 months) was completed and discontinued, those participants with factor V Leiden had a much higher rate of recurrent venous thrombosis than those without. A single-point mutation in the 3' untranslated region of the prothrombin gene (G-to-A transition at nucleotide position 20210) appears to be associated with increased levels of prothrombin (factor II), the precursor of thrombin. In the Physicians' Health Study, the prevalence of the prothrombin gene mutation among control subjects was 3.9%. The G20210A mutation conferred an approximate doubling of the risk of venous thrombosis. Nevertheless, factor V Leiden is more common than all other (identified) inherited hypercoagulable states, including the prothrombin gene mutation, deficiencies in protein C, protein S, antithrombin III, and disorders of plasminogen (Chap. 117). ■

PATHOPHYSIOLOGY

EMBOLIZATION   When venous thrombi become dislodged from their site of formation, they embolize to the pulmonary arterial circulation or, paradoxically, to the arterial circulation through a patent foramen ovale or atrial septal defect. About half of patients with pelvic vein thrombosis or proximal leg deep venous thrombosis (DVT) have PTE, which is usually asymptomatic. Isolated calf vein or upper extremity venous thromboses also pose a risk (albeit lower) of PTE. Isolated calf vein thrombi are the most common source of paradoxical embolism.

PHYSIOLOGY   Pulmonary embolism can have the following effects:

1. *Increased pulmonary vascular resistance* due to vascular obstruction or neurohumoral agents including serotonin
2. *Impaired gas exchange* due to increased alveolar dead space from vascular obstruction and hypoxemia from alveolar hypoventilation in the nonobstructed lung, right-to-left shunting, and impaired carbon monoxide transfer due to loss of gas exchange surface
3. *Alveolar hyperventilation* due to reflex stimulation of irritant receptors
4. *Increased airway resistance* due to bronchoconstriction
5. *Decreased pulmonary compliance* due to lung edema, lung hemorrhage, or loss of surfactant

Right Ventricular Dysfunction   Progressive right heart failure is the usual cause of death from PTE. In the International Cooperative Pulmonary Embolism Registry (ICOPER), the presence of right ventricular dysfunction on baseline echocardiography of PTE patients was associated with a doubling of the 3-month mortality rate. As pulmonary vascular resistance increases, right ventricular wall tension rises and perpetuates further right ventricular dilatation and dysfunction. Consequently, the interventricular septum bulges into and compresses an intrinsically normal left ventricle. Increased right ventricular wall tension also compresses the right coronary artery and may precipitate myocardial ischemia and right ventricular infarction. Underfilling of the left ventricle may lead to a fall in left ventricular output and systemic arterial pressure, thereby provoking myocardial ischemia due to compromised coronary artery perfusion. Eventually, circulatory collapse and death may ensue.

DIAGNOSIS

The clinical setting can be immensely helpful in suggesting the diagnosis of PTE. Patients with prior venous thromboembolism are at increased risk of recurrence (Table 261-1).

CLINICAL SYNDROMES   Patients with *massive PTE* present with systemic arterial hypotension and usually have anatomically widespread thromboembolism. Primary therapy with thrombolysis or embolectomy offers the greatest chance of survival. Those with *moderate to large PTE* have right ventricular hypokinesis on echocardiography but normal systemic arterial pressure. Optimal management is controversial; such patients may benefit from primary therapy to prevent recurrent embolism. Patients with *small to moderate PTE* have both normal right heart function and normal systemic arterial pressure. They have a good prognosis with either adequate anticoagulation or an inferior vena caval filter. The presence of *pulmonary infarction* usually indicates a small PTE, but one that is exquisitely painful, because it lodges near the innervation of pleural nerves.

Nonthrombotic pulmonary embolism may be easily overlooked. Possible etiologies include fat embolism after blunt trauma and long bone fractures, tumor embolism, or air embolism. Intravenous drug users may inject themselves with a wide array of substances, such as hair, talc, or cotton. *Amniotic fluid embolism* occurs when fetal membranes leak or tear at the placental margin. The pulmonary edema seen in this syndrome is probably due primarily to alveolar capillary leakage.

SYMPTOMS AND SIGNS   Dyspnea is the most frequent symptom of PTE, and tachypnea is its most frequent sign. Whereas dyspnea, syncope, hypotension, or cyanosis indicate a massive PTE, pleuritic pain, cough, or hemoptysis often suggest a small embolism located distally near the pleura. On *physical examination*, young and previously healthy individuals may simply appear anxious but otherwise seem deceptively well, even with an anatomically large PTE. They need not have "classic" signs such as tachycardia, low-grade fever, neck vein distention, or an accentuated pulmonic component of the second heart sound. Sometimes, a paradoxical bradycardia occurs.

In older patients who complain of vague chest discomfort, the diagnosis of PTE may not be apparent unless signs of right heart failure are present. Unfortunately, because acute coronary ischemic syndromes are so common, one may overlook the possibility of life-threatening PTE and may inadvertently discharge these patients from the hospital after the exclusion of myocardial infarction with serial cardiac enzyme measurements and electrocardiograms.

DIFFERENTIAL DIAGNOSIS   The differential diagnosis of PTE is broad (Table 261-2). Although PTE is known as "the great masquerader," quite often another illness simulates PTE. For example, when the proposed diagnosis of PTE is supposedly confirmed with a combination of dyspnea, chest pain, and an abnormal lung scan, the correct diagnosis of pneumonia might become apparent 12 h later when an infiltrate blossoms on chest x-ray, purulent sputum is first produced, and high fever and shaking chills develop.

Some patients have PTE and a coexisting illness such as pneumonia or heart failure. In such circumstances, clinical improvement

Table 261-2   Differential Diagnosis of Pulmonary Thromboembolism

Myocardial infarction, unstable angina
Pneumonia, bronchitis, COPD exacerbation
Congestive heart failure
Asthma
Pericarditis
Primary pulmonary hypertension
Rib fracture, pneumothorax
Costochondritis, "musculoskeletal pain," anxiety

NOTE: COPD, chronic obstructive pulmonary disease.

will often fail to occur despite standard medical treatment of the concomitant illness. This situation can serve as a clinical clue to the possible coexistence of PTE.

NONIMAGING DIAGNOSTIC MODALITIES   These are generally safer, less expensive, but also less specific than diagnostic modalities that employ imaging.

Blood Tests   The quantitative *plasma D-dimer enzyme-linked immunosorbent assay (ELISA)* level is elevated (>500 ng/mL) in more than 90% of patients with PTE, reflecting plasmin's breakdown of fibrin and indicating endogenous (though clinically ineffective) thrombolysis. A qualitative latex agglutination D-dimer assay, which is more readily available and less expensive than an ELISA, can be obtained initially; if elevated, the ELISA will also be elevated. However, if the latex agglutination is normal, a D-dimer ELISA should be obtained, because the ELISA is much more sensitive than the latex agglutination D-dimer assay, which cannot be used to exclude PTE. The plasma D-dimer ELISA has a high negative predictive value and can be used to help exclude PTE. However, neither D-dimer assay is specific. Levels increase in patients with myocardial infarction, sepsis, or almost any systemic illness.

Data from the Prospective Investigation of Pulmonary Embolism Diagnosis (PIOPED) indicate that, contrary to classic teaching, *arterial blood gases* lack diagnostic utility for PTE. Among patients suspected of PTE, neither the room air arterial P_{O_2} nor calculation of the alveolar-arterial oxygen gradient can reliably differentiate or triage patients who actually have PTE at angiography.

Electrocardiogram   Classic abnormalities include sinus tachycardia; new-onset atrial fibrillation or flutter; and an S wave in lead I, a Q wave in lead III, and an inverted T wave in lead III (Chap. 226). Often, the QRS axis is greater than 90°. T-wave inversion in leads V_1 to V_4 reflects right ventricular strain.

NONINVASIVE IMAGING MODALITIES   Chest Roentgenography   A normal or near-normal chest x-ray in a dyspneic patient suggests PTE. Well-established abnormalities include focal oligemia (Westermark's sign), a peripheral wedged-shaped density above the diaphragm (Hampton's hump), or an enlarged right descending pulmonary artery (Palla's sign).

Venous Ultrasonography   Confirmed DVT is usually an adequate surrogate for PTE. Ultrasonography of the deep venous system relies upon loss of vein compressibility as the primary criterion for DVT. About one-third of patients with PTE have no imaging evidence of DVT. In these situations, the clot may have already embolized to the lung or is in the pelvic veins, where ultrasonography is usually inadequate. Therefore, the workup for PTE should continue if there is high clinical suspicion, despite a normal ultrasound examination.

Lung Scanning   (See also Chap. 251)   Lung scanning is the principal imaging test for the diagnosis of PTE. Small particulate aggregates of albumin labeled with a gamma-emitting radionuclide are injected intravenously and are trapped in the pulmonary capillary bed. A perfusion scan defect indicates absent or decreased blood flow, possibly due to PTE. Ventilation scans, obtained with radiolabeled inhaled gases such as xenon or krypton, improve the specificity of the perfusion scan. Abnormal ventilation scans indicate abnormal nonventilated lung, thereby providing possible explanations for perfusion defects other than acute PTE. A high probability scan for PTE is defined as having two or more segmental perfusion defects in the presence of normal ventilation (Fig. 261-1).

Lung scanning is particularly useful if the results are normal or near-normal, or if there is a high probability for PTE. The diagnosis of PTE is very unlikely in patients with normal and near-normal scans but, in contrast, is about 90% certain in patients with high-probability scans. Unfortunately, fewer than half of patients with angiographically confirmed PTE have a high-probability scan. Importantly, as many as 40% of patients with high clinical suspicion for PTE and "low-probability" scans do, in fact, have PTE at angiography.

Chest CT   Computed tomography (CT) of the chest with intravenous contrast effectively diagnoses large, central PTE but may fail to detect more peripherally located thrombi that are clinically important. In a comparison with standard contrast pulmonary angiography at Massachusetts General Hospital, the sensitivity of chest CT for PTE was only 60%.

Echocardiography   This technique is useful for rapid triage of acutely ill patients who may have PTE. Bedside echocardiography can usually reliably differentiate among illnesses that have radically different treatment, including acute myocardial infarction, pericardial tamponade, dissection of the aorta, and PTE complicated by right heart failure. Detection of right ventricular dysfunction due to PTE helps to stratify the risk, delineate the prognosis, and plan optimal management.

INVASIVE DIAGNOSTIC MODALITIES   Pulmonary Angiography   Selective pulmonary angiography is the most specific examination available for establishing the definitive diagnosis of PTE and can detect emboli as small as 1 to 2 mm. A definitive diagnosis of PTE depends upon visualization of an intraluminal filling defect in more than one projection. Secondary signs of PTE include abrupt occlusion ("cut-off") of vessels; segmental oligemia or avascularity; a prolonged arterial phase with slow filling; or tortuous, tapering peripheral vessels.

Pulmonary angiography can be carried out safely among properly selected patients at hospitals that perform at least several studies per month. In PIOPED, the procedure resulted in death in five patients (0.5%), two of whom had severe heart failure prior to the procedure. Angiography is most useful when the clinical likelihood of PTE differs substantially from the lung scan result or when the lung scan is of intermediate probability for PTE.

Contrast Phlebography   This technique has been mostly replaced by ultra-

| LPO | POST | RPO |

FIGURE 261-1   These three views of the pulmonary perfusion scan illustrate multiple segmental perfusion defects in both lung fields. The ventilation scan, which is normal, is not shown. The marked mismatch between normal ventilation and abnormal perfusion makes this lung scan *high probability for PTE*. LPO, left posterior oblique; POST, posterior; RPO, right posterior oblique.

sonography. Venography is costly, uncomfortable, and occasionally results in contrast allergy or contrast-induced phlebitis. Contrast phlebography is worthwhile when there is a discrepancy between the clinical suspicion and the ultrasound result. Phlebography is also useful for diagnosing isolated calf vein thrombosis or recurrent DVT. A recently approved nuclear medicine test utilizing a synthetic peptide that binds preferentially to the glycoprotein IIb/IIIa receptors on activated platelets may eventually replace contrast phlebography in clinical practice. This radiopharmaceutical permits scintigraphic imaging of acute DVT and may be especially useful for differentiating acute from chronic DVT.

INTEGRATED DIAGNOSTIC APPROACH We advocate an integrated diagnostic approach to streamline the workup of PTE (Fig. 261-2). This strategy combines the clinical likelihood of PTE with the results of noninvasive testing especially D-dimer ELISA, venous ultrasonography, and lung scanning to determine whether pulmonary angiography is warranted.

℞ TREATMENT Consensus guidelines from the American College of Chest Physicians are summarized as follows.

Primary versus Secondary Therapy Primary therapy consists of clot dissolution with thrombolysis or removal of PTE by embolectomy. Anticoagulation with heparin and warfarin or placement of an inferior vena caval filter constitutes secondary prevention of recurrent PTE rather than primary therapy.

Primary therapy should be reserved for patients at high risk of an adverse clinical outcome. When right ventricular function remains normal, patients typically have good clinical outcomes with anticoagulation alone (Fig. 261-3).

Adjunctive Therapy Important adjunctive measures include pain relief (especially with nonsteroidal anti-inflammatory agents), supplemental oxygenation, and psychological support. Dobutamine—a β-adrenergic agonist with positive inotropic and pulmonary vasolidating effects—may successfully treat right heart failure and cardiogenic shock. Volume loading should be undertaken cautiously because increased right ventricular dilatation can lead to even further reductions in left ventricular forward output.

Heparin Heparin binds to and accelerates the activity of antithrombin III, an enzyme that inhibits the coagulation factors thrombin (factor IIa), Xa, IXa, XIa, and XIIa. Heparin thus prevents additional thrombus formation and permits endogenous fibrinolytic mechanisms to lyse clot that has already formed. After 5 to 7 days of heparin, residual thrombus begins to stabilize in the endothelium of the vein

---

Guidelines for the Treatment of Pulmonary Embolism

1. Treat DVT or PTE with therapeutic levels of unfractionated intravenous heparin, adjusted subcutaneous heparin, or low-molecular-weight heparin for at least 5 days and overlap with oral anticoagulation for at least 4 to 5 days. Consider a longer course of heparin for massive PTE or severe iliofemoral DVT.
2. For most patients, heparin and oral anticoagulation can be started together and heparin discontinued on day 5 or 6 if the INR has been therapeutic for two consecutive days.
3. Continue oral anticoagulant therapy for at least 3 months with a target INR of 2.5 (range 2.0 to 3.0).
4. Patients with reversible or time-limited risk factors can be treated for 3 to 6 months. Patients with a first episode of idiopathic DVT should be treated for at least 6 months. Patients with recurrent venous thrombosis or a continuing risk factor such as cancer, inhibitor deficiency states, or antiphospholipid antibody syndrome should be treated indefinitely.
5. Isolated calf vein DVT should be treated with anticoagulation for at least 3 months.
6. The use of thrombolytic agents continues to be highly individualized, and clinicians should have some latitude in using these agents. Patients with hemodynamically unstable PTE or massive iliofemoral thrombosis are the best candidates.
7. Inferior vena caval filter placement is recommended when there is a contraindication to or failure of anticoagulation, for chronic recurrent embolism with pulmonary hypertension, and with concurrent performance of surgical pulmonary embolectomy or pulmonary endarterectomy.

* Modified from TM Hyers et al: Antithrombotic therapy for venous thromboembolic disease Chest 114:561S, 1998.

---

or pulmonary artery. However, heparin does *not* directly dissolve thrombus that already exists.

Low-molecular-weight heparins These fragments of unfractionated heparin exhibit less binding to plasma proteins and endothelial cells and consequently have greater bioavailability, a more predictable dose response, and a longer half-life than unfractionated heparin. No laboratory monitoring or dose adjustment is needed unless the patient is markedly obese or has renal insufficiency. Therefore, low-molecular-weight heparins are far more convenient to use than unfractionated heparin.

A meta-analysis of more than 3,500 acute DVT patients showed that those treated with low-molecular-weight heparin had an overall 29% reduction in mortality and major bleeding compared with the unfractionated heparin group. *Enoxaparin*, originally approved for prophylaxis, has recently received Food and Drug Administration approval for treatment of PTE in the presence of DVT with a once-daily dose of 1.5 mg/kg subcutaneously. However, it is almost always ad-

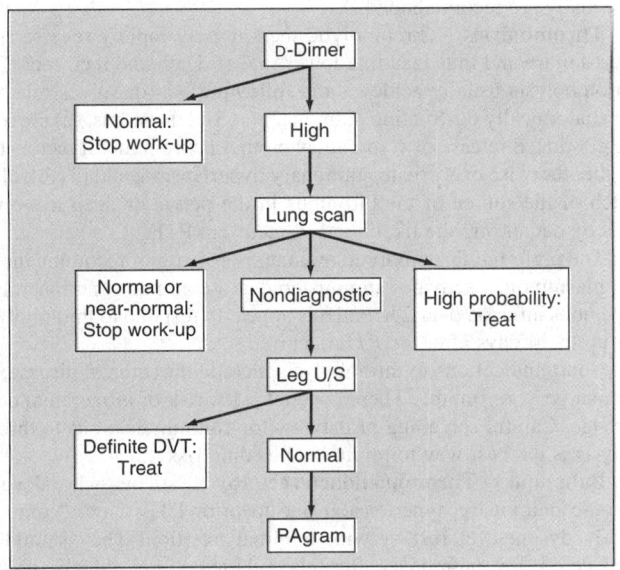

FIGURE 261-2 PTE diagnosis strategy: An integrated diagnostic approach. U/S, ultrasound; PAgram, pulmonary arteriogram.

FIGURE 261-3 Acute PTE management: Risk stratification. RV, right ventricular; IVC, inferior vena cava.

ministered as 1 mg/kg twice daily. *Dalteparin* is approved for prophylaxis but not for treatment of venous thromboembolism.

Dosing   For unfractionated heparin, a typical bolus is 5000 to 10,000 units followed by a continuous infusion of 1000 to 1500 units/h. An activated partial thromboplastin time that is at least twice the control value should provide a therapeutic level of heparin. Nomograms based upon a patient's weight may assist in adjusting the infusion rate of heparin.

Complications   The most important adverse effect of heparin is hemorrhage. For life-threatening or intracranial hemorrhage, protamine sulfate can be administered. Heparin-associated thrombocytopenia and osteopenia are far less common with low-molecular-weight heparins than with unfractionated heparin. Heparin-associated elevations in transaminase levels occur commonly but are rarely associated with clinical toxicity.

Warfarin   This vitamin K antagonist prevents γ carboxylation activation of coagulation factors II, VII, IX, and X. The full effect of warfarin often requires 5 days, even if the prothrombin time, used for monitoring, becomes elevated more rapidly. When warfarin is initiated during an active thrombotic state, the levels of protein C and S decline, thus creating a thrombogenic potential. By overlapping heparin and warfarin for 5 days, the procoagulant effect of unopposed warfarin can be counteracted. Thus, heparin acts as a "bridge" until the full anticoagulant effect of warfarin is obtained.

Dosing   In an average-sized adult, warfarin is usually initiated in a dose of 5 mg. Doses of 7.5 or 10 mg can be used in obese or large framed young patients who are otherwise healthy. Patients who are malnourished or who have received prolonged courses of antibiotics are probably deficient in vitamin K and should receive smaller initial doses of warfarin, such as 2.5 mg. The prothrombin time is standardized by using the International Normalized Ratio (INR) to assess the anticoagulant effect of warfarin (Chap. 118). The target INR should be approximately 2.5–3.0.

Complications   As with heparin, bleeding is the most important and common complication associated with warfarin administration. Life-threatening bleeding can be treated with cryoprecipitate or fresh frozen plasma (usually 2 units) to achieve immediate hemostasis. For less serious bleeding, or an excessively high INR in the absence of bleeding, vitamin K may be administered. An initial dose of 5 to 10 mg subcutaneously will help lower the INR toward the upper portion of the therapeutic range within about 6 h. Reversing excessive INRs with oral rather than subcutaneous vitamin K will facilitate reestablishing a stable dose of warfarin.

Warfarin-induced skin necrosis is a rare complication that may be related to warfarin-induced reduction of protein C. It is usually associated with administration of a high initial dose of warfarin during an acute thrombotic state in which heparin is withheld. During pregnancy, warfarin should be avoided if possible because of warfarin embryopathy, which is most common with exposure during the sixth through twelfth weeks of gestation. However, women can take warfarin postpartum and breast feed safely.

Duration of anticoagulation   After discontinuation of anticoagulation, the risk of recurrent PTE is surprisingly high. Nevertheless, the optimal duration of anticoagulation remains unknown. Schulman and colleagues found that after a 6-month course of anticoagulation, 14% of PTE patients suffered a recurrent venous thromboembolism within the ensuing 2 years. The recurrence rate was twice as high among patients who received only 6 weeks of anticoagulation. It is reasonable to anticoagulate the first episode of PTE for at least 6 months.

Inferior Vena Caval Filters   When anticoagulation cannot be undertaken because of active bleeding, insertion of an inferior vena caval filter is usually necessary. Other indications include recurrent venous thrombosis despite adequate anticoagulation, prevention of recurrent PTE in patients with right heart failure who are not candidates for thrombolysis, or prophylaxis of extremely high risk patients. The

Table 261-3   Prevention of Pulmonary Thromboembolism

Condition	Strategy
Total hip or knee replacement; hip or pelvis fracture	Warfarin (Coumadin) (target INR 2.0–2.5) × 4–6 weeks Low-molecular-weight heparin [e.g., enoxaparin (Lovenox), 30 mg SC twice daily] IPC ± warfarin (Coumadin)
Gynecologic cancer surgery	Warfarin (Coumadin) (target INR 2.0–2.5) ± IPC Unfractionated heparin, 5000 U q8 h ± IPC Dalteparin (Fragmin) 2500 U once daily ± IPC Enoxaparin 40 mg SC once daily
Urologic surgery	Warfarin (Coumadin) (target INR 2.0–2.5) ± IPC
Thoracic surgery	IPC *plus* unfractionated heparin, 5000 U q8 h
High-risk general surgery (e.g., prior VTE, current cancer, or obesity)	IPC *or* graded-compression stockings *plus* unfractionated heparin, 5000 U q8 h Dalteparin (Fragmin) 5000 U SC or Enoxaparin (Lovenox), 40 mg SC once daily
General, gynecologic, or urologic surgery (without prior VTE) for noncancerous conditions	Graded-compression stockings *plus* unfractionated heparin 5000 U q12h Dalteparin 2500 U SC once daily Enoxaparin 40 mg SC once daily IPC alone
Neurosurgery, eye surgery, or other surgery when prophylactic anticoagulation is contraindicated	Graded-compression stockings ± IPC
Medical conditions	Graded-compression stockings ± heparin, 5000 U q8–12h IPC alone Enoxaparin (Lovenox) 40 mg SC once daily

NOTE: IPC, intermittent pneumatic compression; VTE, venous thromboembolism.

Bird's Nest filter infrarenally or, if necessary, a Greenfield filter suprarenally are recommended.

Thrombolysis   Thrombolytic therapy may rapidly reverse right heart failure and thus lead to a lower rate of death and recurrent PTE. Thrombolysis usually achieves the following: (1) dissolves much of the anatomically obstructing pulmonary arterial thrombus; (2) prevents the continued release of serotonin and other neurohumoral factors that might otherwise exacerbate pulmonary hypertension; and (3) dissolves much of the source of the thrombus in the pelvic or deep leg veins, thereby decreasing the likelihood of recurrent PTE.

The preferred thrombolytic regimen is 100 mg of recombinant tissue plasminogen activator administered as a continuous peripheral intravenous infusion over 2 h. Patients appear to respond to thrombolysis for up to 14 days after the PTE occurred.

Contraindications to thrombolysis include intracranial disease, recent surgery, or trauma. There is about a 1% risk of intracranial hemorrhage. Careful screening of patients for contraindications to thrombolysis is the best way to minimize bleeding risk.

Pulmonary Thromboendarterectomy   Patients who develop chronic pulmonary hypertension due to prior PTE may become severely dyspneic at rest or with minimal exertion. They should be considered for pulmonary thromboendarterectomy which, if successful, can markedly reduce and at times even cure pulmonary hypertension.

Prevention Prevention of PTE is of paramount importance because it is both difficult to recognize and expensive to treat. Fortunately, effective mechanical and pharmacologic prophylaxis modalities are widely available and usually effective (Table 261-3).

BIBLIOGRAPHY

DECOUSUS H et al: A clinical trial of vena caval filters in the prevention of pulmonary embolism in patients with proximal deep-vein thrombosis. N Engl J Med 338:409, 1998

FEDULLO PF: Pulmonary thromboembolism, in *Textbook of Respiratory Medicine*, 3d ed. JF Murray, JA Nadel (eds). Philadelphia, Saunders, 2000, pp 1503–1532

GOLDHABER SZ et al: Acute pulmonary embolism: Clinical outcomes in the International Cooperative Pulmonary Embolism Registry (ICOPER). Lancet 353:1386, 1999

GOLDHABER SZ: Contemporary pulmonary embolism thrombolysis. Chest 107:45S, 1995

GOULD MK et al: Low-molecular-weight heparins compared with unfractionated heparin for treatment of acute deep venous thrombosis. A meta-analysis of randomized, controlled trials. Ann Intern Med 130:800, 1999

INDIK JH, ALPERT JS: Detection of pulmonary embolism by D-dimer assay, spiral computed tomography, and magnetic resonance imaging. Progr Cardiovasc Dis 42:261, 2000

KEARON C et al: A comparison of three months of anticoagulation with extended anticoagulation for a first episode of idiopathic venuos thromboembolism. N Engl J Med 340:901, 1999

LUALDI JC, GOLDHABER SZ: Right ventricular dysfunction after acute pulmonary embolism: Pathophysiologic factors, detection, and therapeutic implications. Am Heart J 130:1276, 1995

MULLINS MD et al: The role of spiral volumetric computed tomography in the diagnosis of pulmonary embolism. Arch Intern Med 160:293, 2000

PERRIER A et al: Noninvasive diagnosis of venous thromboembolism in outpatients. Lancet 353:190, 1999

RIDKER P et al: G20210A mutation in prothrombin gene and risk of myocardial infarction, stroke, and venous thrombosis in a large cohort of US Men. Circulation 99:999, 1999

RIDKER PM et al: Mutation in the gene coding for coagulation factor V and risks of future myocardial infarction, stroke, and venous thrombosis in apparently healthy men. N Engl J Med 332:912, 1995

262 Richard W. Light

DISORDERS OF THE PLEURA, MEDIASTINUM, AND DIAPHRAGM

DISORDERS OF THE PLEURA

PLEURAL EFFUSION The pleural space lies between the lung and chest wall and normally contains a very thin layer of fluid, which serves as a coupling system. A pleural effusion is present when there is an excess quantity of fluid in the pleural space.

Etiology Pleural fluid accumulates when pleural fluid formation exceeds pleural fluid absorption. Normally, fluid enters the pleural space from the capillaries in the parietal pleura and is removed via the lymphatics situated in the parietal pleura. Fluid also can enter the pleural space from the interstitial spaces of the lung via the visceral pleura or from the peritoneal cavity via small holes in the diaphragm. The lymphatics have the capacity to absorb 20 times more fluid than is normally formed. Accordingly, a pleural effusion may develop when there is excess pleural fluid formation (from the parietal pleura, the interstitial spaces of the lung, or the peritoneal cavity) or when there is decreased fluid removal by the lymphatics.

Diagnostic Approach When a patient is found to have a pleural effusion, an effort should be made to determine the cause (Fig. 262-1). The first step is to determine whether the effusion is a transudate or an exudate. A *transudative* pleural effusion occurs when *systemic factors* that influence the formation and absorption of pleural fluid are altered. The leading causes of transudative pleural effusions in the United States are left ventricular failure, pulmonary embolism, and cirrhosis. An *exudative* pleural effusion occurs when *local factors* that influence the formation and absorption of pleural fluid are altered. The leading causes of exudative pleural effusions are bacterial pneumonia,

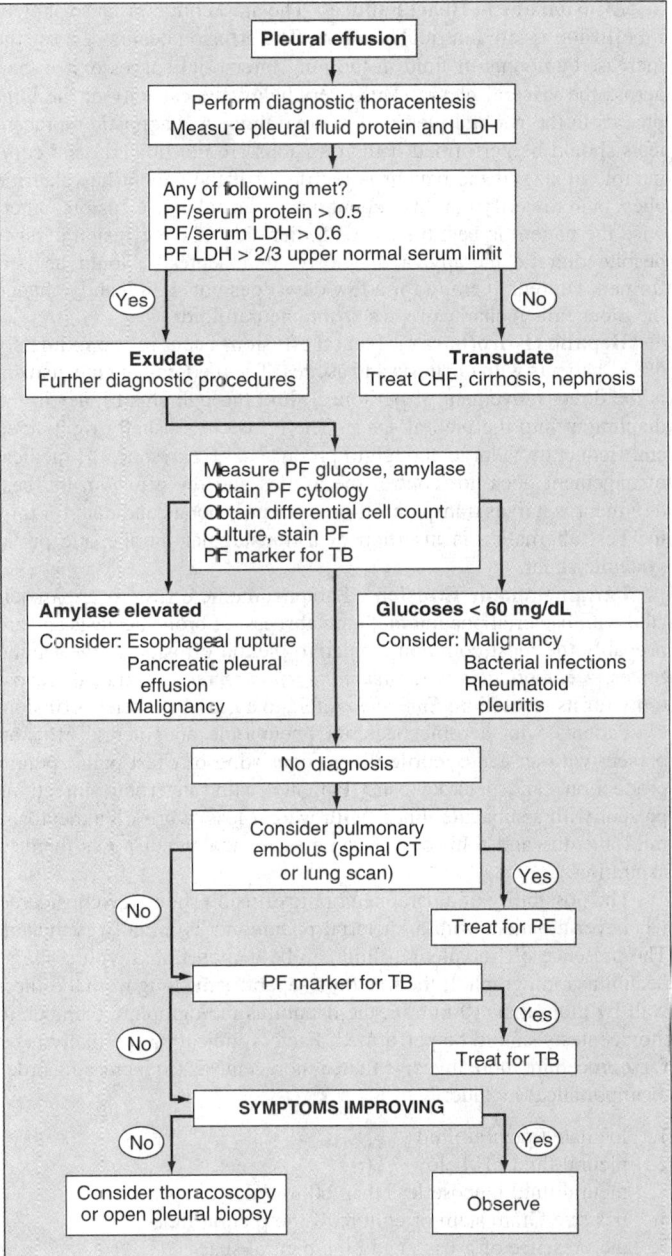

FIGURE 262-1 Approach to the diagnosis of pleural effusions; PF, pleural fluid.

malignancy, viral infection, and pulmonary embolism. The primary reason to make this differentiation is that additional diagnostic procedures are indicated with exudative effusions to define the cause of the local disease.

Transudative and exudative pleural effusions are distinguished by measuring the lactate dehydrogenase (LDH) and protein levels in the pleural fluid. Exudative pleural effusions meet at least one of the following criteria, whereas transudative pleural effusions meet none:

1. pleural fluid protein/serum protein >0.5
2. pleural fluid LDH/serum LDH >0.6
3. pleural fluid LDH more than two-thirds normal upper limit for serum

If a patient has an exudative pleural effusion, the following tests on the pleural fluid should be obtained: description of the fluid, glucose level, amylase level, differential cell count, microbiologic studies, and cytology.

Effusion due to Heart Failure   The most common cause of pleural effusion is left ventricular failure. The effusion occurs because the increased amounts of fluid in the lung interstitial spaces exit in part across the visceral pleura. This overwhelms the capacity of the lymphatics in the parietal pleura to remove fluid. A diagnostic thoracentesis should be performed if the effusions are not bilateral and comparable in size, if the patient is febrile, or if the patient has pleuritic chest pain to verify that the patient has a transudative effusion. Otherwise the patient is best treated with diuretics. If the effusion persists despite diuretic therapy, a diagnostic thoracentesis should be performed. Diuretic therapy for a few days does not significantly change the biochemical characteristics of the pleural fluid.

Hepatic Hydrothorax   Pleural effusions occur in approximately 5% of patients with cirrhosis and ascites. The predominant mechanism is the direct movement of peritoneal fluid through small holes in the diaphragm into the pleural space. The effusion is usually right-sided and frequently is large enough to produce severe dyspnea. If medical management does not control the ascites and the effusion, the best treatment is a liver transplant. If the patient is not a candidate for this, the best alternative is insertion of a transjugular intrahepatic portal systemic shunt.

Parapneumonic Effusion   Parapneumonic effusions are associated with bacterial pneumonia, lung abscess, or bronchiectasis and are probably the most common exudative pleural effusion in the United States. A *complicated parapneumonic effusion* requires tube thoracostomy for its resolution. *Empyema* refers to a grossly purulent effusion.

Patients with aerobic bacterial pneumonia and pleural effusion present with an acute febrile illness consisting of chest pain, sputum production, and leukocytosis. Patients with anaerobic infections present with a subacute illness with weight loss, a brisk leukocytosis, mild anemia, and a history of some factor that predisposes them to aspiration.

The possibility of a parapneumonic effusion should be considered whenever a patient with a bacterial pneumonia is initially evaluated. The presence of free pleural fluid can be demonstrated with a lateral decubitus radiograph. If the free fluid separates the lung from the chest wall by more than 10 mm on the decubitus radiograph, a therapeutic thoracentesis should be performed. Factors indicating the likely need for a procedure more invasive than a thoracentesis (in increasing order of importance) include:

1. loculated pleural fluid
2. pleural fluid pH below 7.20
3. pleural fluid glucose less than 60 mg/dL
4. positive Gram stain or culture of the pleural fluid
5. the presence of gross pus in the pleural space

If the fluid recurs after the initial therapeutic thoracentesis, a repeat thoracentesis should be performed if any of the above characteristics are present. If the fluid recurs a second time, tube thoracostomy should be performed if any of the poor prognostic factors are present. If the fluid cannot be completely removed with the therapeutic thoracentesis, consideration should be given to inserting a chest tube and instilling a thrombolytic (streptokinase, 250,000 units or urokinase, 100,000 units) or performing thoracoscopy with the breakdown of adhesions. Decortication should be considered when the above are ineffective.

Effusion Secondary to Malignancy   Malignant pleural effusions secondary to metastatic disease are the second most common type of exudative pleural effusion. The three tumors that cause approximately 75% of all malignant pleural effusions are lung carcinoma, breast carcinoma, and lymphoma. Most patients complain of dyspnea, which is frequently out of proportion to the size of the effusion. The pleural fluid is an exudate, and its glucose level may be reduced if the tumor burden in the pleural space is high.

The diagnosis is usually made via cytology of the pleural fluid. If the initial cytologic examination is negative, then thoracoscopy is the best next procedure if malignancy is strongly suspected. At the time of thoracoscopy, talc or some similar agent should be instilled into the pleural space to effect a pleurodesis. If thoracoscopy is unavailable, then needle biopsy of the pleura should be performed.

Patients with a malignant pleural effusion are treated symptomatically for the most part, since the presence of the effusion indicates disseminated disease and most malignancies associated with pleural effusion are not curable with chemotherapy. The only symptom that can be attributed to the effusion itself is dyspnea. If the patient's lifestyle is compromised by dyspnea, and if the dyspnea is relieved with a therapeutic thoracentesis, then one of the following procedures should be performed: (1) tube thoracostomy with the instillation of a sclerosing agent such as talc, 5 g in a slurry, or doxycycline, 500 mg; (2) outpatient insertion of a small indwelling catheter; or (3) thoracoscopy with pleural abrasion or the insufflation of talc.

Mesothelioma   Malignant mesotheliomas are primary tumors that arise from the mesothelial cells that line the pleural cavities. Most are related to asbestos exposure. Patients with mesothelioma present with chest pain and shortness of breath. The chest radiograph reveals a pleural effusion, generalized pleural thickening, and a shrunken hemithorax. Thoracoscopy or open pleural biopsy is usually necessary to establish the diagnosis. Various treatment modalities, including radical surgery, chemotherapy, and radiation therapy, have been tried, but none has been proven to be more effective than symptomatic therapy. It is recommended that chest pain be treated with opiates and that shortness of breath be treated with oxygen and/or opiates.

Effusion Secondary to Pulmonary Embolization   The diagnosis most commonly overlooked in the differential diagnosis of a patient with an undiagnosed pleural effusion is pulmonary embolism. Dyspnea is the most common symptom. The pleural fluid can be either transudative or exudative. The diagnosis is suggested by spiral CT scans, perfusion lung scanning and/or pulmonary arteriography (Chap. 261). Treatment of the patient with a pleural effusion secondary to pulmonary embolism is the same as for any patient with pulmonary emboli. If the pleural effusion increases in size after anticoagulation, the patient probably has recurrent emboli or another complication such as a hemothorax or a pleural infection.

Tuberculous Pleuritis   (See also Chap. 169)   In many parts of the world, the most common cause of an exudative pleural effusion is tuberculosis, but this is relatively uncommon in the United States. Tuberculous pleural effusions are thought to be due primarily to a hypersensitivity reaction to tuberculous protein in the pleural space. Patients with tuberculous pleuritis present with fever, weight loss, dyspnea, and/or pleuritic chest pain. The pleural fluid is an exudate with predominantly small lymphocytes. The diagnosis is established by demonstrating high levels of TB markers in the pleural fluid (adenosine deaminase > 45 IU/L, gamma interferon > 140 pg/mL, or positive PCR for tuberculous DNA). Alternatively, the diagnosis can be established by culture of the pleural fluid, needle biopsy of the pleura, or thoracoscopy. The recommended treatment of pleural and pulmonary tuberculosis is identical (Chap. 169).

Effusion Secondary to Viral Infection   Viral infections are probably responsible for a sizable percentage of undiagnosed exudative pleural effusions. In many series, no diagnosis is established for approximately 20% of exudative effusions, and these effusions resolve spontaneously with no long-term residua. The importance of these effusions is that one should not be too aggressive in trying to establish a diagnosis for the undiagnosed effusion, particularly if the patient is improving clinically.

AIDS   Pleural effusions are uncommon in such patients. The most common cause is Kaposi's sarcoma, followed by parapneumonic effusion. Other common causes are tuberculosis, cryptococcosis, and lymphoma. Pleural effusions are very uncommon with *Pneumocystis carinii* infection.

Chylothorax   A chylothorax occurs when the thoracic duct is disrupted and chyle accumulates in the pleural space. The most common cause of chylothorax is trauma, but it also may result from tumors in the mediastinum. Patients with chylothorax present with dyspnea, and a large pleural effusion is present on the chest radiograph. Thoracentesis reveals milky fluid, and biochemical analysis reveals a triglyceride level that exceeds 110 mg/dL. Patients with chylothorax and no obvious trauma should have a lymphangiogram and a mediastinal computed tomographic (CT) scan to assess the mediastinum for lymph nodes. The treatment of choice for most chylothoraces is implantation of a pleuroperitoneal shunt. Patients with chylothoraces should not undergo prolonged tube thoracostomy with chest tube drainage because this will lead to malnutrition and immunologic incompetence.

Hemothorax When a diagnostic thoracentesis reveals bloody pleural fluid, a hematocrit should be obtained on the pleural fluid. If the hematocrit is >50% that of the peripheral blood, the patient has a hemothorax. Most hemothoraces are the result of trauma; other causes include rupture of a blood vessel or tumor. Most patients with hemothorax should be treated with tube thoracostomy, which allows continuous quantification of bleeding. If the bleeding emanates from a laceration of the pleura, apposition of the two pleural surfaces is likely to stop the bleeding. If the pleural hemorrhage exceeds 200 mL/h, consideration should be given to thoracotomy.

Miscellaneous Causes of Pleural Effusion There are many other causes of pleural effusion (Table 262-1). Key features of some of these conditions are as follows: If the pleural fluid amylase level is elevated, the diagnosis of esophageal rupture or pancreatic disease is likely. If the patient is febrile, has predominantly polymorphonuclear cells in the pleural fluid, and has no pulmonary parenchymal abnormalities, an intraabdominal abscess should be considered. The diagnosis of an asbestos pleural effusion is one of exclusion. Benign ovarian tumors can produce ascites and a pleural effusion (Meigs' syndrome), as can the ovarian hyperstimulation syndrome. Several drugs can cause pleural effusion; the associated fluid is usually eosinophilic. Pleural effusions commonly occur following coronary artery bypass surgery. Effusions occurring within the first weeks are typically left-sided and bloody, with large numbers of eosinophils, and respond

Table 262-1 Differential Diagnoses of Pleural Effusions

TRANSUDATIVE PLEURAL EFFUSIONS

1. Congestive heart failure
2. Cirrhosis
3. Pulmonary embolization
4. Nephrotic syndrome
5. Peritoneal dialysis
6. Superior vena cava obstruction
7. Myxedema
8. Urinothorax

EXUDATIVE PLEURAL EFFUSIONS

1. Neoplastic diseases
   a. Metastatic disease
   b. Mesothelioma
2. Infectious diseases
   a. Bacterial infections
   b. Tuberculosis
   c. Fungal infections
   d. Viral infections
   e. Parasitic infections
3. Pulmonary embolization
4. Gastrointestinal disease
   a. Esophageal perforation
   b. Pancreatic disease
   c. Intraabdominal abscesses
   d. Diaphragmatic hernia
   e. After abdominal surgery
   f. Endoscopic variceal sclerotherapy
   g. After liver transplant
5. Collagen-vascular diseases
   a. Rheumatoid pleuritis
   b. Systemic lupus erythematosus
   c. Drug-induced lupus
   d. Immunoblastic lymphadenopathy
   e. Sjögren's syndrome
   f. Wegener's granulomatosis
   g. Churg-Strauss syndrome
6. Post-coronary artery bypass surgery
7. Asbestos exposure
8. Sarcoidosis
9. Uremia
10. Meigs' syndrome
11. Yellow nail syndrome
12. Drug-induced pleural disease
    a. Nitrofurantoin
    b. Dantrolene
    c. Methysergide
    d. Bromocriptine
    e. Procarbazine
    f. Amiodarone
13. Trapped lung
14. Radiation therapy
15. Post-cardiac injury syndrome
16. Hemothorax
17. Iatrogenic injury
18. Ovarian hyperstimulation syndrome
19. Pericardial disease
20. Chylothorax

to one or two therapeutic thoracenteses. Effusions occurring after the first few weeks are typically left-sided and clear yellow, with predominantly small lymphocytes, and tend to recur. Other medical manipulations that induce pleural effusions include abdominal surgery, endoscopic variceal sclerotherapy, radiation therapy, liver or lung transplantation, or the intravascular insertion of central lines.

PNEUMOTHORAX Pneumothorax is the presence of gas in the pleural space. A *spontaneous pneumothorax* is one that occurs without antecedent trauma to the thorax. A *primary spontaneous pneumothorax* occurs in the absence of underlying lung disease, while a *secondary spontaneous pneumothorax* occurs in its presence. A *traumatic pneumothorax* results from penetrating or nonpenetrating chest injuries. A *tension pneumothorax* is a pneumothorax in which the pressure in the pleural space is positive throughout the respiratory cycle.

Primary Spontaneous Pneumothorax Primary spontaneous pneumothoraces are usually due to rupture of apical pleural blebs, small cystic spaces that lie within or immediately under the visceral pleura. Primary spontaneous pneumothoraces occur almost exclusively in smokers, which suggests that these patients have subclinical lung disease. Approximately one-half of patients with an initial primary spontaneous pneumothorax will have a recurrence. The initial recommended treatment for primary spontaneous pneumothorax is simple aspiration. If the lung does not expand with aspiration, or if the patient has a recurrent pneumothorax, thoracoscopy with stapling of blebs and pleural abrasion is indicated. Thoracoscopy or thoracotomy with pleural abrasion is almost 100% successful in preventing recurrences.

Secondary Spontaneous Pneumothorax Most secondary spontaneous pneumothoraces are due to chronic obstructive pulmonary disease, but pneumothoraces have been reported with virtually every lung disease. Pneumothorax in patients with lung disease is more life-threatening than it is in normal individuals because of the lack of pulmonary reserve in these patients. Nearly all patients with secondary spontaneous pneumothorax should be treated with tube thoracostomy and the instillation of a sclerosing agent such as doxycycline or talc. Patients with secondary spontaneous pneumothoraces who have a persistent air leak, an unexpanded lung after 3 days of tube thoracostomy, or a recurrent pneumothorax should be subjected to thoracoscopy with bleb resection and pleural abrasion.

Traumatic Pneumothorax Traumatic pneumothoraces can result from both penetrating and nonpenetrating chest trauma. Traumatic pneumothoraces should be treated with tube thoracostomy unless they are very small. If a hemopneumothorax is present, one chest tube should be placed in the superior part of the hemithorax to evacuate the air, and another should be placed in the inferior part of the hemithorax to remove the blood. Iatrogenic pneumothorax is a type of traumatic pneumothorax which is becoming more common. The leading causes are transthoracic needle aspiration, thoracentesis, and the insertion of central intravenous catheters. The treatment differs according to the degree of distress and can be observation, supplemental oxygen, aspiration, or tube thoracostomy.

Tension Pneumothorax This condition usually occurs during mechanical ventilation or resuscitative efforts. The positive pleural pressure is life-threatening both because ventilation is severely compromised and because the positive pressure is transmitted to the mediastinum, which results in decreased venous return to the heart and reduced cardiac output.

Difficulty in ventilation during resuscitation or high peak inspiratory pressures during mechanical ventilation strongly suggest the diagnosis. The diagnosis is made by the finding of an enlarged hemithorax with no breath sounds and shift of the mediastinum to the contralateral side. Tension pneumothorax must be treated as a medical emergency. If the tension in the pleural space is not relieved, the patient is likely to die from inadequate cardiac output or marked hypoxemia. A large-bore needle should be inserted into the pleural space through the second anterior intercostal space. If large amounts of gas escape from the needle after insertion, the diagnosis is confirmed. The needle should be left in place until a thoracostomy tube can be inserted.

DISORDERS OF THE MEDIASTINUM

The mediastinum is the region between the pleural sacs. It is separated into three compartments. The *anterior mediastinum* extends from the sternum anteriorly to the pericardium and brachiocephalic vessels posteriorly. It contains the thymus gland; the anterior mediastinal lymph nodes; and the internal mammary arteries and veins. The *middle mediastinum* lies between the anterior and posterior mediastina and contains the heart; the ascending and transverse arches of the aorta; the venae cavae; the brachiocephalic arteries and veins; the phrenic nerves; the trachea, main bronchi, and their contiguous lymph nodes; and the pulmonary arteries and veins. The *posterior mediastinum* is bounded by the pericardium and trachea anteriorly and the vertebral column posteriorly. It contains the descending thoracic aorta; esophagus; thoracic duct; azygos and hemiazygos veins; and the posterior group of mediastinal lymph nodes.

MEDIASTINAL MASSES   The first step in evaluating a mediastinal mass lesion is to place it in one of the three mediastinal compartments, since each has different characteristic lesions. The most common lesions in the anterior mediastinum are thymomas, lymphomas, teratomatous neoplasms, and thyroid masses. The most common masses in the middle mediastinum are vascular masses, lymph node enlargement from metastases or granulomatous disease, and pleuropericardial and bronchogenic cysts. In the posterior mediastinum, neurogenic tumors, meningoceles, meningomyeloceles, gastroenteric cysts, and esophageal diverticula are commonly found.

CT scanning is the most valuable imaging technique for evaluating mediastinal masses and is the only imaging technique that should be done in most instances. Barium studies of the gastrointestinal tract are indicated in many patients with posterior mediastinal lesions, since hernias, diverticula, and achalasia are readily diagnosed in this manner. An ^{131}I nuclear medicine scan can efficiently establish the diagnosis of intrathoracic goiter.

A definite diagnosis can be obtained with mediastinoscopy or anterior mediastinotomy in many patients with masses in the anterior or middle mediastinal compartments. A diagnosis can be established without thoracotomy via percutaneous fine-needle aspiration biopsy of mediastinal masses in any of the mediastinal compartments. In many cases the diagnosis can be established and the mediastinal mass removed with video-assisted thoracoscopy.

ACUTE MEDIASTINITIS   Most cases of acute mediastinitis are either due to esophageal perforation or occur after median sternotomy for cardiac surgery. Patients with esophageal rupture are acutely ill with chest pain and dyspnea due to the mediastinal infection. The esophageal rupture can occur spontaneously or as a complication of esophagoscopy or the insertion of a Blakemore tube. Appropriate treatment is exploration of the mediastinum with primary repair of the esophageal tear and drainage of the pleural space and the mediastinum.

The incidence of mediastinitis following median sternotomy is 0.4 to 5.0%. Patients most commonly present with wound drainage. Other presentations include sepsis or a widened mediastinum. The diagnosis is usually established with mediastinal needle aspiration. Treatment includes immediate drainage, debridement, and parenteral antibiotic therapy, but the mortality still exceeds 20%.

CHRONIC MEDIASTINITIS   The spectrum of chronic mediastinitis ranges from granulomatous inflammation of the lymph nodes in the mediastinum to fibrosing mediastinitis. Most cases are due to tuberculosis or histoplasmosis, but sarcoidosis, silicosis, and other fungal diseases are at times causative. Patients with granulomatous mediastinitis are usually asymptomatic. Those with fibrosing mediastinitis usually have signs of compression of some mediastinal structure such as the superior vena cava or large airways, phrenic or recurrent laryngeal nerve paralysis, or obstruction of the pulmonary artery or proximal pulmonary veins. Other than antituberculous therapy for tuberculous mediastinitis, no medical or surgical therapy has been demonstrated to be effective for mediastinal fibrosis.

PNEUMOMEDIASTINUM   In this condition, there is gas in the interstices of the mediastinum. The three main causes are: (1) alveolar rupture with dissection of air into the mediastinum; (2) perforation or rupture of the esophagus, trachea, or main bronchi; and (3) dissection of air from the neck or the abdomen into the mediastinum. Typically, there is severe substernal chest pain with or without radiation into the neck and arms. The physical examination usually reveals subcutaneous emphysema in the suprasternal notch and *Hamman's sign*, which is a crunching or clicking noise synchronous with the heartbeat and best heard in the left lateral decubitus position. The diagnosis is confirmed with the chest radiograph. Usually no treatment is required, but the mediastinal air will be absorbed faster if the patient inspires high concentrations of oxygen. If mediastinal structures are compressed, the compression can be relieved with needle aspiration.

DISORDERS OF THE DIAPHRAGM

DIAPHRAGMATIC PARALYSIS   The presence of bilateral diaphragmatic paralysis almost always causes severe morbidity in adults. The most common causes include high spinal cord injury, thoracic trauma (including cardiac surgery), multiple sclerosis, anterior horn disease, and muscular dystrophy. Most patients with severe diaphragmatic weakness present with hypercapnic respiratory failure, frequently complicated by cor pulmonale and right ventricular failure, atelectasis, and pneumonia.

The degree of diaphragmatic weakness is best quantitated by measuring transdiaphragmatic pressures. The treatment of choice is assisted ventilation for all or part of each day. This is best accomplished without tracheostomy using nasal intermittent positive airway pressure. If the nerve to the diaphragm is intact, diaphragmatic pacing may be a viable alternative. If the paralysis occurs during open heart surgery, recovery frequently occurs, but it may take 6 months or more.

Unilateral paralysis of the diaphragm is much more common than is bilateral paralysis. The most common cause is nerve invasion from malignancy, usually a bronchogenic carcinoma. If the patient does not have malignancy, then usually no cause for the paralysis is found. The diagnosis is suggested by finding an elevated hemidiaphragm on the chest roentgenogram. Confirmation is best established with the "sniff test." When a patient is observed with fluoroscopy while sniffing, the paralyzed diaphragm will move paradoxically upward due to the negative intrathoracic pressure. Patients with a unilateral paralyzed diaphragm are usually asymptomatic. Their vital capacity and total lung capacity are each reduced about 25%. If a patient has a mediastinal mass in conjunction with the diaphragmatic paralysis, further workup should be done. However, if the patient is asymptomatic with a normal chest radiograph, no invasive procedures are warranted.

BIBLIOGRAPHY

GIERADA D et al: Imaging evaluation of the diaphragm. Chest Surg Clin N Am 8:237, 1998

HAMM H et al: Parapneumonic effusion and empyema. Eur Respir J 10:1150, 1997

LIGHT RW et al: Pleural sclerosis for the treatment of pneumothorax and pleural effusion. Lung 175:213, 1997

LIGHT RW, BROADDUS VC: Pleural Effusion, in *Textbook of Respiratory Medicine*, 3d ed, JF Murray, JA Nadel (eds). Saunders, Philadelphia, 2000, pp 2013–2042

SAHN SA, HEFFNER JE: Spontaneous pneumothorax. N Engl J Med 342:868, 2000

STROLLO DC et al: Primary mediastinal tumors. Tumors of the anterior mediastinum. Chest 112:511, 1997

STROLLO DC et al: Primary mediastinal tumors, Part II. Tumors of the middle and posterior mediastinum. Chest 112:1344, 1997

DISORDERS OF VENTILATION

HYPOVENTILATION

DEFINITION AND ETIOLOGY   Alveolar hypoventilation exists by definition when arterial P_{CO_2} (Pa_{CO_2}) increases above the normal range of 37 to 43 mmHg, but in clinically important hypoventilation syndromes Pa_{CO_2} is generally in the range of 50 to 80 mmHg. Hypoventilation disorders can be acute or chronic. The acute disorders, which represent life-threatening emergencies, are discussed in Chap. 265; this chapter deals with chronic hypoventilation syndromes.

Chronic hypoventilation can result from numerous disease entities (Table 263-1), but in all cases the underlying mechanism involves a defect in either the metabolic respiratory control system, the respiratory neuromuscular system, or the ventilatory apparatus. Disorders associated with impaired respiratory drive, defects in the respiratory neuromuscular system, some chest wall disorders such as obesity, and upper airway obstruction produce an increase in Pa_{CO_2}, despite normal lungs, because of a reduction in overall minute volume of ventilation and hence in alveolar ventilation. In contrast, most disorders of the chest wall and disorders of the lower airways and lungs may produce an increase in Pa_{CO_2}, despite a normal or even increased minute volume of ventilation, because of severe ventilation-perfusion mismatching that results in net alveolar hypoventilation.

Several hypoventilation syndromes involve combined disturbances in two elements of the respiratory system. For example, patients with chronic obstructive pulmonary disease may hypoventilate not simply because of impaired ventilatory mechanics but also because of a reduced central respiratory drive, which can be inherent or secondary to a coexisting metabolic alkalosis (related to diuretic and steroid therapy).

PHYSIOLOGIC AND CLINICAL FEATURES   Regardless of cause, the hallmark of all alveolar hypoventilation syndromes is an increase in alveolar P_{CO_2} (PA_{CO_2}) and therefore in Pa_{CO_2} (Fig. 263-1). The resulting respiratory acidosis eventually leads to a compensatory increase in plasma HCO_3^- concentration and a decrease in Cl^- concentration. The increase in PA_{CO_2} produces an obligatory decrease in PA_{O_2}, resulting in hypoxemia. If severe, the hypoxemia manifests clinically as cyanosis and can stimulate erythropoiesis and induce secondary polycythemia. The combination of chronic hypoxemia and hypercapnia may also induce pulmonary vasoconstriction, leading eventually to pulmonary hypertension, right ventricular hypertrophy, and congestive heart failure. The disturbances in arterial blood gases are typically magnified during sleep because of a further reduction in central respiratory drive. The resulting increased nocturnal hypercapnia may cause cerebral vasodilation leading to morning headache; sleep quality may also be severely impaired, resulting in morning fatigue, daytime somnolence, mental confusion, and intellectual impairment. Other clinical features associated with hypoventilation syndromes are related to the specific underlying disease (Table 263-1).

DIAGNOSIS   Investigation of the patient with chronic hypoventilation involves several laboratory tests that will usually localize the disorder to either the metabolic respiratory control system, the neuromuscular system, or the ventilatory apparatus (Fig. 263-2). Defects in the control system impair responses to chemical stimuli, including ventilatory, occlusion pressure, and diaphragmatic electromyographic (EMG) responses. During sleep, hypoventilation is usually more marked, and central apneas and hypopneas are common. However, because the behavioral respiratory control system (which is anatomically distinct from the metabolic control system), the neuromuscular system, and the ventilatory apparatus are intact, such patients can usually hyperventilate voluntarily, generate normal inspiratory and expiratory muscle pressures (PI_{max}, PE_{max}, respectively) against an occluded airway, generate normal lung volumes and flow rates on routine spi-

Table 263-1   **Chronic Hypoventilation Syndromes**

Mechanism	Site of Defect	Disorder
Impaired respiratory drive	Peripheral and central chemoreceptors	Carotid body dysfunction, trauma
		Prolonged hypoxia
		Metabolic alkalosis
	Brainstem respiratory neurons	Bulbar poliomyelitis, encephalitis
		Brainstem infarction, hemorrhage, trauma
		Brainstem demyelination, degeneration
		Chronic drug administration
		Primary alveolar hypoventilation syndrome
Defective respiratory neuromuscular system	Spinal cord and peripheral nerves	High cervical trauma
		Poliomyelitis
		Motor neuron disease
		Peripheral neuropathy
	Respiratory muscles	Myasthenia gravis
		Muscular dystrophy
		Chronic myopathy
Impaired ventilatory apparatus	Chest wall	Kyphoscoliosis
		Fibrothorax
		Thoracoplasty
		Ankylosing spondylitis
		Obesity hypoventilation
	Airways and lungs	Laryngeal and tracheal stenosis
		Obstructive sleep apnea
		Cystic fibrosis
		Chronic obstructive pulmonary disease

SOURCE: From Phillipson, with permission.

rometry, and have normal respiratory system resistance and compliance and a normal alveolar-arterial P_{O_2} [$(A - a)P_{O_2}$] difference. Patients with defects in the respiratory neuromuscular system also have impaired responses to chemical stimuli but in addition are unable to hyperventilate voluntarily or to generate normal static respiratory muscle pressures, lung volumes, and flow rates. However, at least in the early stages of the disease, the resistance and compliance of the respiratory system and the alveolar-arterial oxygen difference are normal.

In contrast to patients with disorders of the respiratory control or neuromuscular systems, patients with disorders of the chest wall, lungs, and airways typically demonstrate abnormalities of respiratory system resistance and compliance and have a widened $(A - a)P_{O_2}$. Because of the impaired mechanics of breathing, routine spirometric tests are abnormal, as is the ventilatory response to chemical stimuli. However, because the neuromuscular system is intact, tests that are independent of resistance and compliance are usually normal, including tests of respiratory muscle strength and of respiratory control that do not involve airflow.

TREATMENT   The management of chronic hypoventilation must be individualized to the patient's particular disorder, circumstances, and needs and should include measures directed toward the underlying disease. Coexistent metabolic alkalosis should be corrected, including elevations of HCO_3^- that are inappropriately high for the degree of chronic hypercapnia. Administration of supplemental oxygen is effective in attenuating hypoxemia, polycythemia, and pulmonary hypertension, but can aggravate CO_2 retention and the associated neurologic symptoms. For this reason, supplemental oxygen must be prescribed judiciously and the results monitored carefully. Pharmacologic agents that stimulate respiration (particularly progesterone) are of benefit in some patients, but generally, results are disappointing.

Most patients with chronic hypoventilation related to impairment of respiratory drive or neuromuscular disease eventually require me-

FIGURE 263-1   Physiologic and clinical features of alveolar hypoventilation. Hb, hemoglobin; PA_{CO_2}, alveolar P_{CO_2}; PA_{O_2}, alveolar P_{O_2}. *(After Phillipson.)*

chanical ventilatory assistance for effective management. When hypoventilation is severe, treatment may be required on a 24-h basis, but in most patients ventilatory assistance only during sleep produces dramatic clinical improvement and lowering of daytime Pa_{CO_2}. In patients with reduced respiratory drive but intact respiratory lower motor neurons, phrenic nerves, and respiratory muscles, diaphragmatic pacing through an implanted phrenic electrode can be very effective. However, for patients with defects in the respiratory nerves and muscles, electrophrenic pacing is contraindicated. Such patients can usually be managed effectively with either intermittent negative-pressure ventilation in a cuirass or intermittent positive-pressure ventilation delivered through a tracheostomy or nose mask. For patients who require ventilatory assistance only during sleep, positive-pressure ventilation through a nose mask is the preferred method because it obviates a tracheostomy and avoids the problem of upper airway occlusion that can arise in a negative-pressure ventilator. Hypoventilation related to restrictive disorders of the chest wall (Table 263-1) can also be man-

aged effectively with nocturnal intermittent positive-pressure ventilation through a nose mask or tracheostomy.

HYPOVENTILATION SYNDROMES

PRIMARY ALVEOLAR HYPOVENTILATION   Primary alveolar hypoventilation (PAH) is a disorder of unknown cause characterized by chronic hypercapnia and hypoxemia in the absence of identifiable neuromuscular disease or mechanical ventilatory impairment. The disorder is thought to arise from a defect in the metabolic respiratory control system, but few neuropathologic studies have been reported in such patients. Recent studies in animals suggest an important role for genetic factors in the pathogenesis of hypoventilation. Isolated PAH is relatively rare, and although it occurs in all age groups, the majority of reported cases have been in males aged 20 to 50 years. The disorder typically develops insidiously and often first comes to attention when severe respiratory depression follows administration of standard doses of sedatives or anesthetics. As the degree of hypoventilation increases, patients typically develop lethargy, fatigue, daytime somnolence, disturbed sleep, and morning headaches; eventually cyanosis, polycythemia, pulmonary hypertension, and congestive heart failure occur (Fig. 263-1). Despite severe arterial blood gas derangements, dyspnea is uncommon, presumably because of impaired chemoreception and ventilatory drive. If left untreated, PAH is usually progressive over a period of months to years and ultimately fatal.

The key diagnostic finding in PAH is a chronic respiratory acidosis in the absence of respiratory muscle weakness or impaired ventilatory mechanics (Fig. 263-2). Because patients can hyperventilate voluntarily and reduce Pa_{CO_2} to normal or even hypocapnic levels, hypercapnia may not be demonstrable in a single arterial blood sample, but the presence of an elevated plasma HCO_3^- level should draw attention to the underlying chronic disturbance. Despite normal ventilatory mechanics and respiratory muscle strength, ventilatory responses to chemical stimuli are reduced or absent (Fig. 263-2), and breath-holding time may be markedly prolonged without any sensation of dyspnea.

Patients with PAH maintain rhythmic respiration when awake, although the level of ventilation is below normal. However, during sleep, when breathing is critically dependent on the metabolic control system, there is typically a further deterioration in ventilation with frequent episodes of central hypopnea or apnea.

PAH must be distinguished from other central hypoventilation

Site of defect	Responses to CO_2, hypoxia			Sleep studies	Voluntary hyperventil.	PI_{max} PE_{max}	Volume flow rates	Resistance, compliance	(A-a) Po_2
	Ventil.	P.1	EMGdi						
Metabolic control system (chemoreceptors, brainstem integrating neurons)	↓	↓	↓	↑ Hypoventil, central apneas	N	N	N	N	N
Respiratory neuromuscular system (brainstem motoneurons, spinal cord, respiratory nerves and muscles)	↓	↓	↓	↑ Hypoventil, central apneas	↓	↓	↓	N	N
Ventilatory apparatus (chest wall, lungs, airways)	↓	N	N	Variable	↓	N	Abnormal	Abnormal	↑

FIGURE 263-2   Pattern of laboratory test results in alveolar hypoventilation syndromes, based on the site of defect. Ventil, ventilation; P.1, mouth pressure generated after 0.1 s of inspiration against an occluded airway; EMGdi, diaphragmatic EMG; PI_{max}, PE_{max}, maximum inspiratory or expiratory pressure that can be generated against an occluded airway; (A − a) P_{O_2}, alveolar-arterial P_{O_2} difference; N, normal. Defects in the metabolic control system impair central respiratory drive in response to chemical stimuli (CO_2 or hypoxia); therefore responses of EMGdi, P.1, and minute volume of ventilation are reduced and hypoventilation during sleep is aggravated. In contrast, tests of voluntary respiratory control, muscle strength, lung mechanics, and gas exchange

[(A − a)P_{O_2}] are normal. Defects in the respiratory neuromuscular system impair muscle strength; therefore all tests dependent on muscular activity (voluntary or in response to metabolic stimuli) are abnormal, but lung resistance, lung compliance, and gas exchange are normal. Defects in the ventilatory apparatus usually impair gas exchange. Because resistance and compliance are also impaired, all tests dependent on ventilation (whether voluntary or in response to chemical stimuli) are abnormal; in contrast, tests of muscle activity or strength that do not involve airflow (i.e., P.1, EMGdi, PI_{max}, PE_{max}) are normal. *(After Phillipson.)*

syndromes that are secondary to underlying neurologic disease of the brainstem or chemoreceptors (Table 263-1). This distinction requires a careful neurologic investigation for evidence of brainstem or autonomic disturbances. Unrecognized respiratory neuromuscular disorders, particularly those that produce diaphragmatic weakness, are often misdiagnosed as PAH. However, such disorders can usually be suspected on clinical grounds (see below) and can be confirmed by the finding of reduced voluntary hyperventilation, as well as PI_{max} and PE_{max}.

Some patients with PAH respond favorably to respiratory stimulant medications and to supplemental oxygen. However, the majority eventually require mechanical ventilatory assistance. Excellent long-term benefits can be achieved with diaphragmatic pacing by electrophrenic stimulation or with negative- or positive-pressure mechanical ventilation. The administration of such treatment only during sleep is sufficient in most patients.

RESPIRATORY NEUROMUSCULAR DISORDERS Several primary disorders of the spinal cord, peripheral respiratory nerves, and respiratory muscles produce a chronic hypoventilation syndrome (Table 263-1). Hypoventilation usually develops gradually over a period of months to years and often first comes to attention when a relatively trivial increase in mechanical ventilatory load (such as mild airways obstruction) produces severe respiratory failure. In some of the disorders (such as motor neuron disease, myasthenia gravis, and muscular dystrophy), involvement of the respiratory nerves or muscles is usually a later feature of a more widespread disease. In other disorders, respiratory involvement can be an early or even isolated feature, and hence the underlying problem is often not suspected. Included in this category are the postpolio syndrome (a form of chronic respiratory insufficiency that develops 20 to 30 years following recovery from poliomyelitis), the myopathy associated with adult acid maltase deficiency, and idiopathic diaphragmatic paralysis.

Generally, respiratory neuromuscular disorders do not result in chronic hypoventilation unless there is significant weakness of the diaphragm. Distinguishing features of bilateral diaphragmatic weakness include orthopnea, paradoxical movement of the abdomen in the supine posture, and paradoxical diaphragmatic movement under fluoroscopy. However, the absence of these features does not exclude diaphragmatic weakness. Important laboratory features are a rapid deterioration of ventilation during a maximum voluntary ventilation maneuver and reduced PI_{max} and PE_{max} (Fig. 263-2). More sophisticated investigations reveal reduced or absent transdiaphragmatic pressures, calculated from simultaneous measurement of esophageal and gastric pressures; reduced diaphragmatic EMG responses (recorded from an esophageal electrode) to transcutaneous phrenic nerve stimulation; and marked hypopnea and arterial oxygen desaturation during rapid eye movement sleep, when there is normally a physiologic inhibition of all nondiaphragmatic respiratory muscles and breathing becomes critically dependent on diaphragmatic activity.

The management of chronic alveolar hypoventilation due to respiratory neuromuscular disease involves treatment of the underlying disorder, where feasible, and mechanical ventilatory assistance as described for the primary alveolar hypoventilation syndrome. However, electrophrenic diaphragmatic pacing is contraindicated in these disorders, except for high cervical spinal cord lesions in which the phrenic lower motor neurons and nerves are intact.

OBESITY-HYPOVENTILATION SYNDROME Massive obesity represents a mechanical load to the respiratory system because the added weight on the rib cage and abdomen serves to reduce the compliance of the chest wall. As a result, the functional residual capacity (i.e., end-expiratory lung volume) is reduced, particularly in the recumbent posture. An important consequence of breathing at a low lung volume is that some airways, particularly those in the lung bases, may be closed throughout part or even all of each tidal breath, resulting in underventilation of the lung bases and widening of the $(A - a)P_{O_2}$. Nevertheless, in the majority of obese individuals, central respiratory drive is increased sufficiently to maintain a normal Pa_{CO_2}. However, a small proportion of obese patients develop chronic hypercapnia, hypoxemia, and eventually polycythemia, pulmonary hypertension, and

right-sided heart failure. Recent studies in mice demonstrate that genetically obese mice lacking circulating leptin also develop chronic hypoventilation that can be reversed by leptin infusions. Those patients who also develop daytime somnolence have been designated as having the *Pickwickian syndrome* (Chap. 27). In many such patients, obstructive sleep apnea is a prominent feature, and even in those patients without sleep apnea, sleep-induced hypoventilation is an important element of the disorder and contributes to its progression. Most patients demonstrate a decrease in central respiratory drive, which may be inherent or acquired, and many have mild to moderate degrees of airflow obstruction, usually related to smoking. Based on these considerations, several therapeutic measures can be of considerable benefit, including weight loss, cessation of smoking, elimination of obstructive sleep apnea, and enhancement of respiratory drive by medications such as progesterone.

HYPERVENTILATION AND ITS SYNDROMES

DEFINITION AND ETIOLOGY Alveolar hyperventilation exists when Pa_{CO_2} decreases below the normal range of 37 to 43 mmHg. *Hyperventilation* is not synonymous with *hyperpnea*, which refers to an increased minute volume of ventilation without reference to Pa_{CO_2}. Although hyperventilation is frequently associated with dyspnea, patients who are hyperventilating do not necessarily complain of shortness of breath; and conversely, patients with dyspnea need not be hyperventilating.

Numerous disease entities can be associated with alveolar hyperventilation (Table 263-2), but in all cases the underlying mechanism involves an increase in respiratory drive that is mediated through either the behavioral or the metabolic respiratory control systems (Fig. 263-3). Thus hypoxemia drives ventilation by stimulating the peripheral chemoreceptors, and several pulmonary disorders and congestive heart failure drive ventilation by stimulating afferent vagal receptors in the lungs and airways. Low cardiac output and hypotension stimulate the peripheral chemoreceptors and inhibit the baroreceptors, both of which increase ventilation. Metabolic acidosis, a potent respiratory stimulant, excites both the peripheral and central chemoreceptors and increases the sensitivity of the peripheral chemoreceptors to coexistent hypoxemia. Hepatic failure can also produce hyperventilation, presumably as a result of metabolic stimuli acting on the peripheral and central chemoreceptors.

Several neurologic and psychological disorders are thought to drive ventilation through the behavioral respiratory control system. Included in this category are psychogenic or anxiety hyperventilation and severe cerebrovascular insufficiency, which may interfere with the inhibitory influence normally exerted by cortical structures on the

Table 263-2 Hyperventilation Syndromes

1. Hypoxemia
   a. High altitude
   b. Pulmonary disease
   c. Cardiac shunts
2. Pulmonary disorders
   a. Pneumonia
   b. Interstitial pneumonitis, fibrosis, edema
   c. Pulmonary emboli, vascular disease
   d. Bronchial asthma
   e. Pneumothorax
   f. Chest wall disorders
3. Cardiovascular disorders
   a. Congestive heart failure
   b. Hypotension
4. Metabolic disorders
   a. Acidosis (diabetic, renal, lactic)
   b. Hepatic failure
5. Neurologic and psychogenic disorders
   a. Psychogenic or anxiety hyperventilation
   b. Central nervous system infection, tumors
6. Drug-induced
   a. Salicylates
   b. Methylxanthine derivatives
   c. β-Adrenergic agonists
   d. Progesterone
7. Miscellaneous
   a. Fever, sepsis
   b. Pain
   c. Pregnancy

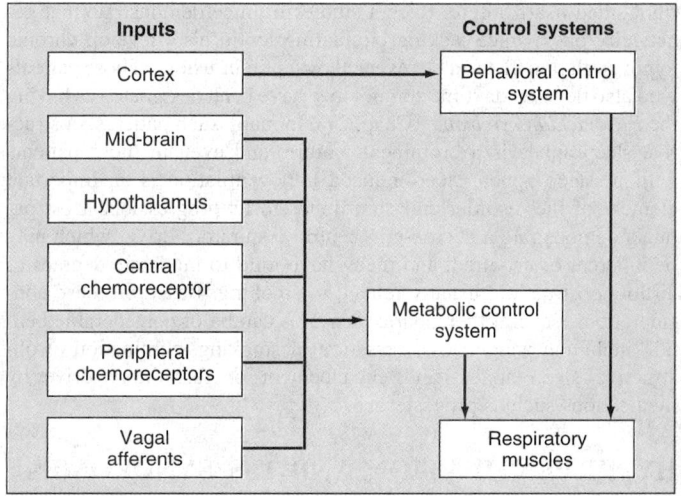

FIGURE 263-3 Schematic diagram of the mechanisms involved in alveolar hyperventilation. *(From Slutsky and Phillipson.)*

brainstem respiratory neurons. Rarely, disorders of the midbrain and hypothalamus induce hyperventilation, and it is conceivable that fever and sepsis also cause hyperventilation through effects on these structures. Several drugs cause hyperventilation by stimulating the central or peripheral chemoreceptors or by direct action on the brainstem respiratory neurons. Chronic hyperventilation is a normal feature of pregnancy and results from the effects of progesterone and other hormones acting on the respiratory neurons.

PHYSIOLOGIC AND CLINICAL FEATURES   Because hyperventilation is associated with increased respiratory drive, muscle effort, and minute volume of ventilation, the most frequent symptom associated with hyperventilation is dyspnea. However, there is considerable discrepancy between the degree of hyperventilation, as measured by Pa_{CO_2}, and the degree of associated dyspnea. From a physiologic standpoint, hyperventilation is beneficial in patients who are hypoxemic, because the alveolar hypocapnia is associated with an increase in alveolar and arterial P_{O_2}. Conversely, hyperventilation can also be detrimental. In particular, the alkalemia associated with hypocapnia may produce neurologic symptoms, including dizziness, visual impairment, syncope, and seizure activity (secondary to cerebral vasoconstriction); parasthesia, carpopedal spasm, and tetany (secondary to decreased free serum calcium); and muscle weakness (secondary to hypophosphatemia). Severe alkalemia can also induce cardiac arrhythmias and evidence of myocardial ischemia. Patients with a primary respiratory alkalosis are also prone to periodic breathing and central sleep apnea (Chap. 264).

DIAGNOSIS   In most patients with a hyperventilation syndrome, the cause is readily apparent on the basis of history, physical examination, and knowledge of coexisting medical disorders (Table 263-2). In patients in whom the cause is not clinically apparent, investigation begins with arterial blood gas analysis, which establishes the presence of alveolar hyperventilation (decreased Pa_{CO_2}) and its severity. Equally important is the arterial pH, which generally allows the disorder to be classified as either a primary respiratory alkalosis (elevated pH) or a primary metabolic acidosis (decreased pH). Also of importance is the Pa_{O_2} and calculation of the $(A - a)P_{O_2}$, since a widened alveolar-arterial oxygen difference suggests a pulmonary disorder as the underlying cause. The finding of a reduced plasma HCO_3^- level establishes the chronic nature of the disorder and points toward an organic cause. Measurements of ventilation and arterial or transcutaneous P_{CO_2} during sleep are very useful in suspected psychogenic hyperventilation, since such patients do not maintain the hyperventilation during sleep.

The disorders that most frequently give rise to unexplained hyperventilation are pulmonary vascular disease (particularly chronic or recurrent thromboembolism) and psychogenic or anxiety hyperventilation. Hyperventilation due to pulmonary vascular disease is associated with exertional dyspnea, a widened $(A - a)P_{O_2}$ and maintenance of hyperventilation during exercise. In contrast, patients with psychogenic hyperventilation typically complain of dyspnea at rest and not during mild exercise and of the need to sigh frequently. They are also more likely to complain of dizziness, sweating, palpitations, and paresthesia. During mild to moderate exercise, their hyperventilation tends to disappear and $(A - a)P_{O_2}$ is normal, but heart rate and cardiac output may be increased relative to metabolic rate.

TREATMENT   Alveolar hyperventilation is usually of relatively minor clinical consequence and therefore is generally managed by appropriate treatment of the underlying cause. In the few patients in whom alkalemia is thought to be inducing significant cerebral vasoconstriction, paresthesia, tetany, or cardiac disturbances, inhalation of a low concentration of CO_2 can be very beneficial. For patients with disabling psychogenic hyperventilation, careful explanation of the basis of their symptoms can be reassuring and is often sufficient. Others have benefited from β-adrenergic antagonists or an exercise program. Specific treatment for anxiety may also be indicated.

BIBLIOGRAPHY

FANBURG BL, SICILIAN L (eds): Respiratory dysfunction in neuromuscular disease. Clin Chest Med 15:(4)607, 1994

KATZ ES et al: Late-onset central hypoventilation with hypothlmic dysfunction: A distinct clinical syndrome. Pediatr Pulmonol 29:62, 2000

O'DONNELL CP et al: Leptin prevents respiratory depression in obesity. Am J Respir Crit Care Med 159:1477, 1999

PHILLIPSON EA, SLUTSKY AS: Hypoventilation and hyperventilation syndromes, in *Textbook of Respiratory Medicine*, 3d ed, JF Murray, JA Nadel (eds). Philadelphia, Saunders, 2000, pp 2139–2152

SLUTSKY AS, PHILLIPSON EA: Hyperventilation syndromes, in *Textbook of Respiratory Medicine*, JF Murray, JA Nadel (eds). Philadelphia, Saunders, 1994, chap 85, pp 2325–2332

TANKERSLEY CG et al: Genetic control of differential baseline breathing pattern. J Appl Physiol 82:874, 1997

264   *Eliot A. Phillipson*

SLEEP APNEA

DEFINITION AND CLASSIFICATION   *Sleep apnea* is defined as an intermittent cessation of airflow at the nose and mouth during sleep. By convention, apneas of at least 10 s duration have been considered important, but in most patients the apneas are 20 to 30 s in duration and may be as long as 2 to 3 min. *Sleep apnea syndrome* refers to a clinical disorder that arises from recurrent apneas during sleep. The clinical importance of sleep apnea arises from the fact that it is one of the leading causes of excessive daytime sleepiness. Indeed, epidemiologic studies have established a prevalence of clinically important sleep apnea of at least 2% in middle-aged women and 4% in middle-aged men.

Sleep apneas can be central or obstructive in type. In central sleep apnea (CSA) the neural drive to all the respiratory muscles is transiently abolished. In contrast, in obstructive sleep apnea (OSA) airflow ceases despite continuing respiratory drive because of occlusion of the oropharyngeal airway.

OBSTRUCTIVE SLEEP APNEA   Pathogenesis   The definitive event in OSA is occlusion of the upper airway usually at the level of the oropharynx. The resulting apnea leads to progressive asphyxia until there is a brief arousal from sleep, whereupon airway patency is restored and airflow resumes. The patient then returns to sleep, and the sequence of events is repeated, often up to 400 to 500 times per night, resulting in marked fragmentation of sleep.

The immediate factor leading to collapse of the upper airway in OSA is the generation of a critical subatmospheric pressure during inspiration that exceeds the ability of the airway dilator and abductor muscles to maintain airway stability. During wakefulness, upper airway muscle activity is greater than normal in patients with OSA, presumably to compensate for airway narrowing (see below) and a high upper airway resistance. Sleep plays a permissive but crucial role by reducing the activity of the muscles and their protective reflex response to subatmospheric airway pressures. Alcohol is frequently an important cofactor because of its selective depressant influence on the upper airway muscles and on the arousal response that terminates each apnea. In most patients the patency of the airway is also compromised structurally and therefore predisposed to occlusion. In a minority of patients the structural compromise is due to obvious anatomic disturbances, such as adenotonsillar hypertrophy, retrognathia, and macroglossia. However, in the majority of patients the structural defect is simply a subtle reduction in airway size that can often be appreciated clinically as "pharyngeal crowding" and that can usually be demonstrated by imaging and acoustic reflection techniques. Obesity frequently contributes to the reduction in size of the upper airways, either by increasing fat deposition in the soft tissues of the pharynx or by compressing the pharynx by superficial fat masses in the neck. More sophisticated studies also demonstrate a high airway compliance—i.e., the airway is "floppy" and therefore prone to collapse.

FIGURE 264-1 The primary sequence of events, physiologic responses, and clinical features of obstructive sleep apnea.

Pathophysiologic and Clinical Features The narrowing of the upper airways during sleep, which predisposes to OSA, inevitably results in snoring. In most patients, snoring antedates the development of obstructive events by many years. However, the majority of snoring individuals do not have an OSA disorder, nor is there definitive evidence that snoring per se is associated with long-term health risks. Hence, in the absence of other symptoms, snoring alone does not warrant an investigation for OSA but does call for preventive counselling, particularly with regard to weight gain and alcohol consumption.

The recurrent episodes of nocturnal asphyxia and of arousal from sleep that characterize OSA lead to a series of secondary physiologic events, which in turn give rise in some patients to the clinical complications of the syndrome (Fig. 264-1). The most common manifestations are neuropsychiatric and behavioral disturbances that are thought to arise from the fragmentation of sleep and loss of slow-wave sleep induced by the recurrent arousal responses. Nocturnal cerebral hypoxia may also play an important role. The most pervasive manifestation is excessive daytime sleepiness. Initially, daytime sleepiness manifests under passive conditions, such as reading or watching television; but as the disorder progresses, sleepiness encroaches into all daily activities and can become disabling and dangerous. Several studies have demonstrated two to seven times more motor vehicle accidents in patients with OSA compared with other drivers. Other related symptoms include intellectual impairment, memory loss, and personality disturbances.

The other major manifestations of OSA are cardiorespiratory in nature and are thought to arise from the recurrent episodes of nocturnal asphyxia and of negative intrathoracic pressure, which increases left ventricular afterload (Fig. 264-1). Many patients demonstrate a cyclical slowing of the heart during the apneas to 30 to 50 beats per minute, followed by a tachycardia of 90 to 120 beats per minute during the ventilatory phase. A small number of patients develop severe bradycardia or dangerous tachyarrhythmias, leading to the notion that OSA may result in sudden death during sleep, but firm corroborative data are lacking. Unlike in healthy subjects, in patients with OSA systemic blood pressure fails to decrease during sleep. In fact, blood pressure typically rises abruptly at the termination of each obstructive event as a result of sympathetic nervous activation and reflex vasoconstriction. Furthermore, over 50% of patients with OSA have systemic hypertension. Several epidemiologic studies have implicated OSA as a risk factor for the development of systemic hypertension, and recent studies in an animal model demonstrate directly that OSA can cause sustained increases in daytime blood pressure. Emerging data also suggest that OSA can precipitate myocardial ischemia in patients with coronary artery disease and can adversely affect left ventricular function, both acutely and chronically, in patients with congestive heart failure. This complication is probably due to the combined effects of increased left ventricular afterload during each obstructive event, secondary to increased negative intrathoracic pressure (Fig. 264-1), recurrent nocturnal hypoxemia, and chronically elevated sympathoadrenal activity. Treatment of OSA in such patients often results in dramatic improvement in left ventricular function and in clinical cardiac status. Finally, up to 20% of patients with OSA develop mild pulmonary hypertension (in the absence of intrinsic lung disease), and a small proportion (<10%) develop pulmonary hypertension, right ventricular failure, polycythemia, and chronic hypercapnia and hypoxemia. All such patients have evidence of sustained daytime hypoxemia in addition to the nocturnal ventilatory disturbance, usually as a result of reduced ventilatory drive and/or diffuse airways obstruction.

Diagnosis Although OSA occurs at any age, and is more prevalent in women than was previously thought, the typical patient is a male aged 30 to 60 years who presents with a history of snoring, excessive daytime sleepiness, nocturnal choking or gasping, witnessed apneas during sleep, moderate obesity, and often mild to moderate hypertension. The definitive investigation for suspected OSA is polysomnography, a detailed overnight sleep study that includes recording of (1) electrographic variables (electroencephalogram, electrooculogram, and submental electromyogram) that permit the identification of sleep and its various stages, (2) ventilatory variables that permit the identification of apneas and their classification as central or obstructive, (3) arterial O_2 saturation by ear or finger oximetry, and (4) heart rate. Continuous measurement of transcutaneous P_{CO_2} (which reflects arterial P_{CO_2}) can also be very useful, particularly in patients with CSA. The key diagnostic finding in OSA is episodes of airflow cessation at the nose and mouth despite evidence of continuing respiratory effort. By the time most patients come to clinical attention they have at least 10 to 15 obstructive events per hour of sleep. However, recent data suggest that a high upper airway resistance during sleep (manifested by snoring) that is accompanied by recurrent arousals from sleep, even in the absence of apneas and hypopneas, can result in a clinically important sleep-related syndrome. Therefore, the absence of outright apneas and hypopneas in a symptomatic patient may not definitely exclude a sleep-related respiratory disorder.

Because polysomnography is a time-consuming and expensive test, there is considerable interest in the role of simplified, unattended, ambulatory sleep monitoring for the investigation of OSA that would allow the patient to be studied at home, rather than in the sleep laboratory. The most useful test in this context is the recording of arterial O_2 saturation by oximetry. However, the reliability of overnight oximetry in the diagnosis of OSA is dependent on the pretest probability of the disorder. In patients with a high pretest probability (based on a history of daytime sleepiness, habitual snoring, nocturnal choking or gasping, and witnessed apneas during sleep), overnight oximetry can be used to *confirm* the diagnosis by demonstrating recurrent episodes of arterial O_2 desaturation (at a rate of at least 10 to 15 events per hour). Such findings obviate the need for full polysomnography and allow initiation of treatment with nasal continuous positive airway pressure (CPAP) during sleep (see "Treatment"). However, negative results in a patient with a high clinical probability of OSA do not exclude the diagnosis but mandate that the patient proceed to polysomnography to investigate the cause of the daytime sleepiness. In contrast, when the pretest probability of OSA is low (such as the patient with only occasional snoring, few witnessed apneas, and no daytime sleepiness), the absence of arterial O_2 desaturation can be used to *exclude* the diagnosis and thereby obviate the need for full polysomnography.

Studies suggest that overnight oximetry can obviate the need for polysomnography in about one-third of clinic patients referred for consideration of OSA, either by *confirming* the diagnosis in patients with a *high* pretest probability of the disorder, or by *excluding* the diagnosis in patients with a *low* pretest probability. In the remaining two-thirds of patients with an intermediate pretest probability of OSA, overnight oximetry alone will not be definitive; hence such patients will require polysomnography.

℞ **TREATMENT** (Table 264-1) Several approaches to treatment of OSA have been advocated, based on an understanding of the mechanisms underlying the disorder. Mild to moderate OSA can often be managed effectively by modest weight reduction, avoidance of alcohol, improvement of nasal patency, and avoidance of sleeping in the supine posture. Intraoral appliances, designed to keep the mandible and tongue forward, are also effective in 55 to 80% of patients. The most widely used treatments in severe OSA are uvulopalatopharyngoplasty and nasal CPAP during sleep. Uvulopalatopharyngoplasty is a surgical procedure designed to increase the pharyngeal lumen by resecting redundant soft tissue. When applied to unselected patients with OSA, it produces long-term cure in fewer than 50% but more discriminating selection of patients yields a higher rate of success. Other surgical approaches, including mandibular advancement and hyoid osteotomy have a more limited application but higher rate of success in selected patients. Nasal CPAP, which prevents upper airway occlusion by splinting the pharyngeal airway with a positive pressure delivered through a nose mask, is currently the most successful long-term approach to treatment, being well tolerated and effective in over 80% of patients, provided that they have received proper training. Patients who are unable to tolerate conventional nasal CPAP may re-

Table 264-1 Management of Obstructive Sleep Apnea (OSA)

Mechanism	Mild to Moderate OSA	Moderate to Severe OSA
↑ Upper airway muscle tone	Avoidance of alcohol, sedatives	—
↑ Upper airway lumen size	Weight reduction	Uvulopalatopharyngoplasty
	Avoidance of supine posture	
	Oral prosthesis	
↓ Upper airway subatmospheric pressure	Improved nasal patency	Nasal continuous positive airway pressure
Bypass occlusion		Tracheostomy

SOURCE: Phillipson, with permission.

spond to newer generation devices that provide more flexibility in adjusting the timing and levels of inspiratory and expiratory pressure cycles. For patients with ischemic heart disease or congestive heart failure who also have OSA, nasal CPAP is the only treatment that has been specifically tested and is considered the treatment of choice. Finally, for the few patients with severe OSA in whom all other treatment approaches have failed, tracheostomy can provide immediate relief, but in most centers is performed only very rarely.

CENTRAL SLEEP APNEA Pathogenesis The definitive event in CSA is transient abolition of central drive to the ventilatory muscles. The resulting apnea leads to a primary sequence of events similar to those of OSA (Fig. 264-1). Several underlying mechanisms can result in cessation of respiratory drive during sleep (Table 264-2). First are defects in the metabolic respiratory control system and respiratory neuromuscular apparatus. Such defects usually produce a chronic alveolar hypoventilation syndrome (in addition to CSA) that becomes more severe during sleep when the stimulatory effect of wakefulness on breathing is abolished. In contrast are CSA disorders that arise from transient instabilities in an otherwise intact respiratory control system. Common to all these disorders is a P_{CO_2} level during sleep that falls transiently below the critical P_{CO_2} required for respiratory rhythm generation. The most frequent instability of this type occurs at sleep onset, because the P_{CO_2} level of wakefulness is often lower than that required for rhythm generation in sleep; hence with loss of the stimulatory effect of wakefulness on breathing (referred to as the *waking neural drive*), an apnea develops at sleep onset until P_{CO_2} rises to the critical level (Fig. 264-2). However, if the central nervous system state fluctuates at sleep onset between "asleep" and "awake," a pattern of periodic breathing develops as respiration follows the changes in state. During each cycle, the waning phase of ventilation includes an hypopnea or outright central apnea (Cheyne-Stokes respiration). In most patients with CSA, the tendency to develop periodic breathing and central apneas during sleep is enhanced by some degree of chronic hyperventilation during wakefulness that

Table 264-2 Mechanisms Underlying Central Sleep Apnea

Underlying Mechanism	Clinical Example
Defects in metabolic control system or respiratory muscles	Primary and secondary central alveolar hypoventilation syndromes
	Respiratory muscle weakness
Transient instabilities in central respiratory drive	Sleep onset
	Hyperventilation-induced hypocapnia
	Idiopathic
	Hypoxia (high altitude, pulmonary disease)
	Cardiovascular disease, pulmonary congestion
	Central nervous system disease
	Prolonged circulation time

SOURCE: Phillipson, with permission.

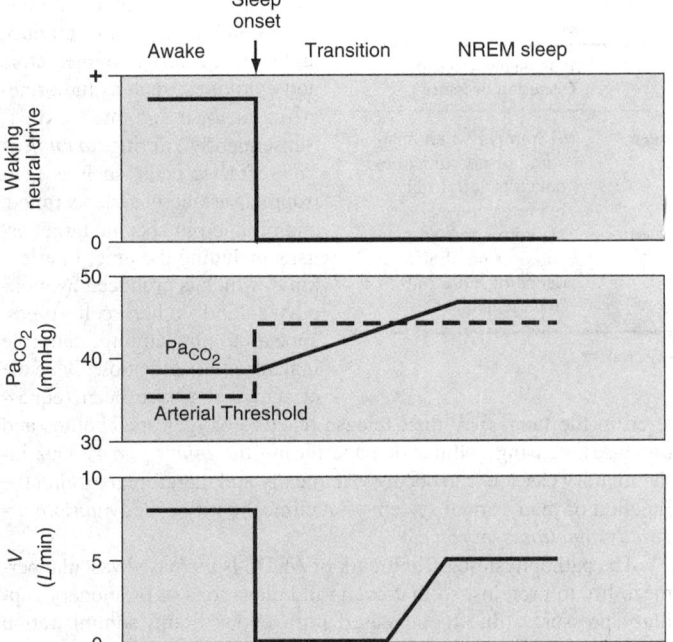

FIGURE 264-2 Schematic diagram of the mechanisms underlying central sleep apnea at sleep onset. With loss of the waking neural drive to breathing, the arterial threshold P_{CO_2} for rhythm generation increases above the Pa_{CO_2} present during wakefulness; ventilation (V) falls to zero and apnea ensues until Pa_{CO_2} rises above the threshold for rhythm generation during sleep. NREM, non-rapid eye movement. (*From TD Bradley, EA Phillipson, Clin Chest Med 13:439, 1992.*)

drives the P_{CO_2} level below the threshold required for rhythm generation during sleep. Such hyperventilation is frequently idiopathic in nature. Hypoxia, whether due to high altitude or to underlying cardiorespiratory disease, also enhances the tendency to periodic breathing and CSA for the same reasons. Periodic breathing and CSA are also common in patients with congestive heart failure. In such patients the decreases in Pa_{CO_2} that trigger transient abolition of central respiratory drive are associated with higher left ventricular end-diastolic volume and filling pressure than in congestive heart failure patients without CSA. The hyperventilation probably results, therefore, from pulmonary congestion and stimulation of pulmonary vagal receptors.

Pathophysiologic and Clinical Features Many healthy individuals demonstrate a small number of central apneas during sleep, particularly at sleep onset and in rapid eye movement sleep. These apneas are not associated with any physiologic or clinical disturbances. In patients with clinically important CSA, the primary sequence of events that characterizes the disorder leads to prominent physiologic and clinical consequences (Fig. 264-1). In those patients whose CSA is a component of an alveolar hypoventilation syndrome, daytime hypercapnia and hypoxemia are usually evident, and the clinical picture is dominated by a history of recurrent respiratory failure, polycythemia, pulmonary hypertension, and right-sided heart failure. Complaints of sleeping poorly, morning headache, and daytime fatigue and sleepiness are also prominent. In contrast, in patients whose CSA results from an instability in respiratory drive, the clinical picture is dominated by features related to sleep disturbance, including recurrent nocturnal awakenings, morning fatigue, and daytime sleepiness. In patients with congestive heart failure, CSA can be an important (and frequently overlooked) cause of daytime sleepiness and fatigue. Recent studies also indicate that CSA can trigger sympathetic nervous activation in patients with heart failure and thereby exert a secondary deleterious effect on the underlying cardiac disorder.

Diagnosis Initially, many patients with CSA are suspected clinically of having OSA because of a history of snoring, sleep disturbance, and daytime sleepiness. However, obesity and hypertension are less prominent in CSA than in OSA. Definitive diagnosis of CSA requires a polysomnographic study, with the *key observation being recurrent apneas that are not accompanied by respiratory effort*. Measurements of transcutaneous P_{CO_2} are particularly useful in CSA. Those patients with a defect in respiratory control or neuromuscular function typically demonstrate an elevated P_{CO_2} that tends to increase progressively during the night, particularly during rapid eye movement sleep. In contrast, patients with instabilities in the respiratory control system typically demonstrate a mild degree of hypocapnia, which is an integral pathogenetic feature of their disorder (see above).

TREATMENT The management of patients whose CSA is a component of an alveolar hypoventilation syndrome is essentially the same as management of the underlying hypoventilation disorder (Chap. 263). Management of patients whose CSA arises from an instability of respiratory drive is more problematic. Patients with hypoxemia usually respond favorably to nocturnal supplemental oxygen. Others have responded to acidification with acetazolamide, and recent reports indicate a good response to nasal CPAP (as for OSA). The mechanism by which CPAP abolishes central apneas probably involves a small increase in Pa_{CO_2} as a result of the added expiratory mechanical load. In patients whose CSA is secondary to congestive heart failure, CPAP is particularly effective in improving sleep quality and daytime cardiac function. In fact, recent randomized trials have demonstrated that CPAP has a beneficial effect on several surrogate markers of mortality in patients with congestive heart failure, including left ventricular ejection fraction, functional mitral regurgitation, and norepinephrine concentrations.

BIBLIOGRAPHY

AMERICAN THORACIC SOCIETY: Indications and standards for use of nasal continuous positive airway pressure (CPAP) in sleep apnea syndromes. Am J Respir Crit Care Med 150:1738, 1994

BRADLEY TD, PHILLIPSON EA: Sleep disorders, in *Textbook of Respiratory Medicine*, 3d ed, JF Murray, JA Nadel (eds). Philadelphia, Saunders, 2000, pp 2153–2170

BROOKS D et al: Obstructive sleep apnea as a cause of systemic hypertension: Evidence from a canine model. J Clin Invest 99:106, 1997

DEEGAN PC, McNICHOLAS WT: Pathophysiology of obstructive sleep apnoea. Eur Respir J 8:1161, 1995

JAVAHERI S et al: Sleep apnea in 81 ambulatory male patients with stable heart failure. Circulation 97:2154, 1998

PHILLIPS BG, SOMERS VK: Neural and humeral mechanisms mediating cardiovascular responses to obstructive sleep apnea. Resp Physiol 119:181, 2000

TERAN-SANTOS J et al: The association between sleep apnea and the risk of traffic accidents. N Engl J Med 340:847, 1999

YOUNG T et al: Population-based study of sleep-disordered breathing as a risk factor for hypertension. Arch Intern Med 157:1746, 1997

265 *Marc Moss, Roland H. Ingram, Jr.*

ACUTE RESPIRATORY DISTRESS SYNDROME

Lung injury in acute respiratory distress syndrome (ARDS) is characterized by increased permeability of the alveolar-capillary membrane, diffuse alveolar damage, and the accumulation of proteinaceous pulmonary edema. This clinical syndrome was first described in the archival literature by military physicians when respiratory failure occurred in battlefield casualties during World Wars I and II. However, it was not until the 1960s, when mechanical ventilation was used for patients with acute respiratory failure, that ARDS was first officially named. Initially the "A" in ARDS stood for "adult" to differentiate this syndrome from the infantile respiratory distress syndrome. With the more recent recognition that ARDS occurs in all age groups, the "A" now stands for "acute."

Table 265-1 Recommended Criteria for Acute Lung Injury (ALI) and Acute Respiratory Distress Syndrome (ARDS)

	Timing	Oxygenation	Chest Radiograph	Pulmonary Arterial Occlusion Pressure
ALI Criteria	Acute onset	$Pa_{O_2}/FI_{O_2} \leq 300$ mmHg (regardless of PEEP level)	Bilateral infiltrates seen on frontal chest radiograph	≤ 18 mmHg when measured or no clinical evidence of left atrial hypertension
ARDS Criteria	Acute onset	$Pa_{O_2}/FI_{O_2} \leq 200$ mmHg (regardless of PEEP level)	Bilateral infiltrates seen on frontal chest radiograph	≤ 18 mmHg when measured or no clinical evidence of left atrial hypertension

NOTE: Pa_{O_2}, arterial oxygen tension; FI_{O_2}, inspiratory O_2 fraction; PEEP, positive end-expiratory pressure.
SOURCE: From Bernard et al.

The diagnostic criteria used to define ARDS have evolved over the past three decades. Originally, most definitions required three general criteria: severe hypoxemia, decreased pulmonary compliance, and diffuse pulmonary infiltrates on chest radiograph. With the increasing utilization of pulmonary arterial catheters in the intensive care unit, ARDS was noted to be a "noncardiogenic" form of pulmonary edema (Chap. 32). Subsequently, some proposed definitions of ARDS required documentation of a normal pulmonary arterial occlusion pressure. However, due to the lack of an established definition and the recognition that ARDS is the severe form of a wide spectrum of lung injury, an American-European Consensus Conference proposed a new definition of ARDS that is now uniformly accepted (Table 265-1). Acute lung injury, which is a mild form of ARDS, was also defined and differs from ARDS based on less severe hypoxemia (Table 265-1).

CLINICAL CHARACTERISTICS Many predisposing factors are associated with the development of ARDS, including conditions that injure the lung directly and those that produce damage through indirect mechanisms via the hematogenous delivery of inflammatory mediators (Table 265-2). The most common of these at-risk conditions are severe sepsis, major trauma, and aspiration of gastric contents. In general, 30 to 40% of individuals with at least one of these diagnoses will eventually develop ARDS. This incidence increases in patients with more than one at-risk condition. A history of chronic alcohol abuse is also associated with an increased risk of developing ARDS in critically ill patients with an at-risk diagnosis.

ARDS occurs within 5 days of the initial at-risk diagnosis in the majority of patients, and over 50% will develop ARDS in the first 24 h. The earliest clinical sign is often an increase in the respiratory frequency, followed by dyspnea. There are no characteristic laboratory abnormalities for ARDS patients except those related to a specific underlying condition, such as leukocytosis in sepsis or an elevated serum amylase level in pancreatitis. Radiographically, the lung fields may be clear initially; diffuse bilateral interstitial or alveolar infiltrates occur as ARDS develops (Fig. 265-1). Though these radiographic changes appear homogeneous on chest radiograph, computed tomography demonstrates a heterogeneous pattern with a predominance of infiltrates in the dependent regions of the lung (Fig. 265-2).

PATHOPHYSIOLOGY ARDS may be the pulmonary manifestation of a systemic process and is the consequence of an overexpression of the normal inflammatory response. This inflammatory cascade has been divided into three overlapping phases—initiation, amplification, and injury. During *initiation*, a precipitating event, such as sepsis, causes both immune and nonimmune cells to produce and release a variety of mediators and cytokines, such as tumor necrosis factor α and interleukin 1. Subsequently, during *amplification*, effector cells, such as neutrophils, are activated, recruited, and retained in specific target organs including the lung. Interleukin 8, which is produced by monocytes and other cell types, appears to play an important role in neutrophil activation. Once the effector cells have been sequestered in the lung, they then release reactive oxygen metabolites and proteases, causing cellular damage during the *injury phase*. This inflammatory cascade can occur systemically and therefore may alter the function of many organ systems—a clinical entity called *multiple organ dysfunction syndrome*.

The pathophysiologic hallmark of ARDS is increased vascular permeability to proteins, so that even mild elevations of pulmonary capillary pressures (due to increased intravenous liquid administration and/or myocardial depression, which may occur in sepsis) greatly increase interstitial and alveolar edema. Alveolar damage is further exaggerated by the quantitative reduction is surfactant synthesis due to injury to type II pneumocytes as well as to further qualitative abnormalities in the size, composition, and metabolism of the remaining surfactant pool, leading to alveolar collapse. Although these atelectatic and liquid-filled regions of the lung contribute to a reduction in the compliance of the lung as a whole, significant regions of nondependent lung have relatively normal mechanical and gas-exchanging properties. However, the decreased overall pulmonary compliance requires large inspiratory pressures to be generated by the respiratory muscles, resulting in an increase in the work of breathing.

Though ARDS is not routinely considered a disease of the airways, airway resistance may be increased due to bronchial wall edema and cytokine-mediated bronchospasm. Pulmonary vascular resistance and pulmonary arterial pressures may also be elevated as a result of in-

Table 265-2 Conditions That May Lead to the Acute Respiratory Distress Syndrome

Direct injury to alveolar epithelium	Indirect lung injury
Aspiration of gastric contents	Sepsis syndrome
Diffuse pulmonary infection	Severe nonthoracic trauma
Near drowning	Hypertransfusion
Pulmonary contusion	Pancreatitis
Toxic inhalation	Cardiopulmonary bypass

FIGURE 265-1 A standard posteroanterior chest radiograph from a patient with acute respiratory distress syndrome secondary to a severe viral pneumonitis. Such a diffuse radiographic change is typical of all conditions listed in Table 265-2 when they are severe enough to cause acute hypoxemic respiratory failure. A similar radiographic picture is also seen in pulmonary edema due to left ventricular failure (Chap. 32).

creased pulmonary vascular smooth-muscle tone, perivascular edema, microvascular thrombosis, and the production of humoral factors such as leukotrienes and thromboxane A_2, which can directly cause vasoconstriction.

PATHOLOGY During the initial exudative phase, covering the first few days after lung injury, the following occur: (1) epithelial cell injury represented by extensive necrosis of type I pneumocytes and a denuded basement membrane, (2) swelling of endothelial cells with the widening of intercellular junctions, (3) the formation of hyaline membranes composed of fibrin and other matrix proteins in alveolar ducts and airspaces, and (4) a neutrophilic inflammation. Fibrin thrombi may be seen in the alveolar capillaries and smaller pulmonary arteries. The second pathologic phase of ARDS is characterized by proliferation of a variety of cells and resolution of the neutrophilic inflammation. Cuboidal type II cells and squamous epithelium cover denuded alveolar basement membranes. Over the ensuing days to weeks, architectural restoration of lung tissue is usually observed in survivors of ARDS. However, interstitial fibrosis and extensive restructuring of the lung parenchyma may occur with cystic and honeycomb changes in some ARDS patients, resulting in chronic pulmonary dysfunction or death.

FIGURE 265-2 Computed tomographic image of a patient with acute respiratory distress syndrome demonstrating marked heterogeneity of pulmonary infiltrates with increased density in dependent regions.

TREATMENT Currently there are no specific therapies that correct the underlying abnormalities in the permeability of the alveolar-capillary membrane or control the activated inflammatory response in patients with ARDS. However, the use of physiologically targeted strategies of mechanical ventilation and intensive care unit management have led to a more favorable outcome for these critically ill patients.

Mechanical Ventilatory Support In the presence of ARDS, adequate oxygenation is not usually maintained when oxygen is supplied through noninvasive measures. Therefore, most ARDS patients require mechanical ventilation during their hospitalization. The primary goal of the ventilatory management in ARDS is to achieve ventilation and oxygenation that are adequate to support organ function. The major complications of mechanical ventilation are oxygen toxicity and barotrauma, which include not only pneumothorax, pneumomedistinum, and subcutaneous emphysema but also primary alveolar damage. As demonstrated on computed tomography images of the lungs in ARDS patients (Fig. 265-2), a large portion of the alveoli are atelectatic or liquid-filled. However, some nondependent regions of the lung remain radiographically unaffected, and due to their greater compliance they receive a greater proportion of the tidal volume. When large tidal volumes (10 to 12 mL/kg of ideal body weight) are forced into these smaller areas, damage may occur in epithelial and endothelial cells. The sequelae of this injury include alterations in lung liquid balance, increases in permeability, and severe alveolar damage. The deleterious effects of these large tidal volumes and subsequent high alveolar pressures has been termed *volutrauma*.

The currently recommended ventilatory strategies for ARDS patients focus on the limitation of airway pressures to a maximum inflation pressure that should not exceed 30 to 35 cmH$_2$O, rather than on strategies that attempt to achieve a normal Pa$_{CO_2}$. Because of the decreased overall lung compliance in ARDS patients, the use of low tidal volumes ($\sim$ 6 mL/kg of ideal body weight) is usually required. The subsequent decrease in minute ventilation may result in hypercapnia and respiratory acidosis. This ventilatory strategy, which emphasizes the limitation of transpulmonary pressures at the expense of hypercapnia, has been termed *permissive hypercapnia*.

After intubation, the inspired oxygen fraction (FI$_{O_2}$) is initially set at 1.0 and then decreased in steps to the lowest FI$_{O_2}$ that will maintain an arterial oxygen tension (Pa$_{O_2}$) of approximately 60 mmHg. If Pa$_{O_2}$ cannot be maintained at 60 mmHg by an FI$_{O_2}$ $\leq$ 0.6, positive end-expiratory pressure (PEEP) may be added (Chap. 266). PEEP improves oxygenation by elevating mean alveolar pressure, thereby recruiting atelectatic alveoli and preventing end-expiratory airway and alveolar closure. In addition, PEEP may prevent alveolar damage by reducing the repetitive and cyclical reopening of closed alveoli during the respiratory cycle. Because PEEP may also overdistend uninvolved alveoli, it should be added cautiously, starting at 5 cmH$_2$O and increasing in increments of 3 to 5 cmH$_2$O to a maximum of 20 to 24 cmH$_2$O. Because airway pressure is transmitted to the pleural space, cardiac output may be adversely affected by the addition of PEEP. In general, the optimal level of PEEP is the amount that achieves an acceptable arterial O$_2$ saturation ($\geq$90%) with nontoxic FI$_{O_2}$ levels ($\leq$0.6) but without significantly compromising cardiac output. The comprehensive ventilatory strategy that combines low tidal volumes with adequate levels of PEEP has been termed a *lung-protective strategy*. ARDS patients ventilated with this technique have improved 28-day survival and require less time on mechanical ventilation when compared with ARDS patients treated with conventional ventilation using large tidal volumes achieving normal Pa$_{CO_2}$ levels.

Several other ventilatory strategies have been examined with the goal of improving oxygenation. However, none of these techniques has definitively been proven to be beneficial for ARDS patients. When turned from a supine to prone position, ARDS patients develop a more uniform distribution of pleural pressures, with an improvement in ventilation/perfusion matching and better postural drainage of secretions. Prone positioning may improve oxygenation in >75% of ARDS patients. However, the turning of these critically ill patients from the supine to the prone position is not without potential complications, such as unplanned extubation and removal of central venous catheters. The term *inverse ratio ventilation* is defined when the inspiratory (I) time exceeds the expiratory (E) time (i.e., > one-half of the respiratory cycle; I:E ratio > 1:1). This mode of ventilation is able to maintain a higher mean airway pressure, a major determinant of oxygenation, with lower peak airway pressures than conventional ventilation. However, due to the decrease in expiratory time, inverse ratio ventilation is potentially associated with dynamic hyperinflation and increases in end-expiratory pressure. Finally, partial liquid ventilation with perfluorocarbon, a radiopaque, inert, colorless liquid that carries a large quantity of O$_2$, and CO$_2$, has been studied in patients with severe ARDS. When perfluorocarbon is administered into the trachea of intubated patients, patients can be safely and adequately oxygenated and ventilated with routine mechanical ventilation.

Intravascular volume management Although pulmonary edema in ARDS patients is a consequence of increased permeability of the alveolar-capillary membrane, elevations in the intravascular hydrostatic pressure may also contribute to the accumulation of alveolar liquid and result in worsening oxygenation. Therefore, the optimal fluid management for patients with ARDS requires a balancing between liquid restriction, which may cause hypotension and decreased perfusion to vital organs, and liquid administration, which may increase oxygen requirements. Small decrements in the intravascular volume with diuretic use produce significant decreases in extravascular lung water. Caution must be exercised in reducing intravascular volume, since vigorous diuresis, especially in the setting of PEEP, may reduce cardiac output and perfusion of critical organs. Ideally, the lowest intravascular hydrostatic pressure that also achieves an adequate cardiac output should be maintained. The placement of a pulmonary arterial catheter may be helpful in monitoring cardiac output and pulmonary arterial occlusion pressure (a measure of intravascular volume) in order to optimize the fluid management of patients with ARDS. However, the placement of a pulmonary arterial catheter and the clinical decisions based upon information derived from the catheter do not appear to improve and may actually worsen the outcome of general intensive care unit patients. Therefore the role of the pulmonary arterial catheter for ARDS patients is presently unclear.

Pharmacologic Therapies   Due to their anti-inflammatory properties, glucocorticoids have been used in patients with ARDS, but when administered in high doses (30 mg/kg intravenously every 6 h for a total of four doses), they are not beneficial in the early course of the disease. In contrast, one small randomized study reported an improvement in mortality when glucocorticoids were given after 7 days of unresolving ARDS. In this study, active surveillance for infection was required before enrollment, and glucocorticoids were administered for up to 32 days. Future recommendations regarding the use of these drugs for ARDS patients will be based upon the results of an ongoing multicenter study.

Patients with ARDS have both quantitative and qualitative abnormalities in surfactant, rendering surfactant-replacement therapy an attractive therapeutic modality. In one large randomized study of sepsis-induced ARDS, the administration of synthetic surfactant in an aerosolized form had no significant effect on outcome. Due to concerns with the efficacy of the delivery technique and the lack of essential surfactant-associated proteins in this particular replacement therapy, further studies of different surfactant preparations and modes of administration are presently ongoing.

When inhaled, nitric oxide vasodilates the pulmonary vasculature adjacent to well-ventilated alveoli, thereby improving ventilation-perfusion mismatching. Because of its subsequent inactivation by hemoglobin, nitric oxide produces a selective pulmonary vasodilation without systemic hemodynamic effects. Though inhaled nitric oxide appears to improve oxygenation initially, it is presently unknown whether this therapy will reduce mortality rates in ARDS patients.

PROGNOSIS   Since the initial descriptions of ARDS, mortality rates have ranged from 50 to 70%, although they may now be declining with optimal therapy. Mortality rates are higher in patients over 65 years of age, in those with an at-risk diagnosis of sepsis, and when associated with dysfunction of other organ systems. The cause of death for patients with ARDS has been traditionally divided into early causes (within 72 h) and late causes (after 3 days). Most early deaths are attributed to the original presenting illness or injury. Secondary infection and sepsis, persistent respiratory failure, and multiple-organ dysfunction are the most common causes of death in those ARDS patients who live at least 3 days.

In survivors of ARDS, abnormalities in pulmonary function normally improve considerably by 3 months and reach maximum levels of correction by 6 months after extubation. Although pulmonary function markedly recovers in many survivors, over 50% of these patients will continue to have abnormalities, including restrictive impairment or decreased diffusing capacity. Patients with severe ARDS, characterized by extreme hypoxemia and a longer duration of illness, usually have more pulmonary dysfunction than individuals with mild ARDS. Survivors of ARDS also have significant reductions in their quality of life, specifically in regard to physical functioning when compared to other previously critically ill patients.

BIBLIOGRAPHY

ABRAHAM E et al: Consensus conference definitions for sepsis, septic shock, acute lung injury, and acute respiratory distress syndrome: Time for a reevaluation. Crit Care Med 28:232, 2000

AMATO MBP et al: Effect of a protective-ventilatory strategy on mortality in the acute respiratory distress syndrome. N Engl J Med 338:347, 1998

BERNARD GR et al: The American-European consensus conference on ARDS: Definitions, mechanisms, relevant outcomes, and clinical trial coordination. Am J Respir Crit Care Med 149:818, 1994

DAVIDSON TA et al: Reduced quality of life in survivors of acute respiratory distress syndrome compared with critically ill control patients. JAMA 281:354, 1999

DREYFUSS D, SAUMON G: Ventilator-induced lung injury: Lessons from experimental studies. Am J Respir Crit Care Med 157:294, 1998

FLICK MR, MATTHAY MA: Pulmonary edema and acute lung injury, in *Textbook of Respiratory Medicine*, 3d ed, JF Murray, JA Nadel (eds). Philadelphia, Saunders, 2000

MILBERG JA et al: Improved survival of patients with acute respiratory distress syndrome (ARDS):1983–1993. JAMA 273:306, 1995

WARE LB, MATTHAY MA: The acute respiratory distress syndrome. N Engl J Med 342:1334, 2000

266   Edward P. Ingenito, Jeffrey M. Drazen

MECHANICAL VENTILATORY SUPPORT

ACMV assist control mode ventilation	NIV noninvasive ventilation
ARDS acute respiratory distress syndrome	OLV open lung ventilation
	PCV pressure-control ventilation
CPAP continuous positive airway pressure	PEEP positive end-expiratory pressure
	PSV pressure-support ventilation
ECMO extracorporeal membrane oxygenation	Sa_{O_2} arterial O_2 saturation
	SIMV synchronized intermittent mandatory ventilation
IRV inverse inspiratory-to-expiratory ratio ventilation	$\dot{V}/\dot{Q}$ ventilation perfusion

Ventilators are specially designed pumps that can support the ventilatory function of the respiratory system and improve oxygenation through application of high oxygen content gas and positive pressure. They are a mainstay of physiologic supportive care and are used to stabilize patients with respiratory failure as the underlying disease process is definitively treated.

INDICATIONS FOR MECHANICAL VENTILATION

Respiratory failure is the primary indication for initiation of mechanical ventilation. There are two basic types of respiratory failure.

Hypoxemic respiratory failure most commonly results from pulmonary conditions such as severe pneumonia, pulmonary edema, pulmonary hemorrhage, and respiratory distress syndrome causing ventilation-perfusion ($\dot{V}/\dot{Q}$) mismatch and shunt. Hypoxemic respiratory failure is present when arterial O_2 saturation (Sa_{O_2}) < 90% is observed despite an inspired O_2 fraction (FI_{O_2}) > 0.6. The goal of ventilator treatment in this setting is to provide adequate Sa_{O_2} through a combination of supplemental O_2 and specific patterns of ventilation that enhance oxygenation.

Hypercarbic respiratory failure results from disease states causing either a decrease in minute ventilation or an increase in physiologic dead space such that, despite adequate total minute ventilation, alveolar ventilation is inadequate to meet metabolic demands. Common clinical conditions associated with hypercarbic respiratory failure include neuromuscular diseases, such as myasthenia gravis, ascending polyradiculopathy, and myopathies, as well as diseases that cause respiratory muscle fatigue due to increased workload, such as asthma, chronic obstructive pulmonary disease, and restrictive lung disease. *Acute* hypercarbic respiratory failure is characterized by arterial P_{CO_2} values of greater than 50 mmHg and an arterial pH above 7.30.

Mechanical ventilation generally should be instituted in acute hypercarbic respiratory failure. In contrast, the decision to institute mechanical ventilation when components of both acute and chronic hypercarbic respiratory failure are present depends on blood gas parameters and clinical evaluation. In particular, if a patient is not in respiratory distress and is not mentally impaired by CO_2 accumulation, it is not mandatory to initiate mechanical ventilation while other forms of treatment are being administered. The goal of ventilator treatment in hypercarbic respiratory failure is to normalize arterial pH through changes in CO_2 tensions. In patients with severe obstructive or restrictive lung disease, elevation in airway pressures may limit tidal volumes to the extent that normalization of pH is not possible, a situation known as *permissive hypercapnia*. Hypoxemic and hypercarbic respiratory failure may coexist in a given individual; in such cases, the indications for and goals of mechanical ventilation are similar to those in these two individual entities.

Accepted therapeutic applications of mechanical ventilation include controlled hyperventilation to reduce cerebral blood flow in patients with increased intracranial pressure or to improve pulmonary hemodynamics in patients with postoperative pulmonary hypertension. Mechanical ventilation also has been used to reduce the work of breathing in patients with congestive heart failure, especially in the presence of myocardial ischemia. Ventilator support is also frequently used in conjunction with endotracheal intubation to prevent aspiration of gastric contents in otherwise unstable patients during gastric lavage for suspected drug overdose or during upper gastrointestinal endoscopy. In the critically ill patient, intubation and mechanical ventilation are indicated before essential diagnostic or therapeutic studies if it appears that respiratory failure may occur during these maneuvers.

PHYSIOLOGIC ASPECTS OF MECHANICAL VENTILATION

Most modern mechanical ventilators function by providing warmed and humidified gas to the airway opening in conformance with various specific volume, pressure, and time patterns. The ventilator serves as the energy source for inspiration, replacing the muscles of the diaphragm and chest wall. Expiration is passive, driven by the recoil of the lungs and chest wall; at the completion of inspiration, internal ventilator circuitry vents the airway to atmospheric pressure or a specified level of positive end-expiratory pressure (PEEP).

PEEP helps maintain alveolar patency in the presence of destabilizing factors and therefore reverses hypoxemia and atelectasis by improving $\dot{V}/\dot{Q}$ matching of ventilation and perfusion. PEEP levels between 0 and 10 cmH_2O are generally safe and effective; higher levels are recommended only in the management of significant refractory hypoxemia unresponsive to increments in $F_{I_{O_2}}$ up to 0.6.

ESTABLISHING AND MAINTAINING AN AIRWAY A cuffed endotracheal tube must be inserted to allow positive-pressure ventilators to deliver conditioned gas, at pressures above atmospheric pressure, to the lungs in a controlled fashion. If neuromuscular paralysis is to be induced during intubation, the use of agents whose mechanism of action includes depolarization at the neuromuscular junction, such as succinylcholine chloride, should be avoided in patients with renal failure, tumor lysis syndrome, crush injuries, medical conditions associated with elevated serum potassium levels, and muscular dystrophy syndromes. Opiates and benzodiazepines can have a deleterious effect on hemodynamics in patients with depressed cardiac function or low systemic vascular resistance and should be used cautiously in this setting. Morphine can promote histamine release from tissue mast cells and may worsen bronchospasm in patients with asthma; fentanyl, sufentanil, and alfentanil are acceptable alternatives to morphine. Ketamine may increase systemic arterial pressure as well as intracranial pressure and has been associated with dramatic hallucinatory responses; it should be used with caution in patients with hypertensive crisis, increased intracranial pressures, or a history of psychiatric disorders.

Patients who require ventilator support for extended periods of

time may be candidates for tracheostomy. Although definitive guidelines for performing a tracheostomy in the ventilated patient have not been established, in current clinical practice patients who are anticipated to require ventilator therapy for more than 3 weeks should be considered for this procedure. While it does not clearly reduce the incidence of laryngeal injury or tracheal stenosis, tracheostomy has been associated with improved patient comfort and enhanced ability to partake in rehabilitation-oriented activities.

VENTILATOR MODES This setting specifies the manner in which ventilator breaths are triggered, cycled, and limited; commonly used modes of mechanical ventilation are given in Table 266-1. The *trigger*, either an inspiratory effort or a time-based signal, defines what the ventilator senses to initiate an assisted cycle. *Cycle* refers to the factors that determine the end of inspiration. For example, in volume-cycled ventilation, inspiration ends when a specific tidal volume is delivered to the patient. Other types of cycling include pressure cycling, time cycling, and flow cycling. *Limiting factors* are operator-specified values, such as airway pressure, that are monitored by transducers internal to the ventilator circuit throughout the respiratory cycle; if the specified values are exceeded, inspiratory flow is immediately stopped, and the ventilator circuit is vented to atmospheric pressure or the specified PEEP.

Assist Control Mode Ventilation (ACMV) An inspiratory cycle is initiated either by the patient's inspiratory effort or, if no patient effort is detected within a specified time window, by a timer signal within the ventilator. Every breath delivered consists of the operator-specified tidal volume. Ventilatory rate is determined either by the patient or by the operator-specified backup rate, whichever is of higher frequency (Fig. 266-1A). ACMV is the recommended mode for initiation of mechanical ventilation because it ensures a backup minute ventilation in the absence of an intact respiratory drive and allows for synchronization of the ventilator cycle with the patient's inspiratory effort.

Problems can arise when ACMV is used in patients with tachypnea due to nonrespiratory or nonmetabolic factors such as anxiety, pain, or airway irritation. Respiratory alkalemia may develop and trigger myoclonus or seizures. Dynamic hyperinflation (so-called auto-PEEP) may occur if the patient's respiratory mechanics are such that inadequate time is available for complete exhalation between inspiratory cycles. Auto-PEEP can limit venous return, decrease cardiac output, and increase airway pressures, predisposing to barotrauma. ACMV is not effective for weaning patients from mechanical ventilation because it provides full ventilator assistance on each patient-initiated breath.

Synchronized Intermittent Mandatory Ventilation (SIMV) The major difference between SIMV and ACMV is that in the former the patient is allowed to breathe spontaneously, i.e., without ventilator assist, between delivered ventilator breaths. However, mandatory breaths are delivered in synchrony with the patient's inspiratory efforts at a frequency determined by the operator. If the patient fails to initiate a breath, the ventilator delivers a fixed-tidal-volume breath and resets the internal timer for the next inspiratory cycle (Fig. 266-1B). SIMV differs from ACMV in that only the preset number of breaths is ventilator-assisted.

SIMV allows patients with an intact respiratory drive to exercise inspiratory muscles between assisted breaths. This characteristic makes SIMV a useful mode of ventilation for both supporting and weaning intubated patients. SIMV may be difficult to use in patients with tachypnea because they may attempt to exhale during the ventilator-programmed inspiratory cycle. When this occurs, the airway pressure may exceed the inspiratory pressure limit, the ventilator-assisted breath will be aborted, and minute volume may drop below that programmed by the operator. In this setting, if the tachypnea is in response to respiratory or metabolic acidosis, a change to ACMV will increase minute ventilation and help normalize the pH while the underlying process is further evaluated.

Continuous Positive Airway Pressure (CPAP) This is not a true support-mode of ventilation, inasmuch as all ventilation occurs

Table 266-1   Clinical Characteristics of Commonly Used Modes of Mechanical Ventilation

Ventilator Mode	Independent Variables (Set by User)	Dependent Variables (Monitored by User)	Trigger/Cycle Limit	Advantages	Disadvantages	Initial Settings
ACMV[a]	FI_{O_2} Tidal volume Ventilator rate Level of PEEP Inspiratory flow pattern Peak inspiratory flow Pressure limit	Peak airway pressure, Pa_{O_2}, Pa_{CO_2} Mean airway pressure I/E ratio	Patient/timer Pressure limit	Timer backup Patient-vent synchrony Patient controls minute ventilation	Not useful for weaning Potential for dangerous respiratory alkalosis	$FI_{O_2} = 1.0^b$ $V_t = 10-15$ mL/kg^a $f = 12-15$/min PEEP = 0-5 cmH$_2$O Inspiratory flow = 60 L/min
SIMV[a]	Same as for ACMV	Same as for ACMV	Same as for ACMV	Timer backup useful for weaning	Potential dysynchrony	Same as for ACMV[a]
CPAP	FI_{O_2} Level of CPAP	Tidal volume Rate, flow pattern Airway pressure Pa_{O_2}, Pa_{CO_2}, I/E ratio	No trigger Pressure limit	Allows assessment of spontaneous function Helps prevent atelectasis	No backup	$FI_{O_2} = 0.5-1.0^b$ CPAP = 5-15 cmH$_2$O
PCV[a]	FI_{O_2} Inspiratory pressure level Ventilator rate Level of PEEP Pressure limit I/E ratio	Tidal volume Flow rate, pattern Minute ventilation Pa_{O_2}, Pa_{CO_2}	Timer/patient Timer/pressure limit	System pressures regulated Useful for barotrauma treatment Timer backup	Requires heavy sedation Not useful for weaning	$FI_{O_2} = 1.0^b$ PC = 20-40 cmH$_2$O^a PEEP = 5-10 cmH$_2$O $f = 12-15$/min I/E = 0.7/1-4/1
PSV	FI_{O_2} Inspiratory pressure level PEEP Pressure limit	Same as for PCV + I/E ratio	Inspiratory flow Pressure limit	Assures synchrony Good for weaning	No timer backup	$FI_{O_2} = 0.5-1.0^b$ PS = 10-30 cmH$_2$O 5 cmH$_2$O usually the level used PEEP = 0-5 cmH$_2$O

[a] Open lung ventilation (OLV) involves the use of any of these specific modes with tidal volumes (or applied pressures) to achieve 5-6 mL/kg, and positive end expiratory pressures achieve maximal alveolar recruitment.

[b] FI_{O_2} is usually set to 1.0 initially, unless there is a specific clinical indication to minimize FI_{O_2}, such as history of chemotherapy with bleomycin. Once adequate oxygenation is documented by blood gas analysis, FI_{O_2} should be decreased in decrements of 0.1-0.2 as tolerated, until the lowest FI_{O_2} required for an Sa_{O_2} >90% is achieved.

ABBREVIATIONS: f, frequency; I/E, inspiration/expiration.

through the patient's spontaneous efforts. The ventilator provides fresh gas to the breathing circuit with each inspiration and charges the circuit to a constant, operator-specified pressure that can range from 0 to 20 cmH$_2$O (Fig. 266-1C). CPAP is used to assess extubation potential in patients who have been effectively weaned and are requiring little ventilator support and in patients with intact respiratory system function who require an endotracheal tube for airway protection.

Pressure-Control Ventilation (PCV)   This form of ventilation is time triggered, time cycled, and pressure limited. During the inspiratory phase, a given pressure is imposed at the airway opening, and the pressure remains at this user-specified level throughout inspiration (Fig. 266-2A). Since inspiratory airway pressure is specified by the operator, tidal volume and inspiratory flow rate are *dependent* rather than *independent* variables and are not user specified. PCV is the preferred mode of ventilation for patients with documented barotrauma, because airway pressures can be limited, and for postoperative thoracic surgical patients, in whom the shear forces across a fresh suture line should be limited. When PCV is used, minute ventilation and tidal volume must be monitored; minute ventilation is altered through changes in rate or in the pressure-control value.

The major practical limitation of PCV is patient-ventilator asynchrony related to its time-cycled and time-triggered characteristics. Because PCV requires that the patient passively accept ventilator breaths, most patients require heavy sedation to be maintained on this ventilatory mode, which may be hazardous in the hemodynamically unstable patient.

PCV with the use of a prolonged inspiratory time is frequently applied to patients with severe hypoxemic respiratory failure. This approach, called inverse inspiratory-to-expiratory ratio ventilation (IRV), increases mean distending pressures without increasing peak airway pressures. It is thought to work in conjunction with PEEP to open collapsed alveoli and improve oxygenation. IRV may be associated with fewer deleterious effects than conventional volume-cycled ventilation, which requires higher peak airway pressures to achieve an equivalent reduction in shunt fraction.

Pressure-Support Ventilation (PSV)   This form of ventilation is patient triggered, flow cycled, and pressure limited; it is specifically designed for use in the weaning process. During PSV, the inspiratory phase is terminated when inspiratory airflow falls below a certain level; in most ventilators this flow rate cannot be adjusted by the operator. When PSV is used, patients receive ventilator assist only when the ventilator detects an inspiratory effort (Fig. 266-2B). PSV also can be used in combination with SIMV to ensure volume-cycled backup for patients whose respiratory drive is depressed either spontaneously or as a result of various therapeutic maneuvers.

PSV is well tolerated by most patients who are being weaned; PSV parameters can be set to provide fully or nearly fully ventilatory support and can be withdrawn slowly over a period of days in a systematic fashion to gradually load the respiratory muscles.

Open Lung Ventilation (OLV)   OLV is not a distinct mode of ventilation, but rather a strategy for applying either volume-cycled or pressure-control ventilation to patients with severe respiratory failure. In OLV, the primary objectives of ventilator support are maintenance of adequate oxygenation and avoidance of cyclic opening and closing of alveolar units by selecting a level of PEEP that allows the majority of units to remain inflated during tidal ventilation. Achievement of eucapnia and normal blood pH through adjustments in ventilator tidal volume and breathing frequency are of lower priority. Clinical and

FIGURE 266-1 *A.* Airway pressure and lung volume versus time profile during ACMV. Assisted breaths are triggered by the patient's effort. Controlled breaths are triggered by the ventilator timer. Every breath, whether triggered by the patient or by the timer, is a complete volume-cycled breath, with airway pressure as a dependent variable. The pressure limit is set above the peak inspiratory pressure. *B.* Airway pressure and lung volume versus time profiles during SIMV. Spontaneous breaths occur between patient-triggered assisted breaths and timer-triggered breaths. The tidal volume of the spontaneous breaths is determined by the patient's effort and lung impedance. Assisted and controlled breaths are volume cycled. *C.* Airway pressure and lung volume versus time profiles during CPAP. Breathing is spontaneous, and no ventilator assist is provided. The spontaneous profile is superimposed on an elevated mean airway pressure that the user specifies. FRC, functional residual capacity.

FIGURE 266-2 *A.* Airway pressure and lung volume versus time profiles during PCV. All breaths are timer triggered, timer cycled, and pressure limited. Peak airway pressure is set by the operator, and tidal volume is a dependent variable. The profiles shown here display the pressure limit as slightly higher than pressure-control level. This need not be the case, but it is appropriate to set the pressure limit only slightly above the pressure-control level when using this mode of ventilation for management of the patient with barotrauma. *B.* Airway pressure and airway flow versus time profiles during PSV. All breaths are patient triggered and flow cycled. Inspiration is cycled off when the inspiratory flow drops below a predetermined threshold internally set in the ventilator circuit. In the example shown, the pressure limit is slightly greater than the pressure-support level. Since each can be set independently, this need not be the case. FRC, functional residual capacity.

experimental observations indicate that high airway pressures and repeated opening and closing of alveoli can cause microstructural lung damage, propagation of lung injury through generation of inflammatory cytokines, and direct barotrauma. Current data suggest that a small tidal volume (i.e., 6 mL/kg) provides adequate ventilatory support with a lower incidence of adverse effects than more conventional tidal volumes of 10-15 mL/kg. These potential complications can have dire consequences in patients with respiratory failure. Alternatively, hypercapnia and consequent respiratory acidosis tend to be well tolerated physiologically, except in patients with significant hemodynamic compromise, ventricular dysfunction, cardiac dysrrhythmias, or increased intracranial pressure. OLV has been used most extensively in the management of patients with hypoxemic respiratory failure due to acute lung injury. Although few randomized clinical trials of OLV have been performed, available data suggest that OLV reduces the morality rate and improves gas exhange in patients with acute lung injury.

Prone Positioning during Mechanical Ventilation Patients with acute respiratory distress syndrome (ARDS) experience hypoxemia as a result of intrapulmonary shunt due to regional atelectasis. Recent studies in patients with ARDS have demonstrated that collapse occurs most extensively in the dependent regions of the lung. Increasing airway pressures to counterbalance the compressive effects of the surrounding lung in these collapsed regions improves gas exchange but may result in potentially dangerous peak airway pressures. Prone positioning, in both experimental and clinical studies, reduces shunt and improves oxygenation by causing regional improvements in transpulmonary distending pressures wtihout overexpanding already patent alveoli. In clinical practice, prone positioning has been used in conjunction with both volume-cycled and pressure-control ventilation with equivalent clinical effectiveness and appears to be a useful adjunct to conventional ventilator support in patients with severe hypoxemic respiratory failure.

Noninvasive Ventilation (NIV) Noninvasive ventilator support through a tight-fitting facemask or nasal mask, traditionally used for treatment of sleep apnea, has recently been used as primary ventilator support in patients with impending respiratory failure. Facemask and nasal devices for administering NIV therapy are most frequently combined with PSV or bi-level positive airway pressure ventilation, inasmuch as both of these modes are well tolerated by the conscious patient and optimize patient-ventilator synchrony. NIV has met with varying degrees of success when applied to patients with acute or chronic respiratory failure. The major limitation to its widespread application has been patient intolerance, because the tight-fitting mask required for NIV can cause both physical and emotional discomfort in patients with dyspnea. In general, centers with experience using NIV have reported clinical success with minimal associated morbidity, whereas centers with less experience have reported more limited success. Aggressive medical therapy directed at the cause of impending respiratory failure, together with an experienced respiratory therapy and physician team, appear to be the keys to successful use of NIV in intensive care units.

Extracorporeal Membrane Oxygenation (ECMO) This nonconventional mode of ventilator support employs a large surface area membrane system connected in series with the patient's circulation to exchange CO_2 and O_2. The lung functions primarily as a passive conduit with gas exchange occurring by diffusion across the membrane. ECMO was first examined in 1970 as an alternative to positive-pressure ventilation in the management of patients with ARDS. Initial studies failed to demonstrate an improvement in survival rates among patients treated with ECMO. Although several uncontrolled trials have since suggested that ECMO does improve outcome among patients with ARDS, a 1993 study comparing survival rates of patients with ARDS treated with ECMO and those treated with conventional ventilator therapy showed no difference in mortality rates, but the morbidity rates and hospital costs were increased among ECMO-treated patients. Presently, the use of ECMO in patients with ARDS is not recommended.

GUIDELINES FOR MANAGING THE VENTILATED PATIENT

Most patients who are started on ventilator support receive ACMV or SIMV, because these modes ensure user-specified backup minute ventilation in the event that the patient fails to initiate respiratory efforts. Once the intubated patient has been stabilized with respect to oxygenation, definitive therapy for the underlying process responsible for respiratory failure is formulated and initiated. Subsequent modifications in ventilator therapy must be provided in parallel with changes in the patient's clinical status. As improvement in respiratory function is noted, the first priorities are to reduce PEEP and supplemental O_2. Once a patient can achieve adequate arterial saturation with an $F_{I_{O_2}} \leq 0.5$ and 5 cmH$_2$O PEEP, attempts should be made to reduce the level of mechanical ventilatory support. Patients previously on full ventilator support should be switched to a ventilator mode that allows for weaning, such as SIMV, PSV, or SIMV combined with PSV. Ventilator therapy can then be gradually removed, as outlined in the section on weaning. Patients whose condition continues to deteriorate after ventilator support is initiated may require increased O_2, PEEP, and alternative modes of ventilation such as IRV.

GENERAL SUPPORT IN THE VENTILATED PATIENT

Patients who are started on mechanical ventilation usually require some form of sedation and analgesia to maintain an acceptable level of comfort. Often, this regimen consists of a combination of a benzodiazepine and opiate administered intravenously. Medications commonly used for this purpose include lorazepam, midazolam, diazepam, morphine, and fentanyl.

Immobilized patients in the intensive care unit on mechanical ventilator support are at increased risk for deep venous thrombosis; accepted practice consists of administering prophylaxis in the form of subcutaneous heparin and/or pneumatic compression boots. Fractionated low molecular weight heparin has also been used for this purpose; it appears to be equally effective and is associated with a decreased incidence of heparin-associated thrombocytopenia.

Prophylaxis against diffuse gastrointestinal mucosal injury is indicated for patients who have suffered a neurologic insult or those with severe respiratory failure in association with ARDS. Histamine receptor antagonists (H$_2$-receptor antagonists), antacids, and cytoprotective agents such as carafate have all been used for this purpose and appear to be effective. Recent data suggest that carafate use is associated with a reduction in the incidence of nosocomial pneumonias, since it does not cause changes in stomach pH and is less likely to permit colonization of the gastrointestinal tract by nosocomial organisms at pH levels near neutral.

Nutrition support by enteral feeding through either a nasogastric or an orogastric tube should be maintained in all intubated patients whenever possible. In those patients with a normal baseline nutritional state, support should be initiated within 7 days. In malnourished patients, nutrition support should be initiated within 72 h. Delayed gastric emptying is common in critically ill patients on sedative medications but often responds to promotility agents such as cisapride or metoclopramide. Parenteral nutrition is an alternative to enteral nutrition in patients with severe gastrointestinal pathology.

COMPLICATIONS OF MECHANICAL VENTILATION

Endotracheal intubation and positive-pressure mechanical ventilation have direct and indirect effects on several organ systems, including the lung and upper airways, the cardiovascular system, and the gastrointestinal system. Pulmonary complications include barotrauma, nosocomial pneumonia, oxygen toxicity, tracheal stenosis, and deconditioning of respiratory muscles. *Barotrauma*, which occurs when high pressures (i.e., > 50 cmH$_2$O) disrupt lung tissue, is clinically manifest by interstitial emphysema, pneumomediastinum, subcutaneous emphysema, or pneumothorax. Although the first three conditions may resolve simply through the reduction of airway pressures, clinically significant pneumothorax, as indicated by hypoxemia, decreased lung compliance, and hemodynamic compromise, requires tube thoracostomy.

Patients intubated for longer than 72 h are at high risk for *nosocomial pneumonia* as a result of aspiration from the upper airways through small leaks around the endotracheal tube cuff; the most common organisms responsible for this condition are enteric gram-negative rods, *Staphylococcus aureus*, and anaerobic bacteria. Because the endotracheal tube and upper airways of patients on mechanical ventilation are commonly colonized with bacteria, the diagnosis of nosocomial pneumonia requires "protected brush" bronchoscopic sampling of airway secretions coupled with quantitative microbiologic techniques to differentiate colonization from infection.

Oxygen toxicity is a potential complication when an $F_{I_{O_2}} \geq 0.6$ is required for more than 72 h. The condition can be prevented in some cases through the use of PEEP to allow for $F_{I_{O_2}}$ values to go below 0.6 while primary therapy for the underlying condition is instituted. Although O_2 toxicity is thought to result from the effects of oxygen free radical on the lung interstitium, the therapeutic use of antioxidants such as superoxide dismutase, catalase, selenium, and vitamin E remains experimental.

Hypotension resulting from elevated intrathoracic pressures with decreased venous return is almost always responsive to intravascular volume repletion. In patients judged to have hypotension or respiratory failure on the basis of alveolar edema, hemodynamic monitoring with a pulmonary arterial catheter may be of value in optimizing O_2 delivery via manipulation of intravascular volume and $F_{I_{O_2}}$ and PEEP levels.

Gastrointestinal effects of positive-pressure ventilation include *stress ulceration* and *mild to moderate cholestasis*. It is common practice to provide prophylaxis with H_2-receptor antagonists or sucralfate for stress-related ulcers. Mild cholestasis (i.e., total bilirubin values ≤ 4.0) attributable to the effects of increased intrathoracic pressures on portal vein pressures is common and generally self-limited. Cholestasis of a more severe degree should not be attributed to a positive-pressure ventilation response and is more likely due to a primary hepatic process.

WEANING FROM MECHANICAL VENTILATION

Removal of mechanical ventilator support requires that a number of criteria be met. Upper airway function must be intact for a patient to remain extubated but is difficult to assess in the intubated patient. Therefore, if a patient can breathe on his or her own through an endotracheal tube but develops stridor or recurrent aspiration once the tube is removed, upper airway dysfunction or an abnormal swallowing mechanism should be suspected and plans for achieving a stable airway developed. An intact cough during suctioning is a good indicator of a patient's ability to mobilize secretions. Respiratory drive and chest wall function are assessed by observation of respiratory rate, tidal volume, inspiratory pressure, and vital capacity. The weaning index, defined as the ratio of breathing frequency to tidal volume (breaths per minute per liter), is both sensitive and specific for predicting the likelihood of successful extubation. When this ratio is less than 105 with the patient breathing without mechanical assistance through an endotracheal tube, successful extubation is likely. An inspiratory pressure of more than -30 cmH_2O and a vital capacity of greater than 10 mL/kg are considered indicators of acceptable chest wall and diaphragm function. Alveolar ventilation is generally adequate when elimination of CO_2 is sufficient to maintain arterial pH in the range of 7.35 to 7.40, and an $Sa_{O_2} > 90\%$ can be achieved with an $F_{I_{O_2}} < 0.5$ and a PEEP ≤ 5 cmH_2O. Although many patients may not meet all criteria for weaning, the likelihood that a patient will tolerate extubation without difficulty increases as more criteria are met.

Many approaches to weaning patients from ventilator support have been advocated. T-piece and CPAP weaning are best tolerated by patients who have undergone mechanical ventilation for brief periods and require little respiratory muscle reconditioning, whereas SIMV and PSV are best for patients who have been intubated for extended periods and require gradual respiratory-muscle reconditioning.

T-piece weaning involves brief spontaneous breathing trials with supplemental O_2. These trials are usually initiated for 5 min/h followed by a 1-h interval of rest. T-piece trials are increased in 5- to 10-min increments until the patient can remain ventilator independent for periods of several hours. Extubation can then be attempted. CPAP weaning is similar to T-piece weaning except that trials of spontaneous breathing are conducted on the ventilator in CPAP mode.

Weaning by means of SIMV involves gradually tapering the mandatory backup rate in increments of 2 to 4 breaths per minute while monitoring blood gas parameters and respiratory rates. Rates of greater than 25 breaths per minute on withdrawal of mandatory ventilator breaths generally indicate respiratory muscle fatigue and the need to combine periods of exercise with periods of rest. Exercise periods are gradually increased until a patient remains stable on SIMV at 4 breaths per minute or less without needing rest at higher SIMV rates. A CPAP or T-piece trial can then be attempted before planned extubation.

PSV, as described in detail above, is used primarily for weaning from mechanical ventilation. PSV is usually initiated at a level adequate for full ventilator support (PSV_{max}); i.e., PSV is set slightly below the peak inspiratory pressures required by the patient during vol-ume-cycled ventilation. The level of pressure support is then gradually withdrawn in increments of 5 cmH_2O until a level is reached at which the respiratory rate increases to 25 breaths per minute. At this point, intermittent periods of higher-pressure support are alternated with periods of lower-pressure support to provide muscle reconditioning without causing diaphragmatic fatigue. Gradual withdrawal of PSV continues until the level of support is just adequate to overcome the resistance of the endotracheal tube (approximately 5 to 10 cmH_2O). Support can be discontinued and the patient extubated.

BIBLIOGRAPHY

AMATO MBP et al: Effect of a protective-ventilation strategy on mortality in the acute respiratory distress syndrome. N Engl J Med 338:347, 1998

ESTEBAN A et al: A comparison of four methods of weaning patients from mechanical ventilation. N Engl J Med 332:345, 1995

HILL LL, PEARL RG: Flow triggering, pressure-triggering, and autotriggering during mechanical ventilation. Crit Care Med 28:579, 2000

HINSON JR, MARINI JJ: Principles of mechanical ventilator use in respiratory failure. Annu Rev Med 43:341, 1992

INGENITO EP, DRAZEN JM: Mechanical ventilators, in *Principles of Critical Care*, 2d ed., JB Hall, GA Schmidt, LDH Wood (eds). New York, McGraw-Hill, 1997, pp 142–154

MACINTYRE NR: Principles of mechanical ventilation, in *Textbook of Respiratory Medicine*, 3d ed, JF Murray, JA Nadel (eds). Philadelphia, Saunders, 2000, pp 2471–2486

MORRIS AH et al: Randomized clinical trial of pressure control inverse ratio ventilation and extracorporeal membrane oxygenation for adult respiratory distress syndrome. Am J Resp Crit Care Med 149:295, 1994

RANIERI VM et al: Physiologic effects of positive end expiratory pressure in patients with chronic obstructive pulmonary disease during acute ventilatory failure and controlled mechanical ventilation. Am Rev Respir Dis 147:5, 1993

YOUNES M: Proportional assist ventilation: A new approach to ventilatory support. Am Rev Respir Dis 45:114, 1992

267 *Janet R. Maurer*

LUNG TRANSPLANTATION

Lung transplantation for end-stage lung disease has been a therapeutic option since the 1980s. Several transplant options are available for carefully selected patients: unilateral lung transplant, bilateral lung transplant, heart-lung transplant (Chap. 233), and living lobar transplant. The first successful type of lung transplant was heart-lung, which was performed for a variety of indications and in increasing numbers until 1989. Beginning in 1989, the numbers of both unilateral and bilateral lung transplants performed increased dramatically and, along with the increasing demand for heart donors, greatly reduced the number of donor organs available for heart-lung procedures. By the mid-1990s, unilateral and bilateral lung transplant numbers also had plateaued because of donor shortages and have remained relatively stable at approximately 1250 operations worldwide per year. Of these, 60% are unilateral lung transplants and 40% are bilateral. Heart-lung transplants have leveled off at between 100 and 150 per year. In its 1999 report, the Registry of the International Society for Heart and Lung Transplantation, in conjunction with the United Network for Organ Sharing, had recorded a cumulative total of 8997 isolated lung transplants and 2350 heart-lung transplants.

INDICATIONS Emphysema, either smoking-induced or secondary to α_1-antitrypsin deficiency, has been the single largest indication for lung transplantation. This diagnosis accounts for about 55% of unilateral lung transplants, 29% of bilateral, and 6% of heart-lung transplants. Other major indications for unilateral lung transplants include idiopathic pulmonary fibrosis (21%) and primary pulmonary hypertension (5%). Patients with cystic fibrosis comprise the largest group of bilateral lung recipients, approximately 34% of the total, followed by patients with emphysema, patients with primary pulmonary hypertension (10%), and those with idiopathic pulmonary fibrosis (7.5%). The major diagnoses among heart-lung recipients are primary and secondary pulmonary hypertension (54%) and cystic fibrosis (16%). With the widespread use of unilateral and bilateral lung transplants, the indications for heart-lung transplant have become very circumscribed, so that now most candidates for this type of transplant have either concomitant left ventricular disease and end-stage lung disease or irreparable congenital heart disease with Eisenmenger's syndrome. Patients receiving living lobar donations have been either children or young adults, and most have suffered from cystic fibrosis. In most of these operations, a lower lobe is donated from each of two adults, who are often, but not always, related to the recipient. Living donation is performed in a limited number of lung transplant programs, and the donor morbidity rate has been acceptable.

RECIPIENT SELECTION Because donor lungs are the scarcest of the common solid organs transplanted, patients with end-stage lung disease undergo extensive evaluation to select the best potential candidates. In 1998, this process was further standardized with the publication of the International Guidelines for the Selection of Lung Transplant Candidates. Approximate age limits of 65 years for unilateral lung, 60 years for bilateral lung, and 55 years for heart-lung transplants were set. Chronic medical conditions that can be adequately controlled and have not resulted in end-organ damage, e.g., systemic hypertension, are acceptable in lung transplant candidates. However, in a case where a chronic illness is often associated with nonpulmonary organ damage, e.g., diabetes mellitus, a careful assessment of target organ function is necessary.

Absolute contraindications to lung transplantation include dysfunction of major organs (other than lung), infection with HIV, active malignancy within 2 years with the exception of basal cell and squamous cell skin cancer, hepatitis B antigen positivity, and hepatitis C with biopsy-proven histologic evidence of liver disease. Conditions that represent relative contraindications include symptomatic osteoporosis; severe musculoskeletal disease affecting the thorax; high-dose corticosteroid use; weight less than 70% or greater than 130% of ideal body weight; alcohol, cigarette, or narcotic abuse/addiction within 6 months before evaluation; psychosocial problems, including noncompliance, that cannot be adequately resolved through pharmacologic treatment or counseling; requirement for invasive ventilation; and colonization with fungi or atypical mycobacteria. Colonization is of particular concern when a unilateral lung transplant is being considered. Disease-specific guidelines (Table 267-1) are chosen to identify candidates who are within the transplant "window"—that is, patients who are ill enough to fit within the category of "end-stage" and have progressive disease, yet are able to survive the pre-transplant waiting and perioperative time periods. In the past few years, increasing experience with large numbers of patients with end-stage disease has made it much easier to estimate life expectancies; however, patients with diagnoses of emphysema and Eisenmenger's type pulmonary hypertension remain problematic in this regard because posttransplant statistical analysis does not show a clear survival benefit for recipients within the first 2 years. In these types of patient, selection usually includes consideration of quality-of-life issues as well as survival rates.

SELECTION OF TRANSPLANT PROCEDURE The only diseases that currently mandate a specific procedure are (1) irreparable congenital cardiac defects with Eisenmenger's syndrome (heart-lung transplant); (2) advanced lung disease with concomitant left ventricular dysfunction (heart-lung transplant); and (3) bronchiectatic lung disease, e.g., cystic fibrosis (bilateral lung transplant or bilobar living donor lung transplant). In essentially all other circumstances unilateral lung transplantation can be performed with acceptable early and midterm results. Bilateral lung transplantation, however, is often preferred if difficulty is anticipated in postoperative management, especially in patients with pulmonary hypertension; if significant bullous disease in

Table 267-1   Disease-specific Selection Guidelines

Emphysema/chronic obstructive pulmonary disease
  $FEV_1 < 25\%$ predicted
  And/or $Pa_{CO_2} \geq 55$ mmHg
  And/or ↑ Pulmonary artery pressures (PAP)
Cystic fibrosis/bronchiectasis
  $FEV_1 < 30\%$ predicted or
  $FEV_1 > 30\%$ predicted and any of the following:
    Rapid decrease in FEV_1
    Massive hemoptysis
    Cachexia
    Frequent hospitalizations
  Useful adjunctive criteria
  $Pa_{CO_2} \geq 50$ mmHg
  $Pa_{O_2} \leq 55$ mmHg
	Idiopathic pulmonary fibrosis
	  Symptomatic, progressive disease despite drug therapy: Reassess every 3 months
	  Rest or exercise desaturation
	  "Symptomatic" often corresponds to
	    VC < 60-70% predicted
	    DLCO < 50-60% predicted
	Pulmonary hypertension
	  Symptomatic, progressive disease despite optimal medical treatment; usually New York Heart Association functional class III or IV; gold standard medical treatment considered to be prostacyclin
	  Useful hemodynamic predictors
	    Cardiac index < 2 L/min/m²
	    Right atrial pressure > 15 mmHg
	    Mean pulmonary artery pressure > 55 mmHg

NOTE: VC, vital capacity; DLCO, lung diffusing capacity measured with carbon monoxide.
SOURCE: Adapted from the Joint Statement of the ASTP/ATS/ERS/ISHCT.

present in emphysema; if a patient is very young; or if there are specific individual recipient considerations. As noted below, the long-term survival rates of bilateral lung recipients may be superior; nevertheless, transplant centers have generally chosen to maximize the donor organ resource by performing unilateral lung transplants whenever possible, rather than opting for potentially slightly increased survival periods.

PROGNOSIS The 1- and 2-year survival rates for unilateral and bilateral lung transplant recipients are 67 and 62%, respectively. Longer term data show a divergence in survival rates by 5 years, with the half-life of bilateral transplant recipients (4.9 years) significantly longer than that of unilateral transplant recipients (3.6 years). Among unilateral graft recipients, patients with emphysema appear to have the best early survival rate (nearly 80% at one year), and patients with idiopathic pulmonary fibrosis and those with pulmonary hypertension have the worst (60 to 65%). Living lobar recipients have early survival rates that are between the rates of these groups, but long-term data are not available for this population.

FUNCTIONAL OUTCOMES Arterial blood gas levels improve markedly in unilateral and bilateral lung transplant recipients by 3 months posttransplant. In both groups, Pa_{CO_2} normalizes; in bilateral lung transplant recipients, Pa_{O_2} also normalizes. Unilateral lung recipients may continue to have mild hypoxemia but rarely require supplemental oxygen. Pulmonary function studies usually reach their maximum values for both groups between 3 and 12 months postoperatively. Unilateral graft recipients who had a preoperative diagnosis of parenchymal lung disease attain 60 to 65% of their predicted FVC and FEV_1 values. The values for bilateral lung recipients often approach normal predicted values, but these patients can have mild restrictive physiology. Diffusing capacities are usually slightly decreased in all groups. Airway hyperresponsiveness without clinically relevant asthma can be demonstrated in the majority of lung transplant recipients.

Exercise capacity has been the most interesting functional outcome observed in lung transplant recipients. With respect to nongraded exercise capacity, usually measured by 6- or 12-min walk studies, unilateral and bilateral graft recipients demonstrate marked and similar improvement in distances covered after transplantation. Typically, transplant recipients can walk 100 to 120 m/min within 6 months of transplant and are generally able to sustain this rate over time. On graded exercise studies, however, both groups achieve only 40 to 60% of predicted maximum values, with bilateral lung recipients usually performing slightly better than unilateral lung recipients. This exercise limitation has been extensively studied particularly in bilateral lung recipients. The limitation appears not to be cardiac or ventilatory but rather related to muscle deconditioning and abnormalities in skeletal muscle oxidative capacity. Rarely is the exercise limitation in these patients enough to impact on their normal daily activities or their quality of life.

POSTTRANSPLANT MANAGEMENT ISSUES **Airway Complications** Technical improvements and surgical experience have greatly reduced significant anastomotic complications in lung transplant recipients. It is not uncommon to see small dehiscences of the airway in the first weeks posttransplant, but these generally heal without significant stricture. Probably fewer than 10% of patients will have stenosis severe enough to require balloon dilatation, laser resection, or a stent. When required, wire stents are most often used and are well tolerated. Late-occurring bronchomalacia, often at the anastomotic site, has also been treated with stents.

Acute Rejection A three-pronged immunosuppressive approach, which is used in most lung transplant programs, includes either cyclosporine or tacrolimus, either azathioprine or mycophenolate mofetil, and prednisone. Cytolytic induction is rarely used in these patients because of the risk of infection. Most lung transplant recipients experience at least one episode of acute rejection, usually within the first 3 months, although episodes have been reported to occur up to several years after transplantation. From 10 to 15% of patients have recurrent acute or persistent acute rejection, which predisposes them to chronic rejection. Symptoms include a general feeling of malaise, dyspnea, and sometimes cough. Findings may include low grade fever, rales, mild hypoxemia, decreasing FVC and FEV_1 values, increased white blood cell count, and ill-defined infiltrates with or without pleural effusion on chest x-ray. If a patient presents early in an episode of acute rejection, as most do, the findings are minimal and the chest radiogram is clear. Histologic diagnosis, which is the "gold standard," is routinely made by transbronchial biopsy, with a sensitivity of about 80% and a specificity approaching 100%. Bronchoscopy is also helpful in this setting to rule out infections that may have similar presentations.

Acute rejection episodes occurring early after transplantation respond in at least 80% of patients to bolus methylprednisolone. Late episodes and recurrent or persistent episodes often require both intensification of immunosuppression and changes in immunosuppressive drugs. Up to 20% of asymptomatic patients have at least one episode of acute rejection detected by surveillance transbronchial biopsy in the first 2 years posttransplant. It is not clear whether asymptomatic rejection requires therapy, as the impact on outcome is unknown. Thus, the use of surveillance bronchoscopy and the treatment of asymptomatic rejection vary considerably from institution to institution, and there are at present no clear guidelines in this area.

Bronchiolitis Obliterans Bronchiolitis obliterans is both the primary manifestation of chronic rejection and the most feared complication in lung transplant recipients. It occurs to some degree in at least 50% of survivors by 5 years posttransplant and is a factor in more than one-third of late deaths. Although it can occur as early as 2 months posttransplant, the onset is more often at least 6 months and the mean onset is from 1 to 2 years after surgery. The precipitating factors and initiating events in bronchiolitis obliterans are topics of intensive research both in transplant recipients and in several animal models. Those factors most consistently associated with the process include the numbers and severity of acute rejection episodes and episodes of cytomegalovirus (CMV) pneumonia, but not clearly CMV infection alone. Other factors with weaker associations include HLA mismatches, other viral infections, and the development of anti-HLA antibodies. Clinically, the onset of this process is often subacute, with a very gradual onset of dyspnea and fatigue or malaise, often accompanied by viral-type symptoms or dry cough. It can also be asymptomatic and detected by routine pulmonary function studies that show, initially, a decrease in the FEF_{25-75}, often followed one to several months later by decreasing FEV_1. This insidious development of small airway obstruction is often well established before it is clinically recognized, and for that reason frequent pulmonary function testing is

recommended for lung transplant recipients. Chest radiograms are usually normal, but even early in the disease expiratory computed tomography (CT) scans show a mottled appearance with peripheral hyperlucency. Transbronchial biopsy is very specific but not sensitive in diagnosis, but patients usually undergo at least one bronchoscopy at the onset of disease to attempt histologic documentation and to rule out possible infections. Because of the difficulty in histologic diagnosis, a typical clinical picture in the absence of other etiology is considered sufficient to establish a diagnosis of *bronchiolitis obliterans syndrome*. The progression of this complication can be very rapid, with early death; but more often it is one of a gradually decreasing FEV_1 over months to years, which in the later stages is frequently accompanied by bronchomalacia, proximal bronchiectasis, and recurrent pseudomonal or other infections.

Effective treatment remains evasive. A few immunosuppressive protocols tried in small numbers of patients have been found to "stabilize" pulmonary function, but improved function is unusual. Likely, by the time the process is recognized in most patients, fibrotic obliteration of the airway is already present; the key to treatment may lie in identifying markers of incipient disease and much earlier intervention.

Infections Infections rank second only to rejection as a cause of morbidity in lung transplant recipients and are the most common cause of mortality, accounting for one-third of all deaths in both the early and the late posttransplant periods. The transplanted lung may be uniquely vulnerable to infection because of impaired mucociliary clearance, loss of cough reflex, and other poorly defined local factors. In addition, the donor lungs are often colonized with organisms that are transmitted directly to the immunosuppressed recipient. Early series reported that at least 60% of lung recipients early in their course develop infections requiring treatment. Now the extensive use of broad antibacterial, antifungal, anti-*pneumocystis*, and antiviral prophylaxis, often maintained for at least 3 months postoperatively, seems to have reduced the early infective morbidity and mortality.

Infections with paramyxoviral organisms, adenovirus, and influenza A have now been well documented and have an overall death rate of about 20%. The role of antiviral therapy is unclear. The most lethal infections are those with invasive fungal organisms, particularly those caused by *Aspergillus* species, which have been reported to colonize in 20 to 50% of recipients. Invasive disease caused by these organisms can vary from ulcerative bronchitis to localized parenchymal infiltrates to empyema to disseminated disease. *Aspergillus* is particularly likely to be problematic when patients require increased immunosuppression or have other complications; one study has reported an increased rate of invasive disease in the native lung of unilateral lung transplant recipients.

The highest risk periods for infection are in the first few months posttransplant and late after transplant if bronchiolitis obliterans or other vital organ dysfunction, e.g., renal failure, develops. Since it may be very difficult to distinguish infection from rejection in the early posttransplant period, bronchoscopy with appropriate biopsies and cultures is often necessary to establish a diagnosis.

Immunosuppressive and Medical Complications Medical complications related to immunosuppression, to the underlying diagnosis, or to aging are major causes of morbidity in long-term survivors of lung transplantation and account for up to 10% of late deaths. Current immunosuppressive regimens with cyclosporine or tacrolimus cause some nephrotoxicity in virtually all patients. Although few progress to renal failure, hypertension and hyperlipidemia are common. Neurotoxicity, including delirium, headaches, seizures, and, occasionally, strokes, has been reported in up to 20% of patients. Osteoporosis occurs in more than half the patients, and vertebral compression fractures are common. Other problems include thromboembolic disease, gastric complications (especially gastroparesis), hyperglycemia, and increased rates of malignancy.

Posttransplant lymphoproliferative disorders associated with Epstein-Barr virus occur in 5 to 10% of lung transplant recipients. Nearly all occur within the first year after transplant. Recent data suggest a much higher incidence of this disease in patients who are Epstein-Barr naïve and who receive an Epstein-Barr positive graft. Treatment for this disorder, reported to have an approximate 50% survival rate, is usually reduced immunosuppression and antiviral and anti-B lymphocyte drugs. Survivors often develop bronchiolitis obliterans.

Recurrence of Underlying Disease   Several different underlying diseases may recur in lung transplant recipients. These diseases include sarcoidosis, lymphangioleiomyomatosis, giant cell interstitial pneumonia, panbronchiolitis, eosinophilic granuloma, bronchoalveolar cell carcinoma, and desquamative interstitial pneumonia.

BIBLIOGRAPHY

BOEHLER A et al: Bronchiolitis obliterans after lung transplantation: A review. Chest 114: 1411, 1998

BOEHLER A, ESTENNE M: Obliterative bronchiolitis after lung transplantation. Curr Opin Pulm Med 6:133, 2000

HOSENPUD JD et al: The Registry of the International Society for Heart and Lung Transplantation. Fifteenth official report–1998. J Heart Lung Transplant 17:656, 1998

JOINT STATEMENT OF THE AMERICAN SOCIETY FOR TRANSPLANT PHYSICIANS (ASTP)/AMERICAN THORACIC SOCIETY (ATS)/EUROPEAN RESPIRATORY SOCIETY (ERS); INTERNATIONAL SOCIETY FOR HEART AND LUNG TRANSPLANTATION (ISHLT): International guidelines for the selection of lung transplant candidates. Am J Respir Crit Care Med 158:335, 1998

MAURER JR (ed): Surgical approaches to end-stage disease: Lung transplantation and volume reduction. Clin Chest Med 18(2), 1997

NOBEL PRIZE IN PHYSIOLOGY OR MEDICINE, 1985

Michael Stuart Brown was born in New York on April 13, 1941, the eldest child of Harry and Evelyn Brown, who moved their family to Elkins Park, Pennsylvania, in 1952. Michael Brown attended high school there and then went to the University of Pennsylvania where he received his B.S. in chemistry in 1962 and his M.D. in 1966 as an honors graduate.

Joseph Leonard Goldstein was born on April 18, 1940, in Sumter, South Carolina, the only child of Isadore and Fannie Goldstein. The family owned a clothing store in Kingstree, South Carolina, a town of five thousand, where Goldstein attended public school. He earned his B.S. in chemistry, graduating *summa cum laude* from Washington and Lee University in Lexington, Virginia, in 1962. He attended medical school at the University of Texas at Dallas where on graduation he received the Outstanding Medical School Graduate Award.

Brown and Goldstein both entered internship in internal medicine at Massachusetts General Hospital in 1966, became good friends, and both went on to the National Institutes of Health (NIH) as Clinical Associates. Brown specialized in digestive and hereditary diseases and worked in Earl Stadtman's Laboratory of Biochemistry; Goldstein worked in Marshall Nirenberg's Laboratory of Biochemical Genetics, where he saw patients with lipid disorders. Goldstein convinced Brown to join the Gastroenterology Division at Texas Southwestern Medical School in 1971. Goldstein arrived at the same institution in 1972 after 2 years in Arno Motulsky's laboratory at the University of Washington in Seattle. Goldstein was appointed head of a new Division of Medical Genetics on his return to Texas Southwestern Medical School, a promise that Donald Seldin, the chair of Internal Medicine, had made to him in 1966 at the time of his graduation from medical school.

Brown and Goldstein decided to combine their laboratories, and

so began one of the most distinguished dual scientific careers in the history of medicine. Goldstein had seen patients at the NIH with familial hypercholesterolemia (FH) who developed skin deposits of cholesterol, atherosclerosis, and heart attacks at a young age. Brown and Goldstein decided to work on this problem, particularly since they had access to some of these patients in Texas. Goldstein then established a culture technique for skin from both normal individuals and patients with FH. The cells were then analyzed biochemically by Brown. In 1973 Brown and Goldstein discovered a key enzyme in cholesterol production, HMG-coenzyme A (CoA) reductase, which could be regulated in normal skin fibroblasts by the amount of low-density lipoprotein (LDL) in the medium. Adding LDL to the normal cells switched off HMG-CoA reductase, and the cells ceased making cholesterol. However, the skin cells from FH patients continued to make cholesterol with even very high levels of LDL in the medium. Because LDL in alcohol entered these normal cells from FH patients and switched off HMG-CoA reductase, Brown and Goldstein concluded that the genetic mutation must involve a receptor that would bind the LDL and facilitate its entry into the cell. In 1976, using radiolabeled LDL and electron microscopy, Brown and Goldstein, along with R.G.W. Anderson, localized the LDL receptor on coated pits in normal skin fibroblasts; the receptors were absent in the FH skin cultures. A further defect relating to impaired internalization of the receptor after LDL binding was then described. Normally the LDL receptor recycled back to the cell surface within 10 min after lysosomal-induced release of the cholesterol and inhibition of HMG-CoA reductase. Drugs were then developed that would inhibit HMG-CoA reductase and thus decrease the cellular production of cholesterol. Lovastatin (mevalin) was the first such drug marketed to block the synthesis of cholesterol in order to decrease the occurrence of heart attacks.

In 1984 the LDL receptor gene was localized on chromosome 19, and the nucleotide sequence of the gene that produces HMG-CoA reductase was established. The human LDL receptor gene was then sequenced, and one domain was shown to be homologous to the gene sequence for epidermal growth factor.

In 1985 Brown and Goldstein received both the Albert D. Lasker Award in Basic Medical Research, and the Nobel Prize in Physiology or Medicine. Their discoveries of the entry process of cholesterol into the cell and the regulation of cellular synthesis of cholesterol were monumental and have implications for millions of people worldwide who have or will have atherosclerotic cardiovascular disease.

REFERENCES

1. Magill FN (ed): *Nobel Prize Winners: Physiology or Medicine*, vol 3. Pasadena, Salem Press, 1993
2. Schrier RW: *A Salute to Nobel Laureates in Physiology and Medicine*, Proceedings of the Association of American Physicians 108(1): Jan 1996

Robert W. Schrier, MD

268

Robert M. Brenner, Barry M. Brenner

DISTURBANCES OF RENAL FUNCTION

Near constancy of the composition of the internal environment, including the volume, tonicity, and compartmental distribution of the body fluids, is essential to survival. With normal day-to-day variations in the intake of food and water, preservation of the internal environment requires the excretion of these substances in amounts that balance the quantities ingested. Although losses from intestines, lungs, and skin contribute to this excretory capacity, the greatest responsibility for solute and water excretion is borne by the kidneys.

The kidneys regulate the composition and volume of the plasma water. This, in turn, determines the composition and volume of the entire *extracellular* fluid compartment. Through the continuous exchange of water and solutes across all cell membranes, the kidneys influence the *intracellular* fluid compartment as well. These functions are served by a variety of physiologic mechanisms that enable individuals to excrete excesses of water and nonmetabolized solutes contained in the diet, as well as the nonvolatile end products of nitrogen metabolism, such as urea and creatinine. Conversely, when faced with deficits of water or solute, excretion of water or specific solute(s) is curtailed via appropriate mechanisms for renal conservation, reducing the likelihood of volume or solute depletion. The purpose of this chapter is to review the excretory functions of the kidney and to examine how these functions are affected by chronic renal disease.

EFFECTS OF NEPHRON LOSS ON RENAL EXCRETORY MECHANISMS

The volume of urine excreted (averaging 1.5 L/d or roughly 1 mL/min) represents the sum of two large, directionally opposite processes—namely, *ultrafiltration* of 180 L/d or more of plasma water (or 125 mL/min) and *reabsorption* of more than 99% of this filtrate by transport processes in the renal tubules. While renal blood flow accounts for about 20% of resting cardiac output, the kidneys comprise only about 1% of total body weight. This disproportionate allocation of cardiac output, greatly exceeding blood flow per gram of brain, heart or liver, is required for the process of ultrafiltration.

GLOMERULAR ULTRAFILTRATION Urine production begins at the glomerulus where an ultrafiltrate of plasma is formed. The rate of glomerular ultrafiltration (glomerular filtration rate, GFR) is governed chiefly by forces favoring filtration on the one hand (hydraulic pressure in the glomerular capillaries) and forces opposing filtration on the other (the sum of hydraulic pressure in Bowman's space and colloid osmotic pressure in the glomerular capillaries). The rate of glomerular plasma flow and the total surface area of the glomerular capillaries are also determinants of GFR. Decreased GFR can therefore be expected when (1) glomerular hydraulic pressure is reduced (as in circulatory shock); (2) tubule (hence Bowman's space) hydraulic pressure is elevated, as in urinary tract obstruction; (3) plasma colloid osmotic pressure rises to high levels (hemoconcentration due to severe volume depletion, myeloma, or other dysproteinemias); (4) renal, and hence glomerular, blood flow is reduced (severe hypovolemia, cardiac failure); (5) permeability is reduced (diffuse glomerular disease); or (6) filtration surface area is diminished, through focal or diffuse nephron loss in progressive renal failure.

The glomerular capillary wall is specially adapted to allow passage of extremely large volumes of water while retaining all but the smallest solute molecules. Molecules the size of inulin (approximately 5200 mol wt) pass freely across the glomerular filtration barrier, appearing at approximately the same concentration in Bowman's space as in plasma. The passage of solutes across the glomerular barrier decreases progressively with increasing molecular size such that, as the molecular weight of albumin is approached, most of the solute is retained in the plasma. Albumin, a polyanionic molecule in plasma, is further retarded at the glomerular filtration barrier by *electrostatic forces* imparted by negatively charged cell-surface molecules on the epithelial foot processes that form the *filtration slits* and the *slit diaphragms*. With disruption of these structural and electrostatic barriers, as in many forms of glomerular injury (Chaps. 273 to 275), large quantities of plasma proteins gain access to the glomerular filtrate.

Glomerular Adaptations to Nephron Loss With loss of nephron mass, the remaining functional (or least injured) nephrons tend to hypertrophy and take on an increased workload so that the overall loss of function is minimized. For example, a patient with a unilateral nephrectomy loses one-half of the nephron mass, resulting in a 50% reduction in GFR at the time of surgery. However, the GFR in the remaining kidney begins to increase after 1 or 2 weeks, and within several months GFR may rise to 80% of the preoperative value. This indicates that the GFR of the individual remaining nephrons has increased above normal, a state known as *hyperfiltration*. Increases in single-nephron GFR may be achieved by renal hemodynamic adjustments (increased glomerular plasma flow and increased glomerular capillary hydraulic pressure), which augment the forces driving ultrafiltration, and by glomerular hypertrophy, which increases the maximum surface area available for filtration. These structural adaptations are evident from the enlargement of glomeruli (and tubules) seen on histologic sections from people with single kidneys. Similar structural changes are observed in kidneys damaged by chronic disease processes; foci of hypertrophied glomeruli and tubules are interspersed with areas of atrophic or scarred parenchyma. Although direct measurements of single-nephron GFR cannot be made in humans, it is reasonable to conclude that focal nephron enlargement as occurs in chronically diseased kidneys generally signifies focally increased single-nephron GFR, and that these dynamic adaptations represent compensatory adjustments for the effects of nephron loss through disease.

Glomerulotubular Balance The close integration of glomerular and tubular functions (*glomerulotubular balance*) seen in chronic renal failure (CRF) supports the notion that progressive nephron obliteration is the usual mode of GFR reduction in CRF. Preservation of glomerulotubular balance until the terminal stages of CRF is fundamental to the *intact-nephron hypothesis*, which states that as CRF advances, kidney function is supported by a diminishing pool of functioning (or hyperfunctioning) nephrons, rather than relatively constant numbers of nephrons, each with diminishing function. This concept has important implications for the mechanisms of disease progression in CRF. A considerable amount of evidence suggests that nephrons subjected to increased excretory burdens for prolonged periods actually sustain injury as a result of these adaptations: thus the cost of these compensatory adaptations to nephron loss may ultimately be relentless destruction of the remaining nephron pool.

The magnitude of the single-nephron hyperfiltration induced by loss of 50% of the total nephron mass usually has no serious adverse clinical consequences, even when sustained over two to three decades. When more than 50% of the total nephron mass is lost, however, as in renal-sparing surgery for bilateral trauma or neoplasm or from a renal disease whose activity has abated, the remaining nephrons are forced to the limits of their compensatory capacity. While these adaptations achieve remarkable short-term success at offsetting the tendency for GFR to fall, over time, proteinuria and focal and segmental glomerulosclerosis develop, the more so where greater amounts of nephrons are lost or removed. As a result, a progressive decline in GFR ensues. Experimental study of the processes that advance glomerular injury show that the adverse long-term consequences of severe nephron deficits are invariably preceded by increases in glomerular capillary hydraulic pressure (glomerular capillary hypertension), glomerular hyperperfusion, and hypertrophy. Interventions directed against these compensatory and maladaptive responses can greatly ameliorate the subsequent development of renal failure. In particular, drugs (e.g., angiotensin-converting enzyme inhibitors and angiotensin II receptor blockers) and other interventions (such as dietary protein restriction) that lower glomerular pressure can slow the rate of progression of experimental and human renal disease. In the absence of such interventions, more and more glomeruli cease to function through advancing glomerulosclerosis and disruption of tubule structure and function, leading eventually to total loss of GFR (i.e., end-stage renal disease). This *final common pathway* for chronic renal injury helps to explain the observed progressive nature of chronic renal failure resulting from many different kidney diseases.

Biologic Consequences of Sustained Reductions in GFR   Although nephron loss can proceed, to some extent, without equivalent loss of GFR due to the compensatory mechanisms described above, determination of the total GFR of both kidneys remains the most reliable clinical index of overall excretory function. The effects of impaired GFR are to reduce the total rate of delivery of solute into the glomerular filtrate. When accompanied by comparably reduced rates of urinary excretion, *retention* and *accumulation* of the unexcreted solute occurs, resulting in increased concentrations of the substance in the plasma and other body fluids.

Figure 268-1 depicts the major types of response to impaired GFR. The degree of reduction in total GFR is plotted on the abscissa, expressed as a percentage of normal (100%). The renal handling of most solutes normally present in glomerular filtrate conforms to one of three patterns. Curve *A* describes the pattern with substances such as cre-

atinine and urea that normally depend largely on glomerular filtration for urinary excretion; i.e., secretion contributes little to overall excretion. Therefore, as illustrated, gradual reductions in GFR are accompanied by progressive increases in plasma levels of creatinine, urea, and other substances normally excreted primarily by filtration.

The clinical course of CRF usually also approximates the pattern described by curve *A*. Patients with CRF usually pass from a long asymptomatic period of "compensation" to a more accelerated and clinically overt terminal phase. In other words, despite chronic injury leading to destruction of more than 50% of nephrons, plasma elevations of creatinine and urea may still lie within the normal limits for these substances. With further nephron loss and reduction in GFR, however, the limits of renal reserve are exceeded and continued accumulations of curve *A*–type solutes lead to abnormally elevated plasma concentrations (Fig. 268-1). Because some of these retained solutes are thought to exert "toxic" effects on all organ systems, clinical manifestations of CRF may now become apparent. Consequently, in patients with substantial reductions in nephron mass but near-normal plasma creatinine, overt uremia may be precipitated by a modest additional decline in GFR.

The accumulation of curve *A*–type solutes with chronic loss of renal function proceeds until external balance is restored, i.e., intake and/or production rates exactly match excretion rates. In the case of creatinine, for example, assuming a constant rate of creatinine production, a 50% reduction in GFR results in an approximate doubling of the plasma creatinine concentration. The latter restores the filtered load of creatinine (i.e., the product of GFR and plasma creatinine concentration) to normal, and the urinary excretion rate once again is equivalent to creatinine production. Since creatinine secretion contributes only slightly, elimination of the retained creatinine is not possible and the plasma concentration remains twice normal. With further loss of GFR, elevations in plasma creatinine are compounded by loss of nephron excretory function and creatinine retained as the result of earlier nephron destruction (Fig. 268-1). *In practice, so long as the net rates of acquisition and production (i.e., liver function and muscle mass) remain reasonably constant, the inverse relationship between plasma concentrations of solutes such as creatinine and urea and GFR is sufficiently reliable to serve as clinical indices of GFR.* However, where muscle mass is low, as with severe weight loss, unremarkable plasma levels of creatinine may belie substantial reductions in GFR.

In contrast to solutes of the curve *A* type, plasma levels of phosphate (PO_4^{3-}), urate, and potassium (K^+) and hydrogen (H^+) ions usually do not rise until the GFR falls to a small percentage of normal. With progressive renal failure this pattern of response (curve *B* in Fig. 268-1) reflects the participation of tubule transport mechanisms in the excretion of these substances. In other words, *as GFR declines, the tubules facilitate greater elimination of these substances, by enhancing secretion and/or by diminishing reabsorption, so that a greater fraction of the filtered load is excreted.* Plasma levels of curve *B*–type solutes, therefore, rise less than those of curve *A* because, with progressive reductions in GFR, *excretion rate per nephron* and therefore *fractional excretion* both increase. Eventually, however, with further loss of GFR, enhanced fractional excretion can no longer mitigate the reduction in net filtered load of these solutes and plasma levels rise (Fig. 268-1). For urate, PO_4^{3-}, and K^+, at least, increased fractional excretion serves to maintain normal plasma levels until GFR falls to less than one-fourth of normal.

Finally, for certain solutes, such as sodium chloride (NaCl), plasma concentrations remain normal throughout the course of CRF, despite unrestricted intake of these substances (curve *C* in Fig. 268-1). The compensatory mechanism required to achieve this represents a fundamental adaptation to chronic renal injury. To illustrate the magnitude of this adaptation, it is useful to compare the excretion of sodium (Na^+) in a normal individual (GFR of 125 mL/min) with that of a patient with advanced renal failure (GFR of 2 mL/min). Both individuals consume a conventional diet containing 7 g/d of salt (120 mmol Na^+). With a normal serum Na^+ concentration of 140 mmol/L, external Na^+ balance is achieved by excreting approximately 0.5% of the filtered

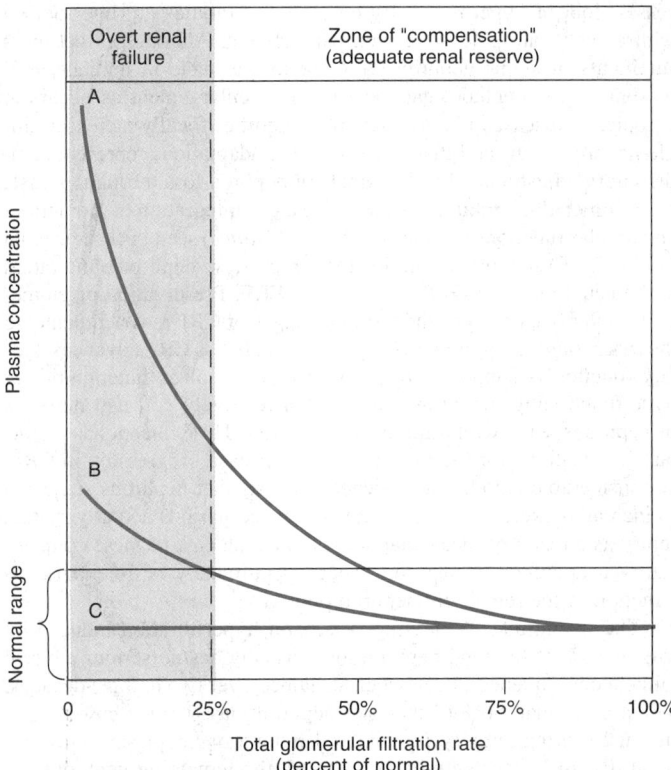

FIGURE 268-1 Representative patterns of adaptation for different types of solutes in body fluids in chronic renal failure. *(After NS Bricker et al, in BM Brenner, 2000.)*

load. By contrast, for external balance to be maintained in the patient with CRF, fractional excretion of Na$^+$ must rise to 30%. In other words, *to maintain external Na$^+$* balance, the same amount of Na$^+$ must be excreted into the urine each day in the patient with CRF as in the normal individual. Given the drastic reduction in GFR in CRF, external balance can only be maintained by marked adaptations in the reabsorptive processes in surviving tubules. In this manner, a progressively larger fraction of the filtered load escapes reabsorption and appears in the final urine. In short, *the rate of excretion of Na$^+$ per surviving nephron increases in inverse proportion to the composite GFR in surviving nephrons.*

ADAPTATIONS IN TUBULE TRANSPORT MECHANISMS IN RESPONSE TO NEPHRON LOSS

Despite progressive nephron loss, many mechanisms that regulate renal solute and water balance differ only quantitatively, and not qualitatively, from those that operate normally. Thus, glomerulotubular balance is maintained. The most important of these mechanisms are considered below.

TUBULAR TRANSPORT OF SODIUM CHLORIDE AND WATER   Most of the filtered water and sodium salts are reabsorbed by the tubules, leaving small and variable amounts, equivalent on average to the quantities ingested, to reach the final urine. About two-thirds of the glomerular ultrafiltrate is reabsorbed in the *proximal tubule* with little change in the osmolality or Na$^+$ concentration of the unreabsorbed fraction (Fig. 268-2). In other words, fluid reabsorption in the proximal tubule is nearly *isosmotic* and is coupled to the active transport of Na$^+$. Since chloride (Cl$^-$) and bicarbonate (HCO$_3^-$) are the primary anions in the extracellular fluid, they constitute the main solutes that accompany Na$^+$ reabsorption in the renal tubules. In the earliest portion of the proximal tubule, bicarbonate is the principal anion that accompanies the reabsorption of Na$^+$. This process occurs via a Na$^+$/H$^+$ exchanger at the luminal brush border and is dependent on the activity of carbonic anhydrase. Glucose, amino acids, and other organic solutes (e.g., lactate) are also extensively reabsorbed in the proximal tubule by cotransport mechanisms that link the cellular entry of these organic molecules with Na$^+$. The coupling of water absorption (i.e., volume) with solute absorption appears to be dependent upon three processes. First, given the remarkably high water permeability of this segment, very small transepithelial osmolality differences, i.e., *luminal hypotonicity* of the order of 2 to 3 mosmol/L produced by solute absorption, could drive water absorption. Second, due to preferential absorption of HCO$_3^-$ and organic solutes in the early portions of the proximal tubule, the concentrations of these substances decrease along the proximal tubule while that of chloride increases. Volume reabsorption would then occur if the diffusion of Na$^+$ and Cl$^-$ down their respective electrochemical gradients across the proximal tubule epithelium occurred more easily than the back-diffusion of sodium bicarbonate into the lumen, creating an *effective osmotic pressure gradient.* Finally, *lateral interstitial space hypertonicity* produced by differences in the rates at which solutes are transported into the spaces or exit them by diffusion may also contribute to the coupling of water and solute reabsorption.

Reabsorption of Fluid from Proximal Convoluted Tubules This is sensitive to *Starling forces*, i.e., the hydraulic and colloid osmotic (or oncotic) pressures acting across the walls of the peritubular capillaries. Because the plasma proteins in glomerular capillaries are concentrated by ultrafiltration, oncotic pressure rises along the glomerular capillary network. This step-up in oncotic pressure is transmitted largely unchanged to the first branches of the peritubular capillaries via the efferent arterioles. These resistance vessels cause a substantial drop in hydraulic pressure, however, so that when the plasma reaches the peritubular capillaries, oncotic pressure greatly exceeds hydraulic pressure. The Starling forces are therefore oriented in an *uptake* mode, in contrast to their configuration at the glomerulus where hydraulic pressure exceeds oncotic pressure, favoring *filtration.*

The extent to which oncotic pressure exceeds hydraulic pressure in the peritubular capillary network modulates the overall rate of fluid absorption by the peritubular capillaries. Therefore, when peritubular capillary oncotic pressure falls, or hydraulic pressure rises, uptake of fluid by these capillaries is reduced. As a result, fluid is retained in the interstitial space, tending to increase hydraulic pressure, ultimately retarding the egress of fluid from the lateral intercellular channels. Without an adequate route of drainage, fluid in the intercellular channels leaks back into the tubule lumen, thereby *diminishing net fluid reabsorption* from this tubule segment. The opposite occurs in states where peritubular oncotic pressure is increased (increased filtration fraction) or hydraulic pressure is decreased (enhanced efferent arteriolar tone). Under these circumstances, peritubular capillary uptake of reabsorbate is augmented, leading ultimately to *enhanced net fluid reabsorption* by the proximal tubule. Although physical factors appear to be the major determinants of fluid reabsorption in the proximal tubule, hormones (e.g., angiotensin II) may also modulate fluid reabsorption directly, by enhancing luminal Na$^+$ entry into proximal tubule cells via an apical Na$^+$/H$^+$ exchanger.

The Limbs of Henle's Loop   In contrast to the proximal tubule, active outward transport of Na has not been established for the *thin ascending limb of Henle's loop*. However, passive outward salt transport does occur, as indicated in Fig. 268-2. In the next nephron segment, the *medullary thick ascending limb of Henle*, the concentration of NaCl is reduced as fluid traverses this segment. Here Cl$^-$ absorption occurs by an active process involving a Na$^+$:K$^+$:2Cl$^-$ cotransport mechanism in the luminal membrane, with one-half of Na$^+$ absorption proceeding passively, driven by the lumen positive transepithelial voltage difference. This cotransporter is the site of action of the powerful loop diuretics and mutations give rise to Bartter's syndrome. Since the ascending limb of Henle is impermeable to water, net NaCl reabsorption generates a hypotonic tubule fluid and gives rise to the high NaCl concentration of the outer medullary interstitium (Fig. 268-2). In certain animals, arginine vasopressin (AVP; also called ADH) enhances NaCl absorption in the medullary portion of the thick ascending limb, but whether this occurs in humans is uncertain.

Distal Tubule   The fluid leaving the thick ascending limb of Henle is normally of low NaCl concentration, a characteristic independent of the organism's hydration or dietary status. In the *distal tubule*, water reabsorption is variable, depending on the state of hydration or, specifically, on the presence or absence of AVP in plasma. In the absence of AVP, this and more distal nephron segments are impermeable to water, so that hypotonic fluid entering this segment is excreted as *dilute urine*. Indeed, continued salt reabsorption along the distal convoluted tubule (DCT) and connecting tubule segments, a process that can be inhibited by the thiazide classes of diuretics, results in further dilution of the urine. In the presence of AVP, the permeability of these nephron segments to water increases. This is made possible by the insertion of proteins known as *aquaporins* into the luminal cell membrane of DCT cells. These proteins facilitate water movement from the low osmolality environment of the DCT lumen into the higher osmolality of the medullary interstitium, thereby contributing to the creation of a concentrated final urine. NaCl continues to be reabsorbed from the tubule lumen against moderately steep chemical and electrical gradients. The reabsorption of NaCl at the collecting tubule is enhanced by *aldosterone*.

Collecting Tubules and Ducts   The *cortical collecting tubule* possesses a low permeability to water in the absence of AVP, whereas permeability increases in the presence of this hormone. The sensitivity of this segment to AVP appears to be more pronounced than that of the DCT. As with the DCT, the cortical collecting tubule is capable of active reabsorption of NaCl and its stimulation by aldosterone.

The terminal segment of the distal nephron is the highly branched *papillary collecting duct*. Continued electrolyte transport in this segment results in the large ion concentration differences that normally exist between urine and plasma. As in the cortical collecting tubule,

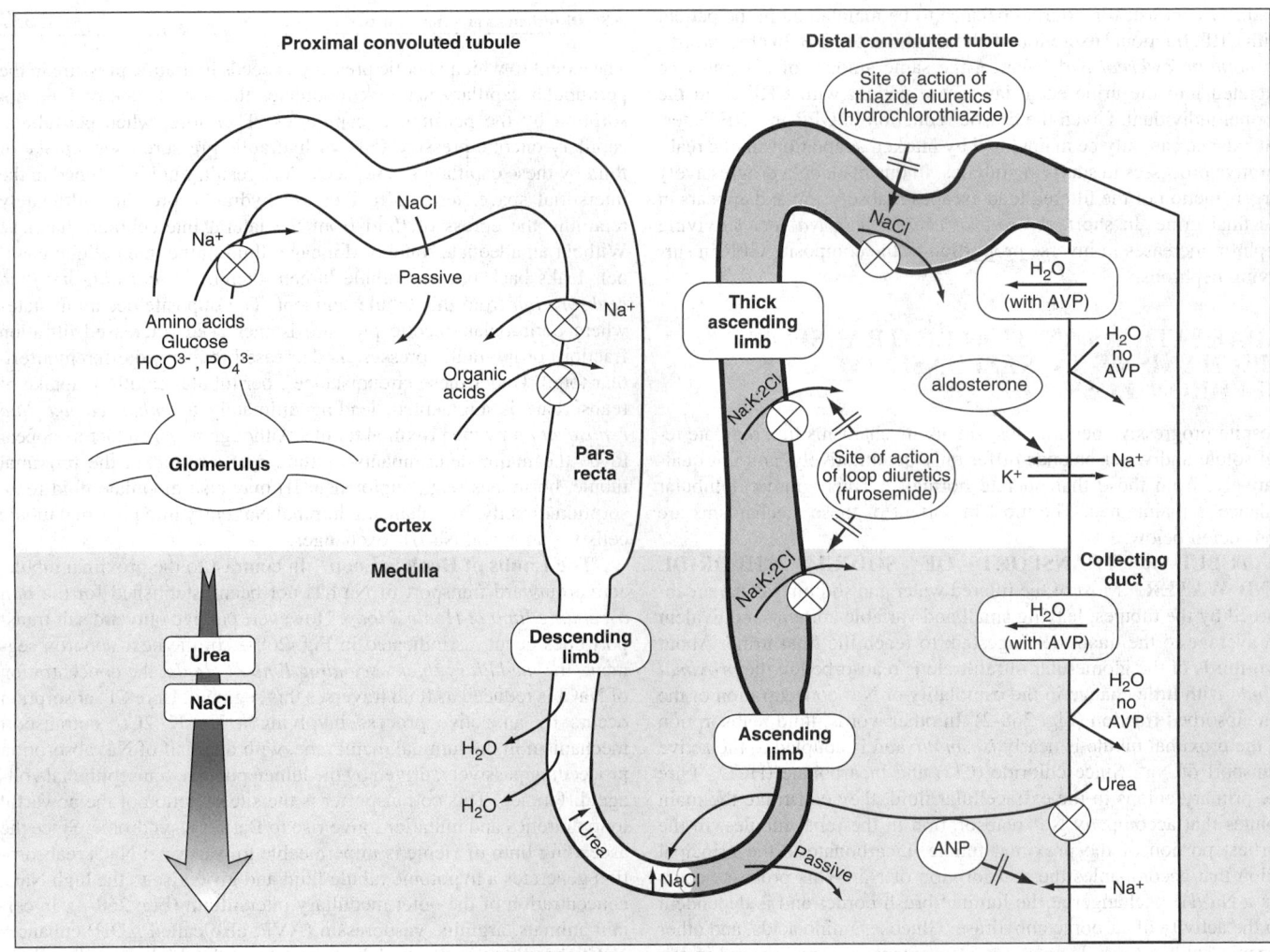

FIGURE 268-2 Transport functions of the various anatomic segments of the mammalian nephron. Fluid reabsorption across the proximal tubule is isosmotic and accounts for reabsorption of approximately two-thirds of the filtered Na^+ and H_2O. The major portions of the filtered HCO_3^-, amino acids, glucose, and phosphate are reabsorbed in the early proximal convoluted tubule. Reabsorption of glucose and amino acids is coupled to Na^+ transport and thereby generates a negative potential difference within the tubule lumen. At the same time, HCO_3^- is reabsorbed by a nonelectrogenic mechanism, via H^+ secretion. The active transport of these solutes results in transepithelial concentration and effective osmotic pressure gradients promoting H_2O flow across the proximal tubule, into the peritubular capillaries. The rise in tubule fluid Cl^- concentration is a necessary reciprocal consequence of the decreased luminal HCO_3^- concentration. The resultant high concentration of Cl^- becomes an important force for the outward passive transport of Cl^- down its concentration gradient, resulting in a lumen-positive potential difference in the late proximal convoluted tubule. The pars recta of the proximal tubule is capable of active electrogenic transport of Na^+ independent of organic solute transport. Under normal conditions, approximately one-third of the glomerular filtrate enters the descending limb of Henle's loop. Because the thin descending limb is incapable of active outward NaCl transport and is characterized by low permeability to Na^+ but high H_2O permeability, H_2O is abstracted passively as the fluid approaches the bend of Henle's loop. Hypertonic fluid with a greater NaCl concentration but lower urea concentration than the surrounding medullary interstitium thus enters the thin ascending limb of Henle, which is largely impermeable to H_2O and urea but highly permeable to NaCl. This permits passive outward diffusion of NaCl. Active Na:K:2Cl transport across the water-impermeable thick ascending limb of Henle allows for separation of solute and water. In consequence, tubule fluid becomes dilute and the medullary interstitium hypertonic. Irrespective of the final osmolality of the urine, the fluid that enters the distal convoluted tubule is always hypoosmotic. This segment exhibits active Na^+ reabsorption. All but the terminal portion of the distal convoluted tubule is water-impermeable, even in the presence of AVP. Aldosterone exerts its effect in this segment by enhancing Na^+ reabsorption, which is variably coupled to K^+ and H^+ secretion. The cortical and papillary portions of the collecting duct are sites where AVP exerts its principal effect. The permeability of these segments to H_2O in the absence of AVP is very low but can be greatly enhanced in the presence of AVP. These segments are also characterized by active Na^+ reabsorption, which appears to depend on the presence of mineralocorticoid. In the absence of AVP, the collecting tubule is water-impermeable so that hypotonic tubule fluid courses through it. However, in the presence of AVP, water is avidly reabsorbed here, resulting in hypertonic final urine. Sites of action of furosemide and thiazide diuretics and of aldosterone and atrial natriuretic peptide (ANP) are shown.

Na^+ transport appears to be active, since reabsorption proceeds against sizeable electrochemical gradients. The rate of Na^+ transport in this segment depends on the load of Na^+ delivered from more proximal segments and is also affected by aldosterone. The permeability to water is also increased markedly in the presence of AVP.

Effects of Nephron Loss on Sodium Chloride Transport in Surviving Nephrons With progressive nephron loss, *maintenance of external balance for NaCl requires that fractional salt excretion increases in concert with the decline in GFR.* Several mechanisms contribute to this adaptive increase in fractional Na^+ excretion. With loss of functioning nephron units, peritubular capillary Starling forces are presumably altered in directions that serve to reduce proximal tubule reabsorption of NaCl and water. For example, a rise in peritubular capillary hydraulic pressure, which tends to inhibit net proximal fluid reabsorption, might be anticipated with systemic hypertension, a common feature of chronic renal failure. Similarly, reductions in peritubular capillary oncotic pressures may be anticipated due to reductions in both filtration fraction and hypoalbuminemia.

Aldosterone, which normally exerts a potent influence on tubule transport, probably does not figure prominently in reducing fractional Na$^+$ excretion, since aldosterone levels are seldom reduced in CRF. Furthermore, external Na$^+$ balance is preserved in bilaterally adrenalectomized dogs on fixed replacement doses of mineralocorticoid. Yet another factor contributing to the suppression of fractional NaCl reabsorption in CRF may relate to the retention of various organic solutes as GFR declines.

Several factors that regulate NaCl transport across tubules under resting conditions are also likely to contribute to the enhanced fractional excretion of salt in renal insufficiency. Atrial natriuretic peptides are released from the heart in response to elevated cardiac (atrial) filling pressures as seen with increased plasma volume or atrial tachyarrhythmias. These peptides affect natriuresis by reducing net Na$^+$ reabsorption through complementary actions on Na$^+$ transport in the collecting duct and by altering Starling forces in the adjacent vasa recta. The vascular actions of natriuretic peptides may also extend to glomerular hemodynamics, with afferent arteriolar vasodilatation contributing to increased single-nephron GFR and hence an increase in the amount of Na$^+$ filtered. Other modulators of tubule transport processes may also contribute to increased single-nephron natriuresis in the setting of reduced renal mass or nephron loss. Vasodilator prostaglandins are present at increased plasma levels in CRF, as are other inhibitors of transport, including inhibitor(s) of the Na$^+$,K$^+$-ATPase. This latter factor has not yet been fully characterized; whether its presence represents a homeostatic adaptation for maintenance of fluid balance or an unregulated accumulation of a toxin remains uncertain.

Serum and urine from patients with uremia contain factors capable of experimentally inhibiting NaCl transport across frog skin, toad bladder, and rat renal tubule. Accumulation of natriuretic factors in uremia may not be without cost; the "trade-off" for maintenance of external Na$^+$ balance is the possibility of generalized abnormalities occurring in Na$^+$ transport across cell membranes, which often occur in advanced renal failure (Chap. 270).

The obligatory high rate of solute excretion per surviving nephron (so-called osmotic diuresis due to urea and other retained solutes) also contributes to enhancing fractional NaCl excretion, much as occurs in normal individuals after the administration of mannitol or other nonreabsorbable solutes. Finally, certain forms of CRF are associated with unusually large losses of salt in the urine. These *salt-wasting nephropathies* include chronic pyelonephritis and other tubulointerstitial diseases (Chap. 277) as well as polycystic and medullary cystic diseases. These disorders have in common greater destruction of medullary and tubulointerstitial, rather than cortical and glomerular, portions of the renal parenchyma. Preferential impairment of tubule reabsorptive function, rather than a primary reduction in glomerular filtration, may, therefore, underlie the salt-losing tendency in these disorders. Clinical derangements that alter renal handling of NaCl in CRF (including hypo- and hypervolemia, hypertension, etc.) are considered in Chap. 270.

EFFECTS OF NEPHRON LOSS ON WATER REABSORPTION IN SURVIVING NEPHRONS As with NaCl, there is a progressive increase in the fractional excretion of water with advancing renal insufficiency, so that external water balance can be maintained even with a total GFR of 5 mL/min or less. The adaptations of water handling by the diseased kidney are of importance in the defects in urinary concentration and dilution and hence the polyuria, nocturia, and tendency to develop water overload encountered in CRF (Chap. 47). To appreciate the mechanisms involved, the responses of a normal and a uremic individual maintaining external water balance need to be considered. Assuming both individuals have the same dietary and fluid intakes, total solute and volume excretion in both should be identical as well. If the *obligatory solute load* to be excreted by each is 600 mmol/d (600 mosmol/d) and the urine osmolality is 300 mmol/kg water (300 mosmol/kg), a urine volume of 2 L/d will be required to

excrete the total solute. If the GFR in normal and uremic individuals totals 180 and 4 L/d, respectively, urinary volume excretion of 2 L/d represents excretion of slightly more than 1% of the total glomerular filtrate in the normal subject compared with 50% in the uremic patient. Since the range of urine osmolalities that the diseased kidney can achieve [250 to 350 mmol/kg (250 to 350 mosmol/kg)] is narrower than in the normal kidney [40 to 1200 mmol/kg (40 to 1200 mosmol/kg)], the individual with normal function is able to excrete the obligatory daily solute load of 600 mmol (600 mosmol) in as little as 500 mL urine per day or as much as 15 L/d, compared with the narrower range in renal insufficiency, from about 1.7 to 2.4 L/d.

In CRF, the limited capacity to concentrate the urine often correlates with other measures of impaired renal function. Isosthenuria (urine of similar osmolality to plasma) is therefore an almost universal finding when the GFR falls below 25 mL/min. At this level of GFR and below, urine osmolality does not rise even when supraphysiologic doses of AVP are administered, suggesting that the concentrating defect relates to impaired concentrating capacity in surviving nephrons. The associated increased fractional excretion per nephron of a variety of solutes produces an obligatory water loss (solute diuresis) at roughly isotonic proportions. Consequently, formation of a concentrated urine is prevented. Disease-induced abnormalities of the architecture of the renal medulla (loops of Henle, vasa recta), aberrations in medullary blood flow, and defective transport of NaCl in the ascending limb of Henle also contribute to this defect in urine concentration.

Since patients with CRF are unable to excrete concentrated or dilute urine, they must have access to adequate, and to some extent, relatively constant amounts of water per day to ensure that they have adequate water to eliminate total daily solute loads. For this reason, restriction of fluid intake may be hazardous in patients with CRF. Likewise, impairment of diluting capacity may prevent many patients from excreting excess ingested fluid. The consequences of the abnormal patterns of water excretion, and the attendant susceptibilities to develop hypo- and hypernatremia, are considered in Chaps. 49 and 270.

TUBULE TRANSPORT OF PHOSPHATE WITH NORMAL AND REDUCED NEPHRON MASS Under normal physiologic conditions, about 80 to 90% of phosphate is reabsorbed, mainly in the proximal tubule. *Parathyroid hormone* (PTH), by augmenting phosphate excretion via inhibition of this proximal reabsorptive process (Chap. 340), plays a central role in phosphate homeostasis. When dietary phosphate intake increases, a *transient* rise in plasma phosphate concentration is usually observed. This results in a similarly transient reduction in the plasma ionized calcium level (due largely to deposition of calcium phosphate in bone), which is sensed by a specific receptor on parathyroid cells, stimulating PTH secretion. By enhancing fractional phosphate excretion, PTH restores external phosphate balance and normophosphatemia. This enables plasma ionized calcium levels to return to normal, thereby removing the stimulus to PTH release and restoring the phosphate control system to the original steady state.

With advancing renal failure and constant dietary intake of phosphate, external phosphate balance is achieved by progressive reduction in fractional phosphate reabsorption. Enhanced PTH secretion is an important determinant of this phosphaturic response. With succeeding decrements in total GFR, the amount of phosphate filtered by surviving glomeruli is reduced, leading to transient phosphate retention and, therefore, a rise (albeit small) in plasma phosphate concentration. This leads to a small, reciprocal decline in plasma levels of ionized calcium and a corresponding increase in PTH secretion. Although the phosphaturic response of surviving tubules to this elevation in circulating PTH restores plasma phosphate and calcium to normal levels (at least in the "compensated" stage of CRF described by curve *B* in Fig. 268-1), the new steady-state conditions are only achieved at the cost of *persistently elevated plasma PTH levels*. With progressive reductions in GFR, the process is repeated, resulting in substantially elevated PTH levels.

Alterations in Vitamin D Metabolism   These alterations also contribute to elevated PTH levels in CRF. The kidney is normally the major site of *conversion of vitamin D to its active metabolites*. As discussed in Chap. 340, vitamin D, synthesized in skin or acquired in the diet, undergoes initial hydroxylation in the liver to form 25-hydroxyvitamin D [25(OH)D]. The kidney is the site of a second important conversion to 1,25-hydroxyvitamin D [1,25(OH$_2$)D]. This active form of vitamin D acts directly on the parathyroid gland to suppress PTH secretion as well as to enhance intestinal absorption of calcium and phosphate resorption and promote resorption of these ions from bone. In addition, 1,25(OH)D$_2$ probably opposes the phosphaturic actions of PTH in the renal tubule by augmenting, rather than diminishing, phosphate reabsorption. With advancing renal disease, nephron loss reduces the renal capacity for vitamin D hydroxylation; phosphate retention also impairs this reaction. Not only are the circulating levels of 1,25(OH)D$_2$ diminished in uremia, but the receptors that mediate its action at the parathyroid gland are also diminished. These two effects remove inhibitory influences on PTH secretion, leading again to increased plasma PTH levels. Reduction in circulating 1,25(OH)D$_2$ levels, by suppressing intestinal calcium absorption, contributes to the development of the hypocalcemia and hyperparathyroidism of CRF (Chap. 270).

Hyperparathyroidism in Chronic Renal Failure   At least two additional processes are thought to contribute to hyperparathyroidism in CRF. One relates to resistance of bone to the calcemic effect of PTH in uremia. This resistance necessitates a higher level of PTH to demineralize bone and maintain the plasma calcium concentration. The other derives from the finding that reductions in renal mass impair the kidneys' capacity to degrade circulating PTH. Ultimately, however, phosphate conforms more to a curve *B*– rather than a curve *C*–type pattern in Fig. 268-1, and phosphate retention occurs when the GFR falls below about 25 mL/min, signifying that these latter forms of adaptation play limited roles.

Since PTH exerts major effects on bone as well as renal tubules, the external balance of phosphate in CRF is achieved at the expense of elevated PTH levels, which, in turn, account for many of the bone changes of renal osteodystrophy (i.e., *secondary hyperparathyroidism*; Fig. 270-1). In support of this *trade-off hypothesis*, when dietary phosphate intake is reduced in proportion to the reduction in GFR in animals with CRF, external balance of phosphate no longer requires augmentation of fractional phosphate excretion in surviving nephrons. Accordingly, circulating levels of PTH no longer rise, and the bone changes of secondary hyperparathyroidism are diminished, if not prevented.

HYDROGEN AND BICARBONATE TRANSPORT WITH NORMAL AND REDUCED RENAL MASS   As discussed in Chap. 50, the pH of extracellular fluid is normally maintained within a narrow range (7.36 to 7.44) despite day-to-day fluctuations in the quantity of acids added to the extracellular fluid from dietary and metabolic sources (approximately 1 mmol H$^+$ per kilogram of body weight per day). These acids consume buffers from both extracellular and intracellular fluid, of which HCO$_3^-$ is the most important in the intracellular compartment. Such buffering minimizes changes in pH. Long-term effectiveness of the HCO$_3^-$ buffer system, however, requires mechanisms for replenishment, otherwise unrelenting acquisition of nonvolatile acids from dietary and metabolic sources would ultimately exhaust buffering capacity, culminating in fatal acidosis. The kidneys normally function to prevent this eventuality by *regenerating* bicarbonate, thereby maintaining plasma concentrations of HCO$_3^-$. In addition, the kidneys also *reclaim* HCO$_3^-$ in the glomerular ultrafiltrate. Reclamation of filtered HCO$_3^-$ takes place largely in the proximal tubule and, under normal circumstances, is virtually complete below a critical plasma HCO$_3^-$ concentration—the threshold concentra-

tion—which in humans is normally about 26 mmol/L, identical to the concentration of HCO$_3^-$ in plasma. As a consequence, HCO$_3^-$ wastage is prevented. Alternatively, when plasma HCO$_3^-$ rises above this threshold, reabsorption becomes less complete, allowing escape of excess HCO$_3^-$ into the final urine, which restores the plasma HCO$_3^-$ towards normal levels. Despite complete reabsorption of HCO$_3^-$, metabolic acidosis would still ensue if HCO$_3^-$ consumed in buffering nonvolatile acids were not constantly regenerated.

The *reabsorption* of filtered HCO$_3^-$ occurs by the following mechanism. Filtered bicarbonate combines with H$^+$ secreted from proximal tubule cells via the Na$^+$/H$^+$ exchange, to form carbonic acid (H$_2$CO$_3$). Dehydration of carbonic acid under the influence of *luminal* carbonic anhydrase yields H$_2$O and CO$_2$, which is free to diffuse from lumen to peritubular blood. In the proximal tubule cell, the OH$^-$ left behind by the H$^+$ secretion reacts with CO$_2$, under the influence of *intracellular* carbonic anhydrase, forming HCO$_3^-$. This ion is transported across the contraluminal proximal tubule cell membrane, via an electrogenic Na/HCO$_3^-$ cotransporter, to reenter the extracellular HCO$_3^-$ pool. The net result is *reclamation of a filtered bicarbonate ion*. Secreted H$^+$ is also free to react with nonbicarbonate buffers [e.g., phosphate or ammonia (NH$_4^+$)] in the tubule lumen, and hydrogen ions are excreted in these forms in the final urine. Again, the OH$^-$ left behind in the proximal tubule cell from H$^+$ secretion reacts with CO$_2$, forming bicarbonate—also representing *regeneration of an HCO$_3^-$ ion*.

Hydrogen ions in the urine are bound to filtered buffers (e.g., phosphate) in amounts equivalent to the amounts of alkali required to titrate the pH of the urine up to the pH of the blood (the so-called titratable acid). It is not usually possible to excrete all the daily acid load in the form of titratable acid due to limits of urinary pH. Metabolism of glutamine by proximal tubule cells to yield ammonium (ammoniagenesis) serves as an additional mechanism for H$^+$ elimination and bicarbonate regeneration. Glutamine metabolism forms not only NH$_4^+$ (i.e., NH$_3$ plus H$^+$) but also HCO$_3^-$, which is transported across the proximal tubule (HCO$_3^-$ regeneration). The NH$_4^+$ must be excreted in the urine for this process to be effective in bicarbonate regeneration. The excretion of ammonium involves secretion by proximal tubule cells (possibly by the Na$^+$/H$^+$ exchanger as Na$^+$/NH$_4^+$), generation of high medullary interstitial NH$_4^+$ concentration by an elaborate countercurrent multiplication/exchange system, and finally, secretion of the interstitial NH$_4^+$ by the collecting duct by a combination of H$^+$ secretion and passive NH$_3$ diffusion. *Ammoniagenesis* is responsive to the acid-base needs of the individual. When faced with an acute acid burden and an increased need for HCO$_3^-$ regeneration, the rate of renal ammonia synthesis increases sharply.

The quantity of hydrogen ions excreted as titratable acid and NH$_4^+$ is equal to the quantity of HCO$_3^-$ regenerated in tubule cells and added to plasma. Under steady-state conditions, the net quantity of acid excreted into the urine (the sum of titratable acid and NH$_4^+$ less HCO$_3^-$) must equal the quantity of acid gained by the extracellular fluid from all sources. Metabolic acidosis and alkalosis result when this delicate balance is perturbed, the former the result of insufficient net acid excretion, and the latter due to excessive acid excretion.

Progressive loss of renal function usually causes little or no change in arterial pH, plasma bicarbonate concentration, or arterial carbon dioxide tension (P$_{CO_2}$) until GFR falls below 25% of normal. Thereafter, all three tend to decline as *metabolic acidosis* ensues. In general, the metabolic acidosis of CRF is not due to overproduction of acids but is rather a reflection of nephron loss, which limits the amount of NH$_3$ (and therefore also HCO$_3^-$) that can be generated. Although surviving nephrons appear to be capable of generating supranormal amounts of NH$_3$ *per nephron*, the diminished nephron population causes overall production to be reduced to an extent that is insufficient to permit adequate buffering of H$^+$ in urine. As a result, although patients with CRF may be able to acidify their urine normally (i.e., urine pH as low as 4.5), the defect in NH$_3$ production limits daily net acid excretion to 30 to 40 mmol, or one-half to two-thirds the quantity of nonvolatile acid added to the extracellular fluid in the same time period. Metabolic acidosis resulting from this daily positive balance of H⁺ is seldom florid in CRF of mild to moderate severity. Relative stability of plasma bicarbonate (albeit at reduced levels of 14 to 18 mmol/L) is maintained at the expense of buffering by bone. Because it contains large reserves of alkaline salts (calcium phosphate and calcium bicarbonate), bone constitutes a major reserve of buffering capacity. Dissolution of these buffers contributes to the osteodystrophy of CRF (Fig. 270-1).

Although the acidosis of CRF is due to loss of tubule mass, it nevertheless depends to a large part on the level of GFR. When GFR is reduced to only a moderate extent (i.e., to about 50% of normal), retention of anions, principally sulfates and phosphates, is not pronounced. Therefore, as the plasma HCO_3^- falls owing to dysfunction or loss of tubules, retention of Cl^- by the kidneys leads to a *hyperchloremic acidosis*. At this stage *the anion gap is normal*. With further reductions in GFR and progressive azotemia, however, the retention of phosphates, sulfates, and other *unmeasured* anions ensues and plasma Cl^- falls to normal levels despite the reduction in plasma HCO_3^- concentration. *An elevated anion gap therefore develops.*

TUBULE POTASSIUM TRANSPORT WITH NORMAL AND REDUCED NEPHRON MASS As with H⁺, the concentration of K⁺ in extracellular fluid is normally maintained within a relatively narrow range, 4 to 5 mmol/L. At least 95% of total-body K⁺ is in the intracellular compartment, where the intracellular concentration is approximately 160 mmol/L. Normal individuals maintain external K⁺ balance by excreting amounts into the urine that equal the intake, less the relatively small losses in stool and sweat. K⁺ is freely filtered at the glomerulus, although the amount excreted usually represents no more than about 20% of the quantity filtered. The great bulk of the K⁺ filtered is reabsorbed in the early portions of the nephron, about two-thirds in the proximal tubule, and an additional 20 to 25% in the loop of Henle. A *K⁺ secretory process* operates in the distal tubule and terminal nephron segments. This process is largely dependent on Na⁺ reabsorption and the accompanying lumen-negative voltage creating an electrical gradient across the tubule wall, favoring K⁺ secretion into the lumen of the distal tubule and collecting duct.

The ability to maintain external K⁺ balance and normal plasma K⁺ concentration until relatively late in the course of CRF is a consequence primarily of a progressive increase in fractional excretion of K⁺. Greatly enhanced rates of K⁺ secretion occur in distal portions of surviving tubules. The augmented secretion rate of aldosterone contributes to enhanced tubule secretion of K⁺. In addition, both the increased distal tubule flow rates in surviving nephrons, due to the osmotic diuresis, and enhanced luminal electronegativity, created by the increased presence of highly impermeable anions such as phosphate and sulfate, enhance K⁺ secretion. Aldosterone also stimulates net entry of K⁺ into the lumen of the colon, a mechanism known to be enhanced in CRF. →*More detailed discussions of abnormal K⁺ homeostasis in acute and chronic forms of renal failure are given in Chaps. 269 and 270.*

ACKNOWLEDGMENT
Harald S. MacKenzie was a co-author of this chapter in the 14th edition and some of the content of that chapter is carried forward to the present edition.

BIBLIOGRAPHY

BRENNER BM: Nephron adaptation to renal injury or ablation. Am J Physiol 249:F324, 1985

——— (ed): *Brenner and Rector's The Kidney*, 6th ed. Philadelphia, Saunders, 2000

——— et al: Diverse biological actions of atrial natriuretic peptides. Physiol Rev 70:665, 1990

BUSHINSKY DA: The contribution of acidosis to renal osteodystrophy. Kidney Int 47: 1816, 1995

KAJI D, KAHN T: Na⁺-K⁺ pump in chronic renal failure. Am J Physiol 252:F785, 1987

PRICE SR, MITCH WE: Metabolic acidosis and uremic toxicity: Protein and amino acid metabolism. Semin Nephrol 14:232, 1994

269 *Hugh R. Brady, Barry M. Brenner*

ACUTE RENAL FAILURE

Acute renal failure (ARF) is a syndrome characterized by rapid decline in glomerular filtration rate (hours to days), retention of nitrogenous waste products, and perturbation of extracellular fluid volume and electrolyte and acid-base homeostasis. ARF complicates approximately 5% of hospital admissions and up to 30% of admissions to intensive care units. Oliguria (urine output < 500 mL/d) is a frequent but not invariable clinical feature (~50%). ARF is usually asymptomatic and is diagnosed when biochemical screening of hospitalized patients reveals a recent increase in plasma urea and creatinine concentrations. It may complicate a wide range of diseases, which for purposes of diagnosis and management are conveniently divided into three categories: (1) diseases that cause renal hypoperfusion without compromising the integrity of renal parenchyma (*prerenal ARF*, prerenal azotemia) (~55%); (2) diseases that directly involve renal parenchyma (*intrinsic renal ARF*, renal azotemia) (~40%); and (3) diseases associated with urinary tract obstruction (*postrenal ARF*, postrenal azotemia) (~5%). Most ARF is reversible, the kidney being relatively unique among major organs in its ability to recover from almost complete loss of function. Nevertheless, ARF is associated with major in-hospital morbidity and mortality, in large part due to the serious nature of the illnesses that precipitate the ARF.

ETIOLOGY AND PATHOPHYSIOLOGY

PRERENAL ARF (PRERENAL AZOTEMIA) Prerenal ARF is the most common form of ARF and represents a physiologic response to mild to moderate renal hypoperfusion. Prerenal ARF is rapidly reversible upon restoration of renal blood flow and glomerular ultrafiltration pressure. Renal parenchymal tissue is not damaged; indeed, kidneys from individuals with prerenal ARF function well when transplanted into recipients with normal cardiovascular function. More severe hypoperfusion may lead to ischemic injury of renal parenchyma and intrinsic renal ARF. Thus, prerenal ARF and intrinsic renal ARF due to ischemia are part of a spectrum of manifestations of renal hypoperfusion. As shown in Table 269-1, prerenal ARF can complicate any disease that induces hypovolemia, low cardiac output, systemic vasodilatation, or selective renal vasoconstriction.

Hypovolemia leads to a fall in mean systemic arterial pressure, which is detected as reduced stretch by arterial (e.g., carotid sinus) and cardiac baroreceptors. Activated baroreceptors trigger a coordinated series of neural and humoral responses designed to restore blood volume and arterial pressure. These include activation of the sympathetic nervous system and renin-angiotensin-aldosterone system and release of arginine vasopressin (AVP; formerly called antidiuretic hormone). Norepinephrine, angiotensin II, and AVP act in concert in an attempt to preserve cardiac and cerebral perfusion by stimulating vasoconstriction in relatively "nonessential" vascular beds, such as the musculocutaneous and splanchnic circulations, by inhibiting salt loss through sweat glands, by stimulating thirst and salt appetite, and by promoting renal salt and water retention. Glomerular perfusion, ultrafiltration pressure, and filtration rate are preserved during mild hypoperfusion through several compensatory mechanisms. Stretch receptors in afferent arterioles, in response to a reduction in perfusion pressure, trigger afferent arteriolar vasodilatation through a local myogenic reflex (autoregulation). Biosynthesis of vasodilator prostaglandins (e.g., prostaglandin F_2 and prostacyclin) is also enhanced, and these compounds preferentially dilate afferent arterioles. In addition, angiotensin II induces preferential constriction of efferent arterioles.

Table 269-1   Classification and Major Causes of Acute Renal Failure (ARF)

PRERENAL ARF

I. Hypovolemia
   A. Hemorrhage, burns, dehydration
   B. Gastrointestinal fluid loss: vomiting, surgical drainage, diarrhea
   C. Renal fluid loss: diuretics, osmotic diuresis (e.g., diabetes mellitus), hypoadrenalism
   D. Sequestration in extravascular space: pancreatitis, peritonitis, trauma, burns, severe hypoalbuminemia
II. Low cardiac output
   A. Diseases of myocardium, valves, and pericardium; arrhythmias; tamponade
   B. Other: pulmonary hypertension, massive pulmonary embolus, positive pressure mechanical ventilation
III. Altered renal systemic vascular resistance ratio
   A. Systemic vasodilatation: sepsis, antihypertensives, afterload reducers, anesthesia, anaphylaxis
   B. Renal vasoconstriction: hypercalcemia, norepinephrine, epinephrine, cyclosporine, FK506, amphotericin B
   C. Cirrhosis with ascites (hepatorenal syndrome)
IV. Renal hypoperfusion with impairment of renal autoregulatory responses
   Cyclooxygenase inhibitors, angiotensin-converting enzyme inhibitors
V. Hyperviscosity syndrome (rare)
   Multiple myeloma, macroglobulinemia, polycythemia

INTRINSIC RENAL ARF

I. Renovascular obstruction (bilateral or unilateral in the setting of one functioning kidney)
   A. Renal artery obstruction: atherosclerotic plaque, thrombosis, embolism, dissecting aneurysm, vasculitis
   B. Renal vein obstruction: thrombosis, compression
II. Disease of glomeruli or renal microvasculature
   A. Glomerulonephritis and vasculitis
   B. Hemolytic uremic syndrome, thrombotic thrombocytopenic purpura, disseminated intravascular coagulation, toxemia of pregnancy, accelerated hypertension, radiation nephritis, systemic lupus erythematosus, scleroderma
III. Acute tubular necrosis
   A. Ischemia: as for prerenal ARF (hypovolemia, low cardiac output, renal vasoconstriction, systemic vasodilatation), obstetric complications (abruptio placentae, postpartum hemorrhage)
   B. Toxins
     1. Exogenous: radiocontrast, cyclosporine, antibiotics (e.g., aminoglycosides), chemotherapy (e.g., cisplatin), organic solvents (e.g., ethylene glycol), acetaminophen, illegal abortifacients
     2. Endogenous: rhabdomyolysis, hemolysis, uric acid, oxalate, plasma cell dyscrasia (e.g., myeloma)
IV. Interstitial nephritis
   A. Allergic: antibiotics (e.g., β-lactams, sulfonamides, trimethoprim, rifampicin), nonsteroidal anti-inflammatory agents, diuretics, captopril
   B. Infection: bacterial (e.g., acute pyelonephritis, leptospirosis), viral (e.g., cytomegalovirus), fungal (e.g., candidiasis)
   C. Infiltration: lymphoma, leukemia, sarcoidosis
   D. Idiopathic
V. Intratubular deposition and obstruction
   Myeloma proteins, uric acid, oxalate, acyclovir, methotrexate, sulphonamides
VI. Renal allograft rejection

POSTRENAL ARF (OBSTRUCTION)

I. Ureteric
   Calculi, blood clot, sloughed papillae, cancer, external compression (e.g., retroperitoneal fibrosis)
II. Bladder neck
   Neurogenic bladder, prostatic hypertrophy, calculi, cancer, blood clot
III. Urethra
   Stricture, congenital valve, phimosis

As a result, intraglomerular pressure is maintained, the fraction of plasma flowing through glomerular capillaries that is filtered is increased (filtration fraction), and glomerular filtration rate (GFR) is preserved. During states of more severe hypoperfusion, these compensatory responses are overwhelmed and GFR falls, leading to prerenal ARF.

Autoregulatory dilatation of afferent arterioles is maximal at mean systemic arterial blood pressures of ~80 mmHg, and hypotension below this level is associated with a precipitous decline in GFR. Lesser degrees of hypotension may provoke prerenal ARF in the elderly and in patients with diseases affecting the integrity of afferent arterioles (e.g., hypertensive nephrosclerosis, diabetic vasculopathy). In addition, drugs that interfere with adaptive responses in the renal microcirculation may convert compensated renal hypoperfusion into overt prerenal ARF or trigger progression of prerenal ARF to ischemic intrinsic renal ARF (see below). Pharmacologic inhibitors of either renal prostaglandin biosynthesis [*cyclooxygenase inhibitors*; nonsteroidal anti-inflammatory drugs (NSAIDs)] or angiotensin-converting enzyme (ACE) activity (ACE inhibitors) are the major culprits and should be used judiciously in the setting of suspected renal hypoperfusion. NSAIDs do not compromise GFR in healthy individuals but may precipitate prerenal ARF in patients with volume depletion or in those with chronic renal insufficiency in whom GFR is maintained, in part, through prostaglandin-mediated hyperfiltration through the remaining functional nephrons. ACE inhibitors can also compromise GFR in individuals with renal hypoperfusion and should be used with special care in patients with bilateral renal artery stenosis or unilateral stenosis in a solitary functioning kidney. Glomerular perfusion and filtration may be exquisitely dependent on the actions of angiotensin II under the latter circumstances. Angiotensin II preserves glomerular filtration pressure distal to stenoses by elevating systemic arterial pressure and by triggering selective constriction of efferent arterioles. ACE inhibitors blunt these responses and precipitate ARF, usually reversible, in ~30% of these patients.

Hepatorenal Syndrome   This is a particularly aggressive form of ARF that frequently complicates hepatic failure due to advanced cirrhosis or other liver diseases, including malignancy, hepatic resection, and biliary obstruction. Intrarenal vasoconstriction and avid sodium retention are early sequelae of these diseases and may be detected before changes in systemic hemodynamics. Patients with advanced liver disease, portal hypertension, and ascites also have increased plasma volume but reduced "effective" arterial blood volume as a consequence of systemic vasodilatation and pooling of blood in the portal circulation. Renal failure typically develops slowly over weeks or months in parallel with deteriorating hepatic function but may accelerate dramatically following a variety of hemodynamic insults, including hemorrhage, paracentesis, and overzealous use of diuretics, vasodilators, or cyclooxygenase inhibitors. In full-blown hepatorenal syndrome, ARF progresses even after optimization of systemic hemodynamics and systemic arterial blood volume and removal of nephrotoxins, probably as a result of ongoing intrarenal vasoconstriction, hypoperfusion, and ischemia triggered by circulating factors or neural impulses originating in the failing liver. Indeed, it must be remembered that patients with liver disease may develop other forms of ARF (e.g., sepsis, nephrotoxic medications), and a diagnosis of hepatorenal syndrome should be made only after exclusion of other possible reversible causes.

INTRINSIC RENAL ARF (INTRINSIC RENAL AZOTEMIA)   Intrinsic renal ARF can complicate many diverse diseases of the renal parenchyma. From a clinicopathologic viewpoint, it is useful to divide the causes of intrinsic renal ARF into (1) diseases of large renal vessels, (2) diseases of the renal microcirculation and glomeruli, (3) ischemic and nephrotoxic ARF, and (4) tubulointerstitial diseases (Table 269-1). Most intrinsic renal ARF is triggered by ischemia (ischemic ARF) or nephrotoxins (nephrotoxic ARF), insults that classically induce acute tubular necrosis (ATN). Accordingly, the terms ARF and ATN are usually used interchangeably in these settings. However, as many as 20 to 30% of patients with ischemic or nephrotoxic ARF do not have clinical (granular or tubular cell urinary casts) or morphologic evidence of tubular necrosis, underscoring the role of sublethal injury to tubular epithelium and injury to other renal cells (e.g., endothelial cells) in the pathophysiology of this syndrome.

Etiology and Pathophysiology of Ischemic ARF Prerenal ARF and ischemic ARF are part of a spectrum of manifestations of renal hypoperfusion. Ischemic ARF differs from prerenal ARF in that the hypoperfusion induces ischemic injury to renal parenchymal cells, particularly tubular epithelium, and recovery typically takes 1 to 2 weeks after normalization of renal perfusion as it requires repair and regeneration of renal cells. In its most extreme form, ischemia leads to bilateral renal cortical necrosis and irreversible renal failure. Ischemic ARF occurs most frequently in patients undergoing major cardiovascular surgery or suffering severe trauma, hemorrhage, sepsis, and/or volume depletion (Table 269-1). Ischemic ARF can also complicate milder forms of true hypovolemia or reduced "effective" arterial blood volume if they occur in the presence of other insults (e.g., nephrotoxins or sepsis) or in patients with compromised autoregulatory defense mechanisms or preexisting renal disease.

The course of ischemic ARF is typically characterized by three phases: the initiation, maintenance, and recovery phases. The *initiation phase* (hours to days) is the initial period of renal hypoperfusion during which ischemic injury is evolving. GFR declines because (1) glomerular ultrafiltration pressure is reduced as a consequence of the fall in renal blood flow, (2) the flow of glomerular filtrate within tubules is obstructed by casts comprising epithelial cells and necrotic debris derived from ischemic tubule epithelium, and (3) there is backleak of glomerular filtrate through injured tubular epithelium (Fig. 269-1). Ischemic injury is most prominent in the terminal medullary portion of the proximal tubule (S_3 segment, pars recta) and the medullary portion of the thick ascending limb of the loop of Henle. Both segments have high rates of active (ATP-dependent) solute transport and oxygen consumption and are located in a zone of the kidney (the outer medulla) that is relatively ischemic, even under basal conditions, by virtue of the unique countercurrent arrangement of the medullary vasculature. Cellular ischemia results in a series of alterations in energetics, ion transport, and membrane integrity that ultimately lead to cell injury and, if severe, cell apoptosis or necrosis. These alterations include depletion of ATP, inhibition of active sodium transport and transport of other solutes, impairment of cell volume regulation and cell swelling, cytoskeletal disruption and loss of cell polarity, cell-cell and cell-matrix attachment, accumulation of intracellular calcium, altered phospholipid metabolism, oxygen free radical formation, and peroxidation of membrane lipids. Importantly, renal injury can be limited by restoration of renal blood flow during this period.

FIGURE 269-1 Overview of the pathophysiology of prerenal ARF and ischemic intrinsic renal ARF: A spectrum of manifestations of renal hypoperfusion (ARF, acute renal failure; AVP, arginine vasopressin; GFR, glomerular filtration rate.)

The initiation phase is followed by a *maintenance phase* (typically 1 to 2 weeks) during which renal cell injury is established, GFR stabilizes at its nadir (typically 5 to 10 mL/min), urine output is lowest, and uremic complications arise (see below). The reasons why the GFR remains low during this phase, despite correction of systemic hemodynamics, are still being defined. Putative mechanisms include persistent intrarenal vasoconstriction and medullary ischemia triggered by dysregulated release of vasoactive mediators from injured endothelial cells (e.g., decreased nitric oxide, increased endothelin-1 and platelet-activating factor), congestion of medullary blood vessels, and reperfusion injury induced by reactive oxygen species and other mediators derived from leukocytes or renal parenchymal cells (Fig. 269-1). In addition, epithelial cell injury per se may contribute to persistent intrarenal vasoconstriction by a process termed *tubuloglomerular feedback*. Specialized epithelial cells in the macula densa region of distal tubules detect increases in distal salt (probably chloride) delivery that occur as a consequence of impaired reabsorption by more proximal nephron segments. Macula densa cells in turn stimulate constriction of adjacent afferent arterioles by a poorly defined mechanism and further compromise glomerular perfusion and filtration, thereby contributing to a vicious cycle. A *recovery phase* is characterized by renal parenchymal cell, particularly tubule epithelial cell, repair and regeneration and a gradual return of GFR to or towards premorbid levels. The recovery phase may be complicated by a marked diuretic phase due to excretion of retained salt and water and other solutes, continued use of diuretics, and/or delayed recovery of epithelial cell function (solute and water reabsorption) relative to glomerular filtration (see below).

Etiology and Pathophysiology of Nephrotoxic ARF   Acute intrinsic renal ARF can complicate exposure to many structurally diverse pharmacologic agents (Table 269-1). With most nephrotoxins, the incidence of ARF is increased in the elderly and in patients with preexisting chronic renal insufficiency, true or "effective" hypovolemia, or concomitant exposure to other toxins.

Intrarenal vasoconstriction is a pivotal event in ARF triggered by *radiocontrast agents* (contrast nephropathy) and *cyclosporine*. In keeping with this pathophysiology, both agents induce ARF that shares features with prerenal ARF: namely, an acute fall in renal blood flow and GFR, a relatively benign urine sediment, and a low fractional excretion of sodium (see below). Severe cases may show clinical or pathologic evidence of ATN. Contrast nephropathy classically presents as an acute (onset within 24 to 48 h) but reversible (peak 3 to 5 days, resolution within 1 week) rise in blood urea nitrogen and creatinine and is most common in individuals with preexisting chronic renal insufficiency, diabetes mellitus, congestive heart failure, hypovolemia, or multiple myeloma. The syndrome appears to be dose-related, and its incidence is only slightly reduced in high-risk individuals by use of more expensive low osmolality, nonionic contrast agents. Endothelin-1, a potent vasoconstrictor peptide released from endothelial cells, is an important mediator of intrarenal vasoconstriction and mesangial cell contraction in this setting. Endothelin-1 has also been implicated as an important mediator of cyclosporine-induced ARF.

Direct toxicity to tubule epithelial cells and/or intratubular obstruction are major pathophysiologic events in ARF induced by many antibiotics and anticancer drugs. Frequent offenders are the antimicrobial agents, such as acyclovir, foscarnet, aminoglycosides, amphotericin B, and pentamidine, and chemotherapeutic agents, such as cisplatin and ifosfamide. ARF complicates 10 to 30% of courses of *aminoglycoside antibiotics*, even in the presence of therapeutic levels. *Amphotericin B* causes dose-related ARF through intrarenal vasoconstriction and direct toxicity to proximal tubule epithelium. Cisplatin, like the aminoglycosides, is accumulated by proximal tubule cells and typically provokes ARF after 7 to 10 days of exposure by inducing mitochondrial injury, inhibition of ATPase activity and solute transport, free radical–mediated injury to cell membranes, apoptosis and/or necrosis.

The most common endogenous nephrotoxins are calcium, myoglobin, hemoglobin, urate, oxalate, and myeloma light chains. Hypercalcemia can compromise GFR, predominantly by inducing intrarenal vasoconstriction. Calcium phosphate deposition within the kidney may also contribute. Both *rhabdomyolysis* and *hemolysis* can induce ARF, particularly in hypovolemic or acidotic individuals. Myoglobinuric ARF complicates approximately 30% of cases of rhabdomyolysis. Common causes of the latter include traumatic crush injury, acute muscle ischemia, seizures, excessive exercise, heat stroke or malignant hyperthermia, intoxications (e.g., alcohol, cocaine), and infectious or metabolic disorders. ARF due to hemolysis is relatively rare and is observed following massive blood transfusion reactions. It has been postulated that myoglobin and hemoglobin or other compounds released from muscle or red blood cells cause ARF via toxic effects on tubule epithelial cells or by inducing intratubular cast formation. Hypovolemia or acidosis may contribute to the pathogenesis of ARF in this setting by promoting intratubular cast formation. In addition, both hemoglobin and myoglobin are potent inhibitors of nitric oxide bioactivity and may trigger intrarenal vasoconstriction and ischemia in patients with borderline renal hypoperfusion. The formation of intratubular casts containing filtered immunoglobulin light chains and other proteins, including Tamm-Horsfall protein produced by thick ascending limb cells, is the major trigger for ARF in patients with *multiple myeloma* (myeloma cast nephropathy). Light chains may also be directly toxic to tubule epithelial cells. Intratubular obstruction may also be an important cause of ARF in patients with severe *hyperuricosuria* or *hyperoxaluria*. Acute uric acid nephropathy typically complicates treatment of lymphoproliferative or myeloproliferative disorders but occasionally occurs in other forms of primary or secondary hyperuricemia if the urine is concentrated.

Pathology of Ischemic and Nephrotoxic ARF   The classic pathologic features of ischemic ARF are patchy and focal necrosis of tubule epithelium with detachment from its basement membrane and occlusion of tubule lumens with casts composed of intact or degenerating epithelial cells, cellular debris, Tamm-Horsfall mucoprotein, and pigments. Leukocyte accumulation is frequently observed in vasa recta; however, the morphology of the glomeruli and renal vasculature is characteristically normal. Necrosis is most severe in the straight portion (pars recta) of proximal tubules but may also affect the medullary thick ascending limb of the loop of Henle.

In nephrotoxic ARF, morphologic changes tend to be most prominent in both the convoluted and straight portions of proximal tubules. Tubule cell necrosis is less pronounced than in ischemic ARF.

Other Causes of Intrinsic Renal ARF   Patients with advanced atherosclerosis can develop ARF after manipulation of the aorta or renal arteries at surgery or angiography, following trauma, or, rarely, spontaneously due to embolization of cholesterol crystals to the renal vasculature (atheroembolic ARF). Cholesterol crystals lodge in small- and medium-sized arteries and incite a giant cell and fibrotic reaction in the vessel wall with narrowing or obstruction of the vessel lumen. Atheroembolic ARF is frequently irreversible. A myriad of structurally diverse pharmacologic agents induce ARF by triggering allergic interstitial nephritis, a disease characterized by infiltration of the tubulointerstitium by granulocytes (typically but not invariably eosinophils), macrophages, and/or lymphocytes and by interstitial edema. The most common offenders are antibiotics (e.g., penicillins, cephalosporins, trimethoprim, sulfonamides, rifampicin) and NSAIDs (Table 269-1).

POSTRENAL ARF   (See also Chap. 281)   Urinary tract obstruction accounts for fewer than 5% of cases of ARF. Since one kidney has sufficient clearance capacity to excrete nitrogenous waste products, ARF from obstruction requires either obstruction to urine flow between the external urethral meatus and bladder neck, bilateral ureteric obstruction, or unilateral ureteric obstruction in a patient with one functioning kidney or preexisting chronic renal insufficiency. Bladder neck obstruction represents the most common cause of postrenal ARF and is usually due to prostatic disease (e.g., hypertrophy, neoplasia, or infection), neurogenic bladder, or therapy with anticholinergic drugs. Less common causes of acute lower urinary tract obstruction include blood clots, calculi, and urethritis with spasm. Ureteric obstruction may result from intraluminal obstruction (e.g., calculi, blood clots, sloughed renal papillae), infiltration of the ureteric wall (e.g., neoplasia), or external compression (e.g., retroperitoneal fibrosis, neoplasia or abscess, inadvertent surgical ligature). During the early stages of obstruction (hours to days), continued glomerular filtration leads to increased intraluminal pressure upstream to the site of obstruction. As a result there are gradual distention of proximal ureter, renal pelvis, and calyces and a fall in GFR. Acute obstruction is initially associated with modest increase in renal blood flow, but arteriolar vasoconstriction soon supervenes, leading to a further decline in glomerular filtration.

CLINICAL FEATURES AND DIFFERENTIAL DIAGNOSIS

Patients presenting with renal failure should be assessed initially to determine if the decline in GFR is acute or chronic. An acute process is easily established if a review of laboratory records reveals a recent rise in blood urea and creatinine levels, but previous measurements are not always available. Findings that suggest chronic renal failure (Chap. 270) include anemia, neuropathy, and radiologic evidence of renal osteodystrophy or small scarred kidneys. However, it should be noted that anemia may also complicate ARF (see below), and renal size may be normal or increased in several chronic renal diseases (e.g., diabetic nephropathy, amyloidosis, polycystic kidney disease). Once a diagnosis of ARF has been established, several issues should be addressed promptly: (1) the identification of the cause of ARF, (2) the elimination of the triggering insult (e.g., nephrotoxin) and/or institution of disease-specific therapies, and (3) the prevention and management of uremic complications.

CLINICAL ASSESSMENT   Clinical clues to *prerenal* ARF are symptoms of thirst and orthostatic dizziness and physical evidence of orthostatic hypotension and tachycardia, reduced jugular venous pressure, decreased skin turgor, dry mucous membranes, and reduced axillary sweating. Case records should be reviewed for documentation of a progressive fall in urine output and body weight and treatment with NSAIDs or ACE inhibitors. Careful clinical examination may reveal stigmata of chronic liver disease and portal hypertension, advanced cardiac failure, sepsis, or other causes of reduced "effective" arterial blood volume (Table 269-1).

Intrinsic renal ARF due to ischemia is likely following severe renal hypoperfusion complicating hypovolemic or septic shock or following major surgery. The likelihood of ischemic ARF is increased further if ARF persists despite normalization of systemic hemodynamics. Diagnosis of nephrotoxic ARF requires careful review of the clinical data and pharmacy, nursing, and radiology records for evidence of recent exposure to nephrotoxic medications or radiocontrast agents or to endogenous toxins (e.g., myoglobin, hemoglobin, uric acid, myeloma protein, or elevated levels of serum calcium).

Although ischemic and nephrotoxic ARF account for more than 90% of cases of intrinsic renal ARF, other renal parenchymal diseases must be considered (Table 269-2). Flank pain may be a prominent symptom following occlusion of a renal artery or vein and with other parenchymal diseases distending the renal capsule (e.g., severe glomerulonephritis or pyelonephritis). Subcutaneous nodules, livido reticularis, bright orange retinal arteriolar plaques, and digital ischemia, despite palpable pedal pulses, are clues to atheroembolization. ARF in association with oliguria, edema, hypertension, and an "active" urine sediment (nephritic syndrome) suggests acute glomerulonephritis or vasculitis. Malignant hypertension is a likely cause of ARF in patients with severe hypertension and evidence of hypertensive injury to other organs (e.g., left ventricular hypertrophy and failure, hypertensive retinopathy and papilledema, neurologic dysfunction). Fever, arthralgias, and a pruritic erythematous rash following exposure to a new drug suggest allergic interstitial nephritis, although systemic features of hypersensitivity are frequently absent.

Postrenal ARF presents with suprapubic and flank pain due to distention of the bladder and of the renal collecting system and capsule, respectively. Colicky flank pain radiating to the groin suggests acute ureteric obstruction. Prostatic disease is likely if there is a history of nocturia, frequency, and hesitancy and enlargement or induration of the prostate on rectal examination. Neurogenic bladder should be suspected in patients receiving anticholinergic medications or with physical evidence of autonomic dysfunction. Definitive diagnosis of postrenal ARF hinges on judicious use of radiologic investigations and rapid improvement in renal function following relief of obstruction.

URINALYSIS   Anuria suggests complete urinary tract obstruction but may complicate severe cases of prerenal or intrinsic renal ARF. Wide fluctuations in urine output raise the possibility of intermittent obstruction, whereas patients with partial urinary tract obstruction can present with polyuria due to impairment of urine concentrating mechanisms.

In prerenal ARF, the sediment is characteristically acellular and contains transparent hyaline casts ("bland," "benign," "inactive" urine sediment). Hyaline casts are formed in concentrated urine from normal constituents of urine—principally Tamm-Horsfall protein, which is secreted by epithelial cells of the loop of Henle. Postrenal ARF may also present with an inactive sediment, although hematuria and pyuria are common in patients with intraluminal obstruction or prostatic disease. Pigmented "muddy brown" granular casts and casts containing tubule epithelial cells are characteristic of ATN and suggest ischemic or nephrotoxic ARF. They are usually found in association with microscopic hematuria and mild "tubular" proteinuria (<1 g/d); the latter reflects impaired reabsorption and processing of filtered proteins by injured proximal tubules. Casts are absent, however, in 20 to 30% of patients with ischemic or nephrotoxic ARF and are not a requisite for diagnosis. In general, red blood cell casts indicate glomerular injury or, less often, acute tubulointerstitial nephritis. White cell casts and nonpigmented granular casts suggest interstitial nephritis, whereas broad granular casts are characteristic of chronic renal disease and probably reflect interstitial fibrosis and dilatation of tubules. Eosinophiluria (>5% of urine leukocytes) is a common finding (~90%) in antibiotic-induced allergic interstitial nephritis when studied using Hansel's stain; however, lymphocytes may predominate in allergic interstitial nephritis induced by NSAIDs. Eosinophiluria is also a feature of atheroembolic ARF. Occasional uric acid crystals (pleomorphic in shape) are common in the concentrated urine of prerenal ARF but suggest acute urate nephropathy if seen in abundance. Oxalate (envelope-shaped) and hippurate (needle-shaped) crystals raise the possibility of ethylene glycol ingestion and toxicity.

Increased urine protein excretion, but <1 g/d, is common in ATN due to failure of injured proximal tubules to reabsorb filtered protein and excretion of cellular debris ("tubular proteinuria"). Proteinuria of >1 g/d suggests injury to the glomerular ultrafiltration barrier ("glomerular proteinuria") or excretion of myeloma light chains. The latter are not detected by conventional dipsticks (which detect albumin) and must be sought by other means (e.g., sulfosalicylic acid test, immunoelectrophoresis). Heavy proteinuria is also a frequent finding (~80%) in patients who develop combined allergic interstitial nephritis and minimal change glomerulopathy when treated with NSAIDs. A similar syndrome can be triggered by ampicillin, rifampicin, or interferon α. Hemoglobinuria or myoglobinuria should be suspected if urine is strongly positive for heme by dipstick, but contains few red cells, and if the supernatant of centrifuged urine is positive for free heme. Bilirubinuria may provide a clue to the presence of hepatorenal syndrome.

RENAL FAILURE INDICES   Analysis of urine and blood biochemistry is particularly useful for distinguishing prerenal ARF from ischemic or nephrotoxic intrinsic renal ARF (Table 269-3). The fractional excretion of sodium (FE_{Na}) is most useful in this regard. The FE_{Na} relates sodium clearance to creatinine clearance. Sodium is reabsorbed avidly from glomerular filtrate in patients with prerenal ARF, in an attempt to restore intravascular volume, but not in patients with ischemic or nephrotoxic intrinsic ARF, as a result of tubular epithelial cell injury. In contrast, creatinine is not reabsorbed in either setting. Consequently, patients with prerenal ARF typically have a FE_{Na} of <1.0% (frequently <0.1%), whereas the FE_{Na} in patients with ischemic or nephrotoxic ARF is usually >1.0%. The *renal failure index* (Table 269-3) provides comparable information, since clinical variations in serum sodium concentration are relatively small. *Urine sodium concentration* is a less sensitive index for distinguishing prerenal ARF from ischemic and nephrotoxic ARF as values overlap between groups. Similarly, indices of urinary concentrating ability such as urine specific gravity, urine osmolality, urine-to-plasma urea ratio, and blood urea-to-creatinine ratio are of limited value in differential diagnosis.

Many caveats apply when interpreting biochemical renal failure indices. FE_{Na} may be >1.0% in prerenal ARF if patients are receiving diuretics or have bicarbonaturia (accompanied by sodium to maintain electroneutrality), preexisting chronic renal failure complicated by salt wasting, or adrenal insufficiency. In contrast, the FE_{Na} is <1.0% in

Cause of Acute Renal Failure	Suggestive Clinical Features	Typical Urinalysis	Some Confirmatory Tests
I. Prerenal ARF	Evidence of true volume depletion (thirst, postural or absolute hypotension and tachycardia, low jugular venous pressure, dry mucous membranes/axillae, weight loss, fluid output > input) or decreased "effective" circulatory volume (e.g., heart failure, liver failure), treatment with NSAIDs or ACE inhibitors	Hyaline casts $FE_{Na} < 1\%$ $U_{Na} < 10$ mmol/L $SG > 1.018$	Occasionally requires invasive hemodynamic monitoring; rapid resolution of ARF upon restoration of renal perfusion
II. Intrinsic renal ARF			
A. Diseases involving large renal vessels			
1. Renal artery thrombosis	History of atrial fibrillation or recent myocardial infarct; flank or abdominal pain	Mild proteinuria Occasionally red cells	Elevated LDH with normal transaminases, renal arteriogram
2. Atheroembolism	Age usually > 50 years, recent manipulation of aorta, retinal plaques, subcutaneous nodules, palpable purpura, livedo reticularis, vasculopathy, hypertension, anticoagulation	Often normal, eosinophiluria, rarely casts	Eosinophilia, hypocomplementemia, skin biopsy, renal biopsy
3. Renal vein thrombosis	Evidence of nephrotic syndrome or pulmonary embolism, flank pain	Proteinuria, hematuria	Inferior vena cavagram and selective renal venogram
B. Diseases of small vessels and glomeruli			
1. Glomerulonephritis/vasculitis	Compatible clinical history (e.g., recent infection) sinusitis, lung hemorrhage, skin rash or ulcers, arthralgias, new cardiac murmur, history of hepatitis B or C infection	Red cell or granular casts, red cells, white cells, mild proteinuria	Low C3, ANCA, anti-GBM Ab, ANA, ASO, anti-DNAse, cryoglobulins, blood cultures, renal biopsy
2. Hemolytic-uremic syndrome/ thrombotic thrombocytopenic purpura	Compatible clinical history (e.g., recent gastrointestinal infection, cyclosporine, anovulants), fever, pallor, ecchymoses, neurologic abnormalities	May be normal, red cells, mild proteinuria, rarely red cell/granular casts	Anemia, thrombocytopenia, schistocytes on blood smear, increased LDH, renal biopsy
3. Malignant hypertension	Severe hypertension with headaches, cardiac failure, retinopathy, neurologic dysfunction, papilledema	Red cells, red cell casts, proteinuria	LVH by echocardiography/ECG, resolution of ARF with control of blood pressure
C. ARF mediated by ischemia or toxins (ATN)			
1. Ischemia	Recent hemorrhage, hypotension (e.g., cardiac arrest), surgery	Muddy brown granular or tubular epithelial cell casts $FE_{Na} > 1\%$ $U_{Na} > 20$ mmol/L $SG < 1.015$	Clinical assessment and urinalysis usually sufficient for diagnosis
2. Exogenous toxins	Recent radiocontrast study, nephrotoxic antibiotics or anticancer agents often coexistent with volume depletion, sepsis, or chronic renal insufficiency	Muddy brown granular or tubular epithelial cell casts $FE_{Na} > 1\%$ $U_{Na} > 20$ mmol/L $SG < 1.015$	Clinical assessment and urinalysis usually sufficient for diagnosis
3. Endogenous toxins	History suggestive of rhabdomyolysis (seizures, coma, ethanol abuse, trauma)	Urine supernatant positive for heme	Hyperkalemia, hyperphosphatemia, hypocalcemia, increased circulating myoglobin, CPK (MM), and uric acid
	History suggestive of hemolysis (blood transfusion)	Urine supernatant pink and positive for heme	Hyperkalemia, hyperphosphatemia, hypocalcemia, hyperuricemia, pink plasma positive for hemoglobin
	History suggestive of tumor lysis (recent chemotherapy), myeloma (bone pain), or ethylene glycol ingestion	Urate crystals, dipstick-negative proteinuria, oxalate crystals, respectively	Hyperuricemia, hyperkalemia, hyperphosphatemia (for tumor lysis); circulating or urinary monoclonal spike (for myeloma); toxicology screen, acidosis, osmolal gap (for ethylene glycol)

(continued)

Cause of Acute Renal Failure	Suggestive Clinical Features	Typical Urinalysis	Some Confirmatory Tests
D. Acute diseases of the tubulo-interstitium			
1. Allergic interstitial nephritis	Recent ingestion of drug, and fever, rash, or arthralgias	White cell casts, white cells (frequently eosinphiluria), red cells, rarely red cell casts, proteinuria (occasionally nephrotic)	Systemic eosinophilia, skin biopsy of rash (leukocytoclastic vasculitis), renal biopsy
2. Acute bilateral pyelonephritis	Flank pain and tenderness, toxic, febrile	Leukocytes, proteinuria, red cells, bacteria	Urine and blood cultures
III. Postrenal ARF	Abdominal or flank pain, palpable bladder	Frequently normal, hematuria if stones, hemorrhage, malignancy, or prostatic hypertrophy	Plain film, renal ultrasound, IVP, retrograde or anterograde pyelography, CT scan

NOTE: NSAIDs, nonsteroidal anti-inflammatory drugs; U_{Na}, urine sodium concentration; SG, specific gravity; LDH, lactate dehydrogenase; C3, complement component; ANCA, antineutrophil cytoplasmic autoantibody; anti-GBM Ab, anti-glomerular basement membrane antibody; ANA, antinuclear antibody; ASO, antistreptolysin O; LVH, left ventricular hypertrophy; ECG, electrocardiogram; CK, creatine kinase; IVP, intravenous pyelogram; CT, computed tomography.

SOURCE: Adapted with permission from Brady et al.

approximately 15% of patients with nonoliguric ischemic or nephrotoxic ARF. The FE_{Na} is often <1.0% in ARF due to urinary tract obstruction, glomerulonephritis, and vascular diseases.

LABORATORY FINDINGS Serial measurements of serum creatinine can provide useful pointers to the cause of ARF. Prerenal ARF is typified by fluctuating levels that parallel changes in hemodynamic function. Creatinine rises rapidly (within 24 to 48 h) in patients with ARF following renal ischemia, atheroembolization, and radiocontrast exposure. Peak creatinine levels are observed after 3 to 5 days with contrast nephropathy and return to baseline after 5 to 7 days. In contrast, creatinine levels typically peak later (7 to 10 days) in ischemic ARF and atheroembolic disease. The initial rise in serum creatinine is characteristically delayed until the second week of therapy with many tubule epithelial cell toxins (e.g., aminoglycosides, cisplatin) and probably reflects the need for accumulation of these agents within cells before GFR falls.

Hyperkalemia, hyperphosphatemia, hypocalcemia, and elevations in serum uric acid and creatine kinase (MM isoenzyme) levels at presentation suggest a diagnosis of rhabdomyolysis. Hyperuricemia

Table 269-3 Urine Diagnostic Indices in Differentiation of Prerenal versus Intrinsic Renal ARF

Diagnostic Index	Typical Findings	
	Prerenal ARF	Intrinsic Renal ARF
Fractional excretion of sodium (%)[a] $$\frac{U_{Na} \times P_{Cr}}{P_{Na} \times U_{Cr}} \times 100$$	<1	>1
Urine sodium concentration (mmol/L)	<10	>20
Urine creatinine to plasma creatinine ratio	>40	<20
Urine urea nitrogen to plasma urea nitrogen ratio	>8	<3
Urine specific gravity	>1.020	~1.010
Urine osmolality (mosmol/kg H_2O)	>500	~300
Plasma BUN/creatinine ratio	>20	<10-15
Renal failure index[a] $$\frac{U_{Na}}{U_{Cr}/P_{Cr}}$$	<1	>1
Urinary sediment	Hyaline casts	Muddy brown granular casts

[a] Most sensitive indices.

NOTE: ARF, acute renal failure; U_{Na}, urine sodium concentration; P_{Cr}, plasma creatinine concentration; P_{Na}, plasma sodium concentration; U_{Cr}, urine creatinine concentration; BUN, blood urea nitrogen.

[>890 μmol/L (>15 mg/dL)] in association with hyperkalemia, hyperphosphatemia, and increased circulating levels of intracellular enzymes such as lactate dehydrogenase may indicate acute urate nephropathy and tumor lysis syndrome following cancer chemotherapy. A wide serum anion and osmolal gap (measured serum osmolality minus the serum osmolality calculated from serum sodium, glucose, and urea concentrations) indicate the presence of an unusual anion or osmole in the circulation and are clues to diagnosis of ethylene glycol or methanol ingestion. Severe anemia in the absence of hemorrhage raises the possibility of hemolysis, multiple myeloma, or thrombotic microangiopathy. Systemic eosinophilia suggests allergic interstitial nephritis but is also a feature of atheroembolic disease and polyangiitis nodosa.

RADIOLOGIC FINDINGS Imaging of the urinary tract by ultrasonography is useful to exclude postrenal ARF. Computed tomography and magnetic resonance imaging are alternative imaging modalities. Whereas pelvicalyceal dilatation is usual with urinary tract obstruction (98% sensitivity), dilatation may be absent immediately following obstruction or in patients with ureteric encasement (e.g., retroperitoneal fibrosis, neoplasia). Retrograde or anterograde pyelography are more definitive investigations in complex cases and provide precise localization of the site of obstruction. A plain film of the abdomen, with tomography if necessary, is a valuable initial screening technique in patients with suspected nephrolithiasis. Doppler ultrasonography and magnetic resonance flow imaging appear promising for assessment of patency of renal arteries and veins in patients with suspected vascular obstruction; however, contrast angiography is usually required for definitive diagnosis.

RENAL BIOPSY Biopsy is reserved for patients in whom prerenal and postrenal ARF have been excluded and the cause of intrinsic renal ARF is unclear. Renal biopsy is particularly useful when clinical assessment and laboratory investigations suggest diagnoses other than ischemic or nephrotoxic injury that may respond to disease-specific therapy. Examples include glomerulonephritis, vasculitis, hemolytic-uremic syndrome, thrombotic thrombocytopenic purpura, and allergic interstitial nephritis.

COMPLICATIONS

ARF impairs renal excretion of sodium, potassium, and water and perturbs divalent cation homeostasis and urinary acidification mechanisms. As a result, ARF is frequently complicated by intravascular volume overload, hyponatremia, hyperkalemia, hyperphosphatemia, hypocalcemia, hypermagnesemia, and metabolic acidosis. In addition, patients are unable to excrete nitrogenous waste products and are prone to develop the uremic syndrome (Chap. 270). The speed of development and the severity of these complications reflect the degree of renal impairment and catabolic state of the patient.

Expansion of extracellular fluid volume is an inevitable consequence of diminished salt and water excretion in oliguric or anuric individuals. Whereas milder forms are characterized by weight gain, bibasilar lung rales, raised jugular venous pressure, and dependent edema, continued volume expansion may precipitate life-threatening pulmonary edema. Hypervolemia may be particularly problematic in patients receiving multiple intravenous medications and enteral or parenteral nutrition. Excessive administration of free water either through ingestion and nasogastric administration or as hypotonic saline or isotonic dextrose solutions (dextrose being metabolized) can induce *hypoosmolality* and *hyponatremia*, which, if severe, lead to cerebral edema and neurologic abnormalities, including seizures.

Hyperkalemia is a frequent complication of ARF. Serum potassium typically rises by 0.5 mmol/L per day in oliguric and anuric patients due to impaired excretion of ingested or infused potassium and potassium released from injured tissue. Coexistent metabolic acidosis may exacerbate hyperkalemia by promoting potassium efflux from cells. Hyperkalemia may be particularly severe, even at the time of diagnosis, in patients with rhabdomyolysis, hemolysis, and tumor lysis syndrome. Mild hyperkalemia (<6.0 mmol/L) is usually asymptomatic. Higher levels are typically associated with electrocardiographic abnormalities and/or increased cardiac excitability (Chap. 226).

Metabolism of dietary protein yields between 50 and 100 mmol/d of fixed nonvolatile acids that are normally excreted by the kidneys. Consequently, ARF is typically complicated by *metabolic acidosis*, often with an increased serum anion gap (Chap. 50). Acidosis can be particularly severe when endogenous production of hydrogen ions is increased by other mechanisms (e.g., diabetic or fasting ketoacidosis; lactic acidosis complicating generalized tissue hypoperfusion, liver disease, or sepsis; metabolism of ethylene glycol or methanol).

Mild *hyperphosphatemia* is an almost invariable complication of ARF. Severe hyperphosphatemia may develop in highly catabolic patients or following rhabdomyolysis, hemolysis, or tumor lysis. Metastatic deposition of calcium phosphate can lead to *hypocalcemia*, particularly when the product of serum calcium (mg/dL) and phosphate (mg/dL) concentrations exceeds 70. Other factors that contribute to hypocalcemia include tissue resistance to the actions of parathyroid hormone and reduced levels of 1,25-dihydroxyvitamin D. Hypocalcemia is often asymptomatic but can cause perioral paresthesias, muscle cramps, seizures, hallucinations and confusion, and prolongation of the QT interval and nonspecific T-wave changes on electrocardiography (Chap. 341).

Anemia develops rapidly in ARF and is usually mild and multifactorial in origin. Contributing factors include impaired erythropoiesis, hemolysis, bleeding, hemodilution, and reduced red cell survival time. Prolongation of the *bleeding time* and *leukocytosis* are also common. Common contributors to the bleeding diathesis include mild thrombocytopenia, platelet dysfunction, and/or clotting factor abnormalities (e.g., factor VIII dysfunction), whereas leukocytosis usually reflects sepsis, a stress response, or other concurrent illness. *Infection* is a common and serious complication of ARF, occurring in 50 to 90% of cases and accounting for up to 75% of deaths. It is unclear whether patients with ARF have a clinically significant defect in host immune responses or whether the high incidence of infection reflects repeated breaches of mucocutaneous barriers (e.g., intravenous cannulae, mechanical ventilation, bladder catheterization). *Cardiopulmonary complications* of ARF include arrhythmias, myocardial infarction, pericarditis and pericardial effusion, pulmonary edema, and pulmonary embolism. Mild *gastrointestinal bleeding* is common (10 to 30%) and is usually due to stress ulceration of gastric or small intestinal mucosa.

Protracted periods of severe ARF are invariably associated with the development of the *uremic syndrome* (Chap. 270).

A *vigorous diuresis* can occur during the recovery phase of ARF (see above) and lead to intravascular volume depletion and delayed recovery of GFR by causing secondary prerenal ARF. *Hypernatremia* can also complicate recovery if water losses via hypotonic urine are not replaced or if losses are inappropriately replaced by relatively hypertonic saline solutions. *Hypokalemia, hypomagnesemia, hypophosphatemia,* and *hypocalcemia* are less common metabolic complications during this period.

TREATMENT **Prevention** Because there are no specific therapies for ischemic or nephrotoxic ARF, prevention is of paramount importance. Many cases of ischemic ARF can be avoided by close attention to cardiovascular function and intravascular volume in high-risk patients, such as the elderly and those with preexisting renal insufficiency. Indeed, aggressive restoration of intravascular volume has been shown to reduce the incidence of ischemic ARF dramatically after major surgery or trauma, burns, or cholera. The incidence of nephrotoxic ARF can be reduced by tailoring the dosage of potential nephrotoxins to body size and GFR; for example, reducing the dose or frequency of administration of drugs in patients with preexisting renal impairment. In this regard, it should be noted that serum creatinine is a relatively insensitive index of GFR and may overestimate GFR considerably in small or elderly patients. For purposes of drug dosing, it is advisable to estimate the GFR using the Cockcroft-Gault formula, which factors in the variables of age and weight (Chap. 47). Adjusting drug dosage according to circulating drug levels also appears to limit renal injury in patients receiving aminoglycoside antibiotics or cyclosporine. Diuretics, cyclooxygenase inhibitors, ACE inhibitors, and other vasodilators should be used with caution in patients with suspected true or "effective" hypovolemia or renovascular disease as they may precipitate prerenal ARF or convert the latter to ischemic ARF. Hypovolemia should be avoided in patients receiving nephrotoxic medications as renal hypoperfusion potentiates the toxicity of most nephrotoxins. Allopurinol and forced alkaline diuresis are useful in patients at high risk for acute urate nephropathy (e.g., cancer chemotherapy in hematologic malignancies) to limit uric acid generation and prevent precipitation of urate crystals in renal tubules. Forced alkaline diuresis may also prevent or attenuate ARF in patients receiving high-dose methotrexate or suffering from rhabdomyolysis. *N*-acetylcysteine limits acetaminophen-induced renal injury if given within 24 h of ingestion. Dimercaprol, a chelating agent, may prevent heavy metal nephrotoxicity. Ethanol inhibits ethylene glycol metabolism to oxalic acid and other toxic metabolites and is an important adjunct to hemodialysis in the emergency management of ethylene glycol intoxication.

Specific Therapies By definition, prerenal ARF is rapidly reversible upon correction of the primary hemodynamic abnormality, and postrenal ARF resolves upon relief of obstruction. To date, there are no specific therapies for established intrinsic renal ARF due to ischemia or nephrotoxicity. Management of these disorders should focus on elimination of the causative hemodynamic abnormality or toxin, avoidance of additional insults, and prevention and treatment of complications. Specific treatment of other causes of intrinsic renal ARF depends on the underlying pathology.

Prerenal ARF The composition of replacement fluids for treatment of prerenal ARF due to hypovolemia must be tailored according to the composition of the lost fluid. Severe hypovolemia due to hemorrhage should be corrected with packed red blood cells, whereas isotonic saline is usually appropriate replacement for mild to moderate hemorrhage or plasma loss (e.g., burns, pancreatitis). Urinary and gastrointestinal fluids can vary greatly in composition but are usually hypotonic. Hypotonic solutions (e.g., 0.45% saline) are usually recommended as initial replacement in patients with prerenal ARF due to increased urinary or gastrointestinal fluid losses, although isotonic saline may be more appropriate in severe cases. Subsequent therapy should be based on measurements of the volume and ionic content of excreted or drained fluids. Serum potassium and acid-base status should be monitored carefully, and potassium and bicarbonate supplemented as appropriate. Cardiac failure may require aggressive management with positive inotropes, preload and afterload reducing agents, antiarrhythmic drugs, and mechanical aids such as intraaortic balloon pumps. Invasive hemodynamic monitoring may be required to guide therapy for complicated conditions in patients in whom clinical assessment of cardiovascular function and intravascular volume proves unreliable.

Fluid management may be particularly difficult in patients with cirrhosis complicated by ascites. In this setting, it is important to distinguish between full-blown hepatorenal syndrome (Chap. 299), which carries a grave prognosis, and reversible ARF due to true or "effective" hypovolemia induced by overzealous use of diuretics or sepsis (e.g., spontaneous bacterial peritonitis). The contribution of hypovolemia to ARF can be definitively assessed only by administration of a fluid challenge. Fluids should be administered slowly and titrated against jugular venous pressure and, if necessary, central venous and pulmonary capillary wedge pressure, abdominal girth, and urine output. Patients with a reversible prerenal component typically have an increase in urine output and fall in serum creatinine, whereas patients with hepatorenal syndrome do not and may suffer increased ascites formation and pulmonary compromise if not monitored closely. Large volumes of ascitic fluid can usually be drained by paracentesis without deterioration in renal function if intravenous albumin is administered simultaneously. Indeed, "large-volume paracentesis" may afford an increase in GFR, possibly by lowering intraabdominal pressure and improving flow in renal veins. Shunting of ascitic fluid from the peritoneum to a central vein (peritoneojugular shunt, LeVeen or Denver shunts) is an alternative approach in refractory cases but has not been shown to improve survival in controlled trials. The efficacy of the newer technique of transjugular intrahepatic portosystemic shunting (TIPS procedure) is currently undergoing rigorous clinical assessment. Shunting can also improve GFR and sodium excretion transiently, probably because the increase in central blood volume stimulates release of atrial natriuretic peptides and inhibits secretion of aldosterone and norepinephrine.

Intrinsic renal ARF Many different approaches have been tested for their ability to attenuate injury or hasten recovery in ischemic and nephrotoxic ARF. These include atrial natriuretic peptide (ANP), low-dose dopamine, loop-blocking diuretics, calcium channel blockers, α-adrenoreceptor blockers, prostaglandin analogues, antioxidants, antibodies against leukocyte adhesion molecules, and insulin-like growth factor. Whereas many of these are beneficial in experimental models of ischemic or nephrotoxic ARF, they have either failed to confer consistent benefit or proved ineffective in humans.

ARF due to other intrinsic renal diseases such as acute glomerulonephritis or vasculitis may respond to glucocorticoids, alkylating agents, and/or plasmapheresis, depending on the primary pathology. Glucocorticoids also hasten remission in some cases of allergic interstitial nephritis. Aggressive control of systemic arterial pressure is of paramount importance in limiting renal injury in malignant hypertensive nephrosclerosis, toxemia of pregnancy, and other vascular diseases. Hypertension and ARF due to scleroderma may be exquisitely sensitive to treatment with ACE inhibitors.

Postrenal ARF Management of postrenal ARF requires close collaboration between nephrologist, urologist, and radiologist. Obstruction of the urethra or bladder neck is usually managed initially by transurethral or suprapubic placement of a bladder catheter, which provides temporary relief while the obstructing lesion is identified and treated definitively. Similarly, ureteric obstruction may be treated initially by percutaneous catheterization of the dilated renal pelvis or ureter. Indeed, obstructing lesions can often be removed percutaneously (e.g., calculus, sloughed papilla) or bypassed by insertion of a ureteric stent (e.g., carcinoma). Most patients experience an appropriate diuresis for several days following relief of obstruction. Approximately 5% of patients develop a transient salt-wasting syndrome that may require administration of intravenous saline to maintain blood pressure.

Supportive Measures (Table 269-4) Following correction of hypovolemia, salt and water intake are tailored to match losses. Hypervolemia can usually be managed by restriction of salt and water

Table 269-4 Management of Ischemic and Nephrotoxic Acute Renal Failure[a]

Management Issue	Therapy
REVERSE CAUSATIVE RENAL INSULT	
Ischemic ARF	Restore systemic hemodynamics and renal perfusion
Nephrotoxic ARF	Eliminate nephrotoxins
	Consider specific measures (e.g., forced alkaline diuresis, chelators: see text)
PREVENTION AND TREATMENT OF COMPLICATIONS	
Intravascular volume overload	Salt (1–2 g/d) and water (usually <1 L/d) restriction
	Diuretics (usually loop blockers ± thiazide)
	Ultrafiltration or dialysis
Hyponatremia	Restriction of enteral free water intake (<1 L/d)
	Avoid hypotonic intravenous solutions (including dextrose solutions)
Hyperkalemia	Restriction of dietary K$^+$ intake (usually <40 mmol/d)
	Eliminate K$^+$ supplements and K$^+$-sparing diuretics
	Potassium-binding ion-exchange resins (e.g., sodium polystyrene sulphonate)
	Glucose (50 mL of 50% dextrose) and insulin (10 units regular)
	Sodium bicarbonate (usually 50–100 mmol)
	Calcium gluconate (10 mL of 10% solution over 5 min)
	Dialysis (with low K$^+$ dialysate)
Metabolic acidosis	Restriction of dietary protein (usually 0.6 g/kg per day of high biologic value)
	Sodium bicarbonate (maintain serum bicarbonate >15 mmol/L or arterial pH >7.2)
	Dialysis
Hyperphosphatemia	Restriction of dietary phosphate intake (usually <800 mg/d)
	Phosphate binding agents (calcium carbonate, aluminum hydroxide)
Hypocalcemia	Calcium carbonate (if symptomatic or if sodium bicarbonate to be administered)
	Calcium gluconate (10–20 mL of 10% solution)
Hypermagnesemia	Discontinue Mg^{2+}-containing antacids
Hyperuricemia	Treatment usually not necessary [if <890 μmol/L (<15 mg/dL)]
Nutrition	Restriction of dietary protein (~0.6 g/kg per day)
	Carbohydrate (~100 g/d)
	Enteral or parenteral nutrition (if recovery prolonged or patient very catabolic)
Indications for dialysis	Clinical evidence (symptoms or signs) of uremia
	Intractable intravascular volume overload
	Hyperkalemia or severe acidosis resistant to conservative measures
	?Prophylactic dialysis when urea >100–150 mg/dL or creatinine >8–10 mg/dL
PRESCRIBING OF MEDICATIONS	
Choice of agents	Avoid other nephrotoxins, ACE inhibitors, cyclooxygenase inhibitors, and radiocontrast unless absolute indication and no alternative agent
Drug dosing	Adjust doses and frequency of administration for degree of renal impairment

[a] These are general recommendations and must be tailored to needs of individual patients.

intake and diuretics. Indeed, there is, as yet, no proven rationale for administration of diuretics in ARF except to treat this complication. High doses of loop-blocking diuretics such as furosemide (up to 200 to 400 mg intravenously) or bumetanide (up to 10 mg intravenously administered as a bolus or by continuous infusion) may promote diuresis in patients who fail to respond to conventional doses. Subpressor doses of dopamine are claimed to promote salt and water excretion by increasing renal blood flow and GFR and by inhibiting tubule sodium reabsorption; however, subpressor ("low-dose," "renal-dose,") dopamine has proved ineffective in clinical trials and may trigger arrythmias and sudden cardiac death in critically ill patients. Ultrafiltration or dialysis is used to treat severe hypervolemia when conservative measures fail. Hyponatremia and hypoosmolality can usually be controlled by restriction of free water intake. Conversely, hypernatremia is treated by administration of water or intravenous hypotonic saline or isotonic dextrose–containing solutions.

→*The management of hyperkalemia is described in Chap. 49.*

Metabolic acidosis is not treated unless serum bicarbonate concentration falls below 15 mmol/L or arterial pH falls below 7.2. More severe acidosis is corrected by oral or intravenous sodium bicarbonate. Initial rates of replacement are guided by estimates of bicarbonate deficit and adjusted thereafter according to serum levels (Chap. 50). Patients are monitored for complications of bicarbonate administration such as hypervolemia, metabolic alkalosis, hypocalcemia, and hypokalemia. From a practical point of view, most patients requiring sodium bicarbonate need emergency dialysis within days. Hyperphosphatemia is usually controlled by restriction of dietary phosphate and by oral aluminum hydroxide or calcium carbonate, which reduce gastrointestinal absorption of phosphate. Hypocalcemia does not usually require treatment unless severe, as may occur with rhabdomyolysis or pancreatitis or following admininstration of bicarbonate. Hyperuricemia is typically mild [<890 μmol/L (< 15 mg/dL)] and does not require intervention.

The objective of *nutritional management* during the maintenance phase of ARF is to provide sufficient calories to avoid catabolism and starvation ketoacidosis, while minimizing production of nitrogenous waste. This is best achieved by restricting dietary protein to approximately 0.6 g/kg per day of protein of high biologic value (i.e., rich in essential amino acids) and to provide most calories as carbohydrate (approximately 100 g daily). Nutritional management is easier in nonoliguric patients and following institution of dialysis. Vigorous parenteral hyperalimentation is claimed to improve prognosis; however, convincing benefit has yet to be demonstrated in controlled trials.

Anemia may necessitate blood transfusion if severe or if recovery is delayed. In contrast to chronic renal failure, recombinant human erythropoietin is rarely used in ARF because bone marrow resistance to erythropoietin is common, more immediate treatment of anemia (if any) is required, and renal failure is usually self-limiting. Uremic bleeding usually responds to correction of anemia, administration of desmopressin or estrogens, or dialysis. Regular doses of antacids appear to reduce the incidence of gastrointestinal hemorrhage significantly and may be more effective in this regard than H$_2$ antagonists, or proton pump inhibitors. Meticulous care of intravenous cannulae, bladder catheters, and other invasive devices is mandatory to avoid infections. Unfortunately, prophylactic antibiotics have not been shown to reduce the incidence of infection in these high-risk patients.

Indications and modalities of dialysis   Dialysis replaces renal function until regeneration and repair restore renal function. Hemodialysis and peritoneal dialysis appear equally effective for management of ARF. Thus, the dialysis modality is chosen according to the needs of individual patients (e.g., peritoneal dialysis may be preferable if the patient is hemodynamically unstable, and hemodialysis after abdominal surgery involving the peritoneum), the expertise of the nephrologist, and the facilities of the institution. Vascular access for conventional intermittent hemodialysis is best achieved by insertion of a temporary double-lumen hemodialysis catheter into the internal jug-

ular vein. The subclavian and femoral veins are alternative access sites. Peritoneal dialysis is achieved by insertion of a single-lumen cuffed catheter into the peritoneal cavity. Absolute indications for dialysis include symptoms or signs of the uremic syndrome and management of refractory hypervolemia, hyperkalemia, or acidosis. Many nephrologists also initiate dialysis empirically for blood urea levels of >100 mg/dL, even in the absence of clinical uremia; however, this approach has yet to be validated in controlled clinical trials. Nor is it clear whether intensive dialysis prescribed to maintain blood urea and creatinine below a certain level is beneficial. The latter are important issues since unnecessary or intensive hemodialysis can exacerbate ATN and delay renal recovery by triggering hypotension and repeated renal hypoperfusion. Moreover, an expanding body of evidence suggests that leukocytes, activated directly by contact with hemodialysis membranes or as a result of membrane-triggered complement activation, then travel to the already-compromised renal microcirculation where they further exacerbate renal injury.

Continuous arteriovenous hemodiafiltration (CAVH) and continuous venovenous hemodiafiltration (CVVH) are alternatives to conventional intermittent hemodialysis techniques for treatment of ARF. They are particularly valuable techniques in patients in whom intermittent hemodialysis fails to control hypervolemia or uremia and for those who do not tolerate intermittent hemodialysis and in whom peritoneal dialysis is not possible. CAVH requires both arterial and venous access. The patient's own blood pressure generates an ultrafiltrate of plasma across a porous biocompatible dialysis membrane. A physiologic crystalloid solution is passed along the other side of the membrane to achieve diffusive clearance. CVVH, in contrast, requires only a double-lumen venous catheter as a blood pump generates ultrafiltration pressure across the dialysis membrane. These newer continuous techniques have not been compared to conventional intermittent hemodialysis in prospective, adequately controlled trials, and the choice of technique is currently tailored to the specific needs of the patient, the resources of the institution, and the expertise of the physician. Potential disadvantages of continuous hemodialysis techniques are the need for prolonged immobilization in bed, systemic anticoagulation, arterial cannulation (in CAVH), and prolonged exposure of blood to synthetic, albeit relatively biocompatible, dialysis membranes.

OUTCOME AND LONG-TERM PROGNOSIS

The mortality rate among patients with ARF approximates 50% and has changed little over the past 30 years. It should be stressed, however, that patients usually die from sequelae of the primary illness that induced ARF and not from ARF itself. Indeed, the kidney is one of the few organs whose function can be replaced artificially (i.e., by dialysis) for protracted periods of time. In agreement with this interpretation, mortality rates vary greatly depending on the cause of ARF: ~15% in obstetric patients, ~30% in toxin-related ARF, and ~60% following trauma or major surgery. Oliguria (<400 mL/d) at time of presentation and a rise in serum creatinine of >265 μmol/L (>3 mg/dL) are associated with a poor prognosis and probably reflect the severity of renal injury and of the primary illness. Mortality rates are higher in older debilitated patients and in those with multiple organ failure. Most patients who survive an episode of ARF recover sufficient renal function to live normal lives. However, 50% have subclinical impairment of renal function or residual scarring on renal biopsy. Approximately 5% of patients never recover function and require long-term renal replacement with dialysis or transplantation. An additional 5% suffer progressive decline in GFR, following an initial recovery phase, probably due to hemodynamic stress and sclerosis of remnant glomeruli (Chap. 273).

BIBLIOGRAPHY

BRADY HR, WILCOX CS (eds): *Therapy in Nephrology and Hypertension*. Philadelphia, Saunders, 1999

——— et al: Acute renal failure, in *Brenner and Rector's The Kidney*, 6th ed., BM Brenner (ed). Philadelphia, Saunders, 2000, pp 1201–1262

DENTON MD et al: "Renal-dose" dopamine for the treatment of acute renal failure: Scientific rationale, experimental studies and clinical trials. Kidney Int 49:4, 1996

HAKIM RM et al: Effect of dialysis membrane in the treatment of patients with acute renal failure. N Engl J Med 334:1338, 1994

HIMMELFARB J et al: Mutlicenter comparison of dialysis membranes in the treatment of acute renal failure requiring dialysis. J Am Soc Nephrol 9:257, 1998

MEYER MM: Renal Replacement therapies. Crit Care Clinics 16:29, 2000

OLSEN S, SOLEZ K: Acute tubular necrosis and toxic renal injury, in *Renal Pathology with Clinical and Functional Correlations*, 2d ed, CC Tisher, BM Brenner (eds). Philadelphia, Lippincott, 1994, pp 769–809

STAR RA: Treatment of acute renal failure. Kidney Int 54:1817, 1998

THADHANI R et al: Acute renal failure. N Engl J Med 334:1448, 1996

Table 270-1   Prevalence and Incidence Counts by Major Etiology for U.S. Medicare–Treated End-Stage Renal Disease for 1997

	Prevalence, $n = 304,083$		Incidence, $n = 79.102$	
	Count	Percent	Count	Percent
Diabetes	100,892	33.2	33,096	41.8
Hypertension	72,961	24.0	20,066	25.4
Glomerulonephritis	52,229	17.2	7,390	9.3
Cystic disease	13,992	4.6	1,772	2.2

SOURCE: From United States Renal Data System 1999 Annual Report Preliminary Data, U.S. Department of Health and Human Services, Health Care Financing Administration (www.med.umich.edu/usrds/).

---

270   *Karl Skorecki, Jacob Green, Barry M. Brenner*

CHRONIC RENAL FAILURE

MECHANISMS OF CHRONIC RENAL FAILURE

DEFINITIONS   *Chronic renal disease (CRD)* is a pathophysiologic process with multiple etiologies, resulting in the inexorable attrition of nephron number and function, and frequently leading to *end-stage renal disease (ESRD)*. In turn, ESRD represents a clinical state or condition in which there has been an irreversible loss of endogenous renal function, of a degree sufficient to render the patient permanently dependent upon renal replacement therapy (dialysis or transplantation) in order to avoid life-threatening *uremia*. Uremia is the clinical and laboratory syndrome, reflecting dysfunction of all organ systems as a result of untreated or undertreated acute or chronic renal failure. Given the capacity of the kidneys to regain function following acute injury (Chap. 269), the vast majority (>90%) of patients with ESRD have reached this state as a result of CRD.

PATHOPHYSIOLOGY OF CRD   The pathophysiology of CRD involves initiating mechanisms specific to the underlying etiology as well as a set of progressive mechanisms that are a common consequence following long-term reduction of renal mass, irrespective of etiology. Such reduction of renal mass causes structural and functional hypertrophy of surviving nephrons. This compensatory hypertrophy is mediated by vasoactive molecules, cytokines, and growth factors and is due initially to adaptive hyperfiltration, in turn mediated by increases in glomerular capillary pressure and flow. Eventually, these short-term adaptations prove maladaptive, in that they predispose to sclerosis of the remaining viable nephron population. This final common pathway for inexorable attrition of residual nephron function may persist even after the initiating or underlying disease process has become inactive. Increased intrarenal activity of the renin-angiotensin axis appears to contribute both to the initial adaptive hyperfiltration and to the subsequent maladaptive hypertrophy and sclerosis. These maladaptive long-term actions of renin-angiotensin axis activation are mediated in part through downstream growth factors such as transforming growth factor β. Interindividual variability in the risk and rate of CRD progression can be explained in part by variations in the genes encoding components of these and other pathways involved in glomerular and tubulointerstitial fibrosis and sclerosis (see "Genetic Considerations in the Progression of CRD," below).

The earliest stage common to all forms of CRD is a loss of renal reserve. When kidney function is entirely normal, glomerular filtration rate (GFR) can be augmented by 20 to 30% in response to the stimulus of a protein challenge. During the earliest stage of loss of renal reserve, basal GFR may be normal or even elevated (hyperfiltration), but the expected further rise in response to a protein challenge is attenuated. This early stage is particularly well documented in diabetic nephropathy. At this stage, the only clue may be at the level of laboratory measurements, which estimate GFR. The most commonly utilized laboratory measurements are the serum urea and creatinine concentrations. By the time serum urea and creatinine concentrations are even mildly elevated, substantial chronic nephron injury has already occurred.

As GFR declines to levels as low as 30% of normal, patients may remain asymptomatic with only biochemical evidence of the decline in GFR, i.e., rise in serum concentrations of urea and creatinine. However, careful scrutiny usually reveals early additional clinical and laboratory manifestations of renal insufficiency. These may include nocturia, mild anemia and loss of energy, decreasing appetite and early disturbances in nutritional status, and abnormalities in calcium and phosphorus metabolism (*moderate renal insufficiency*). As GFR falls to below 30% of normal, an increasing number and severity of uremic clinical manifestations and biochemical abnormalities supervene (*severe renal insufficiency*). At the stages of mild and moderate renal insufficiency, intercurrent clinical stress may compromise renal function still further, inducing signs and symptoms of overt uremia. Such intercurrent clinical conditions to which patients with CRD may be particularly susceptible include infection (urinary, respiratory, or gastrointestinal), poorly controlled hypertension, hyper- or hypovolemia, and drug or radiocontrast nephrotoxicity, among others. When GFR falls below 5 to 10% of normal (ESRD), continued survival without renal replacement therapy becomes impossible.

ETIOLOGY   There has been a dramatic increase in the incidence of ESRD as well as a shift in the relative incidence of etiologies of CRD during the past two decades. Whereas glomerulonephritis was the leading cause of CRD in the past, diabetic and hypertensive nephropathy are now much more frequent underlying etiologies (Table 270-1). This may be a consequence of more effective prevention and treatment of glomerulonephritis or of diminished mortality from other causes among individuals with diabetes and hypertension. Greater overall longevity and diminished premature cardiovascular mortality have also increased the mean age of patients presenting with ESRD. Hypertension is a particularly common cause of CRD in the elderly, in whom chronic renal ischemia due to renovascular disease may be an underrecognized additional contribution to the pathophysiologic process. Many patients present at an advanced stage of CRD, precluding definitive determination of etiology.

GENETIC CONSIDERATIONS   **Progression of CRD**   Disorders with clear-cut monogenic inheritance comprise a small but important component among the etiologies of CRD. Among these, autosomal dominant polycystic kidney disease is the most common on a world-wide basis (Chap. 276). Alport's hereditary nephritis (Chap. 275) is a less common cause of both benign hematuria without progression to CRD and more severe nephron injury with progression to ESRD, and it usually displays an X-linked pattern of inheritance. In contrast, the two most common etiologies of CRD (Table 270-1), namely diabetes mellitus (both types 1 and 2) and essential hypertension, display complex polygenic patterns of inheritance. Both candidate locus and genome-wide strategies have been used to pinpoint genes that contribute to the risks for development of these disorders.

Recent evidence also suggests that reflux nephropathy may have a heritable basis, again involving the contribution of several genetic loci.

Striking interindividual variability in the rate of progression to ESRD is a characteristic feature among patients with either inherited or acquired causes of CRD, irrespective of underlying etiology. This interindividual variability has an important heritable component, clarification of which may help guide therapeutic approaches. A number of genetic loci that contribute to the progression of CRD have been identified. Most extensively studied has been an insertion/deletion polymorphism of the angiotensin-converting enzyme (ACE) gene, previously shown to contribute to cardiovascular disease risk. Studies in a wide variety of disorders, including diabetic nephropathy, glomerulonephritis, polycystic kidney disease, and CRD caused by urologic abnormalities, have revealed an important contribution of this locus to progressive deterioration of renal function. The two different alleles defined by this polymorphism of the ACE gene are associated with corresponding differences in the endogenous activity of the encoded enzyme. The homozygous deletion (D/D) variant is associated with the highest expression of endogenous ACE activity and a greater risk of CRD progression. This finding has important therapeutic implications and leads to the prediction that ACE inhibitor therapy might be most effective in patients who are homozygous for the "at-risk" allele. Similar conclusions have been reached with respect to genes encoding other components of the renin-angiotensin axis, including the angiotensinogen gene, and the angiotensin receptor. These findings are consistent with the important role of intraglomerular hemodynamic perturbations in progressive renal injury. ■

PATHOPHYSIOLOGY AND BIOCHEMISTRY OF UREMIA The uremic syndrome results from functional derangements of many organ systems, although the prominence of specific symptoms varies among patients. *Azotemia* refers to the retention of nitrogenous waste products as renal insufficiency develops. *Uremia* refers to the more advanced stages of progressive renal insufficiency when the complex, multiorgan system derangements become clinically manifest. The term uremia was adopted originally because of the presumption that all of the abnormalities result from retention in the blood of end products of metabolism normally excreted in the urine. The most likely candidates as toxins in uremia are the by-products of protein and amino acid metabolism. Unlike fats and carbohydrates, which are eventually metabolized to carbon dioxide and water—substances readily excreted even in uremic subjects via lungs and skin—the products of protein and amino acid metabolism depend primarily on the kidneys for excretion. Although a number of such products have been identified (Table 270-2), the clinical symptoms of uremia correlate poorly with the blood levels of these products. This is because uremia involves more than renal excretory failure alone. A host of metabolic and endocrine functions normally subserved by the kidney are also impaired, resulting in anemia; malnutrition; impaired metabolism of carbohydrates, fats, and proteins; defective utilization of energy; and metabolic bone disease. Thus, the pathophysiology of the uremic syndrome can be divided into those sets of abnormalities consequent to the accumulation of products of protein metabolism on the one hand, and on the other hand, abnormalities consequent to the loss of other renal functions, such as fluid and electrolyte homeostasis and synthesis of certain hormones [e.g., erythropoietin (EPO), 1.25-dihydroxycholecalciferol].

Although not the major cause of overt uremic toxicity, urea may contribute to some of the clinical abnormalities, including anorexia, malaise, vomiting, and headache. Elevated levels of plasma *guanidinosuccinic acid*, by interfering with activation of platelet factor III by ADP, contribute to the impaired platelet function in CRD. *Creatinine* may cause adverse effects following conversion to metabolites such as sarcosine and methylguanidine. Nitrogenous compounds with a molecular mass of 500 to 12,000 Da (so-called middle molecules) are also

Table 270-2 Uremic "Toxins"

By-products of protein and amino acid metabolism
  Urea—80% of total (excreted nitrogen)
  Guanidino compounds
    Guanidine
    Methylguanidine
    Dimethylguanidine
    Creatinine
    Creatine
    Guanidinosuccinic acid
  Urates and hippurates
  End products of nucleic acid metabolism
  End products of aliphatic amine metabolism
  End products of aromatic amino acid metabolism
    Tryptophan
    Tyrosine
    Phenylalanine
  Other nitrogenous substances
    Polyamines
    Myoinositol
    Phenols
    Benzoates
    Indoles
  Advanced glycation end products
Inhibitors of ligand-protein binding
Glucuronoconjugates and aglycones
Inhibitors of somatomedin and insulin action

retained in CRD and similarly are believed to contribute to morbidity and mortality in uremic subjects. Decreased renal excretion is not the only reason why such middle-sized molecules, along with various cytokines and growth factors, accumulate in uremic plasma. The kidney normally catabolizes a number of circulating plasma proteins and polypeptides; with reduced renal mass, this capacity is impaired. Furthermore, plasma levels of many polypeptide hormones, including parathyroid hormone (PTH) insulin, glucagon, luteinizing hormone, and prolactin, rise with renal failure, not only because of impaired renal catabolism but also because of enhanced glandular secretion. Of these, excessive PTH has been suggested to be an important uremic "toxin" because of its adverse effect of elevating cellular cytosolic Ca^{2+} levels in several tissues and organs.

CLINICAL AND LABORATORY MANIFESTATIONS OF CHRONIC RENAL FAILURE AND UREMIA

Uremia leads to disturbances in the function of every organ system. Chronic dialysis (Chap. 271) reduces the incidence and severity of these disturbances, so that, where modern medicine is practiced, the overt and florid manifestations of uremia have largely disappeared. Unfortunately, as indicated in Table 270-3, even optimal dialysis therapy is not a panacea, because some disturbances resulting from impaired renal function fail to respond fully, while others continue to progress.

FLUID, ELECTROLYTE, AND ACID-BASE DISORDERS (See also Chaps. 49 and 50) **Sodium and Water Homeostasis** When the GFR is normal, >24,000 mmol of Na^+ are filtered per day. An overwhelming fraction of this Na^+ load is reabsorbed by the tubules, leaving only a small fraction (usually <1%) to be excreted. Thus, even when the GFR falls markedly to levels as low as 10% of normal, the filtered load of Na^+ still far exceeds daily requirements for urinary Na^+ excretion. Therefore, any abnormalities in overall Na^+ balance will reflect the relationship between the filtered load and fractional reabsorption (glomerulotubular balance). Progressive nephron injury can be associated with a tendency to Na^+ retention, Na^+ wasting, or maintenance of Na^+ balance, depending in part on the underlying etiology (glomerular vs. tubulointerstitial disease), ongoing diuretic treatment, and comorbid conditions that affect Na^+ balance, such as cardiac failure or cirrhosis. Osmotic regulation of vasopressin release and of thirst are also preserved. Even when tubule response to vasopressin is diminished, normal thirst mechanisms and access to H_2O generally prevent hypernatremia. However, a compromised capacity to excrete a maximally dilute urine with progressive CRD may lead to hyponatremia.

In most patients with stable CRD, the total body contents of Na^+ and H_2O are increased modestly, although this may not be clinically apparent. The underlying etiologic disease process may itself disrupt glomerulotubular balance and promote Na^+ retention (e.g., glomerulonephritis), or excessive Na^+ ingestion may lead to cumulative positive Na^+ balance and attendant extracellular fluid volume (ECFV) expansion. Such ECFV expansion contributes to hypertension, which in turn accelerates further the progression of nephron injury. As long as water intake does not exceed the capacity for free water clearance, the ECFV expansion will be isotonic and the patient will remain normonatremic. On the other hand, hyponatremia will be the consequence of excessive water ingestion. However, in view of the concomitant impairment in urinary concentrating mechanism, severe hyponatremia is not usual in predialysis patients, and water restriction is only necessary when hyponatremia is documented. In such patients, a daily intake of fluid equal to the urine volume per day plus about 500 mL usually maintains the serum Na^+ concentration at normal levels.

Weight gain usually associated with volume expansion may be offset in patients with CRD by concomitant loss of lean body mass. In the CRD patient who is not yet on dialysis but has clear evidence of ECFV expansion, administration of loop diuretics coupled with restriction of salt intake are the mainstays of therapy. It should be noted that resistance to loop diuretics in renal failure often mandates use of higher doses than those usually used when GFR is well preserved. The combination of loop diuretics with metalozone, which inhibits the Na-Cl cotransporter of the distal convoluted tubule, can sometimes overcome diuretic resistance. When the GFR falls to <5 to 10 mL/min, even high doses of combination diuretics are ineffective. ECFV expansion under these circumstances usually means that dialysis is indicated. In dialysis patients with volume expansion, management should include ultrafiltration and restriction of salt and water intake between dialysis treatments.

Patients with CRD also have impaired renal mechanisms for conserving Na^+ and H_2O (Chap. 268). When an *extrarenal* cause for fluid loss is present (e.g., vomiting, diarrhea, sweating, fever), these patients are prone to volume depletion. Depletion of ECFV may compromise residual renal function with resulting signs and symptoms of overt uremia. Because of impaired renal Na^+ and H_2O conservation mechanisms, the usual indices of prerenal azotemia (oliguria, high urine osmolality, low urinary Na^+ concentration, and low fractional excretion of Na^+) are not useful. Cautious volume repletion, usually with normal saline, returns ECFV to normal and usually restores renal function to prior levels.

Potassium Homeostasis (See also Chap. 49) When GFR is normal, the approximate daily filtered load of K^+ is 700 mmol. The ma-

Table 270-3 Clinical Abnormalities in Uremia[a]

Fluid and electrolyte disturbances	Neuromuscular disturbances	Dermatologic disturbances
Volume expansion and contraction (I)	Fatigue (I)[b]	Pallor (I)[b]
Hypernatremia and hyponatremia (I)	Sleep disorders (P)	Hyperpigmentation (I, P, or D)
Hyperkalemia and hypokalemia (I)	Headache (I or P)	Pruritus (P)
Metabolic acidosis (I)	Impaired mentation (I)[b]	Ecchymoses (I)
Hyperphosphatemia (I)	Lethargy (I)[b]	Uremic frost (I)
Hypocalcemia (I)	Asterixis (I)	
	Muscular irritability (I)	Gastrointestinal disturbances
Endocrine-metabolic disturbances	Peripheral neuropathy (I or P)	Anorexia (I)
Secondary hyperparathyroidism (I or P)	Restless legs syndrome (I or P)	Nausea and vomiting (I)
Adynamic osteomalacia (D)	Paralysis (I or P)	Uremic fetor (I)
Vitamin D–deficient osteomalacia (I)	Myoclonus (I)	Gastroenteritis (I)
Carbohydrate intolerance (I)	Seizures (I or P)	Peptic ulcer (I or P)
Hyperuricemia (I or P)	Coma (I)	Gastrointestinal bleeding (I, P, or D)
Hypertriglyceridemia (I or P)	Muscle cramps (D)	Hepatitis (D)
Increased Lp(a) level (P)	Dialysis disequilibrium syndrome (D)	Idiopathic ascites (D)
Decreased high-density lipoprotein level (P)	Myopathy (P or D)	Peritonitis (D)
Protein-calorie malnutrition (I or P)		
Impaired growth and development (P)	Cardiovascular and pulmonary disturbances	Hematologic and immunologic disturbances
Infertility and sexual dysfunction (P)	Arterial hypertension (I or P)	Anemia (I)[b]
Amenorrhea (P)	Congestive heart failure or pulmonary edema (I)	Lymphocytopenia (P)
Hypothermia (I)	Pericarditis (I)	Bleeding diathesis (I or D)[b]
Dialysis-induced β_2-microglobulin Amyloidosis (P)	Cardiomyopathy (I or P)	Increased susceptibility to infection (I or P)
	Uremic lung (I)	Splenomegaly and hypersplenism (P)
	Accelerated atherosclerosis (P or D)	Leukopenia (D)
	Hypotension and arrhythmias (D)	Hypocomplementemia (D)
	Vascular calcification (P or D)	

[a] Virtually all abnormalities in this table are completely reversed in time by successful renal transplantation. The response of these abnormalities to hemodialysis or peritoneal dialysis therapy is more variable. (I) denotes an abnormality that usually improves with an optimal program of dialysis and related therapy; (P) denotes one that tends to persist or even progress, despite an optimal program; (D) denotes one that develops only after initiation of dialysis therapy.
[b] Improves with dialysis and erythropoietin therapy.

jority of this filtered load is reabsorbed in tubule segments prior to the cortical collecting tubule, and most of the K^+ excreted in the final urine reflects events governing K^+ handling at the level of the cortical collecting tubule and beyond. These factors include the flow of luminal fluid and the delivery and reabsorption of Na^+, which generates the lumen-negative electromotive force for K^+ secretion at the aldosterone-responsive distal nephron sites. In CRD, these factors may be well preserved, such that a decline in GFR is not necessarily accompanied by a concomitant and proportionate decline in urinary K^+ excretion. In addition, K^+ excretion in the gastrointestinal tract is augmented in patients with CRD. However, hyperkalemia may be precipitated in a number of clinical situations, including augmented dietary intake, protein catabolism, hemolysis, hemorrhage, transfusion of stored red blood cells, metabolic acidosis, and following the exposure to a variety of medications that inhibit K^+ entry into cells or K^+ secretion in the distal nephron. Most commonly encountered medications in this regard are beta blockers, ACE inhibitors, K^+-sparing diuretics (amiloride, triamterene, spironolactone), and nonsteroidal anti-inflammatory drugs (NSAIDs). In addition, certain etiologies of CRD may be associated with earlier and more severe disruption of K^+ secretory mechanisms in the distal nephron, relative to the reduction in GFR. Most important are conditions associated with hyporeninemic hypoaldosteronism (e.g., diabetic nephropathy and certain forms of distal renal tubular acidosis; Chap. 49).

Most commonly, clinically significant hyperkalemia does not occur until the GFR falls to below 10 mL/min or unless there is exposure to a K^+ load, either endogenous (e.g., hemolysis, trauma, infection) or exogenous (e.g., administration of stored blood, K^+-containing medications, K^+-containing dietary salt substitute). In kidney transplant re-

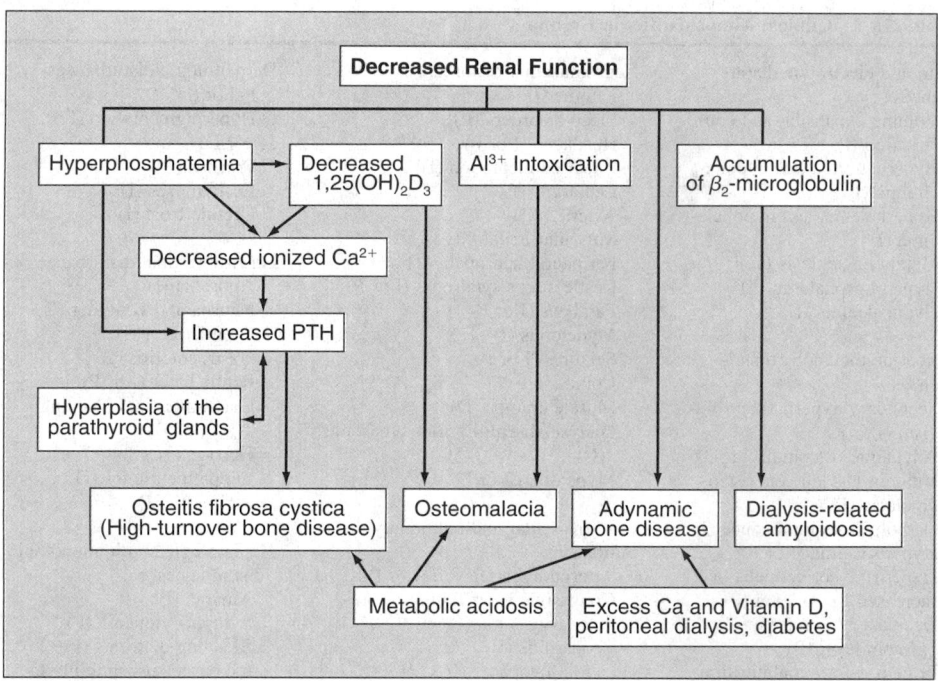

FIGURE 270-1 Flowchart for the development of bone, phosphate, and calcium abnormalities in chronic renal disease. (PTH, parathyroid hormone; PD, peritoneal dialysis.)

cipients, cyclosporine is another common cause of increased plasma K+ concentration. Hyperkalemia in CRD patients may also be induced by abrupt falls in plasma pH, since acidosis is associated with efflux of K+ from the intracellular to the extracellular fluid compartment.

Although total-body K+ is frequently reduced in CRD, *hypokalemia* is uncommon. The occurrence of hypokalemia usually reflects markedly reduced dietary K+ intake, in association with excessive diuretic therapy or gastrointestinal losses. Hypokalemia occurs as a result of primary renal K+ wasting in association with other solute transport abnormalities, as in Fanconi's syndrome, renal tubular acidosis, or other forms of hereditary or acquired tubulointerstitial diseases. However, even under these circumstances, as GFR declines, the tendency to hypokalemia diminishes and hyperkalemia may supervene. Accordingly, K+ supplementation and K+-sparing diuretics should be used with caution as GFR declines.

Metabolic Acidosis (See also Chap. 50) In adults, the metabolism of dietary protein generates approximately 1 mmol/kg per day of H+. The H+ must be excreted, primarily by renal mechanisms, if neutral acid-base balance is to be maintained. Acidosis is a common disturbance during the advanced stages of CRD. Although in a majority of patients with CRD the urine can be acidified normally, these patients have a reduced ability to produce ammonia. In part this is a consequence of limited ATP utilization, resulting from diminished Na+ reabsorption in the proximal tubule. As a result, the use of glutamine as an energy source is limited, which in turn limits proximal tubule ammonia production. Hyperkalemia, when present, further depresses urinary ammonium excretion. The combination of hyperkalemia and hyperchloremic metabolic acidosis (known as type IV renal tubular acidosis or hyporeninemic hypoaldosteronism) is most characteristically seen in patients with diabetes or in those with predominantly tubulointerstitial disease. Treatment of the hyperkalemia frequently improves the acidosis as well.

With advancing renal failure, total urinary net daily acid excretion is usually limited to 30 to 40 mmol; thus, throughout the remainder of their course of CRD, many patients may be in a positive H+ balance of 20 to 40 mmol/d. The retained H+ is buffered by bone salts. In the early stages, the accompanying organic anions are excreted in the urine, and the metabolic acidosis is of the non-anion gap variety. However, with advanced renal failure, a fairly large "anion gap" may develop (to approximately 20 mmol/L) with a reciprocal fall in plasma

HCO_3^- concentration. In most patients, the metabolic acidosis is mild and the pH is rarely less than 7.35. The metabolic acidosis can usually be corrected by treating the patient with 20 to 30 mmol of sodium bicarbonate or sodium citrate daily. However, the concomitant Na+ load mandates careful attention to volume status and the potential need for diuretic agents. Also, citrate enhances aluminum absorption in the large bowel, and citrate-containing antacids should be avoided if aluminum-containing drugs are also administered. As with other abnormalities in CRD, severe symptomatic manifestations of acid-base imbalance occur when the patient is challenged with an excessive endogenous or exogenous acid load or loses excessive alkali (e.g., with diarrhea).

BONE, PHOSPHATE, AND CALCIUM ABNORMALITIES (Fig. 270-1) (See also Chap. 340) Although clinical symptoms of bone disease are present before dialysis in fewer than 10% of patients with ESRD, radiologic and histologic abnormalities are observed in about 35 and 90%, respectively. Two principal types of bone disorders are observed in patients with ESRD: a high-turnover osteodystrophy, known as *osteitis fibrosa cystica*, and a low-turnover state characterized initially by *osteomalacia* and subsequently by *adynamic bone disease*. In osteitis fibrosa, the number and size of the osteoclasts are increased, as are the number and depth of the osteoclastic resorption lacunae. Collagen deposition is less ordered, and the rate of bone turnover is markedly increased. In osteomalacia, the rate of mineralization is slower than that of collagen synthesis, resulting in excessive accumulation of unmineralized osteoid and widened osteoid seams. In adynamic uremic osteodystrophy, a parallel marked reduction in the rate of mineralization and collagen synthesis results in osteoid seams of normal width. While these disorders are often discussed as if they were distinct, they commonly overlap in a given patient with ESRD.

High-Turnover Uremic Osteodystrophy This condition is associated with elevated PTH levels. The hyperparathyroid state is attributable both to hyperplastic growth of the parathyroid glands and to augmented release of hormone from each individual parathyroid cell. The main factors responsible for deranged PTH synthesis in CRD are related to altered metabolism of phosphate, calcitrol $[1,25(OH)_2D_3]$, and Ca^{2+}.

Phosphate (PO_4^{3-}) Hyperphosphatemia is a feature of advanced renal failure. The serum phosphate concentration rises in patients with a GFR < 20 mL/min, but retention of PO_4^{3-} can be documented in balance studies with even less severe declines in GFR. The retained PO_4^{3-} is a major cause of the development of secondary hyperparathyroidism in CRD. PO_4^{3-} exerts indirect effects on PTH secretion by decreasing renal production of calcitrol (see below) and by lowering plasma ionized Ca^{2+}. Recent studies also suggest a direct stimulatory role of PO_4^{3-} at the level of the parathyroid gland, in the absence of changes in serum Ca^{2+} or calcitrol levels. Dietary restriction of PO_4^{3-} as well as gastrointestinal PO_4^{3-} binders may prevent hyperphosphatemia, thereby mitigating the rise in PTH levels.

Calcitrol Under normal conditions, calcitrol exerts negative feedback control on the parathyroid gland through both direct (i.e., diminished transcription of pre-proPTH mRNA) and indirect mechanisms. The latter act through stimulation of intestinal absorption of Ca^{2+} and the skeletal mobilization of Ca^{2+}, thereby increasing plasma Ca^{2+} and inhibiting PTH secretion. Therefore, reduced synthesis of $1,25(OH)_2D_3$ during CRD plays a key role in the pathogenesis of hyperparathyroidism, both directly and through hypocalcemia. The abnormal vitamin D metabolism may be related to the renal disease itself (since the active vitamin D metabolite is normally produced in the proximal tubule) and to the hyperphosphatemia, which has a suppressive effect on the renal 1α-hydroxylase enzyme. Furthermore, a decrease in the number of calcitriol receptors in the parathyroid tissue of uremic patients has been reported by several groups. Recent studies have demonstrated a marked decrease in vitamin D–receptor expression in areas of nodular transformation within hyperplastic parathyroid tissue but revealed no such receptor downregulation in diffuse hyperplastic parathyroid tissue. Since vitamin D also has an antiproliferative effect on parathyroid cells, this phenomenon may provide an explanation for the marked PTH secretion as well as the abnormal glandular growth pattern characteristic of nodular hyperparathyroidism.

Calcium The total plasma Ca^{2+} concentration in patients with CRD is often significantly lower than normal. Patients with CRD tolerate the hypocalcemia quite well; rarely is a patient symptomatic from the decreased Ca^{2+} concentration. This may partly be due to the frequent concomitant acidosis, which offsets some of the neuromuscular effects of hypocalcemia. The hypocalcemia in CRD results from decreased intestinal absorption of Ca^{2+} due to vitamin D deficiency (see above). Also, with the increasing serum PO_4^{3-} level, Ca^{2+} phosphate is deposited in soft tissues and serum Ca^{2+} concentration (both total and ionized) declines. In addition, patients with CRD are resistant to the action of PTH. Hypocalcemia is a potent stimulus to PTH secretion and leads to hyperplasia of the parathyroid gland. Ca^{2+} binds to a specific Ca^{2+}-sensing receptor protein located in the cell membrane. The Ca^{2+}-sensing receptor is linked to several cytoplasmic messenger systems by one or more GTP-binding proteins. These signaling pathways are responsible for either enhanced or suppressed release of PTH during acute hypo- and hypercalcemia, respectively. Several studies have demonstrated the mRNA and protein expression of the Ca^{2+}-sensing receptor to be reduced in primary (adenomas) and secondary hyperparathyroidism (hyperplasia) compared to the expression in normal parathyroid tissue. In secondary hyperparathyroidism, expression of the Ca^{2+}-sensing receptor is often depressed in nodular areas compared with adjacent nonnodular hyperplasia. Thus, decreased Ca^{2+} receptor expression in hyperparathyroidism is compatible with a less efficient control of PTH synthesis and release, in response to varying plasma Ca^{2+} concentration.

In addition to excessive release of PTH from individual parathyroid cells, the size of the glands also increases as renal failure progresses. This abnormal growth of the parathyroid glands may assume one of the following patterns: (1) diffuse hyperplasia (polyclonal growth), (2) nodular growth (monoclonal growth) within diffuse hyperplastic tissue, or (3) diffuse monoclonal hyperplasia ("adenoma," or tertiary autonomous hyperparathyroidism). Patients with monoclonal ("autonomous") hyperplasia are especially prone to develop hypercalcemia following successful kidney transplantation, often necessitating parathyroidectomy.

During the initial phase of CRD, the elevated PTH levels may normalize serum levels of Ca^{2+}, PO_4^{3-}, and vitamin D. Therefore hypocalcemia, hyperphosphatemia, and reduced $1,25(OH)_2D_3$ are observed only as CRD progresses. However, even at the earliest stages of CRD, the elevated PTH levels adversely affect bone metabolism, causing increased osteoclastic and osteoblastic activity (high-turnover bone disease). Additional detrimental factors include the chronic uremic acidosis, which inhibits osteoblastic bone formation and stimulates osteoclastic bone resorption.

Low-Turnover Uremic Osteodystrophy Originally thought to result solely from vitamin D deficiency, *osteomalacia* (Chap. 342) has now been more closely associated with aluminum toxicity. Aluminum was first identified as a presumed cause of dialysis dementia in dialysis patients, and shortly thereafter aluminum deposition in bone was shown to be associated with osteomalacia. The sources of aluminum were phosphate binders and the water used in preparing dialysate. Aluminum is no longer present as a contaminant in dialysate, but it still is widely utilized as a phosphate binder in some settings. Approximately one-third of dialysis and CRD patients ingest at least some aluminum. Aluminum deposition adversely affects mineral deposition at the mineralization front.

Aplastic renal osteodystrophy occurs in many patients who have no evidence of excess aluminum accumulation. These patients have relatively low levels of PTH. The disorder is associated with the use of supraphysiologic Ca^{2+} concentrations in peritoneal dialysate and the excessive use of oral Ca^{2+} and vitamin D preparations in both hemodialysis and peritoneal dialysis patients. These sources of exogenous Ca^{2+} might lower serum PTH to levels that are inadequate for maintaining normal bone turnover.

Yet another type of skeletal lesion that occurs in ESRD patients after many years of dialysis therapy results from *amyloid deposition* related to the accumulation of β_2-microglobulin. This syndrome presents as carpal tunnel syndrome, tenosynovitis of the hands, shoulder arthropathy, bone cysts, cervical spondyloarthropathy, and cervical pseudotumors. It is characterized on x-ray films by cysts in the carpal bones and femoral neck. Amyloid tumoral masses may be best appreciated by ultrasound examination or computed tomography.

With high-turnover osteitis fibrosa cystica, vitamin D–deficient and aluminum-induced osteomalacia, and dialysis-related amyloidosis, ESRD patients are prone to spontaneous fractures, which are slow to heal. The ribs are most commonly involved in the case of osteitis fibrosa cystica. The femoral neck is a frequent site of aluminum-induced osteomalacia and dialysis-related amyloidosis and is also prone to pathologic fractures. Bone pain, even in the absence of fractures, is common. In osteitis fibrosa cystica, a proximal myopathy often coexists, giving rise to gait abnormalities and to impairment of ambulation. Similarly, a myopathy may also accompany amyloid arthropathy. In CRD, there is a tendency to extraosseous or metastatic calcification when the calcium-phosphate product is very high (>70 when expressed as mg/dL). Medium-sized blood vessels; subcutaneous, articular, and periarticular tissues; myocardium; eyes; and lungs are common sites of metastatic calcification. *Calciphylaxis* refers to devastating necrotic extremity soft tissue lesions related to vascular occlusion and metastatic calcification.

The Effect of Uremic Acidosis on Bone Disease As previously noted, in patients with CRD, a decrease in acid excretion leads to unremitting positive H^+ balance. If extracellular fluid HCO_3^- were the only H^+ buffer available, it would become progressively depleted and the concentration of serum HCO_3^-, and thus pH, would fall to levels incompatible with life. However, during CRD, extracellular fluid HCO_3^- and pH remain stable, although reduced, for long periods; thus, either non-HCO_3^- buffers must neutralize the retained hydrogen ions or acid production must decrease. Acid production does not appear to diminish in patients with renal failure; yet such patients excrete only approximately two-thirds of their daily hydrogen ion production. Thus substantial buffering of the retained hydrogen ions almost certainly occurs. Because of its mass and potential buffering capacity, bone is a likely site for the chronic hydrogen ion buffering.

℞ **TREATMENT** *Secondary hyperparathyroidism* and *osteitis fibrosa* are best prevented and treated by reducing serum PO_4^{3-} concentration through the use of a PO_4^{3-} restricted diet as well as oral PO_4^{3-}-binding agents. Calcium carbonate and calcium acetate are the preferred PO_4^{3-} binding agents, but in some rare circumstances a combination of short-term aluminum hydroxide and calcium carbonate is necessary. In such cases, aluminum levels should be monitored, and citrate antacids, which enhance aluminum absorption, should be avoided. Daily oral calcitriol, or intermittent oral or intravenous pulses, appear to exert a direct suppressive effect on PTH secretion, in addition to the indirect effect mediated through raising Ca^{2+} levels. Intravenous pulses are especially convenient for patients on hemodialysis. The use of calcitriol and Ca^{2+} preparations in the predialysis population must take into account potential effects of increased phosphate and Ca^{2+} on the rate of progression of CRD. In the dialysis population, dialysate Ca^{2+}, calcium carbonate, calcium acetate, aluminum hydroxide, and calcitriol must be properly balanced to maintain the serum PO_4^{3-} concentration at approximately 1.4 mmol/L (4.5 mg/dL) and the serum Ca^{2+} at approximately 2.5 mmol/L (10 mg/dL) in an attempt to suppress parathyroid hyperplasia, thus avoiding or reversing osteitis fibrosa cystica, osteomalacia, and myopathy. It is particularly important to maintain the Ca^{2+}-PO_4^{3-} product in the normal range to avoid metastatic calcification. Several analogues of calcitriol are now being evaluated. Such analogues would be beneficial if they had the same effect on PTH mRNA as calcitriol and increased the margin of safety and efficacy by having less hyperphosphatemic and hypercalcemic effects. In this manner, it might be possible to have a greater suppressive effect on PTH transcription because a higher dose could be used safely.

Adynamic bone disease is often a consequence of overzealous treatment of secondary hyperparathyroidism. Therefore, suppression of PTH levels to less than 120 pg/mL in uremic patients may not be desirable. The incidence of aluminum-induced osteomalacia has been greatly reduced with the recognition of aluminum as the principal culprit. Therapy for this disorder is continued avoidance of aluminum, with possible use of a chelating agent such as desferoxamine along with high-flux dialysis. Management of metabolic acidosis should aim to maintain a nearly normal level of plasma HCO_3^-, with the administration of calcium acetate or calcium carbonate in the first instance, and with the addition of $NaHCO_3$ if necessary. Excessive administration of alkali should be avoided to minimize risk of urinary precipitation of calcium phosphate.

At present, there is no good therapy for *dialysis-related amyloidosis*. Local physical therapy, glucocorticoid injections, and NSAIDs constitute current options.

Other Solutes   *Uric acid* retention is a common feature of CRD but rarely leads to symptomatic gout. Treatment of hyperuricemia is not necessary unless recurrent gout becomes a problem. When recurrent symptomatic gout occurs, a reduced dose of allopurinol (100 to 200 mg/d) is usually sufficient to inhibit uric acid synthesis. Hypophosphatemia is rare and, when it occurs, is usually a consequence of overzealous oral administration of phosphate-binding gels. Because serum magnesium levels tend to rise in CRD, magnesium-containing antacids and cathartics should be avoided.

CARDIOVASCULAR AND PULMONARY ABNORMALITIES   Congestive Heart Failure (See also Chap. 232)   Salt and water retention in uremia often result in congestive heart failure and/or pulmonary edema. A unique form of pulmonary congestion and edema may occur even in the absence of volume overload and is associated with normal or mildly elevated intracardiac and pulmonary capillary wedge pressures. This entity, characterized radiologically by peripheral vascular congestion giving rise to a "butterfly wing" distribution, is due to increased permeability of alveolar capillary membranes. This "low-pressure" pulmonary edema as well as cardiopulmonary abnormalities associated with circulatory overload usually respond promptly to vigorous dialysis.

Hypertension and Left Ventricular Hypertrophy (See also Chap. 246)   Hypertension is the most common complication of CRD and ESRD. When it is not found, the patient may have a salt-wasting form of renal disease (e.g., medullary cystic disease, chronic tubulointerstitial disease, or papillary necrosis), may be receiving antihypertensive therapy, or be volume-depleted, the last condition usually due to excessive gastrointestinal fluid losses or overzealous diuretic therapy. Since volume overload is the major cause of hypertension in uremia, the normotensive state can often be restored by appropriate use of diuretics in the predialysis patient or with aggressive ultrafiltration in dialysis patients. Nevertheless, because of hyperreninemia, some patients remain hypertensive despite rigorous salt and water restriction and ultrafiltration. Rarely, patients develop accelerated or malignant hypertension. Intravenous nitroprusside, labetolol, or more re-

cently approved agents such as fenoldopam or urapidil, together with control of ECFV, generally controls such hypertension. Subsequently, such patients usually require more than one oral antihypertensive drug. Enalaprilat or other ACE inhibitors may also be considered, but in the face of bilateral renovascular disease they have the potential to further reduce GFR abruptly. Administration of erythropoietin (EPO) (p. 1557) may raise blood pressure and increase the requirement for antihypertensive drugs. A high percentage of patients with CRD present with left ventricular hypertrophy or dilated cardiomyopathy. These are among the most ominous risk factors for excess cardiovascular morbidity and mortality in patients with CRD and ESRD and are thought to be related primarily to prolonged hypertension and ECFV overload. In addition, anemia and the surgical placement of an arteriovenous anastomosis for future or ongoing dialysis access may generate a high cardiac output state, which also intensifies the burden placed on the left ventricle.

TREATMENT   Management of hypertension in CRD can be considered in terms of two overall goals: to slow the progression of CRD itself and to prevent the extrarenal complications of hypertension, such as cardiovascular disease and stroke. In all patients with CRD, blood pressure should be controlled to at least the level established in the guidelines of the Joint National Commission on Hypertension Detection Education and Follow-up Program (130/80–85 mmHg). In the elderly, levels of 140 mmHg may be a more realistic target. In predialysis patients with proteinuria > 1 g per 24 hr, blood pressure should be further reduced to a mean arterial pressure of 92 mmHg (equivalent to 125/75 mmHg), where possible. Volume control is the mainstay of therapy, with addition of antihypertensive agents as needed when hypertension persists despite achievement of a normovolemic state. When salt retention and hypervolemia contribute to hypertension, salt restriction and diuretics are indicated as initial therapy. The choice of additional agents to slow the progression of CRD based upon reduction of intraglomerular hypertension and proteinuria is considered below. In ESRD patients, considerations related to slowing of nephron injury are less important, and the main goal is to prevent cardiac hypertrophy and stroke. The choice of antihypertensive agents may come from all the major classes, with careful consideration of comorbid conditions. However, powerful direct-acting vasodilators, such as hydralazine or minoxidil, may perpetuate the tendency to cardiac hypertrophy, despite the lowering of blood pressure. Therefore, prolonged use of such agents should be reserved for those very rare patients in whom severe refractory hypertension persists, despite adequate volume reduction and compliance with all other classes of antihypertensives.

Atherosclerotic Coronary and Peripheral Vascular Disease   Hypertension, hyperhomocysteinemia, and lipid abnormalities promote atherosclerosis but are potentially treatable complications of CRD. Ongoing or prior nephrotic syndrome is also associated with hyperlipidemia and hypercoagulability, which increase the risk of occlusive vascular disease. Since diabetes mellitus and hypertension are themselves the two most frequent etiologies of CRD, it is not surprising that cardiovascular disease is the most frequent cause of death in ESRD patients. Therefore, accepted life-style changes and therapeutic measures for cardiac risk reduction (Chap. 242) are especially important in this group of patients. The approach to managing hypertension has been outlined above. Hyperhomocysteinemia may respond to vitamin therapy, which includes folate supplementation to between 1 and 5 mg/d. Hyperlipidemia in patients with CRD and ESRD should be managed aggressively according to the guidelines of the National Cholesterol Education Program (Chaps. 242 and 344). If dietary measures are inadequate, the preferred lipid-lowering medications are gemfibrozil and an HMG-CoA reductase inhibitor. However, these two classes of agents ordinarily should not be combined because of an increased risk of myositis and rhabomyolysis in CRD and ESRD patients.

Abnormalities in Ca^{2+} and PO_4^{3-} metabolism (see above) may lead to metastatic vascular calcification and markedly increase the propensity to coronary, cerebral, and peripheral occlusive vascular disease. By careful attention to the guidelines noted above for the management of divalent ion metabolism and bone disease, avoidance of an elevated Ca^{2+}-PO_4^{3-} product may mitigate this effect.

Pericarditis (See also Chap. 239) With the advent of early initiation of renal replacement therapy, pericarditis is now observed more often in underdialyzed patients than in patients with CRD in whom dialysis has not yet been initiated. Pericardial pain with respiratory accentuation, accompanied by a friction rub, are the hallmarks of uremic pericarditis. The finding of a multicomponent friction rub strongly supports the diagnosis. Furthermore, the usual occurrence of multiple cardiac murmurs, S_3 and S_4 heart sounds, and transmitted bruits from arteriovenous access devices may render precordial auscultation more challenging in this group of patients. Classic electrocardiographic abnormalities include PR-interval shortening and diffuse ST-segment elevation. Pericarditis may be accompanied by the accumulation of pericardial fluid, readily detected by echocardiography, sometimes leading to cardiac tamponade. Pericardial fluid in uremic pericarditis is more often hemorrhagic than in viral pericarditis.

℞ **TREATMENT** Uremic pericarditis is an absolute indication for initiation of dialysis or for intensification of the dialysis prescription in those already on dialysis. Because of the propensity to hemorrhagic pericardial fluid, heparin-free dialysis is indicated. Pericardiectomy should be considered only if more conservative measures fail. Nonuremic causes of pericarditis and pericardial effusion include viral, malignant, and tuberculous pericarditis and pericarditis associated with myocardial infarction; these are also more frequent in patients with ESRD and should be managed according to the dictates of the underlying disease process.

HEMATOLOGIC ABNORMALITIES Anemia of CRD (See also Chap. 105) A normocytic, normochromic anemia is present in the majority of patients with CRD. It is usually observed when the GFR falls below 30 mL/min. When untreated, the anemia of CRD is associated with a number of physiologic abnormalities, including decreased tissue oxygen delivery and utilization, increased cardiac output, cardiac enlargement, ventricular hypertrophy, angina, congestive heart failure, decreased cognition and mental acuity, altered menstrual cycles, and impaired immune responsiveness. In addition, anemia may play a role in growth retardation in children. The primary cause of anemia in patients with CRD is insufficient production of EPO by the diseased kidneys. Additional factors include the following: iron deficiency, either related to or independent of blood loss from repeated laboratory testing, needle punctures, blood retention in the dialyzer and tubing, or gastrointestinal bleeding; severe hyperparathyroidism; acute and chronic inflammatory conditions; aluminum toxicity; folate deficiency; shortened red cell survival; hypothyroidism; and underlying hemoglobinopathies. These potential contributing factors should be considered and addressed.

Before 1989, the EPO-deficient condition characteristic of CRD could only be treated with blood transfusions and anabolic steroids, with limited success and substantial complications. The availability of recombinant human EPO, approved by the U.S. Food and Drug Administration in 1989, has been one of the most significant advances in the care of renal patients in the past decade. Considerable debate continues regarding the optimal target hematocrit in dialysis patients receiving EPO. Mortality and hospitalization studies support the National Kidney Foundation Dialysis Outcomes Quality Initiative target hematocrit range of 33 to 36% as providing the best associated outcomes. EPO can be administered either intravenously or subcutaneously. Most studies have shown that administering EPO by the subcutaneous route has a sparing effect, with the target hematocrit achieved at a lower EPO dose. Management guidelines for the correction of anemia in CRD are as follows:

Management Guidelines—Correction of Anemia in CRD

ERYTHROPOIETIN

SC	80–120 units/kg per week (divided into × 2–3/week)
IV	120–180 units/kg per week (divided into × 3/week)
Target Hct/Hb	33–36%/11–12 g/dL
Optimal rate of correction[a]	Increase Hct by 4–6% over 4-week period (achieve goal values within 2–3 months)

IRON

Monitor iron stores by percent transferrin saturation (TSAT) and serum ferritin.
If patient is iron-deficient [TSAT < 20% ferritin < 100 ng/mL (<100 mg/L)] administer iron 50–100 mg IV twice per week for 5 weeks (or for 10 successive dialysis sessions). If iron indices are still low, repeat the same course.
If iron indices are normal yet Hct/Hb are still inadequate, administer IV iron as outlined above. Monitor Hct/Hb, TSAT, and ferritin.
Withhold iron therapy when TSAT > 50% and/or ferritin > 800 ng/mL (>800 μg/L)

[a] If correction of anemia is inadequate, consider causes for refractoriness as outlined in text.

The iron status of the patient with CRD must be assessed, and adequate iron stores should be available before treatment with EPO is initiated. Iron supplementation is usually essential to ensure an adequate response to EPO in patients with CRD, because the demands for iron by the erythroid marrow frequently exceed the amount of iron that is immediately available for erythropoiesis (as measured by percent transferrin saturation) as well as iron stores (as measured by serum ferritin). In most cases, intravenous iron will be required to achieve and/or maintain adequate iron. However, excessive iron therapy may be associated with a number of complications, including hemosiderosis, accelerated atherosclerosis, increased susceptibility to infection, and possibly an increased propensity to the emergence of malignancies. In addition to iron, an adequate supply of the other major substrates and cofactors for erythrocyte production must be assured, especially vitamin B_{12} and folate. Anemia resistant to recommended doses of EPO in the face of adequate availability of iron and vitamin factors often suggests inadequate dialysis; uncontrolled hyperparathyroidism; aluminum toxicity; chronic blood loss or hemolysis; and associated hemoglobinopathy, malnutrition, chronic infection, multiple myeloma, or another malignancy. Blood transfusions may contribute to suppression of erythropoiesis in CRD; because they increase the risk of hepatitis, hemosiderosis, and transplant sensitization, they should be avoided unless the anemia fails to respond to EPO and the patient is symptomatic.

Abnormal Hemostasis Abnormal hemostasis is common in CRD and is characterized by a tendency to abnormal bleeding and bruising. Bleeding from surgical wounds and spontaneous bleeding into the gastrointestinal tract, pericardial sac, or intracranial vault (in the form of subdural hematoma or intracerebral hemorrhage) are of greatest concern. Prolongation of bleeding time, decreased activity of platelet factor III, abnormal platelet aggregation and adhesiveness, and impaired prothrombin consumption contribute to the clotting defects. The abnormality in platelet factor III correlates with increased plasma levels of guanidinosuccinic acid and can be corrected by dialysis. Prolongation of the bleeding time is common even in well-dialyzed patients. Abnormal bleeding times and coagulopathy in patients with renal failure may be reversed with desmopressin, cryoprecipitate, conjugated estrogens, and blood transfusions, as well as by the use of EPO.

Enhanced Susceptibility to Infection Changes in leukocyte formation and function in uremia lead to enhanced susceptibility to infection. Lymphocytopenia and atrophy of lymphoid structures occur, whereas neutrophil production is relatively unimpaired. Nevertheless, the function of all leukocyte cell types may be affected adversely by uremic serum. Alterations in monocyte, lymphocyte, and neutrophil function cause impairment of acute inflammatory responses, decreased delayed hypersensitivity, and altered late immune function.

There is a tendency for uremic patients to have less fever in response to infection, perhaps because of the effects of uremia on the hypothalamic temperature control center. Leukocyte function may also be impaired in patients with CRD because of coexisting acidosis, hyperglycemia, protein-calorie malnutrition, and serum and tissue hyperosmolarity (due to azotemia). In patients treated with hemodialysis, leukocyte function is disturbed because of the effects of the bioincompatibility of various dialysis membranes. Activation of cytokine and complement cascades likewise occurs when blood comes in contact with dialysis membranes. These substances in turn alter inflammatory and immune responses of the uremic patient. Mucosal barriers to infection may also be defective, and, in dialysis patients, vascular and peritoneal access devices are common portals of entry for pathogens, especially staphylococci. Glucocorticoids and immunosuppressive drugs used for various renal diseases and renal transplantation further increase the risk of infection.

NEUROMUSCULAR ABNORMALITIES Subtle disturbances of central nervous system function, including inability to concentrate, drowsiness, and insomnia, are among the early symptoms of uremia. Mild behavioral changes, loss of memory, and errors in judgment soon follow and may be associated with neuromuscular irritability, including hiccoughs, cramps, and fasciculations/twitching of muscles. Asterixis, myoclonus, and chorea are common in terminal uremia, as are stupor, seizures, and coma. Peripheral neuropathy is also common in advanced CRD. Initially, sensory nerves are involved more than motor nerves, lower extremities more than upper, and distal portions of the extremities more than proximal. The "restless legs syndrome" is characterized by ill-defined sensations of discomfort in the feet and lower legs requiring frequent leg movement. If dialysis is not instituted soon after onset of sensory abnormalities, motor involvement follows, including loss of deep tendon reflexes, weakness, peroneal nerve palsy (foot drop), and, eventually, flaccid quadriplegia. Accordingly, evidence of peripheral neuropathy is a firm indication for the initiation of dialysis or transplantation. Some of the central nervous system and neuromuscular complications of advanced uremia resolve with dialysis, although nonspecific electroencephalographic abnormalities may persist (Table 270-3). Successful transplantation may reverse residual peripheral neuropathy.

Two types of neurologic disturbances are unique to patients on chronic dialysis (Chap. 271). *Dialysis dementia* may occur in patients who have been on dialysis for many years and is characterized by speech dyspraxia, myoclonus, dementia, and eventually seizures and death. Aluminum intoxication is probably the major contributor to this syndrome, but other factors, such as viral infections, may play a role since not all patients with aluminum exposure develop the syndrome. *Dialysis disequilibrium*, which occurs during the first few dialyses in association with rapid reduction of blood urea levels, manifests clinically with nausea, vomiting, drowsiness, headache, and, rarely, seizures. The syndrome has been attributed to cerebral edema and increased intracranial pressure due to the rapid (dialysis-induced) shifts of omsolality and pH between extracellular and intracellular fluids. This complication can often be anticipated and prevented in patients who present with markedly elevated concentrations of plasma urea, by prescribing an initial dialysis regimen that produces slower solute removal.

GASTROINTESTINAL ABNORMALITIES Anorexia, hiccoughs, nausea, and vomiting are common early manifestations of uremia. Protein restriction is useful in diminishing nausea and vomiting late in the course of renal failure. However, protein restriction should not be implemented in patients with early signs of protein-calorie malnutrition. *Uremic fetor*, a uriniferous odor to the breath, derives from the breakdown of urea to ammonia in saliva and is often associated with an unpleasant metallic taste sensation. Mucosal ulcerations leading to blood loss can occur at any level of the gastrointestinal tract in the very late stages of CRD. Peptic ulcer disease is common in uremic patients. Whether this high incidence is related to altered gastric acidity, enhanced colonization by *Helicobacter pylori*, or hypersecretion of gastrin is unknown. Patients with CRD, particularly those with polycystic kidney disease, have an increased incidence of diverticulosis. Pancreatitis and angiodysplasia of the large bowel with chronic bleeding have been noted more commonly in dialysis patients. Hepatitis B antigenemia was very common in the past, but it is much less so now because of the implementation of universal precautions, the use of hepatitis B vaccine, and the diminished need for blood transfusions resulting from the introduction of EPO. There is a higher incidence of hepatitis C virus infection in patients treated with chronic hemodialysis. Unlike hepatitis B, this infection is most often persistent. Although it does not seem to cause significant liver disease in most patients, it is a definite concern in patients who subsequently undergo transplantation and immunosuppression, in whom the incidence of active chronic hepatitis and cirrhosis is considerably higher than in those without hepatitis C infection. →*The role of interferon and antiviral treatment in both hepatitis B and C infections is discussed in Chap. 295.*

ENDOCRINE-METABOLIC DISTURBANCES Disturbances in parathyroid function, protein-calorie and lipid metabolism, and overall nutritional abnormalities of uremia have already been considered.

Glucose metabolism is impaired, as evidenced by a slowing of the rate at which blood glucose levels decline after a glucose load. Fasting blood glucose is usually normal or only slightly elevated, and the mild glucose intolerance related to uremia per se, when present, does not require specific therapy. Because the kidney contributes significantly to insulin removal from the circulation, plasma levels of insulin are slightly to moderately elevated in most uremic subjects, both in the fasting and post-prandial states. However, the response to insulin and glucose utilization is impaired in CRD. Many renal hypoglycemic drugs require dose reduction in renal failure, and some, such as metformin, are contraindicated when GFR has diminished by more than approximately 25 to 50%.

In women, *estrogen levels* are low, and amenorrhea and inability to carry pregnancies to term are common manifestations of uremia. When GFR has declined by approximately 30%, pregnancy may hasten the progression of CRD. In women with ESRD, the reappearance of menses is a sign of efficient renal replacement therapy and is a frequent occurrence after an adequate chronic dialysis regimen has been established. Successful pregnancies are rare. In men with CRD, including those receiving chronic dialysis, impotence, oligospermia, and germinal cell dysplasia are common, as are reduced plasma testosterone levels. Like growth, sexual maturation is often impaired in adolescent children with CRD, even among those treated with chronic dialysis. Many of these abnormalities improve or reverse with successful renal transplantation.

DERMATOLOGIC ABNORMALITIES The skin may show evidence of anemia (pallor), defective hemostasis (ecchymoses and hematomas), calcium deposition and secondary hyperparathyroidism (pruritus, excoriations), dehydration (poor skin turgor, dry mucous membranes), and the general cutaneous consequences of protein-calorie malnutrition. A sallow, yellow cast may reflect the combined influences of anemia and retention of a variety of pigmented metabolites, or *urochromes*. The gray to bronze discoloration of the skin related to transfusional hemochromatosis has now become uncommon with the availability and usage of EPO. In advanced uremia, the concentration of urea in sweat may be so high that, after evaporation, a fine white powder can be found on the skin surface—so-called uremic (urea) frost. Although many of these cutaneous abnormalities improve with dialysis, *uremic pruritus* often remains a problem. The first lines of management are to rule out unrelated skin disorders, to adjust the dialysis prescription so as to ensure adequacy of dialysis, and to control PO_4^{3-} concentration with avoidance of an elevated Ca^{2+}-PO_4^{3-} product. Occasionally, pruritus remains refractory to these measures and to other nonspecific systemic and topical therapies. The latter has itself been reported to improve pruritus. Skin necrosis can occur as part of the calciphylaxis syndrome, which also includes subcutaneous, vascular, joint, and visceral calcification in patients with poorly controlled calcium-phosphate product.

DIAGNOSTIC APPROACH

The most important initial step in the evaluation of a patient presenting de novo with biochemical or clinical evidence of renal failure is to distinguish CRD, which may be first coming to clinical attention, from true acute renal failure. The demonstration of evidence of chronic metabolic bone disease and anemia and the finding of bilaterally reduced kidney size by imaging studies strongly favor a long-standing process consistent with CRD. However, these findings do not rule out the superimposition of an acute and reversible exacerbating factor that has accelerated the decline in GFR (see below). Having established that the patient suffers from CRD, in the early stages it is often possible to establish the underlying etiology. However, when the CRD process is quite advanced, then definitively establishing an underlying etiology becomes less feasible in many cases and also of less therapeutic significance.

ESTABLISHING THE ETIOLOGY Of special importance in establishing the etiology of CRD are a history of hypertension; diabetes; systemic infectious, inflammatory, or metabolic diseases; exposure to drugs and toxins; and a family history of renal and urologic disease. Drugs of particular importance include analgesics (usage frequently underestimated or denied by the patient), NSAIDs, gold, penicillamine, antimicrobials, lithium, and ACE inhibitors. In evaluating the uremic syndrome, questions about appetite, diet, nausea, vomiting, hiccoughing, shortness of breath, edema, weight change, muscle cramps, bone pain, mental acuity, and activities of daily living are especially helpful.

Physical Examination Particular attention should be paid to blood pressure, fundoscopy, precordial examination, examination of the abdomen for bruits and palpable renal masses, extremity examination for edema, and neurologic examination for the presence of asterixis, muscle weakness, and neuropathy. In addition, the evaluation of prostate size in men and potential pelvic masses in women should be undertaken by appropriate physical examination.

Laboratory Investigations These should also focus on a search for clues to an underlying disease process and its continued activity. Therefore, if the history and physical examination warrant, immunologic tests for systemic lupus erythematosus and vasculitis might be considered. Serum and urinary protein electrophoresis should be undertaken in all patients over the age of 40 with unexplained CRD and anemia, to rule out paraproteinemia. Other tests to determine the severity and chronicity of the disease include serial measurements of serum creatinine and blood urea nitrogen, hemoglobin, calcium, phosphate, and alkaline phosphatase to assess metabolic bone disease. Urine analysis may be helpful in assessing the presence of ongoing activity of the underlying inflammatory or proteinuric disease process, and when indicated should be supplemented by a 24-h urine collection for quantifying protein excretion. The latter is particularly helpful in guiding management strategies aimed at ameliorating the progression of CRD. The presence of *broad casts* on examination of the urinary sediment is a nonspecific finding seen with all diverse etiologies and reflects chronic tubulointerstitial scarring and tubular atrophy with widened tubule diameter, usually signifying an advanced stage of CRD.

Imaging Studies The most useful among these is renal sonography. An ultrasound examination of the kidneys verifies the presence of two symmetric kidneys, provides an estimate of kidney size, and rules out renal masses and obstructive uropathy. The documentation of symmetric small kidneys supports the diagnosis of progressive CRD with an irreversible component of scarring. The occurrence of normal kidney size suggests the possibility of an acute rather than chronic process. However, polycystic kidney disease, amyloidosis, and diabetes may lead to CRD with normal-sized or even enlarged kidneys. Documentation of asymmetric kidney size suggests either a unilateral developmental or urologic abnormality or chronic renovascular disease. In the latter case, a vascular imaging procedure, such as duplex Doppler sonography of the renal arteries, radionuclide scintigraphy, or magnetic resonance angiography should be considered. A computed tomographic scan without contrast may be useful in assessing kidney stone activity, in the appropriate clinical context. Voiding cystourethrography to rule out reflux may be indicated in some younger patients with a history of enuresis or with a family history of reflux. However, in most cases, by the time CRD is established, reflux has resolved; even if present, its repair may not stabilize renal function. In any case, imaging studies should avoid exposure to intravenous radiocontrast dye where possible because of its nephrotoxicity.

Differentiation of CRD from Acute Renal Failure The most classic constellation of laboratory and imaging findings that distinguishes progressive CRD from acute renal failure are bilaterally small (<8.5 cm) kidneys, anemia, hyperphosphatemia and hypocalcemia with elevated PTH levels, and a urinary sediment that is inactive or reveals proteinuria and broad casts. Furthermore, integration of a particular constellation of clinical, laboratory, and imaging findings based on the approach noted above strongly supports a particular presumed underlying etiologic disease process. For example, in a patient with insulin-dependent type 1 diabetes mellitus of 15 to 20 years' duration, diabetic retinopathy, and nephrotic-range albuminuria without hematuria, the diagnosis of diabetic nephropathy is likely. The diagnosis of chronic hypertensive nephrosclerosis (Chap. 278) requires a history of long-standing hypertension, in the absence of evidence for another renal disease process, and hence is usually a diagnosis of exclusion. Usually, proteinuria is mild to moderate (<3 g/d) and the urine sediment inactive. In many cases of presumed hypertensive nephrosclerosis, renovascular disease may not only be the cause of hypertension but also may cause ischemic renal damage. Bilateral renovascular ischemic disease may be a greatly underdiagnosed cause of CRD. This is of therapeutic significance from two points of view: (1) documentation of ischemic renal disease may prompt revascularization therapy in some patients, with occasional dramatic stabilization or improvement in renal function; and (2) renovascular ischemic disease is a contraindication to ACE inhibitor therapy in most cases. Analgesic-associated chronic tubulointerstitial nephropathy is also an underdiagnosed cause of CRD. Imaging studies, including computed tomography, often reveal pathognomonic features such as papillary calcification and necrosis. Under such circumstances, cessation of analgesic exposure may dramatically stabilize renal function.

Kidney Biopsy This procedure should be reserved for patients with near-normal kidney size, in whom a clear-cut diagnosis cannot be made by less invasive means, and when the possibility of a reversible underlying disease process remains tenable so that clarification of the underlying etiology may alter management. The extent of tubulointerstitial scarring on kidney biopsy generally provides the most reliable pathologic correlate indicating prognosis for continued deterioration toward ESRD. Contraindications to renal biopsy include bilateral small kidneys, polycystic kidney disease, uncontrolled hypertension, urinary tract or perinephric infection, bleeding diathesis, respiratory distress, and morbid obesity.

℞ TREATMENT This refers to all of the preventive and therapeutic measures that precede and aim to prevent or postpone ESRD and renal replacement therapy.

Specific Therapy   The optimal time for specific therapy aimed at the underlying disease process is usually well before there has been a measurable decline in baseline GFR, and usually well before CRD is established. When kidney size remains well preserved, renal biopsy results may provide an index of chronicity versus disease activity, which might help in guiding therapeutic decisions. In contrast, by the time CRD is established and GFR has irreversibly declined to less than 20 to 30% of normal, the risks of immunomodulatory and other therapies aimed at treating an underlying past or ongoing disease process may outweigh the benefits.

Superimposed Factors   It is of benefit to follow and plot the rate of decline in GFR in patients with CRD. Any acceleration in the rate of decline should prompt a search for a superimposed acute process. The differential diagnosis should be developed in a systematic manner, as for any patient with acute renal failure (Chap. 269). Particular attention should be directed to factors that more commonly lead to an acute and reversible decline in GFR in patients with CRD. These include superimposed volume depletion, accelerated and uncontrolled hypertension, urinary tract infection, superimposed obstructive uropathy (e.g., due to stone disease, papillary necrosis), nephrotoxic effect of medications (e.g., NSAIDs) and radiocontrast agents, and reactivation or flare of the original underlying etiologic disease process.

Measures to Mitigate Hyperfiltration Injury   The two major therapeutic tools currently available in the mitigation of hyperfiltration injury are: (1) dietary protein restriction, and (2) pharmacologic management of intraglomerular hypertension.

Protein Restriction in CRD   Management guidelines for protein restriction in CRD are shown in the following table. In contrast to fat and carbohydrates, protein in excess of the daily requirement is not stored but is degraded to form urea and other nitrogenous wastes, which are principally excreted by the kidney. In addition, protein-rich foods contain hydrogen ions, PO_4^{3-}, sulfates, and other inorganic ions that are also eliminated by the kidney. Therefore, when patients with CRD consume excessive dietary protein, nitrogenous wastes and inorganic ions accumulate, resulting in the clinical and metabolic disturbances characteristic of uremia. Restricting dietary protein can ameliorate many uremic symptoms and may slow the actual rate of nephron injury. The effectiveness of protein restriction in slowing the progression of CRD has been evaluated in a number of controlled clinical trials. The Modification of Diet in Renal Disease (MDRD) Study was the most extensive trial devoted to this question, but it nevertheless yielded an ambiguous result, although positive trends

Management Guidelines—Dietary Protein Restriction in CRD

GFR, mL/min	Protein, g/kg per d	Phosphorus, g/kg per d
>60	Protein restriction not usually recommended	No restriction
25–60	0.6 g/kg per d including ≥0.35 g/kg per d of HBV	≤10
5–25	0.6 g/kg per d including ≥0.35 g/kg per d of HBV *or*	≤10
	0.3 g/kg per d supplemented with EAA or KA	≤9
<60 (nephrotic syndrome)	0.8 g/kg per d (plus 1 g protein/g proteinuria) *or*	≤12
	0.3 g/kg per d supplemented with EAA or KA (plus 1 g protein/g proteinuria)	≤9

NOTE: GFR, glomerular filtration rate; HBV, high biologic value protein; EAA, essential amino acid supplement; KA, ketoanalogue supplement.

emerged when it ended after an average follow-up of only 2.2 years. In a separate study of patients with insulin-dependent diabetic nephropathy, protein restriction was shown to slow progression significantly in one well-controlled study. Two meta-analyses of studies of the effects of protein restriction on progression concluded that low-protein diets slow progression of both diabetic and nondiabetic renal disease.

It is crucial that protein restriction be carried out in the context of an overall dietary program that optimizes nutritional status and avoids malnutrition, especially as patients near dialysis or transplantation. Measurements of urinary nitrogen appearance, anthropometric and biochemical measurements, as well as dietary consultation are mandatory to preempt malnutrition. Among the most readily available and useful indices of malnutrition are plasma concentrations of albumin (<3.8 g/dL), pre-albumin (<18 mg/dL), and transferrin (<180 µg/dL). Metabolic and nutritional studies indicate that protein requirements for patients with CRD are similar to those for normal adults, approximately 0.6 g/kg per day. However, there is a particular requirement in patients with CRD that the composition of dietary protein be higher in essential amino acids, and that this be combined with an overall energy supply sufficient to mitigate a catabolic state. Energy requirements in the range of 35 kcal/kg per day are recommended.

Fortunately, even patients with advanced CRD are able to activate the same adaptive responses to dietary protein restriction as healthy individuals, i.e., a postprandial suppression of whole-body protein degradation and a marked inhibition of amino acid oxidation. After at least 1 year of therapy with a low-protein diet (range 12 to 24 months) these same adaptive responses persist, indicating that the compensatory responses to dietary protein restriction are sustained during long-term therapy. Further evidence that low-protein diets are safe in CRD patients is provided by the finding that nutritional indices remain normal during long-term therapy.

Pharmacologic management of intraglomerular hypertension   In addition to reduction of cardiovascular disease risk, antihypertensive therapy in patients with CRD also aims to slow the progression of nephron injury by ameliorating intraglomerular hypertension and hypertrophy. Progressive renal injury in CRD appears to be most closely related to the height of intraglomerular pressure and/or the extent of glomerular hypertrophy. The MDRD and other studies demonstrated that control of hypertension is as important as dietary protein restriction in slowing the progression of CRD. Furthermore, the target for pharmacologic therapy was highly dependent on the level of proteinuria. Indeed, proteinuria is now considered a risk factor for progressive nephron injury; the prior level of proteinuria correlates with the subsequent rate of GFR decline. Elevated blood pressure increases proteinuria due to the transmission to the glomeruli of the elevated systemic pressure. Conversely, the protective effect of antihypertensive medications is evident through the curtailment of proteinuria. Thus, the more effective a given treatment is in lowering proteinuria, the greater the subsequent impact on protection from GFR decline.

Some antihypertensive agents, particularly the ACE inhibitors, may be superior to others in affording renal protection. The advantage of this pharmacologic class is thought to relate to salutary modulation of intraglomerular hemodynamics over and above effects on systemic blood pressure. Several well-designed studies have now established favorable outcomes for ACE inhibitors in slowing the progression of diabetic nephropathy. ACE inhibitors have been shown to be more effective than diuretics, beta blockers, and calcium antagonists in reducing urinary albumin excretion in both hypertensive and diabetic patients. Furthermore, these drugs have been shown to facilitate the regression of remodeling more generally in the cardiovascular system and to improve endothelial function in resistance arterioles of humans with hypertension. In nondiabetic CRD, the European AIPRI trial documented a 53% additional reduction in the risk of doubling serum creatinine levels with ACE inhibitor therapy compared to conventional regimens that did not include ACE inhibitors. The reduction in the risk was greater in patients with mild renal insufficiency and in those with proteinuria >1g/d. In a recent meta-analysis, information from all the randomized ACE inhibitor trials in patients with nondiabetic renal disease was combined; the conclusion is that ACE inhibitors are more effective than other antihypertensive agents in reducing the development of ESRD. A similar salutary effect on kidney function as observed with ACE inhibitors has been observed recently with the angiotensin II receptor antagonists, which also possess significant antiproteinuric properties.

Among the calcium channel blockers, diltiazem and verapamil appear to exhibit antiproteinuric and renal protective effects not shared by the dihydropyridines. As a group, these drugs do not adversely affect renal function in patients with nondiabetic renal insufficiency, and they may be more effective in preventing or ameliorating progressive renal injury than some other classes of antihypertensive drugs in this group of patients. Thus, it appears that at least two different categories of responses may exist: one in which progression is strongly associated with systemic and intraglomerular hypertension and with proteinuria (e.g., diabetic nephropathy, glomerular diseases) and in which ACE inhibitors and angiotensin-receptor blockers are likely to be the first choice; and the second in which proteinuria is mild or absent (e.g., adult polycystic kidney disease), probably with a less prominent role for intraglomerular hypertension, and which might respond as well to calcium channel blockers. The level of blood pressure lowering is also of crucial importance in achieving a significant renal protective effect. Clinical practice guidelines are summarized below.

Use of Drugs (See also Chaps. 70 and 71)   Although the loading dose of most drugs is not affected by CRD, maintenance doses of many drugs need to be adjusted. One exception is digoxin, whose volume of distribution is decreased in CRD, mandating a concomitant reduction in the loading dose in addition to adjustment of the maintenance dose. For those drugs in which >70% excretion is by a nonrenal (e.g., hepatic or intestinal) route, dosage adjustment may not be needed. Some drugs that should be entirely avoided include meperidine, metformin, and other oral hypoglycemics with a renal route of elimination. Commonly used medications that require either a reduction in dosage or interval include allopurinol, many antibiotics, several hypertensives, and anti-arrhythmics. For a comprehensive detailed and authoritative listing of the recommended dose adjustment for most of the commonly used medications, the reader is referred to the American College of Physicians handbook of "Drug Prescribing in Renal Failure" (see www.acponline.org).

Preparation for Renal Replacement Therapy   Over the past 35 years, renal replacement therapy using dialysis and transplantation has prolonged the lives of hundreds of thousands of patients with ESRD. Renal replacement therapy should *not* be initiated when the patient is totally asymptomatic; however, dialysis and/or transplantation should be started sufficiently early to prevent serious complications of the uremic state. Clear indications for initiation of renal replacement therapy include pericarditis, progressive neuropathy attributable to uremia, encephalopathy, muscle irritability, anorexia and nausea that is not ameliorated by reasonable protein restriction, and fluid and electrolyte abnormalities that are refractory to conservative measures. The latter include volume overload unresponsive to diuretic therapy, hyperkalemia unresponsive to dietary potassium restriction, and progressive metabolic acidosis that cannot be managed with alkali therapy. Clinical clues indicating the imminent development of uremic complications are a history of hiccoughing, intractable pruritus, morning nausea and vomiting, muscle twitching and cramps, and the presence of asterixis on physical examination. In addition, the patient whose follow-up and compliance with conservative management are questionable should be considered for earlier initiation of renal replacement therapy, lest potentially life-threatening uremic complications or electrolyte disturbances supervene.

The correlation of uremic symptoms with renal function varies from patient to patient depending on the cause of renal disease (earlier onset of symptoms in patients with diabetes mellitus), muscle mass (large, muscular patients tolerate high levels of azotemia), diet, nutritional status, and coexisting conditions. Therefore, it is ill-advised to assign a certain "usual" level of blood urea nitrogen, serum creatinine, or GFR to the need to start dialysis. Nevertheless, in the United States, the Health Care Financing Administration has assigned levels of serum creatinine and creatinine clearance to qualify for reimbursement from Medicare for patients receiving dialysis. Serum creatinine must be ≥ 700 μmol/L (≥ 8.0 mg/dL) and the creatinine clearance must be ≤ 0.17 mL/s (≤ 10 mL/min).

Patient education   Social, psychological, and physical preparation for the transition to renal replacement therapy and choice of the optimal initial modality is best accomplished with a gradual approach involving a multidisciplinary team. While conservative measures are being carried out in patients with CRD, it is important to prepare them with an intensive educational program, explaining the likelihood and timing of initiation of renal replacement therapy and the various forms of therapy available. The more knowledgeable patients are concerning hemodialysis, peritoneal dialysis, and transplantation, the easier and more appropriate will be their decisions at a later time. Exploration of social service support resources is of great importance. In those who may perform home dialysis or undergo transplantation, early education of family members for selection and preparation as a home dialysis helper or a related donor for transplantation should occur long before the onset of symptomatic renal failure.

Selection of patients to be treated with various modalities of dialysis or transplantation is a matter of some debate, with considerable variation in different parts of the world. In general, in the United States and some other countries, nearly all patients who have reached ESRD are accepted for dialysis if they or their families desire prolongation of life, irrespective of age.

In terms of dialysis treatment modalities (Chap. 271), large multicenter studies have not shown a consistent or convincing advantage in terms of morbidity or mortality, of one modality over another.

Only kidney transplantation (Chap. 272) offers the potential for nearly complete rehabilitation. This is because dialysis techniques replace only 10 to 15% of normal kidney function at the level of small-solute removal and are even less efficient at the removal of larger solutes. Generally, kidney transplantation follows a prior period of dialysis treatment. All patients in whom an acute reversible component of renal failure has not been completely excluded should be supported with dialysis first, at least for some period of time, to allow for possible return of renal function before consideration of transplantation. Recovery of endogenous renal function in patients treated with dialysis for more than 6 months is a rare occurrence. Usually these are patients in whom the underlying disease process has been acute or subacute—such as one of the thrombotic microangiopathies, rapidly progressive glomerulonephritis, or obstructive uropathy. Patients approaching ESRD in whom a reversible component has been excluded, and who

---

Management Guidelines for BP Control in CRD

• Target BP in CRD	130/80–85 mmHg
• With proteinuria (>1 g/d)	125/75 mmHg (MAP 92 mmHg)
• Recommended medications	• Diuretics to achieve normovolemia
	• In diabetic nephropathy or CRD with proteinuria—ACE inhibitor or angiotensin receptor antagonists alone or in combination with diuretic.
	• In other causes of CRD, calcium entry blocker alpha and beta blockers considered as alternatives

NOTE: MAP, mean arterial pressure.

have a good antigenic match with a willing donor, may occasionally be considered for primary transplantation without intervening dialysis.

ACKNOWLEDGMENT

Dr. J. Michael Lazarus was a co-author of this chapter in the 14th edition, and some of the material in that chapter is carried forward to the present edition.

BIBLIOGRAPHY

ARONOFF GR et al: *Drug Prescribing in Renal Failure,* 4th ed. American College of Physicians, 1999

BAILIE GR et al: Parenteral iron use in the management of anemia in end-stage renal disease patients. Am J Kid Dis 35:1, 2000

BURTON C, HARRIS KP: The role of proteinuria in the progression of chronic renal failure. Am J Kidney Dis 27:765, 1996

BUSHINSKY DA: The contribution of acidosis to renal osteodystrophy. Kidney Int 47: 1816, 1995

HAKIM RM, LAZARUS JM: Initiation of dialysis. J Am Soc Nephrol 6:1319, 1995

LEVEY AS et al: A more accurate method to estimate glomerular filtration rate from serum creatinine: A new prediction equation. Ann Intern Med 130:461, 1999

LEWIS EJ et al: The effect of angiotensin-converting-enzyme inhibition on diabetic nephropathy. N Engl J Med 329:1456, 1993

MASCHIO G et al: Effect of the ACE inhibitor benazepril on the progression of chronic renal insufficiency. N Engl J Med 334:939, 1996

PEDRINI MT et al: The effect of dietary protein restriction on the progression of diabetic and nondiabetic renal diseases: A meta-analysis. Ann Intern Med 124:627, 1996

TOTO RD et al: "Strict" blood pressure control and progression of renal disease in hypertensive nephrosclerosis. Kidney Int 48:851, 1995

WALSER M et al: Should protein intake be restricted in predialysis patients? Kidney Int 55:771, 1999

271

Ajay K. Singh, Barry M. Brenner

DIALYSIS IN THE TREATMENT OF RENAL FAILURE

With the widespread availability of dialysis, the lives of hundreds of thousands of patients with end-stage renal disease (ESRD) have been prolonged. In the United States alone, there are now approximately 300,000 patients with ESRD. The overall incidence of ESRD is 242 cases per million population per year. The incident population of patients with ESRD is increasing at approximately 8% each year. The incidence of ESRD is disproportionately higher in African Americans (758 per million population per year) as compared with white Americans (180 per million population per year). In the United States, the leading cause of ESRD is diabetes mellitus, accounting for more than 40% of newly diagnosed cases of ESRD. The second most common cause is hypertension, which is estimated to cause 30% of ESRD cases. Other causes of ESRD include glomerulonephritis, polycystic kidney disease, and obstructive uropathy.

Dialysis care in the United States is funded through the Medicare End-Stage Renal Dialysis program; the cost was approximately $13.5 billion in 1997. Although the total program expense has increased dramatically, the cost for treating individual patients in inflation-adjusted terms has gone down. In addition, quality and outcomes have improved through better management of dialysis dose, improved nutrition, management of anemia, and control of hypertension. The cost of dialysis, which ranges from $45,000 to $65,000 per year, has been demonstrated to vary according to the presence or absence of diabetes mellitus and whether the treatment modality is hemodialysis or peritoneal dialysis. The mortality of patients with ESRD is lowest in Europe and Japan but is very high in the developing world because of the limited availability of dialysis. In the United States, the mortality rate of patients on dialysis is approximately 18% per year. Deaths are due mainly to cardiovascular diseases and infections (approximately 50% and 15% of deaths, respectively).

TREATMENT OPTIONS FOR ESRD PATIENTS

Commonly accepted criteria for putting patients on dialysis include: the presence of the uremic syndrome; the presence of hyperkalemia unresponsive to conservative measures; extracellular volume expansion; acidosis refractory to medical therapy; a bleeding diathesis; and a creatinine clearance of <10 cc/min per $1.73m^2$. There is emerging consensus that patients with ESRD should be started on dialysis early. Although vigorous protein restriction can maintain the blood urea nitrogen at an acceptable level in these patients, it may come at the price of significant malnutrition, which in turn correlates with mortality on dialysis. In addition to carefully evaluating patients for the onset of uremia (Chap. 270), regular measurement of renal function is important.

Renal function can be assessed by measurement of serum creatinine and blood urea nitrogen or of creatinine and urea clearance, or the direct measurement of glomerular filtration rate (GFR) using a radioisotope such as iothalamate. Creatinine clearance usually over-estimates glomerular filtration rate because a substantial fraction of creatinine excretion in advanced renal failure occurs as a consequence of proximal tubular secretion. On the other hand, urea clearance invariably underestimates GFR because urea is reabsorbed in the distal nephron. Thus, when measurement of GFR by a direct test is not available, the average of the sum of the creatinine and urea clearance, or a cimetidine-blocked creatinine clearance (cimetidine blocks proximal tubular secretion), is recommended. Early referral to a nephrologist for advanced planning and creation of a dialysis access, education about ESRD treatment options, and the aggressive management of the complications of chronic renal failure, including acidosis, anemia, and hyperparathyroidism, are important.

The treatment options available for patients with renal failure depend on whether it is acute or chronic (Fig. 271-1). In acute renal failure, treatments include hemodialysis, continuous renal replacement therapies (see p. 1565), and peritoneal dialysis. In chronic renal failure (ESRD) the options include hemodialysis (in center or at home); peritoneal dialysis, either as continuous ambulatory peritoneal dialysis (CAPD) or continuous cyclic peritoneal dialysis (CCPD); or transplantation (Chap. 272). Although there are geographic variations, hemodialysis remains the most common therapeutic modality for ESRD (>80% of patients in the United States). The choice between hemodialysis and peritoneal dialysis involves the interplay of various factors that include the patient's age, the presence of comorbid conditions, the ability to perform the procedure, and the patient's own conceptions

FIGURE 271-1 Factors in the development of the uremic syndrome and considerations in its treatment.

about the therapy. Peritoneal dialysis is favored in younger patients because of their better manual dexterity and greater visual acuity, and because younger patients prefer the independence and flexibility of home-based peritoneal dialysis treatment. In contrast, larger patients (>80 kg), patients with no residual renal function, and patients who have truncal obesity with or without prior abdominal surgery are more suited to hemodialysis. Larger patients with no residual renal function are more appropriate for hemodialysis because these patients have a large volume of distribution of urea and require significantly higher amounts of peritoneal dialysis, which may be difficult to achieve because of the limited willingness of patients to perform more than four exchanges each day. In some patients, the inability to obtain vascular access predicates a switch from hemodialysis to peritoneal dialysis.

HEMODIALYSIS

This consists of diffusion that occurs bi-directionally across a semipermeable membrane. Movement of metabolic waste products takes place down a concentration gradient from the circulation into the dialysate, and in the reverse direction. The rate of diffusive transport increases in response to several factors, including the magnitude of the concentration gradient, the membrane surface area, and the mass transfer coefficient of the membrane. The latter is a function of the porosity and thickness of the membrane, the size of the solute molecule, and the conditions of flow on the two sides of the membrane. According to the laws of diffusion, the larger the molecule, the slower its rate of transfer across the membrane. A small molecule such as urea (60 Da) undergoes substantial clearance, whereas a larger molecule such as creatinine (113 Da), is cleared much less efficiently. In addition to diffusive clearance, movement of toxic materials such as urea from the circulation into the dialysate may occur as a result of ultrafiltration. Convective clearance occurs because of solvent drag

with solutes getting swept along with water across the semipermeable dialysis membrane.

THE DIALYZER There are three essential components to dialysis: the dialyzer, the composition and delivery of the dialysate, and the blood delivery system (Fig. 271-2). The dialyzer consists of a plastic device with the facility to perfuse blood and dialysate compartments at very high flow rates. The surface area of dialysis membranes in adult patients is usually in the range of 0.8 to 1.2 m².

There are currently two geometric configurations for dialyzers: hollow fiber and flat plate. The hollow fiber dialyzer is the most common in use in the United States. These dialyzers are composed of bundles of capillary tubes through which blood circulates while dialysate travels on the outside of the fiber bundle. In contrast, the less frequently utilized flat plate dialyzers are composed of sandwiched sheets of membrane in a parallel plate configuration. The advantage of the hollow fiber construction is the lower priming volume (60 to 90 mL vs 100 to 120 mL for the flat plate) and easier reprocessing of the filter for reuse in future dialysis treatments.

Recent advances have led to the development of many different types of membrane material. Broadly, there are four categories of dialysis membranes: cellulose, substituted cellulose, cellulosynthetic, and synthetic. Over the past two decades, there has been a gradual switch from cellulose-derived to synthetic membranes, because the latter are more biocompatible. Bioincompatibility may be defined as the ability of the membrane to activate the complement cascade. Cellulosic membranes are bioincompatible because of the presence of free hydroxyl groups on the membrane surface. In contrast, with the substituted cellulose membranes (e.g., cellulose acetate) or the cellulosynthetic membranes, the hydroxyl groups are chemically bonded to either acetate or tertiary amino groups, resulting in limited complement

FIGURE 271-2 Schema for hemodialysis.

activation. Synthetic membranes, such as polysulfone, polymethyl-methacrylate, and polyacrylonitrile membranes are more biocompatible because of the absence of these hydroxyl groups. Polysulfone membranes are now used in over 60% of the dialysis treatments in the United States.

Reprocessing and reuse of hemodialyzers is employed for patients on chronic hemodialysis in nearly 80% of dialysis centers in the United States, in large part because of the expense of individual dialyzers. Evidence also suggests that reuse reduces complement activation, the incidence of anaphylactoid reactions to the membrane (first-use syndrome), and, in some studies, mortality rates among dialysis patients. In most centers, only the dialyzer unit is reprocessed and reused, whereas in the developing world blood lines are also frequently reused. The reprocessing procedure can be either manual or automated. It consists of the sequential rinsing of the blood and dialysate compartments with water, a chemical cleansing step with reverse ultrafiltration from the dialysate to the blood compartment, the testing of the patency of the dialyzer, and, finally, disinfection of the dialyzer. Formaldehyde, peracetic acid–hydrogen peroxide, and glutaraldehyde are the most frequently used reprocessing agents, with peracetic acid–hydrogen peroxide being the most common.

DIALYSATE   The composition of dialysate is listed in Table 271-1. Bicarbonate has replaced acetate as the preferred buffer in the United States. This change has resulted in fewer episodes of hypotension during dialysis. The potassium concentration of dialysate may be varied from 0 to 4 mmol/L depending on the predialysis plasma potassium concentration. The usual dialysate calcium concentration is 1.25 mmol/L (2.5 meq/L). The usual dialysate sodium concentration is 140 mmol/L. Lower dialysate sodium concentrations are associated with a higher frequency of hypotension, cramping, nausea, vomiting, fatigue, and dizziness. In patients who frequently develop hypotension during their dialysis run, sodium modeling to counterbalance urea-related osmolar gradients is now widely used. In this technique, the dialysate sodium concentration is gradually lowered from the range of 148 to 160 meq/L to isotonic levels (140 meq/L) near the end of the dialysis treatment. A dialysate glucose concentration of 200 mg/dL (11 mmol/L) is used to optimize blood glucose concentrations. Because patients are exposed to approximately 120 L of water during each dialysis treatment, untreated water could expose them to a variety of environmental contaminants. Therefore, in 98% of U.S. dialysis centers, water used for the dialysate is subjected to filtration, softening, deionization, and, ultimately, reverse osmosis. During the reverse osmosis process, water is forced through a semipermeable membrane at very high pressure to remove microbiologic contaminants and more than 90% of dissolved ions.

BLOOD DELIVERY SYSTEM   This is composed of the extracorporeal circuit in the dialysis machine and the dialysis access. The dialysis machine consists of a blood pump, dialysis solution delivery system, and various safety monitors. The blood pump, using a roller mechanism, moves blood from the access site, through the dialyzer, and back to the patient. The blood flow rate may range from 250 to 500 mL/min. Negative hydrostatic pressure on the dialysate side can be manipulated to achieve desirable fluid removal, so-called *ultrafil-*

Table 271-1   Composition of Commercial Dialysate for Hemodialysate

Solute	Bicarbonate Dialysate
Sodium (meq/L)	137–143
Potassium (meq/L)	0–4.0
Chloride (meq/L)	100–111
Calcium (meq/L)	0–3.5
Magnesium (meq/L)	0.75–1.5
Acetate (meq/L)	2.0–4.5
Bicarbonate (meq/L)	30–35
Glucose (mg/dL)	0–0.25

tration. Dialysis membranes have different ultrafiltration coefficients (i.e., mL removed/min per mmHg) so that along with hydrostatic changes, fluid removal can be varied. The dialysis solution delivery system dilutes the dialysate concentrate with water, and monitors the temperature, conductivity, and flow of dialysate. The dialysate may be delivered to the dialyzer from a storage tank or a proportioning system that manufactures dialysate online.

Dialysis Access   The fistula, graft, or catheter through which blood is obtained for hemodialysis is often referred to as a *dialysis access.* A native fistula created by the anastomosis of an artery to a vein (e.g., the Cimino-Breschia fistula, in which the cephalic vein is anastomosed to the radial artery) results in arterialization of the vein. This faciliates its subsequent use in the placement of large needles (typically 15 gauge) to access the circulation. Although fistulas have a high patency rate (approximately 80% are patent at 3 years following creation), fistulas are created in only approximately 30% of patients in the United States. In the majority of U.S. dialysis patients, the dialysis access consists of an arteriovenous graft which interposes prosthetic material, such as polytetrafluoroethylene, between an artery and a vein. Such grafts have a 3-year patency rate of only 20%. Reasons for the higher rates of graft placement include the late referral of patients to vascular access surgeons so that by the time surgery is planned, the patient's arm veins have already been obliterated through multiple blood draws; the high prevalence of patients with diabetes mellitus and its associated microvascular disease; and the greater surgical skill required in creating a fistula. The most common access-related complication is thrombosis due to intimal hyperplasia, which results in stenosis proximal to the venous anastomosis.

A double lumen cuffed catheter may be a reasonable alternative to either a native arteriovenous fistula or a graft in selected patients in whom dialysis is required relatively urgently, such as patients who manifest delayed recovery from acute renal failure, or where a further permanent access procedure (e.g., arteriovenous fistula or arteriovenous graft) is not feasible for anatomic reasons. Although double lumen catheters may permit blood flows comparable to a permanent arteriovenous access, these catheters are prone to infection and to occlusion because of thrombosis. Temporary double lumen catheters in either the femoral vein or the internal jugular or subclavian vein are usually employed in patients with acute renal failure. The jugular is preferred to the subclavian vein because, for unclear reasons, a catheter placed in a subclavian vein appears to be associated with a higher rate of venous stenosis. Temporary access can be used for 2 to 3 weeks. Thrombosis, low blood flow, and infection limit the life of the catheter.

GOALS OF DIALYSIS   The hemodialysis procedure is targeted at removing both small and large molecular weight solutes. The procedure consists of pumping heparinized blood through the dialyzer at a flow rate of 300 to 500 mL/min, while dialysate flows in an opposite *counter-current* direction at 500 to 800 mL/min. The clearance of urea ranges from 200 to 350 mL/min, while the clearance of β_2 microglobulin is more modest and ranges from 20 to 25 mL/min. The efficiency of dialysis is determined by blood and dialysate flow through the dialyzer, as well as dialyzer characteristics (i.e., its efficiency in removing solute). The *dose* of dialysis, which is defined as the magnitude of urea clearance during a single dialysis treatment, is further governed by patient size, residual renal function, dietary protein intake, the degree of anabolism or catabolism, and the presence of comorbid conditions. Since the landmark studies of Sargent and Gatch relating the measurement of the dose of dialysis using urea concentration with patient outcome, the *delivered* dose of dialysis has been correlated with morbidity and mortality. This has led to the development of two major models for assessing the adequacy of the dialysis dose. Fundamentally, these two widely used measures of the adequacy of dialysis are calculated from the decrease in the blood urea nitrogen concentration during the dialysis treatment—that is, the urea reduction ratio (URR), and *KT/V*, an index based on the urea clearance rate, *K*, and the size of the urea pool, represented as the urea distribution volume, V. K, which is the sum of clearance by the dialyzer plus renal clearance, is multiplied by the time spent on dialysis, T. Increasingly, KT/V has become the preferred marker for dialysis adequacy. Currently, a URR of 65% and a KT/V of 1.2 per treatment are minimal standards for adequacy; lower levels of dialysis treatment are associated with increased morbidity and mortality.

For the majority of patients with chronic renal failure, between 9 and 12 h of dialysis is required each week, usually divided into three equal sessions. However, the dialysis dose must be individualized. The measurement of dialysis adequacy using KT/V or the URR serve only as a guide; body size, residual renal function, dietary intake, complicating illness, degree of anabolism or catabolism, and the presence of large interdialytic fluid gains are important factors in consideration of the dialysis prescription.

COMPLICATIONS DURING HEMODIALYSIS Hypotension is the most common acute complication of hemodialysis. Numerous factors appear to increase the risk of hypotension, including excessive ultrafiltration with inadequate compensatory vascular filling, impaired vasoactive or autonomic responses, osmolar shifts, food ingestion, impaired cardiac reserve, the use of antihypertensive drugs, and vasodilation due to the use of warm dialysate. Because of the vasodilatory and cardiodepressive effects of acetate, the use of acetate as the buffer in dialysate was once a common cause of hypotension. Since the introduction of bicarbonate-containing dialysate, dialysis-associated hypotension has become common. The management of hypotension during dialysis consists of discontinuing ultrafiltration, the administration of 100 to 250 cc of isotonic saline, and, in patients with hypoalbuminemia, administration of salt-poor albumin. Hypotension during dialysis can frequently be prevented by careful evaluation of the dry weight, holding of antihypertensive medications on the day prior to and on the day of dialysis, and avoiding heavy meals during dialysis. Additional maneuvers include the performance of sequential ultrafiltration followed by dialysis and cooling of the dialysate during dialysis treatment.

Muscle cramps during dialysis are also a common complication of the procedure. However, since the introduction of volumetric controls on dialysis machines and sodium modelling, the incidence of cramps has fallen. The etiology of dialysis-associated cramps remains obscure. Changes in muscle perfusion because of excessively aggressive volume removal, particularly below the estimated dry weight and the use of low sodium containing dialysate, have been proposed as precipitants of dialysis-associated cramps. Strategies that may be used to prevent cramps include reducing volume removal during dialysis, the use of higher concentrations of sodium in the dialysate, and the use of quinine sulfate (260 mg 2 h before treatment).

Anaphylactoid reactions to the dialyzer, particularly on its first use, have been reported most frequently with the bioincompatible cellulosic-containing membranes. With the gradual phasing out of cuprophane membranes in the United States, the first use syndrome has become relatively uncommon. The first use syndrome consists of either an intermediate hypersensitivity reaction due to an IgE mediated reaction to ethylene oxide used in the sterilization of new dialyzers, or a symptom complex of nonspecific chest and back pain, which appears to result from complement activation and cytokine release.

The major cause of death in patients with ESRD receiving chronic dialysis is cardiovascular disease. The rate of death from cardiac disease is higher in patients on hemodialysis as compared to patients on peritoneal dialysis and renal transplantation. The underlying cause of cardiovascular disease is unclear but may be related to the inadequate treatment of hypertension; the presence of hyperlipidemia, homocystinemia and anemia; the calcification of coronary arteries in patients with an elevated calcium-phosphorus product; and perhaps alterations in cardiovascular dynamics during the dialysis treatment. Intensive investigation of the mechanisms and potential interventions that could impact on reducing the mortality from cardiovascular causes is currently underway.

CONTINUOUS RENAL REPLACEMENT THERAPY

Continuous renal replacement therapies (CRRT) have become increasingly prevalent in the intensive care unit setting for management of acute renal failure. The advantages of CRRT over intermittent hemodialysis are that it is usually better tolerated hemodynamically; it facilitates gradual correction of biochemical abnormalities; it is highly effective in removing fluid; and it is technically simple to perform. Clearance of toxic materials (using urea as the marker) can occur with CRRT from convective clearance alone if the ultrafiltration rate is high and with diffusive clearance if dialysis accompanies ultrafiltration. CRRT techniques include continuous arteriovenous hemodiafiltration (CAVH/D) with or without dialysis, and continuous veno-venous hemodiafiltration (CVVH/D) with or without dialysis. Veno-venous therapies differ fundamentally from arteriovenous therapies in that veno-venous therapies do not require arterial access. This allows obtaining less risky and easier vascular access. However, because there is no systemic arterial pressure to drive hemofiltration, veno-venous therapies require a blood pump in the extracorporeal circuit. Veno-venous therapies such as CVVH provide substantial flexibility because changing the blood flow rate in the pump can change the ultrafiltration and clearance rates. In contrast, arterio-venous therapies such as CAVH are associated with variable efficiency because the systemic blood pressure is frequently low or unstable in patients with acute renal failure. Furthermore, low blood flow with CAVH may also result in clotting of the extracorporeal circuit. CAVH often results in clearance rates as low as 10 to 15 mL/min, whereas CVVH may generate clearances in the range of 30 to 40 mL/min. Thus, in light of these advantages of CVVH, many centers have completely switched from arteriovenous to veno-venous therapies in patients with acute renal failure in the ICU setting.

Vascular access in patients on CVVH is usually achieved by the insertion of a double-lumen catheter into the femoral vein. The blood pump is typically set to deliver approximately 150 to 180 mL/min. In automated systems, (e.g., the Cobe Prisma system), the treatment is volumetrically governed by continuously weighing the effluent and replacement solutions and using a servomechanism to drive the replacement fluid pump at a rate computed either to balance the inflow and loss of fluid or to maintain a predetermined rate of fluid loss. Anticoagulation of the extracorporeal circuit is via a heparin infusion (200 to 1600 U/h) through the inflow side of the circuit. Alternatively, citrate can be used to chelate calcium in the extracorporeal circuit to provide regional anticoagulation in selected patients who cannot undergo systemic heparinization. The replacement solution in continuous therapies is designed specifically to replace calcium, magnesium, and bicarbonate. In place of bicarbonate, lactate or citrate is the buffer in the replacement solution. However, bicarbonate-based replacement fluid is the preferred option in patients with liver failure because of the impaired ability of the liver to metabolize either lactate or acetate into bicarbonate.

PERITONEAL DIALYSIS

This consists of infusing 1 to 3 L of a dextrose-containing solution into the peritoneal cavity and allowing the fluid to dwell for 2 to 4 h. As with hemodialysis, toxic materials are removed through a combination of convective clearance generated through ultrafiltration, and diffusive clearance down a concentration gradient. The clearance of solute and water during a peritoneal dialysis exchange depends on the balance between the movement of solute and water into the peritoneal cavity versus absorption from the peritoneal cavity. The rate of diffusion diminishes with time and eventually stops when equilibration between plasma and dialysate is reached. Absorption of solutes and water from the peritoneal cavity occurs across the peritoneal membrane into the peritoneal capillary circulation and via peritoneal lymphatics into the lymphatic circulation. The rate of peritoneal solute transport varies from patient to patient and may be altered by the presence of infection (peritonitis), drugs such as beta blockers and calcium channel blockers, and by physical factors such as position and exercise.

FORMS OF PERITONEAL DIALYSIS Peritoneal dialysis may be carried out as continuous ambulatory peritoneal dialysis (CAPD), continuous cyclic peritoneal dialysis (CCPD), or nocturnal intermittent peritoneal dialysis (NIPD). In CAPD, dialysis solution is manually infused into the peritoneal cavity during the day and exchanged 3 to 4 times daily. A nighttime dwell is frequently instilled at bedtime and remains in the peritoneal cavity through the night. The drainage of spent dialysate (effluence) is performed manually with the assistance of gravity to move fluid out of the abdomen. In CCPD, exchanges are performed in an automated fashion, usually at night; the patient is connected to the automated cycler, which then performs 4 to 5 exchange cycles while the patient sleeps. Peritoneal dialysis cyclers automatically cycle dialysate in and out of the abdominal cavity. In the morning the patient, with the last exchange remaining in the abdomen, is disconnected from the cycler and goes about his regular daily activities. In NIPD, the patient is given approximately 10 h of cycling each night, with the abdomen left dry during the day.

Peritoneal dialysis solutions are available in various volumes ranging from 0.5 to 3.0 L. The electrolyte composition is shown in Table 271-2. Lactate is the preferred buffer in peritoneal dialysis solutions. Acetate in peritoneal dialysis solutions appears to accelerate peritoneal sclerosis, whereas use of bicarbonte results in precipitation of calcium and caramelization of glucose. The most common additives to peritoneal dialysis solutions are heparin and antibiotics during an episode of acute peritonitis. Insulin may also be added in patients with diabetes mellitus.

ACCESS TO THE PERITONEAL CAVITY This is obtained through a peritoneal catheter. These are either *acute* catheters, used to perform acute continuous peritoneal dialysis, usually in an emergency setting, or *chronic* catheters, which have either one or two Dacron cuffs and are tunneled under the skin into the peritoneal cavity. An acute catheter consists of a straight or slightly curved rigid tube with several holes at its distal end. Catheters can be inserted at the bedside by making a small incision in the anterior abdominal wall; the catheter is inserted with the assistance of a guidewire or stylet. Acute catheters are anchored externally with adhesives or sutures and are usually reserved for temporary use because of the risk of infection, which increases after 72 h of use. In contrast, chronic catheters are flexible and made of silicon rubber with numerous side holes at the distal end. These chronic catheters usually have two Dacron cuffs to promote fibroblast proliferation, granulation and invasion of the cuff. The scarring that occurs around the cuffs anchors the catheter and seals it from bacteria tracking from the skin surface into the peritoneal cavity; it also prevents the external leakage of fluid from the peritoneal cavity. The cuffs are placed in the preperitoneal plane and approximately 2 cm from the skin surface. The most common chronic peritoneal dialysis catheter in use is the Tenckhoff catheter, which contains two cuffs.

Table 271-2 Composition of Peritoneal Dialysate

Solute	Dianeal (PD-2)
Sodium (meq/L)	132
Potassium (meq/L)	0
Chloride (meq/L)	96
Calcium (meq/L)	3.5
Magnesium (meq/L)	0.5
D,L-Lactate (meq/L)	40
Glucose (g%)	
1.5	
2.5	
4.25	
pH	5.2

The initial CAPD prescription consists of the infusion of a 2-L volume of a 1.5% dextrose concentration peritoneal dialysis solution into the peritoneal cavity over 10 min and allowing it to dwell for 2.5 h. The effluent solution is then drained over 20 min before the next exchange. Three daytime exchanges are accompanied by a 2 L nighttime dwell as the standard prescription. Because peritoneal membrane characteristics vary from one individual to another, the peritoneal equilibrium test should be employed within 2 months of a patient initiating peritoneal dialysis. This test measures the peritoneal membrane transfer rate for solutes (usually urea and creatinine) based on the ratio of their concentration in dialysate and plasma at specific times during the dialysate dwell. It allows patients to be classified as low, low–average, high–average, and high transporters. Approximately 10 to 17% of patients are high transporters, 50% high–average transporters, 25 to 30% low–average transporters, and 1 to 5% low transporters. Identifying the high transporters early is important, since these patients not only demonstrate excellent solute removal, they also absorb glucose rapidly; maximum ultrafiltration occurs early in the dwell, followed by reabsorption of water back into the circulation over the course of the dwell. Such patients benefit from either NIPD or CAPD without a nighttime dwell.

The dose of peritoneal dialysis required to provide adequate or optimal dialysis as measured by patient outcomes is not known. However, there is emerging consensus that the weekly KT/V should be >2.0 and the creatinine clearance >65 L/week per 1.73 m². The most frequently utilized approach to calculating a weekly KT/V and creatinine clearance is by collecting the spent dialysate and urine over a 24-h period. The peritoneal dialysis prescription can be tailored to improve suboptimal clearance values by either increasing the volume of individual exchanges, increasing the number of exchanges, or by combining the CAPD and CCPD techniques. In combining these techniques, the CAPD patient hooks up to a cycler at night and the machine automatically performs one or two nocturnal exchanges, whereas the CCPD patient makes an additional manual daytime exchange.

ACKNOWLEDGMENT

Dr. J. Michael Lazarus was a co-author of this chapter in the 14th edition; some of his material has been carried forward to the present edition.

BIBLIOGRAPHY

BRENNER BM (ed): *Brenner and Rector's The Kidney*, 6th ed. Philadelphia, Saunders, 2000

BURKART JM: Peritoneal dialysis, in *Brenner and Rector's The Kidney*, 6th ed, BM Brenner (ed). Philadelphia, Saunders, 2000

DENKER BM et al: Hemodialysis, in *Brenner and Rector's The Kidney*, 6th ed, BM Brenner (ed). Philadelphia, Saunders, 2000

DEPNER TA: *Prescribing Hemodialysis: A Guide to Urea Modeling*. Boston, Kluwer Academic, 1991

DIAZ-BUXO JA: Early referral and selection of peritoneal dialysis as a treatment modality. Nephrol Dialy Transplant 15:147, 2000

GOTCH FA, SARGENT JA: A mechanistic analysis of the National Cooperative Dialysis Study (NCDS). Kidney Int 28:526, 1985

HAKIM RM: Clinical implications of hemodialysis membrane bioincompatibility. Kidney Int 44:484, 1993

FORNI LG, HILTON PJ: Current concepts: Continuous hemofiltration in the treatment of acute renal failure. N Engl J Med 336:1303, 1997

KESHAVIAH P: Technology and clinical application of hemodialysis, in *The Principles and Practice of Nephrology*, HR Jacobson et al (eds). St. Louis, Mosby-Year Book, 1995

MEYER MM: Renal replacement therapies. Crit Care Clin 16:29, 2000

PASTAN S, BAILEY J: Dialysis therapy. N Engl J Med 338:1428, 1998

RENAL DATA SYSTEM: USRDS 1997 annual data report. Bethesda, MD, National Institutes of Diabetes and Digestive and Kidney Disease, 1997

SANG GL et al: Sodium ramping in hemodialysis: A study of beneficial and adverse effect. Am J Kidney Dis 29:669 1997

SHULMAN G, JAKIM RM: Complications of hemodialysis, *The Principles and Practice of Nephrology*, HR Jacobson et al (eds.). St. Louis, Mosby-Year Book, p 673, 1995

TASK FORCE ON REUSE OF DIALYZERS, COUNCIL ON DIALYSIS, NATIONAL KIDNEY FOUNDATION: National Kidney Foundation report on dialyzer reuse. Am J Kidney Dis 30:859, 1997

272 | *Charles B. Carpenter, Edgar L. Milford, Mohamed H. Sayegh*

TRANSPLANTATION IN THE TREATMENT OF RENAL FAILURE

Transplantation of the human kidney is frequently the most effective treatment of advanced chronic renal failure. Worldwide, tens of thousands of such procedures have been performed. When azathioprine and prednisone were initially used as immunosuppressive drugs in the 1960s, the results with properly matched familial donors were superior to those with organs from cadaveric donors, namely, 75 to 90% compared with 50 to 60% graft survival rates at 1 year. During the 1970s and 1980s, the success rate at the 1-year mark for cadaveric transplants rose progressively. By the time cyclosporine was introduced in the early 1980s, cadaveric donor grafts had a 70% 1-year survival and reached the 80 to 85% level in the mid 1990s (Fig. 272-1). After the first year, graft survival curves show an exponential decline in numbers of functioning grafts from which a half-life $(t_{1/2})$ in years is calculated (Fig. 272-1). Mortality rates after transplantation are highest in the first year and are age-related: 2% for ages 6 to 45 years, 7% for ages 46 to 60 years, and 10% for ages over 60 years, and lower thereafter. These rates compare favorably to those in the chronic dialysis population, even after risk adjustments for age, diabetes, and cardiovascular status. Occasionally, acute irreversible rejection may occur after many months of good function, especially if the patient neglects to take the immunosuppressive drugs. Most grafts, however, succumb at varying rates to a chronic vascular and interstitial obliterative process termed *chronic rejection*, although its pathogenesis is incompletely understood. Overall, transplantation returns the majority of patients to an improved life-style and an improved life expectancy, as compared to patients on dialysis; however, careful prospective cohort studies have yet to be reported.

RECIPIENT SELECTION Transplantation should be undertaken only when there is a state of irreversible renal failure. When a living donor is available, a period of chronic dialysis may be avoided. When end-stage renal disease is the result of diabetes mellitus, there is special merit in having a transplant before it is necessary to initiate maintenance dialysis in order to minimize progression of cardiovascular complications of diabetes, which are frequently accelerated during chronic dialysis. In patients who must wait for a cadaveric donor kidney, a dialysis program must be established since the waiting time will be in the 3 to 4 year range for most patients. Each candidate must have a careful risk/benefit evaluation. Elderly patients over age 70, patients with metastatic malignancy, or those with advanced cardiopulmonary disease are generally poor operative risks and are also more susceptible to infections in the setting of immunosuppressive medications. Coronary artery revascularization may be indicated in select patients prior to transplantation. Because of the growing shortage of available cadaveric organs in relation to the expanding chronic dialysis population, patients who do not have a life expectancy of at least 5 years are generally not placed on the national waiting list in the United States.

DONOR SELECTION Donors can be cadavers or volunteer living donors. The latter are usually family members selected to have at least partial compatibility for HLA antigens. Living volunteer donors should be normal on physical examination and of the same major ABO blood group, because crossing major blood group barriers prejudices survival of the allograft. It is possible, however, to transplant a kidney of a type O donor into an A, B, or AB recipient. Selective renal arteriography should be performed on donors to rule out the presence of multiple or abnormal renal arteries, because the surgical procedure is difficult and the ischemic time of the transplanted kidney long when vascular abnormalities exist. Cadaveric donors should be free of malignant neoplastic disease, hepatitis, and HIV because of possible transmission to the recipient. Increased risk of graft failure exists when the donor is elderly or has renal failure and when the kidney has a prolonged period of ischemia and storage.

In the United States, there is a coordinated national system (United Network for Organ Sharing) of regulations, allocation support, and outcomes analysis for kidney transplantation. It is now possible to remove cadaver kidneys and to maintain them for up to 48 h on cold pulsatile perfusion or simple flushing and cooling. This permits adequate time for typing, cross-matching, transportation, and selection problems to be solved.

TISSUE TYPING AND CLINICAL IMMUNOGENETICS Matching for antigens of the HLA major histocompatibility gene complex (Chap. 306) is an important criterion for selection of donors for renal allografts. Each mammalian species has a single chromosomal region that encodes the strong, or major, transplantation antigens, and this region on the human sixth chromosome is called *HLA*. HLA antigens have been classically defined by serologic techniques, but methods to define specific nucleotide sequences in genomic DNA are increasingly being used. Other antigens, called "minor," may nevertheless play crucial roles, in addition to the ABH(O) blood groups and endothelial antigens that are not shared with lymphocytes. The Rh system is not expressed on graft tissue. Evidence for designation of HLA as the genetic region encoding major transplantation antigens comes from the success rate in living related donor renal and bone marrow transplantation, with superior results in HLA-identical sibling pairs. Nevertheless, 5% of HLA-identical renal allografts are rejected, often within the first weeks after transplantation. These failures represent states of prior sensitization to non-HLA antigens. Non-HLA antigens are relatively weak when initially encountered and are therefore suppressible by conventional immunosuppressive therapy. Once priming has occurred, however, secondary responses are much more refractory to treatment. ABO incompatibilities are hazardous because

FIGURE 272-1 Graft survival of first cadaveric renal transplant cohorts since 1976. These are registry data from the United States. The upper curve is the actual 1-year graft survival (—□—), which has reached almost 90% for the patients transplanted in 1997. Note the moderate annual rise in the early years up to 1983, when cyclosporine was introduced and 1-year graft survivals increased for 2 years. Since 1985 there has been a slow (1%/year) improvement. The lower curve is a representation of long-term graft survival, expressed as a half-life in years (—◆—) of those grafts functioning at 1 year. With thousands of cases in each cohort and a minimum of 3 years follow-up, an accurate half-life can be determined from a log-linear plot. The last calculated value of 11.6 years, although tentative because of the 2-year follow-up, is close to the historic value for haplotype-matched family donors (Table 272-1). The trend in the rise in half-life during the previous 5 years from 6 to 9 years is certainly meaningful and represents improved clinical management, as well as the introduction of mandatory sharing of HLA-matched cadaveric kidneys through the United Network for Organ Sharing. [*Drawn from data of JM Cecka, in JM Cecka and PI Terasaki (eds): Clinical Transplants, 1997, UCLA Tissue Typing Laboratory Los Angeles, 1998, pp 1–14. Updated from the UNOS web site.*]

of the presence of natural anti-A and anti-B antibodies in recipients and the normal expression of A and B blood group substances on endothelium, resulting in immediate vascular injury.

Living Donors When first-degree relatives are donors, graft survival rates at 1 year are slightly greater than those for cadaver grafts, with the exception of HLA-identical donors where 1-year results are approximately 95%. After the first year, the long-term survival rates as defined by the $t_{1/2}$ still favor the partially matched (one HLA haplotype) family donor over a randomly selected cadaver donor (Table 272-1). In addition, living donors provide the advantage of immediate availability. Waiting lists for cadaveric kidneys have grown faster than the available organ supply, to the point where most new patients with end-stage renal disease wait for more than 4 years. In response to this increasing disparity between cadaver donor supply and patient demand, living unrelated volunteers, usually spouses or close friends, are being accepted as donors in increasing numbers. It is illegal in the United States to purchase organs for transplantation. The results of transplantation using living unrelated donors have been most satisfactory, with initial and long-term survival rates the same as for partial HLA-matched family donors and better than for partially matched cadaveric donors (Table 272-1).

Concern has been expressed regarding the potential risk to a volunteer kidney donor of premature renal failure after several years of increased blood flow and hyperfiltration per nephron in the remaining kidney. There are a few reports of the development of hypertension, proteinuria, and even lesions of focal segmental sclerosis in donors under long-term follow-up. Difficulties in donors followed for 20 or more years are unusual, however, and it may be that having a single kidney becomes significant only when another condition, such as hypertension, is superimposed. It is also desirable to consider the risk of development of type 1 diabetes mellitus in a family member who is a potential donor to a diabetic renal failure patient. Anti-insulin and anti-islet antibodies should be measured, and glucose tolerance tests should be performed in such donors to rule out a prediabetic state.

HLA Matching and Cadaveric Donors The question of whether matching of HLA antigens in unrelated donor-recipient pairs would approximate the high initial success rates and slow rates of subsequent graft loss with HLA-identical sib pairs could not be answered until the late 1980s when reliable class II histocompatibility (DR) typing became widely available. Now that pooled data on tens of thousands of cadaveric renal transplants from all over the world are available, the HLA-matching effect can be clearly seen, especially in the long-term $t_{1/2}$ half-life survival figures. It is shown in Table 272-1 that there is an overall beneficial effect of HLA matching in first cadaveric grafts. When compared with HLA-identical transplants, in which the 1-year graft survival rate is 95% and the subsequent half-life is 25 years, one-HLA-haplotype–matched family donor trans-

plants have 1-year survival rates of 85% with a 12-year half-life (Table 272-1). With increasing numbers of mismatches for cadaveric donors, the half-life decreases from 20 to 7.7 years. The survival rates at the 10-year mark are projected to range from 65 (zero mismatches) to 34% (six mismatches). Many centers now report 1-year graft survival rates in the 85 to 90% range for all renal transplants (Fig. 272-1), possibly the result of heavy initial immunosuppression, but the subsequent half-lives are similar to those above. There is controversy regarding the value of cadaveric organ-sharing rules that are based entirely upon the numbers of HLA mismatches. Avoidance of mismatching for six antigens Table 272-1) is a top priority in the United States, however, and 20% of kidneys are transplanted on this basis. Table 272-1 also shows the interaction of HLA matching and graft ischemia on results; namely, kidneys from HLA-incompatible spousal donors do better than those from similarly mismatched cadaver donors, suggesting that the additional ischemic injury of organ storage is important. When such a cadaveric donor is HLA-compatible, however, ischemia and storage do not impede the matching benefit.

Presensitization A positive cross match of recipient serum with donor T lymphocytes representing anti-HLA class I is usually predictive of an acute vasculitic event termed *hyperacute rejection*. Patients with anti-HLA antibodies can be safely transplanted if careful cross matching of donor blood lymphocytes with recipient serum is performed. Patients sustained by dialysis often show fluctuating antibody titers and specificity patterns. At the time of assignment of a cadaveric kidney, cross matches are performed with at least a current serum. Previously analyzed antibody specificities and additional cross matches are performed accordingly. Techniques for cross matching are not universally standardized; however, at least two techniques are employed in most laboratories. The minimal purpose for the cross match is avoidance of hyperacute rejection mediated by recipient antibodies to donor HLA class I antigens. Sensitive tests, such as the use of flow cytometry, can be useful for avoidance of accelerated, and often untreatable, early graft rejection in patients receiving second or third transplants. Donor T lymphocytes, which express only class I antigens, are used as targets for detection of anti-class I (HLA-A and -B) antibodies. Anti-class II (HLA-DR) antibodies do not contraindicate transplantation, unless present in high titer. B lymphocytes expressing both class I and class II antigens are used in these assays. Non-HLA antigens restricted in expression to endothelium and sometimes monocytes have been described, but clinical relevance is not well established.

Blood Transfusions Exposure to leukocyte HLA antigens during transfusions is a major cause of sensitization that limits transplantation access and increases the risk of early graft rejection. In the 1970s, attempts to avoid all blood exposure in dialysed patients paradoxically increased the risk of graft rejection. The beneficial "transfusion effect" was never fully explained, and it almost disappeared in the 1980s as overall management of patients improved with the use of cyclosporine and more effective means of rejection treatment. Currently, with the use of erythropoietin the need for transfusion is much reduced. It has been noted, however, that nontransfused patients do have more rejection activity.

IMMUNOLOGY OF REJECTION Knowledge of the immunology of tissue transplantation stems largely from animal experimentation. However, enough evidence has accumulated in humans to indicate that the mechanisms are not qualitatively different from those found in other areas of immunology (Chap. 305). Early rejection is associated with activation of T lymphocytes having direct specificity against donor antigens. These may be cytotoxic cells (CD8+ or CD4+) or cells that mediate delayed hypersensitivity (CD4+); however, significant numbers of B lymphocytes, natural killer cells, and macrophages appear in the early infiltrate, and cells capable of mediating antibody-dependent cell-mediated cytotoxicity are also present. Many of the B lymphocytes produce immunoglobulins. The spectrum of cellular and humoral response and graft injury is quite varied, depending on specific genetic differences between donor and recipient and states of presensitization. The greater the degree of presensitization, the more likely it is that one will find antibody-mediated vascular lesions. All

Table 272-1 Effect of HLA-A, -B, -DR Mismatching on Kidney Graft Survival[a]

Donor Mismatches	Half-Life of Graft Survival, years	10-Year Graft Survival, %
Living related donor (HLA-identical sib = none)	24.0	74
Cadaver (none for 6 antigens)	20.3	65
Living related donor (1 haplotype = 3)	12.0	54
Living unrelated donor (average 4)	12.0	54
Cadaver (overall)	9.0	40
Cadaver (1 or 2)	10.4	45
Cadaver (3 or 4)	8.4	38
Cadaver (5 or 6)	7.7	34

[a] HLA antigens are codominantly inherited: each person has two A, two B, and two DR antigens, for a total of six.

the processes shown in Fig. 272-2 are possible, but their relative contribution varies from case to case. Monitoring of peripheral blood lymphocyte subsets utilizing monoclonal antibodies to functionally related surface molecules, such as CD4 (T helper cells) and CD8 (T cytotoxic cells), has been related to the degree of rejection activity in some surveys. Since the principal role of the CD4 molecule is to promote interaction of T cells with class II HLA molecules on antigen-presenting cells and similarly CD8 interacts with class I HLA (Chap. 305), it is not surprising that both types of T cells are usually present. Finally, the cytokine mediators of the cellular immune response [interleukin (IL) 1 to IL-4, IL-6, IL-10, IL-12, tumor necrosis factor (TNF), and interferon γ] are involved in the control and expression of the alloimmune rejection response. For example, T cell production of interferon γ causes increased expression of HLA antigens on endothelial cells. In normal immunobiology this effect may be to promote more efficient presentation of foreign antigen, while in transplantation it enhances the immunogenicity of the vascularized transplant. Also, IL-2, the major growth factor for expansion of effector T cells, is the product of a major subset of CD4 cells (Th1), while other CD4 cells (Th2) produce B cell growth factors, such as IL-4.

The failure of transplanted kidneys after several years of adequate function is said to be due to "chronic rejection." In such kidneys, the development of nephrosclerosis, with proliferation of the vascular intima of renal vessels, and intimal fibrosis, with marked decrease in the lumen of the vessels, takes place (Fig. 272-3). The result is renal ischemia, hypertension, tubular atrophy, interstitial fibrosis, and glomerular atrophy with eventual renal failure. It is not established, however, whether slow deterioration of graft function over years is due to the same mechanisms in all cases. In addition to the established influence of HLA incompatibility, the age, number of nephrons, and ischemic history of a donor kidney may contribute to ultimate progressive renal failure in transplanted patients.

FIGURE 272-2 Recognition pathways for major histocompatibility complex (MHC) antigens. Graft rejection is initiated by CD4 helper T lymphocytes (T_H) having antigen receptors that bind to specific complexes of peptides and MHC class II molecules on antigen-presenting cells (APC). In transplantation, in contrast to other immunologic responses, there are two sets of T cell clones involved in rejection. In the direct pathway the class II MHC of donor allogeneic APCs is recognized by CD4 T_H cells that bind to the intact MHC molecule, and class I MHC allogeneic cells are recognized by CD8 T cells. The latter generally proliferate into cytotoxic cells (T_C). In the indirect pathway, the incompatible MHC molecules are processed into peptides that are presented by the self-APCs of the recipient. The indirect, but not the direct, pathway is the normal physiologic process in T cell recognition of foreign antigens. Once T_H cells are activated, they proliferate, and by secretion of cytokines and direct contact exert strong helper effects on macrophages, T_C, and B cells. *(From Sayegh and Turka, Copyright 1998, Massachusetts Medical Society. All rights reserved.)*

IMMUNOSUPPRESSIVE TREATMENT Immunosuppressive therapy, as presently available, generally suppresses all immune responses, including those to bacteria, fungi, and even malignant tumors. In the 1950s when clinical renal transplantation began, sublethal total-body irradiation was employed. We have now reached the point where sophisticated pharmacologic immunosuppression is available, but it still has the hazard of promoting infection and malignancy. In general, all clinically useful drugs are more selective to primary than to memory immune responses. Agents to suppress the immune response are discussed in the following paragraphs, and those currently in clinical use are listed in Table 272-2.

Drugs *Azathioprine*, an analogue of mercaptopurine, was for two decades the keystone to immunosuppressive therapy in humans. This agent can inhibit synthesis of DNA, RNA, or both. Because cell division and proliferation are a necessary part of the immune response to antigenic stimulation, suppression by this agent may be mediated by the inhibition of mitosis of immunologically competent lymphoid cells, interfering with synthesis of DNA. Alternatively, immunosuppression may be brought about by blocking the synthesis of RNA (possibly messenger RNA), inhibiting processing of antigens prior to lymphocyte stimulation. Therapy with azathioprine in doses of 1.5 to 2.0 mg/kg per day is generally added to cyclosporine as a means of decreasing the requirements for the latter. Because azathioprine is rapidly metabolized by the liver, its dosage need not be varied directly in relation to renal function, even though renal failure results in retention of the metabolites of azathioprine. Reduction in dosage is required because of leukopenia and occasionally thrombocytopenia. Excessive amounts of azathioprine may also cause jaundice, anemia, and alo-

pecia. If it is essential to administer allopurinol concurrently, the azathioprine dose must be reduced, since inhibition of xanthine oxidase delays degradation. This combination is best avoided.

Mycophenolate mofetil is now used in place of azathioprine in many centers. It has a similar mode of action and a mild degree of gastrointestinal toxicity but produces minimal bone marrow suppression. Its advantage is its increased potency in preventing or reversing rejection.

Glucocorticoids are important adjuncts to immunosuppressive therapy. Of all the agents employed, prednisone has effects that are easiest to assess, and in large doses it is usually effective for the reversal of rejection. In general, 200 to 300 mg prednisone is given immediately prior to or at the time of transplantation, and the dosage is reduced to 30 mg within a week. The side effects of the glucocorticoids, particularly impairment of wound healing and predisposition to infection, make it desirable to taper the dose as rapidly as possible in the immediate postoperative period. Customarily, methylprednisolone, 0.5 to 1.0 g intravenously, is administered immediately upon diagnosis of beginning rejection and continued once daily for 3 days. When the drug is effective, the results are usually apparent within 96 h. Such "pulse" doses are not effective in chronic rejection. Most patients whose renal function is stable after 6 months or a year do not require large doses of prednisone; maintenance doses of 10 to 15 mg/d are the rule. Many patients tolerate an alternate-day course of steroids without an increased risk of rejection.

A major effect of steroids is on the monocyte-macrophage system, preventing the release of IL-6 and IL-1. Lymphopenia after large doses of glucocorticoids is primarily due to sequestration of recirculating blood lymphocytes to lymphoid tissue.

FIGURE 272-3 Chronic rejection in a renal allograft (×400). Typical arterial *(left)* and glomerular *(right)* lesions are shown. The arterial lesion, also called graft arteriosclerosis, is similar to that seen in coronary vessels of heart transplant recipients. The main feature is that of myointimal proliferation, mostly of smooth muscle cells (arrow), leading to progressive luminal narrowing (*) with resultant ischemia. The glomerular lesion consists of mesangial proliferation with occlusion of capillary spaces, leading ultimately to glomerulosclerosis (arrow). The net result of these lesions in the vasculature is interstitial atrophy and fibrosis. *(From Sayegh and Turka, Copyright 1998, Massachusetts Medical Society. All rights reserved.)*

Cyclosporine is a fungal peptide with potent immunosuppressive activity. It acts on the calcineurin pathway to block transcription of mRNA for IL-2 and other proinflammatory cytokines, thereby inhibiting T cell proliferation. Although it works alone, cyclosporine is more effective in conjunction with glucocorticoids. Since cyclosporine blocks production of IL-2 by T cells, its combination with steroids is expected to produce a double block in the macrophage → IL-6/IL-1 → T cell → IL-2 sequence. As noted, clinical results with tens of thousands of renal transplants have been impressive. Of its toxic effects (nephrotoxicity, hepatoxicity, hirsutism, tremor, gingival hyperplasia, diabetes), only nephrotoxicity presents a serious management problem and is further discussed below.

Tacrolimus (FK-506) is a fungal macrolide that has the same mode of action, and a similar side effect profile, as cyclosporine. It does not produce hirsutism or gingival hyperplasia, however. De novo induction of diabetes mellitus is more common with tacrolimus. The drug was first used in liver transplantation, and may substitute for cyclosporine entirely, or be tried as an alternative in renal patients whose rejections are poorly controlled by cyclosporine.

Sirolimus (previously called rapamycin) is another fungal macrolide but has a different mode of action: namely, it inhibits T cell growth factor pathways, preventing the response to IL-2 and other cytokines. It shows some promise in clinical trials in combination with cyclosporine.

Antibodies to Lymphocytes When serum from animals made immune to host lymphocytes is injected into the recipient, a marked suppression of cellular immunity to the tissue graft results. The action on cell-mediated immunity is greater than on humoral immunity. A globulin fraction of serum [antilymphocyte globulin (ALG)] is the agent generally employed. For use in humans, peripheral human lymphocytes, thymocytes, or lymphocytes from spleens or thoracic duct fistulas have been injected into horses, rabbits, or goats to produce antilymphocyte serum, from which the globulin fraction is then separated. Monoclonal antibodies against defined lymphocyte subsets offer a more precise and standardized form of therapy. OKT3 is directed to the CD3 molecules that form a portion of the T cell antigen-receptor complex; hence CD3 is expressed on all mature T cells. CD4 or CD8 molecules also form part of the fully activated cluster of molecules, and monoclonal antibodies to these offer the potential for more selective targeting of T cell subsets. Another approach to more selective therapy is to target the 55-kDa alpha chain of the IL-2 receptor, expressed only on T cells that have been recently activated. The problem with such mouse antibodies is the potential for developing human antimouse antibodies (HAMA), an event that limits the effective period of use. Genetically engineered monoclonal antibodies can solve this problem. Two such antibodies to the IL-2 receptor, in which either a chimeric protein has been made between mouse Fab with human Fc (basiliximab) or "humanized" by splicing the combining sites of the mouse into a molecule that is 90% human IgG (daclizumab), have been approved for use, after clinical evidence of reduction of rejection episodes. Their precise clinical role is under study.

CLINICAL COURSE AND MANAGEMENT OF THE RECIPIENT Adequate hemodialysis should be performed within 48 h of surgery, and care should be taken that the serum potassium level is not markedly elevated so that intraoperative cardiac

Table 272-2 Maintenance Immunosuppressive Drugs

Agent	Pharmacology	Mechanisms	Side Effects
Glucocorticoids	Increased bioavailability with hypoalbuminemia and liver disease; prednisone/prednisolone generally used	Binds cytosolic receptors and heat shock proteins. Blocks transcription of IL-1,-2,-3,-6, TNF-α, and IFN-γ	Hypertension, glucose intolerance, dyslipidemia, osteoporosis
Cyclosporine (CsA)	Lipid-soluble polypeptide, variable absorption, microemulsion more predictable	Trimolecular complex with cyclophilin and calcineurin → block in cytokine (e.g., IL-2) production; however, stimulates TGF-β production	Nephrotoxicity, hypertension, dyslipidemia, glucose intolerance, hirsutism/hyperplasia of gums
Tacrolimus (FK506)	Macrolide, well absorbed	Trimolecular complex with FKBP-12 and calcineurin → block in cytokine (e.g., IL-2) production; may stimulate TGF-β production	Similar to CsA, but hirsutism/hyperplasia of gums unusual, and diabetes more likely
Azathioprine	Mercaptopurine analogue	Hepatic metabolites inhibit purine synthesis	Marrow suppression (WBC > RBC > platelets)
Mycophenolate Mofetil (MMF)	Metabolized to mycophenolic acid	Inhibits purine synthesis via inosine monophosphate dehydrogenase	Diarrhea/cramps; dose-related liver and marrow suppression is uncommon
Sirolimus	Macrolide, poor oral bioavailability	Complexes with FKBP-12 and then blocks p70 S6 kinase in the IL-2 receptor pathway for proliferation	Hyperlipidemia, thrombocytopenia

NOTE: IL, interleukin; TNF, tumor necrosis factor; IFN, interferon; TGF, transforming growth factor; FKBP-12, FK506 binding protein 12; WBC, white blood cells; RBC, red blood cells.

arrhythmias can be averted. The diuresis that commonly occurs postoperatively must be carefully monitored; in some instances it may be massive, reflecting the inability of ischemic tubules to regulate sodium and water excretion; with large diureses, massive potassium losses may occur. Most chronically uremic patients have some excess of extracellular fluid, and it is useful to maintain an expanded fluid volume in the immediate postoperative period. Acute tubular necrosis (ATN) may cause immediate oliguria or may follow an initial short period of graft function. ATN is most likely when cadaveric donors have been hypotensive or if the interval between cessation of blood flow and organ harvest (warm ischemic time) is more than a few minutes. Recovery usually occurs within 3 weeks, although periods as long as 6 weeks have been reported. Superimposition of rejection on ATN is common, and the differential diagnosis may be difficult without a graft biopsy. Cyclosporine therapy prolongs ATN, and some patients do not diurese until the dose is drastically reduced. Many centers avoid starting cyclosporine for the first several days, using ALG or a monoclonal antibody along with mycophenolate mofetil and prednisone until renal function is established.

The Rejection Episode Early diagnosis of rejection allows prompt institution of therapy to preserve renal function and prevent irreversible damage. Clinical evidence of rejection is rarely characterized by fever, swelling, and tenderness over the allograft. Rejection may present only with a rise in serum creatinine, with or without a reduction in urine volume. The focus should be on ruling out other causes of functional deterioration.

Arteriography and radioactive iodohippurate sodium renograms of the transplanted kidney may be useful in ascertaining changes in the renal vasculature and in renal blood flow, even in the absence of urinary flow. Thrombosis of the renal vein occurs rarely; it may be reversible if caused by technical factors and intervention is prompt. Diagnostic ultrasound is the procedure of choice to rule out urinary obstruction or to confirm the presence of perirenal collections of urine, blood, or lymph. When renal function has been good initially, a rise in the serum creatinine level is the most sensitive and reliable indicator of possible rejection and may be the only sign.

Calcineurin inhibitors (cyclosporine or tacrolimus) may cause deterioration in renal function in a manner similar to a rejection episode. In fact, rejection processes tend to be more indolent with these inhibitors, and the only way to make a diagnosis may be by renal biopsy. Calcineurin inhibitors have an afferent arteriolar constrictor effect on the kidney and may produce permanent vascular and interstitial injury after sustained high-dose therapy. Addition of angiotensin-converting enzyme (ACE) inhibitors or nonsteroidal anti-inflammatory drugs are likely to raise serum creatinine levels. The former are generally safe to use after the early months, while the latter are best avoided in all renal transplant patients. There is no universally accepted lesion(s) that makes a diagnosis of calcineurin inhibitor toxicity, although interstitial fibrosis, isometric tubular vacuolization, and thickening of arteriolar walls have been noted by some. Basically, if the biopsy does not reveal moderate and active cellular rejection activity, the serum creatinine will most likely respond to a reduction in dose. Blood levels of drug can be useful if very high or very low but do not correlate precisely with renal function, although serial changes in a patient can be useful. If rejection activity is present in the biopsy, appropriate therapy is indicated. The first rejection episode is usually treated with intravenous administration of methylprednisolone, 500 to 1000 mg daily for 3 days. Failure to respond is indication for antibody therapy, usually with OKT3.

OKT3 monoclonal antibody, given intravenously for 10 to 14 days, is effective in more than 90% of first rejections, and less so if methylprednisolone pulses have failed and in cases of severe recurrent rejection activity. A major problem with OKT3 is that severe systemic reactions may be produced during the first day or two of therapy. Chills, fever, hypotension, and headache are the direct result of the antibody effects on the targeted T cells, most likely related to the known potential of OKT3 to activate T cells nonspecifically with release of cytokines, especially TNF-α. If the antibody is administered

to overhydrated oliguric patients, pulmonary edema may be induced. These reactions are not characteristic of other monoclonal antibodies, such as those to the IL-2 receptor. Recurrent or rebound rejection activity may require additional therapy. In such circumstances, methylprednisolone may be effective even though it failed initially. Second courses of OKT3 may be given in spite of HAMA generated in response to the first course if the titers are low and the human antibodies are not directed to the combining-site region (idiotype) of the OKT3.

Management Problems The usual clinical manifestations of infection in the posttransplant period are blunted by immunosuppressive therapy. The major toxic effect of azathioprine is bone marrow suppression, which is less likely with mycophenolate mofetil, while calcineurin inhibitors have no marrow effects. All drugs predispose to unusual opportunistic infections, however. The signs and symptoms of infection may be masked and distorted, and fever without obvious cause is common. Only after days or weeks it may become apparent that it has a viral or fungal origin. Bacterial infections are most common during the first month after transplantation. The importance of blood cultures in such patients cannot be overemphasized, because systemic infection without obvious foci is frequent, although wound infections with or without urinary fistulas are most common. Particularly ominous are rapidly occurring pulmonary lesions, which may result in death within 5 days of onset. When these become apparent, immunosuppressive agents should be discontinued, except for maintenance doses of prednisone. Aggressive diagnostic procedures, including transbronchial and open lung biopsy, are frequently indicated. In the case of *Pneumocystis carinii* (Chap. 209) infection, trimethoprim-sulfamethoxazole is the treatment of choice; amphotericin B has been used effectively in systemic fungal infections. Prophylaxis against *P. carinii* with daily, or alternate day, low-dose trimethoprim-sulfamethoxazole is very effective. Involvement of the oropharynx with *Candida* (Chap. 205) may be treated with local nystatin. Tissue-invasive fungal infections require treatment with systemic agents such as fluconazole. Small doses (a total of 300 mg) of amphotericin given over a period of 2 weeks may be effective in fungal infections refractory to fluconazole. Macrolide antibiotics, especially ketoconazole and erythromycin, and some calcium channel blockers (diltiazem, verapamil) compete with calcineurin inhibitors for P450 catabolism and cause elevated levels of these immunosuppressive drugs. Analeptics, such as phenytoin and carbamazepine, will increase catabolism to result in low levels. *Aspergillus* (Chap. 206), *Nocardia* (Chap. 165), and cytomegalovirus (CMV) (Chap. 185) infections also occur.

CMV is a common and dangerous infection in transplant recipients. It does not generally appear until the end of the first posttransplant month. Active CMV infection is sometimes associated, or occasionally confused, with rejection episodes. Patients at highest risk for severe CMV disease are those without anti-CMV antibodies who receive a graft from a CMV antibody–positive donor (15% mortality). Serial intravenous administration of high-titer CMV immune globulin is effective in reducing this risk. Prophylactic use of ganciclovir is an effective alternative. Early diagnosis in a febrile patient can be made by detecting CMV antigens in the blood. A rise in IgM antibodies to CMV is also diagnostic. Culture of CMV from blood may be less sensitive. Tissue invasion of CMV is common in the gastrointestinal tract and lungs. CMV retinopathy occurs late in the course, if untreated. Treatment of active CMV disease with ganciclovir is always indicated. Many patients immune to CMV can activate the virus after heavy immunosuppression, such as with OKT3. Concurrent treatment with ganciclovir during OKT3 administration appears to be effective for prophylaxis of CMV activation. The complications of glucocorticoid therapy are well known and include gastrointestinal bleeding, impairment of wound healing, osteoporosis, diabetes mellitus, cataract formation, and hemorrhagic pancreatitis. The treatment of unexplained jaundice in transplant patients should include cessation or reduction of immunosuppressive drugs if hepatitis or drug toxicity is suspected. It is surprising that cessation of azathioprine or calcineurin inhibitor therapy in such circumstances often does not result in rejection of a graft, at least for several weeks. Acyclovir is effective in therapy of herpes simplex virus infections.

Antiplatelet agents and anticoagulants, although effective in theory, have not been successful in the prevention of the "chronic rejection" vascular lesions. Persistent elevation of serum creatinine levels above 220 μmol/L (2.5 mg/dL) in patients on calcineurin inhibitor is an indication for dose reduction, particularly if calcineurin inhibitor blood levels are elevated. The risk of long-term cumulative toxicity to the kidney now seems to be low. In general, minimal or no rejection during the first 6 months after transplantation is a predictor of safety in reducing immunosuppression therapy over subsequent months to years, but chronic progressive vasculopathy may still occur.

Despite the potential teratogenic effects of immunosuppressive agents, both women and men have become parents after transplantation. The incidence of congenital abnormalities in the offspring is not increased.

Glomerular Lesions   Glomerular lesions occur in 10 to 15% of allografts, even when the original disease was accidental removal of a solitary kidney. The pathogenesis is related to a chronic rejection process. In some cases the lesions resemble those of the original glomerular disease. In most instances, the recurrence of the original renal lesions represents no threat to the immediate prognosis, and a primary diagnosis of glomerulonephritis is rarely a contraindication to transplantation. Focal segmental glomerulosclerosis may recur up to 30% of the time, with one-third of these patients losing graft function. Hemolytic uremic syndrome also has a high recurrence rate.

Malignancy   The incidence of tumors in patients on immunosuppressive therapy is 5 to 6%, or approximately 100 times greater than that in the general population of the same age range. The most common lesions are cancer of the skin and lips and carcinoma in situ of the cervix, as well as lymphomas, such as non-Hodgkin's lymphomas. The risks are increased in proportion to the total immunosuppressive load administered and time elapsed since transplantation. Surveillance for skin and cervical cancers is necessary.

Other Complications   *Hypercalcemia* after transplantation may indicate failure of hyperplastic parathyroid glands to regress. Aseptic necrosis of the head of the femur is probably due to preexisting hyperparathyroidism, with aggravation by glucocorticoid treatment. With improved management of calcium and phosphorus metabolism during chronic dialysis, the incidence of parathyroid-related complications has fallen dramatically. Persistent hyperparathyroid activity may require subtotal parathyroidectomy.

Hypertension may be caused by (1) native kidneys; (2) rejection activity in the transplant; (3) renal artery stenosis, if an end-to-end anastomosis was constructed with an iliac artery branch; and (4) renal calcineurin inhibitor toxicity. The latter may improve with reduction in dose. Whereas ACE inhibitors may be useful, calcium channel blockers are more frequently used initially. Amelioration of hypertension to the 120–130/70–80 mmHg range should be the goal in all patients.

Chronic hepatitis, particularly when due to hepatitis B virus, can be a progressive, fatal disease over a decade or so. Patients who are persistently hepatitis B surface antigen–positive are at higher risk, according to some studies, but the presence of hepatitis C virus is also a concern when one embarks on a course of immunosuppression in a transplant recipient.

Both chronic dialysis and renal transplant patients have a higher incidence of death from myocardial infarction and stroke than in the population at large, and this is particularly true in diabetic patients. Contributing factors are the use of glucocorticoids, hypertension, and hypertriglyceridemia. Increased low-density lipoprotein cholesterol and depressed high-density lipoprotein cholesterol concentrations may be exaggerated after transplantation and require treatment. Recipients of renal transplants have a high prevalence of coronary artery and peripheral vascular diseases. The percentage of deaths from these

causes has been slowly rising as the numbers of transplanted diabetic patients and the average age of all recipients increase. More than 50% of renal recipient mortality is attributable to cardiovascular disease. In addition to strict control of blood pressure and blood lipid levels, close monitoring of patients for indications of further medical or surgical intervention is an important part of management.

BIBLIOGRAPHY

COSIO FG et al: Relationships between arterial hypertension and renal allograft survival in African-American patients. Am J Kidney Dis 29:419, 1997

MASSY AZ, KASISKE BL: Post-transplant hyperlipidemia: Mechanisms and management. J Am Soc Nephrol 7:971, 1996

MCKAY DB et al: Clinical renal transplantation, in *Brenner and Rector's The Kidney*, 6th ed, B Brenner (ed). Philadelphia, Saunders 2000, pp 2542–2605

PIRSCH J et al: A comparison of tacrolimus (FK506) and cyclosporine for immunosuppression after cadaveric renal transplantation. FK506 Kidney Transplant Study Group. Transplantation 63:977, 1997

SAYEGH MH, TURKA LA: The role of T-cell costimulatory activation pathways in transplant rejection. N Engl J Med 338:1813, 1998

——— et al: Transplantation immunobiology, in *Brenner and Rector's The Kidney*, 6th ed, B Brenner (ed). Philadelphia, Saunders, 2000, pp 2518–2541

STEWART G et al: Ischemic heart disease following renal transplantation. Nephrol Dial Transplant 15:269, 2000

---

273   *Hugh R. Brady, Barry M. Brenner*

PATHOGENESIS OF GLOMERULAR INJURY

The glomerulus is a modified capillary network that delivers an ultrafiltrate of plasma to Bowman's space, the most proximal portion of the renal tubule. Approximately 1.6 million glomeruli are present in two mature kidneys (range 0.5 to 2.4 million) and collectively they produce 120 to 180 L of ultrafiltrate daily. Glomerular filtration rate (GFR) is dependent on glomerular blood flow, ultrafiltration pressure, and surface area. These parameters are tightly regulated through changes in afferent and efferent arteriolar tone (for blood flow and ultrafiltration pressure) and mesangial cell contractility (for filtration surface area). Arteriolar tone and mesangial cell contractility are, in turn, modulated by neurohumoral factors, local myenteric reflexes, and endothelium-derived vasoactive substances, such as nitric oxide, prostacyclin, and endothelins. In health, glomerular endothelium is also antithrombotic and antiadhesive for leukocytes and platelets, thereby preventing inappropriate vascular thrombosis and inflammation during the filtration process. Filtration of most plasma proteins and all blood cells is normally prevented as a consequence of the physiochemical and electrostatic charge characteristics of the glomerular filtration barrier, the latter being composed of fenestrated glomerular endothelium, basement membrane, and the foot processes and slit diaphragms of visceral epithelial cells (podocytes). Parietal epithelium facilitates glomerular filtration by maintaining the integrity of Bowman's space. In keeping with the physiologic functions of the glomerulus outlined above, virtually all glomerular injury results in impairment of glomerular filtration and/or the inappropriate appearance of plasma proteins and blood cells in the urine.

CLINICOPATHOLOGIC CORRELATES IN GLOMERULAR DISEASE

The major glomerulopathies are described in Chap. 274, and major morphologic patterns of glomerular disease and their clinical features are summarized in Table 273-1. These clinicopathologic entities can be induced by a variety of different pathogenetic mechanisms. Thus, prompt diagnosis, optimal management, and accurate prognostication is a multistep process that requires (1) recognition of the presenting clinical syndrome, (2) delineation of the underlying morphologic pat-

Table 273-1 Major Clinicopathologic Presentation of Glomerular Disease

Structural Pattern	Typical Clinical Presentation	Typical Pathology Findings	Most Common Etiologies[a]
Diffuse proliferative GN	Acute nephritic syndrome: Acute renal failure over days to weeks, hypertension, edema, oliguria, active urine sediment, subnephrotic proteinuria	Diffuse increase in cellularity of tufts of most glomeruli due to infiltration by neutrophils and monocytes, and proliferation of glomerular endothelial and mesangial cells	Immune complex GN: idiopathic, postinfectious, SLE, SBE, cryoglobulinemia, HSP Pauci-immune GN and anti-GBM disease (crescentic GN common—see below)
Crescentic GN	Rapidly progressive glomerulonephritis (RPGN): Subacute renal failure over weeks to months, active urine sediment, variable amount of hypertension, edema, oliguria, and proteinuria	Majority of glomeruli contain areas of fibrinoid necrosis and crescents in Bowman's space, composed of proliferating parietal epithelial cells, infiltrating macrophages, and fibrin	Immune complex GN (as above) Pauci-immune GN: Wegener's granulomatosis, microscopic polyarteritis nodosa, renal-limited crescentic GN Anti-GBM disease (Goodpasture's syndrome if lung hemorrhage)
Focal proliferative GN	Mild to moderate glomerular inflammation: Active urine sediment and mild to moderate decline in GFR	Segmental areas of proliferation and necrosis in less than 50% of glomeruli, occasionally with crescent formation	Early and milder forms, or recovery phase of most diseases causing diffuse proliferative and crescentic GN IgA nephropathy/HSP
Mesangial proliferative GN	Chronic glomerular inflammation: Proteinuria, hematuria, hypertension, variable effect on GFR	Proliferation of mesangial cells and matrix	IgA nephropathy/HSP Early and milder forms, or recovery phases of most diseases that cause diffuse proliferative and crescentic GN (see above) In association with minimal change glomerulopathy and FSGS
Membranoproliferative GN	Variable combination of nephritic and nephrotic features: Acute or subacute decline in GFR, active urine sediment, proteinuria often in nephrotic range	Diffuse proliferation of mesangial cells and infiltration of glomeruli by macrophages; increased mesangial matrix and thickening and reduplication of glomerular basement membrane	Immune complex GN (as for diffuse proliferative GN) In association with thrombotic microangiopathies (see below) In association with deposition diseases (see below) Postrenal or -marrow transplantation
Minimal change GN	Nephrotic syndrome: Proteinuria of >3–3.5 g/d, hypoalbuminemia, edema, hyperlipidemia, lipiduria, thrombotic diathesis, slow decline in GFR in 10–30%.	Light microscopy normal, but electron microscopy (EM) shows foot process effacement	Idiopathic In association with drug-induced interstitial nephritis, HIV infection, heroin, Hodgkin's and other lymphomas
Focal segmental glomerulosclerosis	Nephrotic syndrome: Proteinuria of >3–3.5 g/d, hypoalbuminemia, edema, hyperlipidemia, lipiduria, thrombotic diathesis, slow decline in GFR in 10–30%.	Segmental capillary collapse affecting <50% of glomeruli with entrapment of amorphous hyaline material. EM shows foot process effacement	Primary FSGS: idiopathic, HIV, heroin, lysosomal diseases, Charcot-Marie-Tooth Secondary response to reduction in nephron number from any cause (hyperfiltration injury)
Nodular or global sclerosis	Proteinuria and chronic renal failure	Sclerosis of most glomeruli with interstitial fibrosis	Diabetic nephropathy Potential long-term consequence of most glomerulopathies listed above
Membranous GN	Nephrotic syndrome: Proteinuria of >3–3.5 g/d, hypoalbuminemia, edema, hyperlipidemia, lipiduria, thrombotic diathesis, slow decline in GFR in 10–30%	Diffuse thickening of the glomerular basement membrane with subepithelial projections ("spikes") around immune deposits	Idiopathic Infections (e.g., Hepatitis B & C, syphilis, schistasomiasis, malaria, leprosy) Drugs (e.g., gold, penicillamine, captopril) Autoimmune diseases (SLE, rheumatoid arthritis) Paraneoplastic
Deposition diseases	Combination of nephritic and nephrotic features: Renal failure over months to years, proteinuria, hematuria, and hypertension.	Mesangial expansion and thickening of glomerular capillary wall; variable cellular proliferation and crescent formation	Amyloid Cryoglobulinemia Light chain deposition disease Fibrillary/immunotactoid GN

(continued)

tern of glomerular injury, and (3) elucidation of the specific renal-limited or systemic disease that triggered glomerular dysfunction.

NOMENCLATURE The terms *glomerulonephritis* and *glomerulopathy* are usually used interchangeably to denote glomerular injury, although some authorities reserve the former term for injury with evidence of inflammation such as leukocyte infiltration, antibody deposition, and/or complement activation. Glomerular diseases are classified as *primary* when the pathology is confined to the kidney and any

Structural Pattern	Typical Clinical Presentation	Typical Pathology Findings	Most Common Etiologies[a]
Thrombotic microangiopathy	Acute or subacute renal failure: Variable degree of hypertension, edema and proteinuria, urine sediment usually contains red blood cells, but less activity than patients with nephritic syndrome or RPGN	Microthrombi in glomerular capillaries ± endothelial injury	Idiopathic In association with gastrointestinal infections, or drugs such as anovulants, mitomycin C, cyclosporine Other diseases: SLE, scleroderma, toxemia, malignant hypertension
Nonimmune basement membrane abnormalities	Asymptomatic hematuria and variable renal failure	Alport's syndrome—mesangial hypercellularity with focal sclerosis and interstitial fibrosis; splintering of GBM on EM.	Alport's syndrome, Thin basement membrane disease. Nail patella syndrome, Lecithin–cholesterol acyltransferase deficiency

[a] Includes most common etiologies: For complete list, see Chap. 274.
NOTE: Diffuse, affecting ≥50% of glomeruli; focal, affecting <50% of glomeruli; global, affecting ≥50% of glomerular tuft; segmental, affecting <50% of glomerular tuft; GN, glomerulonephritis; FSGS, focal segmental glomerulosclerosis; HSP, Henoch-Schönlein purpura; SLE, systemic lupus erythematosus; SBE, subacute bacterial endocarditis; GBM, glomerular basement membrane; GFR, glomerular filtration rate.

systemic features are a direct consequence of glomerular dysfunction (e.g., pulmonary edema, hypertension, the uremic syndrome). Usually, but not always, the term primary is synonymous with *idiopathic*. Glomerular diseases are classified as *secondary* when part of a multisystem disorder. In general, *acute* refers to glomerular injury occurring over days or weeks, *subacute* or *rapidly progressive* over weeks or a few months, and *chronic* over many months or years. Lesions are classified as *focal* or *diffuse* when they involve the minority (<50%) or majority (≥50%) of glomeruli, respectively. Lesions are termed *segmental* or *global* when they involve part of or almost all of the glomerular tuft, respectively. *Proliferative* is used to describe an increase in glomerular cell number, which can be due to infiltration by leukocytes or proliferation of resident glomerular cells. Proliferation of resident glomerular cells is classified as *intracapillary* or *endocapillary* when referring to endothelial or mesangial cells and *extracapillary* when referring to cells in Bowman's space. A *crescent* is a half-moon-shaped collection of cells in Bowman's space, usually composed of proliferating parietal epithelial cells and infiltrating monocytes. Because crescentic glomerulonephritis is often associated with renal failure that progresses rapidly over week to months, the clinical term *rapidly progressive glomerulonephritis* and pathologic term *crescentic glomerulonephritis* are often used interchangeably. The description *membranous* is applied to glomerulonephritis dominated by expansion of the glomerular basement membrane (GBM) by immune deposits. *Sclerosis* refers to an increase in the amount of homogeneous nonfibrillar extracellular material of the same ultrastructural appearance and chemical composition as GBM and mesangial matrix. This process is distinct from *fibrosis*, which involves deposition of collagens type I and III and is more commonly a consequence of healing of crescents or tubulointerstitial inflammation.

MAJOR CLINICOPATHOLOGIC ENTITIES Most glomerulopathies are still classified and named according to their morphologic features (Table 273-1). The major *inflammatory glomerulopathies* are focal proliferative glomerulonephritis (termed *mesangial proliferative* if the proliferating cells are predominantly mesangial cells), diffuse proliferative glomerulonephritis, and crescentic glomerulonephritis. These diseases typically present with a *nephritic-type* "active" urine sediment characterized by the presence of red blood cells, red blood cell casts, leukocytes, and *subnephrotic* proteinuria of <3 g/24 h. The severity of renal insufficiency varies in proportion to the degree of proliferation and necrosis.

The major morphologic patterns affecting the glomerular filtration barrier for proteins, namely the GBM and visceral epithelial cells, are membranous glomerulopathy, minimal change disease, and focal and segmental glomerulosclerosis. These entities typically present with *nephrotic-range* proteinuria of >3 g/24 h and the presence of few red blood cells, leukocytes, or cellular casts. As a consequence of the heavy proteinuria, nephrotic syndrome is associated with hypoalbuminemia, edema, hyperlipidemia, and lipiduria. Membrano-

proliferative glomerulonephritis, as the name suggests, is a hybrid lesion that presents with a combination of nephritic and nephrotic features.

The *glomerular deposition diseases* are a group of disorders characterized by prominent extravascular deposition of a paraprotein or fibrillar material. These diseases can also trigger nephritic-type and nephrotic-type responses (or a combination of both) and thus show marked clinical and morphologic overlap with the entities described above.

The *thrombotic microangiopathies* are a family of diseases in which the pathologic presentation is dominated by thrombi within the renal microvasculature, often leading to renal insufficiency.

MAJOR DETERMINANTS OF GLOMERULAR INJURY

Important determinants of the severity of glomerular injury include (1) the nature of the primary insult and the secondary mediator systems that it invokes, (2) the site of injury within the glomerulus; and (3) the speed of onset, extent, and intensity of disease.

PRIMARY INSULT Glomeruli are susceptible to a variety of inflammatory, metabolic, hemodynamic, toxic, and infectious insults (Table 273-2). Most human glomerular disease is triggered by immune attack, diabetes mellitus, or hypertension. Diverse insults can induce similar clinicopathologic presentations, suggesting marked overlap among downstream molecular and cellular responses. For example, infections (e.g., streptococcal pharyngitis, bacterial endocarditis) and vasculitides (e.g., Henoch-Schönlein purpura, microscopic polyarteritis) can each trigger acute proliferative glomerulonephritis with the nephritic syndrome. Similarly, metabolic (e.g., diabetes mellitus) and deposition diseases (e.g., amyloid) can each induce glomerulosclerosis with nephrotic syndrome. An important corollary is that pharmacologic agents that inhibit common secondary mediator systems may prove effective in treating glomerular diseases of diverse etiologies (see below).

SITE OF INJURY The consequences of injury at different sites within the glomerulus can be predicted from the physiologic functions of the cells within the local milieu (Table 273-3). The major sequelae of injury to the *endothelium* and *subendothelial aspect of the GBM* are (1) recruitment of leukocytes leading to inflammatory glomerulonephritis, (2) perturbed hemostasis leading to thrombotic microangiopathy, and (3) vasoconstriction and mesangial cell contraction leading to acute renal failure. It is usual for one of these phenotypes to dominate the presentation of specific diseases. *Mesangial* injury is usually immunologic in origin and, being more localized, induces less dramatic impairment of glomerular filtration. Patients typically present with asymptomatic abnormalities of the urinary sediment and mild renal insufficiency. Proteinuria dominates the clinical presentation of injury to the *subepithelial aspect of the GBM* and *visceral epithelial* *cells.* As with mesangial injury, GFR is often only mildly compromised in this setting. The classic pathologic manifestation of *parietal epithelial cell* injury is crescent formation. Crescents can be the dominant morphologic presentation of glomerular disease or complicate proliferative or membranous lesions.

SPEED OF ONSET, INTENSITY, AND EXTENT OF INJURY To illustrate the importance of the speed of onset, extent, and intensity of glomerular injury, it is instructive to compare two forms of immune complex glomerulonephritis, namely, acute postinfectious glomerulonephritis and IgA nephropathy. Postinfectious glomerulonephritis is characterized by rapid and extensive formation of immune complexes throughout the glomerular capillary wall, which often provokes acute renal failure with the classic hallmarks of acute inflammation: complement activation, leukocyte recruitment, lysosomal enzyme release, free radical generation, and perturbation of vascular tone and permeability. In contrast, IgA nephropathy is characterized by slow, but sustained, formation of immune complexes, largely confined to the mesangium; less dramatic activation of complement and other secondary mediator systems; and either stability of GFR or progressive renal insufficiency over 10 to 20 years.

IMMUNOLOGIC GLOMERULAR INJURY

Immune-mediated glomerulonephritis (Chaps. 274 and 275) accounts for a large fraction of acquired renal disease. The majority of cases are associated with the deposition of antibodies, often autoantibodies, within the glomerular tuft, indicating dysregulation of humoral immunity. Cellular immune mechanisms also contribute to the pathogenesis of antibody-mediated glomerulonephritis by modulating antibody production and through antibody-dependent cell cytotoxicity (see below). In addition, cellular immune mechanisms probably play a primary role in the pathophysiology of "pauci-immune" glomerulonephritides, notable for robust glomerular inflammation in the absence of immunoglobulin deposition.

ANTIBODY-MEDIATED INJURY (Fig. 273-1) Most antibody-mediated glomerulonephritis in humans is initiated by reactivity of circulating antibodies with auto- or "planted" antigens within the glomerulus. The major mechanisms of antibody deposition within the glomerulus are (1) reactivity of circulating autoantibodies with intrinsic autoantigens that are components of normal glomerular parenchyma, (2) in situ formation of immune complexes through interaction of circulating antibodies with extrinsic antigens that have been planted within the glomerulus, and (3) intraglomerular trapping of immune complexes that have formed in the systemic circulation. Autoantibodies against neutrophil cytoplasmic antigens in the circulation may represent an additional mechanism of antibody-mediated glomerular injury in patients without discernible immune complexes in the glomerular parenchyma (see below).

Generation of Nephritogenic Antibodies Exposure of the host to a foreign antigen (e.g., a prodromal infection) has been implicated as the trigger for the generation of nephritogenic autoantibodies in several forms of glomerulonephritis. Foreign antigens can provoke autoantibody formation through several mechanisms. First, a foreign antigen, whose structure resembles that of a host glomerular antigen, may stimulate the production of autoantibodies that cross-react with the intrinsic glomerular antigen ("molecular mimickry"). Second, the foreign antigen may trigger aberrant expression of major histocompatibility complex class II molecules on glomerular cells which present previously "invisible" autoantigens to T lymphocytes and thereby generate an autoimmune response. Third, the foreign antigen can trigger polyclonal activation of B lymphocytes, some of which generate nephritogenic antibodies. Alternatively, individuals may suffer a breakdown of immune tolerance through other mechanisms (e.g., genetically programmed). Autoreactive B cells are usually deleted in the thymus during development (clonal deletion) or rendered anergic in peripheral lymphoid tissue (clonal anergy). Similar tolerogenic mechanisms exist for deleting or anergizing autoreactive T helper cells that modulate immunoglobulin production by autoreactive B cells. Perturbation of either of these tolerogenic mechanisms could drive immunoglobulin production in some forms of autoimmune glomerulonephritis. Indeed, defective clonal deletion of autoreactive T cells has been demonstrated in experimental lupus nephritis due to defective synthesis of Fas, a cell-surface receptor that modulates T cell deletion through apoptosis (programmed cell death) within the thymus.

Table 273-2 Primary Mechanisms of Glomerular Injury

Mechanism of Injury	Some Renal Insults/Defects	Glomerular Disease
Immunologic[a]	Immunoglobulin[b]	Immune complex–mediated glomerulonephritis
	Cell-mediated injury[b]	Pauci-immune glomerulonephritis
	Cytokine (or other soluble factor)	Primary focal segmental glomerulosclerosis
	Persistent complement activation	Membranoproliferative glomerulonephritis (type II)
Metabolic[a]	Hyperglycemia[b]	Diabetic nephropathy
	Fabry's disease and sialidosis	Focal segmental glomerulosclerosis
Hemodynamic[a]	Systemic hypertension[b]	Hypertensive nephrosclerosis
	Intraglomerular hypertension[b]	Secondary focal segmental glomerulosclerosis
Toxic	*E. coli*–derived verotoxin	Thrombotic microangiopathy
	Therapeutic drugs (e.g., NSAIDs)	Minimal change disease
	Recreational drugs (heroin)	Focal segmental glomerulosclerosis
Deposition	Amyloid fibrils	Amyloid nephropathy
Infectious	HIV	HIV nephropathy
	Subacute bacterial endocarditis	Immune complex glomerulonephritis
Inherited	Defect in gene for α5 chain of type IV collagen	Alport's syndrome
	Abnormally thin basement membrane	Thin basement membrane disease

[a] Most common categories.
[b] Most common insults within these categories.
NOTE: NSAIDs, nonsteroidal anti-inflammatory drugs.

Table 273-3 Correlation between Site of Glomerular Injury and Clinicopathologic Presentation

Target of Injury	Physiologic Role	Response to Injury	Representative Glomerular Disease
Endothelial cell	Maintains glomerular perfusion	Vasoconstriction	Acute renal failure
	Prevents leukocyte adhesion	Leukocyte infiltration	Focal or diffuse proliferative GN
	Prevents platelet aggregation and clotting	Intravascular microthrombi	Thrombotic microangiopathies
Mesangial cell	Controls glomerular filtration surface area	Proliferation/increased matrix	Mesangioproliferative GN/glomerulosclerosis
Basement membrane	Prevents filtration of plasma proteins	Proteinuria	Membranous nephropathy
Visceral epithelial cell	Prevents filtration of plasma proteins	Proteinuria	Minimal change disease and FSGS
Parietal epithelial cell	Maintains Bowman's space	Crescent formation	Crescentic GN

NOTE: GN, glomerulonephritis; FSGS, focal segmental glomerulosclerosis.

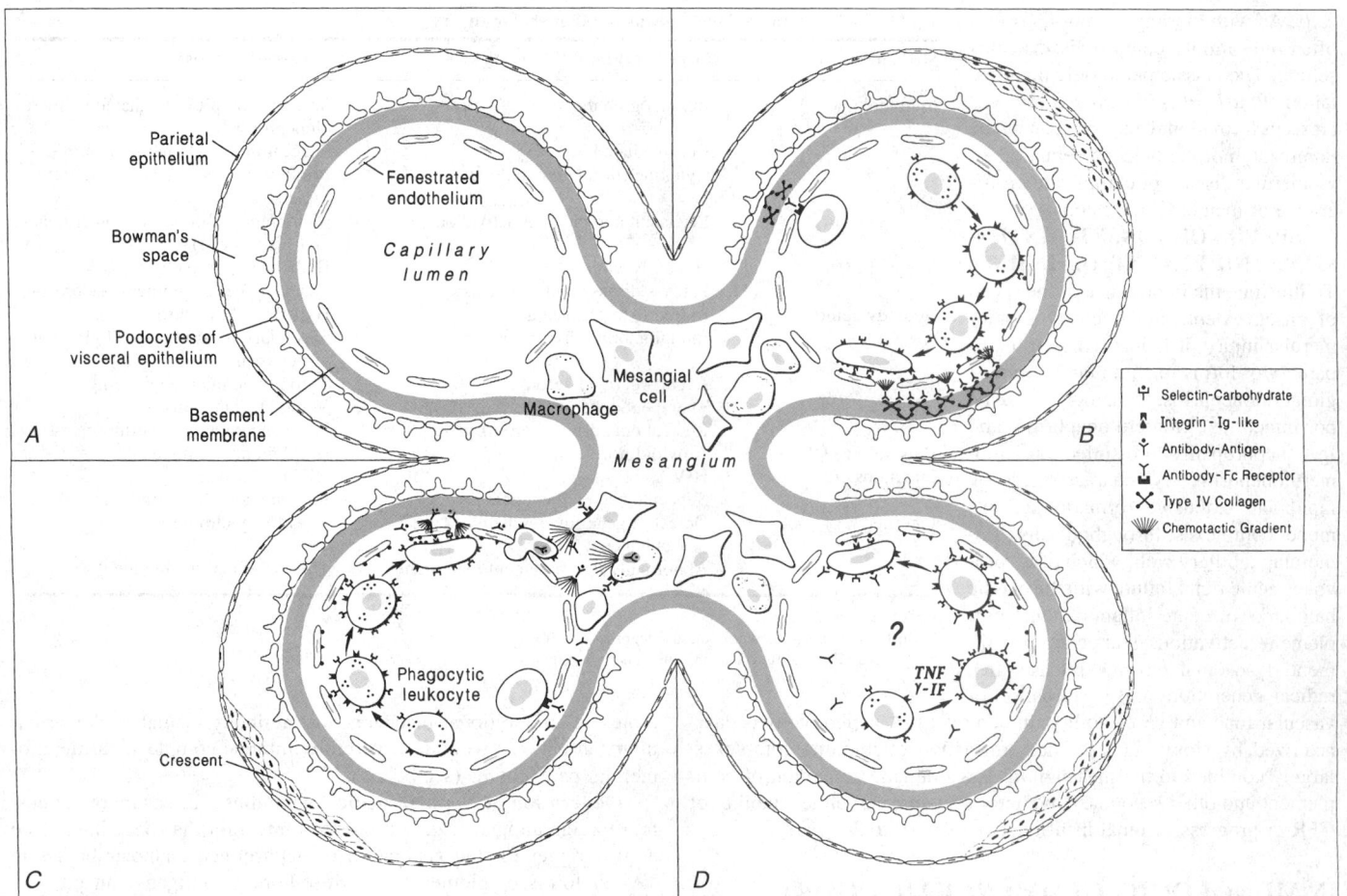

FIGURE 273-1 Major mechanisms of antibody-mediated injury in glomerulonephritis. *A.* Normal glomerulus. Key components of "healthy" glomerular capillary loop. *B.* Antiglomerular basement membrane antibody-mediated glomerulonephritis. Linear deposition of IgG against the Goodpasture antigen. The latter autoantigen is a normal constituent of the noncollagenous domain of α3 chain of type IV collagen, whose "chicken wire"–like structure is essential for maintenance of normal glomerular basement membrane architecture and function. *C.* Immune complex-mediated glomerulonephritis. Immune complexes scattered throughout the glomerular capillary wall, e.g., as can occur in lupus nephritis or postinfectious glomerulonephritis. In mechanisms *B* and *C*, leukocyte chemotaxis is triggered by complement components, chemokines, and other inflammatory mediators. Leukocyte–endothelial cell adhesion is supported by four major classes of adhesion molecules: the selectins and their diverse carbohydrate-bearing ligands, the leukocyte integrins, and immunoglobulin-like molecules such as intercellular adhesion molecule-1. Leukocytes also adhere through binding of their Fc receptors to the Fc domains of immunoglobulin. *D.* Antineutrophil cytoplasmic antibody (ANCA)-associated glomerulonephritis. In diseases such as Wegener's granulomatosis, ANCA are postulated to induce glomerular injury by interacting with neutrophil granule components that have migrated to the cell surface following priming of neutrophils by cytokines, as may occur during a prodromal viral illness. Reactivity of ANCA with neutrophil granule components in vitro triggers neutrophil activation and endothelial cell injury. This mechanism of glomerular injury remains to be established definitively in vivo, however, hence the symbol "?" in the cartoon. Crescents are formed by proliferation of parietal epithelial cells and migration of monocyte-macrophages into the glomerulus from the glomerular capillary lumen and tubulointerstitial space. As they expand, crescents compress the glomerular capillary tuft and are a rich source of mediators that further amplify the inflammatory response. TNF, tumor necrosis factor; γ-IF, interferon-γ.

Deposition of Nephritogenic Antibodies within the Glomerulus (Fig. 273-1) Anti-GBM antibody disease (p. 1583) is the classic nephritis initiated by interaction of autoantibody with intrinsic glomerular antigen. Afflicted patients have a circulating antibody directed at a 28-kDa antigen (Goodpasture antigen) located in the noncollagenous NC1 domain of the α3 chain of type IV collagen. This type of collagen is preferentially expressed in glomerular and pulmonary alveolar basement membranes. Autoantibodies against mesangial cell antigens have been detected in the serum of patients with IgA nephropathy, the most common form of glomerulonephritis in humans; however, the pathogenicity of these autoantibodies has yet to be defined. Poststreptococcal glomerulonephritis and lupus nephritis are examples of glomerulonephritides that are probably initiated by interaction of circulating antibodies with planted antigens. Several streptococcal antigens have been isolated from immune deposits of kidneys with poststreptococcal glomerulonephritis, including nephritis strain–associated antigen and a cytoplasmic protein endostreptosin. In addition, patients with poststreptococcal glomerulonephritis can have circulating antibodies against laminin, type IV collagen, and heparan sulphate proteoglycans, suggesting that molecular mimickry may also contribute. Similar findings have been reported in experimental and human lupus nephritis. Here, circulating anti-DNA antibodies may potentially induce immune complex glomerulonephritis by reacting with DNA bound to GBM or with planted DNA-histone complexes (nucleosomes). However, it should be noted that patients with systemic lupus erythematosus have a variety of circulating autoantibodies, and the pathogenetic culprit(s) in lupus nephritis have yet to be identified definitively. Cryoglobulinemia, due to chronic hepatitis C infection, is an example of glomerulonephritis initiated by trapping of immune complexes. These patients have circulating and intraglomerular immune complexes composed of hepatitis C antigens, polyclonal antihepatitis C IgG, and a second antibody, usually a monoclonal IgM, directed against the IgG. In support of the pathogenicity of circulating cryoglobulins, their injection into laboratory mice induces glomerulonephritis with many of the hallmarks of human disease.

Site of Antibody Deposition The site of antibody deposition within the glomerulus is a critical determinant of the clinicopathologic presentation. Among the factors that determine the site of deposition are the avidity, affinity, and quantity of the antibody; the size, charge, and site of the antigen; the size of the immune complexes; the efficiency of the clearance mechanisms for immune complexes; and local hemodynamic factors. Relatively anionic antigens are repelled by the GBM, which is negatively charged, and tend to be trapped in the subendothelial cell space and mesangium. In contrast, relatively cationic antigens tend to permeate the GBM and deposit within the GBM or in the subepithelial space. Acute deposition of antibody in the subendothelial cell space or mesangium typically triggers a nephritic-type response characterized by rapid recruitment of leukocytes and platelets, probably because inflammatory mediators generated at these sites are strategically positioned to activate endothelial and hematogenous cells. Inflammation is more severe when antibody is deposited in the subendothelial space, as compared with mesangium, at least in part because the mesangium abuts only 25 to 33% of the capillary wall. Antibody deposition in the subepithelial cell space typically induces a nephrotic-type response characterized by proteinuria without a pronounced inflammatory cell infiltrate, probably because the immune complexes are shielded from circulating inflammatory cells by the GBM and because the large fluid flux from blood to Bowman's space minimizes back-diffusion of inflammatory mediators towards the endothelium and vascular lumen.

Recruitment of Inflammatory Cells (Fig. 273-1) Leukocytes and platelets are important mediators of injury in most forms of acute and subacute glomerulonephritis. Immunoglobulin can provoke recruitment of leukocytes through several mechanisms. Many antibody subclasses activate the complement cascade, and complement proteins such as C3a, C5a, and C5b-9 (membrane attack complex) are potent stimuli for leukocyte recruitment, either through their direct effects on leukocytes (C3a, C5a) or by increasing endothelial cell adhesiveness for leukocytes (C5b-9). Complement-independent mechanisms also contribute. Leukocytes express Fc receptors that can directly engage the Fc portion of immunoglobulin. Resident glomerular macrophages, endothelial cells, and mesangial cells also express Fc receptors, engagement of which can trigger release of an array of inflammatory mediators and chemotactic cytokines (chemokines) that promote directed locomotion of leukocytes (chemotaxis), binding of leukocytes to inflamed endothelium through cell surface leukocyte adhesion molecules, and diapedesis of leukocytes to the extravascular space.

The mechanisms of platelet recruitment in glomerulonephritis are less well defined. Potential mechanisms include direct binding of platelet Fc receptors with immunoglobulin, and interactions of platelets with endothelium, trapped leukocytes, collagen, and other components of exposed GBM, and with products of the coagulation cascade such as fibrin.

Mediators of Glomerular Injury (Fig. 273-2) *Nephritic-type antibody-mediated glomerular injury* is a vivid example of host defense gone awry. In normal host defense, leukocytes engulf microorganisms into phagosomes, which then fuse with intracellular lysosomes. Microorganisms are destroyed within phagolysosomes through the actions of free radicals, proteolytic enzymes, and other toxic molecules. This process facilitates killing with relative protection and preservation of host tissue. When host defense is inappropriately activated in autoimmune diseases, the inciting antigens are often fixed to (planted antigens) or are a component of host tissue (autoantigen). As a result, phagocytosis is less efficient ("frustrated phagocytosis"), and there is release of toxic moieties such as oxidants and proteases into the parenchyma where they destroy host cells and matrix components. In addition, cytotoxic T lymphocytes and natural killer cells can damage resident glomerular cells by releasing toxic compounds, such as perforins, a process that is facilitated by binding of these cytotoxic cells to glomerular cells through HLA molecules, Fc portions of immunoglobulin (antibody-dependent cell cytotoxicity), and other immune recognition systems. Platelets promote nephritic injury by promoting leukocyte recruitment and intrarenal vasoconstriction and by triggering microthrombi formation. Cytokines, such as tumor necrosis factor α, interleukin 1β, and interferon γ, play a key role in the amplification and maintenance of glomerular inflammation by induc-

FIGURE 273-2 Mediator systems in acute immune complex–mediated glomerulonephritis: A paradigm of renal inflammation. Abbreviations: LTB$_4$, leukotriene B$_4$; PAF, platelet-activating factor; IL, interleukin; MCP-1, monocyte chemotactic peptide-1; TNF-α, tumor necrosis factor α; Ifγ, interferon γ; RBF, renal blood flow; GFR, glomerular filtration rate.

ing de novo synthesis of leukocyte adhesion molecules, chemokines, and other inflammatory mediators.

Leukocytes play a lesser role in *nephrotic-type antibody-mediated glomerular injury* (Chap. 274). Membranous glomerulopathy is the prototypic entity and is initiated by the formation of subepithelial immune complexes; these provoke production of "spikes" of new basement membrane that eventually encircle and incorporate the immune complexes into the GBM. The antigenic targets in human membranous glomerulopathy have not been determined but may be planted antigens or autoantigens shed from parietal epithelial cells. The frequent association with infections, malignancies, and drugs suggests involvement of planted antigens or molecular mimicry (see above); however, many cases may represent a true loss of tolerance against autoantigens. The membrane attack complex of complement (C5b-9) appears to be a major effector of injury to the glomerular filtration barrier in this setting.

CELL PROLIFERATION AND ACCUMULATION OF EXTRACELLULAR MATRIX A hallmark of the nephritic-type proliferative glomerulopathies is an increase in glomerular cell number. Initially, this hypercellularity is due predominantly to infiltration of the glomerular tuft by leukocytes. Subsequently, resident glomerular cells proliferate in response to growth factors [e.g., epidermal growth factor, platelet-derived growth factor (PDGF), thrombospondin] released into the local inflammatory milieu. The proliferating cells are typically mesangial in mesangioproliferative glomerulonephritis and both endothelial and mesangial cells in diffuse proliferative glomerulonephritis. The visceral epithelial cell is, for the most part, a terminally differentiated cell that does not proliferate rapidly, even when injured.

Whereas acute antibody-mediated glomerulonephritis typically induces acute diffuse proliferative glomerulonephritis and acute renal failure over days to weeks (nephritic syndrome), subacute immune injury often induces the formation of glomerular crescents and renal failure over weeks-to-months (termed *rapidly progressive glomerulonephritis*). As discussed above, crescents are extracapillary proliferations of cells in Bowman's space, composed of infiltrating monocytes, proliferating parietal epithelial cells, and fibrin.

Sustained low level immune complex deposition over months to years can provoke a marked increase in basement membrane or mesangial matrix production. Mild to moderate accumulation of matrix usually manifests as proteinuria due to disruption of the glomerular filtration barrier; however, in its most severe form, matrix accumulation causes glomerulosclerosis and chronic renal insufficiency.

RESOLUTION, REPAIR, AND SCARRING Glomerular inflammation can resolve with complete recovery of renal function or with a variable amount of scarring and chronic renal insufficiency. Acute poststreptococcal glomerulonephritis (p. 1582), for example, usually resolves spontaneously and fully in children, whereas adults are frequently left with residual renal impairment. The resolution process requires cessation of further antibody production and immune complex formation, removal of deposited and circulating immune complexes, inhibition of further recruitment of inflammatory cells, dissipation of the gradients of inflammatory mediators, restoration of normal endothelial adhesiveness and permeability, normalization of vascular tone, and clearance of infiltrating inflammatory cells and proliferating resident glomerular cells (Fig. 273-1).

Unfortunately, the resolution phase of most inflammatory glomerulopathies in adults terminates in some glomerular scarring. This is particularly true in patients with crescentic glomerulopathies who may be left with end-stage renal failure requiring dialysis or transplantation. Transforming growth factor (TGF) β, a cytokine, stimulates production of extracellular matrix by most glomerular cells, inhibits synthesis of tissue proteases that normally degrade matrix proteins, and is a potent stimulus for scar formation immediately following glomerular injury.

Moderate-to-severe glomerulonephritis is usually associated with a variable degree of tubulointerstitial inflammation and scarring in addition to glomerular injury. Indeed, the severity of tubulointerstitial injury usually correlates closely with long-term impairment of renal function. The pathogenesis of tubulointerstitial inflammation in this setting is unclear. Potential mechanisms include: (1) primary involvement of both the glomeruli and the tubulointerstitium in autoimmune disease; (2) induction of tubulointerstitial inflammation by mediators generated by diseased glomeruli which then diffuse into the tubulointerstitium via blood, tubular fluid, or the interstitial space; (3) injury to tubule epithelial cells by excessive filtered proteins ("protein overload" hypothesis); and (4) ischemia to areas of the tubulointerstitium downstream to areas of robust glomerular inflammation or severe glomerulosclerosis.

OTHER MECHANISMS OF ANTIBODY-MEDIATED INJURY Several other autoantibodies have been implicated as mediators of renal injury in patients with glomerulonephritis.

Antineutrophil Cytoplasmic Antibodies (ANCA) Immunoglobulin is not detected in the glomerulus in approximately 40% of patients with rapidly progressive glomerulonephritis ("pauci-immune crescentic glomerulonephritis"). The majority of these patients have Wegener's granulomatosis, microscopic polyangiitis nodosa, or renal-limited crescentic glomerulonephritis and have autoantibodies against neutrophil cytoplasmic antigens in their circulation. When reactive with ethanol-fixed neutrophils isolated from healthy volunteers, ANCA stain results in either a cytoplasmic pattern (c-ANCA) or perinuclear pattern (p-ANCA). In the case of c-ANCA, the neutrophil antigen is usually proteinase-3, a constituent of neutrophil primary granules. In the case of p-ANCA, the antigen is usually myeloperoxidase, another granule constituent that migrates to the perinuclear area upon ethanol fixation. Whereas a greater number of patients with Wegener's granulomatosis have c-ANCA and a greater proportion of patients with renal-limited disease have p-ANCA, the morphologic features, response to treatment, and overall prognosis appear to be similar in patients with either c-ANCA or p-ANCA. ANCA stimulate cytokine-primed human neutrophils to generate reactive oxygen species and injure endothelium in vitro. These findings raise the possibility that ANCA may be pathogenetic in vivo in the presence of circulating cytokines, as may occur following a prodromal infection.

Antiendothelial Cell Antibodies Circulating antibodies against endothelial antigens have been reported in several inflammatory vasculitides and glomerulonephritides. Their titers tend to correlate with disease activity, and some activate endothelial cells and increase their adhesiveness for leukocytes, suggesting a pathogenetic role.

C3 Nephritic Factor Some patients with membranoproliferative glomerulonephritis (Chap. 273) have large deposits of electron-dense material within the GBM that does not stain for immunoglobulin (dense deposit disease; membranoproliferative glomerulonephritis type II). Intriguingly, most of these patients have a circulating IgG, termed the *C3 nephritic factor*, directed at C3bBb (C3 convertase) of the alternative pathway of complement.

CELL-MEDIATED INJURY Although cell-mediated injury is, as yet, less well defined than antibody-mediated glomerular injury, T cells have also been implicated as independent mediators of glomerular injury and as modulators of the production of nephritogenic antibodies. T cells may be particularly important as initiators of injury in pauci-immune glomerulonephritis. T cells interact, through their cell-surface T cell receptor/CD3 complex, with antigens presented in the groove of major histocompatibility complex molecules of resident glomerular endothelial, mesangial, and epithelial cells, a process that is facilitated by cell-cell adhesion and costimulatory molecules. Cytokines and other mediators released by activated T cells are potent stimuli for further leukocyte recruitment, cytotoxicity, and fibrogenesis. CD4 T lymphocytes are important recruiters of macrophages and trigger clonal expansion of autoreactive B cells; they also promote glomerular cell injury by CD8 cytotoxic T lymphocytes and natural killer cells and through antibody-dependent cell cytotoxicity. Soluble factors derived from T cells have also been implicated in the pathogenesis of proteinuria in minimal change disease and primary focal segmental glomerulosclerosis. The identity and molecular characterization of these nonimmunoglobulin circulating permeability factors remain to be determined.

NONIMMUNOLOGIC GLOMERULAR INJURY

METABOLIC Diabetic Nephropathy (See also Chaps. 275 and 333) Nephropathy complicates approximately 30% of cases of type 1 and type 2 diabetes mellitus and is characterized clinically by proteinuria and progressive renal insufficiency. The typical glomerular lesion is glomerulosclerosis due to thickening of the GBM and expansion of the mesangium with extracellular matrix. Factors implicated as triggers for increased matrix production include glomerular hypertension; the direct effects of hyperglycemia on mesangial cells; advanced glycosylation end-products; growth factors such as growth hormone, insulin-like growth factor 1, and angiotensin II; cytokines such as TGF-β; hyperlipidemia; and cell sorbitol accumulation.

Complementary clinical and laboratory approaches suggest a central role for hemodynamic factors. Glomerular hydrostatic pressure and GFR increase within months of the development of hyperglycemia. The mechanism by which diabetes mellitus induces glomerular hypeptide. In this framework, glycosuria triggers increased reabsorption of glucose coupled to sodium in the proximal tubule, thereby increasing total-body sodium and extracellular fluid volume. As a compensatory response, atrial natriuretic peptide is released from cardiac myocytes and induces natriuresis in part by triggering afferent arteriolar dilatation and thereby increasing intraglomerular pressure and GFR. Whereas this compensatory response is appropriate in the short term, sustained glomerular hypertension provokes thickening of the GBM, increased mesangial matrix production, and glomerulosclerosis and disruption of barrier function. In keeping with a central role for intraglomerular pressure in the pathogenesis of diabetic nephropathy, angiotensin-converting enzyme inhibitors, which lower intraglomerular pressure, slow the progression of diabetic nephropathy, even in normotensive patients. It remains to be determined why diabetes mellitus and glomerular hypertension include glomerulosclerosis in some but not all individuals. Epidemiologic studies and studies of disease concordance in identical twins suggest that important, but as yet unidentified, genetic factors may play a role. It is likely that hemodynamic and metabolic factors act in concert to generate the final glomerulosclerotic phenotype in genetically predisposed patients.

Other Metabolic Diseases Several rare inherited lysosomal enzyme defects induce focal segmental glomerulosclerosis, probably by allowing accumulation of toxic metabolites in renal cells. *Fabry's disease* (α-galactosidase deficiency; Chap. 349) and *sialidosis* (N-acetylneuraminic acid hydrolase deficiency; Chap. 349) are the major culprits in this regard. Both tend to induce focal segmental or global glomerulosclerosis by preferentially affecting visceral epithelial cells, probably because these are terminally differentiated cells with a very slow replication rate. *Partial lipodystrophy* is a rare metabolic disorder characterized by lipoatrophy affecting the arms, neck, and chest, often with redistribution of fat to the hips and legs. Approximately one-third of patients develop glomerular disease, usually type II membranoproliferative glomerulopathy (dense deposit disease; Chap. 274).

HEMODYNAMIC GLOMERULAR INJURY High intraglomerular pressure is a major cause of glomerular injury in humans and can result from systemic hypertension or a local change in glomerular hemodynamics (glomerular hypertension).

Systemic Hypertension (See also Chap. 246) Although the kidneys have evolved sophisticated mechanisms for autoregulating glomerular blood flow and pressure, marked or sustained increments in systemic blood pressure can overwhelm these compensatory systems and perturb glomerular morphology and function. In its most dramatic form, namely malignant hypertension, hemodynamic stress causes massive fibrinoid necrosis of afferent arterioles and glomeruli, thrombotic microangiopathy, acute renal failure, and a nephritic urinary sediment. Chronic sustained hypertension typically leads to arteriolar vasoconstriction and sclerosis, which, in turn, cause secondary atrophy and sclerosis of glomeruli and the tubulointerstitium. A variety of molecular signals appear to couple elevations in intravascular pressure to myointimal proliferation and eventually sclerosis of the vessel wall. These include growth factors such as angiotensin II, epidermal growth factor, and PDGF; cytokines such as TGF-β; and activation of stretch activated ion channels and early response genes.

Glomerular Hypertension The pathophysiology of diabetic nephropathy, discussed above, illustrates the importance of intraglomerular pressure as a stimulus for mesangial matrix production and glomerulosclerosis. Glomerular hypertension is also a key factor in the pathogenesis of the progressive glomerulosclerosis and renal failure that complicate the adaptive response of remnant nephrons to increased workload following loss of the other nephrons from any cause, including chronic allograft failure (see below). Importantly, these changes in glomerular hemodynamics and pressure appear to precede the development of systemic hypertension and are independent risk factors for glomerular injury.

TOXIC GLOMERULOPATHIES The renal microvasculature is a relatively uncommon site for toxic injury, by comparison with the tubular interstitium; however, there are a few important exceptions.

Verotoxin, derived from *Escherichia coli* during bouts of infective diarrhea, is directly toxic to renal endothelium and induces the hemolytic-uremic syndrome. In this setting, verotoxin interacts with a specific cell membrane receptor, perturbs the antithrombotic phenotype of endothelium, and triggers the development of thrombotic microangiopathy. Irradiation, mitomycin, cyclosporine, and anovulants can also induce thrombotic microangiopathy through poorly defined mechanisms. Nonsteroidal anti-inflammatory drugs, rifampin, ampicillin, and interferon-α can induce an unusual combination of acute renal failure with nephrotic syndrome. The characteristic pathologic correlates of this syndrome are allergic interstitial nephritis and fusion of the foot processes of the visceral epithelial cells, the latter accounting for the marked proteinuria. How these structurally diverse agents induce epithelial cell injury is unclear.

DEPOSITION DISEASES The glomerular deposition diseases are a group of diverse conditions in which abnormal proteins are deposited in glomeruli, where they provoke an inflammatory reaction and/or glomerulosclerosis. The major glomerular deposition diseases are cryoglobulinemia, amyloidosis, light and heavy chain deposition disease, and fibrillary/immunotactoid glomerulopathy. *Cryoglobulins* (Chap. 317) are immunoglobulins that precipitate in the cold and can be composed of either monoclonal immunoglobulin, usually generated by a lymphoproliferative malignancy (type I); a mixture of polyclonal immunoglobulin (usually IgG) and monoclonal immunoglobulin (usually IgM) directed to epitopes on polyclonal IgG (type II); or a mixture of polyclonal antibodies, one or more having anti-IgG activity (type III). As discussed above, cryoglobulins can induce nephritic-type and nephrotic-type injury depending on the rapidity, severity, and site of immunoglobulin deposition. Most cryoglobulinemic glomerulopathy is associated with type II cryoglobulins, the majority of which are now recognized to be triggered by chronic hepatitis B or C infection. *Glomerular amyloidosis* (Chaps. 275 and 319) is one of the five most common causes of nephrotic syndrome in adults and is characterized by extracellular deposition of amyloid fibrils composed, in part, of fragments of immunoglobulin light chains (AL amyloid) or serum amyloid A, the acute-phase reactant (AA amyloid). In light chain deposition diseases, intact immunoglobulin light chains, usually kappa, are deposited in a granular, rather than fibrillary, pattern. The composition of the deposits in *fibrillary/immunotactoid glomerulopathy* is still being defined and may also include immunoglobulin and/or fibronectin-containing cryoglobulins. These different types of deposits, in addition to directly disrupting glomerular architecture, provoke mesangial matrix production and glomerulosclerosis. Fibrillary/immunotactoid glomerulopathy can also present as acute or subacute glomerular inflammation. How these diverse deposits trigger glomerular matrix production and recruitment of inflammatory cells has yet to be determined.

INFECTIOUS CAUSES OF GLOMERULAR DISEASE Infectious organisms can induce glomerular disease through several different mechanisms: (1) by direct infection of renal cells, (2) by elaborating nephrotoxins such as *E. coli*–derived verotoxin, (3) by inciting intraglomerular deposition of immune complexes (e.g., postinfectious glomerulonephritis) or cryoglobulins (e.g., hepatitis B or C), and (4) by providing a chronic stimulus for amyloid fibril formation, as in AA amyloidosis. Direct infection of glomerular cells is a relatively rare mechanism of injury but has been implicated in the pathogenesis of nephropathy associated with HIV. This entity is characterized histologically by an aggressive form of focal segmental glomerulosclerosis, microcystic tubular dilatation, and interstitial fibrosis. Viral genome and several proteins have been detected in glomerular and tubular cells in this disease, and infection of glomerular cells induces expression of TGF-β, a major stimulus for mesangial matrix production and sclerosis.

INHERITED GLOMERULAR DISEASES *Alport's syndrome* (hereditary nephritis; Chap. 275), the prototypical inherited glomerular disease, is usually transmitted as an X-linked dominant trait, although autosomal recessive forms have been reported. Patients afflicted with the classic X-linked form have a mutation in the COL4A5 gene that encodes the $\alpha5$ chain of type IV collagen located on the X chromosome. As a result, the GBM is irregular with longitudinal layering, splitting, or thickening, and patients develop hematuria, progressive glomerulosclerosis, and renal failure. *Thin basement membrane disease* is another relatively common disorder of the GBM. In contrast to Alport's syndrome, this entity is usually inherited as an autosomal dominant or recessive trait and appears to be relatively benign. As the name suggests, the basement membrane is thin but otherwise ultrastructurally normal. Patients typically experience recurrent benign hematuria. The molecular basis for thin basement membrane disease has yet to be elucidated fully; however, defects in the gene encoding the $\alpha4$ chain of type IV collagen have been reported in some families. Rarer hereditary glomerular diseases include *nail-patella syndrome* (osteoonychodysplasia), which is associated with a relatively benign mottling of the basement membrane with lucent rarefractions; *partial lipodystrophy*, which is associated with type II membranoproliferative glomerulonephritis (dense deposit disease); and *familial lecithin–cholesterol acyltransferase deficiency*, which is associated with distortion of the basement membrane by irregular rounded lucent zones, increased mesangial matrix production, and progressive sclerosis and renal insufficiency.

GLOMERULAR ADAPTATION TO NEPHRON LOSS

Nephron loss, from any cause, is followed by compensatory hyperfiltration in the remaining functional glomeruli. This adaptive response is appropriate in the short-term and maintains GFR. Over years, however, the hyperfiltering remnant nephrons develop focal and segmental glomerulosclerosis, and eventually global sclerosis, that manifests clinically as proteinuria, hypertension, and progressive renal insufficiency. Sustained glomerular capillary hypertension has been implicated as a major stimulus for glomerulosclerosis in this setting. Increased glomerular blood flow and ultrafiltration pressure are early findings in remnant nephrons in most experimental models in which the function of more than 50% of nephron mass has been lost through surgical ablation, immunologic or toxic injury, or other mechanisms. Sustained glomerular hypertension is thought to stimulate the accumulation of extracellular matrix by perturbing the function of visceral epithelial and mesangial cells, either directly or by increasing the flux of circulating macromolecules through the glomerular capillary wall. As with most forms of glomerulosclerosis, TGF-β may be an important regulator of matrix accumulation in remnant nephrons. Angiotensin II, PDGF, and endothelins are other potential modulators of this process. Maneuvers that lower intraglomerular pressure, such as lowprotein diet or treatment with angiotensin-converting enzyme inhibitors, slow the development of glomerulosclerosis and renal failure. Glomerular hypertrophy, intracapillary microthrombi, recruited macrophages, and hyperlipidemia are other potential stimuli for glomerulosclerosis. Indeed, glomerular capillary hypertension and hypertrophy appear to be independent risk factors that could act synergistically to cause progressive renal insufficiency. Intriguingly, angiotensin II may trigger TGF-β production in remnant nephrons, suggesting that angiotensin-converting enzyme inhibitors may be renoprotective through complementary effects on glomerular hemodynamics and matrix production.

BIBLIOGRAPHY

APPEL G, RISHNAM JR: Secondary glomerular diseases, in *Brenner & Rector's The Kidney*, 6th ed, BM Brenner (ed). Philadelphia, Saunders, 2000, pp 1350–1448

BRADY HR: Leukocyte adhesion molecules and kidney diseases. Kidney Int 45:1285, 1994

BERDEN JH: Lupus nephritis. Kidney Int 52:538, 1997

FALK R et al: Primary glomerular diseases, in *Brenner & Rector's The Kidney*, 6th ed, BM Brenner (ed). Philadelphia, Saunders, 2000, pp 1263–1349

HOFFMAN GS, SPECKS U: Antineutrophil cytoplasmic antibodies. Arthritis Rheum 41: 1521, 1998

HOLDSWORTH SR et al: Th1 and Th2 T helper cell subsets affect patterns of injury and outcomes in glomerulonephritis. Kidney Int 55:1198, 1999

KASHTAN CE: Alport syndrome and thin glomerular basement membrane disease. J Am Soc Nephrol 9:1736, 1998

KELLY PT, HAPONIK EF: Goodpasture's syndrome: Molecular and clinical advances. Medicine (Baltimore) 73:171, 1994

KITAMURA M, FINE LH: The concept of glomerular self-defense. Kidney Int 55:1639, 1999

KROWLEWSKI AS: Genetics of diabetic nephropathy: Evidence for major and minor gene effects. Kidney Int 55:1582, 1999

MACKENZIE HS et al: Adaptation to nephron loss, in *Brenner & Rector's The Kidney*, 6th ed, BM Brenner (ed). Philadelphia, Saunders, 2000, pp 1901–1942

SAVIN NJ et al: Circulating factor associated with increased glomerular permeability to albumin in recurrent focal segmental glomerulosclerosis. N Engl J Med 334:878, 1996

STEHMAN-BREEN C, JOHNSON RJ: Hepatitis C virus–associated glomerulonephritis. Adv Intern Med 43:79, 1998

274   Hugh R. Brady, Yvonne M. O'Meara, Barry M. Brenner

THE MAJOR GLOMERULOPATHIES

ACE angiotensin-converting enzyme	MPGN membranoproliferative glomerulonephritis
ANCA antineutrophil cytoplasmic antibody	NSAIDs nonsteroidal anti-inflammatory drugs
ESRD end-stage renal disease	PAS periodic acid–Schiff
FSGS focal and segmental glomerulosclerosis	RPGN rapidly progressive glomerulonephritis
GBM glomerular basement membrane	SLE systemic lupus erythematosus
GFR glomerular filtration rate	TBM thin basement membrane
MCD minimal change disease	

Glomerular injury can arise from diverse renal-limited and systemic diseases and is the major cause of end-stage renal disease (ESRD) requiring dialysis and transplantation. In this chapter, we describe the epidemiology, clinical presentations, pathology, and treatment of the major glomerulopathies. We focus on the *primary glomerulopathies*, glomerular diseases in which the pathologic process is confined to the kidney and in which systemic features are a direct consequence of impaired glomerular filtration (e.g., hypervolemia, hypertension, uremic syndrome). Considered here are the five major clinical presentations of glomerulopathy: acute nephritic syndrome, rapidly progressive glomerulonephritis (RPGN), nephrotic syndrome, asymptomatic abnormalities of the urinary sediment (hematuria, proteinuria), and chronic glomerulonephritis. →*Glomerulopathies associated with systemic diseases (secondary glomerulopathies) are discussed in Chap. 275. The nomenclature pertaining to the classification and clinicopathologic description of glomerular disease and the pathogenetic mechanisms of glomerular injury are reviewed in Chap. 273.*

ACUTE NEPHRITIC SYNDROME AND RAPIDLY PROGRESSIVE GLOMERULONEPHRITIS

CLINICAL FEATURES AND CLINICOPATHOLOGIC CORRELATES   The *acute nephritic syndrome* is the clinical correlate of acute glomerular inflammation. In its most dramatic form, the acute nephritic syndrome is characterized by sudden onset (i.e., over days to weeks) of *acute renal failure* and *oliguria* (<400 mL of urine per day). Renal blood flow and glomerular filtration rate (GFR) fall as a result of obstruction of the glomerular capillary lumen by infiltrating inflammatory cells and proliferating resident glomerular cells. Renal blood flow and GFR are further compromised by intrarenal vasoconstriction and mesangial cell contraction that result from local imbalances of vasoconstrictor (e.g., leukotrienes, platelet-activating factor, thromboxanes, endothelins) and vaso-dilator substances (e.g., nitric oxide, prostacyclin) within the renal microcirculation. *Extracellular fluid volume expansion, edema,* and *hypertension* develop because of impaired GFR and enhanced tubular reabsorption of salt and water. As a result of injury to the glomerular capillary wall, urinalysis typically reveals *red blood cell casts,* dysmorphic red blood cells, leukocytes, and subnephrotic proteinuria of <3.5 g per 24 h ("nephritic urinary sediment"). *Hematuria* is often macroscopic.

The classic pathologic correlate of the nephritic syndrome is *proliferative glomerulonephritis.* The proliferation of glomerular cells is due initially to infiltration of the glomerular tuft by neutrophils and monocytes and subsequently to proliferation of resident glomerular endothelial and mesangial cells (endocapillary proliferation). In its most severe form, the nephritic syndrome is associated with acute inflammation of most glomeruli, i.e., *acute diffuse proliferative glomerulonephritis.* When less vigorous, fewer than 50% of glomeruli may be involved, i.e., *focal proliferative glomerulonephritis.* In milder forms of nephritic injury, cellular proliferation may be confined to the mesangium, i.e., *mesangioproliferative glomerulonephritis.*

RPGN is the clinical correlate of more *subacute glomerular inflammation.* Patients develop renal failure over weeks to months in association with a nephritic urinary sediment, subnephrotic proteinuria and variable oliguria, hypervolemia, edema, and hypertension. The classic pathologic correlate of RPGN is crescent formation involving most glomeruli (*crescentic glomerulonephritis*), crescents being half-moon-shaped lesions in Bowman's space composed of proliferating parietal epithelial cells and infiltrating monocytes (*extracapillary proliferation*). In practice, the clinical term *rapidly progressive glomerulonephritis* and the pathologic term *crescentic glomerulonephritis* are often used interchangeably. In addition to classic crescentic glomerulonephritis, in which crescents dominate the glomerular pathology, crescents can also develop concomitantly with proliferative glomerulonephritis or as a complication of membranous glomerulopathy and other more indolent forms of glomerular inflammation.

The acute nephritic syndrome and RPGN are part of a spectrum of presentations of immunologically mediated proliferative glomerulonephritis. Studies of experimental models suggest that nephritic syndrome and diffuse proliferative glomerulonephritis represent an acute immune response to a sudden large antigen load, whereas RPGN and crescentic glomerulonephritis represent a more subacute immune response to a smaller antigen load in presensitized individuals. At the other end of the spectrum, chronic low-grade immune injury presents with slowly progressive renal insufficiency or asymptomatic hematuria in association with focal proliferative or mesangioproliferative glomerulonephritis. These more indolent forms of immune-mediated glomerulonephritis are discussed later in this chapter.

ETIOLOGY AND DIFFERENTIAL DIAGNOSIS Acute nephritic syndrome and RPGN can result from renal-limited *primary* glomerulopathy or from *secondary* glomerulopathy complicating sys-

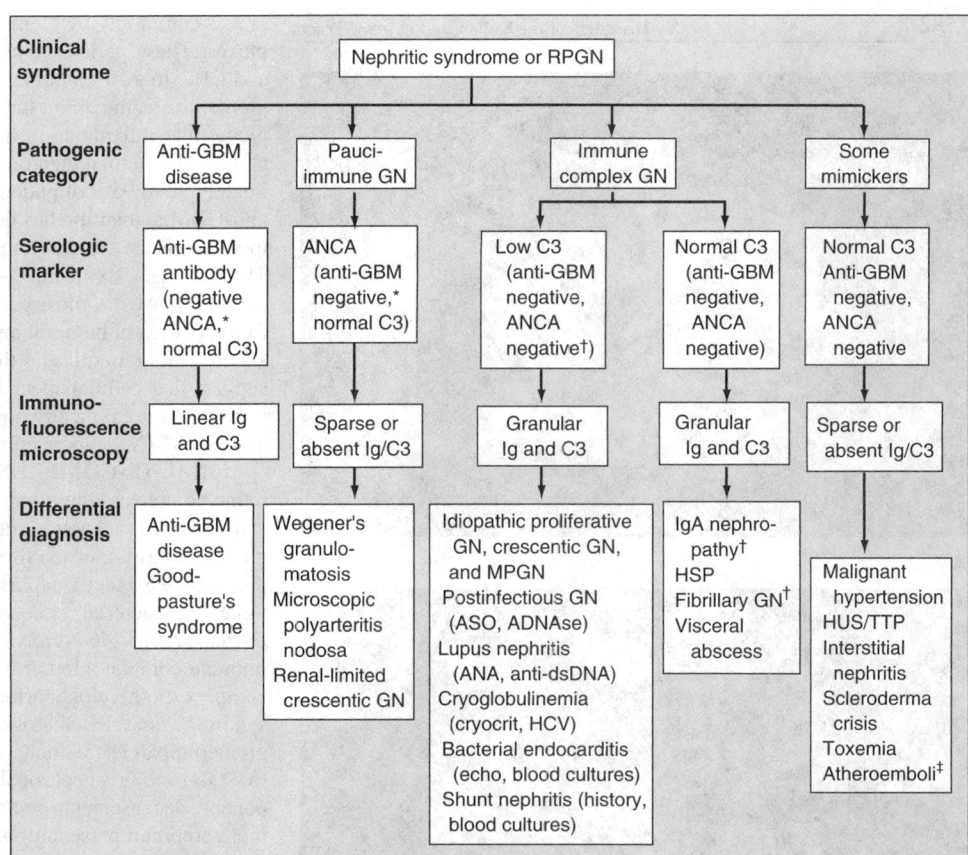

FIGURE 274-1 Differential diagnosis of nephritic syndrome and rapidly progressive glomerulonephritis.

Abbreviations: GN, glomerulonephritis; RPGN, rapidly progressive glomerulonephritis; MPGN, membranoproliferative glomerulonephritis; GBM, glomerular basement membrane; ANCA, antineutrophil cytoplasmic antibodies; Ig, immunoglobulin; C3, third component of complement; ASO, antistreptolysin O antibody titer; ADNAse, anti-deoxyribonuclease antibody titer; ANA, antinuclear antibody; anti-dsDNA, anti-double-stranded DNA antibody; HCV, hepatitis C virus; echo, echocardiogram; HSP, Henoch-Schönlein purpura; HUS, hemolytic-uremic syndrome; TTP, thrombotic thrombocytopenic purpura.

*Approximately 20% of patients with anti-GBM disease have ANCA, which may portend a better prognosis.
†Nephritic syndrome and RPGN are unusual presentations of IgA nephropathy and fibrillary GN.
‡Atheroembolic renal disease may cause transient hypocomplementemia.

temic disease. Figure 274-1 highlights the histopathologic and serologic features that help distinguish among the major causes of nephritic syndrome and RPGN (see also Fig. 274-2). In general, rapid diagnosis and prompt treatment are critical to avoid the development of irreversible renal failure. Renal biopsy remains the "gold standard" for diagnosis. *Immunofluorescence microscopy* is particularly helpful and identifies three major patterns of deposition of immunoglobulin that define three broad diagnostic categories: (1) *granular* deposits of immunoglobulin, a hallmark of *immune-complex glomerulonephritis*; (2) *linear* deposition of immunoglobulin along the glomerular basement membrane (GBM), characteristic of anti-GBM disease; and (3) paucity or absence of immunoglobulin, so-called *pauci-immune glomerulonephritis* (Figs. 273-1 and 274-2). Most patients (>70%) with full-blown acute nephritic syndrome have immune-complex glomerulonephritis. Pauci-immune glomerulonephritis is less common in this setting (<30%) and anti-GBM disease is rare (<1%). Among patients with RPGN, immune-complex glomerulonephritis and pauci-immune glomerulonephritis are equally prevalent (~45% each), whereas anti-GBM disease again accounts for a minority of cases (<10%).

Three *serologic markers* often predict the immunofluorescence microscopy findings in nephritic syndrome and RPGN and may obviate the need for renal biopsy in classic cases. They are the serum C3 level and titers of anti-GBM antibody and antineutrophil cytoplasmic antibody (ANCA) (Fig. 274-1). As discussed in Chap. 273, the kidney is host to immune attack in immune-complex glomerulonephritis, most cases being initiated either by in situ formation of immune complexes

FIGURE 274-2   Typical findings on immunofluorescence microscopy of renal biopsy specimens from patients with anti-glomerular basement membrane antibody disease, immune-complex–mediated glomerulonephritis, and pauci-immune glomerulonephritis. Specimens in the upper and middle panels were stained for immunoglobulin and show the classical linear "ribbon-like" pattern of anti-GBM disease (*A*) and granular pattern of immune-complex–mediated glomerulonephritis (*B*). Immunoglobulin is sparse or absent in patients with pauci-immune glomerulonephritis (not shown); however, abundant fibrin is detected in crescents (*C*). *(Micrographs courtesy of Dr. Helmut Rennke).*

or less commonly by glomerular trapping of circulating immune complexes. These patients typically have hypocomplementemia (low C3 and CH_{50} in 90%) and negative anti-GBM and ANCA serology. The glomerulus is the direct target of immune attack in anti-GBM disease, glomerular inflammation being initiated by an autoantibody directed at a 28-kDa autoantigen on the $\alpha 3$ chain of type IV collagen. Approximately 90 to 95% of patients with anti-GBM disease have circulating anti-GBM autoantibodies detectable by immunoassay; serum complement levels are typically normal, and ANCA are usually not detected. The pathogenesis of pauci-immune glomerulonephritis is still being defined; however, most patients have circulating ANCA, implicating dysregulation of humoral immunity. The presence of mononuclear leukocytes in glomeruli and the paucity of glomerular immune deposits suggest that cellular mechanisms are also involved. Serum complement levels are typically normal, and anti-GBM titers are usually negative in ANCA-associated renal disease.

IMMUNE-COMPLEX   GLOMERULONEPHRITIS   Immune-complex glomerulonephritis may (1) be idiopathic, (2) represent a response to a known antigenic stimulus (e.g., postinfectious glomerulonephritis), or (3) form part of a multisystem immune-complex disorder (e.g., lupus nephritis, Henoch-Schönlein purpura, cryoglobulinemia, bacterial endocarditis; Fig. 274-1). Here, we focus on *postinfectious glomerulonephritis*, the best characterized *primary* immune-complex glomerulonephritis. The major *secondary* immune-complex glomerulonephritides are discussed in Chap. 275. Nephritic syndrome and RPGN occasionally complicate two other primary glomerulopathies, namely, membranoproliferative glomerulonephritis (MPGN) and IgA nephropathy when there is a florid proliferative component. Because nephrotic syndrome and asymptomatic hematuria are more common presentations of MPGN and IgA nephropathy, respectively, these glomerulopathies are discussed in later sections on nephrotic syndrome and asymptomatic urinary abnormalities.

POSTSTREPTOCOCCAL   GLOMERULONEPHRITIS
This is the prototypical postinfectious glomerulonephritis and a leading cause of acute nephritic syndrome. Most cases are sporadic, though the disease can occur as an epidemic. Glomerulonephritis develops, on average, 10 days after pharyngitis or 2 weeks after a skin infection (impetigo) with a nephritogenic strain of group A β-hemolytic streptococcus. The known nephritic strains include M types 1, 2, 4, 12, 18, 25, 49, 55, 57, and 60. Immunity to these strains is type-specific and long-lasting, and repeated infection and nephritis are rare. Epidemic poststreptococcal glomerulonephritis is most commonly encountered in children of 2 to 6 years of age with pharyngitis during the winter months. This entity appears to be decreasing in frequency, possibly due to more widespread and prompt use of antibiotics. Poststreptococcal glomerulonephritis in association with cutaneous infections usually occurs in a setting of poor personal hygiene or streptococcal superinfection of another skin disease.

The classic clinical presentation of poststreptococcal glomerulonephritis is full-blown nephritic syndrome with oliguric acute renal failure; however, most patients have milder disease. Indeed, subclinical cases outnumber overt cases by four- to tenfold during epidemics. Patients with overt disease present with gross hematuria (red or "smoky" urine), headache, and generalized symptoms such as anorexia, nausea, vomiting, and malaise. Swelling of the renal capsule can cause flank or back pain. Physical examination reveals hypervolemia, edema, and hypertension. The urinary sediment is nephritic, with dysmorphic red blood cells, red cell casts, leukocytes, occasionally leukocyte casts, and subnephrotic proteinuria. Fewer than 5% of patients develop nephrotic-range proteinuria. The latter may only manifest as acute nephritis resolves and renal blood flow and GFR recover. Coexistent rheumatic fever is extremely rare.

The serum creatinine is often mildly elevated at presentation. Serum C3 levels and CH_{50} are depressed within 2 weeks in ~90% of cases. C4 levels are characteristically normal, indicating activation of the alternate pathway of complement. Complement levels usually return to normal within 6 to 8 weeks. Persistently depressed levels after this period should suggest another cause, such as the presence of a C3 nephritic factor (see "Membranoproliferative Glomerulonephritis"). The majority of patients (>75%) have transient hypergammaglobulinemia and mixed cryoglobulinemia. The antecedent streptococcal infection may still be evident or may have resolved either spontaneously or in response to antibiotic therapy. Most patients (>90%) have circulating antibodies against streptococcal exoenzymes such as anti-streptolysin O (ASO), anti-deoxyribonuclease B (anti-DNAse B), antistreptokinase (ASKase), anti-nicotinyl adenine dinucleotidase (anti-NADase), and antihyaluronidase (AHase). ASO, anti-DNAse B, anti-NAD, and AHase are most useful after pharyngeal infection, whereas anti-DNAse B and AHase are more sensitive indices of streptococcal skin infection. Antibody titers tend to rise after 7 days, peak after 1 month, and return to normal levels after 3 to 4 months. These tests are relatively specific, with a false-positive rate of <5%. Early antibiotic therapy may prevent the development of an antibody response.

Acute poststreptococcal glomerulonephritis is usually diagnosed on clinical and serologic grounds, without resort to renal biopsy, especially in children with a typical antecedent history. The characteristic lesion on light microscopy is diffuse proliferative glomerulonephritis. Crescents are uncommon, and extraglomerular involvement is usually mild. Immunofluorescence microscopy reveals diffuse granular deposition of IgG and C3, giving rise to a "starry sky" appearance (Fig. 274-2). More extensive immunoglobulin deposition throughout the glomerular capillary wall ("garland pattern") is associated with a worse prognosis. The characteristic finding on electron microscopy is the presence of large electron-dense immune deposits in the subendothelial, subepithelial, and mesangial areas. The acute inflammatory reaction is initiated, in large part, by the subendothelial and mesangial deposits, which activate complement and trigger leukocyte recruitment and glomerular injury. Subepithelial deposits are often more prominent on electron microscopy, however, probably because the subendothelial and mesangial deposits are scavenged more efficiently by invading phagocytes. Extensive subepithelial immune deposits, or "humps," tend to be associated with worse proteinuria, being juxtaposed to the glomerular filtration barrier for protein. →*The pathogenesis of immune-complex glomerulonephritis is discussed extensively in Chap. 273.*

In addition to poststreptococcal glomerulonephritis, the nephritic syndrome and RPGN can complicate acute immune-complex glomerulonephritis due to other viral, bacterial, fungal, and parasitic infections. Several warrant specific mention. Diffuse proliferative immune-complex glomerulonephritis is a well-described complication of acute and subacute bacterial endocarditis and is usually associated with hypocomplementemia. The glomerular lesion typically resolves following eradication of the cardiac infection. *Shunt nephritis* is a syndrome characterized by immune-complex glomerulonephritis secondary to infection of ventriculoatrial shunts inserted for treatment of childhood hydrocephalus. The most common offending organism is coagulase-negative staphylococcus. Renal impairment is usually mild and associated with hypocomplementemia. Nephrotic syndrome complicates 30% of cases. Acute proliferative glomerulonephritis can also complicate *chronic suppurative infections* and *visceral abscesses*. Patients typically present with a fever of unknown origin and an active urine sediment. Although immune deposits containing IgG and C3 are detected on renal biopsy, serum complement levels are usually normal.

℞ **TREATMENT** Treatment of poststreptococcal glomerulonephritis focuses on eliminating the streptococcal infection with antibiotics and providing supportive therapy until spontaneous resolution of glomerular inflammation occurs. Patients are usually confined to bed during the acute inflammatory phase. Diuretics and antihypertensive agents are employed to control extracellular fluid volume and blood pressure. Dialysis is rarely needed to control hypervolemia or the uremic syndrome. Poststreptococcal glomerulonephritis carries an excellent prognosis and rarely causes ESRD. Microscopic hematuria may persist for as long as 1 year after the acute episode but eventually

resolves. Whereas complete recovery is the rule in children, adults may occasionally be left with residual renal impairment.

Antiglomerular Basement Membrane Disease Anti-GBM disease is an autoimmune disease in which autoantibodies directed against type IV collagen induce RPGN and crescentic glomerulonephritis (Figs. 273-1, 274-1, and 274-2). Acute nephritic syndrome is rare. Between 50 and 70% of patients have lung hemorrhage; the clinical complex of anti-GBM nephritis and lung hemorrhage is referred to as *Goodpasture's syndrome*. Anti-GBM disease is a rare disorder of unknown etiology with an annual incidence of 0.5 per million. There is a bimodal peak in incidence. Patients with Goodpasture's syndrome are typically young males (5 to 40 years; male-female ratio of 6:1). In contrast, patients presenting during the second peak in the sixth decade rarely suffer lung hemorrhage and have an almost equal sex distribution. The target antigen is a component of the noncollagenous (NCl) domain of the $\alpha 3$ chain of type IV collagen, the $\alpha 3$ chain being preferentially expressed in glomerular and pulmonary alveolar basement membrane. The trigger(s) for loss of self-tolerance to this Goodpasture antigen has not been well defined. A genetic predisposition is suggested by an association with HLA-DRw2 and occasional occurrence in identical twins. Patients with lung hemorrhage are more likely to be cigarette smokers and to have suffered a recent upper respiratory tract infection or exposure to volatile hydrocarbon solvents. These observations suggest that diverse insults to the alveolar basement membrane may render previously sequestered Goodpasture antigens available for interaction with circulating autoantibodies. It is not clear whether environmental factors also trigger the onset of nephritis. Binding of anti-GBM antibodies to the GBM induces activation of complement, leukocyte recruitment, necrotizing proliferative glomerulonephritis, disruption of the glomerular capillary wall, leakage of fibrin into Bowman's space, and crescent formation (Chap. 273). A similar sequence of events in the lung leads to disruption of the alveolar capillary wall and pulmonary hemorrhage.

Anti-GBM disease commonly presents with hematuria, nephritic urinary sediment, subnephrotic proteinuria, and rapidly progressive renal failure over weeks, with or without pulmonary hemorrhage. When pulmonary hemorrhage occurs, it usually predates nephritis by weeks or months. Hemoptysis can vary from fluffy pulmonary infiltrates on chest x-ray and mild dyspnea on exertion to life-threatening pulmonary hemorrhage. Hypertension is unusual and occurs in fewer than 20% of cases.

The diagnostic serologic marker is circulating anti-GBM antibodies with a specificity for the NCl domain of the $\alpha 3$ chain of type IV collagen (Fig. 274-1). Anti-GBM antibodies are detected in the serum of >90% of patients with anti-GBM nephritis by specific immunoassay. If immunoassays are not available, circulating anti-GBM antibodies can be detected in 60 to 80% of patients by indirect immunofluorescence, i.e., by incubating the patient's serum with stored sections of normal human kidneys. Complement levels are normal. About 20% of patients have low titers of ANCA, usually a perinuclear ANCA (Chap. 275), the pathophysiologic significance of which is unclear. Occasional patients have a positive cytoplasmic ANCA, which may signal the presence of coexistent extraglomerular renal vasculitis. Patients with lung involvement frequently have microcytic, hypochromic, iron-deficiency anemia from alveolar hemorrhage, and abnormal bilateral hilar and basilar interstitial shadowing on chest x-ray that may be difficult to distinguish from pulmonary edema or infection. The diffusion capacity for carbon dioxide is a useful tool for distinguishing among the latter diagnoses, being increased in patients with lung hemorrhage due to uptake of carbon monoxide by alveolar blood, and reduced in patients with infection or pulmonary edema.

Renal biopsy is the gold standard for diagnosis of anti-GBM nephritis. The typical morphologic pattern on light microscopy is diffuse proliferative glomerulonephritis, with focal necrotizing lesions and crescents in >50% of glomeruli (crescentic glomerulonephritis). Immunofluorescence microscopy reveals linear ribbon-like deposition of IgG along the GBM (Fig. 274-2). C3 is present in the same distribution in 70% of patients. Prominent IgG deposition along the tubule basement membrane and tubulointerstitial inflammation is found occasionally. Electron microscopy reveals nonspecific inflammatory changes without immune deposits. Typical features on lung biopsy include alveolar hemorrhage, disruption of alveolar septa, hemosiderin-laden macrophages, and linear staining of IgG along the alveolar capillary basement membrane.

It should be noted that Goodpasture's syndrome is not the only cause of the pulmonary-renal syndrome (i.e., renal failure and lung hemorrhage). Other important causes of this clinical complex include severe cardiac failure complicated by pulmonary edema (often blood-tinged) and prerenal azotemia; renal failure from any cause complicated by hypervolemia and pulmonary edema; immune complex–mediated vasculitides such as systemic lupus erythematosus (SLE), Henoch-Schönlein purpura, and cryoglobulinemia; pauci-immune vasculitides such as Wegener's granulomatosis and polyarteritis nodosa; infections such as Legionnaire's disease; and renal vein thrombosis with pulmonary embolism. In general, these disorders can be differentiated by astute analysis of the clinical, serologic, and histopathologic findings.

℞ **TREATMENT**   Prior to the introduction of immunosuppressive therapy, greater than 80% of patients with anti-GBM nephritis developed ESRD within 1 year, and many patients died from pulmonary hemorrhage or complications of uremia. With early and aggressive use of plasmapheresis, glucocorticoids, cyclophosphamide, and azathioprine, renal and patient survival have improved dramatically. In general, emergency plasmapheresis is performed daily or on alternate days until anti-GBM antibodies are not detected in the circulation (usually 1 to 2 weeks). Prednisone (1 mg/kg per day) is started simultaneously, in combination with either cyclophosphamide (2 to 3 mg/kg per day) or azathioprine (1 to 2 mg/kg per day) to suppress new synthesis of anti-GBM antibodies. The speed of initiation of therapy is a critical determinant of outcome. One-year renal survival approaches 90% if treatment is started before serum creatinine exceeds 442 μmol/L (5 mg/dL) and falls to about 10% if renal failure is more advanced. Patients who require dialysis at presentation rarely recover renal function. Serial anti-GBM titers are monitored to gauge response to therapy. Relapses are not unusual and are often heralded by rising antibody titers. In patients with ESRD, renal transplantation is a viable treatment option. Recurrence of anti-GBM nephritis in the allograft is extremely unusual provided that anti-GBM antibody titers have been consistently negative for 2 to 3 months prior to transplantation. However, in occasional patients with Alport's syndrome, when the allograft presents normal GBM components to the immune system of the recipient for the first time, anti-GBM nephritis can occur de novo in renal allografts.

Pauci-Immune Glomerulonephritis   The major pauci-immune glomerulonephritides are *idiopathic renal-limited crescentic glomerulonephritis, microscopic polyarteritis nodosa,* and *Wegener's granulomatosis* (Fig. 274-1). RPGN is a more common clinical presentation than acute nephritic syndrome, and the usual pathology is necrotizing glomerulonephritis with crescents affecting >50% of glomeruli (crescentic glomerulonephritis). The marked overlap of clinical features and glomerular histopathology, and the presence of circulating ANCA in most patients, suggest that these entities are a spectrum of a single disease. Here, we focus on idiopathic renal-limited crescentic glomerulonephritis. →*The ANCA-associated glomerulopathies with extrarenal features, namely Wegener's granulomatosis, Churg-Strauss syndrome, and microscopic polyarteritis nodosa, are discussed in Chap. 275.*

Idiopathic Renal-Limited Crescentic Glomerulonephritis   This is more common in middle-aged and older patients and shows a slight male preponderance. Patients typically present with RPGN, nephritic syndrome being rare. ANCA, usually a perinuclear ANCA IgG with specificity for myeloperoxidase (Chap. 275), are detected in 70 to 90% of patients (Fig. 274-1). The erythrocyte sedimentation rate and C-reactive protein levels may be elevated; however, C3 levels are typically normal, and circulating immune complexes, cryoglobulins, and anti-GBM antibodies are not detected. Most patients have crescents on light microscopy, often associated with necrotizing glomerulonephritis. Immune deposits are scanty or absent. Immunofluorescence microscopy reveals abundant fibrin deposits within crescents (Fig. 274-2). Most cases are treated aggressively with glucocorticoids, with or without cyclophosphamide or azathioprine (Chap. 275).

NEPHROTIC SYNDROME

GENERAL FEATURES AND COMPLICATIONS   The *nephrotic syndrome* is a clinical complex characterized by a number of renal and extrarenal features, the most prominent of which are proteinuria of >3.5 g per 1.73 m² per 24 h (in practice, >3.0 to 3.5 g per 24 h), hypoalbuminemia, edema, hyperlipidemia, lipiduria, and hypercoagulability. It should be stressed that the key component is *proteinuria*, which results from altered permeability of the glomerular filtration barrier for protein, namely the GBM and the podocytes and their slit diaphragms. The other components of the nephrotic syndrome and the ensuing metabolic complications are all secondary to urine protein loss and can occur with lesser degrees of proteinuria or may be absent even in patients with massive proteinuria.

In general, the greater the proteinuria, the lower the serum albumin level. *Hypoalbuminemia* is compounded further by increased renal catabolism and inadequate, albeit usually increased, hepatic synthesis of albumin. The pathophysiology of *edema* formation in nephrotic syndrome is poorly understood. The *underfilling hypothesis* postulates that hypoalbuminemia results in decreased intravascular oncotic pressure, leading to leakage of extracellular fluid from blood to the interstitium. Intravascular volume falls, thereby stimulating activation of the renin-angiotensin-aldosterone axis and the sympathetic nervous system and release of vasopressin (antidiuretic hormone), and suppressing atrial natriuretic peptide release. These neural and hormonal responses promote renal salt and water retention, thereby restoring intravascular volume and triggering further leakage of fluid to the interstitium. This hypothesis does not, however, explain the occurrence of edema in many patients in whom plasma volume is expanded and the renin-angiotensin-aldosterone axis is suppressed. The latter finding suggests that *primary renal salt and water retention* may also contribute to edema formation in some cases.

Hyperlipidemia is believed to be a consequence of increased hepatic lipoprotein synthesis that is triggered by reduced oncotic pressure and may be compounded by increased urinary loss of proteins that regulate lipid homeostasis. Low-density lipoproteins and cholesterol are increased in the majority of patients, whereas very low density lipoproteins and triglycerides tend to rise in patients with severe disease. Although not proven conclusively, hyperlipidemia may accelerate atherosclerosis and progression of renal disease.

Hypercoagulability is probably multifactorial in origin and is caused, at least in part, by increased urinary loss of antithrombin III, altered levels and/or activity of proteins C and S, hyperfibrinogenemia due to increased hepatic synthesis, impaired fibrinolysis, and increased platelet aggregability. As a consequence of these perturbations, patients can develop spontaneous *peripheral arterial or venous thrombosis, renal vein thrombosis,* and *pulmonary embolism*. Clinical features that suggest acute renal vein thrombosis include sudden onset of flank or abdominal pain, gross hematuria, a left-sided varicocele (the left testicular vein drains into the renal vein), increased proteinuria, and an acute decline in GFR. Chronic renal vein thrombosis is usually asymptomatic. Renal vein thrombosis is particularly common (up to

40%) in patients with nephrotic syndrome due to membranous glomerulopathy, membranoproliferative glomerulonephritis, and amyloidosis.

Other metabolic complications of nephrotic syndrome include *protein malnutrition* and iron-resistant *microcytic hypochromic anemia* due to transferrin loss. *Hypocalcemia* and secondary hyperparathyroidism can occur as a consequence of vitamin D deficiency due to enhanced urinary excretion of cholecalciferol-binding protein, whereas loss of thyroxine-binding globulin can result in *depressed thyroxine levels.* An increased susceptibility to *infection* may reflect low levels of IgG that result from urinary loss and increased catabolism. In addition, patients are prone to unpredictable changes in the *pharmacokinetics* of therapeutic agents that are normally bound to plasma proteins.

ETIOLOGY AND DIFFERENTIAL DIAGNOSIS Proteinuria >150 mg per 24 h is abnormal and can result from a number of mechanisms. *Glomerular proteinuria* results from leakage of plasma proteins through a perturbed glomerular filtration barrier; *tubular proteinuria* results from failure of tubular reabsorption of low-molecular-weight plasma proteins that are normally filtered and then reabsorbed and metabolized by tubular epithelium; *overflow proteinuria* results from filtration of proteins, usually immunoglobulin light chains, that are present in excess in the circulation. Tubular proteinuria virtually never exceeds 2 g per 24 h and thus, by definition, never causes nephrotic syndrome. Overflow proteinuria should be suspected in patients with clinical or laboratory evidence of multiple myeloma or other lymphoproliferative malignancy. Suspicion is heightened when there is a discrepancy between proteinuria detected by dipsticks, which are sensitive to albumin but not light chains, and the sulfosalicylic acid precipitation method, which detects both.

Nephrotic syndrome can complicate any disease that perturbs the negative electrostatic charge or architecture of the GBM and the podocytes and their slit diaphragms. Six entities account for greater than 90% of cases of nephrotic syndrome in adults: minimal change disease (MCD), focal and segmental glomerulosclerosis (FSGS), membranous glomerulopathy, MPGN, diabetic nephropathy, and amyloidosis. Diabetic nephropathy and amyloidosis, being manifestations of systemic diseases, are discussed in Chap. 275. *Renal biopsy* is a valuable tool in adults with nephrotic syndrome for establishing a definitive diagnosis, guiding therapy, and estimating prognosis. Renal biopsy is not required in the majority of children with nephrotic syndrome as most cases are due to MCD and respond to empiric treatment with glucocorticoids.

MINIMAL CHANGE DISEASE This glomerulopathy accounts for about 80% of nephrotic syndrome in children of younger than 16 years and 20% in adults (Table 274-1). The peak incidence is between 6 and 8 years. Patients typically present with nephrotic syndrome and benign urinary sediment. Microscopic hematuria is present in 20 to 30%. Hypertension and renal insufficiency are very rare.

MCD (also called nil disease, lipoid nephrosis, or foot process disease) is so named because glomerular size and architecture are normal by light microscopy. Immunofluorescence studies are typically negative for immunoglobulin and C3. Mild mesangial hypercellularity and sparse deposits of C3 and IgM may be detected. Occasionally, mesangial proliferation is associated with scanty IgA deposits, similar to those found in IgA nephropathy. However, the natural history of

Table 274-1   Major Causes of Minimal Change Disease (Nil Disease, Lipoid Nephrosis)

Idiopathic (majority)
In association with systemic diseases or drugs
   Drug-induced interstitial nephritis induced by NSAIDs, rifampin, interferon α
   Hodgkin's disease and other lymphoproliferative malignancy
   HIV infection

NOTE: NSAIDs, nonsteroidal anti-inflammatory drugs.

this variant and response to therapy resemble classic MCD. Electron microscopy reveals characteristic *diffuse effacement of the foot processes of visceral epithelial cells* (Fig. 274-3). This morphologic finding is referred to as foot process fusion in the older literature.

The etiology of MCD is unknown and the vast majority of cases are idiopathic (Table 274-1). MCD occasionally develops after upper respiratory tract infection, immunizations, and atopic attacks. Patients with atopy and MCD have an increased incidence of HLA-B12, suggesting a genetic predisposition. MCD, often in association with interstitial nephritis, is a rare side effect of nonsteroidal anti-inflammatory drugs (NSAIDs), rifampin, and interferon-α. The occasional association with lymphoproliferative malignancies (such as Hodgkin's lymphoma), the tendency for idiopathic MCD to remit during intercurrent viral infection such as measles, and the good response of idiopathic forms to immunosuppressive agents (see below) suggest an immune etiology. In children, the urine contains albumin principally and minimal amounts of higher molecular weight proteins such as IgG and α_2-macroglobulin. This *selective proteinuria* in conjunction with foot process effacement suggests injury to podocytes and loss of the fixed *negative charge* in the glomerular filtration barrier for protein. Proteinuria is typically nonselective in adults, suggesting more extensive perturbation of membrane permeability.

TREATMENT   MCD is highly steroid-responsive and carries an excellent prognosis. Spontaneous remission occurs in 30 to 40% of childhood cases but is less common in adults. Approximately 90% of children and 50% of adults enter remission following 8 weeks of high-dose oral glucocorticoids. In a typical regimen using prednisone, children receive 60 mg/m² of body surface area daily for 4 weeks, followed by 40 mg/m² on alternate days for an additional 4 weeks; adults receive 1 to 1.5 mg/kg body weight per day for 4 weeks, followed by 1 mg/kg per day on alternate days for 4 weeks. Up to 90% of adults enter remission if therapy is extended for 20 to 24 weeks. Nephrotic syndrome relapses in over 50% of cases following withdrawal of glucocorticoids. Alkylating agents are reserved for the small number of patients who fail to achieve lasting remission. These include patients who relapse during or shortly after withdrawal of steroids (steroid-dependent) and those who relapse more than three times per year (frequently relapsing). In these settings, cyclophosphamide (2 to 3 mg/kg per day) or chlorambucil (0.1 to 0.2 mg/kg per day) is started after steroid-induced remission and continued for 8 to 12 weeks. Cytotoxic agents may also induce remission in occasional steroid-resistant cases. These benefits must be balanced against the risk of infertility, cystitis, alopecia, infection, and secondary malignancies, particularly in children and young adults. Azathioprine has not been proven to be a useful adjunct to steroid therapy. Cyclosporine induces remission in 60 to 80% of patients; it is an alternative to cytotoxic agents and an option in patients who are resistant to cytotoxic agents. Unfortunately, relapse is usual when cyclosporine is withdrawn, and long-term therapy carries the risk of nephrotoxicity and other side effects. Long-term renal and patient survival is excellent in MCD.

FOCAL AND SEGMENTAL GLOMERULOSCLEROSIS WITH HYALINOSIS The pathognomonic morphologic lesion in FSGS is sclerosis with hyalinosis involving portions (segmental) of fewer than 50% (focal) of glomeruli on a tissue section. The incidence of idiopathic (primary) FSGS has increased over the past two decades so that it now accounts for about one-third of cases of nephrotic syndrome in adults and as many as one-half of cases of nephrotic syndrome in blacks. FSGS can complicate a number of systemic diseases and sustained glomerular capillary hypertension following nephron loss from any cause (Table 274-2 and Chap. 273).

Idiopathic FSGS typically presents as nephrotic syndrome (~66%) or subnephrotic proteinuria (~33%) in association with hypertension, mild renal insufficiency, and an abnormal urine sediment that contains

A

B

C

FIGURE 274-3 Typical findings on electron microscopy of renal biopsy specimens from patients with minimal change glomerulopathy, membranous glomerulopathy, and membranoproliferative glomerulonephritis. The pathognomonic feature of minimal change glomerulopathy (*A*) is effacement of foot processes of visceral epithelial cells (podocytes), giving the impression of foot process fusion. Foot process effacement is also evident in focal and segmental glomerulosclerosis (not shown here); in addition, there is typically detachment of podocytes from basement membrane, areas of glomerular capillary collapse, deposits of hyaline material, and sclerosis. Membranous nephropathy (*B*) is characterized by immune complexes in the subepithelial space. These electron-dense immune deposits stimulate production of new GBM, which eventually surrounds and incorporates the immune deposits into the GBM. The hallmarks of type I membranoproliferative glomerulonephritis (*C*) are increased mesangial cellularity and matrix and thickening and reduplication of the GBM. The latter is initiated by formation of electron-dense immune complexes on the subendothelial aspect of the GBM, which are subsequently covered by a new layer of GBM, probably produced by regenerating endothelial cells. (*Micrographs courtesy of Dr. Helmut Rennke.*)

red blood cells and leukocytes. Proteinuria is nonselective in most cases.

Light microscopy of renal biopsy tissue reveals FSGS with entrapment of amorphous hyaline material, a process that shows a predilection for juxtamedullary glomeruli. The sclerotic scars contain areas of glomerular capillary collapse and hyaline material composed of collagen types I, III, and IV. Adhesions occur between areas of capillary collapse and Bowman's capsule. Immunofluorescence studies are usually negative. Electron microscopy reveals evidence of damage to visceral epithelial cells, including swelling and detachment of podocytes from the GBM, effacement of foot processes, transition to foam cells, and overt cell degeneration and necrosis.

The etiology of primary FSGS is unclear (Table 274-2). There is evidence that a circulating nonimmunoglobulin permeability factor triggers FSGS in at least a subgroup of patients. The latter individuals tend to be young and prone to develop early recurrence of FSGS following renal transplantation. Plasmapharesis has been employed with variable success to control the nephrotic syndrome in this group. The overlap of clinical and morphologic features between MCD and FSGS has prompted some authorities to speculate that they are a spectrum of morphologic manifestations of a single pathogenetic process. FSGS is a potential long-term consequence of nephron loss from any cause. It can complicate congenital renal diseases such as congenital oligomeganephronia, in which both kidneys have a reduced complement of nephrons, and congenital unilateral agenesis. In addition, FSGS may develop following acquired loss of nephrons from extensive surgical ablation of renal mass; reflux nephropathy; glomerulonephritis; interstitial nephritis; sickle cell disease; and the combined effects of ischemia, cyclosporine nephrotoxicity, and rejection on renal allograft func-

tion (Table 274-2). It appears that >50% of nephrons must be lost for development of secondary FSGS.

TREATMENT In contrast to MCD, spontaneous remission of primary FSGS is rare and renal prognosis is relatively poor. Proteinuria remits in only 20 to 40% of patients treated with glucocorticoids for 8 weeks. Uncontrolled studies suggest that up to 70% respond

Table 274-2 Etiology of Focal and Segmental Glomerulosclerosis

Idiopathic (majority)
In association with systemic diseases or drugs
   HIV infection
   Diabetes mellitus
   Fabry's disease
   Sialidosis
   Charcot-Marie-Tooth disease
As consequence of sustained glomerular capillary hypertension
   Congenital oligonephropathies
      Unilateral renal agenesis
      Oligomeganephronia
   Acquired nephron loss
      Surgical resection
      Reflux nephropathy
      Glomerulonephritis or tubulointerstitial nephritis
   Other adaptive responses
      Sickle cell nephropathy
      Obesity with sleep apnea syndrome
      Familial dysautonomia
Miscellaneous
   Heroin use

when steroid therapy is prolonged for 16 to 24 weeks. Cyclophospha-mide and cyclosporine, when used at doses described above for MCD, induce partial or complete remission in 50 to 60% of steroid-respon-sive patients but are generally ineffective in steroid-resistant cases. Poor prognostic factors at presentation include hypertension, abnormal renal function, black race, and persistent heavy proteinuria. Renal transplantation is complicated by recurrence of FSGS in the allograft in about 50% of cases and graft loss in about 10%. Factors associated with an increased risk of recurrence include a short time interval be-tween the onset of the FSGS and ESRD, young age at onset, and possibly the presence of mesangial hypercellularity on renal biopsy.

MEMBRANOUS GLOMERULOPATHY
This lesion is a leading cause of idiopathic nephrotic syndrome in adults (30 to 40%) and a rare cause in children (<5%). It has a peak incidence between the ages of 30 to 50 years and a male-female ratio of 2:1 (Table 274-3). Membranous glomerulopathy derives its name from the char-acteristic light-microscopic appearance on renal biopsy, namely dif-fuse thickening of the GBM, which is most apparent upon staining with periodic acid–Schiff (PAS). Most patients (>80%) present with nephrotic syndrome, proteinuria usually being nonselective. Micro-scopic hematuria is present in up to 50% of cases, but red blood cells casts, macroscopic hematuria, and leukocytes are extremely rare. Hy-pertension is documented in only 10 to 30% of patients at the outset but is common later in patients with progressive renal failure. Sero-logic tests such as antinuclear antibody, ANCA, anti-GBM antibody, cryoglobulin titers, and complement levels are normal in the idiopathic form.

Light microscopy of renal biopsy sections reveals diffuse thick-ening of the GBM without evidence of inflammation or cellular pro-liferation. Silver staining demonstrates characteristic *spikes* along the GBM, which represent projections of new basement membrane en-gulfing subepithelial immune deposits. Immunofluorescence reveals granular deposition of IgG, C3, and the terminal components of com-plement (C5b–9) along the glomerular capillary wall. Electron-micro-scopic appearances vary depending on the stage of disease. The earliest finding is the presence of subepithelial immune deposits (Fig. 274-3). As these deposits enlarge, spikes of new basement membrane extend out between the immune deposits and begin to engulf them. With time, the deposits are completely surrounded and incorporated into the base-ment membrane.

The pathogenesis of idiopathic human membranous glomerulop-athy is incompletely understood. The presence of electron-dense im-mune deposits that contain IgG and C3 suggest an immune process. About one-third of adult membranous nephropathy occurs in associ-

Table 274-3   Conditions Associated with Membranous Glomerulopathy

Idiopathic (majority)
In association with systemic diseases or drugs
  Infection
    Hepatitis B and C, secondary and congenital syphilis, malaria, schisto-somiasis, leprosy, hydatid disease, filariasis, enterococcal endocarditis
  Systemic autoimmune diseases
    SLE, rheumatoid disease, Sjögren's syndrome, Hashimoto's disease, Graves' disease, mixed connective tissue disease, primary biliary cirrho-sis, ankylosing spondylitis, dermatitis herpetiformis, bullous pemphi-goid, myasthenia gravis
  Neoplasia
    Carcinoma of the breast, lung, colon, stomach, and esophagus; melanoma; renal cell carcinoma; neuroblastoma; carotid body tumor
  Drugs
    Gold, penicillamine, captopril, NSAIDs, probenecid, trimethadione, chlor-methiazole, mercury
  Miscellaneous
    Sarcoidosis, diabetes mellitus, sickle cell disease, Crohn's disease, Guil-lain-Barré syndrome, Weber-Christian disease, Fanconi's syndrome, α_1 antitrypsin deficiency, angiofollicular lymph node hyperplasia

NOTE: SLE, systemic lupus erythematosus; NSAIDs, nonsteroidal anti-inflammatory drugs.

Table 274-4   Causes of Membranoproliferative (Mesangiocapillary) Glomerulonephritis (MPGN)

Idiopathic	
Type I	With subendothelial and mesangial immune deposits
Type II	With intramembranous dense deposits containing sparse or no Ig; associated with C3 nephritic factor
Type III	Features of type I MPGN and membranous nephropathy
In association with systemic diseases or drugs[a]	
Systemic immune-complex disease	SLE, mixed cryoglobulinemia, Sjögren's syndrome
Chronic infections	Hepatitis B and C, HIV, bacterial endocarditis, ventriculoatrial shunts, visceral abscess
Malignancy	Leukemias, lymphomas
Liver disease	Chronic active hepatitis and cir-rhosis (usually associated with hepatitis B or C)
Miscellaneous	Partial lipodystrophy, heroin use, sarcoidosis, inherited C2 defi-ciency, thrombotic microangiopa-thies

[a] Usual with morphologic features of idiopathic type I MPGN (see above).
NOTE: SLE, systemic lupus erythematosus.

ation with systemic diseases such as SLE, infections such as hepatitis B, malignancy, and drug therapy with gold and penicillamine (Table 274-3).

Nephrotic syndrome remits spontaneously and completely in up to 40% of patients with membranous glomerulopathy. The natural his-tory of another 30 to 40% is characterized by repeated relapses and remissions. The final 10 to 20% suffer a slow progressive decline in GFR that typically culminates in ESRD after 10 to 15 years. Presenting features that predict a poor prognosis include male gender, older age, hypertension, severe proteinuria and hyperlipidemia, and impaired re-nal function. Controlled trials of glucocorticoids have failed to show consistent improvement in proteinuria or renal protection. Cyclophos-phamide, chlorambucil, and cyclosporine have each been shown to reduce proteinuria and/or slow the decline in GFR in patients with progressive disease in small or uncontrolled studies. These observa-tions need to be confirmed in controlled prospective studies. Trans-plantation is a successful treatment option for patients who reach ESRD.

MEMBRANOPROLIFERATIVE GLOMERULONEPHRITIS
This morphologic entity, also known as mesangiocapillary glomeru-lonephritis, is characterized by thickening of the GBM and prolifera-tive changes on light microscopy (Table 274-4). Two major types are identified; both are characterized by a diffuse increase in mesangial cellularity and matrix, and by thickening and reduplication of the GBM such that the lobular pattern of the glomerular tuft is exaggerated. The hallmark of type I MPGN is the presence of subendothelial and mes-angial deposits on electron microscopy that contain C3 and IgG or IgM; rarely, IgA deposits are demonstrated by immunofluorescence microscopy (Fig. 274-3). The hallmark of type II MPGN (dense de-posit disease) is the presence of electron-dense deposits within the GBM and other renal basement membranes (shown by electron mi-croscopy) that stain for C3, but little or no immunoglobulin.

Most patients with type I MPGN present with heavy proteinuria or nephrotic syndrome, active urinary sediment, and normal or mildly impaired GFR. C3 levels are usually depressed, and C1q and C4 levels are borderline or low. Type I MPGN is an immune-complex glomer-ulonephritis and can be associated with a variety of chronic infections (e.g., bacterial endocarditis, HIV, hepatitis B and C), systemic im-mune-complex diseases (e.g., SLE, cryoglobulinemia), and malignan-cies (e.g., leukemias, lymphomas). Type I MPGN is a relatively benign disease, and 70 to 85% of patients survive without clinically significant impairment of GFR. There is no proven therapy for patients with pro-gressive disease beyond eradicating the underlying infection, malignancy, or systemic disease, when possible. The incidence of type I MPGN appears to be falling, possibly because the overall incidence of hepatitis C infection has fallen dramatically in western society over the past decade.

Type II MPGN can also present with proteinuria and nephrotic syndrome; however, some patients present with nephritic syndrome, RPGN, or recurrent macroscopic hematuria. Type II MPGN is an autoimmune disease in which patients have an IgG autoantibody, termed *C3 nephritic factor*, that binds to C3 convertase, the enzyme that metabolizes C3, and renders it resistant to inactivation (Chap. 273). Type II MPGN runs a variable course; the GFR remains stable in some patients and declines gradually to ESRD over 5 to 10 years in others. There is no effective therapy for this disease.

FIBRILLARY-IMMUNOTACTOID GLOMERULOPATHY
This emerging clinicopathologic entity accounts for 1% of diagnoses in most large renal biopsy series. Virtually all patients present with proteinuria, and >50% have nephrotic syndrome. The majority of patients also have hematuria, hypertension, and renal insufficiency. The light-microscopic appearances vary from mesangial expansion and basement membrane thickening with PAS-positive material to proliferative and crescentic glomerulonephritis. On electron microscopy, this PAS-positive material is observed to be composed of randomly arranged (fibrillary glomerulopathy) or organized bundles (immunotactoid glomerulopathy) of microfibrils and microtubules, the compositon of which has yet to be defined. The etiology of fibrillary-immunotactoid glomerulopathy remains to be determined. Patients with the immunotactoid variant have an increased incidence of lymphoproliferative malignancy. There is no proven therapy for fibrillary-immunotactoid glomerulopathy, and many patients progress to ESRD over 1 to 10 years. Transplantation appears to be a viable option in the latter setting.

MESANGIAL PROLIFERATIVE GLOMERULONEPHRITIS
In 5 to 10% of patients with idiopathic nephrotic syndrome, renal biopsy reveals a diffuse increase in glomerular cellularity, predominantly due to proliferation of mesangial and endothelial cells, and infiltration by monocytes. Findings on immunofluorescence microscopy vary and include deposits of IgA, IgG, IgM, and/or complement, or absence of immune reactants. It is likely that this morphologic entity is, in fact, a heterogeneous group of diseases that includes atypical forms of MCD and FSGS and milder or resolving forms of the immune-complex and pauci-immune glomerulopathies described above under nephritic syndrome and RPGN. In keeping with the heterogeneity of this diagnosis, the prognosis is variable. In general, persistent nephrotic-range proteinuria signals a poor prognosis, with many patients progressing to ESRD over 10 to 20 years despite immunosuppressive therapy.

℞ TREATMENT   Nephrotic Syndrome and Complications
The treatment of nephrotic syndrome involves (1) specific treatment of the underlying morphologic entity and, when possible, causative disease (see above); (2) general measures to control proteinuria if remission is not achieved through immunosuppressive therapy and other specific measures; and (3) general measures to control nephrotic complications.

General measures may be warranted to control proteinuria in nephrotic syndrome if patients do not respond to immunosuppressive therapy and other specific measures and suffer progressive renal failure or severe nephrotic complications. Nonspecific measures that may reduce proteinuria include *angiotensin-converting enzyme (ACE) inhibitors*, and *NSAIDs*. The first of these measures aim to reduce proteinuria and slow the rate of progression of renal failure by lowering intraglomerular pressure and preventing the development of hemodynamically mediated focal segmental glomerulosclerosis. There is conclusive evidence that ACE inhibitors are renoprotective in human diabetic nephropathy (Chap. 275) and that ACE inhibitors slow the development of secondary FSGS in experimental animals. Their role

in the treatment of nephrotic syndrome in other settings is unproven. NSAIDs also reduce proteinuria in some patients with nephrotic syndrome, probably by altering glomerular hemodynamics and GBM permeability characteristics. This potential benefit must be balanced against the risk of inducing acute renal failure, hyperkalemia, salt and water retention, and other side effects.

Complications of nephrotic syndrome that may require treatment include edema, hyperlipidemia, thromboembolism, malnutrition, and vitamin D deficiency. Edema should be managed cautiously by moderate *salt restriction*, usually 1 to 2 g/day, and the judicious use of *loop diuretics*. It is unwise to remove >1.0 kg of edema per day as more aggressive diuresis may precipitate intravascular volume depletion and prerenal azotemia. Administration of salt-poor albumin is not recommended as most is excreted within 24 to 48 h. Whereas many nephrologists advocate lowering low-density lipoproteins and cholesterol levels with *lipid-lowering drugs* to prevent accelerated atherosclerosis and slow the rate of decline of GFR, the value of such interventions in this setting has not been conclusively shown. *Anticoagulation* is indicated for patients with deep venous thrombosis, arterial thrombosis, and pulmonary embolism. Patients may be relatively resistant to heparin as a consequence of antithrombin III deficiency. Renal vein and vena caval angiography are probably indicated only when embolization occurs on anticoagulation and insertion of a caval filter is contemplated. There is no consensus regarding the optimal *diet* for patients with nephrotic syndrome. High-protein diets to prevent protein malnutrition are now in disfavor, since protein supplements have little, if any, effect on serum albumin levels and may hasten the progression of renal disease by increasing urinary protein excretion. The potential value of dietary protein restriction for reducing proteinuria must be balanced against the risk of contributing to malnutrition. *Vitamin D* supplementation is advisable in patients with clinical or biochemical evidence of vitamin D deficiency.

ASYMPTOMATIC ABNORMALITIES OF THE URINARY SEDIMENT

HEMATURIA   Most asymptomatic glomerular hematuria is due to *IgA nephropathy* (Berger's disease) or *thin basement membrane (TBM) disease* (benign hematuria). A rarer but more ominous cause of isolated hematuria is *Alport's syndrome*. The latter is the most common form of hereditary nephritis, is usually transmitted as an X-linked dominant trait, and is associated with sensorineural deafness, ophthalmologic abnormalities, and progressive renal insufficiency (Chap. 275). TBM disease is sometimes familial but, in contrast to Alport's syndrome, is usually a benign disorder. Asymptomatic hematuria may also be the presenting feature of indolent forms of most other primary and secondary proliferative glomerulopathies (Fig. 274-1). Glomerular hematuria must be distinguished from a variety of renal parenchymal and extrarenal causes of hematuria. It is particularly important to exclude malignancy of the kidney or urinary tract, particularly in older male patients (Chap. 94). Other potential diagnoses include vascular, cystic, and tubulointerstitial diseases; papillary necrosis; hypercalciuria and hyperuricosuria; benign prostatic hypertrophy; and renal calculi. Important clues to the presence of glomerular hematuria are the presence of urinary red blood cell casts, dysmorphic urinary red blood cells, proteinuria of greater than 2.0 g per 24 h, and clinical or serologic evidence of nephritic syndrome, RPGN, or a compatible systemic disease.

IgA Nephropathy (Berger's Disease)   IgA nephropathy is the most common glomerulopathy worldwide and accounts for 10 to 40% of glomerulonephritis in most series (Table 274-5). The disease is particularly common in southern Europe and Asia and appears to be more common in blacks than whites. Familial clustering has been reported but is rare. No consistent HLA association has emerged, although HLA-B35 appears to be more common in French patients. Most cases are idiopathic. The renal and serologic abnormalities in IgA nephropathy and Henoch-Schönlein purpura (Chap. 275) are indistinguishable, and most authorities consider these to be a spectrum

Table 274-5 Diseases Associated with IgA Nephropathy

Idiopathic (majority)
  Renal-limited or as component of Henoch-Schönlein purpura
In association with systemic diseases or drugs[a]

Liver	Chronic liver disease with involvement of biliary tree
Gastrointestinal	Celiac disease, Crohn's disease, adenocarcinoma
Respiratory	Idiopathic interstitial pneumonitis, obstructive bronchiolitis, adenocarcinoma
Skin	Dermatitis herpetiformis, mycosis fungoides, leprosy
Eyes	Episcleritis, anterior uveitis
Miscellaneous	Ankylosing spondylitis, relapsing polychondritis, Sjögren's syndrome, monoclonal IgA gammopathy, schistosomiasis

[a] Although prominent deposition of IgA has been reported with each of these conditions, significant glomerular inflammation and dysfunction are rare.

of a single disease. Less commonly, IgA nephropathy is found in association with systemic diseases, including chronic liver disease, Crohn's disease, gastrointestinal adenocarcinoma, chronic obstructive bronchiolitis, idiopathic interstitial pneumonia, dermatitis herpetiformis, mycosis fungoides, leprosy, ankylosing spondylitis, relapsing polychondritis, and Sjögren's syndrome. In many of these conditions, IgA is deposited in the glomerulus without inducing inflammation, and this may be a clinically insignificant consequence of perturbed IgA homeostasis.

Patients with IgA nephropathy typically present with gross hematuria, often 24 to 48 h after a pharyngeal or gastrointestinal infection, vaccination, or strenuous exercise. Other cases are diagnosed upon detection of microscopic hematuria during routine physical examinations. Hypertension (20 to 30%) and nephrotic syndrome (~10%) are unusual at presentation. Light microscopy of renal biopsy specimens typically shows mesangial expansion by increased matrix and cells. Diffuse proliferation, cellular crescents, interstitial inflammation, and areas of glomerulosclerosis may be evident in severe cases. The diagnostic finding, for which the disease is named, is mesangial deposition of IgA, detected by immunofluorescence microscopy. C3 is usually detected in the area of immune deposits, and IgG is observed in 50% of cases. Electron microscopy reveals electron-dense deposits in the mesangium and, in severe cases, these extend into the paramesangial subendothelial space. The pathogenesis of IgA nephropathy is incompletely understood.

℞ **TREATMENT** There is no proven therapy for IgA nephropathy. A recent, relatively large randomized controlled trial suggested a benefit of fish oils in patients with progressive disease and heavy proteinuria; however, this experience has not been universal. Some authorities advocate a trial of high-dose glucocorticoids with or without cytotoxic agents in patients with severe nephrotic syndrome and those with nephritic syndrome or RPGN and evidence of active inflammation on renal biopsy.

IgA nephropathy typically smolders for decades, with patients often suffering exacerbations of hematuria and renal impairment during intercurrent infections. As many as 20 to 50% of patients develop ESRD within 20 years. Clinical predictors of a poor prognosis include older age, male sex, hypertension, nephrotic-range proteinuria, and renal insufficiency at presentation. Histologic features that predict an aggressive course include diffuse severe disease, extracapillary proliferation (crescents), extension of immune attack into the paramesangial subendothelial space, glomerulosclerosis, interstitial fibrosis, and arteriolar hyalinosis.

Thin Basement Membrane Disease (Benign Hematuria) This disorder can be heredofamilial or sporadic and is as common as IgA nephropathy in some series of asymptomatic hematuria. When familial, it is usually inherited as an autosomal dominant trait and is due to a defect in the gene encoding the $\alpha 4$ chain of type IV collagen. TBM disease typically manifests in childhood as persistent hematuria. Intermittent hematuria and exacerbation of hematuria during upper res-

piratory tract infections have also been reported. The kidney is normal on light and immunofluorescence microscopy. The GBM is thin (usually <275 nm in children and <300 nm in adults) by comparison with normal subjects. TBM disease is usually a benign condition, and progressive renal impairment or proteinuria should prompt a search for an alternative diagnosis. A small proportion of patients do, however, appear to develop hypertension and focal glomerulosclerosis upon long-term follow-up. The molecular basis for the sporadic form of TBM disease has not been determined.

PROTEINURIA Between 0.5 and 10% of the population have isolated proteinuria, defined as proteinuria in the presence of an otherwise normal urinary sediment, a radiologically normal urinary tract, and the absence of known renal disease. The majority of these patients excrete <2 g of protein per day, and more than 80% have an excellent prognosis (*benign isolated proteinuria*). A minority (10 to 25%) are found to have persistent proteinuria (*persistent isolated proteinuria*), some of whom develop progressive renal insufficiency over 10 to 20 years.

Benign Isolated Proteinuria The major categories of benign isolated proteinuria are idiopathic transient proteinuria, functional proteinuria, intermittent proteinuria, and postural proteinuria. *Idiopathic transient proteinuria* is usually observed in young adults and refers to dipstick-positive proteinuria in an otherwise healthy individual that disappears spontaneously by the next clinic visit. *Functional proteinuria* refers to transient proteinuria during fever, exposure to cold, emotional stress, congestive cardiac failure, or obstructive sleep apnea. This phenomenon is presumed to be mediated through changes in glomerular ultrafiltration pressure and/or membrane permeability. Patients with *intermittent proteinuria* have proteinuria in approximately half of their urine samples in the absence of other renal or systemic abnormalities. *Postural proteinuria* is proteinuria (usually <2.0 g per 24 h) that is evident only in the upright position. This disorder affects 2 to 5% of adolescents and may be transient (~80%) or fixed (~20%). Fixed postural proteinuria resolves within 10 to 20 years in most cases. In each of these conditions, renal biopsy reveals either normal renal parenchyma or mild and nonspecific changes involving podocytes or the mesangium. All carry an excellent prognosis.

Persistent Isolated Proteinuria Isolated proteinuria detected on multiple ambulatory clinic visits in both the recumbent and upright position usually signals a structural renal lesion. Virtually all glomerulopathies that induce nephrotic syndrome (see above) can cause persistent isolated proteinuria. The most common lesion on renal biopsy is mild mesangial proliferative glomerulonephritis with or without focal and segmental glomerulosclerosis (30 to 70%), followed by focal or diffuse proliferative glomerulonephritis (~15%) and interstitial nephritis (~5%). Although this clinical entity carries a worse prognosis than benign isolated proteinuria, the prognosis is still relatively good, with only 20 to 40% of patients developing renal insufficiency after 20 years. Furthermore, progression to ESRD is extremely rare. It is wise to exclude monoclonal gammopathy by urinary electrophoresis in older patients.

CHRONIC GLOMERULONEPHRITIS

This syndrome is characterized by persistent proteinuria and/or hematuria and renal insufficiency that progresses slowly over years. Chronic glomerulonephritis usually comes to light (1) upon routine urinalysis, (2) when routine blood tests reveal unexplained anemia or elevated blood urea nitrogen and creatinine, (3) following discovery of bilateral small kidneys on abdominal imaging, (4) during evaluation for secondary causes of hypertension, or (5) during a clinical exacerbation of glomerulonephritis triggered by pharyngitis (synpharyngitic) or other infections. Chronic glomerulonephritis can be a manifestation of virtually all of the major glomerulopathies. Renal biopsy typically reveals a variable combination of proliferative, membranous, and sclerotic changes, depending on the causative glomerulopathy. Arteriosclerosis, induced by secondary hypertension, is a common finding in the renal vasculature. Tubulointerstitial inflammation and scarring are frequent additional findings and portend a poor prognosis. Glomerular hypertension and hyperfiltration through remnant functioning nephrons can hasten progression to ESRD (Chap. 273). Treatment is directed at lowering systemic and glomerular hypertension, usually with an ACE inhibitor, and controlling extracellular fluid volume, anemia, metabolic abnormalities, and the uremic syndrome through judicious use of diuretics, erythropoietin, and dietary modification (Chap. 270). Some patients develop ESRD and require renal replacement therapy with dialysis or transplantation.

BIBLIOGRAPHY

BOLTON WK: Goodpasture's syndrome. Kidney Int 50:1753, 1996

BRADY HR: Fibrillary glomerulopathy. Kidney Int 53:1421, 1998

———, WILCOX CS (eds): *Therapy in Nephrology and Hypertension*. Philadelphia, Saunders, 1999

COUSER WG: Glomerulonephritis. Lancet 353:1509, 1999

D'AMICO G: Pathogenesis of immunoglobulin A nephropathy. Curr Opin Nephrol Hypertens 7:247, 1998

FALK R et al: Primary glomerular diseases, in *Brenner & Rector's The Kidney*, 6th ed, BM Brenner (ed). Philadelphia, Saunders, 2000, pp 1263–1349

HAAS M et al: Changing etiologies of unexplained adult nephrotic syndrome: A comparison of renal biopsy findings from 1976–1979 and 1995–1997. Am J Kidney Dis 30:621, 1997

HRICIK DE et al: Glomerulonephritis. N Engl J Med 339:889, 1998

JENNETTE C, FALK R: Small-vessel vasculitides. N Engl J Med 337:1512, 1997

MACKENZIE HS et al: Adaptation to nephron loss, in *Brenner & Rector's The Kidney*, 6th ed, BM Brenner (ed). Philadelphia, Saunders, 2000, 1901–1942

ORTH SR, RITZ E: The nephrotic syndrome. N Engl J Med 338:1202, 1998

275   Yvonne M. O'Meara, Hugh R. Brady, Barry M. Brenner

GLOMERULOPATHIES ASSOCIATED WITH MULTISYSTEM DISEASES

AA	amyloid A	HBV	hepatitis B virus
ACE	Angiotensin-converting enzyme	HCV	hepatitis C virus
AL	amyloid L	HIVAN	HIV-associated nephropathy
ANA	antinuclear antibody	LCDD	light chain deposition disease
ANCA	antineutrophil cytoplasmic antibodies	MPGN	membranoproliferative glomerulonephritis
DM	diabetes mellitus	NSAIDs	nonsteroidal anti-inflammatory drugs
EMC	"essential" mixed cryoglobulinemia	PAN	polyarteritis nodosa
ESRD	end-stage renal disease	RPGN	rapidly progressive glomerulonephritis
GBM	glomerular basement membrane	SLE	systemic lupus erythematosus
GFR	glomerular filtration rate		

An array of multisystem diseases can cause glomerular injury, with glomerulopathy being either the dominant presenting feature or a relatively benign and clinically insignificant manifestation that is overshadowed by involvement of other organs. Glomerulopathies associated with multisystem diseases are often classified as *secondary* glomerulopathies to distinguish them from the *primary* glomerulopathies (Chap. 274) in which the pathology is limited to the kidneys. It should be emphasized, however, that most morphologic patterns of glomerular injury (see Table 273-1) can manifest as a renal-limited process (i.e., primary) or as part of a systemic disease (i.e., secondary). The diagnostic approach to glomerular disease involves identifying the presenting clinical syndrome (e.g., nephritic, nephrotic), defining the pathologic features (e.g., proliferative, crescentic, membranous), and attempting to establish the specific disease that provoked glomer-

ular injury [e.g., systemic lupus erythematosus (SLE), Henoch-Schönlein purpura].

In this chapter, we focus on the epidemiology, clinicopathologic features, and management of the major glomerulopathies associated with systemic diseases. →*The pathogenesis of glomerular injury is discussed in Chap. 273, and the overall place of the major glomerulopathies in the differential diagnosis of the major renal syndromes is described in Chap. 274.*

DIABETIC NEPHROPATHY
(See also Chaps. 273 and 333)

Diabetic nephropathy is the leading cause of end-stage renal disease (ESRD) in western societies and accounts for 30 to 35% of patients on renal replacement therapy in North America. Type 1 diabetes mellitus (type 1 DM; formerly, insulin-dependent diabetes mellitus) and type 2 diabetes mellitus (type 2 DM; formerly, non-insulin-dependent diabetes mellitus) affect 0.5 and 4% of the population, respectively. Nephropathy complicates 30% of cases of type 1 DM and approximately 20% of cases of type 2 DM. However, most diabetic patients with ESRD have type 2 DM because of the greater prevalence of type 2 DM worldwide (90% of all individuals with diabetes). Risk factors for the development of diabetic nephropathy include hyperglycemia, systemic hypertension, glomerular hypertension and hyperfiltration, proteinuria, and possibly cigarette smoking, hyperlipidemia, and gene polymorphisms affecting the activity of the renin-angiotensin-aldosterone axis. For reasons that are unclear, ESRD from diabetic nephropathy is more common in blacks with type 2 DM than in whites (4:1 ratio), whereas the reverse is true for type 1 DM.

The pathophysiology, clinical features, and morphology of diabetic nephropathy are similar in type 1 and type 2 DM, although the time course may be condensed in type 2 DM. Glomerular hypertension and hyperfiltration are the earliest renal abnormalities in experimental and human diabetes and are observed within days to weeks of diagnosis. Microalbuminuria, so named because the abnormal albumin excretion of 30 to 300 mg/24 h is below the limits of detection of standard dipsticks, develops after approximately 5 years of sustained glomerular hypertension and hyperfiltration in type 1 DM. Microalbuminuria is the first manifestation of injury to the glomerular filtration barrier and predicts the development of overt nephropathy. Dipstick-positive proteinuria, ultimately reaching nephrotic levels, typically develops 5 to 10 years after the onset of microalbuminuria (i.e., 10 to 15 years after the onset of diabetes) and is associated with hypertension and progressive loss of renal function. In addition, patients can display features of tubulointerstitial disease such as hyperkalemia and type IV renal tubular acidosis. ESRD typically develops 5 to 10 years after the development of overt nephropathy. As noted above, the course of diabetic nephropathy may be shorter in type 2 DM, and many patients present with established nephropathy and hypertension. Diabetic nephropathy is usually diagnosed on clinical grounds without a renal biopsy. Supportive clues are the presence of normal sized or enlarged kidneys, evidence of proliferative diabetic retinopathy, and a bland urinary sediment. Retinopathy is found in 90 and 60% of patients with type 1 and type 2 DM, respectively, who develop nephropathy.

The earliest morphologic abnormalities in diabetic nephropathy are thickening of the glomerular basement membrane (GBM) and expansion of the mesangium due to accumulation of extracellular matrix. With time, matrix accumulation becomes diffuse and is evident as eosinophilic, periodic acid Schiff–positive glomerulosclerosis on renal biopsy. Prominent areas of nodular matrix expansion (nodular glomerulosclerosis, the classic Kimmelstiel-Wilson lesion) are often superimposed on this background. The glomeruli and kidneys are typically normal or increased in size, distinguishing diabetic nephropathy from most other forms of chronic renal insufficiency (renal amyloidosis and polycystic kidney disease being other important exceptions). Immunofluorescence microscopy may reveal deposition of IgG along the GBM in a linear pattern, but this does not appear to be immunopathogenetic as in anti-GBM disease. Immune deposits are not seen.

The renal vasculature typically displays evidence of atherosclerosis, as a consequence of hyperlipidemia, and hypertensive arteriosclerosis.

℞ TREATMENT Therapy is aimed at retarding the progression of nephropathy through control of blood sugar, systemic blood pressure, and glomerular capillary pressure. Glycemic control is achieved through regulation of diet and administration of oral hypoglycemic agents and insulin (Chap. 333). Angiotensin-converting enzyme (ACE) inhibitors are the drugs of choice as they control both systemic hypertension and intraglomerular hypertension by inhibiting the actions of angiotensin II on the systemic vasculature and renal efferent arterioles. ACE inhibitors also attenuate the stimulatory effect of angiotensin II on glomerular cell growth and matrix production. Because ACE inhibitors have been shown conclusively to delay the time to ESRD by 50% in patients with type 1 DM in a large randomized controlled trial and to delay progression significantly in type 2 DM, it is felt that all patients with diabetes should receive an ACE inhibitor on the development of microalbuminuria, even in the absence of systemic hypertension (Fig. 275-1). However, approximately 80% of patients with diabetes require more than one drug to control systemic hypertension, and aggressive lowering of blood pressure in these patients retards not only the rate of progression of nephropathy, but also the rate of progression of other complications of DM.

Diabetic nephropathy is the most common cause of ESRD requiring renal replacement therapy, and patients with diabetes have the highest annual mortality rate (20 to 30%) of any group on dialysis, in large part as a result of accelerated atherosclerosis. The survival rates of younger patients undergoing either peritoneal dialysis or hemodialysis are comparable; however, older patients with diabetes appear to have a higher mortality rate on peritoneal dialysis. Transplantation is the preferred mode of renal replacement therapy in patients who are otherwise medically suitable.

IMMUNOLOGICALLY MEDIATED MULTISYSTEM DISEASES

The glomerulus is a frequent target of injury in a variety of immunologically mediated multisystem diseases, particularly systemic vasculitis and SLE. Systemic vasculitis is usually classified according to the size of the inflamed vessel (Chap. 317). The major *large vessel* vasculitides are Takayasu's disease and giant cell arteritis. Glomerular injury is exceedingly rare in these diseases.

CLASSIC POLYARTERITIS NODOSA(See also Chap. 317) The typical glomerular lesion in classic polyarteritis nodosa (PAN) is ischemic collapse and obsolescence. Characteristic clinical and serologic features are hypertension, a bland urine sediment with subnephrotic proteinuria, slowly progressive renal insufficiency, normal serum complement levels, and absence of antineutrophil cytoplasmic antibodies (ANCA). Treatment with glucocorticoids and immunosuppressive agents, such as cyclophosphamide, affords a 5-year patient survival of approximately 80%, as compared with 10% in untreated cases.

ANCA-ASSOCIATED SMALL-VESSEL VASCULITIS The ANCA-associated small-vessel vasculitides are Wegener's granulomatosis, the microscopic and Churg-Strauss variants of polyarteritis nodosa, and pauci-immune renal-limited glomerulonephritis. These diseases share a number of clinocopathologic and serologic features and may represent a spectrum of manifestations of a single disease. They are more common in whites and older patients (mean age 57 years) and show a slight male preponderance. Their incidence peaks in the winter months, and many patients have a viral-like prodrome, suggesting a pathogenetic role for an infective agent. Patients typically present with nonspecific constitutional symptoms and signs such as lethargy, malaise, anorexia, weight loss, fever, arthralgias, and myalgias. Nonspecific laboratory abnormalities include a rapid sedimentation rate, elevated C-reactive protein, leukocytosis, thrombocytosis, and normochromic, normocytic anemia. Serum complement levels are typically normal.

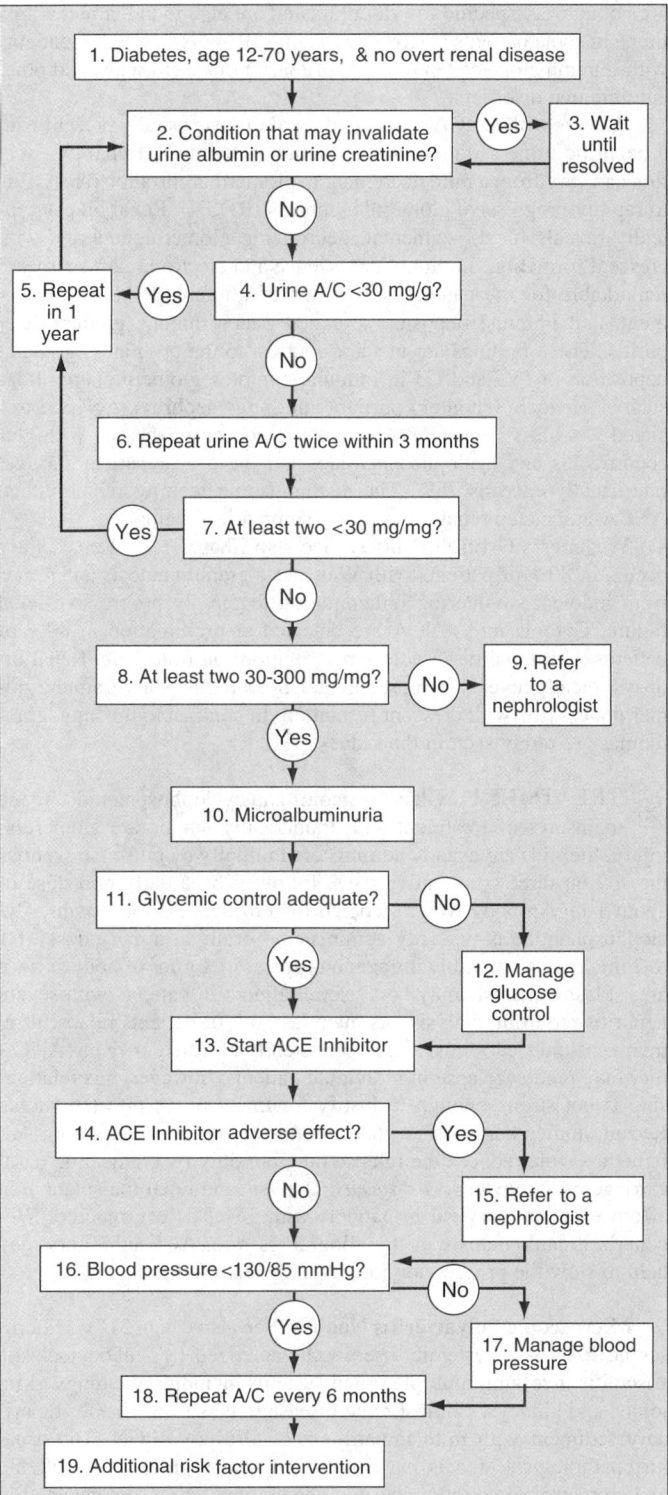

FIGURE 275-1 Algorithm for screening and management of microalbuminuria in patients with diabetes mellitus. A/C, albumin (in mg)/creatinine (in mg) in a spot urine sample. *(Reproduced from Bennett et al, with permission.)*

The majority of patients with these conditions have circulating ANCA. It is not clear whether ANCA are involved in the pathogenesis of vasculitis or merely represent an epiphenomenon of the vasculitic process, and there is debate whether serial ANCA titers are useful for monitoring disease activity and predicting relapse. Some ANCA activate cytokine-primed neutrophils in vitro and provoke them to injure endothelial cells, suggesting a pathogenetic role (Chap. 273). ANCA are not entirely specific for vasculitis and are also found, albeit at low titers, in some patients (~20%) with anti-GBM disease and in patients with inflammatory bowel disease, primary biliary cirrhosis, and other autoimmune disorders.

Patients with ANCA-associated renal disease usually present with a nephritic urine sediment and moderate proteinuria. Renal dysfunction can vary from a mild decrement in glomerular filtration rate (GFR) to rapidly progressive glomerulonephritis (RPGN). Renal biopsy typically reveals focal, segmental, necrotizing glomerulonephritis with crescent formation. Immunofluorescence and electron microscopy are remarkable for the paucity or absence of immunoglobulin, complement, and immune deposits: so-called pauci-immune glomerulonephritis. These findings are in stark contrast to the prominent granular deposition of IgG and C3 in immune-complex glomerulonephritides such as Henoch-Schönlein purpura and lupus nephritis. ANCA-associated vasculitis is usually responsive to combined therapy with glucocorticoids and cyclophosphamide, and the 5-year patient survival rate usually exceeds 75%. The distinguishing features of individual ANCA-associated renal diseases are summarized below.

Wegener's Granulomatosis (See also Chap. 317)   Renal injury occurs in 80% of patients with Wegener's granulomatosis and varies from indolent smoldering inflammation to rapidly progressive renal failure. Cytoplasmic ANCA are detected at presentation in 80% of patients with renal disease and in 10% more on follow-up. Renal biopsy typically reveals focal, segmental, necrotizing pauci-immune glomerulonephritis with crescent formation. In contrast to the lung, granulomas are rarely seen in the kidney.

TREATMENT   Glucocorticoids and cyclophosphamide are the mainstays of treatment and dramatically ameliorate glomerular injury. Steroids are usually administered initially by pulse intravenous therapy on three consecutive days, followed by a daily oral dose of about 1 mg/kg body weight tapered to zero over 3 to 6 months. Cyclophosphamide is typically administered orally at a daily dose of 1 to 2 mg/kg or as monthly intravenous pulses of 1 g/m² of body surface area. Plasmapheresis may be a useful adjunct in patients with severe nephritis requiring dialysis. As many as 30% of patients relapse after treatment-induced remission. A persistently elevated or rising ANCA titer may predict relapse in individual patients; however, this relationship is not strong enough to justify treatment based on titers alone. Recent studies demonstrate that administration of trimethoprim-sulfamethoxazole reduces the relapse rate, possibly by eradicating nasal carriage of *Staphylococcus aureus*. Dialysis and renal transplantation afford excellent survival in patients with ESRD. Recurrence of Wegener's granulomatosis in the allograft is rare. ACE inhibitors may help to slow the progression to end-stage renal failure.

Microscopic Polyarteritis Nodosa (See also Chap. 317)   Microscopic PAN is a systemic disease characterized by leukocytoclastic vasculitis involving multiple organ systems including the lungs, skin, joints, and kidneys. Clinical renal disease ranges from a nephritic urinary sediment with mild impairment of GFR to RPGN. The usual histopathologic lesion is pauci-immune focal segmental necrotizing and crescentic glomerulonephritis. Circulating ANCA are detected in 70 to 80% of patients at presentation, with cytoplasmic and perinuclear ANCA being equally prevalent. The treatment of microscopic PAN involves glucocorticoids and cyclophosphamide, as for Wegener's granulomatosis. Plasmapheresis may benefit patients with severe acute renal failure or massive pulmonary hemorrhage.

Churg-Strauss Syndrome (See also Chap. 317)   Clinical renal involvement in Churg-Strauss syndrome is relatively infrequent and usually limited to mild proteinuria and hematuria. Evolution to chronic renal failure is rare. Renal biopsy most frequently reveals extraglomerular pathology, with involvement of the renal vasculature and tubulointerstitium by granulomatous vasculitis. Focal segmental glomerulonephritis with crescents is also seen. A minority of patients have focal segmental necrotizing glomerulonephritis.

Henoch-Schönlein Purpura (See also Chap. 317)   Extrarenal features of Henoch-Schönlein purpura include a petechial rash on the extremities, arthropathy, and abdominal pain. Nephritis is present in 80% of patients and manifests as a nephritic urine sediment and moderate proteinuria. Macroscopic hematuria and nephrotic-range proteinuria are uncommon. Light-microscopic appearances can vary from mild mesangial proliferation and expansion to diffuse proliferation with glomerular crescents. The glomerular lesion is identical to that found in IgA nephropathy (Berger's disease; see Chap. 274), suggesting that Henoch-Schönlein nephritis and IgA nephropathy are a spectrum of manifestations of a single disease. The *sine qua non* for diagnosis is the presence of mesangial IgA deposition on immunofluorescence microscopy. IgG and C3 are also detected. Electron microscopy reveals mesangial immune deposits. Immune complexes may also be present in the peripheral glomerular capillary wall and paramesangial areas. Biopsy of involved skin reveals dermal IgA deposition and leukocytoclastic vasculitis. IgA deposition is also seen in areas of uninvolved skin.

TREATMENT   Since there is no proven therapy for Henoch-Schönlein nephritis, treatment is supportive. Steroids and/or cytotoxic agents are often tried in patients with severe disease, but without compelling scientific evidence to support their use. The disease typically undergoes clinical exacerbations and remissions in the first year and then enters long-term remission. The prognosis is generally excellent; chronic renal failure and persistent hypertension occur in fewer than 10% of patients.

ESSENTIAL MIXED CRYOGLOBULINEMIA (See also Chap. 317)   Renal involvement is most common with the mixed cryoglobulinemias (types II and III), which are more common in females and usually begin in the sixth decade. Most patients present with a variable combination of leukocytoclastic vasculitis, skin ulcerations, arthralgias, fatigue, and Raynaud's phenomenon. Renal disease is a complication in 50% of patients and usually develops after 12 to 24 months. The typical clinical renal manifestations are nephrotic-range proteinuria, microscopic hematuria, and hypertension. Acute nephritic syndrome occurs in 20 to 30%, and oliguric acute renal failure in about 5% of patients with renal disease. The characteristic morphologic lesions are diffuse mesangial proliferative or membranoproliferative glomerulonephritis. The glomerular capillaries frequently contain eosinophilic hyaline "pseudothrombi" composed of precipitated immunoglobulins. Granular deposition of IgG, IgM, and C3 is usually prominent on immunofluorescence microscopy. Electron microscopy typically reveals subendothelial deposits containing microfibrils and microtubules that display a characteristic "thumbprint" appearance.

Circulating levels of C3, C4, and CH50 are depressed in about 80% of patients with renal involvement, and a transient antinuclear antibody (ANA) (speckled pattern) is sometimes detected. Abnormal liver function tests are found in about 15% of patients at presentation and in up to 50% subsequently. It now appears that most patients with "essential" mixed cryoglobulinemia (EMC) (i.e., idiopathic) are chronically infected with hepatitis C virus (HCV). In keeping with a pathogenetic role for this virus, HCV RNA has been isolated from the serum of patients with EMC, indicating active infection, and anti-HCV antibodies have been detected in both the serum and cryoprecipitates in association with viral antigens.

TREATMENT   Traditionally, glucocorticoids, with or without cyclophosphamide, and plasmapheresis were the standard treatment for EMC. Recent reports indicate that interferon α controls viral replication and stabilizes renal function in most patients infected with EMC and HCV. Unfortunately, most patients relapse when interferon α is discontinued, a major problem given the prohibitive cost of the drug. In general, patient and renal survival are good in EMC, with 75% of patients being alive at 10 years.

SYSTEMIC LUPUS ERYTHEMATOSUS (See also Chap. 311)

Renal involvement is clinically evident in 40 to 85% of patients with SLE; it varies from isolated abnormalities of the urinary sediment to full-blown nephritic or nephrotic syndrome or chronic renal failure. Most glomerular injury is triggered by the formation of immune complexes within the glomerular capillary wall; however, thrombotic microangiopathy may be the dominant reason for renal dysfunction in a small subset of patients with the antiphospholipid antibody syndrome.

Immune-Complex–Mediated Lupus Nephritis The renal biopsy has proven very useful for identifying the different patterns of immune-complex glomerulonephritis in SLE, which are diverse, portend different prognoses, and do not necessarily correlate with the clinical findings. Indeed, clinically silent lupus nephritis is well described in which the urinalysis is virtually normal but renal biopsy demonstrates varying degrees of injury.

The World Health Organization categorizes lupus nephritis into six histologic classes. *Class I* consists of a normal biopsy on light microscopy with occasional mesangial deposits on immunofluorescence microscopy. Patients in this category usually do not have clinical renal disease. Patients with *class II* or mesangial lupus nephritis have prominent mesangial deposits of IgG, IgM, and C3 on immunofluorescence and electron microscopy. Mesangial lupus nephritis is designated as class IIA when the glomeruli are normal by light microscopy and class IIB when there is mesangial hypercellularity. Microscopic hematuria is common with this lesion, and 25 to 50% of patients have moderate proteinuria. Nephrotic syndrome is not seen, and renal survival is excellent (>90% at 5 years). *Class III* describes focal segmental proliferative lupus nephritis with necrosis or sclerosis affecting fewer than 50% of glomeruli. Up to one-third of patients have nephrotic syndrome, and glomerular filtration is impaired in 15 to 25%. In *class IV* or diffuse proliferative lupus nephritis, most glomeruli show cell proliferation, often with crescent formation. Other features on light microscopy include fibrinoid necrosis and "wire loops," which are caused by basement membrane thickening and mesangial interposition between basement membrane and endothelial cells. Deposits of IgG, IgM, IgA, and C3 are evident by immunofluorescence, and crescents stain positive for fibrin. Electron microscopy reveals numerous immune deposits in mesangial, subepithelial, and subendothelial locations. Tubuloreticular structures are frequently seen in endothelial cells. These are not specific for lupus nephritis and also occur in HIV-associated nephropathy. Electron microscopy may also reveal curvilinear parallel arrays of microfibrils, measuring approximately 10 to 15 nm in diameter, with "thumbprinting," similar to those seen in cryoglobulinemia. Nephrotic syndrome and renal insufficiency are present in at least 50% of patients with class IV disease. Diffuse proliferative lupus nephritis is the most aggressive renal lesion in SLE, and as many as 30% of these patients progress to terminal renal failure. *Class V* is termed membranous lupus nephritis because of its similarity to idiopathic membranous glomerulopathy. Thickening of the GBM is evident by light microscopy. Electron microscopy reveals predominant subepithelial deposits in addition to subendothelial and mesangial deposits. Proliferative changes may also be evident, but the predominant pattern is that of membranous glomerulopathy. Most patients present with nephrotic syndrome (90%), but significant impairment of GFR is relatively unusual (10%). Tubulointerstitial changes such as active infiltration by inflammatory cells, tubular atrophy, and interstitial fibrosis are seen to varying degrees in lupus nephritis and are most severe in classes III and IV, especially in patients with long-standing disease. *Class VI* probably represents the end stages of proliferative lupus nephritis and is characterized by diffuse glomerulosclerosis and advanced tubulointerstitial disease. These patients are often hypertensive, may have nephrotic syndrome, and usually have impaired GFR.

Transformation from one class to another is relatively frequent. For example, class III often progresses to class IV spontaneously, and

class IV can transform to class II or class V after treatment. Class II and class V lupus nephritis may predate other manifestations of lupus, whereas class III and class IV usually occur in patients who have systemic features of SLE. A semiquantitative analysis can be performed by using a variety of features on renal biopsy, scored 0 to 3+, to derive indices of disease activity and chronicity. Features that suggest active inflammation include endocapillary proliferation, glomerular leukocyte infiltration, wire loop deposits, cellular crescents, and interstitial inflammation. In contrast, features that suggest chronicity include glomerulosclerosis, fibrous crescents, tubular atrophy, and interstitial fibrosis. In some, but not all, studies, these indices have been useful in predicting response to therapy and renal prognosis.

Patients with active lupus nephritis have a range of serologic abnormalities. Hypocomplementemia is present in 75 to 90% of patients and is most striking with diffuse proliferative glomerulonephritis. ANA are usually detected (95 to 99%), although not specific for SLE. ANA titers tend to fall with treatment, and ANA may not be detected during remissions. Anti-double-stranded DNA (dsDNA) antibodies are highly specific for SLE, and changes in their titers correlate with the activity of lupus nephritis. Almost 100% of patients taking procainamide and 65% of patients taking hydralazine develop ANA; however, overt lupus, including nephritis, occurs in fewer than 10% of these patients, and anti-DNA antibodies are not usually detected. Other antibodies found in patients with SLE include anti-Sm (17 to 30%; highly specific, but not sensitive); anti-RNP, which frequently accompanies anti-Sm in low titer; anti-Ro (35%); anti-La (15%); and anti-histone antibodies (70% of patients with SLE and 95% of patients with drug-induced lupus).

TREATMENT The treatment of lupus nephritis is controversial and based largely on the class of injury and disease activity. Because there is relatively poor correlation between clinical features (urinalysis findings, serum creatinine) and histologic class, the renal biopsy findings are an important guide to therapy. Treatment is not indicated for class I and most cases of class II lupus nephritis, as these histologic patterns portend an excellent prognosis (100% and >90% 5-year survival rates, respectively). Extrarenal manifestations may warrant treatment with glucocorticoids, salicylates, or antimalarials. Glucocorticoids and cyclophosphamide are the mainstays of therapy for patients with proliferative nephritis (classes III and IV). High-dose steroids given as intravenous boluses (pulse therapy) are usually effective at rapidly controlling acute glomerular inflammation. Cyclophosphamide and azathioprine are important adjuncts to steroid therapy and appear to afford better long-term preservation of renal function than steroids alone. Intravenous pulse cyclophosphamide is as efficacious as oral therapy and appears to be less toxic. Most authorities advocate an initial regimen of monthly intravenous boluses of cyclophosphamide for 6 months. Subsequent therapy is tailored to disease activity and typically involves dosing every 3 to 6 months for a total treatment period of 18 to 24 months. The initial dose of cyclophosphamide is 0.5 g/m^2, and the dose is increased gradually to a maximum of 1 g/m^2 unless patients develop leukopenia or other side effects. Steroids are usually started simultaneously at 1 mg/kg per day and are tapered over the first 6 months to a maintenance dose of 5 to 10 mg/d for the duration of cyclophosphamide therapy. Five-year renal survival rates of 60 to 90% have been obtained with this and similar regimens. A large randomized, prospective trial indicated that plasmapheresis does not offer additional benefit in patients with severe proliferative lupus nephritis. Mycophenolate mofetil has recently been used to treat patients with lupus nephritis that is resistant to steroids and cyclophosphamide.

The management of membranous lupus nephritis is less well defined. As with idiopathic membranous glomerulopathy, the incidence of spontaneous remission approaches 50% in membranous lupus nephritis, and the course of the disease is generally indolent, with a 70-

to 90% renal survival rate at 5 years. Some authorities advocate steroids and ACE inhibitors at the time of diagnosis, whereas others reserve them for patients with progressive renal insufficiency or severe nephrotic syndrome. Useful parameters for monitoring the response to therapy and predicting relapse include the activity of the urine sediment, proteinuria, GFR, serum complement levels, and anti-dsDNA titers. Despite maximal immunosuppressive therapy, about 20% of patients with aggressive lupus nephritis develop ESRD requiring dialysis. SLE tends to become quiescent with advanced uremia, and patients rarely develop systemic flares once they commence dialysis. Recurrence of nephritis and systemic flares are also very uncommon after renal transplantation, and allograft survival rates are comparable to those in patients with other causes of ESRD.

ANTIPHOSPHOLIPID ANTIBODY SYNDROME AND THROMBOTIC MICROANGIOPATHY   Patients with this syndrome can develop a variable degree of renal impairment due to thrombotic microangiopathy. The latter typically affects the interlobular arteries, arterioles, and glomerular capillaries and is characterized by intravascular microthrombi and swelling of endothelial cells. Decreased levels of tissue plasminogen activator and increased level of α_2-antiplasmin, both of which would tend to promote thrombosis, have been described in this syndrome. Anticoagulation to maintain the Internalized Normal Ratio (INR) >3.0 may be beneficial in reducing the incidence of recurrent thromboses. There are uncontrolled reports of a benefit of plasmapheresis in the setting of acute renal failure secondary to thrombotic microangiopathy.

RHEUMATOID ARTHRITIS   (See also Chap. 312)   Although extra-articular manifestations are present in 35% of patients with rheumatoid arthritis, direct involvement of the kidney by rheumatoid disease is rare, and glomerular injury is usually secondary to amyloid A (AA) amyloidosis or a side effect of drug therapy. AA amyloidosis is a complication experienced by 10 to 20% of patients with rheumatoid arthritis, and renal involvement is evident clinically in 3 to 10% of these patients (nephrotic syndrome, renal insufficiency). Amyloidosis is more frequent in patients with rheumatoid arthritis of long duration (>10 years), with circulating rheumatoid factor, and with destructive arthropathy. Less frequent glomerular lesions include mesangial proliferative glomerulonephritis and basement membrane thickening by subepithelial immune deposits. Gold and penicillamine may cause nephrotic syndrome by inducing membranous glomerulopathy, whereas nonsteroidal anti-inflammatory drugs (NSAIDs) can trigger the nephrotic syndrome by inducing minimal change nephropathy, usually in association with acute interstitial nephritis (see below).

SJÖGREN'S SYNDROME   (See also Chap. 314)   Tubulointerstitial injury is the most common form of renal involvement in Sjögren's syndrome and usually presents as either Fanconi's syndrome, distal renal tubular acidosis, or impairment of renal concentrating ability. Glomerulonephritis is relatively rare and should prompt a search for evidence of secondary causes. Membranous glomerulopathy and membranoproliferative glomerulonephritis (MPGN) are the most common lesions. Anecdotal reports describe successful therapy with glucocorticoids and cytotoxic agents.

POLYMYOSITIS AND DERMATOMYOSITIS   (See also Chap. 382)   Occasional cases of focal mesangial proliferative glomerulonephritis with mesangial deposition of IgG and complement have been described in polymyositis/dermatomyositis. Membranous glomerulopathy has also been reported, particularly when polymyositis/dermatomyositis is associated with malignancy.

MIXED CONNECTIVE TISSUE DISEASE   (See also Chap. 313)   Mixed connective tissue disease is a syndrome that includes features of SLE, scleroderma, and polymyositis and is associated with high titers of antiribonucleoprotein antibodies and negative antismooth muscle antibodies. Renal involvement occurs in fewer than 15% of patients and manifests as hematuria and subnephrotic proteinuria. The usual pathologic lesion is membranous glomerulopathy or MPGN. The

prognosis is usually excellent, and steroid therapy may be useful in rare patients with progressive renal disease.

GLOMERULAR DEPOSITION DISEASES

The glomerular deposition diseases are characterized by deposition of abnormal proteins, usually immunoglobulins or fragments thereof, within the glomerulus. They include amyloidosis, light and heavy chain deposition disease, cryoglobulinemia, and fibrillary/immunotactoid glomerulonephritis. Here, we focus on amyloidosis and light chain deposition disease (LCDD). Cryoglobulinemic nephropathy is described above in the discussion on systemic vasculitis. →*Fibrillary and immunotactoid glomerulopathy are discussed in Chap. 274.*

AMYLOIDOSIS   (See also Chap. 319)   Amyloidosis is classified according to the major component of its fibrils: for example, immunoglobulin light chains in amyloid L (AL) amyloidosis, serum amyloid A in AA amyloidosis, β_2-microglobulin in dialysis-associated amyloidosis, and amyloid β protein in Alzheimer's disease and Down's syndrome. Amyloid deposits also contain a nonfibrillar component called the P component, a serum α_1 glycoprotein with a high affinity for the fibrillar components of all forms of amyloid. AL and AA amyloidosis frequently involve the kidneys, whereas involvement by other forms of amyloidosis is very rare.

There is substantial overlap in the renal clinicopathologic presentations of AL and AA amyloidosis. Glomeruli are involved in 75 to 90% of patients, usually in association with involvement of other organs. The clinical correlate of glomerular amyloid deposition is nephrotic-range proteinuria. In addition, over 50% of patients have impaired glomerular filtration at diagnosis. Hypertension is present in about 20 to 25%. Renal size is usually normal or slightly enlarged. A minority of patients present with renal failure due to amyloid deposition in the renal vasculature or with Fanconi's syndrome, nephrogenic diabetes insipidus, or renal tubular acidosis due to involvement of the tubulointerstitium. Rectal biopsy and abdominal fat pad biopsy reveal amyloid deposits in about 70% of patients and may obviate the need for renal biopsy.

Renal biopsy gives a very high yield if there is clinical evidence of renal involvement. The earliest pathologic changes are mesangial expansion by amorphous hyaline material and thickening of the GBM. Further amyloid deposition results in the development of large nodular eosinophilic masses. When stained with Congo red, these deposits show apple-green birefringence under polarized light. Immunofluorescence microscopy is usually only weakly positive for immunoglobulin light chains because amyloid fibrils are usually derived from the variable region of light chains. Electron microscopy reveals the characteristic nonbranching extracellular amyloid fibrils of 7.5 to 10 nm in diameter. Tubulointerstitial and vascular deposits of amyloid are also seen and may occasionally be more prominent than glomerular deposits.

R̲x̲   **TREATMENT**   Most patients with renal involvement by AL amyloidosis develop ESRD within 2 to 5 years. No treatment has been shown consistently to improve this prognosis; however, some success has been reported with a combination of melphalan and prednisone. Preliminary studies have reported a benefit of high-dose melphalan with autologous stem cell transplantation. Colchicine delays the onset of nephropathy in patients with familial Mediterranean fever but has not proved useful in patients with established disease or with other forms of amyloid. Remissions may be achieved in AA amyloidosis by eradication of the underlying cause. Renal replacement therapy is offered to patients who reach ESRD; however, the 1-year survival rate on dialysis is low (~66%) by comparison with other causes of ESRD. Most patients die from extrarenal complications, particularly cardiovascular disease. Renal transplantation is a viable option in patients with AA amyloidosis whose primary disease has been eradicated. Transplantation is also an option for patients with AL amyloidosis, although a poor prognosis because of extrarenal organ involvement may preclude them as candidates. Here again, the survival rate is lower by comparison with other causes of ESRD; most of the excess mortality is due to infectious and cardiovascular complications. Recurrence of amyloidosis in the allograft is common but rarely leads to graft loss.

LIGHT CHAIN DEPOSITION DISEASE (See also Chap. 113) Renal involvement is a complication in 90% of patients with LCDD and is often the dominant feature. Nephrotic syndrome and renal impairment are the usual presenting features. Microscopic hematuria occurs in about 20% of patients. Defective hydrogen ion and potassium excretion and urinary concentration may be evident if light chains are deposited predominantly in the tubules. The most common pathologic lesion on renal biopsy is ribbon-like thickening of the tubular basement membrane due to light chain deposition. Mesangial expansion and nodular glomerulosclerosis are found in about 33% of patients. This light-microscopic appearance resembles that of idiopathic MPGN and diabetic nephropathy. Superimposed crescentic change is occasionally seen. Immunofluorescence studies are strongly positive for monoclonal light chains, in contrast to AL amyloid, because the constant region of the immunoglobulin is typically deposited. The tissue deposits in LCDD are granular rather than fibrillar on electron microscopy, appear more amorphous in character, do not stain with Congo red, and seem to have a greater affinity for basement membranes.

The prognosis of LCDD is poor when it is associated with multiple myeloma, and most patients progess rapidly to ESRD. Treatment with melphalan and prednisone has been reported to reduce proteinuria and stabilize renal function in uncontrolled studies. In the absence of myeloma, the prognosis is somewhat more variable, and several patients have undergone successful renal transplantation.

WALDENSTRÖM'S MACROGLOBULINEMIA (See also Chap. 113) This disorder is characterized by monoclonal proliferation of an IgM-secreting clone of plasma cells. The circulating IgM paraprotein frequently gives rise to the hyperviscosity syndrome, which may compromise renal blood flow and GFR. Direct renal involvement is rare and, when present, involves deposition of large amorphous deposits of eosinophilic material in the glomerular capillaries. Renal amyloidosis can also occur.

DRUG-INDUCED GLOMERULAR DISEASE

A variety of drugs damage the glomerular filtration barrier and induce proteinuria and nephrotic syndrome. In contrast, drug-induced proliferative glomerulonephritis is rare. The more common drug-induced glomerulopathies are discussed here. Additional associations are included in Table 275-1 and Table 71-1.

NSAIDs have a variety of renal side effects, including hemodynamically mediated acute renal failure, salt and water retention, hyponatremia, hyperkalemia, papillary necrosis, acute interstitial nephritis, nephrotic syndrome, and ESRD. Nephrotic syndrome and acute renal failure frequently coexist due to a combination of acute interstitial nephritis and a glomerular lesion that is identical to that of minimal change disease. This entity occurs most commonly in patients on propionic acid derivatives such as fenoprofen, ibuprofen, and naproxen but can occur with other NSAIDs, ampicillin, rifampin, and interferon α. Withdrawal of the drug usually results in resolution of renal disease. Membranous nephropathy is also described as an idiosyncratic reaction to NSAIDs.

Gold therapy, administered by injection or orally, induces proteinuria in 5 to 25% of patients with rheumatoid arthritis. Proteinuria develops after 4 to 6 months of therapy, and up to 33% of patients develop full-blown nephrotic syndrome. Renal biopsy typically reveals membranous glomerulopathy, though minimal change disease or mesangial proliferative lesions have also been described. Progressive renal impairment is rare. Nephrotic syndrome is more common in patients who are HLA-B8/DR3 positive, suggesting a genetic susceptibility. Withdrawal of the drug leads to gradual resolution of the proteinuria.

Penicillamine also induces proteinuria in 5 to 30% of patients. As

Table 275-1 Drug-Induced Glomerular Disease

Morphologic Lesion	Causative Agent
Minimal change diseases (usually with interstitial nephritis)	Nonsteroidal anti-inflammatory agents Recombinant interferon α Rifampin Ampicillin
Membranous nephropathy	Penicillamine Gold Mercury Trimethadione Captopril Chlormethiazole
Focal segmental glomerulosclerosis	Heroin
Pauci-immune necrotizing GN	Ciprofloxacin Hydralazine
Proliferative GN with vasculitis	Allopurinol Penicillin Sulfonamides Thiazides Intravenous amphetamines
RPGN	Rifampin Warfarin Carbimazole Amoxicillin Penicillamine

NOTE: GN, glomerulonephritis; RPGN, rapidly progressive glomerulonephritis.

with gold, the underlying glomerular lesion is usually membranous glomerulopathy, and proteinuria gradually resolves after withdrawal of the drug. Acute renal failure secondary to crescentic glomerulonephritis with immune deposits has also been described.

Intravenous heroin use is associated with an increased incidence of focal and segmental glomerulosclerosis (heroin-associated nephropathy). It is not clear whether the nephrotoxin in this setting is heroin itself or a contaminant. Heroin-associated nephropathy occurs predominantly in blacks and is characterized by nephrotic syndrome, hypertension, and a gradual progression to ESRD over a period of 3 to 5 years. The pathologic features are similar to those of idiopathic focal segmental glomerulosclerosis, although mesangial deposition of IgM and C3 may be more prominent. The incidence of this disease appears to be declining steadily. Potential reasons for the decline include increased purity of street heroin and a bias to attribute focal segmental glomerulosclerosis to HIV infection when both risk factors coexist. Intravenous *amphetamine* abuse is a rare cause of systemic necrotizing vasculitis.

HEREDITARY DISEASES WITH GLOMERULAR INVOLVEMENT

ALPORT'S SYNDROME (See also Chap. 351) Alport's syndrome is the most common hereditary nephritis and is usually transmitted as an X-linked dominant trait. The genetic defect resides in the gene for the α5 chain of type IV collagen located on the long arm of the X chromosome; type IV collagen is a major structural component of the GBM. Numerous genetic mutations have been detected, ranging from major deletions to point mutations, and this genetic heterogeneity is reflected in the phenotypic variations of the disease. In the X-linked forms, males usually present with microscopic hematuria, proteinuria (nephrotic-range in 30%), and progressive renal insufficiency. Common extrarenal manifestations include sensorineural hearing loss (~60%), bilateral anterior lenticonus (~15 to 30%), and recurrent corneal erosions. Platelet defects are described but are rare. Female carriers usually have mild disease and do not develop renal insufficiency. Autosomal dominant and recessive forms also exist in which there are mutations in the gene for the $\alpha 3$ chain of type IV collagen, and males and females are equally affected. Genetic analysis to detect mutations in the genes encoding the $\alpha 3$ and $\alpha 5$ chains of type IV collagen may become the diagnostic method of choice.

Typical light-microscopic features on renal biopsy include mesangial hypercellularity, focal and segmental glomerulosclerosis, chronic tubulointerstitial fibrosis, atrophy, and accumulation of foam cells. Electron microscopy reveals thickening, fragmentation, and lamellation of the lamina densa of the GBM. Patchy thinning of the GBM may also be seen, especially early in the course of the disease and in female carriers.

Males with the disease tend to progress to ESRD and are suitable candidates for dialysis and transplantation. About 5% of transplant recipients develop anti-GBM disease in the renal allograft; their immune system recognizes normal GBM of the transplanted kidney as a foreign antigen. These patients can have antibodies against the $\alpha 3$ (Goodpasture antigen) or $\alpha 5$ chains of type IV collagen, probably because defective synthesis of the $\alpha 5$ chain results in defective incorporation or orientation of the $\alpha 3$ chain in the GBM.

SICKLE CELL DISEASE (See also Chap. 106)   Glomerular disease is common (15 to 30%) in homozygotes for sickle cell disease. Glomerular hyperfiltration and hypertrophy occur within the first 5 years of life. Approximately 15 to 30% of patients develop proteinuria in the first three decades, and 5% develop ESRD. The glomerular pathology is usually focal segmental glomerulosclerosis, probably due to sustained glomerular capillary hypertension. MPGN is also seen on occasion. Predictors of chronic renal failure are worsening anemia, proteinuria, nephrotic syndrome, and hypertension. ACE inhibitors may slow the progression of renal disease by lowering systemic and glomerular capillary hypertension.

FABRY'S DISEASE (See also Chap. 349)   In patients with Fabry's disease, renal biopsy reveals accumulation of neutral glycosphingolipids with terminal α-galactosyl moieties in lysosomes of glomerular, tubular, vascular, and interstitial cells. Focal and global glomerulosclerosis are later features. Electron microscopy reveals stacked, concentric lamellar profiles known as "myeloid" bodies, which are characteristic. Renal disease manifests in the late teens to early twenties with lipiduria, proteinuria with minimal hematuria, nephrotic syndrome, hypertension, and progressive renal insufficiency. The most striking systemic manifestations are skin lesions (angiokeratomas), corneal and lens opacities, painful dysesthesias of the extremities, and arthropathy of the terminal interphalangeal joints. The diagnosis of Fabry's disease can often be made by careful physical examination, especially if many of the typical clinical features are present. Measurement of urinary glycosphingolipids and estimation of peripheral leukocyte α-galactosidase levels help confirm the diagnosis. The renal lesion is progressive, and these patients often tolerate hemodynamic changes during dialysis poorly because of progressive vascular disease. Successful renal transplantation has been reported despite recurrence in the allograft.

NAIL-PATELLA SYNDROME   The nail-patella syndrome is a rare hereditary disorder transmitted as an autosomal dominant trait. The abnormal gene is located on the long arm of chromosome 9, and candidate genes include the $\alpha 1$ chain of type V collagen and the LIM homeodomain protein Lmxlb. The phenotype is characterized by multiple osseous abnormalities, primarily affecting the elbows and knees, and nail dysplasia. About 50% of patients have clinically evident nephropathy. The light-microscopic features on renal biopsy include local GBM thickening, tubular atrophy, interstitial fibrosis, and varying degrees of glomerular sclerosis. Electron microscopy reveals irregular thickening of the GBM, with electrolucent areas giving it a "motheaten" appearance. Cross-striated fibrils with the periodicity of collagen can be identified in the mesangium and basement membrane. The disease usually manifests clinically as asymptomatic hematuria and

proteinuria, occasionally in the nephrotic range, but it may be silent. The renal lesion is relatively benign, and progression to ESRD occurs in 10 to 30% of patients.

LIPODYSTROPHY   MPGN type II (dense deposit disease) is the most frequent glomerular lesion in patients with lipodystrophy (80%), whereas MPGN type I affects the remainder (20%). The disease occurs mostly in females between the ages of 5 and 15 years, and the clinical presentation and course are similar to those of idiopathic MPGN, namely nephrotic-range proteinuria and progressive renal insufficiency. Low C3 levels are common in association with C3 nephritic factor (Chap. 274).

LECITHIN-CHOLESTEROL ACYLTRANSFERASE DEFICIENCY (See also Chap. 344)   Renal manifestations of this disease include proteinuria, microscopic hematuria, and progressive renal insufficiency. Renal biopsy typically reveals focal and segmental glomerulosclerosis. Electron-microscopic findings include irregular rounded, lucent lacunae that contain solid or laminated dense structures in the GBM, mesangial matrix, and Bowman's capsular and renal tubular basement membranes. Endothelial cell detachment is also evident, and capillary lumens may be occluded by vacuolated foam cells. Recurrence of the disease has been documented in the renal allograft but without marked impairment of graft function.

GLOMERULAR LESIONS ASSOCIATED WITH INFECTIOUS DISEASES

VIRAL INFECTIONS   Hepatitis B, hepatitis C, and HIV are strongly associated with glomerular disease (Table 275-2). Glomerular lesions associated with *hepatitis B virus* (HBV) infection include

Table 275-2   Glomerular Lesions Associated with Infectious Diseases

Morphologic Lesion	Common Disease or Inciting Organism
Diffuse proliferative glomerulonephritis (classic postinfectious glomerulonephritis)	Streptococcal pharyngitis Acute/subacute bacterial endocarditis Visceral sepsis Typhoid fever Syphilis Leptospirosis (*Mycobacterium leprae*) Toxoplasmosis Falciparum malaria *Plasmodium falciparum* Varicella, mumps, echovirus, coxsackievirus, measles Infectious mononucleosis Hepatitis B and C
Membranoproliferative glomerulonephritis	Subacute bacterial endocarditis Ventriculoatrial shunt infection Visceral sepsis Hepatitis C infection Hepatitis B infection *P. falciparum* Schistosomiasis
Mesangial proliferative glomerulonephritis	Recovery phase of postinfectious glomerulonephritis
Membranous nephropathy	Hepatitis C infection Hepatitis B infection Syphilis Filariasis Hydatid disease Schistosomiasis *Plasmodium malariae* Leprosy Enterococcal endocarditis
Focal segmental glomerulosclerosis	HIV infection Schistosomiasis
Renal amyloidosis	Any chronic infection

membranous glomerulopathy, MPGN, IgA nephropathy, essential mixed cryoglobulinemia, and polyarteritis nodosa. Membranous glomerulopathy is most common. In endemic areas, such as Asia and Africa, 80 to 100% of children and 30 to 45% of adults with membranous glomerulopathy have HBV surface antigenemia. HBV antigens have been identified in renal immune deposits, suggesting in situ immune-complex formation after planting of HBV antigens or trapping of circulating immune complexes containing HBV antigens. Patients typically present with nephrotic syndrome and microscopic hematuria. Hypertension and renal impairment are rare. The most common associated hepatic lesion is chronic persistent or chronic active hepatitis. In nonendemic areas there is a male preponderance, and many patients are intravenous drug users or have other risk factor for acquisition of HBV. The asymptomatic carrier state of HBV is frequently associated with MPGN in endemic areas. Hypertension and azotemia are more common with this morphologic pattern than with membranous glomerulopathy. Children with HBV-associated membranous glomerulonephritis have a good prognosis, and almost two-thirds enter spontaneous remission within 3 years. ESRD is rare. In contrast, 30% of adults develop progressive renal failure within 5 years, with 10% reaching ESRD. Steroids and cytotoxic agents are contraindicated as they may lead to increased viral replication and worsening of liver disease. Interferon α may reduce proteinuria and stabilize renal function in patients with progressive disease.

HCV infection (Chap. 295) should be considered in all patients with cryoglobulinemic proliferative glomerulonephritis, MPGN, and membranous glomerulopathy. These three clinocopathologic entities may represent a spectrum of morphologic manifestations of the same pathogenetic process, namely HCV-induced immune-complex disease. Up to 30% of patients with chronic HCV infection have an abnormal urinary sediment. HCV infection accounts for 10 to 20% of type I MPGN and is a major cause of essential mixed cryoglobulinemia. Renal biopsy reveals typical features of type I MPGN and IgG, IgM, C3, and/or cryoglobulin deposits. Most patients present with nephrotic syndrome and microscopic hematuria and may have red blood cell casts. Liver function tests are usually abnormal, and C3 levels are typically depressed. Anti-HCV antibodies are detected in most patients, and viral RNA has been documented in blood and cryoglobulins. Various treatments have been reported to be useful in HCV-induced renal disease including steroids, cytotoxic agents, and plasmapheresis; however, controlled trials to support their use are lacking. Interferon α has been demonstrated to clear antigenemia, lower cryoglobulin levels, and stabilize renal disease. Unfortunately, relapse is usual once the drug is discontinued.

HIV infection (Chap. 309) has been associated with focal segmental glomerulosclerosis, acute diffuse proliferative glomerulonephritis, and mesangioproliferative glomerulonephritis, including IgA nephropathy, MPGN, and membranous glomerulopathy. The classic and most common HIV-associated glomerulopathy is an aggressive form of focal segmental glomerulosclerosis, an entity that is termed *HIV-associated nephropathy (HIVAN)*. This disease may be the first manifestation of infection in otherwise asymptomatic patients. HIVAN is more common in blacks than in other ethnic groups and is more frequent in intravenous drug abusers with HIV infection than in homosexuals. The disease has been described in all high-risk groups, however, including infants of HIV-positive mothers. Renal biopsy typically reveals visceral epithelial cell swelling, collapse of the glomerular capillary tuft, severe tubulointerstitial inflammation, and microcystic dilatation of renal tubules. Electron microscopy characteristically reveals severe visceral epithelial cell injury and tubuloreticular inclusions in glomerular endothelial cells, tubular cells and infiltrating leukocytes. This constellation of findings has been termed collapsing glomerulopathy, but it should be emphasized that a similar picture can be seen in the absence of HIV infection. The presence of tubuloreticular inclusions and the aggressive clinical course distinguish HIVAN from idiopathic focal segmental glomerulosclerosis. The mechanisms of renal cell injury are still being defined. Viral DNA has been demonstrated in the renal epithelia of HIV-infected patients with and without nephropathy,

suggesting that pathogenetic factors, other than infection of cells, are required for induction of disease. The typical clinical correlates of HIVAN are severe nephrotic syndrome and rapid progression to ESRD, occurring in weeks to months. Despite early reports of poor survival of patients on dialysis, more recent studies indicate improved survival for both asymptomatic patients with HIV and patients with full-blown AIDS. There is no proven therapy for HIVAN. The initial experience with combined highly active antiretroviral therapy (triple therapy) suggests that these regimens have reduced the incidence of nephropathy in HIV-infected patients and improved prognosis in patients with established nephropathy.

BACTERIAL INFECTIONS (Table 275-2) Immune-complex glomerulonephritis is a relatively frequent complication of infective *endocarditis* (Chap. 126). Other mechanisms of renal injury in bacterial endocarditis include embolic renal infarction, septic abscesses, acute tubular necrosis secondary to septicemia and drug therapy, disseminated intravascular coagulation, and antibiotic-induced acute interstitial nephritis. Patients typically present with microscopic hematuria, urinary red blood cell casts, pyuria and modest proteinuria (nephrotic range in 25% of patients), and variable degrees of renal failure. Rheumatoid factor is present in 10 to 70%, and circulating immune complexes in 90%. Serum complement levels are usually depressed. Renal biopsy reveals mild focal proliferative glomerulonephritis with mesangial and capillary wall deposition of IgG and C3 by immunofluorescence microscopy and subendothelial, mesangial, and subepithelial electron-dense deposits by electron microscopy. Occasional patients develop diffuse necrotizing glomerulonephritis with crescent formation and present with nephritic syndrome or RPGN. Endocarditis-associated glomerulonephritis typically has a good prognosis and resolves with eradication of the underlying infection.

Immune-complex glomerulonephritis is a complication in 1 to 4% of patients with *infected ventriculoatrial shunts*. Nephritis can manifest weeks to years after shunt insertion and usually presents with microscopic hematuria. Nephrotic syndrome occurs in 30 to 50%. The usual renal pathology is a membranoproliferative pattern, although diffuse proliferation can also occur. Immunofluorescence reveals IgM and C3 in the capillary wall and mesangial area, while subendothelial deposits and mesangial interposition are seen by electron microscopy. Up to one-third of patients may have residual renal impairment despite removal of the infected shunt and resolution of the infection.

Suppurative infections such as intrathoracic and intraabdominal abscesses, osteomyelitis, and dental abscesses have been associated with glomerulonephritis. The usual presentation is hematuria, urinary red blood cell casts, proteinuria, and acute renal failure. Oliguria and hypertension are common. Pathologic renal lesions include mesangial proliferative, membranoproliferative, and diffuse proliferative glomerulonephritis with crescents. Immunofluorescence reveals mesangial and capillary wall deposition predominantly of C3, although IgG and IgM may also be seen.

Nephrotic syndrome is a complication in 0.3% of patients with secondary *syphilis* and 8% of patients with congenital syphilis. The usual pathology is membranous glomerulopathy; however, mild mesangial and endocapillary proliferation can occur. IgG and IgM are evident in affected regions by immunofluorescence microscopy, and treponemal antigens have been identified in diseased glomeruli. C3 and C4 are typically depressed in congenital syphilis. The treatment consists of penicillin to eradicate the infection.

Leprosy most commonly causes AA amyloidosis; however, a syndrome resembling acute poststreptococcal glomerulonephritis has also been described.

PROTOZOAN AND PARASITIC INFECTIONS   Transient proteinuria (50% of patients) and nephrotic syndrome (<1% of patients) are complications of infection with *Plasmodium falciparum*. Membranoproliferative glomerulonephritis is the usual pathologic lesion and may respond to eradication of infection. *Plasmodium malariae* has been associated with diffuse or focal proliferative glomerulonephritis, membranous glomerulopathy, and minimal change disease. Eradication of the malarial infection does not consistently induce remission of the nephrotic syndrome. *Schistosoma mansoni* causes nephrotic syndrome in 5 to 10% of patients, and progression to ESRD is common. The usual pathology is MPGN or mesangial proliferative glomerulonephritis, although membranous glomerulonephritis and amyloidosis are occasionally seen. *Filiariasis* can trigger membranous glomerulonephritis (*Loa loa*) and occasionally induces proliferative glomerulonephritis (*Onchocerca volvulus*). *Congenital toxoplasmosis* infection occasionally induces immune-complex glomerulonephritis characterized by mesangial and subendothelial immune deposits that contain *Toxoplasma* antigens. Membranous glomerulopathy and proliferative glomerulonephritis are occasional complications of *hydatid disease* and *trichinosis*, respectively.

GLOMERULAR LESIONS ASSOCIATED WITH NEOPLASIA

Glomerulopathies associated with neoplasia include membranous glomerulopathy, minimal change disease, focal segmental glomerulosclerosis, immune-complex glomerulonephritis, fibrillary/immunotactoid glomerulonephritis, LCDD, and amyloidosis. Mild proteinuria is common in patients with *solid tumors*, but overt glomerulonephritis is rare. Occasional patients with solid tumors of the lung, gastrointestinal tract, breast, kidney, and ovary develop full-blown nephrotic syndrome, usually due to a membranous glomerulopathy. Estimates of the incidence of occult malignancy in patients presenting with membranous glomerulopathy range from 0.1 to 10%. Most authorities agree that an extensive search for malignancy is not indicated, unless there are other suggestive clinical features. As many as 35% of patients with renal cell carcinoma have mesangial deposition of IgG and C3 visible on immunofluorescence; however, morphologic abnormalities are detected in only 50% of these patients, and clinically significant glomerulopathy is rare. Glomerular amyloidosis has also been described in association with this tumor.

An array of glomerular disease has been reported in patients with lymphoproliferative malignancy. Nephrotic syndrome is a recognized complication of *Hodgkin's lymphoma*, with 70% of cases due to minimal change disease. The latter may occur concurrently with (40 to 45%), precede (10 to 15%), or follow (40 to 50%) diagnosis of the malignancy. It is postulated that a lymphokine or other mediator released by malignant T lymphocytes perturbs podocyte function and alters glomerular permeability in this setting. Nephrotic syndrome typically resolves with successful treatment and relapses with recurrence of disease. Less frequent associations with Hodgkin's lymphoma include focal segmental glomerulosclerosis, membranous glomerulopathy, MPGN, proliferative glomerulonephritis, and crescentic glomerulonephritis. Minimal change disease, membranous glomerulopathy, MPGN, and crescentic glomerulonephritis have also been reported in patients with *non-Hodgkin's lymphoma*. Glomerulopathy in the context of leukemia is rare. MPGN can complicate *chronic lymphatic leukemia* and related *B cell lymphomas*, particularly when associated with cryoglobulinemia. Other glomerular lesions associated with *paraproteinemia* include primary amyloid, LCDD, proliferative glomerulonephritis induced by cryoglobulinemia, and fibrillary/immunotactoid glomerulopathy. Here again, the renal lesion frequently improves or resolves with successful treatment of the underlying malignancy.

BIBLIOGRAPHY

APPEL G, RISHNAM JR: Secondary glomerular diseases, in *Brenner & Rector's The Kidney*, 6th ed, BM Brenner (ed). Philadelphia, Saunders, 2000, pp 1350–1448

AUSTIN HA: Natural history and treatment of lupus nephritis. Seminar Nephrol 19:2, 1999

BENNETT PH et al: Screening and management of microalbuminuria in patients with diabetes mellitus: Recommendations to the Scientific Advisory Board of the National Kidney Foundation from an ad hoc committee of the Council on Diabetes Mellitus of the National Kidney Foundation. Am J Kidney Dis 25:107, 1995

BRADY HR, WILCOX CS (eds): *Therapy in Nephrology and Hypertension*. Philadelphia, Saunders, 1999

D'AGATI V et al: HIV infection and the kidney. J Am Soc Nephrol 8:139, 1997

DAGHESTANI L et al: Renal manifestations of hepatitis C infection. Am J Med 106:347, 1999

FALK RH, SKINNER M: The systemic amyloidoses: an overview. Adv Intern Med 45:107, 2000

KASHTAN CE: Alport syndrome and thin glomerular basement membrane disease. J Am Soc Nephrol 9:1736, 1998

PARVING HH et al: Diabetic nephropathy, in *Brenner & Rector's The Kidney*, 6th ed, BM Brenner (ed). Philadelphia, Saunders, 2000, pp 1731–1773

STEGALL MD et al: Pancreas transplantation for the prevention of diabetic nephropathy. Mayo Clin Proc 75:49, 2000

STEHMAN-BREEN C, JOHNSON RJ: Hepatitis C virus-associated glomerulonephritis. Adv Intern Med 43:79, 1998

---

276   *John R. Asplin, Fredric L. Coe*

HEREDITARY TUBULAR DISORDERS

The hereditary renal tubular disorders and their morphologic and functional abnormalities, mode of inheritance, and associated abnormalities are summarized in Table 276-1. The individual disorders are discussed in detail below.

AUTOSOMAL DOMINANT POLYCYSTIC KIDNEY DISEASE

ETIOLOGY AND PATHOLOGY   Autosomal dominant polycystic kidney disease (ADPKD) has a prevalence of 1:300 to 1:1000 and accounts for approximately 10% of end-stage renal disease (ESRD) in the United States. Some 90% of cases are inherited as an autosomal dominant trait, and approximately 10% are spontaneous mutations.

GENETIC CONSIDERATIONS   Three forms of ADPKD have been identified. ADPKD-1 accounts for 90% of cases, and the gene has been localized to the short arm of chromosome 16. The gene for ADPKD-2 has been mapped to the long arm of chromosome 4. The protein products of the two genes form the polycystin complex, which may regulate cell-cell or cell-matrix interactions. A defect in either of these proteins interrupts the normal function of the polycystin complex, resulting in the same phenotype for two distinct genetic abnormalities. ADPKD-2 appears to have a later age of onset of symptoms and renal failure than ADPKD-1. A third form has been documented but has not been mapped to a gene at this point. ∎

The kidneys are grossly enlarged, with multiple cysts studding the surface of the kidney. The cysts contain straw-colored fluid that may become hemorrhagic. The cysts are spherical, vary in size from a few millimeters to centimeters, and are distributed evenly throughout the cortex and medulla. Only 1 to 5% of nephrons will develop cysts. Cysts form when a "second hit" causes a somatic mutation in the normal allele of a tubule cell, leading to monoclonal proliferation of the tubular epithelium. The remaining renal parenchyma reveals varying degrees of tubular atrophy, interstitial fibrosis, and nephrosclerosis.

CLINICAL FEATURES   The disease may present at any age but most frequently causes symptoms in the third or fourth decade. Patients may develop chronic flank pain from the mass effect of the enlarged kidneys. Acute pain indicates infection, urinary tract obstruction by clot or stone, or sudden hemorrhage into a cyst. Gross and microscopic hematuria are common, and impaired renal concentrating ability frequently leads to nocturia. Nephrolithiasis occurs in 15 to 20% of patients, calcium oxalate and uric acid stones being most common. Low urine pH, low urine citrate, and urinary stasis from distortion of the collecting system by cysts all play a role in stone formation. Hypertension is found in 20 to 30% of children and up to 75% of adults. It is secondary to intrarenal ischemia from distortion of the renal architecture, leading to activation of the renin-angiotensin system. Patients with hypertension have a much more rapid progression to ESRD. Urinary tract infection is common and may involve the bladder or renal interstitium (pyelonephritis) or infect a cyst (pyocyst). Pyocysts can be difficult to diagnose but are more likely to be present if the patient has positive blood cultures, new renal pain, or failed to improve clinically after a standard course of antibiotic therapy.

Progressive decline in renal function is common, with approximately 50% of patients developing ESRD by age 60. However, there is considerable variation in age of onset of renal failure, even within the same family. Hypertension, recurrent infections, male sex, and early age of diagnosis are related to early onset renal failure. Renal failure usually progresses slowly; if a sudden decrement in kidney function occurs, ureteral obstruction from stone, clot, or compression by a cyst are likely causes. Patients usually have high hematocrits for their level of renal function, as erythropoietin production is high. Fluid overload is uncommon because of a tendency for renal salt wasting.

Extrarenal manifestations of this disease are frequent and underscore the systemic nature of the defect. Hepatic cysts occur in 50 to 70% of patients. Cysts are generally asymptomatic, and liver function

Table 276-1 Renal Tubule Defects

Disease	Renal Morphologic Abnormalities	Renal Functional Abnormalities	Mode of Inheritance	Associated Abnormalities
Autosomal dominant polycystic disease	Cortical and medullary cysts	Chronic renal failure, >20 yr	AD	Hepatic cysts, intracranial aneurysms, colonic diverticula
Autosomal recessive polycystic disease	Distal tubule and collecting duct cysts	Chronic renal failure, <20 yr	AR	Congenital hepatic fibrosis
Tuberous sclerosis	Renal cysts and angiomyolipomas	None	AD	Skin lesions, hamartomas of the central nervous system
Von Hippel–Lindau disease	Renal cysts, increased risk of renal cell cancer	None	AD	Hemangioblastoma of the retina and central nervous system
Medullary sponge kidney	Dilated collecting ducts	Nephrocalcinosis, hematuria	AD, S	None
Juvenile nephronophthisis	Medullary cysts, small kidneys	Chronic renal failure, <20 yr polyuria, salt wasting	AR	Hepatic fibrosis, retinal abnormalities
Medullary cystic disease	Medullary cysts, small kidneys	Chronic renal failure, >20 yr polyuria, salt wasting	AD	None
Liddle's syndrome	None	Hypokalemia, alkalosis, low aldosterone levels	AR	Hypertension
Bartter's syndrome	Juxtaglomerular apparatus hyperplasia	Hypokalemia, alkalosis, high aldosterone levels	AR, S	None
Congenital nephrogenic diabetes insipidus	None	Vasopressin renal concentrating defect	XL, AR	None
Renal tubular acidosis, type 1	Nephrocalcinosis	Impaired proton secretion in distal tubule, non-anion-gap metabolic acidosis	AD, AR, XL, S, ACQ	Rickets, osteomalacia, nephrolithiasis
Renal tubular acidosis, type 2	None	Reduced bicarbonate reabsorption, non-anion-gap metabolic acidosis	AR, AD, XL, ACQ	Fanconi syndrome, rickets
Renal tubular acidosis, type 4	Chronic renal insufficiency	Reduced proton and potassium secretion	ACQ	Renal insufficiency
X-linked hypophosphatemia	None	Reduced phosphate reabsorption	XL	Rickets, osteomalacia, normal serum $1,25(OH)_2D_3$
Vitamin D–dependent rickets, type 1	None	Defective renal $1,25(OH)_2D_3$ production	AR	Rickets, osteomalacia, low serum $1,25(OH)_2D_3$
Vitamin D–dependent rickets, type 2	None	Renal resistance to $1,25(OH)_2D_3$	AR, S	Rickets, osteomalacia, high serum $1,25(OH)_2D_3$
Oncogenic osteomalacia	None	Reduced phosphate reabsorption	ACQ	Osteomalacia, mesenchymal tumors
X-linked recessive nephrolithiasis	Interstitial fibrosis, medullary calcifications	Hypercalciuria, low-molecular-weight proteinuria	XL	Renal failure
Isolated hyperuricemia	None	Reduced urate reabsorption	AR	Variable hypercalciuria
Hartnup disorder	None	Reduced reabsorption of neutral amino acids	AR	Dermatitis, diarrhea, dementia
Cystinuria	Cystine stones	Reduced reabsorption of dibasic amino acids	AR	Short stature
Iminoglycinuria	None	Reduced reabsorption of proline, hydroxyproline, and glycine	AR	None
Fanconi syndrome	Swan neck deformity of proximal tubule	Reduced reabsorption of bicarbonate, glucose, phosphate, uric acid, and amino acids	AR	Rickets, osteomalacia, hypokalemia, metabolic acidosis

NOTE: AD, autosomal dominant; AR, autosomal recessive; XL, X-linked; ACQ, acquired; S, sporadic is normal, though women may develop massive hepatic cystic disease on occasion. Cyst formation has also been observed in the spleen, pancreas, and ovaries. Intracranial aneurysms are present in 5 to 10% of asymptomatic patients, with potential for permanent neurologic injury or death from subarachnoid hemorrhage. Screening of all ADPKD patients for aneurysms is not recommended, but patients with a family history of subarachnoid hemorrhage should be studied noninvasively with magnetic resonance imaging angiography. Colonic diverticular disease is the most common extrarenal abnormality, and patients are more likely to develop perforation than the general population with colonic diverticula. Mitral valve prolapse is found in 25% of patients, and the prevalence of aortic and tricuspid valve insufficiency is increased.

DIAGNOSIS   Ultrasound is the preferred technique for diagnosis of symptomatic patients and for screening asymptomatic family members. The ability to detect cysts increases with the subject's age: 80 to 90% of ADPKD patients over the age of 20 will have detectable cysts, and almost 100% over the age of 30 will have cysts. At least three to five cysts in each kidney is the standard diagnostic criteria for ADPKD. Computed tomography (CT) scan may be more sensitive than ultrasound in detection of small cysts. Genetic linkage analysis is now available for diagnosis of ADPKD but is reserved for cases where radiographic imaging is negative and the need for definitive diagnosis critical, such as screening family members for potential kidney donation.

R̲x̲ TREATMENT   The goals of treatment are to slow the rate of progression of renal disease and minimize symptoms. Hypertension and renal infection should be treated aggressively to maintain renal function. Converting enzyme inhibitors are effective antihypertensive agents, though patients should be closely monitored as some develop renal insufficiency and hyperkalemia. Urinary infection is treated in a standard manner unless a pyocyst is suspected, in which case antibiotics that penetrate cysts should be used, such as trimethoprim-sulfamethoxazole, ciprofloxacin, and chloramphenicol. Chronic pain from cysts can be managed by cyst puncture and sclerosis with ethanol.

AUTOSOMAL RECESSIVE POLYCYSTIC KIDNEY DISEASE

GENETIC CONSIDERATIONS   Autosomal recessive polycystic kidney disease (ARPKD) is a rare genetic disease that has an incidence between 1:10,000 and 1:40,000. The gene for ARPKD has been localized to chromosome 6. In the past, ARPKD was considered to be a family of disorders, categorized as neonatal, infantile, and childhood forms depending on the age of onset and the relative degree of involvement of the kidneys and liver. However, variable clinical presentations within siblings in the same family, as well as the localization of the disease to chromosome 6 in multiple families, support the premise that this is a single genetic disease with variable phenotypic presentation. ■

At birth the kidneys are enlarged with a smooth external surface. The distal tubules and collecting ducts are dilated into elongated cysts that are arranged in a radial fashion. As the patient ages, the cysts may become more spherical and the disease can be confused with ADPKD. Interstitial fibrosis is also seen as renal function deteriorates. Liver involvement includes proliferation and dilation of small intrahepatic bile ducts as well as periportal fibrosis.

CLINICAL FEATURES   The majority of cases are diagnosed in the first year of life, presenting as bilateral abdominal masses. Death in the neonatal period is most commonly due to pulmonary hypoplasia. Hypertension and impaired urinary concentrating ability are common. The time course to ESRD is variable, though many children maintain adequate kidney function for years. Older children present with com-

plications secondary to congenital hepatic fibrosis and generally have less severe kidney disease. Hepatosplenomegaly, portal hypertension, and esophageal varices are frequent complications of ARPKD.

DIAGNOSIS   Ultrasound is the most common technique used to diagnose ARPKD, prenatally and in childhood. Ultrasound examination reveals enlarged kidneys with increased echogenicity. At times spherical cysts may be seen, potentially leading to an incorrect diagnosis of ADPKD. A thorough family history and imaging the kidneys of the parents aids in differentiation from other cystic diseases. The recent mapping of the gene should allow linkage studies to be used in diagnosis.

R̲x̲ TREATMENT   Aggressive treatment of hypertension and urinary tract infection are the major goals of therapy in order to maintain native renal function as long as possible. Dialysis and transplant are appropriate when kidney failure occurs. Hepatic fibrosis may lead to life-threatening variceal hemorrhage, requiring sclerotherapy or portocaval shunting.

TUBEROUS SCLEROSIS

Patients with this multisystem disease most commonly present with skin lesions and benign tumors of the central nervous system (Chap. 370). Renal involvement is common; angiomyolipomas are the most frequent abnormality and are usually bilateral. Renal cysts may be present as well and can give an appearance similar to that of ADPKD. Histologically, the cysts are unique—the cyst lining cells are large with an eosinophilic staining cytoplasm and may form hyperplastic nodules that can fill the cyst space.

GENETIC CONSIDERATIONS   One-third of cases are inherited as an autosomal dominant trait, the rest are due to sporadic mutations. Mutations of tumor-suppression genes have been identified on chromosomes 9 (*TSC1*) and 16 (*TSC2*). Mutations of *TSC2* account for the majority of cases and are more likely to be associated with mental retardation and polycystic kidneys. Tuberous sclerosis may be confused with ADPKD if extrarenal manifestations are minimal. ■

VON HIPPEL–LINDAU DISEASE

This autosomal dominant disease is characterized by hemangioblastomas of the retina and the central nervous system (Chap. 370). Renal cysts occur in the majority of cases and are usually bilateral. The *VHL* gene is a tumor-suppressor gene and has been localized to chromosome 3. It is the same gene that is mutated in sporadic renal cell carcinoma, which may be found in up to 25% of patients with von Hippel–Lindau disease and is frequently multifocal. Yearly screening of adults using CT scans has been recommended in an attempt to diagnose renal cell cancers at an early stage.

MEDULLARY SPONGE KIDNEY

ETIOLOGY AND PATHOLOGY   Medullary sponge kidney (MSK) is a congenital disorder. Although some cases have apparent autosomal dominant inheritance, most are sporadic. It is found in 0.5 to 1% of all intravenous pyelograms. Males and females are affected equally. The pathologic lesion is cystic dilation of the inner medullary and papillary collecting ducts, with collecting diameters ranging from 1 to 5 mm. Bilateral renal involvement is present in 70% of cases, but not all papillae are equally affected. The dilated ducts are lined by cuboidal epithelium with areas of pseudostratified and stratified squamous epithelium. Calculi are frequently found in the dilated collecting ducts.

CLINICAL FEATURES   Patients generally present in the third or fourth decade with kidney stones, infection, or recurrent hematuria. The disease is most commonly diagnosed by intravenous pyelogram,

FIGURE 276-1 *A.* Radiographic appearance of medullary sponge kidney. Abdominal flat plate reveals multiple bilateral calcifications. *B.* Radiographic contrast material accumulates in the dilated and cystic terminal collecting ducts and obscures the calcifications.

which shows linear striations radiating into the renal papillae or small cystic collections of contrast in the dilated ducts (Fig. 276-1). Approximately 60% of patients with MSK have stones, and 12% of all stone formers will have MSK. Hypercalciuria occurs with the same frequency in MSK as it does in random stone formers. Papillary nephrocalcinosis occurs more frequently in patients with MSK than in the random stone former. Proteinuria is minimal, if present at all, and renal function is normally preserved unless there is renal damage from recurrent infection or severe stone disease.

℞ TREATMENT Asymptomatic patients require no specific therapy except to maintain high fluid intake to reduce the risk of nephrolithiasis. If stones are present, standard laboratory evaluation should be done and metabolic abnormalities treated as in any stone former (Chap. 279). Infection should be treated aggressively, and instrumentation of the urinary tract should be minimized to avoid introducing infection.

JUVENILE NEPHRONOPHTHISIS/MEDULLARY CYSTIC DISEASE

ETIOLOGY AND PATHOLOGY Juvenile nephronophthisis (JN) and medullary cystic disease (MCD) have similar pathologic findings but differ in inheritance pattern and age of onset.

GENETIC CONSIDERATIONS JN is inherited as an autosomal recessive disease; linkage studies have shown 70% of the cases to map to a gene (*NPH1*) on the short arm of chromosome 2. MCD is an autosomal dominant disease. Linkage analysis has identified genes on chromosomes 1 and 16 as being associated with MCD. In both conditions, the kidneys tend to be small, with cysts throughout the medulla; the cortex and papilla rarely have cysts. The cysts originate in the collecting ducts, distal convoluted tubules, and loops of Henle and range in size from 1 to 10 mm. Sclerotic glomeruli, tubule atrophy, and interstitial fibrosis are frequent findings on biopsy. ■

CLINICAL FEATURES Patients with JN present during childhood with symptoms of polyuria, growth retardation, anemia, and progressive renal insufficiency. Most patients develop ESRD prior to the age of 20; JN accounts for 2 to 10% of renal failure in children. Hepatic fibrosis and cerebellar ataxia has been reported in association with JN. JN with retinal degeneration is termed the *Senior-Loken syndrome*; it does not link to the *NPH1* gene at chromosome 2. MCD presents in the third or fourth decade, though some cases may be diagnosed in the elderly population. Presenting symptoms in MCD are

the same as in JN except for growth retardation. In addition, MCD does not have extrarenal abnormalities. Severe salt wasting can be seen, though this is usually a transient phase that resolves as the disease progresses to ESRD. Other features of tubule damage are often found, including hyperkalemia and hyperchloremic metabolic acidosis. Proteinuria is mild, and hematuria is rare.

DIAGNOSIS The diagnosis is suggested by a family history of renal disease. The pattern of inheritance and age of onset aid in distinguishing JN/MCD from other inherited diseases. Radiographic studies show small kidneys, loss of the corticomedullary junction, and multiple cysts in the medulla. CT scan is more sensitive than ultrasound in making the diagnosis. Open renal biopsy, including medullary tissue, may be required for diagnosis in some cases.

℞ TREATMENT Treatment is mainly supportive, as there is no specific therapy to prevent loss of renal function. Patients with salt wasting require a large oral intake of salt and water to maintain adequate extracellular volume. Alkali replacement and erythropoietin are required for acidosis and anemia, respectively. Renal transplantation has been performed in numerous patients, and the disease does not recur.

LIDDLE'S SYNDROME

Liddle's syndrome is a rare familial disease with a clinical presentation of hyperaldosteronism, consisting of hypertension, hypokalemia, and metabolic alkalosis. However, aldosterone levels are undetectable in these patients, and a nonaldosterone mineralocorticoid has not been isolated. Increased distal tubule sodium reabsorption, due to activating mutations in the amiloride-sensitive sodium channel, has been described in multiple families. Pharmacologic agents that block distal tubule sodium uptake, such as amiloride and triamterene, are effective in treating the hypertension and electrolyte abnormalities. As expected, spironolactone is ineffective, since the disease is not mediated via the aldosterone receptor.

BARTTER'S SYNDROME

CLINICAL FEATURES Hypokalemia secondary to renal potassium wasting, metabolic alkalosis, and normal to low blood pressure are the clinical features of Bartter's syndrome. Three phenotypes of Bartter's syndrome have now been recognized. *Antenatal Bartter's syndrome* is characterized by polyhydramnios and premature delivery. During infancy, episodes of fever and dehydration are common and can lead to growth retardation. Nephrocalcinosis secondary to hypercalciuria is frequent. The infants also have a characteristic facies consisting of a triangular face with prominent eyes and ears. Prostaglandin E production is very high. Most cases of *classic Bartter's syndrome* present during childhood. Symptoms such as weakness and cramps are secondary to the hypokalemia. Polyuria and nocturia are common due to the hypokalemia-induced nephrogenic diabetes insipidus. Growth retardation may be seen. The *Gitelman's variant of Bartter's syndrome* presents during adolescence or adulthood and generally has a milder course than Bartter's syndrome. The dominant features are fatigue and weakness. It is distinguished from Bartter's syndrome by hypocalciuria, hypomagnesemia with hypermagnesuria, and normal prostaglandin production. All three forms are inherited as autosomal recessive traits. Although rarely required for diagnosis, renal biopsy reveals hyperplasia of the juxtaglomerular apparatus and prominence of medullary interstitial cells, with variable degrees of interstitial fibrosis, though these are not pathognomonic for the syndrome.

PATHOGENESIS   The pathogenesis of Bartter's syndrome has long been a matter of debate as the distinction of the primary disorder from the secondary phenomena induced by volume depletion and hypokalemia is difficult.

GENETIC CONSIDERATIONS   Recently, mutations in several renal tubule transport proteins have been shown to be responsible for the syndrome. In antenatal and classic Bartter's syndrome, impaired Cl^- reabsorption in the thick ascending limb of the loop of Henle is the underlying defect. Inadequate Cl^- reabsorption causes volume depletion and activates the renin-angiotensin system. Distal delivery of NaCl and water are high in the presence of high aldosterone, promoting secretion of K^+ and H^+ ions. Prostaglandin overproduction is mediated by volume depletion, hypokalemia, and high angiotensin II and kallikrein levels. Increased prostaglandin production contributes to the severity of disease by inducing resistance to the pressor effects of angiotensin II and reducing reabsorption in the thick ascending limb of the loop of Henle. Mutations in the bumetanide-sensitive Na:K:2Cl channel, the apical ATP-regulated K^+ channel, and the basolateral Cl^- channel have been described in classic and antenatal Bartter's. All of these mutations would lead to a loss of Cl^- reabsorption in the loop of Henle. In Gitelman's syndrome, mutations have been found in the thiazide-sensitive NaCl transporter. The reduced Na^+ reabsorption in the distal convoluted tubule leads to volume depletion and hypokalemia, though not as severe as would result from a lesion in the loop of Henle. Loss of activity of the thiazide-sensitive transporter increases tubule calcium reabsorption, leading to the classic finding of hypocalciuria in Gitelman's syndrome.   ■

DIAGNOSIS   Hypokalemia, metabolic alkalosis, and normal to low blood pressure are the clinical findings characteristic of Bartter's syndrome. The differential diagnosis includes vomiting, surreptitious diuretic abuse, and magnesium deficiency. Chronic vomiting can be diagnosed by a low urine Cl^- concentration. Magnesium deficiency causes kaluresis and alkalosis, simulating Bartter's syndrome. Serum and urine magnesium will be low in such cases. Diuretic abuse produces metabolic abnormalities indistinguishable from Bartter's syndrome. Urine should be screened for diuretics multiple times before the diagnosis of Bartter's is made in a patient without a family history of the disorder.

TREATMENT   Dietary intake of sodium and potassium should be liberal. Potassium supplements are usually required. Magnesium supplements are needed in patients with Gitelman's syndrome. Spironolactone will reduce potassium wasting. Prostaglandin synthetase inhibitors are useful in patients with antenatal and classic Bartter's syndrome but are of no benefit in Gitelman's syndrome. Angiotensin-converting enzyme inhibitors may be beneficial in some patients.

CONGENITAL NEPHROGENIC DIABETES INSIPIDUS

GENETIC CONSIDERATIONS   This rare genetic disorder is most commonly inherited as an X-linked disease, with full expression in males and variable penetrance in females. Vasopressin acts through two receptors; type 1 receptors are located in the vasculature, while type 2 receptors are found in the collecting ducts of the kidney. In nephrogenic diabetes insipidus (NDI), only the actions requiring type 2 receptors are abnormal. Inactivating mutations of the type 2 vasopressin receptor, located on the long arm of the X chromosome, are responsible for the renal resistance to vasopressin. Less frequently, NDI may be inherited as an autosomal recessive trait, in which mutations in the gene for the water channels in collecting duct cells (aquaporin 2) lead to abnormal cell routing of aquaporin 2.   ■

CLINICAL FEATURES   The clinical presentation is that of persistent polyuria, dehydration, and hypotonic urine in the presence of hypernatremia. Vasopressin levels are appropriately elevated in the hypertonic state, but renal response is lacking. The onset of the disorder is in infancy. The recurrent hypernatremia may lead to seizures or mental retardation. Once old enough to satisfy their thirst, children will be clinically stable though in a chronic state of polyuria and polydypsia. Renal function is normal, and radiographic studies of the urinary system reveal dilated ureters and bladder secondary to the chronically high urine flow. Since the most common form of the disease is X-linked, most patients are male. Heterozygous females generally have mild concentrating defects, though a few have phenotypic expression similar to males due to skewed X-chromosome inactivation. In the autosomal recessive form, males and females are affected equally.

TREATMENT   Treatment is aimed at maintaining adequate hydration. In the infant, low-solute feedings and high water intake are generally adequate. Addition of a thiazide diuretic reduces urine flow by inhibiting sodium reabsorption in the distal convoluted tubule. This lowers free water production and, by causing extracellular volume contraction, increases proximal salt and water reabsorption, reducing delivery to the distal nephron. Administration of vasopressin and its analogues has no role in the management of this disorder.

RENAL TUBULAR ACIDOSIS

Renal tubular acidosis (RTA) is a disorder of renal acidification out of proportion to the reduction in glomerular filtration rate. RTA is characterized by hyperchloremic metabolic acidosis with a normal serum anion gap $[Na^+ - (Cl^- + HCO_3^-)]$. There are multiple forms of RTA, depending on which aspects of renal acid handling have been affected. Defective bicarbonate reabsorption in the proximal tubule, suppressed renal ammoniagenesis, and inadequate distal tublule proton secretion are the abnormalities that produce RTA. Three types of RTA exist (Table 276-2). Types 1 and 2 may be inherited or acquired. Type 4 is acquired and is associated with either hypoaldosteronism or tubular hyporesponsiveness to mineralocorticoids. Type 3 was formerly used to define distal RTA with bicarbonate wasting in children; however, the bicarbonaturia resolves with age and is not truly part of a pathologic process. The term *type 3 RTA* is no longer used.

TYPE 1 (DISTAL) RTA   In this disorder the distal nephron does not lower urine pH normally, either because the collecting ducts permit excessive back-diffusion of hydrogen ions from lumen to blood or because there is inadequate transport of hydrogen ions. Excretion of titratable acid is low, as inadequate proton secretion prevents titration of urinary buffers such as phosphate. Urine ammonium excretion is inappropriately low for the level of acidosis, as the defect in acidification reduces the ion trapping required for ammonium excretion. Urinary concentration and potassium conservation also tend to be impaired.

Chronic acidosis lowers tubule reabsorption of calcium, causing renal hypercalciuria and mild secondary hyperparathyroidism. Buffering of bone by the daily metabolic acid load contributes to hypercalciuria. Urine citrate excretion is low, as acidosis and hypokalemia stimulate proximal tubule reabsorption of citrate. The hypercalciuria, alkaline urine, and low levels of urine citrate, which normally complexes about 40% of urine calcium, cause calcium phosphate stones and nephrocalcinosis. Growth in children is stunted because of rickets; this growth defect responds to amelioration of the acidosis with alkali. In the adult, osteomalacia occurs. In both children and adults, bone diseases may result, in part, from acidosis-induced loss of bone material and inadequate production of 1,25-dihydroxyvitamin D_3 [$1,25(OH)_2D_3$]. Since the kidney does not conserve potassium or concentrate the urine normally, polyuria and hypokalemia occur. With the stress of an intercurrent illness, acidosis and hypokalemia can be life-threatening.

$\math{\S}$ GENETIC CONSIDERATIONS   Type 1 RTA can be familial, with autosomal dominant as the most common form of inheritance. X-linked, autosomal recessive, and sporadic cases have been reported. Mutations in the chloride-bicarbonate exchange gene (*AE1*) have been found in the autosomal dominant form. The cause of the autosomal recessive form is not known at this time. Other hereditary diseases that cause type 1 RTA include galactosemia, Ehler-Danlos syndrome, Fabry's disease, MSK, Wilson's disease, and hereditary elliptocytosis. The majority of cases of type 1 RTA are secondary to a systemic disorder such as Sjögren's syndrome, hypergammaglobulinemia, chronic active hepatitis, or lupus. ■

Diagnosis   The diagnosis of type 1 RTA is suggested by a normal anion gap metabolic acidosis with a simultaneous urine pH greater than 5.5. Osteomalacia or rickets and calcium phosphate stones or nephrocalcinosis support the diagnosis, though they are not present in all cases. Bicarbonaturia is not present, which distinguishes this disorder from type 2 RTA. If acidosis is not severe and urine pH is equivocal, the oral ammonium chloride (NH_4Cl) loading test should be carried out: 0.1 g (1.9 mmol) NH_4Cl per kilogram of body weight is administered, and blood and urine pH are measured repeatedly over the next 6 h. Although systemic acidosis worsens, urine pH does not fall below 5.5. Urinary tract infection must not be present during this test because bacteria may possess urease, which hydrolyzes urea to ammonia and produces an alkaline urine.

Chronic diarrheal states cause normal anion gap acidosis and hypokalemia; urine pH may be >5.5 if ammonium production is very high. The urine anion gap ($Na^+ + K^+ - Cl^-$) can be used to estimate renal ammonium production and distinguish RTA from gastrointestinal bicarbonate loss. Normally the urine anion gap is positive, as unmeasured anions exceed unmeasured cations. If urine ammonium levels are high, urine chloride concentration increases to balance the charge. Unmeasured cation (predominantly ammonium) now exceeds unmeasured anion, and the urine anion gap is negative. During metabolic acidosis, a negative urine anion gap suggests an extrarenal cause of acidosis, whereas a positive urine anion gap suggests RTA. The urine anion gap cannot be used if there are large amounts of unmeasured anions, such as bicarbonate or ketones, in the urine.

$\math{R_x}$ **TREATMENT**   Alkali supplements are the standard therapy. Enough alkali is prescribed to titrate the daily metabolic acid production, usually in the range of 0.5 to 2.0 mmol/kg body weight in four to six divided doses per day. Sodium bicarbonate and Shohl's

Table 276-2   Comparison of Normal Anion-Gap Acidoses

Finding	Type 1 RTA	Type 2 RTA	Type 4 RTA	GI Bicarbonate Loss
Normal anion-gap acidosis	Yes	Yes	Yes	Yes
Minimum urine pH	>5.5	<5.5	<5.5	5 to 6
% filtered bicarbonate excreted	<10	>15	<10	<10
Serum potassium	Low	Low	High	Low
Fanconi syndrome	No	Yes	No	No
Stones/nephrocalcinosis	Yes	No	No	No
Daily acid excretion	Low	Normal	Low	High
Urine anion gap	Positive	Positive	Positive	Negative
Daily bicarbonate replacement needs	<4 mmol/kg	>4 mmol/kg	<4 mmol/kg	Variable

NOTE: RTA, renal tubular acidosis.

solution (1 mmol sodium citrate and 1 mmol citric acid per mL) are common treatments. Potassium alkali salts can be used if hypokalemia is a persistent problem. Citrate requires less frequent dosing than bicarbonate salts as it is metabolized to bicarbonate after absorption. The dose of alkali should be raised until acidosis and hypercalciuria are both eliminated, and the patients should be followed by measurements of serum potassium, chloride, and CO_2 content approximately twice yearly. Requirements for alkali usually rise during intercurrent illnesses but are usually below 4 mmol/kg body weight per day. The relatives of patients with idiopathic type 1 RTA should be screened for this disorder, as timely treatment can prevent growth retardation in children. Incomplete RTA secondary to idiopathic hypercalciuria is best treated using thiazide diuretics in conjunction with potassium citrate (Chap. 279).

TYPE 2 (PROXIMAL) RTA   Type 2 RTA usually occurs as part of a generalized disorder of proximal tubule function, presenting as hyperchloremic acidosis with other features of Fanconi syndrome. Bicarbonate reabsorption in the proximal tubule is defective. At normal concentrations of plasma bicarbonate, large amounts of bicarbonate are delivered to the distal tubule, overwhelming the absorptive capacity of the distal tubule and resulting in bicarbonaturia. As plasma bicarbonate levels fall, the lower filtered load of bicarbonate can be reabsorbed by the proximal tubule, resulting in normal distal delivery of bicarbonate. At this point the distal nephron can acidify the urine normally, resulting in normal excretion of daily metabolic acid production, albeit at a low serum bicarbonate level. Hypophosphatemia and low calcitriol levels are common and may lead to rickets or osteomalacia. Hypercalciuria occurs, but stone formation is unusual since urine citrate levels are normal or high because of reduced proximal tubule citrate reabsorption. Type 2 RTA may be inherited as autosomal dominant, autosomal recessive, or X-linked disorder. It may be acquired in association with other diseases (see "Fanconi Syndrome") or be secondary to drugs that inhibit carbonic anhydrase activity, such as acetazolamide.

Type 2 RTA may be distinguished from type 1 RTA by the ability to normally acidify urine during spontaneous or ammonium chloride–induced acidosis. Correction of acidosis with bicarbonate will result in bicarbonaturia in type 2 RTA but not type 1 RTA. Fractional excretion of bicarbonate is >15% at normal or near-normal serum bicarbonate levels. In distal RTA it is <10%. It is unusual for serum bicarbonate levels to fall below 15 mmol/L in proximal RTA. The urine anion gap will be positive, as ammonium excretion is normal to handle daily acid production but is not elevated as in nonrenal causes of acidosis.

$\math{R_x}$ **TREATMENT**   Children should be treated to prevent growth retardation. Alkali must be given in large amounts daily, 5 to 15 mmol/kg body weight per day, because bicarbonate is rapidly excreted in the urine. A thiazide diuretic can be used in conjunction with a low-salt diet to reduce the amount of bicarbonate required. Potassium supplementation is often required.

TYPE 4 RTA In type 4 RTA, also called *hyperkalemic distal RTA*, distal tubule secretion of both potassium and hydrogen ions is abnormal, resulting in hyperchloremic acidosis with hyperkalemia. Type 4 RTA is an acquired disorder; a moderate degree of renal insufficiency is present in the majority of patients. Patients with type 4 RTA can be differentiated from patients with type 1 since they have an acid urine (pH < 5.5) during periods of acidosis (Table 276-2) and hyperkalemia. They differ from type 2 patients by having a fractional excretion of bicarbonate <10% and a daily bicarbonate requirement of 1 to 3 mmol/kg body weight per day. Because potassium and hydrogen ion excretion are abnormal, such patients are considered to have generalized distal nephron dysfunction due to either insufficient aldosterone production or intrinsic renal disease causing aldosterone resistance. The resulting hyperkalemia reduces proximal tubule ammonia production, in addition to the inadequate proton secretion, leading to inadequate excretion of the daily metabolic proton load. These patients have an acid urine despite reduced proton secretion because there is inadequate ammonia to buffer protons in the distal tubule. If buffer delivery to the distal nephron is increased, urine pH will rise despite persistent acidosis.

Type 4 RTA due to inadequate aldosterone production has multiple etiologies. Hyporeninemic hypoaldosteronism is the most common cause of type 4 RTA. Plasma levels of renin and aldosterone are subnormal, even during extracellular volume depletion, and the most common causes of this are diabetic nephropathy and chronic tubulointerstitial nephropathies. Nonsteroidal anti-inflammatory drugs, angiotensin-converting enzyme inhibitors, trimethoprim, and heparin can reduce aldosterone production and produce a type 4 RTA. Drug-induced type 4 RTA is usually seen in patients with preexisting renal insufficiency. Reduced aldosterone production may be due to adrenal disease, either occurring as an isolated defect or as part of a more generalized adrenal disorder (Chap. 331). Renin levels are normal to high in adrenal disorders.

Patients with tubular resistance to aldosterone present with the same clinical features as those with hyporeninemic hypoaldosteronism. A tubulointerstitial process damages the distal tubule, restricting potassium and hydrogen ion excretion, despite adequate aldosterone levels. Obstructive uropathy and sickle cell disease are the most common causes of acquired tubular resistance to aldosterone. Hyporeninemic hypoaldosteronism can be found in addition to tubular aldosterone resistance in many patients. Spironolactone, a competitive inhibitor of the aldosterone receptor, produces an aldosterone-resistant state. Amiloride and triamterene are diuretics that block sodium transport in the distal nephron, blunting the effect of aldosterone on the distal tubule.

℞ **TREATMENT** This is aimed mainly at reducing serum potassium, as acidosis will usually improve once the hyperkalemic block of ammonium production is removed. All patients should be placed on a low-potassium diet. Any drug that suppresses aldosterone production or blocks aldosterone effect should be discontinued. Mineralocorticoid supplementation with fludrocortisone, 0.1 to 0.2 mg/d, will improve hyperkalemia and acidosis; however, the patients who also have a partial tubule resistance to mineralocorticoid will require a higher dose. Mineralocorticoid replacement may not be appropriate for patients with hypertension or a history of heart failure. In such situations, a loop diuretic with a liberal sodium intake can usually promote adequate potassium excretion. Exchange resins will reduce potassium levels but are usually not tolerated well enough to be used for long-term treatment.

PSEUDOHYPOALDOSTERONISM

𝕊 **GENETIC CONSIDERATIONS** This rare inherited disorder is transmitted as either an autosomal dominant or recessive trait. The autosomal dominant form is caused by mutations in the mineralocorticoid receptor gene; the autosomal recessive disease is caused by inactivating mutations in the amiloride-sensitive epithelial sodium channel. The inability to respond to aldosterone leads to hyperkalemia, metabolic acidosis, salt wasting, and volume depletion, which present during childhood. Plasma renin and aldosterone levels are elevated. Treatment includes salt supplements, alkali, and potassium restriction. ∎

VITAMIN D DISORDERS

X-LINKED HYPOPHOSPHATEMIC RICKETS (See also Chap. 342) This disorder, also called *vitamin D–resistant rickets*, is an X-linked dominant disorder characterized by hypophosphatemia with renal phosphate wasting, rickets, and short stature. Hypophosphatemia is present soon after birth; rachitic bowing of the legs develops when the child begins to walk. Children have growth retardation, which is limited almost entirely to the lower extremities. Dentition is delayed, and skull abnormalities are common. Females generally have less severe disease than males. Presentation in adults ranges from disabling bone pain to no active symptoms, but generally some physical sign of childhood disease, such as short stature or bowed legs, is present. Overgrowth of bone at joints or sites of muscle attachment may reduce the mobility of the joint or cause nerve entrapment.

Hypophosphatemia secondary to reduced renal phosphate reabsorption is the hallmark of the disease. Intestinal phosphate absorption is low, worsening hypophosphatemia. Serum calcium levels are usually normal, with low intestinal absorption and renal excretion of calcium. Serum alkaline phosphatase and osteocalcin levels are elevated. Parathyroid hormone levels are normal, as would be expected with normal serum calcium. $1,25(OH)_2D_3$ levels are usually normal, though in the setting of hypophosphatemia $1,25(OH)_2D_3$ levels should be elevated. Inadequate 1α-hydroxylase activity appears to play some role in the disease. Linkage analysis has localized the gene to the Xp22.1 region of the X chromosome. The gene has been identified and appears to be related to a family of endopeptidase genes.

℞ **TREATMENT** The goal of therapy is to raise serum phosphorous to normal or near-normal levels to improve bone mineralization. Oral neutral phosphate, 1 to 4 g/d in four to six doses, combined with calcitriol is an effective therapy that improves growth rate, reduces bone pain, and leads to radiographically evident improvement of the bone disease. Patients should be closely monitored during therapy as they may develop nephrocalcinosis and renal insufficiency.

VITAMIN D–DEPENDENT RICKETS TYPE I

𝕊 **GENETIC CONSIDERATIONS** This is an autosomal recessive disorder in which $1,25(OH)_2D_3$ levels are very low but 25-hydroxyvitamin D levels are normal. The disease is caused by inactivating mutations in the gene encoding the 1α-hydroxylase enzyme, leading to a clinical syndrome of vitamin D deficiency. ∎

Symptoms usually appear before the age of 2, including rickets and growth retardation. Levels of serum calcium and phosphorous are low, but that of alkaline phosphatase is elevated. Intestinal calcium absorption and urinary calcium excretion are low. Parathyroid hormone is elevated in response to the hypocalcemia, resulting in increased urinary phosphate losses.

℞ **TREATMENT** Calcitriol (0.5 to 1 μg/d) leads to rapid correction of the biochemical abnormalities and resolution of the bone disease. Calcium and phosphorous supplementation are usually not required.

VITAMIN D–DEPENDENT RICKETS TYPE II (See also Chap. 342) End-organ resistance to $1,25(OH)_2D_3$ is the pathogenesis

of this disorder. Serum calcium and phosphate levels are low, secondary hyperparathyroidism is present, and 1,25(OH)$_2$D$_3$ levels are elevated. Inheritance is usually autosomal recessive, though sporadic cases have been reported. Most patients present during childhood with rickets, though some have a milder form of disease not recognized until adulthood. Alopecia is common and tends to be associated with the more severe childhood form of the disease. Multiple defects have been detected in 1,25(OH)$_2$D$_3$ receptor interaction, including absent hormone binding to the receptor, decreased receptor affinity, abnormal hormone-receptor localization, and abnormalities of the DNA-binding domain of the receptor. Pharmacologic doses of calcitriol (5 to 30 μg/d) along with mineral supplementation will improve the biochemical disorders and bone disease, though some patients have no response to massive doses of calcitriol.

ONCOGENIC OSTEOMALACIA This syndrome generally occurs in adults with highly vascular mesenchymal tumors. Patients present with bone pain and muscle weakness. Symptoms may be present for years before the correct diagnosis is made. Over 90% of the tumors are benign, and most are found in the extremities or maxillofacial region. Hypophosphatemia secondary to renal phosphate wasting and low levels of 1,25(OH)$_2$D$_3$ are the major biochemical abnormalities. Serum calcium and parathyroid hormone levels are normal. It appears the tumor produces a humoral agent that reduces proximal tubule phosphate reabsorption and 1α-hydroxylase activity. Removal of the tumor leads to rapid resolution of the disease.

X-LINKED RECESSIVE NEPHROLITHIASIS

This disorder presents as calcium nephrolithiasis in male children and progresses to nephrocalcinosis and renal failure. Low-molecular-weight proteinuria and hypercalciuria are also prominent features of the disease. Kidney biopsy reveals tubular atrophy, interstitial fibrosis, and medullary calcifications. The gene has been mapped to the short arm of the X chromosome and encodes a voltage-gated chloride channel (CLC-5). Dent's disease has been mapped to the same gene and has a similar presentation, except for an increased incidence of rickets.

ISOLATED HYPOURICEMIA (See also Chap. 353)

This disorder is generally inherited as an autosomal recessive trait. Most commonly there is deficient urate reabsorption in the proximal tubule, though some patients have been demonstrated to oversecrete urate. Serum uric acid is usually <120 μmol/L (2 mg/dL) and hyperuricosuria is common, possibly due to decreased intestinal urate excretion. Hypouricemia is usually an incidental finding, as patients with this disorder are asymptomatic except for an increased risk of nephrolithiasis. Other disorders associated with hypouricemia include Fanconi syndrome, Wilson's disease, Hodgkin's disease, and Hartnup disease. No treatment is required except for high fluid intake to prevent kidney stones. Alkali and allopurinol may be used to prevent stones if fluids alone are not sufficient. Hypercalciuria has been associated with isolated hypouricemia in some families.

SELECTED DISORDERS OF AMINO ACID TRANSPORT

HARTNUP DISEASE This disorder is characterized by reduced intestinal absorption and renal reabsorption of neutral amino acids. The defect involves an amino acid transporter on the brush border of the jejunum and the proximal tubule. Intestinal absorption of free amino acids is reduced, though the neutral amino acids can be absorbed when present in di- and tripeptides. Degradation of unabsorbed tryptophan by intestinal bacteria produces indolic acids that are absorbed and subsequently excreted at high levels in the urine of these patients. The disorder is inherited as an autosomal recessive trait, affecting males and females equally. Widespread screening of newborns has estimated an incidence of 1 in 24,000 live births.

The majority of individuals with this disorder are asymptomatic. Approximately 10 to 20% present with clinical symptoms similar to those seen in pellagra, including a photosensitive erythematous scaly rash, intermittent cerebral ataxia, delirium, and diarrhea. Short stature is noted in some patients. The symptoms are thought to be due to deficiency in the essential amino acid tryptophan and resultant inadequate synthesis of nicotinamide. Though the inheritance of the disorder is Mendelian autosomal recessive, the development of symptomatic disease appears to be multifactorial. Diet, environment, and polygenic traits controlling plasma amino acid levels all contribute to development of symptoms.

Clinically affected patients can be differentiated from patients with pellagra by dietary history and the presence of aminoaciduria. Diagnosis is made by the characteristic finding of large amounts of neutral amino acids in the urine. It can easily be distinguished from generalized aminoaciduria by the normal excretion of proline. There are no other renal tubule defects as in Fanconi syndrome. Heterozygotes have normal urinary amino acid excretion.

TREATMENT Symptomatic individuals should receive oral nicotinamide, 40 to 200 mg/d, and a high-protein diet to compensate for the poor amino acid absorption. Some patients who do not respond to nicotinamide may improve with tryptophan ethyl ester, which is lipid soluble and can be absorbed without an active transport system.

FANCONI SYNDROME

GENETIC CONSIDERATIONS Fanconi syndrome is a generalized defect in proximal tubule transport involving amino acids, glucose, phosphate, uric acid, sodium, potassium, bicarbonate, and proteins. Idiopathic Fanconi syndrome may be inherited as an autosomal dominant, autosomal recessive, or X-linked trait. Sporadic cases are also seen. A variety of inherited systemic disorders are also associated with Fanconi syndrome including Wilson's disease, galactosemia, tyrosinemia, cystinosis, fructose intolerance, and Lowe's oculocerebral syndrome. The syndrome may be acquired in multiple myeloma, amyloid, and heavy metal toxicity. ∎

The patients may present with a wide array of laboratory abnormalities including proximal renal tubular acidosis, glucosuria with a normal serum glucose, hypophosphatemia, hypouricemia, hypokalemia, generalized aminoaciduria, and low-molecular-weight proteinuria. Some patients do not have abnormalities in all proximal tubule transporters and may present with only a few of the laboratory findings. Rickets and osteomalacia are common findings secondary to the hypophosphatemia; production of calcitriol may also be abnormal. Metabolic acidosis also contributes to the bone disease. Polyuria, salt wasting, and hypokalemia may be quite severe.

TREATMENT Treatment includes phosphate supplements and calcitriol to heal the bone lesions, alkali for the acidosis, and liberal intake of salt and water. Alkali in the form of potassium salts may be particularly useful in the patient with RTA and hypokalemia. Aminoaciduria, glucosuria, hypouricemia, and low-molecular-weight proteinuria do not require treatment.

BIBLIOGRAPHY

DELIYSKA B et al: Association of Bartter's syndrome with vasculitis. Nephrol Dial Transplant 15:102, 2000

DEVUYST O et al: Intrarenal and subcellular distribution of the human chloride channel CLC-5 reveals a pathophysiologic basis for Dent's disease. Hum Mol Genet 8:247, 1999

DIXON PH et al: Mutational analysis of the PHEX gene in X-linked hypophosphatemia. J Clin Endocrinol Metab 83:3615, 1998

GELLER DS et al: Mutations in the mineralocorticoid receptor gene cause autosomal dominant pseudohypoaldosteronism type 1. Nat Genet 19:279, 1998

KARET FE et al: Mutations in the chloride-bicarbonate exchanger gene AE1 cause autosomal dominant but not autosomal recessive distal renal acidosis. Proc Natl Acad Sci 95:6337, 1998

KONRAD M et al: Familial juvenile nephronophthisis. J Mol Med 76:310, 1998

MONKAWA T et al: Novel mutations in thiazide-sensitive Na-Cl cotransporter gene of patients with Gitelman's syndrome. J Am Soc Nephrol 11:65, 2000

SCHEINMAN SJ et al: Genetic disorders of renal electrolyte transport. N Engl J Med 340: 1177, 1999

VAN ADELSBERG J: Polycystin-1 interacts with E-cadherin and the catenins—clues to the pathogenesis of cyst formation in ADPKD? Nephrol Dial Transplant 15:1, 2000

WANG JT et al: Genetics of vitamin D 1α-hydroxylase deficiency in 17 families. Am J Hum Genet 63:1694, 1998

WARNOCK DG: Liddle syndrome: An autosomal dominant form of human hypertension. Kidney Int 53:18, 1998

277

Alan S. L. Yu, Barry M. Brenner

TUBULOINTERSTITIAL DISEASES OF THE KIDNEY

Primary tubulointerstitial diseases of the kidney, as distinct from the disorders considered in Chaps. 274 and 275, are characterized by histologic and functional abnormalities that involve the tubules and interstitium to a greater degree than the glomeruli and renal vasculature (Table 277-1). Secondary tubulointerstitial disease occurs as a consequence of progressive glomerular or vascular injury. These disorders can be further divided into acute and chronic forms. The chronic group may be due to sustained insults by a factor or factors that initially cause acute disease or to a slower, progressive, cumulative insult without an identifiable acute episode. Morphologically, acute forms of these disorders are characterized by interstitial edema, often associated with cortical and medullary infiltration by both mononuclear cells and polymorphonuclear leukocytes, and patchy areas of tubule cell necrosis. In more chronic forms, interstitial fibrosis predominates, inflammatory cells are typically mononuclear, and abnormalities of the tubules tend to be more widespread, as evidenced by atrophy, luminal dilatation, and thickening of tubule basement membranes. Because of the nonspecific nature of the histology, particularly in chronic tubulointerstitial diseases, biopsy specimens rarely provide a specific diagnosis. The urine sediment is also unlikely to be diagnostic, except in allergic forms of acute tubulointerstitial disease, in which eosinophils may predominate in the urinary sediment.

Defects in renal function often accompany these alterations of tubule and interstitial structure (Table 277-2). Proximal tubule dysfunction may be manifested as selective reabsorptive defects leading to hypokalemia, aminoaciduria, glycosuria, phosphaturia, uricosuria, or bicarbonaturia (proximal or type II renal tubular acidosis; Chap. 276). In combination, these defects constitute the *Fanconi syndrome*. Proteinuria, predominantly of low-molecular-weight proteins, is usually modest, rarely exceeding 2 g/d.

Defects in urinary acidification and concentrating ability often represent the most troublesome of the tubule dysfunctions encountered in patients with tubulointerstitial disease. Hyperchloremic metabolic acidosis often develops at a relatively early stage in the course. Patients with this finding generally elaborate urine of maximal acidity (pH ≤ 5.3). In such patients the defect in acid excretion is usually caused by a reduced capacity to generate and excrete ammonia due to the reduction in renal mass. Preferential damage to the collecting ducts, as in amyloidosis or chronic obstructive uropathy, may also predispose to distal or type I renal tubular acidosis (RTA), characterized by high urine pH (≥5.5) during spontaneous or NH_4Cl-induced metabolic acidosis. Patients with tubulointerstitial diseases affecting predominantly medullary and papillary structures may also exhibit concentrating de-

---

Table 277-1   Principal Causes of Tubulointerstitial Disease of the Kidney

ACUTE INTERSTITIAL NEPHRITIS

Drugs[a]
  Antibiotics (β-lactams, sulfonamides, quinolones, vancomycin, erythromycin, minocycline, rifampin, ethambutol, acyclovir)
  Nonsteroidal anti-inflammatory drugs
  Diuretics (thiazides, furosemide, triamterene)
  Anticonvulsants (phenytoin, phenobarbital, carbamazepine, valproic acid)
  Miscellaneous (captopril, H_2 receptor blockers, omeprazole, mesalazine, indinavir, allopurinol)
Infection
  Bacteria (*Streptococcus, Staphylococcus, Legionella, Salmonella, Brucella, Yersinia, Corynebacterium diphtheriae*)
  Viruses (Epstein-Barr virus, cytomegalovirus, Hantavirus, HIV)
  Miscellaneous (*Leptospira, Rickettsia, Mycoplasma*)
Idiopathic
  Tubulointerstitial nephritis-uveitis syndrome
  Anti-tubule basement membrane disease
  Sarcoidosis

CHRONIC TUBULOINTERSTITIAL DISEASES

Hereditary renal diseases
  Polycystic kidney disease[a] (Chap. 276)
  Medullary cystic disease (Chap. 276)
  Medullary sponge kidney (Chap. 276)
Exogenous toxins
  Analgesic nephropathy[a]
  Lead nephropathy
  Miscellaneous nephrotoxins (e.g. lithium[a], cyclosporine[a], heavy metals, slimming regimens with Chinese herbs)
Metabolic toxins
  Hyperuricemia[a]
  Hypercalcemia
  Miscellaneous metabolic toxins (e.g., hypokalemia, hyperoxaluria, cystinosis, Fabry's disease)
Autoimmune disorders
  Sjögren's syndrome
Neoplastic disorders
  Leukemia
  Lymphoma
  Multiple myeloma[a]
Miscellaneous disorders
  Sickle cell nephropathy
  Chronic pyelonephritis
  Chronic urinary tract obstruction
  Vesicoureteral reflux[a]
  Radiation nephritis
  Balkan nephropathy
  Tubulointerstitial disease secondary to glomerular and vascular disease

[a] Common

Table 277-2   Functional Consequences of Tubulointerstitial Disease

Defect	Cause(s)
Reduced glomerular filtration rate[a]	Obliteration of microvasculature and obstruction of tubules
Fanconi syndrome	Damage to proximal tubular reabsorption of glucose, amino acids, phosphate, and bicarbonate
Hyperchloremic acidosis[a]	1. Reduced ammonia production 2. Inability to acidify the collecting duct fluid (distal renal tubular acidosis) 3. Proximal bicarbonate wasting
Tubular or small-molecular-weight proteinuria[a]	Failure of proximal tubule protein reabsorption
Polyuria, isothenuria[a]	Damage to medullary tubules and vasculature
Hyperkalemia[a]	Potassium secretory defects including aldosterone resistance
Salt wasting	Distal tubular damage with impaired sodium reabsorption

[a] Common

fects, with resultant nocturia and polyuria. Analgesic nephropathy and sickle cell disease are prototypes of this form of injury.

TOXINS

Although the kidneys constitute less than 1% of total body mass, they receive approximately 20% of the cardiac output, and 90% or more of renal blood flow is distributed to the renal cortex. Exposure of tubules and interstitium of the renal cortex to circulating toxins is therefore greater than for most other tissues. Transport processes in renal tubules contribute further to the intrarenal accumulation of toxins, enhancing local concentrations of noxious agents. The urinary concentrating mechanism can also establish high levels of toxins within medullary and papillary portions of the kidney, predisposing these regions to chemical injury. Finally, the relatively acid pH of the fluid within most nephron segments may affect the ionization characteristics of potentially toxic compounds and thereby influence local concentration and solubility. Although these processes render the kidney vulnerable to toxic injury, the role of nephrotoxins in renal damage often goes unrecognized because the manifestations of such injury are usually nonspecific in nature and insidious in onset. Diagnosis largely depends on a history of exposure to a certain toxin. Particular attention should be paid to the occupational history, as well as to an assessment of exposure—current and remote—to drugs, especially antibiotics and analgesics, and to dietary supplements or herbal remedies. The recognition of a potential association between a patient's renal disease and exposure to a nephrotoxin is crucial, because, unlike many other forms of renal disease, progression of the functional and morphologic abnormalities associated with toxin-induced nephropathies may be prevented, and even reversed, by eliminating additional exposure.

EXOGENOUS TOXINS Analgesic Nephropathy A distinct clinicopathologic syndrome has been described in heavy users of analgesic mixtures containing phenacetin in combination with aspirin, acetaminophen, or caffeine. These individuals have an approximately 20-fold increased risk of end-stage renal disease (ESRD). Analgesic nephropathy has been an important cause of chronic renal failure in Australia, Switzerland, Sweden, Belgium, and the southeastern United States.

Morphologically, analgesic nephropathy is characterized by papillary necrosis and tubulointerstitial inflammation. At an early stage, damage to the vascular supply of the inner medulla (vasa recta) leads to a local interstitial inflammatory reaction and, eventually, to papillary ischemia, necrosis, fibrosis, and calcification. The susceptibility of the renal papillae to damage by phenacetin is believed to be related to the establishment of a renal gradient for its acetaminophen metabolite, resulting in papillary tip concentrations tenfold higher than those in renal cortex. Hydration dissipates this gradient and may explain the protective effect of this maneuver in preventing phenacetin-induced papillary necrosis in animals. Aspirin in these analgesic compounds contributes to renal injury by uncoupling oxidative phosphorylation in renal mitochondria and by inhibiting the synthesis of renal prostaglandins, which are potent endogenous renal vasodilator hormones.

Analgesic nephropathy occurs some three to five times more commonly in women than in men. A direct relationship exists between the total amount of analgesic compounds ingested and the degree of renal impairment. The intake of 1.0 g phenacetin per day for 1 to 3 years or the total ingestion of 2 kg phenacetin in combination with other analgesics appears to represent minimum requirements for the development of analgesic nephropathy.

Whether single-ingredient analgesics other than phenacetin, when used alone, cause renal disease is controversial. Recent reports have suggested a two- to threefold increase in the risk of ESRD among regular users of acetaminophen, and perhaps nonsteroidal anti-inflammatory drugs (NSAIDs), but not among regular users of aspirin. Until conclusive evidence is available, physicians should consider screening regular users of acetaminophen and NSAIDs for evidence of renal disease.

In analgesic nephropathy, renal function usually declines gradually, in association with chronic necrosis of papillae and diffuse tubulointerstitial damage to the renal cortex. Occasionally, papillary necrosis may be associated with hematuria and even renal colic owing to obstruction of a ureter by necrotic tissue. More than half of patients with analgesic nephropathy have pyuria, which, if persistently associated with sterile urine, provides an important clue to the diagnosis. Nonetheless, active pyelonephritis may coexist in patients with analgesic nephropathy. Proteinuria, if present, is typically mild (< 1 g/d). Patients with analgesic nephropathy are usually unable to generate maximally concentrated urine, reflecting the underlying medullary and papillary damage. An acquired form of distal RTA may contribute to the development of *nephrocalcinosis*. The occurrence of anemia out of proportion to the degree of azotemia also may provide a clue to the diagnosis of analgesic nephropathy. When analgesic nephropathy has progressed to renal insufficiency, the kidneys usually appear bilaterally shrunken on intravenous pyelography, and the calyces are deformed. A "ring sign" on the pyelogram is pathognomonic of papillary necrosis and represents the radiolucent sloughed papilla surrounded by the radiodense contrast material in the calyx. Renal sonography may reveal papillary calcifications surrounding the central sinus complex in a "garland" pattern. Transitional cell carcinoma may develop in the urinary pelvis or ureters as a late complication of analgesic abuse.

Rx TREATMENT Every effort must be made to convince the patient who ingests excessive amounts of analgesic combinations to discontinue this hazardous practice. When renal damage is at an early stage, cessation of abuse usually arrests the progression of the nephrotoxic process; not infrequently, overall renal function improves with time. With continued abuse, however, progressive renal damage leads invariably to chronic renal failure.

Lead Nephropathy (See also Chap. 395) Lead intoxication may produce a chronic tubulointerstitial renal disease. Children who repeatedly ingest lead-based paints may develop kidney disease as adults. Significant occupational exposure may occur in a diverse variety of workplaces where lead-containing metals or paints are heated to high temperatures, such as battery factories, smelters, salvage yards, and firing ranges. Alcohol, illegally distilled in an apparatus constructed from automobile radiators (so-called moonshine), is another cause of lead poisoning. Environmental lead exposure, particularly in industrial regions, may be great enough to produce changes in renal function.

Tubule transport processes enhance the accumulation of lead within renal cells, particularly in the proximal convoluted tubule, leading to cell degeneration, mitochondrial swelling, and eosinophilic intranuclear inclusion bodies rich in lead. In addition to tubule degeneration and atrophy, lead nephropathy is associated with ischemic changes in the glomeruli, fibrosis of the adventitia of small renal arterioles, and focal areas of cortical scarring. Eventually, the kidneys become atrophic. Urinary excretion of lead, porphyrin precursors such as δ-aminolevulinic acid and coproporphyrin, and urobilinogen, may be increased. Patients with chronic lead nephropathy are characteristically *hyperuricemic*, a consequence of enhanced reabsorption of filtered urate. Acute gouty arthritis (so-called saturnine gout) develops in about 50% of patients with lead nephropathy, in striking contrast to other forms of chronic renal failure in which de novo gout is rare (Chap. 347). Hypertension is also a complication. Therefore, in any patient with slowly progressive renal failure, atrophic kidneys, gout, and hypertension, the diagnosis of lead intoxication should be considered. Features of acute lead intoxication (abdominal colic, anemia, peripheral neuropathy, and encephalopathy) are usually absent.

The diagnosis may be suspected by finding elevated serum levels of lead. However, because blood levels may not be elevated even in the presence of a toxic total-body burden of lead, the quantitation of lead excretion following infusion of the chelating agent calcium disodium edetate is a more reliable indicator of serious lead exposure. While urinary excretion of more than 0.6 mg/d of lead is generally considered to be indicative of overt or potential toxicity, recent evidence suggests that even lead burdens of 0.15 to 0.6 mg/d may cause progressive loss of renal function.

℞ **TREATMENT**   Treatment includes removing the patient from the source of exposure and augmenting lead excretion with a chelating agent such as calcium disodium edetate.

Miscellaneous Nephrotoxins   Use of *lithium salts* for bipolar disorder has been associated with polyuria and polydipsia caused by tubulointerstitial disease. There are only rare reports of chronic renal insufficiency attributable to this agent. Renal function should be followed in patients taking this drug, and caution should be exercised if lithium is employed in patients with underlying renal disease.

The immunosuppressant *cyclosporine* causes both acute and chronic renal injury. The acute injury and the use of cyclosporine in transplantation are discussed in Chap. 272. The chronic injury results in an irreversible reduction in glomerular filtration rate (GFR), with mild proteinuria and arterial hypertension. Hyperkalemia is a relatively common complication and results in part from tubule resistance to aldosterone. Hypomagnesemia due to urinary magnesium wasting is less common but can cause hypocalcemia. The histologic changes in renal tissue include patchy interstitial fibrosis and tubular atrophy. In addition, the intrarenal vasculature often demonstrates hyalinosis, and focal segmental glomerular sclerosis can be present as well. Fibrosis may be the result of a cyclosporine-induced increase in renal collagen production. Vasoconstrictive mediators, such as angiotensin II, or vasoconstriction itself may also play a role in chronic cyclosporine toxicity. In patients receiving this drug for renal transplantation (Chap. 272), chronic rejection and recurrence of the primary disease may coincide with chronic cyclosporine injury, and on clinical grounds, distinction among these may be difficult. Although most patients experience stable, albeit reduced, renal function, progressive renal injury can occur without a progressive reduction in GFR. Dose reduction appears to mitigate cyclosporine-associated renal fibrosis but may increase the risk of rejection and graft loss. The optimal dosage of cyclosporine in renal transplantation remains controversial. Treatment of any associated arterial hypertension may lessen renal injury.

Many agents that commonly lead to acute renal failure are also capable of producing tubulointerstitial injury (Chap. 269). These include antibiotics (e.g., aminoglycosides, amphotericin B), radiographic contrast agents, various hydrocarbons (e.g., carbon tetrachloride), and heavy metals (e.g., mercury, cadmium, and bismuth).

METABOLIC TOXINS   **Acute Uric Acid Nephropathy** (See also Chap. 322)   Acute overproduction of uric acid and extreme hyperuricemia often lead to a rapidly progressive renal insufficiency, so-called acute uric acid nephropathy. This tubulointerstitial disease is usually seen as part of the tumor lysis syndrome in patients given cytotoxic drugs for the treatment of lymphoproliferative or myeloproliferative disorders but may also occur in these patients before such treatment is begun. The pathologic changes are largely the result of deposition of uric acid crystals in the kidneys and their collecting systems, leading to partial or complete obstruction of collecting ducts, renal pelvis, or ureter. Since obstruction is often bilateral, patients typically show the clinical course of acute renal failure, characterized by oliguria and rapidly rising serum creatinine concentration. In the early phase uric acid crystals can be found in urine, usually in association with microscopic or gross hematuria. Hyperuricemia can also be a consequence of renal failure of any etiology. The finding of a urine uric acid–creatinine ratio greater than 1 mg/mg (0.7 mol/mol) distinguishes acute uric acid nephropathy from other causes of renal failure.

Prevention of hyperuricemia in patients at risk by treatment with

allopurinol in doses of 200 to 800 mg/d prior to cytotoxic therapy reduces the danger of acute uric acid nephropathy. Once hyperuricemia develops, however, efforts should be directed to preventing deposition of uric acid within the urinary tract. Increasing urine volume with potent diuretics (furosemide or mannitol) effectively lowers intratubular uric acid concentrations, and alkalinization of the urine to pH 7 or greater with sodium bicarbonate and/or a carbonic anhydrase inhibitor (acetazolamide) enhances uric acid solubility. If these efforts, together with allopurinol therapy, are ineffective in preventing acute renal failure, dialysis should be instituted to lower the serum uric acid concentration as well as to treat the acute manifestations of uremia.

Gouty Nephropathy (See also Chap. 322)   Patients with less severe but prolonged forms of hyperuricemia are predisposed to a more chronic tubulointerstitial disorder, often referred to as *gouty nephropathy*. The severity of renal involvement correlates with the duration and magnitude of the elevation of the serum uric acid concentration. Histologically, the distinctive feature of gouty nephropathy is the presence of crystalline deposits of uric acid and monosodium urate salts in kidney parenchyma. These deposits not only cause intrarenal obstruction but also incite an inflammatory response, leading to lymphocytic infiltration, foreign-body giant cell reaction, and eventual fibrosis, especially of medullary and papillary regions of the kidney. Bacteriuria and pyelonephritis occur in about one-fourth of cases, presumably as complications of intrarenal urinary stasis. Since patients with gout frequently suffer from hypertension and hyperlipidemia, degenerative changes of the renal arterioles may constitute a striking feature of the histologic abnormality, often out of proportion to other morphologic defects. Clinically, gouty nephropathy is an insidious cause of renal insufficiency. Early in its course, GFR may be near normal, often despite focal morphologic changes in medullary and cortical interstitium, proteinuria, and diminished urinary concentrating ability. Whether reducing serum uric acid levels with allopurinol exerts a beneficial effect on the kidney remains to be demonstrated. Although such undesirable consequences of hyperuricemia as gout and uric acid stones respond well to allopurinol, use of this drug in asymptomatic hyperuricemia has not been shown to improve renal function consistently. On the other hand, uricosuric agents such as probenecid, which may increase uric acid stone production, clearly have no role in the treatment of renal disease associated with hyperuricemia.

Hypercalcemic Nephropathy (See also Chap. 341)   Chronic hypercalcemia, as occurs in primary hyperparathyroidism, sarcoidosis, multiple myeloma, vitamin D intoxication, or metastatic bone disease, can cause tubulointerstitial damage and progressive renal insufficiency. The earliest lesion is a focal degenerative change in renal epithelia, primarily in collecting ducts, distal convoluted tubules, and loops of Henle. Tubule cell necrosis leads to nephron obstruction and stasis of intrarenal urine, favoring local precipitation of calcium salts and infection. Dilatation and atrophy of tubules eventually occur, as do interstitial fibrosis, mononuclear leukocyte infiltration, and interstitial calcium deposition (nephrocalcinosis). Calcium deposition also may occur in glomeruli and the walls of renal arterioles.

Clinically, the most striking defect is an inability to concentrate the urine maximally, resulting in polyuria and nocturia. Defective transport of NaCl in the ascending limb of Henle's loop is responsible, at least in part, for this concentrating defect. Additionally, reduced collecting duct responsiveness to vasopressin may contribute. Reductions in GFR and renal blood flow also occur, both in acute severe hypercalcemia and with prolonged hypercalcemia of lesser severity. Distal RTA and sodium and potassium wasting also have been described in these chronic states. Eventually, uncontrolled hypercalcemia leads to severe tubulointerstitial damage and overt renal failure. Abdominal x-rays may demonstrate nephrocalcinosis as well as nephrolithiasis, the latter due to the hypercalciuria that often accompanies hypercalcemia.

℞ **TREATMENT**   This consists of reducing the serum calcium concentration toward normal and correcting the primary abnormality of calcium metabolism. The management of hypercalcemia is discussed in Chap. 341. Prognosis for recovery of renal function depends on the severity of the renal lesion at the time hypercalcemia is corrected. Renal dysfunction of acute hypercalcemia may be completely reversible. Gradual, progressive renal insufficiency related to chronic hypercalcemia, however, may not improve with correction of the calcium disorder. Nonetheless, every effort should be made to return serum calcium concentration to normal to minimize further loss of renal function.

Hypokalemic Nephropathy (See also Chap. 49) Disturbances of renal structure and function occur commonly in patients with moderate to severe potassium depletion of at least several weeks' duration. Histologically, renal epithelial cells are often seen to contain numerous vacuoles, most marked in proximal tubules. Glomeruli are reduced in size and may become sclerotic. Whether prolonged or recurrent potassium deficiency results in irreversible tubulointerstitial fibrosis, scarring, and atrophy is unresolved. Loss of urinary concentrating ability is the most commonly encountered functional defect and may be due to defective operation of the countercurrent multiplier system and elevated intrarenal prostaglandins. Nocturia, polyuria, and polydipsia are frequent symptoms. Urinalysis often reveals no abnormalities except for mild proteinuria. Serum creatinine and urea nitrogen concentrations usually remain within normal limits.

Miscellaneous Metabolic Toxins Urinary oxalate, derived from the metabolism of glycine and, to a variable extent, from ingested oxalate, may deposit as insoluble intratubular calcium oxalate crystals and result in chronic tubulointerstitial damage in patients with hereditary or acquired forms of *hyperoxaluria. Cystinosis* and *Fabry's disease* are other hereditary depositional disorders affecting the renal tubules and interstitium (Chap. 276).

RENAL PARENCHYMAL DISEASE ASSOCIATED WITH EXTRARENAL NEOPLASM

Except for the glomerulopathies associated with lymphomas and several solid tumors (Chap. 275), the renal manifestations of primary extrarenal neoplastic processes are confined mainly to the interstitium and tubules. Although metastatic renal involvement by solid tumors is unusual, the kidneys are often invaded by neoplastic cells in various lymphomas and leukemias and in multiple myeloma. In postmortem studies of patients with *lymphoma*, renal involvement is found in approximately half. The involvement may be focal, in the form of multiple discrete nodules, or diffuse, with lymphomatous infiltration throughout the renal parenchyma. Diffuse infiltration is seen most commonly in lymphomas other than Hodgkin's disease. There may be flank pain related to massive renal infiltration, and x-rays may show enlargement of one or both kidneys. Renal insufficiency occurs in a minority of cases, and overt uremia is rare. Treatment of the primary disease may improve renal function in these cases.

The kidneys are also commonly involved in various forms of *leukemia*. At postmortem examination, bilateral renal involvement is present in approximately 50% of cases. As with lymphoma, uremia is rarely, if ever, a consequence of leukemic infiltration of the kidneys. The kidneys can also be involved in leukemias because of the associated high incidence of hyperuricemia, hypercalcemia, and lysozymuria. The myelogenous leukemias, particularly of the monocytic type, may be complicated by tubule defects involving potassium and magnesium wasting.

PLASMA CELL DYSCRASIAS Several glomerular and tubulointerstitial disorders may occur in association with plasma cell dyscrasias (Table 277-3; Chap. 113). Infiltration of the kidneys with myeloma cells is infrequent. When it occurs, the process is usually focal, so renal insufficiency from this cause is also uncommon. The more usual lesion is *myeloma kidney*, characterized histologically by atrophic tubules, many with eosinophilic intraluminal casts, and numerous multinucleated giant cells within tubule walls and in the interstitium. The frequent occurrence of myeloma kidney in patients with

Table 277-3 Renal Diseases Associated with Plasma Cell Dyscrasias

Disease	Clinical Manifestations
Plasma cell infiltration (Chap. 113)	None
Hypercalcemia[a] (Chap. 341)	Acute renal failure, diabetes insipidus
Myeloma kidney[a] (Chap. 113)	Acute renal failure, Fanconi syndrome, diabetes insipidus
Amyloidosis[a] (Chaps. 275 and 319)	Nephrotic syndrome, distal renal tubular acidosis, diabetes insipidus, renal failure
Light chain deposition disease (Chap. 275)	Nephrotic syndrome, renal failure
Type I/II cryoglobulinemia (Chaps. 273 and 317)	Hematuria, proteinuria, vasculitis, renal failure
Immunotactoid glomerulopathy (Chap. 273)	Nephrotic syndrome, hypertension, renal failure

[a] Common

Bence Jones proteinuria has suggested a causal relation. Bence Jones proteins are thought to cause myeloma kidney through direct toxicity to renal tubule cells. In addition, Bence Jones proteins may precipitate within the distal nephron where the high concentrations of these proteins and the acid composition of the tubule fluid favor intraluminal cast formation and intrarenal obstruction. Occasionally, acute renal failure occurs after intravenous pyelography in patients with multiple myeloma and is believed to result from the further precipitation of Bence Jones proteins induced by dehydration prior to radiographic study. Dehydration of the patient with myeloma in preparation for intravenous pyelography should therefore be avoided. Multiple myeloma may also affect the kidneys indirectly. Hypercalcemia or hyperuricemia may lead to the nephropathies described above. Proximal tubule disorders are also seen occasionally, including type II proximal RTA and the Fanconi syndrome.

AMYLOIDOSIS (See also Chaps. 275 and 319) Glomerular pathology usually predominates and leads to heavy proteinuria and azotemia. However, tubule function may also be deranged, giving rise to a nephrogenic diabetes insipidus and to distal (type I) RTA. In several cases these functional abnormalities correlated with peritubular deposition of amyloid, particularly in areas surrounding vasa rectae, loops of Henle, and collecting ducts. Bilateral enlargement of the kidneys, especially in a patient with massive proteinuria and tubule dysfunction, should raise the possibility of amyloid renal disease.

IMMUNE DISORDERS

ALLERGIC INTERSTITIAL NEPHRITIS An acute diffuse tubulointerstitial reaction may result from hypersensitivity to a number of drugs, including sulfonamides, many penicillins and cephalosporins, the fluoroquinolone antibiotics ciprofloxacin and norfloxacin, and the antituberculous drugs isoniazid and rifampin. Acute tubulointerstitial damage has also occurred after use of thiazide and loop diuretics, antiulcer medications (cimetidine, ranitidine, and omeprazole), and NSAIDs. Of note, the tubulointerstitial nephropathy that develops in some patients taking NSAIDs may be associated with nephrotic-range proteinuria and histologic evidence of either minimal change or membranous glomerulopathy. Grossly, the kidneys are usually enlarged. Histologically, the glomeruli appear normal. The principal pathologic abnormalities are in the interstitium of the kidney, which reveals pronounced edema and infiltration with polymorphonuclear leukocytes, lymphocytes, plasma cells, and, in some cases, large numbers of eosinophils. If the process is severe, tubule cell necrosis and regeneration may also be apparent. Immunofluorescence studies have either been unrevealing or demonstrated a linear pattern of immunoglobulin and complement deposition along tubule basement membranes. In a few cases of methicillin-induced acute tubulointerstitial disease, circulating anti-tubule basement membrane antibodies have also been found, suggesting that autoantibody formation may have been induced by the penicilloyl hapten of methicillin (by conjugation of hapten with tubule basement membrane proteins, thereby altering the native antigenicity of the basement membrane).

Most patients require several weeks of drug exposure before developing evidence of renal injury. Rare cases have occurred after only a few doses or after a year of more of use. Azotemia is usually present; a diagnostic triad of fever, skin rash, and peripheral blood eosinophilia is highly suggestive of acute tubulointerstitial nephritis but is often absent. Examination of the urine sediment reveals hematuria and often pyuria; occasionally, eosinophils may be present. Proteinuria is usually mild to moderate, except in cases of NSAID-induced tubulointerstitial nephritis with minimal change glomerulopathy. The clinical picture may be confused with acute glomerulonephritis, but when acute azotemia and hematuria are accompanied by eosinophilia, skin rash, and a history of drug exposure, a hypersensitivity reaction leading to acute tubulointerstitial nephritis should be regarded as the leading diagnostic possibility. Discontinuation of the drug usually results in complete reversal of the renal injury; rarely, renal damage may be irreversible. Glucocorticoids may accelerate renal recovery, but their value has not been definitively established.

SJÖGREN'S SYNDROME (See also Chap. 314)   When the kidneys are involved in this disorder, the predominant histologic findings are those of chronic tubulointerstitial disease. Interstitial infiltrates are composed primarily of lymphocytes, causing the histology of the renal parenchyma in these patients to resemble that of the salivary and lacrimal glands. Renal functional defects include diminished urinary concentrating ability and distal (type I) RTA. Urinalysis may show pyuria (predominantly lymphocyturia) and mild proteinuria.

TUBULOINTERSTITIAL ABNORMALITIES ASSOCIATED WITH GLOMERULONEPHRITIS   Primary glomerulopathies are often associated with damage to tubules and the interstitium. Occasionally, the primary disorder may affect glomeruli and tubules directly. For example, in more than half of patients with the nephropathy of systemic lupus erythematosus, deposits of immune complexes can be identified in tubule basement membranes, usually accompanied by an interstitial mononuclear inflammatory reaction. Similarly, in many patients with glomerulonephritis associated with anti-glomerular basement membrane antibody, the same antibody is reactive against tubule basement membranes as well. More frequently, tubulointerstitial damage is a secondary consequence of glomerular dysfunction. The extent of tubulointerstitial fibrosis correlates closely with the degree of renal impairment. Potential mechanisms by which glomerular disease might cause tublointerstitial injury include glomerular leak of plasma proteins toxic to epithelial cells, activation of tubule epithelial cells by glomerulus-derived cytokines, reduced peritubular blood flow leading to downstream tubulointerstitial ischemia, and hyperfunction of remnant tubules.

MISCELLANEOUS DISORDERS

VESICOURETERAL REFLUX   (See also Chap. 281) When the function of the ureterovesical junction is impaired, urine may reflux into the ureters due to the high intravesical pressure that develops during voiding. Clinically, reflux is often detected on the voiding and postvoiding films obtained during intravenous pyelography, although voiding cystourethrography may be required for definitive diagnosis. Bladder infection may ascend the urinary tract to the kidneys through incompetent ureterovesical sphincters. Not surprisingly, therefore, reflux is often discovered in patients with acute and/or chronic urinary tract infections. With more severe degrees of reflux, characterized by dilatation of ureters and renal pelves, progressive renal damage often appears, and although active infection may also be present, uncertainty exists as to the necessity of infection in producing the scarred kidney of reflux nephropathy. Substantial proteinuria is often present, and glomerular lesions similar to those of idiopathic

focal glomerulosclerosis (Chap. 274) are often found in addition to the changes of chronic tubulointerstitial disease. Surgical correction of reflux is usually necessary only with the more severe degrees of reflux since renal damage correlates with the extent of reflux. Obviously, if extensive glomerulosclerosis already exists, urologic repair may no longer be warranted.

RADIATION NEPHRITIS   Renal dysfunction can be expected to occur if 23 Gy (2300 rad) or more of x-ray irradiation is administered to both kidneys during a period of 5 weeks or less. Histologic examination of the kidneys reveals hyalinized glomeruli, atrophic tubules, extensive interstitial fibrosis, and hyalinization of the media of renal arterioles. Radiation-induced renal ischemia is believed to be the main pathogenic factor responsible for the tubulointerstitial damage, which may not become evident clinically for months after completion of radiation. The presentation of acute radiation nephritis includes rapidly progressive azotemia, moderate to malignant hypertension, anemia, and proteinuria that may reach the nephrotic range. More than 50% progress to chronic renal failure. A more insidious form is characterized by slower development of azotemia, anemia, and nephrotic syndrome. Malignant hypertension may follow unilateral renal irradiation and resolve with ipsilateral nephrectomy. Radiation nephritis has all but vanished because of heightened awareness of its pathogenesis by radiotherapists.

ACKNOWLEDGMENT
Dr. Elliott Levy and Dr. Thomas H. Hostetter were co-authors of this chapter in the 14th edition and some of the material in that chapter is carried forward to the present edition.

BIBLIOGRAPHY

ADLER SG et al: Hypersensitivity phenomena and the kidney: Role of drugs and environmental agents. Am J Kidney Dis 5:75, 1985

ARANT BS: Reflux nephropathy. Kidney 21:19, 1989

BENNETT WM: Lead nephropathy. Kidney Int 28:218, 1985

————, DEBROE ME: Analgesic nephropathy. A preventable renal disease. N Engl J Med 320:1269, 1989

BOTON R et al: Prevalence, pathogenesis, and treatment of renal dysfunction associated with chronic lithium therapy. Am J Kidney Dis 10:329, 1987

BRUZZI I et al: Role of increased glomerular protein traffic in the progression of renal failure. Kidney Int 52(Suppl 62):S-29, 1997

CAMERON JS: Immunologically mediated interstitial nephritis: Primary and secondary. Adv Nephrol 18:207, 1989

DELZELL E, SHAPIRO S: A review of epidemiologic studies of nonnarcotic analgesics and chronic renal disease. Medicine 77:102, 1998

KELLY CJ, NEILSON EG: Tubulointerstitial diseases, in *Brenner and Rector's The Kidney*, 6th ed, BM Brenner (ed). Philadelphia, Saunders, 2000 pp 1509–1536

KYLE RA: Monoclonal proteins and renal disease. Annu Rev Med 45:71, 1994

LIN J et al: Chelation therapy for patients with elevated body lead burden and progressive renal insufficiency: A randomized, controlled trial. Ann Intern Med 130:7, 1999

MYERS BD et al: The long-term course of cyclosporine-associated chronic nephropathy. Kidney Int 33:590, 1988

278   *Kamal F. Badr, Barry M. Brenner*

VASCULAR INJURY TO THE KIDNEY

ACE	angiotensin-converting enzyme	MRA	magnetic resonance angiography
AST	aspartate aminotransferase	MRI	magnetic resonance imaging
BUN	blood urea nitrogen	PRA	plasma renin activity
FGS	focal segmental sclerosis	RVT	renal vein thrombosis
GFR	glomerular filtration rate	TTP	thrombotic thrombocytopenic purpura
HUS	hemolytic uremic syndrome	VCAM-1	vascular cell adhesion molecule-1
LDH	lactic dehydrogenase		

Adequate delivery of blood to the glomerular capillary network is crucial for glomerular filtration and overall salt and water balance. Thus,

Table 278-1 Clinical Presentations of Ischemic Renal Disease

Acute renal failure
Progressive azotemia in a patient with known renovascular hypertension
  (usually on medical therapy)
Unexplained progressive azotemia in an elderly patient with or without re-
  fractory hypertension
Hypertension and azotemia in a renal transplant patient

in addition to the threat to the viability of renal tissue, vascular injury to the kidney may compromise the maintenance of body fluid volume and composition. Involvement of the renal vessels by atherosclerotic, hypertensive, embolic, inflammatory, and hematologic disorders is usually a manifestation of generalized vascular pathology. The morphologic and clinical responses to these insults and the unique renal vasculopathy associated with the toxemias of pregnancy are considered in this chapter.

THROMBOEMBOLIC DISEASES OF THE RENAL ARTERIES Thrombosis of the major renal arteries or their branches is an important cause of deterioration of renal function, especially in the elderly. It is often difficult to diagnose and therefore requires a high index of suspicion. Thrombosis may occur as a result of intrinsic pathology in the renal vessels (posttraumatic, atherosclerotic, or inflammatory) or as a result of emboli originating in distant vessels, most commonly fat emboli, emboli originating in the left heart (mural thrombi following myocardial infarction, bacterial endocarditis, or aseptic vegetations), or "paradoxical" emboli passing from the right side of the circulation via a patent foramen ovale or atrial septal defect. Renal emboli are bilateral in 15 to 30% of cases.

The clinical presentation is variable, depending on the time course and the extent of the occlusive event. Acute thrombosis and infarction, such as follows embolization, may result in sudden onset of flank pain and tenderness, fever, hematuria, leukocytosis, nausea, and vomiting. If infarction occurs, renal enzymes may be elevated, namely aspartate aminotransferase (AST), lactic dehydrogenase (LDH; most reliable), and alkaline phosphatase, which rise and fall in the order listed. Urinary lactic dehydrogenase and alkaline phosphatase also may increase after infarction. Renal function deteriorates acutely, leading in bilateral thrombosis to acute oliguric renal failure. More gradual (i.e., atherosclerotic) occlusion of a single renal artery may go undetected. A spectrum of clinical presentations lies between these two extremes (Table 278-1). Hypertension usually follows renal infarction and results from renin release in the peri-infarction zone. Hypertension is usually transient but may be persistent. Diagnosis is established by renal arteriography.

℞ **TREATMENT** Management of *acute* renal arterial thrombosis includes surgical intervention, anticoagulant therapy, conservative and supportive therapy, and control of hypertension. The choice of treatment depends mainly on (1) the condition of the patient, in particular the patient's ability to withstand major surgery, and (2) the extent of renovascular occlusion and amount of renal mass at risk of infarction. In general, supportive care and anticoagulant therapy are indicated in unilateral disease. In bilateral thrombosis, medical and surgical therapies yield comparable results. Twenty-five percent of patients die during the acute episode, usually from extrarenal complications. In *chronic* ischemic renal disease, surgical revascularization is more likely to preserve and improve renal function and to control the hypertension (see below).

ATHEROEMBOLIC DISEASE OF THE RENAL ARTERIES Atheroembolic disease typically results from multiple showers of cholesterol-containing microemboli dislodged from atheromatous plaques in large arteries. Such emboli occlude small (150- to 200-μm diameter) vessels in the kidneys and in other organs (retina, brain, pancreas, muscles, skin, and extremities). Atheroembolic disease usually occurs in an elderly individual with atherosclerotic disease elsewhere and usually follows aortic surgery or renal or coronary

arteriography. Spontaneous atheroembolic disease has also been reported. Manifestations include deterioration of renal function (sudden or gradual), mild proteinuria, microscopic hematuria, and leukocyturia. Urine volume may remain normal or fall to oliguric levels depending on severity. Renal ischemia can induce or exacerbate preexisting hypertension. In elderly patients with mild to moderate cholesterol embolization, the remaining nephrons may subsequently undergo injury, likely a result of hyperfiltration, which may lead to nephrotic-range proteinuria. Renal biopsy reveals "focal segmental sclerosis" (FGS). Renal function deteriorates at a slower rate in these individuals than in patients with more substantial embolic burdens, and they would be expected to benefit from angiotensin-converting enzyme (ACE) inhibitor therapy aimed at lowering intraglomerular pressures in remnant nephrons, even if their systemic blood pressure is in the "normal" range.

Antemortem diagnosis of atherosclerotic renal emboli is difficult. The demonstration of cholesterol emboli in the retina is helpful, but a firm diagnosis is established only by demonstration of cholesterol crystals in the smaller arteries and arterioles in renal biopsy or autopsy specimens. These also may be seen in asymptomatic skeletal muscle or skin. No specific treatment is available.

RENAL VEIN THROMBOSIS (RVT) Thrombosis of one or both main renal veins occurs in a variety of settings (Table 278-2). The pathogenesis is not always clear, particularly when it occurs in so-called hypercoagulable states such as may develop in pregnant women, users of oral contraceptives, subjects with nephrotic syndrome, or dehydrated infants. Nephrotic syndrome accompanying membranous glomerulopathy and certain carcinomas seems to predispose to the development of RVT, which occurs in 10 to 50% of patients with these disorders. RVT may exacerbate preexisting proteinuria but is infrequently the cause of the nephrotic syndrome.

The clinical manifestations depend on the severity and abruptness of its occurrence. Acute cases occur typically in children and are characterized by sudden loss of renal function, often accompanied by fever, chills, lumbar tenderness (with kidney enlargement), leukocytosis, and hematuria. Hemorrhagic infarction and renal rupture may lead to hypovolemic shock. In young adults RVT is usually suspected from an unexpected and relatively acute or subacute deterioration of renal function and/or exacerbation of proteinuria and hematuria in the appropriate clinical setting (underlying nephrotic syndrome, trauma, pregnancy, oral contraceptive use). In cases of gradual thrombosis, usually occurring in the elderly, the only manifestation may be recurrent pulmonary emboli or development of hypertension. A Fanconi-like syndrome and proximal renal tubular acidosis have been described.

The definitive diagnosis can only be established through selective renal venography with visualization of the occluding thrombus. Short of angiography, magnetic resonance imaging (MRI) often provides definitive evidence of thrombus.

℞ **TREATMENT** Treatment consists of anticoagulation, the main purpose of which is prevention of pulmonary embolization, although some authors have also claimed improvement in renal function and proteinuria. Encouraging reports have appeared concerning the use of streptokinase. Spontaneous recanalization with clinical improvement also has been observed. Anticoagulant therapy is more rewarding in the acute thrombosis seen in younger individuals. Nephrectomy is

Table 278-2 Conditions Associated with Renal Vein Thrombosis

Trauma
Extrinsic compression (lymph nodes, aortic aneurysm, tumor)
Invasion by renal cell carcinoma
Dehydration (infants)
Nephrotic syndrome
Pregnancy or oral contraceptives

advocated in infants with life-threatening renal infarction. Thrombectomy is effective in some cases.

RENAL ARTERY STENOSIS/ISCHEMIC RENAL DISEASE

Stenosis of the main renal artery and/or its major branches accounts for 2 to 5% of hypertension (see Chap. 246). The common cause in the middle-aged and elderly is an atheromatous plaque at the origin of the renal artery. In a large unselected autopsy series, stenosis producing > 50% renal artery diameter reduction was found in 18% of those between 65 and 74 years of age and in 42% of those older than 75 years. Bilateral involvement was found in half of the affected cases in both age groups. Ischemic renal disease has emerged as an important cause of end-stage renal disease. It should be considered seriously in elderly individuals, particularly in those with evidence of atherosclerotic arterial disease elsewhere. In elderly patients with myocardial infarction or symptomatic peripheral vascular disease, the incidence of renal arterial stenosis can be up to 40%. In younger women, stenosis is due to intrinsic structural abnormalities of the arterial wall caused by a heterogeneous group of lesions termed *fibromuscular dysplasia.*

Renal artery stenosis should be suspected when hypertension develops in a previously normotensive individual over 50 years of age or in the young (under 30 years) with suggestive features: symptoms of vascular insufficiency to other organs, high-pitched epigastric bruit on physical examination, symptoms of hypokalemia secondary to hyperaldosteronism (muscle weakness, tetany, polyuria), and metabolic alkalosis. If renal arterial stenosis is suspected, the best initial screening test is a renal ultrasound, which may reveal unilateral renal hypotrophy (but normal cortical echogenicity). Absence of compensatory hypertrophy in the contralateral kidney should raise the suspicion of bilateral stenosis or superimposed intrinsic (structural) renal disease, most commonly hypertensive or diabetic nephropathy. A positive captopril test, which has a sensitivity and specificity of greater than 95%, constitutes an excellent follow-up procedure to assess the need for more invasive radiographic evaluation. The test relies on the exaggerated increase in plasma renin activity (PRA) after administration of captopril to patients with renovascular hypertension as compared with those with essential hypertension. It is considered positive when all the following criteria are satisfied: stimulated PRA of 12 (μg/L)/h, absolute increase in PRA of 10 (μg/L)/h or more, and increase in PRA of >150% [or 400% if baseline PRA is <3 (μg/L)/h]. Because ACE inhibitors magnify the impairment in renal blood flow and glomerular filtration rate (GFR) caused by functionally significant renal artery stenosis, use of these drugs in association with ^{99m}Tc-DTPA or ^{99m}MAG$_3$ renography greatly enhances the predictive value of radionuclide renography (90% sensitivity and specificity). Magnetic resonance angiography (MRA) has replaced previous modalities as the most sensitive (100%) and specific (95%) test for the diagnosis of renal arterial stenosis. The most definitive diagnostic procedure is bilateral arteriography with repeated bilateral renal vein and systemic renin determinations. If renal vein renin measurements from the two kidneys differ by a factor of 1.5:1 or more (higher value from the affected kidney) in a patient with radiographic unilateral renal artery stenosis, the chance of cure of hypertension by surgical reconstruction or angioplasty is almost 90%, particularly if the renal vein renin level from the unaffected kidney is equal to or less than systemic levels (suppressible). A ratio of less than 1.5:1, however, does not exclude the diagnosis of renovascular hypertension, particularly in the presence of bilateral disease.

℞ **TREATMENT**   The aims of treatment are control of the blood pressure and restoration of perfusion to the ischemic kidney. In general, it is now firmly established that interventional therapy (i.e., surgery or angioplasty) is superior to medical therapy, which, while controlling blood pressure, does little to salvage renal mass lost to ischemic injury. Success rates with percutaneous transluminal angio-

FIGURE 278-1   Bilateral severe ostial renal arterial stenosis prior to and following balloon dilatation and stent placement in a patient with severe hypertension and renal insufficiency.

plasty in young patients with fibromuscular dysplasia are 50% cure and improvement in blood pressure control in another 30%. Angioplasty is best suited for noncalcified, segmental short lesions and is also useful in some elderly patients who are poor surgical risks. About half of elderly individuals with reduced renal function as a result of renal arterial stenosis improve following angioplasty or surgery, even when preintervention arteriography shows little evidence of cortical perfusion. Despite the risks associated with surgery, long-term follow-up studies demonstrate an advantage of surgery over angioplasty both with regard to the incidence of restenosis and to the preservation or improvement in GFR. As with coronary angioplasty, stenting of renal arteries following balloon angioplasty is being used increasingly. Initial results are highly encouraging, with restenosis rates less than 15% at 6 months. Renal functional recovery or stabilization of renal function is seen in approximately 70% of patients. An illustrative example of renal artery stenting is shown in Fig. 278-1.

Renal artery stenosis, particularly if atherosclerotic, is a progressive disease that may lead to gradual and silent loss of renal functional tissue (ischemic renal disease). Progression of ipsilateral atherosclerotic narrowing can be expected in nearly 50% of individuals, resulting in complete occlusion in about 10%. Thus, these patients need careful follow-up of initially nonclinically significant narrowing (<70%) for the possibility of further occlusion or the development of contralateral disease (30%). Compensatory contralateral hypertrophy may maintain renal function until affected by superimposed pathologic processes, at which time azotemia supervenes. Ischemic renal disease is now recognized as a significant cause of end-stage renal disease in patients over 50 years of age (approximately 15%). Even if angioplasty or surgery fail to return blood pressure to normal, these procedures usually render medical therapy easier.

HEMOLYTIC UREMIC SYNDROME (HUS) AND THROMBOTIC THROMBOCYTOPENIC PURPURA (TTP)

(See also Chap. 116) HUS and TTP, consumptive coagulopathies characterized by microangiopathic hemolytic anemia and thrombocytopenia, have a particular predilection for the kidney and the central nervous system, the latter especially in TTP. The kidneys of patients with HUS or TTP often exhibit a "flea-bitten" appearance, the result of multiple cortical hemorrhagic infarcts. The major sites of pathology are the small renal arteries and afferent arterioles, which are nearly occluded as a result of marked intimal hyperplasia (particularly in TTP) and fibrin deposits in the subintimal regions. When the vasoocclusive process is extensive, bilateral cortical necrosis may occur. In addition, arteriolar microaneurysms, glomerular infarction, or nonspecific focal changes may be seen. In keeping with the focal nature of the vascular lesions, patchy areas of interstitial edema, tubular necrosis, and, eventually, fibrosis occur. By immunofluorescence staining, complement components and immunoglobulins may be demonstrated in the arterioles, and fibrinogen deposits are present in arteries, arterioles, and glomerular capillary loops.

Several mechanisms have been implicated in the etiology of the intravascular coagulopathy seen in HUS and TTP, including induction of a generalized Shwartzman phenomenon by microorganisms or endotoxin, genetic predisposition, and deficiency of platelet antiaggregatory substance(s) (e.g., prostacyclin). Some patients improve after exchange transfusion or plasmapheresis, suggesting accumulation of an as yet unidentified toxin.

Renal failure is common in both HUS and TTP, usually manifested by azotemia, mild proteinuria, microscopic and/or gross hematuria, and cylindruria. Patients with HUS have more severe renal failure, often marked by oligoanuria and hypertension and commonly progressing to chronic renal failure. The prognosis in HUS is better in children than in adults. In TTP, the course of which may span days to months, renal failure is usually less severe.

℞ **TREATMENT** In the management of TTP, high-dose glucocorticoids and plasma exchange often provide complete remission or cure. Plasma exchange should be initiated as early as possible, and the treatment cycles can be repeated if thrombocytopenia recurs. Splenectomy and antiplatelet therapy also have been used with varying degrees of success in patients with TTP. The success of plasma exchange in adult HUS is less well established than in TTP.

ARTERIOLAR NEPHROSCLEROSIS

(See also Chaps. 241 and 246) Whether hypertension is "essential" or of known etiology, persistent exposure of the renal circulation to elevated intraluminal pressures results in development of intrinsic lesions of the renal arterioles (hyaline arteriolosclerosis) that eventually lead to loss of function (nephrosclerosis). Nephrosclerosis is divided into two distinct entities: "benign" and "malignant" (or accelerated).

Benign Arteriolar Nephrosclerosis Benign arteriolar nephrosclerosis is seen in patients who are hypertensive for an extended period of time (blood pressure more than 150/90 mmHg) but whose hypertension has not progressed to a malignant form (described below). Such patients, usually in the older age group, are often discovered to be hypertensive on routine physical examination or as a result of nonspecific symptomatology (e.g., headaches, weakness, palpitations).

Kidney size is normal to reduced, with loss of cortical mass leading to a fine granularity. Although the larger arteries may show atherosclerotic changes, the characteristic pathology is in the afferent arterioles, which have thickened walls due to deposition of homogeneous eosinophilic material (hyaline arteriolosclerosis). This material is composed of plasma proteins and fats that have been deposited in the

arteriolar wall due to injury to the endothelium, probably secondary to the elevated intraluminal hydraulic pressure. Narrowing of vascular lumina results, with consequent ischemic injury to glomeruli and tubules.

Nephrosclerosis accompanying long-standing systemic arterial hypertension is only one manifestation of a generalized process affecting the cardiovascular system. Physical examination, therefore, may reveal changes in retinal vessels (arteriolar narrowing and/or flame-shaped hemorrhages), cardiac hypertrophy, and possibly signs of congestive heart failure. Renal disease may manifest as a mild to moderate elevation of serum creatinine concentration, microscopic hematuria, and/or mild proteinuria. In general, clinical evaluation does not reveal significant renal abnormalities. More specialized examination may disclose elevated urinary albumin excretion, tapering and loss of caliber of intrarenal vessels on arteriography, and an exaggerated natriuresis in response to a fluid challenge. Patients with benign nephrosclerosis maintain a near-normal GFR despite a reduction in renal blood flow.

Malignant Arteriolar Nephrosclerosis Patients with long-standing benign hypertension or patients not known to be hypertensive previously may develop malignant hypertension characterized by a sudden (accelerated) elevation of blood pressure (diastolic often above 130 mmHg) accompanied by papilledema, central nervous system manifestations, cardiac decompensation, and acute progressive deterioration of renal function. The absence of papilledema does not rule out the diagnosis in a patient with markedly elevated blood pressure and rapidly declining renal function. The kidneys are characterized by a flea-bitten appearance resulting from hemorrhages in surface capillaries. Histologically, two distinct vascular lesions can be seen. The first, affecting arterioles, is fibrinoid necrosis, i.e., infiltration of arteriolar walls with eosinophilic material including fibrin. There is thickening of vessel walls and, occasionally, an inflammatory infiltrate (necrotizing arteriolitis). The second lesion, involving the interlobular arteries, is a concentric hyperplastic proliferation of the cellular elements of the vascular wall with deposition of collagen to form a hyperplastic arteriolitis (onion-skin lesion). Fibrinoid necrosis occasionally extends into the glomeruli, which also may undergo proliferative changes or total necrosis. Most glomerular and tubular changes are secondary to ischemia and infarction. The sequence of events leading to the development of malignant hypertension is poorly defined. Two pathophysiologic alterations appear central in its initiation and/or perpetuation: (1) increased permeability of vessel walls to invasion by plasma components, particularly fibrin, which activates clotting mechanisms leading to a microangiopathic hemolytic anemia, thus perpetuating the vascular pathology; and (2) activation of the renin-angiotensin-aldosterone system at some point in the disease process, which contributes to the acceleration and maintenance of blood pressure elevation and, in turn, to vascular injury.

Malignant hypertension is most likely to develop in a previously hypertensive individual, usually in the third or fourth decade of life. There is a higher incidence among men, particularly black men. The presenting symptoms are usually neurologic (dizziness, headache, blurring of vision, altered states of consciousness, and focal or generalized seizures). Cardiac decompensation and renal failure appear thereafter. Renal abnormalities include a rapid rise in serum creatinine, hematuria (at times macroscopic), proteinuria, and red and white blood cell casts in the sediment. Nephrotic syndrome may be present. Elevated plasma aldosterone levels cause hypokalemic metabolic alkalosis in the early phase. Uremic acidosis and hyperkalemia eventually obscure these early findings. Hematologic indices of microangiopathic hemolytic anemia (i.e., schistocytes) are often seen.

℞ **TREATMENT** Control of hypertension is the principal goal of therapy for both benign and malignant forms. The time of initiation of therapy, its effectiveness, and patient compliance are crucial factors in arresting the progression of benign nephrosclerosis. Untreated, most of these patients succumb to the extrarenal complications of hypertension. In contrast, malignant hypertension is a medical emergency; its natural course includes a death rate of 80 to 90% within 1 year of onset, almost always due to uremia. Supportive measures should be instituted to control the neurologic, cardiac, and other complications of acute renal failure, but the mainstay of therapy is prompt and aggressive reduction of blood pressure, which, if successful, can reverse all complications in the majority of patients. Presently, 5-year survival is 50%, and some patients have evidence of partial reversal of the vascular lesions and a return of renal function to near-normal levels.

SCLERODERMA (PROGRESSIVE SYSTEMIC SCLEROSIS) (See also Chap. 313)

Renal vascular involvement in scleroderma is characterized by a distinctive lesion of the small arteries (diameters of 150 to 500 μm) consisting of intimal proliferation, medial thinning, and increased collagen deposition in the adventitial layer. Fibrinoid changes in the walls of afferent arterioles and microinfarcts may occur. Glomerular changes are generally nonspecific and secondary to ischemic damage. Tubules are often atrophic. As part of a generalized increase in vasomotor tone, a vasospastic (Raynaud-like) phenomenon at the level of the renal vasculature contributes to the renal insufficiency. Reduction in renal blood flow is the major mechanism underlying the deterioration in kidney function, being present in 80% of patients, even in the absence of other clinical abnormalities. As vascular narrowing progresses, hypertension, azotemia, and proteinuria eventually develop. Plasma renin rises in response to sustained renal ischemia. The resulting hypertension causes further renal injury and may play a role in the ultimate destruction of nephrons. As more and more nephrons are lost to the combined insults of ischemia and hypertension, development of azotemia heralds a particularly grim prognosis. Proteinuria, usually mild, is a consequence of ischemic and hypertensive glomerular injury.

Although most patients with scleroderma present with extrarenal manifestations, renal involvement is eventually manifested in half of patients followed for up to 20 years. Renal involvement can present in one of two ways, depending on whether malignant hypertension is superimposed on the renal pathology: (1) *Persistent urinary abnormalities* with or without hypertension tend to follow an indolent course with mild proteinuria, occasional casts, cellular elements in the urinary sediment, and a propensity for development of hypertension. Azotemia is absent initially, but when it develops, dialysis is required within 1 year. (2) *Scleroderma renal crisis* is a rapid deterioration in renal function, usually accompanied by malignant hypertension, oliguria, fluid retention, microangiopathic hemolytic anemia, and central nervous system involvement. It may occur in patients with previously undemonstrable or slowly progressive renal disease. Untreated, it leads to chronic renal failure within days to months.

The prognosis of scleroderma renal disease is generally poor, particularly following the onset of azotemia. Aggressive antihypertensive therapy may be effective in delaying the progression of renal failure. In scleroderma renal crisis, prompt treatment with beta blockers, minoxidil, and particularly ACE inhibitors may reverse acute renal failure. The effect of these interventions on renal function over the long term is uncertain.

SICKLE CELL NEPHROPATHY (See also Chaps. 106 and 275)

Sickle cell disease causes renal complications that arise mainly as a result of sickling of red blood cells in the microvasculature. The hypertonic and relatively hypoxic environment of the renal medulla, coupled with the slow blood flow in the vasa recta, favors the sickling of red blood cells, with resultant local infarction (papillary necrosis). Functional tubule defects in patients with sickle cell disease are likely the result of partial ischemic injury to the renal tubules.

In addition to the intrarenal microvascular pathology described above, young patients with sickle cell disease are characterized by renal hyperperfusion, glomerular hypertrophy, and hyperfiltration.

Many of these individuals eventually develop a glomerulopathy leading to glomerular proteinuria (present in as many as 30%) and, in some, the nephrotic syndrome. In recent studies, the mechanisms underlying proteinuria in sickle cell nephropathy have been characterized as an early increase in pore radius, followed, as renal failure supervenes, with a reduction in pore number, but the onset of a dramatic loss of size-selectivity. Mild azotemia and hyperuricemia also can develop, but advanced renal failure and uremia are rare. Pathologic examination reveals the typical lesion of "hyperfiltration nephropathy," namely, focal segmental glomerular sclerosis. This finding has led to the suggestion that anemia-induced hyperfiltration in childhood is the principal cause of the adult glomerulopathy. Nephron loss secondary to ischemic injury also contributes to the development of azotemia in these patients.

In addition to the glomerulopathy described above, renal complications of sickle cell disease include the following: *Cortical infarcts* can cause loss of function, persistent hematuria, and perinephric hematomas. *Papillary infarcts*, demonstrated radiographically in 50% of patients with sickle trait, lead to an increased risk of bacterial infection in the scarred renal tissues and functional tubule abnormalities. Painless gross hematuria occurs with a higher frequency in sickle trait than in sickle cell disease and likely results from infarctive episodes in the renal medulla. *Functional tubule abnormalities* such as nephrogenic diabetes insipidus result from marked reduction in vasa recta blood flow, combined with ischemic tubule injury. This concentrating defect places these patients at increased risk of dehydration and, hence, sickling crises. The concentrating defect also occurs in individuals with sickle trait. Other tubule defects involve potassium and hydrogen ion excretion, occasionally leading to hyperkalemic metabolic acidosis and a defect in uric acid excretion which, combined with increased purine synthesis in the bone marrow, results in hyperuricemia.

Management of sickle nephropathy is not separate from that of overall patient management (Chap. 106). In addition, however, the use of ACE inhibitors has been associated with improvement of the hyperfiltration glomerulopathy.

TOXEMIAS OF PREGNANCY (See also Chap. 7)

Renal function is "reset" at a higher level during normal pregnancy. Renal plasma flow and GFR both increase by 30 to 50%. Therefore, serum creatinine levels above 70 μmol/L (0.8 mg/dL) or blood urea nitrogen (BUN) levels above 4.6 mmol/L (13 mg/dL) are abnormal in pregnant women and should be investigated. Systolic and diastolic blood pressures decrease by an average of 10 to 15 mmHg below pregravid values. A diastolic pressure above 75 mmHg during the second trimester or above 85 mmHg during the third trimester is therefore abnormal. Vasodilation in the uterine, renal, and cutaneous beds, vasodilator prostaglandin release from the uteroplacental unit, and a decrease in arteriolar sensitivity to angiotensin II all play a role in the decline of blood pressure during pregnancy.

Preeclampsia-Eclampsia   The toxemia syndrome, usually occurring in the third trimester of primigravidas, includes hypertension, proteinuria, edema, consumptive coagulopathy, sodium retention, hyperreflexia (preeclampsia), and, if uncontrolled, convulsions (eclampsia). In pure preeclampsia (i.e., not superimposed on previously existing hypertensive or renal disease), the primary sites of pathology are the glomerular endothelial cells. These cells show marked swelling due to an increase in cytoplasmic volume with vacuolization (endotheliosis) and encroach on the vascular lumen, rendering the enlarged glomeruli ischemic. The glomerular basement membrane and the extraglomerular blood vessels are intact. The pathogenesis is unknown. Coagulation abnormalities, hormonal factors, uteroplacental ischemia, and immune mechanisms have all been implicated. Increased microvascular reactivity may be a result of endothelial cell damage, which, in turn, alters the balance of endothelium-derived vasodilator/vasoconstrictor autacoids. Recent evidence suggests that preeclampsia may be characterized by selective dysregulation of vascular cell adhesion molecule-1 (VCAM-1) (but not other leukocyte adhesion molecules). This abnormality is not present in non-proteinuric gestational hypertension, and subsides post-partum. Induction of VCAM-1 expression in preeclampsia may contribute to leukocyte-mediated tissue injury in this condition or may reflect perturbation of other, previously unrecognized functions of this molecule in pregnancy. Despite sodium retention, intravascular volume is contracted as compared with pregravid values. An increased sensitivity to angiotensin II is the basis for the "roll-over test" (an increase in diastolic blood pressure of 20 mmHg or more on changing the patient's position from lateral recumbent to supine, presumably due to alterations in circulating angiotensin levels). In the supine position, the reduction in venous return due to compression by the gravid uterus increases circulating levels of angiotensin II. This increase results in a hypertensive response in preeclamptic patients, who are hyperresponsive to angiotensin II, but not in normal women, in whom pregnancy leads to a relative resistance to the pressor effects of this hormone.

A diagnosis of preeclampsia-related hypertension can be made when repeated measurements over a 4- to 6-h period show a blood pressure of 140/85 mmHg or more. The rise in blood pressure tends to be more severe at night. When preeclampsia occurs in a previously hypertensive patient, a rapid acceleration of the blood pressure elevation is accompanied by an increase in proteinuria, oliguria, edema, and coagulopathy. This is a life-threatening syndrome and tends to recur with future pregnancies. In addition to proteinuria, which correlates with the severity of the renal lesion, GFR and renal plasma flow are depressed. In view of the preexisting high levels, however, GFR in preeclamptic women often remains above nonpregnant levels. Uric acid clearance also falls, resulting in hyperuricemia. In the postpartum period, these patients are particularly susceptible to the development of "postpartum renal failure," which is thought to be a form of adult HUS.

Rx TREATMENT Treatment consists of bed rest in a quiet environment and control of neurologic manifestations and blood pressure, the former with magnesium sulfate and the latter usually with vasodilators such as hydralazine and methyldopa. Diuretics are avoided. The ultimate "treatment" is delivery, which should be induced if fetal maturity is adequate or if life-threatening coagulopathy or renal failure occur. The long-term prognosis is generally favorable.

Development of acute renal failure/preeclampsia in a pregnant woman should alert the physician to potential preexisting renal disease and/or hypertension. The latter is particularly likely if systolic blood pressure is greater than 200 mmHg. Hypertension and preexisting proteinuria tend to worsen in 50% of women during pregnancy. In addition, these abnormalities may be unmasked during pregnancy as the first manifestations of an underlying glomerulopathy. Conversely, patients with established underlying renal disease should be followed closely during pregnancy, with monthly measurements of 24-h urinary protein excretion and GFR. Sudden deterioration should raise suspicion of superimposed preeclampsia. There is no convincing evidence that pregnancy has an adverse effect on the long-term outcome of immunologic glomerular diseases or diabetic nephropathy. In all situations, control of blood pressure should be the primary therapeutic goal in view of its established beneficial effects on the progression of renal injury.

Bilateral Cortical Necrosis Acute bilateral cortical necrosis is associated with septic abortions, abruptio placentae, and preeclampsia. Coagulation in cortical vessels and arterioles leads to renal tissue necrosis. Anuria and renal failure ensue and may be irreversible. In other cases, renal function returns partially, but on long-term follow-up most patients slowly progress to uremia.

BIBLIOGRAPHY

CAREY RM et al: Role of the angiotensin type 2 receptor in the regulation of blood pressure and renal function. Hypertension 35:155, 2000

CHATZIANTONIOU C, DUSSAULE JC: Endothelin and renal vascular fibrosis: of mice and men. Curr Opin Nephrol Hypertens 9:31, 2000

GHANIOUS VE et al: Evaluating patients with renal failure for renal artery stenosis with gadolinium-enhanced magnetic resonance angiography. Am J Kidney Dis 33:36, 1999

GREENBERG A et al: Focal segmental glomerulosclerosis associated with nephrotic syndrome in cholesterol atheroembolism. Clinicopathologic correlations. Am J Kidney Dis 29:344, 1997

GRIST TM: Magnetic resonance angiography of renal artery stenosis. Am J Kidney Dis 24:700, 1994

HARDEN RN et al: Effect of renal artery stenting on progression of renovascular renal failure. Lancet 349:1133, 1997

REDMAN CWG: Hypertension in pregnancy, in *Medical Disorders in Obstetric Practice*, M DeSwiet (ed). Oxford, Blackwell Scientific, 1995

SYMPOSIUM ON ISCHEMIC RENAL DISEASE: Am J Kidney Dis 24:614, 1994

TUTTLE KR, RAABE RD: Endovascular stents for renal artery revascularization. Curr Opin Nephrol Hypertens 7:695, 1998

UZO T et al: Prevalence and predictions of renal artery stenosis in patients with myocardial infarction. Am J Kidney Dis 29:733, 1997

YADED M, LLACH F: Vascular complications involving the renal vessels, in *The Kidney*, 6th ed, BM Brenner (ed). Philadelphia, Saunders, 2001

279 *John R. Asplin, Fredric L. Coe, Murray J. Favus*

NEPHROLITHIASIS

TYPES OF STONES

Calcium salts, uric acid, cystine, and struvite ($MgNH_4PO_4$) are the basic constituents of most kidney stones in the western hemisphere. Calcium oxalate and calcium phosphate stones make up 75 to 85% of the total (Table 279-1) and may be admixed in the same stone. Calcium phosphate in stones is usually hydroxyapatite [$Ca_5(PO_4)_3OH$] or, less commonly, brushite ($CaHPO_4 \cdot H_2O$).

Calcium stones are more common in men; the average age of onset is the third decade. Approximately 60% of people who form a single calcium stone eventually form another within the next 10 years. The average rate of new stone formation in patients who have had a previous stone is about one stone every 2 or 3 years. Calcium stone disease is frequently familial.

In the urine, calcium oxalate monohydrate crystals (whewellite) usually grow as biconcave ovals that resemble red blood cells in shape and size but may occur in a larger, "dumbbell" form. In polarized light the crystals appear bright against a dark background, with an intensity that is dependent on orientation, a property known as *birefringence*. Calcium oxalate dihydrate crystals (weddellite) are bipyramidal. Apatite crystals do not exhibit birefringence and appear amorphous because the actual crystals are too small to be resolved by light microscopy.

Uric acid stones (Table 279-1) are radiolucent and are also more common in men. Half of patients with uric acid stones have gout; uric acid lithiasis is usually familial whether or not gout is present. In urine, uric acid crystals are red-orange in color because they absorb the pigment uricine. Anhydrous uric acid produces small crystals that appear amorphous by light microscopy. They are indistinguishable from apatite crystals, except for their birefringence. Uric acid dihydrate tends to form teardrop-shaped crystals as well as flat, rhomboid plates; both are strongly birefringent. Uric acid gravel appears like red dust, and the stones are also orange or red on some occasions. *Cystine stones* are uncommon (Table 279-1), lemon yellow, and sparkle; radiopacity is due to the sulfur content. Cystine crystals appear in the urine as flat, hexagonal plates.

Struvite stones are common (Table 279-1) and potentially dangerous. These stones occur mainly in women or patients who require chronic bladder catheterization and result from urinary tract infection with urease-producing bacteria, usually *Proteus* species. The stones

Table 279-1 Major Causes of Renal Stones

Stone Type and Causes	Percent of all Stones[a]	Percent Occurrence of Specific Causes[a]	Ratio of Males to Females	Etiology	Diagnosis	Treatment
Calcium stones	75–85		2:1 to 3:1			
Idiopathic hyper-calciuria		50–55	2:1	Hereditary (?)	Normocalcemia, unexplained hypercalciuria[b]	Thiazide diuretic agents
Hyperuricosuria		20	4:1	Diet	Urine uric acid >750 mg per 24 h (women), >800 mg per 24 h (men)	Allopurinol or diet
Primary hyperparathyroidism		5	3:10	Neoplasia	Unexplained hypercalcemia	Surgery
Distal renal tubular acidosis		Rare	1:1	Hereditary	Hyperchloremic acidosis, minimum urine pH >5.5	Alkali replacement
Intestinal hyperoxaluria		~1–2	1:1	Bowel surgery	Urine oxalate >50 mg per 24 h	Cholestyramine or oral calcium loading
Hereditary hyperoxaluria		Rare	1:1	Hereditary	Urine oxalate and glycolic or l-glyceric acid increased	Fluids and pyridoxine
Hypocitraturia		15–60	2:1 to 5:1	Hereditary (?), diet	Urine citrate <320 mg per 24 h	Alkali supplements
Idiopathic stone disease		20	2:1	Unknown	None of the above present	Oral phosphate, fluids
Uric acid stones	5–8					
Gout		~50	3:1 to 4:1	Hereditary	Clinical diagnosis	Alkali and allopurinol
Idiopathic		~50	1:1	Hereditary (?)	Uric acid stones, no gout	Alkali and allopurinol if daily urine uric acid above 1000 mg
Dehydration		?	1:1	Intestinal, habit	History, intestinal fluid loss	Alkali, fluids, reversal of cause
Lesch-Nyhan syndrome		Rare	Males only	Hereditary	Reduced hypoxanthine-guanine phosphoribosyltransferase level	Allopurinol
Malignant tumors		Rare	1:1	Neoplasia	Clinical diagnosis	Allopurinol
Cystine stones	1		1:1	Hereditary	Stone type; elevated cystine excretion	Massive fluids, alkali, D-penicillamine if needed
Struvite stones	10–15		2:10	Infection	Stone type	Antimicrobial agents and judicious surgery

[a] Values are percent of patients who form a particular type of stone and who display each specific cause of stones.

[b] Urine calcium above 300 mg per 24 h (men), 250 mg per 24 h (women), or 4 mg/kg per 24 h either sex. Hyperthyroidism, Cushing syndrome, sarcoidosis, malignant tumors, immobilization, vitamin D intoxication, rapidly progressive bone disease, and Paget's disease all cause hypercalciuria and must be excluded in diagnosis of idiopathic hypercalciuria.

can grow to a large size and fill the renal pelvis and calyces to produce a "staghorn" appearance. They are radiopaque and have a variable internal density. In urine, struvite crystals are rectangular prisms said to resemble coffin lids.

MANIFESTATIONS OF STONES

As stones grow on the surfaces of the renal papillae or within the collecting system, they need not produce symptoms. Asymptomatic stones may be discovered during the course of radiographic studies undertaken for unrelated reasons. Stones rank, along with benign and malignant neoplasms, renal cysts, and genitourinary tuberculosis, among the common causes of isolated hematuria. Much of the time, however, stones break loose and enter the ureter or occlude the ureteropelvic junction, causing pain and obstruction.

STONE PASSAGE A stone can traverse the ureter without symptoms, but passage usually produces pain and bleeding. The pain begins gradually, usually in the flank, but increases over the next 20 to 60 min to become so severe that narcotic drugs may be needed for its control. The pain may remain in the flank or spread downward and anteriorly toward the ipsilateral loin, testis, or vulva. Pain that migrates downward indicates that the stone has passed to the lower third of the ureter, but if the pain does not migrate, the position of the stone cannot be predicted. A stone in the portion of the ureter within the bladder wall causes frequency, urgency, and dysuria that may be confused with urinary tract infection. The vast majority of ureteral stones less than 0.5 cm in diameter will pass spontaneously.

It has been standard practice to diagnose acute renal colic by intravenous pyelography; however, helical computed tomography (CT) scan without radiocontrast enhancement is now the preferred procedure. CT has the advantage of detecting uric acid stones in addition to the traditional radioopaque stones, and CT does not expose the patient to the risk of radio-contrast agents.

OTHER SYNDROMES Staghorn Calculi Struvite, cystine, and uric acid stones often grow too large to enter the ureter. They gradually fill the renal pelvis and may extend outward through the infundibula to the calyces themselves.

Nephrocalcinosis Calcium stones grow on the papillae. Most break loose and cause colic, but they may remain in place so that multiple papillary calcifications are found by x-ray, a condition termed *nephrocalcinosis*. Papillary nephrocalcinosis is common in hereditary distal renal tubular acidosis (RTA) and in other types of severe hypercalciuria. In medullary sponge kidney disease (Chap. 276) calcification may occur in dilated distal collecting ducts.

Sludge Sufficient uric acid or cystine in the urine may plug both ureters with precipitate. Calcium oxalate crystals do not do this because less than 100 mg oxalate usually is excreted daily in the urine even in severe hyperoxaluric states, compared with 1000 mg uric acid in patients with hyperuricosuria and 400 to 800 mg cystine in patients with cystinuria. Calcium phosphate crystals can render the urine milky but do not plug the urinary tract.

INFECTION Although urinary tract infection is not a direct consequence of stone disease, it can occur after instrumentation and surgery of the urinary tract, which are frequent in the treatment of stone disease. Stone disease and urinary tract infection can enhance their respective seriousness and interfere with treatment. Obstruction of an infected kidney by a stone may lead to sepsis and extensive damage of renal tissue, since it converts the urinary tract proximal to the obstruction into a closed, or partially closed, space that can become an abscess. Stones may harbor bacteria in the stone matrix, leading to recurrent urinary tract infection. On the other hand, infection due to bacteria that possess the enzyme urease can cause stones composed of struvite.

ACTIVITY OF STONE DISEASE Active disease means that new stones are forming or that preformed stones are growing. Sequential radiographs of the renal areas are needed to document the growth or appearance of new stones and to ensure that passed stones are actually newly formed, not preexistent ones.

PATHOGENESIS OF STONES

Urinary stones usually arise because of the breakdown of a delicate balance. The kidneys must conserve water, but they must excrete materials that have a low solubility. These two opposing requirements must be balanced during adaptation to diet, climate, and activity. The problem is mitigated to some extent by the fact that urine contains substances that inhibit crystallization of calcium salts and others that bind calcium in soluble complexes. These protective mechanisms are less than perfect. When the urine becomes supersaturated with insoluble materials, because excretion rates are excessive and/or because water conservation is extreme, crystals form and may grow and aggregate to form a stone.

SUPERSATURATION In a solution in equilibrium with crystals of calcium oxalate, the product of the chemical activities of the calcium and oxalate ions in the solution is termed the *equilibrium solubility product*. If crystals are removed, and if either calcium or oxalate ions are added to the solution, the activity product increases, but the solution may remain clear; no new crystals form. Such a solution is *metastably supersaturated*. If new calcium oxalate seed crystals are now added, they will grow in size. Ultimately, the activity product reaches a critical value at which a solid phase begins to develop spontaneously. This value is called the *upper limit of metastability*, or the *formation product*. Stone growth in the urinary tract requires a urine that, on average, is above the equilibrium solubility product. Excessive supersaturation is common in stone formation.

Calcium, oxalate, and phosphate form many stable soluble complexes among themselves and with other substances in urine, such as citrate. As a result, their free ion activities are below their chemical concentrations and can be measured only by indirect techniques. Reduction in ligands such as citrate can increase ion activity without changing total urinary calcium. Urine supersaturation can be increased by dehydration or by overexcretion of calcium, oxalate, phosphate, cystine, or uric acid. Urine pH is also important; phosphate and uric acid are weak acids that dissociate readily over the physiologic range of urine pH. Alkaline urine contains more dibasic phosphate, favoring deposits of brushite, and apatite. Below a urine pH of 5.5, uric acid crystals (pK 5.47) predominate, whereas phosphate crystals are rare. The solubility of calcium oxalate, on the other hand, is not influenced by changes in urine pH. Measurements of supersaturation in a pooled 24-h urine sample probably underestimate the risk of precipitation. Transient dehydration, variation of urine pH, and postprandial bursts of overexcretion may cause values considerably above average.

NUCLEATION **Homogeneous Nucleation** In urine that is supersaturated with respect to calcium oxalate, these two ions form clusters. Most small clusters eventually disperse because the internal forces that hold them together are too weak to overcome the random

tendency of ions to move away. Clusters of over 100 ions can remain stable because attractive forces balance surface losses. Once they are stable, nuclei can grow at levels of supersaturation below that needed for their creation. The formation product marks the point at which stable nuclei become frequent enough to create a permanent solid phase.

Heterogeneous Nucleation If a supersaturated urine is seeded with preformed nuclei of a crystal that is similar in structure to calcium oxalate, calcium and oxalate ions in solution will bind to the crystal's surface as they would on a seed crystal of calcium oxalate itself. The seeding of a supersaturated solution by foreign nuclei is called *heterogeneous nucleation*. Cell debris, calcifications on the renal papillae, as well as other urinary crystals, can serve as heterogeneous nuclei that permit calcium oxalate stones to form, even though urine calcium oxalate supersaturation never exceeds the metastable limit for homogenous nucleation.

INHIBITORS OF CRYSTAL FORMATION Stable nuclei must grow and aggregate to produce a stone of clinical significance. Urine contains potent inhibitors of nucleation, growth, and aggregation for calcium oxalate and calcium phosphate but not for uric acid, cystine, or struvite. Inorganic pyrophosphate is a potent inhibitor that appears to affect calcium phosphate more than calcium oxalate crystals. Citrate inhibits crystal growth and nucleation, though most of the stone inhibitory activity of citrate is due to lowering urine supersaturation via complexation of calcium. Other urine components such as glycoproteins inhibit all three processes of calcium oxalate stone formation. Slowing of crystal growth increases the apparent upper limit of metastability because the critical growth of ion clusters into stable nuclei is hindered. As a consequence of the presence of these inhibitors, crystal growth in urine is slow compared with growth in simple salt solutions, and the upper limit of metastability is higher.

EVALUATION AND TREATMENT OF PATIENTS WITH NEPHROLITHIASIS

Most patients with nephrolithiasis have remediable metabolic disorders that cause stones and can be detected by chemical analyses of serum and urine. Adults with recurrent kidney stones and children with even a single kidney stone should be evaluated. A practical outpatient evaluation consists of two or three 24-h urine collections, each with a corresponding blood sample; measurements of serum and urine calcium, uric acid, electrolytes and creatinine, urine pH, volume, oxalate, and citrate should be made. Since stone risks vary with diet, activity, and environment, at least one urine collection should be made on a weekend when the patient is at home and another on a work day. When possible, the composition of kidney stones should be determined because treatment depends on stone type (Table 279-1). No matter what disorders are found, every patient should be counseled to avoid dehydration and to drink sufficient water so that they excrete at least 2 L of urine every day. Since treatment is prolonged, the use of medications must be justified by the activity and severity of stone disease and the importance of protection against new stones.

℞ **TREATMENT** The management of stones already present in the kidneys or urinary tract requires a combined medical and surgical approach. The specific treatment depends on the location of the stone, the extent of obstruction, the function of the affected and unaffected kidney, the presence or absence of urinary tract infection, the progress of stone passage, and the risks of operation or anesthesia given the clinical state of the patient. In general, severe obstruction, infection, intractable pain, and serious bleeding are indications for removal of a stone.

In the past, stones were removed by operation or by passing a flexible basket retrograde up the ureter from the bladder during cystoscopy. There are now three alternatives. *Extracorporeal lithotripsy* causes the in situ fragmentation of stones in the kidney, renal pelvis, or ureter by exposing them to shock waves. The kidney stone is centered at a focal point of parabolic reflectors, and high-intensity shock waves are created by high-voltage discharge. The waves are transmitted to the patient using water as a conduction medium, either by placing the patient in a water tank or by placing water-filled cushions between the patient and the shock wave generators. After multiple discharges, most stones are reduced to powder that moves through the ureter into the bladder. *Percutaneous ultrasonic lithotripsy* requires the passage of a rigid cystoscope-like instrument into the renal pelvis through a small incision in the flank. Stones can be disrupted by a small ultrasound transducer, and fragments can be removed directly. The last method is *laser lithotripsy via a ureteroscope* for removal of ureteral stones. These various forms of lithotripsy have largely replaced pyelolithotomy and ureterolithotomy.

CALCIUM STONES Idiopathic Hypercalciuria (See also Chap. 341) This condition appears to be hereditary, and its diagnosis is straightforward (Table 279-1). In some patients, primary intestinal hyperabsorption of calcium causes transient postprandial hypercalcemia that suppresses secretion of parathyroid hormone. The renal tubules are deprived of the normal stimulus to reabsorb calcium at the same time that the filtered load of calcium is increased. In other patients, reabsorption of calcium by the renal tubules appears to be defective, and secondary hyperparathyroidism is evoked by urinary losses of calcium. Renal synthesis of 1,25-dihydroxyvitamin D is increased, enhancing intestinal absorption of calcium. In the past, the separation of "absorptive" and "renal" forms of hypercalciuria was used to guide treatment. However, these may not be distinct entities but the extremes of a continuum of behavior. Vitamin D overactivity, either through high vitamin D levels or excess vitamin D receptor, is a likely explanation for the hypercalciuria in many of these patients. Hypercalciuria contributes to stone formation by raising urine saturation with respect to calcium oxalate and calcium phosphate.

℞ TREATMENT Thiazide diuretics lower urine calcium in idiopathic hypercalciuria and are effective in preventing the formation of stones. Three 3-year randomized trials have shown a 50% decrease in stone formation in the thiazide-treated group as compared to the placebo-treated controls. The drug effect requires slight contraction of the extracellular fluid volume, and massive use of NaCl reduces its therapeutic effect. Thiazide-induced hypokalemia should be aggressively treated since hypokalemia will reduce urine citrate, increasing urine calcium ion levels.

Hyperuricosuria About 20% of calcium oxalate stone formers are hyperuricosuric, primarily because of an excessive intake of purine from meat, fish, and poultry. The mechanism of stone formation is probably due to salting out calcium oxalate by urate. A low-purine diet is desirable but difficult for many patients to achieve. The alternative is allopurinol, which has been shown to be effective in a randomized controlled trial. A dose of 100 mg bid is usually sufficient.

Primary Hyperparathyroidism (See also Chap. 341) The diagnosis of this condition is established by documenting that hypercalcemia that cannot be otherwise explained is accompanied by inappropriately elevated serum concentrations of parathyroid hormone. Hypercalciuria, usually present, raises the urine supersaturation of calcium phosphate and/or calcium oxalate (Table 279-1). Prompt diagnosis is important because parathyroidectomy should be carried out before renal damage or bone disease occurs.

Distal Renal Tubular Acidosis (See also Chap. 276) The defect in this condition seems to reside in the distal nephron, which cannot establish a normal pH gradient between urine and blood, leading to hyperchloremic acidosis. The diagnosis is suggested by a minimum urine pH in the presence of systemic acidosis above 5.5. If the diagnosis is in doubt because metabolic abnormalities are mild, oral challenge with NH_4Cl, 1.9 mmol/kg of body weight, will not lower urine

pH below 5.5 in patients with distal RTA. Hypercalciuria, an alkaline urine, and a low urine citrate level cause supersaturation with respect to calcium phosphate. Calcium phosphate stones form, nephrocalcinosis is common, and osteomalacia or rickets may occur. Renal damage is frequent, and glomerular filtration rate falls gradually. Treatment with supplemental alkali reverses hypercalciuria and limits the production of new stones. The usual dose of sodium bicarbonate is 0.5 to 2.0 mmol/kg of body weight per day in four to six divided doses. An alternative is potassium citrate supplementation, given at the same dose per day but needing to be given only three to four times per day. In incomplete distal RTA, systemic acidosis is absent, but urine pH cannot be lowered below 5.5 after an exogenous acid load such as ammonium chloride. Incomplete RTA may develop in some patients who form calcium oxalate stones because of idiopathic hypercalciuria; the importance of RTA in producing stones in this situation is uncertain, and thiazide treatment is a reasonable alternative. Some patients with incomplete RTA form calcium phosphate stones because of low urine citrate and an alkaline urine and are best treated with alkali as if RTA were complete.

Hyperoxaluria Overabsorption of dietary oxalate and consequent oxaluria, i.e., so-called intestinal oxaluria, is one consequence of fat malabsorption (Chap. 286). The latter can be caused by a variety of conditions, including bacterial overgrowth syndromes, chronic disease of the pancreas and biliary tract, jejunoileal bypass in treatment of obesity, or ileal resection for inflammatory bowel disease. With fat malabsorption, calcium in the bowel lumen is bound by fatty acids instead of oxalate, which is left free for absorption in the colon. Delivery of unabsorbed fatty acids and bile salts to the colon may injure the colonic mucosa and enhance oxalate absorption. Dietary excess of oxalate in patients with normal intestinal function is a common cause of mild elevation of urine oxalate, but seldom to the level seen in patients with enteric hyperoxaluria. Hereditary hyperoxaluria states are rare causes of severe hyperoxaluria; patients usually present with recurrent calcium oxalate stones during childhood. Type I hereditary hyperoxaluria is inherited as an autosomal recessive trait and is due to a deficiency in the peroxisomal enzyme alanine:glyoxylate aminotransferase. Type II is due to a deficiency of D-glyceric dehydrogenase. Ethylene glycol intoxication and methoxyflurane also can cause oxalate overproduction and hyperoxaluria. Hyperoxaluria from any cause can produce tubulointerstitial nephropathy (Chap. 277) and lead to stone formation.

℞ TREATMENT The oxalate-binding resin cholestyramine at a dose of 8 to 16 g/d, correction of fat malabsorption, and a low-fat, low oxalate diet are effective treatments for oxaluria secondary to intestinal overabsorption. Calcium supplements, given with meals, precipitate oxalate in the gut lumen providing an alternative form of therapy. Treatment for hereditary hyperoxaluria includes a high fluid intake, neutral phosphate, and pyridoxine (25 to 200 mg/d). Citrate supplementation may also have some benefit. Even with aggressive therapy, irreversible renal failure secondary to recurrent stone formation often occurs. Segmental liver transplant, to correct the enzyme defect, combined with a kidney transplant have been successfully utilized in patients with hereditary hyperoxaluria.

Hypocitraturia Urine citrate prevents calcium stone formation by creating a soluble complex with calcium, effectively reducing free urine calcium. Hypocitraturia is found in 15 to 60% of stone formers, either as a single disorder or in combination with other metabolic abnormalities. It can be secondary to systemic disorders, such as RTA, chronic diarrheal illness, or hypokalemia, or it may be a primary disorder, in which case it is called *idiopathic hypocitraturia*.

℞ TREATMENT Treatment is with alkali, which increases urine citrate excretion; generally bicarbonate or citrate salts are used. Potassium salts are preferred as sodium loading increases urinary excretion of calcium, reducing the effectiveness of treatment. A recent randomized, placebo-controlled trial has demonstrated the effectiveness of potassium citrate in idiopathic hypocitraturia.

Idiopathic Calcium Lithiasis Some patients have no metabolic cause for stones despite a thorough metabolic evaluation (Table 279-1). The best treatment appears to be high fluid intake so that the urine specific gravity remains at 1.005 or below throughout the day and night. Oral phosphate at a dose of 2 g phosphorus daily may lower urine calcium and increase urine pyrophosphate and thereby reduce the rate of recurrence. Orthophosphate causes mild nausea and diarrhea initially, but tolerance may improve with continued intake. Thiazide treatment to reduce calcium excretion and allopurinol to diminish uric acid output also may be helpful.

URIC ACID STONES These stones form because the urine becomes supersaturated with undissociated uric acid that is protonated at its N-9 position. In gout, idiopathic uric acid lithiasis, and dehydration, the average pH is usually below 5.4 and often below 5.0. Undissociated uric acid therefore predominates and is soluble in urine only in concentrations of 100 mg/L. Concentrations above this level represent supersaturation that causes crystals and stones to form. Hyperuricosuria, when present, increases supersaturation, but urine of low pH can be supersaturated with undissociated uric acid even though the daily excretion rate is normal. Myeloproliferative syndromes, chemotherapy of malignant tumors, and the Lesch-Nyhan syndrome cause such massive production of uric acid and consequent hyperuricosuria that stones and uric acid sludge form even at a normal urine pH. Plugging of the renal collecting tubules by uric acid crystals can cause acute renal failure.

℞ TREATMENT The two goals of treatment are to raise urine pH and to lower excessive urine uric acid excretion to less than 1 g/d. Supplemental alkali, 1 to 3 mmol/kg of body weight per day, should be given in three or four evenly spaced, divided doses, one of which should be given at bedtime. The form of the alkali may be important. Potassium citrate may reduce the risk of calcium salts crystallizing when urine pH is increased, whereas sodium citrate or sodium bicarbonate may increase the risk. If the overnight urine pH is below 5.5, the evening dose of alkali may be raised or 250 mg acetazolamide added at bedtime. A low-purine diet should be instituted in those uric acid stone formers with hyperuricosuria. Patients who continue to form uric acid stones despite treatment with fluids, alkali, and a low-purine diet should have allopurinol added to their regimen. If hypercalciuria is also present, it should be specifically treated, as alkali alone could lead to calcium phosphate stone formation.

CYSTINURIA AND CYSTINE STONES (See also Chap. 352) In this disorder, proximal tubular and jejunal transport of the dibasic amino acids cystine, lysine, arginine, and ornithine are defective, and excessive amounts are lost in the urine. Clinical disease is due solely to the insolubility of cystine, which forms stones.

Pathogenesis Cystinuria occurs because of defective transport of amino acids by the brush borders of renal tubule and intestinal epithelial cells. Cystine, lysine, arginine, and ornithine appear to share a common renal transport pathway, since infusion of lysine decreases tubular reabsorption of the other three. However, cystine is also transported by a separate transport mechanism, because cystinuria and dibasic aminoaciduria can occur independently. The intestinal defects are not similar in all patients who are homozygous for cystinuria, and the extent of aminoaciduria in individuals who are heterozygous carriers of the defect varies from family to family. Three types of inheritance have been described (Chap. 352). A gene located on chromosome 2 and designated SLC3A1, codes for a dibasic amino acid transporter and has been found to be abnormal in Type I cystinuria. Linkage analysis has mapped Type III cystinuria to chromosome 19.

Diagnosis Cystine stones are formed only by patients with cystinuria, but 10% of stones in cystinuric patients do not contain cystine; therefore, every stone former should be screened for the disease. The sediment from a first morning urine specimen in many patients with homozygous cystinuria reveals typical flat, hexagonal, platelike cystine crystals. Cystinuria also can be detected using the urine sodium nitroprusside test. The test is positive with 75 to 125 mg cystine per gram of creatinine, a concentration lower than that in the urine of patients with cystinuria but above the levels in normal urine. Because the test is sensitive, it is positive in many asymptomatic heterozygotes for cystinuria. A positive nitroprusside test or the finding of cystine crystals in the urine sediment should be evaluated by measurement of daily cystine excretion. Normal adults excrete 40 to 60 mg cystine per gram of creatinine, heterozygotes usually excrete less than 300 mg/g, and homozygotes almost always excrete above 250 mg/g.

℞ TREATMENT This consists of a high fluid intake, even at night. Daily urine volume should exceed 3 L. Raising urine pH with alkali is helpful, provided the urine pH exceeds 7.5. A low-salt diet (100 mmol/d) can reduce cystine excretion up to 40%. Because side effects are frequent, drugs such as penicillamine and tiopronin, which form the soluble disulfide cysteine-drug complexes, should be used only when fluid loading, salt reduction, and alkali therapy are ineffective. Captopril, which has a free sulfhydryl group to bind cysteine, has been used in a limited number of patients with some success. Low-methionine diets have not proved to be practical for clinical use, but patients should avoid protein gluttony.

STRUVITE STONES These stones are a result of urinary infection with bacteria, usually *Proteus* species, which possess urease, an enzyme that degrades urea to NH_3 and CO_2. The NH_3 hydrolyzes to NH_4^+ and raises urine pH to 8 or 9. The CO_2 hydrates to H_2CO_3 and then dissociates to CO_3^{2-} which precipitates with calcium as $CaCO_3$. The NH_4^+ precipitates PO_4^{3-} and Mg^{2+} to form $MgNH_4PO_4$ (struvite). The result is a stone of calcium carbonate admixed with struvite. Struvite does not form in urine in the absence of infection, because NH_4^+ concentration is low in urine that is alkaline in response to physiologic stimuli. Chronic *Proteus* infection can occur because of impaired urinary drainage, urologic instrumentation or surgery, and especially with chronic antibiotic treatment, which can favor the dominance of *Proteus* in the urinary tract.

℞ TREATMENT Complete removal of the stone with subsequent sterilization of the urinary tract is the treatment of choice for patients who can tolerate the procedures. Open surgery is successful in debulking the stone and improving renal function if obstruction is present; however, there is recurrence of stone in 25% of the patients. Irrigation of the renal pelvis and calyces with hemiacidrin, a solution that dissolves struvite, can reduce recurrence after surgery. Newer procedures such as lithotripsy and percutaneous nephrolithotomy, alone or in combination, have largely replaced open surgery. Stone-free rates of 50 to 90% have been reported after these procedures. Antimicrobial treatment is best reserved for dealing with acute infection and for maintenance of a sterile urine after surgery, in the hope of preventing recurrence or minimizing stone growth. Urine cultures and culture of stone fragments removed at surgery should guide the choice of antibiotic. Methenamine mandelate, which lowers urine pH and liberates formaldehyde, can be used for chronic suppression of infection when a stone is present. For patients who are not candidates for surgical removal of stone, acetohydroxamic acid, an inhibitor of urease, can be used. Though effective in treating the stones, acetohydroxamic acid has many side effects, such as headache, tremor, and thrombophlebitis, which limits its use. Lowering urine pH with chronic administration of NH_4Cl may retard stone growth but also may raise urine calcium level and promote the formation of calcium oxalate stones.

BIBLIOGRAPHY

BORGHI L et al: Urinary volume, water and recurrences in idiopathic calcium nephrolithiasis: A 5 year randomized prospective study. J Urol 155:839, 1996

BRUNO M, MARANGELLA M: Cystinuria: Recent advances in pathophysiology and genetics. Contrib Nephrol 122:173, 1997

COE FL, PARKS JH: New insights into the pathophysiology of and treatment of nephrolithiasis: New research venues. J Bone Miner Res 12:522, 1997

CONSENSUS CONFERENCE: Prevention and treatment of kidney stones. JAMA 260:977, 1988

CURHAN GC et al: Comparison of dietary calcium with supplemental calcium and other nutrients as factors affecting the risk of kidney stones in women. Ann Intern Med 126:497, 1997

HEILBERG IP: Update on dietary recommendations and medical treatment of renal stone disease. Nephrol Dial Transplant 15:117, 2000

KRAMER G et al: Role of bacteria in the development of kidney stones. Curr Opin Urol 10:35, 2000

RODMAN JS: Struvite stones. Nephron 81(Suppl 1):50, 1999

SEGURA JW et al: Ureteral Stones Clinical Guidelines Panel summary report on the management of ureteral calculi. J Urol 158:1915, 1997

280   *Walter E. Stamm*

URINARY TRACT INFECTIONS AND PYELONEPHRITIS

DEFINITIONS Acute infections of the urinary tract can be subdivided into two general anatomic categories: lower tract infection (urethritis and cystitis) and upper tract infection (acute pyelonephritis, prostatitis, and intrarenal and perinephric abscesses). Infections at these various sites may occur together or independently and may either be asymptomatic or present as one of the clinical syndromes described below. Infections of the urethra and bladder are often considered superficial (or mucosal) infections, while prostatitis, pyelonephritis, and renal suppuration signify tissue invasion.

From a microbiologic perspective, urinary tract infection (UTI) exists when pathogenic microorganisms are detected in the urine, urethra, bladder, kidney, or prostate. In most instances, growth of more than 10^5 organisms per milliliter from a properly collected midstream "clean-catch" urine sample indicates infection. However, significant bacteriuria is lacking in some cases of true UTI. Especially in symptomatic patients, a smaller number of bacteria (10^2 to 10^4/mL) may signify infection. In urine specimens obtained by suprapubic aspiration or "in-and-out" catheterization and in samples from a patient with an indwelling catheter, colony counts of 10^2 to 10^4/mL generally indicate infection. Conversely, colony counts of $>10^5$/mL of midstream urine are occasionally due to specimen contamination, which is especially likely when multiple species are found.

Infections that recur after antibiotic therapy can be due to the persistence of the originally infecting strain (as judged by species, antibiogram, serotype, and molecular type) or to reinfection with a new strain. "Same-strain" recurrent infections that become evident within 2 weeks of cessation of therapy can be the result of unresolved renal or prostatic infection (termed *relapse*) or of persistent vaginal or intestinal colonization leading to rapid reinfection of the bladder.

Symptoms of dysuria, urgency, and frequency that are unaccompanied by significant bacteriuria have been termed the *acute urethral syndrome*. Although widely used, this term lacks anatomic precision because many cases so designated are actually bladder infections. Moreover, since the causative agent can usually be identified in these patients, the term *syndrome*—implying unknown causation—is inappropriate.

Chronic pyelonephritis refers to chronic interstitial nephritis believed to result from bacterial infection of the kidney (Chap. 277). Many noninfectious diseases also cause an interstitial nephritis that is indistinguishable pathologically from chronic pyelonephritis.

ACUTE UTIs: URETHRITIS, CYSTITIS, AND PYELONEPHRITIS

EPIDEMIOLOGY Epidemiologically, UTIs are subdivided into catheter-associated (or nosocomial) infections and non-catheter-associated (or community-acquired) infections. Infections in either category may be symptomatic or asymptomatic. Acute community-acquired infections are very common and account for more than 7 million office visits annually in the United States. These infections occur in 1 to 3% of schoolgirls and then increase markedly in incidence with the onset of sexual activity in adolescence. The vast majority of acute symptomatic infections involve young women; a prospective study demonstrated an annual incidence of 0.5 to 0.7 infections per patient-year in this group. Acute symptomatic UTIs are unusual in men under the age of 50. The development of asymptomatic bacteriuria parallels that of symptomatic infection and is rare among men under 50 but common among women between 20 and 50. Asymptomatic bacteriuria is more common among elderly men and women, with rates as high as 40 to 50% in some studies.

ETIOLOGY Many different microorganisms can infect the urinary tract, but by far the most common agents are the gram-negative bacilli. *Escherichia coli* causes approximately 80% of acute infections in patients without catheters, urologic abnormalities, or calculi. Other gram-negative rods, especially *Proteus* and *Klebsiella* and occasionally *Enterobacter*, account for a smaller proportion of uncomplicated infections. These organisms, plus *Serratia* and *Pseudomonas*, assume increasing importance in recurrent infections and in infections associated with urologic manipulation, calculi, or obstruction. They play a major role in nosocomial, catheter-associated infections (see below). *Proteus* spp., by virtue of urease production, and *Klebsiella* spp., through the production of extracellular slime and polysaccharides, predispose to stone formation and are isolated more frequently from patients with calculi.

Gram-positive cocci play a lesser role in UTIs. However, *Staphylococcus saprophyticus*—a novobiocin-resistant, coagulase-negative species—accounts for 10 to 15% of acute symptomatic UTIs in young females. Enterococci occasionally cause acute uncomplicated cystitis in women. More commonly, enterococci and *Staphylococcus aureus* cause infections in patients with renal stones or previous instrumentation or surgery. Isolation of *S. aureus* from the urine should arouse suspicion of bacteremic infection of the kidney.

About one-third of women with dysuria and frequency have either an insignificant number of bacteria in midstream urine cultures or completely sterile cultures and have been previously defined as having the urethral syndrome. About three-quarters of these women have pyuria, while one-quarter have no pyuria and little objective evidence of infection. In the women with pyuria, two groups of pathogens account for most infections. Low quantities (10^2 to 10^4 bacteria per milliliter) of typical bacterial uropathogens such as *E. coli*, *S. saprophyticus*, *Klebsiella*, or *Proteus* are found in midstream urine specimens from most of these women. These bacteria are probably the causative agents in these infections because they can usually be isolated from a suprapubic aspirate, are associated with pyuria, and respond to appropriate antimicrobial therapy. In other women with acute urinary symptoms, pyuria, and urine that is sterile (even when obtained by suprapubic aspiration), sexually transmitted urethritis-producing agents such as *Chlamydia trachomatis*, *Neisseria gonorrhoeae*, and herpes simplex virus are etiologically important. These agents are found most frequently in young, sexually active women with new sexual partners.

The causative role of nonbacterial pathogens in UTIs remains poorly defined. *Ureaplasma urealyticum* has frequently been isolated from the urethra and urine of patients with acute dysuria and frequency but is also found in specimens from many patients without urinary symptoms. Ureaplasmas probably account for some cases of urethritis and cystitis. *U. urealyticum* and *Mycoplasma hominis* have been isolated from prostatic and renal tissues of patients with acute prostatitis and pyelonephritis, respectively, and are probably responsible for some of these infections as well. Adenoviruses cause acute hemorrhagic cystitis in children and in some young adults, often in epidemics. Although other viruses can be isolated from urine (e.g., cytomegalovirus), they are thought not to cause UTI. Colonization of the urine of catheterized or diabetic patients by *Candida* and other fungal species is common and sometimes progresses to symptomatic invasive

PATHOGENESIS AND SOURCES OF INFECTION   The urinary tract should be viewed as a single anatomic unit that is united by a continuous column of urine extending from the urethra to the kidney. In the vast majority of UTIs, bacteria gain access to the bladder via the urethra. Ascent of bacteria from the bladder may follow and is probably the pathway for most renal parenchymal infections.

The vaginal introitus and distal urethra are normally colonized by diphtheroids, streptococcal species, lactobacilli, and staphylococcal species but not by the enteric gram-negative bacilli that commonly cause UTIs. In females prone to the development of cystitis, however, enteric gram-negative organisms residing in the bowel colonize the introitus, the periurethral skin, and the distal urethra before and during episodes of bacteriuria. The factors that predispose to periurethral colonization with gram-negative bacilli remain poorly understood, but alteration of the normal vaginal flora by antibiotics, other genital infections, or contraceptives (especially spermicide) appears to play an important role. Loss of the normally dominant H_2O_2-producing lactobacilli in the vaginal flora appears to facilitate colonization by *E. coli*. Small numbers of periurethral bacteria probably gain entry to the bladder frequently, a process that is facilitated in some cases by urethral massage during intercourse. Whether bladder infection ensues depends on interacting effects of the pathogenicity of the strain, the inoculum size, and the local and systemic host defense mechanisms.

Under normal circumstances, bacteria placed in the bladder are rapidly cleared, partly through the flushing and dilutional effects of voiding but also as a result of the antibacterial properties of urine and the bladder mucosa. Owing mostly to a high urea concentration and high osmolarity, the bladder urine of many normal persons inhibits or kills bacteria. Prostatic secretions possess antibacterial properties as well. Polymorphonuclear leukocytes enter the bladder epithelium and the urine soon after infection arises and play a role in clearing bacteriuria. The role of locally produced antibody remains unclear.

Hematogenous pyelonephritis occurs most often in debilitated patients who are either chronically ill or receiving immunosuppressive therapy. Metastatic staphylococcal or candidal infections of the kidney may follow bacteremia or fungemia, spreading from distant foci of infection in the bone, skin, vasculature, or elsewhere.

CONDITIONS AFFECTING PATHOGENESIS   **Gender and Sexual Activity**   The female urethra appears to be particularly prone to colonization with colonic gram-negative bacilli because of its proximity to the anus, its short length (about 4 cm), and its termination beneath the labia. Sexual intercourse causes the introduction of bacteria into the bladder and is temporally associated with the onset of cystitis; it thus appears to be important in the pathogenesis of UTIs in younger women. Voiding after intercourse reduces the risk of cystitis, probably because it promotes the clearance of bacteria introduced during intercourse. In addition, use of spermicidal compounds with a diaphragm or cervical cap or of spermicide-coated condoms dramatically alters the normal introital bacterial flora and has been associated with marked increases in vaginal colonization with *E. coli* and in the risk of UTI.

In males who are <50 years old and who have no history of heterosexual or homosexual rectal intercourse, UTI is exceedingly uncommon, and this diagnosis should be questioned in the absence of clear documentation. An important factor predisposing to bacteriuria in men is urethral obstruction due to prostatic hypertrophy. Homosexuality is also associated with an increased risk of cystitis in men, probably related to rectal intercourse. Men (and women) who are infected with HIV and who have CD4+ T cell counts of <200/μL are at increased risk of both bacteriuria and symptomatic UTI. Finally, lack of circumcision has been identified as a risk factor for UTI in both neonates and young men.

Pregnancy   UTIs are detected in 2 to 8% of pregnant women. Symptomatic upper tract infections, in particular, are unusually common during pregnancy; fully 20 to 30% of pregnant women with asymptomatic bacteriuria subsequently develop pyelonephritis. This predisposition to upper tract infection during pregnancy results from decreased ureteral tone, decreased ureteral peristalsis, and temporary incompetence of the vesicoureteral valves. Bladder catheterization during or after delivery causes additional infections. Increased incidences of low-birth-weight infants, premature delivery, and newborn mortality result from UTIs during pregnancy, particularly those infections involving the upper tract.

Obstruction   Any impediment to the free flow of urine—tumor, stricture, stone, or prostatic hypertrophy—results in hydronephrosis and a greatly increased frequency of UTI. Infection superimposed on urinary tract obstruction may lead to rapid destruction of renal tissue. It is of utmost importance, therefore, when infection is present, to identify and repair obstructive lesions. On the other hand, when an obstruction is minor and is not progressive or associated with infection, great caution should be exercised in attempting surgical correction. The introduction of infection in such cases may be more damaging than an uncorrected minor obstruction that does not significantly impair renal function.

Neurogenic Bladder Dysfunction   Interference with the nerve supply to the bladder, as in spinal cord injury, tabes dorsalis, multiple sclerosis, diabetes, and other diseases, may be associated with UTI. The infection may be initiated by the use of catheters for bladder drainage and is favored by the prolonged stasis of urine in the bladder. An additional factor often operative in these cases is bone demineralization due to immobilization, which causes hypercalciuria, calculus formation, and obstructive uropathy.

Vesicoureteral Reflux   Defined as reflux of urine from the bladder cavity up into the ureters and sometimes into the renal pelvis, vesicoureteral reflux occurs during voiding or with elevation of pressure in the bladder. In practice, this condition is demonstrated by the finding of retrograde movement of radiopaque or radioactive material during a voiding cystourethrogram. An anatomically impaired vesicoureteral junction facilitates reflux of bacteria and thus upper tract infection. However, since a fluid connection between the bladder and the kidney always exists, even in the normal urinary system, some retrograde movement of bacteria probably takes place during infection but is not detected by radiologic techniques.

Vesicoureteral reflux is common among children with anatomic abnormalities of the urinary tract as well as among children with anatomically normal but infected urinary tracts. In the latter group, reflux disappears with advancing age and is probably attributable to factors other than UTI. Long-term follow-up of children with UTI who have reflux has established that renal damage correlates with marked reflux, not with infection.

The routine search for reflux would be aided by the development of noninvasive tests applicable to young children, in whom the need for an effective technique is greatest. In the meantime, it appears reasonable to search for reflux in anyone with unexplained failure of renal growth or with renal scarring, because UTI per se is an insufficient explanation for these abnormalities. On the other hand, it is doubtful that all children who have recurrent UTIs but whose urinary tract appears normal on pyelography should be subjected to voiding cystoureterography merely for the detection of the rare patient with marked reflux not revealed by the intravenous pyelogram.

Bacterial Virulence Factors   Not all strains of *E. coli* are equally capable of infecting the intact urinary tract. Bacterial virulence factors markedly influence the likelihood that a given strain, once introduced into the bladder, will cause UTI. Most *E. coli* strains that cause symptomatic UTIs in noncatheterized patients belong to a small number of specific O, K, and H serogroups. These uropathogenic clones have accumulated a number of virulence genes that are often closely linked on the bacterial chromosome in "virulence islands." Adherence of bacteria to uroepithelial cells is a critical first step in the initiation of infection. For both *E. coli* and *Proteus*, fimbriae (hairlike proteinaceous surface appendages) mediate the attachment of bacteria to specific receptors on epithelial cells. The attachment of bacteria to uroepithelial cells initiates a number of important events in the mucosal epithelial cell, including secretion of interleukin (IL) 6 and IL-8 and induction of both apoptosis and epithelial cell desquamation. Besides fimbriae, uropathogenic *E. coli* strains usually produce hemolysin and aerobactin (a siderophore for scavenging iron) and are resistant to the bactericidal action of human serum. Nearly all *E. coli* strains causing acute pyelonephritis and most of those causing acute cystitis are uropathogenic. In contrast, infections in patients with structural or functional abnormalities of the urinary tract are generally caused by bacterial strains that lack these uropathogenic properties; the implication is that these properties are not needed for infection of the compromised urinary tract.

Genetic Factors   Increasing evidence suggests that host genetic factors influence susceptibility to UTI. A maternal history of UTI is more often found among women who have experienced recurrent UTIs than among controls. The number and type of receptors on uroepithelial cells to which bacteria may attach are at least in part genetically determined. Many of these structures are components of blood group antigens and are present on both erythrocytes and uroepithelial cells. For example, P fimbriae mediate attachment of *E. coli* to P-positive erythrocytes and are found on nearly all strains causing acute uncomplicated pyelonephritis. Conversely, P blood group–negative individuals, who lack these receptors, have a decreased likelihood of pyelonephritis. It has also been demonstrated that nonsecretors of blood group antigens are at increased risk of recurrent UTI; this predisposition may relate to a different profile of genetically determined glycolipids on uroepithelial cells.

LOCALIZATION OF INFECTION   Unfortunately, currently available methods of distinguishing renal parenchymal infection from cystitis are neither reliable nor convenient enough for routine clinical use. Fever or an elevated level of C-reactive protein often accompanies acute pyelonephritis and is found in rare cases of cystitis but may also occur in infections other than pyelonephritis.

CLINICAL PRESENTATION   Cystitis   Patients with cystitis usually report dysuria, frequency, urgency, and suprapubic pain. The urine often becomes grossly cloudy and malodorous, and it is bloody in about 30% of cases. White cells and bacteria can be detected by examination of unspun urine in most cases. However, some women with cystitis have only 10^2 to 10^4 bacteria per milliliter of urine, and in these instances bacteria cannot be seen in a Gram-stained preparation of unspun urine. Physical examination generally reveals only tenderness of the urethra or the suprapubic area. If a genital lesion or a vaginal discharge is evident, especially in conjunction with fewer than 10^5 bacteria per milliliter on urine culture, then pathogens that may cause urethritis, vaginitis, or cervicitis, such as *C. trachomatis, N. gonorrhoeae, Trichomonas, Candida,* and herpes simplex virus, should be considered. Prominent systemic manifestations such as a temperature of >38.3°C (>101°F), nausea, and vomiting usually indicate concomitant renal infection, as does costovertebral angle tenderness. However, the absence of these findings does not ensure that infection is limited to the bladder and urethra.

Acute Pyelonephritis   Symptoms of acute pyelonephritis generally develop rapidly over a few hours or a day and include a fever, shaking chills, nausea, vomiting, and diarrhea. Symptoms of cystitis may or may not be present. Besides fever, tachycardia, and generalized muscle tenderness, physical examination reveals marked tenderness on deep pressure in one or both costovertebral angles or on deep abdominal palpation. In some patients, signs and symptoms of gram-negative sepsis predominate. Most patients have significant leukocytosis and bacteria detectable in Gram-stained unspun urine. Leukocyte casts are present in the urine of some patients, and the detection of these casts is pathognomonic. Hematuria may be demonstrated during the acute phase of the disease; if it persists after acute manifestations of infection have subsided, a stone, a tumor, or tuberculosis should be considered.

Except in individuals with papillary necrosis, abscess formation,

or urinary obstruction, the manifestations of acute pyelonephritis usually respond to therapy within 48 to 72 h. However, despite the absence of symptoms, bacteriuria or pyuria may persist. In severe pyelonephritis, fever subsides more slowly and may not disappear for several days, even after appropriate antibiotic treatment has been instituted.

Urethritis   Approximately 30% of women with acute dysuria, frequency, and pyuria have midstream urine cultures that show either no growth or insignificant bacterial growth. Clinically, these women cannot always be readily distinguished from those with cystitis. In this situation, a distinction should be made between women infected with sexually transmitted pathogens, such as *C. trachomatis, N. gonorrhoeae,* or herpes simplex virus, and those with low-count *E. coli* or staphylococcal infection of the urethra and bladder. Chlamydial or gonococcal infection should be suspected in women with a gradual onset of illness, no hematuria, no suprapubic pain, and >7 days of symptoms. The additional history of a recent sex-partner change, especially if the patient's partner has recently had chlamydial or gonococcal urethritis, should heighten the suspicion of a sexually transmitted infection, as should the finding of mucopurulent cervicitis (Chaps. 132 and 133). Gross hematuria, suprapubic pain, an abrupt onset of illness, a duration of illness of <3 days, and a history of UTIs favor the diagnosis of *E. coli* UTI.

Catheter-Associated UTIs   (See also Chap. 135)   Bacteriuria develops in at least 10 to 15% of hospitalized patients with indwelling urethral catheters. The risk of infection is about 3 to 5% per day of catheterization. *E. coli, Proteus, Pseudomonas, Klebsiella, Serratia,* staphylococci, enterococci, and *Candida* usually cause these infections. Many infecting strains display markedly greater antimicrobial resistance than organisms that cause community-acquired UTIs. Factors associated with an increased risk of catheter-associated UTI include female sex, prolonged catheterization, severe underlying illness, disconnection of the catheter and drainage tube, other types of faulty catheter care, and lack of systemic antimicrobial therapy.

Infection occurs when bacteria reach the bladder by one of two routes: by migrating through the column of urine in the catheter lumen (intraluminal route) or by moving up the mucous sheath outside the catheter (periurethral route). Hospital-acquired pathogens reach the patient's catheter or urine-collecting system on the hands of hospital personnel, in contaminated solutions or irrigants, and via contaminated instruments or disinfectants. Bacteria usually enter the catheter system at the catheter–collecting tube junction or at the drainage bag portal. The organisms then ascend intraluminally into the bladder within 24 to 72 h. Alternatively, the patient's own bowel flora may colonize the perineal skin and periurethral area and reach the bladder via the external surface of the catheter. This route is particularly common in women. Studies have demonstrated the importance of the attachment and growth of bacteria on the surfaces of the catheter in the pathogenesis of catheter-associated UTI. Such bacteria growing in biofilms on the catheter eventually produce encrustations consisting of bacteria, bacterial glycocalyces, host urinary proteins, and urinary salts. These encrustations provide a refuge for bacteria and may protect them from antimicrobial agents and phagocytes.

Clinically, most catheter-associated infections cause minimal symptoms and no fever and often resolve after withdrawal of the catheter. The frequency of upper tract infection associated with catheter-induced bacteriuria is unknown. Gram-negative bacteremia, which follows catheter-associated bacteriuria in 1 to 2% of cases, is the most significant recognized complication of catheter-induced UTIs. The catheterized urinary tract has repeatedly been demonstrated to be the most common source of gram-negative bacteremia in hospitalized patients, generally accounting for about 30% of cases.

Catheter-associated UTIs can sometimes be prevented in patients catheterized for <2 weeks by use of a sterile closed collecting system, by attention to aseptic technique during insertion and care of the catheter, and by measures to minimize cross-infection. Other preventive approaches, including short courses of systemic antimicrobial therapy, topical application of periurethral antimicrobial ointments, use of preconnected catheter–drainage tube units, use of catheters impregnated with antimicrobial agents, and addition of antimicrobial drugs to the drainage bag, have all been protective in at least one controlled trial but are not recommended for general use. Despite precautions, the majority of patients catheterized for >2 weeks eventually develop bacteriuria. The need for treatment as well as the optimal type and duration of treatment for such patients with asymptomatic bacteriuria have not been established. Removal of the catheter in conjunction with a short course of antibiotics to which the organism is susceptible probably constitutes the best course of action and nearly always eradicates bacteriuria. Treatment of asymptomatic catheter-associated bacteriuria may be of greatest benefit to elderly women, who most often develop symptoms if left untreated. If the catheter cannot be removed, antibiotic therapy usually proves to be unsuccessful and may in fact result in infection with a more resistant strain. In this situation, the bacteriuria should be ignored unless the patient develops symptoms or is at high risk of developing bacteremia. In these cases, use of systemic antibiotics or urinary bladder antiseptics may reduce the degree of bacteriuria and the likelihood of bacteremia. Because of spinal cord injury, incontinence, or other factors, some patients in hospitals or nursing homes require long-term or semipermanent bladder catheterization. Measures intended to prevent infection have been largely unsuccessful, and essentially all such chronically catheterized patients develop bacteriuria. If feasible, intermittent catheterization by a nurse or by the patient appears to reduce the incidence of bacteriuria and associated complications in such patients. Treatment should be provided when symptomatic infections arise, but treatment of asymptomatic bacteriuria in such patients has no apparent benefit.

DIAGNOSTIC TESTING Determination of the number and type of bacteria in the urine is an extremely important diagnostic procedure. In symptomatic patients, bacteria are usually present in the urine in large numbers ($\geq 10^5$/mL). In asymptomatic patients, two consecutive urine specimens should be examined bacteriologically before therapy is instituted, and $\geq 10^5$ bacteria of a single species per milliliter should be demonstrable in both specimens. Since the large number of bacteria in the bladder urine is due in part to bacterial multiplication during residence in the bladder cavity, samples of urine from the ureters or renal pelvis may contain $<10^5$ bacteria per milliliter and yet indicate infection. Similarly, the presence of bacteriuria of any degree in suprapubic aspirates or of $\geq 10^2$ bacteria per milliliter of urine obtained by catheterization usually indicates infection. In some circumstances (antibiotic treatment, high urea concentration, high osmolarity, low pH), urine inhibits bacterial multiplication, resulting in relatively low bacterial colony counts despite infection. For this reason, antiseptic solutions should not be used in washing the periurethral area before collection of the urine specimen. Water diuresis or recent voiding also reduces bacterial counts in urine.

Rapid methods of detection of bacteriuria have been developed as alternatives to standard culture methods. These methods detect bacterial growth by photometry, bioluminescence, or other means and provide results rapidly, usually in 1 to 2 h. Compared with urine cultures, these techniques generally exhibit a sensitivity of 95 to 98% and a negative predictive value of >99% when bacteriuria is defined as 10^5 colony-forming units per milliliter. However, the sensitivity of these tests falls to 60 to 80% when 10^2 to 10^4 colony-forming units per milliliter is the standard of comparison.

Microscopy of urine from symptomatic patients can be of great diagnostic value. Microscopic bacteriuria, which is best assessed with Gram-stained uncentrifuged urine, is found in more than 90% of specimens from patients whose infections are associated with colony counts of at least 10^5/mL, and this finding is very specific. However, bacteria cannot usually be detected microscopically in infections with lower colony counts (10^2 to 10^4/mL). The detection of bacteria by urinary microscopy thus constitutes firm evidence of infection, but the absence of microscopically detectable bacteria does not exclude the diagnosis. When carefully sought by means of chamber-count microscopy, pyuria is a highly sensitive indicator of UTI in symptomatic patients. Pyuria is demonstrated in nearly all acute bacterial UTIs, and its absence calls the diagnosis into question. The leukocyte esterase "dipstick" method is less sensitive than microscopy in identifying pyuria but is a useful alternative where microscopy is not feasible. Pyuria in the absence of bacteriuria (sterile pyuria) may indicate infection with unusual bacterial agents such as *C. trachomatis*, *U. urealyticum*, and *Mycobacterium tuberculosis* or with fungi. Alternatively, sterile pyuria may be demonstrated in noninfectious urologic conditions such as calculi, anatomic abnormality, nephrocalcinosis, vesicoureteral reflux, interstitial nephritis, or polycystic disease.

Although many authorities have recommended that urine culture and antimicrobial susceptibility testing be performed for any patient with a suspected UTI, it may be more practical and cost-effective to manage women who have symptoms characteristic of acute uncomplicated cystitis without an initial urine culture. Two approaches to presumptive therapy have generally been used. In the first, treatment is initiated solely on the basis of a typical history and/or typical findings on physical examination. In the second, women with symptoms and signs of acute cystitis and without complicating factors are managed with urinary microscopy (or, alternatively, with a leukocyte esterase test). A positive result for pyuria and/or bacteriuria provides enough evidence of infection to indicate that urine culture and susceptibility testing can be omitted and the patient treated empirically. Urine should be cultured, however, when a woman's symptoms and urine-examination findings leave the diagnosis of cystitis in question. Pretherapy cultures and susceptibility testing are also essential in the management of all patients with suspected upper tract infections and of those with complicating factors, as in these situations any of a variety of pathogens may be involved and antibiotic therapy is best tailored to the individual organism.

TREATMENT The following principles underlie the treatment of UTIs:

1. Except in acute uncomplicated cystitis in women, a quantitative urine culture, a Gram stain, or an alternative rapid diagnostic test should be performed to confirm infection before treatment is begun. When culture results become available, antimicrobial sensitivity testing should be used to direct therapy.
2. Factors predisposing to infection, such as obstruction and calculi, should be identified and corrected if possible.
3. Relief of clinical symptoms does not always indicate bacteriologic cure.
4. Each course of treatment should be classified after its completion as a failure (symptoms and/or bacteriuria not eradicated during therapy or in the immediate posttreatment culture) or a cure (resolution of symptoms and elimination of bacteriuria). Recurrent infections should be classified as same-strain or different-strain and as early (occurring within 2 weeks of the end of therapy) or late.
5. In general, uncomplicated infections confined to the lower urinary tract respond to short courses of therapy, while upper tract infections require longer treatment. After therapy, early recurrences due to the same strain may result from an unresolved upper tract focus of infection but often (especially after short-course therapy for cystitis) result from persistent vaginal colonization. Recurrences >2 weeks after the cessation of therapy nearly always represent reinfection with a new strain or with the previously infecting strain that has persisted in the vaginal and rectal flora.
6. Despite increasing resistance, community-acquired infections, especially initial infections, are usually due to more antibiotic-sensitive strains.
7. In patients with repeated infections, instrumentation, or recent hospitalization, the presence of antibiotic-resistant strains should be suspected.

The anatomic location of a UTI greatly influences the success or failure of a therapeutic regimen. Bladder bacteriuria (cystitis) can usually be eliminated with nearly any antimicrobial agent to which the infecting strain is sensitive; in the past, it was demonstrated that as little as a single dose of 500 mg of intramuscular kanamycin eliminated bladder bacteriuria in most cases. With upper tract infections, however, single-dose therapy fails in the majority of cases, and even a 7-day course is unsuccessful in many instances. Longer periods of treatment (2 to 6 weeks) aimed at eradicating a persistent focus of infection may be necessary in some cases.

In *acute uncomplicated cystitis*, more than 90 to 95% of infections are due to one of two organisms: *E. coli* or *S. saprophyticus*. Although resistance patterns vary geographically and resistance has increased in many areas, most strains are sensitive to many antibiotics. In most parts of the United States, more than one-quarter of *E. coli* strains causing acute cystitis are resistant to amoxicillin, sulfa drugs, and cephalexin, and resistance to trimethoprim (TMP) and trimethoprim-sulfamethoxazole (TMP-SMZ) is now approaching these levels as well.

Many have advocated single-dose treatment for acute cystitis. The advantages of single-dose therapy include less expense, ensured compliance, fewer side effects, and perhaps less intense pressure favoring the selection of resistant organisms in the intestinal, vaginal, or perineal flora. However, more frequent recurrences develop shortly after single-dose therapy than after 3-day treatment, and single-dose therapy does not eradicate vaginal colonization with *E. coli* as effectively as do longer regimens. A 3-day course of therapy with TMP-SMZ, TMP, norfloxacin, ciprofloxacin, or ofloxacin appears to preserve the low rate of side effects of single-dose therapy while improving efficacy (Table 280-1); thus 3-day regimens are currently preferred for acute cystitis. Neither single-dose nor 3-day therapy should be used for women with symptoms or signs of pyelonephritis, urologic abnormalities or stones, or previous infections due to antibiotic-resistant

organisms. Males with UTI often have urologic abnormalities or prostatic involvement and hence are not candidates for single-dose or 3-day therapy. For empirical therapy, they should generally receive a 7- to 14-day course of a fluoroquinolone (Table 280-1).

The choice of treatment for women with acute urethritis depends on the etiologic agent involved. In chlamydial infection, azithromycin (1 g in a single oral dose) or doxycycline (100 mg orally bid for 7 days) should be used. Women with acute dysuria and frequency, negative urine cultures, and no pyuria usually do not respond to antimicrobial agents.

In women, *acute uncomplicated pyelonephritis* without accompanying clinical evidence of calculi or urologic disease is due to *E. coli* in most cases. Although the optimal route and duration of therapy have not been established, a 7- to 14-day course of a fluoroquinolone, an aminoglycoside, or a third-generation cephalosporin is usually adequate. Neither ampicillin nor TMP-SMZ should be used as initial therapy because >25% of strains of *E. coli* causing pyelonephritis are now resistant to these drugs in vitro. For at least the first few days of treatment, antibiotics should probably be given intravenously to most patients, but patients with mild symptoms can be treated for 7 to 14 days with an oral antibiotic (usually ciprofloxacin or ofloxacin), with or without an initial single parenteral dose (Table 280-1). Patients who fail to respond to treatment within 72 h or who relapse after therapy should be evaluated for unrecognized suppurative foci, calculi, or urologic disease.

Complicated UTIs (those arising in a setting of catheterization, instrumentation, urologic anatomic or functional abnormalities, stones, obstruction, immunosuppression, renal disease, or diabetes) are typically due to hospital-acquired bacteria, including *E. coli*, *Klebsiella*, *Proteus*, *Serratia*, *Pseudomonas*, enterococci, and staphylococci. Many of the infecting strains are antibiotic-resistant. Empirical antibiotic therapy ideally provides broad-spectrum coverage against these

Table 280-1   Treatment Regimens for Bacterial Urinary Tract Infections

Condition	Characteristic Pathogens	Mitigating Circumstances	Recommended Empirical Treatment[a]
Acute uncomplicated cystitis in women	*Escherichia coli, Staphylococcus saprophyticus, Proteus mirabilis, Klebsiella pneumoniae*	None	3-Day regimens: oral TMP-SMZ, TMP, quinolone; 7-day regimen: macrocrystalline nitrofurantoin[b]
		Diabetes, symptoms for >7 d, recent UTI, use of diaphragm, age >65 years	Consider 7-day regimen: oral TMP-SMZ, TMP, quinolone[b]
		Pregnancy	Consider 7-day regimen: oral amoxicillin, macrocrystalline nitrofurantoin, cefpodoxime proxetil, or TMP-SMZ[b]
Acute uncomplicated pyelonephritis in women	*E. coli, P. mirabilis, S. saprophyticus*	Mild to moderate illness, no nausea or vomiting; outpatient therapy	Oral[c] quinolone for 7–14 d (initial dose given IV if desired); or single-dose ceftriaxone[d] or gentamicin[d] IV followed by oral TMP-SMZ[b] for 14 d
		Severe illness or possible urosepsis: hospitalization required	Parenteral[d] ceftriaxone, quinolone, gentamicin (± ampicillin), or aztreonam until defervescence; then oral[c] quinolone, cephalosporin, or TMP-SMZ for 14 d
Complicated UTI in men and women	*E. coli, Proteus, Klebsiella, Pseudomonas, Serratia*, enterococci, staphylococci	Mild to moderate illness, no nausea or vomiting: outpatient therapy	Oral[c] quinolone for 10–14 d
		Severe illness or possible urosepsis: hospitalization required	Parenteral[d] ampicillin and gentamicin, quinolone, ceftriaxone, aztreonam, ticarcillin/clavulanate, or imipenem-cilastatin until defervescence; then oral[c] quinolone or TMP-SMZ for 10–21 d

[a] Treatments listed are those to be prescribed before the etiologic agent is known; Gram's staining can be helpful in the selection of empirical therapy. Such therapy can be modified once the infecting agent has been identified. Fluoroquinolones should not be used in pregnancy. TMP-SMZ, although not approved for use in pregnancy, has been widely used. Gentamicin should be used with caution in pregnancy because of its possible toxicity to eighth-nerve development in the fetus.

[b] Multiday oral regimens for cystitis are as follows: TMP-SMZ, 160/800 mg q12h; TMP, 100 mg q12h; norfloxacin, 400 mg q12h; ciprofloxacin, 250 mg q12h; ofloxacin, 200 mg q12h; lomefloxacin, 400 mg/d; enoxacin, 400 mg q12h; macrocrystalline nitrofurantoin, 100 mg qid; amoxicillin, 250 mg q8h; cefpodoxime proxetil, 100 mg q12h.

[c] Oral regimens for pyelonephritis and complicated UTI are as follows: TMP-SMZ, 160/800 mg q12h; ciprofloxacin, 500 mg q12h; ofloxacin, 200–300 mg q12h; lomefloxacin, 400 mg/d; enoxacin, 400 mg q12h; amoxicillin, 500 mg q8h; cefpodoxime proxetil, 200 mg q12h.

[d] Parenteral regimens are as follows: ciprofloxacin, 200–400 mg q12h; ofloxacin, 200–400 mg q12h; gentamicin, 1 mg/kg q8h; ceftriaxone, 1–2 g/d; ampicillin, 1 g q6h; imipenem-cilastatin, 250–500 mg q6-8h; ticarcillin/clavulanate, 3.2 g q8h; aztreonam, 1 g q8–12h.

NOTE: UTI, urinary tract infection; TMP, trimethoprim; TMP-SMZ, trimethoprim-sulfamethoxazole.

pathogens. In patients with minimal or mild symptoms, oral therapy with a fluoroquinolone, such as ciprofloxacin or ofloxacin, can be administered until culture results and antibiotic sensitivities are known. In patients with more severe illness, including acute pyelonephritis or suspected urosepsis, hospitalization and parenteral therapy should be undertaken. Commonly used empirical regimens include imipenem alone, a penicillin or cephalosporin plus an aminoglycoside, and (when the involvement of enterococci is unlikely) ceftriaxone or ceftazidime. When information on the antimicrobial sensitivity pattern of the infecting strain becomes available, a more specific antimicrobial regimen can be selected. Therapy should generally be administered for 10 to 21 days, with the exact duration depending on the severity of the infection and the susceptibility of the infecting strain. Follow-up cultures 2 to 4 weeks after cessation of therapy should be performed to demonstrate cure.

In *pregnancy*, acute cystitis can be managed with 7 days of treatment with amoxicillin, nitrofurantoin, or a cephalosporin. All pregnant women should be screened for asymptomatic bacteriuria during the first trimester and, if bacteriuric, should be treated with one of the regimens listed in Table 280-1. After treatment, a culture should be performed to ensure cure, and cultures should be repeated monthly thereafter until delivery. Acute pyelonephritis in pregnancy should be managed with hospitalization and parenteral antibiotic therapy, generally with a cephalosporin or an extended-spectrum penicillin. Continuous low-dose prophylaxis with nitrofurantoin should be given to women who have recurrent infections during pregnancy.

Asymptomatic bacteriuria is common, especially among elderly patients, but has not been linked to adverse outcomes in most circumstances other than pregnancy (see above). Thus antimicrobial therapy is unnecessary and may in fact promote the emergence of resistant strains in most patients with asymptomatic bacteriuria. High-risk patients with neutropenia, renal transplants, obstruction, or other complicating conditions may require treatment when asymptomatic bacteriuria occurs. Seven days of therapy with an oral agent to which the organism is sensitive should be given initially. If bacteriuria persists, it can be monitored without further treatment in most patients. Longer-term therapy (4 to 6 weeks) may be necessary in high-risk patients with persistent asymptomatic bacteriuria.

UROLOGIC EVALUATION Very few women with recurrent UTIs have correctable lesions discovered at cystoscopy or upon intravenous pyelography, and these procedures should not be undertaken routinely in such cases. Urologic evaluation should be performed in selected instances—namely, in women with relapsing infection, a history of childhood infections, stones or painless hematuria, or recurrent pyelonephritis. Most males with UTI should be considered to have complicated infection and thus should be evaluated urologically. Possible exceptions include young men who have cystitis associated with sexual activity, who are uncircumcised, or who have AIDS. Men or women presenting with acute infection and signs or symptoms suggestive of an obstruction or stones should undergo prompt urologic evaluation, generally by means of ultrasound.

PROGNOSIS In patients with uncomplicated cystitis or pyelonephritis, treatment ordinarily results in complete resolution of symptoms. Lower tract infections in women are of concern mainly because they cause discomfort, morbidity, loss of time from work, and substantial health-care costs. Cystitis may also result in upper tract infection or in bacteremia (especially during instrumentation), but little evidence suggests that renal impairment follows. When repeated episodes of cystitis occur, they are nearly always reinfections, not relapses.

Acute uncomplicated pyelonephritis in adults rarely progresses to renal functional impairment and chronic renal disease. Repeated upper tract infections often represent relapse rather than reinfection, and a vigorous search for renal calculi or an underlying urologic abnormality should be undertaken. If neither is found, 6 weeks of chemotherapy may be useful in eradicating an unresolved focus of infection.

Repeated symptomatic UTIs in children and in adults with obstruc-tive uropathy, neurogenic bladder, structural renal disease, or diabetes progress to chronic renal disease with unusual frequency. Asymptomatic bacteriuria in these groups as well as in adults without urologic disease or obstruction predisposes to increased numbers of episodes of symptomatic infection but does not result in renal impairment in most instances.

PREVENTION Women who experience frequent symptomatic UTIs (≥3 per year on average) are candidates for long-term administration of low-dose antibiotics directed at preventing recurrences. Such women should be advised to avoid spermicide use and to void soon after intercourse. Daily or thrice-weekly administration of a single dose of TMP-SMZ (80/400 mg), TMP alone (100 mg), or nitrofurantoin (50 mg) has been particularly effective. Norfloxacin and other fluoroquinolones have also been used for prophylaxis. Prophylaxis should be initiated only after bacteriuria has been eradicated with a full-dose treatment regimen. The same prophylactic regimens can be used after sexual intercourse to prevent episodes of symptomatic infection in women in whom UTIs are temporally related to intercourse. Other patients for whom prophylaxis appears to have some merit include men with chronic prostatitis; patients undergoing prostatectomy, both during the operation and in the postoperative period; and pregnant women with asymptomatic bacteriuria. All pregnant women should be screened for bacteriuria in the first trimester and should be treated if bacteriuria is demonstrated.

PAPILLARY NECROSIS

When infection of the renal pyramids develops in association with vascular diseases of the kidney or with urinary tract obstruction, renal papillary necrosis is likely to result. Patients with diabetes, sickle cell disease, chronic alcoholism, and vascular disease seem peculiarly susceptible to this complication. Hematuria, pain in the flank or abdomen, and chills and fever are the most common presenting symptoms. Acute renal failure with oliguria or anuria sometimes develops. Rarely, sloughing of a pyramid may take place without symptoms in a patient with chronic UTI, and the diagnosis is made when the necrotic tissue is passed in the urine or identified as a "ring shadow" on pyelography. If renal function deteriorates suddenly in a diabetic individual or a patient with chronic obstruction, the diagnosis of renal papillary necrosis should be entertained, even in the absence of fever or pain. Renal papillary necrosis is often bilateral; when it is unilateral, however, nephrectomy may be a life-saving approach to the management of overwhelming infection.

EMPHYSEMATOUS PYELONEPHRITIS AND CYSTITIS

These unusual clinical entities almost always occur in diabetic patients, often in concert with urinary obstruction and chronic infection. Emphysematous pyelonephritis is usually characterized by a rapidly progressive clinical course, with high fever, leukocytosis, renal parenchymal necrosis, and accumulation of fermentative gases in the kidney and perinephric tissues. Most patients also have pyuria and glucosuria. *E. coli* causes most cases, but occasionally other Enterobacteriaceae are isolated. Gas in tissues can often be seen on plain films and can best be confirmed and localized by computed tomography. Surgical resection of the involved tissue in addition to systemic antimicrobial therapy is usually needed to prevent mortality in emphysematous pyelonephritis.

Emphysematous cystitis also occurs primarily in diabetic patients, usually in association with *E. coli* or other facultative gram-negative rods and often in relation to bladder outlet obstruction. Patients with this condition are generally less severely ill and have less rapidly progressive disease than those with emphysematous pyelonephritis. The patient typically reports abdominal pain, dysuria, frequency, and (in some cases) pneumaturia. Computed tomography shows gas within both the bladder lumen and the bladder wall. Generally, conservative therapy with systemic antimicrobial agents and relief of outlet obstruction are effective, but some patients do not respond to these measures and require cystectomy.

RENAL AND PERINEPHRIC ABSCESS

See Chap. 130.

PROSTATITIS

The term *prostatitis* has been used for various inflammatory conditions affecting the prostate, including acute and chronic infections with specific bacteria and, more commonly, instances in which signs and symptoms of prostatic inflammation are present but no specific organisms can be detected. Patients with acute bacterial prostatitis can usually be identified on the basis of typical symptoms and signs, pyuria, and bacteriuria. To classify a patient with suspected chronic prostatitis correctly, first-void and midstream urine specimens, a prostatic expressate, and a postmassage urine specimen should be quantitatively cultured and evaluated for numbers of leukocytes. On the basis of the results of these studies, patients can be classified as having chronic bacterial prostatitis, chronic nonbacterial prostatitis, or prostatodynia. Patients with suspected chronic prostatitis usually have low back pain, perineal or testicular discomfort, mild dysuria, and lower urinary obstructive symptoms. Microscopic pyuria may be the only objective manifestation of prostatic disease.

ACUTE BACTERIAL PROSTATITIS When it occurs spontaneously, this disease generally affects young men; however, it may also be associated with an indwelling urethral catheter. It is characterized by fever, chills, dysuria, and a tense or boggy, extremely tender prostate. Although prostatic massage usually produces purulent secretions with a large number of bacteria on culture, bacteremia may result from manipulation of the inflamed gland. For this reason and because the etiologic agent can usually be identified by Gram's staining and culture of urine, vigorous prostatic massage should be avoided. In non-catheter-associated cases, the infection is generally due to common gram-negative urinary tract pathogens (*E. coli* or *Klebsiella*). Initially, an intravenous fluoroquinolone, third-generation cephalosporin, or aminoglycoside can be administered if gram-negative rods are visible in urine, and a cephalosporin or nafcillin can be given if gram-positive cocci are detected. Although many of these drugs do not readily diffuse into the noninflamed prostate gland, the response to antibiotics in acute bacterial prostatitis is usually prompt, perhaps because drugs penetrate more readily into the acutely inflamed prostate. In catheter-associated cases, the spectrum of etiologic agents is broader, including hospital-acquired gram-negative rods and enterococci. The urinary Gram stain may be particularly helpful in such cases. Imipenem, an aminoglycoside, a fluoroquinolone, or a third-generation cephalosporin should be used for initial therapy until the organism has been isolated and its susceptibilities have been determined. The long-term prognosis is good, although in some instances acute infection may result in abscess formation, epididymoorchitis, seminal vesiculitis, septicemia, and residual chronic bacterial prostatitis. Since the advent of antibiotics, the frequency of acute bacterial prostatitis has diminished markedly. In many instances, infections diagnosed as acute prostatitis are probably cases of posterior urethritis.

CHRONIC BACTERIAL PROSTATITIS This entity is now infrequent but should be considered in men with a history of recurrent bacteriuria. Symptoms are often lacking between episodes, and the prostate usually feels normal on palpation. Obstructive symptoms or perineal pain develops in some patients. Intermittently, infection spreads to the bladder, producing frequency, urgency, and dysuria. A pattern of relapsing infection in a middle-aged man strongly suggests chronic bacterial prostatitis. Classically, the diagnosis is established by culture of *E. coli*, *Klebsiella*, *Proteus*, or other uropathogenic

bacteria from the expressed prostatic secretion or postmassage urine in higher quantities than are found in first-void or midstream urine. Antibiotics promptly relieve the symptoms associated with acute exacerbations but have been less effective in eradicating the focus of chronic infection in the prostate. The relative ineffectiveness of antimicrobial agents for long-term cure results in part from the poor penetration of the prostate by most of these drugs; the low pH that prevails in this organ precludes the passage of most agents. Fluoroquinolones, including ciprofloxacin and ofloxacin, have been considerably more successful than other antimicrobials, but they must generally be given for at least 12 weeks to be effective. Patients with frequent episodes of acute cystitis in whom attempts at curative therapy fail can be managed with prolonged courses of antimicrobials (usually a sulfonamide, TMP, or nitrofurantoin), with a view toward suppressing symptoms and keeping the bladder urine sterile. Total prostatectomy obviously results in the cure of chronic prostatitis but is associated with considerable morbidity. Transurethral prostatectomy is safer but cures only one-third of patients.

NONBACTERIAL PROSTATITIS Patients who present with symptoms and signs of prostatitis, increased numbers of leukocytes in expressed prostatic secretion and postmassage urine, no bacterial growth in cultures, and no history of recurrent episodes of bacterial prostatitis are classified as having nonbacterial prostatitis. Prostatic inflammation can be considered present when the expressed prostatic secretion and postmassage urine contain at least tenfold more leukocytes than the first-void and midstream urine specimens or when the expressed prostatic secretion contains ≥1000 leukocytes per microliter.

The presumably infectious etiology of this condition remains unidentified. Evidence for a causative role of both *U. urealyticum* and *C. trachomatis* has been presented but is not conclusive. Since most cases of nonbacterial prostatitis occur in young, sexually active men and since many cases follow an episode of nonspecific urethritis, the causative agent may well be sexually transmitted. The effectiveness of antimicrobial agents in this condition remains uncertain. Some patients benefit from a 4- to 6-week course of treatment with erythromycin, doxycycline, TMP-SMZ, or a fluoroquinolone, but controlled trials are lacking.

PROSTATODYNIA Patients who have symptoms and signs of prostatitis but who have no evidence of prostatic inflammation (normal leukocyte counts) and negative urine cultures are classified as having prostatodynia. Despite their symptoms, these patients most likely do not have prostatic infection and should not be given antimicrobial agents.

BIBLIOGRAPHY

AGACE W et al: Host resistance to urinary tract infection, in *Molecular Pathogenesis and Clinical Management*, HLT Mobley, JW Warren (eds). Washington, DC, ASM Press, 1996, pp 221–245

EISENSTADT J, WASHINGTON JA: Diagnostic microbiology for bacteria and yeasts causing urinary tract infections, in *Molecular Pathogenesis and Clinical Management*, HLT Mobley, JW Warren (eds). Washington, DC, ASM Press, 1996, pp 29–67

GRATACOS E et al: Screening and treatment of asymptomatic bacteriuria in pregnancy prevent pyelonephritis. J Infect Dis 169:1390, 1994

GUPTA K et al: Increasing prevalence of antimicrobial resistance among uropathogens causing acute uncomplicated cystitis in women. JAMA 281:736, 1999

HOOTON TM, STAMM WE: Diagnosis and treatment of uncomplicated urinary tract infection. Infect Dis Clin North Am 11:551, 1997

——— et al: Randomized comparative trial and cost analysis of 3-day antimicrobial regimens for treatment of acute cystitis in women. JAMA 273:41, 1995

——— et al: A prospective study of risk factors for symptomatic urinary tract infection in young women. N Engl J Med 335:468, 1996

JOHNSON JR: Treatment and prevention of urinary tract infections, in *Urinary Tract Infections: Molecular Pathogenesis and Clinical Management*, HLT Mobley, JW Warren (eds). Washington, DC, ASM Press, 1996, pp 95–118

SCHAEFFER AJ: Urinary tract infection in men—state of the art. Infection (Suppl 1):S19, 1994

STAMM WE, HOOTON TM: Catheter-associated urinary tract infections: Epidemiology, pathogenesis, prevention. Am J Med 91(Suppl 3B):655, 1991

———, ———: Management of urinary tract infections in adults. N Engl J Med 329:1328, 1993

WARREN JW et al: Guidelines for antimicrobial therapy of uncomplicated acute bacterial cystitis and acute pyelonephritis in women. Clin Infect Dis 29:745, 1999

URINARY TRACT OBSTRUCTION

Obstruction to the flow of urine, with attendant stasis and elevation in urinary tract pressure, impairs renal and urinary conduit functions and is a common cause of acute and chronic renal failure. With early relief of obstruction, the defects in function usually disappear completely. However, chronic obstruction may produce permanent loss of renal mass (renal atrophy) and excretory capability, as well as enhanced susceptibility to local infection and stone formation. Early diagnosis and prompt therapy are therefore essential to minimize the otherwise devastating effects of obstruction on kidney structure and function.

ETIOLOGY Obstruction to urine flow can result from *intrinsic* or *extrinsic mechanical blockade* as well as from *functional defects* not associated with fixed occlusion of the urinary drainage system. Mechanical obstruction can occur at any level of the urinary tract, from the renal calyces to the external urethral meatus. Normal points of narrowing, such as the ureteropelvic and ureterovesical junctions, bladder neck, and urethral meatus, are common sites of obstruction. When blockage is above the level of the bladder, unilateral dilatation of the ureter (*hydroureter*) and renal pyelocalyceal system (*hydronephrosis*) occur; lesions at or below the level of the bladder cause bilateral involvement.

Common forms of obstruction are listed in Table 281-1. In childhood, *congenital malformations*, including marked narrowing of the ureteropelvic junction, anomalous (retrocaval) location of the ureter, and posterior urethral valves, predominate. The latter defect is the most common cause of bilateral hydronephrosis in boys. Children may also have bladder dysfunction secondary to congenital urethral stricture, urethral meatal stenosis, or bladder neck obstruction. In adults, urinary tract obstruction is due mainly to *acquired defects*. Pelvic tumors, calculi, and urethral stricture predominate. Ligation of, or injury to, the ureter during pelvic or colonic surgery can lead to hydronephrosis which, if unilateral, may remain relatively silent and undetected. *Schistosoma haematobium* and genitourinary tuberculosis are infectious causes of ureteral obstruction. Obstructive uropathy may also result from extrinsic neoplastic (carcinoma of cervix or colon, retroperitoneal lymphoma) or inflammatory disorders. One such inflammatory disorder is retroperitoneal fibrosis, a process of unknown cause seen most commonly in middle-aged men, which occasionally leads to bilateral ureteral obstruction. Retroperitoneal fibrosis must be distinguished from other retroperitoneal causes of ureteral obstruction, particularly lymphomas and pelvic neoplasms.

Functional impairment of urine flow usually results from disorders that involve both the ureter and bladder. Common functional lesions include neurogenic bladder, often with adynamic ureter, and vesicoureteral reflux. Reflux of urine from bladder to ureter(s) is more common in children than in adults and may result in severe unilateral or bilateral hydroureter and hydronephrosis. Abnormal insertion of the ureter into the bladder is the most common cause of vesicoureteral reflux in children. Reflux in the absence of urinary tract infection or bladder neck obstruction usually does not lead to renal parenchymal damage and often resolves spontaneously as the child matures. Surgical reinsertion of the ureter into the bladder is indicated if reflux is severe and unlikely to improve spontaneously, if renal function deteriorates, or

if urinary tract infections recur despite chronic antimicrobial therapy. Hydronephrosis, usually more marked on the right than on the left, is common in pregnancy, due both to ureteral compression by the enlarged uterus and to functional effects of progesterone.

CLINICAL FEATURES The pathophysiology and clinical features of urinary tract obstruction are summarized in Table 281-2. *Pain* is the symptom that most commonly provokes the need for medical attention. The pain of urinary tract obstruction is due to distention of the collecting system or renal capsule. The severity of the pain is influenced more by the rate at which distention develops than by the degree of distention. Acute supravesical obstruction, as from a stone lodged in a ureter (Chap. 279), is associated with excruciatingly severe pain, usually called *renal colic*. This pain is relatively steady and continuous, with little fluctuation in intensity, and often radiates to the lower abdomen, testes, or labia. By contrast, more insidious causes of obstruction, such as chronic narrowing of the ureteropelvic junction, may produce little or no pain yet result in total destruction of the affected kidney. Flank pain that occurs only with micturition is pathognomonic of vesicoureteral reflux.

Azotemia develops in urinary tract obstruction when overall excretory function is impaired. This may occur in the setting of bladder outlet obstruction, bilateral renal pelvic or ureteric obstruction, or unilateral disease in a patient with a solitary functioning kidney. Complete bilateral obstruction should be suspected when acute renal failure is accompanied by anuria. Any patient with renal failure otherwise unexplained or with a history of nephrolithiasis, hematuria, diabetes mellitus, prostatic enlargement, pelvic surgery, trauma, or tumor should be evaluated for urinary tract obstruction.

In the acute setting, bilateral obstruction may result in sodium and water retention that may mimic prerenal azotemia. However, with more prolonged obstruction, symptoms of *polyuria* and *nocturia* commonly accompany partial urinary tract obstruction and result from impaired renal concentrating ability. This defect usually does not improve with administration of vasopressin and is therefore a form of acquired nephrogenic diabetes insipidus. Disturbances in sodium chloride transport in the ascending limb of Henle and, in azotemic patients, the

Table 281-1 Common Mechanical Causes of Urinary Tract Obstruction

Ureter	Bladder Outlet	Urethra
CONGENITAL		
Ureteropelvic junction narrowing or obstruction	Bladder neck obstruction	Posterior urethral valves
	Ureterocele	Anterior urethral valves
Ureterovesical junction narrowing or obstruction		Stricture
		Meatal stenosis
Ureterocele		Phimosis
Retrocaval ureter		
ACQUIRED INTRINSIC DEFECTS		
Calculi	Benign prostatic hyperplasia	Stricture
Inflammation	Cancer of prostate	Tumor
Trauma	Cancer of bladder	Calculi
Sloughed papillae	Calculi	Trauma
Tumor	Diabetic neuropathy	Phimosis
Blood clots	Spinal cord disease	
Uric acid crystals	Anticholinergic drugs and α-adrenergic antagonists	
ACQUIRED EXTRINSIC DEFECTS		
Pregnant uterus	Carcinoma of cervix, colon	Trauma
Retroperitoneal fibrosis	Trauma	
Aortic aneurysm		
Uterine leiomyomata		
Carcinoma of uterus, prostate, bladder, colon, rectum		
Lymphoma, pelvic inflammatory disease		
Accidental surgical ligation		

Table 281-2 Pathophysiology of Bilateral Ureteral Obstruction

Hemodynamic Effects	Tubule Effects	Clinical Features
ACUTE		
↑ Renal blood flow	↑ Ureteral and tubule pressures	Pain (capsule distention)
↓ GFR	↑ Reabsorption of Na⁺, urea, water	Azotemia
↓ Medullary blood flow		Oliguria or anuria
↑ Vasodilator prostaglandins		
CHRONIC		
↓ Renal blood flow	↓ Medullary osmolarity	Azotemia
↓ ↓ GFR	↓ Concentrating ability	Hypertension
↑ Vasoconstrictor prostaglandins	Structural damage; parenchymal atrophy	ADH-insensitive polyuria
↑ Renin-angiotensin production	↓ Transport functions for Na⁺, K⁺, H⁺	Natriuresis
		Hyperkalemic, hyperchloremic acidosis
RELEASE OF OBSTRUCTION		
Slow ↑ in GFR (variable)	↓ Tubule pressure	Postobstructive diuresis
	↑ Solute load per nephron (urea, NaCl)	Potential for volume depletion and electrolyte imbalance due to losses of Na⁺, K⁺, PO₄²⁻, Mg²⁺, and water
	Natriuretic factors present	

NOTE: GFR, glomerular filtration rate.

osmotic (urea) diuresis per nephron lead to decreased medullary hypertonicity and hence a concentrating defect. Partial obstruction, therefore, may be associated with increased rather than decreased urine output. Indeed, wide fluctuations in urine output in a patient with azotemia should always raise the possibility of intermittent or partial urinary tract obstruction. If fluid intake is inadequate, severe dehydration and hypernatremia may develop. Hesitancy and straining to initiate the urinary stream, postvoid dribbling, urinary frequency, and (overflow) incontinence are common with obstruction at or below the level of the bladder.

In addition to loss of urinary concentrating ability and azotemia, partial bilateral urinary tract obstruction often results in other derangements of renal function, including *acquired distal renal tubular acidosis*, *hyperkalemia*, and *renal salt wasting*. These defects in tubule function are often accompanied by renal tubulointerstitial damage. Morphologic abnormalities appear early in the course of obstruction; initially the interstitium becomes edematous and infiltrated with mononuclear inflammatory cells. With continued obstruction, the interstitium becomes fibrotic; scarring and atrophy of the papillae and medulla occur and precede these processes in the cortex.

The possibility of urinary tract obstruction must always be considered in patients with urinary tract infections or urolithiasis. Urinary stasis encourages the growth of organisms as well as the formation of crystals, especially magnesium ammonium phosphate (struvite). *Hypertension* is frequent in acute and subacute unilateral obstruction and is usually a consequence of increased release of renin by the involved kidney. Chronic unilateral or bilateral hydronephrosis, in the presence of extracellular volume expansion or other renal disease, may result in significant hypertension. *Erythrocytosis*, an infrequent complication of obstructive uropathy, is probably secondary to increased erythropoietin production by the obstructed kidney.

DIAGNOSIS A history of difficulty in voiding, pain, infection, or changes in urinary volume is common. Evidence for distention of the kidney or urinary bladder can often be obtained by palpation and percussion of the abdomen. A careful rectal examination may reveal enlargement or nodularity of the prostate, abnormal rectal sphincter tone, or a rectal or pelvic mass. The penis should be inspected for evidence of meatal stenosis or phimosis. In the female, vaginal, uterine, and rectal lesions responsible for urinary tract obstruction are usually revealed by inspection and palpation.

Urinalysis and examination of the urine sediment may reveal hematuria, pyuria, and bacteriuria. Often, however, the urine sediment is normal, even when obstruction leads to marked azotemia and extensive structural damage. An abdominal scout film should be obtained to

evaluate the possibility of nephrocalcinosis or a radiopaque stone at any level of the urinary collecting system. As indicated in Fig. 281-1, if urinary tract obstruction is suspected, a bladder catheter should be inserted. If diuresis does not follow, then abdominal ultrasonography should be performed to evaluate renal and bladder size, as well as pyelocalyceal contour. Ultrasonography is approximately 90% specific and sensitive for detection of hydronephrosis. False-positive results are associated with diuresis, renal cysts, or presence of an extrarenal pelvis, a normal congenital variant. Hydronephrosis may be absent on ultrasound when obstruction is associated with volume contraction, staghorn calculi, retroperitoneal fibrosis, or infiltrative renal disease.

In some cases, the intravenous urogram may define the site of obstruction. In the presence of obstruction, the appearance time of the nephrogram is often delayed. Eventually, however, the renal image becomes more dense than normal because of slow tubular fluid flow rate, which results in enhanced water reabsorption by the nephrons and greater concentration of contrast medium within tubules. The kidney involved by an acute obstructive process is usually slightly enlarged, and there is dilatation of the calyces, renal pelvis, and ureter above the obstruction. The ureter, however, is not tortuous, as is the case when the obstruction is chronic. In comparison with the nephrogram, the urogram may be extremely faint, especially if the dilated renal pelvis is voluminous, causing dilution of the contrast medium. The radiographic study

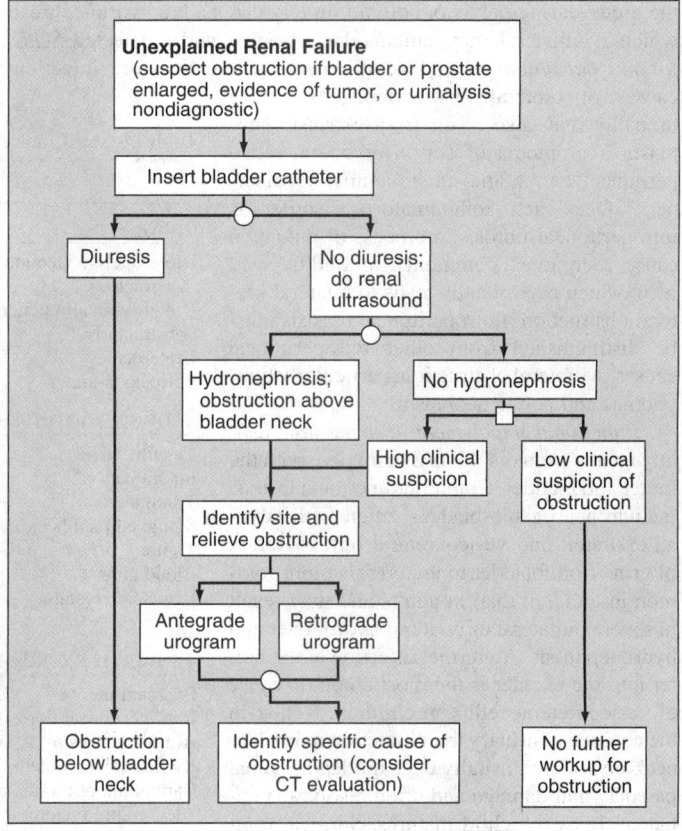

FIGURE 281-1 Diagnostic approach for urinary tract obstruction in unexplained renal failure. Circles represent diagnostic procedures, and squares indicate clinical decisions based on available data. CT, computed tomography.

should be continued until the site of obstruction is determined or the contrast medium is excreted. Radionuclide scans define less anatomic detail than intravenous urography and, like the urogram, are of limited value when renal function is poor. Nonetheless, such scans are sensitive for the detection of obstruction and provide a substitute test in some patients at high risk for reaction to intravenous contrast.

To facilitate visualization of a suspected lesion in a ureter or renal pelvis, *retrograde* or *antegrade urography* should be attempted. These diagnostic studies may be preferable to the intravenous urogram in the azotemic patient, in whom poor excretory function precludes adequate visualization of the collecting system. Furthermore, intravenous urography carries the risk of contrast-induced acute renal failure in patients with proteinuria, renal insufficiency, diabetes mellitus, or multiple myeloma, particularly when performed under conditions of dehydration. The retrograde approach involves catheterization of the involved ureter under cystoscopic control, while the antegrade technique necessitates placement of a catheter into the renal pelvis via a needle inserted percutaneously under ultrasonic or fluoroscopic guidance. While the antegrade approach carries the added advantage of providing immediate decompression of a unilateral obstructing lesion, many urologists initially attempt the retrograde approach and resort to the antegrade method only when attempts at retrograde catheterization are unsuccessful or when cystoscopy or general anesthesia is contraindicated.

Patients suspected of having intermittent ureteropelvic obstruction (whether functional or mechanical) should have radiologic evaluation while they are in pain, since a normal urogram is commonly seen during asymptomatic periods. Hydration often helps to provoke a symptomatic attack. Voiding cystourethrography is of great value in the diagnosis of vesicoureteral reflux and bladder neck and urethral obstructions. Patients with obstruction at or below the level of the bladder exhibit thickening, trabeculation, and diverticula of the bladder wall. Postvoiding films reveal residual urine. If these radiographic studies fail to provide adequate information for diagnosis, endoscopic visualization by the urologist often permits precise identification of lesions involving the urethra, prostate, bladder, and ureteral orifices.

Computed tomography is useful in the diagnosis of specific intraabdominal and retroperitoneal causes of obstruction but is less practical as an initial test to establish the presence of obstruction. Magnetic resonance imaging may also be useful in the identification of specific obstructive causes.

℞ **TREATMENT** An individual with any form of urinary tract obstruction complicated by infection requires relief of obstruction as soon as possible to prevent development of generalized sepsis and progressive renal damage. On a temporary basis, depending on the site of obstruction, drainage is often satisfactorily achieved by nephrostomy; ureterostomy; or ureteral, urethral, or suprapubic catheterization. The patient with acute urinary tract infection and obstruction should be given appropriate antibiotics based on in vitro bacterial sensitivity and ability of the drug to concentrate in the kidney and urine. Treatment may be required for 3 to 4 weeks. Chronic or recurrent infections in an obstructed kidney with poor intrinsic function may necessitate nephrectomy. When infection is not present, immediate surgery often is not required, even in the presence of complete obstruction and anuria (because of the availability of dialysis), at least until acid-base, fluid and electrolyte, and cardiovascular status are restored to normal. Nevertheless, the site of obstruction should be ascertained as soon as feasible, in part because of the possibility that sepsis may occur and necessitate prompt urologic intervention. Elective relief of obstruction is usually recommended in patients with urinary retention, recurrent urinary tract infections, persistent pain, or progressive loss of renal function. Infrequently, mechanical obstruction can be alleviated by nonsurgical means, as with radiation therapy for retroperitoneal lymphoma. Likewise, functional obstruction secondary to neu-

rogenic bladder may be decreased with the combination of frequent voiding and cholinergic drugs. →*The approach to obstruction secondary to renal stones is discussed in Chap. 279.*

PROGNOSIS With relief of obstruction, the prognosis regarding return of renal function depends largely on whether irreversible renal damage has occurred. When obstruction is not relieved, the course will depend mainly on whether the obstruction is complete or incomplete, bilateral or unilateral, and whether urinary tract infection is also present. Complete obstruction with infection can lead to total destruction of the kidney within days. In dogs, relief of complete obstruction of 1 and 2 weeks' duration restores glomerular filtration rate to 60 and 30% of normal, respectively; after 8 weeks of obstruction, recovery does not occur. Nevertheless, in the absence of definitive evidence of irreversibility, every effort should be made to decompress in the hope of restoring renal function at least partially. A renal radionuclide scan, performed after a prolonged period of decompression, may be used to predict reversible renal function.

POSTOBSTRUCTIVE DIURESIS Relief of bilateral, but not unilateral, complete urinary tract obstruction commonly leads to a postobstructive diuresis, characterized by polyuria, which may be massive. The urine is usually hypotonic and may contain large amounts of sodium chloride, potassium, and magnesium. The natriuresis is due, at least in part, to the excretion of retained urea, which acts as a poorly reabsorbable solute and diminishes salt and water reabsorption in the tubules (osmotic diuresis). The increase in intratubular pressure very likely also contributes to the impairment in net sodium chloride reabsorption, especially in the terminal nephron segments. Natriuretic factors (other than urea) may also accumulate during uremia induced by obstruction and depress salt and water reabsorption when urine flow is reestablished. In the majority of patients this diuresis is physiologic, resulting in the *appropriate* excretion of the excesses of salt and water retained during the period of obstruction. When extracellular volume and composition return to normal, the diuresis usually abates spontaneously. Therefore, replacement of urinary losses should serve only to prevent hypovolemia, hypotension, or disturbances in serum electrolyte concentrations. Occasionally, iatrogenic expansion of extracellular volume, secondary to administration of excessive quantities of intravenous fluids, is responsible for, or sustains, the diuresis observed in the postobstructive period. Replacement of no more than two-thirds of urinary volume losses per day is usually effective in avoiding this complication. The loss of electrolyte-free water with urea may result in hypernatremia. Serum and urine sodium and osmolal concentrations should guide the use of appropriate intravenous replacement. Often replacement with 0.45% saline is required. In a rare patient, relief of obstruction may be followed by urinary salt and water losses severe enough to provoke profound dehydration and vascular collapse. In these patients, an intrinsic defect in tubule reabsorptive function is probably responsible for the marked diuresis. Appropriate therapy in such patients includes intravenous administration of salt-containing solutions to replace sodium and volume deficits.

BIBLIOGRAPHY

CURHAN GC et al: Urinary tract obstruction, in *Brenner and Rector's The Kidney*, 6th ed, BM Brenner (ed). Philadelphia, Saunders, 2000, pp 1820–1843

GULMI FA et al: Pathophysiology of urinary tract obstruction, in *Campbell's Urology*, 7th ed, PC Walsh et al (eds). Philadelphia, Saunders, 1998, pp 342–385

KAYE AD, POLLACK HM: Diagnostic imaging approach to the patient with obstructive uropathy. Semin Nephrol 2:55, 1982

KLAHR S: Urinary tract obstruction, in *Diseases of the Kidney*, 6th ed, RW Schrier, CW Gottschalk (eds). Boston, Little, Brown, 1997, pp 709–738

WILSON DR: Renal function during and following obstruction. Annu Rev Med 28:329, 1977

NOBEL PRIZE IN PHYSIOLOGY OR MEDICINE, 1956

Werner Theodor Otto Forssmann was born August 29, 1904, in Berlin, Germany, the son of Julius and Emmy Forssmann. His father was an attorney who was killed in World War I in 1916. Forssmann received a broad liberal arts education early in life and then in 1922 entered Friedrich Wilhelm University in Berlin to study medicine. After graduation in 1929, he received further training by working with surgeons and urologists at several different hospitals. During that time he worked with Richard Schneider in Eberswalde, a small Prussian town north of Berlin. Forssmann had become fascinated with the results of earlier animal work and asked Schneider if he could perform cardiac catheterization in humans. Schneider forbade Forssmann from conducting such experiments either on patients or himself. Nevertheless, Forssmann decided to perform the heart experiment on himself. With local anesthesia, he inserted a needle in his left arm antecubital vein through which he inserted a catheter and then went to the x-ray room where he placed himself in front of the fluoroscope. Forssmann used a mirror and saw that the catheter was at the level of his humerus. Despite the urging to stop by a young colleague who had just entered the room, Forssmann advanced the catheter into the right side of the heart. He then documented his success by taking some x-rays. At first Schneider was furious but then congratulated Forssmann and urged him to publish his results immediately. This paper, entitled "Probing the Right Ventricle of the Heart," was published on November 5, 1929, in *Klinische Wochenschrift*.

To further his research, with the help of Schneider he obtained a position at the "Mecca of German Surgery" with Ferdinand Sauerbruch at Charité Hospital in Berlin. Immediately after publication of his article, Forssmann became a celebrity and was besieged by reporters. Although unfounded, Ernst Unger claimed priority on the basis of his intraarterial therapy. This controversy, combined with professional jealousy that described Forssmann's experiment as a "circus stunt," led Sauerbruch to dismiss him only 3 months after his arrival at Charité. Forssmann then returned to work with Schneider, who encouraged him to continue his work on cardiac catheterization in a systematic manner. He found better x-ray equipment, used contrast material, and worked on dogs that were kept in his mother's apartment. Forssmann also performed further cardiac catheterization experiments on himself, demonstrating the first use of contrast material in humans. Altogether, he performed nine cardiac catheterizations on himself. His contrast medium results were published in the *Münchner Medizinische Wochenschrift*.

Forssmann's experiments had long been forgotten in his own country when André Cournand and Dickinson Richards, over a decade later, began their development of cardiac catheterization at Columbia Physicians and Surgeons Medical School and Bellevue Hospital in New York. In their first journal article they recognized Forssmann's contributions to the development of cardiac catheterization. Unfortunately, because of the events of World War II, Forssmann was unable to participate in this further development of cardiac catheterization in New York City. Nevertheless, because of the courageous experiments on himself, Forssmann demonstrated the safety and potential of cardiac catheterization and contrast radiography and provided the foundation for modern cardiology.

André Frédéric Cournand was born in Paris, France, to Jules and Marguerite Weber Cournand on September 24, 1895. His father was a dentist and inventor who had twenty-five patents. Cournand's early education was at the Lycée Condorcet; he then obtained his baccalauréat at the Faculté des Lettres of the University of Sorbonne in 1913 and a diploma in physics, chemistry, and biology from the Faculté des Sciences in 1914. After his first year in medical school, he volunteered for the French Army and toward the end of World War I was wounded and gassed. He received the Croix de Guerre with three bronze stars. After

the war he completed his thesis and received his medical degree from the University of Paris in 1930. He then traveled to the United States with the intent to spend a year on the chest (tuberculosis) service at Bellevue Hospital in the Columbia University Division. He decided to stay in the United States when he was offered a chief residency and an opportunity to work with Dickinson Richards on the physiology and pathophysiology of respiration. Thus, Cournand and Richards commenced the collaborative research in 1932 that changed the future of cardiology.

Dickinson Woodruff Richards, Jr., was born on October 30, 1895, to Dickinson Woodruff and Sally Lambert Richards. After his early education at Hotchkiss School in Connecticut, where he studied the humanities, Richards entered Yale University and graduated in 1917. He then entered the United States Army as a lieutenant with an artillery unit. After the war, he attended medical school at the College of Physicians and Surgeons at Columbia University, followed, in 1923, by a residency in internal medicine at Presbyterian Hospital. During this time, Lawrence J. Henderson at Harvard University became his mentor, and they published three papers in the area of pulmonary and cardiovascular circulation. Following his residency, he had a fellowship at the National Institute of Medical Research in London from 1927 to 1928 under his other mentor, Henry Hollet Dale. Richards once said, "A man's mind and his actions are chiefly molded by a very few. For me, in the early years, there were Lawrence J. Henderson and Henry Hollet Dale." Richards returned from his fellowship in London and joined the faculty of the College of Physicians and Surgeons at Columbia University. His collaborative research with Cournand began in 1932. In his autobiography, Cournand wrote that "Modesty and greatness seldom harmonize in an individual," but cited Richards as ". . .one of those few in whom these apparently opposite qualities balanced one another."

Cournand and Richards considered themselves primarily as pulmonary rather than cardiac physiologists. They developed a series of pulmonary function tests that were then applied to patients with pulmonary tuberculosis, chronic emphysema, and lung fibrosis. After 4 years of experimental work with dogs and a chimpanzee, they undertook cardiac catheterization in humans in 1940—some 11 years after Forssmann's original publication.

They investigated systemic hypertension, heart failure, and acquired and congenital heart disease. Pulmonary heart disease was characterized as ". . .cardiac hypertrophy and dilatation secondary to disease of the lung." The research of Cournand and Richards was a brilliant demonstration of basic research translated to clinical medicine, including the diagnosis and treatment of disease. On the basis of their research, cardiac surgery for correction of congenital and acquired defects became possible.

REFERENCES

1. Magill FN (ed): *Nobel Prize Winners: Physiology or Medicine*, vol 2. Pasadena, Salem Press, 1993
2. Schrier RW: *A Salute to Nobel Laureates in Physiology and Medicine*, Proceedings of the Association of American Physicians 108(1): Jan 1996
3. Sourkes TL: *Nobel Prize Winners in Medicine and Physiology 1901–1965*. London: Abelard-Schuman, 1967

Robert W. Schrier, MD

PART ELEVEN

DISORDERS OF THE GASTROINTESTINAL SYSTEM

Section 1
DISORDERS OF THE ALIMENTARY TRACT

282 *Daniel K. Podolsky, Kurt J. Isselbacher*

APPROACH TO THE PATIENT WITH GASTROINTESTINAL DISEASE

BIOLOGIC CONSIDERATIONS The mucosal surface of the gastrointestinal (GI) tract is composed of a highly dynamic population of epithelial cells that are specialized for transmembrane absorption and secretion. These secretory and absorptive abilities facilitate digestion and nutrient uptake, which must be accomplished while keeping out potentially harmful pathogens and mutagens in the lumen. The barrier function is accomplished through both the physical integrity of the mucosal surface and the extensive population of resident immune cells.

The intestinal lymphoid system reflects a balance between dampening immune reactivity at the mucosal surface to prevent the constant and unrestrained activation of immune and inflammatory processes and immune response amplification in the underlying lamina propria and submucosa ready to respond when surface defenses have been breached. Derangements in the balance of suppression and stimulation predispose the GI tract to numerous inflammatory conditions.

The epithelial cells of the mucosal surface turn over very rapidly; the entire surface is regenerated every 24 to 72 h. This rapid turnover may permit rapid recovery of function following an acute insult and protect the cells against many mutagens in the lumen. Indeed, the small intestine rarely develops epithelial cancers. The slower turnover of colonic epithelium, the slower movement of the luminal contents, and differences in the mutagens in the luminal contents appear to foster colon cancers. Another fundamental feature of the GI mucosa is the spatial segregation of the proliferative compartment from the terminally differentiated cells, especially in the small intestine, where a gradient of differentiation exists from the depths of the crypts of Lieberkühn to the villus tip. This organization has a strong effect on the histology and pathophysiology of many mucosal disorders, such as celiac sprue.

Diseases of the GI tract produce clinical consequences through physical disruption of the mucosal layer (e.g., blood loss, fluid loss, pathogenic invasion) or nutritional derangements caused by impaired digestion and nutrient absorption. Focal or localized disease processes are more likely to disrupt mucosa; diffuse processes are more likely to alter absorption.

While the essential roles of the GI tract—the absorption of nutrients and the excretion of the products—are accomplished in large part at the luminal surface, GI function also depends on the coordinated propulsion of food through the lumen by smooth-muscle contraction. The local and distant neural and endocrine factors that contribute to the regulation of intestinal motility are complex. Disruption of normal motility is common, with alterations in frequency of bowel movements, abdominal distention, abdominal pain, and nausea, individually or in varying combinations (so-called functional bowel complaints), affecting as many as 15% of adults. Such symptoms may result from dysmotility related to the *direct* effects of an obstructing lesion or to the *indirect* actions of substances released by a primary mucosal disorder (e.g., inflammatory mediators such as arachidonic acid metabolites that also affect smooth-muscle activity).

The spectrum of diseases affecting the GI tract and their clinical manifestations are related to the component organ(s) involved (Table 282-1). Thus, esophageal disorders manifest themselves mainly through their effects on swallowing; gastric disorders are dominated by features relating to acid secretion; and diseases of the small and large intestine demonstrate disruption of nutrition and alterations of bowel movements. The GI tract may also be affected by systemic disorders, including vascular, inflammatory, infectious, and neoplastic conditions leading to focal or diffuse structural lesions. Metabolic and endocrine abnormalities as well as some drugs can disrupt normal bowel motility. When no structural lesion can be identified to explain GI symptoms, the disorder is termed *functional*. Table 282-2 summarizes criteria that may be used to distinguish functional from organic or structural diseases of the GI tract.

CLINICAL CONSIDERATIONS **History** A thorough clinical history is essential in directing the clinician's attention to appropriate diagnostic considerations in the patient with GI symptoms (Table 282-1). The most common complaints include pain and alterations in bowel habit, especially diarrhea or constipation. *Abdominal pain* is the most frequent and variable complaint and may reflect a broad spectrum of problems, from self-limited to urgent (Chap. 14). The intensity should be assessed and an initial distinction should be made between pain of acute onset and more chronic discomfort. Pain of abrupt onset more often reflects serious illness requiring urgent intervention, while a history of chronic discomfort is most often related to an indolent disorder. Dyspepsia, an ill-defined upper abdominal discomfort, is especially common and is often accompanied by varying degrees of nausea, bloating, and distention. Dyspepsia may be associated with peptic ulceration, but non-ulcer dyspepsia (NUD) is more common. A change in the pattern or character of pain may signify disease progression. Ascertaining the location of the pain (upper or lower, localized or diffuse), its character (sharp, burning, cramping), and its relationship to meals will often provide clues into the most important diagnostic considerations. Discomfort while the patient is eating suggests an esophageal disorder. Pain occurring shortly after the meal may signify biliary tract disease or abdominal angina; pain 30 to 90 min later is typical of peptic disease. Pain that is not affected by eating suggests a process outside of the bowel lumen, such as abscess, peritonitis, pancreatitis, and some malignancies. Conversely, factors that relieve the symptom are also helpful. For example, eating or antacid use typically relieves pain in peptic ulcer disease or gastritis. A relationship to bowel movement, especially together with an altered bowel habit, should focus attention on a disorder of the small or large bowel, such as inflammatory bowel disease.

Alterations in bowel habit can result from either disruption of normal intestinal motility or significant structural pathology. The temporal evolution of the change, the nature of the alteration, and the presence of other constitutional symptoms such as weight loss, fever, or anorexia are important. Temporary variation in bowel habit in association with some life stress and in the absence of signs of systemic illness suggests the common "irritable bowel syndrome," especially when the alteration varies between diarrhea and constipation. Small, pellet-like stools associated with symptoms of dyspepsia (bloating, nausea, and "gas") are common. This diagnosis can essentially be made on the basis of a thorough history and physical examination and very limited laboratory testing, to exclude structural disease.

Constipation is a common complaint and may reflect an obstructing process but is more often due to impaired motility; though often

Table 282-1   Overview of Approach to Patients with Common Gastrointestinal Disorders

Site of Disorder	Common Symptoms	Possible Physical Signs	Potential Procedures or Laboratory Studies
Esophagus	Dysphagia Odynophagia Heartburn, chest pain Hematemesis/melena		Esophagoscopy Barium swallow Manometry Bernstein test
Stomach	Nausea and vomiting Epigastric pain Hematemesis/melena Early satiety	Distention Tenderness Succussion splash Mass	Gastroscopy Upper GI x-ray series Nasogastric aspiration Gastric emptying
Small Intestine			
Duodenum	Pain Nausea/vomiting Hematemesis	Tenderness Altered bowel sounds Distention Mass	Duodenoscopy Small bowel follow-through, enteroclysis Kidney-ureter-bladder x-ray series D-Xylose absorption tests
Jejunum	Pain Diarrhea	Altered bowel sounds Distention Mass	CT Stool cultures, stool examination for ova and parasites Small bowel biopsy
Ileum	Pain Diarrhea	Altered bowel sounds Distention Mass	Colonoscopy
Colon	Diarrhea Pain Blood Constipation	Tenderness Mass Distention Altered bowel sounds	Sigmoidoscopy Colonoscopy Barium enema Stool culture, stool examination for ova and parasites *Clostridium difficile* toxin assay
Anus/Rectum	Pain Urgency Hematochezia Pruritus Constipation Incontinence Tenesmus	Tenderness Altered sphincter tone Perianal abnormality	Sigmoidoscopy Anoscopy Anorectal manometry
Nonspecific	Weight loss Fever Anorexia Nausea and vomiting		Complete blood count Erythrocyte sedimentation rate Fecal occult blood test

NOTE: GI, gastrointestinal; CT, computed tomography.

functional in nature, drugs (e.g., anticholinergics), neurologic processes (e.g., Hirschsprung's disease), or smooth-muscle diseases (e.g., scleroderma) may cause decreased motility. The history and physical examination may provide evidence of a more generalized disorder such as hypothyroidism or depression. Pain associated with constipation may suggest an anal or perianal process with stool retention. The his-

Table 282-2   Distinguishing between Functional and Organic/Structural Disease of Gastrointestinal Tract

	Functional	Organic	
		Neoplastic	Inflammatory
Symptoms			
Weight loss	None	Common	Sometimes
Diarrhea	Daytime only	Day ± night	Day and night
Blood loss	None	Frequent	Frequent
Fever	None	Rare	Frequent

Pain	Cramping, relieved by
	  defecation
		Minor to severe	May be localized;
			  may be severe

Bowel habit (diarrhea or
  constipation)
	Alternating diarrhea/con-
	  stipation
		Constipation (rarely
		  diarrhea)
			Diarrhea or normal

	Pellet-like stools	Change in caliber	
Laboratory tests			
Hematocrit	Normal	Often decreased	May be decreased
White blood cell count	Normal	Usually normal	Often elevated
Erythrocyte sedimenta- tion rate	Normal	Usually increased	Usually increased

tory may clarify that "constipation" actually reflects more an unrealized expectation of regularity than significant pathology. In contrast, progressively worsening constipation and weight loss in an adult with previously regular habits suggests the possible presence of an underlying obstructing process, particularly malignancy.

Although *diarrhea* refers to an increased frequency of movements, patients often use the term to describe loose or watery stools. If diarrhea is described, the daily average number of stools, their consistency, their pattern, and the presence of blood should be defined. The occurrence of nocturnal or true bloody diarrhea almost always reflects structural rather than functional bowel disease. A pungent stool odor or the presence of undigested meat in the movement is suggestive of pancreatic insufficiency. An alteration in color can be seen in cholestasis or steatorrhea (light-colored) or hemorrhage (melenic to maroon or bright red). Mucus in the movement is usually a sign of a functional bowel syndrome, while pus suggests infectious or inflammatory disease. Less common but more dramatic are the symptoms of acute GI bleeding, including hematemesis, melena, and hematochezia, which usually lead to prompt seeking of medical attention but should always be enquired after by the clinician.

In the evaluation of male patients, especially those with diarrhea or dysphagia, a tactful inquiry into sexual activity is essential. Homosexual males are at increased risk for a large variety of GI disorders as well as AIDS, which may first manifest itself with GI symptoms. AIDS patients are susceptible to a wide range of infections and neoplastic disorders of the GI tract, liver, and biliary tract (Chap. 308).

Finally, careful attention must be given to a general medical history with an emphasis on present or past use of medications or nonprescription drugs. Thyroid and other metabolic disorders, especially those affecting calcium metabolism, can cause a variety of GI symptoms. Unless asked, patients may forget to mention that they take aspirin almost daily for headache, and this may account for occult blood found in the stool. The use of daily laxatives may explain chronic diarrhea.

Physical Examination, Endoscopy, and Radiology   All of the cardinal methods of examination are helpful in evaluating the patient with GI symptoms (Table 282-1). *Inspection* may disclose signs of cholestasis or nutritional deficiencies. Examination of the abdomen for an abnormal contour or inspection of the perianal region may reveal signs of a mass or a draining fistula. *Auscultation* may elicit a succussion splash in patients with symptoms of gastric outlet obstruction. The absence of bowel sounds or an alteration in pitch can lead to recognition of an evolving ileus or an obstructing process. A bruit may be noted when symptoms of ischemic bowel disease are present. Careful *palpation* of the abdomen is especially important in detecting tenderness and masses, which can lead to the recognition of cholecystitis, Crohn's disease, periappendiceal abscess, and many other disorders. Findings on abdominal palpation will often be complemented by *percussion*, which is essential to assessing liver and spleen size.

Elicitation of *rebound tenderness*, either direct or referred, after abrupt removal of the examining hand provides an important clue to localized or more generalized peritonitis, which may suggest abdominal emergencies, such as a perforated viscus, intraabdominal abscess, or bowel infarction. Typically, the patient will remain immobile to avoid the accentuation of pain that may follow even slight movement or jarring of the abdomen. By contrast, patients with severe pain deriving from visceral disease, such as intestinal ischemia, are sometimes frantic to find a comfortable position. In these disorders, the absence of findings on palpation may be in striking contrast to the evident distress of the patient. Only when the process progresses to tissue destruction (e.g., intestinal infarction) and secondary peritonitis will the abdominal examination prove remarkable, often in concert with striking signs of systemic illness, including hemodynamic instability.

In addition to the examination of the abdomen, a digital rectal examination is also essential. In the patient with complaints of stool incontinence, the integrity of the sphincter can be assessed. Masses intrinsic to the rectum as well as abnormalities in the pelvis or the pouch of Douglas may only be detected by this examination. The presence of frank or occult blood in the stool is always important diagnostic information. Sigmoidoscopy should be viewed as a routine part of the physical examination in the patient with diarrhea, constipation, or frank or occult fecal blood. Sigmoidoscopy performed with either a rigid or a flexible fiberoptic instrument allows for direct inspection of the rectosigmoid mucosa, permitting the detection of cancers and polyps in this lower bowel segment that could be missed by barium x-rays. Inflammatory changes of the mucosa can help identify patients with infectious dysentery or other forms of colitis. Edema, granularity, diffuse friability (easily induced mucosal bleeding), and superficial ulcerations are characteristic of ulcerative colitis. Fresh stool samples for microbiologic studies and superficial mucosal biopsies obtained at the time of sigmoidoscopy can also yield crucial diagnostic information. The presence of polyps is an indication for colonoscopy (Chap. 283).

Many upper and lower GI tract disorders are accessible to inspection via fiberoptic instruments. As a result, endoscopy has supplanted conventional contrast x-ray studies for many clinical problems, both because of its heightened precision for diagnosis and the opportunity in many instances to accomplish meaningful therapeutic intervention. However, it should be emphasized that *no procedure should be considered routine* and used indiscriminately; there must be a rational basis for its use in the individual patient. These techniques are discussed in detail in Chap. 283. Upper GI endoscopy permits evaluation of the esophagus, stomach, duodenum, and, with specially designed instruments, proximal jejunum. Side-viewing scopes permit inspection and cannulation of the ampulla of Vater, facilitating retrograde cholangiopancreatography. Evaluation of some patients will be further benefited by endoscopic ultrasound (US), which can delineate submucosal mass lesions and abnormalities in the pancreas. The colonoscope can be used to visualize the entire colon and often the terminal ileum, resulting in more accurate diagnosis of inflammatory bowel disease and mass lesions. Colonic polyps can almost always be removed at the time of their initial identification.

Endoscopic techniques are relatively precise in defining many

problems, but the limitations of these tools, as well as the continued advantages of x-ray studies in some situations, should be recognized. Endoscopic tools are not useful in assessing GI motility, which may be assessed more accurately by barium studies. In addition, the small intestine remains largely inaccessible to fiberoptic instruments. In hospitals where endoscopy is not feasible, the upper GI series and barium enema remain good diagnostic modalities to evaluate the upper and lower GI tract, especially when air-contrast techniques are employed. However, they should generally be avoided in patients with GI bleeding or suspected bowel obstruction. In addition, the cathartics used to prepare the bowel may markedly worsen the condition of a patient with obstructing lesions or colitis.

Although endoscopy has obviated the need for many conventional GI x-rays, other radiologic imaging modalities, including US, computed tomography (CT), and magnetic resonance imaging (MRI), have assumed a larger role in patients with GI symptoms. Both US and CT are useful in the delineation of abdominal masses. CT, though more expensive, is often more effective in the evaluation of the lower abdomen, where inflammatory masses in patients with Crohn's disease or complications of diverticular disease may be accurately imaged. However, US is an effective and less expensive tool for the evaluation of the right upper quadrant, including the gall bladder and biliary tract. MRI may give exquisitely accurate information on the anatomic extent of invasive rectal cancers and blood flow in patients with vascular disorders, but the full range of its uses in GI disorders remains to be delineated. More sophisticated CT and MRI equipment can actually permit the performance of digital angiography without the invasive catheterization necessary in conventional visceral angiography. CT "virtual colonoscopy," a nonendoscopic method of visualizing the colon, is developing rapidly.

Radionuclide scans can be used to localize a site of bleeding in the GI tract. Radiolabeled technetium can detect a Meckel's diverticulum, which is an occasional source of bleeding.

DIAGNOSTIC APPROACHES (Table 282-1)   **Abdominal Pain** Determining the cause of abdominal pain is frequently a clinical challenge (Chap. 14). Differential diagnostic considerations may encompass diseases extrinsic to the GI tract, such as disorders of the genitourinary tract (e.g., pelvic inflammatory disease) and the peritoneum. The initial goal is to distinguish between an urgent problem and a nonacute disorder. Initial clinical impressions based on the history and physical examination can be further refined through routine laboratory tests such as a complete blood count and differential as well as plain films of the abdomen. Specific features will dictate the appropriateness of urgent US or CT examination or the need to proceed promptly with surgery. In the patient with a long-standing and relatively stable problem, diagnostic evaluation can be more deliberate. A functional basis for the complaint may be established on the strength of the history and physical examination alone. Radiologic contrast studies, other imaging modalities (e.g., US, CT), or endoscopic examination may be appropriate. If these approaches do not determine the cause of the patient's symptoms, more unusual causes of abdominal pain such as acute intermittent porphyria may have to be excluded through specific urine or blood tests (Chap. 346).

Problems of Swallowing Dysphagia nearly always signifies the presence of structural pathology. The approach should be as follows:

1. *Thorough determination of the nature of dysphagia.* Is the difficulty primarily in swallowing liquids, solids, or both? The location of the difficulty from the patient's perspective and presence or absence of accompanying *odynophagia* (pain on swallowing) are important to ascertain. These historic clues are complemented by careful visual and neurologic examination of the oropharynx.

2. *Routine esophageal x-rays* in the upright and lateral or Trendelenburg position. The horizontal views are essential for demonstration of the swallowing mechanism, unaided by gravity, and of the esophagogastric junction. For details of the pharyngoesophageal area, cineradiography is necessary because of the rapidity with which the

contrast medium passes through. Hiatus hernia is extremely common (in 15 to 35% of persons over 50) and is often asymptomatic. Careful attention is usually needed to detect lower esophageal rings or webs, which may be visible as indentations in the barium column only from a limited angle.

3. *Esophagoscopy.* This procedure is desirable to biopsy masses or abnormal mucosa and to obtain washings for exfoliative cytologic study. The diagnoses of peptic esophagitis and Barrett's esophagus are made endoscopically. Endoscopy is the most sensitive technique for identifying esophageal or gastric varices, although they are seldom important in the absence of hemorrhage. Endoscopic instruments with a US probe at the tip (endoscopic ultrasound) are useful diagnostic and staging tools for certain problems of the esophagus (and other sites of the GI tract).

4. *Manometric studies* of the upper esophagus, particularly in conjunction with cineradiography. This procedure offers the best means of differentiating among disorders originating in the central nervous system, primary pharyngeal muscular disease, and cricopharyngeal dystonia. Manometry of the lower esophagus is useful in the diagnosis of diffuse esophageal spasm, achalasia, and infiltrative diseases that alter esophageal motility.

5. *24-Hour monitoring of esophageal pH* may be used to document esophageal reflux.

Peptic or Digestive Disorders   The approaches to these disorders include the following:

1. *Insertion of a nasogastric tube.* This approach is used to establish whether significant gastric retention (more than 75 mL of gastric contents in the fasting state) exists and whether acid, bile, blood, or other materials are present. If pyloric obstruction or gastric atony is present, the tube is used to maintain suction while the patient's electrolyte and fluid balance is restored to normal; the stomach is kept as clean as possible so that diagnostic investigation may be carried out.

2. *Upper gastrointestinal endoscopy* (Chap. 283). This procedure is most helpful in assessing the mucosa in gastritis or, together with biopsy and brushings for cytology, in differentiating between peptic and neoplastic ulcerating lesions. It may identify a specific bleeding site in clinical situations where several potential bleeding sites could exist, as in the patient with portal hypertension. In addition, it may be possible to cauterize or otherwise intervene to control hemorrhage via the endoscope (e.g., by injections of vasoconstricting agents such as epinephrine). *Helicobacter pylori* is a frequent cause of gastritis in patients with peptic ulceration and non-ulcer dyspepsia. Although *H. pylori* infection can be confirmed by endoscopy and biopsy, the diagnosis is more commonly made by breath and serologic tests (Chap. 285). Endoscopy is the diagnostic method of choice in the setting of upper GI bleeding (Chap. 44). Endoscopy can detect a number of potential sources of upper GI bleeding that are often missed by x-ray studies (e.g., erosive gastritis, Mallory-Weiss tear). Gastroscopy is particularly helpful in inspecting the postoperative stomach, especially in detecting stomal ulceration or so-called alkaline reflux gastritis. The first and second portions of the duodenum can also be routinely examined, and important information about ulcers and other lesions can be obtained. Radiologic studies may be useful when endoscopy is not readily available or in the assessment of suspected motility disorders (e.g., gastroparesis). In addition, radiologic examination may be preferred when there are contraindications to safe endoscopy.

3. *Gastric acid secretory studies.* Although not routinely necessary, these studies are useful in the diagnosis of the Zollinger-Ellison syndrome or atrophic gastritis and for determination of completeness of vagotomy. They should not be performed for the routine diagnosis of uncomplicated duodenal ulcer or to influence the choice of surgery for peptic ulcer.

Obstructive and Vascular Disorders of the Small Intestine (See also Chaps. 289 and 290)   The plain x-ray film of the abdomen is the most important diagnostic adjunct to careful physical examination in patients with symptoms of obstruction. Patterns of dilation of individual loops of intestine may be characteristic, as in volvulus or acute pancreatitis; erect and decubitus views will often show fluid levels in the affected segments. Motility disorders of the small intestine (temporary ileus or chronic intestinal pseudoobstruction) may also present with obstructive symptoms and similar x-ray findings but must be managed medically without surgical intervention. Air under the diaphragm is diagnostic of a perforated viscus; air in the portal vein usually results from intestinal necrosis from mesenteric vascular occlusion. The diagnostic accuracy of the plain x-ray film in all types of intestinal obstruction is about 75%. In patients with symptoms of incomplete obstruction, the radiographic small-bowel series will often be diagnostic in defining the site and degree of obstruction. Infrequently, in this setting, all conventional x-ray studies are unremarkable. In such cases, the radiologist may perform a small-bowel enteroclysis study by passing a special tube into the proximal jejunum; the rapid instillation of barium through the tube will distend the intestine and often reveal subtle lesions missed by other tests.

Vascular diseases of the small intestine are among the most difficult diseases to diagnose. In chronic mesenteric ischemia, radiographic, endoscopic, and laboratory tests are usually normal. Early in the course of acute mesenteric ischemia, the plain film of the abdomen may be unremarkable despite complaints of severe abdominal pain. In these settings, prompt mesenteric angiography is essential to confirm the diagnosis of vascular disease.

Inflammatory and Neoplastic Diseases of Small and Large Intestine   Patients with these conditions are usually identified by history, physical examination, and careful examination of the stools for exudate and blood. Examination of fresh stool samples for common bacterial pathogens and parasites by laboratories skilled in these techniques is important in identifying or excluding infectious causes of diarrhea, particularly in the patient with colitis. Sigmoidoscopy is valuable in identifying mucosal and neoplastic lesions of the rectum and distal colon. The mucosal surface of the entire colon and terminal ileum can be examined directly and biopsied through the fiberoptic sigmoidoscope or colonoscope. The radiologic examination of the small intestine is highly reliable in identifying the prestenotic and stenotic lesions of Crohn's disease. In the colon, a single barium enema examination in a well-prepared patient has a diagnostic accuracy of 80 to 85%; the addition of air-contrast technique brings the accuracy up over 90%. Accuracy is greatly limited if the patient is poorly prepared for the examination. Colonoscopy may be preferable because of its greater accuracy and the fact that it enables the operator to remove any polyps that are encountered and to obtain preoperative tissue confirmation in the patient who probably has cancer.

Peroral biopsy of the small intestine (now most often accomplished during endoscopy) and forceps biopsy of the rectosigmoid are of considerable importance in revealing mucosal disease. Rectal biopsy is an excellent means of demonstrating amyloidosis, schistosomiasis, and amebiasis. Submucosal disease is not seen in these superficial biopsies. Hirschsprung's disease is diagnosed histologically by a deep surgical biopsy of the lower part of the rectum.

Malabsorption Syndromes   Malabsorption may be suspected on the basis of history and physical examination and confirmed by examination of the stool. Radiologic examination is helpful to rule out local lesions and to suggest motor and secretory dysfunction, but it is rarely diagnostic unless an abnormal small-bowel mucosa or fistulas between the intestine and stomach are demonstrated.

Microscopic examination of a stool specimen stained with Sudan is a simple screening test for steatorrhea. Chemical analysis of 3-day stool collection for fat, with the patient on a standard diet, is used to establish the diagnosis of steatorrhea. The D-xylose absorption test is about 90% accurate in distinguishing mucosal disease from pancreatic insufficiency. Peroral biopsy of the small intestine via the endoscope or a specialized biopsy device is of value in the diagnosis of celiac disease, and it may show the less common infiltrations of the mucosa by amyloid or bacterial mucoproteins (Whipple's disease). Leakage of protein into the intestinal lumen may cause hypoproteinemia and can be demonstrated by the recovery in stools of the serum protein α_1-antitrypsin or intravenously administrated markers such as iodine- or chromium-labeled isotopes. →*The tests useful in the diagnosis of malabsorption are discussed in Chap. 286.*

GI Bleeding (See also Chap. 44) Acute bleeding in the GI tract is a common clinical problem. The history usually provides a reliable distinction between lower and upper tract sources. Once the patient with upper tract bleeding is hemodynamically stable, a nasogastric tube is placed to confirm the site of blood loss and to empty the stomach. Endoscopy is then performed to define the cause and often to treat it. In patients with acute lower tract bleeding, sigmoidosopy may permit detection of distal sites of bleeding. Colonoscopy may also be of value, but visualization may be limited by active bleeding and poor bowel preparation. Barium studies should be avoided in the acute setting. They are usually nondiagnostic and the persistent contrast may interfere with interpretation of angiographic studies, which can often define a site of bleeding that is otherwise obscure. Radionuclide bleeding scan can locate the bleeding site. A Meckel's scan can be diagnostic when active bleeding arises distal to the duodenum in the absence of an identifiable source in the colon.

BIBLIOGRAPHY

JOHNSON LR et al: *Physiology of the Gastrointestinal Tract,* 3d ed. New York, Raven, 1995

FELDMAN M et al: *Gastrointestinal and Liver Disease,* 6th ed. Philadelphia, Saunders, 1998

YAMADA T et al: *Textbook of Gastroenterology,* 3d ed. Philadelphia, Lippincott Williams & Wilkins, 1999

283   *Mark Topazian*

GASTROINTESTINAL ENDOSCOPY

Gastrointestinal endoscopy has been attempted for over 200 years, but the introduction of semi-rigid gastroscopes in the middle of the twentieth century marked the dawn of the modern endoscopic era. Since then, rapid advances in endoscopic technology have led to dramatic changes in the diagnosis and treatment of many digestive diseases. Innovative endoscopic devices and new endoscopic treatment modalities continue to expand the use of endoscopy in patient care.

Flexible endoscopes provide either an optical image (transmitted over fiberoptic bundles) or an electronic video image (generated by a charge-coupled device in the tip of the endoscope; see **Color Atlas, Section III**). Operator controls permit deflection of the endoscope tip; fiberoptic bundles bring light to the tip of the endoscope; and working channels allow washing, suctioning, and the passage of instruments. Progressive changes in the diameter and stiffness of endoscopes have improved the ease and patient tolerance of endoscopy.

ENDOSCOPIC PROCEDURES

Upper Endoscopy Upper endoscopy, also referred to as esophagogastroduodenoscopy (EGD), is performed by passing a flexible endoscope through the mouth into the esophagus, stomach, bulb, and second duodenum. The procedure is the best method of examining the upper gastrointestinal mucosa. While the upper gastrointestinal radiographic series has similar accuracy for diagnosis of duodenal ulcer, EGD is superior for detection of gastric ulcers and permits directed biopsy and endoscopic therapy, if needed. Topical pharyngeal anesthesia is used, and intravenous conscious sedation is given to most patients in the United States to ease the anxiety and discomfort of the procedure, although in many countries EGD is routinely performed without sedation. The recent development of ultrathin, 5-mm diameter

endoscopes for transnasal, unsedated EGD may decrease the use of sedation for EGD in the United States, also decreasing the costs and risks of the procedure.

Colonoscopy Colonoscopy is performed by passing a flexible colonoscope through the anal canal into the rectum and colon. The cecum is reached in over 95% of cases, and the terminal ileum can often be examined. Colonoscopy is the "gold standard" for diagnosis of colonic mucosal disease. Barium enema is more accurate for evaluation of diverticula and for accurate measurement of colonic strictures, but colonoscopy has greater sensitivity for polyps and cancers. Colonoscopy is more uncomfortable than EGD for most patients, and conscious sedation is usually given before colonoscopy in the United States, although a willing patient and a skilled examiner can complete the procedure without sedation in many cases.

Flexible Sigmoidoscopy Flexible sigmoidoscopy is similar to colonoscopy but visualizes only the rectum and a variable portion of the left colon, typically to 60 cm from the anal verge. This procedure causes abdominal cramping, but it is brief and is almost always performed without sedation. Flexible sigmoidoscopy is primarily used to screen asymptomatic, average-risk patients for colonic polyps and may also be used for evaluation of diarrhea and hematochezia.

Enteroscopy Enteroscopy is the relatively new field of small-bowel endoscopy. Two techniques are currently used. "Push" enteroscopy is performed with a long endoscope similar in design to an upper endoscope. The enteroscope is pushed down the small bowel with the help of a stiffening overtube that extends from the mouth to the duodenum. The mid-jejunum can often be reached; an instrument channel is present for biopsies or endoscopic therapy. "Sonde" enteroscopy uses a very thin, long, flexible endoscope with a weighted tip and no biopsy capability. The sonde enteroscope is passed through the nose, dragged to the duodenum by a standard endoscope, then slowly propelled forward by intestinal peristalsis for several hours. The cecum or distal ileum is reached in most cases. The small-bowel mucosa is examined during sonde enteroscope withdrawal, although parts of the mucosa may be missed when the endoscope is pulled back around turns. The major indication for these procedures is unexplained small-bowel bleeding.

Endoscopic Retrograde Cholangiopancreatography (ERCP) During ERCP, a side-viewing endoscope is passed through the mouth to the duodenum, the ampulla of Vater is identified and cannulated with a thin plastic catheter, and radiographic contrast material is injected into the bile duct and pancreatic duct under fluoroscopic guidance (Fig. 283-1). When indicated, the sphincter of Oddi can be opened using the technique of endoscopic sphincterotomy (Fig. 283-2). Stones can be retrieved from the ducts, and strictures of the ducts can be biopsied, dilated, and stented. ERCP is often performed for therapy but remains an important diagnostic tool, especially for bile duct stones.

Endoscopic Ultrasound (EUS) EUS utilizes high-frequency ultrasound transducers incorporated into the tip of a flexible endoscope. Ultrasound images are obtained of the gut wall and adjacent organs, vessels, and lymph nodes. By sacrificing depth of ultrasound penetration and bringing the ultrasound transducer close to the area of interest via endoscopy, very high resolution images are obtained. EUS provides the most accurate preoperative local staging of esophageal, pancreatic, and rectal malignancies, although it does not detect most distant metastases. Examples of EUS tumor staging are shown in Fig. 283-3. EUS is also highly sensitive for diagnosis of bile duct stones, gallbladder disease, submucosal gastrointestinal lesions, and chronic pancreatitis. Fine-needle aspiration of masses and lymph nodes in the posterior mediastinum, abdomen, and pelvis can be performed under EUS guidance.

RISKS OF ENDOSCOPY

All endoscopic procedures carry some risk of bleeding and gastrointestinal perforation. These risks are quite low with diagnostic upper

FIGURE 283-1 Endoscopic retrograde cholangiopancreatography (ERCP) for bile duct stones with cholangitis. *A.* Faceted bile duct stones are demonstrated in the common bile duct. *B.* After endoscopic sphincterotomy, the stones are extracted with a Dormia basket. A small abscess communicates with the left intrahepatic duct.

endoscopy and colonoscopy (<1:1000 procedures), although the risk is as high as 1:100 when therapeutic procedures such as polypectomy, control of hemorrhage, or stricture dilation are performed. Bleeding and perforation are rare with flexible sigmoidoscopy. The risks for diagnostic EUS are similar to the risks for diagnostic upper endoscopy.

Infectious complications are unusual with most endoscopic procedures. Stricture dilation, variceal sclerotherapy, and ERCP for biliary obstruction all carry a higher incidence of postprocedure bacteremia, and prophylactic antibiotics may be indicated for these procedures in some patients (Table 283-1).

ERCP carries additional risks. Pancreatitis occurs in about 5% of patients undergoing ERCP and is seen in up to 25% of patients with

sphincter of Oddi dysfunction. Post-ERCP pancreatitis is usually mild and self-limited but may infrequently result in prolonged hospitalization, surgery, diabetes, or death. Bleeding occurs after 1% of endoscopic sphincterotomies. Ascending cholangitis, pseudocyst infection, and retroperitoneal perforation and abscess may all occur as a result of ERCP.

The conscious sedation administered during endoscopy may cause respiratory depression or allergic reactions. Percutaneous gastrostomy tube placement during EGD is associated with a 10 to 15% incidence of complications, most often wound infections. Fasciitis, pneumonia, bleeding, and colonic injury may result from gastrostomy placement.

URGENT ENDOSCOPY

ACUTE GASTROINTESTINAL HEMORRHAGE Endoscopy is an important diagnostic and therapeutic technique for patients with acute gastrointestinal hemorrhage. Although most gastrointestinal bleeding stops spontaneously, a minority of patients will have persistent or recurrent hemorrhage that may be life-threatening. Clinical predictors of rebleeding help identify patients most likely to benefit from urgent endoscopy and endoscopic, angiographic, or surgical hemostasis.

Initial Evaluation The initial evaluation of the bleeding patient focuses on the magnitude of hemorrhage as reflected by the postural vital signs, the frequency of hematemesis or melena, and (in some cases) findings on nasogastric lavage. The measured values of hematocrit and hemoglobin lag the clinical course and are not reliable gauges of the magnitude of acute bleeding. This initial evaluation, completed well before the bleeding source is confidently identified, guides immediate supportive care of the patient and helps determine the timing of endoscopy. The magnitude of the initial hemorrhage is probably the most important indication for urgent endoscopy, since a large initial bleed increases the likelihood of ongoing or recurrent bleeding. Patients with resting hypotension, repeated hematemesis, nasogastric aspirate that does not clear with repeated lavage, or those requiring blood transfusions should be considered for urgent endoscopy. In addition, patients with cirrhosis, coagulopathy, or respiratory or renal failure and those over 70 years of age are more likely to have significant rebleeding.

Bedside evaluation also suggests an upper or lower gastrointestinal source of bleeding in most patients. About 90% of patients with melena are bleeding proximal to the ligament of Treitz, and about 90% of patients with hematochezia are bleeding from the colon. It is important to note, however, that melena can result from bleeding in the small bowel or right colon, especially in older patients with slow colonic transit, so colonoscopy should be performed in patients with melena when upper endoscopy is unrevealing. Similarly, a minority of patients with massive hematochezia are bleeding from a duodenal ulcer, with rapid intestinal transit. Hence early upper endoscopy should be considered in patients with massive hematochezia.

Endoscopy should be performed after the patient has been resuscitated with intravenous fluids and transfusions as necessary. Marked coagulopathy or thrombocytopenia is usually treated before endoscopy, since correction of these abnormalities may lead to resolution of bleeding, and techniques for endoscopic hemostasis are limited in such patients. Metabolic derangements should also be addressed. Tracheal intubation for airway protection should be considered before upper endoscopy in patients with repeated hematemesis and suspected variceal hemorrhage.

FIGURE 283-2 Endoscopic sphincterotomy. *A.* A normal-appearing ampulla of Vater. *B.* Sphincterotomy is performed with electrocautery. *C.* Bile duct stones are extracted with a balloon catheter. *D.* Final appearance of the sphincterotomy.

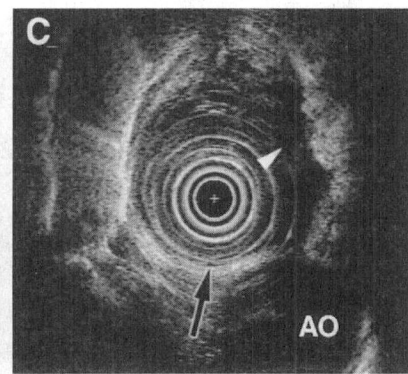

FIGURE 283-3 Local staging of gastrointestinal cancers with endoscopic ultrasound. In each example the white arrowhead marks the primary tumor and the black arrow indicates the muscularis propria (mp) of the intestinal wall. "AO" indicates aorta. *A*. T1 gastric cancer. The tumor does not invade the mp. *B*. T2 esophageal cancer. The tumor invades the mp. *C*. T3 esophageal cancer. The tumor extends through the mp into the surrounding tissue, and focally abuts the aorta.

Most patients with impressive hematochezia can undergo colonoscopy after a rapid colonic purge with a polyethylene glycol solution; the preparation fluid is often administered via a nasogastric tube. In a minority of cases, persistent bleeding and recurrent hemodynamic instability prevent endoscopic visualization of the colonic mucosa, and other techniques (such as bleeding scans, angiography, or emergency subtotal colectomy) must be employed. Even in these cases, however, the anal and rectal mucosa should be visualized endoscopically early in the course, since bleeding lesions in or close to the anal canal are generally amenable to surgical transanal hemostatic techniques; and upper endoscopy should be performed to exclude duodenal ulcer.

Peptic Ulcer The endoscopic appearance of peptic ulcers provides useful prognostic information in patients with acute hemorrhage. When a platelet plug is seen protruding from a vessel wall in the base of an ulcer (a so-called sentinel clot or visible vessel), there is a 40% chance of major rebleeding from the ulcer. This finding often leads to local endoscopic therapy to decrease the rebleeding rate. A clean-based ulcer, on the other hand, is associated with low (3 to 5%) risk of rebleeding; patients with melena and a clean-based duodenal ulcer are often discharged to home from the emergency department or endoscopy suite if they are young, reliable, and otherwise healthy. Other findings have an intermediate risk of rebleeding: flat red or purple spots in the ulcer base have a 10% risk, and large adherent clots covering the ulcer base have a 20% risk. Occasionally, active spurting from an ulcer is seen (with >90% risk of ongoing bleeding). Examples of endoscopic stigmata of recent hemorrhage are shown in Fig. 283-4.

Patients with a visible vessel or active bleeding are usually treated endoscopically, decreasing rebleeding rates by about half. Hemostatic techniques include "coaptive coagulation" of the vessel in the base of the ulcer, using a thermal probe that is pressed against the site of bleeding, or injection of epinephrine or sclerosant into and around the vessel.

Varices Two complementary strategies guide therapy of bleeding varices: local treatment of the bleeding vessel and treatment of underlying portal hypertension. Local therapies (including endoscopic sclerotherapy, endoscopic band ligation, and balloon tamponade with a Sengstaken-Blakemore tube) effectively control acute hemorrhage in most patients and are the mainstay of acute treatment, although therapies that decrease portal pressures (pharmacologic treatment, surgical shunts, or radiologically placed intrahepatic shunts) also play an important role.

Endoscopic band ligation is the preferred local therapy for bleeding esophageal varices. In this technique a varix is suctioned into a cap fitted on the end of the endoscope, and a rubber band is then released from the cap, ligating the varix. Acute hemorrhage can be controlled in up to 90% of patients, and complications (such as sepsis, symptomatic esophageal ulceration, or esophageal stenosis) are uncommon. Endoscopic sclerotherapy is an older technique in which a sclerosing, thrombogenic solution is injected into or next to esophageal varices. Sclerotherapy also controls acute hemorrhage in most patients but has higher complication rates. These techniques are used when varices are actively bleeding during endoscopy or (more commonly) when varices are the only identifiable cause of acute hemorrhage.

After treatment of the acute hemorrhage, an elective course of endoscopic therapy can be undertaken with the goal of eradicating esophageal varices and preventing rebleeding months to years later. This chronic therapy is less successful, preventing long term rebleeding in about 50% of patients. Pharmacologic therapies that decrease portal pressure have similar efficacy, and the two modalities may be combined.

Gastric varices are less amenable to endoscopic therapy and are usually treated with a portal decompressive procedure (surgical portosystemic shunt or radiologic transjugular portosystemic shunt). Endoscopic therapy of gastric varices is usually reserved for actively bleeding varices or for patients with thrombosis of the portal venous system.

Dieulafoy's Lesion This lesion, also called *persistent caliber artery*, is a large-caliber arteriole that runs immediately beneath the gastrointestinal mucosa and bleeds through a pinpoint mucosal erosion. Dieulafoy's lesion is seen most commonly on the lesser curvature of the proximal stomach, causes impressive arterial hemorrhage, and is

Table 283-1 Antibiotic Prophylaxis for Selected Endoscopic Procedures

Patient Condition	Procedure Contemplated	Antibiotic Prophylaxis[a]
Prosthetic valve, history of endocarditis, systemic-pulmonary shunt, Synthetic vascular graft (<1 year old)	High risk[b]	Recommended
	Low risk[c]	Optional (insufficient data)
Rheumatic valvular disease, mitral valve prolapse with insufficiency, congenital cardiac malformations, hypertrophic cardiomyopathy	High risk	Optional (insufficient data)
	Low risk	Not recommended
Pacemakers, implantable defibrillators, Prior coronary artery bypass grafts; prosthetic joints	High or low risk	Not recommended

[a] Acceptable antibiotic regimens for esophageal procedures include amoxicillin, 2 g PO, 1 h before or ampicillin, 2 g IV, 30 min before upper endoscopy; clindamycin, 600 mg PO, may be substituted in penicillin-allergic patients. Acceptable regimens for colonic procedures in high-risk patients include gentamicin, 1.5 mg/kg (not to exceed 120 mg), and ampicillin, 2 g IV, within 30 min of colonoscopy, with amoxicillin, 1 g orally, 6 h later; vancomycin, 1 g IV, may be substituted for penicillins in penicillin-allergic patients. For colonic procedures in moderate-risk patients, amoxicillin, 2 g PO, 1 h before the procedure or vancomycin, 1 g IV, are sufficient.
[b] High-risk endoscopic procedures: stricture dilation, variceal sclerosis, endoscopic retrograde cholangiopancreatography with an obstructed biliary tree.
[c] Low-risk endoscopic procedures: upper endoscopy and colonoscopy with or without biopsy and polyp removal, variceal ligation.
SOURCE: Adapted from *Antibiotic Prophylaxis for Endoscopic Procedures*, American Society for Gastrointestinal Endoscopy, 1998.

1637

FIGURE 283-4 Endoscopic stigmata of recent bleeding in peptic ulcers. *A.* A flat red spot in an ulcer base. *B.* A sentinel clot protruding from an ulcer base. *C.* Coagulation of the sentinel clot shown in (*B*) with a thermal probe. (*Courtesy of American Society for Gastrointestinal Endoscopy.*)

difficult to diagnose; it is often recognized only after repeated endoscopy for recurrent bleeding. Endoscopic therapy with a thermal probe usually controls acute bleeding and successfully ablates the underlying vessel once the bleeding site has been identified. Embolization or surgical oversewing are sometimes required.

Mallory-Weiss Tear A Mallory-Weiss tear is a linear mucosal rent near or across the gastroesophageal junction that is often associated with retching or vomiting. When the tear disrupts a submucosal arteriole, brisk hemorrhage may result. Endoscopy is the best method of diagnosis, and an actively bleeding tear can be treated endoscopically with coaptive coagulation using a thermal probe or by injection of dilute epinephrine. Since Mallory-Weiss tears only rarely rebleed, a sentinel clot in the base of the tear is usually not treated endoscopically.

Vascular Ectasias Vascular ectasias are flat mucosal vascular anomalies best diagnosed by endoscopy. They usually cause slow intestinal blood loss and have several characteristic distributions in the gastrointestinal tract. When limited to the cecum, where they occur as senile lesions, or the gastric antrum (gastric antral vascular ectasias, or "watermelon stomach"), ectasias are often responsive to local endoscopic ablative therapy. Patients with diffuse small-bowel vascular ectasias (associated with chronic renal failure and with hereditary hemorrhagic telangiectasia) often continue to bleed despite endoscopic treatment of accessible lesions and require systemic therapy.

Colonic Diverticula Diverticula form where nutrient arteries penetrate the muscular wall of the colon en route to the colonic mucosa. The artery found in the base of a diverticulum may bleed, causing painless and impressive hematochezia. Colonoscopy is indicated in patients with hematochezia and suspected diverticular hemorrhage, since other causes of bleeding (such as vascular ectasias, colitis, and colonic malignancy) must be excluded. In addition, an actively bleeding diverticulum is occasionally seen and treated during colonoscopy.

GASTROINTESTINAL OBSTRUCTION AND PSEUDO-OBSTRUCTION Endoscopy is useful for evaluation and treatment of some forms of gastrointestinal obstruction. An important exception is small-bowel obstruction, which is generally not diagnosed by endoscopy or amenable to endoscopic therapy. Esophageal, gastroduodenal, and colonic obstruction or pseudoobstruction can all be diagnosed endoscopically and are often managed endoscopically as well.

Acute Esophageal Obstruction Esophageal obstruction by impacted food or an ingested foreign body is a potentially life-threatening event. Left untreated, the patient may develop esophageal ulceration, ischemia, and perforation. Patients with persistent esophageal obstruction often have hypersalivation and are usually unable to swallow water; endoscopy is generally the best initial test in such patients, since endoscopic removal of the obstructing material is usually possible, and the presence of an underlying esophageal stricture can often be determined. Radiographs of the chest and neck should be considered before endoscopy in patients with fever, obstruction for ≥24 h, or ingestion of a sharp object such as a fishbone. Radiographic contrast studies interfere with subsequent endoscopy and are not advisable in patients with a clinical picture of persistent obstruction, unless an esophageal perforation is suspected. Occasionally, sublingual nifedipine or nitrates, or intravenous glucagon, may resolve an esophageal food impaction, but in most patients there is an underlying web, ring, or stricture and endoscopic removal of the obstructing food bolus is necessary.

Gastric Outlet Obstruction Obstruction of the gastric outlet is commonly caused by malignancy of the prepyloric gastric antrum or chronic peptic ulceration with stenosis of the pylorus. Patients vomit partially digested food many hours after eating. Gastric decompression with a nasogastric tube and subsequent lavage for removal of retained material is the first step in treatment. The diagnosis can then be confirmed with a saline load test, if desired. Endoscopy is useful for diagnosis and treatment. Patients with pyloric stenosis may be treated with endoscopic balloon dilation of the pylorus, and a course of endoscopic dilation results in long-term relief of symptoms in about 50% of patients. Malignant pyloric obstruction can be treated with endoscopically placed expandable stents if the patient is deemed a poor surgical candidate.

Colonic Obstruction and Pseudoobstruction These both present with abdominal distention and discomfort; tympany; and a dilated, air-filled colon on plain abdominal radiography. Both conditions may lead to colonic perforation if untreated. Acute colonic pseudoobstruction is a form of colonic ileus that is usually attributable to electrolyte disorders, narcotic and anticholinergic medications, immobility (as after surgery), and retroperitoneal hemorrhage or mass. Multiple causative factors are often present. Either colonoscopy or a water-soluble contrast enema may be used to look for an obstructing lesion and differentiate obstruction from pseudoobstruction. One of these diagnostic studies should be strongly considered if the patient does not have clear risk factors for pseudoobstruction, if radiographs do not show air in the rectum and sigmoid, or if the patient fails to improve when the underlying causes of pseudoobstruction have been addressed. The risk of cecal perforation in pseudoobstruction rises when the cecal diameter exceeds 12 cm, and in such patients decompression of the colon may be achieved using intravenous neostigmine, colonoscopic decompression, or placement of a cecostomy tube. Most patients should receive a trial of conservative therapy (with correction of electrolyte disorders, removal of offending medications, and increased mobilization) before undergoing an invasive decompressive procedure.

Colonic obstruction is an indication for urgent surgery. In poor operative candidates or those with symptomatic partial obstruction from malignancy, a colonoscopically placed expandable stent can relieve obstruction and permit preparation of the bowel for elective surgery.

ACUTE BILIARY OBSTRUCTION The steady, severe pain that occurs when a gallstone acutely obstructs the common bile duct often brings patients to a hospital. The diagnosis of a ductal stone is suspected when the patient is jaundiced or when serum liver tests or pancreatic enzyme levels are elevated, and it is confirmed by direct

FIGURE 283-5 New methods of bile duct imaging. Arrows mark bile duct stones. Arrowheads indicate the common bile duct, and the asterisk marks the portal vein. *A.* Endoscopic ultrasonography (EUS). *B.* Magnetic resonance cholangiography (MRCP). *C.* Helical computed tomography.

cholangiography (performed endoscopically, percutaneously, or during surgery). ERCP is currently the primary means of diagnosing and treating common bile duct stones in most hospitals in the United States.

Bile Duct Imaging While traditional noninvasive imaging tests such as ultrasound and biliary scintigraphy are not sufficiently accurate for reliable diagnosis of bile duct stones, newer imaging modalities such as spiral computed tomography (CT), magnetic resonance cholangiopancreatography (MRCP), and EUS are more accurate and have an emerging role in diagnosis. Examples of these modalities are shown in Fig. 283-5. During MRCP, images are obtained that demonstrate stagnant or slowly flowing fluid and subtract all other tissue. The resulting images of the right upper quadrant are strikingly similar to a direct cholangiogram, although with less resolution. MRCP can be performed rapidly without sedation and does not require any radiographic contrast. When an echo-endoscope is passed into the duodenum, detailed EUS views of the adjacent bile duct are readily obtained. While this procedure requires intravenous sedation, it has a very low incidence of complications, in contradistinction to ERCP. Spiral CT has a sensitivity of 85% for diagnosis of bile duct stones, MRCP has a sensitivity of 85 to 95%, and EUS has a sensitivity of 88 to 98%. EUS is more accurate than ERCP in some hands.

The clinical role of these new imaging techniques is evolving. When a bile duct stone is highly likely and urgent treatment is required (as in a patient with jaundice and biliary sepsis), ERCP is the procedure of choice, since it remains the gold standard for diagnosis and provides immediate treatment. When a persistent bile duct stone is relatively unlikely (as in a patient with gallstone pancreatitis), less-invasive imaging techniques may supplant ERCP or intraoperative cholangiography.

Ascending Cholangitis Charcot's triad of jaundice, abdominal pain, and fever is present in about 70% of patients with ascending cholangitis and biliary sepsis. Initially, such patients are managed with fluid resuscitation and intravenous antibiotics. Abdominal ultrasound is often done early in the course, to look for gallbladder stones and bile duct dilation. The bile duct may not be dilated early in the course of acute biliary obstruction, however. Medical management usually improves the patient's clinical status, providing a window of approximately 24 h during which biliary drainage should be established, typically by ERCP. Undue delay can result in recrudesence of overt sepsis and increased morbidity. If, in addition to Charcot's triad, shock and confusion are present (Reynolds's pentad), urgent attempts to restore biliary drainage are usually indicated.

Gallstone Pancreatitis Gallstones may cause acute pancreatitis as they pass through the ampulla of Vater, where they obstruct the pancreatic duct (and sometimes cause reflux of bile into the pancreas). The occurrence of gallstone pancreatitis usually implies passage of a stone into the duodenum, and only about 20% of patients harbor a persistent stone in the ampulla or the common bile duct. Retained stones are more common in the subset of patients with jaundice, severe pancreatitis, or superimposed ascending cholangitis.

Urgent ERCP decreases the morbidity of gallstone pancreatitis in some subsets of patients, but it remains unclear whether the benefit of ERCP is mainly attributable to treatment and prevention of ascending cholangitis or to relief of pancreatic duct obstruction. ERCP is warranted early in the course of gallstone pancreatitis if ascending cholangitis is also suspected, especially in a jaundiced patient. Urgent ERCP may also be indicated in the minority of patients predicted to have severe pancreatitis using a multifactorial index of severity such as the Glasgow, Ranson's, or Apache II score.

ELECTIVE ENDOSCOPY

Dyspepsia and Reflux Dyspepsia is a burning discomfort in the upper abdomen that may be caused by diverse processes such as gastroesophageal reflux, peptic ulcer disease, and "nonulcer dyspepsia," a heterogeneous category that includes disorders of motility, sensation, and somatization. Gastric and esophageal malignancies are less common causes of dyspepsia. Careful history taking allows accurate differential diagnosis of dyspepsia in only about half of patients. In the remainder, endoscopy can be a useful diagnostic tool, especially in those patients whose symptoms are not resolved by an empirical trial of symptomatic treatment.

Gastroesophageal Reflux Disease (GERD) When classic symptoms of gastroesophageal reflux are present, such as water brash and substernal heartburn, presumptive diagnosis and empirical treatment are often sufficient. Although endoscopy is sensitive for diagnosis of esophagitis, it misses some cases of reflux, since some patients have symptomatic reflux without esophagitis. The most sensitive test for diagnosis of GERD is 24-h ambulatory pH monitoring. Endoscopy is nevertheless indicated in patients with resistant reflux symptoms and in those with recurrent dyspepsia after treatment that is not clearly due to reflux on clinical grounds alone, to assess the esophagus and exclude other diseases. Endoscopy is also advised in a patient with reflux and dysphagia, to look for a stricture or malignancy. Endoscopy is probably also indicated in patients with long-standing (≥10 years) frequent heartburn, who are at sixfold increased risk of Barrett's esophagus compared to a patient with <1 year of reflux symptoms. Patients with Barrett's esophagus usually enter a program of periodic endoscopy with biopsies, to detect dysplasia or early carcinoma.

Peptic Ulcer Peptic ulcer classically causes epigastric gnawing or burning, often occurring nocturnally and promptly relieved by food or antacids. Although endoscopy is the most sensitive diagnostic test for peptic ulcer, immediate endoscopy is not a cost-effective strategy in young patients with ulcer-like dyspeptic symptoms unless endoscopy is available at low cost. Patients with suspected peptic ulcer should be evaluated for *Helicobacter pylori* infection. Serology (which documents past or present infection) and urea breath testing (which demonstrates current infection) are less invasive and costly than endoscopy with biopsy. Patients with ulcer-like symptoms despite treatment should undergo endoscopy to exclude gastric malignancy, and patients with "alarm symptoms" (early satiety or anorexia, early recurrence of symptoms, anemia) should also undergo endoscopy.

Nonulcer Dyspepsia   This may be associated with bloating and, unlike peptic ulcer, tends not to remit and recur. Most patients do not respond to acid-reducing, prokinetic, or anti-*Helicobacter* therapy and are referred for endoscopy to exclude a refractory ulcer. While endoscopy usefully excludes other diagnoses, it generally does little to improve the treatment of patients with nonulcer dyspepsia.

Dysphagia   About 50% of patients with difficulty swallowing have a mechanical obstruction; the remainder have a motor disorder. Careful history taking often suggests a diagnosis and leads to the appropriate use of diagnostic tests. Esophageal strictures typically cause progressive dysphagia, first for solids, then liquids; esophageal motor disorders often cause intermittent dysphagia for both solids and liquids. Some underlying disorders have characteristic historical features: Schatzki's ring causes episodic dysphagia for solids, typically at the beginning of a meal; pharyngeal motor disorders are associated with difficulty initiating deglutition ("transfer dysphagia") and nasal reflux with swallowing; and achalasia may cause nocturnal regurgitation of undigested food particles.

When mechanical obstruction is suspected, endoscopy is a useful initial diagnostic test, since it permits immediate biopsy and dilation of strictures, masses, or rings. Blind or forceful passage of an endoscope may lead to perforation in a patient with stenosis of the cervical esophagus or a Zencker's diverticulum, but gentle passage of an endoscope under direct visual guidance is reasonably safe even in these patients. Endoscopy can miss a subtle stricture or ring in some patients.

When a motor disorder is suspected, esophageal radiography is the best initial diagnostic test. The pharyngeal swallowing mechanism, esophageal peristalsis, and the lower esophageal sphincter can all be assessed. In some disorders, subsequent esophageal manometry may also be important for diagnosis.

Anemia and Occult Blood in the Stool   Iron-deficiency anemia may be attributed to poor iron absorption (as in celiac sprue) or, more commonly, chronic blood loss. Intestinal bleeding should be strongly suspected in men and postmenopausal women with iron-deficiency anemia, and colonoscopy is indicated in such patients, even in the absence of detectable occult blood in the stool. About 30% will have large colonic polyps, 10% will have colorectal cancer, and additional patients will have colonic vascular lesions. When a convincing source of blood loss is not found in the colon, upper gastrointestinal endoscopy should also be performed; if no lesion is found, duodenal biopsies should be obtained to exclude sprue. Evaluation of the small bowel may be appropriate if both EGD and colonoscopy are unrevealing.

Tests for occult blood in the stool detect hemoglobin or the heme moiety and are most sensitive for colonic blood loss, although they will also detect larger amounts of upper gastrointestinal bleeding. Patients with occult blood in normal-appearing stool should undergo colonoscopy to diagnose or exclude colorectal neoplasia. The diagnostic yield is lower than in iron-deficiency anemia. Whether upper endoscopy is also indicated largely depends on the patient's symptoms.

The small intestine may be the source of chronic intestinal bleeding, especially if colonoscopy and upper endoscopy are not diagnostic. The utility of small-bowel evaluation varies with the clinical setting and is most important in patients whose bleeding causes chronic or recurrent anemia. While small-bowel radiography is usually normal, partial or total small-bowel enteroscopy yields a specific diagnosis in

about 50% of such patients. The commonest finding is mucosal vascular ectasias or telangiectasias.

Colorectal Cancer Screening   Most colon cancers develop from preexisting colonic adenomas, and colorectal cancer can be largely prevented by the detection and removal of colonic adenomatous polyps. Screening for polyps and early, asymptomatic cancers can be accomplished both by testing stool specimens for occult blood and by directly examining the colonic mucosa. Since tests for occult blood are insensitive, detecting only about one-fourth of colon cancers and large polyps, visualization of at least a part of the colon is an important component of colorectal cancer screening.

The choice of screening strategy for an asymptomatic patient depends in part on their personal and family history. A past history of inflammatory bowel disease or colorectal polyps, a family history of two or more first-degree family members with adenomatous polyps or cancer, certain familial cancer syndromes, or the finding of occult blood in the stool all place an individual at increased risk and alter screening recommendations. An individual without these factors is generally considered at average risk, and screening flexible sigmoidoscopy every 5 years beginning at age 50 is recommended. Screening strategies for higher risk patients are in Table 283-2. Screening strategies for the patient with one family member with colorectal cancer are debated. When the index case occurred at a young age (<60 years), screening colonoscopy should be offered when the patient is 10 years younger than the affected relative was when diagnosed.

Flexible sigmoidoscopy is an effective screening tool for two reasons: (1) the majority of colorectal cancers have traditionally occurred in the rectum and left colon, and (2) many right-sided colon cancers are associated with synchronous left-sided adenomas. The detection of an adenoma during sigmoidoscopy generally leads to full colonoscopy and detection of right-sided cancers, if present. Over the past several decades, however, there has been a gradual change in the distribution of colon cancers, with proportionally fewer rectal and left-sided can-

Table 283-2 Colorectal Cancer Screening Strategies for Patients at Increased Risk

	Recommendation
PERSONAL HISTORY	
History of colon cancer	Evaluate entire colon around the time of resection, then colonoscopy every 3 to 5 years
History of colonic adenomas	Colonoscopy every 3 to 5 years
Ulcerative pancolitis of 8 years duration, left-sided colitis >15 years' duration	Colonoscopy with biopsies every 1 to 3 years
FAMILY HISTORY	
Familial adenomatous polyposis	Consider genetic testing Annual sigmoidoscopy beginning at age 10 to 12, consider colectomy when polyps develop; if no polyps, annual sigmoidoscopy until age 40, then every 3 to 5 years
Hereditary non-polyposis colorectal cancer (HNPCC)	Consider genetic testing Colonoscopy every 2 years beginning at 25 or when 5 years younger than the youngest affected relative; annual colonoscopy after age 40
Two first-degree relatives with colorectal cancer or adenomas	Colonoscopy every 3 to 5 years, beginning when 10 years younger than the youngest affected relative
One first-degree relative with sporadic colorectal cancer or adenoma before age 60	Same as above

SOURCE: Adapted from *Screening and Surveillance Colonoscopy in Individuals at Increased Risk for Colorectal Cancer*, American Society for Gastrointestinal Endoscopy, 1998.

cers than in the past. This has spurred interest in evaluating the entire colon during a single screening examination. Barium enema has been advocated but requires flexible sigmoidoscopy also, to exclude missed rectal lesions. Large studies of colonoscopy for screening of average-risk individuals are currently underway. In addition, the new imaging technique of "virtual colonoscopy" holds considerable promise. This modality uses data from helical CT to generate a graphical display of a "flight" down the colonic lumen. While this technique is not yet sufficiently sensitive for routine clinical use, further refinement may result in a useful noninvasive screening method.

Diarrhea Most cases of diarrhea are acute, self-limited, and due to infections or medication. Chronic diarrhea (lasting >6 weeks) is more often due to a primary inflammatory or malabsorptive disorder, is less likely to resolve spontaneously, and generally requires diagnostic evaluation. Patients with chronic diarrhea or severe, unexplained acute diarrhea often undergo endoscopy if stool tests for pathogens are unrevealing. The choice of endoscopic test depends on the clinical setting.

Patients with colonic symptoms and findings such as bloody diarrhea, tenesmus, fever, or leukocytes in stool generally undergo sigmoidoscopy or colonoscopy to look for colitis. Sigmoidoscopy is often adequate and is the best initial test in most such patients. On the other hand, patients with symptoms and findings suggesting small-bowel disease such as large-volume watery stools; substantial weight loss; and malabsorption of iron, calcium, or fat may undergo upper endoscopy with duodenal biopsies.

Many patients with chronic diarrhea do not fit either of these patterns. When there is a long-standing history of alternating constipation and diarrhea dating to early adulthood, without findings such as blood in the stool or anemia, a diagnosis of irritable bowel syndrome may be made without direct visualization of the bowel. Steatorrhea and upper abdominal pain may prompt evaluation of the pancreas rather than the gut. Patients whose chronic diarrhea is not easily categorized often undergo initial colonoscopy to examine the entire colon (and terminal ileum) for inflammatory or neoplastic disease.

Minor Hematochezia Bright red blood passed with or on formed brown stool usually has a rectal, anal, or distal sigmoid source. Patients with even trivial amounts of hematochezia should be investigated with flexible sigmoidoscopy to exclude large polyps or cancers in the distal bowel. Patients who report red blood on the toilet tissue only, without blood in the toilet or on the stool, are bleeding from a lesion in the anal canal, and careful external and digital examinations and anoscopy are sufficient for diagnosis in most cases.

Unexplained Pancreatitis About 20% of patients with pancreatitis have no identified cause after routine clinical investigation (including a review of medication and alcohol use, measurement of serum triglyceride and calcium levels, abdominal ultrasonography, and CT). Endoscopic techniques lead to a specific diagnosis in the majority of such patients, often altering clinical management. Endoscopic investigation is particularly appropriate if the patient has had more than one episode of pancreatitis.

Microlithiasis, or the presence of microscopic crystals in bile, is a leading cause of previously unexplained acute pancreatitis and is sometimes seen during abdominal ultrasonography as layering sludge or flecks of floating, echogenic material in the gallbladder. Gallbladder bile can be obtained for microscopic analysis by administering a cholecystokinin analogue during endoscopy, causing contraction of the gallbladder. Bile is suctioned from the duodenum as it drains from the papilla, and the darkest fraction is examined for cholesterol crystals or bilirubinate granules. Alternatively, bile can be aspirated from the bile duct during ERCP or the gallbladder can be examined for sludge or crystals by EUS before administering cholecystokinin. The latter strategy is probably the most sensitive means of diagnosing microlithiasis.

Previously undetected chronic pancreatitis, pancreatic malignancy, or pancreas divisum may be diagnosed by either ERCP or EUS. Although ERCP remains the gold standard imaging test for chronic pancreatitis, EUS has good sensitivity and less risk than ERCP. Sphincter of Oddi dysfunction probably causes some cases of pancreatitis and can be diagnosed by manometric studies performed during ERCP.

OPEN-ACCESS ENDOSCOPY

While gastroenterologists have traditionally seen patients in consultation before arranging an endoscopic procedure, direct scheduling of endoscopic procedures by primary care physicians, or *open-access endoscopy*, is an increasingly common practice. When the indications for endoscopy are clear cut and appropriate, the procedural risks are low, and the patient understands what to expect, open-access endoscopy streamlines patient care and decreases costs.

Patients referred for open-access endoscopy should have a recent history, physical examination, and medication review. A copy of such an evaluation should be available when the patient comes to the endoscopy suite. Patients with unstable cardiovascular or respiratory conditions should not be referred directly for open-access endoscopy. Patients with selected cardiac conditions undergoing certain procedures should be prescribed prophylactic antibiotics prior to endoscopy, as described in Table 283-1. In addition, patients taking anticoagulants may need changes in treatment before endoscopy, as detailed in Table 283-3. While many endoscopists recommend discontinuing aspirin for 5 days before elective endoscopic procedures, most evidence suggests that in the absence of a preexisting bleeding disorder it is safe to perform endoscopic procedures in patients taking aspirin and nonsteroidal anti-inflammatory drugs.

Common indications for open-access EGD include dyspepsia resistant to a trial of appropriate therapy; dysphagia or odynophagia; gastrointestinal bleeding; and persistent vomiting, anorexia, or early satiety. Open-access colonoscopy is often requested in men or postmenopausal women with iron-deficiency anemia, patients with occult blood in the stool, patients with a previous history of colorectal adenomatous polyps or cancer, and for screening in patients with above-average risk for colon cancer, as described in Table 283-2. Flexible sigmoidoscopy is commonly performed as an open-access procedure for cancer screening in asymptomatic persons over 50 and for patients with hematochezia.

Table 283-3 Management of Anticoagulation before Endoscopic Procedures

	High Patient Risk of Thromboembolism[a]	Low Patient Risk of Thromboembolism[b]
High-risk procedure[c]	Stop warfarin 3–5 days before the procedure; consider heparin when INR is below the therapeutic range	Stop warfarin 3–5 days before the procedure; restart warfarin after the procedure
Low-risk procedure[d]	No change in anticoagulation; elective procedures should be delayed while INR is above the therapeutic range	No change in anticoagulation; elective procedures should be delayed while INR is above the therapeutic range

[a] High-risk conditions: atrial fibrillation associated with valvular heart disease, mechanical valve in the mitral position, mechanical valve and prior thromboembolic event.
[b] Low-risk conditions: Uncomplicated or paroxysmal nonvalvular atrial fibrillation, mechanical valve in the aortic position, bioprosthetic valve, deep vein thrombosis.
[c] High-risk procedures: Polypectomy, stricture dilation, treatment of varices, gastrostomy placement, biliary sphincterotomy, endoscopic ultrasound with needle aspiration.
[d] Low-risk procedures: Diagnostic upper endoscopy, colonoscopy, sigmoidoscopy with or without biopsy, diagnostic endoscopic retrograde cholangiopancreatography, endoscopic ultrasound without needle aspiration.
NOTE: INR, international normalized ratio.
SOURCE: Adapted from *The Management of Anticoagulants and Anti-Inflammatory Medications in Patients Undergoing Endoscopic Procedures*, American Society for Gastrointestinal Endoscopy, 1998.

When patients are referred for open-access colonoscopy, the primary care provider may need to choose a colonic preparation. Commonly used oral preparations include polyethelene glycol lavage solution and sodium phosphate. Sodium phosphate may cause fluid and electrolyte abnormalities, especially in patients with renal failure, congestive heart failure, and patients over 70 years of age.

BIBLIOGRAPHY

CALETTI G, FUSAROLI P: Endoscopic ultrasonography. Endoscopy 31:95, 1999

DAJANI AS et al: Prevention of bacterial endocarditis: Recommendations by the American Heart Association. Clin Infect Dis 25:1448, 1997

OFMAN JJ, RABENECK L: The effectiveness of endoscopy in the management of dyspepsia: A qualitative systematic review. Am J Med 106:335, 1999

STANLEY AJ, HAYES PC: Portal hypertension and variceal haemorrhage. Lancet 350:1235, 1997

STEELE RJ: The preprocedural care of the patient with gastrointestinal bleeding. Gastrointest Endosc Clin N Am 7:551, 1997

ZUCCARO G JR: Management of the adult patient with acute lower gastrointestinal bleeding. Am J Gastroenterol 93:1202, 1998

284   Raj K. Goyal

DISEASES OF THE ESOPHAGUS

The two major functions of the esophagus are the transport of the food bolus from the mouth to the stomach and the prevention of retrograde flow of gastrointestinal contents. The transport function is achieved by peristaltic contractions in the pharynx and esophagus associated with relaxation of upper and lower esophageal sphincters (Chap. 40). Retrograde flow is prevented by the two esophageal sphincters, which remain closed between swallows. The upper esophageal sphincter (UES) consists of the cricopharyngeus and inferior pharyngeal constrictor muscles, striated muscles innervated by excitatory somatic lower motor neurons. These muscles exhibit no myogenic tone and receive no inhibitory innervation. The UES remains closed owing to the elastic properties of its wall and to neurogenic tonic contraction of the sphincter muscles. It is opened by central inhibition of the sphincter muscles in concert with forward displacement of the larynx by the suprahyoid muscles. In contrast, the lower esophageal sphincter (LES) is composed of smooth muscle and is innervated by parallel sets of parasympathetic excitatory and inhibitory pathways. It remains closed because of its intrinsic myogenic tone, which is modulated by the excitatory and inhibitory nerves. It opens in response to the activity of the inhibitory nerves. The neurotransmitters of the excitatory nerves are acetylcholine and substance P, and those of the inhibitory nerves are vasoactive intestinal peptide (VIP) and nitric oxide. The function of the LES is supplemented by the striated muscle of the diaphragmatic crura, which surrounds the LES and acts as an external LES. Relaxation of the LES without esophageal contraction occurs during belching and gastric distention. Gastric distention–evoked transient lower esophageal sphincter relaxation (tLESR) is a vasovagal reflex. Fatty meals, smoking, and beverages with a high xanthine content (tea, coffee, cola) also cause a reduction in sphincter pressure. Many hormones and neurotransmitters can modify LES pressure. Muscarinic M_2 and M_3 receptor agonists, α-adrenergic agonists, gastrin, substance P, and prostaglandin $F_{2\alpha}$ cause contraction. Nicotine, β-adrenergic agonists, dopamine, cholecystokinin, secretin, VIP, calcitonin gene–related peptide (CGRP), adenosine, prostaglandin E, and nitric oxide donors such as nitrates reduce sphincter pressure.

SYMPTOMS

DYSPHAGIA See Chap. 40.

ESOPHAGEAL PAIN   *Heartburn*, or pyrosis, is characterized by burning retrosternal discomfort that may move up and down the chest like a wave. When severe, it may radiate to the sides of the chest, the neck, and the angles of the jaw. Heartburn is a characteristic symptom of reflux esophagitis and may be associated with regurgitation or a feeling of warm fluid climbing up the throat. It is aggravated by bending forward, straining, or lying recumbent and is worse after meals. It is relieved by an upright posture, by the swallowing of saliva or water, and, more reliably, by antacids. Heartburn is produced by heightened mucosal sensitivity and can be reproduced by infusion of dilute (0.1 N) hydrochloric acid (Bernstein test) or neutral hyperosmolar solutions into the esophagus.

Odynophagia, or painful swallowing, is characteristic of nonreflux esophagitis, particularly monilial and herpes esophagitis. Odynophagia may occur with peptic ulcer of the esophagus (Barrett's ulcer), carcinoma with periesophageal involvement, caustic damage of the esophagus, and esophageal perforation. Odynophagia is unusual in uncomplicated reflux esophagitis. Crampy chest pain associated with impaction of a food bolus should be distinguished from odynophagia.

Atypical chest pain other than heartburn and odynophagia occurs in reflux esophagitis or esophageal motility disorders such as diffuse esophageal spasm. Spasm may occur spontaneously or during a meal. Chest pain due to periesophageal involvement with carcinoma or peptic ulcer may be constant and agonizing. Sometimes different types of esophageal pains exist together in the same patient, and frequently patients are not able to describe the pain accurately enough to allow its classification. Coronary artery disease should always be excluded before the esophagus is considered as the cause of atypical chest pain. The most frequent esophageal cause of chest pain is reflux esophagitis. Some patients with atypical chest pain have nonspecific esophageal motor abnormalities of uncertain significance. Many of these patients have behavioral abnormalities, psychosomatic disorders, depression, anxiety, panic reactions, and other psychological disorders.

REGURGITATION   *Regurgitation* is the effortless appearance of gastric or esophageal contents in the mouth. In distal esophageal obstruction and stasis, as in achalasia or the presence of a large diverticulum, the regurgitated material consists of tasteless mucoid fluid or undigested food. Regurgitation of sour or bitter-tasting material occurs in severe gastroesophageal reflux and is associated with incompetence of both the UES and the LES. Regurgitation may result in laryngeal aspiration, with spells of coughing and choking that awaken the patient from sleep, and in aspiration pneumonia. Water brash is reflex salivary hypersecretion that occurs in response to peptic esophagitis and should not be confused with regurgitation.

DIAGNOSTIC TESTS

RADIOLOGIC STUDIES   Barium swallow with fluoroscopy and an esophagogram is a widely used test for the diagnosis of esophageal disease and can be used to evaluate both structural and motor disorders. Spontaneous reflux of barium from the stomach into the esophagus suggests gastroesophageal reflux. Esophageal peristalsis is best studied in the recumbent position, because in the upright position barium passage occurs largely by gravity alone. A double-contrast esophagogram, obtained by coating the esophageal mucosa with barium and distending the esophageal lumen with air using effervescent granules, is particularly useful in demonstrating mucosal ulcers and early cancers. A barium-soaked piece of bread or a 13-mm barium tablet is sometimes used to demonstrate an obstructive lesion. Figures 284-1 and 284-2 illustrate the radiographic appearance of some esophageal disorders. Since the oropharyngeal phase of swallowing lasts no more than a second, videofluoroscopy is necessary to permit detection and analysis of abnormalities of oral and pharyngeal function. The pharynx is examined to detect stasis of barium in the valleculae and

FIGURE 284-1 Radiographic appearance of some motor disorders of the pharynx and esophagus. (1) Pharyngeal paralysis with tracheal aspiration (*arrow*). (2) Cricopharyngeal achalasia. Note the prominent cricopharyngeus, which is recognized by its smoothness and location in the posterior wall. (3) Diffuse esophageal spasm. Note typical corkscrew appearance of the lower part of the esophagus. (4) Achalasia, showing a dilated esophageal body with an air-fluid level and a closed lower esophageal sphincter. (5) Muscular (contractile) lower esophageal ring. The asymmetric contraction visible in (5A) has disappeared in (5B), obtained during the same examination. (6) Scleroderma esophagus showing dilated esophagus with a stricture (6A) and reflux of barium from the stomach into the esophagus (6B). *(Courtesy of Dr. Harvey Goldstein.)*

FIGURE 284-2 Selected structural lesions of the esophagus. (1) Carcinoma of the esophagus, with typical annular narrowing with overhanging margins and destruction of the mucosa. (2) Leiomyoma of the esophagus, with a smooth filling defect and right angles of origin from the esophageal wall. (3) Esophageal ulcer in columnar-cell-lined esophagus (Barrett's esophagus). (4) Monilial esophagitis, with irregular plaquelike filling defects. (5) Long stricture secondary to lye ingestion. (6) Peptic stricture, short and tubular, with associated hiatus hernia. (7) Lower esophageal mucosal (Schatzki) ring. A thin, weblike annular constriction at the esophagogastric junction is associated with a small hiatal hernia. *(Courtesy of Dr. Harvey Goldstein.)*

piriform sinuses and regurgitation of barium into the nose and tracheobronchial tree.

ESOPHAGOSCOPY Esophagoscopy is the direct method of establishing the cause of mechanical dysphagia and of identifying mucosal lesions that may not be identified by the usual barium swallow. If the lumen is markedly narrowed, use of a smaller-caliber endoscope may be needed; on occasion a stricture must be dilated before the examination can be completed. Endoscopic biopsies are useful in diagnosing carcinoma, reflux esophagitis, and other mucosal diseases. Cells obtained by a cytology balloon or brushing the mucosa can be evaluated for carcinoma. Endoscopic ultrasonography permits evaluation of intramural masses and staging of esophageal cancer.

ESOPHAGEAL MOTILITY The study of esophageal motility entails simultaneous recording of pressures from different sites in the esophageal lumen with an assembly of pressure sensors positioned 5 cm apart. The UES and LES appear as zones of high pressure that relax on swallowing. The pharynx and esophagus normally show peristaltic waves with each swallow.

Esophageal motility studies are helpful in the diagnosis of esophageal motor disorders (achalasia, spasm, scleroderma) (Fig. 284-3) but

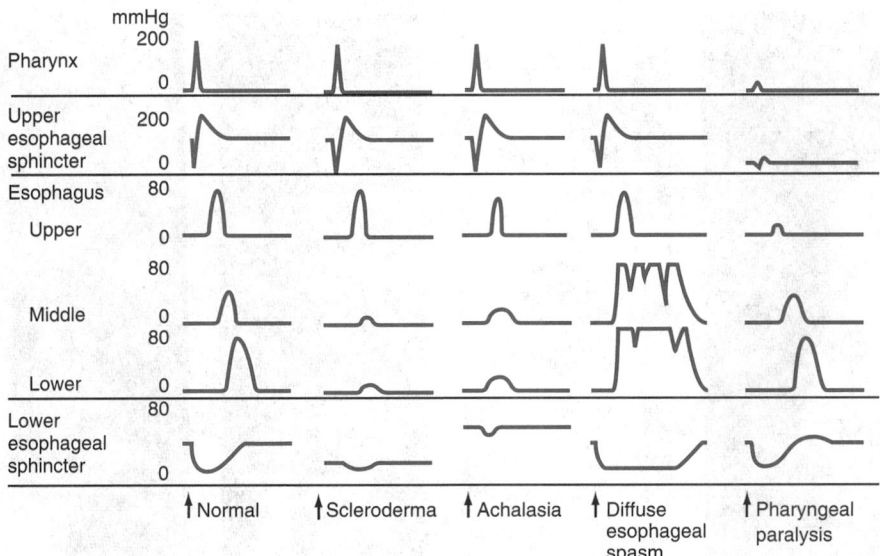

FIGURE 284-3 Motility patterns in selected esophageal and pharyngeal disorders. In normal individuals, the upper and lower esophageal sphincters (UES and LES) appear as zones of high pressure. With a swallow (indicated by ↑), pressure in the sphincters falls and a contraction wave starts in the pharynx and progresses down the esophagus. In scleroderma, the lower part of the esophagus (smooth muscle) shows a reduced amplitude of contractions, which may be peristaltic or simultaneous in onset, and hypotension of the LES. In achalasia, the lower part of the esophagus shows contractions that are reduced in amplitude and simultaneous in onset. In contrast to scleroderma, the LES in achalasia is hypertensive and fails to relax in response to a swallow. In diffuse esophageal spasm, the lower part of the esophagus shows simultaneous-onset, large-amplitude, prolonged, repetitive contractions. In pharyngeal paralysis, the smooth-muscle part of the esophagus is normal. The skeletal muscle part shows a reduced amplitude of contractions. The UES is hypotensive and may not relax normally on swallowing due to associated weakness of the suprahyoid muscles.

are of little value in the diagnosis of mechanical dysphagia. In patients with reflux esophagitis, esophageal manometry is useful in quantitating lower esophageal competence and providing information on the status of the esophageal body motor activity. Manometry provides quantitative data that cannot be obtained by barium swallow or endoscopy. Tests for reflux esophagitis are described later.

MOTOR DISORDERS

STRIATED MUSCLE Oropharyngeal Paralysis Paralysis of oral muscle leads to difficulty initiating swallowing and drooling of food out of the mouth. Pharyngeal paralysis, characterized by dysphagia, nasal regurgitation, and aspiration during swallowing, occurs in a variety of neuromuscular disorders (see Table 40-1). Some of these disorders also involve laryngeal muscles, causing hoarseness. When the suprahyoid muscles are paralyzed, the UES does not open with swallowing, leading to paralytic achalasia of the UES and severe dysphagia.

Videofluoroscopy with barium of various consistencies may reveal difficulties in the oral phase of swallowing. The test may show barium in the valleculae and piriform sinuses, nasal and tracheal aspiration, failure of the upper sphincter to open, and/or abnormal movement of the hyoid bone and the larynx with a swallow (Fig. 284-1). Motility studies demonstrate a reduced amplitude of pharyngeal and upper esophageal contractions and reduced basal upper esophageal sphincter pressure without further relaxation on swallowing (Fig. 284-3). Patients with myasthenia gravis (Chap. 380) and polymyositis (Chap. 382) respond to treatment. Dysphagia resulting from a cerebrovascular accident improves with time, although often not completely. Treatment consists of maneuvers to reduce pharyngeal stasis and enhance airway protection under the direction of a trained swallow therapist. Feeding by a nasogastric tube or an endoscopically placed gastrostomy tube may be necessary for nutritional support; however, these maneuvers do not provide protection against aspiration of salivary secretions. Cricopharyngeal myotomy is sometimes performed, but its usefulness is

unproven. Extensive operative procedures to prevent aspiration are rarely needed. Death is often due to pulmonary complications.

Cricopharyngeal Bar Failure of the cricopharyngeus to relax on swallowing appears as a prominent bar on the posterior wall of the pharynx on barium swallow (Fig. 284-1). A transient cricopharyngeal bar is seen in up to 5% of individuals without dysphagia undergoing upper gastrointestinal studies; it can be produced in normal individuals during a Valsalva maneuver. A persistent cricopharyngeal bar may be caused by fibrosis in the cricopharyngeus. Some of these patients complain of food sticking in their throats. Cricopharyngeal myotomy may be helpful but is contraindicated in the presence of gastroesophageal reflux because it may lead to pharyngeal and pulmonary aspiration.

Globus Pharyngeus A sensation of a constant lump in the throat, but no difficulty in swallowing, occurs especially in individuals with emotional disorders, particularly women. Results of barium studies and manometry are normal. Treatment consists primarily of reassurance. Some patients with globus pharyngeus have associated reflux esophagitis, and they may respond to treatment of the esophagitis.

SMOOTH MUSCLE Achalasia Achalasia is a motor disorder of the esophageal smooth muscle in which the LES does not relax normally with swallowing, and the esophageal body undergoes nonperistaltic contractions.

Pathophysiology The underlying abnormality is the loss of intramural neurons. Inhibitory neurons containing VIP and nitric oxide synthase are predominantly involved, but in advanced disease cholinergic neurons are also affected. Primary idiopathic achalasia accounts for most of the patients seen in the United States. Secondary achalasia may be caused by gastric carcinoma that infiltrates the esophagus, lymphoma, Chagas' disease, certain viral infections, eosinophilic gastroenteritis, and neurodegenerative disorders.

Clinical features Achalasia affects patients of all ages and both sexes. Dysphagia, chest pain, and regurgitation are the main symptoms. Dysphagia appears early, occurs with both liquids and solids, and is worsened by emotional stress and hurried eating. Various maneuvers designed to increase intraesophageal pressure, including the Valsalva maneuver, may aid the passage of the bolus into the stomach. Regurgitation and pulmonary aspiration occur because of retention of large volumes of saliva and ingested food in the esophagus. Patients may complain of difficulty belching. The presence of gastroesophageal reflux argues against achalasia; and in patients with long-standing heartburn, cessation of heartburn and appearance of dysphagia suggest development of achalasia on top of reflux esophagitis. The course is usually chronic, with progressive dysphagia and weight loss over months to years. Achalasia associated with carcinoma is characterized by severe weight loss and a rapid downhill course if untreated.

Diagnosis A chest x-ray shows absence of the gastric air bubble and sometimes a tubular mediastinal mass beside the aorta. An air-fluid level in the mediastinum in the upright position represents retained food in the esophagus. Barium swallow shows esophageal dilation, and in advanced cases the esophagus may become sigmoid. On fluoroscopy, normal peristalsis is lost in the lower two-thirds of the esophagus. The terminal part of the esophagus shows a persistent beak-like narrowing representing the nonrelaxing LES (Fig. 284-1).

Manometry shows the basal LES pressure to be normal or elevated, and swallow-induced relaxation either does not occur or is reduced in degree, duration, and consistency. The esophageal body shows an elevated resting pressure. In response to swallows, primary peristaltic waves are replaced by simultaneous-onset contractions (Fig. 284-3).

These contractions may be of poor amplitude (classic achalasia) or of large amplitude and long duration (vigorous achalasia). Cholecystokinin (CCK), which normally causes a fall in the sphincter pressure, paradoxically causes contraction of the LES (the CCK test). This paradoxical response occurs because, in achalasia, the neurally transmitted inhibitory effect of CCK is absent owing to the loss of inhibitory neurons. Endoscopy is helpful in excluding the secondary causes of achalasia, particularly gastric carcinoma.

℞ **TREATMENT** Treatment with soft foods, sedatives, and anticholinergic drugs is usually unsatisfactory. Nitrates and calcium channel blockers provide short-term benefit, but their use may be limited by side effects. Nitroglycerin, 0.3 to 0.6 mg, is used sublingually before meals and as needed for chest pain. Isosorbide dinitrate, 2.5 to 5 mg sublingually or 10 to 20 mg orally, is used before meals. Nitrates are associated with headache and postural hypotension. The calcium channel blocker nifedipine, 10 to 20 mg orally or sublingually before meals, is also effective. Endoscopic intrasphincteric injection of botulinum toxin is effective over a short period in some patients. Repeated injections may lead to fibrosis, complicating further operative therapy. Botulinum toxin acts by blocking cholinergic excitatory nerves in the sphincter. Balloon dilatation reduces the basal LES pressure by tearing muscle fibers. In experienced hands, this technique is effective in ~85% of patients. Perforation and bleeding are potential complications. Heller's extramucosal myotomy of the LES, in which the circular muscle layer is incised, is equally effective. Laparoscopic myotomy is the procedure of choice. Reflux esophagitis and peptic stricture may follow successful treatment (more often with myotomy than with balloon dilatation).

Diffuse Esophageal Spasm and Related Motor Disorders
These disorders present with clinical symptoms of chest pain and dysphagia and are recognized by their manometric features. In pure form, they all show normal relaxation to swallows. Diffuse esophageal spasm is characterized by nonperistaltic contractions, usually of large amplitude and long duration. An esophageal motility pattern showing hypertensive but peristaltic contractions has been called "nutcracker esophagus."

Pathophysiology Nonperistaltic contractions are due to dysfunction of inhibitory nerves. Histopathologic studies show patchy neural degeneration localized to nerve processes, rather than the prominent degeneration of nerve cell bodies seen in achalasia. Diffuse esophageal spasm may progress to achlasia. Hypertensive peristaltic contractions and hypertensive or hypercontracting LES may represent cholinergic or myogenic hyperactivity.

Clinical features Diffuse spasm and related motor disorders cannot be distinguished clinically. They all present with chest pain, dysphagia, or both. Chest pain is particularly marked in patients with esophageal contractions of large amplitude and long duration. Chest pain usually occurs at rest but may be brought on by swallowing or by emotional stress. The pain is retrosternal; it may radiate to the back, the sides of the chest, both arms, or the sides of the jaw and may last from a few seconds to several minutes. It may be acute and severe, mimicking the pain of myocardial ischemia. Dysphagia for solids and liquids may occur with or without chest pain and is correlated particularly with simultaneous-onset contractions.

Diffuse esophageal spasm and related esophageal motor disorders must be differentiated from other causes of chest pain, particularly ischemic heart disease with atypical angina. A complete cardiac workup should be done before a noncardiac etiology is considered seriously. The presence of dysphagia in association with pain should point to the esophagus as the site of disease. Esophageal motility disorders are an uncommon cause of noncardiac chest pain, which is more commonly due to reflux esophagitis or visceral hypersensitivity.

Diagnosis In diffuse esophageal spasm, barium swallow shows that normal sequential peristalsis below the aortic arch is replaced by uncoordinated simultaneous contractions that produce the appearance of curling or multiple ripples in the wall, sacculations, and pseudodiverticula—the "corkscrew" esophagus (Fig. 284-1). Sometimes an esophageal contraction obliterates the lumen, and barium is pushed away in both directions. The barium swallow is frequently normal in diffuse esophageal spasm and mostly normal in the related disorders.

Diffuse esophageal spasm (Fig. 284-3) and related motor disorders (hypertensive peristaltic contraction, hypertensive LES and hypercontracting LES) are manometric diagnoses. Because these abnormalities may be episodic, the results of manometry may be normal at the time of the study. Several techniques are used to provoke esophageal spasm. Cold swallows produce the chest pain but do not produce spasm on manometric studies. Solid boluses and pharmacologic agents, particularly edrophonium, induce both chest pain and motor abnormalities. However, correlation between induction of pain and motility changes is poor. The usefulness of pharmacologic provocative tests is limited.

℞ **TREATMENT** Anticholinergics are usually of limited value. Agents that relax smooth muscle, such as sublingual nitroglycerin (0.3 to 0.6 mg) or longer-acting agents such as isosorbide dinitrate (10 to 30 mg orally before meals) and nifedipine (10 to 20 mg orally before meals) are helpful. Sublingual forms of these agents can also be used. Reassurance and tranquilizers are helpful in allaying apprehension.

Scleroderma Esophagus The esophageal lesions in systemic sclerosis consist of atrophy of smooth muscle, manifested by weakness in the lower two-thirds of the esophageal body and incompetence of the LES. The esophageal wall is thin and atrophic and may exhibit areas of patchy fibrosis. Patients usually present with dysphagia to solids. Liquids may cause dysphagia when the patient is recumbent. These patients usually also complain of heartburn, regurgitation, and other symptoms of gastroesophageal reflux disease (GERD). Barium swallow shows dilation and loss of peristaltic contractions in the middle and distal portions of the esophagus. The LES is patulous, and gastroesophageal reflux may occur freely (Fig. 284-1). Mucosal changes due to esophageal ulceration and esophageal stricture may be present. Motility studies show a marked reduction in the amplitude of smooth-muscle contractions, which may be peristaltic or nonperistaltic. The resting pressure of the LES is subnormal, but sphincter relaxation is normal (Fig. 284-3). Similar esophageal motor abnormalities are found in other collagen vascular diseases and in Raynaud's syndrome alone. Dietary adjustments with the use of soft foods are helpful in management. GERD and its complications should be treated aggressively.

GASTROESOPHAGEAL REFLUX DISEASE

GERD is one of the most prevalent gastrointestinal disorders. Population-based studies show that up to 15% of individuals have heartburn at least once a week and about 7% have heartburn daily. Symptoms are caused by back flow of gastric acid and other gastric contents into the esophagus due to incompetent barriers at the gastroesophageal junction.

Pathophysiology The normal antireflux mechanisms consist of the LES, the crural diaphragm, and the anatomic location of the gastroesophageal junction below the diaphragmatic hiatus. Reflux occurs only when the gradient of pressure between the LES and the stomach is lost. It can be caused by a sustained or transient decrease in LES tone. A sustained hypotension of the LES may be due to muscle weakness that is often without apparent cause. Secondary causes of LES incompetence include scleroderma-like diseases, myopathy associated with chronic intestinal pseudo-obstruction, pregnancy, smoking, anticholinergic drugs, smooth-muscle relaxants [β-adrenergic agents, aminophylline, nitrates, calcium channel blockers, phosphodiesterase inhibitors that increase cyclic AMP or cyclic GMP (including sildenofil)], surgical destruction of the LES, and esophagitis. tLESR without associated esophageal contraction is due to a vagal reflex in which LES relaxation is elicited by gastric distention. Increased tLESR is associated with GERD. A similar reflex operates during belching. Apart from incompetent barriers, gastric contents are most likely to reflux (1) when gastric volume is increased (after meals, in pyloric obstruction, in gastric stasis, during acid hypersecretion states), (2) when gastric contents are near the gastroesophageal junction (in recumbency, bending down, hiatus hernia), and (3) when gastric pressure is increased (obesity, pregnancy, ascites, tight clothes). Incompetence of the diaphragmatic crural muscle, which surrounds the esophageal hiatus in the diaphragm and functions as an external LES, also predisposes to GERD.

The total exposure of the esophagus to refluxed acid correlates with potential for mucosal damage. Exposure depends on the amount of refluxed material per episode, frequency of episodes, and rate of clearing the esophagus by gravity and peristaltic contractions. When peristaltic contractions are impaired, esophageal clearance is impaired. Acid refluxed into the esophagus is neutralized by saliva. Thus, impaired salivary secretion also increases esophageal exposure time. If the refluxed material extends to the cervical esophagus and breaches the upper sphincter, it can enter the pharynx, larynx, and trachea, causing chronic cough, bronchoconstriction, pharyngitis, laryngitis, or bronchitis.

Reflux esophagitis is a complication of reflux and develops when mucosal defenses are unable to counteract the damage done by acid, pepsin, and bile. *Mild esophagitis* involves microscopic changes of mucosal infiltration with granulocytes or eosinophils, hyperplasia of basal cells, and elongation of dermal pegs. Endoscopic appearance may be normal. *Erosive esophagitis* involves endoscopically apparent mucosal damage, redness, friability, bleeding, superficial, linear ulcers, and exudates. *Peptic stricture* results from fibrosis that causes lumenal constriction. These strictures occur in ~10% of patients with untreated GERD. Short strictures caused by spontaneous reflux are usually 1 to 3 cm long and are present in the distal esophagus near the squamocolumnar junction (Fig. 284-2). Long, tubular peptic strictures can result from persistent vomiting or prolonged nasogastric intubation. Erosive esophagitis may cause bleeding and heal by intestinal metaplasia (*Barrett's esophagus*) that is a risk factor for adenocarcinoma.

Clinical Features　Regurgitation of sour material in the mouth and heartburn are the characteristic symptoms of GERD. Heartburn is produced by the contact of refluxed material with the inflamed or sensitized esophageal mucosa. Angina-like or atypical chest pain occurs in some patients, while others experience no heartburn or chest pain. Persistent dysphagia suggests development of a peptic stricture. Most patients with peptic stricture have a history of several years of heartburn preceding dysphagia. However, in one-third of patients, dysphagia is the presenting symptom. Rapidly progressive dysphagia and weight loss may indicate the development of adenocarcinoma in Barrett's esophagus. Bleeding occurs due to mucosal erosions or Barrett's ulcer. Severe reflux may reach the pharynx and mouth and result in laryngitis, morning hoarseness, and pulmonary aspiration. Recurrent pulmonary aspiration can cause aspiration pneumonia, pulmonary fibrosis, or chronic asthma. By contrast, many patients with GERD remain asymptomatic or self-treated and do not seek attention until severe complications occur.

Diagnosis　The diagnostic approach to GERD can be divided into three categories:

1. documentation of mucosal injury,
2. documentation and quantitation of reflux, and
3. definition of the pathophysiology.

Reflux esophagitis and its complications are documented by the use of barium swallow, esophagoscopy, and mucosal biopsy. The results of barium swallow are usually normal in uncomplicated esophagitis but may reveal a stricture or ulcer. A high esophageal peptic stricture, a deep ulcer, or adenocarcinoma suggest Barrett's esophagus. Uncomplicated Barrett's esophagus is not diagnosed reliably by barium studies. Esophagoscopy may reveal the presence of erosive esoph-

agitis, distal peptic stricture, or a columnar-cell-lined lower esophagus with or without a proximally located peptic stricture, ulcer, or adenocarcinoma. Results of esophagoscopy may be normal in many patients with esophagitis; in such patients, mucosal biopsies and the Bernstein test are helpful. The mucosal biopsies should be performed at least 5 cm above the LES, because the esophageal mucosal changes of chronic esophagitis are quite frequent in the most distal esophagus in otherwise normal individuals. About 10% of biopsies yield a false-positive or false-negative result. The Bernstein test involves the infusion of solutions of 0.1 N HCl and normal saline into the esophagus. It is useful in diagnosing reflux esophagitis that is not endoscopically obvious. In patients with reflux esophagitis, infusion of acid, but not of saline, reproduces the symptoms of heartburn. Infusion of acid in normal individuals usually produces no symptoms. Supraesophageal manifestations are diagnosed by careful otolaryngological exam.

A therapeutic trial with a proton pump inhibitor (such as omeprazole, 40 mg bid) for 1 week provides strong support for the diagnosis of GERD.

Documentation and quantitation of reflux when necessary can be done by ambulatory long-term (24-h) esophageal pH recording. For evaluation of pharyngeal reflux, a system of recording simultaneously from pharyngeal and esophageal sites may be useful. The pH recordings are helpful only in the evaluation of acid reflux. The presence of bile or intestinal alkaline secretions is suggested by the occurrence of reflux symptoms in the absence of gastric acid and demonstration of bile in an aspirate of esophageal reflux fluid. Documentation of reflux is necessary only when the role of reflux in the symptom complex is unclear, particularly in evaluation of supraesophageal symptoms and chest pain without endoscopic evidence of esophagitis.

Definition of pathophysiologic factors in GERD is sometimes indicated for management decisions such as antireflux surgery. Esophageal motility studies may provide useful quantitative information on the competence of the LES and on esophageal motor function.

℞ TREATMENT　The goals of treatment are to decrease gastroesophageal reflux, render the refluxate harmless, improve esophageal clearance, and protect the esophageal mucosa. The management of uncomplicated cases generally includes weight reduction, sleeping with the head of the bed elevated by about 4 to 6 in. with blocks, and elimination of factors that increase abdominal pressure. Patients should not smoke and should avoid consuming fatty foods, coffee, chocolate, alcohol, mint, orange juice, and certain medications (such as anticholinergic drugs, calcium channel blockers, and other smooth-muscle relaxants). They should also avoid ingesting large quantities of fluids with meals. In mild cases, life-style changes and over-the-counter antisecretory agents may be adequate. In moderate cases, H_2 receptor blocking agents (cimetidine, 300 mg; ranitidine, 150 mg bid; famotidine, 20 mg bid; nizatidine 150 mg bid) for 6 to 12 weeks are effective in symptom relief. Higher doses are necessary for healing erosive esophagitis, but proton pump inhibitors (PPIs) are more effective in this setting.

In cases resistant to H_2 receptor blockers and severe cases, rigorous acid suppression with a PPI is recommended. The PPIs are comparably effective: omeprazole (40 mg/d), lansoprazole (30 mg/d), pantoprazole (40 mg/d), and rabeprazole (20 mg/d) for 8 weeks can heal erosive esophagitis in up to 90% of patients. Reflux esophagitis requires prolonged therapy, for 3 to 6 months or longer if the disease recurs quickly. After initial therapy, a lower maintenance dose of PPI is used. Side effects are minimal. Aggressive acid suppression causes hypergastrinemia but does not increase the risk for carcinoid tumors or gastrinomas. Vitamin B_{12} absorption is compromised by the treatment. Patients with reflux esophagitis who have complications, such as Barrett's esophagus with concomitant esophagitis, should be treated vigorously. Patients who have an associated peptic stricture are treated with dilators to relieve dysphagia as well as provided with vigorous treatment for reflux.

Antireflux surgery, in which the gastric fundus is wrapped around the esophagus (fundoplication), increases the LES pressure and should be considered for patients with resistant and complicated reflux esophagitis that does not respond fully to medical therapy or for patients for whom long-term medical therapy is not desirable. Laparoscopic fundoplication is the surgery of choice. Ideal candidates for fundoplication are those in whom motility studies show persistently inadequate LES pressure but normal peristaltic contractions in the esophageal body.

Patients with alkaline esophagitis are treated with general antireflux measures and neutralization of bile salts with cholestyramine, aluminum hydroxide, or sucralfate. Sucralfate is particularly useful in these cases, as it also serves as a mucosal protector.

BARRETT'S ESOPHAGUS The metaplasia of esophageal squamous epithelium to columnar epithelium (Barrett's esophagus) is a complication of severe reflux esophagitis, and it is a risk factor for esophageal adenocarcinoma (Chap. 90). Metaplastic columnar epithelium develops during healing of erosive esophagitis with continued acid reflux because columnar epithelium is more resistant to acid-pepsin damage than squamous epithelium. The metaplastic epithelium is a mosaic of different epithelial types including goblet cells and columnar cells that have features of both secretory and absorptive cells (incomplete or type III metaplasia). Barrett's epithelium progresses through a dysplastic stage before developing into adenocarcinoma. The rate of cancer development is 1 in 200 patient years; those with longer than 2 to 3 cm of intestinal metaplasia have a risk of developing esophageal cancer that is 30 to 125 times the risk of the general population.

Given the natural history, reflux esophagitis should be aggressively treated with drugs, and erosive esophagitis should be treated with drugs and surgery, if necessary, to prevent Barrett's esophagus. The prevalence of intestinal metaplasia is estimated at 4 to 10% of patients with significant heartburn. Barrett's esophagus is more common in men, particularly white men, and prevalence increases with age. A one-time esophagoscopy is recommended in patients with persistent GERD symptoms at age 50. Established metaplasia does not regress with treatment; thus, acid suppression and fundoplication are indicated only when active esophagitis is also present.

The need and frequency of surveillance endoscopies in patients with established Barrett's esophagus are debated. The risk of developing esophageal adenocarcinoma is related to the length of involved esophageal mucosa. People with short segments of Barrett's esophagus (distal 2 to 3 cm) account for up to 25% of unselected patients undergoing endoscopy with or without GERD symptoms and appear to be at low risk. They are not routinely surveyed. However, those with long-segment Barrett's esophagus (>3 cm) are advised to have endoscopic surveillance at 1-year intervals for 2 years and then every 2 to 3 years. The frequency is increased if dysplasia is detected independent of the length of the metaplasia. Optical methods of recognizing dysplasia during the endoscopy (laser-induced fluorescence spectroscopy, optical coherence tomography) are being developed. Once high-grade dysplasia is detected, treatment of choice is esophagectomy of the Barrett's segment. Photodynamic laser or thermocoagulative mucosal ablation and endoscopic mucosal resection are being evaluated as alternatives.

Barrett's esophagus can also lead to chronic peptic ulcer of the esophagus with high (midesophageal) and long strictures.

INFLAMMATORY DISORDERS

INFECTIOUS ESOPHAGITIS Infectious esophagitis can be due to viral, bacterial, fungal, or parasitic organisms. In severely immunocompromised patients, multiple organisms may coexist.

Viral Esophagitis *Herpes simplex virus* (HSV) type 1 occasionally causes esophagitis in immunocompetent individuals, but either HSV type 1 or HSV type 2 may afflict patients who are immunosuppressed (Chap. 182). Patients complain of an acute onset of chest pain, odynophagia, and dysphagia. Bleeding may occur in severe cases; and systemic manifestations such as nausea, vomiting, fever, chills, and mild leukocytosis may be present. Herpetic vesicles on the nose and

lips may provide a clue to the diagnosis. Barium swallow is inadequate to detect early lesions and cannot reliably distinguish HSV infection from other types of infections. Endoscopy shows vesicles and small, discrete, punched-out superficial ulcerations with or without a fibrinous exudate. In later stages, a diffuse erosive esophagitis develops from enlargement and coalescence of the ulcers. Mucosal cells from a biopsy sample taken at the edge of an ulcer or from a cytologic smear show ballooning degeneration, ground-glass changes in the nuclei with eosinophilic intranuclear inclusions (Cowdry type A), and giant cell formation on routine stains. Culture for HSV becomes positive within days and is helpful in diagnosis. In patients with severe odynophagia, intravenous acyclovir, 400 mg five times a day, is usually initiated. Symptoms usually resolve in 1 week, but large ulcerations may take longer to heal. Foscarnet (90 mg/kg intravenously every 8 h) is used if resistance to acyclovir occurs.

Varicella-zoster virus (VZV) (Chap. 183) sometimes produces esophagitis in children with chickenpox and adults with herpes zoster. Esophageal VZV also can be the source of disseminated VZV infection without skin involvement. In an immunocompromised host, VZV esophagitis causes vesicles and confluent ulcers and usually resolves spontaneously, but it may cause necrotizing esophagitis in a severely compromised host. On routine histologic examination of mucosal biopsy samples or cytology specimens, VZV is difficult to distinguish from HSV, but the distinction can be made immunohistologically or by culture. Acyclovir reduces the duration of symptoms in VZV esophagitis.

Cytomegalovirus (CMV) infections (Chap. 185) occur only in immunocompromised patients. CMV is usually activated from a latent stage or may be acquired from blood product transfusions. CMV lesions initially appear as serpiginous ulcers in an otherwise normal mucosa. These may coalesce to form giant ulcers, particularly in the distal esophagus.

Patients present with odynophagia, chest pain, hematemesis, nausea, and vomiting. Diagnosis requires endoscopy and biopsies of the ulcer. Mucosal brushings are not useful. Routine histologic examination shows intranuclear and small intracytoplasmic inclusions in large fibroblasts and endothelial cells. Immunohistology with monoclonal antibodies to CMV and in situ hybridization of CMV DNA on centrifugation culture and are useful for early diagnosis. Ganciclovir, 5 mg/kg every 12 h intravenously, is the treatment of choice. Foscarnet (90 mg/kg every 12 h intravenously) is used in resistant cases. Therapy is continued until healing occurs, which may take 2 to 4 weeks.

HIV (Chap. 309) may be associated with a self-limited syndrome of acute esophageal ulceration associated with oral ulcers and a maculopapular skin rash, which occurs at the time of HIV seroconversion. Some patients with advanced disease have deep, persistent esophageal ulcers requiring treatment with oral glucocorticoids or thalidomide. Some ulcers respond to local steroid injection.

Bacterial Esophagitis *Bacterial esophagitis* is unusual, but esophagitis caused by *Lactobacillus* and β-hemolytic streptococci can occur in the immunocompromised host. In patients with profound granulocytopenia and patients with cancer, bacterial esophagitis is often missed because it is commonly present with other organisms, including viruses and fungi. In patients with AIDS, infection with *Cryptosporidium* or *Pneumocystis carinii* may cause nonspecific inflammation, and *Mycobacterium tuberculosis* infection may cause deep ulcerations of the distal esophagus.

Candida Esophagitis *Candida* species are normal commensals in the throat but become pathogenic and produce esophagitis in immunodeficiency states. *Candida* esophagitis can occur without any predisposing factors. Patients may be asymptomatic or complain of odynophagia and dysphagia. Oral thrush or other evidence of mucocutaneous candidiasis may be absent. Rarely, *Candida* esophagitis is complicated by esophageal bleeding, perforation, and stricture or by systemic invasion. Barium swallow may be normal or show multiple nodular filling defects of various sizes (Fig. 284-2). Large nodular defects may resemble grape clusters. Endoscopy shows small, yellow-white raised plaques with surrounding erythema in mild disease. Confluent linear and nodular plaques reflect extensive disease. Diagnosis is made by demonstration of yeast or hyphal forms in plaque smears and exudate stained with periodic acid–Schiff or Gomori silver stains. Histologic examination is often negative. Culture is not useful in diagnosis but may define the species and the drug sensitivities of the yeast (Chap. 205). Fluconazole (200 mg on the first day, followed by 100 mg daily) is the preferred treatment of esophageal candidiasis because it is effective and its absorption is not affected by high gastric pH. Fluconazole is available in oral and intravenous formulations. Ketoconazole (200 to 400 mg in a single daily oral dose) is also effective treatment, and the higher dose is used in severely immunocompromised hosts; however, its bioavailability is severely reduced at increased gastric pH. Patients who respond poorly are treated with amphotericin, 10 to 15 mg as an intravenous infusion for 6 h daily to a total dose of 300 to 500 mg. Nystatin oral suspension (100,000 units per ml) in doses of 10 to 20 mL every 6 h is effective for oral thrush. In resistant cases, amphotericin lozenges are used for 7 to 10 days followed by nystatin or fluconazole for as long as the host resistance remains low.

OTHER TYPES OF ESOPHAGITIS   *Radiation esophagitis* is a common occurrence during radiation treatment for thoracic cancers. The frequency and severity of esophagitis increase with the amount of radiation delivered and may be enhanced by radiosensitizing drugs like doxorubicin, bleomycin, cyclophosphamide, and cisplatin. Dysphagia and odynophagia may last several weeks to several months after therapy. The esophageal mucosa becomes erythematous, edematous, and friable. Superficial erosions coalesce to form larger superficial ulcers. Submucosal fibrosis and degenerative changes in the blood vessels, muscles, and myenteric neurons may occur. The treatment is relief of pain with viscous lidocaine during the acute phase; indomethacin treatment may reduce radiation damage. Esophageal stricture may develop.

Corrosive esophagitis is caused by the ingestion of caustic agents, such as strong alkali or acid. Severe corrosive injury may lead to esophageal perforation, bleeding, and death. Glucocorticoids are not useful in acute corrosive esophagitis. Healing is usually associated with stricture formation. Caustic strictures are usually long and rigid (Fig. 284-2) and generally require dilatation with dilators passed over a guidewire through the stricture. *Pill-induced esophagitis* is associated with the ingestion of certain types of pills and occurs most often in bedridden patients. Antibiotics such as doxycycline, tetracycline, oxytetracycline, minocycline, penicillin, and clindamycin account for more than half the cases. Nonsteroidal anti-inflammatory agents such as aspirin, indomethacin, and ibuprofen may cause injury. Other commonly prescribed pills that cause esophageal injury include potassium chloride, ferrous sulfate or succinate, quinidine, alprenolol, theophylline, ascorbic acid, pinaverum bromide, alendronate, and pamidronate. Pill esophagitis can be prevented by avoiding the offending agents or by having patients take pills in the upright position and wash them down with copious amounts of fluids.

Sclerotherapy for bleeding esophageal varices usually produces transient retrosternal chest pain and dysphagia; esophageal ulcer, stricture, hematoma, or perforation may occur. Variceal banding causes similar complications but less frequently. *Esophagitis associated with mucocutaneous and systemic diseases* is usually associated with blister and bulla formation, epithelial desquamation, and thin, weblike, or dense esophageal strictures. Pemphigus vulgaris and bullous pemphigoid form intraepithelial and subepithelial bullae, respectively, and can be distinguished by specific immunohistology; both are characterized by sloughing of epithelium or the presence of esophageal casts. Glucocorticoid treatment is usually effective. Cicatricial pemphigoid, Stevens-Johnson syndrome, and toxic epidermolysis bullosa can produce esophageal bullous lesions and strictures requiring gentle dilatation. Graft-versus-host disease occurs in patients who have received allo-geneic bone marrow transplants and is associated with generalized desquamation and esophageal strictures. Behçet's disease and eosinophilic gastroenteritis may involve the esophagus and may respond to glucocorticoid therapy. An erosive lichen planus also can involve the esophagus. Crohn's disease may cause inflammatory strictures, sinus tracts, filiform polyps, and fistulas in the esophagus.

OTHER ESOPHAGEAL DISORDERS

DIVERTICULA   Diverticula are outpouchings of the wall of the esophagus. A *Zenker's diverticulum* appears in the natural zone of weakness in the posterior hypopharyngeal wall (Killian's triangle) and causes halitosis and regurgitation of saliva and food particles consumed several days previously. When it becomes large and filled with food, such a diverticulum can compress the esophagus and cause dysphagia or complete obstruction. Nasogastric intubation and endoscopy should be performed with utmost care in these patients, since they may cause perforation of the diverticulum. A *midesophageal diverticulum* may be caused by traction from old adhesions or by propulsion associated with esophageal motor abnormalities. An *epiphrenic diverticulum* may be associated with achalasia. Small or medium-sized diverticula and midesophageal and epiphrenic diverticula are usually asymptomatic. *Diffuse intramural diverticulosis* of the esophagus is due to dilation of the deep esophageal glands and may lead to chronic candidiasis or to the development of a stricture high up in the esophagus. These patients may present with dysphagia. Symptomatic Zenker's diverticula are treated by cricopharyngeal myotomy with or without diverticulectomy. Very large symptomatic esophageal diverticula are removed surgically. When they are associated with motor abnormalities, distal myotomy is performed. Strictures associated with diffuse intramural diverticulosis are treated with rubber dilators.

WEBS AND RINGS   Weblike constrictions of the esophagus are usually congenital or inflammatory in origin. Asymptomatic hypopharyngeal webs are demonstrated in <10% of normal individuals. When concentric, they cause intermittent dysphagia to solids. The combination of symptomatic hypopharyngeal webs and iron-deficiency anemia in middle-aged women constitutes *Plummer-Vinson syndrome*. The clinical importance of this syndrome is uncertain. Midesophageal webs are rare. A *lower esophageal mucosal ring* (Schatzki ring) is a thin, weblike constriction located at the squamocolumnar mucosal junction at or near the border of the LES (Fig. 284-2). It invariably produces dysphagia when the lumen diameter is <1.3 cm. Dysphagia to solids is the only symptom, and it is usually episodic. Asymptomatic rings may be present in ~10% of normal individuals. A lower esophageal ring is one of the common causes of dysphagia. Symptomatic webs and mucosal lower esophageal rings are easily treated by dilatation. A *lower esophageal muscular ring* (contractile ring) is located proximal to the site of mucosal rings and may represent an abnormal uppermost segment of the LES. These rings can be recognized by the fact that they are not constant in size and shape. They also may cause dysphagia and should be differentiated from peptic strictures, achalasia, and lower esophageal mucosal ring. Muscular rings do not respond well to dilatation.

HIATAL HERNIA   A *hiatal hernia* is a herniation of part of the stomach into the thoracic cavity through the esophageal hiatus in the diaphragm. A *sliding hiatal hernia* is one in which the gastroesophageal junction and fundus of the stomach slide upward. A sliding hernia may result from weakening of the anchors of the gastroesophageal junction to the diaphragm, from longitudinal contraction of the esophagus, or from increased intraabdominal pressure. Small sliding hernias can be demonstrated commonly during barium studies if intraabdominal pressure is increased. Incidence increases with age; in individuals in the sixth decade of life, the prevalence of such hernias is ~60%. Small sliding hiatal hernias alone probably produce no symptoms but can contribute to reflux esophagitis. A *paraesophageal hernia* is one in which the esophagogastric junction remains fixed in its normal location and a pouch of stomach is herniated beside the gastroesophageal junction through the esophageal hiatus. A paraesophageal or mixed paraesophageal and sliding hernia may become incarcerated and strangulate, leading to acute chest pain, dysphagia, and a mediastinal mass and requiring surgery. A herniated gastric pouch may cause dysphagia, develop gastritis, or ulcerate, causing chronic blood loss. Large paraesophageal hernias should be surgically repaired.

MECHANICAL TRAUMA *Esophageal rupture* may be caused by (1) iatrogenic damage from instrumentation of the esophagus or external trauma, (2) increased intraesophageal pressure associated with forceful vomiting or retching (*spontaneous rupture* or *Boerhaave's syndrome*), or (3) diseases of the esophagus such as corrosive esophagitis, esophageal ulcer, and neoplasm. The site of perforation depends on the cause. Instrumental perforation usually occurs in the pharynx or lower esophagus, just above the diaphragm in the posterolateral wall. Esophageal perforation causes severe retrosternal chest pain, which may be worsened by swallowing and breathing. Free air enters the mediastinum and spreads to neighboring structures, causing palpable subcutaneous emphysema in the neck, mediastinal crackling sounds on auscultation, and pneumothorax. With time, secondary infection supervenes, and mediastinal abscess may develop. Esophageal perforation associated with vomiting usually deposits gastric contents in the mediastinum and causes severe mediastinal complications. By contrast, instrumental perforation may be clinically mild and free of severe complications. Spontaneous rupture of the esophagus may mimic myocardial infarction, pancreatitis, or rupture of an abdominal viscus. Symptoms of chest pain may be mild, particularly in the elderly. Mediastinal emphysema may develop late. An x-ray of the chest shows abnormalities in most patients, but computed tomography of the chest is more sensitive in detecting mediastinal air. Fluid from pleural effusions may have a high content of (salivary) amylase. The diagnosis is confirmed by swallow of radiopaque contrast material. Gastrograffin is used initially, and if no leak is found, a small amount of thin barium is used to confirm the diagnosis. Treatment includes esophageal and gastric suction and parenteral broad-spectrum antibiotics. Surgical drainage and repair of the laceration should be performed as soon as possible. In patients with terminal carcinoma, surgical repair may not be feasible, and patients with minor instrumental perforation can be treated conservatively. Extensive corrosive damage may require esophageal diversion and excision of the damaged portion.

Mucosal Tear (Mallory-Weiss Syndrome) This tear is usually caused by vomiting, retching, or vigorous coughing. The tear usually involves the gastric mucosa near the squamocolumnar mucosal junction. Patients present with upper gastrointestinal bleeding, which may be severe. In most patients bleeding ceases spontaneously; continued bleeding may respond to vasopressin therapy or angiographic embolization. Surgery is rarely needed.

Intramural Hematoma Emetogenic injury, particularly in patients with bleeding abnormalities, can cause bleeding between the mucosal and muscle layers of the esophagus. The patients develop sudden dysphagia. The diagnosis is made by barium swallow and computed tomography. Resolution is usually spontaneous.

FOREIGN BODIES Foreign bodies may lodge in the cervical esophagus just beyond the UES, near the aortic arch, or above the LES. Impaction of a bolus of food, particularly a piece of meat or bread, may occur when the esophageal lumen is narrowed due to stricture, carcinoma, or a lower esophageal ring. Acute impaction causes a complete inability to swallow and severe chest pain. Both foreign bodies and food boluses may be removed endoscopically. Use of a meat tenderizer to facilitate passage of a meat bolus is discouraged because of potential esophageal perforation and aspiration pneumonia.

BIBLIOGRAPHY

COOK IJ, KHARILAS PJ: AGA technical review on management of oropharyngeal dysphagia. Gastroenterology 116:455, 1999

GOYAL RK, HAMILTON FA: Columna lined (Barrett's) esophagus: Highlights of the NIDDK/VHA conference. Clinician 17 (6):1, 1999

GOYAL RK, SIVARAO DV: Functional anatomy and physiology of swallowing and esophageal motility, in *The Esophagus*, DO Castell, JE Richter (eds). Philadelphia, Lippincott, Williams and Wilkins, 1999, pp 1–31

HEUDERBERT GR et al: Choice of long-term strategy for the management of patients with severe esophagitis: A cost-utility analysis. Gastroenterology 112:1078, 1997

KIRKENDALL JW: Pill-induced esophageal injury, in *The Esophagus*, DO Castell, JE Richter (eds). Philadelphia, Lippincott, Williams and Wilkins, 1999, pp 527–37

SAMPLINER RE: The Practice Parameters Committee of the American College of Gastroenterology: Practice guidelines on the diagnosis, surveillance, and therapy of Barrett's esophagus. Am J Gastroenterol 93:1028, 1998

SHAKER R (guest ed): First multidisciplinary international symposium on supraesophageal complications of reflux disease. Am J Med 103:1S, 1997

SPECHLER SJ: AGA technical review on treatment of patients with dysphagia caused by benign disorders of the distal esophagus. Gastroenterology 117:233, 1999

285 *John Del Valle*

PEPTIC ULCER DISEASE AND RELATED DISORDERS

PEPTIC ULCER DISEASE

Burning epigastric pain exacerbated by fasting and improved with meals is a symptom complex associated with peptic ulcer disease (PUD). An *ulcer* is defined as disruption of the mucosal integrity of the stomach and/or duodenum leading to a local defect or excavation due to active inflammation. Ulcers occur within the stomach and/or duodenum and are often chronic in nature. Acid peptic disorders are very common in the United States, with 4 million individuals (new cases and recurrences) affected per year. Lifetime prevalence of PUD in the United States is approximately 12% in men and 10% in women. Moreover, an estimated 15,000 deaths per year occur as a consequence of complicated PUD. The financial impact of these common disorders has been substantial, with an estimated burden on health care costs of >\$15 billion per year in the United States.

GASTRIC PHYSIOLOGY Despite the constant attack on the gastroduodenal mucosa by a host of noxious agents (acid, pepsin, bile acids, pancreatic enzymes, drugs, and bacteria), integrity is maintained by an intricate system that provides mucosal defense and repair.

Gastric Anatomy The gastric epithelial lining consists of rugae that contain microscopic gastric pits, each branching into four or five gastric glands made up of highly specialized epithelial cells. The makeup of gastric glands varies with their anatomic location. Glands within the gastric cardia comprise <5% of the gastric gland area and contain mucous and endocrine cells. The majority of gastric glands (75%) are found within the oxyntic mucosa and contain mucous neck, parietal, chief, endocrine, and enterochromaffin cells (Fig. 285-1). Pyloric glands contain mucous and endocrine cells (including gastrin cells) and are found in the antrum.

The parietal cell, also known as the oxyntic cell, is usually found in the neck, or isthmus, or the oxyntic gland. The resting, or unstimulated, parietal cell has prominent cytoplasmic tubulovesicles and intracellular canaliculi containing short microvilli along its apical surface (Fig. 285-2). H^+, K^+-ATPase is expressed in the tubulovesicle membrane; upon cell stimulation, this membrane, along with apical membranes, transforms into a dense network of apical intracellular canaliculi containing long microvilli. Acid secretion, a process requiring high energy, occurs at the apical canalicular surface. Numerous mitochondria (30 to 40% of total cell volume) generate the energy required for secretion.

Gastroduodenal Mucosal Defense The gastric epithelium is under a constant assault by a series of endogenous noxious factors including HCl, pepsinogen/pepsin, and bile salts. In addition, a steady flow of exogenous substances such as medications, alcohol, and bacteria encounter the gastric mucosa. A highly intricate biologic system is in place to provide defense from mucosal injury and to repair any injury that may occur.

The mucosal defense system can be envisioned as a three-level

FIGURE 285-1 Diagramatic representation of the oxyntic gastric gland. *(Adapted from S Ito, RJ Winchester: Cell Biol 16:541, 1963.)*

barrier, composed of preepithelial, epithelial, and subepithelial elements (Fig. 285-3). The first line of defense is a mucus-bicarbonate layer, which serves as a physicochemical barrier to multiple molecules including hydrogen ions. Mucus is secreted in a regulated fashion by gastroduodenal surface epithelial cells. It consists primarily of water (95%) and a mixture of lipids and glycoproteins. Mucin is the constituent glycoprotein that, in combination with phospholipids (also secreted by gastric mucous cells), forms a hydrophobic surface with fatty acids that extend into the lumen from the cell membrane. The mucous gel functions as a nonstirred water layer impeding diffusion of ions and molecules such as pepsin. Bicarbonate, secreted by surface epithelial cells of the gastroduodenal mucosa into the mucous gel, forms a pH gradient ranging from 1 to 2 at the gastric luminal surface and reaching 6 to 7 along the epithelial cell surface. Bicarbonate secretion

FIGURE 285-2 Gastric parietal cell undergoing transformation after secretagogue-mediated stimulation. *(Adapted from SJ Hersey, G Sachs: Physiol Rev 75:155, 1995.)*

is stimulated by calcium, prostaglandins, cholinergic input, and luminal acidification.

Surface epithelial cells provide the next line of defense through several factors, including mucus production, epithelial cell ionic transporters that maintain intracellular pH and bicarbonate production, and intracellular tight junctions. If the preepithelial barrier were breached, gastric epithelial cells bordering a site of injury can migrate to restore a damaged region (*restitution*). This process occurs independent of cell division and requires uninterrupted blood flow and an alkaline pH in the surrounding environment. Several growth factors including epidermal growth factor (EGF), transforming growth factor (TGF) α, and basic fibroblast growth factor (FGF) modulate the process of restitution. Larger defects that are not effectively repaired by restitution require cell proliferation. Epithelial cell regeneration is regulated by prostaglandins and growth factors such as EGF and TGF-α. In tandem with epithelial cell renewal, formation of new vessels (*angiogenesis*) within the injured microvascular bed occurs. Both FGF and vascular endothelial growth factor (VEGF) are important in regulating angiogenesis in the gastric mucosa.

An elaborate microvascular system within the gastric submucosal layer is the key component of the subepithelial defense/repair system. A rich submucosal circulatory bed provides HCO_3^-, which neutralizes the acid generated by parietal cell secretion of HCl. Moreover, this microcirculatory bed provides an adequate supply of micronutrients and oxygen while removing toxic metabolic by-products.

Prostaglandins play a central role in gastric epithelial defense/repair (Fig. 285-4). The gastric mucosa contains abundant levels of prostaglandins. These metabolites of arachidonic acid regulate the release of mucosal bicarbonate and mucus, inhibit parietal cell secretion, and are important in maintaining mucosal blood flow and epithelial cell restitution. Prostaglandins are derived from esterified arachidonic acid, which is formed from phospholipids (cell membrane) by the action of phospholipase A_2. A key enzyme that controls the rate-limiting step in prostaglandin synthesis is cyclooxygenase (COX), which is present in two isoforms (COX-1, COX-2), each having distinct characteristics regarding structure, tissue distribution, and expression. COX-1 is expressed in a host of tissues including the stomach, platelets, kidneys, and endothelial cells. This isoform is expressed in a constitutive manner and plays an important role in maintaining the integrity of renal function, platelet aggregation, and gastrointestinal mucosal integrity. In contrast, the expression of COX-2 is inducible by inflammatory stimuli, and it is expressed in macrophages, leukocytes, fibroblasts, and synovial cells. The beneficial effects of nonsteroidal anti-inflammatory drugs (NSAIDs) on tissue inflammation are due to inhibition of COX-2; the toxicity of these drugs (e.g., gastrointestinal mucosal ulceration and renal dysfunction) is related to inhibition of the COX-1 isoform. The highly COX-2-selective NSAIDs have the potential to provide the beneficial effect of decreasing tissue inflammation while minimizing toxicity in the gastrointestinal tract (see below).

Physiology of Gastric Secretion   Hydrochloric acid and pepsinogen are the two principal gastric secretory products capable of inducing mucosal injury. Acid secretion should be viewed as occurring under basal and stimulated conditions. Basal acid production occurs in a circadian pattern, with highest levels occurring during the night and lowest levels during the morning hours. Cholinergic input via the vagus nerve and histaminergic input from local gastric sources (see below) are the principal contributors to basal acid secretion. Stimulated gastric acid secretion occurs primarily in three phases based on the site where the signal originates (cephalic, gastric, and intestinal). Sight, smell, and taste of food are the components of the cephalic phase, which stimulates gastric secretion via the vagus nerve. The gastric phase is activated once food enters the stomach. This component of secretion is driven by nutrients (amino acids and amines) that directly stimulate the G cell to release gastrin, which in turn activates the parietal cell via direct and indirect mechanisms (see below). Distention of the stomach wall also leads to gastrin release and acid production. The last phase of gastric acid secretion is initiated as food enters the intestine and is mediated by luminal distention and nutrient assimilation. A series of pathways that inhibit gastric acid production are also set into motion during these phases. The gastrointestinal hormone somatostatin is released from endocrine cells found in the gastric mucosa (D cells) in response to HCl. Somatostatin can inhibit acid production by both direct (parietal cell) and indirect mechanisms [decreased histamine release from enterochromaffin-like (ECL) cells and gastrin release from G cells]. Additional neural (central and peripheral) and hormonal (secretin, cholecystokinin) factors play a role in counterbalancing acid secretion. Under physiologic circumstances, these phases are occurring simultaneously.

The acid-secreting parietal cell is located in the oxyntic gland, adjacent to other cellular elements (ECL cell, D cell) important in the gastric secretory process (Fig. 285-5). This unique cell also secretes intrinsic factor. The parietal cell expresses receptors for several stimulants of acid secretion including histamine (H_2), gastrin (cholecystokinin B/gastrin receptor) and acetylcholine (muscarinic, M_3). Each of these are G protein–linked, seven transmembrane–spanning receptors. Binding of histamine to the H_2 receptor leads to activation of adenylate cyclase and an increase in cyclic AMP. Activation of the gastrin and muscarinic receptors results in activation of the protein kinase C/phosphoinositide signaling pathway. Each of these signaling pathways in turn regulates a series of downstream kinase cascades, which control the acid-secreting pump, H^+, K^+-ATPase. The discovery that different ligands and their corresponding receptors lead to activation of different signaling pathways explains the potentiation of acid secretion that occurs when histamine and gastrin or acetylcholine are combined. More importantly, this observation explains why blocking one receptor type (H_2) decreases acid secretion stimulated by agents that activate a different pathway (gastrin, acetylcholine). Parietal cells also express receptors for ligands that inhibit acid production (prostaglandins, somatostatin, and EGF).

The enzyme H^+, K^+-ATPase is responsible for generating the large concentration of H^+. It is a membrane-bound protein that consists of two subunits, α and β. The active catalytic site is found within the α subunit; the function of the β subunit is unclear. This enzyme uses the chemical energy of ATP to transfer H^+ ions from parietal cell cytoplasm to the secretory canaliculi in exchange for K^+. The H^+,K^+-ATPase is located within the secretory canaliculus and in nonsecretory cytoplasmic tubulovesicles. The tubulovesicles are impermeable to K^+, which leads to an inactive pump in this location. The distribution of pumps between the nonsecretory vesicles and the secretory canaliculus varies according to parietal cell activity (Fig. 285-2). Under resting conditions, only 5% of pumps are within the secretory canaliculus, whereas upon parietal cell stimulation, tubulovesicles are immediately transferred to the secretory canalicular membrane, where 60 to 70% of the pumps are activated. Proton pumps are recycled back to the inactive state in cytoplasmic vesicles once parietal cell activation ceases.

The chief cell, found primarily in the gastric fundus, synthesizes and secretes pepsinogen, the inactive precursor of the proteolytic enzyme pepsin. The acid environment within the stomach leads to cleavage of the inactive precursor to pepsin and provides the low pH (<2.0) required for pepsin activity. Pepsin activity is significantly diminished at a pH of 4 and irreversibly inactivated and denatured at a pH of ≥7. Many of the secretagogues that stimulate acid secretion also stimulate pepsinogen release. The precise role of pepsin in the pathogenesis of PUD remains to be established.

PATHOPHYSIOLOGIC BASIS OF PEPTIC ULCER DISEASE PUD encompasses both gastric and duodenal ulcers. Ulcers are defined as a break in the mucosal surface >5 mm in size, with depth to the submucosa. Duodenal (DU) and gastric ulcers (GU) share many common features in terms of pathogenesis, diagnosis, and treatment, but several factors distinguish them from one another.

Epidemiology • *Duodenal ulcers* DUs are estimated to occur in 6 to 15% of the western population. The incidence of DUs declined

FIGURE 285-3 Components involved in providing gastroduodenal mucosal defense and repair.

steadily from 1960 to 1980 and has remained stable since then. The death rates, need for surgery, and physician visits have decreased by >50% over the past 30 years. The reason for the reduction in the frequency of DUs is likely related to the decreasing frequency of *Helicobacter pylori*. Before the discovery of *H. pylori*, the natural history of DUs was typified by frequent recurrences after initial therapy. Eradication of *H. pylori* has greatly reduced these recurrence rates.

Gastric ulcers GUs tend to occur later in life than duodenal lesions, with a peak incidence reported in the sixth decade. More than half of GUs occur in males and are less common than DUs, perhaps due to the higher likelihood of GUs being silent and presenting only after a complication develops. Autopsy studies suggest a similar incidence of DUs and GUs.

Pathology • *Duodenal ulcers* DUs occur most often in the first portion of duodenum (>95%), with ~90% located within 3 cm of the pylorus. They are usually ≤1 cm in diameter but can occasionally reach 3 to 6 cm (giant ulcer). Ulcers are sharply demarcated, with depth at times reaching the muscularis propria. The base of the ulcer often consists of a zone of eosinophilic necrosis with surrounding fibrosis. Malignant duodenal ulcers are extremely rare.

Gastric ulcers In contrast to DUs, GUs can represent a malignancy. Benign GUs are most often found distal to the junction between the antrum and the acid secretory mucosa. This junction is variable, but in general the antral mucosa extends about two thirds of the distance of the lesser curvature and one third the way up the greater curvature. Benign GUs are quite rare in the gastric fundus and are histologically similar to DUs. Benign GUs associated with *H. pylori* are associated with antral gastritis. In contrast, NSAID-related GUs

FIGURE 285-4 Schematic representation of the steps involved in synthesis of prostaglandin E_2 (PGE_2) and prostacyclin (PGI_2). Characteristics and distribution of the cyclooxygenase (COX) enzymes 1 and 2 are also shown. TXA_2, thromboxane A_2.

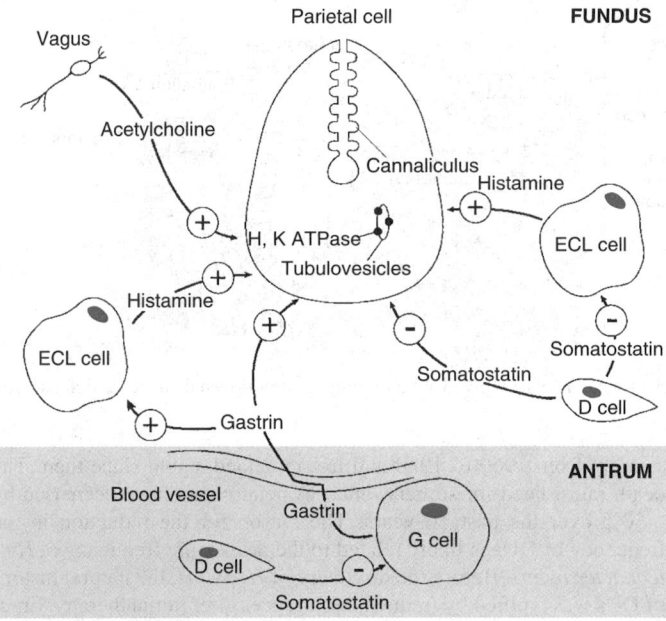

FIGURE 285-5 Regulation of gastric acid secretion at the cellular level. ECL cell, enterochromaffin-like cell.

are not accompanied by chronic active gastritis but may instead have evidence of a chemical gastropathy.

Pathophysiology   It is now clear that *H. pylori* and NSAID-induced injury account for the majority of DUs. Gastric acid contributes to mucosal injury but does not play a primary role.

Duodenal ulcers   Many acid secretory abnormalities have been described in DU patients (Table 285-1). Of these, average basal and nocturnal gastric acid secretion appear to be increased in DU patients as compared to control; however, the level of overlap between DU patients and control subjects is substantial. The reason for this altered secretory process is unclear, but *H. pylori* infection may contribute to this finding. Accelerated gastric emptying of liquids has been noted in some DU patients but is not consistently observed; its role in DU formation, if any, is unclear. Bicarbonate secretion is significantly decreased in the duodenal bulb of patients with an active DU as compared to control subjects. *H. pylori* infection may also play a role in this process.

Gastric ulcer   As in DUs, the majority of GUs can be attributed to either *H. pylori* or NSAID-induced mucosal damage. GUs that occur in the prepyloric area or those in the body associated with a DU or a duodenal scar are similar in pathogenesis to DUs. Gastric acid output (basal and stimulated) tends to be normal or decreased in GU patients. When GUs develop in the presence of minimal acid levels, impairment of mucosal defense factors may be present.

Abnormalities in resting and stimulated pyloric sphincter pressure

Table 285-1 Reported Pathophysiologic Abnormalities in Patients with Duodenal Ulcers

Abnormality	Approximate Frequency, %
↑ Nocturnal acid secretion	70
↓ Duodenal HCO₃ secretion	70
↑ Duodenal acid load	65
↑ Daytime acid secretion	50
↑ Pentagastrin-stimulated MAO	40
↑ Gastrin sensitivity	35–40
↑ Basal gastrin	35–40
↑ Gastric emptying	30
↓ pH inhibition of gastrin release	25
↑ Postprandial gastrin release	25

NOTE: MAO, maximal acid output.

with a concomitant increase in duodenal gastric reflux have been implicated in some GU patients. Although bile acids, lysolecithin, and pancreatic enzymes may injure gastric mucosa, a definite role for these in GU pathogenesis has not been established. Delayed gastric emptying of solids has been described in GU patients but has not been reported consistently. The observation that patients who have undergone disruption of the normal pyloric barrier (pyloroplasty, gastroenterostomy) often have superficial gastritis without frank ulceration decreases enthusiasm for duodenal gastric reflux as an explanation for GU pathogenesis.

H. pylori and acid peptic disorders   Gastric infection with the bacterium *H. pylori* accounts for the majority of PUD. This organism also plays a role in the development of gastric mucosal-associated lymphoid tissue (MALT) lymphoma and gastric adenocarcinoma. Although the entire genome of *H. pylori* has been sequenced, it is still not clear how this organism, which is in the stomach, causes ulceration in the duodenum, or whether its eradication will lead to a decrease in gastric cancer.

THE BACTERIUM   The bacterium, initially named *Campylobacter pyloridis*, is a gram-negative microaerophilic rod found most commonly in the deeper portions of the mucous gel coating the gastric mucosa or between the mucous layer and the gastric epithelium. It may attach to gastric epithelium but under normal circumstances does not appear to invade cells. It is strategically designed to live within the aggressive environment of the stomach. It is S-shaped (~0.5 × 3 μm in size) and contains multiple sheathed flagella. Initially, *H. pylori* resides in the antrum but, over time, migrates towards the more proximal segments of the stomach. The organism is capable of transforming into a coccoid form, which represents a dormant state that may facilitate survival in adverse conditions. The bacterium expresses a host of factors that contribute to its ability to colonize the gastric mucosa and produce mucosal injury. Several of the key bacterial factors include urease (converting urea to NH₃ and water, thus alkalinizing the surrounding acidic environment), catalase, lipase, adhesins, platelet-activating factor, cytotoxin-associated gene protein (Cag A), pic B (induces cytokines), and vacuolating cytotoxin (Vac A). Multiple strains of *H. pylori* exist and are characterized by their ability to express several of these factors (Cag A, Vac A, etc.). It is possible that the different diseases related to *H. pylori* infection can be attributed to different strains of the organism with distinct pathogenic features.

EPIDEMIOLOGY   The prevalence of *H. pylori* varies throughout the world and depends to a great extent on the overall standard of living in the region. In developing parts of the world, 80% of the population may be infected by the age of 20. In contrast, in the United States, this organism is rare in childhood. The overall prevalence of *H. pylori* in the United States is ~30%, with individuals born before 1950 having a higher rate of infection than those born later. About 10% of Americans <30 are colonized with the bacteria. This rate of colonization increases with age, with about 50% of individuals age 50 being infected. Factors that predispose to higher colonization rates include poor socioeconomic status and less education. These factors, not race, are responsible for the rate of *H. pylori* infection in blacks and Hispanic Americans being double the rate seen in whites of comparable age. A summary of risk factors for *H. pylori* infection is shown in Table 285-2.

Transmission of *H. pylori* occurs from person to person, following an oral-oral or fecal-oral route. The risk of *H. pylori* infection is declining in developing countries. The rate of infection in the United States has fallen by >50% when compared to 30 years ago.

Table 285-2 Risk Factors for *H. pylori* Infection

Birth or residence in a developing country
Low socioeconomic status
Domestic crowding
Unsanitary living conditions
Unclean food or water
Exposure to gastric contents of infected individual

PATHOPHYSIOLOGY *H. pylori* infection is virtually always associated with a chronic active gastritis, but only 10 to 15% of infected individuals develop frank peptic ulceration. The basis for this difference is unknown. Initial studies suggested that >90% of all DUs were associated with *H. pylori*, but *H. pylori* is present in only 30 to 60% of individuals with DU and 70% of patients with GU. The pathophysiology of ulcers not associated with *H. pylori* or NSAID ingestion [or the rare Zollinger-Ellison syndrome (ZES)] is unclear.

The particular end result of *H. pylori* infection (gastritis, PUD, gastric MALT lymphoma, gastric cancer) is determined by a complex interplay between bacterial and host factors (Fig. 285-6).

1. *Bacterial factors*: *H. pylori* is able to facilitate gastric residence, induce mucosal injury, and avoid host defense. Different strains of *H. pylori* produce different virulence factors. A specific region of the bacterial genome, the pathogenicity island, encodes the virulence factors Cag A and pic B. Vac A also contributes to pathogenicity, though it is not encoded within the pathogenicity island. These virulence factors, in conjunction with additional bacterial constituents, can cause mucosal damage. Urease, which allows the bacteria to reside in the acidic stomach, generates NH_3, which can damage epithelial cells. The bacteria produce surface factors that are chemotactic for neutrophils and monocytes, which in turn contribute to epithelial cell injury (see below). *H. pylori* makes proteases and phospholipases that break down the glycoprotein lipid complex of the mucous gel, thus reducing the efficacy of this first line of mucosal defense. *H. pylori* expresses adhesins, which facilitate attachment of the bacteria to gastric epithelial cells. Although lipopolysaccharide (LPS) of gram-negative bacteria often plays an important role in the infection, *H. pylori* LPS has low immunologic activity compared to that of other organisms. It may promote a smoldering chronic inflammation.

2. *Host factors*: The host responds to *H. pylori* infection by mounting an inflammatory response, which contributes to gastric epithelial cell damage without providing immunity against infection. The neutrophil response is strong both in acute and chronic infection. In addition, T lymphocytes and plasma cells are components of the chronic inflammatory infiltrate, supporting the involvement of antigen-specific cellular and humoral responses. A number of cytokines are released from both epithelial and immune modulatory cells in response to *H. pylori* infection including the proinflammatory cytokines tumor necrosis factor (TNF)α, interleukin (IL)1α/β, IL-6, interferon (IFN)γ, and granulocyte-macrophage colony stimulating factor. Several chemokines such as IL-8 and growth-regulated oncogene (GRO) α, involved in neutrophil recruitment/activation, and RANTES, which recruits mononuclear cells, have been observed in *H. pylori*-infected mucosa.

The reason for *H. pylori*-mediated duodenal ulceration remains unclear. One potential explanation is that gastric metaplasia in the duodenum of DU patients permits *H. pylori* to bind to it and produce local injury secondary to the host response. Another hypothesis is that *H. pylori* antral infection could lead to increased acid production, increased duodenal acid, and mucosal injury. Basal and stimulated [meal, gastrin-releasing peptide (GRP)] gastrin release are increased in *H. pylori*–infected individuals, and somatostatin-secreting D cells may be decreased. *H. pylori* infection might induce increased acid secretion through both direct and indirect actions of *H. pylori* and proinflammatory cytokines (IL-8, TNF, and IL-1) on G, D, and parietal cells (Fig. 285-7). *H. pylori* infection has also been associated with decreased duodenal mucosal bicarbonate production. Data supporting and contradicting each of these interesting theories have been demonstrated. Thus, the mechanism by which *H pylori* infection of the stomach leads to duodenal ulceration remains to be established.

NSAIDs-induced disease • *EPIDEMIOLOGY* NSAIDs represent one of the most commonly used medications in the United States. More than 30 billion over-the-counter tablets and 70 million prescriptions are sold yearly in the United States alone. The spectrum of NSAID-induced morbidity ranges from nausea and dyspepsia (prevalence reported as high as 50 to 60%) to a serious gastrointestinal complication such as frank peptic ulceration complicated by bleeding or perforation in as many as 3 to 4% of users per year. About 20,000 patients die each year from serious gastrointestinal complications from NSAIDs. Unfortunately, dyspeptic symptoms do not correlate with NSAID-induced pathology. Over 80% of patients with serious NSAID-related complications did not have preceding dyspepsia. In view of the lack of warning signs, it is important to identify patients who are at increased risk for morbidity and mortality related to NSAID usage. A summary of established and possible risk factors is presented in Table 285-3.

PATHOPHYSIOLOGY Prostaglandins play a critical role in maintaining gastroduodenal mucosal integrity and repair. It therefore follows that interruption of prostaglandin synthesis can impair mucosal defense and repair, thus facilitating mucosal injury via a systemic mechanism. A summary of the pathogenetic pathways by which systemically administered NSAIDs may lead to mucosal injury is shown in Fig. 285-8.

FIGURE 285-6 Outline of the bacterial and host factors important in determining *H. pylori*–induced gastrointestinal disease. MALT, mucosal-associated lymphoid tissue.

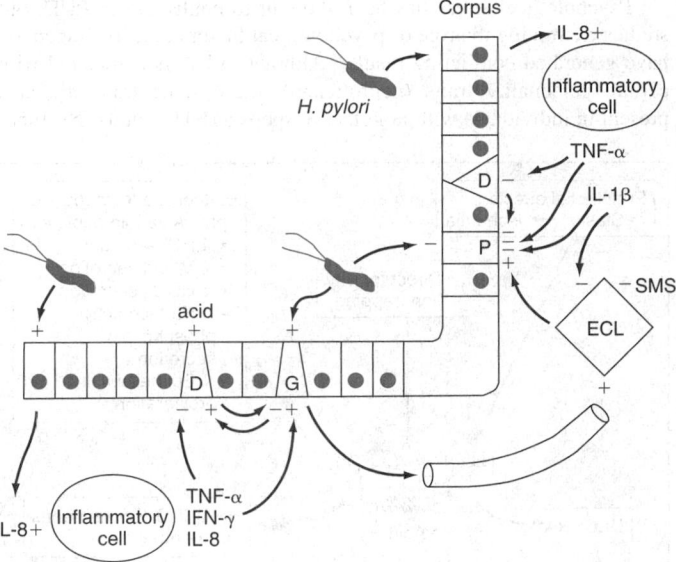

FIGURE 285-7 Summary of potential mechanisms by which *H. pylori* may lead to gastric secretory abnormalities. D, somatostatin cell; ECL, enterochromaffin-like; G, G cell; IFN, interferon; IL, interleukin; P, parietal cell; SMS, somatostatin; TNF, tumor necrosis factor. (*Adapted from J Calam et al: Gastroenterology 113:543, 1997.*)

Table 285-3   Risk Factors for NSAID-Induced Gastroduodenal Ulceration

Established	Possible
Advanced age	Concomitant infection with
History of ulcer	*H. pylori*
Concomitant use of glucocorticoids	Cigarette smoking
High-dose NSAIDs	Alcohol consumption
Multiple NSAIDs	
Concomitant use of anticoagulants	
Serious or multisystem disease	

Injury to the mucosa also occurs as a result of the topical encounter with NSAIDs. Aspirin and many NSAIDs are weak acids that remain in a nonionized lipophilic form when found within the acid environment of the stomach. Under these conditions, NSAIDs migrate across lipid membranes of epithelial cells, leading to cell injury once trapped intracellularly in an ionized form. Topical NSAIDs can also alter the surface mucous layer, permitting back diffusion of H+ and pepsin, leading to further epithelial cell damage.

Miscellaneous pathogenetic factors in acid peptic disease   Cigarette smoking has been implicated in the pathogenesis of PUD. Not only have smokers been found to have ulcers more frequently than do nonsmokers, but smoking appears to decrease healing rates, impair response to therapy, and increase ulcer-related complications such as perforation. The mechanism responsible for increased ulcer diathesis in smokers is unknown. Theories have included altered gastric emptying, decreased proximal duodenal bicarbonate production, and cigarette-induced generation of noxious mucosal free radicals. Acid secretion is *not* abnormal in smokers. Despite these interesting theories, a unifying mechanism for cigarette-induced peptic ulcer diathesis has not been established.

Genetic predisposition has also been considered to play a role in ulcer development. First-degree relatives of DU patients are three times as likely to develop an ulcer; however, the potential role of *H. pylori* infection in contacts is a major consideration. Increased frequency of blood group O and of the nonsecretor status have also been implicated as genetic risk factors for peptic diathesis. However, *H. pylori* preferentially binds to group O antigens. Therefore, the role of genetic predisposition in common PUD has not been established.

Psychological stress has been thought to contribute to PUD, but studies examining the role of psychological factors in its pathogenesis have generated conflicting results. Although PUD is associated with certain personality traits (neuroticism), these same traits are also present in individuals with nonulcer dyspepsia (NUD) and other functional and organic disorders. Although more work in this area is needed, no typical PUD personality has been found.

Diet has also been thought to play a role in peptic diseases. Certain foods can cause dyspepsia, but no convincing studies indicate an association between ulcer formation and a specific diet. This is also true for beverages containing alcohol and caffeine. Specific chronic disorders have been associated with PUD (Table 285-4).

Multiple factors play a role in the pathogenesis of PUD. The two predominant causes are *H. pylori* infection and NSAID ingestion. PUD not related to *H. pylori* or NSAIDs may be increasing. Independent of the inciting or injurious agent, peptic ulcers develop as a result of an imbalance between mucosal protection/repair and aggressive factors. Gastric acid plays an essential role in mucosal injury.

CLINICAL FEATURES   History   Abdominal pain is common to many gastrointestinal disorders, including DU and GU, but has a poor predictive value for the presence of either DU or GU. Up to 10% of patients with NSAID-induced mucosal disease can present with a complication (bleeding, perforation, and obstruction) without antecedent symptoms. Despite this poor correlation, a careful history and physical examination are essential components of the approach to a patient suspected of having peptic ulcers.

Epigastric pain described as a burning or gnawing discomfort can be present in both DU and GU. The discomfort is also described as an ill-defined, aching sensation or as hunger pain. The typical pain pattern in DU occurs 90 min to 3 h after a meal and is frequently relieved by antacids or food. Pain that awakes the patient from sleep (between midnight and 3 A.M.) is the most discriminating symptom, with two-thirds of DU patients describing this complaint. Unfortunately, this symptom is also present in one-third of patients with NUD. The pain pattern in GU patients may be different from that in DU patients, where discomfort may actually be precipitated by food. Nausea and weight loss occur more commonly in GU patients. In the United States, endoscopy detects ulcers in <30% of patients who have dyspepsia. Despite this, 40% of these individuals with typical ulcer symptoms had an ulcer crater, and 40% had gastroduodenitis on endoscopic examination.

The mechanism for development of abdominal pain in ulcer patients is unknown. Several possible explanations include acid-induced activation of chemical receptors in the duodenum, enhanced duodenal sensitivity to bile acids and pepsin, or altered gastroduodenal motility.

Variation in the intensity or distribution of the abdominal pain, as well as the onset of associated symptoms such as nausea and/or vomiting, may be indicative of an ulcer complication. Dyspepsia that becomes constant, is no longer relieved by food or antacids, or radiates to the back may indicate a penetrating ulcer (pancreas). Sudden onset of severe, generalized abdominal pain may indicate perforation. Pain worsening with meals, nausea, and vomiting of undigested food suggest gastric outlet obstruction. Tarry stools or coffee ground emesis indicate bleeding.

Physical Examination   Epigastric tenderness is the most frequent finding in patients with GU or DU. Pain may be found to the right of the midline in 20% of patients. Unfortunately, the predictive value of this finding is rather low. Physical examination is critically important for discovering evidence of ulcer complication. Tachycardia and orthostasis suggest dehydration secondary to vomiting or active gastrointestinal blood loss. A severely tender, boardlike abdomen suggests a perforation. Presence of a succussion splash indicates retained fluid in the stomach, suggesting gastric outlet obstruction.

Table 285-4   Disorders Associated with Peptic Ulcer Disease

Strong association	Possible association
Systemic mastocytosis	Hyperparathyroidism
Chronic pulmonary disease	Coronary artery disease
Chronic renal failure	Polycythemia vera
Cirrhosis	Chronic pancreatitis
Nephrolithiasis	
α Antitrypsin deficiency	

FIGURE 285-8   Mechanisms by which NSAIDs may induce mucosal injury. *(Adapted from J Scheiman et al: J Clin Outcomes Management 3:23, 1996.)*

trointestinal bleeding is the most common complication observed in PUD. It occurs in ~15% of patients and more often in individuals >60 years old. The higher incidence in the elderly is likely due to the increased use of NSAIDs in this group. As many as 20% of patients with ulcer-related hemorrhage bleed without any preceding warning signs or symptoms.

Perforation The second most common ulcer-related complication is perforation, being reported in as many as 6 to 7% of PUD patients. As in the case of bleeding, the incidence of perforation in the elderly appears to be increasing secondary to increased use of NSAIDs. Penetration is a form of perforation in which the ulcer bed tunnels into an adjacent organ. DUs tend to penetrate posteriorly into the pancreas, leading to pancreatitis, whereas GUs tend to penetrate into the left hepatic lobe. Gastrocolic fistulas associated with GUs have also been described.

Gastric outlet obstruction Gastric outlet obstruction is the least common ulcer-related complication, occurring in 1 to 2% of patients. A patient may have relative obstruction secondary to ulcer-related inflammation and edema in the peripyloric region. This process often resolves with ulcer healing. A fixed, mechanical obstruction secondary to scar formation in the peripyloric areas is also possible. The latter requires endoscopic (balloon dilation) or surgical intervention. Signs and symptoms relative to mechanical obstruction may develop insidiously. New onset of early satiety, nausea, vomiting, increase of postprandial abdominal pain, and weight loss should make gastric outlet obstruction a possible diagnosis.

Differential Diagnosis The list of gastrointestinal and nongastrointestinal disorders that can mimic ulceration of the stomach or duodenum is quite extensive. The most commonly encountered diagnosis among patients seen for upper abdominal discomfort is NUD. NUD, also known as *functional dyspepsia* or *essential dyspepsia*, refers to a group of heterogeneous disorders typified by upper abdominal pain without the presence of an ulcer. Dyspepsia has been reported to occur in up to 30% of the U.S. population. Up to 60% of patients seeking medical care for dyspepsia have a negative diagnostic evaluation. The etiology of NUD is not established, and the potential role of *H. pylori* in NUD remains controversial.

Several additional disease processes that may present with "ulcer-like" symptoms include proximal gastrointestinal tumors, gastroesophageal reflux, vascular disease, pancreaticobiliary disease (biliary colic, chronic pancreatitis), and gastroduodenal Crohn's disease.

Diagnostic Evaluation In view of the poor predictive value of abdominal pain for the presence of a gastroduodenal ulcer and the multiple disease processes that can mimic this disease, the clinician is often confronted with having to establish the presence of an ulcer. Documentation of an ulcer requires either a radiographic (barium study) or an endoscopic procedure.

Barium studies of the proximal gastrointestinal tract are still commonly used as a first test for documenting an ulcer. The sensitivity of older single-contrast barium meals for detecting a DU is as high as 80%, with a double-contrast study providing detection rates as high as 90%. Sensitivity for detection is decreased in small ulcers (<0.5 cm), presence of previous scarring, or in postoperative patients. A DU appears as a well-demarcated crater, most often seen in the bulb. A GU may represent benign or malignant disease. Typically, a benign GU also appears as a discrete crater with radiating mucosal folds originating from the ulcer margin. Ulcers >3 cm in size or those associated with a mass are more often malignant. Unfortunately, up to 8% of GUs that appear to be benign by radiographic appearance are malignant by endoscopy or surgery. Radiographic studies that show a GU must be followed by endoscopy and biopsy.

Endoscopy provides the most sensitive and specific approach for examining the upper gastrointestinal tract. In addition to permitting direct visualization of the mucosa, endoscopy facilitates photographic documentation of a mucosal defect and tissue biopsy to rule out malignancy (GU) or *H. pylori*. Endoscopic examination is particularly helpful in identifying lesions too small to detect by radiographic ex-

amination, for evaluation of atypical radiographic abnormalities, or to determine if an ulcer is a source of blood loss.

Although the methods for diagnosing *H. pylori* are outlined in Chap. 154, a brief summary will be included here (Table 285-5). PyloriTek, a biopsy urease test, has a sensitivity and specificity of >90 to 95%. In the interest of making a diagnosis of *H. pylori* without the need for performing endoscopy, several noninvasive methods for detecting this organism have been developed. Three types of studies routinely used include serologic testing, the ^{13}C- or ^{14}C-urea breath test, and the fecal *H. pylori* antigen test.

Occasionally, specialized testing such as serum gastrin and gastric acid analysis or sham feeding may be needed in individuals with complicated or refractory PUD (see "Zollinger-Ellison Syndrome," below). Screening for aspirin or NSAIDS (blood or urine) may also be necessary in refractory, *H. pylori*–negative PUD patients.

℞ **TREATMENT** Before the discovery of *H. pylori*, the therapy of PUD disease was centered on the old dictum by Schwartz of "no acid, no ulcer." Although acid secretion is still important in the pathogenesis of PUD, eradication of *H. pylori* and therapy/prevention of NSAID-induced disease is the mainstay. A summary of commonly used drugs for treatment of acid peptic disorders is shown in Table 285-6.

Acid Neutralizing/Inhibitory Drugs • *Antacids* Before we understood the important role of histamine in stimulating parietal cell activity, neutralization of secreted acid with antacids constituted the main form of therapy for peptic ulcers. They are now rarely, if ever, used as the primary therapeutic agent but instead are often used by patients for symptomatic relief of dyspepsia. The most commonly used agents are mixtures of aluminum hydroxide and magnesium hydroxide. Aluminum hydroxide can produce constipation and phosphate depletion; magnesium hydroxide may cause loose stools. Many of the commonly used antacids (e.g., Maalox, Mylanta) have a combination of both aluminum and magnesium hydroxide in order to avoid these side effects. The magnesium-containing preparation should not be used in chronic renal failure patients because of possible hypermagnesemia, and aluminum may cause chronic neurotoxicity in these patients.

Calcium carbonate and sodium bicarbonate are potent antacids with varying levels of potential problems. The long-term use of calcium carbonate (converts to calcium chloride in the stomach) can lead to milk-alkali syndrome (hypercalcemia, hyperphosphatemia with possible renal calcinosis and progression to renal insufficiency). Sodium bicarbonate may induce systemic alkalosis.

Table 285-5 Tests for Detection of *H. pylori*

Test	Sensitivity/Specificity, %	Comments
INVASIVE (ENDOSCOPY/BIOPSY REQUIRED)		
Rapid urease	80–95/95–100	Simple; false negative with recent use of PPIs, antibiotics, or bismuth compounds
Histology	80–90/>95	Requires pathology processing and staining; provides histologic information
Culture	—/—	Time-consuming, expensive, dependent on experience; allows determination of antibiotic susceptibility
NON-INVASIVE		
Serology	>80/>90	Inexpensive, convenient; not useful for early follow-up
Urea breath test	>90/>90	Simple, rapid; useful for early follow-up; false negative with recent therapy (see rapid urease test)

NOTE: PPI, proton pump inhibitor.

Table 285-6 Drugs Used in the Treatment of Peptic Ulcer Disease

Drug Type/Mechanism	Examples	Dose
Acid-suppressing drugs		
Antacids	Mylanta, Maalox, Tums, Gaviscon	100–140 meq/L 1 and 3 h after meals and hs
H_2 receptor antagonists	Cimetidine	800 mg hs
	Ranitidine	300 mg hs
	Famotidine	40 mg hs
	Nizatidine	300 mg hs
Proton pump inhibitors	Omeprazole	20 mg/d
	Lansoprazole	30 mg/d
	Rabeprazole	20 mg/d
	Pantoprazole	40 mg/d
Mucosal protective agents		
Sucralfate	Sucralfate	1 g qid
Prostaglandin analogue	Misoprostol	200 μg qid
Bismuth-containing compounds	Bismuth subsalicylate (BSS)	See anti-*H. Pylori* regimens (Table 285-7)

H_2 receptor antagonists Four of these agents are presently available (cimetidine, ranitidine, famotidine, and nizatidine), and their structures share homology with histamine (Fig. 285-9). Although each has different potency, all will significantly inhibit basal and stimulated acid secretion to comparable levels when used at therapeutic doses. Moreover, similar ulcer-healing rates are achieved with each drug when used at the correct dosage. Presently, this class of drug is often used for treatment of active ulcers (4 to 6 weeks) in combination with antibiotics directed at eradicating *H. pylori* (see below).

Cimetidine was the first H_2 receptor antagonist used for the treatment of acid peptic disorders. The initial recommended dosing profile for cimetidine was 300 mg four times per day. Subsequent studies have documented the efficacy of using 800 mg at bedtime for treatment of active ulcer, with healing rates approaching 80% at 4 weeks. Cimetidine may have weak antiandrogenic side effects resulting in reversible gynecomastia and impotence, primarily in patients receiving high doses for prolonged periods of time (months to years, as in ZES).

FIGURE 285-9 Structure of H_2 receptor antagonists.

In view of cimetidine's ability to inhibit cytochrome P450, careful monitoring of drugs such as warfarin, phenytoin, and theophylline is indicated with long-term usage. Other rare reversible adverse effects reported with cimetidine include confusion and elevated levels of serum aminotransferases, creatinine, and serum prolactin. Ranitidine, famotidine, and nizatidine are more potent H_2 receptor antagonists than cimetidine. Each can be used once a day at bedtime. Comparable nighttime dosing regimens are ranitidine, 300 mg, famotidine, 40 mg, and nizatidine, 300 mg.

Additional rare, reversible systemic toxicities reported with H_2 receptor antagonists include pancytopenia, neutropenia, anemia, and thrombocytopenia, with a prevalence rate varying from 0.01 to 0.2%. Cimetidine and rantidine (to a lesser extent) can bind to hepatic cytochrome P450, whereas the newer agents, famotidine and nizatidine, do not.

Proton pump (H^+,K^+-ATPase) inhibitors Omeprazole, lansoprazole, and the newest additions, rabeprazole and pantoprazole, are substituted benzimidazole derivatives that covalently bind and irreversibly inhibit H^+,K^+-ATPase. These are the most potent acid inhibitory agents available. Omeprazole and lansoprazole are the proton pump inhibitors (PPIs) that have been used for the longest time. Both are acid labile and are administered as enteric-coated granules in a sustained-release capsule that dissolves within the small intestine at a pH of 6. These agents are lipophilic compounds; upon entering the parietal cell, they are protonated and trapped within the acid environment of the tubulovesicular and canalicular system. These agents potently inhibit all phases of gastric acid secretion. Onset of action is rapid, with a maximum acid inhibitory effect between 2 and 6 h after administration and duration of inhibition lasting up to 72 to 96 h. With repeated daily dosing, progressive acid inhibitory effects are observed, with basal and secretagogue-stimulated acid production being inhibited by >95% after 1 week of therapy. The half-life of PPIs is approximately 18 h, thus it can take between 2 and 5 days for gastric acid secretion to return to normal levels once these drugs have been discontinued. Because the pumps need to be activated for these agents to be effective, their efficacy is maximized if they are administered before a meal (e.g., in the morning before breakfast). Standard dosing for omeprazole and lansoprazole is 20 mg and 30 mg once per day, respectively. Mild to moderate hypergastrinemia has been observed in patients taking these drugs. Carcinoid tumors developed in some animals given the drugs preclinically; however, extensive experience has failed to demonstrate gastric carcinoid tumor development in humans. Serum gastrin levels return to normal levels within 1 to 2 weeks after drug cessation. As with any agent that leads to significant hypochlorhydria, PPIs may interfere with absorption of drugs such as ketoconazole, ampicillin, iron, and digoxin. Hepatic cytochrome P450 can be inhibited by these agents, but the overall clinical significance of this observation is not definitely established. Caution should be taken when using warfarin, diazepam, and phenytoin concomitantly with PPIs.

Cytoprotective Agents • *Sucralfate* Sucralfate is a complex sucrose salt in which the hydroxyl groups have been substituted by aluminum hydroxide and sulfate. This compound is insoluble in water and becomes a viscous paste within the stomach and duodenum, binding primarily to sites of active ulceration. Sucralfate may act by several mechanisms. In the gastric environment, aluminum hydroxide dissociates, leaving the polar sulfate anion, which can bind to positively charged tissue proteins found within the ulcer bed, and providing a physicochemical barrier impeding further tissue injury by acid and pepsin. Sucralfate may also induce a trophic effect by binding growth factors such as EGF, enhance prostaglandin synthesis, stimulate mucous and bicarbonate secretion, and enhance mucosal defense and repair. Toxicity from this drug is rare, with constipation being the most common one reported (2 to 3%). It should be avoided in patients with chronic renal insufficiency to prevent aluminum-induced neurotoxicity. Hypophosphatemia and gastric bezoar formation have also been rarely reported. Standard dosing of sucralfate is 1 g four times per day.

Bismuth-containing preparations Sir William Osler considered bismuth-containing compounds the drug of choice for treating PUD.

The resurgence in the use of these agents is due to their effect against *H. pylori*. Colloidal bismuth subcitrate (CBS) and bismuth subsalicylate (BSS, Pepto-Bismol) are the most widely used preparations. The mechanism by which these agents induce ulcer healing is unclear. Potential mechanisms include ulcer coating; prevention of further pepsin/HCl-induced damage; binding of pepsin; and stimulation of prostaglandins, bicarbonate, and mucous secretion. Adverse effects with short-term usage are rare with bismuth compounds. Long-term usage with high doses, especially with the avidly absorbed CBS, may lead to neurotoxicity. These compounds are commonly used as one of the agents in an anti-*H. pylori* regimen (see below).

Prostaglandin analogues In view of their central role in maintaining mucosal integrity and repair, stable prostaglandin analogues were developed for the treatment of PUD. The prostaglandin E₁ derivative misoprostal is the only agent of this class approved by the U.S. Food and Drug Administration for clinical use in the prevention of NSAID-induced gastroduodenal mucosal injury (see below). The mechanism by which this rapidly absorbed drug provides its therapeutic effect is through enhancement of mucosal defense and repair. Prostaglandin analogues enhance mucous bicarbonate secretion, stimulate mucosal blood flow, and decrease mucosal cell turnover. The most common toxicity noted with this drug is diarrhea (10 to 30% incidence). Other major toxicities include uterine bleeding and contractions; misoprostal is contraindicated in women who may be pregnant, and women of childbearing age must be made clearly aware of this potential drug toxicity. The standard therapeutic dose is 200 μg four times per day.

Miscellaneous drugs A number of drugs aimed at treating acid peptic disorders have been developed over the years. In view of their limited utilization in the United States, if any, they will only be listed briefly. Anticholinergics, designed to inhibit activation of the muscarinic receptor in parietal cells, met with limited success due to their relatively weak acid-inhibiting effect and significant side effects (dry eyes, dry mouth, urinary retention). Tricyclic antidepressants have been suggested by some, but again the toxicity of these agents in comparison to the safe, effective drugs already described, precludes their utility. Finally, the licorice extract carbenoxolone has aldosterone-like side effects with fluid retention and hypokalemia, making it an undesirable therapeutic option.

Therapy of *H. pylori* Extensive effort has been placed into determining who of the many individuals with *H. pylori* infection should be treated. The common conclusion arrived at by multiple consensus conferences (National Institutes of Health Consensus Development, American Digestive Health Foundation International Update Conference, European Maastricht Consensus, and Asia Pacific Consensus Conference) is that *H. pylori* should be eradicated in patients with documented PUD. This holds true independent of time of presentation (first episode or not), severity of symptoms, presence of confounding factors such as ingestion of NSAIDs, or whether the ulcer is in remission. Some have advocated treating patients with a history of documented PUD who are found to be *H. pylori*–positive by serology or breath testing. Over half of patients with gastric MALT lymphoma experience complete remission of the tumor in response to *H. pylori* eradication. Treating patients with NUD or to prevent gastric cancer remains controversial.

Multiple drugs have been evaluated in the therapy of *H. pylori*. No single agent is effective in eradicating the organism. Combination therapy for 14 days provides the greatest efficacy. A short-time course administration (7 to 10 days), although attractive, has not proven as successful as the 14-day regimens. The agents used with the greatest frequency include amoxicillin, metronidazole, tetracycline, clarithromycin, and bismuth compounds.

The physician's goal in treating PUD is to provide relief of symptoms (pain or dyspepsia), promote ulcer healing, and ultimately prevent ulcer recurrence and complications. The greatest impact of understanding the role of *H. pylori* in peptic disease has been the ability to prevent recurrence of what was often a recurring disease. Documented eradication of *H. pylori* in patients with PUD is associated with a dramatic decrease in ulcer recurrence to 4% (as compared to 59%) in GU patients and 6% (compared to 67%) in DU patients. Eradication of the organism may lead to diminished recurrent ulcer bleeding. The impact of its eradication on ulcer perforation is unclear.

Suggested treatment regimens for *H. pylori* are outlined in Table 285-7. Choice of a particular regimen will be influenced by several factors including efficacy, patient tolerance, existing antibiotic resistance, and cost of the drugs. The aim for initial eradication rates should be 85 to 90%. Dual therapy [PPI plus amoxicillin, PPI plus clarithromycin, ranitidine bismuth citrate (Tritec) plus clarithromycin] are not recommended in view of studies demonstrating eradication rates of <80 to 85%. The combination of bismuth, metronidazole, and tetracycline was the first triple regimen found effective against *H. pylori*. The combination of two antibiotics plus either a PPI, H₂ blocker, or bismuth compound has comparable success rates. Addition of acid suppression assists in providing early symptom relief and may enhance bacterial eradication.

Triple therapy, although effective, has several drawbacks, including the potential for poor patient compliance and drug-induced side effects. Compliance is being addressed somewhat by simplifying the regimens so that patients can take the medications twice a day. Simpler (dual therapy) and shorter regimens (7 and 10 days) are not as effective as triple therapy for 14 days. Two anti-*H. pylori* regimens are available in prepackaged formulation: Prevpac (lansoprazole, clarithromycin, and amoxicillin) and Helidac (bismuth subsalicylate, tetracycline, and metronidazole). The contents of the Prevpac are to be taken twice per day for 14 days, whereas Helidac constituents are taken four times per day with an antisecretory agent (PPI or H₂ blocker), also taken for at least 14 days.

Side effects have been reported in up to 20 to 30% of patients on triple therapy. Bismuth may cause black stools, constipation, or darkening of the tongue. The most feared complication with amoxicillin is pseudomembranous colitis, but this occurs in <1 to 2% of patients. Amoxicillin can also lead to antibiotic-associated diarrhea, nausea, vomiting, skin rash, and allergic reaction. Tetracycline has been reported to cause rashes and very rarely hepatotoxicity and anaphylaxis.

One important concern with treating patients who may not need treatment is the potential for development of antibiotic-resistant strains. The incidence and type of antibiotic-resistant *H. pylori* strains vary worldwide. Strains resistant to metronidazole, clarithromycin, amoxicillin, and tetracycline have been described, with the latter two being uncommon. Antibiotic-resistant strains are the most common

Table 285-7 Regimens Recommended for Eradication of *H. pylori* Infection

Drug	Dose
TRIPLE THERAPY	
1. Bismuth subsalicylate *plus*	2 tablets qid
Metronidazole *plus*	250 mg qid
Tetracycline[a]	500 mg qid
2. Ranitidine bismuth citrate *plus*	400 mg bid
Tetracycline *plus*	500 mg bid
Clarithromycin *or* metronidazole	500 mg bid
3. Omeprazole (lansoprazole) *plus*	20 mg bid (30 mg bid)
Clarithromycin *plus*	250 or 500 mg bid
Metronidazole[b] *or*	500 mg bid
Amoxicillin[c]	1 g bid
QUADRUPLE THERAPY	
Omeprazole (lansoprazole)	20 mg (30 mg) daily
Bismuth subsalicylate	2 tablets qid
Metronidazole	250 mg qid
Tetracycline	500 mg qid

[a] Alternative: use prepacked Helidac (see text).
[b] Alternative: use prepacked Prevpac (see text).
[c] Use either metronidazole or amoxicillin, but not both.

cause for treatment failure in compliant patients. Unfortunately, in vitro resistance does not predict outcome in patients. Culture and sensitivity testing of *H. pylori* is not performed routinely. Although resistance to metronidazole has been found in as many as 30% and 95% of isolates in North America and Asia, respectively, triple therapy is effective in eradicating the organism in >50% of patients infected with a resistant strain.

Failure of *H. pylori* eradication with triple therapy is usually due to infection with a resistant organism. Quadruple therapy (Table 285-7) where clarithromycin is substituted for metronidazole (or vice versa) should be the next step. If eradication is still not achieved in a compliant patient, then culture and sensitivity of the organism should be considered.

Reinfection after successful eradication of *H. pylori* is rare in the United States (<1%/year). If recurrent infection occurs within the first 6 months after completing therapy, the most likely explanation is recrudescence as opposed to reinfection, which occurs later in time.

Therapy of NSAID-Related Gastric or Duodenal Injury Medical intervention for NSAID-related mucosal injury includes treatment of an active ulcer and prevention of future injury. Recommendations for the treatment and prevention of NSAID-related mucosal injury are in Table 285-8. Ideally the injurious agent should be stopped as the first step in the therapy of an active NSAID-induced ulcer. If that is possible, then treatment with one of the acid inhibitory agents (H_2 blockers, PPIs) is indicated. Cessation of NSAIDs is not always possible because of the patient's severe underlying disease. Only PPIs can heal GUs or DUs, independent of whether NSAIDs are discontinued.

Prevention of NSAID-induced ulceration can be accomplished by misoprostol (200 μg qid) or a PPI. High-dose H_2 blockers (famotidine, 40 mg bid) have also shown some promise. The use of COX-2-selective NSAIDs may also reduce injury to gastric mucosa. Two highly selective COX-2 inhibitors, celecoxib and rofecoxib, are 100 times more selective inhibitors of COX-2 than standard NSAIDs, leading to gastric or duodenal mucosal injury that is comparable to placebo. However, evaluation of possible drug toxicities, such as altered renal function and induction of thrombosis, requires more data.

Approach and Therapy: Summary Controversy continues regarding the best approach to the patient who presents with dyspepsia (Chap. 41). The discovery of *H. pylori* and its role in pathogenesis of ulcers has added a new variable to the equation. Previously, if a patient <50 presented with dyspepsia and without alarming signs or symptoms suggestive of an ulcer complication or malignancy, an empirical therapeutic trial with acid suppression was commonly recommended. Although this approach is practiced by some today, an approach presently gaining approval for the treatment of patients with dyspepsia is outlined in Fig. 285-10. The referral to a gastroenterologist is for the potential need of endoscopy and subsequent evaluation and treatment if the endoscopy is negative.

Once an ulcer (GU or DU) is documented, then the main issue at stake is whether *H. pylori* or an NSAID is involved. With *H. pylori* present, independent of the NSAID status, triple therapy is recom-

Table 285-8   Recommendations for Treatment of NSAID-Related Mucosal Injury

Clinical Setting	Recommendation
Active ulcer	
NSAID discontinued	H_2 receptor antagonist or PPI
NSAID continued	PPI
Prophylactic therapy	Misoprostol
	PPI
	Selective COX-2 inhibitor
H. pylori infection	Eradication if active ulcer present or there is a past history of peptic ulcer disease

NOTE: PPI, proton pump inhibitor; COX-2, isoenzyme of cyclooxygenase.

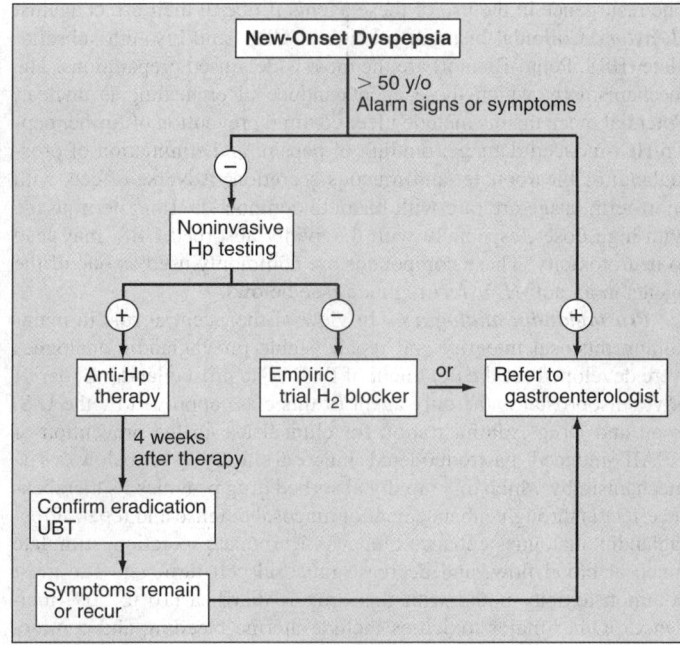

FIGURE 285-10 Overview of new-onset dyspepsia. Hp, *H. pylori*; UBT, urea breath test. *(Adapted from BS Anand and DY Graham: Endoscopy 31: 215, 1999.)*

mended for 14 days, followed by continued acid-suppressing drugs (H_2 receptor antagonist or PPIs) for a total of 4 to 6 weeks. Selection of patients for documentation of *H. pylori* eradication is an area of some debate. The test of choice for documenting eradication is the urea breath test (UBT). The stool antigen study may also hold promise for this purpose and should certainly be performed if UBT is not available. Serologic testing is not useful for the purpose of documenting eradication since antibody titers fall slowly and often do not become undetectable. Two approaches toward documentation of eradication exist: (1) test for eradication only in individuals with a complicated course or in individuals who are frail or with multisystem disease who would do poorly with an ulcer recurrence, and (2) test all patients for successful eradication. Some recommend that patients with complicated ulcer disease or who are frail should be treated with long-term acid suppression, thus making documentation of *H. pylori* eradication a moot point. In view of this discrepancy in practice, it would be best to discuss with the patient the different options available.

Several issues differentiate the approach to a GU versus a DU. GUs, especially of the body and fundus, have the potential of being malignant. Multiple biopsies of a GU should be taken initially; even if these are negative for neoplasm, repeat endoscopy to document healing at 8 to 12 weeks should be performed, with biopsy if the ulcer is still present. About 70% of GUs eventually found to be malignant undergo significant (usually incomplete) healing.

The majority (>90%) of GUs and DUs heal with the conventional therapy outlined above. A GU that fails to heal after 12 weeks and a DU that doesn't heal after 8 weeks of therapy should be considered refractory. Once poor compliance and persistent *H. pylori* infection have been excluded, NSAID use, either inadvertent or surreptitious, must be excluded. In addition, cigarette smoking must be eliminated. For a GU, malignancy must be meticulously excluded. Next, consideration should be given to a gastric hypersecretory state, which can be excluded with gastric acid analysis. Although a subset of patients have gastric acid hypersecretion of unclear etiology as a contributing factor to refractory ulcers, ZES should be excluded with a fasting gastrin or secretin stimulation test (see below). More than 90% of refractory ulcers (either DUs or GUs) heal after 8 weeks of treatment with higher doses of PPI (omeprazole, 40 mg/d). This higher dose is also effective in maintaining remission. Surgical intervention may be a consideration at this point; however, other rare causes of refractory ulcers must be excluded before recommending surgery. Rare etiologies of refractory ulcers that may be diagnosed by gastric or duodenal biopsies include: ischemia, Crohn's disease, amyloidosis, sarcoidosis, lymphoma, eosinophilic gastroenteritis, or infection [cytomegalovirus (CMV), tuberculosis, or syphilis].

Surgical Therapy Surgical intervention in PUD can be viewed as being either elective, for treatment of medically refractory disease, or as urgent/emergent, for the treatment of an ulcer-related complication. Refractory ulcers are an exceedingly rare occurrence. Surgery is more often required for treatment of an ulcer-related complication. Gastrointestinal bleeding (Chap. 44), perforation, and gastric outlet obstruction are the three complications that may require surgical intervention.

Hemorrhage is the most common ulcer-related complication, occurring in ~15 to 25% of patients. Bleeding may occur in any age group but is most often seen in older patients (sixth decade or beyond). The majority of patients stop bleeding spontaneously, but in some, endoscopic therapy (Chap. 283) is necessary. Patients unresponsive or refractory to endoscopic intervention will require surgery (~5% of transfusion-requiring patients).

Free peritoneal perforation occurs in ~2 to 3% of DU patients. As in the case of bleeding, up to 10% of these patients will not have antecedent ulcer symptoms. Concomitant bleeding may occur in up to 10% of patients with perforation, with mortality being increased substantially. Peptic ulcer can also penetrate into adjacent organs, especially with a posterior DU, which can penetrate into the pancreas, colon, liver, or biliary tree.

Pyloric channel ulcers or DUs can lead to gastric outlet obstruction in ~2 to 3% of patients. This can result from chronic scarring or from impaired motility due to inflammation and/or edema with pylorospasm. Patients may present with early satiety, nausea, vomiting of undigested food, and weight loss. Conservative management with nasogastric suction, intravenous hydration/nutrition, and antisecretory agents is indicated for 7 to 10 days with the hope that a functional obstruction will reverse. If a mechanical obstruction persists, endoscopic intervention with balloon dilation may be effective. Surgery should be considered if all else fails.

Specific Operations for Duodenal Ulcers Surgical treatment is designed to decrease gastric acid secretion. Operations most commonly performed include vagotomy and drainage (by pyloroplasty, gastroduodenostomy, or gastrojejunostomy), highly selective vagotomy (which does not require a drainage procedure), and vagotomy with antrectomy. The specific procedure performed is dictated by the underlying circumstances: elective vs. emergency, the degree and extent of duodenal ulceration, and the expertise of the surgeon.

Vagotomy is a component of each of these procedures and is aimed at decreasing acid secretion through ablating cholinergic input to the stomach. Unfortunately, both truncal and selective vagotomy (preserves the celiac and hepatic branches) result in gastric atony despite successful reduction of both basal acid output (BAO, decreased by 85%) and maximal acid output (MAO, decreased by 50%). Drainage procedure through pyloroplasty or gastroduodenostomy is required in an effort to compensate for the vagotomy-induced gastric motility disorder. To minimize gastric dysmotility, highly selective vagotomy (also known as parietal cell, super selective, and proximal vagotomy) was developed. Only the vagal fibers innervating the portion of the stomach that contains parietal cells is transected, thus leaving fibers important for regulating gastric motility intact. Although this procedure leads to an immediate decrease in both BAO and stimulated acid output, acid secretion recovers over time. By the end of the first postoperative year, basal and stimulated acid output are ~30 and 50%, respectively, of preoperative levels. Ulcer recurrence rates are higher with highly selective vagotomy, although the overall complication rates are lower (Table 285-9).

The procedure that provides the lowest rates of ulcer recurrence but has the highest complication rate is vagotomy (truncal or selective) in combination with antrectomy. Antrectomy is aimed at eliminating an additional stimulant of gastric acid secretion, gastrin. Gastrin originates from G cells found in the antrum. Two principal types of reanastomoses are used after antrectomy, gastroduodenostomy (Billroth I) or gastrojejunostomy (Billroth II) (Fig. 285-11). Although Billroth I is often preferred over II, severe duodenal inflammation or scarring may preclude its performance.

Of these procedures, highly selective vagotomy may be the one of choice in the elective setting, except in situations where ulcer recurrence rates are high (prepyloric ulcers and those refractory to H_2 therapy). Selection of vagotomy and antrectomy may be more appropriate in these circumstances.

These procedures have been traditionally performed by standard laparotomy. The advent of laparoscopic surgery has led several surgical teams to successfully perform highly selective vagotomy, truncal vagotomy/pyloroplasty, and truncal vagotomy/antrectomy through this approach. An increase in the number of laparoscopic procedures for treatment of PUD is expected.

Specific Operations for Gastric Ulcers The location and the presence of a concomitant DU dictate the operative procedure performed for a GU. Antrectomy (including the ulcer) with a Billroth I anastomosis is the treatment of choice for an antral ulcer. Vagotomy is performed only if a DU is present. Although ulcer excision with vagotomy and drainage procedure has been proposed, the higher incidence of ulcer recurrence makes this a less desirable approach. Ulcers located near the esophagogastric junction may require a more radical approach, a subtotal gastrectomy with a Roux-en-Y esophagogastrojejunostomy (Csende's procedure). A less aggressive approach including antrectomy, intraoperative ulcer biopsy, and vagotomy (Kelling-Madlener procedure) may be indicated in fragile patients with a high GU. Ulcer recurrence approaches 30% with this procedure.

Surgery-Related Complications Complications seen after surgery for PUD are related primarily to the extent of the anatomical modification performed. Minimal alteration (highly selective vagot-

Table 285-9 Outcome in Patients After Acid-Reducing Gastric Surgery

Operation	Ulcer Recurrence Rates, %	Complication Rates
Vagotomy and antrectomy (Billroth I or II)	1	Highest
Vagotomy and pyloroplasty	10	Intermediate
Highly selective vagotomy	≥10	Lowest

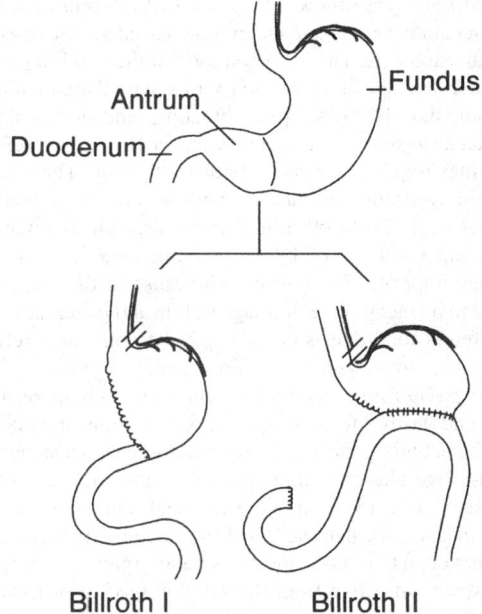

FIGURE 285-11 Schematic representation of Billroth I and II procedures.

omy) is associated with higher rates of ulcer recurrence and less gastrointestinal disturbance. More aggressive surgical procedures have a lower rate of ulcer recurrence but a greater incidence of gastrointestinal dysfunction. Overall, morbidity and mortality related to these procedures are quite low. Morbidity associated with vagotomy and antrectomy or pyloroplasty is ≤5%, with mortality ~1%. Highly selective vagotomy has lower morbidity and mortality rates of 1 and 0.3%, respectively.

In addition to the potential early consequences of any intraabdominal procedure (bleeding, infection, thromboembolism), gastroparesis, duodenal stump leak, and efferent loop obstruction can be observed.

Recurrent ulceration   The risk of ulcer recurrence is directly related to the procedure performed (Table 285-9). Ulcers that recur after partial gastric resection tend to develop at the anastomosis (stomal or marginal ulcer). Epigastric abdominal pain is the most frequent presenting complaint. Severity and duration of pain tend to be more progressive than observed with DUs before surgery.

Ulcers may recur for several reasons including incomplete vagotomy, retained antrum, and, less likely, persistent or recurrent *H. pylori* infection. ZES should have been excluded preoperatively. More recently, surreptitious use of NSAIDs has been found to be a reason for recurrent ulcers after surgery, especially if the initial procedure was done for an NSAID-induced ulcer. Once *H. pylori* and NSAIDs have been excluded as etiologic factors, the question of incomplete vagotomy or retained gastric antrum should be explored. For the latter, fasting plasma gastrin levels should be determined. If elevated, retained antrum or ZES (see below) should be considered. A combination of acid secretory analysis and secretin stimulation (see below) can assist in this differential diagnosis. Incomplete vagotomy can be ruled out by gastric acid analysis coupled with sham feeding. In this test, gastric acid output is measured while the patient sees, smells, and chews a meal (without swallowing). The cephalic phase of gastric secretion, which is mediated by the vagus, is being assessed with this study. An increase in gastric acid output in response to sham feeding is evidence that the vagus nerve is intact.

Medical therapy with H_2 blockers will heal postoperative ulceration in 70 to 90% of patients. The efficacy of PPIs has not been fully assessed in this group, but one may anticipate greater rates of ulcer healing compared to those obtained with H_2 blockers. Repeat operation (complete vagotomy, partial gastrectomy) may be required in a small subgroup of patients who have not responded to aggressive medical management.

Afferent loop syndromes   Two types of afferent loop syndrome can occur in patients who have undergone partial gastric resection with Billroth II anastomosis. The most common of the two is bacterial overgrowth in the afferent limb secondary to stasis. Patients may experience postprandial abdominal pain, bloating, and diarrhea with concomitant malabsorption of fats and vitamin B_{12}. Cases refractory to antibiotics may require surgical revision of the loop. The less common afferent loop syndrome can present with severe abdominal pain and bloating that occur 20 to 60 min after meals. Pain is often followed by nausea and vomiting of bile-containing material. The pain and bloating may improve after emesis. The cause of this clinical picture is theorized to be incomplete drainage of bile and pancreatic secretions from an afferent loop that is partially obstructed. Cases refractory to dietary measures may need surgical revision.

Dumping syndrome   Dumping syndrome consists of a series of vasomotor and gastrointestinal signs and symptoms and occurs in patients who have undergone vagotomy and drainage (especially Billroth procedures). Two phases of dumping, early and late, can occur. Early dumping takes place 15 to 30 min after meals and consists of crampy abdominal discomfort, nausea, diarrhea, belching, tachycardia, palpitations, diaphoresis, light-headedness, and, rarely, syncope. These signs and symptoms arise from the rapid emptying of hyperosmolar gastric contents into the small intestine, resulting in a fluid shift into the gut lumen with plasma volume contraction and acute intestinal distention. Release of vasoactive gastrointestinal hormones (vasoactive intestinal polypeptide, neurotensin, motilin) is also theorized to play a role in early dumping.

The late phase of dumping typically occurs 90 min to 3 h after meals. Vasomotor symptoms (light-headedness, diaphoresis, palpitations, tachycardia, and syncope) predominate during this phase. This component of dumping is thought to be secondary to hypoglycemia from excessive insulin release.

Dumping syndrome is most noticeable after meals rich in simple carbohydrates (especially sucrose) and high osmolarity. Ingestion of large amounts of fluids may also contribute. Up to 50% of postvagotomy and drainage patients will experience dumping syndrome to some degree. Signs and symptoms often improve with time, but a severe protracted picture can occur in up to 1% of patients.

Dietary modification is the cornerstone of therapy for patients with dumping syndrome. Small, multiple (six) meals devoid of simple carbohydrates coupled with elimination of liquids during meals is important. Antidiarrheals and anticholinergic agents are complimentary to diet. The somatostatin analogue octreotide has been successful in diet refractory cases. This drug is administered subcutaneously (50 μg tid), titrated according to clinical response. Recently a long-acting formulation has become available, but its use in dumping syndrome has not been examined.

Postvagotomy diarrhea   Up to 10% of patients may seek medical attention for the treatment of postvagotomy diarrhea. This complication is most commonly observed after truncal vagotomy. Patients may complain of intermittent diarrhea that occurs typically 1 to 2 h after meals. Occasionally the symptoms may be severe and relentless. This is due to a motility disorder from interruption of the vagal fibers supplying the luminal gut. Other contributing factors may include decreased absorption of nutrients (see below), increased excretion of bile acids, and release of luminal factors that promote secretion. Diphenoxylate or loperamide is often useful in symptom control. The bile salt–binding agent cholestyramine may be helpful in severe cases. Surgical reversal of a 10-cm segment of jejunum may yield a substantial improvement in bowel frequency in a subset of patients.

Bile reflux gastropathy   A subset of post-partial gastrectomy patients will present with abdominal pain, early satiety, nausea, and vomiting, who have as the only finding mucosal erythema of the gastric remnant. Histologic examination of the gastric mucosa reveals minimal inflammation but the presence of epithelial cell injury. This clinical picture is categorized as bile or alkaline reflux gastropathy/gastritis. Although reflux of bile is implicated as the reason for this disorder, the mechanism is unknown. Prokinetic agents (cisapride, 10 to 20 mg before meals and at bedtime) and cholestyramine have been effective treatments. Cisapride may cause cardiac arrhythmias. Severe refractory symptoms may require using either nuclear scanning with ^{99m}Tc-HIDA, to document reflux, or an alkaline challenge test, where 0.1 N NaOH is infused into the stomach in an effort to reproduce the patient's symptoms. Surgical diversion of pancreaticobiliary secretions away from the gastric remnant with a Roux-en-Y gastrojejunostomy consisting of a long (50 to 60 cm) Roux limb has been used in severe cases. Bilious vomiting improves, but early satiety and bloating may persist in up to 50% of patients.

Maldigestion and malabsorption   Weight loss can be observed in up to 60% of patients after partial gastric resection. A significant component of this weight reduction is due to decreased oral intake. However, mild steatorrhea can also develop. Reasons for maldigestion/malabsorption include decreased gastric acid production, rapid gastric emptying, decreased food dispersion in the stomach, reduced luminal bile concentration, reduced pancreatic secretory response to feeding, and rapid intestinal transit.

Decreased serum vitamin B_{12} levels can be observed after partial gastrectomy. This is usually not due to deficiency of intrinsic factor (IF), since a minimal amount of parietal cells (source of IF) are removed during antrectomy. Reduced vitamin B_{12} may be due to competition for the vitamin by bacterial overgrowth or inability to split the vitamin from its protein-bound source due to hypochlorhydria.

Iron-deficiency anemia may be a consequence of impaired absorption of dietary iron in patients with a Billroth II gastrojejunotomy. Absorption of iron salts is normal in these individuals; thus a favorable response to oral iron supplementation can be anticipated. Folate deficiency with concomitant anemia can also develop in these patients. This deficiency may be secondary to decreased absorption or diminished oral intake.

Malabsorption of vitamin D and calcium resulting in osteoporosis and osteomalacia is common after partial gastrectomy and gastrojejunostomy (Billroth II). Osteomalacia can occur as a late complication in up to 25% of post-partial gastrectomy patients. Bone fractures occur twice as commonly in men after gastric surgery as in a control population. It may take years before x-ray findings demonstrate diminished bone density. Elevated alkaline phosphatase, reduced serum calcium, bone pain, and pathologic fractures may be seen in patients with osteomalacia. The high incidence of these abnormalities in this subgroup of patients justifies treating them with vitamin D and calcium supplementation indefinitely. Therapy is especially important in females.

Gastric adenocarcinoma The incidence of adenocarcinoma in the gastric stump is increased 15 years after resection. Some have reported a four- to fivefold increase in gastric cancer 20 to 25 years after resection. The pathogenesis is unclear but may involve alkaline reflux, bacterial proliferation, or hypochlorhydria. Endoscopic screening every other year may detect surgically treatable disease.

RELATED CONDITIONS

ZOLLINGER–ELLISON SYNDROME Severe peptic ulcer diathesis secondary to gastric acid hypersecretion due to unregulated gastrin release from a non-β cell endocrine tumor (gastrinoma) defines the components of the ZES. Initially, ZES was typified by aggressive and refractory ulceration in which total gastrectomy provided the only chance for enhancing survival. Today ZES can be cured by surgical resection in up to 30% of patients.

Epidemiology The incidence of ZES varies from 0.1 to 1% of individuals presenting with PUD. Males are more commonly affected than females, and the majority of patients are diagnosed between ages 30 and 50. Gastrinomas are classified into sporadic tumors (more common) and those associated with multiple endocrine neoplasia (MEN) type I (see below).

Pathophysiology Hypergastremia originating from an autonomous neoplasm is the driving force responsible for the clinical manifestations in ZES. Gastrin stimulates acid secretion through gastrin receptors on parietal cells and by inducing histamine release from ECL cells. Gastrin also has a trophic action on gastric epithelial cells. Long-standing hypergastrinemia leads to markedly increased gastric acid secretion through both parietal cell stimulation and increased parietal cell mass. The increased gastric acid output leads to the peptic ulcer diathesis, erosive esophagitis, and diarrhea.

Tumor Distribution Although early studies suggested that the vast majority of gastrinomas occurred within the pancreas, a significant number of these lesions are extrapancreatic. Over 80% of these tumors are found within the hypothetical gastrinoma triangle (confluence of the cystic and common bile ducts superiorly, junction of the second and third portions of the duodenum inferiorly, and junction of the neck and body of the pancreas medially). Duodenal tumors constitute the most common nonpancreatic lesion; up to 50% of gastrinomas are found here. Less common extrapancreatic sites include stomach, bones, ovaries, heart, liver, and lymph nodes. More than 60% of tumors are considered malignant, with up to 30 to 50% of patients having multiple lesions or metastatic disease at presentation. Histologically, gastrin-producing cells appear well differentiated, expressing markers typically found in endocrine neoplasms (chromogranin, neuron-specific enolase).

Clinical Manifestations Gastric acid hypersecretion is responsible for the signs and symptoms observed in patients with ZES. Peptic ulcer is the most common clinical manifestation, occurring in >90% of gastrinoma patients. Initial presentation and ulcer location (duode-

nal bulb) may be indistinguishable from common PUD. Clinical situations that should create suspicion of gastrinoma are ulcers in unusual locations (second part of the duodenum and beyond), ulcers refractory to standard medical therapy, ulcer recurrence after acid-reducing surgery, or ulcers presenting with frank complications (bleeding, obstruction, and perforation). Symptoms of esophageal origin are present in up to two-thirds of patients with ZES, with a spectrum ranging from mild esophagitis to frank ulceration with stricture and Barrett's mucosa.

Diarrhea is the next most common clinical manifestation in up to 50% of patients. Although diarrhea often occurs concomitantly with acid peptic disease, it may also occur independent of an ulcer. Etiology of the diarrhea is multifactorial, resulting from marked volume overload to the small bowel, pancreatic enzyme inactivation by acid, and damage of the intestinal epithelial surface by acid. The epithelial damage can lead to a mild degree of maldigestion and malabsorption of nutrients. The diarrhea may also have a secretory component due to the direct stimulatory effect of gastrin on enterocytes or the cosecretion of additional hormones from the tumor, such as vasoactive intestinal peptide.

Gastrinomas can develop in the presence of MEN I syndrome (Chap. 93) in approximately 25% of patients. This autosomal dominant disorder involves primarily three organ sites: the parathyroid glands (80 to 90%), pancreas (40 to 80%), and pituitary gland (30 to 60%). The genetic defect in MEN I is in the long arm of chromosome 11 (11q11-q13). In view of the stimulatory effect of calcium on gastric secretion, the hyperparathyroidism and hypercalcemia seen in MEN I patients may have a direct effect on ulcer disease. Resolution of hypercalcemia by parathyroidectomy reduces gastrin and gastric acid output in gastrinoma patients. An additional distinguishing feature in ZES patients with MEN I is the higher incidence of gastric carcinoid tumor development (as compared to patients with sporadic gastrinomas). Gastrinomas tend to be smaller, multiple, and located in the duodenal wall more often than is seen in patients with sporadic ZES. Establishing the diagnosis of MEN I is critical not only from the standpoint of providing genetic counseling to the patient and his or her family but also from the surgical approach recommended.

Diagnosis The first step in the evaluation of a patient suspected of having ZES is to obtain a fasting gastrin level. A list of clinical scenarios that should arouse suspicion regarding this diagnosis is shown in Table 285-10. Fasting gastrin levels are usually <150 pg/mL. Virtually all gastrinoma patients will have a gastrin level >150 to 200 pg/mL. Measurement of fasting gastrin should be repeated to confirm the clinical suspicion.

Multiple processes can lead to an elevated fasting gastrin level (Table 285-11), with gastric hypochlorhydria or achlorhydria being the most frequent causes. Gastric acid induces feedback inhibition of gastrin release. A decrease in acid production will subsequently lead to failure of the feedback inhibitory pathway, resulting in net hypergastrinemia. Gastrin levels will thus be high in patients using antisecretory agents for the treatment of acid peptic disorders and dyspepsia. *H. pylori* infection can also cause hypergastrinemia.

Table 285-10 When to Obtain a Fasting Serum Gastrin Level

Multiple ulcers
Ulcers in unusual locations
Ulcers associated with severe esophagitis
Ulcers resistant to therapy, with frequent recurrences
Ulcer patients awaiting surgery
Extensive family history of peptic ulcer disease
Postoperative ulcer recurrence
Basal hyperchlorhydria
Unexplained diarrhea or steatorrhea
Hypercalcemia
Family history of pancreatic islet, pituitary, or parathyroid tumor
Prominent gastric or duodenal folds

Table 285-11   Differential Diagnosis of Hypergastrinemia

Hypochlorhydria or achlorhydria with or without pernicious anemia
Retained gastric antrum
G cell hyperplasia
Gastric outlet obstruction
Renal insufficiency
Massive small-bowel obstruction
Others: rheumatoid arthritis, vitiligo, diabetes, pheochromocytoma

Study	Sensitivity, %	
	Primary Gastrinoma	Metastatic Gastrinoma
Ultrasound	21–28	14
CT scan	35–59	35–72
Selective angiography	35–68	33–86
Portal venous sampling	70–90	N/A
SASI	55–78	41
MRI	30–60	71
Otreoscan	67–86	80–100
EUS	80–100	N/A

NOTE: CT, computed tomography; SASI, selective arterial secretin injection; MRI, magnetic resonance imaging; Octreoscan, imaging with indium-111-labeled pentreotide; EUS, endoscopic ultrasonography.

The next step in establishing a biochemical diagnosis of gastrinoma is to assess acid secretion. Nothing further needs to be done if decreased acid output is observed. In contrast, normal or elevated gastric acid output suggests a need for additional tests. Gastric acid analysis is performed by placing a nasogastric tube in the stomach and drawing samples at 15-min intervals for 1 h during unstimulated or basal state (BAO), followed by continued sampling after administration of intravenous pentagastrin (MAO). Up to 90% of gastrinoma patients may have a BAO of ≥15 meq/h (normal <4 meq/h). Up to 12% of patients with common PUD may have comparable levels of acid secretion. A BAO/MAO ratio >0.6 is highly suggestive of ZES, but a ratio <0.6 does not exclude the diagnosis.

Gastrin provocative tests have been developed in an effort to differentiate between the causes of hypergastrinemia and are especially helpful in patients with indeterminant acid secretory studies. The tests are the secretin stimulation test, the calcium infusion study, and a standard meal test. In each of these, a fasted patient has an indwelling intravenous catheter in place for serial blood sampling and an intravenous line in place for secretin or calcium infusion. The patient receives either secretion (intravenous bolus of 2 μg/kg) or calcium (calcium gluconate, 5 mg/kg body weight over 3 h) or is fed a meal. Blood is then drawn at predetermined intervals (10 min and 1 min before and at 2, 5, 10, 15, 20, and 30 min after injection for secretin stimulation and at 30-min intervals during the calcium infusion). The most sensitive and specific gastrin provocative test for the diagnosis of gastrinoma is the secretin study. An increase in gastrin of ≥200 pg within 15 min of secretin injection has a sensitivity and specificity of >90% for ZES. The calcium infusion study is less sensitive and specific than the secretin test, with a rise of >400 pg/mL observed in ~80% of gastrinoma patients. The lower accuracy, coupled with it being a more cumbersome study with greater potential for adverse effects, makes calcium infusion less useful and therefore rarely, if ever, utilized. Rarely, one may observe increased BAO and hypergastrinemia in a patient who in the past has been categorized as having G cell hyperplasia or hyperfunction. This set of findings may have been due to *H. pylori*. The standard meal test was devised to assist in making the diagnosis of G cell–related hyperactivity, by observing a dramatic increase in gastrin after a meal (>200%). This test is not useful in differentiating between G cell hyperfunction and ZES.

Tumor Localization   Once the biochemical diagnosis of gastrinoma has been confirmed, the tumor must be located. Multiple imaging studies have been utilized in an effort to enhance tumor localization (Table 285-12). The broad range of sensitivity is due to the variable success rates achieved by the different investigative groups. Endoscopic ultrasound (EUS) permits imaging of the pancreas with a high degree of resolution (<5 mm). This modality is particularly helpful in excluding small neoplasms within the pancreas and in assessing the presence of surrounding lymph nodes and vascular involvement. Several types of endocrine tumors express cell-surface receptors for somatostatin. This permits the localization of gastrinomas by measuring the uptake of the stable somatostatin analogue, ^{111}In-pentriotide (*octreoscan*) with sensitivity and specificity rates of >75%.

Up to 50% of patients have metastatic disease at diagnosis. Success in controlling gastric acid hypersecretion has shifted the emphasis of therapy towards providing a surgical cure. Detecting the primary tumor and excluding metastatic disease are critical in view of this paradigm shift. Once a biochemical diagnosis has been confirmed, the patient should first undergo an abdominal computed tomographic scan, magnetic resonance imaging, or octreoscan (depending on availability) to exclude metastatic disease. Once metastatic disease has been excluded, an experienced endocrine surgeon may opt for exploratory laparotomy with intraoperative ultrasound or transillumination. In other centers, careful examination of the peripancreatic area with EUS, accompanied by endoscopic exploration of the duodenum for primary tumors, will be performed before surgery. Selective arterial secretin injection (SASI) may be a useful adjuvant for localizing tumors in a subset of patients.

℞ TREATMENT   Treatment of functional endocrine tumors is directed at ameliorating the signs and symptoms related to hormone overproduction, curative resection of the neoplasm, and attempts to control tumor growth in metastatic disease.

PPIs are the treatment of choice and have decreased the need for total gastrectomy. Initial doses of omeprazole or lansoprazole should be in the range of 60 mg/d. Dosing can be adjusted to achieve a BAO <10 meq/h (at the drug trough) in surgery-naive patients and to <5 meq/h in individuals who have previously undergone an acid-reducing operation. Although the somatostatin analogue has inhibitory effects on gastrin release from receptor-bearing tumors and inhibits gastric acid secretion to some extent, PPIs have the advantage of reducing parietal cell activity to a greater degree.

The ultimate goal of surgery would be to provide a definitive cure. Improved understanding of tumor distribution has led to 10-year disease-free intervals as high as 34% in sporadic gastrinoma patients undergoing surgery. A positive outcome is highly dependent on the experience of the surgical team treating these rare tumors. Surgical therapy of gastrinoma patients with MEN I remains controversial because of the difficulty in rendering these patients disease free with surgery. In contrast to the encouraging postoperative results observed in patients with sporadic disease, only 6% of MEN I patients are disease free 5 years after an operation. Some groups suggest surgery only if a clearly identifiable, nonmetastatic lesion is documented by structural studies. Others advocate a more aggressive approach, where all patients free of hepatic metastasis are explored and all detected tumors in the duodenum are resected; this is followed by enucleation of lesions in the pancreatic head, with a distal pancreatectomy to follow. The outcome of the two approaches has not been clearly defined.

Therapy of metastatic endocrine tumors in general remains suboptimal; gastrinomas are no exception. A host of medical therapeutic approaches including chemotherapy (streptozotocin, 5-fluorouracil, and doxorubicin), IFN-α, and hepatic artery embolization lead to significant toxicity without a substantial improvement in overall survival. Surgical approaches including debulking surgery and liver transplantation for hepatic metastasis have also produced limited benefit. Therefore, early recognition and surgery are the only chances for curing this disease.

The 5- and 10-year survival rates for gastrinoma patients are 62 to

75% and 47 to 53%, respectively. Individuals with the entire tumor resected or those with a negative laparotomy have 5- and 10-year survival rates >90%. Patients with incompletely resected tumors have 5- and 10-year survival of 43% and 25%, respectively. Patients with hepatic metastasis have <20% survival at 5 years. Favorable prognostic indicators include primary duodenal wall tumors, isolated lymph node tumor, and undetectable tumor upon surgical exploration. Poor prognostic indicators include hepatic metastases or the presence of Cushing's syndrome in a sporadic gastrinoma patient.

STRESS-RELATED MUCOSAL INJURY Patients suffering from shock, sepsis, massive burns, severe trauma, or head injury can develop acute erosive gastric mucosal changes or frank ulceration with bleeding. Classified as stress-induced gastritis or ulcers, injury is most commonly observed in the acid-producing (fundus and body) portions of the stomach. The most common presentation is gastrointestinal bleeding, which is usually minimal but can occasionally be life-threatening. Respiratory failure requiring mechanical ventilation and underlying coagulopathy are risk factors for bleeding, which tends to occur 48 to 72 h after the acute injury or insult.

Histologically, stress injury does not contain inflammation or *H. pylori*; thus "gastritis" is a misnomer. Although elevated gastric acid secretion may be noted in patients with stress ulceration after head trauma (Cushing's ulcer) and severe burns (Curling's ulcer), mucosal ischemia and breakdown of the normal protective barriers of the stomach also play an important role in the pathogenesis. Acid must contribute to injury in view of the significant drop in bleeding noted when acid inhibitors are used as a prophylactic measure for stress gastritis.

Improvement in the general management of intensive care unit patients has led to a significant decrease in the incidence of gastrointestinal bleeding due to stress ulceration. The estimated decrease in bleeding is from 20 to 30% to <15%. This improvement has led to some debate regarding the need for prophylactic therapy. The limited benefit of medical (endoscopic, angiographic) and surgical therapy in a patient with hemodynamically compromising bleeding associated with stress ulcer/gastritis supports the use of preventive measures in high-risk patients (mechanically ventilated, coagulopathy, multiorgan failure, or severe burns). Maintenance of gastric pH >3.5 with continuous infusion of H_2 blockers or liquid antacids administered every 2 to 3 h are viable options. Sucralfate slurry (1 g every 4 to 6 h) has also been successful. If bleeding occurs despite these measures, endoscopy, intraarterial vasopressin, or embolization are options. If all else fails, then surgery should be considered. Although vagotomy and antrectomy may be used, the better approach would be a total gastrectomy, which has an exceedingly high mortality rate in this setting.

GASTRITIS The term *gastritis* should be reserved for histologically documented inflammation of the gastric mucosa. Gastritis is *not* the mucosal erythema seen during endoscopy and is *not* interchangeable with "dyspepsia." The etiologic factors leading to gastritis are broad and heterogeneous. Gastritis has been classified based on time course (acute vs. chronic), histologic features, and anatomic distribution or proposed pathogenic mechanism (Table 285-13).

Table 285-13 Classification of Gastritis

I. Acute gastritis	II. Chronic Atrophic Gastritis
A. Acute *H. pylori* infection	A. Type A: Autoimmune,
B. Other acute infectious gastritides	body-predominant
1. Bacterial (other than *H. pylori*)	B. Type B: *H. pylori*–related,
2. *Helicobacter helmanni*	antral predominant
3. Phlegmonous	C. Indeterminant
4. Mycobacterial	III. Uncommon Forms of Gastritis
5. Syphilitic	A. Lymphocytic
6. Viral	B. Eosinophilic
7. Parasitic	C. Crohn's disease
8. Fungal	D. Sarcoidosis
	E. Isolated granulomatous gastritis

The correlation between the histologic findings of gastritis, the clinical picture of abdominal pain or dyspepsia, and endoscopic findings noted on gross inspection of the gastric mucosa is poor. Therefore, there is no typical clinical manifestation of gastritis.

Acute Gastritis The most common causes of acute gastritis are infectious. Acute infection with *H. pylori* induces gastritis. However, *H. pylori* acute gastritis has not been extensively studied. Reported as presenting with sudden onset of epigastric pain, nausea, and vomiting, limited mucosal histologic studies demonstrate a marked infiltrate of neutrophils with edema and hyperemia. If not treated, this picture will evolve into one of chronic gastritis. Hypochlorhydria lasting for up to 1 year may follow acute *H. pylori* infection.

The highly acidic gastric environment may be one reason why infectious processes of the stomach are rare. Bacterial infection of the stomach or phlegmonous gastritis is a rare potentially life-threatening disorder, characterized by marked and diffuse acute inflammatory infiltrates of the entire gastric wall, at times accompanied by necrosis. Elderly individuals, alcoholics, and AIDS patients may be affected. Potential iatrogenic causes include polypectomy and mucosal injection with India ink. Organisms associated with this entity include streptococci, staphylococci, *Escherichia coli*, *Proteus*, and *Haemophilus*. Failure of supportive measures and antibiotics may result in gastrectomy.

Other types of infectious gastritis may occur in immunocompromised individuals such as AIDS patients. Examples include herpetic (herpes simplex) or CMV gastritis. The histologic finding of intranuclear inclusions would be observed in the latter.

Chronic Gastritis Chronic gastritis is identified histologically by an inflammatory cell infiltrate consisting primarily of lymphocytes and plasma cells, with very scant neutrophil involvement. Distribution of the inflammation may be patchy, initially involving superficial and glandular portions of the gastric mucosa. This picture may progress to more severe glandular destruction, with atrophy and metaplasia. Chronic gastritis has been classified according to histologic characteristics. These include superficial atrophic changes and gastric atrophy.

The early phase of chronic gastritis is *superficial gastritis*. The inflammatory changes are limited to the lamina propria of the surface mucosa, with edema and cellular infiltrates separating intact gastric glands. Additional findings may include decreased mucus in the mucous cells and decreased mitotic figures in the glandular cells. The next stage is *atrophic gastritis*. The inflammatory infiltrate extends deeper into the mucosa, with progressive distortion and destruction of the glands. The final stage of chronic gastritis is *gastric atrophy*. Glandular structures are lost; there is a paucity of inflammatory infiltrates. Endoscopically the mucosa may be substantially thin, permitting clear visualization of the underlying blood vessels.

Gastric glands may undergo morphologic transformation in chronic gastritis. Intestinal metaplasia denotes the conversion of gastric glands to a small intestinal phenotype with small-bowel mucosal glands containing goblet cells. The metaplastic changes may vary in distribution from patchy to fairly extensive gastric involvement. Intestinal metaplasia is an important predisposing factor for gastric cancer (Chap. 90).

Chronic gastritis is also classified according to the predominant site of involvement. Type A refers to the body-predominant form (autoimmune) and type B is the central-predominant form (*H. pylori*–related). This classification is artificial in view of the difficulty in distinguishing these two entities. The term *AB gastritis* has been used to refer to a mixed antral/body picture.

Type A Gastritis The less common of the two forms involves primarily the fundus and body, with antral sparing. Traditionally, this form of gastritis has been associated with pernicious anemia (Chap. 107) in the presence of circulating antibodies against parietal cells and intrinsic factor; thus it is also called *autoimmune gastritis*. *H. pylori* infection can lead to a similar distribution of gastritis. The characteristics of an autoimmune picture are not always present.

Antibodies to parietal cells have been detected in >90% of patients with pernicious anemia and in up to 50% of patients with type A gastritis. Anti-parietal cell antibodies are cytotoxic for gastric mucous cells. The parietal cell antibody is directed against H^+,K^+-ATPase. T cells are also implicated in the injury pattern of this form of gastritis.

Parietal cell antibodies and atrophic gastritis are observed in family members of patients with pernicious anemia. These antibodies are observed in up to 20% of individuals over age 60 and in ~20% of patients with vitiligo and Addison's disease. About half of patients with pernicious anemia have antibodies to thyroid antigens, and about 30% of patients with thyroid disease have circulating anti-parietal cell antibodies. Anti-intrinsic factor antibodies are more specific than parietal cell antibodies for type A gastritis, being present in ~40% of patients with pernicious anemia. Another parameter consistent with this form of gastritis being autoimmune in origin is the higher incidence of specific familial histocompatibility haplotypes such as HLA-B8 and -DR3.

The parietal cell–containing gastric gland is preferentially targeted in this form of gastritis, and achlorhydria results. Parietal cells are the source of intrinsic factor, lack of which will lead to vitamin B_{12} deficiency and its sequelae (megaloblastic anemia, neurologic dysfunction).

Gastric acid plays an important role in feedback inhibition of gastrin release from G cells. Achlorhydria, coupled with relative sparing of the antral mucosa (site of G cells), leads to hypergastrinemia. Gastrin levels can be markedly elevated (>500 pg/mL) in patients with pernicious anemia. ECL cell hyperplasia with frank development of gastric carcinoid tumors may result from gastrin trophic effects. The role of gastrin in carcinoid development is confirmed by the observation that antrectomy leads to regression of these lesions. Hypergastrinemia and achlorhydria may also be seen in non-pernicious anemia-associated type A gastritis.

Type B gastritis Type B, or antral-predominant, gastritis is the more common form of chronic gastritis. *H. pylori* infection is the cause of this entity. Although described as "antral-predominant," this is likely a misnomer in view of studies documenting the progression of the inflammatory process towards the body and fundus of infected individuals. The conversion to a pan-gastritis is time-dependent—estimated to require 15 to 20 years. This form of gastritis increases with age, being present in up to 100% of people over age 70. Histology improves after *H. pylori* eradication. The number of *H. pylori* organisms decreases dramatically with progression to gastric atrophy, and the degree of inflammation correlates with the level of these organisms. Early on, with antral-predominant findings, the quantity of *H. pylori* is highest and a dense chronic inflammatory infiltrate of the lamina propria is noted accompanied by epithelial cell infiltration with polymorphonuclear leukocytes (Fig. 285-12).

Multifocal atrophic gastritis, gastric atrophy with subsequent metaplasia, has been observed in chronic *H. pylori*–induced gastritis. This may ultimately lead to development of gastric adenocarcinoma (Fig. 285-13; Chap. 90). *H. pylori* infection is now considered an independent risk factor for gastric cancer. Worldwide epidemiologic studies have documented a higher incidence of *H. pylori* infection in patients with adenocarcinoma of the stomach as compared to control subjects. Seropositivity for *H. pylori* is associated with a three- to sixfold increased risk of gastric cancer. This risk may be as high as ninefold after adjusting for the inaccuracy of serologic testing in the elderly. The mechanism by which *H. pylori* infection leads to cancer is unknown. However, eradication of *H. pylori* as a general preventative measure for gastric cancer is not recommended.

Infection with *H. pylori* is also associated with development of a low grade B cell lymphoma, gastric MALT lymphoma (Chap. 112). The chronic T cell stimulation caused by the infection leads to production of cytokines that promote the B cell tumor. Tumor growth remains dependent upon the presence of *H. pylori* in that its eradication

FIGURE 285-12 Chronic gastritis and *Helicobacter pylori* organisms. *A.* H&E stain of gastric mucosa showing surface foveolar cells, adherent mucus, and scattered bacillary forms within the mucus. *B.* Steiner silver stain of superficial gastric mucosa, showing abundant darkly staining microorganisms layered over the apical portion of the surface epithelium. Note that there is no tissue invasion. *[Courtesy of James M. Crawford, M.D., Ph.D. Reprinted with permission from JM Crawford, in V Kumar et al (eds): Basic Pathology. Philadelphia, Saunders, 1997]*

is often associated with complete regression of the tumor. The tumor may take more than a year to regress after treating the infection. Such patients should be followed by EUS every 2 to 3 months. If the tumor is stable or decreasing in size, no other therapy is necessary. If the tumor grows, it may have become a high-grade B cell lymphoma. When the tumor becomes a high-grade aggressive lymphoma histologically, it loses responsiveness to *H. pylori* eradication.

TREATMENT   Treatment in chronic gastritis is aimed at the sequelae and not the underlying inflammation. Patients with pernicious anemia will require parenteral vitamin B_{12} supplementation on a long-term basis. Eradication of *H. pylori* is not routinely recommended unless PUD or a low-grade MALT lymphoma is present.

Miscellaneous Forms of Gastritis *Lymphocytic gastritis* is characterized histologically by intense infiltration of the surface epithelium with lymphocytes. The infiltrative process is primarily in the body of the stomach and consists of mature T cells and plasmacytes. The etiology of this form of chronic gastritis is unknown. It has been described in patients with celiac sprue, but whether there is a common factor associating these two entities is unknown. No specific symptoms suggest lymphocytic gastritis. A subgroup of patients has thickened folds noted on endoscopy. These folds are often capped by small nodules that contain a central depression or erosion; this form of the disease is called *varioliform gastritis*. *H. pylori* probably plays no significant role in lymphocytic gastritis. Therapy with gluco-corticoids or sodium cromoglycate has obtained unclear results.

Marked eosinophilic infiltration involving any layer of the stomach (mucosa, muscularis propria, and serosa) is characteristic of *eosinophilic gastritis*. Affected individuals will often have circulating eosinophilia with clinical manifestation of systemic allergy. Involvement may range from isolated gastric disease to diffuse eosinophilic gastroenteritis. Antral involvement predominates, with prominent edematous folds being observed on endoscopy. These prominent antral folds can lead to outlet obstruction. Patients can present with epigastric discomfort, nausea, and vomiting. Treatment with glucocorticoids has been successful.

Several systemic disorders may be associated with *granulomatous gastritis*. Gastric involvement has been observed in Crohn's disease. Involvement may range from granulomatous infiltrates noted only on gastric biopsies to frank ulceration and stricture formation. Gastric Crohn's disease usually occurs in the presence of small-intestinal disease. Several rare infectious processes can lead to granulomatous gastritis, including histoplasmosis, candidiasis, syphilis, and tuberculosis. Other unusual causes of this form of gastritis include sarcoidosis, idiopathic granulomatous gastritis, and eosinophilic granulomas involving the stomach. Establishing the specific etiologic agent in this form of gastritis can be difficult, at times requiring repeat endoscopy with biopsy and cytology. Occasionally, a surgically obtained full-thickness biopsy of the stomach may be required to exclude malignancy.

MÉNÉTRIER'S DISEASE Ménétrier's disease is a rare entity characterized by large, tortuous gastric mucosal folds. The differential diagnosis of large gastric folds includes ZES, malignancy, infectious etiologies (CMV, histoplasmosis, syphilis), and infiltrative disorders such as sarcoidosis. The mucosal folds in Ménétrier's disease are often most prominent in the body and fundus. Histologically, massive foveolar hyperplasia (hyperplasia of surface and glandular mucous cells) is noted, which replaces most of the chief and parietal cells. This hyperplasia produces the prominent folds observed. The pits of the gastric glands elongate and may become extremely tortuous. Although the lamina propria may contain a mild chronic inflammatory infiltrate, Ménétrier's disease is *not* considered a form of gastritis. The etiology of this unusual clinical picture is unknown. Overexpression of growth factors such as TGF-α may be involved in the process.

Epigastric pain at times accompanied by nausea, vomiting, anorexia, and weight loss are signs and symptoms in patients with Ménétrier's disease. Occult gastrointestinal bleeding may occur, but overt bleeding is unusual and, when present, is due to superficial mucosal erosions. Between 20 and 100% of patients (depending on time of presentation) develop a protein-losing gastropathy accompanied by hypoalbuminemia and edema. Gastric acid secretion is usually reduced or absent because of the replacement of parietal cells. Large gastric folds are readily detectable by either radiographic (barium meal) or endoscopic methods. Endoscopy with deep mucosal biopsy (and cytology) is required to establish the diagnosis and exclude the other entities that may present in a similar manner. A nondiagnostic biopsy may lead to a surgically obtained full-thickness biopsy to exclude malignancy.

℞ **TREATMENT** Medical therapy with anticholinergic agents, prostaglandins, PPIs, prednisone, and H_2 receptor antagonists has obtained varying results. Anticholinergics decrease protein loss. A high-protein diet should be recommended to replace protein loss in patients with hypoalbuminemia. Ulcers should be treated with a standard approach. Severe disease with persistent and substantial protein loss may require total gastrectomy. Subtotal gastrectomy is performed by some; it may be associated with higher morbidity and mortality secondary to the difficulty in obtaining a patent and long-lasting anastomosis between normal and hyperplastic tissues.

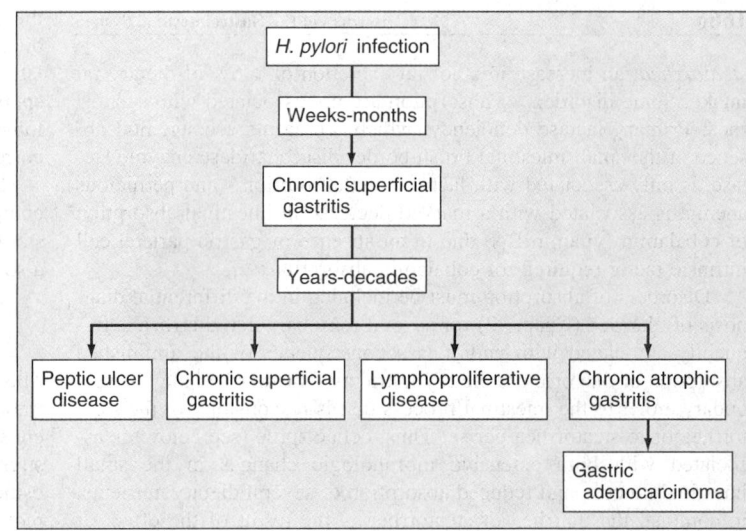

FIGURE 285-13 Potential long-term consequences of *H. pylori* infection.

ACKNOWLEDGMENT
The author acknowledges the contribution of material to this chapter by Dr. Lawrence Friedman and Dr. Walter Peterson from their chapter on this subject in the 14th edition and is grateful to Pamela Glazer for typing this manuscript.

BIBLIOGRAPHY

AGREUS L, TALLEY NJ: Dyspepsia: Current understanding and management. Annu Rev Med 49:475, 1997

BERARDI RR, WELAGE LS: Proton-pump inhibitors in acid-related diseases. Am J Health Syst Pharm 55:2249, 1998

CAPPELL MS, SCHEIN JR: Diagnosis and treatment of nonsteroidal anti-inflammatory drug-associated upper gastrointestinal toxicity. Gastroenterol Clin North Am 29:97, 2000

GRAHAM DY et al: Practical advice on eradicating *Helicobacter pylori* infection. Postgrad Med 105:137, 1999

KALANTAR J et al: Chronic gastritis and nonulcer dyspepsia. Curr Top Microbiol Immunol 241:31, 1999

McCOLL KE et al: Interactions between *H. pylori* infection, gastric acid secretion and antisecretory therapy. Br Med Bull 54:121, 1998

MITCHELL HM: The epidemiology of *Helicobacter pylori*. Curr Top Microbiol Immunol 241:11, 1999

NORTON JA et al: Surgery to cure the Zollinger-Ellison syndrome. N Engl J Med 341: 635, 1999

PEEK RM JR, BLASER MJ: Pathophysiology of *Helicobacter pylori*–induced gastritis and peptic ulcer disease. Am J Med 102:200, 1997

WOLFE MM et al: Gastrointestinal toxicity of nonsteroidal antiinflammatory drugs. N Engl J Med 340:1888, 1999

286   *Henry J. Binder*

DISORDERS OF ABSORPTION

Disorders of absorption represent a broad spectrum of conditions with multiple etiologies and varied clinical manifestations. Almost all of these clinical problems are associated with *diminished* intestinal absorption of one or more dietary nutrients and are often referred to as the *malabsorption syndrome*. This latter term is not ideal as it represents a pathophysiologic state, does *not* provide an etiologic explanation for the underlying problem, and should not be considered an adequate final diagnosis. The only clinical situations in which absorption is *increased* are hemochromatosis and Wilson's disease, in which there is increased absorption of iron and copper, respectively.

Most, but not all, of these clinical conditions are associated with *steatorrhea*, an increase in stool fat excretion of >6% of dietary fat intake. Some disorders of absorption are not associated with steatorrhea: Primary lactase deficiency, which represents a congenital absence of the small intestinal brush border disaccharidase enzyme lactase, is only associated with lactose "malabsorption," and pernicious anemia is associated with a marked decrease in intestinal absorption of cobalamin (vitamin B_{12}) due to an absence of gastric parietal cell intrinsic factor required for cobalamin absorption.

Disorders of absorption must be included in the differential diagnosis of diarrhea (Chap. 42) for several reasons. First, diarrhea is frequently associated with and/or is a consequence of the diminished absorption of one or more dietary nutrients. The diarrhea may be secondary either to the intestinal process that is responsible for the steatorrhea or to steatorrhea per se. Thus, celiac sprue (see below) is associated with both extensive morphologic changes in the small intestinal mucosa and reduced absorption of several dietary nutrients; in contrast, the diarrhea of steatorrhea is the result of the effect of nonabsorbed dietary fatty acids on intestinal, usually colonic, ion transport. For example, oleic acid and ricinoleic acid (a bacterially hydroxylated fatty acid that is also the active ingredient in castor oil, a widely used laxative) induce active colonic Cl secretion, most likely secondary to increasing intracellular Ca. In addition, diarrhea per se may result in mild steatorrhea (<11 g fat excretion while on a 100-g fat diet). Second, as diarrhea is both a symptom and a sign, most patients will indicate that they have diarrhea, not that they have fat malabsorption. Third, many intestinal disorders that have diarrhea as a prominent symptom (e.g., ulcerative colitis, traveler's diarrhea secondary to an enterotoxin produced by *Escherichia coli*) do not necessarily have diminished absorption of any dietary nutrient.

Diarrhea as a *symptom* (i.e., when used by patients to describe their bowel movement pattern) may be either a decrease in stool consistency, an increase in stool volume, an increase in number of bowel movements, or any combination of these three changes. In contrast, diarrhea as a *sign* is a quantitative increase in stool water or weight of >200 to 225 mL, or g per 24 h, when a western-type diet is consumed. Individuals consuming a diet with a higher fiber content may normally have a stool weight of up to 400 g/24 h. Thus, it is essential that the clinician clarify what an individual patient means by diarrhea, especially since 10% of patients referred to gastroenterologists for further evaluation of unexplained diarrhea do not have an increase in stool water when it is determined quantitatively. Such patients may have small, frequent, somewhat loose bowel movements with stool urgency that is indicative of proctitis but do not have an increase in stool weight or volume.

It is also critical to establish whether a patient's diarrhea is secondary to diminished absorption of one or more dietary nutrients, in contrast to diarrhea that is due to small- and/or large-intestinal fluid and electrolyte secretion. The former has often been termed *osmotic diarrhea*, while the latter has been referred to as *secretory diarrhea*. Unfortunately, as there can be both secretory and osmotic elements present simultaneously in the same disorder, this separation is not always precise. Nonetheless, two studies, determination of stool electrolytes, and observation of the effect of a fast on stool output can help make this distinction.

The demonstration of the effect of prolonged (>24 h) fasting on stool output can be very effective in suggesting that a *dietary nutrient* is responsible for the individual's diarrhea. A secretory diarrhea associated with enterotoxin-induced traveler's diarrhea would not be affected by prolonged fasting, as enterotoxin-induced stimulation of intestinal fluid and electrolyte secretion is not altered by eating. In contrast, diarrhea secondary to lactose malabsorption in primary lactase deficiency would undoubtedly cease during a prolonged fast. Thus, a substantial decrease in stool output while fasting during a quantitative stool collection of at least 24 h is presumptive evidence that the diarrhea is related to malabsorption of a dietary nutrient. The persistence of stool output while fasting indicates the likelihood that

the diarrhea is secretory and that the cause of diarrhea is *not* due to a dietary nutrient. Either a luminal (e.g., *E. coli* enterotoxin) or circulating (e.g., vasoactive intestinal peptide) secretogogue could be responsible for the patient's diarrhea persisting unaltered during a prolonged fast. The observed effects of fasting can be compared and correlated with stool electrolyte and osmolality determinations.

Measurement of stool electrolytes and osmolality requires the comparison of stool Na^+ and K^+ concentrations determined in liquid stool to the stool osmolality to determine the presence or absence of a so-called stool osmotic gap. The following formula is used:

$$2 \times (\text{stool } [Na^+] + \text{stool } [K^+]) \geq \text{stool osmolality}$$

The cation concentrations are doubled to estimate stool anion concentrations. The presence of a significant osmotic gap suggests the presence in stool water of a substance(s) other than Na/K/anions that presumably is responsible for the patient's diarrhea. Originally, stool osmolality was measured, but it is almost invariably greater than the required 290 to 300 mosmol/kg H_2O, reflecting bacterial degradation of nonabsorbed carbohydrate either immediately before defecation or in the stool jar while awaiting chemical analysis, even when the stool is refrigerated. As a result, the stool osmolality should be assumed to be 300 mosmol/kg H_2O. When the calculated difference is >50, an osmotic gap is present, suggesting that the diarrhea is due to a nonabsorbed dietary nutrient, e.g., a fatty acid and/or carbohydrate. When this difference is <25 to 50, it is presumed that a dietary nutrient is not responsible for the diarrhea. Since elements of both osmotic (i.e., malabsorption of a dietary nutrient) and secretory diarrhea may be present simultaneously, this separation at times is less clear-cut at the bedside than when used as a teaching example. Ideally, the presence of an osmotic gap will be associated with a marked decrease in stool output during a prolonged fast, while the absence of an osmotic gap will likely be present in an individual whose stool output had not been reduced substantially during a period of fasting.

NUTRIENT DIGESTION AND ABSORPTION

The lengths of the small intestine and colon are ~300 cm and ~80 cm, respectively. However, the effective functional surface area is approximately 600-fold greater than that of a hollow tube as a result of the presence of folds, villi (in the small intestine), and microvilli. The functional surface area of the small intestine is somewhat greater than that of a doubles tennis court. In addition to nutrient digestion and absorption, the intestinal epithelia have several other functions:

1. *Barrier and immune defense.* The intestine is exposed to a large number of potential antigens, enteric and invasive microorganisms, and is extremely effective preventing the entry of almost all these agents. The intestinal mucosa also synthesizes and secretes secretory IgA globulin.
2. *Fluid and electrolyte absorption and secretion.* The intestine absorbs approximately 7 to 8 L of fluid daily, comprising dietary fluid intake (1 to 2 L/d) and salivary, gastric, pancreatic, biliary, and intestinal fluid (6 to 7 L/d). The intestine also responds to several stimuli, especially bacteria and bacterial enterotoxins, that induce fluid and electrolyte secretion, often leading to diarrhea (Chap. 131).
3. *Synthesis and secretion of several proteins.* The intestinal mucosa is a major site for the production of proteins, including apolipoproteins.
4. *Production of several bioactive amines and peptides.* The intestine presents one of the largest endocrine organs in the body and produces several amines and peptides that serve as paracrine and hormonal mediators of intestinal function.

The small and large intestine are anatomically distinct in that villi are present in the small intestine but are absent in the colon and functionally distinct in that nutrient digestion and absorption take place in the small intestine but not in the colon. No precise anatomic characteristics separate duodenum, jejunum, and ileum, although certain nutrients are absorbed exclusively in specific areas of the small intestine. However, villus cells in the small intestine (and surface epithelial cells in the colon) and crypt cells have distinct anatomic and functional characteristics. Intestinal epithelial cells are continuously renewed, with new proliferating epithelial cells at the base of the crypt migrating over 48 to 72 h to the tip of the villus (or surface of the colon), where they are well-developed epithelial cells with digestive and absorptive function. This high rate of cell turnover explains the relatively rapid resolution of diarrhea and other digestive tract side effects during chemotherapy as new cells not exposed to these toxic agents are produced. Equally important is the paradigm of separation of villus/surface cell and crypt cell function: digestive hydrolytic enzymes are present primarily in the brush border of villus epithelial cells. Absorptive and secretory functions are also separated, with villus/surface cells largely being the site for absorptive function, while secretory function is present in crypts of both the small and large intestine.

Nutrients, minerals, and vitamins are absorbed by one or more active transport mechanisms. (The mechanisms of intestinal fluid and electrolyte absorption and secretion are discussed in Chap. 42.) Active transport mechanisms are energy-dependent and mediated by membrane transport proteins. These transport processes will result in the *net* movement of a substance against or in the absence of an electrochemical concentration gradient. Intestinal absorption of amino acids and monosaccharides, e.g., glucose, is also a specialized form of active transport—*secondary active transport*. The movement of these actively transported nutrients against a concentration gradient is Na^+-dependent and is due to a Na^+ gradient across the apical membrane. The Na^+ gradient is maintained by Na^+,K^+-ATPase, the so-called Na^+ pump located on the basolateral membrane, which extrudes Na^+ and maintains a low intracellular [Na] as well as the Na^+ gradient across the apical membrane. As a result, active glucose absorption and glucose-stimulated Na^+ absorption require both the apical membrane transport protein, SGLT, and the basolateral Na^+,K^+-ATPase. In addition to glucose absorption being Na^+-dependent, glucose also stimulates Na^+ and fluid absorption, which is the physiologic basis of oral rehydration therapy for the treatment of diarrhea (Chap. 42).

Although the intestinal epithelial cells are crucial mediators of absorption and ion and water flow, the several cell types in the lamina propria (e.g., mast cells, macrophages, myofibroblasts) and the enteric nervous system interact with the epithelium to regulate mucosal cell function. The function of the intestine is the result of the integrated responses of and interactions between both intestinal epithelial cells and intestinal muscle.

ENTEROHEPATIC CIRCULATION OF BILE ACIDS
Bile acids are not present in the diet but are synthesized in the liver by a series of enzymatic steps that also represent cholesterol catabolism. Indeed, interruption of the enterohepatic circulation of bile acids can reduce serum cholesterol levels by 10% before a new steady state is established. Bile acids are either primary or secondary: primary bile acids are synthesized in the liver from cholesterol, and secondary bile acids are synthesized from primary bile acids in the intestine by colonic bacterial enzymes. The two primary bile acids are cholic acid and chenodeoxycholic acid; the two most abundant secondary bile acids are deoxycholic acid and lithocholic acid. Approximately 500 mg bile acids are synthesized in the liver daily, conjugated to either taurine or glycine to form tauro-conjugated or glyco-conjugated bile acids, respectively, that are secreted into the duodenum in bile. The primary functions of bile acids are (1) to promote bile flow, (2) to solubilize cholesterol and phospholipid in the gall bladder by mixed micelle formation, and (3) to enhance dietary lipid digestion and absorption by forming mixed micelles in the proximal small intestine.

Bile acids are primarily absorbed by an active, Na^+-dependent process that is located exclusively in the ileum, though bile acids can also be absorbed to a lesser extent by non-carrier-mediated transport processes in the jejunum, ileum, and colon. Conjugated bile acids that enter the colon are deconjugated by colonic bacterial enzymes to un-

conjugated bile acids and are rapidly absorbed. Colonic bacterial enzymes also dehydroxylate bile acids to secondary bile acids.

Bile acids absorbed from the intestine return to the liver via the portal vein where they are resecreted (Fig. 286-1). Bile acid synthesis is largely autoregulated by 7α-hydroxylase, the initial enzyme in cholesterol degradation. A decrease in the amount of bile acids returning to the liver from the intestine is associated with an increase in bile acid synthesis/cholesterol catabolism, which helps maintain the bile acid pool size relatively constant. However, there is a relatively limited capacity for an increase in bile acid synthesis—about two to two and one-half times (see below). The bile acid pool size is approximately 4 g and is circulated via the enterohepatic circulation about twice during each meal, or six to eight times during a 24-h period. A relatively small quantity of bile acids is not absorbed and is excreted in stool daily; this fecal loss is matched by hepatic bile acid synthesis.

Defects in any of the steps of the enterohepatic circulation of bile acids can result in a decrease in duodenal concentration of conjugated bile acids and, as a result, steatorrhea. Thus, steatorrhea can be caused by abnormalities in bile acid synthesis and excretion, their physical state in the intestinal lumen, and reabsorption (Table 286-1).

Synthesis Decreased bile acid synthesis and steatorrhea have been demonstrated in chronic liver disease, but steatorrhea is often not a major component of the illness of these patients.

Secretion Although bile acid secretion may be reduced or absent in biliary obstruction, steatorrhea is rarely a significant medical problem in these patients. In contrast, primary biliary cirrhosis represents a defect in canalicular excretion of organic anions, including bile acids, and not infrequently is associated with steatorrhea and its consequences, e.g., chronic bone disease. Thus, the osteomalacia and other chronic bone abnormalities often present in patients with primary biliary cirrhosis and other cholestatic syndromes are secondary to steatorrhea that then leads to calcium and vitamin D malabsorption.

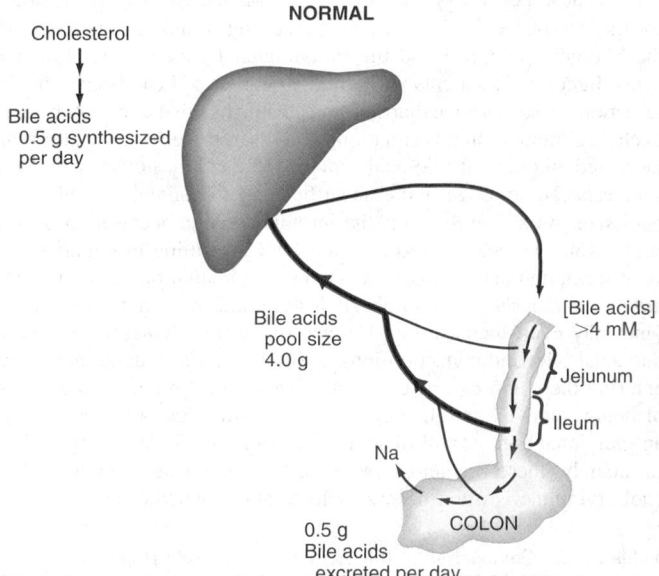

FIGURE 286-1 Schematic representation of the enterohepatic circulation of bile acids. Bile acid synthesis is cholesterol catabolism and occurs in the liver. Bile acids are secreted in bile and are stored in the gall bladder between meals and at night. Food in the duodenum induces the release of cholecystokinin, which is a potent stimulus for gall bladder contraction resulting in bile acid entry into the duodenum. Bile acids are primarily absorbed via a Na-dependent transport process that is located only in the ileum. A relatively small quantity of bile acids (~500 mg) are not absorbed in a 24-h period and are lost in stool. Fecal bile acid losses are matched by bile acid synthesis. The bile acid pool, i.e., the total amount of bile acids in the body at any time, is ~4 g and is circulated twice during each meal or six to eight times in a 24-h period.

Table 286-1   Defects in Enterohepatic Circulation of Bile Acids

Process	Pathophysiologic Defect	Disease Example
Synthesis	Decreased hepatic function	Cirrhosis
Biliary secretion	Altered canalicular function	Primary biliary cirrhosis
Maintenance of conjugated bile acids	Bacterial overgrowth	Jejunal diverticulosis
Reabsorption	Abnormal ileal function	Crohn's disease

Maintenance of Conjugated Bile Acids   In bacterial overgrowth syndromes associated with diarrhea, steatorrhea, and macrocytic anemia, there is an increase in a colonic-type of bacterial flora in the small intestine. The steatorrhea is primarily a result of the decrease in conjugated bile acids secondary to their deconjugation by colonic-type bacteria. Two complementary explanations account for the resulting impairment of micelle formation: (1) unconjugated bile acids are rapidly absorbed in the jejunum by nonionic diffusion resulting in a reduced concentration of duodenal bile acids; and (2) the critical micellar concentration (CMC) of unconjugated bile acids is higher than that of conjugated bile acids, and therefore unconjugated bile acids are less effective than conjugated bile acids in micelle formation.

Reabsorption   Ileal dysfunction caused by either Crohn's disease or surgical resection results in a decrease in bile acid reabsorption in the ileum and an *increase* in the delivery of bile acids to the large intestine. The resulting clinical consequences—diarrhea with or without steatorrhea—is determined by the *degree* of ileal dysfunction and the *response* of the enterohepatic circulation to bile acid losses (Table 286-2). Patients with limited ileal disease or resection will often have diarrhea, but not steatorrhea. The diarrhea, a result of bile acids in the colon stimulating active Cl secretion, has been called *bile acid diarrhea*, or cholorrheic enteropathy, and responds promptly to cholestyramine, an anion-binding resin. Such patients do not develop steatorrhea because hepatic synthesis of bile acids increases to compensate for the rate of fecal bile acid losses resulting in maintenance of both the bile acid pool size and the intraduodenal concentrations of bile acids. In contrast, patients with greater degrees of ileal disease and/or resection will often have diarrhea and steatorrhea that does not respond to cholestyramine. In this situation, ileal disease is also associated with increased amounts of bile acids entering the colon; however, hepatic synthesis can no longer increase sufficiently to maintain the bile acid pool size. As a consequence, the intraduodenal concentration of bile acids is also reduced to less than the CMC, resulting in impaired micelle formation and steatorrhea. This second situation is often called *fatty acid diarrhea*. Although cholestyramine may not be effective (and may even increase the diarrhea by further depleting the intraduodenal bile acid concentration), a low-fat diet to reduce fatty acids entering the colon can be effective. Two clinical features, the length of ileum removed and the degree of steatorrhea, can predict whether an individual patient will or will not respond to cholestyramine. Unfortunately, these predictors are imperfect, and a therapeutic trial of cholestyramine is often necessary to establish whether an individual

Table 286-2   Comparison of Bile Acid and Fatty Acid Diarrhea

	Bile Acid Diarrhea	Fatty Acid Diarrhea
Extent of ileal disease	Limited	Extensive
Ileal bile acid absorption	Reduced	Reduced
Fecal bile acid excretion	Increased	Increased
Fecal bile acid loss compensated by hepatic synthesis	Yes	No
Bile acid pool size	Normal	Reduced
Intraduodenal [bile acid]	Normal	Reduced
Steatorrhea	None or mild	>20 g
Response to cholestyramine	Yes	No
Response to low-fat diet	No	Yes

patient will benefit from cholestyramine. Table 286-2 contrasts the characteristics of bile acid diarrhea (small ileal dysfunction) and fatty acid diarrhea (large ileal dysfunction).

LIPIDS   Steatorrhea is caused by one or more defects in the digestion and absorption of dietary fat. Average intake of dietary fat in the United States is approximately 120 to 150 g/d, and fat absorption is linear to dietary fat intake. The total load of fat presented to the small intestine is considerably greater, as substantial amounts of lipid are secreted in bile each day. (See above for discussion of enterohepatic circulation of bile acids.) Three types of fatty acids compose fats: long-chain fatty acids (LCFAs), medium-chain fatty acids (MCFAs), and short-chain fatty acids (SCFAs) (Table 286-3). Dietary fat is exclusively composed of long-chain triglycerides (LCTs), i.e., glycerol that is bound via ester-linkages to three LCFAs. While the majority of dietary LCFAs have carbon chain lengths of 16 or 18, fatty acids of carbon chain length >12 are metabolized in the same manner; saturated and unsaturated fatty acids are handled identically.

Assimilation of dietary lipid requires several integrated processes that can be divided into (1) an intraluminal, or digestive, phase; (2) a mucosal, or absorptive, phase; and (3) a delivery, or postabsorptive, phase. An abnormality at any site of this process can cause steatorrhea (Table 286-4). Therefore, it is essential that any patient with steatorrhea be evaluated to identify the specific physiologic defect in overall lipid digestion-absorption as therapy will be determined by the specific cause responsible for the steatorrhea.

The digestive phase has two components, *lipolysis* and *micellar formation*. Although dietary lipid is in the form of LCTs, the intestinal mucosa does not absorb triglycerides; they must first be hydrolyzed (Fig. 286-2). The initial step in lipid digestion is the formation of emulsions of finely dispersed lipid, which is accomplished by mastication and gastric contractions. Lipolysis, the hydrolysis of triglycerides to free fatty acids, monoglycerides, and glycerol by lipase, is initiated in the stomach by a gastric lipase that has a pH optimum of 4.5 to 6.0. About 20 to 30% of total lipolysis occurs in the stomach. Lipolysis is completed in the duodenum and proximal jejunal by pancreatic lipase, which is inactivated by pH <7.0. Pancreatic lipolysis is greatly enhanced by the presence of a second pancreatic enzyme, colipase, which facilitates the movement of lipase to the triglyceride.

Impaired lipolysis can lead to steatorrhea and can occur in the presence of pancreatic insufficiency due to chronic pancreatitis in adults or cystic fibrosis in children and adolescents. Normal lipolysis can be maintained by approximately 5% of maximal pancreatic lipase secretion; thus, steatorrhea is a late manifestation of these disorders. A reduction in intraduodenal pH can also result in altered lipolysis as pancreatic lipase is inactivated at pH <7. Thus, ~15% of patients with gastrinoma (Chap. 285) with substantial increases in gastric acid secretion from ectopic production of gastrin (usually from an islet cell

Table 286-3   Comparison of Different Types of Fatty Acids

	Long-Chain	Medium-Chain	Short-Chain
Carbon chain length	>12	8–12	<8
Present in diet	In large amounts	In small amounts	No
Origin	In diet as triglycerides	Only in small amounts in diet as triglycerides	Bacterial degradation in colon of nonabsorbed carbohydrate to fatty acids
Primary site of absorption	Small intestine	Small intestine	Colon
Requires pancreatic lipolysis	Yes	No	No
Requires micelle formation	Yes	No	No
Presence in stool	Minimal	No	Substantial

Table 286-4 Defects in Lipid Digestion and Absorption in Steatorrhea

Phase: Process	Pathophysiologic Defect	Disease Example
Digestive		
Lipolysis formation	Decrease lipase secretion	Chronic pancreatitis
Micelle formation	Decreased intraduodenal [bile acids]	See Table 286-1
Absorptive		
Mucosal uptake and resterification	Mucosal dysfunction	Celiac sprue
Post-absorptive		
Chylomicron formation	Absent betalipoproteins	Abetalipoproteinemia
Delivery from intestine	Abnormal lymphatics	Intestinal lymphangiectasia

adenoma) have diarrhea, and some will have steatorrhea believed secondary to acid-inactivation of pancreatic lipase. Similarly, patients with chronic pancreatitis (who have reduced lipase secretion) often have a decrease in pancreatic bicarbonate secretion, which will also result in a decrease in intraduodenal pH and inactivation of endogenous pancreatic lipase or of therapeutically administered lipase.

Overlying the microvillus membrane of the small intestine is the so-called unstirred water layer, a relatively stagnant aqueous phase that must be traversed by the products of lipolysis that are primarily water-insoluble. Water-soluble mixed micelles provide a mechanism for the water-insoluble products of lipolysis to reach the luminal plasma membrane of villus epithelial cells, the site for lipid absorption. Mixed micelles are molecular aggregates composed of fatty acids, monoglycerides, phospholipids, cholesterol, and conjugated bile acids. Mixed micelles are formed when the concentration of conjugated bile acids is greater than its CMC, which differs among the several bile acids present in the small intestinal lumen. Conjugated bile acids, synthesized in the liver and excreted into the duodenum in bile, are regulated by the enterohepatic circulation (see above). Steatorrhea can result from impaired movement of fatty acids across the unstirred aqueous fluid layer in two situations: (1) an increase in the relative thickness of the unstirred water layer that occurs in bacterial overgrowth syndromes (see below) secondary to functional stasis (e.g., scleroderma), and (2) a decrease in the *duodenal* concentration of conjugated bile acids below its CMC, resulting in impaired micelle formation. Thus, steatorrhea can be caused by one or more defects in the enterohepatic circulation of bile acids.

Uptake and reesterification represent the *absorptive phase* of lipid digestion-absorption. Although passive diffusion has been thought responsible, a carrier-mediated process may mediate fatty acid and monoglyceride uptake. Regardless of the uptake process, fatty acids and monoglycerides are reesterified by a series of enzymatic steps in the endoplasmic reticulum and Golgi to form triglycerides, the form in which lipid exits from the intestinal epithelial cell. Impaired lipid absorption as a result of either mucosal inflammation (e.g., celiac sprue) and/or intestinal resection can also lead to steatorrhea.

The reesterified triglycerides require the formation of *chylomicrons* to permit their exit from the small-intestinal epithelial cell and their delivery to the liver via the *lymphatics.* Chylomicrons are composed of β-lipoprotein and contain triglycerides, cholesterol, cholesterol esters, and phospholipids and enter the lymphatics, not the portal vein. Defects in the *postabsorptive phase* of lipid digestion-absorption can also result in steatorrhea, but these disorders are uncommon. Abetalipoproteinemia, or acanthocytosis, is a rare disorder of impaired synthesis of β-lipoprotein associated with abnormal erythrocytes (acanthocytes), neurologic problems, and steatorrhea. Lipolysis, micelle

formation, and lipid uptake are all normal in patients with abetalipoproteinemia, but the reesterified triglyceride cannot exit from the epithelial cell because of the failure to produce chylomicrons. Small-intestinal biopsies of these rare patients in the postprandial state reveal lipid-laden small-intestinal epithelial cells that become perfectly normal in appearance following a 72- to 96-fast. Similarly, abnormalities of intestinal lymphatics (e.g., intestinal lymphangiectasia) may also be associated with steatorrhea as well as protein loss (see below). Steatorrhea can result from defects at any of the several steps in lipid digestion-absorption. The mechanism of lipid digestion-absorption outlined above is limited to *dietary* lipid that is almost exclusively in the form of LCTs (Table 286-3). Medium-chain triglycerides (MCTs), composed of fatty acids with carbon chain lengths of 8 to 10, are present in large amounts in coconut oil and are used as a nutritional supplement. MCTs can be digested and absorbed by a different pathway from LCTs and at one time held promise as an important treatment of steatorrhea of almost all etiologies. Unfortunately, their therapeutic effects have been less than expected because their use is often not associated with an increase in body weight for reasons that are not completely understood.

MCTs, in contrast to LCTs, do not require pancreatic lipolysis as the triglyceride can be absorbed intact by the intestinal epithelial cell. Further, micelle formation is not necessary for the absorption of MCTs or medium-chain fatty acids, if hydrolyzed by pancreatic lipase. MCTs are absorbed more efficiently than LCTs for the following reasons: (1) the rate of MCT absorption is greater than that of long-chain fatty acids; (2) medium-chain fatty acids following absorption are not reesterified; (3) following absorption, MCTs are hydrolyzed to medium-chain fatty acids; (4) MCTs do not require chylomicron formation for their exit from the intestinal epithelial cells; and (5) their route of exit is via the portal vein and not via lymphatics. Thus, the absorption of MCTs is greater than that of LCTs in pancreatic insufficiency, conditions with reduced intraduodenal bile acid concentrations, small-intestinal mucosal disease, abetalipoproteinemia, and intestinal lymphangiectasia.

SCFAs are not dietary lipids but are synthesized by colonic bacterial enzymes from nonabsorbed carbohydrate and are the anions in highest concentration in stool (between 80 and 130 m*M*). The SCFAs present in stool are primarily acetate, propionate, and butyrate whose carbon chain lengths are 2, 3, and 4, respectively. Butyrate is the primary nutrient for colonic epithelial cells, and its deficiency may be associated with one or more colitides. SCFAs conserve calories and carbohydrate, because carbohydrates not completely absorbed in the small intestine will not be absorbed in the large intestine due to the absence of both disaccharidases and SGLT, the transport protein that

FIGURE 286-2 Schematic representation of lipid digestion and absorption. Dietary lipid is in the form of long-chain triglycerides (LCT). The overall process can be divided into (1) a digestive phase that includes both lipolysis and micelle formation requiring pancreatic lipase and conjugated bile acids, respectively, in the duodenum; (2) an absorptive phase for mucosal uptake and reesterification; and (3) a postabsorptive phase that includes chylomicron formation and exit from the intestinal epithelial cell via lymphatics. *(Courtesy of John M. Dietschy, MD.)*

mediates monosaccharide absorption. In contrast, SCFAs are rapidly absorbed and stimulate colonic Na-Cl and fluid absorption. Most non-*Clostridium difficile* antibiotic-associated diarrhea is due to antibiotic suppression of colonic microflora, with a resulting decrease in SCFA production. As *C. difficile* accounts for about 10 to 15% of all antibiotic-associated diarrhea, a relative decrease in colonic production of SCFAs is the cause of most antibiotic-associated diarrhea.

The clinical manifestations of steatorrhea are a consequence of both the underlying disorder responsible for the development of steatorrhea and steatorrhea per se. Depending on the degree of steatorrhea and the level of dietary intake, significant fat malabsorption may lead to weight loss. Steatorrhea per se can be responsible for diarrhea; if the primary cause of the steatorrhea has not been identified, a low-fat diet can often ameliorate the diarrhea by decreasing fecal fat excretion. Steatorrhea is often associated with fat-soluble vitamin deficiency, which will require replacement with water-soluble preparations of these vitamins.

Disorders of absorption may also be associated with malabsorption of other dietary nutrients, most often carbohydrates, with or without a decrease in dietary lipid digestion and absorption. Therefore, knowledge of the mechanism of the digestion and absorption of carbohydrates, proteins, and other minerals and vitamins is useful in the evaluation of patients with altered intestinal nutrient absorption.

CARBOHYDRATES   Carbohydrates in the diet are present in the form of starch, disaccharides (sucrose and lactose), and glucose. Carbohydrates are absorbed only in the small intestine and only in the form of monosaccharides. Therefore, before their absorption, starch and disaccharides must first be digested by pancreatic amylase and intestinal brush border disaccharidases to monosaccharides. Monosaccharide absorption occurs by a Na-dependent process mediated by the brush border transport protein, SGLT.

Lactose malabsorption is the only clinically important disorder of carbohydrate absorption. Lactose, the disaccharide present in milk, requires digestion by brush border lactase to its two constituent monosaccharides, glucose and galactose. Lactase is present in almost all species in the postnatal period but then disappears throughout the animal kingdom, except in humans. Lactase activity persists in many individuals throughout life. Two different types of lactase deficiency exist—primary and secondary. In *primary lactase deficiency*, a genetically determined decrease or absence of lactase is noted, while all other aspects of both intestinal absorption and brush border enzymes are normal. In a number of non-Caucasian groups, primary lactase deficiency is common in adulthood. Table 286-5 presents the incidence of primary lactase deficiency in several different ethnic groups. Northern European and North American Caucasians are the only population group to maintain small-intestinal lactase activity throughout adult life. It is lactase persistence that is unusual. In contrast, *secondary lactase deficiency* occurs in association with small-intestinal mucosal disease with abnormalities in both structure and function of other brush border enzymes and transport processes. Secondary lactase deficiency is often seen in celiac sprue.

As lactose digestion is rate-limiting compared to glucose/galactose

Table 286-5   Primary Lactase Deficiency in Different Adult Ethnic Groups

Ethnic Group	Prevalence of Lactase Deficiency, %
Northern European	5–15
Mediterranean	60–85
African black	85–100
American black	45–80
American Caucasian	10–25
Native American	50–95
Mexican American	40–75
Asian	90–100

SOURCE: From FJ Simons: Am J Dig Dis 23:963, 1978.

absorption, lactase deficiency is associated with significant lactose malabsorption. Some individuals with lactose malabsorption develop symptoms such as diarrhea, abdominal pain, cramps, and/or flatus. Most individuals with primary lactase deficiency do not have symptoms. Since lactose intolerance may be associated with symptoms suggestive of an irritable bowel syndrome, persistence of such symptoms in an individual with lactose intolerance while on a strict lactose-free diet would suggest that the individual's symptoms were related to irritable bowel syndrome.

Development of symptoms of lactose intolerance is related to several factors:

1. *Amount of lactose in the diet.*
2. *Rate of gastric emptying.* Symptoms are more likely when gastric emptying is rapid than when gastric emptying is slower. Therefore, it is more likely that skim milk will be associated with symptoms of lactose intolerance than whole milk as the rate of gastric emptying following skim milk intake is more rapid. Similarly, the diarrhea observed following subtotal gastrectomy is often a result of lactose intolerance as gastric emptying is accelerated in patients with a gastrojejunostomy.
3. *Small-intestinal transit time.* Although both the small and large intestine contribute to the development of symptoms, many of the symptoms of lactase deficiency are related to the interaction of colonic bacteria and nonabsorbed lactose. More rapid small-intestinal transit makes symptoms more likely.
4. *Colonic compensation by production of SCFAs* from nonabsorbed lactose. Reduced levels of colonic microflora, which can occur following antibiotic use, will also be associated with increased symptoms following lactose ingestion, especially in a lactase-deficient individual.

Glucose-galactose or monosaccharide malabsorption may also be associated with diarrhea and is due to a congenital absence of SGLT. Diarrhea is present when these individuals ingest carbohydrates that contain actively transported monosaccharides (e.g., glucose, galactose) but not monosaccharides that are not actively transported (e.g., fructose). Fructose is absorbed by the brush border transport protein, GLUT 5, a facilitated diffusion process that is not Na-dependent and is distinct from SGLT. In contrast, some individuals develop diarrhea as a result of consuming large quantities of sorbitol, a sugar used in diabetic candy; sorbitol is only minimally absorbed due to the absence of an intestinal absorptive transport mechanism for sorbitol.

PROTEINS   Protein is present in food almost exclusively as polypeptides and requires extensive hydrolysis to di- and tripeptides and amino acids before absorption. Proteolysis occurs in both the stomach and small intestine; it is mediated by pepsin secreted as pepsinogen by gastric chief cells and trypsinogen and other peptidases from pancreatic acinar cells. These proenzymes, pepsinogen and trypsinogen, must be activated to pepsin (by pepsin in the presence of a pH < 5) and trypsin (by the intestinal brush border enzyme, enterokinase, and subsequently by trypsin). Proteins are absorbed by separate transport systems for di- and tripeptides and for different types of amino acids, e.g., neutral, dibasic. Alterations in either protein or amino acid digestion and absorption are rarely observed clinically, even in the presence of extensive small-intestinal mucosal inflammation. However, three rare genetic disorders involve protein digestion-absorption: (1) *enterokinase deficiency* is due to an absence of the brush border enzyme that converts the proenzyme trypsinogen to trypsin and is associated with diarrhea, growth retardation, and hypoproteinemia; (2) *Hartnup syndrome*, a defect in neutral amino acid transport, is characterized by a pellagra-like rash and neuropsychiatric symptoms; and (3) *cystinuria*, a defect in dibasic amino acid transport, is associated with renal calculi and chronic pancreatitis.

EVALUATION OF MALABSORPTION

The clues provided by the history, symptoms, and initial preliminary observations will serve to limit extensive, ill-focused, and expensive patient with symptoms suggestive of malabsorption who recently had extensive small-intestinal resection for mesenteric ischemia should direct the initial assessment almost exclusively to define whether a short-bowel syndrome might explain the entire clinical picture. Similarly, the development of a pattern of bowel movements suggestive of steatorrhea in a patient with long-standing alcohol abuse and chronic pancreatitis should lead toward assessing pancreatic exocrine function.

The classic picture of malabsorption described in textbooks ≥30 years ago is rarely seen today in most parts of the United States. As a consequence, diseases with malabsorption must be suspected in individuals with less severe symptoms and signs and with subtle evidence of the altered absorption of only a *single* nutrient rather than obvious evidence of the malabsorption of multiple nutrients.

Although diarrhea can be caused by changes in fluid and electrolyte movement in either the small or the large intestine, dietary nutrients are absorbed almost exclusively in the small intestine. Therefore, the demonstration of diminished absorption of a dietary nutrient provides unequivocal evidence of small-intestinal disease, although colonic dysfunction may also be present (e.g., Crohn's disease may involve both small and large intestine). Dietary nutrient absorption may be segmental or heterogeneous along the small intestine and is site-specific. Thus, for example, calcium, iron, and folic acid are exclusively absorbed by active transport processes in the proximal small intestine, especially the duodenum; in contrast, the active transport mechanisms for both cobalamin and bile acids are present only in the ileum. Therefore, in an individual who years previously had had an intestinal resection, the details of which are not presently available, a presentation with evidence of calcium, folic acid, and iron malabsorption but without cobalamin deficiency would make it likely that the duodenum and jejunum, but not ileum, had been resected.

Some nutrients, e.g., glucose, amino acids, and lipids, are absorbed throughout the small intestine, though there is evidence that their rate of absorption is greater in the proximal than in the distal segments. However, following segmental resection of the small intestine, the remaining segments will undergo both morphologic and functional "adaptation" to enhance absorption. Such adaptation is secondary to both the presence of luminal nutrients and hormonal stimuli and may not be complete in humans for several months following the resection. Adaptation is critical for individuals who have undergone massive resection of the small intestine and/or colon to help ensure survival.

Establishing the presence of steatorrhea and identifying its specific cause are often quite difficult for several reasons. Despite attempts to develop tests that do *not* require the collection of stool to document the presence of steatorrhea, the "gold standard" still remains a timed, quantitative stool fat determination. On a practical basis, stool collections are invariably difficult and often incomplete as nobody wants to handle stool. A qualitative test—Sudan III stain—has long been available to establish the presence of an increase in stool fat. This test is rapid and inexpensive but, as a qualitative test, does not establish the degree of fat malabsorption and is best used as a preliminary screening study. Many of the blood, breath, and isotopic tests that have been developed either: (1) do not directly measure fat absorption, (2) have excellent sensitivity when steatorrhea is obvious and severe but have poor sensitivity when steatorrhea is mild, or (3) have not survived the transition from their development in a laboratory to commercial utilization and dissemination.

Despite this situation, the use of routine laboratory studies (i.e., complete blood count, prothrombin time, serum protein determination, alkaline phosphatase) may suggest the presence of dietary nutrient depletion, especially iron, folate, cobalamin, and vitamins D and K. Additional studies include measurement of serum carotene, cholesterol, albumin, iron, folate, and cobalamin levels. The serum carotene level can also be reduced if the patient has poor dietary intake of leafy vegetables.

If steatorrhea and/or altered absorption of other nutrients are suspected, the history, clinical observations, and laboratory testing can help detect deficiency of a dietary nutrient, especially the fat-soluble

vitamins A, D, E, or K. Thus, evidence of metabolic bone disease with elevated alkaline phosphatase and/or reduced serum calcium levels would suggest vitamin D malabsorption. A deficiency of vitamin K would be suggested by an elevated prothrombin time in an individual without liver disease who was not taking anticoagulants. Macrocytic anemia would lead to evaluation of whether cobalamin or folic acid malabsorption was present. The presence of iron-deficiency anemia in the absence of occult bleeding from the gastrointestinal tract in either a male or a nonmenstruating female would require evaluation of iron malabsorption and the exclusion of celiac sprue, as iron is absorbed exclusively in the proximal small intestine.

At times, however, a timed (72-h) quantitative stool collection, preferably on a defined diet, must be obtained to determine stool fat content and establish the presence of steatorrhea. The presence of steatorrhea then requires further assessment to establish the pathophysiologic process(es) responsible for the defect in dietary lipid digestion-absorption (Table 286-4). Some of the other studies include the Schilling test, D-xylose test, duodenal mucosal biopsy, small-intestinal radiologic examination, and tests of pancreatic exocrine function.

THE SCHILLING TEST This test is performed to determine the cause for cobalamin malabsorption. Since cobalamin absorption requires multiple steps, including gastric, pancreatic, and ileal processes, the Schilling test can also be used to assess the integrity of these other organs (Chap. 107). Cobalamin is present primarily in meat. Except in strict vegans, *dietary* cobalamin deficiency is exceedingly uncommon. Dietary cobalamin is bound in the stomach to a glycoprotein called *R-binder protein*, which is synthesized in both the stomach and salivary glands. This cobalamin–R binder complex is formed in the acid milieu of the stomach. Cobalamin absorption has an absolute requirement for intrinsic factor, another glycoprotein synthesized and released by gastric parietal cells, to promote its uptake by specific cobalamin receptors on the brush border of ileal enterocytes. Pancreatic protease enzymes split the cobalamin–R binder complex to release cobalamin in the proximal small intestine, where cobalamin is then bound by intrinsic factor.

As a consequence, cobalamin absorption may be abnormal in the following:

1. Pernicious anemia, a disease in which immunologically mediated atrophy of gastric parietal cells leads to an absence of both gastric acid and intrinsic factor secretion.
2. Chronic pancreatitis as a result of deficiency of pancreatic proteases to split the cobalamin–R binder complex. Although 50% of patients with chronic pancreatitis have been reported to have an abnormal Schilling test that was corrected by pancreatic enzyme replacement, the presence of a cobalamin-responsive macrocytic anemia in chronic pancreatitis is extremely rare. Although this probably reflects a difference in the digestion/absorption of cobalamin in food versus that in a crystalline form, the Schilling test can still be used to assess pancreatic exocrine function.
3. Achlorhydria or absence of another factor secreted with acid that is responsible for splitting cobalamin away from the proteins in food to which it is bound can lead to vitamin B_{12} malabsorption. Up to one-third of individuals over >60 years have marginal vitamin B_{12} absorption because of the inability to release cobalamin from food; these people have no defects in absorbing crystalline vitamin B_{12}.
4. Bacterial overgrowth syndromes, which are most often secondary to stasis in the small intestine, produce cobalamin deficiency from bacterial utilization of cobalamin (often referred to as *stagnant bowel syndrome*) (see below).
5. Ileal dysfunction (either as a result of inflammation or prior intestinal resection) due to impaired function of the mechanism of cobalamin–intrinsic factor uptake by ileal intestinal epithelial cells.

The Schilling test is performed by administering [58]Co-labeled cobalamin and collecting urine for 24 h and is dependent upon normal

Table 286-6 Differential Results of Schilling Test in Several Diseases Associated with Cobalamin (Cbl) Malabsorption

	58Co-Cbl	With IF	With Pancreatic Enzymes	After 5 Days of Antibiotics
Pernicious anemia	Reduced	Normal	Reduced	Reduced
Chronic pancreatitis	Reduced	Reduced	Normal	Reduced
Bacterial overgrowth	Reduced	Reduced	Reduced	Normal
Ileal disease	Reduced	Reduced	Reduced	Reduced

NOTE: IF, intrinsic factor.

renal and bladder function. Urinary excretion of cobalamin will reflect cobalamin absorption provided that intrahepatic binding sites for cobalamin are fully occupied. To ensure saturation of hepatic cobalamin binding sites so that all absorbed radiolabeled cobalamin will be excreted in urine, 1 mg cobalamin is administered intramuscularly 1 h following ingestion of the radiolabeled cobalamin. The Schilling test may be abnormal (usually defined as <10% excretion in 24 h) in pernicious anemia, chronic pancreatitis, blind loop syndrome, and ileal disease (Table 286-6). Therefore, whenever an abnormal Schilling test is found, 58Co-labeled cobalamin should be administered on another occasion either bound to intrinsic factor, with pancreatic enzymes, or

following a 5-day course of antibiotics (often tetracycline). A variation of the Schilling test can detect failure to split cobalamin from food proteins. The labeled cobalamin is cooked together with a scrambled egg and administered orally. People with achlorydria will excrete <10% of the labeled cobalamin in the urine. In addition to establishing the etiology for cobalamin deficiency, the Schilling test can be used to help delineate the pathologic process responsible for steatorrhea by assessing ileal, pancreatic, and small-intestinal luminal function.

URINARY D-XYLOSE TEST   The urinary D-xylose test for carbohydrate absorption provides an assessment of proximal small-intestinal mucosal function. D-Xylose, a pentose, is absorbed almost exclusively in the proximal small intestine. The D-xylose test is usually performed by giving 25 g D-xylose and collecting urine for 5 h. An abnormal test (<4.5 g excretion) primarily reflects the presence of duodenal/jejunal mucosal disease. The D-xylose test can also be abnormal in patients with blind loop syndrome (as a consequence primarily of abnormal intestinal mucosa) and, as a false-positive study, in patients with large collections of fluid in a third space (i.e., ascites, pleural fluid). The ease of obtaining a mucosal biopsy of the small intestine by endoscopy and the false-negative rate of the D-xylose test have led to its diminished use. When small-intestinal mucosal disease is suspected, a small-intestinal mucosal biopsy should be performed.

RADIOLOGIC EXAMINATION   Radiologic examination of the small intestine using barium contrast (small-bowel series or study) can provide important information in the evaluation of the patient with presumed or suspected malabsorption. These studies are most often performed in conjunction with the examination of the esophagus, stomach, and duodenal bulb, and insufficient barium is given the patient to permit an adequate examination of the small-intestinal mucosa, especially the ileum. As a result, many gastrointestinal radiologists alter the procedure of a barium contrast examination of the small intestine by performing either a small-bowel series in which a large amount of barium is given by mouth without concurrent examination of the esophagus and stomach or an enteroclysis study in which a large amount of barium is introduced into the duodenum via a fluoroscopically placed tube. In addition, many of the diagnostic features initially described by radiologists to denote the presence of small-intestinal disease (e.g., flocculation, segmentation) are rarely seen with current barium suspensions. Nonetheless, in skilled hands barium contrast examination of the small intestine can yield important information. For example, with extensive mucosal disease, dilatation of intestine can be seen as well as dilution of barium from increased intestinal fluid secretion (Fig. 286-3). A normal barium contrast study does *not* exclude the possibility of small-intestinal disease. However, a small-bowel series remains a very useful examination to assess for the presence of anatomic abnormalities, such as strictures and fistulas (as in Crohn's disease) or blind loop syndrome (e.g., multiple jejunal diverticula), and to define the extent of a previous surgical resection.

BIOPSY OF SMALL-INTESTINAL MUCOSA   A small-intestinal mucosal biopsy is essential in the evaluation of a patient with documented steatorrhea or chronic diarrhea (lasting >3 weeks) (Chap. 42). The

A

B

C

D

FIGURE 286-3 Barium contrast small-intestinal radiologic examinations. *A.* Normal individual. *B.* Celiac sprue. *C.* Jejunal diverticulosis. *D.* Crohn's disease. *(Courtesy of Morton Burrell, MD, Yale University.)*

ready availability of endoscopic equipment to examine the stomach and duodenum has led to their almost uniform use as the preferred method to obtain histologic material of proximal small-intestinal mucosa. The primary indications for a small-intestinal biopsy are (1) evaluation of a patient either with documented or suspected steatorrhea or with chronic diarrhea, and (2) diffuse or focal abnormalities of the small intestine defined on a small-intestinal series. Lesions seen on small-bowel biopsy can be classified into three different categories (Table 286-7): (1) diffuse, specific; (2) patchy, specific; and (3) diffuse, nonspecific.

1. *Diffuse, specific lesions.* There are relatively few diseases associated with altered nutrient absorption that have specific histopathologic abnormalities on small-intestinal mucosal biopsy, and they are uncommon. *Whipple's disease* is characterized by the presence of periodic acid–Schiff (PAS)-positive macrophages in the lamina propria, while the bacilli that are also present may require electron-microscopic examination for identification (Fig. 286-4). *Abetalipoproteinemia* is characterized by a normal mucosal appearance except for the presence of mucosal absorptive cells that contain lipid postprandially and disappear following a prolonged period of either fat-free intake or fasting. *Immune globulin deficiency* is associated with a variety of histopathologic findings on small-intestinal mucosal biopsy. The characteristic feature is the absence or substantial reduction in the number of plasma cells in the lamina propria; the mucosal architecture may be either perfectly normal or flat, i.e., villus atrophy. As patients with immune globulin deficiency are often infected with *Giardia lamblia*, *Giardia* trophozoites may also be seen in the biopsy.

2. *Patchy, specific lesions.* Several diseases are associated with abnormal small-intestinal mucosal biopsies, but the characteristic features that are present have a patchy distribution. As a result, biopsies

Table 286-7   Disease that Can be Diagnosed by Small-Intestinal Mucosal Biopsies

Lesions	Pathologic Findings
Diffuse, specific	
Whipple's disease	Lamina propria contains macrophages containing PAS + material
Agammaglobulinemia	No plasma cells; either normal or absent villi ("flat mucosa");
Abetalipoproteinemia	Normal villi; epithelial cells vacuolated with fat
Patchy, specific	
Intestinal lymphoma	Malignant cells in lamina propria and submucosa
Intestinal lymphangiectasia	Dilated lymphatics; clubbed villi
Eosinophilic gastroenteritis	Eosinophil infiltration of lamina propria and mucosa
Amyloidosis	Amyloid deposits
Crohn's disease	Noncaseating granulomas
Infection by one or more microorganisms (see text)	Specific organisms
Mastocytosis	Mast cell infiltration of lamina propria
Diffuse, nonspecific	
Celiac sprue	Short or absent villi; mononuclear infiltrate; epithelial cell damage; hypertrophy of crypts
Tropical sprue	Similar to celiac sprue
Bacterial overgrowth	Patchy damage to villi; lymphocyte infiltration
Folate deficiency	Short villi; decreased mitosis in crypts; megalocytosis
Vitamin B_{12} deficiency	Similar to folate deficiency
Radiation enteritis	Similar to folate deficiency
Zollinger-Ellison syndrome	Mucosal ulceration and erosion from acid
Protein-calorie malnutrition	Villus atrophy; secondary bacterial overgrowth
Drug-induced enteritis	Variable histology

NOTE: PAS+, periodic acid–Schiff positive.

obtained randomly or in the absence of abnormalities visualized endoscopically may not reveal these diagnostic features. Intestinal *lymphoma* can at times be diagnosed on mucosal biopsy by the identification of malignant lymphoma cells in the lamina propria and submucosa (Chap. 112). The presence of dilated lymphatics in the submucosa and sometimes in the lamina propria indicates the presence of *lymphangiectasia* associated with hypoproteinemia secondary to protein loss into the intestine. *Eosinophilic gastroenteritis* represents a heterogeneous group of disorders with a spectrum of presentations and symptoms with a eosinophilic infiltrate of the lamina propria, with or without peripheral eosinophilia. The patchy nature of the infiltrate as well as its presence in the submucosa often leads to an absence of histopathologic findings on mucosal biopsy. As the involvement of the duodenum in *Crohn's disease* is also submucosal and not necessarily continuous, mucosal biopsies are not the most direct approach to the diagnosis of duodenal Crohn's disease (Chap. 287). Amyloid deposition can be identified by Congo Red stain in some patients with *amyloidosis* involving the duodenum (Chap. 319).

Several microorganisms can be identified on small-intestinal biopsies, establishing a correct diagnosis. Many of these microorganisms are associated with diarrhea that occurs in immunodeficient individuals, especially those with HIV infection, and include *Cryptosporidium*, *Isospora belli*, cytomegalovirus, *Mycobacterium avium intracellulare*, and *G. lamblia*.

3. *Diffuse, nonspecific lesions.* *Celiac sprue* presents with a characteristic mucosal appearance on duodenal/proximal jejunal mucosal biopsy that is not diagnostic of the disease. The diagnosis of celiac sprue is established by clinical, histologic, and immunologic response to a gluten-free diet. *Tropical sprue* is associated with histopathologic findings similar to those of celiac sprue after a tropical or subtropical exposure but does not respond to gluten restriction; most often symptoms improve with antibiotics and folate administration.

Patients with steatorrhea require assessment of *pancreatic exocrine function*, which is often abnormal in chronic pancreatitis. No test assesses pancreatic exocrine function well. Endoscopic approaches provide excellent assessment of pancreatic duct anatomy but do not assess exocrine function (Chap. 303). One noninvasive study (bentiromide test) of pancreatic exocrine function is based on the feeding of a tripeptide containing *p*-aminobenzoic acid (PABA). Following splitting of PABA by pancreatic proteases, PABA is liberated, absorbed, and excreted in urine. Reduced proteolysis results in reduced urinary excretion of PABA. This test is neither sensitive nor specific.

Table 286-8 summarizes the results of the D-xylose test, Schilling test, and small-intestinal mucosal biopsy in patients with five different causes of steatorrhea.

SPECIFIC DISEASE ENTITIES

CELIAC SPRUE   Celiac sprue is a not uncommon cause of malabsorption of one or more nutrients in Caucasians, especially those of European descent. Celiac sprue has had several other names including nontropical sprue, celiac disease (in children), adult celiac disease, and gluten-sensitive enteropathy. The etiology of celiac sprue is not known, but environmental, genetic, and immunologic factors are important. Celiac sprue has protean manifestations, almost all of which are secondary to nutrient malabsorption, and a varied natural history, with the onset of symptoms occurring at ages ranging from the first year of life through the eighth decade.

The hallmark of celiac sprue is the presence of an abnormal small-intestinal biopsy (Fig. 286-4) and the response of both symptoms, evidence of malabsorption and the histopathologic changes on the small-intestinal biopsy, to the elimination of gluten from the diet. The histopathologic changes have a proximal to distal intestinal distribution of severity, which probably reflects the exposure of the intestinal mucosa to varied amounts of dietary gluten; the degree of symptoms is related to the extent of these histopathologic changes.

An *immunologic* component to etiology is suspected for three reasons. First, serum antibodies, IgA antigliadin and antiendomysial antibodies, are present, but it is also not known whether such antibodies are primary or secondary to the tissue damage. The antiendomysial antibody has 90 to 95% sensitivity and 90 to 95% specificity, and the antigen recognized by the antiendomysial antibody test is tissue transglutaminase. The relationship of this autoantibody to pathogenetic mechanism(s) responsible for celiac sprue remains to be established. Nonetheless, this antibody will undoubtedly prove extremely useful in establishing the true prevalence of celiac sprue in the general population and may provide important clues to its etiology. Second, treatment with prednisolone for 4 weeks of a patient with celiac sprue who continues to eat gluten will induce a remission and convert the "flat" abnormal duodenal biopsy to a more normal appearing one. Third, gliadin peptides may interact with gliadin-specific T cells that may either mediate tissue injury or induce the release of one or more cytokines that are responsible for the tissue injury.

Genetic factor(s) also appear to be involved in celiac sprue. The incidence of celiac sprue varies widely in different population groups (high in Caucasians, low in blacks and orientals) and is 10% in first-degree relatives of celiac sprue patients. Furthermore, about 95% of patients with celiac sprue express the HLA-DQ2 allele, though only a minority of all persons expressing DQ2 have celiac sprue.

FIGURE 286-4 Small-intestinal mucosal biopsies. *A.* Normal individual. *B.* Untreated celiac sprue. *C.* Treated celiac sprue. *D.* Intestinal lymphangiectasia. *E.* Whipple's disease. *F.* Lymphoma. *(Courtesy of Marie Robert, MD, Yale University.)*

Diagnosis A small-intestinal biopsy is required to establish a diagnosis of celiac sprue (Fig. 286-4). A biopsy should be performed in patients with symptoms and laboratory findings suggestive of nutrient malabsorption and/or deficiency.

The symptoms of celiac sprue may appear with the introduction of cereals in an infant's diet, although there is frequently a spontaneous remission during the second decade of life that may be either permanent or followed by the reappearance of symptoms over several years. Alternatively, the symptoms of celiac sprue may first become evident at almost any age throughout adulthood. In many patients, frequent spontaneous remissions and exacerbations occur. The symptoms range from significant malabsorption of multiple nutrients with diarrhea, steatorrhea, weight loss, and the consequences of nutrient depletion (i.e., anemia and metabolic bone disease) to the absence of any gastrointestinal symptoms but with evidence of the depletion of a single nutrient (e.g., folate deficiency, osteomalacia, edema from protein loss). Asymptomatic relatives of patients with celiac sprue have been identified as having this disease either by small-intestinal biopsy or by serologic studies (e.g., antiendomysial antibodies).

Etiology The etiology of celiac sprue is not known, but environmental, genetic, and immunologic factors all appear to contribute to the disease.

One *environmental* factor is the clear association of the disease with gliadin, a component of gluten that is present in wheat, barley, rice, and, in smaller amounts, oats. In addition to the role of gluten restriction in treatment, the instillation of gluten into both normal-appearing rectum and distal ileum of patients with celiac sprue results within hours in morphologic changes.

Table 286-8 Results of Diagnostic Studies in Different Causes of Steatorrhea

	D-Xylose Test	Schilling Test	Duodenal Mucosal Biopsy
Chronic pancreatitis	Normal	50% abnormal; if abnormal, normal with pancreatic enzymes	Normal
Bacterial overgrowth syndrome	Normal or only modestly abnormal	Often abnormal; if abnormal, normal after antibiotics	Usually normal
Ileal disease	Normal	Abnormal	Normal
Celiac sprue	Decreased	Normal	Abnormal: probably "flat"
Intestinal lymphangiectasia	Normal	Normal	Abnormal: "dilated lymphatics"

Since the presentation of celiac sprue is often subtle, without overt evidence of malabsorption or nutrient deficiency, it is important to have a relatively low threshold to perform a biopsy. It is more prudent to perform a biopsy than to obtain another test of intestinal absorption, which can never completely exclude or establish this diagnosis.

The diagnosis of celiac sprue requires the presence of characteristic histopathologic changes on small-intestinal biopsy together with a prompt clinical and histopathologic response following the institution of a gluten-free diet. If serologic studies have detected the presence of IgA antiendomysial antibodies, they too should disappear after a gluten-free diet is started. The changes seen on duodenal/jejunal biopsy are restricted to the mucosa and include: (1) absence or reduced height of villi, resulting in a "flat" appearance; (2) increased loss of villus cells in association with increased crypt cell proliferation resulting in crypt hyperplasia and loss of villus structure, with consequent villus, but not mucosal, atrophy; (3) cuboidal appearance and nuclei that are no longer oriented basally in surface epithelial cells and increased intraepithelial lymphocytes; and (4) increased lymphocytes and plasma cells in the lamina propria. Although these histopathologic features are characteristic of celiac sprue, they are *not* diagnostic because a similar appearance can be seen in tropical sprue, eosinophilic enteritis, and milk-protein intolerance in children and occasionally in lymphoma, bacterial overgrowth, Crohn's disease, and gastrinoma with acid hypersecretion. However, the presence of a characteristic histopathologic appearance that reverts to normal following the initiation of a gluten-free diet establishes the diagnosis of celiac sprue. Readministration of gluten with or without an additional small-intestinal biopsy is not necessary.

Failure to Respond to Gluten Restriction The most common cause of persistent symptoms in a patient who fulfills all the criteria of the diagnosis of celiac sprue is continued intake of gluten. Gluten is ubiquitous, and significant effort must be made to exclude all gluten from the diet. Use of rice in place of wheat flour is very helpful, and several support groups provide important aid to patients with celiac sprue and to their families. About 90% of patients who have the characteristic findings of celiac sprue will respond to complete dietary gluten restriction. The remainder represent a heterogeneous group (whose condition is often called *refractory sprue*) that includes some patients who (1) respond to restriction of other dietary protein, e.g., soy; (2) respond to glucocorticoids; (3) are "temporary," i.e., the clinical and morphologic findings disappear after several months or years; or (4) fail to respond to all measures and have a fatal outcome, with or without documented complications of celiac sprue.

Mechanism of Diarrhea The diarrhea in celiac sprue has several pathogenetic mechanisms. Diarrhea may be secondary to (1) steatorrhea, which is primarily a result of the changes in jejunal mucosal function; (2) secondary lactase deficiency, a consequence of changes in jejunal brush border enzymatic function; (3) bile acid malabsorption resulting in bile acid–induced fluid secretion in the colon, in cases with more extensive disease involving the ileum; and (4) endogenous fluid secretion resulting from the crypt hyperplasia. Patients with more severe involvement with celiac sprue may obtain temporary improvement with *dietary lactose and fat restriction* while awaiting the full effects of total gluten restriction, which represents primary therapy.

Associated Diseases Celiac sprue is associated with dermatitis herpetiformis (DH), though the association has not been explained. Patients with DH have characteristic papulovesicular lesions that respond to dapsone. Almost all patients with DH have histopathologic changes in the small intestine consistent with celiac sprue, although usually much milder and less diffuse in distribution. Most patients with DH have mild, or no, gastrointestinal symptoms. In contrast, relatively few patients with celiac sprue have DH.

Celiac sprue is also associated with insulin-dependent diabetes mellitus and IgA globulin deficiency. The clinical importance of the former association is that although severe watery diarrhea without evidence of malabsorption is most often seen in patients with "diabetic diarrhea" (Chap. 333), a small-intestinal biopsy must at times be considered to exclude this association.

Complications The most important complication of celiac sprue is the development of a malignancy. An increased incidence of both gastrointestinal and nongastrointestinal neoplasms as well as intestinal lymphoma exists in patients with celiac sprue. For unexplained reasons the occurrence of lymphoma in patients with celiac sprue is higher in Ireland and the United Kingdom than in the United States. The possibility of lymphoma must be considered whenever a patient with celiac sprue previously doing well on a gluten-free diet is no longer responsive to gluten restriction or a patient who presents with clinical and histopathologic features consistent with celiac sprue does not respond to a gluten-free diet. Other complications of celiac sprue include the development of intestinal ulceration independent of lymphoma and so-called refractory sprue (see above) and collagenous sprue. In *collagenous sprue*, a layer of collagen-like material is present beneath the basement membrane; these patients generally do not respond to a gluten-free diet and often have a poor prognosis.

TROPICAL SPRUE Tropical sprue is a poorly understood syndrome that affects both expatriates and natives in certain but not all tropical areas and is manifested by chronic diarrhea, steatorrhea, weight loss, and nutritional deficiencies, including those of both folate and cobalamin. This disease affects 5 to 10% of the population in some tropical areas.

Chronic diarrhea in a tropical environment is most often caused by infectious agents including *G. lamblia*, *Yersinia enterocolitica*, *C. difficile*, *Cryptosporidium parvum*, and *Cyclospora cayetanensis*, among other organisms. Tropical sprue should not be entertained as a possible diagnosis until the presence of cysts and trophozoites has been excluded in three stool samples. →*Chronic infections of the gastrointestinal tract and diarrhea in patients with or without AIDS are discussed in Chaps. 309 and 131.*

The small-intestinal mucosa in individuals living in tropical areas is not identical to that of individuals who reside in temperate climates. Biopsies reveal a mild alteration of villus architecture with a modest increase in mononuclear cells in the lamina propria, which on occasion can be as severe as that seen in celiac sprue. These changes are observed both in native residents and in expatriates living in tropical regions, are usually associated with mild decreases in absorptive function, but revert to "normal" when an individual moves or returns to a temperate area. Some have suggested that the changes seen in tropical enteropathy and in tropical sprue represent different ends of the spectrum of a single entity, but convincing evidence to support this concept is lacking.

Etiology The etiology of tropical sprue is not known, though because tropical sprue responds to antibiotics, the consensus is that tropical sprue may be caused by one or more infectious agents. Nonetheless, multiple uncertainties regarding the etiology and pathogenesis of tropical sprue exist. First, its occurrence is not evenly distributed in all tropical areas; rather, it is found in specific locations including South India, the Philippines, and several Caribbean islands (e.g., Puerto Rico, Haiti) but is rarely observed in Africa, Jamaica, or Southeast Asia. Second, an occasional individual will not develop symptoms of tropical sprue until long after having left an endemic area. This is the reason why the original term for celiac sprue was *nontropical sprue* to distinguish it from tropical sprue. Third, multiple microorganisms have been identified on jejunal aspirate with relatively little consistency among studies. *Klebsiella pneumoniae*, *Enterobacter cloacae*, or *E. coli* have been implicated in some studies of tropical sprue, while other investigations have favored a role for a toxin produced by one or more of these bacteria. Fourth, the incidence of tropical sprue appears to have decreased substantially during the past decade. One speculation for this reduced occurrence of tropical sprue is the wider use of antibiotics in acute diarrhea especially in travelers to tropical areas from temperate countries. Fifth, the role of folic acid deficiency in the pathogenesis of tropical sprue requires clarification. Folic acid is absorbed exclusively in the duodenum and proximal jejunum, and most patients with tropical sprue have evidence of folate malabsorption and depletion. Although folate deficiency can cause changes in small-intestinal mucosa that are corrected by folate replacement, the several earlier studies reporting that tropical sprue could be cured by folic acid did not provide an explanation for the "insult" that was initially responsible for folate malabsorption.

The clinical pattern of tropical sprue varies in different areas of the world (e.g., India vs. Puerto Rico). Not infrequently, individuals in India initially will report the occurrence of an acute enteritis before the development of steatorrhea and malabsorption. In contrast, in Puerto Rico, a most insidious onset of symptoms and a more dramatic response to antibiotics is seen than in some other locations. Tropical sprue in different areas of the world may not be the same disease; there may be similar clinical entities but with different etiologies.

Diagnosis The diagnosis of tropical sprue is best made by the presence of an abnormal small-intestinal mucosal biopsy in an individual with chronic diarrhea and evidence of malabsorption who is either residing or has recently lived in a tropic country. The small-intestinal biopsy in tropical sprue does not have pathognomonic features but resembles, and can often be indistinguishable from, that seen in celiac sprue (Fig. 286-4). The biopsy in tropical sprue will have less villus architectural alteration and more mononuclear cell infiltrate in the lamina propria. In contrast to celiac sprue, the histopathologic features of tropical sprue are present with a similar degree of severity throughout the small intestine, and a gluten-free diet does not result in either clinical or histopathologic improvement in tropical sprue.

℞ **TREATMENT** Broad-spectrum antibiotics and folic acid are most often curative, especially if the patient leaves the tropical area and does not return. Tetracycline should be used for up to 6 months and may be associated with improvement within 1 to 2 weeks. Folic acid alone will induce a hematologic remission as well as improvement in appetite, weight gain, and some morphologic changes in small intestinal biopsy. Because of the presence of marked folate deficiency, folic acid is most often given together with antibiotics.

SHORT BOWEL SYNDROME This is a descriptive term for the myriad clinical problems that often occur following resection of varying lengths of small intestine. The factors that determine both the type and degree of symptoms include: (1) the specific segment (jejunum vs. ileum) resected, (2) the length of the resected segment, (3) the integrity of the ileocecal valve, (4) whether any large intestine has also been removed, (5) residual disease in the remaining small and/or large intestine (e.g., Crohn's disease, mesenteric artery disease), and (6) the degree of adaptation in the remaining intestine. Short bowel syndrome can occur at any age from neonates through the elderly.

Three different situations in adults demand intestinal resections: (1) mesenteric vascular disease including both atherosclerosis, thrombotic phenomena, and vasculitidies; (2) primary mucosal and submucosal disease, e.g., Crohn's disease; and (3) operations without preexisting small intestinal disease, such as trauma and jejunoileal bypass for obesity.

Following resection of the small intestine, the residual intestine undergoes adaptation of both structure and function that may last for up to 6 to 12 months. Adaptation requires the continued intake of dietary nutrients and calories to stimulate it via direct contact with ileal mucosa, the release of one or more intestinal hormones, and pancreatic and biliary secretions. Thus, enteral nutrition and calorie administration must be maintained, especially in the early postoperative period, even if an extensive intestinal resection requiring total parenteral nutrition (TPN) was required. The subsequent ability of such patients to absorb nutrients will not be known for several months until after adaptation is completed.

Multiple factors besides the absence of intestinal mucosa (required for both lipid and fluid and electrolyte absorption) contribute to the diarrhea and steatorrhea in these patients. Removal of the ileum and especially the ileocecal valve is often associated with more severe diarrhea than jejunal resection. Without part or all of the ileum, diarrhea can be caused by an increase in bile acids entering the colon, leading to their stimulation of colonic fluid and electrolyte secretion. Absence of the ileocecal valve is also associated with a decrease in intestinal transit time and bacterial overgrowth from the colon. Lactose intolerance as a result of the removal of lactase-containing mucosa as well as gastric hypersecretion will also contribute to the diarrhea.

In addition to diarrhea and/or steatorrhea, a range of nonintestinal symptoms are also observed in some patients. A significant increase in renal calcium oxalate calculi is observed in patients with a small-intestinal resection with an intact colon and is due to an increase in oxalate absorption by the large intestine, with subsequent hyperoxaluria. Since oxalate is high in relatively few foods (e.g., spinach, rhubarb, tea), dietary restrictions alone are not adequate treatment. Cholestyramine, an anion-binding resin, and calcium have proved useful in reducing the hyperoxaluria. Similarly, an increase in cholesterol gall stones is seen that is related to a decrease in the bile acid pool size, which results in the generation of cholesterol supersaturation in gall bladder bile. Gastric hypersecretion of acid occurs in many patients following large resections of the small intestine. The etiology is unclear but may be related to either reduced hormonal inhibition of acid secretion or increased gastrin levels due to reduced small-intestinal catabolism of circulating gastrin. The resulting gastric acid secretion may be an important factor contributing to the diarrhea and steatorrhea. A reduced pH in the duodenum can inactivate pancreatic lipase and/or precipitate duodenal bile acids, thereby increasing steatorrhea, and an increase in gastric secretion can create a volume overload relative to the reduced small-intestinal absorptive capacity. Inhibition of gastric acid secretion with either proton pump inhibitors or H_2 receptor antagonists can help in reducing the diarrhea and steatorrhea.

℞ **TREATMENT** Treatment of short bowel syndrome depends on the severity of symptoms and whether the individual is able to maintain caloric and electrolyte balance with oral intake alone. Initial treatment includes judicious use of opiates to reduce stool output and to establish an effective diet. An initial diet should be low-fat, high-carbohydrate to minimize the diarrhea from fatty acid stimulation of colonic fluid secretion. Both MCT (see above), a low-lactose diet, and various fiber-containing diets should also be tried. In the absence of an ileocecal valve, the possibility of bacterial overgrowth must be considered and treated. If gastric acid hypersecretion is contributing to the diarrhea and steatorrhea, a proton pump inhibitor may be helpful. Usually none of these therapeutic approaches will provide an instant solution but will reduce disabling diarrhea.

The patient's vitamin and mineral status must also be monitored, and replacement therapy initiated, if indicated. Fat-soluble vitamins, folate, cobalamin, calcium, iron, magnesium, and zinc are the most critical factors to monitor on a regular basis. If these approaches are not successful, home TPN represents an established therapy that can be maintained for many years. Intestinal transplantation is beginning to become established as a possible approach for individuals with extensive intestinal resection who cannot be maintained without TPN.

BACTERIAL OVERGROWTH SYNDROME Bacterial overgrowth syndrome comprises a group of disorders with diarrhea, steatorrhea, and macrocytic anemia whose common feature is the proliferation of colon-type bacteria within the small intestine. This bacterial proliferation is due to stasis caused by impaired peristalsis (i.e., *functional stasis*), changes in intestinal anatomy (i.e., *anatomic stasis*), or direct communication between the small and large intestine. These conditions have also been referred to as *stagnant bowel syndrome* or *blind loop syndrome*.

Pathogenesis The manifestations of bacterial overgrowth syndromes are a direct consequence of the presence of increased amounts of a colonic-type bacterial flora, such as *E. coli* or *Bacteroides*, in the small intestine. *Macrocytic anemia* is due to cobalamin, not folate, deficiency. Most bacteria require cobalamin for growth, and increasing concentrations of bacteria use up the relatively small amounts of dietary cobalamin. *Steatorrhea* is due to impaired micelle formation as a consequence of a reduced intraduodenal concentration of bile acids and the presence of unconjugated bile acids. Certain bacteria, e.g., *Bacteroides*, deconjugate conjugated bile acids to unconjugated bile acids. In the presence of bacterial overgrowth, unconjugated bile acids will be absorbed more rapidly than conjugated bile acids, and, as a result, the intraduodenal concentration of bile acids will be reduced. In addition, the CMC of unconjugated bile acids is higher than that of conjugated bile acids, resulting in a decrease in micelle formation. *Diarrhea* is due, at least in part, to the steatorrhea, when it is present. However, some patients manifest diarrhea *without* steatorrhea, and it is assumed that the colonic-type bacteria in these patients are producing one or more bacterial enterotoxins that are responsible for fluid secretion and diarrhea.

Etiology The etiology of these different disorders is bacterial proliferation in the small intestinal lumen secondary to either anatomic or functional stasis or to a communication between the relatively sterile small intestine and the colon with its high levels of aerobic and anaerobic bacteria. Several examples of anatomic stasis have been identified: (1) one or more diverticula (both duodenal and jejunal) (Figure 286-3C); (2) fistulas and strictures related to Crohn's disease (Figure 286-3D); (3) a proximal duodenal afferent loop following a subtotal gastrectomy and gastrojejunostomy; (4) a bypass of the intestine, e.g., jejunoileal bypass for obesity; and (5) dilatation at the site of a previous intestinal anastomosis. The common feature of all of these anatomic derangements is the presence of a segment(s) of intestine that is out of continuity of propagated peristalsis, resulting in stasis and bacterial proliferation. Bacterial overgrowth syndromes can also occur in the absence of an anatomic blind loop when functional stasis is present. The best example of impaired peristalsis and bacterial overgrowth in the absence of a blind loop is scleroderma, where motility abnormalities exist in both the esophagus and small intestine (Chap. 313). Functional stasis and bacterial overgrowth can also occur in association with diabetes mellitus and in the small intestine when a direct connection exists between the small and large intestine, including an ileocolonic resection, or occasionally following an enterocolic anastomosis that permits entry of bacteria into the small intestine as a result of bypassing the ileocecal valve.

Diagnosis The diagnosis may be suspected from the combination of a low serum cobalamin level and an elevated serum folate level as enteric bacteria frequently produce folate compounds that will be absorbed in the duodenum. Ideally, the diagnosis of the bacterial overgrowth syndrome is the demonstration of increased levels of aerobic and/or anaerobic colonic-type bacteria in a jejunal aspirate obtained by intubation. This specialized test is rarely available, and bacterial overgrowth is best established by a Schilling test (Table 286-6), which should be abnormal following the administration of ^{58}Co-labeled cobalamin, with or without the administration of intrinsic factor. Following the administration of tetracycline for 5 days, the Schilling test will become normal, confirming the diagnosis of bacterial overgrowth.

℞ **TREATMENT** Primary treatment should be directed, if at all possible, to the surgical correction of an anatomic blind loop. In the absence of functional stasis, it is important to define the anatomic relationships responsible for stasis and bacterial overgrowth. For example, bacterial overgrowth secondary to strictures, one or more diverticula, or a proximal afferent loop can potentially be cured by surgical correction of the anatomic state. In contrast, the functional stasis of scleroderma or certain anatomic stasis states (e.g., multiple jejunal diverticula), cannot be corrected surgically, and these conditions should be treated with broad-spectrum antibiotics. Tetracycline used to be the initial treatment of choice but with increasing resistance, other antibiotics such as metronidazole, amoxicillin/clavulinic acid (Augmentin), and cephalosporin have been employed. The antibiotic should be given for approximately 3 weeks or until symptoms remit. Since the natural history of these conditions is chronic, antibiotics should

not be given continuously, and symptoms usually remit within 2 to 3 weeks of initial antibiotic therapy. Therapy need not be repeated until symptoms recur. In the presence of frequent recurrences several treatment strategies exist, but the use of antibiotics for 1 week per month whether or not symptoms are present is often most effective.

Unfortunately, therapy for bacterial overgrowth syndrome is largely empirical, with an absence of clinical trials on which to base decisions regarding the antibiotic to be used, the duration of treatment, and/or the best approach for treating recurrences. Bacterial overgrowth may also occur as a component of another chronic disease, e.g., Crohn's disease, radiation enteritis, or short bowel syndrome. Treatment of the bacterial overgrowth in these settings will not cure the underlying problem but may be very important in ameliorating a subset of clinical problems that are related to bacterial overgrowth.

WHIPPLE'S DISEASE Whipple's disease is a chronic multisystem disease associated with diarrhea, steatorrhea, weight loss, arthralgia, and central nervous system and cardiac problems that is caused by the bacteria *Tropheryma whippelii*. Until the identification of *T. whippelii* by polymerase chain reaction during the past decade, the hallmark of Whipple's disease had been the presence of PAS-positive macrophages in the small intestine and other organs with evidence of disease. Long before the establishment of *T. whippelii* as the causative agent of Whipple's disease, gram-positive bacilli had been identified both within and outside of macrophages.

Etiology Whipple's disease is caused by a small gram-positive bacillus, *T. whippelii*. The bacillus, an actinobacterium, has low virulence but high infectivity, and relatively minimal symptoms are observed compared to the extent of the bacilli in multiple tissues.

Clinical Presentation The onset of Whipple's disease is insidious and is characterized by diarrhea, steatorrhea, abdominal pain, weight loss, migratory large-joint arthropathy, and fever as well as ophthalmologic and central nervous system symptoms. The development of dementia is a relatively late symptom and is an extremely poor prognostic sign, especially in patients who relapse following the induction of a remission with antibiotics. For unexplained reasons, the disease occurs primarily in middle-aged (50-year-old) Caucasian men. The steatorrhea in these patients is generally believed secondary to both small-intestinal mucosal injury and lymphatic obstruction secondary to the increased number of PAS-positive macrophages in the lamina propria of the small intestine.

Diagnosis The diagnosis of Whipple's disease is suggested by a multisystem disease in a 50-year-old Caucasian male with diarrhea and steatorrhea. Obtaining tissue biopsies from the small intestine and/or other organs that may be involved (e.g., liver, lymph nodes, heart, eyes, central nervous system, or synovial membranes), based on the patient's symptoms, is the primary approach to establish the diagnosis of Whipple's disease. The presence of PAS-positive macrophages containing the characteristic small (0.25×1 to $2\ \mu m$) bacilli is suggestive of this diagnosis. However, Whipple's disease can be confused with the PAS-positive macrophages containing *M. avian* complex, which may be a cause of diarrhea in AIDS. The presence of the *T. whippelii* bacillus outside of macrophages is a more important indicator of active disease than their presence within the macrophages. *T. whippelii* has now been successfully grown in culture.

℞ **TREATMENT** The treatment for Whipple's disease is prolonged use of antibiotics. At the present time the drug of choice is double-strength trimethoprim/sulfamethoxazole for approximately 1 year. PAS-positive macrophages can persist following successful treatment, and the presence of bacilli outside of macrophages is indicative of persistent infection or an early sign of recurrence. Recurrence of disease activity, especially with dementia, is an extremely poor prognostic sign and requires an antibiotic that crosses the blood-brain barrier. If trimethoprim/sulfamethoxazole is not tolerated, chloramphenicol is an appropriate second choice.

PROTEIN-LOSING ENTEROPATHY Protein-losing enteropathy is not a specific disease but rather describes a group of gastrointestinal and nongastrointestinal disorders with hypoproteinemia and edema in the absence of either proteinuria or defects in protein synthesis, e.g., chronic liver disease. These diseases are characterized by excess protein loss into the gastrointestinal tract. Normally, about 10% of the total protein catabolism occurs via the gastrointestinal tract. Evidence of increased protein loss into the gastrointestinal tract has been established in >65 different diseases, which can be classified into three primary groups: (1) mucosal ulceration such that the protein loss primarily represents exudation across damaged mucosa, e.g., ulcerative colitis, gastrointestinal carcinomas, peptic ulcer; (2) nonulcerated mucosa but with evidence of mucosal damage so that the protein loss represents loss across epithelia with altered permeability, e.g., celiac sprue and Ménétrier's disease in the small intestine and stomach, respectively; (3) lymphatic dysfunction, either representing primary lymphatic disease or secondary to partial lymphatic obstruction that may occur as a result of enlarged lymph nodes or cardiac disease.

Diagnosis The diagnosis of protein-losing enteropathy is suggested by the presence of peripheral edema and low serum albumin and globulin levels in the absence of renal and hepatic disease. It is extremely rare for an individual with protein-losing enteropathy to have selective loss of *only* albumin or *only* globulins. Therefore, marked reduction of serum albumin with normal serum globulins should not initiate an evaluation for protein-losing enteropathy but should suggest the presence of renal and/or hepatic disease. Likewise, reduced serum globulins with normal serum albumin levels is more likely a result of reduced globulin synthesis rather than enhanced globulin loss into the intestine. Documentation of an increase in protein loss into the gastrointestinal tract has been established by the administration of one of several radiolabeled proteins and its quantitation in stool during a 24- or 48-h period. Unfortunately, none of these radiolabeled proteins are available for routine clinical use. α_1-Antitrypsin, a protein that represents approximately 4% of total serum proteins and is resistant to proteolysis, can be used to document enhanced rates of serum protein loss into the intestinal tract but cannot be used to assess gastric protein loss due to its degradation in an acid milieu. α_1-Antitrypsin clearance is measured by determining stool volume and both stool and plasma α_1-antitrypsin concentrations. In addition to the loss of protein via abnormal and distended lymphatics, peripheral lymphocytes may also be lost via lymphatics, resulting in a relative lymphopenia. Thus, the presence of lymphopenia in a patient with hypoproteinemia supports the presence of increased loss of protein into the gastrointestinal tract.

Patients with increased protein loss into the gastrointestinal tract from lymphatic obstruction often have steatorrhea and diarrhea. The steatorrhea is a result of altered lymphatic flow as lipid-containing chylomicrons exit from intestinal epithelial cells via intestinal lymphatics (Table 286-4; Fig. 286-4). In the absence of mechanical or anatomic intestinal lymphatic obstruction, instrinsic intestinal lymphatic dysfunction, with or without lymphatic dysfunction in the peripheral extremities, has been named *intestinal lymphangiectasia*. Similarly, about 50% of individuals with intrinsic peripheral lymphatic disease (Milroy's disease) will also have intestinal lymphangiectasia and hypoproteinemia. Other than steatorrhea and enhanced protein loss into the gastrointestinal tract, all other aspects of intestinal absorptive function are normal in intestinal lymphangiectasia.

Other Causes Patients who appear to have idiopathic protein-losing enteropathy without any evidence of gastrointestinal disease should be examined for cardiac disease and especially right-sided valvular disease and chronic pericarditis (Chap. 236). On occasion, hypoproteinemia can be the only presentation for these two types of heart disease. Ménétrier's disease (also called *hypertrophic gastropathy*) is an uncommon entity that involves the body and fundus of the stomach and is characterized by large gastric folds, reduced gastric acid secretion, and, at times, enhanced protein loss into the stomach.

Table 286-9 Classification of Malabsorption Syndromes

Inadequate digestion
  Postgastrectomy[a]
  Deficiency or inactivation of pancreatic lipase
    Exocrine pancreatic insufficiency
      Chronic pancreatitis
      Pancreatic carcinoma
      Cystic fibrosis
      Pancreatic insufficiency—congenital or acquired
  Gastrinoma—acid inactivation of lipase[a]
  Drugs—orlistat

Reduced intraduodenal bile acid concentration/impaired micelle formation
  Liver disease
    Parenchymal liver disease
    Cholestatic liver disease
  Bacterial overgrowth in small intestine:

Anatomic stasis	Functional stasis
Afferent loop stasis/blind loop/strictures/fistulae	Diabetes[a]
	Scleroderma[a]
	Intestinal pseudoobstruction

  Interrupted enterohepatic circulation of bile salts
    Ileal resection
    Crohn's disease[a]
  Drugs (bind or precipitate bile salts)—neomycin, cholestyramine, calcium carbonate

Impaired mucosal absorption/mucosal loss or defect
  Intestinal resection or bypass
  Inflammation, infiltration, or infection:

Crohn's disease[a]	Celiac disease
Amyloidosis	Collagenous sprue
Scleroderma[a]	Whipple's disease
Lymphoma[a]	Radiation enteritis
Eosinophilic enteritis	Folate and vitamin B_{12} deficiency
Mastocytosis	Infections—salmonellosis, giardiasis
Tropical sprue	Graft-vs.-host disease

  Genetic disorders
    Disaccharidase deficiency
    Agammaglobulinemia
    Abetalipoproteinemia
    Hartnup disease
    Cystinuria

Impaired nutrient delivery to and/or from intestine:

Lymphatic obstruction	Circulatory disorders
Lymphoma[a]	Congestive heart failure
Lymphangiectasia	Constrictive pericarditis
	Mesenteric artery atherosclerosis
	Vasculitis

Endocrine and metabolic disorders
  Diabetes[a]
  Hypoparathyroidism
  Adrenal insufficiency
  Hyperthyroidism
  Carcinoid syndrome

[a] Malabsorption caused by more than one mechanism.

TREATMENT As excess protein loss into the gastrointestinal tract is most often secondary to a specific disease, treatment should be directed primarily to the underlying disease process and not to the hypoproteinemia. For example, if significant hypoproteinemia with resulting peripheral edema is present secondary to either celiac sprue or ulceratic colitis, a gluten-free diet or mesalamine, respectively, would be the initial therapy. When enhanced protein loss is secondary to lymphatic obstruction, it is critical to establish the nature of this obstruction. Identification of mesenteric nodes or lymphoma may be possible by imaging studies. Similarly, it is important to exclude cardiac disease as a cause of protein-losing enteropathy either by echosonography or, on occasion, by a right-heart catheterization.

The increased protein loss that occurs in intestinal lymphangiectasia is a result of distended lymphatics associated with lipid malabsorption. Treatment of the hypoproteinemia is accomplished by a low-

Table 286-10 Pathophysiology of Clinical Manifestations of Malabsorption Disorders

Symptom or Sign	Mechanism
Weight loss/malnutrition	Anorexia, malabsorption of nutrients
Diarrhea	Impaired absorption or secretion of water and electrolytes; unabsorbed dihydroxy bile acids and fatty acids
Flatus	Bacterial fermentation of unabsorbed carbohydrate
Glossitis, cheilosis, stomatitis	Deficiency of iron, vitamin B_{12}, folate, and vitamin A
Abdominal pain	Bowel distention or inflammation, pancreatitis
Bone pain	Calcium, vitamin D malabsorption, protein deficiency, osteoporosis
Tetany, paresthesia	Calcium and magnesium malabsorption
Weakness	Anemia, electrolyte depletion (particularly K^+)
Nocturia	Delayed absorption of water, hypokalemia
Azotemia, hypotension	Fluid and electrolyte depletion
Amenorrhea, decreased libido	Protein depletion, decreased calories, secondary hypopituitarism
Anemia	Impaired absorption of iron, folate, vitamin B_{12}
Bleeding	Vitamin K malabsorption, hypoprothrombinemia
Night blindness/xerophthalmia	Vitamin A malabsorption
Peripheral neuropathy	Vitamin B_{12} and thiamine deficiency
Dermatitis	Deficiency of vitamin A, zinc, and essential fatty acid

fat diet and the administration of MCTs (Table 286-3), which do not exit from the intestinal epithelial cells via lymphatics but are delivered to the body via the portal vein.

SUMMARY

A pathophysiologic classification of the many conditions that can produce malabsorption is given in Table 286-9. A summary of the pathophysiology of the various clinical manifestations of malabsorption is given in Table 286-10.

BIBLIOGRAPHY

AMERICAN GASTROENTEROLOGICAL ASSOCIATION: Technical review on the evaluation and management of chronic diarrhea. Gastroenterology 116:1464, 1999

COOK SI, SELLIN JH: Short chain fatty acids in health and disease. Aliment Pharmacol Ther 12:499, 1998

CRAIG RM, EHRENPREIS ED: D-Xylose testing. J Clin Gastroenterol 29:143, 1999

GREENBERGER NJ: Enzymatic therapy in patients with chronic pancreatitis. Gastroenterol Clin North Am 28:687, 1999

HAREWOOD GC, MURRAY JA: Approaching the patient with chronic malabsorption syndrome. Semin Gastrointest Dis 14:138, 1999

RAMAIAH C, BOYNTON RF: Whipple's disease. Gastroenterol Clin North Am 27:683, 1998

SHAW AD, DAVIES GJ: Lactose intolerance: Problems in diagnosis and treatment. J Clin Gastroenterol 28:208, 1999

TRIER JS: Diagnosis of celiac sprue. Gastroenterology 115:211, 1998

287

Sonia Friedman, Richard S. Blumberg

INFLAMMATORY BOWEL DISEASE

Inflammatory bowel disease (IBD) is an idiopathic and chronic intestinal inflammation. Ulcerative colitis (UC) and Crohn's disease (CD) are the two major types of IBD.

EPIDEMIOLOGY

The incidence of IBD varies within different geographic areas. Northern countries, such as the United States, United Kingdom, Nor-

Table 287-1 Epidemiology of IBD

	Ulcerative Colitis	Crohn's Disease
Incidence (U.S.)	11/100,000	7/100,000
Age of onset	15–30 & 60–80	15–30 & 60–80
Ethnicity	Jewish > Non-Jewish Caucasian > African American > Hispanic > Asian	
Male:female ratio	1:1	1.1–1.8:1
Smoking	May prevent disease	May cause disease
Oral contraceptives	No increased risk	Relative risk 1.9
Appendectomy	Not protective	Protective
Monozygotic twins	8% concordance	67% concordance
Dizygotic twins	0% concordance	20% concordance

way, and Sweden, have the highest rates. The incidence rates of UC and CD in the United States are about 11 per 100,000 and 7 per 100,000, respectively (Table 287-1). Countries in southern Europe, South Africa, and Australia have lower incidence rates: 2 to 6.3 per 100,000 for UC, and 0.9 to 3.1 per 100,000 for CD. In Asia and South America, IBD is rare; incidence rates of UC and CD are 0.5 and 0.08 per 100,000, respectively. The highest mortality in IBD patients is during the first years of disease and in long duration disease due to the risk of colon cancer. In a Swedish population study, the standardized mortality ratios for CD and UC were 1.51 and 1.37, respectively.

The peak age of onset of UC and CD is between 15 and 30 years. A second peak occurs between the ages of 60 and 80. The male to female ratio for UC is 1:1 and for CD is 1.1 to 1.8:1. A two- to fourfold increased frequency of UC and CD in Jewish populations has been described in the United States, Europe, and South Africa. Furthermore, disease frequency differs within the Jewish populations. The prevalence of IBD in Ashkenazi Jews is about twice that of Israeli-born, Sephardic, or Oriental Jews. The prevalence decreases progressively in non-Jewish Caucasian, African-American, Hispanic, and Asian populations. Urban areas have a higher prevalence of IBD than rural areas and high socioeconomic classes have a higher prevalence than lower socioeconomic classes.

The effects of cigarette smoking are different in UC and CD. The risk of UC in smokers is 40% that of nonsmokers. Additionally, former smokers have a 1.7-fold increased risk for UC than people who have never smoked. In contrast, smoking is associated with a twofold increased risk of CD. Oral contraceptives are also linked to CD; the relative risk of CD for oral contraceptive users is about 1.9. Appendectomy appears to be protective against UC but further studies are needed.

IBD runs in families. If a patient has IBD, the lifetime risk that a first-degree relative will be affected is ~10%. If two parents have IBD, each child has a 36% chance of being affected. In twin studies, 67% of monozygotic twins are concordant for CD and 20% are concordant for UC, whereas 8% of dizygotic twins are concordant for CD and none are concordant for UC. There is also concordance for anatomic site and clinical type of CD within families.

Additional evidence for genetic predisposition to IBD comes from its association with certain genetic syndromes. UC and CD are both associated with Turner's syndrome, and Hermansky-Pudlak syndrome is associated with a granulomatous colitis. Glycogen storage disease type 1b can present with Crohn's-like lesions of the large and small bowel. Other immunodeficiency disorders, such as hypogammaglobulinemia, selective IgA deficiency, and hereditary angioedema, also exhibit an increased association with IBD.

ETIOLOGY AND PATHOGENESIS

Although IBD has been described as a clinical entity for over 100 years, its etiology and pathogenesis have not been definitively elaborated. Various studies have led to a consensus hypothesis that in genetically predisposed individuals, both exogenous factors (e.g., infectious agents, normal lumenal flora) and host factors (e.g., intestinal epithelial cell barrier function, vascular supply, neuronal activity) together cause a chronic state of dysregulated mucosal immune function that is further modified by specific environmental factors (e.g., smoking). Although it is possible that the chronic activation of the mucosal immune system may represent an appropriate response to a chronic unidentified infectious agent, a search for such an agent has thus far been unrewarding. As such, IBD must currently be considered an inappropriate response to either the endogenous microbial flora within the intestine, with or without some component of autoimmunity. Importantly, the normal intestine contains a significant concentration of immune cells in a chronic state of so-called *physiologic inflammation*, in which the gut is poised for, but actively restrained from, full immunologic responses. During the course of infections in the normal host, full activation of the gut-associated lymphoid tissue occurs but is rapidly superceded by downregulation of the immune response and tissue repair. In IBD this process is not regulated normally.

GENETIC CONSIDERATIONS   IBD is a polygenic disorder that gives rise to multiple clinical subgroups within UC and CD. Genome-wide searches have shown that potential disease-associated loci are present on chromosomes 16, 12, 7, 3, and 1, although their specific gene associations are undefined. HLA alleles may play a role. UC patients disproportionately express DR2-related alleles, whereas in CD an increased use of the DR5 DQ1 haplotype or the DRB*0301 allele has been described. In UC patients with pancolitis undergoing total proctocolectomy, 14.3% versus 3.2% of non-IBD controls express the HLA DRB1*0103 allele. This allele is associated with extensive disease and extraintestinal manifestations such as mouth ulcers, arthritis, and uveitis. Other associations with immunoregulatory genes include the intercellular adhesion molecule R241 allele in UC and CD and the interleukin (IL) 1 receptor antagonist allele 2 in UC patients that is associated with total colonic inflammation. Although not proven at the genetic level, patients with IBD and their first-degree relatives may exhibit diminished intestinal epithelial cell barrier function. ■

DEFECTIVE IMMUNE REGULATION IN IBD   The normal state of the mucosal immune system is one of inhibited immune responses to lumenal contents due to oral tolerance that occurs in the normal individual. When soluble antigens are administered orally rather than subcutaneously or intramuscularly, antigen-specific nonresponsiveness is induced. Multiple mechanisms are involved in the induction of oral tolerance and include deletion or anergy of antigen-reactive T cells or activation of CD4+ T cells that suppress gut inflammation through secretion of inhibitory cytokines (IL-10, TGF-β). Oral tolerance may be responsible for the lack of immune responsiveness to dietary antigens and the commensal flora in the intestinal lumen. In IBD this tightly regulated state of suppression of inflammation is altered, leading to uncontrolled inflammation. The mechanisms that maintain this regulated state of immune suppression are unknown.

Gene knockout (-/-) or transgenic (Tg) mouse models of colitis have revealed that deleting specific cytokines (e.g., IL-2, IL-10, TGF-β) or their receptors, deleting molecules associated with T-cell antigen recognition (e.g., T-cell antigen receptors, MHC class II), or interfering with intestinal epithelial cell barrier function (e.g., blocking N-cadherin, deleting multidrug resistance gene 1a or trefoil factor) leads to colitis. Thus, a variety of specific alterations can lead to unregulated autoimmunity directed at the colon in mice.

In both UC and CD, activated CD4+ T cells present in the lamina propria and peripheral blood secrete inflammatory cytokines. Some directly activate other inflammatory cells (macrophages and B cells) and others act indirectly to recruit other lymphocytes, inflammatory leukocytes, and mononuclear cells from the peripheral vasculature into the gut through interactions between homing receptors on leukocytes (e.g., $\alpha 4\beta 7$ integrin) and addressins on vascular endothelium (e.g., MadCAM1). CD4+ T cells can be subdivided into two major cate-

gories both of which may be associated with colitis in animal models and humans: $T_H 1$ cells (IFN-γ, TNF) and $T_H 2$ cells (IL-4, IL-5, IL-13). $T_H 1$ cells appear to induce transmural granulomatous inflammation that resembles CD, and $T_H 2$ cells appear to induce superficial mucosal inflammation more characteristic of UC. The $T_H 1$ cytokine pathway is initiated by IL-12, a key cytokine in the pathogenesis of experimental models of mucosal inflammation. Thus, use of antibodies to block proinflammatory cytokines (e.g., anti-TNF-α, anti-IL-12) or molecules associated with leukocyte recruitment (e.g., anti-$\alpha 4\beta 7$) or use of cytokines that inhibit inflammation (e.g., IL-10) or promote intestinal barrier function (e.g., IL-11) may be beneficial to humans with colitis.

THE INFLAMMATORY CASCADE IN IBD   Once initiated in IBD, the immune inflammatory response is perpetuated as a consequence of T-cell activation. A sequential cascade of inflammatory mediators acts to extend the response; each step is a potential target for therapy. Inflammatory cytokines, such as IL-1, IL-6, and tumor necrosis factor (TNF) have diverse effects on tissue. They promote fibrogenesis, collagen production, activation of tissue metalloproteinases, and the production of other inflammatory mediators; they also activate the coagulation cascade in local blood vessels (e.g., increased production of von Willebrand's factor). These cytokines are normally produced in response to infection, but are usually turned off or inhibited at the appropriate time to limit tissue damage. In IBD their activity is not regulated, resulting in an imbalance between the proinflammatory and anti-inflammatory mediators. Therapies such as the 5-ASA compounds are potent inhibitors of these inflammatory mediators through inhibition of transcription factors such as NF-κB that regulate their expression.

EXOGENOUS FACTORS   IBD may have an as yet undefined infectious etiology. Three specific agents have received the greatest attention, *Mycobacterium paratuberculosis*, *Paramyxovirus*, and *Helicobacter* species. The immune response to a specific organism could be expressed differently, depending upon the individual's genetic background. Although *M. paratuberculosis* had initially been identified in CD patients, further studies have not confirmed a disease association. In addition, antimycobacterial agents have not been effective in treating CD. A role for the measles virus or paramyxoviruses in the development of CD has been suggested based on an increase in the incidence of CD in England that paralleled use of the measles vaccine. However, studies in the United States have not substantiated this finding. In an animal model of IBD, *Helicobacter hepaticus* has been implicated as a trigger for the inflammatory response; evidence in people is lacking.

Multiple pathogens (e.g., *Salmonella*, *Shigella sp.*, *Campylobacter sp.*) may initiate IBD by triggering an inflammatory response that the mucosal immune system may fail to control. However, in an IBD patient the normal flora is likely perceived as if it were a pathogen. Anaerobic organisms, particularly *Bacteroides* species, may be responsible for the induction of inflammation. Such a notion is supported by the response in patients with CD to agents that alter the intestinal flora, such as metronidazole, ciprofloxacin, and elemental diets. CD also responds to fecal diversion, demonstrating the ability of lumenal contents to exacerbate disease. On the other hand, other bacterial organisms, so-called probiotics such as *Lactobacillus sp.*, downregulate inflammation in animal models and humans.

Psychosocial factors can contribute to clinical exacerbation of symptoms. Major life events such as illness or death in the family, divorce or separation, interpersonal conflict, or other major loss, are associated with an increase in IBD symptoms such as pain, bowel dysfunction, and bleeding. Acute daily stress can exacerbate bowel symptoms even after controlling for major life events. When the *sickness impact profile*, a measurement of overall psychological and physical functioning is used, IBD patients have functional impairment greater than that of a health maintenance organization population but less than that of patients with chronic back pain or amyotrophic lateral sclerosis. IBD patients have been hypothesized to have a characteristic personality that renders them susceptible to emotional stresses. However, emotional dysfunction could also be the result of chronic illness and should be considered when treating these patients.

PATHOLOGY

ULCERATIVE COLITIS: MACROSCOPIC FEATURES

UC is a mucosal disease that usually involves the rectum and extends proximally to involve all or part of the colon. Approximately 40 to 50% of patients have disease limited to the rectum and rectosigmoid, 30 to 40% have disease extending beyond the sigmoid but not involving the whole colon, and 20% have a total colitis. Proximal spread occurs in continuity without areas of uninvolved mucosa. When the whole colon is involved, the inflammation extends 1 to 2 cm into the terminal ileum in 10 to 20% of patients. This is called *backwash ileitis* and has little clinical significance. Although variations in macroscopic activity may suggest skip areas, biopsies from normal-appearing mucosa are usually abnormal. Thus, it is important to obtain multiple biopsies from apparently uninvolved mucosa, whether proximal or distal, during endoscopy.

With mild inflammation, the mucosa is erythematous and has a fine granular surface that looks like sandpaper. In more severe disease, the mucosa is hemorrhagic, edematous, and ulcerated (Fig. 287-1). In long-standing disease, inflammatory polyps (pseudopolyps) may be present as a result of epithelial regeneration. The mucosa may appear normal in remission but in patients with many years of disease it appears atrophic and featureless and the entire colon becomes narrowed and foreshortened. Patients with fulminant disease can develop a toxic colitis or a toxic megacolon where the bowel wall becomes very thin and the mucosa is severely ulcerated, which may lead to perforation.

ULCERATIVE COLITIS: MICROSCOPIC FEATURES

Histologic findings correlate well with the endoscopic appearance and clinical course of UC. The process is limited to the mucosa and superficial submucosa with deeper layers unaffected except in fulminant disease. In UC, two major histologic features are indicative of chronicity and help distinguish it from infectious or acute self-limited colitis. First, the crypt architecture of the colon is distorted; crypts may be bifid and reduced in number, often with a gap between the crypt bases and the muscularis mucosae. Second, some patients have basal plasma cells and multiple basal lymphoid aggregates. Mucosal vascular congestion with edema and focal hemorrhage, and an inflammatory cell infiltrate of neutrophils, lymphocytes, plasma cells, and macrophages may be present. The neutrophils invade the epithelium, usually in the crypts, and give rise to cryptitis and, ultimately, to crypt abscesses (Fig. 287-2). The cryptitis is associated with mucus discharge from goblet cells and increased epithelial cell turnover. His-

FIGURE 287-1 Pan-ulcerative colitis. Mucosa has a lumpy, bumpy appearance because of areas of inflamed but intact mucosa separated by ulcerated areas. *(Courtesy of Dr. EK Rosado and Dr. CA Perkos, Division of Gastrointestinal Pathology, Department of Pathology, Emory University, Atlanta, Georgia.)*

FIGURE 287-2 Characteristic findings of IBD in a case of ulcerative colitis: crypt distortion, cryptitis, and crypt abscess. *(Courtesy of Dr. EK Rosado and Dr. CA Perkos, Division of Gastrointestinal Pathology, Department of Pathology, Emory University, Atlanta, Georgia.)*

tologically, this results in goblet cell depletion. Other chronic changes that are sometimes seen are neuronal hypertrophy and fibromuscular hyperplasia of the muscularis mucosae.

CROHN'S DISEASE: MACROSCOPIC FEATURES

CD can affect any part of the gastrointestinal tract from the mouth to the anus. Some 30 to 40% of patients have small bowel disease alone, 40 to 55% have disease involving both the small and large intestines, and 15 to 25% have colitis alone. In the 75% of patients with small intestinal disease, the terminal ileum is involved in 90%. Unlike UC, which almost always involves the rectum, the rectum is often spared in CD. CD is segmental, with skip areas in the midst of diseased intestine (Fig. 287-3). Perirectal fistulas, fissures, abscesses, and anal stenosis are present in one-third of patients with CD, particularly those with colonic involvement. CD may also involve the liver and the pancreas.

Unlike UC, CD is a transmural process. Endoscopically, aphthous or small superficial ulcerations characterize mild disease; in more ac-

FIGURE 287-3 Portion of colon with stricture in patient with CD. *(Courtesy of Dr. EK Rosado and Dr. CA Perkos, Division of Gastrointestinal Pathology, Department of Pathology, Emory University, Atlanta, Georgia.)*

FIGURE 287-4   Granulomas (arrow) in bowel wall and serosa of colon, CD. *(Courtesy of Dr. EK Rosado and Dr. CA Perkos, Division of Gastrointestinal Pathology, Department of Pathology, Emory University, Atlanta, Georgia.)*

tive disease, stellate ulcerations fuse longitudinally and transversely to demarcate islands of mucosa that frequently are histologically normal. This "cobblestone" appearance is characteristic of CD, both endoscopically and by barium radiography. As in UC, pseudopolyps can form in CD.

Active CD is characterized by focal inflammation and formation of fistula tracts, which resolve by fibrosis and stricturing of the bowel. The bowel wall thickens and becomes narrowed and fibrotic, leading to chronic, recurrent bowel obstructions. Projections of thickened mesentery encase the bowel ("creeping fat") and serosal and mesenteric inflammation promote adhesions and fistula formation.

CROHN'S DISEASE: MICROSCOPIC FEATURES   The earliest lesions are aphthoid ulcerations and focal crypt abscesses with loose aggregations of macrophages, which form noncaseating granulomas in all layers of the bowel wall from mucosa to serosa (Fig. 287-4). Granulomas can be seen in lymph nodes, mesentery, peritoneum, liver, and pancreas. Although granulomas are a pathognomonic feature of CD, only half of cases reveal granulomas on surgical or endoscopic biopsy specimens. Other histologic features of CD include submucosal or subserosal lymphoid aggregates, particularly away from areas of ulceration, gross and microscopic skip areas, and transmural inflammation that is accompanied by fissures that penetrate deeply into the bowel wall and sometimes form fistulous tracts or local abscesses.

CLINICAL PRESENTATION

ULCERATIVE COLITIS   Signs and Symptoms   The major symptoms of UC are diarrhea, rectal bleeding, tenesmus, passage of mucus, and crampy abdominal pain. The severity of symptoms correlates with the extent of disease. Although UC can present acutely, symptoms usually have been present for weeks to months. Occasionally, diarrhea and bleeding are so intermittent and mild that the patient does not seek medical attention.

Patients with proctitis usually pass fresh blood or blood-stained mucus, either mixed with stool or streaked onto the surface of a normal or hard stool. They also have tenesmus, or urgency with a feeling of incomplete evacuation. They rarely have abdominal pain. With proctitis or proctosigmoiditis, proximal transit slows, which may account for the constipation that is commonly seen in patients with distal disease.

When the disease extends beyond the rectum, blood is usually mixed with stool, or grossly bloody diarrhea may be noted. Colonic motility is altered by inflammation with rapid transit through the inflamed intestine. When the disease is severe, patients pass a liquid stool containing blood, pus, and fecal matter. Diarrhea is often nocturnal and/or postprandial. Although severe pain is not a prominent symptom, some patients with active disease may experience vague lower abdominal discomfort or mild central abdominal cramping. Severe cramping and abdominal pain can occur in association with severe attacks of the disease. Other symptoms in moderate to severe disease include anorexia, nausea, vomiting, fever, and weight loss.

Physical signs of proctitis include a tender anal canal and blood on rectal exam. With more extensive disease, patients have tenderness to palpation directly over the colon. Patients with a toxic colitis have severe pain and bleeding, and those with megacolon have hepatic tympany. Both may have signs of peritonitis if a perforation has occurred. The classification of disease activity is shown in Table 287-2.

Laboratory, Endoscopic, and Radiographic Features   Active disease can be associated with a rise in acute phase reactants (C-reactive protein, orosomucoid levels), platelet count, erythrocyte sedimentation rate (ESR) and a decrease in hemoglobin. In severely ill patients, the serum albumin level will fall rather quickly. Leukocytosis may be present but is not a specific indicator of disease activity. Proctitis or proctosigmoiditis rarely causes a rise in C-reactive protein. Diagnosis relies upon the patient's history; clinical symptoms, negative stool examination for bacteria, *Clostridium difficile* toxin, and ova and parasites; sigmoidoscopic appearance; and histology of rectal or colonic biopsy specimens.

Sigmoidoscopy is used to assess disease activity and is often performed before treatment. Histologic features change more slowly than clinical features but can also be used to grade disease activity.

Patients with a severe attack of UC should have a plain, supine film of the abdomen. In the presence of severe disease, the margin of the colon becomes edematous and irregular (Fig. 287-5). Colonic thickening and toxic dilation can both be seen on a plain radiograph.

The earliest radiologic change of UC seen on single-contrast barium enema is a fine mucosal granularity. With increasing severity, the mucosa becomes thickened and superficial ulcers are seen. Deep ulcerations can appear as "collar-button" ulcers, which indicate that the ulceration has penetrated the mucosa. Haustral folds may be normal in mild disease, but as activity progresses they become edematous and thickened. Loss of haustration can occur, especially in patients with long-standing disease. In addition, the colon becomes shortened and narrowed. Polyps in the colon may be postinflammatory polyps or pseudopolyps, adenomatous polyps, or carcinoma.

Computed tomography (CT) scanning is not as helpful as endoscopy and barium enema in making the diagnosis of UC, but typical findings include mild mural thickening (<1.5 cm), inhomogeneous wall density, absence of small bowel thickening, increased perirectal and presacral fat, target appearance of the rectum, and adenopathy.

Complications   Only 15% of patients with UC present initially with catastrophic illness. Massive hemorrhage occurs with severe

Table 287-2   Ulcerative Colitis: Disease Presentation

	Mild	Moderate	Severe
Bowel movements	<4 per day	4–6 per day	>6 per day
Blood in stool	Small	Moderate	Severe
Fever	None	<37.5°C mean	>37.5°C mean
Tachycardia	None	<90 mean pulse	>90 mean pulse
Anemia	Mild	>75%	≤75%
Sedimentation rate	<30 mm		>30 mm
Endoscopic appearance	Erythema, decreased vascular pattern, fine granularity	Marked erythema, coarse granularity, absent vascular markings, contact bleeding, no ulcerations	Spontaneous bleeding, ulcerations

FIGURE 287-5 Barium enema in a patient with acute ulcerative colitis: inflammation of the entire colon. *(Courtesy of Dr. JM Braver, Gastrointestinal Radiology, Department of Radiology, Brigham and Women's Hospital, Boston, Massachusetts.)*

attacks of disease in 1% of patients and treatment for the disease usually stops the bleeding. However, if patients require 6 to 8 units of blood within 24 to 48 h, colectomy is indicated. Toxic megacolon is defined as a transverse colon with a diameter of more than 5.0 cm to 6.0 cm, with loss of haustration in patients with severe attacks of UC. It occurs in about 5% of attacks and can be triggered by electrolyte abnormalities and narcotics. Approximately 50% of acute dilations will resolve with medical therapy alone, but urgent colectomy is required for those that do not improve. Perforation is the most dangerous of the local complications, and the physical signs of peritonitis may not be obvious, especially if the patient is receiving glucocorticoids. Although perforation is rare, the mortality rate for perforation complicating a toxic megacolon is about 15%. In addition, patients can develop a toxic colitis and such severe ulcerations that the bowel may perforate without first dilating.

Obstructions caused by benign stricture formation occur in 10% of patients, with one-third of the strictures occurring in the rectum. These should be surveyed endoscopically for carcinoma. UC patients occasionally develop anal fissures, perianal abscesses, or hemorrhoids but the occurrence of extensive perianal lesions should suggest CD.

CROHN'S DISEASE Signs and Symptoms Although CD usually presents as acute or chronic bowel inflammation, the inflammatory process evolves toward one of two patterns of disease: a fibrostenotic-obstructing pattern or a penetrating-fistulous pattern, each with different treatments and prognoses. The site of disease influences the clinical manifestations.

Ileocolitis Because the most common site of inflammation is the terminal ileum, the usual presentation of ileocolitis is a chronic history of recurrent episodes of right lower quadrant pain and diarrhea. Sometimes the initial presentation mimics acute appendicitis with pronounced right lower quadrant pain, a palpable mass, fever, and leukocytosis. Only at laparotomy, when the appendix is found to be normal, is the ileitis discovered. Pain is usually colicky; it precedes

and is relieved by defecation. A low-grade fever is usually noted. High-spiking fever suggests intraabdominal abscess formation. Weight loss is common—typically 10 to 20% of body weight—and develops as a consequence of diarrhea, anorexia, and fear of eating.

An inflammatory mass may be palpated in the right lower quadrant of the abdomen. The mass is composed of inflamed bowel, adherent and indurated mesentery, and enlarged abdominal lymph nodes. Extension of the mass can cause obstruction of the right ureter or bladder inflammation, manifested by dysuria and fever. Edema, bowel wall thickening, and fibrosis of the bowel wall within the mass account for the radiographic "string sign" of a narrowed intestinal lumen.

Bowel obstruction may take several forms. In the early stages of the disease, bowel wall edema and spasm produce intermittent obstructive manifestations and increasing symptoms of postprandial pain. Over several years, this persistent inflammation gradually progresses to fibrostenotic narrowing and stricture. Diarrhea will decrease and eventually lead to chronic bowel obstruction and obstipation. Acute episodes of obstruction occur as well, precipitated by bowel inflammation and spasm or sometimes by impaction of undigested food. These episodes usually resolve with intravenous fluids and gastric decompression.

Severe inflammation of the ileocecal region may lead to localized wall thinning, with microperforation and fistula formation to the adjacent bowel, the skin, the urinary bladder, or to an abscess cavity in the mesentery. Enterovesical fistulas typically present as dysuria or recurrent bladder infections or less commonly as pneumaturia or fecaluria. Enterocutaneous fistulas follow tissue planes of least resistance, usually draining through abdominal surgical scars. Enterovaginal fistulas are rare and present as dyspareunia or as a feculent or foul-smelling, often painful vaginal discharge. They are unlikely to develop without a prior hysterectomy.

Jejunoileitis Extensive inflammatory disease is associated with a loss of digestive and absorptive surface, resulting in malabsorption and steatorrhea. Nutritional deficiencies can also result from poor intake and enteric losses and protein and other nutrients. Intestinal malabsorption can cause hypoalbuminemia, hypocalcemia, hypomagnesemia, coagulopathy, and hyperoxaluria with nepholithiasis. Vertebral fractures are caused by a combination of vitamin D deficiency, hypocalcemia, and prolonged glucocorticoid use. Pellagra from niacin deficiency has been reported in extensive small bowel disease, and malabsorption of vitamin B12 can lead to a megaloblastic anemia.

Diarrhea is characteristic of active disease; its causes include: (1) bacterial overgrowth in obstructive stasis or fistulization, (2) bile-acid malabsorption due to a diseased or resected terminal ileum, (3) intestinal inflammation with decreased water absorption and increased secretion of electrolytes.

Colitis and Perianal Disease Patients with colitis present with low-grade fevers, malaise, diarrhea, crampy abdominal pain, and sometimes hematochezia. Gross bleeding due to deep colonic ulceration is not as common as in UC and appears in about half of patients with exclusively colonic disease. Only 1 to 2% bleed massively. Pain is caused by passage of fecal material through narrowed and inflamed segments of large bowel. Decreased rectal compliance is another cause for diarrhea in Crohn's colitis patients. Toxic megacolon has been associated with severe inflammation and short-duration disease.

Stricturing can occur in the colon, and patients can develop fibrous strictures with symptoms of bowel obstruction. Also, colonic disease may fistulize into the stomach or duodenum, causing feculent vomiting, or to the proximal or mid small bowel, causing malabsorption by "short circuiting" and bacterial overgrowth. Approximately 10% of women with Crohn's colitis will develop a rectovaginal fistula.

Perianal disease affects about one-third of patients with Crohn's colitis and is manifested by incontinence, large hemorrhoidal tags, anal strictures, anorectal fistulae, and perirectal abscesses. Not all patients with perianal fistula will have endoscopic evidence of colonic inflammation.

Gastroduodenal Disease   Symptoms and signs of upper gastrointestinal tract disease include nausea, vomiting, and epigastric pain. Patients usually have a *H. pylori*-negative gastritis. The second portion of the duodenum is more commonly involved than the bulb. Fistulas involving the stomach or duodenum arise from the small or large bowel and do not necessarily signify the presence of upper gastrointestinal tract involvement. Patients with advanced gastroduodenal CD may develop a chronic gastric outlet obstruction.

Laboratory, Endoscopic, and Radiographic Features   Laboratory abnormalities include elevated sedimentation rate and C-reactive protein. In more severe disease, findings include hypoalbuminemia, anemia, and leukocytosis.

Endoscopic features of CD include rectal sparing, aphthous ulcerations, fistulas, and skip lesions. Endoscopy is useful for biopsy of mass lesions or strictures, or for visualization of filling defects seen on barium enema. Colonoscopy allows examination and biopsy of the terminal ileum, and upper endoscopy is useful in diagnosing gastroduodenal involvement in patients with upper tract symptoms. Ileal or colonic strictures may be dilated with balloons introduced through the colonoscope. Endoscopic appearance correlates poorly with clinical remission; thus, repeated endoscopy is not used to monitor the inflammation.

In CD early radiographic findings in the small bowel include thickened folds and aphthous ulcerations. "Cobblestoning" from longitudinal and transverse ulcerations most frequently involves the small bowel (Fig. 287-6). In more advanced disease, strictures, fistulas (Fig. 287-7), inflammatory masses, and abscesses may be detected. The earliest macroscopic findings of colonic CD are aphthous ulcers. These small ulcers are often multiple and separated by normal intervening mucosa. As more severe disease develops, aphthous ulcers become

FIGURE 287-7   Small bowel series demonstrating distal ileal inflammation and fistulization (arrows) in a patient with CD. *(Courtesy of Dr. JM Braver, Gastrointestinal Radiology, Department of Radiology, Brigham and Women's Hospital, Boston, Massachusetts.)*

enlarged, deeper, and occasionally connected to one another, forming longitudinal stellate, serpiginous, and linear ulcers.

The transmural inflammation of CD leads to decreased luminal diameter and limited distensibility. As ulcers progress deeper, they can lead to fistula formation. The radiographic "string sign" represents long areas of circumferential inflammation and fibrosis, resulting in long segments of luminal narrowing. The segmental nature of CD results in wide gaps of normal or dilated bowel between involved segments.

CT findings include mural thickening >2 cm, homogeneous wall density, mural thickening of small bowel, mesenteric fat stranding, perianal disease, and adenopathy. CT scanning can help identify abscesses, fistulas, and sinus tracts. Magnetic resonance imaging (MRI) may prove superior for demonstrating pelvic lesions such as ischiorectal abscesses.

Complications   Because CD is a transmural process, serosal adhesions develop that provide direct pathways for fistula formation and reduce the incidence of free perforation. Free perforation occurs in 1 to 2% of patients, usually in the ileum but occasionally in the jejunum or as a complication of toxic megacolon. The peritonitis of free perforation, especially colonic, may be fatal. Generalized peritonitis may also result from the rupture of an intraabdominal abscess. Other complications include intestinal obstruction in 40%, massive hemorrhage, malabsorption, and severe perianal disease.

Serologic Markers   Several serologic markers may be used to differentiate between CD and UC and help to predict the course of disease. Two antibodies that can be detected in the serum of IBD patients are perinuclear antineutrophil cytoplasmic antibody (pANCA) and anti-*Saccharomyces cerevisiae* antibodies (ASCA). A distinct set of antineutrophil cytoplasmic antibodies with perinuclear staining by indirect immunofluorescence is associated with UC. The antigens to which these antibodies are directed have not been identified, but they are distinct from those associated with vasculitis and may be related to histones. pANCA positivity is found in about 60 to 70% of UC patients and 5 to 10% of CD patients; 5 to 15% of first-degree relatives

FIGURE 287-6   Crohn's disease: small bowel series demonstrating "cobblestoning" of the terminal ileum (arrows). *(Courtesy of Dr. JM Braver, Gastrointestinal Radiology, Department of Radiology, Brigham and Women's Hospital, Boston, Massachusetts.)*

of UC patients are pANCA positive, whereas only 2 to 3% of the general population is pANCA positive. pANCA may also identify specific disease phenotypes. pANCA positivity is more often associated with pancolitis, early surgery, pouchitis, or inflammation of the pouch after ileal pouch-anal anastamosis (IPAA) and primary sclerosing cholangitis. pANCA in CD is associated with colonic disease that resembles UC.

ASCA antibodies recognize mannose sequences in the cell wall mannan of *S. cerevisiae*; 60 to 70% of CD patients, 10 to 15% of UC patients, and up to 5% of non-IBD controls are ASCA positive. The combined measurement of pANCA and ASCA has been advocated as a valuable diagnostic approach to IBD. In one report, pANCA positivity with ASCA negativity yielded a 57% sensitivity and 97% specificity for UC, whereas pANCA negativity with ASCA positivity yielded a 49% sensitivity and 97% specificity for CD. ASCA was associated with small bowel CD. These antibody tests may help decide whether a patient with indeterminate colitis should undergo an IPAA, because patients with predominant features of CD often have a more difficult postoperative course.

Anti-goblet cell autoantibodies (GABs)—autoantibodies against two target antigens in colonic epithelial cells—are present in 39% of UC patients, 30% of CD patients, 21% of first-degree relatives of UC patients, 19% of first-degree relatives of CD patients, and 2% of healthy controls. An anti-colon antibody is found in 36% of UC patients and 13% of CD patients and healthy controls. In addition, 31% of CD patients and 4% of UC patients have serum antibodies against pancreatic acinar cells or pancreatic autoantibodies (PABs). Antibodies to red cell membrane antigens that cross-react with enteropathogens such as *Campylobacter sp.* may be associated with hemolytic anemia in CD. None of these antibodies are useful in the diagnosis and management of patients with IBD.

DIFFERENTIAL DIAGNOSIS OF UC AND CD

UC and CD have similar features to many other diseases. In the absence of a key diagnostic test, a combination of clinical, laboratory, histopathologic, radiographic, and therapeutic observations is required (Table 287-3). Once a diagnosis of IBD is made, distinguishing between UC and CD is impossible in 10 to 20% of cases. These are termed *indeterminate* colitis.

INFECTIOUS DISEASE Infections of the small intestines and colon can mimic CD or UC. They may be bacterial, fungal, viral, or protozoal in origin (Table 287-4). *Campylobacter* colitis can mimic the endoscopic appearance of severe UC and can cause a relapse of established UC. *Salmonella* can cause watery or bloody diarrhea, nausea, and vomiting. Shigellosis causes watery diarrhea, abdominal pain, and fever followed by rectal tenesmus and by the passage of blood and mucus per rectum. All three are usually self-limited but 1% of patients infected with *Salmonella* become asymptomatic carriers. *Yersinia enterocolitica* infection occurs mainly in the terminal ileum and causes mucosal ulceration, neutrophil invasion, and thickening of the ileal wall. Other bacterial infections that may mimic IBD include *C. difficile*, which presents with watery diarrhea, tenesmus, nausea, and vomiting, and *Escherichia coli*, three categories of which can cause colitis. These are enterohemorrhagic, enteroinvasive, and enteroadherent *E. coli*, all of which can cause bloody diarrhea and abdominal tenderness. Diagnosis of bacterial colitis is made by sending stool specimens for bacterial culture and *C. difficile* toxin analysis. Gonorrhea, *Chlamydia*, and syphilis can also cause proctitis.

Gastrointestinal involvement with mycobacterial infection occurs primarily in the immunosuppressed patient but may occur in patients with normal immunity. Distal ileal and cecal involvement predominates and patients present with symptoms of small bowel obstruction and a tender abdominal mass. The diagnosis is made most directly by colonoscopy with biopsy and culture. *Mycobacterium avium intracellulare* complex infection occurs in advanced stages of HIV infection and in other profoundly immunocompromised states, and usually manifests as a systemic infection with diarrhea, abdominal pain, weight

loss, fever, and malabsorption. Diagnosis is established by acid-fast smear and culture of mucosal biopsies.

Although most of the patients with viral colitis are immunosuppressed, cytomegalovirus (CMV) and herpes simplex proctitis may occur in immunocompetent individuals. CMV occurs most commonly

Table 287-3 Different Clinical, Endoscopic, and Radiographic Features

	Ulcerative Colitis	Crohn's Disease
CLINICAL		
Gross blood in stool	Yes	Occasionally
Mucus	Yes	Occasionally
Systemic symptoms	Occasionally	Frequently
Pain	Occasionally	Frequently
Abdominal mass	Rarely	Yes
Significant perineal disease	No	Frequently
Fistulas	No	Yes
Small intestinal obstruction	No	Frequently
Colonic obstruction	Rarely	Frequently
Response to antibiotics	No	Yes
Recurrence after surgery	No	Yes
ANCA-positive	Frequently	Rarely
ENDOSCOPIC		
Rectal sparing	Rarely	Frequently
Continuous disease	Yes	Occasionally
"Cobblestoning"	No	Yes
Granuloma on biopsy	No	Occasionally
RADIOGRAPHIC		
Small bowel significantly abnormal	No	Yes
Abnormal terminal ileum	Occasionally	Yes
Segmental colitis	No	Yes
Asymmetrical colitis	No	Yes
Stricture	Occasionally	Frequently

NOTE: ANCA, antineutrophil cytoplasm antibody

Table 287-4 Diseases That Mimic IBD

INFECTIOUS ETIOLOGIES

Bacterial	Mycobacterial	Viral
Salmonella	Tuberculosis	Cytomegalovirus
Shigella	*Mycobacterium*	Herpes simplex
Toxigenic *Esche-*	*avium*	HIV
richia coli	**Parasitic**	**Fungal**
Campylobacter	Amebiasis	Histoplasmosis
Yersinia	*Isospora*	Candida
Clostridium diffi-	*Trichuris trichura*	*Aspergillus*
cile	Hookworm	
Gonorrhea	*Strongyloides*	
Chlamydia tracho-		
matis		

NONINFECTIOUS ETIOLOGIES

Inflammatory	Neoplastic	Drugs and
Appendicitis	Lymphoma	**Chemicals**
Diverticulitis	Metastatic carci-	NSAIDs
Diversion colitis	noma	Phosphasoda
Collagenous/lym-	Carcinoma of the	Cathartic colon
phocytic colitis	ileum	Gold
Ischemic colitis	Carcinoid	Oral contraceptives
Radiation colitis/	Familial polyposis	Cocaine
enteritis		Chemotherapy
Solitary rectal ulcer		
Eosinophilc gastro-		
enteritis		
Neutropenic colitis		
Bechet's syndrome		
Graft-versus-host		
disease		

NOTE: NSAIDs, nonsteroidal anti-inflammatory drugs

in the esophagus, colon, and rectum, but may also involve the small intestine. Symptoms include abdominal pain, bloody diarrhea, fever, and weight loss. With severe disease, necrosis and perforation can occur. Diagnosis is made by identification of intranuclear inclusions in mucosal cells on biopsy. Herpes simplex infection of the gastrointestinal tract is limited to the oropharynx, anorectum, and perianal areas. Symptoms include anorectal pain, tenesmus, constipation, inguinal adenopathy, difficulty with urinary voiding, and sacral paresthesias. Diagnosis is made by rectal biopsy. HIV itself can cause diarrhea, nausea, vomiting, and anorexia. Small intestinal biopsies show partial villus atrophy; small bowel bacterial overgrowth and fat malabsorption may also be noted.

Protozoan parasites include *Isospora belli*, which can cause a self-limited infection in healthy hosts but causes a chronic profuse, watery diarrhea and weight loss in AIDS patients. *Entamoeba histolytica* or related species infect about 10% of the world's population; symptoms include abdominal pain, tenesmus, frequent loose stool containing blood and mucus, and abdominal tenderness. Colonoscopy reveals focal punctate ulcers with normal intervening mucosa; diagnosis is made by biopsy or serum amebic antibodies. Fulminant amebic colitis is rare but has a mortality rate of >50%.

Other parasitic infections that may mimic IBD include hookworm (*Necator americanus*), whipworm (*Trichuris trichiura*), and *Strongyloides stercoralis*. In severely immunocompromised patients *Candida* or *Aspergillus* can be identified in the submucosa. Disseminated histoplasmosis can involve the ileocecal area.

NONINFECTIOUS DISEASE   Many diseases may mimic IBD (Table 287-4). Diverticulitis can be confused with CD clinically and radiographically. Both diseases cause fever, abdominal pain, tender abdominal mass, leukocytosis, elevated ESR, partial obstruction, and fistulas. Perianal disease or ileitis on small bowel series favors the diagnosis of CD. Significant endoscopic mucosal abnormalities are more likely in CD than in diverticulitis. Endoscopic or clinical recurrence following segmental resection favors CD. Diverticular-associated colitis is similar to CD, but mucosal abnormalities are limited to the sigmoid and descending colon.

Ischemic colitis is commonly confused with IBD. The ischemic process can be chronic and diffuse as in UC, or segmental as in CD. Colonic inflammation due to ischemia may resolve quickly or may persist and result in transmural scarring and stricture formation. Ischemic bowel disease should be considered in the elderly following abdominal aortic aneurysm repair or when a patient has a hypercoagulable state or a severe cardiac or peripheral vascular disorder. Patients usually present with sudden onset of left lower quadrant pain, urgency to defecate, and the passage of bright red blood per rectum. Endoscopic examination often demonstrates a normal-appearing rectum and a sharp transition to an area of inflammation in the descending colon and splenic flexure.

The effects of radiation therapy on the gastrointestinal tract can be difficult to distinguish from IBD. Acute symptoms can occur within 1 to 2 weeks of starting radiotherapy. When the rectum and sigmoid are irradiated, patients develop bloody, mucoid diarrhea and tenesmus, as in distal UC. With small bowel involvement, diarrhea is common. Late symptoms include malabsorption and weight loss. Stricturing with obstruction and bacterial overgrowth may occur. Fistulas can penetrate the bladder, vagina, or abdominal wall. Flexible sigmoidoscopy reveals mucosal granularity, friability, numerous telangiectasias, and occasionally discrete ulcerations. Biopsy can be diagnostic.

Solitary rectal ulcer syndrome is uncommon and can be confused with IBD. It occurs in mostly young females and may be caused by impaired evacuation and failure of relaxation of the puborectalis muscle. Ulceration may arise from anal sphincter overactivity, higher intrarectal pressures during defecation, and digital removal of stool. Patients complain of constipation with straining and pass blood and mucus per rectum. Other symptoms include abdominal pain, diarrhea, tenesmus, and perineal pain. The ulceration, which can be as large as

5 cm in diameter, is usually seen anteriorly or anteriorlaterally 3 to 15 cm from the anal verge. Biopsies can be diagnostic.

Several types of colitis have been associated with nonsteroidal anti-inflammatory drugs (NSAID), including de novo colitis, reactivation of IBD, and proctitis caused by use of suppositories. Most patients with NSAID-related colitis present with diarrhea and abdominal pain and complications include stricture, bleeding, obstruction, perforation, and fistulization. Withdrawal of these agents is crucial, and in cases of reactivated IBD, standard therapies are indicated.

INDETERMINITE COLITIS   Cases of IBD that cannot be categorized as UC or CD are called *indeterminate* colitis. Long-term follow-up reduces the number of patients labeled indeterminate to about 10%. The disease course of indeterminate colitis is unclear and surgical recommendations are difficult, especially since up to 20% of pouches fail, requiring ileosotomy. A multistage ileal pouch-anal anastamosis (the initial stage consisting of a subtotal colectomy with Hartman pouch) with careful histologic evaluation of the resected specimen to exclude CD is advised. Medical therapy is similar to UC and CD; most clinicians use 5-ASA drugs, glucocorticoids, and immunomodulators as necessary.

THE ATYPICAL COLITIDIES   Two atypical colitides—collagenous colitis and lymphocytic colitis—have completely normal endoscopic appearances. Collagenous colitis has two main histologic components: increased subepithelial collagen deposition and colitis with increased intraepithelial lymphocytes. Female to male ratio is 9:1, and most patients present in the sixth or seventh decades of life. The main symptom is chronic watery diarrhea. Treatments range from sulfasalazine and lomotil to bismuth to glucocorticoids for refractory disease.

Lymphocytic colitis has features similar to collagenous colitis including age at onset and clinical presentation, but it has almost equal incidence in men and women and no subepithelial collagen deposition on pathologic section. However, intraepithelial lymphocytes are increased. Diarrhea stops in the majority of patients treated with sulfasalazine or prednisone.

Diversion colitis is an inflammatory process that arises in segments of the large intestine that are excluded from the fecal stream. It usually occurs in patients with ileostomy or colostomy when a mucus fistula or a Hartman's pouch has been created. Diversion colitis is reversible by surgical reanastamosis. Clinically, patients have mucus or bloody discharge from the rectum. Erythema, granularity, friability, and, in more severe cases, ulceration can be seen on endoscopy. Histopathology shows areas of active inflammation with foci of cryptitis and crypt abscesses. Crypt architecture is normal and this differentiates it from UC. It may be impossible to distinguish from CD. Short-chain fatty acid enemas will help in diversion colitis, but the definitive therapy is surgical reanastamosis.

EXTRAINTESTINAL MANIFESTATIONS

IBD is associated with a variety of extraintestinal manifestations; up to one-third of patients have at least one. Patients with perianal CD are at higher risk for developing extraintestinal manifestations than other IBD patients.

DERMATOLOGIC   Erythema nodosum (EN) occurs in up to 15% of CD patients and 10% of UC patients. Attacks usually correlate with bowel activity; skin lesions develop after the onset of bowel symptoms, and patients frequently have concomitant active peripheral arthritis. The lesions of EN are hot, red, tender nodules measuring 1 to 5 cm in diameter and are found on the anterior surface of the lower legs, ankles, calves, thighs, and arms. Therapy is directed toward the underlying bowel disease.

Pyoderma gangrenosum (PG) is seen in 1 to 12% of UC patients and less commonly in CD colitis. Although it usually presents after the diagnosis of IBD, PG may occur years before the onset of bowel symptoms, run a course independent of the bowel disease, respond poorly to colectomy, and even develop years after proctocolectomy. It is usually associated with severe disease. Lesions are commonly found on the dorsal surface of the feet and legs but may occur on the arms, chest, stoma, and even the face. PG usually begins as a pustule and then spreads concentrically to rapidly undermine healthy skin. Lesions then ulcerate with violaceous edges surrounded by a margin of erythema. Centrally, they contain necrotic tissue with blood and exudates. Lesions may be single or multiple and grow as large as 30 cm. They are sometimes very difficult to treat and often require intravenous antibiotics, intravenous glucocorticoids, dapsone, purinethinol, thalidomide, or intravenous cyclosporine.

Other dermatologic manifestations include pyoderma vegetans that occurs in intertriginous areas, pyostomatitis vegetans that involves the mucous membranes, and metastatic CD, a rare disorder defined by cutaneous granuloma formation. Psoriasis affects 5 to 10% of patients with IBD and is unrelated to bowel activity. Perianal skin tags are found in 75 to 80% of patients with CD, especially those with colonic involvement. Oral mucosal lesions are seen often in CD and rarely in UC and include aphthous stomatitis and "cobblestone" lesions of the buccal mucosa.

RHEUMATOLOGIC Peripheral arthritis develops in 15 to 20% of IBD patients, is more common in CD, and worsens with exacerbations of bowel activity. It is asymmetric, polyarticular, and migratory, and most often affects large joints of the upper and lower extremities. Treatment is directed at reducing bowel inflammation. In severe UC, colectomy frequently cures the arthritis.

Ankylosing spondylitis (AS) occurs in about 10% of IBD patients and is more common in CD than UC. About two-thirds of IBD patients with AS test positive for the HLA-B27 antigen. The activity of AS is not related to bowel activity and does not remit with glucocorticoids or colectomy. It most often affects the spine and pelvis, producing symptoms of diffuse low-back pain, buttock pain, and morning stiffness. The course is continuous and progressive leading to permanent skeletal damage and deformity.

Sacroiliitis is symmetrical, occurs equally in UC and CD, is often asymptomatic, does not correlate with bowel activity, and does not necessarily progress to AS. Other rheumatic manifestations include hypertrophic osteoarthropathy, osteoporosis and osteomalacia secondary to malabsorption of calcium and vitamin D as well as glucocorticoid therapy, pelvic/femoral osteomyelitis, and relapsing polychondritis.

OCULAR The incidence of ocular complications in IBD patients is 1 to 10%. The most common are conjunctivitis, anterior uveitis/iritis, and episcleritis. Uveitis is associated with both UC and CD colitis, may be found during periods of remission, and may develop in patients following bowel resection. Symptoms include ocular pain, photophobia, blurred vision, and headache. Prompt intervention, sometimes with systemic glucocorticoids, is required to prevent scarring and visual impairment. Episcleritis is a benign disorder that presents with symptoms of mild ocular burning. It occurs in 3 to 4% of IBD patients, more commonly in CD colitis, and is treated with topical glucocorticoids.

HEPATOBILIARY Hepatic steatosis is detectable in about half of the abnormal liver biopsies from patients with CD and UC; patients usually present with hepatomegaly. Fatty liver usually results from a combination of chronic debilitating illness, malnutrition, and glucocorticoid therapy. Cholelithiasis is more common in CD than UC and occurs in 10 to 35% of patients with ileitis or ileal resection. Gallstone formation is caused by malabsorption of bile acids resulting in depletion of the bile salt pool and the secretion of lithogenic bile.

Primary sclerosing cholangitis (PSC) is characterized by both intrahepatic and extrahepatic bile duct inflammation and fibrosis, frequently leading to biliary cirrhosis and hepatic failure; 1 to 5% of patients with IBD have PSC, but 50 to 75% of patients with PSC have IBD. Although it can be recognized after the diagnosis of IBD, PSC can be detected earlier or even years after proctocolectomy. Most patients have no symptoms at the time of diagnosis; when symptoms are present they consist of fatigue, jaundice, abdominal pain, fever, anorexia, and malaise. Diagnosis is made by endoscopic retrograde cholangiopancreatography (ERCP), which demonstrates multiple bile duct

strictures alternating with relatively normal segments. The bile acid ursodeoxycholic acid (ursodiol) may reduce alkaline phosphatase and serum aminotransferase levels, but histologic improvement has been marginal and it has no definitive long-term benefit. Endoscopic stenting may be palliative for cholestasis secondary to bile duct obstruction. Patients with symptomatic disease develop cirrhosis and liver failure over 5 to 10 years and eventually require liver transplantation. Ten percent of PSC patients develop cholangiocarcinoma and cannot be transplanted. Pericholangitis is a subset of PSC found in about 30% of IBD patients; it is confined to small bile ducts and is usually benign.

UROLOGIC The most frequent genitourinary complications are calculi, ureteral obstruction, and fistulas. The highest frequency of nephrolithiasis (10 to 20%) occurs in patients with CD following small bowel resection or ileostomy. Calcium oxalate stones develop secondary to hyperoxaluria, which results from increased absorption of dietary oxalate. Normally, dietary calcium combines with luminal oxalate to form insoluble calcium oxalate, which is eliminated in the stool. In patients with ileal dysfunction, however, nonabsorbed fatty acids bind calcium and leave oxalate unbound. The unbound oxalate is then delivered to the colon, where it is readily absorbed, especially in the presence of colonic inflammation.

OTHER The risk of thromboembolic disease increases when IBD becomes active, and patients may present with deep vein thrombosis, pulmonary embolism, cerebrovascular accidents, and arterial emboli. Factors responsible for the hypercoagulable state include reactive thrombocytosis, increased levels of fibrinopeptide A, factor V, factor VIII, fibrinogen, accelerated thromboplastin generation, antithrombin III deficiency secondary to increased gut losses or increased catabolism, and free protein S deficiency. A spectrum of vasculitidies involving small, medium, and large vessels has also been observed in IBD patients.

Patients with IBD have an increased prevalence of osteoporosis secondary to vitamin D deficiency, calcium malabsorption, malnutrition, and corticosteroid use. Deficiencies of vitamin B12 and fat-soluble vitamins may occur after ileal resection or with ileal disease.

More common cardiopulmonary manifestations include endocarditis, myocarditis, pleuropericarditis, and interstitial lung disease. A secondary or reactive amyloidosis can occur in patients with long-standing IBD, especially in patients with CD. Amyloid material is deposited systemically and can cause diarrhea, constipation, and renal failure. The renal disease can be successfully treated with colchicine. Pancreatitis is a rare extra-intestinal manifestation of IBD and results from duodenal fistulas, ampullary CD, gallstones, PSC, drugs such as 6-mercaptopurine or azathioprine, autoimmune pancreatitis, and primary CD of the pancreas.

TREATMENT 5-ASA Agents The mainstay of therapy for mild to moderate UC and CD colitis is sulfasalazine and the other 5-ASA agents. Sulfasalazine was originally developed to deliver both antibacterial (sulfapyridine) and anti-inflammatory (5-aminosalicylic acid, 5-ASA) therapy into the connective tissues of joints and the colonic mucosa. The molecular structure provides a convenient delivery system to the colon by allowing the intact molecule to pass through the small intestine after only partial absorption, and to be broken down in the colon by bacterial azo reductases that cleave the azo bond linking the sulfa and 5-ASA moieties. Sulfasalazine is effective in inducing and maintaining remission in mild to moderate UC and CD ileocolitis and colitis, but its high rate of side effects limits its use. Although sulfasalazine is more effective at higher doses, at 6 or 8 g/d up to 30% of patients experience allergic reactions or intolerable side effects such as headache, anorexia, nausea, and vomiting that are attributable to the sulfapyridine moiety. Hypersensitivity reactions, independent of sulfapyridine levels, include rash, fever, hepatitis, agranulocytosis, hypersensitivity pneumonitis, pancreatitis, worsening of colitis, and reversible sperm abnormalities. Sulfasalazine can also impair folate absorption and patients should be supplemented with folic acid.

Table 287-5 Oral 5-ASA Preparations

Preparation	Formulation	Delivery	Dosing, g/d
AZO-BOND			
Sulfasalazine (500 mg)	Sulfapyridine-5-ASA	Colon	3–6 (acute)
			2–4 (maintenance)
Olsalazine (250 mg)	5-ASA-5-ASA	Colon	1–3
Balsalazide (500–750 mg)	Aminobenzoyl-alanine-5-ASA	Colon	2–6
DELAYED-RELEASE			
Asacol (400 mg)	Eudragit S (pH 7)	Distal ileum-colon	2.4–4.8 (acute)
			0.8–4.8 (maintenance)
Claversal (250–500 mg)	Eudragit L (pH 6)	Ileum-colon	1.5–3 (acute)
			0.75–3 (maintenance)
SUSTAINED-RELEASE			
Pentasa (250 mg)	Ethylcellulose micro-granules	Stomach-colon	2–4 (acute)
			1.5–4 (maintenance)

Newer sulfa-free aminosalicylate preparations deliver increased amounts of the pharmacologically active ingredient of sulfasalazine (5-ASA, mesalamine) to the site of active bowel disease while limiting systemic toxicity. 5-ASA may function through inhibition of NF-κB activity. Sulfa-free aminosalicylate formulations include alternative azo-bonded carriers, 5-ASA dimers, pH-dependent tablets, and continuous-release preparations. Each has the same efficacy as sulfasalazine when equimolar concentrations are used. Olsalazine is composed of two 5-ASA radicals linked by an azo bond which is split in the colon by bacterial reduction and two 5-ASA molecules are released. Olsalazine is similar in effectiveness to sulfasalazine in treating CD and UC, but up to 17% of patients experience non-bloody diarrhea caused by increased secretion of fluid in the small bowel. Balsalazide contains an azo bond binding mesalamine to the carrier molecule 4-amino benzoyl β alanine; it is effective in the colon. Claversal is an enteric-coated form of 5-ASA that consists of mesalamine surrounded by an acrylic-based polymer resin and a cellulose coating that releases mesalamine at pH > 6.0, a level that is present from the mid-jejunum continuously to the distal colon.

The most commonly used drugs besides sulfasalazine in the United States are Asacol and Pentasa. Asacol is also an enteric-coated form of mesalamine, but it has a slightly different release pattern, with 5-ASA liberated at pH > 7.0. The disintegration of Asacol is variable with complete break-up of the tablet occurring in many different parts of the gut ranging from the small intestine to the splenic flexure; it has increased gastric residence when taken with a meal. Asacol is used to induce and maintain remission in UC and in CD ileitis, ileocolitis, and colitis. Appropriate doses of Asacol and the other 5-ASA compounds are shown in (Table 287-5). Some 50 to 75% of patients with mild to moderate UC and CD improve when treated with 2 g/d of 5-ASA; the dose response continues up to at least 4.8 g/d. Doses of 1.5-4 g/d maintain remission in 50 to 75% of patients with UC and CD.

Pentasa is another mesalamine formulation that uses an ethylcellulose coating to allow water absorption into small beads containing the mesalamine. Water dissolves the 5-ASA, which then diffuses out of the bead into the lumen. Disintegration of the capsule occurs in the stomach. The microspheres then disperse throughout the entire gastrointestinal tract from the small intestine through the distal colon in both fasted or fed conditions. Controlled trials of Pentasa and Asacol in active CD demonstrate a 40 to 60% clinical improvement or remission, and meta-analyses demonstrate maintenance of CD remission with 1.5 to 3 g/d of 5-ASA in 68 to 95% of patients. Pentasa at a dose of 2 g/d is more effective than placebo in postoperative prophylaxis of CD.

Topical mesalamine enemas are effective in mild-to-moderate distal UC and CD. Clinical response occurs in up to 80% of UC patients with colitis distal to the splenic flexure. Mesalamine suppositories, which are no longer available in the United States but are available in Canada, at doses of 500 mg twice a day are effective in treating proctitis.

Glucocorticoids The majority of patients with moderate to severe UC benefit from oral or parenteral glucocorticoids. Prednisone is usually started at doses of 40 to 60 mg/d for active UC that is unresponsive to 5-ASA therapy. Parenteral glucocorticoids may be administered as intravenous hydrocortisone 300 mg/d or methylprednisolone 40 to 60 mg/d. Adrenocorticotropic hormone (ACTH) is occasionally preferred for glucocorticoid-naïve patients despite a risk of adrenal hemorrhage. ACTH has equivalent efficacy to intravenous hydrocortisone in both glucocorticoid-naïve and -experienced CD patients.

Topically applied glucocorticoids are also beneficial for distal colitis and may serve as an adjunct in those who have rectal involvement plus more proximal disease. Hydrocortisone enemas or foam may control active disease, although they have no proven role as maintenance therapy. These glucocorticoids are significantly absorbed from the rectum and can lead to adrenal suppression with prolonged administration. The systemic effects of standard glucocorticoid formulations have led to the development of more potent formulations that are less well absorbed and have increased first-pass metabolism. Budesonide is being used in enema form with favorable preliminary results in distal UC.

Glucocorticoids are also effective for treatment of moderate-to-severe CD and induce a 60 to 70% remission rate compared to a 30% placebo response. Controlled ileal-release budesonide has been nearly equal to prednisone for ileocolonic CD at a dose of 9 mg/d.

Glucocorticoids play no role in maintenance therapy in either UC or CD. Once clinical remission has been induced, they should be tapered according to the clinical activity, normally at a rate of no more than 5 mg per week. They can usually be tapered to 20 mg/d within 4 to 5 weeks but often take several months to be discontinued altogether. The side effects are numerous, including fluid retention, abdominal striae, fat redistribution, hyperglycemia, subcapsular cataracts, osteonecrosis, myopathy, emotional disturbances, and withdrawal symptoms. Most of these side effects, aside from osteonecrosis, are related to the dose and duration of therapy.

Antibiotics Despite numerous trials, antibiotics have no role in the treatment of active or quiescent UC. However, pouchitis, which occurs in about a third of UC patients after colectomy and ileal pouch-anal anastamosis, usually responds to treatment with metronidazole or ciprofloxacin.

Metronidazole is effective in active inflammatory, fistulous, and perianal CD and may prevent recurrence after ileal resection. The most effective dose is 15 to 20 mg/kg per day in three divided doses; it is usually continued for several months. Common side effects include nausea, metallic taste, and disulfiram-like reaction. Peripheral neuropathy can occur with prolonged administration (several months) and on rare occasions is permanent despite discontinuation. Ciprofloxacin (500 mg bid) is also beneficial for inflammatory, perianal, and fistulous CD. These two antibiotics should be used as second-line drugs in active CD after 5-ASA agents and as first-line drugs in perianal and fistulous CD.

Azathioprine and 6-Mercaptopurine Azathioprine and 6-mercaptopurine (6-MP) are purine analogues commonly employed in the management of glucocorticoid-dependent IBD. Azathioprine is rapidly absorbed and converted to 6-MP, which is then metabolized to the active end product, thioinosinic acid, an inhibitor of purine ribonucleotide synthesis and cell proliferation. These agents also inhibit the immune response. Efficacy is seen at 3 to 4 weeks. Compliance can be monitored by measuring the level of 6-thioguanine, an end product of 6-MP metabolism. Azathioprine (2.0 to 2.5 mg/kg per day) or 6-MP (1.0-1.5 mg/kg per day) have been employed successfully as glucocorticoid-sparing agents in up to two-thirds of UC and CD patients previously unable to be weaned from glucocorticoids. The role of these immunomodulators as maintenance therapy in UC and CD and for treating active perianal disease and fistulas in CD appears promising. In addition, 6-MP at a dose of 50 mg/d is more effective than Pentasa or placebo for postoperative prophylaxis of CD.

Although azathioprine and 6-MP are usually well tolerated, pancreatitis occurs in 3 to 4% of patients, typically presents within the first few weeks of therapy, and is always completely reversible when the drug is stopped. Other side effects include nausea, fever, rash, and hepatitis. Bone marrow suppression (particularly leukopenia) is dose-related and often delayed, necessitating regular monitoring of the complete blood count. Additionally, 1 in 300 individuals lacks thiopurine methyltransferase, the enzyme responsible for drug metabolism; an additional 11% of the population are heterozygotes with intermediate enzyme activity. Both are at increased risk of toxicity because of increased accumulation of thioguanine metabolites. No increased risk of cancer has been documented in IBD patients taking these medications long-term.

Methotrexate Methotrexate (MTX) inhibits dihydrofolate reductase, resulting in impaired DNA synthesis. Additional anti-inflammatory properties may be related to decreased IL-1 production. Intramuscular or subcutaneous MTX (25 mg per week) is effective in inducing remission and reducing glucocorticoid dosage and 15 mg per week is effective in maintaining remission in active CD. Potential toxicities include leukopenia and hepatic fibrosis, necessitating periodic evaluation of complete blood counts and liver enzymes. The role of liver biopsy in patients on long-term MTX is uncertain. Hypersensitivity pneumonitis is a rare but serious complication of therapy. MTX should only be used when either 6-MP or azathioprine are ineffective or poorly tolerated.

Cyclosporine Cyclosporine (CSA) alters the immune response by acting as a potent inhibitor of T cell-mediated responses. Although CSA acts primarily via inhibition of IL-2 production from T helper cells, it also decreases recruitment of cytotoxic T cells and blocks other cytokines, including IL-3, IL-4, interferon α, and TNF. It has a more rapid onset of action than 6-MP and azathioprine.

CSA is most effective given at 4 mg/kg per day IV in severe UC that is refractory to intravenous glucocorticoids, with 82% of patients responding. CSA can be an alternative to colectomy. The long-term success of oral CSA is not as dramatic, but if patients are started on 6-MP or azathioprine at the time of hospital discharge, remission can be maintained. Intravenous CSA is effective in 80% of patients with refractory fistulas, but 6-MP or azathioprine must be used to maintain remission. Oral CSA alone is only effective at a higher dose (7.5 mg/kg per day) in active disease but is not effective in maintaining remission without 6-MP/azathioprine. Serum levels should be monitored and kept in the range of 200 to 400 ng/mL.

CSA has the potential for significant toxicity, and renal function should be frequently monitored. Hypertension, gingival hyperplasia, hypertrichosis, paresthesias, tremors, headaches, and electrolyte abnormalities are common side effects. Creatinine elevation calls for dose reduction or discontinuation. Seizures may also complicate therapy, especially if serum cholesterol levels are less than 120 mg/dL. Opportunistic infections, most notably *Pneumocystis carinii* pneumonia, have occurred with combination immunosuppressive treatment; prophylaxis should then be given.

Nutritional Therapies Dietary antigens may act as stimuli of the mucosal immune response. Patients with active CD respond to bowel rest, along with total enteral or total parenteral nutrition (TPN). Bowel rest and TPN are as effective as glucocorticoids for inducing remission of active CD but are not as effective as maintenance therapy. Enteral nutrition in the form of elemental or peptide-based preparations are also as effective as glucocorticoids or TPN, but these diets are not palatable. Enteral diets may provide the small intestine with nutrients vital to cell growth and do not have the complications of TPN. In contrast to CD, active UC is not effectively treated with either elemental diets or TPN. Standard medical management of UC and CD is reviewed in (Table 287-6).

Newer Medical Therapies • *Anti-tumor necrosis factor antibody* TNF is a key inflammatory cytokine and mediator of in-

Table 287-6   Medical Management of IBD

Ulcerative Colitis: Active Disease

	Mild	Moderate	Severe	Fulminant
Distal	5-ASA oral and/or enema	5-ASA oral and/or enema Glucocorticoid enema Oral glucocorticoid	5-ASA oral and/or enema Glucocorticoid enema Oral or IV glucocorticoid	Intravenous glucocorticoid Intravenous CSA
Extensive	5-ASA oral or enema	5-ASA oral and/or enema Glucocorticoid enema Oral glucocorticoid	5-ASA oral and/or enema Glucocorticoid enema Oral or IV glucocorticoid	Intravenous glucocorticoid Intravenous CSA

Ulcerative Colitis: Maintenance Therapy

Distal	5-ASA oral and/or enema 6-MP or azathioprine
Extensive	5-ASA oral and/or enema 6-MP or azathioprine

Crohn's Disease: Active Disease

Mild–Moderate	Severe	Perianal or Fistulizing Disease
5-ASA oral or enema Metronidazole and/or ciprofloxacin Oral glucocorticoids Azathioprine or 6-MP Infliximab	5-ASA oral or enema Metronidazole and/or ciprofloxacin Oral or IV glucocorticoids Azathioprine or 6-MP Infliximab TPN or elemental diet Intravenous cyclosporine	Metronidazole and/or ciprofloxacin Azathioprine or 6-MP Infliximab Intravenous CSA

Crohn's Disease: Maintenance Therapy

Inflammatory	Perianal or Fistulizing Disease
5-ASA oral or enema Metronidazole and/or ciprofloxacin Azathioprine or 6-MP	Metronidazole and/or ciprofloxacin Azathioprine or 6-MP

NOTE: CSA, cyclosporine; 6-MP, 6-mercaptopurine; TPN, total parenteral nutrition testinal inflammation. The expression of TNF is increased in IBD. Infliximab is a chimeric mouse-human monoclonal antibody against TNF that is extremely effective in CD. It blocks TNF in the serum and at the cell surface and likely lyses TNF-producing macrophages and T cells through complement fixation and antibody-dependent cytotoxicity. Of active CD patients refractory to glucocorticoids, 6-MP, or 5-ASA, 65% will respond to intravenous infliximab (5 mg/kg); one-third will enter complete remission. Patients who experience an initial response will respond again to repeated infusions of infliximab every 8 weeks up to 44 weeks. Thus infliximab may be also be efficacious in maintaining remission. However, more trials need to be completed on remission maintenance after infliximab therapy.

Infliximab is also effective in CD patients with refractory perianal and enterocutaneous fistulas, with a 68% response rate (50% reduction in fistula drainage) and a 50% complete remission rate. The effects of infliximab for both inflammatory and fistulous disease last 12 weeks on average but longer in some patients.

The incidence of antibodies to infliximab (25% of the molecule is murine) is 13%. One side effect is a lupus-like syndrome, which is rare and reversible after stopping the drug. Anti-double-stranded DNA antibodies occur in 9% but are not associated with clinical lupus.

Among more than 1000 patients treated with infliximab, four developed lymphoma: one patient with CD, two with rheumatoid arthritis, and one with AIDS. Since the risk of lymphoma is already increased in these conditions, it is unclear whether infliximab is the cause. Thus, infliximab is extremely effective in refractory inflammatory and fistulous CD, but should be used only when necessary. Results on the efficacy of infliximab in UC are mixed.

Newer immunosuppressive agents   Tacrolimus has a mechanism of action similar to cyclosporine. It has shown efficacy in children with refractory IBD and in adults with extensive involvement of the small bowel.

Mycophenolate mofetil inhibits the de novo pathway of purine synthesis in lymphocytes, disrupting the conversion of inosine monophosphate to guanosine monophosphate (GMP) by reversible inhibition of inosine monophosphate dehydrogenase. The resulting depletion of intracellular GMP suppresses the generation of cytotoxic T cells and formation of antibodies by activated B cells. Patients with CD or UC who received either 500 mg twice a day or 15 mg/kg per day in two divided doses have tolerated the drug well and have experienced benefit with reduction of glucocorticoid requirements.

Thalidomide has been shown to inhibit TNF production by monocytes and other cells. Thalidomide is effective in glucocorticoid refractory and fistulous CD, but randomized controlled trials still need to be performed.

The anti-inflammatory cytokines   IL-10 is an anti-inflammatory and immunosuppressive cytokine produced by subsets of T and B cells, macrophages, and monocytes. It decreases T_H1 production of IL-2 and interferon γ, and limits production of IL-1, IL-6, IL-8, TNF, IL-12, and granulocyte-macrophage colony-stimulating factor. IL-10 has a moderate benefit in active CD.

IL-11 is a cytokine with thrombopoietic activity and mucosal protective effects that is effective in reducing inflammation in animal models of colitis. It seems to be effective in active CD, but more trials are needed.

Surgical Therapy • *Ulcerative colitis*   Nearly half of patients with extensive chronic UC undergo surgery within the first 10 years of their illness. The indications for surgery are listed in (Table 287-7). Morbidity is about 20% in elective, 30% for urgent, and 40% for emergency proctocolectomy. The risks are primarily hemorrhage, contamination and sepsis, and neural injury. Although single-stage total proctocolectomy with ileostomy has been the operation of choice, newer operations maintain continence while surgically removing the involved rectal mucosa.

The IPAA is the most frequent continence-preserving operation

Table 287-7   Indications for Surgery

Ulcerative Colitis	Crohn's Disease
Intractable disease	CD of Small Intestine
Fulminant disease	Stricture and obstruction unresponsive to medical therapy
Toxic megacolon	
Colonic perforation	Massive hemorrhage
Massive colonic hemorrhage	Refractory fistula
Extracolonic disease	Abscess
Colonic obstruction	CD of Colon and Rectum
Colon cancer prophylaxis	Intractable disease
Colon dysplasia or cancer	Fulminant disease
	Perianal disease unresponsive to medical therapy
	Refractory fistula
	Colonic obstruction
	Cancer prophylaxis
	Colon dysplasia or cancer

performed. Because UC is a mucosal disease, the rectal mucosa can be dissected out and removed down to the dentate line of the anus or about 2 cm proximal to it. The ileum is fashioned into a pouch that serves as a neorectum. This ileal pouch is then sutured circumferentially to the anus in an end-to-end fashion. If performed carefully, this operation preserves the anal sphincter and maintains continence. The overall operative morbidity is 10%, with the major complication being bowel obstruction. Pouch failure necessitating conversion to permanent ileostomy occurs in 5 to 10% of patients. Some inflamed rectal mucosa is usually left behind, and thus endoscopic surveillance is necessary. Primary dysplasia of the ileal mucosa of the pouch has occurred rarely.

Patients with IPAAs usually have about six to eight bowel movements a day. On validated quality of life indices, they report better performance in sports and sexual activities than ileostomy patients. The most frequent late complication of IPAA is pouchitis in about one-third of patients with UC. This syndrome consists of increased stool frequency, watery stools, cramping, urgency, nocturnal leakage of stool, arthralgias, malaise, and fever. Although it usually responds to antibiotics, in 3% of patients it is refractory and requires pouch take-down.

Crohn's disease   Most patients with CD require at least one operation in their lifetime. The need for surgery is related to duration of disease and the site of involvement. Patients with small bowel disease have an 80% chance of requiring surgery. Those with colitis alone have a 50% chance. The indications for surgery are shown in (Table 287-7).

SMALL INTESTINAL DISEASE   Because CD is chronic and recurrent with no clear surgical cure, as little intestine as possible is resected. Current surgical alternatives for treatment of obstructing CD include resection of the diseased segment and strictureplasty. Surgical resection of the diseased segment is the most frequently performed operation, and in most cases primary anastomosis can be done to restore continuity. If much of the small bowel has already been resected and the strictures are short with intervening areas of normal mucosa, strictureplasties should be done to avoid a functionally insufficient length of bowel. The strictured area of intestine is incised longitudinally and the incision sutured transversely, thus widening the narrowed area. Complications of strictureplasty include prolonged ileus, hemorrhage, fistula, abscess, leak, and restricture.

Colorectal disease   A greater percentage of patients with CD colitis require surgery for intractability, fulminant disease, and anorectal disease. Several alternatives are available, ranging from the use of a temporary loop ileostomy to resection of segments of diseased colon or even the entire colon and rectum. For patients with segmental involvement, segmental colon resection with primary anastomosis can be performed. In 20 to 25% of patients with extensive colitis, the rectum is spared sufficiently to consider rectal preservation. Most surgeons believe that an IPAA is contraindicated in CD due to the high incidence of pouch failure. A diverting colostomy may help heal severe perianal disease or rectovaginal fistulas, but disease almost always recurs with reanastomosis. Often, these patients require a total proctocolectomy and ileostomy.

INFLAMMATORY BOWEL DISEASE AND PREGNANCY

When adjusted for patient age, the fertility rate in UC is probably normal. In contrast, fertility is reduced in CD in proportion to disease activity and can be restored when remission is induced. The ovaries and fallopian tubes can be affected by the inflammatory process of CD, especially on the right side because of the proximity of the terminal ileum. In addition, perirectal, perineal, rectovaginal abscesses, and fistulae can result in dyspareunia. Infertility in men can be caused by sulfasalazine but reverses when treatment is stopped.

In UC, fetal outcome approximates that in the normal population. In CD, spontaneous abortions, stillbirths, and developmental defects are increased with increased disease activity, not medications. The courses of CD and UC during pregnancy mostly correlate with disease activity at the time of conception. Most CD patients can deliver vaginally, but cesarean section may be the preferred route of delivery for patients with anorectal and perirectal abscesses and fistulas to reduce the likelihood of fistulas developing or extending into the episiotomy scar.

Sulfasalazine, mesalamine, and olsalazine are safe for use in pregnancy, but folate supplementation must be given with sulfasalazine. No adverse affects have been reported from sulfasalazine in nursing infants. Topical 5-ASA agents are also safe during pregnancy. Glucocorticoids are generally safe for use during pregnancy and are indicated for patients with moderate to severe disease activity. The amount of glucocorticoids received by the nursing infant is minimal. The safest antibiotics to use for CD in pregnancy are ampicillin, cephalosporin, or ciprofloxacin. Flagyl is teratogenic and tumorigenic in high doses, passes into breast milk, and should be avoided.

6-MP and azathioprine pose minimal or no risk during pregnancy, but experience is limited. If the patient cannot be weaned from the drug or has an exacerbation that requires 6-MP/azathioprine during pregnancy, she should continue the drug with informed consent. Their effects during nursing are unknown.

There is little data on cyclosporine in pregnancy. In a small number of patients with severe IBD treated with intravenous cyclosporine during pregnancy, 80% of pregnancies were successfully completed without development of renal toxicity, congenital malformations, or developmental defects. However, because of the lack of data, cyclosporine should probably be avoided unless the patient would otherwise require surgery. Methotrexate is contraindicated in pregnancy and nursing.

Surgery in UC should be performed only for emergency indications, including severe hemorrhage, perforation, and megacolon refractory to medical therapy. Total colectomy and ileostomy carries a 60% risk of postoperative spontaneous abortion. Fetal mortality is also high in CD requiring surgery. Patients with ileostomies and IPAAs tolerate pregnancy well.

INFLAMMATORY BOWEL DISEASE IN THE ELDERLY

The most common presenting symptoms in the elderly are diarrhea, weight loss, and abdominal pain. CD in the elderly is mostly colonic with a distal distribution and occurs predominantly in women. Proctitis has been documented in 50% of elderly patients and the diagnosis is often delayed. Diseases that can mimic CD in the elderly are ischemic colitis, diverticular disease, irritable bowel, infectious colitides, and malignancies, including carcinoma, lymphoma, and carcinoid. The incidence of surgery is high in elderly patients, with up to 50% of patients with ileitis, ileocolitis, or extensive colitis requiring urgent or early surgery for first-time disease. In addition, surgery has a much higher morbidity than in younger patients, although the rate of post-

operative recurrence is less. Most elderly patients respond as well as younger individuals to medical management.

UC in the elderly is more common in men, presents usually with diarrhea and weight loss, and may have a more distal distribution than in younger patients. Most elderly patients have a favorable response to medical therapy, especially 5-ASA agents, and immunosuppressives used in conjunction with low doses of glucocorticoids. Cyclosporine has been used more frequently in the elderly, but the age-related decreases in renal clearance may affect dosing. Glucocorticoid complications such as osteoporosis and hyperglycemia are also increased in the elderly. 6-MP and azathioprine are well tolerated in the elderly. Surgery also has a higher morbidity and mortality in UC, and elderly patients have a longer hospital stay than younger patients. The risk of colon cancer in UC and CD colitis is no greater than that in the general population since the duration of disease is short and the extent of disease is often distal.

CANCER IN INFLAMMATORY BOWEL DISEASE

ULCERATIVE COLITIS Patients with long-standing UC are at increased risk for developing colonic epithelial dysplasia and carcinoma (Fig. 287-8). Several features distinguish sporadic (SCC) and colitis-associated (CAC) colon cancers. First, SCC usually arise from an adenomatous polyp; CAC typically arise from either flat dysplasia or a dysplasia-associated lesion or mass (DALM). Second, multiple synchronous colon cancers occur in 3 to 5% of SCC but in 12% of CAC. Third, the mean age of individuals with SCC is in the sixties; the mean age of those with CAC is in the thirties. Fourth, SCC exhibits a left-sided predominance, whereas CAC is distributed more uniformly

FIGURE 287-8 Low power transition between dysplasia (D) and non-dysplastic (N) mucosa in a case of ulcerative colitis. (*Courtesy of Dr. EK Rosado and Dr. CA Perkos, Division of Gastrointestinal Pathology, Department of Pathology, Emory University, Atlanta, Georgia.*)

throughout the colon. Fifth, mucinous and anaplastic cancers are more common in CAC than SCC. At the molecular level, p53 mutations occur much earlier and *APC* gene mutations much later in CAC than SCC.

The risk of neoplasia in chronic UC increases with duration and extent of disease. For patients with pancolitis, the risk of cancer rises 0.5 to 1% per year after 8 to 10 years of disease. This observed increase in cancer rates has led to the endorsement of surveillance colonoscopies with biopsies for patients with chronic UC as the standard of care. Annual or biennial colonoscopy with multiple biopsies has been advocated for patients with more than 8 to 10 years of pancolitis or 12 to 15 years of left-sided colitis and has been widely employed to screen and survey for subsequent dysplasia and carcinoma.

CROHN'S DISEASE   Risk factors for developing colorectal cancer in CD are a history of colonic (or ileocolonic) involvement and long disease duration. The cancer risks in CD and UC are probably equivalent for similar extent and duration of disease. In patients with extensive colonic involvement, the overall risk is increased 18-fold and the cumulative risk is 8% at 22 years. Thus, the same endoscopic surveillance strategy used for UC is recommended for patients with chronic CD colitis. A pediatric colonoscope can be used to pass narrow strictures in CD patients and impassable strictures can be surveyed with annual barium enemas. A colon resection should be performed if there is evidence of malignancy.

MANAGEMENT OF DYSPLASIA AND CANCER   If high grade dysplasia (HGD) is encountered on colonoscopic surveillance, the usual treatment for UC is colectomy and for CD is either colectomy or segmental resection. If low grade dysplasia (LGD) is found, the management is controversial. Many investigators recommend immediate colectomy, but some repeat the colonoscopy in 1 to 6 months and search for recurrent dysplasia. Polyps in chronic colitis can be removed endoscopically provided that biopsies of the surrounding mucosa are free of dysplasia.

IBD patients are also at greater risk for other malignancies. Patients with CD may have an increased risk of developing non-Hodgkin's lymphoma and squamous cell carcinoma of the skin. Although CD patients have a twelvefold increased risk of developing small bowel cancer, this type of carcinoma is extremely rare.

QUALITY OF LIFE IN INFLAMMATORY BOWEL DISEASE

The assessment of health-related quality of life plays an important role in the evaluation and treatment of IBD patients. Although clinical trials have generally relied upon traditional disease activity indices such as the Crohn's Disease Activity Index (CDAI) to measure therapeutic efficacy, these measures do not reflect quality of life. The Inflammatory Bowel Disease Questionnaire (IBDQ) is a validated, disease-specific instrument that has been used to measure quality of life. It is a 32-item questionnaire that measures global function, systemic and bowel symptoms, functional and social impairment, and emotional function. When compared to the general population, IBD patients have an impaired quality of life in all six categories. The most frequent concerns of UC patients are having an ostomy bag, developing cancer, effects of medication, the uncertain nature of the disease, and having surgery. The most frequent concerns of CD patients are the uncertain nature of the disease, energy level, effects of medication, having surgery, and having an ostomy bag.

BIBLIOGRAPHY

BLUMBERG RS et al: Animal models of mucosal inflammation and their relation to human inflammatory bowel disease. Curr Opin Immunol 111:648, 1999

FEAGAN BG et al: A comparison of methotrexate with placebo for the maintenance of remission in Crohn's disease. N Engl J Med 342:1627, 2000

HANAUER SB, MEYERS S: Management of Crohn's disease in adults. Am J Gastroenterol 92:559, 1997

IRVINE EJ: Quality of life issues in patients with inflammatory bowel disease. Am J Gastroenterol 92:18S, 1997

ITZKOWITZ S: Inflammatory bowel disease and cancer. Gastroenterol Clin North Am 26:129, 1997

KIRSNER JB (ed): *Inflammatory Bowel Disease*, 5th ed. Philadelphia, Saunders, 2000

KORELITZ BI: Inflammatory bowel disease and pregnancy. Gastroenterol Clin North Am 27:213, 1998

KORNBLUTH A, SACHAR DB: Ulcerative colitis practice guidelines in adults. Am J Gastroenterol 92:204, 1997

SHANAHAN F et al: Neutrophil autoantibodies in ulcerative colitis: Familial aggregation and genetic heterogeneity. Gastroenterology 103:456, 1992

TARGAN SR et al: A short-term study of chimeric monoclonal cA2 to tumor necrosis factor alpha for Crohn's disease. N Engl J Med 337:1029, 1997

 288   *Chung Owyang*

IRRITABLE BOWEL SYNDROME

Irritable bowel syndrome (IBS) is a gastrointestinal (GI) disorder characterized by altered bowel habits and abdominal pain in the absence of detectable structural abnormalities. No clear diagnostic markers exist for IBS, so all definitions of the disease are based on the clinical presentation. The Rome criteria for the diagnosis of IBS are summarized in Table 288-1. IBS is one of the most common conditions encountered in clinical practice but one of the least well understood. Until recently, many physicians did not consider IBS to be a disease at all; they viewed it as nothing more than a somatic manifestation of psychological stress. With the availability of better techniques to study colonic and GI motility and visceral sensory function, along with the development of newer concepts about the importance of the brain in regulating gut function, significant progress has been made toward a better understanding of the pathogenesis of IBS. Improved methods of treatment may result from these insights.

CLINICAL FEATURES   IBS is a disorder of young people, with most new cases presenting before age 45. However, some reports suggest that the elderly are troubled by IBS symptoms up to 92% as often as middle-aged persons. Indeed, many of the diagnoses of "painful diverticular disease" given the elderly patients may represent IBS. Women are diagnosed with IBS two to three times as often as men and make up 80% of the population with severe IBS. Patients with IBS may fall into two broad clinical groups. Most commonly, patients have abdominal pain associated with altered bowel habits that include constipation, diarrhea, or both. In the second group, patients have painless diarrhea. This latter group accounts for <20% of patients with IBS; their condition may be a separate entity but is generally considered a variant of IBS.

Abdominal Pain   Abdominal pain in IBS is highly variable in intensity and location. Pain in IBS is localized to the hypogastrum in 25%, the right side in 20%, to the left side in 20%, and the epigastrum in 10% of patients. Pain is frequently episodic and crampy but may be superimposed on a background of constant ache. Pain may be mild enough to be ignored or it may interfere with daily activities. Despite this, malnutrition due to inadequate caloric intake is exceedingly rare with IBS. Sleep deprivation is also unusual because abdominal pain

Table 288-1   Rome Criteria for the Diagnosis of IBS

Abdominal Pain/Discomfort[a]	AND	Two or More at Least 25% of the Time[a]
Relieved with defecation		Change in stool frequency
and/or		Change in consistency
With change in stool frequency		Difficult stool passage
and/or		Sense of incomplete evacuation
With change in stool consistency		Presence of mucus in stool

[a] Symptoms must have been present for > 3 months.

is almost uniformly present only during waking hours. Pain is often exacerbated by eating or emotional stress and relieved by passage of flatus or stools.

Altered Bowel Habits Alteration in bowel habits is the most consistent clinical feature in IBS. Symptoms usually begin in adult life. The most common pattern is constipation alternating with diarrhea, usually with one of these symptoms predominating. At first, constipation may be episodic, but eventually it becomes continuous and increasingly intractable to treatment with laxatives. Stools are usually hard with narrowed caliber, possibly reflecting excessive dehydration caused by prolonged colonic retention and spasm. Most patients also experience a sense of incomplete evacuation, thus leading to repeated attempts at defecation in a short time span. Patients whose predominant symptom is constipation may have weeks or months of constipation interrupted with brief periods of diarrhea. In other patients, diarrhea may be the predominant symptom. Diarrhea resulting from IBS usually consists of small volumes of loose stools, and most patients have stool volumes of <200 mL. Nocturnal diarrhea does not occur in IBS. Diarrhea may be aggravated by emotional stress or eating. Stool may be accompanied by passage of large amounts of mucus; hence, the term *mucous colitis* has been used to describe IBS. This is a misnomer, since inflammation is not present. Bleeding is not a feature of IBS unless hemorrhoids are present, and malabsorption or weight loss does not occur.

Gas and Flatulence Patients with IBS frequently complain of abdominal distention and increased belching or flatulence, all of which they attribute to increased gas. Although some patients with these symptoms actually may have a larger amount of gas, quantitative measurements reveal that most patients who complain of increased gas generate no more than a normal amount of intestinal gas. Most IBS patients develop symptoms even with minimal gut distention, suggesting that the basis of their complaints is reduced tolerance of distention rather than an abnormal quantity of intraluminal gas. In addition, patients with IBS tend to reflux gas from the distal to the more proximal intestine, which may explain the belching.

Upper Gastrointestinal Symptoms Between 25 and 50% of patients with IBS complain of dyspepsia, heartburn, nausea, and vomiting. This suggests that areas of the gut other than the colon may be involved. Prolonged ambulant recordings of small bowel motility in patients with IBS show a high incidence of abnormalities in the small bowel during the waking period; nocturnal motor patterns are no different from those of healthy controls. A characteristic finding is the frequent occurrence of episodes of clustered contractions recurring at 0- to 9-min intervals. These episodes have a mean duration of 46 min and are often associated with transient abdominal pain and discomfort. A similar pattern has been observed in patients with IBS by the application of psychological stressors and by intravenous neostigmine. In addition, temporary abolition of migrating motor complexes is observed in IBS patients under mental stress. Thus, IBS appears to be a paroxysmal motor disorder that may be detected in the small bowel.

PATHOPHYSIOLOGY The pathogenesis of IBS is poorly understood, although roles for abnormal gut motor and sensory activity, central neural dysfunction, psychological disturbances, stress, and luminal factors have been proposed.

Colonic myoelectrical and motor activity under unstimulated conditions are generally normal, but abnormalities are more prominent under stimulated conditions in IBS. IBS patients may exhibit increased rectosigmoid motor activity for up to 3 h after eating. Provocative stimuli also induce exaggerated colonic motor responses in IBS patients compared to healthy volunteers. For example, inflation of rectal balloons both in diarrhea- and constipation-predominant IBS patients leads to marked distention-evoked contractile activity, which may be prolonged.

As with studies of motor activity, IBS patients frequently exhibit exaggerated sensory responses to visceral stimulation. Postprandial pain has been temporally related to entry of food bolus into the cecum in 74% of patients. Exaggerated symptoms can be induced by visceral distention in IBS patients. Rectal balloon inflation produces both non-painful and painful sensations at lower volumes in IBS patients than in healthy controls without altering rectal tension, suggestive of visceral afferent dysfunction in IBS. The visceral hyperalgesia of IBS appears to be selective for mechanoreceptor-activated stimuli, as perception of intestinal mucosal electrical stimulation is normal in IBS. Similar studies show gastric and esophageal hypersensitivity in patients with nonulcer dyspepsia and noncardiac chest pain, raising the possibility that these conditions have a similar pathophysiologic basis. In contrast to their enhanced gut sensitivity, IBS patients do not exhibit heightened sensitivity elsewhere in the body. Thus the afferent pathway disturbances in IBS appear to be selective for visceral innervation, with sparing of somatic pathways. The mechanisms responsible for visceral hypersensitivity are unclear. These exaggerated responses may be due to: (1) increased end organ sensitivity with recruitment of "silent" nociceptors; (2) spinal hyperexcitability with activation of nitric oxide and possibly other neurotransmitters; (3) endogenous (cortical and brainstem) modulation of caudad nociceptive transmission; and (4) over time, the possible development of long-term hyperalgesia due to development of neuroplasticity, resulting in permanent or semipermanent changes in neural responses to chronic or recurrent visceral stimulation.

The role of central nervous system (CNS) factors in the pathogenesis of IBS is strongly suggested by (1) the clinical association of emotional disorders and stress with symptom exacerbation, and (2) the therapeutic response to therapies that act on cerebral cortical sites. Positron emission tomography has shown alterations in regional cerebral blood flow in IBS patients. In healthy individuals, rectal distention increases blood flow in the anterior cingulate cortex, a region with an abundance of opiate receptors, which, when activated, may help to reduce sensory input. In contrast, IBS patients exhibit no increased blood flow in the anterior cingulate gyrus but show activation of the prefrontal cortex, either in response to rectal activation or in anticipation of rectal distention. Activation of the frontal lobes may activate a vigilance network within the brain that increases alertness. The anterior cingulate cortex and the prefrontal cortex appear to have reciprocal inhibitory associations. In patients with IBS, the preferential activation of the prefrontal lobe without activation of the anterior cingulate cortex may represent a form of cerebral dysfunction leading to the increased perception of visceral pain.

Abnormal psychiatric features are recorded in up to 80% of IBS patients; however, no single psychiatric diagnosis predominates. An association between prior sexual or physical abuse and development of IBS has been reported. Forms of sexual abuse associated with IBS include verbal aggression, exhibitionism, sexual harassment, sexual touching, and rape. The pathophysiologic relationship between IBS and sexual or physical abuse is unknown. However, physical and sexual abuse may result in hypervigilence to body sensations at the CNS level and visceral hypersensitivity at the gut level.

Thus patients with IBS frequently demonstrate increased motor reactivity of the colon and small bowel to a variety of stimuli and altered visceral sensation associated with lowered sensation thresholds. These may result from CNS (enteric nervous system) dysregulation.

Approach to the Patient

Because IBS is a disorder for which no pathognomonic abnormalities have been identified, its diagnosis relies on recognition of positive clinical features and elimination of other organic diseases. A careful history and physical examination are frequently helpful in establishing the diagnosis. Clinical features suggestive of IBS include the following: recurrence of lower abdominal pain with altered bowel habits over a period of time without progressive deterioration, onset of symptoms during periods of stress or emotional upset, absence of other systemic symptoms such as fever and weight loss, and small-volume stool without any evidence of blood.

On the other hand, the appearance of the disorder for the first time in old age, progressive course from time of onset, persistent diarrhea after a 48-h fast, and presence of nocturnal diarrhea or steatorrheal stools argue against the diagnosis of IBS.

Because the major symptoms of IBS—abdominal pain, abdominal bloating, and alteration in bowel habits—are common complaints of many GI organic disorders, the list of differential diagnoses is long. The quality, location, and timing of pain may be helpful in suggesting specific disorders. Pain due to IBS that occurs in the epigastric or periumbilical area must be differentiated from biliary tract disease, peptic ulcer disorders, intestinal ischemia, and carcinoma of the stomach and pancreas. If pain occurs mainly in the lower abdomen, the possibility of diverticular disease of the colon, inflammatory bowel disease (including ulcerative colitis and Crohn's disease), and carcinoma of the colon must be considered. Postprandial pain accompanied by bloating, nausea, and vomiting suggests gastroparesis or partial intestinal obstruction. Intestinal infestation with *Giardia lamblia* or other parasites may cause similar symptoms. When diarrhea is the major complaint, the possibility of lactase deficiency, laxative abuse, malabsorption, hyperthyroidism, inflammatory bowel disease, and infectious diarrhea must be ruled out. On the other hand, constipation may be a side effect of many different drugs, such as anticholinergic, antihypertensive, and antidepressant medications. Endocrinopathies such as hypothyroidism and hypoparathyroidism must also be considered in the differential diagnosis of constipation, particularly if other systemic signs or symptoms of these endocrinopathies are present. In addition, acute intermittent porphyria and lead poisoning may present in a fashion similar to IBS, with painful constipation as the major complaint. These possibilities are suspected on the basis of their clinical presentations and are confirmed by appropriate serum and urine tests.

Because IBS is in part a diagnosis of exclusion, certain diagnostic tests should be performed routinely; others may be required depending on the specific presenting symptoms. Factors to be considered when determining the aggressiveness of the diagnostic evaluation include the duration of symptoms, the change in symptoms over time, the age and sex of the patient, the referral status of the patient, prior diagnostic studies, a family history of colorectal malignancy, and the degree of psychosocial dysfunction. Thus a younger individual with mild symptoms requires a minimal diagnostic evaluation, while an older person or an individual with rapidly progressive symptoms should undergo a more thorough exclusion of organic disease. In general most patients should have a complete blood count and sigmoidoscopic examination; in addition, stool specimens should be examined for ova and parasites. In those >40 years, an air-contrast barium enema or colonoscopy should also be done. In patients whose main symptoms are diarrhea and increased gas, the possibility of lactase deficiency should be ruled out with a hydrogen breath test or a lactose-free diet should be prescribed for 3 weeks. In patients with concurrent symptoms of dyspepsia, upper GI radiographs or esophagogastroduodenoscopy may be advisable. In patients with postprandial right upper quadrant pain, ultrasound of the gallbladder should be obtained. Laboratory features that argue against IBS include evidence of anemia, elevated sedimentation rate, presence of leukocytes or blood in stool, and stool volume >200 to 300 mL/d. These findings suggest other diagnostic considerations.

℞ **TREATMENT   Patient Counseling and Dietary Alterations**
Reassurance and careful explanation of the functional nature of the disorder and of how to avoid obvious food precipitants are important first steps in patient counseling and dietary change. Occasionally, a meticulous dietary history may reveal substances (such as coffee, disaccharides, legumes, and cabbage) that aggravate symptoms. As a therapeutic trial, patients should be encouraged to eliminate any foodstuffs that appear to produce symptoms.

Stool Bulking Agents   High-fiber diets and bulking agents, such as bran or hydrophilic colloid, are frequently used in treating IBS. Dietary fiber has multiple effects on colonic physiology. The water-holding action of fibers may contribute to increased stool bulk. Fiber also speeds up colonic transit in most people. In diarrhea-prone patients, whole-colonic transit is faster than average; however, dietary fiber can delay transit. Furthermore, because of their hydrophilic properties, stool-bulking agents bind water and thus prevent both excessive hydration or dehydration of stool. A high-fiber diet relieves diarrhea in some IBS patients. Dietary fiber has also been shown to lower pressures in the sigmoid colon in IBS patients. The effects of fiber on pressure in the rest of the colon are unknown; however, the whole colon is affected by IBS, and the pain of colon spasm often originates from the ascending and transverse segments. Fiber supplementation with psyllium reduces the perception of rectal distention, indicating that fiber may have an effect on visceral afferent function.

The beneficial effects of dietary fiber on colonic physiology suggest that dietary fiber should be an effective treatment for IBS patients, but controlled trials of dietary fiber have produced variable results. IBS is not purely a colonic disorder; many patients may have symptoms originating from the upper gut. Despite the equivocal data regarding efficacy, most gastroenterologists consider stool-bulking agents worth trying in patients with IBS. Patients should be advised to take increasing quantities of bran supplements, such as whole-meal bread, high-bran cereal, or raw bran, until they are passing one or two soft stools daily. Alternatively, psyllium preparations may be used. About 20% of patients, however, complain that a high-fiber diet aggravates such symptoms as bloating and distention. These undesirable effects usually disappear spontaneously after several weeks.

Antispasmodics   Anticholinergic drugs may provide temporary relief for symptoms such as painful cramps related to intestinal spasm. Although controlled clinical trials have produced mixed results, evidence generally supports use of anticholinergic drugs for pain. Meta-analysis of 26 double-blind clinical trials of antispasmodic agents in IBS showed better global improvement (62%) and abdominal pain reduction (64%) compared to placebo (35% and 45%, respectively). The drugs are most effective when prescribed in anticipation of predictable pain. Physiologic studies demonstrate that anticholinergic drugs inhibit the gastrocolic reflex; hence, postprandial pain is best managed by giving antispasmodics 30 min before meals so that effective blood levels are achieved shortly before the anticipated onset of pain. Most anticholinergics contain natural belladonna alkaloids, which may cause xerostomia, urinary hesitancy and retention, blurred vision, and drowsiness. Some physicians prefer to use synthetic anticholinergics, such as dicyclomine, that have less effect on mucous membrane secretions and therefore produce fewer undesirable side effects.

Antidiarrheal Agents   When diarrhea is severe, especially in the painless diarrhea variant of IBS, small doses of diphenoxylate (Lomotil), 2.5 to 5 mg every 4 to 6 h, can be prescribed. These agents are less addictive than paregoric, codeine, or tincture of opium. In general, the intestines do not become tolerant of the antidiarrheal effect of opiates, and increasing doses are not required to maintain antidiarrheal potency. These agents are most useful if taken before anticipated stressful events that are known to cause diarrhea. Treatment with antidiarrheals, however, should be considered only as temporary management; the final goal of treatment is gradual withdrawal of medication with substitution of a high-fiber diet.

Drug Antidepressants   In addition to their mood-elevating effects, antidepressent medications have several physiologic effects that may be beneficial in IBS. In diarrhea-predominant IBS patients, the tricyclic antidepressant imipramine slows jejunal migrating motor complex transit propagation and delays orocecal and whole-gut transit, indicative of a motor inhibitory effect. Tricyclic agents may alter visceral afferent neural function.

Tricyclic antidepressants may be effective in some IBS patients. In a 2-month study of desipramine, abdominal pain improved in 86% of patients compared to 59% given a placebo. Another study of desipramine in 28 IBS patients showed improvement in stool frequency, diarrhea, pain, and depression. Improvements were mainly observed in diarrhea-predominant patients, with no improvement noted in constipated patients. The efficacy of other antidepressant agents is less well evaluated. An uncontrolled review of antidepressant therapy in 138 patients with IBS, including both tricyclic agents and the newer selective serotonin reuptake inhibitors (e.g., fluxetine, paroxetine, and sertraline), reported symptomatic improvement in 89% of individuals, especially those in the pain-predominant subtype. However, no placebo-controlled trials of the selective serotonin inhibitors have been reported in IBS to date.

Antiflatulence Therapy The management of excessive gas is seldom satisfactory, except in cases of obvious aerophagia or disaccharidase deficiency. Patients should be advised to eat slowly; not chew gum or drink carbonated beverages; and avoid artificial sweeteners, legumes, and foods of the cabbage family. Simethicone, antacids, and activated charcoal have all been tried, usually with disappointing results.

FUTURE DIRECTIONS IN MEDICAL TREATMENT OF IBS

Medications that blunt the visceral hyperalgesia of IBS are in development. Such "antiafferent" agents might act via one or more mechanisms, including (1) modification of release of pain-inducing mediators in the gut wall, (2) blockade or activation of peripheral afferent nerve receptors, (3) inhibition of afferent nerve transmission, or (4) modification of afferent activity in the CNS. These include the kappa opioid compounds and serotonin receptor ($5HT_3$) antagonists such as alosetron and octreotide.

Such compounds have been shown to reduce perception of painful mechanical visceral stimulation in patients with IBS. Furthermore, placebo-controlled trials with IBS patients have shown that alosetron or fedotozine, a kappa opioid analogue, reduces both pain and the severity of disease. Additional clinical studies of this group of compounds may lead to new therapeutic approaches for the treatment of IBS.

BIBLIOGRAPHY

BUENO L et al: Mediators and pharmacology of visceral sensitivity: From basic to clinical investigations. Gastroenterology 112:1714, 1997

DROSSMAN DA et al: American Gastroenterological Association technical review on irritable bowel syndrome. Gastroenterology 112:2120, 1997

HASLER WL, OWYANG C: Irritable bowel syndrome, in T Yamada (ed): *Textbook of Gastroenterology*, Philadelphia, Lippincott, Williams & Wilkins, p 1884, 1999

LYNN RB, FRIEDMAN LS: Irritable bowel syndrome. N Engl J Med 329:1940, 1993

MAYER AE, GEDHART GF: Basic and clinical aspects of visceral hyperalgesia. Gastroenterology 107:271, 1994

SILVERMAN DHS et al: Regional cerebral activity in normal and pathologic perception of visceral pain. Gastroenterology 112:64, 1997

289 *Kurt J. Isselbacher, Alan Epstein*

DIVERTICULAR, VASCULAR, AND OTHER DISORDERS OF THE INTESTINE AND PERITONEUM

DIVERTICULAR DISEASE

Diverticula may be either congenital or acquired and may affect either the small or large intestine. Congenital diverticula are herniations of the entire thickness of intestinal wall, while the more common acquired diverticula consist of herniations of the mucosa through the muscularis, generally at the site of a nutrient artery.

SMALL-INTESTINAL DIVERTICULA Diverticula may occur in any portion of the small intestine; however, with the exception of Meckel's diverticulum, the most common locations are in the du-

odenum and jejunum. Most often diverticula are asymptomatic and discovered incidentally on upper gastrointestinal x-rays. On occasion, however, they may cause symptoms either because of their anatomic proximity to other structures or rarely from inflammation or bleeding.

Duodenal diverticula arise singly from the medial surface of the second portion of the duodenum. In most patients they cause no symptoms. Rarely, they may present as acute diverticulitis with abdominal pain, fever, gastrointestinal bleeding, or, most rarely, perforation. Periampullary diverticula are occasionally associated with cholangitis or pancreatitis. Jejunal diverticula, while less common, may also be the site of acute inflammation, bleeding, or perforation with resulting abscess or peritonitis.

Multiple jejunal diverticula may be associated with malabsorption related to bacterial overgrowth within the diverticula, similar to other situations where intestinal stasis (e.g., blind loops) permits bacterial proliferation. →*The consequences of bacterial proliferation with resultant mucosal damage, deconjugation of bile salts, and vitamin B_{12} malabsorption are discussed in Chap. 286.*

Meckel's diverticulum, a persistent omphalomesenteric duct, is the most frequent congenital anomaly of the digestive tract, occurring in ~2% of autopsied adults. The diverticulum is wide-mouthed, about 5 cm long, and arises from the antimesenteric border of the ileum, usually within 100 cm of the ileocecal valve. The sac may be lined with normal ileal mucosa (approximately half) or contain gastric, duodenal, pancreatic, or colonic mucosa. While rarely symptomatic after age 5, Meckel's diverticulum may produce hemorrhage, inflammation, and obstruction in children and teenagers.

Hemorrhage occurs almost exclusively before age 10 and invariably results from peptic ulceration of ileal mucosa adjacent to a Meckel's diverticulum lined with gastric mucosa. The diagnosis may be established by isotope scanning of the abdomen after injection of technetium-99, which is taken up by the ectopic gastric mucosa in the diverticulum. False-negative and false-positive Meckel's scans are not uncommon; thus, other clinical and laboratory features must be assessed carefully before recommending surgery. In older children and young adults, inflammation of the diverticulum may mimic acute appendicitis. Mechanical obstruction may also occur if the diverticulum intussuscepts into the lumen of the bowel or twists on a fibrous remnant of the omphalomesenteric duct that extends from the diverticulum to the abdominal wall. The treatment of any of these complications of Meckel's diverticulum is surgical excision.

COLONIC DIVERTICULA Diverticula of the colon are herniations or saclike protrusions of the mucosa through the muscularis, at the point where a nutrient artery penetrates the muscularis. Diverticula occur most commonly in the sigmoid colon and decrease in frequency in the proximal colon. They increase with age; the incidence is 20 to 50% in western populations over age 50. The exact mechanism for their formation is unknown but may be related to an increase in intraluminal pressure. Thickening of the muscle coat of the colon in most patients with diverticula suggests that herniations of mucosa are caused by increased pressure produced by colonic muscle contractions. The rarity of colonic diverticula in underdeveloped nations has led to the speculation that diverticula result from the highly refined western diet, which is deficient in dietary fiber or roughage. It is proposed that such diets result in decreased fecal bulk, narrowing of the colon, and an increase in intraluminal pressure in order to move the smaller fecal mass. However, the role of dietary fiber in the etiology and treatment of diverticular disease remains to be determined.

Colonic diverticula are usually asymptomatic and are an incidental finding on barium enema or colonoscopy. The major complications of inflammation, both acute and chronic, and hemorrhage occur in only a small percentage of individuals with diverticulosis. Since diverticulosis is quite common in older patients, one must avoid the temptation of attributing pain or bleeding to the diverticula unless other conditions, especially colon cancer, have been excluded.

DIVERTICULITIS Inflammation can occur in or around the diverticular sac. The cause of diverticulitis is probably mechanical, related to retention in the diverticula of undigested food residue and bacteria, which may form a hard mass called a *fecalith*. This compromises the blood supply to the thin-walled sac (made up solely of mucosa and serosa) and renders it susceptible to invasion by colonic bacteria. The inflammatory process may vary from a small intramural or pericolic abscess to generalized peritonitis. Some attacks are accompanied by minimal symptoms and seem to heal spontaneously. Studies of resected specimens indicate that most perforations of the diverticular sac are small and result in inflammation of the sac itself and the adjacent serosal surface. Diverticulitis occurs more often in men than in women and three times as often in the left as in the right colon. This suggests that diverticulitis may be related to the higher intraluminal pressures and the more solid fecal material in the sigmoid and descending colon.

Acute colonic diverticulitis is a disease of variable severity characterized by fever, left lower quadrant abdominal pain, and signs of peritoneal irritation—muscle spasm, guarding, rebound tenderness. Rectal examination may reveal a tender mass if the area of inflammation is close to the rectum. Although constipation may not have been noted before onset of the illness, the inflammation around the colon often results in some degree of acute constipation or obstipation. Rectal bleeding, usually microscopic, is noted in 25% of cases; it is rarely massive. Polymorphonuclear leukocytosis is common. Complications include free perforation, which results in acute peritonitis, sepsis, and shock, particularly in the elderly. The perforation may be walled off by adherent omentum or neighboring structures such as the bladder or small bowel. Abscess formation or fistulas then occur as the inflammatory mass burrows into other organs. Severe pericolitis may cause a fibrous stricture around the bowel, which can be associated with colonic obstruction and may mimic a neoplasm.

Diagnosis During the acute phase of diverticulitis, barium enema and sigmoidoscopy may be hazardous, since contrast material or air under pressure may lead to rupture of an inflamed diverticulum and convert a walled-off inflammatory lesion to a free perforation. These examinations are usually safe after adequate treatment and healing of the diverticulitis. The radiologic findings on barium enema suggestive of diverticulitis are leakage of barium from a diverticular sac, stricture formation, and the presence of a pericolic inflammatory mass. In many patients the distortion caused by inflammation prevents a clear distinction between cancer and diverticulitis. In these cases, colonoscopy or surgical excision may be required for accurate diagnosis. Abdominal computed tomography scan may demonstrate the presence of a pericolic abscess.

℞ **TREATMENT** Most patients with acute diverticulitis require bowel rest, intravenous fluids, and broad-spectrum antibiotics. Repeated attacks of diverticulitis in the same area generally require surgical resection. Severe attacks with acute peritoneal signs, suspected abscess, or perforation require intravenous antibiotics directed against gram-negative anaerobic bacteria, followed by surgical drainage or resection. The usual procedure is a diverting colostomy with resection of the involved colon; reanastomosis is then performed at a second operation.

PAINFUL DIVERTICULAR DISEASE WITHOUT DIVERTICULITIS Some patients with diverticulosis develop recurrent left lower quadrant colicky pain without clinical or pathologic evidence of acute diverticulitis. They often have bouts of alternating constipation and diarrhea; the pain may be relieved by defecation or passage of flatus. These features suggest the coexistence of the irritable bowel syndrome. Examination during a bout of pain reveals tenderness of the sigmoid colon, but signs of peritoneal inflammation such as rebound tenderness, muscle guarding, fever, and leukocytosis are absent. Barium enema shows typical diverticula without evidence of in-flammation and stricture, plus a "sawtooth" irregularity of the lumen, reflecting muscle hypertrophy and spasm. In some patients the pain is severe enough to warrant observation in a hospital and restriction of food, since feeding aggravates the pain by causing colonic contraction. Anticholinergics, which reduce sigmoid contractions, and mild sedation are usually all that is required. After recovery, the patient should be started on a high-residue diet or given a bulk laxative such as hemicellulose, unprocessed bran, or psyllium extract. Surgical excision is usually not indicated unless acute diverticulitis or its complications occur.

HEMORRHAGE FROM DIVERTICULA Massive hemorrhage from colonic diverticula is one of the most common causes of hematochezia in patients over age 60. This complication of diverticulosis is caused by erosion of a vessel by a fecalith within the diverticular sac. The bleeding is painless and not accompanied by signs or symptoms of diverticulitis. Most cases of mild or moderate hemorrhage stop spontaneously with bed rest and blood transfusion. Localization of bleeding can be obtained by bleeding scan or angiography. In patients with severe hemorrhage, mesenteric angiography can be both diagnostic in localizing the bleeding site and therapeutic, since vasoconstrictive drugs or artificial blood clot infused intraarterially can sometimes effectively control hemorrhage. Colonoscopy is also useful in evaluating acute hematochezia, and the endoscopist may be able to cauterize angiodysplasias (Chap. 44). The location of bleeding diverticula is more commonly in the right colon, particularly the ascending colon, in contrast to the sigmoid colon, where diverticula are more numerous.

MOTILITY DISORDERS

Normal intestinal motility involves the delicate interplay of the gut motor system, neural influences of the autonomic and central nervous system, as well as hormonal factors, specifically gut neuropeptides. In addition, many drugs used in the treatment of disease (e.g., opioids, antibiotics) affect and influence intestinal motility directly or indirectly. Table 289-1 lists some of the disorders of the enteric motor and neural system. Only the more clinically relevant ones are discussed.

MEGACOLON Megacolon, or giant colon, is characterized by massive distention of the colon, usually accompanied by severe constipation or obstipation. This condition can be either congenital or acquired and is seen in all age groups. Acute toxic megacolon is a severe complication of ulcerative colitis (Chap. 287).

Aganglionic Megacolon (Hirschsprung's Disease) This is a congenital disorder due to absence of enteric neurons (ganglions) in the distal colon and rectum. This aganglionic segment loses its neural inhibition and remains contracted. Hirschsprung's disease is a heterogeneous genetic disorder—some patients have an autosomal dominant form of the disease with mutations in the *RET* gene; many have an autosomal recessive form with a mutation in the endothelin-B receptor gene. Hirschsprung's disease is a multigenic trait; genes on 9q31 affect the phenotype of the *RET* gene mutations. These defects result in the gestational failure of neural crest cells to migrate to the distal colon. The disease manifests in early infancy, occurring more frequently in males, and is often familial. These infants have massive abdominal distention, absent bowel movements, and impaired nutrition due to chronic obstruction of the colon. In some individuals with less severe symptoms, the disease may not be diagnosed until adolescence or early adulthood. The aganglionic and contracted segment of bowel is unable to relax to permit passage of stool, causing the normal proximal colon to become greatly dilated. On rectal examination the ampulla is empty of feces and the anal sphincter is normal. Barium enema reveals a narrowed segment in the rectosigmoid, with massive dilation above. Diagnosis is made by full-thickness surgical biopsy under anesthesia and demonstration of absent ganglion cells in the diseased segment. In most patients the aganglionic segment is in the rectosigmoid colon. The treatment of choice is a pull-through procedure in which normally innervated colon is anastomosed to the distal rectum just above the

Table 289-1 Some Motility Disorders of the Enteric Nervous System

Disorder	Comment
Intestinal pseudoobstruction	
Visceral neuropathy	Autosomal dominant disorder characterized by dilatation of jejunum and ileum and degeneration and loss of neurons.
Visceral neuropathy with basal ganglia calcifications	Autosomal recessive disorder with dilatation of duodenum and small bowel and mental retardation. Calcification of basal ganglia and degeneration of myenteric plexus.
Megacolon	
Hirschsprung's disease	Congenital disorder characterized by colonic dilatation proximal to an aganglionic, contracted distal colon and rectum. Caused by gestational failure of neural crest cells to migrate to distal colon. An autosomal dominant form is associated with mutations of the *RET* gene, and an autosomal recessive form with mutation of the endothelin, B-receptor gene.
Multiple endocrine neoplasia type 2A (MEN-2A)	Features similar to those of Hirschsprung's disease. Medullary thyroid cancer, parathyroid hyperplasia, and pheochromocytoma are characteristic. ? Mutation of *RET* gene.
Generalized, with hyperganglionosis	
MEN-2B (Sipple's syndrome)	Achalasia and pseudoobstruction reported with ganglioneuromatosis of myenteric and submucosal plexuses. Medullary thyroid cancer, pheochromocytoma, and mucosal neuromas are characteristic. Mutation of *RET* gene reported.
Neurofibromatosis (von Recklinghausen's disease)	Achalasia and megacolon reported, with neuronal dysplasia of the myenteric plexus. Central nervous system tumors, neurofibromas, pigmented iris, hamartomas, café au lait spots, and mental retardation are characteristic.
Generalized, with hypoganglionosis	
Chagas' disease	Achalasia, intestinal, and colonic pseudoobstruction; megaloureter; and myocarditis due to infection with *Trypanosoma cruzi*. Possible autoimmune response to parasitic antigen.
Paraneoplastic syndrome	Achalasia, gastroparesis, and intestinal pseudoobstruction reported in some patients with small-cell lung cancer and carcinoid tumors. Serum antibodies reactive to enteric neurons.
Cytomegalovirus infection	Esophageal dysmotility, delayed gastric emptying, achalasia, and pseudoobstruction reported, with intranuclear neuronal viral inclusions and loss of myenteric neurons.
Myotonic dystrophy	Autosomal dominant disorder with impaired esophageal and gastric transit and intestinal pseudoobstruction, selective loss of substance P– and enkephalin-containing enteric neurons and preservation of neurons containing neuropeptide Y or vasoactive intestinal polypeptide. Myotonia, weakness, cataracts, cardiac abnormalities, gonadal atrophy, and mental retardation are characteristic.
Generalized, other	
Parkinson's disease	Achalasia, pseudoobstruction, and megacolon reported in some patients, with Lewy bodies in the myenteric plexus of the esophagus and colon.
Diabetes mellitus	Gastroparesis and intestinal and colonic dysmotility, with generalized autonomic neuropathy. Myenteric plexus morphologically intact.
Amyloidosis	Achalasia, gastroparesis, and pseudoobstruction, with amyloid deposits in both smooth muscle and the myenteric plexus.
Fabry's disease	Impaired gastric emptying, jejunal and colonic diverticulosis, and malabsorption, with glycolipid deposition in neurons of the myenteric plexus and decreased numbers of enlarged ganglion cells. Cutaneous angiokeratoma, renal insufficiency, and cardiovascular and central nervous system damage are also seen.
Disorders caused by exogenous neural toxins	Intestinal and colonic pseudoobstruction, with increased argyrophilia of the myenteric plexus.

SOURCE: Modified from Goyal and Hirano, with permission.

internal sphincter, thus bypassing the contracted aganglionic segment and restoring normal defecation.

Acquired Megacolon In Central and South America, infection with *Trypanosoma cruzi* (Chagas' disease) can result in destruction of the ganglion cells of the colon, producing a clinical picture similar to congenital megacolon, except that the onset is in adult life rather than in childhood. A number of other diseases are associated with megacolon in adults. Patients with schizophrenia or depression, particularly institutionalized patients, may have obstipation and massive colonic dilatation. Severe neurologic disorders, including cerebral atrophy, spinal cord injury, and parkinsonism, also may cause megacolon. Myxedema, infiltrative diseases such as amyloidosis, and primary systemic sclerosis also can reduce colonic motility and produce marked colonic distention. Narcotic drugs, particularly morphine and codeine, can cause severe constipation, especially when administered to bedridden patients. Digital rectal examination of adults with acquired megacolon reveals a rectum distended with feces, as opposed to the empty rectum in aganglionic megacolon. Treatment is aimed at the underlying disease, as well as the careful use of enemas and cathartics.

Intestinal Pseudoobstruction Intestinal pseudoobstruction is an acute or chronic motility disorder characterized by distention or dilation of the small and large intestine. Abdominal pain, nausea, and vomiting may lead to diagnostic confusion with mechanical obstruction; but as the name of this condition implies, the underlying cause is not obstruction but rather a severe dysmotility resulting in distention. Pseudoobstruction may be primary or secondary and acute or chronic. In primary or idiopathic pseudoobstruction no other contributing condition can be identified, and the motility disorder is attributed to abnormalities of sympathetic innervation or of the muscle layers of the intestine. Secondary pseudoobstruction may result from primary systemic sclerosis, diabetes, amyloidosis, neurologic diseases, drugs, or sepsis.

Chronic or Intermittent Secondary Pseudoobstruction Numerous medical conditions can cause chronic dilation of the large and small bowel. Some of these may involve the intestinal smooth muscle, such as primary systemic sclerosis, amyloidosis, or muscular dystrophy. Endocrine disorders, including myxedema and diabetes mellitus, may result in chronic distention, which in the diabetic patient results from autonomic visceral neuropathy. Chronic neurologic diseases, including Parkinson's disease and stroke, may be complicated by chronic pseudoobstruction; in these patients drugs and relative immobility are contributing features. Finally, institutionalized psychotic patients may suffer from prolonged megacolon.

The symptoms of chronic secondary pseudoobstruction are chronic or intermittent constipation, crampy abdominal pain, anorexia, and bloating. Gastric distention and disordered swallowing may be present. Abdominal x-rays reveal gaseous distention of the large and small bowel and occasionally of the stomach. Air-fluid levels are unusual and should raise the possibility of mechanical obstruction. Upper gastrointestinal series and barium enema do not reveal specific abnormalities of the intestine such as tumor, stricture, or volvulus. The presence of an autoimmune disorder or endocrinopathy may require confirmation by serologic or blood tests; biopsy may be needed as in amyloidosis or muscular dystrophy.

The treatment of chronic intestinal pseudoobstruction is made difficult by the complexity and chronicity of the underlying systemic disease. Patients with primary systemic sclerosis may respond to broad-spectrum antibiotics if intestinal bacterial overgrowth is suspected. Metoclopramide may benefit gastric dysmotility in the diabetic patient. Discontinuation of psychotropic or anti-Parkinson drugs may occasionally result in improvement. Cathartics and enemas may be required to relieve fecal impaction, and the regular use of stool softeners and a high-fiber diet may help prevent recurrences.

Idiopathic Intestinal Pseudoobstruction   This term describes the condition of patients with signs and symptoms of pseudoobstruction in whom no systemic disease can be identified. The typical patient has recurrent attacks of abdominal pain and distention with nausea and vomiting. The small intestine is primarily involved, and chronic constipation is much less frequent than in secondary pseudoobstruction. Steatorrhea secondary to bacterial overgrowth of the small intestine is common and may lead to chronic diarrhea and malnutrition. Many patients exhibit abnormalities of motility in the esophagus and urinary bladder, in addition to the small and large intestine. Neuromuscular defects have been described in patients with this syndrome, including abnormalities of the mesenteric plexus and myopathy of the intestinal and urinary bladder smooth muscle (so-called hollow visceral myopathy). Elevated prostaglandin E levels have been reported in some patients.

Management of idiopathic pseudoobstruction is unsatisfactory. Surgery to relieve "obstruction" is to be avoided, since the condition is often worsened by abdominal surgery. Medical therapy with metoclopramide and cholinergic agents has been unsuccessful. Nutritional support in the form of low-residue elemental diets or parenteral hyperalimentation may be helpful. Unfortunately, the lack of effective therapy and the progressive nature of the illness make the prognosis of idiopathic pseudoobstruction rather poor. Death from malnutrition and steatorrhea are common. The long-term impact of total parenteral nutrition on this disease is not yet clear.

Acute Intestinal Pseudoobstruction   This entity, sometimes referred to as *Ogilvie's syndrome*, is characterized by acute intestinal dilation involving primarily the colon but occasionally also the small intestine. As in other forms of pseudoobstruction, the clinical features are difficult to distinguish from mechanical obstruction. The patient may complain of colicky lower abdominal pain and acute constipation. Examination reveals a distended, tympanitic abdomen, with reduced or absent bowel sounds. Localized tenderness over the distended colon is common, but diffuse abdominal tenderness, rigidity, or rebound tenderness are unusual. Abdominal films reveal massive dilation of the colon and small intestine, occasionally with the presence of air-fluid levels. The cecum, being the most capacious part of the colon, is often massively dilated and tender. The onset of these symptoms usually occurs in patients who have recently undergone severe surgical or medical stress, such as major surgery, myocardial infarction, sepsis, or respiratory failure. Patients with acute pseudoobstruction are frequently on respirators, have received narcotics or sedatives, and have metabolic and electrolyte disturbances. Ogilvie's syndrome may also be due to paraneoplastic obstruction.

Management of acute pseudoobstruction requires careful correction of fluid and electrolyte abnormalities, intubation of the stomach or small intestine for decompression, and avoidance of drugs that depress intestinal motility. Barium enema may be hazardous because of the risk of perforating the already dilated bowel. Decompressive colonoscopy is beneficial in some patients, and cecostomy may be required in some patients with massive cecal dilation. The outcome depends in large part on the prognosis of the associated medical or surgical conditions. Patients who recover from the underlying medical or surgical conditions usually have a return of normal colonic function.

IRRITABLE BOWEL SYNDROME   See Chap. 288.

CHRONIC CONSTIPATION   Chronic constipation is widespread in western society, with ~10% of the population taking laxatives on a regular basis. Most cases of chronic constipation arise from habitual neglect of afferent impulses, failure to initiate defecation, and accumulation of large, dry fecal masses in the rectum. This voluntary suppression of the call to stool may arise during the period of toilet training in childhood or later in life because of a sense of social impropriety, unaccustomed surroundings, uncomfortable toilet facilities, or illnesses that require confinement to bed. Chronic constipation is much more common in women, with onset typically in late adolescence or early adulthood. As constant distention of the rectum with feces becomes chronic, the patient grows less aware of rectal fullness. Bowel movements become progressively more difficult, and painful hemorrhoids or anal fissures reinforce suppression of the urge to defecate. To avoid these problems the patient begins the chronic use of laxatives or enemas, without which defecation becomes impossible. →*The mechanism of defecation is discussed in Chap. 42.*

℞ **TREATMENT**   The physician should make every attempt to educate the patient about the chain of events that has led to chronic constipation. Attempts should be made to alter patterns of many years' duration, and the patient must recognize the importance of responding to, rather than suppressing, the urge to defecate. Defecation should be attempted at a given time each day. In most individuals the call to stool occurs in the morning after breakfast. Physical exercise such as a brisk walk just before attempts at defecation may be helpful. Patients are instructed to increase dietary bulk with foods rich in fiber, such as green vegetables and unprocessed cereal grains, or by the regular use of bulk laxatives, such as hemicellulose, psyllium extract, and powdered unprocessed bran. The success of such a regimen depends to some extent on the duration of symptoms. Elderly patients with long-standing constipation and reliance on enemas or laxatives are more resistant to these measures than younger patients whose bowel patterns are less established. Moreover, poor muscle tone, reduced physical activity, and increased incidence of other medical conditions make the problem more difficult in the older age group. Bedridden elderly patients often develop severe constipation and even fecal impaction unless preventive measures are taken. This applies not only to patients with previous constipation but also to those with regular bowel movements before their confining illness. Regular administration of stool softeners, bulk laxatives, or mild cathartics is necessary until full ambulation and a normal diet are resumed. The onset of fecal impaction in bedridden patients is heralded by a feeling of rectal distention, urgency of defecation, or tenesmus. Occasionally, the fecal impaction will result in low-grade chronic obstruction with dilation and increased fluid content proximal to the impaction; "paradoxical diarrhea" may thus occur as fluid moves past the obstructing fecal mass. This situation will be aggravated if antidiarrheal drugs are given because the underlying constipation will be worsened. The appropriate maneuver is to disimpact the rectum manually or to administer gentle enemas if the impaction is beyond the reach of the finger.

DISORDERS OF THE MESENTERIC CIRCULATION

Ischemia of the intestine is the end result of interruption or reduction of its blood supply. However, the clinical manifestations of intestinal ischemia range from mild chronic symptoms to a catastrophic acute episode, depending on the vascular supply involved, the extent of the occlusion or ischemia, and the rapidity of the process. The clinician should be aware of the spectrum of clinical manifestations (Table 289-2). The gut derives its arterial blood supply from the celiac axis and the superior and inferior mesenteric arteries. The small intestine

Table 289-2 Patterns of Intestinal Ischemia

Condition	Etiology	Clinical Features	Management
Mesenteric artery embolus	Arterial embolus associated with atrial fibrillation or rheumatic heart disease	Acute central abdominal pain, shock, peritonitis	Immediate angiography and embolectomy if possible
Abdominal angina	Atherosclerosis of celiac and superior mesenteric arteries	Chronic postprandial pain, weight loss	Angiography and surgery in selected cases
Ischemic colitis	Low-flow state	Acute lower abdominal pain, rectal bleeding	Sigmoidoscopy; surgery only for peritonitis

FIGURE 289-1 Barium enema showing "thumbprinting" or submucosal edema of the inferior margin of the transverse colon in a patient with acute ischemic colitis.

is supplied by the celiac and superior mesenteric arteries, the colon by branches of the superior and inferior mesenteric arteries. A rich network of anastomotic vessels and the possible development of collateral circulation determine the clinical picture of acute or chronic intestinal arterial insufficiency.

MESENTERIC ISCHEMIA AND INFARCTION Acute intestinal ischemia may be classified as occlusive or nonocclusive. *Occlusion* accounts for about 75% of acute intestinal ischemia and may result from an arterial thrombus (one-third of arterial occlusions) or embolus (two-thirds of arterial occlusions) of the celiac or superior mesenteric arteries, or from venous occlusion (<5% of occlusions) in the same distribution. Arterial embolus occurs most commonly in patients with chronic or recurrent atrial fibrillation, artificial heart valves, or valvular heart disease; arterial thrombosis is usually associated with extensive atherosclerosis or low cardiac output. Venous occlusion is rare; it is occasionally seen in women taking oral contraceptives. Approximately one-fourth of patients with mesenteric ischemia have no definite occlusion of a major vessel, a condition referred to as *nonocclusive ischemia*. The exact cause of nonocclusive disease is obscure; systemic arterial hypotension, cardiac arrhythmias, prolonged heart failure, digitalis therapy, dehydration, and endotoxemia can be contributing factors.

The major clinical feature of acute mesenteric ischemia is severe abdominal pain, often colicky and periumbilical at the onset, later becoming diffuse and constant. Vomiting, anorexia, diarrhea, and constipation are also frequent but of little diagnostic help. Examination of the abdomen may reveal tenderness and distention. Bowel sounds are often normal even in the face of severe infarction. Some patients have a surprisingly normal abdominal examination in spite of severe pain. Mild gastrointestinal bleeding is often detected by examination of stool for occult blood; gross hemorrhage is unusual except in ischemic colitis. Leukocytosis is often present. Late in the course of the disease (24 to 72 h), gangrene of the bowel occurs with diffuse peritonitis, sepsis, and shock. Abdominal plain films in patients with mesenteric ischemia may reveal air-fluid levels and distention. Barium study of the small intestine reveals nonspecific dilation, poor motility, and evidence of thick mucosal folds ("thumbprinting") (Fig. 289-1).

Acute mesenteric ischemia is a grave condition with a high morbidity and mortality. Patients suspected of having acute arterial embolus should undergo immediate celiac and mesenteric angiography to localize the embolus, followed by embolectomy. Restoration of normal circulation may allow complete recovery if performed before irreversible necrosis or gangrene has occurred. Unfortunately, infarction and transmural necrosis are frequently found at surgery, necessitating resection. Arterial or venous thrombosis is not generally amenable to surgical removal of the thrombus, and resection of the affected bowel is required. Similarly, patients with nonocclusive ischemia are not candidates for corrective vascular surgery (as major vessels are patent). These individuals often have extensive necrosis of the small or large intestine because of the widespread nature of the ischemic event. The decision to operate when mesenteric ischemia is suspected is often difficult, because the typical patient is a poor surgical risk owing to

advanced age, dehydration, sepsis, and other serious medical conditions.

Chronic arterial insufficiency may precede acute vascular insufficiency, producing so-called abdominal angina. As in angina pectoris, the pain of chronic mesenteric insufficiency occurs under conditions of increased demand for splanchnic blood flow. The patient complains of intermittent dull or cramping midabdominal pain 15 to 30 min after a meal, lasting for several hours postprandially. Significant weight loss due to decreased food intake may be present. Chronic intestinal ischemia also may produce mucosal damage and malabsorption, which in turn aggravates the weight loss. Since abdominal angina may progress to bowel infarction, arteriographic studies should be performed to confirm the diagnosis in those patients who are candidates for abdominal vascular surgery. The only definitive treatment is vascular surgery or balloon angioplasty to remove the thrombus or the construction of bypass arterial grafts to the ischemic bowel.

A number of systemic conditions are associated with *vasculitis* of the large and small arteries supplying the intestine. Most often these disorders can be recognized by the associated extraintestinal manifestations, as in polyarteritis nodosa, lupus erythematosus, dermatomyositis, Henoch-Schönlein purpura (allergic vasculitis), and rheumatoid vasculitis. When larger arteries are involved, as in polyarteritis nodosa, the picture of acute intestinal infarction is similar to that of embolic or atherosclerotic vascular occlusion. Often the involvement of smaller vessels leads to areas of intramural hemorrhage and edema resulting in abdominal pain, variable degrees of intestinal obstruction, and bleeding. Barium enema may show "thumbprinting" and "spiculation" due to localized edema, hemorrhage, and ulceration (Fig. 289-1). In many instances, treatment of the underlying disorder may lead to regression of symptoms. If signs of an acute abdomen develop, surgical exploration is usually indicated.

Intramural small-intestinal hemorrhage may occur with vasculitis, trauma, or impaired coagulation, especially in patients receiving anticoagulants. The clinical and radiologic features resemble those seen with vasculitis and local mucosal hemorrhage.

ISCHEMIC COLITIS Ischemia of the colon most often affects the elderly because of their greater frequency of vascular disease. Ischemic colitis is almost always nonocclusive. Shunting of blood away from the mucosa may contribute to this condition, but the mechanism of ischemia is not known.

The clinical picture depends on the degree of ischemia and its rate of development. In *acute fulminant ischemic colitis*, the major manifestations are severe lower abdominal pain, rectal bleeding, and hypotension. Dilation of the colon and physical signs of peritonitis are seen in severe cases. Abdominal films may reveal thumbprinting from submucosal hemorrhage and edema (Fig. 289-1). Barium enema is hazardous in the acute situation because of the risk of perforation. Sigmoidoscopy or colonoscopy may detect ulcerations, friability, and bulging folds from submucosal hemorrhage. Angiography is not helpful in the management of patients with presumed ischemic colitis because a remediable occlusive lesion is very rarely found. Surgical resection may be required in some patients with fulminant ischemic colitis to remove gangrenous bowel; others with lesser degrees of ischemia may respond to conservative medical management.

Subacute ischemic colitis is the most common clinical variant of ischemic colonic disease. It produces lesser degrees of pain and bleeding, often occurring over several days or weeks. The left colon may be involved, but the rectum is usually spared because of the collateral blood supply, a feature distinguishing it from acute ulcerative colitis. Barium enema reveals edema, cobblestoning, thumbprinting, and occasionally superficial ulceration. Angiography is not indicated because almost all cases are nonocclusive. Occasionally, *stricture formation* may follow a bout of ischemic colitis or may present de novo without a history of antecedent pain or bloody diarrhea. Most cases of nonocclusive ischemic colitis resolve in 2 to 4 weeks and do not recur. Surgery is not required except for obstruction secondary to postischemic stricture.

ANGIODYSPLASIA OF THE COLON These are vascular ectasias or arteriovenous malformations (AVMs) that occur in the right colon of many older individuals and may cause bleeding (Chap. 44). Angiodysplasia is a degenerative lesion consisting of dilated, distorted, thin-walled vessels lined by vascular endothelium. It may result from partial obstruction of the submucosal venous plexus by the tension generated in the cecal wall during muscular contraction. Grossly, angiodysplasias look similar to spider angiomas of the skin and on colonoscopy appear as star-shaped branching vessels in the submucosa measuring from 2 mm to 1 cm in diameter. The lesions are usually multiple and are found primarily in the cecum and ascending colon, but in some patients they may be distributed from the stomach to rectum.

Cecal angiodysplasia is important because of the likelihood of bleeding, either massively or chronically. In patients over age 60, ~1/4 of colonic bleeding episodes are secondary to angiodysplasia. The diagnosis is easiest to establish by colonoscopy, which allows treatment by laser photocoagulation, electrocautery, or injection with sclerosant. Some patients with massive uncontrolled bleeding or multiple sites of angiodysplasia may require right hemicolectomy. Angiodysplasias may also respond to chronic estrogen-progesterone therapy.

ANORECTAL PROBLEMS

HEMORRHOIDS The internal hemorrhoidal plexus of veins is located in the submucosal space above the valves of Morgagni. The anal canal separates it from the external hemorrhoidal venous plexus, but the two spaces communicate under the anal canal, the submucosa of which is attached to underlying tissue to form the interhemorrhoidal depression. Whenever the internal hemorrhoidal plexus is enlarged, the associated supporting tissue mass is increased, and the resultant venous swelling is called an *internal hemorrhoid*. When veins in the external hemorrhoidal plexus become enlarged or thrombosed, the resultant bluish mass is called an *external hemorrhoid*.

Both types of hemorrhoids are very common and are associated with increased hydrostatic pressure in the portal venous system, such as during pregnancy, straining at stool, or with cirrhosis. When internal hemorrhoids enlarge, pain is not a usual feature until the situation is complicated by thrombosis, infection, or erosion of the overlying mu-

cosal surface. Most persons complain of bright red blood on the toilet tissue or coating the stool, with a feeling of vague anal discomfort. The discomfort is increased when the hemorrhoid enlarges or prolapses through the anus; prolapse is often accompanied by edema and sphincteric spasm. If not treated, prolapse usually becomes chronic as the muscularis stays stretched, and the patient complains of constant soiling of underclothing with very little pain. Prolapsed hemorrhoids may become thrombosed; the overlying mucous membrane may bleed profusely from the trauma of defecation.

Because they lie under the skin, external hemorrhoids are quite often painful, particularly if there is a sudden increase in their mass. These episodes result in a tender blue swelling at the anal verge due to thrombosis of a vein in the external plexus and need not be associated with enlargement of the internal veins. Since the thrombus usually lies at the level of the sphincteric muscles, anal spasm often occurs.

The diagnosis of internal and external hemorrhoids is made by inspection, digital examination, and direct vision through the anoscope and proctoscope. Since such lesions are very common, they must not be regarded as the cause of rectal bleeding or iron deficiency anemia until a thorough investigation has been made of the more proximal gastrointestinal tract. Acute blood loss can occasionally be attributed to internal hemorrhoids. Chronic anemia or occult blood in the stool in the presence of large but not definitely bleeding hemorrhoids requires a search for a polyp, cancer, or ulcer.

℞ **TREATMENT** Most hemorrhoids respond to conservative therapy such as sitz baths or other forms of moist heat, suppositories, stool softeners, and bed rest. Internal hemorrhoids that remain permanently prolapsed are best treated surgically; milder degrees of prolapse or enlargement with pruritus ani or intermittent bleeding can be handled successfully by banding or injection of sclerosing solutions. External hemorrhoids that become acutely thrombosed are treated by incision, extraction of the clot, and compression of the incised area following clot removal. No surgical procedure should be carried out in the presence of acute inflammation of the anus, ulcerative proctitis, or ulcerative colitis. Proctoscopy or colonoscopy should always be performed before a patient undergoes hemorrhoidectomy.

ANAL INFLAMMATION Perianal inflammatory lesions may be primary or may be associated with inflammatory bowel disease or diverticular disease. *Anal fissures* are superficial erosions of the anal canal which usually heal rapidly with conservative therapy. *Anal ulcers* are more chronic and deep and give symptoms largely as the result of painful spasm of the external anal sphincter during and after defecation. Bleeding may occur with either fissure or ulcer; healing of the ulcer is often associated with a hypertrophied anal papilla and some degrees of anal contracture. The spasm associated with chronic anal fissure/ulcer can be managed with oral nifedipine or local botulinum toxin. *Fistula in ano*, a tract leading from the rectal lumen to the perianal skin, usually results from local crypt abscesses. The fistula is a chronically inflamed canal made up of fibrous tissue surrounding granulation tissue, the lumen of which may be difficult to demonstrate. *Perirectal abscesses* often represent the tracking down into the anal area of purulent material escaping from the rectosigmoid; diverticulitis, Crohn's disease, ulcerative colitis, or previous surgery may be the underlying cause. Fistulas between the rectum and vagina or the rectum and bladder represent serious complications of granulomatous, septic, or malignant disorders and require the patient to be hospitalized for definitive diagnostic and therapeutic procedures.

PERITONEAL AND MESENTERIC DISEASES

ACUTE PERITONITIS Peritonitis is a localized or generalized inflammatory process of the peritoneum that may appear in both acute and chronic forms. In the acute form the motor activity of the intestine is decreased, and the intestinal lumen becomes distended with gas and fluid. Fluid accumulates as a result of failure to reabsorb the 7 or 8 L normally secreted daily into the lumen and absorbed from the distal small bowel and colon. Because of accumulation of fluid in the peritoneal cavity as well as decreased oral intake, rapid depletion of the plasma volume with impaired cardiac and renal function may occur.

Etiology *Bacterial peritonitis* may be due to entry of bacteria into the peritoneal cavity from a perforation in the gastrointestinal tract or from an external penetrating wound. *Chemical peritonitis* results from spillage of pancreatic enzymes, gastric acid, or bile as a result of injury or perforation of the intestine or biliary tract. *Sterile peritonitis* occurs in patients with systemic lupus erythematosus, porphyria, and familial Mediterranean fever (FMF) during disease attacks.

The most common causes of bacterial peritonitis are appendicitis; perforations associated with diverticulitis; peptic ulcer; gangrenous gallbladder; and gangrenous obstruction of the small bowel from adhesive bands, incarcerated hernia, or volvulus. Any lesion leading to the escape of intestinal bacteria may be a source, including a perforating carcinoma, foreign body, and ulcerative colitis. The peritoneal cavity is remarkably resistant to contamination, and unless continuing contamination occurs, the peritonitis remains localized. Patients with alcoholic cirrhosis and ascites have an increased susceptibility to *spontaneous bacterial peritonitis*, usually from enteric pathogens. This complication occurs in the absence of recognizable perforation of a viscus and may be due to leakage of bacteria through the intestinal wall (Chap. 299).

Clinical Features The cardinal manifestations of peritonitis are acute abdominal pain and tenderness. The location of the pain and tenderness depends on the underlying cause and whether the inflammation is localized or generalized. In *localized peritonitis*, as seen in uncomplicated appendicitis or diverticulitis, the physical findings are limited to the area of inflammation. With widespread peritoneal inflammation there is *generalized peritonitis* with diffuse abdominal tenderness and rebound. Rigidity of the abdominal wall is a common finding in peritonitis and may be localized or generalized.

Peristalsis may be present initially but usually disappears as the illness progresses and bowel sounds disappear. Hypotension, tachycardia, oliguria, and leukocytosis with cell counts $>20,000/\mu L$, are common, especially in generalized peritonitis. Plain abdominal films may reveal dilation of the large and small bowel with edema of the small-bowel wall, as evidenced by the distance between adjacent loops of gas-filled small intestine. Diagnostic paracentesis is sometimes valuable in determining the nature of the exudate as well as whether bacteria can be demonstrated or cultured.

GONOCOCCAL PERITONITIS This usually involves an extension of gonococcal infection from a primary focus in the female reproductive tract. The signs of inflammation usually are limited to the pelvis, but there may be findings of a mild generalized peritonitis. Occasionally, the patient has right upper quadrant pain and tenderness caused by gonococcal perihepatitis involving the liver capsule and adjacent peritoneum (Fitz-Hugh–Curtis syndrome) (Chap. 147).

STARCH PERITONITIS An acute granulomatous peritonitis can develop in some patients as a foreign-body reaction to cornstarch used to powder surgical gloves. The clinical picture is that of acute abdominal pain and fever 10 to 30 days after an abdominal operation. The diagnosis can be made by paracentesis and demonstration of starch granules in monocytes. However, most patients are reexplored because of the fear of abscess or bacterial peritonitis, with the finding of foreign-body granuloma studding the peritoneum.

PSEUDOMYXOMA PERITONEI This is a rare condition resulting from rupture of a mucocele of the appendix, a mucinous ovarian cyst, or mucin-secreting intestinal or ovarian adenocarcinoma. The abdomen becomes filled with masses of jelly-like mucus. Occasional patients are cured with removal of the mucocele or the ovarian cyst and most of the myxomatous material. In other cases, however, the mucoid material recurs, leading to progressive wasting and eventual

death. Colloid carcinoma arising from the stomach or colon with peritoneal implants may resemble pseudomyxoma at laparotomy. The course of this type of highly malignant tumor is one of rapid cachexia and early death. The diagnosis usually can be made by the appearance of many highly malignant cells in the peritoneal implants.

PNEUMATOSIS CYSTOIDES INTESTINALIS This is a condition in which multiple gas-filled blebs or cysts accumulate in the intestinal wall beneath the serosal surface of the bowel. The exact source of the gas has not been explained satisfactorily. In some instances, this disease is associated with specific ulceration of the intestinal mucosa, in particular peptic ulcer with outlet obstruction. Cysts in the wall of the small bowel are seen as an occasional complication of mesenteric vascular occlusion. In the large bowel, these cysts are usually benign, may be seen with a variety of other disorders, and usually disappear over time.

Physical findings are not specific and the diagnosis is made either by x-ray or at laparotomy. Occasionally, the subserosal cysts may rupture, resulting in pneumoperitoneum.

CHYLOUS ASCITES See Chap. 46.

MESENTERIC LIPODYSTROPHY This is a rare disorder usually affecting middle-aged women and characterized pathologically by infiltration of the mesentery with lipid-laden macrophages and fibrous tissue. These patients present with ill-defined abdominal pain and occasionally an abdominal mass. The diagnosis is made at laparotomy by demonstration of thick fibrofatty masses at the root of the mesentery with retraction and distortion of the bowel loops.

FAMILIAL MEDITERRANEAN FEVER

Familial Mediterranean fever (FMF, familial paroxysmal polyserositis) is an inherited disorder, characterized by recurrent episodes of fever, peritonitis, and/or pleuritis. Arthritis, skin lesions, and amyloidosis are seen in some patients.

FMF occurs predominantly in patients of non-Ashkenazi (Sephardic) Jewish, Armenian, and Arabic ancestry. However, the disease has been seen in patients of Italian, Ashkenazi Jewish, and Anglo-Saxon descent as well as others.

ETIOLOGY FMF is an autosomal recessive trait characterized by mutations in the *MEFV* gene located on 16p. The gene encodes a 781-amino acid protein called *pyrin* expressed in cells of the myeloid lineage. The gene is in the *RoRet* family, and the product appears to function as a transcription factor based on the presence of a nuclear localization signal, a zinc finger, and a coiled-coil domain. Its expression in granulocytes is increased by proinflammatory cytokines and reduced by anti-inflammatory cytokines. Mutations associated with FMF cluster in exon 10. Different mutations appear to be associated with distinct disease manifestations; replacement of methionine 694 by valine is common in patients who have amyloidosis as a feature of the disease. Valine 726 replacement by alanine is rarely associated with amyloidosis. Other as yet unknown genes may modify the phenotype or be responsible for FMF in non-Mediterranean populations.

PATHOLOGY Despite the striking clinical manifestations during an acute attack of FMF, no specific pathologic alterations have been found. At laparotomy there is acute peritoneal inflammation with an exudate that contains a predominance of polymorphonuclear leukocytes. A disproportionately large number of male patients develop gallbladder disease with and without cholelithiasis. Pleural and joint inflammation are also nonspecific.

In the amyloidosis that accompanies FMF, amyloid is deposited in the intima and media of the arterioles, the subendothelial region of venules, the glomeruli, and the spleen. Aside from their vessels, the heart and liver are uninvolved.

MANIFESTATIONS The symptoms of FMF often begin between the ages of 5 and 15, although attacks sometimes commence during infancy and onset has occurred as late as age 50. The duration and frequency of attacks vary greatly in the same patient, and their occurrence follows no set pattern. The usual acute episode lasts 1 to 2 days, but some may be prolonged for 7 to 10 days. The attacks range in frequency from twice weekly to once a year, but 2 to 4 weeks is the most common interval. Spontaneous remissions lasting years have been seen. The severity and frequency of the attacks decrease with age or with development of amyloidosis.

Fever   Fever is a cardinal manifestation and is present during most attacks. Rarely, fever may be present without serositis. The temperature may be preceded by a chill and will peak in 12 to 24 h. Defervescence is often accompanied by diaphoresis. The fever ranges from 38.5° to 40°C but is quite variable.

Abdominal Pain   Abdominal pain occurs in >95% of patients and may vary in severity in the same patient. Minor premonitory discomfort may precede an acute episode by 24 to 48 h. The pain usually starts in one quadrant and then spreads to involve the whole abdomen. The initial site is usually very tender. Tenderness may remain localized with referred pain in other areas, and may radiate to the back. Diaphragmatic irritation may lead to splinting of the chest and pain in one or both shoulders. Nausea and vomiting sometimes occur. The abdomen is usually distended and may become rigid, with decreased or absent bowel sounds. On x-ray the wall of the small intestine may appear edematous, transit of barium is slowed, and fluid levels may be seen. An abdominal operation may precipitate an acute attack of FMF, which may be confused with other postoperative complications.

Chest Pain   Most patients with abdominal attacks have referred chest pain at one time or another, and 75% also develop acute pleuritic pain with or without abdominal symptoms. In 30%, the attacks of pleuritis precede the onset of abdominal attacks by varying periods of time, and a small number of patients never develop abdominal attacks. Chest pain is usually unilateral and is associated with diminished breath sounds, a friction rub, or a transient pleural effusion.

Joint Pain   In Israel, 75% of patients report at least one episode of acute arthritis. Arthritis can be distinct from abdominal or pleural attacks, can be acute or, rarely, chronic, and may involve one or several joints. Effusions are common, with large joints most frequently involved. Radiologic findings are nonspecific. Despite careful search, frank arthritis rarely has been seen in the United States. Some patients have a history of rheumatic fever-like illness in childhood, but in a large series of patients, including 30 from the Middle East, acute arthritis was not observed. Mild arthralgia is common during acute attacks but is nonspecific.

Skin Manifestations   Skin involvement occurs in one-third of patients. These lesions consist of painful, erythematous areas of swelling from 5 to 20 cm in diameter, usually located on the lower legs, the medial malleolus, or the dorsum of the foot. They may occur without abdominal or pleural pain and subside within 24 to 48 h.

Other Signs and Symptoms   Involvement of other serosal membranes has been reported, but pericarditis and meningitis are rare. Hematuria, splenomegaly, and small white dots called *colloid bodies* in the ocular fundus are findings of questionable significance. Rarely, migraine-like headaches accompany acute abdominal attacks, and some patients have become somewhat irrational or show extreme emotional lability during attacks. Whether these are primary manifestations of FMF or secondary effects of pain and fever is unclear.

Complications   Depression and lack of motivation are common, and patients with FMF require considerable support. A striking number of patients have developed gallbladder disease.

Amyloidosis has been reported in Israel, North Africa, and elsewhere in the Middle East, but its occurrence is rare in the United States. These findings are even more striking because there are probably as many known FMF patients in the United States as in Israel. Thus, environmental or nutritional, as well as genetic, factors may play a role in the development of amyloidosis in FMF.

LABORATORY FINDINGS   Polymorphonuclear leukocytosis ranging from 10,000 to 30,000 cells/μL is almost invariable during acute attacks. The erythrocyte sedimentation rate is elevated during attacks but returns to normal between attacks. Plasma fibrinogen, serum haptoglobin, ceruloplasmin, and C-reactive protein increase during the episodes. Plasma lipids are normal, and no consistent abnormalities of hepatic or renal function are seen. When amyloidosis is present, laboratory findings are typical of a nephrotic syndrome followed by renal insufficiency.

DIAGNOSIS   When the typical acute attacks of FMF occur in an individual of appropriate ethnic background with a family history of FMF, the diagnosis is easy. When a patient is seen for the first time, a variety of other febrile illnesses must be excluded, such as acute appendicitis, pancreatitis, porphyria, cholecystitis, intestinal obstruction, and other major abdominal catastrophes.

Some inherited hyperlipidemias may mimic the clinical picture of FMF, but lipid analysis will eliminate them from consideration. The FMF patient is not immune to other diseases, and when an attack differs from the usual pattern or is more prolonged, consideration should be given to other diagnostic possibilities. The pleural form of the disease is sometimes difficult to differentiate from acute pulmonary infection or infarction, but the rapid disappearance of signs and symptoms resolves the problem. The erythema is sometimes difficult to differentiate from superficial thrombophlebitis or cellulitis.

The most difficult diagnostic problem in FMF is the patient who presents with fever alone. In this situation an extensive diagnostic workup for fever of unknown origin may be required. Fortunately, such patients are rare, and all eventually develop serosal involvement. Until specific diagnostic tests for FMF are available, patients with recurrent fever but without signs of inflammation of one of the serosal membranes should not be categorized as having FMF.

PROGNOSIS   Despite the severity of the symptoms during some acute attacks, most patients are remarkably free of debilitation between attacks and are able to lead fairly normal lives. The greatest hazard to patients is prolonged periods of hospitalization due to erroneous diagnoses or failure to understand the disease. In the United States, the prognosis of patients with FMF does not seem to be different from that of patients with other chronic nonfatal illnesses. Death usually results from causes unrelated to the underlying disease.

In the past, ~25% of FMF patients in Israel developed amyloidosis, and this complication usually led to death. However, the widespread use of colchicine has resulted in a dramatic decrease in the incidence of amyloidosis.

TREATMENT   During the past 25 years, the outlook of patients with FMF has been altered dramatically. Chronic administration of colchicine greatly reduces the number of acute attacks of FMF. It is recommended that 0.6 mg colchicine be taken by mouth three times a day. If patients develop gastrointestinal side effects with this dose, it should be reduced to 0.6 mg taken twice a day. Although an occasional patient will respond to 0.6 mg taken only once a day, this amount is less likely to be beneficial. Most FMF patients will respond favorably to colchicine prophylaxis.

BIBLIOGRAPHY

DiLorenzo C: Pseudo-obstruction: Current approaches. Gastroenterology 116:980, 1999

Ferzoco LB et al: Acute diverticulitis. N Engl J Med 338:1521, 1998

Foutch PG: Colonic angiodysplasia. Gastroenterologist 5:148, 1997

Goyal RK, Hirano I: Mechanisms of disease: The enteric nervous system. N Engl J Med 334:1106, 1996

International FMF Consortium: Ancient missense mutations in a new member of the *RoRet* gene family are likely to cause Familial Mediterranean Fever. Cell 90:797, 1997

Jensen DM et al: Urgent colonoscopy for the diagnosis and treatment of severe diverticular hemorrhage. N Engl J Med 342:78, 2000

Kellow JE, Malcolm A: Motility. Curr Opin Gastroenterol 12:134, 1996

Maria R, Brisinda G: Nonoperative management of chronic anal fissure. Dis Colon Rectum 43:721, 2000

McKinsey JF, Gewertz BL: Acute mesenteric ischemia. Surg Clin North Am 77:307, 1997

ACUTE INTESTINAL OBSTRUCTION

ETIOLOGY AND CLASSIFICATION Intestinal obstruction may be *mechanical* or *nonmechanical* (resulting from neuromuscular disturbances that produce either adynamic or dynamic ileus). The causes of mechanical obstruction of the lumen are conveniently divided into (1) lesions *extrinsic* to the intestine, e.g., adhesive bands, internal and external hernias; (2) lesions *intrinsic* to the wall of the intestine, e.g., diverticulitis, carcinoma, regional enteritis; and (3) obturation of the lumen, e.g., gallstone obstruction, intussusception. Clinically, however, it is most useful to consider whether the obstructive mechanism involves the small or large intestine, because the causes, symptoms, and treatments are different (see below). Adhesions and external hernias are the most common causes of obstruction of the small intestine, constituting 70 to 75% of cases of this type. Adhesions, however, almost never produce obstruction of the colon, where carcinoma, sigmoid diverticulitis, and volvulus, in that order, are the most common causes and together account for about 90% of the cases. Primary intestinal pseudoobstruction (Chap. 289) is a chronic motility disorder that frequently mimics mechanical obstruction. Unnecessary operations in such patients should be avoided.

Adynamic ileus is probably the most common overall cause of obstruction. The development of this condition is mediated via the hormonal component of the sympathoadrenal system. Adynamic ileus may occur after any peritoneal insult, and its severity and duration will be dependent to some degree on the type of peritoneal injury. Hydrochloric acid, colonic contents, and pancreatic enzymes are among the most irritating substances, whereas blood and urine are less so. Adynamic ileus occurs to some degree after any abdominal operation. Retroperitoneal hematomas, particularly associated with vertebral fracture, commonly cause severe adynamic ileus, and the latter may occur with other retroperitoneal conditions, such as ureteral calculus or severe pyelonephritis. Thoracic diseases, including lower-lobe pneumonia, fractured ribs, and myocardial infarction, frequently produce adynamic ileus, as do electrolyte disturbances, particularly potassium depletion. Finally, intestinal ischemia, whether the result of vascular occlusion or intestinal distention itself, may perpetuate an adynamic ileus.

Spastic ileus or *dynamic ileus* is very uncommon and results from extreme and prolonged contraction of the intestine. It has been observed in heavy metal poisoning, uremia, porphyria, and extensive intestinal ulcerations.

PATHOPHYSIOLOGY Distention of the intestine is caused by the accumulation of gas and fluid proximal to and within the obstructed segment. Between 70 and 80% of intestinal gas consists of swallowed air, and because this is composed mainly of nitrogen, which is poorly absorbed from the intestinal lumen, removal of air by continuous gastric suction is a useful adjunct in the treatment of intestinal distention. The accumulation of fluid proximal to the obstructing mechanism results not only from ingested fluid, swallowed saliva, gastric juice, and biliary and pancreatic secretions but also from interference with normal sodium and water transport. During the first 12 to 24 h of obstruction, there is a marked depression of flux from lumen to blood of sodium and consequently water in the distended proximal intestine. After 24 h, there is movement of sodium and water into the lumen, contributing further to the distention and fluid losses. Intraluminal pressure rises from a normal of 2 to 4 cmH$_2$O to 8 to 10 cmH$_2$O. During peristalsis, when simple obstruction or a "closed loop" is present, pressures reach 30 to 60 cmH$_2$O. Closed-loop obstruction of the small intestine results when the lumen is occluded at two points by a single mechanism such as a hernial ring or adhesive band, thus producing a closed loop whose blood supply is often obstructed at the same time. Strangulation of the loop itself is thus common in associ-

ation with marked distention proximal to the involved loop. A form of closed-loop obstruction is encountered when complete obstruction of the colon exists in the presence of a competent ileocecal valve (85% of individuals). Although the blood supply of the colon is not entrapped within the obstructing mechanism, distention of the cecum is extreme because of its greater diameter (Laplace's law), and impairment of the intramural blood supply is considerable with consequent gangrene of the cecal wall, usually anteriorly. Necrosis of the small intestine may occur by the same mechanism of interference with intramural blood flow when distention is extreme, but this sequence is uncommon in the small intestine. Once impairment of blood supply occurs, bacterial invasion supervenes, and peritonitis develops. The systemic effects of extreme distention include elevation of the diaphragm with restricted ventilation and subsequent atelectasis. Venous return via the inferior vena cava may also be impaired.

The loss of fluids and electrolytes may be extreme and, unless replacement is prompt, leads to hemoconcentration, hypovolemia, renal insufficiency, shock, and death. Vomiting, accumulation of fluids within the lumen by the mechanisms described above, and the sequestration of fluid into the edematous intestinal wall and peritoneal cavity as a result of impairment of venous return from the intestine all contribute to massive loss of fluid and electrolytes, especially potassium. As soon as significant impedance to venous return is present, the intestine becomes severely congested, and blood begins to seep into the intestinal lumen. Blood loss may reach significant levels when long segments of intestine are involved.

SYMPTOMS *Mechanical small-intestinal obstruction* is characterized by cramping midabdominal pain, which tends to be more severe the higher the obstruction. The pain occurs in paroxysms, and the patient is relatively comfortable in the intervals between the pains. Audible borborygmi are often noted by the patient simultaneously with the paroxysms of pain. The pain may become less severe as distention progresses, probably because motility is impaired in the edematous intestine. When strangulation is present, the pain is usually more localized and may be steady and severe without a colicky component, a fact that often causes delay in diagnosis of obstruction. Vomiting is almost invariable, and it is earlier and more profuse the higher the obstruction. The vomitus initially contains bile and mucus and remains as such if the obstruction is high in the intestine. With low ileal obstruction, the vomitus becomes feculent, i.e., orange-brown in color with a foul odor, which results from the overgrowth of bacteria proximal to the obstruction. Hiccups (singultus) are common. Obstipation and failure to pass gas by rectum are invariably present when the obstruction is complete, although some stool and gas may be passed spontaneously or after an enema shortly after onset of the complete obstruction. Diarrhea is occasionally observed in partial obstruction. Blood in the stool is rare but does occur in cases of intussusception. Other than some minor but inconsistent differences in pain patterns noted above, the symptoms of strangulating obstructions cannot be distinguished from those of nonstrangulating obstructions.

Mechanical colonic obstruction produces colicky abdominal pain similar in quality to that of small-intestinal obstruction but of much lower intensity. Complaints of pain are occasionally absent in stoic elderly patients. Vomiting occurs late, if at all, particularly if the ileocecal valve is competent. Paradoxically, feculent vomitus is very rare. A history of recent alterations in bowel habits and blood in the stool is common because carcinoma and diverticulitis are the most frequent causes. Constipation becomes progressive, and obstipation with failure to pass gas ensues. Acute symptoms may develop over a period of a week. Cecal volvulus more closely resembles obstruction of the small intestine clinically, whereas patients with sigmoid volvulus more typically have the picture of colonic obstruction in which marked distention predominates, with relatively less pain.

In *adynamic ileus*, colicky pain is absent, and only discomfort from distention is evident. Vomiting may be frequent but is rarely profuse. It usually consists of gastric contents and bile and is almost never feculent. Complete obstipation may or may not occur. Singultus (hiccups) is common.

PHYSICAL FINDINGS   *Abdominal distention* is the hallmark of all forms of intestinal obstruction. It is least marked in cases of obstruction high in the small intestine and most marked in colonic obstruction. Early, especially in closed-loop strangulating small-bowel obstruction, distention may be barely perceptible or absent. Tenderness and rigidity are usually minimal; the temperature is rarely above 37.8°C (100°F) in nonstrangulating obstruction of the small and large intestine. Contrary to popular belief, the same is true of strangulating obstruction until very late, a fact that has often resulted in unfortunate delay in treatment. Signs and symptoms of shock also occur *very late* in strangulating obstruction. The appearance of shock, tenderness, rigidity, and fever often means that contamination of the peritoneum with infected intestinal content has occurred. Hernial orifices should always be carefully examined for the presence of a mass. The presence of a palpable abdominal mass usually signifies a closed-loop strangulating small-bowel obstruction because the tense fluid-filled loop is the palpable lesion. Auscultation may reveal loud, high-pitched borborygmi coincident with the colicky pain, but this finding is often absent late in strangulating or nonstrangulating obstruction. A quiet abdomen does not eliminate the possibility of obstruction, nor does it necessarily establish the diagnosis of adynamic ileus.

LABORATORY AND X-RAY FINDINGS   Leukocytosis, with shift to the left, usually occurs when strangulation is present, but a normal white blood cell count does not exclude strangulation. Elevation of the serum amylase level is encountered occasionally in all forms of intestinal obstruction, especially the strangulating variety.

The x-ray is extremely valuable but under certain circumstances may also be misleading. In nonstrangulating complete small-bowel obstruction, x-rays are almost completely reliable. Distention of fluid- and gas-filled loops of small intestine usually arranged in a "stepladder" pattern with air-fluid levels and an absence or paucity of colonic gas are pathognomonic (Fig. 290-1). These findings, however, are absent in slightly over half the cases of strangulating small-bowel obstruction, especially early in the disease. A general haze due to peritoneal fluid and sometimes a "coffee bean"–shaped mass are seen in strangulating obstruction. Occasionally, the films are normal, but when symptoms are consistent with obstruction of the small intestine, a normal film should suggest strangulation. In these circumstances, computed tomography may be very useful. Roentgenographic differentiation of partial mechanical small-bowel obstruction from adynamic ileus may be impossible because gas is present in both the small and large intestines; however, colonic distention is usually more prominent in adynamic ileus. A radiopaque dye given by mouth is useful in making this distinction.

Colonic obstruction with a competent ileocecal valve is easily recognized because distention with gas is mainly confined to the colon. Barium enema, sigmoidoscopy, or colonoscopy, depending on the suspected site of obstruction, is usually advisable to determine the nature of the lesion, except when concomitant perforation is suspected, a rare occurrence. Sigmoidoscopy may be therapeutic in cases of sigmoid volvulus. When the ileocecal valve is incompetent, the films resemble those of partial small-bowel obstruction or adynamic ileus, and barium enema or colonoscopy is necessary to establish the correct diagnosis. Barium given by mouth is perfectly safe when obstruction is in the small intestine, since the barium sulfate does not become inspissated in this location. *Barium should never be given by mouth to a patient with possible colonic obstruction* until that possibility has been excluded by barium enema.

R̲x̲ TREATMENT   Small-Intestinal Obstruction   The overall mortality rate for obstruction of the small intestine is about 10%, even under the most optimal conditions. While the mortality rate for nonstrangulating obstruction is as low as 5 to 8%, that for strangulating obstruction has been reported to be between 20 and 75%. Well over

FIGURE 290-1   Acute mechanical obstruction of small intestine (upright film). Note air-fluid levels, marked distention of bowel loops, and absence of colonic gas.

half the deaths from small-bowel obstruction occur in those with strangulation; however, the latter constitute only one-fourth to one-third of the cases. Careful studies indicate that the clinical, laboratory, and x-ray findings are not reliable in distinguishing strangulating from nonstrangulating obstruction when obstruction is complete. Complete obstruction is suggested when passage of gas or stool per rectum has ceased and when gas is absent in the distal intestine by x-ray. Since strangulating small-bowel obstruction is always complete, operation should always be undertaken in such patients after suitable preparation. Before operation, fluid and electrolyte balance should be restored and decompression instituted by means of a nasogastric tube. Replacement of potassium is especially important because intake is nil and losses in vomitus are large. From 6 to 8 h of preparation may be necessary. During this period, broad-spectrum antibiotics are indicated if strangulation is felt to be likely, but operation should not be delayed unless there is unequivocal clinical and roentgenographic evidence of resolution of the obstruction during the period of preparation. Attempts to pass a long tube into the small intestine usually fail while putting the patient through uncomfortable, unproductive manipulations that delay appropriate fluid replacement and decompression. *There are few, if any, indications for the use of a long intestinal tube.* Procrastination of operation because of improvement in well-being of the patient during resuscitation and gastric decompression usually leads to unnecessary and hazardous delay in proper treatment. Purely nonoperative therapy is safe only in the presence of incomplete obstruction and is best utilized in patients with (1) repeated episodes of partial obstruction, (2) recent postoperative partial obstruction, and (3) partial obstruction following a recent episode of diffuse peritonitis.

Colonic Obstruction   The mortality rate for colonic obstruction is about 20%. As in small-bowel obstruction, nonoperative treatment is contraindicated unless the obstruction is incomplete. Occasionally, but not always, when the obstruction is incomplete, nonoperative therapy may result in sufficient decompression that a definitive operative procedure can be undertaken at a later date. This can usually be accomplished by discontinuation of all oral intake and perhaps by nasogastric suction, although attempts to decompress a *completely* obstructed colon by intubation are almost invariably futile. A long intestinal tube will not decompress an obstructed colon with a competent ileocecal valve. When obstruction is complete, early operation is mandatory, especially when the ileocecal valve is competent; cecal gangrene is likely if the cecal diameter exceeds 10 cm on plain abdominal film. For obstruction on the left side of the colon, the most common site, preliminary operative decompression by cecostomy or transverse colostomy followed by definitive resection of the primary lesion has been the treatment of choice. Recently, primary resection of obstructing left-sided lesions with on-table washout of the colon has been accomplished safely. For a lesion of the right or transverse colon, primary resection and anastomosis can be performed safely because distention of the ileum with consequent discrepancy in size and hazard in suture are not present.

Adynamic Ileus This type of ileus usually responds to nonoperative continuous decompression and adequate treatment of the primary disease. The prognosis is usually good. Successful decompression of severe colonic ileus has been accomplished by colonoscopy, but this should be avoided if tenderness in the right lower quadrant suggests possible cecal gangrene. Neostigmine is effective in cases of colonic ileus that have not responded to other conservative treatment. Rarely, adynamic colonic distention may become so great that cecostomy is required if cecal gangrene is feared. Spastic ileus usually responds to treatment of the primary disease.

BIBLIOGRAPHY

BULKLEY GB et al: Intraoperative determination of small intestinal viability following ischemic injury: Prospective controlled trial of two adjuvant methods (Doppler and fluorescein) compared with standard clinical judgement. Ann Surg 193:628, 1981

DUBOIS A et al: Postoperative ileus: Physiopathology, etiology and treatment. Ann Surg 178:781, 1973

ESKELINEN M et al: Contributions of history-taking, physical examination, and computer assistance to diagnosis of acute small-bowel obstruction. A prospective study of 1333 patients with acute abdominal pain. Scand J Gastroenterol 29:715, 1994

HOFSETTER SR: Acute adhesive obstruction of the small intestine. Surg Gynecol Obstet 152:141, 1981

JACKSON BR: The diagnosis of colonic obstruction. Dis Colon Rectum 25:603, 1982

PESCHIERA JL, BEERMAN SP: Intestinal dysfunction associated with acute thoracolumbar fractures. Orthop Rev 19:284, 1990

PONEC RJ et al: Neostigmine for the treatment of acute colonic pseudo-obstruction. N Engl J Med 341:137, 1999

SILEN W: *Cope's Early Diagnosis of the Acute Abdomen*, 18th ed. London, Oxford, 1991

291 *William Silen*

ACUTE APPENDICITIS

INCIDENCE AND EPIDEMIOLOGY The peak incidence of acute appendicitis is in the second and third decades of life; it is relatively rare at the extremes of age. Males and females are equally affected, except between puberty and age 25, when males predominate in a 3:2 ratio. Perforation is more common in infancy and in the aged, during which periods mortality rates are highest. The mortality rate has decreased steadily in Europe and the United States from 8.1 per 100,000 of the population in 1941 to less than 1 per 100,000 in 1970 and subsequently. The absolute incidence of the disease also decreased by about 40% between 1940 and 1960 but since then has remained unchanged. Although various factors such as changing dietary habits, altered intestinal flora, and better nutrition and intake of vitamins have been suggested to explain the reduced incidence, the exact reasons have not been elucidated. The overall incidence of appendicitis is much lower in underdeveloped countries, especially parts of Africa, and in lower socioeconomic groups.

PATHOGENESIS Luminal obstruction has long been considered the pathogenetic hallmark. However, obstruction can be identified in only 30 to 40% of cases; ulceration of the mucosa is the initial event in the majority. The cause of the ulceration is unknown, although a viral etiology has been postulated. Infection with *Yersinia* organisms may cause the disease, since high complement fixation antibody titers have been found in up to 30% of cases of proven appendicitis. Whether the inflammatory reaction seen with ulceration is sufficient to obstruct the tiny appendiceal lumen even transiently is not clear. Obstruction, when present, is most commonly caused by a fecalith, which results from accumulation and inspissation of fecal matter around vegetable fibers. Enlarged lymphoid follicles associated with viral infections (e.g., measles), inspissated barium, worms (e.g., pinworms, *Ascaris*, and *Taenia*), and tumors (e.g., carcinoid or carcinoma) may also obstruct the lumen. Secretion of mucus distends the organ, which has a capacity of only 0.1 to 0.2 mL, and luminal pressures rise as high as 60 cmH$_2$O. Luminal bacteria multiply and invade the appendiceal wall as venous engorgement and subsequent arterial compromise result from the high intraluminal pressures. Finally, gangrene and perforation occur. If the process evolves slowly, adjacent organs such as the terminal ileum, cecum, and omentum may wall off the appendiceal area so that a localized abscess will develop, whereas rapid progression of vascular impairment may cause perforation with free access to the peritoneal cavity. Subsequent rupture of primary appendiceal abscesses may produce fistulas between the appendix and bladder, small intestine, sigmoid, or cecum. Occasionally, acute appendicitis may be the first manifestation of Crohn's disease.

While chronic infection of the appendix with tuberculosis, amebiasis, and actinomycosis may occur, a useful clinical aphorism states that *chronic appendiceal inflammation is not usually the cause of prolonged abdominal pain of weeks' or months' duration*. In contrast, recurrent acute appendicitis does occur, often with complete resolution of inflammation and symptoms between attacks. Recurrent acute appendicitis may become more frequent as antibiotics are dispensed more freely and if a long appendiceal stump is left after laparoscopic appendectomy.

CLINICAL MANIFESTATIONS The history and sequence of symptoms are important diagnostic features of appendicitis. The initial symptom is almost invariably *abdominal pain* of the visceral type, resulting from appendiceal contractions or distention of the lumen. It is usually poorly localized in the periumbilical or epigastric region with an accompanying urge to defecate or pass flatus, neither of which relieves the distress. This visceral pain is mild, often cramping, and rarely catastrophic in nature, usually lasting 4 to 6 h, but it may not be noted by stoic individuals or by some patients during sleep. As inflammation spreads to the parietal peritoneal surfaces, the pain becomes somatic, steady, and more severe, aggravated by motion or cough, and usually located in the *right lower quadrant*. Anorexia is nearly universal; a hungry patient does not have acute appendicitis. *Nausea* and *vomiting* occur in 50 to 60% of cases, but vomiting is usually self-limited. The development of nausea and vomiting before the onset of pain is extremely rare. Change in bowel habit is of little diagnostic value, since any or no alteration may be observed, although the presence of diarrhea caused by an inflamed appendix in juxtaposition to the sigmoid may cause serious diagnostic difficulties. Urinary frequency and dysuria occur if the appendix lies adjacent to the bladder. The typical sequence of symptoms (poorly localized periumbilical pain followed by nausea and vomiting with subsequent shift of pain to the right lower quadrant) occurs in only 50 to 60% of patients.

Physical findings vary with time after onset of the illness and according to the location of the appendix, which may be situated deep in the pelvic cul-de-sac; in the right lower quadrant in any relation to the peritoneum, cecum, and small intestine; in the right upper quadrant (especially during pregnancy); or even in the left lower quadrant. *The diagnosis cannot be established unless tenderness can be elicited.* While tenderness is sometimes absent in the early visceral stage of the disease, it ultimately always develops and is found in any location corresponding to the position of the appendix. Abdominal tenderness may be completely absent if a retrocecal or pelvic appendix is present, in which case the sole physical finding may be tenderness in the flank or on rectal or pelvic examination. Percussion, rebound tenderness, and referred rebound tenderness are often, but not invariably, present; they are most likely to be absent early in the illness. Flexion of the right hip and guarded movement by the patient are due to parietal peritoneal involvement. Hyperesthesia of the skin of the right lower quadrant and a positive psoas or obturator sign are often late findings and are rarely of diagnostic value. When the inflamed appendix is in close proximity to the anterior parietal peritoneum, muscular rigidity is present yet is often minimal early.

The temperature is usually normal or slightly elevated [37.2 to 38°C (99 to 100.5°F)], but a temperature > 38.3°C (101°F) should suggest perforation. Tachycardia is commensurate with the elevation of the temperature. Rigidity and tenderness become more marked as the disease progresses to perforation and localized or diffuse peritonitis. Distention is rare unless severe diffuse peritonitis has developed. The disappearance of pain and tenderness just before perforation is extremely unusual. A mass may develop if localized perforation has occurred but usually will not be detectable before 3 days after onset. Earlier presence of a mass suggests carcinoma of the cecum or Crohn's disease. Perforation is rare before 24 h after onset of symptoms, but the rate may be as high as 80% after 48 h.

Diagnosis is based primarily on clinical grounds. Although moderate leukocytosis of 10,000 to 18,000 cells/μL is frequent (with a concomitant left shift), the absence of leukocytosis does not rule out acute appendicitis. Leukocytosis of >20,000 cells/μL suggests probable perforation. Anemia and blood in the stool suggest a primary diagnosis of carcinoma of the cecum, especially in elderly individuals. The urine may contain a few white or red blood cells without bacteria if the appendix lies close to the right ureter or bladder. Urinalysis is most useful in excluding genitourinary conditions that may mimic acute appendicitis.

Radiographs are rarely of value except when an opaque fecalith (5% of patients) is observed in the right lower quadrant (especially in children). Consequently, abdominal films are not routinely obtained unless other conditions such as intestinal obstruction or ureteral calculus may be present. In some patients with recurrent or prolonged symptoms, a careful barium enema or computed tomography (CT) scan may reveal an extrinsic defect on the medial wall of the cecum or a calcified fecalith. The value of CT scan in acute appendicitis is being evaluated. The diagnosis may also be established by the ultrasonic demonstration of an enlarged and thick-walled appendix. Ultrasound is most useful to exclude ovarian cysts, ectopic pregnancy, or tuboovarian abscess.

While the typical historic sequence and physical findings are present in 50 to 60% of cases, a wide variety of atypical patterns of disease are encountered, especially at the age extremes and during pregnancy. Infants under 2 years of age have a 70 to 80% incidence of perforation and generalized peritonitis. Any infant or child with diarrhea, vomiting, and abdominal pain is highly suspect. Fever is much more common in this age group, and abdominal distention is often the only physical finding. In the elderly, pain and tenderness are often blunted, and thus the diagnosis is frequently delayed and leads to a 30% incidence of perforation in patients over 70. Elderly patients often present initially with a slightly painful mass (a primary appendiceal abscess) or with adhesive intestinal obstruction 5 or 6 days after a previously undetected perforated appendix.

Appendicitis occurs about once in every 1000 pregnancies and is the most common extrauterine condition requiring abdominal operation. The diagnosis may be missed or delayed because of the frequent occurrence of mild abdominal discomfort and nausea and vomiting during pregnancy. During the last trimester, when the mortality rate from appendicitis is highest, uterine displacement of the appendix to the right upper quadrant and laterally leads to confusion in diagnosis because pain and tenderness are similarly displaced.

DIFFERENTIAL DIAGNOSIS   Appendicitis can be confused with any condition that causes abdominal pain. Diagnostic accuracy is about 75 to 80% for experienced clinicians and must be based solely on the clinical criteria outlined. It is probably better to err slightly in the direction of overdiagnosis, since delay is associated with perforation and increased morbidity and mortality. In unperforated appendicitis, the mortality rate is 0.1%, little more than that associated with general anesthesia; for perforated appendicitis, overall mortality is 3%, (15% in the elderly). In doubtful cases, 4 to 6 h of observation is always more beneficial than harmful. The most common conditions discovered at operation when acute appendicitis is erroneously diagnosed are, in order of frequency, mesenteric lymphadenitis, no organic disease, acute pelvic inflammatory disease, ruptured graafian follicle or corpus luteum cyst, and acute gastroenteritis. In addition, acute cholecystitis, perforated ulcer, acute pancreatitis, acute diverticulitis, strangulating intestinal obstruction, ureteral calculus, and pyelonephritis may present diagnostic difficulties.

Differentiation of *pelvic inflammatory disease* from acute appendicitis on clinical grounds may be virtually impossible. Gram-negative intracellular diplococci on cervical smear are not pathognomonic unless *Neisseria gonorrhoeae* can be cultured. Pain on movement of the cervix is not specific and may occur in appendicitis if perforation has occurred or if the appendix lies adjacent to the uterus or adnexa. *Rupture of a graafian follicle* (mittelschmerz) occurs at midcycle and will spill off blood and fluid to produce pain and tenderness more diffuse and usually of a less severe degree than in appendicitis. Fever and leukocytosis are usually absent. *Rupture of a corpus luteum cyst* is identical clinically to rupture of a graafian follicle but develops about the time of menstruation. The presence of an adnexal mass, evidence of blood loss, and a positive pregnancy test help differentiate *ruptured tubal pregnancy*, but a negative pregnancy test is present when tubal abortion has occurred. *Twisted ovarian cyst* and *endometriosis* are occasionally difficult to distinguish from appendicitis. In all these female conditions, ultrasonography, laparoscopy, and occasionally CT may be of great value.

Acute mesenteric lymphadenitis is the diagnosis usually given when enlarged, slightly reddened lymph nodes at the root of the mesentery and a normal appendix are encountered at operation in a patient who usually has right lower quadrant tenderness. Whether this is a single, discrete entity is unclear, since the causative factor is not known. Some of these patients have infection with *Y. pseudotuberculosis* or *Y. enterocolytica*, in which case the diagnosis can be established by culture of the mesenteric nodes or by serologic titers (Chap. 162). The diagnosis is essentially impossible clinically, although retrospectively these patients may have a higher temperature and more diffuse pain and tenderness. Children seem to be affected more frequently than adults. *Acute gastroenteritis* usually causes profuse watery diarrhea, often with nausea and vomiting, but without localized findings. Between cramps, the abdomen is completely relaxed. In *Salmonella* gastroenteritis, the abdominal findings are similar, although the pain may be more severe and more localized, and fever and chills are common. The occurrence of similar symptoms among other members of the family may be helpful. When the diagnosis of acute pelvic appendicitis with perforation has been missed, gastroenteritis is the most common previous working diagnosis. Persistent abdominal or rectal tenderness should eliminate the diagnosis of gastroenteritis. *Regional enteritis* (Crohn's disease) is usually associated with a more prolonged history, often with previous exacerbations regarded as episodes of gastroenteritis unless the diagnosis has been established previously. *Meckel's diverticulitis* usually cannot be distinguished from acute appendicitis but is very rare.

℞ TREATMENT   Cathartics and enemas should be avoided if appendicitis is under consideration, and antibiotics should not be administered when the diagnosis is in question, since they will only mask the perforation. The treatment is early operation and appendectomy as soon as the patient can be prepared. Appendectomy is increasingly accomplished laparoscopically and may have some benefits over the open technique. Preparation for operation rarely takes more than 1 to 2 h in early appendicitis but may require 6 to 8 h in cases of severe sepsis and dehydration associated with late perforation. The *only* circumstance in which operation is *not* indicated is the presence of a palpable mass 3 to 5 days after the onset of symptoms. Should operation be undertaken at that time, a phlegmon rather than a definitive abscess will be found, and complications from its dissection are frequent. Such patients treated with broad-spectrum antibiotics, parenteral fluids, and rest usually show resolution of the mass and symptoms within 1 week. *Interval appendectomy* should be done safely 3 months later. Should the mass enlarge or the patient become more toxic, drainage of the abscess is necessary. The complications of sub-

phrenic, pelvic, or other intraabdominal abscesses usually follow perforation with generalized peritonitis and can be avoided by early diagnosis of the disease.

BIBLIOGRAPHY

GRONROOS JM, GRONROOS P: Leucocyte count and C-reactive protein in the diagnosis of acute appendicitis. Br J Surg 86:501, 1999

NGUYEN DB et al: Appendectomy in the pre- and postlaparoscopic areas. J Gastrointest Surg 3:67, 1999

RAO P et al: Effect of computed tomography of the appendix on treatment of patients and use of hospital resources. N Engl J Med 338:141, 1998

WADE DS et al: Accuracy of ultrasound in the diagnosis of acute appendicitis compared with the surgeon's clinical impression. Arch Surg 128:1039, 1993

Section 2
LIVER AND BILIARY TRACT DISEASE

292   *Marc Ghany, Jay H. Hoofnagle*

APPROACH TO THE PATIENT WITH LIVER DISEASE

In most instances, a diagnosis of liver disease can be made accurately by a careful history, physical examination, and application of a few laboratory tests. In some instances, radiologic examinations are helpful or, indeed, diagnostic. Liver biopsy is considered the "gold standard" in evaluation of liver disease but is now needed less for diagnosis than for grading and staging disease. This chapter provides an introduction to diagnosis and management of liver disease, briefly reviewing the structure and function of the liver; the major clinical manifestations of liver disease; and the use of clinical history, physical examination, laboratory tests, imaging studies, and liver biopsy.

LIVER STRUCTURE AND FUNCTION The liver is the largest organ of the body, weighing 1 to 1.5 kg and representing 1.5 to 2.5% of the lean body mass. The size and shape of the liver vary and generally match the general body shape—long and lean or squat and square. The liver is located in the right upper quadrant of the abdomen under the right lower rib cage against the diaphragm and projects for a variable extent into the left upper quadrant. The liver is held in place by ligamentous attachments to the diaphragm, peritoneum, great vessels, and upper gastrointestinal organs. It receives a dual blood supply; approximately 20% of the blood flow is oxygen-rich blood from the hepatic artery, and 80% is nutrient-rich blood from the portal vein arising from the stomach, intestines, and spleen.

The majority of cells in the liver are hepatocytes, which constitute two-thirds of the mass of the liver. The remaining cell types are Kupffer cells (members of the reticuloendothelial system), stellate (Ito or fat-storing) cells, endothelial cells and blood vessels, bile ductular cells, and supporting structures. Viewed by light microscopy, the liver appears to be organized in lobules, with portal areas at the periphery and central veins in the center of each lobule. However, from a functional point of view, the liver is organized into acini, with both hepatic arterial and portal venous blood entering the acinus from the portal areas and then flowing through the sinusoids to the terminal hepatic veins. The advantage of viewing the acinus as the physiologic unit of the liver is that it helps to explain the morphologic patterns of many vascular and biliary diseases not explained by the lobular arrangement.

Portal areas of the liver consist of small veins, arteries, bile ducts, and lymphatics organized in a loose stroma of supporting matrix and small amounts of collagen. Blood flowing into the portal areas is distributed through the sinusoids, passing from zone 1 to zone 3 of the acinus and draining into the terminal hepatic veins ("central veins"). The sinusoids are lined by unique endothelial cells that have prominent fenestrae of variable size, allowing the free flow of plasma but not cellular elements. The plasma is thus in direct contact with hepatocytes in the subendothelial space of Disse.

Hepatocytes have distinct polarity. The basolateral side of the hepatocyte lines the space of Disse and is richly lined with microvilli; it demonstrates endocytotic and pinocytotic activity, with passive and active uptake of nutrients, proteins, and other molecules. The apical pole of the hepatocyte forms the cannicular membranes through which bile components are secreted. The canniculi of hepatocytes form a fine network, which fuses into the bile ductular elements near the portal areas. Kupffer cells usually lie within the sinusoidal vascular space and represent the largest group of fixed macrophages in the body. The stellate cells are located in the space of Disse but are not usually prominent unless activated, when they produce collagen and matrix. Red blood cells stay in the sinusoidal space as blood flows through the lobules, but white blood cells can migrate through or around endothelial cells into the space of Disse and from there to portal areas, where they can return to the circulation through lymphatics.

Hepatocytes perform numerous and vital roles in maintaining homeostasis and health. These functions include the synthesis of most essential serum proteins (albumin, carrier proteins, coagulation factors, many hormonal and growth factors), the production of bile and its carriers (bile acids, cholesterol, lecithin, phospholipids), the regulation of nutrients (glucose, glycogen, lipids, cholesterol, amino acids), and metabolism and conjugation of lipophilic compounds (bilirubin, cations, drugs) for excretion in the bile or urine. Measurement of these activities to assess liver function is complicated by the multiplicity and variability of these functions. The most commonly used liver "function" tests are measurements of serum bilirubin, albumin, and prothrombin time. The serum bilirubin level is a measure of hepatic conjugation and excretion, and the serum albumin level and prothrombin time are measures of protein synthesis. Abnormalities of bilirubin, albumin, and prothrombin time are typical of hepatic dysfunction. Frank liver failure is incompatible with life, and the functions of the liver are too complex and diverse to be subserved by a mechanical pump; dialysis membrane; or concoction of infused hormones, proteins, and growth factors.

LIVER DISEASES While there are many causes of liver disease (Table 292-1), they generally present clinically in a few distinct patterns, usually classified as either hepatocellular or cholestatic (obstructive). In *hepatocellular diseases* (such as viral hepatitis or alcoholic liver disease), features of liver injury, inflammation, and necrosis

Table 292-1 Liver Diseases

Inherited hyperbilirubinemia
  Gilbert's syndrome
  Crigler-Najjar syndrome, types I and II
  Dubin-Johnson syndrome
  Rotor syndrome
Viral hepatitis
  Hepatitis A
  Hepatitis B
  Hepatitis C
  Hepatitis D
  Hepatitis E
  Others (mononucleosis, herpes, adenovirus
    hepatitis)
  Cryptogenic hepatitis
Immune and autoimmune liver diseases
  Primary biliary cirrhosis
  Autoimmune hepatitis
  Sclerosing cholangitis
  Overlap syndromes
  Graft-vs-host disease
  Allograft rejection
Genetic liver diseases
  α_1 Antitrypsin deficiency
  Hemochromatosis
  Wilson's disease
  Benign recurrent intrahepatic cholestasis
    (BRIC)
  Familial intrahepatic cholestasis (FIC),
    types I–III
  Others (galactosemia, tyrosinemia, cystic fibrosis,
    Newman-Pick disease, Gaucher's disease)
Alcoholic liver disease
  Acute fatty liver
  Acute alcoholic hepatitis
  Laennec's cirrhosis
Nonalcoholic fatty liver
  Steatosis
  Steatohepatitis
Acute fatty liver of pregnancy

Liver involvement in systemic diseases
  Sarcoidosis
  Amyloidosis
  Glycogen storage diseases
  Celiac disease
  Tuberculosis
  Myobacterium avium intracellulare
Cholestatic syndromes
  Benign postoperative cholestasis
  Jaundice of sepsis
  Total parenteral nutrition (TPN)–induced jaundice
  Cholestasis of pregnancy
  Cholangitis and cholecystitis
  Extrahepatic biliary obstruction (stone, stricture, cancer)
  Biliary atresia
  Caroli's disease
  Cryptosporidiosis
Drug-induced liver disease
  Hepatocellular patterns (isoniazid, acetaminophen)
  Cholestatic patterns (methyltestosterone)
  Mixed patterns (sulfonamides, phenytoin)
  Micro- and macrovesicular steatosis (methotrexate,
    fialuridine)
Vascular injury
  Venoocclusive disease
  Budd-Chiari syndrome
  Ischemic hepatitis
  Passive congestion
  Portal vein thrombosis
  Nodular regenerative hyperplasia
Mass lesions
  Hepatocellular carcinoma
  Cholangiocarcinoma
  Adenoma
  Focal nodular hyperplasia
  Metastatic tumors
  Abscess
  Cysts

predominate. In *cholestatic diseases* (such as gall stone or malignant obstruction, primary biliary cirrhosis, many drug-induced liver diseases), features of inhibition of bile flow predominate. The pattern of onset and prominence of symptoms can rapidly suggest a diagnosis, particularly if major risk factors are considered, such as the age and sex of the patient and a history of exposure or risk behaviors.

Typical presenting symptoms of liver disease include jaundice, fatigue, itching, right upper quadrant pain, abdominal distention, and intestinal bleeding. At present, however, many patients are diagnosed with liver disease who have no symptoms and who have been found to have abnormalities in biochemical liver tests as a part of a routine physical examination or screening for blood donation or for insurance or employment. The wide availability of batteries of liver tests makes it relatively simple to demonstrate the presence of liver injury as well as to rule it out in someone suspected of liver disease.

Evaluation of patients with liver disease should be directed at (1) establishing the etiologic diagnosis, (2) estimating the disease severity (grading), and (3) establishing the disease stage (staging). *Diagnosis* should focus on the category of disease, such as hepatocellular versus cholestatic injury, as well as on the specific etiologic diagnosis. *Grading* refers to assessing the severity or activity of disease—active or inactive, and mild, moderate, or severe. *Staging* refers to estimating the place in the course of the natural history of the disease, whether acute or chronic; early or late; precirrhotic, cirrhotic, or end-stage.

The goal of this chapter is to introduce general, salient concepts in the evaluation of patients with liver disease that help lead to the diagnoses discussed in subsequent chapters.

CLINICAL HISTORY The clinical history should focus on the symptoms of liver disease—their nature, pattern of onset, and progression—and on potential risk factors for liver disease. The symptoms of liver disease include constitutional symptoms such as fatigue, weakness, nausea, poor appetite, and malaise and the more liver-specific symptoms of jaundice, dark urine, light stools, itching, abdominal pain, and bloating. Symptoms can also suggest the presence of cirrhosis, end-stage liver disease, or complications of cirrhosis such as portal hypertension. Generally, the constellation of symptoms and their pattern of onset rather than a specific symptom points to an etiology.

Fatigue is the most common and most characteristic symptom of liver disease. It is variously described as lethargy, weakness, listlessness, malaise, increased need for sleep, lack of stamina, and poor energy. The fatigue of liver disease typically arises after activity or exercise and is rarely present or severe in the morning after adequate rest (afternoon versus morning fatigue). Fatigue in liver disease is often intermittent and variable in severity from hour to hour and day to day. In some patients, it may not be clear whether fatigue is due to the liver disease or to other problems such as stress, anxiety, sleep disturbance, or a concurrent illness.

Nausea occurs with more severe liver disease and may accompany fatigue or be provoked by odors of food or eating fatty foods. Vomiting can occur but is rarely persistent or prominent. Poor appetite with weight loss occurs commonly in acute liver diseases but is rare in chronic disease, except when cirrhosis is present and advanced. Diarrhea is uncommon in liver disease, except with severe jaundice, in which case lack of bile acids reaching the intestine can lead to steatorrhea.

Right upper quadrant discomfort or ache ("liver pain") occurs in many liver diseases and is usually marked by tenderness over the liver area. The pain arises from stretching or irritation of Glisson's capsule, which surrounds the liver and is rich in nerve endings. Severe pain is most typical of gall bladder disease, liver abscess, and severe venoocclusive disease but is an occasional accompaniment of acute hepatitis.

Itching occurs with acute liver disease, appearing early in obstructive jaundice (from biliary obstruction or drug-induced cholestasis) and somewhat later in hepatocellular disease (acute hepatitis). Itching also occurs in chronic liver diseases, typically the cholestatic forms such as primary biliary cirrhosis and sclerosing cholangitis where it is often the presenting symptom, occurring before the onset of jaundice. However, itching can occur in any liver disease, particularly once cirrhosis is present.

Jaundice is the hallmark symptom of liver disease and perhaps the most reliable marker of severity. Patients usually report darkening of the urine before they notice scleral icterus. Jaundice is rarely detectable with a bilirubin level less than 43 μmol/L (2.5 mg/dL). With severe cholestasis there will also be lightening of the color of the stools and steatorrhea. Jaundice without dark urine usually indicates indirect (unconjugated) hyperbilirubinemia and is typical of hemolytic anemia and the genetic disorders of bilirubin conjugation, the common and benign form being Gilbert's syndrome and the rare and severe form being Crigler-Najjar syndrome. Gilbert's syndrome affects up to 5% of the population; the jaundice is more noticeable after fasting and with stress.

Major risk factors for liver disease that should be sought in the clinical history include details of alcohol use, medications (including herbal compounds, birth control pills, and over-the-counter medications), personal habits, sexual activity, travel, exposure to jaundiced or other high-risk persons, injection drug use, recent surgery, remote or recent transfusion with blood and blood products, occupation, accidental exposure to blood or needlestick, and familial history of liver disease.

For assessing the risk of viral hepatitis, a careful history of sexual activity is of particular importance and should include life-time number of sexual partners and, for men, a history of having sex with men. Sexual exposure is a common mode of spread of hepatitis B but is rare for hepatitis C. Maternal-infant transmission occurs with both hepatitis B and C. Vertical spread of hepatitis B can now be prevented by passive and active immunization of the infant at birth. Vertical spread of hepatitis C is uncommon, but there are no known means of prevention. A history of injection drug use, even in the remote past, is of great importance in assessing the risk for hepatitis B and C. Injection drug use is now the single most common risk factor for hepatitis C. Transfusion with blood or blood products is no longer an important risk factor for acute viral hepatitis. However, blood transfusions received before the introduction of sensitive enzyme immunoassays for antibody to hepatitis C virus (anti-HCV) in 1992 is an important risk factor for chronic hepatitis C. Blood transfusion before 1986, when screening for antibody to hepatitis B core antigen (anti-HBc) was introduced, is also a risk factor for hepatitis B. Travel to an underdeveloped area of the world, exposure to persons with jaundice, and exposure to young children in day-care centers are risk factors for hepatitis A. Tattooing and body piercing (for hepatitis B and C) and eating shellfish (for hepatitis A) are frequently mentioned but actually quite rare types of exposure for acquiring hepatitis.

A history of alcohol intake is important in assessing the cause of liver disease and also in planning management and recommendations. In the United States, for example, at least 70% of adults drink alcohol to some degree, but significant alcohol intake is less common; in population-based surveys, only 5% have more than two drinks per day, the average drink representing 11 to 15 g alcohol. Alcohol consumption associated with an increased rate of alcoholic liver disease is probably more than two drinks (22 to 30 g) per day in women and three drinks (33 to 45 g) in men. Most patients with alcoholic cirrhosis have a much higher daily intake and have drunk excessively for 10 years or more before onset of liver disease. In assessing alcohol intake, the history should also focus upon whether alcohol abuse or dependence is present. Alcoholism is usually defined on the behavioral patterns and consequences of alcohol intake, not on the basis of the amount of alcohol intake. *Abuse* is defined by a repetitive pattern of drinking alcohol that has adverse effects on social, family, occupational, or health status. *Dependence* is defined by alcohol-seeking behavior, despite its adverse effects. Many alcoholics demonstrate both dependence and abuse, and dependence is considered the more serious and advanced form of alcoholism. A clinically helpful approach to diagnosis of alcohol dependence and abuse is the use of the CAGE questionnaire (Table 292-2), which is recommended in all medical history taking.

Family history can be helpful in assessing liver disease. Familial causes of liver disease include Wilson's disease; hemochromatosis and α_1-antitrypsin (α_1AT) deficiency; and the more uncommon inherited pediatric liver diseases of familial intrahepatic cholestasis (FIC), benign recurrent intrahepatic cholestasis (BRIC), and Alagille's syndrome. Onset of severe liver disease in childhood or adolescence with a family history of liver disease or neuropsychiatric disturbance should lead to investigation for Wilson's disease. A family history of cirrhosis, diabetes, or endocrine failure and the appearance of liver disease in adulthood should suggest hemochromatosis and lead to investigation of iron status. Patients with abnormal iron studies warrant genotyping of the HFE gene for the C282Y and H63D mutations typical of genetic hemochromatosis. A family history of emphysema should provoke investigation of α_1AT levels and, if low, for Pi genotype.

PHYSICAL EXAMINATION The physical examination rarely demonstrates evidence of liver dysfunction in a patient without symptoms or laboratory findings, nor are most signs of liver disease specific to one diagnosis. Thus, the physical examination usually complements rather than replaces the need for other diagnostic approaches. In many patients, the physical examination is normal unless the disease is acute or severe and advanced. Nevertheless, the physical examination is important in that it can be the first evidence for the presence of hepatic failure, portal hypertension, and liver decompensation. In addition, the physical examination can reveal signs that point to a specific diagnosis, either in risk factors or in associated diseases or findings.

Typical physical findings in liver disease are icterus, hepatomegaly, hepatic tenderness, splenomegaly, spider angiomata, palmar erythema, and excoriations. Signs of advanced disease include muscle-wasting, ascites, edema, dilated abdominal veins, hepatic fetor, asterixis, mental confusion, stupor, and coma.

Icterus is best appreciated by inspecting the sclera under natural light. In fair-skinned individuals, a yellow color of the skin may be obvious. In dark-skinned individuals, the mucous membranes below the tongue can demonstrate jaundice. Jaundice is rarely detectable if the serum bilirubin level is <43 μmol/L (2.5 μg/dL) but may remain detectable below this level during recovery from jaundice (because of protein and tissue binding of conjugated bilirubin).

Spider angiomata and palmar erythema occur in both acute and chronic liver disease and may be especially prominent in persons with cirrhosis, but they can occur in normal individuals and are frequently present during pregnancy. Spider angiomata are superficial, tortuous arterioles and, unlike simple telangiectases, typically fill from the center outwards. Spider angiomata occur only on the arms, face, and upper torso; they can be pulsatile and may be difficult to detect in dark-skinned individuals.

Hepatomegaly is not a very reliable sign of liver disease, because of the variability of the size and shape of the liver and the physical impediments to assessing liver size by percussion and palpation. Marked hepatomegaly is typical of cirrhosis, venooclusive disease, metastatic or primary cancers of the liver, and alcoholic hepatitis. Careful assessment of the liver edge may also demonstrate unusual firmness, irregularity of the surface, or frank nodules. Perhaps the most reliable physical finding in examining the liver is hepatic tenderness. Discomfort on touching or pressing on the liver should be carefully sought with percussive comparison of the right and left upper quadrants.

Splenomegaly occurs in many medical conditions but can be a subtle but significant physical finding in liver disease. The availability of ultrasound (US) assessment of the spleen allows for confirmation of the physical finding.

Signs of advanced liver disease include muscle-wasting and weight loss as well as hepatomegaly, bruising, ascites, and edema. Ascites is best appreciated by attempts to detect shifting dullness by careful percussion. US examination will confirm the finding of ascites in equivocal cases. Peripheral edema can occur with or without ascites. In patients with advanced liver disease, other factors frequently contribute to edema formation, including hypoalbuminemia, venous insufficiency, heart failure, and medications.

Table 292-2 CAGE Questions[a]

Acronym	Question
C	Have you ever felt you ought to *C*ut down on your drinking?
A	Have people *A*nnoyed you by criticizing your drinking?
G	Have you ever felt *G*uilty or bad about your drinking?
E	Have you ever had a drink first thing in the morning to steady your nerves or get rid of a hangover (*E*yeopener)?

[a] One "yes" response should raise suspicion of an alcohol use problem, and more than one is a strong indication that abuse or dependence exists.

Hepatic failure is defined as the occurrence of signs or symptoms of hepatic encephalopathy in a person with severe acute or chronic liver disease. The first signs of hepatic encephalopathy can be subtle and nonspecific—change in sleep patterns, change in personality, irritability, and mental dullness. Thereafter, confusion, disorientation, stupor, and eventually coma supervene. Physical findings include asterixis and flapping tremors of the body and tongue. *Fetor hepaticus* refers to the slightly sweet, ammoniacal odor that is common in patients with liver failure, particularly if there is portal-venous shunting of blood around the liver. Other causes of coma and confusion should be excluded, mainly electrolyte imbalances, sedative use, and renal or respiratory failure. A helpful measure of hepatic encephalopathy is a careful mental status examination and use of the trail-making test, which consists of a series of 20 numbered circles that the patient is asked to connect as rapidly as possible using a pencil. The normal range for the connect-the-dot test is 15 to 30 s; it is considerably delayed in patients with early hepatic encephalopathy. Other tests include drawing abstract objects or comparison of a signature to previous examples.

Other signs of advanced liver disease include umbilical hernia from ascites, prominent veins over the abdomen, and *caput medusa*, which consists of collateral veins seen radiating from the umbilicus and resulting from the recanulation of the umbilical vein. Widened pulse pressure and signs of a hyperdynamic circulation can occur in patients with cirrhosis as a result of fluid and sodium retention, increased cardiac output, and reduced peripheral resistance. Patients with long-standing cirrhosis are prone to develop the hepatopulmonary syndrome with hypoxemia due to pulmonary arteriovenous shunting, characterized by hypoxia that worsens when lying flat.

Several skin disorders and changes occur commonly in liver disease. Hyperpigmentation is typical of advanced chronic cholestatic diseases such as primary biliary cirrhosis and sclerosing cholangitis. In these same conditions, xanthelasma and tendon xanthomata occur as a result of retention and high serum levels of lipids and cholesterol. A slate-gray pigmentation to the skin also occurs with hemochromatosis if iron levels are high for a prolonged period. Mucocutaneous vasculitis with palpable purpura, especially on the lower extremities, is typical of cryoglobulinemia of chronic hepatitis C but can also occur in chronic hepatitis B.

Some physical signs point to specific liver diseases. Kayser-Fleischer rings occur in Wilson's disease and consist of a golden-brown copper pigment deposited at the periphery of the cornea; they are best seen by slit-lamp examination. In metastatic liver disease or primary hepatocellular carcinoma, signs of cachexia and wasting may be prominent, as well as firm hepatomegaly and a hepatic bruit.

LABORATORY TESTING   Diagnosis in liver disease is greatly aided by the availability of reliable and sensitive tests of liver injury and function. Use and interpretation of liver function tests is summarized in Chap. 293. A typical battery of blood tests used for initial assessment of liver disease includes measuring levels of serum alanine and aspartate aminotransferases (ALT and AST), alkaline phosphatase, direct and total serum bilirubin, and albumin and assessing prothrombin time. The pattern of abnormalities generally points to hepatocellular versus cholestatic liver disease and will help to decide whether the disease is acute or chronic and whether cirrhosis and hepatic failure are present. Based on these results, further testing over time may be necessary. Other laboratory tests may be helpful, such as γ-glutamyl transpeptidase (GGT) to define whether alkaline phosphatase elevations are due to liver disease; hepatitis serology to define the type of viral hepatitis; and autoimmune markers to diagnose primary biliary cirrhosis (antimitochondrial antibody; AMA), sclerosing cholangitis (peripheral antineutrophil cytoplasmic antibody; pANCA), autoimmune hepatitis (antinuclear, smooth-muscle, and liver-kidney microsomal antibody). A simple delineation of laboratory abnormalities and common liver diseases is given in Table 292-3.

Table 292-3   Important Diagnostic Tests in Common Liver Diseases

Disease	Diagnostic Test
Hepatitis A	Anti-HAV IgM
Hepatitis B	
Acute	HBsAg and anti-HBc IgM
Chronic	HBsAg and HBeAg and/or HBV DNA
Hepatitis C	Anti-HCV and HCV RNA
Hepatitis D (delta)	HBsAg and anti-HDV
Hepatitis E	Anti-HEV
Autoimmune hepatitis	ANA or SMA, elevated IgG levels, and compatible histology
Primary biliary cirrhosis	Mitochondrial antibody, elevated IgM levels, and compatible histology
Primary sclerosing cholangitis	p-ANCA, cholangiography
Drug-induced liver disease	History of drug ingestion
Alcoholic liver disease	History of excessive alcohol intake and compatible histology
Nonalcoholic steatohepatitis	Ultrasound or CT evidence of fatty liver and compatible histology
α_1 Antitrypsin disease	Reduced α_1 antitrypsin levels, phenotypes PiZZ or PiSZ
Wilson's disease	Decreased serum ceruloplasmin and increased urinary copper; increased hepatic copper level
Hemochromatosis	Elevated iron saturation and serum ferritin; genetic testing for HFE gene mutations
Hepatocellular cancer	Elevated α-fetoprotein level >500; ultrasound or CT image of mass

NOTE: HAV, HBV, HCV, HDV, HEV: hepatitis A, B, C, D, or E virus; HBsAg, hepatitis B surface antigen; HBc, hepatitis B core (antigen); HBeAg, hepatitis e antigen; ANA, antinuclear antibodies; SMA, smooth muscle antibody; p-ANCA, peripheral antineutrophil cytoplasmic antibody; CT, computed tomography.

DIAGNOSTIC IMAGING   There have been great advances made in hepatic imaging, although no method is suitably accurate in demonstrating underlying cirrhosis. There are many modalities available for imaging the liver. US, computed tomography (CT), and magnetic resonance imaging (MRI) are the most commonly employed and are complementary to each other. In general, US and CT have a high sensitivity for detecting biliary duct dilatation and are the first-line options for investigating the patient with suspected obstructive jaundice. Both US and CT can detect a fatty liver, which appears bright on both studies. Endoscopic retrograde cholangiopancreatography (ERCP) is the procedure of choice for visualization of the biliary tree. ERCP also provides several therapeutic options in patients with obstructive jaundice, such as sphincterotomy, stone extraction, and placement of nasobiliary catheters and biliary stents. Doppler US and MRI are used to assess hepatic vasculature and hemodynamics and to monitor surgically or radiologically placed vascular shunts such as transjugular intrahepatic portosystemic shunts (TIPS). CT and MRI are indicated for the identification and evaluation of hepatic masses, staging of liver tumors, and preoperative assessment. With regard to mass lesions, sensitivity of hepatic imaging continues to increase; unfortunately, specificity remains a problem, and often two and sometimes three studies are needed before a diagnosis can be reached. Finally, interventional radiologic techniques allow the biopsy of solitary lesions, insertion of drains into hepatic abscesses, and creation of vascular shunts in patients with portal hypertension. Which modality to use depends on factors such as availability, cost, and experience of the radiologist with each technique.

LIVER BIOPSY   Liver biopsy remains the gold standard in the evaluation of patients with liver disease, particularly in patients with chronic liver diseases. In selected instances, liver biopsy is necessary for diagnosis but is more often useful in assessing the severity (grade) and stage of liver damage, in predicting prognosis, and in monitoring response to treatment.

Diagnosis of Liver Disease   The major causes of liver disease and key diagnostic features are outlined in Table 292-3 (specifics of diagnosis are discussed in later chapters). The most common causes of acute liver disease are viral hepatitis (particularly hepatitis A, B, and C), drug-induced liver injury, cholangitis, and alcoholic liver disease. Liver biopsy is usually not needed in the diagnosis and management of acute liver disease, exceptions being situations where the diagnosis remains unclear despite thorough clinical and laboratory investigation. Liver biopsy can be helpful in the diagnosis of drug-induced liver disease and in establishing the diagnosis of acute alcoholic hepatitis.

The most common causes of chronic liver disease in general order of frequency are chronic hepatitis C, alcoholic liver disease, nonalcoholic steatohepatitis, chronic hepatitis B, autoimmune hepatitis, sclerosing cholangitis, primary biliary cirrhosis, hemochromatosis, and Wilson's disease. Strict diagnostic criteria have not been developed for most liver diseases, but liver biopsy plays an important role in the diagnosis of autoimmune hepatitis, primary biliary cirrhosis, nonalcoholic and alcoholic steatohepatitis, and Wilson's disease (with a quantitative hepatic copper level).

Grading and Staging of Liver Disease Grading refers to an assessment of the severity or activity of liver disease, whether acute or chronic; active or inactive; and mild, moderate, or severe. Liver biopsy is the most accurate means of assessing severity, particularly in chronic liver disease. Serum aminotransferase levels are used as a convenient and noninvasive means to follow disease activity, but aminotransferases are not always reliable in reflecting disease severity. Thus, normal serum aminotransferases in patients with hepatitis B surface antigen (HBsAg) in serum may indicate the inactive HBsAg carrier state or may reflect mild chronic hepatitis B or hepatitis B with fluctuating disease activity. Serum testing for hepatitis B e antigen and hepatitis B virus DNA can help resolve these different patterns, but these markers can also fluctuate and change over time. Similarly, in chronic hepatitis C, serum aminotransferases can be normal despite moderate activity of disease. Finally, in both alcoholic and nonalcoholic steatohepatitis, aminotransferases are quite unreliable in reflecting severity. In these conditions, liver biopsy is helpful in guiding management and recommending therapy, particularly if therapy is difficult, prolonged, and expensive as is often the case in chronic viral hepatitis. There are several well-verified numerical scales for grading activity in chronic liver disease, the most common being the histology activity index and the Ishak histology scale.

Liver biopsy is also the most accurate means of assessing stage of disease as early or advanced, precirrhotic, and cirrhotic. Staging of disease pertains largely to chronic liver diseases in which progression to cirrhosis and end-stage liver disease can occur, but which may require years or decades to develop. Clinical features, biochemical tests, and hepatic imaging studies are helpful in assessing stage but generally become abnormal only in the middle to late stages of cirrhosis. Early stages of cirrhosis are generally detectable only by liver biopsy. In assessing stage, the degree of fibrosis is usually used as its quantitative measure. The amount of fibrosis is generally staged on a 0 to 4+ (histology activity index) or 0 to 6+ scale (Ishak scale).

Cirrhosis can also be staged clinically. A reliable staging system is the modified Child-Pugh classification with a scoring system of 5 to 15: scores of 5 and 6 being Child-Pugh class A (consistent with "compensated cirrhosis"), scores of 7 to 9 indicating class B, and 10 to 15 class C (Table 292-4). This scoring system was initially devised to stratify patients into risk groups prior to undergoing portal decompressive surgery. It is now used to assess prognosis in cirrhosis and provides the standard criteria for listing for liver transplantation (Child-Pugh class B). The Child-Pugh score is a reasonably reliable predictor of survival in many liver diseases and predicts the likelihood of major complications of cirrhosis such as bleeding from varices and spontaneous bacterial peritonitis. Other means of assessing stage and survival have been developed for primary biliary cirrhosis and sclerosing cholangitis (Mayo Risk scores), which are somewhat more accurate but which actually rely mostly on the same measurements as the Child-Pugh score.

Table 292-4 Child-Pugh Classification of Cirrhosis

Factor	1	2	3
Serum bilirubin, μmol/L (mg/dL)	<34(<2.0)	34–51(2.0–3.0)	>51(>3.0)
Serum albumin, g/L(g/dL)	>35(>3.5)	30–35(3.0–3.5)	<30(<3.0)
Ascites	None	Easily controlled	Poorly controlled
Neurologic disorder	None	Minimal	Advanced coma
Prothrombin time (second prolonged) (INR)	0–4 <1.7	4–6 1.7–2.3	>6 >2.3

NOTE: The Child-Pugh score is calculated by adding the scores of the five factors and can range from 5 to 15. Child-Pugh class is either A (a score of 5 to 6), B (7 to 9), or C (10 and above). In general, "decompensation" indicates cirrhosis with a Child-Pugh score of ≥7 (Child-Pugh class B), and this level is an accepted criterion for listing for liver transplantation.

Thus, liver biopsy is helpful not only in diagnosis but also in management of chronic liver disease and assessment of prognosis. Because liver biopsy is an invasive procedure and not without complications, it should be used only when it will contribute materially to management and therapeutic decisions.

BIBLIOGRAPHY

Bacon BR, Di Biscegie AM (eds): *Liver Disease: Diagnosis and Management.* Philadelphia, Churchill Livingstone, 1999

Bellentani S et al: Prevalence of chronic liver disease in the general population of Northern Italy: The Dionysos Study. Hepatology 20:1442, 1994

Bennett WF et al: Review of hepatic imaging and a problem-oriented approach to liver masses. Hepatology 12:761, 1990

Desmet VJ et al: Classification of chronic hepatitis: Diagnosis, grading and staging. Hepatology 19:1513, 1994

Dickson ER et al: Prognosis in primary biliary cirrhosis: Model for decision making. Hepatology 10:1, 1989. Also available at www.mayo.edu/int-med/gi/model/mayomodl.htm

Ewing JA: Detecting alcoholism, the CAGE questionnaire. JAMA 252:1905, 1984

Ishak K et al: Histological grading and staging of chronic hepatitis. J Hepatol 22:696, 1995

Schiff ER et al (eds): *Schiff's Diseases of the Liver,* 8th ed. Philadelphia, Lippincott-Raven, 1999

Zakim D, Boyer TD (eds): *Hepatology: A Textbook of Liver Disease,* 3d ed. Philadelphia, Saunders, 1996

293 *Daniel S. Pratt, Marshall M. Kaplan*

EVALUATION OF LIVER FUNCTION

Several biochemical tests are useful in the evaluation and management of patients with hepatic dysfunction. These tests can be used to (1) detect the presence of liver disease; (2) distinguish among different types of liver disorders; (3) gauge the extent of known liver damage; and (4) follow the response to treatment.

Liver tests have shortcomings. They can be normal in patients with serious liver disease and abnormal in patients with diseases that do not affect the liver. Liver tests rarely suggest a specific diagnosis; rather, they suggest a general category of liver disease, such as hepatocellular or cholestatic, which then further directs the evaluation.

The liver carries out thousands of biochemical functions, most of which cannot be easily measured by blood tests. Laboratory tests measure only a limited number of these functions. In fact, many tests, such as the aminotransferases or alkaline phosphatase, do not measure liver function at all. Rather, they detect liver cell damage or interference

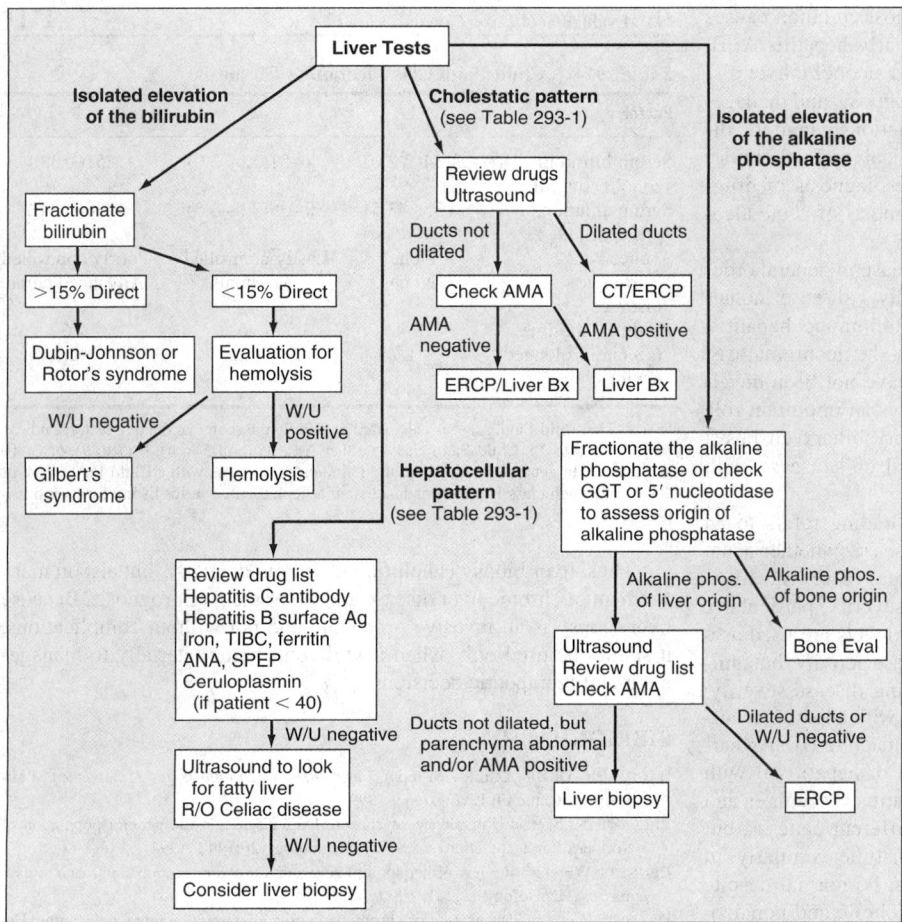

FIGURE 293-1 ERCP, endoscopic retrograde cholangiopancreatography; CT, computerized tomography; AMA, antimitochondrial antibody; ANA, antinuclear antibody; SPEP, serum protein electrophoresis; TIBC, total iron binding capacity; GGT, gamma glutamyl transpeptidase.

with bile flow. Thus, no one test enables the clinician to accurately assess the liver's total functional capacity.

To increase both the sensitivity and the specificity of laboratory tests in the detection of liver disease, it is best to use them as a battery. Those tests usually employed in clinical practice include the bilirubin, aminotransferases, alkaline phosphatase, albumin, and prothrombin time tests. When more than one of these tests provide abnormal findings, or the findings are persistently abnormal on serial determinations, the probability of liver disease is high. When all test results are normal, the probability of missing occult liver disease is low.

When evaluating patients with liver disorders, it is helpful to group these tests into general categories. The classification we have found most useful is given below.

TESTS BASED ON DETOXIFICATION AND EXCRETORY FUNCTIONS **Serum Bilirubin** Bilirubin, a breakdown product of the porphyrin ring of heme-containing proteins, is found in the blood in two fractions—conjugated and unconjugated. The *van den Bergh assay*, or a variation of it, is still used in most clinical chemistry laboratories to determine the total serum bilirubin level and what amount is conjugated or unconjugated bilirubin. In this assay, the direct fraction provides an approximate determination of the conjugated bilirubin in serum. The total serum bilirubin is the amount that reacts after the addition of alcohol. The indirect fraction is the difference between the total and the direct bilirubin and provides an estimate of the unconjugated bilirubin in serum. The unconjugated fraction, also termed the indirect fraction, is insoluble in water and is bound to albumin in the blood. The conjugated (direct) bilirubin fraction is water soluble and can therefore be excreted by the kidney. When measured by the original van den Bergh method, the normal total serum bilirubin concentration is less than 1 mg/dL. Up to 30%, or 0.3 mg/dL, of the total is direct-reacting (or conjugated) bilirubin.

Elevation of the unconjugated fraction of bilirubin is rarely due to liver disease. An isolated elevation of unconjugated bilirubin is seen primarily in hemolytic disorders and in a number of genetic conditions such as Crigler-Najjar and Gilbert's syndromes. *Gilbert's syndrome* is a common, benign condition with a reported incidence in 3 to 7% of the population. It is marked by the impaired conjugation of bilirubin due to reduced bilirubin uridine diphosphate (UDP) glucuronosyltransferase activity. This results in mild unconjugated hyperbilirubinemia, which is marked by considerable fluctuations and is sometimes only identified during periods of fasting. One molecular defect that has been identified in patients with Gilbert's syndrome is in the TATAA element in the 5' promoter region of the bilirubin UDP-glucuronosyltransferase gene upstream of exon 1. This defect alone is not necessarily sufficient for producing the clinical syndrome of Gilbert's, as there are patients who are homozygous for this defect yet do not have the levels of hyperbilirubinemia typically seen in Gilbert's syndrome. Isolated unconjugated hyperbilirubinemia (bilirubin elevated, but less than 15% direct) should prompt a workup for hemolysis (Fig. 293-1). In the absence of hemolysis, an isolated unconjugated hyperbilirubinemia can be attributed to Gilbert's syndrome and no further evaluation is required.

In contrast, conjugated hyperbilirubinemia almost always implies liver or biliary tract disease. The rate-limiting step in bilirubin metabolism is not conjugation of bilirubin, but rather the transport of conjugated bilirubin into the bile canaliculi. Thus, elevation of the conjugated fraction may be seen in any type of liver disease. In most liver diseases, both conjugated and unconjugated fractions of the bilirubin tend to be elevated. Except in the presence of a purely unconjugated hyperbilirubinemia, fractionation of the bilirubin is rarely helpful in determining the cause of jaundice.

Concern may be generated by a slower than expected decline of the serum bilirubin during convalescence from certain liver diseases. This can be attributed to the covalent binding of conjugated bilirubin to serum albumin that occurs when there is a prolonged episode of conjugated hyperbilirubinemia. The serum half-life of the albumin-bilirubin complex (15 days) is much longer than that of conjugated bilirubin and closer to that of albumin.

Urine Bilirubin Unconjugated bilirubin always binds to albumin in the serum and is not filtered by the kidney. Therefore, any bilirubin found in the urine is conjugated bilirubin; the presence of bilirubinuria implies the presence of liver disease. A urine dipstick test can theoretically give the same information as fractionation of the serum bilirubin. This test is almost 100% accurate. Phenothiazines may give a false positive reading with the Ictotest tablet.

Blood Ammonia Ammonia is produced in the body during normal protein metabolism and by intestinal bacteria, primarily those in the colon. The liver plays a role in the detoxification of ammonia by converting it to urea, which is excreted by the kidneys. Striated muscle also plays a role in detoxification of ammonia, which is combined with glutamic acid to form glutamine. Patients with advanced liver disease typically have significant muscle wasting, which likely contributes to hyperammonemia in these patients. Some physicians use the blood ammonia for detecting encephalopathy or for monitoring hepatic synthetic function, although its use for either of these indications has or the degree of acute encephalopathy and elevation of blood ammonia; it can be occasionally useful for identifying the occult liver disease in patients with mental status changes. There is also a poor correlation of the blood serum ammonia and hepatic function. The ammonia can be elevated in patients with severe portal hypertension and portal blood shunting around the liver even in the presence of normal or near normal hepatic function.

Serum Enzymes The liver contains thousands of enzymes, some of which are also present in the serum in very low concentrations. These enzymes have no known function in the serum and behave like other serum proteins. They are distributed in the plasma and in interstitial fluid and have characteristic half-lives, usually measured in days. Very little is known about the catabolism of serum enzymes, although they are probably cleared by cells in the reticuloendothelial system. The elevation of a given enzyme activity in the serum is thought to primarily reflect its increased rate of entrance into serum from damaged liver cells.

Serum enzyme tests can be grouped into three categories: (1) enzymes whose elevation in serum reflects damage to hepatocytes; (2) enzymes whose elevation in serum reflects cholestasis; and (3) enzyme tests that do not fit precisely into either pattern.

Enzymes that reflect damage to hepatocytes The aminotransferases (transaminases) are sensitive indicators of liver cell injury and are most helpful in recognizing acute hepatocellular diseases such as hepatitis. They include the aspartate aminotransferase (AST) and the alanine aminotransferase (ALT). AST is found in the liver, cardiac muscle, skeletal muscle, kidneys, brain, pancreas, lungs, leukocytes, and erythrocytes in decreasing order of concentration. ALT is found primarily in the liver. The aminotransferases are normally present in the serum in low concentrations. These enzymes are released into the blood in greater amounts when there is damage to the liver cell membrane resulting in increased permeability. Liver cell necrosis is not required for the release of the aminotransferases and there is a poor correlation between the degree of liver cell damage and the level of the aminotransferases. Thus, the absolute elevation of the aminotransferases is of no prognostic significance in acute hepatocellular disorders.

Any type of liver cell injury can cause modest elevations in the serum aminotransferases. Levels of up to 300 U/L are nonspecific and may be found in any type of liver disorder. Striking elevations—i.e., aminotransferases >1000 U/L—occur almost exclusively in disorders associated with extensive hepatocellular injury such as (1) viral hepatitis, (2) ischemic liver injury (prolonged hypotension or acute heart failure), or (3) toxin or drug-induced liver injury.

The pattern of the aminotransferase elevation can be helpful diagnostically. In most acute hepatocellular disorders, the ALT is higher than or equal to the AST. An AST:ALT ratio >2:1 is suggestive while a ratio >3:1 is highly suggestive of alcoholic liver disease. The AST in alcoholic liver disease is rarely >300 U/L and the ALT is often normal. A low level of ALT in the serum is due to an alcohol-induced deficiency of pyridoxal phosphate.

The aminotransferases are usually not greatly elevated in obstructive jaundice. One notable exception occurs during the acute phase of biliary obstruction caused by the passage of a gallstone into the common bile duct. In this setting, the aminotransferases can briefly be in the 1,000 to 2,000 U/L range. However, aminotransferase levels decrease quickly and the liver function tests rapidly evolve into one typical of cholestasis.

Enzymes that reflect cholestasis The activities of three enzymes—alkaline phosphatase, 5′-nucleotidase, and gamma glutamyl transpeptidase (GGT)—are usually elevated in cholestasis. Alkaline phosphatase and 5′-nucleotidase are found in or near the bile canalicular membrane of hepatocytes, while GGT is located in the endoplasmic reticulum and in bile duct epithelial cells. Reflecting its more diffuse localization in the liver, GGT elevation in serum is less specific for cholestasis than are elevations of alkaline phosphatase or 5′-nucleotidase. Some have advocated the use of GGT to identify patients

with occult alcohol use. Its lack of specificity makes its use in this setting questionable.

The normal serum alkaline phosphatase consists of many distinct isoenzymes found in the liver, bone, placenta, and, less commonly, small intestine. Patients over age 60 can have a mildly elevated alkaline phosphatase (1 to 1½ times normal), while individuals with blood types O and B can have an elevation of the serum alkaline phosphatase after eating a fatty meal due to the influx of intestinal alkaline phosphatase into the blood. It is also nonpathologically elevated in children and adolescents undergoing rapid bone growth because of bone alkaline phosphatase, and late in normal pregnancies due to the influx of placental alkaline phosphatase.

Elevation of liver-derived alkaline phosphatase is not totally specific for cholestasis and a less than threefold elevation can be seen in almost any type of liver disease. Alkaline phosphatase elevations greater than four times normal occur primarily in patients with cholestatic liver disorders, infiltrative liver diseases such as cancer, and bone conditions characterized by rapid bone turnover (e.g., Paget's disease). In bone diseases, the elevation is due to increased amounts of the bone isoenzymes. In liver diseases, the elevation is almost always due to increased amounts of the liver isoenzyme.

If an elevated serum alkaline phosphatase is the only abnormal finding in an apparently healthy person, or if the degree of elevation is higher than expected in the clinical setting, identification of the source of elevated isoenzymes is helpful (Fig. 293-1). This problem can be approached in several ways. First, and most precise, is the fractionation of the alkaline phosphatase by electrophoresis. The second approach is based on the observation that alkaline phosphatases from individual tissues differ in susceptibility to inactivation by heat. The finding of an elevated serum alkaline phosphatase level in a patient with a heat-stable fraction strongly suggests that the placenta or a tumor is the source of the elevated enzyme in serum. Susceptibility to inactivation by heat increases, respectively, for the intestinal, liver, and bone alkaline phosphatases, bone being by far the most sensitive. The third, best substantiated, and most available approach involves the measurement of serum 5′-nucleotidase or GGT. These enzymes are rarely elevated in conditions other than liver disease.

In the absence of jaundice or elevated aminotransferases, an elevated alkaline phosphatase of liver origin often, but not always, suggests early cholestasis and, less often, hepatic infiltration by tumor or granulomata. Other conditions that cause isolated elevations of the alkaline phosphatase include Hodgkin's disease, diabetes, hyperthyroidism, congestive heart failure, and inflammatory bowel disease.

The level of serum alkaline phosphatase elevation is not helpful in distinguishing between intrahepatic and extrahepatic cholestasis. There is essentially no difference among the values found in obstructive jaundice due to cancer, common duct stone, sclerosing cholangitis, or bile duct stricture. Values are similarly increased in patients with intrahepatic cholestasis due to drug-induced hepatitis, primary biliary cirrhosis, rejection of transplanted livers, and, rarely, alcohol-induced steatonecrosis. Values are also greatly elevated in hepatobiliary disorders seen in patients with AIDS (e.g., AIDS cholangiopathy due to cytomegalovirus or cryptosporidial infection and tuberculosis with hepatic involvement).

TESTS THAT MEASURE BIOSYNTHETIC FUNCTION OF THE LIVER **Serum Albumin** Serum albumin is synthesized exclusively by hepatocytes. Serum albumin has a long half-life: 15 to 20 days, with approximately 4% degraded per day. Because of this slow turnover, the serum albumin is not a good indicator of acute or mild hepatic dysfunction; only minimal changes in the serum albumin are seen in acute liver conditions such as viral hepatitis, drug-related hepatoxicity, and obstructive jaundice. In hepatitis, albumin levels below 3 g/dL should raise the possibility of chronic liver disease. Hypoalbuminemia is more common in chronic liver disorders such as cirrhosis and usually reflects severe liver damage and decreased albumin synthesis. One exception is the patient with ascites

Table 293-1 Liver Test Patterns in Hepatobiliary Disorders

Type of Disorder	Bilirubin	Aminotransferases	Alkaline Phosphatase	Albumin	Prothrombin Time
Hemolysis/Gilbert's syndrome	Normal to 5 mg/dl 85% due to indirect fractions No bilirubinuria	Normal	Normal	Normal	Normal
Acute hepatocellular necrosis (viral and drug hepatitis, hepatotoxins, acute heart failure)	Both fractions may be elevated Peak usually follows aminotransferases Bilirubinuria	Elevated, often >500 IU ALT >AST	Normal to <3 times normal elevation	Normal	Usually normal. If >5X above control and not corrected by parenteral vitamin K, suggests poor prognosis
Chronic hepatocellular disorders	Both fractions may be elevated Bilirubinuria	Elevated, but usually <300 IU	Normal to <3 times normal elevation	Often decreased	Often prolonged Fails to correct with parenteral vitamin K
Alcoholic hepatitis Cirrhosis	Both fractions may be elevated Bilirubinuria	AST:ALT >2 suggests alcoholic hepatitis or cirrhosis	Normal to <3 times normal elevation	Often decreased	Often prolonged Fails to correct with parenteral vitamin K
Intra- and extra-hepatic cholestasis (Obstructive jaundice)	Both fractions may be elevated Bilirubinuria	Normal to moderate elevation Rarely >500 IU	Elevated, often >4 times normal elevation	Normal, unless chronic	Normal If prolonged, will correct with parenteral vitamin K
Infiltrative diseases (tumor, granulomata); partial bile duct obstruction	Usually normal	Normal to slight elevation	Elevated, often > 4 times normal elevation Fractionate, or confirm liver origin with 5′ nucleotidase or gamma glutamyl transpeptidase	Normal	Normal

in whom synthesis may be normal or even increased, but levels are low because of the increased volume of distribution. However, hypoalbuminemia is not specific for liver disease and may occur in protein malnutrition of any cause, as well as protein-losing enteropathies, nephrotic syndrome, and chronic infections that are associated with prolonged increases in serum interleukin-1 and/or tumor necrosis factor levels that inhibit albumin synthesis. Serum albumin should not be measured for screening in patients in whom there is no suspicion of liver disease. A general medical clinic study of consecutive patients in whom no indications were present for albumin measurement showed that while 12% of patients had abnormal test results, the finding was of clinical importance in only 0.4%.

Serum Globulins Serum globulins are a group of proteins made up of gamma globulins (immunoglobulins) produced by B lymphocytes and alpha and beta globulins produced primarily in hepatocytes. Gamma globulins are increased in chronic liver disease, such as chronic hepatitis and cirrhosis. In cirrhosis, the increased serum gamma globulin concentration is due to the increased synthesis of antibodies, some of which are directed against intestinal bacteria. This occurs because the cirrhotic liver fails to clear bacterial antigens that normally reach the liver through the hepatic circulation.

Increases in the concentration of specific isotypes of gamma globulins are often helpful in the recognition of certain chronic liver diseases. Diffuse polyclonal increases in IgG levels are common in autoimmune hepatitis; increases greater than 100% should alert the clinician to this possibility. Increases in the IgM levels are common in primary biliary cirrhosis, while increases in the IgA levels occur in alcoholic liver disease.

Coagulation Factors With the exception of factor VIII, the blood clotting factors are made exclusively in hepatocytes. Their serum half-lives are much shorter than albumin, ranging from 6 hours for factor VII to 5 days for fibrinogen. Because of their rapid turnover, measurement of the clotting factors is the single best acute measure

of hepatic synthetic function and helpful in both the diagnosis and assessing the prognosis of acute parenchymal liver disease. Useful for this purpose is the *serum prothrombin time*, which collectively measures factors II, V, VII, and X. Biosynthesis of factors II, VII, IX, and X depends on vitamin K. The prothrombin time may be elevated in hepatitis and cirrhosis as well as in disorders that lead to vitamin K deficiency such as obstructive jaundice or fat malabsorption of any kind. Marked prolongation of the prothrombin time, >5 s above control and not corrected by parenteral vitamin K administration, is a poor prognostic sign in acute viral hepatitis and other acute and chronic liver diseases.

OTHER DIAGNOSTIC TESTS While tests may direct the physician to a category of liver disease, additional radiologic testing and procedures are often necessary to make the proper diagnosis, as shown in Fig. 293-1. The two most commonly-used ancillary tests are reviewed here.

Percutaneous Liver Biopsy Percutaneous biopsy of the liver is a safe procedure that can be easily performed at the bedside with local anesthesia. Liver biopsy is of proven value in the following situations: (1) hepatocellular disease of uncertain cause; (2) prolonged hepatitis with the possibility of chronic active hepatitis; (3) unexplained hepatomegaly; (4) unexplained splenomegaly; (5) hepatic filling defects by radiologic imaging; (6) fever of unknown origin; (7) staging of malignant lymphoma. Liver biopsy is most accurate in disorders causing diffuse changes throughout the liver and is subject to sampling error in focal infiltrative disorders such as hepatic metastases. Liver biopsy should not be the initial procedure in the diagnosis of cholestasis. The biliary tree should first be assessed for signs of obstruction.

Ultrasonography Ultrasonography is the first diagnostic test to use in patients whose liver tests suggest cholestasis, to look for the presence of a dilated intrahepatic or extrahepatic biliary tree, or to identify gallstones. In addition, it shows space-occupying lesions within the liver, enables the clinician to distinguish between cystic and solid masses, and helps direct percutaneous biopsies. Ultrasound with Doppler imaging can detect the patency of the portal vein, hepatic artery, and hepatic veins and determine the direction of blood flow. This is the first test ordered in patients suspected of having Budd-Chiari syndrome.

USE OF LIVER TESTS   As previously noted, the best way to increase the sensitivity and specificity of laboratory tests in the detection of liver disease is to employ a battery of tests that include the aminotransferases, alkaline phosphatase, bilirubin, albumin, and prothrombin time along with the judicious use of the other tests described in this chapter. Table 293-1 shows how patterns of liver tests can lead the clinician to a category of disease which will direct further evaluation. However, it is important to remember that no single set of liver tests will necessarily provide a diagnosis. It is often necessary to repeat these tests on several occasions over days to weeks for a diagnostic pattern to emerge. Figure 293-1 is an algorithm for the evaluation of chronically abnormal liver tests.

BIBLIOGRAPHY

BOSMA PJ et al: The genetic basis of the reduced expression of bilirubin UDP-glucoronosyltransferase 1 in Gilbert's syndrome. New Engl J Med 333:1171, 1995

BRENSILVER HL, KAPLAN MM: Significance of elevated liver alkaline phosphatase in serum. Gastroenterology 68:1556, 1975

COHEN JA, KAPLAN MM: The SGOT/SGPT ratio: an indicator of alcoholic liver disease. Dig Dis Sci 24:835, 1979

PRATT DS, KAPLAN MM: Laboratory tests, in *Schiff's Diseases of the Liver*, 8th ed, ER Schiff et al (eds). Philadelphia, Lippincott, 1999

WEISS JS et al: The clinical importance of a protein bound fraction of serum bilirubin in patients with hyperbilirubinemia. N Engl J Med 309:147, 1983

294   *Paul D. Berk, Allan W. Wolkoff*

BILIRUBIN METABOLISM AND THE HYPERBILIRUBINEMIAS

BILIRUBIN METABOLISM

SOURCES OF BILIRUBIN   Bilirubin is the end-product of the metabolic degradation of heme, the prosthetic group of hemoglobin, myoglobin, the cytochrome P450s, and various other hemoproteins. The first step in the conversion of heme to bilirubin is the stereospecific oxidative opening of the heme molecule at its α-bridge carbon by the microsomal enzyme *heme oxygenase*, resulting in the formation of equimolar quantities of carbon monoxide and of the green tetrapyrrole biliverdin. Biliverdin is then reduced by a second enzyme, biliverdin reductase, to bilirubin. Between 70 and 90% of bilirubin is derived from degradation of the hemoglobin of senescent or injured circulating red blood cells. The remainder has several sources, including hemoglobin produced during the process of ineffective erythropoiesis within the bone marrow and the turnover of nonhemoglobin hemoproteins in cells throughout the body. Degradation of red-cell hemoglobin occurs principally in the spleen but also throughout the rest of the peripheral reticuloendothelial system, including the Kupffer cells within the liver. Bilirubin produced in the periphery is transported to the liver within the plasma, where, due to its insolubility in aqueous solutions, it is tightly bound to albumin.

The anatomy of the hepatic acinus is highly specialized to facilitate the extraction of such tightly protein-bound compounds (Fig. 294-1). Cuboidal hepatocytes within the hepatic cell plates are immediately adjacent to sinusoids on two surfaces. The endothelial cells of the sinusoids are fenestrated, allowing ready exchange of plasma between the sinusoidal blood and the extracellular space of Disse and affording direct access of the bilirubin-albumin complex to the surface of the hepatocyte, which is greatly expanded by the elaboration of microvilli.

HEPATIC DISPOSITION OF BILIRUBIN   Since bilirubin is a potentially toxic waste product, hepatic handling is designed to

FIGURE 294-1   Hepatocellular bilirubin transport. Albumin-bound bilirubin in sinusoidal blood passes through endothelial cell fenestrae to reach the hepatocyte surface, entering the cell by both facilitated and simple diffusional processes. Within the cell it is bound to glutathione-S-transferases and conjugated by bilirubin-UDP-glucuronosyltransferase (UGT1A1) to mono- and diglucuronides, which are actively transported across the canalicular membrane into the bile. ALB, albumin; UCB, unconjugated bilirubin, UGT1A1, bilirubin-UDP-glucuronosyltransferase; BMG, bilirubin monoglucuronide; GST, glutathione-S-transferase; MRP2, multidrug resistance-associated protein 2; BDG, bilirubin diglucuronide; BT, proposed bilirubin transporter.

eliminate it from the body via the biliary tract. Transfer of bilirubin from blood to bile involves four distinct but interrelated steps, described below (Fig. 294-1).

Hepatocellular Uptake   Bilirubin most likely enters the hepatocyte both by a facilitated transport mechanism and by passive diffusion. While kinetic data suggest that facilitated transport is the predominant process and several putative bilirubin transporters have been identified, none has been cloned successfully. Cloned transporters such as *organic anion transport protein* (OATP) and *sodium taurocholate co-transporting polypeptide* (NTCP), which are responsible for the hepatocellular uptake of other organic substrates, including sulfobromophthalein and bile acids, specifically do not transport bilirubin. Therefore, the precise mechanism of bilirubin uptake remains to be determined.

Intracellular Binding   Having crossed the plasma membrane to enter the cell, bilirubin partitions between the lipid environment of intracellular membranes and the aqueous cytosol, in which it is kept in solution by binding as a nonsubstrate ligand to several of the glutathione-S-transferases, formerly called ligandins.

Conjugation   The aqueous insolubility of bilirubin reflects a rigid, highly ordered molecular structure in which internal hydrogen bonding involving the propionic acid carboxyl groups of one dipyrrolic half of the molecule and the imino and lactam groups of the opposite half blocks solvent access to these polar residues. When the carboxyl groups are esterified by conjugation with glucuronic acid residues, the internal hydrogen bonding is disrupted, rendering the resulting mono- and diglucuronide conjugates highly soluble in aqueous solution.

Bilirubin glucuronidation is catalyzed by a specific UDP-glucuronosyltransferase. The UDP-glucuronosyltransferases have been classified into gene families based on the degree of homology between the various protein isoforms. Those that conjugate bilirubin and certain other substrates have been designated the *UGT1* family and have been shown to be expressed from a single gene complex by alternative splicing. This gene complex contains multiple substrate-specific first exons, designated A1, A2, . . . (Fig. 294-2), each with its own promoter and each encoding the amino-terminal end of a specific isoform, as well as four common exons (exons 2 to 5) that encode the shared carboxyl-terminal end of all of the *UGT1* isoforms. The various first exons encode the specific substrate-binding sites for each isoform, while the shared exons encode common glycosylation, UDP-glucuronic acid-binding, transmembrane, and stop transfer domains. Exon

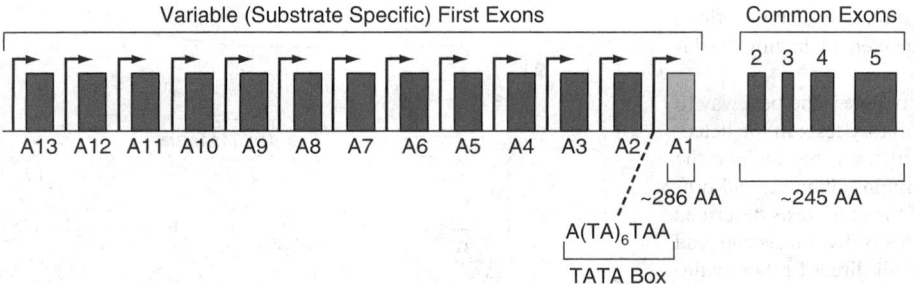

FIGURE 294-2 Structural organization of the human *UGT1* gene complex. This large complex on chromosome 2 contains at least 13 substrate-specific first exons (A1, A2, . . .), each with its own promoter, that encode the amino-terminal substrate-specific 286 amino acids of the various *UGT1* encoded isoforms, and common exons 2 to 5, that encode the 245 carboxyl-terminal amino acids common to all of the isoforms. mRNAs for specific isoforms are assembled by splicing a particular first exon such as the bilirubin-specific exon A1 to exons 2 to 5. The resulting message encodes a complete enzyme, in this particular case bilirubin-UDP-glucuronosyltransferase (UGT1A1). Mutations in a first exon affect only a single isoform. Those in exons 2 to 5 affect all enzymes encoded by the UGT1 complex.

A1 and the four common exons, collectively designated the *UGT1A1* gene (Fig. 294-2), encode the physiologically critical enzyme bilirubin-UDP-glucuronosyltransferase (UGT1A1). A critical corollary of the organization of the *UGT1* gene is that a mutation in one of the first exons will affect only a single enzyme isoform. By contrast, a mutation in exons 2 to 5 will alter all isoforms encoded by the *UGT1* gene complex.

Biliary Excretion Normal bile typically contains less than 5% unconjugated bilirubin, an average of 7% bilirubin monoconjugates, and 90% bilirubin diconjugates. The proportion of monoconjugates increases in the presence of an increased bilirubin load (hemolysis) or a reduced bilirubin-conjugating capacity. Bilirubin mono- and diglucuronides are excreted across the canalicular plasma membrane into the canaliculus by an ATP-dependent transport process mediated by a canalicular membrane protein called *multidrug resistance-associated protein 2* (MRP2). MRP2 is a member of the MRP gene family, other members of which pump certain types of drug conjugates, as well as unmodified anticancer drugs, out of cells. It is also a member of the ATP-binding cassette (ABC) superfamily. Mutations in the rat homologue of MRP2 result in conjugated hyperbilirubinemia in several jaundiced strains that serve as models of the Dubin-Johnson syndrome. It has recently been established that the Dubin-Johnson syndrome in humans also results from mutations in MRP2 (see below).

BILIRUBIN IN PLASMA Although physicians equate the direct-reacting fraction of bilirubin in plasma with conjugated bilirubin and the indirect fraction with unconjugated bilirubin, modern analytical methods document that normal plasma contains virtually no bilirubin conjugates. The 10 to 20% of bilirubin in normal plasma that gives a prompt (direct) diazo reaction is an artifact of the kinetics of the van den Bergh reaction, which, along with various modifications, is the method most commonly used to quantitate bilirubin in clinical laboratories. Indeed, when the direct-reacting fraction is less than 15% of total bilirubin at virtually any total bilirubin concentration, the bilirubin in the sample can be considered as essentially all unconjugated. The canalicular transport mechanism for excretion of bilirubin conjugates is very sensitive to injury. Accordingly, in hepatocellular disease, as well as with either cholestasis or mechanical obstruction to the bile ducts, bilirubin conjugates within the hepatocyte, prevented from taking their normal path into the canaliculi and down the bile ducts, may reflux into the bloodstream, resulting in a mixed or, less often, a truly conjugated hyperbilirubinemia.

EXTRAHEPATIC ASPECTS OF BILIRUBIN DISPOSITION **Bilirubin in the Gut** Following secretion into bile, conjugated bilirubin reaches the duodenum and passes down the gastrointestinal tract without reabsorption by the intestinal mucosa. Although some reaches the feces unaltered, an appreciable fraction is converted to urobilinogen and related compounds by bacterial metabolism within the ileum and colon. Urobilinogen is reabsorbed from these sites, reaches the liver via the portal circulation, and is reexcreted into bile, undergoing an enterohepatic circulation. Urobilinogen not taken up by the liver reaches the systemic circulation, from which some is cleared by the kidneys. Urinary urobilinogen excretion normally does not exceed 4 mg/d. In the presence of hemolysis, which increases the amount of bilirubin entering the gut (and hence the amount of urobilinogen formed and reabsorbed), or in the presence of hepatic disease, which decreases hepatic extraction of urobilinogen, plasma urobilinogen levels rise, as does the amount excreted in the urine. Severe cholestasis, bile duct obstruction, or administration of broad-spectrum antibiotics that eliminate the enteric flora required for the conversion of bilirubin to urobilinogens, markedly decrease formation of urobilinogen and its urinary excretion.

Unconjugated bilirubin ordinarily does not reach the gut except in neonates or, by ill-defined alternative pathways, in the presence of severe unconjugated hyperbilirubinemia (e.g., Crigler-Najjar syndrome type I). In these circumstances, however, unconjugated bilirubin is readily reabsorbed from the gut lumen, amplifying the underlying hyperbilirubinemia.

Renal Excretion of Bilirubin Conjugates Unconjugated bilirubin is not excreted in urine no matter how high its plasma concentration, since it is too tightly bound to albumin for effective glomerular filtration and there is no tubular mechanism for its renal secretion. By contrast, the polar bilirubin conjugates are far less tightly bound to albumin and are readily filtered at the glomerulus. Bilirubin conjugates are not secreted by the renal tubules but may be minimally reabsorbed. Since normal plasma contains virtually exclusively unconjugated bilirubin, no bilirubin normally appears in the urine. Indeed, bilirubinuria indicates the presence of conjugated bilirubin in plasma and, therefore, hepatobiliary dysfunction.

CLINICAL PHYSIOLOGY The plasma concentration of unconjugated bilirubin ([Br]) is determined by the rate at which newly synthesized bilirubin enters the plasma (plasma bilirubin turnover, BrT) and hepatic bilirubin clearance (C_{Br}), according to the following relationship:

$$[Br] = \frac{k \cdot BrT(mg/kg\ body\ weight\ per\ day)}{C_{Br}(mL/min\ per\ kg\ body\ weight)} \quad (1)$$

where k is a constant related to the different units of time employed in the conventional expression of BrT and C_{Br}. BrT closely reflects total bilirubin production; C_{Br}, analogous to the creatinine clearance test widely used to assess kidney function, is a measure of the rate at which bilirubin is extracted from plasma and is a true quantitative test of liver function. While not easily quantified in routine clinical settings, investigative measurements of BrT and C_{Br} have yielded useful pathophysiologic insights into the unconjugated hyperbilirubinemias.

Equation (1) indicates that the unconjugated bilirubin concentration will increase in the presence of either an increase in BrT or a reduction in hepatic C_{Br}. This equation therefore provides a basis for classifying unconjugated hyperbilirubinemias according to pathogenesis. Furthermore, for an individual with a given value for C_{Br}, or for a population in which C_{Br} varies within a narrow range, [Br] will increase as a linear function of BrT, with a slope relating increases in the plasma [Br] to increased BrT equal to k/C_{Br}. For individuals or populations with reduced bilirubin clearance (e.g., in Gilbert's syndrome, see below), this slope will be steeper than in normal individuals. Conversely, for a given BrT, the relationship between [Br] and

C_{Br} is hyperbolic, like the relation between serum creatinine concentration and creatinine clearance. In any patient, if C_{Br} is reduced from its baseline value, [Br] will be increased in consequence, in direct proportion to the extent of the decrease in C_{Br}.

DISORDERS OF BILIRUBIN METABOLISM LEADING TO UNCONJUGATED HYPERBILIRUBINEMIA

INCREASED BILIRUBIN PRODUCTION **Hemolysis** Increased destruction of erythrocytes leads to increased bilirubin turnover and unconjugated hyperbilirubinemia. With normal liver function, the hyperbilirubinemia is usually modest. In particular, since the bone marrow is only capable of a sustained eightfold increase in erythrocyte production in response to a hemolytic stress, hemolysis alone cannot result in a sustained hyperbilirubinemia of more than approximately 68 μmol/L (4 mg/dL). Higher values imply concomitant hepatic dysfunction.

The causes of hemolysis are numerous. Besides specific hemolytic disorders, mild hemolytic processes accompany many acquired systemic diseases. When hemolysis is the only abnormality in an otherwise healthy individual, the result is a purely unconjugated hyperbilirubinemia, with the direct-reacting fraction as measured in a typical clinical laboratory being ≤15% of the total serum bilirubin. In the presence of systemic disease, which may include a degree of hepatic dysfunction, hemolysis may produce a component of conjugated hyperbilirubinemia in addition to an elevated unconjugated bilirubin concentration.

Prolonged hemolysis may lead to the precipitation of bilirubin salts within the gall bladder or biliary tree, resulting in the formation of gallstones in which bilirubin, rather than cholesterol, is the major component. Such pigment stones may lead to acute or chronic cholecystitis, biliary obstruction, or any other biliary tract consequence of calculous disease.

Ineffective Erythropoiesis During erythroid maturation, small amounts of hemoglobin may be lost during nuclear extrusion, and a fraction of developing erythroid cells is destroyed within the marrow. These processes normally account for 10 to 15% of bilirubin produced. In various disorders, including thalassemia major, frankly megaloblastic anemias due to folate or vitamin B_{12} deficiency, congenital erythropoietic porphyria, lead poisoning, and various congenital and acquired dyserythropoietic anemias, the fraction of total bilirubin production derived from ineffective erythropoiesis is increased, reaching as much as 70% of the total, and may be sufficient to produce modest degrees of unconjugated hyperbilirubinemia.

Miscellaneous Degradation of the hemoglobin of extravascular collections of erythrocytes, such as those seen in massive tissue infarctions or large hematomas, may lead transiently to unconjugated hyperbilirubinemia.

DECREASED HEPATIC BILIRUBIN CLEARANCE **Decreased Hepatic Uptake** As noted above, the mechanisms by which bilirubin enters hepatocytes are not fully defined but probably include both diffusion and facilitated transport. Decreased hepatic bilirubin uptake is believed to contribute to the unconjugated hyperbilirubinemia of Gilbert's syndrome (GS), although the molecular basis for this finding remains unclear (see below). Several drugs, including flavispidic acid, novobiocin, and various cholecystographic contrast agents, have been reported to inhibit bilirubin uptake. The resulting unconjugated hyperbilirubinemia resolves with cessation of the medication.

Impaired Conjugation • *Physiologic neonatal jaundice* Bilirubin produced by the fetus is cleared by the placenta and eliminated by the maternal liver. Consequently, bilirubin concentrations in normal neonates at birth are low. The presence of jaundice at birth is pathologic and requires investigation. Immediately after birth, the neonatal liver must assume responsibility for bilirubin clearance and excretion. However, many aspects of hepatic physiology are incompletely developed at birth. Levels of UGT1A1 are low, and alternative pathways allow passage of unconjugated bilirubin into the gut. Since the intes-

tinal flora that converts bilirubin to urobilinogen is also undeveloped, an enterohepatic circulation of unconjugated bilirubin ensues. In consequence, most neonates develop mild unconjugated hyperbilirubinemia between days 2 and 5 after birth. Peak levels are typically less than 85 to 170 μmol/L (5 to 10 mg/dL) and decline to normal adult concentrations within 2 weeks, as mechanisms required for bilirubin disposition mature.

Prematurity, with more profound immaturity of hepatic function, or hemolysis, such as occurs with erythroblastosis fetalis, results in higher levels of unconjugated hyperbilirubinemia. A rapidly rising unconjugated bilirubin concentration, or absolute levels in excess of 340 μmol/L (20 mg/dL), puts the infant at risk for bilirubin encephalopathy, or *kernicterus*, in which bilirubin crosses an immature blood-brain barrier and precipitates in the basal ganglia and other areas of the brain. The consequences range from appreciable neurologic deficits to death. Principal treatment options include phototherapy, which converts bilirubin into photoisomers that are soluble in aqueous media and readily excretable in bile without conjugation, and exchange transfusion.

The canalicular mechanisms responsible for bilirubin excretion are also immature at birth, and their maturation may, on occasion, lag behind that of UGT1A1. This may lead to transient conjugated neonatal hyperbilirubinemia, especially in infants with hemolysis.

Acquired conjugation defects A modest reduction in bilirubin-conjugating capacity may be observed in advanced hepatitis or cirrhosis. However, in this setting, conjugation is better preserved than other aspects of bilirubin disposition, such as canalicular excretion. Various drugs, including pregnanediol, novobiocin, chloramphenicol, and gentamicin, may produce unconjugated hyperbilirubinemia by inhibiting UGT1A1 activity. Finally, certain fatty acids and the progestational steroid $3\alpha,20\beta$-pregnanediol, identified in the breast milk but not the serum of mothers whose infants have excessive neonatal hyperbilirubinemia (*breast milk jaundice*), inhibit bilirubin conjugation. The pathogenesis of breast milk jaundice appears to differ from that of transient familial neonatal hyperbilirubinemia (Lucey-Driscoll syndrome), in which a UGT1A1 inhibitor is found in maternal serum.

HEREDITARY DEFECTS IN BILIRUBIN CONJUGATION Three familial disorders characterized by differing degrees of unconjugated hyperbilirubinemia have long been recognized. The defining clinical features of each are described below (Table 294-1). While these disorders have been recognized for decades to reflect differing degrees of deficiency in the ability to conjugate bilirubin, recent advances in the molecular biology of the *UGT1* gene complex have elucidated their interrelationships and clarified previously puzzling features.

Crigler-Najjar Syndrome, Type I (CN-I) This disorder is characterized by striking unconjugated hyperbilirubinemia of about 340 to 765 μmol/L (20 to 45 mg/dL) that appears in the neonatal period and persists for life. Other conventional hepatic biochemical tests such as serum aminotransferases and alkaline phosphatase are normal, and there is no evidence of hemolysis. Hepatic histology is also essentially normal except for the occasional presence of bile plugs within canaliculi.

Bilirubin glucuronides are markedly reduced or absent from the nearly colorless bile, and there is no detectable constitutive expression of UGT1A1 activity in hepatic tissue. Neither UGT1A1 activity nor the serum bilirubin concentration responds to administration of phenobarbital or other enzyme inducers. In the absence of conjugation, unconjugated bilirubin accumulates in plasma, from which it is eliminated very slowly by alternative pathways that include direct passage into the bile and small intestine. These account for the small amounts of urobilinogen found in feces. No bilirubin is found in the urine.

First described in 1952, the disorder is rare (estimated prevalence of 0.6 to 1.0 per million). Many patients are from geographically or socially isolated communities in which consanguinity is common, and pedigree analyses suggest an autosomal recessive pattern of inheritance. The majority of patients (type IA) exhibit defects in the glu-

| Feature | Crigler-Najjar Syndrome | | Gilbert's Syndrome |
	Type I	Type II	
Total serum bilirubin, μmol/L [mg/dL]	310–755 (usually >345) [18–45 (usually >20)]	100–430 (usually ≤345) [6–25 (usually ≤20)]	Typically ≤70 μmol/L [≤4 mg/dL] in absence of fasting or hemolysis
Routine liver tests	Normal	Normal	Normal
Response to phenobarbital	None	Decreases bilirubin by >25%	Decreases bilirubin to normal
Kernicterus	Usual	Rare	No
Hepatic histology	Normal	Normal	Usually normal; increased lipofuscin pigment in some
Bile characteristics			
Color:	Pale or colorless	Pigmented	Normal dark color
Bilirubin fractions:	>90% unconjugated	Largest fraction (mean:57%) monoconjugates	Mainly diconjugates but monoconjugates increased (mean 23%)
Bilirubin UDP-glucuronosyltransferase activity	Typically absent; traces in some patients.	Markedly reduced: 0 to 10% of normal	Reduced: typically 10–33% of normal
Inheritance (all autosomal)	Recessive	Predominantly recessive	Promoter mutation: recessive Missense mutations: 7 of 8 dominant; 1 reportedly recessive

curonide conjugation of a spectrum of substrates in addition to bilirubin, including various drugs and other xenobiotics. These individuals have mutations in one of the common exons (2 to 5) of the *UGT1* gene (Fig. 294-2). In a smaller subset (type IB), the defect is limited largely to bilirubin conjugation, and the causative mutation is in the bilirubin-specific exon A1. More than 30 different *UGT1A1* mutations responsible for CN-I have been identified, including deletions, frameshifts, alterations in intronic splice donor and acceptor sites, and point mutations that introduce premature stop codons or alter critical aminoacids. Their common feature is that they all encode proteins with absent or, at most, traces of bilirubin-UDP-glucuronosyltransferase enzymatic activity.

Prior to the availability of phototherapy, most patients with CN-I died of bilirubin encephalopathy (kernicterus) in infancy or early childhood. A few lived as long as early adult life without overt neurologic damage, although more subtle testing usually indicated mild but progressive brain damage. In all such cases, in the absence of liver transplantation, death eventually supervened from late-onset bilirubin encephalopathy, which often followed a nonspecific febrile illness. Recent data suggest that the best hope for survival of a neurologically intact patient involves the following regimen: (1) about 12 h/d of phototherapy from birth throughout childhood, perhaps supplemented by exchange transfusion in the immediate neonatal period; (2) use of tinprotoporphyrin to blunt transient episodes of increased hyperbilirubinemia; and (3) early liver transplantation, prior to the onset of brain damage. In a single patient, transplantation with isolated allogeneic hepatocytes produced a clinically significant reduction in serum bilirubin concentration.

Crigler-Najjar Syndrome, Type II (CN-II)   Characterized by marked unconjugated hyperbilirubinemia in the absence of abnormalities of other conventional hepatic biochemical tests, hepatic histology, or hemolysis, this condition was recognized as a distinct entity in 1962. It differs from CN-I in several specific ways (Table 294-1). (1) Although there is considerable overlap, average bilirubin concentrations are lower in CN-II; (2) accordingly, CN-II is only infrequently associated with kernicterus; (3) bile is deeply colored and bilirubin glucuronides are present, with a striking, characteristic increase in monoglucuronides; (4) UGT1A1 in liver is usually present at reduced levels (typically ≤10% of normal) but may be undetectable by less sensitive older assays; (5) while typically detected in infancy, hyperbilirubinemia was not recognized in some cases until later in life, and in one instance, until age 34. As with CN-I, most CN-II cases exhibit abnormalities in the conjugation of other compounds, such as salicylamide and menthol, but in some instances the defect appears limited to bilirubin.

Reduction of serum bilirubin concentrations by more than 25% in response to enzyme inducers such as phenobarbital distinguishes CN-II from CN-I, although this response may not be elicited in early infancy and often is not accompanied by measurable UGT1A1 induction. Bilirubin concentrations during phenobarbital administration do not return to normal but are typically in the range of 51 to 86 μmol/L (3 to 5 mg/dL). Although the incidence of kernicterus in CN-II is low, instances have occurred, not only in infants but in adolescents and adults, often in the setting of an intercurrent illness, fasting, or any other factor that temporarily raises the serum bilirubin concentration above baseline. For this reason, phenobarbital therapy is widely recommended, a single bedtime dose often sufficing to maintain clinically safe plasma bilirubin concentrations.

At least 10 different mutations of *UGT1* associated with CN-II have been identified. Their common feature is that they encode for a bilirubin-UDP-glucuronosyltransferase with markedly reduced but detectable enzymatic activity. The spectrum of residual enzyme activity explains the spectrum of phenotypic severity of the resulting hyperbilirubinemia. Molecular analysis has established that a large majority of CN-II patients are either homozygotes or compound heterozygotes for CN-II mutations and that individuals carrying one mutated and one entirely normal allele have normal bilirubin concentrations. Possible inheritance in one case as a dominant negative mutation remains to be confirmed.

Gilbert's Syndrome   This syndrome is characterized by mild unconjugated hyperbilirubinemia, normal values for standard hepatic biochemical tests, and normal hepatic histology other than a modest increase of lipofuscin pigment in some patients. Serum bilirubin concentrations are most often <51 μmol/L (<3 mg/dL), although both higher and lower values are frequent. The spectrum of hyperbilirubinemia fades into that of CN-II at serum bilirubin concentrations of 86 to 136 μmol/L (5 to 8 mg/dL). At the other end of the scale, the distinction between mild cases of GS and a normal state is often blurred. Bilirubin concentrations may fluctuate substantially in any given individual, and at least 25% of patients will exhibit temporarily normal values during prolonged follow-up. More elevated values are associated with stress, fatigue, alcohol use, reduced caloric intake, and intercurrent illness, while increased caloric intake or administration of enzyme-inducing agents produce lower bilirubin levels. GS is most often diagnosed at or shortly after puberty or in adult life during routine examinations that include multichannel biochemical analyses.

UGT1A1 activity is typically reduced to 10 to 35% of normal, and bile pigments in bile exhibit a characteristic increase in bilirubin monoglucuronides. Studies of radiobilirubin kinetics indicate that hepatic bilirubin clearance is reduced to an average of one-third of normal. Administration of phenobarbital normalizes both the serum bilirubin concentration and hepatic bilirubin clearance. However, failure of UGT1A1 activity to improve in many such instances suggests the pos-bilirubin kinetic data suggests that GS patients have a defect in bilirubin uptake as well as in conjugation. Defect(s) in the hepatic uptake of other organic anions that at least partially share an uptake mechanism with bilirubin, such as sulfobromophthalein and indocyanine green, are observed in some, but not all, patients. The disposition of bile acids, which do not utilize the bilirubin uptake mechanism, is normal.

The magnitude of changes in the plasma bilirubin concentration induced by provocation tests such as 48 h of fasting or the intravenous administration of nicotinic acid have been reported to be of help in separating GS patients from normal individuals. Other studies dispute this assertion. Moreover, on theoretical grounds, the results of such studies should provide no more information than simple measurements of the baseline plasma bilirubin concentration.

Family studies indicate that GS and hereditary hemolytic anemias such as hereditary spherocytosis, glucose-6-phosphate dehydrogenase deficiency, and β-thalassemia trait sort independently. Reports of hemolysis in up to 50% of GS patients are believed to reflect better case finding, since patients with both GS and hemolysis have higher bilirubin concentrations, and are more likely to be jaundiced, than patients with either defect alone.

GS is common, with many series placing its prevalence at 8% or more. Males predominate over females by reported ratios ranging from 1.5:1 to more than 7:1. However, these ratios may have a large artifactual component since normal males have higher mean bilirubin levels than normal females, but the diagnosis of GS is often based on comparison to normal ranges established in men. The high prevalence of GS in the general population may explain the reported frequency of mild unconjugated hyperbilirubinemia in liver transplant recipients.

The disposition of most xenobiotics metabolized by glucuronidation appears to be normal in GS, as is oxidative drug metabolism in the majority of reported studies. The principal exception is the metabolism of the anti-tumor agent irinotecan (CPT-11). Its active metabolite (SN-38) is glucuronidated specifically by bilirubin-UDP-glucuronosyltransferase. Administration of CPT-11 to patients with GS has resulted in several toxicities, including intractable diarrhea and myelosuppression. Some reports also suggest abnormal disposition of menthol, estradiol benzoate, acetaminophen, tolbutamide, and rifamycin SV. Although some of these studies have been disputed, and there have been no reports of clinical complications from use of these agents in GS, prudence should be exercised in prescribing them, or any agents metabolized primarily by glucuronidation, in this condition.

Most older pedigree studies of GS were consistent with autosomal dominant inheritance with variable expressivity. However, studies of the *UGT1* gene in GS have indicated a variety of molecular genetic bases for the phenotypic picture and several different patterns of inheritance. Studies in European and U.S. patients found that the majority of GS patients had normal coding regions for UGT1A1 but were homozygous for an abnormality consisting of an extra TA (i.e., A[TA]$_7$TAA rather than A[TA]$_6$TAA) in the promoter region of the first exon. This appeared to be a necessary but not a sufficient genetic basis for clinically expressed GS, since 15% of normal controls were also homozygous for this variant. While normal by standard criteria, these individuals had somewhat higher bilirubin concentrations than the rest of the controls studied. Heterozygotes for this abnormality had bilirubin concentrations identical to those homozygous for the A[TA]$_6$TAA allele. The prevalence of the A[TA]$_7$TAA allele in a general western population is 30%, in which case 9% would be homozygotes. This is slightly higher than the prevalence of GS based on purely phenotypic parameters. It was suggested that additional variables, such as mild hemolysis or a defect in bilirubin uptake, might be among the factors enhancing phenotypic expression of the defect. Phenotypic expression of GS due solely to the A[TA]$_7$TAA promoter abnormality is inherited as an autosomal recessive trait.

A number of CN-II kindreds have been identified in which there is also an allele containing a normal coding region but the A[TA]$_7$TAA

promoter abnormality. CN-II heterozygotes who have the A[TA]$_6$TAA promoter are phenotypically normal, whereas those with the A[TA]$_7$TAA promoter express the phenotypic picture of GS. GS in such kindreds may also result from homozygosity for the A[TA]$_7$TAA promoter abnormality.

Seven different missense mutations in the *UGT1* gene that reportedly cause GS with dominant inheritance have been found in Japanese individuals. Another Japanese patient with mild unconjugated hyperbilirubinemia was homozygous for a missense mutation in exon 5. GS in her family appeared to be recessive. Missense mutations causing GS have not been reported outside of Japan.

DISORDERS OF BILIRUBIN METABOLISM LEADING TO MIXED OR PREDOMINANTLY CONJUGATED HYPERBILIRUBINEMIA

In hyperbilirubinemia due to acquired liver disease (e.g., acute hepatitis, common bile duct stone), there are usually elevations in the serum concentrations of both conjugated and unconjugated bilirubin. Although biliary tract obstruction or hepatocellular cholestatic injury may present on occasion with a predominantly conjugated hyperbilirubinemia, it is generally not possible to differentiate intrahepatic from extrahepatic causes of jaundice based upon the serum levels or relative proportions of unconjugated and conjugated bilirubin. The major reason for determining the amounts of conjugated and unconjugated bilirubin in the serum is for the initial differentiation of hepatic parenchymal and obstructive disorders (mixed conjugated and unconjugated hyperbilirubinemia) from the inheritable and hemolytic disorders discussed above that are associated with unconjugated hyperbilirubinemia.

FAMILIAL DEFECTS IN HEPATIC EXCRETORY FUNCTION Dubin-Johnson Syndrome This benign, relatively rare disorder is characterized by low-grade, predominantly conjugated hyperbilirubinemia. Total bilirubin concentrations are typically between 34 and 85 μmol/L (2 and 5 mg/dL) but on occasion can be in the normal range or as high as 340 to 430 μmol/L (20 to 25 mg/dL) and can fluctuate widely in any given patient. The degree of hyperbilirubinemia may be increased by intercurrent illness, oral contraceptive use, and pregnancy. As the hyperbilirubinemia is due to a predominant rise in conjugated bilirubin, bilirubinuria is characteristically present. Aside from elevated serum bilirubin levels, other routine laboratory tests are normal. Physical examination is usually normal except for jaundice, although an occasional patient may have hepatosplenomegaly.

Patients with Dubin-Johnson syndrome are usually asymptomatic, although some may have vague constitutional symptoms. These latter patients have usually undergone extensive and often unnecessary diagnostic examinations for unexplained jaundice and have high levels of anxiety. In women, the condition may be subclinical until the patient becomes pregnant or receives oral contraceptives, at which time chemical hyperbilirubinemia becomes frank jaundice. Even in these situations, other routine liver function tests, including serum alkaline phosphatase and transaminase activities, are normal.

A cardinal feature of Dubin-Johnson syndrome is the accumulation in the lysosomes of centrilobular hepatocytes of dark, coarsely granular pigment. As a result, the liver may be grossly black in appearance. This pigment is thought to be derived from epinephrine metabolites that are not excreted normally. The pigment may disappear during bouts of viral hepatitis, only to reaccumulate slowly after recovery.

Biliary excretion of a number of anionic compounds is compromised in Dubin-Johnson syndrome. These include various cholecystographic agents, as well as sulfobromophthalein (Bromsulphalein, BSP), a synthetic dye formerly used in a test of liver function. In this test, the rate of disappearance of BSP from plasma was determined following bolus intravenous administration. BSP is conjugated with glutathione in the hepatocyte; the resulting conjugate is normally excreted rapidly into the canaliculus. Patients with Dubin-Johnson syndrome exhibit a characteristic rise in its plasma concentration at 90 min after injection, due to reflux of conjugated BSP into the circulation from the hepatocyte. Dyes such as indocyanine green (ICG) that are taken up by hepatocytes but are not further metabolized prior to biliary excretion do not show this reflux phenomenon. Continuous BSP infusion studies suggest a reduction in the t_{max} for biliary excretion. Bile acid disposition, including hepatocellular uptake and biliary excretion, are normal in Dubin-Johnson syndrome. These patients have normal serum and biliary bile acid concentrations and do not have pruritus.

By analogy with findings in several mutant rat strains, the selective defect in biliary excretion of bilirubin conjugates and certain other classes of organic compounds, but not of bile acids, that characterizes the Dubin-Johnson syndrome was found to reflect defective expression of MRP2, an ATP-dependent canalicular membrane transporter. Several different mutations in the *MRP2* gene produce the Dubin-Johnson phenotype, which has an autosomal recessive pattern of inheritance. Although MRP2 is undoubtedly important in the biliary excretion of conjugated bilirubin, the fact that this pigment is still excreted in the absence of MRP2 suggests that other, as yet uncharacterized, transport proteins may serve in a secondary role in this process.

Patients with Dubin-Johnson syndrome also have a diagnostic abnormality in urinary coproporphyrin excretion. There are two naturally occurring coproporphyrin isomers, I and III. Normally, approximately 75% of the coproporphyrin in urine is isomer III. In urine from Dubin-Johnson syndrome patients, total coproporphyrin content is normal, but more than 80% is isomer I. Heterozygotes for the syndrome show an intermediate pattern. The molecular basis for this phenomenon remains unclear.

Rotor Syndrome   This benign, autosomal recessive disorder is clinically similar to the Dubin-Johnson syndrome, although it is seen even less frequently. A major phenotypic difference is that the liver in patients with Rotor syndrome has no increased pigmentation and appears totally normal. The only abnormality in routine laboratory tests is an elevation of total serum bilirubin, due to a predominant rise in conjugated bilirubin. This is accompanied by bilirubinuria. Several additional features differentiate Rotor and Dubin-Johnson syndromes. In Rotor syndrome, the gallbladder is usually visualized on oral cholecystography, in contrast to the nonvisualization that is typical of Dubin-Johnson syndrome. The pattern of urinary coproporphyrin excretion also differs. The pattern in Rotor syndrome resembles that of many acquired disorders of hepatobiliary function, in which coproporphyrin I, the major coproporphyrin isomer in bile, refluxes from the hepatocyte back into the circulation and is excreted in urine. Thus, total urinary coproporphyrin excretion is substantially increased in Rotor syndrome, in contrast to the normal levels seen in Dubin-Johnson syndrome. Although the fraction of coproporphyrin I in urine is elevated, it is usually less than 70% of the total, as compared to 80% or more in Dubin-Johnson syndrome. The disorders also can be distinguished by their patterns of BSP excretion. Although clearance of BSP from plasma is delayed in Rotor syndrome, there is no reflux of conjugated BSP back into the circulation as seen in Dubin-Johnson syndrome. Kinetic analysis of plasma BSP infusion studies suggests the presence of a defect in intrahepatocellular storage of this compound. This has never been demonstrated directly, and the molecular basis of Rotor syndrome remains unknown.

Benign Recurrent Intrahepatic Cholestasis (BRIC)   This rare disorder is characterized by recurrent attacks of pruritus and jaundice. The typical episode begins with mild malaise and elevations in serum aminotransferase levels, followed rapidly by rises in alkaline phosphatase and bilirubin and onset of jaundice and itching. The first one or two episodes may be misdiagnosed as acute viral hepatitis. The cholestatic episodes, which may begin in childhood or adulthood, can vary in duration from several weeks to months, following which there is complete clinical and biochemical resolution. Intervals between attacks may vary from several months to years. Between episodes, physical examination is normal, as are serum levels of bile acids, bilirubin, transaminases, and alkaline phosphatase. The disorder is familial and has an autosomal recessive pattern of inheritance. BRIC is considered a benign disorder in that it does not lead to cirrhosis or end-stage liver disease. However, the episodes of jaundice and pruritus can be prolonged and debilitating, and some patients have undergone liver transplantation to relieve the intractable and disabling symptoms. Treatment during the cholestatic episodes is symptomatic; there is no specific treatment to prevent or shorten the occurrence of episodes.

A gene termed *FIC1* was recently identified and found to be mutated in patients with BRIC. Curiously, this gene is expressed strongly in the small intestine but only weakly in the liver. The protein encoded by *FIC1* shows little similarity to genes that have been shown to play a role in bile canalicular excretion of various compounds. Rather, it appears to be a member of a P-type ATPase family that transports aminophospholipids from the outer to the inner leaflet of a variety of cell membranes.

Progressive Familial Intrahepatic Cholestasis (FIC)   This name is applied to three phenotypically related syndromes. Progressive FIC type 1 (Byler disease) presents in early infancy as cholestasis that may be initially episodic. However, in contrast to BRIC, Byler disease progresses to malnutrition, growth retardation, and end-stage liver disease during childhood. This disorder is also a consequence of an FIC1 mutation. The functional relationship of the *FIC1* protein to the pathogenesis of cholestasis in these disorders is unknown. Two other types of progressive FIC (types 2 and 3) have been described. Type 2 is associated with a mutation in the protein named *sister of p-glycoprotein*, which is the major bile canalicular exporter of bile acids. Type 3 has been associated with a mutation of MDR3, a protein that is essential for normal bile canalicular excretion of phospholipids. Although all three types of progressive FIC have similar clinical phenotypes, only type 3 is associated with high serum levels of γ-glutamyltransferase activity. In contrast, activity of this enzyme is normal or only mildly elevated in symptomatic BRIC and progressive FIC types 1 and 2.

BIBLIOGRAPHY

AONO S et al: Analysis of genes for bilirubin UDP-glucuronosyltransferase in Gilbert's syndrome. Lancet 345:959, 1995

BERK PD, NOYER C: Bilirubin metabolism and the hereditary hyperbilirubinemias. Semin in Liver Dis 14:323, 1994

BOSMA P et al: The genetic basis of the reduced expression of bilirubin-UDP-glucuronosyltransferase 1 in Gilbert's syndrome. N Engl J Med 333:1171, 1995

CLARKE DJ et al: Genetic defects of the UDP-glucuronosyltransferase 1 (*UGT1*) gene that cause familial non-haemolytic unconjugated hyperbilirubinaemias. Clin Chim Acta 266:63, 1997

IYANAGI T et al: Biochemical and molecular aspects of genetic disorders of bilirubin metabolism. Biochim Biophys Acta 1407:173, 1998

KARTENBECK J et al: Absence of the canalicular isoform of the *MRP* gene-encoded conjugate export pump from the hepatocytes in the Dubin-Johnson syndrome. Hepatology 23:1061, 1996

PAULUSMA CC et al: A mutation in the human canalicular multispecific organic anion transporter gene causes the Dubin-Johnson syndrome. Hepatology 25:1539, 1997

ROY CHOWDHURY J et al: Hereditary jaundice and disorders of bilirubin metabolism, in *The Metabolic and Molecular Bases of Inherited Disease*, 7th ed. CR Scriver et al (eds.) New York, McGraw-Hill, 1995, pp 2161–2208

ROY CHOWDHURY J et al: Bilirubin metabolism and its disorders, in *Hepatology*, 3d ed. D Zakim, T Boyer (eds.) Philadelphia, Saunders, 1996, pp 323–347

SEPPEN J et al: Discrimination between Crigler-Najjar type I and II by expression of mutant bilirubin uridine diphosphate-glucuronosyltransferase. J Clin Invest 94:2385, 1994

VAN DER VEERE CN et al: Current therapy for Crigler-Najjar syndrome Type 1: Report of a world registry. Hepatology 24:311, 1996

ACUTE VIRAL HEPATITIS

ALT	alanine aminotransferase	HBV	hepatitis B virus
AST	aspartate aminotransferase	HBxAg	hepatitis B x antigen
bDNA	branched-chain	HCV	hepatitis C virus
	complementary DNA	HDV	hepatitis D virus
ELU	enzyme-linked immunoassay	HEV	hepatitis E virus
	units	IG	immune globulin
EMC	essential mixed	LKM	liver-kidney microsomes
	cryoglobulinemia	NS	nonstructural
HAV	hepatitis A virus	PCR	polymerase chain reaction
HBcAg	hepatitis B core antigen	PT	prothrombin time
HBeAg	hepatitis B e antigen	RIBA	recombinant immunoblot
HBIG	hepatitis B immune globulin		assay
HBsAg	hepatitis B surface antigen		

Acute viral hepatitis is a systemic infection affecting the liver predominantly. Almost all cases of acute viral hepatitis are caused by one of five viral agents: hepatitis A virus (HAV), hepatitis B virus (HBV), hepatitis C virus (HCV), the HBV-associated delta agent or hepatitis D virus (HDV), and hepatitis E virus (HEV). Other transfusion-transmitted agents, e.g., "hepatitis G" virus and "TT" virus, have been identified but do not cause hepatitis. All these human hepatitis viruses are RNA viruses, except for hepatitis B, which is a DNA virus. Although these agents can be distinguished by their molecular and antigenic properties, all types of viral hepatitis produce clinically similar illnesses. These range from asymptomatic and inapparent to fulminant and fatal acute infections common to all types, on the one hand, and from subclinical persistent infections to rapidly progressive chronic liver disease with cirrhosis and even hepatocellular carcinoma, common to the bloodborne types (HBV, HCV, and HDV), on the other.

VIROLOGY AND ETIOLOGY **Hepatitis A** Hepatitis A virus is a nonenveloped 27-nm, heat-, acid-, and ether-resistant RNA virus in the hepatovirus genus of the picornavirus family (Fig. 295-1). Its virion contains four capsid polypeptides, designated VP1 to VP4, which are cleaved posttranslationally from the polyprotein product of a 7500-nucleotide genome. Inactivation of viral activity can be achieved by boiling for 1 min, by contact with formaldehyde and chlorine, or by ultraviolet irradiation. Despite nucleotide sequence variation of up to 20% among isolates of HAV, all strains of this virus are immunologically indistinguishable and belong to one serotype. Hepatitis A has an incubation period of approximately 4 weeks. Its replication is limited to the liver, but the virus is present in the liver, bile, stools, and blood during the late incubation period and acute preicteric phase of illness. Despite persistence of virus in the liver, viral shedding in feces, viremia, and infectivity diminish rapidly once jaundice becomes apparent. HAV is the only one of the human hepatitis viruses that can be cultivated reproducibly in vitro.

Antibodies to HAV (anti-HAV) can be detected during acute illness when serum aminotransferase activity is elevated and fecal HAV shedding is still occurring. This early antibody response is predominantly of the IgM class and persists for several months, rarely for 6 to 12 months. During convalescence, however, anti-HAV of the IgG class becomes the predominant antibody (Fig. 295-2). Therefore, the diagnosis of hepatitis A is made during acute illness by demonstrating anti-HAV of the IgM class. After acute illness, anti-HAV of the IgG class remains detectable indefinitely, and patients with serum anti-HAV are im-

mune to reinfection. Neutralizing antibody activity parallels the appearance of anti-HAV, and the IgG anti-HAV present in immune globulin accounts for the protection it affords against HAV infection.

Hepatitis B Hepatitis B virus is a DNA virus with a remarkably compact genomic structure; despite its small, circular, 3200-basepair size, HBV DNA codes for four sets of viral products and has a complex, multiparticle structure. HBV achieves its genomic economy by relying on an efficient strategy of encoding proteins from four overlapping genes: S, C, P, and X (Fig. 295-3), as detailed below. Once thought to be unique among viruses, HBV is now recognized as one of a family of animal viruses, hepadnaviruses (hepatotropic DNA viruses), and is classified as hepadnavirus type 1. Similar viruses infect certain species of woodchucks, ground and tree squirrels, and Pekin ducks, to mention the most carefully characterized. Like HBV, all have the same distinctive three morphologic forms, have counterparts to the envelope and nucleocapsid virus antigens of HBV, replicate in the liver but exist in extrahepatic sites, contain their own endogenous DNA polymerase, have partially double-stranded and partially single-stranded genomes, are associated with acute and chronic hepatitis and hepatocellular carcinoma, and rely on a replicative strategy unique among DNA viruses but typical of retroviruses. Instead of DNA replication directly from a DNA template, hepadnaviruses rely on reverse transcription (effected by the DNA polymerase) of minus-strand DNA from a "pregenomic" RNA intermediate. Then plus-strand DNA is transcribed from the minus-strand DNA template by the DNA-dependent DNA polymerase. Viral proteins are translated by the pregenomic RNA, and the proteins and genome are packaged into virions and secreted from the hepatocyte. Although HBV is difficult to cultivate in vitro in the conventional sense from clinical material, several cell lines have been transfected with HBV DNA. Such transfected cells support in vitro replication of the intact virus and its component proteins.

Viral proteins and particles Three particulate forms of HBV (Table 295-1) can be demonstrated by electron microscopy (Fig. 295-1). The most numerous are the 22-nm particles, which appear as spherical or long filamentous forms; these are antigenically indistinguishable from the outer surface or envelope protein of HBV and are thought to represent excess viral envelope protein. Outnumbered in serum by a factor of 100 or 1000 to 1 compared with the spheres and tubules are large, 42-nm, double-shelled spherical particles, which represent the intact hepatitis B virion. The envelope protein expressed on the outer surface of the virion and on the smaller spherical and tubular structures is referred to as *hepatitis B surface antigen* (HBsAg). The concentration of HBsAg and virus particles in the blood may reach 500 μg/mL and 10 trillion particles per milliliter, respectively. The envelope protein, HBsAg, is the product of the S gene of HBV.

FIGURE 295-1 *A.* Electron micrograph of 27-nm hepatitis A virus particles purified from stool of a patient with acute hepatitis A virus infection and aggregated by hepatitis A antibody. *B.* Electron micrograph of concentrated serum from a patient with hepatitis B infection, demonstrating the 42-nm virions, tubular forms, and spherical 22-nm particles of hepatitis B surface antigen. 132,000×. (Hepatitis D resembles 42-nm virions of hepatitis B but is smaller, 35 to 37 nm; hepatitis E resembles hepatitis A virus but is slightly larger, 32 to 34 nm; hepatitis C has not been visualized definitively.)

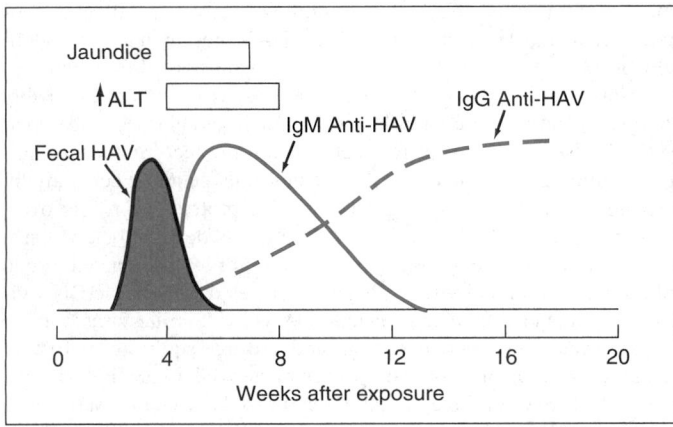

FIGURE 295-2   Scheme of typical clinical and laboratory features of viral hepatitis A.

A number of different HBsAg subdeterminants have been identified. There is a common group-reactive antigen, *a*, shared by all HBsAg isolates. In addition, HBsAg may contain one of several subtype-specific antigens, namely, *d* or *y*, *w* or *r*, as well as other more recently characterized specificities. Hepatitis B isolates fall into one of at least eight subtypes and six genotypes (A–F); however, clinical course and outcome are independent of subtype and genotype [except for an increase in "precore" mutations (see below) in certain genotypes].

Upstream of the S gene are the pre-S genes (Fig. 295-3), which code for pre-S gene products, including receptors on the HBV surface for polymerized human serum albumin and for hepatocyte membrane proteins. The pre-S region actually consists of both pre-S1 and pre-S2. Depending on where translation is initiated, three potential HBsAg

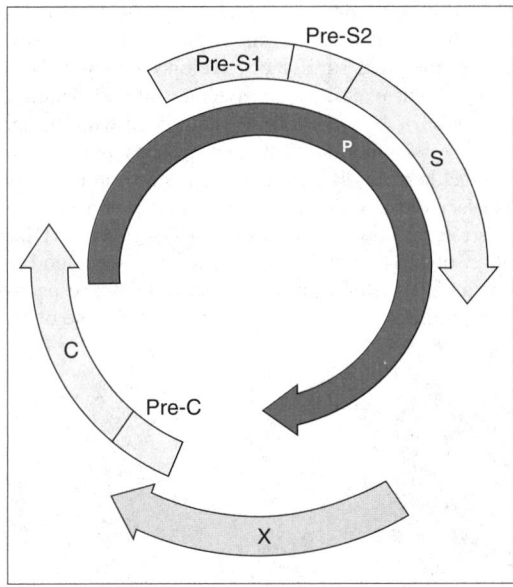

FIGURE 295-3   Its compact genomic structure, with overlapping genes, permits HBV to code for multiple proteins. The S gene codes for the "major" envelope protein, HBsAg. Pre-S1 and pre-S2, upstream of S, combine with S to code for two larger proteins, "middle" protein, the product of pre-S2 + S, and "large" protein, the product of pre-S1 + pre-S2 + S. The largest gene, P, codes for DNA polymerase. The C gene codes for two nucleocapsid proteins, HBeAg, a soluble, secreted protein (initiation from the pre-C region of the gene) and HBcAg, the intracellular core protein (initiation after pre-C). The X gene codes for HBxAg, which can transactivate the transcription of cellular and viral genes; its clinical relevance is not known, but it may contribute to carcinogenesis by binding to p53.

gene products are synthesized. The protein product of the S gene is HBsAg (*major protein*), the product of the S region plus the adjacent pre-S2 region is the *middle protein*, and the product of the pre-S1 plus pre-S2 plus S regions is the *large protein*. Compared with the smaller spherical and tubular particles of HBV, complete 42-nm virions are enriched in the large protein. Both pre-S proteins and their respective antibodies can be detected during HBV infection, and the period of pre-S antigenemia appears to coincide with other markers of virus replication, as detailed below.

The intact 42-nm virion can be disrupted by mild detergents, and the 27-nm nucleocapsid core particle isolated. Nucleocapsid proteins are coded for by the C gene. The antigen expressed on the surface of the nucleocapsid core is referred to as *hepatitis B core antigen* (HBcAg), and its corresponding antibody is anti-HBc. A third HBV antigen is *hepatitis B e antigen* (HBeAg), a soluble, nonparticulate, nucleocapsid protein that is immunologically distinct from intact HBcAg but is a product of the same C gene. The C gene has two initiation codons, a precore and a core region (Fig. 295-3). If translation is initiated at the precore region, the protein product is HBeAg, which has a signal peptide that binds it to the smooth endoplasmic reticulum and leads to its secretion into the circulation. If translation begins with the core region, HBcAg is the protein product; it has no signal peptide, it is not secreted, but it assembles into nucleocapsid particles, which bind to and incorporate RNA and which, ultimately, contain HBV DNA. Also packaged within the nucleocapsid core is a DNA polymerase, which directs replication and repair of HBV DNA. When packaging within viral proteins is complete, synthesis of the incomplete plus strand stops; this accounts for the single-stranded gap and for differences in the size of the gap. HBcAg particles remain in the hepatocyte, where they are readily detectable by immunohistochemical staining, and are exported after encapsidation by an envelope of HBsAg. Therefore, naked core particles do not circulate in the serum. The secreted nucleocapsid protein, HBeAg, provides a convenient, readily detectable, qualitative marker of HBV replication and relative infectivity.

HBsAg-positive serum containing HBeAg is more likely to be highly infectious and to be associated with the presence of hepatitis B virions (and detectable HBV DNA, see below) than HBeAg-negative or anti-HBe-positive serum. For example, HBsAg carrier mothers who are HBeAg-positive almost invariably (>90%) transmit hepatitis B infection to their offspring, whereas HBsAg carrier mothers with anti-HBe rarely (10 to 15%) infect their offspring.

Early during the course of acute hepatitis B, HBeAg appears transiently; its disappearance may be a harbinger of clinical improvement and resolution of infection. Persistence of HBeAg in serum beyond the first 3 months of acute infection may be predictive of the development of chronic infection, and the presence of HBeAg during chronic hepatitis B is associated with ongoing viral replication, infectivity, and inflammatory liver injury.

The third of the HBV genes is the largest, the P gene (Fig. 295-3), which codes for the DNA polymerase; as noted above, this enzyme has both DNA-dependent DNA polymerase and RNA-dependent reverse transcriptase activities. The fourth gene, X, codes for a small, nonparticulate protein that is capable of transactivating the transcription of both viral and cellular genes (Fig. 295-3). Such transactivation may enhance the replication of HBV, leading to the clinical association observed between the expression of the product of the X gene, hepatitis B x antigen (HBxAg), and antibodies to it in patients with severe chronic hepatitis and hepatocellular carcinoma. The transactivating activity can enhance the transcription and replication of other viruses besides HBV, such as HIV. Cellular processes transactivated by X include the human interferon γ gene and class I major histocompatibility genes; potentially, these effects could contribute to enhanced susceptibility of HBV-infected hepatocytes to cytolytic T cells. The expression of X can also induce programmed cell death (apoptosis). The X gene and its protein product, however, are absent in nonmammalian hepadnaviruses; therefore, X is not essential for hepadnavirus replication.

Table 295-1   Nomenclature and Features of Hepatitis Viruses

Hepatitis Type	Virus Particle	Morphology	Genome[a]	Classification	Antigen(s)	Antibodies	Remarks
HAV	27 nm	Icosahedral nonenveloped	7.5-kb RNA, linear, ss, +	Hepatovirus	HAV	anti-HAV	Early fecal shedding Diagnosis: IgM anti-HAV Previous infection: IgG anti-HAV
HBV	42 nm	Double-shelled virion (surface and core) spherical	3.2-kb DNA, circular, ss/ds	Hepadnavirus	HBsAg HBcAg HBeAg	anti-HBs anti-HBc anti-HBe	Bloodborne virus; carrier state Acute diagnosis: HBsAg, IgM anti-HBc Chronic diagnosis: IgG anti-HBc, HBsAg Markers of replication: HBeAg, HBV DNA Liver, lymphocytes, other organs
	27 nm	Nucleocapsid core			HBcAg HBeAg	anti-HBc anti-HBe	Nucleocapsid contains DNA and DNA polymerase; present in hepatocyte nucleus; HBcAg does not circulate; HBeAg (soluble, nonparticulate) and HBV DNA circulate—correlate with infectivity and complete virions
	22 nm	Spherical and filamentous; represents excess virus coat material			HBsAg	anti-HBs	HBsAg detectable in >95% of patients with acute hepatitis B; found in serum, body fluids, hepatocyte cytoplasm; anti-HBs appears following infection—protective antibody
HCV	Approx. 40–60 nm	Enveloped	9.4-kb RNA, linear, ss, +	Flavivirus-like	HCV C100-3 C33c C22-3 NS5	anti-HCV	Bloodborne agent, formerly labeled non-A, non-B hepatitis Acute diagnosis: anti-HCV (C33c, C22-3, NS5), HCV RNA Chronic diagnosis: anti-HCV (C100-3, C33c, C22-3, NS5) and HCV RNA; cytoplasmic location in hepatocytes
HDV	35–37 nm	Enveloped hybrid particle with HBsAg coat and HDV core	1.7-kb RNA, circular, ss, −	Resembles viroids and plant satellite viruses	HBsAg HDV antigen	anti-HBs anti-HDV	Defective RNA virus, requires helper function of HBV (hepadnaviruses); HDV antigen present in hepatocyte nucleus Diagnosis: anti-HDV, HDV RNA; HBV/HDV coinfection—IgM anti-HBc and anti-HDV; HDV superinfection—IgG anti-HBc and anti-HDV
HEV	32–34 nm	Nonenveloped icosahedral	7.6-kb RNA, linear, ss, +	Alphavirus-like	HEV antigen	anti-HEV	Agent of enterically transmitted hepatitis; rare in USA; occurs in Asia, Mediterranean countries, Central America Diagnosis: IgM/IgG anti-HEV (assays being developed); virus in stool, bile, hepatocyte cytoplasm

[a] ss, single-stranded; ss/ds, partially single-stranded, partially double-stranded; −, minus-stranded; +, plus-stranded.

Serologic and virologic markers   After infection with HBV, the first virologic marker detectable in serum is HBsAg (Fig. 295-4). Circulating HBsAg precedes elevations of serum aminotransferase activity and clinical symptoms and remains detectable during the entire icteric or symptomatic phase of acute hepatitis B and beyond. In typical cases, HBsAg becomes undetectable 1 to 2 months after the onset of jaundice and rarely persists beyond 6 months. After HBsAg disappears, antibody to HBsAg (anti-HBs) becomes detectable in serum and remains detectable indefinitely thereafter. Because HBcAg is sequestered within an HBsAg coat, HBcAg is not detectable routinely in the serum of patients with HBV infection. By contrast, anti-HBc is readily demonstrable in serum, beginning within the first 1 to 2 weeks after the appearance of HBsAg and preceding detectable levels of anti-HBs by weeks to months. Because variability exists in the time of appearance of anti-HBs after HBV infection, occasionally a gap of several weeks or longer may separate the disappearance of HBsAg and

the appearance of anti-HBs. During this "gap" or "window" period, anti-HBc may represent serologic evidence of current or recent HBV infection, and blood containing anti-HBc in the absence of HBsAg and anti-HBs has been implicated in the development of transfusion-associated hepatitis B. In part because the sensitivity of immunoassays for HBsAg and anti-HBs has increased, however, this window period is rarely encountered. In some persons, years after HBV infection, anti-HBc may persist in the circulation longer than anti-HBs. Therefore, isolated anti-HBc does not necessarily indicate active virus replication; most instances of isolated anti-HBc represent hepatitis B infection in the remote past. Rarely, however, isolated anti-HBc represents low-level hepatitis B viremia, with HBsAg below the detection threshold; occasionally, isolated anti-HBc represents a cross-reacting or false-positive immunologic specificity. Recent and remote HBV infections can be distinguished by determination of the immunoglobulin class of anti-HBc. Anti-HBc of the IgM class (IgM anti-HBc) predominates

FIGURE 295-4 Scheme of typical clinical and laboratory features of acute viral hepatitis B.

FIGURE 295-5 Scheme of typical laboratory features of chronic viral hepatitis B. HBeAg and HBV DNA can be detected in serum during the *replicative phase* of chronic infection, which is associated with infectivity and liver injury. Seroconversion from the replicative phase to the *nonreplicative phase* occurs at a rate of approximately 10 to 15% per year and is heralded by an acute hepatitis–like elevation of ALT activity; during the nonreplicative phase, infectivity and liver injury are limited.

during the first 6 months after acute infection, whereas IgG anti-HBc is the predominant class of anti-HBc beyond 6 months. Therefore, patients with current or recent acute hepatitis B, including those in the anti-HBc window, have IgM anti-HBc in their serum. In patients who have recovered from hepatitis B in the remote past as well as those with chronic HBV infection, anti-HBc is predominantly of the IgG class. Infrequently, in no more than 1 to 5% of patients with acute HBV infection, levels of HBsAg are too low to be detected; in such cases, the presence of IgM anti-HBc establishes the diagnosis of acute hepatitis B. When isolated anti-HBc occurs in the rare patient with chronic hepatitis B whose HBsAg level is below the sensitivity threshold of contemporary immunoassays (a low-level carrier), the anti-HBc is of the IgG class. Generally, in persons who have recovered from hepatitis B, anti-HBs and anti-HBc persist indefinitely.

The temporal association between the appearance of anti-HBs and resolution of HBV infection as well as the observation that persons with anti-HBs in serum are protected against reinfection with HBV suggest that *anti-HBs is the protective antibody.* Therefore, strategies for prevention of HBV infection are based on providing susceptible persons with circulating anti-HBs (see below). Occasionally, in 10 to 20% of patients with chronic hepatitis B, low-level, low-affinity anti-HBs can be detected. This antibody is directed against a subtype determinant different from that represented by the patient's HBsAg; its presence is thought to reflect the stimulation of a related clone of antibody-forming cells, but it has no clinical relevance and does not signal imminent clearance of hepatitis B.

The other readily detectable serologic marker of HBV infection, HBeAg, appears concurrently with or shortly after HBsAg. Its appearance coincides temporally with high levels of virus replication and reflects the presence of circulating intact virions and detectable HBV DNA. Pre-S1 and pre-S2 proteins are also expressed during periods of peak replication, but assays for these gene products are not routinely available. In self-limited HBV infections, HBeAg becomes undetectable shortly after peak elevations in aminotransferase activity, before the disappearance of HBsAg, and anti-HBe then becomes detectable, coinciding with a period of relatively lower infectivity (Fig. 295-4). Because markers of HBV replication appear transiently during acute infection, testing for such markers is of little clinical utility in typical cases of acute HBV infection. In contrast, markers of HBV replication provide valuable information in patients with protracted infections.

Departing from the pattern typical of acute HBV infections, in chronic HBV infection, HBsAg remains detectable beyond 6 months, anti-HBc is primarily of the IgG class, and anti-HBs is either undetectable or detectable at low levels (see "Laboratory Features," below) (Fig. 295-5). During early chronic HBV infection, HBV DNA can be

detected both in serum and in hepatocyte nuclei, where it is present in free or episomal form. This *replicative stage* of HBV infection is the time of maximal infectivity and liver injury; HBeAg is a qualitative marker and HBV DNA a quantitative marker of this replicative phase, during which all three forms of HBV circulate, including intact virions. Over time, the replicative phase of chronic HBV infection gives way to a relatively *nonreplicative phase.* This occurs at a rate of approximately 10% per year and is accompanied by seroconversion from HBeAg-positive to anti-HBe-positive. In most cases, this seroconversion coincides with a transient, acute hepatitis-like elevation in aminotransferase activity, believed to reflect cell-mediated clearance of virus-infected hepatocytes. In the nonreplicative phase of chronic infection, when HBV DNA is demonstrable in hepatocyte nuclei, it tends to be integrated into the host genome. In this phase, only spherical and tubular forms of HBV, *not intact virions,* circulate, and liver injury tends to subside. Most such patients would be characterized as asymptomatic HBV *carriers.* In reality, the designations *replicative* and *nonreplicative* are only relative; even in the so-called nonreplicative phase, HBV replication can be detected with highly sensitive amplification probes such as the polymerase chain reaction. Still, the distinctions are pathophysiologically and clinically meaningful. Occasionally, nonreplicative HBV infection converts back to replicative infection. Such spontaneous reactivations are accompanied by reexpression of HBeAg and HBV DNA, and sometimes of IgM anti-HBc, as well as by exacerbations of liver injury.

Molecular variants Variation occurs throughout the HBV genome, and clinical isolates of HBV that do not express typical viral proteins have been attributed to mutations in individual or even multiple gene locations. For example, variants have been described that lack nucleocapsid proteins, envelope proteins, or both. Two categories of HBV have attracted the most attention. One of these was identified initially in Mediterranean countries among patients with an unusual serologic-clinical profile. They have severe chronic HBV infection and detectable HBV DNA but with anti-HBe instead of HBeAg. These patients were found to be infected with an HBV mutant that contained an alteration in the precore region rendering the virus incapable of encoding HBeAg. Although several potential mutation sites exist in the pre-C region, the region of the C gene necessary for the expression of HBeAg (see "Virology and Etiology," above), the most commonly encountered in such patients is a single base substitution, from G to A, which occurs in the second to last codon of the pre-C gene at nucleotide 1896. This substitution results in the replacement of the

TGG tryptophan codon by a stop codon (TAG), which prevents the translation of HBeAg. Another mutation in the core promoter region prevents transcription of the coding region for HBeAg and yields an HBeAg-negative phenotype. Patients with such precore mutants that are unable to secrete HBeAg tend to have severe liver disease that progresses rapidly to cirrhosis and that does not respond readily to antiviral therapy. Both "wild-type" HBV and precore mutant HBV can coexist in the same patient, or mutant HBV may arise during wild-type HBV infection. In addition, clusters of fulminant hepatitis B in Israel and Japan have been attributed to common-source infection with a precore mutant. Fulminant hepatitis B in North America and western Europe, however, occurs in patients infected with wild-type HBV, in the absence of precore mutants, and both precore mutants and other mutations throughout the HBV genome occur commonly even in patients with typical, self-limited, milder forms of HBV infection. In areas where chronic HBV infection is common, precore mutations are more frequent and may reflect viral evolution driven by immune selection. Additional investigation is necessary to define the effect of precore mutants on the pathogenicity and natural history of HBV infection.

The second important category of HBV mutants consists of *escape mutants*, in which a single amino acid substitution, from glycine to arginine, occurs at position 145 of the immunodominant *a* determinant common to all subtypes of HBsAg. This change in HBsAg leads to a critical conformational change that results in a loss of neutralizing activity by anti-HBs. This specific HBV/*a* mutant has been observed in two situations, active and passive immunization, in which humoral immunologic pressure may favor evolutionary change ("escape") in the virus—in a small number of hepatitis B vaccine recipients who acquired HBV infection despite the prior appearance of neutralizing anti-HBs and in liver transplant recipients who underwent the procedure for hepatitis B and who were treated with a high-potency human monoclonal anti-HBs preparation. Although such mutants have not been recognized frequently, their existence raises a concern that may complicate vaccination strategies and serologic diagnosis.

Extrahepatic sites Hepatitis B antigens and HBV DNA have been identified in extrahepatic sites, including lymph nodes, bone marrow, circulating lymphocytes, spleen, and pancreas. Although the virus does not appear to be associated with tissue injury in any of these extrahepatic sites, its presence in these "remote" reservoirs has been invoked to explain the recurrence of HBV infection after orthotopic liver transplantation. A more complete understanding of the clinical relevance of extrahepatic HBV remains to be defined.

Hepatitis D The delta hepatitis agent, or HDV, is a defective RNA virus that coinfects with and requires the helper function of HBV (or other hepadnaviruses) for its replication and expression. Slightly smaller than HBV, delta is a formalin-sensitive, 35- to 37-nm virus with a hybrid structure. Its nucleocapsid expresses delta antigen, which bears no antigenic homology with any of the HBV antigens, and contains the virus genome. The delta core is "encapsidated" by an outer envelope of HBsAg, indistinguishable from that of HBV except in its relative compositions of major, middle, and large HBsAg component proteins. The genome is a small, 1700-nucleotide, circular, single-stranded RNA (minus strand) that is nonhomologous with HBV DNA (except for a small area of the polymerase gene) but that has features and the rolling circle model of replication common to genomes of plant satellite viruses or viroids. HDV RNA contains many areas of internal complementarity; therefore, it can fold on itself by internal base pairing to form an unusual, very stable, rodlike structure. HDV RNA replicates via RNA-directed RNA synthesis by transcription of genomic RNA to a complementary antigenomic (plus strand) RNA; the antigenomic RNA, in turn, serves as a template for subsequent genomic RNA synthesis. Between the genomic and antigenomic RNAs of HDV, there are coding regions for nine proteins. Delta antigen, which is a product of the antigenomic strand, exists in two forms, a small, 195-amino-acid species, which plays a role in facilitating HDV RNA replication, and a large, 214-amino-acid species, which appears to suppress replication but is required for assembly of the antigen into viri-

ons. Although complete hepatitis D virions and liver injury require the cooperative helper function of HBV, intracellular replication of HDV RNA can occur without HBV. Genomic heterogeneity among HDV isolates has been described; however, pathophysiologic and clinical consequences of this genetic diversity have not been recognized.

HDV can either infect a person simultaneously with HBV (*coinfection*) or superinfect a person already infected with HBV (*superinfection*); when HDV infection is transmitted from a donor with one HBsAg subtype to an HBsAg-positive recipient with a different subtype, the HDV agent assumes the HBsAg subtype of the recipient, rather than the donor. Because HDV relies absolutely on HBV, the duration of HDV infection is determined by the duration of (and cannot outlast) HBV infection. HDV antigen is expressed primarily in hepatocyte nuclei and is occasionally detectable in serum. During acute HDV infection, anti-HDV of the IgM class predominates, and 30 to 40 days may elapse after symptoms appear before anti-HDV can be detected. In self-limited infection, anti-HDV is low titer and transient, rarely remaining detectable beyond the clearance of HBsAg and HDV antigen. In chronic HDV infection, anti-HDV circulates in high titer, and both IgM and IgG anti-HDV can be detected. HDV antigen in the liver and HDV RNA in serum and liver can be detected during HDV replication.

Hepatitis C Hepatitis C virus, which, before its identification was labeled "non-A, non-B hepatitis," is a linear, single-stranded, positive-sense, 9400-nucleotide RNA virus, the genome of which is similar in organization to that of flaviviruses and pestiviruses; HCV constitutes its own genus in the family Flaviviridae. The HCV genome contains a single large open reading frame (gene) that codes for a virus polyprotein of approximately 3000 amino acids. The 5' end of the genome consists of an untranslated region adjacent to the genes for structural proteins, the nucleocapsid core protein and two envelope glycoproteins, E1 and E2/NS1. The 5' untranslated region and core gene are highly conserved among genotypes, but the envelope proteins are coded for by the hypervariable region, which varies from isolate to isolate and may allow the virus to evade host immunologic containment directed at accessible virus-envelope proteins. The 3' end of the genome contains the genes for nonstructural (NS) proteins. The first reported HCV clone, 5-1-1, and the nucleotide sequence coding for C100-3, the recombinant virus protein used in the first immunoassay for antibodies to HCV, reside within the NS4 gene, and the RNA-dependent RNA polymerase, through which HCV replicates, is encoded by the NS5 region (Fig. 295-6). Because HCV does not rep-

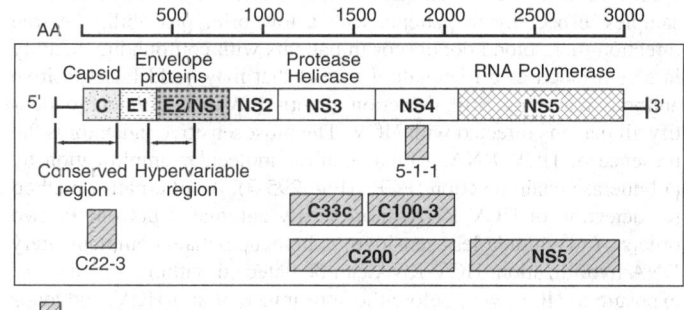

FIGURE 295-6 Organization of the hepatitis C virus genome and its associated proteins. Structural genes at the 5' end include the nucleocapsid region, C, and the envelope regions, E1 and E2. The 5' untranslated region and the C region are highly conserved among isolates, while the envelope domain E2/NS1 contains the hypervariable region. At the 3' end are five nonstructural (NS) regions. Viral proteins included in the first-generation (C100-3), second-generation (C200, a fusion protein of C100-3 and C33c, and C22-3), and third-generation (C22-3, C200, or C33c and C100-3, and NS5) immunoassays and in the recombinant immunoblot assay (5-1-1, C100-3, C33c, C22-3, NS5) are presented below their corresponding genes (AA = amino acid).

licate via a DNA intermediate, it does not integrate into the host genome. Because HCV tends to circulate in very low titer, visualization of virus particles, estimated to be 40 to 60 nm in diameter, has been difficult. Although in vitro HCV replication remains difficult to accomplish convincingly, the chimpanzee has proven to be an invaluable experimental animal model.

At least six distinct genotypes, as well as subtypes within genotypes, of HCV have been identified by nucleotide sequencing. Genotypes differ one from another in sequence homology by ≥30%. Because divergence of HCV isolates within a genotype or subtype, and within the same host, may vary insufficiently to define a distinct genotype, these intragenotypic differences are referred to as *quasispecies* and differ in sequence homology by only a few percent. The genotypic and quasispecies diversity of HCV, resulting from its high mutation rate, interferes with effective humoral immunity. Neutralizing antibodies to HCV have been demonstrated, but they tend to be short-lived; and HCV infection does not induce lasting immunity against reinfection with different virus isolates or even the same virus isolate. Thus, neither *heterologous* nor *homologous* immunity appears to develop after acute HCV infection. Some HCV genotypes are distributed worldwide, while others are more geographically confined. In addition, differences in pathogenicity and responsiveness to antiviral therapy have been reported among genotypes; however, the biologic impact of genotype and quasispecies differences remains incompletely defined.

As noted above, the first assay detected antibodies to C100-3, a recombinant polypeptide derived from the NS4 region of the genome. In most patients with acute hepatitis C, antibody detected with this assay appears between 1 to 3 months after the onset of acute hepatitis but sometimes not for a year or longer. Second-generation assays incorporate recombinant proteins from the nucleocapsid core region, C22-3, and the NS3 region, C33c (expressed in combination with C100-3 as C200); these assays are more sensitive (by approximately 20%) and detect anti-HCV 30 to 90 days earlier, during the period of acute hepatitis. A third-generation immunoassay, which incorporates proteins from the NS5 region and replaces some recombinant proteins with synthetic peptides, may detect anti-HCV even earlier. Because nonspecificity has been encountered in clinical samples tested for anti-HCV, a supplementary recombinant immunoblot assay was introduced. Reactivity in an immunoassay is "confirmed" by incubation with a nitrocellulose strip that contains individual bands of recombinant or synthetic HCV proteins. This approach allows the demonstration of individual antibodies to nonstructural and structural viral proteins and identifies false-positive reactivity associated with nonviral specificities. It is useful to support the validity of anti-HCV-reactive samples, especially in patients with a low prior probability of true infection (e.g., blood donors) or in patients with confounding activity in serum (such as a rheumatoid factor) that may yield false-positive antibody reactivity. Still, detection of anti-HCV is insufficient to identify all persons infected with HCV. The most sensitive indicator is the presence of HCV RNA, which requires molecular amplification by polymerase chain reaction (PCR) (Fig. 295-7). An alternative method for detection of HCV RNA, more easily automated but one or two orders of magnitude less sensitive, is branched-chain complementary DNA hybridization. HCV RNA can be detected within a few days of exposure to HCV, well before the appearance of anti-HCV, and tends to persist for the duration of HCV infection; however, in patients with chronic HCV infection, occasionally, HCV RNA may be detectable only intermittently. Application of sensitive molecular probes for HCV RNA has revealed the presence of replicative HCV in peripheral blood lymphocytes of infected persons; however, as is the case for HBV in lymphocytes, the clinical relevance of HCV lymphocyte infection is not known.

Hepatitis E Previously labeled *epidemic* or *enterically transmitted non-A, non-B hepatitis*, HEV is an enterically transmitted virus that occurs primarily in India, Asia, Africa, and Central America. This agent, with epidemiologic features resembling those of hepatitis A, is

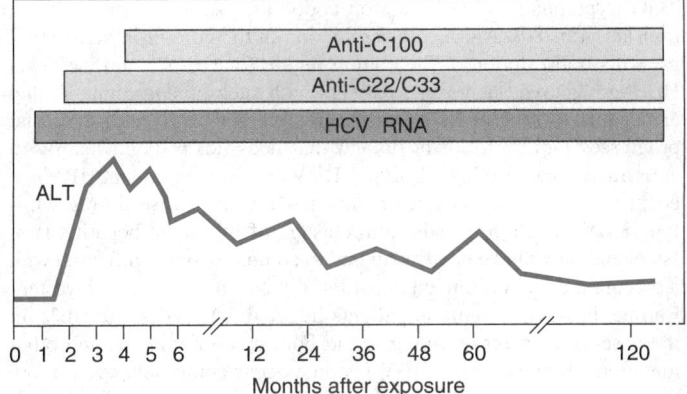

FIGURE 295-7 Scheme of typical laboratory features during acute hepatitis C progressing to chronicity. HCV RNA is the first detectable event, preceding ALT elevation and the appearance of anti-HCV. The appearance of antibody to C100, detectable with first-generation assays, is delayed from 1 to 3 months after the appearance of antibody to C22 and C33, antibodies that are included in second-generation immunoassays. Anti-HCV detectable with second-generation assays appears during acute hepatitis C.

a 32- to 34-nm, nonenveloped, HAV-like virus with a 7600-nucleotide, single-stranded, positive-sense RNA genome. HEV has three open reading frames (genes), the largest of which encodes nonstructural proteins involved in virus replication. A middle-sized gene encodes the nucleocapsid protein, and the smallest, whose function is not known, encodes protein specificities to which antibodies appear in human serum. All HEV isolates appear to belong to a single serotype, despite genomic heterogeneity of up to 25%. There is no genomic or antigenic homology, however, between HEV and HAV or other picornaviruses; and HEV, although resembling calciviruses, appears to be sufficiently distinct from any known agent to merit a new classification of its own within the alphavirus group. The virus has been detected in stool, bile, and liver and is excreted in the stool during the late incubation period; immune responses to viral antigens occur very early during the course of acute infection. Both IgM anti-HEV and IgG anti-HEV can be detected, but both fall rapidly after acute infection, reaching low levels within 9 to 12 months. Currently, serologic testing for HEV infection is not available routinely.

PATHOGENESIS   Under ordinary circumstances, none of the hepatitis viruses is known to be directly cytopathic to hepatocytes. Evidence suggests that the clinical manifestations and outcomes after acute liver injury associated with viral hepatitis are determined by the immunologic responses of the host.

Hepatitis B   Among the viral hepatitides, the immunopathogenesis of hepatitis B has been studied most extensively. Certainly for this agent, the existence of asymptomatic hepatitis B carriers with normal liver histology and function suggests that the virus is not directly cytopathic. The fact that patients with defects in cellular immune competence are more likely to remain chronically infected rather than to clear the virus is cited to support the role of cellular immune responses in the pathogenesis of hepatitis B–related liver injury. The model that has the most experimental support involves cytolytic T cells sensitized specifically to recognize host and hepatitis B viral antigens on the liver cell surface. Recent laboratory observations suggest that nucleocapsid proteins (HBcAg and possibly HBeAg), present on the cell membrane in minute quantities, are the viral target antigens that, with host antigens, invite cytolytic T cells to destroy HBV-infected hepatocytes. Differences in the robustness of cytolytic T cell responsiveness and in the elaboration of antiviral cytokines by T cells have been invoked to explain differences in outcomes between those who recover after acute hepatitis and those who progress to chronic hepatitis or between those with mild and those with severe (fulminant) acute HBV infection.

A recent observation provides further insight into the mechanism of viral clearance in acute hepatitis B. Although a robust cytolytic T cell response occurs and eliminates virus-infected liver cells during acute hepatitis B, more than 90% of HBV DNA has been found in experimentally infected chimpanzees to disappear from the liver and blood before maximal T cell infiltration of the liver and before most of the biochemical and histologic evidence of liver injury. This observation suggests that inflammatory cytokines, independent of cytopathic antiviral mechanisms, participate in early viral clearance; this effect has been shown to represent elimination of HBV replicative intermediates from the cytoplasm and covalently closed circular viral DNA from the nucleus of infected hepatocytes.

Debate continues over the relative importance of viral and host factors in the pathogenesis of HBV-associated liver injury and its outcome. As noted above, precore genetic mutants of HBV have been associated with the more severe outcomes of HBV infection (severe chronic and fulminant hepatitis), suggesting that, under certain circumstances, relative pathogenicity is a property of the virus, not the host. The fact that concomitant HDV and HBV infections are associated with more severe liver injury than HBV infection alone and the fact that cells transfected in vitro with the gene for HDV (delta) antigen express HDV antigen and then become necrotic in the absence of any immunologic influences are also consistent with a viral effect on pathogenicity. Similarly, in patients who undergo liver transplantation for end-stage chronic hepatitis B, occasionally, rapidly progressive liver injury appears in the new liver. This clinical pattern is associated with an unusual histologic pattern in the new liver, *fibrosing cholestatic hepatitis*, which, ultrastructurally, appears to represent a choking of the cell with overwhelming quantities of HBsAg. This observation suggests that under the influence of the potent immunosuppressive agents required to prevent allograft rejection, HBV may have a direct cytopathic effect on liver cells, independent of the immune system.

Although the precise mechanism of liver injury in HBV infection remains elusive, studies of nucleocapsid proteins have shed light on the profound immunologic tolerance to HBV of babies born to mothers with highly replicative (HBeAg-positive), chronic HBV infection. In HBeAg-expressing transgenic mice, in utero exposure to HBeAg, which is sufficiently small to traverse the placenta, induces T cell tolerance to both nucleocapsid proteins. This, in turn, may explain why, when infection occurs so early in life, immunologic clearance does not occur, and protracted, lifelong infection ensues.

Hepatitis C Undoubtedly, cell-mediated immune responses and elaboration by T cells of antiviral cytokines contribute to the containment of infection and pathogenesis of liver injury associated with hepatitis C. Perhaps HCV infection of lymphoid cells plays a role in moderating immune responsiveness to the virus, as well. Intrahepatic HLA class-I-restricted cytolytic T cells directed at nucleocapsid, envelope, and NS viral protein antigens have been demonstrated in patients with chronic hepatitis C. Such virus-specific cytolytic T cell responses, however, do not correlate adequately with the degree of liver injury or with recovery. Several HLA alleles have been linked with self-limited hepatitis C, but such associations do not apply universally. Finally, cross-reactivity between viral and host autoantigens has been invoked to explain the association between hepatitis C and a subset of patients with autoimmune hepatitis and antibodies to liver kidney microsomal antigen (anti-LKM) (Chap. 297).

Extrahepatic Manifestations Immune complex–mediated tissue damage appears to play a pathogenetic role in the extrahepatic manifestations of acute hepatitis B. The occasional prodromal serum sickness–like syndrome observed in acute hepatitis B appears to be related to the deposition in tissue blood vessel walls of circulating immune complexes leading to activation of the complement system. The clinical consequences are urticarial rash, angioedema, fever, and arthritis. During the early prodrome of HBV infection in these patients, HBsAg in high titer in association with small amounts of anti-HBs leads to the formation of soluble, circulating immune complexes (in antigen excess). Complement components in the serum are depressed during the arthritic phase of the illness and are also detectable in the circulating immune complexes, which also contain HBsAg, anti-HBs, IgG, IgM, IgA, and fibrin.

In patients with chronic hepatitis B, other types of immune-complex disease may be seen. Glomerulonephritis with the nephrotic syndrome is occasionally observed; HBsAg, immunoglobulin, and C3 deposition has been found in the glomerular basement membrane. While polyarteritis nodosa develops in considerably fewer than 1% of patients with HBV infection, 20 to 30% of patients with polyarteritis nodosa have HBsAg in serum (Chap. 317). In these patients, the affected small and medium-sized arterioles have been shown to contain HBsAg, immunoglobulins, and complement components. Another extrahepatic manifestation of viral hepatitis, essential mixed cryoglobulinemia (EMC), was reported initially to be associated with hepatitis B. The disorder is characterized clinically by arthritis and cutaneous vasculitis (palpable purpura) and serologically by the presence of circulating cryoprecipitable immune complexes of more than one immunoglobulin class (Chap. 275). Many patients with this syndrome have chronic liver disease, but the association with HBV infection is limited; instead, a substantial proportion have chronic HCV infection. Their circulating immune complexes contain HCV RNA at a concentration that exceeds its serum concentration, favoring a primary role for the virus in the pathogenesis of EMC.

PATHOLOGY The typical morphologic lesions of all types of viral hepatitis are similar and consist of panlobular infiltration with mononuclear cells, hepatic cell necrosis, hyperplasia of Kupffer cells, and variable degrees of cholestasis. Hepatic cell regeneration is present, as evidenced by numerous mitotic figures, multinucleated cells, and "rosette" or "pseudoacinar" formation. The mononuclear infiltration consists primarily of small lymphocytes, although plasma cells and eosinophils occasionally are present. Liver cell damage consists of hepatic cell degeneration and necrosis, cell dropout, ballooning of cells, and acidophilic degeneration of hepatocytes (forming so-called Councilman bodies). Large hepatocytes with a ground glass appearance of the cytoplasm may be seen in chronic but not in acute HBV infection; these cells contain HBsAg and can be identified histochemically with orcein or aldehyde fuchsin. In uncomplicated viral hepatitis, the reticulin framework is preserved.

In hepatitis C, the histologic lesion is often remarkable for a relative paucity of inflammation, a marked increase in activation of sinusoidal lining cells, lymphoid aggregates, the presence of fat, and, occasionally, bile duct lesions in which biliary epithelial cells appear to be piled up without interruption of the basement membrane. Occasionally, microvesicular steatosis occurs in hepatitis D. In hepatitis E, a common histologic feature is marked cholestasis. A cholestatic variant of slowly resolving acute hepatitis A also has been described.

A more severe histologic lesion, *bridging hepatic necrosis*, also termed *subacute* or *confluent necrosis*, is occasionally observed in some patients with acute hepatitis. "Bridging" between lobules results from large areas of hepatic cell dropout, with collapse of the reticulin framework. Characteristically, the bridge consists of condensed reticulum, inflammatory debris, and degenerating liver cells that span adjacent portal areas, portal to central veins, or central vein to central vein. This lesion had been thought to have prognostic significance; in many of the originally described patients with this lesion, a subacute course terminated in death within several weeks to months, or severe chronic hepatitis and postnecrotic cirrhosis developed. More recent investigations have failed to uphold the association between bridging necrosis and such a poor prognosis in patients with acute hepatitis. Although the frequency of bridging may be higher among hospitalized patients with severe acute hepatitis, and although cirrhosis, chronic hepatitis, and even death have occurred in this group, the frequency of bridging necrosis in uncomplicated acute viral hepatitis is probably on the order of 1 to 5%. Prospective studies have failed to demonstrate a difference in prognosis between patients with acute hepatitis who have bridging necrosis and those who do not. Therefore, although demonstration of this lesion in patients with chronic hepatitis has prognostic significance (Chap. 297), its demonstration during acute hepatitis is less meaningful, and liver biopsies to identify this lesion are no longer undertaken routinely in patients with acute hepatitis. In *massive hepatic necrosis* (fulminant hepatitis, acute yellow atrophy), the striking feature at postmortem examination is the finding of a small, shrunken, soft liver. Histologic examination reveals massive necrosis and dropout of liver cells of most lobules with extensive collapse and condensation of the reticulin framework.

Immunofluorescence and immunoperoxidase antibody studies have localized HBsAg to the cytoplasm and plasma membrane of infected liver cells. In contrast, HBcAg predominates in the nucleus, but occasionally, scant amounts are also seen in the cytoplasm and on the cell membrane. Electron-microscopic studies of liver biopsy material have demonstrated the presence of HBsAg particles in the cytoplasm and HBcAg particles in the nucleus of liver cells during hepatitis B infection. These morphologic observations suggest that DNA is synthesized and packaged within core particles in the nucleus, while the envelope is assembled in the cytoplasm, resulting in the formation of intact hepatitis B virus. HDV antigen is localized to the hepatocyte nucleus, while HAV, HCV, and HEV antigens are localized to the cytoplasm.

EPIDEMIOLOGY   Before the availability of serologic tests for hepatitis viruses, all viral hepatitis cases were labeled either as "infectious" or "serum" hepatitis. Modes of transmission overlap, however, and *a clear distinction among the different types of viral hepatitis cannot be made solely on the basis of clinical or epidemiologic features* (Table 295-2). The most accurate means to distinguish the various types of viral hepatitis involves specific serologic testing.

Hepatitis A   *This agent is transmitted almost exclusively by the fecal-oral route.* Person-to-person spread of HAV is enhanced by poor personal hygiene and overcrowding; large outbreaks as well as sporadic cases have been traced to contaminated food, water, milk, frozen raspberries and strawberries, and shellfish. Intrafamily and intrainstitutional spread are also common. Early epidemiologic observations suggested that there is a predilection for hepatitis A to occur in late fall and early winter. In temperate zones, epidemic waves have been recorded every 5 to 20 years as new segments of nonimmune population appeared; however, in developed countries, the incidence of type A hepatitis has been declining, presumably as a function of improved sanitation, and these cyclic patterns are no longer being observed. No HAV carrier state has been identified after acute type A hepatitis; perpetuation of the virus in nature depends presumably on nonepidemic, inapparent subclinical infection.

In the general population, anti-HAV, an excellent marker for previous HAV infection, increases in prevalence as a function of increasing age and of decreasing socioeconomic status. In the 1970s, serologic evidence of prior hepatitis A infection occurred in about 40% of urban populations in the United States, most of whose members never recalled having had a symptomatic case of hepatitis. In subsequent decades, however, the prevalence of anti-HAV has been declining in the United States. In developing countries, exposure, infection, and subsequent immunity are almost universal in childhood. As the frequency of subclinical childhood infections declines in developed countries, a susceptible cohort of adults emerges. Hepatitis A tends to be more symptomatic in adults; therefore, paradoxically, as the frequency of HAV infection declines, the likelihood of clinically apparent, even severe, HAV illnesses increases in the susceptible adult population. Travel to endemic areas is a common source of infection for adults from nonendemic areas. More recently recognized epidemiologic foci of HAV infection include child-care centers, neonatal intensive care units, promiscuous homosexual men, and injection drug users. Although hepatitis A is rarely bloodborne, several outbreaks have been recognized in recipients of clotting factor concentrates.

Hepatitis B   Percutaneous inoculation has long been recognized as a major route of hepatitis B transmission, but the outmoded designation "serum hepatitis" is an inaccurate label for the epidemiologic spectrum of HBV infection recognized today. As detailed below, most of the hepatitis transmitted by blood transfusion is not caused by HBV; moreover, in approximately two-thirds of patients with acute type B hepatitis, there is no history of an identifiable percutaneous exposure. We now recognize that many cases of type B hepatitis result from less obvious modes of nonpercutaneous or covert percutaneous transmis-

Table 295-2   Clinical and Epidemiologic Features of Viral Hepatitis

Feature	HAV	HBV	HCV	HDV	HEV
Incubation (days)	15–45, mean 30	30–180, mean 60–90	15–160, mean 50	30–180, mean 60–90	14–60, mean 40
Onset	Acute	Insidious or acute	Insidious	Insidious or acute	Acute
Age preference	Children, young adults	Young adults (sexual and percutaneous), babies, toddlers	Any age, but more common in adults	Any age (similar to HBV)	Young adults (20–40 years)
Transmission					
Fecal-oral	+++	−	−	−	+++
Percutaneous	Unusual	+++	+++	+++	−
Perinatal	−	+++	±[a]	+	−
Sexual	±	++	±[a]	++	−
Clinical					
Severity	Mild	Occasionally severe	Moderate	Occasionally severe	Mild
Fulminant	0.1%	0.1–1%	0.1%	5–20%[b]	1–2%[e]
Progression to chronicity	None	Occasional (1–10%) (90% of neonates)	Common (50–70% chronic hepatitis; 80–90% chronic infection)	Common[d]	None
Carrier	None	0.1–30%[c]	1.5–3.2%	Variable[f]	None
Cancer	None	+ (neonatal infection)	+	±	None
Prognosis	Excellent	Worse with age, debility	Moderate	Acute, good Chronic, poor	Good
Prophylaxis	IG Inactivated vaccine	HBIG Recombinant vaccine	None	HBV vaccine (none for HBV carriers)	Unknown
Therapy	None	Interferon Lamivudine	Interferon plus ribavirin	Interferon ±	None

[a] Primarily with HIV coinfection and high-level viremia in index case; risk approximately 5%.

[b] Up to 5% in acute HBV/HDV coinfection; up to 20% in HDV superinfection of chronic HBV infection.

[c] Varies considerably throughout the world and in subpopulations within countries; see text.

[d] In acute HBV/HDV coinfection, the frequency of chronicity is the same as that for HBV; in HDV superinfection, chronicity is invariable.

[e] 10–20% in pregnant women.

[f] Common in Mediterranean countries, rare in North America and western Europe.

HBsAg has been identified in almost every body fluid from infected persons, and at least some of these body fluids—most notably semen and saliva—are infectious, albeit less so than serum, when administered percutaneously or nonpercutaneously to experimental animals. Among the nonpercutaneous modes of HBV transmission, oral ingestion has been documented as a potential but inefficient route of exposure. By contrast, the two nonpercutaneous routes considered to have the greatest impact are intimate (especially sexual) contact and perinatal transmission.

In sub-Saharan Africa, intimate contact among toddlers is considered instrumental in contributing to the maintenance of the high frequency of hepatitis B in the population. Perinatal transmission occurs primarily in infants born to HBsAg carrier mothers or mothers with acute hepatitis B during the third trimester of pregnancy or during the early postpartum period. Perinatal transmission is uncommon in North America and western Europe but occurs with great frequency and is the most important mode of HBV perpetuation in the Far East and developing countries. Although the precise mode of perinatal transmission is unknown, and although approximately 10% of infections may be acquired in utero, epidemiologic evidence suggests that most infections occur approximately at the time of delivery and are not related to breast feeding. The likelihood of perinatal transmission of HBV correlates with the presence of HBeAg; 90% of HBeAg-positive mothers but only 10 to 15% of anti-HBe-positive mothers transmit HBV infection to their offspring. In most cases, acute infection in the neonate is clinically asymptomatic, but the child is very likely to become an HBsAg carrier.

The more than 350 million HBsAg carriers in the world constitute the main reservoir of hepatitis B in human beings. Serum HBsAg is infrequent (0.1 to 0.5%) in normal populations in the United States and western Europe. However, a prevalence of up to 5 to 20% has been found in the Far East and in some tropical countries; in persons with Down's syndrome, lepromatous leprosy, leukemia, Hodgkin's disease, polyarteritis nodosa; in patients with chronic renal disease on hemodialysis; and in injection drug users.

Other groups with high rates of HBV infection include spouses of acutely infected persons, sexually promiscuous persons (especially promiscuous homosexual men), health care workers exposed to blood, persons who require repeated transfusions especially with pooled blood product concentrates (e.g., hemophiliacs), residents and staff of custodial institutions for the mentally retarded, prisoners, and, to a lesser extent, family members of chronically infected patients. In volunteer blood donors, the prevalence of anti-HBs, a reflection of previous HBV infection, ranges from 5 to 10%, but the prevalence is higher in lower socioeconomic strata, older age groups, and persons—including those mentioned above—exposed to blood products.

Prevalence of infection, modes of transmission, and human behavior conspire to mold geographically different epidemiologic patterns of HBV infection. In the Far East and Africa, hepatitis B, a disease of the newborn and young children, is perpetuated by a cycle of maternal-neonatal spread. In North America and western Europe, hepatitis B is primarily a disease of adolescence and early adulthood, the time of life when intimate sexual contact as well as recreational and occupational percutaneous exposures tend to occur.

Hepatitis D Infection with HDV has a worldwide distribution, but two epidemiologic patterns exist. In Mediterranean countries (northern Africa, southern Europe, the Middle East), HDV infection is endemic among those with hepatitis B, and the disease is transmitted predominantly by nonpercutaneous means, especially close personal contact. In nonendemic areas, such as the United States and northern Europe, HDV infection is confined to persons exposed frequently to blood and blood products, primarily injection drug users and hemophiliacs. HDV infection can be introduced into a population through drug users or by migration of persons from endemic to nonendemic areas. Thus, patterns of population migration and human behavior facilitating percutaneous contact play important roles in the introduction and amplification of HDV infection. Occasionally, the migrating epidemiology of hepatitis D is expressed in explosive outbreaks of severe hepatitis, such as those that have occurred in remote South American villages as well as in urban centers in the United States. Ultimately, such outbreaks of hepatitis D—either of coinfections with acute hepatitis B or of superinfections in those already infected with HBV—may blur the distinctions between endemic and nonendemic areas.

Hepatitis C Routine screening of blood donors for HBsAg and the elimination of commercial blood sources in the early 1970s reduced the frequency of, but did not eliminate, transfusion-associated hepatitis. During the 1970s, the likelihood of acquiring hepatitis after transfusion of voluntarily donated, HBsAg-screened blood was approximately 10% per patient (up to 0.9% per unit transfused); 90 to 95% of these cases were classified, based on serologic exclusion of hepatitis A and B, as "non-A, non-B" hepatitis. For patients requiring transfusion of pooled products, such as clotting factor concentrates, the risk was even higher, up to 20 to 30%, while for those receiving such products as albumin and immune globulin, because of prior treatment of these materials by heating to 60°C or cold ethanol fractionation, there was no risk of hepatitis.

During the 1980s, voluntary self-exclusion of blood donors with risk factors for AIDS and then the introduction of donor screening for anti-HIV reduced further the likelihood of transfusion-associated hepatitis to under 5%. During the late 1980s and early 1990s, the introduction first of "surrogate" screening tests for non-A, non-B hepatitis [alanine aminotransferase (ALT) and anti-HBc, both shown to identify blood donors with a higher likelihood of transmitting non-A, non-B hepatitis to recipients] and, subsequently, after the discovery of HCV, first-generation immunoassays for anti-HCV reduced the frequency of transfusion-associated hepatitis even further. A prospective analysis of transfusion-associated hepatitis conducted between 1986 and 1990 showed that the incidence of transfusion-associated hepatitis at one urban university hospital fell from a baseline of 3.8% per patient (0.45% per unit transfused) to 1.5% per patient (0.19% per unit) after the introduction of surrogate testing and to 0.6% per patient (0.03% per unit) after the introduction of first-generation anti-HCV assays. The introduction of second-generation anti-HCV assays has reduced the frequency of transfusion-associated hepatitis C to almost imperceptible levels, 1 in 100,000.

In addition to being transmitted by transfusion, hepatitis C can be transmitted by other percutaneous routes, such as self-injection with intravenous drugs. In addition, this virus can be transmitted by occupational exposure to blood, and the likelihood of infection is increased in hemodialysis units. Although the frequency of transfusion-associated hepatitis C fell as a result of blood donor screening, the overall frequency of hepatitis C remained the same until the early 1990s, when the overall frequency fell by 80%, in parallel with a reduction in the number of new cases in injection drug users. After the exclusion of anti-HCV-positive plasma units from the donor pool, rare, sporadic instances have occurred of hepatitis C among recipients of immune globulin preparations for intravenous (but not intramuscular) use.

Serologic evidence for HCV infection occurs in 90% of patients with a history of transfusion-associated hepatitis (almost all occurring before 1992, when second-generation HCV-screening tests were introduced), hemophiliacs and others treated with clotting factors, and injection-drug users; 60 to 70% of patients with sporadic "non-A, non-B" hepatitis who lack identifiable risk factors; 0.5% of volunteer blood donors; and 1.8% of the general population in the United States, which translates into 4 million persons. Comparable frequencies of HCV infection occur in most countries around the world, but extraordinarily high prevalences of HCV infection occur in certain countries, such as Egypt, where more than 20% of the population in some cities is infected. In the United States, African Americans and Mexican Americans have higher frequencies of HCV infection than whites, and 30- to 49-year-old adult males have the highest frequencies of infection. Chronic hepatitis C accounts for 20% of sporadic acute hepatitis and 40% of chronic liver disease, is the most frequent indication for liver transplantation, and is estimated to account for 8000 to 10,000 deaths per year in the United States.

Most asymptomatic blood donors found to have anti-HCV and approximately 40% of persons with reported cases of acute hepatitis C do not fall into a recognized risk group; however, many such blood donors do recall risk-associated behaviors when questioned carefully, and most patients with acute hepatitis C in the absence of clear-cut risk factors tend to be of lower socioeconomic backgrounds. Thorough questioning of anti-HCV-reactive blood donors has identified nasal cocaine inhalation, with shared equipment, as a potential risk factor for acquiring HCV infection.

As a bloodborne infection, HCV potentially can be transmitted sexually and perinatally; however, both of these modes of transmission are inefficient for hepatitis C. Although 10 to 15% of patients with acute hepatitis C report having potential sexual sources of infection, most studies have failed to identify sexual transmission of this agent. The chances of sexual and perinatal transmission have been estimated to be approximately 5%, well below comparable rates for HIV and HBV infections. Moreover, sexual transmission appears to be confined to such subgroups as persons with multiple sexual partners and sexually transmitted diseases; transmission of HCV infection is rare between stable, monogamous sexual partners. Breast feeding does not increase the risk of HCV infection between an infected mother and her infant. Infection of health workers is not dramatically higher than among the general population; however, health workers are more likely to acquire HCV infection through accidental needle punctures, the efficiency of which ranges between 3 and 10%. Infection of household contacts is rare as well.

Other groups with an increased frequency of HCV infection include patients who require hemodialysis and organ transplantation and those who require transfusions in the setting of cancer chemotherapy. In immunosuppressed individuals, levels of anti-HCV may be undetectable, and a diagnosis may require testing for HCV RNA. Although new acute cases of hepatitis C are rare, newly diagnosed cases are common among otherwise healthy persons who experimented briefly with injection drugs two or three decades earlier. Such instances usually remain unrecognized for years, until unearthed by laboratory screening for routine medical examinations, insurance applications, and attempted blood donation.

Hepatitis E   The enteric form of non-A, non-B hepatitis identified in India, Asia, Africa, and Central America resembles hepatitis A in its primarily enteric mode of spread. The commonly recognized cases occur after contamination of water supplies such as after monsoon flooding, but sporadic, isolated cases occur. An epidemiologic feature that distinguishes HEV from other enteric agents is the rarity of secondary person-to-person spread from infected persons to their close contacts. Infections arise in populations that are immune to HAV and favor young adults. It is not known if hepatitis E occurs outside of recognized endemic areas, for example, in the United States, but preliminary studies suggest that HEV does not account for any of the sporadic "non-A, non-B" cases in nonendemic areas. Cases imported from endemic areas have been found in the United States.

CLINICAL AND LABORATORY FEATURES   **Symptoms and Signs**   Acute viral hepatitis occurs after an incubation period that varies according to the responsible agent. Generally, incubation periods for hepatitis A range from 15 to 45 days (mean 4 weeks), for hepatitis B and D from 30 to 180 days (mean 4 to 12 weeks), for hepatitis C from 15 to 160 days (mean 7 weeks), and for hepatitis E from 14 to 60 days (mean 5 to 6 weeks). The *prodromal symptoms* of acute viral hepatitis are systemic and quite variable. Constitutional symptoms of anorexia, nausea and vomiting, fatigue, malaise, arthralgias, myalgias, headache, photophobia, pharyngitis, cough, and coryza may precede the onset of jaundice by 1 to 2 weeks. The nausea, vomiting, and anorexia are frequently associated with alterations in olfaction and taste. A low-grade fever between 38 and 39°C (100 to 102°F) is more often present in hepatitis A and E than in hepatitis B or C,

except when hepatitis B is heralded by a serum sicknesslike syndrome; rarely, a fever of 39.5 to 40°C (103 to 104°F) may accompany the constitutional symptoms. Dark urine and clay-colored stools may be noticed by the patient from 1 to 5 days before the onset of clinical jaundice.

With the onset of *clinical jaundice*, the constitutional prodromal symptoms usually diminish, but in some patients mild weight loss (2.5 to 5 kg) is common and may continue during the entire icteric phase. The liver becomes enlarged and tender and may be associated with right upper quadrant pain and discomfort. Infrequently, patients present with a cholestatic picture, suggesting extrahepatic biliary obstruction. Splenomegaly and cervical adenopathy are present in 10 to 20% of patients with acute hepatitis. Rarely, a few spider angiomas appear during the icteric phase and disappear during convalescence. During the *recovery phase*, constitutional symptoms disappear, but usually some liver enlargement and abnormalities in liver biochemical tests are still evident. The duration of the posticteric phase is variable, ranging from 2 to 12 weeks, and usually is more prolonged in acute hepatitis B and C. Complete clinical and biochemical recovery is to be expected 1 to 2 months after all cases of hepatitis A and E and 3 to 4 months after the onset of jaundice in three-quarters of uncomplicated cases of hepatitis B and C. In the remainder, biochemical recovery may be delayed. A substantial proportion of patients with viral hepatitis never become icteric.

Infection with HDV can occur in the presence of acute or chronic HBV infection; the duration of HBV infection determines the duration of HDV infection. When acute HDV and HBV infection occur simultaneously, clinical and biochemical features may be indistinguishable from those of HBV infection alone, although occasionally they are more severe. As opposed to patients with *acute* HBV infection, patients with *chronic* HBV infection can support HDV replication indefinitely. This can happen when acute HDV infection occurs in the presence of a nonresolving acute HBV infection. More commonly, acute HDV infection becomes chronic when it is superimposed on an underlying chronic HBV infection. In such cases, the HDV superinfection appears as a clinical exacerbation or an episode resembling acute viral hepatitis in someone already chronically infected with HBV. Superinfection with HDV in a patient with chronic hepatitis B often leads to clinical deterioration (see below).

In addition to superinfections with other hepatitis agents, acute hepatitis-like clinical events in persons with chronic hepatitis B may accompany spontaneous HBeAg–to–anti-HBe seroconversion or spontaneous reactivation, i.e., reversion from nonreplicative to replicative infection. Such reactivations can occur as well in therapeutically immunosuppressed patients with chronic HBV infection when cytotoxic-immunosuppressive drugs are withdrawn; in these cases, restoration of immune competence is thought to allow resumption of previously checked cell-mediated cytolysis of HBV-infected hepatocytes. Occasionally, acute clinical exacerbations of chronic hepatitis B may represent the emergence of a precore mutant (see "Virology and Etiology," above).

Laboratory Features   The serum aminotransferases aspartate aminotransferase (AST) and ALT (previously designated SGOT and SGPT) show a variable increase during the prodromal phase of acute viral hepatitis and precede the rise in bilirubin level (Figs. 295-2 and 295-4). The acute level of these enzymes, however, does not correlate well with the degree of liver cell damage. Peak levels vary from 400 to 4000 IU or more; these levels are usually reached at the time the patient is clinically icteric and diminish progressively during the recovery phase of acute hepatitis. The diagnosis of anicteric hepatitis is difficult and requires a high index of suspicion; it is based on clinical features and on aminotransferase elevations, although mild increases in conjugated bilirubin also may be found.

Jaundice is usually visible in the sclera or skin when the serum bilirubin value exceeds 43 μmol/L (2.5 mg/dL). When jaundice appears, the serum bilirubin typically rises to levels ranging from 85 to 340 μmol/L (5 to 20 mg/dL). The serum bilirubin may continue to rise despite falling serum aminotransferase levels. In most instances, the total bilirubin is equally divided between the conjugated and unconjugated fractions. Bilirubin levels above 340 μmol/L (20 mg/dL) extending and persisting late into the course of viral hepatitis are more likely to be associated with severe disease. In certain patients with underlying hemolytic anemia, however, such as glucose-6-phosphate dehydrogenase deficiency and sickle cell anemia, a high serum bilirubin level is common, resulting from superimposed hemolysis. In such patients, bilirubin levels greater than 513 μmol/L (30 mg/dL) have been observed and are not necessarily associated with a poor prognosis.

Neutropenia and lymphopenia are transient and are followed by a relative lymphocytosis. Atypical lymphocytes (varying between 2 and 20%) are common during the acute phase. These atypical lymphocytes are indistinguishable from those seen in infectious mononucleosis. Measurement of the prothrombin time (PT) is important in patients with acute viral hepatitis, for a prolonged value may reflect a severe synthetic defect, signify extensive hepatocellular necrosis, and indicate a worse prognosis. Occasionally, a prolonged PT may occur with only mild increases in the serum bilirubin and aminotransferase levels. Prolonged nausea and vomiting, inadequate carbohydrate intake, and poor hepatic glycogen reserves may contribute to hypoglycemia noted occasionally in patients with severe viral hepatitis. Serum alkaline phosphatase may be normal or only mildly elevated, while a fall in serum albumin is uncommon in uncomplicated acute viral hepatitis. In some patients, mild and transient steatorrhea has been noted as well as slight microscopic hematuria and minimal proteinuria.

A diffuse but mild elevation of the gamma globulin fraction is common during acute viral hepatitis. Serum IgG and IgM levels are elevated in about one-third of patients during the acute phase of viral hepatitis, but the serum IgM level is elevated more characteristically during acute hepatitis A. During the acute phase of viral hepatitis, antibodies to smooth muscle and other cell constituents may be present, and low titers of rheumatoid factor, nuclear antibody, and heterophil antibody also can be found occasionally. In hepatitis C and D, antibodies to liver-kidney microsomes (LKM) may occur; however, the species of LKM antibodies in the two types of hepatitis are different from each other as well as from the LKM antibody species characteristic of autoimmune chronic hepatitis type 2 (Chap. 297). The autoantibodies in viral hepatitis are nonspecific and also can be associated with other viral and systemic diseases. In contrast, virus-specific antibodies, which appear during and after hepatitis virus infection, are serologic markers of diagnostic importance.

As described above, serologic tests are available with which to establish a diagnosis of hepatitis A, B, D, and C. Tests for fecal or serum HAV are not routinely available. Therefore, a diagnosis of type A hepatitis is based on detection of IgM anti-HAV during acute illness (Fig. 295-2). Rheumatoid factor can give rise to false-positive results in this test.

A diagnosis of HBV infection can usually be made by detection of HBsAg in serum. Infrequently, levels of HBsAg are too low to be detected during acute HBV infection, even with the current generation of highly sensitive immunoassays. In such cases, the diagnosis can be established by the presence of IgM anti-HBc.

The titer of HBsAg bears little relation to the severity of clinical disease. Indeed, there may be an inverse correlation between the serum concentration of HBsAg and the degree of liver cell damage. For example, titers are highest in immunosuppressed patients, lower in patients with chronic liver disease (but higher in mild chronic than in severe chronic hepatitis), and very low in patients with acute fulminant hepatitis. These observations suggest that in hepatitis B the degree of liver cell damage and the clinical course are probably related to variations in the patient's immune response to HBV rather than to the amount of circulating HBsAg. In immunocompetent persons, however, there is a correlation between markers of HBV *replication* and liver injury (see below).

Another serologic marker that may be of value in patients with hepatitis B is HBeAg. Its principal clinical usefulness is as an indicator of relative infectivity. Because HBeAg is invariably present during early acute hepatitis B, HBeAg testing is indicated primarily during follow-up of chronic infection.

In patients with hepatitis B surface antigenemia of unknown duration, e.g., blood donors found to be HBsAg-positive and referred to a physician for evaluation, testing for IgM anti-HBc may be useful to distinguish between acute or recent infection (IgM anti-HBc-positive) and chronic HBV infection (IgM anti-HBc-negative, IgG anti-HBc-positive). A false-positive test for IgM anti-HBc may be encountered in patients with high-titer rheumatoid factor.

Anti-HBs is rarely detectable in the presence of HBsAg in patients with *acute* hepatitis B, but 10 to 20% of persons with *chronic* HBV infection may harbor low-level anti-HBs. This antibody is directed not against the common group determinant, *a*, but against the heterotypic subtype determinant (e.g., HBsAg of subtype *ad* with anti-HBs of subtype *y*). In most cases, this serologic pattern cannot be attributed to infection with two different HBV subtypes, and the presence of this antibody is not a harbinger of imminent HBsAg clearance. When such antibody is detected, its presence is of no recognized clinical significance (see "Virology and Etiology," above).

After immunization with hepatitis B vaccine, which consists of HBsAg alone, anti-HBs is the only serologic marker to appear. The commonly encountered serologic patterns of hepatitis B and their interpretations are summarized in Table 295-3. Tests for the detection of HBV DNA in liver and serum are now available. Like HBeAg, serum HBV DNA is an indicator of HBV replication, but tests for HBV DNA are more sensitive and quantitative. Hybridization assays for HBV DNA have a sensitivity of approximately 10^5 to 10^6 virions/mL, a relative threshold below which infectivity and liver injury are limited and HBeAg is usually undetectable. Currently, testing for HBV DNA has shifted from insensitive hybridization assays to amplification assays, e.g., the polymerase chain reaction–based assay, which can detect as few as 100 or 1000 virions/mL. With increased sensitivity,

Table 295-3 Commonly Encountered Serologic Patterns of Hepatitis B Infection

HBsAg	Anti-HBs	Anti-HBc	HBeAg	Anti-HBe	Interpretation
+	−	IgM	+	−	Acute HBV infection, high infectivity
+	−	IgG	+	−	Chronic HBV infection, high infectivity
+	−	IgG	−	+	Late-acute or chronic HBV infection, low infectivity
+	+	+	+/−	+/−	1. HBsAg of one subtype and heterotypic anti-HBs (common)
					2. Process of seroconversion from HBsAg to anti-HBs (rare)
−	−	IgM	+/−	+/−	1. Acute HBV infection
					2. Anti-HBc window
−	−	IgG	−	+/−	1. Low-level HBsAg carrier
					2. Remote past infection
−	+	IgG	−	+/−	Recovery from HBV infection
−	+	−	−	−	1. Immunization with HBsAg (after vaccination)
					2. Remote past infection (?)
					3. False-positive

amplification assays remain reactive well below the threshold for infectivity and liver injury. These markers are useful in following the course of HBV replication in patients with chronic hepatitis B receiving antiviral chemotherapy, e.g., with interferon or lamivudine (Chap. 297). In immunocompetent persons, a general correlation does appear to exist between the level of HBV replication, as reflected by the level of HBV DNA in serum, and the degree of liver injury. High serum HBV DNA levels, increased expression of viral antigens, and necroinflammatory activity in the liver go hand in hand unless immunosuppression interferes with cytolytic T cell responses to virus-infected cells; reduction of HBV replication with antiviral drugs tends to be accompanied by an improvement in liver histology.

In patients with hepatitis C, an episodic pattern of aminotransferase elevation is common. A specific serologic diagnosis of hepatitis C can be made by demonstrating the presence in serum of anti-HCV. When a second- or third-generation immunoassay (that detects antibodies to nonstructural and nucleocapsid proteins) is used, anti-HCV can be detected in acute hepatitis C during the initial phase of elevated aminotransferase activity. This antibody may never become detectable in 5 to 10% of patients with acute hepatitis C, and levels of anti-HCV may become undetectable after recovery from acute hepatitis C. In patients with chronic hepatitis C, anti-HCV is detectable in >95% of cases. Nonspecificity can confound immunoassays for anti-HCV, especially in persons with a low prior probability of infection, such as volunteer blood donors, or in persons with circulating rheumatoid factor, which can bind nonspecifically to assay reagents. A supplementary recombinant immunoblot assay (RIBA), in which serum is incubated with a nitrocellulose strip containing viral protein bands, can be used to establish the specific viral proteins to which anti-HCV is directed (see "Virology and Etiology," above). Such RIBA determinations are used routinely to confirm anti-HCV reactivity in blood donors, but determinations of HCV RNA have supplanted RIBA in many clinical settings. Assays for HCV RNA are the most sensitive tests for HCV infection and represent the "gold standard" in establishing a diagnosis of hepatitis C. HCV RNA can be detected even before acute elevation of aminotransferase activity and before the appearance of anti-HCV in patients with acute hepatitis C. In addition, HCV RNA remains detectable indefinitely, continuously in most but intermittently in some, in patients with chronic hepatitis C (even detectable in some persons with normal liver tests, i.e., asymptomatic carriers). In the small minority of patients with hepatitis C who lack anti-HCV, a diagnosis can be supported by detection of HCV RNA. If all these tests are negative and the patient has a well-characterized case of hepatitis after percutaneous exposure to blood or blood products, a diagnosis of hepatitis caused by another agent, as yet unidentified, can be entertained.

Amplification techniques are required to detect HCV RNA, and two are available. One is a branched-chain complementary DNA (bDNA) assay, in which the detection signal (a colorimetrically detectable enzyme bound to a complementary DNA probe) is amplified. The other is a PCR assay, in which the viral RNA is reverse transcribed to complementary DNA and then amplified by repeated cycles of DNA synthesis and polymerization. Both can be used as quantitative assays and a measurement of relative "viral load"; PCR, with a sensitivity of 10^2 to 10^3 virions per milliliter is more sensitive than bDNA, with a sensitivity of 2×10^5. Determination of viral load is not a reliable marker of disease severity or prognosis but is helpful in predicting relative responsiveness to antiviral therapy. The same is true for determinations of HCV genotype (Chap. 297).

A proportion of patients with hepatitis C have isolated anti-HBc in their blood, a reflection of a common risk in certain populations to multiple bloodborne hepatitis agents. The anti-HBc in such cases is almost invariably of the IgG class and usually represents HBV infection in the remote past, rarely current HBV infection with low-level virus carriage.

The presence of HDV infection can be identified by demonstrating

intrahepatic HDV antigen or, more practically, an anti-HDV seroconversion (a rise in titer of anti-HDV or de novo appearance of anti-HDV). Circulating HDV antigen, also diagnostic of acute infection, is detectable only briefly, if at all. Because anti-HDV is often undetectable once HBsAg disappears, retrospective serodiagnosis of acute self-limited, simultaneous HBV and HDV infection is difficult. Early diagnosis of acute infection may be hampered by a delay of up to 30 to 40 days in the appearance of anti-HDV.

When a patient presents with acute hepatitis and has HBsAg and anti-HDV in serum, determination of the class of anti-HBc is helpful in establishing the relationship between infection with HBV and HDV. Although IgM anti-HBc does not distinguish *absolutely* between acute and chronic HBV infection, its presence is a reliable indicator of recent infection and its absence a reliable indicator of infection in the remote past. In simultaneous acute HBV and HDV infections, IgM anti-HBc will be detectable, while in acute HDV infection superimposed on chronic HBV infection, anti-HBc will be of the IgG class.

Tests for the presence of HDV RNA are useful for determining the presence of ongoing HDV replication and relative infectivity. Currently, probes for this marker are restricted to a limited number of research laboratories. Similarly, diagnostic tests for hepatitis E are confined to a small number of research laboratories.

Liver biopsy is rarely necessary or indicated in acute viral hepatitis, except when there is a question about the diagnosis or when there is clinical evidence suggesting a diagnosis of chronic hepatitis.

A diagnostic algorithm can be applied in the evaluation of cases of acute viral hepatitis. A patient with acute hepatitis should undergo four serologic tests, HBsAg, IgM anti-HAV, IgM anti-HBc, and anti-HCV (Table 295-4). The presence of HBsAg, with or without IgM anti-HBc, represents HBV infection. If IgM anti-HBc is present, the HBV infection is considered acute; if IgM anti-HBc is absent, the HBV infection is considered chronic. A diagnosis of acute hepatitis B can be made in the absence of HBsAg when IgM anti-HBc is detectable. A diagnosis of acute hepatitis A is based on the presence of IgM anti-HAV. If IgM anti-HAV coexists with HBsAg, a diagnosis of simultaneous HAV and HBV infections can be made; if IgM anti-HBc (with or without HBsAg) is detectable, the patient has simultaneous acute hepatitis A and B, and if IgM anti-HBc is undetectable, the patient has acute hepatitis A superimposed on chronic HBV infection. The presence of anti-HCV, if confirmable, supports a diagnosis of acute hepatitis C. Occasionally, testing for HCV RNA or repeat anti-HCV testing later during the illness is necessary to establish the diagnosis. Absence of all serologic markers is consistent with a diagnosis of "non-A, non-B, non-C" hepatitis, if the epidemiologic setting is appropriate.

In patients with chronic hepatitis, initial testing should consist of HBsAg and anti-HCV. Anti-HCV supports and HCV RNA testing establishes the diagnosis of chronic hepatitis C. If a serologic diagnosis

Table 295-4   Simplified Diagnostic Approach in Patients Presenting with Acute Hepatitis

Serologic Tests of Patient's Serum				
HBsAg	IgM Anti-HAV	IgM Anti-HBc	Anti-HCV	Diagnostic Interpretation
+	−	+	−	Acute hepatitis B
+	−	−	−	Chronic hepatitis B
+	+	−	−	Acute hepatitis A superimposed on chronic hepatitis B
+	+	+	−	Acute hepatitis A and B
−	+	−	−	Acute hepatitis A
−	+	+	−	Acute hepatitis A and B (HBsAg below detection threshold)
−	−	+	−	Acute hepatitis B (HBsAg below detection threshold)
−	−	−	+	Acute hepatitis C

of chronic hepatitis B is made, testing for HBeAg and anti-HBe is indicated to evaluate relative infectivity. Testing for HBV DNA in such patients provides a more quantitative and sensitive measure of the level of virus replication and, therefore, is very helpful during antiviral therapy (Chap. 297). In patients with hepatitis B, testing for anti-HDV is useful under the following circumstances: patients with severe and fulminant diseases, patients with severe chronic disease, patients with chronic hepatitis B who have acute hepatitis-like exacerbations, persons with frequent percutaneous exposures, and persons from areas where HDV infection is endemic.

PROGNOSIS Virtually all previously healthy patients with hepatitis A recover completely from their illness with no clinical sequelae. Similarly, in acute hepatitis B, 95 to 99% of previously healthy adults have a favorable course and recover completely. There are, however, certain clinical and laboratory features that suggest a more complicated and protracted course. Patients of advanced age and with serious underlying medical disorders may have a prolonged course and are more likely to experience severe hepatitis. Initial presenting features such as ascites, peripheral edema, and symptoms of hepatic encephalopathy suggest a poorer prognosis. In addition, a prolonged PT, low serum albumin level, hypoglycemia, and very high serum bilirubin values suggest severe hepatocellular disease. Patients with these clinical and laboratory features deserve prompt hospital admission. The case-fatality rate in hepatitis A and B is very low (approximately 0.1%) but is increased by advanced age and underlying debilitating disorders. Among patients ill enough to be hospitalized for acute hepatitis B, the fatality rate is 1%. Hepatitis C occurring after transfusion is less severe during the acute phase than hepatitis B and is more likely to be anicteric; fatalities are rare, but the precise case-fatality rate is not known. In outbreaks of waterborne hepatitis E in India and Asia, the case-fatality rate is 1 to 2% and up to 10 to 20% in pregnant women. Patients with simultaneous acute hepatitis B and hepatitis D do not necessarily experience a higher mortality rate than do patients with acute hepatitis B alone; however, in several recent outbreaks of acute simultaneous HBV and HDV infection among injection drug users, the case-fatality rate has been approximately 5%. In the case of HDV superinfection of a person with chronic hepatitis B, the likelihood of fulminant hepatitis and death is increased substantially. Although the case-fatality rate for hepatitis D has not been defined adequately, in outbreaks of severe HDV superinfection in isolated populations with a high hepatitis B carrier rate, the mortality rate has been recorded in excess of 20%.

COMPLICATIONS AND SEQUELAE A small proportion of patients with hepatitis A experience *relapsing hepatitis* weeks to months after apparent recovery from acute hepatitis. Relapses are characterized by recurrence of symptoms, aminotransferase elevations, occasionally jaundice, and fecal excretion of HAV. Another unusual variant of acute hepatitis A is *cholestatic hepatitis*, characterized by protracted cholestatic jaundice and pruritus. Rarely, liver test abnormalities persist for many months, even up to a year. Even when these complications occur, hepatitis A remains self-limited and does not progress to chronic liver disease. During the prodromal phase of acute hepatitis B, a serum sickness–like syndrome characterized by arthralgia or arthritis, rash, angioedema, and rarely hematuria and proteinuria may develop in 5 to 10% of patients. This syndrome occurs before the onset of clinical jaundice, and these patients are often erroneously diagnosed as having rheumatologic diseases. The diagnosis can be established by measuring serum aminotransferase levels, which are almost invariably elevated, and serum HBsAg. As noted above, EMC is an immune-complex disease that can complicate hepatitis C. Attention has been drawn as well to associations between hepatitis C and such cutaneous disorders as porphyria cutanea tarda and lichen planus. A mechanism for these associations is unknown.

The most feared complication of viral hepatitis is *fulminant hepatitis* (massive hepatic necrosis); fortunately, this is a rare event. Fulminant hepatitis is primarily seen in hepatitis B and D, as well as hepatitis E, but rare fulminant cases of hepatitis A occur primarily in older adults and in persons with underlying chronic liver disease. Hep-

atitis B accounts for more than 50% of fulminant hepatitis cases, a sizable proportion of which are associated with HDV infection. Participation of HDV can be documented in approximately one-third of patients with acute fulminant hepatitis B and two-thirds of patients with fulminant hepatitis superimposed on chronic hepatitis B. Fulminant hepatitis is seen rarely in hepatitis C, but hepatitis E, as noted above, can be complicated by fatal fulminant hepatitis in 1 to 2% of all cases and in up to 20% of cases occurring in pregnant women. Patients usually present with signs and symptoms of encephalopathy that may evolve to deep coma. The liver is usually small and the PT excessively prolonged. The combination of rapidly shrinking liver size, rapidly rising bilirubin level, and marked prolongation of the PT, even as aminotransferase levels fall, together with clinical signs of confusion, disorientation, somnolence, ascites, and edema, indicates that the patient has hepatic failure with encephalopathy. Cerebral edema is common; brainstem compression, gastrointestinal bleeding, sepsis, respiratory failure, cardiovascular collapse, and renal failure are terminal events. The mortality rate is exceedingly high (greater than 80% in patients with deep coma), but patients who survive may have a complete biochemical and histologic recovery. If a donor liver can be located in time, liver transplantation may be life-saving in patients with fulminant hepatitis.

It is particularly important to document the disappearance of HBsAg after apparent clinical recovery from acute hepatitis B. Before laboratory methods were available to distinguish between acute hepatitis and acute hepatitis–like exacerbations (*spontaneous reactivations*) of chronic hepatitis B, observations suggested that approximately 10% of patients remained HBsAg-positive for longer than 6 months after the onset of clinically apparent acute hepatitis B. Half these persons cleared the antigen from their circulations during the next several years, but the other 5% remained chronically HBsAg-positive. More recent observations suggest that the true rate of chronic infection after clinically apparent acute hepatitis B is as low as 1% in normal, immunocompetent, young adults. Earlier, higher estimates may have been biased by inadvertent inclusion of acute exacerbations in chronically infected patients; these patients, chronically HBsAg-positive before exacerbation, were unlikely to seroconvert to HBsAg-negative thereafter. Whether the rate of chronicity is 10 or 1%, such patients have anti-HBc in serum; anti-HBs is either undetected or detected at low titer against the opposite subtype specificity of the antigen (see "Laboratory Features," above). These patients may (1) be asymptomatic carriers, (2) have low-grade, mild chronic hepatitis, or (3) have moderate to severe chronic hepatitis with or without cirrhosis. The likelihood of becoming an HBsAg carrier after acute HBV infection is especially high among neonates, persons with Down's syndrome, chronically hemodialyzed patients, and immunosuppressed patients, including persons with HIV infection.

Chronic hepatitis is an important late complication of acute hepatitis B occurring in a small proportion of patients with acute disease but more common in those who present with chronic infection without having experienced an acute illness (Chap. 297). Certain clinical and laboratory features suggest progression of acute hepatitis to chronic hepatitis: (1) lack of complete resolution of clinical symptoms of anorexia, weight loss, and fatigue and the persistence of hepatomegaly; (2) the presence of bridging or multilobular hepatic necrosis on liver biopsy during protracted, severe acute viral hepatitis; (3) failure of the serum aminotransferase, bilirubin, and globulin levels to return to normal within 6 to 12 months after the acute illness; and (4) the persistence of HBeAg beyond 3 months or HBsAg beyond 6 months after acute hepatitis.

Although acute hepatitis D infection does not increase the likelihood of chronicity of simultaneous acute hepatitis B, hepatitis D has the potential for contributing to the severity of chronic hepatitis B. Hepatitis D superinfection can transform asymptomatic or mild chronic hepatitis B into severe, progressive chronic hepatitis and cirrhosis; it also can accelerate the course of chronic hepatitis B. Some

HDV superinfections in patients with chronic hepatitis B lead to fulminant hepatitis. Although HDV and HBV infections are associated with severe liver disease, mild hepatitis and even asymptomatic carriage have been identified in some patients, and the disease may become indolent beyond the early years of infection. After transfusion-associated acute hepatitis C, at least 50% of patients have abnormal biochemical liver tests for more than a year. In some experiences, the frequency of progression to chronicity after acute hepatitis C is as high as 70%. In most of these patients, liver histology is consistent with moderate to severe chronic hepatitis. Even among those who recover biochemically, the likelihood of retaining circulating HCV RNA is high. Thus, after acute HCV infection, the likelihood of remaining chronically *infected* approaches 85 to 90%. Although many patients with chronic hepatitis C have no symptoms, cirrhosis may develop in as many as 20% within 10 to 20 years of acute illness; in some series of cases, cirrhosis has been reported in as many as 50% of patients with chronic hepatitis C. Although chronic hepatitis C accounts for at least a quarter of cases of chronic liver disease and a quarter of patients undergoing liver transplantation for end-stage liver disease in the United States and Europe, in the majority of patients with chronic hepatitis C, morbidity and mortality are limited during the initial 20 years after the onset of infection. Progression of chronic hepatitis C may be influenced by hepatitis C genotype, age of acquisition, duration of infection, and immunosuppression, as well as by coexisting excessive alcohol use or other hepatitis virus infection. In contrast, neither HAV nor HEV causes chronic liver disease.

Rare complications of viral hepatitis include pancreatitis, myocarditis, atypical pneumonia, aplastic anemia, transverse myelitis, and peripheral neuropathy. *Carriers* of HBsAg, particularly those infected in infancy or early childhood, have an enhanced risk of hepatocellular carcinoma. The risk of hepatocellular carcinoma is increased as well in patients with chronic hepatitis C, almost exclusively in patients with cirrhosis, and almost always after at least several decades, usually after three decades of disease (see Chap. 91). In children, hepatitis B may present rarely with anicteric hepatitis, a nonpruritic papular rash of the face, buttocks, and limbs, and lymphadenopathy (papular acrodermatitis of childhood or Gianotti-Crosti syndrome).

DIFFERENTIAL DIAGNOSIS   Viral diseases such as infectious mononucleosis; those due to cytomegalovirus, herpes simplex, and coxsackieviruses; and toxoplasmosis may share certain clinical features with viral hepatitis and cause elevations in serum aminotransferase and less commonly in serum bilirubin levels. Tests such as the differential heterophile and serologic tests for these agents may be helpful in the differential diagnosis if HBsAg, anti-HBc, IgM anti-HAV, and anti-HCV determinations are negative. Aminotransferase elevations can accompany almost any systemic viral infection; other rare causes of liver injury confused with viral hepatitis are infections with *Leptospira*, *Candida*, *Brucella*, *Mycobacteria*, and *Pneumocystis*. A complete drug history is particularly important, for many drugs and certain anesthetic agents can produce a picture of either acute hepatitis or cholestasis (Chap. 296). Equally important is a past history of unexplained "repeated episodes" of acute hepatitis. This history should alert the physician to the possibility that the underlying disorder is chronic hepatitis. Alcoholic hepatitis also must be considered, but usually the serum aminotransferase levels are not as markedly elevated and other stigmata of alcoholism may be present. The finding on liver biopsy of fatty infiltration, a neutrophilic inflammatory reaction, and "alcoholic hyaline" would be consistent with alcohol-induced rather than viral liver injury. Because acute hepatitis may present with right upper quadrant abdominal pain, nausea and vomiting, fever, and icterus, it is often confused with acute cholecystitis, common duct stone, or ascending cholangitis. Patients with acute viral hepatitis may tolerate surgery poorly; therefore, it is important to exclude this diagnosis, and in confusing cases, a percutaneous liver biopsy may be necessary before laparotomy. Viral hepatitis in the elderly is often misdiagnosed as obstructive jaundice resulting from a common duct stone or carcinoma of the pancreas. Because acute hepatitis in the elderly may be quite severe and the operative mortality high, a thorough evaluation including biochemical tests, radiographic studies of the biliary tree, and even liver biopsy may be necessary to exclude primary parenchymal liver disease. Another clinical constellation that may mimic acute hepatitis is right ventricular failure with passive hepatic congestion or hypoperfusion syndromes, such as those associated with shock, severe hypotension, and severe left ventricular failure. Also included in this general category is any disorder that interferes with venous return to the heart, such as right atrial myxoma, constrictive pericarditis, hepatic vein occlusion (Budd-Chiari syndrome), or venoocclusive disease. Clinical features are usually sufficient to distinguish between these vascular disorders and viral hepatitis. Acute fatty liver of pregnancy, cholestasis of pregnancy, eclampsia, and the HELLP syndrome (hemolysis, elevated liver tests, and low platelets) can be confused with viral hepatitis during pregnancy. Very rarely, malignancies metastatic to the liver can mimic acute or even fulminant viral hepatitis. Occasionally, genetic or metabolic liver disorders (e.g., Wilson's disease, α_1-antitrypsin deficiency) are confused with viral hepatitis.

℞ TREATMENT   Treatment of Acute Attack   Although therapy has been developed for chronic hepatitis B and C (Chap. 297), opportunities for treating acute hepatitis caused by HBV or HCV are limited. In hepatitis B, among previously healthy adults who present with clinically apparent acute hepatitis, recovery occurs in approximately 99%; therefore, antiviral therapy is not likely to improve the rate of recovery and is not required. In rare instances of severe acute hepatitis B, treatment with a nucleoside analogue, such as lamivudine, at the 100-mg/d oral dose used to treat chronic hepatitis B (Chap. 297), has been attempted successfully. However, clinical trials have not been done to establish the efficacy of this approach, severe acute hepatitis B is not an approved indication for therapy, and the duration of therapy has not been determined. In typical cases of acute hepatitis C, recovery is rare, progression to chronic hepatitis is the rule, occurring in 85 to 90% of patients, and meta-analyses of small clinical trials suggest that antiviral therapy with interferon alpha (3 million units subcutaneously three times a week) is beneficial, reducing the rate of chronicity considerably by inducing sustained responses in 40% of patients. The duration of therapy and whether to add the nucleoside analogue ribavirin remain to be determined, but the most reasonable approach is to follow recommendations for treatment of chronic hepatitis C (Chap 297). Because of the marked reduction over the last two decades in the frequency of acute hepatitis C, opportunities to identify and treat patients with acute hepatitis C are rare indeed. Hospital epidemiologists, however, will encounter health workers who sustain hepatitis C-contaminated needle sticks; when monitoring for ALT elevations and HCV RNA after these accidents identifies acute hepatitis C, therapy should be initiated.

Notwithstanding these specific therapeutic considerations, in most cases of typical acute viral hepatitis, specific treatment generally is not necessary. Although hospitalization may be required for clinically severe illness, most patients do not require hospital care. Forced and prolonged bed rest is not essential for full recovery, but many patients will feel better with restricted physical activity. A high-calorie diet is desirable, and because many patients may experience nausea late in the day, the major caloric intake is best tolerated in the morning. Intravenous feeding is necessary in the acute stage if the patient has persistent vomiting and cannot maintain oral intake. Drugs capable of producing adverse reactions such as cholestasis and drugs metabolized by the liver should be avoided. If severe pruritus is present, the use of the bile salt–sequestering resin cholestyramine will usually alleviate this symptom. Glucocorticoid therapy has no value in acute viral hepatitis. Even in severe cases associated with *bridging necrosis*, controlled trials have failed to demonstrate the efficacy of steroids. In fact, such therapy may be hazardous.

Physical isolation of patients with hepatitis to a single room and bathroom is rarely necessary except in the case of fecal incontinence for hepatitis A and E or uncontrolled, voluminous bleeding for hepatitis B (with or without concomitant hepatitis D) and hepatitis C. Because most patients hospitalized with hepatitis A excrete little if any HAV, the likelihood of HAV transmission from these patients during their hospitalization is low. Therefore, burdensome *enteric precautions are no longer recommended.* Although gloves should be worn when the bedpans or fecal material of patients with hepatitis A are handled, these precautions do not represent a departure from sensible procedure for all hospitalized patients. For patients with hepatitis B and hepatitis C, emphasis should be placed on blood precautions, i.e., avoiding direct, ungloved hand contact with blood and other body fluids. Enteric precautions are unnecessary. The importance of simple hygienic precautions, such as hand washing, cannot be overemphasized. Universal precautions that have been adopted for all patients apply to patients with viral hepatitis.

Hospitalized patients may be discharged when there is substantial symptomatic improvement, a significant downward trend in the serum aminotransferase and bilirubin values, and a return to normal of the PT. Mild aminotransferase elevations should not be considered contraindications to the gradual resumption of normal activity.

In *fulminant hepatitis*, the goal of therapy is to support the patient by maintenance of fluid balance, support of circulation and respiration, control of bleeding, correction of hypoglycemia, and treatment of other complications of the comatose state in anticipation of liver regeneration and repair. Protein intake should be restricted, and oral lactulose or neomycin administered. Glucocorticoid therapy has been shown in controlled trials to be ineffective. Likewise, exchange transfusion, plasmapheresis, human cross-circulation, porcine liver cross-perfusion, and hemoperfusion have not been proven to enhance survival. Meticulous intensive care is the one factor that does appear to improve survival. Orthotopic liver transplantation is resorted to with increasing frequency, with excellent results, in patients with fulminant hepatitis (Chap. 301).

PROPHYLAXIS Because application of therapy for acute viral hepatitis is limited, and because antiviral therapy for chronic viral hepatitis is effective in only a proportion of patients (Chap. 297), emphasis is placed on prevention through immunization. The prophylactic approach differs for each of the types of viral hepatitis. In the past, immunoprophylaxis relied exclusively on passive immunization with antibody-containing globulin preparations purified by cold ethanol fractionation from the plasma of hundreds of normal donors. Currently, for hepatitis A and B, active immunization with vaccines is available as well.

Hepatitis A Both passive immunization with immune globulin (IG) and active immunization with a killed vaccine are available. All preparations of IG contain anti-HAV concentrations sufficient to be protective. When administered before exposure or during the early incubation period, IG is effective in preventing clinically apparent hepatitis A. In some cases, IG does not abort infection but, by attenuating it, renders it inapparent. As a result, long-lasting "passive-active" immunity occurs; however, this is now considered to be the exception rather than the rule. For postexposure prophylaxis of intimate contacts (household, institutional) of persons with hepatitis A, the administration of 0.02 mL/kg is recommended as early after exposure as possible; it may be effective even when administered as late as 2 weeks after exposure. Prophylaxis is not necessary for casual contacts (office, factory, school, or hospital), for most elderly persons, who are very likely to be immune, or for those known to have anti-HAV in their serum. In day-care centers, recognition of hepatitis A in children or staff should provide a stimulus for immunoprophylaxis in the center and in the children's family members. By the time most common-source outbreaks of hepatitis A are recognized, it is usually too late in the incubation period for IG to be effective; however, prophylaxis may limit the frequency of secondary cases. For travelers to tropical countries, developing countries, and other areas outside standard tourist routes, IG prophylaxis had been recommended, before a vaccine became available. When such travel lasted less than 3 months, 0.02 mL/kg was given; for longer travel or residence in these areas, a dose of 0.06 mL/

kg every 4 to 6 months was recommended. Administration of plasma-derived globulin is safe; it has not been associated with transmission of AIDS to recipients, and the AIDS virus (HIV) is inactivated by 25% alcohol, to which plasma is subjected during the cold ethanol fractionation process.

Formalin-inactivated vaccines made from strains of HAV attenuated in tissue culture have been shown to be safe, immunogenic, and effective in preventing hepatitis A. Hepatitis A vaccines are approved for use in persons who are at least 2 years old and appear to provide adequate protection 4 weeks after a primary inoculation. If it can be given within 4 weeks of an expected exposure, such as by travel to an endemic area, hepatitis A vaccine is the preferred approach to *preexposure* immunoprophylaxis. If travel is more imminent, IG (0.02 mL/kg) should be administered at a different injection site, along with the first dose of vaccine. Because vaccination provides long-lasting protection (protective levels of anti-HAV should last 20 years after vaccination), persons whose risk will be sustained (e.g., frequent travelers or those remaining in endemic areas for prolonged periods) should be vaccinated, and vaccine should supplant the need for repeated IG injections. Other groups who are candidates for hepatitis A vaccination include military personnel, populations with cyclic outbreaks of hepatitis A (e.g., Alaskan natives), employees of day-care centers, primate handlers, laboratory workers exposed to hepatitis A or fecal specimens, children in communities with a high frequency of hepatitis A, and patients with chronic liver disease. Because of an increased risk of fulminant hepatitis A—observed in some experiences but not confirmed in others—among patients with chronic hepatitis C, patients with chronic hepatitis C have been singled out as candidates for hepatitis A vaccination. Other populations whose recognized risk of hepatitis A is increased should be vaccinated, including men who have sex with men, injection drug users, and persons with clotting disorders who require frequent administration of clotting-factor concentrates. Recommendations for dose and frequency differ for the two approved vaccine preparations; all injections are intramuscular. For the hepatitis A vaccine manufactured by SmithKline Beecham (Havrix), adults (older than 18 years) should receive two 1.0-mL injections containing 1440 enzyme-linked immunoassay units (ELU) 6 to 12 months apart. Children age 2 to 18 years should receive three 0.5-mL injections containing 360 ELU at time zero, 6, and 12 months or two 0.5-mL injections containing 720 ELU 6 to 12 months apart. For the hepatitis A vaccine manufactured by Merck (Vaqta), adults (older than 17 years) should receive two 1.0-mL injections containing 50 units 6 months apart; children age 2 to 17 years should receive two 0.5-mL doses containing 25 units 6 to 18 months apart. Hepatitis A vaccine has been reported to be effective in preventing secondary household cases of acute hepatitis A, but its role in other instances of postexposure prophylaxis remains to be demonstrated.

Hepatitis B Until 1982, prevention of hepatitis B was based on *passive* immunoprophylaxis either with standard IG, containing modest levels of anti-HBs, or hepatitis B immune globulin (HBIG), containing high-titer anti-HBs. The efficacy of standard IG has never been established and remains questionable; even the efficacy of HBIG, demonstrated in several clinical trials, has been challenged, and its contribution appears to be in reducing the frequency of clinical *illness*, not in preventing *infection*. The first vaccine for *active* immunization, introduced in 1982, was prepared from purified, noninfectious 22-nm spherical forms of HBsAg derived from the plasma of healthy HBsAg carriers. In 1987, the plasma-derived vaccine was supplanted by a genetically engineered vaccine derived from recombinant yeast. The latter vaccine consists of HBsAg particles that are nonglycosylated but are otherwise indistinguishable from natural HBsAg; two recombinant vaccines are licensed for use in the United States. Current recommendations can be divided into those for preexposure and postexposure prophylaxis.

For *preexposure* prophylaxis against hepatitis B in settings of frequent exposure (health workers exposed to blood, hemodialysis patients and staff, residents and staff of custodial institutions for the developmentally handicapped, injection drug users, inmates of long-term correctional facilities, promiscuous homosexual men as well as promiscuous heterosexual individuals, persons such as hemophiliacs who require long-term, high-volume therapy with blood derivatives, household and sexual contacts of HBsAg carriers, persons living in or traveling extensively in endemic areas, unvaccinated children under the age of 18, and unvaccinated children who are Alaskan natives, Pacific Islanders, or residents in households of first-generation immigrants from endemic countries), three intramuscular (deltoid, not gluteal) injections of hepatitis B vaccine are recommended at 0, 1, and 6 months. Pregnancy is *not* a contraindication to vaccination. In areas of low HBV endemicity such as the United States, despite the availability of safe and effective hepatitis B vaccines, a strategy of vaccinating persons in high-risk groups has not been effective. The incidence of new hepatitis B cases continued to increase in the United States after introduction of vaccines; fewer than 10% of all targeted persons in high-risk groups have actually been vaccinated, and approximately 30% of persons with sporadic acute hepatitis B do not fall into any high-risk-group category. Therefore, to have an impact on the frequency of HBV infection in an area of low endemicity such as the United States, universal hepatitis B vaccination in childhood has been recommended. For unvaccinated children born after the implementation of universal infant vaccination, vaccination during early adolescence, at age 11 to 12 years, was recommended, and this recommendation has been extended to include all unvaccinated children age 0 to 18 years.

The two available recombinant hepatitis B vaccines are comparable, one containing 10 μg of HBsAg (Recombivax-HB) and the other containing 20 μg of HBsAg (Engerix-B), and recommended doses for each injection vary for the two preparations. For Recombivax-HB, 2.5 μg is recommended for children <11 years of age born to HBsAg-negative mothers, 5 μg for infants born to HBsAg-positive mothers (see below) and for children and adolescents 11 to 19 years of age; 10 μg for immunocompetent adults; and 40 μg for dialysis patients and other immunosuppressed persons. For Engerix-B, 10 μg is recommended for children aged 10 and under, 20 μg for immunocompetent children older than 10 years of age and adults, and 40 μg for dialysis patients and other immunocompromised persons.

For unvaccinated persons sustaining an exposure to HBV, *postexposure* prophylaxis with a combination of HBIG (for rapid achievement of high-titer circulating anti-HBs) and hepatitis B vaccine (for achievement of long-lasting immunity as well as its apparent efficacy in attenuating clinical illness after exposure) is recommended. For *perinatal* exposure of infants born to HBsAg-positive mothers, a single dose of HBIG, 0.5 mL, should be administered intramuscularly in the thigh *immediately after birth*, followed by a complete course of three injections of recombinant hepatitis B vaccine (see doses above) to be started within the first 12 h of life. For those experiencing a direct percutaneous inoculation or transmucosal exposure to HBsAg-positive blood or body fluids (e.g., accidental *needle stick*, other mucosal penetration, or ingestion), a single intramuscular dose of HBIG, 0.06 mL/kg, administered as soon after exposure as possible, is followed by a complete course of hepatitis B vaccine to begin within the first week. For those exposed by *sexual* contact to a patient with acute hepatitis B, a single intramuscular dose of HBIG, 0.06 mL/kg, should be given within 14 days of exposure, to be followed by a complete course of hepatitis B vaccine. When both HBIG and hepatitis B vaccine are recommended, they may be given at the same time but at separate sites.

The precise duration of protection afforded by hepatitis B vaccine is unknown; however, approximately 80 to 90% of immunocompetent vaccinees retain protective levels of anti-HBs for at least 5 years, and 60 to 80% for 10 years. Thereafter and even after anti-HBs becomes undetectable, protection persists against clinical hepatitis B, hepatitis B surface antigenemia, and chronic HBV infection. Currently, *booster* immunizations are not recommended routinely, except in immunosup-

pressed persons who have lost detectable anti-HBs or immunocompetent persons who sustain percutaneous HBsAg-positive inoculations after losing detectable antibody. Specifically, for hemodialysis patients, annual anti-HBs testing is recommended after vaccination; booster doses are recommended when anti-HBs levels fall below 10 mIU/mL.

Hepatitis D Infection with hepatitis D can be prevented by vaccinating susceptible persons with hepatitis B vaccine. No product is available for immunoprophylaxis to prevent HDV superinfection in HBsAg carriers; for them, avoidance of percutaneous exposures and limitation of intimate contact with persons who have HDV infection are recommended.

Hepatitis C IG is ineffective in preventing hepatitis C and is no longer recommended for postexposure prophylaxis in cases of perinatal, needle stick, or sexual exposure. Although a prototype vaccine that induces antibodies to HCV envelope protein has been developed, currently, hepatitis C vaccination is not feasible practically. Genotype and quasispecies viral heterogeneity, as well as rapid evasion of neutralizing antibodies by this rapidly mutating virus, conspire to render HCV a difficult target for immunoprophylaxis with a vaccine. Prevention of transfusion-associated hepatitis C has been accomplished by the following successively introduced measures: Exclusion of commercial blood donors and reliance on a volunteer blood supply; screening donor blood with surrogate markers such as ALT (no longer recommended) and anti-HBc, markers that identify segments of the blood donor population with an increased risk of bloodborne infections; exclusion of blood donors in high-risk groups for AIDS and the introduction of anti-HIV screening tests; and progressively sensitive serologic screening tests for anti-HCV. Chemical and heat treatment of blood products used for large-pool and concentrated blood derivates are being pursued.

In the absence of active or passive immunization, prevention of hepatitis C includes behavior changes and precautions to limit exposures to infected persons. Recommendations designed to identify patients with clinically inapparent hepatitis as candidates for medical management have as a secondary benefit the identification of persons whose contacts could be at risk of becoming infected. A so-called "look-back" program has been recommended to identify persons who were transfused before 1992 with blood from a donor found subsequently to have hepatitis C. In addition, anti-HCV testing is recommended for anyone who received a blood transfusion or a transplanted organ before the introduction of second-generation screening tests in 1992, people who ever used injection drugs, chronically hemodialyzed patients, persons with clotting disorders who received clotting factors made before 1987 from pooled blood products, persons with elevated aminotransferase levels, health workers exposed to HCV-positive blood or contaminated needles, and children born to HCV-positive mothers.

For stable, monogamous sexual partners, sexual transmission of hepatitis C is unlikely, and sexual barrier precautions are not recommended. For persons with multiple sexual partners or with sexually transmitted diseases, the risk of sexual transmission of hepatitis C is increased, and barrier precautions (latex condoms) are recommended. A person with hepatitis C should avoid sharing such items as razors, toothbrushes, and nail clippers with sexual partners and family members. No special precautions are recommended for babies born to mothers with hepatitis C, and breast feeding does not have to be restricted.

Hepatitis E Whether IG prevents hepatitis E remains undetermined. Development of a vaccine is in progress.

BIBLIOGRAPHY

ALTER MJ et al: The epidemiology of viral hepatitis in the United States. Gastroenterol Clin North Am 23:437, 1994

ALTER MJ et al: The prevalence of hepatitis C virus infection in the United States, 1988 through 1994. N Engl J Med 341:556, 1999

BARRERA JM et al: Persistent hepatitis C viremia after acute self-limiting posttransfusion hepatitis C. Hepatology 21:639, 1995

CARMAN W et al: Viral genetic variation: Hepatitis B virus as a clinical example. Lancet 341:349, 1993

CENTERS FOR DISEASE CONTROL AND PREVENTION: Hepatitis B virus: A comprehensive strategy for eliminating transmission in the United States through universal childhood vaccination: Recommendations of the Immunization Practices Advisory Committee (ACIP). MMWR 40 (No. RR-13):1, 1991

————: Update: Recommendations to prevent hepatitis B virus transmission—United States. MMWR 44:574, 1995

————: Prevention of hepatitis A through active or passive immunization: Recommendations of the Advisory Committee on Immunization Practices (ACIP). MMWR 48 (No. RR-12):1, 1999

————: Recommendations for prevention and control of hepatitis C virus (HCV) infection and HCV-related chronic disease. MMWR 47:1, 1998

CONRY-CANTILENA C et al: Routes of infection, viremia, and liver disease in blood donors found to have hepatitis C virus infection. N Engl J Med 334:1691, 1996

CONSENSUS STATEMENT: EASL international consensus conference on hepatitis C. J Hepatol 30:956, 1999

DIENSTAG JL: Non-A, non-B hepatitis. I. Recognition, epidemiology, and clinical features. II. Experimental transmission, putative virus agents and markers, and prevention. Gastroenterology 85:439, 743, 1983

DONAHUE JG et al: The declining risk of post-transfusion hepatitis C virus infection. N Engl J Med 327:369, 1992

FARCI P et al: Lack of protective immunity against reinfection with hepatitis C virus. Science 258:135, 1992

GUIDOTTI LG et al: Viral clearance without destruction of infected cells during acute HBV infection. Science 284:825, 1999

HOOFNAGLE JH: Type D (delta) hepatitis. JAMA 261:1321, 1989

HOUGHTON M et al: Molecular biology of the hepatitis C viruses: Implications for diagnosis, development and control of viral disease. Hepatology 14:381, 1991

HUTIN YJF et al: A multistate, foodborne outbreak of hepatitis A. N Engl J Med 340:595, 1999

KOFF RS: Hepatitis A. Lancet 341:1643, 1998

KRAWCZYNSKI K: Hepatitis E. Hepatology 17:932, 1993

MAJOR ME et al: The molecular virology of hepatitis C. Hepatology 25:1527, 1997

MARGOLIS HS et al: Prevention of hepatitis B virus transmission by immunization: An economic analysis of current recommendations. JAMA 274:1201, 1995

MARINOS G et al: Hepatitis B virus variants with core gene deletions in the evolution of chronic hepatitis B infection. Gastroenterology 111:183, 1996

MARTELL M et al: Hepatitis C virus (HCV) circulates as a population of different but closely related genomes: Quasispecies nature of HCV genome distribution. J Virol 66:3225, 1992

NATIONAL INSTITUTES OF HEALTH CONSENSUS DEVELOPMENT CONFERENCE: Management of hepatitis C. Hepatology 26 (Suppl 1):1S, 1997

OKAMOTO H et al: Superinfection of chimpanzees carrying hepatitis C virus of genotype II/1b with that of genotype III/2a or I/1a. Hepatology 20:1131, 1994

PURCELL RH: Hepatitis viruses: Changing patterns of human disease. Proc Natl Acad Sci USA 91:2401, 1994

REHERMAN B et al: Cytotoxic T lymphocyte responsiveness after resolution of chronic hepatitis B virus infection. J Clin Invest 67:1655, 1996

SATO S et al: Hepatitis B virus strains with mutations in the core promoter in patients with fulminant hepatitis. Ann Intern Med 122:241, 1995

SCHREIBER GB et al: The risk of transfusion-transmitted viral infection. N Engl J Med 334:1685, 1996

SEEFF LB: Natural history of viral hepatitis, type C. Semin Gastrointest Dis 6:20, 1995

———— et al: A serologic follow-up of the 1942 epidemic of post-vaccination hepatitis in the United States Army. N Engl J Med 316:965, 1987

———— et al: Long-term mortality after transfusion-association non-A, non-B hepatitis. N Engl J Med 327:1906, 1992

SHAKIL AO et al: Volunteer blood donors with antibody to hepatitis C virus: Clinical, biochemical, virologic, and histologic features. Ann Intern Med 123:330, 1995

SIMMONDS P: Variability of hepatitis C virus. Hepatology 21:570, 1995

TAKAHASHI M et al: Natural history of chronic hepatitis C. Am J Gastroenterol 88:240, 1993

TONG MJ et al: Clinical outcomes after transfusion-associated hepatitis C. N Engl J Med 332:1463, 1995

VAN DER POEL CL et al: Hepatitis C virus six years on. Lancet 344:1475, 1994

VENTO S et al: Fulminant hepatitis associated with hepatitis A virus superinfection in patients with chronic hepatitis C. N Engl J Med 338:286, 1998

WERZBERGER A et al: A controlled trial of formalin-inactivated hepatitis A vaccine in healthy children. N Engl J Med 327:453, 1992

WILNER IR et al: Serious hepatitis A: An analysis of patients hospitalized during an urban epidemic in the United States. Ann Intern Med 128:111, 1998

296 *Jules L. Dienstag, Kurt J. Isselbacher*

TOXIC AND DRUG-INDUCED HEPATITIS

Liver injury may follow the inhalation, ingestion, or parenteral administration of a number of pharmacologic and chemical agents. These include industrial toxins (e.g., carbon tetrachloride, trichloroethylene, and yellow phosphorus), the heat-stable toxic bicyclic octapeptides of certain species of *Amanita* and *Galerina* (hepatotoxic mushroom poisoning), and, more commonly, pharmacologic agents used in medical therapy. It is essential that any patient presenting with jaundice or altered biochemical liver tests be questioned carefully about exposure to chemicals used in work or at home and drugs taken by prescription or bought "over the counter." Hepatotoxic drugs can injure the hepatocyte directly, e.g., via a free-radical or metabolic intermediate that causes peroxidation of membrane lipids and that results in liver cell injury. Alternatively, the drug or its metabolite can distort cell membranes or other cellular molecules or block biochemical pathways or cellular integrity. Such injuries, in turn, may lead to necrosis of hepatocytes; injure bile ducts, producing cholestasis; or block pathways of lipid movement, inhibit protein synthesis, or impair mitochondrial oxidation of fatty acids, resulting in fat accumulation (steatosis). In general, two major types of chemical hepatotoxicity have been recognized: (1) direct toxic type and (2) idiosyncratic type.

Most drugs, which are water-insoluble, undergo a series of metabolic transformation steps, culminating in a water-soluble form appropriate for renal or biliary excretion. This process begins with oxidation or methylation initially mediated by the mixed-function oxygenases cytochrome P450 (phase I reaction), followed by glucuronidation or sulfation (phase II reaction) or inactivation by glutathione. Most drug hepatotoxicity is mediated by a phase I toxic metabolite, but glutathione depletion, precluding inactivation of harmful compounds by glutathione S-transferase, can contribute as well.

As shown in Table 296-1, direct toxic hepatitis occurs with predictable regularity in individuals exposed to the offending agent and is dose-dependent. The latent period between exposure and liver injury is usually short (often several hours), although clinical manifestations may be delayed for 24 to 48 h. Agents producing toxic hepatitis are generally systemic poisons or are converted in the liver to toxic metabolites. The direct hepatotoxins result in morphologic abnormalities that are reasonably characteristic and reproducible for each toxin. For example, carbon tetrachloride and trichloroethylene characteristically produce a centrilobular zonal necrosis, whereas yellow phosphorus poisoning typically results in periportal injury. The hepatotoxic octapeptides of *Amanita phalloides* usually produce massive hepatic necrosis. The lethal dose of the toxin is about 10 mg, the amount found in a single deathcap mushroom. Tetracycline, when administered in intravenous doses >1.5 g daily, leads to microvesicular fat deposits in the liver. Liver injury, which is often only one facet of the toxicity produced by the direct hepatotoxins, may go unrecognized until jaundice appears.

In idiosyncratic drug reactions the occurrence of hepatitis is usually infrequent and unpredictable, the response is not dose-dependent, and it may occur at any time during or shortly after exposure to the drug. Extrahepatic manifestations of hypersensitivity, such as rash, arthralgias, fever, leukocytosis, and eosinophilia, occur in about one-quarter of patients with idiosyncratic hepatotoxic drug reactions; this observation and the unpredictability of idiosyncratic drug hepatotoxicity contributed to the hypothesis that this category of drug reactions is immunologically mediated. More recent evidence, however, suggests that, in most cases, even idiosyncratic reactions represent direct hepatotoxity but are caused by drug metabolites rather than by the intact compound. Even the prototype of idiosyncratic hepatoxicity re-

Table 296-1 Some Features of Toxic and Drug-Induced Hepatic Injury

| Features | Direct Toxic Effect[a] | | Idiosyncratic[a] | | | Other[a] |
	(Carbon Tetrachloride)	(Acetaminophen)	(Halothane)	(Isoniazid)	(Chlorpromazine)	(Oral Contraceptive Agents)
Predictable and dose-related toxicity	+	+	0	0	0	+
Latent period	Short	Short	Variable	Variable	Variable	Variable
Arthralgia, fever, rash, eosinophilia	0	0	+	0	+	0
Liver morphology	Necrosis, fatty infiltration	Centrilobular necrosis	Similar to viral hepatitis	Similar to viral hepatitis	Cholestasis *with* portal inflammation	Cholestasis *without* portal inflammation, vascular lesions

[a] The drugs listed are typical samples.

actions, halothane hepatitis, and isoniazid hepatotoxicity, associated frequently with hypersensitivity manifestations, are now recognized to be mediated by toxic metabolites that damage liver cells directly. Currently, most idiosyncratic reactions are thought to result from differences in metabolic reactivity to specific agents; host susceptibility is mediated by the kinetics of toxic metabolite generation, which differs among individuals. Occasionally, however, the clinical features of an allergic reaction (prominent tissue eosinophilia, autoantibodies, etc.) are difficult to ignore. In vitro models have been described in which lymphocyte cytotoxicity can be demonstrated against rabbit hepatocytes altered by incubation with the potential offending drug. Furthermore, several instances of drug hepatotoxicity are associated with the appearance of autoantibodies, including a class of antibodies to liver-kidney microsomes, anti-LKM2, directed against a cytochrome P450 enzyme. Similarly, in selected cases, a drug or its metabolite has been shown to bind to a host cellular component forming a hapten; the immune response to this "neoantigen" is postulated to play a role in the pathogenesis of liver injury. Therefore, some authorities subdivide idiosyncratic drug hepatotoxicity into hypersensitivity (allergic) and "metabolic" categories. Several unusual exceptions notwithstanding, true drug allergy is difficult to support in most cases of idiosyncratic drug-induced liver injury.

Idiosyncratic reactions lead to a morphologic pattern that is more variable than those produced by direct toxins; a single agent is often capable of causing a variety of lesions, although certain patterns tend to predominate. Depending on the agent involved, idiosyncratic hepatitis may result in a clinical and morphologic picture indistinguishable from that of viral hepatitis (e.g., halothane) or may simulate extrahepatic bile duct obstruction clinically with morphologic evidence of cholestasis. Drug-induced cholestasis ranges from mild to increasingly severe: (1) bland cholestasis with limited hepatocellular injury (e.g., estrogens, 17, α-substituted androgens); (2) inflammatory cholestasis (e.g., phenothiazines, amoxicillin–clavulanic acid, oxacillin, erythromcyin estolate); (3) sclerosing cholangitis (e.g., after intrahepatic infusion of the chemotherapeutic agent floxuridine for hepatic metastases from a primary colonic carcinoma); (4) disappearance of bile ducts, "ductopenic" cholestasis, similar to that observed in chronic rejection following liver transplantation (e.g., carbamazine, chlorpromazine, tricyclic antidepressant agents). Morphologic alterations may also include bridging hepatic necrosis (e.g., methyldopa), or, infrequently, hepatic granulomas (e.g., sulfonamides). Some drugs result in macrovesicular or microvesicular steatosis or steatohepatitis, which in some cases has been linked to mitochondrial dysfunciton and lipid peroxidation. Severe hepatotoxicity associated with steatohepatitis, most likely a result of mitochondrial toxicity, is being recognized with increasing frequency among patients receiving antiretroviral therapy with reverse transcriptase inhibitors (e.g., zidovudine, didanosine) or protease inhibitors (e.g., indinavir, ritonavir) for HIV infection.

Not all adverse hepatic drug reactions can be classified as either toxic or idiosyncratic in type. For example, oral contraceptives, which combine estrogenic and progestational compounds, may result in impairment of hepatic tests and occasionally in jaundice. However, they do not produce necrosis or fatty change, manifestations of hypersensitivity are generally absent, and susceptibility to the development of oral contraceptive–induced cholestasis appears to be genetically determined. Other instances of genetically determined drug hepatotoxicity have been identified. For example, approximately 10% of the population have an autosomally recessive trait associated with the absence of cytochrome P450 enzyme 2D6 and have impaired debrisoquine-4-hydroxylase enzyme activity. As a result, they cannot metabolize, and are at increased risk of hepatotoxicity resulting from, certain compounds such as desipramine, propranolol, and quinidine.

Because drug-induced hepatitis is often a presumptive diagnosis and many other disorders produce a similar clinicopathologic picture, evidence of a causal relationship between the use of a drug and subsequent liver injury may be difficult to establish. The relationship is most convincing for the direct hepatotoxins, which lead to a high frequency of hepatic impairment after a short latent period. Idiosyncratic reactions may be reproduced, in some instances, when rechallenge, after an asymptomatic period, results in a recurrence of signs, symptoms, and morphologic and biochemical abnormalities. Rechallenge, however, is often ethically unfeasible, because severe reactions may occur.

TREATMENT Treatment of toxic and drug-induced hepatic disease is largely supportive, except in acetaminophen hepatotoxicity (see below). In patients with fulminant hepatitis resulting from drug hepatotoxicity, liver transplantation may be life-saving (Chap. 301). Withdrawal of the suspected agent is indicated at the first sign of an adverse reaction. In the case of the direct toxins, liver involvement should not divert attention from renal or other organ involvement, which may also threaten survival.

In Table 296-2, several classes of chemical agents are listed, together with examples of the pattern of liver injury produced by them. Certain drugs appear to be responsible for the development of chronic as well as acute hepatic injury. For example, oxyphenisatin, methyldopa, and isoniazid have been associated with moderate to severe chronic hepatitis, and halothane and methotrexate have been implicated in the development of cirrhosis. A syndrome resembling primary biliary cirrhosis has been described following treatment with chlorpromazine, methyl testosterone, tolbutamide, and other drugs. Portal hypertension in the absence of cirrhosis may result from alterations in hepatic architecture produced by vitamin A or arsenic intoxication, industrial exposure to vinyl chloride, or administration of thorium dioxide. The latter three agents have also been associated with angiosarcoma of the liver. Oral contraceptives have been implicated in the development of hepatic adenoma and, rarely, hepatocellular carcinoma and occlusion of the hepatic vein (Budd-Chiari syndrome). Another unusual lesion, peliosis hepatis (blood cysts of the liver), has been observed in some patients treated with anabolic steroids. The existence of these hepatic disorders expands the spectrum of liver injury induced by chemical agents and emphasizes the need for a thorough drug history in all patients with liver dysfunction.

Principal Morphologic Change	Class of Agent	Example
Cholestasis	Anabolic steroid	Methyl testosterone
	Anti-inflammatory	Sulindac
	Antithyroid	Methimazole
	Antibiotic	Erythromycin estolate, nitrofurantoin, rifampin, amoxicillin–clavulinic acid, oxacillin
	Oral contraceptive	Norethynodrel with mestranol
	Oral hypoglycemic	Chlorpropamide
	Tranquilizer	Chlorpromazine[b]
	Oncotherapeutic	Anabolic steroids, busulfan, tamoxifen
	Immunosuppressive	Cyclosporine
	Anticonvulsant	Carbamazine
	Calcium channel blocker	Nifedipine, verapamil
Fatty liver	Antibiotic	Tetracycline
	Anticonvulsant	Sodium valproate
	Antiarrhythmic	Amiodarone
	Antiviral	Dideoxynucleosides (e.g., zidovudine) protease inhibitors (e.g., indinavir, ritonavir)
	Oncotherapeutic	Asparaginase, methotrexate
Hepatitis	Anesthetic	Halothane[c]
	Anticonvulsant	Phenytoin, carbamazine
	Antihypertensive	Methyldopa,[c] captopril, enalapril
	Antibiotic	Isoniazid,[c] rifampin, nitrofurantoin
	Diuretic	Chlorothiazide
	Laxative	Oxyphenisatin[c]
	Antidepressant	Iproniazid, amitriptyline, imipramine
	Anti-inflammatory	Ibuprofen, indomethacin, diclofenac, sulindac
	Antifungal	Ketoconazole, fluconazole, itraconazole
	Antiviral	Zidovudine, dideoxy inosine
	Calcium channel blocker	Nifedipine, verapamil, diltiazem
	Antiandrogen	Flutamide
Mixed hepatitis/ cholestatic	Immunosuppressive	Azathioprine
	Lipid-lowering	Nicotinic acid, lovastatin
Toxic (necrosis)	Hydrocarbon	Carbon tetrachloride
	Metal	Yellow phosphorus
	Mushroom	*Amanita phalloides*
	Analgesic	Acetaminophen
	Solvent	Dimethylformamide
Granulomas	Anti-inflammatory	Phenylbutazone
	Antibiotic	Sulfanomides
	Xanthine oxidase inhibitor	Allopurinol
	Antiarrhythmic	Quinidine
	Anticonvulsant	Carbamazine

[a] Several agents cause more than one type of liver lesion and appear under more than one category.
[b] Rarely associated with primary biliary cirrhosis–like lesion.
[c] Occasionally associated with chronic hepatitis or bridging hepatic necrosis or cirrhosis.

The following are the patterns of adverse hepatic reactions for some prototypic agents.

ACETAMINOPHEN HEPATOTOXICITY (DIRECT TOXIN) Acetaminophen has caused severe centrilobular hepatic necrosis when ingested in large amounts in suicide attempts or accidentally by children. A single dose of 10 to 15 g, occasionally less, may produce clinical evidence of liver injury. Fatal fulminant disease is usually (although not invariably) associated with ingestion of 25 g or more. Blood levels of acetaminophen correlate with the severity of hepatic injury (levels >300 μg/mL 4 h after ingestion are predictive of the development of severe damage; levels <150 μg/mL suggest that hepatic injury is highly unlikely). Nausea, vomiting, diarrhea, ab-

dominal pain, and shock are early manifestations occurring 4 to 12 h after ingestion. Then 24 to 48 h later, when these features are abating, hepatic injury becomes apparent. Maximal abnormalities and hepatic failure may not be evident until 4 to 6 days after ingestion, and aminotransferase levels approaching 10,000 units are not uncommon. Renal failure and myocardial injury may be present.

Acetaminophen is metabolized predominantly by a phase II reaction to innocuous sulfate and glucuronide metabolites; however, a small proportion of acetaminophen is metabolized by a phase I reaction to a hepatotoxic metabolite formed from the parent compound by the cytochrome P450 2E1. This metabolite, *N*-acetyl-benzoquinone-imide (NAPQI), is detoxified by binding to "hepatoprotective" glutathione to become harmless, water-soluble mercapturic acid, which undergoes renal excretion. When excessive amounts of NAPQI are formed, or when glutathione levels are low, glutathione levels are depleted and overwhelmed, permitting covalent binding to nucleophilic hepatocyte macromolecules. This process is believed to lead to hepatocyte necrosis; the precise sequence and mechanism are unknown. Hepatic injury may be potentiated by prior administration of alcohol or other drugs, by conditions that stimulate the mixed-function oxidase system, or by conditions such as starvation that reduce hepatic glutathione levels. Cimetidine, which inhibits P450 enzymes, has the potential to reduce generation of the toxic metabolite. Alcohol induces cytochrome P450 2E1; consequently, increased levels of the toxic metabolite NAPQI are produced in chronic alcoholics after acetaminophen ingestion. In addition, alcohol suppresses hepatic glutathione production. Therefore, in chronic alcoholics, the toxic dose of acetaminophen may be as low as 2 g, and alcoholic patients should be warned specifically about the dangers of even standard doses of this commonly used drug. Such "therapeutic misadventures" also occur occasionally in patients with severe, febrile illnesses or pain syndromes; in such a setting, several days of anorexia and near-fasting coupled with regular administration of extra-strength acetaminophen formulations result in a combination of glutathione depletion and relatively high NAPQI levels in the absence of a history of recognized acetaminophen overdose.

R̲x̲ TREATMENT Treatment of acetaminophen overdosage includes gastric lavage, supportive measures, and oral administration of activated charcoal or cholestyramine to prevent absorption of residual drug. Neither of these agents appears to be effective if given more than 30 min after acetaminophen ingestion; if they are used, the stomach lavage should be done before other agents are administered orally. The chances of possible-, probable-, and high-risk hepatotoxicity can be derived from a nomogram plot (see Fig. 396-2), readily available in emergency departments, of acetaminophen plasma levels as a function of hours after ingestion. In patients with high acetaminophen blood levels (>200 μg/mL measured at 4 h or >100 μg/mL at 8 h after ingestion), the administration of sulfhydryl compounds (e.g., cysteamine, cysteine, or *N*-acetylcysteine) appears to reduce the severity of hepatic necrosis. These agents appear to act by providing a reservoir of sulfhydryl groups to bind the toxic metabolites or by stimulating synthesis and repletion of hepatic glutathione. Therapy should be begun within 8 h of ingestion but may be effective even if given as late as 24 to 36 h after overdose. Later administration of sulfhydryl compounds is of uncertain value. Routine use of *N*-acetylcysteine has reduced substantially the occurrence of fatal acetaminophen hepatotoxicity. When given orally, *N*-acetylcysteine is diluted to yield a 5% solution. A loading dose of 140 mg/kg is given, followed by 70 mg/kg every 4 h for 15 to 20 doses. Whenever a patient with potential acetaminophen hepatotoxicity is encountered, a local poison control center should be contacted. Treatment can be stopped when plasma acetaminophen levels indicate that the risk of liver damage is low.

Survivors of acute acetaminophen overdose usually have no evidence of hepatic sequelae. In a few patients, prolonged or repeated administration of acetaminophen in therapeutic doses appears to have led to the development of chronic hepatitis and cirrhosis.

HALOTHANE HEPATOTOXICITY (IDIOSYNCRATIC REACTION) Administration of halothane, a nonexplosive fluorinated hydrocarbon anesthetic agent that is structurally similar to chloroform, results in severe hepatic necrosis in a small number of individuals, many of whom have previously been exposed to this agent. The failure to produce similar hepatic lesions reliably in animals, the rarity of hepatic impairment in human beings, and the delayed appearance of hepatic injury suggest that halothane is not a direct hepatotoxin but rather a sensitizing agent. However, manifestations of hypersensitivity are seen in <25% of cases. A genetic predisposition leading to an idiosyncratic metabolic reactivity has been postulated and appears to be the most likely mechanism of halothane hepatotoxicity. Adults (rather than children), obese people, and women appear to be particularly susceptible. Fever, moderate leukocytosis, and eosinophilia may occur in the first week following halothane administration. Jaundice is usually noted 7 to 10 days after exposure but may occur earlier in previously exposed patients. Nausea and vomiting may precede the onset of jaundice. Hepatomegaly is often mild, but liver tenderness is common. The serum aminotransferase levels are elevated. The pathologic changes at autopsy are indistinguishable from massive hepatic necrosis resulting from viral hepatitis. The case-fatality rate of halothane hepatitis is not known but may vary from 20 to 40% in cases with severe liver involvement. It is strongly suggested that patients in whom unexplained spiking fever, especially delayed fever, or jaundice develops after halothane anesthesia not receive this agent again. Because cross-reactions between halothane and methoxyfluorane have been reported, the latter agent should not be used after halothane reactions. Later-generation halogenated hydrocarbon anesthetics, which have supplanted halothane except in rare instances, are felt to be associated with a lower risk of hepatotoxicity.

METHYLDOPA HEPATOTOXICITY (TOXIC AND IDIOSYNCRATIC REACTION) Minor alterations in liver tests are reported in about 5% of patients treated with this antihypertensive agent. These trivial abnormalities typically resolve despite continued drug administration. In <1% of patients, acute liver injury resembling viral or chronic hepatitis or, rarely, a cholestatic reaction is seen 1 to 20 weeks after methyldopa is started. In 50% of cases the interval is <4 weeks. A prodrome of fever, anorexia, and malaise may be noted for a few days before the onset of jaundice. Rash, lymphadenopathy, arthralgia, and eosinophilia are rare. Serologic markers of autoimmunity are detected infrequently, and <5% of patients have a Coombs-positive hemolytic anemia. In about 15% of patients with methyldopa hepatotoxicity, the clinical, biochemical, and histologic features are those of moderate to severe chronic hepatitis, with or without bridging necrosis and macronodular cirrhosis. With discontinuation of the drug, the disorder usually resolves.

ISONIAZID HEPATOTOXICITY (TOXIC AND IDIOSYNCRATIC REACTION) In approximately 10% of adults treated with the antituberculosis agent isoniazid, elevated serum aminotransferase levels develop during the first few weeks of therapy; this appears to represent an adaptive response to a toxic metabolite of the drug. Whether or not isoniazid is continued, these values (usually <200 units) return to normal in a few weeks. In about 1% of treated patients, an illness develops that is indistinguishable from viral hepatitis; approximately half of these cases occur within the first 2 months of treatment, while in the remainder, clinical disease may be delayed for many months. Liver biopsy reveals morphologic changes similar to those of viral hepatitis or bridging hepatic necrosis. The disease may be severe, with a case-fatality rate of 10%. Important liver injury appears to be age-related, increasing substantially after age 35; the highest frequency is in patients over age 50, the lowest under the age of 20. Even for patients >50 years of age monitored carefully during therapy, hepatotoxicity occurs in only approximately 2%, well below the risk estimate derived from earlier experiences. Isoniazid hepato-

toxicity is enhanced by alcohol and rifampicin. Fever, rash, eosinophilia, and other manifestations of drug allergy are distinctly unusual. A reactive metabolite of acetylhydrazine, a metabolite of isoniazid, may be responsible for liver injury, and patients who are rapid acetylators would be more prone to such injury. A picture resembling chronic hepatitis has been observed in a few patients.

SODIUM VALPROATE HEPATOTOXICITY (TOXIC AND IDIOSYNCRATIC REACTION) Sodium valproate, an anticonvulsant useful in the treatment of petit mal and other seizure disorders, has been associated with the development of severe hepatic toxicity and, rarely, fatalities, predominantly in children but also in adults. Asymptomatic elevations of serum aminotransferase levels have been recognized in as many as 45% of treated patients. These "adaptive" changes, however, appear to have no clinical importance, for major hepatotoxicity is not seen in the majority of patients despite continuation of drug therapy. In those rare patients in whom jaundice, encephalopathy, and evidence of hepatic failure are found, examination of liver tissue reveals microvesicular fat and bridging hepatic necrosis, predominantly in the centrilobular zone. Bile duct injury may also be apparent. It seems likely that sodium valproate is not directly hepatotoxic but that its metabolite, 4-pentenoic acid, may be responsible for hepatic injury.

PHENYTOIN HEPATOTOXICITY (IDIOSYNCRATIC REACTION) Phenytoin, formerly diphenylhydantoin, a mainstay in the treatment of seizure disorders, has been associated in rare instances with the development of severe hepatitis-like liver injury leading to fulminant hepatic failure. In many patients the hepatitis is associated with striking fever, lymphadenopathy, rash (Stevens-Johnson syndrome or exfoliative dermatitis), leukocytosis, and eosinophilia, suggesting an immunologically mediated hypersensitivity mechanism. Despite these observations, there is also evidence that metabolic idiosyncrasy may be responsible for hepatic injury. In the liver, phenytoin is converted by the cytochrome P450 system to metabolites, which include the highly reactive electrophilic arene oxides. These metabolites are normally metabolized further by epoxide hydrolases. A defect (genetic or acquired) in epoxide hydrolase activity could permit covalent binding of arene oxides to hepatic macromolecules, thereby leading to hepatic injury. Regardless of the mechanism, hepatic injury is usually manifest within the first 2 months after beginning phenytoin therapy. With the exception of an abundance of eosinophils in the liver, the clinical, biochemical, and histologic picture resembles that of viral hepatitis. In rare instances, bile duct injury may be the salient feature of phenytoin hepatotoxicity, with striking features of intrahepatic cholestasis. Asymptomatic elevations of aminotransferase and alkaline phosphatase levels have been observed in a sizable proportion of patients receiving long-term phenytoin therapy. These liver changes are believed by some authorities to represent the potent hepatic enzyme–inducing properties of phenytoin and are accompanied histologically by swelling of hepatocytes in the absence of necroinflammatory activity or evidence of chronic liver disease.

CHLORPROMAZINE HEPATOTOXICITY (CHOLESTATIC IDIOSYNCRATIC REACTION) In about 1% of patients receiving chlorpromazine, intrahepatic cholestasis with jaundice develops after 1 to 4 weeks of treatment. In rare instances, jaundice has been reported after a single exposure. Anicteric reactions are frequent. The onset may be abrupt, with fever, rash, arthralgias, lymphadenopathy, nausea, vomiting, and epigastric or right upper quadrant pain. Pruritus may precede the appearance of jaundice, dark urine, and light stools. Eosinophilia with or without mild leukocytosis may be present, and conjugated hyperbilirubinemia, moderately elevated serum alkaline phosphatase, and mildly elevated serum aminotransferase levels (100 to 200 units) are noted. Liver biopsy reveals cholestasis, bile plugs in dilated bile canaliculi, and a dense portal infiltrate of polymorphonuclear, eosinophilic, and mononuclear leukocytes. Occasionally, scattered foci of hepatic parenchymal necrosis may be evident. Jaundice and pruritus usually subside within 4 to 8 weeks following cessation of therapy, without sequelae, and fatalities are rare. Cholestyramine may be of value in relieving severe pruritus. In a small number of patients, jaundice is prolonged for several months to years; rarely, a disorder resembling but distinct from primary biliary cirrhosis may develop.

AMIODARONE HEPATOTOXICITY (TOXIC AND IDIOSYNCRATIC REACTION) Therapy with this potent antiarrhythmic drug is accompanied in 15 to 50% of patients by modest elevations of serum aminotransferase levels that may remain stable or diminish despite continuation of the drug. Such abnormalities may appear days to many months after beginning therapy. A proportion of those with elevated aminotransferase levels have detectable hepatomegaly, and clinically important liver disease develops in <5% of patients. Features that represent a direct effect of the drug on the liver and that are common to the majority of long-term recipients are ultrastructural phospholipidosis, unaccompanied by clinical liver disease, and interference with hepatic mixed-function oxidase metabolism of other drugs. The cationic amphiphilic drug and its major metabolite desethylamiodarone accumulate in hepatocyte lysosomes and mitochondria and in bile duct epithelium. The relatively common elevations in aminotransferase levels are also considered a predictable, dose-dependent, direct hepatotoxic effect. On the other hand, in the rare patient with clinically apparent, symptomatic liver disease, liver injury resembling that seen in alcoholic liver disease is observed. The so-called pseudoalcoholic liver injury can range from steatosis, to alcoholic hepatitis-like neutrophilic infiltration and Mallory's hyaline, to cirrhosis. Electron-microscopic demonstration of phospholipid-laden lysosomal lamellar bodies can help to distinguish amiodarone hepatotoxicity from typical alcoholic hepatitis. This category of liver injury appears to be a metabolic idiosyncracy that allows hepatotoxic metabolites to be generated. Rarely, an acute idiosyncratic hepatocellular injury resembling viral hepatitis or cholestatic hepatitis occurs. Hepatic granulomas have occasionally been observed. Because amiodarone has a long half-life, liver injury may persist for months after the drug is stopped.

ERYTHROMYCIN HEPATOTOXICITY (CHOLESTATIC IDIOSYNCRATIC REACTION) The most important adverse effect associated with erythromycin, more common in children than adults, is the infrequent occurrence of a cholestatic reaction. Although most of these reactions have been associated with erythromycin estolate, other erythromycins may also be responsible. The reaction usually begins during the first 2 or 3 weeks of therapy and includes nausea, vomiting, fever, right upper quadrant abdominal pain, jaundice, leukocytosis, and moderately elevated aminotransferase levels. The clinical picture can resemble acute cholecystitis or bacterial cholangitis. Liver biopsy reveals variable cholestasis; portal inflammation comprising lymphocytes, polymorphonuclear leukocytes, and eosinophils; and scattered foci of hepatocyte necrosis. Symptoms and laboratory findings usually subside within a few days of drug withdrawal, and evidence of chronic liver disease has not been found on follow-up. The precise mechanism remains ill-defined.

ORAL CONTRACEPTIVE HEPATOTOXICITY (CHOLESTATIC REACTION) The administration of oral contraceptive combinations of estrogenic and progestational steroids leads to intrahepatic cholestasis with pruritus and jaundice in a small number of patients weeks to months after taking these agents. Especially susceptible seem to be patients with recurrent idiopathic jaundice of pregnancy, severe pruritus of pregnancy, or a family history of these disorders. With the exception of liver biochemical tests, laboratory studies are normal, and extrahepatic manifestations of hypersensitivity are absent. Liver biopsy reveals cholestasis with bile plugs in dilated canaliculi and striking bilirubin staining of liver cells. In contrast to chlorpromazine-induced cholestasis, portal inflammation is absent. The lesion is reversible on withdrawal of the agent. The two steroid components appear to act synergistically on hepatic function, although the estrogen may be primarily responsible. Oral contraceptives are contraindicated in patients with a history of recurrent jaundice of pregnancy. Primarily benign, but rarely malignant, neoplasms of the liver, hepatic vein occlusion, and peripheral sinusoidal dilatation have also been associated with oral contraceptive therapy.

17,α-ALKYL-SUBSTITUTED ANABOLIC STEROIDS (CHOLESTATIC REACTION) In the majority of patients receiving these agents, used therapeutically mainly in the treatment of bone marrow failure but used surreptitiously and without medical indication by athletes to improve their performance, mild hepatic dysfunction develops. Impaired excretory function is the predominant defect, but the precise mechanism is uncertain. Jaundice, which appears to be dose-related, develops in only a minority of patients and may be the sole clinical manifestation of hepatotoxicity, although anorexia, nausea, and malaise may occur. Pruritus is not a prominent feature. Serum aminotransferase levels are usually <100 units, and serum alkaline phosphatase levels are normal, mildly elevated, or, in <5% of patients, three or more times the upper limit of normal. Examination of liver tissue reveals cholestasis without inflammation or necrosis. Hepatic sinusoidal dilatation and peliosis hepatis have been found in a few patients. The cholestatic disorder is usually reversible on cessation of treatment, although fatalities have been linked to peliosis. An association with hepatic adenoma and hepatocellular carcinoma has been reported.

TRIMETHOPRIM-SULFAMETHOXAZOLE HEPATOTOXICITY (IDIOSYNCRATIC REACTION) This antibiotic combination is used routinely for urinary tract infections in immunocompetent persons and for prophylaxis against and therapy of *Pneumocystis carinii* pneumonia in immunosuppressed persons (transplant recipients, patients with AIDS). With its increasing use, its occasional hepatotoxicity is being recognized with growing frequency. Its likelihood is unpredictable, but when it occurs, trimethoprim-sulfamethoxazole hepatotoxicity follows a relatively uniform latency period of several weeks and is often accompanied by eosinophilia, rash, and other features of a hypersensitivity reaction. Biochemically and histologically, acute hepatocellular necrosis predominates, but cholestatic features are quite frequent. Occasionally, cholestasis without necrosis occurs, and very rarely, a severe cholangiolytic pattern of liver injury is observed. In most cases, liver injury is self-limited, but rare fatalities have been recorded. The hepatotoxicity is attributable to the sulfamethoxazole component of the drug and is similar in features to that seen with other sulfonamides; tissue eosinophilia and granulomas may be seen.

HYDROXYMETHYLGLUTARYL-COENZYME (HMG-COA) REDUCTASE INHIBITORS ("STATINS") (IDIOSYNCRATIC MIXED HEPATOCELLULAR AND CHOLESTATIC REACTION) Between 1 and 2% of patients taking lovastatin, simvastatin, pravastatin, fluvastatin, or one of the newer "statin" drugs for the treatment of hypercholesterolemia experience asymptomatic, reversible elevations (> threefold) of aminotransferase activity. Acute hepatitis-like histologic changes, centrilobular necrosis, and centrilobular cholestasis have been described in several cases. In a larger proportion, minor aminotrasferase elevations appear during the first several weeks of therapy. Careful laboratory monitoring can distinguish between patients with minor, transitory changes, who may continue therapy, and those with more profound and sustained abnormalities, who should discontinue therapy.

TOTAL PARENTERAL NUTRITION (STEATOSIS, CHOLESTASIS) Total parenteral nutrition (TPN) is often complicated by cholestatic hepatitis attributable to either steatosis, cholestasis, or gallstones (or gallbladder sludge). Steatosis or steatohepatitis may result from the excess carbohydrate calories in these nutritional supplements and is the predominant form of TPN-associated liver disorder in adults. The frequency of this complication has been reduced substantially by the introduction of balanced TPN formulas that rely on lipid as an alternative caloric source. Cholestasis and cholelithiasis, caused by the absence of stimulation of bile flow and secretion resulting from the lack of oral intake, is the predominant form of TPN-associated liver disease in infants, especially in premature neonates. Often, cholestasis in such neonates is multifactorial, contributed to by other factors such as sepsis, hypoxemia, and hypotension; occasionally, TPN-induced cholestasis in neonates culminates in chronic liver disease and liver failure. When TPN-associated liver test abnormalities occur in adults, balancing the TPN formula with more lipid is the intervention of first recourse. In infants with TPN-associated cholestasis, the addition of oral feeding may ameliorate the problem. Therapeutic interventions suggested, but not yet shown to be of proven benefit, include CCK, ursodeoxycholic acid, *S*-adenosyl methionine, and taurine.

"ALTERNATIVE MEDICINES" (IDIOSYNCRATIC HEPATITIS, STEATOSIS) The misguided popularity of herbal medications that are of scientifically unproven efficacy and that lack prospective safety oversight by regulatory agencies has resulted in occasional instances of hepatotoxicity. Included among the herbal remedies associated with toxic hepatitis are jin bu huan (Chap. 11), xiao-chai-hu-tang, germander, chaparral, senna, mistletoe, skullcap, gentian, comfrey (containing pyrrolizidine alkaloids), and herbal teas. Recently well characterized are the acute hepatitis-like histologic lesions following jin bu huan use: focal hepatocellular necrosis, mixed mononuclear portal tract infiltration, coagulative necrosis, apoptotic hepatocyte degeneration, tissue eosinophilia, and microvesicular steatosis. Megadoses of vitamin A can injure the liver, as can pyrrolizidine alkaloids, which often contaminate Chinese herbal preparations and can cause a venoocclusive injury leading to sinusoidal hepatic vein obstruction. Given the widespread use of such poorly defined herbal preparations, hepatotoxicity is likely to be encountered with increasing frequency; therefore, a drug history in patients with acute and chronic liver disease should include use of "alternative medicines" and other nonprescription preparations sold in so-called health food stores.

BIBLIOGRAPHY

BLACK M et al: Isoniazid-associated hepatitis in 114 patients. Gastroenterology 69:389, 1975

———— et al: Acetaminophen hepatotoxicity. Ann Rev Med 35:577, 1984

BERSON A et al: Steatohepatitis-inducing drugs cause mitochondrial dysfunction and lipid peroxidation in rat hepatocytes. Gastroenterology 114:764, 1998

FARRELL GC: Drug-induced hepatic injury. J Gastroenterol Hepatol 12(Suppl):S242, 1997

GRIMBERT S et al: Acute hepatitis induced by HMG-CoA reductase inhibitor, lovastatin. Dig Dis Sci 39:2032, 1994

KAPLOWITZ N (ed): Recent advances in drug metabolism and hepatotoxicity. Semin Liver Dis 10:233, 1990

LEE WM: Drug-induced hepatotoxicity. N Engl J Med 333:1118, 1995

LEWIS JH et al: Amiodarone hepatotoxicity: Prevalence and clinicopathologic correlations among 104 patients. Hepatology 9:679, 1989

LUDWIG J, AXELSEN R: Drug effects on the liver: An updated tabular compilation of drugs and drug-related hepatic diseases. Dig Dis Sci 28:651, 1983

MALKIN A et al: A seven year experience of severe acetaminophen-induced hepatotoxicity (1987–1993). Gastroenterology 109:1907, 1995

MORGAN DJ, SMALLWOOD RA: Drug-induced liver disease. Curr Opinion Gastroenterol 12:246, 1996

NOLAN CM et al: Hepatotoxicity associated with isoniazid preventive therapy. JAMA 281:1014, 1999

QUIGLEY EMM et al: Hepatobiliary complications of total parenteral nutrition. Gastroenterology 104:786, 1993

RABINOVITZ M et al: Hepatotoxicity of nonsteroidal anti-inflammatory drugs. Am J Gastroenterol 87:1696, 1992

RUMACK BH et al: Acetaminophen overdose. JAMA 141:380, 1981

SALPETER SR et al: Monitored isoniazid prophylaxis for low-risk tuberculin reactors older than 35 years of age. Ann Intern Med 127:1051, 1997

SCHIODT FV et al: Acetaminophen toxicity in an urban county hospital. N Engl J Med 337:1112, 1997

SEEFF LB et al: Acetaminophen hepatotoxicity in alcoholics: A therapeutic misadventure. Ann Intern Med 104:399, 1986

SMILKSTEIN MJ et al: Efficacy of *N*-acetylcysteine in the treatment of acetaminophen overdose. N Engl J Med 319:1557, 1988

TARAZI EM et al: Sulindac-associated hepatic injury: Analysis of 91 cases reported to the Food and Drug Administration. Gastroenterology 104:569, 1993

WHITCOMB DC et al: Association of acetaminophen hepatotoxicity with fasting and ethanol use. JAMA 272:1845, 1994

WOOLF GM et al: Acute hepatitis associated with the Chinese herbal product Jin Bu Huan. Ann Intern Med 121:729, 1994

ZIMMERMAN HJ: Drug-induced liver disease, in *Schiff's Diseases of the Liver*, 8th ed. E Schiff et al (eds). Philadelphia, Lippincott-Raven, 1999, p 973

————, ISHAK KG: Valproate-induced hepatic injury: Analysis of 23 fatal cases. Hepatology 2:591, 1982

————, MADDREY WC: Acetaminophen (paracetamol) hepatotoxicity with regular intake of alcohol: Analysis of instances of therapeutic misadventure. Hepatology 22:767, 1995

297 *Jules L. Dienstag, Kurt J. Isselbacher*

CHRONIC HEPATITIS

ALT, or SGPT alanine aminotransferase	HBV hepatitis B virus
anti-LKM antibodies to liver-kidney microsomes	HCV hepatitis C virus
	HDV chronic hepatitis D virus
ANA antinuclear antibodies	HCC hepatocellular carcinoma
AST, or SGOT aspartate aminotransferase	HAI histologic activity index
	IFN-α interferon α
HBcAg hepatitis B core antigen	PEG polyethylene glycol
HBeAg hepatitis B e antigen	PCR polymerase chain reaction
HBsAg hepatitis B surface antigen	YMDD tyrosine-methionine-aspartate-aspartate

Chronic hepatitis represents a series of liver disorders of varying causes and severity in which hepatic inflammation and necrosis continue for at least 6 months. Milder forms are nonprogressive or only slowly progressive, while more severe forms may be associated with scarring and architectural reorganization, which, when advanced, lead ultimately to cirrhosis. Several categories of chronic hepatitis have been recognized. These include chronic viral hepatitis (Chap. 295), drug-induced chronic hepatitis (Chap. 296), and autoimmune chronic hepatitis. In many cases, clinical and laboratory features are insufficient to allow assignment into one of these three categories; these "idiopathic" cases are also believed to represent autoimmune chronic hepatitis. Finally, clinical and laboratory features of chronic hepatitis are observed occasionally in patients with such hereditary/metabolic disorders as Wilson's disease (copper overload) and even occasionally in patients with alcoholic liver injury (Chap. 298). Although all types of chronic hepatitis share certain clinical, laboratory, and histopathologic features, chronic viral and chronic autoimmune hepatitis are sufficiently distinct to merit separate discussions.

CLASSIFICATION OF CHRONIC HEPATITIS Common to all forms of chronic hepatitis are histopathologic distinctions based on localization and extent of liver injury. These vary from the milder forms, previously labeled chronic persistent hepatitis and chronic lobular hepatitis, to the more severe form, formerly called chronic active hepatitis. When first defined, these designations were felt to have prognostic implications, which have been challenged by more recent observations. Compared to the time more than two decades ago when the histologic designations chronic persistent, chronic lobular, and chronic active hepatitis were adopted, much more information is currently available about the causes, natural history, pathogenesis, serologic features, and therapy of chronic hepatitis. Therefore, categorization of chronic hepatitis based primarily upon histopathologic features has been replaced by a more informative classification based upon a combination of clinical, serologic, and histologic variables. Classification of chronic hepatitis is based upon (1) its *cause*, (2) its histologic activity, or *grade*, and (3) its degree of progression, or *stage*. Thus, neither clinical features alone nor histologic features—requiring liver biopsy—alone are sufficient to characterize and distinguish among the several categories of chronic hepatitis.

Classification by Cause Clinical and serologic features allow the establishment of a diagnosis of *chronic viral hepatitis*, caused by hepatitis B, hepatitis B plus D, hepatitis C, or potentially other unknown viruses; *autoimmune hepatitis*, including several subcategories,

types 1, 2, and 3, based on serologic distinctions; *drug-associated chronic hepatitis*; and a category of unknown cause, or *cryptogenic* chronic hepatitis (Table 297-1). These are addressed in more detail below.

Classification by Grade Grade, a histologic assessment of necroinflammatory activity, is based upon examination of the liver biopsy. An assessment of important histologic features includes the degree of *periportal necrosis* and the disruption of the limiting plate of periportal hepatocytes by inflammatory cells (so-called *piecemeal necrosis* or *interface hepatitis*); the degree of confluent necrosis that links or forms bridges between vascular structures—between portal tract and portal tract or even more important bridges between portal tract and central vein—referred to as *bridging necrosis*; the degree of hepatocyte degeneration and focal necrosis within the lobule; and the degree of *portal inflammation*. Several scoring systems that take these histologic features into account have been devised, and the most popular is the numerical histologic activity index (HAI), based on the work of Knodell and Ishak (Table 297-2). Technically, the HAI, which is primarily a measure of *grade*, also includes an assessment of fibrosis, which is currently used to categorize *stage* of the disease, as described below. Such precise HAI scoring tends to be used more in measuring disease activity before and after therapy in clinical studies. In clinical practice, more qualitative grading suffices. Based on the presence and degree of these features of histologic activity, chronic hepatitis can be graded as mild, moderate, or severe.

Classification by Stage The stage of chronic hepatitis, which reflects the level of progression of the disease, is based on the degree of fibrosis. When fibrosis is so extensive that fibrous septa surround parenchymal nodules and alter the normal architecture of the liver lobule, the histologic lesion is defined as cirrhosis. Staging is based on the degree of fibrosis as follows:

0 = no fibrosis
1 = mild fibrosis
2 = moderate fibrosis
3 = severe fibrosis, including bridging fibrosis
4 = cirrhosis

Reconciliation between Histologic Classification and New Classification For historical purposes, and to provide the basis for navigating several decades worth of literature on chronic hepatitis, the

Table 297-1 Clinical and Laboratory Features of Chronic Hepatitis

Type of Hepatitis	Diagnostic Test(s)	Autoantibodies	Therapy
Chronic hepatitis B	HBsAg, IgG anti-HBc, HBeAg, HBV DNA	Uncommon	INF-α, lamivudine
Chronic hepatitis C	Anti-HCV (EIA and RIBA), HCV RNA	Anti-LKM1[a]	INF-α plus ribavirin
Chronic hepatitis D	Anti-HDV, HDV RNA, HBsAg, IgG anti-HBc	Anti-LKM3	INF-α (?)
Autoimmune hepatitis	ANA[b] (homogeneous), anti-LKM1(±), hyperglobulinemia	ANA, anti-LKM1, anti-SLA[c]	Prednisone, azathioprine
Drug-associated	—	Uncommon	Withdraw drug
Cryptogenic	All negative	None	Prednisone (?), azathioprine (?)

[a] Antibodies to liver-kidney microsomes type 1 (autoimmune hepatitis type II and some cases of hepatitis C).
[b] Antinuclear antibody (autoimmune hepatitis type I).
[c] Antibodies to soluble liver antigen (autoimmune hepatitis type III).
NOTE: HBsAg, hepatitis B surface antigen; EIA, enzyme immunoassay; RIBA, recombinant immunoblot assay; INF-α, interferon α.

Table 297-2 Histologic Activity Index (Knodell-Ishak Score) in Chronic Hepatitis

Histologic Feature	Severity	Score
1. Periportal necrosis, including piecemeal necrosis (PN), and/or bridging necrosis (BN)	None	0
	Mild PN	1
	Moderate PN	3
	Marked PN	4
	Moderate PN + BN	5
	Marked PN + BN	6
	Multilobular necrosis	10
2. Intralobular necrosis	None	0
	Mild	1
	Moderate	3
	Marked	4
3. Portal inflammation	None	0
	Mild	1
	Moderate	3
	Marked	4
4. Fibrosis	None	0
	Expanding portal tract	1
	Bridging fibrosis	3
	Cirrhosis	4
Maximum score		22

histologic categories of chronic persistent hepatitis, chronic lobular hepatitis, and chronic active hepatitis are worth reviewing and linking with their new-classification counterparts (Table 297-3).

In *chronic persistent hepatitis*, a mononuclear inflammatory infiltrate expands, but is localized to and contained within, portal tracts. The "limiting plate" of periportal hepatocytes is intact, and there is no extension of the necroinflammatory process into the liver lobule. A "cobblestone" arrangement of liver cells, indicative of hepatic regenerative activity, is a common feature, and although minimal periportal fibrosis may be present, *cirrhosis is absent*. As a general rule, patients with chronic persistent hepatitis are asymptomatic or have relatively mild constitutional symptoms (e.g., fatigue, anorexia, nausea); have normal physical findings, except perhaps for liver enlargement, without the usual stigmata of chronic liver disease (see below); and have modest elevations of aminotransferase activities. Progression to more severe lesions (chronic active hepatitis and cirrhosis) was felt to be very unlikely, especially in patients with autoimmune or idiopathic chronic persistent hepatitis; however, progressive disease occurs in patients with chronic persistent *viral* hepatitis and in those with chronic persistent hepatitis following spontaneous or therapeutic remission of autoimmune hepatitis. In the new nomenclature, chronic persistent hepatitis would be classified by *grade* as minimal or mild chronic hepatitis and by *stage* as absent or mild fibrosis.

In patients with *chronic lobular hepatitis*, in addition to portal inflammation, histologic examination of the liver reveals foci of necrosis and inflammation in the liver lobule. Morphologically, chronic lobular hepatitis resembles slowly resolving acute hepatitis. The limiting plate remains intact, periportal fibrosis is absent or limited, lobular architecture is preserved, and progression to chronic active hepatitis and cirrhosis was felt to be rare. Thus chronic lobular hepatitis can be considered a variant of chronic persistent hepatitis with a lobular component, and clinical/laboratory features are comparable. Occasionally, the clinical activity of chronic lobular hepatitis may increase spontaneously; elevation of aminotransferase activity may resemble that seen in acute hepatitis, and transient histologic deterioration can be documented. The same qualifications in prognostic import mentioned above for chronic persistent hepatitis apply to chronic lobular hepatitis. Chronic lobular hepatitis corresponds in the new nomenclature to a mild or moderate *grade* and a *stage* of absent or minimal fibrosis.

Chronic active hepatitis is characterized clinically by continuing hepatic necrosis, portal/periportal and, to a lesser extent, lobular in-

Table 297-3   Correlation Between Earlier and Contemporary Nomenclature of Chronic Hepatitis

	Contemporary Classification	
Old Classification	**Grade (Activity)**	**Stage (Fibrosis)**
Chronic persistent hepatitis	Minimal or mild	None or mild
Chronic lobular hepatitis	Mild or moderate	Mild
Chronic active hepatitis	Mild, moderate, or severe	Mild, moderate, or severe

flammation, and fibrosis. Varying in severity from mild to severe, chronic active hepatitis was recognized to be a progressive disorder that can lead to cirrhosis, liver failure, and death. Morphologic characteristics of chronic active hepatitis include (1) a dense mononuclear infiltrate of the portal tracts, which are substantially expanded into the liver lobule (in the autoimmune type, plasma cells represent a component of the infiltrate); (2) destruction of the hepatocytes at the periphery of the lobule, with erosion of the limiting plate of hepatocytes surrounding the portal triads (piecemeal necrosis or interface hepatitis); (3) connective tissue septa surrounding portal tracts and extending from the portal zones into the lobule, isolating parenchymal cells into clusters and enveloping bile ducts; and (4) evidence of hepatocellular regeneration—"rosette" formation, thickened liver cell plates, and regenerative "pseudolobules." This process may be patchy, with individual liver lobules spared, or it may be diffuse. Histologic evidence of single-cell coagulative necrosis, Councilman or acidophilic bodies, appear in the periportal areas. Piecemeal necrosis is the minimal histologic requirement to establish a diagnosis of chronic active hepatitis, but this change is seen even in mild, relatively nonprogressive forms of chronic active hepatitis. A more severe lesion, *bridging hepatic necrosis* (originally termed *subacute hepatic necrosis*), characterizes a more severe and progressive form of chronic active hepatitis. Although bridging necrosis can be seen occasionally in patients with acute hepatitis, in whom it carries no prognostic importance, in chronic active hepatitis this lesion is associated with progression to cirrhosis. Bridging necrosis is characterized by hepatocellular dropout that spans lobules (i.e., between portal tracts—the periphery of the lobule—or between portal tracts and central veins—the centrizonal part of the lobule). Collapse of the reticulin network is a hallmark of bridging necrosis, and bridging fibrosis follows, leading ultimately to architectural reorganization by nodular regeneration, i.e., cirrhosis. A more extensive and ominous variant of bridging necrosis is multilobular collapse, in which bridging necrosis is widespread throughout the liver and which is associated clinically with rapid deterioration and even acute liver failure.

Although progression to cirrhosis is difficult to demonstrate in patients with chronic active hepatitis who have isolated piecemeal necrosis, in more severe forms of chronic active hepatitis, progression to cirrhosis is common. Among patients with chronic active hepatitis on liver biopsy, 20 to 50% also have cirrhosis, even early during the course of the disease. Ordinarily, chronic active hepatitis is more severe clinically than chronic persistent and lobular hepatitis. Although a sizable proportion of patients with chronic active hepatitis are asymptomatic, the majority tend to have mild to severe constitutional symptoms, especially fatigue. Generally, physical findings associated with chronic liver disease and portal hypertension are more common, aminotransferase levels tend to be higher, and jaundice and hyperbilirubinemia are more frequent in this form of chronic hepatitis.

In the new nomenclature for chronic hepatitis, what used to be called chronic active hepatitis spans the entire spectrum of activity *grade* from minimal, to mild, to severe chronic hepatitis, based on the degree of periportal and piecemeal necrosis, on the degree of lobular inflammation and injury, and on the degree of portal inflammation. Similarly, *stage* in chronic active hepatitis can translate to mild, moderate, or severe fibrosis as well as to cirrhosis.

CHRONIC VIRAL HEPATITIS   Both the enterically transmitted forms of viral hepatitis, hepatitis A and E, are self-limited and do not cause chronic hepatitis (rare reports notwithstanding in which acute hepatitis A serves as a trigger for the onset of autoimmune hepatitis in genetically susceptible patients). In contrast, the entire clinicopathologic spectrum of chronic hepatitis occurs in patients with chronic viral hepatitis B and C as well as in patients with chronic hepatitis D superimposed on chronic hepatitis B.

Chronic Hepatitis B   The likelihood of chronicity after acute hepatitis B varies as a function of age. Infection at birth is associated with a clinically silent acute infection but a 90% chance of chronic infection, while infection in young adulthood in immunocompetent persons is typically associated with clinically apparent acute hepatitis but a risk of chronicity of only approximately 1%. Most cases of chronic hepatitis B among adults, however, occur in patients who never had a recognized episode of clinically apparent acute viral hepatitis. The degree of liver injury (grade) in patients with chronic hepatitis B is variable, ranging from none in asymptomatic carriers, to mild, to severe. Among adults with chronic hepatitis B, histologic features are of prognostic importance. In one long-term study of patients with chronic hepatitis B, investigators found a 5-year survival of 97% for patients with chronic persistent hepatitis (mild chronic hepatitis), of 86% for patients with chronic active hepatitis (moderate to severe chronic hepatitis), and of only 55% for patients with chronic active hepatitis and postnecrotic cirrhosis. The 15-year survival in these cohorts were 77, 66, and 40%, respectively. On the other hand, more recent observations do not allow us to be so sanguine about the prognosis in patients with mild chronic hepatitis; among patients with what used to be labeled chronic persistent hepatitis followed for 1 to 13 years, progression to more severe chronic hepatitis and cirrhosis has been observed in more than a quarter of cases.

Probably more important to consider than histology alone in patients with chronic hepatitis B is the degree of hepatitis B virus (HBV) replication. As reviewed in Chap. 295, chronic hepatitis B can be divided into two phases based on the relative level of HBV replication. The relatively *replicative phase* is characterized by the presence in the serum of markers of HBV replication [hepatitis B e antigen (HBeAg) HBV DNA], by the presence in the liver of detectable intrahepatocyte nucleocapsid antigens [primarily hepatitis B core antigen (HBcAg)], by high infectivity, and by accompanying liver injury; HBV DNA can be detected in the liver but is extrachromosomal. In contrast, the relatively *nonreplicative phase* is characterized by the absence of conventional markers of HBV replication (HBeAg and HBV DNA detectable by hybridization) but an association with anti-HBe, the absence of intrahepatocytic HBcAg, limited infectivity, and minimal liver injury; HBV DNA can be detected in the liver but is integrated into the host genome. Those in the replicative phase tend to have more severe chronic hepatitis, while those in the nonreplicative phase tend to have minimal or mild chronic hepatitis or to be asymptomatic hepatitis B carriers; however, distinctions in HBV replication and in histologic category do not always coincide. The likelihood of converting spontaneously from relatively replicative to nonreplicative chronic HBV infection is approximately 10 to 15% per year. As noted in Chap. 295, the conversion from replicative to nonreplicative chronic hepatitis B is associated with a transient elevation in aminotransferase activity resembling acute hepatitis; occasionally, spontaneous resumptions of replicative activity occur in nonreplicative infection; and occasionally, HBV variants occur in which serologic markers of replication (HBeAg) are absent, despite the presence of replicative infection. Chronic HBV infection, especially when acquired at birth or in early childhood, is associated with an increased risk of hepatocellular carcinoma (Chap. 91). →*A discussion of the pathogenesis of liver injury in patients with chronic hepatitis B appears in Chap. 295.*

The spectrum of *clinical features* of chronic hepatitis B is broad, ranging from asymptomatic infection to debilitating disease or even end-stage, fatal hepatic failure. As noted above, the onset of the disease tends to be insidious in most patients, with the exception of the very few in whom chronic disease follows failure of resolution of clinically ciated with progression from acute to chronic hepatitis B are discussed in Chap. 295. *Fatigue* is a common symptom, and persistent or intermittent *jaundice* is a common feature in severe or advanced cases. Intermittent deepening of jaundice and recurrence of malaise and anorexia, as well as worsening fatigue, are reminiscent of acute hepatitis; such exacerbations may occur spontaneously, often coinciding with evidence of virologic reactivation, may lead to progressive liver injury, and, when superimposed on well-established cirrhosis, may cause hepatic decompensation. Complications of cirrhosis occur in end-stage chronic hepatitis and include ascites, edema, bleeding gastroesophageal varices, hepatic encephalopathy, coagulopathy, or hypersplenism. Occasionally, these complications bring the patient to initial clinical attention. Extrahepatic complications of chronic hepatitis B, similar to those seen during the prodromal phase of acute hepatitis B, are associated with deposition of circulating hepatitis B antigen–antibody immune complexes. These include arthralgias and arthritis, which are common, and the more rare purpuric cutaneous lesions (leukocytoclastic vasculitis), immune-complex glomerulonephritis, and generalized vasculitis (polyarteritis nodosa) (Chaps. 295 and 317).

Laboratory features of chronic hepatitis B do not distinguish adequately between histologically mild and severe hepatitis. Aminotransferase elevations tend to be modest for chronic hepatitis B but may fluctuate in the range of 100 to 1000 units. As is true for acute viral hepatitis B, alanine aminotransferase (ALT, or SGPT) tends to be more elevated than aspartate aminotransferase (AST, or SGOT); however, once cirrhosis is established, AST tends to exceed ALT. Levels of alkaline phosphatase activity tend to be normal or only marginally elevated. In severe cases, moderate elevations in serum bilirubin [51.3 to 171 μmol/L (3 to 10 mg/dL)] occur. Hypoalbuminemia and prolongation of the prothrombin time occur in severe or end-stage cases. Hyperglobulinemia and detectable circulating autoantibodies are distinctly absent in chronic hepatitis B (in contrast to autoimmune hepatitis). →*Viral markers of chronic HBV infection are discussed in Chap. 295.*

℞ **TREATMENT**   Management of chronic hepatitis B depends on the level of virus replication. Although progression to cirrhosis is more likely in severe chronic than in mild or moderate chronic hepatitis B, all forms of chronic viral hepatitis can be progressive. Interferon α (IFN-α) was the first approved therapy for chronic hepatitis B, but the recently approved dideoxynucleoside lamivudine expands the options for treatment. The most common indication for treatment is chronic "replicative" hepatitis B, with detectable HBeAg and HBV DNA (by hybridization assay), elevated ALT activity, and histologic evidence of chronic hepatitis on liver biopsy in an immunocompetent adult. A 16-week course of INF-α given by subcutaneous injection at a daily dose of 5 million units, or three times a week at a dose of 10 million units, results in seroconversion from "replicative" (detectable HBeAg and HBV DNA) to "nonreplicative" (undetectable HBeAg and HBV DNA by hybridization assay) HBV infection in approximately 35% of patients, with a concomitant improvement in liver histologic features. As a result of INF-α therapy, approximately 20% of patients acquire anti-HBe, and in early trials, approximately 8% lost hepatitis B surface antigen (HBsAg). Successful interferon therapy and seroconversion is often accompanied by an acute hepatitis-like elevation in aminotransferase activity, which has been postulated to result from enhanced cytolytic T cell clearance of HBV-infected hepatocytes. Relapse after successful therapy is rare (1 or 2%). The likelihood of responding to interferon is higher in patients with lower levels of HBV DNA and substantial elevations of ALT. Although children can respond as well as adults, interferon therapy has not been effective in very young children infected at birth. Similarly, interferon therapy has not been effective in immunosuppressed persons, Asian patients with minimal-to-mild ALT elevations, patients with pre-core mutant HBV infection (Chap. 295), or in patients with decompensated chronic hepatitis B (in whom such therapy can actually be detrimental, sometimes precipitating decompensation, often associated with severe adverse ef-

fects). Among patients with HBeAg loss during therapy, long-term follow-up has demonstrated that 80% experience eventual loss of HBsAg, i.e., all serologic markers of infection, and normalization of ALT over a 9-year posttreatment period. In addition, improved long-term and complication-free survival as well as a reduction in the frequency of hepatocellular carcinoma have been documented among interferon responders, supporting the conclusion that successful interferon therapy improves the natural history of chronic hepatitis B. Indications for interferon therapy in patients with chronic hepatitis B are summarized in Table 297-4.

Complications of interferon therapy include systemic "flulike" symptoms, marrow suppression, emotional lability (irritability commonly, depression rarely), autoimmune reactions (especially autoimmune thyroiditis), and miscellaneous side effects such as alopecia, rashes, diarrhea, and numbness and tingling of the extremities. With the possible exception of autoimmune thyroiditis, all these side effects are reversible upon dose lowering or cessation of therapy.

In patients with chronic hepatitis B, long-term therapy with glucocorticoids is not only ineffective but also detrimental. Short-term glucocorticoid therapy, however, has been advocated as a potential antiviral approach. Glucocorticoids increase HBV replication and expression in hepatocytes and depress cytolytic T cells. When glucocorticoids are administered for a brief time and then withdrawn abruptly, cytolytic T cells, suppressed while HBV replication was enhanced by the drug, resume their presteroid function. These restored cytolytic T cells attack hepatocytes, the HBV expression of which had been enhanced by the brief pulse of glucocorticoid therapy. An acute hepatitis-like flare of aminotransferase activity follows and may be accompanied by a dramatic drop, or even loss of, HBV replication. Such glucocorticoid "priming" prior to interferon therapy has not been shown to be more effective than interferon alone and has been abandoned.

Several nucleoside analogues active against HBV are being evaluated and developed. Famciclovir and ganciclovir have only limited activity against hepatitis B; however, lamivudine, which inhibits reverse transcriptase activity of both HIV and HBV, is a potent and effective agent for patients with chronic hepatitis B. Lamivudine suppresses HBV DNA by a median of four orders of magnitude at oral daily doses of 100 mg. In clinical trials conducted in Asia, North America, Europe, and Australia, lamivudine therapy for 12 months was associated with almost universal suppression of HBV DNA detectable by hybridization assays; loss of HBeAg in 32 to 33%; HBeAg seroconversion (i.e., conversion from HBeAg-reactive to anti-HBe-reactive) in 16 to 20%; normalization of ALT in approximately 40%; improvement in histology in over 50%; and retardation in fibrosis in 20%. Among patients who experienced HBeAg responses during therapy, 70 to 80% maintained the response over longer than a year of follow-up monitoring. Because maintenance of the response to lamivudine occurs in almost all patients with an HBeAg response, the achievement of an HBeAg response may be a viable stopping point in therapy. If

Table 297-4   **Patients with Chronic Hepatitis B Who Are Candidates for Antiviral Therapy**

	Interferon	Lamivudine
Detectable markers of HBV replication	Yes	Yes
Elevated ALT activity	Yes	Yes
Chronic hepatitis on liver biopsy	Yes	Yes
Immunocompetence	Yes	Yes
Immunosuppression	No	Yes
Acquisition of infection in adulthood (Western)	Yes	Yes
Acquisition of infection in childhood (Asian)	No	Yes
Compensated liver disease	Yes	Yes
Decompensated liver disease	No	Yes
"Wild-type" chronic hepatitis B	Yes	Yes
Pre-core mutant hepatitis B	No	Yes
Prior nonreponse to interferon	No	Yes

HBeAg is unaffected by lamivudine therapy, the current approach is to continue therapy until an HBeAg response occurs, but long-term therapy may be required to suppress HBV replication and, in turn, limit liver injury. Preliminary observations indicate that HBeAg seroconversions can increase to a level of 27% after 2 years and 44% after 3 years of therapy.

Losses of HBsAg have been few during lamivudine therapy, and this observation had been cited as an advantage of interferon over lamivudine; however, in head-to-head comparisons between interferon and lamivudine monotherapy, HBsAg losses were rare in both groups. Trials in which lamivudine and interferon were administered in combination failed to show a benefit of combination therapy over lamivudine monotherapy for either treatment-naive patients or prior interferon nonresponders.

Among patients with HBeAg and HBV DNA but with normal ALT activity, lamivudine suppresses liver injury during therapy but rarely achieves an HBeAg response. In patients with pre-core HBV mutations, who lack HBeAg but who have detectable HBV DNA and liver injury, lamivudine suppresses HBV DNA and normalizes ALT in 65% and improves liver histology in 60%. When therapy is discontinued, reactivation is common, and these patients require long-term therapy.

Clinical and laboratory side effects of lamivudine are negligible, indistinguishable from those observed in placebo recipients. During lamivudine therapy, transient ALT elevations, resembling those seen during interferon therapy and during spontaneous HBeAg-to-anti-HBe seroconversions, occur in a quarter of patients. These ALT elevations may result from restored cytolytic T cell activation permitted by suppression of HBV replication. Similar ALT elevations, however, occur at an identical frequency in placebo recipients, but ALT elevations associated with HBeAg seroconversion are confined to lamivudine-treated patients. When therapy is stopped after a year of therapy, 2- to 3-fold ALT elevations occur in 20 to 30% of lamivudine-treated patients, representing renewed liver-cell injury as HBV replication returns. Although these posttreatment flares are almost always transient and mild, rare severe exacerbations have been observed, mandating close and careful clinical and virologic monitoring after discontinuation of treatment.

Long-term monotherapy with lamivudine is associated with methionine-to-valine or methionine-to-isoleucine mutations in the YMDD (tyrosine-methionine-aspartate-aspartate) motif of HBV DNA polymerase, analogous to mutations that occur in patients with HIV infection treated with this drug. During a year of therapy, YMDD mutations occur in 15 to 30% of patients; the frequency increases at year two to 38% and at year three to almost 50%. Although transient elevations in ALT and HBV DNA levels occur when such variants emerge, YMDD-variant HBV appears to be less replicatively competent and a less robust pathogen. Even after YMDD mutations occur, HBV DNA and ALT levels as well as histologic scores tend to remain lower than baseline levels in immunocompetent patients. In immunosuppressed patients, a proportion of patients with YMDD mutations experience hepatic decompensation. Until other antivirals are developed, the approach to YMDD variants emerging during lamivudine treatment is to continue therapy. Other antiviral drugs, such as the experimental agent adefovir dipivoxil, inhibit YMDD-variant HBV. In the future, combination antiviral therapy will almost invariably become the norm as new agents are introduced.

Because lamivudine monotherapy can result universally in the rapid emergence of YMDD variants in persons with HIV infection, patients with chronic hepatitis B should be tested for anti-HIV prior to therapy; if HIV infection is identified, lamivudine monotherapy at the HBV daily dose of 100 mg is contraindicated. These patients should be treated with triple-drug antiretroviral therapy, including a lamivudine daily dose of 300 mg (Chap. 309). The safety of lamivudine during pregnancy has not been established.

No treatment is indicated or available for asymptomatic "nonreplicative" hepatitis B carriers. Whereas patients with decompensated chronic hepatitis B are not candidates for interferon therapy, they may respond to lamivudine, with reversal of the signs of decompensation.

Table 297-4 summarizes the indications in patients with chronic hepatitis B for antiviral therapy with lamivudine, as compared with interferon. Both drugs are quite comparable in efficacy as first-line therapy for chronic hepatitis B (Table 297-5). Interferon requires only brief-duration therapy, too limited in duration to support viral variants, but requires subcutaneous injections and is associated with a high level of intolerability. Lamivudine requires long-term therapy in most patients and, when used alone, fosters the emergence of viral variants. On the other hand, lamivudine is taken orally, is very well tolerated, leads to improved histology even in the absence of HBeAg responses, and is effective even in patients who fail to respond to interferon. Although some prefer to begin with interferon, most physicians and patients prefer lamivudine as first-line therapy.

For patients with end-stage chronic hepatitis B, liver transplantation is the only potential lifesaving intervention. Reinfection of the new liver is almost universal; however, the likelihood of liver injury associated with hepatitis B in the new liver is variable. The majority of patients become high-level viremic carriers with minimal liver injury. Unfortunately, an unpredictable proportion experience severe hepatitis B–related liver injury, sometimes a fulminant-like hepatitis, sometimes a rapid recapitulation of the original severe chronic hepatitis B (Chap. 301). Prevention of recurrent hepatitis B after liver transplantation has been achieved by *prophylaxis* with hepatitis B immune globulin and with nucleoside analogues such as lamivudine; in addition, nucleoside analogues have been used successfully to *reverse* posttransplantation liver injury associated with recurrent hepatitis B (Chap. 301).

Chronic Hepatitis D (Delta Hepatitis)   The clinical and laboratory features of chronic hepatitis D virus (HDV) infection are summarized in Chap. 295. Chronic hepatitis D may follow acute coinfection with HBV but at a rate no higher than the rate of chronicity of hepatitis B. That is, although HDV coinfection can increase the severity of acute hepatitis B, HDV does not increase the likelihood of progression to chronic hepatitis B. However, when HDV superinfection occurs in a person who is already chronically infected with HBV, long-term HDV infection is the rule and a worsening of the liver disease the expected consequence. Except for severity, chronic hepatitis

Table 297-5   Comparison of Interferon and Lamivudine Therapy for Chronic Hepatitis B

	Interferon	Lamivudine
Route of administration	Injection	Oral
Duration of therapy	4 months	≥1 year
Tolerability	Poorly tolerated	Well tolerated
HBeAg loss	33%	32-33%
HBeAg seroconversion	18-20%	16-20%
Normalization of ALT	Confined to HBeAg responders	>40%
HBsAg loss during therapy	3-8%	2-4%
HBsAg loss after therapy	80% over 9 years	To be determined
Histologic improvement	Confined to HBeAg responders	>50%
Retardation of fibrosis	Not demonstrated	20%
Viral resistance	None	15-30% during 1 year
Natural history	Reduced mortality, decompensation, HCC	To be determined
Pre-core mutant hepatitis B	Limited response	>60% response
Candidate range[a]	Narrow	Broad

[a] See Table 297-4

B plus D has similar clinical and laboratory features to those seen in chronic hepatitis B alone. Relatively severe chronic hepatitis, with or without cirrhosis, is the rule, and mild chronic hepatitis the exception. A distinguishing serologic feature of chronic hepatitis D is the presence in the circulation of antibodies to liver-kidney microsomes (anti-LKM); however, the anti-LKM seen in hepatitis D are designated anti-LKM3, are directed against uridine diphosphate glucuronosyltransferase, and are distinct from anti-LKM1 seen in patients with autoimmune hepatitis and in a subset of patients with chronic hepatitis C (see below).

TREATMENT Management is not well defined. Glucocorticoids are ineffective and are not used. Preliminary experimental trials of interferon α suggested that conventional doses and durations of therapy lower levels of HDV RNA and aminotransferase activity only transiently during treatment but have no impact on the natural history of the disease. Although high-dose IFN-α (9 million units) three times a week for 12 months may be associated with a sustained loss of HDV replication and clinical improvement in up to 50% of patients, ultimately recurrent HDV replication becomes universal after cessation of therapy. Antiviral therapy for chronic hepatitis D remains the subject of experimental trials; early observations suggest that lamivudine is not effective. In patients with end-stage liver disease secondary to chronic hepatitis D, liver transplantation has been effective. If hepatitis D recurs in the new liver without the expression of hepatitis B (an unusual serologic profile in immunocompetent persons, but common in transplant patients), liver injury is limited. In fact, the outcome of transplantation for chronic hepatitis D is superior to that for chronic hepatitis B (Chap. 301).

Chronic Hepatitis C Regardless of the epidemiologic mode of acquisition of hepatitis C virus (HCV) infection, chronic hepatitis follows acute hepatitis C in 50 to 70% of cases; even in those with a return to normal in aminotransferase levels after acute hepatitis C, chronic infection is common, adding up to an 85 to 90% likelihood of chronic HCV infection after acute hepatitis C. Furthermore, in patients with chronic transfusion-associated hepatitis followed for 10 to 20 years, progression to cirrhosis occurs in about 20%. Such is the case even for patients with relatively clinically mild chronic hepatitis, including those without symptoms, with only modest elevations of aminotransferase activity, and with mild chronic hepatitis on liver biopsy. Even in cohorts of well-compensated patients with chronic hepatitis C (no complications of chronic liver disease and with normal hepatic synthetic function), the prevalence of cirrhosis may be as high as 50%. Many cases of hepatitis C are identified in asymptomatic patients who have no history of acute hepatitis C, e.g., those discovered while attempting to donate blood or as a result of routine laboratory screening tests. The source of HCV infection in most of these cases is not defined, although a long-forgotten percutaneous exposure in the remote past can be elicited in a substantial proportion. The natural history of chronic hepatitis C identified under these circumstances remains to be determined. Among asymptomatic persons with anti-HCV, even when aminotransferase levels are normal, between a third and a half have been reported to have chronic hepatitis on liver biopsy, although mild in most cases. In these asymptomatic persons with normal aminotransferase levels, the presence of detectable circulating HCV RNA appears to distinguish those with chronic hepatitis on biopsy from those with normal liver histology.

Despite this substantial rate of progression of chronic hepatitis C, and despite the fact that liver failure can result from end-stage chronic hepatitis C, the long-term prognosis for chronic hepatitis C in a majority of patients is relatively benign. Mortality over 10 to 20 years among patients with transfusion-associated chronic hepatitis C has been shown not to differ from mortality in a matched population of transfused patients in whom hepatitis C did not develop. Although death in the hepatitis group is more likely to result from liver failure, and although hepatic decompensation may occur in approximately 15% of such patients over the course of a decade, the majority (almost

60%) of patients remain asymptomatic and well compensated, with no clinical sequelae of chronic liver disease. Overall, then, chronic hepatitis C tends to be very slowly and insidiously progressive, if at all, in the vast majority of patients, while in approximately a quarter of cases, chronic hepatitis C will progress eventually to end-stage cirrhosis. Referral bias may account for the more severe outcomes described in cohorts of patients reported from tertiary-care centers versus the more benign outcomes in cohorts of patients monitored from initial blood-product-associated acute hepatitis. Still unexplained, however, are the wide ranges in reported progression to cirrhosis, from 2% over 17 years in a population of women with hepatitis C infection acquired from contaminated anti-D immune globulin to 30% over ≤ 11 years in recipients of contaminated intravenous immune globulin.

Progression of liver disease in patients with chronic hepatitis C has been reported to be more likely in patients with older age, longer duration of infection, advanced histologic stage and grade, genotype 1 (especially type 1b), more complex quasispecies diversity, and increased hepatic iron. Among these variables, however, duration of infection appears to be the most important, and many of the others probably reflect disease duration to some extent (e.g., quasispecies diversity, hepatic iron accumulation).

Perhaps the best prognostic indicator in chronic hepatitis C is liver histology. Patients with mild necrosis and inflammation as well as those with limited fibrosis have an excellent prognosis and limited progression to cirrhosis. In contrast, among patients with moderate to severe necroinflammatory activity or fibrosis, including septal or bridging fibrosis, progression to cirrhosis is highly likely over the course of 10 to 20 years. Among patients with compensated cirrhosis associated with hepatitis C, the 10-year survival is close to 80 percent; mortality occurs at a rate of 2 to 6% per year, decompensation at a rate of 4 to 5% per year, and hepatocellular carcinoma at a rate of 1 to 3% per year.

In addition, severity of chronic hepatitis is greater and progression of chronic liver disease is more accelerated in patients who have chronic hepatitis C as well as other liver processes, including alcoholic liver disease, chronic hepatitis B, hemochromatosis, and α_1-antitrypsin deficiency. No other epidemiologic or clinical features of chronic hepatitis C (e.g., severity of acute hepatitis, level of aminotransferase activity, level of HCV RNA, presence or absence of jaundice) are predictive of eventual outcome. Despite the relative benignity of chronic hepatitis C over time, cirrhosis following chronic hepatitis C has been associated with the late development, after several decades, of hepatocellular carcinoma (HCC) (Chap. 91). As noted above, the annual rate of HCC in cirrhotic patients with hepatitis C is 1 to 3%.

Clinical features of chronic hepatitis C are similar to those described above for chronic hepatitis B. Generally, *fatigue* is the most common symptom; jaundice is rare. Immune-complex mediated extrahepatic complications of chronic hepatitis C are less common than in chronic hepatitis B, with the exception of essential mixed cryoglobulinemia (Chap. 295). This is the case despite the fact that assays for immune-complex–like activity are often positive in patients with chronic hepatitis C. In addition, chronic hepatitis C has been associated with extrahepatic complications unrelated to immune-complex injury. These include Sjögren's syndrome, lichen planus, and porphyria cutanea tarda. *Laboratory features* of chronic hepatitis C are similar to those in patients with chronic hepatitis B, but aminotransferase levels tend to fluctuate more (the characteristic episodic pattern of aminotransferase activity) and to be lower, especially in patients with long-standing disease. An interesting and occasionally confusing finding in patients with chronic hepatitis C is the presence of autoantibodies. Rarely, patients with autoimmune hepatitis (see below) and hyperglobulinemia have false-positive enzyme immunoassays for anti-HCV. On the other hand, some patients with serologically confirmable chronic hepatitis C have circulating anti-LKM. These antibodies are anti-LKM1, as seen in patients with autoimmune hepatitis *type 2* (see below), and are directed against a 33-amino-acid sequence of P450

IID6. The occurrence of anti-LKM1 in some patients with chronic hepatitis C may result from the partial sequence homology between the epitope recognized by anti-LKM1 and two segments of the HCV polyprotein. In addition, the presence of this autoantibody in some patients with chronic hepatitis C suggests that autoimmunity may be playing a role in the pathogenesis of chronic hepatitis C. →*Histopathologic features of chronic hepatitis C, especially those that distinguish hepatitis C from hepatitis B, are described in Chap. 295.*

℞ **TREATMENT**   Two approaches to antiviral therapy of chronic hepatitis C have been approved: *monotherapy* with interferon and *combination therapy* with interferon plus ribavirin. According to a National Institutes of Health Consensus Development Conference in March 1997, responses measured at the end of treatment are referred to as end-treatment responses, and responses sustained for at least 6 months after discontinuation of therapy are referred to as sustained responses.

Interferon Monotherapy   Interferon α, administered by subcutaneous injection three times a week for 6 months yields end-treatment biochemical responses (return to normal of ALT levels) as high as approximately 50% and virologic responses (undetectable HCV RNA) by polymerase chain reaction (PCR) of approximately 30%. Unfortunately, because of a relapse rate as high as 90% in end-treatment responders, these responses are not maintained after discontinuation of therapy except in a small minority of patients; after 6 months of interferon monotherapy, the likelihood of a sustained biochemical and virologic response is only approximately 10%. Even in the absence of a biochemical/virologic response, however, end-treatment histologic responses—primarily reductions in periportal and lobular activity—occur in three-fourths of treated patients. Unlike the case in hepatitis B, in chronic hepatitis C successful responses to therapy are not accompanied by transient, acute-hepatitis–like elevations in aminotransferase activity; instead, ALT levels fall precipitously. Between 85 to 90% of responses occur within the first 3 months of therapy; responses thereafter are rare.

In a proportion of cases, markers of HCV replication can be eradicated by interferon therapy, and durable responses with normal ALT, improved histology, and absence of HCV RNA in serum and liver have been documented many years after successful therapy. A small proportion of patients, approximately 10%, experience biochemical "breakthrough" *during* interferon therapy and are classified as nonresponders. In general, they remain refractory to retreatment thereafter; some such breakthroughs are associated with interferon antibodies, while others may reflect mutations in the HCV genome that render HCV nonresponsive to interferon.

Levels of HCV RNA fall in tandem with ALT levels during interferon therapy, but loss of detectable HCV RNA does not preclude relapse. When a patient experiences an apparently sustained biochemical response after discontinuing interferon but continues to remain viremic, as reflected by the persistence of detectable HCV RNA, future biochemical relapse is likely. Patient variables that tend to correlate with *sustained* responsiveness to interferon include a low baseline level of HCV RNA and histologically mild hepatitis. Patients with cirrhosis can respond, but they are less likely to do so and especially unlikely to have a *sustained* response. Patients with HCV genotype 1 are less likely to respond than patients with other genotypes. Other variables reported to correlate with increased responsiveness include brief duration of infection, low HCV quasispecies diversity, immunocompetence, and low liver iron levels. High levels of HCV RNA, more histologically advanced liver disease, and high quasispecies diversity all go hand in hand with advanced duration of infection, which may be the single most important variable determining interferon responsiveness. The ironic fact, then, is that patients whose disease is *least* likely to progress are the ones *most* likely to respond to interferon and vice versa. Finally, among patients with genotype 1b, responsive-

ness to interferon is enhanced in those with amino-acid-substitution mutations in the nonstructural protein 5A gene.

The most effective approach to increasing responsiveness to interferon monotherapy is to increase the duration of therapy to 12 months or longer, a regimen associated with a sustained biochemical and virologic response of approximately 20%. Higher doses of interferon (e.g., 5 to 10 million units) or daily injections increase response rates only marginally and at a substantial cost in intolerability. Thus, if interferon monotherapy is selected, the consensus is that 3 million units for at least 12 months is the preferred regimen. Currently, three types of IFN-α are approved in the United States; for the two recombinant products, the recommended dose is 3 million units, and for the one synthetic consensus interferon (synthesized to represent the amino acids at each position that occur most frequently among the multiple, natural interferon α subspecies), the dose is $9\mu g$. Several other types of INF-α, including lymphoblastoid interferon, are available in Europe and Asia. A review of the different types of INF-α during the NIH Consensus Development Conference in 1997 led to the conclusion that they are all equivalent in efficacy.

Studies of viral kinetics have shown that despite a virion half life in serum of only 2 to 3 h, the level of HCV is maintained by a high replication rate of 10^{12} hepatitis C virions per day. Interferon α blocks virion production or release with an efficacy that increases with increasing drug doses; moreover, the calculated death rate for infected cells during interferon therapy is inversely related to viral load; patients with the most rapid death rate of infected hepatocytes are more likely to achieve undetectable HCV RNA at 3 months; achieving this landmark is predictive of a subsequent sustained response. Therefore, to achieve rapid viral clearance from serum and the liver, *high-dose induction therapy* has been advocated. In practice, high-dose induction therapy has not yielded higher sustained response rates. Other approaches that have been suggested include tapering therapy slowly, rather than discontinuing therapy abruptly, and, because high liver iron levels are associated with nonresponsiveness, the addition of phlebotomy to interferon therapy. None of these approaches has been shown to be effective.

Long-acting interferons bound to polyethylene glycol (PEG) have several advantages. Such "pegylated" interferons, with elimination times seven-fold longer than standard interferons, achieve prolonged concentration peaks and can be administered once, rather than three times, a week. Instead of the frequent drug peaks and troughs associated with frequent administration of short-acting interferons, administration of pegylated interferons results in drug concentrations that are more stable and sustained over time. Preliminary studies suggest that once-a-week injections of pegylated interferons are at least as effective as standard interferons given three times a week and may result in sustained responses comparable to those achieved with combination interferon-ribavirin therapy (see below).

If a patient relapses after a course of interferon monotherapy, repeating a course of interferon monotherapy is unlikely to achieve a sustained response unless the dose or preferably the duration of therapy is increased. Under these circumstances, sustained response rates as high as 40% can be realized. Although a small proportion of interferon nonresponders can respond to a repeat course of interferon monotherapy, and although a 13% sustained response rate has been reported for prior interferon nonresponders treated with high-dose (15 μg) consensus interferon, the likelihood of responding is not increased substantially by retreating interferon nonresponders with interferon monotherapy.

Combination Interferon-Ribavirin Therapy   The most effective way to increase the efficacy of interferon therapy is to add ribavirin, an oral guanoside nucleoside. When used as monotherapy, ribavirin is ineffective and does not reduce HCV RNA levels. In contrast, the combination of interferon at standard doses with ribavirin at doses of 1000 mg (for patients weighing <75 kg) to 1200 mg (for patients weighing ≥75 kg) per day increases both end-treatment responses and sustained responses in previously untreated patients. Large, international, multicenter trials have shown that end-treatment responses at 6 months or 12 months exceed 50% and sustained responses as high as 33% at 6 months and 41% at 12 months have been achieved. Thus, a full year of combination therapy is twice as effective as a year of interferon monotherapy. Sustained responses were more likely in patients with low viral loads (below 2 million copies/mL), genotypes other than 1, minimal fibrosis, age <40, and females. In patients with low viral loads and non-1 genotypes, sustained response rates can be as high as 95%, and combination therapy for 24 weeks suffices, achieving the same end as continuing therapy for a full year. Therefore, for patients with low viral loads and non-1 genotypes, therapy need last only 6 months. Unless contraindications to the use of combination therapy exist (see below), combination interferon-ribavirin is the treatment of choice for chronic hepatitis C (Table 297-6).

For those who relapse after a 6-month course of interferon monotherapy, a 6-month course of combination therapy results in a sustained response rate of 50%, and retreatment of relapsers is another approved indication for combination therapy. Unfortunately, combination therapy has been disappointing in interferon nonresponders.

Side effects of combination therapy are similar to those of interferon monotherapy; however, ribavirin causes hemolysis; a reduction in hemoglobin of up to 2 to 3 gm or in hematocrit of up 5 to 10% can

Table 297-6 Indications and Recommendations for Antiviral Therapy of Chronic Hepatitis C

STANDARD INDICATIONS FOR THERAPY

Elevated ALT activity
Fibrosis or moderate to severe hepatitis on liver biopsy
Detectable HCV RNA

RETREATMENT RECOMMENDED

Relapsers after an initial course of interferon
   A 6-month course of combination interferon-ribavirin or a course of interferon monotherapy longer in duration than the original course

ANTIVIRAL THERAPY NOT RECOMMENDED ROUTINELY BUT MANAGEMENT DECISIONS MADE ON AN INDIVIDUAL BASIS

Children (age <18 years)
Age >60
Mild hepatitis on liver biopsy
Compensated cirrhosis
Patients with HIV infection and normal CD4 counts
Maintenance therapy in repeated relapsers
Nonresponders to a course of recombinant interferon—can be offered a 48-week course of consensus interferon, 15 μg three times a week (clinical trials underway to assess benefit of long-term "suppressive" therapy with other regimens)

LONG-TERM THERAPY RECOMMENDED

Cutaneous vasculitis and glomerulonephritis associated with chronic hepatitis C

ANTIVIRAL THERAPY NOT RECOMMENDED

Decompensated cirrhosis
Normal ALT activity

THERAPEUTIC REGIMENS

First-line treatment: INF-α 3 million units subcutaneously three times a week plus ribavirin 1000 mg/d (weight <75 Kg) to 1200 mg/d (weight ≥75 kg) orally
  Duration of therapy: Genotype 1: 48 weeks
                   Genotypes 2 and 3: 24 weeks
Alternative regimen: INF-α monotherapy 3 million units (of recombinant interferon alfa-2a or alfa-2b or 9 μg of consensus interferon) subcutaneously three times a week for 48 weeks (primarily for patients in whom combination therapy is contraindicated or not tolerated)

FEATURES ASSOCIATED WITH REDUCED RESPONSIVENESS

Advanced histologic lesion (e.g., advanced cirrhosis)
Long-duration disease
Genotype 1
High-level HCV RNA (>2 million copies/mL)
High HCV quasispecies diversity

be anticipated. A small, unpredictable proportion of patients will experience profound, brisk hemolysis, resulting in symptomatic anemia. Therefore, close monitoring of blood counts is crucial, and combination therapy should be avoided in patients with anemia or hemoglobinopathies and in patients with coronary artery disease or cerebrovascular disease, in whom anemia can precipitate an ischemic event. Ribavirin, which is renally excreted, should not be used by patients with renal insufficiency; the drug is teratogenic, precluding its use during pregnancy and mandating the use of efficient contraception during therapy.

Ribavirin therapy has also been characterized by nasal congestion, pruritus, and precipitation of gout; the combination is more difficult to tolerate than interferon monotherapy. In one large clinical trial of combination therapy versus monotherapy among patients treated for a year, 21% of the combination group (but only 14% of the monotherapy group) had to discontinue treatment, while 26% of the combination group (but only 9% of the monotherapy group) required dose reductions.

Indications for Antiviral Therapy Patients with chronic hepatitis C who have elevated ALT levels, detectable HCV RNA, and chronic hepatitis of at least moderate grade and stage are candidates for antiviral therapy with interferon and ribavirin, unless ribavirin is contraindicated (Table 297-6). Preliminary retrospective analyses have shown that interferon treatment improves survival and complication-free survival. One year of combination therapy is standard, but 6 months suffice for patients with non-1 genotypes and low viral loads. For patients treated with interferon monotherapy, 12 months is the standard duration in all cases, regardless of genotype and viral load. According to the NIH Consensus Development Conference in 1997, therapy should be discontinued in patients who have not achieved a normal ALT and an undetectable HCV RNA by month three. Although the vast majority of patients treated with combination therapy who become sustained responders will have achieved an early biochemical and virologic response, a proportion of sustained responders experienced late viral clearance. In addition, even in biochemical and virologic nonresponders, histologic improvement is common. Therefore, recommendations for early cessation of therapy based on interim assessments of biochemical and virologic responsiveness require re-evaluation. Although response rates are lower in patients with certain pretreatment variables, selection for treatment should not be based on symptoms, genotype, viral load, or the mode of acquisition of infection.

Patients who have relapsed after an initial course of interferon monotherapy are candidates for a 6-month course of combination interferon-ribavirin therapy; if they cannot tolerate ribavirin, they should be retreated with interferon monotherapy, but the course should be longer. It remains to be determined whether long-term (even indefinite) maintenance therapy will be necessary or effective in patients who relapse repeatedly whenever therapy is discontinued. For interferon nonresponders, retreatment with interferon monotherapy or combination therapy is unlikely to achieve a sustained response. Clinical trials are in progress to determine whether long-term suppression of virus-induced liver injury with antiviral therapy will be of benefit in this population.

In patients with acute hepatitis C, a course of interferon has been shown to reduce the likelihood of chronicity by one-half (Chapter 295). In patients with normal ALT levels, long-term monitoring studies have shown absence of histologic progression, and clinical trials of antiviral therapy have shown no benefit; therefore, treatment of such patients is not recommended. Because hepatitis C can reactivate in patients with normal ALT levels, laboratory monitoring several times a year should be done, and therapy should be considered for sustained elevations in ALT levels. Patients with mild hepatitis on liver biopsy are not routine candidates for antiviral therapy, but treatment decisions should be individualized between physician and patient. Most authorities would recommend a pretreatment liver biopsy to help in the decision-making about therapy.

Patients with compensated cirrhosis can respond to therapy, although their likelihood of a sustained response is lower than in noncirrhotics. Combination therapy brings sustained response rates in cirrhotics up to the level achieved with interferon monotherapy in noncirrhotics. Retrospective analyses generally have not demonstrated an improvement in survival among interferon-treated cirrhotic patients. Similarly, several studies have suggested that treatment of cirrhotics with hepatitis C reduces the frequency of HCC; however, logistic regression analyses have shown that patient characteristics at the time of therapy (e.g., less advanced disease), not treatment itself, accounted for the reduced frequency of HCC observed in the treated cohort. Patients with decompensated cirrhosis are not candidates for antiviral therapy but should be referred for liver transplantation. After liver transplantation, recurrent hepatitis C is the rule. Most patients who undergo liver transplantation for chronic hepatitis C experience little, if any, morbidity, allograft loss, or mortality associated with recurrent hepatitis C during the early postoperative years (Chapter 301); studies are in progress to determine how best to treat hepatitis C after liver transplantation. The cutaneous and renal vasculitis of HCV-associated essential mixed cryoglobulinemia (Chap. 295) may respond to interferon, but sustained responses are rare after discontinuation of therapy; therefore, prolonged, perhaps indefinite, therapy is recommended in this group.

Anecdotal reports suggest that antiviral therapy may be effective in porphyria cutanea tarda or lichen planus associated with hepatitis C. In patients with HIV infection, responses similar to those seen in other groups have been reported in patients with normal CD4 counts.

AUTOIMMUNE HEPATITIS Definition Autoimmune hepatitis (formerly called autoimmune chronic active hepatitis) is a chronic disorder characterized by continuing hepatocellular necrosis and inflammation, usually with fibrosis, which tends to progress to cirrhosis and liver failure. When fulfilling criteria of severity, this type of chronic hepatitis may have a 6-month mortality of as high as 40%. The prominence of extrahepatic features of autoimmunity as well as seroimmunologic abnormalities in this disorder supports an autoimmune process in its pathogenesis; this concept is reflected in the labels "lupoid," plasma cell, or autoimmune hepatitis. Because autoantibodies and other typical features of autoimmunity do not occur in all cases, however, a broader, more appropriate designation for this type of chronic hepatitis is "idiopathic" or cryptogenic. Cases in which hepatotropic viruses, metabolic/genetic derangements, and hepatotoxic drugs have been excluded merit this designation and probably include a spectrum of heterogeneous liver disorders of unknown cause, a proportion of which have characteristic autoimmune features.

Immunopathogenesis The weight of evidence suggests that the progressive liver injury in patients with idiopathic/autoimmune hepatitis is the result of a cell-mediated immunologic attack directed against liver cells; in all likelihood, predisposition to autoimmunity is inherited, while the liver specificity of this injury is triggered by environmental (e.g., chemical or viral) factors. For example, patients have been described in whom apparently self-limited cases of acute hepatitis A or B led to autoimmune hepatitis, presumably because of genetic susceptibility or predisposition. Evidence to support an autoimmune pathogenesis in this type of hepatitis includes the following: (1) In the liver, the histopathologic lesions are composed predominantly of cytotoxic T cells and plasma cells; (2) circulating autoantibodies (nuclear, smooth muscle, thyroid, etc.; see below), rheumatoid factor, and hyperglobulinemia are common; (3) other autoimmune disorders—such as thyroiditis, rheumatoid arthritis, autoimmune hemolytic anemia, ulcerative colitis, proliferative glomerulonephritis, juvenile diabetes mellitus, and Sjögren's syndrome—occur with increased frequency in patients who have autoimmune hepatitis and in their relatives; (4) histocompatibility haplotypes associated with autoimmune diseases, such as HLA-B1, -B8, -DR3, and -DR4, are common in patients with autoimmune hepatitis; and (5) this type of chronic hepatitis is responsive to glucocorticoid/immunosuppressive therapy, effective in a variety of autoimmune disorders.

Cellular immune mechanisms appear to be important in the pathogenesis of autoimmune hepatitis. In vitro studies have suggested that in patients with this disorder, lymphocytes are capable of becoming sensitized to hepatocyte membrane proteins and of destroying liver cells. Abnormalities of immunoregulatory control over cytotoxic lymphocytes (impaired suppressor cell influences) may play a role as well. Studies of genetic predisposition to autoimmune hepatitis demonstrate that certain haplotypes are associated with the disorder, as enumerated above. The precise triggering factors, genetic influences, and cytotoxic and immunoregulatory mechanisms involved in this type of liver injury remain poorly defined.

Intriguing clues into the pathogenesis of autoimmune hepatitis come from the observation that circulating autoantibodies are prevalent in patients with this disorder. Among the autoantibodies described in these patients are antibodies to nuclei [so-called antinuclear antibodies (ANA), primarily in a homogeneous pattern] and smooth muscle (so-called anti-smooth-muscle antibodies, directed at actin), anti-LKM (see below), antibodies to "soluble liver antigen" (directed at a member of the glutathione S-transferase gene family), as well as antibodies to the liver-specific asialoglycoprotein receptor (or "hepatic lectin") and other hepatocyte membrane proteins. Although some of these provide helpful diagnostic markers, their involvement in the pathogenesis of autoimmune hepatitis has not been established.

Humoral immune mechanisms have been shown to play a role in the extrahepatic manifestations of autoimmune/idiopathic hepatitis. Arthralgias, arthritis, cutaneous vasculitis, and glomerulonephritis occurring in patients with autoimmune hepatitis appear to be mediated by the deposition in affected tissue vessels of circulating immune complexes, followed by complement activation, inflammation, and tissue injury. While specific viral antigen-antibody complexes can be identified in acute and chronic viral hepatitis, the nature of the immune complexes in autoimmune hepatitis has not been defined.

Many of the *clinical features* of autoimmune hepatitis are similar to those described for chronic viral hepatitis. The onset of disease may be insidious or abrupt; the disease may present initially like, and be confused with, acute viral hepatitis; a history of recurrent bouts of what had been labeled acute hepatitis is not uncommon. A subset of patients with autoimmune hepatitis has distinct features. Such patients are predominantly young to middle-aged women with marked hyperglobulinemia and high-titer circulating ANA. This is the group with positive LE preparations (initially labeled "lupoid" hepatitis) in whom other autoimmune features are common. Fatigue, malaise, anorexia, amenorrhea, acne, arthralgias, and jaundice are common. Occasionally, arthritis, maculopapular eruptions (including cutaneous vasculitis), erythema nodosum, colitis, pleurisy, pericarditis, anemia, azotemia, and sicca syndrome (keratoconjunctivitis, xerostomia) occur. In some patients, complications of cirrhosis, such as ascites and edema (associated with hypoalbuminemia), encephalopathy, hypersplenism, coagulopathy, or variceal bleeding may bring the patient to initial medical attention.

The course of autoimmune hepatitis may be variable. In those with mild disease or limited histologic lesions (e.g., piecemeal necrosis without bridging), progression to cirrhosis is limited. In those with severe symptomatic autoimmune hepatitis (aminotransferase levels >10 times normal, marked hyperglobulinemia, "aggressive" histologic lesions—bridging necrosis or multilobular collapse, cirrhosis), the 6-month mortality without therapy may be as high as 40%. Such severe disease accounts for only 20% of cases; the natural history of milder disease is variable, often accentuated by spontaneous remissions and exacerbations. Especially poor prognostic signs include multilobular collapse at the time of initial presentation and failure of the bilirubin to improve after 2 weeks of therapy. Death may result from hepatic failure, hepatic coma, other complications of cirrhosis (e.g., variceal hemorrhage), and intercurrent infection. In patients with established cirrhosis, hepatocellular carcinoma may be a late complication (Chap. 91).

Laboratory features of autoimmune hepatitis are similar to those seen in chronic viral hepatitis. Liver biochemical tests are invariably abnormal but may not correlate with the clinical severity or histopathologic features in individual cases. Many patients with autoimmune hepatitis have normal serum bilirubin, alkaline phosphatase, and globulin levels with only minimal aminotransferase elevations. Serum AST and ALT levels are increased and fluctuate in the range of 100 to 1000 units. In severe cases, the serum bilirubin level is moderately elevated [51 to 171 μmol/L (3 to 10 mg/dL)]. Hypoalbuminemia occurs in patients with very active or advanced disease. Serum alkaline phosphatase levels may be moderately elevated or near normal. In a small proportion of patients, marked elevations of alkaline phosphatase activity occur; in such patients, clinical and laboratory features overlap with those of primary biliary cirrhosis (Chap. 299). The prothrombin time is often prolonged, particularly late in the disease or during active phases.

Hypergammaglobulinemia ($>$2.5 g/dL) is common in autoimmune hepatitis. Rheumatoid factor is common as well. As noted above, circulating autoantibodies are also common. The most characteristic are ANA in a homogeneous staining pattern. Smooth-muscle antibodies are less specific, seen just as frequently in chronic viral hepatitis. Because of the high levels of globulins achieved in the circulation of some patients with autoimmune hepatitis, occasionally the globulins may bind nonspecifically in solid-phase binding immunoassays for viral antibodies. This has been recognized most commonly in tests for antibodies to hepatitis C virus, as noted above. In fact, studies of autoantibodies in autoimmune hepatitis have led to the recognition of new categories of autoimmune hepatitis. *Type I autoimmune hepatitis* is the classic syndrome occurring in young women, associated with marked hyperglobulinemia, lupoid features, and circulating ANA. *Type II autoimmune hepatitis*, often seen in children and more common in Mediterranean populations, is associated not with ANA but with anti-LKM. Actually, anti-LKM represent a heterogeneous group of antibodies. In type II autoimmune hepatitis, the antibody is anti-LKM1, directed against P450 IID6. This is the same anti-LKM seen in some patients with chronic hepatitis C. Anti-LKM2 is seen in drug-induced hepatitis, and anti-LKM3 is seen in patients with chronic hepatitis D. Type II autoimmune hepatitis has been subdivided by some authorities into two categories, one more typically autoimmune and the other associated with viral hepatitis type C. Autoimmune hepatitis type IIa is felt to be autoimmune, is more likely to occur in young women, is associated with hyperglobulinemia, is associated with high-titer anti-LKM1, responds to glucocorticoid therapy, and is seen commonly in western Europe and the United Kingdom. Type IIb autoimmune hepatitis is associated with hepatitis C virus infection, tends to occur in older men, is associated with normal globulin levels and low-titer anti-LKM1, responds to interferon, and occurs most commonly in Mediterranean countries. In addition, another type of autoimmune hepatitis has been recognized, *autoimmune hepatitis type III*. These patients lack ANA and anti-LKM1 and have circulating antibodies to soluble liver antigen, which are directed at hepatocyte cytoplasmic cytokeratins 8 and 18. Most of these patients are women and have clinical features similar to those of patients with type I autoimmune hepatitis.

℞ **TREATMENT** The mainstay of management in autoimmune or idiopathic (nonviral) hepatitis is glucocorticoid therapy. Several controlled clinical trials have documented that such therapy leads to symptomatic, clinical, biochemical, and histologic improvement as well as increased survival. A therapeutic response can be expected in up to 80% of patients. Unfortunately, therapy has not been shown to prevent ultimate progression to cirrhosis. Although some advocate the use of prednisolone (the hepatic metabolite of prednisone), prednisone is just as effective and is favored by most authorities. Therapy may be initiated at 20 mg/d, but a popular regimen in the United States relies on an initiation dose of 60 mg/d. This high dose is tapered successively over the course of a month down to a maintenance level of 20 mg/d. An alternative but equally effective approach is to begin with half the prednisone dose (30 mg/d) along with azathioprine (50 mg/d). With azathioprine maintained at 50 mg/d, the prednisone dose is tapered over the course of a month down to a maintenance level of 10 mg/d. The advantage of the combination approach is a reduction, over the span of an 18-month course of therapy, in serious, life-threatening complications of steroid therapy from 66% down to under 20%. Azathioprine alone, however, is not effective in achieving remission, nor is alternate-day glucocorticoid therapy. Although therapy has been shown to be effective for severe autoimmune hepatitis, therapy is not indicated for mild forms of chronic hepatitis (which used to be labeled chronic persistent hepatitis or chronic lobular hepatitis), and the efficacy of therapy in mild or asymptomatic autoimmune hepatitis has not been established.

Improvement of fatigue, anorexia, malaise, and jaundice tends to occur within days to several weeks; biochemical improvement occurs over the course of several weeks to months, with a fall in serum bilirubin and globulin levels and an increase in serum albumin. Serum aminotransferase levels usually drop promptly, but improvements in AST and ALT alone do not appear to be a reliable marker of recovery in individual patients; histologic improvement, characterized by a decrease in mononuclear infiltration and in hepatocellular necrosis may be delayed for 6 to 24 months. Still, if interpreted cautiously, aminotransferase levels are valuable indicators of relative disease activity, and many authorities do *not* advocate serial liver biopsies to assess therapeutic success or to guide decisions to alter or stop therapy. Therapy should continue for at least 12 to 18 months. After tapering and cessation of therapy, the likelihood of relapse is at least 50%, even if posttreatment histology has improved to show mild chronic hepatitis, and the majority of patients require therapy at maintenance doses indefinitely. Continuing azathioprine alone after cessation of prednisone therapy may reduce the frequency of relapse.

If medical therapy fails, or when chronic hepatitis progresses to cirrhosis and is associated with life-threatening complications of liver decompensation, liver transplantation is the only recourse (Chap. 301). Recurrence of autoimmune hepatitis in the new liver occurs rarely, if at all.

DIFFERENTIAL DIAGNOSIS Early during the course of chronic hepatitis, the disease may resemble typical *acute viral hepatitis*. Without histologic assessment, severe chronic hepatitis cannot be readily distinguished based on clinical or biochemical criteria from mild chronic hepatitis. In adolescence, *Wilson's disease* may present with features of chronic hepatitis long before neurologic manifestations become apparent and before the formation of Kayser-Fleischer rings; in this age group, serum ceruloplasmin and serum and urinary copper determinations plus measurement of liver copper levels will establish the correct diagnosis. *Postnecrotic* or *cryptogenic cirrhosis* and *primary biliary cirrhosis* share clinical features with autoimmune hepatitis; biochemical, serologic, and histologic assessments are usually sufficient to allow these entities to be distinguished from autoimmune hepatitis. Of course, the distinction between autoimmune ("idiopathic") and chronic viral hepatitis is not always straightforward, especially when viral antibodies occur in patients with autoimmune disease or when autoantibodies occur in patients with viral disease. Finally, the presence of extrahepatic features such as arthritis, cutaneous vasculitis, or pleuritis—not to mention the presence of circulating autoantibodies—may cause confusion with *rheumatologic disorders* such as rheumatoid arthritis and systemic lupus erythematosus. The existence of clinical and biochemical features of progressive necroinflammatory liver disease distinguishes chronic hepatitis from these other disorders, which are not associated with severe liver disease.

BIBLIOGRAPHY

ALLEN MI et al: Identification and characterization of mutations in hepatitis B virus resistant to lamivudine. Hepatology 27:1670, 1998

BONI C et al: Lamivudine treatment can restore T cell responsiveness in chronic hepatitis B. J Clin Invest 102:968, 1998

CHAYAMA K et al: Emergence and takeover of YMDD mutant hepatitis B virus during long-term lamivudine therapy and re-takeover by wild type after cessation of therapy. Hepatology 27:1711, 1998

CONSENSUS STATEMENT: EASL international consensus conference on hepatitis C. J Hepatol 30:956, 1999

CZAJA AJ et al: Autoimmune hepatitis: Evolving concepts and treatment strategies. Dig Dis Sci 40:435, 1995

CZAJA AJ et al: Associations between alleles of the major histocompatibility complex and type I autoimmune hepatitis. Hepatology 25:317, 1997

DAVIS GL et al: Interferon alfa-2b alone or in combination with ribavirin for the treatment of relapse of chronic hepatitis C. N Engl J Med 339:1493, 1998

DESMET VJ et al: Classification of chronic hepatitis: Diagnosis, grading, and staging. Hepatology 19:1513, 1994

DI BISCEGLIE AM: Hepatitis C. Lancet 351:351, 1998

DI BISCEGLIE AM (guest editor): Treatment advances in chronic hepatitis C. Semin Liver Dis 19(Suppl 1):1, 1999

DIENSTAG JL et al: Lamivudine as initial treatment for chronic hepatitis B in the United States. N Engl J Med 341:1256, 1999

DONALDSON P et al: The molecular genetics of autoimmune liver disease. Hepatology 20:225, 1994

ENOMOTO N et al: Mutations in the nonstructural protein 5A gene and response to interferon in patients with chronic hepatitis C virus 1b infection. N Engl J Med 334:77, 1996

FARCI P et al: Treatment of chronic hepatitis D with interferon alfa-2a. N Engl J Med 330:88, 1994

FATTOVICH G et al: Morbidity and mortality in compensated cirrhosis type C: A retrospective follow-up study of 384 patients. Gastroenterology 112:463, 1997

HOOFNAGLE JH, DIBISCEGLIE AM: The treatment of chronic viral hepatitis. N Engl J Med 336:347, 1997

HU K-Q et al: The long-term outcomes of patients with compensated hepatitis C virus-related cirrhosis and history of parenteral exposure in the United States. Hepatology 29:1311, 1999

ISHAK K et al: Histologic grading and staging of chronic hepatitis. J Hepatol 22:696, 1995

JOHNSON PJ et al: Meeting report: International autoimmune hepatitis group. Hepatology 18:998, 1993

JOHNSON PJ et al: Azathioprine for long-term maintenance of remission in autoimmune hepatitis. N Engl J Med 333:958, 1995

KENNY-WALSH E et al: Clinical outcomes after hepatitis C infection from contaminated anti-D immune globulin. N Engl J Med 340:1228, 1999

KRAWITT EL: Autoimmune hepatitis. N Engl J Med 334:897, 1996

LAI C-L et al: A one-year trial of lamivudine for chronic hepatitis B. N Engl J Med 339:61, 1998

LAU DT-Y et al: Long-term follow up of patients with chronic hepatitis B treated with interferon alfa. Gastroenterology 113:1660, 1997

LIN S-M et al: Long-term beneficial effect of interferon therapy in patients with chronic hepatitis B virus infection. Hepatology 29:971, 1999

MARCELLIN P et al: Long-term histologic improvement and loss of detectable intrahepatic HCV RNA in patients with chronic hepatitis C and sustained response to interferon alpha therapy. Ann Intern Med 127:875, 1997

MCHUTCHISON JG et al: Interferon alfa-2b alone or in combination with ribavirin as initial treatment for chronic hepatitis C. N Engl J Med 339:1485, 1998

NATIONAL INSTITUTES OF HEALTH CONSENSUS DEVELOPMENT CONFERENCE: Management of hepatitis C. Hepatology 26(Suppl 1):1S, 1997

NATIONAL DIGESTIVE DISEASES INFORMATION CLEARINGHOUSE: Chronic hepatitis C: Current disease management. NIH Publication No. 99-4230, 1999 (www.niddk.nih.gov/health/digest/pubs/chrnhepc.htm)

NEUMANN AU et al: Hepatitis C viral dynamics in vivo and the antiviral efficacy of interferon-α therapy. Science 282:103, 1998

NIEDERAU C et al: Long-term follow-up of HBeAg-positive patients treated with interferon alfa for chronic hepatitis B. N Engl J Med 334:1422, 1996

NIEDERAU C et al: Prognosis of chronic hepatitis C: Results of a large, prospective cohort study. Hepatology 28:1687, 1998

PAYEN J-L et al: Better efficacy of a 12-month interferon alfa-2b retreatment in patients with chronic hepatitis C relapsing after a 6-month treatment: A multicenter, controlled, randomized trial. Hepatology 28:1680, 1998

POYNARD T et al: Natural history of liver fibrosis progression in patients with chronic hepatitis C. Lancet 349:825, 1997

POYNARD T et al: Randomized trial of interferon α2b plus ribavirin for 48 weeks or for 24 weeks versus interferon α2b plus placebo for 48 weeks for treatment of chronic infection with hepatitis C virus. Lancet 352:1426, 1998

ROSENBERG PM et al: Therapy with nucleoside analogues for hepatitis B virus infection. Clin Liver Dis 3:349, 1999

SEEFF LB: Natural history of viral hepatitis, type C. Semin Gastrointest Dis 6:20, 1995

SERFATY L et al: Determinants of outcome of compensated hepatitis C virus-related cirrhosis. Hepatology 27:1435, 1998

TASSOPOULOS NC et al: Efficacy of lamivudine in patients with hepatitis B e antigen-negative/hepatitis B virus DNA-positive (precore mutant) chronic hepatitis B. Hepatology 29:889, 1999

TONG MJ et al: Clinical outcomes after transfusion-associated hepatitis C. N Engl J Med 332:1463, 1995

WESIERSKA-GADEL J et al: Members of the glutathione S-transferase gene family are antigens in autoimmune hepatitis. Gastroenterology 105:1502, 1998

WONG JB et al: Cost-effectiveness of interferon-α2b treatment for hepatitis B e antigen-positive chronic hepatitis B. Ann Intern Med 122:664, 1995

YANO M et al: The long-term pathological evolution of chronic hepatitis C. Hepatology 23:1334, 1996

298   Mark E. Mailliard, Michael F. Sorrell

ALCOHOLIC LIVER DISEASE

Chronic and excessive alcohol ingestion is one of the major causes of liver disease in the western world. Classically, alcoholic liver injury comprises three major forms: (1) fatty liver, (2) alcoholic hepatitis, and (3) cirrhosis. Although cirrhosis is discussed in Chap. 299, it is important to emphasize that rarely does a pure form of liver injury exist by itself. Fatty liver is present in over 90% of binge and heavy drinkers. A much smaller percentage of drinkers progress to alcoholic hepatitis, thought to be a precursor to cirrhosis. Although alcohol is considered a direct hepatotoxin, only 10 to 20% of alcoholics develop alcoholic hepatitis. The explanation for this apparent paradox is unclear but involves complex factors such as gender and heredity.

ETIOLOGY AND PATHOGENESIS   Quantity and duration of alcohol intake are the most important risk factors involved in the development of alcoholic liver disease (Table 298-1). The roles of beverage type and pattern of drinking are less clear. Progress of the hepatic injury beyond the fatty liver stage seems to require additional risk factors that remain incompletely defined. Women are more susceptible to alcoholic liver injury than men; they develop advanced liver disease with substantially less alcohol intake. In general, the time it takes to develop liver disease is directly related to the amount of alcohol consumed. It is useful in estimating alcohol consumption to understand that one beer, four ounces of wine, or one ounce of 80% spirits all contain approximately 12 g of alcohol. The threshold for developing severe alcoholic liver disease in men is an intake of >60 to 80 g/d of alcohol for 10 years, while women are at increased risk for developing similar degrees of liver injury by consuming 20 to 40 g/d. Gender-dependent differences in the gastric and hepatic metabolism of alcohol, in addition to poorly understood hormonal factors, likely contribute to the increased susceptibility of women to alcohol-

Table 298-1   Risk Factors for Alcoholic Liver Disease

Risk Factor	Comment
Quantity	In men, 40–80 g/d of ethanol produces fatty liver; 80–160 g/d for 10–20 years causes hepatitis or cirrhosis. Only 15% of alcoholics develop alcoholic liver disease.
Gender	Women exhibit increased susceptibility to alcoholic liver disease at quantities >20 g/d.
Hepatitis C	HCV infection concurrent with alcoholic liver disease is associated with accelerated disease progression, more advanced histology, and decreased survival rates.
Genetics	The genetics of alcohol dehydrogenase, acetaldehyde dehydrogenase, and polymorphisms of cytochrome P4502E1 need confirmation.
Malnutrition	A common misconception. Alcohol hepatoxicity does not require malnutrition. Patients with alcohol hepatitis should receive aggressive attention to nutritional requirements.

induced liver injury. Social, nutritional, immunologic, and host factors have all been postulated to play a part in the development of the pathogenic process.

Chronic infection with hepatitis C (HCV) (Chap. 297) is an important risk factor in the progression and acceleration of alcoholic liver disease. The presence of HCV in patients with severe alcoholic liver disease is increased five- to tenfold above that in a matched control alcoholic population. Patients with both alcoholic liver injury and HCV develop decompensated liver disease at a younger age and have poorer overall survival rates. As a consequence of the overlapping injurious processes secondary to alcohol abuse and HCV infection, patients can develop an increased liver iron burden and rarely, porphyria cutanea tarda.

Our understanding of the pathogenesis of alcoholic liver injury is incomplete. Alcohol is a direct hepatotoxin, but ingestion of alcohol initiates a variety of metabolic responses that influence the final hepatotoxic response. The initial concept of malnutrition as the major pathogenic mechanism has given way to the present understanding that the metabolism of alcohol by the hepatocyte initiates a cascade of events involving production of protein-aldehyde adducts, lipid peroxidation, immunologic events, and cytokine release (Fig. 298-1). The production of cytokines is in large measure responsible for the systemic manifestations of alcoholic hepatitis, e.g., fever, leukocytosis, and anorexia. The degree of fibrosis stimulated by these complex events determines the extent of architectural derangement of the liver after chronic alcohol ingestion.

PATHOLOGY The liver has a limited repertoire in response to injury. Fatty liver is the initial and most common histologic response to increased alcohol ingestion. The accumulation of fat in the perivenular hepatocytes coincides with the location of alcohol dehydrogenase, the major enzyme responsible for alcohol metabolism. Continuing alcohol ingestion results in fat accumulation throughout the entire hepatic lobule. Despite extensive fatty changes and distortion of the hepatocytes with macrovesicular fat, the cessation of drinking results in normalization of hepatic architecture and fat content in the liver. Alcoholic fatty liver has traditionally been regarded as entirely benign; but similar to the spectrum of non-alcoholic steatohepatitis, certain pathologic features such as giant mitochondria, perivenular fibrosis, and macrovesicular fat may be associated with progressive liver injury.

The transition between fatty liver and the development of alcoholic hepatitis is blurred. The hallmark of alcoholic hepatitis is hepatocyte injury characterized by ballooning degeneration, spotty necrosis, polymorphonuclear infiltration, and fibrosis in the perivenular and perisinusoidal space of Disse. Mallory bodies are often present in florid cases but are neither specific nor necessary to establishing the diagnosis. Alcoholic hepatitis is thought to be a precursor to the development of cirrhosis. However, like fatty liver, it is potentially reversible with cessation of drinking. Cirrhosis is present in up to 50% of patients with biopsy-proven alcoholic hepatitis.

CLINICAL FEATURES The clinical manifestations of alcoholic fatty liver are subtle and characteristically detected as a consequence of the patient's visit for a seemingly unrelated matter. Previously unsuspected hepatomegaly is often the only clinical finding. Occasionally, patients with fatty liver present with right upper quadrant discomfort, tender hepatomegaly, nausea, and jaundice. Differentiation of alcoholic fatty liver from non-alcoholic fatty liver is difficult unless an accurate drinking history is verified. Alcoholism does not respect social and economic class. In every instance where liver disease is present, a thoughtful and sensitive drinking history should be obtained. Alcoholic hepatitis is associated with a wide gamut of clinical features. Fever, spider nevi, jaundice, and abdominal pain simulating an acute abdomen represent the extreme end of the spectrum; but many patients are entirely asymptomatic. Recognition of the clinical features of alcoholic hepatitis is central to the initiation of an effective and appropriate diagnostic and therapeutic strategy.

LABORATORY FEATURES Patients with alcoholic fatty liver are often identified through routine screening tests. The typical laboratory abnormalities are nonspecific and include modest elevations of the aspartate aminotransferase (AST) and alanine aminotransferase (ALT) accompanied by hypertriglyceridemia, hypercholesterolemia, and, occasionally, hyperbilirubinemia. In alcoholic hepatitis and in contrast to other causes of fatty liver, the AST and ALT are usually elevated two- to sevenfold. They rarely are above 400 IU, and the AST/ALT ratio is >1 (Table 298-2). Hyperbilirubinemia is common and is accompanied by modest increases in the alkaline phosphatase. Derangement in hepatocyte synthetic function indicates more serious disease. Hypoalbuminemia and coagulopathy are common in advanced liver injury. The mean corpuscular volume (MCV) and uric acid level are commonly elevated in chronic alcohol abuse. Measurement of the carbohydrate-deficient transferrin (CDT) is superior to the measurement of the gamma-glutamyl transpeptidase (GGTP) or MCV in identifying excessive drinking. Ultrasonography is useful in detecting fatty infiltration of the liver and determining liver size. The demonstration by ultrasound of portal vein flow reversal, ascites, and intra-abdominal collaterals indicates serious liver injury with less potential for complete reversal of liver disease.

PROGNOSIS Critically ill patients with alcoholic hepatitis have short-term mortality rates approaching 70%. Severe alcoholic hepatitis

FIGURE 298-1 Biomedical and cellular pathogenesis of liver injury secondary to chronic ethanol ingestion. MAA, malondialdehyde-acetaldehyde; TNF-α, tumor necrosis factor α; TGF-β, transforming growth factor β; IL, interleukin.

Table 298-2 Laboratory Diagnosis of Alcoholic Fatty Liver and Alcoholic Hepatitis

Test	Comment
AST	Increased two- to seven-fold, less than 400 U/L, greater than ALT
ALT	Increased two- to seven-fold, less than 400 U/L
AST/ALT	Usually > 1
GGT	Not specific to alcohol, easily inducible, elevated in all forms of fatty liver
CDT	Increased in alcoholism, irrespective of liver disease
MCV	Macrocytosis specific, but insensitive marker of alcoholism

FIGURE 298-2   Effect of glucocorticoid therapy of severe alcoholic hepatitis on short-term survival. Prednisolone, solid line; placebo, broken line. *(Adapted from Carithers et al.)*

is heralded by coagulopathy (prothrombin time >5 s), anemia, serum albumin concentrations below 2.5 mg/dL, serum bilirubin levels >8 mg/dL, renal failure, and ascites. A discriminant function calculated as 4.6 × [prothrombin time − control(seconds)] + serum bilirubin (mg/dL) can identify patients with a poor prognosis (discriminant function >32). The presence of ascites, variceal hemorrhage, deep encephalopathy, or hepatorenal syndrome predicts a dismal prognosis. The pathologic stage of the injury can be helpful in predicting prognosis. Liver biopsy should be performed whenever possible to confirm the diagnosis, to establish potential reversibility of the liver disease, and to guide the therapeutic decisions.

℞ TREATMENT   Complete abstinence from alcohol is the cornerstone in the treatment of alcoholic liver disease. Improved survival rates and the potential for reversal of histologic injury regardless of the initial clinical presentation are associated with total avoidance of alcoholic ingestion. Referral of patients to experienced alcohol counselors and/or alcohol treatment programs should be routine in the management of patients with alcoholic liver disease. Attention should be directed to the nutritional and psychosocial states during the evaluation and treatment periods. Because of data suggesting that the pathogenic mechanisms in alcoholic hepatitis involve cytokine release and the perpetuation of injury by immunologic processes, glucocorticoids have been extensively evaluated in the treatment of alcoholic hepatitis. Patients with severe alcoholic hepatitis, defined as a discriminant function >32, were given prednisone, 40 mg/d, or prednisolone, 32 mg/d, for 4 weeks followed by a steroid taper (Fig. 298-2). Exclusion criteria included active gastrointestinal bleeding, sepsis, renal failure, or pancreatitis. Because of inordinate surgical mortality rates and the high rates of recidivism after transplantation, patients with alcoholic hepatitis are not candidates for immediate liver transplantation. The transplant candidacy of these patients should be reevaluated after a defined period of sobriety.

BIBLIOGRAPHY

CARITHERS RL et al: Methylprednisolone therapy in patients with severe alcoholic hepatitis. Ann Intern Med 110:685, 1989

LEEVY CM: Fatty liver: A study of 270 patients with biopsy proven fatty liver and a review of the literature. Medicine 41:249, 1962

SCHIFF ER: Hepatitis C and alcohol. Hepatology 26(3, Suppl 1):395, 1997

TELI MR et al: Determinants of progression to cirrhosis or fibrosis in pure alcoholic fatty liver. Lancet 346:987, 1995

299   *Raymond T. Chung, Daniel K. Podolsky*

CIRRHOSIS AND ITS COMPLICATIONS

ALT alanine aminotransferase	KGDC α-ketoglutarate
AMA antimitochondrial antibody	dehydrogenase complex
AST asparate aminotransferase	PBC primary biliary cirrhosis
BCKDC branched chain–ketoacid	PDC pyruvate dehydrogenase
dehydrogenase complex	complex
CNS central nervous system	SAAG serum-ascites albumin
CREST calcinosis, *Raynaud's*	gradient
phenomenon, *esophageal dysmotility,*	SBC secondary biliary cirrhosis
sclerodactyly, telangiectasia	SBP spontaneous bacterial peritonitis
GABA γ-aminobutyric acid	TIPS transjugular intrahepatic
HBV hepatitis B virus	portosystemic shunt
HCV hepatitis C virus	

Cirrhosis is a pathologically defined entity that is associated with a spectrum of characteristic clinical manifestations. The cardinal pathologic features reflect irreversible chronic injury of the hepatic parenchyma and include extensive fibrosis in association with the formation of regenerative nodules. These features result from hepatocyte necrosis, collapse of the supporting reticulin network with subsequent connective tissue deposition, distortion of the vascular bed, and nodular regeneration of remaining liver parenchyma. The central event leading to hepatic fibrosis is activation of the hepatic stellate cell. Upon activation by factors released by hepatocytes and Kupffer cells, the stellate cell assumes a myofibroblast-like conformation and, under the influence of cytokines such as transforming growth factor β (TGF-β), produces fibril-forming type I collagen. The precise point at which fibrosis becomes irreversible is unclear. The pathologic process should be viewed as a final common pathway of many types of chronic liver injury. Clinical features of cirrhosis derive from the morphologic alterations and often reflect the severity of hepatic damage rather than the etiology of the underlying liver disease. Loss of functioning hepatocellular mass may lead to jaundice, edema, coagulopathy, and a variety of metabolic abnormalities; fibrosis and distorted vasculature lead to portal hypertension and its sequelae, including gastroesophageal varices and splenomegaly. Ascites and hepatic encephalopathy result from both hepatocellular insufficiency and portal hypertension.

Classification of the various types of cirrhosis based on either etiology or morphology alone is unsatisfactory. A single pathologic pattern may result from a variety of insults, while the same insult may produce several morphologic patterns. Nevertheless, most types of cirrhosis may be usefully classified by a mixture of etiologically and morphologically defined entities as follows: (1) alcoholic; (2) cryptogenic and posthepatitic; (3) biliary; (4) cardiac; and (5) metabolic, inherited, and drug-related. This chapter considers the various types of cirrhosis and their complications.

ALCOHOLIC CIRRHOSIS

Definition   *Alcoholic cirrhosis* is only one of many consequences resulting from chronic alcohol ingestion, and it often accompanies other forms of alcohol-induced liver injury, including alcoholic fatty liver and alcoholic hepatitis (Chap. 298). Alcoholic cirrhosis, historically referred to as *Laennec's cirrhosis*, is the most common type of cirrhosis encountered in North America and many parts of western Europe and South America. It is characterized by diffuse fine scarring, fairly uniform loss of liver cells, and small regenerative nodules, and therefore it is sometimes referred to as *micronodular cirrhosis*. However, micronodular cirrhosis may also result from other types of liver injury (e.g., following jejunoileal bypass), and thus alcoholic cirrhosis and micronodular cirrhosis are not necessarily synonymous. Conversely, alcoholic cirrhosis may progress to macronodular cirrhosis with time.

Pathology and Pathogenesis With continued alcohol intake and destruction of hepatocytes, fibroblasts (including activated hepatic stellate cells that have transformed into myofibroblasts with contractile properties) appear at the site of injury and deposit collagen. Weblike septa of connective tissue appear in periportal and pericentral zones and eventually connect portal triads and central veins. This fine connective tissue network surrounds small masses of remaining liver cells, which regenerate and form nodules. Although regeneration occurs within the small remnants of parenchyma, cell loss generally exceeds replacement. With continuing hepatocyte destruction and collagen deposition, the liver shrinks in size, acquires a nodular appearance, and becomes hard as "end-stage" cirrhosis develops. Although alcoholic cirrhosis is usually a progressive disease, appropriate therapy and strict avoidance of alcohol may arrest the disease at most stages and permit functional improvement. In addition, there is strong evidence that concomitant chronic hepatitis C virus (HCV) infection significantly accelerates development of alcoholic cirrhosis.

Clinical Features • Signs and symptoms Alcoholic cirrhosis may be clinically silent, and many cases (10 to 40%) are discovered incidentally at laparotomy or autopsy. In many cases symptoms are insidious in onset, occurring usually after 10 or more years of excessive alcohol use and progressing slowly over subsequent weeks and months. Anorexia and malnutrition lead to weight loss and a reduction in skeletal muscle mass. The patient may experience easy bruising, increasing weakness, and fatigue. Eventually the clinical manifestations of hepatocellular dysfunction and portal hypertension ensue, including progressive jaundice, bleeding from gastroesophageal varices, ascites, and encephalopathy. The abrupt onset of one of these complications may be the first event prompting the patient to seek medical attention. In other cases, cirrhosis first becomes evident when the patient requires treatment of symptoms related to alcoholic hepatitis.

A firm, nodular liver may be an early sign of disease; the liver may be either enlarged, normal, or decreased in size. Other frequent findings include jaundice, palmar erythema, spider angiomas, parotid and lacrimal gland enlargement, clubbing of fingers, splenomegaly, muscle wasting, and ascites with or without peripheral edema. Men may have decreased body hair and/or gynecomastia and testicular atrophy, which, like the cutaneous findings, result from disturbances in hormonal metabolism, including increased peripheral formation of estrogen due to diminished hepatic clearance of the precursor androstenedione. Testicular atrophy may reflect hormonal abnormalities or the toxic effect of alcohol on the testes. In women, signs of virilization or menstrual irregularities may occasionally be encountered. Dupuytren's contractures resulting from fibrosis of the palmar fascia with resulting flexion contracture of the digits are associated with alcoholism but are not specifically related to cirrhosis.

Although the cirrhotic patient may stabilize if drinking is discontinued, over a period of years, the patient may become emaciated, weak, and chronically jaundiced. Ascites and other signs of portal hypertension may become increasingly prominent. Ultimately, most patients with advanced cirrhosis die in hepatic coma, commonly precipitated by hemorrhage from esophageal varices or intercurrent infection. Progressive renal dysfunction often complicates the terminal phase of the illness.

Laboratory findings In advanced alcoholic liver disease, abnormalities of laboratory tests are more common. Anemia may result from acute and chronic gastrointestinal blood loss, coexistent nutritional deficiency (notably of folic acid and vitamin B_{12}), hypersplenism, and a direct suppressive effect of alcohol on the bone marrow. Hemolytic anemia, presumably due to effects of hypercholesterolemia or erythrocyte membranes resulting in unusual spurlike projections (acanthocytosis), has been described in some alcoholics with cirrhosis. Mild or pronounced hyperbilirubinemia may be found, usually in association with varying elevations of serum alkaline phosphatase levels. Levels of serum AST (asparate aminotransferase) are frequently elevated, but levels $>5\mu$kat (300 units) are unusual and should prompt one to look for other coincident or complicating factors. In contrast to viral

hepatitis, the serum AST is usually disproportionately elevated relative to ALT (alanine aminotransferase), i.e., AST/ALT ratio >2. This discrepancy in alcoholic liver disease may result from the proportionally greater inhibition of ALT synthesis by ethanol, which may be partially reversed by pyridoxal phosphate.

The serum prothrombin time is frequently prolonged, reflecting reduced synthesis of clotting proteins, most notably the vitamin K–dependent factors (see "Coagulopathy," below). The serum albumin level is usually depressed, while serum globulins are increased. Hypoalbuminemia reflects in part overall impairment in hepatic protein synthesis, while hyperglobulinemia is thought to result from nonspecific stimulation of the reticuloendothelial system. Elevated blood ammonia levels in patients with hepatic encephalopathy reflect diminished hepatic clearance because of impaired liver function and shunting of portal venous blood around the cirrhotic liver into the systemic circulation (see "Hepatic Encephalopathy," below).

A variety of metabolic disturbances may be detected. Glucose intolerance due to endogenous insulin resistance may be present; however, clinical diabetes is uncommon. Central hyperventilation may lead to respiratory alkalosis in patients with cirrhosis. Dietary deficiency and increased urinary losses lead to hypomagnesemia and hypophosphatemia. In patients with ascites and dilutional hyponatremia, hypokalemia may occur from increased urinary potassium losses due in part to hyperaldosteronism. Prerenal azotemia is also observed in such patients.

Diagnosis Alcoholic cirrhosis should be strongly suspected in patients with a history of prolonged or excessive alcohol intake and physical signs of chronic liver disease. However, since only 10 to 15% of individuals with excessive alcohol intake develop cirrhosis, other causes and types of liver disease may have to be excluded. The clinical features and laboratory findings are usually sufficient to provide reasonable indication of the presence and extent of hepatic injury. Although a percutaneous needle biopsy of the liver is not usually necessary to confirm the typical findings of alcoholic hepatitis or cirrhosis, it may be helpful in distinguishing patients with less advanced liver disease from those with cirrhosis and in excluding other forms of liver injury such as viral hepatitis. Biopsy may also be helpful as a diagnostic tool in evaluating patients with clinical findings suggestive of alcoholic liver disease who deny alcohol intake. In patients with features of cholestasis, ultrasonography may be appropriate to exclude the presence of extrahepatic biliary obstruction. When the clinical status of an otherwise stable cirrhotic patient deteriorates without an obvious explanation, complicating conditions, such as infection, portal vein thrombosis, and hepatocellular carcinoma, should be sought.

Prognosis Abstinence from alcohol as well as early and appropriate medical care can decrease long-term morbidity and mortality and delay or prevent the appearance of further complications. Patients who have had a major complication of cirrhosis and who continue to drink have a 5-year survival of less than 50%. However, those patients who remain abstinent have a substantially better prognosis. In general, the overall outlook in patients with advanced liver disease remains poor; most of these patients eventually die as a result of massive variceal hemorrhage and/or profound hepatic encephalopathy.

TREATMENT Alcoholic cirrhosis is a serious illness that requires long-term medical supervision and careful management. Therapy of the underlying liver disease is largely supportive. Specific treatment is directed at particular complications such as variceal bleeding and ascites (see below). While some studies suggest that administration of glucocorticoids in moderately large doses for 4 weeks is helpful in patients with severe alcoholic hepatitis and encephalopathy, these drugs have no role in the treatment of established alcoholic cirrhosis. While one study suggested a mortality benefit for the antifibrotic agent colchicine in alcoholic cirrhosis, it has not yet been reproduced; thus colchicine cannot be routinely recommended.

The patient should be made to realize that there is no medication that will protect the liver against the effects of further alcohol ingestion. Therefore, alcohol should be absolutely forbidden. An important component of the complete care of such patients is encouragement to become involved in an appropriate alcohol counseling program.

All medicines must be administered with caution in the patient with cirrhosis, especially those eliminated or modified through hepatic metabolism or biliary pathways. In particular, care must be taken to avoid overzealous use of drugs that may directly or indirectly precipitate complications of cirrhosis. For example, vigorous treatment of ascites with diuretics may result in electrolyte abnormalities or hypovolemia, which can lead to coma. Similarly, even modest doses of sedatives can lead to deepening encephalopathy. Aspirin should be avoided in patients with cirrhosis because of its effects on coagulation and gastric mucosa. Acetaminophen should be used with caution and in doses of less than 2 g/day. Patients who drink alcohol are more sensitive to the hepatotoxic effects of acetaminophen, probably due to increased metabolism of the drug to toxic intermediates and decreased glutathione levels.

POSTHEPATIC AND CRYPTOGENIC CIRRHOSIS

Definition   Posthepatitic or postnecrotic cirrhosis represents the final common pathway of many types of chronic liver disease. *Coarsely nodular* and *multilobular cirrhosis* are terms synonymous with posthepatitic cirrhosis. The term *cryptogenic cirrhosis* has been used interchangeably with postpathepatitic cirrhosis, but this designation should be reserved for those cases in which the etiology of cirrhosis is unknown (approximately 10% of all patients with cirrhosis).

Etiology   *Posthepatitic cirrhosis* is a morphologic term referring to a defined stage of advanced chronic liver injury of both specific and unknown (cryptogenic) causes. Epidemiologic and serologic evidence suggest that viral hepatitis (hepatitis B or hepatitis C) may be an antecedent factor in from one-fourth to three-fourths of cases of apparently cryptogenic posthepatitic cirrhosis. In areas where hepatitis B virus (HBV) infection is endemic (e.g., Southeast Asia, sub-Saharan Africa), up to 15% of the population may acquire the infection in early childhood, and cirrhosis may ultimately develop in one-fourth of these chronic carriers. Although HBV infection is much less prevalent in the United States, it is relatively common among certain high-risk groups (e.g., persons with multiple sexual partners, especially men who have sex with men, injection drug users) and contributes to an increased incidence of cirrhosis. In the United States, HCV infection accounts for many cases of cirrhosis following blood transfusions. Before routine screening of blood donors was introduced, hepatitis C occurred in 5 to 10% of blood recipients. Following infection, cirrhosis may ultimately develop in more than 20% of individuals after 20 years. More than half of patients who would previously have been designated as having cryptogenic chronic liver disease have evidence of HCV infection. Increasing recognition of the progressive nature of nonalcoholic steatohepatitis has revealed that a large portion of cases previously designated cryptogenic cirrhosis may be attributable to this disorder (Chap. 300). Posthepatitic cirrhosis may also develop in patients with autoimmune hepatitis (Chap. 297).

The most common causes of cirrhosis in the United States, which ultimately lead to liver transplantation, include chronic HCV infection, alcohol, primary biliary cirrhosis, primary sclerosing cholangitis, and nonalcoholic steatohepatitis (NASH). Less common causes of posthepatitic cirrhosis, including drugs and toxins, are listed in Table 299-1.

Pathology   The posthepatitic liver is typically shrunken in size, distorted in shape, and composed of nodules of liver cells separated by dense and broad bands of fibrosis. The microscopic picture is consistent with the gross impression. Posthepatitic cirrhosis is characterized morphologically by (1) extensive confluent loss of liver cells, (2) stromal collapse and fibrosis resulting in broad bands of connective

Table 299-1   Causes of Cirrhosis and/or Chronic Liver Disease

Infectious Diseases	Drugs and Toxins (Chap. 296)
Brucellosis (Chap. 160)	Alcohol (Chap. 298)
Capillariasis (Chap. 220)	Amioradone
Echinococcosis (Chap. 223)	Arsenicals
Schistosomiasis (Chap. 222)	Oral contraceptives (Budd-Chiari)
Toxoplasmosis (Chap. 217)	Pyrrolidizine alkaloids (venooc-
Viral hepatitis [hepatitis B, C, D;	clusive disease)
cytomegalovirus; Epstein-Barr virus (Chaps. 295, 184, 185)]	**Other Causes**
Inherited and Metabolic Disorders (See Chap. 300)	Biliary obstruction (chronic) (Chap. 302)
α_1-Antitrypsin deficiency (Chap. 300)	Cystic fibrosis (Chap. 257)
Alagille's syndrome (Chap. 292)	Graft-versus-host disease (Chap. 115)
Biliary atresia (Chap. 302)	Jejunoileal bypass (Chap. 43)
Familial intrahepatic cholestasis (FIC) types 1-3 (Chap. 302)	Nonalcoholic steatohepatitis (Chap. 300)
Fanconi's syndrome (Chap. 349)	Primary biliary cirrhosis
Galactosemia (Chap. 350)	Primary sclerosing cholangitis (Chap. 302)
Gaucher's disease (Chap. 349)	Sarcoidosis (Chap. 318)
Glycogen storage disease (Chap. 350)	
Hemochromatosis (Chap. 345)	
Hereditary fructose intolerance (Chap. 350)	
Hereditary tyrosinemia (Chap. 352)	
Wilson's disease (Chap. 348)	

tissue containing the remains of many portal triads, and (3) irregular nodules of regenerating hepatocytes, varying in size from microscopic to several centimeters in diameter.

Clinical Features   In patients with cirrhosis of known etiology in whom there is progression to a posthepatitic stage, the clinical manifestations are an extension of those resulting from the initial disease process. Usually clinical symptoms are related to portal hypertension and its sequelae, such as ascites, splenomegaly, hypersplenism, encephalopathy, and bleeding gastroesophageal varices. The hematologic and liver function abnormalities resemble those seen with other types of cirrhosis. In a few patients with posthepatitic cirrhosis, the diagnosis may be made incidentally at operation, at postmortem, or by a needle biopsy of the liver performed to investigate abnormal liver function tests or hepatomegaly.

Diagnosis and Prognosis   Posthepatitic cirrhosis should be suspected in patients with signs and symptoms of cirrhosis or portal hypertension. Needle or operative liver biopsies confirm the diagnosis, although nonuniformity of the pathologic process may result in sampling errors. The diagnosis of cryptogenic cirrhosis is reserved for those patients in whom no known etiology can be demonstrated. About 75% of patients have progressive disease despite supportive therapy and die within 1 to 5 years from complications, including variceal hemorrhage, hepatic encephalopathy, or superimposed hepatocellular carcinoma.

℞ **TREATMENT**   Management is usually limited to treatment of the complications of portal hypertension, including control of ascites, avoidance of drugs or excessive protein intake that may induce hepatic coma, and prompt treatment of infections (see below). In patients with asymptomatic cirrhosis, expectant management alone is appropriate. In those patients in whom posthepatitic cirrhosis has developed as a result of a treatable condition, therapy directed at the primary disorder may limit further progression (e.g., Wilson's disease, hemochromatosis).

BILIARY CIRRHOSIS

Biliary cirrhosis results from injury to or prolonged obstruction of either the intrahepatic or extrahepatic biliary system. It is associated with impaired biliary excretion, destruction of hepatic parenchyma, and progressive fibrosis. Primary biliary cirrhosis (PBC) is characterized by chronic inflammation and fibrous obliteration of intrahepatic bile ductules. Secondary biliary cirrhosis (SBC) is the result of long-standing obstruction of the larger extrahepatic ducts. Although primary and secondary biliary cirrhosis are separate pathophysiologic entities with respect to the initial insult, many clinical features are similar.

PRIMARY BILIARY CIRRHOSIS **Etiology and Pathogenesis** The cause of PBC remains unknown. Several observations suggest that a disordered immune response may be involved. PBC is frequently associated with a variety of disorders presumed to be autoimmune in nature, such as the syndrome of *c*alcinosis, *R*aynaud's phenomenon, *e*sophageal dysmotility, *s*clerodactyly, *t*elangiectasia (CREST); the sicca syndrome (dry eyes and dry mouth); autoimmune thyroiditis; type 1 diabetes mellitus; and IgA deficiency.

Most important, a circulating IgG antimitochondrial antibody (AMA) is detected in more than 90% of patients with PBC and only rarely in other forms of liver disease. It has been demonstrated that these autoantibodies recognize three to five inner mitochondrial membrane proteins identified as enzymes of the pyruvate dehydrogenase complex (PDC), the branched chain–ketoacid dehydrogenase complex (BCKDC), and the α-ketoglutarate dehydrogenase complex (KGDC). The major autoantigen in PBC (found in 90% of patients) has been identified as the 74-kDa E2 component of the PDC, dihydrolipoamide acetyltransferase. The antibodies are directed to a region essential for binding of a lipoic acid cofactor and inhibit the overall enzymatic activity of the PDC. Other AMA autoantibodies in PNC patients are directed to similar constituents of BCKDC and KGDC and also inhibit their enzymatic function. It remains unclear whether these properties have a direct pathogenetic role in the development of PBC. In addition to AMA, elevated serum levels of IgM and cryoproteins consisting of immune complexes capable of activating the alternative complement pathway are found in 80 to 90% of patients. Aberrant expression of major histocompatibility complex class II molecules has been found on biliary epithelium in association with PBC, suggesting that these cells may serve as antigen-presenting cells in this setting. Lymphocytes are prominent in the portal regions and surround damaged bile ducts. These histologic findings resemble those noted in graft-versus-host disease following bone marrow transplantation and suggest that damage to bile ducts may be immunologically mediated, perhaps reflecting a defect in a suppressor cell population.

Pathology PBC is divided into four stages based on morphologic findings. The earliest recognizable lesion (stage I), termed *chronic nonsuppurative destructive cholangitis*, is a necrotizing inflammatory process of the portal triads. It is characterized by destruction of medium and small bile ducts, a dense infiltrate of acute and chronic inflammatory cells, mild fibrosis, and occasionally, bile stasis. At times, periductal granulomas and lymph follicles are found adjacent to affected bile ducts. Subsequently, the inflammatory infiltrate becomes less prominent, the number of bile ducts is reduced, and smaller bile ductules proliferate (stage II). Progression over a period of months to years leads to a decrease in interlobular ducts, loss of liver cells, and expansion of periportal fibrosis into a network of connective tissue scars (stage III). Ultimately, cirrhosis, which may be micronodular or macronodular, develops (stage IV).

Clinical Features • *Signs and symptoms* Many patients with PBC are asymptomatic, and the disease is initially detected on the basis of elevated serum alkaline phosphatase levels during routine screening. The majority of such patients remain asymptomatic for prolonged periods, although most ultimately develop progressive liver injury.

Among patients with symptomatic disease, 90% are women age 35 to 60. Often the earliest symptom is pruritus, which may be either generalized or limited initially to the palms and soles. In addition, fatigue is commonly a prominent early symptom. After several months or years, jaundice and gradual darkening of the exposed areas of the skin (melanosis) may ensue. Other early clinical manifestations of PBC reflect impaired bile excretion. These include steatorrhea and the

malabsorption of lipid-soluble vitamins. Protracted elevation of serum lipids, especially cholesterol, leads to subcutaneous lipid deposition around the eyes (xanthelasmas) and over joints and tendons (xanthomas). Over a period of months to years, the itching, jaundice, and hyperpigmentation slowly worsen. Eventually, signs of hepatocellular failure and portal hypertension develop and ascites appears. Progression may be quite variable. Whereas a proportion of asymptomatic patients may show no signs of progression for a decade or longer, in others, death due to hepatic insufficiency may occur within 5 to 10 years after the first signs of the illness. Such decompensation is often precipitated by uncontrolled variceal hemorrhage or infection.

Physical examination may be entirely normal in the early phase of the disease, when patients are asymptomatic or pruritus is the sole complaint. Later, there may be jaundice of varying intensity, hyperpigmentation of the exposed skin areas, xanthelasmas and tendinous and planar xanthomas, moderate to striking hepatomegaly, splenomegaly, and clubbing of the fingers. Bone tenderness, signs of vertebral compression, ecchymoses, glossitis, and dermatitis may all be noted. Clinical evidence of the sicca syndrome can be found in as many as 75% of patients, and serologic evidence of autoimmune thyroid disease in 25%. Other conditions encountered with increased frequency include rheumatoid arthritis, CREST syndrome, keratoconjunctivitis sicca, IgA deficiency, type 1 diabetes mellitus, scleroderma, pernicious anemia, and renal tubular acidosis. Bone disease is often a significant problem encountered over the course of the disease. While osteomalacia occurs due to diminished vitamin D absorption, accelerated osteoporosis in this patient population (the majority of whom are postmenopausal women) is even more common.

Laboratory findings PBC is increasingly diagnosed at a presymptomatic stage, prompted by the finding of a twofold or greater elevation of the serum alkaline phosphatase during routine screening. Serum 5′-nucleotidase activity and γ-glutamyl transpeptidase levels are also elevated. In this setting, serum bilirubin is usually normal and aminotransferase levels minimally increased. The diagnosis is supported by a positive AMA test (titer > 1:40). The latter is both relatively specific and sensitive; a positive test is found in over 90% of symptomatic patients and is present in fewer than 5% of patients with other liver diseases. As the disease evolves, the serum bilirubin level rises progressively and may reach 510 μmol/L (30 mg/dL) or more in the final stages. Serum aminotransferase values rarely exceed 2.5 to 3.3 μkat (150 to 200 units). Hyperlipidemia is common, and a striking increase of the serum unesterified cholesterol is often noted. An abnormal serum lipoprotein (lipoprotein X) may be present in PBC but is not specific and appears in other cholestatic conditions. A deficiency of bile salts in the intestine leads to moderate steatorrhea and impaired absorption of the fat-soluble vitamins and hypoprothrombinemia. Patients with PBC have elevated liver copper levels, but this finding is not specific and is found in all disorders in which there is prolonged cholestasis.

Diagnosis PBC should be considered in middle-aged women with unexplained pruritus or an elevated serum alkaline phosphatase and in whom there may be other clinical or laboratory features of protracted impairment of biliary excretion. Although a positive serum AMA determination provides important diagnostic evidence, false-positive results do occur; therefore, liver biopsy should be performed to confirm the diagnosis. Rarely, the AMA test may be negative in patients with histologic features of PBC. Frequently, patients have antibodies to the E2 protein in tests using these specific antigens. In some cases with histologic features of PBC and a negative AMA, antinuclear or smooth-muscle antibodies are present (as in autoimmune hepatitis), and the designation *autoimmune cholangitis* is applied. The natural history of this entity, however, appears to resemble that of PBC. If the AMA test is negative, the biliary tract should be evaluated to exclude primary sclerosing cholangitis and remediable extrahepatic biliary tract obstruction, especially in view of the frequent presence of coexisting cholelithiasis.

℞ **TREATMENT**   While there is no specific therapy for PBC, ursodiol has been shown to improve biochemical and histologic features and might improve survival, particularly liver transplantation–free survival (although this remains unproven). Ursodiol should be given in doses of 10 to 15 mg/kg per day, but lower doses are sometimes just as effective in reducing serum alkaline phosphatase and aminotransferase levels. Ursodiol should be given with food and can be taken in a single dose daily. Side effects are rare: gastrointestinal intolerance (bloating, indigestion) and skin rashes occur but are uncommon. Isolated instances of severe exacerbation of pruritus have been reported in patients with advanced disease. Ursodiol probably works by replacing the endogenously produced hydrophobic bile acids with urosdeoxycholate, a hydrophilic and relatively nontoxic bile acid.

Unfortunately, ursodiol does not prevent ultimate progression of PBC, and the only established "cure" is liver transplantation. Results of liver transplantation for PBC are excellent, survival exceeding that for patients receiving transplantation for most other forms of end-stage liver disease. Recurrence of PBC after liver transplantation has been reported but is uncommon, and the recurrent disease is only slowly progressive. Most patients remain AMA positive after transplantation, and as many as 25% will have histologic features of PBC on liver biopsy after 5 years. Other therapies such as glucocorticoids, colchicine, methotrexate, azathioprine, cyclosporine, and tacrolimus have been reported as effective in small cases series, but none have shown to be effective in adequately controlled trials.

Relief of symptoms is also an important part of management of PBC. As noted, ursodiol may be helpful in controlling symptoms and improving the patient's sense of well-being. Although the mechanism of the protracted pruritus is not entirely clear, cholestyramine, an oral bile salt–sequestering resin, may be helpful in doses of 8 to 12 g/d to decrease both pruritus and hypercholesterolemia. Rifampin, opiate antagonists, ondansetron, plasmapheresis, and ultraviolet light have all been tried for control of pruritus, with varying results. Steatorrhea can be reduced by a low-fat diet and substituting medium-chain triglycerides for dietary long-chain triglycerides. Fat-soluble vitamins A and K should be given by parenteral injection at regular intervals to prevent or correct night blindness and hypoprothrombinemia, respectively. Zinc supplementation may be necessary if night blindness is refractory to vitamin A therapy. An important part of management of PBC and any cholestatic liver disease is assessment and treatment of osteoporosis and osteomalacia. Patients should be screened periodically by bone densitometry and treated as needed with calcium supplements, estrogen, and/or the newer bisphosphonate agents (e.g., alendronate). Progression of PBC leads to the typical complications of advanced liver disease (see below).

SECONDARY BILIARY CIRRHOSIS   Etiology   SBC results from prolonged partial or total obstruction of the common bile duct or its major branches. In adults, obstruction is most frequently caused by postoperative strictures or gallstones, usually with superimposed infectious cholangitis. Chronic pancreatitis may lead to biliary stricture and secondary cirrhosis. SBC is also an important complication of primary sclerosing cholangitis, a progressive immunologic disorder of the intrahepatic and extrahepatic biliary tree (Chap. 302). Patients with malignant tumors of the common bile duct or pancreas rarely survive long enough to develop SBC. In children, congenital biliary atresia and cystic fibrosis are common causes of SBC. Choledochal cysts, if unrecognized, may also be a rare cause of SBC.

Pathology and Pathogenesis   Unrelieved obstruction of the extrahepatic bile ducts leads to (1) bile stasis and focal areas of centrilobular necrosis followed by periportal necrosis, (2) proliferation and dilatation of the portal bile ducts and ductules, (3) sterile or infected cholangitis with accumulation of polymorphonuclear infiltrates around bile ducts, and (4) progressive expansion of portal tracts by edema and fibrosis. Extravasation of bile from ruptured interlobular bile ducts into areas of periportal necrosis leads to the formation of "bile lakes" surrounded by cholesterol-rich pseudoxanthomatous cells. As in other forms of cirrhosis, injury is accompanied by regeneration in residual parenchyma. These changes gradually lead to a finely nodular cirrhosis. In general, at least 3 to 12 months is required for biliary obstruction to result in cirrhosis. Relief of the obstruction is frequently accompanied by biochemical and morphologic improvement.

Clinical Features   The symptoms, signs, and biochemical findings of SBC are similar to those of PBC. Jaundice and pruritus are usually the most prominent features. In addition, fever and/or right upper quadrant pain, reflecting bouts of cholangitis or biliary colic, are typical. The manifestations of portal hypertension are found only in advanced cases. SBC should be considered in any patient with clinical and laboratory evidence of prolonged obstruction to bile flow, especially when there is a history of previous biliary tract surgery or gallstones, bouts of ascending cholangitis, or right upper quadrant pain. Cholangiography (either percutaneous or endoscopic) usually demonstrates the underlying pathologic process. Liver biopsy, although not always necessary from a clinical standpoint, can document the development of cirrhosis.

℞ **TREATMENT**   Relief of obstruction to bile flow, by either endoscopic or surgical means, is the most important step in the prevention and therapy of SBC. Effective decompression of the biliary tract results in a significant improvement in both symptoms and survival, even in patients with established cirrhosis. When obstruction cannot be relieved, as in sclerosing cholangitis, antibiotics may be helpful acutely in controlling superimposed infection or, when administered on a chronic basis, as prophylactic therapy in suppressing recurring episodes of ascending cholangitis. Without relief of obstruction, there is a steady progression to end-stage cirrhosis and its terminal manifestations.

CARDIAC CIRRHOSIS

Definition   Prolonged, severe right-sided congestive heart failure may lead to chronic liver injury and cardiac cirrhosis. The characteristic pathologic features of fibrosis and regenerative nodules distinguish cardiac cirrhosis from both reversible passive congestion of the liver due to acute heart failure and acute hepatocellular necrosis ("ischemic hepatitis" or "shock liver") resulting from systemic hypotension and hypoperfusion of the liver.

Etiology and Pathology   In right-sided heart failure, retrograde transmission of elevated venous pressure via the inferior vena cava and hepatic veins leads to congestion of the liver. Hepatic sinusoids become dilated and engorged with blood, and the liver becomes tensely swollen. With prolonged passive congestion and ischemia from poor perfusion secondary to reduced cardiac output, necrosis of centrilobular hepatocytes ensues and leads to fibrosis in these central areas. Ultimately, centrilobular fibrosis develops, with collagen extending outward in a characteristic stellate pattern from the central vein. Gross examination of the liver shows alternating red (congested) and pale (fibrotic) areas, a pattern often referred to as "nutmeg liver." Improvement in management of cardiac disorders, particularly advances in surgical treatment, has reduced the frequency of cardiac cirrhosis.

Clinical Features   A range of abnormalities of liver function tests may be found, though none is uniformly present. The serum bilirubin is usually only mildly increased and may be predominantly either conjugated or unconjugated. Mild to moderate elevation in alkaline phosphatase level and prothrombin time prolongation are sometimes present. The AST level is typically mildly elevated but may be transiently very high following a period of marked systemic hypotension (shock liver), when the clinical picture can mimic acute viral or drug-induced hepatitis. In cases of tricuspid insufficiency the liver may be pulsatile, but this finding disappears as cirrhosis develops. With prolonged right-sided heart failure the liver becomes enlarged, firm, and usually nontender. The signs and symptoms of heart failure usually overshadow the liver disease. Bleeding from esophageal varices is rare, but chronic encephalopathy may be prominent, with a waxing and failure. Ascites and peripheral edema, often primarily related to the underlying cardiac dysfunction, may be worsened by the superimposed liver disease.

Diagnosis The presence of a firm, enlarged liver with signs of chronic liver disease in a patient with valvular heart disease, constrictive pericarditis, or cor pulmonale of long duration (>10 years) should suggest cardiac cirrhosis. Liver biopsy can confirm the diagnosis but is usually contraindicated because of coagulopathy or ascites. Coexistent chronic heart and liver disease should also raise the possibility of hemochromatosis (Chap. 345), amyloidosis (Chap. 319), or other infiltrative diseases.

Budd-Chiari syndrome resulting from the occlusion of the hepatic veins or inferior vena cava may be confused with acute congestive hepatomegaly. In this condition the liver is grossly enlarged and tender, and severe intractable ascites is present. However, signs and symptoms of heart failure are notably absent. The most common cause is thrombosis of the hepatic veins, often in the setting of polycythemia rubra vera, myeloproliferative syndromes, paroxysmal nocturnal hemoglobinuria, oral contraceptive use, or other hypercoagulable states; it may also result from invasion of the inferior vena cava by tumor, such as renal cell or hepatocellular carcinoma. Idiopathic membranous obstruction of the inferior vena cava is the most common cause of this syndrome in Japan. Hepatic venography or liver biopsy showing centrilobular congestion and sinusoidal dilatation in the absence of right-sided heart failure establishes the diagnosis of Budd-Chiari syndrome. Venocclusive disease affecting the sublobular branches of the hepatic veins and the hepatic venues may result from hepatic irradiation, treatment with certain antineoplastic agents, or ingestion of pyrrolidizine alkaloids present in some herbal teas ("bush tea disease") and can mimic congestive hepatomegaly.

℞ **TREATMENT** Prevention or treatment of cardiac cirrhosis depends on the diagnosis and therapy of the underlying cardiovascular disorder. Improvement in cardiac function frequently results in improvement of liver function and stabilization of the liver disease.

METABOLIC, HEREDITARY, DRUG-RELATED, AND OTHER TYPES OF CIRRHOSIS (See Table 299-1)

Cirrhosis or hepatitis may result from a wide variety of other processes encompassing the spectrum of etiologic factors listed in Table 299-2. Although some of these disorders have distinctive clinical or morphologic features, the manifestations of cirrhosis are largely independent of the underlying pathogenic mechanism.

NONCIRRHOTIC FIBROSIS OF THE LIVER

Several diseases, either congenital or acquired, may be associated with localized or generalized hepatic fibrosis. They are distinguished from cirrhosis by the absence of hepatocellular damage and the lack of nodular regenerative activity. The clinical manifestations in such cases are largely secondary to portal hypertension. The different types of these disorders are indicated in Table 299-2; with the exception of schistosomiasis in some regions of the world, all these conditions are relatively rare.

MAJOR COMPLICATIONS OF CIRRHOSIS

The clinical course of patients with advanced cirrhosis is often complicated by a number of important sequelae that are independent of the etiology of the underlying liver disease. These include portal hypertension and its consequences (e.g., gastroesophageal varices and splenomegaly), ascites, hepatic encephalopathy, spontaneous bacterial peritonitis, hepatorenal syndrome, and hepatocellular carcinoma.

PORTAL HYPERTENSION Definition and Pathogenesis Normal pressure in the portal vein is low (5 to 10 mmHg) because

Table 299-2 Some Causes of Noncirrhotic Hepatic Fibrosis

Idiopathic portal hypertension (noncirrhotic portal fibrosis, Banti's syndrome); three variants:
  Intrahepatic phlebosclerosis and fibrosis
  Portal and splenic vein sclerosis
  Portal and splenic vein thrombosis
Schistosomiasis ("pipe-stem" fibrosis with presinusoidal portal hypertension)
Congenital hepatic fibrosis (may be associated with polycystic disease of liver and kidneys)

vascular resistance in the hepatic sinusoids is minimal. Portal hypertension (>10 mmHg) most commonly results from increased resistance to portal blood flow. Because the portal venous system lacks valves, resistance at any level between the right side of the heart and splanchnic vessels results in retrograde transmission of an elevated pressure. Increased resistance can occur at three levels relative to the hepatic sinusoids: (1) presinusoidal, (2) sinusoidal, and (3) postsinusoidal. Obstruction in the *presinusoidal* venous compartment may be anatomically outside the liver (e.g., portal vein thrombosis) or within the liver itself but at a functional level proximal to the hepatic sinusoids so that the liver parenchyma is not exposed to the elevated venous pressure (e.g., schistosomiasis).

Postsinusoidal obstruction may also occur outside the liver at the level of the hepatic veins (e.g., Budd-Chiari syndrome), the inferior vena cava, or, less commonly, within the liver (e.g., venocclusive disease). When cirrhosis is complicated by portal hypertension, the increased resistance is usually *sinusoidal*. While distinctions between pre-, post-, and sinusoidal processes are conceptually appealing, functional resistance to portal flow in a given patient may occur at more than one level. Portal hypertension may also arise from increased blood flow (e.g., massive splenomegaly or arteriovenous fistulas), but the low outflow resistance of the normal liver makes this a rare clinical problem.

Cirrhosis is the most common cause of portal hypertension in the United States. Clinically significant portal hypertension is present in >60% of patients with cirrhosis. *Portal vein obstruction* is the second most common cause; it may be idiopathic or occur in association with cirrhosis, infection, pancreatitis, or abdominal trauma. Portal vein thrombosis may develop in a variety of hypercoagulable states including polycythemia vera; essential thrombocythemia; deficiencies of protein C, protein S, or antithrombin III; resistance to activated protein C (factor V Leiden); and a mutation of the prothrombin gene (G20210A). Portal vein thrombosis may be idiopathic, though some of these patients may have a subclinical myeloproliferative disorder. Hepatic vein thrombosis (Budd-Chiari syndrome) and hepatic venocclusive disease are relatively infrequent causes of portal hypertension (see above). Portal vein occlusion may result in massive hematemesis from gastroesophageal varices, but ascites is usually found only when cirrhosis is present. Noncirrhotic portal fibrosis (Table 299-2) accounts for only a few cases of portal hypertension.

Clinical Features The major clinical manifestations of portal hypertension include hemorrhage from gastroesophageal varices, splenomegaly with hypersplenism, ascites, and acute and chronic hepatic encephalopathy. These are related, at least in part, to the development of portal-systemic collateral channels. The absence of valves in the portal venous system facilitates retrograde (hepatofugal) blood flow from the high-pressure portal venous system to the lower-pressure systemic venous circulation. Major sites of collateral flow involve the veins around cardioesophageal junction (esophagogastric varices), the rectum (hemorrhoids), retroperitoneal space, and the falciform ligament of the liver (periumbilical or abdominal wall collaterals). Abdominal wall collaterals appear as tortuous epigastric vessels that radiate from the umbilicus toward the xiphoid and rib margins (caput medusae).

A frequent marker of the presence of cirrhosis in a patient being followed for chronic liver disease is a progressive decrease in platelet count. A low-normal platelet count can be the first clue to progression to cirrhosis. Ultimately, a marked decrease in platelets (to 30,000 to 60,000/μL) and white blood cells can occur.

Diagnosis   In patients with known liver disease, the development of portal hypertension is usually revealed by the appearance of spleno-megaly, ascites, encephalopathy, and/or esophageal varices. Con-versely, the finding of any of these features should prompt evaluation of the patient for the presence of underlying portal hypertension and liver disease. Varices are most reliably documented by fiberoptic eso-phagoscopy; their presence lends indirect support to the diagnosis of portal hypertension. Although rarely necessary, portal venous pressure may be measured directly by percutaneous transhepatic "skinny nee-dle" catheterization or indirectly through transjugular cannulation of the hepatic veins. Both free and wedged hepatic vein pressure should be measured. While the latter is elevated in sinusoidal and postsinu-soidal portal hypertension, including cirrhosis, this measurement is usually normal in presinusoidal portal hypertension. In patients in whom additional information is necessary (e.g., preoperative evalua-tion before portal-systemic shunt surgery) or when percutaneous cath-eterization is not feasible, mesenteric and hepatic angiography may be helpful. Particular attention should be directed to the venous phase to assess the patency of the portal vein and the direction of portal blood flow.

℞ **TREATMENT**   Although treatment is usually directed toward a specific complication of portal hypertension, attempts are some-times made to reduce the pressure in the portal venous system. Surgical decompression procedures have been used for many years to lower portal pressure in patients with bleeding esophageal varices (see be-low). However, portal-systemic shunt surgery does not result in im-proved survival rates in patients with cirrhosis. Decompression can now be accomplished without surgery through the percutaneous place-ment of a portal-systemic shunt, termed a *transjugular intrahepatic portosystemic shunt* (TIPS). β-Adrenergic blockade with propranolol or nadolol reduces portal pressure through vasodilatory effects on both the splanchnic arterial bed and the portal venous system in combina-tion with reduced cardiac output. Such therapy has been shown to be effective in preventing both a first variceal bleed and subsequent epi-sodes after an initial bleed. Treatment of patients with clinically sig-nificant sequelae of portal hypertension, especially variceal bleeding, with doses of propranolol titrated to reduce the resting pulse by 25% is reasonable if no contraindications exist.

Vigorous treatment of patients with alcoholic hepatitis and cirrho-sis, chronic active hepatitis, or other liver diseases may lead to a fall in portal pressure and to a reduction in variceal size. In general, how-ever, portal hypertension due to cirrhosis is not reversible. In appro-priately selected patients, hepatic transplantation will be beneficial.

VARICEAL BLEEDING   Pathogenesis   While vigorous hem-orrhage may arise from any portal-systemic venous collaterals, bleed-ing is most common from varices in the region of the gastroesophageal junction. The factors contributing to bleeding from gastroesophageal varices are not entirely understood but include the degree of portal hypertension (>12 mmHg) and the size of the varices.

Clinical Features and Diagnosis   Variceal bleeding often occurs without obvious precipitating factors and usually presents with pain-less but massive hematemesis with or without melena. Associated signs range from mild postural tachycardia to profound shock, de-pending on the extent of blood loss and degree of hypovolemia. Be-cause patients with varices may bleed just as frequently from other gastrointestinal lesions (e.g., peptic ulcer, gastritis), exclusion of other bleeding sources is important even in patients with prior variceal hem-orrhage. Endoscopy is the best approach to evaluate upper gastroin-testinal hemorrhage in patients with known or suspected portal hyper-tension.

℞ **TREATMENT**   (See Fig. 299-1)   Variceal bleeding is a life-threatening emergency. Prompt estimation and vigorous replace-ment of blood loss to maintain intravascular volume are essential and take precedence over diagnostic studies and more specific intervention to stop the bleeding. However, excessive fluid administration can in-crease portal pressure with resultant further bleeding and should there-fore be avoided. Replacement of clotting factors with fresh-frozen plasma is important in patients with coagulopathy. Patients are best managed in an intensive care unit and require close monitoring of central venous or pulmonary capillary wedge pressures, urine output, and mental status. Only when the patient is hemodynamically stable should attention be directed toward specific diagnostic studies (espe-cially endoscopy) and other therapeutic modalities to prevent further or recurrent bleeding.

About half of all episodes of variceal hemorrhage cease without intervention, although the risk of rebleeding is very high. The medical management of acute variceal hemorrhage includes the use of vaso-constrictors (somatostatin/octreotide or vasopressin), balloon tampon-ade, and endoscopic banding of varices or endoscopic sclerosis of varices (sclerotherapy). Intravenous infusion of *vasopressin* at a rate of 0.1 to 0.4 U/min results in generalized vasoconstriction leading to diminished blood flow in the portal venous system. Intravenous infu-sion of vasopressin is as effective as selective intraarterial administra-tion. Control of bleeding can be achieved in up to 80% of cases, but bleeding recurs in more than half after the vasopressin is tapered and discontinued. Furthermore, a number of serious side effects, including cardiac and gastrointestinal tract ischemia, acute renal failure, and hy-ponatremia, may be associated with vasopressin therapy. Concurrent use of venodilators such as nitroglycerin as an intravenous infusion or isosorbide dinitrate sublingually may enhance the effectiveness of vasopressin and reduce complications. *Somatostatin* and its analogue, *octreotide*, are direct splanchnic vasoconstrictors. In some studies so-matostatin, given as an initial 250-μg bolus followed by constant in-fusion (250 μg/h), has been found to be as effective as vasopressin. Octreotide at doses of 50 to 100 μg/h is also effective. These agents are preferable to vasopressin, offering equivalent efficacy with fewer complications. If bleeding is too vigorous or endoscopy is not avail-able, *balloon tamponade* of the bleeding varices may be accomplished

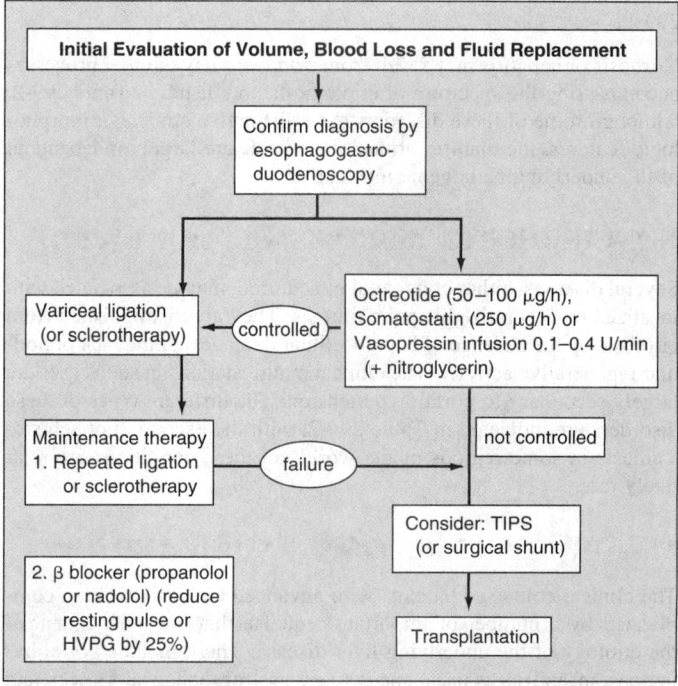

FIGURE 299-1   Approach to the patient with bleeding esophageal varices. Use of a beta blocker is the only intervention demonstrated to offer prophylactic benefit in a patient who has never bled. TIPS, transjugular intrahepatic porto-systemic shunt.

with a triple-lumen (Sengstaken-Blakemore) or four-lumen (Minnesota) tube with esophageal and gastric balloons. Because of the high risk of aspiration, endotracheal intubation should be performed prior to placing one of these tubes. After the tube is introduced into the stomach, the gastric balloon is inflated and pulled back into the cardia of the stomach. If bleeding does not stop, the esophageal balloon is inflated for additional tamponade. Complications occur in 15% or more of patients and include aspiration pneumonitis as well as esophageal rupture.

Where available, *endoscopic intervention* should be employed as the first line of treatment to control bleeding acutely (Chaps. 44 and 283). Over the past 18 years, endoscopic sclerosis of esophageal varices has been extensively employed. In this procedure, the varices are injected with one of several sclerosing agents via a needle-tipped catheter passed through the endoscope. After endoscopic identification of varices as the presumed source of bleeding, sclerotherapy controls acute bleeding in up to 90% of cases. In addition, repeated sclerotherapy can be performed until obliteration of all varices is accomplished in an effort to prevent recurrent bleeding. While available data support the efficacy of sclerotherapy in controlling bleeding acutely and in decreasing rebleeding rates, repeated sclerotherapy has not been documented to prolong survival. Mucosal ulceration resulting from injection of the caustic sclerosant may occur and result in further hemorrhage or stenosis. More recently, endoscopic band ligation, in which esophageal varices are ligated and strangulated with endoscopically placed small elastic O-rings, has gained favor. Band ligation has proven to be at least as effective as sclerotherapy in controlling acute variceal bleeding and preventing rebleeding. Because it has been associated with fewer treatment-related complications, band ligation is recommended for long-term obliteration of varices that have bled. Although prophylactic sclerosis or banding of esophageal varices in the absence of proven bleeding cannot yet be recommended, one report suggests that banding may be more effective than beta-blockade in primary prevention of variceal bleeding in high-risk patients.

The effectiveness of *nonselective β-adrenergic blocking agents* (e.g., propranolol) in the management of acute variceal bleeding is limited due to concomitant hypotension resulting from hypovolemia. However, a number of studies suggest they may be of value in secondary prevention of recurrent variceal hemorrhage. Moreover, prophylactic treatment with nonselective beta blockers (propranolol or nadolol) in patients with large ("high-risk") varices that have never bled appears to decrease the incidence of bleeding and prolong survival. Thus, endoscopic screening for varices in patients with cirrhosis is desirable; some have suggested this should be repeated every other year. Patients with portal hypertension without specific contraindications should be given propranolol in doses that produce a 25% reduction in the resting heart rate or the hepatic venous pressure gradient (HVPG), where available. Propranolol may also prevent recurrent bleeding from severe portal hypertensive gastropathy in patients with cirrhosis. The optimal combination of endoscopic and pharmacologic therapy for prevention of recurrent hemorrhage remains to be established and is the subject of ongoing trials.

Surgical treatment of portal hypertension and variceal bleeding involves the creation of a portal-systemic shunt to permit decompression of the portal system. Two types of portal systemic shunts have been used: *nonselective shunts*, to decompress the entire portal system, and *selective shunts*, intended to decompress only the varices while maintaining blood flow to the liver itself. Nonselective shunts include end-to-side or side-to-side portacaval and proximal splenorenal anastomoses; selective shunts include the distal splenorenal shunt. Nonselective shunts are more likely to be complicated by encephalopathy than selective shunts. Emergency portal-systemic nonselective shunts may control acute hemorrhage, but such surgery is usually used only as a last resort because early operative mortality can be high. The role of portal-systemic shunt surgery after initial control of bleeding by nonoperative means is also uncertain. Surgically created shunts effectively reduce the risk of recurrent hemorrhage, but the overall mortality

of patients undergoing such surgery is comparable to that of unoperated patients. Although patients who have undergone portal-systemic surgery succumb to recurrent bleeding less commonly than unoperated patients, this improvement is counterbalanced by increased morbidity from encephalopathy and death from progressive liver failure. Increasingly, therapeutic portal-systemic shunts have been reserved for patients who experience further bleeding despite serial endoscopic sclerotherapy or band ligation.

In TIPS, a technique developed to create a portal-systemic shunt by a percutaneous approach, an expandable metal stent is advanced to the hepatic veins under angiographic guidance and then through the substance of the liver to create a direct portacaval channel. This technique offers an alternative to surgery for refractory bleeding due to portal hypertension. However, stents frequently undergo stenosis or occlude over a period of months, prompting the need for a second TIPS or an alternative approach. Encephalopathy may be encountered after TIPS just as in the surgical shunts and is especially problematic in the elderly and those patients with preexisting encephalopathy. TIPS should be reserved for those individuals who fail endoscopic or medical management and are poor surgical risks. TIPS may have a useful role as a "bridge" for those patients with end-stage cirrhosis awaiting liver transplantation. Procedures such as esophageal transection have also been advocated for the management of acute variceal bleeding, but their efficacy remains unproven. Even though recent trials found that esophageal transection was as effective as endoscopic sclerotherapy, transection is usually considered a last resort.

The management of bleeding gastric fundal varices, either alone or in conjunction with esophageal varices, is more problematic, since sclerotherapy and banding are generally not effective. Vasoactive pharmacologic therapy should be instituted, but TIPS or shunt surgery should be considered because of high failure and rebleeding rates. For isolated gastric varices, splenic vein thrombosis should be specifically sought, since splenectomy is curative.

Portal Hypertensive Gastropathy Although variceal hemorrhage is the most commonly encountered bleeding complication of portal hypertension, many patients will develop a congestive gastropathy due to the venous hypertension. In this condition, identified by endoscopic examination, the mucosa appears engorged and friable. Indolent mucosal bleeding occurs rather than the brisk hemorrhage typical of a variceal source. β-Adrenergic blockade with propranolol (reducing splanchnic arterial pressure as well as portal pressure) is sometimes effective in ameliorating this condition. H_2 receptor antagonists or other agents useful in the treatment of peptic disease are usually not helpful.

SPLENOMEGALY **Definition and Pathogenesis** Congestive splenomegaly is common in patients with severe portal hypertension. Rarely, massive splenomegaly from nonhepatic disease leads to portal hypertension due to increased blood flow in the splenic vein.

Clinical Features Although usually asymptomatic, splenomegaly may be massive and contribute to the thrombocytopenia or pancytopenia of cirrhosis. In the absence of cirrhosis, splenomegaly in association with variceal hemorrhage should suggest the possibility of splenic vein thrombosis.

TREATMENT Splenomegaly usually requires no specific treatment, although massive enlargement of the spleen may occasionally necessitate splenectomy at the time of shunt surgery. However, it should be noted that splenectomy without an accompanying shunt may actually increase portal pressure, and portal vein thrombosis may result from splenectomy. Splenectomy may also be indicated if splenomegaly is the cause rather than the result of portal hypertension (as in splenic vein thrombosis). Thrombocytopenia alone is rarely severe enough to necessitate removal of the spleen. Splenectomy should be avoided in a patient eligible for liver transplantation.

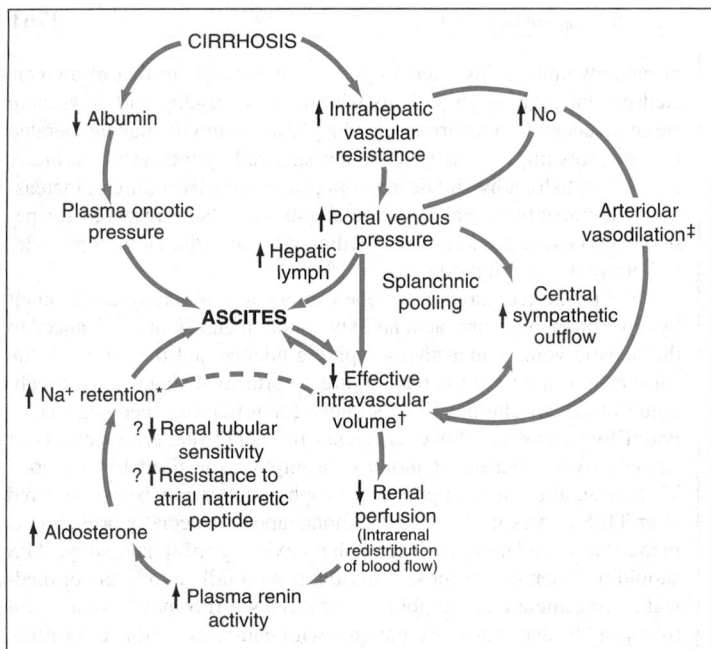

FIGURE 299-2 Multiple factors involved in development of ascites. Current concepts suggest that initiating factor may be primary sodium retention (*"over-flow"), diminished effective intravascular volume (†"underfilling"), or arteriolar vasodilation (‡"vasodilation").

ASCITES   Definition   Ascites is the accumulation of excess fluid within the peritoneal cavity. It is most frequently encountered in patients with cirrhosis and other forms of severe liver disease, but a number of other disorders may lead to either transudative or exudative ascites (Chap. 46).

Pathogenesis   The accumulation of ascitic fluid represents a state of total-body sodium and water excess, but the event that initiates this imbalance is unclear. Three theories have been proposed (Fig. 299-2). The "underfilling" theory suggests that the primary abnormality is inappropriate sequestration of fluid within the splanchnic vascular bed due to portal hypertension and a consequent decrease in effective circulating blood volume. According to this theory, an apparent decrease in intravascular volume (underfilling) is sensed by the kidney, which responds by retaining salt and water. The "overflow" theory suggests that the primary abnormality is inappropriate renal retention of salt and water in the absence of volume depletion. A third and more recent theory, the peripheral arterial vasodilation hypothesis, may unify the earlier theories and accounts for the constellation of arterial hypotension and increased cardiac output in association with high levels of vasoconstrictor substances that are routinely found in patients with cirrhosis and ascites. Again, sodium retention is considered secondary to arterial vascular underfilling and the result of a disproportionate increase of the vascular compartment due to arteriolar vasodilation rather than from decreased intravascular volume. According to this theory, portal hypertension results in splanchnic arteriolar vasodilation, mediated by nitric oxide, and leading to underfilling of the arterial vascular space and baroreceptor-mediated stimulation of renin-angiotensin, sympathetic output, and antidiuretic hormone release.

Regardless of the initiating event, a number of factors contribute to accumulation of fluid in the abdominal cavity (Fig. 299-2). Elevated levels of serum epinephrine and norepinephrine have been well documented. *Increased central sympathetic outflow* is found in patients with cirrhosis and ascites but not in those with cirrhosis alone. Increased sympathetic output results in diminished natriuresis by activation of the renin-angiotensin system and diminished sensitivity to atrial natriuretic peptide. *Portal hypertension* plays an important role in the formation of ascites by raising hydrostatic pressure within the splanchnic capillary bed. *Hypoalbuminemia* and *reduced plasma oncotic pressure* also favor the extravasation of fluid from plasma to the

peritoneal cavity, and thus ascites is infrequent in patients with cirrhosis unless both portal hypertension and hypoalbuminemia are present. Hepatic lymph may weep freely from the surface of the cirrhotic liver due to distortion and obstruction of hepatic sinusoids and lymphatics and contributes to ascites formation. In contrast to the contribution of transudative fluid from the portal vascular bed, hepatic lymph may weep into the peritoneal cavity even in the absence of marked hypoproteinemia because the endothelial lining of the hepatic sinusoids is discontinuous. This mechanism may account for the high protein concentration present in the ascitic fluid of some patients with venoocclusive disease or the Budd-Chiari syndrome.

Renal factors also play an important role in perpetuating ascites. Patients with ascites fail to excrete a water load in a normal fashion. They have increased renal sodium reabsorption by both proximal and distal tubules, the latter due largely to increased plasma renin activity and secondary hyperaldosteronism. Insensitivity to circulating atrial natriuretic peptide, often present in elevated concentrations in patients with cirrhosis and ascites, may be an important contributory factor in many patients. This insensitivity has been documented in those patients with the most severely impaired sodium excretion, who typically also exhibit low arterial pressure and marked overactivity of the renin-aldosterone axis. Renal vasoconstriction, perhaps resulting from increased serum prostaglandin or catecholamine levels, may also contribute to sodium retention. Recently a role for endothelin, a potent vasoconstrictor peptide, has been proposed. While elevated levels have been reported by some, this has not been observed by others.

As discussed in Chap. 46, ascites may arise in a number of clinical settings in addition to cirrhosis and portal hypertension. Although historically ascites was classified as either transudative or exudative, similar to the characterization of pleural fluids, this schema has limitations. Instead, the serum-ascites albumin gradient (SAAG) provides a better classification than total protein content or other parameters. In cirrhosis, the serum albumin concentration is usually at least 10 g/L (1 g/dL) higher than that of the ascitic fluid, thus yielding a high SAAG [≥11 g/L (≥1.1 g/dL)], reflecting indirectly the abnormally high hydrostatic pressure gradient between the portal bed and the ascitic compartment. Conversely, the presence of a low SAAG [<11 g/L (<1.1 g/dL)] will usually exclude cirrhosis and portal hypertension.

Clinical Features and Diagnosis   Usually ascites is first noticed by the patient because of increasing abdominal girth. More pronounced accumulation of fluid may cause shortness of breath because of elevation of the diaphragm. When peritoneal fluid accumulation exceeds 500 mL, ascites may be demonstrated on physical examination by the presence of shifting dullness, a fluid wave, or bulging flanks. Ultrasound examination, preferably with a Doppler study, can detect smaller quantities of ascites and should be performed when physical examination is equivocal or when the cause of the recent onset of ascites is not clear (e.g., exclude Budd-Chiari syndrome or portal vein thrombosis).

℞ TREATMENT (See Fig. 299-3)   A thorough search should be made for precipitating factors in the patient with recent onset of or worsening ascites, e.g., excessive salt intake, medication noncompliance, superimposed infection, worsening liver disease, portal vein thrombosis, or development of hepatocellular carcinoma. When ascites develops in the setting of severe, acute liver disease, resolution of ascites is likely to follow improvement in liver function. More commonly, ascites develops in patients with stable or steadily worsening liver function. Paracentesis should usually be performed with a small-gauge needle at the time of initial evaluation or at the time of any clinical deterioration of a cirrhotic patient with ascites. A small amount of fluid (<200 mL) should be obtained and examined for evidence of infection, tumor, or other possible causes and complications of ascites. Therapeutic intervention is indicated both to prevent potential complications and to control progressive increase in ascites, which may

Initial Evaluation: Identify Precipitants and Correct if Possible

FIGURE 299-3   Approach to the patient with ascites [and spontaneous bacterial peritonitis (SBP)]. PMN, polymorphonuclear leukocytes; TIPS, transjugular intrahepatic portosystemic shunt. *Calculate SAAG [serum ascites albumin gradient = serum albumin − ascites albumin (g/dL)] to confirm high gradient (>1.1 g/dL) in portal hypertension. †If PMN >250/μL but culture is negative = culture negative neutrocytic ascites; begin empirical antibiotic and retap at 48 h; if culture is positive but PMN < 250/μL normal = monomicrobial nonneutrocytic bacterascites; retap; treat if PMN > 250/μL: if polymicrobial infection, exclude secondary peritonitis. U_{Na}, urinary sodium; U_{Ka}, urinary potassium; BUN, blood urea nitrogen.

become pronounced enough to cause physical discomfort. For the patient with a modest accumulation, therapy can be undertaken as an outpatient and should be gentle and incremental (see below). The goal is the loss of no more than 1.0 kg/d if both ascites and peripheral edema are present and no more than 0.5 kg/d in patients with ascites alone. In some patients, particularly those with a large accumulation of fluid, it may be desirable to hospitalize the patient so that daily weights and frequent serum electrolyte levels can be monitored and compliance ensured. Although abdominal girth measurements are frequently used as an index of fluid loss, they tend to be unreliable.

Salt restriction is the cornerstone of therapy. A diet containing 800 mg sodium (2 g NaCl) is often adequate to induce a negative sodium balance and permit diuresis. Response to salt restriction alone is more likely to occur if the ascites is of recent onset, the underlying liver disease is reversible, a precipitating factor can be corrected, or the patient has a high urinary sodium excretion (>25 mmol/d) and normal renal function. Fluid restriction of approximately 1000 mL/d does little to enhance diuresis but may be necessary to correct hyponatremia. If sodium restriction alone fails to result in diuresis and weight loss, diuretics should be prescribed. Because of the role of hyperaldosteronism in sustaining salt retention, spironolactone or other distal tubule–acting diuretics (triamterene, amiloride) are the drugs of choice. These agents are also preferred because of their gentle action and specific potassium-sparing properties. Spironolactone is initially given in a dose of 100 mg a day and is increased as needed by 100 mg/d

every several days to a maximum dose that should rarely exceed 400 mg/d. An indication of the minimum effective dose of spironolactone may be obtained by monitoring urinary electrolyte concentrations for a rise in sodium and fall in potassium levels, reflecting effective competitive inhibition of aldosterone. Conversely, the development of azotemia or hyperkalemia may be dose-limiting or even warrant a reduction in the amount of this medication. In some patients, diuresis cannot be initiated despite maximal doses of distal tubule–acting agents (e.g., 400 mg spironolactone) because of avid proximal tubular sodium absorption. More potent and proximally acting diuretics (furosemide, thiazide, or ethacrynic acid) may then be added cautiously to the regimen. Spironolactone plus furosemide, 40 or 80 mg/d, is usually sufficient to initiate a diuresis in most patients. However, such aggressive therapy must be used with great caution to avoid plasma volume depletion, azotemia, and hypokalemia, which may lead to encephalopathy.

In patients with pronounced ascites, particularly those requiring hospitalization, large-volume paracentesis has proven to be an effective and less costly approach to initial management than prolonged bed rest and conventional diuretic treatment. In this approach, ascitic fluid is removed by peritoneal cannula using strict aseptic techniques and monitoring hemodynamic and renal function. This can be safely accomplished in a single session. The need for concomitant albumin replacement by intravenous infusion remains controversial but may be prudent in the patient without peripheral edema, to avoid depleting the intravascular space and precipitating hypotension. Maintenance diuretic therapy in conjunction with sodium restriction may then be instituted to avoid recurrent ascites.

A minority of patients with advanced cirrhosis has "refractory ascites" or rapidly reaccumulate fluid after control by paracentesis. In some patients, a side-to-side *portacaval shunt* may result in improvement in ascites, although generally these patients are extremely poor surgical risks. In the past, intractable ascites has also been treated with the surgical implantation of a plastic *peritoneovenous shunt*, which has a pressure-sensitive, one-way valve allowing ascitic fluid to flow from the abdominal cavity to the superior vena cava. However, the usefulness of this technique is limited by a high rate of complications such as infection, disseminated intravascular coagulation, and thrombosis of the shunt. More recently, in selected patients TIPS has been used effectively to control refractory ascites, although portal decompression, while mobilizing ascitic fluid, has precipitated severe hepatic encephalopathy in some patients. TIPS remains a promising but unproven treatment for refractory ascites. None of these shunts has been shown to extend life expectancy.

SPONTANEOUS BACTERIAL PERITONITIS (SBP)   Patients with ascites and cirrhosis may develop acute bacterial peritonitis without an obvious primary source of infection. Patients with very advanced liver disease are particularly susceptible to SBP. The ascitic fluid in these patients typically has especially low concentrations of albumin and other so-called opsonic proteins, which normally may provide some protection against bacteria. Although key steps in the pathogenesis of SBP remain to be elucidated, it is clear that most bacteria contributing to SBP derive from the bowel and eventually are spread to ascitic fluid by the hematogenous route after transmigration through the bowel wall and transversing the lymphatics. Clinical features can include abrupt onset of fever, chills, generalized abdominal pain, and, rarely, rebound abdominal tenderness. However, the clinical symptoms *may be minimal*, and some patients manifest only worsening jaundice or encephalopathy in the absence of localizing abdominal complaints. The diagnosis is based on careful examination of the ascitic fluid. An ascitic fluid leukocyte count of >500 cells/L (with a proportion of polymorphonuclear leukocytes of ≥50%) or more than 250 polymorphonuclear leukocytes should suggest the possibility of bacterial peritonitis while results of bacterial cultures of ascitic fluid are pending. Other measurements such as fluid pH or determination of gradients between serum and fluid pH or lactate are generally not necessary. The presence of more than 10,000 leukocytes per liter, multiple organisms, or failure to improve after standard therapy for 48 h suggest that the peritonitis may be secondary to an infection elsewhere in the body.

A variant of SBP, designated *monomicrobial nonneutrocytic bacterascites*, is sometimes seen. In these patients, culture of ascitic fluid yields bacteria, but the neutrophil count is less than 250/L. These patients often have less severe liver disease than those found initially to have typical SBP. While many patients with this variant have cleared the bacterascites at the time of a subsequent paracentesis, nearly 40% will develop typical SBP; thus follow-up paracentesis is usually warranted in this setting.

℞ TREATMENT   Empirical therapy with cefotaxime or ampicillin and an aminoglycoside should be initiated when the diagnosis is first suspected because enteric gram-negative bacilli are found in the majority of cases; less frequently, the infection is caused by pneumococci and other gram-positive bacteria. Cefotaxime is preferable due to the lower rate of renal toxicity. Specific antibiotic therapy can be selected once the specific organism is identified. Therapy is usually administered for 10 to 14 days, although one controlled study has suggested that a 5-day course of intravenous antibiotics may be as effective when repeat paracentesis at 48 h demonstrates a decline in the ascitic polymorphonuclear leukocytes count by more than 50% and negative cultures.

While appropriate antibiotic therapy is usually effective in the treatment of an episode of SBP, recurrent episodes are relatively common; as many as 70% of patients will experience at least one recurrence within a year of the first episode. The risk of recurrence likely reflects the predisposing role of the underlying advanced liver disease that contributed to the development of the first episode of SBP. Recent trials have demonstrated that prophylactic maintenance therapy with norfloxacin (400 mg/d) can reduce the frequency of recurrent SBP. This agent presumably causes selective decontamination of the intestine, eliminating many aerobic gram-negative bacilli. Trimethoprim-sulfamethoxazole given for 5 days a week has also proven effective. Antibiotics may be administered as infrequently as once a week (e.g., ciprofloxacin, 750 mg once weekly). While maintenance therapy reduces the frequency of SBP and need for hospitalization, it is unclear whether this is associated with prolonged survival. Primary prevention of SBP in a subset of high-risk cirrhotic patients [ascitic fluid protein <10 g/L (<1.0 g/dL)] also appears to be warranted, as is prophylaxis for SBP during variceal hemorrhage.

HEPATORENAL SYNDROME   Definition and Pathogenesis   Hepatorenal syndrome is a serious complication in the patient with cirrhosis and ascites and is characterized by worsening azotemia with avid sodium retention and oliguria in the absence of identifiable specific causes of renal dysfunction. The exact basis for this syndrome is not clear, but altered renal hemodynamics appear to be involved. The kidneys are structurally intact; urinalysis and pyelography are usually normal. Renal biopsy, although rarely needed, is also normal, and in fact, kidneys from such patients have been used successfully for renal transplantation. There are indications that an imbalance in certain metabolites of arachidonic acid (prostaglandins and thromboxane) may play a pathogenetic role.

Clinical Features and Diagnosis   Worsening azotemia, hyponatremia, progressive oliguria, and hypotension are the hallmarks of the hepatorenal syndrome. This syndrome, which is distinct from prerenal azotemia, may be precipitated by severe gastrointestinal bleeding, sepsis, or overly vigorous attempts at diuresis or paracentesis; it may also occur without an obvious cause. It is essential to exclude other causes of renal impairment often seen in these patients. These include prerenal azotemia or acute tubular necrosis due to hypovolemia (e.g., secondary to gastrointestinal bleeding or diuretic therapy)

or an increased nitrogen load such as that seen as a result of bleeding. Drug nephrotoxicity is also often a consideration, particularly in the patient who has received agents such as aminoglycosides or contrast dye. The diagnosis rests on the finding of an elevated serum creatinine level [>133 μmol/L (>1.5 g/dL)] that fails to improve with volume expansion or withdrawal of diuretics, together with an unremarkable urine sediment. The diagnosis is supported by the demonstration of avid urinary sodium retention. Typically, the urine sodium concentration is <5 mmol/L, a concentration lower than that generally found in uncomplicated prerenal azotemia.

℞ TREATMENT   Treatment is usually unsuccessful. Although some patients with hypotension and decreased plasma volume may respond to infusions of salt-poor albumin, volume expansion must be undertaken with caution to avoid precipitating variceal bleeding. Vasodilator therapy, including intravenous infusions of low dose dopamine, is not effective. While TIPS has been reported to improve renal function in some patients, its use can not be recommended. In appropriate candidates, the treatment of choice for hepatorenal syndrome is liver transplantation.

HEPATIC ENCEPHALOPATHY   Definition   Hepatic (portal-systemic) encephalopathy is a complex neuropsychiatric syndrome characterized by disturbances in consciousness and behavior, personality changes, fluctuating neurologic signs, asterixis or "flapping tremor," and distinctive electroencephalographic changes. Encephalopathy may be *acute* and reversible or *chronic* and progressive. In severe cases, irreversible coma and death may occur. Acute episodes may recur with variable frequency.

Pathogenesis   The specific cause of hepatic encephalopathy is unknown. The most important factors in the pathogenesis are severe hepatocellular dysfunction and/or intrahepatic and extrahepatic shunting of portal venous blood into the systemic circulation so that the liver is largely bypassed. As a result of these processes, various toxic substances absorbed from the intestine are not detoxified by the liver and lead to metabolic abnormalities in the central nervous system (CNS). *Ammonia* is the substance most often incriminated in the pathogenesis of encephalopathy. Many, but not all, patients with hepatic encephalopathy have elevated blood ammonia levels, and recovery from encephalopathy is often accompanied by declining blood ammonia levels. Other compounds and metabolites that may contribute to the development of encephalopathy include mercaptans (derived from intestinal metabolism of methionine), short-chain fatty acids, and phenol. *False neurochemical transmitters* (e.g., octopamine), resulting in part from alterations in plasma levels of aromatic and branched-chain amino acids, may also play a role. An increase in the permeability of the blood-brain barrier to some of these substances may be an additional factor involved in the pathogenesis of hepatic encephalopathy. Several observations suggest that excessive concentrations of γ-aminobutyric acid (GABA), an inhibitory neurotransmitter, in the CNS are important in the reduced levels of consciousness seen in hepatic encephalopathy. Increased CNS GABA may reflect failure of the liver to extract precursor amino acids efficiently or to remove GABA produced in the intestine. In support of this, there is also evidence to suggest that endogenous benzodiazepines, which act through the GABA receptor, may contribute to the development of hepatic encephalopathy. This evidence includes isolation of 1,4-benzodiazepines from brain tissue of patients with fulminant hepatic failure as well as the partial response observed in some patients and experimental animals after administration of flumazenil, a benzodiazepine antagonist. However, the inconsistent effect of flumazenil in patients with encephalopathy, as well as potential methodologic pitfalls in the measurement of endogenous benzodiazepines, preclude definitive attribution of a role to these substances in the pathogenesis of hepatic encephalopathy. The finding of direct enhancement of GABA receptor activation by ammonia suggests that several of the factors described above may be operating via a final common pathway to produce the neuronal depression of hepatic encephalopathy. Finally, the observation of hyperintensity in the basal ganglia by magnetic resonance imaging in cirrhotic patients suggests that excessive *manganese* deposition may also contribute to the pathogenesis of hepatic encephalopathy. Further studies are needed to determine whether chelation therapy exerts long-term benefit.

In the patient with otherwise stable cirrhosis, hepatic encephalopathy often follows a clearly identifiable precipitating event (Table 299-3). Perhaps the most common predisposing factor is *gastrointestinal bleeding*, which leads to an increase in the production of ammonia and other nitrogenous substances, which are then absorbed. Similarly, *increased dietary protein* may precipitate encephalopathy as a result of increased production of nitrogenous substances by colonic bacteria. *Electrolyte disturbances*, particularly hypokalemic alkalosis secondary to overzealous use of diuretics, vigorous paracentesis, or vomiting, may precipitate hepatic encephalopathy. Systemic alkalosis causes an increase in the amount of nonionic ammonia (NH_3) relative to ammonium ions NH_4^+). Only nonionic (uncharged) ammonia readily crosses the blood-brain barrier and accumulates in the CNS. Hypokalemia also directly stimulates renal ammonia production. Injudicious use of CNS-depressing drugs (e.g., barbiturates, benzodiazepines) and acute infection may trigger or aggravate hepatic encephalopathy, although the mechanisms involved are not clear. Other potential precipitating factors include superimposed acute viral hepatitis, alcoholic hepatitis, extrahepatic bile duct obstruction, constipation, surgery, and other coincidental medical complications.

Hepatic encephalopathy has protean manifestations, and any neurologic abnormality, including focal deficits, may be encountered. In patients with acute encephalopathy, neurologic deficits are completely reversible upon correction of underlying precipitating factors and/or improvement in liver function, but in patients with chronic encephalopathy, the deficits may be irreversible and progressive. Cerebral edema is frequently present and contributes to the clinical picture and overall mortality in patients with both acute and chronic encephalopathy.

The diagnosis of hepatic encephalopathy should be considered when four major factors are present: (1) acute or chronic hepatocellular disease and/or extensive portal-systemic collateral shunts (the latter may be either spontaneous, e.g., secondary to portal hypertension, or surgically created, e.g., portacaval anastomosis); (2) disturbances of awareness and mentation, which may progress from forgetfulness and confusion to stupor and finally coma; (3) shifting combinations of neurologic signs, including asterixis, rigidity, hyperreflexia, extensor plantar signs, and rarely, seizures; and (4) a characteristic (but nonspecific) symmetric, high-voltage, triphasic slow-wave (2 to 5 per second) pattern on the electroencephalogram. Asterixis ("liver flap," "flapping tremor") is a nonrhythmic asymmetric lapse in voluntary sustained position of the extremities, head, and trunk. It is best demonstrated by having the patient extend the arms and dorsiflex the hands. Because elicitation of asterixis depends on sustained voluntary muscle contraction, it is not present in the comatose patient. Asterixis is nonspecific and also occurs in patients with other forms of metabolic brain disease. Disturbances of sleep with reversal of sleep/wake cycles are among the earliest signs of encephalopathy. Alterations in personality, mood disturbances, confusion, deterioration in self-care and

Table 299-3 Common Precipitants of Hepatic Encephalopathy

Increased nitrogen load	Drugs
Gastrointestinal bleeding	Narcotics, tranquilizers, sedatives
Excess dietary protein	Diuretics (see ''Electrolyte imbal-
Azotemia	ance'')
Constipation	Miscellaneous
Electrolyte and metabolic imbal-	Infection
ance	Surgery
Hypokalemia	Superimposed acute liver disease
Alkalosis	Progressive liver disease
Hypoxia	Portal-systemic shunts
Hyponatremia	
Hypovolemia	

Table 299-4 Clinical Stages of Hepatic Encephalopathy

Stage	Mental Status	Asterixis	EEG
I	Euphoria or depression, mild confusion, slurred speech, disordered sleep	+/−	Triphasic waves
II	Lethargy, moderate confusion	+	Triphasic waves
III	Marked confusion, incoherent speech, sleeping but arousable	+	Triphasic waves
IV	Coma; initially responsive to noxious stimuli, later unresponsive	−	Delta activity

handwriting, and daytime somnolence are additional clinical features of encephalopathy. *Fetor hepaticus*, a unique musty odor of the breath and urine believed to be due to mercaptans, may be noted in patients with varying stages of hepatic encephalopathy.

Grading or classifying the stages of hepatic encephalopathy is often helpful in following the course of the illness and assessing response to therapy. One useful classification is shown in Table 299-4.

The diagnosis of hepatic encephalopathy is usually one of exclusion. There are no diagnostic liver function test abnormalities, although an elevated serum ammonia level in the appropriate clinical setting is highly suggestive of the diagnosis. Examination of the cerebrospinal fluid is unremarkable, and computed tomography of the brain shows no characteristic abnormalities until late in stage IV when cerebral edema may supervene. A number of conditions, particularly disorders related to acute and chronic alcoholism, can mimic the clinical features of hepatic encephalopathy. These include acute alcohol intoxication, sedative overdose, delirium tremens, Wernicke's encephalopathy, and Korsakoff's psychosis (Chap. 373). Subdural hematoma, meningitis, and hypoglycemia or other metabolic encephalopathies must also be considered, especially in patients with alcoholic cirrhosis. In young patients with liver disease and neurologic abnormalities, Wilson's disease should be excluded.

℞ TREATMENT (See Fig. 299-4) Early recognition and prompt treatment of hepatic encephalopathy are essential. Patients with acute, severe hepatic encephalopathy (stage IV) require the usual supportive measures for the comatose patient. Specific treatment of hepatic encephalopathy is aimed at (1) elimination or treatment of precipitating factors and (2) lowering of blood ammonia (and other toxin) levels by decreasing the absorption of protein and nitrogenous products from the intestine. In the setting of acute gastrointestinal bleeding, blood in the bowel should be promptly evacuated with laxatives (and enemas if necessary) in order to reduce the nitrogen load. Protein should be excluded from the diet, and constipation should be avoided. Ammonia absorption can be decreased by the administration of lactulose, a nonabsorbable disaccharide that acts as an osmotic laxative. Metabolism of lactulose by colonic bacteria may also result in an acid pH that favors conversion of ammonia to the poorly absorbed ammonium ion. In addition, lactulose may actually diminish ammonia production through its direct effects on bacterial metabolism. Acutely, lactulose syrup can be administered in a dose of 30 to 60 mL every hour until diarrhea occurs; thereafter the dose is adjusted (usually 15 to 30 mL three times daily) so that the patient has two to four soft stools daily. Intestinal ammonia production by bacteria can also be decreased by oral administration of a "nonabsorbable" antibiotic such as neomycin (0.5 to 1.0 g every 6 h). However, despite poor absorption, neomycin may reach sufficient concentrations in the bloodstream to cause renal toxicity. Equal benefits may be achieved with broad-spectrum antibiotics such as metronidazole. The use of agents such as levodopa, bromocriptine, keto analogues of essential amino acids, and intravenous amino acid formulations rich in branched-chain amino acids in the treatment of acute hepatic encephalopathy remains of unproven benefit. Flumazenil, a short-acting benzodiazepine antagonist,

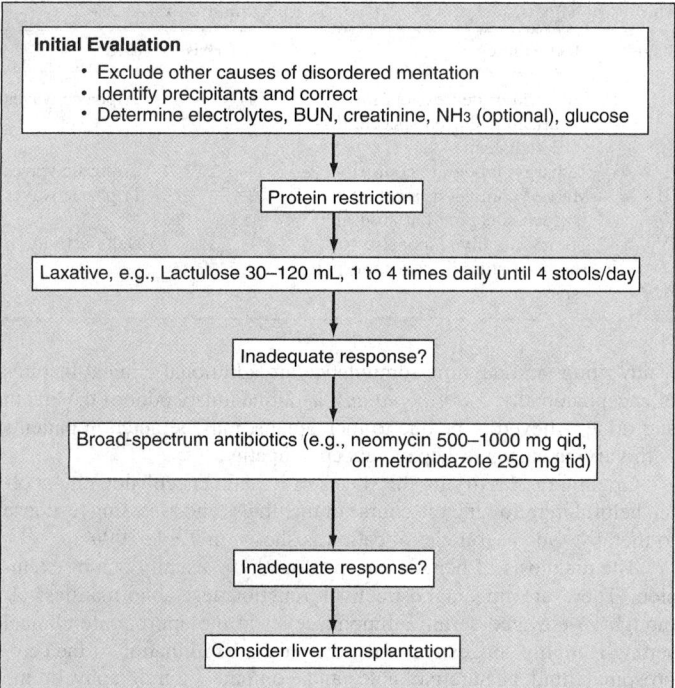

FIGURE 299-4   Approach to the patient with hepatic encephalopathy. BUN, blood urea nitrogen.

may have a role in management of hepatic encephalopathy precipitated by use of benzodiazepines, if there is a need for urgent therapy. Hemoperfusion to remove toxic substances and therapy directed primarily toward coincident cerebral edema in acute encephalopathy are also of unproven value. The efficacy of extracorporeal liver assist devices employing hepatocytes of porcine or human origin to bridge patients to recovery or transplantation is as yet unproven but is currently being studied.

Chronic encephalopathy may be effectively controlled by administration of lactulose. Management of patients with chronic encephalopathy should include dietary protein restriction (usually to 60 g/d) in combination with low doses of lactulose or neomycin. Nephrotoxicity or ototoxicity may be limiting in prolonged usage of neomycin. There are suggestions that vegetable protein may be preferable to animal protein.

OTHER SEQUELAE OF CIRRHOSIS   Coagulopathy   Patients with cirrhosis often demonstrate a variety of abnormalities in both cellular and humoral clotting function. Thrombocytopenia may result from hypersplenism. In the alcoholic patient, there may be direct bone marrow suppression by ethanol. Diminished protein synthesis may lead to reduced production of fibrinogen (factor I), prothrombin (factor II), and factors V, VII, IX, and X. Reduction in levels of all factors except factor V may be worsened by the coincident malabsorption of the fat-soluble cofactor vitamin K due to cholestasis (Chap. 286). Of these, factor VII appears to be pivotal. In cirrhosis, it is the first of the factors to become depleted and, because of its short half-life, replacement with plasma often fails to correct an elevated prothrombin time. Preliminary studies suggest that selective replacement of factor VII can correct the prothrombin time in patients with cirrhosis.

Hepatocellular Carcinoma See Chap. 91.

HYPOXEMIA AND HEPATOPULMONARY SYNDROME   Definition and Pathogenesis   Mild hypoxemia occurs in approximately one-third of patients with chronic liver disease. The hepatopulmonary syndrome is typically manifest by hypoxemia, platypnea, and orthodeoxia. Hypoxemia usually results from right-to-left intrapulmonary shunts through dilatations in intrapulmonary vessels

that can be detected by contrast-enhanced echocardiography or a macroaggregated albumin lung perfusion scan. The mechanisms of shunt formation are unclear, but one animal model suggests that endothelin-1 levels and pulmonary nitric oxide, raised in cirrhosis, correlate with degree of shunting.

TREATMENT   No specific treatment is consistently effective, though large arteriovenous shunts may be embolized. It is now increasingly recognized that liver transplantation may eventually lead to amelioration of the hepatopulmonary syndrome in cases that have not yet been complicated by advanced pulmonary hypertension.

BIBLIOGRAPHY

ALCOHOLIC, POSTNECROTIC, AND CRYPTOGENIC CIRRHOSIS

ARROYO V, GINÉS P: Arteriolar vasodilation and the pathogenesis of the hyperdynamic circulation and renal sodium and water retention in cirrhosis. Gastroenterology 102: 1077, 1992

BACON BR et al: Nonalcoholic steatohepatitis: An expanded clinical entity. Gastroenterology 107:1103, 1994

CALDWELL H et al: Cryptogenic cirrhosis: Clinical characterization and risk factors for underlying disease. Hepatology 29:664, 1999

CARITHERS RL et al: Methylprednisolone therapy in patients with severe alcoholic hepatitis. A randomized multicenter trial. Ann Intern Med 110:685, 1989

FRIEDMAN SL: The cellular basis of hepatic fibrosis. N Engl J Med 328:1828, 1993

MCCULLOUGH AJ, O'CONNOR JFB: Alcoholic liver disease: Recommendations for the American College of Gastroenterology. Am J Gastroenterol 93:2022, 1998

RAMOND M-J et al: A randomized trial of prednisolone in patients with severe alcoholic hepatitis. N Engl J Med 326:507, 1992

SHETH SG et al: Nonalcoholic steatohepatitis. Ann Intern Med 126:137, 1997

BILIARY AND CARDIAC CIRRHOSIS

BEUERS U et al: Ursodeoxycholic acid in cholestasis: Potential mechanisms of action and therapeutic applications. Hepatology 28:1449, 1998

BONNAND AM et al: Clinical significance of serum bilirubin levels under ursodeoxycholic acid therapy in patients with primary biliary cirrhosis. Hepatology 29:39, 1999

COMBES B et al: A randomized, double-blind, placebo-controlled trial of ursodeoxycholic acid in primary biliary cirrhosis. Hepatology 22:759, 1995

KAPLAN MM et al: Medical progress: Primary biliary cirrhosis. N Engl J Med 335:1570, 1996

LOCKE GR III et al: Time course of histological progression in primary biliary cirrhosis. Hepatology 23:52, 1996

METCALF JV et al: Natural history of the early primary biliary cirrhosis. Lancet 348:1399, 1996

POUPON RE et al: Ursodiol for the long-term treatment of primary biliary cirrhosis. N Engl J Med 330:1342, 1994

——— et al: Combined analysis of randomized controlled trials of ursodeoxycholic acid in primary biliary cirrhosis. Gastroenterology 113:884, 1997

WOLFHAGEN FH et al: Oral naltrexone treatment for cholestatic pruritus: A double-blind, placebo-controlled study. Gastroenterology 113:1264, 1997

HEPATIC ENCEPHALOPATHY

BASILE AS, JONES EA: Ammonia and GABAergic neurotransmission: Interrelated factors in the pathogenesis of hepatic encephalopathy. Hepatology 25:1303, 1997

JALAN R et al: Review article: Pathogenesis and treatment of chronic hepatic encephalopathy. Aliment Pharmacol Ther 10:681, 1996

KRIEGER D et al: Manganese and chronic hepatic encephalopathy. Lancet 346:270, 1995

RIORDAN SM, WILLIAMS R: Treatment of hepatic encephalopathy. N Engl J Med 337: 473, 1997

VARICEAL HEMORRHAGE

CELLO JP et al: Endoscopic sclerotherapy compared with percutaneous transjugular intrahepatic portosystemic shunt after initial sclerotherapy in patients with acute variceal hemorrhage. Ann Intern Med 126:858, 1997

GARCIA-VILLARREAL L et al: Transjugular intrahepatic portosystemic shunt versus endoscopic sclerotherapy for the prevention of variceal rebleeding after recent variceal hemorrhage. Hepatology 29:27, 1999

GRACE ND: Diagnosis and treatment of gastrointestinal bleeding secondary to portal hypertension. Am J Gastroenterol 92:1081, 1997

LAINE L et al: Endoscopic ligation compared with sclerotherapy for treatment of esophageal variceal bleeding: A meta-analysis. Ann Intern Med 123:280, 1995

PAGLIARO L et al: Prevention of first bleeding in cirrhosis: A meta-analysis of randomized trials of nonsurgical treatment. Ann Intern Med 117:59, 1992

PLANAS R et al: A prospective randomized trial comparing somatostatin and sclerotherapy in the treatment of acute variceal bleeding. Hepatology 20:370, 1994

SANYAL AJ et al: Transjugular intrahepatic portosystemic shunts compared with endoscopic sclerotherapy for the prevention of recurrent variceal hemorrhage. Ann Intern Med 126:849, 1997

STIEGMANN GV et al: Endoscopic sclerotherapy as compared with endoscopic ligation for bleeding esophageal varices. N Engl J Med 326:1527, 1992

SUNG JJY et al: Octreotide infusion or emergency sclerotherapy for variceal haemorrhage. Lancet 342:637, 1993

PORTAL HYPERTENSION AND ASCITES

CHUNG RT et al: Complications of chronic liver disease. Crit Care Clin 11:431, 1995

D'AMICO G et al: The treatment of portal hypertension: A meta-analytic review. Hepatology 22:332, 1995

GINÉS P et al: Paracentesis with intravenous infusion of albumin as compared wtih peritoneovenous shunting in cirrhosis with refractory ascites. N Engl J Med 325:829, 1991

MARTIN P-Y et al: Nitric oxide as a mediator of hemodynamic abnormalities and salt and water retention in cirrhosis. N Engl J Med 339:533, 1998

OCHS A et al: The transjugular intrahepatic portosystemic stent-shunt procedure for refractory ascites. N Engl J Med 332:1192, 1995

POYNARD T et al: Beta-adrenergic-antagonist drugs in the prevention of gastrointestinal bleeding in patients with cirrhosis and esophageal varices. N Engl J Med 324:1532, 1991

RUNYON BA et al: Management of adult patients with ascites caused by cirrhosis. Hepatology 27:264, 1998

SHIFFMAN ML et al: The role of transjugular intrahepatic portosystemic shunt for treatment of portal hypertension and its complications: A conference sponsored by the National Digestive Diseases Advisory Board. Hepatology 22:1591, 1995

STANLEY AJ et al: Long-term follow of transjugular intrahepatic portosystemic stent shunt (TIPS) for the treatment of portal hypertension: Results in 130 patients. Gut 39:479, 1996

SPONTANEOUS BACTERIAL PERITONITIS

NAVASA M et al: Randomized, comparative study of oral ofloxacin versus intravenous cefotaxime in spontaneous bacterial peritonitis. Gastroenterology 111:1011, 1996

ROLACHON A et al: Ciprofloxacin and long-term prevention of spontaneous bacterial peritonitis: Results of a prospective controlled trial. Hepatology 22:1171, 1995

RUNYON BA et al: Short-course versus long-course antibiotic treatment of spontaneous bacterial peritonitis: A randomized controlled study of 100 patients. Gastroenterology 100:1737, 1991

OTHER COMPLICATIONS OF CIRRHOSIS

ABRAMS GA et al: Use of macroaggregated albumin lung scan to diagnose hepatopulmonary syndrome: A new approach. Gastroenterology 114:305, 1998

BERNSTEIN DE et al: Recombinant factor VIIa corrects prothrombin time in cirrhotic patients: A preliminary study. Gastroenterology 113:1930, 1997

300	*Daniel K. Podolsky*

INFILTRATIVE, GENETIC, AND METABOLIC DISEASES AFFECTING THE LIVER

Many disseminated, systemic, or metabolic diseases involve the liver in a diffuse manner by the infiltration of abnormal cells or the accumulation of chemical substances or metabolites. Chemical accumulation may be extracellular or intracellular and may involve hepatocytes, Kupffer cells, or other elements of the reticuloendothelial system. Although infiltrative diseases may vary widely in cause and extrahepatic manifestations, the findings in the liver may be quite similar. Generalized enlargement and firmness of the liver, gradual and nonspecific deterioration of liver function, and, less often, signs of portal hypertension or ascites are typical features of this group of diseases. Differential diagnosis by clinical means may be difficult on occasion, but in patients in whom ancillary clinical findings do not establish the diagnosis, the diffusely infiltrated liver provides an excellent source of tissue for diagnostic purposes.

HEPATIC STEATOSIS (FATTY LIVER) AND NONALCOHOLIC STEATOHEPATITIS

Slight to moderate enlargement of the liver due to a diffuse accumulation of neutral fat (triglycerides) in hepatocytes is an important clinical and pathologic finding. Imaging techniques such as computed to-

mography (CT), ultrasound, and magnetic resonance imaging (MRI) may each yield alterations suggesting increased fat in the liver. Several mechanisms can contribute to lipid accumulation in the liver. Fatty liver can be separated into two categories based on whether the fat droplets in the hepatocytes are macrovesicular or microvesicular (Table 300-1). In addition, fatty infiltration may be accompanied by necroinflammatory activity, a condition designated *nonalcoholic steatohepatitis (NASH)*.

MACROVESICULAR FATTY LIVER This is the most common type of fatty liver and is seen most frequently in alcoholism or alcoholic liver disease, diabetes mellitus, obesity, and prolonged parenteral nutrition. Hematoxylin and eosin-stained liver sections show hepatocytes with large, empty vacuoles with the nucleus "pushed" to the periphery of the cell. In general, fat in the liver is not damaging per se, and the fat will disappear with improvement or elimination of the predisposing condition.

Etiology The major causes of fatty liver with macrovesicular fat depend on the age, geographic location, and metabolic-nutritional status of the patient population. *Chronic alcoholism* is the most common cause of hepatic steatosis in this country and in other countries with a high alcohol intake. The severity of fatty involvement is roughly proportional to the duration and degree of alcoholic excess. In addition, in western countries NASH is associated with obesity. Many of these patients (up to one-third) have type 2 diabetes and/or hyperlipidemia. Inflammatory activity when present may reflect the combined effects of oxidative stress, subsequent lipid peroxidation and abnormal cytokine expression, especially increased tumor necrosis factor (TNF).

Protein malnutrition, especially in infancy and early childhood, accounts for most cases of severe fatty liver in the tropical zones of Africa, South America, and Asia. The hepatic changes may be associated with other clinical and pathologic features of kwashiorkor. *Jejunoileal bypass* for surgical treatment of morbid obesity was sometimes associated with severe fatty liver and hepatic failure that could be fatal. In patients with Cushing's syndrome and in those receiving large doses of glucocorticoids, fatty infiltration of the liver may occur. In many *chronic illnesses*, especially those complicated by impaired nutrition or malabsorption, increased fat is found in liver cells. For example, patients with severe ulcerative colitis, chronic pancreatitis, or protracted heart failure frequently have moderate hepatic steatosis at the time of death. Patients maintained on prolonged *total parenteral nutrition* also may develop a fatty liver. In some cases, fatty infiltration and steatohepatitis may occur in the absence of an identifiable cause.

Acute fatty liver is caused by a number of hepatotoxins and is frequently accompanied by signs and symptoms of liver failure. Carbon tetrachloride intoxication, DDT poisoning, and ingestion of substances containing yellow phosphorus result in severe hepatic steatosis. Acute and prolonged alcohol ingestion may also be considered in this category and may be associated with a rapidly enlarging and fat-laden liver.

Table 300-1 Causes of Hepatic Steatosis

Macrovesicular (Large Fat Droplets in Hepatocytes)
Alcohol, alcoholic liver disease[a]
Diabetes mellitus[a]
Obesity[a]
Protein-calorie malnutrition
Total parenteral nutrition[a], jejunoileal bypass
Drugs[c], e.g., methotrexate, aspirin, vitamin A, glucocorticoids, amiodarone, and synthetic estrogen, nucleoside analogues (ddI, AZT)

Microvesicular (Small Fat Droplets in Hepatocytes)
Reye's syndrome
Acute fatty liver of pregnancy
Jamaican vomiting sickness
Drugs, e.g., valproic acid, tetracycline, nucleoside analogues

[a] May also be associated with necroinflammatory activity

Clinical Features   The signs and symptoms of hepatic steatosis are related to the degree of fat infiltration, the time course of its accumulation, and the underlying cause. The obese or diabetic patient with a chronic fatty liver is usually asymptomatic and has only mild tenderness over the enlarged liver. The liver function tests are normal or show mild elevations of alkaline phosphatase or aminotransferases. In contrast, the rapid accumulation of fat seen in the setting of hyperalimentation may lead to marked tenderness, presumably resulting from stretching of Glisson's capsule. Similarly, alcoholic patients with acute fatty liver following a bout of heavy drinking may have right upper quadrant pain and tenderness, often with laboratory evidence of cholestasis. The clinical presentation of fatty liver from hepatotoxins is similar to that of fulminant hepatic failure arising from any cause, with evidence of hepatic encephalopathy, marked elevations of prothrombin time and aminotransferases, and variable degrees of jaundice. Although steatohepatitis is generally thought to have a benign clinical course with improvement following elimination of the associated precipitant, in some individuals it may result in significant fibrosis and even cirrhosis. Recent studies indicate that substantial fibrosis or cirrhosis may be present in 15 to 50% of patients with NASH. In the only long-term follow-up study, 30% of patients with fibrosis had cirrhosis after 10 years. It is possible that some cases of "cryptogenic" cirrhosis are due to longstanding NASH and that the fat leaves the liver as endstage liver disease develops.

Diagnosis   The findings of a firm, nontender, and generally enlarged liver with minimal hepatic dysfunction in a patient with chronic alcoholism, malnutrition, poorly controlled diabetes mellitus, or obesity should suggest hepatic steatosis. This can usually be detected by CT, MRI, or ultrasound. Modest elevations of aminotransferases are often found in association with hepatic steatohepatitis. A disproportional elevation in AST leading to an AST/ALT ratio greater than 2 is generally associated with alcoholic hepatitis. When diagnostic uncertainty exists, needle biopsy of the liver will demonstrate the increased fat content, the presence of any fibrosis, and possibly the underlying primary disorder.

℞   **TREATMENT**   Adequate nutritional intake, removal of alcohol or offending toxins, and correction of any associated metabolic disorders usually result in recovery. There is no clinical rationale for the use of lipotropic agents such as choline. When indicated, attention should be directed to abstinence from alcohol, careful control of diabetes, weight loss, or correction of intestinal absorptive defects. In the alcoholic fatty liver, there is gradual disappearance of fat from the liver after 4 to 8 weeks of adequate diet and abstinence from alcohol. Similarly, fatty infiltration usually resolves within 2 weeks after discontinuation of parenteral hyperalimentation. Pilot studies in patients with NASH have suggested benefits from vitamin E and phlebotomy. Troglitazone has shown some benefit in those patients with concomitant insulin resistance.

MICROVESICULAR FATTY LIVER   This is the less common form of fatty liver. On microscopic examination, the fat is present in many small vacuoles. Although the droplets consist of triglycerides in both the macrovesicular and microvesicular forms, the reason for this difference in morphologic appearance is not clear.

Acute fatty liver of pregnancy (AFLP) is a syndrome that occurs late in pregnancy and is often associated with jaundice and hepatic failure. The liver is typically small. AFLP is more common when the mother is carrying a male fetus and may be associated with a deficiency of long-chain-3-hydroxy acyl COH dehydrogenase. Preeclampsia or the HELLP syndrome, which may complicate eclampsia, presents in a similar fashion and progresses to severe liver dysfunction, though typically with a normal size liver. Aminotransferase elevations are typically modest in all of these conditions (generally <500). If diagnosed in time, the disease usually resolves with termination of the pregnancy. Recurrence in subsequent pregnancies is rare.

Microvesicular fat accumulation also may be seen as a toxic reaction to *valproic acid* and with excessive doses of *tetracycline*. It is a typical finding in *Jamaican vomiting sickness*, which is caused by hypoglycin A present in unripened ackee fruit. Lactic acidosis and severe liver injury with microvesicular fat has been described as a complication of nucleoside analogue therapy.

REYE'S SYNDROME (FATTY LIVER WITH ENCEPHALOPATHY)   This acute illness is encountered exclusively in children below 15 years of age. It is characterized clinically by vomiting and signs of progressive central nervous system damage, signs of hepatic injury, and hypoglycemia. Morphologically, there is extensive fatty vacuolization of the liver and renal tubules. There is mitochondrial dysfunction with decreased activity of hepatic mitochondrial enzymes. The cause is unknown, although viral agents and drugs, especially salicylates, have been implicated. Increased aspirin use and much higher serum salicylate levels in children with this illness than in the general population have been described during outbreaks of Reye's syndrome. Recognition of this relationship and reduced aspirin use in this setting may account for the decreasing incidence of Reye's syndrome. However, this illness may occur in the absence of exposure to salicylates. In fatal cases, the liver is enlarged and yellow with striking diffuse fatty microvacuolization of cells. Peripheral zonal hepatic necrosis also has been present in some cases. Fatty changes of the renal tubular cells, cerebral edema, and neuronal degeneration of the brain are the major extrahepatic changes. Electron-microscopic studies show structural alterations of mitochondria in liver, brain, and muscle.

The onset usually follows an upper respiratory tract infection, especially influenza or chickenpox. Within 1 to 3 days, persistent vomiting occurs, together with stupor, which usually progresses rapidly to generalized convulsions and coma. The liver is enlarged, but *jaundice is characteristically absent or minimal*. Elevations in serum aminotransferases and prothrombin time, hypoglycemia, metabolic acidosis, and elevated serum ammonia levels are the major laboratory findings. The mortality rate in Reye's syndrome is approximately 50%. Therapy consists of infusions of 20% glucose and fresh frozen plasma, as well as intravenous mannitol to reduce the cerebral edema. Chronic liver disease has not been reported in survivors.

STORAGE DISEASES

Lipid storage diseases include the hereditary disorders of Gaucher's and Niemann-Pick disease. Other rare diseases associated with increased fat in the liver include abetalipoproteinemia, Tangier disease, Fabry's disease, and types I and V hyperlipoproteinemia (see Chap. 344 for details). Hepatic enlargement caused by distention of liver cells with glycogen is present in some poorly controlled diabetics and frequently in juvenile diabetes. More often, however, hepatomegaly is due to fatty infiltration (see above). Ketoacidosis and vigorous insulin therapy may further enhance hepatic enlargement.

HEPATIC MINERAL ACCUMULATION

WILSON'S DISEASE   This is an uncommon inherited disorder of copper metabolism. Wilson's disease presents clinically in adolescence or young adulthood by which time there is excess copper accumulation in the liver and other tissues. Deficiency of the plasma copper protein ceruloplasmin is a characteristic feature. The accumulation appears to result from impaired copper excretion due to a mutation in a gene that encodes a P-type ATPase copper transporter. Clinically, patients may present in teenage or early adult years with chronic hepatitis, cirrhosis, or their complications. A small number of patients will present with fulminant hepatitis. Liver disease is often accompanied by softening and degeneration of the basal ganglia (hepatolenticular degeneration) due to copper deposition, which results in extrapyramidal neurologic and psychiatric symptoms. Brownish pigmentation of Descemet's membrane in the cornea (Kayser-Fleischer rings) is frequently present. Hemolytic anemia is also common, especially with fulminant disease. Liver biopsy may reveal findings ranging from fulminant hepatitis to chronic hepatitis and macronodular cirrhosis, in addition to excess copper levels. Typically, liver cells are ballooned and show increased glycogen with glycogen vacuolization in the nuclei. All patients under age 40 with unexplained chronic hepatitis or cirrhosis should be evaluated for possible Wilson's disease. Prompt diagnosis is important; treatment, which must be continued throughout life, can prevent progression of end-organ damage. →*For further discussion, see Chap. 348.*

HEMOCHROMATOSIS Hemochromatosis may be the most common genetic disorder of humans; it involves accumulation of abnormal amounts of iron due to inappropriate absorption from the intestine. Between 85 and 95% of patients with genetic hemochromatosis are homozygous for a point mutation (cystine to tyrosine at codon 282:C282). The liver, as a primary site of iron storage, is affected most directly. There is diffuse deposition of excess iron in hepatocytes, in contrast to the characteristic accumulation of iron in the reticuloendothelial compartment typical of secondary iron overload and hemosiderosis. Excess hepatic iron commonly results in hepatomegaly. Although liver function is initially well preserved, if the disease is untreated, progressive impairment is followed by the development of cirrhosis. Prompt diagnosis can permit the institution of effective lifelong therapy to reduce the iron load and halt progression of the disease. → *For further discussion, see Chap. 345.*

OTHER INFILTRATIVE AND METABOLIC DISEASES

α_1-ANTITRYPSIN DEFICIENCY Patients with homozygous deficiency of serum α_1-antitrypsin (α_1AT) are prone to develop emphysema in adult life. The disease is suggested by the absence of alpha$_1$ globulin on serum electrophoresis (α_1AT makes up 90% of this fraction normally) and confirmed by direct measurement of α_1AT. The exact phenotype can then be determined by starch electrophoresis. Although there are approximately 75 recognized alleles, only PiZ and PiS are associated with clinical disease. The molecular bases of these altered products have been related to single nucleic acid substitutions—e.g., PiZ is caused by a G (guanine) to A (adenine) transposition, which results in a substitution of a glutamic acid for lysine at residue 292 in the α_1AT protein. Hepatocytes of some patients with this deficiency contain globules positive with the periodic acid Schiff reaction. Approximately 10% of children with homozygous deficiency (PiZZ phenotype) of α_1AT will develop significant liver disease, including neonatal hepatitis and progressive cirrhosis. It has been suggested that 15 to 20 percent of all chronic liver disease in infancy may be attributed to α_1AT deficiency. In adults, the most common manifestation of α_1AT deficiency is asymptomatic cirrhosis, which may progress from a micronodular to a macronodular state and may be complicated by the development of hepatocellular carcinoma. The occurrence of liver disease in these patients is not dependent on the development of lung disease. →*For further discussion, see Chap. 258.*

HURLER'S SYNDROME This is an uncommon hereditary disease that is characterized by the widespread tissue deposition of mucopolysaccharide (chondroitin sulfate B and heparan sulfate) in many tissues. The liver is frequently enlarged and firm. Microscopically, Kupffer cells and other macrophages are enlarged and filled with metachromatic granular material. Cirrhosis may be a late complication. →*For further discussion, see Chap. 349.*

PORPHYRIAS See Chap. 346.

RETICULOENDOTHELIAL DISORDERS (See also Chaps. 61 and 113)

Moderate to massive hepatomegaly and splenomegaly occur frequently in the various types of *leukemia* and *lymphoma*. Jaundice, when present, is usually slight and results from hemolysis, although cholestasis may occasionally be associated with lymphoma as a para-

neoplastic syndrome. Deep and protracted jaundice is distinctly rare and is caused by obstruction of the intrahepatic or extrahepatic bile ducts by tumor. Liver biopsy specimens reveal portal and sinusoidal infiltrates in most cases of leukemia, but the cellular pattern may be mixed and nonspecific. Liver biopsy is diagnostic in only 5% of patients with *Hodgkin's disease*. This percentage is increased in those with advanced disease or splenomegaly. Directed biopsy at laparoscopy or laparotomy is more likely to be positive than "blind" needle biopsy. Nonspecific histologic changes in the liver have been described in patients with lymphoma and may contribute to the abnormal liver function tests.

Myeloid metaplasia and other myeloproliferative disorders associated with extramedullary hematopoiesis produce hepatomegaly which may reach huge proportions, especially following splenectomy. Serum alkaline phosphatase elevations are often found. Ascites and portal hypertension, resulting from diffuse involvement of portal venules and lymphatics, are rare complications.

GRANULOMATOUS INFILTRATIONS

Perhaps as a result of the large population of mononuclear phagocytes, a number of systemic granulomatous diseases involve the liver, including sarcoidosis, miliary tuberculosis, histoplasmosis, brucellosis, schistosomiasis, berylliosis, and drug reactions (Table 300-2). In addition, isolated granulomas of no diagnostic importance may be found occasionally in patients with various forms of cirrhosis and hepatitis. The liver infiltrated by granulomas may be slightly enlarged and firm, but hepatic dysfunction is usually limited. Increases in serum alkaline phosphatase are common and may range from mild to marked. Occasionally, mild serum elevations in aminotransferases are also present. In a few patients with sarcoidosis or brucellosis, portal hypertension may develop, and extensive postnecrotic scarring or postnecrotic cirrhosis may follow healing of the granulomatous lesions, as in schistosomiasis.

Needle biopsy of the liver often provides the first definite evidence of a systemic or disseminated granulomatous disease. In patients with sarcoidosis who have neither clinical nor laboratory evidence of hepatic involvement, needle biopsy shows sarcoid granulomas in about 80% of cases. In cases of suspected miliary tuberculosis, a portion of the biopsy should be cultured and stained for mycobacteria. The organism can be detected in the majority of cases, particularly when caseating granulomas are present. Serial sections of the biopsy specimen should be examined if granulomas are not apparent. Individual granulomas are rarely specific in their microscopic appearance, and final diagnosis usually requires other clinical, laboratory, or histologic data.

In approximately 20% of patients, it is not possible to identify a

Table 300-2   Some Causes of Hepatic Granulomas

SYSTEMIC DISEASE	
Sarcoidosis	Berylliosis
Hodgkin's and non-Hodgkin's lymphoma	Crohn's disease
	Wegener's granulomatosis
Primary biliary cirrhosis	Granulomatous hepatitis, idiopathic

INFECTIONS	
Bacterial	Parasitic
Tuberculosis	Schistosomiasis
Mycobacterium avium intracellulare	Rickettsial
Brucellosis	Q fever
Leprosy	Spirochetes
Viral	Syphilis
Epstein-Barr virus	Drugs
Cytomegalovirus	Sulfonamides
Chicken pox	Isoniazid
	Allopurinol

cause for the granulomatous infiltration. When these infiltrates are accompanied by fever of unknown origin, the diagnosis of *granulomatous hepatitis* should be considered. This is an uncommon disorder of unknown cause and is diagnosed by exclusion. While granulomatous hepatitis invariably responds to moderate doses of glucocorticoids, relapses are frequent, and such therapy should never be undertaken unless tuberculous disease or other causes of granulomatous infiltration have been excluded. This may include an initial empiric trial of antituberculous therapy.

AMYLOIDOSIS (See also Chap. 319) Systemic amyloidosis, whether primary and idiopathic, familial, or secondary to chronic inflammatory or neoplastic diseases, often involves the liver. Grossly, the liver infiltrated with amyloid is enlarged and pale and rubbery in consistency. Microscopically, the birefringent amyloid deposits appear as homogeneous waxy material within the space of Disse, often being concentrated in the periportal areas and associated with atrophy of adjacent liver cell plates. Selective involvement of the walls of blood vessels, especially of the hepatic arterioles, may be a striking feature of primary amyloidosis. With this possible exception, however, the hepatic lesions are the same in all forms of amyloidosis and are present in 60 to 90% of cases.

An enlarged and firm liver is found in about 60% of patients, and ascites occurs in advanced stages of the disease in about 20%. Jaundice, portal hypertension, and other signs of chronic liver disease are usually absent. Liver function changes, although frequent, correlate poorly with the extent of liver infiltration. Hypoalbuminemia and elevated serum alkaline phosphatase are common. Hypoalbuminemia, however, may be related to the presence of nephrosis; the prothrombin time is usually normal. The diagnosis is established by biopsy of rectum, skin, liver, or other involved organs and demonstration of the characteristic Congo red-staining deposits by polarizing microscopy.

AIDS-RELATED LIVER DISEASE

In AIDS, evidence of liver disease is quite common but is usually mild with minimal morbidity. In these patients, hepatic granulomatous disease is often present and may be caused by opportunistic infections, with *Mycobacterium avium-intracellulare* being the most frequent pathogen. Cytomegalovirus hepatitis and hepatic mycoses are less common. These patients are frequently being treated for *Pneumocystis carinii* infections with sulfonamides, which also may cause hepatic granulomatous disease. AIDS cholangiopathy has become a well recognized entity. It exhibits features similar to those found in primary sclerosing cholangitis and is typically associated with cryptosporidia, microsporidia, and/or cytomegalovirus infection in the biliary tract. Papillary stenosis is frequently present. In addition, AIDS patients are vulnerable to hepatic injury resulting from drugs used to treat HIV, most notably nucleoside analogues.

ACKNOWLEDGMENT
This chapter represents a revised version of a chapter by Dr. Kurt J. Isselbacher and Dr. Daniel K. Podolsky that has appeared in previous editions of this textbook.

BIBLIOGRAPHY

ADAMS PC, CHAKRABARATI S: Genotypic/phenotypic correlations in genetic hemochromatosis: Evolution of diagnostic criteria. Gastroenterology 114:319, 1998

BACON BR et al: Molecular medicine and hemochromatosis: At the crossroads. Gastroenterology 116:193, 1999

CRYSTAL RG: Alpha 1-antitrypsin deficiency, emphysema and liver disease: Genetic basis and strategy for therapy. J Clin Invest 85:1343, 1990

HURWITZ ES et al: Public Health Service Study on Reye's syndrome and medications. N Engl J Med 313:842, 1985

HUTCHISON DC: Natural history of alpha 1-protease inhibitor deficiency. Am J Med 84:3, 1988

JAMES O, DAY C: Non-alcoholic steatohepatitis: Another disease of affluence. Lancet 353:1634, 1999

KNOX TA, OLANS LB: Liver disease in pregnancy. N Engl J Med 335(8):569, 1996

MATTEONI CA: et al: Nonalcoholic fatty liver disease: A spectrum of clinical and pathological severity. Gastroenterology 116:1414, 1999

MINAKAMI H et al: Pre-eclampsia: A microvesicular fat disease of the liver. Am J Obstet Gynecol 159:1043, 1988

PERLMUTTER DH: The cellular basis for liver injury in alpha 1-antitrypsin deficiency. Hepatology 13:172, 1991

SCHIFF ER et al: *Diseases of the Liver*, 8th ed. Philadelphia, Lippincott, 1999

SCRIVER CR et al (eds): *The Metabolic and Molecular Bases of Inherited Disease*, 8th ed. New York, McGraw-Hill, 2001

STEINDL P et al: Wilson's disease in patients with liver disease: A diagnostic challenge. Gastroenterology 113:212, 1997

STERNLIEB I: Perspectives on Wilson's disease. Hepatology 12:1234, 1990

ZAKIM D, BOYER TD: *Hepatology: A Textbook of Liver Disease*, 3d ed. Philadelphia, Saunders, 1996

301 Jules L. Dienstag

LIVER TRANSPLANTATION

Liver transplantation—the replacement of the native, diseased liver by a normal organ (allograft) recovered from a brain-dead donor—has matured from an experimental procedure reserved for desperately ill patients to an accepted, lifesaving operation applied much earlier in the natural history of end-stage liver disease. The preferred and technically most advanced approach is *orthotopic transplantation*, in which the native organ is removed and the donor organ is inserted in the same anatomic location. Pioneered in the 1960s by Starzl at the University of Colorado and, later, at the University of Pittsburgh and by Calne in Cambridge, England, liver transplantation is now performed routinely by dozens of centers throughout North America and western Europe. Success and survival have improved from approximately 30% in the 1970s to >80% today. These improved prospects for prolonged survival, dating back to the early 1980s, resulted from refinements in operative technique (including the introduction of venovenous bypass to allow venous return from the extremities and visceral circulation during clamping of the inferior vena cava), improvements in organ procurement and preservation, advances in immunosuppressive therapy, and, perhaps most influentially, more enlightened patient selection and timing. Despite the perioperative morbidity and mortality, the technical and management challenges of the procedure, and its costs, liver transplantation has become the approach of choice for selected patients whose chronic or acute liver disease is progressive, life-threatening, and unresponsive to medical therapy. Based on the current level of success, the number of liver transplants has continued to grow each year; in 1999, >4000 patients received liver allografts in the United States. Still, the demand for new livers continues to outpace availability; in 1999, >6000 patients in the United States were on a waiting list for a donor liver.

INDICATIONS Potential candidates for liver transplantation are children and adults who, in the absence of contraindications (see below), suffer from severe, irreversible liver disease for which alternative medical or surgical treatments have been exhausted or are unavailable. *Timing of the operation is of critical importance.* Indeed, improved timing and better patient selection are felt to have contributed more to the increased success of liver transplantation in the 1980s and beyond than all the impressive technical and immunologic advances combined. Although the disease should be advanced, and although opportunities for spontaneous or medically induced stabilization or recovery should be allowed, the procedure should be done sufficiently early to give the surgical procedure a fair chance for success. Ideally, transplantation should be considered in patients with end-stage liver disease who are experiencing or have experienced a life-threatening complication of hepatic decompensation, whose quality of life has deteriorated to unacceptable levels, or whose liver disease will result predictably in irreversible damage to the central nervous system

(CNS). If this is done sufficiently early, the patient will not have developed any contraindications or extrahepatic systemic deterioration. Although patients with well-compensated cirrhosis can survive for many years, many patients with quasi-stable chronic liver disease have much more advanced disease than may be apparent. As discussed below, the better the status of the patient prior to transplantation, the higher will be the anticipated success rate of transplantation. The decision about *when* to transplant is complex and requires the combined judgment of an experienced team of hepatologists, transplant surgeons, anesthesiologists, and specialists in support services, not to mention the well-informed consent of the patient and the patient's family.

Transplantation in Children Indications for transplantation in children are listed in Table 301-1. The most common is *biliary atresia*. *Inherited or genetic disorders of metabolism* associated with liver failure constitute another major indication for transplantation in children and adolescents. In Crigler-Najjar disease type I and in certain hereditary disorders of the urea cycle and of amino acid or lactate-pyruvate metabolism, transplantation may be the only way to prevent impending deterioration of CNS function, despite the fact that the native liver is structurally normal. Combined heart and liver transplantation has yielded dramatic improvement in cardiac function and in cholesterol levels in children with homozygous familial hypercholesterolemia; combined liver and kidney transplantation has been successful in patients with hereditary oxalosis. In hemophiliacs with transfusion-associated hepatitis and liver failure, liver transplantation has been associated with recovery of normal factor VIII synthesis.

Transplantation in Adults Liver transplantation is indicated for end-stage *cirrhosis* of all causes (Table 301-1). In sclerosing cholangitis and *Caroli's disease* (multiple cystic dilatations of the intrahepatic biliary tree), recurrent infections and sepsis associated with inflammatory and fibrotic obstruction of the biliary tree may be an indication for transplantation. Because prior biliary surgery complicates, and is a relative contraindication for, liver transplantation, surgical diversion of the biliary tree has been all but abandoned for patients with sclerosing cholangitis. In patients who undergo transplantation for *hepatic vein thrombosis (Budd-Chiari syndrome)*, postoperative anticoagulation is essential; underlying myeloproliferative disorders may have to be treated but are not a contraindication to liver transplantation. If a donor organ can be located quickly, before life-threatening complications—including cerebral edema—set in, patients with *fulminant hepatitis* are candidates for liver transplantation. More controversial as candidates for liver transplantation are patients with *alcoholic cirrhosis*, *chronic viral hepatitis*, and *primary hepatocellular malignancies*. Although all three of these categories are considered to be high risk, liver transplantation can be offered to carefully selected patients. Patients with alcoholic cirrhosis can be consid-

ered as candidates for transplantation if they meet strict criteria for abstinence and reform. Patients with chronic hepatitis C have done as well as any other subset of patients after transplantation, despite the fact that recurrent infection in the donor organ is the rule. In patients with chronic hepatitis B, in the absence of measures to prevent recurrent hepatitis B, survival after transplantation is reduced by approximately 10 to 20%; however, prophylactic use of hepatitis B immune globulin (HBIG) during and after transplantation increases the success of transplantation to a level comparable to that seen in patients with nonviral causes of liver decompensation. Specific antiviral drugs, such as lamivudine, that can be used for both prophylaxis against and treatment of recurrent hepatitis B will facilitate further the management of patients undergoing liver transplantation for end-stage hepatitis B. Issues of disease recurrence are discussed in more detail below. Patients with nonmetastatic primary hepatobiliary tumors—primary hepatocellular carcinoma, cholangiocarcinoma, hepatoblastoma, angiosarcoma, epithelioid hemangioendothelioma, and multiple or massive hepatic adenomata—have undergone liver transplantation; however, for hepatobiliary malignancies, overall survival is significantly lower than that for other categories of liver disease. To minimize the very high likelihood of recurrent tumor after transplantation, some centers are evaluating experimental adjuvant chemotherapy protocols. Some transplantation centers have reported excellent long-term, recurrence-free survival in patients with unresectable hepatocellular carcinoma for single tumors <5 cm in diameter or for three or fewer lesions all <3 cm. Consequently, most centers restrict liver transplanation to patients whose hepatic malignancies are confined to these limits. Because the likelihood of recurrent cholangiocarcinoma is almost universal, this tumor is no longer considered an indication for transplantation.

CONTRAINDICATIONS *Absolute contraindications* for transplantation include life-threatening systemic diseases, uncontrolled extrahepatic bacterial or fungal infections, preexisting advanced cardiovascular or pulmonary disease, multiple uncorrectable life-threatening congenital anomalies, metastatic malignancy, active drug or alcohol abuse, and HIV infection (Table 301-2). Because carefully selected patients in their sixties and even seventies have undergone transplantation successfully, advanced age per se is no longer considered an absolute contraindication; however, in older patients, a more thorough preoperative evaluation should be undertaken to exclude ischemic cardiac disease. Advanced age (>70 years), however, may be considered a *relative contraindication*—that is, a factor to be taken into account with other relative contraindications. Other relative contraindications include highly replicative hepatitis B, portal vein thrombosis, preexisting renal disease not associated with liver disease, intrahepatic or biliary sepsis, severe hypoxemia resulting from right-to-left intrapulmonary shunts, previous extensive hepatobiliary sur-

Table 301-1 Indications for Liver Transplantation

Children	Adults
Biliary atresia	Primary biliary cirrhosis
Neonatal hepatitis	Secondary biliary cirrhosis
Congenital hepatic fibrosis	Primary sclerosing cholangitis
Alagille's disease[a]	Caroli's disease[c]
Byler's disease[b]	Cryptogenic cirrhosis
α_1-Antitrypsin deficiency	Chronic hepatitis with cirrhosis
Inherited disorders of metabolism	Hepatic vein thrombosis
Wilson's disease	Fulminant hepatitis
Tyrosinemia	Alcoholic cirrhosis
Glycogen storage diseases	Chronic viral hepatitis
Lysosomal storage diseases	Primary hepatocellular malignancies
Protoporphyria	Hepatic adenomas
Crigler-Najjar disease type I	
Familial hypercholesterolemia	
Hereditary oxalosis	
Hemophilia	

[a] Arteriohepatic dysplasia, with paucity of bile ducts, and congenital malformations, including pulmonary stenosis.
[b] Intrahepatic cholestasis, progressive liver failure, mental and growth retardation.
[c] Multiple cystic dilatations of the intrahepatic biliary tree.

Table 301-2 Contraindications to Liver Transplantation

Absolute	Relative
Uncontrolled extrahepatobiliary infection	Age >70
Uncorrectable, life-limiting congenital anomalies	Portal vein thrombosis
Active substance or alcohol abuse	HIV seropositivity
Advanced cardiopulmonary disease	Previous extrahepatic malignancy
Extrahepatobiliary malignancy	Severe obesity
Metastatic malignancy to the liver	Severe malnutrition/wasting
Cholangiocarcinoma	Medical noncompliance
AIDS	Renal failure
Life-threatening systemic diseases	Intrahepatic sepsis
	Primary hepatic malignancy
	Prior extensive hepatobiliary surgery
	Severe hypoxemia secondary to right-to-left intrapulmonary shunts
	Uncontrolled psychiatric disorder

gery, and any uncontrolled serious psychiatric disorder. Any one of these relative contraindications is insufficient in and of itself to preclude transplantation. For example, the problem of portal vein thrombosis can be overcome by constructing a graft from the donor liver portal vein to the recipient's superior mesenteric vein.

TECHNICAL CONSIDERATIONS   **Donor Selection**   Donor livers for transplantation are procured primarily from victims of head trauma. Organs from brain-dead donors up to age 60 are acceptable if the following criteria are met: hemodynamic stability; adequate oxygenation; absence of bacterial or fungal infection; serologic exclusion of hepatitis B and C viruses and HIV; absence of abdominal trauma; and absence of hepatic dysfunction. Cardiovascular and respiratory functions are maintained artificially until the liver can be removed. Compatibility in ABO blood group and organ size between donor and recipient are important considerations in donor selection; however, ABO-incompatible or reduced-donor-organ transplants can be performed in emergency or marked donor-scarcity situations. Tissue typing for HLA matching is not required, and preformed cytotoxic HLA antibodies do not preclude liver transplantation. Following perfusion with cold electrolyte solution, the donor liver is removed and packed in ice. The use of University of Wisconsin (UW) solution, rich in lactobionate and raffinose, has permitted the extension of cold ischemic time up to 20 h; however, 12 h may be a more reasonable limit. Improved techniques for harvesting multiple organs from the same donor have increased the availability of donor livers, but the availability of donor livers is far outstripped by the demand. Currently, in the United States, all donor livers are distributed through a nationwide organ-sharing network (United Network of Organ Sharing) designed to allocate available organs based on regional considerations and recipient acuity. Recipients who require the highest level of care (intensive care) have the highest priority, as outlined in Table 301-3.

Surgical Technique   Removal of the recipient's native liver is technically difficult, particularly in the presence of portal hypertension with its associated collateral circulation and extensive varices, and even more so in the presence of scarring from previous abdominal operations. The combination of portal hypertension and coagulopathy (elevated prothrombin time and thrombocytopenia) translates into large blood product transfusion requirements. After the portal vein and infrahepatic and suprahepatic inferior vena cavae are dissected, a pump-driven venovenous bypass system is applied to reroute blood from the portal vein and inferior vena cava, preventing congestion of visceral organs. After the hepatic artery and common bile duct are dissected, the native liver is removed and the donor organ inserted. During the anhepatic phase, coagulopathy, hypoglycemia, hypocalcemia, and hypothermia are encountered and must be managed by the anesthesiology team. Caval, portal vein, hepatic artery, and bile duct anastomoses are performed in succession, the last by end-to-end suturing of the donor and recipient common bile ducts or by choledochojejunostomy to a Roux en Y loop if the recipient common bile duct cannot be used for reconstruction (e.g., in sclerosing cholangitis). A typical transplant operation lasts 8 h, with a range of 6 to 18 h. Because of excessive bleeding, large volumes of blood, blood products, and volume expanders may be required during surgery.

Emerging alternatives to orthotopic liver transplantation include split-liver grafts, in which one donor organ is divided and inserted into two recipients; and living-related-donor procedures, in which the left lobe of the liver is harvested from a living-related donor for transplantation into the recipient. Heterotopic liver transplantation, in which the donor liver is inserted without removal of the native liver, has met with very limited success and acceptance, except in a very small number of centers. To support desperately ill patients until a suitable donor organ can be identified, several transplantation centers are studying extracorporeal perfusion with bioartificial liver cartridges constructed from hepatocytes bound to hollow fiber systems and used as temporary hepatic-assist devices, but their efficacy remains to be established. Areas of research with the potential to overcome the shortage of donor organs include hepatocyte transplantation and xenotransplantation with genetically modified organs of nonhuman origin (e.g., swine).

POSTOPERATIVE COURSE AND MANAGEMENT   **Immunosuppressive Therapy**   The introduction in 1980 of cyclosporine as an immunosuppressive agent contributed substantially to the improvement in survival after liver transplantation. Cyclosporine inhibits early activation of T cells and is specific for T cell functions that result from the interaction of the T cell with its receptor and that involve the calcium-dependent signal transduction pathway. As a result, the activity of cyclosporine leads to inhibition of lymphokine gene activation, blocking interleukins 2, 3, and 4, tumor necrosis factor α, as well as other lymphokines. Cyclosporine also inhibits B cell functions. This process occurs without affecting rapidly dividing cells in the bone marrow, which may account for the reduced frequency of posttransplantation systemic infections. The most common and important side effect of cyclosporine therapy is nephrotoxicity. Cyclosporine causes dose-dependent renal tubular injury and direct renal artery vasospasm. Following renal function, therefore, is important in monitoring cyclosporine therapy, perhaps even a more reliable indicator than blood levels of the drug. Nephrotoxicity is reversible and can be managed by dose reduction. Other adverse effects of cyclosporine therapy include hypertension, hyperkalemia, tremor, hirsutism, glucose intolerance, and gum hyperplasia.

Tacrolimus (originally labeled FK 506) is a macrolide lactone antibiotic isolated from a Japanese soil fungus, *Streptomyces tsukubaensis*. It has the same mechanism of action as cyclosporine but is 10 to 100 times more potent. Initially applied as "rescue" therapy for patients in whom rejection occurred despite the use of cyclosporine, tacrolimus has been shown in two large, multicenter, randomized trials to be associated with a reduced frequency of acute rejection, refractory rejection, and chronic rejection. Although patient and graft survival are the same with these two drugs, the advantage of tacrolimus in minimizing episodes of rejection, reducing the need for additional glucocorticoid doses, and reducing the likelihood of bacterial and cytomegalovirus infection has simplified the management of patients un-

Table 301-3 Liver Transplantation Waiting List Criteria (in Order of Descending Urgency)

Status 1	Fulminant hepatic failure (including primary graft non-function and hepatic artery thrombosis within 7 days after transplantation as well as acute decompensated Wilson's disease)[a]
Status 2A	Chronic liver disease with CTP[b] score ≥10, in intensive care unit, predicted <7 days to live, plus one of following: hepatic encephalopathy ≥ stage III; variceal bleeding; heptorenal syndrome; refractory ascites or hepatic hydrothorax; coagulopathy with ongoing bleeding (cannot have extrahepatic sepsis, high-dose or double pressor dependency, or multiorgan failure)
Status 2B	Chronic liver disease with CTP score ≥ 10 or CTP score ≥7 plus one of following: variceal bleeding; hepatorenal syndrome; history of spontaneous bacterial periotonitis; refractory ascites or hepatic hydrothorax; refractory bleeding
Status 3	CTP score ≥7
Status 7	Inactive

[a] For children < 18 years of age, Status 1 includes acute or chronic liver failure plus hospitalization in an intensive care unit or inborn errors of metabolism.
[b] Child-Turcotte-Pugh score components

Points	1	2	3
Encephalopathy	None	Stages I–II	Stages III–IV
Ascites	Absent	Slight, responsive	Moderate-severe
Bilirubin (mg/dL)	<2	2–3	>3
Albumin (g/dL)	>3.5	2.8–3.5	<2.8
Prothrombin time	<15 s	15–17 s	>17 s

The CTP score is calculated by assigning 1 point for any feature in column 1, 2 points for any feature in column 2, and 3 points for any feature in column 3. Class A = ≤6; Class B = 7–9; Class C = ≥10. For cholestatis disorders, such as primary biliary cirrhosis, primary sclerosing cholangitis, etc., the bilirubin categories are <4, 4–10, and >10.

dergoing liver transplantation. In addition, the oral absorption of tacrolimus is more predictable than that of cyclosporine, especially during the early postoperative period when T-tube drainage interferes with the enterohepatic circulation of cyclosporine. As a result, in most transplantation centers, tacrolimus has now supplanted cyclosporine for primary immunosuppression, and many centers rely on oral, rather than intravenous, administration from the outset. For transplantation centers that prefer cyclosporine, a new, better-absorbed, microemulsion preparation is now available.

Although tacrolimus is more potent than cyclosporine, it is also more toxic and more likely to be discontinued for adverse events. The toxicity of tacrolimus is similar to that of cyclosporine; nephrotoxicity and neurotoxicity are the most commonly encountered adverse effects, and neurotoxicity (tremor, seizures, hallucinations, psychoses, coma) is more likely and more severe in tacrolimus-treated patients. Both drugs can cause diabetes mellitus, but tacrolimus does not cause hirsutism or gingival hyperplasia. Because of overlapping toxicity between cyclosporine and tacrolimus, especially nephrotoxicity, and because tacrolimus reduces cyclosporine clearance, these two drugs should not be used together. Because 99% of tacrolimus is metabolized by the liver, hepatic dysfunction reduces its clearance; in primary graft nonfunction (when, for technical reasons or because of ischemic damage prior to its insertion, the allograft is defective and does not function normally from the outset) tacrolimus doses have to be reduced substantially, especially in children. Both cyclosporine and tacrolimus are metabolized by the cytochrome P450 IIIA system, and, therefore, drugs that induce cytochrome P450 (e.g., phenytoin, phenobarbital, carbamazepine, rifampin) reduce available levels of cyclosporine and tacrolimus; drugs that inhibit cytochrome P450 (e.g., erythromycin, fluconazole, ketoconazole, clotrimazole, itraconazole, verapamil, diltiazem, nicardipine, cimetidine, danazol, metoclopramide, bromocriptine) increase cyclosporine and tacrolimus blood levels. Like azathioprine, cyclosporine and tacrolimus appear to be associated with a risk of lymphoproliferative malignancies (see below), which may occur earlier after cyclosporine or tacrolimus than after azathioprine therapy. Because of these side effects, combinations of cyclosporine or tacrolimus with prednisone and azathioprine—all at reduced doses—are preferable regimens for immunosuppressive therapy.

In patients with pretransplant renal dysfunction or renal deterioration that occurs intraoperatively or immediately postoperatively, tacrolimus or cyclosporine therapy may not be practical; under these circumstances, induction or maintenance of immunosuppression with monoclonal antibodies to T cells, OKT3, may be appropriate. Therapy with OKT3 has been especially effective in reversing acute rejection in the posttransplant period and is the standard treatment for acute rejection that fails to respond to methylprednisolone boluses. Intravenous infusions of OKT3 may be complicated by transient fever, chills, and diarrhea. When this drug is used to induce immunosuppression initially or to provide "rescue" in those who reject despite "conventional" therapy, the incidence of bacterial, fungal, and especially cytomegalovirus infections is increased during and after such therapy. In some centers, ganciclovir antiviral therapy is initiated prophylactically as a routine along with OKT3. Another immunosuppressive drug that is likely to be used in the future for patients undergoing liver transplantation is mycophenolic acid, a nonnucleoside purine metabolism inhibitor derived as a fermentation product from several *Penicillium* species. Mycophenolate has been shown to be better than azathioprine, when used with other standard immunosuppressive drugs, in preventing rejection after renal transplantation and has been approved for use in renal transplantation. Rapamycin, an inhibitor of later events in T cell activation, is yet another drug undergoing experimental evaluation as an immunosuppressive agent.

The most important principle of immunosuppression is that the ideal approach strikes a balance between immunosuppression and immunologic competence. Given sufficient immunosuppression, acute liver allograft rejection is always reversible; however, if the cumulative dose of immunosuppressive therapy is too large, the patient will succumb to opportunistic infection. Therefore, immunosuppressive drugs must be used judiciously, with strict attention to the infectious consequences of such therapy.

Postoperative Complications Complications of liver transplantation can be divided into hepatic and nonhepatic categories (Tables 301-4 and 301-5). In addition, both immediately postoperative and late complications are encountered. Patients who undergo liver transplantation as a rule have been chronically ill for protracted periods and may be malnourished and wasted. The impact of such chronic illness and the multisystem failure that accompanies liver failure continues to require attention in the postoperative period. Because of the massive fluid losses and fluid shifts that occur during the operation, patients may remain fluid overloaded during the immediate postoperative period, straining cardiovascular reserve; this effect can be amplified in the face of transient renal dysfunction and pulmonary capillary vascular permeability. Continuous monitoring of cardiovascular and pulmonary function, measures to maintain the integrity of the intravascular compartment and to treat extravascular volume overload, and scrupulous attention to potential sources of and sites of infection are of paramount importance. Cardiovascular instability may also result from the electrolyte imbalance that may accompany reperfusion of the donor liver. Pulmonary function may be compromised further by paralysis of the right hemidiaphragm associated with phrenic nerve injury. The hyperdynamic state with increased cardiac output that is characteristic of patients with liver failure reverses rapidly after successful liver transplantation.

Other immediate management issues include renal dysfunction; prerenal azotemia, acute kidney injury associated with hypoperfusion (acute tubular necrosis), and renal toxicity caused by antibiotics, tacrolimus, or cyclosporine are frequently encountered in the postoperative period, sometimes necessitating dialysis. Occasionally, postoperative intraperitoneal bleeding may be sufficient to increase intraabdominal pressure, which, in turn, may reduce renal blood flow; this effect is rapidly reversible when abdominal distention is relieved by exploratory laparotomy to identify and ligate the bleeding site and to remove intraperitoneal clot. Anemia also may result from acute upper gastrointestinal bleeding or from transient hemolytic anemia, which may be autoimmune, especially when blood group O livers are transplanted into blood group A or B recipients. This autoimmune hemolytic anemia is mediated by donor intrahepatic lymphocytes that recognize red blood cell A or B antigens on recipient erythrocytes. Transient in nature, this process resolves once the donor liver is repopulated by recipient bone marrow–derived lymphocytes; the hemolysis can be treated by transfusing blood group O red blood cells and/or by administering higher doses of glucocorticoids. Transient thrombocytopenia is also commonly encountered. Aplastic anemia, a late occurrence, is rare but has been reported in almost 30% of patients who underwent liver transplantation for acute, severe hepatitis of unknown cause.

Bacterial, fungal, or viral infections are common and may be life-threatening postoperatively. Early after transplant surgery, common postoperative infections predominate—pneumonia, wound infections, infected intraabdominal collections, urinary tract infections, and intravenous line infections—rather than opportunistic infections; these infections may involve the biliary tree and liver as well. Beyond the first postoperative month, the toll of immunosuppression becomes evident, and opportunistic infections—cytomegalovirus, herpes viruses, fungal infections (*Aspergillus*, *Candida*, cryptococcal disease), mycobacterial infections, parasitic infections (*Pneumocystis*, *Toxoplasma*), bacterial infections (*Nocardia*, *Legionella*, and *Listeria*)—predominate. Rarely, early infections represent those transmitted with the donor liver, either infections present in the donor or infections acquired during procurement processing. De novo viral hepatitis infections acquired from the donor organ or from transfused blood products occur after typical incubation periods for these agents (well beyond the first month). Obviously, infections in an immunosuppressed host demand early recognition and prompt management; prophylactic antibiotic therapy is

Table 301-4   Nonhepatic Complications of Liver Transplantation

Fluid overload	
Cardiovascular instability	Arrhythmias
	Congestive heart failure
	Cardiomyopathy
Pulmonary compromise	Pneumonia
	Pulmonary capillary vascular permeability
	Fluid overload
Renal dysfunction	Prerenal azotemia
	Hypoperfusion injury (acute tubular necrosis)
	Drug nephrotoxicity
	↓ renal blood flow secondary to ↑ intraabdominal pressure
Hematologic	Anemia 2° to gastrointestinal and/or intraabdominal bleeding
	Hemolytic anemia, aplastic anemia
	Thrombocytopenia
Infection	Bacterial: early, common postoperative infections
	Fungal/parasitic: late, opportunistic infections
	Viral: late, opportunistic infections, recurrent hepatitis
Neuropsychiatric	Seizures
	Encephalopathy
	Depression
	Difficult Psychosocial Adjustment
Diseases of donor	Infectious
	Malignant
Malignancy	B-cell lymphoma

administered routinely in the immediate postoperative period. Use of sulfamethoxazole with trimethoprim reduces the incidence of postoperative *Pneumocystis carinii* pneumonia.

Neuropsychiatric complications include seizures (commonly associated with cyclosporine and tacrolimus toxicity), encephalopathy, depression, and difficult psychosocial adjustment. Rarely, diseases are transmitted by the allograft from the donor to the recipient. In addition to viral and bacterial infections, malignancies of donor origin have occurred. Lymphoproliferative malignancies, especially B cell lymphoma, are a recognized complication associated with immunosuppressive drugs such as azathioprine, tacrolimus, and cyclosporine (see above). Epstein-Barr virus has been shown to play a contributory role in some of these tumors, which may regress when immunosuppressive therapy is reduced.

Hepatic Complications   Hepatic dysfunction after liver transplantation is similar to the hepatic complications encountered after major abdominal and cardiothoracic surgery; however, in addition, there may be complications such as primary graft failure, vascular compromise, failure or obstruction of the biliary anastomoses, and rejection. As in nontransplant surgery, postoperative jaundice may result from prehepatic, intrahepatic, and posthepatic sources. *Prehepatic* sources represent the massive hemoglobin pigment load from transfusions, hemolysis, hematomas, ecchymoses, and other collections of blood. *Early intrahepatic* liver injury includes effects of hepatotoxic drugs and anesthesia; hypoperfusion injury associated with hypotension, sepsis, and shock; and benign postoperative cholestasis. *Late intrahepatic* sources of liver injury include posttransfusion hepatitis and exacerbation of primary disease. *Posthepatic* sources of hepatic dysfunction include biliary obstruction and reduced renal clearance of conjugated bilirubin. Hepatic complications unique to liver transplantation include primary graft failure associated with ischemic injury to the organ during harvesting; vascular compromise associated with thrombosis or stenosis of the portal vein or hepatic artery anastomoses; vascular anastomotic leak; stenosis, obstruction, or leakage of the anastomosed common bile duct; recurrence of primary hepatic disorder (see below); and rejection.

Transplant Rejection   Despite the use of immunosuppressive drugs, rejection of the transplanted liver still occurs in a majority of

Table 301-5   Hepatic Complications of Liver Transplantation

HEPATIC DYSFUNCTION COMMON AFTER MAJOR SURGERY

Prehepatic	Pigment load
	Hemolysis
	Blood collections (hematomas, abdominal collections)
Intrahepatic	
Early	Hepatotoxic drugs and anesthesia
	Hypoperfusion (hypotension, shock, sepsis)
	Benign postoperative cholestasis
Late	Transfusion-associated hepatitis
	Exacerbation of primary hepatic disease
Posthepatic	Biliary obstruction
	↓ Renal clearance of conjugated bilirubin (renal dysfunction)

HEPATIC DYSFUNCTION UNIQUE TO LIVER TRANSPLANTATION

Primary graft nonfunction	
Vascular compromise	Portal vein obstruction
	Hepatic artery thrombosis
	Anastomotic leak with intraabdominal bleeding
Bile duct disorder	Stenosis, obstruction, leak
Rejection	
Recurrent primary hepatic disease	

patients, beginning 1 to 2 weeks after surgery. Clinical signs suggesting rejection are fever, right upper quadrant pain, and reduced bile pigment and volume. Leukocytosis may occur, but the most reliable indicators are increases in serum bilirubin and aminotransferase levels. Because these tests lack specificity, distinguishing among rejection and biliary obstruction, primary graft nonfunction, vascular compromise, viral hepatitis, cytomegalovirus infection, drug hepatotoxicity, and recurrent primary disease may be difficult. Radiographic visualization of the biliary tree and/or percutaneous liver biopsy often help to establish the correct diagnosis. Morphologic features of acute rejection include portal infiltration, bile duct injury, and/or endothelial inflammation ("endothelialitis"); some of these findings are reminiscent of graft-versus-host disease and primary biliary cirrhosis. As soon as transplant rejection is suspected, treatment consists of intravenous methylprednisolone in repeated boluses; if this fails to abort rejection, many centers use antibodies to lymphocytes, such as OKT3, or polyclonal antilymphocyte globulin.

Chronic rejection is a relatively rare outcome that may follow repeated bouts of acute rejection or that occurs unrelated to preceding rejection episodes. Morphologically, chronic rejection is characterized by progressive cholestasis, focal parenchymal necrosis, mononuclear infiltration, vascular lesions (intimal fibrosis, subintimal foam cells, fibrinoid necrosis), and fibrosis. This process may be reflected as ductopenia—the vanishing bile duct syndrome. Some of the histologic hallmarks of chronic rejection may be so similar to those of chronic viral hepatitis that differentiation between the two may be difficult. Reversibility of chronic rejection is limited; in patients with therapy-resistant chronic rejection, retransplantation has yielded encouraging results.

OUTCOME   Survival   The survival rate for patients undergoing liver transplantation has improved steadily since 1983. One-year survival rates have increased from approximately 70% in the early 1980s to 80 to 90% in the late 1990s. Currently, the 5-year survival rate exceeds 60%. An important observation is the relation between clinical status before transplantation and outcome. For patients who undergo liver transplantation when their level of compensation is high (e.g., still working or only partially disabled), a 1-year survival rate of 85% is common. For those whose level of decompensation mandates continuous in-hospital care prior to transplantation, the 1-year survival rate is about 70%, while for those who are so decompensated that they require life support in an intensive care unit, the 1-year survival rate is approximately 50%. Indeed, the trend toward transplantation earlier in the natural history of end-stage liver disease is a major factor in the increased success of liver transplantation during the 1980s and 1990s. Another important distinction in survival has been drawn between high-risk and low-risk patient categories. For patients who do not fit any "high-risk" designations, 1-year and 5-year survival rates of 85 and 80%, respectively, have been recorded. In contrast, among patients in high-risk categories—cancer, fulminant hepatitis, hepatitis B, age >65, concurrent renal failure, respirator dependence, portal vein thrombosis, and history of a portacaval shunt or multiple right upper quadrant operations—survival statistics fall into the range of 60% at 1 year and 35% at 5 years. Survival after retransplantation for primary graft nonfunction is approximately 50%. Causes of failure of liver transplantation vary with time. Failures within the first 3 months result primarily from technical complications, postoperative infections, and hemorrhage. Transplant failures after the first 3 months are more likely to result from infection, rejection, or recurrent disease (such as malignancy or viral hepatitis).

Recurrence of Primary Disease The recurrence of autoimmune hepatitis or primary sclerosing cholangitis has not been reported. There have been reports of recurrent primary biliary cirrhosis after liver transplantation; however, the histologic features of primary biliary cirrhosis and acute rejection are virtually indistinguishable and occur as frequently in patients with primary biliary cirrhosis as in patients undergoing transplantation for other reasons. Hereditary disorders such as Wilson's disease and α_1-antitrypsin deficiency have not recurred after liver transplantation; however, recurrence of disordered iron metabolism has been observed in some patients with hemochromatosis. Hepatic vein thrombosis (Budd-Chiari syndrome) may recur; this can be minimized by treating underlying lymphoproliferative disorders and by anticoagulation. Cholangiocarcinoma recurs almost invariably; therefore, few centers now transplant such patients. In patients with hepatocellular carcinoma, tumor recurrence in the liver is common after approximately 1 year, although better success has been reported in patients with an unresectable isolated lesion <5 cm or with three or fewer lesions all <3 cm. Trials are underway to assess the benefit of adjuvant chemotherapy.

Hepatitis A can recur after transplantation for fulminant hepatitis A, but such acute reinfection has no serious clinical sequelae. In fulminant hepatitis B, recurrence is not the rule; however, in the absence of any prophylactic measures, hepatitis B usually recurs after transplantation for end-stage chronic hepatitis B. With sufficient immunosuppressive therapy to prevent allograft rejection, levels of hepatitis B viremia increase markedly, regardless of pretransplantation values. A majority of patients undergoing transplantation for chronic hepatitis B become carriers of hepatitis B virus (HBV) with high levels of virus replication but without liver injury; however, some patients experience a rapid recapitulation of severe injury—severe chronic hepatitis or even fulminant hepatitis—after transplantation. *Fibrosing cholestatic hepatitis* is a histologic feature linked to rapidly progressive liver injury in approximately 10% of patients who undergo liver transplantation for hepatitis B. These patients experience marked hyperbilirubinemia, substantial prolongation of the prothrombin time (both out of proportion to relatively modest elevations of aminotransferase activity), and rapidly progressive liver failure. This lesion has been suggested to represent a "choking off" of the hepatocyte by an overwhelming density of HBV proteins. Complications such as sepsis and pancreatitis have also been observed more frequently in patients undergoing liver transplantation for hepatitis B. Although the risk of recurrent hepatitis B is approximately 20% higher in patients with pretransplantation markers of HBV replication (hepatitis B e antigen and HBV DNA), recurrent hepatitis B occurs in at least 60% of patients whose replicative markers were undetectable prior to transplantation, probably because of the enhancing impact of immunosuppressive drugs on HBV replication. Most transplantation centers will not undertake liver transplantation in patients with hepatitis B unless immunoprophylaxis with HBIG is used. Neither preoperative hepatitis B vaccination, preoperative or postoperative interferon therapy, nor short-term (≤2 months) HBIG prophylaxis has been shown to be effective, but a retrospective analysis of data from several hundred European patients followed for 3 years after transplantation has shown that long-term (≥6 months) prophylaxis with HBIG is associated with a lowering of the risk of HBV reinfection from approximately 75% to 35% and a reduction in mortality from approximately 50 percent to 20%.

As a result of long-term HBIG use following liver transplantation for chronic hepatitis B, similar improvements in outcome have been observed in the United States, with 1-year survival rates between 75 and 90%. Currently, with HBIG prophylaxis, the outcome of liver transplantation for chronic hepatitis B is indistinguishable from that for chronic liver disease unassociated with chronic hepatitis B; essentially, medical concerns regarding liver transplantation for chronic hepatitis B have been eliminated. Passive immunoprophylaxis with HBIG is begun during the anhepatic stage of surgery, repeated daily for the first 6 postoperative days, then continued with infusions that are given either at regular intervals of 4 to 6 weeks or, alternatively, when anti-HBs levels fall below a threshold of 100 mIU/mL. In all likelihood, indefinite HBIG infusions will be required, and, occasionally "breakthrough" HBV infection occurs. This approach is very expensive, approximately $20,000 per year, and involves the intravenous administration of a globulin preparation designed for intramuscular injection. Although this approach is now practiced universally, it has not been approved officially by the U.S. Food and Drug Administration; clinical trials of HBIG preparations produced specifically for intravenous administration are in progress.

An alternative and promising but still experimental approach to the prophylaxis of patients with chronic hepatitis B undergoing liver transplantation is the use of nucleoside analogues such as lamivudine (Chap. 297). Limited evidence available to date suggests that lamivudine can be used to prevent recurrence of HBV infection when administered *prior* to transplantation, to treat hepatitis B that recurs *after* transplantation, including in patients who break through HBIG prophylaxis, and to reverse the course of otherwise fatal fibrosing cholestatic hepatitis. Clinical trials have shown that lamivudine monotherapy reduces the level of HBV replication substantially, sometimes even resulting in clearance of HBsAg; reduces ALT levels; and improves histologic features of necrosis and inflammation. Long-term use of lamivudine is safe and effective, but, after several months, a proportion of patients become resistant to lamivudine, resulting from "YMDD" mutations in the HBV polymerase motif (Chap. 297). In approximately half of such resistant patients, hepatic deterioration may ensue. Perhaps the best results with currently available antiviral approaches can be achieved by combining HBIG and lamivudine. In addition, new nucleoside analogues and related drugs are being assessed as antiviral agents against HBV infection. Some of these are effective against lamivudine-associated YMDD variants of HBV; these novel agents also are likely to be used in patients undergoing liver transplantation. Clinical trials are underway to define the optimal application of these antiviral agents in the management of patients undergoing liver transplantation for chronic hepatitis B.

Patients who undergo liver transplantation for chronic hepatitis B plus D have a better survival rate than patients undergoing transplantation for hepatitis B alone. Accounting for up to 40% of all liver transplantation procedures, the most common indication for liver transplantation is end-stage liver disease resulting from chronic hepatitis C. Recurrence of hepatitis C virus (HCV) after liver transplantation can be documented in almost every patient, if sufficiently sensitive virus markers are used. Although acute and chronic liver injury occur after transplantation in patients with chronic hepatitis C, clinical consequences of recurrent hepatitis C are limited during the first 5 years after transplantation. Nonetheless, despite the relative clinical benignity of recurrent hepatitis C in the early years after liver transplantation, and despite the negligible impact on patient survival during these early years, histologic studies have documented the presence of moderate to severe chronic hepatitis in more than half of all patients and bridging fibrosis or cirrhosis in approximately 10%. Ultimately, such histologic evidence of chronic hepatitis and cirrhosis will be expressed clinically as well, and the expectation is that the 10-year outcome will not be as favorable as the 5-year statistics suggest. In a proportion of patients, even during the early posttransplantation period, recurrent hepatitis C may be sufficiently severe biochemically and histologically to merit antiviral therapy. Treatment with interferon monotherapy, which can *suppress* HCV-associated liver injury in approximately half of patients but rarely leads to *sustained* benefit, has been disappointing. The addition of the nucleoside analogue ribavirin to interferon has resulted in improved responses to antiviral therapy, and many centers have adopted some form of combination therapy for their patients with recurrent chronic hepatitis C; however, the efficacy of such combination therapy remains the subject of clinical trials. Of interest is the preliminary observation that the immunosuppressive agent mycophenolate may have a suppressive effect on HCV. A small number succumb to early HCV-associated liver injury, and a syndrome reminiscent of fibrosing cholestatic hepatitis (see above) has been observed rarely. Because patients with more episodes of rejection receive more immunosuppressive therapy, and because immunosuppressive therapy enhances HCV replication, patients with severe or multiple episodes of rejection are more likely to experience early recurrence of hepatitis C after transplantation. Both HCV genotype 1b and high viral load have been linked to recurrent HCV-induced liver disease and to earlier disease recurrence after transplantation; however, the association between genotype and recurrence of HCV-associated liver injury has not been supported by more recent reports.

Patients who undergo liver transplantation for end-stage alcoholic cirrhosis are at risk of resorting to drinking again after transplantation, a potential source of recurrent alcoholic liver injury. Currently, alcoholic liver disease is one of the more common indications for liver transplantation, accounting for 20 to 25% of all liver transplantation procedures, and most transplantation centers screen candidates carefully for predictors of continued abstinence. Recidivism is more likely in patients whose sobriety prior to transplantation was shorter than 6 months. For abstinent patients with alcoholic cirrhosis, liver transplantation can be undertaken successfully, with outcomes comparable to those for other categories of patients with chronic liver disease, when coordinated by a team approach that includes substance abuse counseling.

Posttransplantation Quality of Life Full rehabilitation is achieved in the majority of patients who survive the early postoperative months and escape chronic rejection or unmanageable infection. Psychosocial maladjustment interferes with medical compliance in a small number of patients, but most manage to adhere to immunosuppressive regimens, which must be continued indefinitely. In one study, 85% of patients who survived their transplants returned to gainful activities. In fact, some women have conceived and carried pregnancies to term after transplantation without demonstrable injury to their infants.

BIBLIOGRAPHY

ARAYA V et al: Hepatitis C after orthotopic liver transplantation. Gastroenterology 112: 575, 1997

BATTS KP: Acute and chronic hepatic allograft rejection: Pathology and classification. Liver Transpl Surg 5(Suppl 1):S21, 1999

BISMUTH H (ed): Consensus conference on indications of liver transplantation. Hepatology 20(Supp):1, 1994

BIZOLLON T et al: Pilot study of the combination of interferon alfa and ribavirin as therapy of recurrent hepatitis C after liver transplantation. Hepatology 26:500, 1997

CHARLTON M et al: Predictors of patient and graft survival following liver transplantation for hepatitis C. Hepatology 28:823, 1998

DAVIES SE et al: Hepatic histological findings after transplantation for chronic hepatitis B virus infection, including a unique pattern of fibrosing cholestatic hepatitis. Hepatology 13:150, 1991

EUROPEAN FK506 MULTICENTRE LIVER STUDY GROUP: Randomised trial comparing tacrolimus (FK506) and cyclosporin in prevention of liver allograft rejection. Lancet 344:423, 1994

FÉRAY C et al: The course of hepatitis C virus infection after liver transplantation. Hepatology 20:1137, 1994

——— et al: Influence of the genotype of hepatitis C virus on the severity of recurrent liver disease after liver transplantation. Gastroenterology 108:1088, 1995

——— et al: European collaborative study on factors influencing outcome after liver transplantation for hepatitis C. Gastroenterology 117:619, 1999

GANE EJ et al: Long-term outcome of hepatitis C infection after liver transplantation. N Engl J Med 334:815, 1996

GRELLIER L et al: Lamivudine prophylaxis against reinfection in liver transplantation for hepatitis B cirrhosis. Lancet 348:1212, 1996

HOOFNAGLE JH et al: Liver transplantation for alcoholic liver disease: Executive statement and recommendations. Liver Transpl Surg 3:347, 1997

MARKOWITZ JS et al: Prophylaxis against hepatitis B recurrence following liver transplantation using combination lamivudine and hepatitis B immune globulin. Hepatology 28:585, 1998

MAZZAFERRO V et al: Liver transplantation for the treatment of small hepatocellular carcinoma in patients with cirrhosis. N Engl J Med 334:693, 1996

OSORIO RW et al: Predicting recidivism after orthotopic liver transplantation for alcoholic liver disease. Hepatology 20:105, 1994

PERRILLO R et al: Multicenter study of lamivudine therapy for hepatitis B after liver transplantation. Hepatology 29:1581, 1999

POTERUCHA JJ et al: Liver transplantation and hepatitis B. Ann Intern Med 126:805, 1997

PRUETT TL: Improved clinical outcomes with liver transplantation for hepatitis B-induced chronic liver failure using passive immunization. Ann Surg 227:841, 1998

SAMUEL D et al: Liver transplantation in European patients with the hepatitis B surface antigen. N Engl J Med 329:1842, 1993

STARZL TE et al: Liver transplantation. N Engl J Med 321:1014, 1989

TIPPLES GA et al: Mutation in HBV RNA-dependent DNA polymerase confers resistance to lamivudine in vivo. Hepatology 24:714, 1996

U.S. MULTICENTER FK506 LIVER STUDY GROUP: A comparison of tacrolimus (FK506) and cyclosporine for immunosuppression in liver transplantation. N Engl J Med 331: 1110, 1994

WADE JJ et al: Bacterial and fungal infections after liver transplantation: An analysis of 284 patients. Hepatology 21:1328, 1995

WRIGHT TL et al: Interferon-α therapy for hepatitis C infection after liver transplantation. Hepatology 20:773, 1994

ZETTERMAN RK (guest ed): Long-term management of the liver transplant patient. Semin Liver Dis 15:123, 1995

---

302 *Norton J. Greenberger, Gustav Paumgartner*

DISEASES OF THE GALLBLADDER AND BILE DUCTS

BSEP bile salt export pump	**OCG** oral cholecystography
CBD common bile duct	**PFIC** progressive familial
CCK cholecystokinin	intrahepatic cholestasis
CDCA chenodeoxycholic acid	**PTHC** percutaneous transhepatic
CT computed tomography	cholangiography
EBS endoscopic biliary	**RUQ** right upper quadrant
sphincterotomy	**UDCA** ursodeoxycholic acid
ERCP endoscopic retrograde	
cholangiopancreatography	

PHYSIOLOGY OF BILE PRODUCTION AND FLOW
Bile Secretion and Composition Bile formed in the hepatic lobules is secreted into a complex network of canaliculi, small bile ductules, and larger bile ducts that run with lymphatics and branches of the portal vein and hepatic artery in portal tracts situated between hepatic lobules. These interlobular bile ducts coalesce to form larger septal bile ducts that join to form the right and left hepatic ducts, which in turn unite to form the common hepatic duct. The common hepatic duct is joined by the cystic duct of the gallbladder to form the common bile duct (CBD), which enters the duodenum (often after joining the main pancreatic duct) through the ampulla of Vater.

Hepatic bile is an isotonic fluid with an electrolyte composition resembling blood plasma. The electrolyte composition of gallbladder bile differs from that of hepatic bile because most of the inorganic anions, chloride and bicarbonate, have been removed by reabsorption across the gallbladder epithelium.

Major components of bile by weight include water (82%), bile acids (12%), lecithin and other phospholipids (4%), and unesterified cholesterol (0.7%). Other constituents include conjugated bilirubin, proteins (IgA, metabolites of hormones, and other proteins metabolized in the liver), electrolytes, mucus, and, often, drugs and their metabolites.

The total daily basal secretion of hepatic bile is approximately 500 to 600 mL. Many substances taken up or synthesized by the hepatocyte are secreted into the bile canalculi. The canalicular membrane forms microvilli and is associated with microfilaments of actin, microtubules, and other contractile elements. Prior to their secretion into the bile, many substances that are taken up into the hepatocyte are conjugated, while others such as phospholipids, a portion of primary bile acids, and some cholesterol are synthesized de novo in the hepatocyte. Three mechanisms are important in regulating bile flow: (1) active transport of bile acids from hepatocytes into the bile canaliculi, (2) active transport of other organic anions, and (3) cholangiocellular secretion. The last is a secretin-mediated and cyclic AMP–dependent mechanism that ultimately results in the secretion of a sodium- and bicarbonate-rich fluid into the bile ducts.

Active vectorial secretion of biliary constituents from the portal blood into the bile canaliculi is driven by a distinct set of polarized transport systems at the basolateral (sinusoidal) and the canalicular plasma membrane domains of the hepatocyte. Two sinusoidal bile salt uptake systems have been cloned in humans, the Na^+/taurocholate co-transporter and the organic anion transporting protein, which also transports a large variety of non-bile salt organic anions. Four ATP-dependent canalicular transport systems ("export pumps") have been identified: a bile salt export pump (BSEP), which was formerly called "sister of P-glycoprotein"; a conjugate export pump (MRP2), also called the canalicular multispecific organic anion transporter, which mediates the canalicular excretion of various amphiphilic conjugates formed by phase II conjugation (e.g., bilirubin diglucuronide); a multidrug export pump (MDR1) for hydrophobic cationic compounds; and a phospholipid export pump (MDR3). The canalicular membrane also contains ATP-independent transport systems such as the Cl^-/HCO_3^- anion exchanger isoform 2 for canalicular bicarbonate secretion. For some of these transporters, genetic defects have been identified that are associated with various forms of cholestasis or defects of biliary excretion. BSEP is defective in progressive familial intrahepatic cholestasis (PFIC) type 2. Mutations of MRP2 cause the Dubin-Johnson syndrome, an inherited form of conjugated hyperbilirubinemia. A defective MDR3 results in PFIC-3. The cystic fibrosis transmembrane regulator located on bile duct epithelial cells is defective in cystic fibrosis, which may be associated with impaired cholangiocellular bile formation and chronic cholestatic liver disease.

The Bile Acids The primary bile acids, cholic acid and chenodeoxycholic acid (CDCA), are synthesized from cholesterol in the liver, conjugated with glycine or taurine, and excreted into the bile. Secondary bile acids, including deoxycholate and lithocholate, are formed in the colon as bacterial metabolites of the primary bile acids. However, lithocholic acid is much less efficiently absorbed from the colon than deoxycholic acid. Another secondary bile acid, found in low concentration is ursodeoxycholic acid (UDCA), a stereoisomer of CDCA. In normal bile, the ratio of glycine to taurine conjugates is about 3:1.

Bile acids are detergents that in aqueous solutions and above a critical concentration of about 2 m*M* form molecular aggregates called *micelles*. Cholesterol alone is poorly soluble in aqueous environments, and its solubility in bile depends on both the total lipid concentration and the relative molar percentages of bile acids and lecithin. Normal ratios of these constituents favor the formation of solubilizing *mixed micelles*, while abnormal ratios promote the precipitation of cholesterol crystals in bile.

In addition to facilitating the biliary excretion of cholesterol, bile acids are necessary for the normal intestinal absorption of dietary fats via a micellar transport mechanism (Chap. 286). Bile acids also serve as a major physiologic driving force for hepatic bile

flow and aid in water and electrolyte transport in the small bowel and colon.

Enterohepatic Circulation Bile acids are efficiently conserved under normal conditions. Unconjugated, and to a lesser degree also conjugated, bile acids are absorbed by *passive diffusion* along the entire gut. Quantitatively much more important for bile salt recirculation, however, is the *active transport* mechanism for conjugated bile acids in the distal ileum (Chap. 286). The reabsorbed bile acids enter the portal bloodstream and are taken up rapidly by hepatocytes, reconjugated, and resecreted into bile (enterohepatic circulation).

The normal bile acid pool size is approximately 2 to 4 g. During digestion of a meal, the bile acid pool undergoes at least one or more enterohepatic cycles, depending on the size and composition of the meal. Normally, the bile acid pool circulates approximately 5 to 10 times daily. Intestinal absorption of the pool is about 95% efficient, so fecal loss of bile acids is in the range of 0.3 to 0.6 g/d. This fecal loss is compensated by an equal daily synthesis of bile acids by the liver, and thus the size of the bile acid pool is maintained. Bile acids returning to the liver suppress de novo hepatic synthesis of primary bile acids from cholesterol by inhibiting the rate-limiting enzyme cholesterol 7α-hydroxylase. While the loss of bile salts in stool is usually matched by increased hepatic synthesis, the maximum rate of synthesis is approximately 5 g/d, which may be insufficient to replete the bile acid pool size when there is pronounced impairment of intestinal bile salt reabsorption.

Gallbladder and Sphincteric Functions In the fasting state, the sphincter of Oddi offers a high-pressure zone of resistance to bile flow from the common bile duct into the duodenum. This tonic contraction serves to (1) prevent reflux of duodenal contents into the pancreatic and bile ducts and (2) promote bile filling of the gallbladder. The major factor controlling the evacuation of the gallbladder is the peptide hormone cholecystokinin (CCK), which is released from the duodenal mucosa in response to the ingestion of fats and amino acids. CCK produces (1) powerful contraction of the gallbladder, (2) decreased resistance of the sphincter of Oddi, (3) increased hepatic secretion of bile, and thus (4) enhanced flow of biliary contents into the duodenum.

Hepatic bile is "concentrated" within the gallbladder by energy-dependent transmucosal absorption of water and electrolytes. Almost the entire bile acid pool may be sequestered in the gallbladder following an overnight fast for delivery into the duodenum with the first meal of the day. The normal capacity of the gallbladder is 30 to 50 mL of bile.

DISEASES OF THE GALLBLADDER

CONGENITAL ANOMALIES Anomalies of the biliary tract may be found in 10 to 20% of the population, including abnormalities in number, size, and shape (e.g., agenesis of the gallbladder, duplications, rudimentary or oversized "giant" gallbladders, and diverticula). Phrygian cap is a clinically innocuous entity in which a partial or complete septum (or fold) separates the fundus from the body. Anomalies of position or suspension are not uncommon and include left-sided gallbladder, intrahepatic gallbladder, retrodisplacement of the gallbladder, and "floating" gallbladder. The latter condition predisposes to acute torsion, volvulus, or herniation of the gallbladder.

GALLSTONES **Pathogenesis** Gallstones are quite prevalent in most western countries. In the United States, autopsy series have shown gallstones in at least 20% of women and in 8% of men over the age of 40. It is estimated that 16 to 20 million persons in the United States have gallstones and that approximately 1 million new cases of cholelithiasis develop each year.

Gallstones are formed by concretion or accretion of normal or abnormal bile constituents. They are divided into three major types; cholesterol and mixed stones account for 80% of the total, with pigment stones comprising the remaining 20%. Mixed and cholesterol gallstones usually contain more than 50% cholesterol monohydrate plus an admixture of calcium salts, bile pigments, proteins, and fatty acids. Pigment stones are composed primarily of calcium bilirubinate; they contain less than 20% cholesterol.

Cholesterol and mixed stones and biliary sludge Cholesterol is essentially water insoluble and requires aqueous dispersion into either micelles or vesicles, both of which require the presence of a second lipid to "liquefy" the cholesterol. Cholesterol and phospholipids are secreted into bile as unilamellar bilayered vesicles, which are converted into mixed micelles consisting of bile acids, phospholipids, and cholesterol by the action of bile acids. If there is an excess of cholesterol in relation to phospholipids and bile acids, unstable cholesterol-rich vesicles remain, which aggregate into large multilamellar vesicles from which cholesterol crystals precipitate (Fig. 302-1).

There are several important mechanisms in the formation of lithogenic (stone-forming) bile. The most important is increased biliary secretion of cholesterol. This may occur in association with obesity, high-caloric and cholesterol-rich diets, or drugs (e.g., clofibrate) and may result from increased activity of HMG-CoA reductase, the rate-limiting enzyme of hepatic cholesterol synthesis, and increased hepatic uptake of cholesterol from blood. In patients with gallstones, dietary cholesterol *increases* biliary cholesterol secretion. This does not occur in non-gallstone patients on high-cholesterol diets. In addition to environmental factors such as high-caloric and cholesterol-rich diets, genetic factors play an important role in cholesterol hypersecretion and gallstone formation. A high prevalence of gallstones is found among first-degree relatives of gallstone carriers and in certain ethnic populations such as American Indians as well as Chilean Indians and Chilean Hispanics. A common genetic trait has been identified for some of these populations by mitochondrial DNA analysis. A genetic defect in the control of cholesterol secretion also exists in certain strains of inbred mice who develop gallstones under a lithogenic diet. In some patients, impaired hepatic conversion of cholesterol to bile acids may also occur, resulting in an increase of the lithogenic cholesterol/bile acid ratio. Lithogenic bile may also result from conditions affecting the enterohepatic circulation of bile acids (e.g., prolonged parenteral alimentation or ileal disease or resection). In addition, most patients with gallstones may have reduced activity of hepatic cholesterol 7α-hydroxylase, the rate-limiting enzyme for primary bile acid synthesis.

Thus an excess of biliary cholesterol in relation to bile acids and phospholipids is primarily due to hypersecretion of cholesterol, but hyposecretion of bile acids may contribute. Two additional disturbances of bile acid metabolism that are likely to contribute to supersaturation of bile with cholesterol are (1) reduction of the bile acid pool and (2) enhanced conversion of cholic acid to deoxycholic acid, with replacement of the cholic acid pool by an expanded deoxycholic acid pool. The first disorder may be caused by more rapid loss of primary bile acid from the small intestine into the colon. The second disturbance may result from enhanced dehydroxylation of cholic acid and increased absorption of newly formed deoxycholic acid. An increased deoxycholate secretion is associated with hypersecretion of cholesterol into bile. While supersaturation of bile with cholesterol is an important prerequisite for gallstone formation, it is not sufficient by itself to produce cholesterol precipitation in vivo. Most people with supersaturated bile do not develop stones because the time required for cholesterol crystals to nucleate and grow is longer than the time bile spends in the gallbladder.

A second important mechanism is *nucleation* of cholesterol monohydrate crystals, which is greatly accelerated in human lithogenic bile; it is this feature rather than the degree of cholesterol supersaturation that distinguishes lithogenic from normal gallbladder bile. Accelerated nucleation of cholesterol monohydrate in bile may be due to either an *excess of pronucleating factors* or a *deficiency of antinucleating factors*. Mucin and certain non-mucin glycoproteins appear to be pronucleating factors, while apolipoproteins AI and AII and other glycoproteins appear to be antinucleating factors. Cholesterol monohydrate

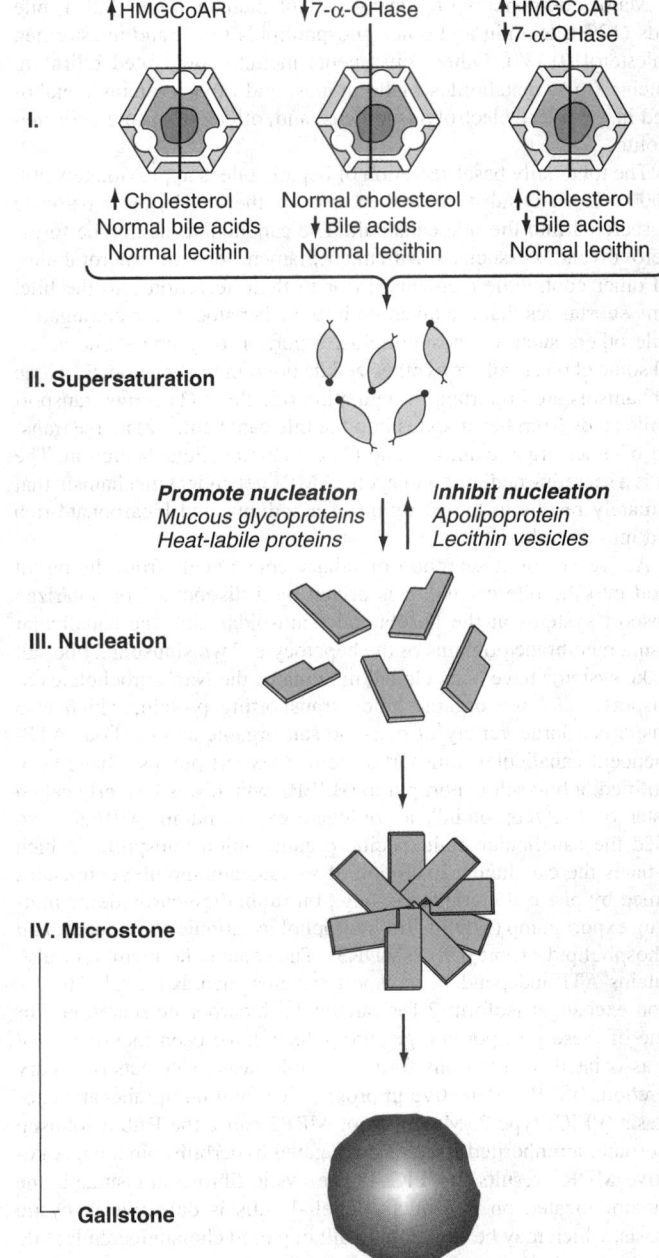

FIGURE 302-1 Scheme showing pathogenesis of gallstone formation. Conditions or factors that increase the ratio of cholesterol to bile acids and lecithin favor gallstone formation (HMG-CoAR, hydroxymethylglutaryl–coenzyme A reductase; 7-α-OHase, cholesterol, 7α-hydroxylase).

crystal nucleation and crystal growth probably occur within the mucin gel layer. Vesicle fusion leads to liquid crystals, which, in turn, nucleate into solid cholesterol monohydrate crystals. Continued growth of the crystals occurs by direct nucleation of cholesterol molecules from supersaturated unilamellar or multilamellar biliary vesicles.

A third important mechanism in cholesterol gallstone formation is *gallbladder hypomotility*. If the gallbladder emptied all supersaturated or crystal-containing bile completely, stones would not be able to grow. A high percentage of patients with gallstones exhibits abnormalities of gallbladder emptying. Ultrasonographic studies show that gallstone patients have an increased gallbladder volume during fasting and also after a test meal (residual volume) and that fractional emptying after gallbladder stimulation is decreased. Gallbladder emptying is a major determinant of gallstone recurrence in patients who underwent biliary lithotripsy. Within 3 years, only 13% of patients with good but 53% of patients with poor gallbladder emptying form recurrent stones.

Cholesterol and Mixed Stones

1. Demographic/genetic factors
   a. Prevalence highest in North American Indians, Chilean Indians, and Chilean Hispanics, greater in Northern Europe and North America than in Asia, lowest in Japan; familial disposition; hereditary aspects
2. Obesity
   a. Normal bile acid pool and secretion but increased biliary secretion of cholesterol
3. Weight loss
   a. Mobilization of tissue cholesterol leads to increased biliary cholesterol secretion while enterohepatic circulation of bile acids is decreased
4. Female sex hormones
   a. Estrogens stimulate hepatic lipoprotein receptors, increase uptake of dietary cholesterol, and increase biliary cholesterol secretion
   b. Natural estrogens, other estrogens, and oral contraceptives lead to decreased bile salt secretion and decreased conversion of cholesterol to cholesteryl esters
5. Ileal disease or resection
   a. Malabsorption of bile acids leads to decreased bile acid pool, and decreased biliary secretion of bile salts
6. Increasing age
   a. Increased biliary secretion of cholesterol, decreased size of bile acid pool, decreased biliary secretion of bile salts
7. Gallbladder hypomotility leading to stasis and formation of sludge
   a. Prolonged parenteral nutrition
   b. Fasting
   c. Pregnancy
   d. Drugs such as octreotide
8. Clofibrate therapy
   a. Increased biliary secretion of cholesterol
9. Decreased bile acid secretion
   a. Primary biliary cirrhosis
   b. Chronic intrahepatic cholestasis
10. Miscellaneous
    a. High-calorie, high-fat diet
    b. Spinal cord injury

Pigment Stones

1. Demographic/genetic factors: Asia, rural setting
2. Chronic hemolysis
3. Alcoholic cirrhosis
4. Chronic biliary tract infection, parasite infestation
5. Increasing age

Biliary sludge is a thick mucous material that upon microscopic examination reveals lecithin-cholesterol crystals, cholesterol monohydrate crystals, calcium bilirubinate, and mucin thread or mucous gels. Biliary sludge typically forms a crescent-like layer in the most dependent portion of the gallbladder and is recognized by characteristic echoes on ultrasonography (see below). The presence of biliary sludge implies two abnormalities: (1) the normal balance between gallbladder mucin secretion and elimination has become deranged and (2) nucleation of biliary solutes has occurred. That biliary sludge may be a precursor form of gallstone disease is evident from several observations. In one study, 96 patients with gallbladder sludge were followed prospectively by serial ultrasound studies. In 18%, biliary sludge disappeared and did not recur for at least 2 years. In 60%, biliary sludge disappeared and reappeared; in 14%, gallstones (8% asymptomatic, 6% symptomatic) developed, and in 6%, severe biliary pain with or without acute pancreatitis occurred. In 12 patients, cholecystectomies were performed, 6 for gallstone-associated biliary pain and 3 in symptomatic patients with sludge but without gallstones who had prior attacks of pancreatitis; the latter did not recur after cholecystectomy. It should be emphasized that biliary sludge can develop with disorders that cause gallbladder hypomotility, i.e., surgery, burns, total parenteral nutrition, pregnancy, and oral contraceptives—all of which are associated with gallstone formation.

Two other conditions are associated with cholesterol stone or biliary sludge formation: pregnancy and very low calorie diet. There appear to be two key changes during pregnancy that contribute to a

"cholelithogenic state." First, the composition of the bile acid pool and the cholesterol-carrying capacity of bile change, with a resultant marked increase in cholesterol saturation during the third trimester. Second, ultrasonographic studies have demonstrated that gallbladder contraction in response to a standard meal is sluggish, resulting in impaired gallbladder emptying. That these changes are related to pregnancy per se is supported by several studies that show reversal of these abnormalities after delivery. During pregnancy, gallbladder sludge develops in 20 to 30% of women and gallstones in 5 to 12%. While biliary sludge is a common finding during pregnancy, it is usually asymptomatic and often resolves spontaneously after delivery. Gallstones, which are less common than sludge and frequently associated with biliary colic, may also disappear after delivery because of spontaneous dissolution related to bile becoming unsaturated with cholesterol post partum.

From 10 to 20% of people having rapid weight reduction through very low calorie dieting develop gallstones. In a study involving 600 patients who completed a 16-week, 520-kcal/d diet, UDCA in a dosage of 600 mg/d proved highly effective in preventing gallstone formation; gallstones developed in only 3% of UDCA recipients compared to 28% of placebo-treated patients.

To summarize, cholesterol gallstone disease occurs because of several defects, which include (1) bile supersaturation with cholesterol, (2) nucleation of cholesterol monohydrate with subsequent crystal retention and stone growth, and (3) abnormal gallbladder motor function with delayed emptying and stasis. Other important factors known to predispose to cholesterol stone formation are summarized in Table 302-1.

Pigment stones   Gallstones composed largely of calcium bilirubinate are much more common in the Far East than in western countries. The presence of increased amounts of unconjugated, insoluble bilirubin in bile results in the precipitation of bilirubin, which may aggregate to form pigment stones or may form the nidus for growth of mixed cholesterol gallstones. In western countries, chronic hemolytic states (with increased conjugated bilirubin in bile) or alcoholic liver disease are associated with an increased incidence of pigment stones. Deconjugation of an excess of soluble bilirubin mono- and diglucuronide may be mediated by endogenous β-glucuronidase but may also occur by spontaneous alkaline hydrolysis. Sometimes, the enzyme is also produced when bile is chronically infected by bacteria. Pigment stone formation is especially prominent in Asians and is often associated with infections in the biliary tree (Table 302-1).

Diagnosis   Procedures of potential use in the diagnosis of cholelithiasis and other diseases of the gallbladder are detailed in Table 302-2. The plain abdominal film may detect gallstones containing sufficient calcium to be radiopaque (10 to 15% of cholesterol and mixed stones and approximately 50% of pigment stones). Plain radiography may also be of use in the diagnosis of emphysematous cholecystitis, porcelain gallbladder, limey bile, and gallstone ileus.

Ultrasonography of the gallbladder is very accurate in the identification of cholelithiasis and has several advantages over oral cholecystography (Fig. 302-2A). The gallbladder is easily visualized with the technique, and in fact, failure to image the gallbladder successfully in a fasting patient correlates well with the presence of underlying gallbladder disease. Stones as small as 2 mm in diameter may be confidently identified provided that firm criteria are used [e.g., acoustic "shadowing" of opacities that are within the gallbladder lumen and that change with the patient's position (by gravity)]. In major medical centers, the false-negative and false-positive rates for ultrasound in gallstone patients are about 2 to 4%. Biliary sludge is material of low echogenic activity that typically forms a layer in the most dependent position of the gallbladder. This layer shifts with postural changes but fails to produce acoustic shadowing; these two characteristics distinguish sludges from gallstones. Ultrasound can also be used to assess the emptying function of the gallbladder.

Oral cholecystography (OCG) is a useful procedure for the diag-

Table 302-2 Diagnostic Evaluation of the Gallbladder

Diagnostic Advantages	Diagnostic Limitations	Comment
PLAIN ABDOMINAL X-RAY		

Low cost
Readily available
	Relatively low yield
	?Contraindicated in pregnancy
		Pathognomonic findings in:
		  Calcified gallstones
		  Limey bile, porcelain GB
		  Emphysematous cholecystitis
		  Gallstone ileus

GALLBLADDER ULTRASOUND		

Rapid
Accurate identification of gallstones
  (>95%)
Simultaneous scanning of GB, liver, bile
  ducts, pancreas
"Real-time" scanning allows assessment
  of GB volume, contractility
Not limited by jaundice, pregnancy
May detect very small stones
	Bowel gas
	Massive obesity
	Ascites
	Recent barium study
		Procedure of choice for detection of stones

RADIOISOTOPE SCANS (HIDA, DIDA, ETC.)		

Accurate identification of cystic duct
  obstruction
Simultaneous assessment of bile ducts
	?Contraindicated in pregnancy
	Serum bilirubin >103–205 μmol/L
	  (6–12 mg/dL)
	Cholecystogram of low resolution
		Indicated for confirmation of suspected acute cholecystitis; less
		sensitive and less specific in chronic cholecystitis; useful in diag-
		nosis of acalculous cholecystopathy, especially if given with CCK
		to assess gallbladder emptying

ORAL CHOLECYSTOGRAM		

Low cost
Readily available
Accurate identification of gallstones
  (90–95%)
Identification of GB anomalies, hyperplastic
  cholecystoses
Identification of chronic GB disease after
  nonvisualization on double dose
	?Contraindicated in pregnancy
	?Contraindicated with history of
	  reaction to iodinated contrast
	Nonvisualization with:
	  Serum bilirubin >34–68 μmol/L
	  (2–4 mg/dL)
	  Failure to ingest or absorb tablets
	  Impaired hepatic excretion
	Very small stones may be undetected
	More time-consuming than GBUS
		Largely replaced by GBUS
		A useful procedure in identification of gallstones if diagnostic limi-
		tations prevent GBUS
		Patency of cystic duct can be evaluated prior to nonsurgical
		therapy

NOTE: GB, gallbladder; CCK, cholecystokinin; GBUS, gallbladder ultrasound.

nosis of gallstones but has been largely replaced by ultrasound. However, OCG is still useful for the selection of patients for nonsurgical
therapy of gallstone disease such as lithotripsy or bile acid dissolution
therapy. In both these settings, OCG is used to assess the patency of
the cystic duct and gallbladder emptying function. Further, OCG can
also delineate the size and number of gallstones and determine whether
they are calcified. Factors that may produce nonvisualization of the
OCG are summarized in Table 302-2.

Radiopharmaceuticals such as ^{99m}Tc-labeled *N*-substituted iminodiacetic acids (HIDA, DIDA, DISIDA, etc.) are rapidly extracted from
the blood and are excreted into the biliary tree in high concentration
even in the presence of mild to moderate serum bilirubin elevations.
Failure to image the gallbladder in the presence of biliary ductal visualization may indicate cystic duct obstruction, acute or chronic cholecystitis, or surgical absence of the organ. Such scans have their greatest application in the diagnosis of acute cholecystitis.

Symptoms of Gallstone Disease Gallstones usually produce
symptoms by causing inflammation or obstruction following their migration into the cystic duct or CBD. The most specific and characteristic symptom of gallstone disease is biliary colic. Obstruction of the
cystic duct or CBD by a stone produces increased intraluminal pressure
and distention of the viscus that cannot be relieved by repetitive biliary
contractions. The resultant visceral pain is characteristically a severe,
steady ache or pressure in the epigastrium or right upper quadrant
(RUQ) of the abdomen with frequent radiation to the interscapular
area, right scapula, or shoulder.

Biliary colic begins quite suddenly and may persist with severe
intensity for 30 min to 5 h, subsiding gradually or rapidly. An episode
of biliary pain is sometimes followed by a residual mild ache or soreness in the RUQ, which may persist for 24 h or so. Nausea and vomiting frequently accompany episodes of biliary colic. An elevated level
of serum bilirubin and/or alkaline phosphatase suggests a common
duct stone. Fever or chills (rigors) with biliary colic usually imply a
complication, i.e., cholecystitis, pancreatitis, or cholangitis. Complaints of vague epigastric fullness, dyspepsia, eructation, or flatulence, especially following a fatty meal, should not be confused with
biliary colic. Such symptoms are frequently elicited from patients with
gallstone disease but are not specific for biliary calculi. Biliary colic
may be precipitated by eating a fatty meal, by consumption of a large
meal following a period of prolonged fasting, or by eating a normal
meal.

Natural History Gallstone disease discovered in an asymptomatic patient or in a patient whose symptoms are not referable to
cholelithiasis is a common clinical problem. The natural history of
"silent" or asymptomatic gallstones has occasioned much debate. A
study of predominantly male silent gallstone patients suggests that the
cumulative risk for the development of symptoms or complications
requiring surgery is relatively low—10% at 5 years, 15% at 10 years,
and 18% at 15 years. Patients remaining asymptomatic for 15 years
were found to be unlikely to develop symptoms during further follow-
up, and most patients who did develop complications from their gallstones experienced *prior* warning symptoms. Similar conclusions apply to diabetic patients with silent gallstones. Decision analysis has
suggested that (1) the cumulative risk of death due to gallstone disease
while on expectant management is small, and (2) prophylactic cholecystectomy is not warranted.

Complications requiring cholecystectomy are much more common
in gallstone patients who have developed symptoms of biliary colic.
Patients found to have gallstones at a young age are more likely to
develop symptoms from cholelithiasis than are patients older than 60
years at the time of initial diagnosis. Patients with diabetes mellitus
and gallstones may be somewhat more susceptible to septic compli-

FIGURE 302-2 Examples of ultrasound and radiologic studies of the biliary tract. *A*. An ultrasound study showing a distended gallbladder containing a single large stone (*arrow*) which casts an acoustic shadow. *B*. Endoscopic retrograde cholangiopancreatogram (ERCP) showing normal biliary tract anatomy. In addition to the endoscope and large vertical gallbladder filled with contrast dye, the common hepatic duct (chd), common bile duct (cbd), and pancreatic duct (pd) are shown. The arrow points to the ampulla of Vater. *C*. Percutaneous transhepatic cholangiogram (PTHC) showing choledocholithiasis. The biliary tract is dilatated and contains multiple radiolucent calculi. *D*. ERCP showing sclerosing cholangitis. The common bile duct shows areas that are strictured and narrowed. (*Reprinted from the Clinical Slide Collection on the Rheumatic Diseases, copyright 1991, 1995, 1997. Used by permission of the American College of Rheumatology.*)

cations, but the magnitude of risk of septic biliary complications in diabetic patients is incompletely defined. In addition, asymptomatic gallstone patients with nonvisualization of the gallbladder on OCG appear to have an increased tendency to develop symptoms and complications.

℞ **TREATMENT** **Surgical Therapy** In asymptomatic gallstone patients, the risk of developing symptoms or complications requiring surgery is quite small (in the range of 1 to 2% per year). Thus a recommendation for cholecystectomy in a patient with gallstones should probably be based on assessment of three factors: (1) the presence of symptoms that are frequent enough or severe enough to interfere with the patient's general routine; (2) the presence of a prior complication of gallstone disease, i.e., history of acute cholecystitis, pancreatitis, gallstone fistula, etc.; or (3) the presence of an underlying condition predisposing the patient to increased risk of gallstone complications (e.g., calcified or porcelain gallbladder and/or a previous attack of acute cholecystitis regardless of current symptomatic status). Patients with very large gallstones (over 2 cm in diameter) and patients having gallstones in a congenitally anomalous gallbladder might also be considered for prophylactic cholecystectomy. Although age under 50 years is a worrisome factor in asymptomatic gallstone patients, few authorities would now recommend routine cholecystectomy in all young patients with silent stones. Laparoscopic cholecystectomy is a minimal-access approach for the removal of the gallbladder together with its stones. Its advantages include a markedly shortened hospital stay as well as decreased cost, and it is the procedure of choice for most patients referred for elective cholecystectomy.

From several studies involving over 4000 patients undergoing laparoscopic cholecystectomy, the following key points emerge: (1) complications develop in about 4% of patients, (2) conversion to laparotomy occurs in 5%, (3) the death rate is remarkably low (i.e., <0.1%), and (4) bile duct injuries are unusual (i.e., 0.2 to 0.5%). These data indicate why laparoscopic cholecystectomy has become the "gold standard" for treating symptomatic cholelithiasis.

Medical Therapy—Gallstone Dissolution UDCA decreases cholesterol saturation of bile and also appears to produce a lamellar liquid crystalline phase in bile that allows a dispersion of cholesterol from stones by physiochemical means. UDCA may also retard cholesterol crystal nucleation. In carefully selected patients with a functioning gallbladder and with radiolucent stones <10 mm in diameter, complete dissolution can be achieved in about 50% of patients within 6 months to 2 years with UDCA at a dose of 8 to 10 mg/kg per day. The highest success rate (i.e., >70%) occurs in patients with small (<5 mm) floating radiolucent gallstones. Probably no more than 10% of patients with *symptomatic* cholelithiasis are candidates for such treatment. However, in addition to the vexing problem of recurrent stones (30 to 50% over 3 to 5 years of follow-up), there is also the factor of taking an expensive drug for an indefinite period of time. The advantages and success of laparoscopic cholecystectomy have largely reduced the role of gallstone dissolution to patients who wish to avoid or are not candidates for elective cholecystectomy.

Gallbladder stones may be fragmented by extracorporeal shock waves. While such shock wave lithotripsy combined with medical litholytic therapy is safe and effective in carefully selected patients with gallbladder calculi (radiolucent, solitary stone <2 cm in well-contracting gallbladder), the procedure is employed infrequently because of the emergence of laparoscopic cholystectomy as the procedure of choice for symptomatic cholelithiasis, the recurrence of gallstones in 30% of patients within 5 years after lithotripsy combined with medical litholytic therapy, and the cost of taking UDCA for a variable period after the procedure.

ACUTE AND CHRONIC CHOLECYSTITIS **Acute Cholecystitis** Acute inflammation of the gallbladder wall usually follows obstruction of the cystic duct by a stone. Inflammatory response can be evoked by three factors: (1) *mechanical inflammation* produced by increased intraluminal pressure and distention with resulting ischemia of the gallbladder mucosa and wall, (2) *chemical inflammation* caused by the release of lysolecithin (due to the action of phospholipase on lecithin in bile) and other local tissue factors, and (3) *bacterial inflammation*, which may play a role in 50 to 85% of patients with acute cholecystitis. The organisms most frequently isolated by culture of gallbladder bile in these patients include *Escherichia coli*, *Klebsiella* spp., group D *Streptococcus*, *Staphylococcus* spp., and *Clostridium* spp.

Acute cholecystitis often begins as an attack of biliary colic that progressively worsens. Approximately 60 to 70% of patients report having experienced prior attacks that resolved spontaneously. As the episode progresses, however, the pain of acute cholecystitis becomes more generalized in the right upper abdomen. As with biliary colic, the pain of cholecystitis may radiate to the interscapular area, right scapula, or shoulder. Peritoneal signs of inflammation such as increased pain with jarring or on deep respiration may be apparent. The patient is anorectic and often nauseated. Vomiting is relatively common and may produce symptoms and signs of vascular and extracellular volume depletion. Jaundice is unusual early in the course of acute cholecystitis but may occur when edematous inflammatory changes involve the bile ducts and surrounding lymph nodes.

A low-grade fever is characteristically present, but shaking chills or rigors are not uncommon. The RUQ of the abdomen is almost invariably tender to palpation. An enlarged, tense gallbladder is palpable in one-quarter to one-half of patients. Deep inspiration or cough during subcostal palpation of the RUQ usually produces increased pain and inspiratory arrest (Murphy's sign). A light blow delivered to the right subcostal area may elicit a marked increase in pain. Localized rebound tenderness in the RUQ is common, as are abdominal distention and hypoactive bowel sounds from paralytic ileus, but generalized peritoneal signs and abdominal rigidity are usually lacking, absent perforation.

The diagnosis of acute cholecystitis is usually made on the basis of a characteristic history and physical examination. The triad of sudden onset of RUQ tenderness, fever, and leukocytosis is highly suggestive. Typically, leukocytosis in the range of 10,000 to 15,000 cells per microliter with a left shift on differential count is found. The serum bilirubin is mildly elevated [<85.5 μmol/L (5 mg/dL)] in 45% of patients, while 25% have modest elevations in serum aminotransferases (usually less than a fivefold elevation). The radionuclide (e.g., HIDA) biliary scan may be confirmatory if bile duct imaging is seen without visualization of the gallbladder. Ultrasound will demonstrate calculi in 90 to 95% of cases.

Approximately 75% of patients treated medically have remission of acute symptoms within 2 to 7 days following hospitalization. In 25%, however, a complication of acute cholecystitis will occur despite conservative treatment (see below). In this setting, prompt surgical intervention is required. Of the 75% of patients with acute cholecystitis who undergo remission of symptoms, approximately one-quarter will experience a recurrence of cholecystitis within 1 year, and 60% will have at least one recurrent bout within 6 years. In view of the natural history of the disease, acute cholecystitis is best treated by early surgery whenever possible.

Acalculous cholecystitis   In 5 to 10% of patients with acute cholecystitis, calculi obstructing the cystic duct are not found at surgery. In over 50% of such cases, an underlying explanation for acalculous inflammation is not found. An increased risk for the development of acalculous cholecystitis is especially associated with serious trauma or burns, with the postpartum period following prolonged labor, and with orthopedic and other nonbiliary major surgical operations in the postoperative period. Other precipitating factors include vasculitis, obstructing adenocarcinoma of the gallbladder, diabetes mellitus, torsion of the gallbladder, "unusual" bacterial infections of the gallbladder (e.g., *Leptospira*, *Streptococcus*, *Salmonella*, or *Vibrio cholerae*), and parasitic infestation of the gallbladder. Acalculous cholecystitis may also be seen with a variety of other systemic disease processes (sarcoidosis, cardiovascular disease, tuberculosis, syphilis, actinomycosis, etc.) and may possibly complicate periods of prolonged parenteral hyperalimentation.

Although the clinical manifestations of acalculous cholecystitis are indistinguishable from those of calculous cholecystitis, the setting of acute gallbladder inflammation complicating severe underlying illness is characteristic of acalculous disease. Ultrasound, computed tomography (CT) scanning, or radionuclide examinations demonstrating a large, tense, static gallbladder without stones and with evidence of poor emptying over a prolonged period may be diagnostically useful in some cases. The complication rate for acalculous cholecystitis exceeds that for calculous cholecystitis. Successful management of acute

acalculous cholecystitis appears to depend primarily on early diagnosis and surgical intervention, with meticulous attention to postoperative care.

Acalculous cholecystopathy   Disordered motility of the gallbladder can produce recurrent biliary pain in patients without gallstones. Infusion of an octapeptide of CCK can be used to measure the gallbladder ejection fraction during cholescintigraphy. In a representative study, CCK cholescintigraphy using ^{99m}Tc-diisopropyl iminodiacetic acid (DIDA) identified 21 patients with an abnormal gallbladder ejection fraction ($<40\%$ at 45 min); 10 of 11 patients who underwent surgery became asymptomatic; all 10 showed abnormalities, i.e., chronic cholecystitis, gallbladder muscle hypertrophy, and/or a markedly narrowed cystic duct. From this and other similar studies, the following criteria can be used to identify patients with acalculous cholecystopathy: (1) recurrent episodes of typical RUQ pain characteristic of biliary tract pain, (2) abnormal CCK cholescintigraphy demonstrating a gallbladder ejection fraction of less than 40%, and (3) infusion of CCK reproduces the patient's pain. An additional clue would be the identification of a large gallbladder on ultrasound examination. Finally, it should be noted that sphincter of Oddi dysfunction can also give rise to recurrent RUQ pain and CCK-scintigraphic abnormalities.

Emphysematous cholecystitis   So-called emphysematous cholecystitis is thought to begin with acute cholecystitis (calculous or acalculous) followed by ischemia or gangrene of the gallbladder wall and infection by gas-producing organisms. Bacteria most frequently cultured in this setting include anaerobes, such as *C. welchii* or *C. perfringens*, and aerobes, such as *E. coli*. This condition occurs most frequently in elderly men and in patients with diabetes mellitus. The clinical manifestations are essentially indistinguishable from those of nongaseous cholecystitis. The diagnosis is usually made on plain abdominal film by the finding of gas within the gallbladder lumen, dissecting within the gallbladder wall to form a gaseous ring, or in the pericholecystic tissues. The morbidity and mortality rates with emphysematous cholecystitis are considerable. Prompt surgical intervention coupled with appropriate antibiotics is mandatory.

Chronic Cholecystitis   Chronic inflammation of the gallbladder wall is almost always associated with the presence of gallstones and is thought to result from repeated bouts of subacute or acute cholecystitis or from persistent mechanical irritation of the gallbladder wall. The presence of bacteria in the bile occurs in more than one-quarter of patients with chronic cholecystitis. Although the presence of infected bile in a patient with *chronic* cholecystitis undergoing elective cholecystectomy probably adds little to the operative risk, intraoperative Gram's staining and routine culturing of bile have been advocated to identify those patients whose gallbladder is colonized with *Clostridium* spp. Appropriate antibiotics intra- and postoperatively are recommended in such patients because colonization with these organisms may be associated with devastating septic complications following surgery. Chronic cholecystitis may be asymptomatic for years, may progress to symptomatic gallbladder disease or to acute cholecystitis, or may present with complications (see below).

Complications of Cholecystitis • *Empyema and hydrops*   Empyema of the gallbladder usually results from progression of acute cholecystitis with persistent cystic duct obstruction to superinfection of the stagnant bile with a pus-forming bacterial organism. The clinical picture resembles that of cholangitis with high fever, severe RUQ pain, marked leukocytosis, and often, prostration. Empyema of the gallbladder carries a high risk of gram-negative sepsis and/or perforation. Emergency surgical intervention with proper antibiotic coverage is required as soon as the diagnosis is suspected.

Hydrops or mucocele of the gallbladder may also result from prolonged obstruction of the cystic duct, usually by a large solitary calculus. In this instance, the obstructed gallbladder lumen is progressively distended, over a period of time, by mucus (mucocele) or by a clear transudate (hydrops) produced by mucosal epithelial cells. A visible, easily palpable, nontender mass sometimes extending from the RUQ into the right iliac fossa may be found on physical examination.

The patient with hydrops of the gallbladder frequently remains asymptomatic, although chronic RUQ pain may also occur. Cholecystectomy is indicated, since empyema, perforation, or gangrene may complicate the condition.

Gangrene and perforation Gangrene of the gallbladder results from ischemia of the wall and patchy or complete tissue necrosis. Underlying conditions often include marked distention of the gallbladder, vasculitis, diabetes mellitus, empyema, or torsion resulting in arterial occlusion. Gangrene usually predisposes to perforation of the gallbladder, but perforation may also occur in chronic cholecystitis without premonitory warning symptoms. *Localized perforations* are usually contained by the omentum or by adhesions produced by recurrent inflammation of the gallbladder. Bacterial superinfection of the walled-off gallbladder contents results in abscess formation. Most patients are best treated with cholecystectomy, but some seriously ill patients may be managed with cholecystostomy and drainage of the abscess. *Free perforation* is less common but is associated with a mortality rate of approximately 30%. Such patients may experience a sudden transient relief of RUQ pain as the distended gallbladder decompresses; this is followed by signs of generalized peritonitis.

Fistula formation and gallstone ileus *Fistulization* into an adjacent organ adherent to the gallbladder wall may result from inflammation and adhesion formation. Fistulas into the duodenum are most common, followed in frequency by those involving the hepatic flexure of the colon, stomach or jejunum, abdominal wall, and renal pelvis. Clinically "silent" biliary-enteric fistulas occurring as a complication of chronic cholecystitis have been found in up to 5% of patients undergoing cholecystectomy. Asymptomatic cholecystoenteric fistulas may sometimes be diagnosed by finding gas in the biliary tree on plain abdominal films. Barium contrast studies or endoscopy of the upper gastrointestinal tract or colon may demonstrate the fistula. Treatment in the symptomatic patient usually consists of cholecystectomy, CBD exploration, and closure of the fistulous tract.

Gallstone ileus refers to mechanical intestinal obstruction resulting from the passage of a large gallstone into the bowel lumen. The stone customarily enters the duodenum through a cholecystoenteric fistula at that level. The site of obstruction by the impacted gallstone is usually at the ileocecal valve, provided that the more proximal small bowel is of normal caliber. The majority of patients do not give a history of either prior biliary tract symptoms or complaints suggestive of acute cholecystitis or fistulization. Large stones over 2.5 cm in diameter are thought to predispose to fistula formation by gradual erosion through the gallbladder fundus. Diagnostic confirmation may occasionally be found on the plain abdominal film (e.g., small-intestinal obstruction with gas in the biliary tree and a calcified, ectopic gallstone) or following an upper gastrointestinal series (cholecystoduodenal fistula with small-bowel obstruction at the ileocecal valve). Laparotomy with stone extraction (or propulsion into the colon) remains the procedure of choice to relieve obstruction. Evacuation of large stones within the gallbladder should also be performed. In general, the gallbladder and its attachment to the intestines should be left alone.

Limey (milk of calcium) bile and porcelain gallbladder Calcium salts may be secreted into the lumen of the gallbladder in sufficient concentration to produce calcium precipitation and diffuse, hazy opacification of bile or a layering effect on plain abdominal roentgenography. This so-called limey bile, or milk of calcium bile, is usually clinically innocuous, but cholecystectomy is recommended because limey bile most often occurs in a hydropic gallbladder. In the entity called *porcelain gallbladder*, calcium salt deposition within the wall of a chronically inflamed gallbladder may be detected on the plain abdominal film. Cholecystectomy is advised in all patients with porcelain gallbladder because in a high percentage of cases this finding appears to be associated with the development of carcinoma of the gallbladder.

℞ **TREATMENT** **Medical Therapy** Although surgical intervention remains the mainstay of therapy for acute cholecystitis and its complications, a period of in-hospital stabilization may be required before cholecystectomy. Oral intake is eliminated, nasogastric suction may be indicated, and extracellular volume depletion and electrolyte abnormalities are repaired. Meperidine or nonsteroidal antiinflammatory drugs (NSAIDs) are usually employed for analgesia because they may produce less spasm of the sphincter of Oddi than drugs such as morphine. Intravenous antibiotic therapy is usually indicated in patients with severe acute cholecystitis even though bacterial superinfection of bile may not have occurred in the early stages of the inflammatory process. Postoperative complications of wound infection, abscess formation, or sepsis are reduced in antibiotic-treated patients. Effective antibiotics include ureidopenicillins, ampicillin, metronidazole, and cephalosporins. Combination with an aminoglycoside or other antibiotics may be considered in diabetic or debilitated patients and in those with signs of gram-negative sepsis (Chap. 134).

Surgical Therapy The optimal timing of surgical intervention in patients with acute cholecystitis depends on stabilization of the patient. The clear trend is toward earlier surgery, and this is due in part to requirements for shorter hospital stays. Urgent (emergency) cholecystectomy or cholecystostomy is probably appropriate in most patients in whom a complication of acute cholecystitis such as empyema, emphysematous cholecystitis, or perforation is suspected or confirmed. In uncomplicated cases of acute cholecystitis, up to 30% of patients fail to resolve their symptoms on appropriate medical therapy, and progression of the attack or a supervening complication leads to the performance of early operation (within 24 to 72 h). The technical complications of surgery are not increased in patients undergoing early as opposed to delayed cholecystectomy. Delayed surgical intervention is probably best reserved for (1) patients in whom the overall medical condition imposes an unacceptable risk for early surgery and (2) patients in whom the diagnosis of acute cholecystitis is in doubt. Early cholecystectomy is the treatment of choice for most patients with acute cholecystitis. Mortality figures for emergency cholecystectomy in most centers approach 3%, while the mortality risk for elective or early cholecystectomy approximates 0.5% in patients under age 60. Of course, the operative risks increase with age-related diseases of other organ systems and with the presence of long- or short-term complications of gallbladder disease. Seriously ill or debilitated patients with cholecystitis may be managed with cholecystostomy and tube drainage of the gallbladder. Elective cholecystectomy may then be done at a later date.

Postcholecystectomy Complications Early complications following cholecystectomy include atelectasis and other pulmonary disorders, abscess formation (often subphrenic), external or internal hemorrhage, biliary-enteric fistula, and bile leaks. Jaundice may indicate absorption of bile from an intraabdominal collection following a biliary leak or mechanical obstruction of the CBD by retained calculi, intraductal blood clots, or extrinsic compression. Routine performance of intraoperative cholangiography during cholecystectomy has helped to reduce the incidence of these early complications.

Overall, cholecystectomy is a very successful operation that provides total or near-total relief of preoperative symptoms in 75 to 90% of patients. The most common cause of persistent postcholecystectomy symptoms is an overlooked extrabiliary disorder (e.g., reflux esophagitis, peptic ulceration, pancreatitis, or—most often—irritable bowel syndrome). In a small percentage of patients, however, a disorder of the extrahepatic bile ducts may result in persistent symptomatology. These so-called postcholecystectomy syndromes may be due to (1) biliary strictures, (2) retained biliary calculi, (3) cystic duct stump syndrome, (4) stenosis or dyskinesia of the sphincter of Oddi, or (5) bile salt–induced diarrhea or gastritis.

Cystic duct stump syndrome In the absence of cholangiographically demonstrable retained stones, symptoms resembling biliary colic or cholecystitis in the postcholecystectomy patient have frequently been attributed to disease in a long (>1 cm) cystic duct remnant (cystic duct stump syndrome). Careful analysis, however, reveals that postcholecystectomy complaints are attributable to other causes in almost all patients in whom the symptom complex was originally thought to result from the existence of a long cystic duct stump. Accordingly, considerable care should be taken to investigate the possible role of other factors in the production of postcholecystectomy symptoms before attributing them to cystic duct stump syndrome.

Papillary dysfunction, papillary stenosis, spasm of the sphincter of Oddi, and biliary dyskinesia   Symptoms of biliary colic accompanied by signs of recurrent, intermittent biliary obstruction may be produced by papillary stenosis, papillary dysfunction, spasm of the sphincter of Oddi, and biliary dyskinesia. Papillary stenosis is thought to result from acute or chronic inflammation of the papilla of Vater or from glandular hyperplasia of the papillary segment. Five criteria have been used to define papillary stenosis: (1) upper abdominal pain, usually RUQ or epigastric; (2) abnormal liver tests; (3) dilatation of the common bile duct upon endoscopic retrograde cholangiopancreatography (ERCP) examination; (4) delayed (>45 min) drainage of contrast material from the duct; and (5) increased basal pressure of the sphincter of Oddi, a finding that may be of only minor significance. An alternative to ERCP is magnetic resonance cholangiography if ERCP and/or biliary manometry are either unavailable or not feasible. In patients with papillary stenosis, quantitative hepatobiliary scintigraphy has revealed delayed transit from the common bile duct to the bowel, ductal dilatation, and abnormal time-activity dynamics. This technique can also be used before and after sphincterotomy to document improvement in biliary emptying. Treatment consists of endoscopic or surgical sphincteroplasty to ensure wide patency of the distal portions of both the bile and pancreatic ducts. The greater the number of the preceding criteria present, the greater the likelihood that a patient does have a degree of papillary stenosis sufficient to justify correction. The factors usually considered as indications for sphincterotomy include (1) prolonged duration of symptoms, (2) lack of response to symptomatic treatment, (3) presence of severe disability, and (4) the patient's choice of sphincterotomy over surgery (given a clear understanding on his or her part of the risks involved in both procedures).

Criteria for diagnosing dyskinesia of the sphincter of Oddi are even more controversial than those for papillary stenosis. Proposed mechanisms include spasm of the sphincter, denervation sensitivity resulting in hypertonicity, and abnormalities of the sequencing or frequency rates of sphincteric contraction waves. When thorough evaluation has failed to demonstrate another cause for the pain, and when cholangiographic and manometric criteria suggest a diagnosis of biliary dyskinesia, medical treatment with nitrites or anticholinergics to attempt pharmacologic relaxation of the sphincter has been proposed. Endoscopic biliary sphincterotomy (EBS) or surgical sphincteroplasty may be indicated in patients who fail to respond to a 2- to 3-month trial of medical therapy, especially if basal sphincter of Oddi pressures are elevated. EBS has become a well-established procedure for removing bile duct stones and for other biliary and pancreatic problems. Approximately 150,000 such procedures are performed annually in the United States. Key findings in a recent study of EBS include: (1) Dysfunction of the sphincter of Oddi was the most frequent patient-related risk factor for complications; (2) pancreatitis was more frequent in young patients; (3) difficulty in cannulating the bile duct and the use of "precut" sphincterotomy were important technique-related risk factors for complications; and (4) experience in the volume of procedures proved to be important; endoscopists who perform more than one EBS per week had lower complication rates than endoscopists who performed a smaller number of procedures.

Bile salt–induced diarrhea and gastritis   Postcholecystectomy patients may develop symptoms and signs of gastritis, which has been attributed to duodenogastric reflux of bile. However, firm data linking an increased incidence of bile gastritis with surgical removal of the gallbladder are lacking. Cholecystectomy induces persistent changes in gut transit, and these changes effect a noticeable modification of bowel habits. Cholecystectomy shortens gut transit time by accel-

erating passage of the fecal bolus through the colon with marked acceleration in the right colon, thus causing an increase in colonic bile acid output and a shift in bile acid composition toward the more diarrheagenic secondary bile acids. Diarrhea that is severe enough, i.e., three or more watery movements per day, can be classified as postcholecystectomy diarrhea, and this occurs in 8 to 12% of patients undergoing elective cholecystectomy. Treatment with a bile acid sequestering agent, such as cholestyramine, is often effective in ameliorating troublesome diarrhea.

THE HYPERPLASTIC CHOLECYSTOSES   The term *hyperplastic cholecystoses* is used to denote a group of disorders of the gallbladder characterized by excessive proliferation of normal tissue components.

Adenomyomatosis is characterized by a benign proliferation of gallbladder surface epithelium with glandlike formations, extramural sinuses, transverse strictures, and/or fundal nodule ("adenoma" or "adenomyoma") formation. Outpouchings of mucosa termed *Rokitansky-Aschoff sinuses* may be seen on oral cholecystography in conjunction with hyperconcentration of contrast medium. Characteristic dimpled filling defects also may be seen.

Cholesterolosis is characterized by abnormal deposition of lipid, especially cholesterol esters, in the lamina propria of the gallbladder wall. In its diffuse form ("strawberry gallbladder"), the gallbladder mucosa is brick red and speckled with bright yellow flecks of lipid. The localized form shows solitary or multiple "cholesterol polyps" studding the gallbladder wall. Cholesterol stones of the gallbladder are found in nearly half the cases. Cholecystectomy is indicated in both adenomyomatosis and cholesterolosis when symptomatic or when cholelithiasis is present.

DISEASES OF THE BILE DUCTS

CONGENITAL ANOMALIES   **Biliary Atresia and Hypoplasia**   Atretic and hypoplastic lesions of the extrahepatic and major intrahepatic bile ducts are the most common biliary anomalies of clinical relevance encountered in infancy. The clinical picture is one of severe obstructive jaundice during the first month of life, with pale stools. The diagnosis is confirmed by surgical exploration with operative cholangiography. Approximately 10% of cases of biliary atresia are treatable with roux-en-Y choledochojejunostomy, with the Kasai procedure (hepatic portoenterostomy) being attempted in the remainder in an effort to restore some bile flow. Most patients, even those having successful biliary-enteric anastomoses, eventually develop chronic cholangitis, extensive hepatic fibrosis, and portal hypertension.

Choledochal Cysts   Cystic dilatation may involve the free portion of the CBD, i.e., choledochal cyst, or may present as diverticulum formation in the intraduodenal segment. In the latter situation, chronic reflux of pancreatic juice into the biliary tree can produce inflammation and stenosis of the extrahepatic bile ducts leading to cholangitis or biliary obstruction. Because the process may be gradual, approximately 50% of patients present with onset of symptoms after age 10. The diagnosis may be made by ultrasound, abdominal CT, or cholangiography. Only one-third of patients show the classic triad of abdominal pain, jaundice, and an abdominal mass. Ultrasonographic detection of a cyst separate from the gallbladder should suggest the diagnosis of choledochal cyst, which can be confirmed by demonstrating the entrance of extrahepatic bile ducts into the cyst. Surgical treatment involves excision of the "cyst" and biliary-enteric anastomosis. Patients with choledochal cysts are at increased risk for the subsequent development of cholangiocarcinoma.

Congenital Biliary Ectasia   Cystic dilatation of the intrahepatic bile ducts may involve either the major intrahepatic radicles (Caroli's disease), the inter- and intralobular ducts (congenital hepatic fibrosis), or both. In Caroli's disease, clinical manifestations include recurrent cholangitis, abscess formation in and around the affected ducts, and, sometimes, gallstone formation within portions of ectatic intrahepatic biliary radicles. The CT scan and cholangiographic patterns are usually diagnostic, and treatment with ongoing antibiotic therapy is usually undertaken in an effort to limit the frequency and severity of recurrent bouts of cholangitis. Progression to secondary biliary cirrhosis with portal hypertension, amyloidosis, extrahepatic biliary obstruction, cholangiocarcinoma, or recurrent episodes of sepsis with hepatic abscess formation is common.

CHOLEDOCHOLITHIASIS **Pathophysiology and Clinical Manifestations** Passage of gallstones into the CBD occurs in approximately 10 to 15% of patients with cholelithiasis. The incidence of common duct stones increases with increasing age of the patient, so that up to 25% of elderly patients may have calculi in the common duct at the time of cholecystectomy. Undetected duct stones are left behind in approximately 1 to 5% of cholecystectomy patients. The overwhelming majority of bile duct stones are cholesterol or mixed stones formed in the gallbladder, which then migrate into the extrahepatic biliary tree through the cystic duct. Primary calculi arising de novo in the ducts are usually pigment stones developing in patients with (1) chronic hemolytic diseases; (2) hepatobiliary parasitism or chronic, recurrent cholangitis; (3) congenital anomalies of the bile ducts (especially Caroli's disease); or (4) dilated, sclerosed, or strictured ducts. Common duct stones may remain asymptomatic for years, may pass spontaneously into the duodenum, or (most often) may present with biliary colic or a complication.

Complications • *Cholangitis* Cholangitis may be acute or chronic, and symptoms result from inflammation, which usually requires at least partial obstruction to the flow of bile. Bacteria are present on bile culture in approximately 75% of patients with acute cholangitis early in the symptomatic course. The characteristic presentation of acute cholangitis involves biliary colic, jaundice, and spiking fevers with chills (Charcot's triad). Blood cultures are frequently positive, and leukocytosis is typical. *Nonsuppurative* acute cholangitis is most common and may respond relatively rapidly to supportive measures and to treatment with antibiotics. In *suppurative* acute cholangitis, however, the presence of pus under pressure in a completely obstructed ductal system leads to symptoms of severe toxicity—mental confusion, bacteremia, and septic shock. Response to antibiotics alone in this setting is relatively poor, multiple hepatic abscesses are often present, and the mortality rate approaches 100% unless prompt endoscopic or surgical relief of the obstruction and drainage of infected bile are carried out. Endoscopic management of bacterial cholangitis is as effective as surgical intervention. ERCP with endoscopic sphincterotomy is safe and the preferred initial procedure for both establishing a definitive diagnosis and providing effective therapy.

Obstructive jaundice Gradual obstruction of the CBD over a period of weeks or months usually leads to initial manifestations of jaundice or pruritus without associated symptoms of biliary colic or cholangitis. Painless jaundice may occur in patients with choledocholithiasis, but this manifestation is much more characteristic of biliary obstruction secondary to malignancy of the head of the pancreas, bile ducts, or ampulla of Vater.

In patients whose obstruction is secondary to choledocholithiasis, associated chronic calculous cholecystitis is very common, and the gallbladder in this setting may be relatively indistensible. The absence of a palpable gallbladder in most patients with biliary obstruction from duct stones is the basis for *Courvoisier's law*, i.e., that the presence of a palpably enlarged gallbladder suggests that the biliary obstruction is secondary to an underlying malignancy rather than to calculous disease. Biliary obstruction causes progressive dilatation of the intrahepatic bile ducts as intrabiliary pressures rise. Hepatic bile flow is suppressed, and regurgitation of conjugated bilirubin into the bloodstream leads to jaundice accompanied by dark urine (bilirubinuria) and light-colored (acholic) stools.

CBD stones should be suspected in any patient with cholecystitis whose serum bilirubin level exceeds 85.5 μmol/L (5 mg/dL). The maximum bilirubin level is seldom over 256.5 μmol/L (15.0 mg/dL) in patients with choledocholithiasis unless concomitant hepatic disease or another factor leading to marked hyperbilirubinemia exists. Serum bilirubin levels of 342.0 μmol/L (20 mg/dL) or more should suggest the possibility of neoplastic obstruction. The serum alkaline phospha-

tase level is almost always elevated in biliary obstruction. A rise in alkaline phosphatase often precedes clinical jaundice and may be the only abnormality in routine liver function tests. There may be a two- to tenfold elevation of serum aminotransferases, especially in association with acute obstruction. Following relief of the obstructing process, serum aminotransferase elevations usually return rapidly to normal, while the serum bilirubin level may take 1 to 2 weeks to return to normal. The alkaline phosphatase level usually falls slowly, lagging behind the decrease in serum bilirubin.

Pancreatitis The most common associated entity discovered in patients with nonalcoholic acute pancreatitis is biliary tract disease. Biochemical evidence of pancreatic inflammation complicates acute cholecystitis in 15% of cases and choledocholithiasis in over 30%, and the common factor appears to be the passage of gallstones through the common duct. Coexisting pancreatitis should be suspected in patients with symptoms of cholecystitis who develop (1) back pain or pain to the left of the abdominal midline, (2) prolonged vomiting with paralytic ileus, or (3) a pleural effusion, especially on the left side. Surgical treatment of gallstone disease is usually associated with resolution of the pancreatitis.

Secondary biliary cirrhosis Secondary biliary cirrhosis may complicate prolonged or intermittent duct obstruction with or without recurrent cholangitis. Although this complication may be seen in patients with choledocholithiasis, it is more common in cases of prolonged obstruction from stricture or neoplasm. Once established, secondary biliary cirrhosis may be progressive even after correction of the obstructing process, and increasingly severe hepatic cirrhosis may lead to portal hypertension or to hepatic failure and death. Prolonged biliary obstruction may also be associated with clinically relevant deficiencies of the fat-soluble vitamins A, D, and K.

Diagnosis and Treatment The diagnosis of choledocholithiasis is usually made by cholangiography (Table 302-3), either preoperatively by ERCP or intraoperatively at the time of cholecystectomy. As many as 15% of patients undergoing cholecystectomy will prove to have CBD stones. With the advent of laparoscopic cholecystectomy, the management of CBD stones in the presence of gallstones is gradually being clarified. Preoperative ERCP with endoscopic papillotomy and stone extraction is the preferred approach. It not only provides stone clearance but also defines the anatomy of the biliary tree in relationship to the cystic duct. ERCP is indicated in gallstone patients who have any of the following risk factors: (1) a history of jaundice or pancreatitis, (2) abnormal tests of liver function, and (3) ultrasonographic evidence of a dilated CBD or stones in the duct. Alternatively, if intraoperative cholangiography reveals retained stones, postoperative ERCP can be carried out. The need for preoperative ERCP is expected to decrease further as laparoscopic techniques improve.

The widespread use of laparoscopic cholecystectomy and ERCP has decreased the incidence of complicated biliary tract disease and the need for choledocholithotomy and T-tube drainage of the bile ducts. EBS followed by spontaneous passage or stone extraction is the treatment of choice in the management of patients with common duct stones, especially in elderly or poor-risk patients.

TRAUMA, STRICTURES, AND HEMOBILIA Benign strictures of the extrahepatic bile ducts result from surgical trauma in approximately 95% of cases and occur in about 1 in 500 cholecystectomies. Strictures may present with bile leak or abscess formation in the immediate postoperative period or with biliary obstruction or cholangitis as long as 2 years or more following the inciting trauma. The diagnosis is established by percutaneous or endoscopic cholangiography. Endoscopic brushing of biliary strictures is an effective way to establish the nature of the lesion and is more accurate than bile cytology alone. When positive exfoliative cytology is obtained, the diagnosis of a neoplastic stricture is established. This procedure is especially important in patients with primary sclerosing cholangitis who are predisposed to the development of cholangiocarcinomas. Successful operative correction by a skillful surgeon with duct-to-bowel anas-

Table 302-3 Diagnostic Evaluation of the Bile Ducts

Diagnostic Advantages	Diagnostic Limitations	Contraindications	Complications	Comment
HEPATOBILIARY ULTRASOUND				
Rapid Simultaneous scanning of GB, liver, bile ducts, pancreas Accurate identification of dilated bile ducts Not limited by jaundice, pregnancy Guidance for fine-needle biopsy	Bowel gas Massive obesity Ascites Barium Partial bile duct obstruction Poor visualization of distal CBD	None	None	Initial procedure of choice in investigating possible biliary tract obstruction
COMPUTED TOMOGRAPHY				
Simultaneous scanning of GB, liver, bile ducts, pancreas Accurate identification of dilated bile ducts, masses Not limited by jaundice, gas, obesity, ascites High-resolution image Guidance for fine-needle biopsy	Extreme cachexia Movement artifact Ileus Partial bile duct obstruction High cost May not be readily available	Pregnancy	Reaction to iodinated contrast, if used	Indicated for evaluation of hepatic or pancreatic masses Procedure of choice in investigating possible biliary obstruction if diagnostic limitations prevent HBUS
MAGNETIC RESONANCE CHOLANGIOPANCREATOGRAPHY				
Useful modality for visualizing pancreatic and biliary ducts Can identify pancreatic duct dilatation or stricture, pancreatic duct stenosis, and pancreas divisum Has excellent sensitivity for bile duct dilatation, biliary stricture, and intraductal abnormalities	Cannot offer therapeutic intervention			
PERCUTANEOUS TRANSHEPATIC CHOLANGIOGRAM				
Extremely successful when bile ducts dilated Best visualization of proximal biliary tract Possible separate visualization of obstructed left ductal system Bile cytology/culture Percutaneous transhepatic drainage	Nondilated or sclerosed ducts	Pregnancy Uncorrectable coagulopathy Massive ascites ? Hepatic abscess	Bleeding Hemobilia Bile peritonitis Bacteremia, sepsis	Usually, initial cholangiogram of choice when bile ducts are dilated
ENDOSCOPIC RETROGRADE CHOLANGIOPANCREATOGRAM				
Simultaneous pancreatography Visualization/biopsy of ampulla and duodenum Best visualization of distal biliary tract Bile or pancreatic cytology Endoscopic sphincterotomy and stone removal Biliary manometry Not limited by ascites, coagulopathy, abscess	Gastroduodenal obstruction ? Roux en Y biliary-enteric anastomosis	Pregnancy ? Acute pancreatitis ? Severe cardiopulmonary disease	Pancreatitis Cholangitis, sepsis Infected pancreatic pseudocyst Perforation (rare) Hypoxemia, aspiration	Cholangiogram of choice in: Absence of dilated ducts ? Pancreatic, ampullary or gastroduodenal disease Prior biliary surgery PTHC contraindicated or failed Endoscopic sphincterotomy a treatment possibility

NOTE: GB, gallbladder; CBD, common bile duct; HBUS, hepatobiliary ultrasound; PTHC, percutaneous transhepatic cholangiogram. Intravenous cholangiography is an obsolete technique because 40% of common duct stones are missed and there is poor resolution even with tomography. There are few indications for its use, especially since other cholangiographic techniques are usually available.

tomosis is usually possible, although mortality rates from surgical complications, recurrent cholangitis, or secondary biliary cirrhosis are high.

Hemobilia may follow traumatic or operative injury to the liver or bile ducts, intraductal rupture of a hepatic abscess or aneurysm of the hepatic artery, biliary or hepatic tumor hemorrhage, or mechanical complications of choledocholithiasis or hepatobiliary parasitism. Diagnostic procedures such as liver biopsy, percutaneous transhepatic cholangiography (PTHC), and transhepatic biliary drainage catheter placement may also be complicated by hemobilia. Patients often present with a classic triad of biliary colic, obstructive jaundice, and melena or occult blood in the stools. The diagnosis is sometimes made by cholangiographic evidence of blood clot in the biliary tree, but selective angiographic verification may be required. Although minor episodes of hemobilia may resolve without operative intervention, surgical ligation of the bleeding vessel is frequently required.

EXTRINSIC COMPRESSION OF THE BILE DUCTS

Partial or complete biliary obstruction may sometimes be produced by extrinsic compression of the ducts. The most common cause of this form of obstructive jaundice is carcinoma of the head of the pancreas. Biliary obstruction may also occur as a complication of either acute or chronic pancreatitis or involvement of lymph nodes in the porta hepatis by lymphoma or metastatic carcinoma. The latter should be distinguished from cholestasis resulting from massive replacement of the liver by tumor.

HEPATOBILIARY PARASITISM Infestation of the biliary tract by adult helminths or their ova may produce a chronic, recurrent pyogenic cholangitis with or without multiple hepatic abscesses, ductal stones, or biliary obstruction. This condition is relatively rare but does occur in inhabitants of southern China and elsewhere in Southeast Asia. The organisms most commonly involved are trematodes or flukes, including *Clonorchis sinensis*, *Opisthorchis viverrini* or *O. felineus*, and *Fasciola hepatica*. The biliary tract also may be involved by intraductal migration of adult *Ascaris lumbricoides* from the duodenum or by intrabiliary rupture of hydatid cysts of the liver produced by *Echinococcus* spp. The diagnosis is made by cholangiography and the presence of characteristic ova on stool examination. When obstruction is present, the treatment of choice is laparotomy under antibiotic coverage, with common duct exploration and a biliary drainage procedure. It should be emphasized that in the Far East, one also sees cholangiohepatitis associated with pigment lithiasis, which may, in fact, be more common than cholangitis due to parasites.

SCLEROSING CHOLANGITIS Primary or idiopathic sclerosing cholangitis is characterized by a progressive, inflammatory, sclerosing, and obliterative process affecting the extrahepatic and/or the intrahepatic bile ducts. The disorder occurs in about 70% in association with inflammatory bowel disease, especially ulcerative colitis. It may also be associated (albeit rarely) with multifocal fibrosclerosis syndromes such as retroperitoneal, mediastinal, and/or periureteral fibrosis; Riedel's struma; or pseudotumor of the orbit. In patients with AIDS, cholangiopancreatography may demonstrate a broad range of biliary tract changes as well as pancreatic duct obstruction and occasionally pancreatitis (Chap. 309). Further, biliary tract lesions in AIDS include infection and cholangiopancreatographic changes similar to primary sclerosing cholangitis. Changes noted include: (1) diffuse involvement of intrahepatic bile ducts alone, (2) involvement of both intra- and extrahepatic bile ducts, (3) ampullary stenosis, (4) stricture of the intrapancreatic portion of the common bile duct, and (5) pancreatic duct involvement. Associated infectious organisms include *Cryptosporidium*, *Mycobacterium avium-intracellulare*, cytomegalovirus, *Microsporidia*, and *Isospora*. In addition, acalculous cholecystitis occurs in up to 10% of patients. ERCP sphincterotomy, while not without risk, provides significant pain reduction in patients with AIDS-associated papillary stenosis. Secondary sclerosing cholangitis may occur as a long-term complication of choledocholithiasis, cholangiocarcinoma, operative or traumatic biliary injury, or contiguous inflammatory processes.

Patients with primary sclerosing cholangitis often present with signs and symptoms of chronic or intermittent biliary obstruction: jaundice, pruritus, RUQ abdominal pain, or acute cholangitis. Late in the course, complete biliary obstruction, secondary biliary cirrhosis, hepatic failure, or portal hypertension with bleeding varices may occur. The diagnosis is usually established by finding multifocal, diffusely distributed strictures with intervening segments of normal or dilated ducts, producing a beaded appearance on cholangiography (Fig. 302-2D). The cholangiographic technique of choice in suspected cases is ERCP, since intrahepatic ductal involvement may make PTHC difficult. When a diagnosis of sclerosing cholangitis has been established, a search for associated diseases, especially for chronic inflammatory bowel disease, should be carried out.

A recent study describes the natural history and outcome for 305 patients of Swedish descent with primary sclerosing cholangitis; 134 (44%) of the patients were asymptomatic at the time of diagnosis and, not surprisingly, had a significantly higher survival rate with a median follow-up time of 63 months. The independent predictors of a bad prognosis were age, serum bilirubin concentration, and liver histologic changes. Cholangiocarcinoma was found in 24 patients (8%). Inflammatory bowel disease was closely associated with primary sclerosing cholangitis and had a prevalence of 81% in this study population.

℞ **TREATMENT** Therapy with cholestyramine may help control symptoms of pruritus, and antibiotics are useful when cholangitis complicates the clinical picture. Vitamin D and calcium supplementation may help prevent the loss of bone mass frequently seen in patients with chronic cholestasis. Glucocorticoids, methotrexate, and cyclosporine have not been shown to be efficacious. UDCA improves serum liver tests, but an effect on survival has not been documented. In cases where complete or high-grade biliary obstruction (dominant strictures) has occurred, balloon dilatation, stenting, or (rarely) surgical intervention may be appropriate. Efforts at biliary-enteric anastomosis or stent placement may, however, be complicated by recurrent cholangitis and further progression of the stenosing process. The role of colectomy in patients with sclerosing cholangitis complicating chronic ulcerative colitis is uncertain. The prognosis is unfavorable, with a median survival of 9 to 12 years following the diagnosis, regardless of therapy. Four variables (age, serum bilirubin level, histologic stage, and splenomegaly) predict survival in patients with primary sclerosing cholangitis and serve as the basis for a risk score. Primary sclerosing cholangitis is one of the most common indications for liver transplantation.

In two large studies involving 627 and 3147 patients, the prevalence of gallbladder polyps was 6.7 and 6.9%, respectively, with a marked male predominance. Few significant changes occurred over a 5-year period in asymptomatic patients in whom gallbladder polyps <10 mm in diameter were found. If polyps >10 mm are present and show rapid growth, cholecystectomy should be considered.

ACKNOWLEDGMENT

This chapter was written by Dr. Norton J. Greenberger and Dr. Kurt J. Isselbacher in the previous edition.

BIBLIOGRAPHY

AFDHAL NH et al: Mucin-vesicle interaction in model bile: Evidence for vesicle aggregation and fusion before cholesterol crystal formation. Hepatology 22:856, 1995

APSETEIN MD, CAREY MC: Pathogenesis of cholesterol gallstones: A parsimonious hypothesis. Eur J Clin Invest 26:343, 1996

BERR F et al: 7-Alpha-dehydroxylating bacteria enhance deoxycholic acid input and cholesterol saturation of bile in patients with gallstones. Gastroenterology 111:1611, 1996

BROOME V et al: Natural history and prognostic factors in 305 Swedish patients with primary sclerosing cholangitis. Gut 38:610, 1996

DICKSON ER: Primary sclerosing cholangitis: Refinement and validation of survival models. Gastroenterology 103:1893, 1992

FORT JM et al: Bowel habit after cholecystectomy: Physiologic changes and clinical implications. Gastroenterology 111:617, 1996

FREEMAN ML et al: Complications of endoscopic biliary sphincterotomy. N Engl J Med 335:909, 1996

GEENEN JE et al: The efficacy of endoscopic sphincterotomy after cholecystectomy in patients with sphincter-of-Oddi dysfunction. N Engl J Med 320:82, 1989

HOLZKNECHT N et al: Breath-hold MR cholangiography using snapshot techniques: A prospective comparison with endoscopic cholangiography. Radiology 206:657, 1998

JOHNSTON DE, KAPLAN MM: Medical progress: Pathogenesis and treatment of gallstones. N Engl J Med 328:412, 1993

MARINGHINI A et al: Gallstones, gallbladder cancer, and other gastrointestinal malignancies: An epidemiologic study in Rochester, Minnesota. Ann Intern Med 107:30, 1987

MAY GR et al: Efficacy of bile acid therapy for gallstone dissolution: A meta-analysis of randomized trials. Aliment Pharmacol Ther 7:139, 1993

MCMAHON AG et al: Laparoscopic versus minilaparotomy cholecystectomy: A randomized trial. Lancet 343:135, 1994

MIQUEL JF et al: Genetic epidemiology of cholesterol cholelithiasis among Chilean Hispanics, American Indians and Maoris. Gastroenterology 115:937, 1998

PAULETZKI J et al: Gallbladder emptying and gallstone formation: A prospective study on gallstone recurrence. Gastroenterology 111:765, 1996

RANSOHOFF DF, GRACIE WA: Treatment of gallstones. Ann Intern Med 119:606, 1993

SARIN SK et al: High familial prevalence of gallstones in the first degree relatives of gallstone patients. Hepatology 22:138, 1995

SHIFFMAN M et al: Prophylaxis against gallstone formation with ursodeoxycholic acid in patients. Ann Intern Med 122:999, 1995

STRASBERG SM: Cholelithiasis and acute cholecystitis. Baillieres Clin Gastroenterol 22: 643, 1997

TRAUNER M et al: Molecular pathogenesis of cholestasis. N Engl J Med 339:1217, 1998

Section 3
DISORDERS OF THE PANCREAS

303   *Phillip P. Toskes, Norton J. Greenberger*

APPROACH TO THE PATIENT WITH PANCREATIC DISEASE

GENERAL CONSIDERATIONS

Inflammatory disease of the pancreas may be acute or chronic. Although good data exist concerning the frequency of acute pancreatitis (about 5000 new cases per year in the United States, with a mortality rate of about 10%), the number of patients who suffer with recurrent acute pancreatitis or chronic pancreatitis is largely undefined. Only one prospective study on the incidence of chronic pancreatitis is available; it showed an incidence of 8.2 new cases per 100,000 per year and a prevalence of 26.4 cases per 100,000. These numbers probably underestimate considerably the true incidence and prevalence, because non-alcohol-induced pancreatitis was largely ignored. At autopsy, the prevalence of chronic pancreatitis ranges from 0.04 to 5%. The relative inaccessibility of the pancreas to direct examination and the nonspecificity of the abdominal pain associated with pancreatitis make the diagnosis of pancreatitis difficult and usually dependent on elevation of blood amylase levels. Many patients with chronic pancreatitis do not have elevated blood amylase levels. Some patients with chronic pancreatitis develop signs and symptoms of pancreatic exocrine insufficiency, and thus objective evidence for pancreatic disease can be demonstrated. However, there is a very large reservoir of pancreatic exocrine function. More than 90% of the pancreas must be damaged before maldigestion of fat and protein is manifested. Even the secretin stimulation test, which is the most sensitive method of assessing pancreatic exocrine function, is probably abnormal only when more than 60% of exocrine function has been lost. Noninvasive, indirect tests of pancreatic exocrine function (bentiromide, serum trypsinogen) are much more likely to give abnormal results in patients with obvious pancreatic disease, i.e., pancreatic calcification, steatorrhea, or diabetes mellitus, than in patients with occult disease. Thus, the number of patients who have subclinical exocrine dysfunction (less than 90% loss of function) is unknown.

The clinical manifestations of acute and chronic pancreatitis and pancreatic insufficiency are protean. Thus, patients may present with hypertriglyceridemia, vitamin B$_{12}$ malabsorption, hypercalcemia, hypocalcemia, hyperglycemia, ascites, pleural effusions, and chronic abdominal pain with normal blood amylase levels. Indeed, if the clinician considers pancreatitis as a possible diagnosis only when presented with a patient having classic symptoms (i.e., severe, constant epigastric pain that radiates through to the back, along with an elevated blood amylase level), only a minority of patients with pancreatitis will be diagnosed correctly.

As emphasized in Chap. 304, the etiologies as well as the clinical manifestations of pancreatitis are quite varied. Although it is well appreciated that pancreatitis is frequently secondary to alcohol abuse and biliary tract disease, it can also be caused by drugs, trauma, and viral infections and is associated with metabolic and connective tissue disorders. In approximately 30% of patients with acute pancreatitis and 25 to 40% of patients with chronic pancreatitis, the etiology is obscure.

TESTS USEFUL IN THE DIAGNOSIS OF PANCREATIC DISEASE

Several tests have proved of value in the evaluation of pancreatic exocrine function. Examples of specific tests and their usefulness in the diagnosis of acute and chronic pancreatitis are summarized in Table 303-1. At most institutions, pancreatic function tests are performed if the diagnosis of pancreatic disease remains a possibility after noninvasive tests [ultrasound, computed tomography (CT)] and invasive tests [endoscopic retrograde cholangiopancreatography (ERCP)] have given normal or inconclusive results. In this regard, tests employing *direct* stimulation of the pancreas are the most sensitive.

PANCREATIC ENZYMES IN BODY FLUIDS   The serum amylase level is widely used as a screening test for acute pancreatitis in the patient with acute abdominal pain or back pain. A value greater than 65 U/L should raise the question of acute pancreatitis. Levels greater than 130 U/L make the diagnosis more likely, and values greater than three times normal virtually clinch the diagnosis if gut perforation or infarction is excluded. In acute pancreatitis, the serum amylase is usually elevated within 24 h of onset and remains so for 1 to 3 days. Levels return to normal within 3 to 5 days unless there is extensive pancreatic necrosis, incomplete ductal obstruction, or pseudocyst formation. Approximately 85% of patients with acute pancreatitis have an elevated serum amylase level. This index may be normal, however, if (1) there is a delay (of 2 to 5 days) before blood samples are obtained, (2) the underlying disorder is chronic pancreatitis rather than acute pancreatitis, or (3) hypertriglyceridemia is present. Patients with hypertriglyceridemia and proven pancreatitis have been found to have spuriously low levels of amylase and lipase activity.

The serum amylase is often elevated in other conditions (Table 303-2), in part because the enzyme is found in many organs in addition to the pancreas (salivary glands, liver, small intestine, kidney, fallopian tube) and can be produced by various tumors (carcinomas of the lung, esophagus, breast, and ovary). Isoenzymes of amylase fall into two general categories: those arising from the pancreas (P isoamylases) and those arising from nonpancreatic sources (S isoamylases). The measurement of serum isoamylases is of clinical importance. In normal serum, about 35 to 45% of the amylase is of pancreatic origin. For example, in patients with acute pancreatitis, the total serum amylase level returns to normal more rapidly than the level of pancreatic isoamylase. Thus, in patients seen after the first day, the pancreatic isoamylase level is a more sensitive indicator of pancreatitis than the total serum amylase level. In the past, elevations in serum amylase seen in certain conditions, such as the postoperative state, acute alcohol intoxication, and diabetic ketoacidosis, were assumed to indicate acute

Table 303-1 Tests Useful in the Diagnosis of Acute and Chronic Pancreatitis and Pancreatic Tumors

Test	Principle	Comment
PANCREATIC ENZYMES IN BODY FLUIDS		
Amylase		
1. Serum	Pancreatic inflammation leads to increased enzyme levels	Simple; 20–40% false negatives and positives; reliable if test results are three times the upper limit of normal
2. Urine	Renal clearance of amylase is increased in acute pancreatitis	May be abnormal when serum levels normal; false negatives and positives
3. Amylase/creatinine clearance ratio (C_{am}/C_{cr})	Renal clearance of amylase greater than clearance of creatinine	No more sensitive than serum amylase; many false positives
4. Ascitic fluid	Disruption of gland or main pancreatic duct leads to increased amylase concentration	Can establish diagnosis of pancreatitis; false positives occur with intestinal obstruction and perforated ulcer
5. Pleural fluid	Exudative pleural effusion with pancreatitis	False positives occur with carcinoma of the lung and esophageal perforation
6. Isoenzymes	P isoamylases arise from the pancreas; S isoamylases are from other sources	More sensitive than total serum amylase in diagnosis of acute pancreatitis; useful in identifying nonpancreatic causes of hyperamylasemia
Serum lipase	Pancreatic inflammation leads to increased enzyme levels	New methods have greatly simplified determination; positive in 70–85% of cases.
Serum trypsinogen	Pancreatic inflammation leads to increased levels	*Elevated* in acute pancreatitis; *decreased* in chronic pancreatitis *with* steatorrhea; normal in chronic pancreatitis *without* steatorrhea and in steatorrhea with normal pancreatic function
Pancreatic polypeptide (PP)	PP confined almost totally to the pancreas; release stimulated by nutrients and hormones; such release parallels pancreatic enzyme secretion	Basal, meal-simulated, and hormone-stimulated (by secretin or CCK) PP levels *decreased* in chronic pancreatitis; a fasting PP level >125 pg/mL argues against chronic pancreatitis and pancreatic cancer; increased levels in pancreatic endocrine tumors
STUDIES PERTAINING TO PANCREATIC STRUCTURE		
Radiologic and radionuclide tests		
1. Plain film of the abdomen	Abnormal in acute and chronic pancreatitis	Simple; normal in >50% of cases of both acute and chronic pancreatitis
2. Upper gastrointestinal x-rays	Abnormally thickened duodenal folds; displacement of stomach or widening of duodenal loop suggests a pancreatic mass (inflammatory, neoplastic, cystic)	Simple; frequently normal; largely superseded by US and CT scanning
3. Ultrasonography (US)	Can provide information on edema, inflammation, calcification, pseudocysts, and mass lesions	Simple, noninvasive; sequential studies quite feasible; useful in diagnosis of pseudocyst
4. CT scan	Permits detailed visualization of pancreas and surrounding structures	Useful in the diagnosis of pancreatic calcification, dilated pancreatic ducts, and pancreatic tumors; may not be able to distinguish between inflammatory and neoplastic mass lesions
5. Selective angiography	Can identify pancreatic neoplasms (1) by sheathing of celiac or superior mesenteric branches by tumor or (2) by tumor staining; displacement of vessels by tumor	Indicated (1) in suspected islet cell tumors and (2) before pancreatic or duodenal resection; most reliable features reflect nonresectable pancreatic cancer
6. Endoscopic retrograde cholangiopancreatography (ERCP)	Cannulation of pancreatic and common bile duct permits visualization of pancreatic-biliary ductal system	Provides diagnostic data in 60–85% of cases; differentiation of chronic pancreatitis from pancreatic carcinoma may be difficult
7. Endoscopic ultrasonography (EUS)	High-frequency transducer employed with EUS can produce very high-resolution images and depict changes in the pancreatic duct and parenchyma with better detail	Exact role of EUS versus ERCP and CT not yet fully defined; sensitivity and specificity under study
8. Magnetic resonance cholangiopancreatography	Three dimensional rendering has been used to produce very good images of the pancreatic duct by a noninvasive technique	May be used to evaluate patients judged to be at high risk for ERCP, such as the elderly; may replace ERCP as a diagnostic test, although large controlled studies need to be done
Pancreatic biopsy with US or CT guidance	Percutaneous biopsy with skinny needle and localization of lesion by US	High diagnostic yield; laparotomy avoided; requires special technical skills
TESTS OF EXOCRINE PANCREATIC FUNCTION		
Direct stimulation of the pancreas with analysis of duodenal contents		
1. Secretin-pancreozymin (CCK) test	Secretin leads to increased output of pancreatic juice and HCO_3^-; CCK leads to increased output of pancreatic enzymes; pancreatic secretory response is related to the functional mass of pancreatic tissue	Sensitive enough to detect occult disease; involves duodenal intubation and fluoroscopy; poorly defined normal enzyme response; overlap in chronic pancreatitis; large secretory reserve capacity of the pancreas

(continued)

Test	Principle	Comment
Indirect stimulation of pancreas with measurement of pancreatic enzymes		
1. Lundh test meal	Test meal (fat, carbohydrate, and protein) causes increased release of CCK, which causes increased enzyme output; trypsin concentration measured	Useful in pancreatic exocrine insufficiency; false negatives with delayed gastric emptying; false positives in primary mucosal disease of the gut and choledocholithiasis; does not measure secretory capacity
2. Benzoyl-tyrosyl-*p*-aminobenzoic acid (Bz-Ty-PABA, bentiromide) test	Synthetic peptide (Bz-Ty-PABA) is specifically cleaved by chymotrypsin, liberating PABA, which is absorbed; PABA metabolite is excreted in the urine	Simple and reliable test of pancreatic exocrine function; measurement of blood PABA level increases sensitivity; not available in the United States
3. Pancreolauryl test	Fluorescein dilaurate is hydrolyzed by pancreatic elastase and absorbed; fluorescein is measured in urine	Sensitivity and specificity similar to those of serum trypsinogen; not available in the United States
Measurement of intraluminal digestion products		
1. Microscopic examination of stool for undigested meat fibers and fat	Lack of proteolytic and lipolytic enzymes causes decreased digestion of meat fibers and triglycerides	Simple, reliable; not sensitive enough to detect milder cases of pancreatic insufficiency
2. Quantitative stool fat determination	Lack of lipolytic enzymes brings about impaired fat digestion	Reliable, reference standard for defining severity of malabsorption; does not distinguish between maldigestion and malabsorption
3. Fecal nitrogen	Lack of proteolytic enzymes leads to impaired protein digestion, resulting in an increase in stool nitrogen	Does not distinguish between maldigestion and malabsorption; low sensitivity
Measurement of pancreatic enzymes in feces		
1. Elastase	Pancreatic secretion of proteolytic enzymes	Excellent specificity; sensitivity similar to that of serum trypsinogen
Miscellaneous tests		
1. Dual-labeled Schilling test	Intrinsic factor [^{57}Co]cobalamin and Hog R protein [^{58}Co]cobalamin are given together. Since proteases are necessary to cleave R protein, the ratio of labeled cobalamin excreted in urine is an index of exocrine dysfunction.	Time-consuming and expensive

pancreatitis. However, the elevation of serum amylase in such conditions has been shown to be due to an elevation of the S isoamylase. Simple tests to distinguish pancreatic from nonpancreatic amylase are no longer readily available, and such tests are often not reliable when the total amylase is minimally to moderately elevated. An assay of serum trypsinogen (performed by several commercial laboratories) is quite helpful in this regard. Since this enzyme is secreted specifically by the pancreas, a normal serum trypsinogen level in a patient with minimal elevation of serum amylase essentially rules out acute pancreatitis. Urinary amylase measurements, including the amylase/creatinine clearance ratio, are no more sensitive or specific than blood amylase levels.

Elevation of ascitic fluid amylase occurs in acute pancreatitis as well as in (1) pancreatogenous ascites due to disruption of the main pancreatic duct or a leaking pseudocyst and (2) other abdominal disorders that simulate pancreatitis (e.g., intestinal obstruction, intestinal infarction, and perforated peptic ulcer). Elevation of pleural fluid amylase occurs in acute pancreatitis, chronic pancreatitis, carcinoma of the lung, and esophageal perforation.

Lipase may now be the single best enzyme to measure for the diagnosis of acute pancreatitis. Improvements in substrates and technology offer clinicians improved options, especially when a turbidimetric assay is used. The newer lipase assays have colipase as a cofactor and are fully automated.

An assay for trypsinogen (or for trypsin-like immunoreactivity) has a theoretical advantage over amylase and lipase determinations in that the pancreas is the only organ that contains this enzyme. The test appears to be useful in the diagnosis of both acute and chronic pancreatitis. Sensitivity and specificity are comparable to those of amylase and lipase determinations. Since trypsinogen is also excreted by the kidney, elevated serum values are found in renal failure, as is the case with serum amylase and lipase levels. *No single blood test is reliable for the diagnosis of acute pancreatitis in patients with renal failure.* Determining whether a patient with renal failure and abdominal pain

has pancreatitis remains a difficult clinical problem. A recent study found that serum amylase levels were elevated in patients with renal dysfunction only when creatinine clearance was less than 50 mL/min.

Table 303-2   Causes of Hyperamylasemia and Hyperamylasuria

PANCREATIC DISEASE

I. Pancreatitis	II. Pancreatic trauma
A. Acute	III. Pancreatic carcinoma
B. Chronic: ductal obstruction	
C. Complications of pancreatitis	
1. Pancreatic pseudocyst	
2. Pancreatogenous ascites	
3. Pancreatic abscess	

NONPANCREATIC DISORDERS

I. Renal insufficiency	IV. Macroamylasemia
II. Salivary gland lesions	V. Burns
A. Mumps	VI. Diabetic ketoacidosis
B. Calculus	VII. Pregnancy
C. Irradiation sialadenitis	VIII. Renal transplantation
D. Maxillofacial surgery	IX. Cerebral trauma
III. "Tumor" hyperamylasemia	X. Drugs: morphine
A. Carcinoma of the lung	
B. Carcinoma of the esophagus	
C. Breast carcinoma, ovarian carcinoma	

OTHER ABDOMINAL DISORDERS

I. Biliary tract disease: cholecystitis, choledocholithiasis
II. Intraabdominal disease
  A. Perforated or penetrating peptic ulcer
  B. Intestinal obstruction or infarction
  C. Ruptured ectopic pregnancy
  D. Peritonitis
  E. Aortic aneurysm
  F. Chronic liver disease
  G. Postoperative hyperamylasemia

In such patients, the serum amylase level was invariably less than 500 IU/L in the absence of objective evidence of acute pancreatitis. In that study, serum lipase and trypsin levels paralleled serum amylase values.

A recent study evaluated the sensitivity and specificity of five assays used to diagnose acute pancreatitis: two for amylase, one for lipase, one for trypsin-like immunoreactivity (TLI), and one for pancreatic isoamylase. The data obtained (1) show that, if the best cutoff level is used, all these assays have similar specificities and (2) suggest that total serum amylase is as good an indicator of acute pancreatitis as any of the alternatives. However, inherent in many such studies is the problem that the recognition and diagnosis of acute pancreatitis hinge on the finding of an elevated serum amylase level. The question arises as to whether any diagnostic test result can be proved superior to the total serum amylase level if hyperamylasemia is required for the diagnosis. In other studies, when "objective" confirmation of the clinical diagnosis of pancreatitis was required (ultrasonography, CT, laparotomy), the sensitivity of the serum amylase has been found to be as low as 68%. With these limitations in mind, the recommended screening tests for acute pancreatitis are *total serum amylase* and *serum lipase activities*. Serum amylase values greater than three times normal are highly specific.

STUDIES PERTAINING TO PANCREATIC STRUCTURE
Radiologic Tests   Plain films of the abdomen provide useful information in 30 to 50% of patients with acute pancreatitis. The most frequent abnormalities include (1) a localized ileus, usually involving the jejunum ("sentinel loop"); (2) a generalized ileus with air-fluid levels; (3) the "colon cutoff sign," which results from isolated distention of the transverse colon; (4) duodenal distention with air-fluid levels; and (5) a mass, which is frequently a pseudocyst. In chronic pancreatitis, an important radiographic finding is pancreatic calcification, which characteristically is localized adjacent to and superimposed on the second lumbar vertebra (see Fig. 304-3A).

Upper gastrointestinal x-rays may reveal displacement of the stomach by the retroperitoneal mass (see Fig. 304-2A) or widening and effacement of the duodenal C loop, which also suggest the presence of a pancreatic mass, which could be inflammatory, cystic, or neoplastic. However, the use of x-ray films has been largely superseded by ultrasound.

Ultrasonography can provide important information in patients with acute pancreatitis, chronic pancreatitis, pancreatic calcification, pseudocyst, and pancreatic carcinoma. Echographic appearances can indicate the presence of edema, inflammation, and calcification (not obvious on plain films of the abdomen), as well as pseudocysts, mass lesions, and gallstones (see Figs. 304-2B and 304-3B). In acute pancreatitis, the pancreas is characteristically enlarged. In pancreatic pseudocyst, the usual appearance is that of an echo-free, smooth, round fluid collection. Pancreatic carcinoma distorts the usual landmarks, and mass lesions greater than 3.0 cm are usually detected as localized, echo-free solid lesions. Ultrasound is often the initial investigation for most patients with suspected pancreatic disease. However, obesity, excess small- and large-bowel gas, and recently performed barium contrast examinations can interfere with ultrasound studies.

CT is the best imaging study for initial evaluation of a suspected chronic pancreatic disorder and for the complications of acute and chronic pancreatitis. It is especially useful in the detection of pancreatic tumors, fluid-containing lesions such as pseudocysts and abscesses, and calcium deposits (see Figs. 304-3C and 304-4A). Most lesions are characterized by (1) enlargement of the pancreatic outline, (2) distortion of the pancreatic contour, and/or (3) a fluid filling that has a different attenuation coefficient than normal pancreas. However, it is occasionally difficult to distinguish between inflammatory and neoplastic lesions. Oral water-soluble contrast agents may be used to opacify the stomach and duodenum during CT scans; this strategy permits more precise delineation of various organs as well as mass lesions. Dynamic CT (using rapid intravenous administration of contrast) is useful in estimating the degree of pancreatic necrosis and in

predicting morbidity and mortality. Spiral (helical) CT provides clear images much more rapidly and essentially negates artifact caused by patient movement (see Fig. 304-2D).

Endoscopic ultrasonography (*EUS*) produces high-resolution images of the pancreatic parenchyma and pancreatic duct with a transducer fixed to an endoscope that can be directed onto the surface of the pancreas through the stomach or duodenum. Although criteria for abnormalities on EUS in severe pancreatic disease have been developed, the true sensitivity and specificity of this procedure has yet to be determined. In particular, it is not clear whether EUS can detect early pancreatic disease before abnormalities appear on more conventional radiograph tests such as ultrasonography or CT. The exact role of EUS versus ERCP and CT has yet to be defined.

Magnetic resonance cholangiopancreatography (*MRCP*) is now being used to view both the bile duct and the pancreatic duct. Non-breath-hold and 3D turbo spin-echo techniques are being utilized to produce superb MRCP images. The main pancreatic duct and common bile duct can be seen well, but there is still a question as to whether changes can be detected consistently in the secondary ducts. MRCP may be particularly useful to evaluate the pancreatic duct in high-risk patients such as the elderly because this is a noninvasive procedure.

Both EUS and MRCP may replace ERCP in some patients. As these techniques become more refined, they may well be the diagnostic tests of choice to evaluate the pancreatic duct. ERCP is still needed to perform therapy of bile duct and pancreatic duct lesions.

Selective catheterization of the celiac and superior mesenteric arteries combined with superselective catheterization of others arteries, such as the hepatic, splenic, and gastroduodenal arteries permits visualization of the pancreas and detection of pancreatic neoplasms and pseudocysts. Pancreatic neoplasms can be identified by the sheathing of blood vessels by a mass lesion (see Fig. 304-1D). Hormone-producing pancreatic tumors are especially likely to exhibit increased vascularity and tumor staining. Angiographic abnormalities are noted in many patients with pancreatic carcinoma but are uncommon in patients without pancreatic disease. Angiography complements ultrasonography and ERCP in the study of patients with a suspected pancreatic lesion and may be carried out if ERCP is either unsuccessful or nondiagnostic.

ERCP may provide useful information on the status of the pancreatic ductal system and thus aid in the differential diagnosis of pancreatic disease (see Figs. 304-1C, 304-3D, and 304-4B). Pancreatic carcinoma is characterized by stenosis or obstruction of either the pancreatic duct or the common bile duct; both ductal systems are often abnormal. In chronic pancreatitis, ERCP abnormalities include (1) luminal narrowing, (2) irregularities in the ductal system with stenosis, dilation, sacculation, and ectasia, and (3) blockage of the pancreatic duct by calcium deposits. The presence of ductal stenosis and irregularity can make it difficult to distinguish chronic pancreatitis from carcinoma. It is important to be aware that ERCP changes interpreted as indicating chronic pancreatitis actually may be due to the effects of aging on the pancreatic duct or to the fact that the procedure was performed within several weeks of an attack of acute pancreatitis. Although aging may cause impressive ductal alterations, it does not affect the results of pancreatic function tests (i.e., the secretin test). Elevated serum and/or urine amylase levels after ERCP have been reported in 25 to 75% of patients, but clinical pancreatitis is uncommon. In a series of 300 patients, pancreatitis occurred in only 5 patients after ERCP. If no lesion is found in the biliary and/or pancreatic ducts in a patient with repeated attacks of acute pancreatitis, manometric studies of the sphincter of Oddi may be indicated. Such studies, however, do increase the risk of post-ERCP/manometry acute pancreatitis. Such pancreatitis appears to be more common in patients with a nondilated pancreatic duct.

Pancreatic Biopsy with Radiologic Guidance   Percutaneous aspiration biopsy of a pancreatic mass often distinguishes a pancreatic inflammatory mass from a pancreatic neoplasm.

TESTS OF EXOCRINE PANCREATIC FUNCTION

Pancreatic function tests (Table 303-1) can be divided into the following:

1. *Direct stimulation of the pancreas* by intravenous infusion of secretin or secretin plus cholecystokinin (CCK) followed by collection and measurement of duodenal contents
2. *Indirect stimulation of the pancreas* using nutrients or amino acids, fatty acids, and synthetic peptides followed by assays of proteolytic, lipolytic, and amylolytic enzymes
3. Study of *intraluminal digestion products*, such as undigested meat fibers, stool fat, and fecal nitrogen
4. *Measurement of fecal pancreatic enzymes* such as elastase

The secretin test, used to detect diffuse pancreatic disease, is based on the physiologic principle that the pancreatic secretory response is directly related to the functional mass of pancreatic tissue. In the standard assay, secretin is given intravenously in a dose of 1 clinical unit (CU) per kilogram, as either a bolus or a continuous infusion. The results will vary with the secretin preparation used, the dose, the mode of administration, and the completeness with which the duodenal contents are collected. Normal values for the standard secretin test are (1) volume output >2.0 mL/kg per hour, (2) bicarbonate (HCO_3^-) concentration >80 meql/L, and (3) HCO_3^- output >10 meq/L in 1 h. The most reproducible measurement, giving the highest level of discrimination between normal subjects and patients with chronic pancreatitis, appears to be the maximal bicarbonate concentration.

The *combined secretin-CCK test* permits measurement of pancreatic amylase, lipase, trypsin, and chymotrypsin. Although there is overlap in the distributions of enzyme output in normal subjects and patients with pancreatitis in response to this test, markedly low enzyme outputs suggest advanced damage and destruction of acinar cells. With frank exocrine pancreatic insufficiency, there is usually an overall reduction in both HCO_3^- concentration and output of several enzymes. However, with lesser degrees of pancreatic damage there may be a dissociation between HCO_3^- concentration and enzyme output. There also may be a dissociation between the results of the secretin test and those of tests of absorptive function. For example, patients with chronic pancreatitis often have abnormally low outputs of HCO_3^- after secretin but have normal fecal fat excretion. Thus the secretin test measures the secretory capacity of ductular epithelium, while fecal fat excretion indirectly reflects intraluminal lipolytic activity. Steatorrhea does not occur until intraluminal levels of lipase are markedly reduced, underscoring the fact that only small amounts of enzymes are necessary for intraluminal digestive activities. An abnormal secretin test result suggests only that chronic pancreatic damage is present; it will not consistently distinguish between chronic pancreatitis and pancreatic carcinoma.

Another test of exocrine pancreatic function is the *bentiromide test*. This test is an indirect measure of pancreatic function and reflects intraluminal chymotrypsin activity. The test has excellent specificity but is not very sensitive. It no longer is available for clinical use in the United States.

The *serum trypsinogen level*, which is determined by radioimmunoassay, also has excellent specificity but is not very sensitive. It is a simple blood test that can detect severe damage to the exocrine pancreas. The normal values are 28 to 58 ng/mL, and any value below 20 ng/mL reflects pancreatic steatorrhea.

Measurement of *intraluminal digestion products*, i.e., undigested muscle fibers, stool fat, and fecal nitrogen, is discussed in Chap. 286. The amount of elastase in stool reflects the pancreatic output of this proteolytic enzyme. Decreased elastase activity in stool has been reported in patients with chronic pancreatitis and cystic fibrosis. →*Tests useful in the diagnosis of exocrine pancreatic insufficiency and the differential diagnosis of malabsorption are also discussed in Chaps. 286 and 304.*

304 *Norton J. Greenberger, Phillip P. Toskes*

ACUTE AND CHRONIC PANCREATITIS

APACHE II acute physiology and chronic health evaluation scoring system	HIDA hepatic 2,6-dimethyliminodiacetic acid
AST aspartate aminotransferase	KUB kidney, ureter, and bladder
CCK cholecystokinin	LDH lactic dehydrogenase
CCK-RF CCK releasing factor	NSAIDs nonsteroidal anti-inflammatory drugs
CECT contrast-enhanced dynamic CT	
CFTR cystic fibrosis transmembrane conductance regulator	PIPIDA *N-p*-isopropylacetanilide-iminodiacetic acid
CT computed tomography	TAP trypsinogen activation peptide
ERCP endoscopic retrograde cholangiopancreatography	VIP vasoactive intestinal peptide

BIOCHEMISTRY AND PHYSIOLOGY OF PANCREATIC EXOCRINE SECRETION

GENERAL CONSIDERATIONS   The pancreas secretes 1500 to 3000 mL of isosmotic alkaline (pH >8.0) fluid per day containing about 20 enzymes and zymogens. The pancreatic secretions provide the enzymes needed to effect the major digestive activity of the gastrointestinal tract and provide an optimal pH for the function of these enzymes.

REGULATION OF PANCREATIC SECRETION   The exocrine pancreas is influenced by intimately interacting hormonal and neural systems. *Gastric acid* is the stimulus for the release of secretin, a peptide with 27 amino acids. Sensitive radioimmunoassay studies for secretin suggest that the pH threshold for its release from the duodenum and jejunum is 4.5. Secretin stimulates the secretion of pancreatic juice rich in *water and electrolytes*. Release of cholecystokinin (CCK) from the duodenum and jejunum is largely triggered by long-chain fatty acids, certain essential amino acids (tryptophan, phenylalanine, valine, methionine), and gastric acid itself. CCK evokes an *enzyme-rich secretion from the pancreas*. Gastrin, although it has the same terminal tetrapeptide as CCK, is a weak stimulus for pancreatic enzyme output. The *parasympathetic nervous system* (via the vagus nerve) exerts significant control over pancreatic secretion. Secretion evoked by secretin and CCK depends on permissive roles of vagal afferent and efferent pathways. This is particularly true for enzyme secretion, whereas water and bicarbonate secretion is heavily dependent on the hormonal effects of secretin and CCK. Also, vagal stimulation effects the release of vasoactive intestinal peptide (VIP), a secretin agonist. Bile salts also stimulate pancreatic secretion, thereby integrating the functions of the biliary tract, pancreas, and small intestine.

Somatostatin acts on multiple sites to induce inhibition of pancreatic secretion. The appropriate roles of other peptides, such as peptide YY, pancreastatin, gastrin-releasing peptide, pituitary adenylate cyclase–activating polypeptide, calcitonin gene–related peptide, and galanin are still being defined. Nitric oxide is an important neurotransmitter in the regulation of pancreatic exocrine secretion, although its mechanism of action has not been fully elucidated.

WATER AND ELECTROLYTE SECRETION   Although sodium, potassium, chloride, calcium, zinc, phosphate, and sulfate are found in pancreatic secretions, *bicarbonate is the ion of primary physiologic importance*. In the acini and in the ducts, secretin causes the cells to add water and bicarbonate to the fluid. In the ducts, an exchange occurs between bicarbonate and chloride. There is a good correlation between the maximal bicarbonate output after stimulation with secretin and the pancreatic mass. The bicarbonate output of 120 to 300 mmol/d helps neutralize gastric acid and creates the appropriate pH for the activity of the pancreatic enzymes.

ENZYME SECRETION   The pancreas secretes amylolytic, lipolytic, and proteolytic enzymes. *Amylolytic enzymes*, such as amylase, hydrolyze starch to oligosaccharides and to the disaccharide maltose. The *lipolytic enzymes* include lipase, phospholipase A, and cholesterol esterase. Bile salts *inhibit* lipase in isolation; but colipase, another constituent of pancreatic secretion, binds to lipase and prevents this inhibition. Bile salts *activate* phospholipase A and cholesterol esterase. *Proteolytic enzymes* include *endopeptidases* (trypsin, chymotrypsin), which act on internal peptide bonds of proteins and polypeptides; *exopeptidases* (carboxypeptidases, aminopeptidases), which act on the free carboxyl- and amino-terminal ends of peptides, respectively; and elastase. The proteolytic enzymes are secreted as inactive precursors (zymogens). Ribonucleases (deoxyribonucleases, ribonuclease) are also secreted. Although pancreatic enzymes usually are secreted in parallel, nonparallel secretion can occur as a result of exocytosis from heterogeneous sources in the pancreas. *Enterokinase*, an enzyme found in the duodenal mucosa, cleaves the lysine-isoleucine bond of trypsinogen to form trypsin. Trypsin then activates the other proteolytic zymogens in a cascade phenomenon. All pancreatic enzymes have pH optima in the alkaline range.

AUTOPROTECTION OF THE PANCREAS Autodigestion of the pancreas is prevented by the packaging of proteases in precursor form and by the synthesis of protease inhibitors. These protease inhibitors are found in the acinar cell, the pancreatic secretions, and the alpha$_1$- and alpha$_2$-globulin fractions of plasma.

Table 304-1 Causes of Acute Pancreatitis

Alcohol ingestion (acute and chronic alcoholism)
Biliary tract disease (gallstones)
Postoperative state (after abdominal or nonabdominal operation)
Endoscopic retrograde cholangiopancreatography (ERCP), especially manometric studies of sphincter of Oddi
Trauma (especially blunt abdominal type)
Metabolic causes
  Hypertriglyceridemia
  Apolipoprotein CII deficiency syndrome
  Hypercalcemia (e.g., hyperparathyroidism), drug-induced
  Renal failure
  After renal transplantation[a]
  Acute fatty liver of pregnancy[b]
Hereditary pancreatitis
Infections
  Mumps
  Viral hepatitis
  Other viral infections (coxsackievirus, echovirus, cytomegalovirus)
  Ascariasis
  Infections with *Mycoplasma*, *Campylobacter*, *Mycobacterium avium* complex, other bacteria
Drugs
  Drugs for which association is definite
    Azathioprine, 6-mercaptopurine
    Sulfonamides
    Thiazide diuretics
    Furosemide
    Estrogens (oral contraceptives)
    Tetracycline
    Valproic acid
    Pentamidine
    Dideoxyinosine (ddI)

Drugs for which association is probable
  Acetaminophen
  Nitrofurantoin
  Methyldopa
  Erythromycin
  Salicylates
  Metronidazole
  Nonsteroidal anti-inflammatory drugs
  Angiotensin-converting enzyme (ACE) inhibitors
Vascular causes and vasculitis
  Vascular
    Ischemic-hypoperfusion state (after cardiac surgery)
    Atherosclerotic emboli
    Aneurysm of celiac axis/hepatic artery
  Connective tissue disorders with vasculitis
    Systemic lupus erythematosus
    Necrotizing angiitis
    Thrombotic thrombocytopenic purpura
Penetrating peptic ulcer
Obstruction of the ampulla of Vater
  Regional enteritis
  Duodenal diverticulum
Pancreas divisum
Causes to be considered in patients having recurrent bouts of acute pancreatitis without an obvious cause
  Occult disease of the biliary tree or pancreatic ducts, especially occult gallstones (microlithiasis, sludge)
  Drugs
  Hypertriglyceridemia
  Pancreas divisum
  Pancreatic cancer
  Sphincter of Oddi dysfunction
  Cystic fibrosis
  Truly idiopathic

[a] Pancreatitis occurs in 3% of renal transplant patients and is due to many factors, including surgery, hypercalcemia, drugs (glucocorticoids, azathioprine, L-asparaginase, diuretics), and viral infections.
[b] Pancreatitis also occurs in otherwise uncomplicated pregnancy and is most often associated with cholelithiasis.

EXOCRINE-ENDOCRINE RELATIONSHIPS Insulin appears to be needed locally for secretin and CCK to promote exocrine secretion; thus, it acts in a permissive role for these two hormones.

ENTEROPANCREATIC AXIS AND FEEDBACK INHIBITION Pancreatic enzyme secretion is controlled, at least in part, by a negative feedback mechanism induced by the presence of active serine proteases in the duodenum. To illustrate, perfusion of the duodenal lumen with phenylalanine causes a prompt increase in plasma CCK levels as well as increased secretion of chymotrypsin. However, simultaneous perfusion with trypsin blunts both responses. Conversely, perfusion of the duodenal lumen with protease inhibitors actually leads to enzyme hypersecretion. The available evidence supports the concept that the duodenum contains a peptide called CCK releasing factor (CCK-RF) that is involved in stimulating CCK release. Two peptides, luminal CCK-RF and diazepam-binding inhibitor, have been found that may be the CCK-RF. Serine proteases inhibit pancreatic secretion by acting on CCK-RF. It appears that serine proteases inhibit pancreatic secretion by acting on a CCK-releasing peptide in the lumen of the small intestine.

ACUTE PANCREATITIS

GENERAL CONSIDERATIONS Pancreatic inflammatory disease may be classified as (1) acute pancreatitis and (2) chronic pancreatitis. The pathologic spectrum of acute pancreatitis varies from *edematous pancreatitis*, which is usually a mild and self-limited disorder, to *necrotizing pancreatitis*, in which the degree of pancreatic necrosis correlates with the severity of the attack and its systemic manifestations. The term *hemorrhagic pancreatitis* is less meaningful in a clinical sense because variable amounts of interstitial hemorrhage can be found in pancreatitis as well as in other disorders such as pancreatic trauma, pancreatic carcinoma, and severe congestive heart failure.

The incidence of pancreatitis varies in different countries and depends on cause, e.g., alcohol, gallstones, metabolic factors, and drugs (Table 304-1). In the United States, for example, acute pancreatitis is related to alcohol ingestion more commonly than to gallstones; in England, the opposite obtains. There are 185,000 new cases of acute pancreatitis per year in the United States.

ETIOLOGY AND PATHOGENESIS There are many causes of acute pancreatitis (Table 304-1), but the mechanisms by which these conditions trigger pancreatic inflammation have not been identified. Alcoholic patients with pancreatitis may represent a special subset, since most alcoholics do not develop pancreatitis. The list of identifiable causes is growing, and it is likely that pancreatitis related to viral infections, drugs, and as yet undefined factors is more common than heretofore recognized.

Approximately 2 to 5% of cases of acute pancreatitis are drug-related (Table 304-1). Drugs cause pancreatitis either by a hypersensitivity reaction or by the generation of a toxic metabolite, although in some cases it is not clear which of these mechanisms is operative.

Autodigestion is one pathogenetic theory, according to which pancreatitis results when proteolytic enzymes (e.g., trypsinogen, chymotrypsinogen, proelastase, and phospholipase A) are activated in the pancreas rather than in the intestinal lumen. A number of factors (e.g., endotoxins, exotoxins, viral infections, ischemia, anoxia, and direct trauma) are believed to activate these proenzymes. Activated proteolytic enzymes, especially trypsin, not only digest pancreatic and peri-pancreatic tissues but also can activate other enzymes, such as elastase and phospholipase. The active enzymes then digest cellular membranes and cause proteolysis, edema, interstitial hemorrhage, vascular damage, coagulation necrosis, fat necrosis, and parenchymal cell necrosis. Cellular injury and death result in the liberation of activated enzymes. In addition, activation and release of bradykinin peptides and vasoactive substances (e.g., histamine) are believed to produce vasodilation, increased vascular permeability, and edema. Thus, a cascade of events culminates in the development of acute necrotizing pancreatitis.

The autodigestion theory has largely eclipsed two older theories. First, according to the "common channel" theory, the existence of a common anatomic channel for pancreatic secretions and bile permits reflux of bile into the pancreatic duct, which results in activation of pancreatic enzymes. (Actually, a common channel with free communication between the common bile duct and the main pancreatic duct is infrequently encountered.) The second theory is that obstruction and hypersecretion are pivotal in the development of pancreatitis. Obstruction of the main pancreatic duct, however, produces pancreatic edema but generally not pancreatitis.

A recent hypothesis to explain the intrapancreatic activation of zymogens is that they become activated by *lysosomal hydrolases* in the pancreatic acinar cell itself. In two different types of experimental pancreatitis, it has been demonstrated that digestive enzymes and lysosomal hydrolases become admixed; as a result, the latter can activate the former in the acinar cell. In vitro, lysosomal enzymes such as cathepsin B can activate trypsinogen, and trypsin can activate the other protease precursors. It is still not clear, however, whether the human acinar cell can provide the pH (about 3.0) necessary for activation of trypsinogen by lysosomal hydrolases. It is now believed that ischemia/hypoperfusion can alone result in activation of trypsinogen and pancreatic injury.

CLINICAL FEATURES *Abdominal pain* is the major symptom of acute pancreatitis. Pain may vary from a mild and tolerable discomfort to severe, constant, and incapacitating distress. Characteristically, the pain, which is steady and boring in character, is located in the epigastrium and periumbilical region and often radiates to the back as well as to the chest, flanks, and lower abdomen. The pain is frequently more intense when the patient is supine, and patients often obtain relief by sitting with the trunk flexed and knees drawn up. Nausea, vomiting, and abdominal distention due to gastric and intestinal hypomotility and chemical peritonitis are also frequent complaints.

Physical examination frequently reveals a distressed and anxious patient. Low-grade fever, tachycardia, and hypotension are fairly common. Shock is not unusual and may result from (1) hypovolemia secondary to exudation of blood and plasma proteins into the retroperitoneal space (a "retroperitoneal burn"); (2) increased formation and release of kinin peptides, which cause vasodilation and increased vascular permeability; and (3) systemic effects of proteolytic and lipolytic enzymes released into the circulation. Jaundice occurs infrequently; when present, it usually is due to edema of the head of the pancreas with compression of the intrapancreatic portion of the common bile duct. Erythematous skin nodules due to subcutaneous fat necrosis may occur. In 10 to 20% of patients, there are pulmonary findings, including basilar rales, atelectasis, and pleural effusion, the latter most frequently left-sided. Abdominal tenderness and muscle rigidity are present to a variable degree, but, compared with the intense pain, these signs may be unimpressive. Bowel sounds are usually diminished or absent. A pancreatic pseudocyst may be palpable in the upper abdomen. A faint blue discoloration around the umbilicus (Cullen's sign) may occur as the result of hemoperitoneum, and a blue-red-purple or green-brown discoloration of the flanks (Turner's sign) reflects tissue catabolism of hemoglobin. The latter two findings, which are uncommon, indicate the presence of a severe necrotizing pancreatitis.

LABORATORY DATA The diagnosis of acute pancreatitis is usually established by the detection of an increased level of serum amylase. Values threefold or more above normal virtually clinch the diagnosis if overt salivary gland disease and gut perforation or infarction are excluded. However, there appears to be no definite correlation between the severity of pancreatitis and the degree of serum amylase elevation. After 48 to 72 h, even with continuing evidence of pancreatitis, total serum amylase values tend to return to normal. However, pancreatic isoamylase and lipase levels may remain elevated for 7 to 14 days. It will be recalled that amylase elevations in serum and urine occur in many conditions other than pancreatitis (see Table 303-2). Importantly, patients with *acidemia* (arterial pH ≤7.32) may have spurious elevations in serum amylase. In one study, 12 of 33 patients with acidemia had elevated serum amylase, but only 1 had an elevated lipase value; in 9, salivary-type amylase was the predominant serum isoamylase. This finding explains why patients with diabetic ketoacidosis may have marked elevations in serum amylase without any other evidence of acute pancreatitis. Serum lipase activity increases in parallel with amylase activity, and measurement of both enzymes increases the diagnostic yield. An elevated serum lipase or trypsin value is usually diagnostic of acute pancreatitis; these tests are especially helpful in patients with nonpancreatic causes of hyperamylasemia (see Table 303-2). Markedly increased levels of peritoneal or pleural fluid amylase [1500 nmol/L (> 5000 U/dL)] are also helpful, if present, in establishing the diagnosis.

Leukocytosis (15,000 to 20,000 leukocytes per microliter) occurs frequently. Patients with more severe disease may show hemoconcentration with hematocrit values exceeding 50% because of loss of plasma into the retroperitoneal space and peritoneal cavity. *Hyperglycemia* is common and is due to multiple factors, including decreased insulin release, increased glucagon release, and an increased output of adrenal glucocorticoids and catecholamines. *Hypocalcemia* occurs in approximately 25% of patients, and its pathogenesis is incompletely understood. Although earlier studies suggested that the response of the parathyroid gland to a decrease in serum calcium is impaired, subsequent observations have failed to confirm this idea. Intraperitoneal saponification of calcium by fatty acids in areas of fat necrosis occurs occasionally, with large amounts (up to 6.0 g) dissolved or suspended in ascitic fluid. Such "soap formation" also may be significant in patients with pancreatitis, mild hypocalcemia, and little or no obvious ascites. *Hyperbilirubinemia* [serum bilirubin >68 μmol/L (> 4.0 mg/dL)] occurs in approximately 10% of patients. However, jaundice is transient, and serum bilirubin levels return to normal in 4 to 7 days. Serum alkaline phosphatase and aspartate aminotransferase (AST) levels are also transiently elevated and parallel serum bilirubin values. Markedly elevated serum lactic dehydrogenase (LDH) levels [>8.5 μmol/L (> 500 U/dL)] suggest a poor prognosis. Serum albumin is decreased to ≤30 g/L (≤3.0 g/dL) in about 10% of patients; this sign is associated with more severe pancreatitis and a higher mortality rate (Table 304-2). *Hypertriglyceridemia* occurs in 15 to 20% of patients, and serum amylase levels in these individuals are often spuriously normal (Chap. 303). Most patients with hypertriglyceridemia and pancreatitis, when subsequently examined, show evidence of an underlying derangement in lipid metabolism which probably antedated the pancreatitis (see below). Approximately 25% of patients have *hypoxemia* (arterial P_{O_2} ≤ 60 mmHg), which may herald the onset of adult respiratory distress syndrome. Finally, the electrocardiogram is occasionally abnormal in acute pancreatitis with ST-segment and T-wave abnormalities simulating myocardial ischemia.

Although one or more radiologic abnormalities are found in over 50% of patients, the findings are inconstant and nonspecific. The chief value of conventional x-rays [chest films; kidney, ureter, and bladder (KUB) studies] in acute pancreatitis is to help exclude other diagnoses, especially a perforated viscus. Upper gastrointestinal tract x-rays have been superseded by ultrasonography and computed tomography (CT). A CT scan may confirm the clinical impression of acute pancreatitis even in the face of normal serum amylase levels. Importantly, CT is quite helpful in indicating the severity of acute pancreatitis and the

Table 304-2 Factors That Adversely Affect Survival in Acute Pancreatitis

Ranson/Imrie criteria
  At admission or diagnosis
    Age >55 years
    Leukocytosis >16,000/μL
    Hyperglycemia >11 mmol/L (>200 mg/dL)
    Serum LDH >400 IU/L
    Serum AST >250 IU/L
  During initial 48 h
    Fall in hematocrit by >10 percent
    Fluid deficit of >4000 mL
    Hypocalcemia [calcium concentration <1.9 mmol/L (<8.0 mg/dL)]
    Hypoxemia (P_{O_2} <60 mmHg)
    Increase in BUN to >1.8 mmol/L (>5 mg/dL) after IV fluid administration
    Hypoalbuminemia [albumin level <32 g/L (<3.2 g/dL)]
Acute physiology and chronic health evaluation (APACHE II) score > 12
Hemorrhagic peritoneal fluid
Obesity [body mass index (BMI) > 29]
Key indicators of organ failure
  Hypotension (blood pressure <90 mmHg) or tachycardia >130 beats per minute
  P_{O_2} <60 mmHg
  Oliguria (<50 mL/h) or increasing blood urea nitrogen (BUN), creatinine
  Metabolic indicators: serum calcium <1.9 mmol/L (<8.0 mg/dL) or serum albumin <32 g/L (<3.2 g/dL)

risk of morbidity and mortality (see below). Sonography and radionuclide scanning [N-p-isopropylacetanilide-iminodiacetic acid (PIPIDA) scan; hepatic 2,6-dimethyliminodiacetic acid (HIDA) scan] are useful in acute pancreatitis to evaluate the gallbladder and biliary tree. →*Radiologic studies useful in the diagnosis of acute pancreatitis are discussed in Chap. 303 and listed in Table 303-1.*

DIAGNOSIS Any severe acute pain in the abdomen or back should suggest acute pancreatitis. The diagnosis is usually entertained when a patient with a possible predisposition to pancreatitis presents with severe and constant abdominal pain, nausea, emesis, fever, tachycardia, and abnormal findings on abdominal examination. Laboratory studies frequently reveal leukocytosis, an abnormal appearance on x-rays of the abdomen and chest, hypocalcemia, and hyperglycemia. The diagnosis is usually confirmed by the finding of an elevated level of serum amylase and/or lipase. Not all the above features have to be present for the diagnosis to be established.

The *differential diagnosis* should include the following disorders: (1) perforated viscus, especially peptic ulcer; (2) acute cholecystitis and biliary colic; (3) acute intestinal obstruction; (4) mesenteric vascular occlusion; (5) renal colic; (6) myocardial infarction; (7) dissecting aortic aneurysm; (8) connective tissue disorders with vasculitis; (9) pneumonia; and (10) diabetic ketoacidosis. A penetrating duodenal ulcer usually can be identified by upper gastrointestinal x-rays and/or endoscopy. A perforated duodenal ulcer is readily diagnosed by the presence of free intraperitoneal air. It may be difficult to differentiate acute cholecystitis from acute pancreatitis, since an elevated serum amylase may be found in both disorders. Pain of biliary tract origin is more right-sided and gradual in onset, and ileus is usually absent; sonography and radionuclide scanning are helpful in establishing the diagnosis of cholelithiasis and cholecystitis. Intestinal obstruction due to mechanical factors can be differentiated from pancreatitis by the history of colicky pain, findings on abdominal examination, and x-rays of the abdomen showing changes characteristic of mechanical obstruction. Acute mesenteric vascular occlusion is usually evident in elderly debilitated patients with brisk leukocytosis, abdominal distention, and bloody diarrhea, in whom paracentesis shows sanguineous fluid and arteriography shows vascular occlusion. Serum as well as peritoneal fluid amylase levels are increased, however, in patients with intestinal infarction. Systemic lupus erythematosus and polyarteritis nodosa may be confused with pancreatitis, especially since pancreatitis may develop as a complication of these diseases. Diabetic ketoacidosis is often accompanied by abdominal pain and elevated total serum am-

ylase levels, thus closely mimicking acute pancreatitis. However, the serum lipase and pancreatic isoamylase levels are not elevated in diabetic ketoacidosis.

COURSE OF THE DISEASE AND COMPLICATIONS It is important to identify patients with acute pancreatitis who have an increased risk of dying. Ranson and Imrie have used multiple prognostic criteria and have demonstrated that there is an increased mortality rate when three or more risk factors are identifiable either at the time of admission to the hospital or during the initial 48 h of hospitalization (Table 304-2). Recent studies indicate that obesity is a major risk factor for severe pancreatitis, presumably because the increased deposits of peripancreatic fat in such patients may predispose them to more extensive pancreatic and peripancreatic necrosis. The acute physiology and chronic health evaluation scoring system (APACHE II) uses the worst values of 12 physiologic measurements plus age and previous health status and provides a good description of illness severity for a wide range of common diseases; this score also correlates with outcome. Prospective studies have compared APACHE II with multiple prognostic criteria, i.e., Ranson and Imrie scores, in predicting the severity of acute pancreatitis. On admission, APACHE II identified approximately two-thirds of severe attacks, and after 48 h, the prognostic accuracy of APACHE II is comparable with that of Ranson and Imrie's scoring system. The drawbacks of APACHE II are (1) its complexity, (2) the requirement of a computer for scoring, and (3) standardization regarding peak values and cutoff scores. McMahon and colleagues have shown that the presence of a "toxic broth" or dark (hemorrhagic) fluid in abdominal pancreatitis is also an important prognostic indicator in acute pancreatitis. These multiple-factor scoring systems are difficult to use and have not been embraced consistently by clinicians. There is a great need for a reliable, simple biochemical test that consistently predicts outcome in patients with acute pancreatitis. Three candidate markers that show great promise are C-reactive protein, serum granulocyte elastase, and urinary trypsinogen activation peptide (TAP). The key indicators of a severe attack of acute pancreatitis are also listed in Table 304-2. Importantly, the presence of any one of these factors is associated with an increased risk of complications, and the presence of any two, with a 20 to 30% mortality rate. The high mortality rate of such severely ill patients is due in large part to infection and warrants intensive radiologic intervention and monitoring and/or a combination of radiologic and surgical means, as discussed in detail below.

The local and systemic complications of acute pancreatitis are listed in Table 304-3. In the first 2 to 3 weeks after pancreatitis patients frequently develop an inflammatory mass, which may be due to pancreatic necrosis (with or without infection) or may represent an abscess or pseudocyst (see below). Systemic complications include pulmonary, cardiovascular, hematologic, renal, metabolic, and central nervous system abnormalities. Pancreatitis and hypertriglyceridemia constitute an association in which cause and effect remain incompletely understood. However, several reasonable conclusions can be drawn. First, hypertriglyceridemia can precede and apparently cause pancreatitis. Second, the vast majority (>80%) of patients with acute pancreatitis do not have hypertriglyceridemia. Third, almost all patients with pancreatitis and hypertriglyceridemia have preexisting abnormalities in lipoprotein metabolism. Fourth, many of the patients with this association have persistent hypertriglyceridemia after recovery from pancreatitis and are prone to recurrent episodes of pancreatitis. Fifth, any factor (e.g., drugs or alcohol) that causes an abrupt increase in serum triglycerides to levels greater than 11 mmol/L (1000 mg/dL) can precipitate a bout of pancreatitis that can be associated with significant complications and even become fulminant. To avert the risk of triggering pancreatitis, a fasting serum triglyceride measurement should be obtained before estrogen replacement therapy is begun in postmenopausal women. Fasting levels less than 300 mg/dL pose no risk, whereas levels greater than 750 mg/dL are associated with a high probability of developing pancreatitis. Finally, patients with a defi-

Table 304-3 Complications of Acute Pancreatitis

LOCAL

Necrosis	Pancreatic ascites
Sterile	Disruption of main pancreatic
Infected	duct
Pancreatic fluid collections	Leaking pseudocyst
Pancreatic abscess	Involvement of contiguous organs
Pancreatic pseudocyst	by necrotizing pancreatitis
Pain	Massive intraperitoneal hemor-
Rupture	rhage
Hemorrhage	Thrombosis of blood vessels
Infection	(splenic vein, portal vein)
Obstruction of gastrointestinal	Bowel infarction
tract (stomach, duodenum, co-	Obstructive jaundice
lon)	

SYSTEMIC

Pulmonary	Renal
Pleural effusion	Oliguria
Atelectasis	Azotemia
Mediastinal abscess	Renal artery and/or renal vein
Pneumonitis	thrombosis
Adult respiratory distress syn-	Acute tubular necrosis
drome	Metabolic
Cardiovascular	Hyperglycemia
Hypotension	Hypertriglyceridemia
Hypovolemia	Hypocalcemia
Hypoalbuminemia	Encephalopathy
Sudden death	Sudden blindness (Purtscher's ret-
Nonspecific ST-T changes in elec-	inopathy)
trocardiogram simulating myo-	Central nervous system
cardial infarction	Psychosis
Pericardial effusion	Fat emboli
Hematologic	Fat necrosis
Disseminated intravascular coagu-	Subcutaneous tissues (erythema-
lation	tous nodules)
Gastrointestinal hemorrhage[a]	Bone
Peptic ulcer disease	Miscellaneous (mediastinum,
Erosive gastritis	pleura, nervous system)
Hemorrhagic pancreatic necrosis	
with erosion into major blood	
vessels	
Portal vein thrombosis, variceal	
hemorrhage	

[a] Aggravated by coagulation abnormalities (disseminated intravascular coagulation).

ciency of apolipoprotein CII have an increased incidence of pancreatitis; apolipoprotein CII activates lipoprotein lipase, which is important in clearing chylomicrons from the bloodstream.

Purtscher's retinopathy, a relatively unusual complication, is manifested by a sudden and severe loss of vision in a patient with acute pancreatitis. It is characterized by a peculiar funduscopic appearance with cotton-wool spots and hemorrhages confined to an area limited by the optic disk and macula; it is believed to be due to occlusion of the posterior retinal artery with aggregated granulocytes.

The two most common causes of acute pancreatitis are alcoholism and biliary tract disease; other causes are listed in Table 304-1. The risk of acute pancreatitis in patients with at least one gallstone smaller than 5 mm in diameter is fourfold greater than that in patients with larger stones. However, after a conventional workup, a specific cause is not identified in about 30% of patients. It is important to note that ultrasound examinations fail to detect gallstones, especially microlithiasis and/or sludge, in 4 to 7% of patients. In one series of 31 patients diagnosed initially as having idiopathic acute pancreatitis, 23 were found to have occult gallstone disease. Thus, approximately two-thirds of patients with recurrent acute pancreatitis without an obvious cause actually have occult gallstone disease due to microlithiasis. Examination of duodenal aspirates in such cases often reveals cholesterol crystals, which confirm the diagnosis. Other diseases of the biliary tree and pancreatic ducts that can cause acute pancreatitis include chole-

dochocele, ampullary tumors, pancreas divisum, and pancreatic duct stones, stricture, and tumor. Approximately 2% of patients with pancreatic carcinoma present with acute pancreatitis.

Pancreatitis in Patients with AIDS The incidence of acute pancreatitis is increased in patients with AIDS for two reasons: (1) the high incidence of infections involving the pancreas, such as infections with cytomegalovirus, *Cryptosporidium*, and the *Mycobacterium avium* complex; and (2) the frequent use by patients with AIDS of medications such as didanosine, pentamidine, and trimethoprim-sulfamethoxazole (Chap. 309).

℞ **TREATMENT** In most patients (approximately 85 to 90%) with acute pancreatitis, the disease is self-limited and subsides spontaneously, usually within 3 to 7 days after treatment is instituted. Conventional measures include (1) analgesics for pain, (2) intravenous fluids and colloids to maintain normal intravascular volume, (3) no oral alimentation, and (4) nasogastric suction to decrease gastrin release from the stomach and prevent gastric contents from entering the duodenum. Recent controlled trials, however, have shown that nasogastric suction offers no clear-cut advantages in the treatment of mild to moderately severe acute pancreatitis. Its use, therefore, must be considered elective rather than mandatory.

It has been demonstrated that CCK-stimulated pancreatic secretion is almost abolished in four different experimental models of acute pancreatitis. This finding probably explains why drugs to block pancreatic secretion in acute pancreatitis have failed to have any therapeutic benefit. For this and other reasons, anticholinergic drugs are not indicated in acute pancreatitis. In addition to nasogastric suction and anticholinergic drugs, other therapies designed to "rest the pancreas" by inhibiting pancreatic secretion have not changed the course of the disease. Although antibiotics have been used in the treatment of acute pancreatitis, randomized, prospective trials have shown no benefit from their use in acute pancreatitis of mild to moderate severity.

However, current experimental evidence favors the use of prophylactic antibiotics in severe acute pancreatitis. Results of four contemporary randomized clinical trials restricted to patients with prognostically severe acute pancreatitis have demonstrated an improved outcome, i.e., reduced rate of infection and/or mortality, associated with the antibiotic treatment. The carbapenem group of antibiotics, including imipenem, has a very broad spectrum including activity against *Pseudomonas*, *Staphylococcus*, and *Enterococcus*; and these agents penetrate well into pancreatic tissue. Furthermore, because secondary infection of necrotic pancreatic tissue (abscess, pseudocyst or obstructed biliary passages, ascending cholangitis complicating choledocholithiasis) contributes to many of the late deaths from pancreatitis, appropriate antibiotic therapy of established infections is quite important.

Several other drugs have been evaluated by prospective controlled trials and found ineffective in the treatment of acute pancreatitis. The list, by no means complete, includes glucagon, H_2 blockers, protease inhibitors such as aprotinin, glucocorticoids, calcitonin, nonsteroidal anti-inflammataory drugs (NSAIDs) and lexiplafant, a platelet-activating factor inhibitor. A recent meta-analysis of somatostatin, octreotide, and the antiprotease gabexate methylate in therapy of acute pancreatitis suggested (1) a reduced mortality rate but no change in complications with octreotide, and (2) no effect on the mortality rate but reduced pancreatic damage with gabexate.

Intraabdominal *Candida* infection during acute necrotizing pancreatitis is increasing in frequency and is associated with an increased mortality rate. In one representatitve trial, intraabdominal *Candida* infection was found in 13 of 37 cases and was associated with a mortality rate fourfold greater than that associated with intraabdominal bacterial infection alone. Given the impact of *Candida* infection on the mortality rate in acute necrotizing pancreatitis and the apparent benefit of prophylactic chemotherapy, these data suggest earlier use of fungicides.

A CT scan, especially a contrast-enhanced dynamic CT (CECT) scan, provides valuable information on the severity and prognosis of acute pancreatitis (Fig. 304-1 and Table 304-4). In particular, a CECT scan allows estimation of the presence and extent of pancreatic necrosis. Recent studies suggest that the likelihood of prolonged pancreatitis or a serious complication is negligible when the CT severity index is 1 or 2 and low with scores of 3 to 6. However, patients with scores of 7 to 10 had a 92% morbidity rate and a 17% mortality rate. Necrosis is present in 20 to 30% of patients. Those with necrosis have a morbidity rate >20%, whereas those without necrosis have a morbidity rate <10% and a negligible mortality rate. A CECT scan is indicated in patients with three or more of Ranson's signs, in all seriously ill patients, and in patients who show evidence of clinical deterioration. The patient with mild to moderate pancreatitis usually requires treatment with intravenous fluids, fasting, and possibly nasogastric suction for 2 to 4 days. A clear liquid diet is frequently started on the third to sixth day, and a regular diet by the fifth to seventh day. The patient with unremitting *fulminant pancreatitis* usually requires inordinate amounts of fluid and close attention to complications such as cardiovascular collapse, respiratory insufficiency, and pancreatic infection. The latter should be managed by a combination of radiologic and surgical means (see below). While earlier uncontrolled studies suggested that *peritoneal lavage* through a percutaneous dialysis catheter was helpful in severe pancreatitis, subsequent studies indicate that this treatment does not influence the outcome of such attacks. Aggressive surgical pancreatic debridement (necrosectomy) should be undertaken soon after confirmation of the presence of infected necrosis, and multiple operations may be required. Since the mortality rate from sterile acute necrotizing pancreatitis is approximately 10%, laparotomy with adequate drainage and removal of necrotic tissue should be considered if conventional therapy does not halt the patient's deterioration. The use of parenteral nutrition makes it possible to give nutritional support to patients with severe, acute, or protracted pancreatitis who are unable to eat normally. Patients with severe gallstone-induced pancreatitis may improve dramatically if papillotomy is carried out within the first 36 to 72 h of the attack. Studies indicate that only those patients with gallstone pancreatitis who are in the very severe group should be considered for urgent endoscopic retrograde cholangiopancreatography (ERCP). Finally, the treatment for patients with hypertriglyceridemia-associated pancreatitis includes (1) weight loss to ideal weight, (2) a lipid-restricted diet, (3) exercise, (4)

Table 304-4 Severity Index in Acute Pancreatitis

	Points
Grade of acute pancreatitis	
A. Normal pancreas	0
B. Pancreatic enlargement alone	1
C. Inflammation compared with pancreas and peripancreatic fat	2
D. One peripancreatic fluid collection	3
E. Two or more fluid collections	4
Degree of pancreatic necrosis	
A. No necrosis	0
B. Necrosis of one-third of pancreas	2
C. Necrosis of one-half of pancreas	4
D. Necrosis of more than one-half of pancreas	6

avoidance of alcohol and of drugs that can elevate serum triglycerides (i.e., estrogens, vitamin A, thiazides, and beta-blockers), and (5) control of diabetes.

INFECTED PANCREATIC NECROSIS, ABSCESS, AND PSEUDOCYST Infected pancreatic necrosis should be differentiated from pancreatic abscess. The former is a diffuse infection of an acutely inflamed, necrotic pancreas occurring in the first 1 to 2 weeks after the onset of pancreatitis. In contrast, a pancreatic abscess is an ill-defined, liquid collection of pus that evolves over a longer period, often 4 to 6 weeks. It tends to be less life-threatening and is associated with a lower rate of surgical mortality. Infected pancreatic necrosis should be treated by surgical debridement because the solid component of the infected pancreas is not amenable to effective radiologically guided percutaneous evacuation. Pancreatic abscess can be treated surgically or, in selected cases, by percutaneous drainage. The necrotic pancreas becomes secondarily infected in 40 to 60% of patients, most frequently with gram-negative bacteria of alimentary origin. Whether infection occurs depends on several factors, including the extent of pancreatic and peripancreatic necrosis, the degree of pancreatic ischemia and hypoperfusion, and the presence of organ or multiorgan failure.

A

B

FIGURE 304-1 Acute pancreatitis: CT evolution. *A.* Contrast-enhanced CT scan of the abdomen performed on admission of a patient with clinical evidence of acute pancreatitis. Note the mildly decreased density of the body of the pancreas to the left of the midline (*arrow*). There are a few linear strands in the peripancreatic fat, suggesting inflammation (*open arrows*). A small amount of fluid is seen in the anterior pararenal space (*arrowhead*). *B.* Nine days after admission, there is a marked worsening with severe inflammation of the pancreas evidenced by anterior displacement of the posterior gastric wall (*arrows*), increased inflammation of the peripancreatic fat, and increased pancreatic effusion in the anterior perirenal space and around the splenic vein (*open arrows*). (*Courtesy of Dr. PR Ros, University of Florida College of Medicine.*)

The early diagnosis of pancreatic infection can be accomplished by CT-guided needle aspiration. In one study, 60 patients, representing 5% of all admissions for acute pancreatitis, were suspected of harboring a pancreatic infection on the basis of fever, leukocytosis, and an abnormal CT scan (pseudocyst or extrapancreatic fluid collection). Importantly, 60% of these patients had a pancreatic infection, and 55% of these infections developed in the first 2 weeks. These findings suggest that only guided aspiration can reliably distinguish sterile from infected pancreatic necrosis. The following are guidelines for patients meeting the above selection criteria: (1) Pseudocysts should be aspirated promptly, because more than half may be infected; (2) extrapancreatic fluid collections need not be aspirated promptly, because most are sterile; (3) if a necrotic pancreas is found initially to be sterile but fever and leukocytosis persist, several days of observation should be allowed to pass before reaspiration is considered, as clinical improvement frequently occurs; and (4) if fever and leukocytosis recur after an interval of well-being, reaspiration should be considered.

Severe pancreatitis with the presence of three or more risk factors, postoperative pancreatitis, early oral feeding, early laparotomy, and perhaps injudicious use of antibiotics predispose to the development of pancreatic abscess, which occurs in 3 to 4% of patients with acute pancreatitis. Pancreatic abscess also may develop because of a communication between a pseudocyst and the colon, inadequate surgical drainage of a pseudocyst, or needling of a pseudocyst. The characteristic signs of abscess are fever, leukocytosis, ileus, and rapid deterioration in a patient previously recovering from pancreatitis. Sometimes, however, the only manifestations are persistent fever and signs of continuing pancreatic inflammation. Drainage of pancreatic abscesses by percutaneous catheter techniques, using CT guidance, has been only moderately successful (resolution in 50 to 60% of patients). Accordingly, laparotomy with radical sump drainage and possibly resection of necrotic tissue is usually required, because the mortality rate for undrained pancreatic abscess approaches 100%. Multiple abscesses are common, and reoperation is frequently necessary.

Pseudocysts of the pancreas are collections of tissue, fluid, debris, pancreatic enzymes, and blood which develop over a period of 1 to 4 weeks after the onset of acute pancreatitis; they form in approximately 15% of patients with acute pancreatitis. In contrast to true cysts, pseudocysts do not have an epithelial lining; their walls consist of necrotic tissue, granulation tissue, and fibrous tissue. Disruption of the pancreatic ductal system is common. However, the subsequent course of this disruption varies widely, ranging from spontaneous healing to continuous leakage of pancreatic juice, which results in tense ascites. Pseudocysts are preceded by pancreatitis in 90% of cases and by trauma in 10%. Approximately 85% are located in the body or tail of the pancreas and 15% in the head. Some patients have two or more pseudocysts. Abdominal pain, with or without radiation to the back, is the usual presenting complaint. A palpable, tender mass may be found in the middle or left upper abdomen. The serum amylase level is elevated in 75% of patients at some point during their illness and may fluctuate markedly.

On x-ray examination, 75% of pseudocysts can be seen to displace some portion of the gastrointestinal tract (Fig. 304-2). Sonography, however, is reliable in detecting pseudocysts. Sonography also permits differentiation between an edematous, inflamed pancreas, which can give rise to a palpable mass, and an actual pseudocyst. Furthermore, serial ultrasound studies will indicate whether a pseudocyst has resolved. CT complements ultrasonography in the diagnosis of pancreatic pseudocyst (Fig. 304-2), especially when the pseudocyst is infected.

In studies with sonography, pseudocysts were seen to resolve in 25 to 40% of patients. Pseudocysts that are greater than 5 cm in diameter and that persist for longer than 6 weeks should be considered for drainage. Recent natural history studies have suggested that noninterventional, expectant management is the best course in selected patients with minimal symptoms and no evidence of active alcohol use in whom the pseudocyst appears mature by radiography and does not resemble a cystic neoplasm. A significant number of these pseudocysts resolve spontaneously more than 6 weeks after their formation. Also, these studies demonstrate that large pseudocyst size is not an absolute indication for interventional therapy and that many peripancreatic fluid collections detected on CT in cases of acute pancreatitis resolve spontaneously. A pseudocyst that does not resolve spontaneously may lead to serious complications, such as (1) pain caused by expansion of the lesion and pressure on other viscera, (2) rupture, (3) hemorrhage, and (4) abscess. Rupture of a pancreatic pseudocyst is a particularly serious complication. Shock almost always supervenes, and mortality rates range from 14% if the rupture is not associated with hemorrhage to over 60% if hemorrhage has occurred. Rupture and hemorrhage are the prime causes of death from pancreatic pseudocyst. A triad of findings—an increase in the size of the mass, a localized bruit over the mass, and a sudden decrease in hemoglobin level and hematocrit without obvious external blood loss—should alert one to the possibility of hemorrhage from a pseudocyst. Thus, in patients who are stable and free of complications and in whom serial ultrasound studies show that the pseudocyst is shrinking, conservative therapy is indicated. Conversely, if the pseudocyst is expanding and is complicated by rupture, hemorrhage, or abscess, the patient should be operated on. With ultrasound or CT guidance, sterile chronic pseudocysts can be treated safely with single or repeated needle aspiration or more prolonged catheter drainage with a success rate of 45 to 75%. The success rate of these techniques for infected pseudocysts is considerably less (40 to 50%). Patients who do not respond to drainage require surgical therapy for internal or external drainage of the cyst.

Pseudoaneurysms develop in up to 10% of patients with acute pancreatitis at sites reflecting the distribution of pseudocysts and fluid collections (Fig. 304-2D). The splenic artery is most frequently involved, followed by the inferior and superior pancreatic duodenal arteries. This diagnosis should be suspected in patients with pancreatitis who develop upper gastrointestinal bleeding without an obvious cause or in whom thin-cut CT scanning reveals a contrast-enhanced lesion within or adjacent to a suspected pseudocyst. Arteriography is necessary to confirm the diagnosis.

PANCREATIC ASCITES AND PANCREATIC PLEURAL EFFUSIONS   Pancreatic ascites is usually due to disruption of the main pancreatic duct, often by an internal fistula between the duct and the peritoneal cavity or a leaking pseudocyst (Chap. 43). This diagnosis is suggested in a patient with an elevated serum amylase level in whom the ascites fluid has both increased levels of albumin [30 g/L (>3.0 g/dL)] and a markedly elevated level of amylase. The fluid in true pancreatic ascites usually has an amylase concentration of >20,000 U/L as a result of the ruptured duct or leaking pseudocyst. Lower amylase elevations may be found in the peritoneal fluid of patients with acute pancreatitis. In addition, ERCP often demonstrates passage of contrast material from a major pancreatic duct or a pseudocyst into the peritoneal cavity. As many as 15% of patients with pseudocysts have concurrent pancreatic ascites. The differential diagnosis should include intraperitoneal carcinomatosis, tuberculous peritonitis, constrictive pericarditis, and Budd-Chiari syndrome.

If the pancreatic duct disruption is posterior, an internal fistula may develop between the pancreatic duct and the pleural space, producing a pleural effusion, which is usually left-sided and often massive. This complication often requires thoracentesis or chest tube drainage.

Treatment usually requires the use of nasogastric suction and parenteral alimentation to decrease pancreatic secretion. In addition, paracentesis is performed to keep the peritoneal cavity free of fluid and, it is hoped, to effect sealing of the leak. The long-acting somatostatin analogue octreotide, which inhibits pancreatic secretion, is useful in cases of pancreatic ascites and pleural effusion. If ascites continues to recur after 2 to 3 weeks of medical management, the patient should

A

B

C

D

FIGURE 304-2 Pseudocyst of pancreas. *A.* Upper gastrointestinal x-ray showing displacement of stomach by pseudocyst. *B.* Sonogram showing pseudocyst (*cyst*). GB, gallbladder; MVP, portal vein. Behind the large pseudocyst is seen the calcified head of the pancreas. A dilated common bile duct (*asterisk*) is noted. *C.* CT scan showing pseudocyst. Note the large, lobulated fluid collection (*arrows*) surrounding the tail of the pancreas (*arrowheads*). Note also the dense, thin rim in the periphery representing the fibrous capsule of the pseudocyst. *D.* Spiral CT showing a pseudocyst (*small arrow*) with a pseudoaneurysm (light area in pseudocyst). Note the demonstration of the main pancreatic duct (*big arrow*), even though this duct is minimally dilated by ERCP. (*A, B courtesy of Dr. CE Forsmark, University of Florida College of Medicine; C, D courtesy of Dr. PR Ros, University of Florida College of Medicine.*)

be operated on after pancreatography to define the anatomy of the abnormal duct. A disrupted main pancreatic duct can also be treated effectively by stenting. Patients in whom ERCP identifies two or more sites of extravasation are unlikely to respond to conservative management and/or stenting.

CHRONIC PANCREATITIS AND PANCREATIC EXOCRINE INSUFFICIENCY

GENERAL AND ETIOLOGIC CONSIDERATIONS Chronic inflammatory disease of the pancreas may present as episodes of acute inflammation in a previously injured pancreas or as chronic damage with persistent pain or malabsorption. The causes of relapsing chronic pancreatitis are similar to those of acute pancreatitis (Table 304-1), except that there is an appreciable incidence of cases of undetermined origin. In addition, the pancreatitis associated with gallstones is predominantly acute or relapsing-acute in nature. A cholecystectomy is almost always performed in patients after the first or second attack of gallstone-associated pancreatitis. Patients with chronic pancreatitis may present with persistent abdominal pain, with or without steatorrhea; some (~15%) present with steatorrhea and no pain.

Patients with chronic pancreatitis in whom there is extensive destruction of the pancreas (less than 10% of exocrine function remaining) have steatorrhea and azotorrhea. Among American adults, alcoholism is the most common cause of clinically apparent pancreatic exocrine insufficiency, while cystic fibrosis is the most frequent cause in children. In up to 25% of American adults with chronic pancreatitis, the cause is not known; that is, they have idiopathic chronic pancreatitis. Mutations of the cystic fibrosis transmembrane conductance regulator (CFTR) gene have been documented in patients with idiopathic chronic pancreatitis. It has been estimated that in patients with idiopathic pancreatitis the frequency of a single CFTR mutation is 11 times the expected frequency and the frequency of two mutant alleles is 80 times the expected frequency. The results of sweat chloride testing are not diagnostic of cystic fibrosis in these patients. However, these patients have functional evidence of a defect in CFTR-mediated ion transport in nasal epithelium. It is suggested that up to 25% of patients with idiopathic chronic pancreatitis may have abnormalities of the CFTR gene. The therapeutic and prognostic implication of these findings remain to be determined. In other parts of the world, severe protein-calorie malnutrition is a common cause. Table 304-5 lists other causes of pancreatic exocrine insufficiency, but they are relatively uncommon.

PATHOPHYSIOLOGY   The events that initiate an inflammatory process in the pancreas are still not well understood, and the many hypotheses will not be reviewed here. In the case of alcohol-induced pancreatitis, it has been suggested that the primary defect may be the precipitation of protein (inspissated enzymes) in the ducts. The resulting ductal obstruction could lead to duct dilation, diffuse atrophy of the acinar cells, fibrosis, and eventual calcification of some of the protein plugs. However, the fact that some alcoholic patients with recurrent acute pancreatitis show no evidence of chronic pancreatitis does not support this hypothesis. In fact, experimental and clinical observations have shown that alcohol has direct toxic effects on the pancreas. While patients with alcohol-induced pancreatitis generally consume large amounts of alcohol, some consume very little (50 g/d or less). Thus prolonged consumption of "socially acceptable" amounts of alcohol is compatible with the development of pancreatitis. In addition, the finding of extensive pancreatic fibrosis in patients who died during their first attack of clinical acute alcohol-induced pancreatitis supports the concept that such patients already have chronic pancreatitis.

CLINICAL FEATURES   Patients with relapsing chronic pancreatitis may present with symptoms identical to those of acute pancreatitis, but pain may be continuous, intermittent, or absent. The pathogenesis of this pain is poorly understood. Although the classic description is of epigastric pain radiating through the back, the pain pattern is often atypical; the pain may be worst in the right or left upper quadrant of the back or may be diffuse throughout the upper abdomen; it may even be referred to the anterior chest or flank. Characteristically it is persistent, deep-seated, and unresponsive to antacids. It often is worsened by ingestion of alcohol or a heavy meal (especially one rich in fat). Often the pain is severe enough to necessitate the frequent use of narcotics.

Weight loss, abnormal stools, and other signs or symptoms suggestive of malabsorption (see Table 286-5) are common in chronic pancreatitis. However, clinically apparent deficiencies of fat-soluble vitamins are surprisingly rare. The physical findings in these patients are usually not impressive, so that there is a disparity between the severity of the abdominal pain and the physical signs (other than some abdominal tenderness and mild temperature elevation).

DIAGNOSTIC EVALUATION   (See also Chap. 303)   In contrast to relapsing acute pancreatitis, the serum amylase and lipase levels are usually not elevated in chronic pancreatitis. Elevations of serum bilirubin and alkaline phosphatase levels may indicate cholestasis secondary to chronic inflammation around the common bile duct (Fig. 304-3). Many patients demonstrate impaired glucose tolerance, and some have an elevated fasting blood glucose level.

The classic triad of pancreatic calcification, steatorrhea, and diabetes mellitus usually establishes the diagnosis of chronic pancreatitis and exocrine pancreatic insufficiency but is found in less than one-third of chronic pancreatitis patients. Accordingly, it is often necessary to perform an intubation test such as the *secretin stimulation test*, which usually gives abnormal results when 60% or more of pancreatic exocrine function has been lost. Approximately 40% of patients with chronic pancreatitis have *cobalamin (vitamin B_{12})* malabsorption, which can be corrected by the administration of oral pancreatic enzymes. There is usually a marked excretion of fecal fat (Chap. 286), which can be reduced by the administration of oral pancreatic enzymes. The serum trypsinogen (Chap. 303) and the D-xylose urinary excretion test are useful in patients with "pancreatic steatorrhea," since the trypsinogen level will be abnormal, and D-xylose excretion usually is normal. A decreased serum trypsinogen level strongly suggests severe pancreatic exocrine insufficiency.

The radiographic hallmark of chronic pancreatitis is the presence of scattered calcification throughout the pancreas (Fig. 304-3). Diffuse pancreatic calcification indicates that significant damage has occurred and obviates the need for a secretin test. While alcohol is by far the most common cause, pancreatic calcification also may be seen in cases of severe protein-calorie malnutrition, hereditary pancreatitis, post-traumatic pancreatitis, hyperparathyroidism, islet cell tumors, and idiopathic chronic pancreatitis. A large prospective study has shown convincingly that pancreatic calcification decreases or even disappears spontaneously in one-third of patients with severe chronic pancreatitis; this outcome may also follow ductal decompression. Pancreatic calcification is a dynamic process that is incompletely understood.

Sonography, CT, and ERCP greatly aid the diagnosis of pancreatic disease. In addition to excluding pseudocysts and pancreatic cancer, sonography and CT may show calcification or dilated ducts associated with chronic pancreatitis (Fig. 304-4). ERCP is the only major technique that provides a direct view of the pancreatic duct. In patients with alcohol-induced pancreatitis, ERCP may reveal a pseudocyst missed by sonography or CT.

COMPLICATIONS OF CHRONIC PANCREATITIS   The complications of chronic pancreatitis are protean. *Cobalamin (vitamin B_{12})* malabsorption occurs in 40% of patients with alcohol-induced chronic pancreatitis and in virtually all with cystic fibrosis. It is consistently corrected by the administration of pancreatic enzymes (containing proteases). It may be due to excessive binding of cobalamin by cobalamin-binding proteins other than intrinsic factor, which ordinarily are destroyed by pancreatic proteases and therefore do not compete with intrinsic factor for cobalamin binding. Although most patients show *impaired glucose tolerance*, diabetic ketoacidosis and coma are uncommon. Similarly, end-organ damage (retinopathy, neu-

Table 304-5   Causes of Pancreatic Exocrine Insufficiency

Alcohol, chronic alcoholism
Idiopathic pancreatitis
Cystic fibrosis
Hypertriglyceridemia
Severe protein-calorie malnutrition with hypoalbuminemia
    Tropical pancreatitis (Africa, Asia)
Pancreatic and duodenal neoplasms
Pancreatic resection
Gastric surgery
    Subtotal gastrectomy with Billroth I anastomosis
    Subtotal gastrectomy with Billroth II anastomosis
    Truncal vagotomy and pyloroplasty
Gastrinoma (Zollinger-Ellison syndrome)
Hereditary pancreatitis
Traumatic pancreatitis
Abdominal radiotherapy
Hemochromatosis
Shwachman's syndrome (pancreatic insufficiency and bone marrow dysfunction)
Trypsinogen deficiency
Enterokinase deficiency
Isolated deficiencies of amylase, lipase, or proteases
α_1-Antitrypsin deficiency

A

B

C

D

FIGURE 304-3 Radiologic abnormalities in chronic pancreatitis. *A.* Pancreatic calcification (*arrows*) and stenosis (tapering) of the intrahepatic portion of the common bile duct demonstrated by percutaneous transhepatic cholangiography. *B.* Pancreatic calcification (*large white arrow*) demonstrated by sonography. Note dilated pancreatic duct (*thin white arrow*) and splenic vein (*open arrow*). *C.* Pancreatic calcification (*vertical arrows*) and dilated pancreatic duct (*horizontal arrow*) demonstrated by CT scan. *D.* Endoscopic retrograde cholangiogram shows grossly dilated pancreatic ducts (*arrows*) in a patient with long-standing pancreatitis.

ropathy, nephropathy) is also uncommon, and the appearance of these complications should raise the question of concomitant genetic diabetes mellitus. A nondiabetic retinopathy, peripheral in location and secondary to vitamin A and/or zinc deficiency, is common in these patients. *Effusions* containing high concentrations of amylase may occur into the pleural, pericardial, or peritoneal space. *Gastrointestinal bleeding* may occur from peptic ulceration, gastritis, a pseudocyst eroding into the duodenum, or ruptured varices secondary to splenic vein thrombosis due to inflammation of the tail of the pancreas. *Icterus* may occur, caused either by edema of the head of the pancreas, which compresses the common bile duct, or by chronic cholestasis secondary to a chronic inflammatory reaction around the intrapancreatic portion of the common bile duct (Fig. 304-3). The chronic obstruction may lead to cholangitis and ultimately to biliary cirrhosis. *Subcutaneous fat necrosis* may appear as tender red nodules on the lower extremities. *Bone pain* may be secondary to intramedullary fat necrosis. Inflammation of the large and small joints of the upper and lower extremities may occur. The incidence of pancreatic carcinoma is increased in patients with chronic pancreatitis who have been followed for 2 or more years. Twenty years after the diagnosis of chronic pancreatitis, the cumulative risk of pancreatic carcinoma is 4%.

Perhaps the most common and troublesome complication is addiction to narcotics.

℞ **TREATMENT** Therapy for patients with chronic pancreatitis is directed toward two major problems—pain and malabsorption. Patients with intermittent attacks of pain are treated essentially like those with acute pancreatitis (see above). Patients with severe and persistent pain should avoid alcohol completely and avoid large meals rich in fat. Since the pain is often severe enough to require frequent use of narcotics (and hence addiction), a number of surgical procedures have been developed for pain relief. ERCP allows the surgeon to plan the operative approach. If there is a stricture of the pancreatic duct, a *local resection* may ameliorate the pain. Unfortunately, isolated localized strictures are not common. In most patients with alcohol-induced disease, the pancreas is diffusely involved, and surgically correctible localized ductal disease is rare. When there is primary ductal obstruction and dilation, ductal decompression may provide effective pain palliation. Short-term pain relief may be achieved in up to 80% of patients, while long-term pain relief occurs in approximately 50%. In some of these patients, however, pain relief can be achieved only by resecting 50 to 95% of the gland. Although pain relief is achieved

A

B

FIGURE 304-4 Chronic pancreatitis and pancreatic calculi: CT scan and ERCP appearance. *A*. In this contrast-enhanced CT scan of the abdomen, there is evidence of an atrophic pancreas with multiple calcifications (*arrows*). Note the markedly dilated pancreatic duct seen in this section through the body and tail (*open arrows*). *B*. ERCP in the same patient demonstrates the dilated pancreatic duct as well as an intrapancreatic duct calculus (*arrows*). These findings correlate nicely with the CT scan appearance.

in three-quarters of these patients, they tend to develop pancreatic endocrine and exocrine insufficiency and must be treated with pancreatic enzyme replacement therapy. It is important to screen patients carefully, for such radical surgery is contraindicated in those who are severely depressed or suicidal or who continue to drink. Procedures such as splanchnicectomy, celiac ganglionectomy, and nerve blocks usually bring only temporary relief and are not recommended. Endoscopic treatment of chronic pancreatitis may involve sphincterotomy of the minor or major pancreatic sphincter, dilatation of strictures, removal of calculi, or stenting of the ventral or dorsal pancreatic duct. Although many of these techniques are technically impressive, none has been subjected to a randomized trial in patients with chronic pancreatitis. In addition, significant complications—acute pancreatitis, pancreatic abscess, damage to the pancreatic duct, and death—have occurred in up to 36% of patients after stent placement.

Three double-blind trials have demonstrated that administration of pancreatic enzymes decreases abdominal pain in selected patients with chronic pancreatitis. In these trials, approximately 75% of the patients evaluated experienced pain relief. The patients most likely to respond are those with mild to moderate exocrine pancreatic dysfunction, as evidenced by an abnormal secretin test, normal fat absorption, and minimal abnormalities on ERCP examination. These clinical observations seem to fit with data from human beings and experimental animals demonstrating a negative feedback regulation for pancreatic exocrine secretion controlled by the amount of proteases within the lumen of the proximal small intestine. It seems reasonable to use the following approach for patients with severe, persistent, or continuous abdominal pain thought to be caused by chronic pancreatitis. After other causes of abdominal pain (peptic ulcer, gallstones, etc.) have been excluded, a pancreatic *sonogram* should be done. If no mass is found, a *secretin test* may be performed, because its results usually are abnormal in cases of chronic pancreatitis with pain. If the results are abnormal (i.e., decreased bicarbonate concentration or volume output), a 3- to 4-week *trial of pancreatic enzyme administration* is appropriate. Eight conventional tablets or capsules are taken at meals and at bedtime. There are a number of studies suggesting that patients may have small-duct chronic pancreatitis and chronic abdominal pain with a normal appearance on radiographic evaluations (ultrasound, CT, ERCP) but abnormal results on hormone stimulation tests (secretin test) and/or abnormal pancreatic histology. Such minimal-change chronic pancreatitis may respond well to pancreatic enzyme therapy (non-enteric-coated) for relief of abdominal pain. If no relief is obtained, and especially if the volume secreted during the secretin test is very low, ERCP should be performed. If a pseudocyst or a localized ductal obstruction is found, surgery should be considered. A patient who has dilated ducts may be a candidate for a surgical ductal decompression procedure. This procedure provides short-term relief in up to 80% of patients, although long-term results are closer to 50%. Some studies have shown octreotide to be effective in decreasing abdominal pain in patients with severe large-duct disease. If no surgically remediable lesion is found and severe pain continues despite abstinence from alcohol, subtotal pancreatic resection may be necessary.

The treatment of malabsorption rests on the use of pancreatic enzyme replacement therapy. Diarrhea and steatorrhea are usually improved by this treatment, although the steatorrhea may not be completely corrected. The major problem is delivering enough active enzyme into the duodenum. Steatorrhea could be abolished if 10% of the normal amount of lipase could be delivered to the duodenum at the proper time. This concentration of lipase cannot be achieved with the current preparations of pancreatic enzymes, even if the latter are given in large doses. The reason for these poor results may be that lipase is inactivated by gastric acid, that food empties from the stomach faster than do the pancreatic enzymes, and that batches of commercially available pancreatic extracts vary in enzyme activity.

For the usual patient, two or three enteric-coated capsules or eight conventional (non-enteric-coated) tablets of a potent enzyme preparation should be administered with meals. Some patients using conventional tablets require adjuvant therapy to improve enzyme replacement treatment. H_2 receptor antagonists, sodium bicarbonate, and proton pump inhibitors are effective adjuvants. Antacids containing calcium carbonate or magnesium hydroxide are not effective and may actually result in increased steatorrhea. Several publications have reported colonic strictures in patients with cystic fibrosis receiving extraordinarily high doses of high-potency pancreatic enzyme preparations. Such lesions have not been reported in adults with chronic pancreatitis.

Supportive measures include diet restriction and pain medications. The diet should be moderate in fat (30%), high in protein (24%), and low in carbohydrate (40%). Restriction of long-chain triglyceride intake can help patients who do not respond satisfactorily to pancreatic enzyme therapy. Use of foods containing mainly medium-chain fatty acids, which do not require lipase for digestion, may be beneficial. Nonnarcotic analgesics should be emphasized. Patients taking narcotic drugs for pain relief often become addicted and continue to have pain.

Table 304-6 Pancreatic Endocrine Tumors

Syndrome	Hormone(s) Produced	Primary Hormone Effects	Pathologic Features	Clinical Features
Zollinger-Ellison	Gastrin	Gastric acid hypersecretion with basal acid outputs usually >15 mmol/h (>15 mEq/h)	Delta cell islet tumors; 10% aberrant (duodenal); 60% malignant	Severe peptic ulcer disease often refractory to therapy; ectopic ulcers; diarrhea; multiple endocrine adenomas (parathyroid, pituitary, adrenal, thyroid)
Insulinoma	Insulin	Hypoglycemia with inappropriately increased serum insulin levels	Beta cell islet tumors; 80–90% benign	Hypoglycemic symptoms
Glucagonoma	Glucagon; pancreatic polypeptide	Hyperglucagonemia → glucose intolerance	Alpha cell islet tumors; 60% malignant	Slow-growing pancreatic tumor; hyperglycemia; eczematoid dermatitis, or necrolytic erythema weight loss; anemia; gastric and intestinal motor abnormalities
Somatostatinoma	Somatostatin; pancreatic polypeptide	Somatostatin inhibits insulin, gastrin, and pancreatic enzyme secretion; decreased bile flow	Delta cell islet tumor	Pancreatic tumor; diarrhea; steatorrhea; gallstones; diabetes mellitus; anemia
Pancreatic cholera	Vasoactive intestinal peptide ? Gastric inhibitory polypeptide ? Prostaglandin E ? Pancreatic peptide	Net secretion of salt and water by gut	? Delta cell tumor; >50% malignant	Pancreatic tumor with severe watery diarrhea; flushing; weight loss; hypokalemia; hypercalcemia; hypochlorhydria; hyperglycemia; inordinate fecal water and electrolyte losses
Carcinoid	Serotonin; prostaglandins	Altered gut motility; diarrhea	Enterochromaffin cells; non-beta-cell islet tumors	Carcinoid syndrome with flushing; wheezing; diarrhea; alcohol intolerance; hepatomegaly

Patients with severe exocrine pancreatic insufficiency secondary to alcohol who continue to drink have a high mortality rate (in one series, 50% of patients who were followed for 5 to 12 years died during this period) and significant morbidity (weight loss, lassitude, vitamin deficiency, and narcotic addiction). Chronic pancreatitis carries significant medical and social costs. A recent study found that pancreatitis led to retirement in 11% of patients with the disease, accounting for 45% of all retirements. In 87% of patients with chronic pancreatitis unable to maintain gainful employment, alcoholism was a contributing factor. Patients with chronic pancreatitis also use substantial medical resources. In 1987 in the United States, this diagnosis accounted for 122,000 recorded outpatient visits and 56,000 hospital admissions. Pain may abate if progressive severe exocrine insufficiency continues. Patients who abstain from alcohol and use vigorous replacement therapy for maldigestion-malabsorption do reasonably well.

HEREDITARY PANCREATITIS Hereditary pancreatitis is a rare disease that is similar to chronic pancreatitis except for an early age of onset and evidence of hereditary factors (involving an autosomal dominant gene with incomplete penetrance). A genome-wide search using genetic linkage analysis identified the hereditary pancreatitis gene on chromosome 7. An R117H mutation in the cationic trypsinogen gene occurs in most of the families with hereditary pancreatitis that have been studied. Molecular modeling predicts the formation of hydrolysis-resistant trypsin that could lead to pancreatic autodigestion. These patients have recurring attacks of severe abdominal pain which may last from a few days to a few weeks. The serum amylase and lipase levels may be elevated during acute attacks but usually are normal. Patients frequently develop pancreatic calcification, diabetes mellitus, and steatorrhea, and, in addition, they have an increased incidence of pancreatic carcinoma. Such patients often require ductal decompression for pain relief. Abdominal complaints in relatives of patients with hereditary pancreatitis should raise the question of pancreatic disease.

PANCREATIC ENDOCRINE TUMORS

→*Pancreatic endocrine tumors are summarized in Table 304-6 and are discussed in Chap. 93.*

OTHER CONDITIONS

ANNULAR PANCREAS When the ventral pancreatic anlage fails to migrate correctly to make contact with the dorsal anlage, the result may be a ring of pancreatic tissue encircling the duodenum. Such an annular pancreas may cause intestinal obstruction in the neonate or the adult. Symptoms of postprandial fullness, epigastric pain, nausea, and vomiting may be present for years before the diagnosis is entertained. The radiographic findings are symmetric dilation of the proximal duodenum with bulging of the recesses on either side of the annular band, effacement but not destruction of the duodenal mucosa, accentuation of the findings in the right anterior oblique position, and lack of change on repeated examinations. The differential diagnosis should include duodenal webs, tumors of the pancreas or duodenum, postbulbar peptic ulcer, regional enteritis, and adhesions. Patients with annular pancreas have an increased incidence of pancreatitis and peptic ulcer. Because of these and other potential complications, the treatment is surgical even if the condition has been present for years. Retrocolic duodenojejunostomy is the procedure of choice, although some surgeons advocate Billroth II gastrectomy, gastroenterostomy, and vagotomy.

PANCREAS DIVISUM Pancreas divisum occurs when the embryologic ventral and dorsal pancreatic anlagen fail to fuse, so that pancreatic drainage is accomplished mainly through the accessory papilla. Pancreas divisum is the most common congenital anatomic variant of the human pancreas. Current evidence indicates that this anomaly does not predispose to the development of pancreatitis in the great majority of patients who harbor it. However, the combination of pancreas divisum and a small accessory orifice could result in dorsal duct obstruction. The challenge is to identify this subset of patients with dorsal duct pathology. Cannulation of the dorsal duct by ERCP is not as easily done as is cannulation of the ventral duct. Patients with pancreatitis and pancreas divisum demonstrated by ERCP should be treated with conservative measures. In many of these patients, pancreatitis is idiopathic and unrelated to the pancreas divisum. Endoscopic or surgical intervention is indicated only when the above methods fail. If marked dilation of the dorsal duct can be demonstrated, surgical ductal decompression should be performed. The appropriate therapy for patients without dilation of the dorsal duct is not yet defined. It should be stressed that the ERCP appearance of pancreas divisum—i.e., a small-caliber ventral duct with an arborizing pattern—may be mistaken as representing an obstructed main pancreatic duct secondary to a mass lesion.

MACROAMYLASEMIA In macroamylasemia, amylase circulates in the blood in a polymer form too large to be easily excreted by the kidney. Patients with this condition demonstrate an elevated serum amylase value, a low urinary amylase value, and a C_{am}/C_{cr} ratio of less than 1%. The presence of macroamylase can be documented by chromatography of the serum. The prevalence of macroamylasemia is 1.5% of the nonalcoholic general adult hospital population. Usually macroamylasemia is an incidental finding and is not related to disease of the pancreas or other organs.

Macrolipasemia has now been documented in a few patients with cirrhosis or non-Hodgkin's lymphoma. In these patients, the pancreas appeared normal on ultrasound and CT examination. Lipase was shown to be complexed with immunoglobulin A. Thus, the possibility of *both* macroamylasemia and macrolipasemia should be considered in patients with elevated blood levels of these enzymes.

ACKNOWLEDGMENT
This chapter represents a revised version of a chapter by Dr. Norton J. Greenberger, Dr. Phillip P. Toskes, and Dr. Kurt J. Isselbacher that was in the previous editions of this textbook.

BIBLIOGRAPHY

ADAMS DB et al: Outcome after lateral pancreaticojejunostomy for chronic pancreatitis. Ann Surg 219:481, 1994

ANDRIULLI A et al: Meta-analysis of somatostatin, octreotide, and gabexate mesilate in the therapy of acute pancreatitis. Aliment Pharmacol Ther 12:237, 1998

BALTHAZAR EJ et al: Acute pancreatitis: Value of CT in establishing prognosis. Radiology 174:331, 1990

BANKS PA et al: CT-guided aspiration of suspected pancreatic infection: Bacteriology and clinical outcome. Int J Pancreatol 18:265, 1995

BASSI C et al: Controlled clinical trial of perfloxicin versus imipenem in severe acute pancreatitis. Gastroenterology 115:1513, 1998

BOZKURT T et al: Comparison of pancreatic morphology and exocrine functional impairment in patients with chronic pancreatitis. Gut 35:1132, 1994

CAVALLINI G et al: Gabexate for the prevention of pancreatic damage related to endoscopic retrograde cholangiopancreatography. N Engl J Med 335:919, 1996

CHEY WY: Neurohormonal control of the exocrine pancreas. Curr Opin Gastroenterol 13: 375, 1997

COHN JA et al: Relation between mutations of the cystic fibrosis gene and idiopathic pancreatitis. N Engl J Med 339:653, 1998

FORSMARK CE, TOSKES PP: What does an abnormal pancreatogram mean? Gastrointest Endosc Clin North Am 5:105, 1995

GELTECK CJ et al: Severe hypertriglyceridemia and pancreatitis when estrogen replacement therapy is given to hypertriglyceridemic women. J Lab Clin Med 123:59, 1994

HOERAUF A et al: Intra-abdominal Candida infection during acute necrotizing pancreatitis has a high prevalence and is associated with increased mortality. Crit Care Med 26: 2010, 1998

JOSEPHSON S, TOSKES PP: Chronic pancreatitis: Medical management. Practical Gastroenterol 20:6, 1996

LEE SP et al: Biliary sludge as a cause of acute pancreatitis. N Engl J Med 326:589, 1992

LOWENFELS AB et al: Prognosis of chronic pancreatitis: An international multi-center study. Am J Gastroenterol 89:1467, 1994

MONTORSI M et al: Efficacy of octreotide in the prevention of pancreatic fistula after elective pancreatic resections: A prospective, controlled randomized clinical trial. Surgery 117:26, 1995

PETTI JJ et al: Pancolonic disease in cystic fibrosis and high dose pancreatic enzyme therapy. J Pediatr 125:587, 1994

POWELL JJ et al: Antibiotic prophylaxis in the initial management of severe acute pancreatitis. Br J Surg 85:582, 1998

SHARER N et al: Mutations of the cystic fibrosis gene in patients with chronic pancreatitis. N Engl J Med 339:645, 1998

SHERMAN S et al: Stent-induced pancreatic ductal and parenchymal changes: Correlation of endoscopic ultrasound with ERCP. Gastrointest Endosc 44:276, 1996

STEER ML et al: Chronic pancreatitis. N Engl J Med 332:1482, 1995

TODD HB, DESIREE EM: Acute necrotizing pancreatitis. N Engl J Med 340:1412, 1999

WALSH TN: Minimal change chronic pancreatitis. Gut 33:1566, 1992

WHITCOMB DC et al: Hereditary pancreatitis is caused by a mutation in the cationic trypsinogen gene. Nat Genet 13:141, 1996

Section 1
DISORDERS OF THE IMMUNE SYSTEM

305

Barton F. Haynes, Anthony S. Fauci

INTRODUCTION TO THE IMMUNE SYSTEM

ADCC antibody-dependent cellular cytotoxicity	MHC major histocompatibility complex
APCs antigen-presenting cells	MIP macrophage inflammatory protein
ATG anti-thymocyte globulin	NK natural killer
BCR B cell receptors	NK-Rs NK receptors
CTLs cytotoxic T lymphocytes	PAMPs pathogen-associated molecular patterns
FDCs follicular dendritic cells	
GM-CSF granulocyte-macrophage colony stimulating factor	PRRs pattern recognition receptors
HEVs high endothelial venules	PTKs protein tyrosine kinases
IDDM insulin-dependent diabetes mellitus	RAG recombinase activating gene
	STAT signal transducers and activators of transcription
IFN interferon	TCR T cell receptor
IL interleukin	TGF transforming growth factor
IVIg intravenous immunoglobulin	TNF tumor necrosis factor
LAK lymphokine-activated killer	X-SCID x-linked form of severe combined immune deficiency syndrome
LGLs large granular lymphocytes	
LPS lipopolysacchride	
MAB monoclonal antibody	
MCP monocyte chemotactic protein	

DEFINITIONS

- *Adaptive immune system*—recently evolved system of immune responses mediated by T and B lymphocytes. Immune responses by these cells are based on specific antigen recognition by clonotypic receptors that are products of genes that rearrange during development and throughout the life of the organism. Additional cells of the adaptive immune system include various types of antigen-presenting cells.
- *Antibody*—B cell–produced molecules encoded by genes that rearrange during B cell development consisting of immunoglobulin heavy and light chains that together form the central component of the B cell receptor for antigen. Antibody can exist as B cell surface antigen-recognition molecules or as secreted molecules in plasma and other body fluids.
- *Antigens*—foreign or self molecules that are recognized by the adaptive and innate immune systems resulting in innate immune cell triggering, T cell activation, and/or B cell antibody production.
- *Antimicrobial peptides*—small peptides <100 amine acids in length that are produced by cells of the innate immune system and have anti-infectious agent activity.
- *B lymphocytes*—bone marrow–derived or bursal-equivalent lymphocytes that express surface immunoglobulin (the B cell receptor for antigen) and secrete specific antibody after interaction with antigen.
- *B cell receptor for antigen*—complex of surface molecules that rearrange during postnatal B cell development, made up of surface immunoglobulin (Ig) and associated Ig $\alpha\beta$ chain molecules that recognize nominal antigen via Ig heavy and light chain variable regions, and signal the B cell to terminally differentiate to make antigen-specific antibody.
- *Complement*—cascading series of plasma enzymes and effector proteins whose function is to lyse pathogens and/or target them to be phagocytized by neutrophils and monocyte/macrophage lineage cells of the reticuloendothelial system.
- *Co-stimulatory molecules*—molecules of antigen-presenting cells (such as B7-1 and B7-2 or CD40) that lead to T cell activation when ligated by ligands on activated T cells (such as CD28 or CD40 ligand).
- *Cytokines*—soluble proteins that interact with specific cellular receptors that are involved in the regulation of the growth and activation of immune cells and mediate normal and pathologic inflammatory and immune responses.
- *Dendritic cells*—myeloid and/or lymphoid lineage antigen-presenting cells of the adaptive immune system. Immature dendritic cells, or dendritic cell precursors, are key components of the innate immune system by responding to infections with production of high levels of cytokines. Dendritic cells are key initiators both of innate immune responses via cytokine production and of adaptive immune responses via presentation of antigen to T lymphocytes.
- *Innate immune system*—ancient immune recognition system of host cells bearing germline encoded pattern recognition receptors (PRRs) that recognize pathogens and trigger a variety of mechanisms of pathogen elimination. Cells of the innate immune system include natural killer (NK) cell lymphocytes, monocytes/macrophages, immature or dendritic cell precursors, neutrophils, basophils, eosinophils, tissue mast cells, and epithelial cells.
- *Large granular lymphocytes*—lymphocytes of the innate immune system with azurophilic cytotoxic granules that have NK cell activity capable of killing foreign and host cells with little or no self major histocompatibility complex (MHC) class I molecules.
- *Natural killer cells*—large granular lymphocytes that kill target cells that express little or no HLA class I molecules, such as malignantly transformed cells and virally infected cells. NK cells express receptors that inhibit killer cell function when self MHC class I is present.
- *Pathogen-associated molecular patterns*—Invariant molecular structures expressed by large groups of microorganisms that are recognized by host cellular PRRs in the mediation of innate immunity.
- *Pattern recognition receptors*—germline-encoded receptors expressed by cells of the innate immune system that recognize pathogen-associated molecular patterns (PAMPs).
- *T cells*—thymus-derived lymphocytes that mediate adaptive cellular immune responses including T helper and cytotoxic T lymphocyte effector cell functions.
- *T cell receptor for antigen*—complex of surface molecules that rearrange during postnatal T cell development made up of clonotypic T cell receptor (TCR) α and β chains that are associated with the CD3 complex composed of invariant γ, δ, ε, ζ, and η chains. The clonotypic TCR α and β chains recognize peptide fragments of protein antigen physically bound in antigen-presenting cell MHC class I or II molecules, leading to signaling via the CD3 complex to mediate effector functions.
- *Tolerance*—recognition of foreign or self antigens by B and T lymphocytes in the absence of expression of antigen-presenting cell co-stimulatory molecules that leads to B and T cell nonresponsiveness to antigens. Active T lymphocyte tolerance can be achieved through blockade of the B7/CD28 co-stimulatory pathway.

INTRODUCTION   The human immune system has evolved over millions of years from both invertebrate and vertebrate organisms to develop sophisticated defense mechanisms highly specific for invading pathogens. Immune systems evolved to protect the host from microbes and their virulence factors. From invertebrates, humans have inherited the innate immune system, an ancient defense system that uses germ line–encoded proteins to recognize pathogens. Cells of the innate immune system, such as macrophages and NK lymphocytes, recognize pathogen molecular motifs that are highly conserved among many microbes (PAMPs) and use a diverse set of receptor molecules (PRRs). Important components of the recognition of microbes by the innate immune system are: (1) recognition by germ line–encoded host molecules, (2) recognition of key microbe virulence factors but not recognition of self molecules, and (3) nonrecognition of benign foreign molecules or microbes. It is particularly important for the innate immune system to not recognize foreign nonpathogenic molecules that are common in the environment, since reaction against them would cause continuous inflammatory disease. Upon contact with pathogens, macrophages and NK cells may kill pathogens directly or may activate a series of events that both slows the infection and recruits the more recently evolved arm of the human immune system, the adaptive immune system.

Adaptive immunity is found only in vertebrates and is based on the generation of antigen receptor T and B lymphocytes by germ-line gene rearrangements that occur during the development of each person. By a complex series of molecular mechanisms of gene rearrangement, individual T or B cells express unique antigen receptors on their surface, such that taken together the pools of adult human T and B lymphocytes contain cells capable of specifically recognizing the diverse antigens of the myriad of infectious agents in the environment. Coupled with finely tuned specific recognition mechanisms that maintain tolerance to self antigen, T and B lymphocytes of the adaptive immune system with their postnatally rearranged clonotypic antigen receptors bring both *specificity* and *immune memory* to vertebrate host defenses.

This chapter describes the cellular components, molecules, and mechanisms that make up the innate and adaptive immune systems and describes how adaptive immunity is recruited to the defense of the host by innate immune responses. An appreciation of the cellular and molecular bases of innate and adaptive immune responses is critical to understanding the pathogenesis of inflammatory, autoimmune, infectious, and immunodeficiency diseases.

THE CD CLASSIFICATION OF HUMAN LYMPHO-CYTE DIFFERENTIATION ANTIGENS   The development of monoclonal antibody technology led to the discovery of a large number of new leukocyte surface molecules. In 1982, the First International Workshop on Leukocyte Differentiation Antigens was held to establish a nomenclature for cell-surface molecules of human leukocytes. From this and subsequent leukocyte differentiation workshops has come the cluster of differentiation (CD) classification of leukocyte antigens (Table 305-1). The data presented in Table 305-1 establish a context to facilitate discussion and study of the complex series of events that transpire during normal and aberrant innate and adaptive human immune responses.

THE INNATE IMMUNE SYSTEM   All multicellular organisms, including humans, have developed the use of a limited number of germ line–encoded molecules that recognize large groups of pathogens. Because of the myriad human pathogens, host molecules of the human innate immune system must recognize PAMPs, the common molecular structures shared by many pathogens. PAMPs must be conserved structures vital to pathogen virulence and survival, such as bacterial endotoxin, so that pathogens cannot mutate molecules of PAMPs to evade human innate immune responses. In addition, one major end product of innate immunity is the destruction of the invading pathogen, thus necessitating that PAMPs recognized by innate immune responses be completely distinct from self molecules. PPRs are host proteins of the innate immune system that recognize PAMPs and are human molecules whose ancestors are evolutionarily ancient (Tables 305-2, 305-3). Thus, recognition of pathogen molecules by hematopoietic and nonhematopoietic cell types leads to activation/production of the complement cascade, cytokines, and antimicrobial peptides as effector molecules.

PATTERN RECOGNITION   Major PRR families of proteins include C-type lectins, leucine-rich proteins, macrophage scavenger receptor proteins, plasma pentraxins, lipid transferase, and integrins (Table 305-3). A major group of PRR collagenous glycoproteins with C-type lectin domains are termed *collectins* and include the serum protein, mannose-binding lectin. Mannose-binding lectin and other collectins, as well as two other protein families—the pentraxins (such as C-reactive protein and serum amyloid P) and macrophage scavenger receptors—all have the property of opsonizing (coating) bacteria for phagocytosis by macrophages and can also activate the complement cascade to lyse bacteria. Integrins are cell-surface adhesion molecules that signal cells after cells bind bacterial lipopolysacchride (LPS) and activate phagocytic cells to ingest pathogens.

A remarkable series of recent discoveries has revealed the mechanisms of connection between the innate and adaptive immune systems; these include (1) the plasma protein, LPS-binding protein, which binds and transfers LPS to the macrophage LPS receptor, CD14; and (2) a human family of proteins called *Toll proteins*, which are associated with CD14, bind LPS, and signal the macrophage to produce cytokines and upregulate cell-surface molecules that signal the initiation of adaptive immune responses (Fig. 305-1, Table 305-3, and Table 305-4). Proteins in the Toll family are expressed on macrophages (Toll 2 and Toll 4) and on dendritic cells and B cells (RP105). Upon ligation these receptors activate a series of intracellular events that lead to the killing of bacteria as well as to the recruitment and ultimate activation of antigen-specific T and B lymphocytes (Fig. 305-1). Importantly, signaling by massive amounts of LPS through Toll receptors leads to the release of large amounts of cytokines that mediate LPS-induced shock. Mutations in Toll proteins in mice protect from LPS shock, and mutations in Toll proteins in humans similarly protect from LPS-induced inflammatory diseases such as LPS-induced asthma.

Cells of invertebrates and vertebrates produce antimicrobial small peptides containing fewer than 100 amino acids that can act as endogenous antibodies (Table 305-2). Some of these peptides are produced by epithelia that line various organs, while others are found in macrophages or neutrophils that ingest pathogens. Antimicrobial peptides have been identified that kill bacteria such as *Pseudomonas* spp., *Escherichia coli*, and *Mycobacterium tuberculosis*.

EFFECTOR CELLS OF INNATE IMMUNITY   Cells of the innate immune system and their roles in the first line of host defense are described in Table 305-4. Equally important as their roles in the mediation of innate immune responses are the roles that each cell type plays in recruiting T and B lymphocytes of the adaptive immune system to engage in specific antipathogen responses.

Monocytes-Macrophages   Monocytes arise from precursor cells within bone marrow (Fig. 305-2) and circulate with a half-life ranging from 1 to 3 days. Monocytes leave the peripheral circulation by marginating in capillaries and migrating into a vast extravascular pool. Tissue macrophages arise from monocytes that have migrated out of the circulation and by in situ proliferation of macrophage precursors in tissue. Common locations where tissue macrophages (and certain of their specialized forms) are found are lymph node, spleen, bone marrow, perivascular connective tissue, serous cavities such as the peritoneum, pleura, skin connective tissue, lung (alveolar macrophage), liver (Kupffer cell), bone (osteoclast), central nervous system (microglia), and synovium (type A lining cell).

In general, monocytes-macrophages are on the first line of defense associated with innate immunity; however, they also play a major role in recruitment of adaptive immune responses by mediation of functions such as binding LPS, the presentation of antigen to T lymphocytes, and the secretion of factors such as interleukin (IL) 1, tumor necrosis factor (TNF), IL-12, and IL-6, which are central to antigen-

Table 305-1 Human Leukocyte Surface Antigens - the CD Classification of Leukocyte Differentiation Antigens

Surface Antigen (Other Names)	Family	Molecular Mass, kDa	Distribution	Ligand(s)	Function
CD1a (T6, HTA-1)	Ig	49	CD, cortical thymocytes	Not known	Possible role in T cell development
CD1b	Ig	45	CD, cortical thymocytes	Not known	Antigen presentation of lipids
CD1c	Ig	43	DC, cortical thymo-cytes, subset of B cells	Not known	Unknown
CD1d	Ig	?	Cortical thymocytes, intestinal epithelium	Not known	Presentation of peptide antigens
CD2 (T12, LFA-2)	Ig	50	T, NK	CD58, CD48, CD59, CD15	Alternative T cell activation, T cell anergy, T cell cytokine produc-tion, T- or NK-mediated cytoly-sis, T cell apoptosis, cell adhesion
CD3 (T3, Leu-4)	Ig	γ:25–28, δ:21–28, ε:20–25, η:21–22, ζ:16	T	Associates with the TCR	T cell activation and function; ζ is the signal transduction compo-nents of the CD3 complex
CD4 (T4, Leu-3)	Ig	55	T, myeloid	MHC-II, HIV, gp120, IL-16, SABP	T cell selection, T cell activation, signal transduction with p56lck, primary receptor for HIV
CD7 (3A1, Leu-9)	Ig	40	T, NK	K-12 (CD7L)	T and NK cell signal transduction and regulation of IFN-γ, TNF-α production
CD8 (T8, Leu-2)	Ig	34	T	MHC-I	T cell selection, T cell activation, signal transduction with p56lck
CD10 (CALLA,	Zn metalloprotease	100	Early T and B precur-sors, G,	Not known	Possible role in B cell develop-ment; Zn metalloprotease
CD11a (LFA-1α, αL integrin)	α Integrin	170–180	All leukocytes	CD54, CD102, CD50	Cell adhesion, co-stimulation
CD11b (αM integrin, Mac-1, CR3)	α Integrin	165–170	G, M, NK, subset of B and T	iC3b, fibrinogen, CD23	Cell adhesion, phagocytosis, ab-sent in Leukocyte Adhesion Defi-ciency-1 patients
CD11c (αX integrin, CR4)	α Integrin	145–150	G, M, NK, subset of B and T	iC3b, fibrinogen, CD23	Cell adhesion, phagocytosis, ab-sent in Leukocyte adhesion defi-ciency (LAD) 1 patients
CD14 (LPS-receptor)	LRG	53–55	M, G (weak), not by myeloid progenitors	Endotoxin (lipopoly-saccharide), lipo-teichoic acid, PI	Endotoxin (LPS) receptor
CD16a (FcγRIIIA, Leu-11)	Ig	50–65	NK, G, M, subset of T	IgG	Low-affinity receptor for IgG, ADCC, activation of cytotoxicity, cytokine production
CD16b (FcγRIIIB)	Ig	50–65	G	IgG	Low-affinity IgG receptor, GPI-linked
CD18 (β2 integrin)	β Integrin	95	All leukocytes	See CD11a, CD11b, CD11c	Associates with CD11a, CD11b, and CD11c; defect in CD18 causes LAD-1
CD19 B4	Ig	95	B (except plasma cells), FDC	Not known	Associates with CD21 and CD81 to form a complex involved in signal transduction in B cell de-velopment, activation, and differentiation
CD20 (B1)	Unassigned	33–37	B (except plasma cells)	Not known	Cell signaling, may be important for B cell activation and proliferation
CD21 (B2, CR2, EBV-R, C3dR)	RCA	145	Mature B, FDC, sub-set of thymocytes	C3d, C3dg, iC3b, CD23, EBV	Associates with CD19 and CD81 to form a complex involved in signal transduction in B cell de-velopment, activation, and differ-entiation; Epstein-Barr virus receptor
CD22 (BL-CAM)	Ig	130–140	Mature B	CDw75	Cell adhesion, signaling through association with p72sky, p53/56lyn, PI3 kinase, SHP1, fLCγ
CD23 (FcεRII, B6, Leu-20, BLAST-2)	C-type lectin	45	B, M, FDC	IgE, CD21, CD11b, CD11c	Regulates IgE synthesis, cytokine release by monocytes
CD27	TNFR	55	T, B, mature thymo-cytes, subset NK	CD70	Co-stimulatory for T cell activation
CD28	Ig	44	T, plasma cells	CD80, CD86	Co-stimulatory for T cell activa-tion; involved in the decision be-tween T cell activation and anergy

(continued)

Surface Antigen (Other Names)	Family	Molecular Mass, kDa	Distribution	Ligand(s)	Function
CD29 (β1 integrin)	β Integrin	130	Broad	See CD49a–f	Associates with CD49a–f to function in cell adhesion
CD30 (Ki-1 antigen)	TNFR	105–120	M; activated T, B, NK; Hodgkin's cells, certain non-hodgkin's lymphomas	CD153	TCR-mediated cell death, activates NfκB, thymocytes negative selection
CD32 (FcγRII)	Ig	40	M, MP, G, B, P, DC, subset EC	IgG	Low-affinity receptor for IgG mediates endocytosis, cytotoxicity, and immunomodulation
CD34	Sialomucin	90	Hematopoietic progenitor cells, endothelium	L-selectin	Cell adhesion
CD35 (CR1, C3bR, C4bR)	RCA	160–255	G, M, E, B, subset T, RBC, FDC, others	C3b, C4b, iC3b, C3dg, iC3, iC4	Binding of C4b/C3b coated particles, removing and processing immune complexes
CD38 (T10)	Unassigned	45	Early B and T, activated B and T, thymocytes, GC B cells, plasma cells	Not known	Co-stimulatory for T cell and B cell activation, ADP ribosyl cyclase activity
CD40	TNFR	48–50	B, DC, EC, thymic epithelium, MP, cancers	CD154	B cell activation, proliferation, and differentiation, formation of GCs, isotype switching, rescue from apoptosis
CD44 (H-CAM, Hermes, In(Lu)-related)	Hyaladherin	85	Broad	Hyaluronan, MIP-1β, osteopontin, ankyrin	Cell adhesion, signaling, activation
CD44R (CD44v)	Hyaladherin	85–250	Epithelia, M, activated leukocytes	Hyaluronan, MIP-1β, bFGF, ostopontin, ankyrin	Unclear, but possibly mediates cell movement through ECM and the metastasis of certain epithelial malignancies
CD45 (LCA, T200, B220)	PTP	180, 200, 210, 220	All leukocytes	Galectin-1, CD2, CD3, CD4	T and B activation, thymocyte development, signal transduction, apoptosis
CD45RA	PTP	210, 220	Subset T, medullary thymocytes, "naive" T	Galectin-1, CD2, CD3, CD4	Isoforms of CD45 containing exon 4 (A), restricted to a subset of T cells
CD45RB	PTP	200, 210, 220	All leukocytes	Galectin-1, CD2, CD3, CD4	Isoforms of CD45 containing exon 5 (B)
CD45RC	PTP	210, 220	Subset T, medullary thymocytes, "naive" T	Galectin-1, CD2, CD3, CD4	Isoforms of CD45 containing exon 6 (C), restricted to a subset of T cells
CD45RO	PTP	180	Subset T, cortical thymocytes, "memory" T	Galectin-1, CD2, CD3, CD4	Isoforms of CD45 containing no differentially spliced exons, restricted to a subset of T cells
CD49a (VLA-1, α1 integrin)	α Integrin	200–210	M, activated T, NK, subset EC, fibroblasts, neuronal cells	Laminin, collagen I, collagen IV	Cell adhesion, associates with β1 integrin (CD29)
CD49b (VLA-2, α2 integrin, GPIa)	α Integrin	155–165	T and B, P, EC, fibroblasts, subset epithelia	Collagen I, II, III, IV; laminin	Cell adhesion, rgulation of matrix metalloproteinase I and collagen I expression, associates with β1 integrin (CD29)
CD49c (VLA-3, α3 integrin)	α Integrin	145–150	B, subset epithelia, fibroblasts	Fibronectin, collagen, laminin	Cell adhesion, associates with β1 integrin (CD29)
CD49d (VLA-4, α4 integrin)	α Integrin	145–150	B, T, M, NK, DC, subset cancers	CD106, MadCAM-1, fibronectin, invasin, thrombospondin	Cell adhesion, lymphocyte migration, associates with β1 integrin (CD29)
CD49e (VLA-5, α5 integrin, FNR-α)	α Integrin	160	T, M, P, EC, fibroblasts, muscle cells, subset epithelia, progenitor cells	L1, fibronectin	Cell adhesion, migration, matrix assembly, associates with β1 integrin (CD29)
CD49f (VLA-6, α6 integrin)	α Integrin	150	T, M, eosinophils, P, epithelia	Laminin	Cell adhesion, spreading and migration, associates with β1 integrin (CD29)
CD54 (ICAM-1)	Ig	75–115	M, activated T and B, activated EC, activated fibroblasts, subset epithelia	CD11a/CD18, CD11b/CD18, rhinovirus	Cell adhesion, receptor for rhinovirus
CD58 (LFA-3)	Ig	40–70	Broad	CD2	Cell adhesion
CD64 (FCRI)	Ig	72	Myeloid cells	IgG	Binds IgG

(continued)

Table 305-5—(continued)

Surface Antigen (Other Names)	Family	Molecular Mass, kDa	Distribution	Ligand(s)	Function
CD70 (CD27L, Ki-24 antigen)	TNF	55–170	Activated T and B, Hodgkin's cells, anaplastic large cell lymphoma	CD27	Antibodies inhibit T cell proliferation in some systems; used for typing lymphomas
CD73 (ecto 5′ nucleotidase)	Unassigned	69–72	Subset of T and B, FDC, EC, epithelia	AMP	Co-stimulatory molecule, may be involved in B-FDC interactions
CD79a	Ig	47	B	Not known	Complexes with sIg to form the BCR
CD79b	Ig	37	B	Not known	Complexes with sIg to form the BCR
CD80 (B7-1, BB1)	Ig	60	Activated B and T, MP, DC	CD28, CD152	Co-regulator of T cell activation; signaling through CD28 stimulates and through CD152 inhibits T cell activation
CD83	Ig	43	DC	Not known	Unknown
CD86 (B7-2, B70)	Ig	80	Subset B, DC, EC, activated T, thymic epithelium	CD28, CD152	Co-regulator of T cell activation; signaling through CD28 stimulates and through CD152 inhibits T cell activation
CD95 (APO-1, Fas)	TNFR	135	Activated T and B	Fas ligand	Mediates apoptosis
CD132 (Common γ chain)	Class I CKR	64–70	T, B, MK, M, G	IL-2, -4, -7, -9, -15	Signal transduction component of the IL-2, -4, -7, -9, and -15 receptors
CD134 (OX40)	TNFR	50	Activated T	gp34	Cell adhesion and T cell co-stimulation
CD152 (CTLA-4)	Ig	30–33	Activated T	CD80, CD86	Inhibits T cell proliferation
CD153 (CD30L)	TNF	38–40	Activated T	CD30	T cell proliferation and cytokine production
CD154 (CD40L)	TNF	33	Activated CD4+ T, subset CD8+ T, NK, M, basophil	CD40	Co-stimulatory for T cell activation, B cell proliferation and differentiation

ABBREVIATIONS: ADCC, antibody-dependent cellular cytotoxicity; AMP, adenosine monophosphate; BL-CAM, B-lymphocyte cell adhesion molecule; BLAST, B cell–specific activation antigen; CALLA, common acute lymphoblastic leukemia antigen; CKR, cytokine receptor; CTLA, cytotoxic T lymphocyte–associated protein; DC, dendritic cells; EBV, Epstein-Barr virus; EC, endothelial cells; ECM, extracellular matrix; FcγRIIIA, low-affinity IgG receptor isoform A; FDC, follicular dendritic cells; G, granulocytes; GC, germinal center; GPI, glycosyl phosphotidylinositol; H-CAM, homing-associated cell adhesion molecule; HTA, human thymocyte antigen; ICAM, intercellular adhesion molecule; IgG, immunoglobulin G; In(Lu), inhibitor lutheran; LCA, leukocyte common antigen; LFA, lymphocyte function antigen; LPS, lipopolysaccharide; LRG, leucine rich repeats; M, monocytes; MAC, macrophage; MadCAM, mucosal addressin cell adhesion molecule; MHC-I, major histocompatibility complex class I; MP, macrophages; Mr, relative molecular mass; NK, natural killer cells; P, platelets; PBT, peripheral blood T cells; PI, phosphotidylinositol; PI3K, phosphotidylinositol 3-kinase; PLC, phospholipase C; PTP, protein tyrosine phosphatase; RBC, red blood cells; SABP, secretory actin binding protein; TCR, T cell receptor; TNF, tumor necrosis factor; TNFR, tumor necrosis factor receptor; VLA, very late activation antigen.

SOURCE: Compiled with permission from T Kishimoto et al (eds): *Leukocyte Typing VI*, New York, Garland Publishing 1997; R Brines et al: Immunology Today 18S:1, 1997; and S Shaw ed: *Protein Reviews on the Web* www.ncbi.nlm.nih.gov/prow.

specific activation of T and B lymphocytes (Fig. 305-1). Although monocytes-macrophages were originally thought to be the major antigen-presenting cells (APCs) of the immune system, it is now clear that dendritic/Langerhans cells are the most potent and effective APCs in the body (see below). Monocytes-macrophages mediate innate immune effector functions such as destruction of antibody-coated bacteria, tumor cells, or even normal hematopoietic cells in certain types of autoimmune cytopenias. Activated macrophages can also mediate antigen-nonspecific lytic activity and eliminate cell types such as tumor cells in the absence of antibody. This activity is largely mediated by cytokines (i.e., TNF-α and IL-1). Monocytes-macrophages express lineage-specific molecules (e.g., the cell-surface LPS receptor, CD14) as well as surface receptors for a number of molecules, including the Fc region of IgG (CD16, CD32, CD64), activated complement components (CD35) (Table 305-1), and various cytokines (Table 305-5). Finally, macrophage secretory products are more diverse than those of any other cell of the immune system. Among monocyte-macrophage-secreted products are hydrolytic enzymes, products of oxidative metabolism, TNF-α, IL-1, -6, -10, -12, -15, -18, and a number of chemoattractant cytokines (chemokines) involved in the orchestration of an immune response in tissues (Table 305-5).

Dendritic/Langerhans Cells Dendritic/Langerhans cells are bone marrow–derived APCs that are distinct from monocytes-macrophages and are derived from both lymphoid and myeloid lineages. They generally lack the standard T, B, NK, and monocyte cell markers but do express CD83 and other molecules that aid in their identification. They can be expanded in culture, and their function is enhanced

by the cytokines granulocyte-macrophage colony stimulating factor (GM-CSF), IL-1, IL-4, and TNF-α. They are distinguished by an exceptional ability to present antigen, by expression of high levels of MHC class II and co-stimulatory molecules, and by dendritic morphology with multiple thin membrane projections (veils).

Dendritic cells are referred to as Langerhans cells when they are present in the skin and beneath the mucosal surface. They comprise the dendritic cells of the blood and the spleen and the veil cells of afferent lymphatics, and they form part of the interdigitating cell network of lymphoid organs. In responses involving the innate immune

Table 305-2   **Major Components of the Innate Immune System**

Pattern recognition receptors (PRR)	C type lectins, leucine-rich proteins, scavenger receptors, pentraxins, lipid transferases, integrins
Antimicrobial peptides	α-Defensins, β-defensins, cathelin, protegrin, granulsyin, histatin, secretory leukoprotease inhibitor, and probiotics
Cells	Macrophages, dendritic cells, NK cells, NK-T cells, neutrophils, eosinophils, mast cells, basophils, and epithelial cells
Complement components	Classic and alternative complement pathway, and proteins that bind complement components
Cytokines	Autocrine, paracrine, endocrine cytokines that mediate host defense and inflammation, as well as recruit, direct, and regulate adaptive immune responses

NOTE: NK cells, natural killer cells.

Table 305-3 Major Pattern Recognition Receptors (PRR) of the Innate Immune System

PRR Protein Family	Sites of Expression	Examples	Ligands (PAMPs)	Functions of PRR
C-type lectins				
Humoral	Plasma proteins	Collectins	Bacterial and viral carbohydrates	Opsonization of bacteria and virus, activation of complement
Cellular	Macrophages, dendritic cell	Macrophage mannose receptor	Terminal mannose	Phagocytosis of pathogens
	Natural killer (NK) cells	NKG2-A	Carbohydrate on HLA molecules	Inhibits killing of host cells expressing HLA+ self peptides
Leucine-rich proteins	Macrophage, epithelial cells	CD14	Lipopolysaccharide (LPS)	Binds LPS and Toll proteins
	Macrophage, many others	Toll proteins (Toll2, Toll4 on macrophages, RP105 on B cells and dendritic cells)	Lipopolysaccharide	Binds LPS and activates the cell to produce cytokines to activate adaptive immunity. Also LPS ligation of Toll or RR105 proteins on macrophages, dendritic cells, or B cell induces B7-1 (CD80) and B7-2 (CD86) co-stimulatory molecules that are required for T and B cell antigen presentation in adaptive immune responses
Scavenger receptors	Macrophage	Macrophage scavenger receptors	Bacterial cell walls	Phagocytosis of bacteria
Pentraxins	Plasma protein	C-creative proteins	Phosphotidyl choline	Opsonization of bacteria, activation of complement
	Plasma protein	Serum amyloid P	Bacterial cell walls	Opsonization of bacteria, activation of complement
Lipid transferases	Plasma protein	LPS binding protein	LPS	Binds LPS, transfers LPS to CD14
Integrins	Macrophages, dendritic cells, NK cells	CD11b,c; CD18	LPS	Signals cells, activates phagocytosis

NOTE: PAMPs, pathogen-associated molecular patterns.
SOURCE: Adapted with permission from Medzhitov and Janeway, 1997a.

system, bacterial LPS binds to dendritic cell RP105 Toll-like protein, upregulating dendritic cell molecules, such as MHC class II, B7-1 (CD80), and B7-2 (CD86), which enhance specific antigen presentation and induce dendritic cell cytokine production.

A critical cell type of the innate immune system is the dendritic cell precursor that, in response to viral infections, produces high levels of interferon (IFN) α. IFN-α in turn activates NK cells to kill virally infected cells and activates monocytes-macrophages and other APCs to recruit antigen-specific T and B cells to respond to viral infections. thus, immature dendritic cells are important components of innate immunity, while mature dendritic cells, as APCs, are important components of adaptive immunity.

Follicular Dendritic Cells Follicular dendritic cells (FDCs) are APCs for B cells and their lineage is distinct from that of dendritic/Langerhans cells, the major APCs for T cells. FDCs are located in the germinal centers of follicles of secondary lymphoid organs. Their main function is to trap and retain antigens in the germinal centers of lymphoid organs and to present these antigens to B cells. Antigen is retained on their membranes in the form of antigen-antibody complexes that bind to the cell via the cellular receptor for C3. FDCs have extensive, thin, finger-like projections that surround the B cells in the germinal centers, allowing for maximal exposure of trapped antigen. The retention of antigen on the surface of FDC membranes is critical for the selection and growth of high-affinity clones of B cells and for the maintenance of B cell memory. Of note, HIV is trapped in large quantities on the processes of FDCs in lymphoid organs, allowing the lymphoid tissue to serve as a reservoir of virus and a source of infection for CD4+ T cells migrating into the area to provide help to B cells in the initiation and propagation of an HIV-specific humoral response (Chap. 309).

Large Granular Lymphocytes/Natural Killer Cells Large granular lymphocytes (LGLs) account for approximately 5 to 10% of peripheral blood lymphocytes. LGLs are nonadherent, nonphagocytic

cells with large azurophilic cytoplasmic granules. LGLs express surface receptors for the Fc portion of IgG (CD16) and for NCAM-I (CD56), and many LGLs express some T lineage markers, particularly CD8, and proliferate in response to IL-2. LGLs arise in both bone marrow and thymic microenvironments (Fig. 305-2).

Functionally, LGLs share features with both monocytes-macrophages and neutrophils in that LGLs mediate both antibody-dependent cellular cytotoxicity (ADCC) and NK activity. ADCC is the binding of an opsonized (antibody-coated) target cell to an Fc receptor–bearing effector cell via the Fc region of antibody, resulting in lysis of the target by the effector cell. NK cell activity is the nonimmune (i.e., effector cell never having had previous contact with the target), MHC-unrestricted, non-antibody-mediated killing of target cells, which are usually malignant cell types, transplanted foreign cells, or virus-infected cells. Thus, LGLs that mediate NK cell activity may play an important role in immune surveillance and destruction of cells that spontaneously undergo malignant transformation in vivo. Subsets of NK cells may play a role in hematopoietic cell engraftment; some subsets stimulate bone marrow stem cells, and others stimulate engraftment. Lymphokine-activated killer (LAK) cells are NK lymphocytes that proliferate in vitro to high concentrations of IL-2 and develop the ability to kill tumor cells more efficiently than unstimulated NK cells. Rare patients with complete absence of NK cells have been described who lack both NK cell activity and CD56+, CD16+ lymphocytes but have normal T and B cell function. NK cell hyporesponsiveness is also observed in patients with the *Chédiak-Higashi syndrome*, an autosomal recessive disease associated with fusion of cytoplasmic granules and defective degranulation of neutrophil lysosomes.

The ability of NK cells to kill target cells is inversely related to target cell expression of MHC class I molecules. Thus, NK cells kill target cells with low or no levels of MHC class I expression and are prevented from killing target cells with high levels of class I expression. Recent studies have demonstrated the presence of NK receptors (NK-Rs) or killer cell inhibitory receptors (KIRs) that bind to either classic MHC class I molecules in a polymorphic way or the MHC-class Ib molecule HLA-E (Fig. 305-3). In every person, NK cells express at least one NK-R that recognizes a self–MHC class I allele. NK-Rs of the Ig superfamily bind specific MHC class I molecules; for example, the NK-R p140 binds HLA-A3, and another NK-R, p70, binds HLA-B27 (Fig. 305-3). A second NK-R of the C-type lectin family of proteins is termed *CD94/NKG2A* and binds the MHC-related protein HLA-E (Fig. 305-3). HLA-E has an MHC class I structure but exclusively binds the leader sequence peptides of classic MHC class I molecules in the HLA-E MHC-like "notch" (see "Molecular Basis of T Cell Recognition of Antigen," below). In this manner, CD94/NKG2A NK cell molecules survey and monitor the total level of classic MHC class I molecules on the surface of host cells. When cell-surface levels of host MHC class I molecules decrease, such as occurs during malignant transformation or viral infection of host cells, the altered host cell with diminished MHC class I expression is recognized by NK-Rs, and the NK cell is activated to kill the host tumor or virally infected cells. The ability of NK-Rs to bind to self-MHC and inhibit NK killing of normal host cells is a key protective mechanism for prevention of NK cell–mediated autoimmune disease.

Some NK cells express CD3 and are termed *NK/T cells.* NK/T cells can also express oligoclonal forms of the TCR for antigen that can recognize lipid molecules of intracellular bacteria when presented in the context of CD1 molecules on APCs. This mode of recognition of intracellular bacteria such as *Listeria monocytogenese* and *M. tuberculosis* by NK/T cells is thought to

FIGURE 305-1 Role of Toll-like receptors (TLR) in the regulation of the response of macrophages to bacterial lipopolysaccharide (LPS). Lipopolysaccharide, a component of the cell wall of gram-negative bacteria, binds with high affinity to CD14, a glycosyl phosphatidylinositol-linked protein expressed on the surface of macrophages, and to TLR4 protein. This leads to activation of the transmembrane TLR4 protein, initiating an intracellular signaling cascade. Signaling by the TLR4 protein to the transcriptional regulatory complex of NF-κB and IκB occurs through the recruitment of MyD88 (a transcription factor) and the interleukin-1 receptor–associated kinase 2 (IRAK2) and involves the adapter tumor necrosis factor receptor–associated factor 6 (TRAF-6) and the NF-κB-inducing kinase (NIK). These kinases phosphorylate IκB, causing its rapid degradation and the release of NF-κB, which then passes into the nucleus. Once in the nucleus, NF-κB binds to specific sequences in the promoter regions of immunomodulatory genes. This leads to the expression of immunomodulatory genes, including cytokines and co-stimulatory molecules. These gene products act on T and B cells to initiate the adaptive immune response. Under pathophysiologic conditions, high levels of immune system activation by bacterial LPS may lead to septic shock. *(With permission from Modlin et al.)*

be an important defense mechanism against these organisms that, via usage of a clonal form of TCRs for antigen, incorporates components of both the innate and adaptive immune systems.

Neutrophils, Eosinophils, and Basophils Granulocytes are present in nearly all forms of inflammation and are amplifiers and effectors of innate immune responses. Unchecked accumulation and activation of granulocytes can lead to host tissue damage, as seen in neutrophil- and eosinophil-mediated *systemic necrotizing vasculitis.* Granulocytes are derived from stem cells in bone marrow (Fig. 305-2). Each type of granulocyte (neutrophil, eosinophil, or basophil) is derived from a different subclass of progenitor cell, which is stimulated to proliferate by colony stimulating factors (Table 305-5). During terminal maturation of granulocytes, class-specific nuclear morphology and cytoplasmic granules appear that allow for histologic identification of granulocyte type.

Neutrophils express Fc receptors for IgG (CD16) and receptors for activated complement components (C3b or CD35) (Table 305-1). Upon interaction of neutrophils with opsonized bacteria or immune complexes, azurophilic granules (containing myeloperoxidase, lysozyme, elastase, and other enzymes) and specific granules (containing lactoferrin, lysozyme, collagenase, and other enzymes) are released, and microbicidal superoxide radicals (O_2^-) are generated at the neutrophil surface. The generation of superoxide leads to inflammation by direct injury to tissue and by alteration of macromolecules such as collagen and DNA.

Eosinophils express Fc receptors for IgG (CD32) and are potent cytotoxic effector cells for various parasitic organisms. Intracytoplasmic contents of eosinophils, such as major basic protein, eosinophil cationic protein, and eosinophil-derived neurotoxin, are capable

of directly damaging tissues and may be responsible in part for the organ system dysfunction in the *hypereosinophilic syndromes* (Chap. 64). Since the eosinophil granule contains anti-inflammatory types of enzymes (histaminase, arylsulfatase, phospholipase D), eosinophils may homeostatically downregulate or terminate ongoing inflammatory responses.

The normal functions of basophils and tissue mast cells are not completely understood; they are potent reservoirs of cytokines such as IL-4. The capacity of basophil cytokines and mediators to increase local delivery of antibodies and complement by increasing vascular permeability is hypothetical. Thus, the basophil is identified principally with allergic reactions and some delayed cutaneous hypersensitivity states. Certainly, the promotion of increased vascular permeability by basophils is important in the genesis of inflammatory lesions in some vasculitis syndromes (Chap. 317). Basophils express high-affinity surface receptors for IgE (FcRI) and, upon cross-linking of basophil-bound IgE by antigen, release histamine, eosinophil chemotactic factor of anaphylaxis, and neutral protease—all mediators of immediate (anaphylaxis) hypersensitivity responses (Table 305-6). In addition, basophils express surface receptors for activated complement components (C3a, C5a), through which mediator release can be directly effected. →*For further discussion of tissue mast cells, see Chap. 310.*

THE COMPLEMENT SYSTEM The complement system, an important soluble component of the innate immune system, is a series of plasma enzymes, regulatory proteins, and proteins that are activated in a cascading fashion, resulting in cell lysis. There are two arms of the complement system (Fig. 305-4). Activation of the classic complement pathway via C1, C4, and C2 and activation of the alter-

Table 305-4   Cells of the Innate Immune System and Their Major Roles in Triggering Adaptive Immunity

Cell Type	Major Role in Innate Immunity	Major Role in Adaptive Immunity
Macrophages	Phagocytose and kill bacteria; produce antimicrobial peptides; bind lipopolysaccharide (LPS); produce inflammatory cytokines	Produce interleukin (IL) 1 and tumor necrosis factor (TNF) α to upregulate lymphocyte adhesion molecules and chemokines to attract antigen-specific lymphocytes; produce IL-12 to recruit T_H1 helper T cell responses; upregulate co-stimulatory and MHC molecules to facilitate T and B lymphocyte recognition and activation; macrophages and dendritic cells, after LPS signaling, upregulate co-stimulatory molecules B7-1 (CD80) and B7-2 (CD86) required for activation of antigen-specific antipathogen T cells; there are also Toll-like proteins on B cells and dendritic cells that after LPS ligation induce CD80 and CD86 on these cells for T cell antigen presentation.
Precursors of dendritic cells or immature dendritic cells	Produce large amounts of interferon (IFN)α, which has antitumor and antiviral activity	IFN-α is a potent activator of macrophage and mature dendritic cells to phagocytose invading pathogens and present pathogen antigens to T and B cells
Natural killer (NK) cells	Kill foreign and host cells that have low levels of MHC+ self peptides. Express NK receptors that inhibit NK function in the presence of high expression of self-MHC.	Produce TNF-α and IFN-γ that recruit T_H1 helper T cell responses
NK-T cells	Lymphocytes with both T cell and NK surface markers that recognize lipid antigens of intracellular bacteria such as *M. tuberculosis* by CD1 molecules and kill host cells infected with intracellular bacteria.	Produce IL-4 to recruit T_H2 helper T cell responses, IgG1 and IgE production
Neutrophils	Phagocytose and kill bacteria, produce antimicrobial peptides	Produce nitric oxide synthase and nitric oxide that inhibit apoptosis in lymphocytes and can prolong adaptive immune responses
Eosinophils	Kill invading parasites	Produce IL-5 that recruits Ig-specific antibody responses
Mast cells and basophils	Release TNF-α, IL-6, IFN-γ in response to a variety of bacterial PAMPs	Produce IL-4 that recruits T_H2 helper T cell responses and recruit IgG1- and IgE-specific antibody responses
Epithelial cells	Produce anti-microbial peptides; tissue specific epithelia produce mediator of local innate immunity, e.g. lung epithelial cells produce surfactant proteins (proteins within the collectin family) that bind and promote clearance of lung invading microbes	Produce TGF-β that triggers IgA-specific antibody responses

NOTE: MHC, major histocompatibility complex; PAMP, pathogen-associated molecular patterns.
SOURCE: Adapted with permission from Medzhitov and Janeway, 1997a.

native complement pathway via factor D, C3, and factor B both lead to cleavage and activation of C3. C3 is a protein whose activation fragments, when bound to target surfaces such as bacteria and other foreign antigens, are critical for opsonization (coating by anti-body and complement) in preparation for phagocytosis.

The protein fragment C3b, split from C3, is necessary for activation of the terminal complement components C5 through C9. These form the membrane attack complex, which, when inserted into cell membranes, brings about osmotic lysis of the cell.

C3b also joins with a cleavage product of factor B (called Bb) to form C3bBb, also known as the *alternative pathway C3 convertase*. Activation of the classic complement pathway results in cleavage of C4 and C2 with a resulting complex of fragments, C4b2a, also called the *classic pathway C3 convertase*. Both the classic pathway C3 convertase (C4b2a) and the alternative pathway C3 convertase (C3bBb) function to cleave C3 to form active C3b, thus driving activation of the C5–9 membrane attack complex. The fact that C3b can combine with Bb to form the alternative pathway C3 convertase gives rise to a potent positive-feedback loop for production of C3b and thus continued activation of terminal complement components.

The classic complement pathway is activated by interaction of antigen and antibody to form immune complexes that bind C1q, a subunit of C1. Immunoglobulin isotypes that bind C1q and activate the classic pathway are IgM, IgG1, IgG2, and IgG3. In contrast, IgA1, IgA2, and IgD activate complement via the alternative pathway. Activation of the complement cascade via the classic pathway by IgG- or IgM-containing immune complexes is a rapid and efficient pathway to activation of terminal complement components. In contrast, activation of the alternative complement pathway via IgA-containing immune complexes or by bacterial endotoxin is a slower and less efficient pathway to terminal component activation. Thus the immunoglobulin isotype composition of immune complexes is a critical factor in determining complement activation and the efficiency of clearance of immune complexes by C3 receptor–bearing cells.

In addition to the role of complement in opsonization of bacteria and cell lysis, several complement fragments are potent mediators of immune cell activation. C3a and C5a bind to receptors on mast cells and basophils, resulting in release of histamine and other mediators of anaphylaxis. C5a is also a potent chemoattractant for neutrophils and monocytes-macrophages (Table 305-7).

CYTOKINES Cytokines are soluble proteins produced by a wide variety of hematopoietic and nonhematopoietic cell types (Table 305-5). They are critical for both normal innate and adaptive immune responses, and their expression may be perturbed in most immune, inflammatory, and infectious disease states.

Cytokines are involved in the regulation of the growth, development, and activation of immune system cells and in the mediation of the inflammatory response. In general, cytokines are characterized by considerable redundancy in that different cytokines have similar functions. In addition, many cytokines are pleiotropic in that they are capable of acting on many different cell types. This pleiotropism results from the expression on multiple cell types of receptors for the same cytokine (see below), leading to the formation of "cytokine networks." The action of cytokines may be: (1) autocrine when the target cell is the same cell that secretes the cytokine, (2) paracrine when the target cell is nearby, and (3) endocrine when the cytokine is secreted into the circulation and acts distal to the source. A number of classifications have been proposed for the grouping of cytokines according to functions; however, these are all imperfect because of the fact that a number of cytokines overlap these groupings. One empirical classification divides the cytokines into the following three groups:

1. Immunoregulatory cytokines involved in the activation, growth, and differentiation of lymphocytes and monocytes, e.g., IL-2, IL-4, IL-10, IFN-γ, and transforming growth factor (TGF) β
2. Proinflammatory cytokines produced predominantly by mononuclear phagocytes in response to infectious agents (e.g., IL-1, TNF-α, and IL-6) and the chemokine family of inflammatory cytokines, within which are included IL-8, monocyte chemotactic protein (MCP)-1, MCP-2, MCP-3, macrophage inflammatory protein (MIP)-1α, MIP-1β, and regulation-upon-activation, normal T expressed and secreted (RANTES) (Chap. 64)

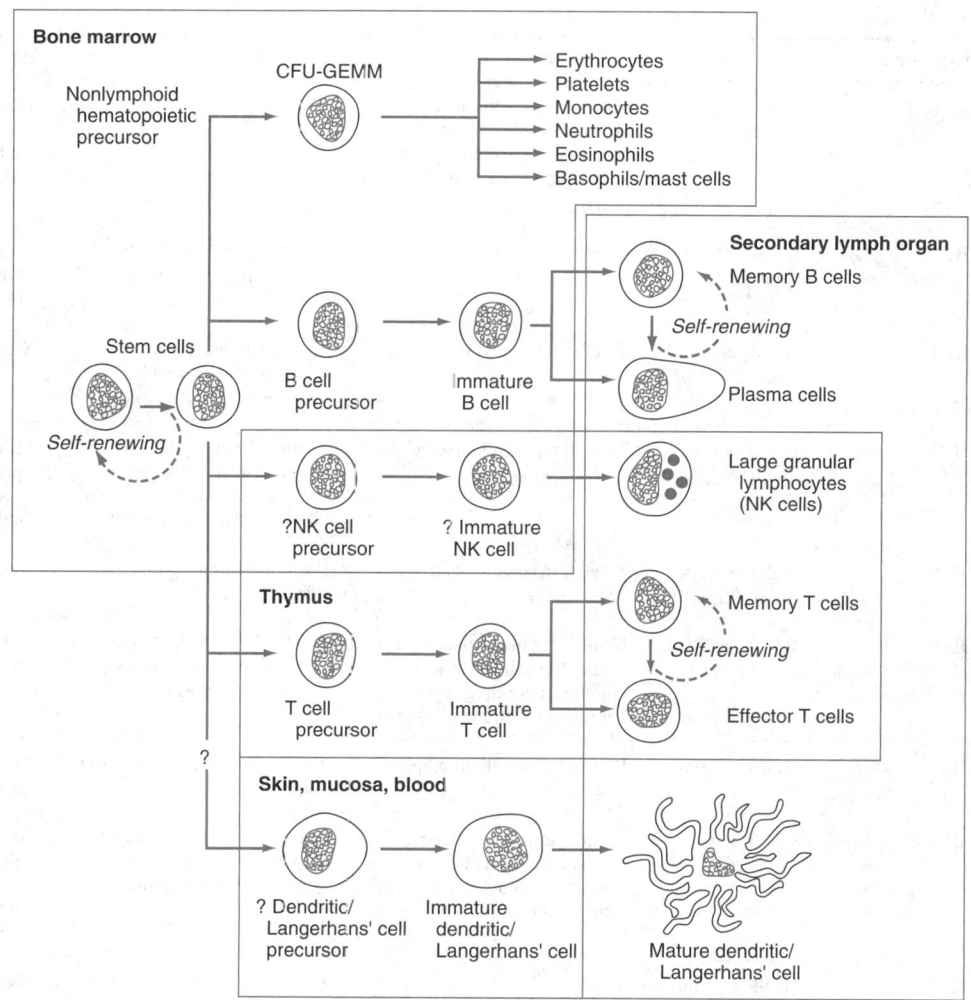

FIGURE 305-2 Hematopoietic stem cell differentiation in bone marrow, thymus, and secondary lymphoid organs. [*After BF Haynes, SM Denning, in G Stamatoyannopoulos et al (eds): The Molecular Basis of Blood Diseases, 2d ed. Philadelphia, Saunders, 1993, with permission*].

3. Cytokines that regulate immature leukocyte growth and differentiation, e.g., IL-3, IL-7, and GM-CSF.

In general, cytokines exert their effects by influencing gene activation that results in cellular activation, growth, differentiation, functional cell-surface molecule expression, and cellular effector function. In this regard, cytokines can have dramatic effects on the regulation of immune responses and the pathogenesis of a variety of diseases. Indeed, T cells have been categorized on the basis of the pattern of cytokines that they secrete that results in either humoral immune response (T_H2) or a cell-mediated immune response (T_H1).

Cytokine receptors can be grouped into five general families based on similarities in their extracellular amino acid sequences and conserved structural domains (Fig. 305-5). The *immunoglobulin (Ig) superfamily* represents a large number of cell-surface and secreted proteins. All members of the Ig superfamily must have at least one common domain in their protein structure. The IL-1 receptors (type 1, type 2) are examples of cytokine receptors with extracellular Ig domains.

The hallmark of the *hematopoietic growth factor (type 1) receptor* family is that the extracellular regions of each receptor contain two conserved motifs. One motif located at the N terminus is rich in cysteine residues. The other motif is located at the C terminus proximal to the transmembrane region and comprises five amino acid residues, tryptophan-serine-X-tryptophan-serine (WSXWS). Cytokine receptors expressing the WSXWS motif are also referred to as "type I family of cytokine receptors." This family can be further grouped on the basis of the number of receptor subunits they have and on the utilization of shared subunits. The shared common receptors often have a critical

role in signal transduction. A number of cytokine receptors, i.e., IL-6, IL-11, IL-12, and leukemia inhibitory factor, are paired with gp130. There is also a common 150-kDa subunit shared by IL-3, IL-5, and GM-CSF receptors. The gamma chain (γ_c) of the IL-2 receptor is common to the IL-2, IL-4, IL-7, IL-9, and IL-15 receptors. Thus, the specific cytokine receptor is responsible for ligand-specific binding, while the subunits such as gp130, the 150-kDa subunit, and γ_c are important in signal transduction. The γ_c gene is on the X chromosome, and mutations in the γ_c protein result in the X-linked form of severe combined immune deficiency syndrome (X-SCID) (Chap. 308).

The members of the *interferon (type II) receptor* family include the receptors for IFN-γ, and -β, which share a similar 210-amino-acid binding domain with conserved cysteine pairs at both the amino and carboxy termini. The receptors for the interferons consist of at least two distinct subunits.

The members of the *TNF (type III) receptor family* share a common binding domain composed of repeated cysteine-rich regions. Members of this family include the p55 and p75 receptors for TNF (TNFR1 and TNFR2, respectively); CD40 antigen, which is an important B cell–surface marker involved in immunoglobulin isotype switching; fas/Apo-1, whose triggering induces apoptosis (programmed cell death); CD27 and CD30, which are found on activated T cells and B cells; and nerve growth factor receptor.

The common motif for the *seven transmembrane helix family* was originally found in receptors linked to GTP-binding proteins. This family includes receptors for chemokines, β-adrenergic receptors, and retinal rhodopsin. It is important to note that two members of the chemokine receptor family, CXC chemokine receptor type 4 (CXCR4)

Table 305-5   Cytokines and Cytokine Receptors

Cytokine	Receptor	Cell Source	Cell Target	Biologic Activity
IL-1α,β	Type 1 IL-1R, type 2 IL-1R	Monocytes/macrophages, B cells, fibroblasts, most epithelial cells including thymic epithelium, endothelial cells	All cells	Upregulates adhesion molecule expression, neutrophil and macrophage emigration; mimics shock, fever; upregulates hepatic acute-phase protein production; facilitates hematopoiesis
IL-2	IL-2R α,β, common γ	T cells	T cells, B cells, NK cells, monocytes/macrophages	T cell activation and proliferation, B cell growth, NK cell proliferation and activation, enhanced monocyte/macrophage cytolytic activity
IL-3	IL-3R, common β	T cells, NK cells, mast cells	Monocytes/macrophages, mast cells, eosinophils, bone marrow progenitors	Stimulation of hematopoietic progenitors
IL-4	IL-4R α, common γ	T cells, mast cells, basophils	T cells, B cells, NK cells, monocytes/macrophages, neutrophils, eosinophils, endothelial cells, fibroblasts	Stimulates $T_H 2$ helper T cell differentiation and proliferation; stimulates B cell Ig class switch to IgG1 and IgE; anti-inflammatory action on T cells, monocytes
IL-5	IL-5R α, common β	T cells, mast cells, and eosinophils	Eosinophils, basophils, murine B cells	Regulates eosinophil migration and activation
IL-6	IL-6R, gp130	Monocytes/macrophages, B cells, fibroblasts, most epithelium including thymic epithelium, endothelial cells	T cells, B cells, epithelial cells, hepatocytes, monocytes/macrophages	Induction of acute-phase protein production, T and B cell differentiation and growth, myeloma cell growth, osteoclast growth and activation
IL-7	IL-7R α, common γ	Bone marrow, thymic epithelial cells	T cells, B cells, bone marrow cells	Differentiation of B, T, and NK cell precursors, activation of T and NK cells
IL-8	CXCR1, CXCR2	Monocytes/macrophages, T cells, neutrophils, fibroblasts, endothelial cells, epithelial cells	Neutrophils, T cells, monocytes/macrophages, endothelial cells, basophils	Induces neutrophil, monocyte, and T cell migration; induces neutrophil adherance to endothelial cells and histamine release from basophils; stimulates angiogenesis; suppresses proliferation of hepatic precursors
IL-9	IL-9R α, common γ	T cells	Bone marrow progenitors, B cells, T cells, mast cells	Induces mast cell proliferation and function, synergizes with IL-4 in IgG and IgE production, T cell growth, activation, and oncogenesis
IL-10	IL-10R	Monocytes/macrophages, T cells, B cells, keratinocytes, mast cells	Monocytes/macrophages, T cells, B cells, NK cells, mast cells	Inhibits macrophage proinflammatory cytokine production; downregulates cytokine class II antigen and B7-1 and B7-2 expression; inhibits differentiation of $T_H 1$ helper T cells; inhibits NK cell function; stimulates mast cell proliferation and function and B cell activation and differentiation
IL-11	IL-11R, gp130	Bone marrow stromal cells	Megakaryocytes, B cells, hepatocytes	Induces megakaryocyte colony formation and maturation; enhances antibody responses; stimulates acute-phase protein production
IL-12 (35-kDa and 40-kDa subunits)	IL-12R	Activated macrophages, dendritic cells, neutrophils	T cells, NK cells	Induces $T_H 1$ T helper cell formation and lymphokine-activated killer cell formation; increases CD8+ CTL activity
IL-13	IL-13/IL-4R	T cells ($T_H 2$)	Monocytes/macrophages, B cells, endothelial cells, keratinocytes	Upregulation of VCAM-1 and C-C chemokine expression on endothelial cells; B cell activation and differentiation; inhibits macrophage proinflammatory cytokine production
IL-14	Unknown	T cells	Normal and malignant B cells	Induces B cell proliferation
IL-15	IL-15R α, common γ, IL-2R β	Monocytes/macrophages, epithelial cells, fibroblasts	T cells, NK cells	T cell activation and proliferation; promotes angiogenesis and NK cells
IL-16	CD4	Mast cells, eosinophils, CD8+ T cells, respiratory epithelium	CD4+ T cells, monocytes/macrophages, eosinophils	Chemoattraction of CD4+ T cells, monocytes, and eosinophils; inhibits HIV replication; inhibits T cell activation through CD3/T cell receptor

(continued)

Table 305-5—(continued)

Cytokine	Receptor	Cell Source	Cell Target	Biologic Activity
IL-17	IL17R	CD4+ T cells	Fibroblasts, endothelium, epithelium	Enhanced cytokine secretion
IL-18	IL-18R (IL-1R-related protein)	Keratinocytes, macrophages	T cells, B cells, NK cells	Upregulated IFN-γ production, enhanced NK cell cytotoxicity
IFN-α	Type I interferon receptor	All cells	All cells	Antiviral activity; stimulates T cell, macrophage, and NK cell activity; direct antitumor effects; upregulates MHC class I antigen expression; used therapeutically in viral and autoimmune conditions
IFN-β	Type I interferon receptor	All cells	All cells	Antiviral activity; stimulates T cell, macrophage, and NK cell activity; direct antitumor effects; upregulates MHC class I antigen expression; used therapeutically in viral and autoimmune conditions
IFN-γ	Type II interferon receptor	T cells, NK cells	All cells	Regulates macrophage and NK cell activation; stimulates immunoglobulin secretion by B cells; induction of class II histocompatibility antigens; T_H1 T cell differentiation
TNF-α	TNF-RI, TNF-RII	Monocytes/macrophages, mast cells, basophils, eosinophils, NK cells, B cells, T cells, keratinocytes, fibroblasts, thymic epithelial cells	All cells except erythrocytes	Fever, anorexia, shock, capillary leak syndrome, enhanced leukocyte cytotoxicity, enhanced NK cell function, acute-phase protein synthesis, proinflammatory cytokine induction
TNF-β	TNF-RI, TNF-RII	T cells, B cells	All cells except erythrocytes	Cell cytotoxicity, lymph node and spleen development
LTβ	LTβR	T cells	All cells except erythrocytes	Cell cytotoxicity, normal lymph node development
G-CSF	G-CSFR; gp130	Monocytes/macrophages, fibroblasts, endothelial cells, thymic epithelial cells, stromal cells	Myeloid cells, endothelial cells	Regulates myelopoiesis; enhances survival and function of neutrophils; clinical use in reversing neutropenia after cytotoxic chemotherapy
GM-CSF	GM-CSFR; common β	T cells, monocytes/macrophages, fibroblasts, endothelial cells, thymic epithelial cells	Monocytes/macrophages, neutrophils, eosinophils, fibroblasts, endothelial cells	Regulates myelopoiesis; enhances macrophage bactericidal and tumoricidal activity; mediator of dendritic cell maturation and function; upregulates NK cell function; clinical use in reversing neutropenia after cytotoxic chemotherapy
M-CSF	M-CSFR (c-*fms* proto-oncogene)	Fibroblasts, endothelial cells, monocytes/macrophages, T cells, B cells, epithelial cells including thymic epithelium	Monocytes/macrophages	Regulates monocyte/macrophage production and function
LIF	LIFR; gp130	Activated T cells, bone marrow stromal cells, thymic epithelium	Megakaryocytes, monocytes, hepatocytes, possibly lymphocyte subpopulations	Induces hepatic acute-phase protein production; stimulates macrophage differentiation; promotes growth of myeloma cells and hematopoietic progenitors; stimulates thromboiesis
OSM	OSMR; LIFR; gp130	Activated monocytes/macrophages and T cells, bone marrow stromal cells, some breast carcinoma cell lines, myeloma cells	Neurons, hepatocytes, monocytes/macrophages, adipocytes, alveolar epithelial cells, embryonic stem cells, melanocytes, endothelial cells, melanocytes, endothelial cells, fibroblasts, myeloma cells	Induces hepatic acute-phase protein production; stimulates macrophage differentiation; promotes growth of myeloma cells and hematopoietic progenitors; stimulates thrombopoiesis; stimulates growth of Kaposi's sarcoma cells.
SCF	SCFR (c-*kit* proto-oncogene)	Bone marrow stromal cells and fibroblasts	Embryonic stem cells, myeloid and lymphoid precursors, mast cells	Stimulates hematopoietic progenitor cell growth, mast cell growth; promotes embryonic stem cell migration

(continued)

Table 305-5 Cytokines and Cytokine Receptors—(*continued*)

Cytokine	Receptor	Cell Source	Cell Target	Biologic Activity
TGF-β (3 isoforms)	Type I, II, III TGF-β receptor	Most cell types	Most cell types	Downregulates T cell, macrophage, and granulocyte responses; stimulates synthesis of matrix proteins; stimulates angiogenesis
Lymphotactin/ SCM-1	Unknown	NK cells, mast cells, double negative thymocytes, activated CD8+ T cells	T cells, NK cells	Chemoattractant for lymphocytes; only known chemokine of C class
MCP-1	CCR2	Fibroblasts, smooth-muscle cells, activated PBMCs	Monocytes/macrophages, NK cells, memory T cells, basophils	Chemoattractant for monocytes, activated memory T cells, and NK cells; induces granule release from CD8+ T cells and NK cells; potent histamine-releasing factor for basophils; suppresses proliferation of hematopoietic precursors; regulates monocyte protease production
MCP-2	CCR1, CCR2	Fibroblasts, activated PBMCs	Monocytes/macrophages, T cells, eosinophils, basophils, NK cells	Chemoattractant for monocytes, memory and naive T cells, eosinophils, ? NK cells; activates basophils and eosinophils; regulates monocyte protease production
MCP-3	CCR1, CCR2	Fibroblasts, activated PBMCs	Monocytes/macrophages, T cells, eosinophils, basophils, NK cells, dendritic cells	Chemoattractant for monocytes, memory and naive T cells, dendritic cells, eosinophils, ? NK cells; activates basophils and eosinophils; regulates monocyte protease production
MCP-4	CCR2, CCR3	Lung, colon, small intestinal epithelial cells, activated endothelial cells	Monocytes/macrophages, T cells, eosinophils, basophils	Chemoattractant for monocytes, T cells, eosinophils, and basophils
Eotaxin	CCR3	Pulmonary epithelial cells, heart	Eosinophils, basophils	Potent chemoattractant for eosinophils and basophils; induces allergic airways disease; acts in concert with IL-5 to activate eosinophils; antibodies to eotaxin inhibit airway inflammation
TARC	CCR4	Thymus, dendritic cells, activated T cells	T cells, NK cells	Chemoattractant for T and NK cells
MDC	CCR4	Monocytes/macrophages, dendritic cells, thymus	Activated T cells	Chemoattractant for activated T cells; inhibits infection with T cell tropic HIV
MIP-1α	CCR1, CCR5	Monocytes/macrophages, T cells	Monocytes/macrophages, T cells, dendritic cells, NK cells, eosinophils, basophils	Chemoattractant for monocytes, T cells, dendritic cells, NK cells; weak chemoattractant for eosinophils and basophils; activates NK cell function; suppresses proliferation of hematopoietic precursors; necessary for myocarditis associated with Coxsackie virus infection; inhibits infection with monocytotropic HIV
MIP-1β	CCR5	Monocytes/macrophages, T cells	Monocytes/macrophages, T cells, NK cells, dendritic cells	Chemoattractant for monocytes, T cells, and NK cells; activates NK cell function; inhibits infection with monocytotropic HIV
RANTES	CCR1, CCR2, CCR5	Monocytes/macrophages, T cells, fibroblasts, eosinophils	Monocytes/macrophages, T cells, NK cells, dendritic cells, eosinophils, basophils	Chemoattractant for monocytes/macrophages, CD4+ CD45RO+ T cells, CD8+ T cells, NK cells, eosinophils, and basophils, induces histamine release from basophils; inhibits infection with monocytotropic HIV
LARC/MIP-3α/Exodus-1	CCR6	Dendritic cells, fetal liver cells, activated T cells	T cells, B cells	Chemoattractant for lymphocytes
ELC/MIP-3β	CCR7	Thymus, lymph node, appendix	Activated T cells and B cells	Chemoattractant for B and T cells; receptor upregulated on EBV-infected B cells and HSV-infected T cells
I-309/TCA-3	CCR8	Activated T cells	Monocytes/macrophages, T cells	Chemoattractant for monocytes; prevents glucocorticoid-induced apoptosis in some T cell lines
SLC/TCA-4/Exodus-2	Unknown	Thymic epithelial cells, lymph node, appendix, and spleen	T cells	Chemoattractant for T lymphocytes; inhibits hematopoiesis

(*continued*)

Table 305-5—(continued)

Cytokine	Receptor	Cell Source	Cell Target	Biologic Activity
DC-CK1/ PARC	Unknown	Dendritic cells in secondary lymphoid tissues	Naive T cells	May have a role in the induction of immune responses
TECK	Unknown	Dendritic cells, thymus, liver, small intestine	T cells, monocytes/macrophages, dendritic cells	Thymic dendritic cell–derived cytokine, possibly involved in T cell development
GRO-α/MGSA	CXCR2	Activated granulocytes, monocytes/macrophages, and epithelial cells	Neutrophils, epithelial cells, ?endothelial cells	Neutrophil chemoattractant and activator; mitogenic for some melanoma cell lines; suppresses proliferation of hematopoietic precursors; angiogenic activity
GROβ/ MIP-2α	CXCR2	Activated granulocytes and monocytes/macrophages	Neutrophils and ?endothelial cells	Neutrophil chemoattractant and activator; angiogenic activity
NAP-2	CXCR2	Platelets	Neutrophils, basophils	Derived from platelet basic protein; neutrophil chemoattractant and activator
IP-10	CXCR3	Monocytes/macrophages, T cells, fibroblasts, endothelial cells, epithelial cells	Activated T cells, tumor-infiltrating lymphocytes, ?endothelial cells, ?NK cells	IFN-γ-inducible protein that is a chemoattractant for T cells; suppresses proliferation of hematopoietic precursors
MIG	CXCR3	Monocytes/macrophages, T cells, fibroblasts	Activated T cells, tumor-infiltrating lymphocytes	IFN-γ-inducible protein that is a chemoattractant for T cells; suppresses proliferation of hematopoietic precursors
SDF-1	CXCR4	Fibroblasts	T cells, dendritic cells, ? basophils, ? endothelial cells	Low-potency, high-efficacy T cell chemoattractant; required for B lymphocyte development; prevents infection of CD4+, CXCR4+ cells by T cell tropic HIV
Fractalkine	CX3CR1	Activated endothelial cells	NK cells, T cells, monocytes/macrophages	Cell surface chemokine/mucin hybrid molecule that functions as a chemoattractant, leukocyte activator, and cell adhesion molecule
PF-4	Unknown	Platelets, megakaryocytes	Fibroblasts, endothelial cells	Chemoattractant for fibroblasts; suppresses proliferation of hematopoietic precursors; inhibits endothelial cell proliferation and angiogenesis

NOTE: CCR, CC-type chemokine receptor; CSF, colony stimulating factor; CXCR, CXC-type chemokine receptor; DC-CK, dendritic cell chemokine; EBV, Epstein-Barr virus; ELC, EBI1 ligand chemokine (MIP-1β); G-CSF, granulocyte CSF; GM-CSF, granulocyte-macrophage CSF; GRO, growth-related peptide; IFN, interferon; IL, interleukin; IP, IFN-γ-inducible protein; LARC, liver and activation-regulated chemokine; LIF, leukemia inhibitory factor; LT, lymphotoxin; MCP, monocyte chemotactic protein; M-CSF, macrophage CSF; MDC, macrophage-derived chemokine; MGSA, melanoma growth-stimulating activity; MHC, major histocompatibility complex; MIG, monoteine induced by IFN-γ; MIP, macrophage inflammatory protein; NAP, neutrophil-activating protein; NK, natural killer; OSM, oncostatin M; PARC, pulmonary and activation-regulated chemokine; PMBC, peripheral blood mononuclear cells; PF, platelet factor; RANTES, regulated on activation, normally T cell expressed and secreted; SCF, stem cell factor; SDF, stromal cell–derived factor; SLC, secondary lymphoid tissue chemokine; TARC, thymus and activation-regulated chemokine; TCA, T cell activation protein; TECK, thymus-express chemokine; TGF, transforming growth factor; TNF, tumor necrosis factor; VCAM, vascular cell adhesion molecule.

SOURCE: From JS Sundy et al, in J Gallin and R Snyderman (eds): *Inflammation, Basic Principles and Clinical Correlates*, 3d ed. Philadelphia, Lippincott Williams & Wilkins, 1999, with permission.

and β chemokine receptor type 5 (CCR5), have recently been found to serve as the two major coreceptors for binding and entry of HIV into CD4-expressing host cells (Chap. 309). Both cytokines and their receptors share similar structures and functions. For example, ligands for the TNF receptor family of receptors regulate and determine activation for programmed cell death (*apoptosis*) and all ligate molecules of the same structural family. Similarly IL-3, IL-5, and GM-CSF are all produced by T helper (T_H) 2 cells, and the receptors of these cytokines share common γ chains. Thus, cytokines and their receptors may have diversified together during evolution.

Significant advances have been made in defining the signaling pathways through which cytokines exert their effects intracellularly. This is particularly true with regard to the diverse family of hematopoietin receptors. The Janus family of protein tyrosine kinases (JAK) is a critical element involved in signaling via the hematopoietin receptors. There are four known JAK kinases, JAK1, JAK2, JAK3, and Tyk2, which preferentially bind different receptor subunits. Cytokine binding to its receptor brings the cytokine receptor subunits into apposition and allows a pair of JAKs to transphosphorylate and activate one another. The JAKs then phosphorylate the receptor on the tyrosine residues and allow signaling molecules to bind to the receptor, where these molecules in turn can become phosphorylated. These signaling molecules can bind the receptor because they have domains (SH2, or

src homology 2 domains) that can bind phosphorylated tyrosine residues. There are a number of these important signaling molecules that bind the receptor, such as the adapter molecule SHC, which can couple the receptor to the activation of the mitogen-activated protein kinase pathway. In addition, a very important class of substrate of the JAKs is the signal transducers and activators of transcription (STAT) family of transcription factors. STATs have SH2 domains that enable them to bind to phosphorylated receptors, where they are then phosphorylated by the JAKs. It appears that different STATs have specificity for different receptor subunits. The STATs then dissociate from the receptor and translocate to the nucleus, bind to DNA motifs that they recognize, and regulate gene expression. The STATs preferentially bind DNA motifs that are slightly different from one another and thereby presumably control transcription of specific genes. The importance of this pathway is particularly relevant to lymphoid development. Mutations of JAK3 itself also result in a disorder identical to X-SCID; however, since JAK3 is found on chromosome 19 and not on the X chromosome, JAK3 deficiency occurs in boys and girls (Chap. 308). In this chapter the cytokines that affect various cell types are discussed in the context of each of the cell types.

THE ADAPTIVE IMMUNE SYSTEM Adaptive immunity is characterized by antigen-specific responses to a foreign antigen or pathogen and, compared to innate immunity which occurs immediately

FIGURE 305-3   A schematic representation of the human natural killer (NK) receptor repertoire. The NK cells of a given individual express clonally distributed NK-Rs for self-HLA class I molecules. In this representative donor (HLA haplotype: HLA-A1, A3; HLA-B7, B27; HLA-Cw3, Cw4), NK cells express at least one inhibitory receptor that interacts with self-HLA alleles. The NK-Rs depicted in white are those belonging to the Ig superfamily that recognize allelic forms of HLA class I molecules. CD94/NKG2A receptors (stippled blue) bind to the MHC class I–like molecules, HLA-E, that present leader sequence peptides of classic MHC class I molecules to CD94/NKG2A molecules. The receptors belonging to the Ig superfamily do not cover the whole set of HLA class I alleles and are not expressed by 100% of NK cells. CD94/NKG2A receptors play important roles in monitoring the total level of MHC class I molecules on viral and malignantly transformed cells. *(Adapted from Moretta A et al, with permission.)*

(1 to 2 days), generally takes several days or longer to materialize. A key feature of adaptive immunity is memory for the antigen such that subsequent antigen exposures lead to more rapid and often more vigorous immune responses. The adaptive immune system consists of dual limbs of cellular and humoral immunity. The principal effectors of cellular immunity are T lymphocytes, while the principal effectors of humoral immunity are B lymphocytes (Table 305-8). Both B and T lymphocytes derive from a common stem cell (Fig. 305-2).

The proportion and distribution of immunocompetent cells in various tissues reflect cell traffic, homing patterns, and functional capa-

FIGURE 305-4   Components of the complement system. *(After Paul, with permission.)*

bilities. Bone marrow is the major site of maturation of B cells, monocytes-macrophages, and granulocytes and contains pluripotent stem cells which, under the influence of various colony stimulating factors, are capable of giving rise to all hematopoietic cell types (Fig. 305-2). T cell precursors also arise from hematopoietic stem cells and home to the thymus for maturation. Mature T lymphocytes, B lymphocytes, monocytes, and dendritic/Langerhans cells enter the circulation and home to peripheral lymphoid organs (lymph nodes, spleen) and the gut-associated lymphoid tissue (tonsil, Peyer's patches, and appendix) as well as the skin and mucous membranes and await activation by foreign antigen.

T CELLS   The pool of effector T cells is established in the thymus early in life and is maintained throughout life both by new T cell production in the thymus and by antigen-driven expansion of virgin peripheral T cells into "memory" T cells that reside in peripheral lymphoid organs. The thymus exports approximately 2% of the total number of thymocytes per day throughout life, with the total number of daily thymic emigrants decreasing by approximately 3% per year during the first four decades of life. Thymic emigrants can be identified

Table 305-6   Mediators Released from Human Mast Cells and Basophils

Mediator	Actions
Histamine	Smooth-muscle contraction, increased vascular permeability
Slow-reacting substance of anaphylaxis (SRSA) (leukotriene C4, D4, E4)	Smooth-muscle contraction
Eosinophil chemotactic factor of anaphylaxis (ECF-A)	Chemotactic attraction of eosinophils
Platelet-activating factor	Activates platelets to secrete serotonin and other mediators; smooth-muscle contraction; induces vascular permeability
Neutrophil chemotactic factor (NCF)	Chemotactic attraction of neutrophils
Leukotactic activity (leukotriene B4)	Chemotactic attraction of neutrophils
Heparin	Anticoagulant
Basophil kallikrein of anaphylaxis (BK-A)	Cleaves kininogen to form bradykinin

Table 305-7   Biologic Activities of Some Complement Components

Component	Activity
C4a weak anaphylatoxin	Evokes histamine release from basophils and mast cells
C3a	Anaphylatoxin; evokes histamine release from basophils and mast cells
C5a	Anaphylatoxin; evokes histamine release from basophils and mast cells; potent chemoattractant for monocytes and neutrophils
C3b, C3bi	Enhancement of phagocytosis by neutrophils and monocytes; promotes immune-complex binding to cells within monocyte-macrophage system, as well as neutrophils; C3b with Bb forms alternative pathway C3 convertase and amplifies alternative pathway; promotes solubilization of immune complexes
C5–9	Membrane attack complex; forms transmembrane channels leading to cell destruction

SOURCE: After S Ruddy, in WN Kelley et al (eds): *Textbook of Rheumatology*, 4th ed. Philadelphia, Saunders, 1993, with permission.

by the expression of certain combinations of T cell surface markers and by the presence in nuclei of excised (deleted) pieces of rearranged TCR DNA, called *T cell receptor excision circles.*

Mature T lymphocytes constitute 70 to 80% of normal peripheral blood lymphocytes (only 2% of the total-body lymphocytes are contained in peripheral blood), 90% of thoracic duct lymphocytes, 30 to 40% of lymph node cells, and 20 to 30% of spleen lymphoid cells. In lymph nodes, T cells occupy deep paracortical areas around B cell germinal centers, and in the spleen, they are located in periarteriolar areas of white pulp (Chap. 63). T cells are the primary effectors of cell-mediated immunity, with subsets of T cells maturing into CD8+ cytotoxic T cells capable of lysis of virus-infected or foreign cells. In general, CD4+ T cells are also the primary regulatory cells of T and B lymphocyte and monocyte function by the production of cytokines and by direct cell contact. In addition, T cells regulate erythroid cell maturation in bone marrow, and through cell contact (CD40 ligand) have an important role in activation of B cells and induction of Ig isotype switching.

Human T cells express cell-surface proteins that mark stages of intrathymic T cell maturation or identify specific functional subpopulations of mature T cells. Many of these molecules mediate or participate in important T cell functions (Table 305-1; Fig. 305-6).

A number of cytokines regulate the process of T cell proliferation and differentiation (Table 305-5). The earliest identifiable T cell precursors in bone marrow are CD34+ pro-T cells (i.e., cells in which TCR genes are neither rearranged nor expressed). In the thymus, CD34+ T cell precursors begin cytoplasmic (c) synthesis of components of the CD3 complex of TCR-associated molecules (Fig. 305-6.) Within T cell precursors, TCR for antigen gene rearrangement begins under the influence of IL-7 and yields two T cell lineages, expressing either TCR$\alpha\beta$ chains or TCR$\gamma\delta$ chains. T cells expressing the TCR$\alpha\beta$ chains comprise the majority of peripheral T cells in blood, lymph node, and spleen and terminally differentiate into either CD4+ or CD8+ cells. Cells expressing TCR$\gamma\delta$ chains circulate as a minor population in blood; their functions, although not fully understood, have been postulated to be those of immune surveillance at epithelial surfaces and cellular defenses against mycobacterial organisms and other intracellular bacteria (see below). Immature cortical thymocytes express, in addition to CD1, both CD4 and CD8 (i.e., they are double positive); however, upon reaching functional maturity, T cell expression of CD1 ceases, and CD4 and CD8 are reciprocally expressed. (i.e., T cells become single positive for either CD4 or CD8).

In the thymus, the recognition of self-peptides on thymic epithelial cells, thymic macrophages, and dendritic cells plays an important role in shaping the T cell repertoire to recognize foreign antigen (*positive selection*) and in eliminating highly autoreactive T cells (*negative selection*). As immature cortical thymocytes begin to express surface TCR for antigen, autoreactive thymocytes are destroyed (negative selection), thymocytes with TCRs capable of interacting with foreign antigen peptides in the context of self–MHC antigens are activated and develop to maturity (positive selection), and thymocytes with TCR that are incapable of binding to self–MHC antigens die of attrition (*no selection*). Mature thymocytes that are positively selected are either CD4+ helper T cells or MHC class II–restricted cytotoxic (killer) T cells, or they are CD8+ T cells destined to become MHC class I–restricted cytotoxic T cells. For T cells to be *MHC class I–* or *class II–restricted* means that T cells recognize antigen peptide fragments

FIGURE 305-5 Cytokine family receptor members. Cytokine receptors have been segregated into several large families based on similarities in the extracellular amino acid sequences and conserved structural domains. There are five cytokine receptor family members. See text for details. (*After Abbas et al, with permission.*)

only when they are presented in the antigen-recognition site of a class I or class II MHC molecule, respectively (see below).

After thymocyte maturation and selection, mature CD4 and CD8 thymocytes leave the thymus and migrate to all sites of the peripheral immune system. It is important to note that the adult thymus continues to function, albeit with decreasing output, well into adult life, with detectable function though age 50. Thus, the thymus continues to be a contributor to the peripheral immune system, both normally and when the peripheral T cell pool is damaged, such as occurs in AIDS and cancer chemotherapy.

MOLECULAR BASIS OF T CELL RECOGNITION OF ANTIGEN The TCR for antigen is a complex of molecules consisting of an antigen-binding heterodimer of either $\alpha\beta$ or $\gamma\delta$ chains noncovalently linked with five CD3 subunits (γ, δ, ϵ, ζ, and η) (Fig. 305-7). The CD3 ζ chains are either disulfide-linked homodimers (CD3-ζ_2) or disulfide-linked heterodimers composed of one ζ chain and one η chain. TCR$\alpha\beta$ or TCR$\gamma\delta$ molecules must be associated with CD3 molecules to be inserted into the T cell surface membrane, TCRα being paired with TCRβ and TCRγ being paired with TCRδ. Molecules of the CD3 complex mediate transduction of T cell activation signals via TCRs, while TCRα and β or γ and δ molecules combine to form the TCR antigen-binding site.

The α, β, γ, and δ TCR for antigen molecules have amino acid sequence homology and structural similarities to immunoglobulin heavy and light chains and are thus members, along with other important molecules of immune cells of the *immunoglobulin gene superfamily* of molecules (e.g., MHC class I or II, CD3, CD4, CD8). The genes encoding the TCR molecules are encoded as clusters of gene segments that rearrange during the course of T cell maturation.

Table 305-8   Components of the Adaptive Immune System

Cellular
Thymus-derived (T) lymphocytes—T cell precursors in the thymus; naive mature T lymphocytes before antigen exposure; memory T lymphocytes after antigen contact; helper T lymphocytes for B and T cell responses; cytotoxic T lymphocytes that kill pathogen-infected target cells

Humoral
Bone-marrow-derived (B) lymphocytes—B cell precursors in bone marrow; naive B cells prior to antigen recognition, memory B cells after antigen contact; plasma cells that secrete specific antibody

Cytokines
Soluble proteins that direct, focus, and regulate specific T versus B lymphocyte immune responses

FIGURE 305-6   Human T cell maturation. sCD3, surface CD3 expression; cCD3, cytoplasmic CD3 expression; TCR, T cell receptor.

This creates an efficient and compact mechanism for housing the diversity requirements of antigen receptor molecules. The TCRα chain is on chromosome 14 and consists of a series of V (variable), J (joining), and C (constant) regions. The TCRβ chain is on chromosome 7 and consists of multiple V, D (diversity), J, and C TCRβ loci. The TCRγ chain is on chromosome 7, and the TCRδ chain is in the middle of the TCRα locus on chromosome 14. Thus, molecules of the TCR for antigen have constant (framework) and variable regions, and the gene segments encoding the α, β, γ, and δ chains of these molecules are recombined and selected in the thymus, culminating in synthesis of the completed molecule. In both T and B cell precursors (see below), DNA rearrangements of antigen receptor genes involves the same enzymes, recombinase activating gene (RAG)1 and RAG2, both DNA-dependent protein kinases.

TCR diversity is created by the different V, (D), and J segments that are possible for each receptor chain by the many permutations of V, D, and J segment combinations, by "N-region diversification" due to the addition of nucleotides at the junction of rearranged gene segments, and the pairing of individual chains to form a TCR dimer. As T cells mature in the thymus, the repertoire of antigen-reactive T cells is modified by selection processes that eliminate many autoreactive T cells, enhance the proliferation of cells that function appropriately with self-MHC molecules and antigen, and allow T cells with nonproductive TCR rearrangements to die. Like B cell antigen receptors (Ig mol-

ecules), TCRs may also undergo affinity maturation by somatic mutation of the receptor, once they leave the thymus.

T cells do not recognize native protein or carbohydrate antigens. Instead, T cells recognize only short (approximately 9 to 13 amino acids) peptide fragments derived from protein antigens taken up or produced in APCs. Foreign antigens may be taken up by endocytosis into acidified intracellar vesicles and degraded into small peptides that associate with MHC class II molecules (exogenous antigen-presentation pathway). Other foreign antigens arise endogenously in the cytosol (such as from replicating viruses) and are broken down into small peptides that associate with MHC class I molecules (endogenous antigen-presenting pathway). Thus, APCs proteolytically degrade foreign proteins and display peptide fragments embedded in the MHC class I or II antigen-recognition site on the MHC molecule surface, where foreign peptide fragments are available to bind to TCR$\alpha\beta$ or TCR$\gamma\delta$ chains of reactive T cells (Fig. 305-8). CD4 molecules act as an adhesive and, by direct binding to MHC class II (DR, DQ, or DP) molecules, stabilize the interaction of TCR with peptide antigen (Fig. 305-7). Similarly, CD8 molecules also act as adhesives to stabilize the TCR-antigen interaction by direct CD8 molecule binding to MHC class I (A, B, or C) molecules.

Antigens that arise in the cytosol and are processed via the endogenous antigen-presentation pathway are cleaved into small peptides by a 28-subunit complex of proteases called the *proteasome*. From the proteasome, antigen peptide fragments are transported from the cytosol into the lumen of the endoplasmic reticulum by a heterodimeric complex termed *transporters associated with antigen processing*, or TAP proteins. There, MHC class I molecules in the endoplasmic reticulum membrane physically associate with processed cytosolic peptides. Following peptide association with class I molecules, peptide–class I complexes are exported to the Golgi apparatus, and then to the cell surface, for recognition by CD8+ T cells.

Antigens taken up from the extracellular space via endocytosis into intracellular acidified vesicles are degraded by vesicle proteases into peptide fragments. Intracellular vesicles containing MHC class II molecules fuse with peptide-containing vesicles, thus allowing peptide fragments to physically bind to MHC class II molecules. Peptide–MHC class II complexes are then transported to the cell surface for recognition by CD4+ T cells.

Whereas it is generally agreed that the TCR$\alpha\beta$ receptor recognizes peptide antigens in the context of MHC class I or class II molecules, recent data suggest that lipids in the cell wall of intracellular bacteria such as *M. tuberculosis* can also be presented to a wide variety of T cells, including subsets of CD4−, CD8− TCR$\alpha\beta$ T cells, TCR$\gamma\delta$ T cells, and a subset of CD8+ TCR$\alpha\beta$ T cells. Importantly, bacterial lipid antigens are not presented in the context of MHC class I or II molecules, but rather are presented in the context of MHC-related CD1 molecules. Some $\gamma\delta$ T cells that recognize lipid antigens via CD1 molecules have very restricted TCR usage, do not need antigen priming to respond to bacterial lipids, and may actually be a form of innate rather than acquired immunity to intracellular bacteria.

Just as foreign antigens are degraded and their peptide fragments presented in the context of MHC class I or class II molecules on APCs, endogenous self-proteins are also degraded and self-peptide fragments are presented to T cells in the context of MHC class I or class II molecules on APCs. In peripheral lymphoid organs, T cells are present that are capable of recognizing self-protein fragments but normally are *anergic* or *tolerant*, i.e., nonresponsive to self-antigenic stimulation, due to lack of self-antigen upregulating APC *co-stimulatory molecules* such as B7-1 and B7-2 (see below).

Once engagement of mature T cell TCR by foreign peptide occurs in the context of self–MHC class I or class II molecules, binding of non-antigen-specific adhesion ligand pairs such as CD54-CD11/CD18 and CD58-CD2 stabilizes MHC peptide–TCR binding and the expression of these adhesion molecules is upregulated (Fig. 305-7). Once antigen ligation of the TCR occurs, the T cell membrane is partitioned into *lipid membrane microdomains*, or *lipid rafts*, that coalesce the key signaling molecules TCR/CD3 complex, CD28, CD2, LAT (linker for activation of T cells), intracellular activated (dephosphorylated) src family protein tyrosine kinases (PTKs), and the key CD3ζ-associated protein-70 (ZAP-70) PTK (Fig. 305-7). Importantly, during T cell activation, the dephosphorylating molecule, CD45, with protein tyrosine phosphatase activity is partitioned away from the TCR complex to allow activating phosphorylation events to occur. The coalescence of signaling molecules of activated T lymphocytes in *microdomains* has suggested that T cell–APC interactions can be considered *immunologic synapses*, analogous in function to neuronal synapses.

After TCR-MHC binding is stabilized, activation signals are transmitted through the cell to the nucleus that lead to the expression of gene products important in mediating the wide diversity of T cell functions such as the secretion of IL-2. The TCR does not have intrinsic signaling activity but is linked to a variety of signaling pathways via immunoreceptor tyrosine-based activation motifs (ITAMs) expressed on the various CD3 chains that bind to proteins that mediate signal transduction. Each of the pathways results in the activation of particular transcription factors that control the expression of cytokine and cytokine receptor genes. Thus, antigen-MHC binding to the TCR induces the activation of the src family of PTKs, fyn and lck (lck is associated with CD4 or CD8 co-stimulatory molecules); phosphorylation of CD3ζ chain; activation of the related tyrosine kinases ZAP-70 and syk; and downstream activation of the calcium-dependent calcineurin pathway, the ras pathway, and the protein kinase C pathway. Each of these pathways leads to activation of specific families of transcription factors (including NF-AT, fos and jun, and rel/NF-κB) that form heteromultimers capable of inducing expression of IL-2, IL-2 receptor, IL-4, TNF-α, and other T cell mediators. The src family kinases require dephosphorylation of an inactivation site by CD45 phosphatase before they can be phosphorylated on an activation site. Furthermore, the activity through the receptor is downregulated by the csk-PEP enzyme, a phosphatase that inactivates the src family kinases.

In addition to the signals delivered to the T cell from the TCR and CD4 and CD8 molecules, co-stimulatory receptors [such as CD28 activated by CD80 (B7-1) and/or CD86 (B7-2)] also deliver important signals that upregulate the function of the T cell. The CD28 signal transduction pathway appears particularly important. CD28 signals through phosphoinositide-3-phosphate kinase; its downstream effects are not completely clear. However, if signal transduction through CD28 does not occur in concert with TCR ligation, or if CD28 is blocked, the T cell becomes inactivated or anergic (nonresponsive or tolerant) rather than activated.

CTLA-4 (CD52) is an Ig superfamily molecule on T cells that, like CD28, is a ligand for B7-1 and B7-2 but has a higher affinity for B7-1 and B7-2 than does CD28. T cell CTLA-4 ligation sends a negative signal to the T cell to become tolerant or nonresponsive to antigen stimulation after TCR-MHC ligation. Blocking of CD28-mediated co-stimulation occurs when a second ligand for B7-1 and B7-2 ligates an APC while the TCR is bound to MHC. Thus, a convergence of molecular and biochemical events involving co-stimulatory molecules is required for normal T cell recognition of antigen and consequent T cell activation. In order to exploit this biology for therapeutic purposes,

FIGURE 305-7 Molecules involved in human T cell recognition of antigen and in human T cell activation. *A.* Schematic arrangement of antigen-presenting cell (APC) molecules (top cell) and T cell molecules (bottom cell) before MHC-peptide binding to T cell receptor (TCR). *B.* The changes that occur in T cell and APC molecules after MHC-peptide binding to TCR. The black triangle at the tip of the αβ chains of MHC class II molecules represents a peptide fragment of "processed" protein antigen. After TCR ligation, src protein tyrosine kinase (PTK) is activated via dephosphorylation and the TCR complex is joined by CD4, CD2, and CD28 as well as the linker for activated T lymphocytes (LAT) in a lipid microdomain area (gray area). Activation signals are mediated via immunoreceptor tyrosine-based activation (ITAM) sequences in LAT and CD3 chains (blue bars) that bind to enzymes and transduce activation signals to the nucleus via the indicated intracellular activation pathways. See text for details of the activation and signal transduction process. *(Adapted from Thomas; from Robey and Allison; and from Weiss and Littman, with permission.)*

one clinical strategy currently being tested is administration of soluble recombinant CTLA-4 protein to patients at the time of organ transplantation in order to induce a cohort of organ transplant–specific tolerant T cells and thereby reduce the rejection of organ allografts. Alternatively, blocking CTLA-4/B7 interactions with soluble CD28 or CTLA-4 monoclonal antibodies might possibly be therapeutically useful to enhance immune responses to human cancers (see "Immunotherapy," below).

T CELL SUPERANTIGENS Conventional antigens bind to MHC class I or II molecules in the groove of the αβ heterodimer and bind to T cells via the V regions of the TCRα and -β chains (Fig. 305-7). In contrast, superantigens bind directly to the lateral portion of the TCRβ chain and MHC class II β chain and stimulate T cells based solely on the Vβ gene segment utilized independent of the D, J, and Vα sequences present. *Superantigens* are protein molecules capable of activating up to 20% of the peripheral T cell pool, whereas conventional antigens activate fewer than 1 in 10,000 T cells. T cell superantigens include staphylococcal enterotoxins, other bacterial products, and certain nonhuman retroviral proteins. Superantigen stimulation of human peripheral T cells occurs in the clinical setting of the *staphylococcal toxic shock syndrome*, leading to massive overproduction of T cell cytokines (Chap. 139).

FIGURE 305-8 Structure of MHC class I and MHC class II molecules. *A* and *B*. Top and schematic side views of an MHC class I molecule. *C* and *D*. Top and schematic side views of an MHC class II molecule. Peptide-binding cleft is the location of short peptide fragments derived from proteolytic cleavage of either foreign or self-proteins. Whereas the peptide-binding cleft of class I comprises the α_1, α_2, and α_3 domains of the class I α chain, the peptide-binding cleft of class II comprises the β_1 and α_1 domains of the class II β and α chains, respectively. *(From Janeway et al, with permission.)*

B CELLS Mature B cells comprise 10 to 15% of human peripheral blood lymphocytes, 50% of splenic lymphocytes, and approximately 10% of bone marrow lymphocytes. B cells express on their surface intramembrane immunoglobulin (Ig) molecules that function as B cell receptors (BCR) for antigen in a complex of Ig-associated α and β signaling molecules with properties similar to those described in T cells (Fig. 305-9). Unlike T cells, which recognize only processed peptide fragments of conventional antigens embedded in the notches of MHC class I and class II antigens of APCs, B cells are capable of recognizing and proliferating to whole unprocessed native antigens via antigen binding to B cell surface Ig (sIg) receptors. B cells also express surface receptors for the Fc region of IgG molecules (CD32) as well as receptors for activated complement components (C3d or CD21, C3b or CD35). The primary function of B cells is to produce antibodies. B cells also serve as APCs and are highly efficient at antigen processing. Their antigen-presenting function is enhanced by a variety of cytokines. Mature B cells are derived from bone marrow precursor cells that arise continuously throughout life (Figs. 305-2, 305-10).

B lymphocyte development can be separated into antigen-independent and antigen-dependent phases. Antigen-independent B cell development occurs in primary lymphoid organs, including fetal liver and bone marrow, and includes all stages of B cell maturation up to the sIg+ mature B cell. Antigen-dependent B cell maturation is driven by the interaction of antigen with the mature B cell sIg, leading to memory B cell induction, Ig class switching, and plasma cell formation. Antigen-dependent stages of B cell maturation occur in secondary lymphoid organs, including lymph node, spleen, and gut Peyer's patches. In contrast to the T cell repertoire that is for the most part

generated intrathymically before contact with foreign antigen, the repertoire of B cells expressing diverse antigen-reactive sites is modified by further alteration of Ig genes after stimulation by antigen—a process called *somatic mutation*—which occurs in lymph node germinal centers.

During B cell development, diversity of the antigen-binding variable region of Ig is generated by an ordered set of Ig gene rearrangements that are similar to the rearrangements undergone by TCR α, β, γ, and δ genes. Heavy chain rearrangements precede those for light chains. For the heavy chain, there is first a rearrangement of D segments to J segments, followed by a second rearrangement between a V gene segment and the newly formed D-J sequence; the C segment is aligned to the V-D-J complex to yield a functional Ig heavy chain gene (V-D-J-C). During later stages, a functional κ or λ light chain gene is generated by rearrangement of a V segment to a J segment, ultimately yielding an intact Ig molecule composed of heavy and light chains.

The process of Ig gene rearrangement is regulated to result in a single antibody specificity produced by each B cell, with each Ig molecule comprising one type of heavy chain and one type of light chain. Although each B cell contains two copies of Ig light and heavy chain genes, only one gene of each type is productively rearranged and expressed in each B cell, a process termed *allelic exclusion*.

There are approximately 300 V_κ genes and 5 J_κ genes, resulting in the pairing of V_κ and J_κ genes to create over 1500 different light chain combinations. The number of distinct κ light chains that can be generated is increased by

FIGURE 305-9 The pre-B cell receptor and B-cell antigen receptor associate with the signal-transducing heterodimer Igα/Igβ. Solid horizontal bars in α and β chains denote the immunoreceptor tyrosine-based activation motif (ITAM). Signals from the antigen receptors are further propagated downstream by other signaling molecules such as the syk and the src family of tyrosine kinases (fyn, lyn, blk, and btk), as well as by the phosphatase, SHP-1. *(Adapted from Lam and Rajewsky, with permission.)*

somatic mutations within the V_κ and J_κ genes, thus creating large numbers of possible specificities from a limited amount of germ-line genetic information. As noted above, in heavy chain Ig gene rearrangement, the VH domain is created by the joining of three types of germ-line genes called V_H, D_H, and J_H, thus allowing for even greater diversity in the variable region of heavy chains than of light chains.

The most immature B cell precursors (early pro-B cells) lack cytoplasmic Ig (cIg) and sIg (Fig. 305-10). The large pre-B cell is marked by the acquisition of the surface pre-BCR composed of μ heavy (H) chains and a pre-B light chain, termed ψLC (Fig. 305-9). ψLC is a surrogate light chain receptor encoded by the nonrearranged V pre-B and the λ5 light chain locus (the pre-BCR). Pro- and pre-B cells are driven to proliferate and mature by signals from bone marrow stroma, in particular, IL-7. Light chain rearrangement occurs in the small pre-B cell stage such that the full BCR is expressed at the immature B cell stage. Immature B cells have rearranged Ig light chain genes and express sIgM. As immature B

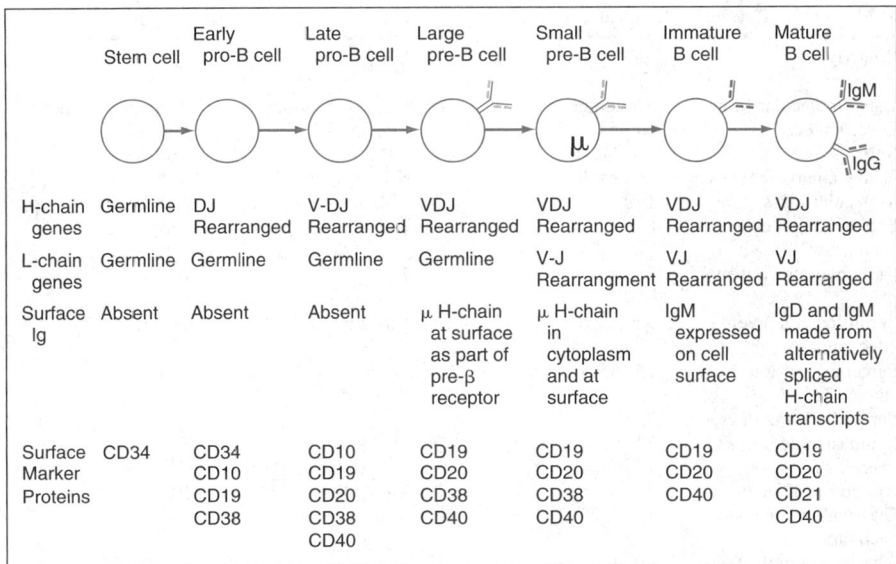

	Stem cell	Early pro-B cell	Late pro-B cell	Large pre-B cell	Small pre-B cell	Immature B cell	Mature B cell
H-chain genes	Germline	DJ Rearranged	V-DJ Rearranged	VDJ Rearranged	VDJ Rearranged	VDJ Rearranged	VDJ Rearranged
L-chain genes	Germline	Germline	Germline	Germline	V-J Rearrangment	VJ Rearranged	VJ Rearranged
Surface Ig	Absent	Absent	Absent	μ H-chain at surface as part of pre-β receptor	μ H-chain in cytoplasm and at surface	IgM expressed on cell surface	IgD and IgM made from alternatively spliced H-chain transcripts
Surface Marker Proteins	CD34	CD34 CD10 CD19 CD38	CD10 CD19 CD20 CD38 CD40	CD19 CD20 CD38 CD40	CD19 CD20 CD38 CD40	CD19 CD20 CD40	CD19 CD20 CD21 CD40

FIGURE 305-10 Developmental stages of B cells. Elements of the developing B cell receptor for antigen (BCR) are shown schematically. The classification into the various stages of B cell development is primarily defined by rearrangement of the immunoglobulin (Ig), heavy (H), and light (L) chain genes and by the absence or presence of specific surface markers. *(Adapted from Janeway et al, with permission.)*

cells develop into mature B cells, sIgD is expressed as well as sIgM. At this point, B lineage development in bone marrow is complete, and B cells exit into the peripheral circulation and migrate to secondary lymphoid organs to encounter specific antigens.

Random rearrangements of Ig genes occasionally generates self-reactive antibodies, and mechanisms must be in place to correct these mistakes. One such mechanism is BCR editing, whereby autoreactive BCRs are mutated to not react with self-antigens. If receptor editing is unsuccessful in eliminating autoreactive B cells, then autoreactive B cells undergo negative selection in the bone marrow through induction of apoptosis after BCR engagement of self-antigen.

After leaving the bone marrow, B cells populate peripheral B cell sites, such as lymph node and spleen, and await contact with foreign antigens that react with each B cell's clonotypic receptor. As antigen-driven B cell activation occurs through the BCR, a process known as *somatic hypermutation* takes place whereby point mutations in rearranged H- and L-genes give rise to mutant sIg molecules, some of which bind antigen better than the original sIg molecules. Somatic hypermutation, therefore, is a process whereby memory B cells in peripheral lymph organs have the best binding, or the highest affinity antibodies. This overall process of generating the best antibodies is called *affinity maturation of antibody*.

Lymphocytes that synthesize IgG, IgA, and IgE are derived from sIgM+, sIgD+ mature B cells. Ig class switching occurs in lymph node and other peripheral lymphoid tissue germinal centers. Pairs of CD40+ B cells and CD40 ligand+ T cells bind and drive B cell Ig switching via T cell–produced cytokines such as IL-4 and TGF-β. IL-1, -2, -4, -5, and -6 synergize to drive mature B cells to proliferate and differentiate into Ig-secreting cells.

Humoral Mediators of Adaptive Immunity: Immunoglobulins
Immunoglobulins are the products of differentiated B cells and mediate the humoral arm of the immune response. The primary functions of antibodies are to bind specifically to antigen and bring about the inactivation or removal of the offending toxin, microbe, parasite, or other foreign substance from the body. The structural basis of Ig molecule function and Ig gene organization has provided insight into the role of antibodies in normal protective immunity, pathologic immune-mediated damage by immune complexes, and autoantibody formation against host determinants.

All immunoglobulins have the basic structure of two heavy and two light chains (Figs. 305-9 and 305-11). Immunoglobulin isotype (i.e., G, M, A, D, E) is determined by the type of Ig heavy chain

present. IgG and IgA isotypes can be divided further into subclasses (G1, G2, G3, G4, and A1, A2) based on specific antigenic determinants on Ig heavy chains. The characteristics of human immunoglobulins are outlined in Table 305-9. The four chains are covalently linked by disulfide bonds. Each chain is made up of a V region and C regions (also called *domains*), themselves made up of units of approximately 110 amino acids. Light chains have one variable (V_L) and one constant (C_L) unit; heavy chains have one variable unit (V_H) and three or four constant (C_H) units, depending on isotype. As the name suggests, the constant, or C, regions of Ig molecules are made up of homologous sequences and share the same primary structure as all other Ig chains of the same isotype and subclass. Constant regions are involved in biologic functions of Ig molecules. The C_{H2} domain of IgG and the C_{H4} units of IgM are involved with the binding of the C1q portion of C1. The C_H region at the carboxy-terminal end of the IgG molecule, the Fc region (Fig. 305-11), binds to surface Fc receptors (CD16, CD32, CD64) of macrophages, LGLs, B cells, neutrophils, and eosinophils.

Variable regions (V_L and V_H) constitute the antibody-binding (Fab) region of the molecule. Within the V_L and V_H regions are hy-

FIGURE 305-11 Schematic structure of the immunoglobulin G (IgG) molecule.

Table 305-9 Physical, Chemical, and Biologic Properties of Human Immunoglobulins

Property	IgG	IgA	IgM	IgD	IgE
Usual molecular form	Monomer	Monomer, dimer	Pentamer, hexamer	Monomer	Monomer
Other chains	None	J chain, SC	J chain	None	None
Subclasses	G1, G2, G3, G4	A1, A2	None	None	None
Heavy chain allotypes	Gm (=30)	No A1, A2m (2)	None	None	None
Molecular mass, kDa	150	160, 400	950, 1150	175	190
Sedimentation constant, Sw20	6.6S	7S, 11S	19S	7S	8S
Carbohydrate content, %	3	7	10	9	13
Serum level in average adult, mg/mL	9.5–12.5	1.5–2.6	0.7–1.7	0.04	0.0003
Percentage of total serum Ig	75–85	7–15	5–10	0.3	0.019
Serum half-life, days	23	6	5	3	2.5
Synthesis rate, mg/kg per day	33	65	7	0.4	0.016
Antibody valence	2	2,4	10,12	2	2
Classical complement activation	+(G1, 2?, 3)	–	++	–	–
Alternate complement activation	+(G4)	+	–	+	–
Binding cells via Fc	Macrophages, neutrophils, large granular lymphocytes	Lymphocytes	Lymphocytes	None	Mast cells, basophils, B cells
Biologic properties	Placental transfer, secondary Ab for most antipathogen responses	Secretory immunoglobulin	Primary Ab responses	Marker for mature B cells	Allergy, antiparasite responses

SOURCE: After L Carayannopoulos and JD Capra, in WE Paul (ed): *Fundamental Immunology*, 2d ed. New York, Raven, 1989, with permission.

pervariable regions (extreme sequence variability) that constitute the antigen-binding site unique to each Ig molecule. The idiotype is defined as the specific region of the Fab portion of the Ig molecule to which antigen binds. Antibodies against the idiotype portion of an antibody molecule are called *anti-idiotype antibodies*. The formation of such antibodies in vivo during a normal B cell antibody response may generate a negative (or "off") signal to B cells to terminate antibody production.

IgG comprises approximately 75 to 85% of total serum immunoglobulin. The four IgG subclasses are numbered in order of their level in serum, IgG1 being found in greatest amounts and IgG4 the least. IgG subclasses have clinical relevance in their varying ability to bind macrophage and neutrophil Fc receptors and to activate complement (Table 305-9). Moreover, selective deficiencies of certain IgG subclasses give rise to clinical syndromes in which the patient is inordinately susceptible to bacterial infections. IgG antibodies are frequently the predominant antibody made after rechallenge of the host with antigen (secondary antibody response).

IgM antibodies normally circulate as a 950-kDa pentamer with 160-kDa bivalent monomers joined by a molecule called the *J chain*, a 15-kDa nonimmunoglobulin molecule that also effects polymerization of IgA molecules. IgM is the first immunoglobulin to appear in the immune response (primary antibody response) and is the initial type of antibody made by neonates. Membrane IgM in the monomeric form also functions as a major antigen receptor on the surface of mature B cells (Fig. 305-9). IgM is an important component of immune complexes in autoimmune diseases. For example, IgM antibodies against IgG molecules (rheumatoid factors) are present in high titers in *rheumatoid arthritis*, other collagen diseases, and some infectious diseases (*subacute bacterial endocarditis*). IgM antibody binds the C1 component of complement via the CH4 domain and thus is a potent activator of the complement cascade.

IgA comprises only 7 to 15% of total serum immunoglobulin but is the predominant class of immunoglobulin in secretions. IgA in secretions (tears, saliva, nasal secretions, gastrointestinal tract fluid, and human milk) is in the form of secretory IgA (sIgA), a polymer consisting of two IgA monomers, a joining molecule, again called the J chain, and a glycoprotein called the *secretory protein*. Of the two IgA

subclasses, IgA1 is primarily found in serum, whereas IgA2 is more prevalent in secretions. IgA fixes complement via the alternative complement pathway and has potent antiviral activity in humans by prevention of virus binding to respiratory and gastrointestinal epithelial cells.

IgD is found in minute quantities in serum and, together with IgM, is a major receptor for antigen on the B cell surface (Table 305-9). IgE, which is present in serum in very low concentrations, is the major class of immunoglobulin involved in arming mast cells and basophils by binding to these cells via the Fc region. Antigen cross-linking of IgE molecules on basophil and mast cell surfaces results in release of mediators of the immediate hypersensitivity response (Table 305-6).

CELLULAR INTERACTIONS IN REGULATION OF NORMAL IMMUNE RESPONSES The net result of activation of the humoral (B cell) and cellular (T cell) arms of the adaptive immune system by foreign antigen is the elimination of antigen directly by specific effector T cells or in concert with specific antibody. In addition, regulatory T cells are activated that modulate effector T cell activation and B cell antibody production. Figure 305-12 is a simplified schematic diagram of the T and B cell responses indicating some of these cellular interactions.

The expression of adaptive immune cell function is the result of a complex series of immunoregulatory events that occur in phases. Both T and B lymphocytes mediate immune functions, and each of these cell types, when given appropriate signals, passes through stages, from activation and induction through proliferation, differentiation, and ultimately effector functions. The effector function expressed may be at the end point of a response, such as secretion of antibody by a differentiated plasma cell, or it might serve a regulatory function that modulates other functions, such as is seen with CD4+ inducer or CD8+ regulatory T lymphocytes, which modulate both differentiation of B cells and activation of CD8+ or CD4+ cytotoxic T cells.

CD4 helper T cells can be subdivided on the basis of cytokines produced (Fig. 305-13). Activated T_H1-type helper T cells secrete IL-2, IFN-γ, IL-3, TNF-α, GM-CSF, and TNF-β, while activated T_H2-type helper T cells secrete IL-3, -4, -5, -6, -10, and -13. T_H1 CD4+ T cells, through elaboration of IFN-γ, have a central role in mediating intracellular killing by a variety of pathogens. T_H1 CD4+ T cells also provide T cell help for generation of cytotoxic T cells and some types of opsonizing antibody, and generally respond to antigens that lead to delayed hypersensitivity types of immune responses for many intracellular viruses and bacteria (such as HIV or *M. tuberculosis*). In contrast, T_H2 cells have a primary role in regulatory humoral immunity and isotype switching. In addition, T_H2 cells, through production of IL-4 and IL-10, have a regulatory role in limiting proinflammatory responses mediated by T_H1 cells (Table 305-5). In addition, T_H2 CD4+ T cells provide help to B cells for specific Ig production and respond to antigens that require high antibody levels for foreign antigen elimination (extracellular encapsulated bacteria such as *Streptococcus pneumoniae* and certain parasite infections). Different cytokines can drive the immune response preferentially towards a T_H1 or a T_H2 response. For example, APC-derived IL-12 induces CD4+ T cell differentiation towards a T_H1 type cell, whereas IL-4 drives differentiation towards a T_H2 type cell (Fig. 305-13).

As shown in Fig. 305-12, upon activation by APCs such as dendritic cells, regulatory T cell subsets that produce IL-2, IL-3, IFN-γ, and/or IL-4, -5, -6, -10, and -13 are generated that exert positive and negative influences on effector T and B cells. For B cells, trophic effects are mediated by a variety of cytokines, particularly T cell–derived IL-3, -4, -5, and -6, which act at sequential stages of B cell maturation, resulting in B cell proliferation, differentiation, and ultimately antibody secretion (Table 305-5). For cytotoxic T cells, trophic factors include inducer T cell secretion of IL-2, IFN-γ, and IL-12 (Table 305-5). In addition, B cells themselves are capable of serving as APCs, processing and presenting antigens to T cells, and secreting TNF-α and IL-6.

Although B cells recognize native antigen via B cell surface Ig receptors, B cells require T cell help to produce high-affinity antibody of multiple isotypes that are the most effective in eliminating foreign antigen. This T cell dependence likely functions in the regulation of B cell responses and in protection against excessive autoantibody production. T cell–B cell interactions that lead to high-affinity antibody production require: (1) processing of native antigen by B cells and expression of peptide fragments on the B cell surface for presentation to T_H cells, (2) the ligation of B cells both by the T cell receptor complex and the CD40 ligand, (3) induction of the process termed *antibody isotype switching* in antigen-specific B cell clones, and (4) induction of the process of *affinity maturation* of antibody in the germinal centers of B cell follicles of lymph node and spleen.

Naive B cells express cell-surface IgD and IgM, and initial contact of naive B cells with antigen is via binding of native antigen to B cell–surface IgM. T cell cytokines, released following T_H2 cell contact with B cells or by a "bystander" effect, induce changes in Ig gene conformation that promote recombination of Ig genes. These events then result in the "switching" of expression of heavy chain exons in a triggered B cell, leading to the secretion of IgG, IgA, or, in some cases, IgE antibody with the same V region antigen specificity as the original IgM antibody, for response to a wide variety of extracellular bacteria, protozoa, and helminths. CD40 ligand expression by activated T cells is critical for induction of B cell antibody isotype switching and for B cell responsiveness to cytokines. Patients with mutations in T cell CD40 ligand have B cells that are unable to undergo isotype switching,

FIGURE 305-12 Schematic model of intercellular interactions of adaptive immune system cells. In this figure the solid arrows denote that cells develop from precursor cells or produce cytokines or antibodies; dotted lines indicate intercellular interactions. Stem cells differentiate into either T cells, antigen-presenting dendritic cells (also called Langerhans cells when located in skin or thymus), or B cells. Foreign antigen is processed by dendritic cells, and peptide fragments of foreign antigen are presented to CD4+ and/or CD8+ T cells. CD8+ T cell activation leads to induction of cytotoxic T lymphocyte (CTL) or killer T cell generation, as well as induction of cytokine-producing CD8+ immunoregulatory cells. For antibody production against the same antigen, active antigen is bound to sIg within the B cell receptor complex and drives B cell maturation into plasma cells that secrete Ig. Regulatory T_H1 or T_H2 CD4+ T cells producing interleukin (IL) 4, IL-5, or interferon (IFN)γ regulate the Ig class switching and determine the type of antibody produced. GM-CSF, granulocyte-macrophage colony stimulating factor; TNF, tumor necrosis factor.

resulting in lack of memory B cell generation and the immunodeficiency syndrome of *X-linked hyper-IgM syndrome* (Chap. 308).

MECHANISMS OF IMMUNE-MEDIATED DAMAGE TO MICROBES OR HOST TISSUES Several responses by the host innate and adaptive immune systems to foreign microbes culminate in rapid and efficient elimination of microbes. In these scenarios, the classic weapons of the adaptive immune system (T cells, B cells) interface with cells (macrophages, dendritic cells, NK cells, neutrophils, eosinophils, basophils) and soluble products (microbial peptides, pentraxins, complement and coagulation systems) of the innate immune system (Chaps. 64 and 310).

There are five general phases of host defenses: (1) migration of leukocytes to sites of antigen localization; (2) antigen nonspecific recognition of pathogens by macrophages and other cells and systems of the innate immune system; (3) specific recognition of foreign antigens mediated by T and B lymphocytes; (4) amplification of the inflammatory response with recruitment of specific and nonspecific effector cells by complement components, cytokines, kinins, arachidonic acid metabolites, and mast cell–basophil products; and (5) macrophage, neutrophil, and lymphocyte participation in destruction of antigen with ultimate removal of antigen particles by phagocytosis (by macrophages or neutrophils) or by direct cytotoxic mechanisms (involving macrophages, neutrophils, and lymphocytes). Under normal circumstances, orderly progression of host defenses through these phases results in a well-controlled immune and inflammatory response that protects the host from the offending antigen. However, dysfunction of any of the host defense systems can damage host tissue and produce clinical disease. Furthermore, for certain pathogens or antigens, the normal immune response itself might contribute substantially to the tissue damage. For example, the immune and inflammatory response in the brain to certain pathogens such as *M. tuberculosis* may be responsible for much of the morbidity of this disease in that organ system (Chap. 169). In addition, the morbidity associated with certain pneumonias

Intracellular bacteria or viruses

Macrophage, or other APC

↓

Activation of T$_H$1 CD4+ T cells

↓

IL-2, IFN-γ, IL-3
TNF-α, TNF-β, GM-CSF → Inhibition of T$_H$2 responses

Induce CD8+ cytotoxic T cells | B cell IgG antibody | Macrophage activation

Kill microbe infected cells | Opsonize microbes for phagocytosis | Kill opsonized microbes

Other bacteria or parasites

Macrophage, dendritic cell, or other APC

↓

Activation of T$_H$2 CD4+ T cells

↓

IL-3, IL-4, IL-5, IL-6
IL-10, IL-13

Inhibition of T$_H$1-Type of responses

Eosinophil | Mast cell basophil | B cell IgM, G, A, and E antibody

Kill parasites | Regulation of vascular permeability; allergic responses | Direct antibody killing of microbes and opsonize for microbal phagocytosis

FIGURE 305-13 CD4+ helper T 1 (T$_H$1) cells and T$_H$2 T cells secrete distinct but overlapping sets of cytokines. T$_H$1 CD4+ cells are frequently activated in immune and inflammatory reactions against intracellular bacteria or viruses, while T$_H$2 CD4+ cells are frequently activated for certain types of antibody production against parasites and extracellular encapsulated bacteria; they are also activated in allergic diseases. APC, antigen-presenting cell; GM-CSF, granulocyte-macrophage colony stimulating factor; IFN, interferon; IL, interleukin; TNF, tumor necrosis factor. *(Adapted from Romagnani, with permission.)*

such as that caused by *Pneumocystis carinii* may be associated more with inflammatory infiltrates than with the tissue destructive effects of the microorganism itself (Chap. 209). Thus, it is important to appreciate how normally protective proinflammatory responses that mediate intracellular killing are regulated. What follows are brief discussions of mechanisms of leukocyte migration to sites of inflammation, immune complex formation, immediate-type hypersensitivity responses, cytotoxic reactions of antibody, delayed cellular types of hypersensitivity responses, and programmed cell death of immune competent cells.

The Molecular Basis of Lymphocyte–Endothelial Cell Interactions The control of lymphocyte circulatory patterns between the bloodstream and peripheral lymphoid organs operates at the level of lymphocyte–endothelial cell interactions to control the specificity of lymphocyte subset entry into organs. Similarly, lymphocyte–endothelial cell interactions regulate the entry of lymphocytes into inflamed tissue. Adhesion molecule expression on lymphocytes and endothelial cells regulates the retention and subsequent egress of lymphocytes within tissue sites of antigenic stimulation, delaying cell exit from tissue and preventing reentry into the circulating lymphocyte pool. All types of lymphocyte migration begin with lymphocyte attachment to specialized regions of vessels, termed *high endothelial venules* (HEVs). An important concept for many of the adhesion molecules listed in Table 305-10 is that the molecules do not generally bind their ligand until a conformational change (ligand activation) occurs in the adhesion molecule that allows ligand binding. Induction of a conformation-dependent determinant on an adhesion molecule can be accomplished by cytokines or via ligation of other adhesion molecules on the cell.

The first stage of lymphocyte–endothelial cell interactions, *attachment and rolling*, occurs when lymphocytes leave the stream of flowing blood cells in a postcapillary venule and roll along venule endothelial cells (Fig. 305-14). Lymphocyte rolling is mediated by the L-selectin molecule (LECAM-1, LAM-1) and slows cell transit time through venules, allowing time for activation of adherent cells.

The second stage of lymphocyte–endothelial cell interactions, *adhesion triggering*, requires stimulation of lymphocytes by chemoattractants or by endothelial cell–derived cytokines. Cytokines thought to participate in adherent cell triggering include members of the IL-8 family, platelet-activation factor, leukotriene B$_4$, and C5a. Following activation by chemoattractants, lymphocytes shed L-selectin from the cell surface and upregulate cell CD11b/18 (MAC-1) or CD11a/18 (LFA-1) molecules, resulting in firm attachment of lymphocytes to HEVs.

Lymphocyte homing to peripheral lymph nodes involves adhesion of L-selectin to carbohydrate of peripheral node HEVs, whereas homing of lymphocytes to intestine Peyer's patches primarily involves adhesion of the α4,β7 integrin to MAdCAM-1 oligosaccharides on the Peyer's patch HEVs. However, for migration to mucosal Peyer's patch lymphoid aggregates, naive lymphocytes primarily use L-selectin, whereas memory lymphocytes use α4,β7 integrin. α4,β1 integrin (CD49d/CD29, VLA-4)–VCAM-1 interactions are important in the initial interaction of memory lymphocytes with HEVs of multiple organs in sites of inflammation.

The third stage of leukocyte emigration in HEVs, *sticking and arrest*, is sticking of the lymphocyte and arrest at the site of sticking, mediated predominantly by ligation of αL,β2 integrin LFA-1 to the integrin ligands ICAM-1 and ICAM-2 on HEVs. While the first three stages of lymphocyte attachment to HEVs takes only a few seconds, the fourth stage of lymphocyte emigration, *transendothelial migration*, takes approximately 10 min. Although the molecular mechanisms that control lymphocyte transendothelial migration are not fully characterized, the HEV CD44 molecule and molecules of the HEV glycocalyx (extracellular matrix) are thought to play important regulatory roles in this process (Fig. 305-14). Finally, expression of matrix metalloproteases capable of di-

Table 305-10 Complement Deficiencies and Associated Diseases

Component	Associated Diseases
CLASSIC PATHWAY	
C1q, C1r, C1s, C4	Immune-complex syndromes,[a] pyogenic infections
C2	Immune-complex syndromes,[a] few with pyogenic infections
C1 inhibitor	Rare immune-complex disease, few with pyogenic infections
C3 AND ALTERNATIVE PATHWAY C3	
C3	Immune-complex syndromes,[a] pyogenic infections
D	Pyogenic infections
Properdin	*Neisseria* infections
I	Pyogenic infections
H	Hemolytic uremic syndrome
MEMBRANE ATTACK COMPLEX	
C5, C6, C7, C8	Recurrent *Neisseria* infections, immune-complex disease
C9	Rare *Neisseria* infections

[a] Immune-complex syndromes include systemic lupus erythematosus (SLE) and SLE-like syndromes, glomerulonephritis, and vasculitis syndromes.
SOURCE: After JA Schifferli and DK Peters, Lancet 88:957, 1983, with permission.

FIGURE 305-14 Lymphocyte emigration in high endothelial venules (HEV). *A.* Lymphocytes circulating in blood initiate contact with high endothelial cells via microvilli. This initial adhesion is transient and is often manifested in rolling of the interacting cells along the HEV endothelium (step 1: attachment and rolling). Activation of lymphocyte adhesiveness (step 2: adhesion triggering) results in firm attachment, which becomes stable to physiologic shear force (step 3: sticking and arrest). Lymphocytes then migrate through endothelial cell junctions and enter lymphoid tissue after crossing the HEV basal lamina (step 4: transendothelial migration). The luminal surface of HEV is coated by a prominent glycocalyx, and this may play an important role in lymphocyte emigration (see text for details). *B.* The initial interaction of lymphocytes with HEV in peripheral lymph nodes (PLNs) is mediated by L-selectin, which recognizes the following HEV mucin-like counter-receptors: CD34 and glycosylation-dependent cell adhesion molecule 1 (GlyCAM-1). Activation of lymphocyte adhesiveness occurs via G protein–coupled receptors, but the local factors involved in physiologic activation of lymphocytes in HEV are not yet characterized. The integrin leukocyte function–associated molecule 1 (LFA-1) (ab;CD11a/CD18) and its HEV counter-receptors intercellular adhesion molecule 1 (ICAM-1) and ICAM-2 play a major role in lymphocyte arrest in PLN HEV. The molecular mechanisms involved in lymphocyte transendothelial migration remain poorly characterized. *(After Girard and Springer, with permission.)*

gesting the subendothelial basement membrane, rich in nonfibrillar collagen, appears to be required for the penetration of lymphoid cells into the extravascular sites.

Abnormal induction of HEV formation and use of the molecules discussed above have been implicated in the induction and maintenance of inflammation in a number of chronic inflammatory diseases. In animal models of insulin-dependent diabetes mellitus (IDDM), MAdCAM–1 and GlyCAM-1 have been shown to be highly expressed on HEVs in inflamed pancreatic islets, and treatment of these animals

with inhibitors of L-selectin and $\alpha 4$ integrin function blocked the development of IDDM (Chap. 333). A similar role for abnormal induction of the adhesion molecules of lymphocyte emigration has been suggested in rheumatoid arthritis (Chap. 312), Hashimoto's thyroiditis (Chap. 330), Graves' disease (Chap. 330), multiple sclerosis (Chap. 371), Crohn's disease (Chap. 287), and ulcerative colitis (Chap. 287).

Immune-Complex Formation Clearance of antigen by immune-complex formation between antigen and antibody is a highly effective mechanism of host defense. However, depending on the level of immune complexes formed and their physicochemical properties, immune complexes may or may not result in host and foreign cell damage. After antigen exposure, certain types of soluble antigen-antibody complexes freely circulate and, if not cleared by the reticulo-endothelial system, can be deposited in blood vessel walls and in other tissues such as renal glomeruli (Chap. 317).

Immediate-Type Hypersensitivity Helper T cells that drive antiallergen IgE responses are usually T_H2-type inducer T cells that secrete IL-4, IL-5, IL-6, and IL-10. Mast cells and basophils have high-affinity receptors for the Fc portion of IgE (FcRI), and cell-bound antiallergen IgE effectively "arms" basophils and mast cells. Mediator release is triggered by antigen (allergen) interaction with Fc receptor–bound IgE; the mediators released are responsible for the pathophysiologic changes of allergic diseases (Table 305-6). Mediators released from mast cells and basophils can be divided into three broad functional types: (1) those that increase vascular permeability and contract smooth muscle (histamine, platelet-activating factor, SRS-A, BK-A), (2) those that are chemotactic for or activate other inflammatory cells (ECF-A, NCF, leukotriene B_4), and (3) those that modulate the release of other mediators (BK-A, platelet-activating factor) (Chap. 310).

Cytotoxic Reactions of Antibody In this type of immunologic injury, complement-fixing (C1-binding) antibodies against normal or foreign cells or tissues (IgM, IgG1, IgG2, IgG3) bind complement via the classic pathway and initiate a sequence of events similar to that initiated by immune-complex deposition, resulting in cell lysis or tissue injury. Examples of antibody-mediated cytotoxic reactions include red cell lysis in *transfusion reactions*, *Goodpasture's syndrome* with anti-glomerular basement membrane antibody formation, and *pemphigus vulgaris* with antiepidermal antibodies inducing blistering skin disease.

Classic Delayed-Type Hypersensitivity Reactions Inflammatory reactions initiated by mononuclear leukocytes and not by antibody alone have been termed *delayed-type hypersensitivity reactions*. The term *delayed* has been used to contrast a secondary cellular response that appears 48 to 72 h after antigen exposure with an *immediate* hypersensitivity response generally seen within 12 h of antigen challenge and initiated by basophil mediator release or preformed antibody. For example, in an individual previously infected with *M. tuberculosis* organisms, intradermal placement of tuberculin purified-protein derivative as a skin test challenge results in an indurated area of skin at 48 to 72 h, indicating previous exposure to tuberculosis.

The cellular events that result in classic delayed-type hypersensitivity responses are centered around T cells (predominantly, though not exclusively, IFN-γ, IL-2, and TNF-α-secreting T_H1-type helper T cells) and macrophages. First, local immune and inflammatory responses at the site of foreign antigen upregulate endothelial cell adhesion molecule expression, promoting the accumulation of lymphocytes at the tissue site. In the general scheme outlined in Fig. 305-12, antigen is processed by dendritic/Langerhans cells or monocytes-macrophages and presented to small numbers of CD4+ T cells expressing a TCR specific for the antigen. IL-12 produced by APCs induces T cells to produce IFN-γ (T_H-1 response). IL-1 and IL-6 secreted by APCs amplify the clonal expansion of antigen-specific T cells, and other cytokines (primarily IL-2, IFN-γ, and TNF-β) are secreted that promote recruitment of diverse populations of T cells and macrophages to the site of the cellular inflammatory response. In particular, CD8+ cytotoxic T cells are induced by IL-2 to become active killer cells. Once recruited, macrophages frequently undergo epithelioid cell transformation and fuse to form multinucleated giant cells. This type of mononuclear cell infiltrate is termed *granulomatous inflammation*. Examples of diseases in which delayed-type hypersensitivity plays a major role are fungal infections (*histoplasmosis*) (Chap. 201), mycobacterial infections (*tuberculosis, leprosy*) (Chaps. 169 and 170), chlamydial infections (*lymphogranuloma venereum*) (Chap. 179), helminth infections (*schistosomiasis*) (Chap. 224), reactions to toxins (*berylliosis*) (Chap. 254), and hypersensitivity reactions to organic dusts (*hypersensitivity pneumonitis*) (Chap. 253). In addition, delayed-type hypersensitivity responses play important roles in tissue damage in autoimmune diseases such as *rheumatoid arthritis, temporal arteritis*, and *Wegener's granulomatosis* (Chaps. 312 and 317).

The Cellular and Molecular Control of Programmed Cell Death (Apoptosis)   The process of apoptosis plays a crucial role in regulating normal immune responses to antigen. In general, a wide variety of stimuli trigger cell surface receptors (e.g., TNF receptor family members or related proteins) or cytoplasmic receptors (e.g., ceramide, glucocorticoids) that activate groups of proteases such as FADD-like IL-1β-converting enzyme (FLICE) or Caspase 8 (Fig. 305-15). These proteases either cleave molecules that lead to cell death themselves or activate other enzymes to cleave molecules that eventuate in cell death (Fig. 305-15). The end stages of this sequence of events lead to cell death characterized by degradation of cytoplasmic (actin) and nuclear cytoskeletal proteins as well as cleavage of DNA at regular intervals (nucleosomes), leading to nuclear disintegration seen on electron microscopy and "laddering" of DNA when analysed

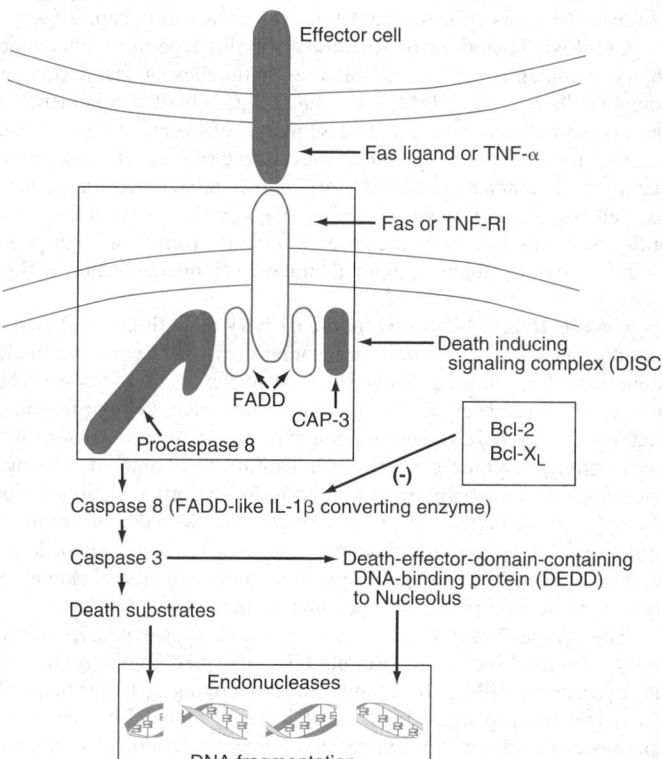

FIGURE 305-15   Intracellular signaling pathways that regulate programmed cell death. Bcl-2 and Bcl-XL are two proteins that inhibit programmed cell death. Caspase activation may result in the translocation of the death-effector-domain containing DNA binding protein (DEDD) that inhibits DNA transcription in the nucleolus. Upon ligation of CD95 by Fas ligand or tumor necrosis factor receptor I (TNF-RI) by TNF-α, a death-inducing signaling complex (DISC) is formed from Procaspase 8, FADD, and Cap-3 proteins. Signaling caspases are activated, eventuating in endonucleases being produced that fragment DNA, leading to cell death. IL, interleukin. (*Adapted with permission from Scaffidi et al.*)

by agarose gel electrophoresis. The level of expression of certain cytosolic proteins, such as Bcl-2 and Bcl-XL, negatively regulates the process of apoptosis by inhibiting activation of cytosolic proteases that induce cell death. For example, T cells that are negatively selected in the thymus are induced to undergo apoptosis and have low levels of proteins such as Bcl-2, whereas medullary thymocytes that have been triggered to proliferate and survive thymocyte selection (positive selection) have high levels of Bcl-2.

Thus, in the immune system, apoptosis is a mechanism induced to remove autoreactive T cells from the thymus during negative selection, to remove autoreactive B and T cells from peripheral lymphoid organs upon contact with antigen or antigen-reactive helper T cells in spleen and lymph node, and to remove virus-infected or malignant cells after contact with antigen-specific CD8+ cytotoxic T lymphocytes. Induction of apoptosis is one of two principal mechanisms of target cell lysis by cytotoxic T lymphocytes, the other consisting of the release of cytotoxic perforin molecules.

CLINICAL EVALUATION OF IMMUNE FUNCTION
Clinical assessment of immunity requires investigation of the four major components of the immune system that participate in host defense and in the pathogenesis of autoimmune diseases: (1) humoral immunity (B cells); (2) cell-mediated immunity (T cells, monocytes); (3) phagocytic cells of the reticuloendothelial system (macrophages), as well as polymorphonuclear leukocytes; and (4) complement. Clinical problems that require an evaluation of immunity include chronic infections, recurrent infection, unusual infecting agents, and certain autoimmune syndromes. The type of clinical syndrome under evaluation can provide information regarding possible immune defects (Chap. 308). Defects in cellular immunity generally result in viral, mycobacterial, and fungal infections. An extreme example of deficiency in cellular immunity is AIDS (Chap. 309). Antibody deficiencies result in recurrent bacterial infections, frequently with organisms such as *S. pneumoniae* and *Haemophilus influenzae* (Chap. 308). Disorders of phagocyte function frequently are manifested by recurrent skin infections, often due to *Staphylococcus aureus* (Chap. 64). Finally, deficiencies of early and late complement components are associated with autoimmune phenomena and recurrent *Neisseria* infections (Table 305-10). →*For further discussion of useful initial screening tests of immune function, see Chap. 308.*

IMMUNOTHERAPY   Most current therapies for autoimmune and inflammatory diseases involve the use of nonspecific immune-modulating or immunosuppressive agents such as glucocorticoids or cytotoxic drugs. The goal of development of new treatments for immune-mediated diseases is to design ways to specifically interrupt pathologic immune responses, leaving nonpathologic immune responses intact. Novel ways to interrupt pathologic immune responses that are under investigation include: the use of anti-inflammatory cytokines or specific cytokine inhibitors as anti-inflammatory agents; the use of monoclonal antibodies against T or B lymphocytes as therapeutic agents; the induction of anergy by administration of soluble CTLA-4 protein, the use of intravenous Ig for certain infections and immune complex–mediated diseases, and the use of specific cytokines to reconstitute components of the immune system (Table 305-11) (Chaps. 64, 308, and 309).

Cytokines and Cytokine Inhibitors   Recently a humanized mouse anti-TNF-α monoclonal antibody (MAB) has been tested in both rheumatoid arthritis and ulcerative colitis. Use of anti-TNF-α antibody therapy has resulted in clinical improvement in patients with these diseases and has opened the way for targeting TNF-α to treat other severe forms of autoimmune and/or inflammatory disease. Anti-TNF-α MAB has been approved for treatment of patients with rheumatoid arthritis.

Other cytokine inhibitors under investigation are recombinant soluble TNF-α receptor (R) fused to human Ig and soluble IL-1 receptor (termed *IL-1 receptor antagonist*, or IL-1 ra). Soluble TNF-αR and IL-1 ra act to inhibit the activity of pathogenic cytokines in rheumatoid arthritis, i.e., TNF-α and IL-1 respectively. Similarly, anti-IL-6, IFN-β, and IL-11 act to inhibit pathogenic proinflammatory cytokines.

Table 305-11 Current Status of Development of Immunomodulatory Agents

Agents	Rationale	Status
CYTOKINES AND CYTOKINE INHIBITORS TO INHIBIT IMMUNE RESPONSES AND INFLAMMATION		
Anti-TNF-α monoclonal antibody	Inhibit TNF-α	FDA approved for rheumatoid arthritis; in trials for Crohn's colitis
Recombinant TNF-receptor-IG fusion protein	Inhibit TNF-α	In trials for rheumatoid arthritis
Recombinant IL-1 receptor antagonist (IL-1Ra)	Inhibit IL-1α and β	In trials for rheumatoid arthritis
Anti-IL-6 monoclonal antibody	Inhibit IL-6	Tested in phase I trial in rheumatoid arthritis
Inferferon-β	Inhibit IL-1, decrease synovial T cells	In trials for use in rheumatoid arthritis
Interferon-γ	Induce monocyte/macrophage activation	Effective in treating monocyte/macrophage phagocytic defects in chronic granulomatous disease
IL-11	Inhibit TNF-α and IL-1 production	In trials for Crohn's colitis
IL-12	Stimulate anti-tumor and anti-viral or bacterial cytotoxic T lymphocyte responses	Trials underway for use in cancer patients; trials planned in humans to prevent/treat severe infections
MONOCLONAL ANTIBODIES AGAINST T OR B CELLS		
Anti-CD3 anti-T cell monoclonal antibody	Inhibit T cell function; Induce T cell lymphopenia	FDA approved for treatment of cardiac and renal allograft rejection
Anti-CD4 monoclonal antibody	Inhibit CD4+ T cell function	In trials for rheumatoid arthritis
Anti-CD40 ligand (CD154) monoclonal antibody	Inhibit CD40-CD40 ligand interaction; induces T cell tolerance	In primate trials for prevention of renal allograft rejection
SOLUBLE T CELL MOLECULE		
Soluble CTLA-4 protein	Inhibit CD28-B7-1 and B7-2 interactions; induce tolerance to organ grafts; inhibit autoimmune T cell reactivity in autoimmune diseases	In trials for preventing GVHD in bone marrow transplantation and for treatment of psoriasis
INTRAVENOUS IMMUNOGLOBULIN		
IVIg	Reticuloendothelial cell blockage; complement inhibition; regulation of idiotype/anti-idiotype antibodies; modulation of cytokine production; modulation of lymphocyte production	FDA approved for Kawasaki's disease and immune thrombocytopenia purpura; treatment of graft versus host disease, multiple sclerosis, myasthenia gravis, Guillain-Barre Syndrome, and chronic inflammatory demyelinating polyneuropathy supported by clinical trials
CYTOKINES FOR IMMUNE RECONSTITUTION		
IL-2	Induce proliferation of peripheral memory CD4+ and CD8+ T cells	In trial for treatment of HIV infection
IL-7	Induce renewed thymopoiesis	Under consideration for treatment of diseases associated with T cell deficiency

Anti-IL-6 inhibits IL-6 activity, while IFN-β and IL-11 decrease IL-1 and TNF-α production.

Recent studies have identified mutations in the IL-12 gene in patients susceptible to severe myobacterial infections. IL-12 is a critical cytokine for induction of IFN-γ and cytotoxic T lymphocytes (CTLs) against intracellular organisms; it is under study for treatment of severe infections such as that caused by *M. tuberculosis* and for treatment of various cancers. In this latter setting, IL-12 is being studied for its ability to enhance antitumor cellular immunity by enhancing the induction of antitumor CTL.

Of particular note has been the successful use of IFN-γ in the treatment of the phagocytic cell defect in *chronic granulomatous disease* (Chap. 64). Intermittent infusions of IL-2 in HIV-infected individuals in the early or intermediate stages of disease have resulted in substantial and sustained increases in CD4+ T cells.

Monoclonal Antibodies to T and B Cells The OKT3 MAB against human T cells has been used for several years as a T cell–specific immunosuppressive agent that can substitute for horse anti-thymocyte globulin (ATG) in the treatment of solid organ transplant rejection. OKT3 produces fewer allergic reactions than ATG but does induce human anti-mouse Ig antibody—thus limiting its use. Anti-CD4 MAB therapy has been used in trials to treat patients with rheumatoid arthritis. While inducing profound immunosuppression, anti-CD4 MAB treatment also induces considerable susceptibility to severe infections. Treatment of patients with a MAB against the T cell molecule CD40 ligand (CD154) is under investigation to induce tolerance to organ transplants, with promising results reported in animal studies.

Tolerance Induction Specific immunotherapy has moved into a new era with the introduction of soluble CTLA-4 protein into clinical trials. Use of this molecule to block T cell activation via TCR/CD28 ligation during organ or bone marrow transplantation has showed promising results in animals and in early human clinical trials. Specifically, treatment of bone marrow with CTLA-4 protein reduces rejection of the graft in HLA-mismatched bone marrow transplantation. In addition, promising results with soluble CTLA-4 have been reported in the downmodulation of autoimmune T cell responses in the treatment of psoriasis.

Intravenous Immunoglobulin (IVIg) IVIg has been successfully used to block reticuloendothelial cell function and immune complex clearance in various immune cytopenias such as immune thrombocytopenia (Chap. 116). In addition, IVIg is useful for prevention of tissue damage in certain inflammatory syndromes such as Kawasaki's disease (Chap. 317) and as Ig replacement therapy for certain types of immunoglobulin deficiencies (Chap. 308). In addition, controlled clinical trials support the use of IVIg in selected patients with graft-versus-host disease, multiple sclerosis, myasthenia gravis, Guillain-Barré syndrome, and chronic demyelinating polyneuropathy (Table 305-11).

Thus, a number of recent insights into immune system function have spawned a new field of interventional immunotherapy and have enhanced the prospect for development of specific and nontoxic therapies for immune and inflammatory diseases.

BIBLIOGRAPHY

ABBAS AK et al (eds): *Cellular and Molecular Immunology*, 2d ed. Philadelphia, Saunders, 1994

ARMITAGE RJ et al: CD40L: A multifunctional ligand. Semin Immunol 5:401, 1993

BENSCHOP RJ, CAMBIER JC: B cell development: Signal transduction by antigen receptors and their surrogates. Curr Opin Immunol 11:143, 1999

DURIE FH et al: The role of CD40 in the regulation of humoral and cell-mediated immunity. Immunol Today 15:406, 1994

FOXWELL BMJ et al: Interleukin-7 can induce the activation of Jak-1, Jak-3, and STAT5 proteins in immune T cells. Eur J Immunol 25:3041, 1995

GEORGE AJT et al: Disease susceptibility, transplantation and the MHC. Immunol Today 16:209, 1995

GIRARD JP, SPRINGER TA: High endothelial venules (HEVs): Specialized endothelium for lymphocyte migration. Immunol Today 16:449, 1995

GLEICH GJ: Eosinophils, basophils and mast cells. J Allergy Clin Immunol 84:1024, 1989

HAYNES BF et al: The role of the thymus in immune reconstitution in aging bone marrow transplantation and AIDS. Ann Rev Immunol, 18:529, 2000

HERMAN A et al: Superantigens: Mechanism of T-cell stimulation and the role in immune responses. Annu Rev Immunol 9:745, 1991

JANEWAY CA et al (eds): *Immunobiology. The Immune System in Health and Disease*, 4th ed. New York, Garland, 1999

JUNE CH et al: The B7 and CD28 receptor families. Immunol Today 15:321, 1994

KELLEY WN et al (eds): *Textbook of Rheumatology*, 4th ed. Philadelphia, Saunders, 1993, chaps. 6, 7, 10, 13, 15, 16

KOPP EB, MEDZHITOV R: The Toll-receptor family and control of innate immunity. Curr Opin Immunol 11:13, 1999

KROEMER G et al: The biochemistry of programmed cell death. FASEB J 9:1277, 1995

LAM K-P, RAJEWSKY K: B cell development, in *Inflammation: Basic Principles and Clinical Correlates*, 3d ed. J Gallin, R Snyderman (eds). Philadelphia, Lippincott Williams & Wilkins, 1999, pp 151–166

MEDZHITOV R, JANEWAY CA Jr.: Innate immunity: Impact on the adaptive immune response. Curr Opin Immunol 9:4, 1997a

———, ———: Innate immunity: The virtues of a nonclonal system of recognition. Cell 91:295, 1997b

MODLIN RL et al: The Toll of innate immunity on microbial pathogens. N Engl J Med 340:1834, 1999

MORETTA A et al: Major histocompatibility complex class I–specific receptors on human natural killer and T lymphocytes. Immunol Rev 155:105, 1997

PAUL WE (ed): *Fundamental Immunology*, 2d ed. New York, Raven, 1989

ROBEY E, ALLISON IP: T-cell activation: Integration of signals from the antigen receptor and costimulatory molecules. Immunol Today 16:306, 1995

ROMAGNANI S: CD4 effector cells, Chapter 12, in *Inflammation: Basic Principles and Clinical Correlates*, 3d ed, J Gallin, R Snyderman, eds. Philadelphia, Lippincott Williams & Wilkins, 1999, pp 177–184

SCAFFIDI C et al: Apoptosis signaling in lymphocytes. Curr Opin Immunol 11:277, 1999

SIEGAL FP et al: The nature of the principal type 1 interferon-producing cells in human blood. Science 284:1835, 1999

SPRINGER TA: Traffic signals for lymphocyte recirculation and leukocyte emigration: The multistep paradigm. Cell 76:301, 1994

SUGITA M et al: Molecule of the month: CD1—a new paradigm for antigen presentation and T cell activation. Clin Immunol Immunopathol 87:8, 1998

THOMAS ML: The regulation of antigen-receptor signaling by protein tyrosine phosphatases: A hole in the story. Curr Opin Immunol 11:270, 1997

WEISS A, LITTMAN DR: Signal transduction by lymphocyte antigen receptor. Cell 76:263, 1995

VAN LEEUWEN JEM, SAMELSON LE: T cell antigen-receptor signal transduction. Curr Opin Immunol 11:242, 1999

306 *Gerald T. Nepom, Joel D. Taurog*

THE MAJOR HISTOCOMPATIBILITY GENE COMPLEX

AS	ankylosing spondylitis	RA	rheumatoid arthritis
CTL	cytolytic T lymphocytes	ReA	reactive arthritis
ER	endoplasmic reticulum	SLE	systemic lupus erythematosus
KIR	killer cell–inhibitory cell receptor	TCRs	T cell receptors
MHC	major histocompatibility complex	TNF	tumor necrosis factor
NK	natural killer		

THE HLA COMPLEX AND ITS PRODUCTS

The human major histocompatibility complex (MHC), commonly called the human leukocyte antigen (HLA) complex, is a 4-megabase (Mb) region on chromosome 6 (6p21.3) that is densely packed with expressed genes. The best known of these genes are the HLA class I and class II genes, whose products are critical for immunologic specificity and transplantation histocompatibility; they play a major role in susceptibility to a number of autoimmune diseases. Many other genes in the HLA region are also essential to the innate and antigen-specific functioning of the immune system. The HLA region shows extensive conservation with the MHC of other mammals in terms of genomic organization, gene sequence, and protein structure and function. Much of our understanding of the MHC has come from investigation of the MHC in mice, where it is termed the *H-2 complex*, and to a lesser degree from other species as well. Nonetheless, in this chapter the discussion will be confined to information applicable to the MHC in humans.

The *HLA class I genes* are located in a 2-Mb stretch of DNA at the telomeric end of the HLA region (Fig. 306-1). The classic (MHC class Ia) HLA-A, -B, and -C loci, the products of which are integral participants in the immune response to intracellular infections, tumors, and allografts, are expressed in all nucleated cells and are highly polymorphic in the population. *Polymorphism* refers to a high degree of allelic variation within a genetic locus that leads to extensive variation between different individuals expressing different alleles. Over 100 alleles at HLA-A, 200 at HLA-B, and 50 at HLA-C have been identified in different human populations. Each of the alleles at these loci encodes a *heavy chain* (also called an α chain) that associates non-covalently with the nonpolymorphic light chain β_2-*microglobulin*, encoded on chromosome 15.

The *nomenclature* of HLA genes and their products reflects the grafting of newer DNA sequence information on an older system based on serology. Among class I genes, alleles of the HLA-A, -B, and -C loci were originally identified in the 1950s, 1960s, and 1970s by alloantisera, derived primarily from multiparous women, who in the course of normal pregnancy produce antibodies against paternal antigens expressed on fetal cells. The serologic allotypes were designated by consecutive numbers, e.g., HLA-A1, HLA-B8. The HLA-C locus alleles were designated HLA-Cw, rather than HLA-C, partly to distinguish them from the HLA-encoded complement loci C2 and C4. With the application of DNA sequence analysis and other molecular techniques in the 1980s, and particularly polymerase chain reaction–based techniques since the late 1980s, most serologically defined specificities were found to include a number of closely related alleles differing by only a few amino acids. These are commonly termed *subtypes* of the parent specificity. Currently, under World Health Organization nomenclature, class I alleles are given a single designation that indicates locus, serologic specificity, and sequence-based subtype. For example, HLA-A*0201 indicates subtype 1 of the serologically defined allele HLA-A2. As new alleles are discovered, they are named and numbered based on sequence homology to known alleles or, in the absence of strong homology, designated as consecutively numbered separate alleles, irrespective of serologic reactivity. Subtypes that differ from each other at the nucleotide but not the amino acid sequence level are designated by an extra numeral; e.g., HLA-B*07021 and HLA-B*07022 are two variants of the HLA-B7 subtype of HLA-B*0702. The nomenclature of class II genes, discussed below, is made more complicated by the fact that both chains of a class II molecule are encoded by closely linked HLA-encoded loci, both of which may be polymorphic, and by the presence of differing numbers of isotypic DRB loci in different individuals. It has become clear that accurate HLA genotyping requires DNA sequence analysis, and the identification of alleles at the DNA sequence level has contributed greatly to the understanding of the role of HLA molecules as peptide-binding ligands, to the analysis of associations of HLA alleles with certain diseases, to the study of the population genetics of HLA, and to a clearer understanding of the contribution of HLA differences in allograft rejection and graft-vs.-host disease. Current databases of HLA class I and class II sequences can be accessed by internet (e.g., from the American Society for Histocompatibility and Immunogenetics, www.swmed.edu/home_pages/ASHI/sequences/seq3.htm), and frequent updates of HLA gene lists are published in several journals.

As shown in Fig. 306-2 and discussed below in detail, a characteristic structural feature of class I and class II HLA molecules is the *peptide-binding groove* that enables these molecules to form highly stable complexes with a wide array of peptide sequences that can be recognized as antigens by T cells. In the case of class I molecules, peptide binding provides a display on the cell surface of peptides derived from intracellular proteins, and this serves as a readout to CD8+ T cells of the proteins being produced within somatic cells. The polymorphism at the loci encoding these molecules predominantly affects the amino acid residues that make up the peptide-binding groove, further amplifying the array of peptides that can be bound by different HLA molecules and generating important functional immune differences and transplantation incompatibility among different individuals.

FIGURE 306-1 Physical map of the HLA region, showing the class I and class II loci, other immunologically important loci, and a sampling of other genes mapped to this region. Gene orientation is indicated by arrowheads. Scale is in kilobase (kb). The approximate genetic distance from DP to A is 3.2 cM. This includes 0.8 cM between A and B (including 0.2 cM between C and B), 0.4 to 0.8 cM between B and DR-DQ, and 1.6 to 2.0 cM between DR-DQ and DP.

The nonclassic, or class Ib, MHC molecules, HLA-E, -F, and -G, are much less polymorphic than MHC Ia and, except for HLA-E, have a more limited tissue distribution. The HLA-E molecule, which has a peptide repertoire restricted to signal peptides cleaved from classic MHC class I molecules, is the major self-recognition target for the natural killer (NK) cell inhibitory receptors NKG2A or NKG2C paired with CD94 (see below and Chap. 305). HLA-G is expressed selectively in extravillous trophoblasts, the fetal cell population directly in contact with maternal tissues. It binds a wide array of peptides, is expressed in six different alternatively spliced forms, and provides inhibitory signals to both NK cells and T cells, presumably in the service of maintaining maternofetal tolerance. The function of HLA-F remains largely unknown. Although HLA-C is considered a classic class I molecule, its degree of polymorphism and level of surface expression are significantly lower than those of HLA-A and HLA-B. Moreover, unlike HLA-A and -B molecules, which function primarily by presenting antigen to CD8+ T cells expressing $\alpha\beta$ T cell receptors (TCRs), the primary function of HLA-C molecules appears to be to serve as targets of NK cell recognition (see below).

Additional class I–like genes have been identified, some HLA-linked and some encoded on other chromosomes, that show only distant homology to the class Ia and Ib molecules but that share the three-dimensional class I structure. Those on chromosome 6p21 include MIC-A and MIC-B, which are encoded centromeric to HLA-B; and HLA-HFE, located 3 to 4 cM (centi-Morgan) telomeric of HLA-F. MIC-A and MIC-B do not bind peptide but are expressed on gut and other epithelium in a stress-inducible manner and serve as activation signals for certain $\gamma\delta$ T cells and NK cells, whereas HLA-HFE encodes the gene defective in hereditary hemochromatosis (Chap. 345). Among the non-HLA, class I–like genes, CD1 refers to a family of molecules that present glycolipids or other nonpeptide ligands to certain T cells, including T cells with NK activity; FcRn binds IgG within lysosomes and protects it from catabolism (Chap. 305); and Zn-α_2-glycoprotein 1 binds a nonpeptide ligand and promotes catabolism of triglycerides in adipose tissue. Like the HLA-A, -B, -C, -E, -F, and -G heavy chains, each of which forms a heterodimer with β_2-microglobulin (Fig. 306-2), the class I–like molecules HLA-HFE, FcRn, and CD1 also bind to β_2-microglobulin, but MIC-A, MIC-B, and Zn-α_2-glycoprotein 1 do not.

The *HLA class II region* is also illustrated in Fig. 306-1. Multiple class II genes are arrayed within the centromeric 1 Mb of the HLA region, forming distinct haplotypes. A *haplotype* refers to an array of alleles at polymorphic loci along a chromosomal segment. In the context of HLA, haplotype can refer either to a large segment of the HLA region encompassing many of the polymorphic HLA loci (also called an *extended haplotype* or to a more restricted segment such as the tightly linked DR and DQ loci. Multiple class II genes are present on a single haplotype, clustered into three major subregions: HLA-DR, -DQ, and -DP. Each of these subregions contains at least one functional alpha (A) locus and one functional beta (B) locus. Together these encode proteins that form the α and β polypeptide chains of a mature class II HLA molecule. Thus, the DRA and DRB genes encode an HLA-DR molecule; products of the DQA1 and DQB1 genes form an HLA-DQ molecule; and the DPA1 and DPB1 genes encode an HLA-DP molecule. There are several DRB genes (DRB1, DRB2, and DRB3, etc.), so that two expressed DR molecules are encoded on most haplotypes by combining the α-chain product of the DRA gene with separate β chains.

The class II region was originally termed the *D-region*. The allelic gene products were first detected by their ability to stimulate lymphocyte proliferation by *mixed lymphocyte reaction*, and were named Dw1, Dw2, etc. Subsequently, serology was used to identify gene products on peripheral blood B cells, and the antigens were termed *DR* (D-related). After additional class II loci were identified, these came to be known as DQ and DP.

The HLA class II DRB and DPB loci are extremely polymorphic, with over 200 DR alleles and over 75 DP alleles, respectively. In the DQ region, both DQA1 and DQB1 are polymorphic, with 20 DQA1 alleles and over 40 DQB1 alleles. The current nomenclature is largely analogous to that discussed above for class I, using the convention "locus*allele." Thus, for example, subtypes of the serologically defined specificity DR4, encoded by the DRB1 locus, are termed DRB1*0401, -0402, etc. In addition to allelic polymorphism, products of different DQA1 alleles can, with some limitations, pair with products of different DQB1 alleles through both *cis* and *trans* pairing to create combinatorial complexity and expand the number of expressed class II molecules. Because of the enormous allelic diversity in the general population, most individuals are heterozygous at all of the class I and class II loci. Thus, most individuals express six classic class I molecules (two each of HLA-A, -B, and -C) and approximately eight class II molecules—two DP, two DR (more in the case of haplotypes with additional functional DRB genes), and up to four DQ (two *cis* and two *trans*).

The localization of polymorphic residues in class II molecules is similar to that for class I, i.e., it is predominantly in sites that affect peptide binding (see below). In the case of class II molecules, the peptides displayed on the cell surface are primarily derived from proteins acquired from the extracellular environment, processed through the endosomal-lysosomal pathway, and presented to CD4+ T cells.

OTHER GENES IN THE MHC Immunologically Relevant Genes In addition to the class I and class II genes themselves,

MHC class I

Peptide-binding cleft

α_2 α_1

N

C

β_2-Microglobulin

α_3

A

MHC class II

Peptide-binding cleft

β_1 α_1

N

C α_2

β_2

B

α_1

Peptide-binding cleft

β Sheet

α Helix

C α_2

α_1

Peptide-binding cleft

β_1

D

FIGURE 306-2 Side (*A, B*) and top (*C, D*) views of the MHC class I and class II molecules. The α_1 and α_2 domains of class I and the α_1 and β_1 domains of class II form a β-sheet platform that forms the floor of the peptide-binding groove, and α helices that form the sides of the groove. The α_3 (*A*) and β_2 domains (*B*) project from the cell surface and form the contact sites for CD8 and CD4, respectively. (*Adapted from C. Janeway et al, Immunobiology Bookshelf, 2d ed., Garland Publishing, New York, 1997, with permission.*)

there are numerous genes interspersed among the HLA loci that have interesting and important immunologic functions. The current concept of the function of MHC genes now encompasses many of these additional genes. As discussed in more detail below, TAP and LMP genes encode molecules that participate in intermediate steps in the HLA class I biosynthetic pathway, and deficiencies of the TAP or LMP genes can markedly alter class I–mediated immune recognition. Another set of HLA genes, DMA and DMB, performs an analogous function for the class II pathway. These genes encode an intracellular molecule that facilitates the proper complexing of HLA class II molecules with antigen (see below). The HLA class III region is a name given to a cluster of genes between the class I and class II complexes, which includes genes for the two closely related cytokines tumor necrosis factor (TNF) α and lymphotoxin (TNF-β); the complement components C2, C4, and Bf; heat shock protein (HSP)70; and the enzyme 21-hydroxylase.

The class I genes HLA-A, -B, and -C are expressed in all nucleated cells, although generally to a higher degree on leukocytes than on other cells. In contrast, the class II genes show a more restricted distribution: HLA-DR and HLA-DP genes are constitutively expressed on most cells of the myeloid cell lineage, whereas all three class II gene families (HLA-DR, -DQ, and -DP) are inducible by certain stimuli provided by inflammatory cytokines such as interferon γ. Within the lymphoid lineage, expression of these class II genes is constitutive on B cells and inducible on human T cells. Most endothelial and epithelial cells in the body, including the vascular endothelium and the intestinal epithelium, are also inducible for class II gene expression. Thus, while these somatic tissues normally express only class I and not class II genes, during times of local inflammation they are recruited by cytokine stimuli to express class II genes as well, thereby becoming active participants in ongoing immune responses. Other HLA genes involved in the immune response, such as TAP and LMP, are also susceptible to upregulation by signals such as interferon γ.

Other Genes and Genetic Elements Large-scale genomic sequencing projects have recently yielded sequence data for the entire HLA region, which can be accessed on the internet (e.g., www.sanger.ac.uk/HGP/Chr6/). As a result, many new genes have been discovered, the functions of which remain to be determined, as well as numerous microsatellite regions and other genetic elements. The gene density of the class II region is high, with approximately one protein encoded every 30 kb; that of the class I and class III regions is even higher, with approximately one protein encoded every 15 kb. It is also of interest that these regions also differ with respect to the GC (guanidine + cytosine) content. Vertebrate genomes have a long-range mosaic structure with regard to relative GC content that is related to chromosome banding. Regions of homogeneous GC content are termed *isochores*. The HLA class I and class III regions belong to the H3 (highest GC) isochore, with 53% GC, whereas the class II region belongs to the L or H1 isochores (low GC), with 40 to 45% GC. An abrupt demarcation between these two isochores occurs near the boundary separating the class II and class III regions.

LINKAGE DISEQUILIBRIUM In addition to extensive polymorphism at the class I and class II loci, another characteristic feature of the HLA complex is *linkage disequilibrium*. This is formally defined as a deviation from Hardy-Weinberg equilibrium for alleles at linked loci. This is reflected in the very low recombination rates between certain loci within the HLA. For example, recombination between DR and DQ loci is almost never observed in family studies, and characteristic haplotypes with particular arrays of DR and DQ alleles are found in every population. Similarly, the complement components C2, C4, and Bf are almost invariably inherited together, and the alleles at these loci are found in characteristic haplotypes. In contrast, there is a recombinational hotspot between DQ and DP, which are separated by 1 to 2 cM of genetic distance, despite their close physical proximity. Certain extended haplotypes encompassing the interval from DQ into the class I region are commonly found, the most notable being the haplotype DR3-B8-A1, which is found, in whole or in part, in 10 to 30% of northern European Caucasians. The genetic mechanisms that account for linkage disequilibrium in HLA have not been determined.

It has been hypothesized that selective pressures may maintain certain haplotypes, but this remains to be demonstrated. As discussed below under HLA and immunologic disease, one consequence of the phenomenon of linkage disequilibrium has been the difficulty it produces in assigning HLA disease associations to a single allele at a single locus.

MHC STRUCTURE AND FUNCTION

Class I and class II molecules display a distinctive structural architecture that contains specialized functional domains responsible for the unique genetic and immunologic properties of the HLA complex. The principal known function of both class I and class II HLA molecules is to bind antigenic peptides in order to present antigen to an appropriate T cell. The ability of a particular peptide to bind to an individual HLA molecule satisfactorily is a direct function of the molecular fit between the amino acid residues on the peptide with respect to the amino acid residues of the HLA molecule. The bound peptide forms a tertiary structure called the *MHC-peptide complex*, which communicates with T lymphocytes through binding to the TCR molecule. The first site of TCR-MHC-peptide interaction in the life of a T cell occurs in the thymus, where self-peptides are presented to developing thymocytes by MHC molecules expressed on thymic epithelium and hematopoietically derived antigen-presenting cells, which are primarily responsible for positive and negative selection, respectively (see Chap. 305 for details of thymic selection of the T cell repertoire). Mature T cells encounter MHC molecules in the periphery both in the maintenance of tolerance (Chap. 305) and in the initiation of immune responses. Because most antibody responses and all T cell responses are T cell dependent (Chap. 305), the MHC-peptide-TCR interaction is the central event in the initiation of most antigen-specific immune responses, since it is the event that actually confers the specificity. Thus, the population of MHC–T cell complexes expressed in the thymus shapes the TCR repertoire. For potentially immunogenic peptides, the ability of a given peptide to be generated and bound by an HLA molecule is a primary determinant of whether or not an immune response to that peptide can be generated; the repertoire of peptides that a particular individual's HLA molecules can bind exerts a major influence over the specificity of that individual's immune response.

When a TCR molecule binds to an HLA-peptide complex, it forms intermolecular contacts with both the antigenic peptide and with the HLA molecule itself. The outcome of this recognition event depends on the density and duration of the binding interaction, accounting for a dual specificity requirement for activation of the T cell. That is, the TCR must be specific both for the antigenic peptide and for the HLA molecule. The polymorphic nature of the presenting molecules, and the influence that this exerts on the peptide repertoire of each molecule, results in the phenomenon of *MHC restriction* of the T cell specificity for a given peptide. The binding of CD8 or CD4 molecules, respectively, to the class I or class II molecule also contributes to the interaction between T cell and the HLA-peptide complex, by providing for the selective activation of the appropriate T cell.

CLASS I STRUCTURE (Fig. 306-2A) As noted above, MHC class I molecules provide a cell-surface display of peptides derived from intracellular proteins; they also provide the signal for self-recognition by NK cells. Surface-expressed class I molecules consist of an MHC-encoded 44-kDa glycoprotein heavy chain, a non-MHC-encoded 12-kDa light chain β_2-microglobulin; and an antigenic peptide, typically 8 to 11 amino acids in length and derived from intracellularly produced protein. The heavy chain contains three domains, termed α_1, α_2, and α_3. The α_1 and α_2 domains form an "intrachain dimer," which together form a peptide-binding groove. In HLA-A and -B molecules, the groove is approximately 3 nm in length by 1-2 nm in maximum width (30 Å × 12 Å), whereas it is apparently somewhat wider in HLA-C. In cell surface–expressed class molecules, each domain contributes four of the eight strands of antiparallel β sheet, the membrane-distal side of which forms the floor of the groove, and one of the pair of α helices, the two coils of which form the walls of the groove (Fig.

306-2A). The membrane-anchored α_3 domain and noncovalently associated β_2-microglobulin chain reside on the membrane-proximal side of the β sheet, each folded in the conformation of an immunoglobulin domain. The peptide is noncovalently bound in an extended conformation within the peptide-binding groove, with both N– and C-terminal ends anchored in pockets within the groove (A and F pockets, respectively) and, in many cases, with a prominent kink, or arch, approximately one-third of the way from the N-terminus that elevates the peptide main chain off the floor of the groove.

A remarkable property of peptide binding by MHC molecules is the ability to form highly stable complexes with a wide array of peptide sequences. This is accomplished by a combination of peptide sequence–independent and –dependent bonding. The former consists of hydrogen bond and van der Waals interactions between conserved residues in the peptide-binding groove and charged or polar atoms along the peptide backbone. The latter are dependent upon the six side pockets that are formed by the irregular surface produced by protrusion of amino acid side chains from within the binding groove. The side chains lining the pockets interact with some of the peptide side chains. The sequence polymorphism among different class I alleles and isotypes predominantly affects the residues that line these pockets, and the interactions of these residues with peptide residues constitute the sequence-dependent bonding that confers a particular sequence "motif" on the range of peptides that can bind any given MHC molecule.

CLASS I BIOSYNTHESIS (Fig. 306-3A) The biosynthesis of the classical MHC class I molecules reflects their role in presenting endogenous peptides. The heavy chain is cotranslationally inserted into the membrane of the endoplasmic reticulum (ER), where it becomes glycosylated and associates sequentially with the chaperone proteins calnexin and ERp57. It then forms a complex with β_2-microglobulin, and this complex associates with the chaperone calreticulin and the MHC-encoded molecule tapasin. Meanwhile, peptides generated within the cytosol from intracellular proteins by the multisubunit, multicatalytic proteasome complex are actively transported into the ER by MHC-encoded TAP (transporter associated with antigen processing) heterodimer. Following association with chaperones and trimming by peptidases within the ER, peptides bind to nascent class I molecules for which they have requisite affinity, to form complete, folded heavy chain–β_2-microglobulin–peptide trimer complexes. These are transported rapidly from the ER, through the *cis*- and *trans*-Golgi, where the N-linked oligosaccharide is further processed, and thence to the cell surface. Other proteins have been implicated in MHC class I assembly, e.g., the chaperones BiP and HSP70, but their roles in the pathway are not clear. The pathways for surface MHC class I degradation are poorly understood. A small proportion of heavy chains within properly assembled MHC class I molecules apparently become unfolded and subsequently degraded in the lysosomal pathway.

Most of the peptides transported by TAP are produced in the cytosol by proteolytic cleavage of intracellular proteins by the multisubunit, multicatalytic proteasome. Inhibitors of the proteasome dramatically reduce expression of class I-presented antigenic peptides, but other proteolytic systems may also generate peptides bound to class I. The MHC-encoded proteasome subunits LMP2 and LMP7 may influence the spectrum of peptides produced, but they are not essential for proteasome function. Under certain circumstances, peptides derived from extracellular proteins in particulate form can become associated with class I molecules, but not necessarily by entering the class I pathway. Peptides are apparently bound to chaperones in the cytosol, including HSP90 and HSP70.

CLASS I FUNCTION **Peptide Antigen Presentation** It is estimated that on any given cell, a given class I allele binds several hundred to several thousand distinct peptide species. The vast majority of these peptides are self peptides to which the host immune system is tolerant by one or more of the mechanisms that maintain tolerance, e.g., clonal deletion in the thymus or clonal anergy or clonal ignorance

FIGURE 306-3 Biosynthesis of class I (*A*) and class II (*B*) molecules. *A.* Nascent heavy chain (HC) becomes associated with β_2-microglobulin (β2m) and peptide through interactions with a series of chaperones. Peptides generated by the proteasome are transported into the endoplasmic reticulum (ER) by TAP. Peptides undergo N-terminal trimming in the ER and become associated with chaperones, including gp96 and PDI. Once peptide binds to HC-β2m, the HC-β2m-peptide trimeric complex exits the ER and is transported by the secretory pathway to the cell surface. In the Golgi, the N-linked oligosaccharide under- goes maturation, with addition of sialic acid residues. Molecules are not nec- essarily drawn to scale. *B.* Pathway of HLA class II molecule assembly and antigen processing. After transport through the Golgi and post-Golgi compart- ment, the class II–invariant chain complex moves to an acidic endosome, where the invariant chain is proteolytically cleaved into fragments and dis- placed by antigenic peptides, facilitated by interactions with the DMA-DMB chaperone protein. This class II molecule–peptide complex is then transported to the cell surface.

in the periphery (Chaps. 305 and 307). However, class I molecules bearing foreign peptides expressed in a permissive immunologic con- text activate CD8 T cells, which, if naïve, will then differentiate into cytolytic T lymphocytes (CTL). These T cells and their progeny, through their $\alpha\beta$ T cell receptors, are then capable of Fas/CD95- and/ or perforin-mediated cytotoxicity and/or cytokine secretion (Chap. 305) upon further encounter with the class I–peptide combination that originally activated it, and also with other combinations of class I molecules plus peptide that present a similar immunochemical stim- ulus to the TCR. As alluded to above, this phenomenon by which T cells recognize foreign antigens in the context of specific MHC alleles is termed *MHC restriction*, and the specific MHC molecule is termed the *restriction element*. The most common source of foreign peptides presented by class I molecules is viral infection, in the course of which peptides from viral proteins enter the class I pathway. The generation of a strong CTL response that destroys virally infected cells represents an important antigen-specific defense against many viral infections (Chap. 305). In the case of some viral infections—hepatitis B, for example—CTL-induced target cell apoptosis is thought to be a more important mechanism of tissue damage than any direct cytopathic ef- fect of the virus itself. The importance of the class I pathway in the defense against viral infection is underscored by the identification of a number of viral products that interfere with the normal class I bio- synthetic pathway and thus block the immunogenetic expression of viral antigens.

Other examples of intracellularly generated peptides that can be presented by class I molecules in an immunogenic manner include peptides derived from nonviral intracellular infectious agents (e.g.,

Listeria, Plasmodium), tumor antigens, minor histocompatibility an- tigens, and presumably certain autoantigens. There are also situations in which cell surface–expressed class I molecules are thought to ac- quire and present exogenously derived peptides.

The role of class I HLA molecules in transplantation and in infec- tious and autoimmune diseases is discussed below.

NK Cell Recognition (See also Chap. 305)   NK cells, which play an important role in innate immune responses, are activated to cyto- toxicity and cytokine secretion by contact with cells that lack MHC class I expression, and NK cell activation is inhibited by cells that express MHC class I. In humans, the recognition of class I molecules by NK cells is carried out by two classes of receptor families, the killer cell–inhibitory cell receptor (KIR) family and the CD94/NKG2 fam- ily. The KIR family, encoded on chromosome 19q13.4, comprises glycoproteins of the immunoglobulin (Ig) superfamily that bind HLA class I molecules and inhibit NK cell–mediated cytotoxicity. An es- timated 40 genes are divided into two subfamilies, KIR2D and KIR3D, which contain either two or three Ig domains, respectively. The KIR2D molecules primarily recognize alleles of HLA-C. The latter all possess either asparagine at position 77 and lysine at position 80, or serine at 77 and asparagine at 80 in the α_1 domain of the heavy chain. Different members of the KIR2D family recognize the alternative forms of this polymorphism as well as other residues of the HLA-C heavy chain. The KIR3D molecules predominantly recognize HLA-B alleles. The latter carry a supertypic polymorphism defined serologically by two allotypes, HLA-Bw4 and -Bw6, that are determined by residues 77 to 83 in the α_1 domain of the heavy chain. It is primarily alleles of the Bw4 supertype that bind KIR3D molecules. Although there is KIR recognition of some HLA-A and -Bw6 alleles, many of these alleles appear not to have a corresponding KIR ligand.

The second family of inhibitory NK receptors for HLA is encoded in the NK complex on chromosome 12p12.3-13.1 and consists of CD94 and four NKG2 genes: A, C, E, and D/F. These molecules are C-type (calcium-binding) lectins and are thought to exist as disulfide-bonded heterodimers between CD94 and the various NKG2 glycoproteins. CD94/NKG2A apparently binds to HLA-E and -G and several alleles of HLA-A, -B, and -C. CD94/NKG2C binds primarily to HLA-E. The specificities of the other NKG2 molecules are not yet established. →*The function of NK cells in immune responses is discussed in Chap. 305.*

CLASS II STRUCTURE   A specialized functional architecture similar to that of the class I molecules can be seen in the example of a class II molecule depicted in Fig. 306-2B, with an antigen-binding cleft arrayed above a supporting scaffold that extends the cleft toward the external cellular environment. However, in contrast to the HLA class I molecular structure, β_2-microglobulin is not associated with class II molecules. Rather, the class II molecule is a heterodimer, composed of a 29-kDa β chain and a 34-kDa α chain. The amino-terminal domains of each chain form the antigen-binding elements, which, like the class I molecule, cradle a bound peptide in a groove bounded by extended α-helical loops, one encoded by the A (α chain) gene and one by the B (β chain) gene. Like the class I groove, the class II antigen-binding groove is punctuated by pockets that contact the side chains of amino acid residues of the bound peptide; unlike the class I groove, it is open at both ends. Therefore, peptides bound by class II molecules vary greatly in length, since both the N- and C-terminal ends of the peptides can extend through the open ends of this groove. Approximately 11 amino acids within the bound peptide form intimate contacts with the class II molecule itself, with backbone hydrogen bonds and specific side chain interactions combining to provide stability and specificity, respectively, to the binding (Fig. 306-4).

The genetic polymorphisms that distinguish different class II genes

FIGURE 306-4   Top view of the HLA-DR1 molecule containing the peptide 306-318 from influenza hemagglutinin. The N terminus of the peptide is at left, and the peptide lies relatively flat within the peptide-binding groove in an extended conformation with a pronounced twist. Some 35% of the peptide surface is potentially available for interaction with the antigen receptor on T cells. Pockets in the peptide-binding site accommodate 5 of the 13 side chains of the bound peptide, manifesting the peptide specificity of HLA-DR1. Twelve hydrogen bonds between conserved HLA-DR1 residues and the main chain of the peptide provide a universal mode of peptide binding. The ends of the binding groove are open, and longer variants of the peptide can extend out from each end. In contrast, peptides bound to class I molecules are anchored into pockets at their N and C termini by conserved residues, and the middle portion of the peptide is typically kinked upwards out of the groove. *(Adapted from LJ Stern et al: Nature 368:215, 1994. Copyright 1994 Macmillan Magazines Ltd, with permission.)*

correspond to changes in the amino acid composition of the class II molecule, and these variable sites are clustered predominantly around the pocket structures within the antigen-binding groove. As with class I, this is a critically important feature of the class II molecule, which explains how genetically different individuals have functionally different HLA molecules.

As noted above, the class I–peptide complex is preferentially recognized by CD8 T cells, and the class II–peptide complex is preferentially recognized by CD4 T cells. These interactions provide an important signal for activation of specific T cell lineages during antigen-recognition events. The CD8 recognition site is located on the α_3 domain of the MHC class I molecule, and the CD4 recognition site is located on the β_2 domain of the class II molecule, in both cases remote from the peptide-binding site.

BIOSYNTHESIS AND FUNCTION OF CLASS II MOLECULES   The intracellular assembly of class II molecules occurs within a specialized compartmentalized pathway that differs dramatically from the class I pathway described above. As illustrated in Fig. 306-3B, the class II molecule assembles in the ER in association with a chaperone molecule, known as the *invariant chain*. The invariant chain performs at least two roles. First, it binds to the class II molecule and blocks the peptide-binding groove, thus preventing antigenic peptides from binding. This role of the invariant chain appears to account for one of the important differences between class I and class II MHC pathways, since it can explain why class I molecules present endogenous peptides from proteins newly synthesized in the ER, but class II molecules generally do not. Second, the invariant chain contains molecular localization signals that direct the class II molecule to traffic into post-Golgi compartments known as *endosomes*, which develop into specialized acidic compartments where proteases cleave the invariant chain, and antigenic peptides can now occupy the class II groove. It is at this stage in the intracellular pathway that the MHC-encoded DM molecule catalytically facilitates the exchange of peptides within the class II groove to help optimize the specificity and stability of the MHC-peptide complex.

Once this MHC-peptide complex is deposited in the outer cell membrane, it becomes the target for T cell recognition via a specific TCR expressed on lymphocytes. Because the endosome environment contains internalized proteins retrieved from the extracellular environment, the class II–peptide complex often contains bound antigens that were originally derived from extracellular proteins. In this way, the class II peptide loading pathway provides a mechanism for immune surveillance of the extracellular space. This appears to be an important feature that permits the class II molecule to bind foreign peptides, distinct from the endogenous pathway of class I–mediated presentation.

ROLE OF HLA IN TRANSPLANTATION   The development of modern clinical transplantation in the decades since the 1950s provided a major impetus for elucidation of the HLA system, as allograft survival is highest when donor and recipient are HLA-identical. Although many molecular events participate in transplantation rejection, allogeneic differences at class I and class II loci play a major role. Class I molecules can promote T cell responses in several different ways. In the cases of allografts in which the host and donor are mismatched at one or more class I loci, host T cells can be activated by classical *direct alloreactivity*, in which the antigen receptors on the host T cells react with the foreign class I molecule expressed on the allograft. In this situation, the response of any given TCR may be dominated by the allogeneic MHC molecule, the peptide bound to it, or some combination of the two. Another type of host antigraft T cell response involves the uptake and processing of donor MHC antigens by host antigen-presenting cells and the subsequent presentation of the resulting peptides by host MHC molecules. This mechanism is termed *indirect alloreactivity*, or *cross-priming*. It appears to play a quantitatively significant role in allograft rejection, although the molecular and cellular basis for the antigen processing remain to be completely elucidated. In the case of class I molecules on allografts that are shared by the host and the donor, a host T cell response may still be triggered because of peptides that are presented by the class I molecules of the graft but not of the host. The most common basis for the existence of these endogenous antigenic peptides, called *minor histocompatibility antigens*, is a genetic difference between donor and host at a non-MHC locus encoding the structural gene for the protein from which the peptide is derived. These loci are termed *minor histocompatibility loci*, and nonidentical individuals typically differ at many such loci, although only a few provide peptides for any given HLA allele. In recent years, the peptides and parent proteins for a number of human and experimental rodent minor histocompatibility antigens have been identified. In many of these cases of allograft rejection, T cell help for the generation of class I–restricted CD8 cells is provided by CD4 T cells reacting to analogous II differences. Moreover, class II differences alone are sufficient to drive allograft rejection.

ASSOCIATION WITH INFECTIOUS DISEASE   It has long been postulated that infectious agents provide the driving force for the allelic diversification seen in the HLA system. This has been difficult to confirm definitively, but one corollary of this hypothesis, namely, that it would be unusual to find HLA alleles strongly associated with susceptibility to any particular infectious disease, has generally been observed. Some modest associations of susceptibility to tuberculosis and leprosy have been found for several subtypes of HLA-DR2 (DRB1*15), and progression of HIV has been associated with several HLA haplotype including HLA-B35, HLA-CW*04, and HLA-A1-B8-DR3 in some studies (Chap. 309). With regard to resistance to infectious disease, the best documented example has been shown for malaria, in which B*5301, DRB1*1302, and DRB1*0101 have been shown to exert varying degrees of protection against severe disease. Slow progression of HIV has been associated with several HLA haplotypes (Chap. 309), and reduced persistence of hepatitis B and C viruses has been associated, respectively, with DRB1*1302 and with DR5.

A polymorphism in the promoter of the TNF-α gene in the HLA class III region, which is associated with quantitative variation in the production of TNF, has recently been shown to have an association with the manifestations of a number of infectious diseases, including cerebral malaria, mucocutaneous leishmaniasis, lepromatous leprosy, scarring trachoma, persistent hepatitis B infection, and fatal meningicoccal meningitis.

ASSOCIATION OF HLA ALLELES WITH SUSCEPTIBILITY TO IMMUNOLOGICALLY MEDIATED DISEASES   Because of the immense polymorphism of HLA loci and strong linkage disequilibrium within the HLA region, it became possible, once a sufficient number of alleles had been defined by the early 1970s, to find associations of particular HLA alleles with certain disease states by comparing allele frequencies in patients with any particular disease and in control populations. A large number of such associations were identified during the 1970s. Most subsequent work in this field has been devoted to refining these associations to molecularly defined alleles and attempting to elucidate the contribution of HLA to disease pathogenesis. Table 306-1 lists the major diseases associated with HLA class I and class II genes. The strength of genetic association is reflected in the term *relative risk*, which is a statistical odds ratio representing the risk of disease in an individual carrying a particular genetic marker compared with the risk in individuals in that population without that marker. The nomenclature shown in Table 306-1 reflects both the HLA serotype (e.g., DR3, DR4) and the HLA genotype (e.g., DRB1*0301, DRB1*0401). Both because of the strong linkage disequilibrium within HLA and because the serologically identified loci represent only a small fraction of the total genes within the region, for many years it could not be established whether the associated alleles themselves participated in disease pathogenesis or were merely markers that were in linkage disequilibrium with the true disease allele. In recent years, it has become clear that it is very likely that the class I and class II alleles themselves are the true disease alleles for most of

these associations. However, as discussed below, because of the extremely strong linkage disequilibrium between the DR and DQ loci, in some cases it has been difficult to determine the specific locus or combination of class II loci involved. At a minimum, different populations with different DR-DQ haplotypes need to be compared.

As might be predicted from the known function of the class I and class II gene products, almost all of the diseases associated with specific HLA alleles have an immunologic component to their pathogenesis. In some cases, as discussed below, specific protein and even peptide antigens have been implicated, but in no case is the molecular and cellular pathogenesis well understood. From a genetic point of view, strong HLA associations with disease (those associations with a relative risk of 10 or greater) are unusual because the implicated HLA alleles are normal, rather than defective, alleles. However, even in diseases with very strong HLA associations such as ankylosing spondylitis (AS) and type I diabetes mellitus, the non-HLA contribution exceeds 50% of the genetic predisposition, and the concordance of disease in monozygotic twins is considerably higher than in HLA-identical dizygotic twins or other sibling pairs. Genome-wide linkage analyses in these two diseases have found that the non-HLA genetic contribution comes from several other regions, although the linkage to HLA is by far the strongest.

Another group of diseases is genetically linked to HLA, not because of the immunologic function of HLA alleles, but rather because they are caused by autosomal dominant or recessive abnormal alleles at loci that happen to reside in or near the HLA region. Examples of these are 21-hydroxylase deficiency, hemochromatosis, and spinocerebellar ataxia (Chaps. 338, 345, and 364, respectively).

CLASS I DISEASE ASSOCIATIONS   Although the associations of human disease with particular HLA alleles or haplotypes predominantly involve the class II region, there are also several prominent disease associations with class I alleles. These include the association of Behçet's disease (Chap. 316) with HLA-B51, psoriasis vulgaris (Chap. 56) with HLA-Cw6, and, most prominently, the spondyloarthropathies (Chap. 315) with HLA-B27. The latter is among the strongest of all HLA associations with disease.

HLA-B27 was originally defined as a serologic determinant. It currently includes a family of 15 HLA-B locus alleles, designated HLA-B*2701-2715, as determined by nucleotide sequencing. HLA-B*2705 is the predominant subtype in Caucasians and most other non-Asian populations, and this subtype has been subjected to the most extensive investigation. All of the subtypes share a common B pocket in the peptide-binding groove, containing characteristic residues His9, Thr24, Glu45, and Cys67, and almost all share adjacent residues Ala69, Lys70, and Ala71. This deep, negatively charged pocket shows a strong preference for binding the arginine side chain, explaining the preference of the B27 binding group for peptides with Arg at P2 (peptide residue 2), as suggested by the crystal structure and confirmed by peptide isolation and sequencing. In addition, B27 is among the most negatively charged of HLA class I heavy chains, and the overall preference is for positively charged peptides. B27 is distinguished among class I alleles as a dominant restricting element for CTL recognition of antigens from a wide variety of viruses, including HIV, and it is associated with prolonged survival in HIV infection (Chap. 309).

HLA-B27 and Disease   HLA-B27 is very highly associated with AS (Chap. 315), both in its idiopathic form and in association with chronic inflammatory bowel disease or psoriasis vulgaris. It is also associated with reactive arthritis (ReA; Chap. 315), with other idiopathic forms of peripheral arthritis (undifferentiated spondyloarthropathy), and with recurrent acute anterior uveitis. B27 is found in 50 to 90% of individuals with these conditions, compared with a prevalence of ~7% in North American Caucasians. The prevalence of B27 in patients with idiopathic AS is 90%, and in AS complicated by iritis or aortic insufficiency is close to 100%. The absolute risk of spondyloarthropathy in unselected B27+ individuals has been variously estimated at 2 to 13% and >20% if a B27+ first-degree relative is affected. The concordance rate of AS in identical twins is very high, approximately 75%. It can be concluded that the B27 molecule itself is involved in disease pathogenesis, based on strong evidence from clinical epidemiology and on the occurrence of a spondyloarthropathy-like disease in HLA-B27 transgenic rats. A well-established association with both AS and ReA exists for subtypes B*2702, -04, and -05, and anecdotal association has been reported for subtypes B*2701, -03, -07, -08, -10, and -11. The propensity of the B27 molecule to induce disease thus presumably derives from one or more unique features of its structure that are shared by several B27 subtypes. It remains a central unanswered question whether the pathogenesis of B27-associated disease derives from the specificity of a particular peptide or family of peptides bound to B27 or whether another mechanism is involved that is independent of the peptide specificity of B27. The first alternative can be further subdivided into mechanisms that involve T cell recognition of B27-peptide complexes, and those that do not. A variety of other roles for B27 in disease pathogenesis have been postulated, including molecular or antigenic mimicry between B27 and certain bacteria and reduced killing of intracellular bacteria in cells expressing B27. However, the most straightforward possibility is the presentation of peptides to CD8 T cells in a way that somehow promotes joint inflammation, i.e., the "arthritogenic peptide" hypothesis. This concept has been supported in ReA by the finding of CD8-restricted antigen-specific T cells, particularly in *Yersinia*-induced ReA. It is of particular interest that the HSP60 molecule from *Y. enterocolitica* has been shown to give rise to dominant antigens recognized by both synovial B27-restricted CD8 and class II–restricted CD4 T cells. This suggests a T cell pathogenesis involving intramolecular help and/or epitope spreading in which a B27-restricted response could well be primary.

In contrast to ReA, there is little direct evidence regarding the molecular role of HLA-B27 in ankylosing spondylitis. However, correlations between disease susceptibility and the peptide-binding specificity of the B27 subtypes have been found that support the "arthritogenic peptide" hypothesis in AS. Specifically, a lack of disease susceptibility has been documented for the subtypes B*2706, found mainly amongst Southeast Asians, and B*2709, found mainly amongst Sardinians. B*2709 differs from B*2705 only at residue 116, carrying His instead of Asp. B*2706 differs from B*2704 at 114 and 116, carrying Asp and Tyr instead of His and Asp. These residues, which lie in the floor of the peptide-binding groove, interact with the C-terminal end of the bound peptide. Unlike the disease-associated subtypes, B*2706 and B*2709 have been found not to carry peptides with C-terminal Tyr. This has led to the hypothesis of a disease-prone B27-bound peptide with C-terminal Tyr.

CLASS II DISEASE ASSOCIATIONS The majority of associations between HLA and disease are with class II alleles (Table 306-1). Several diseases have complex HLA genetic associations.

Celiac Disease In the case of celiac disease (Chap. 286), it is probable that the HLA-DQ genes are the primary basis for the disease association. HLA-DQ genes present on both the celiac-associated DR3 and DR7 haplotypes include the DQB1*0201 gene, and further detailed studies have documented a specific class II αβ dimer encoded

Table 306-1   Significant HLA Class I and Class II Associations with Disease[a]

	Marker	Gene	Strength of Association
SPONDYLOARTHROPATHIES			
Ankylosing spondylitis	B27	B*2702, -04, -05	++++
Reiter's syndrome	B27		++++
Acute anterior uveitis	B27		+++
Reactive arthritis (*Yersinia, Salmonella, Shigella, Chlamydia*)	B27		+++
Psoriatic spondylitis	B27		+++
COLLAGEN-VASCULAR DISEASES			
Juvenile arthritis, pauciarticular	DR8		++
	DR5		++
Rheumatoid arthritis	DR4	DRB1*0401, -04, -05	+++
Sjögren's syndrome	DR3		++
Systemic lupus erythematosus			
Caucasian	DR3		+
Japanese	DR2		++
AUTOIMMUNE GUT AND SKIN			
Gluten-sensitive enteropathy (celiac disease)	DR3	DQA1*0501 DQB1*0201	+++
Chronic active hepatitis	DR3		++
Dermatitis herpetiformis	DR3		+++
Psoriasis vulgaris	Cw6		++
Pemphigus vulgaris	DR4	DRB1*0402	+++
	DR6	DQB1*0503	
AUTOIMMUNE ENDOCRINE			
Type 1 diabetes mellitus	DR4	DQB1*0302	+++
	DR3		++
	DR2	DQB1*0602	—[b]
Hyperthyroidism (Graves')	B8		+
	DR3		+
Hyperthyroidism (Japanese)	B35		+
Adrenal insufficiency	DR3		++
AUTOIMMUNE NEUROLOGIC			
Myasthenia gravis	B8		+
	DR3		+
Multiple sclerosis	DR2	DRB1*1501 DRB5*0101	++
OTHER			
Behçet's disease	B51		++
Congenital adrenal hyperplasia	B47	21-OH (Cyp21B)	+++
Narcolepsy	DR2		++++
Goodpasture's syndrome (anti-GBM)	DR2		++

[a] Various diseases associated with HLA genes are listed, with the HLA serotype or linked marker most frequently found related to disease. Genes are listed for cases where specific alleles have been identified as responsible for this association. The strength of association reflects the likelihood of disease in individuals with the marker compared to individuals who do not carry the marker; ++++, relative risk > 10; +++, relative risk > 5; ++, relative risk > 3; +, relative risk > 1.5.
[b] Strong negative association, i.e., genetic association with protection from diabetes.

by the DQA1*0501 and DQB1*0201 genes, which appears to account for the HLA genetic contribution to celiac disease susceptibility. This specific HLA association with celiac disease may have a straightforward explanation: peptides derived from the wheat gluten component gliadin are bound to the molecule encoded by DQA1*0501 and DQB1*0201 and presented to T cells. A gliadin-derived peptide that has been implicated in this immune activation binds the DQ class II dimer best when the peptide contains a glutamine to glutamic acid substitution. It has been proposed that tissue transglutaminase, an enzyme present at increased levels in the intestinal cells of celiac patients, converts glutamine to glutamic acid in gliadin, creating peptides that are capable of being bound by the DQ2 molecule and presented to T cells.

Pemphigus Vulgaris In the case of pemphigus vulgaris (Chap. 58), there are two HLA haplotypes associated with disease: DRB1*0402-DQB1*0302 and DRB1*1401-DQB1*0503. Peptides derived from epidermal autoantigens have been implicated that preferentially bind to the DRB1*0402-encoded molecule, suggesting that specific peptide binding by this disease-associated class II molecule is important in disease. However, there are no class II genes in common between the disease-associated DR4 and DR14 haplotypes, and there is no evidence for any interaction of the latter haplotype interacting with the epidermal peptides that bind the DRB1*0402-encoded molecule. Thus, the most likely interpretation is that each of these class II associations with pemphigus represents a different pathway to a comparable clinical outcome.

Juvenile Arthritis Pauciarticular juvenile arthritis (Chap. 312) is an autoimmune disease associated with genes at the DRB1 locus and also with genes at the DPB1 locus. Patients with both DPB1*0201 and a DRB1 susceptibility allele (usually DRB1*08 or -*05) have a higher relative risk than expected from the additive effect of those genes alone. In juvenile patients with rheumatoid factor–positive polyarticular disease, heterozygotes carrying both DRB1*0401 and -*0404 have a relative risk >100, reflecting an apparent synergy in individuals inheriting both of these susceptibility genes.

Type 1 Diabetes Mellitus There are several aspects of the genetics of type 1 diabetes (Chap. 333) that illustrate the complex nature of HLA associations with autoimmune diseases. First, type 1 (autoimmune) diabetes mellitus is associated with both DR3 and DR4 serotypes and their corresponding genes. The presence of both the DR3 and DR4 haplotypes in one individual confers the highest known genetic risk for type diabetes, and individuals carrying either of these haplotypes also carry some increased risk. Specific class II genes on each haplotype have been thoroughly studied, and the strongest association is with DQB1*0302, a specific gene on the diabetes-associated DR4 haplotypes. Thus, all DR4 haplotypes that carry a DQB1*0302 gene are associated with type 1 diabetes, whereas related DR4 haplotypes that carry a different DQB1 gene are not. The primary class II determinant of susceptibility, therefore, is HLA-DQB1*0302. However, the relative risk associated with inheritance of this gene can be modified, depending on other HLA genes present either on the same or a second haplotype. For example, just as the presence of a second haplotype containing DR3 is associated with an increased risk of diabetes, the presence of a DR2-positive haplotype containing a DQB1*0602 gene is associated with decreased risk. This gene, DQB1*0602, is considered "protective" for type 1 diabetes. Even some DRB1 genes that can occur on the same haplotype as DQB1*0302 may modulate risk, so that individuals with the DR4 haplotype that contains DRB1*0403 are less susceptible to type 1 diabetes than individuals with other DR4-DQB1*0302 haplotypes.

Although the presence of a DR3 haplotype in combination with the DR4-DQB1*0302 haplotype is a very high risk combination for diabetes susceptibility, the specific gene on the DR3 haplotype that is responsible for this synergy has not yet been identified. This is because the predominant HLA-DR3 haplotype in Caucasians has very tight linkage with other genes within the MHC, including HLA-A1, -B8, -Cw7, and -C4A, as discussed above. Thus, any of a large variety of genes within the HLA region on this DR3 haplotype may be the primary gene(s) responsible for contributing to diabetes susceptibility. An example that more directly implicates other genes linked to DR3 is the association between HLA genes and systemic lupus erythematosus (SLE; Chap. 311). The C4A null alleles that are present on the HLA-DR3 haplotypes in SLE are also often present in patients without DR3, notably those with HLA-DR2. This implies the presence of a C4A silent allele, which is a defective structural gene for the C4 complement component, rather than the expression of any particular class II gene, as a potential susceptibility gene within HLA associated with SLE.

HLA and Rheumatoid Arthritis The HLA genes most highly associated with rheumatoid arthritis (RA) are DRB1*0401 and DRB1*0404 (Chap. 312). These genes encode a distinctive sequence of amino acids from codons 67 to 74 of the DRβ molecule: RA-associated class II molecules carry the sequence LeuLeuGluGlnArg-

ArgAlaAla or LeuLeuGluGlnLysArgAlaAla in this region, while non-RA-associated genes carry one or more differences in this region. These residues form a portion of the molecule that lies in the middle of the α-helical portion of the DRB1-encoded class II molecule, termed the *shared epitope*.

These DR4+ RA-associated alleles are most frequent among patients with more severe, erosive disease. The frequency of these DR4+ alleles is lower among patients with RA who are rheumatoid factor–negative and those with nonerosive forms of the disease. Although the frequency of these DRB1 susceptibility alleles in RA patients is high, the same genes are also prevalent in the unaffected population, and thus the absolute risk associated with these susceptibility alleles is low. The highest risk for susceptibility to RA comes in individuals who carry both a DRB1*0401 and DRB1*0404 gene. Some forms of RA are associated with other HLA genes, such as DRB1*01, -*1001, and -*1402, which also carry the shared epitope sequence, strongly suggesting that this part of the class II molecule contributes directly to disease pathogenesis.

MOLECULAR MECHANISMS FOR HLA DISEASE ASSOCIATIONS As noted above, HLA molecules play a key role in the selection and establishment of the antigen-specific T cell repertoire and a major role in the subsequent activation of those T cells during the initiation of an immune response. Precise genetic polymorphisms characteristic of individual alleles dictate the specificity of these interactions and thereby instruct and guide antigen-specific immune events. These same genetically determined pathways are therefore implicated in disease pathogenesis when specific HLA genes are responsible for autoimmune disease susceptibility.

The fate of developing T cells within the thymus is determined by the affinity of interaction between TCR and HLA molecules bearing self peptides; thus, the particular HLA types of each individual control the precise specificity of the T cell repertoire (Chap. 305). The primary basis for HLA-associated disease susceptibility may well lie within this thymic maturation pathway. The positive selection of potentially autoreactive T cells, based on the presence of specific HLA susceptibility genes, may establish the threshold for disease risk in a particular individual.

At the time of onset of a subsequent immune response, the primary role of the HLA molecule is to bind peptide and present it to antigen-specific T cells. The HLA complex can therefore be viewed as encoding genetic determinants of precise immunologic activation events. Antigenic peptides that bind particular HLA molecules are capable of stimulating T cell immune responses; peptides that do not bind are not presented to T cells and are not immunogenic. This genetic control of the immune response is mediated by the polymorphic sites within the HLA antigen-binding groove that interact with the bound peptides. In autoimmune and immune-mediated diseases, it is likely that specific tissue antigens that are targets for pathogenic lymphocytes are complexed with the HLA molecules encoded by specific susceptibility alleles. In autoimmune diseases with an infectious etiology, it is likely that immune responses to peptides derived from the initiating pathogen are bound and presented by particular HLA molecules to activate T lymphocytes that play a triggering or contributory role in disease pathogenesis. The concept that early events in disease initiation are triggered by specific HLA-peptide complexes offers some prospects for therapeutic intervention, since it may be possible to design compounds that interfere with the formation or function of specific HLA-peptide-TCR interactions.

When considering mechanisms of HLA associations with the immune response and with disease it is well to remember that just as HLA genetics are complex, so are the mechanisms likely to be heterogeneous. Immune-mediated disease is a multistep process in which one of the HLA-associated functions is to establish a repertoire of potentially reactive T cells, while another HLA-associated function is to provide the essential peptide-binding specificity for T cell recognition. For diseases with multiple HLA genetic associations, it is possible that both of these interactions occur and synergize to advance an accelerated pathway of disease.

BIBLIOGRAPHY

BRAUD VM et al: Functions of nonclassical MHC and non-MHC-encoded class I molecules. Curr Opin Immunol 11:100, 1999

BUSCH R, MELLINS ED: Developing and shedding inhibitions: How MHC class II molecules reach maturity. Curr Opin Immunol 8:51, 1996

GODKIN A, JEWELL D: The pathogenesis of celiac disease. Gastroenterology 115:206, 1998

HAMMER J et al: HLA class II peptide binding specificity and autoimmunity. Adv Immunol 66:67, 1997

HILL AV: The immunogenetics of human infectious diseases. Annu Rev Immunol 16:593, 1998

LOPEZ-LARREA C et al: The role of HLA-B27 polymorphism and molecular mimicry in spondyloarthropathy. Mol Med Today 4:540, 1998

NEPOM GT: Major histocompatibility complex–directed susceptibility to rheumatoid arthritis. Adv Immunol 68:315, 1998

———, KWOK WW: Molecular basis for HLA-DQ associations with IDDM. Diabetes 47:1177, 1998

PAMER E, CRESSWELL P: Mechanisms of MHC class I–restricted antigen processing. Annu Rev Immunol 16:323, 1998

STERN LJ, WILEY DC: Antigenic peptide binding by class I and class II histocompatibility proteins. Structure 2(4):245, 1994

TAUROG JD et al: Inflammatory disease in HLA-B27 transgenic rats. Immunol Rev 169:209, 1999

307 Peter E. Lipsky, Betty Diamond

AUTOIMMUNITY AND AUTOIMMUNE DISEASES

One of the classically accepted features of the immune system is the capacity to distinguish self from non-self. Although they are able to recognize and generate reactions to a vast array of foreign materials, most animals do not mount immune responses to self-antigens under ordinary circumstances and thus are tolerant to self. Although recognition of self plays an important role in generating both the T cell and B cell repertoires of immune receptors and plays an essential role in the recognition of nominal antigen by T cells, the development of potentially harmful immune responses to self-antigens is, in general, precluded. Autoimmunity, therefore, represents the end result of the breakdown of one or more of the basic mechanisms regulating immune tolerance.

The presence or absence of pathologic consequences resulting from self-reactivity determines whether autoimmunity leads to the development of an autoimmune disease. The essential feature of an autoimmune disease is that tissue injury is caused by the immunologic reaction of the organism with its own tissues. Autoimmunity, on the other hand, refers merely to the presence of antibodies or T lymphocytes that react with self-antigens and does not necessarily imply that the development of self-reactivity has pathogenic consequences.

Autoimmunity may occur as an isolated event or in the setting of specific clinical syndromes. Autoimmunity may be seen in normal individuals and in higher frequency in normal older people. In addition, autoreactivity may develop during various infectious conditions. The expression of autoimmunity may be self-limited, as occurs with many infectious processes, or persistent. In both circumstances there is a tendency to develop autoreactivity directed against a variety of different tissues or organs. As mentioned above, autoimmunity does not necessarily lead to tissue damage, and even in the presence of organ pathology, it may be difficult to determine whether the damage is mediated by autoreactivity. Thus, the presence of self-reactivity may be either the cause or a consequence of an ongoing pathologic process. Furthermore, when autoreactivity is induced by an inciting event, such as infection or tissue damage from trauma or infarction, there may or may not be ensuing pathology.

MECHANISMS OF AUTOIMMUNITY Since Ehrlich first postulated the existence of mechanisms to prevent the generation of self-reactivity in 1900, ideas concerning the nature of this inhibition

Table 307-1 Mechanisms Preventing Autoimmunity

1. Sequestration of self-antigen
2. Generation and maintenance of tolerance
   a. Central deletion of autoreactive lymphocytes
   b. Peripheral anergy of autoreactive lymphocytes
   c. Receptor replacement by autoreactive lymphocytes
3. Regulatory mechanisms
   a. Anti-idiotype regulation
   b. Regulatory T cells

have developed in parallel with the progressive increase in understanding of the immune system. Burnet's clonal selection theory included the idea that interaction of lymphoid cells with their specific antigens during fetal or early postnatal life would lead to elimination of such "forbidden clones." This idea became untenable, however, when it was shown by a number of investigators that autoimmune diseases could be induced by simple immunization procedures, that autoantigen-binding cells could be demonstrated easily in the circulation of normal individuals, and that self-limited autoimmune phenomena frequently developed during infections. These observations indicated that clones of cells capable of responding to autoantigens were present in the repertoire of antigen-reactive cells in normal adults and suggested that mechanisms in addition to clonal deletion were responsible for preventing their activation.

Currently, three general processes are thought to be involved in the maintenance of selective unresponsiveness to autoantigens (Table 307-1): (1) sequestration of self-antigens, rendering them inaccessible to the immune system; (2) specific unresponsiveness (tolerance or anergy) of relevant T or B cells; and (3) limitation of potential reactivity by regulatory mechanisms. These mechanisms permit the host to respond to the vast universe of foreign antigens but preclude responses to autoantigens that might have pathogenic consequences.

Derangements of these normal processes may predispose to the development of autoimmunity (Table 307-2). In general, these abnormal responses relate to stimulation by exogenous agents, usually bacterial or viral, or endogenous abnormalities in the cells of the immune system. Thus, autoreactivity can result from exogenous stimulation of the immune system in a manner that overcomes the regulated unresponsiveness to self-antigens. Microbial superantigens, such as staphylococcal protein A and staphylococcal enterotoxins, are substances that can stimulate a broad range of T and B cells based upon specific interactions with selected families of immune receptors irrespective of their antigen specificity. If autoantigen reactive T and/or B cells express these receptors, autoimmunity might develop. Alternatively, mo-

Table 307-2 Mechanisms of Autoimmunity

I. Exogenous
   A. Molecular mimicry
   B. Superantigenic stimulation
   C. Microbial adjuvanticity
II. Endogenous
   A. Altered antigen presentation
      1. Loss of immunologic privilege
      2. Presentation of novel or cryptic epitopes (epitope spreading)
      3. Alteration of self-antigen
      4. Enhanced function of antigen-presenting cells
         a. Costimulatory molecule expression
         b. Cytokine production
   B. Increased T cell help
      1. Cytokine production
      2. Costimulatory molecules
   C. Increased B cell function
   D. Apoptotic defects
   E. Cytokine imbalance
   F. Altered immunoregulation
      1. Anti-idiotype regulation
      2. Regulatory T cells

lecular mimicry or cross-reactivity between a microbial product and a self-antigen might lead to activation of autoreactive lymphocytes. One of the best examples of autoreactivity and autoimmune disease resulting from molecular mimicry is rheumatic fever, in which antibodies to the M protein of streptococci cross-react with myosin, laminin, and other matrix proteins. Deposition of these autoantibodies in the heart initiates an inflammatory response. Molecular mimicry between microbial proteins and host tissues has been reported in insulin-dependent diabetes mellitus (IDDM), rheumatoid arthritis, and multiple sclerosis. The capacity of nonspecific stimulation of the immune system to predispose to the development of autoimmunity has been explored in a number of models; one is provided by the effect of adjuvants on the production of autoimmunity. Autoantigens become much more immunogenic when administered with adjuvant. It is presumed that infectious agents may be able to overcome self-tolerance because they possess molecules, such as bacterial endotoxin, that have adjuvant-like effects on the immune system.

Endogenous derangements of the immune system may also contribute to the loss of immunologic tolerance, or anergy, to self-antigens and the development of autoimmunity (Table 307-2). Many autoantigens reside in immunologically privileged sites, such as the brain or the anterior chamber of the eye. These sites are characterized by the inability of engrafted tissue to elicit immune responses. Immunologic privilege results from a number of events, including the limited entry of proteins from those sites into lymphatics, the local production of immunosuppressive cytokines such as transforming growth factor (TGF) β, and the local expression of molecules such as Fas ligand that can induce apoptosis of activated T cells. Lymphoid cells remain in a state of immunologic ignorance (neither activated nor anergized) to proteins expressed uniquely in immunologically privileged sites. If the privileged site is damaged by trauma or inflammation, or if T cells are activated elsewhere, proteins expressed at this site can become the targets of immunologic assault. Such an event may occur in multiple sclerosis and sympathetic ophthalmia, in which antigens uniquely expressed in the brain and eye, respectively, become the target of activated T cells.

Alterations in antigen presentation may also contribute to autoimmunity. This may occur by epitope spreading, in which protein determinants (*epitopes*) not routinely seen by lymphocytes (*cryptic epitopes*) are recognized as a result of immunologic reactivity to associated molecules. For example, animals immunized with one protein component of the spliceosome may be induced to produce antibodies to multiple other spliceosome proteins. Finally, inflammation, drug exposure, or normal senescence may cause a primary chemical alteration in proteins, resulting in the generation of immune responses that cross-react with normal self-proteins. Alterations in the availability and presentation of autoantigens may be important components of immunoreactivity in certain models of organ-specific autoimmune diseases. In addition, these factors may be relevant in understanding the pathogenesis of various drug-induced autoimmune conditions. However, the diversity of autoreactivity manifest in non-organ-specific systemic autoimmune diseases suggests that these conditions might result from a more general activation of the immune system rather than from an alteration in individual self-antigens.

A number of experimental models have suggested that intense stimulation of T lymphocytes can produce nonspecific signals that bypass the need for antigen-specific helper T cells and lead to polyclonal B cell activation with the formation of multiple autoantibodies. For example, antinuclear, antierythrocyte, and antilymphocyte antibodies are produced during the chronic graft-versus-host reaction. In addition, true autoimmune diseases, including autoimmune hemolytic anemia and immune complex–mediated glomerulonephritis, can also be induced in this manner. While it is clear that such diffuse activation of helper T cell activity can cause autoimmunity, nonspecific stimulation of B lymphocytes can also lead to the production of autoanti-

bodies. Thus, the administration of polyclonal B cell activators, such as bacterial endotoxin, to normal mice leads to the production of a number of autoantibodies, including those directed to DNA and IgG (rheumatoid factor).

Primary alterations in the activity of T and/or B cells, cytokine imbalances, or defective immunoregulatory circuits may also contribute to the emergence of autoimmunity. Although the biochemical bases of many of these abnormalities have not been documented, they may contribute to the emergence of autoimmunity either alone or in concert. For example, decreased apoptosis, as can be seen in animals with defects in Fas (CD95) or Fas ligand or in patients with related abnormalities, can be associated with the development of autoimmunity. Similarly, diminished production of tumor necrosis factor (TNF) α and interleukin (IL)10 has been reported to be associated with the development of autoimmunity.

An alternative explanation for the development of autoimmunity is that self-reactivity results not from overstimulation of the immune system but rather from an abnormality of immunoregulatory mechanisms. Observations made in both human autoimmune disease and animal models suggest that defects in the generation and expression of regulatory T cell activity may allow for the production of autoantibodies. The importance of defects in immunoregulatory cells is confirmed by the finding that administration of normal suppressor T cells or factors derived from them can prevent the development of autoimmune disease in rodent models of autoimmunity.

One of the mechanisms that regulates normal humoral immune responses is the production of anti-idiotype antibodies. These are immunoglobulin molecules directed against antigen-binding determinants of the specific antibodies originally elicited by the immunogen. Production of anti-idiotype antibodies may be dependent on helper T cell activity even when the initial immunogen is T cell independent. Therefore, it is possible that abnormalities in the generation of appropriate anti-idiotype antibodies, either at the B or T cell level, are responsible for the development of autoimmunity in certain circumstances.

It should be apparent that no single mechanism can explain all the varied manifestations of autoimmunity. Indeed, it appears likely, especially in systemic autoimmune diseases, that a number of abnormalities may converge to induce the complete syndrome. Moreover, one abnormality may cause a second, which, in concert with the first, facilitates the expression of autoimmunity. This possibility is consistent with recent findings in murine models of IDDM; systemic lupus erythematosus (SLE), rheumatoid arthritis, and multiple sclerosis in which multiple genetic regions, many of which are involved in controlling immune reactivity, appear to contribute to the development of autoimmune disease.

Despite the plethora of immunologic derangements identified in systemic autoimmune diseases such as SLE, the primary abnormality causing the disease remains unclear. In fact, detailed examination of a number of murine strains that spontaneously develop a lupus-like syndrome has failed to demonstrate a common immunologic abnormality. Additional factors that appear to be important determinants in the induction of autoimmunity include age, sex, genetic background, exposure to infectious agents, and environmental contacts. How all of these disparate factors affect the capacity to develop self-reactivity is currently being intensively investigated.

GENETIC CONSIDERATIONS   Evidence in humans that there are susceptibility genes for autoimmunity comes from family studies and especially from studies of twins. Studies in IDDM, rheumatoid arthritis, multiple sclerosis, and SLE have shown that approximately 15 to 30% of pairs of monozygotic twins show disease concordance, compared with <5% of dizygotic twins. The occurrence of different autoimmune diseases within the same family has suggested that certain susceptibility genes may predispose to a variety of autoimmune diseases. In addition to this evidence from humans, certain inbred mouse strains reproducibly develop specific spontaneous or experimentally induced autoimmune diseases, whereas others do not. These findings have led to an extensive search for genes that determine susceptibility to autoimmune disease.

The most consistent association for susceptibility to autoimmune disease has been with the major histocompatibility complex (MHC). Many human autoimmune diseases are associated with particular HLA alleles (Chap. 306). It has been suggested that the association of MHC genotype with autoimmune disease relates to differences in the ability of different allelic variations of MHC molecules to present autoantigenic peptides to autoreactive T cells. An alternative hypothesis involves the role of MHC alleles in shaping the T cell receptor repertoire during T cell ontongeny in the thymus. Additionally, specific MHC gene products themselves may be the source of peptides that can be recognized by T cells. Cross-reactivity between such MHC peptides and peptides derived from proteins produced by common microbes may trigger autoimmunity by molecular mimicry. However, MHC genotype alone does not determine the development of autoimmunity. Identical twins are far more likely to develop the same autoimmune disease than MHC-identical non-twin siblings, suggesting that genetic factors other than the MHC also affect disease susceptibility. Recent studies of the genetics of IDDM, SLE, and multiple sclerosis in humans and mice have shown that there are several independently segregating disease susceptibility loci in addition to the MHC.

There is evidence that several other genes are important in increasing susceptibility to autoimmune disease. In humans, inherited homozygous deficiency of the early proteins of the classic pathway of complement (C1, C4, or C2) is very strongly associated with the development of SLE. In mice and humans, abnormalities in the genes encoding proteins involved in the regulation of apoptosis, including Fas (CD95) and Fas ligand (CD95 ligand), are strongly associated with the development of autoimmunity. There is also evidence that inherited variation in the level of expression of certain cytokines, such as TNF-α or IL-10, may also increase susceptibility to autoimmune disease.

A further important factor in disease susceptibility is the hormonal status of the patient. Many autoimmune diseases show a strong sex bias, which appears in most cases to relate to the hormonal status of women. ■

IMMUNOPATHOGENIC MECHANISMS IN AUTOIMMUNE DISEASES The mechanisms of tissue injury in autoimmune diseases can be divided into antibody-mediated and cell-mediated processes. Representative examples are listed in Table 307-3.

The pathogenicity of autoantibodies can be mediated through several mechanisms, including opsonization of soluble factors or cells, activation of an inflammatory cascade via the complement system, and interference with the physiologic function of soluble molecules or cells.

In autoimmune thrombocytopenic purpura, opsonization of platelets targets them for elimination by phagocytes. Likewise, in autoimmune hemolytic anemia, binding of immunoglobulin to red cell membranes leads to phagocytosis and lysis of the opsonized cell. Goodpastures' syndrome, a disease characterized by lung hemorrhage and severe glomerulonephritis, represents an example of antibody binding leading to local activation of complement and neutrophil accumulation and activation. The autoantibody in this disease binds to the α_3 chain of type IV collagen in the basement membrane. In SLE,

Table 307-3   Mechanisms of Tissue Damage in Autoimmune Disease

Effector	Mechanism	Target	Disease
Autoantibody	Blocking or inactivation	α Chain of the nicotinic acetylcholine receptor	Myasthenia gravis
		Phospholipid–β_2-glycoprotein 1 complex	Antiphospholipid syndrome
		Insulin receptor	Insulin-resistant diabetes mellitus
		Intrinsic factor	Pernicious anemia
	Stimulation	TSH receptor (LATS)	Graves' disease
		Proteinase-3 (ANCA)	Wegener's granulomatosis
		Epidermal cadherin$_1$	
		Desmoglein 3	Pemphigus vulgaris
	Complement activation	α_3 Chain of collagen IV	Goodpastures' syndrome
	Immune-complex formation	Double-stranded DNA	Systemic lupus erythematosus
		Ig	Rheumatoid arthritis
	Opsonization	Platelet GpIIb:IIIa	Autoimmune thrombocytopenic purpura
		Rh antigens, I antigen	Autoimmune hemolytic anemia
	Antibody-dependent cellular cytotoxicity	Thyroid peroxidase, thyroglobulin	Hashimoto's thyroiditis
T cells	Cytokine production	?	Rheumatoid arthritis, Multiple sclerosis, insulin-dependent diabetes mellitus
	Cellular cytotoxicity	?	Insulin-dependent diabetes mellitus

NOTE: ANCA, antineutrophil cytoplasmic antibody; LATS, long-acting thyroid stimulator; TSH, thyroid-stimulating hormone.

activation of the complement cascade at sites of immunoglobulin deposition in renal glomeruli is considered to be a major mechanism of renal damage.

Autoantibodies can also interfere with normal physiologic functions of cells or soluble factors. Autoantibodies against hormone receptors can lead to stimulation of cells or to inhibition of cell function through interference with receptor signaling. For example, long-acting thyroid stimulators (LATS), which are autoantibodies that bind to the receptor for thyroid-stimulating hormone (TSH), are present in Graves' disease and function as agonists, causing the thyroid to respond as if there were an excess of TSH. Alternatively, antibodies to the insulin receptor can cause insulin-resistant diabetes mellitus through receptor blockade. In myasthenia gravis, autoantibodies to the acetylcholine receptor can be detected in 85 to 90% of patients and are responsible for muscle weakness. The exact location of the antigenic epitope, the valence and affinity of the antibody, and perhaps other characteristics determine whether activation or blockade results from antibody binding.

Antiphospholipid antibodies are associated with thromboembolic events in primary and secondary antiphospholipid syndrome and have also been associated with fetal wastage. The major antibody is directed to the phospholipid–β_2-glycoprotein I complex and appears to exert a procoagulant effect. In pemphigus vulgaris, autoantibodies bind to a component of the epidermal cell desmosome, desmoglein 3, and play a role in the induction of the disease. They exert their pathologic effect by disrupting cell-cell junctions through stimulation of the production of epithelial proteases, leading to blister formation. Cytoplasmic antineutrophil cytoplasmic antibody (c-ANCA), found in Wegener's granulomatosis, is an antibody to an intracellular antigen, the 29-kDa serine protease (proteinase-3). In vitro experiments have shown that IgG c-ANCA causes cellular activation and degranulation of primed neutrophils.

It is important to note that autoantibodies of a given specificity may cause disease only in genetically susceptible hosts, as has been shown in experimental models of myasthenia gravis. Finally, some autoantibodies seem to be markers for disease but have as yet no known pathogenic potential.

AUTOIMMUNE DISEASE   Manifestations of autoimmunity are found in a large number of pathologic conditions. However, their presence does not necessarily imply that the pathologic process is an autoimmune disease. A number of attempts to establish formal criteria for the diagnosis of autoimmune diseases have been made, but none is universally accepted. One set of criteria is shown in Table 307-4; however, this should be viewed merely as a guide in consideration of the problem.

To classify a disease as autoimmune, it is necessary to demonstrate that the immune response to a self-antigen causes the observed pathology. Initially, the demonstration that antibodies against the affected tissue could be detected in the serum of patients suffering from various diseases was taken as evidence that these diseases had an autoimmune basis. However, such autoantibodies are also found when tissue damage is caused by trauma or infection, and the autoantibody is secondary to tissue damage. Thus, it is necessary to show that autoimmunity is pathogenic before classifying a disease as autoimmune.

If the autoantibodies are pathogenic, it may be possible to transfer disease to experimental animals by the administration of autoantibodies, with the subsequent development of pathology in the recipient similar to that seen in the patient from whom the antibodies were obtained. This has been shown, for example, in Graves' disease. Some autoimmune diseases can be transferred from mother to fetus and are observed in the newborn babies of diseased mothers. The symptoms of the disease in the newborn usually disappear as the levels of the maternal antibody decrease. An exception is congenital heart block, in which damage to the developing conducting system of the heart as a result of transfer of anti-Ro antibody from the mother results in permanent heart block.

In most situations, the critical factors that determine when the development of autoimmunity results in autoimmune disease have not been delineated. The relationship of autoimmunity to the development of autoimmune disease may relate to the fine specificity of the antibodies or T cells or their specific effector capabilities. In many circumstances a mechanistic understanding of the pathogenic potential of autoantibodies has not been established. In some autoimmune diseases, biased production of cytokines by helper T (T_H) cells may play a role in pathogenesis. In this regard, T cells can differentiate into specialized effector cells that predominantly produce interferon γ (T_H1) or IL-4 (T_H2) (Chap. 305). The former facilitate macrophage activation and classic cell-mediated immunity, whereas the latter are thought to have regulatory functions and are involved in the resolution of normal immune responses and also the development of responses to a variety of parasites. In a number of autoimmune diseases, such as rheumatoid arthritis, multiple sclerosis, IDDM, and Crohn's disease, there appears to be biased differentiation of T_H1 cells, with resultant organ damage.

ORGAN-SPECIFIC VERSUS SYSTEMIC AUTOIMMUNE DISEASES   Autoimmune diseases form a spectrum, from those specifically affecting a single organ to systemic disorders with involvement of many organs (Table 307-5). Hashimoto's autoimmune thyroiditis is probably the best studied example of an organ-specific autoimmune disease (Chap. 330). In this disorder, there is a specific lesion in the thyroid associated with infiltration of mononuclear cells and damage to follicular cells. Antibody to thyroid constituents can be demonstrated in nearly all cases. Other organ- or tissue-specific autoimmune disorders include pemphigus vulgaris, autoimmune hemolytic anemia, idiopathic thrombocytopenic purpura, Goodpasture's syndrome, myasthenia gravis, and sympathetic ophthalmia. One important feature of some organ-specific autoimmune diseases is the tendency for overlap, such that an individual with one specific syndrome is more likely to develop a second syndrome. For example, there is a high incidence of pernicious anemia in individuals with autoimmune thyroiditis. More striking is the tendency for individuals with an organ-specific autoimmune disease to develop multiple other manifestations of autoimmunity without the development of associated organ pathology. Thus, as many as 50% of individuals with pernicious anemia have non-cross-reacting antibodies to thyroid constituents, whereas patients with myasthenia gravis may develop antinuclear antibodies, antithyroid antibodies, rheumatoid factor, antilymphocyte antibodies, and polyclonal hypergammaglobulinemia. Part of the explanation for this may relate to the genetic elements shared by individuals with these different diseases.

SYSTEMIC AUTOIMMUNE DISEASE   Systemic autoimmune diseases differ from organ-specific diseases in that pathologic lesions are found in multiple, diverse organs and tissues. The hallmark of these conditions is the demonstration of associated relevant autoimmune manifestations that are likely to be etiologic in the organ pathology. SLE is the best example of such a disorder. Although a number of other diseases such as Sjögren's syndrome possess certain of the features of a systemic autoimmune disease, SLE represents the prototype of these disorders because of its abundance of autoimmune manifestations.

SLE is a disease of protean manifestations that characteristically involves the kidneys, joints, skin, serosal surfaces, blood vessels, and central nervous system (Chap. 311). The disease is associated with a vast array of autoantibodies whose production appears to be a part of a generalized hyperreactivity of the humoral immune system. Other features of SLE include generalized B cell hyperresponsiveness, polyclonal hypergammaglobulinemia, and increased titers of antibodies to commonly encountered viral antigens.

A number of the autoantibodies found in SLE have clearly been implicated in certain of the pathologic features of the disease. Clas-

Table 307-4   Human Autoimmune Disease: Presumptive Evidence for an Immunologic Pathogenesis

Major Criteria
1. Presence of autoantibodies or evidence of cellular reactivity to self
2. Documentation of relevant autoantibody or lymphocytic infiltrate in the pathologic lesion.
3. Demonstration that relevant autoantibody or T cells can cause tissue pathology
   a. Transplacental transmission
   b. Adaptive transfer into animals
   c. In vitro impact on cellular function

Supportive Evidence
1. Reasonable animal model
2. Beneficial effect from immunosuppressive agents
3. Association with other evidence of autoimmunity
4. No evidence of infection or other obvious cause

Table 307-5   Some Autoimmune Diseases

ORGAN SPECIFIC

Graves' disease	Autoimmune hemolytic anemia
Hashimoto's thyroiditis	Autoimmune thrombocytopenic
Autoimmune polyglandular	purpura
syndrome	Pernicious anemia
Insulin-dependent diabetes mellitus	Myasthenia gravis
Insulin-resistant diabetes mellitus	Multiple sclerosis
Immune-mediated infertility	Guillain-Barré syndrome
Autoimmune Addison's disease	Stiff-man syndrome
Pemphigus vulgaris	Acute rheumatic fever
Pemphigus foliaceus	
Dermatitis herpetiformis	Sympathetic ophthalmia
Autoimmune alopecia	Goodpasture's syndrome
Vitiligo	

ORGAN NONSPECIFIC (SYSTEMIC)

Systemic lupus erythematosus	Wegener's granulomatosis
Rheumatoid arthritis	Antiphospholipid syndrome
Systemic necrotizing vasculitis	Sjögren's syndrome

Table 307-6   Immunopathogenic Mechanisms in Systemic Lupus Erythematosus

Mechanism	Autoantibody	Pathologic Consequence
Inactivation or blocking	Antilymphocyte	Depressed T lymphocyte function
		Inhibition of suppressor T cell function
	Anticoagulants	Inhibition of clotting
	Antineuron	CNS dysfunction
	Antineutrophil	Depressed
	Anti-Ro	phagocytosis
	Antiphospholipid	Congenital heat block Thrombosis
Opsonization	Antierythrocyte	Hemolytic anemia
	Antiplatelet	Thrombocytopenia
	Antilymphocyte	Lymphopenia
	Antineutrophil	Neutropenia
Immune-complex deposition or in situ formation	Anti-DNA	Renal disease
	Antinucleoprotein, Anti-RNP, anti-IgG	

NOTE: CNS, central nervous system.

sically, SLE has been considered a disorder in which immune complexes are the major pathogenic entity. While immune-complex deposition or in situ formation of complexes appears to be a major pathogenic mechanism in lupus renal disease, additional autoimmune processes may be implicated in the pathogenesis of other features of the disease (Table 307-6).

The etiology of SLE remains unknown, and the interplay of a number of factors appears to be involved in its pathogenesis. Race and gender play an important role as evidenced by the increased incidence in young black females. The role of environmental factors is suggested by the high incidence of autoantibodies, especially antilymphocyte antibodies, in nonconsanguineous household contacts of individuals with SLE. The importance of genetic influences is suggested by family studies indicating that first-degree relatives of SLE patients have an increased likelihood of developing autoimmunity and autoimmune disease. The very high concordance rate for SLE and even higher rate for autoimmunity in monozygotic twins supports this concept. Finally, the association of SLE with MHC genes confirms the importance of immunogenetic factors in its pathogenesis. Current hypotheses concerning the immunopathogenesis of SLE suggest that autoantibody formation may result from a combination of exaggerated B cell activation owing either to excessive exogenous stimulation or endogenous hyperactivity and inadequate regulatory T cell or anti-idiotype regulation. Genetic elements may contribute to each of these abnormalities.

BIBLIOGRAPHY

ANDRE I et al: Checkpoints in the progression of autoimmune disease: Lessons from diabetes models. Proc Natl Acad Sci USA 93:2260, 1996

BERNAL A et al: Superantigens in human disease. J Clin Immunol 19:149, 1999

GIANANI R, SARVETNICK N: Viruses, cytokines, antigens, and autoimmunity. Proc Natl Acad Sci USA 93:2257, 1996

MADAIO MP: The role of autoantibodies in the pathogenesis of lupus nephritis. Semin Nephrol 19:48, 1999

McDEVITT HO: The role of MHC class II molecules in susceptibility and resistance to autoimmunity. Curr Opin Immunol 10:677, 1998

MOLLER E: Mechanisms for induction of autoimmunity in humans. Acta Paediatr Suppl 424:16, 1998

O'GARRA A et al: CD4+ T-cell subsets in autoimmunity. Curr Opin Immunol 9:872, 1997

PARISH CR, O'NEILL ER: Dependence of the adaptive immune response on innate immunity: Some questions answered but new paradoxes emerge. Immunol Cell Biol 75:523, 1997

RAY S et al: Pathogenic autoantibodies are routinely generated during the response to foreign antigen: A paradigm for autoimmune disease. Proc Natl Acad Sci USA 93:2019, 1996

RIDWAY WM, FATHMAN CG: The association of MHC with autoimmune disease: Understanding the pathogenesis of autoimmune diabetes. Clin Immunol Immunopathol 86:3, 1998

ROSE NR: The role of infection in the pathogenesis of autoimmune disease. Semin Immunol 10:5, 1998

STEINMAN L, CONLON P: Viral damage and the breakdown of self-tolerance. Nat Med 3:1085, 1997

VANDERLUGT C, MILLER SD: Epitope spreading. Curr Opin Immunol 8:831, 1996

VON HERRATH MG, OLDSTONE MBA: Virus-induced autoimmune disease. Curr Opin Immunol 8:878, 1996

VYSE TJ, TODD JA: Genetic analysis of autoimmune disease. Cell 85:311, 1996

308   Max D. Cooper, Harry W. Schroeder, Jr.

PRIMARY IMMUNE DEFICIENCY DISEASES

ADA	adenosine deaminase	NK	natural killer
AT	ataxia-telangiectasia	PNP	purine nucleoside phosphorylase
Btk	Bruton's tyrosine kinase	PPD	purified protein derivative
EBV	Epstein-Barr virus	SCID	severe combined
IFNGR1	interferon γ receptor 1		immunodeficiency
IFNGR2	interferon γ receptor signal-transducing chain	TCR	T cell receptors
MHC	major histocompatibility complex	WHN	winged-helix-nude

Immunologic functions are mediated by developmentally independent, but functionally interacting, families of lymphocytes. The activities of B and T lymphocytes and their products in host defense are closely integrated with the functions of other cells of the reticuloendothelial system. Dendritic cells, Langerhans' cells in the skin, and macrophages play an important role in the trapping and presentation of antigens to T and B cells to initiate the immune response. Macrophages also become effector cells, especially when activated by cytokine products of lymphocytes. The scavenger activity of macrophages and polymorphonuclear leukocytes is directed and made specific by antibodies in concert with cytokines and the complement system. Natural killer (NK) cells, a population of granular lymphocytes with receptors specific for MHC class I molecules, may spontaneously kill tumor and virus-infected cells, activities that are enhanced by the cytokine products of immune and inflammatory cells. Killing by NK cells can also be targeted by IgG antibodies for which NK cells have cell-surface receptors. The interaction of basophils and tissue mast cells with IgE antibodies in causation of immediate-type hypersensitivity is discussed in Chap. 310. Consideration of these interrelationships is an important part of the analysis of patients with suspected immune deficiency.

DIFFERENTIATION OF T AND B CELLS   The functional deficits that occur in both congenital and acquired immunodeficiencies are usefully viewed as being caused by defects at various points along the differentiation pathways of immunocompetent cells. A subpopulation of hematopoietic stem cells become restricted to lymphoid differentiation prior to migration to the thymus, where T cells are generated, and in the fetal liver and adult bone marrow, where B cell development begins (Fig. 308-1). Immature T and B cells then migrate through the circulation to the spleen, lymph nodes, intestine and other peripheral lymphoid organs. In these sites, they may encounter antigens presented by dendritic cells or macrophages and respond with proliferation, differentiation and mediation of immune responses. Chap. 305 provides a general account of their roles in cellular and humoral immunity.

Differentiation of T or B cells may be arrested at either the primary or secondary stages. Reflecting the complex cellular interactions involved in immune responses and the pivotal role played by T lymphocytes, immune deficiencies primarily involving T cells are usually also associated with abnormal B cell function. Conversely, immuno-

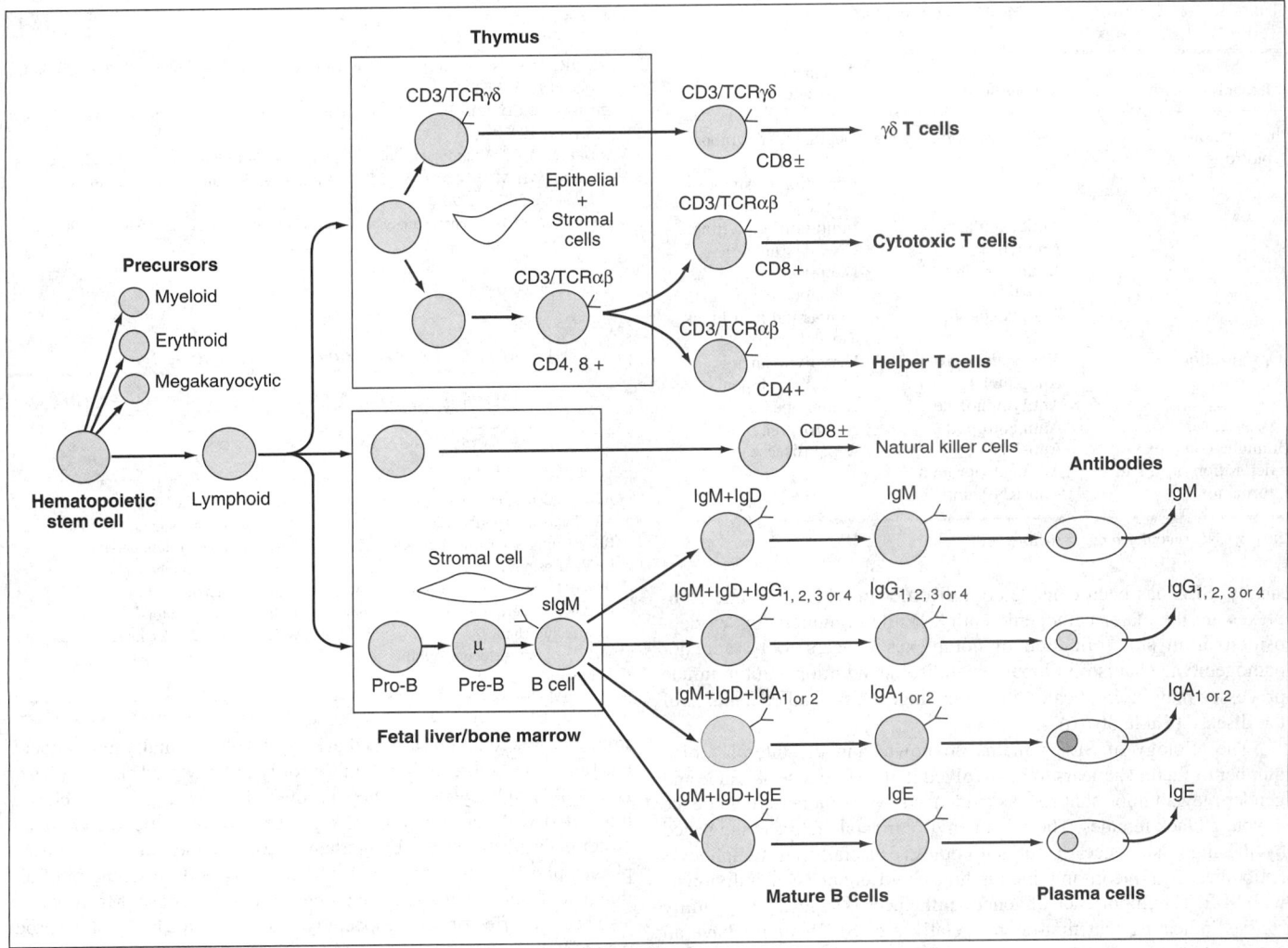

FIGURE 308-1 Hypothetical model outlining the differentiation of hematopoietic stem cells along T, B, and NK cell lineages. The antigen presenting dendritic cells, not shown here, are derived from both lymphoid and myeloid progenitors. Failure to develop T and B cells may result from defective stem cells or from inborn metabolic errors affecting both cell types. Rarely, other hematopoietic cell lines are also absent. Absence of either T or B cells suggests malfunction of central lymphoid tissues, including the thymus and the fetal liver–bone marrow complex. B cell deficiency may result from failure to generate pre-B cells from their stem cell precursors or from failure of pre-B cells to give rise to their B lymphocyte progeny. Similarly, differentiation may be arrested at several levels within the T cell lineage; arrests at the thymocyte level and failure to develop the helper subset have been observed in immunodeficient patients. Agammaglobulinemia and deficiencies of some T cell functions may occur despite the presence of normal numbers of B or T cells in the circulation. Failure of B lymphocytes to differentiate to plasma cells can be due to intrinsic cellular abnormalities or to faulty T cell regulation.

deficiencies manifested primarily by inability to produce antibodies may be caused by T cell defects not associated with abnormal cell-mediated immunity.

CLINICAL DISEASE FEATURES COMMON TO IMMUNE DEFICIENCY Immunodeficiency syndromes, whether congenital, spontaneously acquired, or iatrogenic, are characterized by unusual susceptibility to infection and not infrequently to autoimmune disease and lymphoreticular malignancies. The types of infection often provide the first clue to the nature of the immunologic defect.

Patients with *defects in humoral immunity* have recurrent or chronic sinopulmonary infection, meningitis, and bacteremia, most commonly caused by pyogenic bacteria such as *Haemophilus influenzae*, *Streptococcus pneumoniae*, and staphylococci. These and other pyogenic organisms also cause frequent infections in individuals who have either neutropenia or a deficiency of the pivotal third component of complement (C3). The tripartite collaboration of antibody, complement, and phagocytes in host defense against pyogenic organisms makes it important to assess all three systems in individuals with unusual susceptibility to bacterial infections.

Antibody-deficient patients in whom cell-mediated immunity is intact have an interesting response to viral infections. The clinical course of primary infection with viruses such as varicella zoster or rubeola, unless complicated by bacterial infection, does not differ significantly from that of the normal host. However, long-lasting immunity may not develop, and as a result, multiple bouts of chickenpox and measles may occur. Such observations suggest that intact T cells may be sufficient for control of established viral infections, while antibodies play an important role in limiting the initial dissemination of virus and in providing long-lasting protection. Exceptions to this generalization are becoming more widely recognized. Agammaglobulinemic patients fail to clear hepatitis B virus from their circulation and have a progressive, and often fatal, course. Poliomyelitis has occurred following live-virus vaccination in some patients. Chronic encephalitis, which may progress over a period of months to years, is a particular threat in congenitally agammaglobulinemic boys. Echoviruses and adenoviruses have been isolated from brain, spinal fluid, or other sites in such patients.

The occurrence of an unusually serious infection, for example, *H. influenzae* meningitis in an older child or adult, warrants consideration of humoral immune deficiency. Recurrent bacterial pneumonias also suggest this possibility. Chronic otitis media occurs frequently in patients with hypogammaglobulinemia and is significant because of its relative rarity in normal adults. Pansinusitis, although almost invariably present in immunoglobulin deficiency, is a less helpful finding because it is not rare in apparently normal people. Bacterial infections of the skin or urinary tract are less frequent problems in hypogammaglobulinemic patients.

Infestation with the intestinal parasite *Giardia lamblia* is a frequent cause of diarrhea in antibody-deficient patients.

Abnormalities of cell-mediated immunity predispose to disseminated virus infections, particularly with latent viruses such as herpes simplex (Chap. 182), varicella zoster (Chap. 183), and cytomegalovirus (Chap. 185). In addition, patients so affected almost invariably develop mucocutaneous candidiasis and frequently acquire systemic fungal infections. Pneumonia caused by *Pneumocystis carinii* is also common (Chap. 209). Severe enteritis caused by *Cryptosporidium* infection may extend to the biliary tract to result in sclerosing cholangitis.

T cell deficiency is always accompanied by some abnormality of antibody responses (Fig. 308-1), although this may not be reflected by hypogammaglobulinemia. This explains in part why patients with primary T cell defects are also subject to overwhelming bacterial infection.

The most severe form of immune deficiency occurs in individuals, often infants, who lack both cell-mediated and humoral immune functions. Individuals with severe combined immunodeficiency (SCID) are susceptible to the whole range of infectious agents including organisms not ordinarily considered pathogenic. Multiple infections with viruses, bacteria, and fungi occur, often simultaneously. Because donor lymphocytes cannot be rejected by these recipients, blood transfusions can produce fatal graft-versus-host disease.

EVALUATION OF IMMUNODEFICIENT PATIENTS A careful history and physical examination will usually indicate whether the major problem involves the antibody-complement-phagocyte system or cell-mediated immunity. A history of contact dermatitis due to poison ivy suggests intact cellular immunity. Persistent mucocutaneous candidiasis suggests deficient cell-mediated immunity. Lymphopenia and the absence of palpable lymph nodes may be important findings. However, patients with profound immunodeficiency may have diffuse lymphoid hyperplasia. Most immunodeficiencies may be diagnosed by thoughtful use of tests available in local or regional clinical laboratories. More precise evaluation of immunologic functions and treatment may require referral to specialized centers. Table 308-1 presents a résumé of widely available laboratory investigations.

Humoral Immunity With rare exceptions, deficiency of humoral immunity is accompanied by diminished serum concentration of one or more classes of immunoglobulin. Normal values vary with age, and adult concentrations of IgM (1.0 ± 0.4 g/L) are reached at about 1 year, of IgG (10.0 ± 3.0 g/L) at 5 to 6 years, and of IgA (2.5 ± 1.0 g/L) by puberty (Chap. 305). The wide range of values among normal adults creates difficulty in defining the lower limits of normal. Reasonable estimates for low values are below 0.4 g/L for IgM, 5 g/L for IgG, and 0.5 g/L for IgA. In the presence of borderline hypogammaglobulinemia, assessing the patient's capacity to produce specific antibodies becomes particularly important. Isohemagglutinins, anti-streptolysin O, and "febrile agglutinins" are valuable standard assays, and measurements of pre- and postimmunization titers to tetanus toxoid, diphtheria toxoid, *H. influenzae* capsular polysaccharide, and *S. pneumoniae* serotypes provide a comprehensive assessment of humoral responsiveness.

Estimation of numbers of circulating B and T lymphocytes is of value in determining the pathogenesis of certain types of immune deficiency. B lymphocytes are identified by the presence of membrane-bound immunoglobulins, their associated α- and β-chain units, and other lineage-specific molecules on the B cell surface (Table 308-1), which can be identified and enumerated by specific monoclonal antibodies.

Since antibody deficiency may be mimicked clinically by deficiency of complement components, measurement of total hemolytic complement (CH_{50}) should be a part of the evaluation of host defense. Measurement of C3 alone is inadequate for screening, since deficien-

Table 308-1 Laboratory Evaluation of Host Defense Status

Initial Screening Assays[a]
Complete blood count with differential smear
Serum immunoglobulin levels: IgM, IgG, IgA, IgD, IgE

Other Readily Available Assays
Quantification of blood mononuclear cell populations by immunofluorescence assays employing monoclonal antibody markers[b]

T cells: CD3, CD4, CD8, TCR$\alpha\beta$, TCR$\gamma\delta$
B cells: CD19, CD20, CD21, Ig(μ, δ, γ, α, κ, λ), Ig-associated molecules (α, β)
NK cells: CD16/CD56
Monocytes: CD15
Activation markers: HLA-DR, CD25, CD80 (B cells), CD154 (T cells)

T cell functional evaluation
1. Delayed hypersensitivity skin tests (PPD, *Candida*, histoplasmin, tetanus toxoid)
2. Proliferative response to mitogens (anti-CD3 antibody, phytohemagglutinin, concanavalin A) and allogeneic cells (mixed lymphocyte response)
3. Cytokine production

B cell functional evaluation
1. Natural or commonly acquired antibodies: isohemagglutinins; antibodies to common viruses (influenza, rubella, rubeola) and bacterial toxins (diphtheria, tetanus)
2. Response to immunization with protein (tetanus toxoid) and carbohydrate (pneumococcal vaccine, *H. influenzae B* vaccine) antigens
3. Quantitative IgG subclass determinations

Complement
1. CH_{50} assays (classic and alternative pathways)
2. C3, C4, and other components

Phagocyte function
1. Reduction of nitroblue tetrazolium
2. Chemotaxis assays
3. Bactericidal activity

---

[a] Together with a history and physical examination, these tests will identify more than 95% of patients with primary immunodeficiencies.
[b] The menu of monoclonal antibody markers may be expanded or contracted to focus on particular clinical questions.

cies of both early and late complement components may predispose to bacterial infection (Chap. 305).

Cellular Immunity T lymphocytes may be enumerated by their expression of the TCR/CD3 complex of surface molecules. The CD4 molecule serves as a marker for helper T cells, although macrophages also express this molecule in relatively low levels. Conversely, CD8$\alpha\beta$ heterodimers are expressed by cytotoxic T cells. CD8 is also expressed by some $\gamma\delta$ T cells and by NK cells, although usually as CD8$\alpha\alpha$ homodimeric molecules.

Normal levels of serum immunoglobulins and antibody responsiveness are reliable indices of intact helper T cell function. T lymphocyte function can be measured directly by delayed hypersensitivity skin testing using a variety of antigens to which the majority of older children and adults have been sensitized. A generally useful skin test antigen is a 1:5 dilution of tetanus toxoid injected intradermally, since almost all individuals will have been sensitized. Purified protein derivative (PPD), histoplasmin, mumps antigen, and extracts of *Candida* or *Trichophyton* also may be used.

T lymphocyte function may be estimated in vitro by the capacity of cells to proliferate in response to antigens to which the patient has been sensitized, to lymphocytes from an unrelated donor, to antibodies that cross-link the CD3/TCR complex, or to the T cell mitogens, such as phytohemagglutinin and concanavalin A. The response is usually quantified by measurement of incorporation of radioactive thymidine into newly synthesized DNA. The production of cytokines (or interleukins) by activated T cells, can be measured as can the ability of T cells activated in mixed lymphocyte culture to lyse target cells. Finally, assays exist for detection of defects in T cell surface receptors and specific elements of their signal transduction pathways.

CLASSIFICATION *Primary immunodeficiencies* may be either congenital or manifested later in life and are currently classified according to mode of inheritance and whether the genetic defect affects T cells, B cells, or both (Table 308-2). The following discussion emphasizes three related concepts: (1) that immunodeficiencies are logically viewed as defects of cellular differentiation; (2) that these defects may involve either primary development of T or B cells or the antigen-dependent phase of their differentiation; and (3) that defects of B cell differentiation may in some instances reflect faulty T-B collaboration.

Secondary immunodeficiencies are those not caused by intrinsic abnormalities in development or function of T and B cells. The best known of these is AIDS, which may follow infection with the human immunodeficiency virus (Chap. 309). Other examples are immune deficiency associated with malnutrition, protein-losing enteropathy, and intestinal lymphangiectasia. Also considered secondary are immunodeficiencies resulting from hypercatabolic states such as occur in myotonic dystrophy, immunodeficiency associated with lymphoreticular malignancy, and immunodeficiency resulting from treatment with x-rays, antilymphocyte antibodies, or immunosuppressive drugs.

Incidence As a group, the primary immunodeficiencies are relatively common. The most frequent, isolated IgA deficiency, occurs in approximately 1 in 600 individuals in North America. Common variable immunodeficiency, a related disorder characterized by panhypogammaglobulinemia, is the next most common disorder. Both of these immunodeficiency states often become clinically evident in young adults.

The more severe forms of primary immunodeficiency are relatively rare, have their onset early in life, and all too frequently result in death during childhood. However, patients with congenital hypogammaglobulinemia may survive to middle age and beyond with replacement antibody therapy. In a referral center for patients with immunodeficiency diseases, approximately two-thirds of the immunodeficient patients will be adults.

Severe Combined Immunodeficiency The SCID syndrome is characterized by gross functional impairment of both humoral and cell-mediated immunity and by susceptibility to devastating fungal, bac-

Table 308-2 Classification of Primary Immunodeficiencies

COMBINED IMMUNODEFICIENCIES

Severe combined immunodeficiency (SCID):
Recombinase activating gene (RAG 1/2) deficiency
Adenosine deaminase (ADA) deficiency
Interleukin receptor γ chain (γ_c) deficiency
Janus-associated kinase 3 (JAK3) deficiency
Reticular dysgenesis

Primary T cell immunodeficiency:
DiGeorge syndrome
Nude syndrome
T cell receptor deficiency
MHC class II deficiency
TAP-2 deficiency (MHC class I deficiency)
ZAP70 tyrosine kinase deficiency
Purine nucleotide phosphorylase (PNP) deficiency

PREDOMINANTLY ANTIBODY DEFICIENCIES

X-linked agammaglobulinemia (Bruton's tyrosine kinase deficiency)
Autosomal recessive agammaglobulinemia:
Mu heavy chain deficiency
Surrogate light chain ($\gamma5/14.1$) deficiency
Hyper-IgM syndrome:
X-linked (CD40 ligand deficiency)
Other

Ig heavy chain gene deletions
IgA deficiency
Selective deficiency of IgG subclasses (with or without IgA deficiency)
Common variable immunodeficiency (CVID)
Antibody deficiency with normal immunoglobulins
Transient hypogammaglobulinemia of infancy

OTHER WELL-DEFINED IMMUNODEFICIENCY SYNDROMES

Interferon γ receptor (IFNGR1, IFNGR2) deficiency
Interleukin 12 and interleukin 12 receptor deficiency
Immunodeficiency with thymoma
Wiskott-Aldrich syndrome (WAS protein deficiency)

Ataxia telangiectasia (ATM deficiency)
X-linked lymphoproliferative syndrome (SH2D1A/SAP deficiency)
Hyper IgE syndrome

IMMUNODEFICIENCY ASSOCIATED WITH OR SECONDARY TO OTHER DISEASES

Chromosomal Instability or defective repair:
Bloom syndrome
Xeroderma pigmentosum
Fanconi anemia
ICF syndrome
Nijmegen breakage syndrome
Seckel syndrome
Chromosomal defects:
Down syndrome (Trisomy 21)
Turner syndrome
Deletions or rings of chromosome 18 (18p- and 18q-)
Skeletal abnormalities:
Short-limbed skeletal dysplasia (short-limbed dwarfism)
Cartilage-hair hypoplasia (metaphyseal chondroplasia)
Immunodeficiency with generalized growth retardation:
Schimke immuno-osseous dysplasia
Dubowitz syndrome
Kyphomelic dysplasia with SCID
Mulibrey's nannism
Growth retardation, facial anomalies and immunodeficiency
Progeria (Hutchinson-Gilford syndrome)

Immunodeficiency with dermatologic defects:
Ectrodactyly-ectodermal dysplasia-clefting syndrome
Immunodeficiency with absent thumbs, anosmia and ichthyosis
Partial albinism
Dyskeratosis congenita
Netherton syndrome
Anhidrotic ectodermal dysplasia
Papillon-Lefevre syndrome
Congenital ichthyosis
Hereditary metabolic defects:
Acrodermatitis enteropathica
Transcobalamin 2 deficiency
Type 1 hereditary orotic aciduria
Intractable diarrhea, abnormal facies, trichorrhexis and immunodeficiency
Methylmalonic acidemia
Biotin dependent carboxylase deficiency
Mannosidosis
Glycogen storage disease, type 1b
Chediak-Higashi syndrome
Hypercatabolism of immunoglobulin:
Familial hypercatabolism
Intestinal lymphangiectasia
Other:
Chronic muco-cutaneous candidiasis
Hereditary or congenital hyposplenia or asplenia
Ivermark syndrome

The syndrome has been associated with a diversity of defects in development of immunocompetent cells, which are caused by mutations in genes whose products are necessary for the normal differentiation of T, B, and, sometimes, NK cells.

In one autosomal recessive form of SCID characterized by severe lymphopenia, the failure in T and B cell development is due to *mutations in the RAG-1 or RAG-2 genes*, the combined activities of which are needed for V(D)J recombination. A function-loss *mutation in the DNA-dependent tyrosine kinase gene* in SCID mice may prove to be a cause for SCID in humans as well, since this is another essential enzyme in the V(D)J gene rearrangement process. About half of patients with autosomal recessive SCID are deficient in an enzyme involved in purine metabolism, adenosine deaminase (ADA), due to *mutations in the ADA gene*. The abortive lymphoid differentiation associated with ADA deficiency is due to intracellular accumulation of adenosine and deoxyadenosine nucleotides that interferes with critical metabolic functions, including DNA synthesis.

SCID also may occur with an X-linked inheritance pattern. Aborted thymocyte differentiation and an absence of peripheral T cells and NK cells is seen in *X-linked* SCID. B lymphocytes are present in normal numbers but are functionally defective. The defective gene encodes a common γ chain of the receptors for IL-2, -4, -7, -9, and -15, thus disrupting the action of this important set of lymphokines.

The same T⁻NK⁻B⁺ SCID phenotype seen in X-linked SCID can be inherited as an autosomal recessive disease due to mutations in the gene for *JAK3 protein kinase deficiency*. This enzyme associates with the common γ chain of the receptors for IL-2, -4, -7, -9, and -15 to serve as a key element in their signal transduction pathways.

℞ **TREATMENT** The cellular defects in SCID patients logically rest with the pluripotent hematopoietic stem cells or their lymphoid progenitor progeny. Accordingly, the immunological deficits in all of the different types of SCID patients have been repaired by transplantation of histocompatible bone marrow as a source of stem cells, thereby implying that the stromal microenvironments of these individuals are intact and capable of supporting T and B cell development. However, antibody deficiency requiring immunoglobulin replacement therapy may persist for years in the γc deficient and JAK3 deficient patients, unless the defective B cells are eliminated prior to bone marrow transplantation to allow their replacement with normal B cells of donor origin. In ADA-deficient patients without histocompatible bone marrow donors, the administration of exogenous ADA (conjugated to polyethylene glycol to prolong its half-life) may improve immunological function and clinical status. ADA gene therapy has also been used with limited success in these patients. Treatment of SCID patients should be performed in centers with a strong research interest in this problem. It is crucial that these patients be recognized early and not be given live viral vaccines or blood transfusions, which may cause fatal graft-versus-host disease.

Primary T Cell Immunodeficiency Reflecting the diversity of T cell functions, abnormalities of T cell development may be responsible for a wide spectrum of immune deficiencies, including combined immunodeficiency, selective defects in cell-mediated immunity, and syndromes presenting as antibody deficiency. These defects may be acquired (Chap. 309) as well as congenital.

DiGeorge's syndrome This classic example of isolated T cell deficiency results from maldevelopment of thymic epithelial elements derived from the third and fourth pharyngeal pouches. The gene defect has been mapped to chromosome 22q11 in most patients with DiGeorge's syndrome, and to chromosome 10p in others. Defective development of organs dependent on cells of embryonic neural crest origin includes: congenital cardiac defects, particularly those involving the great vessels; hypocalcemic tetany, due to failure of parathyroid

development; and absence of a normal thymus. Facial abnormalities may include abnormal ears, shortened philtrum, micrognathia, and hypertelorism. Serum immunoglobulin concentrations are frequently normal, but antibody responses, particularly of IgG and IgA isotypes, are usually impaired. T cell levels are reduced, whereas B cell levels are normal. Affected individuals usually have a small, histologically normal thymus located near the base of the tongue or in the neck, allowing most patients to develop functional T cells in numbers that may or may not be adequate for host defense.

The nude syndrome The human disease counterpart to the *nude* mouse is also caused by mutations of the *whn (winged-helix-nude)* gene that result in impairment of hair follicle and epithelial thymic development. The human *nude* phenotype is characterized by congenital baldness, nail dystrophy and severe T cell immunodeficiency.

T cell receptor deficiency Since the expression and function of antigen-specific T cell receptors (TCR) is dependent on their companion CD3γ, δ, ε, and ζ-η chains, defective genes for any of these receptor components can impair T cell development and function. Immunodeficiencies due to inherited CD3γ and CD3ε mutations have been identified. CD3γ mutations result in a selective deficit in CD8 T cells, whereas CD3ε mutations lead to a preferential reduction in CD4 T cells, thus implying differences in the signal transduction roles for each CD3 component.

Major histocompatibility complex (MHC) class II deficiency Because T cells are required for B cell responses to most antigens, any gene defect (or acquired disorder) that interferes with T cell development and cell-mediated immunity will also compromise antibody production and humoral immunity. MHC class II deficiency results in one such immunodeficiency in that the TCRαβ must see protein antigens as peptide fragments held within the α helical grooves of class II and class I molecules encoded by the MHC. Antigen-presenting cells in individuals with this relatively rare disorder fail to express the class II molecules DP, DQ, and DR on their surface. Limited numbers of helper CD4 T cells are therefore generated in the thymus, and they fail to see antigen in the periphery. Affected individuals experience recurrent bronchopulmonary infections, chronic diarrhea, and severe viral infections that usually prove fatal before 4 years of age. The defect is caused by mutations in genes that encode essential transcriptional factors that bind to promoter elements for the MHC class II genes. The class II transactivator gene is mutated in one subgroup of MHC class II deficient patients, whereas mutations in RFX genes encoding additional transcriptional factors for MHC class II genes are responsible for the defective development and function of CD4 T cells in other families: RFXANK in subgroup B, RFX5 in subgroup C, and RFXAP in subgroup D.

Zap70 tyrosine kinase deficiency Recurrent and opportunistic infections begin within the first year of life in individuals with a deficiency in ZAP70 tyrosine kinase, a pivotal component in the TCR/ CD3 signal transduction cascade. The rare inheritance of mutations in both alleles of the ZAP70 gene results in a selective deficiency of CD8 T cells and dysfunction of CD4 T cells, which are present in normal numbers. Severe immunodeficiency is the inevitable consequence.

Purine nucleoside phosphorylation deficiency Function-loss mutations of the purine nucleoside phosphorylase (PNP) gene are associated with an often severe and selective deficiency of T lymphocyte function. This enzyme functions in the same purine salvage pathway as ADA; toxic effects of the PNP deficiency may result from the intracellular accumulation of deoxyguanosine triphosphate.

Ataxia-telangiectasia Ataxia-telangiectasia (AT) is an autosomal recessive genetic disorder characterized by cerebellar ataxia, oculocutaneous telangiectasia, and immunodeficiency. The mutant ATM gene has sequence similarity to the phosphatidyl-inositol-3 kinases that are involved in signal transduction. The ATM gene belongs to a conserved family of genes that monitor DNA repair and coordinate DNA synthesis with cell division. The deleterious effects of the ATM gene are widespread. Truncal ataxia may become evident when walking begins and is progressive. Telangiectasia, primarily represented by dilated blood vessels in the ocular sclera, a butterfly area of the face and on the ears, is an early diagnostic feature. Immunodeficiency may be clinically manifest by recurrent and chronic sinopulmonary infection leading to bronchiectasis, although not all patients have overt immunodeficiency. Ovarian agenesis is a frequent occurrence. Persistence of very high serum levels of oncofetal proteins, including α fetoprotein and carcinoembryonic antigen, may be of diagnostic value. Frequent causes of death are chronic pulmonary disease and malignancy. Lymphomas are most common, although carcinomas also have occurred.

The immunologic abnormalities seem to be related to maldevelopment of the thymus. The markedly hypoplastic thymus is similar in appearance to an embryonic thymus. The peripheral T cell pool is reduced in size, especially in lymphoid tissue compartments. Cutaneous anergy and delayed rejection of skin grafts are common. Although B lymphocyte development is normal, most patients are deficient in serum IgE and IgA, and a smaller number have reduced serum levels of IgG, particularly of the IgG2, IgG4 subclasses.

The defect in DNA repair mechanisms in these patients renders their cells highly susceptible to radiation-induced chromosomal damage and resultant tumor development. AT is a rare disorder, one in 10,000 to 100,000 incidence, but 1% of the population is heterozygous for an AT mutation. This is important because the heterozygous state also predisposes to enhanced cellular radiosensitivity and cancer, especially breast cancer in females (Chap. 364).

℞ TREATMENT Therapeutic options other than symptomatic treatment are limited for this group of patients. Live vaccines and blood transfusions containing viable T cells should be assiduously avoided. Exposure to X-irradiation should also be avoided in patients with AT. Therapeutic intervention in the form of an epithelial thymic transplant should repair the T cell deficiency in patients with the *nude* syndrome and in the most severe cases of DiGeorge's syndrome where T cells are absent. Preventive therapy for *P. carinii* in the form of trimethoprim-sulfamethoxazole should be considered. Immunoglobulin infusions are also recommended for those T cell deficient individuals with severe antibody deficiency reflected by low serum levels of IgG.

Immunoglobulin Deficiency Syndromes • *X-LINKED AGAMMA-GLOBULINEMIA* Males with this syndrome often begin to have recurrent bacterial infections late in the first year of life, when maternally derived immunoglobulins have disappeared. Although B cell progenitors are found in the bone marrow, affected individuals have very few immunoglobulin-bearing B lymphocytes in their circulation and lack primary and secondary lymphoid follicles. The developmental block is evident at the pre-B cell level (Fig. 308-1). Mutations of Bruton's tyrosine kinase (Btk) gene are responsible for X-linked agammaglobulinemia. B cells in heterozygous female carriers exclusively utilize the X chromosome with the normal Btk gene, while T cells and myeloid cells express either X chromosome. *X-linked agammaglobulinemia with growth hormone deficiency* is a rare variant disorder caused by another gene defect that maps to the same region of the X chromosome.

Agammaglobulinemia is a misnomer, since most of these patients synthesize some immunoglobulins. Within the same family, some affected males may have substantial levels of IgM, IgG, and IgA, while others are nearly agammaglobulinemic. Btk-deficient patients typically are very deficient in circulating B lymphocytes. The few B lymphocytes that escape the block in pre-B cell differentiation are impaired in their responsiveness to antigenic stimulation, making antibody replacement therapy essential in these patients.

Sinopulmonary bacterial infections constitute the most frequent clinical problem. Mycoplasma infections also cause arthritis in some

of these patients. Chronic encephalitis of viral etiology, sometimes associated wtih dermatomyositis, can be a fatal complication. These complications are reduced by treatment with intravenous immunoglobulin.

Autosomal recessive agammaglobulinemia This syndrome can result from mutations in a variety of genes whose products are required for B lineage differentiation. For example, signals induced via pre-B receptors are essential for pre-B cell development. Consequently, mutations in any of the genes coding pre-B receptor components—μ heavy chains, surrogate light chains (VpreB and λ5/14.1), Igα and Igβ—can block B lineage differentiation. Congenital absence of B cells, agammaglobulinemia and recurrent bacterial infections have been seen in children with function-loss mutations in both alleles of the μ heavy chain gene or the λ5/14.1 surrogate light chain gene. Disruption of B cell development may also occur as a consequence of mutations in genes coding transcription factors for pre-B receptor genes or for key elements in the pre-B receptor signaling pathway.

Transient hypogammaglobulinemia of infancy This diagnosis is reserved for those rare instances in which normal physiologic hypogammaglobulinemia of infancy is unusually prolonged and severe. IgG levels normally drop to 3.0 to 4.0 g/L between 3 and 6 months of age as maternally derived IgG is catabolized. The IgG levels subsequently rise, reflecting the infants' increased synthetic capacity. Periodic immunologic assessment is needed to differentiate transient hypogammaglobulinemia from other forms of antibody deficiency. Antibody replacement therapy is recommended only in the face of severe or recurrent infections.

IgA deficiency An inability to produce antibodies of the IgA1 and IgA2 subclasses occurs in approximately 1 in 600 individuals of European origin, a much higher incidence than is seen for other primary immunodeficiencies. IgA deficiency is much less common in people of Asian and African origin. In Japan, for example, the incidence is approximately 1 in 18,500. While the precise genetic basis for this difference in incidence is unknown, IgA deficiency is frequently associated with certain MHC haplotypes that are more common in Caucasians.

Individuals with isolated IgA deficiency may appear healthy or present with an increased number of respiratory infections of varying severity, and a few have progressive pulmonary disease leading to bronchiectasis. Chronic diarrheal diseases also occur. Reductions in the IgG2 and IgG4 subclasses are associated with the increased infections in some IgA-deficient individuals. The incidence of asthma and other atopic diseases among IgA-deficient patients is high. Conversely, the incidence of IgA deficiency among atopic children has been found to be more than 20 times that in the normal population. IgA deficiency is also significantly associated with arthritis (Chap. 312) and systemic lupus erythematosus (Chap. 311). IgA-deficient patients frequently produce autoantibodies. Some of them develop significant levels of antibodies to IgA, which may render them vulnerable to severe anaphylactic reactions when transfused with normal blood or blood products.

An accurate picture of the clinical consequences of IgA deficiency requires lifelong study of affected individuals. Among 204 healthy young adults whose IgA deficiency was identified when they served as blood donors, 80% were found to experience episodes of infections, drug allergy, autoimmune disorders, or atopic disease during the next 20 years of their life. They had an increased susceptibility to pneumonia, recurrent episodes of respiratory infections, and a higher incidence of autoimmune diseases, including vitiligo, autoimmune thyroiditis, and possibly rheumatoid arthritis.

IgA deficiency is often familial. It can also occur in association with congenital intrauterine infections, such as toxoplasmosis, rubella, and cytomegalovirus infection, or following treatment with phenytoin, penicillamine, or other medications in genetically susceptible individuals. The pathogenesis of IgA deficiency, whether genetic or triggered by environmental insult, involves a block in B cell differentiation that may reflect defective interaction between T and B cells.

Treatment of IgA deficiency is essentially symptomatic. IgA cannot be effectively replaced by exogenous immunoglobulin or plasma, and use of either can increase the risk of development of antibodies to IgA. IgA-deficient patients in need of transfusion should be screened for the presence of antibodies to IgA and ideally should be given blood only from IgA-deficient donors. Immunoglobulin infusions may benefit the exceptional IgA deficient person in whom IgG2 and IgG4 subclass deficiencies are associated with severe infections, but the risk of anaphylactic reactions to contaminating IgA must always be considered in treating these patients.

IgG subclass deficiencies   Selective deficiencies in one or more of the four IgG subclasses are seen in some patients with repeated infections. The IgG subclass deficiency may easily go undetected when the total serum IgG level is measured, because IgG2, IgG3, and IgG4 together account for only 30 to 40% of the IgG antibodies. Even a deficiency in IgG1 may be masked by increases in the remaining IgG isotypes. However, the availability of subclass-specific monoclonal antibodies allows precise measurement of IgG subclass levels.

Homozygous deletions of genes encoding the constant region of the different γ chains is the basis for the IgG subclass deficiency in some individuals. For example, deletion of the $C_{\alpha1}$, $C_{\gamma2}$, $C_{\gamma4}$, and C_{ϵ} genes in the heavy chain locus on both chromosomes 14 was responsible for one individual's inability to make IgA1, IgG2, IgG4, and IgE. Because other components of their immune system are intact, individuals with this and other patterns of C_H-gene deletions may not have unusual infections.

Most of the IgG subclass–deficient individuals with repeated infections appear to have regulatory defects that prevent normal B cell differentiation. The defect may extend to other isotypes. IgA deficiency may accompany IgG2 and IgG4 subclass deficiencies (see "IgA Deficiency" above); an inability to produce IgM antibodies to polysaccharide antigens often reflects a broader defect in antibody responsiveness. While patients with IgG subclass deficiency may benefit from administration of immunoglobulin, a thorough assessment of humoral immunity is needed to identify the relatively few who need this therapy.

Common variable immunodeficiency   This diagnostic category includes a heterogeneous group of males and females, mostly adults, who have in common the clinical manifestations of deficient production of all the different classes of antibodies. The majority of these hypogammaglobulinemic patients have normal numbers of B lymphocytes that are clonally diverse but phenotypically immature. B lymphocytes in these patients are able to recognize antigens and can proliferate in response, but they largely fail to become mature plasma cells. This abortive differentiation pattern leads to the frequent occurrence of nodular B lymphocyte hyperplasia, resulting in splenomegaly and intestinal lymphoid hyperplasia, sometimes of massive proportion.

It is important to note that common variable immunodeficiency and IgA deficiency represent polar ends of a clinical spectrum due to the same underlying gene defect in a large subset of these patients. The two disorders feature similar B cell differentiation arrests, differing only in the numbers of immunoglobulin classes involved. Over a period of years, IgA deficient patients may progress to the pan-hypogammaglobulinemia phenotype characteristic of common variable immunodeficiency, and vice versa. Both disorders occur frequently within the same family, and the same MHC haplotypes are associated with both immunodeficiency patterns. Family studies suggest an underlying susceptibility gene in the MHC class III region for both disorders.

It is important to consider the diagnosis of common variable immunodeficiency in adults with chronic pulmonary infections, some of whom will present with bronchiectasis. Intestinal diseases—including chronic giardiasis, intestinal malabsorption, and atrophic gastritis with pernicious anemia—are common in this group of patients. Patients with common variable immunodeficiency also may present with signs and symptoms highly suggestive of lymphoid malignancy, including fever, weight loss, anemia, thrombocytopenia, splenomegaly, generalized lymphadenopathy, and lymphocytosis. Histologic examination of lymphoid tissues usually reveals germinal center hyperplasia which may be difficult to distinguish from nodular lymphoma (Chap. 112). Demonstration of a normal distribution of immunoglobulin isotypes and light chain classes for circulating and tissue B lymphocytes can serve to distinguish these patients from those having a monoclonal B cell malignancy with secondary hypogammaglobulinemia. The administration of intravenous immunoglobulin in adequate doses (see below) is an essential part of the prevention and treatment of all these complications.

X-linked immunodeficiency with hyper IgM   In this syndrome, typically the IgG and IgA levels are very low, while IgM levels may be very high, normal, or even low. The development of B lymphocytes bearing IgM and IgD and the absence of IgG and IgA B lymphocytes indicate a defect in isotype switching. The defective gene in these patients encodes a transiently expressed molecule on activated T cells that is the ligand for the CD40 molecule on dendritic cells (DC) and B cells. Gene mutations that preclude normal CD40 ligand expression prevent normal T and B cell cooperation, germinal center formation, V-region diversification by somatic hypermutation, and isotype switching. T cell responses are also compromised in these CD40 ligand deficient patients because their T cells are deprived of an important feedback stimulus as a consequence of the defective T, DC, B cell interactions (Chap. 305). Consequently, these patients experience more severe infections than those occurring with other hypogammaglobulinemic states. In addition to recurrent bacterial infections, pneumonia may be caused by *P. carinii*, cytomegalovirus, *Aspergillus*, *Cryptosporidium*, and other unusual organisms. Enteritis due to cryptosporidial infection may extend into the biliary tract to result in a sclerosing cholangitis and hepatic cirrhosis. Neutropenia is frequent in affected males and increases their vulnerability to infections.

Immunodeficiency with hyper IgM is also seen in patients of both sexes who lack mutations in their CD40 ligand gene. While the phenotype in the non-X-linked form of immunodeficiency with hyper IgM is similar, the clinical course is usually milder than in CD40 ligand deficient patients. Candidate disease genes in this syndrome include the CD40 gene and genes coding signaling elements in the CD40 signaling pathway.

TREATMENT   Replacement therapy with human immunoglobulin is the therapeutic cornerstone for antibody-deficient patients who have recurrent infections and who are deficient in IgG. Maintenance of serum IgG levels above 5.0 g/L will prevent most systemic infections in the patients. These serum levels usually can be achieved by intravenous administration of immunoglobulin, 400 to 500 mg/kg, at 3- to 4-week intervals. In patients with mild to moderate IgG deficiency (3.0 to 5.0 g/L) or isolated IgG subclass deficiencies, the decision to treat should be based on evaluation of clinical symptoms and antibody responses to antigenic challenge. Since immunoglobulin preparations are comprised almost entirely of IgG antibodies, they are of no value for repairing deficiencies of immunoglobulins other than IgG. Infusions of immunoglobulin are also not benign. While HIV transmission has not been reported, previous epidemics of hepatitis C virus infections in hypogammaglobulinemic patients receiving contaminated immunoglobulin preparations have led to improved safety measures for current commercial preparations. Some antibody-deficient patients develop symptoms of diaphoresis, tachycardia, flank pain, and hypotension during immunoglobulin infusion. This reaction may be mediated by aggregates of IgG or other biologically active substances and often is resolved by slowing the rate of immunoglobulin infusion. More serious anaphylactic reactions may occur as a consequence of antibodies produced by the patient against donor immunoglobulins, particularly IgA (Chap. 114). The potential for severe adverse reactions merits administration of the initial immunoglobulin infusion under medical supervision in a hospital or clinic setting.

A heightened index of suspicion of infection is essential for antibody-deficient patients. Identification of infectious agents in order to select appropriate antibiotic, antiparasitic, or antiviral therapy is also very important. Immunoglobulin infusions usually do not suffice to eliminate chronic sinopulmonary infections with *H. influenzae* and other microorganisms, and a prolonged course of antibiotic therapy may be required to effectively treat these infections and prevent progression to pulmonary fibrosis and bronchiectasis. Maintenance of good pulmonary toilet with regular postural drainage can also be especially important in management of these patients. Infestation with *G. lamblia*, a common cause of chronic diarrhea in antibody deficient patients, usually responds to therapy with metronidazole.

Cryptosporidial infections in CD40 ligand deficient patients may respond to long-term treatment with amphotericin B and flucytosine. The neutropenia frequently associated with infections in these patients may or may not resolve with improvement of infections and antibody replacement therapy. Bone marrow transplantation following myeloablative pretransplantation therapy can be curative for boys with this devastating immunodeficiency. This treatment has a much greater chance of success when performed during childhood.

Miscellaneous Immunodeficiency Syndromes   Infection with *Candida albicans* is the almost universal accompaniment of severe deficiencies in cell-mediated immunity. *Chronic mucocutaneous candidiasis* is different because superficial candidiasis is usually the only major manifestation of immunodeficiency in this syndrome. These patients rarely develop systemic infection with *Candida* or other fungal agents and are not unusually susceptible to virus or bacterial disease. No uniformity of immunologic defects has been identified in these patients, although defects of antibody formation have been detected occasionally. Humoral immunity, including ability to make specific anti-*Candida* antibodies, is usually normal. Many patients are anergic, some to a variety of antigens and some only to *Candida*. The syndrome is often congenital and may be associated with single or multiple endocrinopathies as well as iron deficiency. Treatment of associated conditions may lead to improvement or even cure of *Candida* infection. In other patients, intensive treatment with amphotericin B coupled with surgical removal of infected nails has led to sustained improvement. Oral antifungal agents, such as fluconazole and itraconazole, also may be effective.

Interferon γ receptor deficiency   This immunodeficiency is characterized by serious infections caused by bacille Calmette-Guerin vaccine and environmental non-tuberculous mycobacteria. Associated salmonella infections occur in a minority of the cases. This syndrome can be caused by mutations in the interferon γ receptor signal-transducing chain (IFNGR2). Two additional forms of this syndrome are caused by different types of mutations in the interferon γ receptor 1 (IFNGR1) gene that encodes the ligand binding chain of the interferon γ receptor. Null mutations in both IFNGR1 alleles are responsible for a more severe autosomal recessive form. A less severe form, inherited in an autosomal dominant pattern, is caused by IFNGR1 mutations in a small deletional hotspot that result in a truncated receptor chain lacking the cytoplasmic tail. Accumulation of the truncated receptor on the surface of macrophages compromises their response to interferon γ and the killing of ingested mycobacterium.

Interleukin 12 receptor deficiency   Mutations in the gene coding the β_1 subunit of the IL-12 receptor can cause this syndrome. Affected patients suffer from disseminated mycobacterial infections attributable to bacille Calmette-Guerin and nontuberculous mycobacteria, and in some cases non-typhi salmonella infections. Although the clinical manifestations are usually less severe than in patients with complete IFNGR1 deficiency, IL-12 receptor deficiency may predispose individuals to clinical tuberculosis as well. Deficient interferon γ production by the otherwise normal NK and T cells is seen in IL-12 receptor deficient patients, and therapeutic use of interferon γ may cure their mycobacterial infection.

Immunodeficiency with thymoma   The association of hypogammaglobulinemia with spindle cell thymoma usually occurs relatively late in adult life. Bacterial infections and severe diarrhea often reflect the antibody deficiency, whereas fungal and viral infections are infrequent complications. T cell numbers and cell-mediated immunity are usually intact, but these patients are very deficient in circulating B lymphocytes and pre-B cells in the bone marrow. They also frequently have eosinopenia and may develop erythroid aplasia. Complete bone marrow failure sometimes occurs. The relationship between the thymoma and apparent abnormalities of hematopoietic stem cells remains conjectural, and treatment is limited to immunoglobulin administration and symptomatic therapy.

Wiskott-Aldrich syndrome   This X-linked disease characterized by eczema, thrombocytopenia, and repeated infections, is caused by mutations in the WASP gene. The WASP protein is expressed in cells of all hematopoietic lineages. It may serve a cytoskeletal organizing role for signaling elements that are particularly important in platelets and T cells. The platelets are small and have a shortened half-life. Affected male infants often present with bleeding, and most do not survive childhood, dying of complications of bleeding, infection, or lymphoreticular malignancy. The immunologic defects include low serum concentrations of IgM, while IgA and IgG are normal and IgE is frequently increased. The number and class distribution of B lymphocytes are usually normal. Functionally, these patients are unable to make antibodies to polysaccharide antigens normally; responses to protein antigens may also be impaired late in the course of the disease. Most patients eventually acquire T cell deficiencies. Affected boys frequently become anergic, and their T cells do not respond normally to antigenic challenge. This results in vulnerability to overwhelming infections with herpes simplex virus and other infectious agents.

Transplantation of histocompatible bone marrow from a sibling donor following myeloablative therapy can correct both the hematologic and immunologic abnormalities. In patients lacking a suitable donor, intravenous immunoglobulin infusions or splenectomy may improve platelet counts and reduce the risk of serious hemorrhage. Because of the increased risk of pneumococcal bacteremia, splenectomized patients should receive prophylactic penicillin.

X-linked lymphoproliferative syndrome   This disease involves a selective impairment in immune elimination of Epstein-Barr virus (EBV). A fulminant and fatal outcome is the consequence of EBV infection in approximately half of the affected males. Hypogammaglobulinemia is the outcome in 30%, and B cell malignancies are acquired in approximately 25% of EBV-infected patients. The disease may be manifested from early childhood onward, depending on the time of EBV infection. Carrier females handle EBV infections normally. Generation of cytotoxic T cells appears to be the primary mechanism of control of EBV infection in normal persons. In males with the X-linked lymphoproliferative syndrome, this process is impaired as a consequence of mutations in a gene coding for a T cell signaling element called SH2D1A or SAP. Intravenous immunoglobulins should be administered to affected males who develop hypogammaglobulinemia. Bone marrow transplantation from an HLA-matched donor may be curative, especially in younger children with this syndrome. However, myeloablative chemotherapy is a necessary prerequisite to successful bone marrow transplantation, thereby increasing the risk of this procedure.

Hyper-IgE syndrome   The hyper IgE syndrome (Chap. 64) is characterized by recurrent abscesses involving skin, lungs, and other organs and very high IgE levels. IgE levels may decline with time to reach normal levels in approximately 20% of affected adults. Staphylococcal infection is common to all patients, but most have infections with other pyogenic organisms as well. Abnormal neutrophil chemotaxis is an inconsistent finding, and diminished antibody responses to secondary immunization have been noted. Non-immunologic features include impaired shedding of the primary teeth, recurrent bone fractures, hyperextensible joints and scoliosis. Males and females are affected in an inheritance pattern suggesting an autosomal dominant defect with variable penetrance, but the gene defect has not been identified. Prophylaxis with penicillinase-resistant penicillins or cephalosporins is highly recommended to prevent staphylococcal infections. Pneumatoceles, a frequent complication of pneumonias, may require surgical excision.

Metabolic Abnormalities Associated with Immunodeficiency The relation of deficiencies of the purine salvage enzymes adenosine deaminase and purine nucleoside phosphorylase to immunodeficiency was discussed earlier. The syndrome of *acrodermatitis enteropathica* includes severe desquamating skin lesions, intractable diarrhea, bizarre neurologic symptoms, variable combined immunodeficiency, and an often fatal outcome. This disease is apparently caused by an inborn error of metabolism resulting in malabsorption of dietary zinc and can be treated effectively by parenteral or large oral doses of zinc. Zinc deficiency might in part account for the immunodeficiency that accompanies severe malnutrition. Inherited *deficiency of transcobalamin II*, the serum carrier molecule responsible for transport of vitamin B_{12} to tissues, is associated with failure of immunoglobulin production as well as megaloblastic anemia, leukopenia, thrombocytopenia, and severe malabsorption. All abnormalities of this rare disorder are reversed by administration of vitamin B_{12}.

CONCLUSION Defective genes have been identified for most of the primary immunodeficiency diseases that are currently recognized (Table 308-3). It can be anticipated that many different gene mutations will be identified in other individuals with increased susceptibility to infection. Identification of the mutant genes is the first step toward a better understanding of the pathogenesis of immunodeficiency disease and improved therapeutic strategies. Successful gene repair is the ultimate goal for these individuals.

ACKNOWLEDGMENT

This chapter represents a revised version of a chapter by Dr. Max D. Cooper and Dr. Alexander R. Lawton III that has appeared in previous editions of this textbook.

BIBLIOGRAPHY

BUCKLEY RH et al: Hematopoietic stem-cell transplantation for the treatment of severe combined immunodeficiency. N Engl J Med 340:508, 1999

BURROWS PD, COOPER MD: IgA deficiency. Adv Immunol 65:245, 1997

CANDOTTI F, BLAESE RM: Gene therapy of primary immunodeficiencies. Springer Semin Immunopathol 19:493, 1998

CHAPEL HM: Safety and availability of immunoglobulin replacement therapy in relation to potentially transmissable agents. Clin Exp Immunol 118(Suppl 1):29, 1999

DICKLER HB, GELFAND EW: Current perspectives on the use of intravenous immunoglobulin. Adv Int Med 41:641, 1996

FISCHER A, MALISSEN B: Natural and engineered disorders of lymphocyte development. Science 280:237, 1998

GREWAL IS, FLAVELL RA: CD40 and CD154 in cell-mediated immunity. Ann Rev Immunol 16:111, 1998

JOUANGUY E et al: A human IFNGR1 small deletion hotspot associated with dominant susceptibility to mycobacterial infection. Nat Genet 21:370, 1999

KOSKINEN S: Long-term follow-up of health in blood donors with primary selective IgA deficiency. J Clin Immunol 16:165, 1996

MASTERNAK K et al: A gene encoding a novel RFX-associated transactivator is mutated in the majority of MHC class II deficiency patients. Nat Genet 20:273, 1998

OCHS HD et al: *Primary Immunodeficiency Diseases.* New York, Oxford Univ Press, 1999

ROSEN FS et al: Primary immunodeficiency diseases. Report of a WHO Scientific Group. Clin Exp Immunol 109(Suppl 1):1, 1997

SAYOS J et al: The X-linked lymphoproliferative-disease gene product SAP regulated signals induced through the co-receptor SLAM. Nature 395:462, 1998

SCHROEDER HW JR et al: Susceptibility locus for IgA deficiency and Common Variable Immunodeficiency in the HLA-DR3, -B8, -A1 Haplotype. Mol Med 4:72, 1998

Table 308-3 Genes or Genetic Loci Associated with Primary Immunodeficiencies

Disorder	Gene or Locus	Chromosome
Severe combined immunodeficiency (SCID):		
Recombinase activating gene deficiency	RAG1, RAG2	11p13
Adenosine deaminase deficiency	ADA	20q13.11
Interleukin receptor γ chain deficiency	IL2RG	Xq13
Janus-associated kinase 3 deficiency	JAK3	19p13.1
DNA-dependent protein kinase deficiency	PRKDC	8q11
Primary T cell immunodeficiency:		
DiGeorge syndrome	DGCR1	22q11
	DGCR2	10q13
Nude syndrome	WHN	17q11-q12
T cell receptor deficiency:		
CD3γ	CD3G	7q35
CD3ε	CD3E	11q23
MHC class II deficiency:		
MHC class II transactivator (group A)	CIITA	16p13
Regulatory factor X, ankyrin-repeat containing (group B)	RFXANK	19p12
Regulatory factor X, 5 (group C)	RFX5	1q21.1-q21.3
Regulatory factor X-associated protein (group D)	RFXAP	13q14
Transporter, ATP-binding cassette, major histocompatibility complex, 2 deficiency	TAP2	6p21.3
Zeta-chain-associated protein kinase deficiency	ZAP70	2q12
Purine nucleotide phosphorylase deficiency	NP	14q13.1
Predominantly antibody deficiencies:		
X-linked agammaglobulinemia	BTK	Xq21.3-q22
Ig heavy chain deletions	IGHG1	14q32.33
Surrogate light chain deficiency	IGLL5	22q11.21
X-linked hyper-IgM syndrome	HIGM1	Xq26
IgA deficiency/common variable immunodeficiency	MHC class III	6p21.3
Other well-defined immunodeficiency syndromes:		
Interferon γ receptor deficiency	IFNGR1	6q23-q24
	IFNGR2	21q22.1-22.2
Interleukin 12 deficiency	IL12B	5q31-q33
Interleukin 12 receptor deficiency	IL12RB1	19p13.1
Wiskott-Aldrich syndrome	WAS	Xp11.23-p11.22
Ataxia telangiectasia	ATM	11q22.3
X-linked lymphoproliferative syndrome	SH2D1A/SAP	Xq25

309   *Anthony S. Fauci, H. Clifford Lane*

HUMAN IMMUNODEFICIENCY VIRUS (HIV) DISEASE: AIDS AND RELATED DISORDERS

ADCC antibody-dependent cellular cytotoxicity	LIP lymphoid interstitial pneumonitis
CDC Centers for Disease Control and Prevention	MAC *M. avium* complex
	MHC major histocompatibility complex
CIDP chronic inflammatory demyelinating polyneuropathy	MIP macrophage inflammatory protein
CMV cytomegalovirus	MMSE Mini-Mental Status Examination
CNS central nervous system	
CRFs circulating recombinant forms	MRI magnetic resonance imaging
CSF cerebrospinal fluid	NK natural killer
CT computed tomography	NIP nonspecific interstitial pneumonitis
CTLs cytolytic T lymphocytes	
EBV Epstein-Barr virus	PCP *P. carinii* pneumonia
EIA enzyme immunoassay	PCR polymerase chain reaction
ELISA enzyme-linked immunosorbent assay	PML progressive multifocal leukoencephalopathy
FDA Food & Drug Administration	PPD purified protein derivative
FDCs follicular dendritic cells	RT-PCR reverse transcriptase PCR
GM-CSF granulocyte-macrophage colony stimulating factor	SDF stromal cell–derived factor
	SIADH syndrome of inappropriate antidiuretic hormone (vasopressin) secretion
HAART highly active antiretroviral therapy	
HBV hepatitis B virus	SIV simian immunodeficiency virus
HCV hepatitis C virus	STD sexually transmitted disease
HHV human herpesvirus	TAP transporter associated with antigen-presenting
HSV herpes simplex virus	
HTLV human T lymphotropic viruses	TB tuberculosis
ICL idiopathic CD4+ lymphocytopenia	TGF transforming growth factor
	TMP/SMZ trimethoprim/sulfamethoxazole
IDUs injection drug users	
IFN interferon	TNF tumor necrosis factor
IL interleukin	VDRL Venereal Disease Research Laboratory
KS Kaposi's sarcoma	
KSHV Kaposi's sarcoma–associated herpesvirus	WBC white blood cell count

AIDS was first recognized in the United States in the summer of 1981, when the U.S. Centers for Disease Control and Prevention (CDC) reported the unexplained occurrence of *Pneumocystis carinii* pneumonia in five previously healthy homosexual men in Los Angeles and of Kaposi's sarcoma (KS) in 26 previously healthy homosexual men in New York and Los Angeles. Within months, the disease became recognized in male and female injection drug users (IDUs) and soon thereafter in recipients of blood transfusions and in hemophiliacs. As the epidemiologic pattern of the disease unfolded, it became clear that a microbe transmissible by sexual (homosexual and heterosexual) contact and blood or blood products was the most likely etiologic agent of the epidemic.

In 1983, HIV was isolated from a patient with lymphadenopathy, and by 1984 it was demonstrated clearly to be the causative agent of AIDS. In 1985, a sensitive enzyme-linked immunosorbent assay (ELISA) was developed, which led to an appreciation of the scope of

Table 309-1 1993 Revised Classification System for HIV Infection and Expanded AIDS Surveillance Case Definition for Adolescents and Adults[a]

	Clinical Categories		
CD4+ T Cell Categories	A Asymptomatic, Acute (Primary) HIV or PGL[b]	B Symptomatic, Not A or C Conditions	C AIDS-Indicator Conditions
>500/μL	A1	B1	C1
200–499/μL	A2	B2	C2
<200/μL	A3	B3	C3

[a] The shaded areas indicate the expanded AIDS surveillance case definition.
[b] PGL, progressive generalized lymphadenopathy.
SOURCE: MMWR 42(No. RR-17), December 18, 1992.

HIV infection among cohorts of individuals in the United States who admitted to practicing high-risk behavior (see below) as well as among selected populations that had been screened, such as blood donors, military recruits and active-duty military personnel, Job Corps applicants, and patients in selected sentinel hospitals. In addition, seroprevalance studies revealed the enormity of the global pandemic, particularly in developing countries (see below).

The staggering worldwide growth of the HIV pandemic has been matched by an explosion of information in the areas of HIV virology, the pathogenesis (both immunologic and virologic) and treatment of HIV disease, the treatment and prophylaxis of the opportunistic diseases associated with HIV infection, and vaccine development. The information flow related to HIV disease is enormous, and it has become almost impossible for the health care generalist to stay abreast of the literature. The purpose of this chapter is to present the most current information available on the scope of the epidemic; on its pathogenesis, treatment, and prevention; and on prospects for vaccine development. Above all, the aim is to provide a solid scientific basis and practical guidelines for a state-of-the-art approach to the HIV-infected patient.

DEFINITION With the identification of HIV in 1983 and its proof as the etiologic agent of AIDS in 1984, and with the availability of sensitive and specific diagnostic tests for HIV infection, the case definition of AIDS has undergone several revisions over the years. The latest revision took place in 1993; this revised CDC classification system for HIV-infected adolescents and adults categorizes persons on the basis of clinical conditions associated with HIV infection and CD4+ T lymphocyte counts. The system is based on three ranges of CD4+ T lymphocyte counts and three clinical categories and is represented by a matrix of nine mutually exclusive categories (Tables 309-1 and 309-2). Using this system, any HIV-infected individual with a CD4+ T cell count of <200/μL has AIDS by definition, regardless of the presence of symptoms or opportunistic diseases (Table 309-1). The clinical conditions in clinical category C now include pulmonary tuberculosis (TB), recurrent pneumonia, and invasive cervical cancer (Table 309-2). Once individuals have had a clinical condition in category B, their disease cannot again be classified as category A, even if the condition resolves; the same holds true for category C in relation to category B.

While the definition of AIDS is complex and comprehensive, the clinician should not focus on whether AIDS is present but should view HIV disease as a spectrum ranging from primary infection, with or without the acute syndrome, to the asymptomatic stage, to advanced disease (see below). The definition of AIDS was established not for the practical care of patients but for surveillance purposes.

ETIOLOGIC AGENT

The etiologic agent of AIDS is HIV, which belongs to the family of human retroviruses (Retroviridae) and the subfamily of lentiviruses (Chap. 191). Nononcogenic lentiviruses cause disease in other animal species, including sheep, horses, goats, cattle, cats, and monkeys. The

Category A: Consists of one or more of the conditions listed below in an adolescent or adult (>13 years) with documented HIV infection. Conditions listed in categories B and C must not have occurred.

    Asymptomatic HIV infection

    Persistent generalized lymphadenopathy

    Acute (primary) HIV infection with accompanying illness or history of acute HIV infection

Category B: Consists of symptomatic conditions in an HIV-infected adolescent or adult that are not included among conditions listed in clinical category C and that meet at least one of the following criteria: (1) The conditions are attributed to HIV infection or are indicative of a defect in cell-mediated immunity; or (2) the conditions are considered by physicians to have a clinical course or to require management that is complicated by HIV infection. Examples include, but are not limited to, the following:

    Bacillary angiomatosis

    Candidiasis, oropharyngeal (thrush)

    Candidiasis, vulvovaginal; persistent, frequent, or poorly responsive to therapy

    Cervical dysplasia (moderate or severe)/cervical carcinoma in situ

    Constitutional symptoms, such as fever (38.5°C) or diarrhea lasting >1 month

    Hairy leukoplakia, oral

    Herpes zoster (shingles), involving at least two distinct episodes or more than one dermatome

    Idiopathic thrombocytopenic purpura

    Listeriosis

    Pelvic inflammatory disease, particularly if complicated by tuboovarian abscess

    Peripheral neuropathy

Category C: Conditions listed in the AIDS surveillance case definition.

    Candidiasis of bronchi, trachea, or lungs

    Candidiasis, esophageal

    Cervical cancer, invasive[a]

    Coccidioidomycosis, disseminated or extrapulmonary

    Cryptococcosis, extrapulmonary

    Cryptosporidiosis, chronic intestinal (>1 month's duration)

    Cytomegalovirus disease (other than liver, spleen, or nodes)

    Cytomegalovirus retinitis (with loss of vision)

    Encephalopathy, HIV-related

    Herpes simplex: chronic ulcer(s) (>1 month's duration); or bronchitis, pneumonia, or esophagitis

    Histoplasmosis, disseminated or extrapulmonary

    Isosporiasis, chronic intestinal (>1 month's duration)

    Kaposi's sarcoma

    Lymphoma, Burkitt's (or equivalent term)

    Lymphoma, primary, of brain

    Mycobacterium avium complex or *M. kansasii*, disseminated or extrapulmonary

    Mycobacterium tuberculosis, any site (pulmonary[a] or extrapulmonary)

    Mycobacterium, other species or unidentified species, disseminated or extrapulmonary

    Pneumocystis carinii pneumonia

    Pneumonia, recurrent[a]

    Progressive multifocal leukoencephalopathy

    Salmonella septicemia, recurrent

    Toxoplasmosis of brain

    Wasting syndrome due to HIV

---

[a] Added in the 1993 expansion of the AIDS surveillance case definition.
SOURCE: MMWR 42(No. RR-17), December 18, 1992.

---

four recognized human retroviruses belong to two distinct groups: the human T lymphotropic viruses (HTLV) I and HTLV-II, which are transforming retroviruses; and the human immunodeficiency viruses, HIV-1 and HIV-2, which are cytopathic viruses (Chap. 191). The most common cause of HIV disease throughout the world, and certainly in the United States, is HIV-1. HIV-1 comprises several subtypes with different geographic distributions (see below). HIV-2 was first identified in 1986 in West African patients and was originally confined to West Africa. However, a number of cases that can be traced to West Africa or to sexual contacts with West Africans have been identified throughout the world. HIV-2 is more closely related phylogenetically to the simian immunodeficiency virus (SIV) found in sooty mangabeys than it is to HIV-1. In 1999, it was demonstrated that HIV-1 infection in humans was zoonotic and had originated from the *Pan troglodytes troglodytes* species of chimpanzees in whom the virus had co-evolved over centuries. The taxonomic relationship among primate lentiviruses is shown in Fig. 309-1.

MORPHOLOGY OF HIV Electron microscopy shows that the HIV virion is an icosahedral structure (Fig. 309-2A) containing numerous external spikes formed by the two major envelope proteins, the external gp120 and the transmembrane gp41. The virion buds from the surface of the infected cell and incorporates a variety of host proteins, including major histocompatibility complex (MHC) class I and II antigens (Chap. 306), into its lipid bilayer. The structure of HIV-1 is schematically diagrammed in Fig. 309-2B (Chap. 191).

REPLICATION CYCLE OF HIV HIV is an RNA virus whose hallmark is the reverse transcription of its genomic RNA to DNA by the enzyme *reverse transcriptase*. The replication cycle of HIV begins with the high-affinity binding of the gp120 protein via a portion of its V1 region near the N terminus to its receptor on the host cell surface, the CD4 molecule (Fig. 309-3). The CD4 molecule is a 55-kDa protein found predominantly on a subset of T lymphocytes that are responsible for helper or inducer function in the immune system (Chap. 305). It is also expressed on the surface of monocytes/macrophages and dendritic/Langerhans cells. In order for HIV-1 to fuse to and enter its target cell, it must also bind to one of a group of co-receptors. The two major co-receptors for HIV-1 are CCR5 and CXCR4. Both receptors belong to the family of seven-transmembrane-domain G protein–coupled cellular receptors, and the use of one or the other or both receptors by the virus for entry into the cell is an important determinant of the cellular tropism of the virus (see below for details). Following binding, the conformation of the viral envelope changes dramatically, and fusion with the host cell membrane occurs in a coiled-spring fashion via the newly exposed gp41 molecule (Fig. 309-4); the HIV genomic RNA is uncoated and internalized into the target cell (Fig. 309-3). The reverse transcriptase enzyme, which is contained in the infecting virion, then catalyzes the reverse transcription of the genomic RNA into double-stranded DNA. The DNA translocates to the nucleus, where it is integrated randomly into the host cell chromosomes through the action of another virally encoded enzyme, *integrase*. This provirus may remain transcriptionally inactive (latent), or it may manifest varying levels of gene expression, up to active production of virus.

Cellular activation plays an important role in the life cycle of HIV and is critical to the pathogenesis of HIV disease (see below). Following initial binding and internalization of virions into the target cell, incompletely reverse-transcribed DNA intermediates are labile in quiescent cells and will not integrate efficiently into the host cell genome unless cellular activation occurs shortly after infection. Furthermore, some degree of activation of the host cell is required for the initiation of transcription of the integrated proviral DNA into either genomic RNA or mRNA. In this regard, activation of HIV expression from the latent state depends on the interaction of a number of cellular and viral factors. Following transcription, HIV mRNA is translated into proteins that undergo modification through glycosylation, myristylation, phosphorylation, and cleavage. The viral particle is formed by the assembly of HIV proteins, enzymes, and genomic RNA at the plasma membrane of the cells. Budding of the progeny virion occurs through the host cell membrane, where the core acquires its external envelope (Chap. 191). The virally encoded protease then catalyzes the cleavage of the gag-pol precursor to yield the mature virion. Each point in the life cycle of HIV is a real or potential target for therapeutic intervention (see below). Thus far, the reverse transcriptase and protease enzymes have proven to be susceptible to pharmacologic disruption (see below).

HIV GENOME Figure 309-5 illustrates the arrangement of the HIV genome schematically. Like other retroviruses, HIV-1 has genes that encode the structural proteins of the virus: *gag* encodes the proteins that form the core of the virion (including p24 antigen); *pol* encodes the enzymes responsible for reverse transcription and integra-

FIGURE 309-1 A phylogenetic tree, based on the complete genomes of primate immunodeficiency viruses. The scale at the bottom (0.10) indicates a 10% difference at the nucleotide level. *(Prepared by Brian Foley, PhD, of the HIV Sequence Database, Theoretical Biology and Biophysics Group, Los Alamos National Laboratory, from the complete genome alignment available at hiv-web.lanl.gov under the alignments section.)*

tion; and *env* encodes the envelope glycoproteins. However, HIV-1 is more complex than other retroviruses, particularly those of the nonprimate group, in that it also contains at least six other genes (*tat, rev, nef, vif, vpr,* and *vpu*), which code for proteins involved in the regulation of gene expression (Chap. 191). Several of these proteins are felt to play a role in the pathogenesis of HIV disease. For example, Tat, Nef, and Vpu have all been shown to downregulate MHC class I expression; this may be a strategy that the virus employs to evade immune-mediated elimination by CD8+ cytolytic T cells. Nef also downregulates cell surface expression of CD4 by inducing endocytosis and lysosomal degradation. Supernatants from Nef-expressing macrophages have been shown to induce chemotaxis and activation of resting T lymphocytes leading to productive HIV infection. In addition to its primary function as a transcriptional enhancer in infected cells,

Tat may also be secreted and directly activate potential target cells. In addition, in its secreted form Tat has been shown to be immunosuppressive directly as well as indirectly by inducing secretion of interferon (IFN)α from monocytes/macrophages. Flanking these genes are the long terminal repeats (LTRs), which contain regulatory elements involved in gene expression (see below) such as the polyadenylation signal sequence; the TATA promotor sequence; the NF-κB and Sp1 enhancer binding sites; the transactivating response (TAR) sequences, where the Tat protein binds; and the negative regulatory element (NRE), whose deletion increases the level of gene expression (Fig. 309-5). The major difference between the genomes of HIV-1 and HIV-2 is the fact that HIV-2 lacks the *vpu* gene and has a *vpx* gene not contained in HIV-1.

MOLECULAR HETEROGENEITY OF HIV-1 Molecular analyses of various HIV isolates reveal sequence variations over many parts of the viral genome. For example, in different isolates, the degree of difference in the coding sequences of the viral envelope protein ranges from a few percent (very close) to 50%. These changes tend to cluster in hypervariable regions. One such region, called V3, is a target for neutralizing antibodies and contains recognition sites for T cell responses (see below). Variability in this region is likely due to selective pressure from the host immune system. The extraordinary variability of HIV-1 is in marked contrast to the relative genetic stability of HTLV-I and -II.

There are two groups of HIV-1: group M (major), which is responsible for most of the infections in the world; group O (outlier), a relatively rare viral form found originally in Cameroon, Gabon, and France; and a third group (group N) first identified in a Cameroonian woman with AIDS. The M group comprises eight subtypes, or *clades*, designated A, B, C, D, F, G, H, and J, as well as four major circulating recombinant forms (CRFs). These four CRFs are the AE virus, prevalent in southeast Asia and often referred to simply as E, despite the fact that the parental E virus has never been found; AG from west and central Africa; AGI from Cyprus and Greece; and AB from Russia. These 8 subtypes and 4 CRFs create the major branches in the phylogenetic tree that represents the lineage of the M group of HIV-1 (Fig. 309-6; also see hiv-web.lanl.gov/ALIGN_CURRENT/SUBTYPE-REF/Table1.html).

The global patterns of HIV-1 variation likely result from accidents of viral trafficking. Subtype B viruses, which now differ by up to 17% in their *env* coding sequences, are the overwhelmingly predominant viruses seen in the United States, Canada, certain countries in South America, western Europe, and Australia. Other subtypes are also present in these countries to varying degrees. It is thought that, purely by chance, subtype B was seeded into the United States in the late 1970s, thereby establishing an overwhelming founder effect. Subtype C viruses (of the M group) are the most common form worldwide; many countries have cocirculating viral subtypes

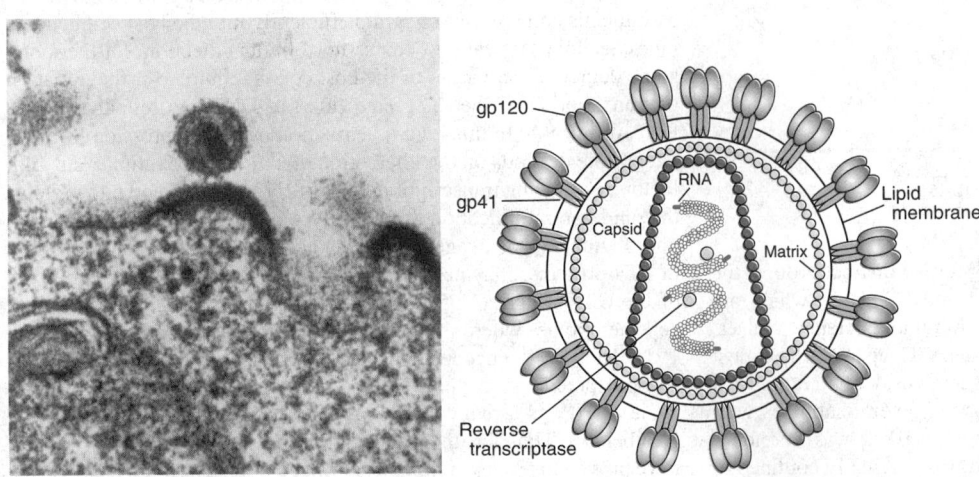

FIGURE 309-2 *A.* Electron micrograph of HIV. Figure illustrates a typical virion following budding from the surface of a CD4+ T lymphocyte, together with two additional incomplete virions in the process of budding from the cell membrane. *B.* Structure of HIV-1, including the gp120 outer membrane, gp41 transmembrane components of the envelope, genomic RNA, enzyme reverse transcriptase, p18(17) inner membrane (matrix), and p24 core protein (capsid). *(Adapted from RC Gallo: Sci Am 256:46, 1987.)*

that are giving rise to CRFs. Figure 309-7 schematically diagrams the worldwide distribution of HIV-1 subtypes by region. The predominant subtype in Europe and the Americas is subtype B. In Africa, >75% of strains recovered to date have been of subtypes A, C, and D, with C being the most common. In Asia, HIV-1 isolates of subtypes E, C, and B predominate. Subtype E accounts for most infections in Southeast Asia, while subtype C is prevalent in India (see "HIV Infections and AIDS Worldwide," below). Sequence analyses of HIV-1 isolates from infected individuals indicate that recombination among viruses of different clades likely occurs as a result of infection of an individual with viruses of more than one clade, particularly in geographic areas where clades overlap.

TRANSMISSION

HIV is transmitted by both homosexual and heterosexual contact; by blood and blood products; and by infected mothers to infants either intrapartum, perinatally, or via breast milk. After approximately 20 years of scrutiny, there is no evidence that HIV is transmitted by casual contact or that the virus can be spread by insects, such as by a mosquito bite.

SEXUAL TRANSMISSION HIV infection is predominantly a sexually transmitted disease (STD) worldwide. Although approximately 42% of new HIV infections in the United States are among men who have sex with men, heterosexual transmission is clearly the most common mode of infection worldwide, particularly in developing countries. Furthermore, the yearly incidence of new cases of AIDS attributed to heterosexual transmission of HIV is steadily increasing in the United States, mainly among minorities, particularly women in minority groups (Fig. 309-8).

HIV has been demonstrated in seminal fluid both within infected mononuclear cells and in the cell-free state. The virus appears to concentrate in the seminal fluid, particularly in situations where there are increased numbers of lymphocytes and monocytes in the fluid, as in genital inflammatory states such as urethritis and epididymitis, conditions closely associated with other STDs (see below). The virus has also been demonstrated in cervical smears and vaginal fluid. There is a strong association of transmission of HIV with receptive anal intercourse, probably because only a thin, fragile rectal mucosal membrane separates the deposited semen from potentially susceptible cells in and beneath the mucosa and trauma may be associated with anal intercourse. Anal douching and sexual practices such as insertion of hard objects or a clenched fist into the rectum ("fisting") traumatize the rectal mucosa, thereby increasing the likelihood of infection during receptive anal intercourse. It is likely that anal intercourse provides at least two modalities of infection: (1) direct inoculation into blood in cases of traumatic tears in the mucosa; and (2) infection of susceptible target cells, such as Langerhans cells, in the mucosal layer in the absence of trauma (see below). Although the vaginal mucosa is several layers thicker than the rectal mucosa and less likely to be traumatized during intercourse, it is clear that the virus can be transmitted to either partner through vaginal intercourse. In a 10-year prospective study in the United States of heterosexual transmission of HIV, male-to-female transmission was approximately eight times more efficient than female-to-male transmission. This difference may be due in part to the prolonged exposure to infected seminal fluid of the vaginal and cervical mucosa, as well as the endometrium (when semen enters through the cervical os). By comparison, the penis and urethral orifice are exposed relatively briefly to infected vaginal fluid. Among various co-

FIGURE 309-3 The replication cycle of HIV. See text for description. *(Adapted from AS Fauci, 1988.)*

FIGURE 309-4 Binding and fusion of HIV-1 with its target cell. HIV-1 binds to its target cell via the CD4 molecule, leading to a conformational change in the gp120 molecule that allows it to bind to the co-receptor CCR5 (for R5-using viruses). The virus then fuses with the host cell membrane in a coiled-spring fashion via the newly exposed gp41 molecule (see text for details). *(Adapted from Doms and Peiper.)*

FIGURE 309-5 The genome of HIV. An expanded version of the 5' long terminal repeat (LTR) is also shown. *(Adapted from WC Greene: N Engl J Med 324:308, 1991, and ZF Rosenberg, AS Fauci: Immunol Today 11: 176, 1990).*

FIGURE 309-6   A phylogenetic tree constructed from HIV-1 M (major), O (outlier), N (first identified in a Cameroonian woman with AIDS), and chimpanzee (CPZ) viral envelope sequences. The scale-bar at the bottom indicates a 10% difference at the nucleotide level. *(Courtesy of Bette Korber, PhD, and Carla Kuiken, PhD, of the HIV database project at Los Alamos National Laboratory, Los Alamos, NM, hiv-web.lanl.gov.)*

FIGURE 309-8   Adult AIDS cases in the United States among heterosexuals and women, 1985 through 1998. *Upper.* Estimated proportion of cases in which infection was acquired by heterosexual transmission; data adjusted for reporting delays and reclassification of cases in which no risk factor was reported or identified. *Lower.* Cases among women. *(Courtesy of the Centers for Disease Control and Prevention.)*

factors examined in this study, a history of STDs (see below) was most strongly associated with HIV transmission. In this regard, there is a close association between genital ulcerations and transmission, from the standpoints of both susceptibility to infection and infectivity. Infections with microorganisms such as *Treponema pallidum* (Chap. 172), *Haemophilus ducreyi* (Chap. 149), and herpes simplex virus (HSV; Chap. 182) are important causes of genital ulcerations linked to transmission of HIV. In addition, pathogens responsible for non-ulcerative inflammatory STDs such as those caused by *Chlamydia trachomatis* (Chap. 179), *Neisseria gonorrhoeae* (Chap. 147), and *Trichomonas vaginalis* (Chap. 218) are also associated with an increased risk of transmission of HIV infection. Bacterial vaginosis, an infection related to sexual behavior, but not strictly an STD, may also be linked to an incresed risk of transmission of HIV infection. Several studies suggest that treating other STDs and genital tract syndromes may help prevent transmission of HIV. In two studies in Africa aimed at decreasing the incidence of HIV infection by empirical treatment of village inhabitants for other STDs, there were divergent results. In Mwanza, Tanzania, empirical treatment for STDs resulted in a decrease in STDs, including HIV infection. In contrast, in the Rakai district of Uganda, empirical treatment of STDs resulted in a decrease in these diseases but not a decrease in HIV infections. The prevalance

of HIV infection in Uganda was considerably greater than that in Tanzania at the time of the studies, and, according to a model of the dynamics of sexual spread of HIV, treatment of other STDs would be expected to have less of an effect on decreasing the transmission of HIV in a population with a higher prevalence than in a population with a lower prevalence of HIV infection. Subsequent studies in Uganda indicated that the chief predictor of heterosexual transmission of HIV was the level of plasma viremia. In some studies the use of oral contraceptives was associated with an increase in incidence of HIV infection over and above that which might be expected by not using a condom for birth control. Finally, lack of circumcision has been

FIGURE 309-7   Geographic distribution of HIV-1 subtypes, 1999. The prevalence of HIV-1 genetic subtypes varies by geographic region. The proportions of subtypes in different regions are indicated by pie charts. *[From the Joint United Nations Programme on HIV/AIDS (UNAIDS).]*

strongly associated with a higher risk of HIV infection in certain cohorts. This difference may be due to increased susceptibility of uncircumcised men to ulcerative STDs, as well as other factors such as microtrauma. In addition, the moist environment under the foreskin may promote the presence or persistence of microbial flora which, via inflammatory changes, may lead to higher concentrations of target cells for HIV in the foreskin. Some studies suggest that only circumcision performed before age 20 is associated with a reduced risk of HIV infection. Thus, in certain cases, these phenomena can also be considered as cofactors for HIV transmission.

Oral sex is a much less efficient mode of transmission of HIV than is receptive anal intercourse. However, there is a misperception by some persons that oral sex, particularly among homosexual men, can be proposed as a form of "safe sex" and a substitute for receptive anal intercourse. This is a dangerous approach, as there have been several reports of documented HIV transmission resulting solely from receptive fellatio and insertive cunnilingus. For example, one study reported that in 12 subjects where the precise date of seroconversion could be identified, 4 individuals reported oral-genital contact as their sole risk factor. There are probably many more cases that go unreported because of the frequent practice of both oral sex and receptive anal intercourse by the same person. The association of alcohol consumption and illicit drug use with unsafe sexual behavior, both homosexual and heterosexual, leads to an increased risk of sexual transmission of HIV.

TRANSMISSION BY BLOOD AND BLOOD PRODUCTS
HIV can be transmitted to individuals who receive HIV-tainted blood transfusions, blood products, or transplanted tissue, as well as to IDUs who are exposed to HIV while sharing injection paraphernalia such as needles, syringes, the water in which drugs are mixed, or the cotton through which drugs are filtered. Parenteral transmission of HIV during injection drug use does not require intravenous puncture; subcutaneous ("skin popping") or intramuscular ("muscling") injections can transit HIV as well, even though these behaviors are sometimes erroneously perceived as low-risk. Among IDUs, the risk of HIV infection increases with the duration of injection drug use; the frequency of needle sharing; the number of partners with whom paraphernalia are shared, particularly in the setting of "shooting galleries" where drugs are sold and large numbers of IDUs may share a limited number of "works"; comorbid psychiatric conditions such as antisocial personality disorder; the use of cocaine in injectable form or smoked as "crack"; and the use of injection drugs in a geographic location with a high prevalence of HIV infection, such as certain inner-city areas in the United States.

From the late 1970s until the spring of 1985, when mandatory testing of donated blood for HIV-1 was initiated, it has been estimated that over 10,000 individuals in the United States were infected through transfusions of blood or blood products (Chap. 114). Approximately 8900 individuals in the United States who survived the illness for which they received HIV-contaminated blood transfusions, blood components, or transplanted tissue have developed AIDS. It is estimated that 90 to 100% of individuals who were exposed to such HIV-contaminated products became infected. Transfusions of whole blood, packed red blood cells, platelets, leukocytes, and plasma are all capable of transmitting HIV infection. In contrast, hyperimmune gamma globulin, hepatitis B immune globulin, plasma-derived hepatitis B vaccine, and Rh$_o$ immune globulin have not been associated with transmission of HIV infection. The procedures involved in processing these products either inactivate or remove the virus.

In addition to the above, several thousand individuals in the United States with hemophilia or other clotting disorders were infected with HIV by receipt of HIV-contaminated fresh frozen plasma or concentrates of clotting factors; approximately 5310 of these individuals have developed AIDS. Currently, in the United States and in most developed countries, the following measures have made the risk of transmission of HIV infection by transfused blood or blood products extremely small: (1) the screening of all blood for p24 antigen and for HIV antibody by ELISA, with a confirmatory western blot where applicable; (2) the self-deferral of donors on the basis of risk behavior;

(3) the screening out of HIV-negative individuals with positive surrogate laboratory parameters of HIV infection, such as hepatitis B and C; and (4) serologic testing for syphilis. It is currently estimated that the risk of infection with HIV in the United States via transfused screened blood is approximately 1 in 676,000 donations. Therefore, among the 12 million donations collected in the United States each year, an estimated 18 infectious donations are available for transfusion. The addition of nucleic acid testing to the blood screening protocol to capture some of these rare HIV antibody–negative units should decrease even further the chances of transmission by transfused blood or blood products. There have been several reports of sporadic breakdowns in routinely available screening procedures in certain countries, where contaminated blood was allowed to be transfused, resulting in small clusters of patients becoming infected. There have been no reported cases of transmission of HIV-2 in the United States via donated blood, and, currently, donated blood is screened for both HIV-1 and HIV-2 antibodies. The chance of infection of a hemophiliac via clotting factor concentrates has essentially been eliminated because of the added layer of safety resulting from heat treatment of the concentrates.

Prior to the screening of donors, a small number of cases of transmission of HIV via semen used in artificial insemination and tissues used in organ transplantation were well documented. At present, donors of such tissues are prescreened for HIV infection.

OCCUPATIONAL TRANSMISSION OF HIV: HEALTH CARE WORKERS AND LABORATORY WORKERS There is a small, but definite, occupational risk of HIV transmission in health care workers and laboratory personnel and potentially in others who work with HIV-infected specimens, particularly when sharp objects are used. An estimated 600,000 to 800,000 health care workers are stuck with needles or other sharp medical instruments in the United States each year. Large, multi-institutional studies have indicated that the risk of HIV transmission following skin puncture from a needle or a sharp object that was contaminated with blood from a person with documented HIV infection is approximately 0.3% (see "HIV and the Health Care Worker," p. 1909). The risk of hepatitis B infection following a similar type of exposure is 6 to 30% in nonimmune individuals; if a susceptible worker is exposed to HBV, postexposure prophylaxis with hepatitis B immune globulin and initiation of HBV vaccine is more than 90% effective in preventing HBV infection. The risk of HCV infection following percutaneous injury is approximately 1.8% (Chap. 295). An increased risk for HIV infection following percutaneous exposures to HIV-infected blood is associated with exposures involving a relatively large quantity of blood, as in the case of a device visibly contaminated with the patient's blood, a procedure that involves a needle placed directly in a vein or artery, or a deep injury. In addition, the risk increases for exposures to blood from patients with advanced-stage disease, probably owing to the higher titer of HIV in the blood as well as to other factors, such as the presence of more virulent strains of virus (see "HIV and the Health Care Worker," p. 1909).

There have been reports of health care workers who became infected through the exposure of mucous membranes or abraded skin to HIV-infected material; however, the risk associated with mucocutaneous exposure has been difficult to quantify, because transmission by this route is extremely rare. Factors that might be associated with mucocutaneous transmission of HIV include exposure to an unusually large volume of blood, prolonged contact, and a potential portal of entry. A prospective study has indicated that the use of antiretroviral drugs as postexposure prophylaxis decreases the risk of infection compared to historic controls in occupationally exposed health care workers. Transmission of HIV through intact skin has not been documented (see "HIV and the Health Care Worker," p. 1909).

Since the beginning of the HIV epidemic, there have been at least three reported instances in which transmission of infection from a health care worker to patients seemed highly probable. The first involved a dentist in Florida who apparently infected six of his patients, most likely through contaminated instruments. Another case involved an orthopedic surgeon in France who apparently infected a patient during placement of a total hip prosthesis. A third case involved the apparent transmission of HIV from a nurse to a surgical patient in France. An additional situation involved the apparent infection of four patients by an HIV-negative general surgeon in Australia during routine outpatient surgery. The cause of the transmission was felt to be a failure on the part of the surgeon to sterilize instruments properly between procedures following prior surgery on an infected patient. Despite these few cases, the risk of transmission from an infected health care worker to patients is extremely low; in fact, too low to be measured accurately. Indeed several epidemiologic studies have been performed tracing thousands of patients of HIV-infected dentists, physicians, surgeons, obstetricians, and gynecologists and no other cases of HIV infection that could be linked to the health care providers were identified. The very occurrence of transmission of HIV as well as hepatitis B and C to and from health care workers in the workplace underscores the importance of the use of universal precautions when caring for all patients (see below and Chap. 134).

MATERNAL-FETAL/INFANT TRANSMISSION HIV infection can be transmitted from an infected mother to her fetus during pregnancy or to her infant during delivery. This is an extremely important form of transmission of HIV infection in developing countries, where the proportion of infected women to infected men is approximately 1:1. Virologic analysis of aborted fetuses indicate that HIV can be transmitted to the fetus as early as the first and second trimester of pregnancy. However, maternal transmission to the fetus occurs most commonly in the perinatal period. This conclusion is based on a number of considerations, including the time frame of identification of infection by the sequential appearance of classes of antibodies to HIV (i.e., the appearance of HIV-specific IgA antibody within 3 to 6 months after birth); a positive viral culture; the appearance of p24 antigenemia weeks to months after delivery, but not at the time of delivery; a polymerase chain reaction (PCR) assay of infant blood following delivery that is negative at birth and positive several months later; the demonstration that the firstborn twin of an infected mother is more commonly infected than is the second twin; and the evidence that cesarean section results in decreased transmission to the infant.

In the absence of prophylactic antiretroviral therapy to the mother during pregnancy, labor, and delivery, and to the fetus following birth (see below), the probability of transmission of HIV from mother to infant/fetus ranges from 15 to 25% in industrialized countries and from 25 to 35% in developing countries. These differences may relate to the adequacy of prenatal care as well as to the stage of HIV disease and the general health of the mother during pregnancy. Higher rates of transmission have been associated with many factors, including high maternal levels of plasma viremia, low maternal CD4+ T cell counts and HIV p24 antibody levels, maternal vitamin A deficiency, a prolonged interval between membrane rupture and delivery, presence of chorioamnionitis at delivery, STDs during pregnancy, cigarette smoking and hard drug use during pregnancy, preterm labor, obstetric procedures such as amniocentesis and amnioscopy, and other factors that may increase the exposure of the infant to the mother's blood. With regard to levels of viremia, several studies indicate that the risk of transmission increases with the maternal plasma HIV RNA level. In one series of 552 singleton pregnancies in the United States, the rate of mother-to-baby transmission was 0% among women with <1000 copies of HIV RNA per milliliter of blood, 16.6% among women with 1000 to 10,000/mL, 21.3% among women with 10,001 to 50,000/mL, 30.9% among women with 50,001 to 100,000/mL, and 40.6% among women with >100,000/mL. However, there may be no lower "threshold" below which transmission never occurs, since other studies have reported transmission by women with viral RNA levels below the level of detectability of 50 copies per milliliter. Finally, it has been speculated that if the mother experiences acute primary infection during pregnancy, there is a higher rate of transmission to the

fetus, owing to the high levels of viremia that occur during primary infection (see below). In the United States and other industrialized countries, zidovudine treatment of HIV-infected pregnant women from the beginning of the second trimester through delivery and of the infant for 6 weeks following birth has dramatically decreased the rate of intrapartum and perinatal transmission of HIV infection from 22.6% in the untreated group to <5%. It is expected that the rate of transmission will decrease even further as more potent combinations of drugs are used in HIV-infected pregnant women (see below).

In developed countries, current recommendations to reduce perinatal transmission of HIV include universal voluntary HIV testing and counseling of pregnant women, zidovudine prophylaxis, obstetric management that attempts to minimize exposure of the infant to maternal blood and genital secretions, and avoidance of breast feeding. It is also recommended that the choice of antiretroviral therapy for pregnant women should be based on the same considerations used for women who are not pregnant, with discussion of the recognized and unknown risks and benefits of such therapy during pregnancy. The cost and logistics of the above protocol are not feasible for developing countries, particularly those in sub-Saharan Africa where the per capita health care delivery allocation is often only a few dollars per year. Studies have demonstrated that truncated regimens of zidovudine alone or in combination with lamivudine given to the mother during the last few weeks of pregnancy or even only during labor and delivery, and to the infant for a week or less, reduced transmission to the infant by 50% compared to placebo. One important study in Uganda demonstrated that a single dose of nevirapine given to the mother at the onset of labor followed by a single dose to the newborn within 72 h of birth decreased transmission to 13% compared to 25% transmission at age 14 to 16 weeks when the mother received multiple doses of zidovudine throughout labor and delivery and the infant received zidovudine daily for a full week following birth. The cost of the nevirapine for the mother and infant was a mere $4.00, which would make this regimen affordable for many developing countries. Approximately 1800 babies are born infected each day throughout the world, and 90% of these are in sub-Saharan Africa; thus, implementation of such a regimen could potentially save 1000 babies per day from becoming infected.

Although most transmission of HIV occurs during pregnancy and at birth, breast feeding may account for 5 to 15% of infants becoming infected after delivery. This is an important modality of transmission of HIV infection in developing countries, particularly where mothers continue to breast feed for prolonged periods. The risk factors for mother-to-child transmission of HIV via breast feeding are not fully understood; factors that increase the likelihood of transmission include detectable levels of HIV in breast milk, the presence of mastitis, low maternal CD4+ T cell counts, and maternal vitamin A deficiency. The risk of HIV infection via breast feeding is highest in the early months of breast feeding. In addition, exclusive breast feeding has been reported to carry a lower risk of HIV transmission than mixed feeding. Certainly, in developed countries breast feeding by an infected mother should be avoided. However, there is disagreement regarding recommendations for breast feeding in certain developing countries, where breast milk is the only source of adequate nutrition as well as immunity against potentially serious infections for the infant. Studies are being conducted to determine whether intermittent administration of nevirapine, which has a relatively long half-life, to uninfected babies born of infected mothers decreases the incidence of infection via breast feeding.

TRANSMISSION BY OTHER BODY FLUIDS There is no convincing evidence that saliva can transmit HIV infection, either through kissing or through other exposures, such as occupationally to health care workers. HIV can be isolated from saliva of only a small proportion of infected individuals, typically in titers that are low compared to those in blood and genital secretions. In addition, saliva contains endogenous antiviral factors; among these factors, HIV-specific immunoglobulins of IgA, IgG, and IgM isotypes are detected readily in salivary secretions of infected individuals. It has been suggested that large glycoproteins such as mucins and thrombospondin-1 sequester HIV into aggregates for clearance by the host. In addition, a number of soluble salivary factors inhibit HIV to various degrees in vitro, probably by targeting host cell receptors rather than the virus itself. Perhaps the best-studied of these, secretory leukocyte protease inhibitor (SLPI), blocks HIV infection in several cell culture systems, and it is found in saliva at levels that approximate those required for inhibition of HIV in vitro. It has also been suggested that submandibular saliva reduces HIV infectivity by stripping gp120 from the surface of virions, and that saliva-mediated disruption and lysis of HIV-infected cells occurs because of the hypotonicity of oral secretions. There have been outlier cases of suspected transmission by saliva, but these have probably been blood-to-blood transmissions. One case was reported of a 91-year-old man who was bitten during a robbery attempt by an HIV-infected person. He seroconverted, and there was no question that the source of the infection was the human bite. However, the individual who bit him had bleeding gums, and it was thought that the infection was actually transmitted via blood. In addition, a most unusual form of HIV transmission from infected children to mothers in the former Soviet Union has been identified. In those cases, the children (infected through transfusion) were said to have bleeding sores in the mouth, and the mothers were said to have lacerations and abrasions on and around the nipples of the breast resulting from trauma from the children's teeth. Breast feeding had been continued until the children were older than is usual in other developed countries.

Although virus can be identified, if not isolated, from virtually any body fluid, there is no evidence that HIV transmission can occur as a result of exposure to tears, sweat, and urine. However, there have been isolated cases of transmission of HIV infection by body fluids that may or may not have been contaminated with blood. Most of these situations occurred in the setting of a close relative providing intensive nursing care for an HIV-infected person without observing universal precautions. These cases underscore the importance of observing universal precautions in the handling of body fluids and wastes from HIV-infected individuals (see below).

EPIDEMIOLOGY

HIV INFECTION AND AIDS WORLDWIDE HIV infection/AIDS is a global pandemic, with cases reported from virtually every country. The current estimate of the number of cases of HIV infection among adults worldwide is approximately 33 million, two-thirds of whom are in sub-Saharan Africa; 47% of cases are women. In addition, an estimated 1.3 million children under 15 are living with HIV/AIDS. The global distribution of these cases is illustrated in Fig. 309-9. According to the Joint United Nations Programme on HIV/AIDS (UNAIDS), in 1999 alone there were an estimated 5.4 million new cases of infection worldwide (more than 15,000 new infections each day) and 2.8 million death from AIDS, making it the fourth leading cause of mortality worldwide. The estimated number of AIDS-re-

FIGURE 309-9 Estimated number of adults and children living with HIV infection as of January 1, 2000. *(From UNAIDS.)*

lated deaths worldwide through the year 2000 is illustrated in Fig. 309-10. The HIV epidemic has occurred in "waves" in different regions of the world, each wave having somewhat different characteristics depending on the demographics of the country and region in question and the timing of the introduction of HIV into the population. As noted above, different subtypes, or clades, of HIV-1 are prevalent in different regions of the world (see above and Fig. 309-7), increasing the difficulty in the development of vaccines and perhaps accounting for different degrees of virulence. It is unlikely that a single vaccine will be applicable to all regions of the world. In this regard, in addition to HIV-1 subtype B, the predominant subtype in the United States, HIV-1 subtypes A, AE, AG, C, D, and O have been detected in individuals in the United States, as might be expected given the degree of international travel that occurs.

Table 309-3 provides the statistics and demographic features of HIV/AIDS in different regions of the world. Although the epidemic was first recognized in the United States and shortly thereafter in western Europe, it very likely began in sub-Saharan Africa (see above), which has been particularly devastated by the epidemic, with the prevalence of infection in many cities in the double digits. According to the United Nations Population Division, by the year 2015 life expectancy in the nine countries in Africa with the highest HIV prevalence rates will fall, on average, 17 years. In certain sub-Saharan African countries such as Zimbabwe and Botswana, available seroprevalence data indicate >25% of the adult population aged 15 to 49 is HIV-

FIGURE 309-10 Estimated/projected annual number of deaths due to AIDS from 1980 through 2000. *(From UNAIDS.)*

Table 309-3 Regional HIV/AIDS Statistics and Features, 1 January 2000

Region	Epidemic Started	Adults and Children Living with HIV/AIDS	Adults and Children Newly Infected with HIV in 1999	Adult Prevalence Rate[a]	HIV-Positive Adult Women, %	Main Mode of Transmission[b] for Adults Living with HIV/AIDS
Sub-Saharan Africa	Late '70s–Early '80s	24.5 million	4.0 million	8.57%	55	Hetero
North Africa & Middle East	Late '80s	220,000	20,000	0.12%	20	IDU, Hetero
South & Southeast Asia	Late '80s	5.6 million	800,000	0.54%	35	Hetero
East Asia & Pacific	Late '80s	530,000	120,000	0.06%	13	IDU, Hetero, MSM
Latin America	Late '70s–Early '80s	1.3 million	150,000	0.49%	25	MSM, IDU, Hetero
Caribbean	Late '70s–Early '80s	360,000	60,000	2.11%	35	Hetero, MSM
Eastern Europe & Central Asia	Early '90s	420,000	130,000	0.21%	25	IDU, MSM
Western Europe	Late '70s–Early '80s	520,000	30,000	0.23%	25	MSM, IDU
North America	Late '70s–Early '80s	900,000	45,000	0.58%	20	MSM, IDU, Hetero
Australia & New Zealand	Late '70s–Early '80s	15,000	500	0.13%	10	MSM, IDU
Total		**34.3 million**	**5.4 million**	**1.07%**	**47**	

[a] The proportion of adults (15 to 49 years of age) living with HIV/AIDS in 1999.
[b] MSM (sexual transmission among men who have sex with men), IDU (transmission through injecting drug use), Hetero (heterosexual transmission).
SOURCE: Joint United Nations Programme on HIV/AIDS (UNAIDS).

infected. In addition, among high-risk individuals (e.g., commercial sex workers, patients attending STD clinics) who live in urban areas of sub-Saharan Africa, seroprevalence is now >50% in many countries. The epidemic in Asian countries, particularly India and Thailand, has lagged temporally behind that in Africa; however, the number of new cases in this region is accelerating rapidly, and the magnitude of the epidemic is projected to exceed that of sub-Saharan Africa in the early part of the twenty-first century. The estimated number of cases in China is still relatively small; however, the potential exists for a major expansion of the epidemic in that nation of over 1 billion people.

The major mode of transmission of HIV worldwide is unquestionably heterosexual sex; this is particularly true and has been so since the begining of the epidemic in developing countries, where the numbers of infected men and women are approximately equal. The epidemic in most developed countries was first introduced among homosexual men and, to a greater or lesser degree (depending on the individual country), among IDUs. In this regard, the total numbers of AIDS cases in those countries still reflect a high proportion of cases among these high-risk groups. However, in most developed countries, including the United States (see below), there has been a gradual shift such that among new cases of AIDS, there is a greater prevalence among heterosexuals and IDUs than among homosexual men.

AIDS IN THE UNITED STATES AIDS has had and will continue to have an extraordinary public health impact in the United States. As of January 1, 2000, >724,600 cumulative cases of AIDS had been reported in adults and adolescents in the United States (Table 309-4) and approximately 425,000 AIDS-related deaths had been reported. It is the fifth leading cause of death among Americans aged 25 to 44 (Fig. 309-11), having dropped from first within the past few years. The death rate from AIDS declined 42% from 1996 to 1997 and 18% from 1997 to 1998. This trend is due to several factors including the improved prophylaxis and treatment of opportunistic infections, the growing experience among health professions in caring for HIV-infected individuals, improved access to health care, and the decrease in infections due to saturational effects and prevention efforts. However, the most influential factor clearly has been the increased use of potent antiretroviral drugs, generally administered in a combination of three or four agents, usually including a protease inhibitor (see below). When one looks at the totality of data collected from the beginning of the epidemic, approximately one-half of cases are among men who have had sex with men. However, over the past few years, the numbers of newly reported cases of AIDS among other groups, including IDUs and heterosexuals, have surpassed the numbers of newly reported cases among men who have had sex with men. The proportion of new cases of AIDS per year attributed to heterosexual contact has increased dramatically over the past 15 years in the United States (Fig. 309-8). Women are increasingly affected; the proportion of AIDS cases in the United States reported among adult and adolescent females has increased from <5% to 24% from 1985 to 1998 (Fig. 309-8). Most cases

Table 309-4 AIDS Cases in Adults/Adolescents in the United States as of 1 January 2000

Exposure Category	White, Not Hispanic No. (%)	Black, Not Hispanic No. (%)	Hispanic No. (%)	Asian/Pacific Islander No. (%)	American Indian/ Alaska Native No. (%)	Total[a] No. (%)
Men who have sex with men	216,564 (68)	74,434 (28)	45,867 (35)	3389 (64)	987 (47)	341,597 (47)
Men who inject drugs	26,856 (8)	68,491 (26)	38,338 (29)	244 (5)	273 (13)	134,356 (19)
Men who have sex with men and inject drugs	23,880 (7)	14,965 (6)	7253 (6)	172 (3)	295 (14)	46,582 (6)
Men with hemophilia/coagulation disorder	3725 (1)	551 (0)	424 (0)	67 (1)	30 (1)	4803 (1)
Men infected through heterosexual contact	5181 (2)	15,121 (6)	5986 (4)	165 (3)	47 (2)	26,530 (4)
Men who received a blood transfusion, blood components, or tissue	3133 (1)	1028 (0)	564 (1)	112 (2)	8 (0)	4863 (1)
Men with unreported or unidentified risk	11,198 (3)	24,658 (9)	9425 (7)	521 (10)	103 (5)	46,112 (6)
Women who inject drugs	11,074 (3)	29,059 (11)	9613 (7)	107 (2)	164 (8)	50,073 (7)
Women with hemophilia/coagulation disorder	102 (0)	108 (0)	53 (0)	5 (0)	2 (0)	272 (0)
Women infected through heterosexual contact	10,528 (3)	25,719 (10)	11,222 (8)	310 (6)	127 (6)	47,946 (7)
Women who received a blood transfusion, blood components, or tissue	1789 (1)	1230 (0)	536 (0)	96 (2)	14 (1)	3668 (1)
Women with unreported or unidentified risk	2805 (1)	12,413 (5)	2407 (2)	111 (2)	51 (2)	17,851 (2)
Total	316,835	267,777	131,698	5299	2101	724,656
% of Total Adult/Adolescent AIDS cases	(44)	(37)	(18)	(<1)	(<1)	(100)

[a] Includes 943 individuals whose race/ethnicity is unknown, and 3 individuals whose sex is unknown.
SOURCE: Centers for Disease Control and Prevention, 2000.

of transmission by injection drug use and heterosexual contact are reported from the northeast and southeast regions of the country, particularly among minorities. HIV infection and AIDS have disproportionately affected minority populations in the United States. The rates of AIDS cases per 100,000 population reported among adults and adolescents in 1999 were 84.2 for African Americans, 34.6 for Hispanics, 9.0 for whites, 11.3 for American Indians/ Alaska Natives, and 4.3 for Asian/Pacific Islanders (Fig. 309-12).

As of January 1, 2000, 8718 cases of AIDS in children <13 years old had been reported, and approximately 60% of these children have died (Table 309-5). Approximately 90% of these children were born to mothers who were HIV-infected or who were at risk for

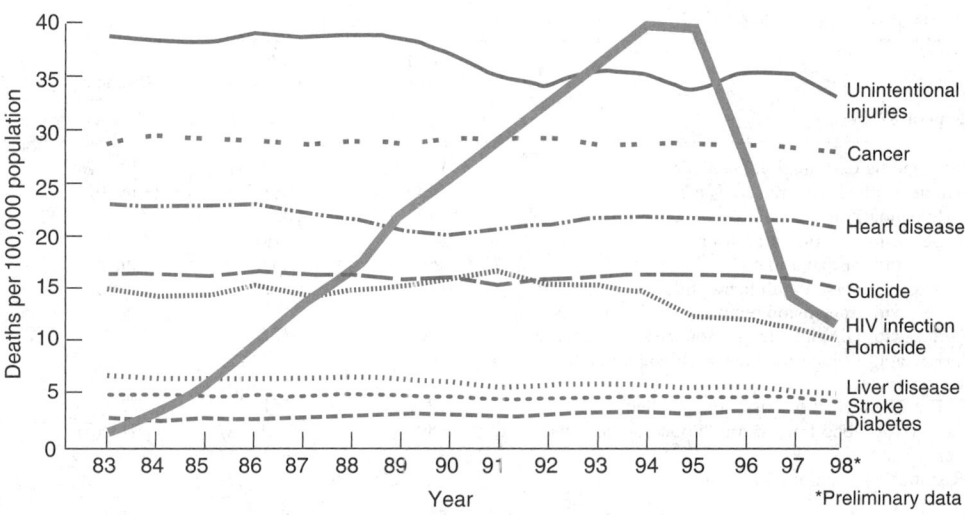

FIGURE 309-11 Death rates from leading causes of death in persons aged 25–44 years in the United States from 1983 through 1998. *(From National Center for Health Statistics.)*

HIV infection and, in approximately 60% of those cases, the mother was either an IDU or the heterosexual partner of an IDU. About 42% of women with AIDS have become infected through injection drug use, compared to 22% of men with AIDS; 40% of women have become infected by heterosexual contact, compared to 4% of men with AIDS. Only 1% of AIDS cases are among hemophiliacs, and 1% are among recipients of blood transfusions, blood products, or transplanted tissue. The relative contribution of the latter groups will gradually decrease, even though individuals infected previously through this mode of transmission will continue to develop AIDS. The risk of additional infections via this mode of transmission in the United States is extremely small (see above). In recent years, the incidence of AIDS has decreased considerably, with ~46,000 new cases in 1999 compared to ~60,000 in 1996. This trend likely reflects both reduced infection rates since the mid-1980s; more widespread use of prophylactic therapies, which delay the onset of AIDS; and the use of highly effective antiretroviral therapy early in the course of HIV infection (see below). Also, the demography of newly infected individuals has changed considerably since the mid-1980s (see below).

HIV PREVALENCE AND INCIDENCE IN THE UNITED STATES It is estimated that between 650,000 and 900,000 adults and adolescents in the United States are living with HIV infection, including 120,000 to 160,000 women. This estimate results in an overall nationwide prevalence of HIV infection of approximately 0.3%. Prevalence is highest among young adults in their late twenties and thirties and among minorities. An estimated 3% of black men and 1% of black women in their thirties are living with HIV infection. The number of new infections per year is estimated to be approximately 40,000, and this number has remained stable for at least 9 years. The estimated proportion of HIV infections has declined among white males, especially those >30, while the proportion of new HIV infections appears to have increased among women and minorities. Among newly infected persons in the United States, ~70% are men and ~30% are women (Fig. 309-13). Of these newly infected individuals, half are <25 years. Of new infections among men, the CDC estimates that ~60% were infected through homosexual sex, 25% through injection drug use, and 15% through heterosexual sex. Of new infections among women, ~75% were infected through heterosexual sex and 25% through injection drug use.

HIV infection and AIDS are widespread in the United States; although the epidemic on the whole is plateauing, it is spreading rapidly among certain populations, stabilizing in others, and decreasing in others. Similar to other STDs, HIV infection will not spread homogeneously throughout the population of the United States. However, it is clear that anyone who practices high-risk behavior is at risk for HIV infection. In addition, the alarming increase in infections and

AIDS cases among heterosexuals (particularly sexual partners of IDUs, women, and adolescents) as well as the spread in certain inner city areas (particularly among underserved minority populations with inadequate access to health care) testifies to the fact that the epidemic of HIV infection in the United States is a public health problem of major proportions.

PATHOPHYSIOLOGY AND PATHOGENESIS

The hallmark of HIV disease is a profound immunodeficiency resulting primarily from a progressive quantitative and qualitative deficiency of the subset of T lymphocytes referred to as *helper T cells*, or *inducer T cells*. This subset of T cells is defined phenotypically by the presence on its surface of the CD4 molecule (Chap. 305), which serves as the primary cellular receptor for HIV. A co-receptor must also be present together with CD4 for efficient fusion and entry of HIV-1 into its target cells (Figs. 309-3 and 309-4). HIV uses two major co-receptors for fusion and entry; these co-receptors are also the primary receptors for certain chemoattractive cytokines termed *chemokines* and belong to the seven-transmembrane-domain G protein–coupled family of receptors. CCR5 and CXCR4 are the major co-receptors used by HIV (see above and below). Although a number of mechanisms responsible for cytopathicity and immune dysfunction of CD4+ T cells have been demonstrated in vitro, particularly direct infection and destruction of these cells by HIV (see below), it remains unclear which mechanisms or combination of mechanisms are primarily responsible for their progressive depletion and functional impairment in vivo. When the number of CD4+ T cells declines below a certain level (see below), the patient is at high risk of developing a variety of opportunistic diseases,

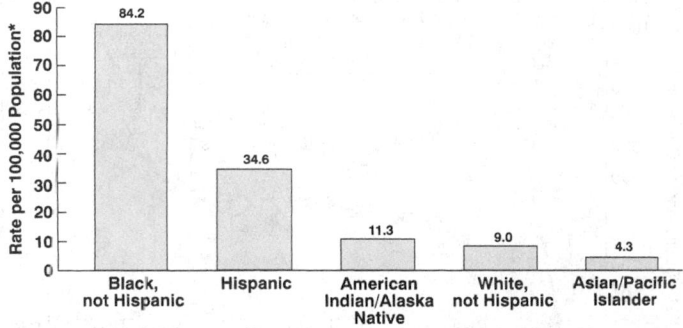

FIGURE 309-12 Rates of adult/adolescent AIDS cases per 100,000 population diagnosed in 1999 in various racial/ethnic groups in the United States. *(From Centers for Disease Control and Prevention, 2000.)*

Exposure Category	White, Not Hispanic No. (%)	Black, Not Hispanic No. (%)	Hispanic No. (%)	Asian/Pacific Islander No. (%)	American Indian/ Alaska Native No. (%)	Total[a] No. (%)
Hemophilia/Coagulation Disorder	158 (10)	34 (1)	38 (2)	3 (6)	2 (7)	235 (3)
Mother with/at Risk for HIV infection	1144 (75)	4881 (96)	1846 (92)	31 (65)	27 (90)	7943 (91)
Injecting drug use	477	1880	737	4	13	3116
Sex with injecting drug user	223	718	489	5	7	1443
Sex with bisexual male	66	63	39	2	—	171
Sex with person with hemophilia	17	7	8	—	—	32
Sex with transfusion recipient with HIV infection	8	8	9	—	—	25
Sex with HIV-infected person, risk not specified	140	777	254	9	3	1185
Receipt of blood transfusion, blood components, or tissue	42	97	33	1	—	153
Has HIV infection, risk not specified	171	1351	277	10	4	1818
Receipt of blood transfusion, blood components, or tissue	189 (12)	89 (2)	91 (5)	10 (21)	— —	379 (4)
Risk not reported or identified	26 (2)	100 (2)	30 (1)	4 (8)	1 (3)	161 (2)
Total	1517	5104	2005	48	30	8718
% of Total Pediatric AIDS Cases	(17)	(58)	(23)	(<1)	(<1)	(100)

[a] Includes 14 children whose race/ethnicity is unknown.
SOURCE: Centers for Disease Control and Prevention, 2000.

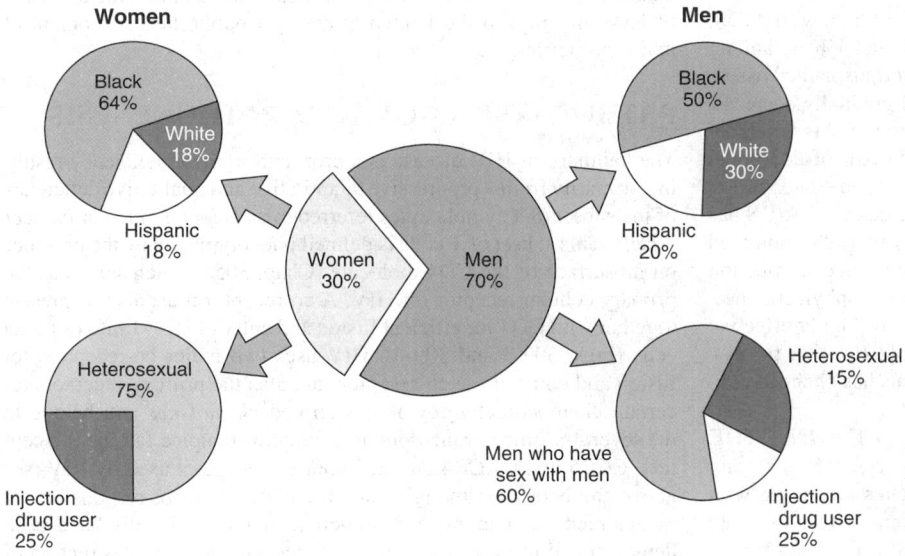

FIGURE 309-13 Estimated new HIV infections by race and risk in the United States in 1998. (*From Centers for Disease Control and Prevention, 1999 National HIV Prevention Conference.*)

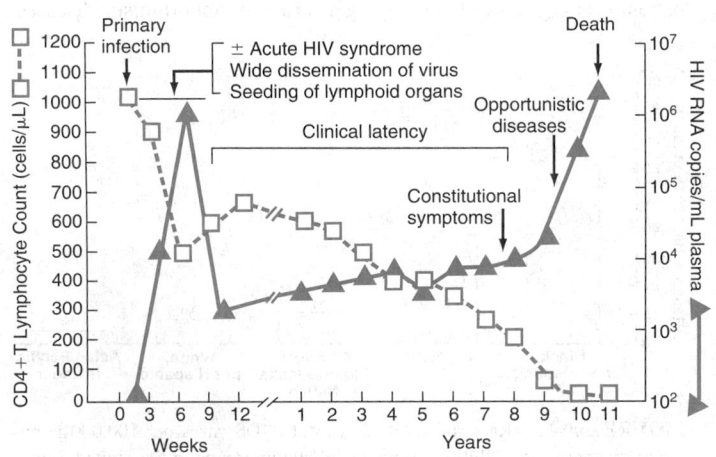

FIGURE 309-14 Typical course of an HIV-infected individual. See text for detailed description. (*From Fauci et al.*)

particularly the infections and neoplasms that are AIDS-defining illnesses. Some features of AIDS, such as KS and neurologic abnormalities (see below), cannot be explained completely by the immunosuppressive effects of HIV, since these complications may occur prior to the development of severe immunologic impairment.

The combination of viral pathogenic and immunopathogenic events that occurs during the course of HIV disease from the moment of initial (primary) infection through the development of advanced-stage disease is complex and varied. It is important to appreciate that the pathogenic mechanisms of HIV disease are multifactorial and multiphasic and are different at different stages of the disease. Therefore, it is essential to consider the typical clinical course of an untreated HIV-infected individual in order to more fully appreciate these pathogenic events (Fig. 309-14).

PRIMARY HIV INFECTION, INITIAL VIREMIA, AND DISSEMINATION OF VIRUS The events associated with primary HIV infection are likely critical determinants of the subsequent course of HIV disease. In particular, the dissemination of virus to lymphoid organs is a major factor in the establishment of a chronic and persistent infection (see below). The initial infection of susceptible cells may vary somewhat with the route of infection. Virus that enters directly into the bloodstream via infected blood or blood products (i.e., transfusions, use of contaminated needles for injecting drugs, sharp-object injuries, maternal-to-fetal transmission either intrapartum or perinatally, or sexual intercourse where there is enough trauma to cause bleeding) is likely cleared from the circulation to the spleen and other lymphoid organs, where it replicates to a critical level and then leads to a burst of viremia that disseminates virus throughout the body. It is uncertain which cell in the blood or lymphoid tissue is the first to actually become infected; however, studies in animal models suggest that dendritic lineage cells may be the initial cells infected. Depending on their stage of maturation, dendritic cells can either be directly infected with virus and pass virus on to CD4+ T cells or physically bring the virus into contact with CD4+ T cells without themselves becoming infected. Studies in the monkey model of mucosal exposure to SIV strongly suggest that the initial cell to become infected at the site of exposure is the Langerhans cell, which is a dendritic lineage cell, and that this cell passes the virus on to CD4+ T cells in the draining lymph nodes. This mechanism likely operates in humans when HIV enters "locally" (as opposed to directly into the blood), via the vagina, rectum, or urethra during intercourse or via the upper gastrointestinal tract from swallowed infected semen, vaginal fluid, or breast milk. Certainly, CD4+ T cells and to a lesser extent cells of monocyte lineage are the major ultimate targets of HIV infection. In primary HIV infection, virus replication in CD4+ T cells intensifies prior to the initiation of an HIV-specific immune response (see below), leading to a burst of viremia (Fig. 309-14) and then to a rapid dissemination of virus to other lymphoid organs, the brain, and other tissues. Individuals who experience the "acute HIV syndrome," which occurs to varying degrees in approximately 50% of individuals with primary infection, have high levels of viremia that last for several weeks (see below). The acute mononucleosis-like symptoms are well correlated with the presence of viremia. Virtually all patients appear to develop some degree of viremia during primary infection, which contributes to virus dissemination, even though they remain asymptomatic or do not recall experiencing symptoms. Careful examination of lymph nodes from more than one site in patients with established HIV infection who did not report symptoms of a primary infection strongly indicate that wide dissemination to lymphoid tissue occurs in most patients. A more detailed description of the role of lymphoid tissue in the immunopathogenesis of HIV disease is given below. It appears that the initial level of plasma viremia in primary HIV infection does not necessarily determine the rate of disease progression; however, the set point of the level of steady-state plasma viremia after approximately 1 year does seem to correlate with the rapidity of disease progression (see below).

ESTABLISHMENT OF CHRONIC AND PERSISTENT INFECTION   Persistent Virus Replication   HIV infection is relatively unique among human viral infections. Despite the robust cellular and humoral immune responses that are mounted following primary infection (see below), once infection has been established the virus is virtually never cleared completely from the body. Rather, a chronic infection develops that persists with varying degrees of virus replication for a median of approximately 10 years before the patient becomes clinically ill (see below). It is this establishment of a chronic, persistent infection that is the hallmark of HIV disease. Throughout the often protracted course of chronic infection, virus replication can almost invariably be detected in untreated patients, both by highly sensitive assays for plasma viremia as well as by demonstration of virus replication in lymphoid tissue. In human viral infections, with very few exceptions, if the host survives, the virus is completely cleared from the body and a state of immunity against subsequent infection develops. HIV infection very rarely kills the host during primary infection. Certain viruses, such as HSV (Chap. 182), are not completely cleared from the body after infection, but instead enter a latent state; in these cases, clinical latency is accompanied by microbiologic latency. This is not the case with HIV infection, in which some degree of virus replication invariably occurs during the period of clinical latency (see below). Chronicity associated with persistent virus replication can also be seen in certain cases of hepatitis B and C infections (Chap. 297); however, in these infections the immune system is not a target of the virus. As mentioned above, HIV usually does not abruptly kill the host; rather it generally succeeds in escaping from a rather vigorous immune response and establishing a state of chronic infection with varying degrees of persistently active virus replication.

Evasion of Immune System Control   Clearly, HIV successfully evades elimination by the immune system in order to establish chronicity. The mechanisms whereby this occurs are not completely clear; however, several have been proposed as playing a role in this phenomenon. HIV has an extraordinary ability to mutate, but this mechanism probably acts mainly after the establishment of chronic infection and contributes to the maintenance of chronicity. Since the transmitted virus and the virus that initially becomes established as a chronic in-

fection are relatively homogeneous, the initial escape from immune system control likely involves mechanisms other than viral mutation. Molecular analysis of clonotypes has demonstrated that clones of CD8+ cytolytic T lymphocytes (CTLs) that expand greatly during primary HIV infection and likely represent the high-affinity clones that would be expected to be most efficient in eliminating virus-infected cells are no longer detectable after their initial burst of expansion. The marked diminution of frequency or disappearance of these HIV-specific cells cannot be explained by mutations in the viral epitope to which they are directed, since virus-sequencing studies indicate that the initial viral epitope is still present when the clones are no longer detected. Furthermore, other, less expanded clones of CD8+ T cells that recognize the same viral epitope persist and likely account for the partial control of virus replication. It is thought that the initially expanded clones may have been deleted owing to the overwhelming exposure to viral antigens during the initial burst of viremia, similar to the exhaustion of CD8+ CTLs that has been reported in the murine model of lymphocytic choriomeningitis virus (LCMV) infection. To compound this phenomenon, virus replication and thus saturation of antigen-presenting cells with viral antigen take place in the lymphoid tissue (see below), which is also the site of generation of HIV-specific CTLs.

Another potential mechanism of HIV escape is related to the fact that, during primary HIV infection and the transition to established chronic infection, both activated HIV-specific CTLs and CTL precursors are preferentially and paradoxically segregated in the peripheral blood, where very little active virus replication takes place, rather than in the lymphoid tissue, which is the main site of virus replication and spread, and the major source of plasma viremia. Finally, the escape of HIV from elimination during primary infection allows the formation of a large pool of latently infected cells that cannot be eliminated by virus-specific CTLs (see below). Thus, despite a potent immune response and the marked downregulation of virus replication following primary HIV infection, HIV succeeds in establishing a state of chronic infection with a variable degree of persistent virus replication. In most cases, during this period the patient makes the clinical transition from acute primary infection to a relatively prolonged state of clinical latency (see below).

Reservoir of Latency Infected Cells   It has been clearly demonstrated that there exists in virtually all HIV-infected individuals a pool of latently infected, resting CD4+ T cells, and that this pool of cells likely serves as at least one component of the persistent reservoir of virus. Such cells manifest postintegration latency in that the HIV provirus integrates into the genome of the cell and can remain in this state until an activation signal drives the expression of HIV transcripts and ultimately replication-competent virus. This form of latency is to be distinguished from preintegration latency, in which HIV enters a resting CD4+ T cell and, in the absence of an activation signal, only a limited degree of reverse transcription of the HIV genome occurs. This period of preintegration latency may last hours to days, and if no activation signal is delivered to the cell, the proviral DNA loses its capacity to initiate a productive infection. If these cells do become activated, reverse transcription proceeds to completion and the virus continues along its replication cycle (see above and Fig. 309-15). The pool of cells that are in the postintegration state of latency are established early during the course of primary HIV infection. Despite the suppression of plasma viremia to below detectable levels (<50 copies of HIV RNA per milliliter) by potent combinations of several antiretroviral drugs for as long as 3 years, this pool of latently infected cells persists and can give rise to replication-competent virus. This persistent pool of latently infected cells is a major obstacle to any goal of eradication of virus from infected individuals.

Viral Dynamics   It was originally thought that very little virus replication occurred during clinical latency. However, studies of lymphoid tissue using PCR analysis for HIV RNA and in situ hybridization for individual virus-expressing cells clearly demonstrated that

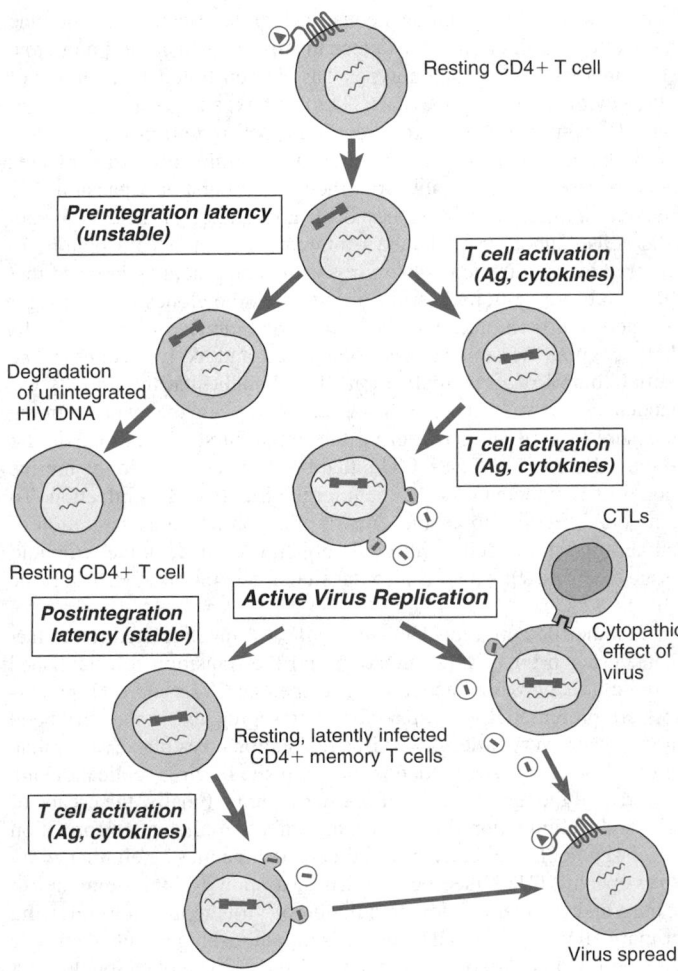

FIGURE 309-15 Generation of latently infected, resting CD4+ T cells in HIV-infected individuals. See text for details; Ag, antigen; CTLs, cytolytic T lymphocytes. *(Courtesy of TW Chun.)*

HIV replication occurs throughout the course of HIV infection, even during clinical latency when it is very difficult to culture virus from unfractionated peripheral blood mononuclear cells. The availability of sensitive PCR techniques led to the demonstration that some degree of plasma viremia is present in virtually all untreated patients at all stages of HIV disease. Subsequently, the dynamics of viral production and turnover were quantified using mathematical modeling in the setting of the administration of reverse transcriptase and protease inhibitors to HIV-infected individuals in clinical studies. Treatment with these drugs resulted in a precipitous decline in the level of plasma viremia, which typically fell by 99% within 2 weeks. The number of CD4+ T cells in the blood increased concurrently, which implies that the killing of CD4+ T cells is linked directly to the levels of replicating virus. However, it is generally agreed that a significant component of the early rise in CD4+ T cell numbers following the initiation of therapy is due to the redistribution of cells into the peripheral blood from other body compartments. It was determined on the basis of the emergence of resistant mutants during therapy that 93 to 99% of the circulating virus originated from recently infected, rapidly turning over CD4+ T cells and that approximately 1 to 7% of circulating virus originated from longer-lived cells, likely monocyte/macrophages. A negligible amount of circulating virus originated from the pool of latently infected cells (see above) (Fig. 309-16). It was also determined that the half-life of a circulating virion was approximately 30 min and that of productively infected cells was 1 day. Given the relatively steady level of plasma viremia and of infected cells, it appears that extremely large amounts of virus (approximately 10^{10} to 10^{11} virions)

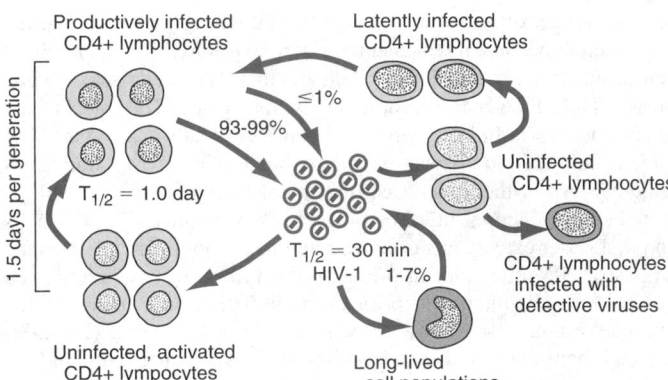

FIGURE 309-16 Dynamics of HIV infection in vivo. See text for detailed description. *(From Perelson et al, 1996.)*

are produced and cleared from the circulation each day. In addition, data suggest that the minimum duration of the HIV-1 replication cycle in vivo averages 1.5 days. Other studies have demonstrated that the decrease in plasma viremia that results from antiretroviral therapy correlates closely with a decrease in virus replication in lymph nodes, further confirming that lymphoid tissue is the main site of HIV replication and the main source of plasma viremia. Using a mathematical formula that assumed a two-phase decay of virus-infected cells, it was originally estimated that virus could be eradicated within 2.3 to 3.1 years from an HIV-infected individual who was receiving antiretroviral therapy that successfully suppressed all virus replication. However, recent data taking into account the pool of latently infected cells (see above) indicate that there is a third, much longer phase of decay that results in a projected time to viral eradication ranging from 10 to 60 years. Concomitant with this finding was the realization that even the most potent combinations of antiretroviral drugs did not completely suppress virus replication, as indicated by the detection of variable degress of cell-associated HIV RNA by sensitive PCR assays in most patients despite the absence of detectable plasma virema. Therefore, it is highly unlikely that virus will be eradicated from HIV-infected individuals with the currently available antiretoviral drugs despite the favorable clinical outcomes that have resulted from such therapy (see below).

The level of steady-state viremia, called the viral *set point*, at approximately 1 year has important prognostic implications for the progression of HIV disease. It has been demonstrated that HIV-infected individuals who have a low set point at 6 months to 1 year progress to AIDS much more slowly than individuals whose set point is very high at that time (Fig. 309-17). Levels of viremia generally increase

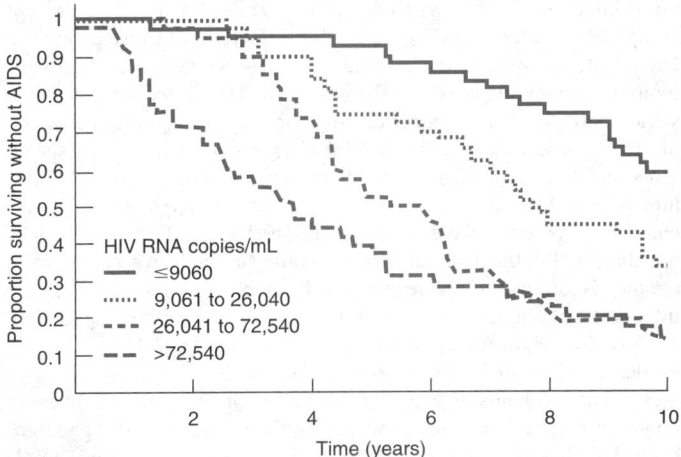

FIGURE 309-17 Relationship between levels of virus and rates of disease progression. Kaplan-Meier curves for AIDS-free survival stratified by baseline HIV-1 RNA categories (copies per milliliter). *(From Mellors et al.)*

as disease progresses. Measurement of the level of viremia is playing an increasingly important role in guiding therapeutic decisions in HIV-infected individuals (see below).

309 HIV: AIDS and Related Disorders **1865**

Immunopathogenic Events during Clinical Latency With few exceptions, the level of CD4+ T cells in the blood decreases gradually and progressively in HIV-infected individuals. The slope of this decline, together with the level of plasma viremia (see above), predict well the pattern of the clinical course and the development of advanced disease. Most patients are entirely asymptomatic while this progressive decline is taking place (see below) and are often described as being in a state of *clinical latency*. However, clinical latency does not mean disease latency, since progression is generally relentless during this period. Furthermore, clinical latency should not be confused with microbiologic latency. Although there are cells present in an infected individual that are latently infected and do not express detectable viral RNA, there is virtually always some degree of ongoing virus replication, even during the early stages of HIV disease.

ADVANCED HIV DISEASE In untreated patients or in patients in whom therapy has not adequately controlled virus replication (see below), after a variable period, usually measured in years, the CD4+ T cell count falls below a critical level (<200 cells per microliter), and the patient becomes highly susceptible to opportunistic disease (Fig. 309-14). For this reason, the CDC case definition of AIDS was modified to include all HIV-infected individuals with CD4+ T cell counts below this level (Table 309-1). Patients may experience constitutional signs and symptoms or may develop an opportunistic disease abruptly without any prior symptoms, although the latter scenario is unusual. The depletion of CD4+ T cells continues to be progressive and unrelenting in this phase. It is not uncommon for CD4+ T cell counts to drop as low as $10/\mu$L or even to zero, yet the patients may survive for months or even for >1 year. This situation has become increasingly common as patients are treated more aggressively and are given prophylaxis against the common life-threatening opportunistic infections (see below). In addition, control of plasma viremia by antiretroviral therapy, even in individuals with extremely low CD4+ T cell counts, has increased survival in these patients despite the fact that their CD4+ T cell counts may not significantly increase as a result of therapy. Ultimately, patients who progress to this severest form of immunodeficiency usually succumb to opportunistic infections or neoplasms (see below).

LONG-TERM SURVIVORS AND LONG-TERM NON-PROGRESSORS The median time from primary HIV infection to the development of AIDS in untreated individuals is approximately 10 years. Treatment with effective combinations of antiretroviral drugs has clearly extended this period; the full extent of this benefit has yet to be realized. The definitions of *long-term survivor* and *long-term nonprogressor* continue to evolve as more data are collected from prospective cohort studies. Predictions from one study that antedated the availability of effective antiretroviral therapy estimated that approximately 13% of homosexual/bisexual men who were infected at an early age may remain free of clinical AIDS for >20 years. Currently, individuals are considered to be long-term survivors if they remain alive for 10 to 15 years after initial infection. In most such individuals the disease has progressed, in that they have significant immunodeficiency, and many have experienced opportunistic diseases. Some of these individuals have CD4+ T cell counts that have decreased to $\leq 200/\mu$L but have remained stable at that level for years. The mechanisms of this stabilization are not entirely clear but may relate to the beneficial effects of antiretroviral therapy and prophylaxis against opportunistic infections. In addition, a number of viral and/or host determinants likely contribute to the long-term survival of these individuals. In some individuals, the virus may either have been less virulent initially or may have mutated to a less virulent form under the influence of antiretroviral therapy. Quantitative and qualitative aspects of the HIV-specific immune response, as well as recognized and unrecognized genetic factors (see below), may also contribute to the long-term survival of these individuals.

Fewer than 5% of HIV-infected individuals are characterized as long-term nonprogressors. All long-term nonprogressors are long-term survivors; however, the reverse is not true. Individuals who have been infected with HIV for a long period ($\geq$10 years), whose CD4+ T cell counts are in the normal range and have remained stable over years, and who have not received antiretroviral therapy are considered to be long-term nonprogressors. These patients are characterized by a low viral burden (low number of HIV-infected cells), low levels of plasma viremia, generally normal immune function according to commonly measured parameters (skin tests, in vitro lymphocyte responses to various mitogens and antigens), and normal-appearing lymphoid tissue architecture as determined on lymph node biopsy. In general, long-term nonprogressors manifest robust HIV-specific immune responses, both humoral (neutralizing antibodies) and cell-mediated (HIV-specific CTLs). However, this may also be true of some individuals early in the course of disease who ultimately progress to advanced disease. Although viremia is consistently very low in long-term nonprogressors, many have persistent viremia as determined by sensitive PCR assays. No qualitative abnormalities in the virus have been detected in most of these patients. However, a small subset of patients do have defective virus; in particular, in one cohort of five long-term nonprogressors, the virus had a defect in the *nef* gene. In another report, a blood donor in Australia who was HIV-infected and a group of seven individuals who were infected by blood or blood products from that donor remained free of HIV-related disease and maintained normal and stable CD4+ T cell counts for several years after infection. Sequence analysis of viruses isolated from the donor and recipients revealed similar deletions in the *nef* gene and the region of overlap of *nef* and the U3 region of the HIV long terminal repeat (Fig. 309-5). However, several of these individuals have now begun to show indications of progressive immunodeficiency, and thus they can no longer be considered nonprogressors. The precise role of host factors in long-term nonprogression remains unclear. There is no obvious and consistent genetic determinant for nonprogression. However, several genetic mutations have been demonstrated to result in a delay in the progression of HIV disease. These include heterozygosity for the *CCR5-Δ32* deletion, heterozygosity for the *CCR2-64I* mutation, homozygosity for the *SDF1-3$'$A* mutation, and heterozygosity for the *RANTES-28G* mutation (see "Genetic Factors in HIV Pathogenesis," below). Since CCR5 is the major co-receptor for R5 or macrophage-tropic strains of HIV and since individuals who are homozygous for the *CCR5-Δ32* deletion are, with rare exceptions, protected against HIV infection, the potential mechanism for slow progression in heterozygotes is clear. In addition, certain single nucleotide polymorphisms in the *CCR5* promoter have been shown to be associated with slower progression of disease. The reason for the slowing of progression of HIV disease in individuals who are heterozygous for the *CCR2-64I* mutation is less clear; however, it has been demonstrated that CXCR4 can dimerize with the CCR2V64I mutant but not with wild-type CCR2. This dimerization may reduce the amount of CXCR4 on the cell surface and as a result inhibit infection with X4 viruses. Homozygosity for the *SDF1-3$'$A* mutation may upregulate the *SDF1* gene enabling SDF-1, which is the natural ligand for CXCR4, to compete more effectively with X4 or T cell tropic virus for the CXCR4 coreceptor. The *RANTES-28G* mutation increases RANTES expression, which is the natural ligand for CCR5 and may thus inhibit infection with R5 viruses. Finally, maximal HLA heterozygosity of class I loci (A, B, and C) has been shown to be associated with delayed progression of HIV disease. Although long-term nonprogressors have robust HIV-specific immune responses as well as competent CD8+ T cell suppressors of HIV replication, it is unclear whether these factors are directly responsible for the state of nonprogression. A substantial proportion of HIV-infected individuals manifest comparable immune responses early in the course of their disease and still experience disease progression. Long-term nonprogressors likely represent a heterogeneous group. The lack of disease progression may be explained in some by a defect in the virus; in others by any of a variety of host factors, including recognized and as yet unrecognized genetic factors; and in others by a combination of both.

ROLE OF LYMPHOID ORGANS IN HIV PATHO-GENESIS Lymphoid tissues are the major anatomic sites for the establishment and propagation of HIV infection (see above). For practical reasons, most studies on the pathogenesis of HIV infection have focused on peripheral blood mononuclear cells. However, lymphocytes in the peripheral blood represent only approximately 2% of the total body lymphocyte pool and so may not always accurately reflect the status of the entire immune system; most of the body's lymphocytes reside in lymphoid organs, such as the lymph nodes, spleen, and gut-associated lymphoid tissue. Furthermore, virus replication occurs mainly in lymphoid tissue and not in blood; the level of plasma viremia reflects virus production in lymphoid tissue. Finally, since HIV disease is an infectious disease of the immune system, it is critical to appreciate the pathogenic events that occur in the lymphoid tissue in HIV infection.

Some patients experience progressive generalized lymphadenopathy (see below) early in the course of the infection; others experience varying degrees of transient lymphadenopathy. Lymphadenopathy reflects the cellular activation and immune response to the virus in the lymphoid tissue, which is generally characterized by follicular or germinal-center hyperplasia. Lymph node involvement is a common denominator of virtually all patients with HIV infection, even those without easily detectable lymphadenopathy.

Simultaneous examination of lymph node and peripheral blood in the same patients during various stages of HIV disease, including the early asymptomatic stage (when CD4+ T cell counts generally are >500/μL), the intermediate stage (when counts are usually 200 to 500/μL) and the advanced stage (when counts are <200/μL) has led to substantial insight into the pathogenesis of HIV disease. Using a combination of PCR techniques for HIV DNA and RNA in tissue and RNA in plasma, in situ hybridization for HIV RNA, and light and electron microscopy, the following picture has emerged. In most untreated patients, early in the course of infection when the viral set point has been reached and prior to significant immunodeficiency (CD4+ T cell counts >500/μL), levels of plasma viremia are variable but generally low; the viral burden (number of infected cells) in the peripheral blood is usually extremely low, and expression of HIV in these cells is minimal or undetectable. Remarkably, at this time copious amounts of extracellular virions are trapped on the processes of the follicular dendritic cells (FDCs) in the germinal centers of the lymph nodes (Fig. 309-18A). In situ hybridization reveals expression of virus in individual cells of the paracortical area and, to a lesser extent, the germinal center (Fig. 309-18B). The number of cells expressing virus is low early in the course of disease and increases as disease progresses. Examination of lymph nodes during primary HIV infection in humans (see above) and SIV infection in macaques indicates that during the transition from primary infection to established chronic infection, germinal centers form and virus is trapped. This trapping, together with the generation of a vigorous HIV-specific immune response, likely contributes to the rapid decrease in plasma viremia seen in most patients following the initial burst of viremia associated with primary infection. A considerable amount of virus can be trapped during the period of high viremia associated with primary infection. The persistence of trapped virus after chronic infection likely reflects a steady state whereby trapped virus turns over and is replaced by fresh virions, which are produced persistently, albeit usually at low levels during the early, clinically latent stage of disease.

During early-stage HIV disease, the architecture of the germinal centers is generally preserved and may even be hyperplastic owing to in situ proliferation of cells (mostly B lymphocytes) and recruitment to the lymph nodes of a number of cell types (B cells, CD4+ and CD8+ T cells). Electron microscopy demonstrates a fine network of FDCs with many long, finger-like processes that envelop virtually every lymphocyte in the germinal center (Fig. 309-18C). Extracellular virions can be seen attached to the processes, yet the FDCs appear to be rel-

atively healthy. The trapping of antigen is a physiologically normal function for the FDCs, which present antigen to B cells and contribute to the generation of B cell memory. However, in the case of HIV, the trapped virions serve as a persistent source of cellular activation, resulting in the secretion of proinflammatory cytokines such as interleukin (IL) 1β, tumor necrosis factor (TNF)α, and IL-6, which can up-regulate virus replication in infected cells (see below). Furthermore, although trapped virus is coated by neutralizing antibodies, it has been demonstrated that these virions remain infectious for CD4+ T cells while attached to the processes of the FDCs. CD4+ T cells that migrate into the germinal center to provide help to B cells in the generation of an HIV-specific immune response thus are susceptible to infection by these trapped virions. Thus, in HIV infection, a normal physiologic function of the immune system, which contributes to the clearance of virus as well as to the generation of a specific immune response, can also have deleterious consequences. It is difficult to demonstrate infection of the FDCs at this point, or even in advanced disease; however, rare examples of virus budding off FDCs have been reported.

As the disease progresses, the architecture of the germinal centers begins to show disruption, and the trapping efficiency of the lymph node diminishes. Electron microscopy reveals swollen organelles, and the FDCs begin to undergo cell death. The mechanisms of FDC death remain unclear; there is no indication by electron microscopy of copious virus replication or budding of virions off the cell in great quantities. At this stage, the level of plasma viremia generally increases. In addition, both the relative number of infected cells in the blood and the expression of virus from these cells increases, approaching the levels in the lymph nodes. As the disease progresses to an advanced stage, there is complete disruption of the architecture of the germinal centers, accompanied by dissolution of the FDC network and massive dropout of FDCs (Fig. 309-18D). The trapping function of the lymph nodes is completely lost, and virus freely spills out into the circulation. Simultaneous PCR analysis of lymph node and peripheral blood mononuclear cells indicates that the relative number of infected cells in the blood and their expression of virus begin to equal the levels in the lymph nodes at this stage. Advanced disease is accompanied by high levels of plasma viremia, which represent a true increase in virus replication, due in part to a further diminution of immune control of virus replication (see below) as well as to the loss of the mechanical trapping function of the lymph nodes. At this point, the lymph nodes are "burnt out." This destruction of lymphoid tissue compounds the immunodeficiency of HIV disease and contributes to the inability to mount adequate immune responses against opportunistic pathogens. The events from primary infection to the ultimate destruction of the immune system are illustrated in Fig. 309-19.

ROLE OF CELLULAR ACTIVATION IN HIV PATHOGENESIS The immune system is normally in a state of homeostasis, awaiting perturbation by foreign antigenic stimuli. Activation of the immune system is an essential component of an appropriate immune response to a foreign antigen. Once the immune response deals with and clears the antigen, the system returns to relative quiescence (Chap. 305). In HIV infection, however, the immune system is chronically activated owing to the chronicity of infection and the persistence of virus replication (see above). This activated state is reflected by hyperactivation of B cells leading to hypergammaglobulinemia; spontaneous lymphocyte proliferation; activation of monocytes; expression of activation markers on CD4+ and CD8+ T cells; lymph node hyperplasia, particularly early in the course of disease (see above); increased secretion of proinflammatory cytokines (see below); elevated levels of neopterin, β_2-microglobulin, acid-labile interferon, and soluble IL-2 receptors; and autoimmune phenomena (see below). Even in the absence of direct infection of a target cell, HIV envelope proteins can interact with cellular receptors (CD4 molecules and chemokine receptors) to deliver potent activation signals resulting in calcium flux, the phosphorylation of certain proteins involved in signal transduction, co-localization of cytoplasmic proteins including those involved in cell trafficking, secretion of certain cytokines, immune dysfunction, and under certain circumstances, apoptosis (see below).

A

B

C

D

FIGURE 309-18 HIV in the lymph nodes of HIV-infected individuals. *A*. Cervical lymph node from an asymptomatic individual with very low levels of plasma viremia. In situ hybridization using a molecular probe for HIV RNA reveals copious virus demarcating the numerous germinal centers (bright areas) of the node. The virus was extracellular and bound to the processes of the follicular dendritic cells (FDCs), which form a matrix within the confines of the germinal centers. Original ×25. *B*. Individual cells infected with HIV. Two cells in the paracortical area of the lymph node are shown expressing HIV RNA by in situ hybridization using a radiolabeled molecular probe. Original ×250. *C*. FDCs in cervical node of an asymptomatic HIV-infected individual.

Electron microscopy reveals an FDC with a prominent nucleolus surrounded by several lymphocytes within the germinal center of the node. Higher magnification of several fields indicates that multiple processes of the FDCs are in contact with several lymphocytes. Original ×1920. *D*. Dissolution of FDCs in the germinal center of a cervical lymph node from a patient with advanced HIV disease. Widespread death of FDCs is associated with a loss of ability of the lymph node to trap virus late in the course of HIV disease. Original ×3744. *(A and B courtesy of Dr. Cecil Fox; C and D courtesy of Dr. Jan Orenstein. Adapted from G Pantaleo et al: N Engl J Med 328:327, 1993.)*

Persistent immune activation may have several deleterious consequences. From a virologic standpoint, although quiescent CD4+ T cells can be infected with HIV, reverse transcription, integration, and virus spread are much more efficient in activated cells. Furthermore, cellular activation induces expression of virus in cells latently infected with HIV (see above). From an immunologic standpoint, chronic exposure of the immune system to a particular antigen over an extended period may ultimately lead to an inability to sustain an adequate immune response to the antigen. Furthermore, the ability of the immune system to respond to a broad spectrum of antigens may be compromised if immune-competent cells are maintained in a state of chronic activation. In addition, activation of the immune system may favor the elimination of cells via programmed cell death (apoptosis) (see below) as well as the secretion of certain cytokines that can induce HIV expression (see below).

Role of Apoptosis *Apoptosis* is a form of programmed cell death that is a normal mechanism for the elimination of effete cells in organogenesis as well as in the cellular proliferation that occurs during a normal immune response (Chap. 305). Apoptosis is strictly dependent on cellular activation. It has been hypothesized that, in HIV infection, sequential activation signals delivered to CD4+ T cells induce apoptosis. Cross-linking of the CD4 molecule by gp120 or gp120/anti-gp120 complexes delivers the first of two signals required for apoptosis. The second signal supposedly leading to cell death is delivered via the T cell receptor by antigen. According to this hypothesis, direct infection of CD4+ T cells is not required for apoptosis to occur, although it has been demonstrated that alterations in tyrosine kinase activity of HIV-infected cells may induce the cell to undergo apoptosis. HIV can trigger both Fas-dependent and Fas-independent pathways of apoptosis. Mechanisms involved in this process include upregulation of Fas and Fas ligand, upregulation of caspase-1 and caspase-8, downregulation of the anti-apoptotic Bcl-2 protein, and activation of cyclin-dependent kinases. Certain viral gene products have been associated with enhanced susceptibility to apoptosis including envelope, Nef, and Vpu. A number of studies, including those examining lymphoid tissue, have demonstrated that the rate of apoptosis is elevated in HIV infection and that apoptosis is seen in "bystander" cells such as CD8+ T cells and B cells as well as in CD4+ T cells.

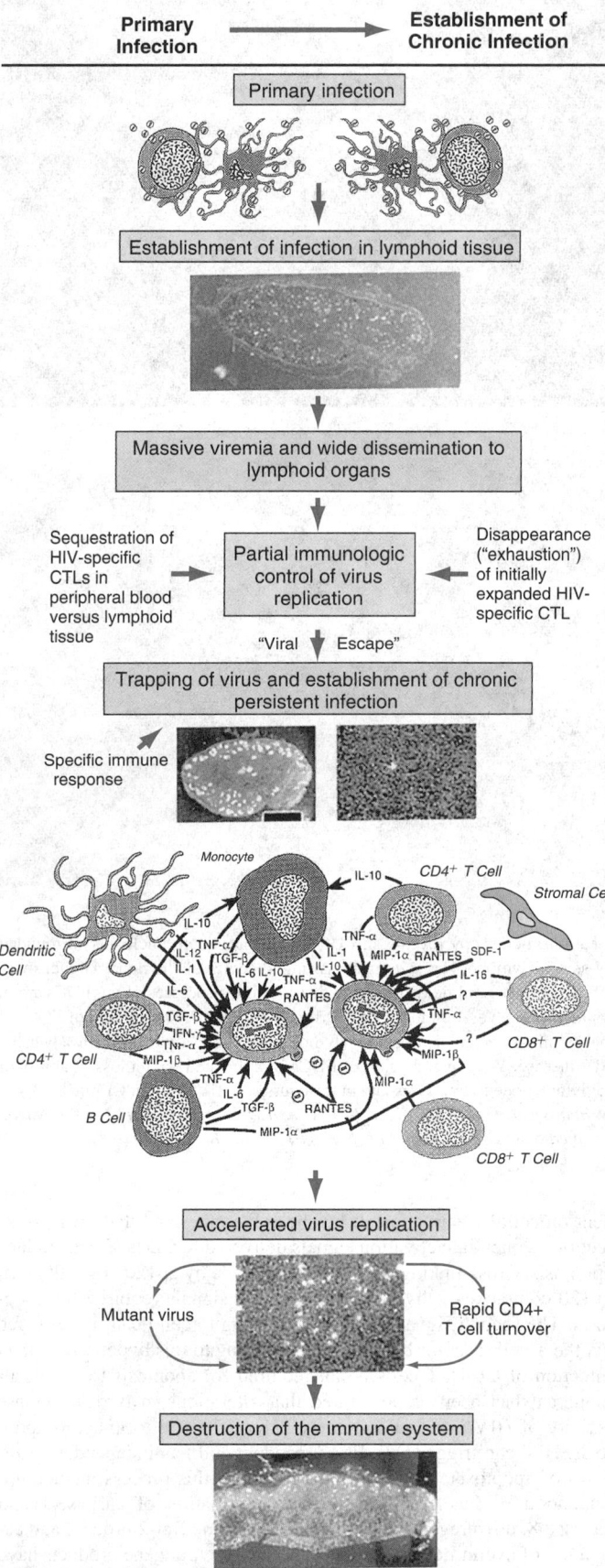

FIGURE 309-19 Events that transpire from primary HIV infection through the establishment of chronic persistent infection to the ultimate destruction of the immune system. See text for details; CTLs, cytolytic T lymphocytes.

Macrophages have been shown to mediate apoptosis of CD8+ T cells by a mechanism involving gp120-induced upregulation of Fas ligand expression on macrophages and enhanced secretion of macrophage-derived TNF-α. The intensity of apoptosis correlates with the general state of activation of the immune system and not with the stage of disease or with viral burden. The potential role of apoptosis in the pathogenesis of HIV disease is underscored by results from animal studies that show an increased frequency of apoptosis in CD4+ T cells in primates infected with pathogenic strains of SIV but not in primates infected with nonpathogenic strains of SIV. It is likely that apoptosis of immune-competent cells contributes to the immune abnormalities in HIV disease; however, this is probably a nonspecific mechanism that merely reflects the aberrant state of immune activation.

Autoimmune Phenomena The autoimmune phenomena that are common in HIV-infected individuals reflect, at least in part, chronic immune system activation as well as molecular mimickry by viral components. Although these phenomena usually occur in the absence of autoimmune disease, a wide spectrum of clinical manifestations that may be associated with autoimmunity have been described (see below). Autoimmune phenomena include antibodies to lymphocytes and, less commonly, to platelets and neutrophils. Antiplatelet antibodies have some clinical relevance, in that they may contribute to the thrombocytopenia of HIV disease (see below). Antibodies to nuclear and cytoplasmic components of cells have been reported, as have antibodies to cardiolipin; CD4 molecules; CD43 molecules, C1q-A; variable regions of the T cell receptor α, β, and γ chains; Fas; denatured collagen; and IL-2. In addition, autoantibodies to a range of serum proteins, including albumin, immunoglobulin, and thyroglobulin, have been reported. There is antigenic cross-reactivity between HIV viral proteins (gp120 and gp41) and MHC class II determinants, and anti-MHC class II antibodies have been reported in HIV infection. These antibodies could potentially lead to the elimination of MHC class II–bearing cells via antibody-dependent cellular cytotoxicity (ADCC) (Chap. 305). In addition, regions of homology exist between HIV envelope glycoproteins and IL-2 as well as MHC class I molecules.

Cofactors Contributing to HIV Pathogenesis Both endogenous and exogenous factors can contribute to HIV pathogenesis by a number of mechanisms; paramount among these is the upregulation of virus expression, a process intimately connected with cellular activation. The main endogenous factors that regulate HIV expression are cytokines (see below). Among exogenous factors, other microbes likely have important effects on HIV replication and HIV pathogenesis. They can thus be considered real or potential *cofactors* in the pathogenesis of HIV disease. Co-infection or simultaneous cotransfection of cells with HIV and other viruses or viral genes has demonstrated that certain viruses, such as HSV type 1, cytomegalovirus (CMV), human herpesvirus (HHV) 6, Epstein-Barr virus (EBV), hepatitis B virus (HBV), adenovirus, pseudorabies virus, and HTLV-I can upregulate HIV expression. Other microbes, such as *Mycoplasma* have been reported to contribute to the induction of HIV expression. *Mycobacterium tuberculosis* is a common opportunistic infection in HIV-infected individuals (see below and Chap. 169). In addition to the fact that HIV-infected individuals are more likely to develop active TB after exposure, it has been demonstrated that active TB can accelerate the course of HIV infection. It has also been shown that levels of plasma viremia are greatly elevated in HIV-infected individuals with active TB, compared to pre-TB levels and levels of viremia after successful treatment of the active TB. In vitro studies demonstrated that virus replication was markedly enhanced in lymphocytes of HIV-infected individuals who were skin test–positive for purified protein derivative (PPD) when PPD antigen was added to culture, resulting in cellular activation. Confirmatory evidence that antigen-induced activation was a major contributor to the accelerated viremia in HIV-infected individuals with active TB was provided by studies in which HIV-infected individuals were immunized with common recall antigens such as tetanus toxoid, influenza, or pneumococcal polysaccharide. Under these circumstances, a transient elevation of plasma viremia accompanied the cellular activation induced by the immunization. A greater degree of induction of virus was seen in those individuals with early stage as opposed to advanced stage HIV disease, and the degree of virus induction correlated with the level of immune system activation.

THE CYTOKINE NETWORK IN HIV PATHOGENESIS

Cytokine Regulation of HIV Expression The immune system is homeostatically regulated by a complex network of immunoregulatory cytokines, which are pleiotropic and redundant and operate in an autocrine and paracrine manner. They are expressed continuously, even during periods of apparent quiescence of the immune system. On perturbation of the immune system by antigenic challenge, the expression of cytokines increases to varying degrees (Chap. 305). Cytokines that are important components of this immunoregulatory network have been demonstrated to play a major role in the regulation of HIV expression in vitro. A number of in vitro model systems of chronically infected monocyte or T cell lines, primary cultures of peripheral blood or lymph node mononuclear cells from HIV-infected individuals, and acutely infected primary cell cultures have been used to demonstrate the role of cytokines in the regulation of HIV expression. Potent modulation of HIV expression has been demonstrated either by manipulating endogenous cytokines or by adding exogenous cytokines to culture. Cytokines that induce HIV expression in one or more of these systems include IL-1, IL-2, IL-3, IL-6, IL-12, TNF-α, and TNF-β, macrophage colony stimulating factor (M-CSF), and granulocyte-macrophage colony stimulating factor (GM-CSF). Among these cytokines, the most consistent and potent inducers of HIV expression are the *proinflammatory cytokines* TNF-α, IL-1β, and IL-6. IFN-α and -β suppress HIV replication, whereas transforming growth factor (TGF) β, IL-4, IL-10, and IFN-γ can either induce or suppress HIV expression, depending on the system involved. The *CC-chemokines* RANTES, macrophage inflammatory protein (MIP) 1α, and MIP-1β (Chap. 305) inhibit infection by and spread of R5 (macrophage-tropic) HIV-1 strains, while *stromal cell–derived factor* (SDF) 1 inhibits infection by and spread of X4 (T cell–tropic) strains (see below). Several of these cytokines act synergistically in regulating HIV infection and replication, and others function in an autocrine and paracrine manner, similar to their physiologic function in the regulation of the immune system. Blocking of endogenous HIV-inducing cytokines or addition of inhibitors of HIV suppressor cytokines in cultures of peripheral blood and lymph node mononuclear cells from HIV-infected individuals has demonstrated that HIV replication is controlled tightly by endogenous cytokines acting in an autocrine and paracrine manner. Indeed, the net level of virus replication in an HIV-infected individual at least in part reflects a balance between inductive and suppressive host factors, mediated mainly by cytokines. An example of this endogenous regulation is the case of IL-10, which inhibits HIV replication in acutely infected monocyte/macrophages by blocking the secretion of the HIV-inducing cytokines TNF-α and IL-6. In addition, IL-4, IL-13, and TGF-β inhibit HIV expression in chronically infected monocytic cell lines stimulated by lipopolysaccharide and GM-CSF by increasing the ratio of expression of endogenous IL-1 receptor antagonist to IL-1β.

The molecular mechanisms of HIV regulation are best understood for TNF-α, which activates NF-κB proteins that function as transcriptional activators of HIV expression. The HIV-inducing effect of IL-1β is thought to occur at the level of viral transcription in an NF-κB-independent manner. IL-6, GM-CSF, and IFN-γ regulate HIV expression mainly by posttranscriptional mechanisms. Elevated levels of TNF-α and IL-6 have been demonstrated in plasma and cerebrospinal fluid (CSF), and increased expression of TNF-α, IL-1β, IFN-γ, and IL-6 has been demonstrated in the lymph nodes of HIV-infected individuals. The mechanisms whereby the CC-chemokines RANTES, MIP-1α, and MIP-1β inhibit infection of R5 strains of HIV very likely involve blocking of the binding of the virus to its co-receptor, the CC-chemokine receptor CCR5 (see above and below). Of note is the fact that CC-chemokines that inhibit infection by R5 strains of virus actually enhance infection by X4 strains of virus by inducing intracellular signal transduction through the CCR5 and CD4 molecules. In addition,

products of bacterial pathogens as well as of certain viruses including HIV-1 itself can induce the expression of CXCR4 and thus potentially favor infection with X4 strains of virus that utilize this co-receptor.

Dysregulation of Cytokines HIV-infected individuals show an imbalance in the T cell limbs of the immune response, which are defined by the patterns of cytokine secretion. T helper (T_H)1 cells are characterized by secretion of IL-2 and IFN-γ and favor cell-mediated immune responses, whereas T_H2 cells are characterized by secretion of IL-4, IL-5, and IL-10 and favor humoral immune responses (Chap. 305). Since several cell types in addition to CD4+ T cells secrete these cytokines, it is more accurate to refer to immune responses that reflect one or the other cytokine pattern as T_H1 or T_H2 type responses. HIV-infected individuals show a decrease in T_H1 type responses relative to T_H2 type cytokine patterns. They manifest a progressive loss in expression of the IL-2 receptor and in the ability to produce the immunoregulatory cytokines IL-2 and IL-12; these cytokines are critical for effective cell-mediated immune responses in that they stimulate proliferation and lytic activity of CTLs and natural killer (NK) cells. Furthermore, IL-12 is important for the stimulation of T_H1 type cytokines such as IL-2 and IFN-γ that favor the development of cell-mediated immune responses. T_H1 type cytokines such as IL-2, IL-12, TNF-α, and IFN-γ upregulate CCR5 expression, while T_H2 type cytokines such as IL-4 and IL-10 upregulate CXCR4 expression and downregulate CCR5 expression. It has also been demonstrated that in vitro apoptosis can be inhibited in T cells from HIV-infected donors by antibodies to IL-4 and IL-10 and enhanced by antibodies to IL-12. Although it has been proposed that a clear-cut switch from a T_H1 type to a T_H2 type of cytokine pattern is a critical step in the pathogenesis of HIV disease, no sharp dichotomy between these two types of cytokine patterns that is directly related to progression of disease has been corroborated. Cytokine dysregulation in HIV infection is complex and cannot be neatly classified in terms of the polarity of T_H1 and T_H2 responses.

CELLULAR TARGETS OF HIV

Although the CD4+ T lymphocytes and CD4+ cells of monocyte lineage are the principal targets of HIV, virtually any cell that expresses the CD4 molecule together with co-receptor molecules (see above and below) can potentially be infected with HIV. Circulating dendritic cells have been reported to express low levels of CD4, and depending on their stage of maturation, these cells can be infected with HIV (see below). Epidermal Langerhans cells express CD4 and have been infected by HIV in vivo. In vitro, HIV has been reported also to infect a wide range of cells and cell lines that express low levels of CD4, no detectable CD4, or only CD4 mRNA; among these are FDCs; megakaryocytes; eosinophils; astrocytes; oligodendrocytes; microglial cells; CD8+ T cells; B cells; NK cells; renal epithelial cells; cervical cells; rectal and bowel mucosal cells such as enterochromaffin, goblet, and columnar epithelial cells; trophoblastic cells; and cells from a variety of organs, such as liver, lung, heart, salivary gland, eye, prostate, testis, and adrenal gland. Since the only cells that have been shown unequivocally to be infected with HIV and to support replication of the virus are CD4+ T lymphocytes and cells of monocyte/macrophage lineage, the relevance of the in vitro infection of these other cell types is questionable.

Of potentially important clinical relevance is the demonstration that thymic precursor cells, which were assumed to be negative for CD3, CD4, and CD8 molecules, actually do express low levels of CD4 and can be infected with HIV in vitro. In addition, human thymic epithelial cells transplanted into an immunodeficient mouse can be infected with HIV by direct inoculation of virus into the thymus. Since these cells may play a role in the normal regeneration of CD4+ T cells, it is possible that their infection and depletion contribute, at least in part, to the impaired ability of the CD4+ T cell pool to completely reconstitute itself in certain infected individuals in whom antiretroviral therapy has suppressed viral replication to below detectable levels (<50 copies of HIV RNA per milliliter; see below). In addition, CD34+ monocyte precursor cells have been shown to be infected in

X4 (T-Tropic) Strain of HIV-1   R5 (M-Tropic) Strain of HIV-1

FIGURE 309-20 Model for the role of co-receptors CXCR4 and CCR5 in the efficient binding and entry of X4 (T cell–tropic) and R5 (macrophage-tropic) strains of HIV-1, respectively, into CD4+ target cells. Blocking of this initial event in the virus life cycle can be accomplished by inhibition of binding to the co-receptor by the normal ligand for the receptor in question. The ligand for CXCR4 is stromal cell–derived factor (SDF-1); the ligands for CCR5 are RANTES, MIP-1α, and MIP-1β.

vivo in patients with advanced HIV disease. It is likely that these cells express low levels of CD4, and therefore it is not essential to invoke CD4-independent mechanisms to explain the infection.

ROLE OF CO-RECEPTORS IN CELL TROPISM OF HIV Different strains of HIV-1 utilize two major co-receptors along with CD4 to bind to, fuse with, and enter target cells; these co-receptors are CCR5 and CXCR4, which are receptors for certain chemokines and belong to the seven-transmembrane-domain G protein–coupled family of receptors (see above). Strains of HIV that utilize CCR5 as a co-receptor are referred to as *R5 viruses*. These viruses were formerly classified as *macrophage tropic viruses* since they readily infect macrophages but not T cell lines. Strains of HIV that utilize CXCR4 are referred to as *X4 viruses*. These viruses are also referred to as *T cell–tropic viruses* since they readily infect T cell lines but not macrophages. In actuality, X4 viruses enter macrophages but do not proceed efficiently along the replication cycle unless an appropriate signal is delivered to the cell. Many virus strains are *dual tropic* in that they utilize both CCR5 and CXCR4; these are referred to as *R5X4 viruses*. Other terminology that has been associated with R5 versus X4 viruses is *non-syncytium-inducing viruses* versus *syncytium-inducing viruses*, respectively, based on the observation that R5 viruses generally do not form syncytia in culture with certain T cell lines, whereas X4 viruses readily form syncytia. In reality, under certain conditions both R5 and X4 viruses are capable of forming syncytia in culture.

The natural chemokine ligands for the major HIV co-receptors can readily block entry of HIV. For example, the CC-chemokines RANTES, MIP-1α, and MIP-1β, which are the natural ligands for CCR5, block entry of R5 viruses, whereas SDF-1, the natural ligand for CXCR4, blocks entry of X4 viruses. The mechanism of inhibition of viral entry is a steric inhibition of binding that is not dependent on signal transduction (Fig. 309-20).

The transmitting virus is almost invariably an R5 virus that predominates during the early stages of HIV disease. In approximately 40% of HIV-infected individuals, there is a transition to a predominantly X4 virus that is associated with a relatively rapid progression of disease. However, at least 60% of infected individuals progress in their disease while maintaining predominance of an R5 virus. Other chemokine receptor family members may function as coreceptors for HIV and SIV entry, but to a much lesser extent than do CCR5 and CXCR4; these include CCR3, BOB/GPR15, Bonzo/STRL33/TYMSTR, CCR2, CCR8, CX$_3$CR1(V28), and GPR1.

The basis for the tropism of different envelope glycoproteins for either CCR5 or CXCR4 relates to the ability of the HIV envelope, particularly the third variable region (V3 loop) of gp120, to interact with these co-receptors. In this regard, binding of gp120 to CD4 induces a conformational change in gp120 that increases its affinity for CCR5. It appears that the interaction of gp120 with CXCR4 is less

dependent on the conformational change induced in gp120 by CD4. In fact, there are X4 strains of HIV that bind to CXCR4 in the absence of surface-bound or soluble CD4. Finally, R5 viruses are more efficient in infecting monocyte/macrophages and microglial cells of the brain (see "Neuropathogenesis," below).

ABNORMALITIES OF MONONU-CLEAR CELLS CD4+ T Cells The range of T cell abnormalities in advanced HIV infection is broad. The defects are both quantitative and qualitative and involve virtually every limb of the immune system (see below), indicating the critical dependence of the integrity of the immune system on the inducer/helper function of CD4+ T cells. Virtually all of the immune defects in advanced HIV disease can ultimately be explained by the quantitative depletion of CD4+ T cells. However, T cell dysfunction (see below) can be demonstrated in patients early in the course of infection, even when the CD4+ T cell count is in the low-normal range. The degree and spectrum of dysfunctions increase as the disease progresses. One of the first abnormalities to be detected is a defect in response to remote recall antigens, such as tetanus toxoid and influenza, at a time when mononuclear cells can still respond normally to mitogenic stimulation. Defects in responses to soluble antigens are followed in time by the loss of T cell proliferative responses to alloantigens, and subsequently to mitogens. Essentially every T cell function has been reported to be abnormal at some stage of HIV infection. These abnormalities include defective T cell cloning and colony-forming efficiencies, impaired expression of IL-2 receptors, defective IL-2 production, and decreased IFN-γ production in response to antigens. The proportion of CD4+ T cells that express CD28, which is a major co-stimulatory molecule necessary for the normal activation of T cells, is reduced during HIV infection. Cells lacking expression of CD28 do not respond to activation signals and may express markers of terminal activation including HLA-DR, CD38, and CD45RO. CD4+ T cells from HIV-infected individuals express abnormally low levels of CD40 ligand, which may explain the dysregulation of B cell function observed in HIV disease.

It is difficult to explain completely the profound immunodeficiency noted in HIV-infected individuals solely on the basis of direct infection and quantitative depletion of CD4+ T cells. This is particularly apparent during the early stages of HIV disease, when CD4+ T cell numbers may be only marginally decreased. Certainly, at the stage of advanced disease when the CD4+ T cell count is in the range of 0 to 50/μL, quantitative depletion alone can explain the immune defects. However, it is likely that CD4+ T cell dysfunction results from a combination of depletion of cells due to direct infection and a number of virus-related but indirect effects on the cell (Table 309-6).

Single-cell killing and the formation of syncytia between infected and uninfected cells have been demonstrated clearly in vitro, although

Table 309-6 Mechanisms of CD4+ T Cell Dysfunction and Depletion

Direct Mechanisms	Indirect Mechanisms
Accumulation of unintegrated viral DNA	Aberrant intracellular signaling events
Interference with cellular RNA processing	Syncytium formation
	Autoimmunity
Intracellular gp120-CD4 autofusion events	Innocent bystander killing of viral antigen–coated cells
Loss of plasma membrane integrity due to viral budding	Apoptosis
Elimination of HIV-infected cells by virus-specific immune responses	Inhibition of lymphopoiesis

the precise mechanisms of cell death in vivo have not been determined. Cytopathicity in an infected cell in vitro may result from a number of mechanisms, including copious budding of virions from the cell surface with resulting disruption of the integrity of the cell membrane; interference with cellular RNA processing or the accumulation of high levels of heterodisperse RNA molecules; disruption of cellular protein synthesis owing to high levels of viral RNA; accumulation of high levels of unintegrated viral DNA in the cell cytoplasm; induction of aberrant patterns of protein tyrosine phosphorylation; and the interaction between HIV gp120 and CD4 intracellularly. Strain differences in single-cell killing are determined largely by gp120 sequences, which supports the importance of the viral envelope in this process. *Syncytia formation* involves fusion of the cell membrane of an infected cell with the cell membranes of variable numbers of uninfected CD4+ cells. Although cell fusion has not been shown to be an important pathogenic process in vivo, a direct relationship between the presence of syncytia and the degree of cytopathic effect has been demonstrated in vitro, and a correlation has been reported between the presence of virus isolates that readily induce syncytia in vitro and a more aggressive clinical course in the patient. Efficient syncytia formation depends on the leukocyte adhesion molecule LFA-1 (Chap. 305) on human CD4+ T cells acutely infected with HIV in vitro.

Humoral and cellular immune responses to HIV may contribute to protective immunity by eliminating virus and virus-infected cells (see below). However, since the main targets of HIV infection are immune-competent cells, these responses may contribute to immune-cell depletion and immunologic dysfunction by eliminating both infected cells and "innocent bystander" cells. Soluble viral proteins, particularly gp120, can bind with high affinity to the CD4 molecules on uninfected T cells and monocytes; in addition, virus and/or viral proteins can bind to dendritic cells or FDCs. HIV-specific antibody can recognize these bound molecules and potentially collaborate in the elimination of the cells by ADCC.

Nonpolymorphic determinants of MHC class I products share a degree of homology with gp120 and gp41 proteins of HIV. Such similarities may lead to the generation of autoantibodies to self-MHC determinants. In fact, anti-HLA-DR antibodies have been demonstrated in the sera of HIV-infected individuals (see "Autoimmune Phenomena," above). These antibodies could contribute to the elimination of HLA-DR–expressing cells by ADCC; in addition, it has been suggested that these antibodies may inhibit certain T cell functions that involve HLA-DR molecules.

HIV envelope glycoproteins gp120 and gp160 manifest high-affinity binding to CD4 as well as to various chemokine receptors (see above). Intracellular signals transduced by gp120 have been associated with a number of immunopathogenic processes including anergy, apoptosis, and abnormalities of cell trafficking. The molecular mechanisms responsible for these abnormalities include dysregulation of the T cell receptor–phosphoinositide pathway, p56lck activation, phosphorylation of focal adhesion kinase, activation of the MAP kinase and ras signaling pathways, and downregulation of the co-stimulatory molecules CD40 ligand and CD80.

Finally, the inexorable decline in CD4+ T cell counts that occurs in most HIV-infected individuals may result in part from the inability of the immune system to regenerate the CD4+ T cell pool rapidly enough to compensate for both HIV-mediated destruction of cells and natural attrition of cells. At least two major mechanisms may contribute to the failure of the CD4+ T cell pool to reconstitute itself adequately over the course of HIV infection. The first is the destruction of lymphoid precursor cells, including thymic and bone marrow progenitor cells (see above); the other is the gradual disruption of the lymphoid tissue microenvironment, which is essential for efficient regeneration of immune-competent cells (see above).

CD8+ T Cells The level of CD8+ T cells varies throughout the course of disease. Following the resolution of acute primary infection, CD8+ T cells generally rebound to higher than normal levels and may remain that way throughout the clinically latent stage of disease. This CD8+ T lymphocytosis may in part reflect the expansion of clones of HIV-specific CD8+ CTLs. During the late stages of HIV infection, there may be a significant reduction in the numbers of CD8+ T cells. HIV-specific CD8+ CTLs have been demonstrated in HIV-infected individuals early in the course of disease (see below). As the disease progresses, this functional capability decreases and may be lost entirely. The cause of this loss of cytolytic activity is unclear. However, it has been demonstrated that, as disease progresses, CD8+ T cells assume an abnormal phenotype characterized by expression of activation markers such as HLA-DR with an absence of expression of the IL-2 receptor (CD25) and a loss of clonogenic potential. It has been reported that the phenotype of CD8+ T cells in HIV-infected individuals may be of prognostic significance. Those individuals whose CD8+ T cells developed a phenotype of HLA-DR+/CD38− following seroconversion had stabilization of their CD4+ T cell counts, whereas those whose CD8+ T cells developed a phenotype of HLA-DR+/CD38+ had a more aggressive course and a poorer prognosis. In addition to the defects in HIV-specific CTLs, functional defects in other MHC-restricted CTLs, such as those directed against influenza and CMV, have been demonstrated. Since the integrity of CD8+ T cell function depends in part on adequate inductive signals from CD4+ T cells, the defect in CD8+ CTLs is likely compounded by the quantitative loss of CD4+ T cells.

B Cells B cells from HIV-infected individuals manifest abnormal activation, which is reflected by spontaneous proliferation and immunoglobulin secretion and by increased spontaneous secretion of TNF-α and IL-6. The enhanced spontaneous in vitro transformation of B cells with EBV is probably due to defective T cell immune surveillance and has as its in vivo counterpart an increase in the incidence of EBV-related B cell lymphomas. Untransformed B cells cannot be infected with HIV. However, HIV or its products can activate B cells directly; portions of the HIV gp41 envelope protein have been reported to induce polyclonal B cell activation. In addition, it has been reported that products of the VH$_3$ genes on the surface of B cells can serve as a receptor for HIV. It is likely that in vivo activation of B cells by virus products accounts at least in part for the spontaneous activation of these cells noted ex vivo. B cells from HIV-infected individuals express abnormally low levels of HLA-DR on their surface and fail to upregulate CD70 normally following stimulation with activated T cells; this latter defect is associated with impaired CD70-dependent immunoglobulin synthesis. In advanced HIV disease, B cells fail to proliferate and differentiate in response to ligation of the B cell antigen receptor and CD40, suggesting a defect in signal transduction. In vivo, this activated state manifests itself by hypergammaglobulinemia and by the presence of circulating immune complexes and autoantibodies (see above). HIV-infected individuals respond poorly to primary and secondary immunizations with protein and polysaccharide antigens. These B cell defects are likely responsible in part for the increase in certain bacterial infections seen in advanced HIV disease in adults, as well as for the important role of bacterial infections in the morbidity and mortality of HIV-infected children, who cannot mount an adequate humoral response to common bacterial pathogens. The absolute number of circulating B cells may be depressed in primary HIV infection; however, this phenomenon is usually transient and likely reflects in part a redistribution of cells out of the circulation and into the lymphoid tissue. In certain patients, the number of circulating B cells decreases in advanced-stage disease.

Monocyte/Macrophages Circulating monocytes are generally normal in number in HIV-infected individuals. Monocytes express the CD4 molecule and several co-receptors for HIV on their surface, including CCR5, CXCR4, and CCR3, and thus are targets of HIV infection. Of note is the fact that the degree of cytopathicity of HIV for cells of the monocyte lineage is low, and HIV can replicate extensively in cells of the monocyte lineage with little cytopathic effect. Hence, monocyte-lineage cells may play a role in the dissemination of HIV in the body and can serve as reservoirs of HIV infection, thus representing an obstacle to the eradication of HIV by antiretroviral drugs.

In vivo infection of circulating monocytes is difficult to demonstrate; however, infection of tissue macrophages and macrophage-lineage cells in the brain (infiltrating macrophages or resident microglial cells) and lung (pulmonary alveolar macrophages) can be demonstrated easily. Infection of monocyte precursors in the bone marrow may directly or indirectly be responsible for certain of the hematologic abnormalities in HIV-infected individuals. A number of abnormalities of circulating monocytes have been reported in HIV-infected individuals, including decreased secretion of IL-1 and IL-12; increased secretion of IL-10; defects in antigen presentation and induction of T cell responses due to decreased MHC class II expression; and abnormalities of Fc receptor function, C3 receptor–mediated clearance, oxidative burst responses, and certain cytotoxic functions such as ADCC, possibly related to low levels of expression of Fc and complement receptors. The mechanisms of the monocyte defects are uncertain but almost certainly cannot be even partly explained by direct infection with HIV. Exposure of monocytes to viral proteins such as gp120 and Tat, as well as to certain cytokines, can cause abnormal activation, and this may play a role in cellular dysfunction (see above).

Dendritic and Langerhans Cells There has been considerable disagreement regarding the HIV infectibility and hence the depletion as well as the dysfunction of circulating dendritic cells. Depending on their state of maturation, dendritic cells express varying levels of CD4 as well as several chemokine receptors. In this regard, it appears that the ability of a dendritic cell to become infected depends in part on its state of maturation. Mature dendritic cells have been demonstrated to be infectable by both R5 and X4 isolates of HIV-1. Immature tissue dendritic cells have been less well studied in their native state. Certain groups have reported infection and dysfunction of dendritic cells from HIV-infected individuals, particularly a decreased ability to present antigen to T cells, and other groups have found little if any HIV infection or functional abnormalities. In this regard, there is general agreement regarding the ability of skin and mucous membrane Langerhans cells to be infected (see above). These latter cells likely play an important role in the initiation and propagation of HIV infection (see above). Even in those dendritic cells in which infection occurs, the efficiency of infection and level of productivity of infection is quite low compared to CD4+ T cells.

Natural Killer Cells The role of NK cells is to provide immunosurveillance against virus-infected cells, certain tumor cells, and allogeneic cells (Chap. 305). Functional abnormalities in NK cells have been observed throughout the course of HIV disease, and the severity of these abnormalities increases as disease progresses. Most studies report that NK cells are normal in number and phenotype in HIV-infected individuals; however, a numerical decrease in the CD16+/CD56+ subpopulation of NK cells has been reported together with an increase in activation markers. The abnormality in NK cell function is thought to result from a defect in postbinding lysis. However, the lytic machinery does not appear to be impaired, since NK cells from HIV-infected individuals mediate ADCC normally. The addition of either IL-2, IL-12, IL-15, or IFN-α to cultures improves the defective in vitro NK cell function of HIV-infected individuals. Enhanced expression of cytolytic inhibitory receptors in HIV-infected individuals may contribute to the abnormalities in NK function. Furthermore, selective HIV-mediated downregulation of HLA-A and -B, but not HLA-C and -D molecules may inhibit NK-mediated killing of HIV-infected target cells. Finally, NK cells serve as important sources of HIV-inhibitory CC-chemokines. NK cells isolated from HIV-infected individuals constitutively produce high levels of MIP-1α, MIP-1β, and RANTES. In addition, high levels of these chemokines are seen when NK cells are stimulated with IL-2 or IL-15 or when CD16 is cross-linked or during the process of lytic killing of target cells.

GENETIC FACTORS IN HIV PATHOGENESIS Several reports have described MHC alleles and other host factors that may influence the pathogenesis and course of HIV disease. These include associations with certain HIV-related manifestations, such as KS and diffuse lymphadenopathy, or with the type of clinical course, such as long-term survival or rapid progression (Table 309-7). A number of mechanisms have been proposed whereby MHC-encoded molecules might predispose an individual either to rapid progression or to nonprogression to AIDS. These proposed mechanisms include the ability to present certain immunodominant HIV T helper or CTL epitopes, leading to a relatively protective immune response against HIV and hence to slow progression of disease. In contrast, certain MHC class I or class II alleles might predispose an individual to an immunopathogenic response against viral epitopes in certain tissues, such as the central nervous system (CNS) or lungs, or against certain HIV-infected cell types, such as macrophages or dendritic cells/Langerhans cells. In addition, certain rare MHC class I and class II alleles might facilitate rapid recognition of HIV-infected cells from the infecting partner in primary HIV infection and promote rejection of these cells by alloreactive responses. Similarly, common MHC alleles could lead to less effective removal of HIV-infected allogeneic cells. It has been clearly demonstrated that maximal *HLA* heterozygosity for class I loci (A, B, and C) is associated with a delayed onset of AIDS among HIV-infected individuals, whereas homozygosity for these loci was associated with a more rapid progression to AIDS and death. This observation is likely due to the fact that individuals heterozygous at *HLA* loci are able to present a greater variety of antigenic peptides to cytotoxic T lymphocytes than are homozygotes resulting in a more effective immune response against a number of pathogens including HIV. Of particular note is the fact that the HLA class I alleles B*35 and Cw*04 were consistently associated with rapid development of AIDS. Other data have indicated that transporter associated with antigen-presenting (TAP) genes play a role in determining the outcome of HIV infection. HLA profiles that reflect certain combinations of MHC-encoded TAP and class I and class II genes are strongly associated with different rates of progression to AIDS.

Rare individuals have been reported who had had repetitive sexual exposure to HIV in high-risk situations but remained uninfected. The peripheral blood mononuclear cells of two such individuals were found to be highly resistant to infection in vitro with R5 strains of HIV-1, but they were readily infected with X4 strains. Genetic analysis revealed that these two individuals inherited a homozygous defect in the gene that codes for CCR5, the cellular co-receptor for R5 strains of HIV-1. The defective *CCR5* allele contained a 32-bp deletion corresponding to the second extracellular loop of the receptor. The encoded protein was severely truncated, and the receptor was nonfunctional, explaining the refractoriness to infection with R5 strains of HIV-1. Population studies revealed that approximately 1% of the Caucasian population of western European ancestry possessed the homozygous defect. Up to 20% of this group had the heterozygous defect. Of note, cohort studies of hundreds of DNA samples originating from western and central Africa and Japan did not reveal a single mutant allele, suggesting that the allele is either absent or extremely rare in Africa and Japan. In a cohort of 1400 HIV-1–infected Caucasian individuals, no subject homozygous for the mutation was found, strongly supporting the concept that the homozygous defect confers protection against infection. This finding is particularly compelling in light of the fact that transmitting viruses are strongly biased towards R5 strains of HIV-1 (see above). Furthermore, there was a higher frequency of individuals heterozygous for the genetic defect among HIV-infected patients who were long-term nonprogressors compared to HIV-infected individuals who progressed more rapidly (see above). Of note, several individuals have been identified who were homozygous for the *CCR5* Δ32 defect who in fact did become infected with HIV. These individuals were found to have an X4 strain of HIV that was associated in some cases with an accelerated course of disease. Slow progression of HIV disease is also seen in individuals who are heterozygous for the *CCR2V64I* mutation; this is felt to be due to dimerization of CXCR4 with the mutated CCR2V64I resulting in a decreased expression of CXCR4 on the cell surface. Individuals who are homozygous for the *SDF1-3'A* mutation manifest slow progression, likely due to the upregulation of SDF-1 and resulting inhibition of binding of X4 viruses

Factor	Association
MAJOR HISTOCOMPATIBILITY LOCI-ENCODED GENES	
B35, C4, DR1, DQ1	Kaposi's sarcoma
DR1	Kaposi's sarcoma
DR2, DR5	Kaposi's sarcoma
DR5	Kaposi's sarcoma
Aw23, Bw49	Kaposi's sarcoma
B62	Fever, skin rash in primary HIV infection
Aw19	HIV seropositivity in individuals multiply exposed to HIV
A1, A24, C7, B8, DR3	Rapid progression to AIDS
DR4, DQB1*0302	Rapid progression to AIDS
DR3, DQ1	Rapid progression to AIDS
B*35	Rapid progression to AIDS
Cw*04	Rapid progression to AIDS
TAP2.1	Promotes HIV progression to AIDS
DR5	Thrombocytopenia and lymphadenopathy in HIV infection
DR5, DR6	Diffuse infiltrative CD8+ lymphocytosis with Sjögren-like syndrome in HIV infection
Bw4	Slow decline in CD4+T cell count
B13, B27, B51, B57, DQB1*0302,0303	Protects from progression to AIDS
B*5701	Strong protection from progression to AIDS
A26, B38, TAP1.4, TAP2.3	Ability to clear HIV infection in transiently infected seronegative individuals
A28, Bw70, Aw69, B18	Protection from HIV infection
A32, B4, C2	Long-term survival in HIV infection
A11, A32, B13, C2, DQA1*0301, DQB1*0302, DRB1*0400, DRB4*0101	Long-term survival in HIV infection
Heterozygosity for Class I loci (A, B, and C)	Delayed onset to AIDS
Homozygosity for Class I loci (A, B, and C)	Rapid onset to AIDS and death
OTHER GENES	
p53 tumor suppressor gene	Controls HIV replicative patterns and determinant of viral latency
CCR5 gene	Homozygous defect involving a 32-bp deletion corresponding to the second extracellular loop of the receptor results in resistance to infection; heterozygous defect appears to result in partial protection against disease progression. Also, several single nucleotide polymorphisms in the CCR5 promoter have been shown to be associated with variable rates of progression in AIDS.
CCR2 gene	Heterozygosity for CCRV641 mutation is associated with delay in progression of HIV disease
CX$_3$CR1 gene	Mutations in I249 and M280 associated with rapid progression to AIDS
RANTES gene	A mutation of the RANTES gene (RANTES-28G) results in increased transcription and expression of RANTES on mononuclear cells with resulting inhibition of infection with R5 strains of HIV and delay of disease progression
SDF1 gene	Homozygosity for SDF1-3′A mutation is associated with a delay in progression of HIV disease
IL-10 gene	Individuals carrying the IL10-5′592A promoter allele were at increased risk for HIV infection and, once infected, progressed more rapidly than homozygotes for the alternative IL10-5′-592 C/C genotype

SOURCES: Adapted from Haynes et al; R Liu et al; Samson et al; Carrington et al; also see Bibliography.

to mononuclear cells. Delayed progression of disease is also seen in those individuals who have any of a number of single nucleotide polymorphisms in the *CCR5* promoter. In addition, individuals who carry a certain allele (IL-10-5′592A) of the IL-10 promoter are at increased risk of infection and, once infected, progress more rapidly than homozygotes for the alternative genotype. The mechanism of this effect is felt to be a downregulation of the inhibitory cytokine IL-10 resulting in facilitation of HIV replication. Finally, individuals with a mutation of the *RANTES* gene (*RANTES-28G*) manifest a delay in disease progression due likely to the increased expression of RANTES and resulting inhibition of infection with R5 viruses (Table 309-7).

NEUROPATHOGENESIS HIV-infected individuals can experience a variety of neurologic abnormalities due either to opportunistic infections and neoplasms (see below) or to direct effects of HIV or its products. With regard to the latter, HIV has been demonstrated in the brain and CSF of infected individuals with and without neuropsychiatric abnormalities. The main cell types that are infected in the brain in vivo are those of the monocyte/macrophage lineage, including monocytes that have migrated to the brain from the peripheral blood as well as resident microglial cells. HIV entry into brain is felt to be due, at least in part, to the ability of virus-infected and immune-activated macrophages to induce adhesion molecules such as E-selectin and vascular cell adhesion molecule-1 (VCAM-1) on brain endothelium. Other studies have demonstrated that HIV gp120 enhances the expression of intercellular adhesion molecule-1 (ICAM-1) in glial cells; this effect may facilitate entry of HIV-infected cells into the CNS and may promote syncytia formation. Virus isolates from the brain are preferentially R5 strains as opposed to X4 strains (see above); in this regard, HIV-infected individuals who are heterozygous for *CCR5Δ32* appear to be relatively protected against the development of HIV encephalopathy compared to wild-type individuals. Distinct HIV envelope sequences are associated with the clinical expression of the AIDS dementia complex (see below). Although there have been reports of infrequent HIV infection of neuronal cells and astrocytes, there is no convincing evidence that brain cells other than those of monocyte/macrophage lineage can be productively infected in vivo. Nonetheless, it has been demonstrated that galactosyl ceramide may be an essential component of the HIV gp120 receptor on neural cells, and antibodies to galactosyl ceramide inhibit entry of HIV into neural cell lines in vitro.

HIV-infected individuals may manifest white matter lesions as well as neuronal loss. Given the relative absence of evidence of HIV infection of neurons either in vivo or in vitro, it is unlikely that direct infection of these cells accounts for their loss. Rather, the HIV-mediated effects on brain tissue are thought to be due to a combination of direct effects, either toxic or function-inhibitory, of gp120 on neuronal cells and effects of a variety of neurotoxins released from infiltrating monocytes, resident microglial cells, and astrocytes. In this regard, it has been demonstrated that both HIV-1 Nef and Tat can induce chemotaxis of leukocytes, including monocytes, into the CNS. Neurotoxins can be released from monocytes as a consequence of infection and/or immune activation. Monocyte-derived neurotoxic factors have been reported to kill neurons via the *N*-methyl-D-aspartate (NMDA) receptor. In addition, HIV gp120 shed by virus-infected monocytes could cause neurotoxicity by antagonizing the function of vasoactive intestinal peptide (VIP), by elevating intracellular calcium levels, and by decreasing nerve growth factor levels in the cerebral cortex. A variety of monocyte-derived cytokines can contribute directly or indirectly to the neurotoxic effects in HIV infection; these include TNF-α, IL-1, IL-6, TGF-β, IFN-γ, platelet-activating factor, and endothelin. Certain studies have correlated levels of CC-chemokines MIP-1α, MIP-1β, and RANTES in CSF with HIV-related encephalopathy. In addition, infection and/or activation of monocyte-lineage cells can result in increased production of eicosanoids, nitric oxide, and quinolinic acid, which may contribute to neurotoxicity. Astrocytes may play diverse roles in HIV neuropathogenesis. Reactive gliosis or astrocytosis has been demonstrated in the brains of HIV-infected individuals, and TNF-α and IL-6 have been shown to induce astrocyte proliferation. In addition, astrocyte-derived IL-6 can induce HIV expression in infected cells in vitro. Furthermore, it has been suggested that astrocytes may downregulate macrophage-produced neurotoxins. It has been reported that HIV-infected individuals with the E4 allele for apolipoprotein E (apo E) are at increased risk for AIDS encephalopathy and peripheral neuropathy. The likelihood that HIV or its products are involved in neuropathogenesis is supported by the observation that neuropsychiatric abnormalities may undergo re-markable and rapid improvement upon the initiation of antiretroviral therapy, particularly in HIV-infected children.

PATHOGENESIS OF KAPOSI'S SARCOMA   KS is an op-portunistic disease in HIV-infected individuals. Unlike opportunistic infections, its occurrence is not strictly related to the level of depres-sion of CD4+ T cell counts (see below). There are at least four distinct epidemiologic forms of Kaposi's sarcoma: (1) the classic form that occurs in older men of predominantly Mediterranean or eastern Eu-ropean Jewish backgrounds with no recognized contributing factors; (2) the equatorial African form that occurs in all ages, also without any recognized precipitating factors; (3) the form associated with or-gan transplantation and its attendant iatrogenic immunosuppressed state; and (4) the form associated with HIV-1 infection. The patho-genesis of KS is complex and has not been fully delineated. KS does not result from a neoplastic transformation of cells in the classic sense and so is not truly a sarcoma. It is a manifestation of excessive pro-liferation of spindle cells that are believed to be of vascular origin and have features in common with endothelial and smooth-muscle cells. In HIV disease the development of KS is dependent on the interplay of a variety of factors including HIV-1 itself, HHV-8, immune acti-vation, and cytokine secretion. A number of epidemiologic and viro-logic studies have clearly linked HHV-8, which is also referred to as *Kaposi's sarcoma–associated herpesvirus* (KSHV), to KS not only in HIV-infected individuals but also in individuals with the other forms of KS. KSHV is a γ-herpesvirus related to EBV and herpesvirus sai-miri. It encodes a homologue to human IL-6 and in addition to KS has been implicated in the pathogenesis of body cavity lymphoma, mul-tiple myeloma, and monoclonal gammopathy of undetermined signif-icance. Sequences of HHV-8 are found universally in the lesions of KS, and patients with KS are virtually all seropositive for HHV-8. HHV-8 DNA sequences can be found in the B cells of 30 to 50% of patients with KS and 7% of patients with AIDS without clinically apparent KS.

Between 1 and 2% of eligible blood donors are positive for anti-bodies to HHV-8, while the prevalence of HHV-8 seropositivity in HIV-infected men is 30 to 35%. The prevalence in HIV-infected women is approximately 4%. This finding is reflective of the lower incidence of KS in women. It has been debated whether HHV-8 is actually the transforming agent in KS; the bulk of the cells in the tumor lesions of KS are not neoplastic cells. However, a recent study has demonstrated that endothelial cells can be transformed in vitro by HHV-8. Despite the complexity of the pathogenic events associated with the development of KS in HIV-infected individuals, it is generally felt that HHV-8 is indeed the etiologic agent of this disease. The ini-tiation and/or propagation of KS requires an activated state and is mediated, at least in part, by cytokines. A number of factors, including TNF-α, IL-1β, IL-6, GM-CSF, basic fibroblast growth factor, and on-costatin M, function in an autocrine and paracrine manner to sustain the growth and chemotaxis of the KS spindle cells. It has been sug-gested that the HIV Tat protein plays a major role in the pathogenesis of KS. In this regard, it has been demonstrated that IFN-γ can induce endothelial cells to proliferate and to invade the extracellular matrix in response to HIV Tat. This occurs as a result of the upregulation by IFN-γ of the expression and activity of the receptors for Tat, which are the integrins $\alpha_5\beta_1$ and $\alpha_v\beta_3$. In addition, the HIV-1 Tat protein has been shown to act synergistically with basic fibroblast growth factor

in the induction of lesions resembling KS lesions in mice. Glucocor-ticoids have been shown to have a stimulatory effect, and human cho-rionic gonadotrophin an inhibitory effect, on KS spindle cells, sug-gesting that modulation of the balance of autocrine factors may have therapeutic potential in KS.

IMMUNE RESPONSE TO HIV

As detailed above and below, following the initial burst of viremia during primary infection, HIV-infected individuals mount a robust im-mune response that usually substantially curtails the levels of plasma viremia and likely contributes to delaying the ultimate development of clinically apparent disease for a median of 10 years. This immune response contains elements of both humoral and cell-mediated im-munity (Table 309-8; Fig. 309-21). It is directed against multiple an-tigenic determinants of the HIV virion as well as against viral proteins expressed on the surface of infected cells. Ironically, those CD4+ T cells with T cell receptors specific for HIV are theoretically those CD4+ T cells most likely to bind to infected cells and themselves be infected and destroyed. Thus, an early consequence of HIV infection may be interference with the generation of an effective immune re-sponse through the elimination of HIV-specific CD4+ T lymphocytes.

Although a great deal of investigation has been directed toward delineating and better understanding the components of this immune response, it remains unclear which of these phenomena are most im-portant in delaying progression of infection and which, if any, play a role in the pathogenesis of HIV disease.

HUMORAL IMMUNE RESPONSE   Antibodies to HIV usu-ally appear within 6 weeks and almost invariably within 12 weeks of primary infection (Fig. 309-22); rare exceptions are individuals who have defects in the ability to produce HIV-specific antibodies. Detec-tion of these antibodies forms the basis of most diagnostic screening tests for HIV infection. The appearance of HIV-binding antibodies detected by ELISA and western blot assays occurs prior to the ap-pearance of neutralizing antibodies; the latter generally appear follow-ing the initial decreases in plasma viremia, which is more closely re-lated to the appearance of HIV-specific CD8+ T lymphocytes. The first antibodies detected are those directed against the structural or gag proteins of HIV, p24 and p17, and the gag precursor p55. The devel-opment of antibodies to p24 is associated with a decrease in the serum levels of free p24 antigen. Antibodies to the gag proteins are followed by the appearance of antibodies to the envelope proteins (gp160, gp120, p88, and gp41) and to the products of the *pol* gene (p31, p51, and p66). In addition, one may see antibodies to the low-molecular-weight regulatory proteins encoded by the HIV genes *vpr, vpu, vif, rev, tat,* and *nef.*

While antibodies to multiple antigens of HIV are produced, the precise functional significance of these different antibodies is unclear. The best studied have been the antibodies directed towards the enve-lope proteins of the virus. As noted above, the envelope of HIV con-

Table 309-8   Elements of the Immune Response to HIV

Humoral immunity
  Binding antibodies
  Neutralizing antibodies
    Type specific
    Group specific
  Antibodies participating in antibody-dependent cellular cytotoxicity
    (ADCC)
    Protective
    Pathogenic (bystander killing)
  Enhancing antibodies
Cell-mediated immunity
  Helper CD4+ T lymphocytes
  Class I MHC–restricted cytotoxic CD8+ T lymphocytes
  CD8+ T cell–mediated inhibition (noncytolytic)
  ADCC
  Natural killer cells

FIGURE 309-21 Schematic representation of the different immunologic effector mechanisms felt to be active in the setting of HIV infection. Detailed descriptions are given in the text. TCR, T cell receptor.

sists of an outer envelope glycoprotein with a molecular mass of 120 kDa and a transmembrane glycoprotein with a molecular mass of 41 kDa. These are initially synthesized as a 160-kDa precursor that is cleaved by cellular proteases. Most of the antienvelope antibodies are directed either toward an epitope in the gp41 region comprising amino acids 579 to 613 or toward a hypervariable region in the gp120 molecule, known as the *V3 loop region*, comprising amino acids 303 through 338. This V3 region is a major site for the development of mutations that lead to variants of HIV that are not well recognized by the immune system.

Antibodies directed toward the envelope proteins of HIV have been characterized both as being protective and as possibly contributing to the pathogenesis of HIV disease. Among the protective antibodies are those that function to neutralize HIV directly and prevent the spread of infection to additional cells, as well as those that participate in ADCC. *Neutralizing antibodies* may be a component of primary HIV infection, and some long-term nonprogressors have been reported to have increased titers of neutralizing antibodies. Neutralizing antibodies appear to be of two forms, type-specific and group-specific. *Type-specific neutralizing antibodies* are generally directed

to the V3 loop region. These antibodies neutralize only viruses of a given strain and are present in low titer in most infected individuals. *Group-specific neutralizing antibodies* are capable of neutralizing a wide variety of HIV isolates. At least two forms of group specific antibodies have been identified: those binding to amino acids 423 to 437 of gp120 and those binding to amino acids 728 to 745 of gp41. The other major class of protective antibodies are those that participate in ADCC, which is actually a form of cell-mediated immunity (Chap. 305) in which NK cells that bear Fc receptors are armed with specific anti-HIV antibodies that bind to the NK cells via their Fc portion. These armed NK cells then bind to and destroy cells expressing HIV antigens. Antibodies to both gp120 and gp41 have been shown to participate in ADCC-mediated killing of HIV-infected cells. The levels of antienvelope antibodies capable of mediating ADCC are highest in the earlier stages of HIV infection. In vitro, IL-2 can augment ADCC-mediated killing.

In addition to playing a role in host defense, HIV-specific antibodies have also been implicated in disease pathogenesis. Antibodies directed to gp41, when present in low titer, have been shown in vitro to be capable of facilitating infection of cells through an Fc receptor–mediated mechanism known as *antibody enhancement*. Thus, the same regions of the envelope protein of HIV that give rise to antibodies capable of mediating ADCC also elicit the production of antibodies that can facilitate infection of cells in vitro. In addition, it has been postulated that anti-gp120 antibodies that participate in the ADCC killing of HIV-infected cells might also kill uninfected CD4+ T cells if the uninfected cells had bound free gp120, a phenomenon referred to as *bystander killing*.

CELLULAR IMMUNE RESPONSE Given the fact that T cell–mediated immunity is known to play a major role in host defense against most viral infections (Chap. 305), it is generally thought to be an important component of the host immune response to HIV. T cell immunity can be divided into two major categories, mediated respectively by the *helper/inducer CD4+ T cells* and the *cytotoxic/immunoregulatory CD8+ T cells*.

It has been difficult to demonstrate the presence of HIV-specific CD4+ T cells in HIV-infected patients directly, particularly in those with advanced disease. This difficulty may be related to the fact that these cells, with their high affinity for binding to HIV-infected cells, may be among the first to be infected and destroyed during HIV infection. CD4+ T lymphocytes with reactivity to the p24 antigen of HIV have been reported to be present in a subset of long-term nonprogressors and in a subset of patients in whom therapy was initiated shortly following infection. While a reverse correlation exists between the presence of these cells and levels of plasma HIV viremia, it is

FIGURE 309-22 Relationship between antigenemia and the development of antibodies to HIV. Antibodies to HIV proteins are generally seen 6 to 12 weeks following infection and 3 to 6 weeks after the development of plasma viremia. Late in the course of illness, antibody levels to p24 decline, generally in association with a rising titer of p24 antigen.

unclear whether or not there is a causal relationship between these parameters. Through the use of computer modeling, several regions of the HIV-1 envelope molecule have been identified that are structurally analogous to other known T cell epitopes by virtue of having structures known as *amphipathic helices*. Peptides from these envelope regions have been used to identify the presence of CD4+ T cells specific for these regions in the peripheral blood of HIV-infected individuals. Other studies have demonstrated that peripheral blood T cells of some healthy, HIV-negative individuals also react to the envelope proteins of HIV. It is unclear whether or not this represents the presence of a degree of protective immunity in these individuals.

MHC class I–restricted, HIV-specific CD8+ T cells have been identified in the peripheral blood of patients with HIV-1 infection. These cells include cytotoxic T cells (CTLs) and T cells that can be induced by HIV antigens to express cytokines such as IFN-γ. CTLs have been identified in the peripheral blood of patients within weeks of HIV infection. These CD8+ T lymphocytes, through their HIV-specific antigen receptors, bind to and cause the lytic destruction of target cells bearing identical MHC class I molecules associated with HIV antigens. Two types of CTL activity can be demonstrated in the peripheral blood or lymph node mononuclear cells of HIV-infected individuals. The first type directly lyses appropriate target cells in culture without prior in vitro stimulation (*spontaneous CTL activity*). The other type of CTL activity reflects the *precursor frequency of CTLs* (CTLp); this type of CTL activity can be demonstrated by stimulation of CD8+ T cells in vitro with a mitogen such as phytohemagglutinin or anti-CD3 antibody. Following primary HIV infection, the qualitative nature of the HIV-specific CTL response is an important predictor of eventual clinical outcome. Patients who mount a broad CD8+ CTL response generally have a more favorable clinical course than do patients who mount a more restricted CTL response. These data are consistent with studies in the SIV model where deletion of CD8+ T cells leads to a more accelerated clinical course.

In addition to CTLs, CD8+ T cells capable of being induced by HIV antigens to express cytokines such as IFN-γ also appear in the setting of HIV-1 infection. It is not clear whether these are the same or different effector pools compared to those cells mediating cytotoxicity; in addition, the relative roles of each in host defense against HIV are not fully understood. It does appear that these CD8+ T cells are driven to in vivo expansion by HIV antigen. There is a direct correlation between levels of CD8+ T cells capable of producing IFN-γ in response to HIV antigens and plasma levels of HIV-1 RNA. Thus, while these cells are clearly induced by HIV-1 infection, their overall ability to control infection remains unclear. Multiple HIV antigens, including Gag, Env, Pol, Tat, Rev, and Nef, can elicit CD8+ T cell responses.

At least three other forms of cell-mediated immunity to HIV have been described: CD8+ T cell–mediated suppression of HIV replication, ADCC, and NK cell activity. *CD8+ T cell–mediated suppression of HIV replication* refers to the ability of CD8+ T cells from an HIV-infected patients to inhibit the replication of HIV in tissue culture in a noncytolytic manner. There is no requirement for HLA compatibility between the CD8+ T cells and the HIV-infected cells. This effector mechanism is thus nonspecific and appears to be mediated by soluble factor(s) including the CC-chemokines RANTES, MIP-1α and MIP-1β (see above). These chemokines are potent suppressors of HIV replication and operate at least in part via blockade of the co-receptor (CCR5) on peripheral blood mononuclear cells for R5 or macrophage-tropic strains of HIV (see above). *ADCC*, as described above in relation to humoral immunity, involves the killing of HIV-expressing cells by NK cells armed with specific antibodies directed against HIV antigens. Finally, *NK cells* alone have been shown to be capable of killing HIV-infected target cells in tissue culture. This primitive cytotoxic mechanism of host defense is directed toward nonspecific surveillance for neoplastic transformation and viral infection through recognition of altered class I MHC molecules.

DIAGNOSIS AND LABORATORY MONITORING OF HIV INFECTION

The establishment of HIV as the causative agent of AIDS and related syndromes early in 1984 was followed by the rapid development of sensitive screening tests for HIV infection. By March, 1985, blood donors in the United States were routinely screened for antibodies to HIV. In June 1996, blood banks in the United States added the p24 antigen capture assay to the screening process to help identify the rare infected individuals who were donating blood in the time (up to 3 months) between infection and the development of antibodies. The development of sensitive assays for monitoring levels of plasma viremia ushered in a new era of being able to monitor the progression of HIV disease more closely. Utilization of these tests, coupled with the measurement of levels of CD4+ T lymphocytes in peripheral blood, is essential in the management of patients with HIV infection.

DIAGNOSIS OF HIV INFECTION The diagnosis of HIV infection depends upon the demonstration of antibodies to HIV and/ or the direct detection of HIV or one of its components. As noted above, antibodies to HIV generally appear in the circulation 2 to 12 weeks following infection.

The standard screening test for HIV infection is the ELISA, also referred to as an enzyme immunoassay (EIA). This solid-phase assay is an extremely good screening test with a sensitivity of >99.5%. Most diagnostic laboratories use a commercial EIA kit that contains antigens from both HIV-1 and HIV-2 and thus are able to detect either. These kits use both natural and recombinant antigens and are continuously updated to increase their sensitivity to newly discovered species, such as group O viruses (Fig. 309-6). EIA tests are generally scored as positive (highly reactive), negative (nonreactive), or indeterminate (partially reactive). While the EIA is an extremely sensitive test, it is not optimal with regard to specificity. This is particularly true in studies of low-risk individuals, such as volunteer blood donors. In this latter population, only 10% of EIA-positive individuals are subsequently confirmed to have HIV infection. Among the factors associated with false-positive EIA tests are antibodies to class II antigens, autoantibodies, hepatic disease, recent influenza vaccination, and acute viral infections. For these reasons, anyone suspected of having HIV infection based upon a positive or inconclusive EIA result must have the result confirmed with a more specific assay.

The most commonly used confirmatory test is the western blot (Fig. 309-23). This assay takes advantage of the fact that multiple HIV antigens of different, well-characterized molecular weights elicit the production of specific antibodies. These antigens can be separated on the basis of molecular weight, and antibodies to each component can be detected as discrete bands on the western blot. A negative western blot is one in which no bands are present at molecular weights corresponding to HIV gene products. In a patient with a positive or indeterminate EIA and a negative western blot, one can conclude with certainty that the EIA reactivity was a false positive. On the other hand, a western blot demonstrating antibodies to products of all three of the major genes of HIV (*gag, pol*, and *env*) is conclusive evidence of infection with HIV. Criteria established by the U.S. Food & Drug Administration (FDA) in 1993 for a positive western blot state that a result is considered positive if antibodies exist to two of the three HIV proteins: p24, gp41, and gp120/160. Using these criteria, approximately 10% of all blood donors deemed positive for HIV-1 infection lacked an antibody band to the *pol* gene product p31. Some 50% of these blood donors were subsequently found to be false positives. Thus, the absence of the p31 band should increase the suspicion that one may be dealing with a false-positive test result. In this setting it is prudent to obtain additional confirmation with an RNA-based test and/or a follow-up western blot. By definition, western blot patterns of reactivity that do not fall into the positive or negative categories are considered "indeterminate." There are two possible explanations for an indeterminate western blot result. The most likely explanation in a low-risk individual is that the patient being tested has antibodies that cross-react with one of the proteins of HIV. The most common patterns of cross-reactivity are antibodies that react with p24 and/or p55. The least likely explanation in this setting is that the individual is infected with HIV and is in the process of mounting a classic antibody response. In either instance, the western blot should be repeated in 1 month to determine whether or not the indeterminate pattern is a pattern in evolution. In addition, one may attempt to confirm a diagnosis of HIV infection with the p24 antigen capture assay or one of the tests for HIV RNA (discussed below). While the western blot is an excellent confirmatory test for HIV infection in patients with a positive or indeterminate EIA, it is a poor screening test. Among individuals with a negative EIA and PCR for HIV, 20 to 30% may show one or more bands on western blot. While these bands are usually faint and represent cross-reactivity, their presence creates a situation in which other diagnostic modalities [such as DNA PCR, RNA PCR, the (b)DNA assay, or p24 antigen capture] must be employed to ensure that the bands do not indicate early HIV infection.

A guideline for the use of these serologic tests in attempting to make a diagnosis of HIV infection is depicted in Fig. 309-24. In patients in whom HIV infection is suspected, the appropriate initial test is the EIA. If the result is negative, unless there is strong reason to suspect early HIV infection (as in a patient exposed within the previous 3 months), the diagnosis is ruled out and retesting should be performed only as clinically indicated. If the EIA is indeterminate or positive, the test should be repeated. If the repeat is negative on two occasions, one can assume that the initial positive reading was due to a technical error in the performance of the assay and that the patient is negative. If the repeat is indeterminate or positive, one should proceed to the HIV-1 western blot. If the western blot is positive, the diagnosis is HIV-1 infection. If the western blot is negative, the EIA can be assumed to have been a false positive for HIV-1 and the diagnosis of HIV-1 infection is ruled out. It would be prudent at this point to perform specific serologic testing for HIV-2 following the same type of algorithm. If the western blot for HIV-1 is indeterminate, it should be repeated in 4–6 weeks; in addition, one may proceed to a p24 antigen capture assay, HIV-1 RNA assay, or HIV-1 DNA PCR and specific serologic testing for HIV-2. If the p24 and HIV RNA assays are negative and there is no progression in the western blot, a diagnosis of HIV-1 is ruled out. If either the p24 or HIV-1 RNA assay is positive and/or the HIV-1 western blot shows progression, a tentative diagnosis of HIV-1 infection can be made and later confirmed with a follow-up western blot demonstrating a positive pattern.

As mentioned above, a variety of laboratory tests are available for the direct detection of HIV or its components (Table 309-9; Fig. 309-25). These tests may be of considerable help in making a diagnosis of HIV infection when the western blot results are indeterminate. In addition, the tests detecting levels of HIV RNA can be used to determine prognosis and to assess the response to antiretroviral therapies. The simplest of the direct detection tests is the *p24 antigen capture assay*. This is an EIA-type assay in which the solid phase consists of antibodies to the p24 antigen of HIV. It detects the viral protein p24 in the blood of HIV-infected individuals where it exists either as free antigen or complexed to anti-p24 antibodies. Overall, approximately 30% of individuals with untreated HIV infection have detectable levels of free p24 antigen. This increases to about 50% when samples are

FIGURE 309-23 *A.* Schematic representation of how a western blot is performed. *B.* Examples of patterns of western blot reactivity. In each instance the western blot strip contains antigens to HIV-1. The sera from the patient immunized to the HIV-1 envelope only contains antibodies to the HIV-1 envelope proteins. The sera from the patient with HIV-2 infection cross-reacts with both *reverse transcriptase* and *gag* gene products of HIV-1.

treated with a weak acid to dissociate antigen-antibody complexes. Throughout the course of HIV infection, an equilibrium exists between p24 antigen and anti-p24 antibodies. During the first few weeks of infection, before an immune response develops, there is a brisk rise in p24 antigen levels (Fig. 309-22). After the development of anti-p24 antibodies, these levels decline. Late in the course of infection, when circulating levels of virus are high, p24 antigen levels also increase, particularly when detected by techniques involving dissociation of antigen-antibody complexes. This assay has its greatest use as a screening test for HIV infection in patients suspected of having the acute HIV syndrome, as high levels of p24 antigen are present prior to the development of antibodies. In addition, it is currently routinely used

FIGURE 309-24 Algorithm for the use of serologic tests in the diagnosis of HIV-1 or HIV-2 infection. * Stable indeterminate western blot 4 to 6 weeks later makes HIV infection unlikely. However, it should be repeated twice at 3-month intervals to rule out HIV infection. Alternatively, one may test for HIV-1 p24 antigen on HIV RNA.

Table 309-9   Characteristics of Tests for Direct Detection of HIV

Test	Technique	Sensitivity	Cost/Test
Immune complex–dissociated p24 antigen capture assay	Measurement of levels of HIV-1 core protein in an ELISA-based format following dissociation of antigen-antibody complexes by weak acid treatment	Positive in 50% of patients; detects down to 15 pg/mL of p24 protein	$1–2
HIV RNA by PCR	PCR amplification of cDNA generated from viral RNA (target amplification)	Positive in >98% of patients; detects down to 40 copies/mL of HIV RNA	$75–150
HIV RNA by bDNA	Measurement of levels of particle-associated HIV RNA in a nucleic acid capture assay employing signal amplification	Positive in 90% of patients; detects down to 50 copies/mL of HIV RNA	$75–150

NOTE: ELISA, enzyme-linked immunosorbent assay; PCR, polymerase chain reaction.

along with the HIV EIA assay to screen blood donors in the United States for evidence of HIV infection. Its utility as an assay is decreasing with the increased use of the reverse transcriptase PCR (RT-PCR) and bDNA technique for direct detection of HIV RNA.

The ability to measure and monitor levels of HIV RNA in the plasma of patients with HIV infection has been of extraordinary value in furthering our understanding of the pathogenesis of HIV infection and in providing a diagnostic tool in settings where measurements of anti-HIV antibodies may be misleading, such as in acute infection and neonatal infection. Two assays are predominantly used for this purpose. They are the *RT-PCR* (Amplicor) and the *bDNA* (Quantiplex). It should be pointed out that the only test approved by the FDA at this time for the measurement of HIV RNA levels is the RT-PCR test. While this approval is limited to the use of the test for determining prognosis, it is the general consensus that this test as well as the bDNA test are also of value for monitoring the effects of therapy and in making a diagnosis of HIV infection. In addition to these two commercially available tests, the *DNA PCR* is also employed by research laboratories for making a diagnosis of HIV infection by amplifying HIV proviral DNA from peripheral blood mononuclear cells. The commercially available RNA detection tests have a sensitivity of 40 to 50 copies of HIV RNA per milliliter of plasma, while the DNA PCR tests can detect proviral DNA at a frequency of one copy per 10,000 to 100,000 cells. Thus, these tests are extremely sensitive. One frequent consequence of a high degree of sensitivity is some loss of specificity, and false-positive results have been reported with each of these techniques. For this reason, a positive EIA with a confirmatory western blot remains the "gold standard" for a diagnosis of HIV infection, and the interpretation of other test results must be done with this in mind.

In the RT-PCR technique, following DNAase treatment, a cDNA copy is made of all RNA species present in plasma. Insofar as HIV is an RNA virus, this will result in the production of DNA copies of the HIV genome in amounts proportional to the amount of HIV RNA present in plasma. This proviral DNA is then amplified and characterized using standard PCR techniques, employing primer pairs that can distinguish genomic cDNA from messenger cDNA. The bDNA assay involves the use of a solid-phase nucleic acid capture system and signal amplification through successive nucleic acid hybridizations to detect small quantities of HIV RNA. Both tests can achieve a tenfold increase in sensitivity to 40 to 50 copies of HIV RNA per milliliter with a preconcentration step in which plasma undergoes ultracentrifugation to pellet the viral particles. In addition to being a diagnostic and prognostic tool, RT-PCR is also useful for amplifying defined areas of the HIV genome for sequence analysis and has become an important technique for studies of sequence diversity and microbial resistance to antiretroviral agents. In patients with a positive or indeterminate EIA test and an indeterminate western blot, and in patients in whom serologic testing may be unreliable (such as patients with hypogammaglobulinemia or advanced HIV disease), these tests provide valuable tools for making a diagnosis of HIV infection. They should only be used for diagnosis when standard serologic testing has failed to provide a definitive result.

LABORATORY MONITORING OF PATIENTS WITH HIV INFECTION The epidemic of HIV infection and AIDS has provided the clinician with new challenges for integrating clinical and laboratory data to effect optimal patient management. The close relationship between clinical manifestations of HIV infection and CD4+ T cell count has made measurement of the latter a routine part of the evaluation of HIV-infected individuals. Determinations of CD4+ T cell counts and measurements of the levels of HIV RNA in serum or plasma provide a powerful set of tools for determining prognosis and monitoring response to therapy. While the CD4+ T cell count provides information on the current immunologic status of the patient, the HIV RNA level predicts what will happen to the CD4+ T cell count in the near future, and hence provides an important piece of prognostic information.

CD4+ T Cell Counts The CD4+ T cell count is the laboratory test generally accepted as the best indicator of the immediate state of immunologic competence of the patient with HIV infection. This measurement, which is the product of the percent of CD4+ T cells (determined by flow cytometry) and the total lymphocyte count [determined by the white blood cell count (WBC) and the differential count] has been shown to correlate very well with the level of immunologic competence. Patients with CD4+ T cell counts <200/μL are at high risk of infection with *P. carinii*, while patients with CD4+ T cell counts <50/μL are at high risk of infection with CMV and mycobacteria of the *M. avium complex* (MAC) (Fig. 309-26). Patients with HIV infection should have CD4+ T cell measurements performed at the time of diagnosis and every 3 to 6 months thereafter. More frequent measurements should be made if a declining trend is noted. According to most guidelines, a CD4 T cell count <500/μL is an indication for consideration of initiating antiretroviral therapy, and a decline in CD4+ T cell count of >25% is an indication for considering a change in

FIGURE 309-25 Comparison of RT-PCR and bDNA assays. *A*. Schematic representation of RT-PCR and bDNA assays. See text for detailed description. *B*. Scatter plot of log₁₀v3 bDNA versus log₁₀ RT-PCR with the line of equity (solid) and the fitted regression line (hatched). The equation for the fitted regression line is given in the lower-right-hand corner. There is good agreement between the two assays. v3, version 3 of the bDNA assay. (*From Highbarger et al.*)

therapy. Once the CD4+ T cell count is <200/μL, patients should be placed on a regimen for *P. carinii* prophylaxis, and once the count is <50/μL, primary prophylaxis for MAC infection is indicated. As with any laboratory measurement, one may wish to obtain two determinations prior to any significant changes in patient management based upon CD4+ T cell count alone.

HIV RNA Determinations Facilitated by highly sensitive techniques for the precise quantitation of small amounts of nucleic acids, the measurement of serum or plasma levels of HIV RNA has become an essential component in the monitoring of patients with HIV infection. As discussed under diagnosis of HIV infection, the two most commonly used techniques are the RT-PCR assay and the bDNA assay. Both assays generate data in the form of number of copies of HIV RNA per milliliter of serum or plasma and, by employing a 1:10 concentration step with ultracentrifugation, can detect as few as 40 to 50 copies of HIV RNA per milliliter of plasma. Although earlier versions of the bDNA assay generated values that were approximately 50% of those of the RT-PCR assay, the

FIGURE 309-26 Relationship between CD4+ T cell counts and the development of opportunistic diseases. Boxplot of the median (line inside the box), first quartile (bottom of the box), third quartile (top of the box), and mean (asterisk) CD4+ lymphocyte count at the time of the development of opportunistic disease. Can, candidal esophagitis; CMV, cytomegalovirus infection; Crp, cryptosporidiosis; Cry, cryptococcal meningitis; DEM, AIDS dementia complex; HSV, herpes simplex virus infection; HZos, herpes zoster; KS, Kaposi's sarcoma; MAC, *Mycobacterium avium* complex bacteremia; NHL, non-Hodgkin's lymphoma; PCP, primary *Pneumocystis carinii* pneumonia; PCP2, secondary *Pneumocystis carinii* pneumonia; PML, progressive multifocal leukoencephalopathy; Tox, *Toxoplasma gondii* encephalitis; WS, wasting syndrome. *(From Moore and Chaisson.)*

more recent versions (version 3 or higher) provide numbers essentially identical to those of the RT-PCR test (Fig. 309-25). While it is common practice to describe levels of HIV RNA below these cut-offs as "undetectable," this is a term that should be avoided as it is imprecise and leaves the false impression that the level of virus is 0. By utilizing more sensitive, nested PCR techniques and by studying tissue levels of virus as well as plasma levels, HIV RNA can be detected in virtually every patient with HIV infection. Measurements of changes in HIV RNA levels over time have been of great value in delineating the relationship between levels of virus and rates of disease progression (Fig. 309-17), the rates of viral turnover, the relationship between immune system activation and viral replication, and the time to development of drug resistance. HIV RNA measurements are greatly influenced by the state of activation of the immune system and may fluctuate greatly in the setting of secondary infections or immunization. For these reasons, decisions based upon HIV RNA levels should never be made on a single determination. Measurements of plasma HIV RNA levels should be made at the time of HIV diagnosis and every 3 to 4 months thereafter in the untreated patient. In general, most guidelines suggest that therapy be initiated in patients with >20,000 copies of HIV RNA per milliliter (see below). Following the initiation of therapy or any change in therapy, plasma HIV RNA levels should be monitored approximately every 4 weeks until the effectiveness of the therapeutic regimen is determined by the development of a new steady-state level of HIV RNA. In most instances of effective therapy this will be <50 copies per milliliter. This level of virus is generally achieved within 6 months of the initiation of effective treatment. During therapy, levels of HIV RNA should be monitored every 3 to 4 months to evaluate the continuing effectiveness of therapy.

HIV Resistance Testing The availability of multiple antiretroviral drugs as treatment options has generated a great deal of interest in the potential for measuring the sensitivity of an individual's HIV virus(es) to different antiretroviral agents. HIV resistance testing can be done through either genotypic or phenotypic measurements. In the genotypic assays, sequence analyses of the HIV genomes obtained from patients are compared to sequences of viruses with known antiretroviral resistance profiles. In the phenotypic assays, the in vivo growth of viral isolates obtained from the patient are compared to the

growth of reference strains of the virus in the presence or absence of different antiretroviral drugs. A modification of this phenotypic approach utilizes a comparison of the enzymatic activities of the reverse transcriptase or protease genes obtained by molecular cloning of patients' isolates to the enzymatic activities of genes obtained from reference strains of HIV in the presence or absence of different drugs targeted to these genes. These tests are quite good in identifying those antiretroviral agents that have been utilized in the past in a given patient. Their clinical value in identifying which antiretroviral regimen is best for an individual patient is still under investigation.

Other Tests A variety of other laboratory tests have been studied as potential markers of HIV disease activity. Among these are quantitative culture of replication-competent HIV from plasma, peripheral blood mononuclear cells, or resting CD4+ T cells; circulating levels of β_2-microglobulin, soluble IL-2 receptor, IgA, acid-labile endogenous interferon, or TNF-α; and the presence or absence of activation markers such as CD38 or HLA-DR on CD8+ T cells. While these measurements have value as markers of disease activity and help to increase our understanding of the pathogenesis of HIV disease, they do not currently play a major role in the monitoring of patients with HIV infection.

CLINICAL MANIFESTATIONS

The clinical consequences of HIV infection encompass a spectrum ranging from an acute syndrome associated with primary infection to a prolonged asymptomatic state to advanced disease. It is best to regard HIV disease as beginning at the time of primary infection and progressing through various stages. As mentioned above, active virus replication and progressive immunologic impairment occur throughout the course of HIV infection in most patients. With the exception of long-term nonprogressors (see above), HIV disease in untreated patients inexorably progresses even during the clinically latent stage.

THE ACUTE HIV SYNDROME It is estimated that 50 to 70% of individuals with HIV infection experience an acute clinical syndrome approximately 3 to 6 weeks after primary infection (Fig. 309-27). Varying degrees of clinical severity have been reported, and although it has been suggested that symptomatic seroconversion lead-

FIGURE 309-27   The acute HIV syndrome. See text for detailed description. *(Adapted from G Pantaleo et al: N Engl J Med 328:327, 1993.)*

ing to the seeking of medical attention indicates an increased risk for an accelerated course of disease, this has not been shown definitively. In fact, there does not appear to be a correlation between the level of the initial burst of viremia in acute HIV infection and the subsequent course of disease. The typical clinical findings are listed in Table 309-10; they occur along with a burst of plasma viremia. The syndrome is typical of an acute viral syndrome and has been likened to acute infectious mononucleosis. Symptoms usually persist for 1 to several weeks and gradually subside as an immune response to HIV develops and the levels of plasma viremia decrease. Opportunistic infections have been reported during this stage of infection, reflecting the immunodeficiency that results from reduced numbers of CD4+ T cells and likely also from the dysfunction of CD4+ T cells owing to crosslinking of the CD4 molecule on the cell surface by viral envelope proteins (see "Mechanisms of CD4+ T Lymphocyte Depletion and Dysfunction," above) associated with the extremely high levels of plasma viremia. A number of immunologic abnormalities accompany the acute HIV syndrome, including multiphasic perturbations of the numbers of circulating lymphocyte subsets. The number of total lymphocytes and T cell subsets (CD4+ and CD8+) are initially reduced. An inversion of the CD4+/CD8+ T cell ratio occurs later because of a rise in the number of CD8+ T cells. In fact, there may be a selective and transient expansion of CD8+ T cell subsets, as determined by T cell receptor analysis (see above). The total circulating CD8+ T cell count may remain elevated or return to normal; however, CD4+ T cell levels usually remain somewhat depressed, although there may be a slight rebound towards normal. Lymphadenopathy occurs in approximately 70% of individuals with primary HIV infection. Most patients recover spontaneously from this syndrome and many are left with only a mildly depressed CD4+ T cell count that remains stable for a variable period before beginning its progressive decline (see below); in some individuals, the CD4+ T cell count returns to the normal range. Approximately 10% of patients manifest a fulminant course of immu-

Table 309-10   Clinical Findings in the Acute HIV Syndrome

General	Neurologic
Fever	Meningitis
Pharyngitis	Encephalitis
Lymphadenopathy	Peripheral neuropathy
Headache/retroorbital pain	Myelopathy
Arthralgias/myalgias	Dermatologic
Lethargy/malaise	Erythematous maculopapular rash
Anorexia/weight loss	Mucocutaneous ulceration
Nausea/vomiting/diarrhea	

SOURCE: From Tindall and Cooper.

nologic and clinical deterioration after primary infection, even after the disappearance of symptoms. In most patients, primary infection with or without the acute syndrome is followed by a prolonged period of clinical latency.

THE ASYMPTOMATIC STAGE—CLINICAL LATENCY
Although the length of time from initial infection to the development of clinical disease varies greatly, the median time for untreated patients is approximately 10 years. As emphasized above, HIV disease with active virus replication is ongoing and progressive during this asymptomatic period. The rate of disease progression is directly correlated with HIV RNA levels. Patients with high levels of HIV RNA in plasma progress to symptomatic disease faster than do patients with low levels of HIV RNA (Fig. 309-17). Some patients referred to as long-term nonprogressors show little if any decline in CD4+ T cell counts over extended periods of time. These patients generally have extremely low levels of HIV RNA. Certain other patients remain entirely asymptomatic despite the fact that their CD4+ T cell counts show a steady progressive decline to extremely low levels. In these patients, the appearance of an opportunistic disease may be the first manifestation of HIV infection. During the asymptomatic period of HIV infection, the average rate of CD4+ T cell decline is approximately 50/μL per year. When the CD4+ T cell count falls to <200/μL, the resulting state of immunodeficiency is severe enough to place the patient at high risk for opportunistic infection and neoplasms, and hence for clinically apparent disease.

SYMPTOMATIC DISEASE   Symptoms of HIV disease can appear at any time during the course of HIV infection. Generally speaking, the spectrum of illness that one observes changes as the CD4+ T cell count declines. The more severe and life-threatening complications of HIV infection occur in patients with CD4+ T cells counts <200/μL. A diagnosis of AIDS is made in anyone with HIV infection and a CD4+ T cell count <200/μL and in anyone with HIV infection who develops one of the HIV-associated diseases considered to be indicative of a severe defect in cell-mediated immunity (category C, Table 309-2). While the causative agents of the secondary infections are characteristically opportunistic organisms such as *P. carinii*, atypical mycobacteria, CMV, and other organisms that do not ordinarily cause disease in the absence of a compromised immune system, they also include common bacterial and mycobacterial pathogens. Approximately 80% of deaths among AIDS patients are as a direct result of an infection other than HIV, with bacterial infections heading the list. Following the widespread use of combination antiretroviral therapy and implementation of guidelines for the prevention of opportunistic infections (Table 309-11), the incidence of secondary infections has decreased dramatically (Fig. 309-28). Overall, the clinical spectrum of HIV disease is constantly changing as patients live longer and new and better approaches to treatment and prophylaxis are developed. In general, it should be stressed that a key element of treatment of symptomatic complications of HIV disease, whether they are primary or secondary, is achieving good control of HIV replication through the use of combination antiretroviral therapy and instituting primary and secondary prophylaxis as indicated.

Disease of the Respiratory System   Acute bronchitis and sinusitis are prevalent during all stages of HIV infection. The most severe cases tend to occur in patients with lower CD4+ T cell counts. Sinusitis presents as fever, nasal congestion, and headache. The diagnosis is made by computed tomography (CT) or magnetic resonance imaging (MRI). The maxillary sinuses are most commonly involved; however, disease is also frequently seen in the ethmoid, sphenoid, and frontal sinuses. While some patients may improve without antibiotic therapy, radiographic improvement is quicker and more pronounced in patients who have received antimicrobial therapy. It is postulated that this high incidence of sinusitis results from an increased frequency of infection with encapsulated organisms such as *H. influenzae* and *Streptococcus pneumoniae*. In patients with low CD4+ T cell counts one may see mucormycosis infections of the sinuses. In contrast to the course of this infection in other patient populations, mucormycosis of the sinuses in patients with HIV infection may progress more slowly. In this set-

Table 309-11 1999 USPHS/IDSA Guidelines for the Prevention of Opportunistic Infections in Persons Infected with HIV

Pathogen	Indications	First Choice(s)	Alternatives
STRONGLY RECOMMENDED AS STANDARD OF CARE FOR PRIMARY AND SECONDARY PROPHYLAXIS			
Pneumocystis carinii	CD4 count <200/μl or Oropharyngeal candidiasis or Unexplained fever >2 weeks Prior bout of PCP	Trimethoprim/sulfamethoxazole (TMP/SMZ), 1 DS tablet qd	Dapsone 50 mg bid PO or 100 mg/d PO Dapsone 50 mg/d PO+ Pyrimethamine 50 mg/wk PO+ Leucovorin 25 mg/wk PO TMP/SMZ, 1 SS tablet qd Dapsone 200 mg PO+ Pyrimethamine 50 mg + Leucovorin 25 mg PO weekly Aerosolized pentamidine, 300 mg qm via Respirgard II nebulizer Atovoquone 1500 mg/d PO TMP/SMZ 1 DS tablet PO 3×/wk
Mycobacterium tuberculosis			
Isoniazid sensitive	Skin test >5 mm or Prior positive test without treatment or Contact with case of active TB	Isoniazid 300 mg PO+ Pyridoxine 500 mg/d PO ×9 mo	Rifabutin 300 mg PO+ Pyrazinamide 20 (mg/kg)/d PO ×2 mo
		Isoniazid 900 mg PO+ Pyridoxine 100 mg PO 2 ×/wk ×9 mo	Rifampin 600 mg/d PO ×4 mo
Isoniazid resistant	Same with high probability of exposure to isoniazid-resistant TB	Rifampin 600 mg PO+ Pyrazinamide 20 (mg/kg)/d PO q ×2 mo	Rifabutin 300 mg PO+ daily Pyrazinamide 20 (mg/kg)/d PO ×2 mo Rifampin 600 mg/d PO ×4 mo Rifabutin 300 mg/d PO ×4 mo
Multidrug resistant	Same with high probability of exposure to multidrug resistant TB	Consult local public health authorities	
Mycobacterium-avium complex	CD4 count <50/μl	Azithromycin 1200 mg weekly PO Clarithromycin 500 mg bid PO	Rifibutin 300 mg/d PO Azithromycin 1200 mg weekly PO+ Rifabutin 300 mg/d PO
	Prior documented disseminated disease	Clarithromycin 500 mg bid PO + Ethambutol 15 (mg/kg)/d PO+/− Rifabutin 300 mg/d PO	Azithromycin 500 mg/d PO+ Ethambutol 15 (mg/kg)/d PO+/− Rifabutin 300 mg/d PO
Toxoplasma gondii	IgG antibody and CD4 count <100/μl	TMP/SMZ 1 DS tablet qd	TMP/SMZ 1 SS tablet qd Dapsone 50 mg PO+ Pyrimethamine 50 mg weekly PO+ Leucovorin 25 mg weekly PO Atovoquone 1500 mg/d PO
	Prior toxoplasmic encephalitis	Sulfadiazine 500–1000 mg qid PO+ Pyrimethamine 25–75 mg/d PO+ Leucovorin 10 mg/d PO	Clindamycin 300–450 mg 16–8h PO+ Pyrimethamine 25–75 mg/d PO+ Leucovorin 10–25 mg/d PO
Varicella zoster virus	Significant exposure to chickenpox or shingles in a patient with no history of immunization or prior exposure to either	Varicella zoster immune globulin 6.25 mL within 96 h	
Cryptococcus neoformans	Prior documented disease	Fluconazole 200 mg/d PO	Amphotericin B 0.6–1.0 mg/kg 3 ×/wk IV Itraconazole 200 mg/d PO
Histoplasma capsulatum	Prior documented disease	Itraconazole 200 mg bid PO	Amphotericin B 1.0 (mg/kg)/wk IV
Coccidioides immitis	Prior documented disease	Fluconazole 400 mg/d PO	Amphotericin B 1.0 (mg/kg)/wk IV Itraconazole 200 mg/d PO
Salmonella species	Prior bacteremia	Ciprofloxacin 500 mg bid PO for several months	
Cytomegalovirus	Prior end-organ disease (any)	Ganciclovir, 5–6 mg/kg 5–7 days/ wk IV Ganciclovir 1000 mg tid PO Foscarnet 90–120 (mg/kg)/d IV	Cidofovir 5 mg/kg every other week IV
	Prior retinitis	Ganciclovir sustained-release implant q6–9mo + ganciclovir 1– 1.5 g tid PO	Fomivirsen, 1 vial injected into the vitreous q2–4wk
IMMUNIZATIONS GENERALLY RECOMMENDED			
Hepatitis B virus	All susceptible (anti-HBc and anti-HBs negative) patients	Hepatitis B vaccine: 3 doses	
Hepatitis A virus	All susceptible (anti-HAV negative) patients with chronic hepatitis C	Hepatitis A vaccine: 2 doses	
Influenza virus	All patients annually	Whole or split virus 1 dose yearly	

(continued)

Table 309-11 1999 USPHS/IDSA Guidelines for the Prevention of Opportunistic Infections in Persons Infected with HIV—*(continued)*

Pathogen	Indications	First Choice(s)	Alternatives
Streptococcus pneumoniae	All patients	Pneumoccal vaccine 0.5 mL IM ×1 if CD4 count >200/μl Reimmunize patients initially immunized at a CD4 count <200/μl whose CD4 count then increases to >200/μl	

RECOMMENDED FOR PREVENTION OF SEVERE OR FREQUENT RECURRENCES

Pathogen	Indications	First Choice(s)	Alternatives
Herpes simplex	Frequent/severe recurrences	Acyclovir 200 mg tid PO Acyclovir 40 mg bid PO Famciclovir 500 mg bid PO	
Candida	Frequent/severe recurrences	Fluconazole 100–200 mg/d PO Itraconazole solution 200 mg/d PO Ketoconazole 200 mg/d PO	

NOTE: DS, double strength; SS, single strength; PCP, *Pneumocystis carinii* pneumonia; TB, tuberculosis

ting aggressive, frequent local debridement in addition to local and systemic amphotericin B may be needed for effective treatment.

Pulmonary disease is one of the most frequent complications of HIV infection. The most common manifestation of pulmonary disease is pneumonia. The two most common causes of pneumonia are bacteria infections and *P. carinii* infection. Other major causes of pulmonary infiltrates include mycobacterial infections, fungal infections, nonspecific interstitial pneumonitis, KS, and lymphoma.

Pneumonia is seen with an increased frequency in patients with HIV infection. Patients with HIV infection appear to be particularly prone to infections with encapsulated organisms. *S. pneumoniae* (Chap. 138) and *H. influenzae* (Chap. 149) are responsible for most cases of bacterial pneumonia in patients with AIDS. This may be a consequence of altered B cell function and/or defects in neutrophil function that may be secondary to HIV disease (see above). Pneumococcal infection may be the earliest serious infection to occur in patients with HIV disease. This can present as pneumonia, sinusitis, and/or bacteremia. Patients with HIV infection have a sixfold increase in the incidence of pneumococcal pneumonia and a 100-fold increase in the incidence of pneumococcal bacteremia. Pneumococcal disease may be seen in patients with relatively intact immune systems. In one study, the baseline CD4+ T cell count at the time of a first episode of pneumococcal pneumonia was ~300/μL. Of interest is the fact that the inflammatory response to pneumococcal infection appears proportional to the CD4+ T cell count. Due to this high risk of pneumococcal disease, immunization with pneumococcal polysaccharide is one of the generally recommended prophylactic measures for patients with HIV infection and CD4+ T cell counts >200/μL. It is less clear if this intervention is of benefit in patients with more advanced disease and high viral loads.

P. carinii pneumonia (PCP), once the hallmark of AIDS, has dramatically declined in incidence following the development of effective prophylactic regimens and the widespread use of combination antiretroviral therapy. The risk of PCP is most common among those who have experienced a previous bout of PCP and those who have CD4+ T cell counts of <200/μL. Overall, 79% of patients with PCP have CD4+ T cell counts <100/μL and 95% of patients have CD4+ T cell counts <200/μL. Recurrent fever, night sweats, thrush, and unexplained weight loss are also associated with an increased incidence of PCP. For these reasons, it is strongly recommended that all patients with CD4+ T cell counts <200/μL (or a CD4 percentage <15) receive some form of PCP prophylaxis. At present the incidence of PCP is approaching zero in patients with known HIV infection receiving appropriate antiretroviral therapy and prophylaxis. Primary PCP is now occurring at a median CD4+ T cell count of 36/μL, while secondary PCP is occurring at a median CD4+ T cell count of 10/μL. Patients with PCP generally present with fever and a cough that is usually nonproductive or productive of only scant amounts of white sputum. They may complain of a characteristic retrosternal chest pain that is worse on inspiration and is described as sharp or burning. HIV-associated PCP may have an indolent course characterized by weeks of vague symptoms and should be included in the differential diagnosis of fever, pulmonary complaints, or unexplained weight loss in any patient with HIV infection and <200 CD4+ T cells/μL. The most common finding on chest x-ray is either a normal film, if the disease is suspected early, or a faint bilateral interstitial infiltrate. The classic finding of a dense perihilar infiltrate is unusual in patients with AIDS. In patients with PCP who have been receiving aerosolized pentamidine for prophylaxis, one may see an x-ray picture of upper lobe cavitary disease, reminiscent of TB. Other less common findings on chest x-ray include lobar infiltrates and pleural effusions. Routine laboratory evaluation is usually of little help in the differential diagnosis of PCP. A mild leukocytosis is common, although this may not be obvious in patients with prior neutropenia. Arterial blood gases may indicate hypoxemia with a decline in Pa_{O_2} and an increase in the arterial-alveolar (a − A) gradient. Arterial blood gas measurements not only aid in making the diagnosis of PCP but also provide important information for staging the severity of the disease and directing treatment. A definitive diagnosis of PCP requires demonstration of the trophozoite or cyst form of the organism in samples obtained from induced sputum, bronchoalveolar lavage, transbronchial biopsy, or open lung biopsy. PCR has been used to detect specific DNA sequences for *P. carinii* in clinical specimens where histologic examinations have failed to make a diagnosis.

In addition to pneumonia, a number of other clinical problems have been reported in HIV-infected patients as a result of infection with *P. carinii*. Otic involvement may be seen as a primary infection, presenting as a polypoid mass involving the external auditory canal. In patients receiving aerosolized penamidine for prophylaxis against PCP one may see a variety of extrapulmonary manifestations of *P. carinii*.

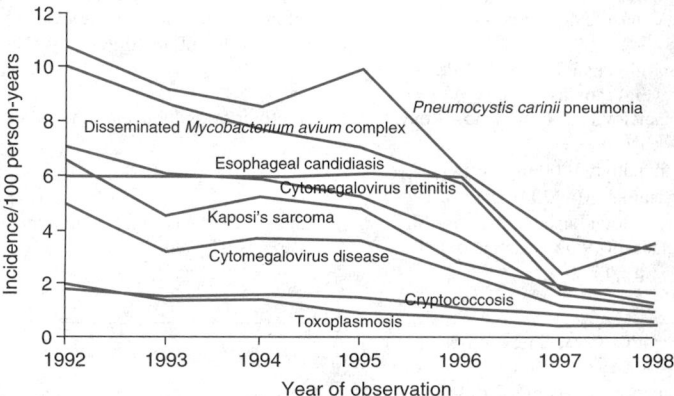

FIGURE 309-28 Decrease in the incidence of opportunistic infections and Kaposi's sarcoma in HIV-infected individuals with CD4+ T cell counts <100/μL from 1992 through 1998. *[Adapted and updated from Palella et al, and JE Kaplan et al: Clin Infect Dis 30(S1):S5, 2000, with permission.]*

These include ophthalmic lesions of the choroid, a necrotizing vasculitis that resembles Burger's disease, bone marrow hypoplasia, and intestinal obstruction. Other organs that have been involved include lymph nodes, spleen, liver, kidney, pancreas, pericardium, heart, thyroid, and adrenals. Organ infection may be associated with cystic lesions that may appear calcified on CT or ultrasound. The standard treatment for PCP or disseminated pneumocystosis is trimethoprim/sulfamethoxazole (TMP/SMZ). A high incidence of side effects, particularly skin rash and bone marrow suppression, is seen with TMP/SMZ in patients with HIV infection. Alternative treatments for mild to moderate PCP include dapsone/trimethoprim and clindamycin/primaquine. Intravenous pentamidine is the treatment of choice for severe disease in the patient unable to tolerate TMP/SMZ. For patients with a Pa_{O_2} <70 mmHg or with an a − A gradient >35 mmHg, adjunct glucocorticoid therapy should be used in addition to specific antimicrobials. Overall, treatment should be for 21 days and followed by secondary prophylaxis. Prophylaxis for PCP is indicated for any HIV-infected individual who has experienced a prior bout of PCP, any patient with a CD4+ T cell count of <200/μL or a CD4 percentage <15, any patient with unexplained fever for >2 weeks, and any patient with a history of oropharyngeal candidiasis. The preferred regimen for prophylaxis is TMP/SMZ, one double-strength tablet daily. This regimen also provides protection against toxoplasmosis and some bacterial respiratory pathogens. For patients who cannot tolerate TMP/SMZ, alternatives include dapsone plus pyrimethamine plus leucovorin, aerosolized pentamidine administered by the Respirgard II nebulizer, and atovaquone. Primary prophylaxis for PCP can be discontinued in those patients treated with combination antiretroviral therapy who maintain good suppression of HIV (<500 copies per milliliter) and CD4+ T cell counts >200/μL for at least 3 to 6 months. There is as yet insufficient information to know if the same recommendation will hold for discontinuation of secondary prophylaxis.

M. tuberculosis, once thought to be on its way to extinction in the United States, experienced a resurgence associated with the HIV epidemic (Chap. 169). Worldwide, approximately one-third of all AIDS-related deaths are associated with TB. In the United States approximately 5% of AIDS patients have active TB. HIV infection increases the risk of developing active tuberculosis by a factor of 15 to 30. For the patient with untreated HIV infection and a positive PPD skin test, the rate of reactivation TB is 7 to 10% per year. Untreated TB can accelerate the course of HIV infection. Levels of plasma HIV RNA increase in the setting of active TB and decline in the setting of successful TB treatment. Active TB is most common in patients 25 to 44 years of age, in African-Americans and Hispanics, in patients in New York City and Miami, and in patients in developing countries. In these demographic groups, 20 to 70% of the new cases of active TB are in patients with HIV infection. The epidemic of TB embedded in the epidemic of HIV infection probably represents the greatest health risk to the general public and the health care profession associated with the HIV epidemic. In contrast to infection with atypical mycobacteria such as MAC, active TB often develops relatively early in the course of HIV infection and may be an early clinical sign of HIV disease. In one study, the median CD4+ T cell count at presentation of TB was 326/μL. The clinical manifestations of TB in HIV-infected patients are quite varied and generally show different patterns as a function of the CD4+ T cell count. In patients with relatively high CD4+ T cell counts, the typical pattern of pulmonary reactivation occurs in which patients present with fever, cough, dyspnea on exertion, weight loss, night sweats, and a chest x-ray revealing cavitary apical disease of the upper lobes. In patients with lower CD4+ T cell counts, disseminated disease is more common. In these patients the chest x-ray may reveal diffuse or lower lobe bilateral reticulonodular infiltrates consistent with miliary spread, pleural effusions, and hilar and/or mediastinal adenopathy. Infection may be present in bone, brain, meninges, gastrointestinal tract, lymph nodes (particularly cervical lymph nodes), and viscera. Approximately 60 to 80% of patients have pulmonary disease, and 30 to 40% have extrapulmonary disease. Respiratory isolation and a negative-pressure room should be used for patients in whom a diagnosis of pulmonary TB is being considered. This approach is critical to limit nosocomial and community spread of infection. Culture of the organism from an involved site provides a definitive diagnosis. Blood cultures are positive in 15% of patients. In the setting of fulminant disease one cannot rely upon the accuracy of a negative PPD skin test to rule out a diagnosis of TB. TB is one of the conditions associated with HIV infection for which cure is possible. Therapy for TB is generally the same in the HIV-infected patient as in the HIV-negative patient (Chap. 169). Due to pharmacokinetic interactions, rifabutin should be substituted for rifampin in patients receiving the HIV protease inhibitors or nonnucleoside reverse transcriptase inhibitors; both drugs should be avoided in patients receiving ritonavir. Treatment is most effective in programs that involve directly observed therapy. Effective prevention of active TB can be a reality if the health care professional is aggressive in looking for evidence of latent TB by making sure that all patients with HIV infection receive a PPD skin test. Anergy testing is not of value in this setting. HIV-infected individuals with a skin test reaction of >5 mm or those who are close household contacts of persons with active TB should receive treatment with 9 months of isoniazid, or 2 months of therapy with rifampin and pyrazinamide, or 2 months of therapy with rifabutin and pyrazinamide.

Atypical mycobacterial infections are also seen with an increased frequency in patients with HIV infection. Infections with at least 12 different mycobacteria have been reported, including *M. bovis* and representatives of all four Runyon groups. The most common atypical mycobacterial infection is with *M. avium* or *M. intracellulare* species, the *M. avium* complex (MAC). Infections with MAC are seen mainly in patients in the United States and are rare in Africa. It has been suggested that prior infection with *M. tuberculosis* decreases the risk of MAC infection. MAC infections probably arise from organisms that are ubiquitous in the environment, including both soil and water. The presumed portals of entry are the respiratory and gastrointestinal tract. MAC infection is a late complication of HIV infection, occurring in patients with CD4+ T cell counts of <50/μL. The average CD4+ T cell count at the time of diagnosis is 10/μL. The most common presentation is disseminated disease with fever, weight loss, and night sweats. At least 85% of patients with MAC infection are mycobacteremic, and large numbers of organisms can often be demonstrated on bone marrow biopsy. The chest x-ray is abnormal in approximately 25% of patients, with the most common pattern being that of a bilateral, lower lobe infiltrate suggestive of miliary spread. Alveolar or nodular infiltrates and hilar and/or mediastinal adenopathy can also occur. Other clinical findings include endobronchial lesions, abdominal pain, diarrhea, and lymphadenopathy. The diagnosis is made by the culture of blood or involved tissue. The finding of two consecutive sputum samples positive for MAC is highly suggestive of pulmonary infection. Cultures may take 2 weeks to turn positive. Therapy consists of a macrolide, usually clarithromycin, with ethambutol. Some physicians elect to add a third drug from among rifabutin, ciprofloxacin, or amikacin in patients with extensive disease. Therapy is generally for life; however, with the advent of highly active antiretroviral therapy (HAART), it may be possible to discontinue therapy in patients with sustained suppression of HIV replication and CD4+ T cell counts >100/μL for >6 months. Primary prophylaxis for MAC is indicated in patients with HIV infection and CD4+ T cell counts <50/μL. This may be discontinued in patients in whom HAART induces a sustained suppression of viral replication and increases in CD4+ T cell counts to >100/μL for 3 to 6 months.

Rhodococcus equi is a gram-positive pleomorphic acid-fast non-spore-forming bacillus that can cause pulmonary and/or disseminated infection in patients with HIV infection. Fever and cough are the most common presenting signs. Radiographically one may see cavitary lesions and consolidation. Blood cultures are often positive. Treatment is based upon antimicrobial sensitivity testing.

Fungal infections of the lung can be seen in patients with AIDS. Patients with pulmonary cryptococcal disease present with fever, cough, dyspnea, and in some cases, hemoptysis. A focal or diffuse interstitial infiltrate is seen on chest x-ray in >90% of patients. In addition, one may see lobar disease, cavitary disease, pleural effusions, and hilar or mediastinal adenopathy. Over half of patients are fungemic, and 90% of patients have concomitant CNS infection. *Coccidioides immitis* is a mold that is endemic in the southwest United States. It can cause a reactivation pulmonary syndrome in patients with HIV infection. Most patients with this condition will have CD4+ T cell counts <250/μL. Patients present with fever, weight loss, cough, and extensive, diffuse reticulonodular infiltrates on chest x-ray. One may also see nodules, cavities, pleural effusions, and hilar adenopathy. While serologic testing is of value in the immunocompetent host, serologies are negative in 25% of HIV-infected patients with coccidioidal infection. Invasive aspergillosis is not an AIDS-defining illness and is generally not seen in patients with AIDS in the absence of neutropenia or administration of glucocorticoids. *Aspergillus* infection may have an unusual presentation in the respiratory tract of patients with AIDS where it gives the appearance of a pseudomembranous tracheobronchitis. Primary pulmonary infection of the lung may be seen with *histoplasmosis*. The most common pulmonary manifestation of histoplasmosis, however, is in the setting of disseminated disease, presumably due to reactivation. In this setting respiratory symptoms are usually minimal, with cough and dyspnea occurring in 10 to 30% of patients. The chest x-ray is abnormal in about 50% of patients, showing either a diffuse interstitial infiltrate or diffuse small nodules.

Two forms of *idiopathic interstitial pneumonia* have been identified in patients with HIV infection: lymphoid interstitial pneumonitis (LIP) and nonspecific interstitial pneumonitis (NIP). LIP, a common finding in children, is seen in about 1% of adult patients with HIV infection. This disorder is characterized by a benign infiltrate of the lung and is felt to be part of the polyclonal activation of lymphocytes seen in the context of HIV and EBV infections. Transbronchial biopsy is diagnostic in 50% of the cases, with an open-lung biopsy required for diagnosis in the remainder of cases. This condition is generally self-limited and no specific treatment is necessary. Severe cases have been managed with brief courses of glucocorticoids. Although rarely a clinical problem since the use of HAART, evidence of NIP may be seen in up to half of all patients with untreated HIV infection. Histologically, interstitial infiltrates of lymphocytes and plasma cells in a perivascular and peribronchial distribution are present. When symptomatic, patients present with fever and nonproductive cough occasionally accompanied by mild chest discomfort. Chest x-ray is usually normal or may reveal a faint interstitial pattern. Similar to LIP, this is a self-limited process for which no therapy is indicated.

Neoplastic diseases of the lung including KS and lymphoma are discussed below in the section on malignancies.

Diseases of the Cardiovascular System While heart disease is a relatively common postmortem finding in HIV-infected patients (25 to 75% in autopsy series), it is less of a problem clinically. The most common clinically significant finding is a dilated cardiomyopathy associated with congestive heart failure referred to as *HIV-associated cardiomyopathy*. This generally occurs as a late complication of HIV infection and, histologically, displays elements of myocarditis. For this reason some have advocated treatment with intravenous Ig. HIV can be directly demonstrated in cardiac tissue in this setting, and there is debate over whether or not it plays a direct role in this condition. Patients present with typical findings of congestive heart failure, namely edema and shortness of breath. Patients with HIV infection may also develop cardiomyopathy as a side effect of IFN-α or nucleoside analogue therapy, which is reversible once therapy is stopped. KS, cryptococcosis, Chagas disease, and toxoplasmosis can involve the myocardium, leading to cardiomyopathy. In one series, most patients with HIV infection and a treatable myocarditis were found to have myocarditis associated with toxoplasmosis. Most of these patients also had evidence of CNS toxoplasmosis. Thus, MRI or double-dose contrast CT scan of the brain should be included in the workup of any patient with advanced HIV infection and cardiomyopathy.

A variety of other cardiovascular problems are found in patients with HIV infection. Pericardial effusions may be seen in the setting of advanced HIV infection. Predisposing factors include TB, congestive heart failure, mycobacterial infection, cryptococcal infection, pulmonary infection, lymphoma, and KS. While pericarditis is quite rare, in one series 5% of patients with HIV disease had pericardial effusions that were considered to be moderate or severe. Tamponade and death have occurred in association with pericardial KS, presumably owing to acute hemorrhage. A high percentage of patients have hypertriglyceridemia and elevations in serum cholesterol, and coronary artery disease has been a relatively frequent finding at autopsy. This problem appears to becoming even more prevalent as a side effect of HAART. While clinically significant ischemic heart disease has not been reported to be occurring with an increased frequency in this patient population, many are concerned that it is just a matter of time before this is the case. Nonbacterial thrombotic endocarditis has been reported and should be considered in patients with unexplained embolic phenomena. Intravenous pentamidine, when given rapidly, can result in hypotension as a consequence of cardiovascular collapse.

Diseases of the Oropharynx and Gastrointestinal System Oropharyngeal and gastrointestinal diseases are common features of HIV infection. They are most frequently due to secondary infections. In addition, oral and gastrointestinal lesions may occur with KS and lymphoma.

Oral lesions, including *thrush, hairy leukoplakia,* and *aphthous ulcers*, are particularly common in patients with untreated HIV infection. Thrush, due to *Candida* infection, and oral hairy leukoplakia, presumed due to EBV, are usually indicative of fairly advanced immunologic decline; they generally occur in patients with CD4+ T cell counts of <300/μL. In one study, 59% of patients with oral candidiasis went on to develop AIDS in the next year. Thrush appears as a white, cheesy exudate, often on an erythematous mucosa in the posterior oropharynx **(see Plate IID-43)**. While most commonly seen on the soft palate, early lesions are often found along the gingival border. The diagnosis is made by direct examination of a scraping for pseudohyphal elements. Culturing is of no diagnostic value, as most patients with HIV infection will have a positive throat culture for *Candida* even in the absence of thrush. Oral hairy leukoplakia presents as white, frondlike lesions, generally along the lateral borders of the tongue and sometimes on the adjacent buccal mucosa **(see Plate IID-42)**. Despite its name, oral hairy leukoplakia is not considered a premalignant condition. Lesions are associated with florid replication of EBV. While usually more disconcerting as a sign of HIV-associated immunodeficiency than a clinical problem in need of treatment, severe cases have been reported to respond to topical podophyllin or systemic therapy with acyclovir. Aphthous ulcers of the posterior oropharynx are also seen with regularity in patients with HIV infection. These lesions are of unknown etiology and can be quite painful and interfere with swallowing. Topical anesthetics provide immediate symptomatic relief of short duration. The fact that thalidomide is an effective treatment for this condition suggests that the pathogenesis may involve the action of tissue-destructive cytokines. Palatal, glossal, or gingival ulcers may also result from cryptococcal disease or histoplasmosis.

Esophagitis (Fig. 309-29) may present with odynophagia and retrosternal pain. Upper endoscopy is generally required to make an accurate diagnosis. Esophagitis may be due to *Candida*, CMV, or HSV. While CMV tends to be associated with a single large ulcer, HSV infection is more often associated with multiple small ulcers. The esophagus may also be the site of KS and lymphoma. Like the oral mucosa, the esophageal mucosa may have large, painful ulcers of unclear etiology that may respond to thalidomide. While achlorhydria is a common problem in patients with HIV infection, other gastric problems are generally rare. Among the conditions involving the stomach are KS and lymphoma. Infections of the small and large intestine leading to diarrhea, abdominal pain, and occasionally fever are among the most significant gastrointestinal problems in the HIV-infected patients. They include infections with bacteria, protozoa, and viruses.

FIGURE 309-29 Barium swallow of a patient with *Candida* esophagitis. The flow of barium along the mucosal surface is grossly irregular.

Bacteria and fungi may be responsible for secondary infections of the gastrointestinal tract. Infections with enteric pathogens such as *Salmonella*, *Shigella*, and *Campylobacter* are more common in homosexual men and are often more severe and more apt to relapse in patients with HIV infection. Patients with untreated HIV have approximately a 20-fold increased risk of infection with *S. typhimurium*. They may present with a variety of nonspecific symptoms including fever, anorexia, fatigue, and malaise of several weeks' duration. Diarrhea is common but may be absent. Diagnosis is made by culture of blood and stool. Long-term therapy with ciprofloxacin is the recommended treatment. HIV-infected patients also have an increased incidence of *S. typhi* infection in areas of the world where typhoid is a problem. *Shigella* spp., particularly *S. flexneri*, can cause severe intestinal disease in HIV-infected individuals. Up to 50% of patients will develop bacteremia. *Campylobacter* infections occur with an increased frequency in patients with HIV infection. While *C. jejuni* is the strain most frequently isolated, infections with many other strains have been reported. Patients usually present with crampy abdominal pain, fever, and bloody diarrhea. Infection may present as proctitis. Stool examination reveals the presence of fecal leukocytes. Systemic infection can occur, with up to 10% of infected patients exhibiting bacteremia. Most strains are sensitive to erythromycin. Abdominal pain and diarrhea may be seen with MAC infection.

Fungal infections may also be a cause of diarrhea in patients with HIV infection. Histoplasmosis, coccidioidomycosis, and penicilliosis have all been identified as a cause of fever and diarrhea in patients with HIV infection. Peritonitis has been seen with *C. immitis*.

Cryptosporidia, microsporidia, and *Isospora belli* (Chap. 218) are the most common opportunistic protozoa that infect the gastrointestinal tract and cause diarrhea in HIV-infected patients. Cryptosporidial infection may present in a variety of ways, ranging from a self-limited or intermittent diarrheal illness in patients in the early stages of HIV infection to a severe, life-threatening diarrhea in severely immunodeficient individuals. In patients with untreated HIV infection and

CD4+ T cell counts of <300/μL, the incidence of cryptosporidiosis is approximately 1% per year. In 75% of cases the diarrhea is accompanied by crampy abdominal pain, and 25% of patients have nausea and/or vomiting. Cryptosporidia may also cause biliary tract disease in the HIV-infected patient, leading to cholecystitis with or without accompanying cholangitis. The diagnosis of cryptosporidial diarrhea is made by stool examination. The diarrhea is noninflammatory, and the characteristic finding is the presence of oocysts that stain with acid-fast dyes. Therapy is predominantly supportive, and marked improvements have been reported in the setting of effective antiretroviral therapy. Treatment with up to 2000 mg/d of nitazoxanide (NTZ) is associated with improvement in symptoms or a decrease in shedding of organisms in about half of patients. Its overall role in the management of this condition remains unclear. Patients can minimize their risk of developing cryptosporidiosis by avoiding contact with human and animal feces and by not drinking untreated water from lakes or rivers.

Microsporidia are small, unicellular, obligate intracellular parasites that reside in the cytoplasm of enteric cells (Chap. 218). The main species causing disease in humans is *Enterocytozoon bieneusi*. The clinical manifestations are similar to those described for Cryptosporidia and include abdominal pain and diarrhea. The small size of the organism may make it difficult to detect; however, with the use of chromotrope-based stains, organisms can be identified in stool samples by light microscopy. Definitive diagnosis generally depends on electron microscopic examination of a stool specimen, intestinal aspirate, or intestinal biopsy specimen. In contrast to cryptosporidia, microsporidia have been noted in a variety of extraintestinal locations, including the eye, muscle, and liver, and have been associated with conjunctivitis and hepatitis. Albendazole, 400 mg bid, has been reported to be of benefit in some patients.

I. belli is a coccidian parasite (Chap. 218) most commonly found as a cause of diarrhea in patients from the Caribbean and Africa. Its cysts appear in the stool as large, acid-fast structures that can be differentiated from those of cryptosporidia on the basis of size, shape, and number of sporocysts. The clinical syndromes of *Isospora* infection are identical to those caused by cryptosporidia. The important distinction is that infection with *Isospora* is generally relatively easy to treat with TMP/SMZ. While relapses are common, a thrice-weekly regimen, similar to that used to provide prophylaxis against PCP, appears adequate to prevent recurrence.

CMV colitis was once seen in 5 to 10% of patients with AIDS. It is much less common with the advent of HAART. CMV colitis presents as diarrhea, abdominal pain, weight loss, and anorexia. The diarrhea is usually nonbloody, and the diagnosis is achieved through endoscopy and biopsy. Multiple mucosal ulcerations are seen at endoscopy, and biopsies reveal characteristic intranuclear inclusion bodies. Bacteremia may result as a consequence of thinning of the bowel wall. Treatment is with either ganciclovir or foscarnet for 3 to 6 weeks. Relapses are common, and maintenance therapy is typically necessary in patients whose HIV infection is poorly controlled. Patients with CMV disease of the gastrointestinal tract should be carefully monitored for evidence of retinitis.

In addition to disease caused by specific secondary infections, patients with HIV infection may also experience a chronic diarrheal syndrome for which no etiologic agent other than HIV can be identified. This entity is referred to as *AIDS enteropathy* or *HIV enteropathy*. It is most likely a direct result of HIV infection in the gastrointestinal tract. Histologic examination of the small bowel in these patients reveals low-grade mucosal atrophy with a decrease in mitotic figures, suggesting a hyporegenerative state. Patients often have decreased or absent small-bowel lactase and malabsorption with accompanying weight loss.

The initial evaluation of a patient with HIV infection and diarrhea should include a set of stool examinations, including culture, examination for ova and parasites, and examination for *Clostridium difficile* toxin. Approximately 50% of the time this workup will demonstrate infection with pathogenic bacteria, mycobacteria, or protozoa. If the initial stool examinations are negative, additional evaluation, including upper and/or lower endoscopy with biopsy, will yield a diagnosis of microsporidial or mycobacterial infection of the small intestine ~30% of the time. In patients for whom this diagnostic evaluation is nonrevealing, a presumptive diagnosis of HIV enteropathy can be made if the diarrhea has persisted for >1 month. An algorithm for the evaluation of diarrhea in patients with HIV infection is given in Fig. 309-30.

Rectal lesions are common in HIV-infected patients, particularly the perirectal ulcers and erosions due to the reactivation of HSV (Fig. 309-31). These may appear quite atypical, as denuded skin without vesicles, and they respond well to treatment with acyclovir, famciclovir, or foscarnet. Other rectal lesions encountered in the patients with HIV infection include condylomata acuminata, KS, and intraepithelial neoplasia.

Hepatobiliary Disease   Diseases of the hepatobiliary system are a major problem in patients with HIV infection. It has been estimated that approximately one-third of the deaths of patients with HIV infection are in some way related to liver disease. While this is predominantly a reflection of the problems encountered in the setting of co-infection with hepatitis B or C, it is also a reflection of the hepatic injury, predominantly in the form of hepatic steatosis, that can be seen in the context of nucleoside analogue antiretroviral therapy.

Over 95% of HIV-infected individuals have evidence of infection with HBV; 5–40% of patients are co-infected with hepatitis C virus (HCV); and co-infection with hepatitis D, E, and/or G viruses is common. HIV infection has a significant impact on the course of hepatitis virus infection. It is associated with approximately a threefold increase in the development of persistent hepatitis B surface antigenemia. Patients infected with both HBV and HIV have decreased evidence of inflammatory liver disease. The presumption that this is due to the immunosuppressive effects of HIV infection is supported by the observations that this situation can be reversed, and one may see the development of more severe hepatitis following the initiation of effective antiretroviral therapy. IFN-α is less successful as a treatment of HBV in patients with HIV co-infection, and lamivudine is the treatment of choice. It is important to remember that lamivudine is also a

FIGURE 309-31   Severe, erosive perirectal herpes simplex in a patient with AIDS.

potent antiretroviral agent in the setting of combination antiretroviral therapy. It should not be used as a single agent in patients with HIV infection, even if it is only being used to treat HBV, in order to avoid the rapid development of lamivudine-resistant quasispecies of HIV. In contrast to the situation with HBV, HCV infection is more severe in the patient with HIV infection. In the setting of HIV and HCV co-infection, levels of HCV are approximately tenfold higher than in the HIV-negative patient with HCV infection. The incidence of HCV-associated liver failure appears to be higher by a similar factor in patients with HIV infection. Hepatitis A virus infection is not seen with an increased frequency in patients with HIV infection. It is recommended that all patients with HIV infection who have not experienced natural infection be immunized with hepatitis A and/or hepatitis B vaccines.

A variety of other infections may also involve the liver. Granulomatous hepatitis may be seen as a consequence of mycobacterial or fungal infections, particularly MAC infection. Hepatic masses may be seen in the context of TB, peliosis hepatis, or fungal infection. Among the fungal opportunistic infection *C. immitis* and *Histoplasma capsulatum* are those most likely to involve the liver. Biliary tract disease in the form of papillary stenosis or sclerosing cholangitis has been reported in the context of cryptosporidiosis, CMV infection, and KS.

Many of the drugs used to treat HIV infection are metabolized by the liver and can cause liver injury. Nucleoside analogues work by inhibiting DNA synthesis. This can result in toxicity to mitochondria, which can lead to disturbances in oxidative metabolism. This may be manifest as hepatic steatosis and, in severe cases, lactic acidosis and fulminant liver failure. It is important to be aware of this condition and to watch for it in patients with HIV infection receiving nucleoside analogues. It is reversible if diagnosed early and the offending agent(s) discontinued. Indinavir may cause mild to moderate elevations in serum bilirubin in 10 to 15% of patients in a syndrome similar to Gilbert's syndrome.

Pancreatic injury is most commonly a consequence of drug toxicity, notably that secondary to pentamidine or dideoxynucleosides.

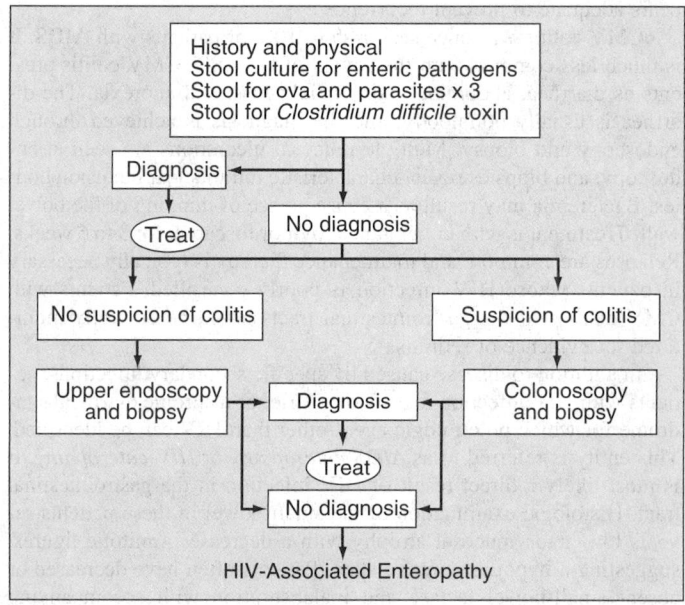

FIGURE 309-30   Algorithm for the evaluation of diarrhea in a patient with HIV infection. HIV-associated enteropathy is a diagnosis of exclusion and can be made only after other, generally treatable, forms of diarrheal illness have been ruled out.

While up to half of patients in some series have biochemical evidence of pancreatic injury, <5% of patients show any clinical evidence of pancreatitis that is not linked to a drug toxicity.

Diseases of the Kidney and Genitourinary Tract Diseases of the kidney or genitourinary tract may be a direct consequence of HIV infection, due to an opportunistic infection or neoplasm, or related to drug toxicity. *HIV-associated nephropathy* was first described in IDUs and was initially thought to be IDU nephropathy in patients with HIV infection; it is now recognized as a true direct complication of HIV infection. HIV-associated nephropathy can be an early manifestation of HIV infection and is also seen in children. Over 90% of reported cases have been in African-American or Hispanic individuals; the disease is not only more prevalent in these populations but also more severe. Proteinuria is the hallmark of this disorder. Overall, microalbuminuria is seen in ~20% of untreated HIV-infected patients; significant proteinuria is seen in closer to 2%. Edema and hypertension are rare. Ultrasound examination reveals enlarged, hyperechogenic kidneys. A definitive diagnosis is obtained through renal biopsy. Histologically, focal segmental glomerulosclerosis is present in 80%, and mesangial proliferation in 10 to 15% of cases. Prior to effective antiretroviral therapy, this disease was characterized by relatively rapid progression to end-stage renal disease. Treatment with prednisone, 60 mg/d, has been reported to be of benefit in some cases. The incidence of this disease in patients receiving adequate antiretroviral therapy has not been well defined; however, the impression is that it has decreased in frequency. It is the leading cause of end-stage renal disease in patients with HIV infection.

Among the drugs commonly associated with renal damage in patients with HIV disease are pentamidine, amphotericin, adefovir, cidofovir, and foscarnet. TMP/SMZ may compete for tubular secretion with creatinine and cause an increase in the serum creatinine level. Sulfadiazine may crystallize in the kidney and result in an easily reversible form of renal shutdown. One of the most common drug-induced renal complications is indinavir-associated renal calculi. This condition is seen in ~10% of patients receiving this HIV protease inhibitor. It may present with a variety of manifestations, ranging from asymptomatic hematuria to renal colic. Adequate hydration is the mainstay of treatment and prevention for this condition.

Genitourinary tract infections are seen with a high frequency in patients with HIV infection; they present with dysuria, hematuria, and/or pyuria and are managed in the same fashion as in patients with HIV infection. Infections with *T. pallidum*, the etiologic agent of *syphilis*, play an important role in the HIV epidemic (Chap. 172). In HIV-negative individuals, genital syphilitic ulcers as well as the ulcers of chancroid are major predisposing factors for heterosexual transmission of HIV infection. While most HIV-infected individuals with syphilis have a typical presentation, a variety of formerly rare clinical problems may be encountered in the setting of dual infection. Among them are *lues maligna*, an ulcerating lesion of the skin due to a necrotizing vasculitis; unexplained fever; nephrotic syndrome; and neurosyphilis. The most common presentation of syphilis in the HIV-infected patient is that of *condylomata lata*, a form of secondary syphilis. Neurosyphilis may be asymptomatic or may present as acute meningitis, neuroretinitis, deafness, or stroke. The rate of neurosyphilis may be as high as 1% in patients with HIV infection. As a consequence of the immunologic abnormalities seen in the setting of HIV infection, diagnosis of syphilis through standard serologic testing may be challenging. On the one hand, a significant number of patients have false-positive Venereal Disease Research Laboratory (VDRL) tests due to polyclonal B cell activation. On the other hand, the development of a new positive VDRL may be delayed in patients with new infections, and the anti-fluorescent treponema antibody (anti-FTA) test may be negative due to immunodeficiency. Thus, dark-field examination of appropriate specimens should be performed in any patient in whom syphilis is suspected, even if the patient has a negative VDRL. Similarly, any patient with a positive serum VDRL test, neurologic findings, and an abnormal spinal fluid examination should be considered to have neurosyphilis, regardless of the CSF VDRL result. In any

setting, patients treated for syphilis need to be carefully monitored to ensure adequate therapy.

Vulvovaginal candidiasis is a common problem in women with HIV infection. Symptoms include pruritus, discomfort, dyspareunia, and dysuria. Vulvar infection may present as a moribilliform rash that may extend to the thighs. Vaginal infection is usually associated with a white discharge, and plaques may be seen along an erythematous vaginal wall. Diagnosis is made by microscopic examination of the discharge for pseudohyphal elements in a 10% potassium hydroxide solution. Mild disease can be treated with topical therapy. More serious disease can be treated with fluconazole. Other causes of vaginitis include *Trichomonas* and mixed bacteria.

Diseases of the Endocrine System and Metabolic Disorders A variety of endocrine and metabolic disorders are seen in the context of HIV infection. Between 33 and 75% of patients with HIV infection receiving HAART develop a syndrome often referred to as *lipodystrophy*, consisting of elevations in plasma triglycerides, total cholesterol, apolipoprotein B, and high-density lipoprotein cholesterol as well as hyperinsulinemia. Many of these patients have been noted to have a characteristic set of body habitus changes associated with fat redistribution, consisting of truncal obesity coupled with peripheral wasting (Fig. 309-32). Truncal obesity is apparent as an increase in abdominal girth related to increases in mesenteric fat, a dorsocervical fat pad ("buffalo hump") reminiscent of patients with Cushing's syndrome, and enlargement of the breasts. The peripheral wasting is particularly noticeable in the face and buttocks and by the prominence of the veins in the legs. Other related problems include insulin-requiring diabetes mellitus and avascular necrosis of the femoral head. These changes may develop at any time ranging from approximately 6 weeks to several years following the initiation of HAART. The syndrome has been reported in association with regimens containing a variety of different drugs, and while initially reported in the setting of protease inhibitor therapy, it appears similar changes can be induced by potent protease-sparing regimens. National Cholesterol Education Program (NCEP) guidelines should be followed in the management of these lipid abnormalities (Chap. 242). Due to concerns regarding drug interactions, the most commonly utilized agents in this setting are gemfibrozil and atorvostatin.

Patients with advanced HIV disease may develop hyponatremia due to the syndrome of inappropriate antidiuretic hormone (vasopressin) secretion (SIADH) as a consequence of increased free water intake and decreased free water excretion. SIADH is usually seen in conjunction with pulmonary or CNS disease. Low serum sodium may also be due to adrenal insufficiency; concomitant high serum potassium should alert one to this possibility. Adrenal gland disease may be due to mycobacterial infections, CMV disease, cryptococcal disease, histoplasmosis, or ketoconazole toxicity.

Thyroid function is generally normal in patients with HIV infection although approximately 2 to 3% of patients may have elevations in thyroid stimulating hormone (TSH). In advanced HIV disease, infection of the thyroid gland may occur with opportunistic pathogens, including *P. carinii*, CMV, mycobacteria, *Toxoplasma gondii*, and *Cryptococcus neoformans*. These infections are generally associated with a nontender, diffuse enlargement of the thyroid gland. Thyroid function is usually normal. Diagnosis is made by fine-needle aspirate or open biopsy.

Advanced HIV disease is associated with *hypogonadism* in approximately 50% of men. While this is generally a complication of underlying illness, testicular dysfunction may also be a side effect of ganciclovir therapy. In some surveys, up to two-thirds of patients report decreased libido and one-third complain of impotence. Androgen replacement therapy should be considered in patients with symptomatic hypogonadism. HIV infection does not seem to have a significant effect on the menstrual cycle outside the setting of advanced disease.

Rheumatologic Diseases Immunologic and rheumatologic disorders are common in patients with HIV infection and range from

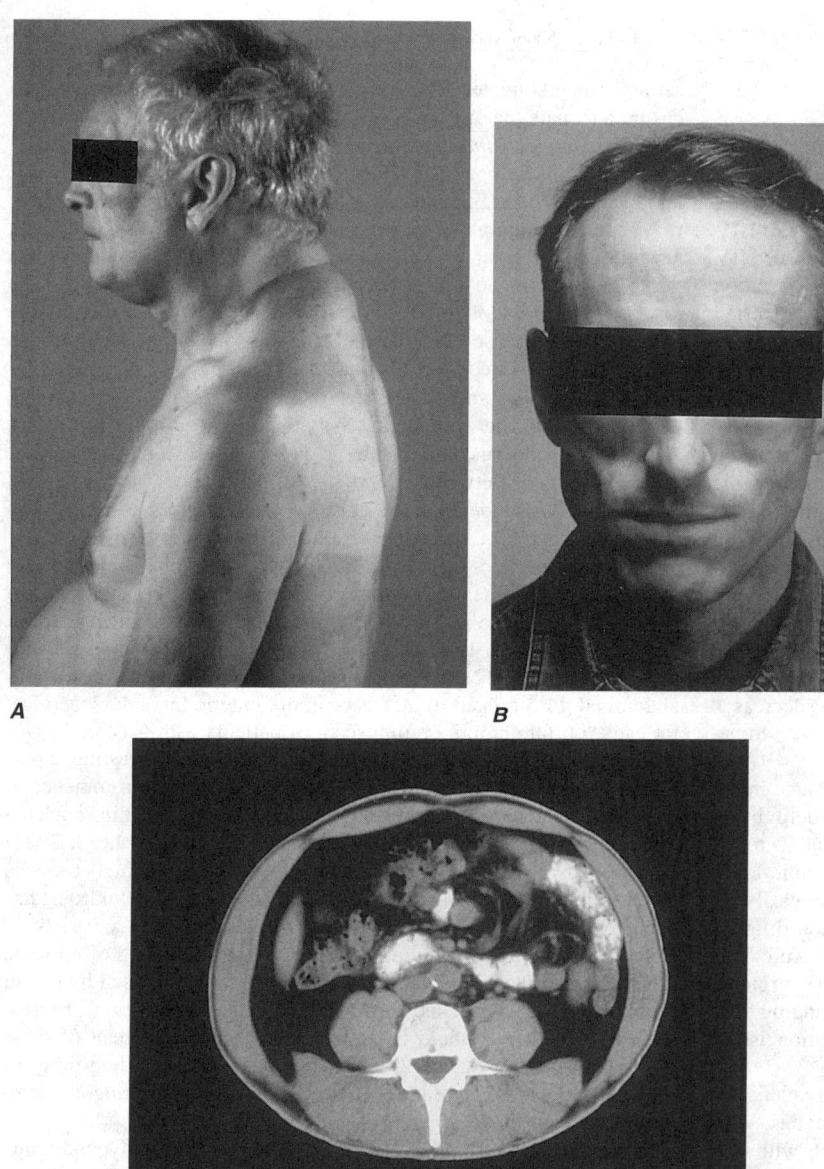

FIGURE 309-32 Characteristics of lipodystrophy. *A*. Truncal obesity and buffalo hump. *B*. Facial wasting. *C*. Accumulation of intraabdominal fat on CT scan.

traindication to future therapy. For other agents, including TMP/SMZ, desensitization regimens are moderatively successful. While the mechanisms underlying these allergic-type reactions remain unknown, patients with HIV infection have been noted to have elevated IgE levels that increase as the CD4+ T cell count declines. The numerous examples of patients with multiple drug reactions suggest that a common pathway is involved.

HIV infection shares many similarities with a variety of autoimmune diseases, including a substantial polyclonal B cell activation that is associated with a high incidence of antiphospholipid antibodies, such as anticardiolipin antibodies, VDRL antibodies, and lupus-like anticoagulants. In addition, HIV-infected individuals have an increased incidence of antinuclear antibodies. Despite these serologic findings, there is no evidence that HIV-infected individuals have an increase in two of the more common autoimmune diseases, i.e., systemic lupus erythematosus and rheumatoid arthritis. In fact, it has been observed that these diseases may be somewhat ameliorated by the concomitant presence of HIV infection, suggesting that an intact CD4+ T cell limb of the immune response plays an integral role in the pathogenesis of these conditions. Similarly, there are anecdotal reports of patients with common variable immunodeficiency (Chap. 308), characterized by hypogammaglobulinemia who have had a normalization of Ig levels following the development of HIV infection, suggesting a possible role for overactive CD4+ T cell immunity in certain forms of that syndrome. The one autoimmune disease that may occur with an increased frequency in patients with HIV infection is a variant of primary Sjögren's syndrome (Chap. 314). Patients with HIV infection may develop a syndrome consisting of parotid gland enlargement, dry eyes, and dry mouth that is associated with lymphocytic infiltrates of the salivary gland and lung. In contrast to Sjögren's syndrome, in which these infiltrates are composed predominantly of CD4+ T cells, in patients with HIV infection the infiltrates are composed predominantly of CD8+ T cells. In addition, while patients with Sjögren's syndrome are mainly women who have autoantibodies to Ro and La and

excessive immediate-type hypersensitivity reactions (Chap. 310) to an increase in the incidence of reactive arthritis (Chap. 315) to conditions characterized by a diffuse infiltrative lymphocytosis. These phenomena occur in an apparent paradox to the profound immunodeficiency and immunosuppression that characterizes HIV infection. In addition, following the initiation of antiretroviral therapy, one may see a variety of exaggerated immune responses to existing opportunistic infections referred to as *immune reactivation syndromes*.

Drug allergies are the most significant allergic reactions occurring in HIV-infected patients and appear to become more common as the disease progresses. They occur in 65% of patients who receive therapy with TMP/SMZ for PCP. In general, these drug reactions are characterized by erythematous, morbilliform eruption that are pruritic, tend to coalesce, and are often associated with fever. Nonetheless, ~33% of patients can be maintained on the offending therapy, and thus these reactions are not an immediate indication to stop the drug. Anaphylaxis is extremely rare in patients with HIV infection, and patients who have a cutaneous reaction during a single course of therapy can still be considered candidates for future treatment or prophylaxis with the same agent. The one exception to this is the nucleoside analogue abacavir, where fatal hypersensitivity reactions have been reported with rechallenge. A hypersensitivity reaction to abacavir is an absolute con-

who frequently have HLA-DR3 or -B8, MHC haplotypes, HIV-infected individuals with this syndrome are usually African-American men who do not have anti-Ro or anti-La and who most often are HLA-DR5. This syndrome appears to be less common with the increased use of effective antiretroviral therapy. The term *diffuse infiltrative lymphocytosis syndrome* (DILS) has been proposed to describe this entity and to distinguish it from Sjögren's syndrome.

Approximately one-third of HIV-infected individuals experience arthralgias; furthermore, 5 to 10% are diagnosed as having some form of reactive arthritis, such as Reiter's syndrome or psoriatic arthritis (Chaps. 315 and 324). These syndromes occur with increasing frequency as the competency of the immune system declines. This association may be related to an increase in the number of infections with organisms that may trigger a reactive arthritis with progressive immunodeficiency. Reactive arthritides in HIV-infected individuals generally respond well to standard treatment; however, therapy with methotrexate has been associated with an increase in the incidence of opportunistic infections and should be used with caution and only in severe cases.

HIV-infected individuals also experience a variety of joint problems without obvious cause that are referred to generically as *HIV- or AIDS-associated arthropathy*. This syndrome is characterized by subacute oligoarticular arthritis developing over a period of 1 to 6 weeks and lasting 6 weeks to 6 months. It generally involves the large joints, predominantly the knees and ankles, and is nonerosive with only a mild inflammatory response. X-rays of the joint are nonrevealing. Nonsteroidal anti-inflammatory drugs are only marginally helpful; however, relief has been noted with the use of intraarticular glucocorticoids. A second form of arthritis also thought to be secondary to HIV infection is called *painful articular syndrome*. This condition, found in as many as 10% of AIDS patients, presents as an acute, severe, sharp pain in the affected joint. It affects primarily the knees, elbows, and shoulders; lasts 2 to 24 h; and may be severe enough to require narcotic analgesics. The cause of this arthropathy is unclear; however, it is thought to result from a direct effect of HIV on the joint. This condition is reminiscent of the fact that other lentiviruses, in particular the caprine arthritis-encephalitis virus, are capable of directly causing arthritis.

A variety of other immunologic or rheumatologic diseases have been reported in HIV-infected individuals, either de novo or in association with opportunistic infections or drugs. Using the criteria of widespread musculoskeletal pain of at least 3 months' duration and the presence of at least 11 of 18 possible tender points by digital palpation, 11% of an HIV-infected cohort containing 55% IDUs were diagnosed as having *fibromyalgia* (Chap. 325). While the incidence of frank arthritis was less in this population than in other studied populations that consisted predominantly of homosexual men, these data support the concept that there are musculoskeletal problems that occur as a direct result of HIV infection. In addition there have been reports of leukocytoclastic vasculitis in the setting of zidovudine therapy. CNS angiitis and polymyositis have also been reported in HIV-infected individuals. Septic arthritis is surprisingly rare, especially given the increased incidence of staphylococcal bacteremias seen in this population. When septic arthritis has been reported, it has usually been due to systemic fungal infections with *C. neoformans*, *Sporothrix schenckii*, or *H. capsulatum*, or systemic mycobacterial infection with *M. haemophilum*.

Following the initiation of effective antiretroviral therapy, a paradoxical worsening of preexisting, untreated opportunistic infections may be noted. These *immune reactivation syndromes* are particularly common in patients with underlying untreated mycobacterial infections. They appear to be related to a phenomenon similar to type IV hypersensitivity reactions and reflect the immediate improvements in immune function that occur as levels of HIV RNA drop and the immunosuppressive effects of HIV infection are controlled. In severe cases the use of immunosuppressive drugs such as glucocorticoids may be required to blunt the inflammatory component of these reactions while specific antimicrobial therapy takes effect.

Diseases of the Hematopoietic System   Disorders of the hematopoietic system including lymphadenopathy, anemia, leukopenia, and/or thrombocytopenia are common throughout the course of HIV infection and may be the direct result of HIV, manifestations of secondary infections and neoplasms, or side effects of therapy (Table 309-12). Direct histologic examination and culture of lymph node or bone marrow tissue are often diagnostic. A significant percentage of bone marrow aspirates from patients with HIV infection have been reported to contain lymphoid aggregates, the precise significance of which is unknown.

Table 309-12   Causes of Bone Marrow Suppression in Patients with HIV Infection

HIV infection	Medications:
Mycobacterial infections	Zidovudine
Fungal infections	Dapsone
B19 parvovirus infection	Trimethoprim/sulfamethoxazole
Lymphoma	Pyrimethamine
	5-Flucytosine
	Ganciclovir
	Interferon-α
	Trimetrexate
	Foscarnet

Some patients, otherwise asymptomatic, may develop *persistent generalized lymphadenopathy* as an early clinical manifestation of HIV infection. This condition is defined as the presence of enlarged lymph nodes (>1 cm) in two or more extrainguinal sites for >3 months without an obvious cause. The lymphadenopathy is due to marked follicular hyperplasia in the node in response to HIV infection. The nodes are generally discrete and freely movable. This feature of HIV disease may be seen at any point in the spectrum of immune dysfunction and is not associated with an increased likelihood of developing AIDS. Paradoxically, a loss in lymphadenopathy or a decrease in lymph node size outside the setting of antiretroviral therapy may be a prognostic marker of disease progression. In patients with CD4+ T cell counts >200/μL, the differential diagnosis of lymphadenopathy includes KS and TB. In patients with more advanced disease, lymphadenopathy may also be due to lymphoma, atypical mycobacterial infection, toxoplasmosis, systemic fungal infection, or bacillary angiomatosis. While indicated in patients with CD4+ T cell counts <200/μL, lymph node biopsy is not indicated in patients with early-stage disease unless there are signs and symptoms of systemic illness, such as fever and weight loss, or unless the nodes begin to enlarge, become fixed, or coalesce.

Anemia is the most common hematologic abnormality in HIV-infected patients. While generally mild, anemia can be quite severe and require chronic blood transfusions. Among the specific reversible causes of anemia in the setting of HIV infection are drug toxicity, systemic fungal and mycobacterial infections, nutritional deficiencies, and parvovirus B19 infections. Zidovudine has a somewhat selective ability to block erythroid maturation, an effect that precedes effects on other marrow elements. A characteristic feature of zidovudine therapy is an elevated mean corpuscular volume (MCV). Another drug used in patients with HIV infection that has a selective effect on the erythroid series is dapsone. This drug can cause a serious hemolytic anemia in patients who are deficient in glucose-6-phosphate dehydrogenase and can create a functional anemia in others through induction of methemoglobinemia. Folate levels are usually normal in HIV-infected individuals; however, vitamin B_{12} levels may be depressed as a consequence of achlorhydria or malabsorption. True autoimmune hemolytic anemia is rare, although ~20% of patients with HIV infection may have a positive direct antiglobulin test as a consequence of polyclonal B cell activation. Infection with parvovirus B19 may also cause anemia. It is important to recognize this possibility given the fact that it responds well to treatment with intravenous immunoglobulin. Erythropoietin levels in patients with HIV infection and anemia are generally less than expected given the degree of anemia. Treatment with erythropoietin at doses of 100 μg/kg three times a week may result in an increase in hemoglobulin levels. An exception to this is a subset of patients with zidovudine-associated anemia in whom erythropoietin levels may be quite high.

During the course of HIV infection, neutropenia may be seen in approximately half of patients. In most instances it is mild; however, it can be severe and can put patients at risk of spontaneous bacterial infections. This is most frequently seen in patients with severely advanced HIV disease and in patients receiving any of a number of potentially myelosuppressive therapies. In the setting of neutropenia, diseases that are not commonly seen in HIV-infected patients, such as aspergillosis or mucormycosis, may occur. The potential role of colony-stimulating factors in the management of patients with HIV infection has undergone extensive evaluation. Both granulocyte colony stimulating factor (G-CSF) and GM-CSF increase neutrophil counts in patients with HIV infection regardless of the cause of the neutropenia. Earlier concerns about the potential of these agents to also increase levels of HIV were not confirmed in controlled clinical trials.

Thrombocytopenia may be an early consequence of HIV infection. Approximately 3% of patients with untreated HIV infection and CD4+ T cell counts ≥400/μL have platelet counts <150,000/μL. For untreated patients with CD4+ T cell counts <400/μL, this incidence increases to 10%. Thrombocytopenia is rarely a serious clinical problem in patients with HIV infection and generally responds well to antiretroviral therapy. Clinically, it resembles the thrombocytopenia seen in patients with idiopathic thrombocytopenic purpura (Chap. 116). Immune complexes containing anti-gp120 antibodies and anti-anti gp120 antibodies have been noted in the circulation and on the surface of platelets in patients with HIV infection. Patients with HIV infection have also been noted to have a platelet-specific antibody directed towards a 25-kDa component of the surface of the platelet. Other data suggest that the thrombocytopenia in patients with HIV infection may be due to a direct effect of HIV on megakaryocytes. Whatever the cause, it is very clear that the most effective medical approach to this problem has been the use of combination antiretroviral therapy. For patients with platelet counts <20,000/μL a more aggressive approach combining intravenous Ig or anti-Rh Ig for an immediate response with antiretroviral therapy for a more lasting response is appropriate. Splenectomy is a rarely needed option and is reserved for patients refractory to medical management. Because of the risk of serious infection with encapsulated organisms, all patients with HIV infection about to undergo splenectomy should be immunized with pneumococcal polysaccharide. It should be noted that, in addition to causing an increase in the platelet count, removal of the spleen will result in an increase in the peripheral blood lymphocyte count, making CD4+ T cell counts unreliable. In this setting, the clinician should rely on the CD4+ T cell percent for making diagnostic decisions with respect to the likelihood of opportunistic infections. A CD4+ T cell percent of 15 is approximately equivalent to a CD4+ T cell count of 200/μL. In patients with early HIV infection, thrombocytopenia has also been reported as a consequence of classic thrombotic thrombocytopenic purpura (Chap. 116). This clinical syndrome, consisting of fever, thrombocytopenia, hemolytic anemia, and neurologic and renal dysfunction, is a rare complication of early HIV infection. As in other settings, the appropriate management is the use of salicylates and plasma exchange. Other causes of thrombocytopenia include lymphoma, mycobacterial infections, and fungal infections.

Dermatologic Diseases   Dermatologic problems occur in >90% of patients with HIV infection. From the macular, roseola-like rash seen with the acute seroconversion syndrome to extensive end-stage KS, cutaneous manifestations of HIV disease can be seen throughout the course of HIV infection. Among the more common nonneoplastic problems are seborrheic dermatitis, eosinophilic pustular folliculitus, and opportunistic infections. Extrapulmonary pneumocystosis may cause a necrotizing vasculitis. Neoplastic conditions are covered below in the section on malignant diseases.

Seborrheic dermatitis occurs in 3% of the general population and in up to 50% of patients with HIV infection. Seborrheic dermatitis increases in prevalence and severity as the CD4+ T cell count declines. In HIV-infected patients, seborrheic dermatitis may be aggravated by concomitant infection with *Pityrosporum*, a yeastlike fungus; use of topical antifungal agents has been recommended in cases refractory to standard topical treatment.

Eosinophilic pustular folliculitis is a rare dermatologic condition that is seen with increased frequency in patients with HIV infection. It presents as multiple, urticarial perifollicular papules that may coalesce into plaquelike lesions. Skin biopsy reveals an eosinophilic infiltrate of the hair follicle, which in certain cases has been associated with the presence of a mite. Patients typically have an elevated serum IgE level and may respond to treatment with topical anthelminthics. Patients with HIV infection have also been reported to develop a severe form of *Norwegian scabies* with hyperkeratotic psoriasiform lesions.

Both *psoriasis* and *ichthyosis*, although they are not reported to be increased in frequency, may be particularly severe when they occur in patients with HIV infection. Preexisting psoriasis may become guttate in appearance and more refractory to treatment in the setting of HIV infection.

Reactivation herpes zoster (*shingles*) is seen in 10 to 20% of patients with HIV infection. This reactivation syndrome of varicella-zoster virus indicates a modest decline in immune function and may be the first indication of clinical immunodeficiency. In one series, patients who developed shingles did so an average of 5 years after HIV infection. In a cohort of patients with HIV infection and localized zoster, the subsequent rate of the development of AIDS was 1% per month. In that study, AIDS was more likely to develop if the outbreak of zoster was associated with severe pain, extensive skin involvement, or involvement of cranial or cervical dermatomes. The clinical manifestations of reactivation zoster in HIV-infected patients, although indicative of immunologic compromise, are not as severe as those seen in other immunodeficient conditions. Thus, while lesions may extend over several dermatomes (**see Plate IID-37**) and frank cutaneous dissemination may be seen, visceral involvement has not been reported. In contrast to patients without a known underlying immunodeficiency state, patients with HIV infection tend to have recurrences of zoster with a relapse rate of approximately 20%. Acyclovir or famciclovir is the treatment of choice. Foscarnet is of value in patients with acyclovir-resistant virus.

Infection with *herpes simplex virus* in HIV-infected individuals is associated with recurrent orolabial, genital, and perianal lesions as part of recurrent reactivation syndromes (Chap. 182). As HIV disease progresses and the CD4+ T cell count declines, these infections become more frequent and severe. Lesions often appear as beefy red, are exquisitely painful, and have a tendency to occur high in the gluteal cleft (Fig. 309-31). Perirectal HSV may be associated with proctitis and anal fissures. HSV should be high in the differential diagnosis of any HIV-infected patient with a poorly healing, painful perirectal lesion. In addition to recurrent mucosal ulcers, recurrent HSV infection in the form of *herpetic whitlow* can be a problem in patients with HIV infection, presenting with painful vesicles or extensive cutaneous erosion. Acyclovir or famciclovir is the treatment of choice in these settings.

Diffuse skin eruptions due to *Molluscum contagiosum* may be seen in patients with advanced HIV infection. These flesh-colored, umbilicated lesions may be treated with local therapy. They tend to regress with effective antiretroviral therapy. Similarly, *condyloma acuminatum* lesions may be more severe and more widely distributed in patients with low CD4+ T cell counts. Atypical mycobacterial infections may present as erythematous cutaneous nodules as may fungal infections, *Bartonella*, *Acanthamoeba*, and KS.

The skin of patients with HIV infection is often a target organ for drug reactions (Chap. 59). Although most skin reactions are mild and not necessarily an indication to discontinue therapy, patients may have particularly severe cutaneous reactions, including erythroderma and *Stevens-Johnson syndrome*, as a reaction to drugs, particularly sulfa drugs, the nonnucleoside reverse transcriptase inhibitors, abacavir, and amprenavir. Similarly, patients with HIV infection are often quite photosensitive and burn easily following exposure to sunlight or as a side effect of radiation therapy (see Chap. 60).

HIV infection and its treatment may be accompanied by cosmetic changes of the skin that are not of great clinical importance but may be troubling to patients. Yellowing of the nails and straightening of the hair, particularly in African-American patients, have been reported as a consequence of HIV infection. Zidovudine therapy has been associated with elongation of the eyelashes and the development of a bluish discoloration to the nails, again more common in African-American patients. Therapy with clofazimine may cause a yellow-orange discoloration of the skin.

Neurologic Diseases   Clinical disease of the nervous system accounts for a significant degree of morbidity in a high percentage of patients with HIV infection (Table 309-13). The neurologic problems that occur in HIV-infected individuals may be either primary to the pathogenic processes of HIV infection or secondary to opportunistic infections or neoplasms (see above). Among the more frequent opportunistic diseases that involve the CNS are toxoplasmosis, cryptococcosis, progressive multifocal leukoencephalopathy, and primary

Opportunistic infections
  Toxoplasmosis
  Cryptococcosis
  Progressive multifocal leukoencephalopathy
  Cytomegalovirus
  Syphilis
  Mycobacterium tuberculosis
  HTLV-I infection
Neoplasms
  Primary CNS lymphoma
  Kaposi's sarcoma
Result of HIV-1 infection
  Aseptic meningitis
  HIV encephalopathy (AIDS dementia complex)
  Myelopathy
    Vacuolar myelopathy
    Pure sensory ataxia
    Paresthesia/dysesthesia
  Peripheral neuropathy
    Acute inflammatory demyelinating polyneuropathy (Guillain-Barré syndrome)
    Chronic inflammatory demyelinating polyneuropathy (CIDP)
    Mononeuritis multiplex
    Distal symmetric polyneuropathy
  Myopathy

CNS lymphoma. Other less common problems include mycobacterial infections; syphilis; and infection with CMV, HTLV-I, or *Acanthamoeba*. Overall, secondary diseases of the CNS occur in approximately one-third of patients with AIDS. These data antedate the widespread use of combination antiretroviral therapy, and this frequency is considerably less in patients receiving effective antiretroviral drugs. Primary processes related to HIV infection of the nervous system are reminiscent of those seen with other lentiviruses, such as the Visna-Maedi virus of sheep. Neurologic problems occur throughout the course of disease and may be inflammatory, demyelinating, or degenerative in nature. While only one of these, the *AIDS dementia complex*, or *HIV encephalopathy*, is considered an AIDS-defining illness, most HIV-infected patients have some neurologic problem during the course of their disease. As noted in the section on pathogenesis, damage to the CNS may be a direct result of viral infection of the CNS macrophages or glial cells or may be secondary to the release of neurotoxins and potentially toxic cytokines such as IL-1β, TNF-α, IL-6, and TGF-β. Virtually all patients with HIV infection have some degree of nervous system involvement with the virus. This is evidenced by the fact that CSF findings are abnormal in approximately 90% of patients, even during the asymptomatic phase of HIV infection. CSF abnormalities include pleocytosis (50 to 65% of patients), detection of viral RNA (~75%), elevated CSF protein (35%), and evidence of intrathecal synthesis of anti-HIV antibodies (90%). It is important to point out that evidence of infection of the CNS with HIV does not imply impairment of cognitive function. The neurologic function of an HIV-infected individual should be considered normal unless clinical signs and symptoms suggest otherwise.

Aseptic meningitis may be seen in any but the very late stages of HIV infection. In the setting of acute primary infection patients may experience a syndrome of headache, photophobia, and meningismus. Rarely, an acute encephalopathy due to encephalitis may occur. Cranial nerve involvement may be seen, predominantly cranial nerve VII but occasionally V and/or VIII. CSF findings include a lymphocytic pleocytosis, elevated protein level, and normal glucose level. This syndrome, which cannot be clinically differentiated from other viral meningitides (Chap. 373), usually resolves spontaneously within 2 to 4 weeks; however, in some patients, signs and symptoms may become chronic. Aseptic meningitis may occur any time in the course of HIV infection; however, it is rare following the development of AIDS. This fact suggests that clinical aseptic meningitis in the context of HIV infection is an immune-mediated disease.

C. neoformans is the leading infectious cause of meningitis in patients with AIDS (Chap. 204). It is the initial AIDS-defining illness in approximately 2% of patients and generally occurs in patients with CD4+ T cell counts <100/μL. Cryptococcal meningitis is particularly common in patients with AIDS in Africa, occurring in ~20% of patients. Most patients present with a picture of subacute meningoencephalitis with fever, nausea, vomiting, altered mental status, headache, and meningeal signs. The incidence of seizures and focal neurologic deficits is low. The CSF profile may be normal or may show only modest elevations in WBC or protein levels. In addition to meningitis, patients may develop cryptococcomas. Approximately one-third of patients also have pulmonary disease. Uncommon manifestations of cryptococcal infection include skin lesions that resemble *molluscum contagiosum*, lymphadenopathy, palatal and glossal ulcers, arthritis, gastroenteritis, myocarditis, and prostatitis. The prostate gland may serve as a reservoir for smoldering cryptococcal infection. The diagnosis of cryptococcal meningitis is made by identification of organisms in spinal fluid with India ink examination or by the detection of cryptococcal antigen. A biopsy may be needed to make a diagnosis of CNS cryptococcoma. Treatment is with intravenous amphotericin B, at a dose of 0.7 mg/kg daily, with flucytosine, 25 mg/kg qid for 2 weeks, followed by fluconazole, 400 mg/d orally for 8 weeks, and then fluconazole, 200 mg/d for life. Other fungi that may cause meningitis in patients with HIV infection are *C. immitis* and *H. capsulatum*. Meningoencephalitis has also been reported due to *Acanthamoeba* or *Naegleria*.

HIV encephalopathy, also called HIV-associated dementia or AIDS dementia complex, consists of a constellation of signs and symptoms of CNS disease that generally occurs late in the course of HIV infection and progresses slowly over months. A major feature of this entity is the development of dementia, defined as a decline in cognitive ability from a previous level. It may present as impaired ability to concentrate, increased forgetfulness, difficulty reading, or increased difficulty performing complex tasks. Initially these symptoms may be indistinguishable from findings of situational depression or fatigue. In contrast to "cortical" dementia (such as Alzheimer's disease), aphasia, apraxia, and agnosia are uncommon, leading some investigators to classify HIV encephalopathy as a "subcortical dementia" (see below). In addition to dementia, patients with HIV encephalopathy may also have motor and behavioral abnormalities. Among the motor problems are unsteady gait, poor balance, tremor, and difficulty with rapid alternating movements. Increased tone and deep tendon reflexes may be found in patients with spinal cord involvement. Late stages may be complicated by bowel and/or bladder incontinence. Behavioral problems include apathy and lack of initiative, with progression to a vegetative state in some instances. Some patients develop a state of agitation or mild mania. These changes usually occur without significant changes in level of alertness. This is in contrast to the finding of somnolence in patients with dementia due to toxic/metabolic encephalopathies.

HIV encephalopathy is the initial AIDS-defining illness in approximately 3% of patients with HIV infection and thus only rarely precedes clinical evidence of immunodeficiency. Clinically significant encephalopathy eventually develops in approximately one-fourth of patients with AIDS. As immunologic function declines, the risk and severity of HIV encephalopathy increases. Autopsy series suggest that 80 to 90% of patients with HIV infection have histologic evidence of CNS involvement. Several classification schemes have been developed for grading HIV encephalopathy; a commonly used clinical staging system is outlined in Table 309-14.

The precise cause of HIV encephalopathy remains unclear, although the condition is thought to be a result of direct effects of HIV on the CNS. HIV has been found in the brains of patients with HIV encephalopathy by Southern blot, in situ hybridization, PCR, and electron microscopy. Multinucleated giant cells, macrophages, and microglial cells appear to be the main cell types harboring virus in the CNS. Histologically, the major changes are seen in the subcortical

Table 309-14   Clinical Staging of HIV Encephalopathy (AIDS Dementia Complex)

Stage	Definition
Stage 0 (normal)	Normal mental and motor function
Stage 0.5 (equivocal/ subclinical)	Absent, minimal, or equivocal symptoms without impairment of work or capacity to perform activities of daily living. Mild signs (snout response, slowed ocular or extremity movements) may be present. Gait and strength are normal.
Stage 1 (mild)	Able to perform all but the more demanding aspects of work or activities of daily living but with unequivocal evidence (signs or symptoms that may include performance on neuropsychological testing) of functional, intellectual, or motor impairment. Can walk without assistance.
Stage 2 (moderate)	Able to perform basic activities of self-care but cannot work or maintain the more demanding aspects of daily life. Ambulatory, but may require a single prop.
Stage 3 (severe)	Major intellectual incapacity (cannot follow news or personal events, cannot sustain complex conversation, considerable slowing of all output) or motor disability (cannot walk unassisted, usually with slowing and clumsiness of arms as well).
Stage 4 (end-stage)	Nearly vegetative. Intellectual and social comprehension and output are at a rudimentary level. Nearly or absolutely mute. Paraparetic or paraplegic with urinary and fecal incontinence.

SOURCE: Adapted from JJ Sidtis, RW Price, Neurology 40:197, 1990.

Table 309-15   Mini-Mental Status Examination

Question	Scoring	Maximum Score
1. Where are you (state, county, city, hospital, clinic)?	1 point for each	5
2. What are the (day, date, month, season, year, time)?	1 point for each	5
3. "Say these three words after me: (yellow, apple, Ohio)"	1 point for each	3
4. Ask patient to begin with 100 and count backwards by 7's. Or, if patient refuses, ask to spell "world" backwards.	Stop after 5, score no. correct Or 1 point for each correct letter	5
5. Recall the three words given in question no. 3.	1 point for each	3
6. Ask the patient to name "watch" then "pencil."	1 point for each	2
7. Ask the patient to repeat "No ifs, ands, or buts."	1 point if correct	1
8. Three-stage command: Take this paper in your right hand, fold it in half, and put it on the floor.	1 point for each correct	3
9. Ask the patient to read silently and obey the command (print in block letters): CLOSE YOUR EYES.	1 point if correct	1
10. Ask the patient to write a sentence.	1 point if it contains a subject and verb and makes sense (ignore spelling and grammar)	1
11. "Draw a clock with numbers and hands showing the time to be 8: 20	2 points if correct	2
12. Have the patient copy this design:	1 point if all sides and angles are preserved and if intersecting sides form a quadrangle	1

areas of the brain and include pallor and gliosis, multinucleated giant cell encephalitis, and vacuolar myelopathy. Less commonly, diffuse or focal spongiform changes occur in the white matter.

There are no specific criteria for a diagnosis of HIV encephalopathy, and this syndrome must be differentiated from a number of other diseases that affect the CNS of HIV-infected patients (Table 309-13). The diagnosis of dementia depends upon demonstrating a decline in cognitive function. This can be accomplished objectively with the use of a Mini-Mental Status Examination (MMSE) (Table 309-15) in patients for whom prior scores are available. For this reason, it is advisable for all patients with a diagnosis of HIV infection to have a baseline MMSE. However, changes in MMSE scores may be absent in patients with mild HIV encephalopathy. Imaging studies of the CNS, by either MRI or CT, often demonstrate evidence of cerebral atrophy (Fig. 309-33). MRI may also reveal small areas of increased density on T2-weighted images. Lumbar puncture is an important element of the evaluation of patients with HIV infection and neurologic abnormalities. It is generally most helpful in ruling out or making a diagnosis of opportunistic infections. In HIV encephalopathy, patients may have the nonspecific findings of an increase in CSF cells and protein level. While HIV RNA can often be detected in the spinal fluid and HIV can be cultured from the CSF, this finding is not specific for HIV encephalopathy. There appears to be no correlation between the presence of HIV in the CSF and the presence of HIV encephalopathy. Elevated levels of β_2-microglobulin, neopterin, and quinolinic acid (a metabolite of tryptophan reported to cause CNS injury) have been noted in the CSF of patients with HIV encephalopathy. These findings suggest that these factors as well as inflammatory cytokines may be involved in the pathogenesis of this syndrome.

Combination antiretroviral therapy is of benefit in patients with HIV encephalopathy. Improvement in neuropsychiatric test scores has been noted for both adult and pediatric patients treated with antiretrovirals. The rapid improvement in cognitive function noted with the initiation of antiretroviral therapy suggests that at least some component of this problem is quickly reversible, again supporting at least a partial role of soluble mediators in the pathogenesis. It should also be noted that these patients have an increased sensitivity to the side effects of neuroleptic drugs. The use of these drugs for symptomatic treatment is associated with an increased risk of extrapyramidal side effects; therefore, patients with HIV encephalopathy who receive these agents must be monitored carefully.

Seizures may be a consequence of opportunistic infections, neoplasms, or HIV encephalopathy (Table 309-16). The seizure threshold is often lower than normal in these patients owing to the frequent presence of electrolyte abnormalities. Seizures are seen in 15 to 40% of patients with cerebral toxoplasmosis, 15 to 35% of patients with primary CNS lymphoma, 8% of patients with cryptococcal meningitis, and 7 to 50% of patients with HIV encephalopathy. Seizures may also be seen in patients with CNS tuberculosis, aseptic meningitis, and progressive multifocal leukoencephalopathy. Seizures may be the presenting clinical symptom of HIV disease. In one study of 100 patients with HIV infection presenting with a first seizure, cerebral mass lesions were the most common cause, responsible for 32 of the 100 new-onset seizures. Of these 32 cases, 28 were due to toxoplasmosis and 4 to lymphoma. HIV encephalopathy accounted for an additional 24 new-onset seizures. Cryptococcal meningitis

FIGURE 309-33 AIDS dementia complex. Postcontrast CT scan through the lateral ventricles of a 47-year old man with AIDS, altered mental status, and dementia. The lateral and third ventricles and the cerebral sulci are abnormally prominent. Mild white matter hypodensity is also seen adjacent to the frontal horns of the lateral ventricles.

was the third most common diagnosis, responsible for 13 of the 100 seizures. In 23 cases, no cause could be found, and it is possible that these cases represent a subcategory of HIV encephalopathy. Of these 23 cases, 16 (70%) had two or more seizures, suggesting that anticonvulsant therapy is indicated in all patients with HIV infection and seizures unless a rapidly correctable cause is found. While phenytoin remains the initial treatment of choice, hypersensitivity reactions to this drug have been reported in >10% of patients with AIDS, and therefore the use of phenobarbital or valproic acid must be considered as alternatives.

Patients with HIV infection may present with *focal neurologic deficits* from a variety of causes. The most common cause are toxoplasmosis, progressive multifocal leukoencephalopathy, and CNS lymphoma. Other causes include cryptococcal infections (discussed above; also Chap. 204), stroke, and reactivation Chagas' disease.

Toxoplasmosis has been one of the most common causes of secondary CNS infections in patients with AIDS, but its incidence is decreasing in the era of HAART. It is most common in patients from the Caribbean and from France. Toxoplasmosis is generally a late complication of HIV infection and usually occurs in patients with CD4+ T cell counts <200/μL. Cerebral toxoplasmosis is thought to represent a reactivation syndrome. It is 10 times more common in patients with antibodies to the organism than in patients who are seronegative. Patients diagnosed with HIV infection should be screened for IgG antibodies to *T. gondii* during the time of their initial workup. Those who are seronegative should be counseled about ways to minimize the risk

Table 309-16 Causes of Seizures in Patients with HIV Infection

Disease	Overall Contribution to First Seizure, %	Fraction of Patients Who Have Seizures, %
HIV encephalopathy	24–47	7–50
Cerebral toxoplasmosis	28	15–40
Cryptococcal meningitis	13	8
Primary central nervous system lymphoma	4	15–30
Progressive multifocal leukoencephalopathy	1	

SOURCE: From Holtzman et al.

of primary infection including avoiding the consumption of undercooked meat and careful hand washing after contact with soil or changing the cat litter box. The most common clinical presentation in patients with HIV infection is fever, headache, and focal neurologic deficits. Patients may present with seizure, hemiparesis, or aphasia as a manifestation of these focal deficits or with a picture more influenced by the accompanying cerebral edema and characterized by confusion, dementia, and lethargy, which can progress to coma. The diagnosis is usually suspected on the basis of MRI findings of multiple lesions in multiple locations, although in come cases only a single lesion is seen. Pathologically, these lesions generally exhibit inflammation and central necrosis and, as a result, demonstrate ring enhancement on contrast MRI (Fig. 309-34) or, if MRI is unavailable or contraindicated, on double-dose contrast CT. There is usually evidence of surrounding edema. In addition to toxoplasmosis, the differential diagnosis of single or multiple enhancing mass lesions in the HIV-infected patient includes primary CNS lymphoma (see below) and, less commonly, TB or fungal or bacterial abscesses. The definitive diagnostic procedure is brain biopsy. However, given the morbidity than can accompany this procedure, it is usually reserved for the patient who has failed 2 to 4 weeks of empirical therapy. If the patient is seronegative for *T. gondii*, the likelihood that a mass lesion is due to toxoplasmosis is <10%. In that setting, one may choose to be more aggressive and perform a brain biopsy sooner. Standard treatment is sulfadiazine and pyrimethamine with leucovorin as needed for a minimum of 4 to 6 weeks. Alternative therapeutic regimens include clindamycin in combination with pyrimethamine; atovaquone plus pyrimethamine; and azithromycin plus pyrimethamine plus rifabutin. Relapses are common, and it is recommended that patients with a history of prior toxoplasmic encephalitis receive maintenance therapy with sulfadiazine, pyrimethamine, and leucovorin. Patients with CD4+ T cell counts <100/μL and IgG antibody to *Toxoplasma* should receive primary prophylaxis for toxoplasmosis. Fortunately, the same daily regimen of a single double-strength tablet of TMP/SMZ used for *P. carinii* prophylaxis provides adequate primary protection against toxoplasmosis. It is likely that future recommendations will allow for discontinuation of prophylaxis for toxoplasmosis in the setting of effective antiretroviral therapy and increases in CD4+ T cell counts to >100/μL for 3 to 6 months.

JC virus, a human papilloma virus that is the etiologic agent of *progressive multifocal leukoencephalopathy* (PML), is an important opportunistic pathogen in patients with AIDS (Chap. 373). While approximately 70% of the general adult population have antibodies to

FIGURE 309-34 CNS toxoplasmosis. A coronal postcontrast T1 weighted MR scan demonstrates a peripheral enhancing lesion in the left frontal lobe, associated with an eccentric nodular area of enhancement (*arrow*); this so-called "eccentric target sign" is typical of toxoplasmosis.

JC virus, indicative of prior infection, <10% of healthy adults show any evidence of ongoing viral replication. PML is the only known clinical manifestation of JC virus infection. It is a late manifestation of AIDS and is seen in ~4% of patients with AIDS. The lesions of PML begin as small foci of demyelination in subcortical white matter that eventually coalesce. The cerebral hemispheres, cerebellum, and brainstem may all be involved. Patients typically have a protracted course with multifocal neurologic deficits, with or without changes in mental status. Ataxia, hemiparesis, visual field defects, aphasia, and sensory defects may occur. MRI typically reveals multiple, nonenhancing white matter lesions that may coalesce and have a predeliction for the occipital and parietal lobes. The lesions show signal hyperintensity on T2-weighted images and diminished signal on T1-weighted images. Prior to the availability of potent antiretroviral combination therapy, the majority of patients with PML died within 3 to 6 months of the onset of symptoms. There is no specific treatment for PML; however, regressions of more than 2.5 years in duration have been reported in patients with PML treated with HAART for their HIV disease. Factors influencing a favorable prognosis include a CD4+ T cell count >100/μL at baseline and the ability to maintain an HIV viral load of <500 copies per milliliter. Baseline viral load does not have independent predictive value of survival. Of note, PML is one of the few opportunistic infections that continue to occur with some frequency despite the widespread use of HAART.

Reactivation American trypanosomiasis may present as acute meningoencephalitis with focal neurologic signs, fever, headache, vomiting, and seizures. In South America, reactivation of *Chagas' disease* is considered to be an AIDS-defining condition and may be the initial AIDS-defining condition. Lesions appear radiographically as single or multiple hypodense areas, typically with ring enhancement and edema. They are found predominantly in the subcortical areas, a feature that differentiates them from the deeper lesions of toxoplasmosis. *Trypanosoma cruzi* amastigotes, or trypanosomes, can be identified from biopsy specimens or CSF. Other CSF findings include elevated protein and a mild (<100 cells/μL) lymphocytic pleocytosis. Organisms can also be identified by direct examination of the blood. Treatment consists of benzimidazole (2.5 mg/kg bid) or nifurtimox (1 mg/kg tid) for at least 60 days, followed by maintenance therapy for life with either drug at a dose of 5 mg/kg three times a week.

Stroke may occur in patients with HIV infection. In contrast to the other causes of focal neurologic deficits in patients with HIV infection, the symptoms of a stroke are sudden in onset. Among the secondary infectious diseases in patients with HIV infection that may be associated with stroke are vasculitis due to cerebral varicella zoster or neurosyphilis and septic embolism in association with fungal infection. Other elements of the differential diagnosis of stroke in the patient with HIV infection include atherosclerotic cerebral vascular disease, thrombotic thrombocytopenic purpura, and cocaine or amphetamine use.

Primary CNS lymphoma is discussed below in the section on neoplastic diseases.

Spinal cord disease, or myelopathy, is present in approximately 20% of patients with AIDS, often as part of HIV encephalopathy. In fact, 90% of the patients with HIV-associated myelopathy have some evidence of dementia, suggesting that similar pathologic processes may be responsible for both conditions. Three main types of spinal cord disease are seen in patients with AIDS. The first of these is a vacuolar myelopathy, as discussed above under HIV encephalopathy. This condition is pathologically similar to subacute combined degeneration of the cord such as occurs with pernicious anemia. Although vitamin B_{12} deficiency can be seen in patients with AIDS, it does not appear to be responsible for the myelopathy seen in the majority of patients. Vacuolar myelopathy is characterized by a subacute onset and often presents with gait disturbances, predominantly ataxia and spasticity; it may progress to include bladder and bowel dysfunction. Physical findings include evidence of increased deep tendon reflexes

and extensor plantar responses. The second form of spinal cord disease involves the dorsal columns and presents as a pure sensory ataxia. The third form is also sensory in nature and presents with paresthesias and dysesthesias of the lower extremities. In contrast to the cognitive problems seen in patients with HIV encephalopathy, these spinal cord syndromes do not respond well to antiretroviral drugs, and therapy is mainly supportive.

One important disease of the spinal cord that also involves the peripheral nerves is a *myelopathy* and *polyradiculopathy* seen in association with CMV infection. This entity is generally seen late in the course of HIV infection and is fulminant in onset, with lower extremity and sacral paresthesias, difficulty in walking, areflexia, ascending sensory loss, and urinary retention. The clinical course is rapidly progressive over a period of weeks. CSF examination reveals a predominantly neutrophilic pleocytosis, and CMV DNA can be detected by CSF PCR. Therapy with ganciclovir or foscarnet can lead to rapid improvement, and prompt initiation of foscarnet or ganciclovir therapy is important in minimizing the degree of permanent neurologic damage. Combination therapy with both drugs should be considered in patients who have been previously treated for CMV disease.→*Other diseases involving the spinal cord in patients with HIV infection include* HTLV-I-associated myelopathy (HAM) (Chap. 191), neurosyphilis (Chap. 172), infection with herpes simplex (Chap. 182) or varicella-zoster (Chap. 183), TB (Chap. 169), and lymphoma (Chap. 112).

Peripheral neuropathies are common in patients with HIV infection. They occur at all stages of illness and take a variety of forms. Early in the course of HIV infection, an acute inflammatory demyelinating polyneuropathy resembling Guillain-Barré syndrome may occur (Chap. 378). In other patients, a progressive or relapsing-remitting inflammatory neuropathy resembling chronic inflammatory demyelinating polyneuropathy (CIDP) has been noted. Patients commonly present with progressive weakness, areflexia, and minimal sensory changes. CSF examination often reveals a mononuclear pleocytosis, and peripheral nerve biopsy demonstrates a perivascular infiltrate suggesting an autoimmune etiology. Plasma exchange or intravenous immunoglobulin has been tried with variable success. Because of the immunosuppressive effects of glucocorticoids, they should be reserved for severe cases of CIDP refractory to other measures. Another autoimmune peripheral neuropathy seen in patients with AIDS is mononeuritis multiplex (Chaps. 378 and 317) due to a necrotizing arteritis of peripheral nerves. The most common peripheral neuropathy in patients with HIV infection is a *distal sensory polyneuropathy* that may be a direct consequence of HIV infection or a side effect of dideoxynucleoside therapy. Two-thirds of patients with AIDS may be shown by electrophysiologic studies to have some evidence of peripheral nerve disease. Presenting symptoms are usually painful burning sensations in the feet and lower extremities. Findings on examination include a stocking-type sensory loss to pinprick, temperature, and touch sensation and a loss of ankle reflexes. Motor changes are mild and are usually limited to weakness of the intrinsic foot muscles. Response of this condition to antiretrovirals has been variable, perhaps because antiretrovirals are responsible for the problem in some instances. When due to dideoxynucleoside therapy, patients with lower extremity peripheral neuropathy may complain of a sensation that they are walking on ice. Other entities in the differential diagnosis of peripheral neuropathy include diabetes mellitus, vitamin B_{12} deficiency, and side effects from metronidazole or dapsone. For distal symmetric polyneuropathy that fails to resolve following the discontinuation of dideoxynucleosides, therapy is symptomatic; gabapentin, carbamazepine, tricyclics, or analgesics may be effective for dysesthesias. Some patients may respond to combination antiretroviral therapy, and preliminary data suggest that nerve growth factor may benefit some cases.

Myopathy may complicate the course of HIV infection; causes include HIV infection itself, zidovudine, and the generalized wasting syndrome. HIV-associated myopathy may range in severity from an asymptomatic elevation in creatine kinase levels to a subacute syndrome characterized by proximal muscle weakness and myalgias.

Quite pronounced elevations in creatine kinase may occur in asymptomatic patients, particularly after exercise. The clinical significance of this as an isolated laboratory finding is unclear. A variety of both inflammatory and noninflammatory pathologic processes have been noted in patients with more severe myopathy, including myofiber necrosis with inflammatory cells, nemaline rod bodies, cytoplasmic bodies, and mitochondrial abnormalities. Profound muscle wasting, often with muscle pain, may be seen after prolonged zidovudine therapy. This toxic side effect of the drug is dose-dependent and is related to its ability to interfere with the function of mitochondrial polymerases. It is reversible following discontinuation of the drug. Red ragged fibers are a histologic hallmark of zidovudine-induced myopathy.

Ophthalmologic Disease   Ophthalmologic problems occur in approximately half of patients with advanced HIV infection. The most common abnormal findings on funduscopic examination are cotton-wool spots. These are hard white spots that appear on the surface of the retina and often have an irregular edge. They represent areas of retinal ischemia secondary to microvascular disease. At times they are associated with small areas of hemorrhage and thus can be difficult to distinguish from CMV retinitis. In contrast to CMV retinitis, however, these lesions are not associated with visual loss and tend to remain stable or improve over time.

One of the most devastating consequences of HIV infection is CMV retinitis. Patients at high risk of CMV retinitis (CD4+ T cell count $<100/\mu L$) should undergo an ophthalmologic examination every 3 to 6 months. The majority of cases of CMV retinitis occur in patients with a CD4+ T cell count $<50/\mu L$. Prior to the availability of HAART, this CMV reactivation syndrome was seen in 25 to 30% of patients with AIDS. CMV retinitis usualy presents as a painless, progressive loss of vision. Patients may also complain of blurred vision, "floaters," and scintillations. The disease is usually bilateral, affecting one eye more than the other. The diagnosis is made on clinical grounds by an experienced ophthalmologist. The characteristic retinal appearance is that of perivascular hemorrhage and exudate (**see Plate III-1**). In situations where the diagnosis is in doubt due to an atypical presentation or an unexpected lack of response to therapy, vitreous or aqueous humor sampling with molecular diagnostic techniques may be of value. CMV infection of the retina results in a necrotic inflammatory process, and the visual loss that develops is irreversible. As a consequence of retinal atrophy in areas or prior inflammation, CMV retinitis may be complicated by rhegmatogenous retinal detachment. Therapy for CMV retinitis consists of intravenous ganciclovir or foscarnet, with cidofovir as an alternative. Combination therapy with ganciclovir and foscarnet has been shown to be slightly more effective than either ganciclovir or foscarnet alone in the patient with relapsed CMV retinitis. A 3-week induction course is followed by maintenance therapy with one of these drugs systemically. While the majority of patients will require intravenous maintenance therapy, a ganciclovir prodrug with better oral bioavailability has shown promise in clinical trials. If CMV disease is limited to the eye, a ganciclovir-releasing intraocular implant, periodic injections of the antisense nucleic acid preparation formivirsen, or intravitreal injections of ganciclovir or foscarnet may be considered; some choose to combine intraocular implants with oral ganciclovir. Intravitreal injections of cidofovir are generally avoided due to the increased risk of uveitis and hypotony. Maintenance therapy is continued until the CD4+ T cell count remains >100 to $150/\mu L$ for >6 months. The majority of patients with HIV infection and CMV disease develop some degree of uveitis with the initiation of antiretroviral therapy. The etiology of this is unknown; however, it has been suggested that this may be due to the generation of an enhanced immune response to CMV. In some instances this has required the use of topical glucocorticoids.

Both HSV and varicella zoster virus can cause a rapidly progressing, bilateral necrotizing retinitis referred to as the *acute retinal necrosis syndrome*. This syndrome, in contrast to CMV retinitis, is associated with pain, keratitis, and iritis. It is often associated with orolabial HSV or trigeminal zoster. Ophthalmologic examination reveals widespread pale gray peripheral lesions. This condition is often complicated by retinal detachment. It is important to recognize and treat this condition with intravenous acyclovir as quickly as possible to minimize the loss of vision.

Several other secondary infections may cause ocular problems in HIV-infected patients. *P. carinii* can cause a lesion of the choroid that may be detected as an incidental finding on ophthalmologic examination. These lesions are typically bilateral, are from half to twice the disc diameter in size, and appear as slightly elevated yellow-white plaques. They are usually asymptomatic and may be confused with cotton-wool spots. Chorioretinitis due to toxoplasmosis can be seen alone or, more commonly, in association with CNS toxoplasmosis.

Additional Disseminated Infections and Wasting Syndrome
Infections with species of the small, gram-negative rickettsia-like organism *Bartonella* (Chap. 163) are seen with increased frequency in patients with HIV infection. While not considered an AIDS-defining illness by the CDC, many experts view infection with *Bartonella* as indicative of a severe defect in cell-mediated immunity. It is usually seen in patients with CD4+ T cell counts $<100/\mu L$. Among the clinical manifestations of *Bartonella* infection are bacillary angiomatosis, cat-scratch disease, and trench fever. *Bacillary angiomatosis* is usually due to infection with *B. henselae*. It is characterized by a vascular proliferation that leads to a variety of skin lesions that have been confused with the skin lesions of KS. In contrast to the lesions of KS, the lesions of bacillary angiomatosis generally blanch, are painful, and typically occur in the setting of systemic symptoms. Infection can extend to the lymph nodes, liver (peliosis hepatis), spleen, bone, heart, CNS, respiratory tract, and gastrointestinal tract. *Cat-scratch disease* generally begins with a papule at the site of inoculation. This is followed several weeks later by the development of regional adenopathy and malaise. Infection with *B. quintana* is transmitted by lice and has been associated with case reports of trench fever, endocarditis, adenopathy, and bacillary angiomatosis. The organism is quite difficult to culture, and diagnosis often relies upon identifying the organism in biopsy specimens using the Warthin-Starry or similar stains. Treatment is with either erythromycin or doxycyline for at least 3 months.

Histoplasmosis is an opportunistic infection that is seen most frequently in patients in the Mississippi and Ohio River valleys, Puerto Rico, the Dominican Republic, and South America. These are all areas in which infection with *H. capsulatum* is endemic (Chap. 201). Because of this limited geographic distribution, the percentage of AIDS cases in the United States with histoplasmosis is only approximately 0.5. Histoplasmosis is generally a late manifestation of HIV infection; however, it may be the initial AIDS-defining condition. In one study, the median CD4+ T cell count for patients with histoplasmosis and AIDS was $33/\mu L$. While disease due to *H. capsulatum* may present as a primary infection of the lung, disseminated disease, presumably due to reactivation, is the most common presentation in HIV-infected patients. Patients usually present with a 4- to 8-week history of fever and weight loss. Hepatosplenomegaly and lymphadenopathy are each seen in about 25% of patients. CNS disease, either meningitis or a mass lesion, is seen in 15% of patients. Bone marrow involvement is common, with thrombocytopenia, neutropenia, and anemia occurring in 33% of patients. Approximately 7% of patients have mucocutaneous lesions consisting of a maculopapular rash and skin or oral ulcers. Respiratory symptoms are usually mild, with chest x-ray showing a diffuse infiltrate or diffuse small nodules in approximately half of cases. Diagnosis is made by culturing the organisms from blood, bone marrow, or tissue. Treatment is typically with amphotericin B, 0.7 to 1.0 mg/kg daily to a total dose of 1 g followed by maintenance therapy with itraconazole. In the setting of mild infection, it may be appropriate to treat with itraconazole alone.

Following the spread of HIV infection to southeast Asia, disseminated infection with *Penicillium marneffei* was recognized as a complication of HIV infection and is considered an AIDS-defining condition in those parts of the world where it occurs. *P. marneffei* is the third most common AIDS-defining illness in Thailand, following TB and cryptococcosis. It is more frequently diagnosed in the rainy than the dry season. Clinical features include fever, generalized lymphadenopathy, hepatosplenomegaly, anemia, thrombocytopenia, and papular skin lesions with central umbilication. Treatment is with amphotericin B followed by itraconazole.

Visceral leishmaniasis (Chap. 215) is recognized with increasing frequency in patients with HIV infection who live in or travel to areas endemic for this protozoal infection transmitted by sandflies. The clinical presentation is one of hepatosplenomegaly, fever, and hematologic abnormalities. Lymphadenopathy and other constitutional symptoms may be present. Organisms can be isolated from cultures of bone marrow aspirates. Histologic stains may be negative, and antibody titers are of little help. Patients with HIV infection usually respond well initially to standard therapy with pentavalent antimony compounds. Eradication of the organism is difficult, however, and relapses are common.

Generalized wasting is an AIDS-defining condition; it is defined as involuntary weight loss of >10% associated with intermittent or constant fever and chronic diarrhea or fatigue lasting >30 days in the absence of a defined cause other than HIV infection. It is the initial AIDS-defining condition in approximately 10% of patients with AIDS in the United States. A constant feature of this syndrome is severe muscle wasting with scattered myofiber degeneration and occasional evidence of myositis. Glucocorticoids may be of some benefit; however, this approach must be carefully weighed against the risk of compounding the immunodeficiency of HIV infection. Androgenic steroids, growth hormone, and total parenteral nutrition have been used as therapeutic interventions with variable success.

Neoplastic Diseases The neoplastic diseases clearly seen with an increased frequency in patients with HIV infection are KS and non-Hodgkin's lymphoma. In addition, there also appears to be an increased incidence of Hodgkin's disease; multiple myeloma; leukemia; melanoma; and cervical, brain, testicular, oral, and anal cancers. Recent years have witnessed a marked reduction in the incidence of KS (Fig. 309-28), felt to be primarily due to the use of potent antiretroviral therapy. Rates of non-Hodgkin's lymphoma have declined as well; however, this decline has not been as dramatic as the decline in rates of KS.

Kaposi's sarcoma is a multicentric neoplasm consisting of multiple vascular nodules appearing in the skin, mucous membranes, and viscera. The course ranges from indolent, with only minor skin or lymph node involvement, to fulminant, with extensive cutaneous and visceral involvement. In the initial period of the AIDS epidemic, KS was a prominent clinical feature of the first cases of AIDS, occurring in 79% of the patients diagnosed in 1981. By 1989 it was seen in only 25% of cases, by 1992 the number had decreased to 9%, and by 1997 the number was <1%. HHV-8 or KSHV has been strongly implicated as a viral cofactor in the pathogenesis of KS (see above).

Clinically, KS has varied presentations and may be seen at any stage of HIV infection, even in the presence of a normal CD4+ T cell count. The initial lesion may be a small, raised reddish-purple nodule on the skin, a discoloration on the oral mucosa, or a swollen lymph node **(see Plate IIB-20)**. Lesions often appear in sun-exposed areas, particularly the tip of the nose, and have a propensity to occur in areas of trauma (Koebner phenomenon). Because of the vascular nature of the tumors and the presence of extravasated red blood cells in the lesions, their color ranges from reddish to purple to brown and often take the appearance of a bruise, with yellowish discoloration and tattooing. Lesions range in size from a few millimeters to several centimeters in diameter and may be either discrete or confluent. KS lesions most commonly appear as raised macules; however, they also can be papular, particularly in patients with higher CD4+ T cell counts. Confluent lesions may give rise to surrounding lymphedema and may be disfiguring when they involve the face and disabling when they involve the lower extremities or the surfaces of joints. Apart from skin, lymph nodes, gastrointestinal tract, and lung are the organ systems

most commonly affected by KS. Lesions have been reported in virtually every organ, including the heart and the CNS. In contrast to most malignancies, in which lymph node involvement implies metastatic spread and a poor prognosis, lymph node involvement may be seen very early in Kaposi's sarcoma and is of no special clinical significance. In fact, some patients may present with disease limited to the lymph nodes. These are generally patients with relatively intact immune function and thus the patients with the best prognosis. Pulmonary involvement with KS generally presents with shortness of breath. Some 80% of patients with pulmonary KS also have cutaneous lesions. The chest x-ray characteristically shows bilateral lower lobe infiltrates that obscure the margins of the mediastinum and diaphragm (Fig. 309-35). Pleural effusions are seen in 70% of cases of pulmonary KS, a fact that is often helpful in the differential diagnosis. Gastrointestinal involvement is seen in 50% of patients and usually takes one of two forms. The first is mucosal involvement, which may lead to bleeding that can be severe. These patients sometimes also develop symptoms of gastrointestinal obstruction if lesions become large. The second gastrointestinal manifestation is due to biliary tract involvement. KS lesions may infiltrate the gallbladder and biliary tree, leading to a clinical picture of obstructive jaundice similar to that seen with sclerosing cholangitis. Several staging systems have been proposed for KS. One in common use was developed by the National Institute of Allergy and Infectious Diseases AIDS Clinical Trials Group; it distinguishes patients on the basis of tumor extent, immunologic function, and presence or absence of systemic disease (Table 309-17).

A diagnosis of KS is based upon biopsy of a suspicious lesion. Histologically one sees a proliferation of spindle cells and endothelial cells, extravasation of red blood cells, hemosiderin-laden macrophages, and, in early cases, an inflammatory cell infiltrate. Included in the differential diagnosis are lymphoma (particularly for oral lesions), bacillary angiomatosis, and cutaneous mycobacterial infections.

Management of KS (Table 309-18) should be carried out in consultation with an expert since definitive treatment guidelines do not exist. In the majority of cases effective antiretroviral therapy will go a long way in achieving control. Indeed, spontaneous regressions have been reported in the setting of HAART. For patients in whom tumor persists or in whom control of HIV replication is not possible, a variety of options exist. In some cases, lesions remain quite indolent, and many of these patients can be managed with no specific treatment. Fewer than 10% of AIDS patients with KS die as a consequence of their malignancy, and death from secondary infections is considerably more common. Thus, whenever possible one should avoid treatment regimens that may further suppress the immune system and increase susceptibility to opportunistic infections. Treatment is indicated under two main circumstances. The first is when a single lesion or a limited

FIGURE 309-35 Chest x-ray of a patient with AIDS and pulmonary Kaposi's sarcoma. The characteristic findings include dense bilateral lower lobe infiltrates obscuring the heart borders and a pleural effusion.

number of lesions are causing significant discomfort or cosmetic problems, such as with prominent facial lesions, lesions overlying a joint, or lesions in the oropharynx that interfere with swallowing or breathing. Under these circumstances, treatment with localized radiation, intralesional vinblastine, or cryotherapy may be indicated. It should be noted that patients with HIV infection are particularly sensitive to the side effects of radiation therapy. This is especially true with respect to the development of radiation-induced mucositis; doses of radiation directed at mucosal surfaces, particularly in the head and neck region, should be adjusted accordingly. The use of systemic therapy, either IFN-α or chemotherapy, should be considered in patients with a large number of lesions or in patients with visceral involvement. The single most important determinant of response appears to be the CD4+ T cell count. This relationship between response rate and baseline CD4+ T cell count is particularly true for IFN-α. The response rate for patients with CD4+ T cell counts >600/μL is approximately 80%, while the response rate for patients with counts <150/μL is <10%. In contrast to the other systemic therapies, IFN-α provides an added advantage of having antiretroviral activity; thus, it may be the appropriate first choice for single-agent systemic therapy for early patients with disseminated disease. A variety of chemotherapeutic agents have also been shown to have activity against KS. Three of them, liposomal daunorubicin, liposomal doxorubicin, and paclitaxel have been approved by the FDA for this indication. Liposomal daunorubicin is approved as first-line therapy for patients with advanced KS. It has fewer side effects than conventional chemotherapy. In contrast, liposomal doxorubicin and paclitaxel are only approved for KS patients who have failed standard chemotherapy. Response rates vary from 23 to 88%, appear to be comparable to what had been achieved earlier with combination chemotherapy regimens, and are greatly influenced by CD4+ T cell count.

Lymphomas occur with an increased frequency in patients with congenital or acquired T cell immunodeficiencies (Chap. 308). AIDS is no exception; at least 6% of all patients with AIDS develop lymphoma at some time during the course of their illness. This is a 120-fold increase in incidence compared to the general population. In contrast to the situation with KS and most opportunistic infections, the incidence of AIDS-associated lymphomas has not experienced as dramatic a decrease as a consequence of the widespread use of effective antiretroviral therapy. Lymphoma occurs in all risk groups, with the highest incidence in patients with hemophilia and the lowest incidence in patients from the Caribbean or Africa with heterosexually acquired infection. Lymphoma is a late manifestation of HIV infection, generally occurring in patients with CD4+ T cell counts of <200/μL. As HIV disease progresses, the risk of lymphoma increases. In contrast to KS, which occurs at a relatively constant rate throughout the course of HIV disease, the attack rate for lymphoma increases exponentially with increasing duration of HIV infection and decreasing level of immunologic function. At 3 years following a diagnosis of HIV infection, the risk of lymphoma is 0.8% per year; by 8 years after infection, it is 2.6% per year. As people with HIV infection live longer as a consequence of improved antiretroviral therapy and better treatment and prophylaxis of opportunistic infections, it is anticipated that the incidence of lymphomas will increase.

Three main categories of lymphoma are seen in patients with HIV infection: grade III or IV immunoblastic lymphoma, Burkitt's lymphoma, and primary CNS lymphoma. Approximately 90% of these lymphomas are B cell in phenotype, and half contain EBV DNA. These tumors may be either monoclonal or oligoclonal in nature and are probably in some way related to the pronounced polyclonal B cell activation seen in patients with AIDS.

Immunoblastic lymphomas account for ~60% of the cases of lymphoma in patients with AIDS. These are generally high grade and would have been classified as diffuse histiocytic lymphomas in earlier classification schemes. This tumor is more common in older patients, increasing in incidence from 0% in HIV-infected individuals <1 year old to >3% in those >50. One variant of immunoblastic lymphoma is body cavity lymphoma. This malignancy presents with lymphomatous pleural, pericardial, and/or peritoneal effusions in the absence of discrete nodal or extranodal masses. The tumor cells do not express surface markers for B cells or T cells. HHV-8 DNA sequences have been found in the genome of the malignant cells (see above).

Small non-cleaved cell lymphoma (Burkitt's lymphoma) accounts for ~20% of the cases of lymphoma in patients with AIDS. It is most frequent in patients 10 to 19 years old and usually demonstrates characteristic c-*myc* translocations from chromosome 8 to chromosomes 14 or 22. Burkitt's lymphoma is not commonly seen in the setting of immunodeficiency other than HIV-associated immunodeficiency, and the incidence of this particular tumor is over 1000-fold higher in the setting of HIV infection than in the general population. In contrast to African Burkitt's lymphoma, where 97% of the cases contain EBV genome, only 50% of HIV-associated Burkitt's lymphomas are EBV-positive.

Primary CNS lymphoma accounts for approximately 20% of the cases of lymphoma in patients with HIV infection. In contrast to HIV-associated Burkitt's lymphoma, primary CNS lymphomas are usually positive for EBV. In one study, the incidence of Epstein-Barr positivity was 100%. This malignancy does not have a predilection for any particular age group. The median CD4+ T cell count at the time of diagnosis is approximately 50/μL. Thus, CNS lymphoma generally presents at a later stage of HIV infection than systemic lymphoma. This fact may at least in part explain the poorer prognosis for this subset of patients.

The clinical presentation of lymphoma in patients with HIV infection is quite varied, ranging from focal seizures to rapidly growing

Table 309-17 National Institute of Allergy and Infectious Diseases AIDS Clinical Trials Group TIS Staging System for Kaposi's Sarcoma

Parameter	Good Risk (stage 0): All of the Following	Poor Risk (stage 1): Any of the Following
Tumor (T)	Confined to skin and/or lymph nodes and/or minimal oral disease	Tumor-associated edema or ulceration Extensive oral lesions Gastrointestinal lesions Nonnodal visceral lesions
Immune system (I) Systemic illness (S)	CD4+ T cell count ≥200/μL No B symptoms[a] Karnofsky performance status >70 No history of opportunistic infection, neurologic disease, lymphoma, or thrush	CD4+ T cell count <200/μL B symptoms[a] present Karnofsky performance status <70 History of opportunistic infection, neurologic disease, lymphoma, or thrush

[a] Defined as unexplained fever, night sweats, >10% involuntary weight loss, or diarrhea persisting for more than 2 weeks.

Table 309-18 Management of AIDS-Associated Kaposi's Sarcoma

Observation and optimization of antiretroviral therapy
Single or limited number of lesions
  Radiation
  Intralesional vinblastine
  Cryotherapy
Extensive disease
  Initial therapy
    Interferon-α (if CD4+ T cells >150/μL)
    Liposomal danorubicin
  Subsequent therapy
    Liposomal doxorubicin
    Paclitaxel
Combination chemotherapy with low-dose doxorubicin, bleomycin, and vinblastine (ABV)
Radiation treatment

mass lesions in the oral mucosa (Fig. 309-36) to persistent unexplained fever. At least 80% of patients present with extranodal disease, and a similar percentage have B-type symptoms of fever, night sweats, or weight loss. Virtually any site in the body may be involved. The most common extranodal site is the CNS, which is involved in approximately one-third of all patients with lymphoma. Approximately 60% of these cases are primary CNS lymphoma. Primary CNS lymphoma generally presents with focal neurologic deficits, including cranial nerve findings, headaches, and/or seizures. MRI or CT generally reveals a limited number (one to three) of 3- to 5-cm lesions (Fig. 309-37). The lesions often show ring enhancement on contrast administration and may occur in any location. Locations that are most commonly involved with CNS lymphoma are deep in the white matter. Contrast enhancement is usually less pronounced than that seen with toxoplasmosis. The main diseases in the differential diagnosis are cerebral toxoplasmosis and cerebral Chagas' disease. In addition to the 20% of lymphomas in HIV-infected individuals that are primary CNS lymphomas, CNS disease is also seen in HIV-infected patients with systemic lymphoma. Approximately 20% of patients with systemic lymphoma have CNS disease in the form of leptomeningeal involvement. This fact underscores the importance of lumbar puncture in the staging evaluation of patients with systemic lymphoma.

Systemic lymphoma is seen at earlier stages of HIV infection than primary CNS lymphoma. In one series the mean CD4+ T cell count was 189/μL. In addition to lymph node involvement, systemic lymphoma may commonly involve the gastrointestinal tract, bone marrow, liver, and lung. Gastrointestinal tract involvement is seen in ~25% of patients. Any site in the gastrointestinal tract may be involved, and patients may complain of difficulty swallowing or abdominal pain. The diagnosis is usually suspected on the basis of CT or MRI of the abdomen. Bone marrow involvement is seen in ~20% of patients and may lead to pancytopenia. Liver and lung involvement are each seen in ~10% of patients. Pulmonary disease may present as either a mass lesion, multiple nodules, or an interstitial infiltrate.

Both conventional and unconventional approaches have been employed in an attempt to treat HIV-related lymphomas. Systemic lymphoma is generally treated by the oncologist with combination chemotherapy. Earlier disappointing figures are being replaced with more optimistic results for the treatment of systemic lymphoma following the availability of more effective combination antiretroviral therapy. As in most situations in patients with HIV disease, those with the higher CD4+ T cell counts tend to do better. Response rates as high as 72% and disease-free intervals >15 months have been reported. Treatment of primary CNS lymphoma remains a significant challenge. Treatment is complicated by the fact that this illness usually occurs in patients with advanced HIV disease. Palliative measures such as ra-

FIGURE 309-37   CNS lymphoma. Postcontrast T1 weighted MR scan with AIDS, an altered mental status, and hemiparesis. Multiple enhancing lesions, some ring-enhancing are present. The left Sylvian lesion shows gyral and subcortical enhancement, and the lesions in the caudate and splenium (*arrowheads*) show enhancement of adjacent ependymal surfaces.

diation therapy provide some relief. The prognosis remains poor in this group, with median survival <1 year.

Evidence of infection with *human papilloma virus*, associated with *intraepithelial dysplasia of the cervix or anus*, is approximately twice as common in HIV-infected individuals as in the general population and can lead to intraepithelial neoplasia and eventually invasive cancer. It is anticipated that both anal and cervical carcinomas will be seen with increased frequency in the HIV-infected population as survival is prolonged with combination antiretroviral therapy. In two separate studies, HIV-infected men without anorectal symptoms were studied for evidence of dysplasia, and Papanicolauo (Pap) smears were found to be abnormal in 40%. These changes were persistent at 1 year follow-up, raising the possibility of a subsequent transition to a more malignant condition. While the incidence of an abnormal Pap smear of the cervix is ~5% in otherwise healthy women, the incidence of abnormal cervical smears in women with HIV infection is 60%. Based on this finding, *invasive cervical cancer* was added to the list of AIDS-defining conditions. Thus far, however, only small increases in the incidence of cervical or anal cancer have been seen as a consequence of HIV infection. However, given this high rate of dysplasia, a comprehensive gynecologic and rectal examination, including Pap smear, is indicated at the initial evaluation and 6 months later for all patients with HIV infection. If these examinations are negative at both time points, the patient should be followed with yearly evaluations. If an initial or repeat Pap smear shows evidence of severe inflammation with reactive squamous changes, the next Pap smear should be performed at 3 months. If, at any time, a Pap smear shows evidence of squamous intraepithelial lesions, colposcopic examination with biopsies as indicated should be performed.

FIGURE 309-36   Diffuse histiocytic lymphoma involving the hard palate of a patient with AIDS.

IDIOPATHIC CD4+ T LYMPHOCYTOPENIA

A syndrome was recognized in 1992 that was characterized by an absolute CD4+ T cell count of <300/μL or <20% of total T cells on more than one occasion; no evidence of HIV-1, HIV-2, HTLV-I, or HTLV-II on testing; and the absence of any defined immunodeficiency or therapy associated with decreased levels of CD4+ T cells. By mid-1993, approximately 100 patients had been described. After extensive multicenter investigations, a series of reports were published in early 1993, which together allowed a number of conclusions. Idiopathic CD4+ lymphocytopenia (ICL) is a very rare syndrome, as determined by studies of blood donors and cohorts of HIV-seronegative homosexual men. Cases were clearly identified as early as 1983, and cases remarkably similar to ICL had been identified decades ago. The definition of ICL based on CD4+ T cell counts coincided with the ready availability of testing for CD4+ T cells in patients suspected of being immunosuppressed. Although, as a result of immune deficiency, certain patients with ICL develop some of the opportunistic diseases (particularly cryptococcosis) seen in HIV-infected patients, the syndrome is demographically, clinically, and immunologically unlike HIV infection and AIDS. Fewer than half of the reported ICL patients had risk factors for HIV infection, and there were wide geographic and age distributions. The fact that a significant proportion of patients did have risk factors probably reflects a selection bias, in that physicians who take care of HIV-infected patients are more likely to monitor CD4+ T cells. Approximately one-third of the patients are women, compared to 16% of women among HIV-infected individuals in the United States. Many patients with ICL remained clinically stable, and their condition did not deteriorate progressively as is common with seriously immunodeficient HIV-infected patients. Certain patients with ICL even experienced spontaneous reversal of the CD4+ T lymphocytopenia. Immunologic abnormalities in ICL are somewhat different from those of HIV infection. ICL patients often also have decreases in CD8+ T cells and in B cells. Furthermore, immunoglobulin levels were either normal or, more commonly, decreased in patients with ICL, compared to the usual hypergammaglobulinemia of HIV-infected individuals. Finally, virologic studies revealed no evidence of HIV-1, HIV-2, HTLV-I, or HTLV-II or of any other mononuclear cell–tropic virus. Furthermore, there was no epidemiologic evidence to suggest that a transmissible microbe was involved. The cases of ICL were widely dispersed, with no clustering. Close contacts and sexual partners who were studied were clinically well and were serologically, immunologically, and virologically negative for HIV. ICL is a heterogeneous syndrome, and it is highly likely that there is no common cause; however, there may be common causes among subgroups of patients that are currently unrecognized.

Patients who present with laboratory data consistent with ICL should be worked up for underlying diseases that could be responsible for the immune deficiency. If no underlying cause is detected, no specific therapy should be initiated. However, if opportunistic diseases occur, they should be treated appropriately (see above). Depending on the level of the CD4+ T cell count, patients should receive prophylaxis for the commonly encountered opportunistic infections.

℞ TREATMENT **General Principles of Patient Management**
The treatment of patients with HIV infection requires not only a comprehensive knowledge of the possible disease processes that may occur but also the ability to deal with the problems of a chronic, potentially life-threatening illness. Great advances have been made in the treatment of patients with HIV infection. The appropriate use of potent combination antiretroviral therapy and other treatment and prophylactic interventions is of critical importance in providing each patient with the best opportunity to live a long and healthy life despite the presence of HIV infection. In contrast to the earlier days of this epidemic, a diagnosis of HIV infection need no longer be equated with an inevitably fatal disease. In addition to medical interventions, the health care provider has a responsibility to provide each patient with appropriate counseling and education concerning their disease as part of a comprehensive care plan. Patients must be educated about the potential transmissibility of their infection and about the fact that while health care providers may refer to levels of the virus as "undetectable" this is more a reflection of the sensitivity of the assay being used to measure

the virus than a comment on the presence or absence of the virus. It is important for patients to be aware and that the virus is still present and capable of being transmitted at all stages of HIV disease. Thus, there needs to be frank discussions concerning sexual practices and the sharing of needles. The treating physician must not only be aware of the latest medications available for patients with HIV infection but must also educate patients concerning the natural history of their illness and listen and be sensitive to their fears and concerns. As with other diseases, therapeutic decisions should be made in consultation with the patient, when possible, and with the patient's proxy if the patient is incapable of making decisions. In this regard, it is recommended that all patients with HIV infection, and in particular those with CD4+ T cell counts $<200/\mu L$, designate a trusted individual with durable power of attorney to make medical decisions on their behalf, if necessary.

No matter how well prepared a patient is for adversity, the discovery of a diagnosis of HIV infection is a devastating event. For this reason, it is recommended that anyone about to undergo testing have "pretest counseling" to prepare him or her at least partially should the results demonstrate the presence of HIV infection. Following a diagnosis of HIV infection, the health care provider should be prepared to activate support systems immediately for the newly diagnosed patient. These should include an experienced social worker or nurse who can spend time talking to the person and ensuring that he or she is emotionally stable. Most communities have HIV crisis centers that can be of great help in these difficult situations.

Following a diagnosis of HIV infection, there are several examinations and laboratory studies that should be performed to help determine the extent of disease and provide baseline standards for future reference (Table 309-19). In addition to routine chemistry and hematology screening panels and chest x-ray, one should also obtain a CD4+ T cell count, two separate plasma HIV RNA levels, a VDRL test, and an anti-*Toxoplasma* antibody titer. A PPD test should be done, and a MMSE performed and recorded. Patients should be immunized with pneumococcal polysaccharide and, if seronegative for these viruses, with hepatitis A and hepatitis B vaccines. In addition, patients should be counseled with regard to sexual practices and needle sharing, and counseling should be offered to those whom the patient knows or suspects may also be infected. Once these baseline activities are performed, short- and long-term medical management strategies should be developed based upon the most recent information available and modified as new information becomes available. The field of HIV medicine is changing rapidly, and it is difficult to remain fully up to date. Fortunately there are a series of excellent sites on the World Wide Web that are frequently updated, and they provide the most recent information on a variety of topics, including consensus panel reports on treatment (Table 309-20).

Antiretroviral Therapy Combination antiretroviral therapy, or HAART, is the cornerstone of management of patients with HIV infection. Following the initiation of widespread use of HAART in the

Table 309-19 Initial Evaluation of the Patient with HIV Infection

History and physical examination
Routine chemistry and hematology
CD4+ T lymphocyte count
Two plasma HIV RNA levels
VDRL test
Anti-*Toxoplasma* antibody titer
PPD skin test
Mini-mental status examination
Serologies for hepatitis A and hepatitis B
Immunization with pneumococcal polysaccharide
Immunization with hepatitis A and hepatitis B if seronegative
Counseling regarding natural history and transmission
Help contacting others who might be infected

NOTE: VDRL, Venereal Disease Research Laboratory; PPD, purified protein derivative.

www.hivatis.org	HIV AIDS Treatment Information Services; posts federally approved treatment guidelines for HIV and AIDS
www.actis.org	AIDS Clinical Trials Information Service (ACTIS); information on federally funded and privately funded clinical trials; CDC information services.
www.cdcnpin.org	Updates on epidemiologic data from the CDC
www.cc.nih.gov/phar/hiv-mgt	Online images of HIV drugs and information regarding dosing

NOTE: CDC, Centers for Disease Control and Prevention.

United States in 1995 to 1996, marked declines have been noted in the incidence of most AIDS-defining conditions (Fig. 309-28). Suppression of HIV replication is an important component in prolonging life as well as improving the quality of life in patients with HIV infection. Unfortunately, many of the most important questions related to the treatment of HIV disease currently lack definitive answers. Among them are the questions of when should therapy be started, what is the best initial regimen, when should a given regimen be changed, and what should it be changed to when a change is made. Notwithstanding these uncertainties, the physician and patient must come to a mutually agreeable plan based upon the best available data. In an effort to facilitate this process, the United States Department of Health and Human Services has published a series of frequently updated guidelines including the *"Principles of Therapy of HIV Infection," "Guidelines for the Use of Antiretroviral Agents in HIV-Infected Adults and Adolescents,"* and *"Guidelines for the Prevention of Opportunistic Infections in Persons Infected with Human Immunodeficiency Virus."* At present, an extensive clinical trials network, involving both clinical investigators and patient advocates, is in place attempting to develop improved approaches to therapy. Consortia comprising representatives of academia, industry, and the federal government are involved in the process of drug development, including clinical trials. As a result, new therapies and new therapeutic strategies are continually emerging. New drugs are often available through expanded access programs prior to official licensure. Given the complexity of this field, decisions regarding antiretroviral therapy are best made in consultation with experts. Currently licensed drugs for the treatment of HIV infection fall into two main categories: those that inhibit the viral reverse transcriptase enzyme (Table 309-21, Fig. 309-3*B*) and those that inhibit the viral protease enzyme. There are numerous drug-drug interactions that one must take into consideration when using these agents (Table 309-22).

The FDA-approved reverse transcriptase inhibitors include the *nucleoside analogues* zidovudine, didanosine, zalcitabine, stavudine, lamivudine, and abacavir and the *nonnucleoside reverse transcriptase inhibitors* nevirapine, delavirdine, and efavirenz (Fig. 309-38; Table 309-21). These were the first class of drugs that were licensed for the treatment of HIV infection. They are indicated for this use as part of combination regimens. It should be stressed that none of these drugs should be used as monotherapy for HIV infection. Thus, when lamivudine is used to treat hepatitis B infection in the setting of HIV infection, one should ensure that the patient is also on additional antiretroviral medication. The reverse transcriptase inhibitors block the HIV replication cycle at the point of RNA-dependent DNA synthesis, the reverse transcription step. While the nonnucleoside reverse transcriptase inhibitors are quite selective for the HIV-1 reverse transcriptase, the nucleoside analogues inhibit a variety of DNA polymerization reactions in addition to those of the HIV-1 reverse transcriptase. For this reason, serious side effects are more common with the nucleoside analogues and include mitochondrial damage that can lead to hepatic steatosis and lactic acidosis as well as peripheral neuropathy and pancreatitis.

Zidovudine (AZT; 3′-azido-2′,3′-dideoxythymidine) was the first drug approved for the treatment of HIV infection and is the prototype nucleoside analogue. These compounds, in which the hydroxyl group in the 3′ position of the ribose moiety is substituted with a hydrogen or other chemical group, act as DNA chain terminators owing to their inability to form a 3′-5′ phosphodiester linkage with another nucleoside. They bind much more avidly to the active site of the RNA-dependent DNA polymerase of HIV (reverse transcriptase) than to the active site of mammalian cell DNA polymerases; this explains their selective effect on HIV replication. Zidovudine also has a relatively high avidity for the DNA polymerase-γ of human mitochondria. This may contribute to the development of the fatty liver and the myopathy sometimes observed in patients taking zidovudine. As with all the nucleoside analogues, the active form of zidovudine is the triphosphate, and the rate of phosphorylation, a thymidine kinase–dependent pathway, may be different in different cells. This may explain why zidovudine is more effective at inhibiting HIV replication in some cells than others. The clinical efficacy of zidovudine was clearly established in 1986 in a phase II, randomized, placebo-controlled trial in patients with advanced HIV disease. However, while treatment of patients with early stages of HIV infection was associated with increases in CD4+ T cell count, it was not associated with a better overall outcome than later intervention. Subsequent trials established the ability of this drug to dramatically decrease the incidence of perinatal transmission of HIV from infected mother to infant. Eventually a series of studies demonstrated the superiority of combination antiretroviral regimens over zidovudine alone, and combination therapy (discussed below) remains the standard of treatment today. Among the side effects of zidovudine at the initiation of therapy are fatigue, malaise, nausea, and headache. These side effects often subside over time. Patients on zidovudine may develop a macrocytic anemia, myopathy, cardiomyopathy, and lactic acidosis associated with fatty infiltration of the liver. As with every antiretroviral drug, HIV has the ability to develop resistance to zidovudine. Zidovudine resistance has been reported to occur ~6 months following the initiation of zidovudine monotherapy. More recently, zidovudine-resistant viruses have been noted in patients with acute infection prior to the initiation of therapy, implying that zidovudine-resistant viruses can be transmitted from person to person. Resistance emerges more rapidly in late-stage patients, presumably as a consequence of a greater degree of viral replication and thus a greater opportunity for mutation. A variety of amino acid changes including substitutions, insertions, and deletions have been reported to confer zidovudine resistance (Fig. 309-39). A combination preparation, Combivir, consists of zidovudine and lamivudine.

Didanosine (ddI; 2′,3′-dideoxyinosine) was the second drug licensed for the treatment of HIV infection, followed shortly thereafter by zalcitabine. Didanosine is metabolized to dideoxyadenosine in vivo. It is best absorbed on an empty stomach at a high pH. For this reason, the current formulations of didanosine contain a buffer, and each dose must be administered in no fewer than two tablets to ensure adequate buffering of stomach acid. The toxicity profile of didanosine is quite different from that of zidovudine. The most common toxicity is a painful sensory peripheral neuropathy that occurs in ~30% of patients receiving >400 mg/d. It generally resolves with discontinuation of the drug and may not recur if the drug is resumed at a reduced dose. At higher doses than are currently used one may see pancreatitis in ~10% of patients. Pancreatitis associated with didanosine therapy can be fatal. Didanosine should be discontinued if a patient experiences abdominal pain consistent with pancreatitis or if an elevated serum amylase or lipase is found in association with an edematous pancreas on ultrasound. Didanosine is contraindicated in patients with a prior history of pancreatitis, regardless of etiology.

Zalcitabine (ddC; 2′,3′-dideoxycytidine) is rarely used today in the management of patients with HIV infection. Among the nucleoside analogues licensed for the treatment of HIV infection, it is probably the weakest. The main toxicity of ddC is pancreatitis.

Stavudine (d4T; 2′,3′-didehydro-3′-deoxythymidine) was the fourth drug licensed for the treatment of HIV infection. Like zidovudine, stavudine is a thymidine analogue. These two drugs are antagonistic in vitro and in vivo and should not be given together. Peripheral neuropathy and hepatic steatosis are the main toxicities of stavudine. It is commonly used with lamivudine as part of an initial treatment regimen.

Lamivudine (3TC; 2′,3′-dideoxy-3′-thiacytidine) is the fifth of the nucleoside analogues to be licensed in the United States. It is licensed for use in combination with zidovudine in situations where zidovudine is indicated. In actual practice, lamivudine, is a frequent element of

many different combination regimens currently in use. It is available either alone or in combination with zidovudine (Combivir). One reason behind the excellent synergy seen between lamivudine and the other nucleoside analogues may be that strains of HIV resistant to lamivudine (M184V substitution) appear to have enhanced sensitivity to other nucleosides, and thus development of dual resistance is quite difficult. In addition, there is a suggestion that 3TC-resistant strains of HIV may

Table 309-21   Antiretroviral Drugs Used in the Treatment of HIV Infection

Drug	Status	Indication	Dose as Monotherapy	Dose in Combination	Supporting Data	Toxicity
REVERSE TRANSCRIPTASE INHIBITORS						
Zidovudine (AZT, azidothymidine, Retrovir, 3′azido-3′-deoxythymidine)	Licensed	Treatment of HIV infection when antiretroviral therapy is indicated	Not indicated	200 mg q8h or 300 mg bid	19 vs 1 death in original placebo-controlled trial in 281 patients with AIDS or ARC. Decreased progression to AIDS in patients with CD4+ T cell counts <500/μL, $n = 2051$	Anemia, granulocytopenia, myopathy, lactic acidosis, hepatomegaly with steatosis, headache, nausea
		Prevention of maternal-fetal HIV transmission	*Mother:* 100 mg 5 ×/d until the start of labor, then 2 mg/kg over 1 h IV, followed by 1 mg/kg per h IV until clamping of umbilical cord; *Infant:* 2 mg/kg q6h PO beginning within 12 h birth, or 1.5 mg/kg q6h IV over 30 min		In pregnant women with CD4+ T cell count ≥200/μL, AZT PO beginning at weeks 14–34 of gestation plus IV drug during labor and delivery plus PO AZT to infant for 6 wk decreased transmission of HIV by 67.5% (from 25.5% to 8.3%), $n = 363$	
Didanosine (Videx, ddI, dideoxyinosine, 2′,3′-dideoxyinosine)	Licensed	For treatment of HIV infection when antiretroviral therapy is warranted	Not indicated	Requires 2 tablets to achieve adequate buffering of stomach acid; should be administered on an empty stomach ≥60 kg: 200 mg bid <60 kg: 125 mg bid 200 mg bid 125 mg bid	Clinically superior to AZT as monotherapy in 913 patients with prior AZT therapy. Clinically superior to AZT and comparable to AZT + ddI and AZT + ddC in 1067 AZT-naive patients with CD4+ T cell counts of 200–500/μL	Pancreatitis, peripheral neuropathy, abnormalities on liver function tests
Zalcitabine (ddC, HIVID, 2′3′-dideoxycytidine)	Licensed	In combination with other antiretroviral agents for the treatment of HIV infection	Not indicated	0.75 mg tid	Clinically inferior to AZT monotherapy as initial treatment. Clinically as good as ddI in advanced patients intolerant to AZT. In combination with AZT, was clinically superior to AZT alone in patients with AIDS or CD4+ T cell count <350/μL	Peripheral neuropathy, pancreatitis, lactic acidosis, hepatomegaly with steatosis, oral ulcers
Stavudine (d4T, Zerit, 2′3′-didehydro-3′-dideoxythymidine)	Licensed	Treatment of HIV-infected patients who have received prolonged prior zidovudine therapy	Not indicated	≥60 kg: 40 mg bid <60 kg: 30 mg bid	Superior to AZT with respect to changes in CD4+ T cell counts in 359 patients who had received ≥24 wk of AZT. Following 12 wk of randomization, the CD4+ T cell count had decreased in AZT-treated controls by a mean of 22/μL, while in stavudine-treated patients, it had increased by a mean of 22/μL	Peripheral neuropathy, pancreatitis

(continued)

Drug	Status	Indication	Dose as Monotherapy	Dose in Combination	Supporting Data	Toxicity
Lamivudine (Epivir, 2'3'-di-deoxy-3'-thiacyti-dine, 3TC)	Licensed	In combination with other anti-retroviral agents for the treatment of HIV infection	Not indicated	150 mg bid	Superior to AZT alone with respect to changes in CD4 counts in 495 patients who were zidovudine-naive and 477 patients who were zido-vudine-experienced. Overall CD4+ T cell counts for the zidovudine group were at baseline by 24 wk, while in the group treated with zido-vudine plus lamivudine, they were 10–50 cells/μL above baseline. 54% decrease in progression to AIDS/death compared to AZT alone	
Abacavir (Ziagen)	Licensed	For treatment of HIV infection in combination with other anti-retroviral agents	Not indicated	300 mg bid	Abacavir + AZT + 3TC equivalent to indinavir + AZT + 3TC with regard to viral load suppression (~60% in each group with <400 HIV RNA copies/mL plasma) and CD4 cell increase (~100/μL in each group) at 24 weeks	Hypersensitivity reaction (can be fatal); fever, rash, nausea, vomiting, malaise or fatigue, and loss of appetite
Delavirdine (Rescrip-tor)	Licensed	For use in combi-nation with ap-propriate anti-retrovirals when treatment is war-ranted	Not indicated	400 mg tid	Delavirdine + AZT superior to AZT alone with regard to viral load suppression at 52 weeks	Skin rash, abnor-malities in liver function tests
Nevirapine (Viramune)	Licensed	In combination with nucleoside analogues for treatment of pro-gressive HIV in-fection	Not indicated	200 mg/d × 14 days then 200 mg bid	Increases in CD4+ T cell count, decrease in HIV RNA when used in combination with nucleosides	Skin rash, abnor-malities in liver function tests
Efavirenz (Sustiva)	Licensed	For treatment of HIV infection in combination with other anti-retroviral agents	Not indicated	600 mg qhs	Efavirenz + AZT + 3TC com-parable to indinavir + AZT + 3TC with regard to viral load suppression (a higher percentage of the efavirenz group achieved viral load <50 copies/mL; however, the discontinuation rate in the indinavir group was unex-pectedly high, accounting for most treatment "failures") and CD4 cell increase (~140/μL in each group) at 24 weeks	Rash, dysphoria, elevated liver function tests

PROTEASE INHIBITORS

Drug	Status	Indication	Dose as Monotherapy	Dose in Combination	Supporting Data	Toxicity
Saquinavir mesylate (Invirase—hard gel capsule)	Licensed	In combination with other anti-retroviral agents when therapy is warranted	Not indicated	600 mg q8h	Increases in CD4+ T cell counts, reduction in HIV RNA most pronounced in combination therapy with ddC. 50% reduction in first AIDS-defining event or death in combination with ddC compared to either agent alone	Diarrhea, nausea, headaches, hy-perglycemia, fat redistribution, lipid abnormali-ties
(Forto-vase—soft gel capsule)	Licensed	For use in combi-nation with other antiretroviral agents when treatment is warranted	Not indicated	1200 mg tid	Reduction in the mortality rate and AIDS-defining events for patients who received hard-gel formulation in combina-tion with ddC	Diarrhea, nausea, abdominal pain, headaches, hy-perglycemia, fat redistribution, lipid abnormali-ties

(continued)

Table 309-21—(continued)

Drug	Status	Indication	Dose as Monotherapy	Dose in Combination	Supporting Data	Toxicity
Ritonavir (Norvir)	Licensed	In combination with nucleoside analogues for treatment of HIV infection when treatment is warranted	Not indicated	600 mg bid	Reduction in the cumulative incidence of clinical progression or death from 34 to 17% in patients with CD4+ T cell count <100/μL treated for a median of 6 months	Nausea, abdominal pain, hyperglycemia, fat redistribution, lipid abnormalities, may alter levels of many other drugs, including saquinavir
Indinavir sulfate (Crixivan)	Licensed	For treatment of HIV infection when antiretroviral treatment is warranted	Not indicated	800 mg q8h	Increase in CD4+ T cell count by 100/μL and 2-log decrease in HIV RNA levels when given in combination with zidovudine and lamivudine. Decrease of 50% in risk of progression to AIDS or death when given with zidovudine and lamivudine compared with zidovudine and lamivudine alone	Nephrolithiasis, indirect hyperbilirubinemia, hyperglycemia, fat redistribution, lipid abnormalities
Nelfinavir mesylate (Viracept)	Licensed	For treatment of HIV infection when antiretroviral therapy is warranted	Not indicated	750 mg tid or 1250 mg bid	2.0-log decline in HIV RNA when given in combination with stavudine	Diarrhea, loose stools, hyperglycemia, fat redistribution, lipid abnormalities
Amprenavir (Agenerase)	Licensed	In combination with other antiretroviral agents for treatment of HIV infection	Not indicated	1200 mg bid	In treatment-naïve patients, amprenavir − AZT + 3TC superior to AZT + 3TC with regard to viral load suppression (53% vs 11% with <400 HIV RNA copies/mL plasma at 24 weeks). CD4+ T cell responses similar between treatment groups. In treatment-experienced patients, amprenavir + NRTIs similar to indinavir + NRTIs with regard to viral load suppression (43% vs 53% with <400 HIV RNA copies/mL plasma at 24 weeks). CD4+ T cell responses superior in the indinavir + NRTIs group	Nausea, vomiting, diarrhea, rash, oral paresthesias, elevated liver function tests, hyperglycemia, fat redistribution, lipid abnormalities
Lopinavir/ ritonavir (Kaletra)	Licensed	For treatment of HIV infection	Not indicated	400 mg/100 mg bid	In treatment of naïve patients, lopinavir/ritonavir + d4T + 3TC superior to nelfinavir + d4T + 3TC with regard to viral load suppression (79% vs 64% with <400 HIV RNA copies/mL at 40 weeks). CD4+ T cell increases similar in both groups.	Diarrhea, hyperglycemia, fat redistribution, lipid abnormalities

NOTE: ARC, AIDS-related complex; NRTIs, nonnucleoside reverse transcriptase inhibitors.

be less virulent and are less able to generate new mutants than are strains of HIV that are 3TC-sensitive. Lamivudine is among the best tolerated and least toxic nucleoside analogues.

Abacavir {(1S,cis)-4-[2-amino-6-(cyclopropylamino)-9H-purin-9-yl]-2-cyclopentene-1-methanol sulfate (salt)(2:1)} is a synthetic carbocyclic analogue of the nucleoside guanosine. It is licensed to be used in combination with other antiretroviral agents for the treatment of HIV-1 infection. Hypersensitivity reactions have been reported in ~5% of patients treated with this drug, and patients developing signs or symptoms of hypersensitivity such as fever, skin rash, fatigue, and gastrointestinal symptoms should discontinue the drug and not restart it. Fatal hypersensitivity reactions have been reported with rechallenge. Abacavir-resistant strains of HIV are typically also resistant to lamivudine, didanosine, and zalcitabine.

Nevirapine, delavirdine, and *efavirenz* are nonnucleoside inhibitors of the HIV-1 reverse transcriptase. They are licensed for use in combination with nucleoside analogues for the treatment of HIV-infected adults. These agents inhibit reverse transcriptase by binding to regions of the enzyme outside the active site and causing conformational changes in the enzyme that render it inactive. Although these agents are active in the nanomolar range, they are also very selective for the reverse transcriptase of HIV-1, have no activity against HIV-2, and, when used as monotherapy, are associated with the rapid emergence of drug-resistant mutants (Table 309-21; Fig. 309-39). Efavirenz is administered once a day, nevirapine twice a day, and delavirdine three times a day. All three drugs are associated with the development of a maculopapular rash, generally seen within the first few weeks of therapy. While it is possible to treat through this rash, it is important

Table 309-22   Drug-Drug Interactions Involving Antiretroviral Agents

Index Drug	Interacting Drug(s)	Mechanism/Effect	Recommendation
Amprenavir	Efavirenz	Induction of metabolism, decreased amprenavir AUC	Consider dosage increase to 1200 mg tid or add ritonavir 200 mg bid
	Indinavir	Inhibition of metabolism—drug levels increased 64%	Combination under investigation
	Ketoconazole	Inhibition of metabolism—drug levels increased 32%	Combination under investigation
	Ritonavir	Inhibition of metabolism—amprenavir AUC increased 2.5-fold	Combination under investigation to optimize amprenavir levels
Amprenavir, indinavir, saquinavir, ritonavir, nelfinavir	Rifampin	Induction of metabolism—marked decrease in protease inhibitor drug levels	Avoid concomitant use
Antiarrhythmics (flecainaide, quinidine, propafenone, amiodarone)	Ritonavir	Inhibition of metabolism—potential for increased levels and toxicity	Use with caution or avoid concomitant use
Atovaquone	Rifampin	Induction of metabolism—decreased drug levels	Concentrations may not be therapeutic—avoid or increase dose
Benzodiazepines (flurazepam, diazepam, midazolam, triazolam)	Protease inhibitors, delavirdine	Inhibition of metabolism—increased drug levels	Monitor for toxicity such as increased sedation, decrease dose, or use temazepam, lorazepam
Cidofovir	Nephrotoxic drugs (aminoglycosides, amphotericin, foscarnet)	Potential for increased side effects	Monitor renal function
Cisapride	Protease inhibitors, azole antifungals, macrolides, delavirdine	Inhibition of metabolism	Cardiotoxic life-threatening effects possible—avoid concomitant use
Clarithromycin	Efavirenz	Induction of metabolism—40% decrease in clarithromycin AUC	Clinical significance unknown, but clarithromycin effectiveness may be altered
	Nevirapine	Induction of metabolism—decrease in clarithromycin AUC by 30%, increase in 14-OH clarithromycin by 58%	No dosage adjustments necessary
	Ritonavir	Inhibition of metabolism—drug levels increased 77%	No adjustment needed in normal renal function
Delavirdine	Adefovir	Decrease in delavirdine AUC by 35–44%	No clinical data, but potential for decreased DLV efficacy
	Agents that increase gastric pH—antacids, H_2 blockers, proton pump inhibitors, didanosine	Delavirdine absorption decreased with increased pH	Avoid concomitant use with H_2 blockers and proton pump inhibitors; separate from antacids by at least 2 h
	Rifabutin	Induction of metabolism—50–60% decrease in delavirdine levels	Clinical significance unknown; may require increased delavirdine dose
	Rifampin	Induction of metabolism—marked decrease in drug levels	Avoid concomitant use
Didanosine (ddl)	Allopurinol	Increased ddl AUC by 2-fold	Clinical significance unknown
	Methadone	Decrease in ddl AUC by 52%	No clinical data, but potential for decreased ddl efficacy
Efavirenz	Fluconazole	Inhibition of metabolism—efavirenz AUC increased 15%	No dosage adjustment necessary
	Indinavir	Induction of hepatic metabolism—indinavir AUC decreased 35%	Consider increasing indinavir dose to 1000 mg q8h
	Nelfinavir	Nelfinavir AUC increased 21%	No dosage adjustment necessary
	Rifampin	Induction of metabolism—significant reduction in efavirenz AUC	Clinical significance unknown; increase in efavirenz dose may be required
	Rifampin	Induction of metabolism—efavirenz AUC decreased 26%	Clinical significance unknown
	Ritonavir	Inhibition of metabolism—efavirenz AUC increased 21%	No dosage adjustment necessary
Ergot alkaloids (ergotamine, dihydroergotamine, ergoloid mesylates)	Protease inhibitors, azole antifungals, macrolides, delavirdine	Inhibition of metabolism—potential for acute toxicity	Use with caution or avoid concomitant use; monitor for toxicity such as peripheral vasoconstriction, nausea and vomiting, and impaired mental status
Ethinyl estradiol	Efavirenz	Inhibition of metabolism—37% increase in estradiol AUC	No dosage adjustment necessary
	Ritonavir, nelfinavir	Induction of metabolism—decreased levels of oral contraceptive	Use alternative methods of contraception
Fluvastatin, lovastatin, simvastatin	Protease inhibitors, azole antifungals, macrolides, delavirdine	Inhibition of metabolism—potential for increased levels and toxicity	Potential for hypolipidemic toxicity (dizziness, headache, GI side effects); monitor patient closely and consider dose reduction or use pravastatin or atorvastatin
Foscarnet	Nephrotoxic drugs (aminoglycosides, amphotericin, cidofovir)	Potential for increased toxicity	Monitor renal function

(continued)

Table 309-21—(continued)

Index Drug	Interacting Drug(s)	Mechanism/Effect	Recommendation
Ganciclovir	Drugs causing bone marrow suppression (i.e., TMP/SMZ, zidovudine)	Potential for increased hematologic toxicity	Monitor for anemia and neutropenia—adjust/change doses and drugs if required; consider supportive therapy with G-CSF
Indinavir, saquinavir, ritonavir, nelfinavir, amprenavir	Anticonvulsants (carbamazepine, phenytoin, phenobarbital)	Induction of metabolism—potential decrease in drug levels	Clinical effects unknown; monitor blood levels, consider dosage increase, or avoid concomitant use
Indinavir	Delavirdine	Increased indinavir levels	Consider reducing indinavir dose to 600 mg q8h
	St. John's wort	Decreased indinavir levels	Avoid use of St. John's wort
	Didanosine, antacids	ddI buffer decreases absorption of indinavir	Separate doses by at least 1 h
	Methadone	Indinavir C_{max} decreased 16–36%; indinavir C_{min} increased by 50–100%	No dosage adjustments necessary
	Nelfinavir	Inhibition of metabolism—indinavir drug levels increased by 51%, nelfinavir drug levels by 83%	Combination currently under evaluation
	Nevirapine	Induction of metabolism—decreased drug levels of indinavir by 30%	Consider increasing indinavir dose to 1000 mg q8h
	Ritonavir	Inhibition of metabolism—indinavir AUC increased 3-7-fold	bid regimens under investigation to optimize indinavir levels—various doses under study including 800 mg indinavir/200 mg ritonavir bid
Meperidine	Ritonavir	Likely induction of metabolism—Decrease in meperidine AUC 67%, increase in normeperidine 47%	Potential for decreased meperidine effectiveness—may require increased dose; caution with chronic dosing
Methadone	Abacavir	Methadone clearance decreased 22%	Low potential for opiate withdrawal; monitor closely and increase methadone dose as required to control symptoms
	Fluconazole	Inhibition of metabolism—drug levels increased 30%	Monitor for methadone toxicity such as respiratory depression, drop in blood pressure, and mental status changes; consider dosage adjustment
	Nevirapine	Induction of metabolism—substantial decrease in methadone levels	Potential for opiate withdrawal; monitor closely and increase methadone dose as required to control symptoms
Nelfinavir	Ritonavir	Inhibition of metabolism—increased drug levels of nelfinavir by 152%	Currently under investigation
Pentamidine	Drugs that cause pancreatitis (didanosine, zalcitabine)	Increased risk of pancreatitis	Monitor amylase, lipase
Quinolone antibiotics (ciprofloxacin, levofloxacin, ofloxaxin, etc)	Didanosine, antacids, iron products, calcium products, sucralfate	Chelation resulting in marked decrease in quinolone drug levels	Administer cation preparations at least 2 h after quinolone
Rifabutin	Amprenavir, ritonavir, indinavir, nelfinavir	Inhibition of metabolism—marked increase in rifabutin drug levels	Use 150 mg qd with indinavir, nelfinavir, emprenavir, Use 150 mg every other day with ritonavir
	Fluconazole	Inhibition of metabolism—marked increase in rifabutin drug levels	Monitor for rifabutin toxicity such as uveitis, nausea, neutropenia
Saquinavir	Nevirapine	Induction of metabolism—drug levels decreased 27%	Clinical significance unknown—consider dosage increase of saquinavir or add ritonavir
	Ritonavir	Inhibition of metabolism—3-fold or higher increase in saquinavir drug levels	Various combinations used to optimize saquinavir therapy including 400 mg saquinavir/400 mg ritonavir
	Efavirenz	Induction of metabolism—saquinavir AUC decreased 62%	Avoid concomitant use unless saquinavir is administered with ritonavir
Sildenafil	Ritonavir	Inhibition of metabolism—sildenafil AUC increased 11-fold	Use 25-mg sildenafil dose and do not repeat for 48 h
	Saquinavir, indinavir	Inhibition of metabolism—sildenafil AUC increased 3–4-fold	Use 25-mg sildenafil dose
Terfenadine, astemizole	Protease inhibitors, azole antifungals, macrolides, delavirdine	Inhibition of metabolism	Cardiotoxic life-threatening effects possible—avoid concomitant use
Theophylline	Ritonavir	Induction of metabolism—decreased blood levels	Monitor theophylline levels
Tipranavir	Ritonavir	Inhibition of metabolism—tipranavir AUC increased 7–45-fold	Combination under investigation to optimize tipranavir levels
TMP/SMZ	Rifampin	TMP AUC decreased 63%, SMZ AUC decreased 23%	Clinical significance unknown
Zalcitabine, stavudine, didanosine	Drugs that cause peripheral neuropathy—INH, d4T, ddI, ddC	Potential for increased risk of peripheral neuropathy	Monitor for signs and symptoms such as numbness and tingling in extremities
Zidovudine	Drugs causing bone marrow suppression (i.e., TMP/SMZ, ganciclovir, sulfadiazine)	Increased bone marrow suppression	Monitor for anemia, neutropenia—may require supportive therapy (EPO, G-CSF)

NOTE: AUC, area under the curve; C, concentration; EPO, erythropoietin; G-CSF, granulocyte colony stimulating factor; TMP/SMZ, trimethoprim/sulfamethoxazole.

FIGURE 309-38 Molecular structures of antiretroviral agents.

to be sure that one is not dealing with a more severe eruption such as Stevens-Johnson syndrome by looking carefully for signs of mucosal involvement, significant fever, or painful lesions with desquamation. In addition to skin rash, many patients treated with efavirenz note a feeling of light-headedness, dizziness, or out of sorts following the initiation of therapy. Some complain of vivid dreams. These symptoms tend to disappear after several weeks of therapy. Aside from difficulties with dreams, taking efavirenz at bedtime may minimize the side effects. Nevirapine and efavirenz are both commonly used as part of initial treatment regimens in combination with two nucleoside analogues. Another common use of these drugs is as part of salvage regimens in patients whose current regimen is inadequate.

The introduction of the HIV-1 protease inhibitors (saquinavir, indinavir, ritonavir, nelfinavir, and amprenavir) to the therapeutic armamentarium of antiretrovirals has had a profound impact on the efficacy of antiretroviral therapy. When used as part of initial regimens in combination with reverse transcriptase inhibitors, these agents have been shown to be capable of suppressing levels of HIV replication to under 50 copies per milliliter in the majority of patients for a minimum of 3 years. As in the case of reverse transcriptase inhibitors, resistance to protease inhibitors can develop rapidly in the setting of monotherapy, and thus these agents should be used as part of combination therapeutic regimens. A summary of known resistance mutations

for reverse transcriptase and protease inhibitors is shown in Fig. 309-39.

Saquinavir was the first of the HIV-1 protease inhibitors to be licensed. Initially provided as a hard gel (Invirase) with poor bioavailability, the current soft-get formulation (Fortavase) provides good plasma levels of drug, particularly when administered in conjunction with ritonavir. Saquinavir is metabolized by the cytochrome P450 system, and ritonavir therapy results in inhibition of cytochrome P450 action. Thus, when both drugs are administered together there is the potential for increases in saquinavir levels. The use of low doses of ritonavir to provide pharmacodynamic boosting of other agents has become a fairly common strategy in HIV therapy. Saquinavir is perhaps the best-tolerated protease inhibitor and the one with the fewest side effects.

Ritonavir was the first protease inhibitor for which clinical efficacy was demonstrated. In a study of 1090 patients with CD4+ T cell counts $<100/\mu L$ who were randomized to receive either placebo or ritonavir in addition to any other licensed medications, patients receiving ritonavir had a reduction in the cumulative incidence of clinical progression or death from 34% to 17%. Mortality decreased from 10.1% to 5.8%. At full doses, ritonavir is poorly tolerated. Among the main side effects are nausea, diarrhea, abdominal pain, and circumoral paresthesia. Ritonavir has a high affinity for several isoforms of cytochrome

P450, and its use can result in large increases in the plasma concentrations of drugs metabolized by this pathway. Among the agents affected in this manner are saquinavir, indinavir, macrolide antibiotics, R-warfarin, ondansetron, rifampin, most calcium channel blockers, glucocorticoids, and some of the chemotherapeutic agents used to treat KS. In addition, ritonavir may increase the activity of glucuronyltransferases, thus decreasing the levels of drugs metabolized by this pathway. Overall, great care must be taken when prescribing additional drugs to patients taking ritonavir. As mentioned above, the pharmacodynamic boosting property of ritonavir, seen with doses as low as 100 to 200 mg twice a day, is often used in the setting of HIV infection to derive more convenient regimens. For example, when given with low-dose ritonavir, saquinavir and indinavir can both be given on twice-a-day schedules and taken with food.

Indinavir is among the best studied of the HIV-1 protease inhibitors. It was the first protease inhibitor used in combination with dual nucleoside therapy. The combination of zidovudine, lamivudine, and indinavir was the first "triple combination" shown to have a profound effect on HIV replication. The main side effects of indinavir are nephrolithiasis (seen in 4% of patients) and asymptomatic indirect hyperbilirubinemia (seen in 10%). Indinavir is predominantly metabolized by the liver. The dose should be lowered in patients with cirrhosis. Indinavir shares metabolic pathways with terfenadine, astemizole, cisapride, triazolam, and midazolam. To avoid the potential for cardiac arrhythmias or prolonged sedation, these drugs should not be administered to patients taking indinavir. Levels of indinavir are decreased during concurrent therapy with rifabutin or nevirapine and increased during concurrent therapy with ketoconazole, delavirdine, efavirenz, or ritonavir. Dosages should be modified appropriately in these circumstances (Table 309-22).

Nelfinavir was approved in 1997 and *amprenavir* was approved in 1999 for the treatment of adult or pediatric HIV infection when antiretroviral therapy is warranted. As with most of the newer antiretroviral agents, these approvals were based on randomized, controlled trials that demonstrated decreases in plasma HIV RNA levels and increases in CD4+ T cell counts. Both agents have unique resistance profiles. Nelfinavir resistance is associated with a D30N substitution in the protease gene. Viruses harboring this single mutation retain sensitivity to other protease inhibitors, and it has been suggested that for this reason nelfinavir is a good initial protease inhibitor. It is not clear, however, whether this theoretical consideration will be borne out in the results of clinical trials. Protease inhibitor resistance typically involves multiple amino acid substitutions and reduced susceptibility across the class. Amprenavir resistance is associated with a unique substitution at amino acid 50 (I50V), and it has been suggested that amprenavir may be of particular value in salvage regimens. This assumption also awaits verification in controlled clinical trials. Nel-

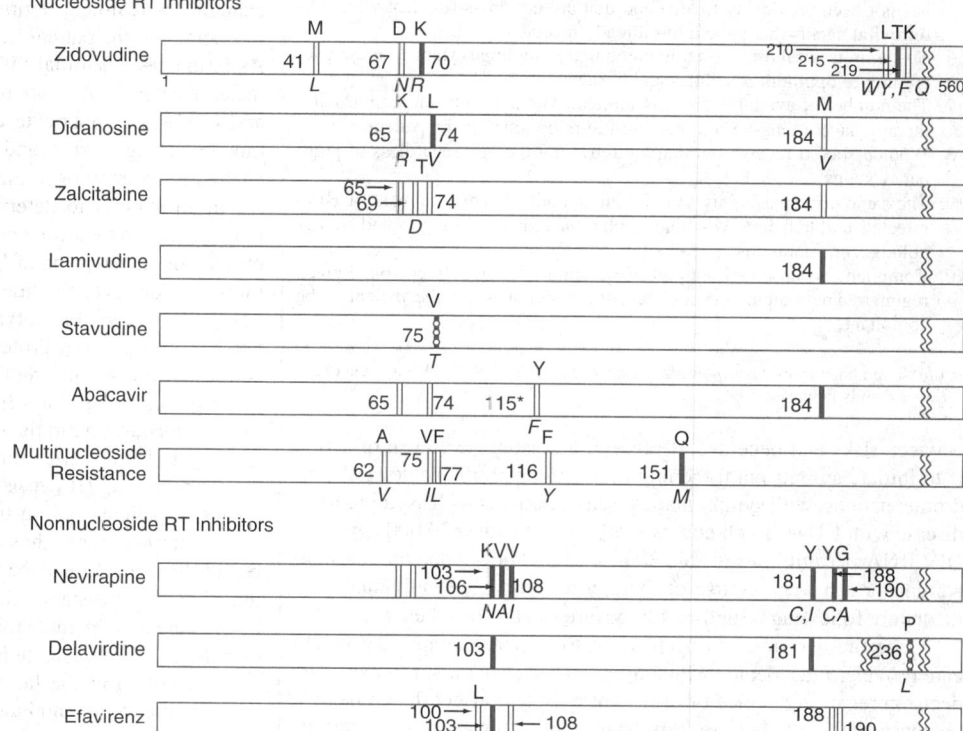

FIGURE 309-39 Amino acid substitutions conferring resistance to antiretroviral drugs. The most common HIV-1 mutations selected by protease inhibitors *(A)*, and nucleoside and nonnucleoside reverse transcriptase inhibitors *(B)*. For each amino acid residue listed, the letter above the listing indicates the amino acid associated with the wild-type virus. The italicized letter below the residue indicates the substitution that confers drug resistance. *(From Hirsch et al.)*

finavir and amprenavir are both associated with gastrointestinal side effects. About 1% of patients receiving amprenavir have experienced severe and life-threatening skin reactions. An additional disadvantage of amprenavir is that the current formulation requires the patient to take 8 large capsules twice a day.

One of the main problems that has been encountered with the widespread use of HAART therapy has been a syndrome of hyperlipidemia and fat distribution often referred to as *lipodystrophy syndrome* (discussed above under metabolic abnormalities).

The principles of therapy for HIV infection have been articulated by a panel sponsored by the U.S. Department of Health and Human Services and the Henry J. Kaiser Family Foundation. These principles are summarized in Table 309-23. However, *one element of HIV disease not currently covered by these principles is that eradication of HIV infection has not yet been possible.* Treatment decisions must take into account the fact that one is dealing with a chronic infection. While early therapy is generally the rule in infectious diseases, immediate treatment of every HIV-infected individual upon diagnosis may not be prudent, and therapeutic decisions must take into account the balance

Table 309-23 Principles of Therapy of HIV Infection

1. Ongoing HIV replication leads to immune system damage and progression to AIDS.
2. Plasma HIV RNA levels indicate the magnitude of HIV replication and the rate of CD4+ T cell destruction. CD4+ T cell counts indicate the current level of competence of the immune system.
3. Rates of disease progression differ among individuals, and treatment decisions should be individualized based upon plasma HIV RNA levels and CD4+ T cell counts.
4. Maximal suppression of viral replication is a goal of therapy; the greater the suppression the less likely the appearance of drug-resistance quasispecies.
5. The most effective therapeutic strategies involve the simultaneous initiation of combinations of effective anti-HIV drugs with which the patient has not been previously treated and that are not cross-resistant with antiretroviral agents that patient has already received.
6. The antiretroviral drugs used in combination regimens should be used according to optimum schedules and dosages.
7. The number of available drugs is limited. Any decisions on antiretroviral therapy have a long-term impact on future options for the patient.
8. Women should receive optimal antiretroviral therapy regardless of pregnancy status.
9. The same principals apply to children and adults. The treatment of HIV-infected children involves unique pharmacologic, virologic, and immunologic considerations.
10. Compliance is an important part of ensuring maximal effect from a given regimen. The simpler the regimen, the easier it is for the patient to be compliant.

SOURCE: Modified from, *Principles of Therapy of HIV Infection*, USPHS and the Henry J. Kaiser Family Foundation.

between risks and benefits. At present, a reasonable course of action is to initiate antiretroviral therapy in anyone with the acute HIV syndrome; patients with symptomatic disease; patients with asymptomatic disease with CD4+ T cell counts <500/μL or with >20,000 copies of HIV RNA per milliliter (Table 309-24). In addition, one may wish to administer a 6-week course of therapy to uninfected individuals immediately following a high-risk exposure to HIV (see below).

Once the decision has been made to initiate therapy, the health care provider must decide which drugs to use as the first regimen. The decision regarding choice of drugs not only will affect the immediate response to therapy but also will have implications regarding options for future therapeutic regimens. The initial regimen is usually the most effective insofar as the virus has yet to develop significant resistance. The two options for initial therapy most commonly in use today are two different three-drug regimens. The first regimen utilizes two nucleoside analogues (one of which is usually lamivudine) and a protease inhibitor. The second regimen utilizes two nucleoside analogues and a nonnucleoside reverse transcriptase inhibitor. Unfortunately there are no clear data at present on which to base distinctions between these two approaches. Following the initiation of therapy one should expect a 1 log (tenfold) reduction in plasma HIV RNA levels within 1 to 2 months and eventually a decline in plasma HIV RNA levels to <50 copies per milliliter. During this same time there should be a rise in

Table 309-24 Indications for the Initiation of Antiretroviral Therapy in Patients with HIV Infection

I. Acute infection syndrome
II. Chronic infection
    A. Symptomatic disease
    B. Asymptomatic diseases[a]
        1. CD4+ T cell count <500/μL or decreasing
        2. HIV RNA >20,000 copies per milliliter or increasing
III. Postexposure prophylaxis

[a] This is the area of greatest controversy. Some experts would wait until the CD4 cell count declines to 200/μl, whereas others would treat everyone regardless of CD4+ T cell count.
SOURCE: *Guidelines for the Use of Antiretroviral Agents in HIV-Infected Adults and Adolescents.* USPHS.

the CD4+ T cell count of 100 to 150/μL that is particularly brisk during the first month of therapy. Many clinicians feel that failure to achieve this endpoint is an indication for a change in therapy. Other reasons for a change in therapy include a persistently declining CD4+ T cell count, clinical deterioration, or drug toxicity (Table 309-25). As in the case of initiating therapy, changing therapy may have a lasting impact on future therapeutic options. When changing therapy because of treatment failure (clinical progression or worsening laboratory parameters), it is important to attempt to provide a regimen with at least two new drugs. In the patient in whom a change is made for reasons of drug toxicity, a simple replacement of one drug is reasonable. It should be stressed that in attempting to sort out a drug toxicity it may be advisable to hold all therapy for a period of time to distinguish between drug toxicity and disease progression. Drug toxicity will usually begin to show signs of reversal within 1 to 2 weeks. Prior to changing a treatment regimen because of drug failure, it is important to ensure that the patient has been adherent to the prescribed regimen. As in the case of initial therapy, the simpler the therapeutic regimen, the easier it is for the patient to be compliant. Plasma HIV RNA levels and CD4+ T lymphocyte counts should be monitored every 3 to 4 months during therapy and more frequently if one is contemplating a change in regimen or immediately following a change in regimen.

In an attempt to determine an optimal therapeutic regimen, one may attempt to measure antiretroviral drug susceptibility through genotyping or phenotyping of HIV quasispecies. Genotyping may be done through dideoxynucleotide sequencing, DNA chip hybridization, or line probe assays. Phenotypic assays measure the performance of reverse transcriptase or protease in the presence or absence of different concentrations of different drugs. These assays will generally detect quasispecies present at a frequency of at least 10%. The precise role of resistance testing in the management of patients with HIV infection is not yet clear. While randomized studies have suggested that information regarding HIV resistance profiles may improve therapeutic outcomes in patients failing their current antiretroviral regimen, the degree of improvement thus far has been small and the duration of the benefit limited. Resistance testing may be of particular value in distinguishing drug-resistant virus from poor patient compliance; it may also be of value to help guide initial therapy in a setting where transmission of a drug-resistant isolate is felt to be likely.

In addition to the licensed medications discussed above, a large number of experimental agents are being evaluated as possible therapies for HIV infection. Therapeutic strategies are being developed that interfere with virtually every step of the replication cycle of the virus (Fig. 309-3). In addition, as more is discovered about the role of the immune system in controlling viral replication, additional strategies, generically referred to as "immune-based therapies," are being developed as a complement to antiviral therapy. Among the antiviral agents in early clinical trials are additional nucleoside analogues, nucleotide analogues, additional protease inhibitors including nonpeptidomimetic compounds, integrase inhibitors, antisense nucleic acids, and fusion inhibitors. Among the immune-based therapies being evaluated are IFN-α, bone marrow transplantation, adoptive transfer of lymphocytes

Table 309-25 Indications for Changing Antiretroviral Therapy in Patients with HIV Infection[a]

Less than a 1-log drop in plasma HIV RNA by 4 weeks following the initiation of therapy
A reproducible significant increase (defined as 3-fold or greater) from the nadir of plasma HIV RNA level not attributable to intercurrent infection, vaccination, or test methodology
Persistently declining CD4+ T cell numbers
Clinical deterioration
Side effects

[a] Generally speaking, a change should involve the initiation of at least 2 drugs felt to be effective in the given patient. The exception to this is when change is being made to manage toxicity, in which case a single substitution is reasonable.
SOURCE: *Guidelines for the Use of Antiretroviral Agents in HIV-Infected Adults and Adolescents.* USPHS.

genetically modified to resist infection or enhance HIV-specific immunity, active immunotherapy with inactivated HIV, and IL-2.

HIV AND THE HEALTH CARE WORKER

Health care workers, especially those who deal with large numbers of HIV-infected patients, have a small but definite risk of becoming infected with HIV as a result of professional activities. As of January 1, 2000, 56 health care workers in the United States had been documented as having seroconverted to HIV following occupational exposure; 25 have developed AIDS. The individuals who seroconverted include 19 laboratory workers (16 of whom were clinical laboratory workers), 23 nurses, 6 physicians, 2 surgical technicians, 1 dialysis technician, 1 respiratory therapist, 1 health aide, 1 embalmer/morgue technician, and 2 housekeeper/maintenance workers. The exposures included 48 percutaneous (puncture/cut injury), 5 mucocutaneous (mucous membrane and/or skin), 2 both percutaneous and mucocutaneous, and 1 unknown route of exposure. Fifty exposures were to HIV-infected blood, three to concentrated virus in a laboratory, one to visibly bloody fluid, and one to unspecified fluid. As of January 1, 2000, there had been 136 other cases of HIV infection or AIDS among health care workers who have not reported other risk factors for HIV infection and who report a history of exposure to blood, body fluids, or HIV-infected laboratory material, but for whom seroconversion after exposure was not documented. The number of these workers who actually acquired their infection through occupational exposures is not known. Taken together, the data from several large studies suggest that the risk of HIV infection following a percutaneous injury with an HIV-contaminated hollow-bore needle (in contrast to a solid-bore needle, i.e., a suture needle) is approximately 0.3%. A seroprevalence survey of 3420 orthopedic surgeons, 75% of whom practiced in an area with a relatively high prevalence of HIV infection and 39% of whom reported percutaneous exposure to patient blood, usually through an accident involving a suture needle, failed to reveal any cases of possible occupational infection, suggesting that the risk of infection with a suture needle may be considerably less than that with a blood-drawing needle.

Most cases of health care worker seroconversion occur as a result of needle-stick injuries. When one considers the circumstances that result in needle-stick injuries, it is immediately obvious that adhering to the standard guidelines for dealing with sharp objects would result in a significant decrease in this type of accident. In one study, 27% of needle-stick injuries resulted from improper disposal of the needle (over half of these were due to recapping the needle), 23% occurred during attempts to start an intravenous line, 22% occurred during blood drawing, 16% were associated with an intramuscular or subcutaneous injection, and 12% were associated with giving an intravenous infusion.

Recommendations regarding postexposure prophylaxis must take into account that several circumstances determine the risk of transmission of HIV following occupational exposure. In this regard, five factors have been associated with an increased risk for occupational transmission of HIV infection: deep injury, the presence of visible blood on the instrument causing the exposure, injury with a device that had been placed in the vein or artery of the source patient, terminal illness in the source patient, and lack of postexposure antiretroviral therapy in the exposed health care worker. Other important considerations include pregnancy in the health care worker and the possibility of exposure to drug-resistant virus. Regardless of the decision to use postexposure prophylaxis, the wound should be cleansed immediately and antiseptic applied. If a decision is made to offer postexposure prophylaxis, U.S. Public Health Service guidelines recommend (1) a combination of two nucleoside analogue reverse transcriptase inhibitors given for 4 weeks for routine exposures, or (2) a combination of two nucleoside analogue reverse transcriptase inhibitors plus a protease inhibitor given for 4 weeks for high-risk or otherwise complicated exposures, although most clinicians administer the latter regimen in all cases in which a decision is made to treat. Further details are available from the U.S. Public Health Service *Guidelines for the Management*

of Health-Care Worker Exposures to HIV and Recommendations for Postexposure Prophylaxis (CDC, 1998).

Health care workers can minimize their risk of occupational HIV infection by following the CDC guidelines of July 1991, which include adherence to universal precautions, refraining from direct patient care if one has exudative lesions or weeping dermatitis, and disinfecting and sterilizing reusable devices employed in invasive procedures. The premise of universal precautions is that every specimen should be handled as if it came from someone infected with a bloodborne pathogen. All samples should be double-bagged, gloves should be worn when drawing blood, and spills should be immediately disinfected with bleach.

In attempting to put this small but definite risk to the health care worker in perspective, it is important to point out that approximately 200 health care workers die each year as a result of occupationally acquired hepatitis B infection. The tragedy in this instance is that these infections and deaths due to HBV could be greatly decreased by more extended use of the HBV vaccine. The risk of HBV infection following a needle-stick injury from a hepatitis antigen–positive patient is much higher than the risk of HIV infection (see "Transmission," above). There are multiple examples of needle-stick injuries where the patient was positive for both HBV and HIV and the health care worker became infected only with HBV. For these reasons, it is advisable, given the high prevalence of HBV infection in HIV-infected individuals, that all health care workers dealing with HIV-infected patients be immunized with the HBV vaccine.

TB is another infection common to HIV-infected patients that can be transmitted to the health care worker. For this reason, all health care workers should know their PPD status, have it checked yearly, and receive one year of isoniazid treatment if their skin test converts to positive. In addition, all patients in whom a diagnosis of TB is being entertained should be placed immediately in respiratory isolation, pending results of the diagnostic evaluation. The emergence of drug-resistant organisms has made TB an increasing problem for health care workers. This is particularly true for the health care worker with pre-existing HIV infection.

One of the most charged issues ever to come between health care workers and patients is that of transmission of infection from HIV-infected health care workers to their patients. This is discussed under "Occupational Transmission of HIV: Health Care Workers and Laboratory Workers," p. 1857. Theoretically, the same universal precautions that are used to protect the health care worker from the HIV-infected patient will also protect the patient from the HIV-infected health care worker.

VACCINES

Historically, vaccines have provided a safe, cost-effective, and efficient means of preventing illness, disability, and death from infectious diseases. Given the fact that human behavior, especially human sexual behavior, is extremely difficult to change, the best hope for preventing the spread of HIV infection rests with the development of a safe and effective vaccine. This task is problematic for a number of reasons, including the high mutability of the virus, the fact that the infection can be transmitted by cell-free or cell-associated virus, the likely need for the development of effective mucosal immunity, and the fact that it has been difficult to establish the precise correlates of protective immunity to HIV infection. Some HIV-infected individuals are long-term nonprogressors (see above), and a number of individuals have been exposed to HIV multiple times but remain uninfected; these facts suggest that there are protective elements of an HIV-specific immune response. In addition, studies using animal models, specifically SIV in the monkey and HIV-1 in the chimpanzee, have been encouraging and suggest that an HIV vaccine is possible. It should be pointed out that while the ideal goal of an HIV vaccine is to prevent infection, a vaccine given to an uninfected individual that significantly alters the

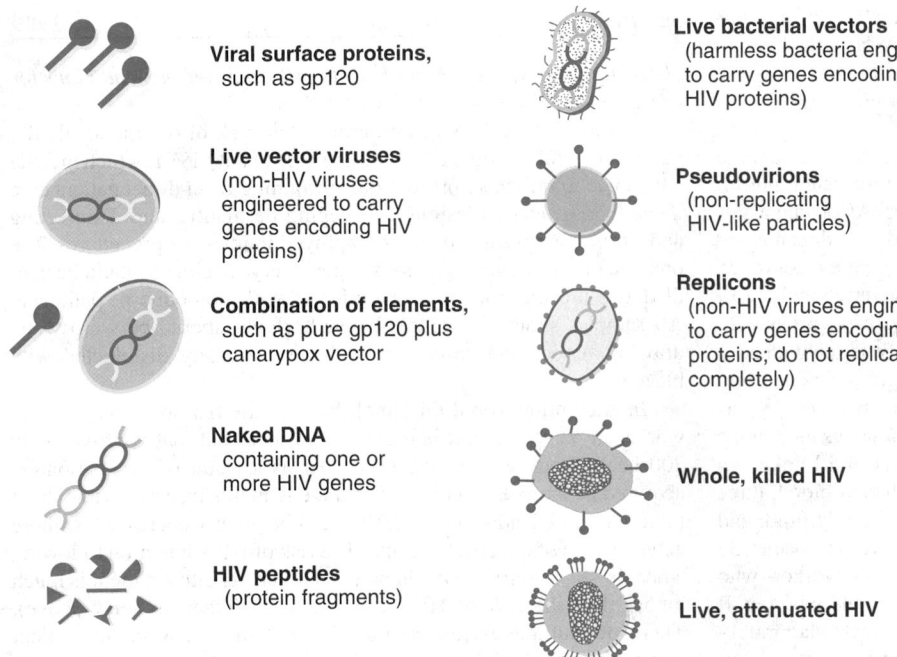

FIGURE 309-40 Candidate HIV vaccines. See text for detailed discussion. *(Adapted from Baltimore and Heilman, 1998.)*

course of disease or the infectivity of the individual, should that person become infected, could have an impact not only on the individual in question but also on the spread of infection in the community.

A number of clinical trials ranging from several small phase I trials to determine safety, to fewer intermediate-sized phase II trials to determine safety and immunogenicity, to a single phase III trial to determine efficacy have been or are currently being conducted in humans. The single phase III trial is testing a bivalent gp 120 protein; this product has been shown to induce antibodies but not cytolytic T cells responses in phase I and II trials. The furthest advanced among phase II trials involves a combination approach using a live canarypox vector expressing one or multiple HIV epitopes given together with gp120 or using the gp120 as a boost. This approach has resulted in neutralizing antibodies in virtually all recipients and HIV-specific cytolytic T cells in approximately 30% of individuals at any given time during the course of the trial.

Other approaches currently being tested in phase I and/or phase II trials in humans include naked DNA; vaccines employing vectors such as modified vaccinia Ankara (MVA), salmonella, Venezuela equine encephalitis (VEE) virus, among others; peptide and subunit vaccines; and pseudovirions (Fig. 309-40). Live attenuated HIV vaccines have not proceeded into human trials at this time because of safety concerns. It is clear that it will take several years of clinical trials to establish the efficacy or lack thereof of a candidate vaccine for HIV.

PREVENTION

Education, counseling, and behavior modification are the cornerstones of an HIV prevention strategy. Widespread voluntary testing of individuals who have practiced or are practicing high-risk behavior, together with counseling of infected individuals, is recommended. Information gathered from such an approach should serve as the basis for behavior-modification programs, both for infected individuals who may be unaware of their HIV status and who could infect others and for uninfected individuals practicing high-risk behavior. The practice of "safer sex" is the most effective way for sexually active uninfected individuals to avoid contracting HIV infection and for infected individuals to avoid spreading infection. Abstinence from sexual relations is the only absolute way to prevent sexual transmission of HIV infection. However, this may not be feasible, and there are a number of

relatively safe practices that can markedly decrease the chances of transmission of HIV infection. Partners engaged in monogamous sexual relationships who wish to be assured of safety should both be tested for HIV antibody. If both are negative, it must be understood that any divergence from monogamy puts both partners at risk; open discussion of the importance of honesty in such relationships should be encouraged. When the HIV status of either partner is not known, or when one partner is positive, there are a number of options. Use of condoms can markedly decrease the chance of HIV transmission. It should be remembered that condoms are not 100% effective in preventing transmission of HIV infection, and there is an ~10% failure rate of condoms used for contraceptive purposes. Most condom failures result from breakage or improper usage, such as not wearing the condom for the entire period of intercourse. Latex condoms are preferable, since virus has been shown to leak through natural skin condoms. Petroleum-based gels should never be used for lubrication of the condom, since they increase the likelihood of condom rupture. There has been a tendency among homosexual men to practice fellatio as a "minimal risk" activity compared to receptive anal intercourse. It should be emphasized that receptive oral fellatio is definitely not safe sex, and there has been clear-cut documentation of transmission of HIV where receptive fellatio was the only sexual act performed (see "Transmission," above). Topical microbicides for vaginal and anal use are being pursued actively as a means by which individuals could avoid infection when the insertive partner cannot be relied on to use a condom. Kissing is considered safe, although there is a theoretical possibility of transmission via virus in saliva. The low concentration of virus in saliva of infected individuals, as well as the presence in saliva of HIV-inhibitory proteins (see above), lessens any risk of transmission by kissing.

The most effective way to prevent transmission of HIV infection among IDUs is to stop the use of injectable drugs. Unfortunately, that is extremely difficult to accomplish unless the individual enters a treatment program. For those who will not or cannot participate in a drug treatment program and who will continue to inject drugs, the avoidance of sharing of needles and other paraphernalia ("works") is the next best way to avoid transmission of infection. The cultural and social factors that contribute to the sharing of paraphernalia are complex and difficult to overcome. In addition, needles and syringes may be in short supply. Under these circumstances, paraphernalia should be cleaned after each usage with a virucidal solution, such as undiluted sodium hypochlorite (household bleach). Data from a number of studies have indicated that programs that provide sterile needles to addicts in exchange for used needles have resulted in a decrease in HIV transmission without increasing the use of injection drugs. It is important for IDUs to be tested for HIV infection and counseled, to avoid transmission to their sexual partners. Secondary and tertiary spread of HIV infection by the heterosexual route within settings of a high level of injection drug use has increased greatly in the United States (see above).

Transmission of HIV via transfused blood or blood products has been decreased dramatically by a combination of screening of all blood donors for HIV infection by assays for both HIV antibody and p24 antigen and self-deferral of individuals at risk for HIV infection. In addition, clotting factor concentrates are heat-treated, essentially eliminating the risk to hemophiliacs who require these products. Autologous transfusions are preferable to transfusions from another individual. However, logistic constraints as well as the unpredictability of the need for most transfusions limit the feasibility of this approach. At present the risk of becoming HIV-infected from a contaminated blood transfusion is approximately 1 in 676,000 donations.

HIV can be transmitted via breast milk and colostrum. The avoidance of breast feeding may not be practical in developing countries, where nutritional concerns override the risk of HIV transmission. However, it is becoming appreciated that from 5 to 15% of infants who were born of HIV-infected mothers and who were fortunate enough not to have been infected intrapartum or peripartum become infected via breast feeding. Therefore, even in developing countries, breast feeding from an infected mother should be avoided if at all possible. Unfortunately, this is rarely the case, and given the disadvantages of withholding breast feeding in developing countries (see above), health authorities in most developing countries continue to recommend breast feeding despite the potential for HIV transmission. In developed countries such as the United States, where bottled formula and milk are readily accessible, breast feeding is absolutely contraindicated when a mother is HIV positive.

BIBLIOGRAPHY

ALKHATIB G et al: CC CKR5: A RANTES, MIP-1α, MIP-1β receptor as a fusion cofactor for macrophage-tropic HIV-1. Science 272:1955, 1996

ANTMAN K, CHANG Y: Kaposi's sarcoma. N Engl J Med 342:1027, 2000

BALOTTA C et al: Identification of two distinct subsets of long-term nonprogressors with divergent viral activity by stromal-derived factor 1 chemokine gene polymorphism analysis. J Infect Dis 180:285, 1999

BALTIMORE D, HEILMAN C: HIV vaccines: Prospects and challenges. Sci Am 279:98, 1998

BERGER JR, MAJOR EO: Progressive multifocal leukoencephalopathy. Semin Neurol 19:193, 1999

BLEUL CC et al: The lymphocyte chemoattractant SDF-1 is a ligand for LESTR/fusin and blocks HIV-1 entry. Nature 382:829, 1996

BREAM JH et al: CCR5 promoter alleles and specific DNA binding factors. Science 284:223a, 1999

CAMERON DW et al: Randomised placebo-controlled trial of ritonavir in advanced HIV-1 disease. Lancet 351:543, 1998

CAO Y et al: Virologic and immunologic characterization of long-term survivors of human immunodeficiency virus type-1 infection. N Engl J Med 332:201, 1995

CARDO DM et al: A case-control study of HIV seroconversion in health care workers after percutaneous exposure. N Engl J Med 337:1485, 1997

CARR A et al: Pathogenesis of HIV-1 protease inhibitor–associated peripheral lipodystrophy, hyperlipidemia and insulin resistance. Lancet 351:1881, 1998

CARRINGTON M et al: HLA and HIV-1: Heterozygote advantage and B*35-cw*04 disadvantage. Science 283:1, 1999

CENTERS FOR DISEASE CONTROL AND PREVENTION: Human immunodeficiency virus transmission in household settings—United States. MMWR 347:353, 1994

———: Public Health Service guidelines for the management of health-care worker exposures to HIV and recommendations for postexposure prophylaxis. MMWR 47(RR-7):1, 1998

———: Diagnosis and reporting of HIV and AIDS in states with integrated HIV and AIDS surveillance—United States, January 1994–June 1997. MMWR 47:309, 1998

———: Guidelines for the use of antiretroviral agents in HIV-infected adults and adolescents. MMWR 47(RR-5):43, 1998 (See updates at www.hivatis.org)

———: Public Health Service Task Force recommendations for the use of antiretroviral drugs in pregnant women infected with HIV-1 for maternal health and for reducing perinatal HIV-1 transmission in the United States. MMWR 47(RR-2):1, 1998 (See updates at www.hivatis.org)

———: HIV/AIDS surveillance report, 1999; 11(No. 2):1, 2000

———: 1999 USPHS/IDSA guidelines for the prevention of opportunistic infections in persons infected with human immunodeficiency virus. U.S. Public Health Service (USPHS) and Infectious Diseases Society of America (IDSA). MMWR 48(RR-10):1, 1999

CHOE H et al: The β-chemokine receptors CCR3 and CCR5 facilitate infection by primary HIV-1 isolates. Cell 85:1135, 1996

CHUN TW, FAUCI AS: Latent reservoirs of HIV: Obstacles to the eradication of virus. Proc Natl Acad Sci USA 96:10958, 1999

——— et al: Presence of an inducible HIV-1 latent reservoir during highly active antiretroviral therapy. Proc Natl Acad Sci USA 94:13193, 1997

——— et al: Re-emergence of HIV after stopping therapy. Nature 401:874, 1999

———: Relationship between preexisting viral reservoirs and the reemergence of plasma viremia after discontinuation of highly active anti-retroviral therapy. Nat Med 6:757, 2000

CLIFFORD DB et al: HAART improves prognosis in HIV-associated progressive multifocal leukoencephalopathy. Neurology 52:623, 1999

COCCHI F et al: Identification of RANTES, MIP-1α, and MIP-1β as the major HIV-suppressive factors produced by CD8+ T cells. Science 270:1811, 1995

COHEN GB et al: The selective downregulation of class 1 major histocompatibility complex proteins by HIV-1 protects HIV-infected cells from NK cells. Immunity 10:661, 1999

COHEN OJ et al: The immunology of human immunodeficiency virus infection, in: Principles and Practice of Infectious Diseases, 5th ed, GL Mandell, JE Bennett, and R Dolin (eds.). Philadelphia, Churchill Livingstone, pp 1374–1397, 2000

———, FAUCI AS: Benchmarks for antiretroviral therapy [comment]. J Clin Invest 105:709, 2000

CONNORS M et al: HIV infection induces changes in CD4+ T cell phenotype and depletions within the CD4+ T cell repertoire that are not immediately restored by antiviral or immune-based therapies. Nature Med 3:533, 1997

CORDER EH et al: HIV-infected subjects with the E4 allele for APOE have excess dementia and peripheral neuropathy. Nat Med 4:1182, 1998

COUTSOUDIS A et al: Influence of infant-feeding patterns on early mother-to-child transmission of HIV-1 in Durban, South Africa: A prospective cohort study. Lancet 354:471, 1999

DAVEY RT JR et al: HIV-1 and T cell dynamics after interruption of highly active antiretroviral therapy (HAART) in patients with a history of sustained viral suppression. Proc Natl Acad Sci USA 21:96,15109, 1999

——— et al: Immunologic and virologic effects of subcutaneous interleukin 2 in combination with antiretroviral therapy: A randomized controlled trial. JAMA 284:183, 2000

DENG HK et al: Identification of a major co-receptor for primary isolates of HIV-1. Nature 381:661, 1996

DEPARTMENT OF ECONOMIC AND SOCIAL AFFAIRS OF THE UNITED NATIONS SECRETARIAT: The Demographic Impact of HIV/AIDS. New York, 1999

DOMS RW, PEIPER SC: Unwelcomed guests with master keys: How HIV uses chemokine receptors for cellular entry. Virology 235:179, 1997

DONOVAN B, ROSS MW: Preventing HIV: Determinants of sexual behaviour. Lancet 355:1897, 2000

DONG KL et al: Changes in body habitus and serum lipid abnormalities in HIV-positive women on highly active antiretroviral therapy. J Acquir Immune Defic Syndr 21:107, 1999

DORANZ BJ et al: A dual-tropic primary HIV-1 isolate that uses fusin and the β-chemokine receptors CKR-5, CKR-3, and CKR-2b as fusion cofactors. Cell 85:1149, 1996

DOUEK D et al: Changes in thymic function with age and during treatment of HIV infection. Nature 396:690, 1999

DRAGIC T et al: HIV-1 entry into CD4+ cells is mediated by the chemokine receptor CC-CKR-5. Nature 381:667, 1996

EMERY S, LANE HC: Immune reconstitution in HIV infection. Curr Opin Immunol 9:568, 1997

FAUCI AS: The AIDS epidemic—considerations for the 21st century. N Engl J Med 341:1046, 1999

———: The human immunodeficiency virus: Infectivity and mechanisms of pathogenesis. Science 239:617, 1988

———: CD4+ T lymphocytopenia without HIV infection—no lights, no camera, just facts. N Engl J Med 328:429, 1993

———: Multifactorial nature of human immunodeficiency virus disease: Implications for therapy. Science 262:1011, 1993

———: An HIV vaccine: Breaking the paradigms. Proc Assoc Am Physicians 108:6, 1996

———: Host factors and the pathogenesis of HIV-induced disease. Nature 384:529, 1996

———: The AIDS epidemic—considerations for the 21st century. N Engl J Med 341:1046, 1999

——— et al: Immunopathogenic mechanisms of HIV infection. Ann Intern Med 124:654, 1996

FAUKE S et al: Rapid progression to AIDS in HIV⁺ individuals with a structural variant of the chemokine receptor CX₃CR1. Science 287:2274, 2000

FIORELLI V et al: IFN-γ induces endothelial cells to proliferate and to invade the extracellular matrix in response to the HIV-1 tat protein: Implications for AIDS–Kaposi's sarcoma pathogenesis. J Immunol 162:1165, 1999

FLEXNER C: HIV-protease inhibitors. N Engl J Med 338:1281, 1998

FLORE O et al: Transformation of primary human endothelial cells by Kaposi's sarcoma–associated herpesvirus. Nature 394:588, 1998

GALLO R: The enigmas of Kaposi's sarcoma. Science 282:1837, 1998

GAO F et al: Origin of HIV-1 in the chimpanzee Pan troglodytes troglodytes. Nature 397:436, 1999

GARCIA P et al: Maternal level of plasma human immunodeficiency virus type 1 RNA and the risk of perinatal transmission. N Engl J Med 341:394, 1999

GERBERDING J: Provider-to-patient HIV transmission: How to keep it exceedingly rare. Ann Intern Med 130:64, 1999

GILKS CF et al: Invasive pneumococcal disease in a cohort of predominantly HIV-1 infected female sex-workers in Nairobi, Kenya. Lancet 347:718, 1996

GOEDERT JJ et al: Spectrum of AIDS-associated malignant disorders. Lancet 351:1833, 1998

GUAY LA et al: Intrapartum and neonatal single-dose nevirapine compared with zidovudine for prevention of mother-to-child transmission of HIV-1 in Kampala, Uganda: HIVNET 012 randomised trial. Lancet 354:795, 1999

GULICK RM et al: Treatment with indinavir, zidovudine and lamivudine in adults with human immunodeficiency virus infection and prior antiretroviral therapy. N Engl J Med 337:734, 1997

HALPERIN DT, BAILEY RC: Male circumcision and HIV infection: 10 years and counting. Lancet 354:1813, 1999

HAYNES BF et al: Toward an understanding of the correlates of protective immunity to HIV infection. Science 271:324, 1996

HIGHBARGER HC et al: Comparison of the quantiplex version 3.0 assay and a sensitized amplicor monitor assay for measurement of human immunodeficiency virus type 1 RNA levels in plasma samples. J Clin Microbiol 37:3612, 1999

HIRSCH MS et al: Antiretroviral drug resistance testing in adults with HIV infection: Implications for clinical management. International AIDS Society—USA Panel. JAMA 279:1984, 1998

HITCHCOCK P, FRANSEN L: Preventing HIV infection: Lessons from Mwanza and Rakai. Lancet 353:513, 1999

HO DD et al: Rapid turnover of plasma virions and CD4 lymphocytes in HIV infection. Nature 373:123, 1995

HOLTZMAN DM et al: New-onset seizures associated with human immunodeficiency virus infection: Causation and clinical features in 100 cases. Am J Med 87:173, 1989

JACOBSEN H et al: In vivo resistance to human immunodeficiency virus type 1 proteinase inhibitor: Mutations, kinetics and frequencies. J Infect Dis 173:1379, 1996

JACOBSON JM et al: Thalidomide for the treatment of oral aphthous ulcers in patients with human immunodeficiency virus infection. N Engl J Med 336:1487, 1997

JOINT UNITED NATIONS PROGRAMME ON HIV/AIDS (UNAIDS): Report on the Global HIV/AIDS Epidemic, June 2000. Geneva, 2000

KAHN JO, WALKER BD: Acute human immunodeficiency virus type 1 infection. N Engl J Med 339:33, 1998

KAPLAN JE et al: 14-year followup of HIV-infected homosexual men with lymphadenopathy syndrome. J Acquired Immune Defic Syndr Hum Retrovirol 11:206, 1996

KASLOW RA et al: Influence of combinations of human major histocompatibility complex genes on the course of HIV-1 infection. Nat Med 2:405, 1996

KEDES D et al: The seroepidemiology of human herpesvirus 8 (Kaposi's sarcoma–associated herpesvirus): Distribution of infection in KS risk groups and evidence for sexual transmission. Nat Med 2:918, 1996

KEET I et al: Consistent associations of HLA class I and II and transporter gene products with progression of human immunodeficiency virus type 1 infection in homosexual men. J Infect Dis 180:299, 1999

KIRCHHOFF F et al: Brief report: Absence of intact *nef* sequences in a long-term survivor with nonprogressive HIV-1 infection. N Engl J Med 332:228, 1995

KLEIN RS et al: Chemokine receptor expression and signaling in macaque and human fetal neurons and astrocytes: Implications for the neuropathogenesis of AIDS. J Immunol 163:1636, 1999

KLEINMAN S et al: False-positive HIV-1 test results in a low-risk screening setting of voluntary blood donation. JAMA 280:1080, 1998

KODEL U et al: HIV type 1 nef protein is a viral factor for leukocyte recruitment into the central nervous system. J Immunol 163:1245, 1999

KOVACS JA, MASUR H: Prophylaxis against opportunistic infections in patients with human immunodeficiency virus infection. N Engl J Med 342:1416, 2000

LACKRITZ EM et al: Estimated risk of HIV transmission by screened blood in the United States. N Engl J Med 333:1721, 1995

LANDESMAN SH et al: Obstetrical factors and the transmission of human immunodeficiency virus type 1 from mother to child. N Engl J Med 334:1617, 1997

LEARMONT JC et al: Immunologic and virologic status after 14 to 18 years of infection with an attenuated strain of HIV-1. A report from the Sydney Blood Bank Cohort. N Engl J Med 340:1715, 1999

LETENDRE S et al: Cerebrospinal fluid β chemokine concentrations in neurocognitively impaired individuals infected with human immunodeficiency virus type 1. J Infect Dis 180:310, 1999

LITTMAN D: Chemokine receptors: Keys to AIDS pathogenesis? Cell 93:677, 1998

LIU H et al: Polymorphism in RANTES chemokine promoter affects HIV-1 disease progression. Proc Nat Acad Sci USA 96:4581, 1999

LIU R et al: Homozygous defect in HIV-1 coreceptor accounts for resistance of some multiply exposed individuals to HIV-1 infection. Cell 86:367, 1996

LOT F et al: Probable transmission of HIV from an orthopedic surgeon to a patient in France. Ann Intern Med 130:1, 1999

MAIMAN M et al: Cervical cancer as an AIDS-defining illness. Obstet Gynecol 89:76, 1997

MANNHEIMER SB, SOAVE R: Protozoal infections in patients with AIDS. Cryptosporidiosis, isosporiasis, cyclosporiasis, and microsporidiosis. Infect Dis Clin North Am 8: 483, 1994

MARTIN JA et al: *Births and Deaths: Preliminary Data for 1998*. National Vital Statistics Reports, vol 27, no. 25. Hyattsville, MD, National Center for Health Statistics, 1999

MELLADO M et al: Chemokine control of HIV-1 infection. Nature 400:723, 1999

MELLORS JW et al: Prognosis in HIV-1 infection predicted by the quantity of virus in plasma. Science 272:1167, 1996

MIGUELES SA et al: HLAB*5701 is highly associated with restriction of virus replication

in a subgroup of HIV-infected long term nonprogressors. Proc Nat Acad Sci USA 97:2709, 2000

MILLER KD et al: Visceral abdominal fat accumulation associated with the use of indinavir. Lancet 351:871, 1998

MIOTTI P et al: HIV transmission through breastfeeding: A study in Malawi. JAMA 282: 744, 1999

MOFENSON LM et al: Risk factors for perinatal transmission of human immunodeficiency virus type 1 in women treated with zidovudine. N Engl J Med 334:385, 1999

———, MCINTYRE JA: Advances and research directions in the prevention of mother-to-child HIV-1 transmission. Lancet 355:2237, 2000

MOORE PS, CHANG Y: Detection of herpesvirus-like DNA sequences in Kaposi's sarcoma in patients with and those without HIV infection. N Engl J Med 332:1181, 1995

MOORE RD, CHAISSON RE: Natural history of opportunistic diseases in an HIV-infected urban clinical cohort. Ann Intern Med 124:633, 1996

NATIONAL INSTITUTE FOR OCCUPATIONAL SAFETY AND HEALTH, CENTERS FOR DISEASE CONTROL AND PREVENTION: *Preventing Needlestick Injuries in Health Care Settings*, 1999

OBERLIN E et al: The CXC chemokine receptor SDF-1 is the ligand for LESTR/fusin and prevents infection by T-cell-line-adapted HIV-1. Nature 382:833, 1996

O'BRIEN SJ: AIDS: A role for host genes. Hosp Pract (Off Ed) 33:53, 1998

———, DEAN M: In search of AIDS-resistance genes. Sci Am 277:44, 1997

O'BRIEN WA et al: Changes in plasma HIV-1 RNA and CD4+ lymphocyte count and the risk of progression to AIDS. N Engl J Med 334:426, 1996

——— et al: Changes in plasma HIV RNA levels and CD4+ T lymphocyte counts predict both response to antiretroviral therapy and therapeutic failure. Ann Intern Med 126: 939, 1997

OGG GS et al: Quantitation of HIV-1 specific cytotoxic T-lymphocytes and plasma load of viral RNA. Science 279:2103, 1998

PADIAN NS et al: Heterosexual transmission of human immunodeficiency virus (HIV) in northern California: Results from a ten-year study. Am J Epidemiol 146:350, 1997

PAGANO MA et al: Cerebral tumor-like American trypanosomiasis in acquired immunodeficiency syndrome. Ann Neurol 45:403, 1999

PALELLA FJ et al: Declining morbidity and mortality among patients with advanced human immunodeficiency virus infection. N Engl J Med 338:853, 1998

PANTALEO G, FAUCI AS: HIV infection is active and progressive in lymphoid tissue during the clinically latent stage of disease. Nature 362:355, 1993

———, ———: New concepts in the pathogenesis of HIV infection. Annu Rev Immunol 13:487, 1995

——— et al: Studies in subjects with long-term nonprogressive human immunodeficiency virus infection. N Engl J Med 332:209, 1995

PECKHAM C, GIBB D: Mother-to-child transmission of the human immunodeficiency virus. N Engl J Med 333:298, 1995

PERELSON AS et al: HIV-1 dynamics in vivo: Virion clearance rate, infected cell lifespan, and viral generation time. Science 271:1582, 1996

——— et al: Decay characteristics of HIV-1 infected compartments during combination therapy. Nature 386:188, 1997

PRICE RW: Neurological complications of HIV infection. Lancet 348:445, 1996

QUINN TC et al: Viral load and heterosexual transmission of human immunodeficiency virus type 1. Rakai Project Study Group. N Engl J Med 342:921, 2000

RETTIG MB et al: Kaposi's sarcoma–associated herpesvirus infection of bone marrow dendritic cells from multiple myeloma patients. Science 276:1851, 1997

RICH JD et al: Misdiagnosis of HIV infection by HIV-1 plasma viral load testing: A case series. Ann Intern Med 130:37, 1999

RICHMAN DD: Normal physiology and HIV pathophysiology of human T-cell dynamics [In Process Citation]. J Clin Invest 105:565, 2000

ROBERTSON DL et al: Recombination in HIV-1. Nature 374:124, 1995

ROSENBERG ES: Vigorous HIV-1 specific CD4+ T cell responses associated with control of viremia. Science 278:1447, 1997

SAMSON M et al: Resistance to HIV-1 infection in Caucasian individuals bearing mutant alleles of the CCR-5 chemokine receptor gene. Nature 382:722, 1996

SCHMITZ JE et al: Control of viremia in simian immunodeficiency virus infection by CD8 lymphocytes. Science 283:852, 1999

SEWANKAMBO N et al: HIV-1 infection associated with abnormal vaginal flora morphology and bacterial vaginosis. Lancet 350:546, 1997

SILVA-CARDOSO J et al: Pericardial involvement in human immunodeficiency virus infection. Chest 115:418, 1999

SIMON F et al: Identification of a new human immunodeficiency virus type distinct from group M and group O. Nat Med 4:1032, 1998

SMITH KJ et al: Cutaneous findings in HIV-1 positive patients: A 42-month prospective study. J Am Acad Dermatol 31:746, 1994

SOTO-RAMIREZ LE et al: HIV-1 Langerhans' cell tropism associated with heterosexual transmission of HIV. Science 271:1291, 1996

SPARANO JA: Treatment of AIDS-related lymphomas. Curr Opin Oncol 7:442, 1995

SPIRA AI et al: Cellular targets of infection and route of viral dissemination after an intravaginal inoculation of simian immunodeficiency virus into rhesus macaques. J Exp Med 183:215, 1996

STANSELL JD et al: Predictors of *Pneumocystis carinii* pneumonia in HIV-infected persons. Am J Respir Crit Care Med 155:60, 1997

SULLIVAN PS et al: Persistently negative HIV-1 antibody enzyme immunoassay screening results for patients with HIV-1 infection and AIDS: Serologic, clinical, and virologic results. AIDS 13:89, 1999

Swingler S et al: HIV-1 nef mediates lymphocyte chemotaxis and activation by infected macrophages. Nat Med 5:997, 1999

Tavel JA et al: Guide to major clinical trials of antiretroviral therapy in human immunodeficiency virus-infected patients: Protease inhibitors, non-nucleoside reverse transcriptase inhibitors, and nucleotide reverse transcriptase inhibitors. Clin Infect Dis 28:643, 1999

Tindall B, Cooper DA: Primary HIV infection. Host responses and intervention strategies. AIDS 5:1, 1991

Vanhems P et al: Comprehensive classification of symptoms and signs reported among 218 patients with acute HIV-1 infection. J Acquir Immune Defic Syndr 21:99, 1999

Vittinghoff E et al: Per-contact risk of human immunodeficiency virus transmission between male sexual partners. Am J Epidemiol 150:306, 1999

Walker CM et al: CD8+ lymphocytes can control HIV infection in vitro by suppressing virus replication. Science 234:1563, 1986

Wei X et al: Viral dynamics in human immunodeficiency virus type 1 infection. Nature 373:117, 1995

Weiss JM et al: HIV-1 tat induces monocyte chemoattractant protein-1 mediated monocyte transmigration across a model of the human blood-brain barrier and up-regulates CCR5 expression on human monocytes. J Immunol 163:2953, 1999

Whalen C et al: Accelerated course of human immunodeficiency virus infection after tuberculosis. Am J Respir Crit Care Med 151:129, 1995

World Health Organization: The World Health Report 1999: Making a Difference. Geneva, 1999

Section 2
DISORDERS OF IMMUNE-MEDIATED INJURY

| 310 | K. Frank Austen |

ALLERGIES, ANAPHYLAXIS, AND SYSTEMIC MASTOCYTOSIS

BPL benzylpenicilloyl-polylysine	IP$_3$ inositol-1,4,5-triphosphate
C1INH C1 inhibitor	ITAMs immunoreceptor tyrosine-based activation motifs
CPA carboxypeptidase A	LT leukotriene
1,2-DAGs 1,2-diacylglycerols	MDM minor determinant mixture
ELISA enzyme-linked immunosorbent assays	MHC major histocompatibility complex
FLAP 5-lipoxygenase activating protein	PAF platelet-activating factor
GM-CSF granulocyte-macrophage colony-stimulating factor	PG prostaglandin
IFN interferon	SCF stem cell factor
IL interleukin	TCR T cell receptor
	TNF-α tumor necrosis factor α

The term *atopic allergy* implies a familial tendency to manifest such conditions as asthma, rhinitis, urticaria, and eczematous dermatitis (atopic dermatitis) alone or in combination. However, individuals without an atopic background may also develop hypersensitivity reactions, particularly urticaria and anaphylaxis, associated with the same class of antibody, IgE, found in atopic individuals. Inasmuch as the mast cell is the key effector cell of the biologic response in allergic rhinitis, urticaria, anaphylaxis, and systemic mastocytosis, the introduction to these clinical problems will consider the developmental biology, activation pathway, product profile, and target tissues for this cell type.

The fixation of IgE to human mast cells and basophils, a process termed *sensitization*, prepares these cells for subsequent antigen-specific activation. The interaction of the high-affinity Fc receptor for IgE, designated FcϵRI, upregulates the cellular expression of the receptor, possibly by ligand-mediated stabilization. FcϵRI is composed of one α, one β, and two disulfide-linked γ chains, which together cross the plasma membrane seven times. The α chain is solely responsible for IgE binding, and the β and γ chains are responsible for signal transduction that results from the aggregation of the tetrameric receptors by polymeric antigen.

The interaction of specific multivalent antigen with receptor-bound IgE results in clustering of the receptors to initiate signal transduction through the action of a *src* family–related tyrosine kinase, termed *Lyn*, that is constitutively associated with the β chain. Lyn transphosphorylates the canonical immunoreceptor tyrosine-based activation motifs (ITAMs) of the β and γ chains of the receptor, resulting in recruitment of more active Lyn to the β chain and of the Syk/zap-70 family ty-

rosine kinases. The two phosphorylated tyrosines in the ITAMs function as binding sites for the tandem *src* homology two (SH2) domains within these kinases. It appears that Syk activates not only phospholipase Cγ but also phosphatidylinositol-3-kinase to provide phosphatidyl-3,4,5-triphosphate, which allows membrane targeting of the Tec family kinases (Btk and Itk) and their activation by Lyn. The resulting Tec kinase–dependent phosphorylation of phospholipase Cγ with cleavage of its phospholipid membrane substrate provides inositol-1,4,5-triphosphate (IP$_3$) and 1,2-diacylglycerols (1,2-DAGs) so as to mobilize intracellular calcium and activate protein kinase C. The subsequent opening of calcium-regulated activated channels provides the sustained elevations of intracellular calcium required to recruit the mitogen-activated protein kinases, JNK and p38 (serine/threonine kinases), which provide cascades to augment arachidonic acid release and to mediate nuclear translocation of transcription factors for various cytokines. The calcium ion–dependent activation of phospholipases cleaves membrane phospholipids to generate lysophospholipids, which, like 1,2-DAG, are fusogenic and may facilitate the fusion of the secretory granule perigranular membrane with the cell membrane, a step that releases the membrane-free granule containing the preformed or primary mediators of mast cell effects.

The secretory granule of the human mast cell has a crystalline structure, unlike mast cells of lower species, and IgE-dependent cell activation can be characterized morphologically by solubilization and swelling of the granule contents within the first minute of receptor perturbation; this reaction is followed by the ordering of intermediate filaments about the swollen granule, movement toward the cell surface, and fusion of the perigranular membrane with that of other granules and with the plasmalemma to form extracellular channels for mediator release while maintaining cell viability.

In addition to exocytosis, aggregation of FcϵRI initiates two other pathways for generation of bioactive products, namely, lipid mediators and cytokines. The biochemical steps involved in expression of such cytokines as tumor necrosis factor α (TNF-α), interleukin (IL) 6, IL-4, IL-5, granulocyte-macrophage colony-stimulating factor (GM-CSF), and others have not been specifically defined for mast cells. Nonetheless, inhibition studies of cytokine production (IL-1β, TNF-α, and IL-6) in mouse mast cells with cyclosporine or FK506 reveal binding to the ligand-specific immunophilin and attenuation of the calcium ion- and calmodulin-dependent serine/threonine phosphatase, calcineurin.

Lipid mediator generation (Fig. 310-1) involves translocation of calcium ion–dependent cytosolic phospholipase A$_2$ to the perinuclear membrane, with subsequent release of arachidonic acid for metabolic processing by the distinct prostanoid and leukotriene pathways. The constitutive prostaglandin endoperoxide synthase (PGHS-1/cyclooxygenase-1) and the de novo inducible PGHS-2 (cyclooxygenase-2)

FIGURE 310-1 Pathways for biosynthesis and release of membrane-derived lipid mediators from mast cells. In the 5-lipoxygenase pathway leukotriene A_4 (LTA_4) is the intermediate from which the terminal-pathway enzymes generate the distinct final products, leukotriene C_4 (LTC_4) and leukotriene B_4 (LTB_4), which leave the cell by separate saturable transport systems. Gamma glutamyl transpeptidase and a dipeptidase then cleave glutamic acid and glycine from LTC_4 to form LTD_4 and LTE_4, respectively, for which there appears to be a common receptor. The only mast cell product of the cyclooxygenase system is PGD_2.

convert released arachidonic acid to the sequential intermediates prostaglandin (PG) G_2 and PGH_2. The glutathione-dependent hematopoietic PGD_2 synthase then converts PGH_2 to PGD_2, the predominant mast cell prostanoid.

For processing by the leukotriene pathway, the released arachidonic acid is translocated to an integral perinuclear membrane protein, the 5-lipoxygenase activating protein (FLAP). The calcium ion–dependent activation of 5-lipoxygenase involves translocation to the perinuclear membrane, which allows conversion of the arachidonic acid to the sequential intermediates, 5-hydroperoxyeicosatetraenoic acid and leukotriene (LT) A_4. LTA_4 is conjugated with reduced glutathione by LTC_4 synthase, an integral membrane protein with significant homology to FLAP. Intracellular LTC_4 is released by a carrier-specific export step for extracellular conversion to the receptor-active cysteinyl leukotrienes LTD_4 and LTE_4 by sequential removal of glumatic acid and glycine. A cytosolic LTA_4 hydrolase converts some LTA_4 to the dihydroxy leukotriene LTB_4, which then undergoes specific export for extracellular receptor–mediated actions. The lysophospholipid formed during release of arachidonic acid from 1-O-alkyl-2-acyl-sn-glyceryl-3-phosphorylcholine can be acetylated in the second position to form platelet-activating factor (PAF).

Unlike other cells of bone marrow origin, mast cells leave the marrow and circulate as committed progenitors lacking their definitive secretory granules. These committed progenitors express the receptor, c-kit, for stem cell factor (SCF) before the expression of FcεRI. Whereas c-kit is lost or markedly diminished in expression by other cell types, it is retained by mature, differentiated mast cells and is an absolute requirement for the development of constitutive tissue mast cells residing in skin and connective tissue sites and for the T cell–dependent mast cells residing in mucosal surfaces or undergoing reactive hyperplasia. Indeed, in clinical T cell deficiencies, mast cells are absent from the intestinal mucosa but are present in the submucosa. It is thus assumed that unrecognized mast cell progenitors enter the tissue and undergo regulated proliferation, differentiation, and maturation. Based on the immunodetection of secretory granule neutral proteases, mast cells in the lung parenchyma and intestinal mucosa selectively express tryptase; those in the intestinal and airway submucosa, skin, lymph nodes, and breast parenchyma express tryptase, chymase, and carboxypeptidase A (CPA); and occasional mast cells in intestinal submucosa express chymase and CPA but not tryptase. The secretory granules of mast cells selectively positive for tryptase in lung and intestinal mucosa exhibit closed scrolls with a periodicity suggestive of a crystalline structure by electron microscopy; whereas the secretory granules of mast cells with mutiple proteases residing in skin, lymph nodes, breast parenchyma, and submucosa of airways and intestine are scroll-poor, with an amorphous or latticelike appearance.

Mast cells are distributed at cutaneous and mucosal surfaces and in deeper tissues about venules and could regulate the entry of foreign substances by their rapid response capability (Fig. 310-2). Upon stimulus-specific activation in vitro, histamine and secretory granule–associated acid hydrolases are solubilized, whereas the neutral proteases, which are cationic, remain largely complexed to the anionic proteoglycans, heparin and chrondroitin sulfate E. The macromolecular complex serves to deliver the neutral proteases so that the endo- and exoproteases can function in concert at the substrate site to clear damaged tissue and facilitate repair. Histamine and the various lipid mediators (PGD_2, LTD_4/E_4, PAF) alter venular permeability, thereby allowing influx of plasma proteins such as complement and immunoglobulins, whereas LTB_4 mediates leukocyte–endothelial cell adhesion with subsequent directed migration (chemotaxis). The accumulation of leukocytes and opsonins would facilitate defense of the microenvironment. The cysteinyl leukotrienes constrict both vascular and nonvascular smooth muscle and are much more potent than histamine in constricting human airway smooth muscle when administered by aerosol.

The cellular component of the inflammatory response elicited by preformed secretory granule–associated and membrane-

FIGURE 310-2 Bioactive mediators of three categories generated by IgE-dependent activation of murine mast cells can elicit common but sequential target cell effects leading to acute and sustained inflammatory responses.

derived lipid mediators would be augmented and sustained by the addition of cytokines of mast cell or T cell origin to the microenvironment. Activation of human skin mast cells in situ elicits TNF-α production and release, which in turn induces endothelial cell responses favoring leukocyte adhesion. Activation of purified human lung mast cells in vitro results in substantial production of IL-5 and lesser quantities of IL-4. Bronchial biopsies of patients with bronchial asthma reveal that mast cells are immunohistochemically positive for IL-4 and IL-5, but that the predominant localization of IL-4, IL-5, and GM-CSF is to T cells, defined as T_H2 by this profile. It is speculated that IL-4 modulates the T cell phenotype to the T_H2 subtype, and that IL-5 or GM-CSF converts infiltrating eosinophils to an activated, autoaggressive phenotype with augmented capacity for cytotoxicity and generation of O_2^- and the cysteinyl leukotrienes.

The view of immediate and late cellular phase of allergic inflammation is supported by the response of the skin, nose, or lung of allergic humans to local allergen challenge; greater quantities of allergen are needed to elicit the cellular phase. In the immediate phase of a local challenge, there is pruritus and watery discharge from the nose, bronchospasm and mucous secretion in the lungs, and a wheal-and-flare response with pruritus in the skin. The reduced nasal patency, reduced pulmonary function, or evident erythema with swelling at the skin site in a late-phase response at 6 to 8 h are associated with biopsy findings of infiltrating and activated T_H2 type T cells, eosinophils, basophils, and even some neutrophils. This allergic inflammation proceeding from early mast cell activation to late cellular infiltration is believed to promote end-organ hyperresponsivity, as would be characteristic of perennial rhinitis or bronchial asthma; for attenuation, it requires introduction of an anti-inflammatory agent such as a glucocorticoid. The particular chemokines responsible for directed migration of eosinophils and T cells after their integrin-dependent endothelial cell adhesion are not yet defined, although eotaxin is a likely contributor since both cell types, as well as basophils, express the selective receptor CCR-3.

Consideration of the mechanism of immediate type hypersensitivity diseases in the human has focused largely on the IgE-dependent recognition of otherwise nontoxic substances. A region of chromosome 5 (5q23-31) contains genes implicated in the control of IgE levels including IL-4 and IL-13, as well as IL-3 and IL-9 involved in reactive mast cell hyperplasia and IL-5 and GM-CSF central to eosinophil development and their enhanced tissue viability. Genes with linkage to the specific IgE response to particular allergens include those encoding the major histocompatibility complex (MHC) and certain chains of the T cell receptor (TCR-$\alpha\delta$). The complexity of atopy and the associated diseases is such that susceptibility, severity, and therapeutic responses most likely relate not only to specific IgE but also to constitutive target tissue reactivity and the superimposed effects of the local inflammatory response mediated by T_H2 cells, mast cells, basophils, and eosinophils.

The induction of allergic disease requires sensitization of a predisposed individual to specific allergen. This sensitization can occur anytime in life, although the greatest propensity for the development of allergic disease appears to occur in childhood and early adolescence. Exposure of a susceptible individual to an allergen results in processing of the allergen by antigen-presenting cells, including macrophage-like cells located throughout the body at surfaces that contact the outside environment, such as the nose, lungs, eyes, skin, and intestine. These antigen-presenting cells process the allergen protein and present the epitope-bearing peptides via their MHC to particular T cell subsets. The T cell response depends both on cognate recognition through various ligand/receptor interactions and on the cytokine microenvironment, with IL-4 directing a T_H2 response and interferon (IFN)γ a T_H1 profile. T cells can potentially induce several responses to an allergen, including those typical of contact dermatitis, known as the T_H1 type response, and those mediated by IgE, known as the T_H2 allergic response. The T_H2 response is associated with activation of specific B cells that transform into plasma cells. Synthesis and release into the serum of allergen-specific IgE by plasma cells result in sensitization

of IgE Fc receptor–bearing cells including mast cells and basophils, which subsequently are capable of becoming activated upon exposure to the specific allergen. In certain diseases, including those associated with atopy, the monocyte and eosinophil populations can express a trimeric high-affinity receptor, FcϵRI, which lacks the β chain, and yet respond to its aggregation.

ANAPHYLAXIS

DEFINITION The life-threatening anaphylactic response of a sensitized human appears within minutes after administration of specific antigen and is manifested by respiratory distress often followed by vascular collapse or by shock without antecedent respiratory difficulty. Cutaneous manifestations exemplified by pruritus and urticaria with or without angioedema are characteristic of such systemic anaphylactic reactions. Gastrointestinal manifestations include nausea, vomiting, crampy abdominal pain, and diarrhea.

PREDISPOSING FACTORS AND ETIOLOGY There is no convincing evidence that age, sex, race, occupation, or geographic location predisposes a human to anaphylaxis except through exposure to some immunogen. According to most studies, atopy does not predispose individuals to anaphylaxis from penicillin therapy or venom of a stinging insect but is a risk factor for allergens in food or latex.

The materials capable of eliciting the systemic anaphylactic reaction in humans include the following: heterologous proteins in the form of hormones (insulin, vasopressin, parathormone), enzymes (trypsin, chymotrypsin, penicillinase, streptokinase), pollen extracts (ragweed, grass, trees), nonpollen extracts (dust mites, dander of cats, dogs, horses, and laboratory animals), food (milk, eggs, seafood, nuts, grains, beans, gelatin in capsules), antiserum (antilymphocyte gamma globulin), occupation-related proteins (latex rubber products), and Hymenoptera venom (yellow jacket, yellow and baldfaced hornets, paper wasp, honey bee, imported fire ants); polysaccharides such as dextran and thiomerosal as a vaccine preservative; and most commonly drugs such as protamine and antibiotics (penicillins, cephalosporins, amphotericin B, nitrofurantoin, quinolones), local anesthetics (procaine, lidocaine), muscle relaxants (suxamethonium, gallamine, pancuronium), vitamins (thiamine, folic acid), diagnostic agents (sodium dehydrocholate, sulfobromophthalein), and occupation-related chemicals (ethylene oxide), which are considered to function as haptens that form immunogenic conjugates with host proteins. The conjugating hapten may be the parent compound, a nonenzymatically derived storage product, or a metabolite formed in the host.

PATHOPHYSIOLOGY AND MANIFESTATIONS Individuals differ in the time of appearance of symptoms and signs, but the hallmark of the anaphylactic reaction is the onset of some manifestation within seconds to minutes after introduction of the antigen, generally by injection or less commonly by ingestion. There may be upper or lower airway obstruction or both. Laryngeal edema may be experienced as a "lump" in the throat, hoarseness, or stridor, while bronchial obstruction is associated with a feeling of tightness in the chest and/or audible wheezing. Patients with bronchial asthma are predisposed to severe involvement of the lower airways. A characteristic feature is the eruption of well-circumscribed, discrete cutaneous wheals with erythematous, raised, serpiginous borders and blanched centers. These urticarial eruptions are intensely pruritic and may be localized or disseminated. They may coalesce to form giant hives, and they seldom persist beyond 48 h. A localized, nonpitting, deeper edematous cutaneous process, angioedema, may also be present. It may be asymptomatic or cause a burning or stinging sensation.

In fatal cases with clinical bronchial obstruction, the lungs show marked hyperinflation on gross and microscopic examination. The microscopic findings in the bronchi, however, are limited to luminal secretions, peribronchial congestion, submucosal edema, and eosinophilic infiltration, and the acute emphysema is attributed to intractable bronchospasm that subsides with death. The angioedema resulting in death by mechanical obstruction occurs in the epiglottis and larynx, but the process is also evident in the hypopharynx and to some extent in the trachea; on microscopic examination there is wide separation of the collagen fibers and the glandular elements; vascular congestion and eosinophilic infiltration are also present. Patients dying of vascular collapse without antecedent hypoxia from respiratory insufficiency have visceral congestion with a presumptive loss of intravascular blood volume. The associated electrocardiographic abnormalities, with or without infarction, noted in some patients may reflect a primary cardiac event or be secondary to a critical reduction in blood volume.

The angioedematous and urticarial manifestations of the anaphylactic syndrome have been attributed to release of endogenous histamine. A role for the cysteinyl leukotrienes in altering pulmonary mechanics by causing marked bronchiolar constriction seems likely. Vascular collapse without respiratory distress in response to experimental challenge with the sting of a hymenopteran was associated not only with marked and prolonged elevations in blood histamine but also with evidence of intravascular coagulation and kinin generation. The findings that patients with systemic mastocytosis and episodic hypotension proceeding to vascular collapse excrete large amounts of PGD_2 metabolites in addition to histamine and that these events are controlled by administration of a nonsteroidal agent but not by antihistamines alone suggest that PGD_2 is also of importance in the hypotensive anaphylactic reactions. The cysteinyl leukotrienes may be involved in the pathobiologic process in patients with myocardial ischemia without or with infarction.

DIAGNOSIS   The diagnosis of an anaphylactic reaction depends largely on an accurate history revealing the onset of the appropriate symptoms and signs within minutes after the responsible material is encountered. When only a portion of the full syndrome is present, such as isolated urticaria, sudden bronchospasm in a patient with asthma, or vascular collapse after intravenous administration of an agent, it may be appropriate to consider a complement-mediated immune complex reaction, an idiosyncratic response to any of the nonsteroidal anti-inflammatory agents, or the direct effect of certain drugs or diagnostic agents on mast cells. Intravenous administration of a chemical mast cell–degranulating agent, including opiate derivatives and radiographic contrast media, may elicit generalized urticaria, angioedema, and a sensation of retrosternal oppression with or without clinically detectable bronchoconstriction or hypotension. Aspirin and other nonsteroidal anti-inflammatory agents such as indomethacin, aminopyrine, and mefenamic acid may precipitate a life-threatening episode of obstruction of upper or lower airways, especially in patients with asthma, that is clinically reminiscent of anaphylaxis but is not associated with a detectable IgE response. This syndrome, which is commonly associated with nasal polyposis, is due to inhibition of PGHS-1 with corresponding unregulated, amplified generation of the cysteinyl leukotrienes via the 5-lipoxygenase/LTC_4 synthase pathway. In the transfusion anaphylactic reaction that occurs in patients with IgA deficiency, the responsible specificity resides in IgG or IgE anti-IgA; the mechanism of the reaction mediated by IgG anti-IgA is presumed to be complement activation with secondary mast cell participation.

The presence of specific IgE in the heart blood of patients dying of systemic anaphylaxis has been demonstrated at postmortem by passive transfer of the serum intradermally into a normal recipient, followed in 24 h by antigen challenge into the same site, with subsequent development of a wheal and flare, the Prausnitz-Küstner reaction. To avoid the hazards of transferring hepatitis or other infections to a recipient, it is preferable to use the serum to seek passive sensitization of a human leukocyte suspension enriched with basophils for subsequent antigen-induced histamine release. Furthermore, radioimmunoassays have demonstrated specific IgE antibodies in patients with anaphylactic reactions, but such approaches require purified antigens. Elevations of β-tryptase levels in serum implicate mast cell activation in an adverse systemic reaction and are particularly informative with

episodes of hypotension during general anesthesia or when there has been a fatal outcome.

℞ **TREATMENT**   Early recognition of an anaphylactic reaction is mandatory, since death occurs within minutes to hours after the first symptoms. Mild symptoms such as pruritus and urticaria can be controlled by administration of 0.2 to 0.5 mL of 1:1000 epinephrine subcutaneously, with repeated doses as required at 20-min intervals for a severe reaction. If the antigenic material was injected into an extremity, the rate of absorption may be reduced by prompt application of a tourniquet proximal to the reaction site, administration of 0.2 mL of 1:1000 epinephrine into the site, and removal without compression of an insect stinger, if present. An intravenous infusion should be initiated to provide a route for administration of 2.5 mL epinephrine, diluted 1:10,000, at 5- to 10-min intervals, volume expanders such as normal saline, and vasopressor agents such as dopamine if intractable hypotension occurs. Replacement of intravascular volume due to postcapillary venular leakage may require several liters of saline. Epinephrine provides both α- and β-adrenergic effects, resulting in vasoconstriction, bronchial smooth-muscle relaxation, and attenuation of enhanced venular permeability. Beta blockers are relatively contraindicated in persons at risk for anaphylactic reactions, especially those sensitive to Hymenoptera venom or those undergoing immunotherapy for respiratory system allergy. When epinephrine fails to control the anaphylactic reaction, hypoxia due to airway obstruction or related to a cardiac arrhythmia, or both, must be considered. Oxygen via a nasal catheter or intermittent positive-pressure breathing of oxygen with 0.5 mL isoproterenol diluted 1:200 in saline may be helpful, but either endotracheal intubation or a tracheostomy is mandatory for oxygen delivery if progressive hypoxia develops. Ancillary agents such as the antihistamine diphenhydramine, 50 to 100 mg intramuscularly or intravenously, and aminophylline, 0.25 to 0.5 g intravenously, are appropriate for urticaria-angioedema and bronchospasm, respectively. Intravenous glucocorticoids are not effective for the acute event but may alleviate later recurrence of bronchospasm, hypotension, or urticaria. Furthermore, in a syndrome termed *idiopathic anaphylaxis* with recurrent angioedema of the upper airways, glucocorticoid administration may be beneficial by reducing the frequency of attacks and/or the severity of episodes.

PREVENTION   Prevention of anaphylaxis must take into account the sensitivity of the recipient, the dose and character of the diagnostic or therapeutic agent, and the effect of the route of administration on the rate of absorption. If there is a definite history of a past anaphylactic reaction, even though mild, it is advisable to select another agent or procedure. A knowledge of cross-reactivity among agents is critical since, for example, cephalosporins share a common β-lactam ring with the penicillins. A skin test should be performed before the administration of certain materials that are likely to elicit anaphylactic reactions, such as allergenic extracts, or when the nature of the past adverse reaction is unknown. A scratch test should precede an intradermal test in very sensitive patients. With regard to penicillin, two-thirds of patients with a positive reaction history and positive skin tests to benzylpenicilloyl-polylysine (BPL) and/or the minor determinant mixture (MDM) of benzylpenicillin products experience allergic reactions with treatment, and these are almost uniformly of the anaphylactic type in those patients with minor determinant reactivity. Even patients without a history of previous clinical reactions have a 2 to 6 percent incidence of positive skin tests to the two test materials, and about 3 per 1000 with a negative history experience anaphylaxis with therapy, with a mortality of about 1 per 100,000. Skin testing for antibiotics should be performed only on patients with a positive clinical history consistent with an IgE-mediated reaction and in imminent need of the antibiotic in question; skin testing is of no value for non-IgE-mediated eruptions. Desensitization with most antibiotics can proceed by the intravenous, subcutaneous, or oral route. Typically, graded quantities of the antibiotic are given by the selected route using double doses until a therapeutic dosage is achieved. Due to the risk of systemic anaphylaxis during the course of desensitization, such a procedure should be performed only in a setting in which resuscitation equipment is at hand and an intravenous line is in place. It is critical to give the therapeutic agent at regular intervals to prevent the reestablishment of a sensitized cell pool of large size.

A different form of protection involves the development of blocking antibody of the IgG class, which is protective against Hymenoptera venom–induced anaphylaxis by interacting with antigen so that less reaches the sensitized tissue mast cells; to be effective, this immunotherapy requires the use of specific or cross-reacting Hymenoptera venom. Because sensitization can be transient, the maximal risk for systemic anaphylactic reactions in persons with Hymenoptera sensitivity occurs in association with a currently positive skin test. Although there is only low-grade cross-reactivity between honey bee and yellow jacket venoms, there is a high degree of cross-reactivity between yellow jacket venom and the rest of the vespid venoms (yellow or bald-faced hornets and wasps). Prevention involves modification of outdoor activities to exclude bare feet, wearing perfumed toiletries, eating in areas attractive to insects, clipping hedges or grass, and hauling away trash or fallen fruit. As with each anaphylactic sensitivity, the individual should wear an informational bracelet and have immediate access to an unexpired epinephrine kit. The limitations of lifestyle and the psychological duress can be addressed by venom immunotherapy to achieve a venom-specific IgG titer. Although it has been recommended that venom therapy be continued indefinitely or until the skin and specific serum IgE tests are unremarkable, there is evidence that 5 years of treatment induces a state of resistance to sting reactions that is independent of serum levels of specific IgG or IgE. This contrasts with the definite relation of sting immunity to specific IgG earlier in the treatment regime. For children with a systemic reaction limited to skin, the likelihood of progression to more serious respiratory or vascular manifestations is low, and thus immunotherapy is not recommended.

URTICARIA AND ANGIOEDEMA

DEFINITION Urticaria and angioedema may appear separately or together as cutaneous manifestations of localized nonpitting edema; a similar process may occur at mucosal surfaces of the upper respiratory or gastrointestinal tract. *Urticaria* involves only the superficial portion of the dermis, presenting as well-circumscribed wheals with erythematous raised serpiginous borders with blanched centers that may coalesce to become giant wheals. *Angioedema* is a well-demarcated localized edema involving the deeper layers of the skin, including the subcutaneous tissue. Recurrent episodes of urticaria and/or angioedema of less than 6 weeks' duration are considered acute, whereas attacks persisting beyond this period are designated chronic.

PREDISPOSING FACTORS AND ETIOLOGY The occurrence of urticaria and angioedema is probably more frequent than usually described because of the evanescent, self-limited nature of such eruptions, which seldom require medical attention when limited to the skin. Although persons in any age group may experience acute or chronic urticaria and/or angioedema, these lesions increase in frequency after adolescence, with the highest incidence occurring in persons in the third decade of life; indeed, one survey of college students indicated that 15 to 20% had experienced a pruritic wheal reaction.

The classification of urticaria-angioedema presented in Table 310-1 focuses on the different mechanisms for eliciting clinical disease and can be useful for differential diagnosis; nonetheless, most cases of chronic urticaria are idiopathic. Urticaria and/or angioedema occurring during the appropriate season in patients with seasonal respiratory allergy or as a result of exposure to animals or molds is attributed to inhalation or physical contact with pollens, animal dander, and mold spores, respectively. However, urticaria and angioedema secondary to inhalation are relatively uncommon compared to urticaria and angioedema elicited by ingestion of fresh fruits, shellfish, fish, milk products, chocolate, legumes including peanuts, and various

Table 310-1 Classification of Urticaria and/or Angioedema

1. IgE-dependent
   a. Specific antigen sensitivity (pollens, foods, drugs, fungi, molds, Hymenoptera venom, helminths)
   b. Physical: dermographism, cold, solar, cholinergic, vibratory, exercise-related
2. Complement-mediated
   a. Hereditary angioedema: type 1, type 2
   b. Acquired angioedema: type 1, type 2
   c. Necrotizing vasculitis
   d. Serum sickness
   e. Reactions to blood products
3. Nonimmunologic
   a. Direct mast cell–releasing agents: opiates, antibiotics, curare, D-tubocurarine, radiocontrast media
   b. Agents that alter arachidonic acid metabolism: aspirin and nonsteroidal anti-inflammatory agents, azo dyes, and benzoates
4. Idiopathic

drugs that may elicit not only the anaphylactic syndrome with prominent gastrointestinal complaints but also chronic urticaria.

Additional etiologies include physical stimuli such as cold, heat, solar rays, exercise, and mechanical irritation. The physical urticarias can be distinguished by the precipitating event and other aspects of the clinical presentation. *Dermographism*, which occurs in 1 to 4% of the population, is defined by the appearance of a linear wheal at the site of a brisk stroke with a firm object or by any configuration appropriate to the eliciting event. Dermographism has a prevalence that peaks in the second to third decades. It is not influenced by an atopic diathesis and has a duration generally of less than 5 years. *Pressure urticaria*, which often accompanies dermographism or chronic idiopathic urticaria, presents in response to a sustained stimulus such as a shoulder strap or belt, running (feet), or manual labor (hands). *Cholinergic urticaria* is distinctive in that the pruritic wheals are of small size (1 to 2 mm) and are surrounded by a large area of erythema; attacks are precipitated by fever, a hot bath or shower, or exercise and are presumptively attributed to a rise in core body temperature. *Exercise-related anaphylaxis* can be limited to erythema and pruritic urticaria but may progress to angioedema of the face, oropharynx, larynx, or intestine or to vascular collapse; it is distinguished from cholinergic urticaria by presenting with wheals of conventional size and by not occurring with fever or a hot bath. *Cold urticaria*, either acquired or hereditary, is local at body areas exposed to low ambient temperature or cold objects (ice cube) but can progress to vascular collapse with immersion in cold water (swimming). *Solar urticaria* is subdivided into three groups by the response to specific portions of the light spectrum. *Vibratory angioedema* may occur after years of occupational exposure or can be idiopathic; it may be accompanied by cholinergic urticaria. Other rare forms of physical allergy, always defined by stimulus-specific elicitation, include *local heat urticaria, aquagenic urticaria* from contact with water of any temperature (sometimes associated with polycythemia vera), and *contact urticaria* from direct interaction with some chemical substance.

Angioedema without urticaria occurs with C1 inhibitor (C1INH) deficiency that may be inborn as an autosomal dominant characteristic or may be acquired. The urticaria and angioedema associated with classic serum sickness or with hypocomplementemic cutaneous necrotizing angiitis are believed to be immune-complex diseases. The drug reactions to mast cell granule–releasing agents and to nonsteroidal anti-inflammatory drugs may be systemic, resembling anaphylaxis, or limited to cutaneous sites.

PATHOPHYSIOLOGY AND MANIFESTATIONS Urticarial eruptions are distinctly pruritic, involve any area of the body from the scalp to the soles of the feet, and appear in crops of 24- to 72-h duration, with old lesions fading as new ones appear. The most common sites for urticaria are the extremities and face, with angioedema often being periorbital and in the lips. Although self-limited in duration, angioedema of the upper respiratory tract may be life-threatening due to laryngeal obstruction, while gastrointestinal involvement may present with abdominal colic, with or without nausea and vomiting, and may precipitate unnecessary surgical intervention. No residual discoloration occurs with either urticaria or angioedema unless there is an underlying process leading to superimposed extravasation of erythrocytes.

The pathology of urticaria and angioedema is usually characterized by edema of the dermis in urticaria and of the subcutaneous tissue as well as the dermis in angioedema. Collagen bundles in affected areas are widely separated, and the venules are sometimes dilated. The perivenular infiltrate may consist of lymphocytes, eosinophils, and neutrophils that are present in varying combination and number throughout the dermis.

Perhaps the best-studied example of IgE- and mast cell–mediated urticaria and angioedema is *cold urticaria*. Cryoglobulins may be recognized, but not in the majority of patients. Immersion of an extremity in an ice bath precipitates angioedema of the distal portion with urticaria at the air interface within minutes of the challenge. Histologic studies reveal marked mast cell degranulation with associated edema of the dermis and subcutaneous tissues. The venous effluent of the cold-challenged and angioedematous extremity reveals a marked rise in plasma content of histamine, whereas the venous effluent of the contralateral normal extremity contains none of this mediator. Elevated levels of histamine have been found in the plasma of venous effluent and in the fluid of suction blisters at experimentally induced lesional sites in patients with dermographism, pressure urticaria, vibratory angioedema, light urticaria, and heat urticaria. By ultrastructural analysis, the pattern of mast cell degranulation in cold urticaria resembles an IgE-mediated response with solubilization of granule contents, fusion of the perigranular and cell membranes, and discharge of granule contents, whereas in a dermographic lesion there is an additional superimposed zonal (piecemeal) degranulation. Elevations of plasma histamine levels with biopsy-proven mast cell degranulation have also been demonstrated with systemic attacks of *cholinergic urticaria* and *exercise-related anaphylaxis* precipitated experimentally in subjects exercising on a treadmill while wearing a wet suit; however, only in cholinergic urticaria is there a concomitant decrease in pulmonary function.

DIAGNOSIS The rapid onset and self-limited nature of urticarial and angioedematous eruptions are distinguishing features. Additional characteristics are the occurrence of the urticarial crops in various stages of evolution and the asymmetric distribution of the angioedema. Urticaria and/or angioedema involving IgE-dependent mechanisms are often appreciated by historic considerations implicating specific allergens or physical stimuli, by seasonal incidence, and by exposure to certain environments. Direct reproduction of the lesion with physical stimuli is particularly valuable because it so often establishes the cause of the lesion. The diagnosis of an environmental allergen based on the clinical history can be confirmed by skin testing or assay for allergen-specific IgE in serum. IgE-mediated urticaria and/or angioedema may or may not be associated with an elevation of total IgE or with peripheral eosinophilia. Fever, leukocytosis, and an elevated sedimentation rate are absent.

The classification of urticarial and angioedematous states noted in Table 310-1 in terms of possible mechanisms necessarily includes some differential diagnostic points. Hypocomplementemia is not observed in IgE-mediated mast cell disease and may reflect either an acquired abnormality generally attributed to the formation of immune complexes or a genetic deficiency of C1INH. Chronic recurrent urticaria, generally in females, associated with arthralgias, an elevated sedimentation rate, and normo- or hypocomplementemia suggests an underlying cutaneous necrotizing angiitis. Vasculitic urticaria typically persists longer than 72 h, whereas conventional urticaria often has a duration of less than 24 to 48 h. Confirmation depends on a biopsy that reveals cellular infiltration, nuclear debris, and fibrinoid necrosis

of the venules. The same pathobiologic process accounts for the urticaria in association with such diseases as systemic lupus erythematosus or viral hepatitis with or without an associated arteritis. Serum sickness per se or a similar clinical entity due to drugs includes not only urticaria but also pyrexia, lymphadenopathy, myalgia, and arthralgia or arthritis. Urticarial reactions to blood products or intravenous administration of immunoglobulin are defined by the event and generally are not progressive unless the recipient is IgA-deficient in the former case or the reagent is aggregated in the latter.

Hereditary angioedema is an autosomal dominant disease due to a deficiency of antigenic and/or functional C1INH. The diagnosis is suggested not only by family history but also by the lack of pruritus and of urticarial lesions, the prominence of recurrent gastrointestinal attacks of colic, and episodes of laryngeal edema. Laboratory diagnosis depends on demonstrating a deficiency of C1INH antigen (type 1) in most kindreds, but some kindreds have an antigenically intact nonfunctional protein (type 2) and require a functional assay to establish the diagnosis. The natural substrates of uninhibited C1 protease, C4 and C2, are chronically depleted but fall further during attacks due to the activation of additional C1. Because the C1INH protein also regulates the Hageman factor–initiated activation of kallikrein and of plasmin, the vasoactive peptides responsible for the angioedema are likely some combination of bradykinin and a plasmin-derived fragment of C1-cleaved C2. An acquired form of C1INH deficiency, associated with lymphoproliferative disorders, has the same clinical manifestations but differs in the lack of a familial element; in the reduction of C1 function and C1q protein as well as C1INH, C4, and C2; and in the presence of an anti-idiotypic antibody to the monoclonal immunoglobulin expressed on the B cells. A second acquired form of C1INH deficiency with angioedema due to the appearance of IgG anti-C1INH may be associated with systemic lupus erythematosus.

Urticaria and angioedema must be differentiated from contact sensitivity, a vesicular eruption that progresses to chronic thickening of the skin with continued allergenic exposure. They must also be differentiated from atopic dermatitis, a condition that may present as erythema, edema, papules, vesiculation, and oozing proceeding to a subacute and chronic stage in which vesiculation is less marked or absent and scaling, fissuring, and lichenification predominate in a distribution that characteristically involves the flexor surfaces. In cutaneous mastocytosis, the reddish brown macules and papules, characteristic of urticaria pigmentosa, urticate with pruritus upon trauma; and in systemic mastocytosis, without or with urticaria pigmentosa, there is an episodic systemic flushing with or without urticaria but no angioedema.

TREATMENT Identification of the etiologic factor(s) and their elimination provide the most satisfactory therapeutic program; this approach is feasible to varying degrees with IgE-mediated reactions to allergens or physical stimuli. For most forms of urticaria, H1 antihistamines such as chlorpheniramine or diphenhydramine, and including the nonsedating class such as loratadine or cetirizine, are effective in attenuating both urtication and pruritus. Cyproheptadine and especially hydroxyzine have proven effective when H1 antihistamines have been inadequate. Doxepin, a dibenzoxepin tricyclic compound with both H1 and H2 receptor antagonist activity, is yet another alternative. Topical glucocorticoids are of no value in the management of urticaria and/or angioedema. Systemic glucocorticoids are generally avoided in idiopathic, allergen-induced, or physical urticarias due to their long-term toxicity. However, systemic glucocorticoids are useful in the management of patients with pressure urticaria, with vasculitic urticaria (especially with eosinophil prominence), with idiopathic angioedema with or without urticaria, or with chronic urticaria that responds poorly to conventional treatment. With persistent vasculitic urticaria, hydroxychloroquine or colchicine may be added to the regimen after hydroxyzine and before or along with systemic glucocorticoids.

The therapy of inborn C1INH deficiency has been simplified by the finding that attenuated androgens correct the biochemical defect and afford prophylactic protection. Since the affected individuals are heterozygous, with the depletion of C1INH being due to deficient synthesis and consequent excessive utilization of the limited amount available, the efficacy of the attenuated androgens is attributed to production by the normal gene of an amount of functional C1INH sufficient to control the spontaneous activation of C1 to C1 protease. Since the use of such agents for children and pregnant women is not yet accepted, the antifibrinolytic agent ϵ-aminocaproic acid may be used occasionally to control spontaneous attacks or for preoperative prophylaxis in some patients. This agent should not be used in patients with thrombotic tendencies or ischemia due to arterial athrosclerosis. Infusion of isolated C1INH protein appears useful in prophylaxis and to ameliorate an attack but is not yet widely available.

SYSTEMIC MASTOCYTOSIS

DEFINITION *Systemic mastocytosis* is defined by mast cell hyperplasia that in most instances is indolent and nonneoplastic. Since human mast cells originate from pluripotent bone marrow cells (CD34+), circulate as nonmetachromatically staining, c-*kit*-positive mononuclear cells, and undergo tissue-specific proliferation and maturation, the hyperplasia is generally recognized only in bone marrow and in the normal peripheral distribution sites of the cells, such as skin, gastrointestinal mucosa, liver, and spleen. Mastocytosis occurs at any age and has a slight preponderance in males. The prevalence of systemic mastocytosis is not known, a familial occurrence has not been established, and atopy is not increased.

CLASSIFICATION, PATHOPHYSIOLOGY, AND CLINICAL MANIFESTATIONS A recent consensus classification for systemic mastocytosis recognizes four forms (Table 310-2). The form designated as *indolent* accounts for the majority of patients and is not known to alter life expectancy. When a patient is classified as having indolent systemic mastocytosis, the concomitant clinical findings must be carefully noted, since they define the complications and directions for management. In systemic mastocytosis *associated with hematologic disorders*, the prognosis is determined by the nature of that disorder, which can range from dysmyelopoiesis to leukemia. In *aggressive* systemic mastocytosis, mast cell proliferation in parenchymal organs such as liver, spleen, and lymph nodes is marked and in a subset of patients is associated with prominent eosinophilia in affected organs or peripheral blood; the prognosis is poor due to widespread tissue infiltration. *Mast cell leukemia* is the rarest form of the disease and is invariably fatal at present; in contrast to the other forms, the peripheral blood contains circulating, metachromatically staining, atypical mast cells. In types II and IV systemic mastocytosis there is a point mutation of the c-*kit* tyrosine kinase in the leukocytes and mast cells, respectively; this mutation can also be detected in lesional tissue such as the small, reddish brown macules or papules, termed *urticaria pigmentosa*, at skin sites of patients with type I. The most common mutation, a substitution of valine for aspartate in codon 816 (V816D), leads to constitutively activated c-*kit*, which then drives proliferation independently of SCF. More than half of the cases of type II systemic mastocytosis with a V816D mutation exhibit cytogenetic abnormalities on routine karyotyping. In types I and III there is excessive production of the c-*kit* ligand (SCF) in the microenvironment of the mast cells, and this may be autocrine in type III. In infants and children (type I) with

Table 310-2 Classification of Systemic Mastocytosis

Type	Description
I	*Indolent* with cutaneous manifestations, vascular collapse, ulcer disease, malabsorption, skeletal disease, hepatosplenomegaly, or lymphadenopathy
II	*Concomitant hematologic disorder*, either myelodysplastic or myeloproliferative
III	*Aggressive* per se or lymphadenopathic mastocytosis with eosinophilia
IV	*Mastocytic leukemia*

cutaneous manifestations, namely, urticaria pigmentosa or bullous lesions, visceral involvement is usually lacking, and resolution is common because there are no mutations to activate the tyrosine kinase. The clinical manifestations of systemic mastocytosis, particularly types I and II, distinct from a leukemic complication, are due to tissue occupancy by the mast cell mass, the tissue response to that mass, and the release of bioactive substances acting at both local and distal sites. The pharmacologically induced manifestations are pruritus, flushing, palpitations and vascular collapse, gastric distress, lower abdominal crampy pain, and recurrent headache. The increase in cell burden is evidenced by the lesions of urticaria pigmentosa at skin sites, but it also contributes to bone pain and malabsorption. The mast cell–mediated fibrotic changes are limited to liver, spleen, and bone marrow and presumably relate to the functional characteristics of mast cells developing at those sites, as opposed to those at sites without fibrosis, such as the gastrointestinal tissue or skin. Immunofluorescent analysis of bone marrow and skin lesions in indolent mastocytosis and of spleen, lymph node, and skin in aggressive systemic mastocytosis has revealed only one mast cell phenotype, namely, scroll-poor cells expressing tryptase, chymase, and CPA.

The cutaneous lesions of urticaria pigmentosa respond to trauma with urtication and erythema (Darier's sign). The apparent incidence of these lesions is 90 percent or greater in patients with indolent systemic mastocytosis. Approximately 1 percent of patients with indolent mastocytosis have skin lesions that appear as tan-brown macules with striking patchy erythema and associated telangiectasia (telangiectasia macularis eruptiva perstans). In the upper gastrointestinal tract, histamine-mediated hypersecretion is the most common problem, with resultant gastritis and peptic ulcer. In the lower intestinal tract, the occurrence of diarrhea and abdominal pain is attributed to increased motility due to mast cell mediators, and this can be aggravated by malabsorption with secondary nutritional insufficiency and osteomalacia. The periportal fibrosis associated with mast cell infiltration and a prominence of eosinophils may lead to portal hypertension and ascites. In some patients, flushing and recurrent vascular collapse are markedly aggravated by an idiosyncratic response to a minimal dosage of nonsteroidal anti-inflammatory agents. The neuropsychiatric disturbances are clinically most evident as impaired recent memory, decreased attention span, and "migraine-like" headaches. Patients in every category of systemic mastocytosis may experience exacerbation of a specific clinical sign or symptom with alcohol ingestion, use of mast cell–interactive narcotics, or ingestion of nonsteroidal anti-inflammatory agents.

DIAGNOSIS Although the diagnosis is generally suspected on the basis of the clinical history and physical findings, the contention can be strengthened by certain laboratory procedures and established only by a tissue diagnosis. A 24-h urine collection for measurement of histamine, histamine metabolites, or metabolites of PGD_2 is currently the most common noninvasive approach. A convenient alternative is to measure blood levels of the mast cell–derived neutral protease tryptase. The α form of tryptase is elevated in more than one-half of patients with type I systemic mastocytosis and in virtually all those with types II and III, whereas the β form is increased in patients undergoing an anaphylactic reaction. Additional studies directed by the presentation include a bone scan or skeletal survey; contrast studies of the upper gastrointestinal tract with small-bowel follow-through, computed tomography scan, or endoscopy; and a neuropsychiatric evaluation, including an electroencephalogram. The tissue diagnosis is straightforward if there are lesions of urticaria pigmentosa, but the diagnosis of systemic mastocytosis requires involvement of other organs and is most frequently established by bone marrow biopsy and aspiration. The bone marrow lesions consist of focal and paratrabecular aggregates of spindle-shaped mast cells, often mixed with eosinophils, lymphocytes, and, on occasion, plasma cells, histiocytes, and fibroblasts.

The differential diagnosis requires the exclusion of other flushing disorders. The 24-h urine assessment of 5-hydroxy-indoleacetic acid and metanephrines should exclude a carcinoid tumor or a pheochromocytoma. Most patients with recurrent anaphylaxis, including the idiopathic group, present with angioedema and/or wheezing, which are not manifestations of systemic mastocytosis.

℞ TREATMENT   The management of systemic mastocytosis uses a stepwise and symptom/sign–directed approach that includes an H_1 antihistamine for flushing and pruritus, an H_2 antihistamine or proton pump inhibitor for gastric acid hypersecretion, oral cromolyn sodium for diarrhea and abdominal pain, and a nonsteroidal anti-inflammatory agent for severe flushing associated with vascular collapse despite use of H_1 and H_2 antihistamines to block biosynthesis of PGD_2. Systemic glucocorticoids appear to alleviate the malabsorption. Headaches are generally managed with tricyclic antidepressants and other neurotransmitter-modifying agents. Ketotifen has been used to alleviate flushing in patients with gastric intolerance to nonsteroidal anti-inflammatory agents and in patients with bone pain or intractable headaches. The efficacy of IFN-α in aggressive systemic mastocytosis is controversial, and this may relate to the difficulty in achieving the necessary dosage in some patients due to the attendant side effects. Treatment with hydroxyurea to reduce the mast cell lineage progenitors may have merit in type III systemic mastocytosis. Chemotherapy is appropriate for the frank leukemias in types II and IV.

ALLERGIC RHINITIS

DEFINITION   Allergic rhinitis is characterized by sneezing; rhinorrhea; obstruction of the nasal passages; conjunctival, nasal, and pharyngeal itching; and lacrimation, all occurring in a temporal relationship to allergen exposure. Although commonly seasonal due to elicitation by airborne pollens, it can be perennial in an environment of chronic exposure. The incidence of allergic rhinitis in North America is about 7%, with the peak occurring in childhood and adolescence.

PREDISPOSING FACTORS AND ETIOLOGY   Allergic rhinitis generally presents in atopic individuals, i.e., in persons with a family history of a similar or related symptom complex and a personal history of collateral allergy expressed as eczematous dermatitis, urticaria, and/or asthma (Chap. 252). Symptoms generally appear before the fourth decade of life and tend to diminish gradually with aging, although complete spontaneous remissions are uncommon. A relatively small number of weeds that depend on wind rather than insects for cross-pollination, as well as certain grasses and trees, produce sufficient quantities of pollen suitable for wide distribution by air currents to elicit seasonal allergic rhinitis. The dates of pollination of these species generally vary little from year to year in a particular locale but may be quite different in another climate. In the temperate areas of North America, trees typically pollinate from March through May, grasses in June and early July, and ragweed from mid-August to early October. Molds, which are widespread in nature because they occur in soil or decaying organic matter, may propagate spores in a pattern dependent on climatic conditions. Perennial allergic rhinitis occurs in response to allergens that are present throughout the year such as in desquamating epithelium in animal dander or cockroach-derived proteins, the processed materials or chemicals utilized in an industrial setting, or the dust accumulating at work or at home. Dust has a diverse allergen content including *Dermatophagoides farinae* and *D. pteronyssinus*, which may be present alone or together in house dust. Dust mites are scavengers of flecks of human skin and coat the digestate with mite-specific protein for subsequent excretion as part of a fecal ball. In up to two-thirds of patients with perennial rhinitis, no clearcut allergen can be demonstrated. The ability of allergens to cause rhinitis rather than lower respiratory symptoms may be attributed to their size, 10 to 100 μm, and retention within the nose.

PATHOPHYSIOLOGY AND MANIFESTATIONS   Episodic rhinorrhea, sneezing, obstruction of the nasal passages with lac-

rimation, and pruritus of the conjunctiva, nasal mucosa, and oropharynx are the hallmarks of allergic rhinitis. The nasal mucosa is pale and boggy, the conjunctiva congested and edematous, and the pharynx is generally unremarkable. Swelling of the turbinates and mucous membranes with obstruction of the sinus ostia and eustachian tubes precipitates secondary infections of the sinuses and middle ear, respectively, commonly in perennial but rarely in seasonal disease. Nasal polyps, representing mucosal protrusions containing edema fluid with variable numbers of eosinophils, arise concurrently with edema and/or infection within the sinuses and increase obstructive symptoms.

The nose presents a large mucosal surface area through the folds of the turbinates and serves to adjust the temperature and moisture content of inhaled air and to filter out particulate materials above 10 μm in size by impingement in a mucous blanket; ciliary action moves the entrapped particles toward the pharynx. Entrapment of pollen and digestion of the outer coat by mucosal enzymes such as lysozymes release protein allergens generally of 10,000 to 40,000 molecular weight. The initial interaction occurs between the allergen and intraepithelial mast cells and then proceeds to involve deeper perivenular mast cells, both of which are sensitized with specific IgE. During the symptomatic season when the mucosae are already swollen and hyperemic, there is enhanced adverse reactivity to the seasonal pollen as well as to antigenically unrelated pollens for which there is underlying hypersensitivity due to improved penetration of the allergens. Biopsy specimens of nasal mucosa during seasonal rhinitis show submucosal edema with infiltration by eosinophils, along with some basophils and neutrophils.

The mucosal surface fluid contains IgA that is present because of its secretory piece and also IgE, which apparently arrives by diffusion from plasma cells in proximity to mucosal surfaces. IgE fixes to mucosal and submucosal mast cells, and the intensity of the clinical response to inhaled allergens is quantitatively related to the naturally occurring pollen dose. Specific IgE is distributed also to circulating basophilic leukocytes; patients with more severe clinical disease have basophils that release histamine in response to lesser concentrations of allergen in vitro than do cells from patients with milder disease. In sensitive individuals, the introduction of allergen into the nose is associated with sneezing, "stuffiness," and discharge, and the fluid contains histamine, PGD_2, and leukotrienes. Thus the mast cells of the nasal mucosa and submucosa generate and release mediators through IgE-dependent reactions that are capable of producing tissue edema and eosinophilic infiltration.

DIAGNOSIS   The diagnosis of seasonal allergic rhinitis depends largely on an accurate history of occurrence coincident with the pollination of the offending weeds, grasses, or trees. The continuous character of perennial allergic rhinitis due to contamination of the home or place of work makes historic analysis difficult, but there may be a variability in symptoms that can be related to exposure to animal dander, dust mite and/or cockroach allergens, or work-related allergens such as latex. Patients with perennial rhinitis commonly develop the problem in adult life, are more often women than men, and manifest nasal polyps and thickening of the sinus membranes demonstrated by radiography. The term *vasomotor rhinitis* designates a condition of enhanced reactivity of the nasopharynx in which a symptom complex resembling perennial allergic rhinitis occurs with nonspecific stimuli. Other entities to be excluded are structural abnormalities of the nasopharynx; exposure to irritants; upper respiratory infection; pregnancy with prominent nasal mucosal edema; prolonged topical use of α-adrenergic agents in the form of nose drops (rhinitis medicamentosa); and the use of certain therapeutic agents such as rauwolfia, β-adrenergic antagonists, or estrogens.

The nasal secretions of allergic patients are rich in eosinophils, and peripheral eosinophilia is a common feature. Local or systemic neutrophilia implies infection. Total serum IgE is frequently elevated, but the demonstration of immunologic specificity for IgE is critical to an etiologic diagnosis. A skin test by the epicutaneous route (scratch or prick) with the allergens of interest provides a rapid and reliable approach to identifying allergen-specific IgE that has sensitized cutaneous mast cells. An intradermal test may follow if indicated by history when the epicutaneous test is negative, but it is less reliable due to the

310 Allergies, Anaphylaxis, and Systemic Mastocytosis **1921**

ous mast cells. An intradermal test may follow if indicated by history when the epicutaneous test is negative, but it is less reliable due to the reactivity of some asymptomatic individuals at the test dose. Skin testing by scratch or prick for food allergens is controversial but does seem to have predictive value for the absence of specific IgE sensitivity. A double-blind, placebo-controlled challenge may document a food allergy, but such a procedure does bear the risk of an anaphylactic reaction. An elimination diet is safer but is tedious and less definitive. Food allergy is uncommon as a cause of allergic rhinitis.

Newer methodology for detecting total IgE, including the development of enzyme-linked immunosorbent assays (ELISA) employing anti-IgE bound to either a solid-phase or a liquid-phase paramagnetic particle, provides rapid and cost effective determinations. Measurements of specific anti-IgE in serum are obtained by its binding to a solid-phase allergen and quantitation by subsequent uptake of radio-labeled anti-IgE. This radioallergosorbent technique correlates with the bioassay of specific IgE by skin test, which is mast cell–dependent, and by histamine release from peripheral blood leukocytes, which is basophil-dependent. As compared to the skin test, the assay of specific IgE in serum is less sensitive but has high specificity. Furthermore, ELISA utilizing reactions that generate visible light or fluorescence have replaced the radioimmunoassays, and newer chemiluminescent tracers provide additional sensitivity for detection of minute quantities of allergen-specific IgE.

PREVENTION Avoidance of exposure to the offending allergen is the most effective means of controlling allergic diseases; removal of pets from the home to avoid animal danders, utilization of air filtration devices to minimize the concentrations of airborne pollens, elimination of cockroach-derived proteins by chemical destruction of the pest and careful food storage, travel to nonpollinating areas during the critical periods, and even a change of domicile to eliminate a mold spore problem may be necessary. Control of dust mites by allergen avoidance includes use of plastic-lined covers for mattresses, pillows, and comforters, and elimination of carpets and drapes.

TREATMENT Management with pharmacologic agents represents the standard approach to seasonal or perennial allergic rhinitis. Antihistamines of the H_1 class are effective for nasopharyngeal itching, sneezing, and watery rhinorrhea and for such ocular manifestations as itching, tearing, and erythema, but they are not efficacious for the nasal congestion. The older antihistamines are sedating, and their anticholinergic (muscarinic) effects include visual disturbance, urinary retention, and even arrhythmias. Because the newer H_1 antihistaminics such as loratadine and cetirizine are less lipophilic, their ability to cross the blood-brain barrier is reduced, and thus their sedating and anticholinergic side effects are minimized. Because life-threatening ventricular arrhythmias with some fatalities have been caused by prolongation of the QT interval resulting from inhibition of the metabolism of terfenadine and astemizole by their interactions with macrolide antibiotics, these agents have been subtantially replaced by loratadine, fexofenadine, and cetirizine. α-Adrenergic agents such as phenylephrine or oximetazoline are generally used topically to alleviate nasal congestion and obstruction, but the duration of efficacy is limited because of rebound rhinitis and such systemic responses as insomnia, irritability, and hypertension. The latter are more frequent with use of oral α-adrenergic agonists, which nonetheless are useful in relieving nasal congestion and diminishing the sedating effects of conventional antihistamines. Cromolyn sodium, a nasal spray, is essentially without side effects and is used prophylactically on a continuous basis during the season to attenuate allergen activation of nasal mast cells. The clinical efficacy of cromolyn sodium and that of nonsedating antihistamines are roughly equivalent. Intranasal high-potency glucocorticoids are the most potent drugs available for the relief of established rhinitis, seasonal or perennial, and even vasomotor rhinitis; they provide efficacy with substantially reduced side effects as compared with this same class of agent administered orally. Their most frequent side effect is local irritation, with *Candida* overgrowth being a rare occurrence. The topical-to-systemic activity of flunisolide or budesonide is significantly greater than for beclomethasone or triamcinolone with much less systemic absorption. For patients who do not benefit adequately from a full dosage of a nonsedating H_1 antihistamine and a maintenance dosage of cromolyn sodium, an α-adrenergic agent for short-term relief should be replaced by high-potency topical glucocorticoids. For systemic symptoms not related to the nasopharynx, such as allergic conjunctivitis, treatment may be local.

Immunotherapy, often termed *hyposensitization*, consists of repeated subcutaneous injections of gradually increasing concentrations of the allergen(s) considered to be specifically responsible for the symptom complex. Controlled studies of ragweed, grass, dust mite, and cat dander allergens administered for treatment of allergic rhinitis have demonstrated at least partial relief of symptoms and signs. The duration of such immunotherapy is 3 to 5 years, with discontinuation being based on minimal symptoms over two consecutive seasons of exposure. Clinical benefit appears related to the administration of a high dose of allergen at weekly or biweekly intervals. Patients should remain at the treatment site for at least 20 min after allergen administration so that any anaphylactic consequence can be managed. Local reactions with erythema and induration are not uncommon and may persist for 1 to 3 days. Immunotherapy is contraindicated in patients with significant cardiovascular disease or unstable asthma and should be conducted with particular caution in any patient requiring β-adrenergic blocking therapy because of the difficulty in managing an anaphylactic complication. The immunologic characteristics of a response include a rise in antibodies of the IgG class, a small increase in specific IgE early in the treatment course followed by a plateau or decline, and a decline in the percentage of histamine released from peripheral blood basophilic leukocytes challenged with a fixed concentration of the allergen. The antibodies of the IgG class might well reduce or neutralize the quantity of allergen available for interaction with the tissue mast cells but, more important, could modify the seasonal booster response in specific IgE synthesis. None of the individual parameters of the response to immunotherapy correlates well with the assessments of clinical efficacy, suggesting that benefit is derived from a complex of effects that likely includes a reduction in T cell cytokine production. Immunotherapy should be reserved for clearly documented seasonal or perennial rhinitis, clinically related to defined allergen exposure with confirmation by the presence of allergen-specific IgE, which has failed management by allergen avoidance and pharmacotherapy due to lack of efficacy or side effects. A sequence for the management of allergic or perennial rhinitis based on an allergen-specific diagnosis and stepwise management as required for symptom control would include the following: (1) identification of the offending allergen(s) by history with confirmation of the presence of allergen-specific IgE by skin test (epicutaneous) and/or serum assay; (2) avoidance of the offending allergen; (3) for mild symptoms, prophylactic management with topical cromolyn sodium or treatment with a single bedtime dose of chlorpheniramine (if the latter is associated with undue side effects, substitute a second-generation nonsedating antihistamine); combination with an oral decongestant such as pseudoephedrine can be beneficial; (4) for prominent symptoms, utilization of topical beclomethasone, budesonide, fluticasone, momestasone, or triamcinalone may be needed for a satisfactory clinical outcome; and (5) for management failures despite avoidance and pharmacotherapy, progression to immunotherapy.

BIBLIOGRAPHY

Austen KF, Metcalfe DD: Anaphylactic syndrome, in *Immunological Diseases*, 5th ed, M Frank et al (eds). Boston, Little, Brown, 1995

Bingham CO, Austen KF: The molecular and cellular biology of the mast cell, in *Fitzpatrick's Dermatology in General Medicine*, 5th ed, IM Freedberg et al (eds). New York, McGraw-Hill, 1999, pp 414–423

Ewan PW: Anaphylaxis. BMJ 316:1442, 1997

Metcalfe DD: The mastocytosis syndrome, in *Fitzpatrick's Dermatology in General Medicine*, 5th ed, IM Freedberg et al (eds). New York, McGraw-Hill, 1999, pp 1902–1908

O'HOLLAREN MT: Update in allergy and immunology. Ann Intern Med 129:1036, 1998

PENROSE JF et al: Leukotrienes: Biosynthetic pathways, release, and receptor-mediated actions with relevance to disease states, in *Inflammation: Basic Principles and Clinical Correlates*, 3rd ed, JI Gallin and R Snyderman (eds). Philadelphia, Lippincott Williams & Wilkins, 1999

SOTER NA: Urticaria and angioedema, in *Fitzpatrick's Dermatology in General Medicine*, 5th ed, IM Freedberg et al (eds). New York, McGraw-Hill, 1999, pp 1409–1419

VALENTINE MD: Insect venom allergy, in *Immunological Diseases*, 5th ed, M Frank et al (eds). Boston, Little, Brown, 1995

311 *Bevra Hannahs Hahn*

SYSTEMIC LUPUS ERYTHEMATOSUS

aCL anticardiolipin	LA lupus anticoagulant
ANA antinuclear antibody	MCP metacarpophalangeal
CNS central nervous system	MRI magnetic resonance imaging
CSF cerebrospinal fluid	NSAIDs nonsteroidal anti-inflammatory
CT computed tomography	drugs
DEJ dermal-epidermal junction	PIP proximal interphalangeal
DLE discoid lupus erythematosus	SCLE subacute cutaneous lupus
ERT estrogen replacement therapy	erythematosus
GI gastrointestinal	SLE systemic lupus erythematosus
GN glomerulonephritis	UV ultraviolet

DEFINITION AND PREVALENCE Systemic lupus erythematosus (SLE) is a disease of unknown etiology in which tissues and cells are damaged by pathogenic autoantibodies and immune complexes. Ninety percent of cases are in women, usually of child-bearing age, but children, men, and the elderly can be affected. In the United States, the prevalence of SLE in urban areas varies from 15 to 50 per 100,000 population; it is more common in blacks than in whites. Hispanic and Asian populations are also susceptible.

PATHOGENESIS AND ETIOLOGY SLE results from tissue damage caused by pathogenic subsets of autoantibodies and immune complexes. The abnormal immune responses include (1) polyclonal and antigen-specific T and B lymphocyte hyperactivity, and (2) inadequate regulation of that hyperactivity. These abnormal immune responses probably depend upon interactions between susceptibility genes and environment. Evidence for genetic predisposition includes increased concordance for disease in monozygotic (24 to 58%) compared with dizygotic (0 to 6%) twins, a $\lambda_s > 10$, and a 10 to 15% frequency of patients with more than one affected family member. Studies of association, linkage, and genome scanning show complex genetic susceptibility. Most people with homozygous deficiencies of early components of complement (C1q, C2, C4) have SLE or similar disease (accounting for <5% of SLE patients), suggesting that these genes are major predisposing factors. Most patients must inherit multiple susceptibility genes, and probably experience environmental stimuli as well, to develop clinical disease. A defective or deleted class III allele, C4AQO, is the most common genetic marker associated with SLE in many ethnic groups (40 to 50% of patients compared with 15% of healthy controls). One extended haplotype, B8.DR3.DQw2.C4AQO, predisposes to SLE in populations with Northern European heritage. SLE is associated with HLA-DR2 or -DR3 in many groups, and single-gene associations occur between HLA class II (especially DQ_β) and autoantibodies that associate with clinical subsets of lupus. For example, antibodies to Ro/La (SS-A/SS-B) are associated with subacute cutaneous lupus and certain DQA and DQB genes that are usually inherited with DR3. Normal alleles of FcγRIIA or of FcγRIIIA that bind IgG2 or IgG1 and IgG3, respectively, less efficiently than other alleles are associated with SLE, particularly with nephritis. FcγRIIA predisposes to SLE in African Amer-

icans and South Koreans; FcγRIIIA predisposes across different ethnic groups. Such alleles might account for impaired clearing of autoantibodies and immune complexes, thus predisposing to their deposition in tissues. Genome scanning from several laboratories has shown two regions of chromosome 1 that link to disease in sibpairs or multiplex families. One region, 1q23, contains the FcγRIIA gene; the other, 1q41-42, contains poly (ADP-ribosyl) polymerase (PARP), which may be another predisposing gene that plays a role in DNA repair and apoptosis. Other results of genome scanning suggest that at least 10 other regions on various chromosomes, in addition to HLA and the two regions on chromosome 1 discussed above, participate in susceptibility. Some genes may be "autoimmunity" genes common to different autoimmune diseases across different ethnic groups; others are likely to be restricted to a single disease and/or a single ethnic group. Family studies suggest that females are more likely than males to express the autoimmune manifestations of their genotypes.

Environmental factors that cause flares of SLE are largely unknown, with the exception of ultraviolet (UV)-B (and sometimes UV-A) light. As many as 70% of patients are photosensitive. Other factors, such as ingested alfalfa sprouts, and chemicals, such as hydrazines, have been implicated. Searches for viral/retroviral disease inducers have been inconclusive. Although some drugs can induce lupus-like disease, there are notable clinical and autoantibody differences between drug-induced and spontaneous lupus. Femaleness is clearly a susceptibility factor, since the prevalence in women of child-bearing years is seven to nine times higher than in men, whereas the female: male ratio is 3:1 in pre- and postmenopausal years. Metabolism of estrogenic and androgenic hormones may be abnormal in lupus patients. Sex hormones also influence immune tolerance.

Abnormal immune responses permit sustained production of pathogenic subsets of autoantibodies and immune complexes. Some autoantibodies, such as anti-DNA, can bind to tissue via charge or cross-reactivity, or in immune complexes, and cause complement-mediated damage. Some subsets of anti-DNA and anti-RNP can bind and enter living cells, altering their function. Other autoantibodies cause damage by direct binding to cell membranes (erythrocytes, platelets) that cause those cells to be phagocytized and destroyed. T cell help is critical to development of full-blown disease; cells of CD4+CD8−, CD4−CD8+, and CD4− CD8− phenotypes all help autoantibody production in SLE. The abnormalities that permit hyperactivated self-reactive B and T cells to dominate immune repertoires in murine and human SLE are multiple and include defects in cell activation, tolerance, apoptosis, idiotypic networks, immune complex clearance, and generation of regulatory cells. The structure of antigens that stimulate autoantibodies is under investigation. Some are clearly derived from self (nucleosomes, ribonucleoprotein, erythrocyte and lymphocyte surface antigens); others may be from the external environment and mimic self (e.g., components of vesicular stomatitis virus mimic peptides in Sm antigen). Many DNA/protein and RNA/protein antigens may be presented to the immune system in surface blebs of apoptotic cells. Since UV light induces apoptosis in skin cells, this might be a mechanism for flaring disease. Autoantibodies characteristic of SLE are listed in Table 311-1.

In summary, some individuals are genetically predisposed to SLE. Under the influence of multiple genes, possibly triggered by environmental challenges and highly influenced by sex, they may develop a number of different clinical syndromes that fulfill diagnostic criteria for SLE. The etiology of these syndromes is complex and probably differs between patients.

CLINICAL MANIFESTATIONS At onset, SLE may involve only one organ system (additional manifestations occur later) or may be multisystemic. Clinical manifestations are listed in Table 311-2; those that fulfill American Rheumatism Association (currently the American College of Rheumatology) updated criteria for a diagnosis of SLE are listed in Table 311-3. Autoantibodies are detectable at disease onset. Severity varies from mild and intermittent to persistent and fulminant. Most patients experience exacerbations interspersed with periods of relative quiescence. True remissions with no symptoms and requiring no therapy occur in up to 20% but are usually not permanent. Systemic symptoms are usually prominent and include fatigue, malaise, fever, anorexia, and weight loss.

Musculoskeletal Manifestations Almost all patients experience arthralgias and myalgias; most develop intermittent arthritis. Pain is often out of proportion to physical findings. Symmetric fusiform swelling in joints [most frequently proximal interphalangeal (PIP) and metacarpophalangeal (MCP) joints of the hands, wrists, and knees], diffuse puffiness of hands and feet, and tenosynovitis can be seen. Joint deformities are unusual, with 10% of patients developing swan-neck deformities of fingers and ulnar drift at MCP joints. Erosions are rare; subcutaneous nodules occur. Myopathy can be inflammatory (during periods of active disease), or secondary to treatment (hypokalemia, glucocorticoid myopathy, hydroxychloroquine myopathy). Ischemic necrosis of bone is a common cause of hip, knee, or shoulder pain in patients receiving glucocorticoids.

Cutaneous Manifestations The malar ("butterfly") rash is a photosensitive, fixed erythematous rash, flat or raised, over the cheeks and bridge of the nose, often involving the chin and ears. Scarring is absent; telangiectases may develop. A more diffuse maculopapular rash, predominant in sun-exposed areas, is also common and usually indicates disease flare. Loss of scalp hair is usually patchy but can be extensive; hair often regrows in SLE lesions but not in lesions of discoid lupus erythematosus (DLE). DLE occurs in about 20% of pa-

Table 311-1 Autoantibodies in Patients with SLE

	Incidence, %	Antigen Detected	Clinical Importance
Antinuclear antibodies	98	Multiple nuclear	Human cell substrates are more sensitive than murine. Repeatedly negative tests make SLE unlikely.
Anti-DNA	70	DNA (ds)	Anti-dsDNA is relatively disease-specific; anti-ssDNA is not. High titers are associated with nephritis and clinical activity in some patients.
Anti-Sm	30	Protein complexed to 6 species of small nuclear RNA	Specific for SLE.
Anti-RNP	40	Protein complexed to U1RNA	High titer in syndromes with features of polymyositis, lupus, scleroderma, and mixed connective tissue disease. If present in SLE without anti-DNA, risk for nephritis is low.
Anti-Ro (SS-A)	30	Protein complexed to y_1–y_5 RNA	Associated with Sjögren's syndrome, subacute cutaneous lupus, inherited C' deficiencies, ANA-negative lupus, lupus in the elderly, neonatal lupus, congenital heart block. Can cause nephritis.
Anti-La (SS-B)	10	Phosphoprotein	Always associated with anti-Ro. Risk for nephritis is low if present. Associated with Sjögren's syndrome.
Antihistone	70	Histones	More frequent in drug-induced LE (95%) than in spontaneous SLE.
Antiphospholipid	50	Phospholipids	Three types—lupus anticoagulant (LA), anticardiolipin (aCL), and false-positive test for syphilis (BFP). The LA and aCL (particular high-titer IgG) are associated with clotting, fetal loss, thrombocytopenia, and valvular heart disease. Antibodies to β_2-glycoprotein I are part of this group.
Antierythrocyte	60	Erythrocyte	A small proportion of these patients develop overt hemolysis.
Antiplatelet	30	Platelet surface + cytoplasm	Associated with thrombocytopenia in 15% of patients.
Antilymphocyte	70	Lymphocyte surface	Probably associated with leukopenia and abnormal T cell function.
Antineuronal	60	Neuronal and lymphocyte surface	In some series, high titers of IgG correlate with diffuse CNS lupus.
Antiribosomal P	20	Ribosomal P protein	In some series, antibody in serum correlates with psychosis or depression due to CNS SLE.

tients with SLE and can be disfiguring, since the lesions have central atrophy and scarring, with permanent loss of appendages. DLE lesions are circular with an erythematous raised rim, scaliness, follicular plugging, and telangiectasia. They occur over the scalp, ears, face, and sun-exposed areas of the arms, back, and chest. Only 5% of patients with DLE subsequently develop SLE. Less frequent SLE skin lesions include urticaria, bullae, erythema multiforme, lichen planus–like lesions, and panniculitis ("lupus profundus").

Patients with subacute cutaneous lupus erythematosus (SCLE) are a distinct subset with recurring extensive dermatitis. Arthritis and fatigue are frequent; central nervous system and renal involvement are not. Some patients are antinuclear antibody (ANA)–negative. Most have antibodies to Ro (SS-A) or to single-stranded (ss) DNA. Skin lesions are photosensitive and either annular or papulosquamous psoriasiform; they occur over the arms, trunk, and face but do not scar.

Patients with SLE, DLE, or SCLE can develop vasculitic skin lesions. These include purpura, subcutaneous nodules, nail fold infarcts, ulcers, vasculitic urticaria, panniculitis, and gangrene of digits. Shallow, slightly painful ulcers in the mouth and nose are frequent in patients with SLE.

Renal Manifestations Most patients with SLE have immunoglobulins deposited in glomeruli, but only one-half have clinical nephritis, defined by proteinuria. Early in the disease most are asymptomatic, although some develop the edema of nephrotic syndrome. Urinalysis shows hematuria, cylindruria, and proteinuria. Most patients with mesangial or mild focal proliferative nephritis (see discus-

sion under "Pathology," below) maintain good renal function. Patients with diffuse proliferative nephritis develop renal failure if untreated. Because severe nephritis requires aggressive immunosuppression with high-dose glucocorticoids and cytotoxic drugs and mild lesions do not, renal biopsy may provide information that affects therapy. Patients with rapidly deteriorating renal function and active urine sediment require prompt, aggressive therapy; biopsy is not necessary unless they fail to respond. However, patients with a slow rise in serum creatinine to levels >265 μmol/L (3 mg/dL) should be biopsied; a high proportion of sclerotic glomeruli on biopsy suggests that these patients are unlikely to respond to immunosuppressive therapies and are candidates for dialysis or transplantation. Patients with persistently abnormal urinalyses, high titers of anti-dsDNA, and/or hypocomplementemia are at risk for severe nephritis; kidney biopsy may guide therapy.

Nervous System Any region of the brain can be involved in SLE, as can the meninges, spinal cord, and cranial and peripheral nerves. Central nervous system (CNS) events may be single or multiple and often occur when SLE is active in other organ systems. Mild cognitive dysfunction is the most frequent manifestation. Headaches are common and may be migraine-like or nonspecific. Seizures of any type may occur. Less frequent manifestations include psychosis, acute confusional states, demyelinating disorders, cerebrovascular disease, movement disorders, aseptic meningitis, myelopathy, mononeuropathy or polyneuropathy of cranial or peripheral nerves, autonomic dysfunction, acute demyelinating polyneuropathy (Guillain-Barré), mood disorders, optic neuritis, subarachnoid hemorrhage, pseudotumor cer-

Table 311-2 Clinical Manifestations of SLE

	Percent of Patients Positive during Course of Disease		Percent of Patients Positive during Course of Disease
Systemic	95	Neurologic (Continued)	
Fatigue, malaise, fever, anorexia, nausea, weight loss		Aseptic meningitis	<1
		Myelopathy	<1
		Other (see text)	5
Musculoskeletal	95	Cardiopulmonary	60
Arthralgias/myalgias	95	Pleurisy	50
Nonerosive polyarthritis	60	Pericarditis	30
Hand deformities	10	Myocarditis	10
Myopathy/myositis	40/5	Endocarditis (Libman-Sacks)	10
Ischemic necrosis of bone	15	Valvular insufficiency	2
Cutaneous	80		
Malar rash	50	Coronary artery disease	8
Discoid rash	15		
Photosensitivity	70	Pleural effusions	30
Oral ulcers	40	Lupus pneumonitis	10
Other rashes—maculo-papular, urticarial, bul-lous, subacute cutaneous lupus	40	Interstitial fibrosis	5
		Pulmonary hypertension	<5
Alopecia	40	ARDS/hemorrhage	<5
Vasculitis	20	Renal	50
Panniculitis	5	Proteinuria >500 mg/24 h	50
Hematologic	85	Cellular casts	50
Anemia (of chronic disease)	70	Nephrotic syndrome	25
Hemolytic anemia	10	Renal failure	5–10
Leukopenia (<4000/mm³)	65	Gastrointestinal	45
Lymphopenia (<1500/mm³)	50	Nonspecific (anorexia, nausea, mild pain, diarrhea)	30
Thrombocytopenia (<100,000/mm³)	15	Vasculitis with bleeding or perforation	5
Circulating anticoagulant	10–20	Ascites	<5
Splenomegaly	15	Abnormal liver enzymes	40
Lymphadenopathy	20	Thrombosis	15
Neurologic	60	Venous	10
Cognitive dysfunction	50	Arterial	5
Mood disorder	40	Fetal loss	30 (of pregnancies)
Headache	25		
Seizures	20	Ocular	15
Mono- or polyneuropathy	15	Retinal vasculitis	5
Cerebrovascular disease	10	Conjunctivitis/episcleritis	10
Demyelinating syndrome	8		
Acute confusional state	5	Sicca syndrome	15
Movement disorder	2		

ebri, and hypothalamic dysfunction with inappropriate secretion of vasopressin. Depression and anxiety are frequent.

Laboratory diagnosis of CNS lupus can be difficult. Abnormal electroencephalograms occur in about 70% of patients with neurologic complaints and usually show diffuse slowing or focal abnormalities. Cerebrospinal fluid (CSF) shows elevated protein levels in 50% and increased mononuclear cells in 30% of patients; oligoclonal bands and increased Ig synthesis may be found. Lumbar puncture is recommended when the diagnosis of CNS lupus is in doubt or when infection is a possible cause of symptoms. Magnetic resonance imaging (MRI) with contrast is the most sensitive radiographic technique to detect acute and chronic lesions of SLE; changes are often nonspecific. Patients with focal neurologic lesions are more likely to have positive MRI scans than those with diffuse manifestations. Computed tomography (CT) scans are useful to rule out bleeding or mass lesions, if indicated. Angiograms can detect vasculitis and vascular occlusions or emboli; they cannot visualize vessels smaller than 50 μm; lupus vasculitis usually involves smaller vessels. Laboratory measures of disease activity often do not correlate with neurologic manifestations. Neurologic problems (with the exception of deficits resulting from large infarcts) usually improve with immunosuppressive therapy and/or time; recurrences are seen in approximately one-third of patients.

Vascular System Thrombosis in vessels of any size can be a major problem. Although vasculitis may underly thrombosis, there is increasing evidence that antibodies against phospholipids [lupus anticoagulant (LA), anti-cardiolipin (aCL)] are associated with clotting without inflammation. The source of cerebral emboli may be the lesions of Libman-Sacks endocarditis. In addition, degenerative vascular changes after years of exposure of blood vessels to circulating immune complexes and hyperlipidemia from glucocorticoid therapy predispose to degenerative cerebral and coronary artery disease in lupus patients. Therefore, anticoagulation is more appropriate than immunosuppression in some patients.

Hematologic Manifestation Anemia of chronic disease occurs in most patients when lupus is active. Hemolysis occurs in a small proportion of those with positive Coombs' tests; it is usually responsive to high-dose glucocorticoids; resistant cases may respond to splenectomy. Leukopenia (usually lymphopenia) is common but is rarely associated with recurrent infections and does not require treatment. Mild thrombocytopenia is common; severe thrombocytopenia with bleeding and purpura occurs in 5% of patients and should be treated with high-dose glucocorticoids. Short-term improvement can be achieved by administration of intravenous gamma globulin. If the platelet count fails to reach acceptable levels in 2 weeks, addition of cytotoxic drugs, cyclosporine, danazole, and/or splenectomy should be considered.

The LA belongs to a family of antiphospholipid antibodies. It is recognized by prolongation of the partial thromboplastin time and failure of added normal plasma to correct the prolongation. More sensitive tests include the Russell viper venom time. aCL are detected in enzyme-linked immunosorbent assays. Clinical manifestations of LA and aCL include thrombocytopenia, recurrent venous or arterial clotting, recurrent fetal loss, and valvular heart disease. If the LA is associated with hypoprothrombinemia or thrombocytopenia, bleeding may occur. Less commonly, antibodies to clotting factors (VIII, IX) arise; they cause bleeding. Bleeding syndromes usually respond to glucocorticoids; clotting syndromes do not.

Cardiopulmonary System Pericarditis is the most frequent manifestation of cardiac lupus; effusions can occur and occasionally lead to tamponade; constrictive pericarditis is rare. Myocarditis can cause arrhythmias, sudden death, and/or heart failure. Valvular insufficiency (usually aortic or mitral) can occur, with or without Libman-Sacks endocarditis. Lesions on valves are best detected by transesophageal echocardiography. Myocardial infarcts usually result from degenerative disease, although they can result from vasculitis.

Pleurisy and pleural effusions are common manifestations of SLE. Lupus pneumonitis causes fever, dyspnea, and cough; x-rays show

Table 311-3 The 1982 Criteria for Classification of Systemic Lupus Erythematosus, Updated 1997

1. Malar rash	Fixed erythema, flat or raised, over the malar eminences
2. Discoid rash	Erythematous raised patches with adherent keratotic scaling and follicular plugging; atrophic scarring may occur
3. Photosensitivity	Exposure to UV light causes rash
4. Oral ulcers	Includes oral and nasopharyngeal, observed by physician
5. Arthritis	Nonerosive arthritis involving two or more peripheral joints, characterized by tenderness, swelling, or effusion
6. Serositis	Pleuritis or pericarditis documented by ECG or rub or evidence of pericardial effusion
7. Renal disorder	Proteinuria > 0.5 g/d or > 3+, or cellular casts
8. Neurologic disorder	Seizures without other cause or psychosis without other cause
9. Hematologic disorder	Hemolytic anemia or leukopenia (< 4000/μL) or lymphopenia (< 1500/μL) or thrombocytopenia (< 100,000/μL) in the absence of offending drugs
10. Immunologic disorder	Anti-dsDNA, anti-Sm, and/or anti-phospholipid
11. Antinuclear antibodies	An abnormal titer of ANAs by immunofluorescence or an equivalent assay at any point in time in the absence of drugs known to induce ANAs

If four of these criteria are present at any time during the course of disease, a diagnosis of systemic lupus can be made with 98% specificity and 97% sensitivity.

SOURCE: Criteria published by EM Tan et al, Arthritis Rheum 25:1271, 1982; updated by MC Hochberg, Arthritis Rheum 40:1725, 1997.

fleeting infiltrates and/or areas of platelike atelectasis; this syndrome responds to glucocorticoids. However, *the most common cause of pulmonary infiltrates in patients with SLE is infection.* Interstitial pneumonitis leading to fibrosis occurs occasionally; the inflammatory phase may respond to treatment; the fibrosis does not. Pulmonary hypertension is an uncommon, grave manifestation of SLE. Infrequent pulmonary manifestations with high mortality rates include adult respiratory distress syndrome and massive intraalveolar hemorrhage.

Gastrointestinal System Common gastrointestinal (GI) symptoms include nausea, diarrhea, and vague discomfort. Symptoms may result from lupus peritonitis and may herald a flare of SLE. Vasculitis of the intestine is the most dangerous manifestation, presenting with acute crampy abdominal pain, vomiting, and diarrhea. Intestinal perforation can occur and usually requires immediate surgery. Patients with pseudoobstruction have abdominal pain; x-rays show dilated loops of small bowel which may be edematous; surgery should be avoided unless frank obstruction is present. Glucocorticoid therapy is useful for all these GI syndromes. Some patients have GI motility disorders similar to those in scleroderma; they are not benefited by steroids. Acute pancreatitis occurs and can be severe, resulting from active SLE or from therapy with glucocorticoids or azathioprine. Elevated amylase levels may reflect pancreatitis, salivary gland inflammation, or macroamylasemia. Elevated serum transaminase levels are common in patients with active SLE but are not associated with significant hepatic damage; they return to normal as the disease is treated.

Ocular Manifestation Retinal vasculitis is a serious manifestation; blindness can develop over a few days, and aggressive immunosuppression should be instituted. Examination shows areas of sheathed, narrow retinal arterioles and cytoid bodies (white exudates) adjacent to vessels. Other ocular abnormalities include conjunctivitis, episcleritis, optic neuritis, and the sicca syndrome.

PATHOLOGY **Cutaneous Lesions** Lesions of acute SLE, DLE, and SCLE show similar histopathology, with degeneration of the basal layer of the epidermis, disruption of the dermal-epidermal junction (DEJ), and mononuclear infiltrates around vessels and appendages in the upper dermis. In DLE, follicular plugging and hyper-

keratosis are prominent. Deposits of Ig and C' are seen in the DEJ in 80 to 100% of lesional and 50% of nonlesional skin in active SLE; the proportions are lower during remissions. Only 50% of SCLE lesions are positive for Ig and C' deposits. Ig deposition in the DEJ is not specific for SLE. Vasculitic skin lesions usually show leukocytoclastic angiitis.

Renal Lesions Glomerulonephritis (GN) is caused by deposition of circulating immune complexes or in situ complex formation in mesangium and glomerular basement membrane. Renal biopsy should be considered when results would affect therapy. Information regarding location of immune deposits, histologic pattern of renal damage, and activity and chronicity of lesions are all useful in predicting prognosis and selecting appropriate treatment. In mild GN unlikely to lead to renal failure, Ig deposits are confined to the mesangium, and histology shows no changes or mesangial proliferation. If Ig and C' are deposited outside the mesangium in capillary glomerular basement membrane, prognosis worsens. Histologic changes that should be treated with aggressive immunosuppression include focal proliferative, membranoproliferative, and diffuse proliferative GN (Chap. 275). Progression from focal to diffuse lesions can occur. Membranous changes without proliferation are uncommon but have a better prognosis than proliferative GN. Activity and chronicity scores indicate severity and reversibility of lesions. *Reversible "active" lesions* associated with high risk of progression to renal failure are glomerular necrosis, cellular epithelial crescents, hyaline thrombi, interstitial inflammatory infiltrates, and necrotizing vasculitis. *Irreversible changes unlikely to respond to immunosuppression* and highly associated with renal failure include glomerular sclerosis, fibrous crescents, interstitial fibrosis, and tubular atrophy. In patients with high chronicity scores, treatment of lupus should be determined by extrarenal disease.

LABORATORY MANIFESTATIONS The presence of characteristic antibodies (Table 311-1) confirms the diagnosis of SLE. ANAs are the best screening test. If the test substrate contains human nuclei (WIL-2 or HEP-2 cells), more than 95% of lupus patients will be positive. A positive ANA test is not specific for SLE; ANAs occur in some normal individuals (usually in low titer); the frequency increases with aging. Other autoimmune diseases, viral infections, chronic inflammatory processes, and several drugs induce ANAs. Therefore, a positive ANA test supports the diagnosis of SLE but is not specific; a negative ANA test makes the diagnosis unlikely but not impossible. Antibodies to double-stranded DNA (dsDNA) and to Sm are relatively specific for SLE; other autoantibodies listed in Table 311-1 are not. However, determining the complete autoantibody profile of each patient helps predict clinical subsets. High serum levels of ANAs and anti-dsDNA and low levels of complement usually reflect disease activity, especially in patients with nephritis. Total functional hemolytic complement (CH_{50}) levels are the most sensitive measure of complement activation but are also most subject to laboratory error. Quantitative levels of C3 and C4 are widely available. Very low levels of CH_{50} with normal levels of C3 suggest inherited deficiency of a complement component, which is highly associated with SLE and with ANA negativity.

Hematologic abnormalities include anemia (usually normochromic normocytic but occasionally hemolytic), leukopenia, lymphopenia, and thrombocytopenia. The Westergren erythrocyte sedimentation rate correlates with disease activity in some patients.

Urinalysis should be performed and serum creatinine levels should be measured periodically in patients with SLE. With active nephritis, the urinalysis usually shows proteinuria, hematuria, and cellular or granular casts. Urinary protein excretion measured over 24 h increases during periods of activity. (See the discussion under "Pathology" for a description of renal biopsy.)

PREGNANCY Fertility rates are normal in patients with SLE, but spontaneous abortion and stillbirths are frequent (10 to 30%), especially in women with LA and/or aCL. The treatment of choice for pregnant women with prior fetal loss and antiphospholipid antibodies

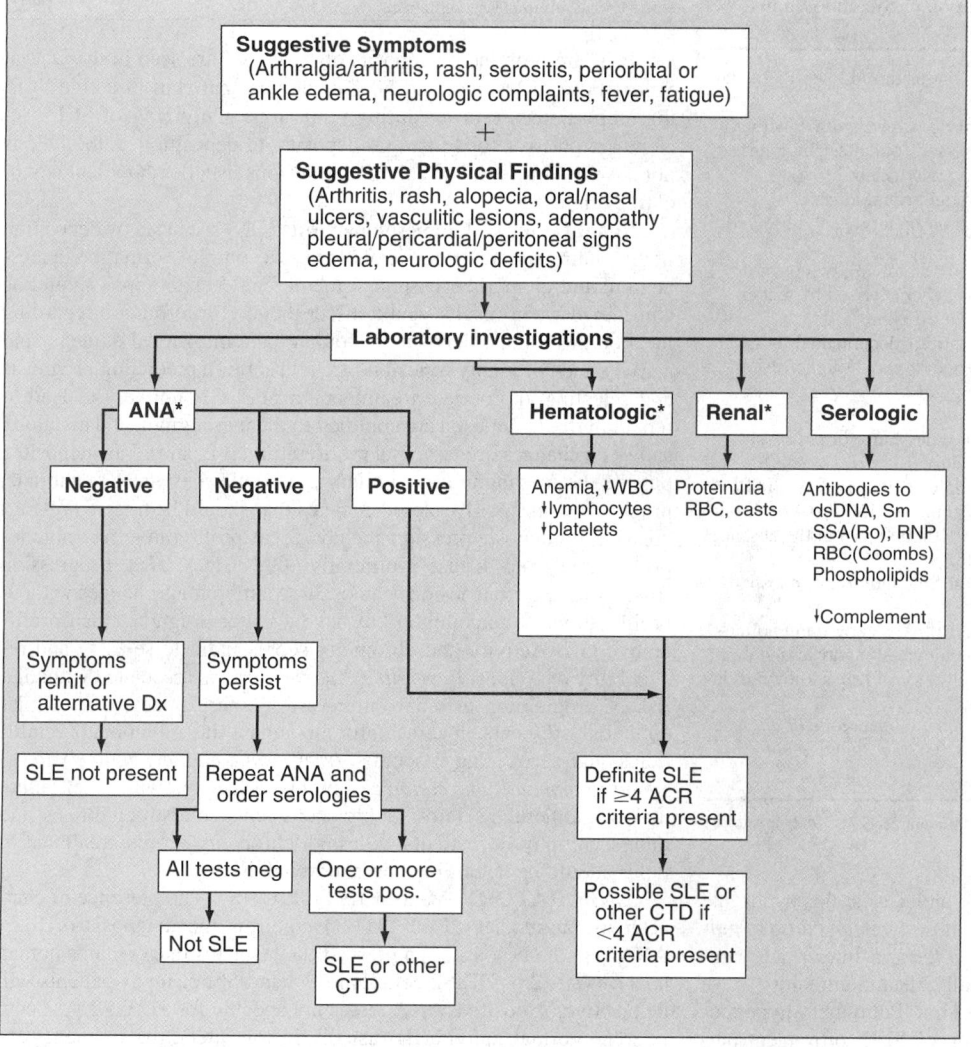

FIGURE 311-1 Algorithm for the diagnosis of SLE. ANA, antinuclear antibody; ACR, American College of Rheumatology; CTD, connective tissue disease; WBC, white blood cell count; RBC, red blood cell count, *, recommended in initial evaluation.

of SLE, rheumatoid arthritis, polymyositis, and scleroderma, accompanied by high titers of anti-ribonucleoprotein antibodies (Chap. 313); patients have a low incidence of nephritis and CNS disease and a high incidence of pulmonary manifestations and evolution into scleroderma. The possibility of drug-induced lupus should always be considered. Figure 311-1 presents an algorithm for diagnosis of SLE.

DRUG-INDUCED LUPUS Several drugs can cause a syndrome resembling SLE, including procainamide, hydralazine, isoniazid, chlorpromazine, D-penicillamine, practolol, methyldopa, quinidine, interferon α, and possibly hydantoin, ethosuximide, and oral contraceptives. The syndrome is rare with all but procainamide, the most frequent offender, and hydralazine. There is genetic predisposition to drug-induced lupus, partly determined by drug acetylation rates. Procainamide induces ANA in 50 to 75% of individuals within a few months; hydralazine induces ANA in 25 to 30%. Between 10 and 20% of ANA-positive individuals develop lupus-like symptoms. Most common are systemic complaints and arthralgias; polyarthritis and pleuropericarditis occur in 25 to 50%. Renal and CNS involvement are rare. All patients have ANA and most have antibodies to histones. Antibodies to dsDNA and hypocomplementemia are rare—a helpful point in distinguishing drug-induced from idiopathic lupus. Anemia, leukopenia, LA, aCL, thrombocytopenia, cryoglobulins, rheumatoid factors, false-positive VDRL, and positive direct Coombs' tests can occur. The initial therapeutic approach is withdrawal of the offending drug; most patients improve in a few weeks. If symptoms are severe, a short course (2 to 10 weeks) of glucocorticoids is indicated. Symptoms rarely persist more than 6 months; ANA may persist for years. Most lupus-inducing drugs can be used safely in patients with idiopathic SLE.

PROGNOSIS Survival in patients with SLE is 90 to 95% at 2 years, 82 to 90% at 5 years, 71 to 80% at 10 years, and 63 to 75% at 20 years. The following factors have been associated with poor prognosis (approximately 50% mortality in 10 years): high serum creatinine levels [>124 μmol/L(>1.4 mg/dL)], hypertension, nephrotic syndrome (24-h urine protein excretion >2.6 g), anemia [hemoglobin < 124 g/L(<12.4g/dL)], hypoalbuminemia and hypocomplementemia at the time of diagnosis, and low socioeconomic status. Other factors associated with a poor prognosis in most studies include thrombocytopenia, serious CNS involvement, antibodies to phospholipids, and African American race. Disability in SLE patients is common. However, approximately 20% of patients experience disease remissions (usually transient), and the likelihood of remission increases with each decade after diagnosis. Infections and active SLE, especially renal failure, are the leading causes of death in the first decade of disease. Thromboembolic events are frequent causes of death in the second decade.

℞ **TREATMENT** There is no cure for SLE. Complete sustained remissions are rare. Therefore, patient and physician should plan to control acute, severe flares and to develop maintenance strategies

is low-dose heparin, e.g., 5000 units subcutaneously twice a day. This may be associated with maternal bone loss. If there are contraindications to heparin therapy, low-dose aspirin or low- to moderate-dose glucocorticoids may be used.

Pregnancy has varied effects on SLE activity. Disease flares in a small proportion, especially during the 6 weeks postpartum. If severe renal or cardiac disease is absent and SLE activity is controlled, most patients complete pregnancy safely and deliver normal infants. Glucocorticoids (except dexamethasone and betamethasone) are inactivated by placental enzymes and do not cause fetal abnormalities in humans; they should be used to suppress disease activity. Neonatal lupus, caused by transmission of maternal anti-Ro across the placenta, consists of transient skin rash and (rarely) permanent heart block. Transient thrombocytopenia from maternal antiplatelet antibodies also occurs.

DIFFERENTIAL DIAGNOSIS The American Rheumatism Association published diagnostic criteria for SLE (Table 311-3) which were updated in 1997. Any four of the manifestations listed establish a diagnosis of SLE. Early disease confined to a few systems is more difficult to classify; it may take several years for a patient to fulfill criteria. Disorders with which SLE can be confused include rheumatoid arthritis; various forms of dermatitis; neurologic disorders such as epilepsy, multiple sclerosis, and psychiatric disorders; and hematologic diseases such as idiopathic thrombocytopenic purpura. Many autoimmune disorders have overlapping features so that exact classification may be difficult. Mixed connective tissue disease has features in which symptoms are suppressed to an acceptable level, usually at the cost of some drug side effects. Approximately 25% of SLE patients have mild disease with no life-threatening manifestations, although pain and fatigue may be disabling. These patients should be managed without glucocorticoids. Arthralgias, arthritis, myalgias, fever, and mild serositis may improve on nonsteroidal anti-inflammatory drugs (NSAIDs) including salicylates. However, NSAID toxicities such as elevated serum transaminases, aseptic meningitis, and renal impairment are especially frequent in SLE. The role of NSAIDs, which are primarily COX-2 inhibitors, in treatment of SLE has not been studied; they are likely to be useful. The dermatitides of SLE, fatigue, and lupus arthritis may respond to antimalarials. Doses of 400 mg hydroxychloroquine daily may improve skin lesions in a few weeks. Side effects are uncommon and include retinal toxicity, rash, myopathy, and neuropathy. Regular ophthalmologic examinations should be performed at least annually, since retinal toxicity is related to cumulative dose. Other therapies include sunscreens (an SPF rating ≥ 15 is recommended), topical or intralesional glucocorticoids, quinacrine, retinoids, and dapsone. Recent studies suggest that daily oral doses of dihydroepiandrosterone may lower disease activity in patients with mild SLE. Systemic glucocorticoids should be reserved for patients with disabling disease unresponsive to these conservative measures.

Life-threatening, severely disabling manifestations of SLE that are responsive to immunosuppression should be treated with high doses of *glucocorticoids* (1 to 2 mg/kg per day). When disease is active, glucocorticoids should be given in divided doses every 8 to 12 h. After the disease is controlled, therapy should be consolidated to one morning dose; thereafter the daily dose should be tapered as rapidly as clinical disease permits. Ideally, patients should be slowly converted to alternate-day therapy with a single morning dose of short-acting glucocorticoid (prednisone, prednisolone, methylprednisolone) to minimize side effects. However, the disease may flare on the day off steroids, in which case the lowest single daily dose that suppresses disease should be used. Acutely ill lupus patients, including those with proliferative GN, can be treated with 3 to 5 days of 1000 mg intravenous "pulses" of methylprednisolone, followed by maintenance daily or alternate-day glucocorticoids. Disease flares are probably controlled more rapidly by this approach, but it is unclear whether long-term outcome is changed.

Undesirable effects of chronic glucocorticoid therapy include cushingoid habitus, weight gain, hypertension, infection, capillary fragility, acne, hirsutism, accelerated osteoporosis, ischemic necrosis of bone, cataracts, glaucoma, diabetes mellitus, myopathy, hypokalemia, irregular menses, irritability, insomnia, and psychosis. Prednisone doses of 15 mg daily (or less) given before noon usually do not suppress the hypothalamic-pituitary axis. Some side effects can be minimized; sustained hyperglycemia, hypertension, edema, and hypokalemia should be treated; infections should be identified and treated early; immunizations with influenza and pneumococcal vaccines are safe if disease is stable. To minimize osteoporosis, supplemental calcium (1000 mg daily) should be added in most patients; in those with 24-h urinary calcium excretion <120 mg, vitamin D, 50,000 units one to three times weekly, can be added (monitor for hypercalcemia). Estrogen replacement therapy (ERT) should be considered at menopause. There is debate regarding the ability of oral contraceptives or ERT to cause flares of SLE in some patients; these therapies should be withheld from patients with a history of thrombosis. Calcitonin and bisphosphonates (alendronate, didronel, or acetonel) are also useful in preventing and treating osteoporosis.

The use of *cytotoxic agents* (azathioprine, chlorambucil, cyclophosphamide, methotrexate, mycophenolate mofetil) in SLE is probably beneficial in controlling active disease, reducing the rate of disease flares, and reducing steroid requirements. Patients with lupus nephritis have significantly less renal failure and better survival if treated with combinations of glucocorticoids plus intravenous cyclophosphamide; azathioprine as the second drug is less beneficial but is also effective in preventing renal failure. Open trials suggest that mycophenolate, and possibly methotrexate, are also effective second

FIGURE 311-2 Algorithm for the treatment of SLE. GC, glucocorticoids; high-dose GC, methylprednisolone 1000 mg, IV, qd × 3, then 1 to 2 mg/kg prednisone per day orally, or 1 to 2 mg/kg prednisone per day orally; cytotox, cytotoxic drugs such as cyclophosphamide (Cy) and azathioprine (Aza); qod, alternate day therapy; NSAIDs, nonsteroidal anti-inflammatory agents.

drugs and sometimes benefit patients who fail to respond to cyclophosphamide plus glucocorticoids. Undesirable side effects of cytotoxic drugs include bone marrow suppression, increased infection with opportunistic organisms such as herpes zoster, irreversible ovarian failure, hepatotoxicity (azathioprine, methotrexate, and mycophenolate), bladder toxicity (cyclophosphamide), alopecia, and increased risk for malignancy. Azathioprine is the least toxic; recommended doses are 2 to 3 mg/kg per day orally. Cyclophosphamide is the most effective and the most toxic. Intravenous pulse doses (10 to 15 mg/kg) once every 4 weeks have less urinary bladder toxicity than daily oral doses. Cyclophosphamide can also be used in daily oral doses (1.5 to 2.5 mg/kg per day of each). Mycophenolate can be given orally (1 to 2.5 g a day in divided doses) or methotrexate (5 to 20 mg once a week, orally or subcutaneously). After disease activity has been controlled for a few months, tapering of cytotoxic agents and attempts to discontinue them are appropriate. Figure 311-2 presents an algorithm for treatment of SLE.

Some manifestations of SLE do not respond to immunosuppression, including clotting disorders, some behavioral abnormalities, and end-stage GN. Anticoagulation is the therapy of choice for prevention of clotting; chronic warfarin therapy in relatively high doses (maintaining INR at 2.5 to 3.0) is effective in preventing venous and arterial clotting in patients with antiphospholipid syndromes; the effects of aspirin, ticlopidine, and heparin on arterial thrombosis are unclear. Psychoactive drugs should be used when appropriate. "Pure" membranous GN may not respond to immunosuppression; several weeks of therapy can be tried but should be abandoned if improvement is not obvious. With regard to renal transplantation, patients with SLE have about twice the rate of allograft failure as do patients with renal failure due to other diseases; the 5-year rate of allograft loss is about 50%. However, overall patient survival is good, >90% at 5 years.

Alternatives to therapy with glucocorticoids plus cytotoxic agents for patients who do not respond to or cannot tolerate these regimens include addition of high-dose intravenous pulse therapy with methylprednisolone, which is ultimately converted to daily prednisone, plus cyclophosphamide, and combinations of cytotoxic drugs; there is some evidence for efficacy of high-dose intravenous glucocorticoids plus intravenous cyclophosphamide and of azathioprine plus cyclophosphamide. All of these regimens increase infection rates. Less well studied, but effective in some patients, are plasmapheresis (which must be accompanied by cytotoxic treatment to prevent rebound of undesirable autoantibodies), cyclosporine, and intravenous immunoglobulin. Experimental therapies in progress include studies of efficacy of inducing tolerance to DNA, interruption of T and B cell second signals with antibodies to CD40L, and immunoablation with high-dose cyclophosphamide with or without autologous stem cell transplantation.

BIBLIOGRAPHY

AMERICAN COLLEGE OF RHEUMATOLOGY: Ad Hoc Committee on Neuropsychiatric Lupus Nomenclature: The American College of Rheumatology nomenclature and case definitions for neuropsychiatric lupus syndromes. Arthritis Rheum 42:599, 1999. [For definitions: Internet: www.rheumatology.org Click on Arthritis Rheum. Click on Appendix A: Case definitions for neuropsychiatric syndromes in SLE.]

AUSTIN HA, BALOW JE: Natural history and treatment of lupus nephritis. Semin Nephrol 19:2, 1999

BANSAL VK, BETO JA: Treatment of lupus nephritis: A meta-analysis of clinical trials. Am J Kidney Dis 29:193, 1997

BOUMPAS DT et al: Systemic lupus erythematosus: Emerging concepts. Part 1: Renal, neuropsychiatric, cardiovascular, pulmonary and hematologic disease. Part 2: Dermatologic and joint disease, the antiphospholipid antibody syndrome, pregnancy and hormonal therapy, morbidity and mortality, and pathogenesis. Ann Intern Med 123: 42, 940, 1995

COWCHOCK S: Treatment of antiphospholipid syndrome in pregnancy. Lupus 7(Suppl 2): S95, 1998

HAHN BH: Mechanisms of disease: Antibodies to DNA. N Engl J Med 338:1359, 1998

HARLEY JB et al: The genetics of human systemic lupus erythematosus. Curr Opin Immunol 10:690, 1998

KIMBERLY RP: Glucocorticoids. Curr Opin Rheumatol 6:273, 1994

QUISMORIO FP JR: Clinical application of serologic abnormalities in systemic lupus erythematosus, in Dubois' Lupus Erythematosus, 5th ed, DJ Wallace, BH Hahn (eds). Baltimore, Williams & Wilkins, 1997, pp. 925–942

STONE JH et al: Outcome of renal transplantation in ninety-seven cyclosporine-era patients with systemic lupus erythematosus and matched controls. Arthritis Rheum 41:1438, 1998

TUMLIN JA: Lupus nephritis: Novel immunosuppressive modalities and future directions. Semin Nephrol 19:67, 1999

WARD MM et al: Long-term survival in systemic lupus erythematosus: Patient characteristics associated with poorer outcomes. Arthritis Rheum 38:274, 1995

WERTH VP et al: Pathogenetic mechanisms and treatment of cutaneous lupus erythematosus. Curr Opin Rheumatol 9:400, 1997

RHEUMATOID ARTHRITIS

Cox cyclooxygenase	IFN interferon
CSIs Cox-2-specific inhibitors	IL interleukin
DMARDs disease-modifying antirheumatic drugs	NSAIDs nonsteroidal anti-inflammatory drugs
EBV Epstein-Barr virus	RA rheumatoid arthritis
GM-CSF granulocyte-macrophage colony stimulating factor	TGF-β transforming growth factor β
	TNF tumor necrosis factor

Rheumatoid arthritis (RA) is a chronic multisystem disease of unknown cause. Although there are a variety of systemic manifestations, the characteristic feature of RA is persistent inflammatory synovitis, usually involving peripheral joints in a symmetric distribution. The potential of the synovial inflammation to cause cartilage destruction and bone erosions and subsequent changes in joint integrity is the hallmark of the disease. Despite its destructive potential, the course of RA can be quite variable. Some patients may experience only a mild oligoarticular illness of brief duration with minimal joint damage, whereas others will have a relentless progressive polyarthritis with marked functional impairment.

EPIDEMIOLOGY AND GENETICS   The prevalence of RA is approximately 0.8% of the population (range 0.3 to 2.1%); women are affected approximately three times more often than men. The prevalence increases with age, and sex differences diminish in the older age group. RA is seen throughout the world and affects all races. However, the incidence and severity seem to be less in rural sub-Saharan Africa and in Caribbean blacks. The onset is most frequent during the fourth and fifth decades of life, with 80% of all patients developing the disease between the ages of 35 and 50. The incidence of RA is more than six times as great in 60- to 64-year-old women compared to 18- to 29-year-old women.

Family studies indicate a genetic predisposition. For example, severe RA is found at approximately four times the expected rate in first-degree relatives of individuals with disease associated with the presence of the autoantibody, rheumatoid factor; approximately 10% of patients with RA will have an affected first-degree relative. Moreover, monozygotic twins are at least four times more likely to be concordant for RA than dizygotic twins, who have a similar risk of developing RA as nontwin siblings. Only 15 to 20% of monozygotic twins are concordant for RA, however, implying that factors other than genetics play an important etiopathogenic role. Of note, the highest risk for concordance of RA is noted in twins who have two HLA-DRB1 alleles known to be associated with RA. The class II major histocompatibility complex allele HLA-DR4. (DRB1*0401) and related alleles are known to be major genetic risk factors for RA. Early studies showed that as many as 70% of patients with classic or definite RA express HLA-DR4 compared with 28% of control individuals. An association with HLA-DR4 has been noted in many populations, including North American and European whites, Chippewa Indians, Japanese, and native populations in India, Mexico, South America, and southern China. In a number of groups, including Israeli Jews, Asian Indians, and Yakima Indians of North America, however, there is no association between the development of RA and HLA-DR4. In these individuals, there is an association between RA and HLA-DR1 in the former two groups and HLA-Dw16 in the latter. Molecular analysis of HLA-DR antigens has provided insight into these apparently disparate findings. The HLA-DR molecule is composed of two chains, a nonpolymorphic α chain and a highly polymorphic β chain. Allelic variations in the HLA-DR molecule reflect differences in the amino acids of the β chain, with the major amino acid changes occurring in the three hypervariable regions of the molecule. Each of the HLA-DR molecules that is associated with RA has the same or a very similar sequence of amino acids in the third hypervariable region of the β chain of the molecule. Thus the β chains of the HLA-DR molecules associated with RA, including HLA-Dw4 (DRβ1*0401), HLA-Dw14 (DRβ1*0404), HLA-Dw15 (DRβ1*0405), HLA-DR1 (DRβ1*0101), and HLA-Dw16 (DRβ1*1402), contain the same amino acids at positions 67 through 74, with the exception of a single change of one basic amino acid for another (arginine $\rightarrow$ lysine) in position 71 of HLA-Dw4. All other HLA-DR β chains have amino acid changes in this region that alter either their charge or hydrophobicity. These results indicate that a particular amino acid sequence in the third hypervariable region of the HLA-DR molecule is a major genetic element conveying susceptibility to RA, regardless of whether it occurs in HLA-DR4, HLA-Dw16, or HLA-DR1. It has been estimated that the risk of developing RA in a person with HLA-Dw4 (DRβ1*0401) or HLA-Dw14 (DRβ1*0404) is 1 in 35 and 1 in 20, respectively, whereas the presence of both alleles puts persons at an even greater risk. The lack of association of HLA-DR4 and RA in certain populations is explained by the major member of the DR4 family found in that population. HLA-DR4 is a family of closely related, serologically defined molecules, including HLA-Dw4, -Dw10, -Dw13, and -Dw15. Different members of the HLA-DR family of molecules are found to predominate in different ethnic groups. Thus, in HLA-DR4–positive North American whites, HLA-Dw4 and -Dw14 are the most frequent, whereas HLA-Dw15 is most frequent in Japanese and southern Chinese. Each of these is associated with RA. By contrast, HLA-Dw10, which is not associated with RA and contains nonconservative amino acid changes in positions 70 and 71 of the β chain, is most common in Israeli Jews. Therefore, HLA-DR4 is not associated with RA in this population. In certain groups of patients, there does not appear to be a clear association between HLA-DR4–related epitopes and RA. Thus, nearly 75% of African American RA patients do not have this genetic element. Moreover, there is an association with HLA-DR10 (DRB1*1001) in Spanish and Italian patients, with HLA-DR9 (DRB1*0901) in Chileans, and with HLA-DR3 (DRB1*0301) in Arab populations.

Additional genes in the HLA-D complex may also convey altered susceptibility to RA. Certain HLA-DR alleles, including HLA-DR5 (DRB1*1101), HLA-DR2 (DRB1*1501), HLA-DR3 (DRB1*0301), and HLA-DR7 (DRB1*0701), may protect against the development of RA in that they tend to be found at lower frequency in RA patients than in controls. Moreover, the HLA-DQ alleles, DQB1*0301 and DQB1*0302, that are in linkage disequilibrium with HLA-DR4 and DQB1*0501, have also been associated with RA. This has raised the possibility that HLA-DQ alleles may represent the actual RA susceptibility genes, whereas specific HLA-DR alleles may convey protection. In this model, the complement of HLA-DR and DQ alleles determines RA susceptibility. Disease manifestations have also been associated with HLA phenotype. Thus, early aggressive disease and extraarticular manifestations are more frequent in patients with DRB1*0401 or DRB1*0404, and more slowly progressive disease in those with DRB1*0101. The presence of both DRB1*0401 and DRB1*0404 appears to increase the risk for both aggressive articular and extraarticular disease. It has been estimated that HLA genes contribute only a portion of the genetic susceptibility to RA. Thus genes outside the HLA complex also contribute. These include genes controlling the expression of the antigen receptor on T cells and both immunoglobulin heavy and light chains. Moreover, polymorphisms in the tumor necrosis factor (TNF) α and the interleukin (IL) 10 genes are also associated with RA, as is a region on chromosome 3 (3q13).

Genetic risk factors do not fully account for the incidence of RA, suggesting that environmental factors also play a role in the etiology of the disease. This is emphasized by epidemiologic studies in Africa that have indicated that climate and urbanization have a major impact on the incidence and severity of RA in groups of similar genetic background.

ETIOLOGY The cause of RA remains unknown. It has been suggested that RA might be a manifestation of the response to an infectious agent in a genetically susceptible host. Because of the worldwide distribution of RA, it has been hypothesized that if an infectious agent is involved, the organism must be ubiquitous. A number

of possible causative agents have been suggested, including *Mycoplasma*, Epstein-Barr virus (EBV), cytomegalovirus, parvovirus, and rubella virus, but convincing evidence that these or other infectious agents cause RA has not emerged. The process by which an infectious agent might cause chronic inflammatory arthritis with a characteristic distribution also remains a matter of controversy. One possibility is that there is persistent infection of articular structures or retention of microbial products in the synovial tissues which generates a chronic inflammatory response. Alternatively, the microorganism or response to the microorganism might induce an immune response to components of the joint by altering its integrity and revealing antigenic peptides. In this regard, reactivity to type II collagen and heat shock proteins has been demonstrated. Another possibility is that the infecting microorganism might prime the host to cross-reactive determinants expressed within the joint as a result of "molecular mimicry." Recent evidence of similarity between products of certain gram-negative bacteria and EBV and the HLA-DR4 molecule itself has supported this possibility. Finally, products of infecting microorganisms might induce the disease. Recent work has focused on the possible role of "superantigens" produced by a number of microorganisms, including staphylococci, streptococci and *M. arthritidis*. Superantigens are proteins with the capacity to bind to HLA-DR molecules and particular V_β segments of the heterodimeric T cell receptor and stimulate specific T cells expressing the V_β gene products (Chap. 305). The role of superantigens in the etiology of RA remains speculative. Of all the potential environmental triggers, the only one clearly associated with the development of RA is cigarette smoking.

PATHOLOGY AND PATHOGENESIS Microvascular injury and an increase in the number of synovial lining cells appear to be the earliest lesions in rheumatoid synovitis. The nature of the insult causing this response is not known. Subsequently, an increased number of synovial lining cells is seen along with perivascular infiltration with mononuclear cells. Before the onset of clinical symptoms, the perivascular infiltrate is predominantly composed of myeloid cells, whereas in symptomatic arthritis, T cells can also be found, although their number does not appear to correlate with symptoms. As the process continues, the synovium becomes edematous and protrudes into the joint cavity as villous projections.

Light-microscopic examination discloses a characteristic constellation of features, which include hyperplasia and hypertrophy of the synovial lining cells; focal or segmental vascular changes, including microvascular injury, thrombosis, and neovascularization; edema; and infiltration with mononuclear cells, often collected into aggregates around small blood vessels (Fig. 312-1). The endothelial cells of the rheumatoid synovium have the appearance of high endothelial venules of lymphoid organs and have been altered by cytokine exposure to facilitate entry of cells into tissue. Rheumatoid synovial endothelial cells express increased amounts of various adhesion molecules involved in this process. Although this pathologic picture is typical of RA, it can also be seen in a variety of other chronic inflammatory arthritides. The mononuclear cell collections are variable in composition and size. The predominant infiltrating cell is the T lymphocyte. CD4+ T cells predominate over CD8+ T cells and are frequently found in close proximity to HLA-DR+ macrophages and dendritic cells. Increased numbers of a separate population of T cells expressing the $\gamma\delta$ form of the T cell receptor have also been found in the synovium, although they remain a minor population there and their role in RA has not been delineated. The major population of T cells in the rheumatoid synovium is composed of CD4+ memory T cells that form the majority of cells aggregated around postcapillary venules. Scattered throughout the tissue are CD8+ T cells. Both populations express the early activation antigen, CD69. Besides the accumulation of T cells, rheumatoid synovitis is also characterized by the infiltration of variable numbers of B cells and antibody-producing plasma cells. In advanced disease, structures similar to germinal centers of secondary lymphoid organs may be observed in the synovium. Both polyclonal immuno-

FIGURE 312-1 Histology of rheumatoid synovitis. *A.* The characteristic features of rheumatoid inflammation with hyperplasia of the lining layer *(arrow)* and mononuclear infiltrates in the sublining layer *(double arrow)*. *B.* A higher magnification of the largely CD4+ T cell infiltrate around postcapillary venules *(arrow)*.

globulin and the autoantibody rheumatoid factor are produced within the synovial tissue, which leads to the local formation of immune complexes. Finally, the synovial fibroblasts in RA manifest evidence of activation in that they produce a number of enzymes such as collagenase and cathepsins that can degrade components of the articular matrix. These activated fibroblasts are particularly prominent in the lining layer and at the interface with bone and cartilage. Osteoclasts are also prominent at sites of bone erosion.

The rheumatoid synovium is characterized by the presence of a number of secreted products of activated lymphocytes, macrophages, and fibroblasts. The local production of these cytokines and chemokines appears to account for many of the pathologic and clinical manifestations of RA. These effector molecules include those that are derived from T lymphocytes such as interleukin IL-2, interferon (IFN) γ, IL-6, IL-10, granulocyte-macrophage colony stimulating factor (GM-CSF), TNF-α, transforming growth factor β (TGF-β); IL-13, IL-16, and IL-17; those originating from activated myeloid cells, including IL-1, TNF-α, IL-6, IL-8, IL-10, IL-12, GM-CSF, macrophage CSF, platelet-derived growth factor, insulin-like growth factor, and TGF-β; as well as those secreted by other cell types in the synovium, such as fibroblasts and endothelial cells, including IL-1, IL-6, IL-8, GM-CSF, IL-15, IL-16, IL-18, and macrophage CSF. The activity of these chemokines and cytokines appears to account for many of the features of rheumatoid synovitis, including the synovial tissue inflammation, synovial fluid inflammation, synovial proliferation, and cartilage and bone damage, as well as the systemic manifestations of RA. In addition to the production of effector molecules that propagate the inflammatory process, local factors are produced that tend to slow the inflammation, including specific inhibitors of cytokine action and additional cytokines, such as TGF-β, which inhibits many of the features of rheumatoid synovitis including T cell activation and proliferation, B cell differentiation, and migration of cells into the inflammatory site.

These findings have suggested that the propagation of RA is an immunologically mediated event, although the original initiating stimulus has not been characterized. One view is that the inflammatory process in the tissue is driven by the CD4+ T cells infiltrating the synovium. Evidence for this includes (1) the predominance of CD4+ T cells in the synovium; (2) the increase in soluble IL-2 receptors, a product of activated T cells, in blood and synovial fluid of patients with active RA; and (3) amelioration of the disease by removal of T cells by thoracic duct drainage or peripheral lymphapheresis or suppression of their function by drugs, such as cyclosporine or nonde-

pleting monoclonal antibodies to CD4. In addition, the association of RA with certain HLA-DR or -DQ alleles, whose only known functions are to shape the repertoire of CD4+ T cells during ontogeny in the thymus and bind and present antigenic peptides to CD4+ T cells in the periphery, strongly implies a role for CD4+ T cells in the pathogenesis of the disease. Finally, patients with established RA who become infected with HIV also have been noted to improve, although this has not been a uniform finding. Within the rheumatoid synovium, the CD4+ T cells differentiate predominantly into Th1-like effector cells producing the proinflammatory cytokine IFN-γ and appear to be deficient in differentiation into Th2-like effector cells capable of producing the anti-inflammatory cytokine IL-4. As a result of the ongoing secretion of IFN-γ without the regulatory influences of IL-4, macrophages are activated to produce the proinflammatory cytokines IL-1 and TNF-α and also increase expression of HLA molecules. Moreover, T lymphocytes express surface molecules such as CD154 (CD40 ligand) and also produce a variety of cytokines that promote B cell proliferation and differentiation into antibody-forming cells and therefore also may promote local B cell stimulation. The resultant production of immunoglobulin and rheumatoid factor can lead to immune-complex formation with consequent complement activation and exacerbation of the inflammatory process by the production of the anaphylatoxins, C3a and C5a, and the chemotactic factor C5a. The tissue inflammation is reminiscent of delayed type hypersensitivity reactions occurring in response to soluble antigens or microorganisms, although it has become clear that the number of T cells producing cytokines such as IFN-γ is less than is found in typical delayed type hypersensitivity reactions, perhaps owing to the large amount of reactive oxygen species produced locally in the synovium that can dampen T cell function. It remains unclear whether the persistent T cell activity represents a response to a persistent exogenous antigen or to altered autoantigens such as collagen, immunoglobulin, or one of the heat shock proteins, or perhaps both. Alternatively, it could represent persistent responsiveness to activated autologous cells such as might occur as a result of EBV infection or persistent response to a foreign antigen or superantigen in the synovial tissue. Finally, rheumatoid inflammation could reflect persistent stimulation of T cells by synovial-derived antigens that cross-react with determinants introduced during antecedent exposure to foreign antigens or infectious microorganisms.

Overriding the chronic inflammation in the synovial tissue is an acute inflammatory process in the synovial fluid. The exudative synovial fluid contains more polymorphonuclear leukocytes than mononuclear cells. A number of mechanisms play a role in stimulating the exudation of synovial fluid. Locally produced immune complexes can activate complement and generate anaphylatoxins and chemotactic factors. Local production, by a variety of cells, of chemokines and cytokines with chemotactic activity as well as inflammatory mediators such as leukotriene B4 and products of complement activation can attract neutrophils. Moreover, many of these same agents can also stimulate the endothelial cells of postcapillary venules to become more efficient at binding circulating cells. The net result is the enhanced migration of polymorphonuclear leukocytes into the synovial site. In addition, vasoactive mediators such as histamine produced by the mast cells that infiltrate the rheumatoid synovium may also facilitate the exudation of inflammatory cells into the synovial fluid. Finally, the vasodilatory effects of locally produced prostaglandin E2 may also facilitate entry of inflammatory cells into the inflammatory site. Once in the synovial fluid, the polymorphonuclear leukocytes can ingest immune complexes, with the resultant production of reactive oxygen metabolites and other inflammatory mediators, further adding to the inflammatory milieu. Locally produced cytokines and chemokines can additionally stimulate polymorphonuclear leukocytes. The production of large amounts of cyclooxygenase and lipoxygenase pathway products of arachidonic acid metabolism by cells in the synovial fluid and tissue further accentuates the signs and symptoms of inflammation.

The precise mechanism by which bone and cartilage destruction occurs has not been completely resolved. Although the synovial fluid contains a number of enzymes potentially able to degrade cartilage, the majority of destruction occurs in juxtaposition to the inflamed synovium, or pannus, that spreads to cover the articular cartilage. This vascular granulation tissue is composed of proliferating fibroblasts, small blood vessels, and a variable number of mononuclear cells and produces a large amount of degradative enzymes, including collagenase and stromelysin, that may facilitate tissue damage. The cytokines IL-1 and TNF-α play an important role by stimulating the cells of the pannus to produce collagenase and other neutral proteases. These same two cytokines also activate chondrocytes in situ, stimulating them to produce proteolytic enzymes that can degrade cartilage locally and also inhibiting synthesis of new matrix molecules. Finally, these two cytokines may contribute to the local demineralization of bone by activating osteoclasts that accumulate at the site of local bone resorption. Prostaglandin E_2 produced by fibroblasts and macrophages may also contribute to bone demineralization. The common final pathway of bone erosion is likely to involve the activation of osteoclasts that are present in large numbers at these sites. Systemic manifestations of RA can be accounted for by release of inflammatory effector molecules from the synovium. These include IL-1, TNF-α, and IL-6, which account for many of the manifestations of active RA, including malaise, fatigue, and elevated levels of serum acute-phase reactants. The importance of TNF-α in producing these manifestations is emphasized by the prompt amelioration of symptoms following administration of a monoclonal antibody to TNF-α or a soluble TNF-α receptor Ig construct to patients with RA. In addition, immune complexes produced within the synovium and entering the circulation may account for other features of the disease, such as systemic vasculitis.

As shown in Fig. 312-2, the pathology of RA evolves over the duration of this chronic disease. The earliest event appears to be a nonspecific inflammatory response initiated by an unknown stimulus and characterized by accumulation of macrophages and other mononuclear cells within the sublining layer of the synovium. The activity of these cells is demonstrated by the increased appearance of macrophage-derived cytokines, including TNF-α, IL-1β, and IL-6. Subsequently, activation of CD4+ T cells is induced, presumably in response to antigenic peptides displayed by a variety of antigen-presenting cells in the synovial tissue. The activated T cells are capable of producing cytokines, especially IFN-γ, which amplify and perpetuate the inflammation. The presence of activated T cells expressing CD154 (CD40 ligand) can induce polyclonal B cell stimulation and the local production of rheumatoid factor. The cascade of cytokines produced in the synovium activates a variety of cells in the synovium, bone, and cartilage to produce effector molecules that can cause tissue damage characteristic of chronic inflammation. It is important to emphasize that there is no current way to predict the progress from one stage of inflammation to the next, and once established, each can influence the other. Important features of this model include the following: (1) the major pathologic events vary with time in this chronic disease; (2) the time required to progress from one step to the next may vary in different patients and the events, once established, may persist simultaneously; (3) once established, the major pathogenic events operative in an individual patient may vary at different times; and (4) the process is chronic and reiterative, with successive events stimulating progressive amplification of inflammation. These considerations have important implications with regard to appropriate treatment.

FIGURE 312-2 The progression of rheumatoid synovitis. This figure depicts the evolution of the pathogenic mechanisms and ultimate pathologic changes involved in the development of rheumatoid synovitis. The stages of rheumatoid arthritis are proposed to be an initiation phase of nonspecific inflammation, followed by an amplification phase resulting from T cell activation, and finally a stage of chronic inflammation with tissue injury. A variety of stimuli may initiate the initial phase of nonspecific inflammation, which may last for a protracted period of time with no or moderate symptoms. When activation of memory T cells in response to a variety of peptides presented by antigen-presenting cells occurs in genetically susceptible individuals, amplification of inflammation occurs with the promotion of local rheumatoid factor production and enhanced capacity to mediate tissue damage.

CLINICAL MANIFESTATIONS Onset Characteristically, RA is a chronic polyarthritis. In approximately two-thirds of patients, it begins insidiously with fatigue, anorexia, generalized weakness, and vague musculoskeletal symptoms until the appearance of synovitis becomes apparent. This prodrome may persist for weeks or months and defy diagnosis. Specific symptoms usually appear gradually as several joints, especially those of the hands, wrists, knees, and feet, become affected in a symmetric fashion. In approximately 10% of individuals, the onset is more acute, with a rapid development of polyarthritis, often accompanied by constitutional symptoms, including fever, lymphadenopathy, and splenomegaly. In approximately one-third of patients, symptoms may initially be confined to one or a few joints. Although the pattern of joint involvement may remain asymmetric in a few patients, a symmetric pattern is more typical.

Signs and Symptoms of Articular Disease Pain, swelling, and tenderness may initially be poorly localized to the joints. Pain in affected joints, aggravated by movement, is the most common manifestation of established RA. It corresponds in pattern to the joint involvement but does not always correlate with the degree of apparent inflammation. Generalized stiffness is frequent and is usually greatest after periods of inactivity. Morning stiffness of greater than 1-h duration is an almost invariable feature of inflammatory arthritis and may serve to distinguish it from various noninflammatory joint disorders. Notably, however, the presence of morning stiffness may not reliably distinguish between chronic inflammatory and noninflammatory arthritides, as it is also found frequently in the latter. The majority of patients will experience constitutional symptoms such as weakness, easy fatigability, anorexia, and weight loss. Although fever to 40°C occurs on occasion, temperature elevation in excess of 38°C is unusual and suggests the presence of an intercurrent problem such as infection.

Clinically, synovial inflammation causes swelling, tenderness, and limitation of motion. Warmth is usually evident on examination, especially of large joints such as the knee, but erythema is infrequent. Pain originates predominantly from the joint capsule, which is abundantly supplied with pain fibers and is markedly sensitive to stretching or distention. Joint swelling results from accumulation of synovial fluid, hypertrophy of the synovium, and thickening of the joint capsule. Initially, motion is limited by pain. The inflamed joint is usually held in flexion to maximize joint volume and minimize distention of the capsule. Later, fibrous or bony ankylosis or soft tissue contractures lead to fixed deformities.

Although inflammation can affect any diarthrodial joint, RA most often causes symmetric arthritis with characteristic involvement of certain specific joints such as the proximal interphalangeal and metacarpophalangeal joints. The distal interphalangeal joints are rarely involved. Synovitis of the wrist joints is a nearly uniform feature of RA and may lead to limitation of motion, deformity, and median nerve entrapment (carpal tunnel syndrome). Synovitis of the elbow joint often leads to flexion contractures that may develop early in the disease. The knee joint is commonly involved with synovial hypertrophy, chronic effusion, and frequently ligamentous laxity. Pain and swelling behind the knee may be caused by extension of inflamed synovium into the popliteal space (Baker's cyst). Arthritis in the forefoot, ankles, and subtalar joints can produce severe pain with ambulation as well as a number of deformities. Axial involvement is usually limited to the upper cervical spine. Involvement of the lumbar spine is not seen, and lower back pain cannot be ascribed to rheumatoid inflammation. On occasion, inflammation from the synovial joints and bursae of the upper cervical spine leads to atlantoaxial subluxation. This usually presents as pain in the occiput but on rare occasions may lead to compression of the spinal cord.

With persistent inflammation, a variety of characteristic joint changes develop. These can be attributed to a number of pathologic events, including laxity of supporting soft tissue structures; damage or weakening of ligaments, tendons, and the joint capsule; cartilage degradation; muscle imbalance; and unopposed physical forces associated with the use of affected joints. Characteristic changes of the hand include (1) radial deviation at the wrist with ulnar deviation of the digits, often with palmar subluxation of the proximal phalanges ("Z" deformity); (2) hyperextension of the proximal interphalangeal joints, with compensatory flexion of the distal interphalangeal joints (swanneck deformity); (3) flexion contracture of the proximal interphalangeal joints and extension of the distal interphalangeal joints (boutonnière deformity); and (4) hyperextension of the first interphalangeal joint and flexion of the first metacarpophalangeal joint with a consequent loss of thumb mobility and pinch. Typical joint changes may also develop in the feet, including eversion at the hindfoot (subtalar joint), plantar subluxation of the metatarsal heads, widening of the forefoot, hallux valgus, and lateral deviation and dorsal subluxation of the toes.

Extraarticular Manifestations RA is a systemic disease with a variety of extraarticular manifestations. Although these occur frequently, not all of them have clinical significance. However, on occasion, they may be the major evidence of disease activity and source of morbidity and require management per se. As a rule, these manifestations occur in individuals with high titers of autoantibodies to the Fc component of immunoglobulin G (rheumatoid factors).

Rheumatoid nodules develop in 20 to 30% of persons with RA. They are usually found on periarticular structures, extensor surfaces, or other areas subjected to mechanical pressure, but they can develop elsewhere, including the pleura and meninges. Common locations include the olecranon bursa, the proximal ulna, the Achilles tendon, and the occiput. Nodules vary in size and consistency and are rarely symptomatic, but on occasion they break down as a result of trauma or become infected. They are found almost invariably in individuals with circulating rheumatoid factor. Histologically, rheumatoid nodules consist of a central zone of necrotic material including collagen fibrils, noncollagenous filaments, and cellular debris; a midzone of palisading macrophages that express HLA-DR antigens; and an outer zone of granulation tissue. Examination of early nodules has suggested that

the initial event may be a focal vasculitis. In some patients, treatment with methotrexate can increase the number of nodules dramatically.

Clinical weakness and atrophy of skeletal muscle are common. Muscle atrophy may be evident within weeks of the onset of RA and is usually most apparent in musculature approximating affected joints. Muscle biopsy may show type II fiber atrophy and muscle fiber necrosis with or without a mononuclear cell infiltrate.

Rheumatoid vasculitis (Chap. 317), which can affect nearly any organ system, is seen in patients with severe RA and high titers of circulating rheumatoid factor. Rheumatoid vasculitis is very uncommon in African Americans. In its most aggressive form, rheumatoid vasculitis can cause polyneuropathy and mononeuritis multiplex, cutaneous ulceration and dermal necrosis, digital gangrene, and visceral infarction. While such widespread vasculitis is very rare, more limited forms are not uncommon, especially in white patients with high titers of rheumatoid factor. Neurovascular disease presenting either as a mild distal sensory neuropathy or as mononeuritis multiplex may be the only sign of vasculitis. Cutaneous vasculitis usually presents as crops of small brown spots in the nail beds, nail folds, and digital pulp. Larger ischemic ulcers, especially in the lower extremity, may also develop. Myocardial infarction secondary to rheumatoid vasculitis has been reported, as has vasculitic involvement of lungs, bowel, liver, spleen, pancreas, lymph nodes, and testes. Renal vasculitis is rare.

Pleuropulmonary manifestations, which are more commonly observed in men, include pleural disease, interstitial fibrosis, pleuropulmonary nodules, pneumonitis, and arteritis. Evidence of pleuritis is found commonly at autopsy, but symptomatic disease during life is infrequent. Typically, the pleural fluid contains very low levels of glucose in the absence of infection. Pleural fluid complement is also low compared with the serum level when these are related to the total protein concentration. Pulmonary fibrosis can produce impairment of the diffusing capacity of the lung. Pulmonary nodules may appear singly or in clusters. When they appear in individuals with pneumoconiosis, a diffuse nodular fibrotic process (Caplan's syndrome) may develop. On occasion, pulmonary nodules may cavitate and produce a pneumothorax or bronchopleural fistula. Rarely, pulmonary hypertension secondary to obliteration of the pulmonary vasculature occurs. In addition to pleuropulmonary disease, upper airway obstruction from cricoarytenoid arthritis or laryngeal nodules may develop.

Clinically apparent heart disease attributed to the rheumatoid process is rare, but evidence of asymptomatic pericarditis is found at autopsy in 50% of cases. Pericardial fluid has a low glucose level and is frequently associated with the occurrence of pleural effusion. Although pericarditis is usually asymptomatic, on rare occasions death has occurred from tamponade. Chronic constrictive pericarditis may also occur.

RA tends to spare the central nervous system directly, although vasculitis can cause peripheral neuropathy. *Neurologic manifestations* may also result from atlantoaxial or midcervical spine subluxations. Nerve entrapment secondary to proliferative synovitis or joint deformities may produce neuropathies of median, ulnar, radial (interosseous branch), or anterior tibial nerves.

The rheumatoid process involves the *eye* in fewer than 1% of patients. Affected individuals usually have long-standing disease and nodules. The two principal manifestations are episcleritis, which is usually mild and transient, and scleritis, which involves the deeper layers of the eye and is a more serious inflammatory condition. Histologically, the lesion is similar to a rheumatoid nodule and may result in thinning and perforation of the globe (scleromalacia perforans). From 15 to 20% of persons with RA may develop Sjögren's syndrome with attendant keratoconjunctivitis sicca.

Felty's syndrome consists of chronic RA, splenomegaly, neutropenia, and, on occasion, anemia and thrombocytopenia. It is most common in individuals with long-standing disease. These patients frequently have high titers of rheumatoid factor, subcutaneous nodules, and other manifestations of systemic rheumatoid disease. Felty's syndrome is very uncommon in African Americans. It may develop after joint inflammation has regressed. Circulating immune complexes are often present, and evidence of complement consumption may be seen. The leukopenia is a selective neutropenia with polymorphonuclear leukocyte counts of <1500 cells per microliter and sometimes <1000 cells per microliter. Bone marrow examination usually reveals moderate hypercellularity with a paucity of mature neutrophils. However, the bone marrow may be normal, hyperactive, or hypoactive; maturation arrest may be seen. Hypersplenism has been proposed as one of the causes of leukopenia, but splenomegaly is not invariably found and splenectomy does not always correct the abnormality. Excessive margination of granulocytes caused by antibodies to these cells, complement activation, or binding of immune complexes may contribute to granulocytopenia. Patients with Felty's syndrome have increased frequency of infections usually associated with neutropenia. The cause of the increased susceptibility to infection is related to the defective function of polymorphonuclear leukocytes as well as the decreased number of cells.

Osteoporosis secondary to rheumatoid involvement is common and may be aggravated by glucocorticoid therapy. Glucocorticoid treatment may cause significant loss of bone mass, especially early in the course of therapy, even when low doses are employed. Osteopenia in RA involves both juxtaarticular bone and long bones distant from involved joints. RA is associated with a modest decrease in mean bone mass and a moderate increase in the risk of fracture. Bone mass appears to be adversely affected by functional impairment and active inflammation, especially early in the course of the disease.

RA in the Elderly The incidence of RA continues to increase past age 60. It has been suggested that elderly-onset RA might have a poorer prognosis, as manifested by more persistent disease activity, more frequent radiographically evident deterioration, more frequent systemic involvement, and more rapid functional decline. Aggressive disease is largely restricted to those patients with high titers of rheumatoid factor. By contrast, elderly patients who develop RA without elevated titers of rheumatoid factor (seronegative disease) generally have less severe, often self-limited disease.

LABORATORY FINDINGS No tests are specific for diagnosing RA. However, rheumatoid factors, which are autoantibodies reactive with the Fc portion of IgG, are found in more than two-thirds of adults with the disease. Widely utilized tests largely detect IgM rheumatoid factors. The presence of rheumatoid factor is not specific for RA. Rheumatoid factor is found in 5% of healthy persons. The frequency of rheumatoid factor in the general population increases with age, and 10 to 20% of individuals over 65 years old have a positive test. In addition, a number of conditions besides RA are associated with the presence of rheumatoid factor. These include systemic lupus erythematosus, Sjögren's syndrome, chronic liver disease, sarcoidosis, interstitial pulmonary fibrosis, infectious mononucleosis, hepatitis B, tuberculosis, leprosy, syphilis, subacute bacterial endocarditis, visceral leishmaniasis, schistosomiasis, and malaria. In addition, rheumatoid factor may appear transiently in normal individuals after vaccination or transfusion and may also be found in relatives of individuals with RA.

The presence of rheumatoid factor does not establish the diagnosis of RA as the predictive value of the presence of rheumatoid factor in determining a diagnosis of RA is poor. Thus fewer than one-third of unselected patients with a positive test for rheumatoid factor will be found to have RA. Therefore, the rheumatoid factor test is not useful as a screening procedure. However, the presence of rheumatoid factor can be of prognostic significance because patients with high titers tend to have more severe and progressive disease with extraarticular manifestations. Rheumatoid factor is uniformly found in patients with nodules or vasculitis. In summary, a test for the presence of rheumatoid factor can be employed to confirm a diagnosis in individuals with a suggestive clinical presentation and, if present in high titer, to designate patients at risk for severe systemic disease. A number of additional autoantibodies may be found in patients with RA, including antibodies to filaggrin, citrulline, calpastatin, components of the spliceosome (RA-33), and an unknown antigen, Sa. Some of these may be useful in diagnosis in that they may occur early in the disease before

rheumatoid factor is present or may be associated with aggressive disease.

Normochromic, normocytic anemia is frequently present in active RA. It is thought to reflect ineffective erythropoiesis; large stores of iron are found in the bone marrow. In general, anemia and thrombocytosis correlate with disease activity. The white blood cell count is usually normal, but a mild leukocytosis may be present. Leukopenia may also exist without the full-blown picture of Felty's syndrome. Eosinophilia, when present, usually reflects severe systemic disease.

The erythrocyte sedimentation rate is increased in nearly all patients with active RA. The levels of a variety of other acute-phase reactants including ceruloplasmin and C-reactive protein are also elevated, and generally such elevations correlate with disease activity and the likelihood of progressive joint damage.

Synovial fluid analysis confirms the presence of inflammatory arthritis, although none of the findings is specific. The fluid is usually turbid, with reduced viscosity, increased protein content, and a slightly decreased or normal glucose concentration. The white cell count varies between 5 and 50,000/μL; polymorphonuclear leukocytes predominate. A synovial fluid white blood cell count >2000/μL with more than 75% polymorphonuclear leukocytes is highly characteristic of inflammatory arthritis, although not diagnostic of RA. Total hemolytic complement, C3, and C4 are markedly diminished in synovial fluid relative to total protein concentration as a result of activation of the classic complement pathway by locally produced immune complexes.

RADIOGRAPHIC EVALUATION Early in the disease, roentgenograms of the affected joints are usually not helpful in establishing a diagnosis. They reveal only that which is apparent from physical examination, namely, evidence of soft tissue swelling and joint effusion. As the disease progresses, abnormalities become more pronounced, but none of the radiographic findings is diagnostic of RA. The diagnosis, however, is supported by a characteristic pattern of abnormalities, including the tendency toward symmetric involvement. Juxtaarticular osteopenia may become apparent within weeks of onset. Loss of articular cartilage and bone erosions develop after months of sustained activity. The primary value of radiography is to determine the extent of cartilage destruction and bone erosion produced by the disease, particularly when one is monitoring the impact of therapy with disease-modifying drugs or surgical intervention. Other means of imaging bones and joints, including ^{99m}Tc bisphosphonate bone scanning and magnetic resonance imaging, may be capable of detecting early inflammatory changes that are not apparent from standard radiography but are rarely necessary in the routine evaluation of patients with RA.

CLINICAL COURSE AND PROGNOSIS The course of RA is quite variable and difficult to predict in an individual patient. Most patients experience persistent but fluctuating disease activity, accompanied by a variable degree of joint abnormalities and functional impairment. After 10 to 12 years, fewer than 20% of patients will have no evidence of disability or joint abnormalities. Within 10 years, approximately 50% of patients will have work disability. A number of features are correlated with a greater likelihood of developing joint abnormalities or disabilities. These include the presence of more than 20 inflamed joints, a markedly elevated erythrocyte sedimentation rate, radiographic evidence of bone erosions, the presence of rheumatoid nodules, high titers of serum rheumatoid factor, the presence of functional disability, persistent inflammation, advanced age at onset, the presence of comorbid conditions, low socioeconomic status or educational level, or the presence of HLA-DRB1*0401 or -DRB*0404. The presence of one or more of these implies the presence of more aggressive disease with a greater likelihood of developing progressive joint abnormalities and disability. Persistent elevation of the erythrocyte sedimentation rate, disability, and pain on longitudinal follow-up are good predictors of work disability. Patients who lack these features have more indolent disease with a slower progression to joint abnormalities and disability. The pattern of disease onset does not appear to predict the development of disabilities. Approximately 15% of patients with RA will have a short-lived inflammatory process that remits without major disability. These individuals tend to lack the aforementioned features associated with more aggressive disease.

Several features of patients with RA appear to have prognostic significance. Remissions of disease activity are most likely to occur during the first year. White females tend to have more persistent synovitis and more progressively erosive disease than males. Persons who present with high titers of rheumatoid factor, C-reactive protein, and haptoglobin also have a worse prognosis, as do individuals with subcutaneous nodules or radiographic evidence of erosions at the time of initial evaluation. Sustained disease activity of more than 1 year's duration portends a poor outcome, and persistent elevation of acute-phase reactants appears to correlate strongly with radiographic progression. A large proportion of inflamed joints manifest erosions within 2 years, whereas the subsequent course of erosions is highly variable; however, in general, radiographic damage appears to progress at a constant rate in patients with RA. Foot joints are affected more frequently than hand joints. Despite the decrease in the rate of progressive joint damage with time, functional disability, which develops early in the course of the disease, continues to worsen at the same rate, although the most rapid rate of functional loss occurs within the first 2 years of disease.

The median life expectancy of persons with RA is shortened by 3 to 7 years. Of the 2.5-fold increase in mortality rate, RA itself is a contributing feature in 15 to 30%. The increased mortality rate seems to be limited to patients with more severe articular disease and can be attributed largely to infection and gastrointestinal bleeding. Drug therapy may also play a role in the increased mortality rate seen in these individuals. Factors correlated with early death include disability, disease duration or severity, glucocorticoid use, age at onset, and low socioeconomic or educational status.

DIAGNOSIS The mean delay from disease onset to diagnosis is 9 months. This is often related to the nonspecific nature of initial symptoms. The diagnosis of RA is easily made in persons with typical established disease. In a majority of patients, the disease assumes its characteristic clinical features within 1 to 2 years of onset. The typical picture of bilateral symmetric inflammatory polyarthritis involving small and large joints in both the upper and lower extremities with sparing of the axial skeleton except the cervical spine suggests the diagnosis. Constitutional features indicative of the inflammatory nature of the disease, such as morning stiffness, support the diagnosis. Demonstration of subcutaneous nodules is a helpful diagnostic feature. Additionally, the presence of rheumatoid factor, inflammatory synovial fluid with increased numbers of polymorphonuclear leukocytes, and radiographic findings of juxtaarticular bone demineralization and erosions of the affected joints substantiate the diagnosis.

The diagnosis is somewhat more difficult early in the course when only constitutional symptoms or intermittent arthralgias or arthritis in an asymmetric distribution may be present. A period of observation may be necessary before the diagnosis can be established. A definitive diagnosis of RA depends predominantly on characteristic clinical features and the exclusion of other inflammatory processes. The isolated finding of a positive test for rheumatoid factor or an elevated erythrocyte sedimentation rate, especially in an older person with joint pains, should not itself be used as evidence of RA.

In 1987, the American College of Rheumatology developed revised criteria for the classification of RA (Table 312-1). These criteria demonstrate a sensitivity of 91 to 94% and a specificity of 89% when used to classify patients with RA compared with control subjects with rheumatic diseases other than RA. Although these criteria were developed as a means of disease classification for epidemiologic purposes, they can be useful as guidelines for establishing the diagnosis. Failure to meet these criteria, however, especially during the early stages of the disease, does not exclude the diagnosis. Moreover, in

Table 312-1 The 1987 Revised Criteria for the Classification of Rheumatoid Arthritis

1. Guidelines for classification
   a. Four of seven criteria are required to classify a patient as having rheumatoid arthritis (RA).
   b. Patients with two or more clinical diagnoses are not excluded.
2. Criteria[a]
   a. Morning stiffness: Stiffness in and around the joints lasting 1 h before maximal improvement.
   b. Arthritis of three or more joint areas: At least three joint areas, observed by a physician simultaneously, have soft tissue swelling or joint effusions, not just bony overgrowth. The 14 possible joint areas involved are right or left proximal interphalangeal, metacarpophalangeal, wrist, elbow, knee, ankle, and metatarsophalangeal joints.
   c. Arthritis of hand joints: Arthritis of wrist, metacarpophalangeal joint, or proximal interphalangeal joint.
   d. Symmetric arthritis: Simultaneous involvement of the same joint areas on both sides of the body.
   e. Rheumatoid nodules: Subcutaneous nodules over bony prominences, extensor surfaces, or juxtaarticular regions observed by a physician.
   f. Serum rheumatoid factor: Demonstration of abnormal amounts of serum rheumatoid factor by any method for which the result has been positive in less than 5% of normal control subjects.
   g. Radiographic changes: Typical changes of RA on posteroanterior hand and wrist radiographs that must include erosions or unequivocal bony decalcification localized in or most marked adjacent to the involved joints.

---

[a] Criteria a–d must be present for at least 6 weeks. Criteria b–e must be observed by a physician.
SOURCE: From FC Arnett et al: Arthritis Rheum 31:315, 1988.

patients with early arthritis, the criteria do not discriminate effectively between patients who subsequently develop persistent, disabling, or erosive disease and those who do not.

℞ TREATMENT General Principles The goals of therapy of RA are (1) relief of pain, (2) reduction of inflammation, (3) protection of articular structures, (4) maintenance of function, and (5) control of systemic involvement. Since the etiology of RA is unknown, the pathogenesis is not completely delineated, and the mechanisms of action of many of the therapeutic agents employed are uncertain, therapy remains largely empirical. None of the therapeutic interventions is curative, and therefore all must be viewed as palliative, aimed at relieving the signs and symptoms of the disease. The various therapies employed are directed at nonspecific suppression of the inflammatory or immunologic process in the hope of ameliorating symptoms and preventing progressive damage to articular structures.

Management of patients with RA involves an interdisciplinary approach, which attempts to deal with the various problems that these individuals encounter with functional as well as psychosocial interactions. A variety of physical therapy modalities may be useful in decreasing the symptoms of RA. Rest ameliorates symptoms and can be an important component of the total therapeutic program. In addition, splinting to reduce unwanted motion of inflamed joints may be useful. Exercise directed at maintaining muscle strength and joint mobility without exacerbating joint inflammation is also an important aspect of the therapeutic regimen. A variety of orthotic and assistive devices can be helpful in supporting and aligning deformed joints to reduce pain and improve function. Education of the patient and family is an important component of the therapeutic plan to help those involved become aware of the potential impact of the disease and make appropriate accommodations in life-style to maximize satisfaction and minimize stress on joints.

Medical management of RA involves five general approaches. The first is the use of aspirin and other nonsteroidal anti-inflammatory drugs (NSAIDs) and simple analgesics to control the symptoms and signs of the local inflammatory process. These agents are rapidly effective at mitigating signs and symptoms, but they appear to exert minimal effect on the progression of the disease. Recently, specific inhibitors of the isoform of cyclooxygenase (Cox) that is upregulated at inflammatory sites (Cox-2) have been developed. Cox-2-specific inhibitors (CSIs) have been shown to be as effective as classic NSAIDs, which inhibit both isoforms of Cox, but to cause significantly less gastroduodenal ulceration. The second line of therapy involves use of low-dose oral glucocorticoids. Although low-dose glucocorticoids have been widely used to suppress signs and symptoms of inflammation, recent evidence suggests that they may also retard the development and progression of bone erosions. Intraarticular glucocorticoids can often provide transient symptomatic relief when systemic medical therapy has failed to resolve inflammation. The third line of agents includes a variety of agents that have been classified as the disease-modifying or slow-acting antirheumatic drugs. These agents appear to have the capacity to decrease elevated levels of acute-phase reactants in treated patients and, therefore, are thought to modify the inflammatory component of RA and thus its destructive capacity. Recently, combinations of disease-modifying antirheumatic drugs (DMARDs) have shown promise in controlling the signs and symptoms of RA. A fourth group of agents are the TNF-α neutralizing agents, which have been shown to have a major impact on the signs and symptoms of RA. A fifth group of agents are the immunosuppressive and cytotoxic drugs that have been shown to ameliorate the disease process in some patients. Additional approaches have been employed in an attempt to control the signs and symptoms of RA. Substituting omega-3 fatty acids such as eicosapentaenoic acid found in certain fish oils for dietary omega-6 essential fatty acids found in meat has also been shown to provide symptomatic improvement in patients with RA. A variety of nontraditional approaches have also been claimed to be effective in treating RA, including diets, plant and animal extracts, vaccines, hormones, and topical preparations of various sorts. Many of these are costly, and none has been shown to be effective. However, belief in their efficacy ensures their continued use by some patients.

Drugs • _Nonsteroidal anti-inflammatory drugs_ Besides aspirin, many NSAIDs are available to treat RA. As a result of the capacity of these agents to block the activity of the Cox enzymes and therefore the production of prostaglandins, prostacyclin, and thromboxanes, they have analgesic, anti-inflammatory, and antipyretic properties. In addition, the agents may exert other anti-inflammatory effects. These agents are all associated with a wide spectrum of toxic side effects. Some, such as gastric irritation, azotemia, platelet dysfunction, and exacerbation of allergic rhinitis and asthma, are related to the inhibition of cyclooxygenase activity, whereas a variety of others, such as rash, liver function abnormalities, and bone marrow depression, may not be. None of the NSAIDs has been shown to be more effective than aspirin in the treatment of RA. However, these nonaspirin drugs are associated with a lower incidence of gastrointestinal intolerance. None of the newer NSAIDs appears to show significant therapeutic advantages over the other available agents. In addition, there is no consistent advantage of any of these newer agents over the others with respect to the incidence or severity of toxic manifestations. Recent evidence indicates that two separate enzymes, Cox-1 and -2, are responsible for the initial metabolism of arachidonic acid into various inflammatory mediators. The former is constitutively present in many cells and tissues, including the stomach and the platelet, whereas the latter is specifically induced in response to inflammatory stimuli. Inhibition of Cox-2 accounts for the anti-inflammatory effects of NSAIDs, whereas inhibition of Cox-1 induces much of the mechanism-based toxicity. As the currently available NSAIDs inhibit both enzymes, therapeutic benefit and toxicity are intertwined. CSIs have now been approved for the treatment of RA. Clinical trials have shown that CSIs suppress the signs and symptoms of RA as effectively as classic Cox-nonspecific NSAIDs but are associated with a significantly reduced incidence of gastroduodenal ulceration. This suggests that CSIs might be considered instead of classic Cox-nonspecific NSAIDs, especially in persons with increased risk of NSAID-induced major upper gastrointestinal side effects, including persons over 65, those with a history of peptic ulcer disease, persons receiving glucocorticoids or anticoagulants, or those requiring high doses of NSAIDs.

Disease-modifying antirheumatic drugs Clinical experience has delineated a number of agents that appear to have the capacity to alter the course of RA. This group of agents includes methotrexate, gold compounds, D-penicillamine, the antimalarials, and sulfasalazine. Despite having no chemical or pharmacologic similarities, in practice these agents share a number of characteristics. They exert minimal direct nonspecific anti-inflammatory or analgesic effects, and therefore NSAIDs must be continued during their administration, except in a few cases when true remissions are induced with them. The appearance of benefit from DMARD therapy is usually delayed for weeks or months. As many as two-thirds of patients develop some clinical improvement as a result of therapy with any of these agents, although the induction of true remissions is unusual. In addition to clinical improvement, there is frequently an improvement in serologic evidence of disease activity, and titers of rheumatoid factor and C-reactive protein and the erythrocyte sedimentation rate frequently decline. Moreover, emerging evidence suggests that DMARDs actually retard the development of bone erosions or facilitate their healing. Furthermore, developing evidence suggests that early aggressive treatment with DMARDs may be effective at slowing the appearance of bone erosions.

Which DMARD should be the drug of first choice remains controversial, and trials have failed to demonstrate a consistent advantage of one over the other. Despite this, methotrexate has emerged as the DMARD of choice because of its relatively rapid onset of action, its capacity to effect sustained improvement with ongoing therapy, and the high level of patient retention on therapy. Each of the DMARDs is associated with considerable toxicity, and therefore careful patient monitoring is necessary. Toxicity of the various agents also becomes important in determining the drug of first choice. Of note, failure to respond or development of toxicity to one DMARD does not preclude responsiveness to another. Thus, a similar percentage of RA patients who have failed to respond to one DMARD will respond to another when it is given as the second disease-modifying drug.

No characteristic features of patients have emerged that predict responsiveness to a DMARD. Moreover, the indications for the initiation of therapy with one of these agents are not well defined, although recently the trend has been to begin DMARD therapy early in the course of the disease, and data have begun to emerge to support the conclusion that this approach may slow the development of bone erosions, although this remains controversial.

The folic acid antagonist methotrexate, given in an intermittent low dose (7.5 to 30 mg once weekly), is currently a frequently utilized DMARD. Most rheumatologists recommend use of methotrexate as the initial DMARD, especially in individuals with evidence of aggressive RA. Recent trials have documented the efficacy of methotrexate and have indicated that its onset of action is more rapid than other DMARDs, and patients tend to remain on therapy with methotrexate longer than they remain on other DMARDs because of better clinical responses and less toxicity. Long-term trials have indicated that methotrexate does not induce remission but rather suppresses symptoms while it is being administered. Maximal improvement is observed after 6 months of therapy, with little additional improvement thereafter. Major toxicity includes gastrointestinal upset, oral ulceration, and liver function abnormalities that appear to be dose-related and reversible and hepatic fibrosis that can be quite insidious, requiring liver biopsy for detection in its early stages. Drug-induced pneumonitis has also been reported. Liver biopsy is recommended for individuals with persistent or repetitive liver function abnormalities. Concurrent administration of folic acid or folinic acid may diminish the frequency of some side effects without diminishing effectiveness.

Glucocorticoid Therapy Systemic glucocorticoid therapy can provide effective symptomatic therapy in patients with RA. Low-dose ($<$7.5 mg/d) prednisone has been advocated as useful additive therapy to control symptoms. Moreover, recent evidence suggests that low-dose glucocorticoid therapy may retard the progression of bone erosions. Monthly pulses with high-dose glucocorticoids may be useful-

FIGURE 312-3 Algorithm for the medical management of rheumatoid arthritis. NSAID, nonsteroidal antiinflammatory drug; CSI, Cox-2 specific inhibitor; DMARD, disease-modifying antirheumatic drug; TNF-α, tumor necrosis factor α.

in some patients and may hasten the response when therapy with a DMARD is initiated.

TNF-α neutralizing agents Recently, biologic agents that bind and neutralize TNF-α have become available. One of these is a TNF-α type II receptor fused to IgG1 (etanercept), and the second is a chimeric mouse/human monoclonal antibody to TNF-α (infliximab). Clinical trials have shown that parenteral administration of either TNF-α neutralizing agent is remarkably effective at controlling signs and symptoms of RA in patients who have failed DMARD therapy. Repetitive therapy with these agents is effective with or without concomitant methotrexate. Although these agents are notably effective in persistently controlling signs and symptoms of RA in a majority of patients, their impact on the progression of bone erosions has not been proven. Side effects include the potential for an increased risk of serious infections and the development of anti-DNA antibodies, but with no associated evidence of signs and symptoms of systemic lupus erythematosus. Although these side effects are uncommon, their occurrence mandates that TNF-α neutralizing therapy be supervised by physicians with experience in their use.

Immunosuppressive Therapy The immunosuppressive drugs azathioprine, leflunomide, cyclosporine, and cyclophosphamide have been shown to be effective in the treatment of RA and to exert therapeutic effects similar to those of the DMARDs. However, these agents appear to be no more effective than the DMARDs. Moreover, they cause a variety of toxic side effects, and cyclophosphamide appears to predispose the patient to the development of malignant neoplasms. Therefore, these drugs have been reserved for patients who have clearly failed therapy with DMARDs. On occasion, extraarticular disease such as rheumatoid vasculitis may require cytotoxic immunosuppressive therapy.

Surgery Surgery plays a role in the management of patients with severely damaged joints. Although arthroplasties and total joint replacements can be done on a number of joints, the most successful procedures are carried out on hips, knees, and shoulders. Realistic goals of these procedures are relief of pain and reduction of disability. Reconstructive hand surgery may lead to cosmetic improvement and some functional benefit. Open or arthroscopic synovectomy may be useful in some patients with persistent monarthritis, especially of the knee. Although synovectomy may offer short-term relief of symptoms, it does not appear to retard bone destruction or alter the natural history of the disease. In addition, early tenosynovectomy of the wrist may prevent tendon rupture.

Approach to the Patient

An approach to the medical management of patients with RA is depicted in Fig. 312-3. The principles underlying care of these patients reflect the variability of the disease, the frequent persistent nature of the inflammation and its potential to cause disability, the relationship between sustained inflammation and bone erosions, and the need to reevaluate the patient frequently for symptomatic response to therapy, progression of disability and joint damage, and side effects of treatment. At the onset of disease it is difficult to predict the natural history of an individual patient's illness. Therefore, the usual approach is to attempt to alleviate the patient's symptoms with NSAIDs or CSIs. Some patients may have mild disease that requires no additional therapy.

At some time during most patients' course, the possibility of initiating DMARD therapy and/or low-dose oral glucocorticoids is entertained. With aggressive disease this might occur sooner, often within 1 to 3 months of diagnosis, whereas in patients with more indolent disease, smoldering activity may not require such therapy for many years. The development of bone erosions or radiographic evidence of cartilage loss is clear-cut evidence of the destructive potential of the inflammatory process and indicates the need for DMARD therapy. The other indications as outlined above, including persistent pain, joint swelling, or functional impairment, are much more subjective, however. As persistent inflammation, involvement of multiple joints, elevated levels of acute-phase reactants, and rheumatoid factor titers correlate with the development of disability and/or bony erosions, some have advocated the use of these prognostic indicators of aggressive disease in the decision to employ DMARDs early in the course of RA. The decision to begin use of a DMARD and/or low-dose oral glucocorticoids requires experience and clinical judgment as well as the ability to assess joint swelling and functional activity and the patient's pain tolerance and expectation of therapy accurately. In this setting, the fully informed patient must play an active role in the decision to begin DMARD and/or low-dose oral glucocorticoid therapy, after careful review of the therapeutic and toxic potential of the various drugs.

If a patient responds to a DMARD, therapy is continued with careful monitoring to avoid toxicity. All DMARDs provide a suppressive effect and therefore require prolonged administration. Even with successful therapy, local injection of glucocorticoids may be necessary to diminish inflammation that may persist in a limited number of joints. In addition, NSAIDs or CSIs may be necessary to mitigate symptoms. Even after inflammation has totally resolved, symptoms from loss of cartilage and supervening degenerative joint disease or altered joint function may require additional treatment. Surgery may also be necessary to relieve pain or diminish the functional impairment secondary to alterations in joint function. Recently an alternative approach to treat patients with RA has been suggested. This involves the initiation of therapy with multiple agents early in the course of disease in an attempt to control inflammation, followed by maintenance on one or more agents as necessary to control disease activity. The effectiveness of this therapeutic alternative has not been proved.

BIBLIOGRAPHY

ABU-SHAKRA M et al: Clinical and radiographic outcomes of rheumatoid arthritis patients not treated with disease-modifying drugs. Arthritis Rheum 41:1190, 1998

BUCHT A et al: Expression of interferon-gamma (IFN-γ), IL-10, IL-12 and transforming growth factor-beta (TGF-β) mRNA in synovial fluid cells from patients in the early and late phases of Rheumatoid arthritis (RA). Clin Exp Immunol 103:357, 1996

GOUGH A et al: Osteoclastic activation is the principal mechanism leading to secondary osteoporosis in rheumatoid arthritis. J Rheumatol 25:1282, 1998

GRAUDAL NA et al: Radiographic progression in rheumatoid arthritis. Arthritis Rheum 41:1470, 1998

HARRISON BJ et al: The performance of the 1987 ARA classification criteria for rheumatoid arthritis in a population-based cohort of patients with early inflammatory polyarthritis. J Rheumatol 25:2324, 1998

KAARELA K, KAUTIAINEN H: Continuous progression of radiological destruction in seropositive rheumatoid arthritis. J Rheumatol 24:1285, 1997

KANIK KS et al: Distinct patterns of cytokine secretion characterize new onset synovitis versus chronic rheumatoid arthritis. J Rheumatol 25:16, 1998

KIM H-J et al: Plasma cell development in synovial germinal centers in patients with rheumatoid and reactive arthritis. J Immunol 162:3053, 1999

KOTAKE S et al: IL-17 in synovial fluids from patients with rheumatoid arthritis is a potent stimulator of osteoclastogenesis. J Clin Invest 103:1345, 1999

KRAAN MC et al: Asymptomatic synovitis precedes clinically manifest arthritis. Arthritis Rheum 41:1481, 1998

KWOH CK et al: American College of Rheumatology Guidelines for the Management of Rheumatoid Arthritis. Arthritis Rheum 39:713, 1996

LAWRENCE RC et al: Estimates of the prevalence of arthritis and selected musculoskeletal disorders in the United States. Arthritis Rheum 41:778, 1998

LIPSKY PE, DAVIS LS: The central involvement of T cells in rheumatoid arthritis. Immunologist 6:121, 1998

MACDONALD KPA et al: Functional CD40 ligand is expressed by T cells in rheumatoid arthritis. J Clin Invest 100:2404, 1997

MAINI RN et al: Therapeutic efficacy of multiple intravenous infusions of anti-tumor necrosis factor α monoclonal antibody combined with low-dose weekly methotrexate in rheumatoid arthritis. Arthritis Rheum 41:1552, 1998

MORELAND LW et al: Treatment of rheumatoid arthritis with a recombinant human necrosis factor receptor (p75)-Fc fusion protein. N Engl J Med 337:141, 1997

MORITA Y et al: Expression of interleukin-12 in synovial tissue from patients with rheumatoid arthritis. Arthritis Rheum 41:306, 1998

MU H et al: Tumor necrosis factor α microsatellite polymorphism is associated with rheumatoid arthritis severity through an interaction with the HLA-DRB1 shared epitope. Arthritis Rheum 42:438, 1999

PLANT MJ et al: Patterns of radiological progression in early rheumatoid arthritis: Results of an 8-year prospective study. J Rheumatol 25:417, 1998

RAU R et al: Long-term combination therapy of refractory and destructive rheumatoid arthritis with methotrexate (MTX) and intramuscular gold or other disease-modifying antirheumatic drugs compared to MTX monotherapy. J Rheumatol 25:1485, 1998

SCHULZE-KOOPS H et al: Reduction of Th1 cell activity in the peripheral circulation of patients with rheumatoid arthritis after treatment with a non-depleting humanized monoclonal antibody to CD4. J Rheumatol 25:2065, 1998

SHARIF M et al: Changes in biochemical markers of joint tissue metabolism in a randomized controlled trial of glucocorticoid in early rheumatoid arthritis. Arthritis Rheum 41:1203, 1998

SIMMS RW et al: American College of Rheumatology Guidelines for Monitoring Drug Therapy in Rheumatoid Arthritis. Arthritis Rheum 39:723, 1996

SIMON LS et al: Preliminary study of the safety and efficacy of SC-58635, a novel cyclooxygenase 2 inhibitor. Arthritis Rheum 41:1591, 1998

SMOLEN JS et al: Efficacy and safety of leflunomide compared with placebo and sulphasalazine in active rheumatoid arthritis: A double-blind, randomised, multicentre trial. Lancet 353:259, 1999

STEIN CM et al: Combination treatment of severe rheumatoid arthritis with cyclosporine and methotrexate for forty-eight weeks. Arthritis Rheum 40:1843, 1997

SYMMONS DPM et al: Long-term mortality outcome in patients with rheumatoid arthritis: Early presenters continue to do well. J Rheumatol 25:1072, 1998

THOMAS R, LIPSKY PE: Could endogenous self-peptides presented by dendritic cells initiate rheumatoid arthritis? Immunol Today 17:559, 1996

VINCENT C et al: Immunoblotting detection of autoantibodies to human epidermis filaggrein: A new diagnostic test for rheumatoid arthritis. J Rheumatol 25:838, 1998

WAGNER U et al: HLA markers and prediction of clinical course and outcome in rheumatoid arthritis. Arthritis Rheum 40:341, 1997

WEINBLATT WE et al: Long-term prospective study of methotrexate in rheumatoid arthritis: Conclusion after 132 months of therapy. J Rheumatol 25:238, 1998

——— et al: A trial of etanercept, a recombinant tumor necrosis factor receptor: Fc fusion protein, in patients with rheumatoid arthritis receiving methotrexate. N Engl J Med 340:253, 1999

WEYAND DM et al: The influence of sex on the phenotype of rheumatoid arthritis. Arthritis Rheum 41:817, 1998

WOLFE F, HAWLEY D: The long-term outcomes of rheumatoid arthritis: Work disability: A prospective 18-year study of 823 patients. J Rheumatol 25:2108, 1998

———, SHARP JT: Radiographic outcome of recent-onset rheumatoid arthritis. Arthritis Rheum 41:1571, 1998

313 Bruce C. Gilliland

SYSTEMIC SCLEROSIS (SCLERODERMA)

EMS	eosinophilia-myalgia syndrome	PDGF	platelet-derived growth factor
GVHD	graft-versus-host disease		
ICAM-1	intercellular adhesion molecule-1	RNP	ribonucleoprotein
		SLE	systemic lupus erythematosus
IL	interleukin	SSc	systemic sclerosis
MCTD	mixed connective tissue disease	TGF	transforming growth factor

DEFINITION Systemic sclerosis (SSc) is a chronic multisystem disorder of unknown etiology characterized clinically by thickening of the skin caused by accumulation of connective tissue and by involvement of visceral organs, including the gastrointestinal tract, lungs, heart, and kidneys. Classification of SSc and sclerodermal-like disorders is shown in (Table 313-1). Vascular abnormalities, especially of the microvasculature are a prominent feature of SSc. The degree and rate of skin and internal organ involvement vary among patients.

Table 313-1 Classification of Scleroderma/Systemic Sclerosis and Scleroderma-Like Disorders

Systemic sclerosis
    Limited cutaneous disease
    Diffuse cutaneous disease
    Sine scleroderma
    Undifferentiated connective tissue disease
    Overlap syndromes
Localized scleroderma
    Morphea
    Linear scleroderma
    En coup de sabre
Chemically induced scleroderma-like disorders
    Toxic-oil syndrome
    Vinyl chloride–induced disease
    Bleomycin-induced fibrosis
    Pentazocine-induced fibrosis
    Epoxy- and aromatic hydrocarbons–induced fibrosis
    Eosinophilia-myalgia syndrome
Other scleroderma-like disorders
    Scleredema adultorum of Buschke
    Scleromyxedema
    Chronic graft-vs.-host disease
    Eosinophilic fasciitis
    Digital sclerosis in diabetes
    Primary amyloidosis and amyloidosis associated with multiple myeloma

Two subsets, however, can be identified, even though there is some overlap (Table 313-2). One subset is referred to as *diffuse cutaneous scleroderma* and is characterized by the rapid development of symmetric skin thickening of proximal and distal extremities, face, and trunk. These patients are at greater risk for developing kidney and other visceral disease early in their course. The other subset is *limited cutaneous scleroderma*, which is defined by symmetric skin thickening limited to distal extremities and face. This subset frequently has features of the *CREST syndrome*, standing for *c*alcinosis, *R*aynaud's phenomenon, *e*sophageal dysmotility, *s*clerodactyly, and *t*elangiectasia. The prognosis in limited cutaneous scleroderma is better except for those patients who, after many years, develop pulmonary arterial hypertension or biliary cirrhosis. Involvement of visceral organs may also occur in the absence of any skin involvement, which is referred to as *systemic sclerosis sine scleroderma*. Survival is determined by the severity of visceral disease, especially involving the lungs, heart, and/or kidneys.

Preliminary criteria for the classification of systemic sclerosis were developed by the American Rheumatism Association (now called the American College of Rheumatology) for the purpose of uniformity in clinical studies. A major criterion was the presence of sclerodermatous skin changes of the fingers of both hands plus involvement at any location proximal to the metacarpal phalangeal joints, entire extremity, face, neck, chest, and abdomen. Minor criteria were sclerodactyly, digital pitting scars or tissue loss of the volar pads of the fingertips, and bibasilar pulmonary fibrosis. The diagnosis of SSc was based on the presence of the major criterion or two or more minor criteria. The sensitivity of these criteria was 97%, and the specificity 98%. These criteria are not, however, applicable to clinical practice as many patients have SSc who do not meet these criteria. Scleroderma can also occur in a localized form limited to the skin, subcutaneous tissue, and muscle and without systemic involvement. Localized scleroderma occurs most often in children and young women but can affect any age group. The two localized forms are *morphea*, which occurs as single or multiple plaques of skin induration, and *linear scleroderma*, which involves an extremity or face. Linear scleroderma of one side of the forehead and scalp produces a disfiguration referred to as *en coup de sabre* because it resembles a wound from a sword. It may be associated with hemiatrophy of the same side of the face.

SSc also occurs in association with features of other connective tissue diseases. The term *overlap syndrome* has been used to describe such patients. Undifferentiated connective tissue disease has been suggested as a designation for patients who do not have diagnostic criteria for any one connective tissue disease. *Mixed connective tissue disease* (MCTD), a syndrome involving features of systemic lupus erythematosus (SLE), SSc, polymyositis, and rheumatoid arthritis and very high titers of circulating antibody to nuclear ribonucleoprotein (RNP) antigen, will be discussed later in the chapter. *Eosinophilic fasciitis*

and the *eosinophilia-myalgia syndrome* (EMS) associated with contaminated L-tryptophan ingestion (Chap. 382) are scleroderma-like illnesses and will also be discussed in this chapter.

EPIDEMIOLOGY SSc has a worldwide distribution and affects all races. The onset of disease is unusual in childhood and young men. The incidence increases with age, peaking in the third to fifth decade. Women overall are affected approximately three times as often as men and even more often during the late childbearing years (≥8:1). SSc is more frequent and severe in young black women. The annual incidence has been estimated to be 19 cases per million population. The reported prevalence of SSc is between 19 and 75 per 100,000 persons. An exceptionally high prevalence of SSc (472 per 100,000 persons) has been noted in the Choctaw Native Americans in Oklahoma—the highest found to date in any ethnic group. Both incidence and prevalence may be underestimated because patients with early and atypical disease may be overlooked in surveys. The role of heredity has not been clarified. Several examples of familial SSc have been reported, and the finding of other connective tissue diseases and antinuclear antibodies in relatives of involved patients suggests a hereditary predisposition. However, spouses of SSc patients also have an increased incidence of antinuclear antibodies, suggesting environmental factors. Discordance of SSc in identical twins speaks against a significant genetic predisposition to disease. Immunogenetic studies have not shown strong associations between the major histocompatibility complex and susceptibility to SSc. Some studies have shown an association of SSc with HLA-A1, -B8, -DR3, or with DR3/DR52. C4A null alleles (C4AQ0) and HLA-DQA2 have been reported by some investigators to be markers for disease susceptibility. A more consistent relationship has been found between certain HLA types and the occurrence of specific autoantibodies in SSc patients. Anticentromere antibodies have been shown to be associated with HLA-DQB1*05 allele and, less often, with -DQB1*0301, -*0401, or -*0402. Antitopoisomerase 1 antibodies, on the other hand, are associated most frequently with HLA-DQB1*0301 in several populations, including Caucasians and African Americans.

Several environmental factors have been associated with the development of SSc and scleroderma-like illnesses. SSc appears to be more common in coal and gold miners, especially in those with more extensive exposure, suggesting that silica dust may be a predisposing factor. Workers exposed to polyvinyl chloride may develop Raynaud's phenomenon, acroosteolysis, scleroderma-like skin lesions, pulmonary fibrosis, and nail fold capillary abnormalities similar to those observed in SSc. These workers may also develop hepatic fibrosis and angiosarcoma. The observation that individuals exposed to similar amounts of vinyl chloride do not develop the same degree of disease suggests that a genetic factor may determine susceptibility and disease severity. The development of scleroderma has also been associated with exposure to epoxy resins and aromatic hydrocarbons such as benzine, toluene, and trichloroethylene. In 1981, in Spain, a multisystem disease resembling scleroderma occurred following the ingestion of aniline-adulterated cooking oil (rapeseed oil). Approximately 20,000 people were affected. The patients initially developed interstitial pneumonitis, eosinophilia, arthralgias, arthritis, and myositis, followed subsequently by joint contractures, skin thickening, Raynaud's phenomenon, pulmonary hypertension, sicca syndrome, and resorption of the distal fingertips. Extensive sclerosis of the dermis and subcutaneous tissue has been noted in patients receiving pentazocine, a nonnarcotic analgesic agent. Bleomycin, an anticancer agent, produces fibrotic skin nodules, linear hyperpigmentation, alopecia, Raynaud's phenomenon, gangrene of fingers, and pulmonary fibrosis affecting mainly the lower lobes. Scleroderma and other connective tissue diseases have been reported in women who have had silicone breast implants. Recent studies have not shown that women with these implants carry an increased risk for developing scleroderma or other connective tissue diseases. Localized fibrosis, however, can occur around the implant. While environmental factors or undefined infectious agents may be of etiologic significance, the cause of SSc remains unknown.

Table 313-2 Subsets of Systemic Sclerosis

	Diffuse	Limited[a]
Skin involvement	Distal and proximal extremities, face, trunk	Distal to elbows, face
Raynaud's phenomenon	Onset within 1 year or at time of skin changes	May precede skin disease by years
Organ involvement	Pulmonary (interstitial fibrosis); renal (renovascular hypertensive crisis); gastrointestinal; cardiac	Gastrointestinal; pulmonary arterial hypertension after 10–15 years of disease in <10% of patients; biliary cirrhosis
Nail fold capillaries	Dilatation and dropout	Dilatation without significant dropout
Antinuclear antibodies	Antitopoisomerase 1	Anticentromere

[a] Also referred to as CREST (*c*alcinosis, *R*aynaud's, *e*sophageal dysmotility, *s*clerodactyly, *t*elangiectasia).

PATHOGENESIS The outstanding feature of SSc is overproduction and accumulation of collagen and other extracellular matrix proteins, including fibronectin, tenascin, and glycosaminoglycans, in skin and other organs. The disease process involves immunologic mechanisms, vascular endothelial cell activation and/or injury, and activation of fibroblasts resulting in production of excessive collagen.

An early event in SSc that precedes fibrosis is vascular injury involving small arteries, arterioles, and capillaries in the skin, gastrointestinal tract, kidneys, heart, and lungs. Raynaud's phenomenon, the initial symptom of SSc in the majority of patients, is a clinical expression of the abnormal regulation of blood flow resulting from vascular injury. Injury to endothelial cells and basal lamina occurs early and is followed by thickening of the intima, narrowing of the lumen, and eventual obliteration of the vessel. As vascular damage progresses, the microvascular bed in the skin and other sites is diminished, producing a state of chronic ischemia. Vascular abnormalities can be observed in the nail folds by wide-field microscopy, which shows dropout of capillaries with dilatation and tortuosity of remaining ones. In the skin, remaining capillaries may proliferate and dilate to become visible telangiectasia. Endothelial cell damage is reflected in elevated levels of factor VIII/von Willebrand factor in the sera of some patients with SSc.

Several mechanisms for endothelial injury or activation have been proposed in SSc. Any or all of these mechanisms may be involved in a given patient; some evidence for each exists. A cytotoxic factor for endothelium has been identified in some patients that degrades the basal lamina, releasing fragments of type IV collagen and laminin. This factor, a type IV collagenase, is secreted by activated T cells and is referred to as *granzyme 1* because of its location in cytolytic T cells. Type IV collagen and laminin fragments may stimulate an immune response to the basal lamina. Both antibodies and cell-mediated immunity to type IV collagen and laminin have been observed in some SSc patients and may be involved in endothelial injury or may be an epiphenomenon. Anti-endothelial cell antibodies (AECA) may be another mechanism for microvascular damage. In 25% of SSc patients, AECA have been shown to mediate antibody-dependent cell cytotoxicity against human endothelial cells. Circulating AECA in general have been reported in the sera of SSc patients in amounts ranging from 21 to 85%. This wide variation reflects patient selection, type of assay, and the source of endothelium. These antibodies are not specific for SSc and are found in other connective tissue diseases. The frequency of AECA is higher in patients with diffuse cutaneous SSc. They have also been shown to be associated with digital infarcts, pulmonary hypertension, and impaired alveolocapillary diffusion. Studies have show that AECA initiate programmed cell death (apoptosis), which may be an important event in the pathogenesis of SSc. These antibodies also induce expression of vascular cell adhesion molecule-1 (VCAM-1), intercellular adhesion molecule-1 (ICAM-1), E-selectin, and P-selectin on endothelial cells in SSc and stimulate the production of chemoattractants [interleukin (IL) 1, IL-8, monocyte chemotactic protein], leading to the binding of lymphocytes to the endothelium and their migration into the perivascular tissue. Elevated serum levels of VCAM-1, ICAM-1, and P-selectin are observed in early stages of SSc.

The injury to the endothelium leads to a state favoring vasoconstriction and ischemia. The damaged endothelium produces decreased amounts of prostacylin, which is an important vasodilator and inhibitor of platelet aggregation. Platelets are activated on binding to the damaged endothelium and release thromboxane, a potent vasoconstrictor. Activated platelets also release platelet-derived growth factor (PDGF), which is chemotactic and mitogenic for both smooth-muscle cells and fibroblasts, and transforming growth factor (TGF)β, which stimulates fibroblast collagen synthesis. These and other cytokines stimulate intimal fibrosis and, with their passage through the injured endothelium, may produce adventitial and perivascular fibrosis. Endothelin-1, a vasoconstricting factor released from endothelial cells on cold exposure, is also increased in SSc patients. In addition, it stimulates fibroblasts and smooth-muscle cells. The vasoconstriction action of endothelin-1 is normally opposed by endothelium-derived relaxation factor (EDRF,

nitric oxide), also secreted by endothelial cells. The normal compensatory increase in EDRF is not seen in some patients with SSc, suggesting impairment of its synthesis. A deficiency of vasodilatory neuropeptides resulting from sensory system nerve damage may also produce a condition favoring vasoconstriction. Vasoconstriction itself also contributes to endothelial damage through a mechanism of reperfusion injury, resulting in vascular occlusion and fibrosis.

Existing evidence indicates that cell-mediated immunity plays a central role in the development of fibrosis in SSc. T cells, macrophages, endothelial cells, and other cells along with cytokines and growth factors interact in a complex manner to stimulate fibrosis. The vascular endothelium has been proposed as a target for cell-mediated immunity. Laminin and type IV collagen, components of the subendothelial basement membrane, induce in vitro transformation of lymphocytes from SSc patients. In the early stages of SSc, a mononuclear cell infiltrate consisting predominantly of activated helper-inducer T cells surrounds small blood vessels in the dermis. Subsequently, mononuclear cell infiltrates are found in macroscopically normal-appearing skin adjacent to areas of fibrosis. T cell hyperactivity is reflected by increased serum levels of CD4+ T cells. The ratio of CD4+ to CD8+ T cells is also increased. Elevated circulating levels of IL-2, a product of activated T cells, and IL-2 receptors have been shown to be associated with active fibrosis. In addition, serum levels of IL-4 are increased in SSc patients. IL-4, a product of activated T cells, stimulates fibroblast chemotaxis and proliferation and collagen production. In a recent study, CD8+ T cells isolated from bronchoalveolar lavage fluid from SSc patients made IL-4 and/or IL-5 mRNA. SSc patients with these type 2 cytokines were more likely to have alveolitis and a lower forced vital capacity. Although larger studies are needed, the findings suggest that these cytokines are involved in the pathogenesis of interstitial pulmonary fibrosis. Another cytokine, interferon γ, is produced by activated T cells and stimulates macrophages but inhibits collagen synthesis by fibroblasts. Reduced serum levels of interferon γ are found in some SSc patients. In vitro stimulation of T cells from SSc patients did not show an increased production of interferon γ compared to normal individuals, suggesting an inability in SSc patients to suppress fibrosis normally.

Macrophages are present in increased numbers in the infiltrates of SSc lesions, including the pulmonary alveoli. Activated macrophages secrete several important products involved in the pathogenesis of SSc including IL-1, IL-6, tumor necrosis factor (TNF) α, TGF-β, and PDGF. IL-1 has been shown to stimulate fibroblast proliferation and collagen synthesis. The important role for IL-6 may be in stimulating the local release of tissue inhibitor of metalloproteinase (TIMP) by fibroblasts and thereby limiting the breakdown of collagen. TNF-α, in conjunction with interferon γ, can cause endothelial cell cytolysis and also induces the expression of endothelial cell adhesion molecules (see above), which are responsible for the binding of T cells and subsequent vascular injury. The role of TGF-β and PDGF secreted by macrophages and other cells is discussed below. In addition to the above cytokines, macrophages secrete *fibronectin*, a large matrix protein that is increased in SSc lesions. Fibronectin is also secreted by fibroblasts. Fibronectin interacts with collagen in the SSc lesions where it binds fibroblasts and mononuclear cells through receptors called *integrins*. Fibronectin functions as a chemoattractant and mitogen for fibroblasts.

Additional support for involvement of cell-mediated immunity in the pathogenesis of SSc is the appearance of scleroderma-like lesions in patients with graft-versus-host disease (GVHD) after bone marrow transplantation and in a murine model of chronic GVHD, conditions known to be associated with activated T cells. GVHD and SSc are both associated with progressive skin induration, joint contractures, and gastrointestinal and pulmonary involvement and are frequently accompanied by Sjögren's syndrome. Antinuclear antibodies are present in both diseases. Raynaud's phenomenon and kidney involvement are infrequent in GVHD.

Mast cells may also be involved in the development of fibrosis.

Increased numbers of mast cells are found in the dermis in both involved and uninvolved skin. Mast cell degranulation has been noted in skin that subsequently became fibrosed. Interaction with T cells may be one mechanism for mast cell degranulation resulting in release of products that stimulate fibroblast collagen synthesis. Release of histamine from mast cells may also contribute to edema observed in early disease.

Fibroblast growth and synthesis of collagen, fibronectin, and glycosaminoglycans are increased in SSc. Fibroblasts from SSc appear to have aberrant regulation of growth compared with fibroblasts from normal persons. When fibroblasts from affected SSc skin are removed and cultured in vitro, they continue to produce excessive quantities of collagen. The collagen is biochemically normal, and the proportion of type I to type III is the same as in normal skin. Fibroblasts from SSc patients appear to be in a state of permanent activation, most likely as a result of stimulation by cytokines. These activated cells are thought to represent an expanded subpopulation of fibroblasts that inherently express increased matrix genes. Studies have revealed a subpopulation of SSc fibroblasts that produces two to three times more collagen than other cells from the same tissue. Fibroblasts expressing elevated levels of mRNA for types I and III collagen have been demonstrated by in situ hybridization, particularly around dermal blood vessels in affected SSc skin. Collagen deposition is also initially perivascular in other organs including myocardium, muscle, and kidney. A small number of fibroblasts express increased levels of mRNA for types VI and VII collagen. Type VII collagen is normally found at the dermal-epidermal basement membrane zone and is the major component of anchoring fibrils that act to stabilize the attachment of the basement membrane to the underlying dermis. In SSc patients, type VII collagen is found throughout the dermis and may account for the indurated, tightly bound skin in this disease. PDGF receptors are expressed on SSc fibroblasts not only from affected areas but also from macroscopically normal-appearing skin. Fibroblasts from normal persons lack expression of these receptors. TGF-β has been shown to upregulate the expression of these receptors in SSc fibroblasts but not in normal cells and, in conjunction with PDGF, stimulates SSc fibroblast proliferation. Macrophages and fibroblasts are capable of secreting PDGF and TGF-β, and activated T cells release TGF-β. TGF-β also induces the autocrine production of PDGF-related peptides, referred to as connective tissue growth factor (CTGF), by fibroblasts. TGF-β interacts with CTGF on fibroblasts to stimulate fibroblast proliferation and collagen synthesis. Serum levels of CTGF have been found to be elevated in SSc and correlate with the degree of dermal and pulmonary fibrosis.

Fibroblasts may activate T cells to release cytokines that stimulate fibrosis. Fibroblasts in SSc patients have been shown to have increased expression of an adhesion molecule, ICAM-1, which binds to specific integrins on T cells. This binding allows interaction between T cell antigen receptor and class II molecules and antigen on fibroblasts, resulting in T cell activation and cytokine release. T cells may also be activated by their interaction with extracellular matrix molecules including collagen, fibronectin, and laminin.

Recent studies have suggested that microchimerism may be involved in the pathogenesis of SSc. Microchimerism in SSc is of interest because of the clinical similarities between SSc and GVHD after allogeneic bone marrow transplantation. Also relevant are the predilection for women in SSc and the increased incidence of SSc in women after the childbearing years. Fetal progenitor cells can persist in the serum of normal women for many years after childbirth. Compared to normal controls, both the quantity and frequency of fetal cells have been found to be increased in the serum of SSc patients. Microchimerism can also occur in nulligravid women and in men with SSc as non-host cells may come from blood transfusion, engraftment of cells from a twin, or from maternal cells in utero. Two-directional traffic of cells occurs during pregnancy. The mechanism by which microchimerism is involved in the pathogenesis is not known, but it is conceivable that these small numbers of non-host cells interfere with immune regulation, leading to autoimmunity.

Chromosomal abnormalities have been noted in >90% of SSc patients. These acquired abnormalities include chromatid breaks, acentric fragments, and ring chromosomes and are found in ~30% of mitotic cells. A chromosomal breakage factor has been found in the serum of SSc patients and their first-degree relatives. The significance of these chromosomal abnormalities is unknown.

PATHOLOGY   Skin   In the skin, a thin epidermis overlies compact bundles of collagen that lie parallel to the epidermis. Finger-like projections of collagen extend from the dermis into the subcutaneous tissue and bind the skin to the underlying tissue. Dermal appendages are atrophied, and rete pegs are lost. In early stages of disease, a mononuclear cell infiltrate of predominantly T cells surrounds small dermal blood vessels. Increased numbers of T cells, monocytes, plasma cells, and mast cells are found, particularly in the lower dermis of involved skin.

Gastrointestinal Tract   In the lower two-thirds of the esophagus, the histologic findings consist of a thin mucosa and increased collagen in the lamina propria, submucosa, and serosa. The degree of fibrosis is less than in the skin. Atrophy of the muscularis in the esophagus and throughout the involved portions of the gastrointestinal tract is more prominent than the amount of fibrotic replacement of muscle. Ulceration of the mucosa is often present and may be due to either SSc or superimposed peptic esophagitis. Chronic esophageal reflux can lead to metaplasia of the lower esophagus (Barrett's esophagus), which is a premalignant lesion. Striated muscles in the upper third of the esophagus are relatively spared. Similar changes may be found throughout the gastrointestinal tract, especially in the second and third portions of the duodenum, in the jejunum, and in the large intestine. Atrophy of the muscularis of the large intestine may lead to the development of large-mouth diverticula. In the later stages of the disease, the involved portions of the gastrointestinal tract become dilated. Infiltration of lymphocytes and plasma cells in the lamina propria is also present.

Lung   With pulmonary involvement, diffuse interstitial fibrosis, thickening of the alveolar membrane, and peribronchial and pleural fibrosis are observed. Bronchiolar epithelial proliferation accompanies the pulmonary fibrosis. Rupture of septa produces small cysts and areas of bullous emphysema. Small pulmonary arteries and arterioles show intimal thickening, fragmentation of the elastica, and muscular hypertrophy; this may occur without interstitial pulmonary fibrosis and produce pulmonary hypertension, particularly in a subset of patients with limited cutaneous SSc.

Musculoskeletal System   The synovium in patients with arthritis is similar to that seen in early rheumatoid arthritis and shows edema with infiltration of lymphocytes and plasma cells. A characteristic finding is a thick layer of fibrin overlying and within the synovium. Later in the disease the synovium may become fibrotic. Fibrinous deposits appear on the surfaces of tendon sheaths and in the overlying fascia and may lead to audible creaking over moving tendons.

Histologic features of primary myopathy consist of interstitial and perivascular lymphocytic infiltrations, degeneration of muscle fibers, and interstitial fibrosis. Arterioles may be thickened, and capillaries may be decreased in number. Pathologic and electrophysiologic findings of polymyositis in proximal muscles are present in the few patients who are considered to have the overlap syndrome of SSc and polymyositis.

Heart   Cardiac involvement consists of degeneration of myocardial fibers and irregular areas of interstitial fibrosis that are most prominent around blood vessels. Intermittent spasm of blood vessels may result in contraction band necrosis, similar to change observed in myocardial infarction in patients with atherosclerotic coronary artery disease. Fibrosis also involves the conduction system, leading to atrioventricular conduction defects and arrhythmias. The wall of smaller coronary arteries may be thickened. Fibrinous pericarditis and pericardial effusions are found in some patients.

Kidney   Renal involvement is found in over half the patients and consists of intimal hyperplasia of the interlobular arteries; fibrinoid necrosis of the afferent arterioles, including the glomerular tuft; and thickening of the glomerular basement membrane. Small cortical infarctions and glomerulosclerosis may be present. The renal pathologic change is often indistinguishable from that observed in malignant hypertension. Renal vascular lesions, however, may be present in the absence of hypertension. Immunofluorescence studies of kidney have shown IgM, complement components, and fibrinogen in the walls of affected vessels. Angiographic renal studies in patients with SSc may show constriction of the intralobular arteries, a finding that simulates the vasospasm of the digital arteries observed in Raynaud's phenomenon. Cold-induced Raynaud's phenomenon has been shown to decrease renal blood flow.

Other Organs Primary liver involvement is not common. Primary biliary cirrhosis occurs in some patients, particularly in those with the limited cutaneous form of SSc. Fibrosis of the thyroid gland may develop in the presence or absence of autoimmune thyroiditis.

Thickening of the periodontal membrane with replacement of the lamina dura is demonstrated radiographically as widening of the periodontal space and may cause gingivitis and loosening of the teeth. The decreased oral aperture and mucosal dryness make eating and oral hygiene difficult.

CLINICAL MANIFESTATIONS (See Table 313-3) **Raynaud's Phenomenon** SSc usually begins insidiously; the first symptoms are frequently Raynaud's phenomenon and puffy fingers. Some 95% of patients will experience Raynaud's phenomenon, which is defined as episodic vasoconstriction of small arteries and arterioles of fingers, toes, and sometimes the tip of the nose and earlobes. Episodes are brought on by cold exposure, vibration, or emotional stress. Patients experience pallor and/or cyanosis followed by rubor on rewarming. Pallor and/or cyanosis are usually associated with coldness and numbness of fingers and/or toes, and rubor with pain and tingling. Not all patients appreciate the three color phases. A history of digit pallor appears to be the most reliable symptom for the presence of Raynaud's phenomenon. Raynaud's phenomenon may precede skin changes by several months or even years in those patients who subsequently develop the limited cutaneous form of SSc. In diffuse cutaneous SSc, skin changes are seen typically within a year of the onset of Raynaud's phenomenon. After 2 or more years of Raynaud's phenomenon, few patients who have this as their only symptom will subsequently develop SSc.

Skin Features In early disease, fingers and hands are swollen. Swelling may also involve forearms, feet, lower legs, and face. However, lower extremities are relatively spared. This edematous phase may last for a few weeks, months, or even longer. The edema may be pitting or nonpitting and accompanied by erythema. The skin changes begin distally in the extremities and advance proximally. The skin gradually becomes firm, thickened, and eventually tightly bound to underlying subcutaneous tissue (indurative phase). In patients with diffuse cutaneous scleroderma, skin changes will become generalized, involving initially the extremities, followed by the face and trunk over

a period of time, varying from months to a few years. In some patients, the skin changes may develop gradually over several years. Rapid progression of these changes over a 1- to 3-year period is associated with a greater risk of visceral disease, particularly of the lungs, heart, or kidneys. Also in diffuse cutaneous SSc, the skin changes usually peak in 3 to 5 years and then slowly improve. On the other hand, patients with limited cutaneous scleroderma will usually have a more gradual progression of skin changes, which are restricted to fingers or distal extremity and face and may continue to worsen. In both subsets of SSc, skin thickening is usually greater in the distal extremity. After many years of disease, the skin may soften and return to normal thickness or become thin and atrophic.

In the extremities, the taut skin over fingers gradually limits full extension, and flexion contractures develop. Ulcers may appear on the volar pads of the fingertips and over bony prominences such as elbows, malleoli, and the extensor surface of the proximal interphalangeal joints of the hands. These ulcers may become secondarily infected. The volar pads of the fingertips develop pitting scars and lose soft tissue. In some instances, resorption of the terminal phalanges occurs. Skin over the extremities, face, and trunk may become darkly pigmented, even without exposure to the sun. Hyperpigmentation of the skin may occur over superficial blood vessels and tendons. Areas of hypopigmentation may also develop, similar to vitiligo, involving the eyebrows, scalp, and trunk. The sparing of pigment around hair follicles gives the skin a "salt-and-pepper" appearance. Other patients may develop a diffuse tanning of the skin. The skin loses hair, oil, and sweat glands and so becomes dry and coarse. Vaginal dryness occurs and may cause dyspareunia.

In some patients, particularly those with the limited cutaneous form of disease, calcific deposits develop in intracutaneous and subcutaneous tissue. The sites commonly involved are periarticular tissue, digital pads, olecranon and prepatellar bursae, and skin along the extensor surface of the forearms. The overlying skin may break down, with drainage of calcific material. Involvement of the face results in thinning of the lips, loss of skin wrinkles and facial expression, as well as microstomia, which may make eating and dental hygiene difficult. The nose takes on a pinched or beaklike appearance. Wrinkles appear around the mouth perpendicular to the lips. Small telangiectatic mats may appear on the fingers, face, lips, tongue, and buccal mucosa after several years. They are seen more frequently in patients with limited cutaneous SSc but are also observed in patients with long-standing diffuse cutaneous SSc. The capillary beds of nail folds of the fingers may show enlargement of capillaries with little or no capillary loss, usually indicative of limited cutaneous scleroderma. In diffuse cutaneous scleroderma, there is disorganization of the capillary beds with dilated capillaries interspersed with areas where capillaries have disappeared. These capillary changes, which are observed by wide-angle microscopy or with an ophthalmoscope used as a magnifier, are not found in patients who have only Raynaud's phenomenon.

Musculoskeletal Features More than half the patients with SSc complain of pain, swelling, and stiffness of the fingers and knees. A symmetric polyarthritis resembling rheumatoid arthritis may be seen. In more advanced stages of the disease, leathery crepitation can be palpated over moving joints, especially the knee. Extensive fibrotic thickening of the tendon sheaths in the wrist can produce a carpal tunnel syndrome. Muscle weakness is usually present in patients with severe skin involvement and, in most cases, is due to disuse atrophy. There is a distinctive histologic myopathy that accompanies SSc that is not associated with muscle enzyme abnormalities. A few patients develop a myositis characterized by proximal muscle weakness and muscle enzyme elevations that are identical to polymyositis (overlap syndrome). In addition to terminal phalanges, resorption of bone may involve ribs, clavicle, and angle of mandible.

Gastrointestinal Features The majority of patients from both subsets of SSc have gastrointestinal involvement. Symptoms attributable to esophageal involvement are present in >50% of patients and

Table 313-3 Clinical Features of Systemic Sclerosis

Clinical Feature	Percent of Patients with Clinical Feature during Course of Disease	
	Limited[a]	Diffuse[a]
Raynaud's phenomenon	95–100	90–95
Skin thickening	98[b]	100
Subcutaneous calcinosis	50	10
Telangiectasia	85	40
Arthralgias/arthritis	40	70
Myopathy	5	50
Esophageal dysmotility	80	80
Pulmonary fibrosis	35	40
Isolated pulmonary arterial hypertension	<10	<1
Congestive heart failure	<1	30
Renal crisis	<1	15

[a] Limited cutaneous and diffuse cutaneous subsets of SSc.
[b] 2% or fewer of patients have SSc sine scleroderma.

include epigastric fullness, burning pain in the epigastric or retrosternal regions, and regurgitation of gastric contents. These symptoms, most noticeable when the patient is lying flat or bending over, are due to the reduced tone of the gastroesophageal sphincter and to dilatation of the distal esophagus. Peptic esophagitis frequently occurs and may lead to strictures and narrowing of the lower esophagus. However, it seldom results in bleeding. Barrett's metaplasia may develop, but transition to adenocarcinoma is uncommon. Dysphagia, particularly of solid foods, may occur independent of other esophageal symptoms and is caused by loss of esophageal motility due to neuromuscular dysfunction. Manometry or cineradiography reveals decreased amplitude or disappearance of peristaltic waves in the lower two-thirds of the esophagus. Raynaud's phenomenon in the absence of a connective tissue disease is also associated with esophageal dysmotility. Later in the course of the illness, dilatation and atony of the lower portion of the esophagus as well as reflux are seen. With gastric involvement, barium studies show dilatation, atony, and delayed gastric emptying. Patients may complain of early satiety. Gastric outlet obstruction can also occur.

Hypomotility of the small intestine produces symptoms of bloating and abdominal pain and may suggest an intestinal obstruction or paralytic ileus (pseudoobstruction). Malabsorption syndrome with weight loss, diarrhea, and anemia is due to bacterial overgrowth in the atonic intestine or possibly to obliteration of lymphatics by fibrosis. Roentgenographic features of the second and third portions of the duodenum and of the jejunum include dilatation, loss of the usual feathery pattern, and delayed disappearance of barium. Pneumatosis intestinalis occasionally occurs and appears as radiolucent cysts or linear streaks within the wall of the small intestine. Benign pneumoperitoneum may result from the rupture of these cysts. Involvement of the large intestine may cause chronic constipation and fecal impaction with episodes of bowel obstruction. A segment of atonic bowel may act as a fulcrum for intussusception to occur. Barium studies of the large intestine may show dilatation, atony, and large-mouth diverticula. Laxity of the anal sphincter may cause incontinence or rarely anal prolapse. Some patients may have gastrointestinal features of SSc with little or no cutaneous or other organ involvement, referred to as *SSc sine scleroderma*. Vascular ectasia may develop in the stomach and intestine and can be the source of gastrointestinal bleeding. These dilated submucosal capillaries in the stomach appear on endoscopy as broad stripes—hence the term "watermelon stomach."

Pulmonary Features   Pulmonary involvement occurs in at least two-thirds of SSc patients and is now the leading cause of death in SSc, replacing renal disease, which can usually be treated effectively. The most common symptom is exertional dyspnea, often accompanied by a dry, nonproductive cough. Bilateral basilar rales may be present. In the majority of patients, symptoms usually correlate with radiologic evidence of pulmonary fibrosis and with restrictive lung disease on pulmonary function tests.

Pulmonary function tests are frequently abnormal and show a reduction in vital capacity and decreased lung compliance. Impairment of gas exchange is reflected by a low diffusing capacity and low P_{O_2} with exercise. These abnormalities may be present even when the chest radiograph is normal. Chest film may show a pattern of linear densities, mottling, and honeycombing involving most prominently the lower two-thirds of the lung. Early interstitial pulmonary disease can be detected by high-resolution computed tomography (HRCT) and bronchoalveolar lavage (BAL). Active inflammatory alveolitis gives a "ground glass" appearance on HRCT. The recovery by BAL of increased numbers of cells, mostly alveolar macrophages accompanied by neutrophils or eosinophils, is evidence for alveolitis.

Both interstitial fibrosis and vascular lesions are found in the lungs of patients with SSc. Interstitial pulmonary fibrosis may be the predominant lesion in patients with diffuse or limited cutaneous SSc. Patients with diffuse cutaneous involvement who have antitopoisomerase 1 antibodies are particularly at risk of developing severe pul-

monary fibrosis. In the absence of significant interstitial fibrosis, a severe form of pulmonary arterial hypertension may develop after many years of disease in a subset of patients with limited cutaneous SSc. Fewer than 10% of patients will develop this complication, which is caused by narrowing and obliteration of pulmonary arteries and arterioles by intimal fibrosis and medial hypertrophy. Pulmonary hypertension is manifested initially by exertional dyspnea and eventually by the appearance of right-sided heart failure. Pulmonary artery pressure can be measured noninvasively by two-dimensional echocardiography. The prognosis is extremely poor with the development of pulmonary hypertension; the mean duration of survival is approximately 2 years.

A less common pulmonary problem is aspiration pneumonia resulting from gastric reflux due to lower esophageal atony. Restriction of chest movement caused by extensive fibrotic skin involvement of the thorax rarely occurs. Superimposed bacterial or viral infection can be a serious complication in patients with pulmonary fibrosis. An increased frequency of alveolar cell and bronchogenic carcinoma is seen in patients with pulmonary fibrosis.

Cardiac Features   Primary cardiac involvement in SSc includes pericarditis with or without effusions, heart failure, and varying degrees of heart block or arrhythmias. The majority of patients with diffuse cutaneous SSc have cardiac abnormalities. Cardiomyopathy attributable to myocardial fibrosis appears in <10% of patients and involves primarily those patients with diffuse cutaneous scleroderma. Radionuclide studies have shown abnormalities of left ventricular function due to myocardial fibrosis. Cold-induced vasospasm of the hands produces defects in myocardial thallium perfusion. The characteristic pathologic feature of contraction band necrosis results from cardiac muscle damage caused by intermittent vasospasm of coronary vessels. Patients may experience angina pectoris even though coronary angiograms are normal. Patients can also develop left ventricular failure secondary to systemic hypertension or cor pulmonale secondary to pulmonary arterial hypertension.

Renal Features   Renal failure was the leading cause of death in SSc until the advent of effective treatment. Significant renal disease occurs mostly in those patients with diffuse cutaneous scleroderma. A high risk of renal crisis is present in those patients who have rapidly progressive widespread skin thickening in their first 2 to 3 years of disease. Renal crisis is characterized by malignant hypertension, which can progress rapidly to renal failure. These patients manifest hypertensive encephalopathy, severe headache, retinopathy, seizures, and left ventricular failure. Hematuria and proteinuria are followed by oliguria and renal failure. The mechanism for the hypertensive crisis is activation of the renin-angiotensin system. Before the advent of effective antihypertensive drugs, the majority of these patients died within 6 months. A small number of patients may develop renal crises in the absence of hypertension. Renal failure can also develop insidiously later in the course of disease in the setting of mild to moderate hypertension and proteinuria. In these patients or those with clinically unrecognized renal disease, reduction of renal plasma flow secondary to heart failure or volume depletion resulting from overdiuresis may precipitate renal crisis. An indicator of impending renal failure is microangiopathic anemia, which may occur in a normotensive patient. The presence of a large chronic pericardial effusion may also herald subsequent renal failure.

Other Features   Symptoms of dry eyes and/or dry mouth are frequently present in patients with SSc. Lip biopsy may show lymphocytic infiltration of minor salivary glands characteristic of Sjögren's syndrome or intraglandular or periglandular fibrosis secondary to SSc. Antibodies to SS-A (Ro) and/or SS-B (La) are found in those patients with lip biopsies consistent with Sjögren's syndrome (overlap syndrome-SSc and Sjögren's syndrome) and not in those with salivary gland fibrosis.

Hypothyroidism occurs in a significant number of patients and may be associated with high levels of antithyroid antibodies. Fibrosis of the thyroid gland may be present but also occurs in the absence of autoimmune thyroiditis. Other manifestations of SSc include trigeminal neuralgia and male impotence secondary to decreased penile tumescence. These men have normal serum levels of testosterone and gonadotropins. Pathogenesis of this abnormality has been considered to be caused by vascular and/or autonomic nervous system abnormalities. Biliary cirrhosis is occasionally observed in patients with limited cutaneous SSc.

LABORATORY FINDINGS The erythrocyte sedimentation rate may be elevated. Hypoproliferative anemia related to chronic inflammation is the most common cause of anemia in SSc. Anemia may also be caused by iron deficiency secondary to gastrointestinal bleeding. Bacterial overgrowth due to atony of the small bowel may lead to vitamin B_{12} and/or folic acid–deficiency anemia. Microangiopathic hemolytic anemia is most often associated with renal involvement and is caused by the presence of intravascular fibrin in renal arterioles. Polyclonal hypergammaglobulinemia, consisting mostly of IgG, is found in approximately half the patients. Rheumatoid factor, in low titer, is present in 25% of patients. Cryoglobulins may be present in the serum. Antinuclear antibodies detected by using a cultured human laryngeal carcinoma cell line (HEp-2) substrate are present in 95% of patients (Table 313-4). Antinuclear antibodies that have a high specificity for SSc are antitopoisomerase 1 (Scl-70), antinucleolar, and anticentromere. Antitopoisomerase 1, originally called anti-Scl-70, recognizes the nuclear enzyme DNA topoisomerase 1, a nuclear enzyme involved in the unwinding of DNA for replication and RNA transcription. These antibodies are found in ~20% of all SSc patients and in ~40% of those with diffuse cutaneous SSc. They are associated with diffuse cutaneous involvement, interstitial pulmonary disease, and renal and other visceral organ involvement. A very high frequency of these antibodies has been reported in Choctaw Native Americans in association with diffuse cutaneous SSc. They are seldom present in other disorders or in conjunction with anticentromere antibodies. Anticentromere antibodies react with protein antigens located in the kinetochore region of chromosomes and are present in 40 to 80% of patients with limited cutaneous scleroderma or CREST syndrome. Anticentromere antibodies are found in only about 2 to 5% of patients with diffuse cutaneous scleroderma and rarely in other connective tissue diseases. They are found occasionally in patients with only Raynaud's phenomenon and may indicate subsequent development of limited cutaneous disease. Antinucleolar antibodies are relatively specific for SSc and are present in ~20 to 30% of patients. Several antinucleolar antibodies have been associated with SSc: Anti-RNA polymerases I, II, and III are found in patients with diffuse cutaneous SSc who have a higher prevalence of renal and cardiac involvement. Anti-Th RNP has been found in patients with limited cutaneous SSc, and anti-PM-Scl, formerly referred to as anti-PM1, along with anti-Ku, may be found in a subset of patients with overlapping features of limited cutaneous SSc and polymyositis. Anti-U_3 RNP (anti-fibrillarin) is also highly specific for SSc and may be associated with skeletal muscle disease, bowel involvement, and pulmonary arterial hypertension. Anti-U_1 RNP is found in ~5 to 10% of SSc patients and in 95 to 100% of those patients with the overlap syndrome of MCTD. The titers in MCTD are usually high (see below). Anti-SS-A (Ro) and/or anti-SS-B (La) are present in those patients with overlap syndrome of SSc and Sjögren's syndrome.

DIAGNOSIS The diagnosis of SSc presents no difficulty in the presence of Raynaud's phenomenon, with typical skin lesions and visceral involvement. Although Raynaud's phenomenon may be the first symptom of SSc, most patients with Raynaud's phenomenon alone do not develop a connective tissue disease. Other causes of Raynaud's phenomenon include thoracic outlet (scalenus anticus and cervical rib) syndromes, shoulder-hand syndrome, trauma (jackhammer or vibratory machine operators), previous cold injury, vinyl chloride exposure, and circulating cryoglobulins or cold agglutinins. Linear scleroderma and morphea are localized forms of scleroderma that can usually be distinguished clinically. In early disease, SSc may initially be confused with rheumatoid arthritis, SLE, or polymyositis when articular or muscle involvement is prominent. SSc without cutaneous involvement should be considered in patients with unexplained pulmonary fibrosis, pulmonary hypertension, cardiomyopathies, heart block, dysphagia, or malabsorption syndrome. Several conditions have scleroderma-like features but lack the visceral involvement. Scleredema (scleredema adultorum of Buschke) occurs predominantly in children and is characterized by painless edematous induration involving the face, scalp, neck, trunk, and proximal portions of the extremities. Involvement of the hands and feet usually does not occur. Scleredema may be associated with previous streptococcal infection and is usually self-limited, resolving in 6 to 12 months. Histology reveals accumulation of mucopolysaccharides in the dermis and skeletal muscle. A rare entity, scleromyxedema is manifested by yellowish or pale red papules in association with diffuse skin thickening that may involve the face and hands. Acid mucopolysaccharide deposits are found in the dermis. Monoclonal IgG may be detected in some of these patients. Patients with insulin-dependent diabetes mellitus may develop digital sclerosis and contractures (prayer hand deformity). Primary amyloidosis and amyloidosis associated with multiple myeloma may involve the skin of the extremities and face diffusely to give the appearance of scleroderma. Biopsy will clearly differentiate these entities.

COURSE AND PROGNOSIS The course of SSc is quite variable. Until the disease differentiates into recognizable subsets, prognosis in early disease is difficult to predict. Patients with limited cutaneous scleroderma, especially those with anticentromere antibodies, have a good prognosis, with the notable exception of those few patients, <10%, who after ≥10 to 20 years develop pulmonary arterial hypertension. Malabsorption syndrome and primary biliary cirrhosis are the causes of morbidity and mortality in some patients with limited cutaneous disease. On the other hand, the prognosis is generally worse in patients with diffuse cutaneous disease, particularly when the onset occurs at an older age. In addition, males have a worse prognosis. Renal and other visceral organ disease may develop early in the course of those patients with rapidly progressive generalized skin thickening. Death occurs most often from pulmonary, cardiac, and renal involvement. With the advent of effective therapy for renal crisis along with renal dialysis for those patients with renal failure, survival has greatly improved. In patients with diffuse cutaneous disease, the 5-year cumulative survival rate is ~70% and the 10-year is ~55%. In limited cutaneous disease the 5-year is ~90% and the 10-year is ~75%.

Skin may spontaneously soften after years of disease. Softening occurs in the reverse order of original skin involvement, beginning with the trunk and followed by the proximal and then the distal extremities. Sclerodactyly and flexion contractures may persist. Skin thickness may eventually approach normal; however, the skin may be atrophic.

TREATMENT Even though SSc cannot be cured, treatment of involved organ systems can relieve symptoms and improve function. The doctor-patient relationship is extremely important in caring for patients with this chronic debilitating illness. Once the diagnosis of SSc has been made, the patient and family should be instructed about this disorder. The patient will need repeated explanations and reassurances throughout his or her illness. Depending on the severity

Table 313-4 Autoantibodies in Systemic Sclerosis

Autoantibody	Clinical Association	Percent[a]
Antitopoisomerase 1	Diffuse cutaneous SSc	40
Anticentromere	Limited cutaneous SSc	60–80
Anti-RNA polymerase I, II, III	Diffuse cutaneous SSc	5–40
Anti-Th RNP	Limited cutaneous SSc	14
Anti-U_1 RNP	Limited cutaneous SSc	5–10
	Mixed connective tissue disease	95–100
Anti-PM/Scl	Overlap (SSc, polymyositis)	25

[a] Approximate percentages for the predominant clinical association.

of illness, the patient will require monitoring of blood pressure, blood counts, urinalysis, and monitoring of renal and pulmonary function on a regular basis.

Effectiveness of drug therapy in SSc is difficult to evaluate because of the variable course and severity of the disease. Many drugs have been used in the treatment of SSc without any consistent or prolonged benefit. In uncontrolled studies, D-penicillamine has been reported to reduce skin thickening and prevent development of significant organ involvement when compared to similar historic controls. Five-year cumulative survival rates of 80% have been reported in D-penicillamine-treated patients. This drug interferes with inter- and intramolecular cross-linking of collagen and is also immunosuppressive. Its immunosuppressive activity may also lead to decreased collagen production. Penicillamine is better tolerated when started at a low dose, usually 250 mg/d, and then increased at 1- to 3-month intervals up to 1.5 g/d as tolerated. Although a few patients can tolerate higher doses, most patients are maintained on a dose between 0.5 and 1 g/d. For optimal absorption, it is important to give this drug 1 h before or 2 h after a meal. This drug can be quite toxic; its more serious complications include glomerulonephritis with nephrotic syndrome, aplastic anemia, leukopenia, thrombocytopenia, and myasthenia gravis. Other side effects are fever, rash, anorexia, nausea, and loss of taste. Patients should have monthly complete blood counts (including platelet count) and urinalyses. The results of a 2-year double-blind randomized study comparing high-dose D-penicillamine (750 to 1000 mg/d) with low-dose D-penicillamine (125 mg every other day) in patients with early diffuse cutaneous SSc were recently reported. The degree of skin thickening and the occurrence of renal crises and other organ involvement as well as mortality were not significantly different between the high- and low-dose treated groups. This study suggested that there was no advantage in using doses >125 mg every other day. Azathioprine, methotrexate, cyclophosphamide, and other immunosuppressives have also been used in SSc and should be reserved for those patients with rapidly progressive disease. Control studies are lacking. Trials of treatment with recombinant interferon γ, 5-fluorouracil, and extracorporeal photochemotherapy have shown improvement in some disease parameters. No therapy, however, has been clearly demonstrated in a controlled, prospective study to suppress or reverse the disease process of SSc. Because of the poor prognosis in SSc patients who have a rapid onset of diffuse cutaneous disease and early visceral organ involvement (pulmonary, cardiac, or renal), clinical trials are under way using high-dose immunosuppressive therapy followed by autologous stem cell transplantation. The rationale is that high doses of an immunosuppressive drug such as cyclophosphamide may reverse or modify the disease course. The autologous stem cell transplantation permits the rapid reconstitution of hematopoiesis.

Antiplatelet therapy may play a role in the treatment of SSc, since the biologic products of platelets affect blood vessels. Low doses of aspirin block the formation of thromboxane A_2, a powerful vasoconstrictor and platelet aggregator. In addition, dipyridamole, 200 to 400 mg in divided daily doses, also decreases platelet adhesion to damaged vessel walls. While these drugs have a reasonable therapeutic rationale, a 2-year double-blind study did not show any benefit from their use. Reports of beneficial effects of colchicine or chlorambucil have not been documented in controlled studies.

Glucocorticoids are indicated in those patients with inflammatory myositis or pericarditis. The initial dose is 40 to 60 mg/d and is tapered based on clinical improvement (see below). They should not be used for the indolent primary form of muscle disease of SSc. Prednisone in the range of 20 to 40 mg/d may decrease edema associated with the edematous phase of early skin involvement. Glucocorticoids are not otherwise indicated in the long-term treatment of SSc. High doses of glucocorticoids may play a role in precipitating acute renal failure. A retrospective case-control study in patients with early diffuse cutaneous SSc showed a significant association between prior high-dose glucocorticoids (prednisone $\geq$ 15 mg/d) and the development of scleroderma renal crisis. Based on these observations, immunosuppressive drugs (e.g. methotrexate, azathioprine, or cyclophosphamide) should be considered in treating the inflammatory myositis, pericarditis, or early inflammatory skin disease.

The management of Raynaud's phenomenon is directed at control of vasospasm. Patients should be advised to dress warmly and wear mittens and socks, not to smoke, to remove causes of external stress, and to avoid drugs such as amphetamine and ergotamine. Cold drafts should be avoided. Air-conditioned rooms in warm climates can also be a problem for patients with Raynaud's phenomenon. Beta-blocking drugs may make Raynaud's phenomenon worse. Warmth of the central body induces peripheral vasodilatation. Drugs that block sympathetic vasoconstriction, such as reserpine, α-methyldopa, phenoxybenzamine, and prazosin, may be useful in the treatment of Raynaud's phenomenon, but their side effects often curtail extended use. The calcium channel blockers nifedipine, diltiazem, and the longer acting amlodipine can be effective in alleviating Raynaud's phenomenon, but side effects of light-headedness and palpitations may limit their use. The sustained-release form of nifedipine is better tolerated; the dose is 30 mg/d up to 60 or 90 mg/d as required to control symptoms. Nitroglycerine paste, applied to an affected digit, may improve local blood flow. In a 12-week pilot study, losartan, a specific nonpeptide angiotensen II type 1 receptor antagonist, reduced the severity and frequency of Raynaud's phenomenon episodes. Ketanserin, an oral serotonin antagonist, also has been shown to be effective. Selective serotonin reuptake inhibitors (e.g., fluoxetine) may be beneficial in some patients. These drugs decrease platelet 5-hydroxytryptamine, which is thought to play a role in the pathogenesis of Raynaud's phenomenon. Studies with intravenous iloprost, a prostacyclin analogue, have shown a decrease in frequency and severity of Raynaud's phenomenon and healing of digital ulcers in some patients. Iloprost is still not available in the United States for general use. Intravenous alprostadil, a prostaglandin, can be effective in treating severe Raynaud's phenomenon with digital ulcers. Epoprostenol (prostacyclin), used in the treatment of pulmonary hypertension, also improves Raynaud's phenomenon. Pentoxifylline may also improve perfusion by increasing the deformability of the red cell plasma membranes. Techniques of biofeedback have also been used with variable success for teaching patients to control the temperature of their hands. Stellate ganglion blockage may be useful in temporarily alleviating severe ischemic pain in the fingers. Surgical sympathectomy usually provides only temporary improvement, and it, along with other forms of therapy, does not prevent progression of the vascular lesion. Digital sympathectomy can be effective in some patients. The response to any therapy for Raynaud's phenomenon is limited by the degree of existing structural narrowing of digital arteries. In patients with severe Raynaud's phenomenon and refractory digital ulcers, distal ulnar artery occlusion should be considered. A positive Allen test is suggestive, and the diagnosis is confirmed by angiography. When ulnar artery occlusion is present, revascularization and a digital sympathectomy may be beneficial. Gangrene of distal digits may occur and require surgical amputation.

Numerous drugs have been claimed to soften the hidebound skin, but documentation in controlled studies is lacking. These drugs include D-penicillamine, colchicine, p-aminobenzoic acid, and vitamin E. In a recent randomized, double-blind, placebo-controlled trial, recombinant human relaxin given by continuous subcutaneous infusion for 24 weeks was associated with reduced skin thickening and improved mobility in patients with moderate to severe diffuse cutaneous scleroderma. Relaxin, a hormone associated with pregnancy, has been shown to have antifibrotic properties. Dryness of the skin may be reduced by avoiding frequent use of detergent soaps and by regularly applying hydrophilic ointments and bath oils. Regular exercise helps to maintain flexibility of extremities and pliability of skin. Massaging the skin several times a day may also be beneficial. Fingertip ulcerations can be protected by applying a guard or cage over the end of the finger. The use of an occlusive dressing, such as the hydrocolloid duo-DERM or other membranes, over a noninfected ulcer may promote healing and protect the finger. Skin ulcers should be kept clean by soaking or by surgical or chemical debridement. Sympatholytic drugs or local nitroglycerine paste applied to or adjacent to the ulcer may be beneficial in promoting healing. Infected ulcers can usually be treated with topical antibiotics but may require systemic antibiotics, especially when there is a question of underlying osteomyelitis. The development of calcinosis cannot be prevented, nor can deposits be dissolved. Warfarin has been reported to reduce calcinosis in a few patients.

In patients experiencing dry mouth, frequent sips of water help to relieve symptoms. Pilocarpine hydrochloride tablets may increase salivary secretions in some patients. Patients with dry eyes should use artificial tears regularly.

Patients with reflux esophagitis are treated with small, frequent meals, antacids between meals, and elevation of the head of the bed. Patients should be advised not to lie down for a few hours after a meal and to avoid coffee, tea, alcohol, peppermint, and chocolate, which reduce the pressure of the lower esophageal sphincter. Fatty foods and late-evening snacks should be avoided. Cimetidine, ranitidine or other newer H_2 blockers may be beneficial. Gastric acid (proton) pump inhibitors are more effective in treating erosive esophagitis than are H_2 blockers. Metoclopramide and cisapride increase gastrointestinal motility but do not significantly improve esophageal motility. They both increase lower esophageal sphincter tone and can be of help in some patients. Cisapride is no longer available (as of July 2000) because it caused life-threatening arrhythmias. Nifedipine and, to a lesser extent, diltiazem reduce lower esophageal sphincter tone resulting in esophageal reflux. Patients with dysphagia should be instructed to chew their food thoroughly and wash it down with fluids. Malabsorption syndrome due to duodenal hypomotility and bacterial overgrowth causes bloating and diarrhea, which may improve with intermittent use of appropriate antibiotics. Antibiotics are rotated every 2 weeks. Commonly used antibiotics are metronidazole, vancomycin, erythromycin, ciprofloxacin, neomycin, and tetracycline. Patients with severe debilitating malabsorption may benefit from parenteral hyperalimentation. Patients with chronic intestinal pseudoobstruction might respond to octreotide. Stool softeners and mild laxatives are usually adequate for treating constipation caused by hypomotility of the colon.

Articular symptoms are treated with nonsteroidal anti-inflammatory agents. Low-dose prednisone (≤ 10 mg/d) may improve symptoms in those not responding to these agents. Physical therapy may help to reduce the loss of joint mobility that occurs in SSc.

In patients with diffuse cutaneous SSc, the early recognition of alveolitis as previously described (see "Pulmonary Features") may allow treatment that might slow or prevent the development of pulmonary fibrosis. Cyclophosphamide has been reported in uncontrolled studies to be beneficial, and a controlled study is presently being done. The role of glucocorticoids in preventing progression of interstitial lung disease is not clear but may be of benefit in early disease. Pulmonary fibrosis is not reversible, and therefore treatment is directed at symptoms or complications. Pulmonary infection requires prompt treatment with antibiotics. Hypoxia necessitates giving low concentrations of oxygen. Patients should receive polyvalent pneumoccal vaccine (Pneumovax) and yearly influenza immunizations.

For patients with limited cutaneous SSc who develop isolated pulmonary arterial hypertension, treatment is limited. The usual treatment is supplemental oxygen, anticoagulation, and the administration of a vasodilator. A calcium channel blocker such as nifedipine lowers pulmonary arterial resistance and improves cardiac function, but in most patients this is only for a short period of time. Few patients survive more than 5 years. Heart-lung or single-lung transplantation may be a therapeutic option only in those patients without other significant systemic involvement. Current reports of intravenous epoprostenol (prostacyclin) in the treatment of SSc-associated pulmonary hypertension have been encouraging. Epoprostenol is infused continuously via a central line with a portable pump. Improvement in symptoms of right heart failure and exercise tolerance occurred. Also hemodynamic tests showed a decrease in the pulmonary vascular resistance and pulmonary artery pressure both in the short term and in a few patients after 1 or 2 years.

Recognition of early signs of renal hypertensive crisis is important in order to preserve renal function and prevent hypertensive encephalopathy. Renal involvement is often accompanied by hypertension and mild to moderate proteinuria. An occasional patient may be normotensive. Antihypertensive agents are often effective in lowering blood pressure and stabilizing or reversing renal failure. These drugs include propranolol, clonidine, and minoxidil. Particularly effective are the angiotensin-converting enzyme inhibitors, which include captopril, enalapril, and lisinopril. Dialysis may be required in patients with progressive renal failure. Some patients, however, have a slow return of renal function after several months and may no longer require dialysis. Patients are usually not candidates for kidney transplantation because of the other systemic manifestations of SSc.

Patients with cardiac failure require careful monitoring of digitalis and diuretic administration. Noninflammatory pericardial effusions may also improve with diuretics. Care should be taken to avoid overdiuresis, which may lead to decreased renal blood flow, decreased cardiac output, and renal failure.

MIXED CONNECTIVE TISSUE DISEASE MCTD is an overlap syndrome characterized by combinations of clinical features of SLE (Chap. 311), SSc, polymyositis (Chap. 382), and rheumatoid arthritis (Chap. 312) and the presence of very high titers of circulating autoantibodies to nuclear RNP antigen. This antibody in high titer, now referred to as *anti-U₁ RNP*, has been a justification for considering MCTD as a distinct clinical entity. MCTD has been challenged as a distinct disorder by those who consider it as a subset of SLE or scleroderma. Others prefer to classify MCTD as an undifferentiated connective tissue disease. MCTD occurs worldwide and in all races. The peak onset of disease is in the second and third decades, but MCTD is seen in children and the elderly. Women are predominantly affected. The pathogenic mechanisms in MCTD reflect the disorders making up this syndrome.

Clinical Features The presenting symptoms of MCTD are most often Raynaud's phenomenon, puffy hands, arthralgias, myalgias, and fatigue. Occasionally, patients may present with the acute onset of high fever, polymyositis, arthritis, and neurologic features such as trigeminal neuralgia and aseptic meningitis. The various features of the connective tissue disorders making up MCTD develop over months and years.

The fingers as well as the entire hand may be puffy, followed later by sclerodactyly. Sclerodermal changes are usually limited to the distal extremities and sometimes the face but spare the trunk. Telangiectasia and calcinosis may develop. Some patients have mucocutaneous features of SLE including a classic malar rash, photosensitivity, discoid lesions, alopecia, and painful oral ulcerations. An erythematous rash over the knuckles, elbows, and knees and heliotropic eyelids, typical of dermatomyositis, are uncommon.

Joint pain, stiffness, and swelling involving the peripheral joints occur frequently. Deformities of the hands similar to those of rheumatoid arthritis may develop but usually without bony erosions. A destructive polyarthritis is occasionally observed. Myalgias are a frequent symptom. Some patients develop typical symptoms of polymyositis with proximal muscle weakness, abnormal electromyographic findings, elevated levels of muscle enzymes, and inflammatory changes on muscle biopsy.

Approximately 85% of patients have pulmonary involvement, which is often asymptomatic. Diffusing capacity for carbon monoxide may be the only abnormality. Pleurisy commonly occurs but is seldom associated with large pleural effusions. Some patients develop interstitial lung disease. Pulmonary arterial hypertension is the most common cause of death in MCTD.

Approximately 25% of patients develop renal disease. Membranous glomerulonephritis is most common and usually mild but can cause nephrotic syndrome. Diffuse proliferative glomerulonephritis is unusual in MCTD, perhaps because of the protective role believed to be played by the high titers of anti-U$_1$ RNP. Renal crisis secondary to malignant renovasculature hypertension, as occurs in scleroderma, is seen in a few patients.

Gastrointestinal involvement is seen in ~70% of patients. The most common manifestations are esophageal dysmotility, lower esophageal sphincter laxity, and gastroesophageal reflux. Bowel manifestations mimic those of scleroderma bowel disease.

Pericarditis occurs in 30% of patients. Other cardiac features include myocarditis, arrhythmia, conduction disturbances, and mitral valve prolapse. Other clinical features of MCTD include trigeminal neuropathy, peripheral neuropathy, aseptic meningitis, lymphadenopathy, and Sjögren's syndrome. The majority of patients have developed, or will develop within 5 years of presentation, diagnostic clinical criteria for one of the overlapping connective tissue diseases, most often SLE or SSc.

Laboratory Findings   Anemia of chronic inflammation is seen in the majority of patients. A positive direct Coombs' test is found in many patients, but hemolytic anemia is unusual. Leukopenia, thrombocytopenia, or both are present in some patients. Hypergammaglobulinemia is common, and rheumatoid factor is present in 50% of patients.

All patients, by definition of MCTD, have antibodies to U$_1$ RNP. The specificity of this antibody is to the 70-kDa protein complexed to small nuclear RNA. The anti-U$_1$ RNP antibodies are associated with HLA-DR4 but not with -DR2 and -DR3 as found in SLE. Molecular mimicry has been demonstrated between U$_1$ RNP and retroviral antigens by some laboratories.

℞ **TREATMENT**   The treatment of MCTD is essentially the same as would be indicated for the respective connective tissue diseases defining this syndrome. More than half the patients have a favorable course. The 10-year survival rate overall is approximately 80% but varies depending on the connective tissue disease that may eventually develop.

EOSINOPHILIC FASCIITIS   Eosinophilic fasciitis is a scleroderma-like syndrome of unknown cause characterized by inflammation followed later by sclerosis of the dermis, subcutis, and deep fascia. The disease affects adults and often occurs after strenuous physical activity. Patients do not have Raynaud's phenomenon or internal organ involvement. Several immunologic abnormalities have been associated with eosinophilic fasciitis and include aplastic anemia, myelodysplastic syndrome, and thrombocytopenia. Patients usually have the abrupt onset of symmetric tenderness and swelling of the extremities, rapidly followed by induration of the skin and subcutaneous tissue. The skin takes on a cobblestone or puckered appearance. Carpal tunnel syndrome appears early in the course, and flexion contractures develop later. A low-grade myositis is often present, but creatinine kinase levels are usually normal. A marked eosinophilia is found in the early stage of disease and subsequently decreases. Increased levels of polyclonal IgG and immune complexes are often present in the serum. A full-thickness biopsy consisting of skin, fascia, and superficial muscle shows perivascular infiltration of histiocytes, eosinophils, lymphocytes, and plasma cells. Biopsies later in the course show sclerosis. Spontaneous improvement and occasionally complete remission may occur after 2 to 5 years of disease. Some patients have persistent disease, while others are left with flexion contractures. Administration of glucocorticoids may provide symptomatic improvement and will decrease the eosinophilia. Improvement has been reported with the use of the H$_2$ blocker cimetidine.

EOSINOPHILIA-MYALGIA SYNDROME   In 1989, reports of patients with scleroderma-like skin changes, myalgias, and eosinophilia dramatically increased. Most, but not all, of these cases were associated with ingestion of L-tryptophan manufactured by a single Japanese company. Batches of L-tryptophan implicated in EMS were found to contain trace amounts of a contaminant identified as a dimer

of L-tryptophan that appeared in 1988 after changes were made in the method of manufacturing this drug. It is not clear whether this chemical contaminant is the etiologic agent or whether another unidentified substance is responsible. *L-Tryptophan products were taken off the market in 1990.* The onset of EMS can be either abrupt or insidious. In the early phases of the disease, clinical manifestations include low-grade fever, fatigue, dyspnea, cough, arthralgias/arthritis, evanescent erythematous rashes, muscle cramping, and severe myalgias. Pulmonary infiltrates may be present. Over the next 2 to 3 months, scleroderma-like skin changes appear. Some patients develop a peripheral neuropathy, which may persist. An ascending polyneuropathy may lead to paralysis and respiratory failure requiring ventilatory assistance. Cognitive dysfunction with impairment of memory and concentration has been recognized in this syndrome. Myocarditis and cardiac arrhythmias occur in some patients, and a few patients develop pulmonary hypertension. Approximately a third of patients have features of eosinophilic fasciitis. EMS most closely resembles toxic oil syndrome; however, Raynaud's phenomenon does not occur, and there is a lower prevalence of pulmonary hypertension and thromboembolic disease. The peripheral eosinophil count is >1000/μL in most patients. The histologic findings on biopsy of skin, fascia, and superficial muscle are similar to those found in eosinophilic fasciitis. The clinical features of EMS may persist after L-tryptophan has been discontinued. EMS may run a chronic course, and response to therapy has been variable. Treatment has included glucocorticoids, antimalarial drugs, immunosuppressive drugs, and plasmapheresis. Prednisone was beneficial during the acute inflammatory phase of the disease in the majority of patients and resulted in resolution of pulmonary infiltrates, peripheral edema, and eosinophilia. In the later phase of the illness, no treatment was found to be of particular value. The pathogenesis of this disease is not known. A follow-up of patients 2 years after their onset of illness showed that most symptoms and physical findings had resolved or improved except for cognitive dysfunction, which became worse in approximately one-third of the patients, and peripheral neuropathy, which remained unchanged (Chap. 382).

BIBLIOGRAPHY

ARNETT FC: HLA and autoimmunity in scleroderma (systemic sclerosis). Int Rev Immunol 12:107, 1995

BENNETT RM: Mixed connective tissue disease and other overlap syndromes, in *Textbook of Rheumatology*, 5th ed, WN Kelley et al (eds). Philadelphia, Saunders, 1997, p 1065

BLACK CM: Systemic sclerosis: Management, in *Rheumatology*, 2 ed, JH Klippel, PA Dieppe (eds). London, Mosby International, 1998, 7:11.1

BOLSTER MB, SILVER RM: Assessment and management of scleroderma lung disease. Curr Opin Rheumatol 11:508, 1999

BORDRON A et al: The binding of some human antiendothelial cell antibodies induces endothelial cell apoptosis. J Clin Invest 101:2029, 1998

CARPENTIER PH, MARICQ HR: Microvasculature in systemic sclerosis. Rheum Dis Clin North Am 16:75, 1990

CLEMENTS PJ, FURST DE: Choosing appropriate patients with systemic sclerosis for treatment by autologous stem cell transplantation. J Rheumatol 24(Suppl 48):85, 1997

———— et al: High-dose versus low-dose D-penicillamine in early diffuse systemic sclerosis: Analysis of a two-year, double-blind, randomized, controlled clinical trial. Arthritis Rheum 42:1194, 1999

EVANS PC et al: Long-term fetal microchimerism in peripheral blood mononuclear cell subsets in healthy women and women with scleroderma. Blood 93:2033, 1999

HARVEY GR, MCHUGH NJ: Serologic abnormalities in systemic sclerosis. Curr Opin Rheumatol 11:495, 1999

HERTZMAN PA et al: The eosinophilia-myalgia syndrome: Status of 205 patients and results of treatment 2 years after onset. Ann Intern Med 122:851, 1995

KAHALEH B, MATUCCI-CERINIC M: Raynaud's phenomenon and scleroderma: Dysregulated neuroendothelial control of vascular tone. Arthritis Rheum 38:1, 1995

KLINGS ES et al: Systemic sclerosis–associated pulmonary hypertension: Short- and long-term effects of epoprostenol (prostacyclin). Arthritis Rheum 42:2638, 1999

LAKHANPAL S et al: Eosinophilic fasciitis: Clinical spectrum and therapeutic response in 52 cases. Semin Arthritis Rheum 17:221, 1988

LEROY EC: Pathogenesis of systemic sclerosis (scleroderma), in *Arthritis and Allied Conditions*, 13th ed, WJ Koopman (ed). Baltimore, Williams & Wilkins, 1997, p 1481

———— et al: Systemic sclerosis (scleroderma): Classification, subsets and pathogenesis. J Rheumatol 15:202, 1988

MCSWEENEY PA: High-dose immunosuppressive therapy for rheumatoid arthritis: Some answers, more questions. Arthritis Rheum 42:2269, 1999

MEDSGER TA JR: Systemic sclerosis (scleroderma), Clinical aspects, in *Arthritis and Allied Conditions*, 13th ed, WJ Koopman (ed). Baltimore, Williams & Wilkins, 1997, p 1433

NELSON JL: Microchimerism and the pathogenesis of systemic sclerosis. Curr Opin Rheumatol 10:564, 1998

POSTLETHWAITE AE: Role of T cells and cytokines in effecting fibrosis. Int Rev Immunol 12:247, 1995

REICHLIN M: Undifferentiated connective tissue diseases, overlap syndromes, and mixed connective tissue disease, in *Arthritis and Allied Conditions*, 13th ed, WJ Koopman (ed). Baltimore, Williams & Wilkins, 1997, p 1309

RENAUDINEAU Y et al: Anti-endothelial cell antibodies in systemic sclerosis. Clin Diagn Lab Immunol 6:156, 1999

ROSE S et al: Gastrointestinal manifestations of scleroderma. Gastroenterol Clin North Am 27:563, 1998

SATO S et al: Serum levels of connective tissue growth factor are elevated in patients with SSc: Association with extent of skin sclerosis and severity of pulmonary fibrosis. J Rheumatol 27:149, 2000

SEIBOLD JR: Scleroderma, in *Textbook of Rheumatology*, 5th ed, WN Kelley et al (eds). Philadelphia, Saunders, 1997, p 1133

SEIBOLD JR et al: Recombinant human relaxin in the treatment of scleroderma, a randomized, double-blind, placebo-controlled trial. Ann Intern Med 132:871, 2000

SILVER RM: Variant forms of scleroderma, in *Arthritis and Allied Conditions*, 13th ed, WJ Koopman (ed). Baltimore, Williams & Wilkins, 1997, p 1465

——— et al: Trytophan metabolism via the kyurenine pathway in patients with the esoinophilia myalgia syndrome. Arthritis Rheum 35:1097, 1992

STEEN VD: Renal involvement in systemic sclerosis. Clin Dermatol 12:253, 1994

———, MEDSGER TA: Case-control study of corticosteroids and other drugs that either precipitate or protect from the development of scleroderma renal crisis. Arthritis Rheum 41:1613, 1998

——— et al: Therapy for severe interstitial lung disease in systemic sclerosis. A retrospective study. Arthritis Rheum 37:1290, 1994

SUBCOMMITTEE FOR SCLERODERMA CRITERIA OF THE AMERICAN RHEUMATISM ASSOCIATION DIAGNOSTIC AND THERAPEUTIC CRITERIA COMMITTEE: Preliminary criteria for the classification of systemic sclerosis (scleroderma). Arthritis Rheum 23:581, 1980

TAN FK et al: Association of microsatellite markers near the fibrillin 1 gene on human chromosome 15q with scleroderma in a Native American population. Arthritis Rheum 41:1729, 1998

VARGA J, BASHEY RI: Regulation of connective tissue synthesis in systemic sclerosis. Int Rev Immunol 12:187, 1995

V'AZQUEZ AD, ROTHFIELD NF: Autoantibodies in systemic sclerosis. Int Rev Immunol 12:145, 1995

314 *Haralampos M. Moutsopoulos*

SJÖGREN'S SYNDROME

DEFINITION Sjögren's syndrome is a chronic, slowly progressive autoimmune disease characterized by lymphocytic infiltration of the exocrine glands resulting in xerostomia and dry eyes. Approximately one-third of patients present with systemic manifestations. A small but significant number of the patients may develop malignant lymphoma. The disease can be seen alone (primary Sjögren's syndrome) or in association with other autoimmune rheumatic diseases (secondary Sjögren's syndrome) (Table 314-1).

INCIDENCE AND PREVALENCE The disease affects predominantly middle-aged women (female-to-male ratio 9:1), although it occurs in all ages, including childhood. The prevalence of primary Sjögren's syndrome is approximately 0.5 to 1.0%. In addition, 30% of patients with autoimmune rheumatic diseases suffer from secondary Sjögren's syndrome.

PATHOGENESIS Sjögren's syndrome is characterized by lymphocytic infiltration of the exocrine glands and B lymphocyte hyperreactivity, as illustrated by circulating autoantibodies. The latter is accompanied by an oligomonoclonal B cell process, which is characterized by serum and urine monoclonal light chains and cryoprecipitable monoclonal immunoglobulins.

Sera of patients with Sjögren's syndrome often contain a number of autoantibodies directed against non-organ-specific antigens such as immunoglobulins (rheumatoid factors) and extractable nuclear and cy-

Table 314-1   Association of Sjögren's Syndrome with Other Autoimmune Diseases

Rheumatoid arthritis	Primary biliary cirrhosis
Systemic lupus erythematosus	Vasculitis
Scleroderma	Chronic active hepatitis
Mixed connective tissue disease	

toplasmic antigens (Ro/SS-A, La/SS-B). Ro/SS-A autoantigen consists of three polypeptide chains (52, 54, and 60 kDa) in conjunction with RNAs, whereas the 48-kDa La/SS-B protein is bound to RNA III polymerase transcripts. The presence of autoantibodies to Ro/SS-A and La/SS-B antigens in Sjögren's syndrome is associated with earlier disease onset, longer disease duration, salivary gland enlargement, severity of lymphocytic infiltration of minor salivary glands, and certain extraglandular manifestations such as lymphadenopathy, purpura, and vasculitis. Antibodies to α-fordin (120 kDa), a salivary gland–specific protein, have recently been found in sera of patients with Sjögren's syndrome but not in sera of patients with other connective tissue diseases.

Phenotypic and functional studies have shown that the predominant cell infiltrating the affected exocrine glands is the helper/inducer T cell with characteristics of memory cells. Both B and T infiltrating lymphocytes are activated, as illustrated by production of immunoglobulins with autoantibody activity, spontaneous release of interleukin 2, and expression on the T cell surface of activation markers such as class II HLA as well as costimulatory molecules and lymphocyte function–associated antigen 1. Macrophages and natural killer cells are rarely detected in infiltrates, while epithelial cells of the affected glands inappropriately express class II molecules and possess messages for c-*myc* protooncogene and proinflammatory cytokines. All these phenomena suggest that the epithelial cell of the exocrine glands in Sjögren's syndrome may act as an antigen-presenting cell. In contrast to infiltrating lymphocytes, these cells undergo apoptotic death, resulting in exocrine gland dysfunction.

Immunogenetic studies have demonstrated that HLA-B8, -DR3, and -DRw52 are prevalent in patients with primary Sjögren's syndrome as compared with the normal control population. Molecular analysis of HLA class II genes has revealed that patients with Sjögren's syndrome, regardless of their ethnic origin, are highly associated with the HLA DQA1*0501 allele.

CLINICAL MANIFESTATIONS The majority of the patients with Sjögren's syndrome have symptoms related to diminished lacrimal and salivary gland function. In most patients, the primary syndrome runs a slow and benign course. The initial manifestations can be mucosal dryness or nonspecific, and 8 to 10 years elapse from the initial symptoms to full-blown development of the disease.

The principal oral symptom of Sjögren's syndrome is dryness (xerostomia). Patients complain of difficulty in swallowing dry food, inability to speak continuously, a burning sensation, increase in dental caries, and problems in wearing complete dentures. Physical examination shows a dry, erythematous, sticky oral mucosa. There is atrophy of the filiform papillae on the dorsum of the tongue, and saliva from the major glands is either not expressible or is cloudy. Enlargement of the parotid or other major salivary glands occurs in two-thirds of patients with primary Sjögren's syndrome but is uncommon in those with the secondary syndrome. Diagnostic tests include sialometry, sialography, and scintigraphy. The labial minor salivary gland biopsy permits histopathologic confirmation of the focal lymphocytic infiltrates.

Ocular involvement is the other major manifestation of Sjögren's syndrome. Patients usually complain of dry eyes, with a sandy or gritty feeling under the eyelids. Other symptoms include burning, accumulation of thick strands at the inner canthi, decreased tearing, redness, itching, eye fatigue, and increased photosensitivity. These symptoms are attributed to the destruction of corneal and bulbar conjunctival epithelium, defined as keratoconjunctivitis sicca. Diagnostic evaluation of keratoconjunctivitis sicca includes measurement of tear flow by Schirmer's I test and tear composition as assessed by the tear breakup time or tear lysozyme content. Slit-lamp examination of the cornea and conjunctiva after rose Bengal staining reveals punctate corneal ulcerations and attached filaments of corneal epithelium.

Involvement of other exocrine glands occurs less frequently and includes a decrease in mucous gland secretions of the upper and lower respiratory tree, resulting in dry nose, throat, and trachea (xerotrachea), and diminished secretion of the exocrine glands of the gastrointestinal tract, leading to esophageal mucosal atrophy, atrophic gastritis, and subclinical pancreatitis. Dyspareunia due to dryness of the external genitalia and dry skin also may occur.

Extraglandular (systemic) manifestations are seen in one-third of patients with Sjögren's syndrome (Table 314-2), while they are very rare in patients with Sjögren's syndrome associated with rheumatoid arthritis. These patients complain more often of easy fatigability, low-grade fever, Raynaud's phenomenon, myalgias, and arthralgias. Most patients with primary Sjögren's syndrome experience at least one episode of nonerosive arthritis during the course of their disease. Manifestations of pulmonary involvement are frequent but rarely important clinically. Dry cough is the major manifestation that is attributed to small airway disease. Renal involvement includes interstitial nephritis, clinically manifested by hypostenuria and renal tubular dysfunction with or without acidosis. Untreated acidosis may lead to nephrocalcinosis. Glomerulonephritis is a rare finding that occurs in patients with systemic vasculitis, cryoglobulinemia, or systemic lupus erythematosus overlapping with Sjögren's syndrome. Vasculitis affects small and medium-sized vessels. The most common clinical features are purpura, recurrent urticaria, skin ulcerations, glomerulonephritis, and mononeuritis multiplex. Sensorineural hearing loss was found in one-half of patients with Sjögren's syndrome and correlated with the presence of anticardiolipin antibodies.

It has been suggested that primary Sjögren's syndrome with vasculitis also may present with multifocal, recurrent, and progressive nervous system disease, such as hemiparesis, transverse myelopathy, hemisensory deficits, seizures, and movement disorders. Aseptic meningitis and multiple sclerosis also have been reported in these patients.

Lymphoma is a well-known manifestation of Sjögren's syndrome that usually presents later in the illness. Persistent parotid gland enlargement, lymphadenopathy, cutaneous vasculitis, peripheral neuropathy, lymphopenia, and cryoglobulinemia are manifestations suggesting the development of lymphoma. Most lymphomas are extranodal, marginal zone B cell, and low grade. Salivary glands are the most common site of involvement.

Routine laboratory tests reveal mild normochromic, normocytic anemia. An elevated erythrocyte sedimentation rate is found in approximately 70% of patients.

DIAGNOSIS AND DIFFERENTIAL DIAGNOSIS   A European multicenter study has developed diagnostic criteria of Sjögren's syndrome (Table 314-3), which have been validated and present high

Table 314-2   Incidence of Extraglandular Manifestations in Primary Sjögren's Syndrome

Clinical Manifestation	Percent
Arthralgias/arthritis	60
Raynaud's phenomenon	37
Lymphadenopathy	14
Lung involvement	14
Vasculitis	11
Kidney involvement	9
Liver involvement	6
Lymphoma	6
Splenomegaly	3
Peripheral neuropathy	2
Myositis	1

Table 314-3   Diagnostic Criteria for Sjögren's Syndrome[a]

Criteria	Definitions
1. Ocular symptoms	Dry eyes every day for more than 3 months, recurrent sensation of sand or gravel in the eyes, or use of tear substitutes more than three times a day
2. Oral symptoms	Daily feeling of dry mouth for more than 3 months, recurrent or persistently swollen salivary glands, or use of liquids to aid in swallowing dry food
3. Ocular signs	Positive Schirmer's I test (<5 mm in 5 min), or a rose Bengal score of ≥4 according to van Bijsterveld's scoring system
4. Histopathology	Focus score 1 in a minor salivary gland biopsy
5. Salivary gland involvement	Positive result in one of the following tests: salivary scintigraphy, parotid sialography, salivary flow (≤1.5 mL in 15 min)
6. Autoantibodies	Antibodies to Ro(SS-A) or La(SS-B), antinuclear antibodies, or rheumatoid factor

[a] Probable Sjögren's syndrome: three items are present.
  Definite Sjögren's syndrome: four or more items are present.

specificity and sensitivity. A diagnostic algorithm is depicted in Fig. 314-1.

The differential diagnosis of Sjögren's syndrome includes other conditions that may cause dry mouth or eyes or parotid salivary gland enlargement (Table 314-4). Infections with HIV and hepatitis C virus (Chap. 309) and sarcoidosis (Chap. 318) appear to produce a clinical picture indistinguishable from that of Sjögren's syndrome (Table 314-5).

℞ TREATMENT   Sjögren's syndrome remains fundamentally an incurable disease. Hence treatment is aimed at symptomatic relief and limiting the damaging local effects of chronic xerostomia and keratoconjunctivitis sicca by substitution of the missing secretions.

The sicca complex is treated with fluid replacement supplied as often as necessary. To replace deficient tears, there are several readily available ophthalmic preparations (Tearisol; Liquifilm; 0.5% methylcellulose; Hypo Tears). It may be necessary for severely affected patients to use these preparations as often as every 30 min. If corneal ulceration is present, eye patching and boric acid ointments are recommended. Certain drugs that may increase lacrimal and salivary hy-

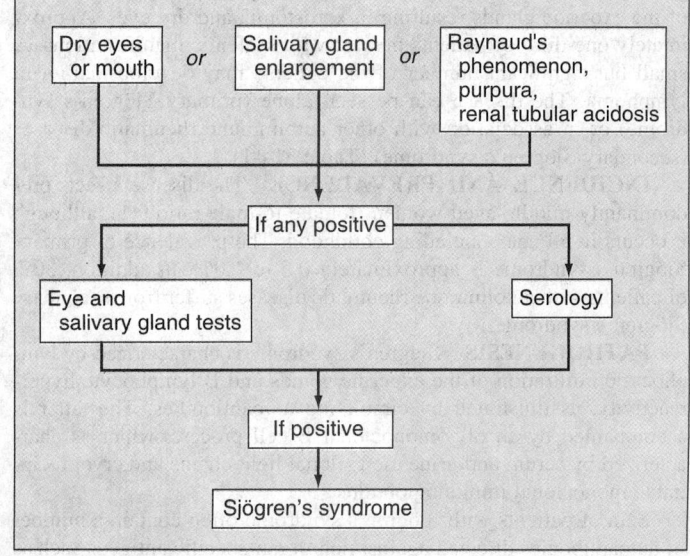

FIGURE 314-1   Algorithm for the diagnosis of Sjögren's syndrome.

Table 314-4 Differential Diagnosis of Sicca Symptoms

Xerostomia	Dry Eye	Bilateral Parotid Gland Enlargement
Viral infections	Inflammation	Viral infections
Drugs	Stevens-Johnson	Mumps
Psychotherapeutic	syndrome	Influenza
Parasympatholytic	Pemphigoid	Epstein-Barr
Antihypertensives	Chronic conjuncti-	Coxsackievirus A
Psychogenic	vitis	Cytomegalovirus
Irradiation	Chronic blepharitis	HIV
Diabetes mellitus	Sjögren's syn-	Sarcoidosis
Trauma	drome	Amyloidosis
Sjögren's	Toxicity	Sjögren's syndrome
syndrome	Burns	Metabolic
	Drugs	Diabetes mellitus
	Neurologic condi-	Hyperlipoproteinemias
	tions	Chronic pancreatitis
	Impaired lacrimal	Hepatic cirrhosis
	gland function	Endocrine
	Impaired eyelid	Acromegaly
	function	Gonadal hypofunction
	Miscellaneous	
	Trauma	
	Hypovitaminosis A	
	Blink abnormality	
	Lid scarring	
	Anesthetic cornea	
	Epithelial irregu-	
	larity	

Table 314-5 Differential Diagnosis of Sjögren's Syndrome with HIV Infection

HIV Infection and Sicca Syndrome	Sjögren's Syndrome	Sarcoidosis
Predominant in young males	Predominant in middle-aged women	Invariable
Lack of autoantibodies to Ro/SS-A and/or La/SS-B	Presence of autoanti-bodies	Lack of autoantibodies to Ro/SS-A and/or La/SS-B
Lymphoid infiltrates of salivary glands by CD8+ lymphocytes	Lymphoid infiltrates of salivary glands by CD4+ lymphocytes	Granulomas in salivary glands
Association with HLA-DR5	Association with HLA-DR3 and -DRw52	Unknown
Positive serologic tests for HIV	Negative serologic tests for HIV	Negative serologic tests for HIV

pofunction such as diuretics, antihypertensive drugs, and antidepressants should be avoided. Propionic acid gels may be used to treat vaginal dryness.

Pilocarpine (5 mg thrice daily) given orally appears to improve sicca manifestations. Hydroxychloroquine (200 mg/day) is helpful for arthralgias. Glucocorticoids (1 mg/kg per day) or other immunosuppressive agents (i.e., cyclophosphamide) are indicated for the treatment of extraglandular manifestations, particularly when renal or severe pulmonary involvement and systemic vasculitis have been documented.

BIBLIOGRAPHY

DAFNI UG et al: Prevalence of Sjögren's syndrome in a closed rural community. Ann Rheum Dis 56:521, 1997

HANEJI N et al: Identification of alpha-fodrin as a candidate autoantigen in primary Sjögren's syndrome. Science 276:604, 1997

MANOUSSAKIS MN et al: Expression of B7 costimulatory molecules by salivary gland epithelial cells in patients with Sjögren's syndrome. Arthritis Rheum 42:229, 1999

PAPIRIS SA et al: Lung involvement in Sjögren's syndrome. Semin Respir Crit Care Med 20, 179, 1999

POLIHRONIS M et al: Modes of epithelial cell death and repair in Sjögren's syndrome. Clin Exp Immunol 114:485, 1998

TUMIATI B et al: Hearing loss in the Sjögren syndrome. Ann Intern Med 126:450, 1997

TZIOUFAS AG, MOUTSOPOULOS HM: Sjögren's syndrome, in *Rheumatology*, JH Klippel, PA Dieppe (eds). London, Mosby, 1998

315

Joel D. Taurog, Peter E. Lipsky

ANKYLOSING SPONDYLITIS, REACTIVE ARTHRITIS, AND UNDIFFERENTIATED SPONDYLOARTHROPATHY

The spondyloarthropathies are a group of disorders that share certain clinical features and an association with the HLA-B27 allele. These disorders include ankylosing spondylitis, Reiter's syndrome, reactive arthritis, psoriatic arthritis and spondylitis, enteropathic arthritis and spondylitis, juvenile-onset spondyloarthropathy, and undifferentiated spondyloarthropathy. The similarities in clinical manifestations and genetic predisposition suggest that these disorders share pathogenic mechanisms. Specific definitions and diagnostic criteria for the individual conditions will be provided in subsequent sections of this chapter.

ANKYLOSING SPONDYLITIS

Ankylosing spondylitis (AS) is an inflammatory disorder of unknown cause that primarily affects the axial skeleton; peripheral joints and extraarticular structures may also be involved. The disease usually begins in the second or third decade; the prevalence in men is approximately three times that in women. It is considered the prototype of the spondyloarthropathies. Older names include *Marie-Strümpell disease* or *Bechterew's disease*.

EPIDEMIOLOGY AS shows a striking correlation with the histocompatibility antigen HLA-B27 and occurs worldwide roughly in proportion to the prevalence of this antigen (Chap. 306). In North American Caucasians, the general prevalence of B27 is 7%, whereas over 90% of patients with AS have inherited this antigen. The association with B27 is independent of disease severity.

In population surveys, 1 to 6% of adults inheriting B27 have been found to have AS. In contrast, in families of patients with AS, the prevalence is 10 to 30% among adult first-degree relatives inheriting B27. The concordance rate in identical twins is estimated to exceed 65%. It is currently believed that susceptibility to AS is determined almost entirely by genetic factors, with as yet unidentified allelic genes in addition to B27 comprising about two-thirds of the genetic component and B27 itself comprising about one-third. AS is strongly associated with inflammatory bowel disease (IBD), including both ulcerative colitis and Crohn's disease. IBD is a risk factor for AS independent of HLA-B27, although 50 to 75% of patients with both AS and IBD are B27 positive. →*See also Chap. 287.*

PATHOLOGY The *enthesis*, the site of ligamentous attachment to bone, is thought to be the primary site of pathology in AS, particularly in the lesions around the pelvis and spine. Enthesitis is associated with prominent edema of the adjacent bone marrow and is often characterized by erosive lesions that eventually undergo ossification.

Sacroiliitis is usually one of the earliest manifestations of AS, with features of both enthesitis and synovitis. The early lesions consist of subchondral granulation tissue containing lymphocytes, plasma cells, mast cells, macrophages, and chondrocytes; infiltrates of lymphocytes and macrophages in ligamentous and periosteal zones; and subchondral bone marrow edema. Synovitis follows and may progress to pannus formation. Islands of new bone formation can be found within the inflammatory infiltrates. Usually, the thinner iliac cartilage is eroded before the thicker sacral cartilage. The irregularly eroded, sclerotic margins of the joint are gradually replaced by fibrocartilage regeneration and then by ossification. Ultimately, the joint may be totally obliterated. This progression is evident by imaging techniques (see below).

In the spine, early in the process there is inflammatory granulation tissue at the junction of the annulus fibrosus of the disk cartilage and the margin of vertebral bone. The outer annular fibers are eroded and eventually replaced by bone, forming the beginning of a bony excrescence called a *syndesmophyte*, which then grows by continued enchondral ossification, ultimately bridging the adjacent vertebral bodies. Ascending progression of this process leads to the "bamboo spine" observed radiographically. Other lesions in the spine include diffuse osteoporosis, erosion of vertebral bodies at the disk margin, "squaring" of vertebrae, and inflammation and destruction of the disk-bone border. Inflammatory arthritis of the apophyseal joints is common, with erosion of cartilage by pannus, often followed by bony ankylosis.

Bone mineral density is significantly diminished in the spine and proximal femur early in the course of the disease, before the advent of significant immobilization. The mechanism for this is not known.

Peripheral arthritis in AS can show synovial hyperplasia, lymphoid infiltration, and pannus formation, but the process lacks the exuberant synovial villi, fibrin deposits, ulcers, and accumulations of plasma cells seen in rheumatoid arthritis (Chap. 312). Central cartilaginous erosions caused by proliferation of subchondral granulation tissue are common in AS but rare in rheumatoid arthritis.

Acute anterior uveitis (iritis) occurs in at least 20% of patients with AS. Few cases have been studied histologically, none at an early stage. After recurrent attacks, the iris shows nonspecific inflammatory changes, scarring, increased vascularity, and pigment-laden macrophages. Pupillary synechiae and cataract formation are common sequelae.

Aortic insufficiency develops in a small percentage of cases. There is thickening of the aortic valve cusps and the aorta near the sinuses of Valsalva, with dense adventitial scar tissue and intimal fibrous proliferation. The scar tissue can extend into the ventricular septum with resultant heart block.

Microscopic inflammatory lesions of the colon and ileocecal valve have been found in 25 to 50% of patients with AS, even in those lacking any clinical evidence of IBD. IgA nephropathy has been reported with increased frequency.

PATHOGENESIS The pathogenesis of AS is incompletely understood. A number of features of the disease implicate immune-mediated mechanisms, including elevated serum levels of IgA and acute-phase reactants, inflammatory histology, and close association with HLA-B27. The inflamed sacroiliac joint is infiltrated with CD4+ and CD8+ T cells and macrophages and shows high levels of tumor necrosis factor α. Transforming growth factor β is detectable near the sites of new bone formation. No specific event or exogenous agent that triggers the onset of disease has been identified, although overlapping features with reactive arthritis and IBD suggest that enteric bacteria may play a role. Elevated serum titers of antibodies to certain enteric bacteria, particularly *Klebsiella pneumoniae*, are common in AS patients, but no role for these antibodies in the pathogenesis of AS has been identified. Evidence that B27 plays a direct role is provided by the finding that rats transgenic for B27 spontaneously develop spondylitis, along with colitis, peripheral arthritis, and other lesions characteristic of the spondyloarthropathies (see below).

Some evidence has accumulated for autoimmunity to the cartilage proteoglycan aggrecan, and particularly its G1 globulin domain and link protein. AS patients have been found to have cellular immunity to these molecules, and mice immunized with the G1 domain develop spondylitis and discitis. Sharing of proteoglycan antigenic epitopes among the pathologic sites in the skeleton, uveal tract, and aorta in AS suggests a possible explanation for the distribution of pathologic sites in AS.

CLINICAL MANIFESTATIONS The symptoms of the disease are usually first noticed in late adolescence or early adulthood; the median age in western countries is 23 in both genders. In 5% of patients, symptoms begin after age 40. The initial symptom is usually dull pain, insidious in onset, felt deep in the lower lumbar or gluteal region, accompanied by low-back morning stiffness of up to a few

hours' duration that improves with activity and returns following periods of inactivity. Within a few months of onset, the pain has usually become persistent and bilateral. Nocturnal exacerbation of pain that forces the patient to rise and move around may be frequent.

In some patients bony tenderness may accompany back pain or stiffness, while in others it may be the predominant complaint. Common sites include the costosternal junctions, spinous processes, iliac crests, greater trochanters, ischial tuberosities, tibial tubercles, and heels. Occasionally, bony chest pain is the presenting complaint. Arthritis in the hips and shoulders ("root" joints) occurs in 25 to 35% of patients, in many cases early in the disease course. Arthritis of peripheral joints other than the hips and shoulders, usually asymmetric, occurs in up to 30% of patients and can occur at any stage of the disease. Neck pain and stiffness from involvement of the cervical spine are usually relatively late manifestations. Occasional patients, particularly in the older age group, present with predominantly constitutional symptoms such as fatigue, anorexia, fever, weight loss, or night sweats.

AS often has a juvenile onset in developing countries. In these individuals, peripheral arthritis and enthesitis usually predominate, with axial symptoms supervening in late adolescence.

The most common extraarticular manifestation is acute anterior uveitis, which can antedate the spondylitis. Attacks are typically unilateral, causing pain, photophobia, and increased lacrimation. These tend to recur, often in the opposite eye. Cataracts and secondary glaucoma are not uncommon sequelae. Aortic insufficiency, sometimes producing symptoms of congestive heart failure, occurs in a few percent of patients, occasionally early in the course of the spinal disease. Third-degree heart block may occur alone or together with aortic insufficiency. The block is in the atrioventricular node in 95% of cases. Up to half the patients have inflammation in the colon or ileum. This is usually asymptomatic, but in 5 to 10% of patients with AS, frank IBD will develop.

Initially, physical findings mirror the inflammatory process. The most specific findings involve loss of spinal mobility, with limitation of anterior and lateral flexion and extension of the lumbar spine and of chest expansion. Limitation of motion is usually out of proportion to the degree of bony ankylosis, reflecting muscle spasm secondary to pain and inflammation. Pain in the sacroiliac joints may be elicited either with direct pressure or with maneuvers that stress the joints, but these techniques are unreliable in discriminating inflammatory sacroiliitis. In addition, there is commonly tenderness upon palpation at the sites of symptomatic bony tenderness and paraspinous muscle spasm.

The Schober test is a useful measure of flexion of the lumbar spine. The patient stands erect, with heels together, and marks are made directly over the spine 5 cm below and 10 cm above the lumbosacral junction (identified by a horizontal line between the posterosuperior iliac spines.) The patient then bends forward maximally, and the distance between the two marks is measured. The distance between the two marks increases 5 cm or more in the case of normal mobility and less than 4 cm in the case of decreased mobility. Chest expansion is measured as the difference between maximal inspiration and maximal forced expiration in the fourth intercostal space in males or just below the breasts in females. Normal chest expansion is 5 cm or greater.

Limitation or pain with motion of the hips or shoulders is usually present if either of these joints is involved. Careful examination is also necessary to detect inflammatory disease of peripheral joints. It should be emphasized that early in the course of mild cases, symptoms may be subtle and nonspecific, and the physical examination may be completely normal.

The course of the disease is extremely variable, ranging from the individual with mild stiffness and radiographically equivocal sacroiliitis to the patient with a totally fused spine and severe bilateral hip arthritis, possibly accompanied by severe peripheral arthritis and extraarticular manifestations. Pain tends to be persistent early in the disease and then to become intermittent, with alternating exacerbations and quiescent periods. In a typical severe untreated case with progression of the spondylitis to syndesmophyte formation, the patient's posture undergoes characteristic changes. The lumbar lordosis is obliterated with accompanying atrophy of the buttocks. The thoracic kyphosis is accentuated. If the cervical spine is involved, there may be a forward stoop of the neck. Hip involvement with ankylosis may lead to flexion contractures, compensated by flexion at the knees. The progression of the disease may be followed by measuring the patient's height, chest expansion, Schober test, and occiput-to-wall distance when the patient stands erect with the heels and back flat against the wall. Occasional individuals are encountered with advanced physical findings suggestive of long-standing AS who report having never had significant symptoms.

In some but not all studies, onset of the disease in adolescence correlates with a worse prognosis, but there is general agreement that early severe hip involvement is an indication of progressive disease. The disease in women tends to progress less frequently to total spinal ankylosis, although there is some evidence for an increased prevalence of isolated cervical ankylosis and peripheral arthritis in women. In industrialized countries, peripheral arthritis (distal to hips and shoulders) occurs overall in about 25% of patients, usually as a late manifestation, whereas in developing countries, the prevalence is much higher, with onset typically early in the disease course. Pregnancy has no consistent effect on AS, with symptoms improving, remaining the same, or deteriorating in about one-third of pregnant patients, respectively.

The most serious complication of the spinal disease is spinal fracture, which can occur with even minor trauma to the rigid, osteoporotic spine. The cervical spine is most commonly involved. These fractures are often displaced and cause spinal cord injury. Cauda equina syndrome and slowly progressive upper pulmonary lobe fibrosis are rare complications of long-standing AS. The prevalence of aortic insufficiency and of cardiac conduction disturbances, including third-degree heart block, increases with prolonged disease. Subclinical pulmonary lesions and cardiac dysfunction may be relatively common. Prostatitis has been reported to have an increased prevalence in men with AS. Amyloidosis is only rarely associated (Chap. 319).

Several validated measures of disease activity and functional outcome have recently been developed for AS. Despite the persistence of the disease, most patients remain gainfully employed. The effect of AS on survival is controversial. Some, but not all, studies have suggested that AS shortens life span, compared with the general population. Mortality attributable to AS is largely the result of spinal trauma, aortic insufficiency, respiratory failure, amyloid nephropathy, or complications of therapy such as upper gastrointestinal hemorrhage.

LABORATORY FINDINGS   No laboratory test is diagnostic of AS. In most ethnic groups, the HLA-B27 gene is present in approximately 90% of patients with AS. Most, but not all, patients with active disease have an elevated erythrocyte sedimentation rate and an elevated level of C-reactive protein. A mild normochromic, normocytic anemia may be present. Patients with severe disease may show an elevated alkaline phosphatase level. Elevated serum IgA levels are common. Rheumatoid factor and antinuclear antibodies are largely absent unless caused by a coexistent disease. Synovial fluid from inflamed peripheral joints in AS is not distinctly different from that of other inflammatory joint diseases. In cases with restriction of chest wall motion, decreased vital capacity and increased functional residual capacity are common, but airflow measurements are normal and ventilatory function is usually well maintained.

RADIOGRAPHIC FINDINGS   Radiographically demonstrable sacroiliitis is usually present in AS. The earliest changes in the sacroiliac joints demonstrable by standard radiography are blurring of the cortical margins of the subchondral bone, followed by erosions and sclerosis. Progression of the erosions leads to "pseudowidening" of the joint space; as fibrous and then bony ankylosis supervene, the joints may become obliterated radiographically. The changes and progression of the lesions are usually symmetric.

Roentgenographic abnormalities generally appear in the sacroiliac joints before appearing elsewhere in the spine. In the lumbar spine, progression of the disease leads to straightening, caused by loss of

lordosis, and reactive sclerosis, caused by osteitis of the anterior corners of the vertebral bodies with subsequent erosion, leading to "squaring" of the vertebral bodies. Progressive ossification of the superficial layers of the annulus fibrosus leads to eventual formation of marginal syndesmophytes, visible on plain films as bony bridges connecting successive vertebral bodies anteriorly and laterally.

In mild cases, years may elapse before unequivocal sacroiliac abnormalities are evident on plain radiographs. Computed tomography (CT) and magnetic resonance imaging (MRI) can detect abnormalities reliably at an earlier stage than plain radiography. MRI has emerged as a highly sensitive and specific technique for identifying early intra-articular inflammation, cartilage changes, and underlying bone marrow edema in sacroiliitis (Fig. 315-1). In suspected cases in which conventional radiography does not reveal definite sacroiliac abnormalities or is undesirable (e.g., in young women or children), dynamic MRI is the procedure of choice for establishing a diagnosis of sacroiliitis.

Reduced bone mineral density can be detected by dual-energy x-ray absorptiometry of the femoral neck and the lumbar spine. Falsely elevated readings related to spinal ossification can be avoided by using a lateral projection of the L3 vertebral body.

DIAGNOSIS   The diagnosis of early AS before the development of irreversible deformity can be difficult to establish. Currently, modified New York criteria (1984) are widely used for diagnosis. These consist of the following: (1) a history of inflammatory back pain (see below); (2) limitation of motion of the lumbar spine in both the sagittal and frontal planes; (3) limited chest expansion, relative to standard values for age and sex; and (4) definite radiographic sacroiliitis. Using these criteria, the presence of radiographic sacroiliitis plus any one of the other three criteria is sufficient for a diagnosis of definite AS. These

FIGURE 315-1   Early sacroiliitis of ankylosing spondylitis. Magnetic resonance imaging of the sacroiliac joints of a 23-year-old woman with progressive right-sided inflammatory back pain of 6 months' duration. Conventional radiographs were normal. A fat-suppressed image employing a short tau inversion recovery (STIR) sequence shows acute sacroiliitis on the right side, with edema in the juxtaarticular bone marrow (*asterisks*), in the region of the synovium and joint capsule (*thin arrow*), and in the region of the interosseous ligaments (*thick arrow*). Early chronic changes, including cortical erosions and joint space widening, were evident in the right sacroiliac joint in T1-, contrast-enhanced T1-, and T2*-weighted images (not shown). The patient subsequently developed radiographically evident bilateral sacroiliitis fulfilling the criteria for ankylosing spondylitis. (*Photo provided by Dr. Jürgen Braun, Freie Universität Berlin; previously published in Zeitschrift für Rheumatologie 58:61, 1999. Reproduced with permission.*)

criteria may need to be further modified to include sacroiliitis demonstrated by MRI to increase their sensitivity.

The presence of B27 is neither necessary nor sufficient for the diagnosis, but the B27 test can be helpful in patients with suggestive clinical findings who have not yet developed radiographic sacroiliitis. Moreover, the absence of B27 in a typical case of AS significantly increases the probability of coexistent IBD.

AS must be differentiated from numerous other causes of low-back pain, some of which are far more common than AS. The inflammatory back pain of AS is usually distinguished by the following five features: (1) age of onset below 40, (2) insidious onset, (3) duration greater than 3 months before medical attention is sought, (4) morning stiffness, and (5) improvement with exercise or activity. The most common causes of back pain other than AS are primarily mechanical or degenerative rather than inflammatory and do not show these features. Less common metabolic, infectious, and malignant causes of back pain also must be differentiated from AS. Ochronosis can produce a phenotype that is clinically and radiographically similar to AS.

Marked calcification and ossification of paraspinous ligaments occur in *diffuse idiopathic skeletal hyperostosis* (DISH). Although DISH is often categorized as a variant of osteoarthritis, diarthrodial joints are not involved. Ligamentous calcification and ossification are usually most prominent in the anterior spinal ligament and give the appearance of "flowing wax" on the anterior bodies of the vertebrae. However, a radiolucency may be seen between the newly deposited bone and the vertebral body, differentiating DISH from the marginal osteophytes in spondylosis. Intervertebral disk spaces are preserved, and sacroiliac and apophyseal joints appear normal, helping to differentiate DISH from spondylosis and from AS, respectively.

DISH occurs in the middle-aged and the elderly and is more common in men than in women. Patients are frequently asymptomatic but may have stiffness. Radiographic changes are generally much more severe than might be predicted from the mild symptoms caused by DISH.

℞ TREATMENT   There is no definitive treatment for AS. The principal goal of management is the conscientious participation by the patient in an exercise program designed to maintain functional posture and to preserve range of motion. There is evidence that exercise increases mobility and improves function. The proportion of patients wtih severe deformity has decreased markedly in recent decades, probably because of earlier diagnosis and widespread use of physical therapy. Smoking has been associated with a poor outcome and should be emphatically discouraged. Most patients require anti-inflammatory agents to achieve sufficient symptomatic relief to be able to remain functional and carry out the exercise program. It is not known whether drug treatment alone can alter the progression of the disease.

Several nonsteroidal anti-inflammatory drugs (NSAIDs) have proved effective in reducing the pain and stiffness of AS and are commonly used. Indomethacin is particularly effective as a 75-mg slow-release preparation taken once or twice daily. Although phenylbutazone, at doses of 200 to 400 mg/d, has been considered the most effective anti-inflammatory agent in AS, because of its greater potential for serious side effects such as aplastic anemia and agranulocytosis, its use in the United States is confined to patients with very severe disease whose symptoms do not respond at all to other agents. Recent controlled trials suggest that sulfasalazine,[1] in doses of 2 to 3 g/d, is useful in reducing peripheral joint symptoms as well as reversing laboratory evidence of inflammation. Some studies have not shown it to benefit axial arthritis, and its effect on natural progression of the disease is unproven. The peripheral arthritis may also respond to the folic acid antagonist methotrexate.[1] No therapeutic role for gold, pen-

icillamine, immunosuppressive drugs, or oral glucocorticoids has been documented in AS. Occasionally, intralesional or intraarticular glucocorticoid injections may be beneficial in patients with persistent enthesopathy or synovitis unresponsive to anti-inflammatory agents. Recent studies have suggested that symptomatic benefit can be achieved from CT-guided glucocorticoid injections into the sacroiliac joints, but the effects are not sustained. Anecdotal benefit has been reported for diverse agents such as pamidronate, thalidomide, pulse intravenous methylprednisolone, and tumor necrosis factor α antagonists. Controlled trials of these and other agents are needed, since for many patients current therapy is inadequate even for control of pain and stiffness.

The most common indication for surgery in patients with AS is severe hip joint arthritis, the pain and stiffness of which are usually dramatically relieved by total hip arthroplasty. A small number of patients may benefit from surgical correction of extreme flexion deformities of the spine or of atlantoaxial subluxation.

Attacks of iritis are usually effectively managed with local glucocorticoid administration in conjunction with mydriatic agents, although systemic glucocorticoids or even immunosuppressive drugs may be required in some cases. Coexistent cardiac disease may require pacemaker implantation and/or aortic valve replacement.

REACTIVE ARTHRITIS AND UNDIFFERENTIATED SPONDYLOARTHROPATHY

Reactive arthritis (ReA) refers to acute nonpurulent arthritis complicating an infection elsewhere in the body. In recent years, the term has been used primarily to refer to spondyloarthropathies following enteric or urogenital infections and occurring predominantly in individuals with the histocompatibility antigen HLA-B27. Included in this category is the constellation of clinical findings formerly commonly called *Reiter's syndrome. →Other forms of reactive and infection-related arthritis not associated with B27 and showing a different spectrum of clinical features, such as rheumatic fever or Lyme disease, are discussed in Chaps. 235 and 176.*

HISTORIC BACKGROUND   The association of acute arthritis with episodes of diarrhea or urethritis has been recognized for centuries. A large number of cases during World Wars I and II focused attention on the triad of arthritis, urethritis, and conjunctivitis, which became known as Reiter's syndrome, often occurring with additional mucocutaneous lesions.

The identification of bacterial species capable of triggering the clinical syndrome and the finding that up to 85% of the patients possess the B27 antigen have led to the unifying concept of ReA as a clinical syndrome triggered by specific etiologic agents in a genetically susceptible host. A similar spectrum of clinical manifestations can be triggered by enteric infection with any of several *Shigella, Salmonella, Yersinia,* and *Campylobacter* species, by genital infection with *Chlamydia trachomatis*; and possibly by other agents as well. Although Reiter's syndrome can be said to represent one part of the spectrum of the clinical manifestations of ReA, particularly that induced by *Shigella* or *Chlamydia*, the term is now largely of historic interest only. Since most patients with spondyloarthropathy do not have the classic features of Reiter's syndrome, it has become customary to employ the term *reactive arthritis*, regardless of whether or not there is evidence for a triggering infection. For the purposes of this chapter, the use of ReA will be restricted to those cases of spondyloarthropathy in which there is at least presumptive evidence for a related antecedent infection. Patients with clinical features of ReA who lack both evidence of an antecedent infection and the classic findings of Reiter's syndrome (urethritis, arthritis, conjunctivitis) will be considered to have *undifferentiated spondyloarthropathy*, which is discussed at the end of this chapter.

EPIDEMIOLOGY   Like AS, ReA occurs predominantly in individuals who have inherited the B27 gene; in most series, 60 to 85% of patients are B27 positive. In epidemics of arthritogenic bacterial

---

[1]Azathioprine, methotrexate, and sulfasalazine have not been approved for this purpose by the U.S. Food and Drug Administration at the time of publication.

infection, e.g., *S. flexneri*, it has been estimated that ReA develops in ~20% of exposed B27-positive individuals. In families with multiple cases of AS or ReA, the two conditions have been said to "breed true," i.e., to be uncommonly found together within an individual family. Whether this is caused by genetic or environmental factors is not known. The disease is most common in individuals 18 to 40 years of age, but it can occur both in children over 5 years of age and in older adults.

The sex ratio in ReA following enteric infection is nearly 1:1, whereas venereally acquired ReA is predominantly confined to men. The overall prevalence and incidence of ReA are difficult to assess because of the variable prevalence of the triggering infections and genetic susceptibility factors in different populations. For example, in Olmsted County, MN, the incidence was estimated as 3.5 cases per 100,000 population per year. In contrast, in a population with a high rate of genitourinary and/or gastrointestinal infections such as urban homosexual and bisexual men, the prevalence may approach 1 per 1000.

A particularly severe form of peripheral spondyloarthropathy has been described in patients with AIDS (Chap. 309). Most of these patients are HLA-B27 positive, but HIV infection per se is not an independent risk factor for spondyloarthropathy.

PATHOLOGY Synovial histology is similar to that of other inflammatory arthropathies. Enthesitis is a common clinical finding in ReA; the histology of this lesion resembles that of AS. Microscopic histopathologic evidence of inflammation has occasionally been noted in the colon and ileum of patients with postvenereal ReA, but much less commonly than in postenteric ReA. The skin lesions of keratoderma blenorrhagica, which is associated mainly with venereally acquired ReA, are histologically indistinguishable from psoriatic lesions.

ETIOLOGY AND PATHOGENESIS The first bacterial infection noted to be causally related to ReA was *S. flexneri*. An outbreak of shigellosis among Finnish troops in 1944 resulted in numerous cases of ReA. Of the four species *S. sonnei*, *S. boydii*, *S. flexneri*, and *S. dysenteriae*, *S. flexneri* has most often been implicated in cases of ReA, both sporadic and epidemic. *S. sonnei*, although responsible for the majority of cases of shigellosis in the United States, has only rarely been implicated in cases of ReA.

Other bacteria that have been definitively identified as triggers of ReA include several *Salmonella* spp., *Y. enterocolitica*, *C. jejuni*, and *C. trachomatis*. There is suggestive evidence implicating several other microorganisms, including *Y. pseudotuberculosis*, *Clostridium difficile*, and *Ureaplasma urealyticum*. *Chlamydia pneumoniae*, a respiratory pathogen, has also recently been implicated in triggering ReA. There are also numerous isolated reports of acute arthritis preceded by other bacterial, viral, or parasitic infections, but whether the microorganisms involved are actual triggers of ReA remains to be determined.

It has not been determined whether ReA occurs by the same pathogenic mechanism following infection with each of these microorganisms, nor has the mechanism been fully elucidated in the case of any one of the known bacterial triggers. Most, if not all, of the triggering organisms produce lipopolysaccharide (LPS) and share a capacity to attack mucosal surfaces, to invade host cells, and survive intracellularly. Antigens from *Chlamydia*, *Yersinia*, *Salmonella*, and *Shigella* have been shown to be present in the synovium and/or synovial fluid leukocytes of patients with ReA for long periods following the acute attack. In ReA triggered by *Y. enterocolitica*, bacterial LPS and heat shock protein antigens have been found in peripheral blood cells years after the triggering infection. In the case of *C. trachomatis*, synovial persistence of microbial DNA and RNA suggests the presence of viable organisms, despite uniform failure to culture the organism from these specimens. There is thus evidence that ReA, at least in some cases, may be a form of chronic infection, rather than solely "reactive." T cells that specifically respond to antigens of the inciting organism are typically found in inflamed synovium but not in peripheral blood of patients with ReA. These T cells are predominantly CD4+, but CD8+ B27-restricted bacteria-specific cytolytic T cells have also been

isolated in *Yersinia*- and *C. trachomatis*-induced ReA. Specific peptide antigens from these organisms have been identified as dominant T cells epitopes. Unlike the synovial CD4 T cells in rheumatoid arthritis, which are predominantly of the T_H1 phenotype, those in ReA also show a T_H2 phenotype. It is likely that antigen-specific T cells play an important role in the pathogenesis of ReA, but the precise mechanisms remain to be determined.

The role of HLA-B27 in ReA also remains to be determined. Transgenic rats with high expression of B27 spontaneously develop a multiple organ system inflammatory disease affecting the gut, peripheral and axial joints, male genital tract, and skin that resembles these human conditions clinically and histologically. When raised in a germ-free environment, the B27 rats do not develop gut or joint inflammation, but the skin and genital lesions are not prevented. These findings suggest that bacteria are necessary, and normal gut bacteria are sufficient, to induce B27-related joint inflammation. In both the rat and human diseases, it remains to be determined whether the primary process is an autoimmune response against host tissues or an immune response against antigens of the triggering organism that have disseminated to the target tissues, and the specific role of B27 itself remains to be determined. A potentially very informative converse observation, in which humans develop a disease process resembling one first described in rats, is the recent finding that 0.4 to 0.8% of individuals treated with intravesicular bacillus Calmette-Guérin for bladder cancer develop reactive arthritis, and 60% of these patients are B27 positive. The process closely mimics adjuvant-induced arthritis in rats given complete Freund's adjuvant, first described over 40 years ago, which is currently thought to be mediated by CD4+ T cells specific for mycobacterial heat shock protein.

An intriguing in vitro finding indicates that the presence of HLA-B27 significantly prolongs the intracellular survival of *Y. enterocolitica*, and *S. enteritides* in human and mouse cell lines. A unifying hypothesis suggests that prolonged intracellular bacterial survival, promoted by B27, other factors, or both, permits trafficking of infected leukocytes from the site of primary infection to joints, where a T cell response to persistent bacterial antigens promotes arthritis. Evidence exists supporting each step of this scheme.

CLINICAL FEATURES The clinical manifestations of ReA constitute a spectrum that ranges from an isolated, transient monarthritis to severe multisystem disease. In the majority of cases, a careful history will elicit some evidence of an antecedent infection 1 to 4 weeks before the onset of symptoms of the reactive disease. However, in a sizable minority, no clinical or laboratory evidence of an antecedent infection can be found. In many cases of presumed venereally acquired reactive disease, there is a history of a recent new sexual partner, even in the absence of laboratory evidence of infection.

Constitutional symptoms are common, including fatigue, malaise, fever, and weight loss. The musculoskeletal symptoms are usually acute in onset. Arthritis is usually asymmetric and additive, with involvement of new joints occurring over a period of a few days to 1 to 2 weeks. The joints of the lower extremities, especially the knee, ankle, and subtalar, metatarsophalangeal, and toe interphalangeal joints, are the most common sites of involvement, but the wrist and fingers can be involved as well. The arthritis is usually quite painful, and tense joint effusions are not uncommon, especially in the knee. Dactylitis, or "sausage digit," a diffuse swelling of a solitary finger or toe, is a distinctive feature of both ReA and psoriatic arthritis (Chap. 324). It is not specific, however, in that it is also seen in polyarticular gout and sarcoidosis. Tendinitis and fasciitis are particularly characteristic lesions, producing pain at multiple insertion sites, especially the Achilles insertion, the plantar fascia, and sites along the axial skeleton. Spinal and low-back pain are quite common and may be caused by insertional inflammation, muscle spasm, acute sacroiliitis, or, presumably, arthritis in intervertebral articulations.

Urogenital lesions may occur throughout the course of the disease. In males, urethritis may be marked or relatively asymptomatic and may be either an accompaniment of the triggering infection or a result of the reactive phase of the disease. Prostatitis is also common. Similarly, in females, cervicitis or salpingitis may be caused either by the infectious trigger or by the sterile reactive process.

Ocular disease is common, ranging from transient, asymptomatic conjunctivitis to an aggressive anterior uveitis that occasionally proves refractory to treatment and may result in blindness.

Mucocutaneous lesions are frequent. Oral ulcers tend to be superficial, transient, and often asymptomatic. The characteristic skin lesions, *keratoderma blenorrhagica*, consist of vesicles that become hyperkeratotic, ultimately forming a crust before disappearing. They are most common on the palms and soles but may occur elsewhere as well. In patients with HIV infection, these lesions are often extremely severe and extensive, to the point of dominating the clinical picture (Chap. 309). Lesions on the glans penis, termed *circinate balanitis*, are common; these consist of vesicles that quickly rupture to form painless superficial erosions, which in circumcised individuals can form crusts similar to those of keratoderma blenorrhagica. Nail changes are common and consist of onycholysis, distal yellowish discoloration, and/or heaped-up hyperkeratosis.

Less frequent or rare manifestations of ReA include cardiac conduction defects, aortic insufficiency, central or peripheral nervous system lesions, and pleuropulmonary infiltrates.

Long-term follow-up studies suggest that some joint symptoms persist in 30 to 60% of patients with ReA. Recurrences of the acute syndrome are common, and as many as 25% of patients either become unable to work or are forced to change occupations because of persistent joint symptoms. Chronic heel pain is often a particularly distressing symptom. Some aspects of ankylosing spondylitis are also common sequelae (see below). In some but not all studies, HLA-B27-positive patients have shown a worse outcome than B27-negative patients. The extent to which the long-term prognosis varies with different inciting agents is not known. However, patients with *Yersinia*-induced arthritis appear to have less chronic disease than those whose initial episode follows epidemic shigellosis.

LABORATORY AND RADIOGRAPHIC FINDINGS   The erythrocyte sedimentation rate is usually elevated during the acute phase of the disease. Mild anemia may be present, and acute-phase reactants tend to be increased. Synovial fluid is nonspecifically inflammatory, showing an elevated white cell count with a predominance of neutrophils. In most ethnic groups, 50 to 75% of the patients are B27 positive. It is unusual for the triggering infection to persist at the site of primary mucosal infection through the time of onset of the reactive disease, but it may occasionally be possible to culture the organism, e.g., in the case of *Yersinia*- or *Chlamydia*-induced disease. Serologic evidence of a recent infection may be present, such as a marked elevation of antibodies to *Yersinia*, *Salmonella*, or *Chlamydia*.

In early or mild disease, radiographic changes may be absent or confined to juxtaarticular osteoporosis. With long-standing persistent disease, marginal erosions and loss of joint space can be seen in affected joints. Periostitis with reactive new bone formation is characteristic of the disease, as it is with all the spondyloarthropathies. Spurs at the insertion of the plantar fascia are common.

Sacroiliitis and spondylitis may be seen as late sequelae. The sacroiliitis is more commonly asymmetric than in AS, and the spondylitis, rather than ascending symmetrically from the lower lumbar segments, can begin anywhere along the lumbar spine. The syndesmophytes may be coarse and nonmarginal, arising from the middle of a vertebral body, a pattern rarely seen in primary AS. Progression to spinal fusion as a sequela of ReA is uncommon.

DIAGNOSIS   ReA is a clinical diagnosis, there being no definitively diagnostic laboratory test or radiographic finding. The diagnosis should be entertained in any patient with an acute inflammatory, asymmetric, additive arthritis or tendinitis. The evaluation of such a patient should include careful questioning regarding possible antecedent triggering events such as an episode of diarrhea or dysuria. On physical

examination, careful attention must be paid to the distribution of the joint and tendon involvement and to possible sites of extraarticular involvement, such as the eyes, mucous membranes, skin, nails, and genitalia. Synovial fluid aspiration and analysis may be helpful in excluding septic or crystal-induced arthritis. Culture or serology may help to identify a triggering infection. The role of molecular methods of microbial detection has not been established (see below).

Although typing for B27 is not needed to secure the diagnosis in clear-cut cases, it may have prognostic significance in terms of severity, chronicity, and the propensity for spondylitis and uveitis. Furthermore, it can be helpful diagnostically in atypical cases, a positive test increasing and a negative test decreasing the probability of ReA.

It is particularly important to differentiate ReA from disseminated gonococcal disease, both of which can be venereally acquired and associated with urethritis (Chap. 147). Gonococcal arthritis and tenosynovitis tend to involve both upper and lower extremities equally, whereas in ReA lower extremity symptoms usually predominate. Back pain is common in ReA but is not a feature of gonococcal disease, whereas the vesicular skin lesions characteristic of disseminated gonococcal disease are not found in ReA. A positive gonococcal culture from the urethra or cervix does not exclude a diagnosis of ReA; however, culturing gonococci from blood, skin lesion, or synovium establishes the diagnosis of disseminated gonococcal disease. Polymerase chain reaction (PCR) technology has recently been used in the diagnosis of infections with *Neisseria gonorrheae* and with *C. trachomatis*. Occasionally, the only definitive way to distinguish the two is through a therapeutic trial of antibiotics.

ReA shares many features in common with psoriatic arthropathy, including the asymmetry of the arthritis, a propensity for "sausage digits" and nail involvement, an association with uveitis, and skin lesions of similar histology (Chap. 324). However, psoriatic arthritis is usually gradual in onset, the arthritis tends to affect primarily the upper extremities, and there is less associated periarthritis. Psoriatic arthritis is not associated with mouth ulcers or urethritis, or, usually, with bowel symptoms. Although psoriatic arthropathy shows some distinctive radiographic features that are not found in ReA, these occur only late in the disease and are of little help diagnostically. Only psoriatic spondylitis, not the peripheral arthritis, is associated with B27, about 50% of patients being positive. Occasional patients, usually B27 positive, following what appears to be a typical episode of ReA, will develop typical psoriasis and persistent arthritis such that the two entities become indistinguishable.

Undifferentiated spondyloarthropathy, or simply "spondyloarthropathy," is diagnosed in patients who lack evidence of an antecedent infection that might trigger ReA and who do not meet criteria for AS but who show clinical features of these disorders.

℞ TREATMENT   Most patients with ReA are benefitted to some degree by NSAIDs, although rarely are symptoms of the acute arthritis completely ameliorated, and some patients fail to respond at all. Indomethacin, 75 to 150 mg/d in divided doses, is the initial treatment of choice. Other NSAIDs may be tried, with phenylbutazone, 100 mg tid or qid, being the NSAID of last resort, to be used only in severe, refractory cases because of its potentially serious side effects.

It is unclear whether antibiotics have a role in the therapy of ReA. One controlled study suggested that prolonged administration of a long-acting tetracycline may accelerate recovery from *Chlamydia*-induced ReA, but subsequent results have been less encouraging, and therapy for other bacterial triggers of ReA has shown little or no benefit. However, there is evidence that prompt, appropriate antibiotic treatment of acute chlamydial urethritis may prevent subsequent ReA. Currently, expert opinion supports the use of antibiotic therapy in established urogenital ReA but not in gastrointestinal ReA.

Two recent multicenter trials have suggested that sulfasalazine, up to 3 g/d in divided doses, may be beneficial to patients with persistent ReA.[1] Patients with debilitating symptoms refractory to NSAID and sulfasalazine therapy may respond to immunosuppressive agents such as azathioprine, 1 to 2 mg/kg per day, or to methotrexate, 7.5 to

15 mg per week. Systemic glucocorticoids are not generally recommended but in rare instances may be helpful in mobilizing a severely affected bedridden patient. Antimalarials, gold, and penicillamine are not useful in the treatment of ReA. Trials of new agents proven useful in rheumatoid arthritis, such as COX-2 inhibitors, leflunomide, and tumor necrosis factor α inhibitors, remain to be implemented.

Tendinitis and other enthesitic lesions occasionally may benefit from intralesional glucocorticoids. Uveitis may require aggressive treatment with glucocorticoids to prevent serious sequelae. Skin lesions ordinarily require only symptomatic treatment. In patients with HIV infection and ReA, many of whom have severe skin lesions, the skin lesions in particular appear to respond to systemic treatment with anti-retroviral agents (Chap. 309). Cardiac complications are managed conventionally; management of neurologic complications is symptomatic.

Patients need to be educated about the nature of the disease and the factors that predispose to its recurrence. Comprehensive management includes counseling of patients in the avoidance of sexually transmitted disease and exposure to enteropathogens, as well as appropriate use of physical therapy, vocational counseling, and continued surveillance for long-term complications such as ankylosing spondylitis.

FIGURE 315-2   Algorithm for diagnosis of the spondyloarthropathies.

UNDIFFERENTIATED AND JUVENILE-ONSET SPONDYLOARTHROPATHY

It is not uncommon for clinicians to encounter patients, usually young adults, who do not have IBD or psoriasis, lack evidence of an antecedent triggering infection, and do not have the classic triad of Reiter's syndrome or meet criteria for ankylosing spondylitis, who nonetheless present with some features of one or more of the spondyloarthropathies discussed above. For example, a patient may present with inflammatory synovitis of one knee, Achilles tendinitis, and dactylitis of one digit ("sausage digit"), or sacroiliitis in the absence of other criteria for AS. It is now common to consider such patients as having *undifferentiated spondyloarthropathy*, or simply *spondyloarthropathy*. Other terms for this condition have included *seronegative oligoarthritis*, *undifferentiated oligoarthritis*, and the now-outmoded *incomplete Reiter's syndrome*. There is strong evidence that some, perhaps most, of these patients have ReA in which the triggering infection remains clinically silent. In some other cases, the patient subsequently develops IBD or psoriasis or the process eventually meets criteria for ankylosing spondylitis. Approximately half the patients with undifferentiated spondyloarthropathy are HLA-B27 positive, and thus the absence of B27 is not useful in establishing or excluding the diagnosis.

In *juvenile-onset spondyloarthropathy*, which begins most commonly in boys (60 to 80%) between ages 7 and 16, an asymmetric, predominantly lower extremity oligoarthritis and enthesitis without extraarticular features is the typical mode of presentation. The prevalence of B27 in this condition, which has been termed the *SEA syndrome* (*s*eronegative, *e*nthesopathy, *a*rthropathy), is approximately 80%. Many, but not all, of these patients go on to develop typical ankylosing spondylitis in late adolescence or adulthood.

Management of undifferentiated spondyloarthropathy is similar to that of the other spondyloarthropathies, with NSAIDs and physical therapy forming the mainstays of treatment. Textbooks of pediatrics should be consulted for information on management of juvenile-onset spondyloarthropathy. An algorithm for the diagnosis of the spondyloarthropathies in adults is presented in Fig. 315-2.

BIBLIOGRAPHY

BERGFELDT L: HLA-B27-associated cardiac disease. Ann Intern Med 127:621, 1997

BRAUN J et al: Prevalence of spondylarthropathies in HLA-B27 positive and negative blood donors. Arthritis Rheum 41:58, 1998

——— et al: Radiologic diagnosis and pathology of spondyloarthropathies. Rheum Dis Clin North Am 24:697, 1998

BROWN MA et al: Susceptiblity to ankylosing spondylitis in twins: The role of genes, HLA, and the environment. Arthritis Rheum 40:1823, 1997

CALIN A, TAUROG JD (eds): *The Spondyloarthritides*. Oxford, Oxford Univ Press, 1998

DOUGADOS M et al: Spondylarthropathy treatment: Progress in medical treatment, physical therapy and rehabilitation. Baillieres Clin Rheumatol 12:717, 1998

GLADMAN DD: Psoriatic arthritis. Rheum Dis Clin North Am 24:829, 1998

LEE YS et al: Skeletal status of men with early and late ankylosing spondylitis. Am J Med 103:233, 1997

POWER WJ et al: Outcomes in anterior uveitis associated with the HLA-B27 haplotype. Ophthalmology 105:1646, 1998

BEHÇET'S SYNDROME

DEFINITION   Behçet's syndrome is a multisystem disorder presenting with recurrent oral and genital ulcerations as well as ocular involvement. Internationally agreed diagnostic criteria have been proposed (Table 316-1).

PREVALENCE, PATHOGENESIS, AND PATHOLOGY
The disease has a worldwide distribution. The prevalence of Behçet's syndrome ranges from 1:10,000 in Japan to 1:500,000 in North America and Europe. It affects mainly young adults, with males having more severe disease than females.

The etiology and pathogenesis of this syndrome remain obscure; vasculitis is the main pathologic lesion with a tendency to venous thrombus formation, and circulating autoantibodies to human oral mucous membrane are found in approximately 50% of the patients. Familial occurrence has been sporadically reported; and in patients from eastern Mediterranean countries and Japan, the disease appears to be linked to HLA-B5 (B51) alloantigens.

CLINICAL FEATURES   The recurrent aphthous ulcerations are a sine qua non for the diagnosis. The ulcers are usually painful, shallow or deep with a central yellowish necrotic base, appear singly or in crops, and are located anywhere in the oral cavity. The ulcers persist for 1 to 2 weeks and subside without leaving scars. The genital ulcers resemble the oral ones.

Skin involvement includes folliculitis, erythema nodosum, an acne-like exanthem, and infrequently vasculitis. Nonspecific skin inflammatory reactivity to any scratches or intradermal saline injection (pathergy test) is a common and specific manifestation.

Eye involvement is the most dreaded complication, since it occasionally progresses rapidly to blindness. The eye disease is usually present at the onset but also may develop within the first few years. In addition to iritis, posterior uveitis, retinal vessel occlusions, and optic neuritis can be seen in some patients with the syndrome. Hypopyon uveitis, which is considered the hallmark of Behçet's syndrome, is in fact a rare manifestation.

The arthritis of Behçet's syndrome is not deforming and affects the knees and ankles.

Superficial or deep peripheral vein thrombosis is seen in one-fourth of the patients. Pulmonary emboli are a rare complication. The superior vena cava is obstructed occasionally, producing a dramatic clinical picture. Arterial involvement occurs infrequently and presents with aortitis or peripheral arterial aneurysm and arterial thrombosis. Pulmonary artery vasculitis presenting with dyspnea, cough, chest pain, hemoptysis, and infiltrates on chest roentgenograms has been reported recently in 5% of patients.

Central nervous system involvement is found more frequently in patients from northern Europe and the United States. The most common lesions are benign intracranial hypertension, a multiple sclerosis–like picture, pyramidal involvement, and psychiatric disturbances.

Gastrointestinal involvement is reported in patients from Japan and includes mucosal ulcerations of the gut.

Laboratory findings are mainly nonspecific indices of inflammation such as leukocytosis and elevated erythrocyte sedimentation rate

as well as C-reactive protein levels; antibodies to human oral mucosa are also found.

TREATMENT   The severity of the syndrome usually abates with time. Apart from the patients with neurologic complications, the life expectancy seems to be normal, and the only serious complication is blindness.

Mucous membrane involvement may respond to topical glucocorticoids in the form of mouthwash or paste. In more serious cases thalidomide (100 mg/d) is effective. Thrombophlebitis is treated with aspirin, 325 mg/d. Colchicine or interferon α can be beneficial for the arthritis of the syndrome. Uveitis and central nervous system involvement require systemic glucocorticoid therapy (prednisone, 1 mg/kg per day) and azathioprine, 2 to 3 mg/kg per day, or cyclosporine, 5 to 10 mg/kg per day. Early initiation of azathioprine tends to favorably affect the long-term prognosis of Behçet's syndrome.

BIBLIOGRAPHY

HAMURYUDAN V et al: Systemic interferon α2b treatment in Behçet's syndrome. J Rheumatol 21:1098, 1994

—— et al: Azathioprine in Behçet's syndrome: Effects on long-term prognosis. Arthritis Rheum 40:769, 1997

—— et al: Thalidomide in the treatment of the mucocutaneous lesions of the Behçet syndrome. A randomized double-blind, placebo-controlled trial. Ann Intern Med 128: 443, 1998

INTERNATIONAL STUDY GROUP FOR BEHÇET'S DISEASE: Criteria of diagnosis of Behçet's disease. Lancet 335:1078, 1990

MASUDA K et al: Double masked trial of cyclosporin in Behçet's disease. Lancet 1:1093, 1989

PAPIRIS SA, MOUTSOPOULOS HM: Rare rheumatic disorders: Behçet's disease. Baillieres Clin Rheumatol 7:173, 1993

SAKANE T et al: Behçet's disease. N Engl J Med 341:1284, 1999

YAZICI H et al: Behçet's syndrome. Curr Opin Rheumatol 11:53, 1999

THE VASCULITIS SYNDROMES

AIL angiocentric immunoproliferative lesions	IFN interferon
ANCA antineutrophil cytoplasmic antibodies	IL interleukin
	PAN classic polyarteritis nodosa
ELAM-1 endothelial-leukocyte adhesion molecule 1	TNF tumor necrosis factor
	VCAM-1 vascular cell adhesion molecule 1
ESR erythrocyte sedimentation rate	WBC white blood count

DEFINITION   *Vasculitis* is a clinicopathologic process characterized by inflammation of and damage to blood vessels. The vessel lumen is usually compromised, and this is associated with ischemia of the tissues supplied by the involved vessel. A broad and heterogeneous group of syndromes may result from this process, since any type, size, and location of blood vessel may be involved. Vasculitis and its consequences may be the primary or sole manifestation of a disease; alternatively, vasculitis may be a secondary component of another primary disease. Vasculitis may be confined to a single organ such as the skin, or it may simultaneously involve several organ systems.

CLASSIFICATION OF VASCULITIC SYNDROMES   A major feature of the vasculitic syndromes as a group is the fact that there is a great deal of heterogeneity at the same time as there is considerable overlap among them. This has led to both difficulty and confusion with regard to the categorization of these diseases. The classification scheme listed in Table 317-1 takes into account this heterogeneity and overlap and will serve as a matrix to emphasize the fact that certain syndromes are predominantly systemic in nature and almost invariably lead to irreversible organ system dysfunction and even

Table 316-1   Diagnostic Criteria of Behçet's Disease

Recurrent oral ulceration plus two of the following:
  Recurrent genital ulceration
  Eye lesions
  Skin lesions
  Pathergy test

Table 317-1   Classification of the Vasculitis Syndromes

I. Systemic necrotizing vasculitis
   A. Polyarteritis nodosa (PAN)
      1. Classic PAN
      2. Microscopic polyangiitis
   B. Allergic angiitis and granulomatosis of Churg-Strauss
   C. Polyangiitis overlap syndrome
II. Wegener's granulomatosis
III. Temporal arteritis
IV. Takayasu's arteritis
V. Henoch-Schönlein purpura
VI. Predominantly cutaneous vasculitis (hypersensitivity vasculitis)
   A. Exogenous stimuli proven or suspected
      1. Drug-induced vasculitis
      2. Serum sickness and serum sickness–like reactions
      3. Vasculitis associated with infectious diseases
   B. Endogenous antigens likely involved
      1. Vasculitis associated with neoplasms (particularly lymphoid malignancies)
      2. Vasculitis associated with connective tissue diseases
      3. Vasculitis associated with other underlying diseases
      4. Vasculitis associated with congenital deficiencies of the complement system
VII. Other vasculitic syndromes
   A. Kawasaki disease
   B. Isolated central nervous system vasculitis
   C. Thromboangiitis obliterans (Buerger's disease)
   D. Behçet's syndrome
   E. Miscellaneous vasculitides

death if untreated, while others are usually localized to the skin and rarely result in irreversible dysfunction of vital organs. The distinguishing and overlapping features of the diseases listed in Table 317-1, which justify this classification scheme, will be discussed below.

PATHOPHYSIOLOGY AND PATHOGENESIS Generally, most of the vasculitic syndromes are assumed to be mediated at least in part by immunopathogenic mechanisms (Table 317-2). However, evidence to this effect is for the most part indirect and may reflect epiphenomena as opposed to true causality.

Pathogenic Immune-Complex Formation Vasculitis is generally considered within the broader category of *immune-complex diseases* that include serum sickness and certain of the connective tissue diseases of which systemic lupus erythematosus (Chap. 311) is the prototype. Although deposition of immune complexes in vessel walls is the most widely accepted pathogenic mechanism of vasculitis, the causal role of immune complexes has not been clearly established in most of the vasculitic syndromes. Circulating immune complexes need not result in deposition of the complexes in blood vessels with ensuing vasculitis, and many patients with active vasculitis do not have demonstrable circulating or deposited immune complexes. The actual antigen contained in the immune complex has only rarely been iden-

Table 317-2   Potential Mechanisms of Vessel Damage in Vasculitis Syndromes

Pathogenic immune complex formation and/or deposition
   Henoch-Schönlein purpura
   Vasculitis associated with collagen vascular diseases
   Serum sickness and cutaneous vasculitis syndromes
   Hepatitis C–associated essential mixed cryoglobulinemia
   Hepatitis B–associated polyarteritis nodosa
Production of antineutrophilic cytoplasmic autoantibodies
   Wegener's granulomatosis
   Churg-Strauss syndrome
   Microscopic polyangiitis
Pathogenic T lymphocye responses and granuloma formation
   Temporal arteritis
   Takayasu's arteritis
   Wegener's granulomatosis
   Churg-Strauss syndrome
   Kawasaki disease

SOURCE: Adapted from MC Sneller, AS Fauci: Med Clin North Am 81:221, 1997.

tified in vasculitic syndromes. In this regard, hepatitis B antigen has been identified in both the circulating and deposited immune complexes in a subset of patients with systemic vasculitis, most notably within the polyarteritis nodosa group (see below). Essential mixed cryoglobulinemia has been associated with hepatitis C virus infection; hepatitis C virions and hepatitis C virus antigen-antibody complexes have been identified in the cryoprecipitates of these patients. An association between persistent parvovirus B19 infection and certain vasculitides has been reported; however, the pathogenic mechanisms related to this association are unclear.

The mechanisms of tissue damage in immune complex–mediated vasculitis resemble those described for serum sickness. In this model, antigen-antibody complexes are formed in antigen excess and are deposited in vessel walls whose permeability has been increased by vasoactive amines such as histamine, bradykinin, and leukotrienes released from platelets or from mast cells as a result of IgE-triggered mechanisms. The deposition of complexes results in activation of complement components, particularly C5a, which is strongly chemotactic for neutrophils. These cells then infiltrate the vessel wall, phagocytose the immune complexes, and release their intracytoplasmic enzymes, which damage the vessel wall. As the process becomes subacute or chronic, mononuclear cells infiltrate the vessel wall. The common denominator of the resulting syndrome is compromise of the vessel lumen with ischemic changes in the tissues supplied by the involved vessel.

Antineutrophil Cytoplasmic Antibodies (ANCA) ANCA are antibodies directed against certain proteins in the cytoplasm of neutrophils. They are present in a high percentage of patients with systemic vasculitis, particularly Wegener's granulomatosis, as well as in patients with microscopic polyangiitis and in patients with necrotizing and crescentic glomerulonephritis. There are two major categories of ANCA based on different targets for the antibodies. The terminology of *cytoplasmic* (c) *ANCA* refers to the diffuse, granular cytoplasmic staining pattern observed by immunofluorescence microscopy when serum antibodies bind to indicator neutrophils. Proteinase-3, the 29-kDa neutral serine proteinase present in neutrophil azurophilic granules is the major c-ANCA antigen. More than 90% of patients with typical Wegener's granulomatosis and active glomerulonephritis have a positive c-ANCA titer. The terminology of *perinuclear* (p) *ANCA* refers to the more localized perinuclear or nuclear staining pattern of the indicator neutrophils. The major target for p-ANCA is the enzyme myeloperoxidase; other targets of p-ANCA include elastase, cathepsin G, lactoferrin, lysozyme, and bactericidal/permeability-increasing protein. p-ANCA have been reported to occur in variable percentages of patients with microscopic polyangiitis, polyarteritis nodosa, Churg-Strauss syndrome, crescentic glomerulonephritis, and Goodpasture's syndrome as well as in association with nonvasculitic entities such as certain rheumatic and nonrheumatic autoimmune diseases, inflammatory bowel disease, certain drugs, and infections such as endocarditis and bacterial airway infections in patients with cystic fibrosis.

It is unclear why patients with these vasculitis syndromes develop ANCA, whereas ANCA are rare in other inflammatory diseases. However, once ANCA are present, there are a number of in vitro observations that suggest feasible mechanisms whereby these antibodies can contribute to the pathogenesis of the vasculitis syndromes. When neutrophils are in the resting state, proteinase-3 exists in the azurophilic granules of the cytoplasm, apparently inaccessible to serum antibodies. However, when neutrophils are primed by tumor necrosis factor (TNF)α or interleukin (IL)1, proteinase-3 translocates to the cell membrane where it can interact with extracellular ANCA. The neutrophils then degranulate and produce reactive oxygen species that can cause tissue damage. Endothelial cells also translocate their cytoplasmic proteinase-3 to the cell membrane upon priming with TNF-α, IL-1, or interferon (IFN)γ, thus rendering them susceptible to interaction with ANCA and leading possibly to tissue damage due to complement-mediated cytotoxicity or antibody-dependent cellular cytotoxicity. Despite the attractiveness of these in vitro data, there is no conclusive evidence that ANCA are directly involved in the pathogenesis of the vasculitis syndromes, and they may represent merely an epiphenomenon; in fact, a number of clinical and laboratory observations argue against a primary pathogenic linkage. Patients may have vasculitis in the absence of ANCA; the absolute height of the antibody titers does not correlate well with disease activity; and patients with vasculitis, particularly Wegener's granulomatosis, in remission may continue to have high c-ANCA titers for years. Thus, their role in the pathogenesis of systemic vasculitis remains an open question.

Pathogenic T Lymphocyte Responses and Granuloma Formation In addition to the classic immune complex–mediated mechanisms of vasculitis as well as ANCA, other immunopathogenic mechanisms may be involved in damage to vessels. The most prominent of these are delayed hypersensitivity and cell-mediated immune injury as reflected in the histopathologic feature of granulomatous vasculitis. However, immune complexes themselves may induce granulomatous responses. Vascular endothelial cells can express HLA class II molecules following activation by cytokines such as IFN-γ. This allows these cells to participate in immunologic reactions such as interaction with CD4+ T lymphocytes in a manner similar to antigen-presenting macrophages. Endothelial cells can secrete IL-1 which may activate T lymphocytes and initiate or propagate in situ immunologic processes within the blood vessel. In addition, IL-1 and TNF-α are potent inducers of endothelial-leukocyte adhesion molecule 1 (ELAM-1) and vascular cell adhesion molecule 1 (VCAM-1), which may enhance the adhesion of leukocytes to endothelial cells in the blood vessel wall. Other mechanisms such as direct cellular cytotoxicity or antibody directed against vessel components or antibody-dependent cellular cytotoxicity have been suggested in certain types of vessel damage. However, there is no convincing evidence to support their causal contribution to the pathogenesis of any of the recognized vasculitic syndromes.

It is unknown why certain individuals develop vasculitis in response to certain antigenic stimuli, whereas others do not. However, it is likely that a number of factors are involved in the ultimate expression of a vasculitic syndrome. These include the genetic predisposition and the regulatory mechanisms associated with immune response to certain antigens. When immune complexes are involved in the pathogenic process, the ability of the reticuloendothelial system to clear circulating complexes from the blood, the size and physicochemical properties of immune complexes, the relative degree of turbulence of blood flow, the intravascular hydrostatic pressure in different vessels, and the preexisting integrity of the vessel endothelium likely explain why only certain types of immune complexes cause vasculitis and why the vasculitic process is selective for only certain vessels in individual patients.

Approach to the Patient

Given the heterogeneous nature of the vasculitis syndromes, workup of a patient with suspected vasculitis should follow a series of progressive steps that establish the diagnosis of vasculitis, determine where possible the category of the vasculitis syndrome (Table 317-1), and determine the pattern and extent of disease activity. This information should then be utilized to determine the choice of therapeutic options (Fig. 317-1). This approach is of considerable importance since several of the vasculitis syndromes require aggressive therapy with glucocorticoids and immunosuppressive agents, while other syndromes usually resolve spontaneously and require symptomatic treatment only. Vasculitis is often suspected on clinical and laboratory grounds (see individual syndromes below). Depending on the individual category of vasculitis, measurement of ANCA titers may be helpful in this regard. However, a diagnosis of a vasculitis syndrome should not be made nor should treatment be initiated on the basis of a positive ANCA titer alone. The definitive diagnosis of vasculitis is made upon biopsy of involved tissue. The yield of "blind" biopsies of organs with

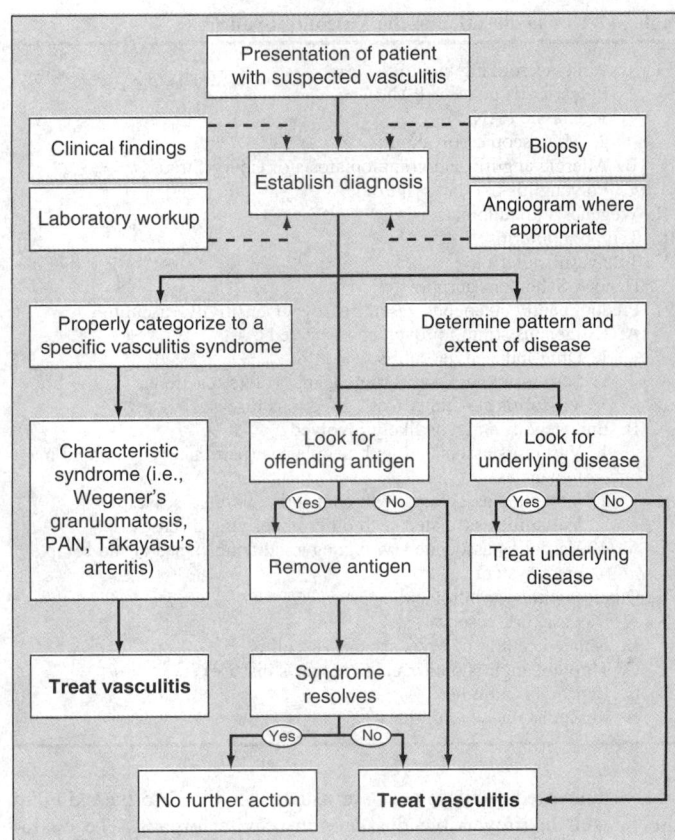

FIGURE 317-1 Algorithm for the approach to a patient with suspected diagnosis of vasculitis.

no subjective or objective evidence of involvement is very low and should be avoided. When syndromes such as classic polyarteritis nodosa, Takayasu's arteritis, or the polyangiitis overlap syndrome are suspected, angiogram of organs with suspected involvement should be performed. However, angiograms should not be performed routinely when patients present with localized cutaneous vasculitis with no clinical indication of visceral involvement.

The constellation of clinical, laboratory, biopsy, and radiographic findings usually allows proper categorization to a specific syndrome, and therapy where appropriate should be initiated according to this information (see individual syndromes below). If an offending antigen that precipitates the vasculitis is recognized, the antigen should be removed where possible. If the syndrome resolves, no further action should be taken. If disease activity continues, treatment should be initiated. If the vasculitis is associated with an underlying disease such as an infection, neoplasm, or connective tissue disease, the underlying disease should be treated. If the syndrome resolves, no further action should be taken. If the syndrome does not resolve or if there is no recognizable underlying disease and the vasculitis persists, treatment should be initiated according to the category of the vasculitis syndrome. Treatment options will be considered under the individual syndromes, and general principles of therapy will be considered at the end of the chapter.

SYSTEMIC NECROTIZING VASCULITIS

POLYARTERITIS NODOSA AND MICROSCOPIC POLYANGIITIS Definition *Classic polyarteritis nodosa* (PAN) was described in 1866 by Kussmaul and Maier. It is a multisystem, necrotizing vasculitis of small and medium-sized muscular arteries in which involvement of the renal and visceral arteries is characteristic. Classic PAN does not involve pulmonary arteries, although bronchial vessels may be involved; granulomas, significant eosinophilia, and an allergic diathesis are not part of the classic syndrome. The term *mi-*

croscopic polyangiitis (microscopic polyarteritis) was introduced into the literature by Davson in 1948. The Chapel Hill Consensus Conference on the Nomenclature of Systemic Vasculitis held in 1992 officially adopted the term to connote a necrotizing vasculitis with few or no immune complexes (pauci-immune) affecting small vessels (capillaries, venules, or arterioles). Since necrotizing arteritis involving small and medium-sized arteries may also be present, it shares features with classic PAN except that glomerulonephritis is very common in microscopic polyangiitis, and pulmonary capillaritis often occurs.

Incidence and Prevalence It is difficult to establish an accurate incidence of these diseases because of the fact that many reports of PAN actually have included both classic PAN and microscopic polyangiitis as well as other related vasculitides. Both diseases are uncommon, but classic PAN is felt to be more uncommon than microscopic polyangiitis. The mean age of onset of both PAN and microscopic polyangiitis is approximately 50 years of age, and males are slightly more frequently affected than females in both diseases.

Pathophysiology and Pathogenesis The vascular lesion in classic PAN is a necrotizing inflammation of small and medium-sized muscular arteries. The lesions are segmental and tend to involve bifurcations and branchings of arteries. They may spread circumferentially to involve adjacent veins. However, involvement of venules is not seen in classic PAN and, if present, suggests microscopic polyangiitis or the polyangiitis overlap syndrome (see below). In the acute stages of disease, polymorphonuclear neutrophils infiltrate all layers of the vessel wall and perivascular areas, which results in intimal proliferation and degeneration of the vessel wall. Mononuclear cells infiltrate the area as the lesions progress to the subacute and chronic stages. Fibrinoid necrosis of the vessels ensues with compromise of the lumen, thrombosis, infarction of the tissues supplied by the involved vessel, and, in some cases, hemorrhage. As the lesions heal, there is collagen deposition, which may lead to further occlusion of the vessel lumen. Aneurysmal dilatations up to 1 cm in size along the involved arteries are characteristic of classic PAN. Granulomas and substantial eosinophilia with eosinophilic tissue infiltrations are not characteristically found and suggest allergic angiitis and granulomatosis (see below).

Multiple organ systems are involved, and the clinicopathologic findings reflect the degree and location of vessel involvement and the resulting ischemic changes. As mentioned above, pulmonary arteries are not involved in classic PAN, and bronchial artery involvement is uncommon, whereas pulmonary capillaritis occurs frequently in microscopic polyangiitis. The pathology in the kidney in classic PAN is predominantly that of arteritis without glomerulonephritis. In contrast, glomerulonephritis is very common in microscopic polyangiitis. In patients with significant hypertension, typical pathologic features of glomerulosclerosis may be seen alone or superimposed on lesions of glomerulonephritis. In addition, pathologic sequelae of hypertension may be found elsewhere in the body.

The presence of hepatitis B antigenemia in approximately 20 to 30% of patients with systemic vasculitis, particularly of the classic PAN type, together with the isolation of circulating immune complexes composed of hepatitis B antigen and immunoglobulin, and the demonstration by immunofluorescence of hepatitis B antigen, IgM, and complement in the blood vessel walls, strongly suggest the role of immunologic phenomena in the pathogenesis of this disease. Hepatitis C infection has been reported in approximately 5% of patients with PAN; however, its pathogenic role in the vasculitis is unclear at present. Hairy cell leukemia can be associated with classic PAN; the pathogenic mechanisms of this association are unclear.

Clinical and Laboratory Manifestations Nonspecific signs and symptoms are the hallmarks of classic PAN. Fever, weight loss, and malaise are present in over one-half of cases. Patients usually present with vague symptoms such as weakness, malaise, headache, abdominal pain, and myalgias. Specific complaints related to the vascular involvement within a particular organ system may also dominate the presenting clinical picture as well as the entire course of the illness (Table 317-3). In classic PAN, renal involvement most commonly

Table 317-3 Clinical Manifestations Related to Organ System Involvement in Classic Polyarteritis Nodosa

Organ System	Percent Incidence	Clinical Manifestations
Renal	60	Renal failure, hypertension
Musculoskeletal	64	Arthritis, arthralgia, myalgia
Peripheral nervous system	51	Peripheral neuropathy, mononeuritis multiplex
Gastrointestinal tract	44	Abdominal pain, nausea and vomiting, bleeding, bowel infarction and perforation, cholecystitis, hepatic infarction, pancreatic infarction
Skin	43	Rash, purpura, nodules, cutaneous infarcts, livedo reticularis, Raynaud's phenomenon
Cardiac	36	Congestive heart failure, myocardial infarction, pericarditis
Genitourinary	25	Testicular, ovarian, or epididymal pain
Central nervous system	23	Cerebral vascular accident, altered mental status, seizure

SOURCE: From TR Cupps, AS Fauci: *The Vasculitides*. Philadelphia, Saunders, 1981.

manifests as hypertension, renal insufficiency, or hemorrhage due to microaneurysms. In microscopic polyangiitis acute glomerulonephritis is the characteristic renal lesion.

There are no diagnostic serologic tests for classic PAN. In over 75% of patients, the leukocyte count is elevated with a predominance of neutrophils. Eosinophilia is seen only rarely and, when present at high levels, suggests the diagnosis of allergic angiitis and granulomatosis. The anemia of chronic disease may be seen, and an elevated erythrocyte sedimentation rate (ESR) is almost always present. Other common laboratory findings reflect the particular organ involved. Hypergammaglobulinemia may be present, and up to 30% of patients have a positive test for hepatitis B surface antigen. Positive ANCA titers (usually of the p-ANCA type) are found in a low percentage (<20%) of patients with classic PAN. Microscopic polyangiitis is strongly associated with ANCA that are usually of the p-ANCA type, but c-ANCA have also been reported. In contrast, the ANCA in Wegener's granulomatosis (see below) are almost always of the c-ANCA type. Arteriograms may demonstrate characteristic abnormalities such as aneurysms in the small and medium-sized muscular arteries of the kidneys and abdominal viscera in classic PAN.

Diagnosis The diagnosis of classic PAN is based on the demonstration of characteristic findings of vasculitis on biopsy material of involved organs. In the absence of easily accessible tissue for biopsy, the angiographic demonstration of involved vessels, particularly in the form of aneurysms of small and medium-sized arteries in the renal, hepatic, and visceral vasculature, is sufficient to make the diagnosis. Aneurysms of vessels are not pathognomonic of classic PAN; furthermore, aneurysms need not always be present, and angiographic findings may be limited to stenotic segments and obliteration of vessels. Biopsy of symptomatic organs such as nodular skin lesions, painful testes, and muscle groups provides the highest diagnostic yields, while blind biopsy of asymptomatic organs is frequently negative. The presence of small vessel vasculitis, particularly in the setting of glomerulonephritis and pulmonary capillaritis distinguishes microscopic polyangiitis from classic PAN. In this regard, biopsy of the kidney or lung may establish the diagnosis of microscopic polyangiitis.

Prognosis The prognosis of untreated classic PAN as well as that of microscopic polyangiitis is extremely poor. The usual clinical course is characterized either by fulminant deterioration or by relentless progression associated with intermittent acute flare-ups. In classic PAN, death usually results from renal failure; from gastrointestinal complications, particularly bowel infarcts and perforation; and from cardiovascular causes. In microscopic polyangiitis, death usually results from renal failure or pulmonary hemorrhage. Intractable hypertension often compounds dysfunction in other organ systems, such as the kidneys, heart, and central nervous system, leading to additional late morbidity and mortality in classic PAN. The 5-year survival rate of untreated patients has been reported to be between 10 and 20% for both diseases; this rate has increased substantially as a result of treatment (see below).

℞ **TREATMENT**   Extremely favorable therapeutic results have been reported in classic PAN with the combination of prednisone, 1 mg/kg per day, and cyclophosphamide, 2 mg/kg per day (see "Wegener's Granulomatosis" for a detailed description of this therapeutic regimen). This regimen has been reported to result in up to a 90% long-term remission rate even following the discontinuation of therapy. In less severe cases of classic PAN, glucocorticoids alone have resulted in disease remission. In addition, long-term remissions have been reported in PAN associated with hepatitis B virus antigenemia using the antiviral agent vidarabine in combination with plasma exchange with and without glucocorticoids. Favorable results have also been reported in the treatment of PAN related to hepatitis B virus with IFN-α and plasma exchange. Careful attention to the treatment of hypertension can lessen the acute and late morbidity and mortality associated with renal, cardiac, and central nervous system complications of PAN. The treatment regimen for microscopic polyangiitis is similar to that for Wegener's granulomatosis (see below), particularly if glomerulonephritis is present.

ALLERGIC ANGIITIS AND GRANULOMATOSIS (CHURG-STRAUSS DISEASE)

Definition   *Allergic angiitis and granulomatosis* was described in 1951 by Churg and Strauss and is a disease characterized by granulomatous vasculitis of multiple organ systems, particularly the lung. It is characterized by vasculitis of blood vessels of various types or sizes (including veins and venules), intra- and extravascular granuloma formation together with eosinophilic tissue infiltration, and a strong association with severe asthma and peripheral eosinophilia.

Incidence and Prevalence   Allergic angiitis and granulomatosis is an uncommon disease whose exact incidence, similar to classic PAN, is difficult to determine due to the grouping of multiple types of vasculitic syndromes in many reported series. The disease can occur at any age with the possible exception of infants. The mean age of onset is 44 years, with a male-to-female ratio of 1.3:1.

Pathophysiology and Pathogenesis   The vasculitis of allergic angiitis and granulomatosis involves small and medium-sized muscular arteries, capillaries, veins, and venules. The characteristic histopathologic features of allergic angiitis and granulomatosis are granulomatous reactions that may be present in the tissues or even within the walls of the vessels themselves. These are usually associated with infiltration of the tissues with eosinophils. This process can occur in any organ in the body; lung involvement is predominant, with skin, cardiovascular system, kidney, peripheral nervous system, and gastrointestinal tract also commonly involved. Although the precise pathogenesis of this disease is uncertain, its strong association with asthma and its clinicopathologic manifestations including eosinophilia, granulomata, and vasculitis, which strongly suggest hypersensitivity phenomena, point to aberrant immunologic phenomena.

Clinical and Laboratory Manifestations   Patients with allergic angiitis and granulomatosis exhibit nonspecific manifestations such as fever, malaise, anorexia, and weight loss, which are characteristic of a multisystem disease. The pulmonary findings in allergic angiitis and granulomatosis clearly dominate the clinical picture with severe asthmatic attacks and the presence of pulmonary infiltrates. Clinically recognizable heart disease occurs in approximately one-third of patients. Heart involvement is seen at autopsy in 62% of cases and is the cause of death in 23% of patients. Skin lesions occur in approximately 70% of patients and include purpura in addition to cutaneous and subcu-

taneous nodules. The renal disease in allergic angiitis and granulomatosis is less common and generally less severe than that of classic PAN and microscopic polyangiitis.

The characteristic laboratory finding in virtually all patients with allergic angiitis and granulomatosis is a striking eosinophilia, which reaches levels greater than 1000 cells/μL in more than 80% of patients. The other laboratory findings are similar to those of classic PAN and microscopic polyangiitis and reflect the organ systems involved. Allergic angiitis and granulomatosis is associated with p-ANCA.

Diagnosis   The diagnosis of allergic angiitis and granulomatosis is made by biopsy in a patient with the characteristic clinical manifestations (see above). Granulomatous vasculitis with eosinophilic tissue involvement together with peripheral eosinophilia are typical.

Prognosis   The prognosis of untreated allergic angiitis and granulomatosis is poor, with a reported 5-year survival of 25%. The cause of death is likely to be related to pulmonary and cardiac disease.

℞ **TREATMENT**   Glucocorticoid therapy has been reported to increase the 5-year survival to more than 50%. In certain patients, the disease may be quite mild and may remit spontaneously or with short courses of glucocorticoids. In glucocorticoid failures or in patients who present with fulminant multisystem disease, the treatment of choice is a combined regimen of cyclophosphamide and alternate-day prednisone, which has resulted in a high rate of complete remission (see "Wegener's Granulomatosis" for a detailed description of this therapeutic regimen).

POLYANGIITIS OVERLAP SYNDROME   Many patients with systemic vasculitis manifest clinicopathologic characteristics that do not fit precisely into any classification but have overlapping features of classic PAN, allergic angiitis and granulomatosis, Wegener's granulomatosis, Takayasu's arteritis, and the hypersensitivity group of vasculitides. This subgroup has been referred to as the *polyangiitis overlap syndrome* and is part of the major grouping of systemic necrotizing vasculitis. This entity has been designated with a distinct classification in order to avoid confusion in attempting to fit such overlap syndromes into one or other of the more classic vasculitic syndromes. This subgroup is truly a systemic vasculitis with the same potential for resulting in irreversible organ system dysfunction as the other systemic necrotizing vasculitides. The diagnostic and therapeutic considerations as well as the prognosis for this subgroup are the same as those for classic PAN, microscopic polyangiitis, and allergic angiitis and granulomatosis.

WEGENER'S GRANULOMATOSIS

DEFINITION   *Wegener's granulomatosis* is a distinct clinicopathologic entity characterized by granulomatous vasculitis of the upper and lower respiratory tracts together with glomerulonephritis. In addition, variable degrees of disseminated vasculitis involving both small arteries and veins may occur.

INCIDENCE AND PREVALENCE   Wegener's granulomatosis is an uncommon disease whose true incidence is difficult to determine. It is extremely rare in blacks compared with whites; the male-to-female ratio is 1:1. The disease can be seen at any age; approximately 15% of patients are less than 19 years of age, but only rarely does the disease occur before adolescence; the mean age of onset is approximately 40 years.

PATHOPHYSIOLOGY AND PATHOGENESIS   The histopathologic hallmarks of Wegener's granulomatosis are necrotizing vasculitis of small arteries and veins together with granuloma formation, which may be either intravascular or extravascular (Fig. 317-2). Lung involvement typically appears as multiple, bilateral, nodular cavitary infiltrates (Fig. 317-3), which on biopsy almost invariably reveal the typical necrotizing granulomatous vasculitis. Endobronchial disease, either in its active form or as a result of fibrous scarring, may lead to obstruction with atelectasis. Upper airway lesions, particularly

FIGURE 317-2 Lung biopsy in a patient with Wegener's granulomatosis. Biopsy revealed necrotizing vasculitis with granuloma formation. This section demonstrates several well-formed multinucleated giant cells in an area of granulomatous inflammation.

those in the sinuses and nasopharynx, typically reveal inflammation, necrosis, and granuloma formation with or without vasculitis.

In its earliest form, renal involvement is characterized by a focal and segmental glomerulitis that may evolve into a rapidly progressive crescentic glomerulonephritis. Granuloma formation is only rarely seen on renal biopsy. In addition to the classic triad of upper and lower

FIGURE 317-3 Computed tomography scan of a patient with Wegener's granulomatosis. The patient developed multiple, bilateral, and cavitary infiltrates.

respiratory tracts and kidney disease, virtually any organ can be involved with vasculitis, granuloma, or both.

The immunopathogenesis of this disease is unclear, although the involvement of upper airways and lungs with granulomatous vasculitis suggests an aberrant hypersensitivity response to an exogenous or even endogenous antigen that enters through or resides in the upper airway. Chronic nasal carriage of *Staphylococcus aureus* has been reported to be associated with a higher relapse rate of Wegener's granulomatosis; however, there is no evidence for a role of this organism in the pathogenesis of the disease.

Peripheral blood mononuclear cells obtained from patients with Wegener's granulomatosis manifest increased secretion of IFN-γ but not of IL-4, IL-5, or IL-10 compared to normal controls. The increased IFN-γ production is inhibited by exogenous IL-10. In addition, TNF-α production from peripheral blood mononuclear cells and CD4+ T is elevated. Furthermore, monocytes from patients with Wegener's granulomatosis produce increased amounts of IL-12. These findings indicate an unbalanced Th1-type T cell cytokine pattern in this disease that may have pathogenic and perhaps ultimately therapeutic implications.

A high percentage of patients with Wegener's granulomatosis develop ANCA; c-ANCA are the predominant ANCA in this disease. As with the other categories of vasculitis, there is no clear evidence that ANCA play a primary role in the pathogenesis of Wegener's granulomatosis.

CLINICAL AND LABORATORY MANIFESTATIONS

A typical patient presents with severe upper respiratory tract findings such as paranasal sinus pain and drainage and purulent or bloody nasal discharge with or without nasal mucosal ulceration (Table 317-4). Nasal septal perforation may follow, leading to saddle nose deformity. Serous otitis media may occur as a result of eustachian tube blockage.

Pulmonary involvement may be manifested as asymptomatic infiltrates or may be clinically expressed as cough, hemoptysis, dyspnea, and chest discomfort. It is present in 85 to 90% of patients. Subglottic stenosis resulting from active disease or scarring occurs in approximately 16% of patients and may result in severe airway obstruction.

Eye involvement (52% of patients) may range from a mild conjunctivitis to dacryocystitis, episcleritis, scleritis, granulomatous sclerouveitis, ciliary vessel vasculitis, and retroorbital mass lesions leading to proptosis.

Skin lesions (46% of patients) appear as papules, vesicles, palpable purpura, ulcers, or subcutaneous nodules; biopsy reveals vasculitis, granuloma, or both. Cardiac involvement (8% of patients) manifests as pericarditis, coronary vasculitis, or, rarely, cardiomyopathy. Nervous system manifestations (23% of patients) include cranial neuritis, mononeuritis multiplex, or, rarely, cerebral vasculitis and/or granuloma.

Renal disease (77% of patients) generally dominates the clinical picture and, if left untreated, accounts directly or indirectly for most of the mortality in this disease. Although it may smolder in some cases as a mild glomerulitis with proteinuria, hematuria, and red blood cell casts, it is clear that once clinically detectable renal functional impairment occurs, rapidly progressive renal failure usually ensues unless appropriate treatment is instituted.

While the disease is active, most patients have nonspecific symptoms and signs such as malaise, weakness, arthralgias, anorexia, and weight loss. Fever may indicate activity of the underlying disease but more often reflects secondary infection, usually of the upper airway.

Characteristic laboratory findings include a markedly elevated ESR, mild anemia and leukocytosis, mild hypergammaglobulinemia (particularly of the IgA class), and mildly elevated rheumatoid factor. Thrombocytosis may be seen as an acute-phase reactant. In typical Wegener's granulomatosis with granulomatous vasculitis of the respiratory tract and glomerulonephritis, approximately 90% of patients have a positive c-ANCA. However, in the absence of renal disease, the sensitivity drops to approximately 70%.

Table 317-4 Wegener's Granulomatosis: Frequency of Clinical Manifestations in 158 Patients Studied at the National Institutes of Health

Manifestation	Percent at Disease Onset	Percent Throughout Course of Disease
Kidney		
Glomerulonephritis	18	77
Ear/nose/throat	73	92
Sinusitis	51	85
Nasal disease	36	68
Otitis media	25	44
Hearing loss	14	42
Subglottic stenosis	1	16
Ear pain	9	14
Oral lesions	3	10
Lung	45	85
Pulmonary infiltrates	25	66
Pulmonary nodules	24	58
Hemoptysis	12	30
Pleuritis	10	28
Eyes		
Conjunctivitis	5	18
Dacryocystitis	1	18
Scleritis	6	16
Proptosis	2	15
Eye pain	3	11
Visual loss	0	8
Retinal lesions	0	4
Corneal lesions	0	1
Iritis	0	2
Other[a]		
Arthralgias/arthritis	32	67
Fever	23	50
Cough	19	46
Skin abnormalities	13	46
Weight loss (greater than 10% body weight)	15	35
Peripheral neuropathy	1	15
Central nervous system disease	1	8
Pericarditis	2	6
Hyperthyroidism	1	3

[a] Fewer than 1% had parotid, pulmonary artery, breast, or lower genitourinary (urethra, cervix, vagina, testicular) involvement.
SOURCE: Hoffman et al.

DIAGNOSIS The diagnosis of Wegener's granulomatosis is a clinicopathologic one made by the demonstration of necrotizing granulomatous vasculitis on biopsy of appropriate tissue in a patient with the clinical findings of upper and lower respiratory tract disease together with evidence of glomerulonephritis. Pulmonary tissue, preferably obtained by open thoracotomy, offers the highest diagnostic yield, almost invariably revealing granulomatous vasculitis. Biopsy of upper airway tissue usually reveals granulomatous inflammation with necrosis but may not show vasculitis. Renal biopsy confirms the presence of glomerulonephritis.

The specificity of a positive c-ANCA titer for Wegener's granulomatosis is very high, especially if active glomerulonephritis is present. However, the presence of c-ANCA should be adjunctive and, with very rare exceptions, should not substitute for a tissue diagnosis. False-positive ANCA titers have been reported in certain infectious and neoplastic diseases.

In its typical presentation, the classic clinicopathologic complex of Wegener's granulomatosis usually provides ready differentiation from other disorders. However, if all the typical features are not present at once, it needs to be differentiated from the other vasculitides, particularly allergic angiitis and granulomatosis, Goodpasture's syndrome (Chap. 275), tumors of the upper airway or lung, and infectious diseases such as histoplasmosis (Chap. 201), mucocutaneous leishmaniasis (Chap. 215), and rhinoscleroma (Chap. 30) as well as noninfectious granulomatous diseases.

Of particular note is the differentiation from *midline granuloma* and *upper airway neoplasms*, which are part of the spectrum of *midline destructive diseases*. These diseases lead to extreme tissue destruction and mutilation localized to the midline upper airway structures including the sinuses; erosion through the skin of the face commonly occurs, a feature that is extremely rare in Wegener's granulomatosis. Although blood vessels may be involved in the intense inflammatory reaction and necrosis, primary vasculitis is seen rarely. When systemic involvement occurs, it usually declares itself as a neoplastic process. In this regard, it is likely that midline granuloma is part of the spectrum of *angiocentric immunoproliferative lesions* (AIL). The latter are considered to represent a spectrum of postthymic T cell proliferative lesions and should be treated as such (Chap. 112). The term *idiopathic* has been applied to midline granuloma when extensive diagnostic workup including multiple biopsies has failed to reveal anything other than inflammation and necrosis. Under these circumstances, it is possible that the tumor cells were masked by the intensive inflammatory response. Such cases have responded to local irradiation with 50 Gy (5000 rad). Upper airway lesions should never be irradiated in Wegener's granulomatosis.

Wegener's granulomatosis must also be differentiated from *lymphomatoid granulomatosis*, the latter also being a part of the spectrum of AIL. Lymphomatoid granulomatosis is characterized by lung, skin, central nervous system, and kidney involvement in which atypical lymphocytoid and plasmacytoid cells infiltrate tissue in an angioinvasive manner. In this regard, it clearly differs from Wegener's granulomatosis in that it is not an inflammatory vasculitis in the classic sense but an infiltration of vessels with atypical mononuclear cells; granuloma may be present in involved tissues. Approximately 50% of patients develop a true malignant lymphoma. The presence of c-ANCA in Wegener's granulomatosis proves extremely helpful in the differentiation from all the preceding diseases.

℞ TREATMENT Wegener's granulomatosis was formerly universally fatal, usually within a few months after the onset of clinically apparent renal disease. Glucocorticoids alone led to some symptomatic improvement, with little effect on the ultimate course of the disease. It has been well established that the most effective therapy in this disease is cyclophosphamide given in doses of 2 mg/kg per day orally together with glucocorticoids. The leukocyte count should be monitored closely during therapy, and the dosage of cyclophosphamide should be adjusted in order to maintain the count above 3000/μL, which generally maintains the neutrophil count at approximately 1500/μL. With this approach, clinical remission can usually be induced and maintained without causing severe leukopenia with its associated risk of infection. Cyclophosphamide should be continued for 1 year following the induction of complete remission and gradually tapered and discontinued thereafter.

At the initiation of therapy, glucocorticoids should be administered together with cyclophosphamide. This can be given as prednisone, 1 mg/kg per day initially (for the first month of therapy) as a daily regimen, with gradual conversion to an alternate-day schedule followed by tapering and discontinuation after approximately 6 months.

Using the above regimen, the prognosis of this disease is excellent; marked improvement is seen in more than 90% of patients, and complete remissions are achieved in 75% of patients. A number of patients who developed irreversible renal failure but who achieved subsequent remission on appropriate therapy have undergone successful renal transplantation.

Despite the dramatic remissions induced by the therapeutic regimen described above, long-term follow-up of patients has revealed that approximately 50% of remissions are later associated with one or more relapses. Reinduction of remission is almost always achieved; however, a high percentage of patients ultimately have some degree of morbidity from irreversible features of their disease, such as varying degrees of renal insufficiency, hearing loss, tracheal stenosis, saddle nose deformity, and chronically impaired sinus function. In evaluating patients for relapse, the ANCA titer can be misleading. Many patients who achieve remission continue to have elevated titers for years. In addition, over 40% of patients who were in remission and had a four-fold increase in c-ANCA titer did not have a relapse in disease. In this regard, therapy should not be reinstituted or increased on the basis of a rise in the ANCA titer alone; however, such a finding should prompt the clinician to examine the patient carefully for any objective evidence of active disease and to monitor that patient more closely.

Certain types of morbidity are related to toxic side effects of treatment. Since the preceding therapeutic regimen calls for conversion to alternate-day glucocorticoid therapy within 3 months and ultimate discontinuation within 6 to 12 months, glucocorticoid-related side effects such as diabetes mellitus, cataracts, life-threatening infectious disease complications, serious osteoporosis, and severe cushingoid features are infrequently encountered except in those patients requiring prolonged courses of daily glucocorticoids. However, cyclophosphamide-related toxicities are more frequent and severe. Cystitis to varying degrees occurs in 50% of patients, bladder cancer in 6%, and myelodysplasia in 2%.

Some reports have indicated therapeutic success with less frequent and severe toxic side effects using intermittent boluses of intravenous cyclophosphamide (1 g/m² per month) in place of daily drug administered orally. However, we and others have found an increased rate of relapse with bolus intravenous cyclophosphamide. We therefore strongly recommend that the drug be given as daily oral therapy.

Despite concerns regarding toxicity, a regimen of daily cyclophosphamide and glucocorticoids is clearly the treatment of choice in patients with immediately life-threatening disease such as rapidly progressive glomerulonephritis. However, methotrexate together with glucocorticoids may be considered as an alternative for initial therapy for certain patients whose disease is not immediately life-threatening or as a switch regimen in those patients who have experienced significant cyclophosphamide toxicity. In one study, patients in this category were given oral prednisone as described above, and methotrexate was administered orally starting at a dosage of 0.3 mg/kg, with a maximum of 15 mg/week. If the treatment was well tolerated after 1 to 2 weeks, the dosage was increased by 2.5 mg weekly up to a dosage of 20 to 25 mg/week and maintained at that level. Remissions were achieved in 33 of 42 patients (79%). Nineteen patients relapsed; 15 of these 19 relapses occurred when patients were receiving 15 mg or less of methotrexate per week; 13 of these 19 were treated with a second course of methotrexate and prednisone and 10 of 13 achieved a second remission. Toxicities of methotrexate included elevated transaminase levels (24%), leukopenia (7%), opportunistic infection (9.5%), methotrexate pneumonitis (7%), and stomatitis (2%).

Azathioprine, in doses of 1 to 2 mg/kg per day, has proven effective in some patients, particularly in maintaining remission in those in whom remission was induced by cyclophosphamide. The drug should be administered together with the glucocorticoid regimen described above. Although certain reports have indicated that trimethoprim-sulfamethoxazole may be of benefit in the treatment of Wegener's granulomatosis, there are no firm data to substantiate this, particularly in patients with serious renal and pulmonary disease. In a study examining the effect of trimethoprim-sulfamethoxazole on relapse, decreased relapses were shown only with regard to upper airway disease, and no differences in major organ relapses were observed. Trimethoprim-sulfamethoxazole alone should never be used to treat active Wegener's granulomatosis outside of the upper airway.

TEMPORAL ARTERITIS

DEFINITION *Temporal arteritis*, also referred to as *cranial arteritis* or *giant cell arteritis*, is an inflammation of medium- and large-sized arteries. It characteristically involves one or more branches of the carotid artery, particularly the temporal artery; hence the name. However, it is a systemic disease that can involve arteries in multiple locations.

INCIDENCE AND PREVALENCE The incidence of temporal arteritis varies widely in different studies and in different geographic regions. A high incidence has been found in Scandanavia and in regions of the United States with large Scandanavian populations, compared to a lower incidence in southern Europe. The annual incidence rates in individuals 50 years of age and older range from 0.49 to 23.3 per 100,000 population. It occurs almost exclusively in individuals older than 55 years; however, well-documented cases have occurred in patients 40 years old or younger. It is more common in women than in men and is rare in blacks. Familial aggregation has been reported, as has an association with HLA-DR4. In addition, genetic linkage studies have demonstrated an association of temporal arteritis with alleles at the HLA-DRB1 locus, particularly HLA-DRB1*04 variants. The disease is closely associated with *polymyalgia rheumatica*, which is more common than temporal arteritis. In Olmsted County, Minnesota, the annual incidence of polymyalgia rheumatica in individuals 50 years of age and older is 52.5 per 100,000 population.

PATHOPHYSIOLOGY AND PATHOGENESIS Although the temporal artery is most frequently involved in this disease, patients often have a systemic vasculitis of multiple medium- and large-sized arteries, which may go undetected. Histopathologically, the disease is a panarteritis with inflammatory mononuclear cell infiltrates within the vessel wall with frequent giant cell formation. There is proliferation of the intima and fragmentation of the internal elastic lamina. Pathophysiologic findings in organs result from the ischemia related to the involved vessels. Distinct cytokine patterns as well as T lymphocytes expressing specific antigen receptors have been described suggesting the involvement of immunopathogenic mechanisms in temporal arteritis. IL-6 and IL-1β expression has been detected in a majority of circulating monocytes of patients with temporal arteritis and polymyalgia rheumatica. T cells recruited to vasculitic lesions in patients with temporal arteritis produce predominantly IL-2 and IFN-γ, and the latter has been suggested to be involved in the progression to overt arteritis. Sequence analysis of the T cell receptor of tissue-infiltrating T cells in lesions of temporal arteritis indicates restricted clonal expansion, suggesting that an antigen residing in the arterial wall is recognized by a small fraction of T cells.

CLINICAL AND LABORATORY MANIFESTATIONS The disease is characterized clinically by the classic complex of fever, anemia, high ESR, and headaches in an elderly patient. Other manifestations include malaise, fatigue, anorexia, weight loss, sweats, and arthralgias. The polymyalgia rheumatica syndrome is characterized by stiffness, aching, and pain in the muscles of the neck, shoulders, lower back, hips, and thighs.

In patients with involvement of the temporal artery, headache is the predominant symptom and may be associated with a tender, thickened, or nodular artery, which may pulsate early in the disease but become occluded later. Scalp pain and claudication of the jaw and tongue may occur. A well-recognized and dreaded complication of temporal arteritis, particularly in untreated patients, is ocular involvement due primarily to ischemic optic neuropathy, which may lead to serious visual symptoms, even sudden blindness in some patients. However, most patients have complaints relating to the head or eyes for months before objective eye involvement. Attention to such symptoms with institution of appropriate therapy (see below) will usually avoid this complication. Claudication of the extremities, strokes, myocardial infarctions, and infarctions of visceral organs have been reported. Of note, temporal arteritis is associated with a markedly increased risk of aortic aneurysm, which is usually a late complication and may lead to dissection and death.

Characteristic laboratory findings in addition to the elevated ESR include a normochromic or slightly hypochromic anemia. Liver function abnormalities are common, particularly increased alkaline phosphatase levels. Increased levels of IgG and complement have been reported. Levels of enzymes indicative of muscle damage such as serum creatine kinase are not elevated.

DIAGNOSIS The diagnosis of temporal arteritis and its associated clinicopathologic syndrome can often be made clinically by the demonstration of the classic picture of fever, anemia, and high ESR with or without symptoms of polymyalgia rheumatica in an elderly patient. The diagnosis is confirmed by biopsy of the temporal artery. Since involvement of the vessel may be segmental, the diagnosis may be missed on routine biopsy; serial sectioning of biopsy specimens is recommended. When the temporal arteries appear clinically normal, but temporal arteritis is strongly suspected, a biopsy segment of a few centimeters may be required to establish the diagnosis. Ultrasonography of the temporal artery has been reported to be helpful in diagnosis. A temporal artery biopsy should be obtained as quickly as possible in the setting of ocular signs and symptoms, and under these circumstances therapy should not be delayed pending a biopsy. In this regard, it has been reported that temporal artery biopsies may show vasculitis even after more than 14 days of glucocorticoid therapy. A dramatic clinical response to a trial of glucocorticoid therapy can confirm the diagnosis.

℞ **TREATMENT**   Temporal arteritis and its associated symptoms are exquisitely sensitive to glucocorticoid therapy. Treatment should begin with prednisone, 40 to 60 mg per day for approximately 1 month, followed by a gradual tapering to a maintenance dose of 7.5 to 10 mg per day. In order to lessen glucocorticoid side effects in elderly individuals, conversion to alternate-day therapy may be attempted, but only after the disease has been put into remission with daily therapy. When ocular signs and symptoms occur, it is important that therapy be initiated or adjusted to control them. Because of the possibility of relapse, therapy should be continued for at least 1 to 2 years. The ESR can serve as a useful indicator of inflammatory disease activity in monitoring and tapering therapy and can be used to judge the pace of the tapering schedule. However, minor increases in the ESR can occur as glucocorticoids are being tapered and do not necessarily reflect an exacerbation of arteritis, particularly if the patient remains symptom free. Under these circumstances, the tapering should continue with caution. If one attempts to maintain a normal ESR throughout the tapering period, glucocorticoid toxicity will almost surely occur. The prognosis is generally good, and most patients achieve complete remission that is often maintained after withdrawal of therapy.

TAKAYASU'S ARTERITIS

DEFINITION   *Takayasu's arteritis* is an inflammatory and stenotic disease of medium- and large-sized arteries characterized by a strong predilection for the aortic arch and its branches. For this reason, it is often referred to as the *aortic arch syndrome.*

INCIDENCE AND PREVALENCE   Takayasu's arteritis is an uncommon disease, much less common than temporal arteritis. It is most prevalent in adolescent girls and young women. Although it is more common in the Orient, it is neither racially nor geographically restricted.

PATHOPHYSIOLOGY AND PATHOGENESIS   The disease involves medium- and large-sized arteries, with a strong predilection for the aortic arch and its branches; the pulmonary artery may also be involved. The most commonly affected arteries seen by angiography are listed in Table 317-5. The involvement of the major branches of the aorta is much more marked at their origin than distally. The disease is a panarteritis with inflammatory mononuclear cell infiltrates and occasionally giant cells. There are marked intimal proliferation and fibrosis, scarring and vascularization of the media, and disruption and degeneration of the elastic lamina. Narrowing of the lumen occurs with or without thrombosis. The vasa vasorum are frequently involved. Pathologic changes in various organs reflect the compromise of blood flow through the involved vessels.

Immunopathogenic mechanisms, the precise nature of which is uncertain, are suspected in this disease. As with several of the vasculitis syndromes, circulating immune complexes have been demonstrated, but their pathogenic significance is unclear.

Table 317-5   Frequency of Arteriographic Abnormalities and Potential Clinical Manifestations of Arterial Involvement in Takayasu's Arteritis

Artery	Percent of Arteriographic Abnormalities	Potential Clinical Manifestations
Subclavian	93	Arm claudication, Raynaud's phenomenon
Common carotid	58	Visual changes, syncope, transient ischemic attacks, stroke
Abdominal aorta[a]	47	Abdominal pain, nausea, vomiting
Renal	38	Hypertension, renal failure
Aortic arch or root	35	Aortic insufficiency, congestive heart failure
Vertebral	35	Visual changes, dizziness
Coeliac axis[a]	18	Abdominal pain, nausea, vomiting
Superior mesenteric[a]	18	Abdominal pain, nausea, vomiting
Iliac	17	Leg claudication
Pulmonary	10–40	Atypical chest pain, dyspnea
Coronary	<10	Chest pain, myocardial infarction

[a] Arteriographic lesions at these locations are usually asymptomatic but may potentially cause these symptoms.
SOURCE: Kerr et al.

CLINICAL AND LABORATORY MANIFESTATIONS   Takayasu's arteritis is a systemic disease with generalized as well as local symptoms. The generalized symptoms include malaise, fever, night sweats, arthralgias, anorexia, and weight loss, which may occur months before vessel involvement is apparent. These symptoms may merge into those related to pain over the involved vessels, followed by symptoms of ischemia in organs supplied by the compromised vessels. Pulses are commonly absent in the involved vessels, particularly the subclavian artery. The frequency of arteriographic abnormalities and the potentially associated clinical manifestations are listed in Table 317-5.

The clinical course may be fulminant, may progress gradually, or may stabilize. Complications are related to the distribution of the involved vessels. Death usually occurs from congestive heart failure or cerebrovascular accidents.

Characteristic laboratory findings include an elevated ESR, mild anemia, and elevated immunoglobulin levels.

DIAGNOSIS   The diagnosis of Takayasu's arteritis should be suspected strongly in a young woman who develops a decrease or absence of peripheral pulses, discrepancies in blood pressure, and arterial bruits. The diagnosis is confirmed by the characteristic pattern on arteriography, which includes irregular vessel walls, stenosis, poststenotic dilatation, aneurysm formation, occlusion, and evidence of increased collateral circulation. Complete aortic arteriography should be obtained, unless this is renally contraindicated, in order to fully delineate the distribution and degree of arterial disease. Histopathologic demonstration of inflamed vessels adds confirmatory data; however, tissue is rarely readily available for examination.

℞ **TREATMENT**   The course of the disease is variable, and spontaneous remissions may occur. Reported mortality statistics range from less than 10 to 75%. Although glucocorticoid therapy in doses of 40 to 60 mg prednisone per day alleviates symptoms, there are no convincing studies that indicate that they alone increase survival. The combination of glucocorticoid therapy for acute signs and symptoms and an aggressive surgical and/or angioplastic approach to stenosed vessels has markedly improved survival and decreased morbidity by lessening the risk of stroke, correcting hypertension due to renal artery stenosis, and improving blood flow to ischemic viscera and limbs. Unless it is urgently required, surgical correction of stenosed arteries should be undertaken only when the vascular inflammatory process is well controlled with medical therapy. Most recent mortality figures using this therapeutic approach are less than 10%. In individuals who are refractory to glucocorticoids, methotrexate in doses up to 25 mg per week has yielded encouraging results; however, long-term studies will be needed to confirm this.

DEFINITION *Henoch-Schönlein purpura*, also referred to as *anaphylactoid purpura*, is a distinct systemic vasculitis syndrome that is characterized by palpable purpura (most commonly distributed over the buttocks and lower extremities), arthralgias, gastrointestinal signs and symptoms, and glomerulonephritis. It is a small vessel vasculitis.

INCIDENCE AND PREVALENCE Henoch-Schönlein purpura is usually seen in children; most patients range in age from 4 to 7 years; however, the disease may also be seen in infants and adults. It is not a rare disease; in one series it accounted for between 5 and 24 admissions per year at a pediatric hospital. The male-to-female ratio is 1.5:1. A seasonal variation with a peak incidence in spring has been noted.

PATHOPHYSIOLOGY AND PATHOGENESIS The presumptive pathogenic mechanism for Henoch-Schönlein purpura is immune-complex deposition. A number of inciting antigens have been suggested including upper respiratory tract infections, various drugs, foods, insect bites, and immunizations. IgA is the antibody class most often seen in the immune complexes and has been demonstrated in the renal biopsies of these patients.

CLINICAL AND LABORATORY MANIFESTATIONS In pediatric patients, presenting symptoms related to the skin, gut, and joints are present in 50% of cases. In adults, presenting symptoms related to the skin are seen in over 70% of patients, while initial complaints related to the gut or the joints are noted in fewer than 20% of cases. The typical palpable purpura is seen in virtually all patients; most patients develop polyarthralgias in the absence of frank arthritis. Gastrointestinal involvement, which is seen in almost 70% of pediatric patients, is characterized by colicky abdominal pain usually associated with nausea, vomiting, diarrhea, or constipation and is frequently accompanied by the passage of blood and mucus per rectum; bowel intussusception may occur rarely. The renal involvement is usually characterized by mild glomerulonephritis leading to proteinuria and microscopic hematuria, with red blood cell casts in the majority of patients (Chap. 275); it usually resolves spontaneously without therapy. Rarely, a progressive glomerulonephritis will develop. Renal failure is the most common cause of death in the rare patient who dies of Henoch-Schönlein purpura. Although certain studies have found that renal disease is more severe in adults, this has not been a consistent finding. However, the course of renal disease in adults may be more insidious and thus requires close follow-up. Myocardial involvement can occur in adults but is rare in children.

Routine laboratory studies generally show a mild leukocytosis, a normal platelet count, and occasionally eosinophilia. Serum complement components are normal, and IgA levels are elevated in about one-half of patients.

TREATMENT The prognosis of Henoch-Schönlein purpura is excellent. Most patients recover completely, and some do not require therapy. Treatment is similar for adults and children. When glucocorticoid therapy is required, prednisone in doses of 1 mg/kg per day and tapered according to clinical response has been shown to be useful in decreasing tissue edema, arthralgias, and abdominal discomfort; however, it has not proven beneficial in the treatment of skin or renal disease and does not appear to shorten the duration of active disease or lessen the chance of recurrence. Patients with rapidly progressive glomerulonephritis have been anecdotally reported to benefit from intensive plasma exchange combined with immunosuppressive drugs.

PREDOMINANTLY CUTANEOUS VASCULITIS

DEFINITION The term *predominantly cutaneous vasculitis* has been used interchangeably with the terms *hypersensitivity vasculitis* and *cutaneous leukocytoclastic vasculitis*. Due to the heterogeneity of this group of disorders, none of these terms is totally adequate. The common denominator of this group of diseases is the involvement of small vessels of the skin. The syndrome is presumed to be associated with an aberrant hypersensitivity reaction to an antigen such as an infectious agent, a drug, or other foreign or endogenous substances. In most instances, however, an antigen is never identified and the disease remains idiopathic. The term *hypersensitivity vasculitis* is a misleading term since most of the other groups of vasculitis syndromes are probably also associated with some form of hypersensitivity or aberrant immunologic reaction to as yet unidentified antigens. The term *cutaneous leukocytoclastic vasculitis* is a better term; however, not all of these vasculitides are truly leukocytoclastic in nature. We have elected to use the term *"predominantly" cutaneous vasculitis* since skin involvement generally dominates the clinical picture, but the skin is not always the exclusive organ involved. Indeed, any organ system can be involved with this type of vasculitis; however, the extracutaneous involvement is usually much less severe than that of the systemic necrotizing vasculitides.

INCIDENCE AND PREVALENCE Although the exact incidence of this group of vasculitis syndromes is uncertain, it is clearly more common than the systemic necrotizing vasculitis group. The disease can occur at any age and in both sexes; however, different subgroups have a higher incidence in certain age groups, and some are more common in males than females, or vice versa.

PATHOPHYSIOLOGY AND PATHOGENESIS The typical histopathologic feature of the predominantly cutaneous vasculitides is the presence of vasculitis of small vessels. Postcapillary venules are the most commonly involved vessels; capillaries and arterioles may be involved less frequently. This vasculitis is characterized by a *leukocytoclasis*, a term that refers to the nuclear debris remaining from the neutrophils that have infiltrated in and around the vessels during the acute stages. In the subacute or chronic stages, mononuclear cells predominate; in certain subgroups, eosinophilic infiltration is seen. Erythrocytes often extravasate from the involved vessels, leading to palpable purpura.

Immune-complex deposition is generally considered to be the immunopathogenic mechanism of this type of vasculitis; however, formal proof that this is the case has not been established for all subgroups (see above). The predominantly cutaneous vasculitides can be broken down empirically into two major categories depending on the type of putative antigen involved in the hypersensitivity reaction. In the originally described group, the antigen was foreign to the host, i.e., a drug, microbe, or foreign protein. In this regard, essential mixed cryoglobulinemia has been associated with hepatitis C virus infection. In the second category, the antigen is felt to be endogenous to the host. Examples of these are the "self" proteins such as DNA or immunoglobulin, which form immune complexes with their respective antibodies and lead to vasculitic complications in systemic lupus erythematosus and rheumatoid arthritis, respectively; other examples are the recognized and putative tumor antigens that form immune complexes with antibody and lead to vasculitis associated with certain neoplasms. Certain lymphoid malignancies may also secrete cytokines that contribute to the pathogenic process.

CLINICAL AND LABORATORY MANIFESTATIONS The hallmark of this broad group of vasculitides is the predominance of skin involvement. Skin lesions may appear typically as palpable purpura; however, other cutaneous manifestations of the vasculitis may occur, including macules, papules, vesicles, bullae, subcutaneous nodules, ulcers, and recurrent or chronic urticaria. Despite the fact that skin lesions predominate, other organ systems may be involved to varying degrees, and the extent to which this occurs may define a relatively distinct subgroup. Even in patients with isolated cutaneous involvement, the disease may be characterized by systemic signs and symptoms such as fever, malaise, myalgia, and anorexia. The skin lesions may be pruritic or even quite painful, with a burning or stinging sensation. Lesions most commonly occur in the lower extremities in ambulatory patients or in the sacral area in bedridden patients due to the effects of hydrostatic forces on the postcapillary venules. Edema may accompany certain lesions, and hyperpigmentation often occurs in areas of recurrent or chronic lesions.

There are no specific laboratory tests diagnostic of this category of vasculitis. A mild leukocytosis with or without eosinophilia is characteristic, as is an elevated ESR. Cryoglobulins and rheumatoid factor may be seen in certain cases, and serum complement levels follow no definite pattern. Laboratory abnormalities related to specific organ dysfunction reflect the involvement of these organs in the particular syndrome in question.

Drug-Induced Vasculitis Cutaneous drug reactions take a number of forms, and vasculitis is only one of these (Chaps. 57 and 59). Vasculitis associated with drug reactions usually presents as palpable purpura that may be generalized or limited to the lower extremities or other dependent areas; however, urticarial lesions, ulcers, and hemorrhagic blisters may also occur (Chap. 59). Signs and symptoms may be limited to the skin, although systemic manifestations such as fever, malaise, and polyarthralgias may occur. Although the skin is the predominant organ involved, systemic vasculitis may result from drug reactions. Drugs that have been implicated in vasculitis include allopurinol, thiazides, gold, sulfonamides, phenytoin, and penicillin (Chap. 59).

Serum Sickness and Serum Sickness–Like Reactions These reactions are characterized by the occurrence of fever, urticaria, polyarthralgias, and lymphadenopathy 7 to 10 days after primary exposure and 2 to 4 days after secondary exposure to a heterologous protein (classic serum sickness) or a nonprotein drug such as penicillin or sulfa (serum sickness–like reaction). Most of the manifestations are not due to a vasculitis; however, occasional patients will have typical cutaneous venulitis that may progress rarely to a systemic vasculitis.

Vasculitis Associated with Other Underlying Primary Diseases A number of diseases have vasculitis as a secondary manifestation of the underlying primary process. Foremost among these are the connective tissue diseases, particularly *systemic lupus erythematosus* (Chap. 311), *rheumatoid arthritis* (Chap. 312), and *Sjögren's syndrome* (Chap. 314). The most common form of vasculitis in these conditions is the small vessel venulitis isolated to the skin and clinically indistinguishable from the predominantly cutaneous vasculitides noted in response to an exogenous antigen. However, certain patients may develop a fulminant systemic necrotizing vasculitis indistinguishable from the PAN group.

Cryoglobulinemia may be seen in a number of the diverse vasculitic syndromes. *Essential mixed cryoglobulinemia* (Chap. 275) may present as a predominantly cutaneous vasculitis. However, typically, it is associated with glomerulonephritis, arthralgias, hepatosplenomegaly, and lymphadenopathy in addition to skin involvement.

Vasculitis can be associated with certain *malignancies*, particularly lymphoid or reticuloendothelial neoplasms. Leukocytoclastic venulitis confined to the skin is the most common finding; however, widespread systemic vasculitis may occur. Of particular note is the association of *hairy cell leukemia* (Chap. 112) with classic PAN.

A leukocytoclastic vasculitis predominantly involving the skin with occasional involvement of other organ systems may be a minor component of many other diseases. These include *subacute bacterial endocarditis, Epstein-Barr virus infection, HIV infection, chronic active hepatitis,* as well as a number of other infections; *ulcerative colitis, congenital deficiencies of various complement components, retroperitoneal fibrosis,* and *primary biliary cirrhosis.* Association of predominantly cutaneous vasculitis with α_1-*antitrypsin deficiency, intestinal bypass surgery,* and *relapsing polychondritis* has been reported.

DIAGNOSIS The diagnosis of this category of vasculitis is made by the demonstration of vasculitis on biopsy. Given the predominance of cutaneous involvement, biopsy material is generally readily available. An important principle in the diagnostic approach to patients with presumed isolated cutaneous vasculitis is to search for an etiology of the vasculitis—be it an exogenous agent such as a drug or an infection or an endogenous condition such as an underlying disease (Fig. 317-1). In addition, a careful physical and laboratory examination should be performed to rule out the possibility of systemic disease. This should start with the least invasive diagnostic approach and proceed to the more invasive only if clinically indicated.

℞ TREATMENT Most cases of predominantly cutaneous vasculitis resolve spontaneously, and others remit and relapse before finally remitting completely. In those patients in whom persistent cutaneous disease evolves or in whom extracutaneous organ system involvement occurs, a variety of therapeutic regimens have been tried with variable results. In general, the treatment of this type of vasculitis has not been satisfactory. Fortunately, since the disease is generally limited to the skin, this lack of consistent response to therapy usually does not lead to a life-threatening situation. When an antigenic stimulus is recognized as the precipitating factor in the vasculitis, it should be removed; if this is a microbe, appropriate antimicrobial therapy should be instituted. If the vasculitis is associated with another underlying disease, treatment of the latter often results in resolution of the former. In situations where disease is apparently self-limited, no therapy, except possibly symptomatic therapy, is indicated. When disease persists and when there is no evidence of an inciting agent, an associated disease, or an underlying systemic vasculitis, the decision to treat should be based on weighing the balance between the degree of symptoms and the risk of treatment. If the decision is made to treat, glucocorticoid therapy should be instituted, usually as prednisone, 1 mg/kg per day, in a regimen aimed at rapid tapering where possible, either directly to discontinuation or by conversion to an alternate-day regimen followed by ultimate discontinuation. In cases that prove refractory to glucocorticoids, a trial of an immunosuppressive agent may be indicated. Patients with chronic vasculitis isolated to cutaneous venules rarely respond dramatically to any therapeutic regimen, and immunosuppressive agents should be used only as a last resort in these patients. Methotrexate and azathioprine have been used in such situations in anecdotal reports (see above for specific regimens). Although cyclophosphamide is the most effective therapy for the systemic vasculitides, it should almost never be used for predominantly cutaneous vasculitis because of the potential toxicity. Plasmapheresis has been used with some success in fulminant cases. Dapsone has been tried in a number of patients with isolated cutaneous vasculitis with rare anecdotal reports of success. However, this drug has been consistently beneficial as therapy for cutaneous vasculitis only in patients with erythema elevatum diutinum (see below).

KAWASAKI DISEASE

Kawasaki disease (mucocutaneous lymph node syndrome) is an acute, febrile, multisystem disease of children. It is characterized by unresponsiveness to antibiotics, nonsuppurative cervical adenitis, and changes in the skin and mucous membranes such as edema; congested conjunctivae; erythema of the oral cavity, lips, and palms; and desquamation of the skin of the fingertips. Although the disease is generally benign and self-limited, it is associated with coronary artery aneurysms in approximately 25% of cases, with an overall case fatality rate of 0.5 to 2.8%. These complications usually occur between the third and fourth weeks of illness during the convalescent stage. Vasculitis of the coronary arteries is seen in almost all the fatal cases that have been autopsied. There is typical intimal proliferation and infiltration of the vessel wall with mononuclear cells. Beadlike aneurysms and thromboses may be seen along the artery. Most investigators agree that many of the cases of PAN formerly reported in children were actually arteritic complications of unrecognized Kawasaki disease. Other manifestations include pericarditis, myocarditis, myocardial ischemia and infarction, and cardiomegaly.

It is likely that immune-mediated injury to blood vessel endothelium is involved in the pathogenesis of this disease. Patients with Kawasaki disease have been demonstrated to have evidence of increased immune activation characterized by increased activated helper T cells and monocytes, elevated serum-soluble IL-2 receptor levels, elevated levels of spontaneous IL-1 production by peripheral blood mononuclear cells, anti-endothelial cell antibodies, and increased cytokine-inducible activation antigens on their vascular endothelium. A strong association has been reported between a novel form of *S. aureus* that releases toxic shock syndrome toxin 1 and Kawasaki disease, suggesting that this was the causative organism and was acting as a superantigen similar to the superantigen effect in toxic shock syndrome. However, analysis of the T cell receptor repertoire of patients with Kawasaki disease has yielded conflicting data as to whether the T cell response is driven by a superantigen or by a conventional antigen.

Apart from the up to 2.8% of patients who develop fatal complications, the prognosis of this disease for uneventful recovery is excellent. High-dose intravenous γ globulin (2 g/kg as a single infusion over 10 h) together with aspirin (100 mg/kg per day for 14 days followed by 3 to 5 mg/kg per day for several weeks) have been shown to be effective in reducing the prevalence of coronary artery abnormalities when administered early in the course of the disease.

ISOLATED VASCULITIS OF THE CENTRAL NERVOUS SYSTEM

Isolated vasculitis of the central nervous system is an uncommon clinicopathologic entity characterized by vasculitis restricted to the vessels of the central nervous system without other apparent systemic vasculitis. Although the arteriole is most commonly affected, vessels of any size can be involved. The inflammatory process is usually composed of mononuclear cell infiltrates with or without granuloma formation. Cases have been associated with cytomegalovirus, syphilis, pyogenic bacterial, and varicella-zoster infections, as well as with Hodgkin's disease and amphetamine abuse; however, in most cases no underlying disease process has been identified.

Patients may present with severe headaches, altered mental function, and focal neurologic defects. Systemic symptoms are generally absent. Devastating neurologic abnormalities may occur depending on the extent of vessel involvement. The diagnosis is generally made by demonstration of characteristic vessel abnormalities on arteriography and confirmed by biopsy of the brain parenchyma and leptomeninges. In the absence of a brain biopsy, care should be taken not to misinterpret as true primary vasculitis angiographic abnormalities that might actually be vessel spasm related to another cause. The prognosis of this disease is poor; however, in certain patients the disease may remit spontaneously, and some reports indicate that glucocorticoid therapy alone or together with cyclophosphamide in steroid-resistant patients administered as described above for the systemic vasculitides has induced sustained clinical remissions in a small number of patients.

THROMBOANGIITIS OBLITERANS (BUERGER'S DISEASE)

Thromboangiitis obliterans is an inflammatory occlusive peripheral vascular disease of unknown etiology that affects arteries and veins. Thrombosis of the vessels is likely the primary event, and so this disease is not a classic vasculitis. However, it is considered among the vasculitides because of the intense inflammatory response within the thrombus and the fact that there is often a vasculitis of the vasa vasorum in the arterial wall. →*The disease is discussed in detail in Chap. 248.*

BEHÇET'S SYNDROME

Behçet's syndrome is a clinicopathologic entity characterized by recurrent episodes of oral and genital ulcers, iritis, and cutaneous lesions. The underlying pathologic process is a leukocytoclastic venulitis, although vessels of any size and in any organ can be involved. →*This disorder is described in detail in Chap. 316.*

MISCELLANEOUS VASCULITIDES

A variety of disorders, many of which are uncommon, are characterized by varying degrees of inflammatory responses involving blood vessels. *Cogan's syndrome* is a disease characterized by nonsyphilitic interstitial keratitis together with vestibuloauditory symptoms. It may be associated with a systemic vasculitis involving vessels of different sizes as well as the aortic valve.

Erythema elevatum diutinum is a rare chronic skin disorder of unknown etiology characterized by persistent red, purple, and yellowish papules, plaques, and nodules usually distributed symmetrically over the extensor surface of the limbs; on biopsy, they demonstrate a leukocytoclastic venulitis together with a marked dermal inflammatory infiltrate. An association with streptococcal infections has been reported. The disease responds dramatically to dapsone therapy.

Certain *infections* may directly trigger an inflammatory vasculitic process. For example, rickettsias can invade and proliferate in the endothelial cells of small blood vessels causing a vasculitis (Chap. 177). In addition, the inflammatory response around blood vessels associated with certain systemic fungal diseases such as histoplasmosis (Chap. 201) may mimic a primary vasculitic process.

PRINCIPLES OF TREATMENT

Once a diagnosis of vasculitis has been established, a decision regarding therapeutic strategy must be made (Fig. 317-1). The vasculitis syndromes represent a wide spectrum of diseases with varying degrees of severity. Some require immediate and aggressive therapy with glucocorticoids and immunosuppressive agents, while others should be treated conservatively and symptomatically, usually with nonsteroidal anti-inflammatory drugs. Since the potential toxic side effects of certain therapeutic regimens may be substantial, the risk-versus-benefit ratio of any therapeutic approach should be weighed carefully. Specific therapeutic regimens are discussed above for the individual vasculitis syndromes; however, certain general principles regarding therapy should be considered. On the one hand, glucocorticoids and/or immunosuppressive therapy should be instituted immediately in diseases where irreversible organ system dysfunction and high morbidity and mortality have been clearly established. Wegener's granulomatosis is the prototype of a severe systemic vasculitis requiring such a therapeutic approach (see above). On the other hand, when feasible, aggressive therapy should be avoided for vasculitic manifestations that rarely result in irreversible organ system dysfunction and that usually do not respond to such therapy. For example, isolated cutaneous vasculitis usually resolves with symptomatic treatment, and prolonged courses of glucocorticoids uncommonly result in clinical benefit. Immunosuppressive agents have not proven to be beneficial in isolated cutaneous vasculitis, and their toxic side effects generally outweigh any potential beneficial effects. Glucocorticoids should be initiated in those systemic vasculitides that cannot be specifically categorized or for which there is no established standard therapy; immunosuppressive therapy should be added in these diseases only if an adequate response does not result or if remission can only be achieved and maintained with an unacceptably toxic regimen of glucocorticoids. When remission is achieved, one should continually attempt to taper glucocorticoids to an alternate-day regimen and discontinue when possible. When using immunosuppressive regimens, one should taper and discontinue the drug as soon as is feasible upon induction of remission (see below).

When glucocorticoids are used, prednisone is generally the formulation of choice and is administered as 1 mg/kg per day orally, first in divided doses and then converted to a single daily dose. After clinical improvement is noted (usually within a month), the regimen is gradually converted to an alternate-day schedule, followed by tapering and discontinuation after approximately 6 months or as the clinical response dictates. When an immunosuppressive agent is required, cyclophosphamide is the drug of choice and its efficacy has been clearly established in Wegener's granulomatosis and the severe systemic vasculitides (see above). It should be given in doses of 2 mg/kg per day orally. It is recommended that the drug be taken as a single dose in the morning together with large amounts of fluid. Dose adjustments should be based on the leukocyte count, which should be maintained above 3000/μL. Leukocyte counts at any given time will reflect the dosage of cyclophosphamide taken the previous week. Of note, neutropenia may become more pronounced as glucocorticoids are tapered. The regimen that has proven successful in Wegener's granulomatosis (see above) and that should be followed for the other severe systemic vasculitides has called for continuation of cyclophosphamide for approximately 1 year following the induction of complete remission, with gradual tapering (by 25-mg decrements of the daily dose) over several months until discontinuation. No other drug has proven to be as effective as cyclophosphamide for severe life-threatening vasculitis. However, immediate and long-range toxic side effects may be severe. Alternative immunosuppressive regimens may be instituted where indicated in those patients who cannot tolerate cyclophosphamide due to unacceptable side effects or who do not wish to take cyclophosphamide because of the potential side effects, particularly infertility or sterility in individuals of child-bearing age. Methotrexate has been shown to be an acceptable alternative to cyclophosphamide when the latter drug cannot be used. Methotrexate is administered as a single weekly dose initially at a dosage of 0.3 mg/kg, not to exceed 15 mg/week. If the treatment is well tolerated after 1 to 2 weeks, the dosage should be increased by 2.5 mg weekly up to a dosage of 20 to 25 mg/week and maintained at that level. Azathioprine at a dosage of 2 mg/kg per day orally has also been employed as an alternative to cyclophosphamide in severe systemic vasculitis with less favorable results. In unusual cases in which none of the above regimens have resulted in remission of the vasculitis, certain experimental approaches have been used, such as plasmapheresis together with immunosuppressive drugs, with anecdotal reports of limited success. In addition, other immunosuppressive agents such as cyclosporine have been employed with minimal success.

Physicians should be thoroughly aware of the toxic side effects of therapeutic agents employed (Table 317-6). Side effects of glucocorticoid therapy are markedly decreased in frequency and duration in patients on alternate-day regimens compared to daily regimens. When cyclophosphamide is administered chronically in doses of 2 mg/kg per day for substantial periods of time (one to several years), the incidence of cystitis as defined by nonglomerular hematuria is approximately 50% and the incidence of bladder cancer is 6%. Bladder cancer can occur several years after discontinuation of cyclophosphamide therapy; therefore, monitoring for bladder cancer should continue indefinitely in patients who have received prolonged courses of daily cyclophosphamide. Significant alopecia is unusual in the chronically administered, low-dose regimen. When patients are receiving low-dose cyclophosphamide, the white blood count (WBC) is maintained above 3000/μL, and the patient is not receiving daily glucocorticoids, the incidence of life-threatening opportunistic infections is very low. However, the WBC is not an accurate predictor of risk of opportunistic infections in patients receiving methotrexate; infections with *Pneumocystis carinii* and certain fungi can be seen in the face of WBC that are within normal limits. All vasculitis patients who are not allergic to sulfa and who are receiving daily glucocorticoids in combination with an immunosuppressive drug should receive trimethoprim-sulfamethoxazole as prophylaxis against *P. carinii* infection.

Finally, it should be emphasized that each patient is unique and requires individual decision-making. The above outline should serve

Table 317-6   Major Toxic Side Effects of Drugs Commonly Used in the Treatment of Systemic Vasculitis

GLUCOCORTICOIDS

Osteoporosis	Growth suppression in children
Cataracts	Hypertension
Glaucoma	Avascular necrosis of bone
Diabetes mellitus	Myopathy
Electrolyte abnormalities	Alterations in mood
Metabolic abnormalities	Psychosis
Suppression of inflammatory and immune responses leading to opportunistic infections	Pseudotumor cerebri
	Peptic ulcer diathesis
	Pancreatitis
Cushingoid features	

CYCLOPHOSPHAMIDE

Bone marrow suppression	Hypogammaglobulinemia
Cystitis	Pulmonary fibrosis
Bladder carcinoma	Myelodysplasia
Gonadal suppression	Oncogenesis
Gastrointestinal intolerance	

METHOTREXATE

Gastrointestinal intolerance	Pneumonitis
Stomatitis	Teratogenicity
Neutropenia	Opportunistic infections
Hepatotoxicity (may lead to fibrosis or cirrhosis)	

as a framework to guide therapeutic approaches; however, flexibility should be practiced in order to provide maximal therapeutic efficacy with minimal toxic side effects in each patient.

BIBLIOGRAPHY

FAUCI AS et al: Wegener's granulomatosis: Prospective clinical and therapeutic experience with 85 patients for 21 years. Ann Intern Med 98:76, 1983

GUILLEVIN L et al: Treatment of polyarteritis nodosa related to hepatitis B virus with interferon-alpha and plasma exchanges. Ann Rheum Dis 53:334, 1994

—— et al: Microscopic polyangiitis. Clinical and laboratory findings in eighty-five patients. Arthritis Rheum 42:421, 1999

HOFFMAN GS, SPECKS U: Antineutrophil cytoplasmic antibodies. Arthritis Rheum 41:1521, 1998

—— et al: Wegener's granulomatosis: An analysis of 158 patients. Ann Intern Med 116:488, 1992

HUNDER GG: Giant cell arteritis and polymyalgia rheumatica. Med Clin North Am 81:195, 1997

JENNETTE JC et al: Nomenclature of systemic vasculitis. Proposal of an international consensus conference. Arthritis Rheum 37:187, 1994

KERR G et al: Takayasu arteritis. Ann Intern Med 120:919, 1994

LANGFORD CA et al: Use of cytotoxic agents and cyclosporine in the treatment of autoimmune disease. Part 2: Inflammatory bowel disease, systemic vasculitis, and therapeutic toxicity. Ann Intern Med 129:49, 1998

LEUNG DYM et al: The immunopathogenesis and management of Kawasaki syndrome. Arthritis Rheum 41:1538, 1998

LUDVIKSSON BR et al: Active Wegener's granulomatosis is associated with HLA-DR+ CD4+ T cells exhibiting an unbalanced Th-1 type T cell cytokine pattern: Reversal with IL-10. J Immunol 160:3602, 1998

SNELLER MC, FAUCI AS: Pathogenesis of vasculitis syndromes. Adv Rheumatol 81:221, 1997

—— et al: An analysis of forty-two Wegener's granulomatosis patients treated with methotrexate and prednisone. Arthritis Rheum 38:608, 1995

SOMER T, FINEGOLD SM: Vasculitis associated with infections, immunization, and antimicrobial drugs. Clin Infect Dis 20:1010, 1995

TALAR-WILLIAMS C et al: Cyclophosphamide-induced cystitis and bladder cancer in patients with Wegener's granulomatosis. Ann Intern Med 124:477, 1996

WEYLAND CM et al: Distinct vascular lesions in giant cell arteritis share identical T cell clonotypes. J Exp Med 179:951, 1994

—— et al: Tissue cytokine patterns in patients with polymyalgia rheumatica and giant cell arteritis. Ann Intern Med 121:484, 1994

SARCOIDOSIS

DEFINITION Sarcoidosis is a chronic, multisystem disorder of unknown cause characterized in affected organs by an accumulation of T lymphocytes and mononuclear phagocytes, noncaseating epithelioid granulomas, and derangements of the normal tissue architecture. Although there are usually skin anergy and depressed cellular immune processes in the blood, sarcoidosis is characterized at the sites of disease by exaggerated T helper 1 (T_H1) lymphocyte immune processes. All parts of the body can be affected, but the organ most frequently affected is the lung. Involvement of the skin, eye, liver, and lymph nodes is also common. The disease is often acute or subacute and self-limiting, but in many individuals it is chronic, waxing and waning over many years.

ETIOLOGY The cause of sarcoidosis is unknown. Various infectious and noninfectious agents have been implicated, but there is no proof that any specific agent is responsible. However, all available evidence is consistent with the concept that the disease results from an exaggerated cellular immune response (acquired, inherited, or both) to a limited class of persistent antigens or self-antigens.

INCIDENCE AND PREVALENCE Sarcoidosis is a relatively common disease affecting individuals of both sexes and almost all ages, races, and geographic locations. Females appear to be slightly more susceptible than males. Cases of sarcoidosis have been described in all of the major races, and the disease is found throughout the world. It has been suggested that sarcoidosis is more common in certain geographic areas such as the southeastern part of the United States, but when case-matched controls have been used, these geographic differences are less convincing. There is a remarkable diversity of the prevalence of sarcoidosis among certain ethnic and racial groups, with a range of <1 to 64 per 100,000 worldwide. The prevalence of sarcoidosis is from 10 to 40 per 100,000 in the United States and Europe. In the United States, most patients are black, with a ratio of blacks to whites ranging from 10:1 to 17:1. In Europe, however, the disease affects mostly whites. Furthermore, while the prevalence per 100,000 in Sweden is 64, in France it is 10, in Poland 3, yet for Irish females living in London it is 200. In contrast, the disease is very rare among Inuit, Canadian Indians, New Zealand Maoris, and Southeast Asians.

Most patients present with sarcoidosis between the ages of 20 and 40, but the disease can occur in children and in the elderly. Several hundred kindred groups with familial sarcoidosis have been described, and the disease has been observed in twins, more commonly in monozygotic than in dizygotic pairs. There also have been several instances of husband-wife pairs identified, and geographic foci of sarcoidosis among unrelated individuals living closely within a community, arguing for some environmental factors in the pathogenesis of the disease. Although the disease is believed to result from exaggerated cellular immune responses to a limited class of antigens, no clear patterns in any HLA locus have emerged. Unlike many diseases in which the lung is involved, sarcoidosis favors nonsmokers.

PATHOPHYSIOLOGY AND IMMUNOPATHOGENESIS The first manifestation of the disease is an accumulation of mononuclear inflammatory cells, mostly CD4+ T_H1 lymphocytes and mononuclear phagocytes, in affected organs. This inflammatory process is followed by the formation of granulomas, aggregates of macrophages and their progeny, epithelioid cells, and multinucleated giant cells. The typical sarcoid granuloma is a compact structure composed of an aggregate of mononuclear phagocytes surrounded by a rim of CD4+ T lymphocytes and, to a far lesser extent, B lymphocytes. The overall structure is relatively discrete and is interspersed with fine collagen fibrils, presumably remnants of the underlying connective tissue matrix. The giant cells within the granuloma can be of the Langhans' or foreign-body variety and often contain inclusions such as Schaumann bodies (conchlike structures), asteroid bodies (stellate-like structures), and residual bodies (refractile calcium-containing inclusions).

Together the accumulated T cells, mononuclear phagocytes, and granulomas represent the active disease. Other than the fact that they take up space and thus their bulk modifies the local architecture, for all except late stage cases, there is no evidence that the mononuclear inflammatory cells dispersed in the tissue or in the granuloma injure the affected organ by releasing mediators that damage the normal parenchymal cells or the extracellular matrix. Rather, organ dysfunction in sarcoidosis results mostly from the accumulated inflammatory cells distorting the architecture of the affected tissue; if a sufficient number of structures vital to the function of the tissue are involved, the disease becomes clinically apparent in that organ. Thus, while autopsy series show that, to some extent, sarcoidosis involves most organs in the majority of patients, the disease manifests clinically only in organs where it affects function (such as the lung and eye) or in organs where it is readily observed (such as the skin or, by x-ray, the hilar nodes). For example, in the lung, the inflammatory cells and granulomas distort the walls of the alveoli, bronchi, and blood vessels (Fig. 318-1*A*), thus altering the intimate relationships between air and blood necessary for normal gas exchange. When a sufficient amount of pulmonary tissue is involved, it is sensed by the individual as dyspnea. In contrast, most individuals with sarcoidosis have granulomatous mononuclear cell inflammation in the liver but usually do not have symptoms or significant functional derangements referable to that organ, likely because the disease process does not modify the local structures sufficiently to affect function.

If the disease is suppressed, either spontaneously or with therapy, the mononuclear inflammation is reduced in intensity and the number of granulomas is reduced. The granulomas resolve either by dispersion of the cells or by centripetal proliferation of fibroblasts from the periphery of the granuloma inward, to form a small scar. In chronic cases, the mononuclear cell inflammation persists for years. If the intensity of the inflammation is sufficiently high for a sufficiently long period, the derangements to the affected tissues result in extensive damage, the development of fibrosis, and permanent loss of organ function.

All available evidence suggests that active sarcoidosis results from an exaggerated cellular immune response to a variety of antigens or self-antigens, in which the process of T lymphocyte triggering, proliferation, and activation is skewed in the direction of CD4+ T_H1 lymphocyte processes (Fig. 318-1*B*). The result is an exaggerated T_H1 T lymphocyte response and thus the accumulation of large numbers of activated T_H1 cells in the affected organs. Since the activated T_H1 lymphocyte releases mediators that attract and activate mononuclear phagocytes, it is likely that the process of granuloma formation is a secondary phenomenon that is a consequence of the exaggerated T_H1 cell process. In this context, the current hypotheses of the cause of sarcoidosis, not mutually exclusive, include the following: (1) The disease is caused by a class of persistent antigens, nonself or self, that trigger only the T_H1 cell arm of the immune response; (2) the disease results from an inadequate suppressor arm of the immune response, such that T_H1 cell processes cannot be shut down in a normal fashion; or (3) the disease results from inherited (and/or acquired) differences in immune response genes, such that the response to a variety of antigens is an exaggerated, T_H1 cell process.

Independent of the inciting agent(s) or the reason why there is an exaggerated T_H1 cell response, there is a general understanding of the processes responsible for the maintenance of the inflammation and the development of the granuloma. The T_H1 lymphocytes accumulate at the sites of disease, at least in part, because they proliferate in these sites at an exaggerated rate. This T cell proliferation is maintained by the spontaneous release of interleukin (IL) 2, the T cell growth factor, by activated T_H1 cells in the local milieu. In this regard, sarcoidosis is a remarkable example of compartmentalization of the immune system and a dramatic illustration of why disease activity of sarcoidosis cannot be assessed by evaluating the immune system only in the blood.

Whereas the T_H1 cells in the involved organs are releasing IL-2 and proliferating at an enhanced rate, the T cells in other sites, such as blood, are quiescent. Furthermore, while there is a marked enhancement of the number of T_H1 cells at the sites of disease, the numbers of T_H1 cells in the blood are normal or slightly reduced. In the involved organs, the ratio of CD4+ to CD8+ T cells may be as high as 10:1 compared to the ratio of 2:1 found in normal tissues or in the blood of affected individuals.

In addition to driving other T_H1 cells in the affected organs to proliferate, the T_H1 cells at the sites of disease are activated and release mediators that both recruit and activate mononuclear phagocytes. The activated T_H1 cells accomplish this by releasing a variety of mediators (lymphokines) including proteins capable of recruiting blood monocytes to the local milieu of the activated T cells and interferon γ, a protein that, among its many actions, activates mononuclear phagocytes. Together with cytokines such as interleukin (IL)-12 and others released locally, these mediators recruit blood monocytes to the affected organs and activate them, providing the building blocks for the formation of the granuloma.

In addition to these exaggerated cellular immune processes, active sarcoidosis is also characterized by hyperglobulinemia. Included among the immunoglobulins are antibodies against a variety of infectious agents as well as IgM anti-T cell antibodies. However, there is no evidence that any of these antibodies plays a role in the pathogenesis of the disease, and they are thought to result from the nonspecific polyclonal stimulation of B cells by the activated T cells at the site of disease.

If the damage in the affected organs is sufficiently extensive that the remaining parenchymal cells cannot reestablish the normal tissue architecture, the usual result is fibrosis, the proliferation of mesenchymal cells, and deposition of their connective tissue products. There is convincing evidence that the fibroblast proliferation is directed by tissue macrophages spontaneously releasing growth signals for fibroblasts, including platelet-derived growth factor, fibronectin, and insulin-like growth factor 1. It is not known, however, why this fibrotic process occurs only in a relatively small proportion of individuals with sarcoidosis.

CLINICAL MANIFESTATIONS   Sarcoidosis is a systemic disease, and thus the clinical manifestations may be generalized or focused on one or more organs. However, because the lung is almost always involved, most patients have symptoms referable to the respiratory system. Independent of the site, the clinical manifestations of the disease relate directly to the exaggerated T_H1 lymphocyte–mononuclear phagocyte granulomatous inflammatory process itself or to the sequelae resulting from the permanent damage caused by this process.

Sarcoidosis is occasionally discovered in a completely asymptomatic individual, but more commonly it presents abruptly over 1 to 2 weeks or the affected individual develops symptoms insidiously over several months. Independent of the mode of presentation, ~75% of all cases present in individuals younger than 40 years.

The asymptomatic form is usually detected by a routine examination, such as a chest film. In the United States, this form represents about 10 to 20% of all cases, but in countries where chest films are mandatory in preemployment screening programs, the proportion of asymptomatic patients is higher.

So-called acute or subacute sarcoidosis develops abruptly over a period of a few weeks and represents 20 to 40% of all cases. These individuals usually have constitutional symptoms such as fever, fa-

FIGURE 318-1   Pathogenesis of sarcoidosis. *A.* Histologic abnormalities. Normal alveoli (*top*) and alveoli in active sarcoidosis (*bottom*). The latter are distorted by the accumulated CD4+ T_H1 lymphocytes, alveolar macrophages, and macrophages aggregated into granulomas. There is mild damage to alveolar epithelial and endothelial cells. *B.* The exaggerated processes of T_H1 lymphocytes in affected organs result in the accumulation of these cells along with macrophages and macrophages aggregated into granulomas. The trigger for the T_H1 lymphocytes is unknown. It may be a limited class of antigens or self-antigens presented in the context of class II HLA surface molecules by mono-

nuclear phagocytes to the T_H1 lymphocyte. The antigen class II HLA complex is identified by the T cell antigen receptor, and the T cell is activated. Consequent to this process the immune response is exaggerated and skewed to produce activated T_H1 lymphocytes that release IL-2, which drives the accumulation of more T lymphocytes. The activated T_H1 lymphocytes also release interferon γ (INF-γ). Together with cytokines such as IL-12, macrophage inflammatory protein 1α and granulocyte-macrophage colony stimulating factor released in the local milieu, there is recruitment and activation of blood monocytes and subsequent granuloma formation.

tigue, malaise, anorexia, or weight loss. These symptoms are usually mild, but in approximately 25% of the acute cases the constitutional complaints are extensive. Many patients have respiratory symptoms, including cough, dyspnea, a vague retrosternal chest discomfort and/or polyarthritis. Two syndromes have been identified in the acute group. Löfgren's syndrome, frequent in Scandinavian, Irish, and Puerto Rican females, includes the complex of erythema nodosum **(Plate IIE-70)** and x-ray findings of bilateral hilar adenopathy, often accompanied by joint symptoms, including arthritis at the ankles, knees, wrists, or elbows. The Heerfordt-Waldenström syndrome describes individuals with fever, parotid enlargement, anterior uveitis, and facial nerve palsy.

The insidious form of sarcoidosis develops over months and is associated usually with respiratory complaints without constitutional symptoms. In the United States, 40 to 70% of all patients with sarcoidosis patients are in this category. About 10% of these individuals have symptoms referable to organs other than the lung. It is the individuals who present with the insidious form of sarcoidosis who most commonly go on to develop chronic sarcoidosis, with permanent damage to the lung and other organs.

Despite the fact that sarcoidosis is a systemic disease and some evidence of inflammation can be detected in most organs in the ma-

jority of patients, sarcoidosis is important clinically because of the pulmonary abnormalities and, to a lesser extent, lymph node, skin, liver, and eye involvement. Far less commonly, other organs are involved significantly.

Lung Of individuals with sarcoidosis, 90% have abnormal findings on chest x-ray at some time during their course (Fig. 318-2A). Overall, ~50% develop permanent pulmonary abnormalities, and 5 to 15% have progressive fibrosis of the lung parenchyma. Sarcoidosis of the lung is primarily an interstitial lung disease (Chap. 259) in which the inflammatory process involves the alveoli, small bronchi, and small blood vessels. These individuals typically have symptoms of dyspnea, particularly with exercise, and a dry cough. In acute and subacute cases, physical examination usually reveals dry rales. Hemoptysis is rare, as is production of sputum. Occasionally, the large airways are involved to a degree sufficient to cause dysfunction. Distal atelectasis can result from endobronchial sarcoidosis or from external compression from enlarged intrathoracic nodes. Rarely, wheezing is heard, incorrectly suggesting asthma. Large-vessel pulmonary granulomatous arteritis is common, but it rarely causes major problems. If it dominates the pulmonary lesions, it is sometimes called *necrotizing sarcoidal granulomatosis*. The pleura is involved in 1 to 5% of cases, almost always manifesting as a unilateral pleural effusion with characteristics of an exudate containing lymphocytes. The effusions usually clear within a few weeks, but chronic pleural thickening can result. Pneumothorax is very rare.

Lymph Nodes Lymphadenopathy is very common in sarcoidosis. Intrathoracic nodes are enlarged in 75 to 90% of all patients; usually this involves the hilar nodes, but the paratracheal nodes are commonly involved (Fig. 318-2A). Less frequently, there is enlargement of subcarinal, anterior mediastinal, or posterior mediastinal nodes. Peripheral lymphadenopathy is very common, particularly involving the cervical, axillary, epitrochlear, and inguinal nodes. The nodes in the retroperitoneal area and in the mesenteric chain also can enlarge. All these nodes are nonadherent, with a firm, rubbery texture. Palpation causes no pain. Unlike nodes in tuberculosis, the nodes do not ulcerate. The lymphadenopathy rarely causes a problem for the affected individual; however, if it is massive, it can be disfiguring and can impinge on other organs and lead to functional impairment.

FIGURE 318-2 Common laboratory findings of sarcoidosis. *A.* Schematic view of the abnormal findings on the chest x-ray. Shown are changes observed with the average frequency of occurrence. *B.* Typical gallium-67 scan of an individual with active sarcoidosis. The isotope has accumulated in the lung parenchyma (LP), liver (L), spleen (S), parotid (P), hilar nodes (HN), and pelvic nodes (PN). *C.* Cells recovered by bronchoalveolar lavage of an individual with active pulmonary sarcoidosis. The lavage analysis reflects the inflammation in the tissue. Shown are alveolar macrophages (*large cells*) and lymphocytes (*small cells*). The cell population is dominated by the T_H1 subset of CD4+ lymphocytes, in contrast to normal individuals, in whom lymphocytes represent <20% of the cell population.

Skin Sarcoidosis involves the skin in ~25% of patients. The most common lesions are erythema nodosum **(Plate IIE-70)**, plaques, maculopapular eruptions, subcutaneous nodules, and lupus pernio. Erythema nodosum, comprising bilateral, tender red nodules on the anterior surface of the legs, is not specific for sarcoidosis but is common, particularly in acute sarcoidosis, in combination with systemic symptoms and polyarthralgias. Treatment is not required, since the lesions resolve spontaneously in 2 to 4 weeks. Erythema nodosum is much more common among patients with sarcoidosis in Europe than in the United States. Skin plaques associated with sarcoidosis are purple, indolent lesions, often raised, and usually occur on the face, buttocks, and extremities. The maculopapular eruptions occur on the face around the eyes and nose, on the back, and on the extremities. These are elevated lesions <1 cm in diameter with a flat, waxy top. Subcutaneous nodules are most common on the trunk and extremities. Lupus pernio is characterized by indurated blue-purple, swollen, shiny lesions on the nose, cheeks, lips, ears, fingers, and knees. The lesions on the tip of the nose cause a bulbous appearance, sometimes associated with varicosities. The nasal mucosa is usually involved, and underlying bone can be destroyed. Sarcoidosis also can involve old surgical scars and tattoos. Although it may be disfiguring, cutaneous sarcoidosis rarely causes major problems. Clubbing of the fingers is occasionally observed in sarcoidosis, usually in association with extensive pulmonary fibrosis.

Eye Eye involvement occurs in ~25% of patients with sarcoidosis, and it can cause blindness. The usual lesions involve the uveal tract, iris, ciliary body, and choroid. Of those patients with eye involvement, ~75% have anterior uveitis and 25 to 35% have posterior uveitis. There is blurred vision, tearing, and photophobia. The uveitis can develop rapidly and may clear spontaneously over a 6- to 12-month period. It also can develop insidiously and be chronic. Conjunctival involvement is also common, usually with small, yellow nodules. When the lacrimal gland is involved, a keratoconjunctivitis sicca syndrome, with dry, sore eyes, can result.

Upper Respiratory Tract The nasal mucosa is involved in up to 20% of patients, usually presenting with nasal stuffiness. Any of the structures of the mouth can be involved, particularly the tonsils. Sarcoidosis involves the larynx in ~5% of patients. The epiglottis and areas around the true vocal cords are usually involved, but the cords themselves are not. These individuals are usually hoarse, and they have dyspnea, wheezing, and stridor; complete obstruction can occur.

Bone Marrow and Spleen Sarcoidosis of the marrow is reported in 15 to 40% of patients, but it rarely causes hematologic abnormalities other than a mild anemia, neutropenia, eosinophilia, and occasionally, thrombocytopenia. Although splenomegaly occurs in only 5 to 10% of patients, celiac angiography or splenic biopsy reveals involvement in 50 to 60% of patients. The presentation and complications of splenomegaly in sarcoidosis are similar to those of splenomegaly in general.

Liver Although liver biopsy reveals liver involvement in 60 to 90% of patients, liver dysfunction is usually not important clinically. Sarcoidosis involves generally the periportal areas. Isolated granulomatous hepatitis can occur. Approximately 20 to 30% have hepatomegaly and/or biochemical evidence of liver involvement. Usually these changes reflect a cholestatic pattern and include an elevated alkaline phosphatase level; the bilirubin and aminotransferase levels are only mildly elevated, and jaundice is rare. Rarely, portal hypertension can develop, as can intrahepatic cholestasis with cirrhosis.

Kidney Clinically apparent primary renal involvement in sarcoidosis is rare, although tubular, glomerular, and renal artery diseases have been reported. More commonly, but still in only 1 to 2% of all patients, there is a disorder of calcium metabolism with hypercalciuria, with or without hypercalcemia. If chronic, nephrocalcinosis and nephrolithiasis can result. It is believed that the calcium abnormalities are associated with enhanced calcium absorption in the gut, which is related to an abnormally high level of circulating 1,25-dihydroxyvitamin D produced by mononuclear phagocytes in the granulomas.

Nervous System All components of the nervous system can be involved in sarcoidosis. Neurologic findings are observed in about 5% of patients. Seventh nerve involvement with unilateral facial paralysis is most common. It occurs suddenly and is usually transient. Other common manifestations of neurosarcoid include optic nerve dysfunction, papilledema, palate dysfunction, hearing abnormalities, hypothalamic and pituitary abnormalities, chronic meningitis, and, occasionally, space-occupying lesions. Psychiatric disturbances have been described, and seizures can occur. Rarely, multiple lesions occur that mimic multiple sclerosis, spinal cord abnormalities, and peripheral neuropathy.

Musculoskeletal System The bones, joints, and/or muscles can be involved in sarcoidosis. Bone lesions are observed in 5% of patients and include variable-sized cysts in areas of expanded bone; well-defined, round, punched-out lesions; or lattice-like changes. Hand and foot bones are the common sites, but most bones can be involved. Occasionally, the bone lesions are tender and painful. Joint involvement is more common, with an incidence of 25 to 50% in known cases of sarcoidosis. Arthralgias and frank arthritis occur mostly in large joints; they can be migratory and are usually transient, but they can be chronic and result in deformities. Although muscle biopsy frequently demonstrates granulomatous inflammation, muscle dysfunction is rare. However, nodules, polymyositis, and chronic myopathy have been described.

Heart Approximately 5% of patients have significant heart involvement, with clinical evidence of cardiac dysfunction. Left ventricular wall involvement is common. Arrhythmias are frequent, and serious conduction disturbances, including complete heart block, can occur. Papillary muscle dysfunction, pericarditis, and congestive heart failure are also observed. Cor pulmonale secondary to chronic pulmonary fibrosis may occur but is uncommon.

Endocrine and Reproductive System The hypothalamic-pituitary axis is the part of the endocrine system most commonly involved; this condition usually presents as diabetes insipidus. Anterior pituitary dysfunction is also seen, manifesting as a deficiency in one or more pituitary hormones. Complete hypopituitarism is rare. Much less frequently, sarcoidosis can cause primary dysfunction of other endocrine glands. Adrenal cortical involvement resulting in Addison's syndrome has been described. The reproductive organs may be involved, but infertility is rare. Pregnancy is not affected by sarcoidosis, and common with sarcoidosis who become pregnant usually improve during pregnancy. However, the disease may flare post partum; presumably this variation results from fluctuations in endogenous glucocorticoid production.

Exocrine Glands Parotid enlargement is a classic feature of sarcoidosis, but clinically apparent parotid involvement occurs in <10% of patients. Bilateral involvement is the rule. The gland is usually nontender, firm, and smooth. Xerostomia can occur; other exocrine glands are affected only rarely.

Gastrointestinal Tract Although sarcoidosis involvement of the gastrointestinal tract is found occasionally at autopsy, it rarely has clinical importance. Occasionally, patients have esophageal or gastric symptoms.

COMPLICATIONS The respiratory tract abnormalities cause most of the morbidity and mortality associated with sarcoidosis. The major problems are those characteristic of interstitial lung disease (Chap. 259), particularly dyspnea and insufficient oxygen delivery to vital organs. Respiratory failure with carbon dioxide retention is rare. In some patients, lung destruction results in formation of bullae that may harbor mycetomas, which are usually aspergillomas; erosion into the parenchyma can result in massive bleeding. The most common complications apart from the lung are associated with the eye; however, with therapy, blindness is rare. Complications of other organs include a gamut of abnormalities. The most serious are central nervous system (CNS) lesions or cardiac involvement leading to congestive heart failure or sudden death.

LABORATORY ABNORMALITIES Common abnormalities in the blood include lymphocytopenia, an occasional mild eosinophilia, an increased erythrocyte sedimentation rate, hyperglobulinemia, and an elevated level of angiotensin-converting enzyme (ACE). False-positive tests for rheumatoid factor or antinuclear antibodies can be observed. Hypercalcemia is rare. Other serum abnormalities relate to involvement of specific organs such as liver, kidney, or endocrine glands.

Because the lung is involved so commonly, the routine chest film is almost always abnormal (Fig. 318-2A). The three classic x-ray patterns of pulmonary sarcoidosis are type I—bilateral hilar adenopathy with no parenchymal abnormalities; type II—bilateral hilar adenopathy with diffuse parenchymal changes; and type III—diffuse parenchymal changes without hilar adenopathy. The type III pattern is sometimes split into two categories, with films that show fibrosis and upper lobe retraction classified separately. Although patients with type I x-ray patterns tend to have the acute or subacute, reversible form of the disease while those with types II and III often have the chronic, progressive disease, these patterns do not represent consecutive "stages" of sarcoidosis. Thus, except for epidemiologic purposes, this x-ray categorization is mostly of historic interest. The hilar adenopathy is almost always bilateral, but unilateral node enlargement can be seen. Nodes are also common in the paratracheal region. The diffuse parenchymal changes are typically reticulonodular infiltrates, but an acinar pattern is observed occasionally. Large nodules, similar to those of metastatic disease, are unusual but can occur. When there is massive fibrosis, the hila are pulled upward and there are conglomerate masses in the midlung zones. Some of the unusual chest x-ray findings in sarcoidosis include "egg shell" calcification of hilar nodes, pleural effusions, cavitation, atelectasis, pulmonary hypertension, pneumothorax, and cardiomegaly. Computed tomography of the chest is rarely helpful for either diagnosis or prognosis but can identify early fibrosis, and a "ground-glass" appearance is thought to be consistent with an active alveolitis.

The lung function abnormalities of sarcoidosis are typical for interstitial lung disease (Chap. 259) and include decreased lung volumes and diffusing capacity with a normal or supernormal ratio of the forced expiratory volume in 1 s to the forced vital capacity. Occasionally there is evidence of airflow limitation. There is usually mild hypoxemia and a mild, compensated hypocarbia.

The gallium-67 lung scan is usually abnormal, showing a pattern of diffuse uptake. If present, enlarged nodes are detected in these scans, as is inflammation in a variety of extrathoracic sites that usually have no clinical importance (Fig. 318-2B). Bronchoalveolar lavage typically demonstrates an increased proportion of lymphocytes, most of which are members of the activated T_H1 subset of CD4+ T lymphocytes (Fig. 318-2C). The remaining cells are mostly alveolar macrophages. In patients with significant fibrosis, a few neutrophils are also found. Eosinophils are rare.

The other laboratory features of sarcoidosis depend on the specific organ involved.

DIAGNOSIS For a typical case, the diagnosis of sarcoidosis is made by a combination of clinical, radiographic, and histologic findings (Fig. 318-3A). In a young adult with constitutional complaints, respiratory symptoms, erythema nodosum, blurred vision, and bilateral hilar adenopathy, the diagnosis is almost always sarcoidosis. Commonly, however, the findings are more subtle. Furthermore, because sarcoidosis can occur in almost any place in the body, like tuberculosis or syphilis, it can be confused with many other disorders. In this context, the differential diagnosis of sarcoidosis must cover a wide range. However, it is confused most commonly with neoplastic diseases such as lymphoma or with disorders characterized also by a mononuclear

FIGURE 318-3 Diagnostic and therapeutic algorithms relevant to sarcoidosis. *A.* Diagnosis of sarcoidosis. If the history and physical examination suggest sarcoidosis, the diagnosis is made by a combination of history, physical examination, and diagnostic test. No tests are definitive for sarcoidosis; the diagnosis is made by a combination of findings. The major diagnostic tests carry the most weight, with biopsy and histologic assessment of the relevant organ the most important. Assessment of function of the organ systems that appear to be affected help with diagnosis and decisions about therapy. *B.* Therapy of sarcoidosis. Once the definitive diagnosis is made, the decision to not treat or to institute treatment with glucocorticoids is based on the presence or absence of disabling symptoms, organ dysfunction, organ derangement, and results of various tests of disease activity. Any organ can be threatened by sarcoidosis, but lung, eye, heart, liver, and central nervous system are at greatest risk. The disease can wax and wane, and periodic assessments at 3- to 6-month intervals are used to reevaluate decisions regarding therapy.

cell granulomatous inflammatory process, such as the mycobacterial and fungal disorders.

The presence of skin anergy is typical but not diagnostic of sarcoidosis. Individuals with sarcoidosis who develop active tuberculosis react strongly to skin tests with purified protein derivative. The Kveim-Siltzbach skin test, the intradermal injection of a heat-treated suspension of a sarcoidosis spleen extract which is biopsied 4 to 6 weeks later, yields sarcoidosis-like lesions in 70 to 80% of individuals with sarcoidosis, with <5% false-positive results. However, the material is not widely available, and with the use of the transbronchial biopsy to obtain lung parenchyma for diagnostic purposes, the Kveim-Siltzbach test is not in general use.

No blood findings are diagnostic of the disease. Serum levels of ACE are elevated in approximately two-thirds of patients with sarcoidosis. Approximately 5% of all positive tests are not sarcoidosis and are seen in a variety of disorders, including asbestosis, silicosis, berylliosis, fungal infection, granulomatous hepatitis, hypersensitivity pneumonitis, leprosy, lymphoma, and tuberculosis. Hypercalcemia or an elevated 24-h urine calcium level is consistent with the diagnosis but is not specific.

The chest x-ray cannot be used as the sole criterion for the diagnosis of sarcoidosis. While the finding of bilateral hilar adenopathy is the hallmark of this disease, a similar pattern is occasionally observed in lymphoma, tuberculosis, coccidioidomycosis, brucellosis, and bronchogenic carcinoma.

The pattern of the gallium-67 scan is not diagnostic for sarcoidosis, nor is the finding of an increased proportion of lymphocytes among the cells recovered by bronchoalveolar lavage. However, the typical patterns of these tests (Fig. 318-2*B* and *C*) put the diagnosis in the general category of granulomatous lung disorders.

Whether or not the presentation is "classic," biopsy evidence of a mononuclear cell granulomatous inflammatory process is mandatory to make a definitive diagnosis of sarcoidosis. Because the lung is involved so frequently, it is the most common site to be biopsied, usually through a fiberoptic bronchoscope. Less common, but acceptable, sites for biopsy are the hilar nodes (by mediastinoscopy), the skin, conjunctiva, or lip. Rarely, the spleen, intraabdominal nodes, muscle, parotid or other salivary glands, upper respiratory tract, or the heart is biopsied for diagnostic purposes. At any of these sites, the findings must include the typical noncaseating granulomas. However, although histologic evidence is mandatory for a definitive diagnosis of sarcoidosis, the histologic findings are not sufficiently specific to make the diagnosis by themselves, since noncaseating granulomas are found in a number of other diseases, including infections and malignancy. Furthermore, although the liver or scalene nodes often reveal "positive" biopsies in cases of sarcoidosis, noncaseating granulomas from other causes are so frequent in these sites that they are not considered acceptable sites for establishing the diagnosis. Thus the definitive diagnosis of sarcoidosis is based on the biopsy in the context of the history, physical examination, blood tests, x-ray, lung function, and, if available, gallium-67 scan and bronchoalveolar lavage. Patients with HIV infection commonly have lymphocytopenia, chest x-ray abnormalities, positive gallium-67 chest scans, and increased proportions of lavage lymphocytes (early in the course of the disease), and they can have lung granulomas; thus, serologic testing for HIV infection should always be done in individuals suspected of having sarcoidosis.

PROGNOSIS   Overall, the prognosis in sarcoidosis is good. Most individuals who present with the acute disease are left with no significant sequelae. Approximately half of all patients have some permanent organ dysfunction, but for most this is mild, stable, and progresses rarely. In ~15 to 20% of patients, the disease remains active or recurs intermittently. Death is attributable directly to the disease in ~10% of all those affected.

℞ **TREATMENT**   The therapy of choice for sarcoidosis is glucocorticoids (Fig. 318-3*B*), Various other drugs have been tried, including indomethacin, oxyphenbutazone, chloroquine, hydroxychloroquine, methotrexate, *p*-aminobenzoate, allopurinol, levamisole, azothioprine, and cyclophosphamide; but there is no evidence, apart from anecdotal, uncontrolled reports, to support their efficacy. Cyclosporine is ineffective for the pulmonary manifestations of the disease; anecdotal reports suggest that it may be useful in extrathoracic sarcoid not responding to glucocorticoids.

The major problem in treating sarcoidosis is in deciding when to treat. Because the disease clears spontaneously in ~50% of patients, and because the permanent organ derangements often do not improve with glucocorticoid treatment, there is controversy among clinicians as to the criteria for treatment. However, there is no question that glucocorticoids suppress effectively the activated T_H1 lymphocyte processes occurring at the sites of disease. Thus, the major problem in making decisions concerning therapy in sarcoidosis is to determine the extent and activity of the inflammatory process in the organs at greatest risk, such as the lung, eye, heart, and CNS.

For the lung, this is based on a combination of history, physical findings, chest x-ray, and pulmonary function tests. Centers that see large numbers of these individuals sometimes use criteria based on gallium-67 lung scans and bronchoalveolar lavage findings. The serum

level of ACE has been suggested as a criterion for disease activity, but it is not specific for the lung. Unless the respiratory impairment is devastating, active pulmonary sarcoidosis is observed usually without therapy for 2 to 3 months; if the inflammation does not subside spontaneously, therapy is instituted. For the eye, decisions concerning therapy are based on slit-lamp examination and tests for visual acuity. For the heart and CNS, decisions are based on an estimate of the severity of the involvement; patients with minor dysfunction are usually observed, while patients with significant cardiac or neurologic abnormalities are treated. Usually, it is not necessary to treat the systemic symptoms, but occasionally the extent of the fevers, fatigue, and/or weight loss necessitate therapy.

The usual therapy for sarcoidosis is prednisone, 1 mg/kg, for 4 to 6 weeks, followed by a slow taper over 2 to 3 months. This regimen is repeated if the disease again becomes active. Alternate-day therapy is used by some clinicians, but there is no evidence that it is as effective. High-dose bolus intravenous glucocorticoids are used occasionally but are probably not as effective as oral therapy. There is no evidence that inhaled glucocorticoids are efficacious. Mild ocular disease responds usually to local therapy, but suppression of the uveitis often requires systemic glucocorticoids.

BIBLIOGRAPHY

BAUGHMAN RP, LOWER EE: Alternatives to corticosteroids in the treatment of sarcoidosis. Sarcoidosis Vasc Diffuse Lung Dis 14:121, 1997

CONSENSUS CONFERENCE: Activity of sarcoidosis. Third WASOG Meeting. Eur Respir J 7:624, 1994

CRYSTAL RG: Interstitial lung disease of unknown etiology: Disorders characterized by chronic inflammation of the lower respiratory tract. N Engl J Med 310:154, 235, 1984

DU BOIS RM: Corticosteroids in sarcoidosis: Friend or foe? Eur Respir J 7:1203, 1994

DU BOIS RM: Granulomatous processes, in *The Lung: Scientific Foundations*, 2d ed, RG Crystal et al (eds). Philadelphia, Lippincott-Raven, 1996, pp 2395–2409

FANBURG BL, PITT EA: Sarcoidosis, in *Textbook of Respiratory Medicine*, JF Murray, JA Nadel (eds). Philadelphia, Saunders, 1988, pp 1486–1500

JAMES DG (ed): *Sarcoidosis and Other Granulomatous Disorders*, New York, Marcel Dekker, 1994

JOHNS CJ, MICHELE TM: The clinical management of sarcoidosis. A 50-year experience at the Johns Hopkins Hospital. Medicine 78:65, 1999

JUDSON MA et al: Defining organ involvement in sarcoidosis: The ACCESS proposed instrument. Sarcoidosis Vasc Diffuse Lung Dis 16:75, 1999

MOLLER DR: T-cell receptor genes in sarcoidosis. Sarcoidosis Vasc Diffuse Lung Dis 15: 158, 1998

———: Cells and cytokines involved in the pathogenesis of sarcoidosis. Sarcoidosis Vasc Diffuse Lung Dis 16:24, 1999

NAGAI S, IZUMI T: Pulmonary sarcoidosis: Population differences and pathophysiology. South Med J 88:1001, 1995

PINKSTON P et al: Spontaneous release of interleukin-2 by lung T-lymphocytes in active pulmonary sarcoidosis. N Engl J Med 208:793, 1983

ROBINSON BWS et al: Gamma interferon is spontaneously released by alveolar macrophages and lung T-lymphocytes in patients with pulmonary sarcoidosis. J Clin Invest 75:1488, 1985

ROBINSON DS et al: Granulomatous processes, in *The Lung: Scientific Foundations*, 2d ed, RG Crystal et al (eds). Philadelphia, Lippincott-Raven, 1996, pp 2395–2410

SHARMA OP: Pulmonary sarcoidosis and corticosteroids. Am Rev Resp Dis 147:1598, 1993

| 319 | *Jean D. Sipe, Alan S. Cohen* |

AMYLOIDOSIS

AD	Alzheimer's disease	IDOX	iododoxorubicin
AβPP	amyloid β-precursor protein	IL	interleukin
FAP	familial amyloid polyneuropathies	SAP	serum amyloid P
FHF	familial Hibernian fever	TNF	tumor necrosis factor
FMF	familial Mediterranean fever	TTR	transthyretin

DEFINITION AND CLASSIFICATION   *Amyloidosis* results from the deposition of insoluble, fibrous amyloid proteins, mainly in the extracellular spaces of organs and tissues. Named by Virchow in 1854 on the basis of color after staining with iodine and sulfuric acid, all amyloid fibrils share an identical secondary structure, the β-pleated sheet conformation, and a unique ultrastructure. All amyloid deposits contain an identical nonfibrillar component, the pentraxin serum amyloid P (SAP), and are associated with glycosaminoglycans. Abnormal protein folding and assembly can also result in protein deposition (e.g., in brain or kidney) that lacks the classic fibrillar morphology of amyloid and the presence of SAP. Depending upon the biochemical nature of the amyloid precursor protein, amyloid fibrils can be deposited locally or may involve virtually every organ system of the body. Amyloid fibril deposition may have no apparent clinical consequences or may lead to severe pathophysiologic changes. Often the disease falls between these two extremes. Regardless of etiology, the clinical diagnosis of amyloidosis is usually not made until the disease is far advanced.

Although the fibril precursors differ in their amino acid sequences, the polypeptide backbones of these protein precursors assume similar fibrillar morphologies that render them resistant to proteolysis.

Table 319-1   Amyloid Fibril Proteins and Their Precursors in Humans

Amyloid Protein	Precursor	Systemic (S) or Localized (L)	Syndrome or Involved Tissues
AL	Immunoglobulin light chain	S, L	Primary
			Myeloma-associated
AH	Immunoglobulin heavy chain	S, L	Primary
			Myeloma-associated
ATTR	Transthyretin	S	Familial (prototype Portuguese, Japanese, Swedish)
			Senile systemic
		L?	Tenosynovium
AA	(Apo)serum AA	S	Secondary, reactive
Aβ_2M	β_2-microglobulin	S	Chronic hemodialysis
		L?	Joints
AApoAI	Apolipoprotein AI	S	Familial
		L	Aortic
AGel	Gelsolin	S	Familial (prototype Finnish)
ALys	Lysozyme	S	Familial
AFib	Fibrinogen α-chain	S	Familial
ACys	Cystatin C	S	Familial (protype Icelandic)
Aβ	Aβ protein precursor (AβPP)	L	Alzheimer's disease, aging
			Familial (prototype Dutch)
APrP^{sc}	Prion protein	L	Spongiform encephalopathies
ACal	(Pro)calcitonin	L	C cell thyroid tumors
AIAPP	Islet amyloid polypeptide	L	Islets of Langerhans
			Insulinomas
AANF	Atrial natriuretic factor	L	Cardiac atria
APro	Prolactin	L	Aging pituitary
			Prolactinomas
AIns	Insulin	L	Iatrogenic
ALac^a	Lactoferrin	L	Cornea

^{a} Preliminary, awaiting for confirmation.
SOURCE: From P Westermark et al: Amyloid Int J Exp Clin Invest 6:63, 1999, reprinted with permission.

The amyloidoses are classified according to the biochemical nature of the fibril-forming protein (Table 319-1). *Systemic amyloidoses* include biochemically distinct forms that are neoplastic, inflammatory, genetic, or iatrogenic in origin, while *localized* or *organ-limited amyloidoses* are associated with aging and diabetes and occur in isolated organs, often endocrine, without evidence of systemic involvement.

Despite their biochemical and clinical differences, the various amyloidoses share common pathophysiologic features: (1) an amyloidogenic precursor in appropriate concentration; (2) appropriate host genetic background; (3) abnormalities in proteolysis of fibril precursors and nascent amyloid fibrils; and (4) alterations in extracellular matrix constituents such as glycosaminoglycans, including the presence of amyloid-enhancing factor and Apo E. The guidelines for nomenclature and classification of amyloid and amyloidosis were updated in 1998 by the Nomenclature Committee of the International Society for Amyloidosis (Table 319-1). Amyloid deposits should be classified using the capital letter A as the first letter of designation followed by the protein designation without any open space; for example, AL for amyloidosis involving immunoglobulin light chains.

ETIOLOGY AND PATHOGENESIS   Light Chain Amyloidosis (AL) The most common form of systemic amyloidosis seen in current clinical practice is AL (primary idiopathic amyloidosis, or that associated with multiple myeloma) resulting from fibril formation by monoclonal antibody light chains in primary amyloidosis and in some cases of multiple myeloma (Chap. 113). Fewer than 20% of patients with AL have myeloma. The rest have other monoclonal gammopathies, light chain disease, or even agammaglobulinemia (producing light chains, but not intact immunoglobulin). About 15 to 20% of patients with myeloma have amyloidosis. A monoclonal population of bone marrow plasma cells is present and consistently produces either small lambda or kappa fragments or immunoglobulins that are processed (cleaved) in an abnormal fashion by macrophage enzymes to produce the partially degraded light chains responsible for AL amyloidosis. Lambda chain class predominates over kappa in AL by a 2:1 ratio, whereas in multiple myeloma and normal immunoglobulin synthesis, the reverse is true. Indeed, almost all lambda VI family chains have been associated with amyloid. The primary structure of each amyloid-forming light chain is unique, reflecting the features of the B cell clone that produced it. In patients with multiple myeloma, light chains can be deposited as casts in kidney tubules or as punctate deposits on basement membranes. Also, nonfibrillar deposition diseases have been described; thus there are three forms of human light chain–associated renal and systemic diseases: AL amyloidosis, cast nephropathy, and light chain deposition disease. Rarely, heavy chain amyloid deposition has been reported.

Amyloid A Amyloidosis (AA) AA amyloidosis (secondary, reactive, or acquired amyloidosis) occurs most frequently as a complication of chronic inflammatory disease. Effective treatment of the underlying inflammatory condition has reduced incidence in developed countries. In the past in the United States, tuberculosis (Chap. 169), osteomyelitis (Chap. 129), and leprosy (Chap. 170) were the most common precipitating diseases, and they remain so in developing countries. During inflammation, proinflammatory cytokines such as interleukin (IL) 1, IL-6, and tumor necrosis factor (TNF) stimulate the synthesis in liver of serum amyloid A, an injury-specific component of high-density lipoprotein. Thus, effective treatment of the underlying inflammatory disorder blocks the stimulus for precursor synthesis. Familial deposition of the AA protein occurs in some groups of patients with familial Mediterranean fever (FMF) and Familial Hibernian Fever (FHF) (Chap. 289). Colchicine treatment has been very effective both in blocking attacks of FMF and in reducing the incidence of AA amyloidosis in association with FMF. FMF is an autosomal recessive disorder subdivided into phenotype I, with irregularly occurring fever and abdominal, chest, or joint pain, preceding or accompanying renal amyloid; and phenotype II, in which renal amyloidosis is the first or only manifestation of the disease (Chap. 289). FMF is caused by mutations (16 identified to date) in the gene designated *MEFV* that encodes a 781-amino-acid protein named *pyrin* that appears to be a transcription factor. There is a strong correlation between the M694V mutation in MEFV and development of amyloidosis. FHF is an autosomal dominant disorder characterized by missense mutations in the TNF receptor.

Heredofamilial Amyloidoses   Heredofamilial amyloidoses other than the AA form associated with FMF and FHF primarily involve the nervous system, and their mode of inheritance is autosomal dominant. Familial amyloid polyneuropathies (FAP) are dominant hereditary diseases affecting kinships originating in Portugal, Japan, Sweden, Finland, Greece, Italy, and elsewhere. FAP can be subclassified based on clinical symptoms and the biochemical nature of the fibrils; in nearly all cases the fibrils are variants of transthyretin (TTR), apolipoprotein AI, gelsolin, cystatin C, and rarely the α chain of fibrinogen A or lysozyme. The mutant proteins, although present from birth, are associated with a delayed onset of disease symptoms, usually after three to seven decades of life. The FAP transthyretin prototype is the lower limb neuropathy first described in Portugal. It has a poor prognosis and is characterized by progressively severe neuropathy, including marked autonomic nervous system involvement. In some of these individuals, bilateral "scalloped" pupils are pathognomonic of the disease.

ATTR   The most frequently occurring form of FAP involves TTR, a 14-kDa protein originally described as prealbumin, that transports thyroxine and retinol-binding protein in the blood. The first mutation to be identified in Portuguese families and in families of Swedish origin was a single amino acid substitution, methionine for valine at position 30. To date, more than 60 TTR variants have been defined, several of which are nonamyloidogenic. Variant TTR gene carriers exhibit clinically heterogeneous amyloidoses according to the position and nature of the amino acid substitution. Substitution of proline for leucine at position 55 results in an early onset and rapidly progressing disease, whereas substitution of methionine for threonine at position 119 appears to protect against amyloid fibril formation. In Denmark, patients with a methionine substitution for leucine at position 111 have a severe cardiopathy. Nonpathogenic TTR mutants such as the substitution of serine for glycine at position 6 also exist, and several are associated with changes in association with retinol-binding protein.

AApoAI   Deposition of one of five apolipoprotein AI variants (G26R, W50R, L60R, L90P, and deletion of residues 61-7 with VT inserts) can be associated with peripheral neuropathy that is clinically similar to the type of familial amyloidosis that is caused by variants of TTR. In some kindreds, the clinical presentation is renal failure without neurologic symptoms.

AGel   A unique form of hereditary systemic amyloidosis has been reported primarily in Finland but also in patients of Japanese and Dutch backgrounds. Fibrils of gelsolin fragments, a calcium-binding protein that binds to and fragments actin filaments, are deposited in blood vessels and basement membranes, leading to clinical manifestations of lattice corneal dystrophy and cranial neuropathy, followed by peripheral neuropathy, dystrophic skin changes, and involvement of other organs. Two mutations at position 187, within the actin-binding domain of gelsolin, are associated with the disease.

ALys   Hereditary nonneuropathic systemic amyloidosis has been described in English families in which lysozyme is the major fibril protein. Two mutations have been described—I56T and D67H.

AFib   Hereditary nonneuropathic renal amyloidosis has been described in families with one of three mutations in the fibrinogen A α chains, R524L, E526V, or R554L.

Aβ_2M   In long-term hemodialysis, amyloidosis is now well recognized as a serious bone and joint complication. β_2-microglobulin is the major constituent of the amyloid fibrils, and formation of advanced glycation end products of β_2-microglobulin has been implicated in the pathogenesis of Aβ_2M.

Localized or Organ-Limited Amyloidoses   Depending upon the biochemical nature of the amyloid fibril protein, instead of systemic deposition involving the cardiovascular and gastrointestinal systems along with lymph nodes, spleen, liver, kidneys, and adrenals, amyloid deposition may be limited to a single organ such as the pan-creas, brain, or heart. Recently, lactoferrin has been found to occur as amyloid fibrils in a rare form of corneal amyloidosis, and amyloid fibrils of prolactin have been identified in the pituitary gland and in a prolactin-producing tumor.

Polypeptide hormone–derived amyloidosis   Amyloid deposits are common in polypeptide hormone–producing tissues and tumors. Calcitonin is deposited in the hereditary amyloid syndrome, medullary carcinoma of the thyroid (ACal) (Chap. 330). Also AANF (atrial natriuretic factor–derived) amyloid deposits are found in the sarcolemma of ~80% of persons over 80 years of age. AIAPP (islet amyloid polypeptide–derived, or amylin) is deposited as amyloid fibrils in 90% of individuals with type 2 diabetes (Chap. 333), in endocrine tumors (Chap. 93), and in insulinoma (Chap. 93). It is produced in β cells of the pancreas and stored and released together with insulin. Human insulin does not naturally form amyloid fibrils, although fibrils of porcine insulin, AIns, are sometimes found as subcutaneous nodules at sites of insulin injection in diabetic individuals.

Amyloidosis associated with Alzheimer's disease   A novel protein, β-amyloid protein (Aβ), is the major fibril protein in the amyloid deposits of the cerebrovascular walls and the cores of the neuritic plaques of Alzheimer's disease (AD) patients and also in individuals with Down's syndrome (Chap. 66). The intracellular neurofibrillary tangles are composed of paired helical filaments arranged in a twisted conformation and have as their major component an abnormally phosphorylated τ-protein, a microtubule-associated protein whose semantic relation to the Aβ of AD is arguable. Aβ varies in length from 39 to 43 amino acids and is derived from a large transmembrane glycoprotein called amyloid β-precursor protein (AβPP). Mutations in AβPP are associated with familial AD and also with a different type of amyloidosis, hereditary cerebral hemorrhage with amyloidosis (Dutch type). Other forms of familial AD are associated with mutations in genes that encode presenilin proteins.

Prion diseases   Prions are a unique class of infectious proteins associated with a group of neurodegenerative diseases, the transmissible spongiform encephalopathies. In humans, these diseases include kuru, Creutzfeldt-Jakob disease, Gerstmann-Straussler-Scheinker syndrome, and fatal familial insomnia (Chap. 373); in animals, scrapie and bovine spongiform encephalopathy (mad cow disease). PrP^{Sc} is a pathogenic, transmissible spongiform encephalopathy–specific form of the host-encoded prion protein (PrP); PrP^{Sc} differs from PrP in that it contains a high amount of β-pleated sheet structure and is insoluble and resistant to proteolytic enzymes. PrP^{Sc} deposits either consist of or can be readily converted to amyloid fibrils. APrP is similar to Aβ and ATTR in that both familial and sporadic forms occur. In addition, infectious prior diseases have resulted from the transmission of PrP^{Sc} by ritualistic cannibalism, corneal transplantation, treatment with cadaveric human growth hormone, and a variety of neurosurgical procedures. It has been suggested that the earlier onset familial forms of amyloidosis are due to accelerated fibril formation from mutant precursors, whereas in sporadic cases, amyloid fibrils are formed more slowly from normal precursor molecules. The mutant PrP molecules are nearer the threshold for transition to the amyloidogenic PrP^{Sc} than are the normal. The transition from normal to amyloidogenic PrP^{Sc} is irreversible but very slow. The disease progresses because, once formed, amyloidogenic PrP^{Sc} can seed the conversion of normal molecules into an amyloidogenic form.

CLINICAL MANIFESTATIONS   The clinical manifestations of amyloidosis are varied and depend entirely on the biochemical nature of the fibril protein and thus the area of the body that is involved (Table 319-2). The diagnosis of amyloidosis is usually not made until after the point of irreversible organ damage. Proteinuria is often the first symptom associated with systemic amyloidosis, particularly of the AA and AL type; peripheral neuropathies are associated with FAP, and dementia and cognitive dysfunction with amyloid deposits in brain. Organ enlargement, especially of the liver, kidney, spleen, and heart, may be prominent; however, this does not occur in FAP, AD, or PrP diseases.

Table 319-2   Clinical Presentation of Systemic Amyloidosis

Disease	Symptoms

AL (primary)	Monoclonal immunoglobulin in urine or serum plus any of the following:
	    Unexplained nephrotic syndrome
	    Hepatomegaly
	    Carpal tunnel syndrome
	    Macroglossia
	    Malabsorption or unexplained diarrhea or constipation
	    Peripheral neuropathy
	    Cardiomyopathy

AA (secondary)	Chronic infection (osteomyelitis, tuberculosis) or chronic inflammation (rheumatoid arthritis, granulomatous ileitis) plus development of any of the following:
	    Proteinuria
	    Hepatomegaly
	    Unexplained gastrointestinal disease

Hereditary amyloidosis	Family history of neuropathy plus any of the following:
	    Early sensorimotor disassociation
	    Vitreous opacities
	    Renal disease
	    Autonomic nervous system symptoms
	    Cardiovascular disease
	    Gastrointestinal disease

Kidney   Renal involvement may consist of mild proteinuria or frank nephrosis. In some cases, the urinary sediment may show a few red blood cells. The renal lesion is usually not reversible and in time leads to progressive azotemia and death. The prognosis does not appear to be related to the degree of the proteinuria; when azotemia finally develops, the prognosis is grave. Treatment by peritoneal or hemodialysis or kidney transplantation improves the prognosis considerably. Hypertension is rare, except in long-standing amyloidosis. Renal tubular acidosis or renal vein thrombosis may occur. Localized accumulation of amyloid may be noted in the ureter, bladder, or other parts of the genitourinary tract.

Heart   Cardiac amyloidosis can present as intractable heart failure. Electrocardiographic abnormalities include a low-voltage QRS complex and abnormalities in atrioventricular and intraventricular conduction, often resulting in varying degrees of heart block. Owing to their propensity to develop conduction defects and arrhythmias, patients with cardiac amyloidosis appear to be especially sensitive to digitalis, and this drug should be used with caution.

With respect to systemic amyloidoses, cardiac amyloidosis is common in primary (AL) and heredofamilial amyloidosis and very rare in the secondary (AA) form. With respect to localized amyloidosis, cardiac amyloidosis of the wild type or nonvariant TTR type is common after 80 years of age; also atrial natriuretic factor may be present in the atria. In systemic amyloidosis, cardiac manifestations consist primarily of congestive failure and cardiomegaly (with or without murmurs) and a variety of arrhythmias and are comparable in AL and FAP, the predominant forms with cardiomyopathy (Chap. 238). Although these manifestations predominantly reflect diffuse myocardial amyloid, the endocardium, valves, and pericardium may also be involved. Pericarditis with effusion is rare, although the differential diagnosis of constrictive pericarditis versus restrictive cardiomyopathy frequently arises. Echocardiography has demonstrated symmetric thickening of the left ventricular wall, hypokinesia and decreased systolic contraction and thickening of the interventricular septum and left ventricular posterior wall, and left ventricular cavities of small to normal size. Two-dimensional echocardiography produces the characteristic findings of thickened right and left ventricles, a normal left ventricular cavity, and, especially, a diffuse hyperrefractile "granular sparkling" appearance. Hearts that are heavily infiltrated with amyloid may or may not show an enlarged silhouette. Fluoroscopy usually shows decreased mobility of the ventricular wall; angiographic studies usually demonstrate thickened ventricular wall, decreased ventricular mobility, and absence of rapid ventricular filling in early diastole.

Liver   While hepatic involvement is common except in heredofamilial amyloidosis of the TTR type, liver function abnormalities are minimal and occur late in the disease. Portal hypertension occurs but is uncommon. Intrahepatic cholestasis has been noted in about 5% of patients with AL (primary) amyloidosis. Hepatomegaly is common, and AL hepatic amyloid is usually accompanied by the nephrotic syndrome and congestive heart failure with poor prognosis. Amyloidosis of the spleen characteristically is not associated with leukopenia and anemia.

Skin   Involvement of the skin is one of the most characteristic manifestations of primary (AL) amyloidosis (Chap. 57). Other forms of amyloidosis such as lichen amyloidosis are thought to involve forms of keratin. In AL amyloidosis, the usually nonpruritic lesions may consist of slightly raised, waxy papules or plaques that are usually clustered in the folds of the axillae, anal, or inguinal regions; the face and neck; or mucosal areas such as ear or tongue. Periorbital ecchymoses ("black eye" or "raccoon syndrome") have been reported.

Gastrointestinal Tract   Gastrointestinal symptoms are common in all systemic types of amyloidosis either from direct involvement of the gastrointestinal tract at any level or from infiltration of the autonomic nervous system with amyloid. Symptoms include obstruction, ulceration, malabsorption, hemorrhage, protein loss, and diarrhea (Chap. 286). Infiltration of the tongue is characteristic of primary amyloidosis (AL) or amyloidosis accompanying multiple myeloma and occasionally leads to macroglossia. When not enlarged, the tongue may become stiffened and firm to palpation. Gastrointestinal bleeding may occur from any of a number of sites, notably the esophagus, stomach, or large intestine, and may be severe. Amyloid infiltration of the esophagus may lead to an incompetent or nonrelaxing lower esophageal sphincter, nonspecific motility disorders of the esophageal body, or rarely achalasia. Small-bowel lesions may lead to clinical and x-ray changes of obstruction. A malabsorption syndrome is common. Amyloidosis (AA or secondary) may also develop in association with other entities involving the gastrointestinal tract, especially tuberculosis (Chap. 169), granulomatous enteritis (Chap. 287), lymphoma (Chap. 112), and Whipple's disease (Chap. 286); differentiation of these conditions, which give rise to secondary amyloidosis, from diffuse primary amyloidosis of the small bowel may be difficult. Similarly, amyloidosis of the stomach may closely mimic gastric carcinoma, with obstruction, achlorhydria, and the radiologic appearance of tumor masses.

Nervous System   Neurologic manifestations, especially prominent in the heredofamilial amyloidoses may include peripheral neuropathy, postural hypotension, inability to sweat, Adies's pupil, hoarseness, and sphincter incompetence. The cranial nerves are generally spared, except in the Finnish hereditary amyloidosis. Carpal tunnel syndrome may be caused by several amyloidoses, especially primary (AL) and chronic hemodialysis ($A\beta_2M$) amyloid. Peripheral neuropathy is frequent in the former type. $A\beta$ amyloid occurs in the central nervous system as a component of senile plaques and in blood vessels ("congophilic angiopathy"). The protein concentration in the cerebrospinal fluid may be increased. Infiltrates of the cornea or vitreous body may be present in hereditary amyloid syndromes. Certain of these syndromes (advanced FAP) are characterized by a bilateral scalloping appearance of the pupil.

Endocrine   Amyloid may infiltrate the thyroid or other endocrine glands but rarely causes endocrine dysfunction. Local amyloid deposits almost invariably accompany medullary carcinoma of the thyroid. Amyloid is often found in the adrenal gland, pituitary gland, and pancreas. Pancreatic islet amyloid as a complication of type 2 diabetes is especially prominent and is caused by the β cell peptide islet amyloid polypeptide. Little if any clinical dysfunction is present unless there is massive replacement of the gland by amyloid.

Joints and Muscles   Amyloid can directly, although rarely, involve articular structures by its presence in the synovial membrane and synovial fluid or in the articular cartilage. In these cases it is almost always of the AL type and associated with multiple myeloma. Amyloid arthritis can mimic a number of the rheumatic diseases because it can present as a symmetric arthritis of small joints with nodules, morning stiffness, and fatigue (Chap. 320). The synovial fluid usually has a low white blood cell count, a good to fair mucin clot, a predominance of mononuclear cells, and no crystals. Studies of surgical specimens suggest a significant incidence of amyloid in cartilage, capsule, and synovium in osteoarthritis (Chap. 321). Amyloid infiltration of muscle may lead to a pseudomyopathy. Shoulder muscle infiltration can produce the "shoulder pad" sign. Amyloid is found in muscle inclusion body disease, where $A\beta$ and/or PrP have been identified.

Deposition of β_2-microglobulin as amyloid fibrils in the musculoskeletal systems is a serious complication of long-term hemodialysis.

Table 319-3   Diagnosis of Amyloidosis

BIOPSY	APPROPRIATE STAIN
Common sites	Congo red, viewed by polarization microscopy
Subcutaneous abdominal fat	
aspirate	Thioflavin (less specific)
Rectum	Potassium permanganate pretreatment,
Skin	then Congo red stain
Gingiva	Other:
Occasional sites	Cotton dyes (comparable with Congo
Small intestine	red)
Muscle	Crystal violet (less sensitive)
Nerve	**PROTEIN OR DNA STUDIES**
Rare sites	
Kidney	Mutant protein identification
Liver	Immunocytochemistry: immunofluorescent or immunoperoxidase stains with
Bone marrow	specific antisera
Synovium	
Spleen	

$A\beta_2M$ presents as the carpal tunnel syndrome, cystic bone lesions, and even destructive spondyloarthropathy.

Respiratory System   The nasal sinuses, larynx, and trachea may be involved by accumulation of AL amyloid, which blocks the ducts, in the case of the sinuses, or the air passages. Amyloidosis of the lung involves the bronchi and alveolar septa diffusely. The lower respiratory tract is affected most frequently in primary (AL) amyloidosis and in the disease associated with dysproteinemia. Pulmonary symptoms attributable to amyloid are present in about 30% of cases. Amyloid may be localized in the bronchi or pulmonary parenchyma and may resemble a neoplasm. In these cases, local excision should be attempted and, when successful, may be followed by prolonged remissions.

Hematopoietic System   Hematologic changes may include fibrinogenopenia, increased fibrinolysis, and selective deficiency of clotting factors. Deficient factor X seems to be due to nonspecific calcium-dependent binding to the polyanionic amyloid fibrils. Splenectomy in the patient with such a factor X deficiency can relieve the deficiency and the associated bleeding disorder, since factor X has been shown to bind to the large masses of splenic amyloid. Endothelial damage together with the clotting abnormalities lead to a propensity toward abnormal bleeding.

DIAGNOSIS   Amyloid fibrils are identified in biopsy or necropsy tissue sections (Table 319-3). The systemic amyloidoses offer a choice of biopsy sites; abdominal fat aspirates or renal or rectal biopsies are often performed. Microscopically, amyloid deposits stain pink with the hematoxylin-eosin stain and show metachromasia with crystal violet. The widely used and useful Congo red stain imparts a unique green birefringence when stained tissue sections are viewed using the polarizing microscope (Fig. 319-1). Fluorescent dyes such as thioflavin are sensitive screening stains for amyloid deposits in brain and other tissues; however, specificity should be confirmed. After amyloid has been identified by staining, it can be chemically classified by genomic DNA and protein studies and by immunohistochemistry. In the case of FAP, the presence of mutant TTR (or gelsolin, Apo AI, etc.) establishes the specific diagnosis of the disease. Isoelectric focusing is used as a simple screening test for variant transthyretins associated with familial TTR amyloidosis. In order to establish the relationship of immunoglobulin-related amyloid to multiple myeloma, electrophoretic and immunoelectrophoretic studies on serum and urine should be performed when the biopsy reveals amyloid deposition. Most of these patients will have only relatively small paraprotein components, and only a few will have frank multiple myeloma.

PROGNOSIS   Generalized amyloidosis is usually a slowly progressive disease that leads to death in several years, but in some instances, prognosis is improving. The average survival in most large series of AL amyloid is ~12 months and in FAP is ~7 to 15 years. A number of individuals with amyloid have been followed 5 to 10 years and longer. The course of amyloidosis is difficult to document, because dating the time of origin of the disease is rarely possible. When amyloidosis develops in patients with rheumatoid arthritis, it seldom becomes evident when the arthritis is of less than 2 years' duration. When amyloidosis develops in patients with multiple myeloma, manifestations leading to initial hospitalization are more apt to

FIGURE 319-1   Microscopic tissue appearance of amyloid. *A.* Congo red stained section of amyloidotic kidney. *B.* Polarization microscopy of section *A* showing green birefringence of glomeruli and blood vessels. *C.* Congo red–stained section of uterus. *D.* Polarization microscopy of section *C* showing the vascular amyloid as well as amyloid in the muscle wall.

be related to amyloid disease than to myeloma. In these cases, prognosis is very poor, and life expectancy is usually less than 6 months.

℞ **TREATMENT** Rational therapy should be directed at (1) reducing precursor production, (2) inhibiting the synthesis and extracellular deposition of amyloid fibrils, and (3) promoting lysis or mobilization of existing amyloid deposits. There are new specific therapies for the various amyloidoses. In certain of the heredofamilial amyloidoses, genetic counseling is an important aspect of treatment, and the removal of the site of synthesis of the mutant protein by liver transplantation has proven remarkably successful. Liver transplantation has been carried out since 1990 for FAP patients in Sweden, the United States, Portugal, Spain, and other countries. It appears that disease progression is halted and that there is some improvement in autonomic nervous system function. The utilization of chronic hemodialysis and of kidney transplantation has clearly improved the prognosis of renal amyloid.

In the case of AL amyloid, the fact that immunoglobulin light chain is made by plasma cells has led to the use of alkylating agents. However, these agents are toxic and not very effective. The most effective form of treatment currently is stem cell transplantation and immunosuppressive drugs (melphalan). Several long-term remissions have been reported, but serious complications, even death, can occur. A novel anthracycline, iododoxorubicin (IDOX), has been shown to bind to AL amyloid (similar to Congo red) in vivo and promote amyloid resorption. A subset of AL patients responds transiently to this experimental agent; and it is thought that IDOX may prove useful in combination with other forms of treatment. Cardiac tranplantation in selected cases of AL or FAP amyloidosis has its advocates and has been successful.

Colchicine has been shown to be effective in preventing acute attacks and amyloidosis in patients with FMF (Chap. 289).

The major causes of death are heart disease and renal failure. Sudden death, presumably due to arrhythmias, is common. Occasionally, gastrointestinal hemorrhage, respiratory failure, intractable heart failure, and superimposed infections are the terminal events.

BIBLIOGRAPHY

BENSON MD, UEMICHI T: Transthyretin amyloidosis. Amyloid Int J Exp Clin Invest 3:44, 1996

COHEN AS: Amyloidosis. Bull Rheum Dis 40:1, 1991

———, JONES LA: Advances in amyloidosis. Curr Opin Rheumatol 5:62, 1993

———, SIPE JD: Amyloidosis, in *Clinical Immunology*, RR Rich et al (eds). St. Louis, Mosby Year Book, 1995, pp 1264–1272

FALK RH et al: The systemic amyloidoses. N Engl J Med 337:898, 1997

GLENNER GG, MURPHY MA: Amyloidosis of the nervous system. J Neurol Soc 94:1, 1989

HUSBY G et al: Serum amyloid A (SAA): Biochemistry, genetics and the pathogenesis of AA amyloidosis. Amyloid Int J Exp Clin Invest 1:119, 1994

LEWIS WD, SKINNER M: Liver transplantation for familial amyloidotic polyneuropathy: A potentially curative treatment. Amyloid Int J Exp Clin Invest 1:143, 1994

PRUSINER SB, DEARMOND SJ: Prion protein amyloid and neurodegeneration. Amyloid Int J Exp Clin Invest 2:39, 1995

SIPE JD: Amyloidosis. Crit Rev Clin Lab Sci 31:325, 1994

ZEMER D et al: Colchicine in the prevention and treatment of the amyloidosis of familial Mediterranean fever. N Engl J Med 314:1001, 1986

Section 3
DISORDERS OF THE JOINTS

320

John J. Cush, Peter E. Lipsky

APPROACH TO ARTICULAR AND MUSCULOSKELETAL DISORDERS

Musculoskeletal complaints account for more than 315,000,000 outpatient visits per year. Many of the musculoskeletal complaints that cause patients to seek medical attention are related to self-limited conditions requiring minimal evaluation and only symptomatic therapy and reassurance. However, some patients with similar symptoms have a more serious condition that requires further evaluation or additional laboratory testing to confirm the suspected diagnosis or determine the extent and nature of the pathologic process. A primary objective is to determine if a "red flag" or urgent rheumatologic condition is present and, if not, to formulate a differential diagnosis that leads to accurate diagnosis and timely therapy while avoiding excessive diagnostic testing and unnecessary treatment (Table 320-1) There are several urgent conditions that must be diagnosed promptly to avoid significant morbid or mortal sequelae. These red flag diagnoses include septic arthritis, acute crystal-induced arthritis (e.g., gout), and fracture. Each of these may be suspected by an acute onset with a monoarticular or focal presenting complaint (see below).

Individuals with musculoskeletal complaints should be evaluated in a uniform, logical manner by means of a thorough history, a comprehensive physical examination, and, if appropriate, laboratory testing. The goals of the initial encounter are to determine whether the musculoskeletal complaint is (1) *articular* or *nonarticular* in origin, (2) *inflammatory* or *noninflammatory* in nature, (3) *acute* or *chronic* in duration, and (4) *localized* or *widespread* (*systemic*) in distribution.

With such an approach and an understanding of the pathophysiologic processes that underlie musculoskeletal complaints, an adequate diagnosis can be made in the vast majority of individuals. However, some patients will not fit immediately into an established diagnostic category. Many musculoskeletal disorders resemble each other at the outset, and some take weeks or months to evolve into a readily recognizable diagnostic entity. This consideration should temper the desire always to establish a definitive diagnosis at the first encounter.

ARTICULAR VERSUS NONARTICULAR The musculoskeletal evaluation must discriminate the anatomic site(s) of origin of the patient's complaint. For example, ankle pain can result from a variety of pathologic conditions involving disparate anatomic structures, including gonococcal arthritis, calcaneal fracture, Achilles tendinitis, cellulitis, and peripheral neuropathy. Articular structures include the synovium, synovial fluid, articular cartilage, intraarticular ligaments, joint capsule, and juxtaarticular bone. Nonarticular (or periarticular) structures, such as supportive extraarticular ligaments, tendons, bursae, muscle, fascia, bone, nerve, and overlying skin, may be

Table 320-1 Evaluation of Patients with Musculoskeletal Complaints

Goals
  Accurate diagnosis
  Timely provision of therapy
  Avoidance of unnecessary diagnostic testing
Approach
  Anatomic localization of complaint (articular vs. nonarticular)
  Determination of the nature of the pathologic process (inflammatory vs. noninflammatory)
  Determination of the extent of involvement (monarticular, polyarticular, focal, widespread)
  Determination of chronology (acute vs. chronic)
  Formulation of a differential diagnosis

FIGURE 320-1 Algorithm for the diagnosis of musculoskeletal complaints. An approach to formulating a differential diagnosis (shown in italics). (ESR, erythrocyte sedimentation rate; CRP, C-reactive protein; DIP, distal interphalangeal; CMC, carpometacarpal; PIP, proximal interphalangeal; MCP, metacarpophalangeal; MTP, metatarsophalangeal; PMR, polymyalgia rheumatica; SLE, systemic lupus erythematosus; JA, juvenile arthritis.)

primary objective is to identify the nature of the underlying pathologic process. Musculoskeletal disorders are generally classified as inflammatory or noninflammatory. Inflammatory disorders may be infectious (infection with *Neisseria gonorrhoea* or *Mycobacterium tuberculosis*), crystal-induced (gout, pseudogout), immune-related [rheumatoid arthritis (RA), systemic lupus erythematosus (SLE)], reactive (rheumatic fever, Reiter's syndrome), or idiopathic. Inflammatory disorders may be identified by the presence of some or all of the four cardinal signs of inflammation (erythema, warmth, pain, and swelling), by systemic symptoms (prolonged morning stiffness, fatigue, fever, weight loss), or by laboratory evidence of inflammation (elevated erythrocyte sedimentation rate or C-reactive protein level, thrombocytosis, anemia of chronic disease, or hypoalbuminemia). Articular stiffness is common in chronic musculoskeletal disorders. However, the chronology and magnitude of stiffness may be diagnostically important. Morning stiffness related to inflammatory disorders (such as RA) is precipitated by prolonged rest, often lasts several hours, and may improve with activity and anti-inflammatory medications. By contrast, intermittent stiffness associated with noninflammatory conditions, such as osteoarthritis, is precipitated by brief periods of rest, usually lasts less than 60 min, and is exacerbated by activity. Noninflammatory disorders may be related to trauma (rotator cuff tear), ineffective repair (osteoarthritis), cellular overgrowth (pigmented villonodular synovitis), or pain amplification (fibromyalgia). They are often characterized by pain without swelling or warmth, the absence of inflammatory or systemic features, little or no morning stiffness, and normal laboratory findings.

Identification of the nature of the underlying process and the site of the complaint will enable the examiner to narrow the diagnostic considerations and to assess the need for immediate diagnostic or therapeutic intervention or for continued observation. Figure 320-1 presents a logical approach to the evaluation of patients with musculoskeletal complaints.

CLINICAL HISTORY Additional historic features may be helpful in establishing the nature and extent of the pathologic process and may provide important clues to the diagnosis. When evaluating patients with musculoskeletal complaints, the clinician should always consider the most common conditions (e.g., low back pain, osteoarthritis) seen in the general population (Fig. 320-2). Aspects of the patient profile, including age, sex, race, and family history, can provide important information. Certain diagnoses are more frequent in specific age groups. SLE, rheumatic fever, and Reiter's syndrome are more common in the young, whereas fibromyalgia and RA are most common in middle age, and osteoarthritis and polymyalgia rheumatica in the elderly. Some diseases are more common in a particular gender or race. Gout and the spondyloarthropathies (e.g., ankylosing spondylitis,

involved in the pathologic process. Pain from nonarticular structures may mimic true articular pain because of their proximity to the joint. Distinguishing between articular and nonarticular disease requires a careful and detailed examination. Articular disorders may be characterized by deep or diffuse joint pain, limited range of motion on active and passive movement, swelling caused by synovial proliferation or effusion or bony enlargement, crepitation, instability, locking, or deformity. By contrast, nonarticular disorders tend to be painful on active but not passive range of motion, demonstrate point or focal tenderness in regions distinct from articular structures, and have physical findings remote from the joint capsule. Moreover, nonarticular disorders seldom demonstrate crepitus, instability, deformity, or swelling.

INFLAMMATORY VERSUS NONINFLAMMATORY In the course of a musculoskeletal evaluation, the examiner should elicit symptoms and signs that will narrow or establish the diagnosis. A

1980

Reiter's syndrome) are more common in men, whereas SLE, RA, and fibromyalgia are more common in women. Polymyalgia rheumatica, giant cell arteritis, and Wegener's granulomatosis preferentially affect whites, whereas sarcoidosis and SLE are more common in blacks. *Familial aggregation* occurs in some disorders, such as ankylosing spondylitis, gout, RA, and Heberden's nodes of osteoarthritis.

The chronology of the complaint (*onset*, *evolution*, and *duration*) is an important diagnostic feature. The onset of disorders such as septic arthritis and gout tends to be abrupt, whereas osteoarthritis, RA, and fibromyalgia may develop more indolently. In terms of evolution, disorders are classified as acute (e.g., septic arthritis), chronic (e.g., osteoarthritis), intermittent (e.g., gout), migratory (e.g., rheumatic fever, gonococcal or viral arthritis), or additive (e.g., RA, Reiter's syndrome). Musculoskeletal disorders typically are called *acute* if they last less than 6 weeks and *chronic* if they last longer. Acute and intermittent arthropathies tend to be infectious, crystal-induced, or reactive. Noninflammatory and immune-related arthritides, such as osteoarthritis and RA, respectively, are often chronic. The duration of the patient's complaints may alter the diagnostic considerations. For example, the musculoskeletal signs and symptoms of hepatitis B virus infection may be identical with those of early RA at the onset but rarely persist beyond 3 weeks.

The *number and distribution* of involved articulations should be noted. Articular disorders are classified as *monarticular* (one joint involved), *oligoarticular* or *pauciarticular* (two to three joints involved), or *polyarticular* (more than three joints involved). Nonarticular disorders can be classified as either *focal* or *widespread*. Complaints secondary to trauma and gout are typically focal or monarticular, whereas polymyositis, RA, and fibromyalgia are more diffuse or polyarticular. Joint involvement tends to be symmetric in RA but is often asymmetric in the spondyloarthropathies and in gout. The upper extremities are frequently involved in RA, whereas lower extremity arthritis is characteristic of Reiter's syndrome and gout at their onset. Involvement of the axial skeleton is common in osteoarthritis and ankylosing spondylitis but infrequent in RA, with the notable exception of the cervical spine.

The clinical history should also identify *precipitating events*, such as trauma, drug administration (Table 320-2), or antecedent or intercurrent illnesses, that may have contributed to the patient's complaint. Last, a thorough *rheumatic review of systems* may disclose associated features outside the musculoskeletal system and provide useful diagnostic information. A variety of musculoskeletal disorders may be associated with systemic features such as fever (SLE, infection), rash (SLE, Reiter's syndrome, dermatomyositis), myalgias, weakness (polymyositis, polymyalgia rheumatica), and morning stiffness (inflammatory arthritis). In addition, some conditions are associated with involvement of other organ systems, including the eyes (Behçet's disease, sarcoidosis, Reiter's syndrome), gastrointestinal tract (scleroderma, inflammatory bowel disease), genitourinary tract (Reiter's syndrome, gonococcemia, Behçet's disease), and nervous system (Lyme disease, SLE, vasculitis).

PHYSICAL EXAMINATION The goal of the physical examination is to ascertain the structures involved, the nature of the underlying pathology, the extent and functional consequences of the process, and the presence of systemic or extraarticular manifestations. A knowledge of topographic anatomy is necessary to identify the primary site(s) of involvement and differentiate articular from nonarticular disorders. The musculoskeletal examination depends largely on careful inspection, palpation, and a variety of specific physical maneuvers to elicit diagnostic signs (Table 320-3). Although most artic-

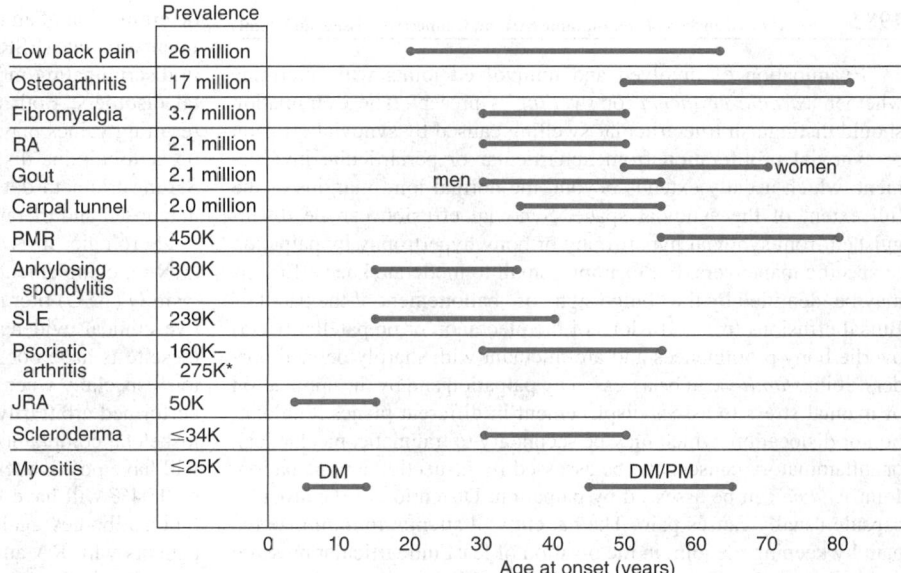

FIGURE 320-2 Age at onset for common rheumatic conditions; ranked by prevalance estimates in the United States in 1998. *Estimates vary.

Table 320-2   Drug-Induced Musculoskeletal Conditions

Arthralgias   Quinidine, amphotericin B, cimetidine, quinolones, chronic acyclovir, interferon, IL-2, nicardipine, vaccines, rifabutin
Myalgias/myopathy   Glucocorticoids, penicillamine, hydroxychloroquine, AZT, lovastatin, simvastatin, pravastatin, clofibrate, interferon, IL-2, alcohol, cocaine, taxol, docetaxel, colchicine, quinolones
Gout   Diuretics, aspirin, cytotoxics, cyclosporine, alcohol, moonshine, ethambutol
Drug-induced lupus   Hydralazine, procainamide, quinidine, phenytoin, methyldopa, isoniazid, chlorpromazine, lithium, penicillamine, tetracycline, infliximab
Osteonecrosis   Glucocorticoids, alcohol, radiation
Osteopenia   Glucocorticoids, chronic heparin, phenytoin, methotrexate
Scleroderma   Vinyl chloride, bleomycin, pentazocine, organic solvents, carbidopa, tryptophan, rapeseed oil
Vasculitis   Allopurinol, amphetamines, cocaine, thiazides, penicillamine, propylthiouracil

---

NOTE: IL-2, interleukin 2.

Table 320-3   Glossary of Musculoskeletal Terms

Crepitus   A palpable (less commonly audible) vibratory or crackling sensation elicited with joint motion; fine joint crepitus is common and often insignificant in large joints; coarse joint crepitus indicates advanced cartilaginous and degenerative changes (as in osteoarthritis).
Subluxation   Alteration of joint alignment such that articulating surfaces incompletely approximate each other
Dislocation   Abnormal displacement of articulating surfaces such that the surfaces are not in contact
Range of motion   For diarthrodial joints, the arc of measurable movement through which the joint moves in a single plane
Contracture   Loss of full movement resulting from a fixed resistance due either to tonic spasm of muscle (reversible) or to fibrosis of periarticular structures (permanent)
Deformity   Abnormal shape or size of a structure; may result from bony hypertrophy, malalignment of articulating structures, or damage to periarticular supportive structures
Enthesitis   Inflammation of the entheses (tendinous or ligamentous insertions on bone)
Epicondylitis   Infection or inflammation involving an epicondyle

---

ulations of the appendicular skeleton can be examined in this manner, adequate inspection and palpation are not possible for many axial (e.g., zygapophyseal) and inaccessible (e.g., sacroiliac or hip) joints. For such joints, there is a greater reliance on specific maneuvers and imaging for assessment.

Examination of involved and uninvolved joints will determine whether *warmth*, *erythema*, or *swelling* is present. The examination should distinguish true articular swelling caused by synovial effusion or synovial proliferation from nonarticular or periarticular involvement, which usually extends beyond the normal joint margins or the full extent of the synovial space. Synovial effusion can be distinguished from synovial hypertrophy or bony hypertrophy by palpation or specific maneuvers. For example, small to moderate knee effusions may be identified by the "bulge sign" or "ballottement of the patella." Bursal effusions (e.g., effusions of the olecranon or prepatellar bursa) overlie bony prominences and are fluctuant with sharply defined borders. Joint *stability* can be assessed by palpation and by the application of manual stress to assess displacement in different planes. Subluxation or dislocation, which may be secondary to traumatic, mechanical, or inflammatory causes, can be assessed by inspection and palpation. Joint *volume* can be assessed by palpation. Distention of the articular capsule usually causes pain. The patient will attempt to minimize the pain by keeping the joint in the position of least intraarticular pressure and greatest volume, usually partial flexion. Clinically, joint distention may be detected as obvious swelling, voluntary or fixed flexion deformities, or diminished range of motion—especially on extension, which decreases joint volume. Active and passive *range of motion* should be assessed in all planes, with contralateral comparison. Serial evaluations of joint motion may be made using a goniometer to quantify the arc of movement. Each joint should be passively manipulated through its full range of motion (including, as appropriate, flexion, extension, rotation, abduction, adduction, inversion, eversion, supination, pronation, and medial or lateral deviation or bending). Limitation of motion is frequently caused by effusion, pain, deformity, or contracture. *Contractures* may reflect antecedent synovial inflammation or trauma. Joint *crepitus* may be felt during palpation or maneuvers and may be prominent or coarse in osteoarthritis. Joint *deformity* usually indicates a long-standing or aggressive pathologic process. Deformities may result from ligamentous destruction, soft tissue contracture, bony enlargement, ankylosis, erosive disease, or subluxation. Examination of the musculature will permit assessment of strength and reveal atrophy, pain, or spasm. The examiner should look carefully for nonarticular or periarticular involvement, especially when articular complaints are not supported by objective findings referable to the joint capsule. The identification of musculoskeletal pain of soft tissue origin (nonarticular pain) will prevent unwarranted and often expensive additional evaluations. Specific maneuvers may reveal nonarticular abnormalities, such as a carpal tunnel syndrome (which can be identified by Tinel's or Phalen's sign). Other examples of soft tissue abnormalities include olecranon bursitis, epicondylitis (tennis elbow), enthesitis (e.g., Achilles tendinitis), and trigger points associated with fibromyalgia.

LABORATORY INVESTIGATIONS The vast majority of musculoskeletal disorders can be diagnosed easily by a complete history and physical examination. An additional objective of the initial encounter is to determine whether additional investigations or immediate therapy are required. A number of features indicate the need for additional evaluation. *Monarticular* conditions require additional evaluation, as do *traumatic* or *inflammatory* conditions and conditions accompanied by *neurologic changes* or *systemic manifestations* of serious disease. Finally, individuals with *chronic* symptoms (lasting more than 6 weeks), especially when there has been a lack of response to symptomatic measures, are candidates for additional evaluation. The extent and nature of the additional investigation should be dictated by the clinical features and suspected pathologic process. Laboratory tests should be used to confirm a specific clinical diagnosis and not be used as a tool to screen or evaluate patients with vague rheumatic complaints. Indiscriminate use of broad batteries of diagnostic tests and radiographic procedures are rarely useful or cost-effective.

Besides a complete blood count, including a white blood cell (WBC) and differential count, the routine evaluation should include determination of an acute-phase indicator, such as the erythrocyte sedimentation rate (ESR) or C-reactive protein (CRP), which can be useful in discriminating inflammatory from noninflammatory musculoskeletal disorders. Both tests are inexpensive and easily performed; the resulting values may be elevated with infections, inflammatory arthritis, autoimmune disorders, neoplasia, pregnancy, and advanced age. Serum uric acid determinations are only useful when gout has been diagnosed and therapy contemplated.

Serologic tests for rheumatoid factor, antinuclear antibodies (ANA), complement levels, Lyme disease antibodies, or antistreptolysin O (ASO) titer should be carried out only when there is substantive clinical evidence suggesting a relevant associated diagnosis, as these tests have poor predictive value when used in a screening fashion, especially when the pretest probability is low. They should not be performed arbitrarily in patients with minimal or nonspecific musculoskeletal complaints. For example, 4 to 5% of the general population will have positive tests for rheumatoid factor and ANAs, yet only 1% or 0.04% will have RA or SLE, respectively. IgM rheumatoid factor (autoantibodies against the Fc portion of IgG) is found in 80% of patients with RA and may also be seen in low titers in patients with chronic infections (tuberculosis, leprosy); other autoimmune diseases (SLE, Sjögren's syndrome); or chronic pulmonary, hepatic, or renal diseases. ANAs are found in nearly all patients with SLE and may also be seen in patients with other autoimmune diseases (polymyositis, scleroderma, antiphospholipid syndrome), drug-induced lupus (resulting from hydralazine, procainamide, or quinidine administration), or chronic hepatitic or renal disorders. The interpretation of a positive ANA determination may depend on the titer and on the pattern observed by immunofluorescence microscopy. Diffuse and speckled patterns are most common but least specific, whereas a peripheral, or rim, pattern is highly specific and is suggestive of autoantibodies against double-stranded (native) DNA. This pattern is seen only in patients with SLE.

Aspiration and analysis of synovial fluid are always indicated in acute monarthritis or when an infectious or crystal-induced arthropathy is suspected. Synovial fluid analysis may be crucial in distinguishing between noninflammatory and inflammatory processes. This distinction can be made on the basis of the appearance, viscosity, and cell count of the synovial fluid. Tests for synovial fluid glucose, protein, lactate dehydrogenase, lactic acid, or autoantibodies are not recommended, as they are insensitive or have little discriminatory value. Normal synovial fluid is clear or a pale straw color and is viscous, primarily because of the high levels of hyaluronate. Noninflammatory synovial fluid is clear, viscous, and amber-colored, with a WBC count of $<2000/\mu L$ and a predominance of mononuclear cells. The viscosity of synovial fluid is assessed by expressing fluid from the syringe one drop at a time. Normally there is a stringing effect, with a long tail behind each drop. Effusions due to osteoarthritis or trauma usually have normal viscosity. Inflammatory fluid is turbid and yellow, with an increased WBC (2000 to $50,000/\mu L$) and a predominance of polymorphonuclear leukocytes. Inflammatory fluid has a reduced viscosity, diminished hyaluronate, and little or no tail following each drop of synovial fluid. Such effusions are found in RA, gout, other inflammatory arthritides, and septic arthritis. Infectious fluid is turbid and opaque, with a WBC count usually $>50,000/\mu L$, a predominance of polymorphonuclear leukocytes ($>75\%$), and low viscosity. Such effusions are typical of septic arthritis, but they occur rarely with sterile inflammatory arthritides such as RA or gout. In addition, hemorrhagic synovial fluid may be seen with trauma, hemarthrosis, or neuropathic arthritis. An algorithm for synovial fluid aspiration and analysis is shown in Fig. 320-3. Synovial fluid should be analyzed immediately for appearance, viscosity, and cell count. Cellularity and the presence of crystals may be assessed by light or polarizing microscopy, respectively. Monosodium urate crystals, seen in gouty effusions, are long, needle-shaped, negatively birefringent, and usually intracellular, whereas calcium pyrophosphate dihydrate crystals, found in chondrocalcinosis and pseudogout, are usually short, rhomboid-shaped, and positively birefringent. Whenever infection is suspected, synovial fluid

FIGURE 320-3 Algorithmic approach to the use and interpretation of synovial fluid aspiration and analysis.

should be Gram-stained and cultured appropriately. If gonococcal arthritis is suspected, immediate plating of the fluid on appropriate culture medium is indicated. Synovial fluid from chronic monarthritis patients should also be cultured for *M. tuberculosis* and fungi. Last, it should be noted that crystal-induced arthritis and infection occasionally occur together in the same joint.

DIAGNOSTIC IMAGING IN JOINT DISEASES   Conventional radiography has been a valuable tool in the diagnosis and staging of articular disorders. Plain x-rays are most appropriate when there is a history of trauma, suspected chronic infection, progressive disability, or monarticular involvement; when therapeutic alterations are considered; or when a baseline assessment is desired for what appears to be a chronic process. However, in most inflammatory disorders, early radiography is rarely helpful in establishing a diagnosis and may only reveal soft tissue swelling or juxtaarticular demineralization. As the disease progresses, calcification (of soft tissues, cartilage, or bone), joint space narrowing, erosions, bony ankylosis, new

bone formation (sclerosis, osteophyte formation, or periostitis), or subchondral cysts may develop and suggest specific clinical entities. Consultation with a radiologist will help define proper technique and positioning and prevent the need for further studies.

Additional imaging techniques may possess greater diagnostic sensitivity and facilitate early diagnosis in a limited number of articular disorders and are indicated in selected circumstances when conventional radiography is not adequate (Table 320-4). *Ultrasonography* is useful in the detection of soft tissue abnormalities that cannot be appreciated fully by clinical examination. Although ultrasonography is inexpensive and easily performed, only in a limited number of circumstances is it the preferred method of evaluation. The foremost application of ultrasound is in the diagnosis of synovial (Baker's) cysts, although rotator cuff tears and various tendon injuries may be evaluated with ultrasound by an experienced operator. *Radionuclide scintigraphy* provides useful information regarding the metabolic status of bone and, along with radiography, is well suited for total-body assessment of the extent and distribution of musculoskeletal involvement. It is a very sensitive but poorly specific means of detecting inflammatory or metabolic alterations in bone or periarticular soft tissue structures. The limited tissue resolution of scintigraphy may obscure the distinction between bony and periarticular processes and may necessitate the use of additional imaging modalities. Scintigraphy, using ^{99m}Tc, ^{67}Ga, or WBCs labeled with ^{111}In, has been applied to a variety of articular disorders with variable success (Table 320-4). [^{99m}Tc]pertechnetate or [^{99m}Tc]diphosphonate scintigraphy may be useful in identifying infection, neoplasia, inflammation, increased blood flow, bone remodeling, heterotopic bone formation, or avascular necrosis (Fig. 320-4). However, the poor specificity of ^{99m}Tc scanning has limited its use to investigational and serial assessments of joint or bone involvement, assessment of inflammatory or infectious processes, and surveys for bone metastases. ^{67}Ga binds to serum and cellular transferrin and lactoferrin and is preferentially taken up by neutrophils, macrophages, bacteria, and tumor tissue (e.g., lymphoma) and is useful in the identification of infection and malignancies. Scanning with ^{111}In-labeled WBCs has been used to detect both infectious and inflammatory arthritis. Although both have been used with success, ^{111}In-labeled WBC scanning is superior to ^{67}Ga in the early diagnosis of osteomyelitis and infected prosthetic joints. Prior treatment with antibiotics may reduce the diagnostic sensitivity of both ^{67}Ga and ^{111}In-labeled WBC scintigraphy.

Computed tomography (CT) provides rapid reconstruction of sagittal, coronal, and axial images and thus of the spatial relationships among anatomic structures. It has proved most useful in the assessment of the axial skeleton because of its ability to visualize in the axial plane. Articulations that are difficult to visualize by conventional radiography, such as the zygapophyseal, sacroiliac, sternoclavicular, and hip joints, can be evaluated effectively using CT. CT has been demonstrated to be useful in the diagnosis of low back pain syndromes, sacroiliitis, osteoid osteoma, tarsal coalition, osteomyelitis, intraarticular osteochondral fragments, and advanced osteonecrosis.

Magnetic resonance imaging (MRI) has significantly advanced the ability to image musculoskeletal structures. MRI can provide multiplanar images with fine anatomic detail and contrast resolution (Fig. 320-5). Other advantages are the absence of ionizing radiation and adverse effects and the superior ability to visualize bone marrow and soft tissue periarticular structures. However, the high cost and long procedural time of MRI limit its use in the evaluation of musculoskeletal disorders. MRI should be used only when it will provide necessary information that cannot be obtained by less expensive and noninvasive means.

MRI can image fascia, vessels, nerve, muscle, cartilage, ligaments, tendons, pannus, synovial effusions, cortical bone, and bone marrow. Visualization of particular structures can be enhanced by altering the pulse sequence to produce either T1-weighted or T2-weighted spin echo, gradient echo, or inversion recovery [including short tau inver-

Table 320-4   Diagnostic Imaging Techniques for Musculoskeletal Disorders

Method	Imaging Time, h	Cost[a]	Current Indications
Ultrasound[b]	<1	+	Synovial cysts Rotator cuff tears Tendon injury
Radionuclide scintigraphy			
^{99m}Tc	1–4	++	Metastatic bone survey Evaluation of Paget's disease Quantitative joint assessment Acute infection Acute and chronic osteomyelitis
^{111}In-WBC	24	+++	Acute infection Prosthetic infection Acute osteomyelitis
^{67}Ga	24–48	++++	Acute and chronic infection Acute osteomyelitis
Computed tomography	<1	+++	Herniated intervertebral disk Sacroiliitis Spinal stenosis Spinal trauma Osteoid osteoma Tarsal coalition
Magnetic resonance imaging	1/2–2	+++++	Avascular necrosis Osteomyelitis Intraarticular derangement and soft tissue injury Derangements of axial skeleton and spinal cord Herniated intervertebral disk Pigmented villonodular synovitis Inflammatory and metabolic muscle pathology

[a] Relative cost for imaging study.
[b] Results depend on operator.

FIGURE 320-4 [^{99m}Tc]diphosphonate scintigraphy of the feet of a 33-year-old black male with Reiter's syndrome, manifested by sacroiliitis, urethritis, uveitis, asymmetric oligoarthritis, and enthesitis. This bone scan demonstrates increased uptake indicative of enthesitis involving the insertions of the left Achilles tendon, plantar aponeurosis, and right tibialis posterior tendon as well as arthritis of the right first interphalangeal joint.

sion recovery (STIR) images. Because of its sensitivity to changes in marrow fat, MRI is a sensitive although nonspecific means of detecting osteonecrosis and osteomyelitis (Fig. 320-5). Because of its enhanced soft tissue resolution, MRI is more sensitive than arthrography or CT for the diagnosis of soft tissue injuries (e.g., meniscal and rotator cuff tears), intraarticular derangements, and spinal cord damage following injury, subluxation, or synovitis of the vertebral facet joints.

RHEUMATOLOGIC EVALUATION OF THE ELDERLY

Musculoskeletal disorders in elderly patients are often not diagnosed because the signs and symptoms may be insidious or chronic in these patients. In addition, the nature of the problem is often obscured by the presence of multiple interacting factors, including other medical conditions and therapies. These difficulties are compounded by the diminished reliability of laboratory testing in the elderly, who often manifest nonpathologic abnormal results. For example, erythrocyte sedimentation rates may be misleadingly elevated and low titer positive tests for rheumatoid factor and ANAs may be seen in up to 15% of elderly patients. Although nearly all rheumatic disorders can afflict the elderly, certain diseases and drug-induced disorders (Table 320-2) are more common in this age group. The elderly should be approached in the same manner as other patients with musculoskeletal complaints but with additional inquiries to exclude common geriatric musculoskeletal disorders. An emphasis on identifying the rheumatic consequences of intercurrent medical conditions and therapies is extremely important. Osteoarthritis, gout, polymyalgia rheumatica, drug-induced lupus erythematosus, and chronic salicylate toxicity are all more common in the elderly than in other individuals. The physical examination should identify the nature of the musculoskeletal complaint, as well as coexisting diseases that may influence the diagnosis and choice of treatment.

Approach to the Patient

Regional Rheumatic Complaints Although all patients should be evaluated in a logical and thorough manner, many cases of focal musculoskeletal complaints are caused by commonly encountered disorders that exhibit a predictable pattern of onset, evolution, and localization and that can often be diagnosed immediately on the basis of limited historic information and selected maneuvers or tests. Although nearly every joint can be approached in this manner, the evaluation of four commonly involved anatomic regions—the hand, shoulder, hip, and knee—are reviewed here.

Hand pain Focal or unilateral hand pain may result from trauma, overuse, infection, or a reactive or crystal-induced arthritis. By contrast, bilateral hand complaints suggest a degenerative (e.g., osteoarthritis), systemic, or inflammatory/immune etiology. Patterns of joint involvement are highly suggestive of certain disorders. The distribution of affected joints in the hand may provide important diagnostic information (Fig. 320-6). Thus, osteoarthritis (or degenerative arthritis) may manifest as distal interphalangeal (DIP) and proximal interphalangeal (PIP) joint pain with bony hypertrophy sufficient to produce Heberden's and Bouchard's nodes, respectively. Pain, with or without bony swelling, involving the base of the thumb (first carpometacarpal joint) is also highly suggestive of osteoarthritis. By contrast, RA tends to involve the PIP, metacarpophalangeal, intercarpal, and carpometacarpal joints (wrist) with pain, prolonged stiffness, and palpable synovial tissue hypertrophy. Psoriatic arthritis may also involve the DIP and PIP joints and the carpus with inflammatory pain, stiffness, and synovitis. Moreover, the diagnosis of psoriatic arthritis can be suggested by nail pitting or onycholysis. Soft tissue swelling may also be noted over the dorsum of the hand and wrist and may suggest an inflammatory extensor tendon tenosynovitis, possibly caused by gonococcal infection, gout, or inflammatory arthritis. The diagnosis of tenosynovitis may be suggested by local warmth and edema and is confirmed when pain is induced by maintaining the wrist in a fixed, neutral position and flexing the digits distal to the metacarpophalangeal joints to stretch the extensor tendon sheaths.

Focal wrist pain localized to the radial aspect may be caused by DeQuervain's tenosynovitis resulting from inflammation of the tendon sheath(s) involving the abductor pollicis longus or extensor pollicis brevis (Fig. 320-6). This condition commonly results from overuse or

FIGURE 320-5 Superior sensitivity of magnetic resonance imaging in the diagnosis of osteonecrosis of the femoral head. A 45-year-old woman receiving high-dose glucocorticoids developed right hip pain. Conventional x-rays (*top*) demonstrated only mild sclerosis of the right femoral head. T1-weighted MRI (*bottom*) demonstrated low-density signal in the right femoral head, diagnostic of osteonecrosis.

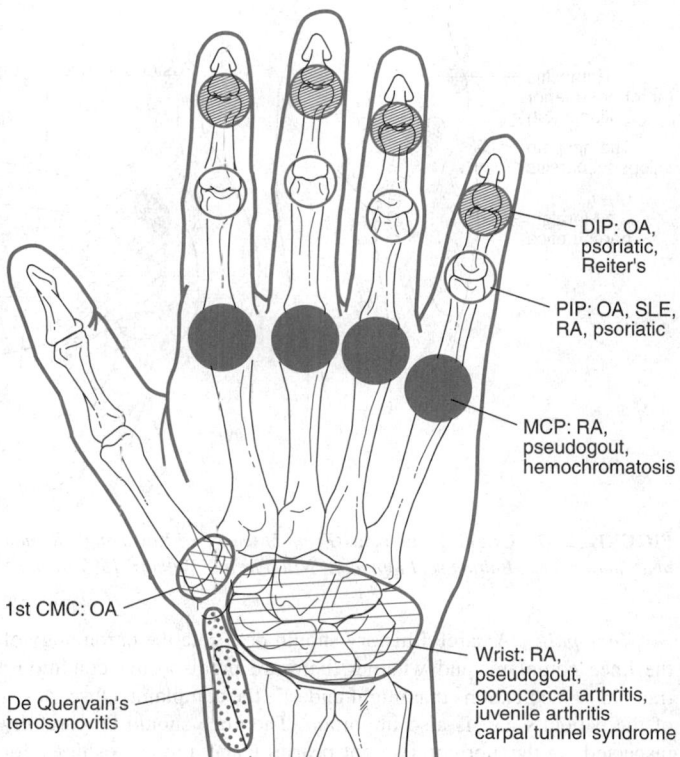

FIGURE 320-6 Sites of hand or wrist involvement and their potential disease associations. (DIP, distal interphalangeal; OA, osteoarthritis; PIP, proximal interphalangeal; SLE, systemic lupus erythematosus; RA, rheumatoid arthritis; MCP, metacarpophalangeal; CMC, carpometacarpal.) *(From JJ Cush, AF Kavanaugh, Rheumatology: Diagnosis and Therapeutics, Baltimore, Lippincott, Williams and Wilkins, 1999, with permission.)*

develops after pregnancy and may be diagnosed with Finkelstein's test. A positive result in Finkelstein's test is present when local wrist pain is induced after the thumb is flexed across the palm and placed inside a clenched fist and the patient actively moves the hand downward with ulnar deviation at the wrist. Carpal tunnel syndrome is another common disorder of the upper extremity and results from compression of the median nerve within the carpal tunnel. Manifestations include paresthesias in the thumb and the second, third, and radial half of the fourth fingers, and sometimes, atrophy of thenar musculature. Carpal tunnel syndrome is commonly associated with pregnancy, edema, trauma, osteoarthritis, inflammatory arthritis, and infiltrative disorders (e.g., amyloidosis). The diagnosis is suggested by a positive Tinel's or Phalen's sign. With each test, paresthesia in a median nerve distribution is induced or increased by either "thumping" the volar aspect of the wrist (Tinel's sign) or pressing the extensor surfaces of the two flexed wrists against each another (Phalen's sign).

Shoulder pain During the evaluation of shoulder disorders, the examiner should carefully note any history of trauma, infection, inflammatory disease, occupational hazards, or previous cervical disease. In addition, the patient should be questioned as to the activities or movement(s) that elicit shoulder pain. Shoulder pain is frequently referred from the cervical spine, but it may also be referred from intrathoracic lesions (e.g., a Pancoast tumor) or from gallbladder, hepatic, or diaphragmatic disease. The shoulder should be put through its full range of motion both actively and passively (with examiner assistance): forward flexion, extension, abduction, adduction, and rotation. Manual inspection of the periarticular structures will often provide important diagnostic information. The examiner should apply direct manual pressure over the subacromial bursa, which lies lateral to and immediately beneath the acromion. Subacromial bursitis is a fre-

quent cause of shoulder pain. Anterior to the subacromial bursa, the bicipital tendon traverses the bicipital groove. This tendon is best identified by palpating it in its groove as the patient rotates the humerus internally and externally. Direct pressure over the tendon may reveal pain indicative of bicipital tendinitis. Palpation of the acromioclavicular joint may disclose local pain, bony hypertrophy, or synovial swelling. Whereas osteoarthritis and RA commonly affect the acromioclavicular joint, osteoarthritis seldom involves the glenohumeral joint, unless there is a traumatic or occupational cause. The glenohumeral joint is best palpated anteriorly by placing the thumb over the humeral head (just medial and inferior to the coracoid process) and having the patient rotate the humerus internally and externally. Pain localized to this region is indicative of glenohumeral pathology. Synovial effusion or tissue is seldom palpable but, if present, may suggest infection, RA, or an acute tear of the rotator cuff.

Rotator cuff tendinitis or tear is a very common cause of shoulder pain. The rotator cuff is formed by the tendons of the supraspinatus, infraspinatus, teres minor, and subscapularis muscles. Rotator cuff tendinitis is suggested by pain on active abduction (but not passive abduction), pain over the lateral deltoid muscle, night pain, and evidence of the impingement sign. This maneuver is performed by the examiner raising the patient's arm into forced flexion while stabilizing the scapula and preventing it from rotating. A positive sign is present if pain develops before 180° of forward flexion. A complete tear of the rotator cuff, which often results from trauma, may manifest in the same manner but is less common than tendinitis. The diagnosis is suggested by the drop arm test, in which the patient is asked to maintain the arm outstretched after it has been passively abducted. If the patient is unable to hold the arm up once 90° of abduction is reached, the test is positive. Tendinitis or tear of the rotator cuff can be confirmed by MRI or ultrasonography.

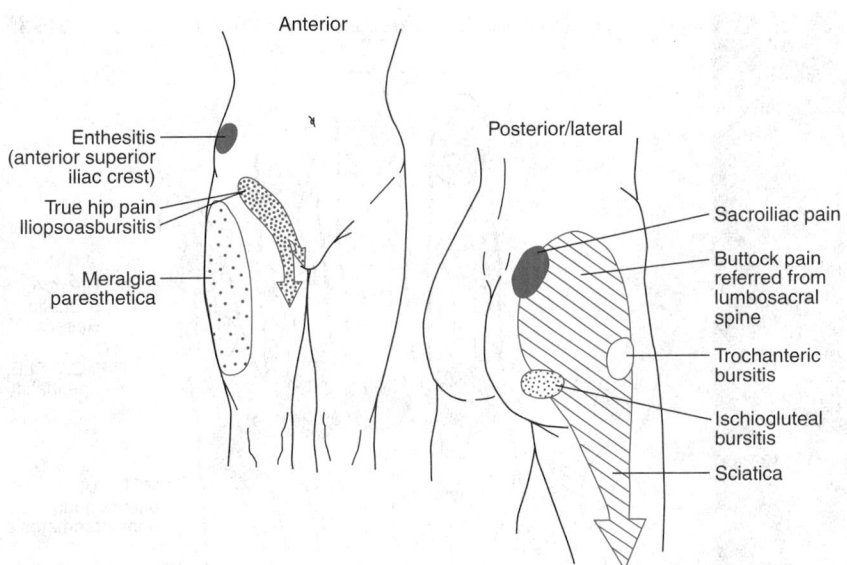

FIGURE 320-7 Origins of hip pain. *(From JJ Cush, AF Kavanaugh, Rheumatology: Diagnosis and Therapeutics, Baltimore, Lippincott, Williams and Wilkins, 1999, with permission.)*

Knee pain   A careful history should delineate the chronology of the knee complaint and whether there are predisposing conditions, trauma, or medications that might underlie the complaint. Observation of the patient's gait is also important. The knee should be carefully inspected in the upright (weight-bearing) and prone positions for swelling, erythema, contusion, laceration, and malalignment. The most common form of malalignment in the knee is genu varum (bow-legs) and genu valgum (knock-knees). Bony swelling of the knee joint commonly results from hypertrophic osseous changes seen with disorders such as osteoarthritis and neuropathic arthropathy. Swelling caused by hypertrophy of intrasynovial structures (synovial enlargement or effusion) may manifest as a fluctuant, ballotable, or soft tissue enlargement in the suprapatellar pouch (superior reflection of the synovial cavity) or lateral and medial to the patella. Synovial effusions may also be detected by balloting the patella downward toward the femoral groove or by eliciting a bulge sign. To elicit this sign, the examiner positions the knee in extension and manually compresses or milks synovial fluid down from the suprapatellar pouch and lateral to the patellae. Manual pressure lateral to the patella may cause an observable shift in synovial fluid (bulge) to the medial aspect. This maneuver is only effective for detecting small to moderate effusions (<100 mL). Inflammatory disorders such as RA, gout, and Reiter's syndrome may involve the knee joint and produce significant pain, stiffness, swelling, or warmth. A popliteal or *Baker's cyst* is best palpated with the knee partially flexed and is best seen with the patient standing with knees fully extended to visualize popliteal swelling or fullness from a posterior view.

Anserine bursitis is an often missed cause of knee pain in adults. The pes anserine bursa underlies the semimembranosus tendon and may become inflamed or painful owing to trauma, overuse, or inflammation. Anserine bursitis manifests primarily as point tenderness inferior and medial to the patella and overlying the medial tibial plateau. Swelling and erythema may not be present. Other forms of bursitis may also present as knee pain. The prepatellar bursa is superficial and is located over the inferior portion of the patella. The infrapatellar bursa is deeper and lies beneath the patellar ligament before its insertion on the tibial tubercle.

Internal derangement of the knee may result from trauma or degenerative processes. Damage to the meniscal cartilage (medial or lateral) frequently presents as chronic or intermittent knee pain. Such an injury should be suspected when there is a history of trauma or athletic activity and when the patient relates symptoms of locking, clicking, or "giving way" of the joint. Pain may be detected during direct palpation over the medial or lateral joint line. The diagnosis may also be suggested by ipsilateral joint-line pain when the knee is stressed laterally or medially. A positive McMurray test may indicate a meniscal tear. To perform this test, the knee is first flexed at 90°, and the leg is then extended while simultaneously the lower extremity is torqued medially or laterally. A painful click during inward rotation may indicate a lateral meniscus tear, and pain during outward rotation may indicate a tear in the medial meniscus. Finally, damage to the cruciate ligaments should be suspected if there is pain of acute onset, possibly with swelling, a history of trauma, or a synovial fluid aspirate that is grossly bloody. Examination of the cruciate ligaments is best accomplished by eliciting a drawer sign. With the patient recumbent, the knee should be partially flexed and the foot stabilized on the examining surface. The examiner should manually attempt to displace the tibia anteriorly or posteriorly with respect to the femur. If anterior movement is detected, then anterior cruciate ligament damage is likely. Conversely, significant posterior movement may indicate posterior cruciate damage. Contralateral comparison will assist the examiner in detecting significant anterior or posterior movement.

Hip pain   The hip is best evaluated by observing the patient's gait and assessing range of motion. The vast majority of patients reporting "hip pain" localize their pain unilaterally to the posterior or gluteal musculature (Fig. 320-7). Such pain may or may not be associated with low back pain and tends to radiate down the posterolateral aspect of the thigh. This presentation frequently results from degenerative arthritis of the lumbosacral spine and commonly follows a dermatomal distribution with involvement of nerve roots between L5 and S1. Some individuals instead localize their "hip pain" laterally to the area overlying the trochanteric bursa. Because of the depth of this bursa, swelling and warmth are usually absent. Diagnosis of trochanteric bursitis can be confirmed by inducing point tenderness over the trochanteric bursa. Range of movement may be limited by pain. Pain in the hip joint is less common and tends to be located anteriorly, over the inguinal ligament; it may radiate medially to the groin or along the anteromedial thigh. Uncommonly, iliopsoas bursitis may mimic true hip joint pain. Diagnosis of iliopsoas bursitis may be suggested by a history of trauma or inflammatory arthritis. Pain associated with an iliopsoas bursitis is localized to the groin or anterior thigh and tends to worsen with hyperextension of the hip; many patients prefer to flex and externally rotate the hip to reduce the pain from a distended bursa.

BIBLIOGRAPHY

BEESON PB: Age and sex associations of 40 autoimmune diseases. Am J Med 96:457, 1994

BROWER AC: Imaging techniques and modalities, in *Arthritis in Black and White*, 2d ed., AC Brower (ed). Philadelphia, Saunders, 1996, p 1

CUSH JJ et al: Evaluation of musculoskeletal complaints, in *Rheumatology: Diagnosis and Therapeutics*. JJ Cush, AF Kavanaugh (eds). Williams & Wilkins, Baltimore, 1998, pp 1–15

LAWRENCE RC et al: Estimates of the prevalence of arthritis and selected musculoskeletal disorders in the United States. Arthritis Rheum 41:778, 1998

LIPSKY PE et al: Algorithms for the diagnosis and management of musculoskeletal complaints. Am J Med 103:49S, 1997

SHMERLING RH et al: Synovial fluid tests: What should be ordered? JAMA 264:1009, 1990

WARD MW: Laboratory testing for systemic rheumatic diseases. Postgrad Med 103:93, 1998

WERNICK R: Avoiding laboratory test misinterpretation. Geriatrics 44:61, 1989

321

Kenneth D. Brandt

OSTEOARTHRITIS

Cox cyclooxygenase	NSAID nonsteroidal anti-
CSIs Cox-2-specific inhibitors	inflammatory drug
DISH diffuse idiopathic skeletal	OA osteoarthritis
hyperostosis	PAI-1 plasminogen activator
GI gastrointestinal	inhibitor-1
IGF-1 insulin-like growth factor-1	PGs proteoglycans
IL interleukin	TGF-β transforming growth factor β
MMPs matrix metallopro-	TIMP tissue inhibitor of
teinases	metalloproteinase

Osteoarthritis (OA), also erroneously called degenerative joint disease, represents failure of the diarthrodial (movable, synovial-lined) joint. In idiopathic (primary) OA, the most common form of the disease, no predisposing factor is apparent. Secondary OA is pathologically indistinguishable from idiopathic OA but is attributable to an underlying cause (Table 321-1).

EPIDEMIOLOGY AND RISK FACTORS   OA is the most common joint disease of humans. Among the elderly, knee OA is the leading cause of chronic disability in developed countries; some 100,000 people in the United States are unable to walk independently from bed to bathroom because of OA of the knee or hip.

Under the age of 55 years the joint distribution of OA in men and women is similar; in older individuals, hip OA is more common in men, while OA of interphalangeal joints and the thumb base is more common in women. Similarly, radiographic evidence of knee OA and, especially *symptomatic* knee OA, is more common in women than in men (Table 321-2).

Racial differences exist in both the prevalence of OA and the pattern of joint involvement. The Chinese in Hong Kong have a lower incidence of hip OA than whites; OA is more frequent in native Americans than in whites. Interphalangeal joint OA and, especially, hip OA are much less common in South African blacks than in whites in the same population. Whether these differences are genetic or are due to differences in joint usage related to life-style or occupation is unknown.

In some cases, the relation of heredity to OA is less ambiguous. Thus, the mother and sister of a woman with distal interphalangeal joint OA (Heberden's nodes) are, respectively, twice and thrice as likely to exhibit OA in these joints as the mother and sister of an unaffected woman. Point mutations in the cDNA coding for articular cartilage collagen have been identified in families with chondrodysplasia and polyarticular secondary OA.

Age is the most powerful risk factor for OA. In a radiographic survey of women less than 45 years old, only 2% had OA; between the ages of 45 to 64 years, however, the prevalence was 30%, and for those older than 65 years it was 68%. In males, the figures were similar but somewhat lower in the older age groups.

Major trauma and repetitive joint use are also important risk factors for OA. Anterior cruciate ligament insufficiency or meniscus damage (and meniscectomy) may lead to knee OA. Although damage to the articular cartilage may occur at the time of injury or subsequently, with use of the affected joint, even normal cartilage will degenerate if the joint is unstable. A person with a trimalleolar fracture will almost certainly develop ankle OA.

The pattern of joint involvement in OA is influenced by prior vocational or avocational overload. Thus, while ankle OA is common in ballet dancers, elbow OA in baseball pitchers, and metacarpophalangeal joint OA in prize fighters, OA is not very common at any of these sites in the general population.

Table 321-1   Classification of OA

I. Idiopathic
  A. Localized OA
    1. Hands: Heberden's and Bouchard's nodes (nodal), erosive interphalangeal arthritis (nonnodal), 1st carpometacarpal joint
    2. Feet: hallux valgus, hallux rigidus, contracted toes (hammer/cock-up toes), talonavicular
    3. Knee:
      a. Medial compartment
      b. Lateral compartment
      c. Patellofemoral compartment
    4. Hip:
      a. Eccentric (superior)
      b. Concentric (axial, medial)
      c. Diffuse (coxae senilis)
    5. Spine:
      a. Apophyseal joints
      b. Intervertebral joints (disks)
      c. Spondylosis (osteophytes)
      d. Ligamentous (hyperostosis, Forestier's disease, diffuse idiopathic skeletal hyperostosis
    6. Other single sites, e.g., glenohumoral, acromioclavicular, tibiotalar, sacroiliac, temporomandibular
  B. Generalized OA includes 3 or more of the areas listed above (Kellgren-Moore)
II. Secondary
  A. Trauma
    1. Acute
    2. Chronic (occupational, sports)
  B. Congenital or developmental
    1. Localized diseases: Legg-Calvé-Perthes, congenital hip dislocation, slipped epiphysis
    2. Mechanical factors: unequal lower extremity length, valgus/varus deformity, hypermobility syndromes
    3. Bone dysplasias: epiphyseal dysplasia, spondyloepiphyseal dysplasia, osteonychodystrophy
  C. Metabolic
    1. Ochronosis (alkaptonuria)
    2. Hemochromatosis
    3. Wilson's disease
    4. Gaucher's disease
  D. Endocrine
    1. Acromegaly
    2. Hyperparathyroidism
    3. Diabetes mellitus
    4. Obesity
    5. Hypothyroidism
  E. Calcium deposition diseases
    1. Calcium pyrophosphate dihydrate deposition
    2. Apatite arthropathy
  F. Other bone and joint diseases
    1. Localized: fracture, avascular necrosis, infection, gout
    2. Diffuse: rheumatoid (inflammatory) arthritis, Paget's disease, osteopetrosis, osteochondritis
  G. Neuropathic (Charcot joints)
  H. Endemic
    1. Kashin-Beck
    2. Mseleni
  I. Miscellaneous
    1. Frostbite
    2. Caisson's disease
    3. Hemoglobinopathies

SOURCE: From Mankin et al.

Table 321-2   Risk Factors for OA

Age	Repetitive stress, e.g., vocational[a]
Female sex	Obesity[a]
Race	Congenital/developmental defects[a]
Genetic factors	Prior inflammatory joint disease
Major joint trauma[a]	Metabolic/endocrine disorders

[a] Potentially modifiable
SOURCE: Adapted from M Hochberg: J Rheumatol 18: 1438, 1991.

FIGURE 321-1 *A.* Normal articular cartilage. Note the intact surface and even distribution of chondrocytes. Mitotic figures are not present in normal adult articular cartilage. *B.* Osteoarthritic cartilage. Note the disruption of surface integrity, with vertical fissures (fibrillation) and irregular distribution of cells. Many of the chondrocytes have replicated and exist in clusters. Stained with safranin-O, which binds to the sulfated glycosaminoglycan chains of proteoglycans. Note patchy areas of diminished staining (pale extracellular matrix) due to proteoglycan depletion.

Given the growing participation of the population of this country in cardiovascular fitness programs, it is important to note that there are no convincing data to support an association between specific athletic activities and arthritis if major trauma is excluded. Neither long-distance running nor jogging has been shown to cause OA. This apparent lack of association may, however, be due to the lack of good long-term studies, the difficulty of retrospective assessment of activities, and selection bias, i.e., early discontinuation of the activity by those incurring joint damage. In contrast, vocational activities, such as those performed by jackhammer operators, cotton mill and shipyard workers, and coal miners, may lead to OA in the joints exposed to repetitive occupational use. Men whose jobs required knee bending and at least medium physical demands had a higher rate of radiographic evidence of knee OA, and more severe radiographic changes, than men whose jobs required neither.

Obesity is a risk factor for knee OA and hand OA. For those in the highest quintile for body mass index at baseline examination, the relative risk for developing knee OA in the ensuing 36 years was 1.5 for men and 2.1 for women. For *severe* knee OA, the relative risk rose to 1.9 for men and 3.2 for women, suggesting that obesity plays an even larger role in the etiology of the most serious cases of knee OA. Furthermore, obese individuals who have not yet developed OA can reduce their risk: A weight loss of only 5 kg was found to be associated with a 50% reduction in the odds of developing symptomatic knee OA.

The correlation between the pathologic severity of OA and symptoms is poor. Many individuals with radiographic changes of advanced OA have no symptoms. The risk factors for *pain* and *disability* in affected individuals are poorly understood. Disability in those with knee OA is more strongly associated with quadriceps muscle weakness than with either joint pain or radiographic severity of the disease. For the same degree of pathologic severity, women are more likely to be symptomatic than men, those on welfare more likely than those who are working, and those who are divorced more likely than those who are married. For individuals with OA who had poor social support, periodic telephone calls from a trained lay interviewer were as effective as a nonsteroidal anti-inflammatory drug (NSAID) in reducing joint pain, emphasizing the importance of psychosocial factors as determinants of pain.

PATHOLOGY Although the cardinal pathologic feature of OA is a progressive loss of articular cartilage, OA is not a disease of any single tissue but a disease of an *organ*, the synovial joint, in which all of the tissues are affected: the subchondral bone, synovium, meniscus, ligaments, and supporting neuromuscular apparatus as well as the cartilage.

The most striking morphologic changes in OA are usually seen in load-bearing areas of the articular cartilage. In the early stages the cartilage is thicker than normal, but with progression of OA the joint surface thins, the cartilage softens, the integrity of the surface is breached, and vertical clefts develop (fibrillation) (Fig. 321-1). Deep cartilage ulcers, extending to bone, may appear. Areas of fibrocartilaginous repair may develop, but the repair tissue is inferior to pristine hyaline articular cartilage in its ability to withstand mechanical stress. All of the cartilage is metabolically active, and the chondrocytes replicate, forming clusters (clones). Later, however, the cartilage becomes hypocellular.

Remodeling and hypertrophy of bone are also major features of OA. Appositional bone growth occurs in the subchondral region, leading to the bony "sclerosis" seen radiographically. The abraded bone under a cartilage ulcer may take on the appearance of ivory (eburnation). Growth of cartilage and bone at the joint margins leads to osteophytes (spurs), which alter the contour of the joint and may restrict movement. A patchy chronic synovitis and thickening of the joint capsule may further restrict movement. Periarticular muscle wasting is common and may play a major role in symptoms and, as indicated above, in disability.

PATHOGENESIS The main load on articular cartilage—the major target tissue in OA—is produced by contraction of the muscles that stabilize or move the joint. Although cartilage is an excellent shock absorber in terms of its bulk properties, at most sites it is only 1 to 2 mm thick—too thin to serve as the sole shock-absorbing structure in the joint. Additional protective mechanisms are provided by subchondral bone and periarticular muscles.

Articular cartilage serves two essential functions within the joint, both of which are mechanical. First, it provides a remarkably smooth bearing surface, so that, with joint movement, the bones glide effortlessly over each other. With synovial fluid as lubricant, the coefficient of friction for cartilage rubbed against cartilage, even under physiologic loading, is 15 times lower than that of two ice cubes passed across each other! Second, articular cartilage prevents the concentration of stresses, so the bones do not shatter when the joint is loaded.

OA develops in either of two settings: (1) the biomaterial properties of the articular cartilage and subchondral bone are normal, but excessive loading of the joint causes the tissues to fail, or (2) the applied load is reasonable, but the material properties of the cartilage or bone are inferior.

Although articular cartilage is highly resistant to wear under conditions of repeated oscillation, repetitive impact loading soon leads to joint failure. This fact accounts for the high prevalence of OA at specific sites related to vocational or avocational overloading. In general, the earliest changes occur at the sites in the joint that are subject to the greatest compressive loads. Some cases of "idiopathic" OA of the hip may be due to subtle congenital or developmental defects, such as congenital subluxation/dislocation, acetabular dysplasia, Legg-Calvé-Perthes disease, or slipped capital femoral epiphysis, which increase joint congruity and concentrate the dynamic load.

Clinical conditions that reduce the ability of the cartilage or subchondral bone to deform are associated with development of OA. In ochronosis, for example, accumulation of homogentisic acid polymers leads to stiffening of the cartilage; in osteopetrosis, stiffness of the subchondral trabeculae occurs. In both conditions, severe generalized

OA is usually apparent by the age of 40. If the subchondral bone is stiffened experimentally, repetitive impact loading soon leads to breakdown of the overlying cartilage. Conversely, osteoporosis, in which the bone is abnormally soft, may protect against OA.

The Extracellular Matrix of Normal Articular Cartilage Articular cartilage is composed of two major macromolecular species: proteoglycans (PGs), which are responsible for the compressive stiffness of the tissue and its ability to withstand load, and collagen, which provides tensile strength and resistance to shear. Although lysomal proteases (cathepsins) have been demonstrated within the cells and matrix of normal articular cartilage, their low pH optimum makes it likely that the proteoglycanase activity of these enzymes will be confined to intracellular sites or the immediate pericellular area. However, cartilage also contains a family of matrix metalloproteinases (MMPs), including stromelysin, collagenase, and gelatinase, which can degrade all the components of the extracellular matrix at neutral pH. Each is secreted by the chondrocyte as a latent proenzyme that must be activated by proteolytic cleavage of its N-terminal sequence. The level of MMP activity in the cartilage at any given time represents the balance between activation of the proenzyme and inhibition of the active enzyme by tissue inhibitors. It has recently become apparent that much of the total tissue pool of aggrecan, the major PG in articular cartilage, is degraded by a proteinase that cleaves the protein core of the molecule at a site distinct from that at which the MMPs are active. The enzyme responsible for this cleavage is referred to as "aggrecanase" but has not been clearly identified.

The turnover of normal cartilage is effected through a degradative cascade, for which many investigators consider the driving force to be interleukin (IL) 1, a cytokine produced by mononuclear cells (including synovial lining cells) and synthesized by chondrocytes. IL-1 stimulates the synthesis and secretion of the latent MMPs and of tissue plasminogen activator. Plasminogen, the substrate for the latter enzyme, may be synthesized by the chondrocyte or may enter the cartilage from the synovial fluid. Both plasminogen and stromelysin may play a role in activation of the latent MMPs. In addition to its catabolic effect on cartilage, IL-1, at concentrations even lower than those needed to stimulate cartilage degradation, suppresses PG synthesis by the chondrocyte, inhibiting matrix repair (see below).

The balance of the system lies with at least two inhibitors, tissue inhibitor of metalloproteinase (TIMP) and plasminogen activator inhibitor-1 (PAI-1), which are synthesized by the chondrocyte and limit the degradative activity of MMPs and plasminogen activator, respectively. If TIMP or PAI-1 is destroyed or is present in concentrations that are insufficient relative to those of active enzymes, stromelysin and plasmin are free to act on matrix substrates. Stromelysin can degrade the protein core of the PG and activate latent collagenase. Conversion of latent stromelysin to an active, highly destructive protease by plasmin provides a second mechanism for matrix degradation.

Polypeptide mediators, e.g., insulin-like growth factor-1 (IGF-1) and transforming growth factor β (TGF-β), stimulate biosynthesis of PGs. They regulate matrix metabolism in normal cartilage and may play a role in matrix repair in OA. Notably, these growth factors modulate catabolic as well as anabolic pathways of chondrocyte metabolism; by down-regulating chondrocyte receptors for IL-1, they may decrease PG degradation.

In addition to its responsiveness to cytokines and a variety of other biologic mediators, chondrocyte metabolism in normal cartilage can be modulated directly by mechanical loading. Whereas static loading and prolonged cyclic loading inhibit synthesis of PGs and protein, loads of relatively brief duration may stimulate matrix biosynthesis.

Pathophysiology of Cartilage Changes in OA Most investigators feel that the primary changes in OA begin in the cartilage. A change in the arrangement and size of the collagen fibers is apparent. Biochemical data are consistent with the presence of a defect in the collagen network of the matrix, perhaps due to disruption of the "glue" that binds adjacent fibers. This is among the earliest matrix changes observed and appears to be irreversible.

Although "wear" may be a factor in the loss of cartilage, strong evidence supports the concept that lysosomal enzymes and MMPs account for much of the loss of cartilage matrix in OA. Whether their synthesis and secretion are stimulated by IL-1 or by other factors (e.g., mechanical stimuli), MMPs, plasmin, and cathepsins all appear to be involved in the breakdown of articular cartilage in OA. TIMP and PAI-1 may work to stabilize the system, at least temporarily, while growth factors, such as IGF-1, TGF-β, and basic fibroblast growth factor, are implicated in repair processes that may heal the lesion or, at least, stabilize the process. A stoichiometric imbalance exists between the levels of active enzyme and the level of TIMP, which may be only modestly increased.

Of current interest is the possible role of nitric oxide (NO) in articular cartilage damage in OA, since NO has been shown to stimulate synthesis of MMPs by chrondrocytes. Chondrocytes are a major source of NO, the synthesis of which is stimulated by IL-1 and tumor necrosis factor and by shear stresses on the tissue. In an experimental model of OA, treatment with a selective inhibitor of inducible NO synthase reduced the severity of cartilage damage.

The chondrocytes in OA cartilage undergo active cell division and are very active metabolically, producing increased quantities of DNA, RNA collagen, PG, and noncollagenous proteins. (For this reason, it is inaccurate to call OA a *degenerative* joint disease). Prior to cartilage loss and PG depletion, this marked biosynthetic activity may lead to an increase in PG concentration, which may be associated with thickening of the cartilage and a stage of homeostasis referred to as "compensated" OA. These mechanisms may maintain the joint in a reasonably functional state for years. The repair tissue, however, often does not hold up as well under mechanical stresses as normal hyaline cartilage and eventually, at least in some cases, the rate of PG synthesis falls off and "end-stage" OA develops, with full-thickness loss of cartilage.

CLINICAL FEATURES The joint pain of OA is often described as a deep ache and is localized to the involved joint. Typically, the pain of OA is aggravated by joint use and relieved by rest, but, as the disease progresses, it may become persistent. Nocturnal pain, interfering with sleep, is seen particularly in advanced OA of the hip and may be enervating. Stiffness of the involved joint upon arising in the morning or after a period of inactivity (e.g., an automobile ride) may be prominent but usually lasts less than 20 min. Systemic manifestations are not a feature of primary OA.

Because articular cartilage is aneural, the joint pain in OA must arise from other structures (Table 321-3). In some cases it may be due to stretching of nerve endings in the periosteum covering osteophytes; in others, to microfractures in subchondral bone or from medullary hypertension caused by distortion of blood flow by thickened subchondral trabeculae. Joint instability, leading to stretching of the joint capsule, and muscle spasm may also be sources of pain.

In some patients with OA, joint pain may be due to synovitis. In advanced OA, histologic evidence of synovial inflammation may be as marked as that in the synovium of a patient with rheumatoid arthritis. Synovitis in OA may be due to phagocytosis of shards of cartilage and bone from the abraded joint surface (wear particles), to release from the cartilage of soluble matrix macromolecules, or to crystals of calcium pyrophosphate or hydroxyapatite. In other cases, immune complexes, containing antigens derived from cartilage matrix, may be sequestered in collagenous tissue of the joint, leading to low-

Table 321-3 Causes of Joint Pain in Patients with OA

Source	Mechanism
Synovium	Inflammation
Subchondral bone	Medullary hypertension, microfractures
Osteophyte	Stretching of periosteal nerve endings
Ligaments	Stretch
Capsule	Inflammation, distention
Muscle	Spasm

grade chronic synovitis. In contrast, in the earlier stages of OA, even in the patient with chronic joint pain, synovial inflammation may be absent, suggesting that the joint pain is due to one of the other factors mentioned above.

Physical examination of the OA joint may reveal localized tenderness and bony or soft tissue swelling. Bony crepitus (the sensation of bone rubbing against bone, evoked by joint movement) is characteristic. Synovial effusions, if present, are usually not large. Palpation may reveal some warmth over the joint. Periarticular muscle atrophy may be due to disuse or to reflex inhibition of muscle contraction. In the advanced stages of OA, there may be gross deformity, bony hypertrophy, subluxation, and marked loss of joint motion. The notion that OA is inexorably progressive, however, is incorrect. In many patients the disease stabilizes; in some, regression of joint pain and even of radiographic changes occurs.

Although the diagnosis of OA is often straightforward because of the high prevalence of radiographic changes of OA in asymptomatic individuals, it is important to ensure that joint pain in a patient with radiographic evidence of OA is not due to some other cause, such as soft tissue rheumatism (e.g., anserine bursitis at the knee, trochanteric bursitis at the hip), radiculopathy, referral of pain from another joint (e.g., 25% of patients with hip disease have pain referred to the knee), entrapment neuropathy, vascular disease (claudication), or some other type of arthritis (e.g., crystal-induced synovitis, septic arthritis). These are all common pitfalls in the diagnosis of OA. It is usually not difficult to differentiate OA from a systemic rheumatic disease, such as rheumatoid arthritis, because, in the latter diseases, joint involvement is usually symmetric and polyarticular, with arthritis in wrists and metacarpophalangeal joints (which are generally not involved in OA), and there are also constitutional features such as prolonged morning stiffness, fatigue, weight loss, or fever.

LABORATORY AND RADIOGRAPHIC FINDINGS   The diagnosis of OA is usually based on clinical and radiographic features. In the early stages, the radiograph may be normal, but joint space narrowing becomes evident as articular cartilage is lost. Other characteristic radiographic findings include subchondral bone sclerosis, subchondral cysts, and osteophytosis. A change in the contour of the joint, due to bony remodeling, and subluxation may be seen. Although tibiofemoral joint space narrowing has been considered to be a radiographic surrogate for articular cartilage thinning, in patients with early OA who do not have radiographic evidence of bony changes (e.g., subchondral sclerosis or cysts, osteophytes), joint space narrowing alone does not accurately indicate the status of the articular cartilage. Similarly, osteophytosis alone, in the absence of other radiographic features of OA, may be due to aging rather than to OA.

As indicated above, there is often great disparity between the severity of radiographic findings, the severity of symptoms, and functional ability in OA. Thus, while more than 90% of persons over the age of 40 have some radiographic changes of OA in weight-bearing joints, only 30% of these persons are symptomatic.

No laboratory studies are diagnostic for OA, but specific laboratory testing may help in identifying one of the underlying causes of secondary OA (Table 321-1). Because primary OA is not systemic, the erythrocyte sedimentation rate, serum chemistry determinations, blood counts, and urinalysis are normal. Analysis of synovial fluid reveals mild leukocytosis (<2000 white blood cells per microliter), with a predominance of mononuclear cells. Synovial fluid analysis is of particular value in excluding other conditions, such as calcium pyrophosphate dihydrate deposition disease (Chap. 322), gout (Chap. 322), or septic arthritis (Chap. 323).

Prior to the appearance of radiographic changes, the ability to diagnose OA clinically without an invasive procedure (e.g., arthroscopy) is limited. Approaches such as magnetic resonance imaging (MRI) and ultrasonography have not been sufficiently validated to justify their routine clinical use for diagnosis of OA or monitoring of disease progression.

OA AT SPECIFIC JOINT SITES   Interphalangeal Joints

Heberden's nodes, bony enlargements of the distal interphalangeal joints, are the most common form of idiopathic OA (Fig. 321-2). A similar process at the proximal interphalangeal joints leads to Bouchard's nodes. Often, these nodes develop gradually, with little or no discomfort. However, they may present acutely with pain, redness, and swelling, sometimes triggered by minor trauma. Gelatinous dorsal cysts filled with hyaluronic acid may develop at the insertion of the digital extensor tendon into the base of the distal phalanx.

Erosive OA   In erosive OA distal and/or proximal interphalangeal joints of the hands are most prominently affected. Erosive OA is more destructive than typical nodal OA; x-ray evidence of collapse of the subchondral plate is characteristic, and bony ankylosis may occur. Joint deformity and functional impairment may be severe. Pain and tenderness are commonly episodic. The synovium is much more extensively infiltrated with mononuclear cells than in other forms of OA.

Generalized OA   Generalized OA is characterized by involvement of three or more joints or groups of joints (distal interphalangeal and proximal interphalangeal joints are counted as one group each). Heberden's and Bouchard's nodes are prominent. Symptoms may be episodic, with "flare-ups" of inflammation marked by soft tissue swelling, redness, and warmth. The erythrocyte sedimentation rate may be elevated, but serum rheumatoid factor tests are negative.

Thumb Base   The second most frequent area of involvement in OA is the thumb base. Swelling, tenderness, and crepitus on movement of the joint are typical. Osteophytes may lead to a "squared" appearance of the thumb base (Fig. 321-3). In contrast to Heberden's nodes, which usually do not interfere significantly with function, thumb base OA frequently causes loss of motion and strength. Pain with pinch leads to adduction of the thumb and contracture of the first web space, often resulting in compensatory hyperextension of the first metacarpophalangeal joint and swan-neck deformity of the thumb.

The Hip   Congenital or developmental defects (e.g., acetabular dysplasia, Legg-Calvé-Perthes disease, slipped capital epiphysis) can lead to cases of hip OA. Some 20% of patients will develop bilateral involvement. Pain from hip OA is generally referred to the inguinal area but may be referred to the buttock or proximal thigh. Less commonly, hip OA presents as knee pain. Pain can be evoked by putting the involved hip through its range of motion. Flexion may be painless initially, but internal rotation will exacerbate pain. Loss of internal rotation occurs early, followed by loss of extension, adduction, and flexion due to capsular fibrosis and/or buttressing osteophytes.

The Knee   OA of the knee may involve the medial or lateral femorotibial compartment and/or the patellofemoral compartment. Palpation may reveal bony hypertrophy (osteophytes) and tenderness.

FIGURE 321-2   Nodal osteoarthritis. Note bony enlargement of distal and proximal interphalangeal joints (Heberden's nodes and Bouchard's nodes, respectively). *(Reprinted from the Clinical Slide Collection on the Rheumatic Diseases, © 1991, 1995. Reproduced with permission of the American College of Rheumatology.)*

FIGURE 321-3 Osteoarthritis of the first carpometacarpal joint. Note the squared appearance of the thumb base, due to bony enlargement and remodeling of the joint.

Effusions, if present, are generally small. Joint movement commonly elicits bony crepitus. OA in the medial compartment may result in a varus (bow-leg) deformity; in the lateral compartment it may produce a valgus (knock-knee) deformity. A positive "shrug" sign (pain when the patella is compressed manually against the femur during quadriceps contraction) may be a sign of patellofemoral OA.

Chondromalacia patellae, which also is characterized by anterior knee pain and a positive shrug sign, is a syndrome of patellofemoral pain, often bilateral, in teenagers and young adults. It is more common in females than in males. It may be caused by a variety of factors (e.g., abnormal quadriceps angle, patella alta, trauma). Although exploration of the knee may reveal softening and fibrillation of cartilage on the posterior aspect of the patella, this change is usually not progressive; chondromalacia patellae is usually not a precursor of OA. In most cases, analgesics or NSAIDs and physical therapy are effective; in some, pain may be relieved by surgical correction of patellar malalignment.

The Spine Degenerative disease of the spine can involve the apophyseal joint, intervertebral disks, and paraspinous ligaments. *Spondylosis* refers to degenerative *disk* disease. The diagnosis of spinal OA should be reserved for patients with involvement of the apophyseal joints and not only disk degeneration. Symptoms of spinal OA include localized pain and stiffness. Nerve root compression by an osteophyte blocking a neural foramen, prolapse of a degenerated disk, or subluxation of an apophyseal joint may cause radicular pain and motor weakness.

Marked calcification and ossification of paraspinous ligaments occur in *diffuse idiopathic skeletal hyperostosis* (DISH). Although DISH is often categorized as a variant of OA, diarthrodial joints are not involved. Ligamentous calcification and ossification in the anterior spinal ligaments give the appearance of "flowing wax" on the anterior vertebral bodies. However, a radiolucency may be seen between the newly deposited bone and the vertebral body, differentiating DISH from the marginal osteophytes in spondylosis. Intervertebral disk spaces are preserved, and sacroiliac and apophyseal joints appear normal, helping to differentiate DISH from spondylosis and from ankylosing spondylitis, respectively. DISH occurs in the middle-aged and elderly and is more common in men than in women. Patients are frequently asymptomatic but may have musculoskeletal stiffness. The radiographic changes are generally much more severe than might be predicted from the mild symptoms.

℞ TREATMENT Treatment of OA is aimed at reducing pain, maintaining mobility, and minimizing disability. The vigor of the therapeutic intervention should be dictated by the severity of the condition in the individual patient. For those with only mild disease, reassurance, instruction in joint protection, and an occasional analgesic

may be all that is required; for those with more severe OA, especially of the knee or hip, a comprehensive program comprising a spectrum of nonpharmacologic measures supplemented by an analgesic and/or NSAID is appropriate.

Nonpharmacologic Measures • *Reduction of joint loading* OA may be caused or aggravated by poor body mechanics. Correction of poor posture and a support for excessive lumbar lordosis can be helpful. Excessive loading of the involved joint should be avoided. Patients with OA of the knee or hip should avoid prolonged standing, kneeling, and squatting. Obese patients should be counseled to lose weight. In patients with medial-compartment knee OA, a wedged insole may decrease joint pain.

Rest periods during the day may be of benefit, but complete immobilization of the painful joint is rarely indicated. In patients with unilateral OA of the hip or knee, a cane, held in the contralateral hand, may reduce joint pain by reducing the joint contact force. Bilateral disease may necessitate use of crutches or a walker.

Physical therapy Application of heat to the OA joint may reduce pain and stiffness. A variety of modalities are available; often, the least expensive and most convenient is a hot shower or bath. Occasionally, better analgesia may be obtained with ice than with heat.

It is important to note that patients with OA of weight-bearing joints are less active and tend to be less fit with regard to musculoskeletal and cardiovascular status than normal controls. An exercise program should be designed to maintain range of motion, strengthen periarticular muscles, and improve physical fitness. The benefits of aerobic exercise include increases in aerobic capacity, muscle strength, and endurance; less exertion with a given workload; and weight loss. Those who exercise regularly live longer and are healthier than those who are sedentary. Patients with hip or knee OA can participate safely in conditioning exercises to improve fitness and health without increasing their joint pain or need for analgesics or NSAIDs.

Disuse of the OA joint because of pain will lead to muscle atrophy. Because periarticular muscles play a major role in protecting the articular cartilage from stress, strengthening exercises are important. In individuals with knee OA, strengthening of the periarticular muscles may result, within weeks, in a decrease in joint pain as great as that seen with NSAIDs.

Drug Therapy of OA Therapy for OA today is palliative; no pharmacologic agent has been shown to prevent, delay the progression of, or reverse the pathologic changes of OA in humans. Although claims have been made that some NSAIDs have a "chondroprotective effect," adequately controlled clinical trials in humans with OA to support this view are lacking. In management of OA pain, pharmacologic agents should be used as adjuncts to nonpharmacologic measures, such as those described above, which are the keystone of OA treatment.

Although NSAIDs often decrease joint pain and improve mobility in OA, the magnitude of this improvement is generally modest—on average, about 30% reduction in pain and 15% improvement in function. In a double-blinded, controlled trial in patients with symptomatic knee OA, an anti-inflammatory dose of ibuprofen (2400 mg/d) was no more effective than a low (i.e., essentially analgesic) dose of ibuprofen (1200 mg/d) or than acetaminophen (4000 mg/d), a drug with essentially no anti-inflammatory effect. Other studies confirm that an analgesic dose of ibuprofen may be as effective as anti-inflammatory doses of other NSAIDs, including the potent agent, phenylbutazone (400 mg/d), in symptomatic treatment of OA. Even in the presence of clinical signs of inflammation (e.g., synovial effusion, tenderness), relief of joint pain by acetaminophen may be as effective as that achieved with an NSAID. Nonetheless, if simple analgesics are inadequate, it is reasonable to cautiously prescribe an NSAID for a patient with OA.

It should be recognized that concern over the use of NSAIDs in OA has grown in recent years because of side effects of these agents, especially those related to the gastrointestinal (GI) tract. Those at greatest risk for OA, i.e., the elderly, appear also to be at greater risk than younger individuals for GI symptoms, ulceration, hemorrhage, and death as a result of NSAID use. The annual rate of hospitalization for peptic ulcer disease among elderly current NSAID users was 16 per 1000—four times greater than that for persons not taking an NSAID. Among those age 65 and older, as many as 30% of all hospitalizations and deaths related to peptic ulcer disease have been attributed to NSAID use. In addition to age, risk factors for hemorrhage and other ulcer complications associated with NSAID use include a history of peptic ulcer disease or of upper GI bleeding, concomitant use of glucocorticoids or anticoagulants, and, possibly, smoking and alcohol consumption (Table 321-4).

In patients who carry risk factors for an NSAID-associated GI catastrophe, a cyclooxygenase (Cox)-2–specific NSAID may be preferable to even a low dose of a nonselective Cox inhibitor. In contrast to the NSAIDs available to date—all of which inhibit Cox-1 as well as Cox-2—two Cox-2-specific inhibitors (CSIs), celecoxib and rofecoxib, are now available. Both appear to be comparable in efficacy to the nonselective NSAIDs. Endoscopic studies have shown that both agents are associated with an incidence of gastroduodenal ulcer lower than that of comparator NSAIDs and comparable to that of placebo. Of additional advantage with respect to the issue of upper GI bleeding, CSIs do not have a clinically significant effect on platelet aggregation or bleeding time, suggesting that CSIs may be especially advantageous in patients at high risk for incurring an NSAID-associated GI catastrophe. Long-term studies are now in progress that are designed to ascertain whether clinically important differences exist between CSIs and nonselective NSAIDs with respect to major GI clinical outcomes.

Systemic glucocorticoids have no place in the treatment of OA. However, intra- or periarticular injection of a depot glucocorticoid preparation may provide marked symptomatic relief for weeks to months. Because studies in animal models have suggested that glucocorticoids may produce cartilage damage, and frequent injections of large amounts of steroids have been associated with joint breakdown in humans, the injection should generally not be repeated in a given joint more often than every 4 to 6 months.

Intraarticular injection of hyaluronic acid has been approved recently for treatment of patients with knee OA who have failed a program of nonpharmacologic therapy and simple analgesics. Because the duration of benefit following treatment may exceed by months the synovial half-life of exogenous hyaluronic acid, the mechanism of action is unclear. The placebo response to intraarticular injection of hyaluronic acid is often large and sustained. Although relief of knee pain is achieved more slowly after hyaluronic acid injection than after intraarticular glucocorticoid injection, the effect may last much longer after hyaluronic acid injection than after glucocorticoid injection.

Capsaicin cream, which depletes local sensory nerve endings of substance P, a neuropeptide mediator of pain, may reduce joint pain and tenderness when applied topically by patients with hand or knee OA, even when used as monotherapy, i.e., without NSAIDs or systemic analgesics.

A Rational Approach to the Nonsurgical Management of OA Nonpharmacologic management is the foundation of treatment of OA pain and is as important as—and often more important than—drug treatment, which should play an adjunctive or complementary role in the management of this disease. Nonpharmacologic measures may comprise instruction of the patient in principles of joint protection; thermal modalities; exercises to strengthen periarticular muscles;

Table 321-4   Risk Factors for Upper Gastrointestinal Adverse Events in Patients Taking NSAIDs

Increasing age	History of upper gastrointestinal bleeding
Comorbidity (poor or fair general health)	Anticoagulation
Oral glucocorticoids	Combination NSAID therapy
History of peptic ulcer disease	Increasing NSAID dose

weight reduction, if the patient is obese; avoidance of excessive loading of the arthritic hip or knee joint by use of shoes with well-cushioned soles and a cane or walker, when appropriate; and prescription of orthotics for the patient with varus or valgus knee deformity. Medial taping of the patella may reduce knee pain in patients with patellofemoral OA. In patients with painful knee OA, if the above measures are ineffective, tidal irrigation of the joint with a large quantity of saline or Ringer's lactate warrants consideration (see below). A health education program designed to assist the patient with self-management can reduce pain and decrease health care costs; the benefits may persist for years. At any point in the course of OA, if acute joint pain and effusion develop, intraarticular injection of glucocorticoids may be indicated once joint infection is excluded by synovial fluid analysis.

Figure 321-4 provides an algorithm that might be applied to treatment of a newly diagnosed patient with knee OA. The progressive levels of treatment are associated with increasing cost, decreasing convenience for the patient, and increasing risk of side effects. The scheme should not be interpreted dogmatically as a fixed progression of steps; rather, treatment of OA must be individualized. The treatment program should be flexible. For example, in some patients it may be reasonable to institute patellar taping or prescribe a wedged insole on the initial visit, or an intraarticular glucocorticoid injection on a later visit. As indicated above, maintaining regular contact with the patient, e.g., via periodic telephone calls, may reduce joint pain to a level beyond what can be achieved with an NSAID alone, and this, or some surrogate measure, warrants incorporation into the treatment program (Fig. 321-4).

Because of its low cost, excellent safety profile, and an efficacy in many patients comparable to that of NSAIDs, when an analgesic is required for treatment of OA pain it is reasonable to prescribe acetaminophen initially, in a dose up to 4000 mg/d. If this does not control joint symptoms within a reasonable period of time, a *low dose* of NSAID (e.g., ibuprofen, 1200 mg/d; naproxen, 500 mg/d) may be substituted for, or added to, the acetaminophen. If a nonselective NSAID is used, even in a low dose, it is reasonable to recommend coadministration of a gastroprotective agent, such as misoprostol, or a proton pump inhibitor, such as famotidine or omeprazole, which have been shown by endoscopy to be effective in treating and preventing NSAID gastropathy. Because the risk of an NSAID-associated GI catastrophe is dose-dependent, the lowest effective dose of NSAID should be employed. Salsalate and other nonacetylated salicylates, which have only a minimal effect on prostaglandin synthase, are as effective as other NSAIDs and have a lower rate of serious GI side effects. However, phototoxicity and central nervous system toxicity may limit their use.

If the above approach does not provide adequate symptomatic relief, tramadol, a weak opioid, for which the risks of tolerance and addiction appear to be minimal, may be prescribed. Mean daily doses have typically been in the range of 200 to 300 mg. Side effects (e.g., nausea and vomiting, constipation, and drowsiness) are common, but their frequency may be reduced by initiating treatment with a dose of only 25 mg/d, which is then gradually increased over the next several days. If this is not effective or opioids are contraindicated, an anti-inflammatory dose of a CSI or of a nonselective NSAID may be prescribed, with coadministration of a gastroprotective agent in the latter instance.

When NSAIDs are required, they may be prescribed on an "as needed" basis, rather than in a fixed daily dose; pain control has been shown to be comparable and the risk of toxicity will be reduced. Once treatment with an NSAID or simple analgesic is initiated, the need for continuation of that treatment requires ongoing assessment. For many patients with OA, it will be possible eventually to reduce the dose of drug or to use the agent only intermittently, during exacerbations of joint pain.

Tidal Irrigation   Copious irrigation of the OA knee to flush out fibrin, cartilage shards, and other debris may provide months of comfort for the patient whose joint pain has been refractory to analgesics, NSAIDs, and intraarticular glucocorticoid injections. It should be rec-

FIGURE 321-4 Algorithm for management of a newly diagnosed patient with knee OA. CSI, Cox-2-specific inhibitor; TF, tibiofemoral; PF, patellofemoral; PPI, proton pump inhibitor; d/c, discontinue *(Modified from Brandt, 1996, with permission.)*

ognized, however, that invasive procedures such as this are accompanied by a large placebo effect, and studies that include a sham lavage control group have not yet been reported.

Orthopedic Surgery Joint replacement surgery should be reserved for patients with advanced OA in whom aggressive medical management has failed. In such cases total joint arthroplasty may be remarkably effective in relieving pain and increasing mobility. Osteotomy, which is surgically more conservative, can eliminate concentrations of peak dynamic loading and may provide effective pain relief in patients with hip or knee OA. It is of greatest benefit when the disease is only moderately advanced. Arthroscopic removal of loose cartilage fragments can prevent locking and relieve pain. Chondroplasty (abrasion arthroplasty) has also had some popularity as treatment for OA, but well-controlled studies of its efficacy are lacking, and the fibrocartilage that resurfaces the abraded bone is inferior to normal hyaline cartilage in its ability to withstand mechanical loads. In patients who had undergone tibial osteotomy for medial compart-

ment knee OA, knee pain and function were not related to the extent of cartilage regeneration 2 years later.

Autologous chondrocyte transplantation and attempts at cartilage repair using mesenchymal stem cells and autologous osteochondral plugs are currently being used experimentally for repair of focal chondral defects, but have not proved to be effective in treatment of OA.

ACKNOWLEDGMENT
Kathie Lane provided exemplary secretarial assistance during the preparation of this manuscript.

BIBLIOGRAPHY

ANDERSON JJ, FELSON DT: Factors associated with osteoarthritis of the knee in the first national health and nutrition examination survey (HANES I). Evidence for an association with overweight, race, and physical demands of work. Am J Epidemiol 128: 179, 1988

BRADLEY JD et al: Comparison of an anti-inflammatory dose of ibuprofen, an analgesic dose of ibuprofen, and acetaminophen in the treatment of patients with osteoarthritis of the knee. N Engl J Med 325:87, 1991

—— et al: Treatment of knee osteoarthritis: Relationship of clinical features of joint inflammation to the response to a nonsteroidal antiinflammatory drug or pure analgesic. J Rheumatol 19:1950, 1992

BRANDT KD: Nonsurgical management of osteoarthritis with an emphasis on nonpharmacologic measures. Arch Fam Med 4:1057, 1995

——: *Diagnosis and Nonsurgical Management of Osteoarthritis.* Caddo, OK, Professional Communications, 1996, pp 1–225

——: Management of osteoarthritis, in *Textbook of Rheumatology,* 6th ed, WN Kelley et al (eds). Philadelphia, Saunders, 2000

——, FLUSSER D: Osteoarthritis, in *Prognosis in the Rheumatic Diseases,* N Bellamy (ed). Lancaster, UK, Kluwer Academic, 1991, pp 11–35

——, RADIN E: The physiology of articular stress: Osteoarthrosis. Hospital Pract 22: 103, 1987

FELSON DT: Epidemiology of osteoarthritis, in *Osteoarthritis,* KD Brandt et al (eds). Oxford, Oxford University Press, 1998, pp 13–22

GRIFFIN MR et al: Practical management of osteoarthritis: Integration of pharmacologic and nonpharmacologic measures. Arch Fam Med 4:1049, 1995

HOCHBERG MC et al: Guidelines for the medical management of osteoarthritis: Part I. Arthritis Rheum 38:1535, 1995

—— et al: Guidelines for the medical management of osteoarthritis: Part II. Arthritis Rheum 38:1541, 1995

MANKIN HJ: Clinical features of osteoarthritis, in *Textbook of Rheumatology,* 4th ed, WN Kelley et al (eds). Philadelphia, Saunders, 1993, pp 1374–1384

——, BRANDT KD: Pathogenesis of osteoarthritis, in *Textbook of Rheumatology,* 6th ed, WN Kelley et al (eds). Philadelphia, Saunders, 2000

—— et al: Workshop on Etiopathogenesis of Osteoarthritis. J Rheumatol 13:1127, 1986

MINOR MA: Exercise in the treatment of osteoarthritis. Rheum Dis Clin North Am 25: 397, 1999

PELLETIER JP et al: Reduced progression of experimental osteoarthritis in vivo by selective inhibition of inducible nitric oxide synthase. Arthritis Rheum 41:1275, 1998

RENÉ J et al: Reduction of joint pain in patients with knee osteoarthritis who have received monthly telephone calls from lay personnel and whose medical treatment regimens have remained stable. Arthritis Rheum 35:511, 1992

322   *Antonio J. Reginato*

GOUT AND OTHER CRYSTAL ARTHROPATHIES

"GOUT" CRYSTALLOGRAPHY AND ARTHRITIS   The use of polarizing microscopy during synovial fluid analysis and the application of other crystallographic techniques, such as electron microscopy, energy-dispersive elemental analysis, and x-ray diffraction, have established the role of different microcrystals, including monosodium urate (MSU), calcium pyrophosphate dihydrate (CPPD), calcium hydroxyapatite (HA), and calcium oxalate (CaOx), in inducing acute or chronic arthritis or periarthritis. In spite of differences in crystal morphology, chemistry, and physical properties, the clinical events that result from deposition of MSU, CPPD, HA, and CaOx may be indistinguishable (Table 322-1). Prior to the use of crystallographic techniques in rheumatology, much of what was considered to be MSU gouty arthritis in fact was not. Simkin has suggested that the generic term *gout* be used to describe the whole group of crystal-induced arthritides (MSU gout, CPPD gout, HA gout, and CaOx gout). This concept further emphasizes the identical clinical presentations of these entities (Table 322-1) and the need to perform synovial fluid analysis

Table 322-1   Musculoskeletal Manifestations of Crystal-Induced Arthritis

Acute mono- or polyarthritis	Destructive arthropathies
Bursitis	Pseudo-rheumatoid arthritis
Tendinitis	Pseudo-ankylosing spondylitis
Enthesitis	Spinal stenosis
Tophaceous deposits	Carpal tunnel syndrome
Peculiar type of osteoarthritis	Tendon rupture
Synovial osteochondromatosis	

to distinguish the type of crystal involved. In the setting of acute articular or periarticular inflammation, aspiration and analysis of effusions are most important to assess the possibility of infection and to identify the type of crystals present. Polarization microscopy alone can identify most typical crystals and allow diagnosis. HA, however, is an exception. Apart from the identification of specific microcrystalline materials or organisms, synovial fluid characteristics are nonspecific, and synovial fluid can be inflammatory or noninflammatory.

MONOSODIUMURATE GOUT   MSU gout is a metabolic disease most often affecting middle-aged to elderly men. It is typically associated with an increased uric acid pool, hyperuricemia, episodic acute and chronic arthritis, and deposition of MSU crystals in connective tissue tophi and kidneys (Chap. 347).

Acute and Chronic Arthritis   Acute arthritis is the most frequent early clinical manifestation of MSU gout. Usually, only one joint is affected initially, but polyarticular acute gout is also seen in male hypertensive patients with ethanol abuse as well as in postmenopausal women. The metatarsophalangeal joint of the first toe is often involved, but tarsal joints, ankles, and knees are also commonly affected. In elderly patients, finger joints may be inflamed. Inflamed Heberden's or Bouchard's nodes may be a first manifestation of gouty arthritis. The first episode of acute gouty arthritis frequently begins at night with dramatic joint pain and swelling. Joints rapidly become warm, red, and tender, and the clinical appearance often mimics a cellulitis. Early attacks tend to subside spontaneously within 3 to 10 days, and most of the patients do not have residual symptoms until the next episode. Several events may precipitate acute gouty arthritis: dietary excess, trauma, surgery, excessive ethanol ingestion, adrenocorticotropic hormone (ACTH) and glucocorticoid withdrawal, hypouricemic therapy, and serious medical illnesses such as myocardial infarction and stroke.

After many acute mono- or oligoarticular attacks, a proportion of gouty patients may present with a chronic nonsymmetric synovitis, causing potential confusion with rheumatoid arthritis (Chap. 312). Less commonly, chronic gouty arthritis will be the only manifestation and, more rarely, the disease will manifest as inflamed or noninflamed periarticular tophaceous deposits in the absence of chronic synovitis (Table 322-1). Women represent only 5 to 17% of all patients with gout. Premenopausal gout is a rare occurrence and accounts for only about 17% of all women with gout; it is seen mostly in individuals with a strong family history of gout. A few kindreds of precocious gout in young females caused by decreased renal urate clearance and renal insufficiency have been described. Most women with gouty arthritis are postmenopausal and elderly, have arterial hypertension causing mild renal insufficiency, and are usually receiving diuretics. Also, most of these patients have underlying degenerative joint disease, and inflamed tophaceous deposits may be seen on Heberden's and Bouchard's nodes.

Laboratory diagnosis   Even if the clinical appearance strongly suggests gout, the diagnosis should be confirmed by needle aspiration of acutely or chronically inflamed joints or tophaceous deposits. Acute septic arthritis, several of the other crystalline-associated arthropathies, palindromic rheumatism, and psoriatic arthritis may present with similar clinical features. During acute gouty attacks, strongly birefringent needle-shaped MSU crystals with negative elongation are largely intracellular (Fig. 322-1). Synovial fluid cell counts are elevated from 2000 to 60,000/μL. Effusions appear cloudy due to leukocytes, and large amounts crystals occasionally produce a thick pasty or chalky joint fluid. Bacterial infection can coexist with urate crystals in synovial fluid; if there is any suspicion of septic arthritis, joint fluid must also be cultured. MSU crystals can often be demonstrated in the first metatarsophalangeal (MTP) joint and in knees not acutely involved with gout. Arthrocentesis of these joints is a useful technique to establish the diagnosis of gout between attacks. Serum uric acid levels can be normal or low at the time of the acute attack, since lowering of uric acid with hypouricemic therapy or other medications limits the value of serum uric acid determinations for the diagnosis of gout. Despite these limitations, serum uric acid is almost always elevated at some time and can be used to follow the course of hypouricemic therapy. A 24-h urine collection for uric acid is valuable in assessing the risk of stones, in elucidating overproduction or underexcretion of uric acid, and in deciding which hypouricemic regimen to use (Chap. 347). Excretion of more than 800 mg of uric acid per 24 h on a regular diet suggests that causes of overproduction of purine should be considered. Urinalysis, blood urea nitrogen, serum creatinine, white blood cell (WBC) count, and serum lipids should be monitored because of possible pathologic sequelae of gout and other associated diseases requiring treatment.

Radiographic features Cystic changes, well-defined erosions described as punched-out lytic lesions with overhanging bony edges (Martel's sign), associated with soft tissue calcified masses are characteristic radiographic features of chronic tophaceous gout. However, similar radiographic signs can also be observed in erosive osteoarthritis, destructive apatite arthropathies, and rheumatoid arthritis.

FIGURE 322-1 Extracellular and intracellular monosodiun urate crystals, as seen in a fresh preparation of synovial fluid, illustrate needle- and rod-shaped strongly negative birefringent crystals (compensated polarized light microscopy; 400×).

℞ **TREATMENT** **Acute Gouty Arthritis**
The mainstay of treatment during an acute attack is the administration of an anti-inflammatory drug such as colchicine, nonsteroidal anti-inflammatory drugs (NSAIDs), or glucocorticoids depending on the age of the patient and comorbid conditions. Both colchicine and NSAIDs may be quite toxic in the elderly, particularly in the presence of renal insufficiency and gastrointestinal disorders. In elderly patients, one may favor the use of intraarticular glucocorticoid injections for attacks involving one or two larger joints or cool applications along with lower oral doses of colchicine for gouty synovitis affecting small joints. Colchicine given orally is a traditional and effective treatment, if used early in the attack, in at least 85% of patients. One tablet (0.6 mg) is given every hour until relief of symptoms or gastrointestinal toxicity occurs, or a total of four to eight tablets have been taken in accordance with the age of the patient. The drug must be stopped promptly at the first sign of loose stools, and symptomatic treatment must be given for the diarrhea. Intravenous colchicine is sometimes used and can reduce, though not eliminate, the gastrointestinal side effects. Intravenous colchicine is most reliable for pre- or postoperative prophylaxis in 1- to 2-mg doses when patients cannot take medications orally. Life-threatening colchicine toxicity and sudden death have been described with the administration of more than 4 mg/d intravenously. The intravenous dose for acute gouty arthritis is 1 to 2 mg given slowly through an established venous line over 10 min in a soluset, and two additional doses of 1 mg each may be given at 6-h intervals, but the total dose should never exceed 4 mg. NSAIDs are affective in about 90% of patients, and the resolution of signs and symptoms usually occurs in 5 to 7 days. The most effective drugs are those with a short half-life and include indomethacin, 25 to 50 mg tid, ibuprofen, 800 mg tid, or diclofenac, 50 mg tid. Cyclooxigenase-2-specific inhibitors are probably equally effective but with less short-term gastrointestinal toxicity. Oral glucocorticoids such as prednisone, 30 to 50 mg/d as the initial dose and tapered over 5 to 7 days, a single intravenous dose of methylprednisolone, 7 mg of betametasone, or 60 mg of triamcinolone acetonide have been equally effective. ACTH as an intramuscular injection of 40 to 80 IU in a single dose or every 12 h for 1 to 2 days is effective in patients with acute polyarticular refractory gout or with a contraindication for using colchicine or NSAIDs.

Hypouricemic Therapy Attempts to normalize serum uric acid to <300 μmol/L (5.0 mg/dL) to prevent recurrent gouty attacks and eliminate tophaceous deposits entail a commitment to long-term hypouricemic regimens and medications that generally are required for life. Hypouricemic therapy should be considered when the hyperuricemia cannot be corrected by simple means (control of body weight, low-purine diet, increase in liquid ingestion, limitation of ethanol intake, and avoidance of diuretic use). The decision to initiate hypouricemic therapy is usually made taking into consideration the number of acute attacks, family history of gout, presence of MSU tophaceous deposits, uric acid excretion >800 mg per 24 hours, presence of uric acid stones, and risk for acute uric acid nephropathy during chemotherapy for myeloproliferative disorders. Uricosuric agents, such as probenecid, can be used in patients with good renal function who underexcrete uric acid, with <600 mg in a 24-hour urine sample. Urine volume must be maintained by ingestion of 1500 mL of water every day. Probenecid can be started at a dosage of 200 mg twice daily and increased gradually as needed up to 2 g in order to maintain a serum uric acid level <300 μmol/L (5 mg/dL). Probenecid is the drug of choice to treat elderly patients with hypertension and thiazide dependence; however, probenecid is not effective with a renal creatinine clearance <1 mL/s. These patients may require allopurinol or benzbromarone (not available in the United States), which is another uricosuric drug that is effective in patients with renal failure and who are receiving diuretics. Allopurinol is the best drug to lower serum urate in overproducers, stone formers, and patients with advanced renal failure. It can be given in a single morning dose, 300 mg initially and increasing up to 800 mg if needed. In most patients, it is not necessary to start at a lower dose; however, in patients with renal failure, the dosage should be adjusted depending on the serum creatinine concentration in order to minimize side effects. Patients with frequent acute attacks may require lower initial doses to prevent exacerbations. Toxicity of allopurinol has been recognized increasingly in patients with renal failure who use thiazide diuretics and in those patients allergic to penicillin and ampicillin. The most serious side effects include skin rash with progression to life-threatening toxic epidermal necrolysis, systemic vasculitis, bone marrow suppression, granulomatous hepatitis, and renal failure. Urate-lowering drugs should not be initiated during acute attacks. This is especially important in patients who have refractory acute arthritis or who had a flare-up previously with hypouricemic drugs. Colchicine prophylaxis in doses of 0.6 mg one to two times daily is usually continued, along with hypouricemic therapy, until the patient is normouricemic and without gouty attacks for 3 months. However, prophylactic colchicine treatment may be necessary as long as tophi are present.

CPPD DEPOSITION DISEASE **Pathogenesis** The deposition of CPPD crystals in articular tissues is most common in the elderly, affecting 10 to 15% of persons 65 to 75 years old and 30 to

60% of those more than 85 years old. In most cases this process is asymptomatic, and the cause of CPPD deposition is uncertain. Because over 80% of patients are more than 60 years old and 70% have preexisting joint damage from other conditions, it is likely that biochemical changes in aging cartilage favor crystal nucleation. Examples of such chemical alterations include the following. There is an increased production of inorganic pyrophosphate and decreased levels of pyrophosphatases in cartilage extracts from patients with CPPD arthritis. The increase in pyrophosphate production appears to be related to enhanced activity of ATP pyrophosphohydrolase and $5'$-nucleotidase, which catalyze the reaction of ATP to adenosine and pyrophosphate. This pyrophosphate could combine with calcium to form CPPD crystals in matrix vesicles or on collagen fibers. There is a diminution in the levels of cartilage glycosaminoglycans that normally inhibit and regulate crystal nucleation. These deficiencies may lead to increased crystal deposition. In vitro studies have demonstrated that transforming growth factor $\beta 1$ and epidermal growth factor both stimulate the production of pyrophosphate by articular cartilage and thus may contribute to the deposition of CPPD crystals. The release of CPPD crystals into the joint space is followed by the phagocytosis of these crystals by neutrophils, which respond by releasing inflammatory substances. In addition, neutrophils release a glycopeptide that is chemotactic for other neutrophils, thus augmenting the inflammatory events. The same substance is present in MSU gout.

A minority of patients with CPPD arthropathy have metabolic abnormalities or hereditary CPPD disease (Table 322-2). These associations suggest that a variety of different metabolic products may enhance CPPD deposition. Included among these conditions are the "four H's" of hyperparathyroidism, hemochromatosis, hypophosphatasia, and hypomagnesemia. Hemochromatosis and hyperparathyroidism are good examples. Ferrous ions and hypercalcemia may either directly alter cartilage or inhibit inorganic pyrophosphatases, leading to enhanced susceptibility to CPPD deposition. The presence of CPPD arthritis in individuals less than 50 years old should lead to consideration of these metabolic disorders and inherited forms of disease, including those identified in a variety of ethnic groups (Table 322-2). Genomic DNA studies performed on four different kindreds have shown a possible location of the genetic defects on chromosome 8q in one, and on chromosome 5p in the other three. Identification of these genes will help elucidate the pathogenesis of both the familial and the more common sporadic form of the disease. Investigation should include inquiry for evidence of familial aggregation and evaluation of serum calcium, phosphorus, alkaline phosphatase, magnesium, serum ferritin, and transferritin saturation.

Clinical Manifestations CPPD arthropathy may be asymptomatic, acute, subacute, or chronic or cause acute synovitis superimposed on chronically involved joints. Acute CPPD arthritis was originally termed *pseudogout* by McCarty and coworkers because of its striking similarity to MSU gout. Other clinical manifestations of CPPD deposition include (1) induction or enhancement of peculiar forms of osteoarthritis; (2) induction of severe destructive disease that may radiographically mimic neuropathic arthritis; (3) production of symmetric proliferative synovitis, clinically similar to rheumatoid arthritis and frequently seen in familial forms with early onset; (4) intervertebral disk and ligament calcification with restriction of spine mobility, mimicking ankylosing spondylitis (also seen in hereditary forms); and (5) rarely spinal stenosis (most commonly seen in the elderly (Table 322-1).

The knee is the joint most frequently affected in CPPD arthropathy. Other sites include the wrist, shoulder, ankle, elbow, and hands. Rarely, the temporomandibular joint and ligamentum flavum of the spinal canal are involved. Clinical and radiographic evidence indicates that CPPD deposition is polyarticular in at least two-thirds of patients. When the clinical picture resembles that of slowly progressive osteoarthritis, diagnosis may be more difficult. Joint distribution may provide important clues suggesting CPPD disease. For example, primary osteoarthritis rarely involves a metacarpophalangeal, wrist, elbow, shoulder, or ankle joint. If radiographs reveal punctate and/or linear radiodense deposits in fibrocartilaginous joint menisci or articular hyaline cartilage (chondrocalcinosis), the diagnostic certainty of CPPD is further enhanced. *Definitive diagnosis* requires demonstration of typical crystals in synovial fluid or articular tissue (Fig. 322-2). In the absence of joint effusion or indications to obtain a synovial biopsy, chondrocalcinosis is presumptive of CPPD deposition. One exception is chondrocalcinosis due to CaOx in some patients with chronic renal failure.

Acute attacks of CPPD arthritis may be precipitated by trauma, arthroscopy, or hyaluronate injections. Rapid diminution of serum calcium concentration, as may occur in severe medical illness or after surgery (especially parathyroidectomy), can also lead to pseudogout attacks.

In as many as 50% of cases, CPPD gout is associated with low-grade fever and, on occasion, temperatures as high as 40°C. Whether or not radiographic proof of chondrocalcinosis is evident in the involved joint(s), synovial analysis with microbial cultures is essential to rule out the possibility of infection. In fact, infection in a joint with any microcrystalline deposition process can lead to crystal shedding and subsequent synovitis from both crystals and microorganisms. Synovial fluid in acute CPPD gout has inflammatory qualities. The WBC count can range from several thousand cells to 100,000 cells/μL, the

Table 322-2   Conditions Associated with Calcium Pyrophosphate Dihydrate Disease

Aging
Disease-associated
  Primary hyperparathyroidism
  Hemochromatosis
  Hypophosphatasia
  Hypomagnesemia
  Chronic tophaceous gout
  Post-meniscectomy
Epiphyseal dysplasias
Hereditary: Slovakian-Hungarian, Spanish, Spanish-American (Argentian, Colombian, and Chilean), French, Swedish, Dutch, Canadian, Mexican-American, Italian-American, German-American, Japanese, Tunisian, Jewish, English

FIGURE 322-2   Intracellular and extracellular calcium pyrophosphate dihydrate crystals, as seen in a fresh preparation of synovial fluid, illustrate rectangular, rod-shaped, and rhomboid weakly positive birefringent crystals (compensated polarized light microscopy; 400×).

mean being about 24,000 cells/μL and the predominant cell being the neutrophil. Polarization microscopy usually reveals rhomboid crystals with weak positive birefringence inside fibrim and in neutrophils (Fig. 322-2).

℞ **TREATMENT** Untreated acute attacks may last a few days to as long as a month. Treatment by joint aspiration and NSAIDs, or colchicine, or intraarticular glucocorticoid injection may result in return to prior status in 10 days or less. For patients with frequent recurrent attacks of CPPD gout, daily prophylactic treatment with low doses of colchicine may be helpful in decreasing the frequency of the attacks. Severe polyarticular attacks usually require short courses of glucocorticoids. Unfortunately, there is no effective way to remove CPPD deposits from cartilage and synovium. Uncontrolled studies suggest that radioactive synovectomy (with yttrium 90) or the administration of antimalarial agents may be helpful in controlling persistent synovitis. Patients with progressive destructive large-joint arthropathy usually require joint replacement.

FIGURE 322-3 *A*. Cytoplasmic round inclusions inside synovial fluid cells represent aggregates of apatite crystals (fresh preparation, ordinary light microscopy; 288×). *B*. An electron micrograph demonstrates a cluster of dark apatite crystals within a synovial fluid mononuclear cell (21,600×).

CALCIUM HYDROXYAPATITE DEPOSITION DISEASE

Pathogenesis HA is the primary mineral of bone and teeth. Abnormal accumulation can occur in areas of tissue damage (dystrophic calcification), in hypercalcemic or hyperparathyroid states (metastatic calcification), and in certain conditions of unknown cause (Table 322-3). In chronic renal failure, hyperphosphatemia enhances HA deposition both in and around joints.

HA may be released from exposed bone and cause the acute synovitis occasionally seen in chronic stable osteoarthritis (e.g., "hot" Heberden's nodes). HA deposition is also an important factor in an extremely destructive chronic arthropathy of the elderly that occurs most often in knees and shoulders (Milwaukee shoulder). Joint destruction is associated with attenuation or rupture of supporting structures, leading to instability and deformity. Progression tends to be indolent, and synovial fluid WBC counts are usually less than 1000/μL. Symptoms range from minimal to severe pain and disability that may lead to joint replacement surgery. Whether severely affected patients merely represent an extreme synovial tissue response to the HA crystals that are so common in osteoarthritis is uncertain. Synovial

Table 322-3 Conditions Associated with Hydroxyapatite Deposition Disease

Aging
Osteoarthritis
Hemorrhagic shoulder effusions in the elderly (Milwaukee shoulder)
Destructive arthropathy
Tendinitis, bursitis
Tumoral calcinosis (sporadic cases)
Disease-associated
  Hyperparathyroidism
  Milk alkali syndrome
  Renal failure/long-term dialysis
  Connective tissue diseases (e.g., progressive systemic sclerosis, CREST syndrome, idiopathic myositis, SLE)
  Heterotopic calcification following neurologic catastrophes (e.g., stroke, spinal cord injury)
Hereditary
  Bursitis, arthritis
  Tumoral calcinosis
  Fibrodysplasia ossificans progressiva

NOTE: CREST, calcinosis cutis, Raynaud's phenomenon, esophageal dysmotility, sclerodactyly, telangiectasia; SLE, systemic lupus erythematosus.

membrane tissue cultures exposed to HA (or CPPD) crystals markedly increased the release of collagenases and neutral proteases, underscoring the destructive potential of abnormally stimulated synovial lining cells.

Clinical Manifestations Periarticular and articular deposits may coexist and be associated with acute and/or chronic damage to the joint capsule, tendons, bursa, or articular surfaces. The most common sites of HA deposition include bursae and tendons in and/or around the knees, shoulders, hips, and fingers. Clinical manifestations include asymptomatic radiographic abnormalities, acute synovitis, bursitis, tendinitis, and chronic destructive arthropathy. Most patients with HA arthropathy are elderly. Although the true incidence of HA arthritis is not known, 30 to 50% of patients with osteoarthritis have HA microcrystals in their synovial fluid. Such crystals can frequently be identified in clinically stable osteoarthritic joints, but they are more likely to come to attention in persons experiencing acute or subacute worsening of joint pain and swelling. The synovial fluid WBC count in HA arthritis is usually low (<2000/μL) but may at times have as many as 50,000/μL. Most synovial fluid analyses reveal a predominance of mononuclear cells. Occasionally, neutrophils may dominate.

Diagnosis Radiographic findings in HA arthropathy are not diagnostic. Intra- and/or periarticular calcifications with or without erosive, destructive, or hypertrophic changes may be present.

Definitive diagnosis of HA arthropathy depends on identification of crystals from synovial fluid or tissue (Fig. 322-3). Individual crystals are very small, nonbirefringent, and can only be seen by electron microscopy. Clumps of crystals may appear as 1- to 20-μm shiny intra- or extracellular globules that stain purplish with Wright's stain and bright red with alizarin red S. Absolute identification depends on electron microscopy with energy-dispersive elemental analysis, x-ray diffraction, or infrared spectroscopy.

℞ **TREATMENT** Treatment of HA arthritis is nonspecific. Acute attacks of bursitis or synovitis may be self-limiting, resolving in from days to several weeks. Aspiration of effusions and the use of either NSAIDs or oral colchicine for 2 weeks or intra- or periarticular injection of glucocorticoid salts appear to shorten the duration and intensity of symptoms. In patients with underlying severe destructive articular changes, response to medical therapy is usually less rewarding.

CaOx DEPOSITION DISEASE **Pathogenesis** *Primary oxalosis* is a rare hereditary metabolic disorder (Chap. 352). Enhanced production of oxalic acid may result from at least two different enzyme defects, leading to hyperoxalemia and deposition of calcium oxalate crystals in tissues. Nephrocalcinosis, renal failure, and death usually

FIGURE 322-4   Bipyramidal and small polymorphic calcium oxalate crystals (ordinary light microscopy; 400×).

occur before age 20. Acute and/or chronic CaOx arthritis and periarthritis may complicate primary oxalosis during later years of illness.

Secondary oxalosis is more common than the primary disorder. It is one of the many metabolic abnormalities that complicate end-stage renal disease (ESRD). In ESRD, calcium oxalate deposits have long been recognized in visceral organs, blood vessels, bones, and even cartilage. However, it was not until 1982 that such deposits were demonstrated to be one of the causes of arthritis in chronic renal failure. Thus far, reported patients have been dependent on long-term hemodialysis or peritoneal dialysis (Chap. 272), and many had received ascorbic acid supplements. Ascorbic acid is metabolized to oxalate, which is inadequately cleared in uremia and by dialysis. Such supplements are now usually avoided in dialysis programs because of the risk of enhancing hyperoxalosis and its sequelae.

Clinical Manifestations and Diagnosis   As was noted for the other calcium salts, CaOx aggregates can be found in bone, articular cartilage, synovium, and periarticular tissues. From these sites, crystals may be shed, causing acute synovitis. Persistent aggregates of CaOx may, like HA and CPPD, stimulate synovial proliferation and enzyme release, resulting in progressive articular destruction. Deposits have been documented in fingers, wrists, elbows, knees, ankles, and feet.

Each of the known microcrystalline arthropathies may be a complication of ESRD, and rare patients have more than one type of crystal present in a joint effusion. The advent of crystallographic techniques has made it clear that most arthritic problems in ESRD are not, as was once believed, due to MSU gout. Clinical features of acute CaOx arthritis may not be distinguishable from those due to sodium urate, CPPD, or HA. Radiographs may reveal chondrocalcinosis, a feature of either CPPD or CaOx deposition. CaOx-induced synovial effusions are usually noninflammatory, with fewer than 2000 leukocytes/μL. Neutrophils or mononuclear cells have predominated. CaOx crystals have a variable shape and variable birefringence to polarized light. The most easily recognized forms are bipyramidal and have strong positive birefringence (Fig. 322-4).

℞ **TREATMENT**   Treatment of CaOx arthropathy with NSAIDs, colchicine, intraarticular glucocorticoids, and/or an increased frequency of dialysis has produced only slight improvement. In primary oxalosis, liver transplantation has induced a significant reduction in crystal deposits (Chap. 352).

BIBLIOGRAPHY

ANDREW LJ et al: Refinement of the chromosome 5p locus for familial calcium pyrophosphate dihydrate deposition disease. Am J Med Genet 64:136, 1999

BENHAMOU CL et al: Bone involvement in primary oxalosis (study of 20 cases). Rev Rhum Mal Osteoartic 58:763, 1991

DIEPPE PA et al: Apatite deposition disease: A new arthropathy. Lancet 1:266, 1976

DOHERTY M et al: Inorganic pyrophosphate in metabolic diseases predisposing to calcium pyrophosphate dihydrate crystal deposition. Arthritis Rheum 34:1297, 1991

EMERSON BE: The management of gout. N Engl J Med 334:445, 1996

GEORGE T, MANDEL B: Gout in the transplant patients. J Clin Rheumatol 1:328, 1995

MASUDA I et al: Inorganic pyrophosphate metabolism, in *Gout, Hyperuricemia and Other Crystal-Associated Arthropathies*, Ch J Smyth, VM Holers (eds). New York, Marcel Dekker, 1999, pp 359–367

PEREZ RUIZ F et al: Treatment of chronic gout in patients with renal function impairment. An open, randomized, actively controlled study. J Clin Rheumatol 5:49, 1999

REGINATO AJ, FALASCA GF: Calcium oxalate and other miscellaneous crystal-related arthropathies, in *Gout, Hyperuricemia and Other Crystal-Associated Arthropathies*, ChJ Smyth, VM Holers (eds). New York, Marcel Dekker, 1999, pp 370–393

———, SCHUMACHER HR: Apatite crystals in joint fluid: Clinical relevance and search for a simple and accurate diagnostic test. Rheumatol Rev 3:9, 1994

——— et al: Familial calcium pyrophosphate crystal deposition disease or calcium pyrophosphate gout. Rev Rheum [Engl Ed] 62:376, 1995

ROSENTHAL AK, RYAN LM: Treatment of refractory crystal-associated arthritis. Rheum Dis Clin North Am 21:151, 1995

SIMKIN PA: Oxalate crystals and the taxonomy of gout. JAMA 260:1285, 1988

---

323   *Scott J. Thaler, James H. Maguire*

INFECTIOUS ARTHRITIS

INTRODUCTION AND APPROACH TO THE PATIENT

While *Staphylococcus aureus, Neisseria gonorrhoeae*, and other bacteria are the most common causes of infectious arthritis, various mycobacteria, spirochetes, fungi, and viruses also infect joints. Since acute bacterial infection can rapidly destroy articular cartilage, all inflamed joints must be evaluated without delay to exclude noninfectious processes and to determine appropriate antimicrobial therapy and drainage procedures. For more detailed information on infectious arthritis due to specific organisms, the reader is referred to the chapters on those organisms.

Acute bacterial infection typically involves a single joint or a few joints. Subacute or chronic monarthritis or oligoarthritis suggests mycobacterial or fungal infection; episodic inflammation is seen in syphilis, Lyme disease, and the reactive arthritis that follows enteric infections and chlamydial urethritis (Table 323-1). Acute polyarticular inflammation occurs as an immunologic reaction during the course of endocarditis, rheumatic fever, disseminated neisserial infection, and acute hepatitis B. Bacteria and viruses occasionally infect multiple joints, the former most commonly in persons with rheumatoid arthritis.

Aspiration of synovial fluid, an essential element in the evaluation of potentially infected joints, can be performed without difficulty in most cases by the insertion of a large-bore needle into the site of maximal fluctuation or tenderness or by the route of easiest access. Ultrasonography or fluoroscopy may be used to guide aspiration of difficult-to-localize effusions of the hip and, occasionally, the shoulder and other joints. Normal synovial fluid contains <180 cells (predominantly mononuclear cells) per microliter. Synovial cell counts averaging 100,000/μL (range, 25,000 to 250,000/μL), with >90% neutrophils, are characteristic of acute bacterial infections. Crystal-induced, rheumatoid, and other noninfectious inflammatory arthritides are usually associated with <30,000 to 50,000 cells/μL; cell counts of 10,000 to 30,000/μL, with 50 to 70% neutrophils and the remainder lymphocytes, are common in mycobacterial and fungal infections. Definitive diagnosis of an infectious process relies on identification of the pathogen in stained smears of synovial fluid, isolation of the pathogen from cultures of synovial fluid and blood, or detection of microbial nucleic acids and proteins by polymerase chain reaction (PCR)–based assays and immunologic techniques.

ACUTE BACTERIAL ARTHRITIS Pathogenesis   Bacteria enter the joint from the bloodstream, from a contiguous site of infection in bone or soft tissue, or by direct inoculation during surgery, injection, or trauma. In hematogenous infection, bacteria escape from synovial capillaries, which have no limiting basement membrane, and within hours provoke neutrophilic infiltration of the synovium. Neutrophils and bacteria enter the joint space; later, bacteria adhere to articular cartilage. Degradation of cartilage begins within 48 h as a result of increased intraarticular pressure, release of proteases and cytokines from chondrocytes and synovial macrophages, and invasion of the cartilage by bacteria and inflammatory cells. Histologic studies reveal bacteria lining the synovium and cartilage as well as abscesses extending into the synovium, cartilage, and—in severe cases—subchondral bone. Synovial proliferation results in the formation of a pannus over the cartilage, and thrombosis of inflamed synovial vessels develops. Bacterial factors that appear important in the pathogenesis of infective arthritis include various surface-associated adhesins in *S. aureus* that permit adherence to cartilage and endotoxins that promote chondrocyte-mediated breakdown of cartilage.

Microbiology The hematogenous route of infection is the most common route in all age groups. In infants, group B streptococci, gram-negative enteric bacilli, and *S. aureus* are the usual pathogens. Since the advent of the *Haemophilus influenzae* vaccine, *S. aureus*, *Streptococcus pyogenes* (group A *Streptococcus*), and (in some centers) *Kingella kingae* have predominated among children <5 years of age. Among young adults and adolescents, *N. gonorrhoeae* is the most commonly implicated organism. *S. aureus* accounts for most nongonococcal isolates in adults of all ages; gram-negative bacilli, pneumococci, and β-hemolytic streptococci—particularly groups A and B, but also groups C, G, and F—are involved in up to one-third of cases in older adults, especially those with underlying comorbid illnesses.

Infections following surgical procedures or penetrating injuries are due most often to *S. aureus* and occasionally to other gram-positive bacteria or gram-negative bacilli. Infections with coagulase-negative staphylococci are unusual except after the implantation of prosthetic joints or arthroscopy. Anaerobic organisms, often in association with aerobic or facultative bacteria, are found after human bites and when decubitus ulcers or intraabdominal abscesses spread into adjacent joints. Polymicrobial infections complicate traumatic injuries with extensive contamination. Cat bites or scratches may introduce *Pasteurella multocida* into joints.

Nongonococcal Bacterial Arthritis • *Epidemiology* Although hematogenous infections with virulent organisms such as *S. aureus*, *H. influenzae*, and pyogenic streptococci occur in healthy persons, there is an underlying host predisposition in many cases of septic arthritis. Patients with rheumatoid arthritis have the highest incidence of infective arthritis, most often secondary to *S. aureus*, because of chronically inflamed joints, glucocorticoid therapy, and frequent breakdown of rheumatoid nodules, vasculitic ulcers, and skin overlying deformed joints. Diabetes mellitus, glucocorticoid therapy, hemodialysis, and malignancy all carry an increased risk of infection with *S. aureus* and gram-negative bacilli. Pneumococcal infections complicate alcoholism, deficiencies of humoral immunity, and hemoglobinopathies. Pneumococci, *Salmonella*, and *H. influenzae* cause septic arthritis in persons infected with HIV. Persons with primary immunoglobulin deficiency are at risk for mycoplasmal arthritis, which results in permanent joint damage if treatment with tetracycline and intravenous immunoglobulin replacement is not administered promptly. Intravenous drug users acquire staphylococcal and streptococcal infections from their own flora and acquire pseudomonal and other gram-negative infections from drugs and injection paraphernalia.

Clinical manifestations Some 90% of patients present with involvement of a single joint: most commonly the knee, less frequently

Table 323-1 Differential Diagnosis of Arthritis Syndromes

Acute Monarticular Arthritis	Chronic Monarticular Arthritis	Polyarticular Arthritis
Staphylococcus aureus	*Mycobacterium tuberculosis*	*Neisseria meningitidis*
Streptococcus pneumoniae	Nontuberculous mycobacteria	*N. gonorrhoeae*
β-Hemolytic streptococci	*Borrelia burgdorferi*	Nongonococcal bacterial arthritis
Gram-negative bacilli	*Treponema pallidum*	Bacterial endocarditis
Neisseria gonorrhoeae	*Candida* species	*Candida* species
Candida species	*Sporothrix schenckii*	Poncet's disease (tuberculous rheumatism)
Crystal-induced arthritis	*Coccidioides immitis*	Hepatitis B virus
Fracture	*Blastomyces dermatitidis*	Parvovirus B19
Hemarthrosis	*Aspergillus* species	HIV
Foreign body	*Cryptococcus neoformans*	Human T lymphotropic virus type I
Osteoarthritis	*Nocardia* species	Rubella virus
Ischemic necrosis	*Brucella* species	Arthropod-borne viruses
Monarticular rheumatoid arthritis	Legg-Calvé-Perthes disease	Sickle cell disease flare
	Osteoarthritis	Reactive arthritis
		Serum sickness
		Acute rheumatic fever
		Inflammatory bowel disease
		Systemic lupus erythematosus
		Rheumatoid arthritis/Still's disease
		Other vasculitides
		Sarcoidosis

the hip, and still less often the shoulder, wrist, or elbow. Small joints of the hands and feet are more likely to be affected after direct inoculation or a bite. Among intravenous drug users, infections of the spine, sacroiliac joints, or sternoclavicular joints are more common than infections of the appendicular skeleton. Polyarticular infection is most common among patients with rheumatoid arthritis and may resemble a flare of the underlying disease.

The usual presentation consists of moderate to severe pain that is uniform around the joint, effusion, muscle spasm, and decreased range of motion. Fever in the range of 38.3 to 38.9°C (101 to 102°F) and sometimes higher is common but may be lacking, especially in persons with rheumatoid arthritis, renal or hepatic insufficiency, or conditions requiring immunosuppressive therapy. The inflamed, swollen joint is usually evident on examination except in the case of a deeply situated joint, such as the hip, shoulder, or sacroiliac joint. Cellulitis, bursitis, and acute osteomyelitis, which may produce a similar clinical picture, should be distinguished from septic arthritis by their greater range of motion and less-than-circumferential swelling. A focus of extraarticular infection, such as a boil or pneumonia, should be sought. Peripheral-blood leukocytosis with a left shift and elevation of the erythrocyte sedimentation rate or C-reactive protein are common findings.

Plain radiographs show evidence of soft tissue swelling, joint-space widening, and displacement of tissue planes by the distended capsule. Narrowing of the joint space and bony erosions indicate advanced infection and a poor prognosis. Ultrasound is useful for detecting effusions in the hip, and computed tomography or magnetic resonance imaging can demonstrate infections of the sacroiliac joint, sternoclavicular joint, and the spine very well.

Laboratory findings Specimens of peripheral blood and synovial fluid should be obtained before antibiotics are administered. Blood cultures are positive in up to 50% of *S. aureus* infections but are less frequently positive in infections due to other organisms. The synovial fluid is turbid, serosanguineous, or frankly purulent. Gram-stained smears confirm the presence of large numbers of neutrophils. Levels of total protein and lactate dehydrogenase in synovial fluid are elevated, and the glucose level is depressed; however, these findings are not specific for infection, and measurement of these levels is not necessary to make the diagnosis. The synovial fluid should be examined for crystals, because gout and pseudogout can resemble septic arthritis clinically, and infection and crystal-induced disease occasionally occur together. Organisms are seen on synovial fluid smears in nearly three-quarters of infections with *S. aureus* and streptococci and in 30 to 50% of infections due to gram-negative and other bacteria. Cultures of synovial fluid are positive in >90% of cases. Inoculation of synovial fluid into bottles containing liquid media for blood cultures increases the yield of culture, especially if the pathogen is a fastidious organism or the patient is taking an antibiotic. Although not yet widely available, PCR-based assays for bacterial DNA will also be useful for the diagnosis of partially treated or culture-negative bacterial arthritis.

℞ **TREATMENT**   Prompt administration of systemic antibiotics and drainage of the involved joint can prevent destruction of cartilage, postinfectious degenerative arthritis, joint instability, or deformity. Once samples of blood and synovial fluid have been obtained for culture, empirical antibiotics should be given that are directed against bacteria visualized on smears or against the pathogens that are likely, given the patient's age and risk factors. Initial therapy should consist of the intravenous administration of bactericidal agents; direct instillation of antibiotics into the joint is not necessary to achieve adequate levels in synovial fluid and tissue. An intravenous third-generation cephalosporin such as cefotaxime (1 g every 8 h) or ceftriaxone (1 to 2 g every 24 h) will provide adequate empirical coverage for most community-acquired infections in adults when smears show no organisms. Either oxacillin or nafcillin (2 g every 4 h) is used if there are gram-positive cocci on the smear. If methicillin-resistant *S. aureus* is a possible pathogen, as in hospitalized patients, intravenous vancomycin (1 g every 12 h) should be given. In addition, an aminoglycoside should be given to intravenous drug users or other patients in whom *Pseudomonas aeruginosa* may be the responsible agent.

Definitive therapy is based on the identity and antibiotic susceptibility of the bacteria isolated in culture. Infections due to staphylococci are treated with oxacillin, nafcillin, or vancomycin for 4 weeks. Pneumococcal and streptococcal infections due to penicillin-susceptible organisms respond to 2 weeks of therapy with penicillin G (2 million units intravenously every 4 h); infections caused by *H. influenzae* and by strains of *S. pneumoniae* that are resistant to penicillin are treated with cefotaxime or ceftriaxone for 2 weeks. Most enteric gram-negative infections can be cured in 3 to 4 weeks by a second- or third-generation cephalosporin given intravenously or by a fluoroquinolone, such as levofloxacin (500 mg intravenously or orally every 24 h). *P. aeruginosa* infection should be treated for at least 2 weeks with a combination regimen of an aminoglycoside plus either an extended-spectrum penicillin, such as mezlocillin (3 g intravenously every 4 h), or an antipseudomonal cephalosporin, such as ceftazidime (1 g intravenously every 8 h). If tolerated, this regimen is continued for an additional 2 weeks; alternatively, a fluoroquinolone, such as ciprofloxacin (750 mg orally bid), is given by itself or with the penicillin or cephalosporin in place of the aminoglycoside.

Timely drainage of pus and necrotic debris from the infected joint is required for a favorable outcome. Needle aspiration of readily accessible joints such as the knee may be adequate if loculations or particulate matter in the joint does not prevent its thorough decompression. Arthroscopic drainage and lavage may be employed initially or within several days if repeated needle aspiration fails to relieve symptoms, decrease the volume of the effusion and the synovial white cell count, and clear bacteria from smears and cultures. In some cases, arthrotomy is necessary to remove loculations and debride infected synovium, cartilage, or bone. Septic arthritis of the hip is best managed with arthrotomy, particularly in young children, in whom infection threatens the viability of the femoral head. Septic joints do not require immobilization except for pain control before symptoms are alleviated by treatment. Weight bearing should be avoided until signs of inflammation have subsided, but frequent passive motion of the joint is indicated to maintain full mobility. While addition of glucocorticoids to antibiotic treatment improves the outcome of *S. aureus* arthritis in experimental animals, no clinical trials have yet evaluated this approach in humans.

Gonococcal Arthritis • Epidemiology   Gonococcal arthritis, accounting for 70% of episodes of infectious arthritis in persons <40

years of age, results from bacteremia arising from gonococcal infection or, more frequently, from asymptomatic gonococcal mucosal colonization of the urethra, cervix, or pharynx. Women are at greatest risk during menses or during pregnancy and overall are two to three times more likely than men to develop disseminated gonococcal infection and arthritis. Persons with complement deficiencies, especially of the terminal components, are prone to recurrent episodes of gonococcemia. Strains of gonococci that are most likely to cause disseminated infection include those that produce transparent colonies in culture, have the type IA outer-membrane protein, or are of the AUH-auxotroph type.

Clinical manifestations and laboratory findings   The most common manifestation of disseminated gonococcal infection is a syndrome of fever, chills, rash, and articular symptoms. Small numbers of papules that progress to hemorrhagic pustules develop on the trunk and the extensor surfaces of the distal extremities. Migratory arthritis and tenosynovitis of the knees, hands, wrists, feet, and ankles are prominent. The cutaneous lesions and articular findings are believed to be the consequence of an immune reaction to circulating gonococci and immune-complex deposition in tissues. Thus, cultures of synovial fluid are consistently negative, and blood cultures are positive in <45% of patients. Synovial fluid may be difficult to obtain from inflamed joints and usually contains only 10,000 to 20,000 leukocytes/μL.

True gonococcal septic arthritis is less common than the disseminated gonococcal infection syndrome and always follows disseminated infection, which is unrecognized in one-third of patients. A single joint, such as the hip, knee, ankle, or wrist, is usually involved. Synovial fluid, which contains >50,000 leukocytes/μL, can be obtained with ease; the gonococcus is only occasionally evident in gram-stained smears, and cultures of synovial fluid are positive in <40% of cases. Blood cultures are almost always negative.

Because it is difficult to isolate gonococci from synovial fluid and blood, specimens for culture should be obtained from potentially infected mucosal sites. Cultures and gram-stained smears of skin lesions occasionally are positive. All specimens for culture should be plated onto Thayer-Martin agar directly or in special transport media at the bedside and transferred promptly to the microbiology laboratory in an atmosphere of 5% CO_2, as generated in a candle jar. PCR-based assays are extremely sensitive in detecting gonococcal DNA in synovial fluid. A dramatic alleviation of symptoms within 12 to 24 h after the initiation of appropriate antibiotic therapy supports a clinical diagnosis of the disseminated gonococcal infection syndrome if cultures are negative.

℞ **TREATMENT**   Initial treatment consists of ceftriaxone (1 g intravenously or intramuscularly every 24 h) to cover possible penicillin-resistant organisms. Once local and systemic signs are clearly resolving, the 7-day course of therapy can be completed with an oral agent such as cefixime (400 mg bid) or ciprofloxacin (500 mg bid) or, if penicillin-susceptible organisms are isolated, amoxicillin (500 mg tid). Suppurative arthritis usually responds to needle aspiration of involved joints and 7 to 14 days of antibiotic treatment. Arthroscopic lavage or arthrotomy is rarely required.

It is noteworthy that arthritis symptoms similar to those seen in disseminated gonococcal infections occur in meningococcemia. A dermatitis-arthritis syndrome, purulent monarthritis, and reactive polyarthritis have been described. All respond to treatment with intravenous penicillin.

SPIROCHETAL ARTHRITIS Lyme Disease   Lyme disease due to infection with the spirochete *Borrelia burgdorferi* causes arthritis in up to 70% of persons who are not treated. Intermittent arthralgias and myalgias, but not arthritis, occur within days or weeks of inoculation of the spirochete by the *Ixodes* tick. Later, there are three patterns of joint disease: (1) Fifty percent of untreated persons experience intermittent episodes of monarthritis or oligoarthritis involving the knee and/or other large joints. The symptoms wax and wane without treatment over months, and each year 10 to 20% of patients report loss of joint symptoms. (2) Twenty percent of untreated persons develop a pattern of waxing and waning arthralgias. (3) Ten percent of patients develop chronic inflammatory synovitis resulting in erosive lesions and destruction of the joint. Serologic tests for IgG antibodies to *B. burgdorferi* are positive in >90% of persons with Lyme arthritis, and a PCR-based assay detects *Borrelia* DNA in 85%.

℞ **TREATMENT** Lyme arthritis generally responds well to therapy. A regimen of oral doxycycline (100 mg bid for 30 days), oral amoxicillin (500 mg qid for 30 days), or parenteral ceftriaxone (2 g/d for 2 to 4 weeks) is recommended. Patients who do not respond to a total of 2 months of oral therapy or 1 month of parenteral therapy are unlikely to benefit from additional antibiotic therapy and are treated with anti-inflammatory agents or synovectomy. Failure of therapy is associated with host features such as the HLA-DR4 genotype, persistent reactivity to OspA (outer-surface protein A), and the presence of hLFA-1 (human leukocyte function–associated antigen-1), which cross-reacts with OspA.

Syphilitic Arthritis Articular manifestations occur in different stages of syphilis. In early congenital syphilis, periarticular swelling and immobilization of the involved limbs (Parrot's pseudoparalysis) complicate osteochondritis of long bones. Clutton's joint, a late manifestation of congenital syphilis that typically develops between the ages of 8 and 15 years, is caused by chronic painless synovitis with effusions of large joints, particularly the knees and elbows. Secondary syphilis may be associated with arthralgias; symmetric arthritis of the knees and ankles and occasionally of the shoulders and wrists; and sacroiliitis. The arthritis follows a subacute to chronic course with a mixed mononuclear and neutrophilic synovial-fluid pleocytosis (typical cell counts, 5000 to 15,000/μL). Immunologic mechanisms may contribute to the arthritis, and symptoms usually improve rapidly with penicillin therapy. In tertiary syphilis, Charcot's joint is a result of sensory loss due to tabes dorsalis. Penicillin is not helpful in this setting.

MYCOBACTERIAL ARTHRITIS Tuberculous arthritis accounts for ~1% of all cases of tuberculosis and for 10% of extrapulmonary cases. The most common presentation is chronic granulomatous monarthritis. An unusual syndrome, Poncet's disease, is a reactive symmetric form of polyarthritis that affects persons with visceral or disseminated tuberculosis. No mycobacteria are found in the joints, and symptoms resolve with antituberculous therapy.

Unlike tuberculous osteomyelitis, which typically involves the thoracic and lumbar spine (50% of cases), tuberculous arthritis primarily involves the large weight-bearing joints, in particular the hips, knees, and ankles, and only occasionally involves smaller non-weight-bearing joints. Progressive monarticular swelling and pain develop over months to years, and systemic symptoms are seen in only half of all cases. Tuberculous arthritis occurs as part of a disseminated primary infection or through late reactivation, often in persons with HIV infection or other immunocompromised hosts. Coexistent active pulmonary tuberculosis is unusual.

Aspiration of the involved joint yields fluid with an average cell count of 20,000/μL, with ~50% neutrophils. Acid-fast staining of the fluid yields positive results in fewer than one-third of cases, and cultures are positive in 80%. Culture of synovial tissue taken at biopsy is positive in ~90% of cases and shows granulomatous inflammation in most. DNA amplification methods such as PCR can shorten the time to diagnosis to 1 or 2 days. Radiographs reveal peripheral erosions at the points of synovial attachment, periarticular osteopenia, and eventually joint-space narrowing. Therapy for tuberculous arthritis is the same as that for tuberculous pulmonary disease, requiring the administration of multiple agents for 6 to 9 months. Therapy is more prolonged in immunosuppressed individuals, such as those infected with HIV.

Various atypical mycobacteria found in water and soil may cause chronic indolent arthritis. Such disease results from trauma and direct inoculation associated with farming, gardening, or aquatic activities.

Smaller joints, such as the digits, wrists, and knees, are usually involved. Involvement of tendon sheaths and bursae is typical. The mycobacterial species involved include *Mycobacterium marinum*, *M. avium-intracellulare*, *M. terrae*, *M. kansasii*, *M. fortuitum*, and *M. chelonae*. In persons who have HIV infection or are receiving immunosuppressive therapy, hematogenous spread to the joints has been reported for *M. kansasii*, *M. avium-intracellulare*, and *M. haemophilum*. Diagnosis usually requires biopsy and culture, and therapy is based on antimicrobial susceptibility patterns.

FUNGAL ARTHRITIS Fungi are an unusual cause of chronic monarticular arthritis. Granulomatous articular infection with the endemic dimorphic fungi *Coccidioides immitis*, *Blastomyces dermatitidis*, and (less commonly) *Histoplasma capsulatum* results from hematogenous seeding or direct extension from bony lesions in persons with disseminated disease. Joint involvement is an unusual complication of sporotrichosis (infection with *Sporothrix schenckii*) among gardeners and other persons who work with soil or sphagnum moss. Articular sporotrichosis is six times more common among men than among women, and alcoholics and other debilitated hosts are at risk for polyarticular infection.

Candida infection involving a single joint, usually the knee, hip, or shoulder, results from surgical procedures, intraarticular injections, or (among critically ill patients with debilitating illnesses such as diabetes mellitus or hepatic or renal insufficiency and patients receiving immunosuppressive therapy) hematogenous spread. *Candida* infections in intravenous drug users typically involve the spine, sacroiliac joints, or other fibrocartilaginous joints. Unusual cases of arthritis due to *Aspergillus* species, *Cryptococcus neoformans*, *Pseudallescheria boydii*, and the dematiaceous fungi have also resulted from direct inoculation or disseminated hematogenous infection in immunocompromised persons.

The synovial fluid in fungal arthritis usually contains 10,000 to 40,000 cells/μL, with ~70% neutrophils. Stained specimens and cultures of synovial tissue often confirm the diagnosis of fungal arthritis when studies of synovial fluid give negative results. Treatment consists of drainage and lavage of the joint and systemic administration of amphotericin B, fluconazole, or itraconazole (the exact drug depending on the species involved). The doses and duration of therapy are the same as for disseminated disease (see Part Seven, Section 15). Intraarticular instillation of amphotericin B has been used in addition to intravenous therapy.

VIRAL ARTHRITIS Viruses produce arthritis by infecting synovial tissue during systemic infection or by provoking an immunologic reaction that involves joints. As many as 50% of women report persistent arthralgias and 10% frank arthritis within 3 days of the rash that follows natural infection with *rubella virus* and within 2 to 6 weeks after receipt of live virus vaccine. Episodes of symmetric inflammation of fingers, wrists, and knees uncommonly recur for longer than a year, but syndrome of chronic fatigue, low-grade fever, headaches, and myalgias can persist for months or years. Intravenous immunoglobulin has been helpful in selected cases. Self-limited monarticular or migratory polyarthritis may develop within 2 weeks of the parotitis of *mumps*; this sequela is more common in men than in women. Approximately 10% of children and 60% of women develop arthritis after infection with *parvovirus B19*. In adults, arthropathy sometimes occurs without fever or rash. Pain and stiffness, with less prominent swelling (primarily of the hands but also of the knees, wrists, and ankles), usually resolve within weeks, although a small proportion of patients develop chronic arthropathy.

About 2 weeks before the onset of jaundice, up to 10% of persons with acute *hepatitis B* develop an immune complex–mediated, serum sickness–like reaction with maculopapular rash, urticaria, fever, and arthralgias. Less common developments include symmetric arthritis involving the hands, wrists, elbows, or ankles and morning stiffness that resembles a flare of rheumatoid arthritis. Symptoms resolve at the time jaundice develops. Approximately one-third of persons with chronic hepatitis C infection report persistent arthralgia or arthritis, both in the presence and in the absence of cryoglobulinemia. Painful arthritis involving larger joints often accompanies the fever and rash of several arthropod-borne viral infections, including those caused by *chikungunya*, *O'nyong-nyong*, *Ross River*, *Mayaro*, and *Barmah Forest* viruses. Symmetric arthritis involving the hands and wrists may occur during the convalescent phase of infection with *lymphocytic choriomeningitis virus*. Patients infected with an *enterovirus* frequently report arthralgias, and *echovirus* has been isolated from patients with acute polyarthritis.

Several arthritis syndromes are associated with *HIV* infection. Reiter's syndrome with painful lower-extremity oligoarthritis often follows an episode of urethritis in HIV-infected persons. HIV-associated Reiter's syndrome appears to be extremely common among persons with the HLA-B27 haplotype, but sacroiliac joint disease is unusual and is seen mostly in the absence of HLA-B27. Up to one-third of HIV-infected persons with psoriasis develop psoriatic arthritis. Painless monarthropathy and persistent symmetric polyarthropathy occasionally complicate HIV infection. Chronic persistent oligoarthritis of the shoulders, wrists, hands, and knees occurs in women infected with human T lymphotropic virus type I. Synovial thickening, destruction of articular cartilage, and leukemic-appearing atypical lymphocytes in synovial fluid are characteristic, but progression to T cell leukemia is unusual.

PARASITIC ARTHRITIS Arthritis due to parasitic infection is rare. The guinea worm *Dracunculus medinensis* may cause destructive joint lesions in the lower extremities as migrating gravid female worms invade joints or cause ulcers in adjacent soft tissues that become secondarily infected. Hydatid cysts infect bones in 1 to 2% of cases of infection with *Echinococcus granulosus*. The expanding destructive cystic lesions may spread to and destroy adjacent joints, particularly the hip and pelvis. In rare cases, chronic synovitis has been associated with the presence of schistosomal eggs in synovial biopsies. Monarticular arthritis in children with lymphatic *filariasis* appears to respond to therapy with diethylcarbamazine even in the absence of microfilariae in synovial fluid. Reactive arthritis has been attributed to *hookworm*, *Strongyloides*, *Cryptosporidium*, and *Giardia* infection in case reports, but confirmation is required.

POSTINFECTIOUS OR REACTIVE ARTHRITIS Reiter's syndrome, a reactive polyarthritis, develops several weeks after ~1% of cases of nongonococcal urethritis and 2% of enteric infections, particularly those due to *Yersinia enterocolitica*, *Shigella flexneri*, *Campylobacter jejuni*, and *Salmonella* species. Only a minority of these patients have the other findings of classic Reiter's syndrome, including urethritis, conjunctivitis, uveitis, oral ulcers, and rash. Studies have identified microbial DNA or antigen in synovial fluid or blood, but the pathogenesis of this condition is poorly understood.

Reiter's syndrome is most common among young men (except after *Yersinia* infection) and has been linked to the HLA-B27 locus as a potential genetic predisposing factor. Patients report painful, asymmetric oligoarthritis affecting mainly the knees, ankles, and feet. Low-back pain is common, and radiographic evidence of sacroiliitis is found in patients with long-standing disease. Most patients recover within 6 months, but prolonged recurrent disease is more common in cases following chlamydial urethritis. Anti-inflammatory agents help to relieve symptoms, but the role of prolonged antibiotic therapy in eliminating microbial antigen from the synovium is controversial.

Migratory polyarthritis and fever constitute the usual presentation of acute rheumatic fever in adults. This presentation is distinct from that of poststreptococcal reactive arthritis, which also follows infections with group A β-hemolytic *Streptococcus* but is not migratory, lasts beyond the typical 3-week maximum of acute rheumatic fever, and responds poorly to aspirin.

INFECTIONS IN PROSTHETIC JOINTS Infection complicates 1 to 4% of total joint replacements. The majority of infections are acquired intraoperatively or immediately postoperatively as a result of wound breakdown or infection; less commonly, these joint infections develop later after joint replacement and are the result of hematogenous spread or direct inoculation. The presentation may be acute, with fever, pain, and local signs of inflammation, especially in infections due to *S. aureus*, pyogenic streptococci, and enteric bacilli. Alternatively, infection may persist for months or years without causing constitutional symptoms when less virulent organisms, such as coagulase-negative staphylococci or diphtheroids, are involved. Such indolent infections are usually acquired during joint implantation and are discovered during evaluation of chronic unexplained pain or after a radiograph shows loosening of the prosthesis; the erythrocyte sedimentation rate and C-reactive protein are usually elevated in such cases.

The diagnosis is best made by needle aspiration of the joint; accidental introduction of organisms during aspiration must be meticulously avoided. Synovial fluid pleocytosis with a predominance of polymorphonuclear leukocytes is highly suggestive of infection, since other inflammatory processes uncommonly affect prosthetic joints. Culture and Gram's stain usually yield the responsible pathogen. Use of special media for unusual pathogens such as fungi, atypical mycobacteria, and *Mycoplasma* may be necessary if routine and anaerobic cultures are negative.

℞ **TREATMENT** Treatment includes surgery and high doses of parenteral antibiotics, which are given for 4 to 6 weeks because bone is usually involved. In most cases, the prosthesis must be replaced to cure the infection. Implantation of a new prosthesis is best delayed for several weeks or months because relapses of infection occur most commonly within this time frame. In some cases, reimplantation is not possible, and the patient must manage without a joint, with a fused joint, or even with amputation. Cure of infection without removal of the prosthesis is occasionally possible in cases that are due to streptococci or pneumococci and that lack radiologic evidence of loosening of the prosthesis. In these cases, antibiotic therapy must be initiated within several days of the onset of infection, and the joint should be drained vigorously either by open arthrotomy or arthroscopically. A high cure rate with retention of the prosthesis has been reported when the combination of oral rifampin and ciprofloxacin is given for 3 to 6 months to persons with staphylococcal prosthetic joint infection of short duration. This approach, which is based on the ability of rifampin to kill organisms adherent to foreign material and in the stationary growth phase, requires confirmation in prospective trials.

Prevention To avoid the disastrous consequences of infection, candidates for joint replacement should be selected with care. Rates of infection are particularly high among patients with rheumatoid arthritis, persons who have undergone previous surgery on the joint, and persons with medical conditions requiring immunosuppressive therapy. Perioperative antibiotic prophylaxis, usually with cefazolin, and measures to decrease intraoperative contamination, such as laminar flow, have lowered the rates of perioperative infection to <1% in many centers. After implantation, measures should be taken to prevent or rapidly treat extraarticular infections that might give rise to hematogenous spread to the prosthesis. The effectiveness of prophylactic antibiotics for the prevention of hematogenous infection following dental procedures has not been demonstrated; in fact, viridans streptococci and other components of the oral flora are extremely unusual causes of prosthetic joint infection. Accordingly, the American Dental Association and the American Academy of Orthopaedic Surgeons do not recommend antibiotic prophylaxis for most dental patients with total joint replacements. They do, however, recommend prophylaxis for patients who may be at high risk of hematogenous infection, including those with inflammatory arthropathies, immunosuppression, type 1 diabetes mellitus, joint replacement within 2 years, previous prosthetic joint infection, malnourishment, or hemophilia. The recommended regimen is amoxicillin (2 g orally) 1 h before dental procedures associated with a high incidence of bacteremia. Clindamycin (600 mg orally) is suggested for patients allergic to penicillin.

BERMAN A et al: Human immunodeficiency virus infection associated arthritis: Clinical characteristics. J Rheumatol 26:1158, 1999

CUCURULL E, ESPINOZA LR: Gonococcal arthritis. Rheum Dis Clin North Am 24:305, 1998

CUNNINGHAM R et al: Clinical and molecular aspects of the pathogenesis of *Staphylococcus aureus* bone and joint infections. J Med Microbiol 44:157, 1996

DONATTO KC: Orthopedic management of septic arthritis. Rheum Dis Clin North Am 24:275, 1998

GILLESPIE WJ: Prevention and management of infection after total joint replacement. Clin Infect Dis 25:1310, 1997

GOLDENBERG DL: Septic arthritis. Lancet 351:197, 1998

HARRINGTON JT: Mycobacterial and fungal arthritis. Curr Opin Rheumatol 10:335, 1998

WUORELA M, GRANFORS K: Infectious agents as triggers of reactive arthritis. Am J Med Sci 316:264, 1998

YTTERBERG SR: Viral arthritis. Curr Opin Rheumatol 11:275, 1999

ZIMMERLI W et al: Role of rifampin for treatment of orthopedic implant–related staphylococcal infections: A randomized controlled trial. Foreign-Body Infection (FBI) Study Group. JAMA 279:1537, 1998

324 *Peter H. Schur*

PSORIATIC ARTHRITIS AND ARTHRITIS ASSOCIATED WITH GASTROINTESTINAL DISEASE

PSORIATIC ARTHRITIS

Psoriatic arthritis (PsA) is a chronic inflammatory arthritis that affects 5 to 42% of people with psoriasis.

ETIOLOGY AND PATHOGENESIS   To date, the cause and pathogenesis of PsA are unknown. Indirect evidence has suggested that interactions of infections, trauma, increased humoral and cellular immunity (e.g., to streptococci), cytokines (including TH1 and TH2), adhesion molecules, and abnormal fibroblast, dendritic cell, keratinocyte, and polymorphonuclear leukocyte (PMN) function are involved. Polyarthritis has developed in patients with psoriasis and hepatitis treated with interferon α. Most studies have observed an increased frequency of HLA-B17, CW6, and/or B27 in patients with psoriatic spondylitis, while B27, B38, B39, and DR7 have been noted in association with peripheral arthritis in different studies. Fulminant disease should make one suspect HIV disease (Chap. 309).

CLINICAL MANIFESTATIONS   Three major types of PsA are generally recognized: asymmetric inflammatory arthritis, symmetric arthritis, and psoriatic spondylitis. A mean of 47% of patients (range, 16 to 70%) have an asymmetric inflammatory arthritis. Disease appears equally in men and women. Psoriasis tends to precede the arthritis by years. Many patients complain of morning stiffness. The proximal interphalangeal (PIP) and distal interphalangeal (DIP) joints are commonly involved [with characteristic sausage-shaped digits (dactylitis)], while knees, hips, ankles, temporomandibular joints, and wrists are less frequently involved. Most patients have onychodystrophy (onycholysis, ridging and pitting of nails), the course of which does not parallel that of the synovitis. The prognosis is good, with only one-fourth of the patients developing progressive destructive disease; one-third develop inflammatory ocular complications (conjunctivitis, iritis, episcleritis).

A mean of 25% of patients (range, 15 to 39%) develop symmetric arthritis resembling rheumatoid arthritis (Chap. 312). This disease occurs twice as frequently in women. Psoriasis and inflammatory arthritis usually develop simultaneously; most patients experience morning stiffness. The DIP, PIP, metacarpophalangeal (MCP), metatarsophalangeal (MTP), sternoclavicular, and, in particular, large peripheral joints are involved. Practically all patients have onychodystrophy, which helps distinguish them from patients with rheumatoid arthritis. Over half of the patients in this group go on to develop destructive arthritis, including arthritis mutilans. Eye complications are uncom-

mon. Subcutaneous nodules are not present, but one-fourth of patients have rheumatoid factors. Unilateral upper limb edema has been described.

A mean of 23% of the patients (range 5 to 40%) have psoriatic "spondylitis," with or without peripheral joint involvement. Psoriasis tends to precede the arthritis by a few years, and low back pain with morning stiffness is common. Psoriatic spondylitis is more common in men. About half the patients in this group have spondylitis and the other half have sacroiliitis. The back disease is usually slowly progressive, with little clinical deterioration as compared with ankylosing spondylitis; the peripheral disease also tends not to be destructive except for the occasional patient with arthritis mutilans. Enthesopathy, i.e., inflammation of tendons and ligamentous attachments to bone, is characteristic, for example, of the Achilles tendon or of the plantar fascia causing heel pain. Many patients have onychodystrophy, but few have inflammatory ocular complications. Gut inflammation occurs in 30% (no gut inflammation was noted in patients with only peripheral arthritis).

Some authors have described additional subsets of psoriatic arthritis: predominant DIP joint involvement, arthritis mutilans, peripheral enthesitis, juvenile PsA, and SAPHO (synovitis, acne, pustulosis, hyperostosis, osteomyelitis).

The pathology of PsA is similar to that seen in rheumatoid arthritis: synoviocytic hyperplasia, early PMN infiltration and later mononuclear cell infiltration, cartilage erosion, and pannus formation. However, in PsA, the synovium is more vascular and there are fewer macrophages and less expression of endothelial cell leukocyte adhesion molecule-1 (ELAM-1). Fibrosis of the joint capsule and marrow is prominent in many patients.

LABORATORY FINDINGS   There are few laboratory abnormalities. Elevated erythrocyte sedimentation rates, C-reactive proteins, and complement levels reflect inflammation. Rheumatoid factors are uncommon and are more likely to be observed in those with symmetric arthritis. Immunoglobulin levels, especially IgA levels, may be elevated (IgA antibodies to cytokeratins and antienterobacteria antibodies are elevated). Uric acid levels may be elevated; sodium urate crystals in joint fluids suggest gout.

Radiologic investigation reveals findings similar to those of rheumatoid arthritis: soft tissue swelling, loss of the cartilage space, erosions, bony ankylosis of fingers, subluxations, and subchondral cysts; of note, there is less demineralization. However, more unique and suggestive of psoriatic arthritis are erosions at DIP joints, expansion of the base of the terminal phalanx, tapering of the proximal phalanx and cuplike erosions and bony proliferation of the distal terminal phalanx ("pencil-in-cup" appearance), proliferation of bone near osseous erosions, terminal phalangeal osteolysis, bone proliferation and periostitis (especially of phalanges), and telescoping of one bone into its neighbor, leading to the "opera-glass" deformity (Fig. 324-1). The axial skeleton shows asymmetric or unilateral sacroiliitis, often asymptomatic paravertebral ossification, including cervical involvement, and large asymmetric nonmarginal syndesmophytes. Echocardiographic abnormalities resemble those of ankylosing spondilitis.

DIAGNOSIS   The diagnosis of PsA should be considered in individuals with arthritis and psoriasis. Psoriasis should be distinguished from seborrheic dermatitis and eczema. Psoriatic lesions may be quite small peripherally and are often hidden in the scalp, umbilicus, and gluteal folds. Fungal infection of nails can be distinguished from psoriasis, for the latter will demonstrate pitting and onycholysis. Furthermore, onychodystrophy is uncommon (20% of cases) in uncomplicated psoriasis. It is often difficult to distinguish Reiter's syndrome (Chap. 315) from PsA, since both manifest dactylitis. Reiter's syndrome usually presents in younger individuals, especially males; is less frequently progressive or destructive; and is more likely to be associated with characteristic skin lesions (keratoderma blenorrhagica—which may, however, resemble pustular psoriasis), urethritis, and conjunctivitis. Gout can be distinguished by the presence of intraar-

FIGURE 324-1   X-ray of hands of a patient with severe psoriatic arthritis characterized by destructive phalangeal changes (see text).

ticular sodium urate crystals (Chap. 322). Psoriasis in association with Heberden's nodes or Bouchard's nodes of the DIP and PIP joints, respectively, rather suggests osteoarthritis (Chap. 321). PsA differs from rheumatoid arthritis by the relative lack of rheumatoid factors; the tendency to asymmetry, dactylitis, iritis, enthesopathy, and onychodystrophy; the high frequency of HLA-B27, especially in patients with axial skeletal involvement; and characteristic radiologic features.

℞   **TREATMENT**   The treatment of PsA begins with patient education and physical and occupational therapy to maintain muscle strength and joint and muscle function. Orthotics and occasional intraarticular glucocorticoids for isolated acutely and severely inflamed joints may be added as needed (Fig. 324-2). The mainstay, however, is the use of nonsteroidal anti-inflammatory drugs (NSAIDs), which reduce inflammation and alleviate pain for most patients. For patients with more severe involvement, a disease-modifying antirheumatic drug should be used. While hydroxychloroquine is often successful in

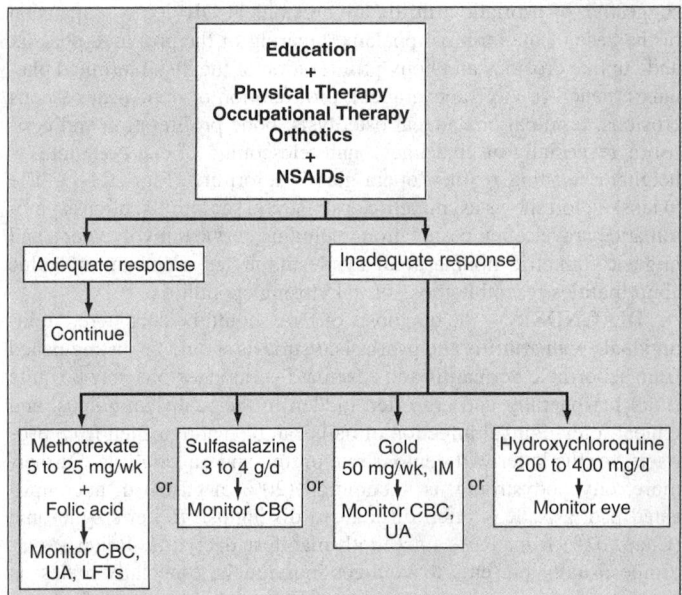

FIGURE 324-2   Algorithm for the treatment of psoriatic arthritis. See text for detailed description. NSAID, nonsteroidal anti-inflammatory drugs; CBC, complete blood count; UA, urinalysis; LFTs, liver function tests.

producing either amelioration or remission, it carries a significant risk of exacerbation of psoriasis and exfoliation. Sulfasalizine (2 to 4 g/d) has well-demonstrated efficacy for PsA. For more severe cases, especially with extensive skin involvement, 5 to 25 mg methotrexate per week is recommended. Most patients respond well with respect to both skin lesions and arthritis. Patients who are resistant to oral therapy may respond to parenteral therapy. Folic acid (1 mg/d) is recommended to prevent hematologic complications. Renal and liver function tests and a complete blood count should be performed every 6 to 8 weeks, and any abnormalities should suggest modification of the dosage. Liver biopsies are recommended after a total of 1.5 g methotrexate have been given and then every 2 years to identify the rare patient with fibrosis and cirrhosis, which necessitate withdrawal of the drug. Patients are advised to avoid nephrotoxic and hepatotoxic (e.g., ethanol) drugs. Patients with HIV infection may have worsening of their disease when treated with methotrexate. Intramuscular gold, cyclosporine (2 to 5 mg/kg per day), etretinate (0.5 mg/kg per day), and azathioprine have also proved successful. The arthritis may also respond to heliotherapy.

ARTHRITIS ASSOCIATED WITH GASTROINTESTINAL DISEASE

INFLAMMATORY BOWEL DISEASE   Peripheral arthritis occurs in 9 to 30% of patients with inflammatory bowel disease (IBD) (e.g., ulcerative colitis or Crohn's disease; Chap. 287), and arthralgia is more common. Arthritis is somewhat more likely to occur in patients with large-bowel disease and in those patients with complications such as abscesses, pseudomembranous polyposis, perianal disease, massive hemorrhage, erythema nodosum, stomatitis, uveitis, and pyoderma gangrenosum. Males and females are affected equally. The arthritis tends to be acute, is associated with a flare-up of the bowel disease, occurs early in the course of the bowel disease, is self-limiting (90% of cases resolve within 6 months), and does not result in destruction. Most patients have a symmetric, migratory polyarthritis affecting primarily large joints of the lower extremity. Rheumatoid factors are not present. There is some association with HLA-BW62. Synovial fluids have 5000 to 12,000 white blood cells per microliter, mostly PMNs. Radiographs demonstrate soft tissue swelling and effusions without erosions or destruction. Pathologic examination of synovial biopsy specimens reveals only nonspecific inflammation. The peripheral arthritis responds to successful treatment of the bowel disease, such as colectomy (for ulcerative colitis), or administration of glucocorticoids, anti-tumor necrosis factor α therapy, or sulfasalazine. NSAIDs relieve pain and inflammation but should be used with caution because of possible gastrointestinal side effects.

Spondylitis occurs in 1.1 to 43% of patients with IBD (while gut inflammation develops in 68% of patients with spondyloarthropathies). Spondylitis often precedes IBD; their clinical courses are often strongly related. Males are affected more frequently. Patients typically complain of stiffness in the back and/or buttocks in the morning or after rest. The stiffness and associated pain are often relieved by exercise. Gastrointestinal infection/inflammation is thought to play a role in exacerbation of spondylitis. Physical examination reveals limitation of spinal flexion and reduced chest expansion. Some patients may have peripheral arthritis, especially of the hips and/or shoulders. Uveitis is a frequent complication. Radiographs of the back show the typical findings of ankylosing spondylitis and bilateral sacroiliitis. HLA-B27 is found in 53 to 75% of these patients. Treatment includes physical therapy, NSAIDs, glucocorticoids, and sulfasalazine. NSAIDs should be used with caution lest they exacerbate the IBD. The axial disease progresses slowly in a manner akin to that of ankylosing spondylitis.

Asymptomatic sacroiliitis detected by radiography occurs in 4 to 32% of patients with IBD. By contrast, 52% of patients with IBD have abnormalities on technetium pyrophosphate bone scans of the sacroiliac joint. There is no increased frequency of HLA-B27 in these patients. This "disease" does not necessarily progress to spondylitis.

Other complications of chronic IBD include (1) finger clubbing (observed in 4 to 13% of patients with Crohn's disease, especially those with small-bowel involvement), which may regress after surgery; (2) development of amyloid, especially in association with Crohn's disease; and (3) osteoporosis resulting from inactivity, malabsorption, and/or treatment with glucocorticoids. Osteomalacia can result from malabsorption. In this setting, with acutely increased back pain, one should suspect compression fracture.

INTESTINAL BYPASS ARTHRITIS Intestinal bypass surgery was developed for the treatment of obesity in 1952; 11 years later arthritis was recognized as a postoperative complication. Polyarthralgia, tenosynovitis, and sometimes arthritis occur weeks, even years, after surgery in 8 to 36% of patients. There is often an associated urticarial, vesicular, pustular, macular, or nodular eruption. X-rays generally show no joint damage. Tests for rheumatoid factors, antinuclear antibodies, and HLA-B27 are usually negative, while immune complexes (and cryoglobulins) are often present. They contain bacterial antigens, the corresponding antibodies, IgA secretory component, and complement components. These observations suggest that the syndrome has the following pathogenesis: Bacteria proliferate in intestinal blind loops; bacterial antigens are absorbed; and antibodies to these antigens develop and combine with them to form immune complexes, which deposit in synovial tissue to cause arthritis. NSAIDs and glucocorticoids can relieve the joint symptoms, but more lasting results can be achieved by tetracycline therapy to decrease the bacterial load; even better is reanastomosis of the bowel or resection of the blind loop.

WHIPPLE'S DISEASE (INTESTINAL LIPODYSTROPHY) Whipple's disease is rare and occurs mostly in middle-aged Caucasian males, who develop arthritis, prolonged diarrhea, malabsorption, and weight loss as a result of infection with the actinomyocete, *Tropheryma whippelii*. The organism has been found in waste water. Up to 90% of patients with the disease develop arthritis, usually prior to other symptoms. Knees and ankles and, to a lesser extent, fingers, hips, shoulders, elbows, and wrists are involved. The arthritis is acute in onset, migratory, usually lasts just a few days, and is rarely chronic or a cause of permanent joint damage. Associated symptoms may include fever (54%), edema, serositis (pleurisy, pericarditis, endocarditis), pneumonia, hypotension, lymphadenopathy (54%), hyperpigmentation (54%), subcutaneous nodules, clubbing, and uveitis. Central nervous system involvement may develop (80%), with cognitive changes, headache, diplopia, and papilledema, and may be appreciated by abnormalities in magnetic resonance images of the brain. Oculomasticatory myorhythmia and oculo-facial-skeletal myorhythmia are felt to be pathognomonic and are found in 20% of patients; they are always accompanied by supranuclear vertical gaze palsy. Laboratory abnormalities include anemia (75%), low serum levels of carotene (95%), and albumin (93%). The presence of HLA-B27 (8 to 30%) occurs in those patients with axial arthritis. Synovial fluids have been reported to contain 450 to 36,000 white blood cells per microliter (30 to 95% neutrophils) or a mild monocytosis. Joint x-rays rarely show erosions but may show a sacroiliitis in the occasional patients who have axial skeletal symptoms; abdominal computed tomographic scans may reveal lymphadenopathy. The lamina propria and/or foamy macrophages in small intestine contain PAS-staining bacterial remnants, presumably of *T. whippelii*. These inclusion-containing foamy macrophages have also been detected in the synovium, lymph nodes, and other tissues. Diagnosis is often established by polymerase chain reaction of the 165 ribosomal gene sequences of these bacteria in biopsied tissue, usually the duodenum. The syndrome responds best to therapy with penicillin (or ceftriaxone) and streptomycin for 2 weeks followed by trimethoprim-sulfamethoxazole for 1 to 2 years. However, central nervous system relapse may develop, which has been treated with cefixime.

REACTIVE ARTHRITIS A Reiter's-like syndrome of arthritis can develop 2 to 3 weeks following diarrhea caused by *Shigella*, *Salmonella*, *Yersinia*, *Chlamydia trachomatis*, or *Campylobacter* organisms. →*This condition is described in Chap. 315.*

BIBLIOGRAPHY

Bos JD, De Rie MA: The pathogenesis of psoriasis: Immunological facts and speculations. Immunol Today 20:40, 1999

Bruckle W et al: Treatment of psoriatic arthritis with auranofin and gold sodium thiomalate. Clin Rheumatol 13:209, 1994

Clegg DO et al: Comparison of sulfasalazine and placebo in the treatment of psoriatic arthritis. A Department of Veterans Affairs Cooperative Study. Arthritis Rheum 39:2013, 1996

Cuellar ML, Espinoza LR: Methotrexate use in psoriasis and psoriatic arthritis. Rheum Dis Clin North Am 23:797, 1997

De Keyser F et al: Bowel inflammation and the spondyloarthropathies. Rheum Dis Clin North Am 24:785, 1998

Durand F et al: Whipple disease. Clinical review of 52 cases. The SNFMI Research Group on Whipple Disease. Societé Nationale Francaise de Medecine Interne. Medicine 76:170, 1997

Espinoza LR et al: Insights into the pathogenesis of psoriasis and psoriatic arthritis. Am J Med Sci 316:271, 1998

Gladman DD: Psoriatic arthritis. Rheum Dis Clin North Am 24:829, 1998

Jones G et al: Psoriatic arthritis: A quantitative overview of therapeutic options. The Psoriatic Arthritis Meta-Analysis Study Group. Br J Rheumatol 36:95, 1997

Kahn MF, Chamot AM: Sapho syndrome. Rheum Dis Clin North Am 18:225, 1992

Katz JP, Lichtenstein GR: Rheumatologic manifestations of gastrointestinal diseases. Gastroenterol Clin North Am 27:533, 1998

Louis ED et al: Diagnostic guidelines in central nervous system Whipple's disease. Ann Neurol 40:561, 1996

Mahrle G et al: Low-dose short-term cyclosporine versus etretinate in psoriasis: Improvement of skin, nail, and joint involvement. J Am Acad Dermatol 32:78, 1995

McGonagle D et al: Psoriatic arthritis. A unified concept twenty years on. Arthritis Rheum 42:1080, 1999

Porter GG: Psoriatic arthritis. Plain radiology and other imaging techniques. Baillieres Clin Rheumatol 8:465, 1994

Ramzan NN et al: Diagnosis and monitoring of Whipple disease by polymerase chain reaction. Ann Intern Med 126:520, 1997

325

Bruce C. Gilliland

RELAPSING POLYCHONDRITIS AND OTHER ARTHRITIDES

RELAPSING POLYCHONDRITIS

Relapsing polychondritis is an uncommon inflammatory disorder of unknown cause characterized by an episodic and generally progressive course affecting predominantly the cartilage of the ears, nose, and laryngotracheobronchial tree. Other manifestations include scleritis, neurosensory hearing loss, polyarthritis, vasculitis, cardiac abnormalities, skin lesions, and glomerulonephritis. The peak age of onset is between the ages of 40 to 50 years but relapsing polychondritis may affect children and the elderly. It is found in all races, and both sexes are equally affected. No familial tendency is apparent. A significantly higher frequency of HLA-DR4 has been found in patients with relapsing polychondritis than in normal individuals. A predominant subtype allele(s) of HLA-DR4 was not found. Approximately 30% of patients with relapsing polychondritis will have another rheumatologic disorder, the most frequent being systemic vasculitis, followed by rheumatoid arthritis, systemic lupus erythematosus (SLE), or Sjögren's syndrome. Nonrheumatic disorders associated with relapsing polychondritis include inflammatory bowel disease, primary biliary cirrhosis, and myelodysplastic syndrome.

Diagnostic criteria were suggested several years ago by McAdam et al. and modified by Damiani and Levine a few years later. These criteria continue to be generally used in clinical practice. McAdam et al. proposed the following: (1) recurrent chondritis of both auricles; (2) nonerosive inflammatory arthritis; (3) chondritis of nasal cartilage; (4) inflammation of ocular structures including conjunctivitis, keratitis, scleritis/episcleritis, and/or uveitis; (5) chondritis of the laryngeal and/or tracheal cartilages; and (6) cochlear and/or vestibular damage manifested by neurosensory hearing loss, tinnitus, and/or vertigo. The diagnosis is certain when three or more of these features were present with biopsy confirmation. Damiana and Levine later suggested that the diagnosis could be made when one or more of the above features and a positive biopsy were present, when two or more separate sites of cartilage inflammation were present that responded to glucocorticoids or dapsone, or when three or more of the above features were present. A biopsy is not necessary in most patients with clinically evident disease.

PATHOLOGY AND PATHOPHYSIOLOGY The earliest abnormality of cartilage noted histologically is a focal or diffuse loss of basophilic staining indicating depletion of proteoglycan from the cartilage matrix. Inflammatory infiltrates are found adjacent to involved cartilage and consist predominantly of mononuclear cells and occasional plasma cells. In acute disease, polymorphonuclear white cells may also be present. Destruction of cartilage begins at the outer edges and advances centrally. There is lacunar breakdown and loss of chondrocytes. Degenerating cartilage is replaced by granulation tissue and later by fibrosis and focal areas of calcification. Small loci of cartilage regeneration may be present. Immunofluorescence studies have shown immunoglobulins and complement at sites of involvement. Fine granular material observed in the degenerating cartilage matrix by electron microscopy has been interpreted to be enzymes or immunoglobulins.

Immunologic mechanisms play a role in the pathogenesis of relapsing polychondritis. Immunoglobulin and complement deposits are found at sites of inflammation. In addition, antibodies to type II collagen and to matrilin-1 and immune complexes are detected in the sera of some patients. The possibility that an immune response to type II collagen may be important in the pathogenesis is supported experimentally by the occurrence of auricular chondritis in rats immunized with type II collagen. Antibodies to type II collagen are found in the sera of these animals, and immune deposits are detected at sites of ear inflammation. Cell-mediated immunity may also be operative in causing tissue injury, since lymphocyte transformation can be demonstrated when lymphocytes of patients are exposed to cartilage extracts. Humoral and cellular immune responses to type IX and type XI collagen have been demonstrated in some patients. In a recent study, rats immunized with cartilage matrix protein (matrilin-1) were found to develop severe inspiratory stridor and swelling of the nasal septum. Cartilage matrix protein is a noncollagenous protein present in the extracellular matrix in cartilage. It is present in high concentrations in the trachea and is also present in the nasal septum but not in articular cartilage. The immunized rats had severe inflammation in the larynx close to the epiglottis, which was characterized by increased numbers of CD 4+ and CD 8+ T cells. All had IgG antibodies to cartilage matrix protein. The inflammation was believed to have been largely mediated by T cells. The results of the study suggest that immune responses to various cartilage proteins play a role in the pathogenesis of relapsing polychondritis.

Dissolution of cartilage matrix can be induced by the intravenous injection of crude papain, a proteolytic enzyme, into young rabbits, which results in collapse of their normally rigid ears within 4 h. Reconstitution of the matrix occurs in about 7 days. In relapsing polychondritis, loss of cartilage matrix also most likely results from action of proteolytic enzymes released from chondrocytes, polymorphonuclear white cells, and monocytes that have been activated by inflammatory mediators.

CLINICAL MANIFESTATIONS The onset of relapsing polychondritis is frequently abrupt with the appearance of one or two sites of cartilagenous inflammation. Fever, fatigue, and weight loss occur and may precede the clinical signs of relapsing polychondritis by several weeks. Relapsing polychondritis may go unrecognized for several months or even years in patients who only initially manifest intermittent joint pain and/or swelling, or who have unexplained eye inflammation, hearing loss, valvular heart disease, or pulmonary symptoms. The pattern of cartilagenous involvement and the frequency of episodes vary widely among patients.

Auricular chondritis is the most frequent presenting manifestation of relapsing polychondritis in 40% of patients and eventually affects about 85% of patients (Table 325-1). One or both ears are involved, either sequentially or simultaneously. Patients experience the sudden onset of pain, tenderness, and swelling of the cartilaginous portion of the ear. Earlobes are spared because they do not contain cartilage. The overlying skin has a beefy red or violaceous color. Prolonged or recurrent episodes result in a flabby or droopy ear as a sequela of cartilage destruction. Swelling may close off the eustachian tube (causing otitis media) or the external auditory meatus, either of which can impair hearing. Inflammation of the internal auditory artery or its cochlear branch produces hearing loss, vertigo, ataxia, nausea, and vomiting. The cartilage of the nose becomes inflamed during the first or subsequent attacks. Approximately 50% of patients will eventually have nose involvement. Patients may experience nasal stuffiness, rhinorrhea, and epistaxis. The bridge of the nose becomes red, swollen, and tender and may collapse, producing a saddle deformity. In some patients, the saddle deformity develops insidiously without overt inflammation. Saddle nose is observed more frequently in younger patients, especially in women.

Arthritis is the presenting manifestation in relapsing polychondritis in approximately one-third of patients and may be present for several months before other features appear. Eventually, more than half the patients will have arthritis. The arthritis is usually asymmetric and oligo- or polyarticular, and involves both large and small peripheral joints. An episode of arthritis lasts from a few days to several weeks and resolves spontaneously without residual joint deformity. Attacks of arthritis may not be temporally related to other manifestations of relapsing polychondritis. The joints are warm, tender, and swollen. Joint fluid has been reported to be noninflammatory. In addition to peripheral joints, inflammation may involve the costochondral, sternomanubrial, and sternoclavicular cartilages. Destruction of these cartilages may result in a pectus excavatum deformity or even a flail anterior chest wall. Relapsing polychondritis may occur in patients with preexisting rheumatoid arthritis, Reiter's syndrome, psoriatic arthritis, or ankylosing spondylitis.

Eye manifestations occur in more than half of patients and include conjunctivitis, episcleritis, scleritis, iritis, and keratitis. Ulceration and perforation of the cornea may occur and cause blindness. Other manifestations include eyelid and periorbital edema, proptosis, cataracts, optic neuritis, extraocular muscle palsies, retinal vasculitis, and renal vein occlusion.

Laryngotracheobronchial involvement occurs in ~50% of patients. Symptoms include hoarseness, a nonproductive cough, and tenderness over the larynx and proximal trachea. Mucosal edema, strictures, and/or collapse of laryngeal or tracheal cartilage may cause stridor and life-threatening airway obstruction necessitating tracheostomy. Collapse of cartilage in bronchi leads to pneumonia and, when extensive, to respiratory insufficiency.

Aortic regurgitation occurs in about 5% of patients and is due to progressive dilation of the aortic ring or to destruction of the valve

Table 325-1 Clinical Manifestations of Relapsing Polychondritis

Clinical Feature	Frequency, %	
	Presenting	Cumulative
Auricular chondritis	40	85
Hearing loss	10	30
Nasal chondritis	25	55
Saddle nose deformity	20	30
Ocular deformities	20	50
Respiratory disease	25	50
Arthritis	35	50
Aortic regurgitation	—	5
Vasculitis	3	10

SOURCE: Modified from Isaak et al: Ophthalmology 93:681, 1986.

cusps. Mitral and other heart valves are less often affected. Other cardiac manifestations include pericarditis, myocarditis, and conduction abnormalities. Aneurysms of the proximal, thoracic, or abdominal aorta may occur and occasionally rupture.

Systemic vasculitis may occur in association with relapsing polychondritis. Vasculitides include leukocytoclastic vasculitis, polyarteritis, temporal arteritis, and Takayasu's arteritis (Chap. 317). Neurologic abnormalities usually occur as a result of underlying vasculitis, manifesting as seizures, strokes, ataxia, and peripheral and cranial nerve neuropathies. Cranial nerves VI and VII are most often involved. Approximately 25% of patients have skin lesions, none of which is characteristic for relapsing polychondritis. These include purpura, erythema nodosum, erythema multiforme, angioedema/urticaria, livedo reticularis, and panniculitis. Segmental necrotizing glomerulonephritis with crescent formation has been noted in some patients in the absence of systemic vasculitis.

The course of disease is highly variable, with episodes lasting from a few days to several weeks and then subsiding spontaneously. Attacks may recur at intervals varying from weeks to months. In other patients, the disease has a chronic, smoldering course. In a few patients, the disease may be limited to one or two episodes of cartilage inflammation. In one study, the 5-year estimated survival rate was 74% and the 10-year survival rate 55%. In contrast to earlier series, only about half the deaths could be attributed to relapsing polychondritis or complications of treatment. Pulmonary complications accounted for only 10% of all fatalities. In general, patients with more widespread disease have a worse prognosis.

LABORATORY FINDINGS Mild leukocytosis and normocytic, normochromic anemia are often present. The erythrocyte sedimentation rate is usually elevated. Rheumatoid factor and antinuclear antibody tests are occasionally positive in low titers. Antibodies to type II collagen are present in most patients, but they are not specific. Circulating immune complexes may be detected, especially in patients with early active disease. Elevated levels of γ globulin may be present. Antineutrophil cytoplasmic antibodies (ANCA), either cytoplasmic (C-ANCA) or perinuclear (P-ANCA), are found in some patients with active disease. The upper and lower airways can be evaluated by imaging techniques such as linear tomography, laryngotracheography, and computed tomography, and by bronchoscopy. Bronchography is performed to demonstrate bronchial narrowing. Intrathoracic airway obstruction can also be evaluated by inspiratory-expiratory flow studies. The chest film may show narrowing of the trachea and/or the main bronchi, widening of the ascending or descending aorta due to an aneurysm, and cardiomegaly when aortic insufficiency is present. Radiographs may show calcification at previous sites of cartilage damage involving ear, nose, larynx, or trachea.

DIAGNOSIS Diagnosis is based on recognition of the typical clinical features. Biopsies of the involved cartilage from the ear, nose, or respiratory tract will confirm the diagnosis but are only necessary when clinical features are not typical. Patients with Wegener's granulomatosis may have a saddle nose and pulmonary involvement but can be distinguished by the absence of auricular involvement and the presence of granulomatous lesions in the tracheobronchial tree. Patients with Cogan's syndrome have interstitial keratitis and vestibular and auditory abnormalities, but this syndrome does not involve the respiratory tract or ears. Reiter's syndrome may initially resemble relapsing polychondritis because of oligoarticular arthritis and eye involvement, but it is distinguished in time by the appearance of urethritis and typical mucocutaneous lesions and the absence of nose or ear cartilage involvement. Rheumatoid arthritis may initially suggest relapsing polychondritis because of arthritis and eye inflammation. The arthritis in rheumatoid arthritis, however, is erosive and symmetric. In addition, rheumatoid factor titers are usually high compared with those in relapsing polychondritis. Bacterial infection of the pinna may be mistaken for relapsing polychondritis but differs by usually involving only one ear, including the earlobe. Auricular cartilage may also be damaged by trauma or frostbite.

Relapsing polychondritis may develop in patients with a variety of autoimmune disorders, including SLE, rheumatoid arthritis, Sjögren's syndrome, and vasculitis. In most cases, these disorders antedate the appearance of polychondritis, usually by months or years. It is likely that these patients have an immunologic abnormality that predisposes them to development of this group of autoimmune disorders.

℞ TREATMENT In patients with active chondritis or associated vasculitis, prednisone, 40 to 60 mg/d, is often effective in suppressing disease activity; it is tapered gradually once disease is controlled. In some patients, prednisone can be stopped, while in others low doses in the range of 10 to 15 mg/d are required for continued suppression of disease. Immunosuppressive drugs such as methotrexate, cyclophosphamide, or azathioprine should be reserved for patients who fail to respond to prednisone or who require high doses for control of disease activity. Methotrexate has been found by some investigators to be very effective in treating relapsing polychondritis. Dapsone and cyclosporine have been reported to be beneficial in a few patients. Patients with significant ocular inflammation often require intraocular steroids as well as high doses of prednisone. Heart valve replacement or repair of an aortic aneurysm may be necessary. In patients with early subglottic disease, intralesional injection of glutocorticoids may be beneficial. When obstruction is severe, tracheostomy is required. Stents may be necessary in patients with tracheobronchial collapse.

OTHER ARTHRITIDES

NEUROPATHIC JOINT DISEASE Neuropathic joint disease (Charcot's joint) is a progressive destructive arthritis associated with loss of pain sensation, proprioception, or both. In addition, normal muscular reflexes that modulate joint movement are decreased. Without these protective mechanisms, joints are subjected to repeated trauma, resulting in progressive cartilage and bone damage. Neuropathic arthropathy was first described by Jean-Martin Charcot in 1868 in patients with tabes dorsalis. The term *Charcot joint* is commonly used interchangeably with *neuropathic joint*. Today, diabetes mellitus is the most frequent cause of neuropathic joint disease. A variety of other disorders are associated with neuropathic arthritis including leprosy, yaws, syringomyelia, meningomyelocoele, congenital indifference to pain, peroneal muscular atrophy (Charcot-Marie-Tooth disease), and amyloidosis. An arthritis resembling neuropathic joint disease is seen in patients who have received frequent intraarticular glucocorticoid injections into a weight-bearing joint and in patients with calcium pyrophosphate dihydrate crystal deposition disease. The distribution of joint involvement depends on the underlying neurologic disorder (Table 325-2). In tabes dorsalis, knees, hips, and ankles are most commonly affected; in syringomyelia, the glenohumeral joint, elbow, and wrist; and in diabetes mellitus, the tarsal and tarsometatarsal joints.

Pathology and Pathophysiology The pathologic changes in the neuropathic joint are similar to those found in the severe osteoarthritic joint. There is fragmentation and eventual loss of articular cartilage with eburnation of the underlying bone. Osteophytes are found at the joint margins. With more advanced disease, erosions are present on the joint surface. Fractures, devitalized bone, and intraarticular loose bodies may be present. Microscopic fragments of cartilage and bone are seen in the synovial tissue.

At least two underlying mechanisms are believed to be involved in the pathogenesis of neuropathic arthritis. An abnormal autonomic

Table 325-2 Disorders Associated with Neuropathic Joint Disease

Diabetes mellitus	Amyloidosis
Tabes dorsalis	Leprosy
Meningomyelocele	Congenital indifference to pain
Syringomyelia	Peroneal muscular atrophy

nervous system is thought to be responsible for the increased blood flow to the joint and subsequent resorption of bone. Loss of bone, particularly in the diabetic foot, may be the initial manifestation. With the loss of deep pain, proprioception, and protective neuromuscular reflexes, the joint is subjected to repeated injuries including ligamental tears and bone fractures. The mechanism of injury that occurs following frequent intraarticular glucocorticoid injections is thought to be due to the analgesic effect of glucocorticoids leading to overuse of an already damaged joint, which results in accelerated cartilage damage. It is not understood why only a few patients with neuropathies develop neuropathic arthritis.

Clinical Manifestations Neuropathic joint disease usually begins in a single joint and then progresses to involve other joints, depending on the underlying neurologic disorder. The involved joint progressively becomes enlarged from bony overgrowth and synovial effusion. Loose bodies may be palpated in the joint cavity. Joint instability, subluxation, and crepitus occur as the disease progresses. Neuropathic joints may develop rapidly, and a totally disorganized joint with multiple bony fragments may evolve in a patient within weeks or months. The amount of pain experienced by the patient is less than would be anticipated based on the degree of joint involvement. Patients may experience sudden joint pain from intraarticular fractures of osteophytes or condyles.

Neuropathic arthritis is encountered most often in patients with diabetes mellitus, with the incidence estimated in the range of 0.5%. The usual age of onset is ≥50 years following several years of diabetes, but exceptions occur. The tarsal and tarsometatarsal joints are most often affected, followed by the metatarsophalangeal and talotibial joints. The knees and spine are occasionally involved. In about 20%, neuropathic arthritis may be present in both feet. Patients often attribute the onset of foot pain to antecedent trauma such as twisting their foot. Neuropathic changes may develop rapidly following a foot fracture or dislocation. Swelling of the foot and ankle are often present. Downward collapse of the tarsal bones leads to convexity of the sole, referred to as a "rocker foot." Large osteophytes may protrude from the top of the foot. Calluses frequently form over the metatarsal heads and may lead to infected ulcers and osteomyelitis. Radiographs may show resorption and tapering of the distal metatarsal bones. The term *Lisfranc fracture-dislocation* is sometimes used to describe the destructive changes at the tarsometatarsal joints.

Diagnosis The diagnosis of neuropathic arthritis is based on the clinical features and characteristic radiographic findings in a patient with an underlying sensory neuropathy. The differential diagnosis of neuropathic arthritis includes osteomyelitis, osteonecrosis, advanced osteoarthritis, stress fractures, and calcium pyrophosphate dihydrate (CPDD) deposition disease. Radiographs in neuropathic arthritis initially show changes of osteoarthritis with joint space narrowing, subchondral bone sclerosis, osteophytes, and joint effusions followed later by marked destructive and hypertrophic changes. Soft tissue swelling, bone resorption, fractures, large osteophytes, extraarticular bone fragments, and subluxation are present with advanced arthropathy. The radiographic findings of neuropathic arthritis may be difficult to differentiate from those of osteomyelitis, especially in the diabetic foot. The joint margins in a neuropathic joint tend to be distinct, while in osteomyelitis, they are blurred. Imaging studies and cultures of fluid and tissue from the joint are often required to exclude osteomyelitis. Magnetic resonance imaging is helpful in differentiating these disorders. Another useful study is a bone scan using indium 111–labeled white blood cells or indium 111–labeled immunoglobulin G, which will show an increased uptake in osteomyelitis but not in a neuropathic joint. A technetium bone scan will not distinguish osteomyelitis from neuropathic arthritis as increased uptake is observed in both. The joint fluid in neuropathic arthritis is noninflammatory; may be xanthochromic or even bloody; and may contain fragments of synovium, cartilage, and bone. The finding of CPPD crystals suggests the diagnosis of a crystal associated neuropathic-like arthropathy. In the absence of CPPD crystals, the presence of increased number of leukocytes may indicate osteomyelitis.

℞ **TREATMENT** The primary focus of treatment is to provide stabilization of the joint. Treatment of the underlying disorder, even if successful, does not usually alter the joint disease. Braces and splints are helpful. Their use requires close surveillance, since patients may be unable to appreciate pressure from a poorly adjusted brace. In the diabetic patient, early recognition and treatment of a Charcot's foot by prohibiting weight bearing of the foot for at least 8 weeks may possibly prevent severe disease from developing. Fusion of a very unstable joint may improve function, but nonunion is frequent, especially when immobilization of the joint is inadequate.

HYPERTROPHIC OSTEOARTHROPATHY AND CLUBBING Hypertrophic osteoarthropathy (HOA) is characterized by clubbing of digits and, in more advanced stages, by periosteal new bone formation and synovial effusions. HOA occurs in primary and familial forms and usually begins in childhood. The secondary form of HOA is associated with intrathoracic malignancies, suppurative lung disease, congenital heart disease, and a variety of other disorders and is more common in adults. Clubbing is almost always a feature of HOA but can occur as an isolated manifestation (Fig. 325-1). The presence of clubbing in isolation is generally considered to represent either an early stage or an element in the spectrum of HOA. The presence of only clubbing in a patient usually has the same clinical significance as HOA.

Pathology and Pathophysiology In HOA, the bone changes in the distal extremities begin as periostitis followed by new bone formation. At this stage, a radiolucent area may be observed between the new periosteal bone and subjacent cortex. As the process progresses, multiple layers of new bone are deposited, which become contiguous with the cortex and result in cortical thickening. The outer portion of bone is laminated in appearance, with an irregular surface. Initially, the process of periosteal new bone formation involves the proximal and distal diaphyses of the tibia, fibula, radius, and ulna and, less frequently, the femur, humerus, metacarpals, metatarsals, and phalanges. Occasionally, scapulae, clavicles, ribs, and pelvic bones are also affected. In long-standing disease, these changes extend to involve metaphyses and musculotendinous insertions. The adjacent interosseous membranes may become ossified. The distribution of the bone manifestations is usually bilateral and symmetric. The soft tissue overlying the distal third of the arms and legs may be thickened. Mononuclear cell infiltration may be present in the adjacent soft tissue. Proliferation of connective tissue occurs in the nail bed and volar pad of digits, giving the distal phalanges a clubbed appearance. Small blood vessels in the clubbed digits are dilated and have thickened walls. In addition, the number of arteriovenous anastomoses is increased. The synovium of involved joints shows edema, varying degrees of synovial

FIGURE 325-1 Clubbing of fingers. *(Reprinted from the Clinical Slide Collection on the Rheumatic Diseases, Copyright 1991, 1995. Used by permission of the American College of Rheumatology.)*

cell proliferation, thickening of the subsynovium, vascular congestion, vascular obliteration with thrombi, and small numbers of lymphocyte infiltrates.

Several theories have been suggested for the pathogenesis of HOA. Most have either been disproved or have not explained the development in all clinical disorders associated with HOA. Previously proposed neurogenic and humoral theories are no longer considered likely explanations for HOA. The neurogenic theory was based on the observation that vagotomy resulted in symptomatic improvement in a small number of patients with lung tumors and HOA. It was postulated that vagal stimuli from the tumor site led via a neural reflex to efferent nerve impulses to the distal extremities, resulting in HOA. This theory, however, did not explain HOA in conditions where vagal stimulation did not occur, as in cyanotic congenital heart disease or arterial aneurysms. The humoral theory postulated that soluble substances that are normally inactivated or removed during passage through the lung reached the systemic circulation in an active form and stimulated the changes of HOA. Substances proposed included prostaglandins, ferritin, bradykinin, estrogen, and growth hormone. These substances seemed unlikely candidates, since their blood levels in HOA patients overlapped those in individuals without HOA. Furthermore, these substances did not explain the development of localized HOA associated with arterial aneurysms or infected arterial grafts.

Recent studies have suggested a role for platelets in the development of HOA. It has been observed that megakaryocytes and large platelet particles, present in venous circulation, were fragmented in their passage through normal lung. In patients with cyanotic congenital heart disease and in other disorders associated with right-to-left shunts, these large platelet particles may bypass the lung and reach the distal extremities, where they can interact with endothelial cells. Platelet clumps have been demonstrated to form on an infected heart valve in bacterial endocarditis, in the wall of arterial aneurysms, and on infected arterial grafts. These platelet particles may also reach the distal extremities and interact with endothelial cells. Platelet-endothelial activation in the distal portion of extremities would then result in the release of platelet-derived growth factor (PDGF) and other factors leading to the proliferation of connective tissue and periosteum. Stimulation of fibroblasts by PDGF and transforming growth factor β (TGF-β) results in cell growth and collagen synthesis. Elevated plasma levels of von Willebrand factor antigen have been found in patients with both primary and secondary forms of HOA, indicating endothelial activation or damage. Abnormalities of collagen synthesis have been demonstrated in the involved skin of patients with primary HOA. Fibroblasts from affected skin were shown to have increased collagen synthesis, increased $\alpha 1$(I) procollagen mRNA, and evidence for upregulation of collagen transcription. Other factors are undoubtedly involved in the pathogenesis of HOA, and further studies are needed to better understand this disorder.

Clinical Manifestations   Primary HOA, also referred to as *pachydermoperiostitis* or *Touraine-Solente-Golé syndrome*, usually begins insidiously at puberty. In a smaller number of patients, the onset is in the first year of life. The disorder is inherited as an autosomal dominant trait with variable expression and is nine times more common in boys than in girls. Approximately one-third of patients have a family history of primary HOA.

Primary HOA is characterized by clubbing, periostitis, and unusual skin features. A small number of patients with this syndrome do not express clubbing. The skin changes and periostitis are prominent features of this syndrome. The skin becomes thickened and coarse. Deep nasolabial folds develop, and the forehead may become furrowed. Patients may have heavy-appearing eyelids and ptosis. The skin is often greasy, and there may be excessive sweating of the hands and feet. Patients may also experience acne vulgaris, seborrhea, and folliculitis. In a few patients, the skin over the scalp becomes very thick and corrugated, a feature that has been descriptively termed *cutis verticis gyrata*. The distal extremities, particularly the legs, become thickened owing to proliferation of new bone and soft tissue; when the process is extensive, the distal lower extremities resemble those of an elephant.

The periostitis is usually not painful, as it may be in secondary HOA. Clubbing of the fingers may be extensive, producing large, bulbous deformities and clumsiness. Clubbing also affects the toes. Patients may experience articular and periarticular pain, especially in the ankles and knees, and joint motion may be mildly restricted owing to periarticular bone overgrowth. Noninflammatory effusions occur in the wrists, knees, and ankles. Synovial hypertrophy is not found. Associated abnormalities observed in patients with primary HOA include hypertrophic gastropathy, bone marrow failure, female escutcheon, gynecomastia, and cranial suture defects. In patients with primary HOA, the symptoms disappear when adulthood is reached.

HOA secondary to an underlying disease occurs more frequently than primary HOA. It accompanies a variety of disorders and may precede clinical features of the associated disorder by months. Clubbing is more frequent than the full syndrome of HOA in patients with associated illnesses. Because clubbing evolves over months and is usually asymptomatic, it is often recognized first by the physician and not the patient. Patients may experience a burning sensation in their fingertips. Clubbing is characterized by widening of the fingertips, enlargement of the distal volar pad, convexity of the nail contour, and the loss of the normal 15° angle between the proximal nail and cuticle. The thickness of the digit at the base of the nail is greater than the thickness at the distal interphalangeal joint. An objective measurement of finger clubbing can be made by determining the diameter at the base of the nail and at the distal interphalangeal joint of all 10 digits. Clubbing is present when the sum of the individual digit ratios is >10. At the bedside, clubbing can be appreciated by having the patient place the dorsal surface of the fourth fingers together. Normally, an open area is visible between the opposing fingers; when clubbing is present, this open space is no longer visible. The base of the nail feels spongy when compressed, and the nail can be easily rocked on its bed. Marked periungual erythema is usually present. When clubbing is advanced, the finger may have a drumstick appearance, and the distal interphalangeal joint can be hyperextended. Periosteal involvement in the distal extremities may produce a burning or deep-seated aching pain. The pain can be quite incapacitating and is aggravated by dependency and relieved by elevation of the affected limbs. The overlying soft tissue may be swollen, and the skin slightly erythematous. Pressure applied over the distal forearms and legs may be quite painful.

Patients may also experience joint pain, most often in the ankles, wrists, and knees. Joint effusions may be present; usually they are small and noninflammatory. The small joints of the hands are rarely affected. Severe joint or bone pain may be the presenting symptom of an underlying lung malignancy and may precede the appearance of clubbing. In addition, the progression of HOA tends to be more rapid when associated with malignancies, most notably bronchogenic carcinoma. Unlike primary HOA, excessive sweating and oiliness of the skin and thickening of the facial skin are uncommon in secondary HOA.

HOA occurs in 5 to 10% of patients with intrathoracic malignancies, the most common being bronchogenic carcinoma and pleural tumors (Table 325-3). Lung metastases infrequently cause HOA. HOA is also seen in patients with intrathoracic infections, including lung abscesses, empyema, bronchiectasis, chronic obstructive lung disease, and, uncommonly, pulmonary tuberculosis. HOA may also accompany chronic interstitial pneumonitis, sarcoidosis, and cystic fibrosis. In the latter, clubbing is more common than the full syndrome of HOA. Other causes of clubbing include congenital heart disease with right-to-left shunts, bacterial endocarditis, Crohn's disease, ulcerative colitis, sprue, and neoplasms of the esophagus, liver, and small and large bowel. In patients with congenital heart disease with right-to-left shunts, clubbing alone occurs more often than the full syndrome of HOA.

Unilateral clubbing has been found in association with aneurysms of major extremity arteries, infected arterial grafts, and with arteriovenous fistulas of brachial vessels. Clubbing of the toes but not fingers

Table 325-3   Disorders Associated with Hypertrophic Osteoarthropathy

Pulmonary	Cardiovascular
Bronchogenic carcinoma and other neoplasms	Cyanotic congenital heart disease
Lung abscesses, empyema, bronchiectasis	Subacute bacterial endocarditis
	Infected arterial grafts[a]
Chronic interstitial pneumonitis	Aortic aneurysm[b]
Cystic fibrosis	Aneurysm of major extremity artery[a]
Chronic obstructive lung disease	Patent ductus arteriosus[b]
Sarcoidosis	Arteriovenous fistula of major extremity vessel[a]
Gastrointestinal	
Inflammatory bowel disease	Thyroid (thyroid acropachy)
Sprue	Hyperthyroidism (Graves' disease)
Neoplasms: esophagus, liver, bowel	

[a] Unilateral involvement.
[b] Bilateral lower extremity involvement.

has been associated with an infected abdominal aortic aneurysm and patent ductus arteriosus. Clubbing of a single digit may follow trauma and has been reported in tophaceous gout and sarcoidosis. While clubbing occurs more commonly than the full syndrome in most diseases, periostitis in the absence of clubbing has been observed in the affected limb of patients with infected arterial grafts.

Hyperthyroidism (Graves' disease), treated or untreated, is occasionally associated with clubbing and periostitis of the bones of the hands and feet. This condition is referred to as *thyroid acropachy*. Periostitis is asymptomatic and occurs in the midshaft and diaphyseal portion of the metacarpal and phalangeal bones. The long bones of the extremities are seldom affected. Elevated levels of long-acting thyroid stimulator (LATS) are found in the serum of these patients.

Laboratory Findings   The laboratory abnormalities reflect the underlying disorder. The synovial fluid of involved joints has <500 white cells per microliter, and the cells are predominantly mononuclear. Radiographs show a faint radiolucent line beneath the new periosteal bone along the shaft of long bones at their distal end. These changes are observed most frequently at the ankles, wrists, and knees. The ends of the distal phalanges may show osseous resorption. Radionuclide studies show pericortical linear uptake along the cortical margins of long bones that may be present before any radiographic changes.

℞ **TREATMENT**   The treatment of HOA is to identify the associated disorder and treat it appropriately. The symptoms and signs of HOA may disappear completely with removal or effective chemotherapy of a tumor or with antibiotic therapy and drainage of a chronic pulmonary infection. Vagotomy or percutaneous block of the vagus nerve leads to symptomatic relief in some patients. Aspirin, other nonsteroidal anti-inflammatory drugs (NSAIDs), or analgesics may help control symptoms of HOA.

FIBROMYALGIA   Fibromyalgia is a commonly encountered disorder characterized by widespread musculoskeletal pain, stiffness, paresthesia, nonrestorative sleep, and easy fatigability along with multiple tender points which are widely and symmetrically distributed. Fibromyalgia affects predominantly women in a ratio of 8 or 9 to 1 compared to men. This disorder is found in most countries, in most ethnic groups, and in all types of climates. The prevalence of fibromyalgia in the general population of a community in the United States using the 1990 American College of Rheumatology (ACR) classification criteria was reported to be 3.4% in women and 0.5% in men. Contrary to some previous reports, fibromyalgia was not found to be present mainly in young women but, rather, to be most prevalent in women ≥50 years. The prevalence increased with age, being 7.4% in women between the ages of 70 and 79. Although not common, fibromyalgia also occurs in children. The reported prevalence of fibromyalgia in some rheumatology clinics has been as high as 20%.

Pathogenesis   Several causative mechanisms for fibromyalgia have been postulated. Disturbed sleep has been implicated as a factor in the pathogenesis. Nonrestorative sleep or awakening unrefreshed has been observed in most patients with fibromyalgia. Sleep electroencephalographic studies in patients with fibromyalgia have shown disruption of normal stage 4 sleep [non–rapid eye movement (NREM) sleep] by many repeated α-wave intrusions. The idea that stage 4 sleep deprivation has a role in causing this disorder was supported by the observation that symptoms of fibromyalgia developed in normal subjects whose stage 4 sleep was disrupted artificially by induced α-wave intrusions. This sleep disturbance, however, has been demonstrated in healthy individuals; in emotionally distressed individuals; and in patients with sleep apnea, fever, osteoarthritis, or rheumatoid arthritis. Low levels of serotonin metabolites have been reported in the cerebrospinal fluid of patients with fibromyalgia, suggesting that a deficiency of serotonin, a neurotransmitter that regulates pain and NREM sleep, might also be involved in the pathogenesis of fibromyalgia. Drugs that affect serotonin metabolism have not had a dramatic effect on fibromyalgia, however. Since patients experience pain from muscle and musculotendinous sites, many studies have been done to examine muscle, both structurally and physiologically. Inflammation or diagnostic muscle abnormalities have not been found. Evidence indicates deconditioning of muscles, and patients experience a greater degree of postexertional pain than do unaffected persons. Fibromyalgia patients as a group have been reported by some investigators to have reduced levels of growth hormone, which is important for muscle repair and strength. Growth hormone is secreted normally during stage 4 sleep, which is disturbed in patients with fibromyalgia. The reduction of growth hormone may explain the extended periods of muscle pain following exertion in these patients. The level of the neurotransmitter substance P has been reported to be increased in the cerebrospinal fluid of fibromyalgia patients and may play a role in spreading muscle pain. Patients with fibromyalgia have a decreased cortisol response to stress. Low urinary free cortisol and a diminished cortisol response to corticotropin-releasing hormone suggest an abnormal hypothalamic-pituitary-adrenal axis. Disturbances of the autonomic and peripheral nervous systems may account for the cold sensitivity and Raynaud's-like symptoms seen in patients with fibromyalgia.

Many patients with fibromyalgia have psychological abnormalities; there has been disagreement as to whether some of these abnormalities represent reactions to the chronic pain or whether the symptoms of fibromyalgia are a reflection of psychiatric disturbance. Many patients fit a psychiatric diagnosis, the most common being depression, anxiety, somatization, and hypochondriases. Studies have also shown a high prevalence of sexual and physical abuse and eating disorders. However, fibromyalgia also occurs in patients without significant psychiatric problems. Patients with fibromyalgia may have a lower pain threshold than usual, although not all investigators in the field agree on this point. A better understanding of fibromyalgia awaits further studies.

Clinical Manifestations   Symptoms are generalized aching and stiffness of the trunk, hip, and shoulder girdles. Other patients complain of generalized muscle aching and weakness. Patients may complain of low back pain, which may radiate into the buttocks and legs. Others complain of pain and tightness in the neck and across the upper posterior shoulders. Patients complain of muscle pain after even mild exertion. Some degree of pain is always present. The pain has been described as a burning or gnawing pain or as soreness, stiffness, or aching. While pain may begin in one region, such as the shoulders, neck, or lower back, it eventually becomes widespread. Patients may complain of joint pain and perceive that their joints are swollen; however, joint examination yields normal findings. Stiffness is usually present on arising in the morning; usually it improves during the day, but in some patients it lasts all day. Patients may complain of numbness of their hands and feet. They may also feel colder overall than others in the home, and some may experience Raynaud's-like phe-

ing fatigued and exhausted and wake up tired. They also awaken frequently at night and have trouble falling back to sleep. Symptoms are
made worse by stress or anxiety, cold, damp weather, and overexertion. Patients often feel better during warmer weather and vacations.

The characteristic feature on physical examination is the demonstration of specific tender points, which are exclusively more tender
or painful than adjacent areas. The ACR Criteria for Fibromyalgia
defines 18 tender points (Fig. 325-2). These points of tenderness are
remarkably constant in location. A moderate degree of pressure should
be used in digital palpation of these tender points. Some workers recommend that the tender site be palpated using a rolling motion, which
may be more effective in eliciting the tenderness. The tender sites can
also be examined using a dolorimeter, which is a spring-loaded pressure gauge. Digital palpation appears to be as effective and accurate
for the diagnosis of fibromyalgia as dolorimetry. The amount of pressure applied by the examiner introduces variability in the interpretation, however. If too much pressure is applied, the pain will be produced even in normal subjects. Likewise, tenderness will not be
appreciated if too little pressure is applied or the site is missed on
palpation. Some investigators have quantitated their response, but the
number of tender point sites is more diagnostic. Some patients are
tender all over and not just at the specific tender point sites. These
patients are still more tender over the specific tender point sites, however. Sites where there is usually no tenderness and which can be used
as controls are the dorsum of the third digit between the proximal
interphalangeal and distal interphalangeal joints, the medial third of
the clavicle, the medial malleolus, and the forehead. If tenderness at
these sites is also present, the diagnosis of fibromyalgia should be
questioned and possible psychiatric disorders investigated. Whether
such patients can be diagnosed as also having fibromyalgia is debatable.

Skinfold tenderness may be present, particularly over the upper

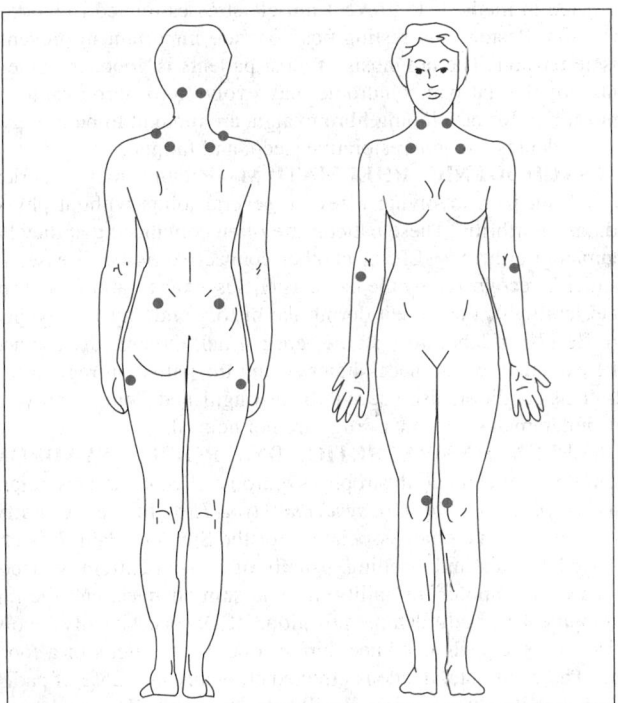

FIGURE 325-2 Tender points in fibromyalgia. Suboccipital muscle insertion
at base of skull; anterior aspect of intertransverse process spaces at C5–7;
midpoint of upper border of trapezius muscle; above scapular spine near medial
border of scapula; second costochondral junction; lateral epicondyle; upper
outer quadrant of buttocks; posterior aspect of trochanteric prominence; medial
fat pad of knee (all bilateral). *(From the brochure "Fibromyalgia," Arthritis
Information, Advise and Guidance, Disease Series. Used by permission of the
Arthritis Foundation.)*

scapular region. Subcutaneous nodules may be felt at sites of tenderness. Nodules in similar locations are present in normal persons but
are not tender.

Fibromyalgia may be triggered by emotional stress, medical illness, surgery, hypothyroidism, and trauma. It has appeared in some
patients with human immunodeficiency virus (HIV) infection, parvovirus B19 infection, or Lyme disease. In the latter situation, fibromyalgia persisted despite adequate antibiotic treatment for Lyme disease. Disorders commonly associated with fibromyalgia include
irritable bowel syndrome, irritable bladder, headaches (including
migraine headaches), dysmenorrhea, premenstrual syndrome, restless legs syndrome, temporomandibular joint pain, and sicca
syndrome.

The course of fibromyalgia is variable. Symptoms wax and wane
in some patients, while in others pain and fatigue are persistent regardless of therapy. Studies from tertiary medical centers indicate a
poor prognosis for most patients. The prognosis may be better in com-
munity-treated patients. In a community-based study reported after 2
years of treatment, 24% of patients were in remission, and 47% no
longer fulfilled the ACR criteria for fibromyalgia.

Diagnosis Fibromyalgia is diagnosed by a history of widespread
pain and the demonstration of at least 11 of the 18 tender point sites
on digital palpation (Fig. 325-2). The ACR criteria are useful for standardizing the diagnosis; however, not all patients with fibromyalgia
meet these criteria (Table 325-4). Some patients have fewer tender
sites and more regional pain and may be considered to have probable
fibromyalgia.

Results of joint and muscle examinations are normal in fibromyalgia patients, and there are no laboratory abnormalities. Fibromyalgia may occur in patients with rheumatoid arthritis, other connective tissue diseases, or other medical illness. A distinction is no
longer made between primary and secondary fibromyalgia (concomitant with other disease), as the signs and symptoms are similar. Fibromyalgia and chronic fatigue syndrome have many similarities (Chap.
384). Both are associated with fatigue, abnormal sleep, musculoskeletal pain, and psychiatric conditions such as less severe forms of de-

**Table 325-4 The American College of Rheumatology 1990 Criteria for
the Classification of Fibromyalgia**[a]

1. History of widespread pain. Pain is considered widespread when all of the
   following are present:
   a. Pain in the left side of the body
   b. Pain in the right side of the body
   c. Pain above the waist
   d. Pain below the waist
   e. Axial skeletal pain (cervical spine or anterior chest or thoracic spine or
      low back)
2. Pain on digital palpation in at least 11 of the following 18 tender point sites
   (see Fig. 325-2):
   a. Occiput: bilateral, at the suboccipital muscle insertion
   b. Low cervical: bilateral, at the anterior aspect of the intertransverse spaces
      at C5–7
   c. Trapezius: bilateral, at the midpoint of the upper border
   d. Supraspinatus: bilateral, at the origin, above the scapular spine near the
      medial border
   e. Second rib: bilateral, at the second costochondral junction, just lateral to
      the junction on the upper surface
   f. Lateral epicondyle: bilateral, 2 cm distal to the epicondyle
   g. Gluteal: bilateral, in the upper outer quadrant of the buttock
   h. Greater trochanter: bilateral, posterior to the trochanteric prominence
   i. Knee: bilateral, at the medial fat pad proximal to the joint line

Digital palpation should be performed with a moderate degree of pressure.
For a tender point to be considered positive, the subject must state that the
palpation was painful. "Tender" is not to be considered painful.

[a] For purposes of classification, patients will be said to have fibromyalgia if both criteria
are satisfied. Widespread pain must have been present for at least 3 months. The presence
of a second clinical disorder does not exclude the diagnosis of fibromyalgia.
SOURCE: Modified from F Wolfe et al: Arthritis Rheum 33:171, 1990.

pression and anxiety. Patients with chronic fatigue syndrome, however, are more likely to have symptoms suggesting a viral illness. These include mild fever, sore throat, and pain in the axillary and anterior and posterior cervical lymph nodes. The onset of chronic fatigue syndrome is usually sudden; patients are usually able to date the onset. Patients also have impaired memory and concentration. While many patients with chronic fatigue syndrome have tender points, the diagnosis does not require their presence. Polymyalgia rheumatica is distinguished from fibromyalgia in an elderly patient by the presence of more proximal muscle stiffness and pain and an elevated erythrocyte sedimentation rate. Patients should be evaluated for hypothyroidism, which may have symptoms similar to fibromyalgia or may accompany fibromyalgia.

The diagnosis of fibromyalgia has taken on a more complex significance in regard to labor and industry issues. This has become a significant issue since it has been reported that 10 to 25% of patients are not able to work in any capacity, while others require modification of their work. Disability evaluation in fibromyalgia is controversial. The diagnosis of fibromyalgia is not accepted by all. It is hard to evaluate patients' perceptions of their inability to function. The determination of tender points can also be subjective, on the part of both the physician and the patient, particularly when issues of compensation are pending. Patients also encounter difficulty in having their illness recognized as a disability. Physicians have been placed in the inappropriate role of assessing the patient's disability. Physicians are not in a position to quantitate disability at the workplace; that is better done by a work evaluation specialist. Better instruments are clearly needed for measuring disability, particularly in patients with fibromyalgia.

℞ **TREATMENT**   Patients should be informed that they have a condition that is not crippling, deforming, or degenerative, and that treatment is available. Salicylates or other NSAIDs only partially improve symptoms. Glucocorticoids have been of little benefit and should not be used in these patients. Opiate analgesics should be avoided. Local measures such as heat, massage, injection of tender sites with steroids or lidocaine, and acupuncture provide only temporary relief of symptoms. Other therapies that may help to varying degrees including biofeedback, behavioral modification, hypnotherapy, and stress management and relaxation response training. The use of tricyclics such as amitriptyline (10 to 50 mg) and doxepin (10 to 25 mg) or a pharmacologically similar drug, cyclobenzaprine (10 to 40 mg), 1 to 2 h before bedtime will give the patient restorative sleep (stage 4 sleep), resulting in clinical improvement. Patients should be started on a low dose, which is increased gradually as needed. Side effects of these tricyclics and cyclobenzoprine limit their use; these include constipation, dry mouth, weight gain, drowsiness, and difficulty thinking. Depression and anxiety should be treated with appropriate drugs and, when indicated, with psychiatric counseling. Alprazolam and lorazepam can be used for anxiety, while trazodone, sertraline, fluoxetine, paroxetine or other newer selective serotonin reuptake inhibitors can be used as antidepressants. Patients may also benefit by regular aerobic exercises. Exercise should be of a low-impact type and begun at a low level. Eventually, the patient should be exercising 20 to 30 min 3 to 4 days a week. Regular stretching exercises are also very important. Life stresses should be identified and discussed with the patient, and the patient should be provided with help on how to cope with these stresses. Patients may benefit from a multidisciplinary team approach involving a mental health professional, a physical therapist, and a physical medicine and rehabilitation specialist. Group therapy may be beneficial. Patients should be well educated about their disorder and taught the importance of self help. There are patient support groups in many communities. While treatment of fibromyalgia is effective in some patients, others continue to have chronic disease, which is relieved only partially if at all.

MYOFASCIAL PAIN SYNDROME   Myofascial pain syndrome is characterized by localized musculoskeletal pain and tenderness in association with trigger points. The pain is deep and aching and may be accompanied by a burning sensation. Myofascial pain may follow trauma, overuse, or prolonged static contraction of a muscle or muscle group, which may occur when reading or writing at a desk or working at a computer. In addition, this syndrome may be associated with underlying osteoarthritis of the neck or low back. Trigger points are a diagnostic feature of this syndrome. Pain is referred from trigger points to defined areas distant from the original tender points. Palpation of the trigger point reproduces or accentuates the pain. The trigger points are usually located in the center of a muscle belly, but they can occur at other sites, such as costosternal junctions, the xyphoid process, ligamentous and tendinous insertions, fascia, and fatty areas. Trigger point sites in muscle have been described as feeling indurated and taut, and palpation may cause the muscle to twitch. These findings, however, have been shown not to be unique for myofascial pain syndrome, since in a controlled study they were also present in fibromyalgia patients and normal subjects. Myofascial pain most often involves the posterior neck, low back, shoulders, and chest. Chronic pain in the muscles of the posterior neck may involve referral of pain from the trigger point in the erector neck muscle or upper trapezius to the head, leading to persistent headaches which may last for days. Trigger points in the paraspinal muscles of the low back may refer pain to the buttock. Pain may be referred down the leg from a trigger point in the gluteus medius and can mimic sciatica. A trigger point in the infraspinatus muscle may produce local and referred pain over the lateral deltoid and down the outside of the arm into the hand. Injection of a local anesthetic such as 1% lidocaine into the trigger point site often results in pain relief. Another useful technique is first to spray from the trigger point toward the area of referred pain with an agent such as ethyl chloride and then to stretch the muscle. This maneuver may need to be repeated several times. Massage and application of ultrasound to the affected area may also be beneficial. Patients should be instructed in methods to prevent muscle stresses related to work and recreation. Posture and resting positions are important in preventing muscle tension. The prognosis in most patients is good. In some patients, myofascial pain syndrome may evolve into fibromyalgia. Patients at risk for developing fibromyalgia are thought to be those with anxiety, depression, nonrestorative sleep, and fatigue.

PSYCHOGENIC RHEUMATISM   Patients may experience severe joint pain involving a few to several joints without physical findings of arthritis. These patients are often convinced that they have rheumatoid arthritis, SLE, or another connective tissue disease. This disorder is recognized by the inconsistencies, exaggerations, and emotional lability of the patient during the history and physical examination. Results of laboratory studies are normal. Organic disease needs to be excluded, which necessitates seeing the patient at regular intervals. This condition also needs to be distinguished from fibromyalgia. Anti-inflammatory or other drugs are not helpful.

REFLEX SYMPATHETIC DYSTROPHY SYNDROME
The reflex sympathetic dystrophy syndrome (RSDS) is now referred to as *complex regional pain syndrome, type 1,* by the new Classification of the International Association for the Study of Pain. It is characterized by pain and swelling, usually of a distal extremity, accompanied by vasomotor instability, trophic skin changes, and the rapid development of bony demineralization. RSDS occasionally involves an isolated site such as a knee, hip, or one or two digits of a foot or hand. The contralateral side is affected clinically in ~25% of patients and may be involved in virtually all patients with RSDS, as shown by scintigraphic studies. A precipitating event can be identified in at least two-thirds of cases. These events include trauma, such as fractures and crush injuries; myocardial infarction; strokes; peripheral nerve injury; and use of certain drugs, including barbiturates, anti-tuberculous drugs, and, more recently, cyclosporine administered to patients undergoing renal transplantation. The pathogenesis of RSDS is poorly understood and is thought to involve abnormal activity of the sympathetic nervous system following a precipitating event.

RSDS evolves through three clinical phases. The first phase is characterized by an intense burning pain and swelling of a distal extremity. The involved extremity is warm, edematous, and very tender, especially around joints. Sweating and hair growth are increased. Light touch causes pain, which may continue after the stimulus is removed. Passive or active motion of joints is very painful, and the joints are stiff. In the first phase, especially when both sides are involved, the clinical findings may suggest early rheumatoid arthritis. Redness and swelling over a distal extremity such as an ankle or wrist may also mimic inflammatory arthritis, or even an infectious arthritis. In 3 to 6 months, the skin gradually becomes thin, shiny, and cool. This is the second phase of the disease. The clinical features of the first and second phases often overlap. In another 3 to 6 months (third phase), the skin becomes atrophic and dry, and irreversible flexion contractures, palmar fibromatosis, and Dupuytren's contractures develop, resulting in a clawlike hand deformity. Similar changes occur in the feet. When RSDS occurs in the upper extremity, motion of the shoulder on the affected side may be painful and restricted, a condition referred to as *shoulder-hand syndrome* (see "Adhesive Capsulitis," below). →*Reflex sympathetic dystrophy syndrome, including its treatment, is covered in greater detail in Chap. 366.*

TIETZE'S SYNDROME AND COSTOCHONDRITIS Tietze's syndrome is manifested by painful swelling of one or more costochondral articulations. The age of onset is usually before 40, and both sexes are affected equally. In most patients only one joint is involved, usually the second or third costochondral joint. The onset of anterior chest pain may be sudden or gradual. The pain may radiate to the arms or shoulder and is aggravated by sneezing, coughing, deep inspirations, or twisting motions of the chest. The term *costochondritis* is often used interchangeably with *Tietze's syndrome*, but some workers restrict the former term to pain of the costochondral articulations without swelling. Costochondritis is observed in patients over age 40; tends to affect the third, fourth, and fifth costochondral joints; and occurs more often in women. Both syndromes may mimic cardiac or upper abdominal causes of pain. Rheumatoid arthritis, ankylosing spondylitis, and Reiter's syndrome may involve costochondral joints but are distinguished easily by their other clinical features. Other skeletal causes of anterior chest wall pain are xiphoidalgia and the slipping rib syndrome, which usually involves the tenth rib. Malignancies such as breast cancer, prostate cancer, plasma cell cytoma, and sarcoma can invade the ribs, thoracic spine, or chest wall and produce symptoms suggesting Tietze's syndrome. They should be easily distinguishable by radiographs and biopsy. Analgesics, anti-inflammatory drugs, and local glucocorticoid injections usually relieve symptoms.

MUSCULOSKELETAL DISORDERS ASSOCIATED WITH HYPERLIPIDEMIA (See also Chap. 344) Musculoskeletal manifestations may be the first indication of a hereditary disorder of lipoprotein metabolism. Patients with familial hypercholesterolemia (previously referred to as type II hyperlipoproteinemia) may have recurrent migratory polyarthritis involving knees and other large peripheral joints and, to a lesser degree, peripheral small joints. In a few patients, the arthritis is monarticular. Fever may accompany the arthritis. Pain ranges from moderate to very severe to incapacitating. The involved joints can be warm, erythematous, swollen, and tender. Arthritis usually has a sudden onset, lasts from a few days to 2 weeks, and does not cause joint damage. Episodes may suggest acute gout attacks. Several attacks occur a year. Synovial fluid from involved joints is not inflammatory and contains few white cells and no crystals. Joint involvement may actually represent inflammatory periarthritis or peritendinitis and not intraarticular disease. The recurrent, transient nature of the arthritis may suggest rheumatic fever, especially since patients with lipoproteinemia have an elevated erythrocyte sedimentation rate, and a falsely elevated antistreptolysin O titer. Patients may also experience Achilles tendinitis, which can be very painful. Attacks of tendinitis come on gradually and last only a few days. Fever is not present. Patients may be asymptomatic between attacks. During an attack the Achilles tendon is warm, erythematous, swollen, and tender

to palpation. Achilles tendinitis and other joint manifestations often precede the appearance of xanthomas and may be the first clinical indication of hyperlipoproteinemia. Attacks of tendinitis may occur following treatment with a lipid-lowering drug. Patients also have tendinous xanthomas in the Achilles, patellar, and extensor tendons of the hands over the knuckles and feet. Xanthomas have also been reported in the peroneal tendon, the plantar aponeurosis, and the periosteum overlying the distal tibia. These xanthomas are located within tendon fibers. Tuberous xanthomas are soft subcutaneous masses located over the extensor surfaces of the elbows, knees, and hands, as well as on the buttocks. They appear in childhood in homozygous patients and after the age of 30 in heterozygous patients. Patients with elevated plasma levels of very low density lipoprotein (VLDL) and triglyceride (previously referred to as type IV hyperlipoproteinemia) may also have a mild inflammatory arthritis affecting large and small peripheral joints, usually in an asymmetric pattern with only a few joints involved at a time. The onset of arthritis is usually in middle age. Arthritis may be persistent or recurrent, with episodes lasting a few days to weeks. Joint pain is severe in some patients. Patients may experience morning stiffness. Joint tenderness and periarticular hyperesthesia may also be present, as may synovial thickening. Joint fluid is usually noninflammatory and without crystals, but may have increased white blood cell counts with predominantly mononuclear cells. The fluid is occasionally lactescent. Radiographs may show juxtaarticular osteopenia and cystic lesions. Large bone cysts have been noted in a few patients. Xanthoma and bone cysts are also observed in other lipoprotein disorders. The pathogenesis of arthritis in patients with familial hypercholesterolemia or with elevated levels of VLDL and triglyceride is not well understood. Salicylates, other NSAIDs, or analgesics usually provide relief of symptoms. Clinical improvement also may occur in patients treated with lipid lowering agents. Patients, however, treated with a HMG CoA reductase agent may experience myalgias and a few patients may develop polymysitis or even rhabdomyolysis (Chap. 382).

ARTHROPATHY OF ACROMEGALY Acromegaly is the result of excessive production of growth hormone by an adenoma in the anterior pituitary gland (Chap. 328). Middle-aged persons are most often affected. The excessive secretion of growth hormone along with insulin-like growth factor I stimulates proliferation of cartilage, periarticular connective tissue, and bone, resulting in several musculoskeletal abnormalities, including osteoarthritis, back pain, muscle weakness, and carpal tunnel syndrome.

An arthropathy resembling osteoarthritis is a common feature, affecting most often the knees, shoulders, hips, and hands. Single or multiple joints may be affected. The overgrowth of cartilage initially produces widening of the joint space. The newly synthesized cartilage is not developed in an organized manner, making it susceptible to fissuring, ulceration, and destruction. Ligamental laxity of the joint resulting from the growth of connective tissue also contributes to the development of osteoarthritis. With breakdown and loss of cartilage, the joint space narrows, and subchondral sclerosis and osteophytes appear on radiographs. Joint examination reveals marked crepitus and hypermobility. Joint fluid is noninflammatory. Calcium pyrophosphate dihydrate crystals are found in the cartilage in some cases of acromegaly arthropathy and, when shed into the joint, can produce attacks of pseudogout. Chondrocalcinosis may also be observed radiographically. Approximately half of the patients with acromegaly experience back pain, which is predominantly lumbosacral. Hypermobility of the spine may be a contributing factor in back pain. Radiograph of the spine shows normal or increased intervertebral disk spaces, hypertrophic anterior osteophytes, and ligamental calcification. These changes are similar to those observed in patients with diffuse idiopathic skeletal hyperostosis. Dorsal kyphosis in conjunction with elongation of the ribs contributes to the development of the barrel chest seen in acromegalic patients. The hands and feet become enlarged owing to soft tissue proliferation. The fingers are thickened and have spadelike distal tufts. One-third of patients have a thickened heel pad. Approximately 25% of patients have Raynaud's phenomenon.

Carpal tunnel syndrome occurs in about half of patients. The median nerve is compressed by the excessive growth of connective tissue in the carpal tunnel. The median nerve also becomes enlarged. Patients with acromegaly also develop proximal muscle weakness, which is thought to be caused by the effect of growth hormone on muscle. Results of muscle enzyme assays and electromyography are normal. Muscle biopsy specimens show muscle fibers of varying size and no inflammatory changes.

ARTHROPATHY OF HEMOCHROMATOSIS   Hemochromatosis is a disorder of iron storage. Excessive amounts of iron are absorbed from the intestine, leading to iron deposition in parenchymal cells, which results in tissue damage and impairment of organ function (Chap. 345). Symptoms of hemochromatosis usually begin between the ages of 40 and 60 but can occur earlier. Arthritis, which occurs in 20 to 40% of patients, usually begins after the age of 50 and may be the first clinical feature of hemochromatosis. The arthropathy is an inflammatory osteoarthritis-like disorder affecting the small joints of the hands, followed later by larger joints such as knees, ankles, shoulders, and hips. The second and third metacarpophalangeal joints of both hands are often the first joints affected; they can provide an important clue to the possibility of hemochromatosis. Patients experience stiffness and pain. Morning stiffness usually lasts less than half an hour. The affected joints are enlarged and mildly tender. Synovial tissue is not appreciatively increased. Radiographs show irregular narrowing of the joint space, subchondral sclerosis, and subchondral cysts. There is juxtaarticular proliferation of bone, with frequent hooklike osteophytes. The synovial fluid is noninflammatory. The synovium shows mild to moderate proliferation of lining cells, fibrosis, and a low number of inflammatory cells, which are mononuclear. In approximately half of patients, there is evidence of calcium pyrophosphate deposition disease. Iron can be demonstrated in the lining cells of the synovium and also in chondrocytes.

Iron may damage the articular cartilage in several ways. Promotion by iron of superoxide-dependent lipid peroxidation may play a role in joint damage. In animal models, ferric iron has been shown to interfere with collagen formation. Iron has also been shown to increase the release of lysosomal enzymes from cells in the synovial membrane. Iron may also play a role in the development of chondrocalcinosis. Iron inhibits synovial tissue pyrophosphatase in vitro and, therefore, may inhibit pyrophosphatase in vivo, resulting in chondrocalcinosis. Iron in synovial cells may also inhibit the clearance of calcium pyrophosphate from the joint.

℞ **TREATMENT**   The treatment of hemochromatosis is repeated phlebotomy. Unfortunately, this treatment has little effect on the arthritis, which, along with chondrocalcinosis, usually continues to progress. Treatment of the arthritis consists of administration of acetaminophen and NSAIDs. Placement of a hip or knee prosthesis has been successful in advanced disease.

HEMOPHILIC ARTHROPATHY   Hemophilia is a sex-linked recessive genetic disorder characterized by the absence or deficiency of factor VIII (hemophilia A, or classic hemophilia) or factor IX (hemophilia B, or Christmas disease) (Chap. 117). Hemophilia A is by far the more common type, constituting 85% of cases. Spontaneous hemarthrosis is a common problem with both types of hemophilia and can lead to a chronic deforming arthritis. The frequency and severity of hemarthrosis are related to the degree of clotting factor deficiency. Hemarthrosis is not common in other inherited disorders of coagulation, such as von Willebrand's disease or factor V deficiency.

Hemarthrosis becomes evident after 1 year of age, when the child begins to walk and run. In order of frequency, the joints most commonly affected are the knees, ankles, elbows, shoulders, and hips. Small joints of the hands and feet are occasionally involved.

In the initial stage of arthropathy, hemarthrosis produces a warm, tensely swollen, and painful joint. The patient holds the affected joint in flexion and guards against any movement. Blood in the joint remains liquid because of the absence of intrinsic clotting factors and the absence of tissue thromboplastin in the synovium. The blood in the joint space is resorbed over a period of a week or longer, depending on the size of the hemarthrosis. Joint function usually returns to normal or baseline in about 2 weeks.

Recurrent hemarthrosis leads to the development of a chronic arthritis. The involved joints remain swollen, and flexion deformities develop. In the later stages of arthropathy, joint motion is restricted and function is severely limited. Joint ankylosis, subluxation, or laxity are features of end-stage disease.

Bleeding into muscle and soft tissue also causes musculoskeletal disorders. When bleeding into the iliopsoas muscle occurs, the hip is held in flexion because of the pain, resulting in a hip flexion contracture. Rotation of the hip is preserved, which distinguishes this problem from intraarticular hemorrhage. Expansion of the hematoma may place pressure on the femoral nerve, resulting in a femoral neuropathy. Another problem is shortening of the heel cord secondary to bleeding into the gastrocnemius. Hemorrhage into a closed compartment space, such as the volar compartment in the forearm, can result in muscle necrosis and flexion deformities of the wrist and fingers. When bleeding involves periosteum or bone, a pseudotumor forms. These occur distal to the elbows or knees in children and improve with treatment of the hemophilia. Surgical removal is indicated if the pseudotumor continues to enlarge. In adults, they occur in the femur and pelvis and are usually refractory to treatment. When bleeding occurs in muscle, cysts may develop within the muscle. Needle aspiration of a cyst is contraindicated because it can induce bleeding.

Septic arthritis can occur in hemophilia and is difficult at times to distinguish from acute hemarthrosis. Whenever there is suspicion of an infected joint, the joint should be aspirated immediately, the fluid cultured, and the patient started on a broad-spectrum antibiotic. The patient should be infused with the deficient clotting factor before the joint is tapped to decrease the risk of further bleeding.

Radiographs of joints reflect the stage of disease. In early stages there is only capsule distention; later, juxtaarticular osteopenia, marginal erosions, and subchondral cysts develop. In late disease, the joint space is narrowed and there is bony overgrowth. The changes are similar to those observed in osteoarthritis. Unique features of hemophilic arthropathy are widening of the femoral intercondylar notch, enlargement of the proximal radius, and squaring of the distal end of the patella.

Recurrent hemarthrosis produces synovial hyperplasia and hypertrophy. A pannus covers the cartilage. Cartilage is damaged by collagenase and other degradative enzymes released by mononuclear cells in the overlying synovium. Hemosiderin is found in synovial lining cells, the subsynovium, and chondrocytes and may also play a role in cartilage destruction.

℞ **TREATMENT**   The treatment of hemarthrosis is initiated with the immediate infusion of factor VIII or IX at the first sign of joint or muscle hemorrhage. The patient is placed at bed rest, with the involved joint in as much extension as the patient can tolerate. Analgesic NSAIDs and local icing may help with the pain. NSAIDs can be given safely for short periods even though they have a stabilizing effect on platelets. Studies have shown no significant abnormalities in platelet function or bleeding time in hemophiliacs receiving ibuprofen. The new cyclooxygenase-2 inhibitors celecoxib and rofecoxib do not interfere with platelet function and can be safely given for pain. Synovectomy, open or arthroscopic, may be indicated in patients with chronic synovial proliferation and recurrent hemarthrosis. Hypertrophied synovium is very vascular and subject to bleeding. Both types of synovectomy reduce the number of hemarthroses and slow the roentgenographic progression of hemophilic arthropathy. Open surgical synovectomy, however, is associated with some loss of range of motion. Radiosynovectomy with either yttrium 90 silicate or phosphorus 31 colloid has also been effective and may be a useful alternative when surgical synovectomy is not practical. Total joint replacement is indicated for severe joint destruction and incapacitating pain. Because of the young age of hemophilic patients, total-joint prostheses may need to be replaced more than once during their lives.

ARTHROPATHIES ASSOCIATED WITH HEMOGLOBINOPATHIES Sickle Cell Disease

Sickle cell disease (Chap. 106) is associated with several musculoskeletal abnormalities (Table 325-5). Children under the age of 5 may develop diffuse swelling, tenderness, and warmth of the hands and feet lasting from 1 to 3 weeks. The condition, referred to as *sickle cell dactylitis* or *hand-foot syndrome* has also been observed in sickle cell disease and sickle cell thalassemia. Dactylitis is believed to result from infarction of the bone marrow and cortical bone leading to periostitis and soft tissue swelling. Radiographs show periosteal elevation, subperiosteal new bone formation, and areas of radiolucency and increased density involving the metacarpals, metatarsals, and proximal phalanges. These bone changes disappear after several months. The syndrome leaves little or no residual damage. Because hematopoiesis ceases in the small bones of hands and feet with age, the syndrome is rarely seen after age 4 or 5 and does not occur in adults.

Sickle cell crisis is often associated with periarticular pain and joint effusions. The joint and periarticular area are warm and tender. Knees and elbows are most often affected, but other joints can be involved. Joint effusions are noninflammatory, with white cell counts <1000/μL; mononuclear cells predominate. There have been a few reports of sterile inflammatory effusion with high cell counts consisting of mostly polymorphonuclear white cells. Synovial biopsies have shown mild lining cell proliferation and microvascular thrombosis. Scintigraphic studies have shown decreased marrow uptake adjacent to the involved joint. The joint effusion and periarticular pain are considered to be the result of ischemia and infarction of the synovium and adjacent bone and bone marrow. The treatment is that for sickle cell crisis (Chap. 106).

Patients with sickle cell disease may also develop osteomyelitis, which commonly involves the long tubular bones (Chap. 129). These patients are particularly susceptible to bacterial infections, especially *Salmonella* infections, which are found in more than half of cases (Chap. 156). Radiographs of the involved site show periosteal elevation initially, followed by disruption of the cortex. Treatment of the infection results in healing of the bone lesion. Sickle cell disease is also associated with bone infarction resulting from thrombosis secondary to the sickling of red cells. Bone infarction also occurs in hemoglobin S-C disease and sickle cell thalassemia (Chap. 106). The bone pain in sickle cell crisis is due to bone and bone marrow infarction. In children, infarction of the epiphyseal growth plate interferes with normal growth of the affected extremity. Radiographically, infarction of the bone cortex results in periosteal elevation and irregular thickening of the bone cortex. Infarction in the bone marrow leads to lysis, fibrosis, and new bone formation.

Avascular necrosis of the head of the femur is seen in ~5% of patients. It also occurs in the humeral head and less commonly in the distal femur, tibial condyles, distal radius, vertebral bodies, and other juxtaarticular sites. The mechanism for avascular necrosis is most likely the same as for bone infarction. Subchondral hemorrhage may play a role in the deterioration of articular cartilage. Irregularity of the femoral head or of other bone surfaces affected by avascular necrosis eventually results in degenerative joint disease. Radiograph of the affected joint may show patchy radiolucency and density followed by

flattening of the bone. Magnetic resonance imaging is a sensitive technique for detecting early avascular necrosis as well as bone infarction elsewhere. Total hip replacement and placement of prostheses in other joints may improve function and relieve pain in those patients with severe joint destruction.

Septic arthritis is occasionally encountered in sickle cell disease (Chap. 323). Multiple joints may be infected. Joint infection may result from hematogenous spread or from spread of contiguous osteomyelitis. Microorganisms identified include staphylococcus, *Streptococcus*, *Escherichia coli*, and *Salmonella*. The latter is not seen as frequently in septic arthritis as it is in osteomyelitis. Acute gouty arthritis is uncommon in sickle cell disease, even though 40% of patients are hyperuremic. Hyperuricemia is due to overproduction of uric acid secondary to increased red cell turnover. Attacks may be polyarticular.

The bone marrow hyperplasia in sickle cell disease results in widening of the medullary cavities, thinning of the cortices, and coarse trabeculations and central cupping of the vertebral bodies. These changes are also seen to a lesser degree in hemoglobin S-C disease and sickle cell thalassemia. In normal individuals, red marrow is located mostly in the axial skeletal, but in sickle cell disease, red marrow is found in the bones of the extremities and even in the tarsal and carpal bones. Vertebral compression may lead to dorsal kyphosis, and softening of the bone in the acetabulum may result in protrusio acetabuli.

Thalassemia β-Thalassemia is a congenital disorder of hemoglobin synthesis characterized by impaired production of β chains (Chap. 106). Bone and joint abnormalities occur in β-thalassemia, being most common in the major and intermedia groups. In one study, approximately 50% of patients with β-thalassemia had evidence of symmetric ankle arthropathy, characterized by a dull aching pain aggravated by weight bearing. The onset was most often in the second or third decade of life. The degree of ankle pain in these patients varied. Some patients experienced self-limited ankle pain, which occurred only after strenuous physical activity and lasted several days to weeks. Other patients had chronic ankle pain, which became worse with walking. Symptoms eventually abated in a few patients. Compression of the ankle, calcaneus, or forefoot was painful in some patients. Synovial fluid from two patients was noninflammatory. Radiographs of ankle showed osteopenia, widened medullary spaces, thin cortices, and coarse trabeculations. These findings were largely the result of bone marrow expansion. The joint space was preserved. Specimens of bone from three patients revealed osteomalacia, osteopenia, and microfractures. Increased osteoblasts as well as increased foci of bone resorption were present on the bone surface. Iron staining was found in the bone trabeculae, in osteoid, and in the cement line. Synovium showed hyperplasia of lining cells which contained deposits of hemosiderin. This arthropathy was considered to be related to the underlying bone pathology. The role of iron overload or abnormal bone metabolism in the pathogenesis of this arthropathy is not known. The arthropathy was treated with analgesics and splints. Patients were also transfused to decrease hematopoiesis and bone marrow expansion.

Patients with β-thalassemia major and intermedia also have involvement of other joints, including the knees, hips, and shoulders. Acquired hemochromatosis with arthropathy has been described in a patient with thalassemia. Gouty arthritis and septic arthritis can occur. Avascular necrosis is not a feature of thalassemia because there is no sickling of red cells leading to thrombosis and infarction.

β-Thalassemia minor (trait) is also associated with joint manifestations. Chronic seronegative oligoarthritis affecting predominantly ankles, wrists, and elbows has been described. These patients had mild persistent synovitis without large effusions. Joint erosions were not seen. Recurrent episodes of an acute asymmetric arthritis also have been reported; episodes last less than a week and may affect knees, ankles, shoulders, elbows, wrists, and metacarpal phalangeal joints. The mechanism for this arthropathy is unknown. Treatment with nonsteroidal drugs was not particularly effective.

Table 325-5 **Musculoskeletal Abnormalities in Sickle Cell Disease**

Sickle cell dactylitis	Avascular necrosis
Joint effusions in sickle cell crises	Bone changes secondary to marrow hyperplasia
Osteomyelitis	
Infarction of bone	Septic arthritis
Infarction of bone marrow	Gouty arthritis

TUMORS OF JOINTS Primary tumors and tumor-like disorders of synovium are uncommon but should be considered in the differential diagnosis of monarticular joint disease. In addition, metastases to bone and primary bone tumors adjacent to a joint may produce joint symptoms. →*For further discussion, see Chap. 98.*

Pigmented villonodular synovitis is characterized by the slowly progressive, exuberant, benign proliferation of synovial tissue, usually involving a single joint. The most common age of onset is in the third decade, and women are affected slightly more often than men. The cause of this disorder is unknown.

The synovium has a brownish color and numerous large, finger-like villi that fuse to form pedunculated nodules. There is marked hyperplasia of synovial cells in the stroma of the villi. Hemosiderin granules and lipids are found in the cytoplasm of macrophages and in the interstitial tissue. Multinucleated giant cells may be present. The proliferative synovium grows into the subsynovial tissue and invades adjacent cartilage and bone.

The clinical picture of pigmented villonodular synovitis is characterized by the insidious onset of swelling and pain in one joint, most commonly the knee. Other joints affected include the hips, ankles, calcaneocuboid joints, elbows, and small joints of the fingers or toes. The disease may also involve the common flexor sheath of the hand or fingers. Less commonly, tendon sheaths in the wrist, ankle, or foot may be involved. Symptoms may be mild and intermittent and may be present for years before the patient seeks medical attention. Radiographs may show joint space narrowing, erosions, and subchondral cysts. The joint fluid contains blood and is dark red or almost black in color. Lipid-containing macrophages may be present in the fluid. The joint fluid may be clear if hemorrhages have not occurred.

The treatment of pigmented villonodular synovitis is complete synovectomy. With incomplete synovectomy, the villonodular synovitis recurs, and the rate of tissue growth may be faster than originally. Irradiation of the involved joint has been successful in some patients.

Synovial chondromatosis is a disorder characterized by multiple focal metaplastic growths of normal-appearing cartilage in the synovium or tendon sheath. Segments of cartilage break loose and continue to grow as loose bodies. When calcification and ossification of loose bodies occur, the disorder is referred to as *synovial osteochondromatosis.* The disorder is usually monarticular and affects young to middle-aged individuals. The knee is most often involved, followed by hip, elbow, and shoulder. Symptoms are pain, swelling, and decreased motion of the joint. Radiographs may show several rounded calcifications within the joint cavity. Treatment is synovectomy; however, the tumor may recur.

Hemangiomas occur in synovium and in tendon sheaths. The knee is affected most commonly. Recurrent episodes of joint swelling and pain usually begin in childhood. The joint fluid is bloody. Treatment is excision of the lesion. *Lipomas* occur most often in the knee, originating in the subsynovial fat on either side of the patellar tendon. Lipomas also appear in tendon sheaths of the hands, wrists, feet, and ankles. In some instances, surgical removal is necessary.

Synovial sarcoma is a malignant neoplasm often found near a large joint of both upper and lower extremities, being more common in the lower extremity. It seldom arises within the joint itself. Synovial sarcomas comprise 10% of sarcomas. The tumor is believed to arise from primitive mesenchymal tissue which differentiates into epithelial cells and/or spindle cells. Small foci of calcification may be present in the tumor mass. It occurs most often in young adults and is more common in men. The tumor presents as a slowly growing deep seated mass near a joint, without much pain. The area of the knee is the most common site, followed by the foot, ankle, elbow, and shoulder. Other primary sites include the buttocks, abdominal wall, retioperitoneum and mediastinum. The tumor spreads along tissue planes. The most common site of visceral metastasis is lung. The diagnosis is made by biopsy. Treatment is wide resection of the tumor including adjacent muscle and regional lymph nodes, followed by chemotherapy and radiation therapy. Currently used chemotherapeutic agents are doxorubicin, ifosfamide, and cisplatin. Amputation of the involved distal extremity may be required. Chemotherapy may be beneficial in some patients with metastatic disease. Isolated pulmonary mitostasis can be surgically removed. The 5-year survival with treatment has been reported as high as 88%.

BIBLIOGRAPHY

ALTMAN RD, TENENBAUM J: Hypertrophic osteoarthropathy, in *Textbook of Rheumatology*, 5th ed, WN Kelley et al (eds). Philadelphia, Saunders, 1997, pp 1514–1520

ARMAN MI et al: Brief report. Frequency and features of rheumatic findings in thalassaemia minor: A blind controlled study. Br J Rheumatol 31:197, 1992

BENNETT RM: The fibromyalgia syndrome, in *Textbook of Rheumatology*, 5th ed, WN Kelley et al (eds). Philadelphia, Saunders, 1997, pp 511–519

———: Emerging concepts in the neurobiology of chronic pain: Evidence of abnormal sensory processing in fibromyalgia. May Clin Proc 74:385, 1999

CANOSO JJ: Tumors of joints and related structures, in *Arthritis and Allied Conditions*, 13th ed, WJ Koopman (ed.). Baltimore, Williams & Wilkins, 1997, pp 1867–1886

CARELESS DJ, COHEN MG: Rheumatic manifestations of hyperlipidemia and antihyperlipidemia drug therapy. Semin Arthritis Rheum 23:90, 1993

CRONIN ME: Rheumatic aspects of endocrinopathies, in *Arthritis and Allied Conditions*, 13th ed, WJ Koopman (ed). Baltimore, Williams & Wilkins, 1997, pp 2233–2249

ELLMAN MH: Neuropathic joint disease (Charcot joints), in *Arthritis and Allied Conditions*, 13th ed, WJ Koopman (ed). Baltimore, Williams & Wilkins, 1997, pp 1641–1659

GOLDENBERG DL: Fibromyalgia syndrome a decade later: What have we learned? Arch Intern Med 159:777, 1999

HECK LW JR: Arthritis associated with hematologic disorders, storage diseases, disorders of lipid metabolism, and dysproteinemias, in *Arthritis and Allied Conditions*, 13th ed, WJ Koopman (ed). Baltimore, Williams & Wilkins, 1997, pp 1697–1717

LAMBERT RE, McGUIRE JL: Iron storage disease, in *Textbook of Rheumatology*, 5th ed, WN Kelley et al (eds). Philadelphia, Saunders, 1997, pp 1423–1429

MARTINEZ-LAVIN M: Hypertrophic osteoarthropathy, in *Rheumatology*, JF Klippel, PA Dieppe (eds). St. Louis, Mosby, 1998, section 8, chap 46, pp 1–4

ROSENBERG EA, SCHILLER AC: Tumors and tumor-like lesions of joints and related structures, in *Textbook of Rheumatology*, 5th ed, WN Kelley et al (eds). Philadelphia, Saunders, 1997, pp 1593–1617

SCHUMACHER RH JR: Hemoglobinopathies and arthritis, in *Textbook of Rheumatology*, 5th ed, WN Kelley et al (eds). Philadelphia, Saunders, 1997, pp 1493–1498

UPCHURCH KS, BRETTLER DB: Hemophilic arthropathy, in *Textbook of Rheumatology*, 5th ed, WN Kelley et al (eds). Philadelphia, Saunders, 1997, pp 1485–1492

WOLFE F et al: The prevalence and characteristics of fibromyalgia in the general population. Arthritis Rheum 38:19, 1995

326 *Bruce Gilliland*

PERIARTICULAR DISORDERS OF THE EXTREMITIES

A number of periarticular disorders have become increasingly common over the past two to three decades, due in part to greater participation in recreational sports by individuals of a wide range of ages. This chapter discusses some of the more common periarticular disorders of the extremities.

BURSITIS Bursitis is inflammation of a bursa, which is a thin-walled sac lined with synovial tissue. The function of the bursa is to facilitate movement of tendons and muscles over bony prominences. Excessive frictional forces, trauma, systemic disease (e.g., rheumatoid arthritis, gout), or infection may cause bursitis. *Subacromial bursitis* (subdeltoid bursitis) is the most common form of bursitis. The subacromial bursa, which is contiguous with the subdeltoid bursa, is located between the undersurface of the acromion and the humeral head, and is covered by the deltoid muscle. Bursitis is caused by repetitive overhead motion and often accompanies rotator cuff tendinitis. Another frequently encountered form is *trochanteric bursitis*, which involves the bursa around the insertion of the gluteus medius onto the greater trochanter of the femur. Patients experience pain over the lateral aspect of the hip and upper thigh and have tenderness over the posterior aspect of the greater trochanter. External rotation and resisted abduction of the hip elicit pain. *Olecranon bursitis* occurs over the posterior elbow, and when the area is acutely inflamed, infection should be excluded by aspirating and culturing fluid from the bursa. *Achilles bursitis* involves the bursa located above the insertion of the tendon to the calcaneus and results from overuse and wearing tight shoes. *Retrocalcaneal bursitis* involves the bursa that is located between the calcaneus and posterior surface of the Achilles tendon. The pain is experienced at the back of the heel, and swelling appears on the medial and/or lateral side of the tendon. It occurs in association with spondyloarthropathies, rheumatoid arthritis, gout, or trauma. *Ischial bursitis* (weaver's bottom) affects the bursa separating the gluteus medius from the ischial tuberosity and develops from prolonged sitting and pivoting on hard surfaces. *Iliopsoas bursitis* affects the bursa that lies between the iliopsoas muscle and hip joint and is lateral to the femoral vessels. Pain is experienced over this area and is made worse by hip extension and flexion. Bursitis results from trauma or overuse but can also be seen in patients with rheumatoid arthritis. *Anserine bursitis* is an inflammation of the sartorius bursa located over the medial side of the tibia just below the knee and under the conjoint tendon and is manifested by pain on climbing stairs. Tenderness is present over the insertion of the conjoint tendon of the sartorius, gracilis, and semitendinosus. *Prepatellar bursitis* (housemaid's knee) occurs in the bursa situated between the patella and overlying skin and is caused by kneeling on hard surfaces. Treatment of bursitis consists of prevention of the aggravating situation, rest of the involved part, administration of a nonsteroidal anti-inflammatory drug (NSAID), or local glucocorticoid injection.

ROTATOR CUFF TENDINITIS AND IMPINGEMENT SYNDROME Tendinitis of the rotator cuff is the major cause of a painful shoulder and is currently thought to be caused by inflammation of the tendon(s). The rotator cuff consists of the tendons of the supraspinatus, infraspinatus, subscapularis, and teres minor muscles, and inserts on the humeral tuberosities. Of the tendons forming the rotator cuff, the supraspinatus tendon is the most often affected, probably because of its repeated impingement (impingement syndrome) between the humeral head and the undersurface of the anterior third of the acromion and coracoacromial ligament above as well as the reduction in its blood supply that occurs with abduction of the arm (Fig. 326-1). The tendon of the infraspinatus or the long head of the biceps is less commonly involved. The process begins with edema and hemorrhage of the rotator cuff, which evolves to fibrotic thickening and eventually to rotator cuff degeneration with tendon tears and bone

spurs. Subacromial bursitis also accompanies this syndrome. Symptoms usually appear after injury or overuse, especially with activities involving elevation of the arm with some degree of forward flexion. Impingement syndrome occurs in persons participating in baseball, tennis, swimming, or occupations that require repeated elevation of the arm. Those over age 40 are particularly susceptible. Patients complain of a dull aching in the shoulder, which may interfere with sleep. Severe pain is experienced when the arm is actively abducted into an overhead position. The arc between 60 and 120° is especially painful. Tenderness is present over the lateral aspect of the humeral head just below the acromion. NSAIDs, local glucocorticoid injection, and physical therapy may relieve symptoms.

Patients may tear the supraspinatus tendon acutely by falling on an outstretched arm or lifting a heavy object. Symptoms are pain, along with weakness of abduction and external rotation of the shoulder. Atrophy of the supraspinatus muscles develops. The diagnosis is established by arthrogram or ultrasound. Surgical repair may be necessary in patients who fail to respond to conservative measures. In patients with moderate to severe tears and functional loss, surgery is indicated.

CALCIFIC TENDINITIS This condition is characterized by deposition of calcium salts, primarily hydroxyapatite, within a tendon. The exact mechanism of calcification is not known but may be initiated by ischemia or degeneration of the tendon. The supraspinatus tendon is most often affected because it is frequently impinged on and has a reduced blood supply when the arm is abducted. The condition usually develops after age 40. Calcification within the tendon may evoke acute inflammation, producing sudden and severe pain in the shoulder. However, it may be asymptomatic or not related to the patient's symptoms.

BICIPITAL TENDINITIS AND RUPTURE Bicipital tendinitis, or tenosynovitis, is produced by friction on the tendon of the long head of the biceps as it passes through the bicipital groove. When the inflammation is acute, patients experience anterior shoulder pain that radiates down the biceps into the forearm. Abduction and external rotation of the arm are painful and limited. The bicipital groove is very tender to palpation. Pain may be elicited along the course of the tendon by resisting supination of the forearm with the elbow at 90° (Yergason's supination sign). Acute rupture of the tendon may occur with vigorous exercise of the arm and is often painful. In a young patient, it should be repaired surgically. Rupture of the tendon in an older person may be associated with little or no pain and is recognized by the presence of persistent swelling of the biceps ("Popeye" muscle) produced by the retraction of the long head of the biceps. Surgery is usually not necessary in this setting.

ADHESIVE CAPSULITIS Often referred to as "frozen shoulder," adhesive capsulitis is characterized by pain and restricted movement of the shoulder, usually in the absence of intrinsic shoulder disease. Adhesive capsulitis, however, may follow bursitis or tendinitis of the shoulder or be associated with systemic disorders such as chronic pulmonary disease, myocardial infarction, and diabetes mellitus. Prolonged immobility of the arm contributes to the development of adhesive capsulitis, and reflex sympathetic dystrophy is thought to be a pathogenic factor. The capsule of the shoulder is thickened, and a mild chronic inflammatory infiltrate and fibrosis may be present.

Adhesive capsulitis occurs more commonly in women after age 50. Pain and stiffness usually develop gradually over several months to a year but progress rapidly in some patients. Pain may interfere with sleep. The shoulder is tender to palpation, and both active and passive movement are restricted. Radiographs of the shoulder show osteopenia. The diagnosis is confirmed by arthrography, in that only a limited amount of contrast material, usually <15 mL, can be injected under pressure into the shoulder joint.

In most patients, the condition improves spontaneously 1 to 3 years after onset, but some have permanent restriction of movement. Early mobilization of the arm following an injury to the shoulder may prevent the development of this disease. Slow but forceful injection of contrast material into the joint may lyse adhesions and stretch the

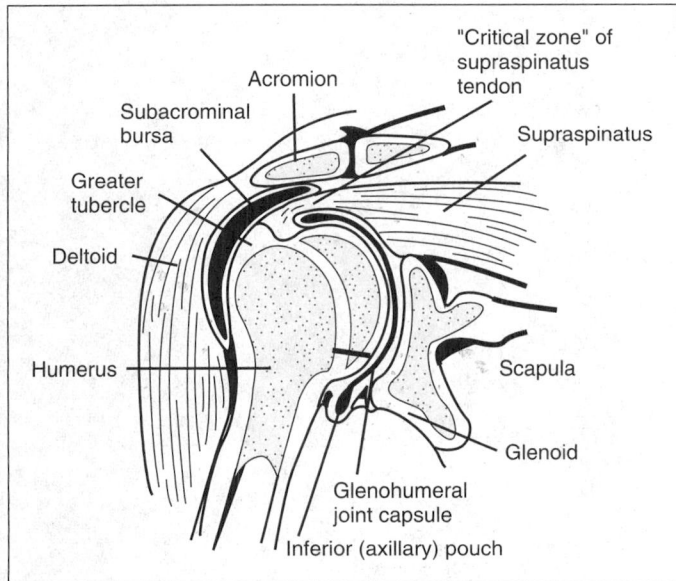

FIGURE 326-1 Coronal section of the shoulder illustrating the relationships of the glenohumeral joint, the joint capsule, the subacromial bursa, and the rotator cuff (supraspinatus tendon). *(From Kozin, with permission.)*

capsule, resulting in improvement of shoulder motion. Manipulation under anesthesia may be helpful in some patients. Once the disease is established, therapy may have little effect on its natural course. Local injections of glucocorticoids, NSAIDs, and physical therapy may provide relief of symptoms.

LATERAL EPICONDYLITIS (TENNIS ELBOW)   Lateral epicondylitis, or tennis elbow, is a painful condition involving the soft tissue over the lateral aspect of the elbow. The pain originates at or near the site of attachment of the common extensors to the lateral epicondyle and may radiate into the forearm and dorsum of the wrist. This painful condition is thought to be caused by small tears of the extensor aponeurosis resulting from repeated resisted contractions of the extensor muscles. The pain usually appears after work or recreational activities involving repeated motions of wrist extension and supination against resistance. Most patients with this disorder injure themselves in activities other than tennis, such as pulling weeds, carrying suitcases or briefcases, or using a screwdriver. The injury in tennis usually occurs when hitting a backhand with the elbow flexed. Shaking hands and opening doors can reproduce the pain. Striking the lateral elbow against a solid object may also induce pain.

The treatment is usually rest along with administration of an NSAID. Ultrasound, icing, and friction massage may also help relieve pain. When pain is severe, the elbow is placed in a sling or splinted at 90° of flexion. When the pain is acute and well localized, injection of a glucocorticoid using a small-gauge needle may be effective. Following injection, the patient should be advised to rest the arm for at least 1 month and avoid activities that would aggravate the elbow. Once symptoms have subsided, the patient should begin rehabilitation to strengthen and increase flexibility of the extensor muscles before resuming physical activity involving the arm. A forearm band placed 2.5 to 5.0 cm (1 to 2 in) below the elbow may help to reduce tension on the extensor muscles at their attachment to the lateral epicondyle. The patient should be advised to restrict activities requiring forcible extension and supination of the wrist. Improvement may take several months. The patient may continue to experience mild pain but, with care, can usually avoid the return of debilitating pain. In an occasional patient, surgical release of the extensor aponeurosis may be necessary.

MEDIAL EPICONDYLITIS   Medial epicondylitis is an overuse syndrome resulting in pain over the medial side of the elbow with radiation into the forearm. The cause of this syndrome is considered to be repetitive resisted motions of wrist flexion and pronation, which lead to microtears and granulation tissue at the origin of the pronator teres and forearm flexors, particularly the flexor carpi radialis. This overuse syndrome is usually seen in patients >35 years and is much less common than lateral epicondylitis. It occurs most often in work-related repetitive activities but also occurs with recreational activities such as swinging a golf club (golfer's elbow) or throwing a baseball. On physical examination, there is tenderness just distal to the medial epicondyle over the origin of the forearm flexors. Pain can be reproduced by resisting wrist flexion and pronation with the elbow extended. Radiographs are usually normal. The differential diagnosis of patients with medial elbow symptoms include tears of the pronator teres, acute medial collateral ligament tear, and medial collateral ligament instability. Ulnar neuritis has been found in 25 to 50% of patients with medial epicondylitis and is associated with tenderness over the ulnar nerve at the elbow as well as hypesthesia and paresthesia on the ulnar side of the hand.

The initial treatment of medial epicondylitis is conservative, involving rest, NSAIDs, friction massage, ultrasound, and icing. Some patients may require splinting. Injections of glucocorticoids at the painful site may also be effective. Patients should be instructed to rest at least 1 month. Also, patients should be started on physical therapy once the pain has subsided. In patients with chronic debilitating medial epicondylitis that remains unresponsive after at least a year of treatment, surgical release of the flexor muscle at its origin may be necessary and is often successful.

BIBLIOGRAPHY

KOZIN F: Painful shoulder and the reflex sympathetic dystrophy syndrome, in *Arthritis and Allied Conditions*, 13th ed, WJ Koopman (ed). Baltimore, Williams & Wilkins, 1997, pp 1887–1922

LINTNER SA et al: Sports medicine, in *Textbook of Rheumatology*, 5th ed, WN Kelley et al (eds). Philadelphia, Saunders, 1997, pp 546–563

MATSEN FA III, ARNTZ CT: Subacromial impingement, in *The Shoulder*, L Reines (ed). Philadelphia, Saunders, 1990, pp 623–646

NEER CS II: Impingement lesions. Clin Orthop 173:70, 1983

Section 1
ENDOCRINOLOGY

327

J. Larry Jameson

PRINCIPLES OF ENDOCRINOLOGY

CRH	corticotropin-releasing hormone	POMC	proopiomelanocortin
EGF	epidermal growth factor	PTHrP	parathyroid hormone–related peptide
GHRH	growth hormone–releasing hormone	SERMs	selective estrogen response modulators
GnRH	gonadotropin-releasing hormone	SHBG	sex hormone–binding globulin
GPCRs	G protein–coupled receptors	STAT	signal transduction and activators of transcription
hCG	human chorionic gonadotropin		
HPA	hypothalamic-pituitary-adrenal		
IGF	insulin-like growth factor	TBG	thyroxine-binding globulin
MEN	multiple endocrine neoplasia	TRH	thyrotropin-releasing hormone

The management of endocrine disorders requires an understanding of such disparate areas as intermediary metabolism, reproductive physiology, bone metabolism, and growth. Accordingly, the practice of endocrinology is intimately linked to a conceptual framework for understanding hormone secretion, hormone action, and principles of feedback control systems. The endocrine system is investigated primarily by measuring hormone concentrations, thereby arming the clinician with valuable diagnostic information. Most disorders of the endocrine system are amenable to effective treatment, once the correct diagnosis is determined. Endocrine deficiency disorders are treated with physiologic hormone replacement; hormone excess conditions, usually due to benign glandular adenomas, are managed by removing tumors surgically or by reducing hormone levels medically.

SCOPE OF ENDOCRINOLOGY

The specialty of endocrinology encompasses the study of glands and the hormones they produce. The term *endocrine* was coined by Starling to contrast the actions of hormones secreted internally (endocrine) with those secreted externally (*exocrine*) or into a lumen, such as the gastrointestinal tract. The term *hormone*, derived from a Greek phrase meaning "to set in motion," aptly describes the dynamic actions of these circulating substances as they elicit cellular responses and regulate physiologic processes through feedback mechanisms.

Unlike certain other specialties in medicine, it is not possible to define endocrinology strictly along anatomic lines. The classic endocrine glands—pituitary, thyroid, parathyroid, pancreatic islets, adrenal, and gonads—communicate broadly with other organs through the nervous system, hormones, cytokines, and growth factors. In addition to its traditional synaptic functions, the brain produces a vast array of peptide hormones, spawning the discipline of neuroendocrinology. Through the production of hypothalamic releasing factors, the central nervous system exerts a major regulatory influence over pituitary hormone secretion (Chap. 328). The peripheral nervous system modulates adrenal medulla and pancreatic islet hormone production. The immune and endocrine systems are also intimately intertwined. The adrenal glucocorticoid, cortisol, is a powerful immunosuppressant. Cytokines and interleukins (ILs) have profound effects on the functions of the pituitary, adrenal, thyroid, and gonads. Common endocrine diseases, such as autoimmune thyroid disease and type 1 diabetes mellitus, are caused by dysregulation of immune surveillance and tolerance. Less common diseases such as polyglandular failure, Addison's disease, and lymphocytic hypophysitis also have an immunologic basis.

The interdigitation of endocrinology with physiologic processes in other specialties sometimes blurs the role of hormones. For example, hormones play an important role in maintenance of blood pressure, intravascular volume, and peripheral resistance in the cardiovascular system. The heart is the principal source of atrial natriuretic peptide, which acts in classic endocrine fashion to induce natriuresis at a distant target organ (the kidney). Vasoactive substances such as catecholamines, angiotensin II, endothelin, and nitric oxide are involved in dynamic changes of vascular tone, in addition to their multiple roles in other tissues. Erythropoietin, a traditional circulating hormone, is made in the kidney and stimulates erythropoiesis in the bone marrow (Chap. 104). The kidney is also integrally involved in the renin-angiotensin axis (Chap. 331) and is a primary target of several hormones including parathyroid hormone (PTH), mineralocorticoids, and vasopressin. The gastrointestinal tract produces a surprising number of peptide hormones such as cholecystokinin, gastrin, secretin, and vasoactive intestinal peptide, among many others. Carcinoid and islet tumors can secrete excessive amounts of these hormones, leading to specific clinical syndromes (Chap. 93). Many of these gastrointestinal hormones are also produced in the central nervous system, where their functions remain poorly understood. As new hormones such as inhibin, ghrelin, and leptin are discovered, they become integrated into the science and practice of medicine on the basis of their functional roles rather than through their structures or mechanisms of action.

Characterization of hormone receptors frequently reveals unexpected relationships to factors in nonendocrine disciplines. The growth hormone (GH) receptor, for example, is a member of the cytokine receptor family. The G protein–coupled receptors (GPCRs), which mediate the actions of many peptide hormones, are used in numerous physiologic processes including vision, smell, and neurotransmission.

It is apparent that hormones and growth factors play an important functional role in all organ systems. Though endocrinologists are not usually involved in the administration of the hormones or growth factors used to treat diseases in other specialties (e.g., cardiology, hematology), the principles of endocrinology can be applied in these cases, thus emphasizing the impact of endocrinology across multiple disciplines.

NATURE OF HORMONES

Hormones can be divided into five major classes: (1) *amino acid derivatives* such as dopamine, catecholamines, and thyroid hormone; (2) *small neuropeptides* such as gonadotropin-releasing hormone (GnRH), thyrotropin-releasing hormone (TRH), somatostatin, and vasopressin; (3) *large proteins* such as insulin, luteinizing hormone (LH), and PTH produced by classic endocrine glands; (4) *steroid hormones* such as cortisol and estrogen that are synthesized from cholesterol-based precursors; and (5) *vitamin derivatives* such as retinoids (vitamin A) and vitamin D. A variety of *peptide growth factors*, most of which act locally, share actions with hormones. As a rule, amino acid derivatives and peptide hormone interact with cell-surface membrane receptors. Steroids, thyroid hormones, vitamin D, and retinoids are lipid-soluble and interact with intracellular nuclear receptors.

HORMONE AND RECEPTOR FAMILIES Many hormones and receptors can be grouped into families, reflecting their

Table 327-1   Membrane Receptor Families and Signaling Pathways

Receptors	Effectors	Signaling Pathways
G protein–coupled seven-transmembrane (GPCR)		
β-Adrenergic	$G_s\alpha$, adenylate cyclase	Stimulation of cyclic AMP production, protein kinase A Calmodulin, Ca^{2+}-dependent kinases
LH, FSH, TSH	Ca^{2+} channels	
Glucagon		
PTH, PTHrP		
ACTH, MSH		
GHRH, CRH		
α-Adrenergic	$G_i\alpha$	Inhibition of cyclic AMP production
Somatostatin		Activation of K^+, Ca^{2+} channels
TRH, GnRH	G_q, G_{11}	Phospholipase C, diacylglycerol, IP_3, protein kinase C, Voltage-dependent Ca^{2+} channels
Receptor tyrosine kinase		
Insulin, IGF-I	Tyrosine kinases, IRS-1 to IRS-4	MAP kinases, PI 3-kinase, RSK
EGF, NGF	Tyrosine kinases, ras	Raf, MAP kinases, RSK
Cytokine receptor–linked kinase		
GH, PRL	JAK, tyrosine kinases	STAT, MAP kinase, PI 3-kinase, IRS-1, IRS-2
Serine Kinase		
Activin, TGF-β, MIS	Serine kinase	Smads

NOTE: IP_3, inositol triphosphate; IRS, insulin receptor substrates; MAP, mitogen-activated protein; MIS, müllerian-inhibiting substance; MSH, melanocyte-stimulating hormone; NGF, nerve growth factor; PI, phosphatylinositol; RSK, ribosomal S6 kinase; TGF-β, transforming growth factor β. For all other abbreviations, see text.

structural similarities (Table 327-1). The evolution of these families generates diverse but highly selective pathways of hormone action. Recognizing these relationships allows extrapolation of information gleaned from one hormone or receptor to other family members.

The glycoprotein hormone family, consisting of thyroid-stimulating hormone (TSH), follicle-stimulating hormone (FSH), LH, and human chorionic gonadotropin (hCG), illustrates many features of related hormones. The glycoprotein hormones are heterodimers that share the α subunit in common; the β subunits are distinct and confer specific biologic actions. The overall three-dimensional architecture of the β subunits is similar, reflecting the locations of conserved disulfide bonds that restrain protein conformation. The cloning of the β-subunit genes from multiple species suggests that this family arose from a common ancestral gene, probably by gene duplication and subsequent divergence to evolve new biologic functions.

As the hormone families enlarge and diverge, their receptors must co-evolve, if new biologic functions are to be derived. Related GPCRs, for example, have evolved for each of the glycoprotein hormones. These receptors are structurally similar, and each is coupled to the $G_s\alpha$ signaling pathway. However, there is minimal overlap of hormone binding. For example, TSH binds with high specificity to the TSH receptor but interacts weakly with the LH or the FSH receptor. Nonetheless, there can be subtle physiologic consequences of hormone cross-reactivity with other receptors. Very high levels of hCG during pregnancy stimulate the TSH receptor and increase thyroid hormone levels.

Insulin, insulin-like growth factor (IGF) I, and IGF-II share structural similarities that are most apparent when precursor forms of the proteins are compared. In contrast to the high degree of specificity seen with the glycoprotein hormones, there is moderate cross-talk among the members of the insulin/IGF family. High concentrations of an IGF-II precursor produced by certain tumors (e.g., sarcomas) can cause hypoglycemia, partly because of binding to insulin and IGF-I receptors (Chap. 334). High concentrations of insulin also bind to the IGF-I receptor, perhaps accounting for some of the clinical manifestations seen in severe insulin resistance.

Another important example of receptor cross-talk is seen with PTH and parathyroid hormone–related peptide (PTHrP) (Chap. 341). PTH is produced by the parathyroid glands, whereas PTHrP is expressed at high levels during development and by a variety of tumors. These hormones share amino acid sequence similarity, particularly in their amino-terminal regions. Both hormones bind to a single PTH receptor that is expressed in bone and kidney. Hypercalcemia and hypophosphatemia may therefore result from excessive production of either hormone, making it difficult to distinguish hyperparathyroidism from hypercalcemia of malignancy solely on the basis of serum chemistries. However, sensitive and specific assays for PTH now allow these disorders to be separated more readily.

Based on their specificities for DNA binding sites, the nuclear receptor family can be subdivided into type 1 receptors (GR, MR, AR, ER, PR) that bind steroids and type 2 receptors (TR, VDR, RAR, PPAR) that bind thyroid hormone, vitamin D, retinoic acid, or lipid derivatives. Certain functional domains in nuclear receptors, such as the zinc finger DNA-binding domains, are highly conserved. However, selective amino acid differences within this domain confer DNA sequence specificity. The hormone-binding domains are more variable, providing great diversity in the array of small molecules that can bind to different nuclear receptors. With few exceptions, hormone binding is highly specific for a single type of nuclear receptor. One exception involves the highly related glucocorticoid and mineralocorticoid receptors. Because the mineralocorticoid receptor also binds glucocorticoids with high affinity, an enzyme (11β-hydroxysteroid dehydrogenase) located in renal tubular cells inactivates glucocorticoids, allowing selective responses to mineralocorticoids such as aldosterone. However, when very high glucocorticoid concentrations occur, as in Cushing's syndrome, the glucocorticoid degradation pathway becomes saturated, allowing excessive cortisol levels to exert mineralocorticoid effects (sodium retention, potassium wasting). This phenomenon is particularly pronounced in ectopic adrenocorticotropic hormone (ACTH) syndromes (Chap. 331). Another example of relaxed nuclear receptor specificity involves the estrogen receptor, which can bind an array of compounds, some of which share little structural similarity to the high-affinity ligand estradiol. This feature of the estrogen receptor makes it susceptible to activation by "environmental estrogens" such as resveratrol, octylphenol, and many other aromatic hydrocarbons. On the other hand, this lack of specificity provides an opportunity to synthesize a remarkable series of clinically useful antagonists (e.g., tamoxifen) and selective estrogen response modulators (SERMs), such as raloxifene. These compounds generate distinct conformations that alter receptor interactions with components of the transcription machinery (see below), thereby conferring their unique actions.

HORMONE SYNTHESIS AND PROCESSING The synthesis of peptide hormones and their receptors occurs through a classic pathway of gene expression: transcription → mRNA → protein → posttranslational protein processing → intracellular sorting, membrane integration, or secretion (Chap. 65). Though endocrine genes contain regulatory DNA elements similar to those found in many other genes, their exquisite control by other hormones also necessitates the presence of specific hormone response elements. For example, the TSH genes are repressed directly by thyroid hormones acting through the thyroid hormone receptor, a member of the nuclear receptor family. Steroidogenic enzyme gene expression requires specific transcription factors such as steroidogenic factor-1 (SF-1), acting in conjunction with signals transmitted by trophic hormones (e.g., ACTH or LH). For some hormones, substantial regulation occurs at the level of translational efficiency. Insulin biosynthesis, while requiring ongoing gene transcription, is regulated primarily at the translational level in response to elevated levels of glucose or amino acids.

Many hormones are embedded within larger precursor polypeptides that are proteolytically processed to yield the biologically active hormone. Examples include: proopiomelanocortin (POMC) $\rightarrow$ ACTH; proglucagon $\rightarrow$ glucagon; proinsulin $\rightarrow$ insulin; pro-PTH $\rightarrow$ PTH, among others. In many cases, such as POMC and proglucagon, these precursors generate multiple biologically active peptides. It is provocative that hormone precursors are typically inactive, presumably adding an additional level of regulatory control. This is true not only for peptide hormones but also for certain steroids (testosterone $\rightarrow$ dihydrotestosterone) and thyroid hormone ($T_4 \rightarrow T_3$).

Hormone precursor processing is intimately linked to intracellular sorting pathways that transport proteins to appropriate vesicles and enzymes, resulting in specific cleavage steps, followed by protein folding and translocation to secretory vesicles. Hormones destined for secretion are translocated across the endoplasmic reticulum under the guidance of an amino-terminal signal sequence that is subsequently cleaved. Cell-surface receptors are inserted into the membrane via short segments of hydrophobic amino acids that remain embedded within the lipid bilayer. During translocation through the Golgi and endoplasmic reticulum, hormones and receptors are also subject to a variety of posttranslational modifications, such as glycosylation and phosphorylation, which can alter protein conformation, modify circulating half-life, and alter biologic activity.

Synthesis of most steroid hormones is based on modifications of the precursor, cholesterol. Multiple regulated enzymatic steps are required for the synthesis of testosterone (Chap. 335), estradiol (Chap. 336), cortisol (Chap. 331), and vitamin D (Chap. 340). This large number of synthetic steps predisposes to multiple genetic and acquired disorders of steroidogenesis (see below).

HORMONE SECRETION, TRANSPORT, AND DEGRADATION The circulating level of a hormone is determined by its rate of secretion and its circulating half-life. After protein processing, peptide hormones (GnRH, insulin, GH) are stored in secretory granules. As these granules mature, they are poised beneath the plasma membrane for imminent release into the circulation. In most instances, the stimulus for hormone secretion is a releasing factor or neural signal that induces rapid changes in intracellular calcium concentrations, leading to secretory granule fusion with the plasma membrane and release of its contents into the extracellular environment and blood stream. Steroid hormones, in contrast, diffuse into the circulation as they are synthesized. Thus, their secretory rates are closely aligned with rates of synthesis. For example, ACTH and LH induce steroidogenesis by stimulating the activity of *s*teroidogenic *a*cute *r*egulatory (StAR) protein (transports cholesterol into the mitochondrion) along with other rate-limiting steps (e.g., cholesterol side-chain cleavage enzyme, CYP11A1) in the steroidogenic pathway.

Hormone transport and degradation dictate the rapidity with which a hormonal signal decays. Some hormonal signals are evanescent (e.g., somatostatin), whereas others are longer lived (e.g., TSH). Because somatostatin exerts effects in virtually every tissue, a short half-life allows it concentrations and actions to be controlled locally. Structural modifications that impair somatostatin degradation have been useful for generating long-acting therapeutic analogues, such as octreotide (Chap. 328). On the other hand, the actions of TSH are highly specific for the thyroid gland. Its prolonged half-life accounts for relatively constant serum levels, even though TSH is secreted in discrete pulses.

An understanding of circulating hormone half-life is important for achieving physiologic hormone replacement, as the frequency of dosing and the time required to reach steady state are intimately linked to rates of hormone decay. T_4, for example, has a plasma half-life of 7 days. Consequently, >1 month is required to reach a new steady state, but single daily doses are sufficient to achieve constant hormone levels. T_3, in contrast, has a half-life of 1 day. Its administration is associated with more dynamic serum levels and it must be administered two to three times per day. Similarly, synthetic glucocorticoids vary

widely in their half-lives; those with longer half-lives (e.g., dexamethasone) are associated with greater suppression of the hypothalamic-pituitary-adrenal (HPA) axis. Most protein hormones [e.g., ACTH, GH, prolactin (PRL); PTH, LH] have relatively short half-lives (<20 min), leading to sharp peaks of secretion and decay. The only accurate way to profile the pulse frequency and amplitude of these hormones is to measure levels in frequently sampled blood (every 10 min) over long durations (8 to 24 h). Because this is not practical in a clinical setting, an alternative strategy is to pool three to four samples drawn at about 30-min intervals, recognizing that pulsatile secretion makes it difficult to establish a narrow normal range. Rapid hormone decay is useful in certain clinical settings. For example, the short half-life of PTH allows the use of intraoperative PTH determinations to confirm successful removal of an adenoma. This is particularly valuable diagnostically when there is a possibility of multicentric disease or parathyroid hyperplasia, as occurs with multiple endocrine neoplasia (MEN) or renal insufficiency.

Many hormones circulate in association with serum-binding proteins. Examples include: (1) T_4 and T_3 binding to thyroxine-binding globulin (TBG), albumin, and thyroxine-binding prealbumin (TBPA); (2) cortisol binding to cortisol-binding globulin (CBG); (3) androgen and estrogen binding to sex hormone–binding globulin (SHBG) (also called testosterone-binding globulin, TeBG); (4) IGF-I and -II binding to multiple IGF-binding proteins (IGFBPs); (5) GH interactions with GH-binding protein (GHBP), a circulating fragment of the GH receptor extracellular domain; and (6) activin binding to follistatin. These interactions provide a hormonal reservoir, prevent otherwise rapid degradation of unbound hormones, restrict hormone access to certain sites (e.g., IGFBPs), and modulate the unbound, or "free," hormone concentrations. Although a variety of binding protein abnormalities have been identified, most have little clinical consequence, aside from creating diagnostic problems. For example, TBG deficiency can greatly reduce total thyroid hormone levels, but the free concentrations of T_4 and T_3 remain normal. Liver disease and certain medications can also influence binding protein levels (e.g., estrogen increases TBG) or cause displacement of hormones from binding proteins (e.g., salsalate displaces T_4 from TBG). Only free hormone is available to bind receptors and thereby elicit a biologic response. Short-term perturbations in binding proteins change the free hormone concentration, which in turn induces compensatory adaptations through feedback loops. SHBG changes in women are an exception to this self-correcting mechanism. When SHBG decreases because of insulin resistance or androgen excess, the free testosterone concentration is increased, potentially leading to hirsutism (Chap. 53). The increased free testosterone levels does not result in an adequate compensatory feedback correction because estrogen, and not testosterone, is the primary regulator of the reproductive axis.

HORMONE ACTION THROUGH RECEPTORS

Receptors for hormones are divided into two major classes—membrane and nuclear. *Membrane receptors* primarily bind peptide hormones and catecholamines. *Nuclear receptors* bind small molecules that can diffuse across the cell membrane, such as thyroid hormone, steroids, and vitamin D. Certain general principles apply to hormone-receptor interactions, regardless of the class of receptor. Hormones bind to receptors with specificity and a high affinity that generally coincides with the dynamic range of circulating hormone concentrations. Low concentrations of free hormone (usually 10^{-12} to 10^{-9} M) rapidly associate and dissociate from receptors in a bimolecular reaction, such that the occupancy of the receptor at any given moment is a function of hormone concentration and the receptor's affinity for the hormone. Receptor numbers vary greatly in different target tissues, providing one of the major determinants of specific cellular responses to circulating hormones. For example, ACTH receptors are located almost exclusively in the adrenal cortex, and FSH receptors are found only in the gonads. In contrast, insulin and thyroid hormone receptors are widely distributed, reflecting the need for metabolic responses in all tissues.

MEMBRANE RECEPTORS   Membrane receptors for hormones can be divided into several major groups: (1) seven transmembrane GPCRs, (2) tyrosine kinase receptors, (3) cytokine receptors, and (4) serine kinase receptors (Fig. 327-1). The *seven transmembrane GPCR* family binds a remarkable array of hormones including large proteins (e.g., LH, PTH), small peptides (e.g., TRH, somatostatin), catecholamines (epinephrine, dopamine), and even minerals (e.g., calcium). The extracellular domains of GPCRs vary widely in size and are the major binding site for large hormones. The transmembrane-spanning regions are composed of hydrophobic α-helical domains that traverse the lipid bilayer. Like some channels, these domains are thought to circularize and form a hydrophobic pocket into which certain small ligands fit. Hormone binding induces conformational changes in these domains, transducing structural changes to the intracellular domain, which is a docking site for G proteins.

The large family of *G proteins*, so named because they bind guanine nucleotides (GTP, GDP), provides great diversity for coupling to different receptors. G proteins form a heterotrimeric complex that is composed of various α and $\beta\gamma$ subunits. The α subunit contains the guanine nucleotide–binding site and hydrolyzes GTP $\rightarrow$ GDP. The $\beta\gamma$ subunits are tightly associated and modulate the activity of the α subunit, as well as mediating their own effector signaling pathways. G protein activity is regulated by a cycle that involves GTP hydrolysis and dynamic interactions between the α and $\beta\gamma$ subunits. Hormone binding to the receptor induces GDP dissociation, allowing Gα to bind GTP and dissociate from the $\beta\gamma$ complex. Under these conditions, the Gα subunit is activated and mediates signal transduction through various enzymes such as adenylate cyclase or phospholipase C. GTP hydrolysis to GDP allows reassociation with the $\beta\gamma$ subunits and restores the inactive state. As described below, a variety of endocrinopathies result from G protein mutations or from mutations in receptors that modify their interactions with G proteins.

There are more than a dozen isoforms of the Gα subunit. G$_s\alpha$ stimulates, whereas G$_i\alpha$ inhibits adenylate cyclase, an enzyme that generates the second messenger, cyclic AMP, leading to activation of protein kinase A (Table 327-1). G$_q$ subunits couple to phospholipase C, generating diacylglycerol and inositol triphosphate, leading to activation of protein kinase C and the release of intracellular calcium.

The *tyrosine kinase receptors* transduce signals for insulin and a variety of growth factors, such as IGF-I, epidermal growth factor (EGF), nerve growth factor, platelet-derived growth factor, and fibroblast growth factor. The cysteine-rich extracellular ligand-binding domains contain growth factor binding sites. After ligand binding, this class of receptors undergoes autophosphorylation, inducing interactions with intracellular adaptor proteins such as Shc and insulin receptor substrates 1 to 4. In the case of the insulin receptor, multiple kinases are activated including the Raf-Ras-MAPK and the Akt/protein kinase B pathways. The tyrosine kinase receptors play a prominent role in cell growth and differentiation as well as in intermediary metabolism.

The GH and PRL receptors belong to the *cytokine receptor* family (Chap. 305). Analogous to the tyrosine kinase receptors, ligand binding induces receptor binding to intracellular kinases—the Janus kinases (JAKs), which phosphorylate members of the signal transduction and activators of transcription (STAT) family—as well as other signaling pathways (Ras, PI3-K, MAPK). The activated STAT proteins translocate to the nucleus and stimulate expression of target genes (Chap. 328).

The *serine kinase receptors* mediate the actions of activins, transforming growth factor β, müllerian-inhibiting substance (MIS, also known as anti-müllerian hormone, AMH), and bone morphogenic proteins (BMPs). This family of receptors (consisting of type I and II subunits) signal through proteins termed *smads* (fusion of terms for *Caenorhabditis elegans* sma + mammalian mad). Like the STAT proteins, the smads serve a dual role of transducing the receptor signal and acting as transcription factors. The pleomorphic actions of these growth factors dictate that they act primarily in a local (paracrine or autocrine) manner. Binding proteins, such as follistatin (which binds activin and other members of this family), function to inactivate the growth factors and restrict their distribution.

NUCLEAR RECEPTORS   The family of nuclear receptors has grown to nearly 100 members, many of which are still classified as orphan receptors because their ligands, if they exist, remain to be identified (Fig. 327-2). Otherwise, most nuclear receptors are classified based on the nature of their ligands. Though all nuclear receptors ultimately act to increase or decrease gene transcription, some (e.g., glucocorticoid receptor) reside primarily in the cytoplasm, whereas others (e.g., thyroid hormone receptor) are always located in the nucleus. After ligand binding, the cytoplasmically localized receptors translocate to the nucleus.

The structures of nuclear receptors have been extensively studied, including by x-ray crystallography. The DNA binding domain, consisting of two zinc fingers, contacts specific DNA recognition sequences in target genes. Most nuclear receptors bind to DNA as dimers. Consequently, each monomer recognizes an individual DNA motif, referred to as a "half-site." The steroid receptors, including the glucocorticoid, estrogen, progesterone, and androgen receptors, bind to DNA as homodimers. Consistent with this twofold symmetry, their DNA recognition half-sites are palindromic. The thyroid, retinoid, PPAR, and vitamin D receptors bind to DNA preferentially as heterodimers in combination with retinoid X receptors (RXRs). Their DNA half-sites are arranged as direct repeats. Receptor specificity for DNA sequences is determined by (1) the sequence of the half-site, (2) the orientation of the half-sites (palindromic, direct repeat), and (3) the spacing between the half-sites. For example, vitamin D, thyroid and retinoid receptors recognize similar tandemly repeated half-sites (TAAGTCA), but these DNA repeats are spaced by three, four, and five nucleotides, respectively.

The carboxy-terminal hormone-binding domain mediates transcriptional control. For type II receptors, such as TR and RAR, co-repressor proteins bind to the receptor in the absence of ligand and silence gene transcription. Hormone binding induces conformational changes, triggering the release of co-repressors and inducing the recruitment of coactivators that stimulate transcription. Thus, these receptors are capable of mediating dramatic changes in the level of gene activity. Certain disease states are associated with defective regulation of these events. For example, mutations in the thyroid hormone receptor prevent co-repressor dissociation, resulting in a dominant form of hormone resistance (Chap. 330). In promyelocytic leukemia, fusion of RARα to other nuclear proteins causes aberrant gene silencing and prevents normal cellular differentiation. Treatment with retinoic acid reverses this repression and allows cellular differentiation and apoptosis to occur (Chap. 111). Type 1 steroid receptors do not interact

FIGURE 327-1   Membrane receptor signaling. For abbreviations, see text.

with co-repressors, but ligand binding still mediates interactions with an array of coactivators. X-ray crystallography shows that various SERMs induce distinct receptor conformations. The tissue-specific responses caused by these agents in breast, bone, and uterus appear to reflect distinct interactions with coactivators. The receptor-coactivator complex stimulates gene transcription by several pathways including (1) recruitment of enzymes (histone acetyl transferases) that modify chromatin structure, (2) interactions with additional transcription factors on the target gene, and (3) direct interactions with components of the general transcription apparatus to enhance the rate of RNA polymerase II–mediated transcription.

FIGURE 327-2 Nuclear receptor signaling. ER, estrogen receptor; AR, androgen receptor; PR, progesterone receptor; GR, glucocorticoid receptor; TR, thyroid hormone receptor; VDR, vitamin D receptor; RAR, retinoic acid receptor; PPAR, peroxisome proliferator activated receptor; SF-1, steroidogenic factor-1; DAX, *d*osage sensitive sex-reversal; *a*drenal hypoplasia congenita, *X*-chromosome; HNF4α, hepatic nuclear factor 4α

FUNCTIONS OF HORMONES

The functions of individual hormones are described in detail in subsequent chapters. Nonetheless, it is useful to illustrate how most biologic responses require integration of several different hormonal pathways. The physiologic functions of hormones can be divided into three general areas: (1) growth and differentiation, (2) maintenance of homeostasis, and (3) reproduction.

GROWTH Multiple hormones and nutritional factors mediate the complex phenomenon of growth (Chap. 328). Short stature may be caused by GH deficiency, hypothyroidism, Cushing's syndrome, precocious puberty, malnutrition or chronic illness, or genetic abnormalities that affect the epiphyseal growth plates (e.g., *FGFR3* or *SHOX* mutations). Many factors (GH, IGF-I, thyroid hormone) stimulate growth, whereas others (sex steroids) lead to epiphyseal closure. Understanding these hormonal interactions is important in the diagnosis and management of growth disorders. For example, delaying exposure to high levels of sex steroids may enhance the efficacy of GH treatment.

MAINTENANCE OF HOMEOSTASIS Though virtually all hormones affect homeostasis, the most important among these are the following:

1. Thyroid hormone—controls about 25% of basal metabolism in most tissues (Chap. 330)
2. Cortisol—exerts a permissive action for many hormones in addition to its own direct effects (Chap. 331)
3. PTH—regulates calcium and phosphorus levels (Chap. 341)
4. Vasopressin—regulates serum osmolality by controlling renal free water clearance (Chap. 329)
5. Mineralocorticoids—control vascular volume and serum electrolyte (Na⁺, K⁺) concentrations (Chap. 331)
6. Insulin—maintains euglycemia in the fed and fasted states (Chap. 333)

The defense against hypoglycemia is an impressive example of integrated hormone action (Chap. 334). In response to the fasted state and falling blood glucose, insulin secretion is suppressed, resulting in decreased glucose uptake and enhanced glycogenolysis, lipolysis, proteolysis, and gluconeogenesis to mobilize fuel sources. If hypoglycemia develops (usually from insulin administration or sulfonylureas), an orchestrated counterregulatory response occurs—glucagon and epinephrine rapidly stimulate glycogenolysis and gluconeogenesis, whereas GH and cortisol act over several hours to raise glucose levels and antagonize insulin action.

Although free water clearance is primarily controlled by vasopressin, cortisol and thyroid hormone are also important for facilitating renal tubular responses to vasopressin effects (Chap. 329). PTH and vitamin D function in an interdependent manner to control calcium metabolism (Chap. 340). PTH stimulates renal synthesis of 1,25 dihydroxyvitamin D, which increases calcium absorption in the gastrointestinal tract and enhances PTH action in bone. Increased calcium, along with vitamin D, feeds back to suppress PTH, thereby maintaining calcium balance.

Depending on the severity of a given stress and whether it is acute or chronic, multiple endocrine and cytokine pathways are activated to mount an appropriate physiologic response (Chap. 328). In severe acute stress such as trauma or shock, the sympathetic nervous system is activated and catecholamines are released, leading to increased cardiac output and a primed musculoskeletal system. Catecholamines also increase mean blood pressure and stimulate glucose production (Chap. 72). Multiple stress-induced pathways converge on the hypothalamus, stimulating several hormones including vasopressin and corticotropin-releasing hormone (CRH). These hormones, in addition to cytokines (tumor necrosis factor α, IL-2, IL-6), increase ACTH and GH production. ACTH stimulates the adrenal gland, increasing cortisol, which in turn helps to sustain blood pressure and dampen the inflammatory response. Increased vasopressin acts to conserve free water.

REPRODUCTION The stages of reproduction include: (1) sex determination during fetal development (Chap. 338); (2) sexual maturation during puberty (Chap. 8); (3) conception, pregnancy, lactation, and child-rearing (Chap. 336), and (4) cessation of reproductive capability at menopause. Each of these stages involves an orchestrated interplay of multiple hormones, a phenomenon well illustrated by the dynamic hormonal changes that occur during each 28-day menstrual cycle. In the early follicular phase, pulsatile secretion of LH and FSH stimulate the progressive maturation of the ovarian follicle. This results in a gradual increase of estrogen and progesterone leading to enhanced pituitary sensitivity to GnRH, which, when combined with accelerated GnRH secretion, triggers the LH surge and rupture of the mature follicle. Inhibin, a protein produced by the granulosa cells, enhances follicular growth and feeds back to the pituitary to selectively suppress FSH, without affecting LH. Growth factors, such as EGF and IGF-I modulate follicular responsiveness to gonadotropins. Vascular endothelial growth factor and prostaglandins play a role in follicle vascularization and rupture.

During pregnancy, the increased production of prolactin, in combination with placentally derived steroids (e.g., estrogen and progesterone), prepares the breast for lactation (Chap. 337). Estrogens induce the production of progesterone receptors, allowing for increased responsiveness to progesterone. In addition to these and other hormones involved in lactation, the nervous system and oxytocin mediate the suckling response and milk release.

HORMONAL FEEDBACK REGULATORY SYSTEMS

Feedback control, both negative and positive, is a fundamental feature of endocrine systems. Each of the major hypothalamic-pituitary-hormone axes is governed by negative feedback, a process that maintains hormone levels within a relatively narrow range (Chap. 328). Examples of hypothalamic-pituitary negative feedback include (1) thyroid hormones on the TRH-TSH axis, (2) cortisol on the CRH-ACTH axis, (3) gonadal steroids on the GnRH-LH/FSH axis, and (4) IGF-I on the growth hormone–releasing hormone (GHRH)-GH axis (Fig. 327-3). These regulatory loops include both positive (e.g., TRH, TSH) and negative components (e.g., T_4, T_3), allowing for exquisite control of hormone levels. As an example, a small reduction of thyroid hormone triggers a rapid increase of TRH and TSH secretion, resulting in thyroid gland stimulation and increased thyroid hormone production. When the thyroid hormone reaches a normal level, it feeds back to suppress TRH and TSH, and a new steady state is attained. Feedback regulation also occurs for endocrine systems that do not involve the pituitary gland, such as calcium feedback on PTH, glucose inhibition of insulin secretion, and leptin feedback on the hypothalamus. An understanding of feedback regulation provides important insights into endocrine testing paradigms (see below).

Positive feedback control also occurs but is not well understood. The primary example is estrogen-mediated stimulation of the midcycle LH surge. Though chronic low levels of estrogen are inhibitory, gradually rising estrogen levels stimulate LH secretion. This effect, which is illustrative of an endocrine rhythm (see below), involves activation of the hypothalamic GnRH pulse generator. In addition, estrogen-primed gonadotropes are extraordinarily sensitive to GnRH, leading to a 10- to 20-fold amplification of LH release.

PARACRINE AND AUTOCRINE CONTROL The aforementioned examples of feedback control involve classic endocrine pathways in which hormones are released by one gland and act on a distant target gland. However, local regulatory systems, often involving growth factors, are increasingly recognized. *Paracrine regulation* refers to factors released by one cell that act on an adjacent cell in the same tissue. For example, somatostatin secretion by pancreatic islet δ cells inhibits insulin secretion from nearby β cells. *Autocrine regulation* describes the action of a factor on the same cell from which it is produced. IGF-I acts on many cells that produce it, including chondrocytes, breast epithelium, and gonadal cells. Unlike endocrine actions, paracrine and autocrine control are difficult to document because local growth factor concentrations cannot be readily measured.

Anatomic relationships of glandular systems also greatly influence hormonal exposure—the physical organization of islet cells enhances their intercellular communication; the portal vasculature of the hypothalamic-pituitary system exposes the pituitary to high concentrations of hypothalamic releasing factors; testicular seminiferous tubules gain exposure to high testosterone levels produced by the interdigitated Leydig cells; the pancreas receives nutrient information from the gastrointestinal tract; and the liver is the proximal target of insulin action because of portal drainage from the pancreas.

HORMONAL RHYTHMS The feedback regulatory systems described above are superimposed on hormonal rhythms that are used for adaptation to the environment. Seasonal changes, the daily occurrence of the light-dark cycle, sleep, meals, and stress are examples of the many environmental events that affect hormonal rhythms. The *menstrual cycle* is repeated on average every 28 days, reflecting the time required to follicular maturation and ovulation (Chap. 336). Essentially all pituitary hormone rhythms are entrained to sleep and the *circadian cycle*, generating reproducible patterns that are repeated approximately every 24 h. The HPA axis, for example, exhibits characteristic peaks of ACTH and cortisol production in the early morning, with a nadir in the afternoon and evening. Recognition of these rhythms is important for endocrine testing and treatment. Patients with Cushing's syndrome characteristically exhibit increased midnight cortisol levels when compared to normal individuals (Chap. 331). In contrast, morning cortisol levels are similar in these groups, as cortisol is normally high at this time of day in normal individuals. The HPA axis is more susceptible to suppression by glucocorticoids administered at night as they blunt the early morning rise of ACTH. Understanding these rhythms allows glucocorticoid replacement that mimics diurnal production by administering larger doses in the morning than in the afternoon (Chap. 331).

Other endocrine rhythms occur on a more rapid time scale. Many peptide hormones are secreted in discrete bursts every few hours. LH and FSH secretion are exquisitely sensitive to GnRH pulse frequency. Intermittent pulses of GnRH are required to maintain pituitary sensitivity, whereas continuous exposure to GnRH causes pituitary gonadotrope desensitization. This feature of the hypothalamic-pituitary-gonadotrope (HPG) axis forms the basis for using long-acting GnRH agonists to treat central precocious puberty or to decrease testosterone levels in the management of prostate cancer.

It is important to be aware of the pulsatile nature of hormone secretion and the rhythmic patterns of hormone production when relating serum hormone measurements to normal values. For some hormones, integrated markers have been developed to circumvent hormonal fluctuations. Examples include 24-h urine collections for cortisol, IGF-I as a biologic marker of GH action, and HbA1c as an index of long-term (weeks to months) blood glucose control.

Often, one must interpret endocrine data only in the context of other hormonal results. For example, parathyroid hormone levels are typically assessed in combination with serum calcium concentrations. A high serum calcium level in association with elevated PTH is suggestive of hyperparathyroidism, whereas a suppressed PTH in this situation is more likely to be caused by hypercalcemia of malignancy or other causes of hypercalcemia. Similarly, TSH should be elevated when T_4 and T_3 concentrations are low, reflecting reduced feedback inhibition. When this is not the case, it is important to consider other abnormalities in the hormonal axis, such as secondary hypothyroidism, which is caused by a defect at the level of the pituitary.

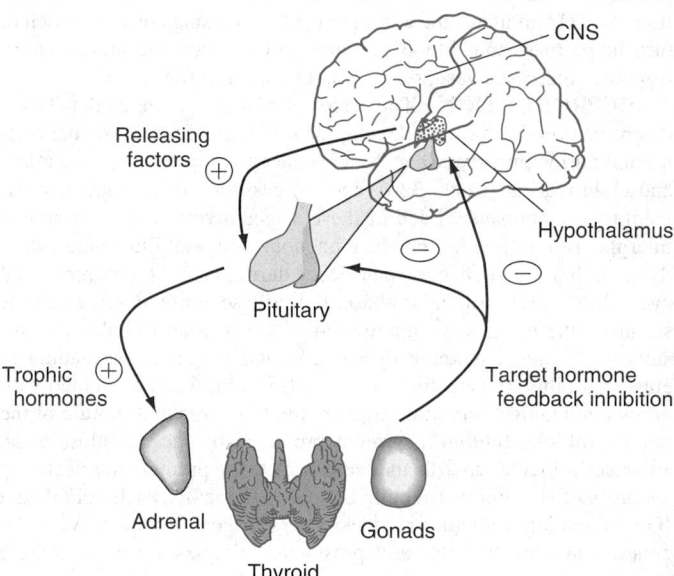

FIGURE 327-3 Feedback regulation of endocrine axes. CNS, central nervous system.

Endocrine diseases can be divided into three major types of conditions: (1) hormone excess, (2) hormone deficiency, and (3) hormone resistance (Table 327-2).

CAUSES OF HORMONE EXCESS   Syndromes of hormone excess can be caused by neoplastic growth of endocrine cells, autoimmune disorders, and excess hormone administration. Benign endocrine tumors, including parathyroid, pituitary, and adrenal adenomas, often retain the capacity to produce hormones, perhaps reflecting the fact that they are relatively well differentiated. Many endocrine tumors exhibit relatively subtle defects in their "set points" for feedback regulation. For example, in Cushing's disease, impaired feedback inhibition of ACTH secretion is associated with autonomous function. However, the tumor cells are not completely resistant to feedback, as revealed by the fact that ACTH is ultimately suppressed by higher doses of dexamethasone (e.g., high-dose dexamethasone test) (Chap. 331). Similar set point defects are also typical of parathyroid adenomas and autonomously functioning thyroid nodules.

The molecular basis of some endocrine tumors, such as the MEN syndromes (MEN-1, -2A, -2B), have provided important insights into tumorigenesis (Chap. 339). MEN-1 is characterized primarily by the triad of parathyroid, pancreatic islet, and pituitary tumors. MEN-2 predisposes to medullary thyroid carcinoma, pheochromocytoma, and hyperparathyroidism. The *MEN1* gene, located on chromosome 11q13, encodes a putative tumor-suppressor gene. Analogous to the paradigm first described for retinoblastoma, the affected individual inherits a mutant copy of the *MEN1* gene, and tumorigenesis ensues after a somatic "second hit" leads to loss of function of the normal *MEN1* gene (through deletion or point mutations).

In contrast to inactivation of a tumor-suppressor gene, as occurs in MEN-1 and most other inherited cancer syndromes, MEN-2 is caused by activating mutations in a single allele. In this case, activating mutations of the *RET* proto-oncogene, which encodes a receptor tyrosine kinase, leads to thyroid C-cell hyperplasia in childhood before the development of medullary thyroid carcinoma. Elucidation of the pathogenic mechanism has allowed early genetic screening for *RET* mutations in individuals at risk for MEN-2, permitting identification of those who may benefit from prophylactic thyroidectomy and biochemical screening for pheochromocytoma and hyperparathyroidism.

Mutations that activate hormone receptor signaling have been identified in several GPCRs (Table 327-3). For example, activating mutations of the LH receptor causes a dominantly transmitted form of male-limited precocious puberty, reflecting premature stimulation of testosterone synthesis in Leydig cells (Chap. 335). Activating mutations in these GPCRs are located primarily in the transmembrane domains and induce receptor coupling to $G_s\alpha$, even in the absence of hormone. Consequently, adenylate cyclase is activated and cyclic AMP levels increase in a manner that mimics hormone action. A similar phenomenon results from activating mutations in $G_s\alpha$. When these occur early in development, they cause McCune-Albright syndrome. When they occur only in somatotropes, the activating $G_s\alpha$ mutations cause GH-secreting tumors and acromegaly (Chap. 328).

In autoimmune Graves' disease, antibody interactions with the TSH receptor mimic TSH action, leading to hormone overproduction (Chap. 330). Analogous to the effects of activating mutations of the TSH receptor, these stimulating autoantibodies induce conformational changes that release the receptor from a constrained state, thereby triggering receptor coupling to G proteins.

CAUSES OF HORMONE DEFICIENCY   Most examples of hormone deficiency states can be attributed to glandular destruction caused by autoimmunity, surgery, infection, inflammation, infarction, hemorrhage, or tumor infiltration (Table 327-2). Autoimmune damage to the thyroid gland (Hashimoto's thyroiditis) and pancreatic islet β cells (type 1 diabetes mellitus) are prevalent causes of endocrine disease. Mutations in a number of hormones, hormone receptors, transcription factors, enzymes, and channels can also lead to hormone deficiencies (Table 327-3).

HORMONE RESISTANCE   Most severe hormone resistance syndromes are due to inherited defects in membrane receptors, nuclear receptors, or in the pathways that transduce receptor signals (Table 327-3). These disorders are characterized by defective hormone action, despite the presence of increased hormone levels. In complete androgen resistance, for example, mutations in the androgen receptor cause genetic (XY) males to have a female phenotypic appearance, even though LH and testosterone levels are increased (Chap. 338). In addition to these relatively rare genetic disorders, more common acquired forms of functional hormone resistance include insulin resistance in type 2 diabetes mellitus, leptin resistance in obesity, and GH resistance in catabolic states. The pathogenesis of functional resistance involves receptor downregulation and postreceptor desensitization of signaling pathways; functional forms of resistance are generally reversible.

Table 327-2   Causes of Endocrine Dysfunction

Type of Endocrine Disorder	Examples
Hyperfunction	
Neoplastic	
Benign	Pituitary adenomas, hyperparathyroidism, autonomous thyroid or adrenal nodules, pheochromocytoma
Malignant	Adrenal cancer, medullary thyroid cancer, carcinoid
Ectopic	Ectopic ACTH, SIADH secretion
Multiple endocrine neoplasia	MEN-1, MEN-2
Autoimmune	Graves' disease
Iatrogenic	Cushing's syndrome, hypoglycemia
Infectious/Inflammatory	Subacute thyroiditis
Activating receptor mutations	LH, TSH, Ca^{2+} and PTH receptors, $G_s\alpha$ (see Table 327-3)
Hypofunction	
Autoimmune	Hashimoto's thyroiditis, type 1 diabetes mellitus, Addison's disease, polyglandular failure
Iatrogenic	Radiation-induced hypopituitarism, hypothyroidism, surgical
Infectious/inflammatory	Adrenal insufficiency, hypothalamic sarcoidosis
Hormone mutations	GH, LHβ, FSHβ, vasopressin (see Table 327-3)
Enzyme defects	21-Hydroxylase deficiency (see Table 327-3)
Developmental defects	Kallmann syndrome, Turner syndrome, transcription factors (see Table 327-3)
Nutritional/vitamin deficiency	Vitamin D deficiency, iodine deficiency
Hemorrhage/infarction	Sheehan's syndrome, adrenal insufficiency
Hormone Resistance	
Receptor mutations	
Membrane	GH, vasopressin, LH, FSH, ACTH, GnRH, GHRH, PTH, leptin, Ca^{2+} (see Table 327-3)
Nuclear	AR, TR, VDR, ER, GR, PPAR$_\gamma$ (see Table 327-3)
Signaling pathway mutations	Albright's hereditary osteodystrophy
Postreceptor	Type 2 diabetes mellitus, leptin resistance

NOTE: AR, androgen receptor; ER, estrogen receptor; GR, glucocorticoid receptor; SIADH, syndrome of inappropriate antidiuretic hormone; TR, thyroid hormone receptor; VDR, vitamin D receptor. For all other abbreviations, see text.

_____ *Approach to the Patient* _____

Because endocrinology interfaces with numerous physiologic systems, there is no standard endocrine history and examination. Moreover,

Table 327-3   Examples of Genetic Endocrine Diseases

Endocrine Mutation	Disorder[a]	Mode of Inheritance	Chromosome Location	Types of Mutation
Hormone Mutations				
Insulin	Hyperproinsulinemia	AR	11p15.5	P
Growth hormone	GH deficiency; dwarfism	AR,AD	17q22-q24	D,P
POMC	Adrenal insufficiency; obesity	AR	2p23.3	P
Parathyroid hormone	Hypoparathyroidism	AD	11p15.3-15.1	P
Thyroid-stimulating hormone	TSH deficiency; hypothyroidism	AR	1p22	D,P
Thyroglobulin	Hypothyroidism; goiter	AR	8q24.2-q24.3	P
Luteinizing hormone	LH deficiency; hypogonadism	AR	19q13.32	P
Follicle-stimulating hormone	FSH deficiency; hypogonadism	AR	11p13	P
Vasopressin/neurophysin II	Neurohypophyseal diabetes insipidus (DI)	AD	20p12.21	P
Anti-müllerian hormone	Retained müllerian ducts	AR	19p13.3-p13.2	P
Leptin	Obesity	AR	7q31.3	P
Binding Protein Mutations				
Thyroxine-binding globulin	Euthyroid hypothyroxinemia	XL	Xq21-22	D,P
Transthyretin	Euthyroid hyperthyroximemia	AD	18q11.2-12.1	P
Albumin	Euthyroid hyperthyroximemia	AD	4q11-q13	P
Membrane Receptor Mutations				
Insulin receptor	Insulin resistance	AR, AD	19p13.3-13	P
GnRH receptor	Hypogonadotropic hypogonadism	AR	4q21.2	P
GHRH receptor	GH deficiency; dwarfism	AR	7p15-p14	P
TRH receptor	Hypothalamic hypothyroidism	AR	8q23	P
Growth hormone receptor	Laron dwarfism	AR	5p13-p12	P
TSH receptor (inactive)	TSH resistance	AR	14q31	P
TSH receptor (activating)	Hyperthyroidism	AD, S	14q31	P
LH receptor (inactive)	Hypogonadism	AR	2p21	P
LH receptor (activating)	Male precocious puberty	AD,S	2p21	P
FSH receptor (inactivating)	Ovarian failure; ↓ spermatogenesis	AR	2p21-p16	P
PTH receptor (inactivating)	Blomstrand chondrodysplasia	AR	3p22-p21.1	P
PTH receptor (activating)	Jansen chondrodysplasia	AD	3p22-p21.1	P
ACTH receptor	Adrenal insufficiency	AR	18p11.2	P
Vasopressin V₂ receptor	Nephrogenic DI	XL	Xq27-q28	P
Calcium receptor (inactive)	Hypocalciuric hypercalcemia	AD,AR	3q21-q24	P
Calcium receptor (activating)	Hypoparathyroidism	AD	3q21-q24	P
MIS receptor	Retained müllerian ducts	AR	12q13	P
Leptin receptor	Obesity	AR	1p31	P
Melanocortin 4 receptor	Obesity	AD	18q22	P
$G_s\alpha$	Acromegaly	S	20q13.2-13.3	P
$G_s\alpha$	Albright osteodystrophy	AD; imprinting	20q13.2-13.3	P
$G_s\alpha$	McCune-Albright	Mosaic	20q13.2-13.3	P
Nuclear Receptor Mutations				
Vitamin D	Type II vitamin D–resistant rickets (VDRR)	AR	12q12-q14	P
Thyroid hormone	Thyroid hormone resistance	AD	3p24.3	P,D
Glucocorticoid	Glucocorticoid resistance	AR	5q31	P
Mineralocorticoid	Pseudohypoaldosteronism type 1	AD	4q31.1	P
Androgen	Androgen resistance	XL,S	Xcen-q13	P,D
Estrogen	Estrogen resistance	AR,S	6p25.1	P
PPAR γ2	Obesity; insulin resistance	AD	3p25	P
Steroidogenic factor 1	XY sex-reversal; adrenal insufficiency	AD	9q33	P
DAX1	Adrenal hypoplasia congenita	XL	Xp21.3-p21.2	P,D
HNF 4α	MODY 1	AD	20q12-q13.1	P
Transcription Factor Mutations				
HNF 1α	MODY 3	AD	12q24.2	P
HNF 1β	MODY 5	AD	17cen-q21.3	P
Insulin promoter factor 1	MODY 4	AD	13q12.1	P
Pit1	GH, PRL, TSH deficiency	AR, AD	3p11	D,P
Prop1	GH, PRL, TSH, LH, FSH deficiency	AR	5q	P
Thyroid transcription factor 1	Congenital hypothyroidism	Unknown	14q13	Low expression
Thyroid transcription factor 2	Congenital hypothyroidism	AR	9q22	P
PAX-8	Congenital hypothyroidism	AR	2q12-q14	P
SRY translocation	XX male	XL	Ypter	Translocation
SRY mutation	XY female	YL	Ypter	P
SOX-9	XY female; campomelic dysplasia	AD	17q24.3-q25.1	P
Wilms' tumor	Frasier syndrome; Denys-Drash	AD	11p13	P
DAZ (RNA-binding protein)	Azoospermia	YL	Yq11	D
Endocrine Syndromes				
Kallmann	Hypogonadotropic hypogonadism	XL, AR, AD	Xp22.3	D,P,translocation
Prader-Willi	Hypogonadism, obesity, short stature	AD; imprint	15q11	D
Von Hippel–Lindau	Pheochromocytoma; renal Ca	AD	3p26-p25	D,P

(continued)

Table 327-3—(continued)

Endocrine Mutation	Disorder[a]	Mode of Inheritance	Chromosome Location	Types of Mutation
MEN-1	Neoplasia: Pit, pancreas, parathyroid	AD	11q13	P
MEN-2 (activating *ret* mutations)	Neoplasia: Parathyroid, pheo, MTC	AD	10q11.2	P
MEN-2b	MEN-2 and neurofibromas	AD	10q11.2	P
Carney complex	Cushing's; acromegaly, myxomas	AD	2p16	Unknown
Pendred syndrome	Goiter; deafness	AR	7q31	P,D
DiGeorge syndrome	Hypoparathyroidism; cardiac abn.	AD	22q11	D
Prohormone convertase 1	ACTH, GnRH, insulin deficiency	AR	5q15-q21	P
Polyglandular failure type 1	Polyglandular failure	AR	21q22.3	P
Enzyme and Channel Mutations				
Glucokinase	MODY 2	AD	7p15-p13	P
Sulfonylurea receptor	Nesidioblastosis	AR	11p15.1-p14	P
Potassium channel KCNJ11	Nesidioblastosis	AR	11p15.1	P
Sodium iodide symporter	Goiter, hypothyroidism	AR	19p12-13.2	P
Thyroid peroxidase	Goiter, hypothyroidism	AR	2pter-12	P
21-hydroxylase	CAH, androgen excess	AR	6p21	P,D
17α-Hydroxylase	Androgen deficiency, HTN	AR	10q24.3	P
17,20-Lyase activity	XY ambiguous genitalia	AR	10q24.3	P
11β-Hydroxylase	Androgen excess, HTN	AR	8q21	P
3β-Hydroxysteroid dehydrog.	CAH; Androgen deficiency	AR	1p13.1	P
Steroidogenic acute regulatory	Lipoid CAH	AR	8p11.2	P
5α-Reductase type 2	Male pseudohermaphroditism	AR	2p23	D,P
Aldosterone synthase	Glucocorticoid remediable HTN	AD	8q21	D, translocation
Amiloride sensitive Na channel	Liddle syndrome; HTN	AD	16p13-p12	P
Aquaporin 2	Nephrogenic DI	AR	12q13	P
PEX	Hypophosphatemic VDRR	XL	Xp22.2-pp22.1	P
1α Hydroxylase	Type 1 VDRR	AR	12q14	P

NOTE: AD, autosomal dominant; AR, autosomal recessive; CAH, congenital adrenal hyperplasia; D, deletion, HNF, hepatic nuclear factor; HTN, hypertension; MODY, maturity onset diabetes of the young; MTC, medullary thyroid carcinoma; P, point mutation; S, somatic cell mutation; XL, X-linked; YL, Y-linked. For other abbreviations, see text. SOURCE: Adapted from DeGroot and Jameson, with permission.

because most glands are relatively inaccessible, the examination usually focuses on the manifestations of hormone excess or deficiency, as well as direct examination of palpable glands, such as the thyroid and gonads. For these reasons, it is important to evaluate patients in the context of their presenting symptoms, review of systems, family and social history, and exposure to medications that may affect the endocrine system. Astute clinical skills are required to detect subtle symptoms and signs suggestive of underlying endocrine disease. For example, a patient with Cushing's syndrome may manifest specific findings, such as central fat redistribution, striae, and proximal muscle weakness, in addition to features seen commonly in the general population, such as obesity, plethora, hypertension, and glucose intolerance. Similarly, the insidious onset of hypothyroidism—with mental slowing, fatigue, dry skin, and other features—can be difficult to distinguish from similar, nonspecific findings in the general population. Clinical judgment, based on knowledge of pathophysiology and experience, is required to decide when to embark on more extensive evaluation of these disorders. As described below, laboratory testing plays an essential role in endocrinology by allowing quantitative assessment of hormone levels and dynamics. Radiologic imaging tests, such as CT scan, MRI, thyroid scan, and ultrasound, are also used for the diagnosis of endocrine disorders. However, these tests are generally employed only after a hormonal abnormality has been established by biochemical testing.

Hormone Measurements and Endocrine Testing Radioimmunoassays are the most important diagnostic tool in endocrinology, as they allow sensitive, specific, and quantitative determination of steady-state and dynamic changes in hormone concentrations. Radioimmunoassays use antibodies to detect specific hormones. For many peptide hormones, these measurements are now configured as immunoradiometric assays (IRMAs), which use two different antibodies to increase binding affinity and specificity. There are many variations of these assays—a common format involves using one antibody to capture the antigen (hormone) onto an immobilized surface and a second antibody, labeled with a fluorescent or radioactive tag, to detect the antigen. These assays are sensitive enough to detect plasma hormone concentrations in the picomolar to nanomolar range, and they can read-

ily distinguish structurally related proteins, such as PTH from PTHrP. A variety of other techniques are used to measure specific hormones, including mass spectroscopy, various forms of chromatography, and enzymatic methods; bioassays are now used rarely.

Most hormone measurements are based on plasma or serum samples. However, urinary hormone determinations remain useful for the evaluation of some conditions. Urinary collections over 24 h provide an integrated assessment of the production of a hormone or metabolite, many of which vary during the day. It is important to assure complete collections of 24-h urine samples; simultaneous measurement of creatinine provides an internal control for the adequacy of collection and can be used to normalize some hormone measurements. A 24-h urine free cortisol measurement largely reflects the amount of unbound cortisol, thus providing a reasonable index of biologically available hormone. Other commonly used urine determinations include: 17-hydroxycorticosteroids, 17-ketosteroids, vanillylmandelic acid (VMA), metanephrine, catecholamines, 5-hydroxyindoleacetic acid (5-HIAA), and calcium.

The value of quantitative hormone measurements lies in their correct interpretation in a clinical context. The normal range for most hormones is relatively broad, often varying by a factor of two- to tenfold. The normal ranges for many hormones are gender- and age-specific. Thus, using the correct normative database is an essential part of interpreting hormone tests. The pulsatile nature of hormones and factors that can affect their secretion, such as sleep, meals, and medications, must also be considered. Cortisol values increase fivefold between midnight and dawn; reproductive hormone levels vary dramatically during the female menstrual cycle.

For many endocrine systems, much information can be gained from basal hormone testing, particularly when different components of an endocrine axis are assessed simultaneously. For example, low testosterone and elevated LH levels suggest a primarily gonadal problem, whereas a hypothalamic-pituitary disorder is likely if both LH and testosterone are low. Because TSH is a sensitive indicator of thyroid function, it is generally recommended as a first-line test for thyroid disorders. An elevated TSH level is almost always the result of primary hypothyroidism, whereas a low TSH is most often caused by thyro-

Table 327-4 Examples of Prevalent Endocrine and Metabolic Disorders in the Adult

Disorder	Approx. Prevalence in Adults[a]	Screening/Testing Recommendations[b]	Specific Guidelines	Chapter
Obesity	23% BMI > 30 50% BMI > 25	Calculate BMI Measure waist circumference Exclude secondary causes Consider comorbid complications	NHLBI Clinical Guidelines on the Identification, Evaluation, and Treatment of Overweight and Obesity	77

Type 2 diabetes mellitus	>6%	Test every 3 years or more often in high-risk groups:
		    Fasting plasma glucose (FPG) > 126 mg/dL
		    Random plasma glucose > 200 mg/dL
		An elevated HbA1c
		Consider comorbid complications
			Expert Committee on the Diagnosis and Classification of Diabetes Mellitus	333

Hyperlipidemia	5–10%	Cholesterol screening at least every 5 years; more often in high-risk groups Lipoprotein analysis (LDL, HDL) for increased cholesterol, CAD, diabetes Consider secondary causes	Expert Panel of the National Cholesterol Education Program (NCEP)	344
Hypothyroidism	5–10%, women 0.5–2%, men	TSH; confirm with free T_4		330
Graves' disease	1–3%, women 0.1%, men	TSH, free T_4		330
Thyroid nodules and neoplasia	5%	Physical examination of thyroid Fine-needle aspiration biopsy	American Thyroid Association	330
Osteoporosis	5%, women 1%, men	Bone mineral density measurements in individuals at risk Exclude secondary causes	World Health Organization	342
Hyperparathyroidism	0.1–0.5%, women > men	Serum calcium PTH, if calcium is elevated Assess comorbid conditions	NIH Consensus Conference on Diagnosis and Management of Asymptomatic Primary Hyperparathyroidism	341
Infertility	10%, couples	Investigate male and female member of couple Semen analysis in male Assess ovulatory cycles in female Specific tests as indicated		54
Polycystic ovarian syndrome	4–7% women	Free testosterone, DHEAS Consider comorbid conditions		336
Hirsutism	Variable	Free testosterone, DHEAS Exclude secondary causes Additional tests as indicated		53
Menopause	Median age, 51	FSH		336
Hyperprolactinemia	Common in women with amenorrhea or galactorrhea	PRL level MRI, if not medication-related		328
Erectile dysfunction	10–15%	PRL, testosterone Consider secondary causes (e.g., diabetes)		51
Gynecomastia	Common in older men	Often, no tests are indicated Consider Klinefelter syndrome Consider medications, hypogonadism, liver disease		337
Klinefelter syndrome	0.2%, men	Karyotype Testosterone		338
Turner syndrome	0.03%, women	Karyotype Consider comorbid conditions		338

[a] The prevalence of most disorders varies among ethnic groups and with aging.
[b] See individual chapters for additional information on evaluation and treatment. Early testing is indicated in patients with signs and symptoms of disease or in those at increased risk.

NOTE: BMI, body mass index; CAD, coronary artery disease; DHEAS, dehydroepiandrosterone; HDL, high-density lipoprotein; LDL, low-density lipoprotein; MRI, magnetic resonance imaging. For other abbreviations, see text.

toxicosis. These predictions can be confirmed by determining the free thyroxine level. Elevated calcium and PTH levels suggest hyperparathyroidism, whereas PTH is suppressed in hypercalcemia caused by malignancy or granulomatous diseases. A suppressed ACTH in the setting of hypercortisolemia, or increased urine free cortisol, is seen with hyperfunctioning adrenal adenomas.

It is not uncommon, however, for baseline hormone levels associated with pathologic endocrine conditions to overlap with the normal range. In this circumstance, dynamic testing is useful to further separate the two groups. There are a multitude of dynamic endocrine tests, but all are based on principles of feedback regulation, and most responses can be remembered based on the pathways that govern endocrine axes. *Suppression tests* are used in the setting of suspected endocrine hyperfunction. An example is the dexamethasone suppression test used to evaluate Cushing's syndrome (Chaps. 328 and 331). *Stimulation tests* are generally used to assess endocrine hypofunction. The ACTH stimulation test, for example, is used to assess the adrenal gland response in patients with suspected adrenal insufficiency. Other stimulation tests use hypothalamic-releasing factors such as TRH, GnRH, CRH, and GHRH to evaluate pituitary hormone reserve (Chap. 328). Insulin-induced hypoglycemia evokes pituitary ACTH and GH responses. Stimulation tests based on reduction or inhibition of endogenous hormones are less commonly used. Examples include metyrapone inhibition of cortisol synthesis and clomiphene inhibition of estrogen feedback.

Screening and Assessment of Common Endocrine Disorders Because many endocrine disorders are prevalent in the adult population (Table 327-4), most are diagnosed and managed by general internists, family practitioners, or other primary health care providers. The high prevalence and clinical impact of certain endocrine diseases justifies vigilance for features of these disorders during routine physical examinations; laboratory screening is indicated in selected high-risk populations.

BIBLIOGRAPHY

CANAFF L et al: Peptide hormone precursor processing: Getting sorted? Mol Cell Endocrinol 156:1, 1999

CARTER-SU C, SMIT LS: Signaling via JAK tyrosine kinases: Growth hormone receptor as a model system. Recent Prog Horm Res 53:61, 1998

CZEISLER CA, KLERMAN EB: Circadian and sleep-dependent regulation of hormone release in humans. Recent Prog Horm Res 54:97, 1999

DEGROOT LJ, JAMESON JL: *Endocrinology*, 4th ed. Philadelphia, Saunders, 2001 (in press)

GETHER U: Uncovering molecular mechanisms involved in activation of G protein–coupled receptors. Endocr Rev 21:90, 2000

GIGUERE V: Orphan nuclear receptors: From gene to function. Endocr Rev 20:689, 1999

JAMESON JL: *Hormone Resistance Syndromes*. Totowa, NJ, Humana, 1999

MARX SJ et al: Multiple endocrine neoplasia type 1: Clinical and genetic features of the hereditary endocrine neoplasias. Recent Prog Horm Res 54:397, 1999

MCKENNA NJ et al: Nuclear receptor coregulators: Cellular and molecular biology. Endocr Rev 20:321, 1999

VIRKAMAKI A et al: Protein-protein interaction in insulin signaling and the molecular mechanisms of insulin resistance. J Clin Invest 103:931, 1999

WILSON JD et al: *William's Textbook of Endocrinology*, 9th ed. Philadelphia, Saunders, 1998

328 *Shlomo Melmed*

DISORDERS OF THE ANTERIOR PITUITARY AND HYPOTHALAMUS

ACTH adrenocorticotropin hormone	hMG human menopausal gonadotropin
AGHD adult GH deficiency	
AVP arginine vasopressin	HPA hypothalamo-pituitary-adrenal
CNS central nervous system	IGFBPs IGF-binding proteins
CRH corticotropin-releasing hormone	IGF insulin-like growth factor
CSF cerebrospinal fluid	IL interleukin
CT computed tomography	JAK Janus kinase
FSH follicle-stimulating hormone	LH luteinizing hormone
GH growth hormone	LOH loss of heterozygosity
GHBP GH binding protein	MAP mitogen activated protein
GHRH growth hormone–releasing hormone	MRI magnetic resonance imaging
GHRPs growth hormone–releasing peptides	POMC proopiomelanocortin
	PRL prolactin
GnRH gonadotropin-releasing hormone	STAT signal transduction and activators of transcription
GPCR G protein–coupled receptor	TNF tumor necrosis factor
	TRH thyrotropin-releasing hormone
hCG human chorionic gonadotropin	TSH thyroid-stimulating hormone

The anterior pituitary is often referred to as the "master gland" because, together with the hypothalamus, it orchestrates the complex regulatory functions of multiple other endocrine glands. The anterior pituitary gland produces six major hormones: (1) prolactin (PRL), (2) growth hormone (GH), (3) adrenocorticotropin hormone (ACTH), (4) luteinizing hormone (LH), (5) follicle-stimulating hormone (FSH), and (6) thyroid-stimulating hormone (TSH) (Table 328-1). Pituitary hormones are secreted in a pulsatile manner, reflecting stimulation by an array of specific hypothalamic releasing factors. Each of these pituitary hormones elicits specific responses in peripheral target tissues. The hormonal products of these peripheral glands, in turn, exert feedback control at the level of the hypothalamus and pituitary to modulate pituitary function (Fig. 328-1). Pituitary tumors cause characteristic hormone excess syndromes. Hormone deficiency may be inherited or acquired. Fortunately, efficacious treatments exist for the various pituitary hormone excess and deficiency syndromes. Nonetheless, these diagnoses are often elusive, emphasizing the importance of recognizing subtle clinical manifestations and performing the correct laboratory diagnostic tests. →*For discussion of disorders of the posterior pituitary, or neurohypophysis, see Chap. 329.*

ANATOMY AND DEVELOPMENT **Anatomy** The pituitary gland weighs ~600 mg and is located within the sella turcica ventral to the diaphragma sella; it comprises anatomically and functionally distinct anterior and posterior lobes. The sella is contiguous to vascular and neurologic structures, including the cavernous sinuses, cranial nerves, and optic chiasm. Thus, expanding intrasellar pathologic processes may have significant central mass effects in addition to their endocrinologic impact.

Hypothalamic neural cells synthesize specific releasing and inhibiting hormones that are secreted directly into the portal vessels of the pituitary stalk. Blood supply of the pituitary gland is derived from the superior and inferior hypophyseal arteries (Fig. 328-2). The hypothalamic-pituitary portal plexus provides the major blood source for the anterior pituitary, allowing reliable transmission of hypothalamic peptide pulses without significant systemic dilution; consequently, pituitary cells are exposed to sharp spikes of releasing factors and in turn release their hormones as discrete pulses (Fig. 328-3).

The posterior pituitary is supplied by the inferior hypophyseal arteries. In contrast to the anterior pituitary, the posterior lobe is directly innervated by hypothalamic neurons (supraopticohypophyseal and tuberohypophyseal nerve tracts) via the pituitary stalk (Chap. 329).

Table 328-1 Anterior Pituitary Hormone Expression and Regulation

Cell	Corticotrope	Somatotrope	Lactotrope	Thyrotrope	Gonadotrope
Tissue-specific transcription factor	PTX-1, CUTE	Prop I, Pit-I	Prop I, Pit I	Prop I, Pit 1, TEF	SF-1, DAX-1
Fetal appearance	6 weeks	8 weeks	12 weeks	12 weeks	12 weeks
Hormone	POMC	GH	PRL	TSH	FSH LH
Chromosomal locus	2 p	17q	6	α −6q; β-1p	β-11p; β-19q
Protein	Polypeptide	Polypeptide	Polypeptide	Glycoprotein α, β subunits	Glycoprotein α, β subunits
Amino acids	266 (ACTH 1–39)	191	199	211	210 204
Stimulators	CRH, AVP, gp-130 cytokines	GHRH, GHRP	Estrogen, TRH, VIP	TRH	GnRH, activins, estrogen
Inhibitors	Glucocorticoids	Somatostatin, IGF-I	Dopamine	T_3, T_4, dopamine, somatostatin, glucocorticoids	Sex steroids, inhibin
Target gland	Adrenal	Liver, other tissues	Breast, other tissues	Thyroid	Ovary, testis
Trophic effect	Steroid production	IGF-I production, growth induction, insulin antagonism	Milk production	T_4 synthesis and secretion	Sex steroid production, follicle growth germ cell maturation
Normal range	ACTH, 4–22 pg/L	<0.5 μg/L[a]	M < 15; F <20 μg/L	0.1–5 mU/L	M, 5–20 IU/L, F (basal), 5–20 IU/L

[a] Hormone secretion integrated over 24 h.
NOTE: M, male; F, female. For other abbreviations, see text.
SOURCE: Adapted from I Shimon, S Melmed, in P Conn, S Melmed (eds): *Endocrinology: Basic and Clinical Principles*. Totowa, NJ, Humana, 1996.

the proopiomelanocortin (POMC) gene, requires corticotropin upstream transcription element (CUTE) and the PTX-1 transcription factor. Abnormalities of pituitary development caused by mutations of Pit-1, Prop-1, SF-1, and DAX-1 result in a series of rare, selective or combined, pituitary hormone deficits.

HYPOTHALAMIC AND ANTERIOR PITUITARY INSUFFICIENCY

Hypopituitarism results from impaired production of one or more of the anterior pituitary trophic hormones. Reduced pituitary function can result from inherited disorders; more commonly, it is acquired and reflects the mass effects of tumors or the consequences of inflammation or vascular damage. These processes may also impair synthesis or secretion of hypothalamic hormones, with resultant pituitary failure (Table 328-2).

Thus, posterior pituitary production of vasopressin (antidiuretic hormone; ADH) and oxytocin is particularly sensitive to neuronal damage by lesions that affect the pituitary stalk or hypothalamus.

Pituitary Development The embryonic differentiation and maturation of anterior pituitary cells have been elucidated in considerable detail. Pituitary development from Rathke's pouch involves a complex interplay of lineage-specific transcription factors expressed in pluripotential stem cells and gradients of locally produced growth factors (Table 328-1). The transcription factor Pit-1 determines cell-specific expression of GH, PRL, and TSH in somatotropes, lactotropes, and thyrotropes. Expression of high levels of estrogen receptors in cells that contain Pit-1 favors PRL expression, whereas thyrotrope embronic factor (TEF) induces TSH expression. Pit-1 binds to GH, PRL, and TSH gene regulatory elements, as well as to recognition sites on its own promoter, providing a mechanism for perpetuating selective pituitary phenotypic stability. The transcription factor Prop-1 induces the pituitary development of Pit-1-specific lineages, as well as gonadotropes. Gonadotrope cell development is further defined by the cell-specific expression of the nuclear receptors, steroidogenic factor (SF-1) and DAX-1. Development of corticotrope cells, which express

DEVELOPMENTAL AND GENETIC CAUSES OF HYPO-PITUITARISM Pituitary Dysplasia Pituitary dysplasia may result in aplastic, hypoplastic, or ectopic pituitary gland development. Because pituitary development requires midline cell migration from the nasopharyngeal Rathke's pouch, midline craniofacial disorders, such as cleft lip and palate, basal encephalocele, hypertelorism, and optic nerve hypoplasia, may be associated with pituitary dysplasia. Acquired pituitary failure in the newborn can also be caused by birth trauma, including cranial hemorrhage, asphyxia, and breech delivery.

Septo-optic dysplasia Hypothalamic dysfunction and hypopituitarism may result from dysgenesis of the septum pellucidum or corpus callosum. Affected children have mutations in the *HESX1* gene, which is involved in early development of the ventral prosencephalon. These children exhibit cleft palate, syndactyly, ear deformities, hypertelorism, optic atrophy, micropenis, and anosmia. Pituitary dysfunction leads to diabetes insipidus, GH deficiency and short stature, and, occasionally, TSH deficiency.

Tissue-Specific Factor Mutations Several pituitary cell–specific transcription factors, such as Pit-1 and Prop-1, are critical for determining the development and function of specific anterior pituitary

FIGURE 328-1 Diagram of pituitary axes. Hypothalamic hormones regulate anterior pituitary trophic hormones that, in turn, determine target gland secretion. Peripheral hormones feedback to regulate hypothalamic and pituitary hormones. For abbreviations, see text.

FIGURE 328-2 Diagram of hypothalamic-pituitary vasculature: The hypothalamic nuclei produce hormones that traverse the portal system and impinge on anterior pituitary cells to regulate pituitary hormone secretion. Posterior pituitary hormones are derived from direct neural extensions.

cell lineages. Autosomal dominant or recessive Pit-1 mutations cause combined GH, PRL, and TSH deficiencies. These patients present with growth failure and varying degrees of hypothyroidism. The pituitary may appear hypoplastic on magnetic resonance imaging (MRI).

Prop-1 is expressed early in pituitary development and appears to be required for Pit-1 function. Familial and sporadic *PROP1* mutations result in combined GH, PRL, TSH, and gonadotropin deficiency, with preservation of ACTH. Over 80% of these patients have growth retardation and, by adulthood, all are deficient in TSH and gonadotropins. Because of gonadotropin deficiency, they do not enter puberty spontaneously (Fig. 328-4).

Developmental Hypothalamic Dysfunction • *Kallmann syndrome* This syndrome results from defective hypothalamic gonadotropin-releasing hormone (GnRH) synthesis and is associated with anosmia or hyposmia due to olfactory bulb agenesis or hypoplasia (Chap. 335). The syndrome may also be associated with color blindness, optic atrophy, nerve deafness, cleft palate, renal abnormalities, cryptorchidism, and neurologic abnormalities such as mirror movements. Defects in the *KAL* gene, which maps to chromosome Xp22.3, prevent embryonic migration of GnRH neurons from the hypothalamic olfactory placode to the hypothalamus. Genetic abnormalities, in addition to *KAL* mutations, can also cause isolated GnRH deficiency, as autosomal recessive and dominant modes of transmission have been described. GnRH deficiency prevents progression through puberty. Males present with delayed puberty and pronounced hypogonadal features, including micropenis, probably the result of low testosterone levels during infancy (Chap. 335). Female patients present with primary amenorrhea and failure of secondary sexual development.

Kallmann syndrome and other causes of congenital GnRH defi-

Table 328-2 Etiology of Hypopituitarism[a]

Development/structural
  Transcription factor defect
  Pituitary dysplasia/aplasia
  Congenital CNS mass, encephalocele
  Primary empty sella
  Congenital hypothalamic disorders (septo-optic dysplasia, Prader-Willi syndrome, Laurence-Moon-Biedl syndrome, Kallmann syndrome)
Traumatic
  Surgical resection
  Radiation damage
  Head injuries
Neoplastic
  Pituitary adenoma
  Parasellar mass (meningioma, germinoma, ependymoma, glioma)
  Rathke's cyst
  Craniopharyngioma
  Hypothalamic hamartoma, gangliocytoma
  Pituitary metastases (breast, lung, colon carcinoma)
  Lymphoma and leukemia
  Meningioma
Infiltrative/inflammatory
  Hemochromatosis
  Lymphocytic hypophysitis
  Sarcoidosis
  Histiocytosis X
  Granulomatous hypophysitis
Vascular
  Pituitary apoplexy
  Pregnancy-related (infarction with diabetes; postpartum necrosis)
  Sickle cell disease
  Arteritis
Infections
  Fungal (histoplasmosis)
  Parasitic (toxoplasmosis)
  Tuberculosis
  Pneumocystis carinii

[a] Trophic hormone failure associated with pituitary compression or destruction usually occurs sequentially GH > FSH > LH > TSH > ACTH. During childhood, growth retardation is often the presenting feature, and in adults hypogonadism is the earliest symptom.

ciency are characterized by low LH and FSH levels and low concentrations of sex steroids (testosterone or estradiol). In sporadic cases of isolated gonadotropin deficiency, the diagnosis is often one of exclusion after eliminating other causes of hypothalamic-pituitary dysfunction. Repetitive GnRH administration restores normal pituitary gonadotropin responses, pointing to a hypothalamic defect.

Long-term treatment of males with human chorionic gonadotropin

FIGURE 328-4 Gradual development of anterior pituitary hormone deficiencies in 35 patients with *PROP1* gene mutations. Combined pituitary hormone deficiency develops gradually. By adulthood, all patients have growth hormone (GH, ●), thyroid-stimulating hormone (TSH, □), and gonadotropin (LH, luteinizing hormone; FSH, follicle-stimulating hormone, ■) deficiency. (*Adapted from Deladoey et al, 1999.*)

FIGURE 328-3 Hypothalamic gonadotropin-releasing hormone (GnRH) pulses induce secretory pulses of luteinizing hormone (LH).

(hCG) or testosterone restores pubertal development and secondary sex characteristics; females can be treated with cyclic estrogen and progestin. Fertility may also be restored by the administration of subcutaneous, pulsatile GnRH using a portable infusion pump.

Laurence-Moon-Bardet-Biedl syndrome   This rare autosomal recessive disorder is characterized by mental retardation; obesity; and hexadactyly, brachydactyly, or syndactyly. Central diabetes insipidus may or may not be associated. GnRH deficiency occurs in 75% of males and half of affected females. Retinal degeneration begins in early childhood, and most patients are blind by age 30.

Fröhlich syndrome (adipose genital dystrophy)   A broad spectrum of hypothalamic lesions may be associated with hyperphagia, obesity, and central hypogonadism. Decreased GnRH production in these patients results in attenuated pituitary FSH and LH synthesis and release.

Prader-Willi syndrome   Chromosome 15q deletions are associated with hypogonadotropic hypogonadism, hyperphagia-obesity, chronic muscle hypotonia, mental retardation, and adult-onset diabetes mellitus (Chap. 66). Multiple somatic defects also involve the skull, eyes, ears, hands, and feet. Diminished hypothalamic oxytocin- and vasopressin-producing nuclei have been reported. Deficient GnRH synthesis is suggested by the observation that chronic GnRH treatment restores pituitary LH and FSH release.

ACQUIRED HYPOPITUITARISM   Hypopituitarism may be caused by accidental or neurosurgical trauma; vascular events such as apoplexy; pituitary or hypothalamic neoplasms such as pituitary adenomas, craniopharyngiomas, or metastatic deposits; inflammatory disease such as lymphocytic hypophysitis; infiltrative disorders such as sarcoidosis, hemochromatosis (Chap. 345), and tuberculosis; or irradiation. It is often difficult to localize the site of hormonal dysfunction as many processes, including hemochromatosis and radiation, may affect both hypothalamic and pituitary function.

Hypothalamic Infiltration Disorders   These disorders—including those associated with sarcoidosis, histiocytosis X, amyloidosis, and hemochromatosis—frequently involve both hypothalamic and pituitary neuronal and neurochemical tracts. Consequently, diabetes insipidus occurs in half of patients with these disorders. Growth retardation is seen if attenuated GH secretion occurs before pubertal epiphyseal closure. Hypogonadotropic hypogonadism and hyperprolactinemia are also common.

Inflammatory Lesions   Pituitary damage and subsequent dysfunction can be seen with chronic infections such as tuberculosis, opportunistic fungal infections associated with AIDS, and in tertiary syphilis. Other inflammatory processes, such as granulomas or sarcoidosis, may mimic a pituitary adenoma. These lesions may cause extensive hypothalamic and pituitary damage, leading to trophic hormone failure.

Cranial Irradiation   Cranial irradiation may result in long-term hypothalamic and pituitary dysfunction, especially in children and adolescents who are more susceptible to damage following whole-brain or head and neck therapeutic irradiation. The development of hormonal abnormalities correlates strongly with irradiation dosage and the time interval after completion of radiotherapy. Up to two-thirds of patients ultimately develop hormone insufficiency afer a median dose of 50 Gy (5000 rad) directed at the skull base. The development of hypopituitarism occurs over 5 to 15 years and usually reflects hypothalamic damage rather than absolute destruction of pituitary cells. Though the pattern of hormone loss is variable, GH deficiency is most commonly followed by gonadotropin and ACTH deficiency. When deficiency of one or more hormones is documented, the possibility of diminished reserve of other hormones is likely. Accordingly, anterior pituitary function should be evaluated over the long term in previously irradiated patients, and replacement therapy instituted when appropriate (see below).

Lymphocytic Hypophysitis   This occurs mainly in pregnant or post-partum women; it usually presents with hyperprolactinemia and MRI evidence of a prominent pituitary mass resembling an adenoma, with mildly elevated PRL levels. Pituitary failure caused by diffuse lymphocytic infiltration may be transient or permanent but requires immediate evaluation and treatment. Rarely, isolated pituitary hormone deficiencies have been described, suggesting a selective autoimmune process targeted to specific cell types. Most patients manifest symptoms of progressive mass effects with headache and visual disturbance. The erythrocyte sedimentation rate is often elevated. As the MRI image may be indistinguishable from that of a pituitary adenoma, hypophysitis should be considered in a post-partum woman with a newly diagnosed pituitary mass before embarking on unnecessary surgical intervention. The inflammatory process often resolves after several months of glucocorticoid treatment, and pituitary function may be restored, depending on the extent of damage.

Pituitary Apoplexy   Acute intrapituitary hemorrhagic vascular events can cause substantial damage to the pituitary and surrounding sellar structures. Pituitary apoplexy may occur spontaneously in a preexisting adenoma (usually nonfunctioning); postpartum (Sheehan's syndrome); or in association with diabetes, hypertension, sickle cell anemia, or acute shock. The hyperplastic enlargement of the pituitary during pregnancy increases the risk for hemorrhage and infarction. Apoplexy is an endocrine emergency that may result in severe hypoglycemia, hypotension, central nervous system (CNS) hemorrhage, and death. Acute symptoms include severe headache with signs of meningeal irritation, bilateral visual changes, ophthalmoplegia that varies, and, in severe cases, cardiovascular collapse and loss of consciousness. Pituitary computed tomography (CT) or MRI may reveal signs of intratumoral or sellar hemorrhage, with deviation of the pituitary stalk and compression of pituitary tissue.

Patients with no evident visual loss or impaired consciousness can be observed and managed conservatively with high-dose glucocorticoids. Those with significant or progressive visual loss or loss of consciousness require urgent surgical decompression. Visual recovery after surgery is inversely correlated with the length of time after the acute event. Therefore, severe ophthalmoplegia or visual deficits are indications for early surgery. Hypopituitarism is very common after apoplexy.

Empty Sella   A partial or apparently totally empty sella is usually an incidental MRI finding. These patients usually exhibit normal pituitary function, implying that the surrounding rim of pituitary tissue is fully functional. Hypopituitarism, however, may develop insidiously. Pituitary masses may undergo clinically silent infarction with development of a partial or totally empty sella by cerebrospinal fluid (CSF) filling the dural herniation. Rarely, functional pituitary adenomas may arise within the rim of pituitary tissue, and these are not always visible on MRI.

PRESENTATION AND DIAGNOSIS   The clinical manifestations of hypopituitarism depend on which hormones are lost and the extent of the hormone deficiency. GH deficiency causes growth disorders in children and leads to abnormal body composition in adults (see below). Gonadotropin deficiency causes menstrual disorders and infertility in women and decreased sexual function, infertility, and loss of secondary sexual characteristics in men. TSH and ACTH deficiency usually develop later in the course of pituitary failure. TSH deficiency leads to growth retardation in children and features of hypothyroidism in children and in adults. The secondary form of adrenal insufficiency caused by ACTH deficiency leads to hypocortisolism with relative preservation of mineralocorticoid production. PRL deficiency causes failure of lactation. When lesions involve the posterior pituitary tracts, polyuria and polydipsia reflect loss of vasopressin secretion. Epidemiologic studies have documented an increased mortality rate in patients with longstanding pituitary damage, primarily from increased cardiovascular and cerebrovascular disease.

LABORATORY INVESTIGATION   Biochemical diagnosis of pituitary insufficiency is made by demonstrating low levels of trophic hormones in the setting of low target hormone levels. For example, low free thyroxine in the setting of a low or inappropriately normal TSH level suggests secondary hypothyroidism. Similarly, a

Table 328-3 Tests of Pituitary Insufficiency

Hormone	Test	Blood Samples	Interpretation
Growth hormone	Insulin tolerance test: Regular insulin (0.05–0.15 U/kg IV)	−30, 0, 30, 60, 120 min for glucose and GH	Glucose < 40 mg/dL; GH should be >3 μg/L
	GHRH test: 1 μg/kg IV	0, 15, 30, 45, 60, 120 min for GH	Normal response is GH >3 μg/L
	L-Arginine test: 30 g IV over 30 min	0, 30, 60, 120 min for GH	Normal response is GH >3 μg/L
	L-dopa test: 500 mg PO	0, 30, 60, 120 min for GH	Normal response is GH >3 μg/L
Prolactin	TRH test: 200–500 μg IV	0, 20, and 60 min for TSH and PRL	Normal prolactin is >2 μg/L and increase >200% of baseline
ACTH	Insulin tolerance test: Regular insulin (0.05–0.15 U/kg IV)	−30, 0, 30, 60, 90 min for glucose and coritsol	Glucose <40 mg/dL Cortisol should increase by >7 μg/dL or to >20 μg/dL
	CRH test: 1 μg/kg ovine CRH IV at 0800 h	0, 15, 30, 60, 90, 120 min for ACTH and cortisol	Basal ACTH increases 2- to 4-fold and peaks at 20–100 pg/mL Cortisol levels >20–25 μg/dL
	Metyrapone test: Metyrapone (30 mg/kg) at midnight	Plasma 11-deoxycortisol and cortisol at 8 A.M.; ACTH can also be measured	Plasma cortisol should be <4 μg/dL to assure an adequate response Normal response is 11-deoxycortisol >7.5 μg/dL or ACTH >75 pg/mL
	Standard ACTH stimulation test: ACTH 1-24 (Cosyntropin), 0.25 mg IM or IV	0, 30, 60 min for cortisol and aldosterone	Normal response is cortisol >21 μg/dL and aldosterone response of >4 ng/dL above baseline
	Low-dose ACTH test: ACTH 1-24 (Cosyntropin), 1 μg IV	0, 30, 60 min for cortisol	Cortisol should be >21 μg/dL
	3-day ACTH stimulation test consists of 0.25 mg ACTH 1-24 given IV over 8 h each day		Cortisol >21 μg/dL
TSH	Basal thyroid function tests: T$_4$, T$_3$, TSH	Basal tests	Low free thyroid hormone levels in the setting of TSH levels that are not appropriately increased
	TRH test: 200–500 μg IV	0, 20, 60 min for TSH and PRL	TSH should increase by >5 mU/L unless thyroid hormone levels are increased
LH, FSH	LH, FSH, testosterone, estrogen	Basal tests	Basal LH and FSH should be increased in postmenopausal women Low testosterone levels in the setting of low LH and FSH
	GnRH test: GnRH (100 μg) IV	0, 30, 60 min for LH and FSH	In most adults, LH should increase by 10 IU/L and FSH by 2 IU/L Normal responses are variable
Multiple hormones	Combined anterior pituitary test: GHRH (1 μg/kg), CRH (1 μg/kg), GnRH (100 μg), TRH (200 μg) are given IV	−30, 0, 15, 30, 60, 90, 120 min for GH, ACTH, cortisol, LH, FSH, and TSH	Combined or individual releasing hormone responses must be elevated in the context of basal target gland hormone values and may not be diagnostic (see text)

low testosterone level without elevation of gonadotropins suggests hypogonadotropic hypogonadism. Provocative tests may be required to assess pituitary reserve (Table 328-3). GH responses to insulin-induced hypoglycemia, arginine, L-dopa, growth hormone–releasing hormone (GHRH), or growth hormone–releasing peptides (GHRPs) can be used to assess GH reserve. PRL and TSH responses to thyrotropin-releasing hormone (TRH) reflect lactotrope and thyrotrope function. Corticotropin-releasing hormone (CRH) administration induces ACTH release, and administration of synthetic ACTH (cortrosyn) evokes adrenal cortisol release as an indirect indicator of pituitary ACTH reserve (Chap. 331). ACTH reserve is most reliably assessed during insulin-induced hypoglycemia. However, this test should be performed cautiously in patients with suspected adrenal insufficiency because of increased risk of hypoglycemia and hypotension.

℞ **TREATMENT** Hormone replacement therapy, including glucocorticoids, thyroid hormone, sex steroids, growth hormone, and vasopressin, is usually free of complications. Treatment regimens that mimic physiologic hormone production allow for maintenance of satisfactory clinical homeostasis. Effective dosage schedules are outlined in Table 328-4. Patients in need of glucocorticoid replacement require careful dose adjustments during stressful events such as acute illness, dental procedures, trauma, and acute hospitalization (Chap. 331).

HYPOTHALAMIC, PITUITARY, AND OTHER SELLAR MASSES

PITUITARY TUMORS Pituitary adenomas are the most common cause of pituitary hormone hypersecretion and hyposecretion syndromes in adults. They account for ~10% of all intracranial neoplasms. At autopsy, up to a quarter of all pituitary glands harbor an unsuspected microadenoma (<10 mm diameter). Similarly, pituitary imaging detects small pituitary lesions in at least 10% of normal individuals.

Pathogenesis Pituitary adenomas are benign neoplasms that arise from one of the five anterior pituitary cell types. The clinical and biochemical phenotype of pituitary adenomas depend on the cell type from which they are derived and are described in detail below. Thus, tumors arising from lactotrope (PRL), somatotrope (GH), corticotrope (ACTH), thyrotrope (TSH), or gonadotrope (LH, FSH) cells hypersecrete their respective hormones (Table 328-5). Plurihormonal tumors that express combinations of GH, PRL, TSH, ACTH, and the glycoprotein hormone α subunit may be diagnosed by careful immunocytochemistry or may, in fact, present with mixed clinical features of these hormonal hypersecretory syndromes. Morphologically, these tumors may arise from a single polysecreting cell type or consist of cells with mixed function within the same tumor.

Hormonally active tumors are characterized by autonomous hor-

Table 328-4   Hormone Replacement Therapy for Adult Hypopituitarism[a]

Trophic Hormone Deficit	Hormone Replacement
ACTH	Hydrocortisone (10–20 mg A.M.; 10 mg P.M.)
	Cortisone acetate (25 mg A.M.; 12.5 mg P.M.)
	Prednisone (5 mg A.M.; 2.5 mg P.M.)
TSH	L-Thyroxine (0.075–0.15 mg daily)
FSH/LH	Males
	Testosterone enanthate (200 mg IM every 2 weeks)
	Testosterone skin patch (5 mg/d)
	Females
	Conjugated estrogen (0.65–1.25 mg qd for 25 days)
	Progesterone (5–10 mg qd) on days 16–25
	Estradiol skin patch (0.5 mg, every other day)
	For fertility: Menopausal gonadotropins, human chorionic gonadotropins
GH	Adults: Somatotropin (0.3–1.0 mg SC qd)
	Children: Somatotropin [0.02–0.05 (mg/kg/day)]
Vasopressin	Intranasal desmopressin (5–20 μg twice daily)
	Oral 300–600 μg qd

[a] All doses shown should be individualized for specific patients and should be reassessed during stress, surgery, or pregnancy. Male and female fertility requirements should be managed as discussed in Chap. 54.

mone secretion with diminished responsiveness to the normal physiologic pathways of inhibition. Hormone production does not always correlate with tumor size. Small hormone-secreting adenomas may cause significant clinical perturbations, whereas larger adenomas that produce less hormone may be clinically silent and remain undiagnosed (if no central compressive effects occur). About one-third of all adenomas are clinically nonfunctioning and produce no distinct clinical hypersecretory syndrome. Most arise from gonadotrope cells and may secrete α- and β-glycoprotein hormone subunits or, very rarely, intact circulating gonadotropins. True pituitary carcinomas with documented extracranial metastases are exceedingly rare.

Almost all pituitary adenomas are monoclonal in origin, implying the acquisition of one or more somatic mutations that confer a selective growth advantage. In addition to direct studies of oncogene mutations, this idea is supported by X-chromosomal inactivation analyses of tumors in female patients heterozygous for X-linked genes. Consistent with their clonal origin, complete surgical resection of small pituitary adenomas usually cures hormone hypersecretion. Nevertheless, hypothalamic hormones, such as GHRH or CRH, also enhance the mitotic activity of their respective pituitary target cells, in addition to

Table 328-5   Classification of Pituitary Adenomas[a]

Adenoma Cell Origin	Hormone Product	Clinical Syndrome
Lactotrope	PRL	Hypogonadism, galactorrhea
Gonadotrope	FSH, LH, subunits	Silent or hypogonadism
Somatotrope	GH	Acromegaly/gigantism
Corticotrope	ACTH	Cushing's disease
Mixed growth hormone and prolactin cell	GH, PRL	Acromegaly, hypogonadism, galactorrhea
Other plurihormonal cell	Any	Mixed
Acidophil stem cell	PRL, GH	Hypogonadism, galactorrhea acromegaly
Mammosomatotrope	PRL, GH	Hypogonadism, galactorrhea acromegaly
Thyrotrope	TSH	Thyrotoxicosis
Null cell	None	Pituitary failure
Oncocytoma	None	Pituitary failure

[a] Hormone-secreting tumors are listed in decreasing order of frequency. All tumors may cause local pressure effects, including visual disturbances, cranial nerve palsy, and headache.

SOURCE: Adapted from S Melmed, in JL Jameson (ed): *Principles of Molecular Medicine*, Totowa, Humana Press, 1998.

their role in pituitary hormone regulation. Thus, patients harboring rare abdominal or chest tumors elaborating ectopic GHRH or CRH may present with somatotrope or corticotrope hyperplasia.

Several etiologic genetic events have been implicated in the development of pituitary tumors. The pathogenesis of sporadic forms of acromegaly has been particularly informative as a model of tumorigenesis. GHRH, after binding to its G protein–coupled somatotrope receptor, utilizes cyclic AMP as a second messenger to stimulate GH secretion and somatotrope proliferation. A subset (~35%) of GH-secreting pituitary tumors contain mutations in Gsα (Arg 201 → Cys or His; Gln 227 → Arg). These mutations inhibit intrinsic GTPase activity, resulting in constitutive elevation of cyclic AMP, Pit-1 induction, and activation of cyclic AMP response element binding protein (CREB), thereby promoting somatotrope cell proliferation.

Characteristic loss of heterozygosity (LOH) in various chromosomes has been documented in large or invasive macroadenomas, suggesting the presence of putative tumor suppressor genes at these loci. LOH of chromosome region on 11q13, 13, and 9 is present in up to 20% of sporadic pituitary tumors including GH-, PRL-, and ACTH-producing adenomas and in some nonfunctioning tumors.

Compelling evidence also favors growth factor promotion of pituitary tumor proliferation. Basic fibroblast growth factor (bFGF) is abundant in the pituitary and has been shown to stimulate pituitary cell mitogenesis. Other factors involved in initiation and promotion of pituitary tumors include loss of negative-feedback inhibition (as seen with primary hypothyroidism or hypogonadism) and estrogen-mediated or paracrine angiogenesis. Growth characteristics and neoplastic behavior may also be influenced by several activated oncogenes, including *RAS* and pituitary tumor transforming gene (*PTTG*).

Genetic Syndromes Associated with Pituitary Tumors   Several familial syndromes are associated with pituitary tumors, and the genetic mechanisms for some of these have been unraveled (Table 328-6).

Multiple endocrine neoplasia (MEN) 1 is an autosomal dominant syndrome characterized primarily by a genetic predisposition to parathyroid, pancreatic islet, and pituitary adenomas (Chap. 339). MEN-1 is caused by inactivating germline mutations in *MENIN*, a constitutively expressed tumor-suppressor gene located on chromosome 11q13. Loss of heterozygosity, or a somatic mutation of the remaining normal *MENIN* allele, leads to tumorigenesis. About half of affected patients develop prolactinomas; acromegaly and Cushing's syndrome are less commonly encountered.

Carney syndrome is characterized by spotty skin pigmentation, myxomas, and endocrine tumors including testicular, adrenal, and pituitary adenomas. Acromegaly occurs in about 20% of patients. This autosomal dominant syndrome is associated with microsatellite alterations on chromosome 2p16.

McCune-Albright syndrome consists of polyostotic fibrous dysplasia, pigmented skin patches, and a variety of endocrine disorders, including GH-secreting pituitary tumors, adrenal adenomas, and autonomous ovarian function (Chap. 343). Hormonal hypersecretion is due to constitutive cyclic AMP production caused by inactivation of the GTPase activity of Gsα. The Gsα mutations occur postzygotically, leading to a mosaic pattern of mutant expression.

Familial acromegaly is a rare disorder in which family members may manifest either acromegaly or gigantism. The disorder is associated with LOH at a chromosome 11q13 locus distinct from that of *MENIN*.

OTHER SELLAR MASSES   *Craniopharyngiomas* are derived from Rathke's pouch. They arise near the pituitary stalk and commonly extend into the suprasellar cistern. These tumors are often large, cystic, and locally invasive. Many are partially calcified, providing a characteristic appearance on skull x-ray and CT images. More than half of all patients present before age 20, usually with signs of increased intracranial pressure, including headache, vomiting, papilledema, and hydrocephalus. Associated symptoms include visual field abnormalities, personality changes and cognitive deterioration, cranial nerve damage, sleep difficulties, and weight gain. Anterior pituitary dysfunction and diabetes insipidus are common. About half of affected children present with growth retardation.

Treatment usually involves transcranial or transsphenoidal surgical resection followed by postoperative radiation of residual tumor. This approach can result in long-term survival and ultimate cure, but most patients require lifelong pituitary hormone replacement. If the pituitary stalk is uninvolved and can be preserved at the time of surgery, the incidence of subsequent anterior pituitary dysfunction is significantly diminished.

Developmental failure of Rathke's pouch obliteration may lead to *Rathke's cysts*, which are small (<5 mm) cysts entrapped by squamous epithelium; these cysts are found in about 20% of individuals at autopsy. Although Rathke's cleft cysts do not usually grow and are often diagnosed incidentally, about a third present in adulthood with compressive symptoms, diabetes insipidus, and hyperprolactinemia due to stalk compression. Rarely, internal hydrocephalus develops. The diagnosis is suggested preoperatively by visualizing the cyst wall on MRI, which distinguishes these lesions from craniopharyngiomas. Cyst contents range from CSF-like fluid to mucoid material. *Arachnoid cysts* are rare and generate an MRI image isointense with cerebrospinal fluid.

Sella chordomas usually present with bony clival erosion, local invasiveness, and, on occasion, calcification. Normal pituitary tissue may be visible on MRI, distinguishing chordomas from aggressive pituitary adenomas. Mucinous material may be obtained by fine-needle aspiration.

Meningiomas arising in the sellar region may be difficult to distinguish from nonfunctioning pituitary adenomas. On MRI they may be asymmetric, and on CT they may show evidence of bony erosion. Meningiomas may cause compressive symptoms.

Histiocytosis X comprises a variety of syndromes associated with foci of eosinophilic granulomas. Diabetes insipidus, exophthalmos, and punched-out lytic bone lesions (*Hand-Schüller-Christian disease*) are associated with granulomatous lesions visible on MRI, as well as a characteristic axillary skin rash. Rarely, the pituitary stalk may be involved.

Pituitary metastases occur in ~3% of cancer patients. Blood-borne metastatic deposits are found almost exclusively in the posterior pituitary. Accordingly, diabetes insipidus can be a presenting feature of lung, gastrointestinal, breast, and other pituitary metastases. About half of pituitary metastases originate from breast cancer; about 25% of patients with breast cancer have such deposits. Rarely, pituitary stalk involvement results in anterior pituitary insufficiency. The MRI diagnosis of a metastatic lesion may be difficult to distinguish from an aggressive pituitary adenoma; the diagnosis may require histologic examination of excised tumor tissue. Primary or metastatic lymphoma, leukemias, and plasmacytomas also occur within the sella.

Hypothalamic hamartomas and *gangliocytomas* may arise from astrocytes, oligodendrocytes, and neurons with varying degrees of differentiation. These tumors may overexpress hypothalamic neuropeptides including GnRH, GHRH, or CRH. In GnRH-producing tumors, children present with precocious puberty, psychomotor delay, and laughing-associated seizures. Medical treatment of GnRH-producing hamartomas with long-acting GnRH analogues effectively suppresses gonadotropin secretion and controls pubertal development. Rarely, hamartomas are also associated with craniofacial abnormalities; imperforate anus; cardiac, renal, and lung disorders; and pituitary failure (*Pallister-Hall syndrome*). Hypothalamic hamartomas are often con-

Table 328-6 Genetic Syndromes Associated with Pituitary Tumors

Syndrome	Clinical Features	Chromosomal Location	Gene	Protein	Proposed Function/Defect
Multiple endocrine neoplasia type I (MEN-I)	Parathyroid, endocrine pancreas, anterior pituitary (mostly prolactinomas) tumors	11q13	*MEN1*	Menin	Nuclear, unknown
Familial acromegaly	GH-cell adenomas, acromegaly/gigantism	11q13 and other loci	Not *MEN1*	—	—
McCune-Albright syndrome	Polyostic fibrous dysplasia, pigmented skin patches; Endocrine abnormalities: precocious puberty, GH-cell adenomas, acromegaly/gigantism	20q13.2 (mosaic)	*GNAS1* (*gsp*)	Gsα	Signal transduction/inactive Inactive GTPase results in constitutive cyclic AMP elevation, independent of GHRH
Carney syndrome	Skin and cardiac myxomas, Cushing's syndrome, acromegaly	2p16	—	—	Telomere alteration?

SOURCE: Adapted from T Prezant, S Melmed, in S Webb (ed): *Pituitary Tumours*: Epidemiology, Pathogenesis, and Management. BioScientifica, Bristol, UK 1998.

tiguous with the pituitary, and preoperative MRI diagnosis may not be possible. Histologic evidence of hypothalamic neurons in tissue resected at transsphenoidal surgery may be the first indication of a primary hypothalamic lesion.

Hypothalamic gliomas and *optic gliomas* occur mainly in childhood and usually present with visual loss. Adults have more aggressive tumors; about a third are associated with neurofibromatosis.

Brain germ-cell tumors may arise within the sellar region. These include *dysgerminomas*, which are associated with diabetes insipidus and visual loss and rarely metastasize. *Germinomas*, *embryonal carcinomas*, *teratomas*, and *choriocarcinomas* may arise in the parasellar region and produce hCG. These germ-cell tumors present with precocious puberty, diabetes insipidus, visual field defects, and thirst disorders. Many patients are GH-deficient with short stature.

METABOLIC EFFECTS OF HYPOTHALAMIC LESIONS The hypothalamus is subject to injury from mass lesions, granulomatous disorders, infections, and hemorrhage. Lesions involving the anterior and preoptic hypothalamic regions cause paradoxical vasoconstriction, tachycardia, and hyperthermia. Acute hyperthermia is usually due to a hemorrhagic insult, but poikilothermia may also occur. Central disorders of thermoregulation result from posterior hypothalamic damage. The *periodic hypothermia syndrome* comprises episodic attacks of rectal temperatures <30°C, sweating, vasodilation, vomiting, and bradycardia (Chap. 20). Damage to the ventromedial nuclei by craniopharyngiomas, hypothalamic trauma, or inflammatory disorders may be associated with *hyperphagia* and *obesity*. This region appears to contain an energy-satiety center where melanocortin receptors are influenced by leptin, insulin, POMC products, and gastrointestinal peptides (Chap. 77). Median eminence involvement results in diabetes insipidus in about 50% of patients. Hypothalamic gliomas in early childhood may be associated with a diencephalic syndrome characterized by progressive severe emaciation and growth failure. Polydipsia or hypodipsia are associated with damage to central osmoreceptors located in preoptic nuclei (Chap. 329). Slow-growing hypothalamic lesions can cause increased somnolence and disturbed sleep cycles as well as obesity, hypothermia, and emotional outbursts. Lesions of the central hypothalamus may stimulate sympathetic neurons, leading to elevated serum catecholamine and cortisol levels.

These patients are predisposed to cardiac arrhythmias, hypertension, and gastric erosions.

EVALUATION   Local Mass Effects   Clinical manifestations of sellar lesions vary, depending on the anatomic location of the mass and direction of its extension (Table 328-7). The dorsal roof of the sella presents the least resistance to soft tissue expansion from within the confines of the sella; consequently, pituitary adenomas frequently extend in a suprasellar direction. Bony invasion may ultimately occur as well.

Headaches are common features of small intrasellar tumors, even with no demonstrable suprasellar extension. Because of the confined nature of the pituitary, small changes in intrasellar pressure stretch the dural plate; however, the severity of the headache correlates poorly with adenoma size or extension.

Suprasellar extension can lead to visual loss by several mechanisms, the most common being compression of the optic chiasm, but direct invasion of the optic nerves or obstruction of CSF flow leading to secondary visual disturbances also occur. Pituitary stalk compression by a hormonally active or inactive intrasellar mass may compress the portal vessels, disrupting pituitary access to the hypothalamic hormones and dopamine; this results in hyperprolactinemia and concurrent loss of other pituitary hormones. This "stalk section" phenomenon may also be caused by trauma, whiplash injury with posterior clinoid stalk compression, or skull base fractures. Lateral mass invasion may impinge on the cavernous sinus and compress its neural contents, leading to cranial nerve III, IV, and VI palsies as well as effects on the ophthalmic and maxillary branches of the fifth cranial nerve (Chap. 367). Patients may present with diplopia, ptosis, ophthalmoplegia, and decreased facial sensation, depending on the extent of neural damage. Extension into the sphenoid sinus indicates that the pituitary mass has eroded through the sellar floor. Aggressive tumors may also invade the palate roof and cause nasopharyngeal obstruction, infection, and, rarely, CSF leakage. Both temporal and frontal lobes may be invaded, leading to uncinate seizures, personality disorders, and anosmia. Direct hypothalamic encroachment by an invasive pituitary mass may cause important metabolic sequelae, precocious puberty or hypogonadism, diabetes insipidus, sleep disturbances, dysthermia, and appetite disorders.

MRI   Sagittal and coronal T1-weighted spin-echo MRI imaging, before and after administration of gadolinium, allow precise visualization of the pituitary gland with clear delineation of the hypothalamus, pituitary stalk, pituitary tissue and surrounding suprasellar cisterns, cavernous sinuses, sphenoid sinus, and optic chiasm. Pituitary gland height ranges from 6 mm in children to 8 mm in adults; during pregnancy and puberty, the height may reach 10 to 12 mm. The upper aspect of the adult pituitary is flat or slightly concave, but in adolescent and pregnant individuals, this surface may be convex, reflecting physiologic pituitary enlargement. The stalk should be vertical. CT scan is indicated to define the extent of bony erosion or the presence of calcification.

The soft tissue consistency of the pituitary gland is slightly heterogeneous on MRI. Anterior pituitary signal intensity resembles that of brain matter on T1-imaging (Fig. 328-5). Adenoma density is usually lower than that of surrounding normal tissue on T1-weighted imaging, and the signal intensity increases with T2-weighted images. The high phospholipid content of the posterior pituitary results in a bright enhancing signal.

Sellar masses are commonly encountered as incidental findings on MRI, and most of these are pituitary adenomas (incidentalomas). This finding is consistent with the observation that clinically silent pituitary microadenomas can be identified in up to 25% of pituitaries in autopsy series. In the absence of hormone hypersecretion, these small lesions can be safely monitored by MRI, which is performed annually and then less often if there is no evidence of growth. Resection should be considered for incidentally discovered macroadenomas, as about one-third become invasive or cause local pressure effects. If hormone hypersecretion is evident, specific therapies are indicated. When larger masses (>1 cm) are encountered, they should also be distinguished from nonadenomatous lesions. Meningiomas are often associated with bony hyperostosis; craniopharyngiomas may be calcified and are usually hypodense, whereas gliomas are hyperdense on T2-weighted images.

Ophthalmologic Evaluation   Because optic tracts may be contiguous to an expanding pituitary mass, reproducible visual field assessment that uses perimetry techniques should be performed on all patients with sellar mass lesions that abut the optic chiasm. Loss of red perception is an early sign of optic tract pressure. Bitemporal hemianopia or superior bitemporal defects are classically observed, reflecting the location of these tracts within the inferior and posterior part of the chiasm. Early diagnosis reduces the risk of blindness, scotomas, or other visual disturbances.

Table 328-7   Features of Sellar Mass Lesions[a]

Impacted Structure	Clinical Impact
Pituitary	Hypogonadism
	Hypothyroidism
	Growth failure and adult hyposomatotropism
	Hypoadrenalism
Optic tract	Loss of red perception
	Bitemporal hemianopia
	Superior or bitemporal field defect
	Scotoma
	Blindness
Hypothalamus	Temperature dysregulation
	Appetite and thirst disorders
	Obesity
	Diabetes insipidus
	Sleep disorders
	Behavioral dysfunction
	Autonomic dysfunction
Cavernous sinus	Opthalmoplegia ± ptosis or diplopia
	Facial numbness
Frontal lobe	Personality disorder
	Anosmia
Brain	Headache
	Hydrocephalus
	Psychosis
	Dementia
	Laughing seizures

[a] As the intrasellar mass expands, it first compresses intrasellar pituitary tissue, then usually invades dorsally through the dura to lift the optic chiasm or laterally to the cavernous sinuses. Bony erosion is rare, as is direct brain compression. Microadenomas may present with headache.

FIGURE 328-5   Pituitary adenoma. Coronal T1-weighted postcontrast MR image shows a homogeneously enhancing mass (arrowheads) in the sella turcica and suprasellar region compatible with a pituitary adenoma; the small arrows outline the carotid arteries.

Laboratory Investigation The presenting clinical features of functional pituitary adenomas (e.g., acromegaly, prolactinomas, or Cushing's disease) should guide the laboratory studies (see below). However, for a sellar mass with no obvious clinical features of hormone excess, laboratory studies are geared towards determining the nature of the tumor and assessing the possible presence of hypopituitarism. When a pituitary adenoma is suspected based on MRI, initial hormonal evaluation usually includes: (1) basal PRL; (2) insulin-like growth factor (IGF) I; (3) 24-h urinary free cortisol (UFC) and/or overnight oral dexamethasone (1 mg) suppression test; (4) α-subunit, FSH, and LH levels; and (5) thyroid function tests. Additional hormonal evaluation may be indicated based on the results of these tests. Pending more detailed assessment of hypopituitarism, a menstrual history, testosterone level, 8 A.M. cortisol, and thyroid function tests usually identify patients with pituitary hormone deficiencies that require hormone replacement before further testing or surgery.

Histologic Evaluation Immunohistochemical staining of pituitary tumor specimens obtained at transsphenoidal surgery confirm clinical and laboratory studies and provide a histologic diagnosis when hormone studies are equivocal and in cases of clinically nonfunctioning tumors. Occasionally, ultrastructural assessment by electron microscopy is required for diagnosis.

℞ **TREATMENT** **Overview** Successful management of sellar masses requires accurate diagnosis as well as selection of optimal therapeutic modalities. Most pituitary tumors are benign and slow-growing. Clinical features result from local mass effects and hormonal hypo- or hypersecretion syndromes caused directly by the adenoma or as a consequence of treatment. Thus, lifelong management and follow-up are necessary for these patients.

Improved MRI technology with gadolinium enhancement for pituitary visualization, new advances in transsphenoidal surgery and in stereotactic radiotherapy (including gamma-knife radiotherapy), and novel therapeutic agents have improved pituitary tumor management. The goals of pituitary tumor treatment include normalization of excess pituitary secretion, amelioration of symptoms and signs of hormonal hypersecretion syndromes, and shrinkage or ablation of large tumor masses with relief of adjacent structure compression. Residual anterior pituitary function should be preserved and can sometimes be restored by removing tumor mass. Ideally, adenoma recurrence should be prevented.

Transsphenoidal Surgery Transsphenoidal rather than transfrontal resection is the desired surgical approach for pituitary tumors, except for the rare invasive suprasellar mass surrounding the frontal or middle fossa, the optic nerves, or invading posteriorly behind the clivus. Intraoperative microscopy facilitates visual distinction between adenomatous and normal pituitary tissue, as well as microdissection of small tumors that may not be visible by MRI (Fig. 328-6). Transsphenoidal surgery also avoids the cranial invasion and manipulation of brain tissue required by subfrontal surgical approaches. Endoscopic techniques with three-dimensional intraoperative localization have improved visualization and access to tumor tissue. The endoscopic approach is also less traumatic, as the technique is endonasal and does not require a transsphenoidal retractor.

In addition to correction of hormonal hypersecretion, pituitary surgery is indicated for mass lesions that impinge on surrounding structures. Surgical decompression and resection are required for an expanding pituitary mass accompanied by pesistent headache, progressive visual field defects, cranial nerve palsies, internal hydrocephalus, and, occasionally, intrapituitary hemorrhage and apoplexy. Repeat surgery may be required for persistent postoperative CSF leakage. Transsphenoidal surgery is sometimes used for pituitary tissue biopsy and histologic diagnosis.

Whenever possible, the pituitary mass lesion should be selectively excised; normal tissue should be manipulated or resected only when critical for effective dissection. Nonselective hemihypophysectomy or total hypophysectomy may be indicated if no mass lesion is clearly discernible, multifocal lesions are present, or the remaining nontu-

FIGURE 328-6 Transsphenoidal resection of pituitary mass via the endonasal approach. *(Adapted from Fahlbusch R: Endocrinol Metab Clin 21:669, 1992.)*

morous pituitary tissue is obviously necrotic. This strategy increases the likelihood of hypopituitarism and the need for lifelong hormonal replacement.

Preoperative local compression signs, including visual field defects or compromised pituitary function, may be reversed by surgery, particularly when these deficits are not long-standing. For large and invasive tumors, it is necessary to determine the optimal balance between maximal tumor resection and preservation of anterior pituitary function, especially for preserving growth and reproductive function in younger patients. Similarly, tumor invasion outside of the sella is rarely amenable to surgical cure; the surgeon must judge the risk:benefit ratio of extensive tumor resection.

Side effects Tumor size and the degree of invasiveness largely determine the incidence of surgical complications. Operative mortality is about 1%. Transient diabetes insipidus and hypopituitarism occur in up to 20% of patients. Permanent diabetes insipidus, cranial nerve damage, nasal septal perforation, or visual disturbances may be encountered in up to 10% of patients. CSF leaks occur in 4% of patients. Less common complications include carotid artery injury, loss of vision, hypothalamic damage, and meningitis. Permanent side effects are rarely encountered after surgery for microadenomas.

Radiation Radiation is used either as a primary therapy for pituitary or parasellar masses or, more commonly, as an adjunct to surgery or medical therapy. Focused megavoltage irradiation is achieved by precise MRI localization, using a high-voltage linear accelerator and accurate isocentric rotational arcing. A major determinant of accurate irradiation is to reproduce the patient's head position during multiple visits and to maintain absolute head immobility. A total of <50 Gy (5000 rad) is given as 180-cGy (180 rad) fractions split over about 6 weeks. Stereotactic radiosurgery delivers a large single high-energy dose from a cobalt 60 source (gamma knife), linear accelerator, or cyclotron. Long-term effects of gamma-knife surgery are as yet unknown.

The role of radiation therapy in pituitary tumor management depends on multiple factors including the nature of the tumor, age of the patient, and the availability of surgical and radiation expertise. Because of its relatively slow onset of action, radiation therapy is usually reserved for postsurgical management. As an adjuvant to surgery, radiation is used to treat residual tumor and in an attempt to prevent regrowth. Irradiation offers the only effective means for ablating significant residual tumor tissue derived from nonfunctioning tumors. PRL-, GH-, and ACTH-secreting tumor tissues are also amenable to medical therapy.

Side effects   In the short term, radiation may cause transient nausea and weakness. Alopecia and loss of taste and smell may be more long-lasting. Failure of pituitary hormone synthesis is common in patients who have undergone head and neck or pituitary-directed irradiation. More than 50% of patients develop failure of GH, ACTH, TSH, and/or gonadotropin secretion within 10 years, usually due to hypothalamic damage. Lifelong follow-up with testing of anterior pituitary hormone reserve is therefore necessary after radiation treatment. Optic nerve damage with impaired vision due to optic neuritis is reported in about 2% of patients who undergo pituitary irradiation. Cranial nerve damage is uncommon now that radiation doses are ≤2 Gy (200 rad) at any one treatment session and the maximum dose is <50 Gy (5000 rad). The advent of stereotactic radiotherapy may reduce damage to adjacent structures. The cumulative risk of developing a secondary tumor after conventional radiation is 1.3% after 10 years and 1.9% after 20 years.

Medical   Medical therapy for pituitary tumors is highly specific and depends on tumor type. For prolactinomas, dopamine agonists are the treatment of choice. For acromegaly and TSH-secreting tumors, somatostatin analogues and, occasionally, dopamine agonists are indicated. ACTH-secreting tumors and nonfunctioning tumors are generally not responsive to medication and require surgery and/or irradiation.

PROLACTIN

SYNTHESIS   PRL consists of 198 amino acids and has a molecular mass of 21,500 kDa; it is weakly homologous to GH and human placental lactogen (hPL), reflecting the duplication and divergence of a common GH-PRL-hPL precursor gene on chromosome 6. PRL is synthesized in lactotropes, which comprise about 20% of anterior pituitary cells. Lactotropes and somatotropes are derived from a common precursor cell that may give rise to a tumor secreting both PRL and GH. Marked lactotrope cell hyperplasia develops during the last two trimesters of pregnancy and the first few months of lactation. These transient adaptive changes in the lactotrope population are induced by estrogen.

SECRETION   Fetal PRL synthesis begins at 12 weeks' gestation (about 4 weeks after GH). Normal adult serum PRL levels are about 10 to 25 μg/L in women and 10 to 20 μg/L in men. PRL secretion is pulsatile, with the highest secretory peaks occurring during rapid eye movement sleep. Peak serum PRL levels (up to 30 μg/L) occur between 4:00 and 6:00 A.M. The circulating half-life of PRL is about 50 min.

PRL is unique among the pituitary hormones in that the predominant central control mechanism is inhibitory, reflecting dopamine-mediated suppression of PRL release. This regulatory pathway is exemplified by the spontaneous PRL hypersecretion that occurs after pituitary stalk section, often a consequence of mass lesions at the skull base.

Dopamine action is mediated by multiple receptor subtypes, each a member of the seven-transmembrane G protein–coupled receptor

(GPCR) superfamily. In the pituitary, dopamine type 2 (D_2) receptors are predominant and mediate PRL inhibition. Targeted disruption (gene knockout) of the murine D_2 receptor results in hyperprolactinemia and lactotrope proliferation. Activation of D_2 receptors inhibits the cyclic AMP pathway, causing membrane hyperpolarization and closing of voltage-gated calcium channels; these events block secretory granule exocytosis by reducing intracellular free calcium. Because of the potent PRL inhibitory effects of dopamine, physiologic, pharmacologic, or pathologic alterations in dopamine action increase PRL levels. As discussed below, dopamine agonists play a central role in the management of hyperprolacinemic disorders.

TRH (pyro Glu-His-Pro-NH2) is a hypothalamic tripeptide that releases prolactin within 15 to 30 min after intravenous injection. The physiologic relevance of TRH for PRL regulation is unclear, as it appears to primarily regulate TSH (Chap. 330). *Vasoactive intestinal peptide* (VIP) also induces PRL release, whereas glucocorticoids and thyroid hormone suppress PRL secretion.

Serum PRL levels rise after exercise, meals, sexual intercourse, minor surgical procedures, general anesthesia, acute myocardial infarction, and other forms of acute stress. PRL levels also increase significantly (~tenfold) during pregnancy and decline rapidly within 2 weeks of parturition. If breastfeeding is initiated, basal PRL levels remain elevated; suckling stimulates reflex increases in PRL levels that last for about 30 to 45 min. Breast suckling activates neural afferent pathways in the hypothalamus that induce PRL release. With time, the suckling-induced responses diminish and interfeeding PRL levels return to normal.

ACTION   The PRL receptor is a member of the type I cytokine receptor family that also includes GH and interleukin (IL) 6 receptors. Ligand binding leads to receptor dimerization followed by intracellular signaling mediated by the Janus kinase (JAK) pathway, which phosphorylates components of the signal transduction and activators of transcription (STAT) family. The STAT proteins translocate to the nucleus, where they act as transcription factors on target genes. In the breast, the lobuloalveolar epithelium proliferates in response to PRL, placental lactogens, elevated progesterone, and local paracrine growth factors; lactogenesis occurs as a result of complex multihormonal interactions (Chap. 337).

PRL acts to induce and maintain lactation, decrease reproductive function, and suppress sexual drive. These functions are geared towards ensuring that maternal lactation is sustained and not interrupted by pregnancy. PRL inhibits reproductive function at multiple levels, including suppression of hypothalamic GnRH and pituitary gonadotropin secretion, as well as impairing gonadal steroidogenesis in both female and male subjects. In the hypothalamus, PRL-mediated suppression of GnRH leads to loss of pulsatile LH secretion and abrogation of the preovulatory LH surge. In the ovary, PRL blocks folliculogenesis and inhibits granulosa cell aromatase activity, leading to hypoestrogenism and anovulation. PRL also has a luteolytic effect, generating a shortened, or inadequate, luteal phase of the menstrual cycle. In males, attenuated LH secretion leads to low testosterone levels and decreased spermatogenesis. These hormonal changes decrease libido and reduce fertility in patients with hyperprolactinemia (Chap. 54).

PRL exerts widespread metabolic effects to ensure maintenance of sustained lactation. Gastrointestinal calcium absorption is increased, bone calcium is mobilized, bile acids are elevated, and pancreatic β cell growth is induced by PRL. Centrally, PRL acts on brain centers involved in parenting behavior, appetite stimulation, and analgesia. Concomitant with these effects, maintenance of bone mineral density is abrogated; hyperprolactinemia is associated with enhanced risk for bone loss and the long-term development of osteoporosis. PRL receptors are abundant in the osteoblasts of developing bone, and the accompanying hypoestrogenemia contributes to accelerated bone loss in hyperprolactinemic women.

HYPERPROLACTINEMIA   Etiology   Hyperprolactinemia is the most common pituitary hormone hypersecretion syndrome in both males and females. PRL-secreting pituitary adenomas (prolactinomas) are the most common cause of PRL levels >100 μg/L (see below). Less pronounced PRL elevation can also be caused by microprolactinomas but is more commonly caused by drugs, pituitary stalk compression, hypothyroidism, or renal failure (Table 328-8).

Pregnancy and lactation are the important physiologic causes of hyperprolactinemia. Sleep-associated hyperprolactinemia reverts to normal within an hour of awakening. Nipple stimulation and sexual orgasm may also cause acute PRL increases. Chest wall stimulation or trauma (including chest surgery and herpes zoster) invoke the reflex suckling arc with resultant hyperprolactinemia. Chronic renal failure elevates PRL by decreasing peripheral PRL clearance. Primary hypothyroidism is associated with mild hyperprolactinemia, probably because of enhanced TRH secretion.

Lesions of the hypothalamic-pituitary region that disrupt hypothalamic dopamine synthesis, portal vessel delivery, or lactotrope responses are associated with hyperprolactinemia. Thus, hypothalamic tumors, cysts, infiltrative disorders, and radiation-induced damage cause elevated PRL levels, usually in the range of 30 to 100 μg/L. Plurihormonal adenomas (including GH and ACTH tumors) may directly hypersecrete PRL. Clinically nonfunctioning pituitary tumors commonly cause stalk pressure and hyperprolactinemia.

Drug-induced inhibition or disruption of dopaminergic receptor function results in hyperprolactinemia (Table 328-8). Thus, many antipsychotics and antidepressants cause hyperprolactinemia. Methyldopa inhibits dopamine synthesis and verapamil blocks dopamine release, also leading to hyperprolactinemia. Hormonal agents that induce PRL include estrogens, antiandrogens, and TRH.

Presentation and Diagnosis Amenorrhea, galactorrhea, and infertility are the hallmarks of hyperprolactinemia in women. If hyperprolactinemia develops prior to the menarche, primary amenorrhea results. More commonly, hyperprolactinemia develops later in life and leads to oligomenorrhea and, ultimately, to amenorrhea. Patients present with infertility, vaginal dryness, dyspareunia, and loss of libido. If hyperprolactinemia is sustained, vertebral bone mineral density can be reduced compared to age-matched controls, particularly when associated with pronounced hypoestrogenemia. Galactorrhea is present in up to 80% of hyperprolactinemic women. Though usually

bilateral and spontaneous, it may be unilateral or only expressed manually. Patients may also complain of weight gain and mild hirsutism.

In men with hyperprolactinemia, diminished libido or visual loss (from optic nerve compression) are the usual presenting symptoms. Gonadotropin suppression leads to reduced testosterone, impotence, and oligospermia. True galactorrhea is uncommon in men with hyperprolactinemia. If the disorder is longstanding, secondary effects of hypogonadism are evident, including osteopenia, reduced muscle mass, and decreased beard growth.

The diagnosis of idiopathic hyperprolactinemia is made by exclusion of known causes of hyperprolactinemia in the setting of a normal pituitary MRI. Some of these patients may have small microadenomas below MRI sensitivity (~2 mm).

Laboratory Investigation Basal, fasting morning PRL levels (normally <20 μg/L) should be measured to assess hypersecretion. Because hormone secretion is pulsatile and levels vary widely in some individuals with hyperprolactinemia, it may be necessary to measure levels on several different occasions when clinical suspicion is high. Both false-positive and false-negative results may be encountered. In patients with markedly elevated PRL levels (>1000 μg/L), results may be falsely lowered because of assay artifacts; sample dilution is required to assess these high values accurately. Falsely elevated values may be caused by aggregated forms of circulating PRL, which are biologically inactive (macroprolactinemia). Hypothyroidism should be excluded by measuring TSH and T$_4$ levels.

℞ **TREATMENT** Treatment of hyperprolactinemia depends on the cause of elevated PRL levels. Regardless of the etiology, however, treatment should be aimed at normalizing PRL levels to alleviate suppressive effects on gonadal function, halt the galactorrhea, and preserve bone mineral density. Dopamine agonists are effective for many different causes of hyperprolactinemia (see "Treatment" for "Prolactinoma," below).

If the patient is taking a medication known to cause hyperprolactinemia, the drug should be withdrawn, if possible. For psychiatric patients who require neuroleptic agents, dose titration or the addition of a dopamine agonist can help restore normoprolactinemia and alleviate reproductive symptoms. However, dopamine agonists sometimes worsen the underlying psychiatric condition, especially at high doses. Hyperprolactinemia usually resolves after adequate thyroid hormone replacement in hypothyroid patients or after renal transplantation in patients or dialysis. Resection of hypothalamic or sellar mass lesions can reverse hyperprolactinemia caused by reduced dopamine tone. Granulomatous infiltrates rarely respond to glucocorticoid administration. In patients with irreversible hypothalamic damage, no treatment may be warranted. In up to 30% of patients with hyperprolactinemia—with or without a visible pituitary microadenoma—the condition resolves spontaneously.

PROLACTINOMA **Etiology and Prevalence** Tumors arising from lactotrope cells account for about half of all functioning pituitary tumors, with an annual incidence of ~3/100,000 population. Mixed tumors secreting combinations of GH and PRL, ACTH and PRL, and rarely TSH and PRL, are also seen. These plurihormonal tumors are usually recognized by immunohistochemistry, without apparent clinical manifestations from the production of additional hormones. Microadenomas are classified as <1 cm in diameter and do not usually invade the parasellar region. Macroadenomas are >1 cm in diameter, are locally invasive, and may impinge on adjacent structures. The female:male ratio for microprolactinomas is 20:1, whereas the gender ratio is near 1:1 for macroadenomas. Tumor size generally correlates directly with PRL concentrations; values >100 μg/L are usually associated with macroadenomas. Males tend to present with larger tumors than females, possibly because the features of hypogonadism are less readily evident. PRL levels remain stable in most patients, reflecting the slow growth of these tumors. About 5% of

Table 328-8 Etiology of Hyperprolactinemia^a

I. Physiologic hypersecretion	IV. Systemic disorders
A. Pregnancy	A. Chronic renal failure
B. Lactation	B. Hypothyroidism
C. Chest wall stimulation	C. Cirrhosis
D. Sleep	D. Pseudocyesis
E. Stress	E. Epileptic seizures
II. Hypothalamic–pituitary stalk damage	V. Drug-induced hypersecretion
A. Tumors	A. Dopamine receptor blockers
1. Craniopharyngioma	1. Phenothiazines: chlorpromazine, perphenazine
2. Suprasellar pituitary mass extension	2. Butyrophenones: haloperidol
3. Meningioma	3. Thioxanthenes
4. Dysgerminoma	4. Metoclopramide
5. Metastases	B. Dopamine synthesis inhibitors
B. Empty sella	1. α-methyldopa
C. Lymphocytic hypophysitis	C. Catecholamine depletors
D. Adenoma with stalk compression	1. Reserpine
E. Granulomas	D. Opiates
F. Rathke's cyst	E. H$_2$ antagonists
G. Irradiation	1. Cimetidine, ranitidine
H. Trauma	F. Imipramines
1. Pituitary stalk section	1. Amitriptyline, amoxapine
2. Suprasellar surgery	G. Serotonin-reuptake inhibitors
III. Pituitary hypersecretion	1. Fluoxetine
A. Prolactinoma	H. Calcium channel blockers
B. Acromegaly	1. Verapamil
	I. Hormones
	1. Estrogens
	2. Antiandrogens

NOTE: Hyperprolactinemia >100 μg/L almost invariably is indicative of a prolactin-secreting pituitary adenoma. Physiologic causes, hypothyroidism, and drug-induced hyperprolactinemia should be excluded before extensive evaluation.

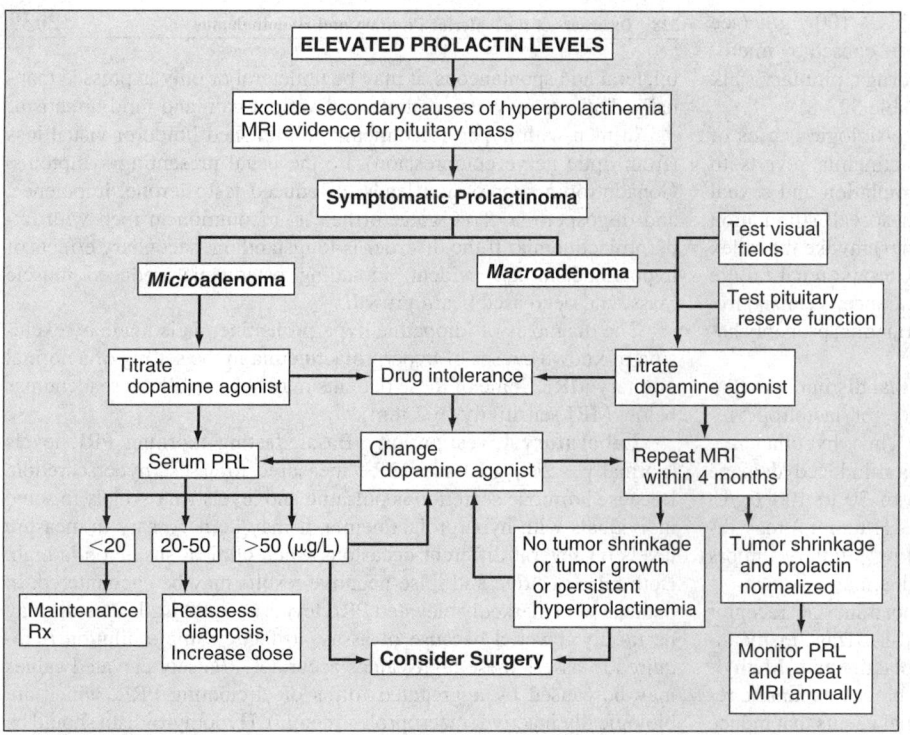

FIGURE 328-7 Management of prolactinoma. (MRI, magnetic resonance imaging; PRL, prolactin.)

ELEVATED PROLACTIN LEVELS → Exclude secondary causes of hyperprolactinemia MRI evidence for pituitary mass → **Symptomatic Prolactinoma**

Microadenoma and **Macroadenoma**

For Macroadenoma: Test visual fields; Test pituitary reserve function

Microadenoma: Titrate dopamine agonist → Serum PRL → <20 / 20-50 / >50 (μg/L)
- <20 → Maintenance Rx
- 20-50 → Reassess diagnosis, Increase dose

Drug intolerance → Change dopamine agonist

Macroadenoma: Titrate dopamine agonist → Repeat MRI within 4 months
- No tumor shrinkage or tumor growth or persistent hyperprolactinemia → Consider Surgery
- Tumor shrinkage and prolactin normalized → Monitor PRL and repeat MRI annually

---

microadenomas progress in the long term to macroadenomas. Hyperprolactinemia resolves spontaneously in about 30% of microadenomas.

Presentation and Diagnosis Women usually present with amenorrhea, infertility, and galactorrhea. If the tumor extends outside of the sella, visual field defects or other mass effects may be seen. Men often present with impotence, loss of libido, infertility, or signs of central CNS compression including headaches and visual defects. Assuming that known physiologic and medication-induced causes of hyperprolactinemia are excluded (Table 328-8), the diagnosis of prolactinoma is likely with a PRL level >100 μg/L. PRL levels <100μg/L may be caused by microadenomas, other sellar lesions that decrease dopamine inhibition, or nonneoplastic causes of hyperprolactinemia. For this reason, an MRI should be performed in all patients with hyperprolactinemia. It is important to remember that hyperprolactinemia caused by the mass effects of nonlactotrope lesions is also corrected by treatment with dopamine agonists. Consequently, PRL suppression by dopamine agonists does not necessarily indicate that the lesion is a prolactinoma.

℞ TREATMENT As microadenomas rarely progress to become macroadenomas, no treatment may be needed if fertility is not desired. Estrogen replacement is indicated to prevent bone loss and other consequences of hypoestrogenemia and does not appear to increase the risk of tumor enlargement. These patients should be monitored by regular serial PRL and MRI measurements.

For symptomatic microadenomas, therapeutic goals include control of hyperprolactinemia, reduction of tumor size, restoration of menses and fertility, and improvement of galactorrhea. Dopamine agonists should be titrated to achieve maximal PRL suppression and restoration of reproductive function (Fig. 328-7). A normalized PRL level does not assure reduced tumor size. However, tumor shrinkage is not usually seen in those who do not respond with lowered PRL levels. For macroadenomas, formal visual field testing should be performed before initiating dopamine agonists. MRI and visual fields should be assessed at 6- to 12-month intervals until the mass shrinks and annually thereafter until maximum size reduction has occurred.

Medical Oral dopamine agonists (cabergoline or bromocriptine) are the mainstay of therapy for patients with micro- or macroprolactinomas. Dopamine agonists suppress PRL secretion and synthesis as well as lactotrope cell proliferation.

Bromocriptine The ergot alkaloid bromocriptine mesylate is a dopamine receptor agonist that suppresses prolactin secretion by binding directly to lactotrope D_2 dopamine receptors. Bromocriptine is used as initial therapy for both micro- and macroprolactinomas. In microadenomas the drug rapidly lowers serum prolactin levels to normal in up to 70% of patients, decreases tumor size, and restores gonadal function. In patients with macroadenomas, prolactin levels are also normalized in 70% of patients and tumor mass shrinkage (≥50%) is achieved in up to 40% of patients. Mass effect symptoms, including headaches and visual disorders, usually improve dramatically within days after bromocriptine initiation; improvement of sexual function requires several weeks of treatment but may occur before complete normalization of prolactin levels. Drug withdrawal usually results in recurrent hyperprolactinemia and tumor reexpansion, with the risk of visual compromise. After initial control of PRL levels has been achieved, bromocriptine should be reduced to the lowest effective maintenance dose. In ~5% of treated patients, hyperprolactinemia may resolve and not recur when bromocriptine is discontinued after long-term treatment.

Therapy is initiated by administering a low bromocriptine dose (0.625 to 1.25 mg) at bedtime with a snack, followed by gradually increasing the dose. Most patients are successfully controlled with a daily dose of ≤7.5 mg (2.5 mg tid). About 20% of patients are resistant to dopaminergic treatment; they may have decreased D_2 dopamine receptor numbers or a postreceptor defect. D_2 receptor gene mutations in the pituitary have not been reported.

Nausea, vomiting, and postural hypotension with faintness may occur in ~25% of patients after the initial dose. These symptoms may persist in some patients. Other side effects include constipation, nasal stuffiness, dry mouth, nightmares, insomnia, and vertigo; decreasing the dose usually alleviates these problems. For the approximately 15% of patients who cannot tolerate oral bromocriptine, intravaginal administration of tablets is often efficacious.

Auditory hallucinations, delusions, and mood swings have been reported in up to 5% of patients and may be due to the dopamine agonist properties or to the lysergic acid derivative of the compound. Rare reports of leukopenia, thrombocytopenia, pleural fibrosis, cardiac arrhythmias, and hepatitis have been described.

Cabergoline An ergoline derivative, cabergoline is a long-acting dopamine agonist with high D_2 receptor affinity. The drug effectively suppresses PRL for >14 days after a single oral dose and induces prolactinoma shrinkage in most patients. Cabergoline (0.5 to 1.0 mg twice weekly) achieves normoprolactinemia and resumption of normal gonadal function in ~80% of patients with microadenomas; galactorrhea improves or resolves in 90% of patients. Cabergoline normalizes PRL and shrinks ~70% of macroprolactinomas. It may also be effective in patients resistant to bromocriptine. Adverse effects and drug intolerance are encountered less commonly than with bromocriptine.

Other dopamine agonists These include *pergolide mesylate*, an ergot derivative with dopaminergic properties; *lisuride*, an ergot derivative; and *quinagolide* (CV 205-502, Norprolac), a nonergot oral dopamine agonist with specific D_2 receptor activity.

Surgery Indications for surgical debulking include dopamine resistance or intolerance and the presence of an invasive macroadenoma with compromised vision that fails to improve rapidly after drug treatment. Initial PRL normalization is achieved in about 70% of microprolactinomas after surgical resection, but only 30% of macroadenomas can be successfully resected. However, follow-up studies have shown that recurrence of hyperprolactinemia occurs in up to 20% of patients within the first year after surgery; long-term recurrence rates exceed 50% for macroadenomas. Radiotherapy for prolactinomas is reserved for patients with aggressive tumors that do not respond to maximally tolerated dopamine agonists and/or surgery.

Pregnancy The pituitary increases in size during pregnancy, reflecting the stimulatory effects of estrogen and perhaps other growth factors. About 5% of microadenomas significantly increase in size, but 15 to 30% of macroadenomas may grow during pregnancy. Bromocriptine has been used for over 25 years to restore fertility in women with hyperprolactinemia, without evidence of untoward teratogenic effects. Nonetheless, most authorities recommend strategies to minimize fetal exposure to the drug. For women taking bromocriptine who desire pregnancy, mechanical contraception should be used through three regular menstrual cycles to allow for conception timing. When pregnancy is confirmed, bromocriptine should be discontinued and PRL levels followed serially, especially if headaches or visual symptoms occur. For women harboring macroadenomas, regular visual field testing is recommended, and the drug should be reinstituted if tumor growth is apparent. Although pituitary MRI may be safe during pregnancy, this procedure should be reserved for symptomatic patients with severe headache and/or visual field defects. Alternatively, surgical decompression may be indicated if vision is threatened. Though comprehensive data support the efficacy and relative safety of bromocriptine-facilitated fertility, patients should be advised of potential unknown deleterious effects and the risk of tumor growth during pregnancy. At present, the experience with cabergoline is too limited to recommend its routine use when fertility is desired.

GROWTH HORMONE

SYNTHESIS GH is the most abundant anterior pituitary hormone and is expressed early in fetal life (at 8 weeks' gestation). GH-secreting somatotrope cells constitute up to 50% of the total anterior pituitary cell population. Mammosomatotrope cells, which coexpress PRL with GH, can be identified using double immunostaining techniques. Somatotrope development is determined by expression of the cell-specific Pit-1 nuclear transcription factor. In addition to controlling cell differentiation, it also enhances GH gene expression. Five distinct genes on chromosome 17q22 encode GH and related proteins. The pituitary GH gene (hGH-N) produces two alternatively spliced products that give rise to 22-kDa GH (191 amino acids) and a less abundant, 20-kDa GH molecule, with similar biologic activity. Placental syncytiotrophoblast cells express a GH variant (hGH-V) gene; the related hormone human chorionic somatotropin (HCS) is expressed by distinct members of the gene cluster. HCS shares high homology with GH yet exhibits minimal growth-promoting properties.

SECRETION GH secretion is controlled by complex hypothalamic and peripheral factors. *GHRH* is a 44 amino acid hypothalamic peptide that stimulates GH synthesis and release. Synthetic agonists of the *GHRP* receptor stimulate GHRH and also directly stimulate GH release, but putative endogenous agonists remain incompletely characterized. *Somatostatin* (SRIF) is synthesized in the medial preoptic area of the hypothalamus and inhibits GH secretion. GHRH is secreted as discrete spikes that elicit GH pulses, whereas SRIF sets basal GH tone. SRIF is also expressed in many extrahypothalamic tissues, including the CNS, gastrointestinal system, and pancreas, where it also acts to inhibit the hormone secretion. *IGF-I*, the peripheral target hormone for GH, feeds back to inhibit GH; estrogens induce GH (Chap. 8), whereas glucocorticoid excess suppresses GH release.

Two distinct surface receptors on the somatotrope regulate GH synthesis and secretion. The GHRH receptor is a GPCR that signals through the intracellular cyclic AMP pathway. Activation of this receptor stimulates somatotrope cell proliferation as well as hormone production. Inactivating mutations of the GHRH receptor cause profound dwarfism (see below). A distinct surface receptor for GHRP has also been identified. This receptor is expressed in the hypothalamus and pituitary. A natural ligand, termed *ghrelin*, binds to the GHRP receptor; it is produced in large amounts in the stomach, though its

physiologic role remains unknown. Hypothalamic somatostatin binds to five distinct receptor subtypes (SSTR1 to SSTR5) that are widely expressed in different tissues, including in the pituitary. SSTR2 and SSTR5 subtypes preferentially suppress GH (and TSH) secretion.

GH secretion is pulsatile, with greater levels at night generally correlating with the onset of sleep. GH secretory rates decline markedly with age so that hormone production in middle age is about 15% of production during puberty. These changes are paralleled by an age-related decline in lean muscle mass. GH secretion is also reduced in obese individuals, though IGF-I levels are preserved, suggesting a change in the setpoint for feedback control. Elevated GH levels occur within an hour of deep sleep onset as well as after exercise, physical stress, trauma, and during sepsis. Integrated 24-h GH secretion is higher in women and is also enhanced by estrogen replacement. Using assays in common clinical use, random GH measurements are undetectable in ~50% of daytime samples obtained from healthy subjects and are undetectable in most obese and elderly subjects. Thus, single random GH measurements do not distinguish patients with adult GH deficiency from normal persons.

GH secretion is profoundly influenced by nutritional factors. Using newer ultrasensitive chemiluminescence-based GH assays with a sensitivity of 0.002 μg/L, a glucose load can be shown to suppress GH to <0.7 μg/L in female and to <0.07 μg/L in male subjects. Increased GH pulse frequency and peak amplitudes occur with chronic malnutrition or prolonged fasting. GH is stimulated by high-protein meals and by L-arginine. GH secretion is induced by dopamine and apomorphine (a dopamine receptor agonist), as well as by α-adrenergic pathways. β-Adrenergic blockage induces basal GH and enhances GHRH- and insulin-evoked GH release.

ACTION The pattern of GH secretion may affect tissue responses. The higher GH pulsatility observed in males, as compared to the relatively continuous GH secretion in females, may be an important biologic determinant of linear growth patterns and liver enzyme induction.

The 70-kD peripheral GH receptor protein shares structural homology with the cytokine/hematopoietic superfamily. A fragment of the receptor extracellular domain generates a soluble GH binding protein (GHBP) that interacts with GH in the circulation. The liver contains the greatest number of GH receptors. GH binding induces receptor dimerization by making distinct contact through two separate binding domains of the hormone. The dimerized receptor interacts with members of the JAK/STAT family. The activated STAT proteins translocate to the nucleus, where they modulate expression of GH-regulated target genes. GH analogues that bind to the receptor, but are incapable of mediating receptor dimerization, are potent antagonists of GH action and are being investigated for potential use in the treatment of acromegaly and diabetic microangiopathy.

GH induces protein synthesis and nitrogen retention and impairs glucose tolerance by antagonizing insulin action. GH also stimulates lipolysis, leading to increased circulating fatty acid levels, reduced omental fat mass, and enhanced lean body mass. GH promotes sodium, potassium, and water retention and elevates serum levels of inorganic phosphate. Linear bone growth occurs as a result of complex hormonal and growth factor actions, including those of IGF-I. GH stimulates epiphyseal prechondrocyte differentiation. These precursor cells produce IGF-I locally and are also responsive to the growth factor.

INSULIN-LIKE GROWTH FACTORS Though GH exerts direct effects in target tissues, many of its physiologic effects are mediated indirectly through IGF-I, a potent growth and differentiation factor. The major source of circulating IGF-I is hepatic in origin. Peripheral tissue IGF-I exerts local paracrine actions that appear to be both dependent and independent of GH. Thus, GH administration induces circulating IGF-I level as well as stimulating IGF-I expression in multiple tissues.

Both IGF-I and -II are bound to one of six high-affinity circulating IGF-binding proteins (IGFBPs) that regulate IGF bioactivity. Levels of IGFBP3 are GH-dependent, and it serves as the major carrier protein for circulating IGF-I. GH deficiency and malnutrition are associated with low IGFBP3 levels. IGFBP1 and -2 regulate local tissue IGF action but do not bind appreciable amounts of circulating IGF-I.

Serum IGF-I concentrations are profoundly affected by various physiologic factors. Levels increase during puberty, peak at 16 years, and subsequently decline by >80% during the aging process. IGF-I concentrations are higher in females than in males. Because GH is the major determinant of hepatic IGF-I synthesis, abnormalities of GH synthesis or action (e.g., pituitary failure, GHRH receptor defect, or GH receptor defect) reduce IGF-I levels. Hypocaloric states are associated with GH resistance; IGF-I levels are therefore low with cachexia, malnutrition, and sepsis. In acromegaly, IGF-I levels are invariably high and reflect a log-linear relationship with GH concentrations.

IGF-I Physiology   Though IGF-I is not an approved drug, investigational studies provide insight into its physiologic effects. High doses of injected IGF-I (100 μg/kg) induce hypoglycemia, primarily because of actions through the insulin receptor. Low IGF-I doses improve insulin sensitivity in patients with severe insulin resistance and diabetes. In cachectic subjects, IGF-I infusion (12 μg/kg per hour) enhances nitrogen retention and lowers cholesterol levels. Longer-term subcutaneous IGF-I injections exert a marked anabolic effect with enhanced protein synthesis. The impact of long-term IGF-I administration on bone mineral content is as yet unclear. Although bone formation markers are induced, bone turnover may also be stimulated by IGF-I.

Side effects of IGF-I are dose-dependent. An acute overdose may result in hypoglycemia and hypotension. Fluid retention, temporomandibular jaw pain, and increased intracranial pressure are reversible. Avascular necrosis of the femoral head has been reported. Chronic excess IGF-I would presumably result in features of acromegaly.

DISORDERS OF GROWTH AND DEVELOPMENT
Skeletal Maturation and Somatic Growth   Linear growth is a function of endochrondral bone formation whereby cartilage is converted into bony skeleton in the long bones and vertebrae (Chap. 340). Ossification occurs within central diaphyseal and peripheral epiphyseal centers. A cartilaginous growth plate forms between the two centers, and chondrocytes proliferate within the growth plate. Linear bone growth ceases when this cartilage layer ossifies and fuses with epiphyseal and diaphyseal bone.

The growth plate is dependent on a variety of hormonal stimuli including GH, IGF-I, sex steroids, thyroid hormones, paracrine growth factors, and cytokines. GH directly stimulates prechondrocyte differentiation and clonal expansion, resulting in chondrocytes that express both IGF-I receptors and IGF-I protein. The growth-promoting process also requires caloric energy, amino acids, vitamins, and trace metals and consumes about 10% of normal energy production. Malnutrition impairs chondrocyte activity and reduces circulating IGF-I and IGFBP3 levels.

Bone age is delayed in patients with all forms of true GH deficiency or GH receptor defects that result in attenuated GH action. Rarely, GH excess accelerates growth, particularly in the setting of delayed bone age from concomitant hypogonadism. Thyroid hormone is permissive for GH synthesis and secretion as well as for maintaining normal circulating IGF-I and binding protein levels. Bone age is delayed by thyroid hormone deficiency. Consequently, congenital or acquired hypothyroidism is associated with stunted growth, which is partially reversed by thyroid hormone replacement (Chap. 330). Elevated pubertal sex steroid levels (especially estrogen) induce the GHRH-GH-IGF-I axis and also directly stimulate epiphyseal growth. High doses of estrogen lead to epiphyseal closure. A mutation of the estrogen receptor α prevented epiphyseal closure, confirming the important role of this pathway in bone maturation. Several pathologic conditions accompanied by increased levels of sex steroids, including precocious puberty, androgen exposure (exogenous or endogenous),

congenital adrenal hyperplasia, and obesity, are associated with accelerated bone maturation. Thus, children with these conditions have accelerated early growth, but end up with reduced final height. In contrast to sex steroids, glucocorticoid excess inhibits linear growth. Glucocorticoids also stimulate SRIF and inhibit peripheral GH and IGF-I receptor signaling.

Linear bone growth rates are very high in infancy and are pituitary-dependent. Mean growth velocity is ~6 cm/year in later childhood and is usually maintained within a given range on a standardized percentile chart. Peak growth rates occur during midpuberty when bone age is 12 (girls) or 13 (boys) (Chap. 8). Secondary sexual development is associated with elevated sex steroids that cause progressive epiphyseal growth plate closure.

Short stature may occur as a result of constitutive intrinsic growth defects or because of acquired extrinsic factors that impair growth (Table 328-9). Genetic disorders, including pituitary transcription factor defects, mutations in growth-related genes, and pituitary hypoplasia syndromes, may all be associated with growth delay and short stature. In general, delayed bone age in a child with short stature is suggestive of a hormonal or systemic disorder, whereas normal bone age in a short child is more likely to be caused by a genetic growth plate disorder (Chap. 351). Other bone and cartilage dysplasia syndromes are associated with specific limb-body proportion phenotypes, and some involve associated calcium disorders (Chap. 343).

Intrauterine growth retardation results in short stature and may be caused by specific congenital anomalies (e.g., IGF-I deficiency, *Russell-Silver syndrome*, chromosomal disomy) or maternal factors such as diabetes mellitus, infections, hypoxia, drug addiction, or placental dysfunction. Long-term responses of these children to GH treatment are currently being evaluated.

Turner syndrome is caused by loss of all, or part, of an X chromosome in females (XO). It is characterized by short stature, in addition to gonadal dysgenesis and other characteristic features (Chap. 338). Short stature may be improved with a combination of GH and an anabolic steroid (oxandrolone); estrogen is required to induce and sustain sexual development. *Noonan syndrome* resembles Turner syndrome phenotypically, but patients have apparently normal sex chromosomes. These patients have delayed pubertal development but not primary gonadal failure.

GH Deficiency in Children • *GH deficiency*   Isolated GH deficiency is characterized by short stature, micropenis, increased fat, high-pitched voice, and a propensity to hypoglycemia. The etiology of GH deficiency is not identifiable in most children with the disorder. Familial modes of inheritance are seen in one-third of these individuals and may be autosomal dominant, recessive, or X-linked, indicating that multiple genetic abnormalities can lead to GH deficiency. About 10% of children with growth hormone deficiency have mutations in the GH-N gene. These include gene deletions and a wide range of point mutations, including some that function in a dominant negative manner (heterozygous mutations) to impair the synthesis or function of GH expressed from the normal allele. Mutations in transcription factors Pit-1 and Prop-1, which control somatotrope development, cause GH deficiency in combination with other pituitary hormone deficiencies. The diagnosis of *idiopathic GH deficiency* (IGHD) should be made only after known molecular defects have been excluded.

GHRH receptor mutations   Recessive mutations of the GHRH receptor gene have been described in several unrelated families with severe proportionate dwarfism. The low basal GH levels in these patients cannot be stimulated by exogenous GHRH, GHRP, or insulin-induced hypoglycemia, confirming the importance of the GHRH receptor for somatotrope cell proliferation and hormonal responsiveness.

Growth hormone insensitivity   This is caused by defects of GH receptor structure or signaling. Homozygous or heterozygous exonic and intronic mutations of the GH receptor occur mainly in the extracellular ligand-binding domain and are associated with partial or complete GH insensitivity and growth failure (*Laron syndrome*). The diagnosis of this syndrome is based on normal or high GH levels, with decreased circulating GHBP, and low IGF-I levels. Very rarely, defective IGF-I, IGF-I receptor, or IGF-I signaling defects are also encountered.

Nutritional short stature Caloric deprivation and malnutrition, uncontrolled diabetes, and chronic renal failure represent secondary causes of abrogated GH receptor function. These conditions also stimulate the production of proinflammatory cytokines, including tumor necrosis factor (TNF) α and ILs, which can block GH-mediated signal transduction. Children with these conditions typically exhibit features of acquired short stature with elevated GH and low IGF-I levels. Circulating GH receptor antibodies may rarely cause peripheral GH insensitivity.

Psychosocial short stature Emotional and social deprivation lead to growth retardation accompanied by delayed speech, discordant hyperphagia, and attenuated response to administered GH. A nurturing environment restores growth rates.

Presentation and Diagnosis Short stature is commonly encountered in clinical practice, but the criteria for biochemical diagnosis of true GH deficiency have been difficult to define. The decision to evaluate these children requires clinical judgement in association with auxologic data and family history. Short stature should be comprehensively evaluated if a patient's height is >3 SD below the mean for age or if the growth rate has decelerated. Skeletal maturation is best evaluated by measuring a radiologic bone age, which is based mainly on the degree of growth plate fusion. Final height can be predicted using standardized scales (Bayley-Pinneau or Tanner-Whitehouse) or estimated by adding 6.5 cm (boys) or subtracting 6.5 cm (girls) from the midparental height.

Laboratory Investigation Because GH secretion is pulsatile, GH deficiency is best assessed by examining the response to provocative stimuli. Random GH measurements do not distinguish normal children from those with true GH deficiency. Adequate adrenal and thyroid hormone replacement should be assured before testing. Provocative stimuli such as exercise, insulin-induced hypoglycemia, and other pharmacologic tests normally increase GH to >7 μg/L in children. Insulin-induced hypoglycemia testing requires the blood sugar nadir to be <50% of baseline levels. This test should be performed under close supervision and is contraindicated in children with seizure disorders. IGF-I levels are not sufficiently sensitive or specific to make the diagnosis but can be useful to confirm GH deficiency; they must be controlled

Table 328-9 Etiology and Diagnosis of Short Stature

	Representative Conditions	Clinical and Laboratory Features
Genetic		
Normal variants	Familial intrinsic short stature	Family short stature, normal bone age; no clinical or laboratory abnormalities
	Constitutional delay in growth	Family history of delayed growth, delayed bone age; no clinical or laboratory abnormalities
Genetic disorders	Turner syndrome	Short, gonadal dysgenesis, variable phenotype, karyotype required
Chromosomal Aneuploidy		
SHOX mutations	Leri-Weill syndrome SHOX: short stature homeobox-containing gene Xp22, Yp11.3	Short stature with variable osteochondrosteosis, mesomelic dysplasia, and Madelung deformity; GH levels normal
Bone dysplasias	Achondroplasia	Abnormal body proportions, macrocephaly, short limbs, low nasal bridge, occasional hydrocephalus
Dysmorphic syndrome	Noonan's syndrome	Similar to Turner, normal karyotype, and present in both sexes
	Prader-Willi syndrome	Obesity, hypogonadism, hypotonia, intellectual and behavioral deficits, chromosome 15 abnormalities
	Pseudohypoparathyroidism (type 1A)	Hypocalcemia, moon facies, brachydactyly, mental retardation, abnormal Gsα
Intrauterine		
Growth retardation	Small for gestational age	Ongoing growth failure in a minority of nonsyndromic cases; diverse maternal, placental, and fetal disorders
	Russell-Silver syndrome	IUGR, relative macrocephaly, small triangular face, asymmetry
Nutritional		
Inadequate intake	Starvation Psychosocial feeding problems Anorexia due to chronic disease	Weight generally depressed more than height
Vitamin/mineral deficiency	Rickets	Nutritional deficiency in vitamin D is most common cause
Nutrient loss	Malabsorption Chronic vomiting	Gastrointestinal, liver, respiratory, or pancreatic disease Gastrointestinal obstruction, achalasia of esophagus, electrolyte disturbances, increased intracranial pressure
Metabolic disorders	Uncontrolled diabetes mellitus Hyperthyroidism	High glycohemoglobin, hepatomegaly Goiter, eye signs, elevated T$_4$ levels
Hormonal		
GH/IGF-I deficiency		
Congenital		May have neonatal hypoglycemia, midline defects; may have only short stature
Acquired		May have history of trauma, CNS insult, or abnormal CNS examination
Psychosocial deprivation		May show abnormal behavior, hyperphagia; may mimic panhypopituitarism; growth improves with better environment
Hypothyroidism		Growth failure may be only symptom; low T$_4$
Glucocorticoid excess		Supraphysiologic levels attenuate growth; often associated with obesity
Sex steroid deficiency		Deficiency after 10–11 years of age impairs growth
Chronic illness		May have features of chronic condition or short stature may be presenting feature; weight often impaired more than height

NOTE: GH, growth hormone; IGF, insulin-like growth factor; CNS, central nervous system; IUGR, intrauterine growth rate.
SOURCE: Adapted from RL Rosenfeld, L Cuttler, in LJ De Groot, JL Jameson (eds): *Somatic Growth and Maturation in Endocrinology*, 4th ed. Philadelphia, Saunders, 2000, with permission.

for age and gender. Pituitary MRI may reveal pituitary mass lesions or structural defects.

℞ TREATMENT Replacement therapy with recombinant GH (0.02 to 0.05 mg/kg per day subcutaneously) restores growth velocity in GH-deficient children to ~10 cm/year. If pituitary insufficiency is documented, other associated hormone deficits should be corrected—especially adrenal steroids. GH treatment is also moderately effective for accelerating growth rates in patients with Turner syndrome and chronic renal failure.

In patients with GH insensitivity and growth retardation due to mutations of the GH receptor, treatment with IGF-I bypasses the dysfunctional GH receptor. Growth rates have been maintained for several years, and this therapy now portends improved final adult stature in this group of patients.

ADULT GH DEFICIENCY (AGHD) This disorder is usually caused by hypothalamic or pituitary somatotrope damage. Acquired pituitary hormone deficiency follows a typical sequential pattern whereby loss of adequate GH reserve foreshadows subsequent hormone deficits. The sequential order of hormone loss is usually GH → FSH/LH → TSH → ACTH. The presence of documented central hypogonadism, hypothyroidism, and/or hypoadrenalism invariably assures the presence of GH deficiency. Conversely, ~40% of patients with incipient preclinical pituitary insufficiency already manifest GH deficiency, if rigorously tested.

Presentation and Diagnosis The clinical features of AGHD include changes in body composition, lipid metabolism, and quality of life and cardiovascular dysfunction (Table 328-10). Body composition changes are common and include reduced lean body mass, increased fat mass with selective deposition of intraabdominal visceral fat, and increased waist-to-hip ratio. Hyperlipidemia, left ventricular dysfunction, hypertension, and increase plasma fibrinogen levels may also be present. Bone mineral content is reduced, with resultant increased fracture rates. Patients may exhibit social isolation, depression, and difficulty in maintaining gainful employment. Adult hypopituitarism is associated with a three-fold increased cardiovascular mortality rate in comparison to age- and sex-matched controls, and this may be due to GH deficiency.

Laboratory Investigation AGHD is rare, and in light of the nonspecific nature of associated clinical symptoms, patients appropriate for testing should be carefully selected on the basis of well-defined criteria. With few exceptions, testing should be restricted to patients with the following predisposing factors: (1) pituitary surgery, (2) pituitary or hypothalamic tumor or granulomas, (3) cranial irradiation, (4) radiologic evidence of a pituitary lesion, (5) childhood requirement for GH replacement therapy, or, rarely, (6) unexplained low age- and sex-matched IGF-I level. The transition of the GH-deficient adolescent to adulthood requires retesting to document adult GH deficiency. Up to 20% of patients treated for childhood-onset GH deficiency are found to be GH-sufficient on repeat testing as adults.

A significant proportion (~25%) of truly GH-deficient adults have low-normal IGF-I levels. Thus, as in the evaluation of GH deficiency in children, valid age- and gender-matched IGF-I measurements provide a useful index of therapeutic responses but are not sufficiently sensitive for diagnostic purposes. AGHD is diagnosed by demonstrating a subnormal GH response (<3 μg/L) to a standard provocative test. None of the available stimulation tests provides standardized GH responses that clearly discriminate normal subjects from truly GH-deficient adults. The age-related decline of GH blurs this distinction further in elderly individuals. The most validated test to distinguish pituitary-sufficient patients from those with AGHD is insulin-induced (0.05 to 0.1 U/kg) hypoglycemia. After glucose reduction to ~40 mg/dL, most individuals experience neuroglycopenic symptoms (Chap. 334), and peak GH release occurs at 60 min and remains elevated for up to 2 h. About 90% of healthy adults exhibit GH responses >5 μg/L; AGHD is defined by a peak GH response to hypoglycemia of <3 μg/L. An attenuated GH response is observed in patients with pituitary damage, obesity, untreated hypothyroidism, depression, or chronic renal failure. Although an *insulin tolerance test* (ITT) is safe when performed under appropriate supervision, it is contraindicated in patients with diabetes, ischemic heart disease, cerebrovascular disease, or epilepsy and in elderly patients. Alternative stimulatory tests include L-dopa (500 mg orally) and intravenous arginine (30 g), GHRH (1 μg/kg), and GHRP-6 (90 μg). Combinations of these tests may evoke GH secretion in subjects not responsive to a single test.

℞ TREATMENT Once the diagnosis of AGHD is unequivocally established, replacement of GH may be indicated. Contraindications to therapy include the presence of an active neoplasm, intracranial hypertension, or uncontrolled diabetes and retinopathy. The starting dose of 0.15 to 0.3 mg/d should be titrated (up to a maximum of 1.25 mg/d) to maintain IGF-I levels in the mid-normal range for age- and gender-matched controls (Fig. 328-8). Women require higher doses than men, and elderly patients require less GH. Long-term GH maintenance sustains normal IGF-I levels and is associated with persistent body composition changes (e.g., enhanced lean body mass and lower body fat). High-density lipoprotein cholesterol increases, but total cholesterol and insulin levels do not change significantly. Lumbar spine bone mineral density increases, but this response is gradual (>1 year). Many patients note significant improvement in quality of life when evaluated by standardized questionnaires. The effect of GH replacement on mortality rates in GH-deficient patients is currently the subject of long-term prospective investigation.

About 30% of patients exhibit reversible dose-related fluid retention, joint pain, and carpal tunnel syndrome, and up to 40% exhibit myalgias and paresthesias. Patients receiving insulin require careful monitoring for dosing adjustments, as GH is a potent counterregulatory hormone for insulin action. Patients with type 2 diabetes mellitus initially develop further insulin resistance. However, glycemic control improves with the sustained loss of abdominal fat associated with long-term GH replacement. Headache, increased intracranial pressure, hypertension, atrial fibrillation, and tinnitus occur rarely. Prevalence of pituitary tumor regrowth and potential progression of skin lesions are currently being assessed in long-term surveillance programs. To date, development of these potential side effects does not appear significant. For some patients, the expense of long-term GH replacement is prohibitive.

Table 328-10 Features of Adult Growth Hormone Deficiency

Clinical	Imaging
Impaired quality of life	Pituitary: Mass or structural damage
Decreased energy and drive	Bone: Reduced bone mineral density
Poor concentration	Abdomen: Excess omental adiposity
Low self esteem	**Laboratory**
Social isolation	Evoked GH <3 ng/ml
Body composition changes	IGF-I and IGFBP3 low or normal
Increased body fat mass	Increased LDL-cholesterol
Central fat deposition	Concomitant gonadotropin, TSH,
Increased waist-hip ratio	and/or ACTH reserve deficits may
Decreased lean body mass	be present
Reduced exercise capacity	
Reduced maximum O_2 uptake	
Impaired cardiac function	
Reduced muscle mass	
Cardiovascular risk factors	
Impaired cardiac structure and	
function	
Abnormal lipid profile	
Decreased fibrinolytic activity	
Atherosclerosis	
Omental obesity	

NOTE: GH, growth hormone; IGF, insulin-like growth factor; IGFBP, IGF-binding proteins; LDL, low-density lipoprotein; TSH, thyroid-stimulating hormone; ACTH, adrenocorticotropin.

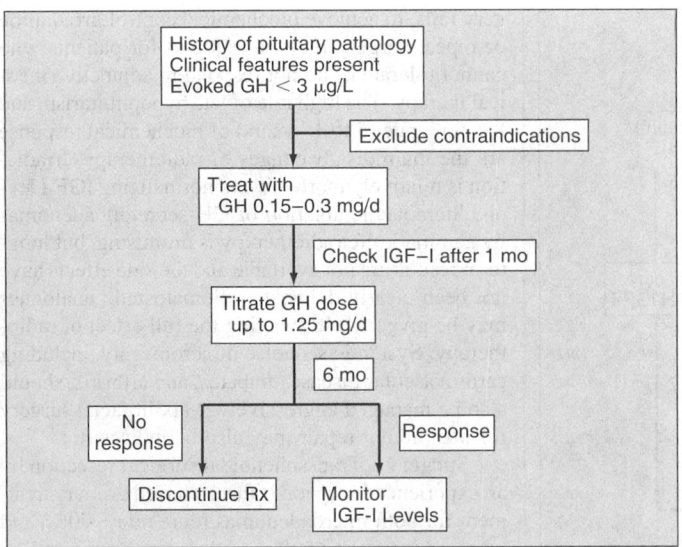

FIGURE 328-8 Management of adult growth hormone (GH) deficiency. (IGF, insulin-like growth factor.)

Table 328-11 Causes of Acromegaly

	Prevalence, %
Excess growth hormone secretion	
Pituitary	98
Densely or sparsely granulated GH cell adenoma	60
Mixed GH cell and PRL cell adenoma	25
Mammosomatrope cell adenoma	10
Plurihormonal adenoma	
GH cell carcinoma or metastases	
Multiple endocrine neoplasia-1 (GH cell adenoma)	
McCune-Albright syndrome	
Ectopic sphenoid or parapharyngeal sinus pituitary adenoma	
Extrapituitary tumor	
Pancreatic islet cell tumor	<1
Excess growth hormone–releasing hormone secretion	
Central	<1
Hypothalamic hamartoma, choristoma, ganglioneuroma	<1
Peripheral	<1
Bronchial carcinoid, pancreatic islet cell tumor, small cell lung cancer, adrenal adenoma, medullary thyroid carcinoma, pheochromocytoma	

SOURCE: Adapted from S Melmed: N Engl J Med 322:966, 1990. Copyright © 1990, Massachusetts Medical Society. All rights reserved.

ACROMEGALY Etiology GH hypersecretion is usually the result of somatotrope adenomas but is also rarely caused by extrapituitary lesions (Table 328-11). In addition to typical GH-secreting somatotrope adenomas, mixed mammosomatotrope tumors and acidophilic stem-cell adenomas can secrete both GH and PRL. In patients with acidophilic stem-cell adenomas, features of hyperprolactinemia (hypogonadism and galactorrhea) predominate over the less clinically evident signs of acromegaly. Occasionally, mixed plurihormonal tumors are encountered that secrete ACTH, the glycoprotein hormone α subunit, or TSH, in addition to GH. Patients with partially empty sella may present with GH hypersecretion due to a small GH-secreting adenoma within the compressed rim of pituitary tissue; some of these may reflect the spontaneous necrosis of tumors that were previously larger. GH-secreting tumors rarely arise from ectopic pituitary tissue remnants in the nasopharynx or midline sinuses.

There are case reports of ectopic GH secretion by tumors of pancreatic, ovarian, or lung origin. Excess GHRH production may cause acromegaly because of chronic stimulation of somatotropes. These patients present with classic features of acromegaly, elevated GH levels, pituitary enlargement on MRI, and pathologic characteristics of pituitary hyperplasia. The most common cause of GHRH-mediated acromegaly is a chest or abdominal carcinoid tumor. Although these tumors usually express positive GHRH immunoreactivity, clinical features of acromegaly are evident in only a minority of patients with carcinoid disease. Excessive GHRH may also be elaborated by hypothalamic tumors, usually choristomas or neuromas.

Presentation and Diagnosis

Protean manifestations of GH and IGF-I hypersecretion are indolent and often are not clinically diagnosed for 10 years or more. Acral bony overgrowth results in frontal bossing, increased hand and foot size, mandibular enlargement with prognathism, and widened space between the lower incisor teeth. In children and adolescents, initiation of GH hypersecretion prior to epiphyseal long bone closure is associated with the development of pituitary gigantism (Fig. 328-9). Soft tissue swelling results in increased heel pad thickness, increased shoe or glove size, ring tightening, characteristic coarse facial features, and a large fleshy nose. Other commonly encountered clinical features include hyperhidrosis, deep and hollow-sounding voice, oily skin, arthropathy, kyphosis, carpal tunnel syndrome, proximal muscle weakness and fatigue, acanthosis nigricans, and skin tags. Generalized visceromegaly occurs, including cardiomegaly, macroglossia, and thyroid gland enlargement.

FIGURE 328-9 Features of acromegaly/gigantism. A 22-year-old man with gigantism due to excess growth hormone is shown to the left of his identical twin. The increased height and prognathism (A) and enlarged hand (B) and foot (C) of the affected twin are apparent. Their clinical features began to diverge at the age of approximately 13 years. (*Reproduced from R Gagel, IE McCutcheon: N Engl J Med 324:524, 1999, with permission.*)

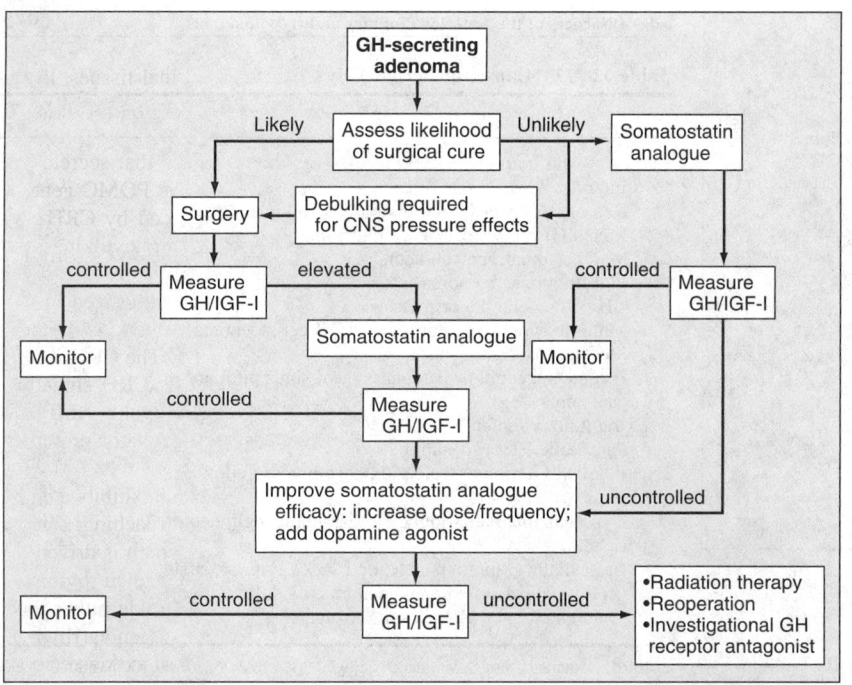

FIGURE 328-10 Management of acromegaly. (GH, growth hormone; CNS, central nervous system; IGF, insulin-like growth factor.) *(Adapted from Melmed et al.)*

The most significant clinical impact of GH excess occurs with respect to the cardiovascular system. Coronary heart disease, cardiomyopathy with arrhythmias, left ventricular hypertrophy, decreased diastolic function, and hypertension occur in about 30% of patients. Upper airway obstruction with sleep apnea occurs in about 60% of patients and is associated with both soft tissue laryngeal airway obstruction and central sleep dysfunction. Diabetes mellitus develops in 25% of patients with acromegaly, and most patients are intolerant of a glucose load (as GH counteracts the action of insulin). Acromegaly is associated with an increased risk of colon polyps and colonic malignancy; polyps are diagnosed in up to one-third of acromegalic patients. Overall mortality is increased about three-fold and is due primarily to cardiovascular and cerebrovascular disorders, malignancy, and respiratory disease. Unless GH levels are controlled, survival is reduced by an average of 10 years compared with an age-matched control population.

Laboratory Investigation Age- and gender-matched serum IGF-I levels are invariably elevated in acromegaly. Consequently, an IGF-I level provides a useful laboratory screening measure when clinical features raise the possibility of acromegaly. Due to the pulsatility of GH secretion, measurement of a single random GH level is not useful for the diagnosis or exclusion of acromegaly and does not correlate with disease severity. The diagnosis of acromegaly is confirmed by demonstrating the failure of GH suppression to $< 1 \mu g/L$ within 1 to 2 h of an oral glucose load (75 g). About 20% of patients exhibit a paradoxical GH rise after glucose. About 60% of patients with GH-secreting tumors may exhibit paradoxical GH responses to TRH administration. PRL should be measured as it is elevated in ~25% of patients with acromegaly. Thyroid function, gonadotropins, and sex steroids may be attenuated because of tumor mass effects. Because most patients will undergo surgery with glucocorticoid coverage, tests of ACTH reserve in asymptomatic patients are more efficiently deferred until after surgery.

℞ **TREATMENT** Surgical resection of GH-secreting adenomas is the initial treatment for most patients (Fig. 328-10). Somatostatin analogues are used as adjuvant treatment for preoperative shrinkage of large invasive macroadenomas, immediate relief of debilitating symptoms, and reduction of GH hypersecretion, in elderly patients experiencing morbidity, in patients who decline surgery, or, when sur-

gery fails, to achieve biochemical control. Irradiation or repeat surgery may be required for patients who cannot tolerate or do not respond to adjunctive medical therapy. The high rate of late hypopituitarism and the slow rate (5 to 15 years) of biochemical response are the main disadvantages of radiotherapy. Irradiation is relatively ineffective in normalizing IGF-I levels. Stereotactic ablation of GH-secreting adenomas by gamma-knife radiotherapy is promising, but long-term results are not available and the side effects have not been clearly delineated. Somatostatin analogues may be given while awaiting the full effect of radiotherapy. Systemic sequelae of acromegaly, including cardiovascular disease, diabetes, and arthritis, should also be managed aggressively. Maxillofacial surgery for mandibular repair may also be indicated.

Surgery Transsphenoidal surgical resection by an experienced surgeon is the preferred primary treatment for both microadenomas (cure rate ~70%) and macroadenomas (<50% cured). Soft tissue swelling improves immediately after tumor resection. GH levels return to normal within an hour, and IGF-I levels are normalized within 3 to 4 days. In ~10% of patients, acromegaly may recur several years after apparently successful surgery; hypopituitarism develops in up to 15% of patients.

Somatostatin Analogues Somatostatin analogues exert their therapeutic effects through SSTR2 and -5 receptors, both of which are expressed by GH-secreting tumors. Octreotide acetate is an 8-amino-acid synthetic somatostatin analogue. In contrast to native somatostatin, the analogue is relatively resistant to plasma degradation. It has a 2-h serum half-life and possesses at least 40-fold greater potency than native somatostatin to suppress GH. These properties often allow effective pharmacologic control of GH hypersecretion without prior surgery or radiotherapy. Octreotide is administered by subcutaneous injection, beginning with 50 μg tid; the dose can be gradually increased up to 1500 $\mu g/d$. Fewer than 10% of patients do not respond to the analogue. Octreotide suppresses integrated GH levels to <5 $\mu g/L$ in ~70% of patients and to <2 $\mu g/L$ in up to 60% of patients. It normalizes IGF-I levels in ~75% of treated patients (Fig. 328-11). Prolonged use of the analogue is not associated with desensitization, even after ≥10 years of treatment. Rapid relief of headache and soft tissue swelling occurs in ~75% of patients within days to weeks of treatment initiation. Subjective clinical benefits of octreotide therapy occur more frequently than biochemical remission, and most patients report symptomatic improvement, including amelioration of headache, perspiration, obstructive apnea, and cardiac failure. Modest pituitary tumor size reduction occurs in about 40% of patients, but this effect is reversed when treatment is stopped.

Two long-acting somatostatin depot formulations, octreotide and lanreotide, are becoming the preferred medical treatment for acrome-

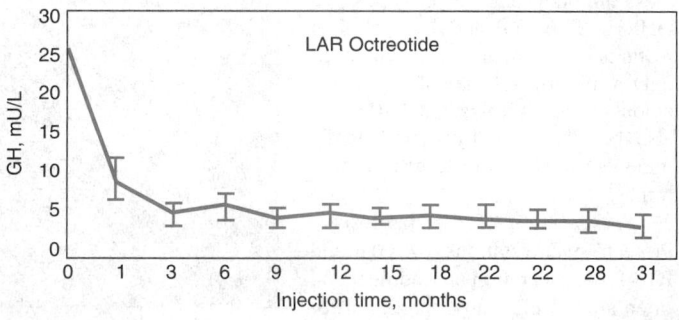

FIGURE 328-11 Medical therapy of acromegaly. Serum growth hormone (GH) levels in acromegaly following monthly LAR octreotide injections in 12 patients for 1 year, and 8 patients for 31 months. *(Reproduced from PH Davies, et al: Clin Endocrinol 48:311, 1998.)*

galic patients. *Sandostatin-LAR* is a sustained-release, long-acting formulation of octreotide incorporated into microspheres that sustain drug levels for several weeks after intramuscular injection. GH suppression occurs for as long as 6 weeks after a 30-mg injection; long-term monthly treatment sustains GH and IGF-I suppression and reduction of pituitary tumor size. *Lanreotide*, a slow-release depot somatostatin preparation, is a cyclic somatostatin octapeptide analogue that suppresses GH and IGF-I hypersecretion for 10 to 14 days after a 30-mg intramuscular injection. Long-term administration controls GH hypersecretion in two-thirds of treated patients and improves patient compliance because of the long interval required between drug injections.

Side effects Somatostatin analogues are well tolerated in most patients. Adverse effects are short-lived and mostly relate to drug-induced suppression of gastrointestinal motility and secretion. Nausea, abdominal discomfort, fat malabsorption, diarrhea, and flatulence occur in one-third of patients, though these symptoms usually remit within 2 weeks. Octreotide suppresses postprandial gallbladder contractility and delays gallbladder emptying; up to 30% of patients treated long-term develop echogenic sludge or asymptomatic cholesterol gallstones. Other side effects include mild glucose intolerance due to transient insulin suppression, asymptomatic bradycardia, hypothyroxinemia, and local pain at the injection site. The cost of chronic treatment may be prohibitive.

Dopamine Agonists Bromocriptine may suppress GH secretion in some acromegalic patients, particularly those with cosecretion of PRL. High doses ($\geq$20 mg/d), administered as three to four daily doses, are usually required to lower GH, and therapeutic efficacy is modest. GH levels are suppressed to <5 μg/L in ~20% of patients, and IGF-I levels are normalized in only 10% of patients. Cabergoline also suppresses GH and decreases adenoma size when given at a relatively high dose of 0.5 mg/d. Combined treatment with octreotide and bromocriptine induces additive biochemical control compared to either drug alone.

GH Antagonists Investigational GH analogues antagonize endogenous GH action by blocking peripheral GH binding to its receptor. Consequently, serum IGF-I levels are suppressed, potentially reducing the deleterious effects of excess endogenous GH.

Radiation External radiation therapy or high-energy stereotactic techniques are used as adjuvant therapy for acromegaly. An advantage of radiation is that patient compliance with long-term treatment is not required. Tumor mass is reduced, and GH levels are attenuated over time. However, 50% of patients require at least 8 years for GH levels to be suppressed to <5 μg/L; this suboptimal level of GH reduction is achieved in about 90% of patients after 18 years. Patients may require interim medical therapy for several years prior to attaining maximal radiation benefits. Most patients also experience hypothalamic-pituitary damage, leading to gonadotropin, ACTH, and/or TSH deficiency within 10 years of therapy.

In summary, surgery is the preferred primary treatment for GH-secreting microadenomas (Fig. 328-10). The high frequency of GH hypersecretion after macroadenoma resection usually necessitates adjuvant or primary medical therapy for these larger tumors. Patients unable to receive or respond to medical treatment can be offered radiation.

ADRENOCORTICOTROPIN HORMONE
(See also Chap. 331)

SYNTHESIS ACTH-secreting corticotrope cells constitute about 20% of the pituitary cell population. ACTH (39 amino acids) is derived from the POMC precursor protein (266 amino acids) that also generates several other peptides, including β-lipotropin, β-endorphin, met-enkephalin, α melanocyte-stimulating hormone (MSH), and corticotropin-like intermediate lobe protein (CLIP). The POMC gene is located on chromosome 2 and possesses at least three different promoter regions that account for pituitary and peripheral tissue–specific POMC expression. A proximal promoter mediates POMC expression

in corticotropes. The gonads, placenta, gastrointestinal tissues, liver, kidney, adrenal medulla, lung, and lymphocytic tissue express shorter POMC transcripts derived from a downstream promoter region. Tumors arising from peripheral neuroendocrine tissues that secrete ectopic ACTH express the longer form of POMC. The POMC gene is powerfully suppressed by glucocorticoids and induced by CRH, arginine vasopressin (AVP), and gp 130 proinflammatory cytokines, including IL-6, and leukemia inhibitory factor.

CRH, a 41-amino-acid hypothalamic peptide synthesized in the paraventricular nucleus as well as in higher brain centers, is the predominant stimulator of ACTH synthesis and release. The CRH receptor is a GPCR that is expressed on the corticotrope. CRH signaling induces POMC transcription and is mediated by cyclic AMP, as well as mitogen activated protein (MAP) kinase–activator protein-1 (AP-1) cascades.

SECRETION ACTH secretion is pulsatile and exhibits a characteristic circadian rhythm, peaking at 6 A.M. and reaching a nadir about midnight. Adrenal glucocorticoid secretion, which is driven by ACTH, follows a parallel diurnal pattern. ACTH circadian rhymicity is determined by variations in secretory pulse amplitude rather than changes in pulse frequency. Superimposed on this endogenous rhythm, ACTH levels are increased by AVP, physical stress, exercise, acute illness, and insulin-induced hypoglycemia.

Loss of cortisol feedback inhibition, as occurs in primary adrenal failure, results in extremely high ACTH levels. Glucocorticoid-mediated negative regulation of the hypothalamo-pituitary-adrenal (HPA) axis occurs as a consequence of both hypothalamic CRH suppression and direct attenuation of pituitary POMC gene expression and ACTH release. Hypothalamic AVP stimulates the protein kinase C pathway and acts synergistically with CRH to enhance ACTH production.

Acute inflammatory or septic insults activate the HPA axis through the integrated actions of proinflammatory cytokines, bacterial toxins, and neural signals. The overlapping cascade of ACTH-inducing cytokines (TNF; IL-1, -2, and -6; and leukemia inhibitory factor) activates hypothalamic CRH and AVP secretion, pituitary POMC gene expression, and local paracrine pituitary cytokine networks. The resulting cortisol elevation restrains the inflammatory response and provides host protection. Concomitantly, cytokine-mediated central glucocorticoid receptor resistance impairs glucocorticoid suppression of the HPA. Thus, the neuroendocrine stress response reflects the net result of highly integrated hypothalamic, intrapituitary, and peripheral hormone and cytokine signals.

ACTION The major function of the HPA axis is to maintain metabolic homeostasis and to mediate the neuroendocrine stress response. Peripheral and central afferent signals, which are integrated by the pituitary corticotrope cell, ultimately affect the pattern and quantity of adrenal cortisol secretion. ACTH induces cortical steroidogenesis by maintaining adrenal cell proliferation and function. The receptor for ACTH, designated *melanocortin-2 receptor*, is a GPCR that activates cyclic AMP and MAP kinase pathways; it induces steroidogenesis by stimulating a cascade of steroidogenic enzymes (Chap. 331).

ACTH DEFICIENCY **Presentation and Diagnosis** Secondary adrenal insufficiency occurs as a result of pituitary ACTH deficiency. It is characterized by fatigue, weakness, anorexia, nausea, vomiting, and, occasionally, hypoglycemia (due to diminished insulin counterregulation). In contrast to primary adrenal failure, hypocortisolism associated with pituitary failure is not usually accompanied by pigmentation changes or mineralocorticoid deficiency. ACTH deficiency is commonly due to glucocorticoid withdrawal following treatment-associated suppression of the HPA axis. Isolated ACTH deficiency may occur after surgical resection of an ACTH-secreting pituitary adenoma that has suppressed the HPA axis; this phenomenon is suggestive of a surgical cure. The mass effects of other pituitary adenomas or sellar lesions may lead to ACTH deficiency, but usually in combination with other pituitary hormone deficiencies. Partial

ACTH deficiency may be unmasked in the presence of an acute medical or surgical illness, when clinically significant hypocortisolism reflects diminished ACTH reserve.

Laboratory Diagnosis Inappropriately low ACTH levels in the setting of low cortisol levels are characteristic of diminished ACTH reserve. Low basal serum cortisol levels are associated with blunted cortisol responses to ACTH provocative stimulation and impaired cortisol response to insulin-induced hypoglycemia, or testing with metyrapone or CRH. →*For description of provocative ACTH tests, see "Tests of Pituitary-Adrenal Responsiveness" in Chap. 331.*

℞ **TREATMENT** Glucocorticoid replacement therapy improves most features of ACTH deficiency. The total daily dose of hydrocortisone replacement should not exceed 30 mg daily, divided into two or three doses. Prednisone (5 mg each morning; 2.5 mg each evening) is longer acting and has fewer mineralocorticoid effects than hydrocortisone. Some authorities advocate lower maintenance doses in an effort to avoid cushingoid side effects. Doses should be increased several-fold during periods of acute illness or stress.

CUSHING'S DISEASE (ACTH-PRODUCING ADENOMA) (See also Chap. 331)

Etiology and Prevalence Pituitary corticotrope adenomas account for 70% of patients with endogenous causes of Cushing's syndrome. However, it should be recalled that iatrogenic hypercortisolism is the most common cause of cushingoid features. Ectopic tumor ACTH production, cortisol-producing adrenal adenomas, carcinoma, and hyperplasia account for the other causes; rarely, ectopic tumor CRH production is encountered.

ACTH-producing adenomas account for about 10 to 15% of all pituitary tumors. Because the clinical features of Cushing's syndrome often lead to early diagnosis, most ACTH-producing pituitary tumors are relatively small microadenomas. However, macroadenomas are also seen, and some ACTH-secreting adenomas are clinically silent. Cushing's disease is 5 to 10 times more common in women than in men. These pituitary adenomas exhibit unrestrained ACTH secretion, with resultant hypercortisolemia. However, they retain partial suppressibility in the presence of high doses of administered glucocorticoids, providing the basis for dynamic testing to distinguish pituitary and nonpituitary causes of Cushing's syndrome.

Presentation and Diagnosis The diagnosis of Cushing's syndrome presents two great challenges: (1) to distinguish patients with pathologic cortisol excess from those with physiologic or other disturbances of cortisol production; and (2) to determine the etiology of cortisol excess, which can include iatrogenic administration of glucocorticoids, adrenal adenomas or carcinomas, pituitary adenomas, and ectopic sources of ACTH and CRH.

Typical features of chronic cortisol excess include thin, brittle skin, central obesity, hypertension, plethoric moon facies, purple striae and easy bruisability, glucose intolerance or diabetes mellitus, gonadal dysfunction, osteoporosis, proximal muscle weakness, signs of hyperandrogenism (acne, hirsutism), and psychologic disturbances (depression, mania, and psychoses) (Table 328-12). Hematopoietic features of hypercortisolism include leukocytosis, lymphopenia, and eosinopenia. Immune suppression includes delayed hypersensitivity. The protean manifestations of hypercortisolism make it challenging to decide which patients mandate formal laboratory evaluation. Certain features make pathologic causes of hypercortisolism more likely—these include characteristic central redistribution of fat, thin skin with striae and bruising, and proximal muscle weakness. In children and in young females, early osteoporosis may be particularly prominent. The primary cause of death is cardiovascular disease, but infections and risk of suicide are also increased.

Rapid development of features of hypercortisolism associated with skin hyperpigmentation and severe myopathy suggests the possibility of ectopic sources of ACTH. Hypertension, hypokalemic alkalosis, glucose intolerance, and edema are also more pronounced in these

Table 328-12 Clinical Features of Cushing's Syndrome (All Ages)

Symptoms/Signs	Frequency, %
Obesity or weight gain (>115% ideal body weight)	80
Thin skin	80
Moon facies	75
Hypertension	75
Purple skin striae	65
Hirsutism	65
Abnormal glucose tolerance	55
Impotence	55
Menstrual disorders (usually amenorrhea)	60
Plethora	60
Proximal muscle weakness	50
Truncal obesity	50
Acne	45
Bruising	45
Mental changes	45
Osteoporosis	40
Edema of lower extremities	30
Hyperpigmentation	20
Hypokalemic alkalosis	15
Diabetes mellitus	15

SOURCE: Adapted from MA Magiokou et al, in ME Wierman (ed), *Diseases of the Pituitary.* Totowa, NJ, Humana, 1997.

patients. Serum potassium levels <3.3 mmol/L are evident in ~70% of patients with ectopic ACTH secretion but are seen in <10% of patients with pituitary-dependent Cushing's disease.

Laboratory Investigation The diagnosis of Cushing's syndrome is based on laboratory documentation of endogenous hypercortisolism. Measurements of 24-h urine free cortisol (UFC) is a precise and cost-effective screening test. Alternatively, the failure to suppress plasma cortisol after an overnight 1-mg dexamethasone suppression test can be used to identify patients with hypercortisolism. As nadir levels of cortisol occur at night, elevated midnight samples of cortisol are suggestive of Cushing's syndrome. Basal plasma ACTH levels often distinguish patients with ACTH-independent (adrenal or exogenous glucocorticoid) from those with ACTH-dependent (pituitary, ectopic ACTH) Cushing's disease. Mean basal ACTH levels are about eight-fold higher in patients with ectopic ACTH secretion compared to those with pituitary ACTH-secreting adenomas. However, extensive overlap of ACTH levels in these two disorders precludes using ACTH to make the distinction. Instead, dynamic testing, based on differential sensitivity to glucocorticoid feedback, or ACTH stimulation in response to CRH or cortisol reduction is used to discriminate ectopic versus pituitary sources of excess ACTH (Table 328-13). Very rarely, circulating CRH levels are elevated, reflecting ectopic tumor-derived secretion of CRH and often ACTH. →*For discussion of dynamic testing for Cushing's syndrome, see Chap. 331.*

Most ACTH-secreting pituitary tumors are <5 mm in diameter, and about half are undetectable by sensitive MRI. The high prevalence of incidental pituitary microadenomas diminishes the ability to distinguish ACTH-secreting pituitary tumors accurately by MRI.

Inferior petrosal venous sampling Because pituitary MRI with gadolinium enhancement is insufficiently sensitive to distinguish small (<2 mm) pituitary ACTH-secreting adenomas from ectopic ACTH-secreting tumors that may have similar clinical and biochemical characteristics, bilateral inferior petrosal sinus ACTH sampling before and after CRH administration may be required. Simultaneous assessment of ACTH concentrations in each inferior petrosal vein and in the peripheral circulation provides a strategy for confirming and localizing pituitary ACTH production. Sampling is performed at baseline and 2, 5, and 10 min after intravenous ovine CRH (1 μg/kg) injection. An increased ratio (>2) of inferior petrosal:peripheral vein ACTH confirms pituitary Cushing's disease. After CRH injection, peak petrosal:peripheral ACTH ratios of ≥3 confirm the presence of a pituitary ACTH-secreting tumor. The sensitivity of this test is 99%, with very rare false-positive results. False-negative results may be encountered in patients with aberrant venous anatomic drainage. Petrosal sinus

Table 328-13 Differential Diagnosis of ACTH-Dependent Cushing's Syndrome[a]

	ACTH-Secreting Pituitary Tumor	Ectopic ACTH Secretion
Etiology	Pituitary corticotrope adenoma	Bronchial, abdominal carcinoid
	Plurihormonal adenoma	Small cell lung cancer
		Thymoma
Gender	F > M	M > F
Clinical features	Slow onset	Rapid onset
		Pigmentation
		Severe myopathy
Serum potassium <3.3 μg/L	<10%	75%
24-h urinary free cortisol (UFC)	High	High
Basal ACTH level	Inappropriately high	Very high
Dexamethasone suppression 1 mg overnight		
Low dose (0.5 mg q6h)	Cortisol >5 μg/dL	Cortisol >5 μg/dL
High dose (2 mg q6h)	Cortisol >5 μg/dL	Cortisol >5 μg/dL
UFC > 80% suppressed	Microadenomas: 90%	10%
	Macroadenomas: 50%	
Inferior petrosal sinus sampling (IPSS) Basal		
IPSS: peripheral	>2	<2
CRH-induced		
IPSS: peripheral	>3	<3

[a] ACTH-independent causes of Cushing's syndrome are diagnosed by suppressed ACTH levels and an adrenal mass in the setting of hypercortisolism. Iatrogenic Cushing's syndrome is excluded by history.

NOTE: ACTH, adrenocorticotropin hormone; F, female; M, male; CRH, corticotropin-releasing hormone.

catheterizations are technically difficult, and about 0.05% of patients develop neurovascular complications. The procedure should not be performed in patients with hypertension or in the presence of a well-visualized pituitary adenoma on MRI.

℞ **TREATMENT** Selective transsphenoidal resection is the treatment of choice for Cushing's disease (Fig. 328-12). The remission rate for this procedure is ~80% for microadenomas but <50% for macroadenomas. After successful tumor resection, most patients experience a postoperative period of adrenal insufficiency that lasts for up to 12 months. This usually requires low-dose cortisol replacement, as patients experience steroid withdrawal symptoms as well as having a suppressed HPA axis. Biochemical recurrence occurs in approximately 5% of patients in whom surgery was initially successful.

When initial surgery is unsuccessful, repeat surgery is sometimes indicated, particularly when a pituitary source for ACTH is well documented. In older patients in whom growth and fertility are no longer important, hemi- or total hypophysectomy may be necessary if an adenoma is not recognized. Pituitary irradiation may be used after unsuccessful surgery, but it cures only about 15% of patients. Because radiation is slow and only partially effective in adults, steroidogenic inhibitors are used in combination with pituitary irradiation to block the adrenal effects of persistently high ACTH levels.

Mitotane (*o*,*p*′-DDD) suppresses cortisol hypersecretion by inhibiting 11β-hydroxylase and cholesterol side-chain cleavage enzymes and by destroying adrenocortical cells. Side effects of mitotane include gastrointestinal symptoms, dizziness, gynecomastia, hyperlipidemia, skin rash, and hepatic enzyme elevation. It may also lead to hypoaldosteronism. *Ketoconazole*, an imidazole derivative antimycotic agent, inhibits several P450 enzymes and effectively lowers cortisol in most patients with Cushing's disease when administered twice daily (600 to 1200 mg/d). Elevated hepatic transaminases, gynecomastia, impotence, gastrointestinal upset, and edema are common side effects.

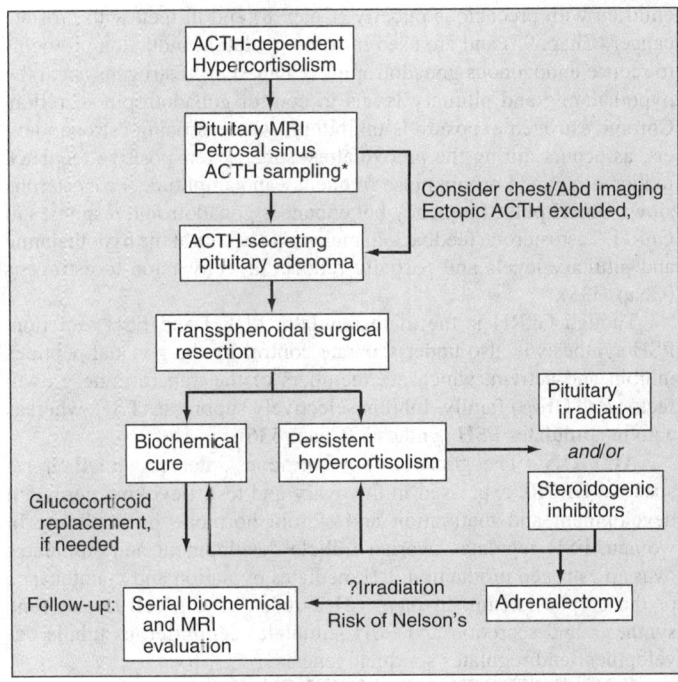

FIGURE 328-12 Management of Cushing's disease. (ACTH, adrenocorticotropin hormone; MRI, magnetic resonance imaging.) *, Not usually required.

Metyrapone (2 to 4 g/d) inhibits 11β-hydroxylase activity and normalizes plasma cortisol in up to 75% of patients. Side effects include nausea and vomiting, rash, and exacerbation of acne or hirsutism. Other agents include *aminoglutethimide* (250 mg tid), *trilostane* (200 to 1000 mg/d), *cyproheptadine* (24 mg/d), and IV *etomidate* (0.3 mg/kg per hour). Glucocorticoid insufficiency is a potential side effect of agents used to block steroidogenesis.

The use of steroidogenic inhibitors has decreased the need for bilateral adrenalectomy. Removal of both adrenal glands corrects hypercortisolism but may be associated with significant morbidity and necessitates permanent glucocorticoid and mineralocorticoid replacement. Adrenalectomy in the setting of residual corticotrope adenoma tissue predisposes to the development of *Nelson's syndrome*, a disorder characterized by rapid pituitary tumor enlargement and increased pigmentation secondary to high ACTH levels. Radiation therapy may be indicated to prevent the development of Nelson's syndrome after adrenalectomy.

GONADOTROPINS: FSH AND LH

SYNTHESIS AND SECRETION Gonadotrope cells comprise about 10% of anterior pituitary cells and produce two gonadotropins—LH and FSH. Like TSH and hCG, LH and FSH are glycoprotein hormones consisting of α and β subunits. The α subunit is common to these glycoprotein hormones; specificity is conferred by the β subunits, which are expressed by separate genes.

Gonadotropin synthesis and release are dynamically regulated. This is particularly true in females, in whom the rapidly fluctuating gonadal steroid levels vary throughout the menstrual cycle. Hypothalamic GnRH, a 10-amino-acid peptide synthesized in the preoptic region, regulates the synthesis and secretion of both LH and FSH. GnRH is secreted in discrete pulses every 60 to 120 min, which in turn elicit LH and FSH pulses (Fig. 328-3). GnRH acts through a GPCR to stimulate phospholipase C, protein kinase C, and calcium signaling pathways. The pulsatile mode of GnRH input is essential to its action; pulses prime gonadotrope responsiveness, whereas continuous GnRH exposure induces desensitization. Based on this phenomenon, long-acting GnRH agonists are used to suppress gonadotropin levels in children with precocious puberty (Chap. 8) and in men with prostate cancer (Chap. 95) and are used in some ovulation-induction protocols to reduce endogenous gonadotropins (Chap. 336). Estrogens act at the hypothalamic and pituitary levels to control gonadotropin secretion. Chronic estrogen exposure is inhibitory, whereas rising estrogen levels, as occurs during the preovulatory surge, exert positive feedback to increase gonadotropin pulse frequency and amplitude. Progesterone slows GnRH pulse frequency but enhances gonadotropin responses to GnRH. Testosterone feedback in males also occurs at the hypothalamic and pituitary levels and partially reflects its conversion to estrogens (Chap. 335).

Though GnRH is the main regulator of LH and FSH secretion, FSH synthesis is also under separate control by the gonadal peptides inhibin and activin, which are members of the transforming growth factor β (TGF-β) family. Inhibin selectively suppresses FSH, whereas activin stimulates FSH synthesis (Chap. 336).

ACTION   The gonadotropin hormones interact with their respective GPCRs expressed in the ovary and testis, evoking germ-cell development and maturation and steroid hormone biosynthesis. In women, FSH regulates ovarian follicle development and stimulates ovarian estrogen production. LH mediates ovulation and maintenance of the corpus luteum. In men, LH induces Leydig cell testosterone synthesis and secretion and FSH stimulates seminiferous tubule development and regulates spermatogenesis.

GONADOTROPIN DEFICIENCY   Hypogonadism is the most common presenting feature of adult hypopituitarism, even when other pituitary hormones are also deficient. It is often a harbinger of hypothalamic or pituitary diseases that impair GnRH production or delivery through the pituitary stalk. As noted above, hypogonadotropic hypogonadism is a common presenting feature of hyperprolactinemia.

A variety of inherited and acquired disorders are associated with *isolated hypogonadotropic hypogonadism* (IHH) (Chap. 335). Hypothalamic defects associated with GnRH deficiency include two X-linked disorders, Kallmann syndrome (see above) and mutations in the *DAX1* gene. GnRH receptor mutations and inactivating mutations of the LH β and FSH β subunit genes are rare causes of selective gonadotropin deficiency. Acquired forms of GnRH deficiency leading to hypogonadotropism are seen in association with anorexia nervosa (Chap. 78), stress, starvation, and extreme exercise, but may also be idiopathic. Hypogonadotropic hypogonadism in these disorders is reversed by removal of the stressful stimulus.

Presentation and Diagnosis   In premenopausal women, hypogonadotropic hypogonadism presents as diminished ovarian function leading to oligomenorrhea or amenorrhea, infertility, decreased vaginal secretions, decreased libido, and breast atrophy. In hypogonadal adult males, secondary testicular failure is associated with decreased libido and potency, infertility, decreased muscle mass with weakness, reduced beard and body hair growth, soft testes, and characteristic fine facial wrinkles. Osteoporosis occurs in both untreated hyogonadal females and males.

Laboratory Investigation   Central hypogonadism is associated with low or inappropriately low serum gonadotropin levels and low sex hormone concentrations (testosterone in males, estradiol in females). Three pooled serum samples drawn 20 min apart are used for accurate measurement of serum LH and FSH levels, thus allowing for the effects of hormone secretory pulses. Male patients have abnormal semen analysis.

Intravenous GnRH (100 μg) stimulates gonadotropes to secrete LH (which peaks within 30 min) and FSH (which plateaus during the ensuing 60 min). Normal responses vary according to menstrual cycle stage, age, and sex of the patient. Generally, LH levels increase about threefold, whereas FSH responses are less pronounced. In the setting of gonadotropin deficiency, a normal gonadotropin response to GnRH indicates intact gonadotrope function and suggests a hypothalamic abnormality. An absent response, however, cannot reliably distinguish pituitary from hypothalamic causes of hypogonadism. For this reason,

GnRH testing usually adds little to the information gained from baseline evaluation of the hypothalamic-pituitary-gonadotrope axis, except in cases of isolated GnRH deficiency (e.g., Kallmann syndrome).

MRI examination of the sellar region and assessment of other pituitary functions are usually indicated in patients with documented central hypogonadism.

TREATMENT   In males, testosterone replacement is necessary to achieve and maintain normal growth and development of the external genitalia, secondary sex characteristics, male sexual behavior, and androgenic anabolic effects including maintenance of muscle function and bone mass. Testosterone may be administered by intramuscular injections every 1 to 4 weeks or using patches that are replaced daily (Chap. 335). Gonadotropin injections [hCG or human menopausal gonadotropin (hMG)] over 12 to 18 months are used to restore fertility. Pulsatile GnRH therapy (25 to 150 ng/kg every 2 h), administered by a subcutaneous infusion pump, is also effective for treatment of hypothalamic hypogonadism when fertility is desired.

In premenopausal women, cyclical replacement of estrogen and progesterone maintains secondary sexual characteristics and genitourinary tract integrity and prevents premature osteoporosis and possibly coronary artery disease (Chap. 336). Gonadotropin therapy is used for ovulation induction. Follicular growth and maturation are initiated using hMG or recombinant FSH; hCG is subsequently injected to induce ovulation. As in men, pulsatile GnRH therapy can be used to treat hypothalamic causes of gonadotropin deficiency.

NONFUNCTIONING AND GONADOTROPIN-PRODUCING PITUITARY ADENOMAS   **Etiology and Prevalence** Nonfunctioning pituitary adenomas include those that secrete little or no pituitary hormones, as well as tumors that produce too little hormone to result in recognizable clinical features. They are the most common type of pituitary adenoma and are usually macroadenomas at the time of diagnosis because clinical features are inapparent until tumor mass effects occur. Based on immunohistochemistry, most clinically nonfunctioning adenomas can be shown to originate from gonadotrope cells. These tumors typically produce small amounts of intact gonadotropins (usually FSH) as well as uncombined α and LH β and FSH β subunits. Tumor secretion may lead to elevated α and FSH β subunits and, rarely, to increased LH β subunit levels. Some adenomas express α subunits without FSH or LH. TRH administration often induces an atypical increase of tumor-derived gonadotropins or subunits.

Presentation and Diagnosis   Clinically nonfunctioning tumors may present with optic chiasm pressure and other symptoms of local expansion or be incidentally discovered on an MRI performed for another indication. Menstrual disturbances or ovarian hyperstimulation rarely occur in women with large tumors that produce FSH and LH. More commonly, adenoma compression of the pituitary stalk or surrounding pituitary tissue leads to attenuated LH and features of hypogonadism. Prolactin levels are usually slightly increased, also because of stalk compression. It is important to distinguish this circumstance from true prolactinomas, as most nonfunctioning tumors respond poorly to treatment with dopamine agonists.

Laboratory Investigation   The goal of laboratory testing in clinically nonfunctioning tumors is to classify the type of the tumor, to identify hormonal markers of tumor activity, and to detect possible hypopituitarism. Free α subunit levels may be elevated in 10 to 15% of patients with nonfunctioning tumors. In female patients, peri- or postmenopausal basal FSH concentrations are difficult to distinguish from tumor-derived FSH elevation. Premenopausal women have cycling FSH levels, also preventing clear-cut diagnostic distinction from tumor-derived FSH. In men, gonadotropin-secreting tumors may be diagnosed because of slightly increased gonadotropins (FSH > LH) in the setting of a pituitary mass. Testosterone levels are usually low, despite the normal or increased LH level, perhaps reflecting reduced LH bioactivity or the loss of normal LH pulsatility. Because this pattern of hormone tests is also seen in primary gonadal failure and, to some extent, with aging (Chap. 335), the increased gonadotropins alone are insufficient for the diagnosis of a gonadotropin-secreting tumor. In the majority of patients with gonadotrope adenomas, TRH administration stimulates LH β subunit secretion; this response is not seen in normal individuals. GnRH testing is not helpful for making the diagnosis. For nonfunctioning and gonadotropin-secreting tumors, the diagnosis usually rests on immunohistochemical analyses of resected tumor tissue, as the mass effects of these tumors usually necessitate resection.

Although acromegaly or Cushing's syndrome usually presents with unique clinical features, clinically inapparent somatotrope or corticotrope adenomas can be excluded by a normal IGF-I value and normal 24-h urinary free cortisol levels. If PRL levels are <100 μg/L in a patient harboring a pituitary mass, a nonfunctioning adenoma causing pituitary stalk compression should be considered.

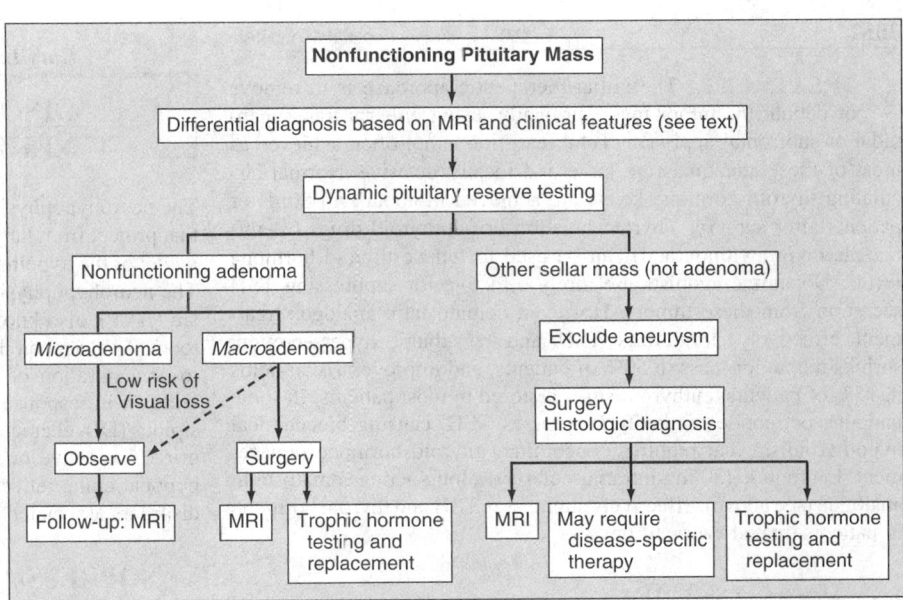

FIGURE 328-13 Management of a nonfunctioning pituitary mass.

℞ **TREATMENT** Asymptomatic small nonfunctioning adenomas with no threat to vision may be followed with regular MRI and visual field testing without immediate intervention. However, for larger macroadenomas, transsphenoidal surgery is the only effective way to reduce tumor size and relieve mass effects (Fig. 328-13). Although it is not usually possible to remove all adenoma tissue surgically, vision improves in 70% of patients with preoperative visual field defects. Preexisting hypopituitarism that results from tumor mass effects commonly improves or may resolve completely. Early postoperative complications include diabetes insipidus and/or inappropriate antidiuretic hormone secretion. Beginning about 6 months postoperatively, MRI scans should be performed yearly to detect tumor regrowth. Within 5 to 6 years following successful surgical resection, ~15% of nonfunctioning tumors recur. When substantial tumor remains after transsphenoidal surgery, adjuvant radiotherapy may be indicated to prevent tumor growth. Radiotherapy may be deferred if no postoperative residual mass is evident.

Nonfunctioning pituitary tumors respond poorly to dopamine agonist treatment, with modest tumor shrinkage occurring in <10% of patients. Although SSTR subtypes 2 and 5 have been identified on nonfunctioning pituitary adenomas, octreotide does not shrink these tumors and only modestly suppresses gonadotropin and α subunit levels. Visual improvement sometimes occurs without evident reduction of tumor size by MRI, presumably reflecting relief of pressure on the optic tracts. The selective GnRH antagonist, Nal-Glu GnRH, suppresses FSH hypersecretion but has no effect on adenoma size.

THYROID-STIMULATING HORMONE

SYNTHESIS AND SECRETION TSH-secreting thyrotrope cells comprise 5% of the anterior pituitary cell population. TSH is structurally related to LH and FSH. It shares a common α subunit with these hormones but contains a specific TSH β subunit. TRH is a hypothalamic tripeptide (pyroglutamyl histidylprolinamide) that acts through a GPCR to stimulate phospholipase C, protein kinase C, and calcium pathways. TRH stimulates TSH synthesis and secretion; it also stimulates the lactotrope cell to secrete PRL. TSH secretion is stimulated by TRH, whereas thyroid hormones, dopamine, SRIF, and glucocorticoids suppress TSH by overriding TRH induction.

The thyrotrope is stimulated when TSH is released from the negative feedback inhibition of thyroid hormones. Thus, thyroid damage, including surgical thyroidectomy, radiation-induced hypothyroidism, chronic thyroiditis, or prolonged goitrogen exposure, are associated with increased TSH. Long-standing untreated hypothyroidism can lead to thyrotrope hyperplasia and pituitary enlargement, which may be evident on MRI.

ACTION TSH is secreted in pulses, though the excursions are modest in comparison to other pituitary hormones because of the relatively low amplitude of the pulses and the relatively long half-life of TSH. Consequently, single determinations of TSH suffice to assess its circulating levels. TSH binds to a GPCR on thyroid follicular cells to stimulate thyroid hormone synthesis and release (Chap. 330).

TSH DEFICIENCY Features of central hypothyroidism, due to TSH deficiency, mimic those seen with primary hypothyroidism but are generally less severe. Pituitary hypothyroidism is characterized by low basal TSH levels in the setting of low free thyroid hormone. In contrast, patients with hypothyroidism of hypothalamic origin (presumably due to a lack of endogenous TRH) may exhibit normal or even slightly elevated TSH levels. There is evidence that the TSH produced in this circumstance has reduced biologic activity because of altered glycosylation.

TRH (200 μg) injected intravenously causes a two- to threefold increase in TSH (and PRL) levels within 30 min. Although TRH testing can be used to assess TSH reserve, abnormalities of the thyroid axis can usually be detected based on basal free T_4 and TSH levels, without the need for TRH testing.

Thyroid-replacement therapy should be initiated after establishing adequate adrenal function. Dose adjustment is based on thyroid hormone levels and clinical parameters rather than the TSH level.

TSH-SECRETING ADENOMAS TSH-producing macroadenomas are rare but are often large and locally invasive when they occur. Patients usually present with thyroid goiter and hyperthyroidism, reflecting overproduction of TSH. Diagnosis is based on demonstrating elevated serum free T_4 levels, inappropriately normal or high TSH secretion, and MRI evidence of a pituitary adenoma. An elevated free α subunit level occurs in about half of patients and supports the diagnosis of a TSH-secreting adenoma.

It is important to exclude other causes of inappropriate TSH secretion, such as resistance to thyroid hormone, an autosomal dominant disorder caused by mutations in the thyroid hormone β receptor (Chap. 330). The presence of a pituitary mass and elevated α subunit levels are suggestive of a TSH-secreting tumor. Dysalbuminemic hyperthyroxinemia syndromes, caused by various mutations in serum thyroid hormone binding proteins, are also characterized by elevated thyroid hormone levels, but with normal rather than suppressed TSH levels. However, free thyroid hormone levels are normal in these disorders, most of which are familial.

℞ **TREATMENT**   The initial therapeutic approach is to remove or debulk the tumor mass surgically, using either a transsphenoidal or subfrontal approach. Total resection is not often achieved as most of these adenomas are large and locally invasive. Normal circulating thyroid hormone levels are achieved in about two-thirds of patients after surgery. Thyroid ablation or antithyroid drugs (methimazole or propylthiouracil) can be used to reduce thyroid hormone levels. Dopamine agonists are rarely effective for suppressing TSH secretion from these tumors. However, somatostatin analogue treatment effectively normalizes TSH and α subunit hypersecretion, shrinks the tumor mass in 50% of patients, and improves visual fields in 75% of patients; euthyroidism is restored in most patients. In some patients, octreotide markedly suppresses TSH, causing biochemical hypothyroidism that requires concomitant thyroid hormone replacement. Lanreotide (30 mg intramuscularly), a long-acting somatostatin analogue (see above), effectively suppresses TSH and thyroid hormone in patients treated every 14 days.

DIABETES INSIPIDUS

→See Chap. 329 for diagnosis and treatment of diabetes insipidus.

BIBLIOGRAPHY

BRUCKER-DAVIS F et al: Thyrotropin-secreting pituitary tumors: Diagnostic criteria, thyroid hormone sensitivity, and treatment outcome in 25 patients followed at the National Institutes of Health. J Clin Endocrinol Metab 84:476, 1999

Consensus guidelines for the diagnosis and treatment of adults with growth hormone deficiency: Summary statement of the Growth Hormone Research Society workshop on adult growth hormone deficiency. J Clin Endocrinol Metab 83:379, 1998

DELADOEY J et al: "Hot spot" in the PROP1 gene responsible for combined pituitary hormone deficiency. J Clin Endocrinol Metab 84:1645, 1999

GREENMAN Y, MELMED S: Diagnosis and management of nonfunctioning pituitary tumors. Ann Rev Med 47:95, 1996

HONEGGER J et al: Surgical treatment of craniopharyngiomas: Endocrinological results. J Neurosurg 90:251, 1999

KOJIMA M et al: Ghrelin is a growth-hormone-releasing acylated peptide from stomach. Nature 402:656, 1999

MELMED S et al: Current treatment guidelines for acromegaly. J Clin Endocrinol Metab 83:2646, 1998

MOLITCH ME: Diagnosis and treatment of prolactinomas. Adv Intern Med 44:117, 1999

NEWELL-PRICE J et al: The diagnosis and differential diagnosis of Cushing's syndrome and pseudo-Cushing's states. Endocr Rev 19:647, 1998

NEWMAN CB et al: Medical therapy of acromegaly. Endocrinol Metab Clin North Am 28:171, 1999

NIEMAN LK: Cushing's syndrome. Curr Ther Endocrinol Metab 6:161, 1997

SHALET SM et al: The diagnosis of growth hormone deficiency in children and adults. Endocr Rev 19:203, 1998

SHIMON I, MELMED S: Genetic basis of endocrine disease: Pituitary tumor pathogenesis. J Clin Endocrin Metab 82:1675, 1997

SHIN J et al: Cystic lesions of the pituitary: Clinicopathological features distinguishing craniopharyngioma, Rathke's cleft cyst, and arachnoid cyst. J Clin Endocrinol Metab 84:3972, 1999

SNYDER PJ: Gonadotrope adenomas. Curr Ther in Endocrinol Metab 6:56, 1997

SONINO N, BOSCARO M: Medical therapy for Cushing's disease. Endocrinol Metab Clin North Am 28:211, 1999

TREIER M et al: Multistep signaling requirements for pituitary organogenesis in vivo. Genes Dev 12:1691, 1998

TSIGOS C: Differential diagnosis and management of Cushing's syndrome. Ann Rev Med 47:443, 1996

WEBSTER J: A comparative review of the tolerability profiles of dopamine agonists in the treatment of hyperprolactemia and inhibition of lactation. Drug Safety 14:118, 1998

329   *Gary L. Robertson*

DISORDERS OF THE NEUROHYPOPHYSIS

The neurohypophysis, or posterior pituitary gland, is formed by axons that project from large cell bodies in the supraoptic and paraventricular nuclei of the hypothalamus to the posterior portion of the sella turcica. The neurohypophysis produces two hormones: (1) arginine vasopressin (AVP), also known as antidiuretic hormone (ADH); and (2) oxytocin. AVP acts on the renal tubules to induce water retention, leading to concentration of the urine. Oxytocin stimulates postpartum milk letdown in response to suckling. AVP deficiency causes diabetes insipidus (DI), characterized by the production of large amounts of dilute urine. Excessive or inappropriate production of AVP predisposes to hyponatremia, reflecting water retention. There are no known clinical disorders associated with oxytocin deficiency or excess.

VASOPRESSIN

ACTION   AVP is a nonapeptide composed of a six-membered disulfide ring and a tripeptide tail on which the C-terminal carboxy group is amidated (Fig. 329-1). The most important, if not the only, physiologic action of AVP is to influence the rate of water excretion by promoting concentration of urine. This antidiuretic effect is achieved by increasing the hydroosmotic permeability of cells that line the distal tubule and medullary collecting ducts of the nephron. In the absence of AVP, these cells are impermeable to water and reabsorb little, if any, of the relatively large volume of dilute filtrate that enters from the cortical nephron. Low AVP concentration results in the production of large amounts of urine (as much as 0.2 mL/kg per minute) that is maximally dilute (specific gravity and osmolality ~1.000 and 50 mmol/L, respectively), a condition known as a *water diuresis*. In the presence of AVP, the luminal surface of the cells lining the terminal collecting duct becomes selectively permeable to water, allowing it to diffuse back down the osmotic gradient created by the hypertonic renal medulla. As a result, the dilute fluid passing through the tubules is concentrated and the rate of urine flow decreases. The magnitude of this antidiuretic effect varies in direct proportion to the plasma AVP concentration. It is mediated via binding of AVP to G protein–coupled V_2 receptors on the serosal surface of the cell, activation of adenyl cyclase, and insertion into the luminal surface of water channels composed of a protein known as *aquaporin 2* (Fig. 329-2). The genes encoding the V_2 receptors and aquaporin 2 have been cloned and appear to be expressed exclusively in the distal and collecting tubules of the kidney. Nonpeptide, as well as peptide, AVP analogues with potent agonist or antagonist actions at human V_2 receptors have been developed for treating disorders of water metabolism caused by deficient or excessive production of AVP (see below).

At high concentrations, AVP also has several other actions, including contraction of smooth muscle in blood vessels in the skin and gastrointestinal tract, glycogenolysis in the liver, and potentiation of adrenocorticotropic hormone (ACTH) release by corticotropin-releasing factor (CRF). These effects are mediated by V_{1a} or V_{1b} receptors that are coupled to phospholipase C. The genes that encode these receptors have also been cloned and sequenced and are expressed in

FIGURE 329-1   Primary structures of arginine vasopressin (AVP), oxytocin, and desamino-D-arginine-8 vasopressin (DDAVP).

many organs, including blood vessels, the anterior and posterior pituitary, and certain other areas of brain. Their role, if any, in human physiology/pathophysiology is still uncertain.

SYNTHESIS AVP is synthesized via a polypeptide precursor that includes a binding protein known as *neurophysin II* and a glycosylated peptide called *copeptin*. The gene encoding the AVP precursor is located on chromosome 20 and has three exons. It is expressed in distinct subpopulations of magno- and parvocellular neurons in the supraoptic and paraventricular nuclei. Like other peptide hormones destined for secretion, newly synthesized AVP–neurophysin II precursor is translocated from the cytosol to the endoplasmic reticulum, where the signal peptide is removed and the prohormone folds and oligomerizes before moving through the Golgi apparatus to the neurosecretory vesicles; there it is transported down the axons and further cleaved to AVP, neurophysin II, and copeptin. Stimulation of the neurons results in an influx of calcium, fusion of the neurosecretory vesicle with the cell membrane, and extrusion of its contents into the systemic circulation.

SECRETION The secretion of AVP is regulated primarily by the "effective" osmotic pressure of body fluids. This control is mediated by specialized cells, known as *osmoreceptors*, which appear to be located in the anteromedial hypothalamus near the supraoptic nucleus. These osmoreceptors are extremely sensitive to small changes in the plasma concentration of sodium and certain other effective solutes such as mannitol but show little or no response to other solutes such as urea or glucose. They appear to have inhibitory as well as stimulatory components that function in concert to regulate AVP secretion around a specific set point. Thus, when plasma osmolality/sodium are depressed to a certain minimum or threshold level of ~280 mosmol/kg or 135 meq/L, respectively, plasma AVP is suppressed to low or undetectable levels and a water diuresis ensues. Conversely, when plasma osmolality/sodium rise above this "threshold," plasma AVP rises steeply in direct proportion, reaching a concentration sufficient to produce a maximum antidiuresis when plasma osmolality/sodium reach ~295 mosmol/kg and 143 meq/L. However, the exact "set" and "sensitivity" of this osmoregulatory system vary appreciably from person to person, apparently as a result of genetic influences, and change during pregnancy, the menstrual cycle, and normal aging; they can also be altered or disrupted by various pathologic conditions.

AVP secretion can also be influenced by acute changes in blood volume or pressure. This baroregulation is mediated largely by neuronal afferents that originate in transmural pressure receptors of the cardiac atria, aorta, and carotid arteries; project via the vagus and glossopharyngeal nerves to the nucleus tractus solitarius of the brain stem; and then ascend to the paraventricular and supraoptic nucleii of the hypothalmus. These pathways regulate AVP release by maintaining a tonic inhibitory tone that decreases when blood volume or pressure falls by >10 to 20%. This baroregulatory system is probably of minor importance in the physiology of AVP secretion because the hemodynamic changes required to affect it are larger than those usually occurring in the course of normal activities. Moreover, moderate he-

FIGURE 329-2 Antidiuretic effect of AVP in the regulation of urine volume. In a typical 70-kg adult, the kidney filters about 180 L /d of plasma. Of this, approximately 144 L (80%) is reabsorbed isosmotically in the proximal tubule and another 8 L (4 to 5%) is reabsorbed without solute in the descending limb of Henle's loop. The remainder is diluted to an osmolality of about 60 mmol/kg by selective reabsorption of sodium and chloride in the ascending limb. In the absence of AVP, the urine issuing from the loop passes largely unmodified through the distal tubules and collecting ducts, resulting in a maximum water diuresis. In the presence of AVP, solute-free water is reabsorbed osmotically through the principal cells of the collecting ducts, resulting in the excretion of a much smaller volume of concentrated urine. This antidiuretic effect is mediated via a G protein–coupled V_2 receptor that increases intracellular cyclic AMP, thereby inducing translocation of aquaporin 2 (AQP2) water channels into the apical membrane. The resultant increase in permeability permits an influx of water that diffuses out of the cell through AQP3 and AQP4 water channels on the basal-lateral surface. The net rate of flux across the cell is determined by the number of AQP2 water channels in the apical membrane and the strength of the osmotic gradient between tubular fluid and the renal medulla. Tight junctions on the lateral surface of the cells serve to prevent unregulated water flow.

modynamic stimuli do not disrupt or override the osmoregulatory system but do lower its threshold or set point by an amount proportional to the magnitude of the hypovolemia or hypotension. However, the baroregulatory system undoubtedly plays an important role in AVP secretion in patients with large, acute disturbances of hemodynamic function.

AVP secretion can also be stimulated by a variety of other nonosmotic variables including nausea, acute hypoglycemia, glucocorticoid deficiency, smoking, and, possibly, hyperangiotensinemia. The emetic stimuli are extremely potent since they typically elicit immediate, 50- to 100-fold increases in plasma AVP, even when the nausea is transient and unassociated with vomiting or other symptoms. They appear to act via the emetic center in the medulla and can be completely blocked by treatment with antiemetics such as fluphenazine. There is no evidence that pain or other noxious stresses have any affect on AVP unless they elicit a vasovagal reaction with its associated nausea and hypotension.

METABOLISM From the venous circulation, AVP distributes rapidly into a space roughly equal in size to the extracellular fluid volume. It is cleared irreversibly from this space with a $t_{1/2}$ of 10 to 30 min. Most AVP clearance is due to degradation in the liver and kidneys. Urinary clearance of the hormone is normally much less than creatinine clearance but can vary as much as tenfold, depending on individual differences and changes in total solute clearance. Therefore, measurement of urinary AVP excretion rates are not always a reliable indicator of changes in secretion or plasma levels of the hormone. During pregnancy, the metabolic clearance of AVP is increased three- to fourfold due to placental production of an N-terminal peptidase.

Table 329-1 Causes of Diabetes Insipidus

Pituitary diabetes insipidus	Nephrogenic diabetes insipidus
Acquired	Acquired
Head trauma (closed and penetrating)	Drugs
Neoplasms	Lithium
Primary	Demeclocycline
Craniopharyngioma	Methoxyflurane
Pituitary adenoma (suprasellar)	Amphotericin B
Dysgerminoma	Aminoglycosides
Meningioma	Cisplatin
Metastatic (lung, breast)	Rifampin
Hematologic (lymphoma, leukemia)	Foscarnet
Granulomas	Metabolic
Neurosarcoid	Hypercalcemia, hypercalciuria
Histiocytosis	Hypokalemia
Xanthoma disseminatum	Obstruction (ureter or urethra)
Infectious	Vascular
Chronic meningitis	Sickle cell disease and trait
Viral encephalitis	Ischemia (acute tubular necrosis)
Toxoplasmosis	Granulomas
Inflammatory	Neurosarcoid
Lymphocytic infundibuloneurohypophysitis	Neoplasms
Wegener's granulomatosis	Sarcoma
Lupus erythematosus	Infiltration
Scleroderma	Amyloidosis
Chemical toxins	Pregnancy
Tetrodotoxin	Idiopathic
Snake venom	Genetic
Vascular	X-linked recessive (AVP receptor-2 gene)
Sheehan's syndrome	Autosomal recessive (aquaporin-2 gene)
Aneurysm (internal carotid)	Autosomal dominant (aquaporin-2 gene)
Aortocoronary bypass	**Primary polydipsia**
Hypoxic encephalopathy	Acquired
Pregnancy (vasopressinase)	Psychogenic
Idiopathic	Schizophrenia
Congenital malformations	Obsessive-compulsive disorder
Septooptic dysplasia	Dipsogenic (abnormal thirst)
Midline craniofacial defects	Granulomas
Holoprosencephaly	Neurosarcoid
Hypogensis, ectopia of pituitary	Infectious
Genetic	Tuberculous meningitis
Autosomal dominant (AVP-neurophysin gene)	Head trauma (closed and penetrating)
Autosomal recessive (AVP-neurophysin gene)	Demyelination
Autosomal recessive-Wolfram-(4p − WFS 1 gene)	Multiple sclerosis
X-linked recessive (Xq28)	Drugs
Deletion chromosome 7q	Lithium
	Carbamazepine
	Idiopathic
	Iatrogenic

THIRST Though AVP regulates the effective osmotic pressure of body fluids by varying the rate of urinary free-water excretion, it cannot reduce insensible or urinary water output below a certain minimum obligatory level. Thus, an additional mechanism—thirst—is essential to prevent hypertonic dehydration. Like AVP, thirst is regulated primarily by an osmostat that is located in the anteromedial hypothalamus and is able to detect very small changes in the plasma concentration of sodium and certain other effective solutes. It functions like the AVP osmostat except that it appears to be "set" slightly higher. This arrangement ensures that thirst, polydipsia, and dilution of body fluids do not occur until dehydration and the resultant rise in plasma osmolality start to exceed the defensive capacity of the antidiuretic mechanism.

OXYTOCIN

Oxytocin is also a nonapeptide and differs from AVP only at positions 3 and 8 (Fig. 329-1). However, it has relatively little antidiuretic effect and seems to act mainly on mammary ducts to facilitate milk letdown during nursing (Chap. 337). It may also help to initiate or facilitate labor by stimulating contraction of uterine smooth muscle, but it is not yet clear if this action is physiologic or necessary for normal delivery. Both the mammary and uterine effects are mediated by a G protein–coupled receptor that is linked to phospholipase C. Antagonists for this receptor have been developed and tested in humans for possible use in treating premature labor.

Oxytocin is also synthesized via a macromolecular precursor that is encoded by a gene located on chromosome 20, very near the AVP gene. However, it differs in orientation and size and encodes only a signal peptide, the hormone, and its associated neurophysin. Oxytocin is also expressed in different magnocellular neurons than AVP and, in humans, is not subject to any of the same regulatory influences. Indeed, with the possible exception of nipple stimulation in the postpartum period, no other stimuli are known to consistently induce release of the hormone in humans. Plasma oxytocin is not increased during pregnancy or at the initiation of labor, although the latter condition may be facilitated by upregulation of oxytocin receptors. The distribution and clearance of oxytocin are similar to those of AVP. Oxytocin is also degraded by the liver and kidneys and an N-terminal peptidase produced by the placenta.

DEFICIENCIES OF VASOPRESSIN SECRETION AND ACTION

DIABETES INSIPIDUS **Clinical Characteristics** Decreased secretion or action of AVP usually manifests as DI, a syndrome characterized by the production of abnormally large volumes of dilute urine. The 24-h urine volume is >50 mL/kg body weight and the osmolality is <300 mmol/kg. The polyuria produces symptoms of urinary frequency, enuresis, and/or nocturia, which may disturb sleep and cause mild daytime fatigue or somnolence. It is also associated with thirst and a commensurate increase in fluid intake (polydipsia). Clinical signs of dehydration are uncommon unless fluid intake is impaired.

Etiology Deficient secretion of AVP can be primary or secondary. The primary form usually results from agenesis or irreversible destruction of the neurohypophysis and is variously referred to as *neurohypophyseal DI, neurogenic DI, pituitary DI, cranial DI,* or *central DI.* It can be caused by a variety of congenital, acquired, or genetic disorders but almost half the time it is idiopathic (Table 329-1). The genetic form of neurohypophyseal DI is usually transmitted in an autosomal dominant mode and is caused by diverse mutations in the coding region of the AVP–neurophysin II gene. The mutant precursor cannot be processed properly or efficiently and eventually destroys the neuron, thereby accounting for the dominant mode of transmission and the delayed onset of the disorder. An X-linked recessive form also occurs. A primary deficiency of plasma AVP can also result from increased metabolism by an N-terminal aminopeptidase produced by the placenta. It is referred to as *gestational DI* since the signs and symptoms manifest during pregnancy and usually remit several weeks after delivery. However, a subclinical deficiency in AVP secretion can often be demonstrated in the nonpregnant state in these individuals, indicating that damage to the neurohypophysis may also contribute to the AVP deficiency. Finally, a primary deficiency of AVP can also result from malformation or destruction of the neurohypophysis by a variety of diseases or toxins (Table 329-1).

Secondary deficiencies of AVP result from inhibition of secretion by excessive intake of fluids. They are referred to as *primary polydip-*

sia and can be divided into three subcategories. One of them, called *dipsogenic DI*, seems to be caused by an inappropriate increase in thirst caused by a reduction in the "set" of the osmoregulatory mechanism. It sometimes occurs in association with multifocal diseases of the brain such as neurosarcoid, tuberculous meningitis, or multiple sclerosis but is often idiopathic. The second subtype, called *psychogenic polydipsia*, is not associated with thirst, and the polydipsia seems to be a feature of psychosis. The third subtype, which may be referred to as *iatrogenic polydipsia*, results from recommendations of health professionals or the popular media to increase fluid intake for its presumed preventive or therapeutic benefits for other disorders.

Primary deficiencies in the antidiuretic action of AVP result in *nephrogenic DI* (Table 329-1). It can be genetic, acquired, or caused by exposure to various drugs. The genetic form is usually transmitted in an X-linked mode and is caused by mutations in the coding region of the V_2 receptor gene. An autosomal recessive form is caused by mutations in the gene encoding the aquaporin protein that forms the water channels in the distal nephron.

Secondary deficiencies in the antidiuretic response to AVP result from polyuria per se. They appear to be caused by washout of the medullary concentration gradient and/or suppression of aquaporin function. They usually resolve 24 to 48 h after the polyuria is corrected but often complicate interpretation of certain acute tests commonly used for differential diagnosis.

Pathophysiology   When the net secretion or antidiuretic effect of AVP is decreased by >80 to 85%, the amount of hormone produced under basal conditions is insufficient to concentrate the urine and the rate of output increases exponentially to symptomatic levels. If the AVP defect is primary (e.g., the patient has pituitary, gestational, or nephrogenic DI), the polyuria results in a small (1 to 2%) decrease in body water and a commensurate increase in plasma osmolality and sodium concentration that stimulate thirst and a compensatory increase in water intake. As a result, *overt physical or laboratory signs of dehydration do not develop unless the patient also has a defect in thirst* (see below) *or fails to drink for some other reason.*

The severity of the defect in antidiuretic function varies markedly among patients with pituitary, gestational, or nephrogenic DI. In some, the deficiencies in AVP secretion or action are so severe that basal urine output approximates the maximum (10 to 15 mL/min); even an intense stimulus such as nausea or severe dehydration does not increase plasma AVP enough to concentrate the urine. In others, however, the deficiency in AVP secretion or action is less pronounced, and a modest stimulus such as a few hours of fluid deprivation, smoking, or a vasovagal reaction increases plasma AVP sufficiently to produce a profound antidiuresis. The maximum urine osmolality achieved in these patients is usually less than normal, largely because their maximal concentrating capacity is temporarily impaired by chronic polyuria per se. However, in a few patients with partial pituitary or nephrogenic DI, it can reach levels as high as 800 mosmol/kg (Fig. 329-3).

In primary polydipsia, the pathogenesis of the polydipsia and polyuria is the reverse of that in neurohypophyseal, nephrogenic, and gestational DI. Thus, the excessive intake of fluids slightly increases body water, thereby reducing plasma osmolality, AVP secretion, and urinary concentration. The latter results in a compensatory increase in urinary free-water excretion that varies in direct proportion to intake. Therefore, clinically appreciable overhydration is uncommon unless the compensatory water diuresis is impaired by a drug or disease that stimulates or mimics endogenous AVP.

FIGURE 329-3   Urine osmolality under basal conditions of *ad libitum*/fluid intake, during fluid deprivation, and after the administration of AVP or DDAVP in patients with primary polydipsia (*left*), pituitary DI (*middle*), or nephrogenic DI (*right*). Normal ranges are depicted by shaded regions. DI, diabetes insipidus.

In the dipsogenic form of primary polydipsia, fluid intake is excessive because the osmotic threshold for thirst appears to be reset to the left, often well below that for AVP release. As a result, thirst is abnormally increased and cannot be completely relieved because plasma AVP is suppressed and an offsetting water diuresis develops before plasma osmolality is reduced sufficiently to eliminate the dipsogenic stimulus. Typically, therefore, patients with dipsogenic DI present with complaints of chronic thirst, polydipsia, and polyuria indistinguishable from those in patients with pituitary, gestational, or nephrogenic DI. When deprived of fluids or subjected to some other acute osmotic or nonosmotic stimulus, they invariably increase plasma AVP normally, but the resultant increase in urine concentration is usually subnormal because their renal capacity to concentrate the urine is also blunted by chronic polyuria. Thus, their antidiuretic response to these stimuli may be indistinguishable from that in patients with partial pituitary, partial gestational, or partial nephrogenic DI (Fig. 329-3).

Differential Diagnosis   When symptoms of urinary frequency, enuresis, nocturia, and/or persistent thirst are present, causes other than polyuria should be excluded. A 24-h urine output > 50 mL/kg per day (>3500 mL in a 70-kg man) is suspicious for DI. If the osmolality of the 24-h urine is >300 mosmol/kg, the patient has a solute diuresis and should be evaluated for uncontrolled diabetes mellitus or other less common causes of excessive solute excretion. However, if the 24-h urine osmolality is <300 mosmol/kg, the patient has a water diuresis and should be evaluated further to determine which type of DI is present.

In differentiating between the various types of DI, the history, physical examination, and routine laboratory tests may be helpful but are rarely sufficient because few, if any, of the findings are pathognomonic. Except in the rare patient who is clearly dehydrated under basal conditions of *ad libitum* fluid intake, this evaluation should begin with a *fluid deprivation test*. To minimize patient discomfort, avoid excessive dehydration, and maximize the information obtained, the test should be started in the morning and water balance should be monitored closely with hourly measurements of body weight, plasma osmolality and/or sodium concentration, and urine volume and osmolality.

If fluid deprivation does not result in urine concentration (osmolality >300 mosmol/kg, specific gravity >1.010) before body weight decreases by 5% or plasma osmolality/sodium exceed the upper limit of normal, primary polydipsia and a partial defect in AVP secretion or action are largely excluded (Fig. 329-3). In these patients, severe pituitary or nephrogenic DI can usually be distinguished by administering desmopressin (DDAVP, 0.03 μg/kg subcutaneously or intravenously) and repeating the measurement of urine osmolality 1 to 2 h

FIGURE 329-4 Relationship of plasma AVP to urine osmolality (*left*) and plasma osmolality (*right*) before and during fluid deprivation-hypertonic saline infusion test in patients with primary polydipsia (●), partial (□) or severe (■) pituitary diabetes insipidus (DI), or partial (△) or severe (▲) nephrogenic DI.

later. An increase of >50% indicates severe pituitary DI, whereas a smaller or absent response is strongly suggestive of nephrogenic DI.

However, these indirect criteria are not useful for diagnosis in patients who concentrate their urine during fluid deprivation, because the changes in urine osmolality are remarkably similar in primary polydipsia and partial pituitary and partial nephrogenic DI (Fig. 329-3). In this situation, the safest and most reliable way to differentiate these conditions is to measure plasma or urine AVP collected before and during the fluid deprivation test and analyze the result in relation to the concurrent plasma or urine osmolality (Fig. 329-4). This approach invariably differentiates partial nephrogenic DI from partial pituitary DI and primary polydipsia. It also differentiates pituitary DI from primary polydipsia if the hormone is measured when plasma osmolality or sodium is clearly above the normal range. However, the requisite level of hypertonic dehydration is difficult to produce by fluid deprivation alone when urine concentration occurs. Therefore, it is usually necessary to add an infusion of hypertonic (3%) saline and repeat the AVP measurements when plasma osmolality rises to >300 mmol/kg ($Na^+ > 145$ mmol/L). This endpoint is usually reached within 30 to 120 min if the hypertonic saline is infused at a rate of 0.1 mL/kg per minute and the fluid deprivation is maintained.

The differential diagnosis of DI may also be facilitated by magnetic resonance imaging (MRI) of the pituitary and hypothalamus. In most healthy adults and children, the posterior pituitary emits a hyperintense signal in T1 weighted mid-saggital images. This "bright spot" is almost invariably absent or abnormally small in patients with pituitary DI but is present in 80 to 90% of those with primary polydipsia. Thus, the presence of a normal bright spot virtually excludes pituitary DI, whereas its absence supports but does not prove this diagnosis. Therefore, the MRI findings must be interpreted with caution and only in conjunction with other diagnostic studies based on assays of AVP or the differential responses to treatment.

℞ **TREATMENT** The signs and symptoms of uncomplicated pituitary DI can be eliminated completely by treatment with DDAVP (Fig. 329-5). It is a synthetic analogue of AVP (Fig. 329-1) that acts selectively at V_2 receptors to increase urine concentration and decrease urine flow in a dose-dependent manner. However, it is more resistant to degradation than AVP and has a three- to fourfold longer duration of action. This property makes it particularly useful in the treatment of gestational DI or pituitary DI during pregnancy. DDAVP can be given by intravenous or subcutaneous injection, nasal inhalation, or oral tablet. The doses required to control pituitary DI completely vary widely, depending on the patient and the route of administration. However, they usually range from 1 to 2 μg qd or bid by

injection, 10 to 20 μg bid or tid by nasal spray, and 100 to 400 μg bid or tid orally. The onset of action is rapid, ranging from as little as 15 min after injection to 60 min after oral administration. When given in doses sufficient to completely normalize urinary osmolality and flow, DDAVP produces a slight (1 to 3%) increase in total-body water and a commensurate decrease in plasma osmolality and sodium concentration that rapidly eliminates thirst and polydipsia. Consequently, water balance is maintained and hyponatremia does not develop unless the patient has an associated abnormality in the osmoregulation of thirst or ingests/receives excessive amounts of fluid for some other reason. Fortunately, abnormal thirst occurs in <10% of patients with pituitary DI, and the other causes of excessive intake can usually be eliminated by educating the patient about the risks of drinking for reasons other than thirst. Therefore, most patients with pituitary DI can take desmopressin in doses sufficient to maintain a normal urine output continuously and do not need to endure the inconvenience and discomfort of allowing intermittent escape to prevent water intoxication.

Pituitary DI can also be treated with chlorpropamide (Diabinese). The mechanism of its antidiuretic action is uncertain but may involve potentiation of the effect of small amounts of AVP or direct activation of the V_2 receptor. In patients with severe as well as partial pituitary DI, doses of chlorpropamide similar to those used in the treatment of diabetes mellitus (125 to 500 mg once daily) increase urine concentration and decrease urine flow, thirst, and polydipsia in a manner similar to DDAVP. The antidiuresis is usually less rapid and smaller than that produced by DDAVP but is almost always sufficient to re-

FIGURE 329-5 Effect of DDAVP therapy on water balance in patient with uncomplicated pituitary diabetes insipidus. Note that treatment rapidly reduces thirst and fluid intake as well as urine output to normal, with only a slight increase in body water (weight) and decrease in plasma osmolality/sodium. [*From Endocrinology and Metabolism, 4th e, P Felig, L Frohman (eds). New York, McGraw-Hill, 2001, with permission.*]

duce urine output by 30 to 70%. Moreover, its antidiuretic effect can be enhanced appreciably by cotreatment with a thiazide diuretic. The ability of water loading to reduce the antidiuretic effect of chlorpropamide makes it particularly useful in the treatment of patients who have pituitary DI and abnormal thirst since it is less likely than DDAVP to produce water intoxication. However, unlike DDAVP, chlorpropamide can have other side effects including hypoglycemia, which can be precipitated by severe reductions in caloric intake or heavy exercise, and it exhibits a disulfuram (Antabuse)-like reaction to ethanol. Chlorpropamide is contraindicated in the treatment of gestational DI because its teratogenicity is unknown.

Primary polydipsia cannot be treated with DDAVP in the usual way because a sustained inhibition of the compensatory water diuresis almost invariably results in the development of water intoxication within 24 to 48 h. This complication can also be caused by administration of a thiazide diuretic, smoking, or other nonosmotic stimuli to endogenous AVP secretion. Iatrogenic polydipsia can often be corrected by patient counseling; however, there is no effective treatment for either psychogenic or dipsogenic DI. In the latter, nocturia or nocturnal enuresis can often be controlled safely by administering a single small dose of DDAVP at bedtime. If the dose is adjusted carefully to provide no more than 8 to 10 h of antidiuresis, it will not result in water intoxication, because patients with dipsogenic, as well as other forms of DI, tend to drink less fluid at night than during the day. Family or other caregivers of patients with psychogenic or dipsogenic DI should also be warned about the hazards of water intoxication caused by a variety of diseases or drugs that can stimulate or mimic the antidiuretic effects of endogenous AVP (see below).

The symptoms and signs of nephrogenic DI are not affected by treatment with DDAVP or chlorpropamide but may be reduced by treatment with a thiazide diuretic and/or amiloride in conjunction with a low-sodium diet. Inhibitors of prostaglandin synthesis (e.g., indomethacin) are also effective in many patients.

ADIPSIC HYPERNATREMIA   **Clinical Characteristics**
Adipsic hypernatremia is characterized by chronic or recurrent hypertonic dehydration and a deficient AVP response to osmotic stimulation. Despite their dehydration, the patients have little or no thirst and may even resist efforts to increase their oral intake of fluids. The hypernatremia varies in severity and is associated with commensurate signs of hypovolemia such as tachycardia, postural hypotension, azotemia, hyperuricemia, and hypokalemia. Muscle weakness, pain, rhabdomyolysis, hyperglycemia, hyperlipidemia, and acute renal failure may also occur. Most patients remain conscious unless they have severe hyperglycemia and/or hypertonicity or go on to develop hyponatremia as a result of excessive rehydration.

Etiology   Adipsic hypernatremia is caused by agenesis or destruction of the hypothalamic osmoreceptors that normally regulate thirst and AVP secretion. The osmoreceptor deficiency can usually be traced to an identifiable congenital or acquired disease in the hypothalamus but is sometimes idiopathic (Table 329-2). The neurohypophysis and its other regulatory afferents are usually spared; an MRI typically shows a normal posterior pituitary bright spot, and the AVP response to nonosmotic stimuli is also normal. Occasionally, the neurohypophysis is also affected, resulting in a combined defect in water balance that is particularly severe and difficult to manage.

Pathophysiology   Lack of thirst and failure to drink enough water to replenish renal and extrarenal losses decrease total-body water and increase plasma osmolality/sodium. Plasma renin activity and aldosterone secretion also increase, and plasma potassium falls due to increased urinary excretion. The severity, frequency, and speed with which hypertonic dehydration develops vary markedly from patient to patient, or from time to time in the same patient, owing largely to differences in the rate of insensible and/or renal loss.

The osmoregulation of AVP secretion is also impaired in nearly all patients with adipsic hypernatremia (Fig. 329-6). This deficiency is obvious when the hormone is measured in the presence of hypertonic dehydration but is rarely severe enough to produce DI. During rehy-

Table 329-2   Causes of Adipsic Hypernatremia

Acquired
  Vascular: Occlusion anterior communicating artery
  Tumors
    Primary
      Craniopharyngioma
      Pinealoma, germinoma
      Meningioma
      Glioma
    Metastatic (lung, breast)
  Granulomas: Neurosarcoid
          Histocytosis
  Trauma: Closed
        Penetrating (pituitary-hypothalamic surgery)
  Psychogenic: Psychotic depression
  Other: Hydrocephalus
      Neurodegenerative
      AIDS, cytomegalovirus encephalitis
  Idiopathic
Congenital
  Midline malformation (septum and corpus callosum)
  Microcephaly
  Genetic: Autosomal recessive (Schinzel-Giedion syndrome)

dration, however, some patients exhibit a further decrease in their plasma AVP and develop DI before their hypernatremia is fully corrected. In other patients, the osmoregulatory deficiency appears to be complete because basal plasma AVP remains relatively fixed, irrespective of whether plasma osmolality and sodium are above, within, or below the normal range. Thus, if overhydrated, these patients do not mount a compensatory water diuresis and quickly develop a hyponatremic syndrome that is clinically and biochemically indistinguishable from acute syndrome of inappropriate antidiuretic hormone, which is commonly referred to as SIADH (see below). In all but a few patients, the abnormality of AVP secretion is limited to the osmoregulatory system since the hormone responds normally to all nonosmotic stimuli, such as nausea.

Differential Diagnosis   Adipsic hypernatremia should be distinguished from the hypernatremia that results from various other causes. These distinctions can usually be made from the history, physical examination, and routine laboratory tests. If a conscious patient denies thirst and/or does not drink vigorously in the presence of significant hypernatremia, the diagnosis of hypodipsia or adipsia can be made with confidence. This diagnosis is supported by laboratory evidence of hypovolemia (azotemia, hypokalemia, hyperuricemia, hyperreninemia) and a relative deficiency of plasma AVP. Close monitoring of these variables and urine osmolality during rehydration is useful for differentiating the patients who develop DI or SIADH in response to forced hydration. If the patient is obtunded or otherwise unable to answer questions or drink at the time of presentation, the possibility of adipsic hypernatremia can be evaluated after treatment by assessing the thirst and plasma AVP response to a controlled fluid deprivation–hypertonic saline infusion test similar to that described for evaluation of DI.

℞ **TREATMENT**   Adipsic hypernatremia should be treated by administering water by mouth, if the patient is alert, or 0.45% saline by vein, if the patient is obtunded or uncooperative. The number of liters of free water that will be required to correct the deficit (ΔFW) can be estimated from body weight in kg (BW) and the serum sodium concentration in mmol/L (S_{Na}) by the formula $\Delta FW = 0.5BW \times [(S_{Na} - 140)/140]$. If serum glucose ($S_{Glu}$) is elevated, the measured S_{Na} should be corrected (S_{Na}^*) by the formula $S_{Na}^* = S_{Na} + [(S_{Glu} - 90)/36]$. This amount plus an allowance for continuing insensible and urinary losses should be given over a 24- to 48-h period. If DI is present or develops during rehydration, DDAVP should also be given in standard doses to minimize urinary losses. If hyperglycemia and/or hypokalemia are present, insulin and/or potassium supplements should

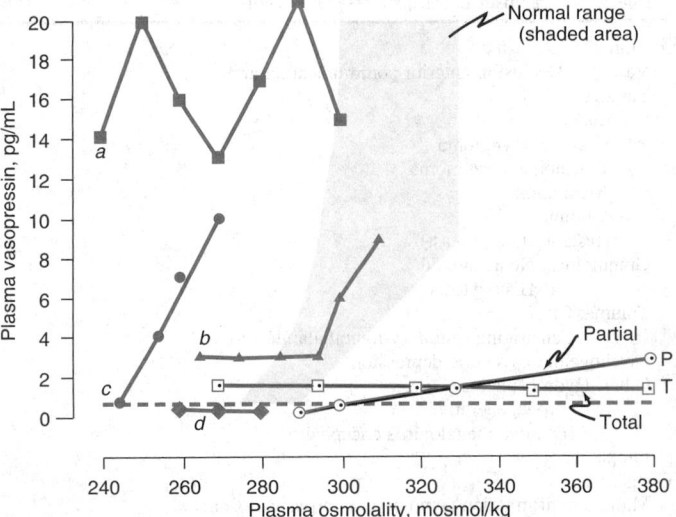

FIGURE 329-6 Heterogeneity of osmoregulatory dysfunction in adipsic hypernatremia (AH) and the syndrome of inappropriate antidiuretic hormone (SIADH). Each line depicts schematically the relationship of plasma AVP to plasma osmolality during water loading and/or infusion of 3% saline in a different patient with either AH (open symbols) or SIADH (closed symbols). The shaded area indicates the normal range of the relationship. The horizontal broken line indicates the plasma AVP level below which the hormone is undetectable and urinary concentration usually does not occur. Lines P and T represent patients with a selective deficiency in the osmoregulation of thirst and AVP that is either partial (○) or total (□). In the latter, plasma AVP does not change in response to increases or decreases in plasma osmolality but remains within a range sufficient to concentrate the urine even if overhydration produces hypotonic hyponatremia. In contrast, if the osmoregulatory deficiency is partial (○), rehydration of the patient suppresses plasma AVP to levels that result in urinary dilution and polyuria before plasma osmolality and sodium are reduced to normal. Lines a–d represent different defects in the osmoregulation of plasma AVP observed in patients with SIADH. In a (■), plasma AVP is markedly elevated and fluctuates widely without relation to changes in plasma osmolality, indicating complete loss of osmoregulation. In b (▲), plasma AVP remains fixed at a slightly elevated level until plasma osmolality reaches the normal range at which point it begins to rise appropriately, indicating a selective defect in the inhibitory component of the osmoregulatory mechanism. In c (●), plasma AVP rises in close correlation with plasma osmolality before the latter reaches the normal range, indicating downward resetting of the osmostat. In d (♦), plasma AVP appears to be osmoregulated normally, suggesting that the inappropriate antidiuresis is caused by some other abnormality.

be given. These variables plus urine output and plasma urea/creatinine should be monitored closely during treatment for signs of emerging DI, SIADH, or acute renal failure.

Once the acute fluid and electrolyte imbalances are corrected, an MRI of the brain and tests of anterior pituitary function should be performed. A long-term management plan to prevent or minimize recurrence of the fluid and electrolyte imbalance should also be developed, including a practical method that the patient can use to regulate fluid intake in accordance with day-to-day variations in water balance. The most effective way to accomplish these objectives is to prescribe DDAVP or chlorpropamide to completely control DI, if it is present, and teach the patient how to use day-to-day changes in body weight as a guide for adjusting fluid intake. Prescribing a constant fluid intake is less satisfactory because it does not take into account the large, uncontrolled variations in insensible loss that inevitably occur.

EXCESS VASOPRESSIN SECRETION AND ACTION

HYPONATREMIA (See also Chap. 49)   **Clinical Characteristics**   Excessive secretion or action of AVP results in the produc-

tion of decreased volumes of more highly concentrated urine. If not accompanied by a commensurate reduction in fluid intake, the reduced suppressibility of AVP results in water retention and a decrease in plasma osmolality/sodium. If the hyponatremia develops gradually or has been present for more than a few days, it may be asymptomatic. However, if it develops acutely, it is almost always accompanied by symptoms and signs of water intoxication that may include mild headache, confusion, anorexia, nausea, vomiting, coma, and convulsions. Severe hyponatremia may be lethal. Depending on the cause of the increased antidiuresis, osmotically inappropriate thirst and/or fluid intake and other disturbances of fluid and electrolyte balance may also be present.

Etiology   Osmotically inappropriate antidiuresis can be caused by a primary defect in AVP secretion or action or can be secondary to a recognized nonosmotic stimulus such as hypovolemia, hypotension, or glucocorticoid deficiency (Table 329-3). The primary forms are generally referred to as SIADH or euvolemic (type III) hyponatremia. They have many different causes, including ectopic production of AVP by lung cancer or other neoplasms, eutopic release by various diseases or drugs, and exogenous administration of AVP, DDAVP, or large doses of oxytocin. The ectopic forms result from abnormal and presumably unregulated expression of the AVP-NPII gene by primary or metastatic malignancies. They do not usually remit unless the ectopic source is eliminated. The eutopic forms manifest most often in patients with acute infections or strokes, but the mechanisms by which these diseases disrupt osmoregulation are not known. A form of acute or chronic hyponatremia very similar to SIADH can also result from stimulation of AVP secretion by protracted nausea or isolated glucocorticoid deficiency. In these patients the excess AVP secretion can be corrected quickly and completely by specific treatments (antiemetics or glucocorticoids) that are not useful in other forms of SIADH.

The secondary forms of osmotically inappropriate antidiuresis are usually divided into two groups: type I (hypervolemic) and type II (hypovolemic) hyponatremia. Type I occurs in sodium-retaining, edema-forming states such as congestive heart failure, cirrhosis, or nephrosis and is thought to be due to a reduction in "effective" blood volume. Type II occurs in sodium-depleted states such as severe gas-

Table 329-3   Causes of Syndrome of Inappropriate Antidiuretic Hormone (SIADH)

Neoplasms	**Neurologic**
Carcinomas	Guillain-Barré syndrome
Lung	Multiple sclerosis
Duodenum	Delerium tremens
Pancreas	Amytrophic lateral sclerosis
Ovary	Hydrocephalus
Bladder, ureter	Psychosis
Other neoplasms	Peripheral neuropathy
Thymoma	Congenital malformations
Mesothelioma	Agenesis corpus callosum
Bronchial adenoma	Cleft lip/palate
Carcinoid	Other midline defects
Gangliocytoma	**Metabolic**
Ewing's sarcoma	Acute intermittent porphyria
Head trauma (closed and penetrating)	**Pulmonary**
Infections	Asthma
Pneumonia, bacterial or viral	Pneumothorax
Abscess, lung or brain	Positive-pressure respiration
Cavitation (aspergillosis)	**Drugs**
Tuberculosis, lung or brain	Vasopressin or DDAVP
Meningitis, bacterial or viral	Chlorpropamide
Encephalitis	Oxytocin, high dose
AIDS	Vincristine
Vascular	Carbamazepine
Cerebrovascular occlusions, hemorrhage	Nicotine
Cavernous sinus thrombosis	Phenothiazines
	Cyclophosphamide
	Tricyclic antidepressants
	Monoamine oxidase inhibitors
	Serotonin reuptake inhibitors

troenteritis, diuretic abuse, or mineralocorticoid deficiency and is probably due to a reduction in blood volume and/or pressure.

Pathophysiology In SIADH, interference with the osmotic suppression of AVP results in significant expansion and dilution of body fluids only if water intake exceeds the rate of insensible and urinary output. These abnormalities in water intake often result from an associated defect in the osmoregulation of thirst but can also be due to psychogenic or iatrogenic factors, including the administration of intravenous fluids.

In SIADH, the defect in the osmoregulation of antidiuretic function can take any of four distinct forms (Fig. 329-6). In one of them, AVP secretion remains fully responsive to changes in plasma osmolality/sodium, but the threshold or set point of the osmoregulatory system is abnormally low. Patients with this kind of downward resetting of the osmostat differ from those with the other types of osmoregulatory defect in that they are able to maximally suppress plasma AVP and dilute their urine if their fluid intake is high enough to reduce their plasma osmolality/sodium to the new set point. Another, smaller subgroup (about 10% of the total) do not have a demonstrable defect in the osmoregulation of AVP (Fig. 329-6). Thus, their inappropriate antidiuresis may be due to other abnormalities such as enhanced renal sensitivity to the antidiuretic effect of normally low levels of AVP or activation of aquaporin 2 water channels by a mechanism that is independent of AVP and V_2 receptors.

The extracellular volume expansion that results from excessive retention of water in SIADH also produces an increase in atrial natriuretic hormone, suppression of plasma renin activity, and a compensatory increase in urinary sodium excretion that serves to reduce the hypervolemia but aggravates the hyponatremia. Thus, hyponatremia is due to a decrease in total-body sodium as well as an increase in total-body water. The acute retention of water and fall in plasma sodium also cause a rise in intracellular volume. The resultant brain swelling increases intracranial pressure and probably causes the acute symptoms of water intoxication. After several days, this intracellular volume expansion may be reduced by inactivation or elimination of intracellular solutes, resulting in the remission of symptoms that often occur with hyponatremia of this duration.

In type I (edematous) or type II (hypovolemic) hyponatremia, the osmotic inhibition of AVP and urine concentration is counteracted by a hemodynamic stimulus that results from a substantial reduction in effective or absolute blood volume. In both cases, the inadequate suppression of AVP appears to be due to downward resetting of the osmostat. The resultant antidiuresis is usually enhanced by decreased distal delivery of filtrate that results from increased reabsorption of sodium in proximal nephrons secondary to the hypovolemia. If it is not associated with a commensurate reduction in water intake, the marked reduction in urine output that ensues also leads to expansion and dilution of body fluids with symptoms of hyponatremia. This attenuates, but does not completely eliminate, the antidiuresis because the amount of water retained is usually insufficient to fully correct the effective or absolute hypovolemia. Unlike SIADH, therefore, plasma renin activity is elevated, causing secondary hyperaldosteronism and hypokalemia. The disturbance in salt and water balance that underlies the hyponatremia also differs from SIADH in that total-body sodium as well as water is increased in type I, whereas both are decreased in type II.

Differential Diagnosis When unexplained symptoms or signs consistent with water intoxication are present, serum sodium should be measured. If it is low and the reduction cannot be accounted for by an increase in plasma glucose or other solutes such as mannitol (e.g., plasma osmolality is also low), the type of hypotonic hyponatremia present can be determined by estimating extracellular fluid volume from the history, physical examination, and routine chemistries. If these findings are ambiguous or contradictory, measuring the rate of urinary sodium excretion or plasma renin activity may be helpful. These measurements can be misleading, however, if SIADH is stable or resolving or if the patient has type II hyponatremia due to a primary defect in renal conservation of sodium, surreptitious diuretic abuse, or

hyporeninemic hypoaldosteronism. The latter may be suspected if serum potassium is elevated instead of low as is usually seen in types I and II hyponatremia. Measurements of plasma AVP are currently of no diagnostic value since they exhibit the same wide variation in abnormalities in all three types of hyponatremia. In patients who fulfill the clinical criteria for SIADH, plasma cortisol should also be measured to rule out unsuspected secondary adrenal insufficiency. If this is normal and there is no other obvious cause for SIADH, a careful search for occult lung cancer should also be undertaken.

℞ TREATMENT In acute SIADH, the keystone to treatment of hyponatremia is to restrict total fluid intake to less than the sum of insensible losses and urinary output. Total intake should include the water derived from food (300 to 500 mL/d). Because insensible losses in adults usually approximate 500 mL/d total discretionary intake (all water in liquid form) should be at least 500 mL less than urinary output. If achieved, this deficit usually reduces body water and increases serum sodium by about 1 to 2% per day. If more rapid correction of the hyponatremia is desired to eliminate severe symptoms or signs, the fluid restriction can be supplemented by intravenous infusion of hypertonic (3%) saline. This treatment has the advantage of correcting the sodium deficiency that is partly responsible for the hyponatremia as well as producing a solute diuresis that serves to remove some of the excess water. However, if the hyponatremia has been present for more than 24 to 48 h and is corrected too rapidly, the saline infusion also has the potential to produce central pontine myelinolysis, an acute, potentially fatal neurologic syndrome characterized by quadriparesis, ataxia, and abnormal extraocular movements (Chap. 376). The following guidelines appear to minimize, if not eliminate, the risk of this complication: the 3% saline should be infused a rate ≤0.05 mL/kg body weight per minute; the effect should be monitored continuously by STAT measurements of serum sodium at least once every hour; and the infusion should be stopped as soon as serum sodium increases by 12 mmol/L or to 130 mmol/L, whichever comes first. Urinary output should also be monitored continuously since spontaneous remission of the SIADH can result in an acute water diuresis that greatly accelerates the rate of rise in serum sodium produced by fluid restriction and 3% saline infusion.

In chronic SIADH, the hyponatremia can be minimized or eliminated by treatment with demeclocycline, 150 to 300 mg orally three or four times a day, or fludrocortisone, 0.05 to 0.2 mg orally twice a day. The effect of the demeclocycline manifests in 7 to 14 days and is due to production of a reversible form of nephrogenic DI. Potential side effects include phototoxicity and azotemia. The effect of fludrocortisone also manifests in 1 to 2 weeks and is partly due to increased retention of sodium and possibly inhibition of thirst. It also increases urinary potassium excretion, which may require replacement through dietary adjustments or supplements. Fludrocortisone may induce hypertension, occasionally necessitating discontinuation of the treatment.

One or more nonpeptide AVP antagonists that block the antidiuretic effect of AVP may soon be approved for use in the United States. Preliminary studies with these antagonists in acute or chronic SIADH indicate that they produce a dose-dependent increase in urinary free-water excretion, which, if combined with a modest restriction of fluid intake, gradually reduces body water and corrects the hyponatremia without any recognized adverse effect. Thus, they may become the treatment of choice for those forms of SIADH in which there is inappropriate secretion of AVP that cannot be corrected by other, more specific therapy such as antiemetics or glucocorticoids.

When an SIADH-like syndrome is due to protracted nausea and vomiting or isolated glucocorticoid deficiency, all abnormalities can be corrected quickly and completely by giving an antiemetic or hydrocortisone. As with other treatments, care must be taken to ensure that serum sodium does not rise too quickly or too far.

In type I hyponatremia, the only treatment currently available is severe fluid restriction, administration of urea or mannitol to produce a solute diuresis, and/or administration of cardiotonics or serum albumin to correct the effective hypovolemia. None of these treatments is particularly effective, and some (e.g., administration of mannitol or albumin) carry significant risks. Infusion of hypertonic saline is contraindicated because it worsens the sodium retention and edema and may precipitate cardiovascular decompensation. However, preliminary studies indicate that the AVP antagonists may be almost as effective and safe in type I hyponatremia as they are in SIADH. Thus, they may become the treatment of choice for this form of hyponatremia also.

In type II hyponatremia, the defect in AVP secretion and water balance can usually be corrected easily and quickly by stopping the loss of sodium and water and/or replacing the deficits by mouth or intravenous infusion of normal or hypertonic saline. As with the treatment of other forms of hyponatremia, care must be taken to ensure that plasma sodium does not increase too rapidly. Fluid restriction or administration of AVP antagonists is contraindicated as they would only aggravate the underlying volume depletion and could result in cardiovascular decompensation.

BIBLIOGRAPHY

BICHET DG: Vasopressin receptors in health and disease. Kidney Int 49:1706, 1996

————, FUJIWARA TM: Diversity of nephrogenic diabetes insipidus mutations and importance of early recognition and treatment. Clin Exp Nephrol 2:253, 1998

DRINCIC A, ROBERTSON GL: Treatment of diabetes insipidus, in *Hormone Replacement Therapy for Contemporary Endocrinology*, AW Miekle (ed). Totowa, NJ, Humana Press, 1999, pp 21–38

HANSEN LK et al: The genetic basis of familial neurohypophyseal diabetes insipidus. Trends Endocrinol Metab 8:363, 1997

KNEPPER MA: Molecular physiology of urinary concentrating mechanism: Regulation of aquaporin water channels by vasopressin. Am J Physiol 272:F3, 1997

KOVACS L, ROBERTSON GL: Syndrome of inappropriate antidiuresis. Endocrinol Metab Clin North Am 21:859, 1992

OHNISHI A et al: Potent aquaretic agent: A novel nonpeptide selective vasopressin 2 antagonist (OPC-31260) in men. J Clin Invest 92:2653, 1993

ROBERTSON GL: Disorders of thirst in man, in *Thirst: Physiological and Psychological Aspects*, D Ramsey (ed). London, Springer, 1991, pp 453–475

————: The use of vasopressin assays in vasopressin physiology and pathophysiology. Semin Nephrol 14:368, 1994

VERBALIS JG: Hyponatremia: Epidemiology, pathophysiology, and therapy. Curr Opin Nephrol Hypertens 2:636, 1993

330

J. Larry Jameson, Anthony P. Weetman

DISORDERS OF THE THYROID GLAND

AIT	amiodarone-induced thyrotoxicosis	RTH	resistance to thyroid hormone
ATC	anaplastic thyroid cancer	RXRs	retinoic acid X receptors
CT	computed tomography	SES	sick euthyroid syndrome
ESR	erythrocyte sedimentation rate	SLE	systemic lupus erythematosus
FNA	fine-needle aspiration	TBG	thyroxine-binding globulin
FTC	follicular thyroid cancer	TBII	TSH-binding inhibiting immunoglobulins
GPCR	G protein–coupled receptor	Tg	thyroglobulin
hCG	human chorionic gonadotropin	TPO	thyroid peroxidase
IFN	interferon	TRH	thyrotropin-releasing hormone
ILs	interleukins	TRs	thyroid hormone receptors
IRMAs	immunoradiometric assays	TSH	thyroid-stimulating hormone
MEN	multiple endocrine neoplasia	TSH-R	thyroid-stimulating hormone receptor
MNG	multinodular goiter	TSI	thyroid-stimulating immunoglobulins
MRI	magnetic resonance imaging	TTF	thyroid transcription factor
MTC	medullary thyroid cancer	TTR	transthyretin
NIS	sodium iodide symporter		
PTC	papillary thyroid cancer		

The thyroid gland produces two related hormones, thyroxine (T_4) and triiodothyronine (T_3) (Fig. 330-1). These hormones play a critical role in cell differentiation during development and help to maintain thermogenic and metabolic homeostasis in the adult. Thyroid hormones act through nuclear hormone receptors to modulate gene expression. Disorders of the thyroid gland result primarily from autoimmune processes that either stimulate the overproduction of thyroid hormones (*thyrotoxicosis*) or cause glandular destruction and underproduction of thyroid hormones (*hypothyroidism*). In addition, neoplastic processes in the thyroid gland can lead to benign nodules and various forms of thyroid cancer.

ANATOMY AND DEVELOPMENT

The thyroid gland is located in the neck, anterior to the trachea, between the cricoid cartilage and the suprasternal notch. The thyroid (Greek *thyreos*, shield, plus *eidos*, form) consists of two lobes that are connected by an isthmus. It is normally 12 to 20 g in size, highly vascular, and soft in consistency. Four parathyroid glands, which produce parathyroid hormone (Chap. 341), are located in the posterior region of each pole of the thyroid. The recurrent laryngeal nerves traverse the lateral borders of the thyroid gland and must be identified during thyroid surgery to avoid vocal cord paralysis.

The thyroid gland develops from the floor of the primitive pharynx during the third week of gestation. The gland migrates from the foramen cecum, at the base of the tongue, along the thyroglossal duct to reach its final location in the neck. This feature accounts for the rare ectopic location of thyroid tissue at the base of the tongue (lingual thyroid), as well as for the presence of thyroglossal duct cysts along this developmental tract. Thyroid hormone synthesis normally begins at about 11 weeks' gestation.

The parathyroid glands migrate from the third (inferior glands) and fourth (superior glands) pharyngeal pouches before becoming embedded in the thyroid gland. Neural crest derivatives from the ultimobranchial body give rise to thyroid medullary C cells that produce calcitonin, a calcium-lowering hormone. The C cells are interspersed throughout the thyroid gland, although their density is greatest in the juncture of the upper one-third and lower two-thirds of the gland.

Thyroid gland development is controlled by a series of developmental transcription factors. Thyroid transcription factor (TTF) 1 (also known as NKX2A), TTF-2 (also known as FKHL15), and paired homeobox-8 (PAX-8) are expressed selectively, but not exclusively, in the thyroid gland. In combination, they orchestrate thyroid cell development and the induction of thyroid-specific genes such as thyroglobulin (Tg), thyroid peroxidase (TPO), the sodium iodide symporter (NIS), and the thyroid-stimulating hormone receptor (TSH-R). Mutations in these developmental transcription factors or their downstream target genes are rare causes of thyroid agenesis or dyshormonogenesis and can cause congenital hypothyroidism (Table 330-1). Congenital hypothyroidism is common enough (approximately 1 in 3000 to 4000 newborns) that neonatal screening is now performed in most industrialized countries (see below). Though the underlying causes of most cases of congenital hypothyroidism are unknown, early treatment with thyroid hormone replacement precludes potentially severe developmental abnormalities.

The mature thyroid gland contains numerous follicles composed of thyroid follicular cells that surround secreted colloid, a proteinaceous fluid that contains large amounts of thyroglobulin, the protein precursor of thyroid hormones (Fig. 330-2). The thyroid follicular cells are polarized—the basolateral surface is apposed to the bloodstream and an apical surface faces the follicular lumen. Increased demand for thyroid hormone, usually signaled by thyroid-stimulating hormone (TSH) binding to its receptor on the basolateral surface of the follicular cells, leads to Tg reabsorption from the follicular lumen and proteolysis within the cell to yield thyroid hormones for secretion into the bloodstream.

REGULATION OF THE THYROID AXIS

TSH, secreted by the thyrotrope cells of the anterior pituitary, plays a pivotal role in control of the thyroid axis and serves as the most useful physiologic marker of thyroid hormone action. TSH is a 31-kDa hormone composed of α and β subunits; the α subunit is common to the other glycoprotein hormones [luteinizing hormone, follicle-stimulating hormone, human chorionic gonadotropin (hCG)], whereas the TSH β subunit is unique to TSH. The extent and nature of carbohydrate modification are modulated by thyrotropin-releasing hormone (TRH) stimulation and influence the biologic activity of the hormone. TSH has been produced recombinantly and is approved for use in the detection of residual thyroid cancer (see "Follow-up Whole-Body Scanning and Thyroglobulin Determinations," below).

The thyroid axis is a classic example of an endocrine feedback loop. Hypothalamic TRH stimulates pituitary production of TSH, which, in turn, stimulates thyroid hormone synthesis and secretion. Thyroid hormones feed back negatively to inhibit TRH and TSH production (Fig. 330-2). The "set-point" in this axis is established by TSH, the level of which is a sensitive and specific marker of thyroid function. TRH is the major positive regulator of TSH synthesis and secretion. TRH acts through a seven-transmembrane G protein–coupled receptor (GPCR) that activates phospholipase C to generate phosphatidylinositol turnover and the release of intracellular calcium. Peak TSH secretion occurs ~15 min after administration of exogenous TRH. Dopamine, glucocorticoids, and somatostatin suppress TSH but are not of major physiologic importance except when these agents are administered in pharmacologic doses. Reduced levels of thyroid hormone increase basal TSH production and enhance TRH-mediated stimulation of TSH. High thyroid hormone levels rapidly and directly suppress TSH and inhibit TRH-mediated stimulation of TSH, indicating that thyroid hormones are the dominant regulator of TSH production. Like other pituitary hormones, TSH is released in a pulsatile manner and exhibits a diurnal rhythm; its highest levels occur at night. However, these TSH excursions are modest in comparison to those of other pituitary hormones, in part because TSH has a relatively long plasma half-life (50 min). Consequently, single measurements of TSH are adequate for assessing its circulating level. TSH is measured using immunoradiometric assays that are highly sensitive and specific. These assays are capable of distinguishing between normal and suppressed TSH values, thus allowing TSH to be used for the diagnosis of hyperthyroidism (low TSH) as well as hypothyroidism (high TSH).

THYROID HORMONE SYNTHESIS, METABOLISM, AND ACTION

THYROID HORMONE SYNTHESIS Thyroid hormones are derived from Tg, a large iodinated glycoprotein. After secretion into the thyroid follicle, Tg is iodinated on selected tyrosine residues that are subsequently coupled via an ether linkage. Reuptake of Tg into the thyroid follicular cell allows proteolysis and the release of T_4 and T_3.

Iodine Metabolism and Transport Iodide uptake is a critical first step in thyroid hormone synthesis. Ingested iodine is bound to serum proteins, particularly albumin. Unbound iodine is excreted in the urine. The thyroid gland extracts iodine from the circulation in a highly efficient manner. For example, 10 to 25% of radioactive tracer (e.g., ^{123}I) is taken up by the normal thyroid gland over 24 h; this value can rise to 70 to 90% in Graves' disease.

Iodide uptake is mediated by the Na^+/I^- symporter (NIS), which is expressed at the basolateral membrane of thyroid follicular cells. NIS is most highly expressed in the thyroid gland but is also expressed at low levels in the salivary glands, lactating breast, and placenta. The iodide transport mechanism is highly regulated, allowing adaptation to variations in dietary supply. Low iodine levels increase the amount of NIS and stimulate uptake, whereas high iodine levels suppress NIS expression and uptake. The selective expression of the NIS in the thyroid allows isotopic scanning, treatment of hyperthyroidism, and ablation of thyroid cancer with radioisotopes of iodine, without significant effects on other organs. Mutation of the *NIS* gene is a rare cause of congenital hypothyroidism, underscoring its importance in thyroid hormone synthesis.

Iodine deficiency is prevalent in many mountainous regions and in central Africa, central South America, and northern Asia. In areas of relative iodine deficiency, there is an increased prevalence of goiter and, when deficiency is severe, hypothyroidism and cretinism. *Cretinism* is characterized by mental and growth retardation and occurs when children who live in iodine-deficient regions are not treated with iodine or thyroid hormone to restore normal thyroid hormone levels during early childhood. These children are often born to mothers with iodine deficiency, suggesting that maternal thyroid hormone deficiency worsens the condition. Concomitant selenium deficiency may also contribute to the neurologic manifestations of cretinism. Iodine supplemen-

FIGURE 330-1 Structures of thyroid hormones. Thyroxine (T_4) contains four iodine atoms. Deiodination leads to production of the potent hormone, triiodothyronine (T_3), or the inactive hormone, reverse T_3.

Thyroxine (T4)
3,5,3′,5′-Tetraiodothyronine

Deiodinase 1 or 2
(5′-Deiodination)

Deiodinase 3 > 2
(5-Deiodination)

Tri-iodothyronine (T3)
3,5,3′-Triiodothyronine

Reverse T3 (rT3)
3,3′,5′-Triiodothyronine

Table 330-1 Genetic Causes of Congenital Hypothyroidism

Defective Gene Protein	Inheritance	Consequences
PROP-1	Autosomal recessive	Combined pituitary hormone deficiencies with preservation of ACTH
PIT-1	Autosomal recessive Autosomal dominant	Combined deficiencies of growth hormone, prolactin, thyroid-stimulating hormone (TSH)
TSHβ	Autosomal recessive	TSH deficiency
TTF-2	Autosomal recessive	Thyroid agenesis, choanal atresia, spiky hair
PAX-8	Autosomal dominant	Thyroid dysgenesis
TSH-receptor	Autosomal recessive	Resistance to TSH
$G_{s\alpha}$ (Albright hereditary osteodystrophy)	Autosomal dominant	Resistance to TSH
Na^+/I^- symporter	Autosomal recessive	Inability to transport iodide
Thyroid peroxidase	Autosomal recessive	Defective organification of iodide
Thyroglobulin	Autosomal recessive	Defective synthesis of thyroid hormone
Pendrin (anion transporter)	Autosomal recessive	Pendred's syndrome: sensorineural deafness and partial organification defect in thyroid
Dehalogenase	Autosomal recessive	Loss of iodide reutilization

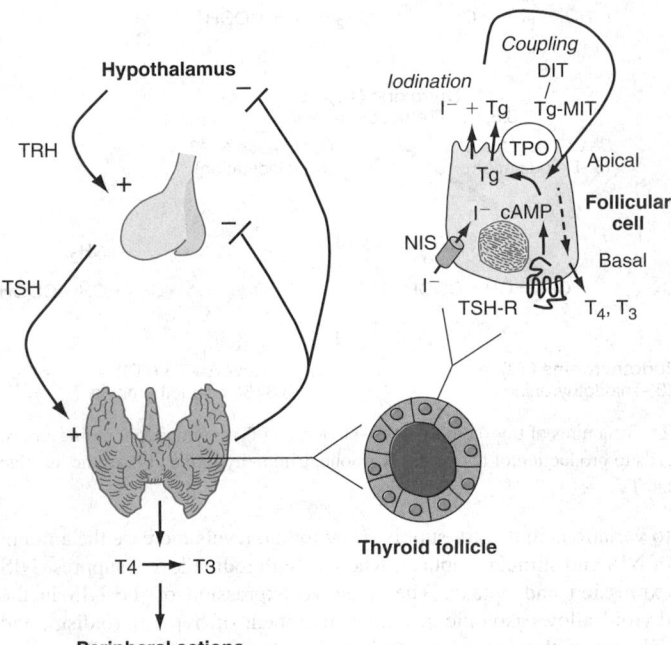

FIGURE 330-2   Regulation of thyroid hormone synthesis. *Left.* Thyroid hormones T_4 and T_3 feed back to inhibit hypothalamic production of thyrotropin-releasing hormone (TRH) and pituitary production of thyroid-stimulating hormone (TSH). TSH stimulates thyroid gland production of T_4 and T_3. *Right.* Thyroid follicles are formed by thyroid epithelial cells surrounding proteinaceous colloid, which contains thyroglobulin. Follicular cells, which are polarized, synthesize thyroglobulin and carry out thyroid hormone biosynthesis (see text for details). TSH-R, thyroid-stimulating hormone receptor; Tg, thyroglobulin; NIS, sodium-iodide symporter; TPO, thyroid peroxidase; DIT, di-iodotyrosine; MIT, monoiodotyrosine

tation of salt, bread, and other food substances has markedly reduced the prevalence of cretinism. Unfortunately, however, iodine deficiency remains the most common cause of preventable mental deficiency, often because of resistance to the use of food additives or the cost of supplementation. In addition to overt cretinism, mild iodine deficiency can lead to subtle reduction of IQ. Iodine intake is assessed by determination of excretion in a 24-h urine collection. Oversupply of iodine, through supplements or foods enriched in iodine (e.g., shellfish, kelp), is associated with an increased incidence of autoimmune thyroid disease. The recommended average daily intake of iodine is 150 μg/d for adults, 90 to 120 μg/d for children, and 200 μg/d for pregnant women.

Organification, Coupling, Storage, Release   After iodide enters the thyroid, it is trapped and transported to the apical membrane of thyroid follicular cells where it is oxidized in an organification reaction that involves TPO and hydrogen peroxide. The reactive iodine atom is added to selected tyrosyl residues within Tg, a large (660 kDa) dimeric protein consisting of 2769 amino acids. The iodotyrosines in Tg are then coupled via an ether linkage in a reaction that is also catalyzed by TPO. Either T_4 or T_3 can be produced by this reaction, depending on the number of iodine atoms present in the iodotyrosines. After coupling, Tg is taken back into the thyroid cell where it is processed in lysosomes to release T_4 and T_3. Uncoupled mono- and diiodotyrosines (MIT, DIT) are deiodinated by the enzyme dehalogenase, thereby recycling any iodide that is not converted into thyroid hormones.

Disorders of thyroid hormone synthesis are rare causes of congenital hypothyroidism. The vast majority of these disorders are due to recessive mutations in TPO or Tg, but defects have also been identified in the TSH-R, NIS, the pendrin anion transporter, hydrogen peroxide generation, and in dehalogenase. Because of the biosynthetic defect, the gland is incapable of synthesizing adequate amounts of hormone, leading to increased TSH and a large goiter.

TSH Action   TSH regulates thyroid gland function through the TSH-R, a seven-transmembrane GPCR. The TSH-R is coupled to the α subunit of stimulatory G protein ($G_{s\alpha}$) and activates adenylyl cyclase, leading to increased production of cyclic AMP. TSH also stimulates phosphatidylinositol turnover by activating phospholipase C. The functional role of the TSH-R has been underscored by naturally occurring mutations. Recessive loss-of-function mutations are a rare cause of thyroid hypoplasia and congenital hypothyroidism. Dominant gain-of-function mutations cause sporadic or familial nonautoimmune hyperthyroidism that is characterized by goiter, thyroid cell hyperplasia, and autonomous function. Most of these activating mutations involve in amino acid substitutions in the transmembrane domain of the receptor. They are thought to mimic conformational changes in the receptor similar to those induced by TSH binding or the interactions of thyroid-stimulating immunoglobulins (TSI) in Graves' disease. Activating TSH-R mutations also occur as somatic events and lead to clonal selection and expansion of the affected thyroid follicular cell (see below).

Factors that Influence Hormone Synthesis and Release   TSH is the dominant hormonal regulator of thyroid gland growth and function. However, a variety of growth factors, most produced locally in the thyroid gland, also influence thyroid hormone synthesis. These include insulin-like growth factor I (IGF-I), epidermal growth factor, transforming growth factor β (TGF-β), endothelins, and various cytokines. The quantitative roles of these factors are not well understood, but they are important in selected disease states. In acromegaly, for example, increased levels of growth hormone and IGF-I are associated with goiter and predisposition to multinodular goiter. Certain cytokines and interleukins (ILs) produced in association with autoimmune thyroid disease induce thyroid growth, whereas others lead to apoptosis. As noted above, iodine is an important regulator of thyroid function. For example, iodine deficiency increases thyroid blood flow and stimulates uptake by the NIS. Excess iodide transiently inhibits thyroid iodide organification, a phenomenon known as the *Wolff-Chaikoff effect*. In individuals with a normal thyroid, the gland escapes from this inhibitory effect and iodide organification resumes; the suppressive action of high iodide may persist, however, in patients with underlying autoimmune thyroid disease.

THYROID HORMONE TRANSPORT AND METABOLISM   **Serum Binding Proteins** T_4 is secreted from the thyroid gland in at least 20-fold excess over T_3 (Table 330-2). Both hormones circulate bound to plasma proteins, including thyroxine-binding globulin (TBG), transthyretin (TTR, formerly known as thyroxine-binding prealbumin, or TBPA), and albumin. The functions of serum-binding proteins are to increase the pool of circulating hormone, delay hormone clearance, and perhaps to modulate hormone delivery to selected tissue sites. The concentration of TBG is relatively low (1 to 2 mg/dL), but because of its high affinity for thyroid hormones ($T_4 > T_3$), it carries about 80% of the bound hormones. Albumin has relatively low affinity for thyroid hormones but has a high plasma concentration ($\sim$3.5 g/dL), and it binds up to 10% of T_4 and 30% of T_3. TTR also carries about 10% of T_4 but little T_3.

Table 330-2   Characteristics of Circulating T_4 and T_3

Hormone Property	T_4	T_3
Serum concentrations		
Total hormone	8 μg/dL	0.14 μg/dL
Fraction of total hormone in the free form	0.02%	0.3%
Free hormone	21×10^{-12} M	6×10^{-12} M
Serum half-life	7 d	0.75 d
Fraction directly from the thyroid	100%	20%
Production rate, including peripheral conversion	90 μg/d	32 μg/d
Intracellular hormone fraction	$\sim$20%	$\sim$70%
Relative metabolic potency	0.3	1
Receptor binding	10^{-10} M	10^{-11} M

When the effects of the various binding proteins are combined, approximately 99.98% of T_4 and 99.7% of T_3 are protein-bound. Because T_3 is less tightly bound than T_4, the amount of free T_3 is greater than free T_4, even though there is less total T_3 in the circulation. The unbound, or free, concentrations of the hormones are $\sim 2 \times 10^{-11}\ M$ for T_4 and $\sim 6 \times 10^{-12}\ M$ for T_3, which roughly correspond to the thyroid hormone receptor binding constants for these hormones (see below). Only the free hormone is biologically available to tissues. Therefore, homeostatic mechanisms that regulate the thyroid axis are directed towards maintenance of normal concentrations of free hormones.

Dysalbuminemic Hyperthyroxinemia A number of inherited and acquired abnormalities affect thyroid hormone binding proteins. X-linked TBG deficiency is associated with very low levels of total T_4 and T_3. However, because free hormone levels are normal, patients are euthyroid and TSH levels are normal. The importance of recognizing this disorder is to avoid efforts to normalize total T_4 levels, as this leads to thyrotoxicosis and is futile because of rapid hormone clearance in the absence of TBG. TBG levels are elevated by estrogen because of increased sialylation and delayed TBG clearance. Consequently, in women who are pregnant or taking estrogen-containing contraceptives, elevated TBG increases total T_4 and T_3 levels; however, free T_4 and T_3 levels are normal. Mutations in TBG, TTR, and albumin that increase binding affinity for T_4 and/or T_3 cause disorders known as *euthyroid hyperthyroxinemia* or *familial dysalbuminemic hyperthyroxinemia* (FDH) (Table 330-3). These disorders are usually

Table 330-3 Conditions Associated with Euthyroid Hyperthyroxinemia

Disorder	Cause	Transmission	Characteristics
Familial dysalbuminemic hyperthyroxinemia (FDH)	Albumin mutations, usually R218H	AD	Increased T_4 Normal free T_4 Rarely increased T_3
TBG			
Familial excess	Increased TBG production	XL	Increased total T_4, T_3 Normal free T_4, T_3
Acquired excess	Medications (estrogen), pregnancy, cirrhosis, hepatitis	Acquired	Increased total T_4, T_3 Normal free T_4, T_3
Transthyretin[a]			
Excess	Islet tumors	Acquired	Usually normal T_4, T_3
Mutations	Increased affinity for T_4 or T_3	AD	Increased total T_4, T_3 Normal free T_4, T_3
Medications: propranolol, ipodate, iopanoic acid, amiodarone	Decreased $T_4 \rightarrow T_3$ conversion	Acquired	Increased T_4 Decreased T_3 Normal or increased TSH
Sick-euthyroid syndrome	Acute illness, especially psychiatric disorders	Acquired	Transiently increased free T_4 Decreased TSH T_4 and T_3 may also be decreased (see text)
Resistance to thyroid hormone (RTH)	Thyroid hormone receptor β mutations	AD	Increased free T_4, T_3 Normal or increased TSH Some patients clinically thyrotoxic

[a] Also known as thyroxine-binding prealbumin, TBPA.
NOTE: AD, autosomal dominant; TBG, thyroxine-binding globulin; TSH, thyroid-stimulating hormone; XL, X-linked.

dominantly transmitted and result in increased total T_4 and/or T_3, but free hormone levels are normal. The familial nature of the disorders, and the fact that TSH levels are normal rather than suppressed, should suggest the diagnosis. Free hormone levels (ideally measured by dialysis) are normal in FDH. The diagnosis can be confirmed, if necessary, by using tests that measure the affinities of radiolabeled hormone binding to specific transport proteins or by performing DNA sequence analyses of the abnormal transport protein genes.

Certain medications, such as salicylates and salsalate, can displace thyroid hormones from circulating binding proteins. Though these drugs transiently perturb the thyroid axis by increasing free thyroid hormone levels, TSH is suppressed until a new steady state is reached, thereby restoring euthyroidism. Circulating factors associated with acute illness may also displace thyroid hormone from binding proteins (see "Sick Euthyroid Syndrome," below).

Deiodinases In many respects, T_4 may be thought of as a precursor for the more potent T_3. T_4 is converted to T_3 by the deiodinase enzymes (Fig. 330-1). Type I deiodinase, which is located primarily in thyroid, liver, and kidney, has a relatively low affinity for T_4. Type II deiodinase has a higher affinity for T_4 and is found primarily in the pituitary gland, brain, brown fat, and thyroid gland. The presence of type II deiodinase allows it to regulate T_3 concentrations locally, a property that may be important in the context of levothyroxine (T_4) replacement. Type II deiodinase is also regulated by thyroid hormone—hypothyroidism induces the enzyme, resulting in enhanced $T_4 \rightarrow T_3$ conversion in tissues such as brain and pituitary. $T_4 \rightarrow T_3$ conversion may be impaired by fasting, systemic illness or acute trauma, oral contrast agents, and a variety of medications (e.g., propylthiouracil, propranolol, amiodarone, glucocorticoids). Type III deiodinase inactivates T_4 and T_3 and is the most important source of reverse T_3 (rT_3).

THYROID HORMONE ACTION **Nuclear Thyroid Hormone Receptors** Thyroid hormones act by binding to nuclear receptors, termed *thyroid hormone receptors* (TRs) α and β. Both TRα and TRβ are expressed in most tissues, but their relative levels of expression vary among organs; TRα is particularly abundant in brain, kidney, gonads, muscle, and heart, whereas TRβ expression is relatively high in the pituitary and liver. Both receptors are variably spliced to form unique isoforms. The TRβ2 isoform, which has a unique amino terminus, is selectively expressed in the hypothalamus and pituitary, where it appears to play a role in feedback control of the thyroid axis. The TRα2 isoform contains a unique carboxy terminus that prevents thyroid hormone binding; it may function to block the action of other TR isoforms.

The TRs contain a central DNA-binding domain and a C-terminal ligand-binding domain. They bind to specific DNA sequences, termed *thyroid response elements* (TREs), in the promoter regions of target genes (Fig. 330-3). The activated receptor can either stimulate gene transcription (e.g., myosin heavy chain α) or inhibit transcription (e.g., TSH β-subunit gene), depending on the nature of the regulatory elements in the target gene. The receptors bind as homodimers or as heterodimers with retinoic acid X receptors (RXRs) (Chap. 327).

Thyroid hormones bind with similar affinities to TRα and TRβ. However, T_3 is bound to its receptors with about 10 to 15 times greater affinity than T_4, which explains its increased hormonal potency. Though T_4 is produced in excess of T_3, receptors are occupied mainly by T_3, reflecting $T_4 \rightarrow T_3$ conversion by peripheral tissues, greater T_3 bioavailability in the plasma, and receptors' greater affinity for T_3. After binding to TRs, thyroid hormone induces conformational changes in the receptors that modify its interactions with accessory transcription factors. In the absence of thyroid hormone binding, the aporeceptors bind to corepressor proteins that inhibit gene transcription. Hormone binding dissociates the corepressors and allows the recruitment of coactivators that enhance transcription. The discovery of TR interactions with corepressors explains the fact that TR silences gene expression in the absence of hormone binding. Consequently,

FIGURE 330-3 Mechanism of thyroid hormone receptor action. The thyroid hormone receptor (TR) and retinoid X receptor (RXR) form heterodimers that bind specifically to thyroid hormone response elements (TRE) in the promoter regions of target genes. In the absence of hormone, TR binds corepressor (CoR) proteins that silence gene expression. The numbers refer to a series of ordered reactions that occur in response to thyroid hormone: (1) T_4 or T_3 enters the nucleus; (2) T_3 binding dissociates CoR from TR; (3) Coactivators (CoA) are recruited to the T_3-bound receptor; (4) gene expression is altered.

hormone deficiency has a profound effect on gene expression because it causes active gene repression as well as loss of hormone-induced stimulation. This concept has been corroborated by the finding that targeted deletion of the TR genes in mice has a less pronounced phenotypic effect than hormone deficiency.

Thyroid Hormone Resistance Resistance to thyroid hormone (RTH) is an autosomal dominant disorder characterized by elevated free thyroid hormone levels and inappropriately normal or elevated TSH. Individuals with RTH do not, in general, exhibit signs and symptoms that are typical of hypothyroidism, apparently because hormone resistance is compensated by increased levels of thyroid hormone. The clinical features of RTH can include goiter, attention deficit disorder, mild reduction in IQ, delayed skeletal maturation, tachycardia, and impaired metabolic responses to thyroid hormone.

The disorder is caused by mutations in the TRβ receptor gene. These mutations, located in restricted regions of the ligand-binding domain, cause loss of receptor function. However, because the mutant receptors retain the capacity to dimerize with RXRs, bind to DNA, and recruit corepressor proteins, they function as antagonists of the remaining, normal TRβ and TRα receptors. This property, referred to as "dominant negative" activity, explains the autosomal dominant mode of transmission. The diagnosis is suspected when free thyroid hormone levels are increased without suppression of TSH. Similar hormonal abnormalities are common in other affected family members, though the TRβ mutation arises de novo in about 20% of patients. DNA sequence analysis of the TRβ gene provides a definitive diagnosis. RTH must be distinguished from other causes of euthyroid hyperthyroxinemia (e.g., familial dysalbuminemic hyperthyroxinemia) and inappropriate secretion of TSH by TSH-secreting pituitary adenomas (Chap. 328). In most patients, no treatment is indicated; the importance of making the diagnosis is to avoid inappropriate treatment of mistaken hyperthyroidism and to provide genetic counseling.

PHYSICAL EXAMINATION

In addition to the examination of the thyroid itself, the physical examination should include a search for signs of abnormal thyroid function and the extrathyroidal features of ophthalmopathy and dermopathy (see below). Examination of the neck begins by inspecting the

seated patient from the front and side, and noting any surgical scars, obvious masses, or distended veins. The thyroid can be palpated with both hands from behind or the examiner can face the patient, using the thumbs to palpate each lobe. Most often it is best to use a combination of these methods, especially in cases of doubt or when there are small nodules. The patient's neck should be slightly flexed to relax the neck muscles. After locating the cricoid cartilage, the isthmus can be identified and followed laterally to locate either lobe (the right lobe is normally slightly larger than the left). By asking the patient to swallow sips of water, thyroid consistency can be better appreciated as the gland moves beneath the examiner's fingers.

Features to be noted include thyroid size, consistency, nodularity, and any tenderness or fixation. An estimate of thyroid size (normally 12 to 20 g) should be made, and a drawing is often the best way to record findings. However, ultrasound is the method of choice when it is important to determine thyroid size accurately. The size, location, and consistency of any nodules should also be depicted. A bruit over the gland indicates increased vascularity, as occurs in hyperthyroidism. If the lower borders of the thyroid lobes are not clearly felt, a goiter may be retrosternal. Large retrosternal goiters can cause venous distention over the neck and difficulty breathing, especially when the arms are raised (Pemberton's sign). With any central mass above the thyroid, the patient should be asked to stick out his or her tongue, as thyroglossal cysts then move upward. The thyroid examination is not complete without assessment for lymphadenopathy in the supraclavicular and cervical regions of the neck.

LABORATORY EVALUATION

MEASUREMENT OF THYROID HORMONES The enhanced sensitivity and specificity of *TSH assays* have greatly improved laboratory assessment of thyroid function. Because TSH levels change dynamically in response to alterations of free T_4 and T_3, a logical approach to thyroid testing is to determine first whether TSH is suppressed, normal, or elevated. With rare exceptions (see below), a normal TSH level excludes a primary abnormality of thyroid function. This strategy depends on the use of immunoradiometric assays (IRMAs) for TSH that are sensitive enough to discriminate between the lower limit of the reference range and the suppressed values that occur with thyrotoxicosis. Extremely sensitive (fourth generation) assays can detect TSH levels ≤ 0.004 mU/L, but for practical purposes assays sensitive to ≤ 0.1 mU/L are sufficient. The widespread availability of the TSH IRMA has rendered the TRH stimulation test virtually obsolete, as the failure of TSH to rise after an intravenous bolus of 200 to 400 μg TRH has the same implications as a suppressed basal TSH measured by IRMA.

The finding of an abnormal TSH level must be followed by measurements of circulating thyroid hormone levels to confirm the diagnosis of hyperthyroidism (suppressed TSH) or hypothyroidism (elevated TSH). Radioimmunoassays are widely available for serum *total T_4* and *total T_3*. T_4 and T_3 are highly protein-bound, and numerous factors (illness, medications, genetic factors) can influence protein binding. It is useful, therefore, to measure the free or unbound hormone levels, which correspond to the biologically available hormone pool. Two direct methods are used to measure *free thyroid hormones*: (1) free thyroid hormone competition with radiolabeled T_4 (or an analogue) for binding to a solid-phase antibody, and (2) physical separation of the free hormone fraction by ultracentrifugation or equilibrium dialysis. Though early free hormone immunoassays suffered from artifacts, newer assays agree well with the results of the more technically demanding and expensive physical separation methods. An indirect method to estimate free thyroid hormone levels is to calculate the free T_3 or free T_4 index from the total T_4 or T_3 concentration and the *thyroid hormone binding ratio* (THBR). The latter is derived from the *T_3-resin uptake test*, which determines the distribution of radiolabeled T_3 between an absorbent resin and the unoccupied thyroid hormone binding proteins in the sample. The binding of the labeled T_3 to the resin is increased when there is reduced unoccupied protein binding sites (e.g., TBG deficiency) or increased total thyroid hormone in the sample; it is decreased under the opposite circumstances. The product of THBR and total T_3 or T_4 provides the *free T_3 or T_4 index*. In effect, the index corrects for anomalous total hormone values caused by abnormalities in hormone-protein binding.

Total thyroid hormone levels are elevated when TBG is increased due to estrogens (pregnancy, oral contraceptives, hormone replacement therapy, tamoxifen), and decreased when TBG binding is decreased (androgens, the nephrotic syndrome). Genetic disorders and acute illness can also cause abnormalities in thyroid hormone binding proteins, and various drugs (phenytoin, carbamazepine, salicylates, and nonsteroidal anti-inflammatory drugs) can interfere with thyroid hormone binding. Because free thyroid hormone levels are normal and the patient is euthyroid in all of these circumstances, assays that measure free hormone are preferable to those for total thyroid hormones.

For most purposes, the free T_4 level is sufficient to confirm thyrotoxicosis, but 2 to 5% of patients have only an elevated T_3 level (T_3 toxicosis). Thus, free T_3 levels should be measured in patients with a suppressed TSH but normal free T_4 levels. Free T_3 levels are normal in about 25% of patients with hypothyroidism and provide little useful information in this setting.

There are several clinical conditions in which the use of TSH as a screening test may be misleading, particularly without simultaneous free T_4 determinations. Any severe nonthyroidal illness can cause abnormal TSH levels (see below). Although hypothyroidism is the most common cause of an elevated TSH level, rare causes include a TSH-secreting pituitary tumor (Chap. 328), thyroid hormone resistance, and assay artifact. Conversely, a suppressed TSH level, particularly <0.1 mU/L, usually indicates thyrotoxicosis but may also be seen during the first trimester of pregnancy (due to hCG secretion), after treatment of hyperthyroidism (because TSH remains suppressed for several weeks), and in response to certain medications (e.g., high doses of glucocorticoids or dopamine). Importantly, secondary hypothyroidism, caused by hypothalamic-pituitary disease, is associated with a variable (low to high-normal) TSH level, which is inappropriate for the low free T_4 level. Thus, *TSH should not be used to assess thyroid function in patients with suspected or known pituitary disease.*

Tests for the end-organ effects of thyroid hormone excess or depletion, such as estimation of basal metabolic rate, tendon reflex speed, or serum cholesterol, are not useful as clinical determinants of thyroid function.

TESTS TO DETERMINE THE ETIOLOGY OF THYROID DYSFUNCTION Autoimmune thyroid disease is detected most easily by measuring circulating antibodies against TPO and Tg. As antibodies to Tg alone are rare, it is reasonable to measure only TPO antibodies. About 5 to 15% of euthyroid women and up to 2% of euthyroid men have thyroid antibodies; such individuals are at increased risk of developing thyroid dysfunction. Almost all patients with autoimmune hypothyroidism, and up to 80% of those with Graves' disease, have TPO antibodies, usually at high levels.

TSI are antibodies that stimulate the TSH-R in Graves' disease. They can be measured in bioassays or indirectly in assays that detect antibody binding to the receptor. The main use of these assays is to predict neonatal thyrotoxicosis caused by high maternal levels of TSI in the last trimester of pregnancy.

Serum Tg levels are increased in all types of thyrotoxicosis except thyrotoxicosis factitia. The main role for Tg measurement, however, is in the follow-up of thyroid cancer patients. After total thyroidectomy and radioablation, Tg levels should be undetectable; measurable levels (>1 to 2 ng/mL) suggest incomplete ablation or recurrent cancer.

RADIOIODINE UPTAKE AND THYROID SCANNING The thyroid gland selectively transports radioisotopes of iodine (^{123}I, ^{125}I, ^{131}I) and ^{99m}Tc pertechnetate, allowing thyroid imaging and quantitation of radioactive tracer fractional uptake.

Graves' disease is characterized by an enlarged gland and increased tracer uptake that is distributed homogeneously. Toxic adenomas appear as focal areas of increased uptake, with suppressed tracer uptake in the remainder of the gland. In toxic multinodular goiter, the gland is enlarged—often with distorted architecture—and there are multiple areas of relatively increased or decreased tracer uptake. Subacute thyroiditis is associated with very low uptake because of follicular cell damage and TSH suppression. *Thyrotoxicosis factitia*, caused by self-administration of thyroid hormone, is also associated with low uptake.

Although the use of fine-needle aspiration (FNA) biopsy has diminished the use of thyroid scans in the evaluation of solitary thyroid nodules, the functional features of thyroid nodules have some prognostic significance. So-called cold nodules, which have diminished tracer uptake, are usually benign. However, these nodules are more likely to be malignant (~5 to 10%) than so-called hot nodules, which are almost never malignant.

Thyroid scanning is also used in the follow-up of thyroid cancer. After thyroidectomy and ablation using ^{131}I, there is diminished radioiodine uptake in the thyroid bed, allowing the detection of metastatic thyroid cancer deposits that retain the ability to transport iodine. Whole-body scans using 111 to 185 MBq (3 to 5 mCi) ^{131}I are typically performed after thyroid hormone withdrawal to raise the TSH level or after the administration of recombinant human TSH.

THYROID ULTRASOUND Ultrasonography is used increasingly to assist in the diagnosis of nodular thyroid disease, a reflection of the limitations of the physical examination and improvements in ultrasound technology. Using 10-MHz instruments, spatial resolution and image quality are excellent, allowing the detection of nodules and cysts >3 mm. In addition to detecting thyroid nodules, ultrasound is useful for monitoring nodule size, for guiding FNA biopsies, and for the aspiration of cystic lesions. Ultrasound is also used in the evaluation of recurrent thyroid cancer, including possible spread to cervical lymph nodes.

AUTOIMMUNE BASIS OF THYROID DISEASE

PREVALENCE Thyroid autoimmunity can cause several forms of thyroiditis and may lead to hypothyroidism as well as Graves' disease. Focal thyroiditis is present in 20 to 40% of autopsy cases and is associated with serologic evidence of autoimmunity, particularly the presence of TPO antibodies. These antibodies are 4 to 10 times more common in otherwise healthy women than men. About 5% of women experience self-limited *postpartum (silent) thyroiditis* in the months after pregnancy, often with transient clinical symptoms. This condition is associated with the presence of TPO antibodies ante-partum. Up to 20% of women with an episode of postpartum thyroiditis develop permanent hypothyroidism 5 to 10 years after delivery. Autoimmune-mediated hypothyroidism affects about 5 to 10% of middle-aged and elderly women, depending on diagnostic criteria and geographic location. Graves' disease is about one-tenth as common as hypothyroidism and tends to occur in younger individuals. Although seemingly diverse, these disorders have many pathophysiologic features in common, and patients may progress from one state to the other as the autoimmune process changes.

SUSCEPTIBILITY FACTORS As with most autoimmune disorders, susceptibility is determined by a combination of genetic and environmental factors. The concordance rate for Graves' disease in monozygotic twins is 20 to 30%. The risk of autoimmune thyroid disease is increased among siblings, who may exhibit features of either Graves' disease or autoimmune hypothyroidism. The autoimmune polyglandular syndrome type 2 (Chap. 339) involves the occurrence of autoimmune thyroid dysfunction with other autoimmune diseases (type 1 diabetes mellitus, Addison's disease, pernicious anemia, vitiligo). Shared genetic factors are likely in this group of autoimmune disorders.

HLA-DR3 is the best documented genetic risk factor for Graves' disease and autoimmune hypothyroidism in Caucasians, though different HLA associations exist for other racial groups, such as the Japanese and Chinese. A weak association with polymorphisms in the T cell regulatory gene CTLA-4 has been found in several racial groups. Other loci, including a region on chromosome 18q21, may be linked to Graves' disease as well as to several other autoimmune disorders such as type 1 diabetes mellitus, rheumatoid arthritis, and systemic lupus erythematosus (SLE). The female preponderance of thyroid autoimmunity is most likely due to the influence of sex steroids. Some studies suggest an association between antecedent major life events and Graves' disease, but a causal role for stress in the autoimmune process remains to be clearly established. Smoking is a minor risk factor for Graves' disease but a major risk factor for the development of ophthalmopathy. There is no convincing evidence for a role of infection in susceptibility, except for the congenital rubella syndrome, which is associated with a high frequency of autoimmune hypothyroidism. Viral thyroiditis does not induce subsequent autoimmune thyroid disease.

HUMORAL FACTORS   The thyrotoxicosis of Graves' disease is caused by TSH-R-stimulating immunoglobulins that bind to the receptor and mimic the action of TSH. These TSI can cross the placenta and cause *transient neonatal thyrotoxicosis*, a phenomenon that complicates 1 to 2% of pregnancies in women with active or previous Graves' disease. However, the autoimmune response against the TSH-R can also result in antibodies that block TSH function, causing hypothyroidism. Stimulating and blocking antibodies bind to separate epitopes on the receptor. TSH-R blocking antibodies are found in about 20% of Asian patients with autoimmune hypothyroidism and are associated with thyroid atrophy; blocking antibodies are less common in Caucasians. Patients may have a mixture of TSH-R antibodies, and thyroid function can oscillate between hyperthyroidism and hypothyroidism as stimulating or blocking antibodies become dominant. Predicting the course of disease in such individuals is difficult, and close monitoring of thyroid function is required. Assays that measure the binding of antibodies to the receptor by competition with radiolabeled TSH [TSH-binding inhibiting immunoglobulins (TBII)] provide no information about functional effects and are used primarily to demonstrate the presence of TSH-R antibodies in atypical patients. Bioassays measure antibody-mediated stimulation of cyclic AMP production in cultured thyroid cells or cells transfected with the TSH-R. The use of these assays does not generally alter clinical management.

Antibodies to Tg and TPO, readily measured by immunofluorescence, hemagglutination, enzyme-linked immunosorbent assay, or radioimmunoassay, are clinically useful markers of thyroid autoimmunity, as discussed above. Any pathogenic effect is likely to be restricted to a secondary role in amplifying an ongoing autoimmune response. For instance, T cell– or cytokine-mediated injury to thyroid follicles could expose the enzyme on the apical border of follicles to TPO antibodies, which may then bind to the autoantigen and fix complement. There is evidence for intrathyroidal complement activation in both Graves' disease and autoimmune hypothyroidism. Tg antibodies do not fix complement, but could be involved in antibody-dependent, natural killer cell-mediated cytotoxicity. The NIS is also a target of autoantibody production in up to one-third of patients with autoimmune thyroid disease, but the functional consequences, if any, have not been established.

CELL-MEDIATED FACTORS   Activated circulating T cells are increased in autoimmune thyroid disease, and the gland is infiltrated with CD4+ and CD8+ T cells. The latter are believed to mediate perforin-dependent cytotoxicity, leading ultimately to thyroid cell destruction. In addition, thyroid cells undergo apoptosis through cytokine-mediated upregulation of Fas and possibly Fas ligand. Cytokines produced by the infiltrating immune cells also induce expression of thyroid cell-surface molecules that lead to: (1) engagement by immune cells (e.g., adhesion molecules, HLA class I and II molecules); (2) induction of cytokine secretion by the thyroid cells themselves; (3) production of nitric oxide; and (4) reduction of thyroid hormone production through inhibition of TSH-R, TPO, and Tg synthesis. Administration of high concentrations of cytokines for therapeutic purposes

[especially interferon (IFN)α] is associated with increased autoimmune thyroid disease, presumably via mechanisms similar to those that occur in sporadic autoimmune disease.

Cytokines appear to play a major role in thyroid-associated ophthalmopathy. There is infiltration of the extraocular muscles by activated T cells; the release of cytokines results in fibroblast activation and increased synthesis of glycosaminoglycans that trap water, thereby leading to characteristic muscle swelling. Late in the disease, there is fibrosis and only then do the muscle cells show evidence of injury. Orbital fibroblasts may be uniquely sensitive to cytokines, perhaps explaining the anatomic localization of the immune response. Though the pathogenesis of thyroid-associated ophthalmopathy remains unclear, there is mounting evidence that expression of the TSH-R may provide an important orbital autoantigen. In support of this idea, injection of TSH-R into certain strains of mice induces autoimmune hyperthyroidism, as well as features of ophthalmopathy. A variety of autoantibodies against orbital muscle and fibroblast antigens have been detected in patients with ophthalmopathy, but these antibodies most likely arise as a secondary phenomenon, dependent on T cell–mediated autoimmune responses.

HYPOTHYROIDISM

Iodine deficiency remains the most common cause of hypothyroidism worldwide. In areas of iodine sufficiency, autoimmune disease (Hashimoto's thyroiditis) and iatrogenic causes (treatment of hyperthyroidism) are most common (Table 330-4).

CONGENITAL HYPOTHYROIDISM   **Prevalence**   Hypothyroidism occurs in about 1 in 3000 to 4000 newborns. It may be transient, especially if the mother has TSH-R blocking antibodies or has received antithyroid drugs, but permanent hypothyroidism occurs in the majority. Neonatal hypothyroidism is due to thyroid gland dysgenesis in 85%, inborn errors of thyroid hormone synthesis in 10 to 15%, and is TSH-R antibody-mediated in 5% of affected newborns. The developmental abnormalities are twice as common in girls. Mutations that cause congenital hypothyroidism are being increasingly recognized, but the vast majority remain idiopathic (Table 330-1).

Clinical Manifestations   The majority of infants appear normal at birth, and <10% are diagnosed based on clinical features, which include prolonged jaundice, feeding problems, hypotonia, enlarged tongue, delayed bone maturation, and umbilical hernia. Importantly, permanent neurologic damage results if treatment is delayed. Typical features of adult hypothyroidism may also be present (Table 330-5).

Table 330-4   Causes of Hypothyroidism

Primary
  Autoimmune hypothyroidism: Hashimoto's thyroiditis, atrophic thyroiditis
  Iatrogenic: ^{131}I treatment, subtotal or total thyroidectomy, external irradiation of neck for lymphoma or cancer
  Drugs: iodine excess (including iodine-containing contrast media and amiodarone), lithium, antithyroid drugs, p-aminosalicyclic acid, interferon-α and other cytokines, aminoglutethimide
  Congenital hypothyroidism: absent or ectopic thyroid gland, dyshormonogenesis, TSH-R mutation
  Iodine deficiency
  Infiltrative disorders: amyloidosis, sarcoidosis, hemochromatosis, scleroderma, cystinosis, Riedel's thyroiditis
Transient
  Silent thyroiditis, including postpartum thyroiditis
  Subacute thyroiditis
  Withdrawal of thyroxine treatment in individuals with an intact thyroid
  After ^{131}I treatment or subtotal thyroidectomy for Graves' disease
Secondary
  Hypopituitarism: tumors, pituitary surgery or irradiation, infiltrative disorders, Sheehan's syndrome, trauma, genetic forms of combined pituitary hormone deficiencies
  Isolated TSH deficiency or inactivity
  Bexarotene treatment
  Hypothalamic disease: tumors, trauma, infiltrative disorders, idiopathic

NOTE: TSH, thyroid-stimulating hormone; TSH-R, TSH receptor.

Symptoms	Signs
Tiredness, weakness	Dry coarse skin; cool peripheral extremities
Dry skin	
Feeling cold	Puffy face, hands and feet (myxedema)
Hair loss	
Difficulty concentrating and poor memory	Diffuse alopecia
	Bradycardia
Constipation	Peripheral edema
Weight gain with poor appetite	Delayed tendon reflex relaxation
Dyspnea	Carpal tunnel syndrome
Hoarse voice	Serous cavity effusions
Menorrhagia (later oligomenorrhea or amenorrhea)	
Paresthesias	
Impaired hearing	

Diagnosis and Treatment Because of the severe neurologic consequences of untreated congenital hypothyroidism, neonatal screening programs have been established in developed countries (Chap. 68). These are generally based on measurement of TSH or T_4 levels in heel-prick blood specimens. When the diagnosis is confirmed, T_4 is instituted at a dose of 10 to 15 μg/kg per day and the dosage is adjusted by close monitoring of TSH levels. T_4 requirements are relatively great during the first year of life, and a high circulating T_4 level is usually needed to normalize TSH. Early treatment with T_4 results in normal IQ levels, but subtle neurodevelopmental abnormalities may be detected in those with the most severe hypothyroidism at diagnosis or when treatment is suboptimal.

AUTOIMMUNE HYPOTHYROIDISM Classification
Autoimmune hypothyroidism may be associated with a goiter (Hashimoto's, or *goitrous thyroiditis*) or, at the later stages of the disease, minimal residual thyroid tissue (*atrophic thyroiditis*). Because the autoimmune process gradually reduces thyroid function, there is a phase of compensation during which normal thyroid hormone levels are maintained by a rise in TSH. Though some patients may have minor symptoms, this state is called *subclinical hypothyroidism*. Later, free T_4 levels fall and TSH levels rise further; symptoms become more readily apparent at this stage (usually TSH > 10 mU/L), which is referred to as *clinical hypothyroidism* (*overt hypothyroidism*).

Prevalence The mean annual incidence rate of autoimmune hypothyroidism is up to 4 per 1000 women and 1 per 1000 men. It is more common in certain populations, such as the Japanese, probably as a consequence of genetic factors and chronic exposure to a high-iodine diet. The mean age at diagnosis is about 60 years, and the prevalence of overt hypothyroidism increases with age. Subclinical hypothyroidism is found in 6 to 8% of women (10% over the age of 60) and 3% of men. The annual risk of developing clinical hypothyroidism is about 4% when subclinical hypothyroidism is associated with positive TPO antibodies.

Pathogenesis In Hashimoto's thyroiditis, there is a marked lymphocytic infiltration of the thyroid with germinal center formation, atrophy of the thyroid follicles accompanied by oxyphil metaplasia, absence of colloid, and mild to moderate fibrosis. In atrophic thyroiditis, the fibrosis is much more extensive, lymphocyte infiltration is less pronounced, and thyroid follicles are almost completely absent. Atrophic thyroiditis likely represents the end stage of Hashimoto's thyroiditis rather than a distinct disorder. Autoimmune features are similar in both types of hypothyroidism, though TSH-R blocking antibodies may be more frequent in Asian patients with atrophic thyroiditis. The mechanisms that result in thyroid follicular destruction are predominantly T cell mediated, but antibodies may also contribute to thyroid dysfunction by complement fixation or inhibition of thyroid cell function (see "Autoimmune Basis of Thyroid Disease," above).

Clinical Manifestations The main clinical features of hypothyroidism are summarized in Table 330-5. The onset is usually insidious, and the patient may become aware of symptoms only when euthy-

roidism is restored. Patients with Hashimoto's thyroiditis may present because of goiter rather than symptoms of hypothyroidism. The goiter may not be large but is usually irregular and firm in consistency. It is often possible to palpate a pyramidal lobe, normally a vestigial remnant of thyroglossal duct. Rarely, uncomplicated Hashimoto's thyroiditis is associated with pain.

Patients with atrophic thyroiditis, or the late stage of Hashimoto's thyroiditis, present with symptoms and signs of hypothyroidism. The skin is dry, and there is decreased sweating, thinning of the epidermis, and hyperkeratosis of the stratum corneum. Increased dermal glycosaminoglycan content traps water, giving rise to skin thickening without pitting (*myxedema*). Typical features include a puffy face with edematous eyelids and nonpitting pretibial edema (Fig. 330-4). There is pallor, often with a yellow tinge due to carotene accumulation. Nail growth is retarded, and hair is dry, brittle, difficult to manage, and falls out easily. In addition to diffuse alopecia, there is thinning of the outer third of the eyebrows.

Other common features include constipation and weight gain (despite a poor appetite). In contrast to popular perception, the weight gain is usually modest and due mainly to fluid retention in the myxedematous tissues. Libido is decreased in both sexes, and there may be oligomenorrhea or amenorrhea in long-standing disease, but menorrhagia is also common. Fertility is reduced and the incidence of miscarriage is increased. Prolactin levels are often modestly increased (Chap. 328) and may contribute to alterations in libido and fertility as well as causing galactorrhea.

Myocardial contractility and pulse rate are reduced, leading to a reduced stroke volume and bradycardia. Increased peripheral resistance may be accompanied by hypertension, particularly diastolic. Blood flow is diverted from the skin, producing the cool extremities. Pericardial effusions occur in up to 30% of patients but rarely compromise cardiac function. Though alterations in myosin heavy chain isoform expression have been documented, cardiomyopathy is unusual. Fluid may also accumulate in other serous cavities and in the middle ear, giving rise to conductive deafness. Pulmonary function is generally normal, but dyspnea may be due to pleural effusion, impaired respiratory muscle function, diminished ventilatory drive, or sleep apnea.

Carpal tunnel and other entrapment syndromes are common, as is impairment of muscle function with stiffness, cramps, and pain. On examination, there may be slow relaxation of tendon reflexes and pseudomyotonia. Memory and concentration are impaired. Rare neurologic problems include reversible cerebellar ataxia, dementia, psychosis, and myxedema coma. *Hashimoto's encephalopathy* is a rare and distinctive syndrome associated with myoclonus and slow-wave activity on electroencephalography, which can progress to confusion, coma, and

FIGURE 330-4 Facial appearance in hypothyroidism. Note puffy eyes and thickened, pale skin.

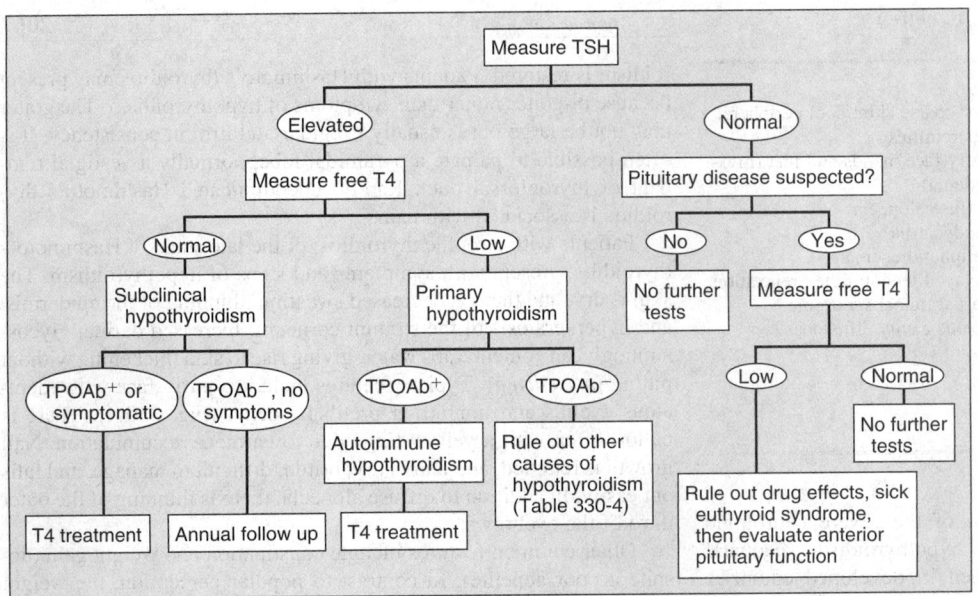

FIGURE 330-5 Evaluation of hypothyroidism. TPOAB⁺, thyroid peroxidase antibodies present; TPOAB⁻, thyroid peroxidase antibodies not present.

death. It is steroid-responsive and may occur in the presence of auto-immune thyroiditis, without hypothyroidism. The hoarse voice and occasionally clumsy speech of hypothyroidism are due to fluid accumulation in the vocal cords and tongue.

The features described above are due to a shortage of thyroid hormone. However, autoimmune hypothyroidism may be associated with signs or symptoms of other autoimmune diseases, particularly vitiligo, pernicious anemia, Addison's disease, alopecia areata, and type 1 diabetes mellitus. Less common associations include celiac disease, dermatitis herpetiformis, chronic active hepatitis, rheumatoid arthritis, SLE, and Sjögren's syndrome. Thyroid-associated ophthalmopathy, which usually occurs in Graves' disease (see below), occurs in about 5% of patients with autoimmune hypothyroidism.

Autoimmune hypothyroidism is uncommon in children and usually presents with slow growth and delayed facial maturation. The appearance of permanent teeth is also delayed. Myopathy, with muscle swelling, is more common than in adults. In most cases, puberty is delayed, but precocious puberty sometimes occurs. There may be intellectual impairment if the onset is before 3 years and the hormone deficiency is severe.

Laboratory Evaluation A summary of the investigations used to determine the existence and cause of hypothyroidism is provided in Fig. 330-5. A normal TSH level excludes primary (but not secondary) hypothyroidism. If the TSH is elevated, a free T_4 level is needed to confirm the presence of clinical hypothyroidism, but free T_4 is inferior to TSH when used as a screening test, as it will not detect subclinical or mild hypothyroidism. Circulating free T_3 levels are normal in about 25% of patients, reflecting adaptive responses to hypothyroidism. T_3 measurements are therefore not indicated.

Once clinical or subclinical hypothyroidism is confirmed, the etiology is usually easily established by demonstrating the presence of TPO antibodies, which are present in 90 to 95% of patients with autoimmune hypothyroidism. TBII can be found in 10 to 20% of patients, but these determinations are not needed routinely. If there is any doubt about the cause of a goiter associated with hypothyroidism, FNA biopsy can be used to confirm the presence of autoimmune thyroiditis. Other abnormal laboratory findings in hypothyroidism may include increased creatine phosphokinase, elevated cholesterol and triglycerides, and anemia (usually normocytic or macrocytic). Except when accompanied by iron deficiency, the anemia and other abnormalities gradually resolve with thyroxine replacement.

Differential Diagnosis An asymmetric goiter in Hashimoto's thyroiditis may be confused with a multinodular goiter or thyroid carcinoma, even when thyroid antibodies are present. Ultrasound can be used to show the presence of a solitary lesion or a multinodular goiter, rather than the heterogeneous thyroid enlargement typical of Hashimoto's thyroiditis. FNA biopsy is useful in the investigation of focal nodules. Other causes of hypothyroidism are discussed below but rarely cause diagnostic confusion (Table 330-4).

OTHER CAUSES OF HYPO-THYROIDISM *Iatrogenic hypothyroidism* is a common cause of hypothyroidism and can often be detected by screening before symptoms develop. In the first 3 to 4 months after radioiodine treatment, transient hypothyroidism may occur due to reversible radiation damage rather than to cellular destruction. Low-dose thyroxine treatment can be withdrawn if recovery occurs. Because TSH levels are suppressed by hyperthyroidism, free T_4 levels are a better measure of thyroid function than TSH in the months following radioiodine treatment. Mild hypothyroidism after subtotal thyroidectomy may also resolve after several months, as the gland remnant is stimulated by increased TSH levels.

Iodine deficiency is responsible for endemic goiter and cretinism but is an uncommon cause of adult hypothyroidism unless the iodine intake is very low or there are complicating factors, such as the consumption of thiocyanates in cassava or selenium deficiency. Though hypothyroidism due to iodine deficiency can be treated with thyroxine, public health measures to improve iodine intake should be advocated to eliminate this problem. Iodized salt or bread or the use of a single bolus of oral or intramuscular iodized oil have all been used successfully.

Paradoxically, chronic iodine excess can also induce goiter and hypothyroidism. The intracellular events that account for this effect are unclear, but individuals with autoimmune thyroiditis are especially susceptible. Iodine excess is responsible for the hypothyroidism that occurs in up to 13% of patients treated with amiodarone (see below). Other drugs, particularly lithium, may also cause hypothyroidism.

Secondary hypothyroidism is usually diagnosed in the context of other anterior pituitary hormone deficiencies; isolated TSH deficiency is very rare (Chap. 328). TSH levels may be low, normal, or even slightly increased in secondary hypothyroidism; the latter is due to secretion of immunoactive but bioinactive forms of TSH. The diagnosis is confirmed by detecting a low free T_4 level. The goal of treatment is to maintain free T_4 levels in the upper half of the reference range, as TSH levels cannot be used to monitor therapy.

TREATMENT **Clinical Hypothyroidism** If there is no residual thyroid function, the daily replacement dose of levothyroxine is usually 1.5 μg/kg body weight (typically 100 to 150 μg). In many patients, however, lower doses suffice until residual thyroid tissue is destroyed. In patients who develop hypothyroidism after the treatment of Graves' disease, there is often underlying autonomous function, necessitating lower replacement doses (typically 75 to 125 μg/d).

Adult patients under 60 without evidence of heart disease may be started on 50 to 100 μg levothyroxine (T_4) daily. The dose is adjusted on the basis of TSH levels, with the goal of treatment being a normal TSH, ideally in the lower half of the reference range. TSH responses are gradual and should be measured about 2 months after instituting treatment or after any subsequent change in levothyroxine dosage. The clinical effects of levothyroxine replacement are often slow to appear.

Patients may not experience full relief from symptoms until 3 to 6 months after normal TSH levels are restored. Adjustment of levothyroxine dosage is made in 12.5- or 25-μg increments if the TSH is high; decrements of the same magnitude should be made if the TSH is suppressed. Patients with a suppressed TSH of any cause, including T$_4$ overtreatment, have an increased risk of atrial fibrillation and reduced bone density.

Although dessicated animal thyroid preparations (thyroid extract USP) are available, they are not recommended as potency and composition vary between batches. Interest in using levothyroxine combined with liothyronine (triiodothyronine, T$_3$) has been revived, based on studies suggesting that patients feel better when taking the T$_4$/T$_3$ combination compared to T$_4$ alone. However, a long-term benefit from this combination is not established. There is no place for liothyronine alone as long-term replacement, because the short half-life necessitates three or four daily doses and is associated with fluctuating T$_3$ levels.

Once full replacement is achieved and TSH levels are stable, follow-up measurement of TSH is recommended at annual intervals and may be extended to every 2 to 3 years, if a normal TSH is maintained over several years. It is important to ensure ongoing compliance, however, as patients do not feel any difference after missing a few doses of levothyroxine, sometimes leading to self-discontinuation.

In patients of normal body weight who are taking $\geq$200 μg of levothyroxine per day, an elevated TSH level is often a sign of poor compliance. This is also the likely explanation for fluctuating TSH levels, despite a constant levothyroxine dosage. Such patients often have normal or high free T$_4$ levels, despite an elevated TSH, because they remember to take medication for a few days before testing; this is sufficient to normalize T$_4$ but not TSH levels. It is important to consider variable compliance, as this pattern of thyroid function tests is otherwise suggestive of disorders associated with inappropriate TSH secretion (Table 330-3). Because T$_4$ has a long half-life (7 days), patients who miss doses can be advised to take up to three doses of the skipped tablets at once. Other causes of increased levothyroxine requirements must be excluded, particularly malabsorption (e.g., celiac disease, small-bowel surgery) and drugs that interfere with T$_4$ absorption or clearance such as cholestyramine, ferrous sulfate, calcium supplements, lovastatin, aluminum hydroxide, rifampicin, amiodarone, carbamazepine, and phenytoin.

Subclinical Hypothyroidism By definition, subclinical hypothyroidism refers to biochemical evidence of thyroid hormone deficiency in patients who have few or no apparent clinical features of hypothyroidism. There are no generally accepted guidelines for the treatment of subclinical hypothyroidism. As long as excessive treatment is avoided, there is little risk in correcting a slightly increased TSH, and some patients likely derive modest clinical benefit from treatment. Moreover, there is some risk that patients will progress to overt hypothyroidism, particularly when TPO antibodies are present. Treatment is administered by starting with a low dose of levothyroxine (25 to 50 μg/d) with the goal of normalizing TSH.

Special Treatment Considerations Rarely, levothyroxine replacement is associated with pseudotumor cerebri in *children*. Presentation appears to be idiosyncratic and occurs months after treatment is begun. Women with a history or high risk of hypothyroidism should ensure that they are euthyroid prior to conception and during early pregnancy as maternal hypothyroidism may adversely affect fetal neural development. TSH and free T$_4$ levels should be measured once pregnancy is confirmed and at the beginning of the second and third trimesters. The dose of levothyroxine may need to be increased by $\geq$50% during pregnancy and returned to previous levels after delivery. In the *elderly*, especially patients with known coronary artery disease, the starting dose of levothyroxine is 12.5 to 25 μg/d with similar increments every 2 to 3 months until TSH is normalized. In some patients it may be impossible to achieve full replacement, despite optimal antianginal treatment. *Emergency surgery* is generally safe in patients with untreated hypothyroidism, although routine surgery in a hypothyroid patient should be deferred until euthyroidism is achieved.

Myxedema coma still has a high mortality rate, despite intensive treatment. Clinical manifestations include reduced level of consciousness, sometimes associated with seizures, as well as the other features of hypothyroidism (Table 330-5). Hypothermia can reach 23°C (74°F). There may be a history of treated hypothyroidism with poor compliance, or the patient may be previously undiagnosed. Myxedema coma almost always occurs in the elderly and is usually precipitated by factors that impair respiration, such as drugs (especially sedatives, anesthetics, antidepressants), pneumonia, congestive heart failure, myocardial infarction, gastrointestinal bleeding, or cerebrovascular accidents. Sepsis should also be suspected. Exposure to cold may also be a risk factor. Hypoventilation, leading to hypoxia and hypercapnia, plays a major role in pathogenesis; hypoglycemia and dilutional hyponatremia also contribute to the development of myxedema coma.

Levothyroxine can initially be administered as a single intravenous bolus of 500 μg, which serves as a loading dose. Although further levothyroxine is not strictly necessary for several days, it is usually continued at a dose of 50 to 100 μg/d. If a suitable intravenous preparation is not available, the same initial dose of levothyroxine can be given by nasogastric tube (though absorption may be impaired in myxedema). An alternative is to give liothyronine (T$_3$) intravenously or via nasogastric tube, in doses ranging from 10 to 25 μg every 8 to 12 h. This treatment has been advocated because T$_4$ $\rightarrow$ T$_3$ conversion is impaired in myxedema coma. However, excess liothyroxine has the potential to provoke arrhythmias. Another commonly used option is to combine levothyroxine (200 μg) and liothyronine (25 μg) as a single, initial intravenous bolus followed by daily treatment with levothyroxine (50 to 100 μg/d) and liothyronine (10 μg every 8 h).

Supportive therapy should be provided to correct any associated metabolic disturbances. External warming is indicated only if the temperature is <30°C, as it can result in cardiovascular collapse (Chap. 17). Space blankets should be used to prevent further heat loss. Parenteral hydrocortisone (50 mg every 6 h) should be administered, as there is impaired adrenal reserve in profound hypothyroidism. Any precipitating factors should be treated, including the early use of broad-spectrum antibiotics, pending the exclusion of infection. Ventilatory support with regular blood gas analysis is usually needed during the first 48 h. Hypertonic saline or intravenous glucose may be needed if there is hyponatremia or hypoglycemia; hypotonic intravenous fluids should be avoided because they may exacerbate water retention secondary to reduced renal perfusion and inappropriate vasopressin secretion. The metabolism of most medications is impaired, and sedatives should be avoided if possible or used in reduced doses. Blood levels should be monitored, when available, to guide medication dosage.

THYROTOXICOSIS

Thyrotoxicosis is defined as the state of thyroid hormone excess and is not synonymous with *hyperthyroidism*, which is the result of excessive thyroid function. However, the major etiologies of thyrotoxicosis are hyperthyroidism caused by Graves' disease, toxic multinodular goiter, and toxic adenomas. Other causes are listed in Table 330-6.

GRAVES' DISEASE Epidemiology Graves' disease accounts for 60 to 80% of thyrotoxicosis, though the prevalence varies among populations, depending mainly on iodine intake (high iodine intake is associated with an increased prevalence of Graves' disease). Graves' disease occurs in up to 2% of women but is one-tenth as frequent in men. The disorder rarely begins before adolescence and typically occurs between 20 and 50 years of age, though it also occurs in the elderly.

Pathogenesis The hyperthyroidism of Graves' disease is caused by TSI that are directed to the TSH-R (see "Autoimmune Basis of Thyroid Disease," below). Other thyroid autoimmune responses coexist in these patients, and therefore there is no direct correlation between the levels of TSI and thyroid hormones. The extrathyroidal manifestations of Graves' disease—i.e., ophthalmopathy and dermo-

Table 330-6   Causes of Thyrotoxicosis

Primary hyperthyroidism
  Graves' disease
  Toxic multinodular goiter
  Toxic adenoma
  Functioning thyroid carcinoma metastases
  Activating mutation of the TSH receptor (autosomal dominant)
  Struma ovarii
  Drugs: iodine excess (Jod-Basedow phenomenon)
Thyrotoxicosis without hyperthyroidism
  Subacute thyroiditis
  Silent thyroiditis
  Other causes of thyroid destruction: amiodarone, radiation, infarction of
    adenoma
  Ingestion of excess thyroid hormone (thyrotoxicosis factitia) or thyroid
    tissue
Secondary hyperthyroidism
  TSH-secreting pituitary adenoma
  Thyroid hormone resistance syndrome: occasional patients may have fea-
    tures of thyrotoxicosis
  Chorionic gonadotropin-secreting tumors[a]
  Gestational thyrotoxicosis[a]

---

[a] Circulating TSH levels are low in these forms of secondary hyperthyroidism.
NOTE: TSH, thyroid-stimulating hormone.

---

pathy—are due to immunologically mediated activation of fibroblasts in the extraocular muscles and skin, with accumulation of glycosaminoglycans, leading to the trapping of water and edema. Later, fibrosis becomes prominent. The fibroblast activation is caused by cytokines (IFN-γ, tumor necrosis factor, IL-1) derived from locally infiltrating T cells and macrophages.

Clinical Manifestations   Signs and symptoms include features that are common to any cause of thyrotoxicosis (Table 330-7) as well as those specific for Graves' disease. The clinical presentation depends on the severity of thyrotoxicosis, the duration of the disease, individual susceptibility to excess thyroid hormone, and the age of the patient. In the elderly, features of thyrotoxicosis may be subtle or masked, and patients may present mainly with fatigue and weight loss, leading to *apathetic hyperthyroidism.*

Thyrotoxicosis may cause unexplained weight loss, despite an enhanced appetite, and is due to the increased metabolic rate. Weight gain occurs in 5 to 10% of patients, however, as a result of increased food intake. Other prominent features include hyperactivity, nervousness, and irritability, ultimately leading to a sense of easy fatiguability in some patients. Insomnia and impaired concentration are common; apathetic thyrotoxicosis may be mistaken for depression in the elderly. Fine tremor is a very frequent finding, best elicited by asking patients to stretch out the fingers and feeling the fingertips with the palm. Common neurologic manifestations include hyperreflexia, muscle wasting, and proximal myopathy without fasciculation. Chorea is a rare feature. Thyrotoxicosis is sometimes associated with a form of hypokalemic periodic paralysis; this disorder is particularly common in Asian males with thyrotoxicosis.

Table 330-7   Signs and Symptoms of Thyrotoxicosis
(Descending Order of Frequency)

Symptoms	Signs[a]
Hyperactivity, irritability, dysphoria	Tachycardia; atrial fibrillation in the elderly
Heat intolerance and sweating	Tremor
Palpitations	Goiter
Fatigue and weakness	Warm, moist skin
Weight loss with increased appetite	Muscle weakness, proximal myopathy
Diarrhea	Lid retraction or lag
Polyuria	Gynecomastia
Oligomenorrhea, loss of libido	

---

[a] Excludes the signs of ophthalmopathy and dermopathy specific for Graves' disease.

The most common cardiovascular manifestation is sinus tachycardia, often associated with palpitations and sometimes due to supraventricular tachycardia. The high cardiac output produces a bounding pulse, widened pulse pressure, and an aortic systolic murmur, and can lead to worsening of angina or heart failure in the elderly or those with preexisting heart disease. Atrial fibrillation is more common in patients >50. Treatment of the thyrotoxic state alone reverts atrial fibrillation to normal sinus rhythm in fewer than half of patients, suggesting the existence of an underlying cardiac problem in the remainder.

The skin is usually warm and moist, and the patient complains of sweating and heat intolerance, particularly during warm weather. Palmar erythema; onycholysis; and, less commonly, pruritus, urticaria, and diffuse hyperpigmentation may be evident. Hair texture may become fine, and a diffuse alopecia occurs in up to 40% of patients, persisting for months after restoration of euthyroidism. Gastrointestinal transit time is decreased, leading to increased stool frequency, often with diarrhea and occasionally mild steatorrhea. Women frequently experience oligomenorrhea or amenorrhea; in men there may be impaired sexual function and, rarely, gynecomastia. The direct effect of thyroid hormones on bone resorption leads to osteopenia in long-standing thyrotoxicosis; mild hypercalcemia occurs in up to 20% of patients, but hypercalcuria is more common. There is a small increase in fracture rate in patients with a previous history of thyrotoxicosis.

In Graves' disease the thyroid is usually diffusely enlarged to two to three times its normal size. The consistency is firm, but less so than in multinodular goiter. There may be a thrill or bruit due to the increased vascularity of the gland and the hyperdynamic circulation.

Lid retraction, causing a staring appearance, can occur in any form of thyrotoxicosis and is the result of sympathetic overactivity. However, Graves' disease is associated with specific eye signs that comprise *Graves' ophthalmopathy* (Fig. 330-6A). This condition is also called *thyroid-associated ophthalmopathy*, as it occurs in the absence of Graves' disease in 10% of patients. Most of these individuals have autoimmune hypothyroidism or thyroid antibodies. The onset of Graves' ophthalmopathy occurs within the year before or after the diagnosis of thyrotoxicosis in 75% of patients but can sometimes precede or follow thyrotoxicosis by several years, accounting for some cases of euthyroid ophthalmopathy.

Many patients with Graves' disease have little clinical evidence of ophthalmopathy. However, the enlarged extraocular muscles typical of the disease, and other subtle features, can be detected in almost all patients when investigated by ultrasound or computed tomography (CT) imaging of the orbits. Unilateral signs are found in up to 10% of patients. The earliest manifestations of ophthalmopathy are usually a sensation of grittiness, eye discomfort, and excess tearing. About a third of patients have proptosis, best detected by visualization of the sclera between the lower border of the iris and the lower eyelid, with the eyes in the primary position. Proptosis can be measured using an exophthalmometer. In severe cases, proptosis may cause corneal exposure and damage, especially if the lids fail to close during sleep. Periorbital edema, scleral injection, and chemosis are also frequent. In 5 to 10% of patients, the muscle swelling is so severe that diplopia results, typically but not exclusively when the patient looks up and laterally. The most serious manifestation is compression of the optic nerve at the apex of the orbit, leading to papilledema, peripheral field defects, and, if left untreated, permanent loss of vision.

Many scoring systems have been used to gauge the extent and activity of the orbital changes in Graves' disease. The NO SPECS scheme is an acronym derived from the following classes of eye change:

0 = No signs or symptoms
1 = Only signs (lid retraction or lag), no symptoms
2 = Soft tissue involvement (periorbital edema)
3 = Proptosis (>22 mm)
4 = Extraocular muscle involvement (diplopia)
5 = Corneal involvement
6 = Sight loss

Although useful as a mnemonic, the NO SPECS scheme is inadequate to describe the eye disease fully, and patients do not necessarily progress from one class to another. When Graves' eye disease is active and severe, referral to an ophthalmologist is indicated and objective measurements are needed, such as lid fissure width; corneal staining with fluorescein; and evaluation of extraocular muscle function (e.g., Hess chart), intraocular pressure and visual fields, acuity, and color vision.

Thyroid dermopathy occurs in <5% of patients with Graves' disease (Fig. 330-6*B*), almost always in the presence of moderate or severe ophthalmopathy. Although most frequent over the anterior and lateral aspects of the lower leg (hence the term *pretibial myxedema*), skin changes can occur at other sites, particularly after trauma. The typical lesion is a noninflamed, indurated plaque with a deep pink or purple color and an "orange-skin" appearance. Nodular involvement can occur, and the condition can rarely extend over the whole lower leg and foot, mimicking elephantiasis. *Thyroid acropachy* refers to a form of clubbing found in <1% of patients with Graves' disease (Fig. 330-6*C*). It is so strongly associated with thyroid dermopathy that an alternative cause of clubbing should be sought in a Graves' patient without coincident skin and orbital involvement.

FIGURE 330-6 Features of Graves' disease. *A.* Facial appearance in Graves' disease; lid retraction, periorbital edema, and proptosis are marked. *B.* Thyroid dermopathy over the lateral aspects of the shins. *C.* Thyroid acropachy.

Laboratory Evaluation Investigations used to determine the existence and cause of thyrotoxicosis are summarized in Fig. 330-7. In Graves' disease, the TSH level is suppressed and free and total thyroid hormone levels are increased. In 2 to 5% of patients (and more in areas of borderline iodine intake), only T_3 is increased (T_3 toxicosis). The converse state of T_4 toxicosis, with elevated total and free T_4 and normal T_3 levels, is occasionally seen when hyperthyroidism is induced by excess iodine, providing surplus substrate for thyroid hormone synthesis. Measurement of TPO antibodies is useful in differential diagnosis, but assays for TSH-R antibodies are not usually needed. Associated abnormalities that may cause diagnostic confusion in thyrotoxicosis include elevation of bilirubin, liver enzymes, and ferritin. Microcytic anemia and thrombocytopenia occur less often.

Differential Diagnosis Diagnosis of Graves' disease is straightforward in a patient with biochemically confirmed thyrotoxicosis, diffuse goiter on palpation, ophthalmopathy, positive TPO antibodies, and often a personal or family history of autoimmune disorders. For patients with thyrotoxicosis who lack these features, the most reliable diagnostic method is a radionuclide (^{99m}Tc, ^{123}I, or ^{131}I) scan of the thyroid, which will distinguish the diffuse, high uptake of Graves' disease from nodular thyroid disease, destructive thyroiditis, ectopic thyroid tissue, and factitious thyrotoxicosis. In secondary hyperthyroidism due to a TSH-secreting pituitary tumor, there is also a diffuse goiter. The presence of a nonsuppressed TSH level, and the finding of a pituitary tumor on CT or magnetic resonance imaging (MRI) scan readily identify such patients.

Clinical features of thyrotoxicosis can mimic certain aspects of other disorders including panic attacks, mania, pheochromocytoma, and the weight loss associated with malignancy. The diagnosis of thyrotoxicosis can be easily excluded if the TSH level is normal. A normal TSH also excludes Graves' disease as a cause of diffuse goiter.

Clinical Course Clinical features generally worsen without treatment; mortality was 10 to 30% before the introduction of satisfactory therapy. Some patients with mild Graves' disease experience spontaneous relapses and remissions. Rarely, there may be fluctuation between hypo- and hyperthyroidism due to changes in the functional activity of TSH-R antibodies. About 15% of patients who enter remission after treatment with antithyroid drugs develop hypothyroidism 10 to 15 years later as a result of the destructive autoimmune process. The clinical course of ophthalmopathy does not follow that of the thyroid disease. Ophthalmopathy typically worsens over the initial 3 to 6 months, followed by a plateau phase over the next 12 to 18 months, with spontaneous improvement, particularly in the soft tissue changes. However, the course is more fulminant in up to 5% of patients, requiring intervention in the acute phase if there is optic nerve compression or corneal ulceration. Diplopia may appear late in the disease due to fibrosis of the extraocular muscles. Some studies suggest that radioiodine treatment for hyperthyroidism worsens the eye disease in a small proportion of patients (especially smokers). Antithyroid drugs or surgery have no adverse effects on the clinical course of ophthalmopathy. Thyroid dermopathy, when it occurs, usually appears 1 to 2 years after the development of Graves' hyperthyroidism; it may improve spontaneously.

TREATMENT The *hyperthyroidism* of Graves' disease is treated by reducing thyroid hormone synthesis, using antithyroid drugs, or by reducing the amount of thyroid tissue with radioiodine (^{131}I) treatment or subtotal thyroidectomy. Antithyroid drugs are the predominant therapy in many centers in Europe and Japan, whereas radioiodine is more often the first line of treatment in North America. These differences reflect the fact that no single approach is optimal and that patients may require multiple treatments to achieve remission.

The main *antithyroid drugs* are the thionamides, such as propyl-

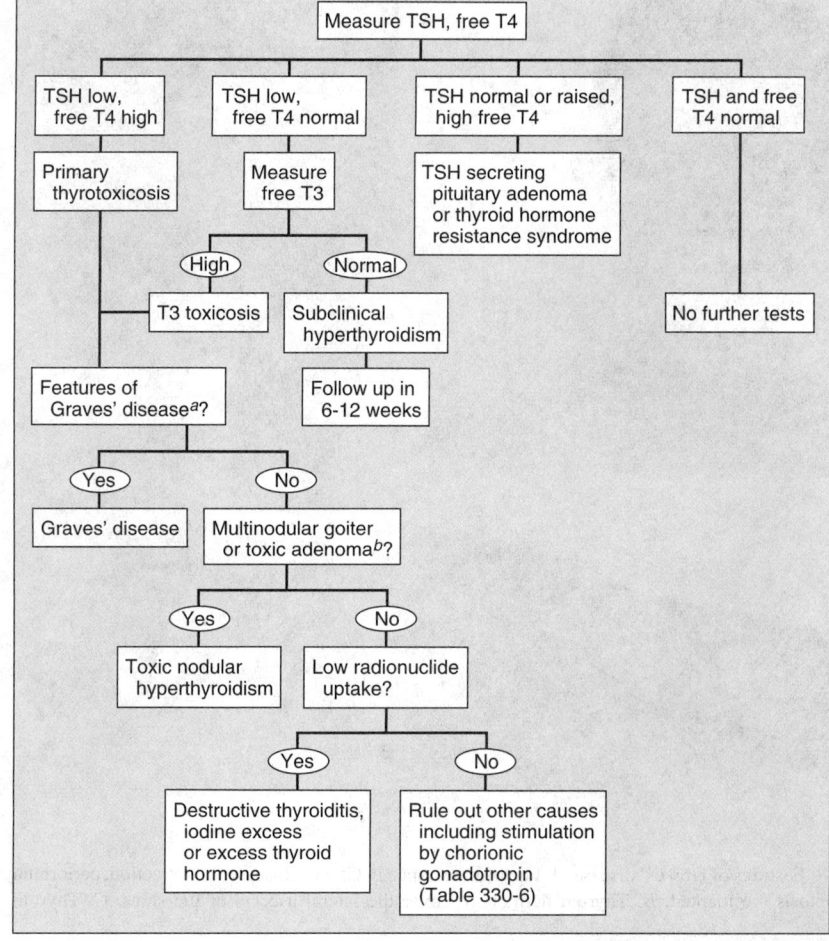

FIGURE 330-7 Evaluation of thyrotoxicosis. [a]Diffuse goiter, positive TPO antibodies, ophthalmopathy, dermopathy; [b] can be confirmed by radionuclide scan.

Flowchart content:

Measure TSH, free T4

- TSH low, free T4 high → Primary thyrotoxicosis
- TSH low, free T4 normal → Measure free T3
- TSH normal or raised, high free T4 → TSH secreting pituitary adenoma or thyroid hormone resistance syndrome
- TSH and free T4 normal → No further tests

Measure free T3:
- High → T3 toxicosis
- Normal → Subclinical hyperthyroidism → Follow up in 6-12 weeks

T3 toxicosis / Primary thyrotoxicosis → Features of Graves' disease[a]?
- Yes → Graves' disease
- No → Multinodular goiter or toxic adenoma[b]?
  - Yes → Toxic nodular hyperthyroidism
  - No → Low radionuclide uptake?
    - Yes → Destructive thyroiditis, iodine excess or excess thyroid hormone
    - No → Rule out other causes including stimulation by chorionic gonadotropin (Table 330-6)

thiouracil, carbimazole, and the active metabolite of the latter, methimazole. All inhibit the function of TPO, reducing oxidation and organification of iodide. These drugs also reduce thyroid antibody levels by mechanisms that remain unclear, and they appear to enhance rates of remission. Propylthiouracil inhibits deiodination of $T_4 \rightarrow T_3$. However, this effect is of minor benefit, except in the most severe thyrotoxicosis, and is offset by the much shorter half-life of this drug (90 min) compared to methimazole (6 h).

There are many variations of antithyroid drug regimens. The initial dose of carbimazole or methimazole is usually 10 to 20 mg every 8 or 12 h, but once-daily dosing is possible after euthyroidism is restored. Propylthiouracil is given at a dose of 100 to 200 mg every 6 to 8 h, and divided doses are usually given throughout the course. Lower doses of each drug may suffice in areas of low iodine intake. The starting dose of antithyroid drugs can be gradually reduced (titration regimen) as thyrotoxicosis improves. Alternatively, high doses may be given combined with levothyroxine supplementation (block-replace regimen) to avoid drug-induced hypothyroidism. Initial reports suggesting superior remission rates with the block-replace regimen have not been reproduced in several other trials. The titration regimen is often preferred to minimize the dose of antithyroid drug and provide an index of treatment response.

Thyroid function tests and clinical manifestations are reviewed 3 to 4 weeks after starting treatment, and the dose is titrated based on free T_4 levels. Most patients do not achieve euthyroidism until 6 to 8 weeks after treatment is initiated. TSH levels often remain suppressed for several months and therefore do not provide a sensitive index of treatment response. The usual daily maintenance doses of antithyroid drugs in the titration regimen are 2.5 to 10 mg of carbimazole or methimazole and 50 to 100 mg of propylthiouracil. In the block-re-

place regimen, the initial dose of antithyroid drug is held constant and the dose of levothyroxine is adjusted to maintain normal free T_4 levels.

Maximum remission rates (up to 30 to 50% in some populations) are achieved by 18 to 24 months. For unclear reasons, remission rates appear to vary in different geographic regions. Patients with severe hyperthyroidism and large goiters are most likely to relapse when treatment stops, but outcome is difficult to predict. All patients should be followed closely for relapse during the first year after treatment and at least annually thereafter.

The common side effects of antithyroid drugs are rash, urticaria, fever, and arthralgia (1 to 5% of patients). These may resolve spontaneously or after substituting an alternative antithyroid drug. Rare but major side effects include hepatitis, an SLE-like syndrome, and, most importantly, agranulocytosis (<1%). It is essential that antithyroid drugs are stopped and not restarted if a patient develops major side effects. Patients should be given written instructions regarding the symptoms of possible agranulocytosis (e.g., sore throat, fever, mouth ulcers) and the need to stop treatment pending a complete blood count to confirm that agranulocytosis is not present. Management of agranulocytosis is described in Chap. 109. Most physicians do not prospectively monitor blood counts, as the onset of agranulocytosis is idiosyncratic and abrupt.

Propranolol (20 to 40 mg every 6 h) or longer acting beta blockers, such as atenolol, may be useful to control adrenergic symptoms, especially in the early stages before antithyroid drugs take effect. Anticoagulation with warfarin should be considered in all patients with atrial fibrillation. If digoxin is used, increased doses are often needed in the thyrotoxic state.

Radioiodine causes progressive destruction of thyroid cells and can be used as initial treatment or for relapses after a trial of antithyroid drugs. There is a small risk of thyrotoxic crisis (see below) after radioiodine, which can be avoided by pretreatment with antithyroid drugs for at least a month before treatment. Antecedent treatment with antithyroid drugs should be considered in all elderly patients, or in those with cardiac problems, to deplete thyroid hormone stores before administration of radioiodine. Antithyroid drugs must be stopped 3 to 5 days before radioiodine administration to achieve optimum iodine uptake.

Efforts to calculate an optimal dose of radioiodine that achieves euthyroidism, without a high incidence of relapse or progression to hypothyroidism, have not been successful. Some patients inevitably relapse after a single dose because the biologic effects of radiation vary between individuals, and hypothyroidism cannot be uniformly avoided even using accurate dosimetry. A practical strategy is to give a fixed dose based on clinical features, such as the severity of thyrotoxicosis, the size of the goiter (increases the dose needed), and the level of radioiodine uptake (decreases the dose needed). [131]I dosage generally ranges between 185 MBq (5 mCi) to 555 MBq (15 mCi). Incomplete treatment or early relapse is more common in males and in patients <40 years of age. Many authorities favor an approach aimed at thyroid ablation (as opposed to euthyroidism), given that levothyroxine replacement is straightforward and most patients ultimately progress to hypothyroidism over 5 to 10 years anyway, frequently with some delay in the diagnosis of hypothyroidism.

Certain radiation safety precautions are necessary in the first few days after radioiodine treatment, but the exact guidelines vary depending on local protocols. In general, patients need to avoid close, prolonged contact with children and pregnant women for several days because of possible transmission of residual isotope and excessive exposure to radiation emanating from the gland. Rarely there may be mild pain due to radiation thyroiditis 1 to 2 weeks after treatment.

Hyperthyroidism can persist for 2 to 3 months before radioiodine takes full effect. For this reason, β-adrenergic blockers or antithyroid drugs can be used to control symptoms during this interval. Persistent hyperthyroidism can be treated with a second dose of radioiodine, usually 6 months after the first dose. The risk of hypothyroidism after radioiodine depends on the dosage but is at least 10 to 20% in the first year and 5% per year thereafter. Patients should be informed of this possibility before treatment and require close follow-up during the first year and annual thyroid function testing thereafter.

Pregnancy and breast feeding are absolute contraindications to radioiodine treatment, but patients can conceive safely 6 to 12 months after treatment. The presence of severe ophthalmopathy requires caution, and some authorities advocate the use of prednisone, 40 mg/d, at the time of radioiodine treatment, tapered over 2 to 3 months to prevent exacerbation of ophthalmopathy. The overall risk of cancer after radioiodine treatment in adults is not increased, but many physicians avoid radioiodine in children and adolescents because of the theoretical risks of malignancy.

Subtotal thyroidectomy is an option for patients who relapse after antithyroid drugs and prefer this treatment to radioiodine. Some experts recommend surgery in young individuals, particularly when the goiter is very large. Careful control of thyrotoxicosis with antithyroid drugs, followed by potassium iodide (3 drops SSKI orally tid) is needed prior to surgery to avoid thyrotoxic crisis and to reduce the vascularity of the gland. The major complications of surgery—i.e., bleeding, laryngeal edema, hypoparathyroidism, and damage to the recurrent laryngeal nerves—are unusual when the procedure is performed by highly experienced surgeons. Recurrence rates in the best series are <2%, but the rate of hypothyroidism is only slightly less than that following radioiodine treatment.

The titration regimen of antithyroid drugs should be used to manage Graves' disease in *pregnancy*, as blocking doses of these drugs produce fetal hypothyroidism. Propylthiouracil is usually used because of relatively low transplacental transfer and its ability to block $T_4 \rightarrow T_3$ conversion. Also, carbimazole and methimazole have been associated with rare cases of fetal *aplasia cutis*. The lowest effective dose of propylthiouracil should be given, and it is often possible to stop treatment in the last trimester since TSH-R antibodies tend to decline in pregnancy. Nonetheless, the transplacental transfer of these antibodies rarely causes *fetal thyrotoxicosis* or *neonatal thyrotoxicosis*. Poor intrauterine growth, a fetal heart rate of >160 beats/min, and high levels of maternal TSH-R antibodies should suggest this complication. Antithyroid drugs given to the mother can be used to treat the fetus and may be needed for 1 to 3 months after delivery, until the maternal antibodies disappear from the baby's circulation. The postpartum period is a time of major risk for relapse of Graves' disease. Breast feeding is safe with low doses of antithyroid drugs. Graves' disease in *children* is best managed with antithyroid drugs, often given as a prolonged course of the titration regimen. Surgery may be indicated for severe disease. Radioiodine can also be used in children, though most experts defer this treatment until adolescence or later.

Thyrotoxic crisis, or *thyroid storm*, is rare and presents as a life-threatening exacerbation of hyperthyroidism, accompanied by fever, delirium, seizures, coma, vomiting, diarrhea, and jaundice. The mortality rate due to cardiac failure, arrhythmia, or hyperthermia is ~30%, even with treatment. Thyrotoxic crisis is usually precipitated by acute illness (e.g., stroke, infection, trauma, diabetic ketoacidosis), surgery (especially on the thyroid), or radioiodine treatment of a patient with partially treated or untreated hyperthyroidism. Management requires intensive monitoring and supportive care, identification and treatment of the precipitating cause, and measures that reduce thyroid hormone synthesis. Large doses of propylthiouracil (600-mg loading dose and 200 to 300 mg every 6 h) should be given orally or by nasogastric tube or per rectum; the drug's inhibitory action on $T_4 \rightarrow T_3$ conversion makes it the agent of choice. One hour after the first dose of propylthiouracil, stable iodide is given to block thyroid hormone synthesis via the Wolff-Chaikoff effect (the delay allows the antithyroid drug to prevent the excess iodine from being incorporated into new hormone).

A saturated solution of potassium iodide (5 drops SSKI every 6 h), or ipodate or iopanoic acid (0.5 mg every 12 h), may be given orally. (Sodium iodide, 0.25 g intravenously every 6 h is an alternative but is not generally available.) Propranolol should also be given to reduce tachycardia and other adrenergic manifestations (40 to 60 mg orally every 4 h; or 2 mg intravenously every 4 h). Although other β-adrenergic blockers can be used, high doses of propranolol have been documented to decrease $T_4 \rightarrow T_3$ conversion, and the doses can be easily adjusted. Caution is needed to avoid acute negative inotropic effects, but controlling the heart rate is important, as some patients develop a form of high-output heart failure. Additional therapeutic measures include glucocorticoids (e.g., dexamethasone, 2 mg every 6 h), antibiotics if infection is present, cooling, and intravenous fluids.

Ophthalmopathy requires no active treatment when it is mild or moderate, as there is usually spontaneous improvement. General measures include meticulous control of thyroid hormone levels, advice about cessation of smoking, and an explanation of the natural history of ophthalmopathy. Discomfort can be relieved with artificial tears (e.g., 1% methylcellulose) and the use of dark glasses with side frames. Periorbital edema responds to a more upright sleeping position. Corneal exposure during sleep can be avoided by taping the eyelids shut. Minor degrees of diplopia improve with prisms fitted to spectacles. Severe ophthalmopathy, with optic nerve involvement or chemosis resulting in corneal damage, is an emergency requiring joint management with an ophthalmologist. Short-term benefit can be gained in about two-thirds of patients by the use of high-dose glucocorticoids (e.g., prednisone, 40 to 80 mg daily), sometimes combined with cyclosporine. Glucocorticoid doses are tapered by 5 mg every 1 to 2 weeks, but the taper often results in reemergence of congestive symptoms. Pulse therapy with intravenous methylprednisolone (1 g of methylprednisolone in 250 mL of saline infused over 2 h daily for 1 week) followed by an oral regimen is also used. Once the eye disease has stabilized, surgery may be indicated for relief of diplopia and correction of the appearance of the eyes. Orbital decompression can be achieved by removing bone from any wall of the orbit, thereby allowing displacement of fat and swollen extraocular muscles. The transantral route is used most often, as it requires no external incision. Proptosis recedes an average of 5 mm, but there may be residual or even worsened diplopia. Alternatively, retroorbital tissue can be decompressed without removal of bony tissue. External beam radiotherapy of the orbits has been used for many years, but the objective evidence that this therapy is beneficial remains equivocal.

Thyroid dermopathy does not usually require treatment but can cause cosmetic problems or interfere with the fit of shoes. Surgical removal is not indicated. Treatment consists of topical, high-potency glucocorticoid ointment under an occlusive dressing. Octreotide may be beneficial.

OTHER CAUSES OF THYROTOXICOSIS Destructive thyroiditis (subacute or silent thyroiditis) typically presents with a short thyrotoxic phase due to the release of preformed thyroid hormones and catabolism of Tg (see "Subacute Thyroiditis," below). True hyperthyroidism is absent, as demonstrated by a low radionuclide uptake. Circulating Tg and IL-6 levels are usually increased. Other causes of thyrotoxicosis with low or absent thyroid radionuclide uptake include *thyrotoxicosis factitia*; iodine excess and, rarely, ectopic thyroid tissue, particularly teratomas of the ovary (*struma ovarii*); and functional metastatic follicular carcinoma. Whole-body radionuclide studies can demonstrate ectopic thyroid tissue, and thyrotoxicosis factitia can be distinguished from destructive thyroiditis by the clinical features and low levels of Tg. Amiodarone treatment is associated with thyrotoxicosis in up to 10% of patients, particularly in areas of low iodine intake.

TSH-secreting pituitary adenoma is a rare causes of thyrotoxicosis. It can be identified by the presence of an inappropriately normal or increased TSH level in a patient with hyperthyroidism, diffuse goiter, and elevated free T_4 and T_3 levels (Chap. 328). Elevated levels of the α subunit of TSH, released by the TSH-secreting adenoma, support this diagnosis, which can be confirmed by demonstrating the pituitary tumor on CT or MRI scan. A combination of transsphenoidal surgery, sella irradiation, and octreotide may be required to normalize TSH, as many of these tumors are large and locally invasive at the time of diagnosis. Radioiodine or antithyroid drugs can be used to control thyrotoxicosis.

Thyrotoxicosis caused by *toxic multinodular goiter* and *hyperfunctioning solitary nodules* is discussed below.

THYROIDITIS

A clinically useful classification of thyroiditis is based on the onset and duration of disease (Table 330-8).

ACUTE THYROIDITIS   Acute thyroiditis is rare and is due to suppurative infection of the thyroid. In children and young adults, the most common cause is the presence of a piriform sinus, a remnant of the fourth branchial pouch that connects the oropharynx with the thyroid. Such sinuses are predominantly left sided. A long-standing goiter and degeneration in a thyroid malignancy are risk factors in the elderly. The patient presents with thyroid pain, often referred to the throat or ears, and a small, tender goiter that may be asymmetric. Fever, dysphagia, and erythema over the thyroid are common, as are systemic symptoms of a febrile illness and lymphadenopathy.

The differential diagnosis of *thyroid pain* includes subacute or, rarely, chronic thyroiditis, hemorrhage into a cyst, malignancy including lymphoma, and, rarely, amiodarone-induced thyroiditis or amyloidosis. However, the abrupt presentation and clinical features of acute thyroiditis rarely cause confusion. The erythrocyte sedimentation rate (ESR) and white cell count are usually increased, but thyroid function is normal. FNA biopsy shows infiltration by polymorphonuclear leukocytes; culture of the sample can identify the organism. Caution is needed in immunocompromised patients as fungal or *Pneumocystis* thyroiditis can occur in this setting. Antibiotic treatment is guided initially by Gram stain and subsequently by cultures of the FNA biopsy. Surgery may be needed to drain an abscess, which can be localized by CT scan or ultrasound. Tracheal obstruction, septicemia, retropharyngeal abscess, mediastinitis, and jugular venous thrombosis may complicate acute thyroiditis but are uncommon with prompt use of antibiotics.

SUBACUTE THYROIDITIS   This is also termed *de Quervain's thyroiditis*, *granulomatous thyroiditis*, or *viral thyroiditis*. Many viruses have been implicated, including mumps, coxsackie, influenza, adenoviruses, and echoviruses, but attempts to identify the virus in an individual patient are often unsuccessful and do not influence management. The diagnosis of subacute thyroiditis is often overlooked because the symptoms can mimic pharyngitis. The peak incidence oc-

curs at 30 to 50 years, and women are affected three times more frequently than men.

Pathophysiology   The thyroid shows a characteristic patchy inflammatory infiltrate with disruption of the thyroid follicles and multinucleated giant cells within some follicles. The follicular changes progress to granulomas accompanied by fibrosis. Finally, the thyroid returns to normal, usually several months after onset. During the initial phase of follicular destruction, there is release of Tg and thyroid hormones, leading to increased circulating free T_4 and T_3 and suppression of TSH (Fig. 330-8). During this destructive phase, radioactive iodine uptake is low or undetectable. After several weeks, the thyroid is depleted of stored thyroid hormone and a phase of hypothyroidism typically occurs, with low free T_4 (and sometimes T_3) and moderately increased TSH levels. Radioactive iodine uptake returns to normal or is even increased as a result of the rise in TSH. Finally, thyroid hormone and TSH levels return to normal as the disease subsides.

Clinical Manifestations   The patient usually presents with a painful and enlarged thyroid, sometimes accompanied by fever. There may be features of thyrotoxicosis or hypothyroidism, depending on the phase of the illness. Malaise and symptoms of an upper respiratory tract infection may precede the thyroid-related features by several weeks. In other patients, the onset is acute, severe, and without obvious antecedent. Though the patient typically complains of a sore throat, examination reveals a small goiter that is exquisitely tender, and asymmetry is common. Pain is often referred to the jaw or ear. Complete resolution is the usual outcome, but permanent hypothyroidism can occur, particularly in those with coincidental thyroid autoimmunity. A prolonged course over many months, with one or more relapses, occurs in a small percentage of patients.

Laboratory Evaluation   As depicted in Fig. 330-8, thyroid function tests characteristically evolve through three distinct phases over about 6 months: (1) thyrotoxic phase, (2) hypothyroid phase, and (3) recovery phase. In the thyrotoxic phase, T_4 and T_3 levels are increased, reflecting their discharge from the damaged thyroid cells, and TSH is suppressed. The T_4/T_3 ratio is greater than in Graves' disease or thyroid autonomy, in which T_3 is often disproportionately increased. The diagnosis is confirmed by a high ESR and low radioiodine uptake. Serum IL-6 levels increase during the thyrotoxic phase. The white blood cell count may be increased, and thyroid antibodies are negative. If the diagnosis is in doubt, FNA biopsy may be useful, particularly to distinguish unilateral involvement from bleeding into a cyst or neoplasm.

R_x **TREATMENT**   Relatively large doses of aspirin (e.g., 600 mg every 4 to 6 h) or nonsteroidal anti-inflammatory drugs are suf-

Table 330-8   Causes of Thyroiditis

Acute
  Bacterial infection: especially *Staphylcoccus*, *Streptococcus*, and
    Enterobacter
  Fungal infection: *Aspergillus*, *Candida*, *Coccidioides*, *Histoplasma*, and
    Pneumocystis
  Radiation thyroiditis after ^{131}I treatment
  Amiodarone (may also be subacute or chronic)
Subacute
  Viral (or granulomatous) thyroiditis
  Silent thyroiditis (including postpartum thyroiditis)
  Mycobacterial infection
Chronic
  Autoimmunity: focal thyroiditis, Hashimoto's thyroiditis, atrophic
    thyroiditis
  Riedel's thyroiditis
  Parasitic thyroiditis: echinococcosis, strongyloidiasis, cysticercosis
  Traumatic: after palpation

FIGURE 330-8   Clinical course of subacute thyroiditis. The release of thyroid hormones is initially associated with a thyrotoxic phase and suppressed TSH. A hypothyroid phase then ensues, with low T_4 and TSH levels that are initially low but gradually increase. During the recovery phase, increased TSH levels combined with resolution of thyroid follicular injury leads to normalization of thyroid function, often several months after the beginning of the illness.

ficient to control symptoms in most cases. If this treatment is inadequate, or if the patient has marked local or systemic symptoms, glucocorticoids should be given. The usual starting dose is 40 to 60 mg prednisone, depending on severity. The dose is gradually tapered over 6 to 8 weeks, in response to improvement in symptoms and the ESR. If a relapse occurs during glucocorticoid withdrawal, treatment should be started again and withdrawn more gradually. In these patients, it is useful to wait until the radioactive iodine uptake normalizes before stopping treatment. Thyroid function should be monitored every 2 to 4 weeks using TSH and free T_4 levels. Symptoms of thyrotoxicosis improve spontaneously but may be ameliorated by β-adrenergic blockers; antithyroid drugs play no role in treatment of the thyrotoxic phase. Levothyroxine replacement may be needed if the hypothyroid phase is prolonged, but doses should be low enough (50 to 100 μg daily) to allow TSH-mediated recovery.

SILENT THYROIDITIS *Painless thyroiditis*, or *"silent"* thyroiditis, occurs in patients with underlying autoimmune thyroid disease. It has a clinical course similar to that of subacute thyroiditis, except that there is little or no thyroid tenderness. The condition occurs most frequently 3 to 6 months after pregnancy and is then termed *postpartum thyroiditis*. Typically, patients have a brief phase of thyrotoxicosis, lasting 2 to 4 weeks, followed by hypothyroidism for 4 to 12 weeks, and then resolution; often, however, only one phase is apparent. As in subacute thyroiditis, the radioactive iodine uptake is initially suppressed. In addition to the painless goiter, silent thyroiditis can be distinguished from subacute thyroiditis by the normal ESR and the presence of TPO antibodies. Glucocorticoid treatment is not indicated for silent thyroiditis. Severe thyrotoxic symptoms can be managed with a brief course of propranolol, 20 to 40 mg three or four times daily. Thyroxine replacement may be needed for the hypothyroid phase but should be withdrawn after 6 to 9 months, as recovery is the rule. Annual follow-up thereafter is recommended, as a proportion of these individuals develop permanent hypothyroidism.

DRUG-INDUCED THYROIDITIS Patients receiving IFN-α, IL-2, or amiodarone may develop painless thyroiditis. INF-α, which is used to treat chronic hepatitis B or C, causes thyroid dysfunction in up to 5% of treated patients. It has been associated with painless thyroiditis, hypothyroidism, and Graves' disease. IL-2, which has been used to treat various malignancies, has also been associated with thyroiditis and hypothyroidism, though fewer patients have been studied. For discussion of amiodarone, see "Amiodarone Effects on Thyroid Function," below.

CHRONIC THYROIDITIS The most common cause of chronic thyroiditis is *Hashimoto's thyroiditis*, an autoimmune disorder that often presents as a firm or hard goiter of variable size (see above). *Riedel's thyroiditis* is a rare disorder that typically occurs in middle-aged women. It presents with an insidious, painless goiter with local symptoms due to compression of the esophagus, trachea, neck veins, or recurrent laryngeal nerves. Dense fibrosis disrupts normal gland architecture and can extend outside the thyroid capsule. Despite these extensive histologic changes, thyroid dysfunction is uncommon. The goiter is hard, nontender, often asymmetric and fixed, leading to suspicion of a malignancy. Diagnosis requires open biopsy as FNA biopsy is usually unhelpful. Treatment is surgical and directed to relief of compressive symptoms. There is an association between Riedel's thyroiditis and idiopathic fibrosis at other sites (retroperitoneum, mediastinum, biliary tree, lung, and orbit).

SICK EUTHYROID SYNDROME

Any acute, severe illness can cause abnormalities of circulating TSH or thyroid hormone levels in the absence of underlying thyroid disease, making these measurements potentially misleading. The major cause of these hormonal changes is the release of cytokines. Unless a thyroid disorder is strongly suspected, the routine testing of thyroid function should be avoided in acutely ill patients.

The most common hormone pattern in sick euthyroid syndrome

(SES) is a decrease in total and free T_3 levels (low T_3 syndrome) with normal levels of T_4 and TSH. The magnitude of the fall in T_3 correlates with the severity of the illness. T_4 conversion to T_3 via peripheral deiodination is impaired, leading to increased reverse T_3 (rT_3). Despite this effect, decreased clearance rather than increased production is the major basis for increased rT_3. Also, T_4 is alternately metabolized to the hormonally inactive T_3 sulfate. It is generally assumed that this low T_3 state is adaptive, as it can be induced in normal individuals by fasting. Teleologically, the fall in T_3 may provide a mechanism for limiting catabolism in starved or ill patients.

Very sick patients may have a fall in total T_4 and T_3 levels (low T_4 syndrome). This state has a poor prognosis. A key factor in the fall in T_4 levels is altered binding to TBG. Free T_4 assays usually demonstrate a normal free T_4 level in such patients, depending on the assay method used. Fluctuation in TSH levels also creates challenges in the interpretation of thyroid function in sick patients. TSH levels may range from <0.1 to >20 mU/L; these alterations reverse after recovery, confirming the absence of underlying thyroid disease. A rise in cortisol or administration of glucocorticoids may provide a partial explanation for decreased TSH levels. However, the exact mechanisms underlying the subnormal TSH seen in 10% of sick patients and the increased TSH seen in 5% remain unclear.

Any severe illness can induce changes in thyroid hormone levels, but certain disorders exhibit a distinctive pattern of abnormalities. Acute liver disease is associated with an initial rise in total (but not free) T_3 and T_4 levels, due to TBG release; these levels become subnormal with progression to liver failure. A transient increase in total and free T_4 levels, usually with a normal T_3 level, is seen in 5 to 30% of acutely ill psychiatric patients. TSH values may be transiently low, normal, or high in these patients. In the early stage of HIV infection, T_3 and T_4 levels rise, even if there is weight loss. T_3 levels fall with progression to AIDS, but TSH levels usually remain normal. Renal disease is often accompanied by low T_3 concentrations, but with normal rather than increased rT_3 levels, due to an unknown factor that increases uptake of rT_3 into the liver.

The diagnosis of the SES is challenging. Historic information may be limited, and patients often have multiple metabolic derangements. Useful features to consider include previous history of thyroid disease and thyroid function tests, evaluation of the severity and time course of the patient's acute illness, documentation of medications that may affect thyroid function or thyroid hormone levels, and measurements of rT_3 together with free thyroid hormones and TSH. The diagnosis of SES is frequently presumptive, given the clinical context and pattern of laboratory values; only resolution of the test results with clinical recovery can clearly establish this disorder. Treatment of SES with thyroid hormone (T_4 and/or T_3) is controversial, but most authorities recommend monitoring the patient's thyroid function tests during recovery, without administering thyroid hormone, unless there is historic or clinical evidence suggestive of hypothyroidism. Sufficiently large randomized controlled trials using thyroid hormone are unlikely to resolve this therapeutic controversy in the near future, because clinical presentations and outcomes are highly variable.

AMIODARONE EFFECTS ON THYROID FUNCTION

Amiodarone is a commonly used type III antiarrhythmic agent (Chap. 230). It is structurally related to thyroid hormone and contains 39% iodine by weight. Thus, typical doses of amiodarone (200 mg/d) are associated with very high iodine intake, leading to >40-fold increases in plasma and urinary iodine levels. Moreover, because amiodarone is stored in adipose tissue, high iodine levels persist for >6 months after discontinuation of the drug. Amiodarone inhibits deiodinase activity, and its metabolites function as weak antagonists of thyroid hormone action. Amiodarone has the following multiple effects on thyroid function: (1) acute, transient changes in thyroid function; (2) hypothyroidism in patients susceptible to the inhibitory effects of a high iodine load; and (3) thyrotoxicosis that may be caused by at least three mechanisms—a Jod-Basedow effect from the iodine load in the setting of multinodular goiter, a thyroiditis-like condition, and possibly induction of autoimmune Graves' disease.

The initiation of amiodarone treatment is associated with a transient decrease of T_4 levels, reflecting the inhibitory effect of iodine on T_4 release. Soon thereafter, most individuals escape from iodide-dependent suppression of the thyroid (Wolff-Chaikoff effect), and the inhibitory effects on deiodinase activity and thyroid hormone receptor action become predominant. These events lead to the following pattern of thyroid function tests: increased T_4, decreased T_3, increased rT_3, and a transient increase of TSH (up to 20 mU/L). TSH levels normalize or are slightly suppressed after about 1 to 3 months.

The incidence of hypothyroidism from amiodarone varies geographically, apparently correlating with iodine intake. Hypothyroidism occurs in up to 13% of amiodarone-treated patients in iodine-replete countries, such as the United States, but is less common (<6% incidence) in areas of lower iodine intake, such as Italy or Spain. The pathogenesis appears to involve an inability of the thyroid to escape from the high iodine load. Consequently, amiodarone-associated hypothyroidism is more common in women and individuals with positive TPO antibodies. It is usually unnecessary to discontinue amiodarone for this side effect, as levothyroxine can be used to normalize thyroid function. TSH levels should be monitored, because T_4 levels are often increased for the reasons described above.

The management of amiodarone-induced thyrotoxicosis (AIT) is complicated by the fact that there are several causes of thyrotoxicosis and because the increased thyroid hormone levels exacerbate underlying arrhythmias and coronary artery disease. Amiodarone treatment causes thyrotoxicosis in 10% of patients living in areas of low iodine intake and in 2% of patients in regions of high iodine intake. There are two major forms of AIT. Type 1 AIT is associated with an underlying thyroid abnormality (preclinical Graves' disease or nodular goiter). Thyroid hormone synthesis becomes excessive as a result of increased iodine exposure (Jod-Basedow phenomenon). Type 2 AIT occurs in individuals with no intrinsic thyroid abnormalities and is the result of drug-induced lysosomal activation leading to destructive thyroiditis with histiocyte accumulation in the thyroid. Mild forms of type 2 AIT can resolve spontaneously or can occasionally lead to hypothyroidism. Color-flow doppler thyroid scanning shows increased vascularity in type 1 but decreased vascularity in type 2 AIT; IL-6 levels are markedly raised in type 2 but only slightly increased in type 1 AIT. Thyroid scans are difficult to interpret in this setting, because the high endogenous iodine levels diminish tracer uptake. However, the presence of normal or increased uptake favors type 1 AIT.

In amiodarone-induced thyrotoxicosis the drug should be stopped, if possible, though this is often impractical because of the underlying cardiac disorder. Discontinuation of amiodarone will not have an acute effect because of its storage and prolonged half-life. High doses of antithyroid drugs can be used in type 1 AIT but are often ineffective. Potassium perchlorate, 200 mg every 6 h, has been used to reduce thyroidal iodide content. Perchlorate treatment has been associated with agranulocytosis, though the risk appears relatively low with short-term use. Glucocorticoids, administered as for subacute thyroiditis, are beneficial in type 2 AIT. Lithium blocks thyroid hormone release and can provide modest benefit. Near-total thyroidectomy rapidly decreases thyroid hormone levels and may be the most effective long-term solution, if the patient can undergo the procedure safely.

THYROID FUNCTION IN PREGNANCY

Three factors alter thyroid function in pregnancy: (1) the transient increase in hCG during the first trimester, which stimulates the TSH-R; (2) the estrogen-induced rise in TBG during the first trimester, which is sustained during pregnancy; and (3) increased urinary iodide excretion, which can cause impaired thyroid hormone production in areas of marginal iodine sufficiency. Women with a precarious iodine intake (<50 μg/d) are most at risk of developing a goiter during pregnancy, and iodine supplementation should be considered to prevent maternal and fetal hypothyroidism and the development of neonatal goiter.

The rise in circulating hCG levels during the first trimester is accompanied by a reciprocal fall in TSH that persists into the middle of pregnancy. This appears to reflect weak binding of hCG, which is present at very high levels, to the TSH-R. Rare individuals have been described with variant TSH-R sequences that enhance hCG binding and TSH-R activation. Occasionally these hCG-induced changes in thyroid function result in transient gestational hyperthyroidism and/or *hyperemesis gravidarum*, a condition characterized by severe nausea and vomiting and risk of volume depletion. Antithyroid drugs are rarely needed, and parenteral fluid replacement usually suffices until the condition resolves.

Maternal hypothyroidism occurs in 2 to 3% of women of childbearing age and is associated with increased risk of developmental delay in the offspring. Thyroid hormone requirements are increased by 25 to 50 μg/d during pregnancy.

GOITER AND NODULAR THYROID DISEASE

Goiter refers to an enlarged thyroid gland. Biosynthetic defects, iodine deficiency, autoimmune disease, and nodular diseases can each lead to goiter, though by different mechanisms. Biosynthetic defects and iodine deficiency are associated with reduced efficiency of thyroid hormone synthesis, leading to increased TSH, which stimulates thyroid growth as a compensatory mechanism to overcome the block in hormone synthesis. Graves' disease and Hashimoto's thyroiditis are also associated with goiter. In Graves' disease, the goiter results mainly from the TSH-R-mediated effects of TSI. The goitrous form of Hashimoto's thyroiditis occurs because of acquired defects in hormone synthesis, leading to elevated levels of TSH and its consequent growth effects. Lymphocytic infiltration and immune system–induced growth factors also contribute to thyroid enlargement in Hashimoto's thyroiditis. Nodular disease is characterized by the disordered growth of thyroid follicles, often combined with the gradual development of fibrosis. The management of goiter differs in patients depending on the etiology, and the detection of thyroid enlargement on physical examination should prompt further evaluation to identify its cause.

Nodular thyroid disease is common, occurring in about 3 to 7% of adults when assessed by physical examination. Using more sensitive techniques, such as ultrasound, it is present in >25% of adults. Thyroid nodules may be solitary or multiple, and they may be functional or nonfunctional.

DIFFUSE NONTOXIC (SIMPLE) GOITER **Etiology and Pathogenesis** When diffuse enlargement of the thyroid occurs in the absence of nodules and hyperthyroidism, it is referred to as a *diffuse nontoxic goiter*. This is sometimes called *simple goiter*, because of the absence of nodules, or *colloid goiter*, because of the presence of uniform follicles that are filled with colloid. Worldwide, diffuse goiter is most commonly caused by iodine deficiency and is termed *endemic goiter* when it affects >5% of the population. In nonendemic regions, *sporadic goiter* occurs, and the cause is usually unknown. Thyroid enlargement in teenagers is sometimes referred to as *juvenile goiter*. In general, goiter is more common in women than men, probably because of the greater prevalence of underlying autoimmune disease and the increased iodine demands associated with pregnancy.

In *iodine-deficient areas*, thyroid enlargement reflects a compensatory effort to trap iodide and produce sufficient hormone under conditions in which hormone synthesis is relatively inefficient. Somewhat surprisingly, TSH levels are usually normal or only slightly increased, suggesting increased sensitivity to TSH or activation of other pathways that lead to thyroid growth. Iodide appears to have direct actions on thyroid vasculature and may indirectly affect growth through vasoactive substances such as endothelins and nitric oxide. Endemic goiter is also caused by exposure to environmental *goitrogens* such as cassava root, which contains a thiocyanate, vegetables of the Cruciferae family (e.g., brussels sprouts, cabbage, and cauliflower), and milk from regions where goitrogens are present in grass. Though relatively rare, inherited defects in thyroid hormone synthesis also lead to a diffuse nontoxic goiter. These involve abnormalities at each step in hormone synthesis including iodide transport (NIS), Tg synthesis, organification and coupling (TPO), and the regeneration of iodide (dehalogenase).

Clinical Manifestations and Diagnosis If thyroid function is preserved, most goiters are asymptomatic. Spontaneous hemorrhage into a cyst or nodule may cause the sudden onset of localized pain and swelling. Examination of a diffuse goiter reveals a symmetrically enlarged, nontender, generally soft gland without palpable nodules. Goiter is defined, somewhat arbitrarily, as a lateral lobe with a volume greater than the thumb of the individual being examined. If the thyroid is markedly enlarged, it can cause tracheal or esophageal compression. These features are unusual, however, in the absence of nodular disease and fibrosis. *Substernal goiter* may obstruct the thoracic inlet. *Pemberton's sign* refers to symptoms of faintness with evidence of facial congestion and external jugular venous obstruction when the arms are raised above the head, a maneuver that draws the thyroid into the thoracic inlet. Respiratory flow measurements and CT or MRI should be used to evaluate substernal goiter in patients with obstructive signs or symptoms.

Thyroid function tests should be performed in all patients with goiter to exclude thyrotoxicosis or hypothyroidism. It is not unusual, particularly in iodine deficiency, to find a low total T_4, with normal T_3 and TSH, reflecting enhanced $T_4 \rightarrow T_3$ conversion. A low TSH, particularly in older patients, suggests the possibility of thyroid autonomy or undiagnosed Graves' disease, causing subclinical thyrotoxicosis. TPO antibodies may be useful to identify patients at increased risk of autoimmune thyroid disease. Low urinary iodine levels (<100 μg/L) support a diagnosis of iodine deficiency. Thyroid scanning is not generally necessary but will reveal increased uptake in iodine deficiency and most cases of dyshormonogenesis. Ultrasound is not generally indicated in the evaluation of diffuse goiter, unless a nodule is palpable on physical examination.

℞ **TREATMENT** Iodine or thyroid hormone replacement induces variable regression of goiter in iodine deficiency, depending on how long it has been present and the degree of fibrosis that has developed. For other causes of nontoxic diffuse goiter, levothyroxine can be used in an attempt to reduce goiter size. Because of the possibility of underlying thyroid autonomy, caution should be exercised when instituting suppressive thyroxine therapy, particularly if the baseline TSH is in the low-normal range. In younger patients, the dose can be started at 100 μg/d and adjusted to suppress the TSH into the low-normal but detectable range. Treatment of elderly patients should be initiated at 50 μg/d. The efficacy of suppressive treatment is greater in younger patients and in those with soft goiters. Significant regression is usually seen within 3 to 6 months of treatment; after this time it is unlikely to occur. In older patients, and in those with some degree of nodular disease or fibrosis, fewer than one-third demonstrate significant shrinkage of the goiter. Surgery is rarely indicated for diffuse goiter. Exceptions include documented evidence of tracheal compression or obstruction of the thoracic inlet, which are more likely to be associated with substernal multinodular goiters (see below). Subtotal or near-total thyroidectomy for these or cosmetic reasons should be performed by an experienced surgeon to minimize complication rates, which occur in up to 10% of cases. Surgery should be followed by mild suppressive treatment with levothyroxine to prevent regrowth of the goiter. Radioiodine reduces goiter size by about 50% in the majority of patients. It is rarely associated with transient acute swelling of the thyroid, which is usually inconsequential unless there is severe tracheal narrowing. If not treated with levothyroxine, patients should be followed after radioiodine treatment for the possible development of hypothyroidism.

NONTOXIC MULTINODULAR GOITER

Etiology and Pathogenesis Depending on the geographic region and the sensitivity of the methods used to detect the disorder, multinodular goiter (MNG) is common, occurring in between 1 and 12% of the population. MNG is more common in women than men and increases in prevalence with age. It is more common in iodine-deficient regions but also occurs in regions of iodine sufficiency, reflecting multiple genetic, autoimmune, and environmental influences on the pathogenesis.

Individual patients exhibit wide variation in nodule size. Histology reveals a spectrum of morphologies ranging from hypercellular regions to cystic areas filled with colloid. Fibrosis is often extensive, and areas of hemorrhage or lymphocytic infiltration may be seen. Using molecular techniques, most nodules within a MNG are polyclonal in origin, suggesting a hyperplastic response to locally produced growth factors and cytokines. TSH, which is usually not elevated, may play a permissive or contributory role. Monoclonal lesions also occur within a MNG, reflecting mutations in genes that confer a selective growth advantage to the progenitor cell.

Clinical Manifestations Most patients with nontoxic MNG are asymptomic and, by definition, euthyroid. MNG typically develops over many years and is detected on routine physical examination or because an individual notices an enlargement in the neck. If the goiter is large enough, it can ultimately lead to compressive symptoms including difficulty swallowing, respiratory distress (tracheal compression), or plethora (venous congestion), but these symptoms are uncommon. Symptomatic MNGs are usually extraordinarily large and/or develop fibrotic areas that cause compression. Sudden pain in a MNG is often caused by hemorrhage into a nodule but should raise the possibility of invasive malignancy. Hoarseness, reflecting laryngeal nerve involvement, also suggests malignancy.

Diagnosis On examination, thyroid architecture is distorted and multiple nodules of varying size can be appreciated. Substernal goiter is suggested by Pemberton's sign. Because many nodules are deeply embedded in thyroid tissue or reside in posterior or substernal locations, it is not possible to palpate all nodules. A TSH level should be measured to exclude subclinical hyper- or hypothyroidism, but thyroid function is usually normal. Tracheal deviation is common, but compression must usually exceed 70% of the tracheal diameter before there is significant airway compromise. Pulmonary function testing can be used to assess the functional effects of compression and to detect tracheomalacia, which characteristically causes inspiratory stridor. CT or MRI can be used to evaluate the anatomy of the goiter and the extent of substernal extension, which is often much greater than is apparent on physical examination. A barium swallow may reveal the extent of esophageal obstruction. MNG does not appear to predispose to thyroid carcinoma or to more aggressive carcinoma. For this reason, and because it is not possible to biopsy all nodular lesions, thyroid biopsies should only be performed if malignancy is suspected because of a dominant or enlarging nodule.

℞ **TREATMENT** Most nontoxic MNGs can be managed conservatively. T_4 suppression is rarely effective for reducing goiter size and introduces the risk of thyrotoxicosis, if there is underlying autonomy or if it develops during treatment. If levothyroxine is used, it should be started at low doses (50 μg) and advanced gradually while monitoring the TSH level to avoid excessive suppression. Contrast agents and other iodine-containing substances should be avoided because of the risk of inducing the *Jod-Basedow effect*, characterized by enhanced thyroid hormone production by autonomous nodules. Radioiodine is being used with increasing frequency because it often decreases goiter size and may selectively ablate regions of autonomy. Dosage of ^{131}I depends on the size of the goiter and radioiodine uptake but is usually about 3.7 MBq (0.1 mCi) per gram of tissue, corrected for uptake [typical dose, 370 to 1070 Mbq (10 to 29 mCi)]. Repeat treatment may be needed. It is possible to achieve a 40 to 50% reduction in goiter size in most patients. Earlier concerns about radiation-induced thyroid swelling and tracheal compression have diminished as recent studies have shown this complication to be rare. When acute compression occurs, glucocorticoid treatment or surgery may be needed. Radiation-induced hypothyroidism is less common than occurs after treatment for Graves' disease. However, posttreatment autoimmune thyrotoxicosis may occur in up to 5% of patients treated for nontoxic MNG. Surgery remains highly effective but is not without risk, particularly in older patients with underlying cardiopulmonary disease.

TOXIC MULTINODULAR GOITER   The pathogenesis of toxic MNG appears to be similar to that of nontoxic MNG, the major difference being the presence of functional autonomy in toxic MNG. The molecular basis for autonomy in toxic MNG remains unknown. As in nontoxic goiters, many nodules are polyclonal, while others are monoclonal and vary in their clonal origins. Genetic abnormalities known to confer functional autonomy, such as activating TSH-R or $G_{s\alpha}$ mutations (see below), are not usually found in the autonomous regions of toxic MNG goiter.

In addition to features of goiter, the clinical presentation of toxic MNG includes subclinical hyperthyroidism or mild thyrotoxicosis. The patient is usually elderly and may present with atrial fibrillation or palpitations, tachycardia, nervousness, tremor, or weight loss. Recent exposure to iodine, from contrast dyes or other sources, may precipitate or exacerbate thyrotoxicosis. The TSH level is low. The T_4 level may be normal or minimally increased; T_3 is often elevated to a greater degree than T_4. Thyroid scan shows heterogeneous uptake with multiple regions of increased and decreased uptake; 24-h uptake of radioiodine may not be increased.

℞ TREATMENT   The management of toxic MNG is challenging. Antithyroid drugs, often in combination with beta blockers, can normalize thyroid function and address clinical features of thyrotoxicosis. This treatment, however, often stimulates the growth of the goiter, and, unlike in Graves' disease, spontaneous remission does not occur. Radioiodine can be used to treat areas of autonomy, as well as to decrease the mass of the goiter. Usually, however, some degree of autonomy remains, presumably because multiple autonomous regions emerge as soon as others are treated. Nonetheless, a trial of radioiodine should be considered before subjecting patients, many of whom are elderly, to surgery. Surgery provides definitive treatment of underlying thyrotoxicosis as well as goiter. Patients should be rendered euthyroid using antithyroid drugs before operation.

HYPERFUNCTIONING SOLITARY NODULE   A solitary, autonomously functioning thyroid nodule is referred to as *toxic adenoma*. The pathogenesis of this disorder has been unraveled by demonstrating the functional effects of mutations that stimulate the TSH-R signaling pathway. Most patients with solitary hyperfunctioning nodules have acquired somatic, activating mutations in the TSH-R (Fig. 330-9). These mutations, located primarily in the receptor transmembrane domain, induce constitutive receptor coupling to $G_{s\alpha}$, increasing cyclic AMP levels and leading to enhanced thyroid follicular cell proliferation and function. Less commonly, somatic mutations are identified in $G_{s\alpha}$. These mutations, which are similar to those seen in McCune-Albright syndrome (Chap. 336) or in a subset of somatotrope adenomas (Chap. 328), impair GTP hydrolysis, also causing constitutive activation of the cyclic AMP signaling pathway. In most series, activating mutations in either the TSH-R or the $G_{s\alpha}$ subunit genes are identified in >90% of patients with solitary hyperfunctioning nodules.

Thyrotoxicosis is usually mild. The disorder is suggested by the presence of the thyroid nodule, which is generally large enough to be palpable, and by the absence of clinical features suggestive of Graves' disease or other causes of thyrotoxicosis. A thyroid scan provides a definitive diagnostic test, demonstrating focal uptake in the hyper-

TSH-R

Extracellular domain

Transmembrane domains

Activating mutations

$G_{s\alpha}$

AC

↑ **Cell growth, differentiation**
↑ **Hormone synthesis**

← cyclic AMP

FIGURE 330-9   Activating mutations of the TSH-R. Mutations (*) that activate the thyroid-stimulating hormone receptor (TSH-R) reside mainly in transmembrane 5 and intracellular loop 3, though mutations have occurred in a variety of different locations. The effect of these mutations is to induce conformational changes that mimic TSH binding, thereby leading to coupling to stimulatory G protein ($G_{s\alpha}$) and activation of adenylate cyclase (AC), an enzyme that generates cyclic AMP (cAMP).

functioning nodule and diminished uptake in the remainder of the gland, as activity of the normal thyroid is suppressed.

℞ TREATMENT   Radioiodine ablation is usually the treatment of choice. Because normal thyroid function is suppressed, ^{131}I is concentrated in the hyperfunctioning nodule with minimal uptake and damage to normal thyroid tissue. Relatively large radioiodine doses [e.g., 370 to 1110 MBq (10 to 29.9 mCi)^{131}I] have been shown to correct thyrotoxicosis in about 75% of patients within 3 months. Hypothyroidism occurs in <10% of patients over the next 5 years. Surgical resection is also effective and is usually limited to enucleation of the adenoma or lobectomy, thereby preserving thyroid function and minimizing risk of hypoparathyroidism or damage to the recurrent laryngeal nerves. Medical therapy using antithyroid drugs and beta blockers can normalize thyroid function but is not an optimal long-term treatment. Ethanol injection under ultrasound guidance has been used successfully in some centers to ablate hyperfunctioning nodules. Repeated injections (often more than 5 sessions) are required but reduce nodule size. Normal thyroid function can be achieved in most patients using this technique.

BENIGN NEOPLASMS

The various types of benign thyroid nodules are listed in Table 330-9. These lesions are common (5 to 10% adults) and often multiple, particularly when assessed by sensitive techniques such as ultrasound. The risk of malignancy is very low for *macrofollicular adenomas* and *normofollicular adenomas. Microfollicular, trabecular, and Hürthle cell variants* raise greater concern, partly because the histology is more difficult to interpret. About one-third of palpable nodules are *thyroid cysts*. These may be recognized by their ultrasound appearance or based on aspiration of large amounts of pink or straw-colored fluid (colloid). Many are mixed cystic/solid lesions, in which case it is desirable to aspirate cellular components under ultrasound or harvest cells after cytospin of cyst fluid. Cysts frequently recur, even after repeated aspiration, and may require surgical excision if they are large or if the cytology is suspicious. Sclerosis has been used with variable

Table 330-9   Classification of Thyroid Neoplasms

	Approximate Prevalence, %
Benign	
Follicular epithelial cell adenomas	
Macrofollicular (colloid)	
Normofollicular (simple)	
Microfollicular (fetal)	
Trabecular (embryonal)	
Hürtle cell variant (oncocytic)	
Malignant	
Follicular epithelial cell	
Well-differentiated carcinomas	
Papillary carcinomas	80–90
Pure papillary	
Follicular variant	
Diffuse sclerosing variant	
Tall cell, columnar cell variants	
Follicular carcinomas	5–10
Minimally invasive	
Widely invasive	
Hürthle cell carcinoma (oncocytic)	
Insular carcinoma	
Undifferentiated (anaplastic) carcinomas	
C cell (calcitonin-producing)	
Medullary thyroid cancer	10
Sporadic	
Familial	
MEN-2	
Other malignancies	
Lymphomas	1–2
Sarcomas	
Metastases	
Others	

NOTE: MEN, multiple endocrine neoplasia.

success but is often painful and may be complicated by infiltration of the sclerosing agent.

The treatment approach for benign nodules is similar to that for MNG. TSH suppression with levothyroxine decreases the size of about 30% of nodules and may prevent further growth. The TSH level should be suppressed into the low-normal range, assuming there are no contraindications; alternatively, nodule size can be monitored without suppression. If a nodule has not decreased in size after 6 to 12 months of suppressive therapy, treatment should be discontinued as little benefit is likely to accrue from long-term treatment.

THYROID CANCER

Thyroid carcinoma is the most common malignancy of the endocrine system. Malignant tumors derived from the follicular epithelium are classified according to histologic features. Differentiated tumors, such as papillary thyroid cancer (PTC) or follicular thyroid cancer (FTC), are often curable, and the prognosis is good for patients identified with early-stage disease. In contrast, anaplastic thyroid cancer (ATC) is aggressive, responds poorly to treatment, and is associated with a bleak prognosis.

The incidence of thyroid cancer (~9/100,000 per year) increases with age, plateauing after about age 50 (Fig. 330-10). Age is also an important prognostic factor—thyroid cancer at young age (<20) or in older persons (>65) is associated with a worse prognosis. Thyroid cancer is twice as common in women as men, but male sex is associated with a worse prognosis. Additional important risk factors include a history of childhood head or neck irradiation, large nodule size (≥4 cm), evidence for local tumor fixation or invasion into lymph nodes, and the presence of metastases (Table 330-10).

Several unique features of thyroid cancer facilitate its management: (1) thyroid nodules are readily palpable, allowing early detection and biopsy by FNA; (2) iodine radioisotopes can be used to diagnose

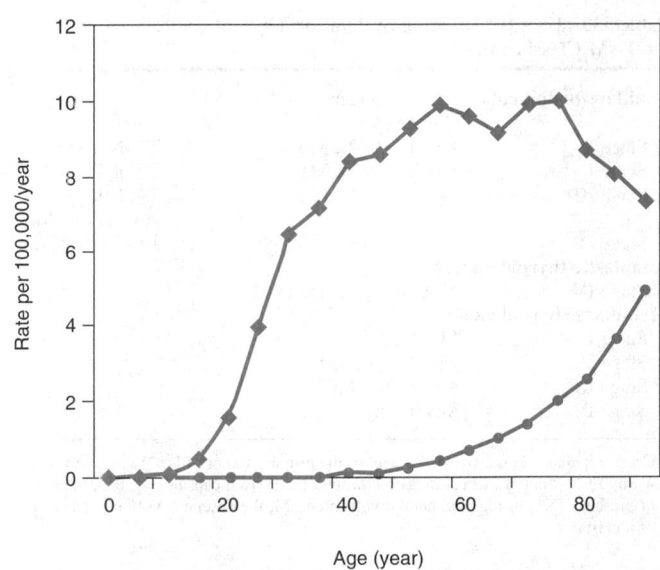

FIGURE 330-10 Age-associated incidence (◆—) and mortality (●—) rates for invasive thyroid cancer. *(Adapted from LAG Ries et al (eds): SEER Cancer Statistics Review, 1973–1996, Bethesda, National Cancer Institute, 1999.)*

(^{123}I) and treat (^{131}I) differentiated thyroid cancer, reflecting the unique uptake of this anion by the thyroid gland; and (3) serum markers allow the detection of residual or recurrent disease, including the use of Tg levels for PTC and FTC and calcitonin for medullary thyroid cancer (MTC).

CLASSIFICATION   Thyroid neoplasms can arise in each of the cell types that populate the gland, including thyroid follicular cells, calcitonin-producing C cells, lymphocytes, and stromal and vascular elements, as well as metastases from other sites (Table 330-9). The American Joint Committee on Cancer (AJCC) has designated a staging system using the TNM classification (Table 330-11). Several other classification and staging systems are also widely used, some of which place greater emphasis on histologic features or risk factors such as age or gender.

PATHOGENESIS AND GENETIC BASIS   **Radiation** Early studies of the pathogenesis of thyroid cancer focused on the role of external radiation, which predisposes to chromosomal breaks, presumably leading to genetic rearrangements and loss of tumor-suppressor genes. External radiation of the mediastinum, face, head, and neck region was administered in the past to treat an array of conditions including acne and enlargement of the thymus, tonsils, and adenoids. Radiation exposure increases the risk of benign and malignant thyroid nodules, is associated with multicentric cancers, and shifts the incidence of thyroid cancer to an earlier age group. Radiation from nuclear fallout also predisposes to thyroid cancer. Children seem more predisposed to the effects of radiation than adults. Of note, radiation derived from ^{131}I therapy appears to contribute little, if any, increased risk of thyroid cancer.

TSH and Growth Factors   Thyroid growth is regulated primarily by TSH but also by a variety of growth factors and cytokines. Many

Table 330-10   Risk Factors for Thyroid Carcinoma in Patients with a Thyroid Nodule

History of head and neck irradiation	Family history of thyroid cancer or MEN-2
Age <20 or >70 years	Vocal cord paralysis, hoarse voice
Increased nodule size (>4 cm)	Nodule fixed to adjacent structures
New or enlarging neck mass	Suspected lymph node involvement
Male gender	Iodine deficiency (follicular cancer)

NOTE: MEN, multiple endocrine neoplasia.

Table 330-11   AJCC Staging System for Thyroid Cancers Using the TNM Classification[a]

Papillary or follicular thyroid cancers

	<45 years	>45 years
Stage I	Any T, any N, M0	T1, N0, M0
Stage II	Any T, any N, M1	T2 or T3, N0, M0
Stage III	—	T4, N0, M0
		Any T, N1, M0
Stage IV	—	Any T, any N, M1

Anaplastic thyroid cancer

Stage IV	All cases are stage IV

Medullary thyroid cancer

Stage I	T1, N0, M0
Stage II	T2–T4, N0, M0
Stage III	Any T, N1, M0
Stage IV	Any T, any N, M1

[a] Criteria include: T, the size and extent of the primary tumor (T1 ≤ 1 cm; 1 cm < T2 ≤ 4 cm; T3 > 4 cm; T4 direct invasion through the thyroid capsule); N, the absence (N0) or presence (N1) of regional node involvement; M, the absence (M0) or presence (M1) of metastases.

differentiated thyroid cancers express TSH receptors and, therefore, remain responsive to TSH. This observation provides the rationale for T_4 suppression of TSH in patients with thyroid cancer. Residual expression of TSH receptors also allows TSH-stimulated uptake of ^{131}I therapy (see below).

Oncogenes and Tumor-Suppressor Genes   Thyroid cancers are monoclonal in origin, consistent with the idea that they originate as a consequence of mutations that confer a growth advantage to a single cell. In addition to increased rates of proliferation, some thyroid cancers exhibit impaired apoptosis and features that enhance invasion, angiogenesis, and metastasis (Chap. 83). By analogy with the model of multistep carcinogenesis proposed for colon cancer (Chap. 81), thyroid neoplasms have been analyzed for a variety of genetic alterations, but without clear evidence of an ordered acquisition of somatic mutations as they progress from the benign to the malignant state. On the other hand, certain mutations are relatively specific for thyroid neoplasia, some of which correlate with histologic classification (Table 330-12). For example, activating mutations of the TSH-R and the $G_{s\alpha}$ subunit are associated with autonomously functioning nodules. Though these mutations induce thyroid cell growth, this type of nodule is almost always benign. A variety of rearrangements involving the *RET* gene on chromosome 10 bring this receptor tyrosine kinase under the control of other promoters, leading to receptor overexpression. *RET* rearrangements occur in 20 to 40% of PTCs in different series and were observed with increased frequency in tumors developing after the Chernobyl radiation disaster. Rearrangements in PTC have also been observed for another tyrosine kinase gene, *TRK1*, which is located on chromosome 1. To date, the identification of PTC with *RET* or *TRK1* rearrangements has not proven useful for predicting prognosis or treatment responses. *RAS* mutations are found in about 20 to 30% of thyroid neoplasms, including adenomas as well as PTC and FTC, suggesting that these mutations do not strongly affect tumor phenotype. Loss of heterozygosity (LOH), consistent with deletions of tumor-suppressor genes, is particularly common in FTC, often involving chromosomes 3p or 11q. Mutations of the tumor suppressor, p53, appear to play an important role in the development of ATC. Because p53 plays a role in cell cycle surveillance, DNA repair, and apoptosis,

Table 330-12   Genetic Alterations in Thyroid Neoplasia

Gene/Protein	Type of Gene	Chromosomal Location	Genetic Abnormality	Tumor
TSH receptor	GPCR receptor	14q31	Point mutations	Toxic adenoma, differentiated carcinomas
$G_{s\alpha}$	G protein	20q13.2	Point mutations	Toxic adenoma, differentiated carcinomas
RET/PTC	Receptor tyrosine kinase	10q11.2	Rearrangements PTC1: (inv(10)q11.2q21) PTC2: (t(10;17)(q11.2;q23)) PTC3: ELE1/TK	PTC
RET	Receptor tyrosine kinase	10q11.2	Point mutations	MEN-2, medullary thyroid cancer
TRK	Receptor tyrosine kinase	1q23-24	Rearrangements	Multinodular goiter, papillary thyroid cancer
RAS	Signal transducing p21	Hras 11p15.5 Kras 12p12.1; Nras 1p13.2	Point mutations	Differentiated thyroid carcinoma, adenomas
p53	Tumor suppressor, cell cycle control, apoptosis	17p13	Point mutations Deletion, insertion	Anaplastic cancer
APC	Tumor suppressor, adenomatous polyposis coli gene	5q21-q22	Point mutations	Anaplastic cancer, also associated with familial polyposis coli
p16 (MTS1, CDKN2A)	Tumor suppressor, cell cycle control	9p21	Deletions	Differentiated carcinomas
p21/WAF	Tumor suppressor, cell cycle control	6p21.2	Overexpression	Anaplastic cancer
MET	Receptor tyrosine kinase	7q31	Overexpression	Follicular thyroid cancer
c-MYC	Receptor tyrosine kinase	8q24.12.-13	Overexpression	Differentiated carcinoma
PTEN	Phosphatase	10q23	Point mutations	PTC in Cowden's syndrome (multiple hamartomas, breast tumors, gastrointestinal polyps, thyroid tumors)
Loss of heterozygosity (LOH)	?Tumor suppressors	3p; 11q13 Other loci	Deletions	Differentiated thyroid carcinomas, anaplastic cancer
PAX8-PPARγ1	Transcription factor Nuclear receptor fusion	t(2;3)(q13;p25)	Translocation	Follicular carcinoma

NOTE: TSH, thyroid-stimulating hormone; $G_{s\alpha}$, G-protein stimulating α-subunit; RET, rearranged during transfection proto-oncogene; PTC, papillary thyroid cancer; TRK, tyrosine kinase receptor; RAS, rat sarcoma proto-oncogene; p53, p53 tumor suppressor gene; MET, met proto-oncogene (hepatocyte growth factor receptor); c-MYC, cellular homologue of myelocytomatosis virus proto-oncogene; PTEN, phosphatase and tensin homologue; APC, adenomatous polyposis coli; MTS, multiple tumor suppressor; CDKN2A, cyclin-dependent kinase inhibitor 2A; P21, p21 tumor suppressor; WAF, wild-type p53 activated fragment; GPCR, G protein–coupled receptor; ELE1/TK, ret-activating gene ele1/tyrosine kinase; MEN-2, multiple endocrine neoplasia-2; PAX8, Paired domain transcription factor; PPARγ1, Peroxisome-proliferator activated receptor 81.
SOURCE: Adapted with permission from P Kopp, JL Jameson, in JL Jameson (ed): *Principles of Molecular Medicine*. Totowa, NJ, Humana Press, 1998.

its loss may contribute to the rapid acquisition of genetic instability as well as poor treatment responses (Chap. 82). The role of other tumor-suppressor genes in thyroid cancer is under investigation (Table 330-12).

MTC, when associated with multiple endocrine neoplasia (MEN) type 2, harbors an inherited mutation of the *RET* gene. Unlike the rearrangements of *RET* seen in PTC, the mutations in MEN-2 are point mutations that induce constitutive activity of the tyrosine kinase (Chap. 339). MTC is preceded by hyperplasia of the C cells, raising the likelihood that as-yet-unidentified "second hits" lead to cellular transformation. A subset of sporadic MTC contain somatic mutations that activate *RET*.

WELL-DIFFERENTIATED THYROID CANCER

Papillary PTC is the most common type of thyroid cancer, accounting for 70 to 90% of well-differentiated thyroid malignancies. Microscopic PTC is present in as many 25% of thyroid glands at autopsy, but most of these lesions are very small (several millimeters) and are not clinically significant. Characteristic cytologic features of PTC help make the diagnosis by FNA or after surgical resection; these include psammoma bodies, cleaved nuclei with an "orphan-Annie" appearance caused by large nucleoli, and the formation of papillary structures.

PTC tends to be multifocal and to invade locally within the thyroid gland as well as through the thyroid capsule and into adjacent structures in the neck. It has a propensity to spread via the lymphatic system but can metastasize as well, particularly to bone and lung. Because of the relatively slow growth of the tumor, a significant burden of pulmonary metastases may accumulate, sometimes with remarkably few symptoms. The prognostic implication of lymph node spread is debated. Lymph node involvement by thyroid cancer can be remarkably well tolerated but probably increases the risk of recurrence and mortality, particularly in older patients. The staging of PTC by the TNM system is outlined in Table 330-11. Most papillary cancers are identified in the early stages (>80% stages I or II) and have an excellent prognosis, with survival curves similar to expected survival (Fig. 330-11A). Mortality is markedly increased in stage IV disease (distant metastases), but this group comprises only about 1% of patients. The treatment of PTC is described below.

Follicular The incidence of FTC varies widely in different parts of the world; it is more common in iodine-deficient regions. FTC is difficult to diagnose by FNA because the distinction between benign and malignant follicular neoplasms rests largely on evidence of invasion into vessels, nerves, or adjacent structures. FTC tends to spread by hematogenous routes leading bone, lung, and central nervous system metastases. Mortality rates associated with FTC are less favorable than for PTC, in part because a larger proportion of patients present with stage IV disease (Fig. 330-11B). Poor prognostic features include distant metastases, age >50 years, primary tumor size >4 cm, Hürthle cell histology, and the presence of marked vascular invasion.

℞ **TREATMENT** **Surgery** All well-differentiated thyroid cancers should be surgically excised. In addition to removing the primary lesion, surgery allows accurate histologic diagnosis and staging, and multicentric disease is commonly found in the contralateral lobe. Lymph node spread can also be assessed at the time of surgery, and involved nodes can be removed. Recommendations about the extent of surgery vary for stage I disease, as survival rates are similar for lobectomy and near-total thyroidectomy. Lobectomy is associated with a lower incidence of hypoparathyroidism and injury to the recurrent laryngeal nerves. However, it is not possible to monitor Tg levels or to perform whole-body ^{131}I scans in the presence of the residual lobe. Moreover, if final staging or subsequent follow-up indicates the need for radioiodine scanning or treatment, repeat surgery is necessary to remove the remaining thyroid tissue. The authors favor near-total thyroidectomy in almost all patients; complication rates are acceptably low if the surgeon is highly experienced in the procedure. This approach, in combination with postsurgical radioablation of the remnant

FIGURE 330-11 Survival rates in patients with differentiated thyroid cancer. *A.* Papillary cancer, cohort of 1851 patients. I, 1107 (60%), II, 408 (22%), III, 312 (17%), IV, 24 (1%); *n* = 1185. *B.* Follicular cancer, cohort of 153 patients. I, 42 (27%), II, 82 (54%), III, 6 (4%); IV, 23 (15%); *n* = 153. *(Adapted from Larsen et al.)*

thyroid tissue, facilitates the use of radioiodine scanning and Tg determinations to assess disease recurrence.

TSH Suppression Therapy As most tumors are still TSH-responsive, levothyroxine suppression of TSH is a mainstay of thyroid cancer treatment. Though TSH suppression clearly provides therapeutic benefit, there are no prospective studies that identify the optimal level of TSH suppression. A reasonable goal is to suppress TSH to as low as possible without subjecting the patient to unnecessary side effects from excess thyroid hormone, such as atrial fibrillation, osteopenia, anxiety, and other manifestations of thyrotoxicosis. For patients at low risk of recurrence, TSH should be suppressed into the low but detectable range (0.1 to 0.5 IU/L). For patients at high risk of recurrence, or with known metastatic disease, complete TSH suppression is indicated, if there are no strong contraindications to mild thyrotoxicosis. In this instance, free T_4 or free T_3 levels must also be monitored to avoid excessive treatment.

Radioiodine Treatment Well-differentiated thyroid cancer still incorporates radioiodine, though less efficiently than normal thyroid follicular cells. Radioiodine uptake is determined primarily by expression of the NIS and is stimulated by TSH, requiring expression of the TSH-R. The retention time for radioactivity is influenced by the extent to which the tumor retains differentiated functions such as iodide trapping and organification. After near-total thyroidectomy, substantial thyroid tissue remains, particularly in the thyroid bed and surrounding the parathyroid glands. Consequently, ^{131}I ablation is necessary to eliminate remaining normal thyroid tissue and may treat residual tumor cells.

Indications The use of therapeutic doses of radioiodine remains an area of controversy in thyroid cancer management. Postoperative thyroid ablation and radiodine treatment of known residual PTC or FTC reduce recurrence rates. [131]I ablation of remaining normal thyroid tissue also facilitates the detection of recurrent disease, using either whole-body iodine scanning or measurements of Tg. For tumors that take up iodine, ^{131}I treatment can reduce or eliminate residual disease with relatively little associated toxicity. However, it is not clear that prophylactic radioiodine treatment reduces mortality for patients at relatively low risk. Most patients with stage 1 PTC with primary tumors <1.5 cm in size can usually be managed safely with thyroxine suppression, without radiation treatment, as the risk of recurrence and mortality is very low. For patients with larger papillary tumors, spread to the adjacent lymph nodes, FTC, or evidence of metastases, thyroid ablation and radioiodine treatment are generally indicated.

[131]I thyroid ablation and treatment   As noted above, the decision to use ^{131}I for thyroid ablation should be coordinated with the surgical approach, as radioablation is much more effective when there is minimal remaining normal thyroid tissue. A typical strategy is to treat the patient for several weeks postoperatively with liothyronine (25 μg bid or tid), followed by thyroid hormone withdrawal. Ideally, the TSH level should increase to >50 IU/L over about 3 to 4 weeks. The level to which TSH rises is dictated largely by the amount of normal thyroid tissue remaining postoperatively. A scanning dose of [131]I [usually 148 to 185 MBq (4 to 5 mCi)] will reveal the amount of residual tissue and provides guidance about the dose needed to accomplish ablation. A maximum outpatient dose of 1110 MBq (29.9 mCi) [131]I can be administered in the United States, though ablation is often more complete using greater doses [1850 to 2775 MBq (50 to 75 mCi)]. In patients with known residual cancer, the larger doses ensure thyroid ablation and may destroy remaining tumor cells. A whole-body scan following the high-dose radioiodine treatment is useful to identify possible metastatic disease.

Follow-up whole-body thyroid scanning and thyroglobulin determinations   An initial whole-body scan should be performed about 6 months after surgery and thyroid ablation. The strategy for follow-up management of thyroid cancer has been altered by the availability of recombinant human TSH (rhTSH) to stimulate ^{131}I uptake and by the improved sensitivity of Tg assays to detect residual or recurrent disease. A scheme for using either rhTSH or thyroid hormone withdrawal for thyroid scanning is summarized in Fig. 330-12. After thyroid ablation, rhTSH can be used to stimulate ^{131}I uptake without subjecting patients to thyroid hormone withdrawal and its associated symptoms of hypothyroidism and the risk of prolonged TSH-stimulated tumor growth. This approach is recommended for patients predicted to be at low risk of disease recurrence, since rhTSH is not currently approved for use in conjunction with therapeutic doses of [131]I. Alternatively, in patients who are likely to require ^{131}I treatment, the traditional approach of thyroid hormone withdrawal can be used to increase TSH. This involves switching patients from levothyroxine (T$_4$) to the more rapidly cleared hormone, liothyronine (T$_3$), thereby allowing TSH to increase more quickly. If residual disease is detected on the initial whole-body scan [148 to 185 MBq (4 to 5 mCi)], a larger treatment dose, usually between 2775 and 5550 MBq (75 and 150 mCi), can be administered depending on the degree of residual uptake and assessment of cancer risk. Because TSH stimulates Tg levels, Tg measurements should be obtained after administration of rhTSH or when TSH levels have risen after thyroid hormone withdrawal. If the initial whole-body scan is negative and Tg levels are low, a repeat scan should be performed 1 year later. If still negative, the patient can be managed with suppressive therapy and measurements of Tg every 6 to 12 months. If a second follow-up scan is negative, no further scanning may be necessary if the patient is at low risk and there is no clinical or laboratory evidence of recurrence. Many authorities advocate radioiodine treatment for scan-negative, Tg-positive (Tg >5 to 10 ng/mL) patients, as many derive therapeutic benefit from a large dose of [131]I.

In addition to radioiodine, external beam radiotherapy is also used

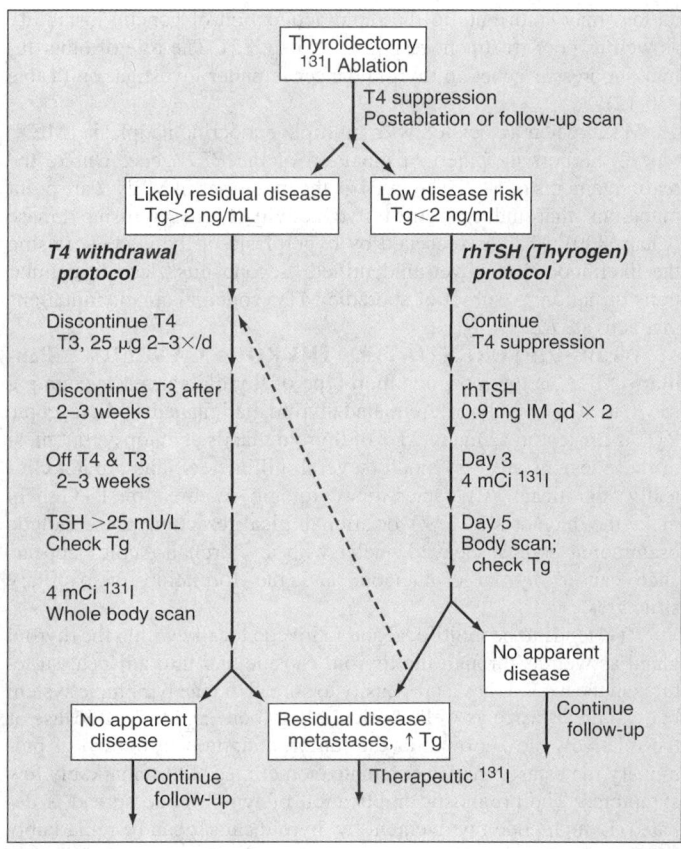

FIGURE 330-12   Use of recombinant thyroid-stimulating hormone (TSH) in the follow-up of patients with thyroid cancer.

to treat specific metastatic lesions, particularly when they cause bone pain or threaten neurologic injury (e.g., vertebral metastases).

ANAPLASTIC AND OTHER FORMS OF THYROID CANCER Anaplastic Thyroid Cancer As noted above, ATC is a poorly differentiated and aggressive cancer. The prognosis is poor, and most patients die within 6 months of diagnosis. Because of the undifferentiated state of these tumors, radioiodine uptake is usually negligible but can be used therapeutically if there is residual uptake. Chemotherapy has been attempted with multiple agents, including anthracyclines and paclitaxel, but is usually futile. External radiation therapy can be attempted and continued if tumors are responsive.

Thyroid Lymphoma Lymphoma in the thyroid gland often arises in the background of Hashimoto's thyroiditis. A rapidly expanding thyroid mass should suggest the possibility of this diagnosis. Diffuse large cell lymphoma is the most common type in the thyroid. Biopsies reveal sheets of lymphoid cells that can be difficult to distinguish from small cell lung cancer or ATC. These tumors are often highly sensitive to external radiation. Surgical resection should be avoided as initial therapy because it may spread disease that is otherwise localized to the thyroid. If staging indicates disease outside of the thyroid, treatment should follow guidelines used for other forms of lymphoma (Chap. 112).

MEDULLARY THYROID CARCINOMA MTC can be sporadic or familial and accounts for about 5 to 10% of thyroid cancers. There are three familial forms of MTC: MEN-2A, MEN-2B, and familial MTC without other features of MEN (Chap. 339). In general, MTC is more aggressive in MEN-2B than in MEN-2A, and familial MTC is more aggressive than sporadic MTC. Elevated serum calcitonin provides a marker of residual or recurrent disease. It is reasonable to test all patients with MTC for *RET* mutations, as genetic counseling and testing of family members can be offered to those individuals who test positive for mutations.

The management of MTC is primarily surgical. Unlike tumors derived from thyroid follicular cells, these tumors do not take up radioiodine. External radiation treatment and chemotherapy may provide palliation in patients with advanced disease (Chap. 339).

_____ *Approach to the Patient* _____

Palpable thyroid nodules are found in about 5% of adults, though the prevalence varies considerably worldwide. Given this high prevalence rate, it is common for the practitioner to identify and evaluate thyroid nodules. The main goal of this evaluation is to identify, in a cost-effective manner, the small subgroup of individuals with malignant lesions.

As described above, nodules are more common in iodine-deficient areas, in women, and with aging. Most palpable nodules are >1 cm in diameter, but the ability to feel a nodule is influenced by its location within the gland (superficial versus deeply embedded), the anatomy of the patient's neck, and the experience of the examiner. More sensitive methods of detection, such as thyroid ultrasound and pathologic studies, reveal thyroid nodules in >20% of glands. These findings have led to much debate about how to detect nodules and which nodules to investigate further. Most authorities still rely on physical examination to detect thyroid nodules, reserving ultrasound for monitoring nodule size or as an aid in thyroid biopsy.

It is important to distinguish whether a patient presents with a solitary thyroid nodule or a prominent nodule in the context of a MNG, as the incidence of malignancy is greater in solitary nodules. An approach to the evaluation of a solitary nodule is outlined in Fig. 330-13. Most patients with thyroid nodules have normal thyroid function tests. Nonetheless, thyroid function should be assessed by measuring a TSH level, which may be suppressed by one or more autonomously functioning nodules. If the TSH is suppressed, a radionuclide scan is indicated to determine if the identified nodule is "hot," as lesions with increased uptake are almost never malignant and FNA is unnecessary. Otherwise, FNA biopsy should be the first step in the evaluation of a thyroid nodule. FNA has good sensitivity and specificity when performed by physicians familiar with the procedure and when the results are interpreted by experienced cytopathologists. The technique is particularly accurate for detecting PTC. The distinction of benign and malignant follicular lesions is often not possible using cytology alone.

In several large studies, FNA biopsies yield the following findings: 70% benign, 10% malignant or suspicious for malignancy, and 20% nondiagnostic or yielding insufficient material for diagnosis. Characteristic features of malignancy mandate surgery. A diagnosis of follicular neoplasm also warrants surgery, as benign and malignant lesions cannot be distinguished based on cytopathology or frozen section. The management of patients with benign lesions is more variable. Many authorities advocate TSH suppression, whereas others monitor nodule size without suppression. With either approach, thyroid nodule size should be monitored, either by palpation or ultrasound. Repeat FNA is indicated if a nodule enlarges, and most authorities recommend a second biopsy within 2 to 5 years to confirm the benign status of the nodule.

Nondiagnostic biopsies occur for many reasons, including a fibrotic reaction with relatively few cells available for aspiration, a cystic lesion in which cellular components reside along the cyst margin, or a nodule that may be too small for accurate aspiration. For these reasons, ultrasound-guided FNA is useful when the FNA is repeated. Ultrasound is also increasingly used for initial biopsies in an effort to enhance nodule localization and the accuracy of sampling.

The evaluation of a thyroid nodule is stressful for most patients. They are concerned about the possibility of thyroid cancer, whether verbalized or not. It is constructive, therefore, to review the diagnostic approach and to reassure patients when malignancy is not found. When a suspicious lesion or thyroid cancer is identified, an explanation of the generally favorable prognosis and available treatment options should be provided.

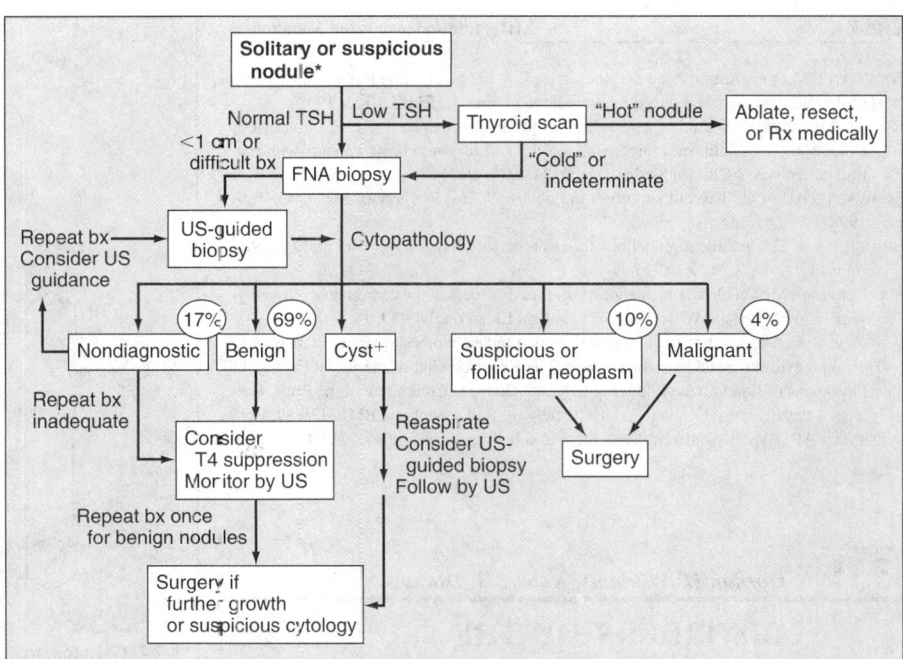

FIGURE 330-13 Approach to the patient with a thyroid nodule. *There are many exceptions to the suggested options. See text and references for details. †About one-third of nodules are cystic or mixed solid-cystic. US, ultrasound.

BIBLIOGRAPHY

ALLAHABADIA A et al: Age and gender predict the outcome of treatment for Graves' hyperthyroidism. J Clin Endocrinol Metab 85:1038, 2000

AMERICAN JOINT COMMITTEE ON CANCER: *Thyroid gland: AJCC Cancer Staging Manual,* 5th ed. Philadelphia, Lippincott-Raven, 1997, pp 59–64

BARTALENA L et al: Management of Graves' ophthalmopathy: Reality and perspectives. Endocr Rev 21:168, 2000

BRUCKER-DAVIES F et al: Thyrotropin-secreting pituitary tumors: Diagnostic criteria, thyroid hormone sensitivity, and treatment outcome in 25 patients followed at the National Institutes of Health. J Clin Endocrinol Metab 84:476, 1999

BUNEVICIUS R et al: Effects of thyroxine as compared with thyroxine plus triiodothyronine in patients with hypothyroidism. N Engl J Med 340:424, 1999

DELANGE F: Risks and benefits of iodine supplementation. Lancet 351:923, 1998

DEGROOT LJ et al: Thyroid gland (Part III), in *Endocrinology,* 4th ed, LJ DeGroot, JL Jameson (eds). Philadelphia, Saunders, 2000

FERRETTI E et al: Evaluation of the adequacy of levothyroxine replacement therapy in patients with central hypothyroidism. J Clin Endocrinol Metab 84:924, 1999

GHARIB H: Changing concepts in the diagnosis and management of thyroid nodules. Endocrinol Metab Clin North Am 26:777, 1997

HAUGEN BR et al: A comparison of recombinant human thyrotropin and thyroid hormone withdrawal for the detection of thyroid remnant or cancer. J Clin Endocrinol Metab 84:3877, 1999

KOPP P: Pendred's syndrome and genetic defects in thyroid hormone synthesis. Rev Endocrinol Metabol Dis 1:109, 2000

KOUTRAS DA: Subclinical hyperthyroidism. Thyroid 9:311, 1999

KROLL TG et al: PAX8-PPARγl fusion oncogene in human thyroid carcinoma. Science 289:1357, 2000

LARSEN PR et al: Thyroid, in *William's Textbook of Endocrinology,* 9th ed, JD Wilson et al (eds). Philadelphia, Saunders, 1998, pp 389–515

LAURBERG P et al: Guidelines for TSH-receptor antibody measurements in pregnancy: Results of an evidence-based symposium organized by the European Thyroid Association. Eur J Endocrinol 139:584, 1998

LEECH NJ, DAYAN CM: Controversies in the management of Graves' disease. Clin Endocrinol 49:273, 1998

LINDSAY RS, TOFT AD: Hypothyroidism. Lancet 349:413, 1997

MACCHIA PE: Recent advances in understanding the molecular basis of primary congenital hypothyroidism. Mol Med Today 6:36, 2000

MASIUKIEWICZ US, BURROW GN: Hyperthyroidism in pregnancy: Diagnosis and treatment. Thyroid 9:647, 1999

NEWMAN CM et al: Amiodarone and the thyroid: A practical guide to the management of thyroid dysfunction induced by amiodarone therapy. Heart 79:121, 1998

RINGEL MD et al: Quantitative reverse transcription–polymerase chain reaction of circulating thyroglobulin messenger ribonucleic acid for monitoring patients with thyroid carcinoma. J Clin Endocrinol Metab 84:4037, 1999

SCHWARTZ AE et al: Thyroid surgery—the choice. J Clin Endocrinol Metab 83:1097, 1998

SINGER PA et al: Treatment guidelines for patients with hyperthyroidism and hypothyroidism. JAMA 273:806, 1995

VANDERPUMP MPJ et al: The incidence of thyroid disorders in the community: A twenty-year follow-up of the Whickham Survey. Clin Endocrinol 43:55, 1995

——— et al: Consensus statement for good practice and audit measures in the management of hypothyroidism and hyperthyroidism. The Research Unit of the Royal College of Physicians of London, the Endocrinology and Diabetes Committee of the Royal College of Physicians of London, and the Society for Endocrinology. BMJ 313:539, 1996

WEETMAN AP: Hypothyroidism: Screening and subclinical disease. BMJ 314:1175, 1997

FIGURE 331-1 Basic steroid structure and nomenclature.

331

Gordon H. Williams, Robert G. Dluhy

DISORDERS OF THE ADRENAL CORTEX

ACE	angiotensin-converting enzyme	IL	interleukin
ACTH	adrenocorticotropic hormone	LDL	low-density lipoprotein
AVP	arginine vasopressin	β-LPT	β-lipotropin
CAH	congenital adrenal hyperplasia	MIF	migration-inhibiting factor
CBG	cortisol-binding globulin	MR	mineralocorticoid receptor
CMV	cytomegalovirus	MRI	magnetic resonance imaging
CRH	corticotropin-releasing hormone	PHA-I	pseudohypoaldosteronism type I
CT	computed tomography		
DHEA	dehydroepiandrosterone	POMC	pro-opiomelanocortin
GABA	γ-aminobutyric acid	PRA	plasma renin activity
GR	glucocorticoid receptor	STAR	steroidogenic acute regulatory
GRA	glucocorticoid-remediable aldosteronism	TNF	tumor necrosis factor
11β-HSD	hydroxysteroid dehydrogenase		

BIOCHEMISTRY AND PHYSIOLOGY

The adrenal cortex produces three major classes of steroids: (1) glucocorticoids, (2) mineralocorticoids, and (3) adrenal androgens. Consequently, normal adrenal function is important for modulating intermediary metabolism and immune responses through glucocorticoids; blood pressure, vascular volume, and electrolytes through mineralocorticoids; and secondary sexual characteristics (in females) through androgens. The adrenal axis plays an important role in the stress response by rapidly increasing cortisol levels. Adrenal disorders include hyperfunction (Cushing's syndrome) and hypofunction (adrenal insufficiency) as well as a variety of genetic abnormalities of steroidogenesis.

STEROID NOMENCLATURE Steroids contain as their basic structure a cyclopentenoperhydrophenanthrane nucleus consisting of three 6-carbon hexane rings and a single 5-carbon pentane ring (Fig. 331-1). The carbon atoms are numbered in a sequence beginning with ring A. Adrenal steroids contain either 19 or 21 carbon atoms. The C_{19} steroids have methyl groups at C-18 and C-19. C_{19} steroids with a ketone group at C-17 are termed *17-ketosteroids*; C_{19} steroids have predominantly androgenic activity. The C_{21} steroids have a 2-carbon side chain (C-20 and C-21) attached at position 17 and methyl groups at C-18 and C-19; C_{21} steroids with a hydroxyl group at position 17 are termed *17-hydroxycorticosteroids*. The C_{21} steroids have either glucocorticoid or mineralcorticoid properties.

BIOSYNTHESIS OF ADRENAL STEROIDS Cholesterol, derived from the diet and from endogenous synthesis, is the substrate for steroidogenesis. Uptake of cholesterol by the adrenal cortex is me-

diated by the low-density lipoprotein (LDL) receptor. With long-term stimulation of the adrenal cortex by adrenocorticotropic hormone (ACTH), the number of LDL receptors increases. The three major adrenal biosynthetic pathways lead to the production of glucocorticoids (cortisol), mineralocorticoids (aldosterone), and adrenal androgens (dehydroepiandrosterone). Separate zones of the adrenal cortex synthesize specific hormones (Fig. 331-2). This zonation is accompanied by the selective expression of the genes encoding the enzymes unique to the formation of each type of steroid: aldosterone synthase is normally expressed only in the outer (glomerulosa) cell layer, whereas 17-hydroxylase is expressed only in the (inner) faciculata-reticularis cell layers, which are the sites of cortisol and androgen biosynthesis, respectively.

STEROID TRANSPORT Cortisol occurs in the plasma in three forms: free cortisol, protein-bound cortisol, and cortisol metabolites. *Free cortisol* is physiologically active hormone that is not protein-bound and, can act therefore, directly on tissue sites. Normally, <5% of circulating cortisol is free. Only the unbound cortisol and its metabolites are filterable at the glomerulus. Increased quantities of free steroid are excreted in the urine in states characterized by hypersecretion of cortisol, because the unbound fraction of plasma cortisol rises. Plasma has two cortisol-binding systems. One is a high-affinity, low-capacity α_2-globulin termed *transcortin* or *cortisol-binding globulin* (CBG), and the other is a low-affinity, high-capacity protein, *albumin*. The binding affinity of CBG for cortisol is reduced in areas of inflammation, thus increasing the local concentration of free cortisol. When the concentration of cortisol exceeds 700 nmol/(25 μg/dL), part of the excess binds to albumin, and a greater proportion than usual circulates unbound. The CBG level is increased in high-estrogen states (e.g., pregnancy, oral contraceptive administration). The rise in CBG is accompanied by a parallel rise in *protein-bound cortisol*, with the result that the plasma cortisol concentration is elevated. However, the free cortisol level probably remains normal, and manifestations of glucocorticoid excess are absent. Most synthetic glucocorticoid analogues bind less efficiently to CBG (~70% binding). This may explain the propensity of some synthetic analogues to produce cushingoid effects at low doses. *Cortisol metabolites* are biologically inactive and bind only weakly to circulating plasma proteins.

Aldosterone is bound to proteins to a smaller extent than cortisol, and an ultrafiltrate of plasma contains as much as 50% of the circulating concentration of aldosterone.

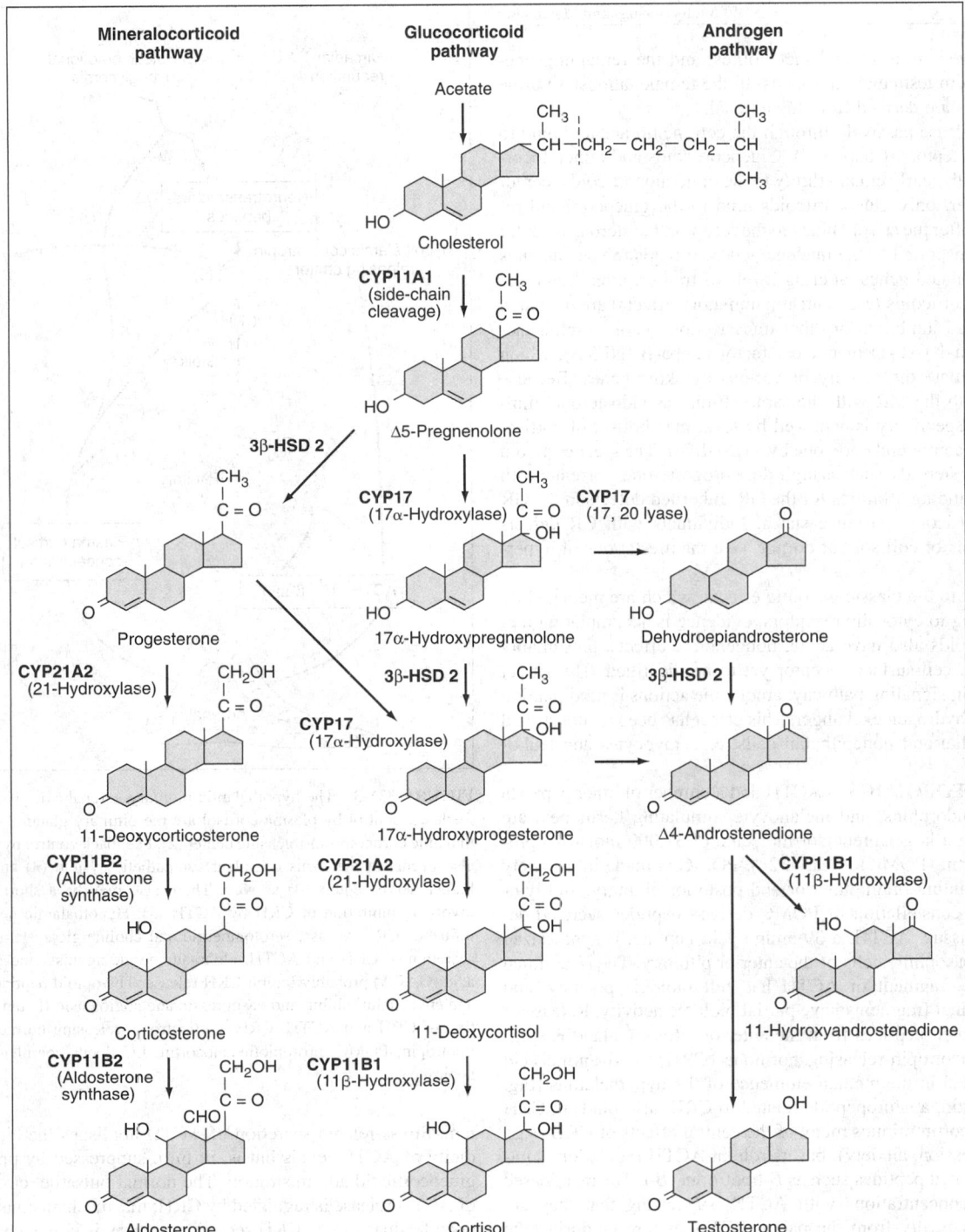

FIGURE 331-2 Biosynthetic pathways for adrenal steroid production; major pathways to mineralocorticoids, glucocorticoids, and androgens. 3β-HSD, 3β-hydroxysteroid dehydrogenase.

STEROID METABOLISM AND EXCRETION **Glucocorticoids** The daily secretion of cortisol ranges between 40 and 80 μmol (15 and 30 mg, 8–10 mg/m²), with a pronounced circadian cycle. The plasma concentration of cortisol is determined by the rate of secretion, the rate of inactivation, and the rate of excretion of free cortisol. The liver is the major organ responsible for steroid inactivation. A major enzyme regulating cortisol metabolism is 11β-hydroxysteroid dehydrogenase (11β-HSD). There are two isoforms: 11β-HSD I is primarily expressed in the liver and acts as a reductase, converting the inactive cortisone to the active glucocorticoid, cortisol; the 11β-HSD II isoform is expressed in a number of tissues and converts cortisol to the inactive metabolite cortisone. The oxidative reaction of IIβ-HSD I is increased in hyperthyroidism.

Mineralocorticoids In normal individuals with a normal salt intake, the average daily secretion of aldosterone ranges between 0.1 and 0.7 μmol (50 and 250 μg). During a single passage through the liver, >75% of circulating aldosterone is normally inactivated by ring A reduction and conjugation with glucuronic acid because it is only weakly bound to proteins. However, under certain conditions, such as congestive failure, this rate of inactivation is reduced.

Adrenal Androgens The major androgen secreted by the adrenal is dehydroepiandrosterone (DHEA) and its sulfuric acid ester (DHEAS). From 15 to 30 mg of these compounds is secreted daily. Smaller amounts of androstenedione, 11β-hydroxyandrostenedione, and testosterone are secreted. DHEA is the major precursor of the urinary 17-ketosteroids. Two-thirds of the urine 17-ketosteroids in the male are derived from adrenal metabolites, and the remaining one-third comes from testicular androgens. In the female, almost all urine 17-ketosteroids are derived from the adrenal.

Steroids diffuse passively through the cell membrane and bind to intracellular receptors (Chap. 327). Glucocorticoids and mineralocorticoids bind with nearly equal affinity to the mineralocorticoid receptor (MR). However, only glucocorticoids bind to the glucocorticoid receptor (GR). After the steroid binds to the receptor, the steroid-receptor complex is transported to the nucleus, where it binds to specific sites on steroid-regulated genes, altering levels of transcription. Some actions of glucocorticoids (e.g., anti-inflammatory effects) are mediated by GR-mediated inhibition of other transcription factors, such as activating protein-1 (AP-1) or nuclear factor kappa-B (NFKB), which normally stimulate the activity of various cytokine genes. Because cortisol binds to the MR with the same affinity as aldosterone, mineralocorticoid specificity is achieved by local metabolism of cortisol to the inactive compound cortisone by 11β-HSDII. The glucocorticoid effects of other steroids, such as high-dose progesterone, correlate with their relative binding affinities for the GR. Inherited defects in the GR cause glucocorticoid resistance states. Individuals with GR defects have high levels of cortisol but do not have manifestations of hypercortisolism.

In addition to the classic genomic effects, which are mediated by steroids binding to cytosolic receptors, evidence is accumulating that mineralocorticoids also have acute, nongenomic effects, presumably by activating a cell-surface receptor yet to be identified. This effect uses a G-protein signaling pathway; among the actions is modification of the sodium-hydrogen exchanger. This effect has been demonstrated in both epithelial and nonepithelial cells, e.g., myocytes and leukocytes.

ACTH PHYSIOLOGY   ACTH and a number of other peptides (lipotropins, endorphins, and melanocyte-stimulating hormones) are processed from a larger precursor molecule of 31,000 mol wt—pro-opiomelanocortin (POMC) (Chap. 328). POMC is made in a variety of tissues, including brain, anterior and posterior pituitary, and lymphocytes. The constellation of POMC-derived peptides secreted depends on the tissue. ACTH, a 39-amino acid peptide, is synthesized and stored in basophilic cells of the anterior pituitary. The N-terminal 18-amino acid fragment of ACTH has full biologic potency, and shorter N-terminal fragments have partial biologic activity. Release of ACTH and related peptides from the anterior pituitary gland is stimulated by corticotropin-releasing hormone (CRH), a 41-amino acid peptide produced in the median eminence of the hypothalamus (Fig. 331-3). Urocortin, a neuropeptide related to CRH, also binds to CRH receptors. Urocortin mimics many of the central effects of CRH (e.g., appetite suppression, anxiety), but its role in ACTH regulation is unclear. Some related peptides such as β-lipotropin (β-LPT) are released in equimolar concentrations with ACTH, suggesting that they are cleaved enzymatically from the parent POMC before or during the secretory process. However, β-endorphin levels may or may not correlate with circulating levels of ACTH, depending on the nature of the stimulus. The functions and regulation of secretion of the related peptides derived from POMC are poorly understood.

The major factors controlling ACTH release include CRH, the free cortisol concentration in plasma, stress, and the sleep-wake cycle (Fig. 331-3). The plasma level of ACTH varies during the day as a result of its pulsatile secretion, and it follows a circadian pattern with a peak just prior to waking and a nadir before sleeping. If a new sleep-wake cycle is adopted, the pattern changes over several days to conform to it. ACTH and cortisol levels also increase in response to eating. Stress (e.g., pyrogens, surgery, hypoglycemia, exercise, and severe emotional trauma) causes the release of CRH and arginine vasopressin (AVP) and activation of the sympathetic nervous system. These changes in turn enhance ACTH release, acting individually or in concert. For example, AVP release acts synergistically with CRH to amplify ACTH secretion; CRH also stimulates the locus coeruleus/sympathetic sys-

FIGURE 331-3 The hypothalamic-pituitary-adrenal axis. The main sites for feedback control by plasma cortisol are the pituitary gland (1) and the hypothalamic corticotropin-releasing center (2). Feedback control by plasma cortisol also occurs at the locus coeruleus/sympathetic system (3) and may involve higher nerve centers (4) as well. There also may be a short feedback loop involving inhibition of CRH by ACTH (5). Hypothalamic neurotransmitters influence CRH release; serotoninergic and cholinergic systems stimulate the secretion of CRH and ACTH; alpha-adrenergic agonists and γ-aminobutyric acid (GABA) probably inhibit CRH release. The opioid peptides β-endorphin and enkephalin inhibit, and vasopressin and angiotensin II augment, the secretion of CRH and ACTH. CRH, corticotropin-releasing hormone; β-LPT, β-lipotropin; POMC, pro-opiomelanocortin; LC, locus coeruleus; NE, norepinephrine.

tem. Stress-related secretion of ACTH abolishes the circadian periodicity of ACTH levels but is, in turn, suppressed by prior high-dose glucocorticoid administration. The normal pulsatile, circadian pattern of ACTH release is regulated by CRH; this mechanism is the so-called open feedback loop. CRH secretion, in turn, is influenced by hypothalamic neurotransmitters. For example, serotoninergic and cholinergic systems stimulate the secretion of CRH and ACTH; there is contradictory evidence regarding the inhibitory effects of α-adrenergic agonists and γ-aminobutyric acid (GABA) on CRH release. In addition, there may be direct pituitary effects of these neurotransmitters. There is also evidence for peptidergic regulation of ACTH release. For example, β-endorphin and enkephalin inhibit the secretion of ACTH, whereas vasopressin and angiotensin II augment it. The immune system also influences the hypothalamic-pituitary-adrenal axis (Fig. 331-4). For example, inflammatory cytokines [tumor necrosis factor (TNF)-α, interleukin (IL)-1α, IL-1β, and IL-6] produced by monocytes increase ACTH release by stimulating secretion of CRH and/or AVP. Finally, ACTH release is regulated by the level of free cortisol in plasma. Cortisol decreases the responsiveness of pituitary corticotropic cells to CRH; the response of the POMC mRNA to CRH is also inhibited by glucocorticoids. In addition, glucocorticoids inhibit the locus coeruleus/sympathetic system and CRH release. The latter ser-

Immune-adrenal axis

FIGURE 331-4 The immune-adrenal axis. Cortisol has anti-inflammatory properties that include effects on the microvasculature, cellular actions, and the suppression of inflammatory cytokines (the so-called immune-adrenal axis). A stress such as sepsis increases adrenal secretion, and cortisol in turn suppresses the immune response via this system. −, suppression; +, stimulation; CRH, corticotropin-releasing hormone; ACTH, adrenocorticotropin; IL, interleukin; TNF, tumor necrosis factor; PAF, platelet activating factor.

vomechanism establishes the primacy of cortisol in the control of ACTH secretion. The inhibition of ACTH occurs in two phases: (1) an early fast feedback, mediated via the MR, which lasts <10 min and depends on both the rate of increase of glucocorticoid levels and the specific glucocorticoid administered; and (2) a time-dependent, delayed feedback, likely mediated by the GR, which is probably due to inhibition of synthesis of the precursor protein. The suppression of ACTH secretion that results in adrenal atrophy following *prolonged* glucocorticoid therapy is caused primarily by suppression of hypothalamic CRH release, as exogenous CRH administration in this circumstance produces a rise in plasma ACTH. Cortisol also exerts feedback effects on higher brain centers (hippocampus, reticular system, and septum) and perhaps on the adrenal cortex (Fig. 331-4).

The biologic half-life of ACTH in the circulation is <10 min. The action of ACTH is also rapid; within minutes of its release, the concentration of steroids in the adrenal venous blood increases. ACTH stimulates steroidogenesis via activation of the membrane-bound adenyl cyclase. Adenosine-3′,5′-monophosphate (cyclic AMP), in turn, activates protein kinase enzymes, thereby resulting in the phosphorylation of proteins that activate steroid biosynthesis.

RENIN-ANGIOTENSIN PHYSIOLOGY (See also Chap. 246) Renin is a proteolytic enzyme that is produced and stored in the granules of the juxtaglomerular cells surrounding the afferent arterioles of glomeruli in the kidney. Renin exists in both active and inactive forms. Whether the inactive form is a precursor ("prorenin") or is a product formed after release is uncertain. Renin acts on the basic substrate angiotensinogen (a circulating α_2-globulin made in the liver) to form the decapeptide angiotensin I (Fig. 331-5). Angiotensin I is then enzymatically

transformed by angiotensin-converting enzyme (ACE), which is present in many tissues (particularly the pulmonary vascular endothelium), to the octapeptide angiotensin II by the removal of the two C-terminal amino acids. Angiotensin II is a potent pressor agent and exerts its action by a direct effect on arteriolar smooth muscle. In addition, angiotensin II stimulates production of aldosterone by the zona glomerulosa of the adrenal cortex; the heptapeptide angiotensin III may also stimulate aldosterone production. The two major classes of angiotensin receptors are termed *AT1* and *AT2*; AT1 may exist as two subtypes α and β. Most of the effects of angiotensins II and III are mediated by the AT1 receptor. Angiotensinases rapidly destroy angiotensin II (half-life, approximately 1 min), while the half-life of renin is more prolonged (10 to 20 min). In addition to circulating renin-angiotensin, many tissues have a local renin-angiotensin system and the ability to produce angiotensin II. These tissues include the uterus, placenta, vascular tissue, heart, brain, and, particularly, the adrenal cortex and kidney. Although the role of locally generated angiotensin II is not established, it may be involved in the growth and modulation of function of the adrenal cortex and vascular smooth muscle.

The amount of renin released reflects the combined effects of four interdependent factors. The *juxtaglomerular cells*, which are specialized myoepithelial cells that cuff the afferent arterioles, act as miniature pressure transducers, sensing renal perfusion pressure and corresponding changes in afferent arteriolar perfusion pressures. For example, under conditions of a reduction in circulating blood volume, there is a corresponding reduction in renal perfusion pressure and, therefore, in afferent arteriolar pressure (Fig. 331-5). This change is perceived by the juxtaglomerular cells as a decreased stretch exerted on the afferent arteriolar walls. The juxtaglomerular cells then release more renin into the renal circulation. This results in the formation of angiotensin I, which is converted in the kidney and peripherally to angiotensin II by ACE. Angiotensin II influences sodium homeostasis via two major mechanisms: it changes renal blood flow so as to maintain a constant glomerular filtration rate, thereby changing the filtration fraction of sodium, and it stimulates the adrenal cortex to release aldosterone. Increasing plasma levels of aldosterone enhance renal sodium retention and thus result in expansion of the extracellular fluid volume, which, in turn, dampens the stimulus for renin release. In this context, the renin-angiotensin-aldosterone system regulates volume by modifying renal hemodynamics and tubular sodium transport.

A second control mechanism for renin release is centered in the *macula densa* cells, a group of distal convoluted tubular epithelial cells directly apposed to the juxtaglomerular cells. They may function as chemoreceptors, monitoring the sodium (or chloride) load presented to the distal tubule, and such information may be conveyed to the juxtaglomerular cells, where appropriate modifications in renin release take place. Under conditions of increased delivery of filtered sodium

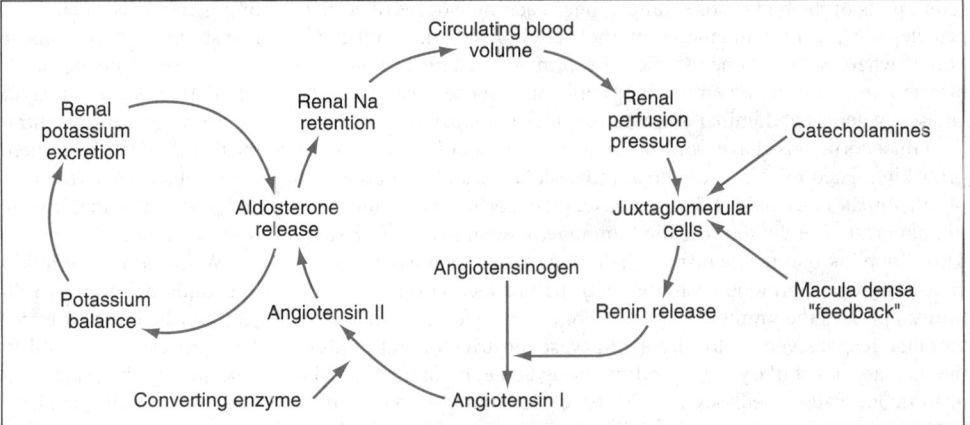

FIGURE 331-5 The interrelationship of the volume and potassium feedback loops on aldosterone secretion. Integration of signals from each loop determines the level of aldosterone secretion.

to the macula densa, increasing release of renin decreases the glomerular filtration rate, thereby reducing the filtered load of sodium.

The *sympathetic nervous system* regulates the release of renin in response to assumption of the upright posture. The mechanism is either a direct effect on the juxtaglomerular cell to increase adenyl cyclase activity or an indirect effect on either the juxtaglomerular or the macula densa cells via vasoconstriction of the afferent arteriole.

Finally, circulating factors influence renin release. Increased dietary intake of *potassium* decreases, and decreased potassium intake increases, renin release. The significance of these effects is unclear. *Angiotensin II* exerts negative feedback control on renin release that is independent of alterations in renal blood flow, blood pressure, or aldosterone secretion. *Atrial natriuretic peptides* also inhibit renin release. Thus, the control of renin release involves both *intrarenal* (pressor receptor and macula densa) and *extrarenal* (sympathetic nervous system, potassium, angiotensin, etc.) mechanisms. Steady-state renin levels reflect all these factors, with the intrarenal mechanism predominating.

GLUCOCORTICOID PHYSIOLOGY   The division of adrenal steroids into glucocorticoids and mineralocorticoids is arbitrary in that most glucocorticoids have some mineralocorticoid-like properties. The descriptive term *glucocorticoid* is used for adrenal steroids whose predominant action is on intermediary metabolism. Their overall actions are directed at enhancing the production of the high-energy fuel, glucose, and reducing all other metabolic activity not directly involved in that process. Sustained activation, however, results in a pathophysiologic state, e.g., Cushing's syndrome. The principal glucocorticoid is cortisol (hydrocortisone). The effect of glucocorticoids on intermediary metabolism is mediated by the GR. Physiologic effects of glucocorticoids include the regulation of protein, carbohydrate, lipid, and nucleic acid metabolism. Glucocorticoids raise the blood glucose level by acting as an insulin antagonist and by suppressing the secretion of insulin, thereby inhibiting peripheral glucose uptake, which promotes hepatic glucose synthesis (gluconeogenesis) and increases hepatic glycogen content. The actions on protein metabolism are mainly catabolic in effect, resulting in an increase in protein breakdown and nitrogen excretion. In large part, these actions reflect a mobilization of glycogenic amino acid precursors from peripheral supporting structures, such as bone, skin, muscle, and connective tissue, due to protein breakdown and inhibition of protein synthesis and amino acid uptake. Hyperaminoacidemia also facilitates gluconeogenesis by stimulating glucagon secretion. Glucocorticoids act directly on the liver to stimulate the synthesis of certain enzymes, such as tyrosine aminotransferase and tryptophan pyrrolase. Glucocorticoids regulate fatty acid mobilization by enhancing the activation of cellular lipase by lipid-mobilizing hormones (e.g., catecholamines and pituitary peptides).

The actions of cortisol on protein and adipose tissue vary in different parts of the body. For example, pharmacologic doses of cortisol can deplete the protein matrix of the vertebral column (trabecular bone), whereas long bones (which are primarily compact bone) are affected only minimally; similarly, peripheral adipose tissue mass decreases, whereas abdominal and interscapular fat expand.

Glucocorticoids have anti-inflammatory properties, which are probably related to effects on the microvasculature and to suppression of inflammatory cytokines. In this sense, glucocorticoids modulate the immune response via the so-called immune-adrenal axis (Fig. 331-4). This "loop" is one mechanism by which a stress, such as sepsis, increases adrenal hormone secretion, and the elevated cortisol level in turn suppresses the immune response. For example, cortisol maintains vascular responsiveness to circulating vasoconstrictors and opposes the increase in capillary permeability during acute inflammation. Glucocorticoids cause a leukocytosis due to release from the bone marrow of mature cells as well as to inhibition of their egress through the capillary wall. Glucocorticoids produce a depletion of circulating eosinophils and of lymphoid tissue, specifically T cells, by causing a

redistribution from the circulation into other compartments. Thus, cortisol impairs cell-mediated immunity. Glucocorticoids also inhibit the production and action of the mediators of inflammation, such as the lymphokines and prostaglandins. These actions occur via the GR and are blocked by inhibitors of RNA and protein synthesis. Glucocorticoids inhibit the production and action of interferon by T lymphocytes and the production of IL-1 and IL-6 by macrophages. The antipyretic action of glucocorticoids may be explained by the effect on IL-1, which appears to be an endogenous pyrogen (Chap. 17). Glucocorticoids also inhibit the production of T cell growth factor (IL-2) by T lymphocytes. Glucocorticoids reverse macrophage activation and antagonize the action of migration-inhibiting factor (MIF), leading to reduced adherence of macrophages to vascular endothelium. Glucocorticoids inhibit prostaglandin and leukotriene production by inhibiting the activity of phospholipase A_2, thus blocking release of arachidonic acid from phospholipids. Finally, glucocorticoids inhibit the production and inflammatory effects of bradykinin, platelet-activating factor, and serotonin. It is probably only at pharmacologic dosages that antibody production is reduced and lysosomal membranes are stabilized, the latter effect suppressing the release of acid hydrolases.

Cortisol levels respond within minutes to stress, whether physical (trauma, surgery, exercise), psychological (anxiety, depression), or physiologic (hypoglycemia, fever). The reasons why elevated glucocorticoid levels protect the organism under stress are not understood, but in conditions of glucocorticoid deficiency, such stresses may cause hypotension, shock, and death. Consequently, in individuals with adrenal insufficiency, glucocorticoid administration should be increased during stress.

Cortisol has major effects on body water. It helps regulate the extracellular fluid volume by retarding the migration of water into cells and by promoting renal water excretion, the latter effect mediated by suppression of vasopressin secretion, by an increase in the rate of glomerular filtration, and by a direct action on the renal tubule. The consequence is to prevent water intoxication by increasing solute-free water clearance. Glucocorticoids also have weak mineralocorticoid-like properties, and high doses promote renal tubular sodium reabsorption and increased urine potassium excretion. Glucocorticoids also can influence behavior; emotional disorders may occur with either an excess or a deficit of cortisol. Last, cortisol suppresses the secretion of pituitary POMC and its derivative peptides (ACTH, β-endorphin, and β-LPT) and the secretion of hypothalamic CRH and vasopressin.

MINERALOCORTICOID   PHYSIOLOGY   Mineralocorticoids are major regulators of extracellular fluid volume and the major determinant of potassium metabolism. These effects are mediated by the binding of aldosterone to the MR in target tissues, primarily the kidney. Volume is regulated through a direct effect on the collecting duct, where aldosterone causes an increase in sodium retention and an increase in potassium excretion. The reabsorption of sodium ions causes a fall in the transmembrane potential, thus enhancing the flow of positive ions, such as potassium, out of the cell into the lumen. The reabsorbed sodium ions are transported out of the tubular epithelium into the renal interstitial fluid and from there into the renal capillary circulation. Water passively follows the transported sodium.

Because the concentration of hydrogen ion is greater in the lumen than in the cell, hydrogen ion is also actively secreted. Mineralocorticoids also act on the epithelium of the salivary ducts, sweat glands, and gastrointestinal tract to cause reabsorption of sodium in exchange for potassium.

When normal individuals are given aldosterone, an initial period of sodium retention is followed by natriuresis, and sodium balance is reestablished after 3 to 5 days. As a result, edema does not develop. This process is referred to as the *escape phenomenon*, signifying an "escape" by the renal tubules from the sodium-retaining action of aldosterone. While renal hemodynamic factors may play a role in the escape, the level of atrial natriuretic peptide also increases. However, it is important to realize that there is no escape from the potassium-losing effects of mineralocorticoids.

There are additional nonclassic effects of mineralocorticoids, primarily on nonepithelial cells. These effects are likely genomic and therefore mediated through activation of the cytosolic MR, but they do not include a modification of sodium-potassium homeostasis. They are probably mediated by mineralocorticoids modifying the expression of several collagen genes and/or genes controlling tissue growth factors, e.g., transforming growth factor β (TGF-β) and plasminogen activator inhibitor (PAI-1). The resultant effects lead to microangiopathy, necrosis (acutely), and fibrosis in a variety of tissues, e.g., heart, kidney, and vasculature. Increased levels of aldosterone are not necessary to produce this damage; rather, an imbalance between the level of aldosterone and the volume and/or sodium balance state appears to be the critical factor.

Three primary mechanisms control aldosterone release—the renin-angiotensin system, potassium, and ACTH (Table 331-1). The renin-angiotensin system controls extracellular fluid volume via regulation of aldosterone secretion (Fig. 331-5). In effect, the renin-angiotensin system maintains the circulating blood volume constant by causing aldosterone-induced sodium retention during volume deficiency and by decreasing aldosterone-dependent sodium retention when volume is ample.

Potassium ion directly stimulates aldosterone secretion, independent of the circulating renin-angiotensin system, which it suppresses (Fig. 331-5). In addition to potassium's direct effect, it also modifies aldosterone secretion indirectly by activating the local renin-angiotensin system in the zona glomerulosa. This effect can be blocked by the administration of ACE inhibitors that reduce the local production of angiotensin II and thereby reduce the acute aldosterone response to potassium. An increase in serum potassium of as little as 0.1 mmol/L increases plasma aldosterone levels under certain circumstances. Oral potassium loading therefore increases aldosterone secretion, excretion, and plasma levels.

Physiologic amounts of ACTH stimulate aldosterone secretion acutely, but this action is not sustained unless ACTH is administered in a pulsatile fashion. Most studies relegate ACTH to a minor role in the control of aldosterone. For example, subjects receiving high-dose glucocorticoid therapy, and with presumed complete suppression of ACTH, have normal aldosterone secretion in response to sodium restriction.

Prior dietary intake of both potassium and sodium can alter the magnitude of the aldosterone response to acute stimulation. This effect results from a change in the expression and activity of aldosterone synthase. Increasing potassium intake or decreasing sodium intake sensitizes the response of the glomerulosa cells to acute stimulation by ACTH, angiotensin II, and/or potassium. Thus, regulation of aldosterone secretion occurs both early and late in its synthetic pathway.

Neurotransmitters (dopamine and serotonin) and some peptides, such as atrial natriuretic peptide, γ-melanocyte-stimulating hormone (γ-MSH), and β-endorphin, also participate in the regulation of al-

Table 331-1 Factors Regulating Aldosterone Biosynthesis

Factor	Effect
Renin-angiotensin system	Stimulation
Sodium ion	Inhibition (?physiologic)
Potassium ion	Stimulation
Neurotransmitters	
Dopamine	Inhibition
Serotonin	Stimulation
Pituitary hormones	
ACTH	Stimulation
Non-ACTH pituitary hormones (e.g., growth hormone)	Permissive (for optimal response to sodium restriction)
β-Endorphin	Stimulation
γ-Melanocyte-stimulating hormone	Permissive
Atrial natriuretic peptide	Inhibition
Ouabain-like factors	Inhibition
Endothelin	Stimulation

dosterone secretion (Table 331-1). Thus, the control of aldosterone secretion involves both stimulatory and inhibitory factors.

ANDROGEN PHYSIOLOGY Androgens regulate male secondary sexual characteristics and can cause virilizing symptoms in women (Chap. 53). Adrenal androgens have a minimal effect in males whose sexual characteristics are predominately determined by gonadal steroids (testosterone). In females, however, several androgen-like effects, e.g., sexual hair, are largely mediated by adrenal androgens. The principal adrenal androgens are DHEA, androstenedione, and 11-hydroxyandrostenedione. DHEA and androstenedione are weak androgens and exert their effects via conversion to the potent androgen testosterone in extraglandular tissues. DHEA also has poorly understood effects on the immune and cardiovascular systems. Adrenal androgen formation is regulated by ACTH, not by gonadotropins. It follows that adrenal androgens are suppressed by exogenous glucocorticoid administration.

LABORATORY EVALUATION OF ADRENOCORTICAL FUNCTION

A basic assumption is that measurements of the plasma or urinary level of a given steroid reflects the rate of adrenal *secretion* of that steroid. However, urine *excretion* values may not truly reflect the secretion rate because of improper collection or altered metabolism. Plasma levels reflect the level of secretion only at the time of measurement. The plasma level (PL) depends on two factors: the secretion rate (SR) of the hormone and the rate at which it is metabolized, i.e., its metabolic clearance rate (MCR). These three factors can be related as follows:

$$PL = \frac{SR}{MCR} \quad \text{or} \quad SR = MCR \times PL$$

BLOOD LEVELS Peptides The plasma levels of ACTH and angiotensin II can be measured by immunoassay techniques. Basal ACTH secretion shows a circadian rhythm, with lower levels in the early evening than in the morning. However, ACTH is secreted in a pulsatile manner, leading to rapid fluctuations superimposed on this circadian rhythm. Angiotensin II levels also vary diurnally and are influenced by dietary sodium and potassium intakes and posture. Both upright posture and sodium restriction elevate angiotensin II levels.

Most clinical determinations of the renin-angiotensin system, however, involve measurements of peripheral *plasma renin activity* (PRA) in which the renin activity is gauged by the generation of angiotensin I during a standardized incubation period. This method depends on the presence of sufficient angiotensinogen in the plasma as substrate. The generated angiotensin I is measured by radioimmunoassay. The PRA depends on the dietary sodium intake and on whether the patient is ambulatory. In normal humans, the PRA shows a diurnal rhythm characterized by peak values in the morning and decreases in activity in the afternoon. An alternative approach is to measure plasma active renin, which is easier and not dependent on endogenous substrate concentration. PRA and active renin correlate very well on low-sodium diets ($r = 0.85$ to 0.9) but less well on high-sodium diets.

Steroids Cortisol and aldosterone are both secreted episodically, and levels generally vary during the day, with peak values in the morning and low levels in the evening. In addition, the plasma level of aldosterone, but not of cortisol, is increased by dietary potassium loading, by sodium restriction, or by assumption of the upright posture. Measurement of the sulfate conjugate of DHEA may be a useful index of adrenal androgen secretion, as little DHEA sulfate is formed in the gonads and because the half-life of DHEA sulfate is 7 to 9 h. However, DHEA sulfate levels reflect both DHEA production and sulfatase activity.

URINE LEVELS For the assessment of glucocorticoid secretion, the urine *17-hydroxycorticosteroid* assay has been replaced by measurement of urinary free cortisol. Elevated levels of urinary free cortisol correlate with states of hypercortisolism, reflecting changes in the levels of unbound, physiologically active circulating cortisol. Normally, the rate of excretion is higher in the daytime (7 A.M. to 7 P.M.) than at night (7 P.M. to 7 A.M.).

Urinary *17-ketosteroids* originate in either the adrenal gland or the gonad. In normal women, 90% of urinary 17-ketosteroids is derived from the adrenal, and in men 60 to 70% is of adrenal origin. Urine 17-ketosteroid values are highest in young adults and decline with age.

A carefully timed urine collection is a prerequisite for all excretory determinations. Urinary creatinine should be measured simultaneously to determine the accuracy and adequacy of the collection procedure.

STIMULATION TESTS   Stimulation tests are useful in the diagnosis of hormone deficiency states.

Tests of Glucocorticoid Reserve   Within minutes after administration of ACTH, cortisol levels increase. This responsiveness can be used as an index of the functional reserve of the adrenal gland for production of cortisol. Under maximal ACTH stimulation, cortisol secretion increases tenfold, to 800 μmol/d (300 mg/d), but maximal stimulation can be achieved only with prolonged ACTH infusions.

A screening test (the so-called rapid ACTH stimulation test) involves the administration of 25 units (0.25 mg) of cosyntropin intravenously or intramuscularly and measurement of plasma cortisol levels before and 30 and 60 min after administration; the test can be performed at any time of the day. The most clear-cut criterion for a normal response is a stimulated cortisol level of >500 nmol/L (>18 μg/dL), and the minimal stimulated normal increment of cortisol is >200 nmol/L (>7 μg/dL) above baseline. Severely ill patients with elevated basal cortisol levels may show no further increases following acute ACTH administration.

Tests of Mineralocorticoid Reserve and Stimulation of the Renin-Angiotensin System   Stimulation tests use protocols designed to create a programmed volume depletion, such as sodium restriction, diuretic administration, or upright posture. A simple, potent test consists of severe sodium restriction and upright posture. After 3 to 5 days of a 10-mmol/d sodium intake, rates of aldosterone secretion or excretion should increase two- to threefold over the control values. Supine morning plasma aldosterone levels are usually increased three- to sixfold, and they increase a further two- to fourfold in response to 2 to 3 h of upright posture.

When the dietary sodium intake is normal, stimulation testing requires the administration of a potent diuretic, such as 40 to 80 mg furosemide, followed by 2 to 3 h of upright posture. The normal response is a two- to fourfold rise in plasma aldosterone levels.

SUPPRESSION TESTS   Suppression tests to document hypersecretion of adrenal hormones involve measurement of the target hormone response after standardized suppression of its tropic hormone.

Tests of Pituitary-Adrenal Suppressibility   The ACTH release mechanism is sensitive to the circulating glucocorticoid level. When blood levels of glucocorticoid are increased in normal individuals, less ACTH is released from the anterior pituitary and less steroid is produced by the adrenal gland. The integrity of this feedback mechanism can be tested clinically by giving a glucocorticoid and judging the suppression of ACTH secretion by analysis of urine steroid levels and/or plasma cortisol and ACTH levels. A potent glucocorticoid such as dexamethasone is used, so that the agent can be given in an amount small enough not to contribute significantly to the pool of steroids to be analyzed.

The best *screening* procedure is the overnight dexamethasone suppression test. This involves the measurement of plasma cortisol levels at 8 A.M. following the oral administration of 1 mg dexamethasone the previous midnight. The 8 A.M. value for plasma cortisol in normal individuals should be <140 nmol/L (5 μg/dL).

The definitive test of adrenal suppressibility consists in administering 0.5 mg dexamethasone every 6 h for two successive days while collecting urine over a 24-h period for determination of creatinine and free cortisol and/or measuring plasma cortisol levels. In a patient with a normal hypothalamic-pituitary ACTH release mechanism, a fall in the urine free cortisol to <80 nmol/d (30 μg/d) or of plasma cortisol to <140 nmol/L (5 μg/dL) is seen on the second day of administration.

A normal response to either suppression test implies that the glucocorticoid regulation of ACTH and its control of the adrenal glands is physiologically normal. However, an isolated abnormal result, particularly to the overnight suppression test, does not in itself imply pituitary and/or adrenal disease.

Tests of Mineralocorticoid Suppressibility   These tests rely on an expansion of extracellular fluid volume, which should decrease circulating plasma renin activity and decrease the secretion and/or excretion of aldosterone. Various tests differ in the rate at which extracellular fluid volume is expanded. One convenient suppression test involves the intravenous infusion of 500 mL/h of normal saline solution for 4 h, which normally suppresses plasma aldosterone levels to <220 pmol/L (<8 ng/dL) on a sodium-restricted diet or to <140 pmol/L (<5 ng/dL) on a normal sodium intake. Alternatively, a high-sodium diet can be administered for 3 days with 0.2 mg fludrocortisone twice daily. Aldosterone excretion is measured on the third day and should be <28 nmol/d (10 μg/d). These tests should not be performed in potassium-depleted individuals since they carry a risk of precipitating hypokalemia.

TESTS OF PITUITARY-ADRENAL RESPONSIVENESS   Stimuli such as insulin-induced hypoglycemia, AVP, and pyrogens cause the release of ACTH from the pituitary by an action on higher neural centers or on the pituitary itself. Insulin-induced hypoglycemia is particularly useful, because it stimulates the release of both growth hormone and ACTH. In this test, regular insulin (0.05 to 0.1 U/kg body weight) is given intravenously as a bolus to reduce the fasting glucose level to at least 50% below basal. The normal cortisol response is a rise to more than 500 nmol/L (18 μg/dL).

One of the best ways to test the integrity of the pituitary-adrenal axis is the metyrapone test. Metyrapone inhibits 11β-hydroxylase in the adrenal. As a result, the conversion of 11-deoxycortisol (compound S) to cortisol is impaired, causing 11-deoxycortisol to accumulate in the blood and the blood level of cortisol to decrease (Fig. 331-2). The hypothalamic-pituitary axis responds to the declining cortisol blood levels by releasing more ACTH. Note that assessment of the response depends on both an intact hypothalamic-pituitary axis and an intact adrenal gland.

Although modifications of the original metyrapone test have been described, we believe the best involves administering 750 mg of the drug by mouth every 4 h over a 24-h period and comparing the control and postmetyrapone plasma levels of 11-deoxycortisol, cortisol, and ACTH. In normal individuals, plasma 11-deoxycortisol levels should exceed 210 nmol/L (7 μg/dL) and ACTH levels should exceed 17 pmol/L (75 pg/mL) following metyrapone administration. The metyrapone test does not accurately reflect ACTH reserve if subjects are ingesting exogenous glucocorticoids or drugs that accelerate the metabolism of metyrapone (e.g., phenytoin).

A direct and selective test of the pituitary corticotrophs can be achieved with CRH. The bolus injection of ovine CRH (corticorelin, ovine triflutate; 1 μg/kg body weight) stimulates secretion of ACTH and β-LPT in normal human subjects within 15 to 60 min. In normal individuals, the mean increment in ACTH is 9 pmol/L (40 pg/mL). However, the magnitude of the ACTH response is less than that produced by the insulin tolerance test, which implies that additional factors (such as vasopressin) augment stress-induced increases in ACTH secretion.

Although the rapid ACTH stimulation test is useful for the diagnosis of primary adrenal insufficiency, normal cortisol responsiveness may be seen in some patients with a partial ACTH deficit and absence of adrenal atrophy. These patients have an inadequate pituitary ACTH reserve and fail to increase ACTH secretion in response to a stress such as surgery or hypoglycemia. Because the use of a bolus of exogenous ACTH does not invariably exclude a diagnosis of secondary adrenocortical insufficiency, direct tests of pituitary ACTH reserve (metyrapone test, insulin tolerance testing) may be required in the appropriate clinical setting. Alternatively, ACTH at a physiologic dose (1 μg), the so-called low-dose ACTH test, may be used. Abnormal response is similar to the rapid ACTH test. However, levels need to be measured at 30 min, and the ACTH needs to be injected directly intravenously because it can be absorbed to plastic tubing. On the other hand, the rapid ACTH test can distinguish between primary and secondary adrenal insufficiency, because aldosterone secretion is preserved in secondary adrenal failure by the renin-angiotensin system and potassium. Cosyntropin (25 units) is given intravenously or intramuscularly, and plasma cortisol and aldosterone levels are measured before and 30 and 60 min after administration. The cortisol response is abnormal in both groups, but patients with secondary insufficiency show an increase in aldosterone levels by at least 140 pmol/L (5 ng/dL). No aldosterone response is seen in patients in whom the adrenal cortex is destroyed.

HYPERFUNCTION OF THE ADRENAL CORTEX

Excess cortisol is associated with Cushing's syndrome; excess aldosterone causes aldosteronism; and excess adrenal androgens cause adrenal virilism. These syndromes do not always occur in the "pure" form but may have overlapping features.

CUSHING'S SYNDROME Etiology Cushing described a syndrome characterized by truncal obesity, hypertension, fatigability and weakness, amenorrhea, hirsutism, purplish abdominal striae, edema, glucosuria, osteoporosis, and a basophilic tumor of the pituitary. As awareness of this syndrome has increased, the diagnosis of Cushing's syndrome has been broadened into the classification shown in Table 331-2. Regardless of etiology, all cases of endogenous Cushing's syndrome are due to increased production of cortisol by the adrenal. In most cases the cause is *bilateral adrenal hyperplasia* due to hypersecretion of pituitary ACTH or ectopic production of ACTH by a nonpituitary source. The incidence of pituitary-dependent adrenal hyperplasia is three times greater in women than in men, and the most frequent age of onset is the third or fourth decade. Most evidence indicates that the primary defect is the de novo development of a pituitary adenoma, as tumors are found in >90% of patients with pituitary-dependent adrenal hyperplasia. Alternatively, the defect may occasionally reside in the hypothalamus or in higher neural centers, leading to release of CRH inappropriate to the level of circulating cortisol. The consequence would be that a higher level of cortisol is required to reduce ACTH secretion to normal. This primary defect leads to hyperstimulation of the pituitary, resulting in hyperplasia or tumor formation. In surgical series, most individuals with hypersecretion of pituitary ACTH are found to have a microadenoma (<10 mm in diameter; 50% are ≤5 mm in diameter), but a pituitary macroadenoma (>10 mm) or diffuse hyperplasia of the corticotropic cells may be found. In some studies, the recurrence rate is >20%. Unfortunately, it may be difficult to distinguish between recurrence and inadequate primary therapy. Traditionally, only an individual who has an ACTH-producing pituitary tumor is defined as having *Cushing's disease*.

Nonpituitary tumors may secrete polypeptides that are biologically, chemically, and immunologically indistinguishable from either ACTH or CRH and that cause bilateral adrenal hyperplasia (Chap. 100). The ectopic production of CRH results in clinical, biochemical, and radiologic features indistinguishable from those caused by hypersecretion of pituitary ACTH. The typical signs and symptoms of Cushing's syndrome may be absent or minimal with ectopic ACTH production, and hypokalemic alkalosis is a prominent manifestation. Most of these cases are associated with the primitive small cell (oat cell) type of bronchogenic carcinoma or with tumors of the thymus, pancreas, or ovary; medullary carcinoma of the thyroid; or bronchial adenomas. The onset of Cushing's syndrome may be sudden, particularly in patients with carcinoma of the lung, and this feature accounts in part for the failure of these patients to exhibit the classic manifestations. On the other hand, patients with carcinoid tumors or pheochromocytomas have longer clinical courses and usually exhibit the typical cushingoid features. The ectopic secretion of ACTH is also accompanied by the accumulation of ACTH fragments in plasma and by elevated plasma levels of ACTH precursor molecules. Because such tumors may produce large amounts of ACTH, baseline steroid values are usually markedly elevated, and increased skin pigmentation may be present. Indeed, hyperpigmentation in patients with Cushing's syndrome almost always points to an extraadrenal tumor, either in an extracranial location or within the cranium.

Approximately 20 to 25% of patients with Cushing's syndrome have an adrenal neoplasm. These tumors are usually unilateral, and about half are malignant. Occasionally, patients have biochemical features both of pituitary ACTH excess and of an adrenal adenoma. These individuals usually have *nodular hyperplasia* of both adrenal glands often the result of prolonged ACTH stimulation in the absence of a pituitary adenoma. Two additional entities cause nodular hyperplasia: a familial disorder in children or young adults (so-called pigmented micronodular dysplasia; see below) and an abnormal cortisol response to gastric inhibitory polypeptide or luteinizing hormone, probably secondary to expression of receptors for these hormones in the adrenal cortex.

The most common cause of Cushing's syndrome is *iatrogenic* administration of steroids for a variety of reasons. Although the clinical features bear some resemblance to those seen with adrenal tumors, these patients are usually distinguishable on the basis of history and laboratory studies.

Clinical Signs, Symptoms, and Laboratory Findings Many of the signs and symptoms of Cushing's syndrome follow logically from the known action of glucocorticoids (Table 331-3). Mobilization of

Table 331-2 Causes of Cushing's Syndrome

Adrenal hyperplasia
  Secondary to pituitary ACTH overproduction
    Pituitary-hypothalamic dysfunction
    Pituitary ACTH-producing micro- or macroadenomas
  Secondary to ACTH or CRH-producing nonendocrine tumors (bronchogenic carcinoma, carcinoid of the thymus, pancreatic carcinoma, bronchial adenoma)
Adrenal macronodular hyperplasia
Adrenal micronodular dysplasia
  Sporadic
  Familial (Carney's syndrome)
Adrenal neoplasia
  Adenoma
  Carcinoma
Exogenous, iatrogenic causes
  Prolonged use of glucocorticoids
  Prolonged use of ACTH

NOTE: CRH, corticotropin-releasing hormone.

Table 331-3 Frequency of Signs and Symptoms in Cushing's Syndrome

Sign or Symptom	Percent of Patients
Typical habitus (centripetal obesity)[a]	97
Increased body weight	94
Fatigability and weakness	87
Hypertension (blood pressure >150/90)	82
Hirsutism[a]	80
Amenorrhea	77
Broad violaceous cutaneous striae[a]	67
Personality changes	66
Ecchymoses[a]	65
Proximal myopathy[a]	62
Edema	62
Polyuria, polydipsia	23
Hypertrophy of clitoris	19

[a] Features more specific for Cushing's syndrome.

peripheral supportive tissue causes muscle weakness and fatigability, osteoporosis, broad violaceous cutaneous striae, and easy bruisability. The latter signs are secondary to weakening and rupture of collagen fibers in the dermis. Osteoporosis may cause collapse of vertebral bodies and pathologic fractures of other bones. Decreased bone mineralization is particularly pronounced in children. Increased hepatic gluconeogenesis and insulin resistance can cause impaired glucose tolerance. Overt diabetes mellitus occurs in <20% of patients, who probably are individuals with a predisposition to this disorder. Hypercortisolism promotes the deposition of adipose tissue in characteristic sites, notably the upper face (producing the typical "moon" facies), the interscapular area (producing the "buffalo hump"), and the mesenteric bed (producing "truncal" obesity) (Fig. 331-6). Rarely, episternal fatty tumors and mediastinal widening secondary to fat accumulation occur. The reason for this peculiar distribution of adipose tissue is not known, but it is associated with insulin resistance and/or elevated insulin levels. The face appears plethoric, even in the absence of any increase in red blood cell concentration. Hypertension is common, and emotional changes may be profound, ranging from irritability and emotional lability to severe depression, confusion, or even frank psychosis. In women, increased levels of adrenal androgens can cause acne, hirsutism, and oligomenorrhea or amenorrhea. Some signs and symptoms in patients with hypercortisolism—i.e., obesity, hypertension, osteoporosis, and diabetes—are nonspecific and therefore are less helpful in diagnosing the condition. On the other hand, easy bruising, typical striae, myopathy, and virilizing signs (although less frequent) are, if present, more suggestive of Cushing's syndrome (Table 331-3).

Except in iatrogenic Cushing's syndrome, plasma and urine cortisol levels are variably elevated. Occasionally, hypokalemia, hypochloremia, and metabolic alkalosis are present, particularly with ectopic production of ACTH.

Diagnosis   The diagnosis of Cushing's syndrome depends on the demonstration of increased cortisol production and failure to suppress cortisol secretion normally when dexamethasone is administered (Chap. 328). Once the diagnosis is established, further testing is designed to determine the etiology (Fig. 331-7 and Table 331-4).

FIGURE 331-6   A woman with Cushing's syndrome due to a right adrenal cortical adenoma. *A.* Two years prior to surgery, age 18. *B.* One month prior to surgery, age 20. *C.* One year after surgery, age 21.

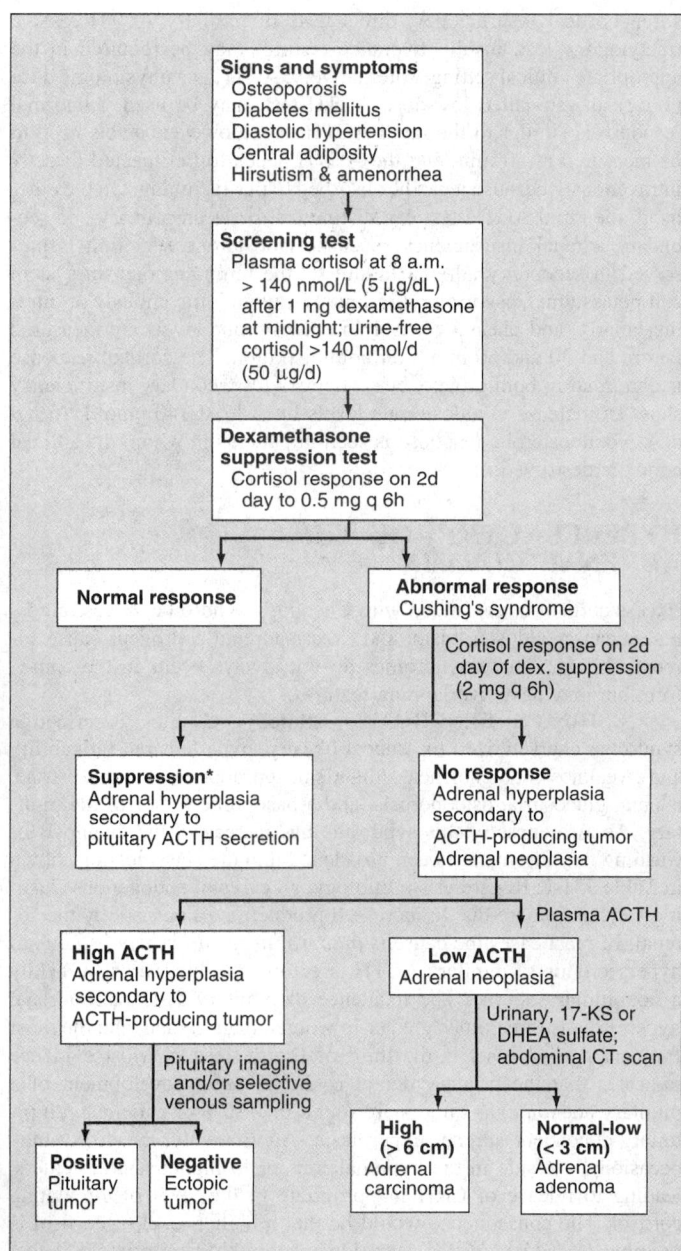

FIGURE 331-7   Diagnostic flowchart for evaluating patients suspected of having Cushing's syndrome. *This group probably includes some patients with pituitary-hypothalamic dysfunction and some with pituitary microadenomas. In some instances, a microadenoma may be visualized by pituitary MRI scanning. 17-KS, 17-ketosteroids; DHEA, dehydroepiandrosterone.

For initial screening, the overnight dexamethasone suppression test is recommended (see above). In difficult cases (e.g., in obese patients), measurement of a 24-h urine free cortisol also can be used as a screening test. A level >140 nmol/d (50 μg/d) is suggestive of Cushing's syndrome. The definitive diagnosis is then established by failure of urinary cortisol to fall to less than <25 nmol/d (10 μg/d) or of plasma cortisol to fall to <140 nmol/L (5 μg/dL) after a standard low-dose dexamethasone suppression test (0.5 mg every 6 h for 48 h). Owing to circadian variability, plasma cortisol and, to a certain extent, ACTH determinations are not meaningful when performed in isolation, but the absence of the normal fall of plasma cortisol at midnight is consistent with Cushing's syndrome.

The task of determining the etiology of Cushing's syndrome is complicated by the fact that all the available tests lack specificity and by the fact that the tumors producing this syndrome are prone to spontaneous and often dramatic changes in hormone secretion (periodic

Test	Pituitary Macroadenoma	Pituitary Microadenoma	Ectopic ACTH or CRH Production	Adrenal Tumor
Plasma ACTH level	↑ to ↑↑	N to ↑	↑ to ↑↑↑	↓
Percent who respond to high-dose dexamethasone	<10	95	<10	<10
Percent who respond to CRH	>90	>90	<10	<10

NOTE: CRH, corticotropin-releasing hormone; N, normal; ↑, elevated; ↓, decreased. See text for definition of a response.

hormonogenesis). No test has a specificity >95%, and it may be necessary to use a combination of tests to arrive at the correct diagnosis. A useful step to distinguish patients with an ACTH-secreting pituitary microadenoma or hypothalamic-pituitary dysfunction from those with other forms of Cushing's syndrome is to determine the response of cortisol output to administration of high-dose dexamethasone (2 mg every 6 h for 2 days). An alternative 8-mg, overnight high-dose dexamethasone test has been developed; however, this test has a lower sensitivity and specificity than the standard test. When the diagnosis of Cushing's syndrome is clear-cut on the basis of baseline urinary and plasma assays, the high-dose dexamethasone suppression test may be used without performing the preliminary low-dose suppression test. The high-dose suppression test provides close to 100% specificity if the criterion used is suppression of urinary free cortisol by >90%. Occasionally, in individuals with bilateral nodular hyperplasia and/or ectopic CRH production, steroid output is also suppressed. Failure of low- and high-dose dexamethasone administration to suppress cortisol production (Table 331-4) is usual in patients with adrenal hyperplasia secondary to an ACTH-secreting pituitary macroadenoma or an ACTH-producing tumor of nonendocrine origin and in those with adrenal neoplasms.

Plasma ACTH levels can be useful in distinguishing the various causes of Cushing's syndrome, particularly in separating ACTH-dependent from ACTH-independent causes. In general, measurement of plasma ACTH is useful in the diagnosis of ACTH-independent etiologies of the syndrome, since most adrenal tumors cause low or undetectable ACTH levels [<2 pmol/L (10 pg/mL)]. Furthermore, ACTH-secreting pituitary macroadenomas and ACTH-producing nonendocrine tumors usually result in elevated ACTH levels. In the ectopic ACTH syndrome, ACTH levels may be elevated to >110 pmol/L (500 pg/mL), and in most patients the level is >40 pmol/L (200 pg/mL). In Cushing's syndrome as the result of a microadenoma or pituitary-hypothalamic dysfunction, ACTH levels range from 6 to 30 pmol/L (30 to 150 pg/mL) [normal, <14 pmol/L (<60 pg/mL)], with half of values falling in the normal range. However, the main problem with the use of ACTH levels in the differential diagnosis of Cushing's syndrome is that ACTH levels may be similar in individuals with hypothalamic-pituitary dysfunction, pituitary microadenomas, ectopic CRH production, and ectopic ACTH production (especially carcinoid tumors) (Table 331-4).

Because of these difficulties, several additional tests have been advocated, such as the metyrapone and CRH infusion tests. The rationale underlying these tests is that steroid hypersecretion by an adrenal tumor or the ectopic production of ACTH will suppress the hypothalamic-pituitary axis so that inhibition of pituitary ACTH release can be demonstrated by either test. Thus, most patients with pituitary-hypothalamic dysfunction and/or a microadenoma have an increase in steroid or ACTH secretion in response to metyrapone or CRH administration, whereas most patients with ectopic ACTH-producing tumors do not. Most pituitary macroadenomas also respond to CRH, but their response to metyrapone is variable. However, false-positive and -negative CRH tests can occur in patients with ectopic ACTH and pituitary tumors.

The main diagnostic dilemma in Cushing's syndrome is to distinguish those instances due to microadenomas of the pituitary and/or pituitary-hypothalamic dysfunction from those due to tumors (e.g., carcinoids or pheochromocytoma) that produce CRH and/or ACTH ectopically. The clinical manifestations are similar unless the ectopic tumor produces other symptoms, such as diarrhea and flushing from a carcinoid tumor or episodic hypertension from a pheochromocytoma. Sometimes, one can distinguish between ectopic and pituitary ACTH production by using metyrapone or CRH tests, as noted above. In these situations, computed tomography (CT) of the pituitary gland is usually normal. Magnetic resonance imaging (MRI) with the enhancing agent gadolinium may be better than CT for this purpose but demonstrates pituitary microadenomas in only half of patients with Cushing's disease. In subjects with negative imaging studies, selective petrosal sinus venous sampling for ACTH is employed in some centers. Demonstration of an ACTH gradient between the petrosal sinus and peripheral blood localizes the source of ACTH overproduction to the pituitary gland but does not distinguish pituitary-dependent adrenal hyperplasia from pituitary hyperplasia secondary to a tumor producing CRH. CRH levels should be measured in the peripheral blood prior to petrosal sinus sampling. In centers where petrosal sinus sampling is performed frequently, it has proved useful for distinguishing pituitary and nonpituitary sources of ACTH excess. However, the catheterization procedure is technically difficult, and complications have occurred.

The diagnosis of a *cortisol-producing adrenal adenoma* is suggested by disproportionate elevations in baseline urine free-cortisol levels with only modest changes in urinary 17-ketosteroids or plasma DHEA sulfate. Adrenal androgen secretion is usually reduced in these patients owing to the cortisol-induced suppression of ACTH and subsequent involution of the androgen-producing zona reticularis.

The diagnosis of *adrenal carcinoma* is suggested by a palpable abdominal mass and by *markedly* elevated baseline values of *both* urine 17-ketosteroids and plasma DHEA sulfate. Plasma and urine cortisol levels are variably elevated. Adrenal carcinoma is usually resistant to both ACTH stimulation and dexamethasone suppression. Elevated adrenal androgen secretion often leads to virilization in the female. Estrogen-producing adrenocortical carcinoma usually presents with gynecomastia in men and dysfunctional uterine bleeding in women. These adrenal tumors secrete increased amounts of androstenedione, which is converted peripherally to the estrogens estrone and estradiol (Chap. 337). Adrenal carcinomas that produce Cushing's syndrome are often associated with elevated levels of the intermediates of steroid biosynthesis (especially 11-deoxycortisol), suggesting inefficient conversion of the intermediates to the final product. This feature also accounts for the characteristic increase in 17-ketosteroids. Approximately 20% of adrenal carcinomas are not associated with endocrine syndromes and are presumed to be nonfunctioning or to produce biologically inactive steroid precursors. In addition, the excessive production of steroids is not always clinically evident (e.g., androgens in adult men).

Differential Diagnosis • *Pseudo-Cushing's Syndrome* Problems in diagnosis include patients with obesity, chronic alcoholism, depression, and acute illness of any type. Extreme *obesity* is uncommon in Cushing's syndrome; furthermore, with exogenous obesity, the adiposity is generalized, not truncal. On adrenocortical testing, abnormalities in patients with exogenous obesity are usually modest. Basal urine steroid excretion levels in obese patients are also either normal or slightly elevated. Some patients have elevated conversion of secreted cortisol into excreted metabolites. Urinary and blood cortisol levels are usually normal, and the diurnal pattern in blood and urine levels is normal. Patients with *chronic alcoholism* and those with *depression* share similar abnormalities in steroid output: modestly elevated urine cortisol, blunted circadian rhythm of cortisol levels, and resistance to suppression using the overnight dexamethasone test. In contrast to alcoholic subjects, depressed patients do not have signs and

FIGURE 331-8 Computed tomography is the preferred method for visualizing the adrenal glands (*arrows*). *A.* The normal right adrenal gland is adjacent to the inferior vena cava (V) where it emerges from the liver. Approximately 90% of right adrenal glands appear as linear structures extending posteriorly from the inferior vena cava into the space between the right lobe of the liver and the crus of the diaphragm. The normal left adrenal gland is lateral to the left crus of the diaphragm and below the stomach. Most left adrenal glands are shaped like an inverted V or Y. *B.* Adrenal CT scan of a patient with ectopic ACTH production. Both adrenal glands (*arrows*) are enlarged (compare with *A*). In contrast, only 50% of patients with bilateral adrenal hyperplasia secondary to pituitary ACTH hypersecretion show enlargement of the adrenals when imaged by CT scan. *C.* CT scan of a patient with Cushing's syndrome with biochemical evidence only of cortisol overproduction. The left adrenal has been replaced by a racquet-shaped 2-cm tumor (*arrow*). Attenuation of the tumor is low because of its high lipid content. *D.* CT scan in a patient with Cushing's syndrome and biochemical evidence of an adrenal carcinoma. In contrast to the tumor in *C*, the right-sided mass in this patient is large and has a heterogeneous appearance—usual characteristics of an adrenal carcinoma.

Radiologic Evaluation for Cushing's Syndrome The preferred radiologic study for visualizing the adrenals is a CT scan of the abdomen (Fig. 331-8). CT is of value both for localizing adrenal tumors and for diagnosing bilateral hyperplasia. All patients believed to have hypersecretion of pituitary ACTH should have a pituitary MRI scan with the contrast agent gadolinium. Even with this technique, small microadenomas may be undetectable; alternatively, false-positive masses due to cysts or nonsecretory lesions of the normal pituitary may be imaged. In patients with ectopic ACTH production, chest CT is a useful first step.

Evaluation of Asymptomatic Adrenal Masses With abdominal CT scanning, many incidental adrenal masses (so-called incidentalomas) are discovered. This is not surprising, since 10 to 20% of subjects at autopsy have adrenocortical adenomas. The first step in evaluating such patients is to determine whether the tumor is functioning by means of appropriate screening tests, e.g., measurement of 24-h urine catecholamines and metabolites and serum potassium and assessment of adrenal cortical function by dexamethasone-suppression testing. However, 90% of incidentalomas are nonfunctioning. If an extraadrenal malignancy is present, there is a 30 to 50% chance that the adrenal tumor is a metastasis. If the primary tumor is being treated and there are no other metastases, it is prudent to obtain a fine-needle aspirate of the adrenal mass to establish the diagnosis. In the absence of a known malignancy the next step is unclear. The probability of adrenal carcinoma is <0.01 percent, the vast majority of adrenal masses being benign adenomas. Features suggestive of malignancy include large size (a size >4 to 6 cm suggests carcinoma); irregular margins; and inhomogeneity, soft tissue calcifications visible on CT (Fig. 331-8), and findings characteristic of malignancy on a chemical-shift MRI image. If surgery is not performed, a repeat CT scan should be obtained in 3 to 6 months. Fine needle aspiration is not useful to distinguish between benign and malignant primary adrenal tumors.

℞ **TREATMENT Adrenal Neoplasm** When an adenoma or carcinoma is diagnosed, adrenal exploration is performed with excision of the tumor. Adenomas may be resected using laparoscopic techniques. Because of the possibility of atrophy of the contralateral adrenal, the patient is treated pre- and postoperatively as if for total adrenalectomy, even when a unilateral lesion is suspected, the routine being similar to that for an Addisonian patient undergoing elective surgery (see Table 331-8).

Despite operative intervention, most patients with adrenal carcinoma die within 3 years of diagnosis. Metastases occur most often to liver and lung. The principal drug for the treatment of adrenocortical carcinoma is mitotane (*o,p'*-DDD), an isomer of the insecticide DDT. This drug suppresses cortisol production and decreases plasma and urine steroid levels. Although its cytotoxic action is relatively selective for the glucocorticoid-secreting zone of the adrenal cortex, the zona glomerulosa may also be inhibited. Because mitotane also alters the extraadrenal metabolism of cortisol, plasma and urinary cortisol levels

symptoms of Cushing's syndrome. Following discontinuation of alcohol and/or improvement in the emotional status, results of steroid testing usually return to normal. One or more of three tests have been used to differentiate mild Cushing's syndrome and pseudo-Cushing's syndrome. The serum cortisol level following the standard 2-day low-dose dexamethasone test has very high sensitivity and specificity. While the CRH test alone is less useful, in combination with the low-dose dexamethasone test, there is nearly complete discrimination between these two conditions. Finally, a midnight cortisol level obtained in awake patients may have similar predictive value as the low-dose dexamethasone test if a cut-off of 210 nmol/L (7.5 μg/dL) is used. Patients with *acute illness* often have abnormal results on laboratory tests and fail to exhibit pituitary-adrenal suppression in response to dexamethasone, since major stress (such as pain or fever) interrupts the normal regulation of ACTH secretion. *Iatrogenic Cushing's syndrome*, induced by the administration of glucocorticoids or other steroids such as megestrol that bind to the glucocorticoid receptor, is indistinguishable by physical findings from endogenous adrenocortical hyperfunction. The distinction can be made, however, by measuring blood or urine cortisol levels in a basal state; in the iatrogenic syndrome these levels are low secondary to suppression of the pituitary-adrenal axis. The severity of iatrogenic Cushing's syndrome is related to the total steroid dose, the biologic half-life of the steroid, and the duration of therapy. Also, individuals taking afternoon and evening doses of glucocorticoids develop Cushing's syndrome more readily and with a smaller total daily dose than do patients taking morning doses only. The enzymatic disposition and binding of administered steroids differ among patients.

must be assessed to titrate the effect. The drug is usually given in divided doses three to four times a day, with the dose increased gradually to tolerability (usually <6 g daily). At higher doses, almost all patients experience side effects, which may be gastrointestinal (anorexia, diarrhea, vomiting) or neuromuscular (lethargy, somnolence, dizziness). All patients treated with mitotane should receive long-term glucocorticoid maintenance therapy, and, in some, mineralocorticoid replacement is appropriate. In approximately one-third of patients, both tumor and metastases regress, but long-term survival is not altered. In many patients, mitotane only inhibits steroidogenesis and does not cause regression of tumor metastases. Osseous metastases are usually refractory to the drug and should be treated with radiation therapy. Mitotane can also be given as adjunctive therapy after surgical resection of an adrenal carcinoma, although there is no evidence that this improves survival. Because of the absence of a long-term benefit with mitotane, alternative chemotherapeutic approaches based on platinum therapy have been used. However, there are no data presently available indicating a prolongation of life.

Bilateral hyperplasia   Patients with hyperplasia have a relative or absolute increase in ACTH levels. Since therapy would logically be directed at reducing ACTH levels, the ideal primary treatment for ACTH- or CRH-producing tumors, whether pituitary or ectopic, is surgical removal. Occasionally (particularly with ectopic ACTH production) surgical excision is not possible because the disease is far advanced. In this situation, "medical" or surgical adrenalectomy may correct the hypercortisolism.

Controversy exists as to the proper treatment for bilateral adrenal hyperplasia when the source of the ACTH overproduction is not apparent. In some centers, these patients (especially those who suppress after the administration of a high-dose dexamethasone test) undergo surgical exploration of the pituitary via a transsphenoidal approach in the expectation that a microadenoma will be found. However, in most circumstances selective petrosal sinus venous sampling is recommended, and the patient is referred to an appropriate center if the procedure is not available locally. If a microadenoma is not found at the time of exploration, total hypophysectomy may be needed. Complications of transsphenoidal surgery include cerebrospinal fluid rhinorrhea, diabetes insipidus, panhypopituitarism, and optic or cranial nerve injuries.

In other centers, total adrenalectomy is the treatment of choice. The cure rate with this procedure is close to 100%. The adverse effects include the certain need for lifelong mineralocorticoid and glucocorticoid replacement and a 10 to 20% probability of a pituitary tumor developing over the next 10 years (Nelson's syndrome; Chap. 328). Many of these tumors require surgical therapy. It is uncertain whether they arise de novo in these patients or were present prior to adrenalectomy but were too small to be detected. Periodic radiologic evaluation of the pituitary gland by MRI as well as serial ACTH measurements should be performed in all individuals after bilateral adrenalectomy for Cushing's disease. Such pituitary tumors may become locally invasive and impinge on the optic chiasm or extend into the cavernous or sphenoid sinuses.

Except in children, pituitary irradiation is rarely used as primary treatment, being reserved rather for postoperative tumor recurrences. In some centers, high levels of gamma radiation can be focused on the desired site with less scattering to surrounding tissues by using stereotactic techniques. Side effects of radiation include ocular motor palsy and hypopituitarism. There is a long lag time between treatment and remission, and the remission rate is usually <50%.

Finally, in occasional patients in whom a surgical approach is not feasible, "medical" adrenalectomy may be indicated (Table 331-5). Inhibition of steroidogenesis may also be indicated in severely cushingoid subjects prior to surgical intervention. Chemical adrenalectomy may be accomplished by the administration of the inhibitor of steroidogenesis ketoconazole (600 to 1200 mg/d). In addition, mitotane (2 or 3 g/d) and/or the blockers of steroid synthesis aminoglutethimide (1 g/d) and metyrapone (2 or 3 g/d) may be effective either alone or in combination. Mitotane is slow to take effect (weeks). Mifepristone,

Table 331-5   Treatment Modalities for Patients with Adrenal Hyperplasia Secondary to Pituitary ACTH Hypersecretion

Treatments to reduce pituitary ACTH production
   Transsphenoidal resection of microadenoma
   Radiation therapy
Treatments to reduce or eliminate adrenocortical cortisol secretion
   Bilateral adrenalectomy
   Medical adrenalectomy (metyrapone, mitotane, aminoglutethimide, ketoconazole)[a]

---

[a] Not curative but effective as long as chronically administered in selected patients.

a competitive inhibitor of the binding of glucocorticoid to its receptor, may be a treatment option. Adrenal insufficiency is a risk with all these agents, and replacement steroids may be required.

ALDOSTERONISM   Aldosteronism is a syndrome associated with hypersecretion of the mineralocorticoid aldosterone. In *primary* aldosteronism the cause for the excessive aldosterone production resides within the adrenal gland; in *secondary* aldosteronism the stimulus is extraadrenal.

Primary Aldosteronism   In the original case of excessive and inappropriate aldosterone production, the disease was the result of an *aldosterone-producing adrenal adenoma* (Conn's syndrome). Most cases involve a unilateral adenoma, which is usually small and may occur on either side. Rarely, primary aldosteronism is due to an adrenal carcinoma. Aldosteronism is twice as common in women as in men, usually occurs between the ages of 30 and 50, and is present in approximately 1% of unselected hypertensive patients. However, the prevalence may be as high as 10%, depending on the criteria and study population. Most of this difference is not secondary to the prevalence of patients with an aldosteronoma but rather because of the inclusion of those with bilateral hyperplasia. In many patients with clinical and biochemical features of primary aldosteronism, a solitary adenoma is not found at surgery. Instead, these patients have *bilateral cortical nodular hyperplasia*. In the literature, this disease is also termed *idiopathic hyperaldosteronism*, and/or *nodular hyperplasia*. The cause is unknown.

Signs and symptoms   Hypersecretion of aldosterone increases the renal distal tubular exchange of intratubular sodium for secreted potassium and hydrogen ions, with progressive depletion of body potassium and development of hypokalemia. Most patients have diastolic hypertension, which may be very severe, and headaches. The hypertension is probably due to the increased sodium reabsorption and extracellular volume expansion. *Potassium depletion* is responsible for the muscle weakness and fatigue and is due to the effect of potassium depletion on the muscle cell membrane. The polyuria results from impairment of urinary concentrating ability and is often associated with polydipsia.

Electrocardiographic and roentgenographic signs of left ventricular enlargement are, in part, secondary to the hypertension. However, the left ventricular hypertrophy is disproportionate to the level of blood pressure when compared to individuals with essential hypertension, and regression of the hypertrophy occurs even if blood pressure is not reduced after removal of an aldosteronoma. Electrocardiographic signs of potassium depletion include prominent U waves, cardiac arrhythmias, and premature contractions. In the absence of associated congestive heart failure, renal disease, or preexisting abnormalities (such as thrombophlebitis), edema is characteristically absent. However, structural damage to the cerebral circulation, retinal vasculature, and kidney occurs more frequently than would be predicted based on the level and duration of the hypertension. Proteinuria may occur in as many as 50% of patients with primary aldosteronism, and renal failure occurs in up to 15%. Thus, it is probable that excess aldosterone production induces cardiovascular damage independent of its effect on blood pressure.

Laboratory findings Laboratory findings depend on both the duration and the severity of potassium depletion. An overnight concentration test often reveals impaired ability to concentrate the urine, probably secondary to the hypokalemia. Urine pH is neutral to alkaline because of excessive secretion of ammonium and bicarbonate ions to compensate for the metabolic alkalosis.

Hypokalemia may be severe (<3 mmol/L) and reflects body potassium depletion, usually >300 mmol. In mild forms of primary aldosteronism, potassium levels may be normal. *Hypernatremia* is due to sodium retention, a concomitant water loss from polyuria, and a resetting of the osmostat. Metabolic alkalosis and elevation of serum bicarbonate are a result of hydrogen ion loss into the urine and migration into potassium-depleted cells. The alkalosis is perpetuated by potassium deficiency, which increases the capacity of the proximal convoluted tubule to reabsorb filtered bicarbonate. If hypokalemia is severe, serum magnesium levels are also reduced.

Diagnosis The diagnosis is suggested by persistent hypokalemia in a nonedematous patient with a normal sodium intake who is not receiving potassium-wasting diuretics (furosemide, ethacrynic acid, thiazides). If hypokalemia occurs in a hypertensive patient taking a potassium-wasting diuretic, the diuretic should be discontinued and the patient should be given potassium supplements. After 1 to 2 weeks, the potassium level should be remeasured, and if hypokalemia persists, the patient should be evaluated for a mineralocorticoid excess syndrome (Fig. 331-9).

The criteria for the diagnosis of primary aldosteronism are (1) diastolic hypertension without edema, (2) hyposecretion of renin (as judged by low plasma renin activity levels) that fails to increase appropriately during volume depletion (upright posture, sodium depletion), and (3) hypersecretion of aldosterone that does not suppress appropriately in response to volume expansion.

Patients with primary aldosteronism characteristically *do not have edema*, since they exhibit an "escape" phenomenon from the sodium-retaining aspects of mineralocorticoids. Rarely, pretibial edema is present in patients with associated nephropathy and azotemia.

The estimation of plasma renin activity is of limited value in separating patients with primary aldosteronism from those with hypertension of other causes. Although failure of plasma renin activity to rise normally during volume-depletion maneuvers is a criterion for a diagnosis of primary aldosteronism, suppressed renin activity also occurs in about 25% of patients with essential hypertension.

Although a renin measurement alone lacks specificity, the ratio of serum aldosterone to plasma renin activity is a very useful screening test. A high ratio (>30), when aldosterone is expressed as ng/dL and plasma renin activity as ng/mL per hour, strongly suggests autonomy of aldosterone secretion. Aldosterone levels need to be >500 pmol/L (>15 ng/dL) and the salt intake not be restricted in making this assessment. Ultimately, it is necessary to demonstrate a lack of aldosterone suppression to diagnose primary aldosteronism (Fig. 331-9). The autonomy exhibited in these patients refers only to the resistance to suppression of secretion during volume expansion; aldosterone can and does respond in a normal or above-normal fashion to the stimulus of potassium loading or ACTH infusion.

Once hyposecretion of renin and failure of aldosterone secretion suppression are demonstrated, aldosterone-producing adenomas should be localized by abdominal CT scan, using a high-resolution scanner as many aldosteronomas are <1 cm in size. If the CT scan is negative, percutaneous transfemoral bilateral adrenal vein catheterization with adrenal vein sampling may demonstrate a two- to threefold increase in plasma aldosterone concentration on the involved side. In cases of hyperaldosteronism secondary to cortical nodular hyperplasia, no lateralization is found. It is important for samples to be obtained simultaneously if possible and for cortisol levels to be measured to ensure that false localization does not reflect dilution or an ACTH- or stress-induced rise in aldosterone levels. In a patient with an adenoma, the aldosterone/cortisol ratio lateralizes to the side of the lesion.

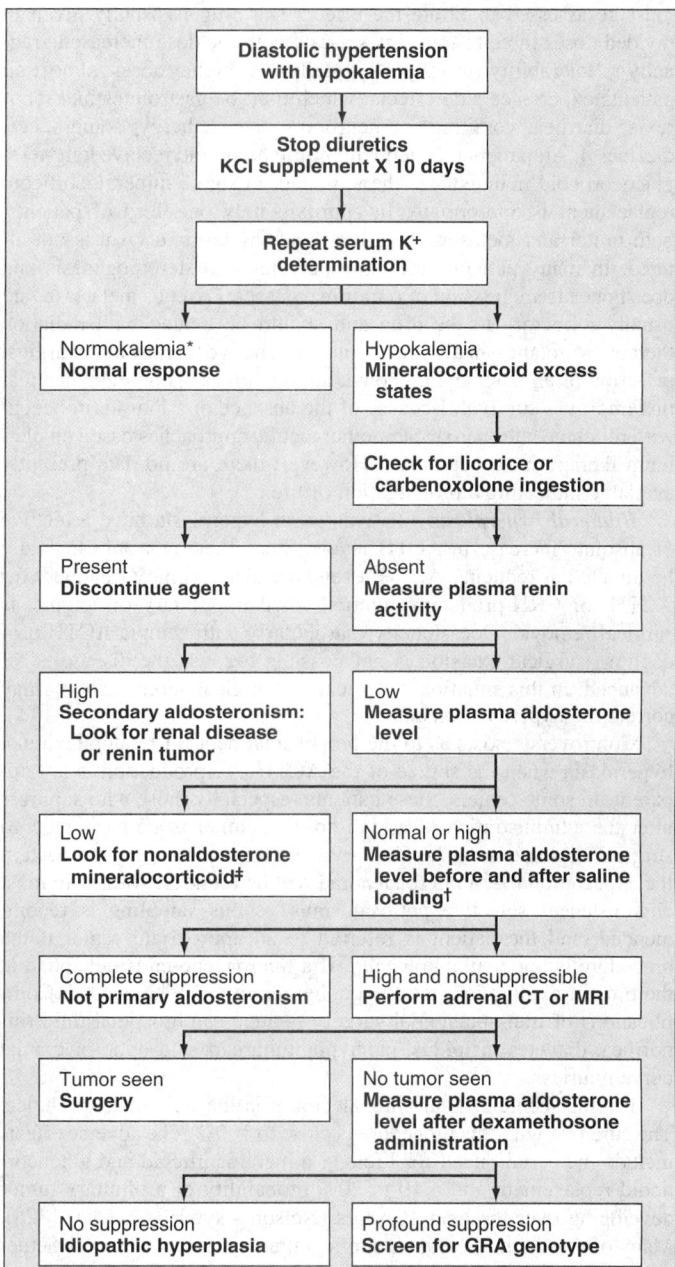

FIGURE 331-9 Diagnostic flowchart for evaluating patients with suspected primary aldosteronism. *Serum K+ may be normal in some patients with hyperaldosteronism who are taking potassium-sparing diuretics (spironolactone, triamterene) or who have a low sodium intake and a high potassium intake. †This step should not be taken if hypertension is severe (diastolic pressure >115 mmHg) or if cardiac failure is present. Also, serum potassium levels should be corrected before the infusion of saline solution. Alternative methods that produce comparable suppression of aldosterone secretion include oral sodium loading (200 mmol/d) and the administration of fludrocortisone, 0.2 mg BID, for 3 days. (GRA, glucocorticoid-remediable aldosteronism.) ‡For example, Liddle's syndrome, apparent mineralocorticoid excess syndrome, or a deoxycorticosterone-secreting tumor.

Differential diagnosis Patients with hypertension and hypokalemia may have either primary or secondary hyperaldosteronism (Fig. 331-10). A useful maneuver to distinguish between these conditions is the measurement of plasma renin activity. Secondary hyperaldosteronism in patients with accelerated hypertension is due to elevated plasma renin levels; in contrast, patients with primary aldosteronism have suppressed plasma renin levels. Indeed, in patients with a serum potassium concentration of <2.5 mmol/L, a high ratio of plasma aldosterone to plasma renin activity in a random sample is usually suf-

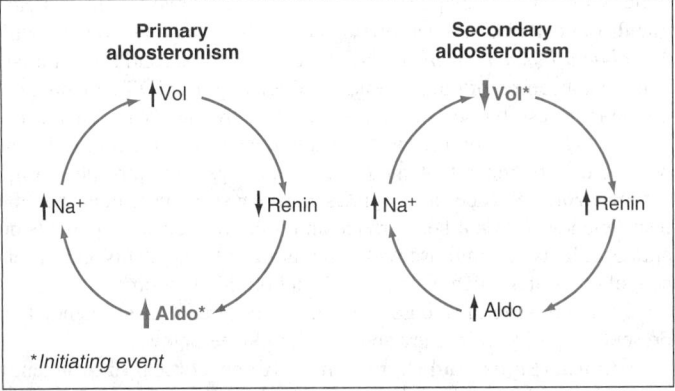

FIGURE 331-10 Responses of the renin-aldosterone volume control loop in primary versus secondary aldosteronism.

ficient to establish the diagnosis of primary aldosteronism without additional testing.

Primary aldosteronism must also be distinguished from other *hypermineralocorticoid states*. Nonaldosterone mineralocorticoid states will have suppressed plasma renin activity but low aldosterone levels. The most common problem is to distinguish between hyperaldosteronism due to an adenoma and that due to idiopathic bilateral nodular hyperplasia. This distinction is of importance because hypertension associated with idiopathic hyperplasia is usually not benefited by bilateral adrenalectomy, whereas hypertension associated with aldosterone-producing tumors is usually improved or cured by removal of the adenoma. Although patients with idiopathic bilateral nodular hyperplasia tend to have less severe hypokalemia, lower aldosterone secretion, and higher plasma renin activity than do patients with primary aldosteronism, differentiation is impossible solely on clinical and/or biochemical grounds. An anomalous postural decrease in plasma aldosterone and elevated plasma 18-hydroxycorticosterone levels are present in most patients with a unilateral lesion. However, these tests are also of limited diagnostic value in the individual patient, because some adenoma patients have an increase in plasma aldosterone with upright posture, so-called renin-responsive aldosteronoma. A definitive diagnosis is best made by radiographic studies, including bilateral adrenal vein catheterization, as noted above.

In a few instances, hypertensive patients with hypokalemic alkalosis have adenomas that secrete deoxycorticosterone (DOC). Such patients have reduced plasma renin activity levels, but aldosterone levels are either normal or reduced, suggesting the diagnosis of mineralocorticoid excess due to a hormone other than aldosterone. Several inherited disorders have clinical features similar to those of primary aldosteronism (see below).

℞ TREATMENT Primary aldosteronism due to an adenoma is usually treated by surgical excision of the adenoma. Where possible a laparoscopic approach is favored. However, dietary sodium restriction and the administration of an aldosterone antagonist, e.g., spironolactone, are effective in many cases. Hypertension and hypokalemia are usually controlled by doses of 25 to 100 mg spironolactone every 8 h. In some patients medical management has been successful for years, but chronic therapy in men is usually limited by side effects of spironolactone such as gynecomastia, decreased libido, and impotence.

When idiopathic bilateral hyperplasia is suspected, surgery is indicated only when significant, symptomatic hypokalemia cannot be controlled with medical therapy, e.g., by spironolactone, triamterene, or amiloride. Hypertension associated with idiopathic hyperplasia is usually not benefited by bilateral adrenalectomy.

Secondary Aldosteronism *Secondary aldosteronism* refers to an appropriately increased production of aldosterone in response to activation of the renin-angiotensin system (Fig. 331-10). The production rate of aldosterone is often higher in patients with secondary al-

dosteronism than in those with primary aldosteronism. Secondary aldosteronism usually occurs in association with the accelerated phase of hypertension or on the basis of an underlying edema disorder. Secondary aldosteronism in pregnancy is a normal physiologic response to estrogen-induced increases in circulating levels of renin substrate and plasma renin activity and to the antialdosterone actions of progestogens.

Secondary aldosteronism in hypertensive states is due either to a primary overproduction of renin (primary reninism) or to an overproduction of renin secondary to a decrease in renal blood flow and/or perfusion pressure (Fig. 331-10). Secondary hypersecretion of renin can be due to a narrowing of one or both of the major renal arteries by atherosclerosis or by fibromuscular hyperplasia. Overproduction of renin from both kidneys also occurs in severe arteriolar nephrosclerosis (malignant hypertension) or with profound renal vasoconstriction (the accelerated phase of hypertension). The secondary aldosteronism is characterized by hypokalemic alkalosis, moderate to severe increases in plasma renin activity, and moderate to marked increases in aldosterone levels (Chap. 246).

Secondary aldosteronism with hypertension can also be caused by rare renin-producing tumors (primary reninism). These patients have the biochemical characteristics of renal vascular hypertension, but the primary defect is renin secretion by a juxtaglomerular cell tumor. The diagnosis can be made by demonstration of normal renal vasculature and/or demonstration of a space-occupying lesion in the kidney by radiographic techniques and documentation of a unilateral increase in renal vein renin activity. Rarely, these tumors arise in tissues such as the ovary.

Secondary aldosteronism is present in many forms of *edema*. The rate of aldosterone secretion is usually increased in patients with edema caused by either cirrhosis or the nephrotic syndrome. In congestive heart failure, elevated aldosterone secretion varies depending on the severity of cardiac failure. The stimulus for aldosterone release in these conditions appears to be *arterial hypovolemia* and/or hypotension. Thiazides and furosemide often exaggerate secondary aldosteronism via volume depletion; hypokalemia and, on occasion, alkalosis can then become prominent features. On occasion secondary hyperaldosteronism occurs without edema or hypertension (Bartter's and Gitelman's syndromes, see below).

SYNDROMES OF ADRENAL ANDROGEN EXCESS Adrenal androgen excess results from excess production of DHEA and androstenedione, which are converted to testosterone in extraglandular tissues; elevated testosterone levels account for most of the virilization. Adrenal androgen excess may be associated with the secretion of greater or smaller amounts of other adrenal hormones and may, therefore, present as "pure" syndromes of virilization or as "mixed" syndromes associated with excessive glucocorticoids and Cushing's syndrome. →*For further discussion of hirsutism and virilization, see Chap. 53.*

HYPOFUNCTION OF THE ADRENAL CORTEX

Cases of adrenal insufficiency can be divided into two general categories: (1) those associated with primary inability of the adrenal to elaborate sufficient quantities of hormone, and (2) those associated with a secondary failure due to inadequate ACTH formation or release (Table 331-6).

PRIMARY ADRENOCORTICAL DEFICIENCY (ADDISON'S DISEASE) The original description of Addison's disease—"general languor and debility, feebleness of the heart's action, irritability of the stomach, and a peculiar change of the color of the skin"—summarizes the dominant clinical features. Advanced cases are usually easy to diagnose, but recognition of the early phases can be a real challenge.

Incidence Primary insufficiency is relatively rare, may occur at any age, and affects both sexes equally. Because of the common ther-

Table 331-6   Classification of Adrenal Insufficiency

PRIMARY ADRENAL INSUFFICIENCY

Anatomic destruction of gland (chronic or acute)
  ''Idiopathic'' atrophy (autoimmune, adrenoleukodystrophy)
  Surgical removal
  Infection (tuberculous, fungal, viral—especially in AIDS patients)
  Hemorrhage
  Invasion: metastatic
Metabolic failure in hormone production
  Congenital adrenal hyperplasia
  Enzyme inhibitors (metyrapone, ketoconazole, aminoglutethimide)
  Cytotoxic agents (mitotane)
ACTH-blocking antibodies
Mutation in ACTH receptor gene
Adrenal hypoplasia congenita

SECONDARY ADRENAL INSUFFICIENCY

Hypopituitarism due to hypothalamic-pituitary disease
Suppression of hypothalamic-pituitary axis
  By exogenous steroid
  By endogenous steroid from tumor

apeutic use of steroids, secondary adrenal insufficiency is relatively common.

Etiology and Pathogenesis   Addison's disease results from progressive destruction of the adrenals, which must involve >90% of the glands before adrenal insufficiency appears. The adrenal is a frequent site for chronic granulomatous diseases, predominantly tuberculosis but also histoplasmosis, coccidioidomycosis, and cryptococcosis. In early series, tuberculosis was responsible for 70 to 90% of cases, but the most frequent cause now is *idiopathic* atrophy, and an autoimmune mechanism is probably responsible. Rarely, other lesions are encountered, such as adrenoleukodystrophy, bilateral hemorrhage, tumor metastases, HIV, cytomegalovirus (CMV), amyloidosis, adrenomyelo-neuropathy, familial adrenal insufficiency, or sarcoidosis.

Although half of patients with idiopathic atrophy have circulating adrenal antibodies, autoimmune destruction is probably secondary to cytotoxic T lymphocytes. Specific adrenal antigens to which autoantibodies may be directed include 21-hydroxylase (CYP21A2) and side chain cleavage enzyme but the significance of these antibodies in the pathogenesis of adrenal insufficiency is unknown. Some antibodies cause adrenal insufficiency by blocking the binding of ACTH to its receptors. Some patients also have antibodies to thyroid, parathyroid, and/or gonadal tissue (Chap. 339). There is also an increased incidence of chronic lymphocytic thyroiditis, premature ovarian failure, type 1 diabetes mellitus, and hypo- or hyperthyroidism. The presence of two or more of these autoimmune endocrine disorders in the same person defines the polyglandular autoimmune syndrome type II. Additional features include pernicious anemia, vitiligo, alopecia, nontropical sprue, and myasthenia gravis. Within families, multiple generations are affected by one or more of the above diseases. Type II polyglandular syndrome is the result of a mutant gene on chromosome 6 and is associated with the HLA alleles B8 and DR3.

The combination of parathyroid and adrenal insufficiency and chronic mucocutaneous moniliasis constitutes type I polyglandular autoimmune syndrome. Other autoimmune diseases in this disorder include pernicious anemia, chronic active hepatitis, alopecia, primary hypothyroidism, and premature gonadal failure. There is no HLA association; this syndrome is inherited as an autosomal recessive trait. It is caused by mutations in *a*utoimmune *p*olyendocrinopathy *c*andidiasis *e*ctodermal *d*ystrophy (APECED) located on chromosome 21q22.3. The gene encodes a transcription factor thought to be involved in lymphocyte function. The type I syndrome usually presents during childhood, whereas the type II syndrome is usually manifested in adulthood.

Clinical suspicion of adrenal insufficiency should be high in patients with AIDS (Chap. 309). CMV regularly involves the adrenal glands (so-called CMV necrotizing adrenalitis), and involvement with *Mycobacterium avium-intracellulare*, *Cryptococcus*, and Kaposi's sarcoma has been reported. Adrenal insufficiency in AIDS patients may not be manifest, but tests of adrenal reserve frequently give abnormal results. When interpreting tests of adrenocortical function, it is important to remember that medications such as rifampin, phenytoin, ketoconazole, megace, and opiates may cause or potentiate adrenal insufficiency. Adrenal hemorrhage and infarction occur in patients on anticoagulants and in those with circulating anticoagulants and hypercoagulable states, such as the antiphospholipid syndrome.

There are several rare genetic causes of adrenal insufficiency that present primarily in infancy and childhood (see below).

Clinical Signs and Symptoms   Adrenocortical insufficiency caused by gradual adrenal destruction is characterized by an insidious onset of fatigability, weakness, anorexia, nausea and vomiting, weight loss, cutaneous and mucosal pigmentation, hypotension, and occasionally hypoglycemia (Table 331-7). Depending on the duration and degree of adrenal hypofunction, the manifestations vary from mild chronic fatigue to fulminating shock associated with acute destruction of the glands, as described by Waterhouse and Friderichsen.

Asthenia is the cardinal symptom. Early it may be sporadic, usually most evident at times of stress; as adrenal function becomes more impaired, the patient is continuously fatigued, and bed rest is necessary.

Hyperpigmentation may be striking or absent. It commonly appears as a diffuse brown, tan, or bronze darkening of parts such as the elbows or creases of the hand and of areas that normally are pigmented such as the areolae about the nipples. Bluish-black patches may appear on the mucous membranes. Some patients develop dark freckles, and irregular areas of vitiligo may paradoxically be present. As an early sign, tanning following sun exposure may be persistent.

Arterial hypotension with postural accentuation is frequent, and blood pressure may be in the range of 80/50 or less.

Abnormalities of gastrointestinal function are often the presenting complaint. Symptoms vary from mild anorexia with weight loss to fulminating nausea, vomiting, diarrhea, and ill-defined abdominal pain, which may be so severe as to be confused with an acute abdomen. Patients may have personality changes, usually consisting of excessive irritability and restlessness. Enhancement of the sensory modalities of taste, olfaction, and hearing is reversible with therapy. Axillary and pubic hair may be decreased in women due to loss of adrenal androgens.

Laboratory Findings   In the early phase of gradual adrenal destruction, there may be no demonstrable abnormalities in the routine laboratory parameters, but adrenal reserve is decreased—that is, while basal steroid output may be normal, a subnormal increase occurs after stress. Adrenal stimulation with ACTH uncovers abnormalities in this stage of the disease, eliciting a subnormal increase of cortisol levels or no increase at all. In more advanced stages of adrenal destruction, serum sodium, chloride, and bicarbonate levels are reduced, and the

Table 331-7   Frequency of Symptoms and Signs in Adrenal Insufficiency

Sign or Symptom	Percent of Patients
Weakness	99
Pigmentation of skin	98
Weight loss	97
Anorexia, nausea, and vomiting	90
Hypotension (<110/70)	87
Pigmentation of mucous membranes	82
Abdominal pain	34
Salt craving	22
Diarrhea	20
Constipation	19
Syncope	16
Vitiligo	9

serum potassium level is elevated. The hyponatremia is due both to loss of sodium into the urine (due to aldosterone deficiency) and to movement into the intracellular compartment. This extravascular sodium loss depletes extracellular fluid volume and accentuates hypotension. Elevated plasma vasopressin and angiotensin II levels may contribute to the hyponatremia by impairing free water clearance. Hyperkalemia is due to a combination of aldosterone deficiency, impaired glomerular filtration, and acidosis. Basal levels of cortisol and aldosterone are subnormal and fail to increase following ACTH administration. Mild to moderate hypercalcemia occurs in 10 to 20% of patients for unclear reasons. The electrocardiogram may show nonspecific changes, and the electroencephalogram exhibits a generalized reduction and slowing. There may be a normocytic anemia, a relative lymphocytosis, and a moderate eosinophilia.

Diagnosis The diagnosis of adrenal insufficiency should be made only with ACTH stimulation testing to assess adrenal reserve capacity for steroid production (see above for ACTH test protocols). In brief, the best screening test is the cortisol response 60 min after 250 μg of cosyntropin given intramuscularly or intravenously. Cortisol levels should exceed 495 nmol/L (18 μg/dL). If the response is abnormal, then primary and secondary adrenal insufficiency can be distinguished by measuring aldosterone levels from the same blood samples. In secondary, but not primary, adrenal insufficiency the aldosterone increment will be normal [≥150 pmol/l (5 ng/dL)]. Furthermore, in primary adrenal insufficiency, plasma ACTH and associated peptides (β-LPT) are elevated because of loss of the usual cortisol-hypothalamic-pituitary feedback relationship, whereas in secondary adrenal insufficiency, plasma ACTH values are low or "inappropriately" normal (Fig. 331-11).

Differential Diagnosis Since weakness and fatigue are common, diagnosis of early adrenocortical insufficiency may be difficult. However, the combination of mild gastrointestinal distress, weight loss, anorexia, and a suggestion of increased pigmentation makes it mandatory to perform ACTH stimulation testing to rule out adrenal insuf-

FIGURE 331-11 Diagnostic flowchart for evaluating patients with suspected adrenal insufficiency. Plasma ACTH levels are low in secondary adrenal insufficiency. In adrenal insufficiency secondary to pituitary tumors or idiopathic panhypopituitarism, other pituitary hormone deficiencies are present. On the other hand, ACTH deficiency may be isolated, as seen following prolonged use of exogenous glucocorticoids. Because the isolated blood levels obtained in these screening tests may not be definitive, the diagnosis may need to be confirmed by a continuous 24-h ACTH infusion. Normal subjects and patients with secondary adrenal insufficiency may be distinguished by insulin tolerance or metyrapone testing.

ficiency, particularly before steroid treatment is begun. Weight loss is useful in evaluating the significance of weakness and malaise. Racial pigmentation may be a problem, but a *recent* and progressive *increase* in pigmentation is usually reported by the patient with gradual adrenal destruction. Hyperpigmentation is usually absent when adrenal destruction is rapid, as in bilateral adrenal hemorrhage. The fact that hyperpigmentation occurs with other diseases may also present a problem, but the appearance and distribution of pigment in adrenal insufficiency are usually characteristic. When doubt exists, measurement of ACTH levels and testing of adrenal reserve with the infusion of ACTH provide clear-cut differentiation.

℞ **TREATMENT** All patients with adrenal insufficiency should receive specific hormone replacement. Like diabetics, these patients require careful education about the disease. Replacement therapy should correct both glucocorticoid and mineralocorticoid deficiencies. Hydrocortisone (cortisol) is the mainstay of treatment. The dose for most adults (depending on size) is 20 to 30 mg/d. Patients are advised to take glucocorticoids with meals or, if that is impractical, with milk or an antacid, because the drugs may increase gastric acidity and exert direct toxic effects on the gastric mucosa. To simulate the normal diurnal adrenal rhythm, two-thirds of the dose is taken in the morning, and the remaining one-third is taken in the late afternoon. Some patients exhibit insomnia, irritability, and mental excitement after initiation of therapy; in these, the dosage should be reduced. Other situations that may necessitate smaller doses are hypertension and diabetes mellitus. Obese individuals and those on anticonvulsive medications may require increased dosages. Measurements of plasma ACTH or cortisol or of urine cortisol levels do not appear to be useful in determining optimal glucocorticoid dosages.

Since the replacement dosage of hydrocortisone does not replace the mineralocorticoid component of the adrenal hormones, mineralocorticoid supplementation is usually needed. This is accomplished by the administration of 0.05 to 0.1 mg fludrocortisone per day by mouth. Patients should also be instructed to maintain an ample intake of sodium (3 to 4 g/d).

The adequacy of mineralocorticoid therapy can be assessed by measurement of blood pressure and serum electrolytes. Blood pressure should be normal and without postural changes; serum sodium, potassium, creatinine, and urea nitrogen levels should also be normal. Measurement of plasma renin levels may also be useful in titrating the dose.

In female patients with adrenal insufficiency, androgen levels are also low. Thus, some physicians believe that daily replacement with 25 to 50 mg of DHEA orally may improve quality of life and skeletal density.

Complications of glucocorticoid therapy, with the exception of gastritis, are *rare* at the dosages recommended for treatment of adrenal insufficiency. Complications of mineralocorticoid therapy include hypokalemia, hypertension, cardiac enlargement, and even congestive heart failure due to sodium retention. Periodic measurements of body weight, serum potassium level, and blood pressure are useful. All patients with adrenal insufficiency should carry medical identification, should be instructed in the parenteral self-administration of steroids, and should be registered with a medical alerting system.

Special Therapeutic Problems During periods of intercurrent illness, especially in the setting of fever, the dose of hydrocortisone should be doubled. With severe illness it should be increased to 75 to 150 mg/d. When oral administration is not possible, parenteral routes should be employed. Likewise, before surgery or dental extractions, supplemental glucocorticoids should be administered. Patients should also be advised to increase the dose of fludrocortisone and to add salt to their otherwise normal diet during periods of strenuous exercise with sweating, during extremely hot weather, and with gastrointestinal upsets such as diarrhea. A simple strategy is to supplement the diet

Table 331-8 Steroid Therapy Schedule for a Patient with Adrenal Insufficiency Undergoing Surgery[a]

	Hydrocortisone Infusion, Continuous, mg/h		Hydrocortisone (Orally)		Fludrocortisone (Orally), 8 A.M.
			8 A.M.	4 P.M.	
Routine daily medication			20	10	0.1
Day before operation			20	10	0.1
Day of operation	10				
Postoperative					
Day 1	5–7.5				
Day 2	2.5–5				
Day 3	2.5–5	*or*	40	20	0.1
Day 4	2.5–5	*or*	40	20	0.1
Day 5			40	20	0.1
Day 6			20	20	0.1
Day 7			20	10	0.1

[a] All steroid doses are given in milligrams. An alternative approach is to give 100 mg hydrocortisone as an intravenous bolus injection every 8 h on the day of the operation (see text).

one to three times daily with salty broth (1 cup of beef or chicken bouillon contains 35 mmol of sodium). For a representative program of steroid therapy for the patient with adrenal insufficiency who is undergoing major surgery, see Table 331-8. This schedule is designed so that on the day of surgery it will mimic the output of cortisol in normal individuals undergoing prolonged major stress (10 mg/h, 250 to 300 mg/d). Thereafter, if the patient is improving and is afebrile, the dose of hydrocortisone is tapered by 20 to 30% daily. Mineralocorticoid administration is unnecessary at hydrocortisone doses >100 mg/d because of the mineralocorticoid effects of hydrocortisone at such dosages.

SECONDARY ADRENOCORTICAL INSUFFICIENCY
ACTH deficiency causes *secondary* adrenocortical insufficiency; it may be a selective deficiency, as is seen following prolonged administration of excess glucocorticoids, or it may occur in association with deficiencies of multiple pituitary hormones (panhypopituitarism) (Chap. 328). Patients with secondary adrenocortical hypofunction have many symptoms and signs in common with those having primary disease but are *characteristically not hyperpigmented*, since ACTH and related peptide levels are low. In fact, plasma ACTH levels distinguish between primary and secondary adrenal insufficiency, since they are elevated in the former and decreased to absent in the latter. Patients with total pituitary insufficiency have manifestations of multiple hormone deficiencies. An additional feature distinguishing primary adrenocortical insufficiency is the *near-normal level of aldosterone secretion* seen in pituitary and/or isolated ACTH deficiencies (Fig. 331-11). Patients with pituitary insufficiency may have hyponatremia, which can be dilutional or secondary to a subnormal increase in aldosterone secretion in response to severe sodium restriction. However, severe *dehydration*, *hyponatremia*, and *hyperkalemia* are characteristic of severe mineralocorticoid insufficiency and favor a diagnosis of primary adrenocortical insufficiency.

Patients receiving long-term steroid therapy, despite physical findings of Cushing's syndrome, develop adrenal insufficiency because of prolonged pituitary-hypothalamic suppression and adrenal atrophy secondary to the loss of endogenous ACTH. These patients have two deficits, a loss of adrenal responsiveness to ACTH and a failure of pituitary ACTH release. They are characterized by low blood cortisol and ACTH levels, a low baseline rate of steroid excretion, and abnormal ACTH and metyrapone responses. Most patients with steroid-induced adrenal insufficiency eventually recover normal hypothalamic-pituitary-adrenal responsiveness, but recovery time varies from days to months. The rapid ACTH test provides a convenient assessment of recovery of hypothalamic-pituitary-adrenal function. Because the plasma cortisol concentrations after injection of cosyntropin and during insulin-induced hypoglycemia are usually similar, the rapid ACTH test assesses the integrated hypothalamic-pituitary-adrenal function (see "Tests of Pituitary-Adrenal Responsiveness," above). Some investigators suggest using the low-dose (1 μg) ACTH test for suspected secondary ACTH deficiency. Additional tests to assess pituitary ACTH reserve include the standard metyrapone and insulin-induced hypoglycemia tests.

Glucocorticoid therapy in patients with secondary adrenocortical insufficiency does not differ from that for the primary disorder. Mineralocorticoid therapy is usually not necessary, as aldosterone secretion is preserved.

ACUTE ADRENOCORTICAL INSUFFICIENCY Acute adrenocortical insufficiency may result from several processes. On the one hand, *adrenal crisis* may be a rapid and overwhelming intensification of chronic adrenal insufficiency, usually precipitated by sepsis or surgical stress. Alternatively, acute hemorrhagic destruction of both adrenal glands can occur in previously well subjects. In children, this event is usually associated with septicemia with *Pseudomonas* or meningococcemia (Waterhouse-Friderichsen syndrome). In adults, anticoagulant therapy or a coagulation disorder may result in bilateral adrenal hemorrhage. Occasionally, bilateral adrenal hemorrhage in the newborn results from birth trauma. Hemorrhage has been observed during pregnancy, following idiopathic adrenal vein thrombosis, and as a complication of venography (e.g., infarction of an adenoma). The third and most frequent cause of acute insufficiency is the rapid withdrawal of steroids from patients with adrenal atrophy owing to chronic steroid administration. Acute adrenocortical insufficiency may also occur in patients with congenital adrenal hyperplasia or those with decreased adrenocortical reserve when they are given drugs capable of inhibiting steroid synthesis (mitotane, ketoconazole) or of increasing steroid metabolism (phenytoin, rifampin).

Adrenal Crisis The long-term survival of patients with adrenocortical insufficiency depends largely on the prevention and treatment of adrenal crisis. Consequently, the occurrence of infection, trauma (including surgery), gastrointestinal upsets, or other stresses necessitates an immediate increase in hormone. In untreated patients, preexisting symptoms are intensified. Nausea, vomiting, and abdominal pain may become intractable. Fever may be severe or absent. Lethargy deepens into somnolence, and hypovolemic vascular collapse ensues. In contrast, patients previously maintained on chronic glucocorticoid therapy may not exhibit dehydration or hypotension until they are in a preterminal state, since mineralocorticoid secretion is usually preserved. In all patients in crisis, a precipitating cause should be sought.

℞ **TREATMENT** Treatment is directed primarily toward repletion of circulating glucocorticoids and replacement of the sodium and water deficits. Hence an intravenous infusion of 5% glucose in normal saline solution should be started with a bolus intravenous infusion of 100 mg hydrocortisone followed by a continuous infusion of hydrocortisone at a rate of 10 mg/h. An alternative approach is to administer a 100-mg bolus of hydrocortisone intravenously every 6 h. However, only continuous infusion maintains the plasma cortisol constantly at stress levels [830 nmol/L (30 μg/dL)]. Effective treatment of hypotension requires glucocorticoid replacement and repletion of sodium and water deficits. If the crisis was preceded by prolonged nausea, vomiting, and dehydration, several liters of saline solution may be required in the first few hours. Vasoconstrictive agents (such as dopamine) may be indicated in extreme conditions as adjuncts to volume replacement. With large doses of steroid, e.g., 100 to 200 mg hydrocortisone, the patient receives a maximal mineralocorticoid effect, and supplementary mineralocorticoid is superfluous. Following improvement, the steroid dosage is tapered over the next few days to maintenance levels, and mineralocorticoid therapy is reinstituted if needed (Table 331-8).

Isolated aldosterone deficiency accompanied by normal cortisol production occurs in association with hyporeninism, as an inherited biosynthetic defect, postoperatively following removal of aldosterone-secreting adenomas, during protracted heparin or heparinoid administration, in pretectal disease of the nervous system, and in severe postural hypotension.

The feature common to all forms hypoaldosteronism is the inability to increase aldosterone secretion appropriately in response to salt restriction. Most patients have unexplained hyperkalemia, which often is exacerbated by restriction of dietary sodium intake. In severe cases, urine sodium wastage occurs at a normal salt intake, whereas in milder forms, excessive loss of urine sodium occurs only with salt restriction.

Most cases of isolated hypoaldosteronism occur in patients with a deficiency in renin production (so-called hyporeninemic hypoaldosteronism), most commonly in adults with diabetes mellitus and mild renal failure and in whom hyperkalemia and metabolic acidosis are out of proportion to the degree of renal impairment. Plasma renin levels fail to rise normally following sodium restriction and postural changes. The pathogenesis is uncertain. Possibilities include renal disease (the most likely), autonomic neuropathy, extracellular fluid volume expansion, and defective conversion of renin precursors to active renin. Aldosterone levels also fail to rise normally after salt restriction and volume contraction; this effect is probably related to the hyporeninism, since biosynthetic defects in aldosterone secretion usually cannot be demonstrated. In these patients, aldosterone secretion increases promptly after ACTH stimulation, but it is uncertain whether the magnitude of the response is normal. On the other hand, the level of aldosterone appears to be subnormal in relationship to the hyperkalemia.

Hypoaldosteronism can also be associated with high renin levels and low or elevated levels of aldosterone (see below). Severely ill patients may also have hyperreninemic hypoaldosteronism; such patients have a high mortality rate (80%). Hyperkalemia is not present. Possible explanations for the hypoaldosteronism include adrenal necrosis (uncommon) or a shift in steroidogenesis from mineralocorticoids to glucocorticoids, possibly related to prolonged ACTH stimulation.

Before the diagnosis of isolated hypoaldosteronism is considered for a patient with hyperkalemia, "pseudohyperkalemia" (e.g., hemolysis, thrombocytosis) should be excluded by measuring the *plasma* potassium level. The next step is to demonstrate a normal cortisol response to ACTH stimulation. Then, the response of renin and aldosterone levels to stimulation (upright posture, sodium restriction) should be measured. Low renin and aldosterone levels establish the diagnosis of hyporeninemic hypoaldosteronism. A combination of high renin levels and low aldosterone levels is consistent with an aldosterone biosynthetic defect or a selective unresponsiveness to angiotensin II. Finally, there is a condition that clinically and biochemically mimics hypoaldosteronism with elevated renin levels. However, the aldosterone levels are not low but high—so-called pseudohypoaldosteronism. This inherited condition is caused by a mutation in the epithelial sodium channel (see below).

℞ **TREATMENT**   The treatment is to replace the mineralocorticoid deficiency. For practical purposes, the oral administration of 0.05 to 0.15 mg fludrocortisone daily should restore electrolyte balance if salt intake is adequate (e.g., 150 to 200 mmol/d). However, patients with hyporeninemic hypoaldosteronism may require higher doses of mineralocorticoid to correct hyperkalemia. This need poses a potential risk in patients with hypertension, mild renal insufficiency, or congestive heart failure. An alternative approach is to reduce salt intake and to administer furosemide, which can ameliorate acidosis and hyperkalemia. Occasionally, a combination of these two approaches is efficacious.

GENETIC CONSIDERATIONS   Glucocorticoid Diseases •
Congenital adrenal hyperplasia   Congenital adrenal hyperplasia (CAH) is the consequence of recessive mutations that cause one of several distinct enzymatic defects (see below). Because cortisol is the principal adrenal steroid regulating ACTH elaboration and because ACTH stimulates adrenal growth and function, a block in cortisol synthesis may result in the enhanced secretion of adrenal androgens and/or mineralocorticids depending on the site of the enzyme block. In severe congenital virilizing hyperplasia, the adrenal output of cortisol may be so compromised as to cause adrenal deficiency despite adrenal hyperplasia.

CAH is the most common adrenal disorder of infancy and childhood (Chap. 338). Partial enzyme deficiencies can be expressed after adolescence, predominantly in women with hirsutism and oligomenorrhea but minimal virilization. Late-onset adrenal hyperplasia may account for 5 to 25% of cases of hirsutism and oligomenorrhea in women, depending on the population.

ETIOLOGY   Enzymatic defects have been described in 21-hydroxylase (CYP21A2), 17α-hydroxylase/17,20-Lyase (CYP17), 11β-hydroxylase (CYP11B1), and in (3β-HSD2) (Fig. 331-2). Although the cDNAs for these enzymes have been cloned, the diagnosis of specific enzyme deficiencies with genetic techniques is not practical for routine use. CYP21A2 deficiency is closely linked to the HLA-B locus of chromosome 6 so that HLA typing and/or DNA polymorphism can be used to detect the heterozygous carriers and to diagnose affected individuals in some families (Chap. 306). The clinical expression in the different disorders is variable, ranging from virilization of the female (CYP2/A2) to feminization of the male (3β-HSD2) (Chap. 338).

Adrenal virilization in the female at birth is associated with ambiguous external genitalia (*female pseudohermaphroditism*). Virilization probably begins after the fifth month of intrauterine development. At birth there may be enlarged genitalia in the male infant and enlargement of the clitoris, partial or complete fusion of the labia, and sometimes a urogenital sinus in the female. If the labial fusion is nearly complete, the female infant has external genitalia resembling a penis with hypospadias. In the *postnatal* period, CAH is associated with virilization in the female and isosexual precocity in the male. The excessive androgen levels result in accelerated growth, so that bone age exceeds chronologic age. Because epiphyseal closure is hastened by excessive androgens, growth stops, but truncal development continues, the characteristic appearance being a short child with a well-developed trunk.

The most common form of CAH (95% of cases) is a result of impairment of CYP21A2. In addition to cortisol deficiency, aldosterone secretion is decreased in approximately one-third of the patients. Thus, with CYP21A2 deficiency, adrenal virilization occurs with or without a salt-losing tendency due to aldosterone deficiency (Fig. 331-2).

CYP11B1 deficiency causes a "hypertensive" variant of CAH. Hypertension and hypokalemia occur because of the impaired conversion of 11-deoxycorticosterone to corticosterone, resulting in the accumulation of 11-deoxycorticosterone, a potent mineralocorticoid. The degree of hypertension is variable. Increased shunting again occurs into the androgen pathway.

CYP17 deficiency is characterized by hypogonadism, hypokalemia, and hypertension. This rare disorder causes decreased production of cortisol and shunting of precursors into the mineralocorticoid pathway with hypokalemic alkalosis, hypertension, and suppressed plasma renin activity. Usually, 11-deoxycorticosterone production is elevated. Because CYP17 hydroxylation is required for biosynthesis of both adrenal androgens and gonadal testosterone and estrogen, this defect is associated with sexual immaturity, high urinary gonadotropin levels, and low urinary 17-ketosteroid excretion. Female patients have primary amenorrhea and lack of development of secondary sexual characteristics. Because of deficient androgen production, male patients have either ambiguous external genitalia or a female phenotype (*male pseudohermaphroditism*). Exogenous glucocorticoids can correct the hypertensive syndrome, and treatment with appropriate gonadal steroids results in sexual maturation.

With 3β-HSD2 deficiency, conversion of pregnenolone to progesterone is impaired, so that the synthesis of both cortisol and aldosterone is blocked, with shunting into the adrenal androgen pathway via 17α-hydroxypregnenolone and DHEA. Because DHEA is a weak androgen, and because this enzyme deficiency is also present in the gonad, the genitalia of the male fetus may be incompletely virilized or feminized. Conversely, in the female, overproduction of DHEA may produce partial virilization.

DIAGNOSIS The diagnosis of CAH should be considered in infants having episodes of acute adrenal insufficiency or salt-wasting or with hypertension. The diagnosis is further suggested by the finding of hypertrophy of the clitoris, fused labia, or a urogenital sinus in the female or of isosexual precocity in the male. In infants and children with a CYP21A2 defect, increased urine 17-ketosteroid excretion and increased plasma DHEA sulfate levels are typically associated with an increase in the blood levels of 17-hydroxyprogesterone and the excretion of its urinary metabolite pregnanetriol. Demonstration of elevated levels of 17-hydroxyprogesterone in amniotic fluid at 14 to 16 weeks of gestation allows prenatal detection of affected female infants.

The diagnosis of a *salt-losing form* of CAH due to defects in CYP21A2 is suggested by episodes of acute adrenal insufficiency with hyponatremia, hyperkalemia, dehydration, and vomiting. These infants and children often crave salt and have laboratory findings indicating deficits in both cortisol and aldosterone secretion.

With the *hypertensive form* of CAH due to CYP11B1 deficiency, 11-deoxycorticosterone and 11-deoxycortisol accumulate. The diagnosis is confirmed by demonstrating increased levels of 11-deoxycortisol in the blood or increased amounts of tetrahydro-11-deoxycortisol in the urine. Elevation of 17-hydroxyprogesterone levels does not imply a coexisting CYP21A2 deficiency.

Very high levels of urine DHEA with low levels of pregnanetriol and of cortisol metabolites in urine are characteristic of children with 3β-HSD2 deficiency. Marked salt-wasting may also occur.

Adults with *late-onset adrenal hyperplasia* (partial deficiency of CYP21A2, CYP11B1, or 3β-HSD2) are characterized by normal or moderately elevated levels of urinary 17-ketosteroids and plasma DHEA sulfate. A high basal level of a precursor of cortisol biosynthesis (such as 17-hydroxyprogesterone, 17-hydroxypregnenolone, or 11-deoxycortisol), or elevation of such a precursor after ACTH stimulation, confirms the diagnosis of a partial deficiency. Measurement of steroid precursors 60 min after bolus administration of ACTH is usually sufficient. Adrenal androgen output is easily suppressed by the standard low-dose (2 mg) dexamethasone test. ∎

℞ **TREATMENT** Patients with CAH have a fundamental defect of cortisol deficiency with resultant excessive ACTH secretion, producing hyperplasia of the adrenal glands and causing additional shunting into the precursor steroid pathways. Therapy in these patients consists of daily administration of glucocorticoids to suppress pituitary ACTH secretion. Because of its cost and intermediate half-life, prednisone is the drug of choice except in infants, in whom hydrocortisone is usually used. In adults with late-onset adrenal hyperplasia, the smallest single bedtime dose of a long- or intermediate-acting glucocorticoid that suppresses pituitary ACTH secretion should be administered. The amount of steroid required by children with CAH is approximately 1 to 1.5 times the normal cortisol production rate of 27 to 35 μmol (10 to 13 mg) of cortisol per square meter of body surface per day and is given in divided doses two or three times per day. The dosage schedule is governed by repetitive analysis of the urinary 17-ketosteroids, plasma DHEA sulfate, and/or precursors of cortisol biosynthesis. Skeletal growth and maturation must also be monitored closely, as overtreatment with glucocorticoid replacement therapy retards linear growth.

Receptor Mutations Much less common than CAH are three syndromes secondary to mutation(s) in a key receptor involved in adrenal function. *Isolated glucocorticoid deficiency* is a rare autosomal recessive disease secondary to a mutation in the ACTH receptor. Usually mineralocorticoid function is normal. Adrenal insufficiency is manifest within the first 2 years of life usually as hyperpigmentation, convulsions, and/or frequent episodes of hypoglycemia. In some patients the adrenal insufficiency is associated with achalasia and alacrima—Allgrove's, or triple A, syndrome. However, in some triple A syndrome patients, no mutation in the ACTH receptor has been identified, suggesting that a distinct genetic abnormality causes this syndrome. *Adrenal hypoplasia congenita* is a rare X-linked disorder caused by a mutation in the *DAX1* gene located on the X chromosome. This gene encodes an orphan nuclear receptor that plays an important role in the development of the adrenal cortex and also the hypothalamic-pituitary-gonadal axis. Thus, patients present with signs and symptoms secondary to deficiencies of all three major adrenal steroids—cortisol, aldosterone, and adrenal androgens—as well as gonadotropin deficiency. Finally a rare cause of hypercortisolism without cushingoid stigmata is *primary cortisol resistance* due to mutations in the glucocorticoid receptor. The resistance is incomplete because patients do not exhibit signs of adrenal insufficiency. Thus, these three rare inherited disorders have in common an elevated ACTH. However, the clinical manifestations range from no evidence of adrenal insufficiency to only cortisol deficiency (similar to secondary adrenal insufficiency) to a clinical picture indistinguishable from classic Addison's disease.

Miscellaneous Conditions Adrenoleukodystrophy causes severe demyelination and early death in children, and adrenomyeloneuropathy is associated with a mixed motor and sensory neuropathy with spastic paraplegia in adults; both disorders are associated with elevated circulating levels of very long chain fatty acids and cause adrenal insufficiency. Autosomal recessive mutations in the *s*teroidogenic *a*cute *r*egulatory (STAR) protein gene cause congenital lipoid adrenal hyperplasia (Chap. 338), which is characterized by adrenal insufficiency and defective gonadal steroidogenesis. Because STAR mediates cholesterol transport into the mitochondrion, mutations in the protein cause massive lipid accumulation in steroidogenic cells, ultimately leading to cell toxicity. Thus, these three rare inherited disorders have in common an elevated ACTH. However, the clinical manifestations range from no evidence of adrenal insufficiency to only cortisol deficiency (similar to secondary adrenal insufficiency) to a clinical picture indistinguishable from classic Addison's disease.

MINERALOCORTICOID DISEASES Some forms of CAH have a mineralocorticoid component (see above). Others are caused by a mutation in other enzymes or ion channels important in mediating or mimicking aldosterone's action.

Hypermineralocorticoidism • *Low plasma renin activity* Rarely, hypermineralocorticoidism is due to a defect in cortisol biosynthesis, specifically 11- or 17-hydroxylation. ACTH levels are increased, with a resultant increase in the production of the mineralocorticoid 11-deoxycorticosterone. Hypertension and hypokalemia can be corrected by glucocorticoid administration. The definitive diagnosis is made by demonstrating an elevation of precursors of cortisol biosynthesis in the blood or urine or by direct demonstration of the genetic defect.

Glucocorticoid administration can also ameliorate hypertension or produce normotension even though a hydroxylase deficiency cannot be identified (Fig. 331-9). These patients have normal to slightly elevated aldosterone levels that do not suppress in response to saline but do suppress in response to 2 days of dexamethasone (2 mg/d). The condition is inherited as an autosomal dominant trait and is termed *glucocorticoid-remediable aldosteronism* (GRA). This entity is secondary to a chimeric gene duplication whereby the 11-β hydroxylase gene promoter (which is under the control of ACTH) is fused to the aldosterone synthase coding sequence. Thus, aldosterone synthase activity is ectopically expressed in the zona fasciculata and is regulated by ACTH, in a fashion similar to the regulation of cortisol secretion. Screening for this defect is best performed by assessing the presence or absence of the chimeric gene. Because the abnormal gene may be present in the absence of hypokalemia, its frequency as a cause of hypertension is unknown. Individuals with suppressed plasma renin levels and juvenile-onset hypertension or a history of early-onset hypertension in first-degree relatives should be screened for this disorder. Early hemorrhagic stroke also occurs in GRA-affected individuals.

Glucocorticoid-remediable hyperaldosteronism documented by genetic analysis may be treated with glucocorticoid administration or antimineralocorticoids, e.g., spironolactone, triamterene, or amiloride. Glucocorticoids should be used only in small doses to avoid inducing iatrogenic Cushing's syndrome. A combination approach is often necessary.

High plasma renin activity Bartter's syndrome is characterized by severe hyperaldosteronism (hypokalemic alkalosis) with moderate to marked increases in renin activity and hypercalciuria, but normal blood pressure and no edema; this disorder usually begins in childhood. Renal biopsy shows juxtaglomerular hyperplasia. The pathogenesis involves a defect in the renal conservation of sodium or chloride. The renal loss of sodium is thought to stimulate renin secretion and aldosterone production. Hyperaldosteronism produces potassium depletion, and hypokalemia further elevates prostaglandin production and plasma renin activity. In some cases, the hypokalemia may be potentiated by a defect in renal conservation of potassium. Increased production of prostaglandins is probably not a primary abnormality, since administration of inhibitors of prostaglandin synthesis reverses the features only temporarily (Chap. 276). Bartter's syndrome is caused by a mutation in the renal Na-K-2Cl co-transporter gene.

Gitelman's syndrome is an autosomal recessive trait characterized by renal salt wasting and as a result, as in Bartter's syndrome, activation of the renin-angiotensin-aldosterone system. As a consequence affected individuals have low blood pressure, low serum potassium, low serum magnesium, and high serum bicarbonate. In contrast to Bartter's syndrome, urinary calcium excretion is reduced. Gitelman's syndrome results from loss-of-function mutations of the renal thiazide-sensitive Na-Cl co-transporter.

Increased Mineralocorticoid Action Liddle's syndrome is a rare autosomal dominant disorder that mimicks hyperaldosteronism. The defect is in the genes encoding the β or γ subunits of the epithelial sodium channel. Both renin and aldosterone levels are low, owing to the constitutively activated sodium channel and the resulting excess sodium reabsorption in the renal tubule.

A rare autosomal recessive cause of hypokalemia and hypertension is 11β-HSD II deficiency, in which cortisol cannot be converted to cortisone and hence binds to the MR and acts as a mineralocorticoid. This condition, also termed *apparent mineralocorticoid excess syndrome*, is caused by a defect in the gene encoding the renal isoform of this enzyme, 11β-HSD II. Patients can be identified either by documenting an increased ratio of cortisol to cortisone in the urine or by genetic analysis. Patients with the 11β-HSD deficiency syndrome can be treated with small doses of dexamethasone. Although dexamethasone is a potent glucocorticoid that suppresses ACTH and endogenous cortisol production, it binds less well to the mineralocorticoid receptor than does cortisol.

The ingestion of candies or chewing tobacco containing certain forms of licorice produces a syndrome that mimics primary aldosteronism. The component of such agents that causes sodium retention is glycyrrhizinic acid, which inhibits the 11β-HSD II and hence allows cortisol to act as a mineralocorticoid and cause sodium retention, expansion of the extracellular fluid volume, hypertension, depressed plasma renin levels, and suppressed aldosterone levels. The diagnosis is established or excluded by a careful history.

Decreased Mineralocorticoid Production or Action In patients with these conditions, disorders of aldosterone biosynthesis or action are associated with high renin levels, salt wasting, and hyperkalemia. The aldosterone levels may be low or elevated. In patients with a deficiency in aldosterone biosynthesis, the transformation of corticosterone into aldosterone is impaired, owing to a mutation in the aldosterone synthase (CYP11B2) gene. These patients have low to absent aldosterone secretion, elevated plasma renin levels, and elevated levels of the intermediates of aldosterone biosynthesis (corticosterone and 18-hydroxycorticosterone).

Pseudohypoaldosteronism type I (PHA-I) is an autosomal recessive disorder that is seen in the neonatal period and is characterized by salt wasting, hypotension, hyperkalemia, and high renin and aldosterone levels. In contrast to the gain-of-function mutations in the epithelial sodium channel (ENaC) in Liddle's syndrome, mutations in PHA-I result in loss of ENaC function.

NONSPECIFIC CLINICAL USE OF ADRENAL STEROIDS

The widespread use of glucocorticoids emphasizes the need for a thorough understanding of the metabolic effects of these agents. Before adrenal hormone therapy is instituted, the expected gains should be weighed against undesirable effects.

HOW SERIOUS IS THE DISORDER? In a patient who has unexplained shock or in whom other measures have failed, the physician need not hesitate to employ high-dose steroid therapy. In contrast, one should exercise restraint in administering steroids to a patient with early rheumatoid arthritis for whom physiotherapy, anti-inflammatory agents, disease-modifying agents, and general medical care have not been tried (Chap. 312).

HOW LONG WILL GLUCOCORTICOID THERAPY BE REQUIRED? The use of intravenous steroids for 24 to 48 h for a life-threatening situation such as status asthmaticus or pseudotumor cerebri has few or no contraindications, in contrast to the initiation of chronic steroid therapy for asthma, arthritis, or psoriasis. In the latter instances, the almost certain development of some degree of Cushing's syndrome must be weighed against the potential benefit. These side effects should be minimized by a careful choice of steroid preparations, alternate-day or interrupted therapy; the use of topical steroids, e.g., inhaled, intranasal, or dermal, whenever possible; and the judicious use of supplementary adjuvants.

WHICH PREPARATION IS BEST? Several considerations should be taken into account in deciding which steroid preparation to use.

1. *The biologic half-life.* The rationale behind alternate-day therapy is to decrease the metabolic effects of the steroids for a significant part of each 48 h period while still producing a pharmacologic effect durable enough to be effective. Too long a half-life would defeat the first purpose, and too short a half-life would defeat the second. In general, the more potent the steroid, the longer its biologic half-life.

2. *The importance of the mineralocorticoid effects of the steroid.* Most synthetic steroids have less mineralocorticoid effect than hydrocortisone (Table 331-9).

3. *The biologically active form of the steroid.* Cortisone and prednisone have to be converted to biologically active metabolites before anti-inflammatory effects can occur. Because of this, in a condition for which steroids are known to be effective and when an adequate dose has been given without response, one should consider substituting hydrocortisone or prednisolone for cortisone or prednisone.

4. *The cost of the medication.* This is a serious consideration if chronic administration is planned. Prednisone is the least expensive of available steroid preparations.

5. *The type of formulation.* Topical steroids have the distinct advantage over oral steroids in reducing the likelihood of systemic side effects. In addition, some inhaled steroids have been designed to minimize side effects by increasing their hepatic inactivation if they are swallowed (Chap. 252). However, all topical steroids can be absorbed into the systemic circulation.

EVALUATION OF PATIENTS PRIOR TO INITIATING STEROID THERAPY (See Table 331-10)   **Chronic Infection** Three issues demand attention: (1) Any active infection, particularly

Table 331-9   Glucocorticoid Preparations

Commonly Used Name[a]	Estimated Potency[b]	
	Glucocorticoid	Mineralocorticoid
SHORT-ACTING		
Hydrocortisone	1	1
Cortisone	0.8	0.8
INTERMEDIATE-ACTING		
Prednisone	4	0.25
Prednisolone	4	0.25
Methylprednisolone	5	<0.01
Triamcinolone	5	<0.01
LONG-ACTING		
Paramethasone	10	<0.01
Betamethasone	25	<0.01
Dexamethasone	30–40	<0.01

[a] The steroids are divided into three groups according to the duration of biologic activity. Short-acting preparations have a biologic half-life <12 h; long-acting, >48 h; and intermediate, between 12 and 36 h. Triamcinolone has the longest half-life of the intermediate-acting preparations.

[b] Relative milligram comparisons with hydrocortisone, setting the glucocorticoid and mineralocorticoid properties of hydrocortisone as 1. Sodium retention is insignificant for commonly employed doses of methylprednisolone, triamcinolone, paramethasone, betamethasone, and dexamethasone.

tuberculosis, should be identified. (2) If tuberculosis is present, steroid therapy should be employed only in conjunction with antituberculous chemotherapy. The chest film and tuberculin test provide baseline information for future comparison. Since high-dose steroids may impair the tuberculin reaction, serial chest roentgenograms may be necessary. (3) Infection due to opportunistic pathogens should be constantly considered in patients on steroid therapy, especially when combined with other immunosuppressive agents.

Diabetes Mellitus   Prolonged glucocorticoid therapy may unmask or aggravate diabetes mellitus. The presence of diabetes mellitus or the demonstration of impaired glucose tolerance may affect the decision to institute glucocorticoid therapy.

Osteoporosis   Patients receiving long-term steroid therapy are at risk for osteoporosis. Indeed, osteoporosis with vertebral fractures or compression is a dreaded complication for patients at high risk (postmenopausal women, elderly men, patients with restricted physical activity, and especially organ transplant patients who are maintained on high doses to prevent rejection). Alternate-day or interrupted steroid therapy does not prevent the risk of this complication (Table 331-11). Adjunctive therapies with antiresorptive agents, such as parenteral or oral bisphosphonates, have been shown to be effective in treating the osteoporosis (Chap. 342). Bone mineral density should be assessed periodically with dual-energy X-ray absorptiometry (DEXA) scans.

Peptic Ulcer, Gastric Hypersecretion, or Esophagitis   In conventional doses (equivalent to ≤15 mg prednisone per day), glucocorticoids probably do not cause peptic ulceration; whether higher doses cause ulcer disease is not established and probably depends on duration, dose of treatment, and predisposing factors such as hypoalbuminemia or cirrhosis and also whether subjects are concomitantly ingesting nonsteroidal anti-inflammatory agents (NSAIDs). However,

Table 331-10   A Checklist for Use Prior to the Administration of Glucocorticoids in Pharmacologic Doses

Presence of tuberculosis or other chronic infection (chest x-ray, tuberculin test)
Evidence of glucose intolerance or history of gestational diabetes mellitus
Evidence of preexisting osteoporosis (bone density assessment in organ transplant recipients or postmenopausal patients)
History of peptic ulcer, gastritis, or esophagitis (stool guaiac test)
Evidence of hypertension or cardiovascular disease
History of psychological disorders

Table 331-11   Supplementary Measures to Minimize Undesirable Metabolic Effects of Glucocorticoids

Monitor caloric intake to prevent weight gain.
Restrict sodium intake to prevent edema and minimize hypertension and potassium loss.
Provide supplementary potassium if necessary.
Provide antacid, H_2 receptor antagonist, and/or H^+,K^+-ATPase inhibitor therapy.
Institute alternate-day steroid schedule if possible. Patients receiving steroid therapy over a prolonged period should be protected by an appropriate increase in hormone level during periods of acute stress. A rule of thumb is to *double* the maintenance dose.
Minimize osteopenia by
  Administering gonadal hormone replacement therapy: 0.625–1.25 mg conjugated estrogens given cyclically with progesterone, unless the uterus is absent; testosterone replacement for hypogonadal men
Ensuring high calcium intake (should be approximately 1200 mg/d)
Administering supplemental vitamin D if blood levels of calciferol or $1,25(OH)_2$ vitamin D are reduced
Administering bisphosphonate prophylactically, orally or parenterally, in high-risk patients

even at conventional doses, patients with a history of ulcer may experience aggravation of symptoms while receiving glucocorticoids. Consequently, all individuals with a positive history or with known risk factors should be managed with a vigorous antiulcer program (antacids, H_2 receptor antagonists, or ATPase inhibitors) along with glucocorticoids. *The development of anemia in a patient receiving glucocorticoids should suggest gastrointestinal bleeding as a cause.*

Hypertension or Cardiovascular Disease   The capacity of many adrenal steroid preparations to promote sodium retention makes it necessary to exercise caution when using them in patients with preexisting hypertension or cardiovascular or renal disease. The use of preparations with minimal sodium-retaining activity, restriction of dietary sodium intake, and the use of diuretic agents and supplementary potassium salts minimize the mineralocorticoid effects of steroids. However, hypertension may be exacerbated by steroid-induced increases in renin substrate and angiotensin II levels and by reduction in vasodilator prostaglandin production. Steroids also accelerate atherogenesis by induction of hypertension, glucose intolerance, and unfavorable lipid profiles. Glucocorticoid-associated lipid abnormalities include hypertriglyceridemia, hypercholesterolemia, and increased LDL cholesterol levels.

Psychological Difficulties   Steroid therapy may cause psychological disturbances. In general, these disturbances correlate better with the patient's personality than with the dose of hormone, although larger doses cause more serious reactions. There is no reliable method of predicting the psychological reaction to steroid therapy; moreover, previous tolerance of steroids does not necessarily ensure the safety of subsequent courses. Likewise, untoward psychological reactions on one occasion do not invariably mean that the patient will respond unfavorably to a second course. However, patients with depressive symptoms during a first course of steroids may benefit from prophylactic treatment prior to a second course.

Sleeplessness is common and can be minimized by using the shorter-acting steroids and by prescribing the total daily amount as a single early-morning dose.

ALTERNATE-DAY STEROID THERAPY   The most effective way to minimize the cushingoid effects of glucocorticoids is to administer the total 48-h dose as a *single* dose of *intermediate-acting steroid* in the morning, *every other day*. If symptoms of the underlying disorder can be controlled by this technique, it offers distinct advantages. Three considerations deserve mention: (1) The alternate-day schedule may be approached through transition schedules that allow the patient to adjust gradually; (2) supplementary nonsteroid medications may be needed on the "off" day to minimize symptoms of the underlying disorder; and (3) many symptoms that occur during the off day (e.g., fatigue, joint pain, muscle stiffness or tenderness, and fever) may represent relative adrenal insufficiency rather than exacerbation of the underlying disease.

The alternate-day approach capitalizes on the fact that cortisol secretion and plasma levels normally are highest in the early morning and lowest in the evening. The normal pattern is mimicked by administering an intermediate-acting steroid in the morning (7 to 8 A.M.) (Table 331-9).

Initially, the steroid program often requires daily or more frequent doses of steroid to achieve the desired anti-inflammatory or immunity-suppressing action. *Only after this desired effect is achieved is an attempt made to switch to an alternate-day program.* A number of schedules can be used for transferring from a daily to an alternate-day program. The key points to be considered are flexibility in arranging a program and the use of supportive measures on the off day. One may attempt a gradual transition to the alternate-day schedule rather than an abrupt changeover. One approach is to keep the steroid dose constant on one day and gradually reduce it on the alternate day. Alternatively, the steroid dose can be increased on one day and reduced on the alternate day. In any case, it is important to anticipate that some increase in pain or discomfort may occur in the 36 to 48 h following the last dose.

WITHDRAWAL OF GLUCOCORTICOIDS FOLLOWING LONG-TERM USE It is possible to reduce gradually and eventually to discontinue a daily steroid dose, but under most circumstances withdrawal of steroids should be initiated by first implementing an alternate-day schedule. Patients who have been on an alternate-day program for a month or more experience less difficulty during termination regimens. The dosage is gradually reduced and finally discontinued after a replacement dosage has been reached (e.g., 5 to 7.5 mg prednisone). Complications rarely ensue unless undue stress is experienced, and patients should understand that for 1 year or longer after withdrawal from long-term high-dose steroid therapy, supplementary hormone should be given in the event of a serious infection, operation, or injury. A useful strategy in patients with symptoms of adrenal insufficiency on a tapering regimen is to measure plasma cortisol levels prior to the steroid dose. A level <140 nmol/L (5 μg/dL) indicates continuing suppression of the pituitary-adrenal axis and implies that a more cautious tapering of steroids is indicated.

In patients on high-dose daily steroid therapy, it is advised to reduce dosage to approximately 20 mg prednisone daily as a single morning dose before beginning the transition to alternate-day therapy. If a patient cannot tolerate an alternate-day program, consideration should be given to the possibility that the patient has developed primary adrenal insufficiency.

BIBLIOGRAPHY

AZZIZ R et al: Nonclassic adrenal hyperplasia: Current concepts. Clinical review 56. J Clin Endocrinol Metab 78:810, 1994

BARZON L et al: Risk factors and long-term follow-up of adrenal incidentalomas. J Clin Endocrinol Metab 84:520, 1999

BORNSTEIN SR et al: Adrenocortical tumors: Recent advances in basic concepts and clinical management. Ann Intern Med 130:579, 1999

BRAND E et al: Structural analysis and evaluation of the aldosterone synthase gene in hypertension. Hypertension 32:198, 1998

CONLIN PR et al: Disorders of the renin-angiotensin-aldosterone system, in *Renal and Electrolyte Disorders*, 5th ed, RW Schrier (ed). Boston, Little, Brown, 1997

DLUHY RG et al: Glucocorticoid-remediable aldosteronism. Endocrinol Metab Clin North Am 23:385, 1994

GANGULY A: Primary aldosteronism. N Engl J Med 339:1828, 1998

GHOSE R et al: Medical management of aldosterone-producing adenomas. Ann Intern Med 131:105, 1999

HABIBY RL et al: Adrenal hypoplasia congenita with hypogonadotropic hypogonadism: Evidence that DAX-1 mutations lead to combined hypothalamic and pituitary defects in gonadotropin production. J Clin Invest 98:1055, 1996

INVITTI C et al: Diagnosis and management of Cushing's syndrome: Results of an Italian multicentre study. J Clin Endocrinol Metab 84:440, 1999

JORGE P et al: X-linked adrenoleukodystrophy in patients with idiopathic Addison disease. Eur J Pediatr 153:594, 1994

KALTSAS GA et al: A critical analysis of the value of simultaneous inferior petrosal sinus sampling in Cushing's disease and the occult ectopic adrenocorticotropin syndrome. J Clin Endocrinol Metab 84:487, 1999

KEREM E et al: Pulmonary epithelial sodium-channel dysfunction and excess airway liquid in pseudohypoaldosteronism. N Engl J Med 341:156, 1999

KJELLMAN M et al: Molecular genetics of adrenal cortical tumors. Curr Opin Endocrinol Diabetes 6:70, 1999

KONG MF et al: Eighty-six cases of Addison disease. Clin Endocrinol 41:757, 1994

LIPWORTH B et al: Systemic adverse effects of inhaled corticosteroid therapy. Arch Intern Med 159:941, 1999

MORTENSEN RM, WILLIAMS GH: Aldosterone action (physiology), in *Endocrinology*, 4th ed, LJ DeGroot et al (eds). Philadelphia, Saunders, 2001

NEW M: Steroid 21-hydroxylase deficiency (congenital adrenal hyperplasia). Am J Med 98:2S, 1995

NEWELL-PRICE J et al: Diagnosis and management of Cushing's syndrome. Lancet 353:2087, 1999

PAPANICOLAOU DA et al: A single midnight serum cortisol measurement distinguishes Cushing's syndrome from pseudo-Cushing's states. J Clin Endocrinol Metab 83:1163, 1998

ROGOFF D et al: The codon 213 of the 11beta-hydroxysteroid dehydrogenase type 2 gene is a hot spot for mutations in apparent mineralocorticoid excess. J Clin Endocrinol Metab 83:4391, 1998

SAMBROOK P et al: Prevention of corticosteroid osteoporosis. A comparison of calcium, calcitriol, and calcitonin. N Engl J Med 328:1747, 1993

SHIMKET RA et al: Liddle's syndrome: Heritable human hypertension caused by mutations in the beta subunit of the epithelial sodium channel. Cell 79:407, 1994

SWEARINGEN B et al: Long-term mortality after transsphenoidal surgery for Cushing's disease. Ann Intern Med 130:821, 1999

YOUNG MJ et al: Mineralocorticoids, salt hypertension: Effects on the heart. Steroids 61:233, 1996

332 *Lewis Landsberg, James B. Young*

PHEOCHROMOCYTOMA

Pheochromocytomas produce, store, and secrete catecholamines. They are usually derived from the adrenal medulla but may develop from chromaffin cells in or about sympathetic ganglia (extraadrenal pheochromocytomas or paragangliomas). Related tumors that secrete catecholamines and produce similar clinical syndromes include chemodectomas derived from the carotid body and ganglioneuromas derived from the postganglionic sympathetic neurons.

The clinical features are due predominantly to the release of catecholamines and, to a lesser extent, to the secretion of other substances. Hypertension is the most common sign, and hypertensive paroxysms or crises, often spectacular and alarming, occur in over half the cases.

Pheochromocytoma occurs in approximately 0.1% of the hypertensive population but is, nevertheless, an important correctable cause of high blood pressure. Indeed, it is usually curable if properly diagnosed and treated, but it may be fatal if undiagnosed or mistreated. Postmortem series indicate that most pheochromocytomas are unsuspected clinically, even when the tumor is related to the fatal outcome.

PATHOLOGY   Location and Morphology In adults, approximately 80% of pheochromocytomas are unilateral and solitary, 10% are bilateral, and 10% are extraadrenal. In children, a fourth of tumors are bilateral, and an additional fourth are extraadrenal. Solitary lesions inexplicably favor the right side. Although pheochromocytomas may grow to large size (over 3 kg), most weigh less than 100 g and are less than 10 cm in diameter. The tumors are highly vascular.

The tumors are made up of large, polyhedral, pleomorphic chromaffin cells. Less than 10% of these tumors are malignant. As with other endocrine tumors, malignancy cannot be determined from the histologic appearance; tumors that contain large numbers of aneuploid or tetraploid cells, as determined by flow cytometry, are more likely to recur. Local invasion of surrounding tissues or distant metastases indicate malignancy.

Extraadrenal pheochromocytomas Extraadrenal pheochromocytomas usually weigh 20 to 40 g and are <5 cm in diameter. Most are located within the abdomen in association with the celiac, superior mesenteric, and inferior mesenteric ganglia. Approximately 10% are in the thorax, 1% are within the urinary bladder, and <3% are in the neck, usually in association with the sympathetic ganglia or the extracranial branches of the ninth or tenth cranial nerves.

Catecholamine Synthesis, Storage, and Release Pheochromocytomas synthesize and store catecholamines by processes resembling those of the normal adrenal medulla (Chap. 72). Little is known about the mechanisms of catecholamine release from pheochromocytomas, but changes in blood flow and necrosis within the tumor may be the cause in some instances. These tumors are not innervated, and catecholamine release does not result from neural stimulation. Pheochromocytomas also store and secrete a variety of peptides, including endogenous opioids, adrenomedullin, endothelin, erythropoietin, parathyroid hormone–related protein, neuropeptide Y, and chromagranin A (Chap. 72). These peptides contribute to the clinical manifestations in selected cases, as noted below.

Epinephrine, norepinephrine, and dopamine Most pheochromocytomas contain and secrete both norepinephrine and epinephrine, and the percentage of norepinephrine is usually greater than in the normal adrenal. Most extraadrenal pheochromocytomas secrete norepinephrine exclusively. Rarely, pheochromocytomas produce epinephrine alone, particularly in association with multiple endocrine neoplasia (MEN). Although epinephrine-producing tumors may cause a preponderance of metabolic and beta-receptor effects, in general the major catecholamine secreted cannot be predicted from the clinical presentation. Increased production of dopamine and homovanillic acid (HVA) is uncommon with benign lesions but may occur with malignant pheochromocytoma.

FAMILIAL PHEOCHROMOCYTOMA In approximately 5% of cases, pheochromocytoma is inherited as an autosomal dominant trait either alone or in combination with other abnormalities such as MEN type 2a (Sipple's syndrome) or type 2b (mucosal neuroma syndrome) (Chap. 339), von Hippel–Lindau's retinal cerebellar hemangioblastomosis, or von Recklinghausen's neurofibromatosis. Bilateral adrenal pheochromocytomas are common in the familial syndromes; within MEN kindreds, over half of pheochromocytomas are bilateral. A familial syndrome should be suspected in any patient with bilateral pheochromocytomas.

§ **GENETIC CONSIDERATIONS** Several molecular genetic abnormalities have been identified in the familial pheochromocytoma syndromes. The MEN 2A and B syndromes are associated with abnormalities in the RET protooncogene located in pericentromeric region of chromosome 10 (Chap. 339). These mutations result in the constitutive activation of the receptor tyrosine kinase exposing adrenal medullary chromaffin cells and parafollicular C cells to hyperplasia and rendering them susceptible to malignant transformation. The RET mutations are located in the extracellular domain in MEN 2A and in the intracellular portion of the receptor in families with the MEN 2B syndrome. Interestingly, mutations at specific sites in the RET protooncogene are highly predictive of pheochromocytoma. The different phenotypic manifestations of the syndrome in different families, therefore, reflect differences in the specific mutations.

In the von Hippel–Landau (VHL) syndrome, mutation of one copy of the VHL tumor suppressor gene is associated with the development of tumors characteristic of the syndrome including pheochromocytomas. Loss of function of the VHL tumor suppressor gene promotes tumor formation by mechanisms that are incompletely understood but may involve mRNA transcript elongation. In the VHL syndrome, the frequency of pheochromocytoma varies considerably in different kindreds. As in the MEN 2 syndromes, certain VHL mutations are highly associated with the development of pheochromocytoma. Of further interest is the recent finding that the VHL mutation has been identified in some kindreds with familial pheochromocytoma as the sole manifestation without other clinical evidence of the VHL syndrome. Missense mutations, as opposed to deletions, insertions, or non-sense mutations, appear to be more commonly associated with pheochro-

mocytoma. There is also a high incidence of germ-line VHL mutations in patients with thoracic extraadrenal pheochromocytomas.

Interestingly, neither the RET protooncogene nor the VHL mutation occurs commonly as a somatic mutation in sporadic pheochromocytomas. Screening apparently sporadic cases, however, may uncover a germ-line mutation and lead to the identification of an involved family that was unsuspected on clinical grounds. ■

CLINICAL FEATURES Pheochromocytoma occurs at all ages but is most common in young to midadult life. Some series show a slight female preponderance. Most patients come to medical attention as a result of hypertensive crisis, paroxysmal symptoms suggestive of seizure disorder or anxiety attacks, or hypertension that responds poorly to conventional treatment. Less commonly, unexplained hypotension or shock in association with surgery or trauma will suggest the diagnosis. Most patients have hypertension in association with headaches, excessive sweating, and/or palpitations.

Hypertension Hypertension is the most common manifestation. In approximately 60% of cases the hypertension is sustained, although significant blood pressure lability is usually present, and half of patients with sustained hypertension have distinct crises or paroxysms. The other 40% have blood pressure elevations only during an attack. The hypertension is often severe, occasionally malignant, and may be resistant to treatment with standard antihypertensive drugs.

Paroxysms or Crises The paroxysm or crisis occurs in over half of patients. In an individual patient, the symptoms are often similar with each attack. The paroxysms may be frequent or sporadic, occurring at intervals as long as weeks or months. With time, the paroxysms usually increase in frequency, duration, and severity.

The attack usually has a sudden onset. It may last from a few minutes to several hours or longer. Headache, profuse sweating, palpitations, and apprehension, often with a sense of impending doom, are common. Pain in the chest or abdomen may be associated with nausea and vomiting. Either pallor or flushing may occur during the attack. The blood pressure is elevated, often to alarming levels, and the elevation is usually accompanied by tachycardia.

The paroxysm may be precipitated by any activity that displaces the abdominal contents. In some cases a particular stimulus may induce an attack in a characteristic fashion, but in others no clearly defined precipitating event can be found. Although anxiety may accompany the attacks, mental or psychological stress does not usually provoke a crisis.

Other Distinctive Clinical Features Symptoms and signs of an increased metabolic rate, such as profuse sweating and mild to moderate weight loss, are common. Orthostatic hypotension is a consequence of diminished plasma volume and blunted sympathetic reflexes. Both these factors predispose the patient with unsuspected pheochromocytoma to hypotension or shock during surgery or trauma. Secretion of the hypotensive peptide adrenomedullin may contribute to the hypotension in some patients.

Cardiac manifestations Sinus tachycardia, sinus bradycardia, supraventricular arrhythmias, and ventricular premature contractions all have been noted. Angina and acute myocardial infarction may occur even in the absence of coronary artery disease. A catecholamine-induced increase in myocardial oxygen consumption and, perhaps, coronary spasm may play a role in these ischemic events. Electrocardiographic changes, including nonspecific ST-T wave changes, prominent U waves, left ventricular strain patterns, and right and left bundle branch blocks may be present in the absence of demonstrable ischemia or infarction. Cardiomyopathy, either congestive with myocarditis and myocardial fibrosis or hypertrophic with concentric or asymmetric hypertrophy, may be associated with heart failure and cardiac arrhythmias. Multiorgan system failure with noncardiogenic pulmonary edema may be the presenting manifestation. Elevated levels of amylase originating from damaged pulmonary endothelium and abdominal pain may suggest acute pancreatitis, although serum lipase levels are normal.

Carbohydrate intolerance Over half of patients have impaired carbohydrate tolerance due to suppression of insulin and stimulation of hepatic glucose output. The impaired glucose tolerance rarely requires treatment with insulin and disappears after removal of the tumor.

332 Pheochromocytoma   **2107**

Hematocrit   The elevated hematocrit is secondary to diminished plasma volume. Rarely, production of erythropoietin by the tumor may cause a true erythrocytosis.

Other manifestations   Hypercalcemia has been attributed to the ectopic secretion of parathyroid hormone–related protein. Fever and an elevated erythrocyte sedimentation rate have been reported in association with the production of interleukin 6. Elevated temperature more commonly reflects catecholamine-mediated increases in metabolic rate and diminished heat dissipation secondary to vasoconstriction. Polyuria is an occasional finding, and rhabdomyolysis with myoglobinuric renal failure may result from extreme vasoconstriction with muscle ischemia.

Pheochromocytoma of the urinary bladder   Pheochromocytoma in the wall of the urinary bladder may result in typical paroxysms in relation to micturition. The location in the bladder wall is responsible for the occurrence of symptoms while the tumors are quite small, and, consequently, catecholamine excretion may be normal or minimally elevated. Hematuria is present in over half of patients, and the tumor can often be visualized at cystoscopy.

Adverse Drug Interactions   Severe and occasionally fatal paroxysms have been induced by opiates, histamine, adrenocorticotropin, saralasin, and glucagon. These agents appear to release catecholamines directly from the tumor. Indirect-acting sympathomimetic amines, including methyldopa (when administered intravenously), may cause an increase in blood pressure by releasing catecholamines from the augmented stores within nerve endings. Drugs that block neuronal uptake of catecholamines, such as tricyclic antidepressants or guanethidine, may enhance the physiologic effects of circulating catecholamines. Indeed, all medications should be considered carefully and administered cautiously in patients with known or suspected pheochromocytoma.

Associated Diseases   Pheochromocytoma is associated with medullary carcinoma of the thyroid in the MEN syndrome types 2a and 2b and with hyperparathyroidism in MEN 2a (Chap. 339). Hypercalcemia, resolving after tumor resection, also has been described in the absence of parathyroid disease, as described above. Individuals at risk for MEN 2a and 2b should be screened periodically for pheochromocytoma by assay of a 24-h urine sample for catecholamines, including measurement of epinephrine. Pheochromocytoma should be excluded or removed before thyroid or parathyroid surgery.

The association of pheochromocytoma and neurofibromatosis is not common. Nevertheless, since incomplete forms of neurofibromatosis may be associated with pheochromocytoma, minor manifestations such as café au lait spots, vertebral abnormalities, or kyphoscoliosis should increase the suspicion of pheochromocytoma in a patient with hypertension. The incidence of pheochromocytoma in some kindreds with von Hippel–Lindau disease may be as high as 10 to 25%. Many of these are unsuspected clinically and diagnosed on a computed tomography (CT) scan or at postmortem.

The incidence of cholelithiasis is 15 to 20%. Cushing's syndrome is a rare association, usually a consequence of ectopic secretion of adrenocorticotropic hormone by the pheochromocytoma or, less commonly, by a coexistent medullary carcinoma of the thyroid.

Diagnosis   The diagnosis is established by the demonstration of increased excretion of catecholamines or catecholamine metabolites. The diagnosis can usually be made by the analysis of a single 24-h urine sample, provided the patient is hypertensive or symptomatic at the time of collection.

Biochemical Tests   The assays employed include those for vanillylmandelic acid (VMA), the metanephrines, and unconjugated or "free" catecholamines (Chap. 72). The VMA assay is both less sensitive and less specific than assays of metanephrines or catecholamines. Accuracy of diagnosis is improved when two of three determinations are employed. The following considerations apply to all the urinary tests: (1) Despite claims for the adequacy of determinations made on random urine samples, analysis of a full 24-h urine sample is preferable. Creatinine should also be determined to assess the ade-

quacy of collection. (2) Where possible, the collection should be made when the patient is at rest, on no medication, and without recent exposure to radiographic contrast media. When it is not practical to discontinue all medications, drugs known specifically to interfere with these assays (as noted below) should be avoided. (3) The urine should be acidified and refrigerated during and after collection. (4) With high-quality assays, dietary restrictions are minimal and should be specified by the laboratory performing the analyses. (5) Although most patients with pheochromocytoma excrete increased amounts of catecholamines and catecholamine metabolites at all times, the yield is increased in patients with paroxysmal hypertension if a 24-h urine collection is initiated during a crisis.

Free catecholamines   The upper limit of normal for total urinary catecholamines is between 590 and 885 nmol (100 and 150 μg) per 24 h. In most patients with pheochromocytoma, values in excess of 1480 nmol (250 μg) per day are obtained. Measurement of epinephrine is often of value, since increased epinephrine excretion [over 275 nmol (50 μg) per 24 h] is usually due to an adrenal lesion and may be the only abnormality in cases associated with MEN. False-positive increases in catecholamine excretion result from exogenous catecholamines and related drugs such as methyldopa, levodopa, labetalol, and sympathomimetic amines, which may elevate catecholamine excretion for up to 2 weeks. Endogenous catecholamines from stimulation of the sympathoadrenal system also may increase urinary catecholamine excretion. Relevant clinical situations that cause such increases include hypoglycemia, strenuous exertion, central nervous system disease with increased intracranial pressure, severe hypoxia, and clonidine withdrawal.

Metanephrines and VMA   In most laboratories, the upper limit of normal is 7 μmol (1.3 mg) of total metanephrines and 35 μmol (7.0 mg) of VMA excretion per 24 h. In most patients with pheochromocytoma, the increase in these urinary metabolites is considerable, often to more than three times the normal range. Metanephrine excretion is increased by exogenous and endogenous catecholamines and by treatment with monoamine oxidase inhibitors; propranolol may cause a spurious increase in metanephrine excretion, since a propranolol metabolite interferes in the commonly used spectrophotometric assay. VMA is less affected by endogenous and exogenous catecholamines but is spuriously increased by a variety of drugs, including carbidopa. VMA excretion is decreased by monoamine oxidase inhibitors.

Plasma catecholamines   Measurement of plasma catecholamines has a limited application. The care required in obtaining basal levels (Chap. 72) and the satisfactory results with urinary determinations make measurement of plasma catecholamines unnecessary in most cases. Plasma catecholamine levels are affected by the same drugs and physiologic perturbations that increase urinary catecholamine excretion. In addition, α- and β-adrenergic receptor blocking agents may elevate plasma catecholamines by impairing clearance.

When the clinical features suggest pheochromocytoma and the urinary assay results are borderline, measurement of plasma catecholamines may be worthwhile. Markedly elevated basal levels of total catecholamines support the diagnosis, although approximately one-third of patients with pheochromocytoma have normal or slightly elevated basal values. The usefulness of plasma catecholamine determinations may be increased by agents that suppress sympathetic nervous system activity. Clonidine and ganglionic blocking agents (Chap. 72) reduce plasma catecholamine levels in normal subjects and in patients with essential hypertension. These drugs have little effect on catecholamine levels in patients with pheochromocytoma. In patients with elevated or borderline basal catecholamine values, failure to suppress plasma or urinary levels with clonidine supports the diagnosis of pheochromocytoma.

Pharmacologic Tests   Reliable methods for the measurement of catecholamines and catecholamine metabolites in urine have rendered obsolete both the provocative and adrenolytic tests, which are nonspecific and entail considerable risk. A modified version of the adrenolytic test may be of some use, however, as a therapeutic trial in a patient in hypertensive crisis with features suggestive of pheochromocytoma. A positive response to phentolamine (5-mg bolus following a test dose of 0.5 mg) is a reduction in blood pressure of at least 35/25 mmHg that peaks after 2 min and persists for 10 to 15 min. The pharmacologic response is never diagnostic, and biochemical confirmation is essential. Provocative tests in normotensive patients are potentially dangerous and rarely indicated. However, a glucagon provocative test may be of use in patients with paroxysmal hypertension and nondiagnostic basal catecholamine levels. Glucagon has a negligible effect on blood pressure or plasma catecholamine levels in normal or hypertensive subjects. In patients with pheochromocytoma, on the other hand, glucagon may increase both blood pressure and circulating catecholamine levels. The elevation in plasma catecholamine concentration, moreover, may occur without a blood pressure response. It must be emphasized, however, that life-threatening pressor crises have occurred after administration of glucagon to patients with pheochromocytoma, so the test should never be performed casually. Careful continuous monitoring of the blood pressure is required, intravenous access must be adequate, and phentolamine must be at hand to terminate the test if a significant pressor reaction ensues.

Differential Diagnosis   Since the manifestations of pheochromocytoma can be protean, the diagnosis must be considered and excluded in many patients with suggestive clinical features. In patients with essential hypertension and "hyperadrenergic" features such as tachycardia, sweating, and increased cardiac output, and in patients with anxiety attacks associated with blood pressure elevations, analysis of a 24-h urine collection is usually decisive in excluding the diagnosis. Repeated determinations on urine collected during attacks may be necessary, however, before the diagnosis can be excluded with certainty. The clonidine suppression and glucagon stimulation tests may be helpful in excluding the diagnosis in difficult cases. Pressor crises associated with clonidine withdrawal and the use of cocaine or monoamine oxidase inhibitors (Chap. 72) may mimic the paroxysms of pheochromocytoma. Factitious crises may be produced by self-administration of sympathomimetic amines in psychiatrically disturbed patients.

Intracranial lesions, particularly posterior fossa tumors or subarachnoid hemorrhage, may cause hypertension and increased excretion of catecholamines or catecholamine metabolites. While this is most common in patients with an obvious neurologic catastrophe, the possibility of subarachnoid or intracranial hemorrhage secondary to pheochromocytoma should be considered. Diencephalic or autonomic epilepsy may be associated with paroxysmal spells, hypertension, and increased plasma catecholamine levels. This rare entity may be difficult to distinguish from pheochromocytoma, but an aura, an abnormal electroencephalogram, and a beneficial response to anticonvulsant medications will often suggest the proper diagnosis.

℞ **TREATMENT   Preoperative Management**   The induction of stable α-adrenergic blockade is the basis of preoperative management and provides the foundation for successful surgical treatment. Once the diagnosis is established, the patient should be placed on phenoxybenzamine to induce a long-lived, noncompetitive α-receptor blockade. The usual initial dose is 10 mg every 12 h with increments of 10 to 20 mg added every few days until the blood pressure is controlled and the paroxysms disappear. Because of the long duration of action, the therapeutic effects are cumulative, and the optimal dose must be achieved gradually with careful monitoring of supine and upright blood pressures. Most patients require between 40 and 80 mg phenoxybenzamine per day, although 200 mg or more may be necessary. Phenoxybenzamine should be administered for at least 10 to 14 days prior to surgery. Over this time, the combination of α-receptor blockade and a liberal salt intake will restore the contracted plasma volume to normal. Before adequate α-adrenergic blockade with phen-

oxybenzamine is achieved, paroxysms may be treated with oral prazosin or noncompetitive intravenous phentolamine. Selective α_1 antagonists have been employed for preoperative preparation, but their role in preparative management should be limited to the treatment of individual paroxysms. They may be useful as antihypertensive agents in patients with suspected pheochromocytoma while workup is in progress, since they are usually better tolerated than phenoxybenzamine and will prevent serious pressor crises if pheochromocytoma is present. Nitroprusside, calcium channel blocking agents, and possibly angiotensin-converting enzyme inhibitors reduce blood pressure in patients with pheochromocytoma. Nitroprusside may also be useful in the treatment of pressor crises.

β-Adrenergic receptor blocking agents should be given only after alpha blockade has been induced, since administration of such agents by themselves may cause a paradoxic increase in blood pressure by antagonizing beta-mediated vasodilation in skeletal muscle. Beta blockade is usually initiated when tachycardia develops during the induction of α-adrenergic blockade. Low doses often suffice, and a reasonable starting dose is 10 mg propranolol three to four times per day, increased as needed to control the pulse rate. Beta blockade is effective for catecholamine-induced arrhythmias, particularly those potentiated by anesthetic agents.

Preoperative Localization of the Tumor   Surgical removal of pheochromocytoma is facilitated if the location of the tumor or tumors can be established preoperatively. Once pheochromocytoma is diagnosed, localization should be undertaken while the patient is being prepared for surgery. CT or magnetic resonance imaging (MRI) of the adrenals is usually successful in identifying intraadrenal lesions. Extraadrenal tumors within the chest can frequently be identified by conventional chest films or CT. MRI is useful in identifying extraadrenal tumors in the abdomen. If these studies are negative, abdominal aortography (once α-adrenergic blockade is complete) may identify extraadrenal pheochromocytomas in the abdomen, since these lesions are often supplied by a large aberrant artery. If aortography, CT, and MRI fail to localize the lesion, venous sampling at different levels of the inferior and superior vena cava may reveal catecholamine gradients in the region drained by the tumor; this area may then be restudied by selective angiography or scanning by CT or MRI. An additional localization technique involves a radionuclide scintiscan after administration of the radiopharmaceutical [131I]metaiodobenzylguanidine (MIBG). This agent is concentrated by the amine uptake process and produces an external scintigraphic image at the site of the tumor. This type of scanning may be useful in characterizing lesions discovered by CT when biochemical confirmation is indeterminate, as well as in localizing extraadrenal pheochromocytomas. Percutaneous fine-needle aspiration of chromaffin tumors is contraindicated; indeed, pheochromocytoma should be considered before any adrenal lesions are aspirated.

Surgery   Surgical treatment of pheochromocytoma is best performed in centers with experience in the preoperative, anesthetic, and intraoperative management of pheochromocytoma. In experienced hands, surgical mortality is <2 or 3%.

Monitoring during the surgical procedure should include continuous recording of arterial pressure and central venous pressure as well as electrocardiography; in the presence of cardiac disease or if congestive failure has been present, pulmonary capillary wedge pressure should be monitored. Adequate fluid replacement is crucial. Intraoperative hypotension responds better to volume replacement than to vasoconstrictors. Hypertension and cardiac arrhythmias are most likely during induction of anesthesia, intubation, and manipulation of the tumor. Intravenous phentolamine is usually sufficient to control the blood pressure, but nitroprusside may be required. Propranolol may be given in the treatment of tachycardia or ventricular ectopy.

Pheochromocytoma in pregnancy   Spontaneous labor and vaginal delivery in unprepared patients are usually disastrous for mother and fetus. In early pregnancy, the patient should be prepared with phenoxybenzamine, and the tumor should be removed as soon as the diagnosis is confirmed. The pregnancy need not be terminated, but the operative procedure itself may result in spontaneous abortion. In the third trimester, treatment with adrenergic blocking agents should be undertaken; when the fetus is of sufficient size, cesarean section may be followed by extirpation of the tumor. Although the safety of adrenergic blocking drugs in pregnancy is not established, these agents have been administered in several cases without obvious adverse effect. Antepartum diagnosis and treatment lowers the maternal death rate to that approaching nonpregnant pheochromocytoma patients; fetal death rate, however, remains elevated.

Unresectable and malignant tumors In cases of metastatic or locally invasive tumor in patients with intercurrent illness that precludes surgery, long-term medical management is required. When the manifestations cannot be adequately controlled by adrenergic blocking agents, the concomitant administration of metyrosine may be required. This agent inhibits tyrosine hydroxylase, diminishes catecholamine production by the tumor, and often simplifies chronic management. Malignant pheochromocytoma frequently recurs in the retroperitoneum, and it metastasizes most commonly to bone and lung. Although these malignant tumors are resistant to radiotherapy, combination chemotherapy has had limited success in controlling them. Use of ^{131}I-MIBG has had limited success in the treatment of malignant pheochromocytoma, due to poor uptake of the radioligand.

PROGNOSIS AND FOLLOW-UP The 5-year survival rate after surgery is usually over 95%, the recurrence rate is <10%. After successful surgery, catecholamine excretion returns to normal in about 2 weeks and should be measured to ensure complete tumor removal. Catecholamine excretion should be assessed at the reappearance of suggestive symptoms or yearly if the patient remains asymptomatic. For malignant pheochromocytoma, the 5-year survival rate is <50%.

Complete removal cures the hypertension in approximately three-fourths of patients. In the remainder, hypertension recurs but is usually well controlled by standard antihypertensive agents. In this group, either underlying essential hypertension or irreversible vascular damage induced by catecholamines may cause the persistence of the hypertension.

BIBLIOGRAPHY

AVERBUCH SD et al: Malignant pheochromocytoma: Effective treatment with a combination of cyclophosphamide, vincristine, and dacarbazine. Ann Intern Med 109:267, 1988

BERNHARD BU et al: Functioning thoracic paraganglioma: Association with von Hippel–Landau syndrome. J Clin Endocrinol Metab 82:3356, 1997

DALY PA, LANDSBERG L: Phaeochromocytoma: Diagnosis and management. Baillieres Clin Endocrinol Metab 6:143, 1992

ENG C et al: Mutations in the RET proto-oncogene and the von Hippel–Landau disease tumor suppressor gene in sporadic and syndromic pheochromocytomas. J Med Genet 32:934, 1995

FRANK-RAUE K et al: Diagnosis and management of pheochromocytomas in patients with multiple endocrine neoplasis type 2: Relevance of specific mutations in the RET proto-oncogene. Eur J Endocrinol 135:222, 1996

GARCIA A et al: Molecular diagnosis of von Hippel–Landau disease in a kindred with a predominance of familial phaeochromocytoma. Clin Endocrinol 46:359, 1997

GRAHAM PE et al: Laboratory diagnosis of pheochromocytoma: Which analyses should we measure? Ann Clin Biochem 30:129, 1993

KREMPF M et al: Use of m-(^{131}I) iodobenzylguanidine in the treatment of malignant pheochromocytoma. J Clin Endocrinol Metab 72:455, 1991

LANDSBERG L: Pheochromocytoma complicating pregnancy. Eur J Endocrinol 130:215, 1994

MACDOUGALL IC et al: Overnight clonidine suppression test in the diagnosis and exclusion of pheochromocytoma. Am J Med 84:993, 1988

MCCORKELL SJ, NILES NL: Fine-needle aspiration of catecholamine-producing adrenal masses: A possibly fatal mistake. Am J Roentgenol 145:113, 1985

MERIGIAN KS et al: Adrenergic crisis from crack cocaine ingestion: Report of five cases. J Emerg Med 12:485, 1994

NEUMANN HPH et al: Pheochromocytomas, multiple endocrine neoplasia type 2, and von Hippel-Lindau disease. N Engl J Med 329:1531, 1993

PANG L-C et al: Flow cytometric DNA analysis for the determination of malignant potential in adrenal and extra-adrenal pheochromocytomas or paragangliomas. Arch Pathol Lab Med 117:1142, 1993

REINIG JW, DOPPMAN JL: Magnetic resonance imaging of the adrenal. Radiologe 26:186, 1986

SHEMIN D et al: Pheochromocytoma presenting as rhabdomyolysis and acute myoglobinuric renal failure. Arch Intern Med 150:2384, 1990

STEWART AF et al: Hypercalcemia in pheochromocytoma. Ann Intern Med 102:776, 1985

333 *Alvin C. Powers*

DIABETES MELLITUS

Diabetes mellitus (DM) comprises a group of common metabolic disorders that share the phenotype of hyperglycemia. Several distinct types of DM exist and are caused by a complex interaction of genetics, environmental factors, and life-style choices. Depending on the etiology of the DM, factors contributing to hyperglycemia may include reduced insulin secretion, decreased glucose usage, and increased glucose production. The metabolic dysregulation associated with DM causes secondary pathophysiologic changes in multiple organ systems that impose a tremendous burden on the individual with diabetes and on the health care system. In the United States, DM is the leading cause of end-stage renal disease, nontraumatic lower extremity amputations, and adult blindness. With an increasing incidence worldwide, DM will likely continue to be a leading cause of morbidity and mortality for the foreseeable future.

CLASSIFICATION

Recent advances in the understanding of the etiology and pathogenesis of diabetes have led to a revised classification (Table 333-1). Although all forms of DM are characterized by hyperglycemia, the pathogenic mechanisms by which hyperglycemia arises differ widely. Some forms of DM are characterized by an absolute insulin deficiency or a genetic defect leading to defective insulin secretion, whereas other forms share insulin resistance as their underlying etiology. Recent changes in classification reflect an effort to classify DM on the basis of the pathogenic process that leads to hyperglycemia, as opposed to criteria such as age of onset or type of therapy (Fig. 333-1).

The two broad categories of DM are designated type 1 and type 2. Type 1A DM results from autoimmune beta cell destruction, which usually leads to insulin deficiency. Type 1B DM is also characterized by insulin deficiency as well as a tendency to develop ketosis. However, individuals with type 1B DM lack immunologic markers indicative of an autoimmune destructive process of the beta cells. The mechanisms leading to beta cell destruction in these patients are unknown. Relatively few patients with type 1 DM fall into the type 1B idiopathic category; many of these individuals are either African-American or Asian in heritage.

Type 2 DM is a heterogeneous group of disorders usually characterized by variable degrees of insulin resistance, impaired insulin secretion, and increased glucose production. Distinct genetic and metabolic defects in insulin action and/or secretion give rise to the common phenotype of hyperglycemia in type 2 DM (see below). The identification of distinct pathogenic processes in type 2 DM has important potential therapeutic implications, as pharmacologic agents that target specific metabolic derangements become available.

Two features of the current classification of DM diverge from previous classifications. First, the terms *insulin-dependent diabetes mellitus* (IDDM) and *noninsulin-dependent diabetes mellitus* (NIDDM)

Table 333-1   Etiologic Classification of Diabetes Mellitus

I. Type 1 diabetes (β-cell destruction, usually leading to absolute insulin deficiency)
   A. Immune-mediated
   B. Idiopathic
II. Type 2 diabetes (may range from predominantly insulin resistance with relative insulin deficiency to a predominantly insulin secretory defect with insulin resistance)
III. Other specific types of diabetes
   A. Genetic defects of β-cell function characterized by mutations in:
      1. Hepatocyte nuclear transcription factor (HNF) 4α (MODY 1)
      2. Glucokinase (MODY 2)
      3. HNF-1α (MODY 3)
      4. Insulin promoter factor (IPF) 1 (MODY 4)
      5. HNF-1β (MODY 5)
      6. Mitochondrial DNA
      7. Proinsulin or insulin conversion
   B. Genetic defects in insulin action
      1. Type A insulin resistance
      2. Leprechaunism
      3. Rabson-Mendenhall syndrome
      4. Lipoatrophic diabetes
   C. Diseases of the exocrine pancreas—pancreatitis, pancreatectomy, neoplasia, cystic fibrosis, hemochromatosis, fibrocalculous pancreatopathy
   D. Endocrinopathies—acromegaly, Cushing's syndrome, glucagonoma, pheochromocytoma, hyperthyroidism, somatostatinoma, aldosteronoma
   E. Drug- or chemical-induced—Vacor, pentamidine, nicotinic acid, glucocorticoids, thyroid hormone, diazoxide, β-adrenergic agonists, thiazides, phenytoin, α-interferon, protease inhibitors, clozapine, beta blockers
   F. Infections—congenital rubella, cytomegalovirus, coxsackie
   G. Uncommon forms of immune-mediated diabetes—"stiff-man" syndrome, anti-insulin receptor antibodies
   H. Other genetic syndromes sometimes associated with diabetes—Down's syndrome, Klinefelter's syndrome, Turner's syndrome, Wolfram's syndrome, Friedreich's ataxia, Huntington's chorea, Laurence-Moon-Biedl syndrome, myotonic dystrophy, porphyria, Prader-Willi syndrome
IV. Gestational diabetes mellitus (GDM)

NOTE: MODY, maturity onset of diabetes of the young.
SOURCE: Adapted from American Diabetes Association, 2000

are obsolete. These previous designations reflected the observation that most individuals with type 1 DM (previously IDDM) have an absolute requirement for insulin treatment, whereas many individuals with type 2 DM (previously NIDDM) do not require insulin therapy to prevent ketoacidosis. However, because many individuals with type 2 DM eventually require insulin treatment for control of glycemia, the use of the latter term generated considerable confusion.

A second difference is that age is no longer used as a criterion in the new classification system. Although type 1 DM most commonly develops before the age of 30, an autoimmune beta cell destructive process can develop at any age. In fact, it is estimated that between 5 and 10% of individuals who develop DM after age 30 have type 1A DM. Likewise, although type 2 DM more typically develops with increasing age, it also occurs in children, particularly in obese adolescents.

OTHER TYPES OF DM   Other etiologies for DM include specific genetic defects in insulin secretion or action, metabolic abnormalities that impair insulin secretion, and a host of conditions that impair glucose tolerance (Table 333-1). *Maturity onset diabetes of the young* (MODY) is a subtype of DM characterized by autosomal dominant inheritance, early onset of hyperglycemia, and impairment in insulin secretion (discussed below). Mutations in the insulin receptor cause a group of rare disorders characterized by severe insulin resistance.

DM can result from pancreatic exocrine disease when the majority of pancreatic islets (>80%) are destroyed. Several endocrinopathies

can lead to DM as a result of excessive secretion of hormones that antagonize the action of insulin. Notable within this group are acromegaly and Cushing's disease, both of which may present with DM. Viral infections have been implicated in pancreatic islet destruction, but are an extremely rare cause of DM. Congenital rubella greatly increases the risk for DM; however, most of these individuals also have immunologic markers indicative of autoimmune beta cell destruction.

GESTATIONAL DIABETES MELLITUS (GDM)   Glucose intolerance may develop and first become recognized during pregnancy. Insulin resistance related to the metabolic changes of late pregnancy increases insulin requirements and may lead to hyperglycemia or impaired glucose tolerance. GDM is seen in approximately 4% of pregnancies in the United States; most women revert to normal glucose tolerance post-partum but have a substantial risk (30 to 60%) of developing DM later in life.

EPIDEMIOLOGY

The worldwide prevalence of DM has risen dramatically over the past two decades. It is projected that the number of individuals with DM will continue to increase in the near future. Between 1976 and 1994, for example, the prevalence of DM among adults in the United States increased from 8.9% to 12.3%. These findings, based on national epidemiologic data, include individuals with a diagnosis of DM and those with undiagnosed DM (based on identical diagnostic criteria). Likewise, prevalence rates of impaired fasting glucose (IFG) increased from 6.5% to 9.7% over the same period. Although the prevalence of both type 1 and type 2 DM is increasing worldwide, the prevalence of type 2 DM is expected to rise more rapidly in the future because of increasing obesity and reduced activity levels.

There is considerable geographic variation in the incidence of both type 1 and type 2 DM. For example, Scandinavia has the highest rate of type 1 DM (in Finland, incidence is 35/100,000 per year). The

Type of Diabetes	Normal glucose tolerance	Hyperglycemia		
		Impaired fasting glucose or impaired glucose tolerance	Diabetes Mellitus		
			Not insulin requiring	Insulin required for control	Insulin required for survival
Type 1					
Type 2					
Other specific types					
Gestational Diabetes					
Time (years)					
FPG (mg/dL)	<110	110–125	≥126		
2-h PG (mg/dL)	<140	140–199	≥200		

FIGURE 333-1   Spectrum of glucose homeostasis and diabetes. The spectrum from normal glucose tolerance to diabetes in type 1 diabetes, type 2 diabetes, other specific types of diabetes, and gestational diabetes is shown from left to right. In most types of diabetes, the individual traverses from normal glucose tolerance to impaired glucose tolerance to frank diabetes. Arrows indicate that changes in glucose tolerance may be bi-directional in some types of diabetes. For example, individuals with type 2 diabetes may return to the impaired glucose tolerance category with weight loss; in gestational diabetes, diabetes may revert to impaired glucose tolerance or even normal glucose tolerance after delivery. The fasting plasma glucose (FPG) and 2-h plasma glucose (PG), after a glucose challenge for the different categories of glucose tolerance, are shown at the lower part of the figure (as defined by recent consensus panels—see text). These values do not apply to the diagnosis of gestational diabetes. Some types of diabetes may or may not require insulin for survival, hence the dotted line. (Conventional units are used in the figure.) *(Adapted from American Diabetes Association: Clinical Practice Guidelines, 2000)*

Pacific Rim has a much lower rate (in Japan and China, incidence is 1 to 3/100,000 per year) of type 1 DM; Northern Europe and the United States share an intermediate rate (8 to 17/100,000 per year). Much of the increased risk of type 1 DM is believed to reflect the frequency of high-risk HLA alleles among ethnic groups in different geographic locations.

The prevalence of type 2 DM and its harbinger, impaired glucose tolerance (IGT), is highest in certain Pacific islands, intermediate in countries such as India and the United States, and relatively low in Russia and China. This variability is likely due to both genetic and environmental factors. There is also considerable variation in DM prevalence among different ethnic populations within a given country.

In 1998, approximately 16 million individuals in the United States met the diagnostic criteria for DM. This represents ~6% of the population. About 800,000 individuals in the United States develop DM each year. The vast majority of these (>90%) have type 2 DM. The number of people with DM increases with the age of the population, ranging from an incidence of ~1.5% in individuals from 20 to 39 years to ~20% of individuals >75 years. The incidence of DM is similar in men and women throughout most age ranges but is slightly greater in men >60 years. The prevalence of DM is approximately twofold greater in African Americans, Hispanic Americans, and Native Americans than in non-Hispanic whites, and the onset of type 2 DM occurs, on average, at an earlier age in the former groups than in the non-Hispanic white population. The incidence of type 2 DM in these ethnic groups is rapidly increasing. The reasons for these differences are not yet clear.

DIAGNOSIS

Revised criteria for diagnosing DM have been issued by consensus panels of experts from the National Diabetes Data Group and the World Health Organization (Table 333-2). The revised criteria reflect new epidemiologic and metabolic evidence and are based on the following premises: (1) the spectrum of fasting plasma glucose (FPG) and the response to an oral glucose load varies in normal individuals, and (2) DM defined as the level of glycemia at which diabetes-specific complications are noted and not on the level of glucose tolerance from a population-based viewpoint. For example, the prevalence of retinopathy in Native Americans (Pima Indian population) begins to increase at a FPG > 6.4 mmol/L (116 mg/dL) (Fig. 333-2).

Glucose tolerance is classified into three categories based on the FPG: (1) FPG < 6.1 mmol/L (110 mg/dL) is considered normal; (2) FPG ≥ 6.1 mmol/L (110 mg/dL) but < 7.0 mmol/L (126 mg/dL) is defined as IFG; and (3) FPG ≥ 7.0 mmol/L (126 mg/dL) warrants the diagnosis of DM. IFG is a new diagnostic category defined by the Expert Committee on the Diagnosis and Classification of Diabetes Mellitus. It is analogous to IGT, which is defined as plasma glucose levels between 7.8 and 11.1 mmol/L (140 and 200 mg/dL) 2 h after a 75-g oral glucose load (Table 333-2). Individuals with IFG or IGT are at substantial risk for developing type 2 DM and cardiovascular disease in the future, though they may not meet the criteria for DM.

Table 333-2 Criteria for the Diagnosis of Diabetes Mellitus

- Symptoms of diabetes plus random blood glucose concentration ≥11.1 mmol/L (200 mg/dL)[a]

  or
- Fasting plasma glucose ≥7.0 mmol/L (126 mg/dL)[b]

  or
- Two-hour plasma glucose ≥11.1 mmol/L (200 mg/dL) during an oral glucose tolerance test[c]

In the absence of unequivocal hyperglycemia and acute metabolic decompensation, these criteria should be confirmed by repeat testing on a different day.

[a] Random is defined as without regard to time since the last meal.
[b] Fasting is defined as no caloric intake for at least 8 h.
[c] The test should be performed using a glucose load containing the equivalent of 75 g anhydrous glucose dissolved in water; not recommended for routine clinical use.

SOURCE: Adapted from American Diabetes Association, 2000.

FIGURE 333-2 Relationship of diabetes-specific complication and glucose tolerance. This figure shows the incidence of retinopathy in Pima Indians as a function of the fasting plasma glucose (FPG), the 2-h plasma glucose after a 75-g oral glucose challenge (2hPG), or glycated hemoglobin (HbA1c). Note that the incidence of retinopathy greatly increases at a fasting plasma glucose >116 mg/dL, or a 2-h plasma glucose of 185 mg/dL, or a HbA1c >6.0%. (Conventional units are used in the figure.) *(From American Diabetes Association: Clinical Practice Guidelines, 2000, as adapted from McCance et al: BMJ 308:1323, 1994)*

The revised criteria for the diagnosis of DM emphasize the FPG as the most reliable and convenient test for diagnosing DM in asymptomatic individuals. A random plasma glucose concentration ≥11.1 mmol/L (200 mg/dL) accompanied by classic symptoms of DM (polyuria, polydipsia, weight loss) is sufficient for the diagnosis of DM (Table 333-2). Oral glucose tolerance testing, although still a valid mechanism for diagnosing DM, is not recommended as part of routine screening.

Some investigators have advocated the hemoglobin A1c (HbA1c) as a diagnostic test for DM. Though there is a strong correlation between elevations in the plasma glucose and the HbA1c (discussed below), the relationship between the FPG and the HbA1c in individuals with normal glucose tolerance or mild glucose intolerance is less clear, and the test is not universally standardized or available.

The diagnosis of DM has profound implications for an individual from both a medical and financial standpoint. Thus, the health care provider must be certain that these criteria are completely satisfied before assigning the diagnosis of DM to an individual. The revised criteria also allow for the diagnosis of DM to be withdrawn in situations where the FPG no longer exceeds these criteria. Abnormalities on screening tests for diabetes should be repeated before making a definitive diagnosis of DM, unless acute metabolic derangements or a markedly elevated plasma glucose are present (Table 333-2).

SCREENING Widespread use of the FPG as a screening test for type 2 DM is strongly encouraged because: (1) a large number of individuals who meet the current criteria for DM are unaware that they have the disorder, (2) epidemiologic studies suggest that type 2 DM may be present for up to a decade before diagnosis, and (3) as many as 50% of individuals with type 2 DM have one or more diabetes-specific complications at the time of their diagnosis. The Expert Committee suggests screening all individuals >45 years every 3 years and screening asymptomatic individuals with additional risk factors (Table 333-3) at an earlier age. In contrast to type 2 DM, it is rare for an individual to have a long asymptomatic period of hyperglycemia prior to the diagnosis of type 1 DM. A number of immunologic markers for type 1 DM are becoming available (discussed below), but their use is currently discouraged pending the identification of clinically beneficial interventions for individuals at high risk for developing type 1 DM.

Table 333-3   **Risk Factors for Type 2 Diabetes Mellitus**

- Family history of diabetes (i.e., parent or sibling with type 2 diabetes)
- Obesity (i.e., $\geq 20\%$ desired body weight or BMI ≥ 27 kg/m^2)
- Age ≥ 45 years
- Race/ethnicity (e.g., African American, Hispanic American, Native American, Asian American, Pacific Islander)
- Previously identified IFG or IGT
- History of GDM or delivery of baby over 9 lbs
- Hypertension (blood pressure $\geq 140/90$ mm Hg)
- HDL cholesterol level ≤ 0.90 mmol/L (35 mg/dL) and/or a triglyceride level ≥ 2.82 mmol/L (250 mg/dL)
- Polycystic ovary syndrome

NOTE: BMI, body mass index; IFG, impaired fasting glucose; IGT, impaired glucose tolerance; GDM, gestational diabetes mellitus; HDL, high-density lipoprotein.
SOURCE: Adapted from American Diabetes Association, 2000.

INSULIN BIOSYNTHESIS, SECRETION, AND ACTION

BIOSYNTHESIS   Insulin is produced in the beta cells of the pancreatic islets. It is initially synthesized as a single-chain 86-amino-acid precursor polypeptide, preproinsulin. Subsequent proteolytic processing removes the aminoterminal signal peptide, giving rise to proinsulin. Proinsulin is structurally related to insulin-like growth factors I and II, which bind weakly to the insulin receptor (Chap. 327). Cleavage of an internal 31-residue fragment from proinsulin generates the C peptide and the A (21 amino acids) and B (30 amino acids) chains of insulin, which are connected by disulfide bonds. The mature insulin molecule and C peptide are stored together and cosecreted from secretory granules in the beta cells. Because the C peptide is less susceptible than insulin to hepatic degradation, it is a useful a marker of insulin secretion and allows discrimination of endogenous and exogenous sources of insulin in the evaluation of hypoglycemia (Chap. 334). Human insulin is now produced by recombinant DNA technology; structural alterations at one or more residues are useful for modifying its physical and pharmacologic characteristics (see below).

SECRETION   Glucose is the key regulator of insulin secretion by the pancreatic beta cell, although amino acids, ketones, various nutrients, gastrointestinal peptides, and neurotransmitters also influence insulin secretion. Glucose levels >3.9 mmol/L (70 mg/dL) stimulate insulin synthesis, primarily by enhancing protein translation and processing, as well as inducing insulin secretion. Glucose stimulates insulin secretion through a series of regulatory steps that begin with transport into the beta cell by the GLUT2 glucose transporter (Fig. 333-3). Glucose phosphorylation by glucokinase is the rate-limiting step that controls glucose-regulated insulin secretion.

Further metabolism of glucose-6-phosphate via glycolysis generates ATP, which inhibits the activity of an ATP-sensitive K$^+$ channel. This channel is a complex of two separate proteins, one of which is the receptor for certain oral hypoglycemics (e.g., sulfonylureas, meglitinides); the other subunit is an inwardly rectifying K$^+$ channel protein. Inhibition of this K$^+$ channel induces beta cell membrane depolarization, opening of voltage-dependent calcium channels (leading to an influx of calcium), and stimulation of insulin secretion. Careful studies of insulin secretory profiles reveal pulsatile pattern of hormone release, with small secretory bursts occurring about every 10 min, superimposed upon greater amplitude oscillations of about 80 to 150 min. Meals or other major stimuli of insulin secretion induce large (four- to fivefold increase versus baseline) bursts of insulin secretion that usually last for 2 to 3 h before returning to baseline. Derangements in these normal secretory patterns are one of the earliest signs of beta cell dysfunction in DM (see below).

ACTION   Once insulin is secreted into the portal vein, ~50% is removed and degraded by the liver. Unextracted insulin enters the systemic circulation and binds to its receptor in target sites. The insulin receptor belongs to the tyrosine kinase class of membrane-bound receptors (Chap. 327). Insulin binding to the receptor stimulates intrinsic

FIGURE 333-3   Diabetes and abnormalities in glucose-stimulated insulin secretion. Glucose and other nutrients regulate insulin secretion by the pancreatic beta cell. Glucose is transported by the GLUT2 glucose transporter; subsequent glucose metabolism by the beta cell alters ion channel activity, leading to insulin secretion. The SUR receptor is the binding site for oral hypoglycemic agents. Mutations in the events or proteins underlined are a cause of maturity onset diabetes of the young (MODY) or other forms of diabetes. SUR, sulfonylurea receptor; ATP, adenosine triphosphate; ADP, adenosine diphosphate. *(Adapted from Lowe, 1998.)*

tyrosine kinase activity, leading to receptor autophosphorylation and the recruitment of intracellular signaling molecules, such as insulin receptor substrates (IRS) 1 and 2 (Fig. 333-4). These and other adaptor proteins initiate a complex cascade of phosphorylation and dephosphorylation reactions, ultimately resulting in the widespread metabolic and mitogenic effects of insulin. As an example, activation of the phosphatidylinositol-3′-kinase (PI-3 kinase) pathway stimulates translocation of glucose transporters (e.g., GLUT4) to the cell surface, an event that is crucial for glucose uptake by skeletal muscle and fat. Activation of other insulin receptor signaling pathways induces glycogen synthesis, protein synthesis, lipogenesis, and regulation of various genes in insulin-responsive cells.

Glucose homeostasis reflects a precise balance between hepatic glucose production and peripheral glucose uptake and utilization. Insulin is the most important regulator of this metabolic equilibrium, but the effects of other pathways including neural input, metabolic signals, and hormones (e.g., glucagon) result in integrated control of glucose supply and utilization (Chap. 334; Fig. 334-1). In the fasting state, low insulin levels promote hepatic gluconeogenesis and glycogenolysis to prevent hypoglycemia. Low insulin levels decrease glycogen synthesis, reduce glucose uptake in insulin-sensitive tissues, and promote mobilization of stored precursors. Reduced insulin levels are also permissive in allowing glucagon to stimulate glycogenolysis and gluconeogenesis by the liver and renal medulla. These processes are of critical importance to ensure an adequate glucose supply for the brain. Postprandially, a large glucose load elicits a rise in insulin and fall in glucagon, leading to a reversal of these processes. The major portion of postprandial glucose is utilized by skeletal muscle. Other tissues, most notably the brain, utilize glucose in an insulin-independent fashion.

PATHOGENESIS

TYPE 1 DM   Type 1A DM develops as a result of the synergistic effects of genetic, environmental, and immunologic factors that ultimately destroy the pancreatic beta cells. The temporal development of type 1A DM is shown schematically as a function of beta cell mass in Fig. 333-5. Individuals with a genetic susceptibility have normal beta cell mass at birth but begin to lose beta cells secondary to autoimmune destruction that occurs over months to years. This autoimmune process is thought to be triggered by an infectious or environmental stimulus and to be sustained by a beta cell–specific molecule. In the majority of individuals, immunologic markers appear after the triggering event but before diabetes becomes clinically overt. Beta cell mass then begins to decline, and insulin secretion becomes progressively impaired, although normal glucose tolerance is maintained. The rate of decline in beta cell mass varies widely among individuals, with some patients progressing rapidly to clinical diabetes and others evolving more slowly. Features of diabetes do not become evident until a majority of beta cells are destroyed (~80%). At this point, residual functional beta cells still exist but are insufficient in number to maintain glucose tolerance. The events that trigger the transition from glucose intolerance to frank diabetes are often associated with increased insulin requirements, as might occur during infections or puberty. Following the initial clinical presentation of type 1A DM, a "honeymoon" phase may ensue during which time glycemic control is achieved with modest doses of insulin or, rarely, insulin is not needed. However, this fleeting phase of endogenous insulin production from residual beta cells disappears as the autoimmune process destroys the remaining beta cells, and the individual becomes completely insulin deficient.

FIGURE 333-4 Insulin signal transduction pathway. The insulin receptor has intrinsic tyrosine kinase activity and interacts with insulin receptor substrates (IRS and Shc) proteins. A number of "docking" proteins bind to these cellular proteins and initiate the metabolic actions of insulin [GrB-2, SOS, SHP-2, p65, p110, and phosphoinositol phosphate 3-kinase (PI 3-kinase)]. Insulin increases glucose transport through PI 3-kinase, which promotes the translocation of intracellular vesicles containing GLUT4 glucose transporter to the plasma membrane. *(Adapted from Lowe, 1998; Virkamaki et al, 1999)*

GENETIC CONSIDERATIONS

The genetic contributions to type 1A DM involve multiple genes. The development of the disease appears to require inheritance of a sufficient complement of genes to confer susceptibility to the disorder. The concordance of type 1A DM in identical twins ranges between 30 and 70%, indicating that additional modifying factors must be involved in determining whether diabetes develops. The major susceptibility gene for type 1A DM is located in the HLA region on chromosome 6. Polymorphisms in the HLA complex appear to account for 40 to 50% of the genetic risk of developing type 1A DM. This region contains genes that encode the class II MHC molecules, which present antigen to helper T cells and thus are involved in initiating the immune response (Chaps. 305, 306, 307). The ability of class II MHC molecules to present antigen is dependent on the amino acid composition of their antigen-binding sites. Amino acid substitutions may influence the specificity of the immune response by altering the binding affinity of different antigens for the class II molecules.

Most individuals with type 1A DM have the HLA DR3 and/or DR4 haplotype. Refinements in genotyping of HLA loci have shown that the haplotypes DQA1*0301, DQB1*0302 and DQA1*501, DQB1*0201 have the strongest association with type 1A DM. These haplotypes are present in 40% of children with type 1A DM as compared to 2% of the normal U.S. population.

In addition to MHC class II associations, at least 17 different genetic loci may contribute susceptibility to type 1A DM. For example, polymorphisms in the promoter region of the insulin gene appear to account for ~10% of the predisposition to type 1A DM. Genes that confer protection against the development of the disease also exist. For example, the haplotype DQA1*0102, DQB1*0602 is present in 20% of the U.S. population but is extremely rare in individuals with type 1A DM (<1%).

Although type 1A DM is clearly associated with certain predisposing genotypes, most individuals with these haplotypes do not develop diabetes. In addition, most individuals with type 1A DM do not have a first-degree relative with this disorder. Nevertheless, the risk of developing type 1A DM for relatives of individuals with the disease is considerably higher compared to the risk for the general population. ■

Autoimmune Factors Although other islet cell types [alpha cells (glucagon-producing), delta cells (somatostatin-producing) or PP cells (pancreatic polypeptide-producing)] are functionally and embryologically similar to beta cells and express most of the same proteins as beta cells, they are inexplicably spared from the autoimmune process. Pathologically, the pancreatic islets are infiltrated with lymphocytes (in a process termed *insulitis*). After all beta cells are destroyed,

FIGURE 333-5 Temporal model for development of type 1 diabetes. Individuals with a genetic predisposition are exposed to an immunologic trigger that initiates an autoimmune process, resulting in a gradual decline in beta cell mass. The downward slope of the beta cell mass varies among individuals. This progressive impairment in insulin release results in diabetes when ~80% of the beta cell mass is destroyed. A "honeymoon" phase may be seen in the first 1 or 2 years after the onset of diabetes and is associated with reduced insulin requirements. *(Adapted from Medical Management of Type 1 Diabetes, 3d ed, JS Skyler (ed). Alexandria, VA, American Diabetes Association, 1998)*

the inflammatory process abates, the islets become atrophic, and immunologic markers disappear. Studies of the insulitis and autoimmune process in humans and animal models of type 1A DM (NOD mouse and BB rat) have identified the following abnormalities in both the humoral and cellular arms of the immune system: (1) islet cell autoantibodies; (2) activated lymphocytes in the islets, peripancreatic lymph nodes, and systemic circulation; (3) T lymphocytes that proliferate when stimulated with islet proteins; and (4) release of cytokines within the insulitis. Beta cells seem to be particularly susceptible to the toxic effect of some cytokines (tumor necrosis factor α, interferon γ, and interleukin 1). The precise mechanisms of beta cell death are not known but may involve formation of nitric oxide metabolites, apoptosis, and direct CD8+ T cell cytotoxicity. Islet autoantibodies are not thought to be involved in the destructive process, as these antibodies do not generally react with the cell surface of islet cells and are not capable of transferring diabetes mellitus to animals.

Pancreatic islet molecules targeted by the autoimmune process include insulin, glutamic acid decarboxylase (GAD; the biosynthetic enzyme for the neurotransmitter GABA), ICA-512/IA-2 (homology with tyrosine phosphatases), and phogrin (insulin secretory granule protein). Other less clearly defined autoantigens include an islet ganglioside and carboxypeptidase H. With the exception of insulin, none of the autoantigens are beta cell specific, which raises the question of how the beta cells are selectively destroyed. Current theories favor initiation of an autoimmune process directed at one beta cell molecule, which then spreads to other islet molecules as the immune process destroys beta cells and creates a series of secondary autoantigens. The beta cells of individuals who develop type 1A DM do not differ from beta cells of normal individuals, since transplanted islets are destroyed by a recurrence of the autoimmune process of type 1A DM.

Immunologic Markers Islet cell autoantibodies (ICAs) are a composite of several different antibodies directed at pancreatic islet molecules such as GAD, insulin, IA-2/ICA512, and an islet ganglioside and serve as a marker of the autoimmune process of type 1A DM. Testing for ICAs can be useful in classifying the type of DM as type IA and in identifying nondiabetic individuals at risk for developing type 1A DM. ICAs are present in the majority of individuals (>75%) diagnosed with new-onset type 1A DM, in a significant minority of individuals with newly diagnosed type 2 DM, and occasionally in individuals with GDM (<5%). ICAs are present in 3 to 4% of first-degree relatives of individuals with type 1A DM. In conjunction with impaired insulin secretion on intravenous glucose tolerance testing, they predict a >50% risk of developing type 1A DM within 5 years. Without this impairment in insulin secretion, the presence of ICAs predicts a 5-year risk of <25%. Based on these data, the risk of a first-degree relative developing type 1A DM is relatively low, and even ICA-positive individuals are not destined to develop diabetes. At present, the ICAs are used predominantly as a research tool and not in clinical practice, in part because of the technically demanding nature of the assay but also because no treatments have been proven to prevent the occurrence or progression of type 1A DM.

Environmental Factors Numerous environmental events have been proposed to trigger the autoimmune process in genetically susceptible individuals; however, none have been conclusively linked to diabetes. Identification of an environmental trigger has been difficult because the event may precede the onset of DM by several years (Fig. 333-5). Putative environmental triggers include viruses (coxsackie and rubella most prominently), early exposure to bovine milk proteins, and nitrosourea compounds. Epidemiologic studies have noted an association between bovine milk intake and type 1A DM; studies are ongoing to investigate a possible relationship between exposure to bovine milk and the autoimmune process of type 1A DM.

Prevention of Type 1A DM A number of interventions have successfully delayed or prevented diabetes in animal models. Some interventions have targeted the immune system directly (immunosuppression, selective T cell subset deletion, induction of immunologic tolerance to islet proteins), whereas others have prevented islet cell death by blocking cytotoxic cytokines or increasing islet resistance to the destructive process. Though results in animal models are promising, most of these interventions have not been successful in preventing type 1A DM in humans. Clinical trials of several interventions are underway in the United States and Europe. The Diabetes Prevention Trial—type 1 is being conducted to determine whether administering insulin to individuals at high risk for developing type 1A DM can induce immune tolerance and alter the autoimmune process of type 1A DM.

TYPE 2 DM Type 2 DM is a heterogeneous disorder with a complex etiology that develops in response to genetic and environmental influences. Central to the development of type 2 DM are insulin resistance and abnormal insulin secretion. Although controversy remains regarding the primary defect, most studies support the view that insulin resistance precedes insulin secretory defects.

GENETIC CONSIDERATIONS Type 2 DM has a strong genetic component. Although the major genes that predispose to this disorder have yet to be identified, it is clear that the disease is polygenic and multifactorial. Various genetic loci contribute to susceptibility, and environmental factors (such as nutrition and physical activity) further modulate phenotypic expression of the disease. The concordance of type 2 DM in identical twins is between 70 and 90%. Individuals with a parent with type 2 DM have an increased risk of diabetes; if both parents have type 2 DM, the risk in offspring may reach 40%. Insulin resistance, as demonstrated by reduced glucose utilization in skeletal muscle, is present in many nondiabetic, first-degree relatives of individuals with type 2 DM. However, definition of the genetic abnormalities of type 2 DM remains a challenge because the genetic defect in insulin secretion or action may not manifest itself unless an environmental event or another genetic defect, such as obesity, is superimposed.

The identification of individuals with mutations in various molecules involved in insulin action (e.g., the insulin receptor and enzymes involved in glucose homeostasis) has been useful for characterizing key steps in insulin action. However, mutations in these molecules account for a very small fraction of type 2 DM. Likewise, genetic defects in proteins involved in insulin secretion have not been found in most individuals with type 2 DM. Genome-wide scanning for mutations or polymorphisms associated with type 2 DM is being used in an effort to identify genes associated with type 2 DM. ■

Pathophysiology Type 2 DM is characterized by three pathophysiologic abnormalities: impaired insulin secretion, peripheral insulin resistance, and excessive hepatic glucose production. Obesity, particularly visceral or central, is very common in type 2 DM. Insulin resistance associated with obesity augments the genetically determined insulin resistance of type 2 DM. Adipocytes secrete a number of biologic products (leptin, tumor necrosis factor α, free fatty acids) that modulate processes such as insulin secretion, insulin action, and body weight and may contribute to the insulin resistance. In the early stages of the disorder, glucose tolerance remains normal, despite insulin resistance, because the pancreatic beta cells compensate by increasing insulin output. As insulin resistance and compensatory hyperinsulinemia progress, the pancreatic islets become unable to sustain the hyperinsulinemic state. IGT, marked by elevations in postprandial glucose, then develops. A further decline in insulin secretion and an increase in hepatic glucose production lead to overt diabetes with fasting hyperglycemia. Ultimately, beta cell failure may ensue.

Metabolic Abnormalities • Insulin resistance This is caused by the decreased ability of insulin to act effectively on peripheral target tissues (especially muscle and liver) and is a prominent feature of type 2 DM. This resistance is relative, since supernormal levels of circulating insulin will normalize the plasma glucose. Insulin dose-response curves exhibit a rightward shift, indicating reduced sensitivity, and a reduced maximal response, indicating an overall decrease in maximum glucose utilization (30 to 60% lower than normal individuals). Resistance to the action of insulin impairs glucose utilization by insulin-sensitive tissues and increases hepatic glucose output—both effects contributing to the hyperglycemia of diabetes. Increased hepatic glucose output predominantly accounts for increased FPG levels, whereas decreased peripheral glucose usage results in postprandial hyperglycemia. In skeletal muscle, there is a greater impairment in nonoxidative glucose usage (glycogen formation) than in oxidative glucose metabolism through glycolysis. Glucose usage in insulin-independent tissues is not decreased in type 2 DM.

The precise molecular mechanism of insulin resistance in type 2 DM has yet to be elucidated. Insulin receptor levels and tyrosine kinase activity in skeletal muscle are reduced, but these alterations are most likely secondary to hyperinsulinemia and are not a primary defect. Therefore, postreceptor defects are believed to play the predominant role in insulin resistance (Fig. 333-4). Polymorphisms in IRS-1 may be associated with glucose intolerance, raising the possibility that polymorphisms in various postreceptor molecules may combine to create an insulin-resistant state.

A current focus for the pathogenesis of insulin resistance focuses on a PI-3 kinase signaling defect, which causes reduced translocation of GLUT4 to the plasma membrane, among other abnormalities. Of note, not all insulin signal transduction pathways are resistant to the effects of insulin (e.g., those controlling cell growth and differentiation). Consequently, hyperinsulinemia may actually increase the insulin action through these pathways.

Another emerging theory proposes that elevated levels of free fatty acids, a common feature of obesity, may contribute to the pathogenesis of type 2 DM in several different ways. Free fatty acids can impair glucose utilization in skeletal muscle, promote glucose production by the liver, and impair beta cell function.

Impaired insulin secretion Insulin secretion and sensitivity are interrelated (Fig. 333-6). In type 2 DM, insulin secretion initially increases in response to insulin resistance in order to maintain normal glucose tolerance. Initially, the insulin secretory defect is mild and selectively involves glucose-stimulated insulin secretion. The response to other nonglucose secretagogues, such as arginine, is preserved. Eventually, the insulin secretory defect progresses to a state of grossly inadequate insulin secretion. Some endogenous insulin production continues, but the amount secreted is less than the amount secreted by normal individuals at the same plasma glucose concentration.

The reason(s) for the decline in insulin secretory capacity in type 2 DM is unclear. Despite the assumption that a second genetic defect—superimposed upon insulin resistance—leads to beta cell failure, intense genetic investigation has so far excluded mutations in islet candidate genes. Islet amyloid polypeptide or amylin is cosecreted by the beta cell and likely forms the amyloid fibrillar deposit found in the islets of individuals with longstanding type 2 DM. Whether such islet amyloid deposits are a primary or secondary event is not known. The metabolic environment may also impact islet function negatively. For example, chronic hyperglycemia paradoxically impairs islet function ("glucose toxicity") and leads to a worsening of hyperglycemia. Improvement in glycemic control is often associated with improved islet function. In addition, elevation of free fatty acid levels ("lipotoxicity") also worsens islet function.

Increased hepatic glucose production The liver maintains plasma glucose during periods of fasting through glycogenolysis and gluconeogenesis using substrates derived from skeletal muscle and fat (alanine, lactate, glycerol, and fatty acids). Insulin promotes the storage of glucose as hepatic glycogen and suppresses gluconeogenesis. In type 2 DM, insulin resistance in the liver arises from the failure of hyperinsulinemia to suppress gluconeogenesis, which results in fasting hyperglycemia and decreased glucose storage by the liver in the postprandial state. Increased hepatic glucose production occurs early in the course of diabetes, though likely after the onset of insulin secretory abnormalities and insulin resistance in skeletal muscle.

Insulin Resistance Syndromes It is likely that the insulin resistance condition comprises a spectrum of disorders, with hyperglycemia representing one of the most readily diagnosed features. *Syndrome X* is a term used to describe a constellation of metabolic derangements

FIGURE 333-6 Metabolic changes during the development of type 2 diabetes. *A.* The mean plasma insulin and insulin-mediated glucose uptake during an oral glucose tolerance test (OGTT). *B.* The mean plasma glucose during an OGTT. On the x-axis are groups of: control individuals, obese individuals, obese and glucose intolerant individuals, obese individuals with diabetes and high insulin, and obese individuals with diabetes and low insulin. *(From RA DeFronzo: Lilly lecture. The triumvirate: Beta-cell, muscle, liver: A collusion responsible for NIDDM. Diabetes 37:667, 1998, with permission.)*

that includes insulin resistance, hypertension, dyslipidemia, central or visceral obesity, endothelial dysfunction, and accelerated cardiovascular disease. Epidemiologic evidence supports hyperinsulinemia as a marker for coronary artery disease risk, though an etiologic role has not been demonstrated.

A number of forms of severe insulin resistance may be associated with a phenotype similar to that in type 2 DM or IGT (Table 333-1). *Acanthosis nigricans* and signs of hyperandrogenism (hirsutism, acne, and oligomenorrhea) are common physical features. In addition to rare genetic syndromes seen in early childhood, two distinct syndromes of severe insulin resistance have been described in adults: (1) type A, which affects young women and is characterized by severe hyperinsulinemia, obesity, and features of hyperandrogenism; and (2) type B, which affects middle-aged women and is characterized by severe hyperinsulinemia, features of hyperandrogenism, and autoimmune disorders. Individuals with the type A insulin resistance syndrome have an undefined defect in the insulin signaling pathway; individuals with the type B insulin resistance syndrome have autoantibodies directed at the insulin receptor. These receptor autoantibodies may block insulin binding or may stimulate the insulin receptor, leading to intermittent hypoglycemia.

Polycystic ovary syndrome (PCOS) is a common disorder that affects premenopausal women and is characterized by chronic anovulation and hyperandrogenism. Insulin resistance is seen in a significant subset of women with PCOS, and the disorder substantially increases the risk for type 2 DM, independent of the effects of obesity. Both metformin and thiazolidinediones may attenuate hyperinsulinemia, ameliorate hyperandrogenism, and induce ovulation, but are not approved for this indication.

Prevention　Because type 2 DM is preceded by a period of IGT, a number of life-style modifications and pharmacologic agents have been suggested to prevent or delay its onset. Individuals with a strong family history or those at high risk for developing DM should be strongly encouraged to maintain a normal body mass index and to engage in regular physical activity. Beyond this general advice, however, there are no specific interventions proven to prevent type 2 DM. Clinical trials of various interventions in individuals with IGT or early DM are underway in the United States and worldwide.

MODY: GENETICALLY DEFINED, MONOGENIC FORMS OF DIABETES MELLITUS

Several monogenic forms of DM have recently been identified. MODY comprises a phenotypically and genetically heterogeneous subtype of DM. Onset of the disease typically occurs between the ages of 10 and 25. Five different variants of MODY, due to mutations in genes encoding islet cell transcription factors or glucokinase (Fig. 333-3), have been identified so far, and all are transmitted as autosomal dominant disorders (Table 333-1). MODY 2, the most common variant, is caused by mutations in the glucokinase gene. Glucokinase catalyzes the formation of glucose-6-phosphate from glucose, a reaction that is important for glucose sensing by the beta cells and for glucose utilization by the liver. As a result of glucokinase mutations, higher glucose levels are required to elicit insulin secretory responses, thus altering the set point for insulin secretion. MODY 1, MODY 3, and MODY 5 are caused by mutations in the hepatocyte nuclear transcription factors HNF-4α, HNF-1α, and HNF-1β, respectively. As their names imply, these transcription factors are expressed in the liver but also in other tissues, including the pancreatic islets. The mechanisms by which such mutations lead to DM is not well understood, but it is likely that these factors affect islet development or the transcription of genes that are important in stimulating insulin secretion. MODY 4 is a rare variant caused by mutations in the insulin promoter factor (IPF-1), which is a transcription factor that regulates both pancreatic development and insulin gene transcription. Homozygous inactivating mutations lead to pancreatic agenesis, whereas heterozygous mutations result in early-onset DM. Studies of populations with type 2 DM suggest that mutations in the glucokinase gene and various islet cell transcription factors do not account for ordinary type 2 DM. Nevertheless, elucidation of the molecular genetics underlying these rare forms of DM has been important in identifying critical steps in the control of pancreatic beta cell function.

COMPLICATIONS OF DM

ACUTE COMPLICATIONS　Diabetic ketoacidosis (DKA) and nonketotic hyperosmolar state (NKHS) are acute complications of diabetes. DKA is seen primarily in individuals with type 1 DM, and NKHS is seen in individuals with type 2 DM. Both disorders are associated with absolute or relative insulin deficiency, volume depletion, and altered mental status. DKA and NKHS exist along a continuum of hyperglycemia, with or without ketosis. The metabolic similarities and differences in DKA and NKHS are highlighted in Table 333-4. Both disorders are associated with potentially serious complications if not promptly diagnosed and treated.

DIABETIC KETOACIDOSIS　**Clinical Features**　The symptoms and physical signs of DKA are listed in Table 333-5. DKA may be the initial symptom complex that leads to a diagnosis of type 1 DM, but more frequently it occurs in individuals with established diabetes. Nausea and vomiting are often prominent, and their presence in an individual with diabetes warrants laboratory evaluation for DKA. Abdominal pain may be severe and sometimes suggests acute pancreatitis or ruptured viscous. Hyperglycemia leads to glucosuria, volume depletion, tachycardia, and possibly hypotension. Kussmaul respirations and an acetone odor on the patient's breath (both secondary to metabolic acidosis) are classic signs of the disorder. Lethargy and central nervous system depression may evolve into coma with severe DKA. Cerebral edema, an extremely serious complication of DKA, is seen most frequently in children. Signs of infection, which may precipitate DKA, should be sought on physical examination, even in the absence of fever.

Pathophysiology　DKA results from insulin deficiency combined with counterregulatory hormone excess (glucagon, catecholamines, cortisol, and growth hormone). Both insulin deficiency and glucagon excess, in particular, are necessary for DKA to develop. The hyperglycemia of DKA results from increased hepatic glucose production (gluconeogenesis and glycogenolysis) and impaired peripheral glucose utilization. The decreased ratio of insulin to glucagon promotes gluconeogenesis, glycogenolysis, and ketone body formation in the liver, as well as increasing substrate delivery from fat and muscle (free fatty acids, amino acids) to the liver.

The combination of insulin deficiency and hyperglycemia reduces the hepatic level of fructose-2,6-phosphate, which alters the activity of phosphofructokinase and fructose-1,6-bisphosphatase. Glucagon excess decreases the activity of pyruvate kinase, whereas insulin deficiency increases the activity of phosphoenolpyruvate carboxykinase. These hepatic changes shift the handling of pyruvate toward glucose synthesis and away from glycolysis. Glycogenolysis is promoted by the increased levels of glucagon and catecholamines in the face of low insulin levels. Insulin deficiency also reduces levels of the GLUT4 glucose transporter, which impairs glucose uptake into skeletal muscle and fat and reduces intracellular glucose metabolism (Fig. 333-4).

Ketosis results from a marked increase in free fatty acid release from adipocytes, with a resulting shift toward ketone body synthesis in the liver. Reduced insulin levels, in combination with elevations in catecholamines and growth hormone, lead to an increase in lipolysis and release of free fatty acids. Normally, these free fatty acids are converted to triglycerides or very low density lipoproteins (VLDL) in the liver, but in DKA, hyperglucagonemia alters hepatic metabolism to favor ketone body formation, through activation of the enzyme carnitine palmitoyltransferase I. This enzyme is crucial for regulating fatty acid transport into

Table 333-4　Laboratory Values in Diabetic Ketoacidosis (DKA) and Nonketotic Hyperosmolar States (NKHS) (Representative Ranges at Presentation)

	DKA	NKHS
Glucose,[a] mmol/L (mg/dL)	16.7–33.3 (300–600)	33.3–66.6 (600–1200)
Sodium, meq/L	125–135	135–145
Potassium,[a] meq/L	Normal to ↑[b]	Normal
Magnesium [a]	Normal[b]	Normal
Chloride[a]	Normal	Normal
Phosphate[a]	↓	Normal
Creatinine, μmol/L (mg/dL)	Slightly ↑	Moderately ↑
Osmolality, mOsm/mL	300–320	330–380
Plasma ketones[a]	++++	+/−
Serum bicarbonate,[a] meq/L	<15 meq/L	Normal to slightly ↓
Arterial pH	6.8–7.3	>7.3
Arterial P_{CO_2}, mmHg	20–30	Normal
Anion gap[a] [Na − (Cl + HCO$_3$)], meq/L	↑	Normal to slightly ↑

[a] Large changes occur during treatment of DKA.

[b] Although plasma levels may be normal or high at presentation, total-body stores are usually depleted.

Table 333-5 Manifestations of Diabetic Ketoacidosis

Symptoms	Physical findings
Nausea/vomiting	Tachycardia
Thirst/polyuria	Dry mucous membranes/reduced
Abdominal pain	skin turgor
Altered mental function	Dehydration / hypotension
Shortness of breath	Tachypnea / Kussmaul respira-
Precipitating events	tions/respiratory distress
Inadequate insulin administration	Abdominal tenderness (may re-
Infection (pneumonia/UTI/gas-	semble acute pancreatitis or sur-
troenteritis/sepsis)	gical abdomen)
Infarction (cerebral, coronary,	Fever
mesenteric, peripheral)	Lethargy /obtundation / cerebral
Drugs (cocaine)	edema / possibly coma

NOTE: UTI, urinary tract infection.

the mitochondria, where beta oxidation and conversion to ketone bodies occurs. At physiologic pH, ketone bodies exist as ketoacids, which are neutralized by bicarbonate. As bicarbonate stores are depleted, metabolic acidosis ensues. Increased lactic acid production also contributes to the acidosis. The increased free fatty acids result in increased triglyceride production and increased hepatic production of VLDL. VLDL clearance is also reduced because the activity of insulin-sensitive lipoprotein lipase is decreased. Hypertriglyceridemia may be severe enough to cause pancreatitis.

DKA can be precipitated by inadequate levels of plasma insulin for a variety of reasons (Table 333-5). Most commonly, DKA is precipitated when relatively insufficient insulin is available when insulin requirements increase, as might occur during a concurrent illness. Failure to augment insulin therapy appropriately by the patient or health care team compounds the problem. Occasionally, complete omission of insulin by the patient or health care team (in a hospitalized patient with type 1 DM) precipitates DKA. Patients using insulin infusion devices with short-acting insulin have a greater potential for DKA, since even a brief interruption in insulin delivery (e.g., mechanical malfunction) quickly leads to insulin deficiency.

Laboratory Abnormalities and Diagnosis The timely diagnosis of DKA is crucial and allows for prompt initiation of therapy. DKA is characterized by hyperglycemia, ketosis, and metabolic acidosis (increased anion gap) along with a number of secondary metabolic derangements (Table 333-4)). Serum bicarbonate is frequently <10 mmol/L, and arterial pH ranges between 6.8 and 7.3, depending on the severity of the acidosis. Despite a total-body potassium deficit, the serum potassium at presentation is typically at the high end of the normal range or mildly elevated, secondary to the acidosis. Total-body stores of sodium, chloride, phosphorous, and magnesium are also reduced in DKA, but are not accurately reflected by their levels in the serum. Elevated blood urea nitrogen (BUN) and serum creatinine levels reflect intravascular volume depletion. Interference from acetoacetate may falsely elevate the serum creatinine measurement. Leukocytosis, hypertriglyceridemia, and hyperlipoproteinemia are commonly found as well. Hyperamylasemia may suggest a diagnosis of pancreatitis, especially when accompanied by abdominal pain. However, in DKA the amylase is usually of salivary origin and thus is not diagnostic of pancreatitis.

The measured serum sodium is reduced as a consequence of the hyperglycemia [1.6 meq (1.6 mmol/L) reduction in serum sodium for each 100 mg/dL (5.6 mmol/L) rise in the serum glucose]. A normal serum sodium in the setting of DKA indicates a more profound water deficit. In "conventional" units, the calculated serum osmolality [2 × (serum sodium + serum potassium) + plasma glucose (mg/dL)/18 + BUN/2.8] is mildly to moderately elevated, though to a lesser degree than that found in NKHS hyperosmolar state (see below).

In DKA, the ketone body, β-hydroxybutyrate, is synthesized at a threefold greater rate than acetoacetate; however, the latter ketone body is preferentially detected by a commonly used ketosis detection reagent (nitroprusside). Serum ketones are present at significant levels (usually positive at serum dilution of 1:8 or greater). The nitroprusside

tablet, or stick, is often used to detect urine ketones; certain medications such as captopril or penicillamine may cause false-positive reactions. Serum or plasma assays for β-hydroxybutyrate more accurately reflect the true ketone body level.

The metabolic derangements of DKA exist along a spectrum, beginning with mild acidosis with moderate hyperglycemia evolving into more severe findings. The degree of acidosis and hyperglycemia do not necessarily correlate closely, as a variety of factors determine the level of hyperglycemia (oral intake, urinary glucose loss). Ketonemia is a consistent finding in DKA and distinguishes it from simple hyperglycemia.

℞ **TREATMENT** The management of DKA is outlined in Table 333-6. After initiating intravenous fluid replacement and insulin therapy, the agent or event that precipitated the episode of DKA should be sought and aggressively treated. If the patient is vomiting or has altered mental status, a nasogastric tube should be inserted to prevent aspiration of gastric contents. Central to successful treatment of DKA is careful patient monitoring and frequent reassessment to ensure that the patient and the metabolic derangements are improving. A comprehensive flow sheet should record chronologic changes in vital signs, fluid intake and output, and laboratory values as a function of insulin administered.

After the initial bolus of normal saline, replacement of the sodium and free water deficit is carried out over the next 24 h (fluid deficit is often 3 to 5 L). When hemodynamic stability and adequate urine output are achieved, intravenous fluids should be switched to 0.45% saline at a rate of 200 to 300 mL/h, depending on the calculated volume deficit. The change to 0.45% saline helps reduce the trend toward hyperchloremia later in the course of DKA. Alternatively, initial use of lactated Ringer's intravenous solution may reduce the hyperchloremia that commonly occurs with normal saline.

A bolus of intravenous or intramuscular insulin (10 to 20 units) should be administered immediately (Table 333-6)), and subsequent treatment should provide continuous and adequate levels of circulating insulin. Intravenous administration is preferred, because it assures

Table 333-6 Management of Diabetic Ketoacidosis

1. Confirm diagnosis (↑ plasma glucose, positive serum ketones, metabolic acidosis).
2. Admit to hospital; intensive-care setting may be necessary for frequent monitoring or if pH < 7.00 or unconscious.
3. Assess: Serum electrolytes (K^+, Na^+, Mg^{2+}, Cl^-, bicarbonate, phosphate)
   Acid-base status—pH, HCO_3^-, P_{CO_2}
   Renal function (creatinine, urine output)
4. Replace fluids: 2–3 L 0.9% saline over first 1–3 h (5–10 mL/kg per hour); subsequently, 0.45% saline at 150–300 mL/h; change to 5% glucose and 0.45% saline at 100–200 mL/h when plasma glucose reaches 14 mmol/L (250 mg/dL).
5. Administer regular insulin: 10–20 units IV or IM, then 5–10 units/h by continuous IV infusion; increase 2- to 10-fold if no response by 2–4 h.
6. Assess patient: What precipitated the episode (noncompliance, infection, trauma, infarction, cocaine)? Initiate appropriate workup for precipitating event [cultures, chest x-ray, electrocardiogram (ECG)]
7. Measure capillary glucose every 1–2 h; measure electrolytes (especially K^+, bicarbonate, phosphate) and anion gap every 4 h for first 24 h.
8. Monitor blood pressure, pulse, respirations, mental status, fluid intake and output every 1–4 h.
9. Replace K^+: 10 meq/h when plasma K^+ < 5.5 meq/L, ECG normal, urine flow, and normal creatinine documented; administer 40–80 meq/h when plasma K^+ < 3.5 meq/L or if bicarbonate is given.
10. Continue above until patient is stable; glucose goal is 8.3–13.9 mmol/L (150–250 mg/dL), until acidosis is resolved. Insulin infusion may be decreased to 1–4 units/h.
11. Administer intermediate or long-acting insulin as soon as patient is eating. Allow for overlap in insulin infusion and subcutaneous insulin injection.

SOURCE: Adapted from M Sperling, in *Therapy for Diabetes Mellitus and Related Disorders*, 1998.

rapid distribution and allows adjustment of the infusion rate as the patient responds to therapy. Intravenous insulin should be continued until the acidosis resolves and the patient is metabolically stable. As the acidosis and insulin resistance associated with DKA resolve, the insulin infusion rate can be decreased (to 1 to 4 units/h). Intermediate or long-acting insulin, in combination with subcutaneous regular insulin, should be administered as soon as the patient resumes eating, as this facilitates transition to an outpatient insulin regimen and reduces length of hospital stay. It is crucial to continue the insulin infusion until adequate insulin levels are achieved by the subcutaneous route. Even relatively brief periods of inadequate insulin administration in this transition phase may allow for DKA relapse.

Hyperglycemia usually improves at a rate of 4.2 to 5.6 mmol/L (75 to 100 mg/dL per hour) as a result of insulin-mediated glucose disposal, reduced hepatic glucose release, and rehydration. The latter reduces catecholamines, increases urinary glucose loss, and expands the intravascular volume. The decline in the plasma glucose within the first 1 to 2 h may be more rapid and is mostly related to volume expansion. When the plasma glucose reaches 13.9 mmol/L (250 mg/dL), glucose should be added to the 0.45% saline infusion to maintain the plasma glucose in the 11.1 to 13.9 mmol/L (200 to 250 mg/dL) range, and the insulin infusion should be continued. Ketoacidosis begins to resolve as insulin reduces lipolysis, increases peripheral ketone body use, suppresses hepatic ketone body formation, and promotes bicarbonate regeneration. However, the acidosis and ketosis resolve at a slower rate than does the hyperglycemia. As ketoacidosis improves, β-hydroxybutyrate is converted to acetoacetate. Ketone body levels may appear to increase if measured by laboratory assays that use the nitroprusside reaction, which only detects acetoacetate and acetone levels. The improvement in acidosis and anion gap, a result of bicarbonate regeneration and decline in ketone bodies, is reflected by a rise in the serum bicarbonate level and the arterial pH. Depending on the rise of serum chloride, the anion gap (but not bicarbonate) will normalize. A hyperchloremic acidosis [serum bicarbonate of 15 to 18 mmol/L (15 to 18 meq/L)] often follows successful treatment and is minimized by the use of hypotonic intravenous solutions. This gradually resolves as the kidney regenerates bicarbonate and excretes chloride.

Potassium stores are depleted in DKA [estimated deficit 3 to 5 mmol/kg (3 to 5 meq/kg)], but the serum potassium may be normal or even elevated at the time of presentation. During treatment with insulin and fluids, various factors contribute to the development of hypokalemia. These include insulin-mediated potassium transport into cells, resolution of the acidosis (which also promotes potassium entry into cells), and urinary loss of potassium salts of organic acids. Thus, potassium repletion should commence as soon as adequate urine output and a normal serum potassium are documented. If the initial serum potassium level is elevated, then potassium repletion should be delayed until the potassium falls into the normal range. Inclusion of 20 to 40 meq of potassium in each liter of intravenous fluid is reasonable, but additional potassium supplements may also be required. To reduce the amount of chloride administered, potassium phosphate or acetate can be substituted for the chloride salt. The goal is to maintain the serum potassium >3.5 mmol/L (3.5 meq/L).

Despite a bicarbonate deficit, bicarbonate replacement is not usually necessary or advisable. In fact, theoretical arguments suggest that bicarbonate administration and rapid reversal of acidosis may impair cardiac function, impair tissue oxygenation, and promote hypokalemia. The results of most clinical trials do not support the routine use of bicarbonate replacement. In the presence of severe acidosis (arterial pH < 7.0 or hypotension unresponsive to fluid resuscitation), some physicians administer bicarbonate [50 to 150 mmol/L (meq/L) of sodium bicarbonate in 250 mL of 0.45% saline over 1 to 2 h until the serum bicarbonate rises to approximately 10 mmol/L (meq/L)]. Hypophosphatemia may result from increased glucose usage, but randomized clinical trials have not demonstrated that phosphate replacement is beneficial in DKA. If the serum phosphate is < 0.32 mmol/L (1.0 mg/dl), then phosphate supplement should be considered and the serum calcium monitored. Hypomagnesemia may develop during DKA therapy and may also require supplementation.

With appropriate therapy, the mortality of DKA is low (<5%) and is related more to the underlying or precipitating event, such as infection or myocardial infarction. The major nonmetabolic complication of DKA therapy is cerebral edema, which most often develops in children as DKA is resolving. The etiology and optimal therapy for cerebral edema are not well established, but overreplacement of free water should be avoided. Venous thrombosis and adult respiratory distress syndrome occasionally complicate DKA.

Following successful treatment of DKA, the physician and patient should review the sequence of events that led to DKA to prevent future recurrences. Foremost is patient education about the symptoms of DKA, its precipitating factors, and the management of diabetes during a concurrent illness. During illness or when oral intake is compromised, patients should: (1) frequently measure the capillary blood glucose; (2) measure urinary ketones when the serum glucose >16.5 mmol/L (300 mg/dL); (3) drink fluids to maintain hydration; (4) continue or increase insulin; and (5) seek medical attention if dehydration, persistent vomiting, or uncontrolled hyperglycemia develop. In this way, early DKA can be detected and treated appropriately on an outpatient basis.

NONKETOTIC HYPEROSMOLAR STATE   Clinical Features   NKHS is most commonly seen in elderly individuals with type 2 DM. Its most prominent features include polyuria; orthostatic hypotension; and a variety of neurologic symptoms that include altered mental status, lethargy, obtundation, seizure, and possibly coma. The prototypical patient is a mildly diabetic, elderly individual with a several week history of polyuria, weight loss, and diminished oral intake that culminates in mental confusion, lethargy, or coma. The physical examination reflects profound dehydration and hyperosmolality and reveals hypotension, tachycardia, and altered mental status. Notably absent are symptoms of nausea, vomiting, and abdominal pain and the Kussmaul respirations characteristic of DKA. NKHS is often precipitated by a serious, concurrent illness such as myocardial infarction or stroke. Sepsis, pneumonia, and other serious infections are frequent precipitants and should be sought thoroughly. In addition, a debilitating condition (prior stroke or dementia) or social situation that compromises water intake may contribute to the development of the disorder. Finally, the development of NKHS can be associated with the use of certain medications (thiazide diuretics, glucocorticoids, phenytoin).

Pathophysiology   Insulin deficiency and inadequate fluid intake are the underlying causes of NKHS. Insulin deficiency increases hepatic glucose production (through glycogenolysis and gluconeogenesis) and impairs glucose utilization in skeletal muscle (see above discussion under DKA). Hyperglycemia induces an osmotic diuresis that leads to profound intravascular volume depletion, which is exacerbated by inadequate fluid replacement. The absence of ketosis in NKHS is not completely understood. Presumably, the insulin deficiency is only relative and less severe than in DKA. Lower levels of counterregulatory hormones and free fatty acids have been found in NKHS than in DKA in some studies. It is also possible that the liver is less capable of ketone body synthesis or that the insulin/glucagon ratio does not favor ketogenesis.

Laboratory Abnormalities and Diagnosis   The laboratory features in NKHS are summarized in Table 333-4. Most notable are the marked hyperglycemia [plasma glucose may be >55.5 mmol/L (1000 mg/dL)], hyperosmolality (>350 mosmol/L), and prerenal azotemia. The measured serum sodium may be normal or slightly low despite the marked hyperglycemia. The corrected serum sodium is usually increased [add 1.6 meq to measured sodium for each 5.6 mmol/L (100 mg/dL) rise in the serum glucose]. In contrast to DKA, acidosis and ketonemia are absent or mild. A small anion gap metabolic acidosis may be present secondary to increased lactic acid. Moderate ketonuria, if present, is secondary to starvation.

℞ **TREATMENT** Volume depletion and hyperglycemia are prominent features of both NKHS and DKA. Consequently, therapy of these disorders involves several shared elements (Table 333-6). In both disorders, careful monitoring of the patient's fluid status, laboratory values, and insulin infusion rate is crucial. Underlying or precipitating problems should be aggressively sought and treated. In NKHS, the volume depletion, free water deficit, and hyperosmolality are greater than in DKA. The patient with NKHS is usually older, more likely to have mental status changes, and thus more likely to have a life-threatening precipitating event with accompanying comorbidities. Even with proper treatment, NKHS has a substantially higher mortality than DKA (up to 50% in some clinical series).

Fluid replacement should initially stabilize the hemodynamic status of the patient (1 to 3 L of 0.9% normal saline over the first 2 to 3 h). Because the fluid deficit in NKHS is accumulated over a period of days to weeks, the rapidity of reversal of the hyperosmolar state must balance the need for free water repletion and the observation that too rapid a reversal may worsen neurologic function. If the serum sodium is >150mmol/L (150 meq/L), 0.45% saline should be used. After hemodynamic stability is achieved, the intravenous fluid administration is directed at reversing the free water deficit using hypotonic fluids (0.45% saline initially then 5% dextrose in water, D_5W). The calculated free water deficit (which averages 9 to 10 L) should be reversed over the next 1 to 2 days (infusion rates of 200 to 300 mL/h of hypotonic solution). Potassium repletion is usually necessary and should be dictated by repeated measurements of the serum potassium. In patients taking diuretics, the potassium deficit can be quite large and may be accompanied by magnesium deficiency. Hypophosphatemia may occur during therapy and can be improved by using KPO_4 and beginning nutrition.

As in DKA, rehydration and volume expansion lower the plasma glucose initially, but insulin is eventually required. In NKHS, patients tend to be more sensitive to insulin than in DKA and dose requirements are not usually as large. A reasonable regimen for NKHS begins with an intravenous insulin bolus of 5 to 10 units followed by intravenous insulin at a constant infusion rate (3 to 7 units/h). As in DKA, glucose should be added to intravenous fluid when the plasma glucose falls to 13.9 mmol/L (250 mg/dL), and the insulin infusion rate should be decreased to 1 to 2 units/h. The insulin infusion should be continued until the patient has resumed eating and can be transferred to a subcutaneous insulin regimen. The patient should be discharged from the hospital on insulin, though some patients can later undergo a trial of oral glucose-lowering agents.

CHRONIC COMPLICATIONS The chronic complications of DM affect many organ systems and are responsible for the majority of morbidity and mortality associated with the disease. Chronic complications can be divided into vascular and nonvascular complications (Table 333-7). The vascular complications of DM are further subdivided into microvascular (retinopathy, neuropathy, nephropathy) and macrovascular complications (coronary artery disease, peripheral vascular disease, cerebrovascular disease). Nonvascular complications include problems such as gastroparesis, sexual dysfunction, and skin changes. This division is rather arbitrary since it is likely that multiple pathogenic processes are involved in all forms of complications.

The risk of chronic complications increases as a function of the duration of hyperglycemia; they usually become apparent in the second decade of hyperglycemia. Since type 2 DM may have a long asymptomatic period of hyperglycemia, many individuals with type 2 DM have complications at the time of diagnosis.

The microvascular complications of both type 1 and type 2 DM result from chronic hyperglycemia. Randomized, prospective clinical trials involving large numbers of individuals with type 1 or type 2 DM have conclusively demonstrated that a reduction in chronic hyperglycemia prevents or reduces retinopathy, neuropathy, and nephropathy. Other incompletely defined factors also modulate the development of complications. For example, despite longstanding DM, some individuals never develop nephropathy or retinopathy. Many of these patients

Table 333-7 Chronic Complications of Diabetes Mellitus

Microvascular	Macrovascular
Eye disease	Coronary artery disease
Retinopathy (nonproliferative/ proliferative)	Peripheral vascular disease
Macular edema	Cerebrovascular disease
Cataracts	Other
Glaucoma	Gastrointestinal (gastroparesis, diarrhea)
Neuropathy	Genitourinary (uropathy/sexual dysfunction)
Sensory and motor (mono- and polyneuropathy)	Dermatologic
Autonomic	
Nephropathy	

have glycemic control that is indistinguishable from those who develop microvascular complications. Because of these observations, it is suspected that a genetic susceptibility for developing particular complications exists. However, the genetic loci responsible for these susceptibilities have not yet been identified.

Evidence implicating a causative role for chronic hyperglycemia in the development of macrovascular complications is less conclusive, but some results suggest a role for chronic hyperglycemia in the development of macrovascular disease. For example, coronary heart disease events and mortality are two to four times greater in patients with type 2 DM. These events correlate with fasting and postprandial plasma glucose levels as well as with the HbA1c. Other factors (dyslipidemia and hypertension) also play important roles in macrovascular complications.

MECHANISMS OF COMPLICATIONS Although chronic hyperglycemia is an important etiologic factor leading to complications of DM, the mechanism(s) by which it leads to such diverse cellular and organ dysfunction is unknown. Three major theories, which are not mutually exclusive, have been proposed to explain how hyperglycemia might lead to the chronic complications of DM (Fig. 333-7).

One hypothesis is that increased intracellular glucose leads to the formation of advanced glycosylation end products (AGEs) via the nonenzymatic glycosylaton of cellular proteins. Nonenzymatic glycosylation results from the interaction of glucose with amino groups on proteins. AGEs have been shown to cross-link proteins (e.g., collagen, extracellular matrix proteins), accelerate atherosclerosis, promote glomerular dysfunction, reduce nitric oxide synthesis, induce endothelial dysfunction, and alter extracellular matrix composition and structure. The serum level of AGEs correlates with the level of glycemia, and these products accumulate as glomerular filtration rate declines.

A second hypothesis proposed to explain how chronic hyperglycemia leads to complications of DM is based on the observation that hyperglycemia increases glucose metabolism via the sorbitol pathway. Intracellular glucose is predominantly metabolized by phosphorylation and subsequent glycolysis, but when intracellular glucose is increased, some glucose is converted to sorbitol by the enzyme aldose reductase. Increased sorbitol concentrations affect several aspects of cellular physiology (decreased myoinositol, altered redox potential) and may lead to cellular dysfunction. However, testing of this theory in humans, using aldose reductase inhibitors, has not demonstrated beneficial effects on clinical endpoints of retinopathy, neuropathy, or nephropathy.

A third hypothesis proposes that hyperglycemia increases the formation of diacylglycerol leading to activation of certain isoforms of protein kinase C (PKC), which, in turn, affect a variety of cellular events that lead to DM-related complications. For example, PKC activation by glucose alters the transcription of genes for fibronectin, type IV collagen, contractile proteins, and extracellular matrix proteins in endothelial cells and neurons in vitro. Growth factors appear to play an important role in DM-related complications. Vascular endothelial growth factor (VEGF) is increased locally in diabetic proliferative ret-

FIGURE 333-7 Possible molecular mechanisms of diabetes-related complications. AGEs, advanced glycation end products; PKC, protein kinase C; DAG, diacylglycerol; cPLA$_2$, phospholipase A$_2$; Na,K-ATPase, sodium-potassium ATPase.

inopathy and decreases after laser photocoagulation. Transforming growth factor β (TGF-β) is increased in diabetic nephropathy and appears to stimulate basement membrane production of collagen and fibronectin by mesangial cells. Other growth factors, such as platelet-derived growth factor, epidermal growth factor, insulin-like growth factor I, growth hormone, basic fibroblast growth factor, and even insulin, have been suggested to play a role in DM-related complications.

Although hyperglycemia serves as the initial trigger for complications of diabetes, it is still unknown whether the same pathophysiologic processes are operative in all complications or whether certain processes predominate in certain organs. Finally, oxidative stress and free radical generation, as a consequence of the hyperglycemia, may also promote the development of complications.

GLYCEMIC CONTROL AND COMPLICATIONS The Diabetes Control and Complications Trial (DCCT) provided definitive proof that reduction in chronic hyperglycemia can prevent many of the early complications of type 1 DM. This large multicenter clinical trial randomized over 1400 individuals with type 1 DM to either intensive or conventional diabetes management, and then evaluated the development of retinopathy, nephropathy, and neuropathy. Individuals in the intensive diabetes management group received multiple administrations of insulin each day along with intense educational, psychological, and medical support. Individuals in the conventional diabetes management group received twice daily insulin injections and quarterly nutritional, educational, and clinical evaluation. The goal in the former group was normoglycemia; the goal in the latter group was prevention of symptoms of diabetes. Individuals in the intensive diabetes management group achieved a substantially lower HbA1c (7.2%) than individuals in the conventional diabetes management group (HbA1c of 9.0%).

Results from the DCCT demonstrated that improvement of glycemic control reduced nonproliferative and proliferative retinopathy (47% reduction), microalbuminuria (39% reduction), clinical nephropathy (54% reduction), and neuropathy (60% reduction). Improved glycemic control also slowed the progression of early diabetic complications. There was a nonsignificant trend in reduction of macrovascular events. The results of the DCCT predicted that individuals in the intensive diabetes management group would gain 7.7 additional years of sight, 5.8 additional years free from end-stage renal disease (ESRD), and 5.6 years free from lower extremity amputations. If all complications of DM were combined, individuals in the intensive diabetes management group would experience 15.3 more years of life

without significant microvascular or neurologic complications of DM as compared to individuals who received standard therapy. This translates into an additional 5.1 years of life expectancy for individuals in the intensive diabetes management group. The benefit of the improved glycemic control during the DCCT persisted even after the study concluded and glycemic control worsened.

The benefits of an improvement in glycemic control occurred over the entire range of HbA1c values (Fig. 333-8), suggesting that at any HbA1c level, an improvement in glycemic control is beneficial. Therefore, there is no threshold beneath which the HbA1c can be reduced and the complications of DM prevented. The clinical implication of this finding is that the goal of therapy is to achieve an HbA1c level as close to normal as possible, without subjecting the patient to excessive risk of hypoglycemia.

Considerable debate has emerged as to whether the DCCT findings are applicable to individuals with type 2 DM, in whom insulin resistance, hyperinsulinemia, and obesity predominate. Concerns have been raised that therapies associated with weight gain and additional insulin therapy may worsen underlying insulin resistance and hyperinsulinemia. Despite these concerns, most available data support extrapolation of the results of the DCCT to individuals with type 2 DM.

The United Kingdom Prospective Diabetes Study (UKPDS) studied the course of >5000 individuals with type 2 DM for >10 years. This complex and important study utilized multiple treatment regimens and monitored the effect of intensive glycemic control and risk factor treatment on the development of diabetic complications. Newly diagnosed individuals with type 2 DM were randomized to (1) intensive management using various combinations of insulin, a sulfonylurea, or metformin; or (2) conventional therapy using dietary modification and pharmacotherapy with the goal of symptom prevention. In addition, individuals were randomly assigned to different antihypertensive regimens. Individuals in the intensive treatment arm achieved an HbA1c of 7.0%, compared to a 7.9% HbA1c in the standard treatment group. The UKPDS demonstrated that each percentage point reduction in HbA1c was associated with a 35% reduction in microvascular complications, a 25% reduction in DM-related deaths, and a 7% reduction in all-cause mortality. As in the DCCT, there was a continuous relationship between glycemic control and development of complications. Although there was no statistically significant effect of

FIGURE 333-8 Relationship of glycemic control and diabetes duration to diabetic retinopathy. The progression of retinopathy in individuals in the Diabetes Control and Complications Trial is graphed as a function of the length of follow-up with different curves for different HbA1c values. (*Adapted from The Diabetes Control and Complications Trial Research Group, Diabetes 44: 968, 1995*)

One of the major findings of the UKPDS was the observation that strict blood pressure control significantly reduced both macro- and microvascular complications. In fact, the beneficial effects of blood pressure control were greater than the beneficial effects of glycemic control. Lowering blood pressure to moderate goals (144/82 mmHg) reduced the risk of DM-related death, stroke, microvascular end points, retinopathy, and heart failure (risk reductions between 32 and 56%). Improved glycemic control did not conclusively reduce (nor worsen) cardiovascular mortality but was associated with improvement with lipoprotein risk profiles, such as reduced triglycerides and increased high-density lipoprotein (HDL).

Similar reductions in the risks of retinopathy and nephropathy were also seen in a small trial of lean Japanese individuals with type 2 DM randomized to either intensive glycemic control or standard therapy with insulin (Kumamoto study). These results demonstrate the effectiveness of improved glycemic control in individuals of different ethnicity with a presumably different etiology of DM (i.e., phenotypically different from those in the DCCT and UKPDS).

The findings of the DCCT, UKPDS, and Kumamoto study support the idea that chronic hyperglycemia plays a causative role in the pathogenesis of diabetic microvascular complications. These landmark studies prove the value of metabolic control and emphasize the importance of (1) intensive glycemic control in all forms of DM, and (2) early diagnosis and strict blood pressure control in type 2 DM.

OPHTHALMOLOGIC COMPLICATIONS OF DIABETES MELLITUS

DM is the leading cause of blindness between the ages of 20 and 74 in the United States. The gravity of this problem is highlighted by the finding that individuals with DM are 25 times more likely to become legally blind than individuals without DM. Blindness is primarily the result of progressive diabetic retinopathy and clinically significant macular edema. Diabetic retinopathy is classified into two stages: nonproliferative and proliferative. *Nonproliferative diabetic retinopathy* usually appears late in the first decade or early in the second decade of the disease and is marked by retinal vascular microaneurysms, blot hemorrhages, and cotton wool spots (**see Plate IV-15**). Mild nonproliferative retinopathy progresses to more extensive disease, characterized by changes in venous vessel caliber, intraretinal microvascular abnormalities, and more numerous microaneurysms and hemorrhages. The pathophysiologic mechanisms invoked in nonproliferative retinopathy include loss of retinal pericytes, increased retinal vascular permeability, alterations in retinal blood flow, and abnormal retinal microvasculature, all of which lead to retinal ischemia.

The appearance of neovascularization in response to retinal hypoxia is the hallmark of *proliferative diabetic retinopathy*. These newly formed vessels may appear at the optic nerve and/or macula and rupture easily, leading to vitreous hemorrhage, fibrosis, and ultimately retinal detachment. Not all individuals with nonproliferative retinopathy develop proliferative retinopathy, but the more severe the nonproliferative disease, the greater the chance of evolution to proliferative retinopathy within 5 years. This creates a clear opportunity for early detection and treatment of diabetic retinopathy (discussed below). In contrast, *clinically significant macular edema* may appear when only nonproliferative retinopathy is present. Fluorescein angiography is often useful to detect macular edema, which is associated with a 25% chance of moderate visual loss over the next 3 years.

Duration of DM and degree of glycemic control are the best predictors of the development of retinopathy. Nonproliferative retinopathy is found in almost all individuals who have had DM for >20 years (25% incidence with 5 years, and 80% incidence with 15 years of type 1 DM). Although there is genetic susceptibility for retinopathy, it confers less influence on the development of retinopathy than either the duration of DM or the degree of glycemic control.

℞ **TREATMENT** The most effective therapy for diabetic retinopathy is prevention. Intensive glycemic control will greatly delay the development or slow the progression of retinopathy in individ-

uals with either type 1 or type 2 DM. Paradoxically, during the first 6 to 12 months of improved glycemic control, established diabetic retinopathy may transiently worsen. Fortunately, this progression is temporary, and in the long term, improved glycemic control is associated with less diabetic retinopathy. Individuals with known retinopathy should be considered candidates for prophylactic photocoagulation when initiating intensive therapy. Once advanced retinopathy is present, improved glycemic control imparts less benefit, though adequate ophthalmologic care can prevent most blindness.

Equally as important as glycemic control are regular, comprehensive eye examinations for all individuals with DM. Most diabetic eye disease can be successfully treated if detected early. Routine, nondilated eye examinations by the primary care provider or diabetes specialist are *inadequate* to detect diabetic eye disease properly. The treatment of diabetic eye disease requires an ophthalmologist experienced in these disorders. Laser photocoagulation is very successful in preserving vision. Proliferative retinopathy is usually treated with panretinal laser photocoagulation, whereas macular edema is treated with focal laser photocoagulation. Although exercise has not been conclusively shown to worsen proliferative diabetic retinopathy, most ophthalmologists advise individuals with advanced diabetic eye disease to limit physical activities associated with repeated Valsalva maneuvers. Aspirin therapy (650 mg/d) does not appear to influence the natural history of diabetic retinopathy, but studies of other antiplatelet agents are under way.

RENAL COMPLICATIONS OF DIABETES MELLITUS

Diabetic nephropathy is the leading cause of ESRD in the United States and a leading cause of DM-related morbidity and mortality. Proteinuria in individuals with DM is associated with markedly reduced survival and increased risk of cardiovascular disease. Individuals with diabetic nephropathy almost always have diabetic retinopathy also.

Like other microvascular complications, the pathogenesis of diabetic nephropathy is related to chronic hyperglycemia (Fig. 334-7). The mechanisms by which chronic hyperglycemia leads to ESRD, though incompletely defined, involve the following: interaction of soluble factors (growth factors, angiotensin II, endothelin, AGEs), hemodynamic alterations in the renal microcirculation (glomerular hyperfiltration, increased glomerular capillary pressure), and structural changes in the glomerulus (increased extracellular matrix, basement membrane thickening, mesangial expansion, fibrosis). Some of these effects may be mediated through angiotensin receptors. Smoking accelerates the decline in renal function.

The natural history of diabetic nephropathy is shown schematically in Fig. 333-9 and is characterized by a fairly predictable pattern of events. Although this sequence of events was defined for individuals with type 1 DM, a similar pattern is also likely in type 2 DM. Glomerular hyperfusion and renal hypertrophy occur in the first years after the onset of DM and are reflected by an increased glomerular filtration rate (GFR). During the first 5 years of DM, thickening of the glomerular basement membrane, glomerular hypertrophy, and mesangial volume expansion occur as the GFR returns to normal. After 5 to 10 years of type 1 DM, ~40% of individuals begin to excrete small amounts of albumin in the urine (microalbuminuria). *Microalbuminuria* is defined as 30 to 300 mg/d in a 24-h collection or 30 to 300 μg/mg creatinine in a spot collection. The appearance of microalbuminuria (incipient nephropathy) in type 1 DM is a very important predictor of progression to overt proteinuria (>300 mg/d). Blood pressure may rise slightly at this point but usually remains in the normal range. Once overt proteinuria is present, there is a steady decline in GFR, and ~50% of individuals reach ESRD in 7 to 10 years. The early pathologic changes and albumin excretion abnormalities are reversible with normalization of plasma glucose. However, once nephropathy becomes overt, the pathologic changes are likely irreversible.

The nephropathy that develops in type 2 DM differs from that of

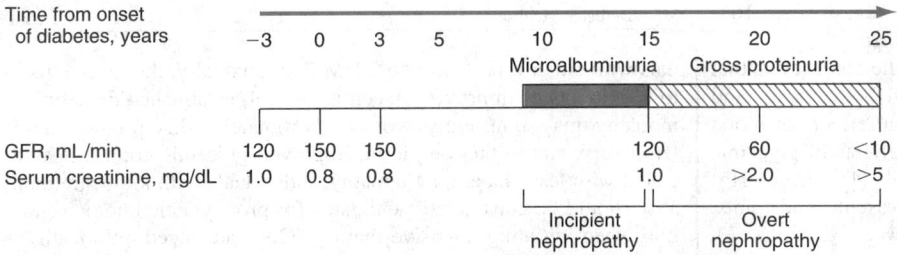

Time from onset of diabetes, years	−3	0	3	5	10	15	20	25

Microalbuminuria   Gross proteinuria

| GFR, mL/min | 120 | 150 | 150 | | 120 | 60 | <10 |
| Serum creatinine, mg/dL | 1.0 | 0.8 | 0.8 | | 1.0 | >2.0 | >5 |

Incipient nephropathy   Overt nephropathy

FIGURE 333-9 Time course of development of diabetic nephropathy. The relationship of time from onset of diabetes, the glomerular filtration rate (GFR), and the serum creatinine are shown. *(Adapted from DeFronzo RA, in Therapy for Diabetes Mellitus and Related Disorders, 1998)*

type 1 DM in the following respects: (1) microalbuminuria or overt nephropathy may be present when type 2 DM is diagnosed, reflecting its long asymptomatic period; (2) hypertension more commonly accompanies microalbuminuria or overt nephropathy in type 2 DM; and (3) microalbuminuria may be less predictive of progression to overt nephropathy in type 2 DM. Finally, it should be noted that albuminuria in type 2 DM may be secondary to factors unrelated to DM, such as hypertension, congestive heart failure, prostate disease, or infection.

Other renal problems may also occur in individuals with DM. Type IV renal tubular acidosis (hyporeninemic hypoaldosteronism) occurs in many individuals with DM. These individuals develop a propensity to hyperkalemia, which may be exacerbated by medications [especially angiotensin-converting enzyme (ACE) inhibitors]. Patients with DM are predisposed to radiocontrast-induced nephrotoxicity. Individuals with DM undergoing radiographic procedures with contrast dye should be well hydrated before and after dye exposure, and the serum creatinine should be monitored for several days following the procedure.

℞ **TREATMENT** The optimal therapy for diabetic nephropathy is prevention. As part of comprehensive diabetes care, microalbuminuria should be detected at an early stage when effective therapies can be instituted. The recommended strategy for detecting microalbuminuria is outlined in Fig. 333-10. Interventions effective in slowing progression from microalbuminuria to overt nephropathy include: (1) near normalization of glycemia, (2) strict blood pressure control, and (3) administration of ACE inhibitors.

Improved glycemic control reduces the rate at which microalbuminuria appears and progresses in both type 1 and type 2 DM. However, once overt nephropathy exists, it is unclear whether improved glycemic control will slow progression of renal disease. During the

FIGURE 333-10 Screening for microalbuminuria. *(Adapted from DeFronzo RA, in Therapy for Diabetes Mellitus and Related Disorders, 1998)*

phase of declining renal function, insulin requirements may fall as the kidney is a site of insulin degradation. Furthermore, glucose-lowering medications (sulfonylureas and metformin) may accumulate and are contraindicated in renal insufficiency.

Many individuals with type 1 or type 2 DM develop hypertension. Numerous studies in both type 1 and type 2 DM demonstrate the effectiveness of strict blood pressure control in reducing albumin excretion and slowing the decline in renal function. Blood pressure should be maintained at <130/85 mmHg in diabetic individuals without proteinuria. A slightly lower blood pressure (120/80) should be targeted for individuals with microalbuminuria or overt nephropathy. Treatment of hypertension is discussed below.

ACE inhibitors reduce the progression of overt nephropathy in individuals with type 1 or type 2 DM and should be prescribed in individuals with type 1 or type 2 DM and microalbuminuria. After 2 to 3 months of therapy, measurement of proteinuria should be repeated and the drug dose increased until either the albuminuria disappears or the maximum dose is reached. If an ACE inhibitor has an unacceptable side-effect profile (hyperkalemia, cough, and renal insufficiency), angiotensin II receptor blockers and calcium channel blockers (phenylalkylamine class) are alternatives. However, their efficacy in slowing the fall in glomerular filtration rate is not proven. Blood pressure control with any agent is extremely important, but a drug-specific benefit in diabetic nephropathy, independent of blood pressure control, has been shown only for ACE inhibitors.

A consensus panel of the American Diabetes Association (ADA) suggests modest restriction of protein intake in diabetic individuals with microalbuminuria (0.8 g/kg per day, which is the adult Recommended Daily Allowance, and about 10% of the daily caloric intake). Protein intake should be restricted further in individuals with overt diabetic nephropathy (0.6 g/kg per day), though conclusive proof of the efficacy of protein restriction is lacking.

Nephrology consultation should be considered after the diagnosis of early nephropathy. Once overt nephropathy ensues, the likelihood of ESRD is very high. As compared to nondiabetic individuals, hemodialysis in patients with DM is associated with more frequent complications, such as hypotension (autonomic neuropathy, loss of reflex tachycardia), more difficult vascular access, and accelerated progression of retinopathy. Survival after the onset of ESRD is shorter in the diabetic population compared to nondiabetics with similar clinical features. Atherosclerosis is the leading cause of death in diabetic individuals on dialysis, and hyperlipidemia should be aggressively treated. Renal transplantation from a living-related donor is the preferred therapy but requires chronic immunosuppression. Combined pancreas-kidney transplant offers the promise of normoglycemia but requires substantial expertise.

NEUROPATHY AND DIABETES MELLITUS Diabetic neuropathy occurs in approximately 50% of individuals with long-standing type 1 and type 2 DM. It may manifest as polyneuropathy, mononeuropathy, and/or autonomic neuropathy. As with other complications of DM, the development of neuropathy correlates with the duration of diabetes and glycemic control. Because the clinical features of diabetic neuropathy are similar to those of other neuropathies, the diagnosis of *diabetic* neuropathy should be made only after other possible etiologies are excluded (Chap. 378).

Polyneuropathy/Mononeuropathy The most common form of diabetic neuropathy is distal symmetric *polyneuropathy*. It most frequently presents with distal sensory loss. Hyperesthesia, parathesia, and pain also occur. Any combination of these symptoms may develop as neuropathy progresses. Physical examination reveals sensory loss, loss of ankle reflexes, and abnormal position sense. Parethesia is characteristically perceived as a sensation of numbness, tingling, sharpness, or burning that begins in the feet and spreads proximally. Neuropathic pain develops in some of these individuals, occasionally preceded by improvement in their glycemic control. Pain typically involves the lower extremities, is usually present at rest, and worsens at night. Both an acute (lasting <12 months) and a chronic form of painful diabetic neuropathy have been described. As diabetic neuropathy progresses, the pain subsides and eventually disappears, and a sensory deficit in the lower extremities persists.

Diabetic polyradiculopathy is a syndrome characterized by severe disabling pain in the distribution of one or more nerve roots. It may be accompanied by motor weakness. Intercostal or truncal radiculopathy causes pain over the thorax or abdomen. Involvement of the lumbar plexus or femoral nerve may cause pain in the thigh or hip and may be associated with muscle weakness in the hip flexors or extensors (diabetic amyotrophy). Fortunately, diabetic polyradiculopathies are usually self-limited and resolve over 6 to 12 months.

Mononeuropathy (dysfunction of isolated cranial or peripheral nerves) is less common than polyneuropathy in DM and presents with pain and motor weakness in the distribution of a single nerve. A vascular etiology is favored, but the pathogenesis is unknown. Involvement of the third cranial nerve is most common and is heralded by diplopia. Physical examination reveals ptosis and opthalmoplegia with normal papillary constriction to light. Sometimes cranial nerves IV, VI, or VII (Bell's palsy) are affected. Peripheral mononeuropathies or simultaneous involvement of more than one nerve (mononeuropathy multiplex) may also occur.

Autonomic Neuropathy Individuals with long-standing type 1 or 2 DM may develop signs of autonomic dysfunction involving the cholinergic, noradrenergic, and peptidergic (peptides such as pancreatic polypeptide, substance P, etc.) systems. DM-related autonomic neuropathy can involve multiple systems, including: the cardiovascular, gastrointestinal, genitourinary, sudomotor, and metabolic systems. Autonomic neuropathies affecting the cardiovascular system cause a resting tachycardia and orthostatic hypotension. Reports of sudden death have also been attributed to autonomic neuropathy. Gastroparesis and bladder-emptying abnormalities are also likely related to the autonomic neuropathy seen in DM (discussed below). Hyperhidrosis of the upper extremities and anhidrosis of the lower extremities result from sympathetic nervous system dysfunction. Anhidrosis of the feet can promote dry skin with cracking, which increases the risk of skin ulceration. Autonomic neuropathy may reduce counterregulatory hormone release, leading to an inability to sense hypoglycemia appropriately (*hypoglycemia unawareness*; Chap. 334), thereby subjecting the patient to the risk of severe hypoglycemia and complicating efforts to improve glycemic control.

R̲x̲ **TREATMENT** Treatment of diabetic neuropathy is less than satisfactory. Improved glycemic control should be pursued and will improve nerve conduction velocity, but the symptoms of diabetic neuropathy may not necessarily improve. Efforts to improve glycemic control may be confounded by autonomic neuropathy and hypoglycemia unawareness. Avoidance of neurotoxins (alcohol), supplementation with vitamins for possible deficiencies (B_{12}, B_6, folate; Chap. 75), and symptomatic treatment are the mainstays of therapy. Aldose reductase inhibitors do not currently offer significant symptomatic relief. Loss of sensation in the foot places the patient at risk for ulceration and its sequelae; consequently, prevention of such problems is of paramount importance. Since the pain of acute diabetic neuropathy may resolve over the first year, analgesics may be discontinued as progressive neuronal damage from DM occurs. Chronic, painful diabetic neuropathy is difficult to treat but may respond to tricyclic antidepressants (amitriptyline, desipramine, nortriptyline), gabapentin, nonsteroidal anti-inflammatory agents (avoid in renal dysfunction), and other agents (mexilitine, phenytoin, carbamazepine, capsaicin cream). Referral to a pain management center may be necessary.

Therapy of orthostatic hypotension secondary to autonomic neuropathy is difficult. A variety of agents have limited success (fludrocortisone, midodrine, clonidine, octreotide, and yohimbine) but have

significant side effects. Nonpharmacologic maneuvers (adequate salt intake, avoidance of dehydration and diuretics, and lower extremity support hose) may offer some benefit.

GASTROINTESTINAL/GENITOURINARY DYSFUNCTION Long-standing type 1 and 2 DM may affect the motility and function of gastrointestinal (GI) and genitourinary systems. The most prominent GI symptoms are delayed gastric emptying (gastroparesis) and altered small- and large-bowel motility (constipation or diarrhea). *Gastroparesis* may present with symptoms of anorexia, nausea, vomiting, early satiety, and abdominal bloating. Nuclear medicine scintigraphy after ingestion of a radiolabeled meal is the best study to document delayed gastric emptying, but noninvasive "breath tests" following ingestion of a radiolabeled meal are under development. Though parasympathetic dysfunction secondary to chronic hyperglycemia is important in the development of gastroparesis, hyperglycemia itself also impairs gastric emptying. Nocturnal diarrhea, alternating with constipation, is a common feature of DM-related GI autonomic neuropathy. In type 1 DM, these symptoms should also prompt evaluation for celiac sprue because of its increased frequency. Esophageal dysfunction in long-standing DM is common but usually asymptomatic.

Diabetic autonomic neuropathy may lead to genitourinary dysfunction including cystopathy, erectile dysfunction, and female sexual dysfunction (reduced sexual desire, dyspareunia, reduced vaginal lubrication). Symptoms of diabetic cystopathy begin with an inability to sense a full bladder and a failure to void completely (Chap. 48). As bladder contractility worsens, bladder capacity and the postvoid residual increase, leading to symptoms of urinary hesitancy, decreased voiding frequency, incontinence, and recurrent urinary tract infections. Diagnostic evaluation includes cystometry and urodynamic studies.

Erectile dysfunction and retrograde ejaculation are very common in DM and may be one of the earliest signs of diabetic neuropathy. Erectile dysfunction, which increases in frequency with the age of the patient and the duration of diabetes, may occur in the absence of other signs of diabetic autonomic neuropathy.

R̲x̲ **TREATMENT** Current treatments for these complications of DM are inadequate. Improved glycemic control should be a primary goal, as some aspects (neuropathy, gastric function) may improve as near-normoglycemia is achieved. Smaller, more frequent meals that are easier to digest (liquid) and low in fat and fiber may minimize symptoms of gastroparesis. Cisapride (10 to 20 mg before each meal) is probably the most effective medication but has been removed from use in the U.S. market except under special circumstances. Other agents with some efficacy include dopamine agonists (metoclopramide, 5 to 10 mg, and domperidone, 10 to 20 mg, before each meal) and bethanechol (10 to 20 mg before each meal). Erythromycin interacts with the motilin receptor and may promote gastric emptying. Diabetic diarrhea in the absence of bacterial overgrowth is treated symptomatically with loperamide but may respond to clonidine at higher doses (0.6 mg tid) or octreotide (50 to 75 μg tid subcutaneously). Treatment of bacterial overgrowth with antibiotics is sometimes useful (Chap. 286).

Diabetic cystopathy should be treated with timed voiding or self-catherization. Medications (bethanechol) are inconsistently effective. The drug of choice for erectile dysfunction is sildenafil, but the efficacy in individuals with DM is slightly lower than in the nondiabetic population (Chap. 51). Sexual dysfunction in women may be improved with use of vaginal lubricants, treatment of vaginal infections, and systemic or local estrogen replacement.

CARDIOVASCULAR MORBIDITY AND MORTALITY Cardiovascular disease is increased in individuals with type 1 or type 2 DM. The Framingham Heart Study revealed a marked increase in several cardiovascular diseases in DM including peripheral vascular disease, congestive heart failure, coronary artery disease, myocardial infarction, and sudden death (risk increase from one- to fivefold). The American Heart Association recently designated DM as a major risk factor for cardiovascular disease (same category as smoking, hypertension, and hyperlipidemia). Because of the extremely high frequency of underlying cardiovascular disease in individuals with diabetes (especially in type 2 DM), evidence of atherosclerotic vascular disease should be sought in the individual with diabetes who has symptoms suggestive of cardiac ischemia, peripheral or carotid arterial disease, a resting electrocardiogram indicative of prior infarction, plans to initiate an exercise program, proteinuria, or two other cardiac risk factors (ADA recommendations). The absence of chest pain ("silent ischemia") is common in individuals with diabetes, and a thorough cardiac evaluation is indicated in individuals undergoing major surgical procedures.

The increase in morbidity and mortality appears to relate to the synergism of hyperglycemia with other cardiovascular risk factors. For example, after controlling for all known cardiovascular risk factors, type 2 DM increases the cardiovascular death rate by twofold in men and fourfold in women. Risk factors for macrovascular disease in diabetic individuals include dyslipidemia, hypertension, obesity, reduced physical activity, and cigarette smoking. Additional risk factors specific to the diabetic population include microalbuminuria, gross proteinuria, an elevation in serum creatinine, and altered platelet function. Insulin resistance, as reflected by elevated serum insulin levels, is associated with an increased risk of cardiovascular complications in individuals with and without DM. Individuals with insulin resistance and type 2 DM have elevated levels of plasminogen activator inhibitors (especially PAI-1) and fibrinogen, which enhances the coagulation process and impairs fibrinolysis, thus favoring the development of thrombosis.

Despite proof that improved glycemic control reduces microvascular complications in DM, it is possible that macrovascular complications may be unaffected or even worsened by such therapy. Concerns about the anabolic and atherogenic potential of insulin remain, since in nondiabetic individuals, higher serum insulin levels (indicative of insulin resistance) are associated with a greater risk of cardiovascular morbidity and mortality. In the DCCT, the number of cardiovascular events did not differ between the standard and intensively treated groups. However, the duration of DM in these individuals was relatively short, and the total number of events was very low. An improvement in the lipid profile of individuals in the intensive group [lower total and low-density lipoprotein (LDL) cholesterol, lower triglycerides] suggested that intensive therapy may reduce the risk of cardiovascular morbidity and mortality associated with DM. In the UKPDS, improved glycemic control did not conclusively reduce cardiovascular mortality. Importantly, treatment with insulin and the sulfonylureas did not appear to increase the risk of cardiovascular disease in individuals with type 2 DM, refuting prior claims about the atherogenic potential of these agents.

In addition to coronary artery disease, cerebrovascular disease is increased in individuals with DM (threefold increase in stroke). Individuals with DM have an increased incidence of congestive heart failure (diabetic cardiomyopathy). The etiology of this abnormality is probably multifactorial and includes factors such as myocardial ischemia from atherosclerosis, hypertension, and myocardial cell dysfunction secondary to chronic hyperglycemia.

℞ **TREATMENT** In general, the treatment of coronary disease is no different in the diabetic individual (Chap. 244), though overall prognosis after myocardial infarction is worse in the diabetic population. Revascularization procedures for coronary artery disease, including percutaneous transluminal coronary angioplasty (PTCA) and coronary artery bypass grafting (CABG), are less efficacious in the diabetic individual. Initial success rates of PTCA in diabetic individuals are similar to those in the nondiabetic population, but diabetic

patients have higher rates of restenosis and lower long-term patency and survival rates. Perioperative mortality from CABG is not altered in DM, but both short- and long-term survival are reduced. Recent trials indicate that diabetic individuals with multivessel coronary artery disease or who recently suffered a Q-wave myocardial infarction have better long-term survival with CABG than PTCA.

Results of studies investigating the effect of intensive diabetes management on survival rates and cardiovascular events after myocardial infarction have been conflicting. In the face of conflicting data, the ADA has emphasized the importance of glycemic control and aggressive cardiovascular risk modification in all individuals with DM. Despite past trepidation about using beta blockers in individuals who have diabetes, these agents clearly benefit diabetic patients after myocardial infarction, analogous to the benefit in nondiabetic individuals. ACE inhibitors may also be particularly beneficial in reducing mortality after myocardial infarction in patients with DM.

Antiplatelet therapy reduces cardiovascular events in individuals with DM who have coronary artery disease. Current recommendations by the ADA suggest the use of aspirin as secondary prevention of additional coronary events. Although data demonstrating efficacy in primary prevention of coronary events are lacking, antiplatelet therapy should be considered, especially in diabetic individuals with other coronary risk factors such as hypertension, smoking, or hyperlipidemia. The aspirin dose (81 to 325 mg) is the same as that in nondiabetic individuals. Aspirin therapy does not have detrimental effects on renal function or hypertension, nor does it influence the course of diabetic retinopathy or maculopathy.

Cardiovascular Risk Factors • *Dyslipidemia* Individuals with DM may have several forms of dyslipidemia (Chap. 344). Because of the additive cardiovascular risk of hyperglycemia and hyperlipidemia, lipid abnormalities should be aggressively detected and treated as part of comprehensive diabetes care (Fig. 333-11). The most common pattern of dyslipidemia is hypertriglyceridemia and reduced HDL cholesterol levels. DM itself does not increase levels of LDL, but the small dense LDL particles found in type 2 DM are more atherogenic because they are more easily glycated and susceptible to oxidation.

According to guidelines of the ADA and the American Heart Association, the lipid profile in diabetic individuals without cardiovascular disease (primary prevention) should be: LDL < 3.4 mmol/L (130 mg/dL); HDL > 0.9 mmol/L (35 mg/dL) in men and >1.2 mmol/L

FIGURE 333-11 Dyslipidemia management in diabetes. *Triglycerides increased but <400 mg/dL. †Second line treatment: fibric acid derivative or bile acid–binding resin. ‡Alternative treatment: high dose HMG CoA reductase inhibitor. The level of HDL in women should be 10 mg/dl higher.

(45 mg/dL) in women; and triglycerides < 2.3 mmol/L (200 mg/dL). In diabetic individuals with cardiovascular disease, the LDL goal is < 2.6 mmol/L (100 mg/dL). Because of the risk of cardiovascular disease in diabetic individuals, many authorities recommend that optimal lipid levels for all individuals with DM (with or without cardiovascular disease) should be: LDL < 2.6 mmol/L (100 mg/dL), HDL > 1.15 mmol/L (45 mg/dL) in men and > 1.41 mmol/L (55 mg/dL) in women; and triglycerides < 2.3 mmol/L (200 mg/dL). The ADA recommends dietary modification in diabetic individuals without cardiovascular disease and a LDL cholesterol of 2.6 to 3.3 mmol/L (100 to 129 mg/dL). If multiple cardiovascular risk factors are present, the goal should be a LDL < 2.6 mmol/L (100 mg/dL) even without known cardiovascular disease.

Almost all studies of diabetic dyslipidemia have been performed in individuals with type 2 DM because of the greater frequency of dyslipidemia in this form of diabetes. Interventional studies have shown that the beneficial effects of LDL reduction are similar in the diabetic and nondiabetic populations. Large prospective trials of primary and secondary intervention for coronary heart disease have included a small number of individuals with type 2 DM, and subset analyses have consistently found that reductions in LDL reduce cardiovascular events and morbidity in individuals with DM. Most clinical trials used HMG CoA reductase inhibitors, although a fibric acid derivative was also beneficial in one trial. No prospective studies have addressed similar questions in individuals with type 1 DM.

Based on the guidelines provided by the ADA and the American Heart Association, the order of priorities in the treatment of hyperlipidemia is: (1) lower the LDL cholesterol, (2) raise the HDL cholesterol, and (3) decrease the triglycerides. A treatment strategy depends on the pattern of lipoprotein abnormalities (Fig. 333-11). Initial therapy for all forms of dyslipidemia should include dietary changes, as well as the same life-style modifications recommended in the nondiabetic population (smoking cessation, control of blood pressure, weight loss, increased physical activity). The dietary recommendations for individuals with DM are similar to those advocated by the National Cholesterol Education Program (Chap. 344) and include an increase in monounsaturated fat and carbohydrates and a reduction in saturated fats and cholesterol. Though viewed as important, the response to dietary alterations is often modest [<0.6-mmol/L (<25-mg/dL) reduction in the LDL]. Improvement in glycemic control will lower triglycerides and have a modest beneficial effect on raising HDL. Most medications that improve glycemic control are useful in lowering triglycerides and may raise the HDL slightly. Though fibric acid derivatives have some efficacy and are well tolerated, nicotinic acid may worsen glycemic control and increase insulin resistance; thus, niacin is relatively contraindicated in diabetic patients on oral glucose-lowering agents. As noted above, HMG CoA reductase inhibitors have proven benefit in patients with DM, even with modest elevations in LDL. Combination therapy with an HMG CoA reductase inhibitor and fibric acid derivative may be useful but increases the possibility of myositis. Bile acid–binding resins should not be used if hypertriglyceridemia is present.

Hypertension Hypertension can accelerate other complications of DM, particularly cardiovascular disease and nephropathy. Hypertension therapy should first emphasize life-style modifications such as weight loss, exercise, stress management, and sodium restriction (Chap. 35). Antihypertensive agents should be selected based on the advantages and disadvantages of the therapeutic agent in the context of an individual patient's risk factor profile. ACE inhibitors are glucose- and lipid-neutral and thus positively impact the cardiovascular risk profile. For example, captopril actually improves insulin resistance, reduces LDL slightly, and increases HDL slightly. In one study of nondiabetic individuals, the ACE inhibitor ramipril reduced the risk of developing type 2 DM. Other effective agents include α-adrenergic blockers (prazocin, terazosin, doxazosin), calcium channel blockers, beta blockers (both β_1 selective and nonselective), thiazide diuretics (hydrochlorothiazide and its derivatives), central adrenergic antago-

nists (clonidine, methyldopa), and vasodilators (minoxidil, hydralazine). DM-related considerations include the following:

1. α-Adrenergic blockers slightly improve insulin resistance and positively impact the lipid profile, whereas beta blockers and thiazide diuretics can increase insulin resistance, negatively impact the lipid profile, and slightly increase the risk of developing type 2 diabetes.
2. Beta blockers, often questioned because of the potential masking of hypoglycemic symptoms, are effective agents and hypoglycemic events are rare when cardioselective (β_1) agents are used.
3. Central adrenergic antagonists and vasodilators are lipid- and glucose-neutral.
4. Sympathetic inhibitors and α-adrenergic blockers may be associated with orthostatic hypotension in the diabetic individual with autonomic neuropathy.
5. Calcium channel blockers are glucose- and lipid-neutral, and some evidence suggests that they reduce cardiovascular morbidity and mortality in type 2 DM, particularly in elderly patients with systolic hypertension.

If microalbuminuria or overt albuminuria is present, the optimal antihypertensive agent is an ACE inhibitor. If albumin excretion is normal, then an ACE inhibitor or other antihypertensive agent may be used. Low-dose diuretics and beta blockers are sometimes preferred as initial agents because of their clear efficacy in the nondiabetic population. Since hypertension is often difficult to control with a single agent (especially in type 2 DM), multiple antihypertensive agents are usually required when blood pressure goals (<130/85 mmHg) are not achieved. In this setting, long-acting calcium channel antagonists should be considered as additional, or second-line, agents, as these drugs appear to provide protection against cardiovascular events. ACE inhibitors are contraindicated in pregnant diabetic patients and those anticipating pregnancy. Because of the high prevalence of atherosclerotic disease in individuals with DM, the possibility of renovascular hypertension should be considered when the blood pressure is not readily controlled.

LOWER EXTREMITY COMPLICATIONS   DM is the leading cause of nontraumatic lower extremity amputation in the United States. Foot ulcers and infections are also a major source of morbidity in individuals with DM. The reasons for the increased incidence of these disorders in DM are complex and involve the interaction of several pathogenic factors: neuropathy, abnormal foot biomechanics, peripheral vascular disease, and poor wound healing. The peripheral sensory neuropathy interferes with normal protective mechanisms and allows the patient to sustain major or repeated minor trauma to the foot, often without knowledge of the injury. Disordered proprioception causes abnormal weight bearing while walking and subsequent formation of callus or ulceration. Motor and sensory neuropathy leads to abnormal foot muscle mechanics and to structural changes in the foot (hammer toe, claw toe deformity, prominent metatarsal heads). Autonomic neuropathy results in anhidrosis and altered superficial blood flow in the foot, which promote drying of the skin and fissure formation. Peripheral vascular disease and poor wound healing impede resolution of minor breaks in the skin, allowing them to enlarge and to become infected.

Approximately 15% of individuals with DM develop a foot ulcer, and a significant subset of those individuals will at some time undergo amputation (14 to 24% risk with that ulcer or subsequent ulceration). Risk factors for foot ulcers or amputation include: male sex, diabetes >10 years' duration, peripheral neuropathy, abnormal structure of foot (bony abnormalities, callus, thickened nails), peripheral vascular disease, smoking, and history of previous ulcer or amputation. Glycemic control is also a risk factor—each 2% increase in the HbA1c increases the risk of a lower extremity ulcer by 1.6 times and the risk of lower extremity amputation by 1.5 times.

℞ **TREATMENT**   The optimal therapy for foot ulcers and amputations is prevention through identification of high-risk patients, education of the patient, and institution of measures to prevent ulceration. High-risk patients should be identified during the routine foot examination performed on all patients with DM (see "Ongoing Aspects of Comprehensive Diabetes Care," below). Patient education should emphasize: (1) careful selection of footwear, (2) daily inspection of the feet to detect early signs of poor-fitting footwear or minor trauma, (3) daily foot hygiene to keep the skin clean and moist, (4) avoidance of self-treatment of foot abnormalities and high-risk behavior (e.g., walking barefoot), and (5) prompt consultation with a health care provider if an abnormality arises. Patients at high risk for ulceration or amputation may benefit from evaluation by a foot care specialist. Interventions directed at risk factor modification include orthotic shoes and devices, callus management, nail care, and prophylactic measures to reduce increased skin pressure from abnormal bony architecture. Attention to other risk factors for vascular disease (smoking, dyslipidemia, hypertension) and improved glycemic control are also important.

Despite preventive measures, foot ulceration and infection are common and represent a potentially serious problem. Due to the multifactorial pathogenesis of lower extremity ulcers, management of these lesions must be multidisciplinary and often demands expertise in orthopedics, vascular surgery, endocrinology, podiatry, and infectious diseases. The plantar surface of the foot is the most common site of ulceration. Cellulitis without ulceration is also frequent and should be treated with antibiotics that provide broad-spectrum coverage, including anaerobes (see below).

An infected ulcer is a clinical diagnosis, since superficial culture of any ulceration will likely find multiple possible bacterial pathogens. The infection surrounding the foot ulcer is often the result of multiple organisms (gram-positive and -negative cocci and anaerobes), and gas gangrene may develop in the absence of clostridial infection. Cultures taken from the debrided ulcer base or from purulent drainage are most helpful. Wound depth should be determined by inspection and probing with a blunt-tipped sterile instrument. Plain radiographs of the foot should be performed to assess the possibility of osteomyelitis in chronic ulcers that have not responded to therapy. Nuclear medicine bone scans may be helpful, but overlying subcutaneous infection is often difficult to distinguish from osteomyelitis. Indium-labeled white cell studies are more useful in determining if the infection involves bony structures or only soft tissue, but they are technically demanding. Magnetic resonance imaging of the foot may be the most specific modality, although distinguishing bony destruction due to osteomyelitis from destruction secondary to Charcot arthropathy is difficult. If surgical debridement is necessary, bone biopsy and culture usually provide the answer.

Osteomyelitis is best treated by a combination of prolonged antibiotics and debridement of infected bone. The possible contribution of vascular insufficiency should be considered in all patients. Noninvasive blood-flow studies are often unreliable in DM, and angiography may be required, recognizing the risk of contrast-induced nephrotoxicity. Peripheral vascular bypass procedures are often effective in promoting wound resolution and in decreasing the need for amputation of the ischemic limb.

A growing number of possible treatments for diabetic foot ulcers exist, but they have yet to demonstrate clear efficacy in prospective, controlled trials. A recent consensus statement from the ADA identified six interventions with demonstrated efficacy in diabetic foot wounds: (1) off-loading, (2) debridement, (3) wound dressings, (4) appropriate use of antibiotics, (5) revascularization, and (6) limited amputation. Off-loading is the complete avoidance of weight bearing on the ulcer, which removes the mechanical trauma that retards wound healing. Bed rest and a variety of orthotic devices limit weight bearing on wounds or pressure points. Surgical debridement of neuropathic wounds is important and effective, but clear efficacy of other modalities for wound cleaning (enzymes, soaking, whirlpools) is lacking. Dressings promote wound healing by creating a moist environment and protecting the wound. Antiseptic agents and topical antibiotics should be avoided. Referral for physical therapy, orthotic evaluation, and rehabilitation may be useful once the infection is controlled.

Mild or non-limb-threatening infections can be treated with oral antibiotics (cephalosporin, clindamycin, amoxicillin/clavulanate, and fluoroquinolones), surgical debridement of necrotic tissue, local wound care (avoidance of weight bearing over the ulcer), and close surveillance for progression of infection. More severe ulcers may require intravenous antibiotics as well as bed rest and local wound care. Urgent surgical debridement may be required. Intravenous antibiotics should provide broad-spectrum coverage directed toward *Staphylococcus aureus*, streptococci, gram-negative aerobes, and anaerobic bacteria. Initial antimicrobial regimens include cefotetan, ampicillin/sulbactam, or the combination of clindamycin and a fluoroquinolone. Severe infections, or infections that do not improve after 48 h of antibiotic therapy, require expansion of antimicrobial therapy to treat methicillin-resistant *S. aureus* (e.g., vancomycin) and *Pseudomonas aeruginosa*. If the infection surrounding the ulcer is not improving with intravenous antibiotics, reassessment of antibiotic coverage and reconsideration of the need for surgical debridement or revascularization are indicated. With clinical improvement, oral antibiotics and local wound care can be continued on an outpatient basis with close follow-up. As infection improves, a comprehensive assessment of modifiable risk factors for foot ulceration should be performed and should involve health professionals with expertise in podiatry, orthotics, vascular surgery, and orthopedics.

New information about wound biology has led to a number of new technologies (e.g., living skin equivalents and growth factors such as basic fibroblast growth factor) that may prove useful. Recombinant platelet-derived growth factor has some benefit and complements the basic therapies of off-loading, debridement, and antibiotics. Hyperbaric oxygen has been used, but rigorous proof of efficacy is lacking.

INFECTIONS   Individuals with DM exhibit a greater frequency and severity of infection. The reasons for this increase include incompletely defined abnormalities in cell-mediated immunity and phagocyte function associated with hyperglycemia, as well as diminished vascularization secondary to long-standing diabetes. Hyperglycemia likely aids the colonization and growth of a variety of organisms (*Candida* and other fungal species). Many common infections are more frequent and severe in the diabetic population, whereas several rare infections are seen almost exclusively in the diabetic population. Examples of this latter category includes rhinocerebral mucormycosis and malignant otitis externa, which is usually secondary to *P. aeruginosa* infection in the soft tissue surrounding the external auditory canal. Malignant otitis externa begins with pain and discharge and may progress rapidly to osteomyelitis and meningitis. These infections should be sought, in particular, in patients presenting with NKHS.

Pneumonia, urinary tract infections, and skin and soft tissue infections are all more common in the diabetic population. In general, the organisms that cause pulmonary infections are similar to those found in the nondiabetic population; however, gram-negative organisms, *S. aureus*, and *Mycobacterium tuberculosis* are more frequent pathogens. Urinary tract infections (either lower tract or pyelonephritis) are the result of common bacterial agents such as *Escherichia coli*, though several yeast species (*Candida* and *Torulopsis glabrata*) are commonly observed. Complications of urinary tract infections include emphysematous pyelonephritis and emphysematous cystitis. Bacteriuria occurs frequently in individuals with diabetic cystopathy. Susceptibility to furunculosis, superficial candidal infections, and vulvovaginitis is increased. Poor glycemic control is a common denominator in individuals with these infections. Diabetic individuals have an increased rate of colonization of *S. aureus* in the skin folds and nares. Diabetic patients also have a greater risk of postoperative wound infections.

DERMATOLOGIC MANIFESTATIONS   The most common skin manifestations of DM are protracted wound healing and skin ulcerations. Diabetic dermopathy, sometimes termed *pigmented pretibial papules*, or "diabetic skin spots," begins as an erythematous area and evolves into an area of circular hyperpigmentation. These lesions result from minor mechanical trauma in the pretibial region and are more common in elderly men with DM. Bullous diseases (shallow ulcerations or erosions in the pretibial region) are also seen. *Necrobiosis lipoidica diabeticorum* is a rare disorder of DM that predominantly affects young women with type 1 DM, neuropathy, and retinopathy. It usually begins in the pretibial region as an erythematous plaque or papules that gradually enlarge, darken, and develop irregular margins, with atrophic centers and central ulceration. They may be painful. *Acanthosis nigricans* (hyperpigmented velvety plaques seen on the neck or extensor surfaces) is sometimes a feature of severe insulin resistance and accompanying diabetes. Generalized or localized *granuloma annulare* (erythematous plaques on the extremities or trunk) and *scleredema* (areas of skin thickening on the back or neck at the site of previous superficial infections) are more common in the diabetic population. *Lipoatrophy* and *lipohypertrophy* can occur at insulin injection sites but are unusual with the use of human insulin. Xerosis and pruritus are common and are relieved by skin moisturizers.

Approach to the Patient

DM and its complications produce a wide range of symptoms and signs; those secondary to acute hyperglycemia may occur at any stage of the disease, whereas those related to chronic complications begin to appear during the second decade of hyperglycemia. Individuals with previously undetected type 2 DM may present with chronic complications of DM at the time of diagnosis. The history and physical examination should assess for symptoms or signs of acute hyperglycemia and should screen for the chronic complications and conditions associated with DM.

History A complete medical history should be obtained with special emphasis on DM-relevant aspects such as weight, family history of DM and its complications, risk factors for cardiovascular disease, prior medical conditions, exercise, smoking, and ethanol use. Symptoms of hyperglycemia include polyuria, polydipsia, weight loss, fatigue, weakness, blurry vision, frequent superficial infections (vaginitis, fungal skin infections), and slow healing of skin lesions after minor trauma. Metabolic derangements relate mostly to hyperglycemia (osmotic diuresis, reduced glucose entry into muscle) and to the catabolic state of the patient (urinary loss of glucose and calories, muscle breakdown due to protein degradation and decreased protein synthesis). Blurred vision results from changes in the water content of the lens and resolves as the hyperglycemia is controlled.

In a patient with established DM, the initial assessment should also include special emphasis on prior diabetes care, including the type of therapy, prior HbA1c levels, self-monitoring blood glucose results, frequency of hypoglycemia, presence of DM-specific complications, and assessment of the patient's knowledge about diabetes. The chronic complications may afflict several organ systems, and an individual patient may exhibit some, all, or none of the symptoms related to the complications of DM (see above). In addition, the presence of DM-related comorbidities should be sought (cardiovascular disease, hypertension, dyslipidemia).

Physical Examination In addition to a complete physical examination, special attention should be given to DM-relevant aspects such as weight or body mass index, retinal examination, orthostatic blood pressure, foot examination, peripheral pulses, and insulin injection sites. Careful examination of the lower extremities should seek evidence of peripheral neuropathy, calluses, superficial fungal infections, nail disease, and foot deformities (such as hammer or claw toes and Charcot foot) in order to identify sites of potential skin ulceration. Vibratory sensation (128-MHz tuning fork at the base of the great toe) and the ability to sense touch with a monofilament (5.07, 10-g monofilament) are useful to detect moderately advanced diabetic neuropathy. Since dental disease is more frequent in DM, the teeth and gums should also be examined.

Classification of DM in an Individual Patient The etiology of diabetes in an individual with new-onset disease can usually be assigned on the basis of clinical criteria. Individuals with type 1 DM tend to have the following characteristics: (1) onset of disease prior to age 30; (2) lean body habitus; (3) requirement of insulin as the initial therapy; (4) propensity to develop ketoacidosis; and (5) an increased risk of other autoimmune disorders such as autoimmune thyroid disease, adrenal insufficiency, pernicious anemia, and vitiligo. In contrast, individuals with type 2 DM often exhibit the following features: (1) develop diabetes after the age of 30; (2) are usually obese (80% are obese, but elderly individuals may be lean); (3) may not require insulin therapy initially; and (4) may have associated conditions such as insulin resistance, hypertension, cardiovascular disease, dyslipidemia, or polycystic ovary syndrome. In type 2 DM, insulin resistance is often associated with abdominal obesity (as opposed to hip and thigh obesity) and hypertriglyceridemia. Although most individuals diagnosed with type 2 DM are older, the age of diagnosis appears to be declining in some ethnic groups, and there is a marked increase among overweight teenagers. On the other hand, some individuals (<10%) with the phenotypic appearance of type 2 DM do not have absolute insulin deficiency but have autoimmune markers suggestive of type 1 DM. Thus, despite the revised classification of DM, it is remains difficult to categorize some patients unequivocally. Individuals who deviate from the clinical profile of type 1 and type 2 DM, or who have other associated defects such as deafness, pancreatic exocrine disease, and other endocrine disorders, should be classified accordingly (Table 333-1).

Laboratory Assessment The laboratory assessment should first determine whether the patient meets the diagnostic criteria for DM (Table 333-2) and should then assess the degree of glycemic control (HbA1c, discussed below). In addition to the standard laboratory evaluation, the patient should be screened for DM-associated conditions (e.g., microalbuminuria, dyslipidemia, thyroid dysfunction). Individuals at high risk for cardiovascular disease should be screened for asymptomatic coronary artery disease by appropriate cardiac stress testing, when indicated.

The classification of the type of DM does not usually require laboratory assessments. Serum insulin or C-peptide measurements do not clearly distinguish type 1 from type 2 DM at the time of diabetes onset; a low C-peptide level merely confirms a patient's need for insulin. Conversely, many individuals with new-onset type 1 DM retain some C-peptide production. Measurement of islet cell antibodies at the time of diabetes onset may be useful if the type of DM is not clear based on the characteristics discussed above, but this knowledge does not usually alter therapy, which is based primarily on empirical metabolic features.

LONG-TERM TREATMENT

OVERALL PRINCIPLES The goals of therapy for type 1 or type 2 DM are to: (1) eliminate symptoms related to hyperglycemia, (2) reduce or eliminate the long-term microvascular and macrovascular complications of DM, and (3) allow the patient to achieve as normal a life-style as possible. To reach these goals, the physician should identify a target level of glycemic control for each patient, provide the patient with the educational and pharmacologic resources necessary to reach this level, and monitor/treat DM-related complications. Symptoms of diabetes usually resolve when the plasma glucose is <11.1 mmol/L (200 mg/dL), and thus most DM treatment focuses on achieving the second and third goals.

The care of an individual with either type 1 or type 2 DM requires a multidisciplinary team. Central to the success of this team are the patient's participation, input, and enthusiasm, all of which are essential for optimal diabetes management. Members of the health care team include the primary care provider and/or the endocrinologist or diabetologist, a certified diabetes educator, and a nutritionist. In addition, when the complications of DM arise, subspecialists (including neurologists, nephrologists, vascular surgeons, cardiologists, ophthalmologists, and podiatrists) with experience in DM-related complications are essential.

A number of names are sometimes applied to different approaches to diabetes care, such as intensive insulin therapy, intensive glycemic control, and "tight control." The current chapter, however, will use the term *comprehensive diabetes care* to emphasize the fact that optimal diabetes therapy involves more than plasma glucose management. Though glycemic control is central to optimal diabetes therapy, comprehensive diabetes care of both type 1 and type 2 DM should also detect and manage DM-specific complications and modify risk factors for DM-associated diseases.

In addition to assessing the physical aspects of the patient with DM, the physician and members of the diabetes management team should consider social, family, financial, cultural, and employment-related issues that may have an impact on diabetes care. With this information, the physician can work with the patient and his or her family to establish therapeutic goals and design a comprehensive and feasible plan for optimal diabetes care.

EDUCATION OF THE PATIENT ABOUT DM, NUTRITION, AND EXERCISE Patient participation is an essential component of comprehensive diabetes care. The patient with type 1 or type 2 DM should receive education about nutrition, exercise, care of diabetes during illness, and medications to lower the plasma glucose. Along with improved compliance, patient education allows individuals with DM to assume greater responsibility for their care. Patient education should be viewed as a continuing process with regular visits for reinforcement; it should *not* be a process that is completed after one or two visits to a nurse educator or nutritionist.

Diabetes Education The diabetes educator is a health care professional (nurse, dietician, or pharmacist) with specialized patient education skills who is certified in diabetes education (indicating demonstrated skills in diabetes knowledge and education and certification by the American Association of Diabetes Educators). The educator is a vital member of the comprehensive diabetes care program and educates the patient about a number of issues important for optimal diabetes care, including self-monitoring of blood glucose; urine ketone monitoring (type 1 DM); insulin administration; guidelines for diabetes management during illnesses; management of hypoglycemia; foot and skin care; diabetes management before, during, and after exercise; and risk factor–modifying activities.

Nutrition *Medical nutrition therapy* (MNT) is a term used by the ADA to describe the optimal coordination of caloric intake with other aspects of diabetes therapy (insulin, exercise, weight loss). Historically, nutrition has imposed restrictive, complicated regimens on the patient. Current practices have greatly changed, though many patients and health care providers still view the diabetic diet as monolithic and static. For example, modern MNT now includes foods with sucrose and seeks to modify other risk factors such as hyperlipidemia and hypertension rather than focusing exclusively on weight loss in individuals with type 2 DM. Like other aspects of DM therapy, MNT must be adjusted to meet the goals of the individual patient. Furthermore, MNT education is an important component of comprehensive diabetes care and should be reinforced by regular patient education. In general, the components of optimal MNT are similar for individuals with type 1 or type 2 DM (Table 333-8).

The goal of MNT in the individual with type 1 DM is to coordinate and match the caloric intake, both temporally and quantitatively, with the appropriate amount of insulin. MNT in type 1 DM and self-monitoring of blood glucose must be integrated to define the optimal insulin regimen. MNT must be flexible enough to allow for exercise, and the insulin regimen must allow for deviations in caloric intake. An important component of MNT in type 1 DM is to minimize the weight gain often associated with intensive diabetes management.

Table 333-8 Nutritional Recommendations for All Persons with Diabetes

- Protein to provide ~10–20% of kcal/d (~10% for those with nephropathy)
- Saturated fat to provide <10% of kcal/d (<7% for those with elevated LDL)
- Polyunsaturated fat to provide ≤10% of kcal
- Remaining calories to be divided between carbohydrate and monounsaturated fat, based on medical needs and personal tolerance
- Use of caloric sweeteners, including sucrose, is acceptable. Sugars must be accounted for so that the insulin demand they create is matched to available insulin
- Fiber (20–35 g/d) and sodium (≤3000 mg/d) levels as recommended for the general healthy population
- Cholesterol intake ≤300 mg/d
- The same precautions regarding alcohol use in the general population also apply to individuals with diabetes. In addition, alcohol may increase risk for hypoglycemia and therefore should be taken with food.

NOTE: LDL, low-density lipoprotein.
SOURCE: Adapted from Farkas-Hirsch, 1998.

The goals of MNT in type 2 DM are slightly different and address the greatly increased prevalence of cardiovascular risk factors (hypertension, dyslipidemia, obesity) and disease in this population. The majority of these individuals are obese, and weight loss is still strongly encouraged and should remain an important goal. Medical treatment of obesity is a rapidly evolving area and is discussed in Chap. 77. Hypocaloric diets and modest weight loss often result in rapid and dramatic glucose lowering in individuals with new-onset type 2 DM. Nevertheless, numerous studies document that long-term weight loss is uncommon. Therefore, current MNT for type 2 DM should emphasize modest caloric reduction, increased physical activity, and reduction of hyperlipidemia and hypertension. Increased consumption of soluble, dietary fiber may improve glycemic control in individuals with type 2 DM.

Exercise Exercise is an integral component of comprehensive diabetes care that can have multiple positive benefits (cardiovascular benefits, reduced blood pressure, maintenance of muscle mass, reduction in body fat, weight loss, etc.). For individuals with type 1 or type 2 DM, exercise is also useful for lowering plasma glucose (during and following exercise) and increasing insulin sensitivity.

Despite its benefits, exercise presents several challenges for individuals with DM because they lack the normal glucoregulatory mechanisms. Skeletal muscle is a major site for metabolic fuel consumption in the resting state, and the increased muscle activity during vigorous, aerobic exercise greatly increases fuel requirements. Individuals with type 1 DM are prone to either hyperglycemia or hypoglycemia during exercise, depending on the preexercise plasma glucose, the circulating insulin level, and the level of exercise-induced catecholamines. If the insulin level is too low, the rise in catecholamines may increase the plasma glucose excessively, promote ketone body formation, and possibly lead to ketoacidosis. Conversely, if the circulating insulin level is excessive, this relative hyperinsulinemia may reduce hepatic glucose production (decreased glycogenolysis, decreased gluconeogenesis) and increase glucose entry into muscle, leading to hypoglycemia.

To avoid exercise-related hyper- or hypoglycemia, individuals with type 1 DM should: (1) monitor blood glucose before, during, and after exercise; (2) delay exercise if blood glucose is >14 mmol/L (250 mg/dL), <5.5 mmol/L (100 mg/dL), or if ketones are present; (3) eat a meal 1 to 3 h before exercise and take supplemental carbohydrate feedings at least every 30 min during vigorous or prolonged exercise; (4) decrease insulin doses (based on previous experience) before exercise and inject insulin into a nonexercising area; and (5) learn individual glucose responses to different types of exercise and increase food intake for up to 24 h after exercise, depending on intensity and duration of exercise. In individuals with type 2 DM, exercise-related hypoglycemia is less common but can occur in individuals taking either insulin or sulfonylureas.

Because asymptomatic cardiovascular disease appears at a younger age in both type 1 and type 2 DM, formal exercise tolerance testing may be warranted in diabetic individuals with any of the following: age ≥35 years, long-standing type 1 DM (>20 to 25 years' duration), microvascular complications of DM (retinopathy, microalbuminuria, or nephropathy), peripheral vascular disease, other risk factors of coronary artery disease, or autonomic neuropathy. Untreated proliferative retinopathy is a relative contraindication to vigorous exercise, since this may lead to vitreous hemorrhage or retinal detachment.

MONITORING THE LEVEL OF GLYCEMIC CONTROL Optimal monitoring of glycemic control involves plasma glucose measurements by the patient and an assessment of long-term control by the physician (measurement of HbA1c and review of the patient's self-measurements of plasma glucose). These measurements are complementary: the patient's measurements provide a picture of short-term glycemic control, whereas the HbA1c reflects average glycemic control over the previous 2 to 3 months. Integration of both measurements provides an accurate assessment of the glycemic control achieved.

Self-Monitoring of Blood Glucose Self-monitoring of blood glucose (SMBG) is the standard of care in diabetes management and allows the patient to monitor his or her blood glucose at any time. In SMBG, a small drop of blood and an easily detectable enzymatic reaction allow measurement of the capillary plasma glucose. By combining glucose measurements with diet history, medication changes, and exercise history, the physician and patient can improve the treatment program.

The frequency of SMBG measurements must be individualized and adapted to address the goals of diabetes care as defined by the patient and the health care provider. Individuals with type 1 DM should routinely measure their plasma glucose four to eight times per day to estimate and select mealtime boluses of short-acting insulin and to modify long-acting insulin doses. Most individuals with type 2 DM require less frequent monitoring, though the optimal frequency of SMBG has not been clearly defined. Individuals with type 2 DM who are on oral medications should utilize SMBG as a means of assessing the efficacy of their medication and diet. Since plasma glucose levels fluctuate less in these individuals, one to two SMBG measurements per day (or fewer) may be sufficient. Individuals with type 2 DM who are on insulin should utilize SMBG more frequently than those on oral agents.

Two devices for continuous blood glucose monitoring have been recently approved by the U.S. Food and Drug Administration (FDA). The Glucowatch uses iontophoresis to assess glucose in interstitial fluid, whereas the Minimed device uses an indwelling subcutaneous catheter to monitor interstitial fluid glucose. Both devices utilize immobilized glucose oxidase to generate electrons in response to changing glucose levels. Though clinical experience with these devices is limited, they perform well in clinical trials and appear to provide useful short-term information about the patterns of glucose changes as well as an enhanced ability to detect hypoglycemic episodes.

Although urine glucose testing does not provide an accurate assessment of glycemic control, urine ketones are a sensitive indicator of early diabetic ketoacidosis and should be measured in individuals with type 1 DM when the plasma glucose is consistently 16.7 mmol/L (300 mg/dL); during a concurrent illness; or with symptoms such as nausea, vomiting, or abdominal pain.

Assessment of Long-Term Glycemic Control Measurement of glycated hemoglobin is the standard method for assessing long-term glycemic control. When plasma glucose is consistently elevated, there is an increase in nonenzymatic glycation of hemoglobin; this alteration reflects the glycemic history over the previous 2 to 3 months, since erythrocytes have an average life span of 120 days. There are numerous laboratory methods for measuring the various forms of glycated hemoglobin, and these have significant interassay variations. Because of its superior specificity and reliability, the HbA1c assay performed by the high-performance liquid chromatography (HPLC) method has become the standard reference method for most glycated hemoglobin measurements. Since glycated hemoglobin measurements are usually compared to prior measurements, it is essential for the assay results to

be comparable. Depending on the assay methodology for HbA1c, hemoglobinopathies, hemolytic anemia, and uremia may interfere with the HbA1c result.

Glycated hemoglobin or HbA1c should be measured in all individuals with DM during their initial evaluation and as part of their comprehensive diabetes care. As the primary predictor of long-term complications of DM, the HbA1c should mirror, to a certain extent, the short-term measurements of SMBG. These two measurements are complementary in that recent intercurrent illnesses may impact the SMBG measurements but not the HbA1c. Likewise, postprandial and nocturnal hyperglycemia may not be detected by the SMBG of fasting and preprandial capillary plasma glucose but will be reflected in the HbA1c. When measured by HPLC, the HbA1c approximates the following mean plasma glucose values: an HbA1c of 6% is 6.6 mmol/L (120 mg/dL), 7% is 8.3 mmol/L (150 mg/dL), 8% is 10.0 mmol/L (180 mg/dL), etc. [A 1% rise in the HbA1c translates into a 1.7-mmol/L (30 mg/dL) increase in the mean glucose.] The degree of glycation of other proteins, such as albumin, has been used as an alternative indicator of glycemic control when the HbA1c is inaccurate (hemolytic anemia, hemoglobinopathies). The fructosamine assay (using albumin) is an example of an alternative measurement of glycemic control and reflects the glycemic status over the 2 to 4 prior weeks. Current consensus statements do not favor the use of alternative assays of glycemic control, as there are no studies to indicate whether such assays accurately predict the complications of DM.

℞ TREATMENT Establishment of a Target Level of Glycemic Control Because the complications of DM are related to glycemic control, normoglycemia or near normoglycemia is the desired, but often elusive, goal for most patients. However, normalization of the plasma glucose for long periods of time is extremely difficult, as demonstrated by the DCCT. Regardless of the level of hyperglycemia, improvement in glycemic control will lower the risk of diabetes complications (Fig. 333-8).

The target for glycemic control (as reflected by the HbA1c) must be individualized, and the health care provider should establish the goals of therapy in consultation with the patient after considering a number of medical, social, and life-style issues. Some important factors to consider include the patient's age, ability to understand and implement a complex treatment regimen, presence and severity of complications of diabetes, ability to recognize hypoglycemic symptoms, presence of other medical conditions or treatments that might alter the response to therapy, life-style and occupation (e.g., possible consequences of experiencing hypoglycemia on the job), and level of support available from family and friends.

The ADA has established suggested glycemic goals based on the premise that glycemic control predicts development of DM-related complications. In general, the target HbA1c should be <7.0% (Table 333-9). Other consensus groups (such as the Veterans Administration) have suggested HbA1c goals that take into account the patient's life expectancy at the time of diagnosis and the presence of microvascular complications. Such recommendations strive to balance the financial and personal costs of glycemic therapy with anticipated benefits (reduced health care costs, reduced morbidity). One limitation to this approach is that the onset of hyperglycemia in type 2 DM is difficult to ascertain and likely predates the diagnosis. Furthermore, though the life expectancy can be predicted for a patient population, the physician must treat an individual patient; consequently, the target HbA1c must be individualized to accommodate these other considerations.

Type 1 Diabetes Mellitus • General aspects Comprehensive diabetes care should be instituted in all individuals with type 1 DM and should involve attention to nutrition, exercise, and risk factor management in addition to insulin administration. The ADA recommendations for fasting and bedtime glycemic goals and HbA1c targets are summarized in Table 333-9. The goal is to design and implement insulin regimens that mimic physiologic insulin secretion. Because in-

Table 333-9 Ideal Goals for Glycemic Control[a]

Index	Normal Range	Goal	Additional Action Suggested
Average preprandial glucose, mmol/L (mg/dL)	<5.5 (100)	4.4–6.7 (80–120)	<4.4 (80) or >7.8 (140)
Average bedtime glucose, mmol/L (mg/dL)	<6.1 (110)	5.5–7.8 (100–140)	<5.5 (100) or >8.8 (160)
HbA1c, %	<6	<7	>8

[a] These values are for whole blood measurements, and home glucose-monitoring devices may report either whole blood or plasma glucose values. Plasma glucose values are 10–15% higher than whole blood values. The upper limit of the HbA1c reference range is 6.0% (mean 5.0%, with a standard deviation of 0.5%). These goals must be individualized for each patient and must consider the patient's age and other medical conditions.
SOURCE: Adapted from American Diabetes Association, 2000.

dividuals with type 1 DM lack endogenous insulin production, administration of basal, exogenous insulin is essential for regulating glycogen breakdown, gluconeogenesis, lipolysis, and ketogenesis. Likewise, postprandial insulin replacement should be appropriate for the carbohydrate intake and promote normal glucose utilization and storage.

Intensive management Intensive diabetes management is defined by the ADA as ". . . a mode of treatment for the person with DM that has the goal of achieving euglycemia or near-normal glycemia using all available resources to accomplish this goal." These resources include thorough and continuing patient education, comprehensive recording of plasma glucose measurements and nutrition intake by the patient, and a variable insulin regimen that matches glucose intake and insulin dose. Insulin regimens usually include multiple-component insulin regimens, multiple daily injections (MDI), or insulin infusion devices (all discussed below).

The benefits of intensive diabetes management and improved glycemic control include a reduction in the microvascular complications of DM and a possible delay or reduction in the macrovascular complications of DM. From a psychological standpoint, the patient experiences greater control over his or her diabetes and often notes an improved sense of well-being, greater flexibility in the timing and content of meals, and the capability to alter insulin dosing with exercise. In addition, intensive diabetes management in pregnancy reduces fetal malformation and morbidity. Intensive diabetes management is also strongly encouraged in newly diagnosed patients with type 1 DM because it may prolong the period of C-peptide production, which may result in better glycemic control and a reduced risk of serious hypoglycemia.

Although intensive management confers impressive benefits, it is also accompanied by significant personal and financial costs and is therefore not appropriate for all individuals. It requires a combination of dedication, persistence, and motivation on the part of the patient, as well as medical, educational, nursing, nutritional, and psychological expertise on the part of the diabetes management team. Circumstances in which intensive diabetes management should be strongly considered are listed in Table 333-10.

Insulin preparations Current insulin preparations are generated by recombinant DNA technology and consist of the amino acid se-

Table 333-10 Indications for Intensive Diabetes Management

- Otherwise healthy adults with either type 1 or type 2 diabetes (selected adolescents and older children)
- Purposeful, therapeutic attempt to avoid or lessen microvascular complications
- All pregnant women with diabetes; all women with diabetes who are planning pregnancy
- Management of labile diabetes
- Availability of health care professionals with appropriate expertise
- Patients who have had kidney transplantation for diabetic nephropathy

SOURCE: Adapted from Farkas-Hirsch, 1998.

quence of human insulin. Animal insulin (beef or pork) is no longer used. Human insulin has been formulated with distinctive pharmacokinetics to mimic physiologic insulin secretion (Table 333-11). In the United States, all insulin is formulated as U-100 (100 units/mL), whereas in some other countries it is available in other units (e.g., U-40 = 40 units/mL). One short-acting insulin formulation, lispro, is an insulin analogue in which the 28th and 29th amino acids (lysine and proline) on the insulin B chain have been reversed by recombinant DNA technology. This insulin analogue has full biologic activity but less tendency toward subcutaneous aggregation, resulting in more rapid absorption and onset of action and a shorter duration of action. These characteristics are particularly advantageous for allowing entrainment of insulin injection and action to rising plasma glucose levels following meals, although improvement in HbA1c values have not been found consistently. The shorter duration of action also appears to be associated with a decreased number of hypoglycemic episodes, primarily because the decay of lispro action corresponds better to the decline in plasma glucose after a meal. Insulin glargine is a long-acting biosynthetic human insulin that differs from normal insulin in that asparagine is replaced by glycine at amino acid 21, and two arginine residues are added to the C-terminus of the B chain. Compared to NPH insulin, the onset of insulin glargine action is later, the duration of action is longer (~24 h), and there is no pronounced peak. A lower incidence of hypoglycemia, especially at night, was reported in one trial with insulin glargine when compared to NPH insulin. Since glargine has only recently approved, clinical experience is limited. Additional insulin analogues are currently under development.

Basal insulin requirements are provided by intermediate (NPH or lente) or long-acting (ultralente or glargine) insulin formulations. These are usually combined with short-acting insulin in an attempt to mimic physiologic insulin release with meals. Although mixing of intermediate and short-acting insulin formulations is common practice, this mixing may alter the insulin absorption profile (especially those of short-acting insulins). For example, the absorption of regular insulin is delayed when mixed for even short periods of time (<5 min) with lente or ultralente insulin, but not when mixed with NPH insulin. Lispro absorption is delayed by mixing with NPH but not ultralente. Insulin glargine should not be mixed with other insulins. The miscibility of human regular and NPH insulin allows for the production of combination insulins that contain 75% NPH and 25% regular (75/25), 70% NPH and 30% regular (70/30), or equal mixtures of NPH and regular. These combinations of insulin are more convenient for the patient but prevent adjustment of only one component of the insulin formulation. The alteration in insulin absorption when the patient mixes different insulin formulation should not discourage the patient from mixing insulin. However, the following guidelines should be followed: (1) mix the different insulin formulations in the syringe immediately before injection (inject within 2 min after mixing); (2) if possible, do not store insulin as a mixture; and (3) follow the same routine in terms of insulin mixing and administration to standardize the physiologic response to injected insulin.

Insulin regimens Representations of the various insulin regimens that may be utilized in type 1 DM are illustrated in Fig. 333-12. Although the insulin profiles are depicted as "smooth," symmetric curves, there is considerable patient-to-patient variation in the peak and duration. In all regimens, long-acting insulins (NPH, lente, ultralente, or glargine insulin) supply basal insulin, whereas prandial insulin is provided by either regular or lispro insulin. Lispro should be injected just before a meal; regular insulin is given 30 to 45 min prior to a meal.

A shortcoming of current insulin regimens is that injected insulin immediately enters the systemic circulation, whereas endogenous insulin is secreted into the portal vein. Thus, exogenous insulin administration exposes the liver to subphysiologic insulin levels. No insulin regimen reproduces the precise insulin secretory pattern of the pancreatic islet. However, the most physiologic regimens entail more frequent insulin injections, greater reliance on short-acting insulin, and more frequent capillary plasma glucose measurements. In general, individuals with type 1 DM require 0.5 to 1.0 U/kg per day of insulin divided into multiple doses. Initial insulin-dosing regimens should be conservative; approximately 40 to 50% of the insulin should be given as basal insulin. A single daily injection of insulin is not appropriate therapy in type 1 DM.

Table 333-11 **Pharmacokinetics of Insulin Preparations**

Preparation	Time of Action			
	Onset, h	Peak, h	Effective Duration, h	Maximum Duration, h
Short-acting				
Lispro	<0.25	0.5–1.5	3–4	4–6
Regular	0.5–1.0	2–3	3–6	6–8
Intermediate-acting				
NPH	2–4	6–10	10–16	14–18
Lente	3–4	6–12	12–18	16–20
Long-acting				
Ultralente	6–10	10–16	18–20	20–24
Glargine	4	–[a]	24	>24
Combinations				
75/25–75% NPH, 25% regular	0.5–1	Dual	10–16	14–18
70/30–70% NPH, 30% regular	0.5–1	Dual	10–16	14–18
50/50–50% NPH, 50% regular	0.5–1	Dual	10–16	14–18

[a] Glargine has minimal peak activity.
SOURCE: Adapted from JS Skyler, in *Therapy for Diabetes Mellitus and Related Disorders*, 1998

One commonly used regimen consists of twice-daily injections of an intermediate insulin (NPH or lente) mixed with a short-acting insulin before the morning and evening meal (Fig. 333-12A). Such regimens usually prescribe two-thirds of the total daily insulin dose in the morning (with about two-thirds given as intermediate-acting insulin and one-third as short-acting) and one-third before the evening meal (with approximately one-half given as intermediate-acting insulin and one-half as short-acting). The drawback to such a regimen is that it enforces a rigid schedule on the patient, in terms of daily activity and the content and timing of meals. Although it is simple and effective at avoiding severe hyperglycemia, it does not generate near-normal glycemic control in most individuals with type 1 DM. Moreover, if the patient's meal pattern or content varies or if physical activity is increased, hyperglycemia or hypoglycemia may result. Moving the intermediate insulin from before the evening meal to bedtime may avoid nocturnal hypoglycemia and provide more insulin as glucose levels rise in the early morning (so-called dawn phenomenon). The insulin dose in such regimens should be adjusted based on SMBG results with the following general assumptions: (1) the fasting glucose is primarily determined by the prior evening intermediate-acting insulin; (2) the pre-lunch glucose is a function of the morning short-acting insulin; (3) the pre-supper glucose is a function of the morning intermediate-acting insulin; and (4) the bedtime glucose is a function of the pre-supper, short-acting insulin.

Multiple-component insulin regimens refer to the combination of basal insulin; preprandial short-acting insulin; and changes in short-acting insulin doses to accommodate the results of frequent SMBG, anticipated food intake, and physical activity. Sometimes also referred to as *multiple daily injections*, such regimens offer the patient maximal flexibility in terms of life-style and the best chance for achieving near

normoglycemia. One such regimen, shown in Fig. 333-12B, consists of a basal insulin with ultralente twice a day and preprandial lispro. The lispro dose is based on individualized algorithms that integrate the preprandial glucose and the anticipated carbohydrate intake. An alternative multiple-component insulin regimen consists of bedtime intermediate insulin, a small dose of intermediate insulin at breakfast (20 to 30% of bedtime dose), and preprandial short-acting insulin. There are numerous variations of these regimens that can be optimized for individual patients. Frequent SMBG (four to 8 times per day) is absolutely essential for these types of insulin regimens.

Continuous subcutaneous insulin infusion (CSII) is another multiple-component insulin regimen (Fig. 333-12C). Sophisticated insulin infusion devices are now available that can accurately deliver small doses of insulin (microliters per hour). For example, multiple basal infusion rates can be programmed to: (1) accommodate nocturnal versus daytime basal insulin requirement, (2) alter infusion rate during periods of exercise, or (3) select different waveforms of insulin infusion. A preprandial insulin ("bolus") is delivered by the insulin infusion device based on instructions from the patient, which follow individualized algorithms that account for preprandial plasma glucose and anticipated carbohydrate intake. These devices require a health professional with considerable experience with insulin infusion devices and very frequent patient interactions with the diabetes management team. Insulin infusion devices present unique challenges, such as infection at the infusion site, unexplained hyperglycemia because the infusion set becomes obstructed, or diabetic ketoacidosis if the pump becomes disconnected. Since most physicians use lispro insulin in CSII, the extremely short half-life of this insulin quickly leads to

FIGURE 333-12 Representative insulin regimens for the treatment of diabetes. For each panel, the y-axis shows the amount of insulin effect and the x-axis shows the time of day. B, breakfast; L, lunch; S, supper; HS, bedtime; CSII, continuous subcutaneous insulin infusion. The time of insulin injection is shown with a vertical arrow. The type of insulin is noted above each insulin curve. A. The injection of two shots of intermediate-acting insulin (NPH or lente) and short-acting insulin (lispro or regular). Only one formulation of short-acting insulin is used. B: A multiple-component insulin regimen consisting of two shots of ultralente each day to provide basal insulin coverage and three shots of Lispro to provide glycemic coverage for each meal. The ultralente doses are usually 10 to 12 h apart. C: Insulin administration by insulin infusion device is shown with the basal insulin and a bolus injection at each meal. The basal insulin rate is decreased during the evening and increased slightly prior to the patient awakening in the morning. (*Adapted from Intensive Diabetes Management, 2d ed, R. Farkas-Hirsch (ed). Alexandria, VA, American Diabetes Association, 1998*)

insulin deficiency if the delivery system is interrupted. Essential to the safe use of infusion devices is thorough patient education about pump function and frequent SMBG.

Type 2 Diabetes Mellitus · *General aspects* The goals of therapy for type 2 DM are similar to those in type 1: improved glycemic control with near normalization of the HbA1c. While glycemic control tends to dominate the management of type 1 DM, the care of individuals with type 2 DM must also include attention to the treatment of conditions associated with type 2 DM (obesity, hypertension, dyslipidemia, cardiovascular disease) and detection/management of DM-related complications (Fig. 333-13). DM-specific complications may be present in up to 20 to 50% of individuals with newly diagnosed type 2 DM. Reduction in cardiovascular risk is of paramount importance as this is the leading cause of mortality in these individuals.

Diabetes management should begin with MNT (discussed above). An exercise regimen to increase insulin sensitivity and promote weight loss should also be instituted. After MNT and increased physical activity have been instituted, glycemic control should be reassessed; if the patient's glycemic target is not achieved after 3 to 4 weeks of MNT, pharmacologic therapy is indicated. Pharmacologic approaches to the management of type 2 DM include both oral glucose-lowering agents and insulin; most physicians and patients prefer oral glucose-lowering agents as the initial choice. Any therapy that improves glycemic control reduces "glucose toxicity" to the islet cells and improves endogenous insulin secretion.

Glucose-lowering agents Recent advances in the therapy of type 2 DM have generated considerable enthusiasm for oral glucose-lowering agents that target different pathophysiologic processes in type 2 DM. Based on their mechanisms of action, oral glucose-lowering agents are subdivided into agents that increase insulin secretion, reduce glucose production, or increase insulin sensitivity (Table 333-12). Oral glucose-lowering agents (with the exception of α-glucosidase inhibitors) are ineffective in type 1 DM and should not be used for glucose management of severely ill individuals with type 2 DM. Insulin is sometimes the initial glucose-lowering agent.

INSULIN SECRETAGOGUES Insulin secretagogues stimulate insulin secretion by interacting with the ATP-sensitive potassium channel on the beta cell (Fig. 333-1). These drugs are most effective in individuals with type 2 DM of relatively recent onset (<5 years), who have endogenous insulin production and tend to be obese. At maximum doses, first-generation sulfonylureas are similar in potency to second-generation agents but have a longer half-life, a greater incidence of hypoglycemia, and more frequent drug interactions (Table 333-13). Thus, second-generation sulfonylureas are generally preferred. An advantage to a more rapid onset of action is better coverage of the postprandial glucose rise, but the shorter half-life of such agents requires more than once-a-day dosing. Sulfonylureas reduce both fasting and postprandial glucose and should be initiated at low doses and increased at 1- to 2-week intervals based on SMBG. In general, sulfonylureas increase insulin acutely and thus should be taken shortly before a meal; with chronic therapy, though, the insulin release is more sustained. Replaglinide is not a sulfonylurea but also interacts with the ATP-sensitive potassium channel. Because of its short half-life, it is usually given with or immediately before each meal to reduce meal-related glucose excursions.

Insulin secretagogues are well tolerated in general. All of these agents, however, have the potential to cause profound and persistent hypoglycemia, especially in elderly individuals. Hypoglycemia is usually related to delayed meals, increased physical activity, alcohol intake, or renal insufficiency. Individuals who ingest an overdose of these agents develop prolonged and serious hypoglycemia and should be monitored closely in the hospital (Chap. 334). Most sulfonylureas are metabolized in the liver to compounds that are cleared by the kidney. Thus, their use in individuals with significant hepatic or renal dysfunction is not advisable. Weight gain, a common side effect of sulfonylurea therapy, results from the increased insulin levels and improvement in glycemic control. Some sulfonylureas have significant drug interactions with other medications such as alcohol, warfarin, aspirin, ketoconazole, α-glucosidase inhibitors, and fluconazole. Despite prior concerns that use of sulfonylureas might increase cardiovascular risk, recent trials have refuted this claim.

BIGUANIDES Metformin is representative of this class of agents. It reduces hepatic glucose production through an undefined mechanism and may improve peripheral glucose utilization slightly (Table 333-12). Metformin reduces fasting plasma glucose and insulin levels, improves the lipid profile, and promotes modest weight loss. The initial starting dose of 500 mg once or twice a day can be increased to 850 mg tid or 1000 mg bid. Because of its relatively slow onset of action and gastrointestinal symptoms with higher doses, the dose should be escalated every 2 to 3 weeks based on SMBG measurements. The major toxicity of metformin, lactic acidosis, can be prevented by careful patient selection. Metformin should not be used in patients with renal insufficiency [serum creatinine >133 μmol/L (1.5 mg/dL) in men or >124 μmol/L (1.4 mg/dL) in women, with adjustments for age], any form of acidosis, congestive heart failure, liver disease, or severe hypoxia. Metformin should be discontinued in patients who are seriously ill, in patients who can take nothing orally, and in those receiving radiographic contrast material. Insulin should be used until metformin can be restarted. Though well tolerated in general, some individuals develop gastrointestinal side effects (diarrhea, anorexia, nausea, and metallic taste) that can be minimized by gradual dose escalation. Because the drug is metabolized in the liver, it should not be used in patients with liver disease or heavy ethanol intake.

α-GLUCOSIDASE INHIBITORS α-Glucosidase inhibitors (acarbose and miglitol) reduce postprandial hyperglycemia by delaying glucose absorption; they do not affect glucose utilization or insulin secretion (Table 333-12). Postprandial hyperglycemia, secondary to impaired hepatic and peripheral glucose disposal, contributes significantly to the hyperglycemic state in type 2 DM. These drugs, taken just before each meal, reduce glucose absorption by inhibiting the enzyme that cleaves oligosaccharides into simple sugars in the intestinal lumen. Therapy should be initiated at a low dose (25 mg of acarbose or miglitol) with the evening meal and may be increased to a maximal dose over weeks to months (50 to 100 mg for acarbose or 50 mg for miglitol with each meal). The major side effects (diarrhea, flatulence, abdominal distention) are related to increased delivery of oligosaccharides to the large bowel and can be reduced somewhat by gradual upward dose titration. α-Glucosidase inhibitors may increase levels of sulfonylureas and increase the incidence of hypoglycemia. Simultaneous treatment with bile acid resins and antacids should be avoided. These agents should not be used in individuals with inflammatory bowel disease, gastroparesis, or a serum creatinine >177 μmol/L (2.0 mg/dL). This class of agents is not as potent as other oral agents in lowering the HbA1c but is unique in that it reduces the postprandial glucose rise even in individuals with type 1 DM.

THIAZOLIDINEDIONES Thiazolidinediones represent a new class of agents that reduce insulin resistance. These drugs bind to a nuclear receptor (peroxisome proliferator-activated receptor, PPAR-γ) that regulates gene transcription. The PPAR-γ receptor is found at highest

FIGURE 333-13 Essential elements in comprehensive diabetes care of type 2 diabetes.

Table 333-12   Oral Glucose-Lowering Therapies in Type 2 DM

	Mechanism of Action	Examples	Anticipated Reduction in HbA1c, %	Agent-Specific Advantages	Agent-Specific Disadvantages	Contraindications
Insulin secretagogues	↑ Insulin		1–2			
Sulfonylureas		See Table 333-13		Lower fasting blood glucose	Hypoglycemia weight gain, hyperinsulinemia	Renal/liver disease
Meglitinide		Repaglinide		Short onset of action, lower postprandial glucose	Hypoglycemia	Liver disease
Biguanides	↓ Hepatic glucose production, weight loss, ↑ glucose utilization	Metformin	1–2	Weight loss, improved lipid profile, no hypoglycemia	Lactic acidosis, diarrhea, nausea, possible increased cardiovascular mortality	Serum creatinine >1.5 mg/dL (men), >1.4 mg/dL (women), radiographic contrast studies, seriously ill patients, acidosis
α-Glucosidase inhibitors	↓ Glucose absorption	Acarbose, miglitol	0.5–1.0	No risk of hypoglycemia	GI flatulence, ↑ liver function tests	Liver/renal disease
Thiazolidinediones	↓ Insulin resistance, ↑ glucose utilization	Rosiglitazone, pioglitazone	1–2	↓ Insulin and sulfonylurea requirements, ↓ triglycerides	Frequent hepatic monitoring for idiosyncratic hepatocellular injury (see text)	Liver disease, congestive heart failure
Medical nutrition therapy and physical activity	↓ Insulin resistance	Low-calorie, low-fat diet, exercise	1–2	Other health benefits	Compliance difficult, long-term success low	

levels in adipocytes but is expressed at lower levels in many other insulin-sensitive tissues. Agonists of this receptor promote adipocyte differentiation and may reduce insulin resistance in skeletal muscle indirectly. Thiazolidinediones reduce the fasting plasma glucose by improving peripheral glucose utilization and insulin sensitivity (Table 333-12). Circulating insulin levels decrease with use of the thiazolidinediones, indicating a reduction in insulin resistance. Although direct comparisons are not available, the two currently available thiazolidinediones appear to have similar efficacy; the therapeutic range for pioglitazone is 15 to 45 mg/d in a single daily dose and for rosiglitazone is 2 to 8 mg/d—once a day at lower doses and bid at higher doses. The ability of thiazolidinediones to influence other features of the insulin resistance syndrome is under investigation.

The prototype of this class of drugs, troglitazone, was withdrawn

Table 333-13   Characteristics of Agents that Increase Insulin Secretion

Generic Name	Approved Daily Dosage Range, mg	Duration of Action, h	Clearance
Sulfonylurea			
First generation			
Chlorpropamide	100–500	>48	Renal
Tolazamide	100–1000	12–24	Hepatic, renal
Tolbutamide	500–3000	6–12	Hepatic
Second generation			
Glimepiride	1–8	24	Hepatic, renal
Glipizide	2.5–40	12–18	Hepatic
Glipizide (extended release)	5–10	24	Hepatic
Glyburide	1.25–20	12–24	Hepatic, renal
Glyburide (micronized)	0.75–12	12–24	Hepatic, renal
Meglitinide			
Repaglinide	0.5–16	2–6	Hepatic

SOURCE: Adapted from Zimmerman, 1998.

from the U.S. market after reports of hepatotoxicity and an association with an idiosyncratic liver reaction that sometimes led to hepatic failure. The two other thiazolidinediones, rosiglitazone and pioglitazone, thus far do not appear to induce the liver abnormalities seen with troglitazone. However, long-term experience with the newer agents is limited. Consequently, the FDA recommends measurement of liver function tests prior to initiating therapy with a thiazolidinedione and at regular intervals (every two months for the first year and then periodically). The thiazolidinediones raise LDL and HDL slightly and lower triglycerides by 10 to 15%, but the clinical significance of these changes is not known. Thiazolidinediones are associated with minor weight gain (1 to 2 kg), a small reduction in the hematocrit, and a mild increase in plasma volume. Cardiac function is not affected, but the incidence of peripheral edema is increased. They are contraindicated in patients with liver disease or congestive heart failure (class III or IV). Thiazolidinediones have been shown to induce ovulation in premenopausal women with polycystic ovary syndrome (see "Insulin Resistance Syndromes," above). Women should be warned about the risk of pregnancy, since the safety of thiazolidinediones in pregnancy is not established.

INSULIN THERAPY IN TYPE 2 DM   Modest doses of insulin are quite efficacious in controlling hyperglycemia in newly diagnosed type 2 DM. Insulin should be considered as the initial therapy in type 2 DM, particularly in lean individuals or those with severe weight loss, in individuals with underlying renal or hepatic disease that precludes oral glucose-lowering agents, or in individuals who are hospitalized or acutely ill. Insulin therapy is ultimately required by a substantial number of individuals with type 2 DM because of the progressive nature of the disorder and the relative insulin deficiency that develops in patients with long-standing diabetes.

Because endogenous insulin secretion continues and is capable of providing some coverage of mealtime caloric intake, insulin is usually initiated in a single dose of intermediate-acting insulin (0.3 to 0.4 U/

kg per day), given either before breakfast or just before bedtime (or ultralente at bedtime). Since fasting hyperglycemia and increased hepatic glucose production are prominent features of type 2 DM, bedtime insulin is more effective in clinical trials than a single dose of morning insulin. Some physicians prefer a relatively low, fixed starting dose of intermediate-acting insulin (~15 to 20 units in the morning and 5 to 10 units at bedtime) to avoid hypoglycemia. The insulin dose may then be adjusted in 10% increments as dictated by SMBG results. Both morning and bedtime intermediate insulin may be used in combination with oral glucose-lowering agents (biguanides, α-glucosidase inhibitors, or thiazolidinediones).

CHOICE OF INITIAL GLUCOSE-LOWERING AGENT Though insulin is an effective primary therapy for type 2 DM, most patients and physicians currently prefer oral glucose-lowering drugs as the initial pharmacologic approach. The level of hyperglycemia should influence the initial choice of therapy. Assuming maximal benefit of MNT and increased physical activity has been realized, patients with mild to moderate hyperglycemia [fasting plasma glucose <11.1 to 13.9 mmol/L (200 to 250 mg/dL)] often respond well to a single oral glucose-lowering agent. Patients with more severe hyperglycemia [fasting plasma glucose >13.9 mmol/L (250 mg/dL)] may respond partially but are unlikely to achieve normoglycemia with oral monotherapy. Nevertheless, many physicians prefer a stepwise approach that starts with a single agent and adds a second agent to achieve the glycemic target (see "Combination Therapy," below). Some physicians begin insulin in individuals with severe hyperglycemia [fasting plasma glucose >13.9 to 16.7 mmol/L (250 to 300 mg/dL)]. This approach is based on the rationale that more rapid glycemic control will reduce "glucose toxicity" to the islet cells, improve endogenous insulin secretion, and possibly allow oral glucose-lowering agents to be more effective. If this occurs, the insulin may be discontinued.

Insulin secretagogues, biguanides, α-glucosidase inhibitors, thiazolidinediones, and insulin are approved for monotherapy of type 2 DM. Although each class of oral glucose-lowering agents has unique advantages and disadvantages, certain generalizations apply: (1) insulin secretagogues, biguanides, and thiazolidinediones improve glycemic control to a similar degree (1 to 2% reduction in HbA1c) and are more effective than α-glucosidase inhibitors; (2) assuming a similar degree of glycemic improvement, no clinical advantage to one class of drugs has been demonstrated, and any therapy that improves glycemic control is beneficial; (3) insulin secretagogues and α-glucosidase inhibitors begin to lower the plasma glucose immediately, whereas the glucose-lowering effects of the biguanides and thiazolidinediones are delayed by several weeks to months; (4) not all agents are effective in all individuals with type 2 DM (primary failure); (5) biguanides, α-glucosidase inhibitors, and thiazolidinediones do not directly cause hypoglycemia; and (6) most individuals will eventually require treatment with more than one class of oral glucose-lowering agents, reflecting the progressive nature of type 2 DM.

Considerable clinical experience exists with sulfonylureas and metformin because they have been available for several decades. It is assumed that the α-glucosidase inhibitors and thiazolidinediones, which are newer classes of oral glucose-lowering drugs, will reduce DM-related complications by improving glycemic control, although long-term data are not yet available. The thiazolidinediones are theoretically attractive because they target a fundamental abnormality in type 2 DM, namely insulin resistance. However, these agents are currently more costly than others and require liver function monitoring.

A reasonable treatment algorithm for initial therapy proposes either a sulfonylurea or metformin as initial therapy because of their efficacy, known side-effect profile, and relatively low cost (Fig. 333-14). Metformin has the advantage that it promotes mild weight loss, lowers insulin levels, improves the lipid profile slightly, and may have a lower secondary failure rate. However, there is no difference in response rate or degree of glycemic control when metformin and

FIGURE 333-14 Glycemic management of type 2 diabetes. See text for discussion. *See text about use as monotherapy. The broken line indicates that biguanides or insulin secretagogues, but not α glucosidase inhibitors or thiazolidinediones, are preferred for initial therapy.

sulfonylureas are compared in randomized, prospective clinical trials. Based on SMBG results and the HbA1c, the dose of either the sulfonylurea or metformin should be increased until the glycemic target is achieved. α-Glucosidase inhibitors and thiazolidinediones are alternative, initial agents (Fig. 333-14).

When used as monotherapy, approximately one-third of individuals will reach their target glycemic goal with either a sulfonylurea or metformin. Approximately 25% of individuals will not respond to sulfonylureas or metformin; under these circumstances, the drug usually should be discontinued. Some individuals respond to one agent but not the other. The remaining individuals treated with either sulfonylureas or metformin alone will exhibit some improvement in glycemic control but will not achieve their glycemic target and should be considered for combination therapy.

COMBINATION THERAPY WITH GLUCOSE-LOWERING AGENTS A number of combinations of therapeutic agents are successful in type 2 DM, and the dosing of agents in combination is the same as when the agents are used alone. Because mechanisms of action of the first and second agents are different, the effect on glycemic control is usually additive. Commonly used regimens include: (1) insulin secretagogue with metformin or thiazolidinedione, (2) sulfonylurea with α-glucosidase inhibitor, and (3) insulin with metformin or thiazolidinedione. The combination of metformin and a thiazolidinedione is also effective and complementary. If adequate control is not achieved with two oral agents, bedtime insulin or a third oral agent may be added stepwise. However, long-term experience with any triple combination is lacking, and experience with two-drug combinations is relatively limited.

Insulin becomes required as type 2 DM enters the phase of relative insulin deficiency (as seen in long-standing DM) and is signaled by inadequate glycemic control on one or two oral glucose-lowering agents. Insulin can be used in combination with any of the oral agents in patients who fail to reach the glycemic target. For example, a single dose of intermediate-acting insulin at bedtime is effective in combination with metformin. As endogenous insulin production falls further, multiple injections of intermediate-acting and short-acting insulin regimens are necessary to control postprandial glucose excursions. These combination regimens are identical to the intermediate- and short-acting combination regimens discussed above for type 1 DM. Since the hyperglycemia of type 2 DM tends to be more "stable," these regimens can be increased in 10% increments every 2 to 3 days using SMBG results. The daily insulin dose required can become quite large (1 to 2 units/kg per day) as endogenous insulin production falls and insulin resistance persists. Individuals who require >1 unit/kg per day of intermediate-acting insulin should be considered for combination therapy with metformin or a thiazolidinedione. The addition of a thiazolidinedione can reduce insulin requirements in some individuals with type 2 DM, while maintaining or even improving glycemic control.

Intensive diabetes management (Table 333-10) is a treatment option in type 2 patients who cannot achieve optimal glycemic control and are capable of implementing such regimens. A recent study from the Veterans Administration found that intensive diabetes management is not associated with a greater degree of side effects (hypoglycemia, weight gain) than standard insulin therapy. The effect of higher insulin levels associated with intensive diabetes management on the prognosis of diseases commonly associated with type 2 DM (cardiovascular disease, hypertension) is still debated. In selected patients with type 2 DM, insulin pumps improve glycemic control and are well tolerated.

Emerging Therapies Whole pancreas transplantation (conventionally performed concomitantly with a renal transplant) may normalize glucose tolerance and is an important therapeutic option in type 1 diabetes, though it requires substantial expertise and is associated with the side effects of immunosuppression. Pancreatic islet transplantation has been plagued by limitations in pancreatic islet isolation and graft survival, but recent advances in specific immunomodulation have greatly improved the results. Islet transplantation is an area of active clinical investigation.

Advances in molecular biology and new insights into normal mechanisms of glucose homeostasis have led to a number of emerging therapies for diabetes and its complications. For example, glucagon-like peptide 1, a potent insulin secretagogue, may be efficacious in type 2 DM. Inhaled insulin and additional insulin analogues are in advanced stages of clinical trials. Aminoguanidine, an inhibitor of the formation of advanced glycosylation end products, and inhibitors of protein kinase C may reduce the complications of DM. Closed-loop pumps that infuse the appropriate amount of insulin in response to changing glucose levels are potentially feasible now that continuous glucose-monitoring technology has been developed.

COMPLICATIONS OF THERAPY FOR DIABETES MELLITUS

As with any therapy, the benefits of efforts directed towards glycemic control must be weighed against the risks of treatment. Side effects of intensive treatment include an increased frequency of serious hypoglycemia, weight gain, increased economic costs, and greater demands on the patient. In the DCCT, quality of life was very similar in the intensive therapy and standard therapy groups. The most serious complication of therapy for DM is hypoglycemia (Chap. 334). Weight gain occurs with most (insulin, insulin secretagogues, thiazolidinediones) but not all (metformin and α-glucosidase inhibitors) therapies that improve glycemic control due to the anabolic effects of insulin and the reduction in glucosuria. In the DCCT, individuals with the greatest weight gain exhibited increases in LDL cholesterol and triglycerides as well as increases in blood pressure (both systolic and diastolic) similar to those seen in individuals with type 2 DM and insulin resistance. These effects could increase the risk of cardiovascular disease in intensively managed patients. As discussed previously, improved glycemic control is sometimes accompanied by a transient worsening of diabetic retinopathy or neuropathy.

ONGOING ASPECTS OF COMPREHENSIVE DIABETES CARE

The morbidity and mortality of DM-related complications can be greatly reduced by timely and consistent surveillance procedures (Table 333-14). These screening procedures are indicated for all individ-

Table 333-14 Guidelines for Ongoing Medical Care for Patients with Diabetes

- Self-monitoring of blood glucose (individualized frequency)
- HbA1c testing (2–4 times/year)
- Patient education in diabetes management (annual)
- Medical nutrition therapy and education (annual)
- Eye examination (annual)
- Foot examination (1–2 times/year by physician; daily by patient)
- Screening for diabetic nephropathy (annual; see Fig. 333-13)
- Blood pressure measurement (quarterly)
- Lipid profile (annual)

uals with DM, but numerous studies have documented that most individuals with diabetes do not receive comprehensive diabetes care. Screening for dyslipidemia and hypertension should be performed annually. In addition to routine health maintenance, individuals with diabetes should also receive the pneumococcal and tetanus vaccines (at recommended intervals) and the influenza vaccine (annually).

An annual comprehensive eye examination should be performed by a qualified optometrist or ophthalmologist. If abnormalities are detected, further evaluation and treatment require an ophthalmologist skilled in diabetes-related eye disease. Because many individuals with type 2 DM have had asymptomatic diabetes for several years before diagnosis, a consensus panel from the ADA recommends the following ophthalmologic examination schedule: (1) individuals with onset of DM at <29 years should have an initial eye examination within 3 to 5 years of diagnosis, (2) individuals with onset of DM at >30 years should have an initial eye examination at the time of diabetes diagnosis, and (3) women with DM who are contemplating pregnancy should have an eye examination prior to conception and during the first trimester.

An annual foot examination should: (1) assess blood flow, sensation, and nail care; (2) look for the presence of foot deformities such as hammer or claw toes and Charcot foot; and (3) identify sites of potential ulceration. Calluses and nail deformities should be treated by a podiatrist; the patient should be discouraged from self-care of even minor foot problems.

An annual microalbuminuria measurement is advised in individuals with type 1 or type 2 DM and no protein on a routine urinalysis (Fig. 333-10). If the urinalysis detects proteinuria, the amount of protein should be quantified by standard urine protein measurements. If the urinalysis was negative for protein in the past, microalbuminuria should be the annual screening examination. Routine urine protein measurements do not detect low levels of albumin excretion. Screening should commence 5 years after the onset of type 1 DM and at the time of onset of type 2 DM.

SPECIAL CONSIDERATIONS IN DIABETES MELLITUS

PSYCHOSOCIAL ASPECTS As with any chronic, debilitating disease, the individual with DM faces a series of challenges that affect all aspects of daily life. The individual with DM must accept that he or she may develop complications related to DM. Even with considerable effort, normoglycemia can be an elusive goal, and solutions to worsening glycemic control may not be easily identifiable. The patient should view him- or herself as an essential member of the diabetes care team and not as someone who is cared for by the diabetes team. Emotional stress may provoke a change in behavior so that individuals no longer adhere to a dietary, exercise, or therapeutic regimen. This can lead to the appearance of either hyper- or hypoglycemia. Depression and eating disorders (in women) are more common in individuals with type 1 or type 2 DM (Chap. 78).

MANAGEMENT IN THE HOSPITALIZED PATIENT Virtually all medical and surgical subspecialties may be involved in the care of hospitalized patients with diabetes. General anesthesia, surgery, and concurrent illness raise the levels of counterregulatory hormones (cortisol, growth hormone, catecholamines, and glucagon), and infection may lead to transient insulin resistance. These factors increase insulin requirements by increasing glucose production and impairing glucose utilization and thus may worsen glycemic control. On the other hand, the concurrent illness or surgical procedure may prevent the patient with DM from eating normally and may promote hypoglycemia. Glycemic control should be assessed (with HbA1c) and, if feasible, should be optimized prior to surgery. Electrolytes, renal function, and intravascular volume status should be assessed as well. The extremely high prevalence of asymptomatic cardiovascular disease in individuals with DM (especially in type 2 DM) may require preoperative cardiovascular evaluation.

The goals of diabetes management during hospitalization are avoidance of hypoglycemia, optimization of glycemic control, and transition back to the outpatient diabetes treatment regimen. Attention to each stage in this process requires integrating information regarding the plasma glucose, diabetes treatment regimen, and clinical status of the patient. For example, some surgical procedures utilizing local anesthesia or epidural anesthesia may have minimal effects on glycemic control. If the patient is eating soon after the procedure and there is no disruption of the patient's regular meal plans, then glycemic control is usually maintained.

The physician caring for an individual with diabetes in the perioperative period, during times of infection or serious physical illness, or simply when fasting for a diagnostic procedure must monitor the plasma glucose vigilantly, adjust the diabetes treatment regimen, and provide glucose infusion as needed. Several different treatment regimens (intravenous or subcutaneous insulin regimens) can be employed successfully. Individuals with type 1 DM require continued insulin administration to maintain the levels of circulating insulin necessary to prevent DKA. Prolongation of a surgical procedure or delay in the recovery room is not uncommon and may result in periods of insulin deficiency. Even relatively brief periods without insulin may lead to mild DKA. Individuals with type 1 DM who are undergoing general anesthesia and surgery, or who are seriously ill, should receive continuous insulin, either through an intravenous insulin infusion or by subcutaneous administration of a reduced dose of long-acting insulin. Short-acting insulin alone is insufficient.

Individuals with type 2 DM can be managed with either insulin infusion or a reduced dose of subcutaneous insulin. Oral glucose-lowering agents are discontinued at the time a combined insulin/glucose infusion is started. Oral agents such as sulfonylureas, metformin, acarbose, and thiazolidinediones are not useful in regulating the plasma glucose in clinical situations where the insulin requirements and glucose intake are changing rapidly. Moreover, these oral agents may be dangerous if the patient is fasting (e.g., hypoglycemia with sulfonylureas). Metformin should be withheld when radiographic contrast media will be given or if severe congestive heart failure, acidosis, or declining renal function is present.

Insulin infusions can effectively control plasma glucose in the perioperative period and when the patient is unable to take anything by mouth. The absorption of subcutaneous insulin may be variable in such situations because of changes in blood flow. The physician must consider carefully the clinical setting in which an insulin infusion will be utilized, including whether adequate ancillary personnel are available to monitor the plasma glucose frequently and whether they can adjust the insulin infusion rate, either based on an algorithm or in consultation with the physician. The initial rate for an insulin infusion may range from 0.5 to 5 units/h, depending on the degree of insulin resistance and the clinical situation. Based on hourly capillary glucose measurements, the insulin infusion rate is adjusted to maintain the plasma glucose within the desired range [5.6 to 11.1 mmol/L (100 to 200 mg/dL)]. Glucose infusion, initiated at the time the patient begins fasting,

should be adjusted to deliver the equivalent of 50 to 150 mL of $D_5W/$h until the patient is reliably taking nutrition orally. The insulin infusion can be temporarily discontinued if hypoglycemia occurs and may be resumed at a lower infusion rate once the plasma glucose exceeds 5.6 mmol/L (100 mg/dL).

Insulin infusion is the preferred method for managing patients with type 1 DM in the perioperative period or when serious concurrent illness is present. Individuals with type 2 DM can be managed with an insulin infusion, but subcutaneous insulin in reduced doses can be used effectively as well. If the diagnostic or surgical procedure is brief and performed under local or regional anesthesia, a reduced dose of subcutaneous, long-acting insulin may suffice. This approach facilitates the transition back to the long-acting insulin after the procedure. The dose of long-acting insulin should be reduced by 30 to 40%, and short-acting insulin is either held or, likewise, reduced by 30 to 40%. Glucose should be infused to prevent hypoglycemia.

Total Parenteral Nutrition (See Chap. 76)   Total parenteral nutrition (TPN) greatly increases insulin requirements. In addition, individuals not previously known to have DM may become hyperglycemic during TPN and require insulin treatment. Intravenous insulin infusion is the preferred treatment for hyperglycemia, and rapid titration to the required insulin dose is done most efficiently using a separate insulin infusion. After the total insulin dose has been determined, insulin may be added directly to the TPN solution. Often, individuals receiving either TPN or enteral nutrition receive their caloric loads continuously and not at "meal times"; consequently, subcutaneous insulin regimens must be adjusted.

GLUCOCORTICOIDS   Glucocorticoids increase insulin resistance, decrease glucose utilization, increase hepatic glucose production, and impair insulin secretion. These changes lead to a worsening of glycemic control in individuals with DM and may precipitate diabetes in other individuals ("steroid-induced diabetes"). The effects of glucocorticoids on glucose homeostasis are dose-related, usually reversible, and most pronounced in the postprandial period. If the fasting plasma glucose is near the normal range, oral diabetes agents (sulfonylureas and acarbose) may be sufficient to reduce hyperglycemia. If the fasting plasma glucose >11.1 mmol/L (200 mg/dL), oral agents are usually not efficacious and insulin therapy is required. Short-acting insulin may be required to supplement long-acting insulin in order to control postprandial glucose excursions.

REPRODUCTIVE ISSUES   Reproductive capacity in either men or women with DM appears to be normal. Menstrual cycles may be associated with alterations in glycemic control in women with DM. Pregnancy is associated with marked insulin resistance; the increased insulin requirements often precipitate DM and lead to the diagnosis of GDM. Glucose, which at high levels is a teratogen to the developing fetus, readily crosses the placenta, but insulin does not. Thus, hyperglycemia or hypoglycemia from the maternal circulation may stimulate insulin secretion in the fetus. The anabolic and growth effects of insulin may result in macrosomia. GDM complicates approximately 4% of pregnancies in the United States. The incidence of GDM is greatly increased in certain ethnic groups, including African Americans and Hispanic Americans, consistent with a similar increased risk of type 2 DM. Current recommendations advise screening for glucose intolerance between weeks 24 and 28 of pregnancy in women with high risk for GDM (≥25 years; obesity; family history of DM; member of an ethnic group such as Hispanic American, Native American, Asian American, African American, or Pacific Islander). Therapy for GDM is similar to that for individuals with pregnancy-associated diabetes and involves MNT and insulin, if hyperglycemia persists. Oral glucose-lowering agents have not been approved for use during pregnancy. With current practices, the morbidity and mortality of the mother with GDM and the fetus are no different from those in the nondiabetic population. Individuals who develop GDM are at marked increased risk for developing type 2 DM in the future and should be screened periodically for DM. After delivery, glucose homeostasis should be reassessed in the mother. Most individuals with GDM revert to normal glucose tolerance, but some will continue to have overt diabetes or impairment of glucose tolerance. In addition, children of women with GDM appear to be at risk for obesity and glucose intolerance and have an increased risk of diabetes beginning in the later stages of adolescence.

Pregnancy in individuals with known DM requires meticulous planning and adherence to strict treatment regimens. Intensive diabetes management and normalization of the HbA1c are the standard of care for individuals with existing DM who are planning pregnancy. The crucial period of glycemic control is extremely early following fertilization. The risk of fetal malformations is increased 4 to 10 times in individuals with uncontrolled DM at the time of conception. The goals are normal plasma glucose during the preconception period and throughout the periods of organ development in the fetus.

LIPODYSTROPHIC DM (See also Chap. 354) Lipodystrophy, or the loss of subcutaneous fat tissue, may be generalized in certain genetic conditions such as leprechaunism. Generalized lipodystrophy is associated with severe insulin resistance and is often accompanied by acanthosis nigricans and dyslipidemia. Localized lipodystrophy associated with insulin injections has been reduced considerably by the use of human insulin.

Protease Inhibitors and Lipodystrophy Protease inhibitors used in the treatment of HIV disease (Chap. 309) have been associated with a centripetal accumulation of fat (visceral and abdominal area), accumulation of fat in the dorsocervical region, loss of extremity fat, decreased insulin sensitivity (elevations of the fasting insulin level and reduced glucose tolerance on intravenous glucose tolerance testing), and dyslipidemia. Although many aspects of the physical appearance of these individuals resemble Cushing's syndrome, derangements in cortisol secretion have not been found consistently and do not appear to account for this appearance. Although some individuals have IGT, diabetes is not a common feature. The possibility remains that this is related to HIV infection by some undefined mechanism, since some features of the syndrome were observed before the introduction of protease inhibitors. Therapy for HIV-related lipodystrophy is not well established.

BIBLIOGRAPHY

GENERAL

ALBERTI KG, ZIMMET PZ: Definition, diagnosis and classification of diabetes mellitus and its complications. Part 1: Diagnosis and classification of diabetes, provisional report of a WHO Consultation. Diabet Med 15:539, 1997

AMERICAN DIABETES ASSOCIATION: Diabetes Care 23(Suppl 1), 2000

CARTER JS et al: Non-insulin-dependent diabetes mellitus in minorities in the United States. Ann Intern Med 125:221, 1996

HARRIS MI et al: Prevalence of diabetes, impaired fasting glucose, and impaired glucose tolerance in U.S. adults. The Third National Health and Nutrition Examination Survey, 1988–1994. Diabetes Care 21:518, 1998

REPORT OF THE EXPERT COMMITTEE ON THE DIAGNOSIS AND CLASSIFICATION OF DIABETES MELLITUS. Diabetes Care 20:1183, 1997

ROSENBLOOM AL et al: Emerging epidemic of type 2 diabetes in youth. Diabetes Care 22:345, 1999

GENETICS/PATHOGENESIS

CLINE GW et al: Impaired glucose transport as a cause of decreased insulin-stimulated muscle glycogen synthesis in type 2 diabetes. N Engl J Med 341:240, 1999

DEFRONZO RA: Pathogenesis of type 2 diabetes. Diabetes Rev 5:177, 1997

FROGUEL P, VELHO G: Molecular genetics of maturity-onset diabetes of the young. Trends Endocrinol Metab 10:142, 1999

GERICH JE: The genetic basis of type 2 diabetes mellitus: Impaired insulin secretion versus impaired insulin sensitivity. Endocr Rev 19:491, 1998

LOWE WL: Genetics of diabetes, in Principles of Molecular Medicine, JL Jameson (ed). Totowa, NJ, Humana, 1998, pp 433–442

PUGLIESE A: Unraveling the genetics of insulin-dependent type 1A diabetes: The search must go on. Diabetes Rev 7:39, 1999

SCHRANZ DB, LERNMARK A: Immunology in diabetes: An update. Diabetes Metab Rev 14:3, 1998

SHEPHERD PR, KAHN BB: Glucose transporters and insulin action—implications for insulin resistance and diabetes mellitus. N Engl J Med 341:248, 1999

SHULMAN GI: Cellular mechanisms of insulin resistance in humans. Am J Cardiol 84:3J, 1999

TRITOS NA, MANTZOROS CS: Syndromes of severe insulin resistance. J Clin Endocrinol Metab 83:3025, 1998

VIRKAMAKI A et al: Protein-protein interaction in insulin signaling and the molecular mechanisms of insulin resistance. J Clin Invest 103:931, 1999

COMPLICATIONS OF DIABETES

AIELLO LP et al: Diabetic retinopathy. Diabetes Care 21:143, 1998

CHEN YDI, REAVEN GM: Insulin resistance and atherosclerosis. Diabetes Rev 5:331, 1997

Consensus development conference on diabetic foot wound care. Diabetes Care 22:1354, 1999

DETRE KM et al: The effect of previous coronary-artery bypass surgery on the prognosis of patients with diabetes who have acute myocardial infarction. N Engl J Med 342:989, 2000

DIABETES CONTROL AND COMPLICATIONS TRIAL RESEARCH GROUP: The relationship of glycemic exposure (HbAlC) to the risk of development and progression of retinopathy in the diabetes control and complications trial. Diabetes 44:968, 1995

GRUNDY SM et al: Diabetes and cardiovascular disease: A statement for healthcare professionals from the American Heart Association. Circulation 100:1134, 1999

MOGENSEN CE: Preventing end-stage renal disease. Diabet Med 15(Suppl 4):S51, 1998

RITZ E, ORTH SR: Nephropathy in patients with type 2 diabetes. N Engl J Med 341:1127, 1999

THERAPY

ABRAIRA C et al: Cardiovascular events and correlates in the Veterans Affairs diabetes feasibility trial: Veterans Affairs diabetes cooperative study on glycemic control and complication in type II diabetes. Arch Intern Med 157:181, 1997

AMERICAN DIABETES ASSOCIATION: Therapy for Diabetes Mellitus and Related Disorders, 3d ed, HS Lebovitz (ed). Alexandria, VA, American Diabetes Association, 1998

———: Clinical Practice Guidelines 2000. Diabetes Care 23(Suppl):S1, 2000

BUSE JB: Overview of current therapeutic options in type 2 diabetes. Rationale for combining oral agents with insulin therapy. Diabetes Care 22(Suppl 3):C65, 1999

DAVIDSON MB, PETERS AL: An overview of metformin in the treatment of type 2 diabetes mellitus. Am J Med 102:99, 1997

DEFRONZO RA: Pharmacologic therapy for type 2 diabetes mellitus. Ann Intern Med 131:281, 1999

DIABETES CONTROL AND COMPLICATIONS TRIAL RESEARCH GROUP: The effect of intensive treatment of diabetes on the development and progression of long-term complications in insulin-dependent diabetes mellitus. N Engl J Med 329:977, 1993

ESTACIO RO et al: The effect of nisoldipine as compared with enalapril on cardiovascular outcomes in patients with non-insulin-dependent diabetes and hypertension. N Engl J Med 338:645, 1998

FARKAS-HIRSCH R (ed): Intensive Diabetes Management, 2d ed. Alexandria VA, American Diabetes Association, 1998

JACOBER SJ, SOWERS JR: An update on perioperative management of diabetes. Arch Intern Med 159:2405, 1999

KREISBERG RA: Diabetic dyslipidemia. Am J Cardiol 82:67U, 1998

MARSHALL SM: Blood pressure control, microalbuminuria and cardiovascular risk in Type 2 diabetes mellitus. Diabet Med 16:358, 1999

OHKUBO Y et al: Intensive insulin therapy prevents the progression of diabetic microvascular complications in Japanese patients with non-insulin-dependent diabetes mellitus: A randomized prospective 6-year study. Diabetes Res Clin Pract 28:103, 1995

SKYLER JS (ed): Medical Management of Type 1 Diabetes, 3d ed. Alexandria VA, American Diabetes Association, 1998

TUOMILEHTO et al: Effects of calcium-channel blockade in older patients with diabetes and systolic hypertension. Systolic Hypertension in Europe Trial Investigators. N Engl J Med 340:677, 1999

UK PROSPECTIVE DIABETES STUDY GROUP: Intensive blood-glucose control with sulphonylureas or insulin compared with conventional treatment and risk of complications in patients with type 2 diabetes (UKPDS 33). Lancet 352:837, 1998

———: Effect of intensive blood-glucose control with metformin on complications in overweight patients with type 2 diabetes (UKPDS 34). Lancet 352:854, 1998

———: Tight blood pressure control and risk of macrovascular and microvascular complications in type 2 diabetes: UKPDS 38. BMJ 317:708, 1999

UMPIERREZ GE et al: Review: Diabetic ketoacidosis and hyperglycemic hyperosmolar nonketotic syndrome. Am J Med Sci 311:225, 1996

VETERANS HEALTH ADMINISTRATION: Clinical guidelines for management of patients with diabetes mellitus. www.VA.gov/health/diabetes, 1997

YKI-JARVINEN H et al: Comparison of bedtime insulin regimens in patients with type 2 diabetes mellitus: A randomized, controlled trial. Ann Intern Med 130:389, 1999

ZIMMERMAN BR (ed): Medical Management of Type 2 Diabetes, 4d ed. Alexandria VA, American Diabetes Association, 1998

334   *Philip E. Cryer*

HYPOGLYCEMIA

Hypoglycemia occurs most commonly as a result of treating patients with diabetes mellitus. However, a number of other disorders, including insulinoma, large mesenchymal tumors, end-stage organ failure, alcoholism, endocrine deficiencies, postprandial reactive hypoglycemic conditions, and inherited metabolic disorders, are also associated with hypoglycemia (Table 334-1). Hypoglycemia is sometimes defined as a plasma glucose level <2.5 to 2.8 mmol/L (<45 to 50 mg/dL). However, as discussed below, the glucose thresholds for hypoglycemia-induced symptoms and physiologic responses vary widely, depending on the clinical setting. Therefore, *Whipple's triad* provides an important framework for making the diagnosis of hypoglycemia: (1) symptoms consistent with hypoglycemia, (2) a low plasma glucose concentration, and (3) relief of symptoms after the plasma glucose level is raised. Hypoglycemia can cause significant morbidity and can be lethal, if severe or prolonged; it should be considered in any patient who presents with confusion, altered level of consciousness, or seizures.

SYSTEMIC GLUCOSE BALANCE AND COUNTERREGULATION

Glucose is an obligate metabolic fuel for the brain under physiologic conditions. By contrast, other organs can use fatty acids, in addition to glucose, to generate energy. The brain cannot synthesize glucose and stores only a few minutes' supply as glycogen. It therefore requires a continuous supply of glucose, which is delivered by facilitated diffusion from arterial blood. As the plasma glucose concentration falls below the physiologic range, blood-to-brain glucose transport becomes

Table 334-1   Causes of Hypoglycemia

Drugs
   Especially insulin, sulfonylureas, ethanol
   Sometimes pentamidine, quinine
   Rarely salicylates, sulfonamides, and others
Endogenous hyperinsulinism
   Insulinoma
   Other β cell disorders
   Secretagogue (sulfonylurea)
   Autoimmune (autoantibodies to insulin, insulin receptor, β cell?)
   Ectopic insulin secretion
Critical illnesses
   Hepatic, renal, or cardiac failure
   Sepsis
   Starvation and inanition
Endocrine deficiencies
   Cortisol, growth hormone
   Glucagon and epinephrine (type 1 diabetes)
Non-β-cell tumors
   Fibrosarcoma, mesothelioma, rhabdomyosarcoma, liposarcoma, other
      sarcomas
   Hepatoma, adrenocortical tumors, carcinoid
   Leukemia, lymphoma, melanoma, teratoma
Disorders of infancy or childhood
   Transient intolerance of fasting
   Infants of diabetic mothers (hyperinsulinism)
   Persistent hyperinsulinemic hypoglycemia of infancy
   Inherited enzyme defects
Postprandial
   Reactive (after gastric surgery)
   Ethanol-induced
   Autonomic symptoms without true hypoglycemia
Factitious
   Insulin, sulfonylureas

insufficient for adequate brain energy metabolism and functioning. It is therefore not surprising that redundant physiologic mechanisms prevent or rapidly correct hypoglycemia.

Plasma glucose levels are maintained within a narrow range, usually between 3.3 and 8.3 mmol/L (60 and 150 mg/dL), despite wide variation in food intake and activity level. This delicate balance requires dynamic regulation of glucose influx into the circulation as glucose utilization in various tissues can change rapidly. The diet is normally a major source of glucose. However, between meals or during fasting, serum glucose levels are maintained primarily by the breakdown of glycogen in the liver and by gluconeogenesis (Fig. 334-1). In most people, hepatic glycogen stores are sufficient to maintain plasma glucose levels for 8 to 12 h, but this time period can be shorter if glucose demand is increased by exercise or if glycogen stores are depleted by illness or starvation.

As glycogen stores are depleted, glucose is generated by gluconeogenesis, which occurs primarily in the liver but also in the kidney. Gluconeogenesis requires a coordinated supply of precursors from liver, muscle, and adipose tissue. Muscle provides lactate, pyruvate, alanine, and other amino acids; triglycerides in adipose tissue are broken down into glycerol, which is a precursor for gluconeogenesis, and free fatty acids, which generate acetyl CoA for gluconeogenesis and provide an alternative fuel source to tissues other than brain.

The balance of glucose production and its uptake and utilization in peripheral tissues is exquisitely regulated by a network of hormones, neural pathways, and metabolic signals (Chap. 333). Among the factors that control glucose production and utilization, insulin plays a dominant and pivotal role. In the fasting state, insulin is suppressed, allowing increased gluconeogenesis in the liver and the kidney and enhancing glucose generation by the breakdown of liver glycogen. Low insulin levels also reduce glucose uptake and utilization in peripheral tissues and allow lipolysis and proteolysis to occur, leading to the release of precursors for gluconeogenesis and providing alternative energy sources. In the fed state, insulin release from the pancreatic β cells reverses these processes. Glycogenolysis and gluconeogenesis are inhibited, thereby reducing hepatic and renal glucose output; peripheral glucose uptake and utilization are enhanced; lipolysis and proteolysis are restrained; and energy storage is promoted by the conversion of substrates into glycogen, triglycerides, and proteins. Other hormones including glucagon, epinephrine, growth hormone, and cortisol play less important roles in the control of glucose flux during normal physiologic circumstances. However, as described below, these hormones are critically important in the response to hypoglycemia.

As glucose levels approach, and ultimately enter, the hypoglycemic range, a characteristic sequence of *counterregulatory hormone responses* occurs. Glucagon is the first and most important of these responses. It promotes glycogenolysis and gluconeogenesis. Epineph-

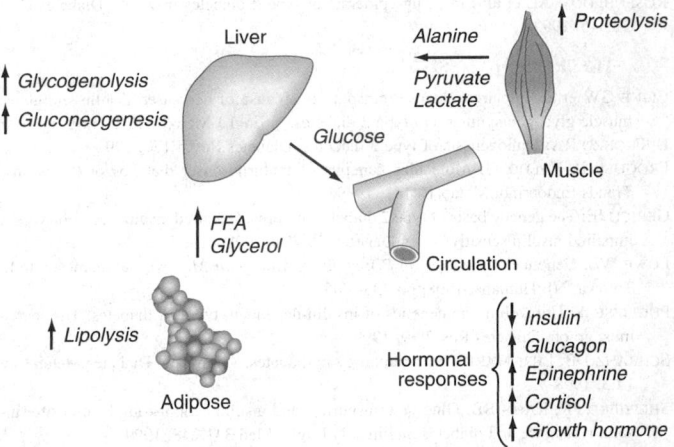

FIGURE 334-1 Overview of glucose metabolism and pathways of counterregulatory responses to fasting and hypoglycemia.

rine can also play an important role in the acute response to hypoglycemia, particularly when glucagon is insufficient. It, too, stimulates glycogenolysis and gluconeogenesis as well as limiting glucose utilization by insulin-sensitive tissues. When hypoglycemia is prolonged, growth hormone and cortisol also reduce glucose utilization and support its production.

The glucose thresholds at which various counterregulatory hormone responses occur are quite similar in healthy subjects (Table 334-2). Nonetheless, these thresholds are dynamic and can be influenced by recent metabolic events. A person with poorly controlled diabetes can have symptoms of hypoglycemia at higher-than-normal glucose levels. Recurrent hypoglycemia, as may occur in individuals with diabetes or in the setting of an insulinoma, shifts thresholds for symptoms and counterregulatory responses to lower glucose levels.

Table 334-2 Physiologic Responses to Decreasing Plasma Glucose Concentrations

Response	Glycemic Threshold, mmol/L (mg/dL)	Physiologic Effects	Role in the Prevention or Correction of Hypoglycemia (Glucose Counterregulation)
↓ Insulin	4.4–4.7 (80–85)	↑ R_a (↓ R_d)	Primary glucose regulatory factor/first defense against hypoglycemia
↑ Glucagon	3.6–3.9 (65–70)	↑ R_a	Primary glucose counterregulatory factor
↑ Epinephrine	3.6–3.9 (65–70)	↑ R_a, ↓ R_d	Involved, critical when glucagon is deficient
↑ Cortisol and growth hormone	3.6–3.9 (65–70)	↑ R_a, ↓ R_d	Involved, not critical
Symptoms	2.8–3.1 (50–55)	↑ Exogenous glucose	Prompt behavioral defense (food ingestion)
↓ Cognition	< 2.8 (< 50)	—	(Compromises behavioral defense)

NOTE: R_a, rate of glucose appearance, glucose production by the liver and kidneys; R_d, Rate of glucose disappearance, glucose utilization by insulin-sensitive tissues such as skeletal muscle, and by the central nervous system (where glucoregulatory hormones have no direct effect on glucose utilization).

CLINICAL MANIFESTATIONS

Symptoms of hypoglycemia can be divided into two categories, neuroglycopenic and neurogenic (or autonomic) responses. Neuroglycopenic symptoms are the direct result of central nervous system neuronal glucose deprivation. They include behavioral changes, confusion, fatigue, seizure, loss of consciousness, and, if hypoglycemia is severe and prolonged, death. Hypoglycemia-induced autonomic responses include adrenergic symptoms such as palpitations, tremor, and anxiety as well as cholinergic symptoms such as sweating, hunger, and paresthesia. Adrenergic symptoms are mediated by norepinephrine released from sympathetic postganglionic neurons and the release of epinephrine from the adrenal medullae. Increased sweating is mediated by cholinergic sympathetic nerve fibers. Patients with diabetes mellitus learn to recognize the characteristic symptoms of hypoglycemia, but these are less familiar to individuals with other causes of hypoglycemia. Symptoms may be less pronounced with repeated hypoglycemic episodes (see below).

Common signs of hypoglycemia include pallor and diaphoresis. Heart rate and the systolic blood pressure are typically raised, but these findings may not be prominent. The neuroglycopenic manifestations are valuable, albeit nonspecific, signs. Transient focal neurologic deficits occur occasionally.

CAUSES

Hypoglycemia is traditionally classified as *postprandial* or *fasting*. However, in the clinical setting, hypoglycemia most commonly results from the treatment of diabetes. This topic is therefore addressed before considering the other causes of hypoglycemia.

HYPOGLYCEMIA IN DIABETES Frequency and Impact Were it not for hypoglycemia, diabetes would be rather easy to treat by administering enough insulin (or any effective drug) to lower plasma glucose concentrations to, or below, the normal range. Because of imperfections in all current insulin-replacement regimens, individuals with type 1 diabetes are at ongoing risk for periods of relative hyperinsulinemia with resultant hypoglycemia. Those attempting to achieve near-normal glycemic control may experience several episodes of asymptomatic or symptomatic hypoglycemia each week. Plasma glucose levels may be <2.8 mmol/L (<50 mg/dL) as much as 10% of the time. At least 25% of such patients suffer an episode of severe, temporarily disabling hypoglycemia, often with seizure or coma, in a given year. Although seemingly complete recovery from the latter is the rule, the possibility of persistent cognitive deficits has been raised, but permanent neurologic defects are rare. About 2 to 4% of deaths associated with type 1 diabetes are estimated to result from

hypoglycemia. Fear of hypoglycemia also can lead to disabling psychosocial morbidity.

Hypoglycemia is a less frequent problem in type 2 diabetes but occurs nevertheless in those treated with insulin or sulfonylureas. Transient, mild hypoglycemia may be seen with the shorter-acting sulfonylureas and repaglinide, which also acts by enhancing insulin secretion. Patients taking the long-acting sulfonylureas, chlorpropamide and glyburide, occasionally experience episodes of severe hypoglycemia that may last up to 24 to 36 h.

Conventional Risk Factors Insulin excess is the primary determinant of risk from iatrogenic hypoglycemia. Relative or absolute insulin excess occurs when: (1) insulin (or oral agent) doses are excessive, ill timed, or of the wrong type; (2) the influx of exogenous glucose is reduced, as during an overnight fast or following missed meals or snacks; (3) insulin-independent glucose utilization is increased, as during exercise; (4) insulin sensitivity is increased, as occurs with effective intensive therapy, in the middle of the night, late after exercise, or with increased fitness or weight loss; (5) endogenous glucose production is reduced, as following alcohol ingestion; and (6) insulin clearance is reduced, as in renal failure. However, analyses of the Diabetes Control and Complications Trial (DCCT) indicate that these conventional risk factors explain only a minority of episodes of severe iatrogenic hypoglycemia and that other causes are involved in the majority of episodes.

Hypoglycemia-Associated Autonomic Failure It is now clear that inadequate physiologic counterregulatory and behavioral responses greatly compound the problem of hypoglycemia caused by insulin excess. Hypoglycemia-associated autonomic failure has two main components: (1) reduced counterregulatory hormone responses, which result in impaired glucose generation; and (2) hypoglycemia unawareness, which precludes appropriate behavioral responses, such as eating.

Defective glucose counterregulation The counterregulatory hormone response is fundamentally altered in all people with established (e.g., absent C peptide) type 1 diabetes. As the patient becomes totally insulin-deficient over the first few months or years of the disease, circulating insulin levels are no longer tightly coordinated with glucose levels and are a passive function of administered insulin. Thus, insulin levels do not always decline as glucose levels fall; the first defense against hypoglycemia is lost. Over the same time frame, the glucagon response to falling glucose levels diminishes, and the second defense against hypoglycemia is lost. The cause of defective glucagon production by the pancreatic islet α cells is unknown, but it is tightly linked to the loss of insulin production by the β cells. It is a functional abnormality rather than an absolute deficiency of glucagon, as responses to stimuli other than hypoglycemia are intact. The third defense against hypoglycemia is compromised when the epinephrine response to hypoglycemia is reduced. In contrast to the absent glucagon response, epinephrine deficiency is a threshold abnormality; an epinephrine response can still be elicited, but a lower plasma glucose concentration is required. This threshold shift is largely the result of recent antecedent hypoglycemia, although an additional anatomic component may be present as well in patients affected by classic diabetic autonomic neuropathy. The development of a reduced epinephrine response is a critical pathophysiologic event. Prospective studies have shown that patients with combined deficiencies of glucagon and epinephrine suffer severe hypoglycemia at rates 25-fold or greater than individuals with absent glucagon but intact epinephrine responses.

Hypoglycemia unawareness   Hypoglycemia unawareness refers to loss of the warning symptoms of hypoglycemia that normally alert individuals to the presence of hypoglycemia and prompt them to eat to abort the episode. Under these circumstances, the first manifestation of hypoglycemia is neuroglycopenia, and it is often too late for patients to treat themselves. Like defective counterregulation, the presence of hypoglycemia unawareness has been shown in prospective studies to be associated with a high frequency of severe hypoglycemia.

The interplay of factors involved in hypoglycemia-associated autonomic failure in type 1 diabetes, and consequent hypoglycemia unawareness, is summarized in Fig. 334-2. Periods of relative or absolute therapeutic insulin excess, in the setting of absent glucagon responses, lead to episodes of iatrogenic hypoglycemia. These episodes, in turn, cause reduced autonomic (including adrenomedullary) responses to falling glucose concentrations. These impaired autonomic responses result in reduced symptoms of impending hypoglycemia (e.g., hypoglycemia unawareness) and, because epinephrine responses are reduced in the setting of absent glucagon responses, impaired physiologic defense against developing hypoglycemia. Thus, a vicious cycle of recurrent hypoglycemia is created and perpetuated. The syndrome of hypoglycemia unawareness and the reduced epinephrine component of defective glucose counterregulation are reversible after as little as 2 weeks of scrupulous avoidance of hypoglycemia. This involves a shift of glycemic thresholds back to higher plasma glucose concentrations.

Hypoglycemia Risk Factor Reduction   It is possible to minimize the risk of hypoglycemia by applying the principles of modern therapy—patient education and empowerment, frequent self-monitoring of blood glucose, flexible insulin (and other drug) regimens, rational glycemic goals, and ongoing professional guidance and support. With respect to the latter, the issue of hypoglycemia needs to be addressed in every patient contact. If hypoglycemia is a recognized problem, first consider each of the conventional risk factors summarized earlier and recommend the appropriate adjustments of medications, diet, and life-style. Nonselective beta blockers may attenuate the recognition of hypoglycemia and they impair glycogenolysis; a relatively selective β_1-antagonist (e.g., metoprolol or atenolol) is preferable when a beta blocker is indicated. One should consider the issue of compromised glucose counterregulation. Although it is possible to test for this abnormality using a low-dose insulin infusion test, this is not practical. A diagnosis of hypoglycemia unawareness can usually be made from the history. It should be remembered that hypoglycemia unawareness implies that previous episodes of hypoglycemia have occurred, whether these are documented or not. If low glucose levels are not apparent from the patient's self-monitoring log, one should suspect hypoglycemia during the night. The presence of clinical hypoglycemia unawareness makes defective glucose counterregulation quite likely. A 2 to 3 week period of conscientious avoidance of hypoglycemia is advisable.

REACTIVE HYPOGLYCEMIA   The postprandial (reactive) hypoglycemias occur only after meals, and hypoglycemia is self-limited. Postprandial hypoglycemia occurs in children with certain rare enzymatic defects in carbohydrate metabolism such as hereditary fructose intolerance and galactosemia (Chap. 350). Reactive hypoglycemia also occurs in some individuals who have undergone gastric surgery that results in the rapid passage of food from the stomach to the small intestine. This type of *alimentary hypoglycemia* causes a rapid postprandial rise in plasma glucose levels and the release of gut incretins, which induce an exuberant insulin response and subsequent hypoglycemia. Administration of an α-glucosidase inhibitor, which delays carbohydrate digestion and thus glucose absorption from the intestine, can be considered for treatment of reactive hypoglycemia, although its efficacy remains to be established in controlled trials.

If postprandial symptoms occur as an idiopathic disorder, caution should be exercised before labeling a person with the diagnosis of hypoglycemia. Indeed, a self-diagnosis of hypoglycemia has often been reinforced by the finding of a "low" venous glucose concentration late after glucose ingestion. An oral glucose tolerance test should not be used in this setting. Plasma glucose falls as low as 2.4 mmol/L (43 mg/dL) after a 100-g glucose load in 5% of normal asymptomatic individuals, making it difficult to identify hypoglycemia based on the results of this test. The diagnosis of postprandial hypoglycemia requires documentation of Whipple's triad after a typical mixed meal. The cause of repetitive postprandial symptoms in certain individuals is unknown, but they may be particularly sensitive to the normal autonomic responses that follow ingestion of a meal.

FASTING HYPOGLYCEMIA   There are many causes of fasting hypoglycemia (Table 334-1). In addition to insulin and sulfonylureas used in the treatment of diabetes, ethanol use is a relatively common cause of hypoglycemia. Sepsis and renal failure are often complicated by hypoglycemia, but it is less common in other critical illnesses. Endocrine deficiencies, non-β-cell tumors, and endogenous hyperinsulinemia (including that caused by an insulinoma) are rare causes of hypoglycemia. Enzymatic metabolic errors that cause hypoglycemia are also rare but are being recognized more frequently in infants and children (Chaps. 350 and 352).

Drugs   In contrast to the sulfonylureas and benzoic acid derivatives (e.g., repaglinide), other oral hypoglycemic agents—biguanides (e.g., metformin), α-glucosidase inhibitors (e.g., acarbose, miglitol), and thiazolidinediones (e.g., troglitazone, rosiglitazone, pioglitazone)—do not act by stimulating insulin secretion. Therefore, with these agents, insulin levels usually decrease appropriately as plasma glucose levels fall. Nonetheless, these drugs can contribute to hypoglycemia in other ways. Treatment with an α-glucosidase inhibitor alters the management of hypoglycemia; pure glucose should be used rather than ingestion of complex carbohydrates. Thiazolidinediones, as well as metformin, can predispose to hypoglycemia in patients receiving combined treatment with insulin or an insulin secretagogue. Ethanol blocks gluconeogenesis but not glycogenolysis. Thus, al-

FIGURE 334-2 Hypoglycemia-associated autonomic failure and hypoglycemia unawareness in type 1 diabetes. (*Modified from PE Cryer: Diabetes 41: 255, 1992, with permission.*)

cohol-induced hypoglycemia typically occurs after a several-day ethanol binge during which the person eats little food, thereby causing
glycogen depletion. Hypoglycemia in this setting can be profound,
with mortality rates as high as 10%. Blood ethanol levels correlate
poorly with plasma glucose concentrations at the time of diagnosis, as
hypoglycemia occurs late in the sequence and often precludes further
alcohol consumption.

Pentamidine, which is used to treat *Pneumocystis* pneumonia and
other parasitic infections, is toxic to the pancreatic β cell. It causes
insulin release initially, with hypoglycemia in about 10% of treated
patients, and predisposes to the development of diabetes mellitus later.
Quinine also stimulates insulin secretion. However, the relative contribution of hyperinsulinemia to the pathogenesis of hypoglycemia in
quinine-treated patients who are critically ill with malaria is debated.
Salicylates and sulfonamides can cause hypoglycemia but do so rarely.
There are reports of hypoglycemia attributed to nonselective β-adre-
nergic antagonists (e.g., propranolol) and a variety of other drugs.

Critical Illness Rapid and extensive hepatic destruction (e.g.,
severe toxic hepatitis) causes fasting hypoglycemia because the liver
is the major site of endogenous glucose production. The mechanism
of hypoglycemia reported in patients with cardiac failure is unknown
but likely involves hepatic congestion. Although the kidneys are a
source of glucose production, it is perhaps too simplistic to attribute
hypoglycemia in people with renal failure to this mechanism alone.
The clearance of insulin is reduced substantially in renal failure, and
reduced mobilization of gluconeogenic precursors has been reported.

Sepsis is sometimes complicated by hypoglycemia, which is multifactorial in origin. There is impaired endogenous glucose production,
perhaps the result of hepatic hypoperfusion, and increased glucose
utilization, which is induced by cytokines in macrophage-rich tissues
such as the liver, spleen, and ileum and in muscle. Nutrition is also
often inadequate in the setting of sepsis. Hypoglycemia can be seen
with prolonged starvation, perhaps as a result of the loss of whole-
body fat stores and the subsequent depletion of gluconeogenic precursors (e.g., amino acids), which necessitate increased glucose utilization.

Endocrine Deficiencies Neither cortisol nor growth hormone is
critical to the prevention of acute hypoglycemia, at least in adults.
Nonetheless, hypoglycemia can occur with prolonged fasting in patients with untreated primary adrenocortical failure (Addison's disease) or hypopituitarism. Anorexia and weight loss are typical features
of chronic cortisol deficiency and likely result in glycogen depletion
with increased reliance on gluconeogenesis. Cortisol deficiency is associated with low levels of gluconeogenic precursors, suggesting that
substrate-limited gluconeogenesis, in the setting of glycogen depletion, is the cause of the impaired ability to tolerate fasting in cortisol-
deficient individuals. Growth hormone deficiency can cause hypoglycemia in young children. In addition to extended fasting, high rates of
glucose utilization (e.g., during exercise, pregnancy) or low rates of
glucose production (e.g., following alcohol ingestion) can precipitate
hypoglycemia in adults with hypopituitarism. Cortisol and growth hormone secretion should be evaluated in patients with fasting hypoglycemia when the history suggests pituitary or adrenal disease and when
other causes of hypoglycemia are not apparent.

As discussed earlier, the combined loss of counterregulatory glucagon and epinephrine responses plays a central role in the pathogenesis of hypoglycemia in diabetes mellitus. However, hypoglycemia is
not a feature of the epinephrine-deficient state that results from bilateral adrenalectomy when glucocorticoid replacement is adequate, nor
does it occur during pharmacologic adrenergic blockage when other
glucoregulatory systems are intact. There are case reports of fasting
hypoglycemia attributed to isolated glucagon or epinephrine deficiency, although hyperinsulinemia was not excluded convincingly in
the neonatal cases and other counterregulatory defects may have contributed in the adults. Thus, the regular assessment of glucagon and
epinephrine secretion is not warranted.

Non-β-Cell Tumors Fasting hypoglycemia, often termed *non-
islet cell tumor hypoglycemia*, occurs in some patients with large mes-

enchymal or other tumors (e.g., hepatoma, adrenocortical tumors,
carcinoids). The glucose kinetic patterns resemble those of hyperinsulinism, but insulin secretion is suppressed appropriately during hypoglycemia. In most instances, hypoglycemia is due to overproduction
of an incompletely processed form of insulin-like growth factor
(IGF)II. Although total IGF-II levels are not consistently elevated,
circulating free IGF-II levels are high. Hypoglycemia may result from
IGF-II actions through the insulin or IGF-I receptors. Because of negative-feedback suppression of growth hormone secretion, IGF-I levels
tend to be low, causing an increased IGF-II to IGF-I ratio.

Endogenous Hyperinsulinism Hypoglycemia due to excessive
endogenous insulin secretion can be caused by: (1) a primary pancreatic islet β cell disorder, typically a β cell tumor (insulinoma), sometimes multiple insulinomas, or, especially in infants or young children,
a functional β cell disorder without an anatomic correlate; (2) a β cell
secretagogue, often a sulfonylurea, and, theoretically, a β cell–stimulating autoantibody; (3) an autoantibody to insulin; or (4) perhaps
ectopic insulin secretion. None of these disorders is common. Endogenous hyperinsulinism is more likely in an overtly well individual
without other apparent causes of hypoglycemia such as a relevant drug
history, critical illness, endocrine deficiencies, or a non-β-cell tumor.
Accidental, surreptitious, or even malicious administration of a
sulfonylurea or insulin should also be considered in such individuals.

The fundamental pathophysiologic feature of endogenous hyperinsulinism is the failure of insulin secretion to fall to very low rates
during hypoglycemia. This is assessed by measuring insulin, proinsulin, and C peptide, which is derived from the processing of proinsulin. The critical diagnostic findings are a plasma insulin concentration ≥ 36 pmol/L (≥ 6 μU/mL) and a plasma C-peptide concentration
≥ 0.2 mmol/L (≥ 0.6 ng/mL) when the plasma glucose concentration
is ≤ 2.5 mmol/L (≤ 45 mg/dL) in the fasting state with symptoms of
hypoglycemia. Insulin and C-peptide levels do not need to be absolutely high (e.g., relative to euglycemic normal values) but only inappropriately high in the setting of fasting hypoglycemia. Plasma
proinsulin concentrations are also inappropriately high, particularly in
patients with an insulinoma. Sulfonylureas, because they stimulate insulin secretion, result in a pattern of glucose, insulin, and C-peptide
levels that is indistinguishable from that produced by a primary β cell
disorder. The measurement of sulfonylureas in plasma or urine distinguishes these conditions. Antibodies to insulin produce *autoimmune
hypoglycemia* following the transition from the postprandial to the
postabsorptive state, as insulin slowly dissociates from the antibodies.
Total and free plasma insulin concentrations are inappropriately high.
The distinguishing finding is the presence of circulating antibodies to
insulin, but the need to measure these routinely is debated, since autoimmune hypoglycemia appears to be rare. Autoantibodies to the insulin receptor are another rare cause of hypoglycemia and usually occur in the context of other autoimmune diseases. A few cases of
apparent ectopic secretion of insulin (from a non-β-cell tumor) have
been reported.

Insulinoma and other primary β cell disorders Insulinomas are
rare, but because approximately 90% are benign, they are a treatable
cause of potentially fatal hypoglycemia. The yearly incidence is estimated to be 1 in 250,000. About 60% of cases occur in women. The
median age at presentation is 50 years in sporadic cases, but it usually
presents in the third decade when associated with multiple endocrine
neoplasia type 1 (Chap. 339). Insulinomas arise within the substance
of the pancreas in >99% of cases and are usually small (1 to 2 cm).
About 5 to 10% of insulinomas are malignant, as evidenced by the
presence of metastases.

Insulinomas almost always come to clinical attention because of
hypoglycemia rather than mass effects. As noted earlier, unusually low
plasma glucose concentrations may be required to produce symptoms
and signs of hypoglycemia because recurrent hypoglycemia shifts the
glycemic thresholds. Although symptomatic hypoglycemia can be
seen after an overnight fast, it often follows exercise. Rarely, symp-

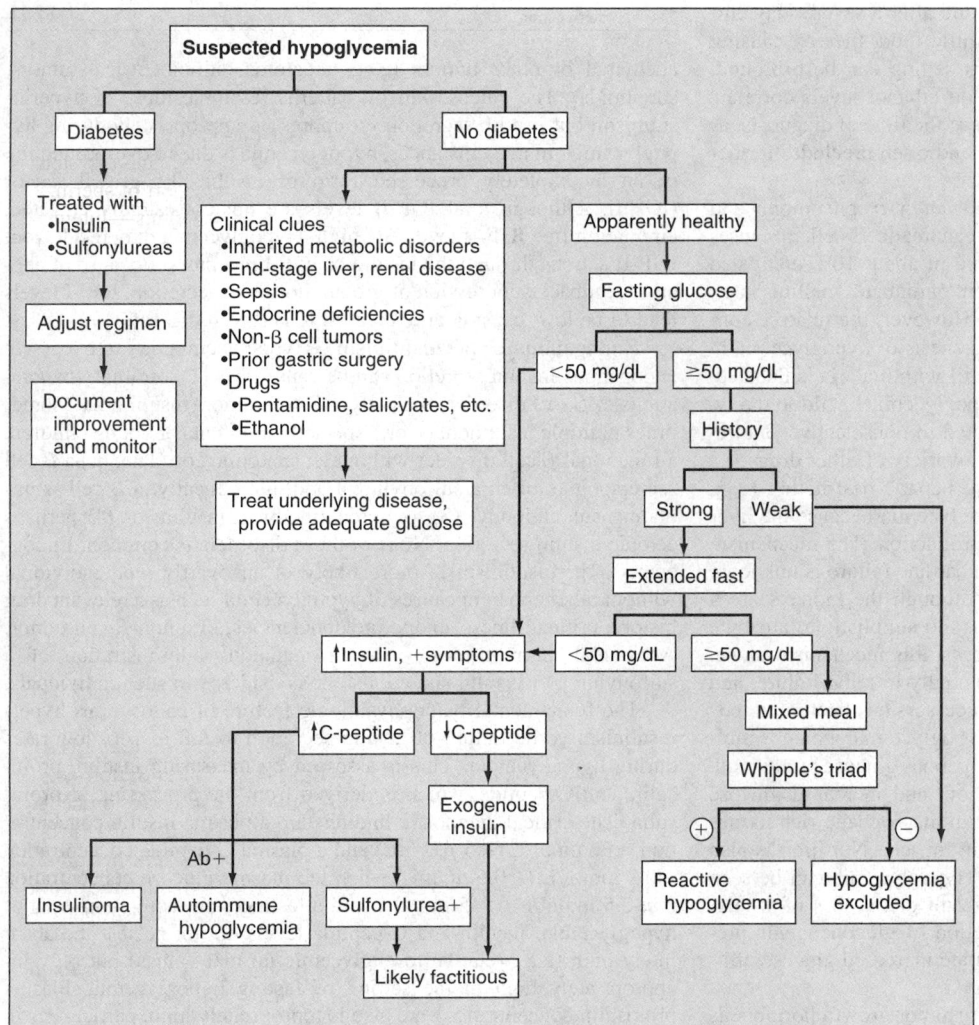

FIGURE 334-3   Diagnostic approach to a patient with suspected hypoglycemia based on a history of symptoms, a low plasma glucose concentration, or both.

patient requiring a fasting test for hypoglycemia. In addition to laboratory tests, observing the behavior of the patient may help make this diagnosis.

Approach to the Patient

In addition to recognition and documentation of hypoglycemia, and often urgent treatment, diagnosis of the hypoglycemic mechanism is critical for choosing a treatment that prevents, or at least minimizes, recurrent hypoglycemia. A diagnostic algorithm is shown in Fig. 334-3.

Recognition and Documentation
Urgent treatment is often necessary in patients with suspected hypoglycemia. Nevertheless, blood should be drawn, whenever possible, before the administration of glucose to allow documentation of the plasma glucose level. Convincing documentation of hypoglycemia requires the fulfillment of Whipple's triad. Thus, *the ideal time to test the plasma glucose is during an episode associated with hypoglycemic symptoms.* A normal plasma glucose concentration measured when the patient is free of symptoms does not exclude hypoglycemia at the time of earlier symptoms. When the cause of hypoglycemia is obscure, additional assays should include glucose, insulin, C peptide, sulfonylurea levels, cortisol, and ethanol.

Hypoglycemia is sometimes detected serendipitously. A distinctly low plasma glucose measurement in a person without a history of corresponding symptoms raises the possibility of a laboratory error caused by ongoing metabolism of glucose by the formed elements of the blood after the sample is drawn. This type of artifactually low glucose level is particularly likely when leukocyte, erythrocyte, or platelet counts are abnormally high, but it can also occur if separation of the plasma or serum from the formed elements is delayed.

Diagnosis of the Hypoglycemic Mechanism   In an adult patient with documented hypoglycemia, a plausible hypoglycemic mechanism and further diagnostic evaluation can be guided by the history, physical examination, and available laboratory data (Fig. 334-3). Relevant historic elements include: drug history, particularly hypoglycemic agents or alcohol use; relevant critical illness (hepatic, renal, or cardiac failure, sepsis, or inanition); previous gastric surgery associated with postprandial hypoglycemia; features suggestive of cortisol or growth hormone deficiency; inherited enzyme deficiencies associated with hypoglycemia; or features of a non-β-cell tumor. Absent these, one must consider medication error, endogenous hyperinsulinism, or surreptitious sulfonylurea or insulin administration. In the absence of documented spontaneous hypoglycemia, overnight fasting, or food deprivation during observation in the outpatient setting, will sometimes elicit hypoglycemia and allow diagnostic evaluation. If these maneuvers do not reveal hypoglycemia, and there is a high degree of clinical suspicion, an extended fast lasting up to 72 h is often required to make these diagnoses. This procedure should be performed in the hospital with careful supervision and should be terminated if the plasma glucose drops to <2.5 mmol/L (<45 mg/dL) and the patient has symptoms. It is essential to draw blood samples for appropriate tests before administering glucose or allowing the patient to eat.

tomatic hypoglycemia occurs following meals, but most such patients have evidence of fasting hypoglycemia as well.

Octreotide scans localize about half of insulinomas. Arteriography has been used extensively in the past, but false-negative and false-positive results occur, and it is generally preferable to use less invasive computed tomography (CT) or magnetic resonance imaging (MRI) scans, which detect 45 to 75% of tumors. Preoperative ultrasound is of value in some patients. Intraoperative ultrasonography has high sensitivity and may localize tumors not identified by palpation. Surgical resection of a solitary insulinoma is generally curative. Diazoxide, which inhibits insulin secretion, and the somatostatin analogue, octreotide, can be used to treat hypoglycemia in patients with unresectable insulinomas.

Factitious Hypoglycemia   Factitious hypoglycemia, caused by malicious or self-administration of insulin or ingestion of a sulfonylurea, shares many clinical and laboratory features with insulinoma. It is most common among health care workers, patients with diabetes or their relatives, and people with a history of other factitious illnesses. When this diagnosis is suspected, it is useful to seek previous medical records, which may reveal admissions for similar episodes as well as relevant laboratory data. In individuals taking exogenous insulin, factitious hypoglycemia can be distinguished from insulinoma by the presence of high insulin levels without a concomitant increase in the C-peptide level, which is suppressed by the exogenous insulin. As noted above, sulfonylureas stimulate endogenous insulin and can therefore be detected only by measuring drug levels in plasma or urine. Factitious or surreptitious hypoglycemia should be considered in every

Urgent Treatment   Oral treatment with glucose tablets or glucose-containing fluids, candy, or food is appropriate if the patient is able and willing to take these. A reasonable initial dose is 20 g of glucose. If neuroglycopenia precludes oral feedings, parenteral therapy is necessary. Intravenous glucose (25 g) should be given using a 50% solution followed by a constant infusion of 5 or 10% dextrose. If intravenous therapy is not practical, subcutaneous or intramuscular glucagon can be used, particularly in people with type 1 diabetes mellitus. Because it acts primarily by stimulating glycogenolysis, glucagon is ineffective in glycogen-depleted individuals (e.g., those with alcohol-induced hypoglycemia). These treatments raise plasma glucose concentrations only transiently, and patients should be encouraged to eat as soon as practical in order to replete glycogen stores.

Prevention of Recurrent Hypoglycemia   Prevention of recurrent hypoglycemia requires an understanding of the hypoglycemic mechanism. Offending drugs can be discontinued or their doses reduced. It should be remembered that hypoglycemia caused by sulfonylureas may recur after a period of many hours or days. Underlying critical illnesses can often be treated. Cortisol and growth hormone can be replaced, if deficient. Surgical, radiotherapeutic, or chemotherapeutic reduction of a non-β-cell tumor can alleviate hypoglycemia, even if the tumor cannot be cured; glucocorticoid or growth hormone administration may also reduce hypoglycemic episodes in such patients. Surgical resection of an insulinoma is often curative; medical therapy with diazoxide or octreotide can be used if resection is not possible and in patients with a nontumor primary β cell disorder. The treatment of autoimmune hypoglycemia (e.g., with a glucocorticoid) is more problematic, but this disorder is often self-limited. Failing these treatments, frequent feedings and avoidance of fasting may be required. Uncooked cornstarch at bedtime or an overnight infusion of intragastric glucose may be necessary in some patients.

BIBLIOGRAPHY

CRYER PE: *Hypoglycemia: Pathophysiology, Diagnosis and Treatment.* New York, Oxford Univ Press, 1997

FRIER BM, FISHER BM: *Hypoglycaemia in Clinical Diabetes.* Chichester, Wiley, 1999

THE DIABETES CONTROL AND COMPLICATIONS TRIAL RESEARCH GROUP: Adverse events and their association with treatment regimens in the Diabetes Control and Complications Trial. Diabetes Care 18:1415, 1995

THE UNITED KINGDOM PROSPECTIVE DIABETES STUDY GROUP: UKPDS 24: A 6-year, randomized, controlled trial comparing sulfonylurea, insulin and metformin therapy in patients with newly diagnosed type 2 diabetes that could not be controlled with diet therapy. Ann Intern Med 128:165, 1998

SERVICE FJ: Hypoglycemic disorders. Endocrinol Metab Clin North Am 28:467, 1999

---

335   *James E. Griffin, Jean D. Wilson*

DISORDERS OF THE TESTES

The testes produce sperm and the steroid hormones that regulate male sexual function. Both processes are under complex feedback control by the hypothalamic-pituitary system so that the testes have biosynthetic and regulatory features similar to those of the ovary and the adrenal. Testicular hormones are also responsible for the formation of the basic male phenotype during embryogenesis (Chap. 338). Disorders that affect testicular function are common. Infertility occurs in about 5% of men; Klinefelter syndrome (XXY) occurs in 1 in 500 men and often escapes diagnosis; and various disorders cause hypogonadism, a condition that can be treated by hormone replacement. The testes are also a site of malignancies, most of which are highly responsive to radiation and/or chemotherapy (Chap. 96).

PHYSIOLOGY AND REGULATION OF TESTICULAR FUNCTION

The testis consists of two components—clusters of interstitial or Leydig cells, where androgenic steroids are synthesized, and a system of spermatogenic tubules for the production and transport of sperm. The components are regulated by the pituitary gonadotropins—luteinizing hormone (LH), which stimulates Leydig cell function, and follicle-stimulating hormone (FSH), which controls Sertoli cell function and spermatogenesis (Fig. 335-1).

GONADOTROPIN REGULATION AND TESTICULAR FUNCTION   Gonadotropin-releasing hormone (GnRH), also called luteinizing hormone–releasing hormone (LHRH), regulates the production of the gonadotropins, LH and FSH (Chap. 328). Because hypothalamic GnRH is secreted in discrete pulses, the plasma concentrations of LH, FSH, and testosterone are not constant, but fluctuate in a pulsatile pattern that mirrors the secretion of GnRH (Fig. 335-2). Pulsatile secretion is most apparent for LH because it has a relatively short plasma half-life by comparison to FSH; pulsatile secretion of testosterone in response to LH is also apparent, although the pulses are dampened because of the need to stimulate steroid synthesis and secretion by the Leydig cell. In contrast to women, in whom the frequency and amplitude of LH pulses vary during the menstrual cycle, the frequency of LH pulses in adult men is relatively constant at about one pulse every 1 to 2 h.

Testosterone secretion is regulated primarily by pituitary LH. FSH may augment testosterone secretion by stimulating a Sertoli-cell derived factor that enhances testosterone production. Testosterone feeds back to regulate the hypothalamic-pituitary production of LH. It decreases hypothalamic GnRH pulse frequency and diminishes pituitary sensitivity to GnRH, leading to lower LH levels. Although the pituitary can convert testosterone to dihydrotestosterone and to estrogens, testosterone itself is the primary regulator of gonadotropin secretion by the pituitary. Under ordinary circumstances, LH secretion is exquisitely sensitive to the feedback effects of testosterone, with almost complete suppression after the administration of amounts of exogenous

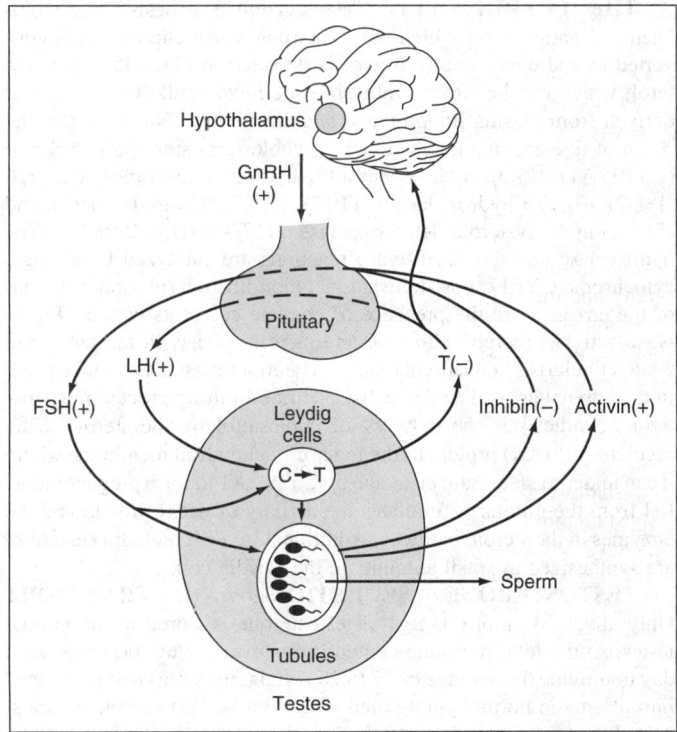

FIGURE 335-1   Regulation of testosterone and sperm production by LH and FSH. C, cholesterol; T, testosterone.

FIGURE 335-2 The 24-h pattern of plasma LH and testosterone in a normal man as samples every 20 min. *(From Griffin and Wilson.)*

androgen that approximate the normal daily secretory rate of testosterone (~20 μmol or 6 mg). However, prolonged elevation of plasma LH (as in testicular deficiency) renders the pituitary less sensitive to negative feedback control by androgen.

FSH is regulated by GnRH and also by the gonadal peptides—inhibins and activins. Inhibins A and B are heterodimeric proteins (composed of α-$β_A$ or α-$β_B$ subunits) that selectively suppress FSH without affecting LH; activins are homodimeric proteins (composed of $β_A$ or $β_B$ subunits) that selectively stimulate FSH production. Inhibin B, which is the major form of inhibin in the male, is produced by the Sertoli cell and provides feedback control of FSH production. Activins, which are produced in the pituitary as well as the gonad, stimulate FSH production through an autocrine-paracrine mechanism.

The interlocking system in which two pituitary hormones (LH and FSH) regulate testicular function provides a precise dual-control mechanism in which hormonal signals from Leydig cells and the spermatogenic tubules feed back on the hypothalamic-pituitary system to regulate their own function (Fig. 335-1).

THE LEYDIG CELL   Testosterone Synthesis   The biochemical pathway by which the 27-carbon sterol cholesterol is converted to androgens and estrogens is depicted in Fig. 335-3. Cholesterol, which can be either synthesized de novo in the Leydig cell or derived from plasma lipoproteins, is converted to testosterone as the result of five enzymatic reactions: (1) cholesterol side chain cleavage (CYP11A1); (2) 3β-hydroxysteroid dehydrogenase/isomerase 2 (3β-HSD2); (3) 17α-hydroxylase (CYP17); (4) 17,20-lyase (CYP17); and (5) 17β-hydroxysteroid dehydrogenase 3 (17β-HSD3). Both the 17α-hydroxylase and the 17,20-lyase reactions are catalyzed by a single cytochrome CYP17; post-translational modification (phosphorylation) of the enzyme and the presence of enzyme cofactors confers 17,20-lyase activity, thereby allowing androgen synthesis in the testis and zona reticularis of the adrenal gland. The first four reactions take place in the adrenal as well as the testis. The rate-limiting process in testosterone synthesis is the delivery of cholesterol by the steroid acute regulatory (StAR) protein to the inner mitochondrial membrane where it can undergo side chain cleavage by CYP11A1 to form pregnenolone. LH from the pituitary stimulates the activity of StAR protein and the enzymes in the steroid pathway. Additional steroids including estradiol are synthesized in small amounts in the Leydig cell.

TESTOSTERONE   SECRETION   AND   TRANSPORT   Only about 70 nmol (20 μg) of testosterone is stored in the normal testes, so the total hormone content turns over about 200 times each day to provide the average of 17 to 20 μmol (5 to 6 mg) that is secreted into plasma in normal young men (Fig. 335-4). Testosterone is transported in plasma bound to protein, largely to albumin and to a specific transport protein, sex hormone–binding globulin (SHBG), also called testosterone-binding globulin (TeBG). The bound and unbound

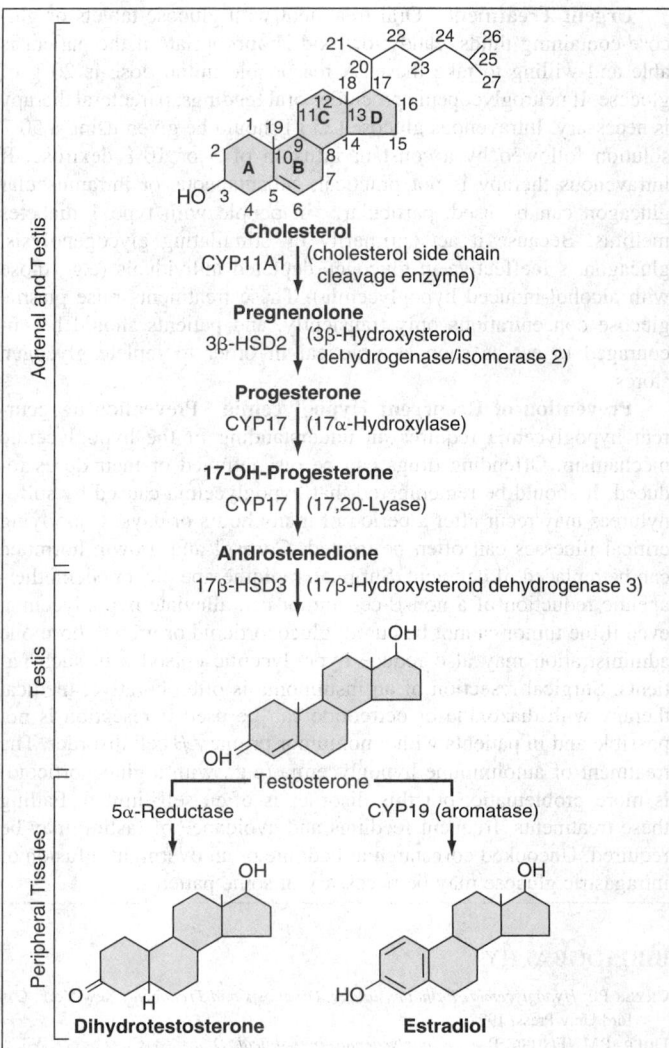

FIGURE 335-3 The biochemical pathway in the conversion of 27-carbon sterol cholesterol to androgens and estrogens.

fractions in plasma are in dynamic equilibrium, only ~1 to 3% being unbound. Because of rapid dissociation from albumin, the fraction of circulating testosterone available for entry into tissues (bioavailable testosterone) approximates the sum of the free and albumin-bound fractions or about half the total plasma level.

Peripheral Metabolism of Androgens   Testosterone serves as a circulating precursor (or prohormone) for the formation of two other hormones that mediate many of the physiologic processes involved in androgen action (Fig. 335-3). Testosterone can be 5α-reduced to dihydrotestosterone, which is responsible for many of the differentiative, growth-promoting, and functional aspects of male sexual differentiation and virilization. Circulating testosterone (and androstenedione) also can be converted to estrogens by aromatase (CYP19) in extraglandular tissues (Fig. 335-4). All estrone production [averaging about 240 nmol (66 μg) per day] can be accounted for by formation from circulating precursors. The mean estradiol production is approximately 170 nmol (45 μg) per day; ~35% is derived from circulating testosterone, 50% is derived from the estrone, and 15% is secreted directly by the testes. When gonadotropin levels are elevated, estradiol secretion by the testes increases. Thus, the physiologic effects of testosterone are the result of the combined actions of testosterone itself plus those of the active androgen and estrogen metabolites of the parent molecule.

The 5α-reduced and estrogenic metabolites can exert local (paracrine) actions in the tissues in which they are formed or enter the circulation and act as hormones at other sites. Circulating dihydrotes-

FIGURE 335-4 Androgen and estrogen production in normal young men. The average production of androstenedione and testosterone is shown in the top boxes, and the mean daily production of esterone and estradiol is shown in the lower boxes. Estrogen is formed by extraglandular aromatization (*braces*) or is secreted directly by the testes. *Vertical arrows* indicate the rates of extraglandular aromatization of androgens, and *horizontal arrows* indicate the interconversion of androgen and estrogens by 17β-hydroxysteroid dehydrogenase. Thus, estradiol arises from plasma testosterone, from estrone, and by direct secretion by the testes. *(Adapted from MacDonald et al.)*

tosterone is formed principally in the androgen target tissues; estrogen formation takes place in many tissues, the most significant being adipose tissue. The overall rate of extraglandular estrogen formation increases with age and with increased mass of adipose tissue.

Testosterone and its active metabolites are catabolized in the liver and excreted predominantly in the urine, approximately half in the form of urinary 17-ketosteroids (primarily androsterone and etiocholanolone) and half as polar metabolites (diols, triols, and conjugates).

Androgen Action The major functions of androgen are formation of the male phenotype during sexual differentiation, regulation of LH secretion, and induction of sexual maturation at puberty. The cellular process by which androgens perform these functions is schematized in Fig. 335-5. Testosterone enters the cell by passive diffusion and can be converted to dihydrotestosterone by either steroid 5α-reductase 1 or 2; 5α-reductase 2 is responsible for dihydrotestosterone formation in most androgen target tissues. Testosterone or dihydrotestosterone is then bound to the androgen-receptor protein in the nucleus. The hormone-receptor complex binds to specific DNA sequences to regulate the transcription of messenger RNA and, ultimately, the synthesis of cellular proteins. The androgen receptor, which is encoded by a gene on the long arm of the X chromosome, contains 917 amino acids and has a molecular mass of about 110 kDa. A polymorphic region in the amino terminus of the receptor, which contains a variable number of glutamine repeats, appears to modify the activity of the receptor. The androgen receptor is similar in structure to other steroid hormone receptors and has distinct hormone-binding, DNA-binding, and transcriptional regulatory domains (Chap. 327). Estradiol acts by a similar mechanism but has its own distinct estrogen receptors α and β (Chap. 336).

Although testosterone and dihydrotestosterone bind to the same receptor, their physiologic roles differ. The testosterone-receptor complex regulates gonadotropin secretion, spermatogenesis, and the virilization of the wolffian ducts during sexual differentiation (Chap. 338), whereas the dihydrotestosterone-receptor complex is responsible for

external virilization during embryogenesis and for most androgen actions during sexual maturation and adult sexual life. The mechanism by which two hormones can interact with the same receptor but have different physiologic effects is not well understood. However, dihydrotestosterone binds to the receptor much more tightly than does testosterone, and hence its formation serves to amplify the hormonal signal.

THE SEMINIFEROUS TUBULES AND SPERMATOGENESIS Spermatogenesis is dependent on both pituitary FSH and androgen production by the adjacent Leydig cells (Fig. 335-1). The function of FSH in gametogenesis has been clarified by rare, naturally occurring mutations in the *FSHβ* gene and in the FSH receptor. Females with these mutations are hypogonadal and infertile because ovarian follicles do not mature, whereas males with mutations in the FSH pathway exhibit variable degrees of impaired spermatogenesis. Thus, while FSH is not absolutely required for spermatogenesis, it increases the number and maturation of sperm. The major site of FSH action is the Sertoli cell, which regulates germ cell proliferation and maturation in the seminiferous tubules. Androgen, which reaches very high concentrations locally in the testis, appears to be essential for spermatogenesis, acting through receptors located in the seminiferous tubules. Several cytokines and growth factors are also involved in the regulation of spermatogenesis by paracrine and autocrine mechanisms. The normal adult testes produce >100 million sperm per day.

The Sertoli cell cannot synthesize steroid hormones de novo but can convert testosterone that diffuses from adjacent Leydig cells to estradiol and to dihydrotestosterone. The Sertoli cell also produces inhibin B. Damage to the seminiferous tubules (e.g., by radiation) reduces inhibin B production, causing a selective increase in FSH.

ASSESSMENT OF TESTICULAR FUNCTION

LEYDIG CELL FUNCTION **History and Physical Examination** The assessment of Leydig cell function and androgen status should include inquiry about the presence of developmental abnormalities of the urogenital tract; the timing and extent of sexual maturation at puberty; the rate of beard growth; and the current libido, sexual function, strength, and energy. Inadequate Leydig cell function or androgen action during embryogenesis may cause hypospadias, cryptorchidism, or microphallus. If Leydig cell failure occurs before puberty, sexual maturation will not occur, and the individual will develop the features termed *eunuchoidism*, including an infantile amount and distribution of body hair, poor development of skeletal muscles, and delayed closure of the epiphyses, so that the arm span is more than 5 cm greater than the height and the lower body segment (heel to pubic bone) is more than 5 cm longer than the upper body segment (pubic bone to crown). Detection of postpubertal Leydig cell failure requires a high index of suspicion and appropriate laboratory assessment because some functions that require androgens for initiation continue unabated when Leydig cell failure occurs, and functions that

FIGURE 335-5 The mechanism of androgen action.

eventually regress may do so very slowly. For example, the frequency of shaving may not decrease for months or years because of slow decline in the rate of beard growth once established. Furthermore, decreased sexual function in adult men may be caused by nonendocrine as well as endocrine factors (Chap. 51).

Plasma Testosterone and Dihydrotestosterone Levels Plasma testosterone is measured by immunoassay. Testosterone is secreted into plasma in a pulsatile fashion every 60 to 90 min (Fig. 335-2). A single random testosterone sample provides a result within ±20% of the true mean value only two-thirds of the time; a pool of three samples spaced 15 to 20 min apart provides a more accurate assessment. The plasma testosterone level in normal adult men ranges from 10 to 35 nmol/L (3 to 10 ng/mL). However, in some normal men with long interpulse intervals of LH, testosterone levels can transiently fall below this normal range, emphasizing the importance of using pooled or repeated samples before making a diagnosis of testosterone deficiency. In adult men, plasma testosterone levels also vary somewhat throughout the day and at different times of the year. In young adult men the plasma testosterone level is ~30% higher in the morning than in the evening. Estimation of SHBG concentration by radioimmunoassay is sometimes useful in the interpretation of total plasma testosterone levels. Bioavailable testosterone in plasma can be estimated by measuring the non-SHBG-bound fraction of testosterone.

The plasma testosterone level is slightly higher in prepubertal boys than in girls, ranging in both from 0.2 to 0.7 nmol/L (0.05 to 0.2 ng/mL). The rise in plasma testosterone level at the start of male puberty begins as a result of sleep-related nocturnal gonadotropin surges, so that levels of plasma testosterone and LH are initially higher at night than during the day. Random daytime levels of plasma testosterone increase gradually as puberty progresses and reach adult levels at about age 17.

Dihydrotestosterone is also measured by immunoassay. In young men the plasma dihydrotestosterone level is about one-tenth the value for testosterone, averaging ~2 nmol/L (0.6 ng/mL). In older men with benign prostatic hyperplasia, plasma dihydrotestosterone levels average ~3 nmol/L (0.9 ng/mL).

Urinary 17-Ketosteroids The measurement of urinary 17-ketosteroids is not a valid way to assess testicular function because testosterone contributes only ~40% of urinary 17-ketosteroids in men, the bulk being derived from adrenal androgens.

Plasma LH Plasma LH is also measured by immunoassay. Dual-site immunometric assays have largely replaced radioimmunoassays. Because LH is secreted in a pulsatile fashion, assay of a pool of three samples drawn 15 to 20 min apart, as described above, provides a value approaching the true mean. In early puberty, plasma LH secretion increases only during sleep, but in the adult the pulsatile secretion is of similar magnitude during sleep and waking periods. The normal plasma LH values should be established for a given laboratory with an appropriate reference standard. A low plasma testosterone level can be interpreted correctly only if plasma LH is measured simultaneously, and, likewise, the "appropriateness" of a given plasma LH value must be interpreted in relation to the plasma testosterone level. For example, a low plasma testosterone level coupled with a low LH level implies hypothalamic or pituitary disease, whereas the finding of a low plasma testosterone level and a high LH level suggests primary testicular insufficiency.

Response to Gonadotropin Stimulation Leydig cell function is difficult to assess before puberty, when both LH and testosterone levels are low, but it is possible to measure response of plasma testosterone to gonadotropin stimulation as an index of Leydig cell capacity. Normal prepubertal boys respond to 3 to 5 days of injection of 1000 to 2000 IU of human chorionic gonadotropin (hCG) with an increase in the plasma testosterone level to ~7 nmol/L (2 ng/mL); the response increases with the initiation of puberty and peaks in early puberty.

Response to GnRH Before puberty, there is minimal response of plasma LH and FSH to the administration of GnRH because the

pituitary has not been "primed" by previous exposure to GnRH or gonadal steroids. After pubertal development, the LH response to acute administration of GnRH increases, while the FSH response is less robust. The amount of LH released after acute administration of GnRH probably reflects the amount of stored hormone in the pituitary. When 100 μg GnRH is given subcutaneously or intravenously to normal men, LH levels usually increase four- to fivefold, with the peak level at 30 min. However, the range of response is broad, and some normal men exhibit less than a doubling of LH levels. In primary testicular failure, measurement of basal LH is usually sufficient, and assessment of GnRH response is of little aid in diagnosis. Since men with either pituitary or hypothalamic disease can have a normal or an abnormal LH response to acute administration of GnRH, a normal response does not clearly distinguish these causes of gonadal deficiency. A subnormal response is, however, of value in establishing that an abnormality exists, even though the site of the defect is not clearly determined. If pulsatile GnRH or daily infusions of GnRH for a week lead to the development of a normal acute LH response, a hypothalamic etiology is likely.

SEMINIFEROUS TUBULE FUNCTION **Examination of the Testes** Evaluation of the testes is an essential portion of the physical examination. The prepubertal testis measures about 2 cm in length and 2 mL in volume and grows during puberty to reach the adult proportions by age 16. When damage to the seminiferous tubules occurs before puberty, the testes are small and firm, whereas the testes are usually soft after postpubertal damage (the capsule, once enlarged, does not contract to its previous size). Testes in adult men average 4.6 cm in length (range, 3.5 to 5.5 cm), corresponding to a volume of 12 to 25 mL, and the seminiferous tubules account for ~60% of testicular mass. Advanced age does not influence testicular size, so the significance of small testes in the adult is the same at all ages. Asian men have smaller testes than western Europeans, independent of differences in body size. Because of its possible causal role in infertility, the presence of varicocele should be sought by palpation with the patient standing.

Semen Analysis Seminal fluid is analyzed on samples obtained by masturbation into a glass container after 24 to 36 h of abstinence. Analysis should be performed within an hour of collection. The normal ejaculate volume is 2 to 6 mL. Immediately after ejaculation, the seminal fluid coagulates, followed in 15 to 30 min by liquefaction. Motility should be assessed in undiluted seminal fluid; >60% of the sperm should be motile and of normal morphology. The normal range for sperm density is generally considered to be >20 million per milliliter, with a total count of >60 million per ejaculate, but the definition of a minimally adequate ejaculate is not clear. Some men with low sperm counts are nevertheless fertile. This uncertainty as to the lower level of sperm density, percent motility, and percent normal forms in fertile semen stems from two issues. First, the seminal fluid is routinely evaluated by tests that do not assess the functional capacity of sperm. Second, many factors produce temporary aberrations in sperm count; in men with semen of equivocal quality, it is necessary to examine three or more ejaculates to determine whether the abnormal findings are permanent.

Plasma FSH Plasma FSH, as measured by immunoassay, usually correlates inversely with spermatogenesis. When damage to the germinal epithelium is severe, plasma levels of inhibin B fall and plasma levels of FSH increase.

Testicular Biopsy Testicular biopsy is useful in some patients with oligospermia and azoospermia both as an aid in diagnosis and as an indication of the feasibility of treatment. For example, normal findings on testicular biopsy and a normal FSH level in an azoospermic man suggest obstruction of the vas deferens, which may be correctable surgically. In some men with severe oligospermia, testicular biopsy allows retrieval of sperm for intracytoplasmic sperm injections (ICSI) into oocytes (Chap. 54).

ESTROGENIC FUNCTION **Examination of the Breasts** Breast enlargement (gynecomastia) is the most consistent feature of feminizing states in men (Chap. 337). Gynecomastia is due to an increase in both glandular and adipose tissue. The presence of gyneco-mastia should be sought by examining the sitting patient, using the fingers to grasp glandular tissue. Early or minimal breast enlargement may be missed if the breast is palpated with the flat of the hand while the patient is supine. In obese men it is important to try to define the rim of the glandular tissue where it meets the adipose tissue of the chest wall.

Plasma Estrogen As discussed above, most of the estradiol and all of the estrone produced in normal men is formed by extraglandular aromatization of circulating androgens. The plasma level of estradiol usually is <180 pmol/L (50 pg/mL) in normal men; the plasma estrone level is somewhat higher but usually is <300 pmol/L (80 pg/mL). Elevations in estrogen production and estrogen plasma levels can be due to increases in plasma precursors (liver or adrenal disease), to increased extraglandular aromatization (obesity), or to increased production by the testes (testicular tumors, androgen resistance, gonadotropin stimulation).

PHASES OF NORMAL TESTICULAR FUNCTION

The phases of male sexual life can be defined in terms of the plasma testosterone value (Fig. 335-6). In the male embryo the production of testosterone by the testes commences at about 7 weeks of gestation and is stimulated in part by placental hCG. Shortly thereafter, plasma testosterone attains a high level that is maintained until late in gestation. The level then falls so that at the time of birth the plasma testosterone level is only slightly higher in males than in females. Shortly after birth, a transient increase of pituitary gonadotropins raises the plasma testosterone level in the male infant for ~3 months, before hormone levels again decrease to low levels by age 6 months to 1 year. The significance of the rise in plasma testosterone level during the first year of life is not certain. However, in other primates neonatal activation of the hypothalamic-pituitary-testicular axis is important for subsequent normal pubertal development. The testosterone concentration then remains low (but slightly higher in boys than in girls) until the onset of puberty, when it begins to rise in boys, reaching adult levels by about age 17. The level of bioavailable testosterone remains constant until the 40s when it begins to decline at a rate of ~1.2% per year; the level of SHBG increases by ~1.2% per year so that there is little decline in total testosterone until the later decades of life. During the third, or adult, phase of male sexual life, sperm production becomes sufficient to allow reproduction to take place. The physiologic events during these various phases differ, as do the pathologic consequences of derangements in testicular function. Male sexual differentiation during embryogenesis is considered in Chap. 338.

ABNORMALITIES OF TESTICULAR FUNCTION

PUBERTY The control of puberty is poorly understood and may reside in the hypothalamic-pituitary system, the testes, or the adrenals (Chap. 8). Before the onset of puberty, gonadotropin secretion by the pituitary is low, but prepubertal castration causes a rise in plasma gonadotropin levels. This finding suggests that before puberty the negative feedback control of gonadotropin secretion is exquisitely sensitive to the small amount of circulating testosterone. The onset of puberty is heralded by sleep-associated surges in gonadotropin secretion. Later in puberty the rises in LH and FSH levels persist throughout the day. Thus, with maturation, the hypothalamic-pituitary system becomes less sensitive to negative feedback control, and the consequences are higher mean plasma levels of testosterone and gonadotropins, maturation of the testes, and the onset of spermatogenesis. The rise in gonadotropin secretion is the consequence of an increase both in GnRH secretion and in the sensitivity of the pituitary to GnRH.

The somatic changes at the time of puberty are secondary to the rise in plasma testosterone, which induces the growth of the accessory organs of male reproduction (the penis, the prostate, the seminal vesicles, and the epididymides). Accelerated linear growth is accompanied by growth of muscle and connective tissue, which account for the major portion of nitrogen retention at puberty. The principal androgen-sensitive muscles are those of the pectoral region and the shoulder. The characteristic hair growth of male puberty involves development of mustache and beard; regression of the scalp line; appearance of body, extremity, and perianal hair; and extension of the pubic hair upward into a diamond-shaped pattern. Growth of axillary and pubic hair is initiated under the control of adrenal androgens and is promoted by testicular androgens. The larynx enlarges, and the vocal cords thicken, resulting in a lowering of the pitch of the voice. Hemoglobin levels increase by ~1 g/dL. These various androgen-mediated growth and maturation processes reach some limiting value, so that once puberty is completed, the administration of pharmacologic doses of androgen has no further effect. The entire process is heralded by testicular enlargement beginning at age 11 to 12 and is usually completed within 5 years, although some aspects of virilization, such as growth of the chest hair, may continue over a decade or more.

The events of normal male puberty are variable in onset, duration, and sequence. The central issue in dealing with disorders of puberty is separating true absence or precocity from the extremes of normal variation. The use of staging criteria that correlate developmental and anatomic landmarks with chronologic age is useful in making this distinction (Chap. 8).

Sexual Precocity Premature development of sexual characteristics that are phenotypically appropriate—i.e., virilization in boys—is termed *isosexual precocity. Heterosexual precocity* refers to feminizing syndromes in boys.

Isosexual precocity Sexual development before age 9 in boys is generally considered abnormal. *True precocious puberty* or *complete isosexual precocity* occurs when both virilization and spermatogenesis are premature. *Precocious pseudopuberty* or *incomplete isosexual precocity* refers to virilization unaccompanied by spermatogenesis. This distinction is blurred in practice, because pure virilizing syndromes may cause activation of gonadotropin secretion secondarily and thus be followed by development of spermatogenesis. Furthermore, local androgen production in the testis, as in Leydig cell tumors, can cause local areas of spermatogenesis and limited sperm production around the tumor. We therefore prefer a two-part classification: virilizing syndromes (in which hypothalamic-pituitary activity is appropriate for age) and premature activation of the hypothalamic-pituitary system.

Virilizing syndromes can result from Leydig cell tumors, hCG-secreting tumors, adrenal tumors, congenital adrenal hyperplasia (most commonly 21-hydroxylase deficiency), androgen administration, or Leydig cell hyperplasia. In these disorders plasma testosterone levels are inappropriately elevated for the age. Leydig cell tumors are rare in children but should be suspected when the testes are asymmetric in size (Chap. 96). Virilizing adrenal tumors mainly secrete androstenedione and dehydroepiandrosterone, some of which is converted to testosterone; consequently, they cause increased 17-ketosteroid excre-

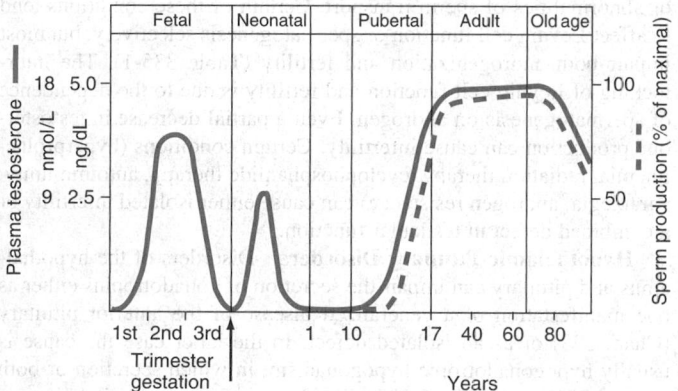

FIGURE 335-6 Phases of male sexual life. (*From Griffin and Wilson.*)

tion. Glucocorticoid administration does not reduce 17-ketosteroid excretion to normal in patients with testicular or adrenal tumors, in contrast to the prompt decrease that occurs after such treatment in patients with congenital adrenal hyperplasia. Congenital adrenal hyperplasia leads to elevated 17-hydroxyprogesterone levels and, as a consequence, elevated androgen levels (Chaps. 331 and 338). When this disorder is treated with glucocorticoids, true precocious puberty can then result if the increased androgen levels have caused sufficient hypothalamic maturation.

Gonadotropin-independent sexual precocity in boys may occur as a result of autonomous Leydig cell hyperplasia in the absence of a Leydig cell tumor. The disorder can occur sporadically or can be inherited as a male-limited autosomal disorder either from affected fathers or from mothers who are unaffected carriers. It is due to point mutations in the LH receptor that cause constitutive activation of the receptor in the absence of LH. Virilization usually begins by age 2. Testosterone levels are elevated, often to the adult male range; however, immunoreactive and bioactive LH levels and the LH response to GnRH are prepubertal. In the past many of these boys were mistakenly thought to have true precocious puberty because spermatogenesis may be present.

Premature activation of the hypothalamic-pituitary system Central precocious puberty may be "idiopathic" or due to central nervous system (CNS) tumors, infections, or injuries. Early hypothalamic-pituitary activation typically is associated with features of normal puberty, i.e., sleep-related gonadotropin secretion, elevated plasma bioactive LH, and enhanced gonadotropin response to GnRH. Since the diagnosis of idiopathic true precocious puberty is one of exclusion, patients may later prove to have been misclassified and to have a CNS abnormality. With improved means of diagnosis, such as magnetic resonance imaging, delays in diagnosis will probably be less frequent.

Management of sexual precocity due to steroid- or gonadotropin-producing tumors, congenital adrenal hyperplasia, or CNS abnormality is directed toward the primary disease. In boys with Leydig cell hyperplasia, attempts have been made to lower plasma testosterone with medroxyprogesterone acetate or ketoconazole, or to blunt hormone action with spironolactone, but treatment remains suboptimal. Idiopathic true precocious puberty and true precocious puberty due to inoperable CNS lesions are treated with long-acting GnRH analogue therapy, which inhibits gonadotropin production and testosterone synthesis, reversing pubertal maturation and decreasing the rate of skeletal development.

Heterosexual precocity Feminization in prepubertal boys can result from absolute or relative increases in estrogen due to a variety of causes (Chap. 337).

Delayed or Incomplete Puberty Separating failure of puberty from variants of normal development is one of the most difficult problems in endocrinology. Some boys fail to show the normal spurt of growth and sexual development at the usual time but eventually commence puberty by age 16 or older. Adolescence may then either progress rapidly, or slow pubertal development and growth may continue until age 20 to 22. Many men with delayed onset of puberty attain heights within the normal adult range. The history may reveal that a parent or sibling had a similar pattern of development. Panhypopituitarism and hypothyroidism can cause pubertal failure (Chaps. 328 and 330). Absent puberty also can result from primary testicular disease; this diagnosis is suspected on the basis of low plasma testosterone levels and elevated FSH and LH levels. Hereditary androgen resistance (in which plasma testosterone and LH levels are both high) usually causes male pseudohermaphroditism but in mild form may be manifested by absent or incomplete puberty (Chap. 338).

Most boys with absent puberty have low plasma levels of both testosterone and gonadotropins; in these boys it is necessary to distinguish delayed puberty from isolated gonadotropin deficiency or idiopathic *hypogonadotropic hypogonadism (Kallman syndrome)*. The

manifestations of isolated gonadotropin deficiency vary from boys with eunuchoidal features and testes of prepubertal size to those with partial LH and/or FSH deficiency and some degree of testicular enlargement and pubertal development. Ansomia or hyposmia is caused by abnormal development of the olfactory tracts (which share progenitor cells with GnRH neurons) and is characteristically seen in Kallmann syndrome. X-linked *adrenal hypoplasia congenita (AHC)* is characterized by primary adrenal insufficiency, which usually presents in infancy, and hypogonadotropic hypogonadism, caused by deficient GnRH production and abnormal gonadotrope function. Congenital hypogonadotropic hypogonadism is frequently associated with cryptorchidism and a prepubertal manifestation can be microphallus, in which the size of the penis is below the fifth percentile for the age.

The pathogenesis of hypogonadotropic hypogonadism can involve several distinct abnormalities of GnRH formation or action. Some cases are inherited as an X-linked recessive trait associated with defects in a neural cell adhesion molecule (KAL) involved in the migration of GnRH neurons into the olfactory bulb. Other causes involve autosomal dominant disorders with variable expressivity; rare autosomal recessive cases are due to mutations that impair the GnRH receptor. Serum FSH and LH levels are usually below the normal male range, and plasma testosterone levels are low for age. The secretion of other pituitary hormones is normal. The administration of pulsatile GnRH corrects the endocrine abnormalities and initiates spermatogenesis in patients with GnRH deficiency; all patients respond to gonadotropin replacement. If untreated, these patients usually remain in the prepubertal state indefinitely.

It is particularly difficult to distinguish hypogonatropic hypogonadism from delayed puberty in boys of early or midpubertal age; the presence of microphallus, anosmia, or a family history may suggest the diagnosis. In the absence of such evidence, observation through the teenage years may be required before it becomes clear whether a patient has delayed puberty or a permanent form of hypogonadotropic hypogonadism. Since delayed puberty is associated with a decreased bone mass, therapy should not be delayed too long. In some cases the response of plasma LH to GnRH stimulation may be helpful in suggesting that puberty is imminent.

ADULTHOOD At the completion of puberty, plasma testosterone levels reach the adult level of 10 to 35 nmol/L (3 to 10 ng/mL) throughout the day, plasma gonadotropins are in the normal adult range, and sperm production is sufficient to allow reproduction. The adult pattern of hypothalamic-pituitary-gonadal regulation is sustained in the normal man for more than 40 years. However, the system is subject to a variety of influences, at the level of both the testes and the hypothalamic-pituitary system. Spermatogenesis is exquisitely sensitive to alterations in scrotal temperature, and brief increases in either systemic or local temperature (as in a hot bath) can be followed by temporary decreases in sperm production. The system also is influenced by diet, drugs, alcohol, environmental agents, and psychological stress, any of which may cause temporary decreases in sperm count.

Persistent abnormalities of testicular function in adult men can be due to hypothalamic-pituitary disorders (Chap. 328), testicular defects, or abnormalities of sperm transport. Certain of these conditions tend to affect Leydig cell function or spermatogenesis selectively, but most impair both androgenization and fertility (Table 335-1). The interlocking of Leydig cell function and fertility is due to the dependence of spermatogenesis on androgen. Even a partial decrease in testosterone production can cause infertility. Certain conditions (hyperprolactinemia, radiation therapy, cyclophosphamide therapy, autoimmunity, paraplegia, androgen resistance) can cause either isolated infertility or a combined defect in testicular function.

Hypothalamic-Pituitary Disorders Disorders of the hypothalamus and pituitary can impair the secretion of gonadotropins either as one manifestation of a generalized disease of the anterior pituitary (Chap. 328) or as an isolated defect. In the latter case the cause is usually hypogonadotropic hypogonadism, in which secretion of both LH and FSH are impaired. This disorder usually is congenital but may be acquired. Alternatively, gonadotropin secretion can be altered by

Infertility with Underandrogenization	Infertility with Normal Virilization
HYPOTHALAMIC-PITUITARY	
Panhypopituitarism	
Isolated gonadotropin deficiency	Isolated FSH deficiency
Adrenal hypoplasia congenita	Congenital adrenal hyperplasia
Cushing's syndrome	Hyperprolactinemia
Hyperprolactinemia	Androgen use
Hemochromatosis	
TESTICULAR	
Developmental and structural defects	
Klinefelter's syndrome[a]	AZF mutations of the Y chromo-
XX male	some
	Germinal cell aplasia
	Cryptorchidism
	Varicocele
	Immotile cilia syndrome
Acquired defects	
Viral orchitis*	*Mycoplasma* infection
Trauma	
Radiation	Radiation
Drugs (spironolactone, alcohol, ke-	Drugs (cyclophosphamide)
toconazole, cyclophosphamide)	
Environmental toxins	Environmental toxins
Autoimmunity	Autoimmunity
Granulomatous disease	
Associated with systemic diseases	
Liver disease	Febrile illness
Renal failure	Celiac disease
Sickle cell disease	
Immune disease (AIDS, rheumatoid	
arthritis)	
Neurologic disease (myotonic dys-	Neurologic disease (paraplegia)
trophy, spinobulbar muscular atro-	
phy, and paraplegia)	
Androgen resistance	Androgen resistance
SPERM TRANSPORT	
	Obstruction of the epididymis or
	vas deferens (cystic fibrosis, di-
	ethylstilbesterol exposure, con-
	genital absence)

[a] The common testicular causes of underandrogenization and infertility in adults—Klinefelter's syndrome and viral orchitis—are associated with small testes.

factors other than hypothalamic-pituitary pathology. For example, elevation of plasma cortisol, as in the *Cushing syndrome*, can depress LH secretion independent of a space-occupying lesion of the pituitary. Critical illness also suppresses plasma gonadotropin levels. Some patients with uncontrolled *congenital adrenal hyperplasia* have elevated levels of adrenal androgens, suppressed gonadotropin secretion, and consequent infertility. Likewise, the use of *androgens* for purposes other than replacement therapy can inhibit gonadotropin secretion and impair sperm production (see below). *Hyperprolactinemia* (as the consequence either of pituitary adenomas or of drugs such as phenothiazines) can cause combined Leydig cell and seminiferous tubule dysfunction, presumably due to inhibition of LH and FSH secretion by prolactin. Occasionally, impaired fertility in hyperprolactinemia is associated with normal gonadotropin and androgen levels and is presumed to result from direct inhibition of spermatogenesis by prolactin. *Hemochromatosis* usually impairs testicular function as the result of effects on the pituitary; less often it affects the testis directly (Chap. 345). In some conditions, testosterone levels may be decreased in association with normal LH levels, and the mechanism is less clear. Men with massive obesity have decreased levels of SHBG and of total and bioavailable testosterone, which return toward normal with weight loss. Obesity may also contribute to the decreased testosterone levels in the subset of such men with Pickwickian syndrome (Chap. 263). Some men with temporal lobe seizures also have hypogonadotropic hypogonadism.

Testicular Defects Abnormalities of testicular function in the adult man can be grouped into several categories: developmental and structural defects of the testes, acquired testicular defects, and disorders secondary to systemic disease.

Developmental abnormalities The *Klinefelter syndrome* (*XXY*, both the classic and the mosaic forms) and the *XX male syndrome* are usually not recognized until after the time of expected puberty (Chap. 338). Some developmental defects cause infertility in the presence of normal androgen production. These include varicocele, germinal cell aplasia, deletions or mutations of the azoospermia factor (*AZF*) genes on the Y chromosome, and cryptorchidism. *Varicocele* may be of etiologic importance in as much as one-third of all cases of male infertility. It is caused by retrograde flow of blood into the internal spermatic vein that eventuates in progressive, often palpable dilation of the peritesticular pampiniform plexus of veins. Varicocele occurs in ~10 to 15% of men in the general population and in 20 to 40% of men with infertility. It is thought to result from incompetence of the valve between the internal spermatic vein and the renal vein and is more common on the left side (85%). Unilateral varicocele increases the blood flow and the temperature of both testes as a result of the extensive anastomoses of the venous systems. The increased scrotal (and testicular) temperature is believed to be the cause of the poor-quality semen and infertility (the testes no longer are 2°C cooler than the abdominal cavity). The findings on semen analysis are usually nonspecific, with all parameters showing some abnormality. Surgical repair of varicocele results in fertility in about half of men, with the best results (70% pregnancy rate) in those whose preoperative sperm counts are >10 million per milliliter.

Some patients with *germinal cell aplasia* (the Sertoli cell-only syndrome) have a positive family history and may constitute a specific group in whom the germinal epithelium is missing with resulting azoospermia; plasma testosterone and LH values are normal, and plasma FSH levels are elevated. Other patients with identical histologic and clinical findings have androgen resistance or a history of viral orchitis or cryptorchidism; microdeletions of one or more genes (e.g., *Deleted in Azoospermia, DAZ*) on the Y chromosome have been documented in 10 to 20% of men with azoospermia or oligospermia (many of whom have germinal cell aplasia), depending on the criteria used for selection.

Unilateral *cryptorchidism*, even when corrected before puberty, is associated with abnormal semen in many individuals, indicating that the testes can be bilaterally abnormal even in unilateral cryptorchidism.

The *immotile cilia syndrome* is an autosomal recessive defect characterized by immotility or poor motility of the cilia of the airways and of the sperm. Kartagener's syndrome is a subgroup of the immotile cilia syndrome associated with situs inversus, chronic sinusitis, and bronchiectasis (Chap. 256). The structural abnormality leading to impaired motility of cilia can usually be defined by the electron-microscopic appearance showing defects in the dynein arms, spokes, or microtubule doublets. Cilia from epithelia and sperm tails exhibit the same defects, but the pulmonary manifestations may be minor. Other less well understood structural defects can cause immotility of sperm without involvement of cilia in the lung.

Acquired testicular defects Acquired testicular failure in the adult man can be due to *viral orchitis*. The responsible viruses include mumps virus, echovirus, lymphocytic choriomeningitis virus, and group B arboviruses. The orchitis is due to actual infection of the tissue by virus rather than to indirect effects of infection. Orchitis occurs in as many as one-fourth of adult men with mumps; in about two-thirds the orchitis is unilateral, and in the remainder it is bilateral. Orchitis usually develops a few days after the onset of parotitis but may precede it. The testis may return to normal size and function or undergo atrophy. Atrophy is believed to be due both to direct effects of the virus on the seminiferous tubules and to ischemia secondary to pressure and edema within the taut tunica albuginea. Semen analysis returns to normal in three-fourths of men with unilateral involvement and in only one-third of men with bilateral orchitis. Atrophy is usually perceptible within 1 to 6 months after the acute illness, and the degree of atrophy is not necessarily proportional to the severity of the acute orchitis. Unilateral atrophy occurs in about one-third of patients, and bilateral atrophy occurs in about one-tenth.

Trauma, including torsion, can also cause secondary atrophy of the testes. The exposed position of the testes in the scrotum renders them susceptible to both thermal and physical trauma—particularly in men with hazardous occupations.

The testes are sensitive to *radiation damage*; decreased secretion of testosterone appears to be a consequence of diminished testicular blood flow. Doses >200 mGy (20 rad) cause increases in plasma FSH and LH levels and damage to the spermatogonia. After about 800 mGy (80 rad), oligospermia or azoospermia develops, and higher doses may obliterate the germinal epithelium, except for occasional stem and Sertoli cells. Fractionated radiation may have a more profound effect than single-dose radiation. Recovery of sperm density occurs in a dose-related fashion, and complete recovery of sperm density may require as long as 5 years. Permanent infertility can occur after radiation therapy for malignant lymphoma despite shielding of the testes. Permanent androgen deficiency in adult men is uncommon after therapeutic radiation; however, most boys given direct testicular radiation therapy for acute lymphoblastic leukemia have permanently low plasma testosterone levels. Sperm banking should be considered in patients before they undergo radiation treatment or chemotherapy.

In general, *drugs* interfere with testicular function in one of four ways—inhibition of testosterone synthesis, blockade of androgen action, enhancement of estrogen levels, or direct inhibition of spermatogenesis. Spironolactone and ketoconazole block the synthesis of androgen by interfering with the late steps in androgen biosynthesis. Spironolactone and cimetidine compete with androgen for binding to the androgen receptor and thus block androgen action in target cells. Testosterone levels may be low, and estradiol levels may be elevated in persons using marijuana, heroin, or methadone, although the exact reasons are unclear. Alcohol, when consumed in excess for prolonged periods, causes decreased plasma testosterone levels, independent of liver disease or malnutrition. Elevated plasma estradiol and decreased plasma testosterone levels may occur in men taking digitalis.

Antineoplastic and chemotherapeutic agents commonly interfere with spermatogenesis. Cyclophosphamide causes azoospermia or extreme oligospermia within a few weeks after the initiation of therapy. Cessation of therapy is followed by a return of spermatogenesis within 3 years in about half of patients. Combination chemotherapy for acute leukemia, Hodgkin's disease, and other malignancies also may impair Leydig cell function. In pubertal boys this impairment is manifested by decreased serum testosterone and elevated LH levels; in adult men testosterone levels do not decline, and the impaired Leydig cell function may be detected only as an enhanced LH response to GnRH. The alkylating agents in the chemotherapeutic regimens seem to be responsible for Leydig cell toxicity.

Because of the toxic effects of many physical and chemical agents on spermatogenesis, the occupational and recreational history should be carefully evaluated in all men with infertility. Known environmental hazards include microwaves, ultrasound, and chemicals such as the nematocide dibromochloropropane, cadmium, and lead. In some populations, sperm density is said to have declined by as much as 40% in the past 50 years, and it has been postulated that environmental estrogens or antiandrogens may be responsible.

Testicular failure also occurs as a part of *polyglandular autoimmune insufficiency* (Chap. 339). Sperm antibodies can cause isolated male infertility. In some instances these antibodies are secondary phenomena resulting from duct obstruction or vasectomy. *Granulomatous diseases* can destroy the testes, and testicular atrophy occurs in 10 to 20% of men with lepromatous leprosy owing to direct invasion of the tissue by the mycobacteria. The tubules are involved initially, followed by endarteritis and destruction of Leydig cells.

Testicular abnormalities associated with systemic disease   In *cirrhosis of the liver*, a combined testicular and pituitary abnormality leads to decreased testosterone production independent of the direct toxic effects of ethanol. Although the plasma LH level is elevated, the level may be below the expected range given the degree of androgen deficiency. This situation most likely results from the inhibition of LH secretion by estrogen in patients with chronic liver disease. Increased estrogen production results from impaired hepatic extraction of adrenal androstenedione and subsequent increased extraglandular conversion to estrone and estradiol. In effect, estrogen precursors are shunted to sites of extraglandular aromatization. Testicular atrophy and gynecomastia are present in about half of men with cirrhosis, and many such men are impotent. Successful liver transplantation reverses the effects of cirrhosis on the pituitary-testicular axis.

In chronic *renal failure*, androgen synthesis and sperm production decrease despite elevated plasma gonadotropins. The elevated LH level is due to increased production and reduced clearance but does not restore normal testosterone production. In addition, about one-fourth of men with renal failure have hyperprolactinemia; the role of hyperprolactinemia in decreasing testosterone production is unclear. Low testosterone coupled with normal or increased plasma estrogen levels cause gynecomastia in about half of men on chronic hemodialysis, and about half of men on dialysis have decreased libido and/or impotence. Improvement in testosterone production with hemodialysis is incomplete, but successful transplantation may return testicular function to normal.

Men with *sickle cell anemia* usually have impaired secondary sexual development, and testicular atrophy is present in one-third of them. The defect may be at either the testicular or the hypothalamic-pituitary level. Abnormalities in Leydig cell function, frequently accompanied by decreased sperm density, have been noted in a variety of chronic systemic diseases, including protein-energy *malnutrition*, advanced *Hodgkin's disease* and *cancer* before chemotherapy, and *amyloidosis*. Most of these disorders cause a lowered plasma testosterone level coupled with a normal to increased plasma LH level, suggesting combined hypothalamic-pituitary and testicular defects. Similar hormone changes occur after *surgery*, *myocardial infarction*, and severe *burns* and thus may be a nonspecific effect of illness.

In HIV-infected men, elevation of gonadotropins (a compensated state of hypogonadism) may precede the development of overt hypogonadism, but 35 to 50% of men with AIDS eventually develop low testosterone levels. Elevation of SHBG levels may partially mask the fall in testosterone. Some of the hormonal changes in this disorder are likely nonspecific and related to severe illness. Whether testosterone deficiency contributes to the muscle wasting and weight loss characteristic of this disorder is unclear, but androgen replacement therapy may increase muscle and lean body mass.

Sperm density can decrease temporarily after *acute febrile illness* in the absence of a change in testosterone production. Infertility in men with *celiac disease* is associated with a hormonal pattern typical of androgen resistance, namely, elevated testosterone and LH levels. *Neurologic* diseases associated with altered testicular function include myotonic dystrophy, spinobulbar muscular atrophy, and paraplegia. In myotonic dystrophy, small testes may be associated with impairment of both spermatogenesis and Leydig cell function. Spinobulbar muscular atrophy is caused by an expansion of the glutamine repeat sequences in the amino-terminal region of the androgen receptor; this expansion impairs function of the androgen receptor, but it is unclear how the alteration is related to the neurologic manifestations. Men with spinobulbar muscular atrophy often have as a late manifestation underandrogenization and infertility and the hormonal features of androgen resistance (Chap. 338). *Spinal cord lesions* that cause paraplegia lead to a temporary decrease in testosterone levels and may cause persistent defects in spermatogenesis; some patients retain the capacity for penile erection and ejaculation.

Androgen resistance   Defects of the androgen receptor cause resistance to the action of androgen, usually associated with defective male phenotypic development, infertility, and underandrogenization

(Chap. 338). Mutations of the androgen receptor that cause mild androgen resistance can cause infertility due to oligo- or azoospermia in otherwise phenotypically normal men.

Impairment of Sperm Transport Disorders of sperm transport may cause infertility in as many as 6% of infertile men with normal virilization. Obstruction of the ejaculatory system may be unilateral or bilateral, congenital or acquired. In men with unilateral obstruction, infertility may result from antisperm antibodies. Congenital defects of the vas deferens can occur as an isolated abnormality associated with absence of the seminal vesicles (and consequently absence of fructose in the ejaculate), in men whose mothers received *diethylstilbestrol* during pregnancy, and in men with *cystic fibrosis*. Furthermore, congenital bilateral absence of the vas deferens can be due to mutations in the cystic fibrosis conductance regulator (*CFTR*) gene; some of these mutations are distinct from those associated with the more typical pulmonary and gastrointestinal manifestations of cystic fibrosis. Acquired obstructive azoospermia can occur at the level of the epididymis in association with chronic infections of the paranasal sinuses and lungs and with tuberculosis, leprosy, and gonorrhea.

Empirical Therapy of Male Infertility Disorders for which there are logical or effective treatments (genital tract obstruction, sperm autoimmunity, gonadotropin deficiency) account for only 10% of infertile men, and pregnancies are infrequent when the male partner has genital tract obstruction or sperm autoimmunity. Severe oligospermia/azoospermia from other causes accounts for about one-fourth of cases of male infertility and has largely been considered untreatable. The other two-thirds of infertile men have a partial reduction in semen parameters and subfertility of a variable degree, and in this group spontaneous fertility may occur in untreated men (as high as 25% in one year). In the past various empirical therapies (e.g., testosterone rebound, gonadotropins, antiestrogens) have been tried without success. The only successful empirical therapy for men with mild to moderate defects in semen quality is in vitro fertilization. However, standard in vitro fertilization does not provide a good outcome in the presence of severe semen abnormalities, such as a sperm density of <5 million per milliliter, poor motility, and many abnormal forms. For such men the technique of intracytoplasmic sperm injection (ICSI) has been a major advance; indeed fertilization and pregnancy rates with this technique are similar to those for standard in vitro techniques in couples with fallopian tube pathology, e.g., a 50 to 70% fertilization rate and a 30% pregnancy rate per cycle. This technique is sometimes successful with spermatozoa recovered from testicular biopsies in men with azoospermia. →*The management of male infertility is discussed in Chap. 54.*

Fertility Control in Men (See also Chap. 54) A variety of approaches to fertility control in men have been tried, including use of the condom as an effective barrier that also prevents sexually transmitted diseases. Vasectomy, which involves transection or ligation of the vas deferens, has a high success rate and can be performed on an outpatient basis. The time required for azoospermia to occur after the operation depends on the number of sperm in the terminal vas deferens and ejaculatory ducts at the time of surgery, but it is usually less than 40 days. Azoospermia should be documented in each case to prove effectiveness. No deleterious effects on either testosterone production or the hypothalamic-pituitary axis have been documented. Despite reports of immune-complex–associated accelerated atherosclerosis in vasectomized nonhuman primates, there does not appear to be any association between vasectomy and atherosclerosis in men. Vasectomy should be recommended only for men requesting permanent sterilization. Only about 30 to 40% of men subjected to vasovasostomy for reanastomosis of the vas subsequently achieve fertility. Suppression of gonadotropins with long-acting GnRH analogues or GnRH antagonists causes marked reduction in sperm counts but requires concomitant androgen replacement. The efficacy and acceptance of this approach to male contraception remain to be established.

GONADAL FUNCTION DURING AGING Beginning at about age 40, mean plasma bioavailable testosterone concentrations decline gradually; about 40% of elderly men have low bioavailable testosterone levels. Although statistically lower than the levels in young men, the concentrations of total testosterone usually remain within the normal range, even in elderly men. The cause of the reduced testosterone level is likely a decreased number of Leydig cells. In older men seminiferous tubule function and sperm production also usually decline. Plasma LH and FSH levels are often slightly elevated, consistent with a decline in gonadal function. An increase in the conversion of androgen to estrogen in peripheral tissues results in a decrease in the effective ratio of androgen to estrogen. These latter hormonal changes may play a role in the development of prostatic hyperplasia and in the development of gynecomastia in aging men (Chaps. 95 and 337). Male sexual function gradually declines after early adulthood, but there is no convincing evidence that hormonal changes have any direct bearing on changes in sexual function with age in healthy men.

Prostatic Hyperplasia See Chap. 95.

Cancer of the Prostate See Chap. 95.

DISORDERS OF ALL AGES **Testicular Tumors** (See also Chap. 96) Low levels of hCG are present in normal testes may be elevated in persons with testicular tumors. Indeed, an elevated plasma level of the β subunit of hCG (hCG-β) is a sensitive and specific marker of tumor activity in some men with germ cell tumors. Plasma levels of hCG-β are elevated in all men with choriocarcinoma, in one-third of those with embryonal carcinomas and teratocarcinomas, and rarely in those with seminomas. Changes in hCG-β levels correlate with response to therapy.

Testicular tumors can cause elevated estradiol and testosterone levels by at least two mechanisms: (1) Trophoblastic, Leydig, and Sertoli cell tumors produce both hormones autonomously; pituitary gonadotropin secretion and hormone production by the uninvolved portions of the testes are depressed, and azoospermia is common; (2) hCG secretion by the tumors can increase estradiol and testosterone production in the unaffected areas of the testes; azoospermia is uncommon with such tumors. When estrogens and androgens are formed (directly or indirectly) by the tumors, feminization, virilization, or no obvious change may result, depending on the hormones produced and the age of the patient. α-Fetroprotein can provde another cellular marker of testicular tumor activity.

Gynecomastia See Chap. 337.

℞ **TREATMENT** **Androgens • *Pharmacologic preparations*** When testosterone is taken by mouth, it is absorbed into the portal blood and degraded promptly by the liver, so that only insignificant amounts reach the systemic circulation; when administered parenterally, testosterone is rapidly absorbed from the injection vehicle and rapidly degraded. As a consequence, effective androgen therapy requires the administration of either a slowly absorbed form of testosterone (dermal patches or micronized oral testosterone) or modified analogues. Chemical modifications either retard absorption or catabolism, or enhance the androgenic potency, so that full effects can be achieved at a lower blood level of drug. Three types of modification have had widespread clinical application (Fig. 335-7): (1) esterification of the 17β-hydroxyl group, (2) alkylation at the 17α position, and (3) alteration of the ring structure, particularly by substitutions at the 2, 9, and 11 positions. Most pharmacologic agents actually have combinations of ring structure alterations and either 17α-alkylation or esterification of the 17β-hydroxyl group. Esterification decreases the polarity of the molecule so that the steroid is more soluble in the fat vehicles used for injection, leading to slower release into the circulation. Most esters must be injected parenterally. The larger the acid esterified, the slower the release and the more prolonged the action. Esters such as testosterone cypionate and testosterone enanthate can be injected every 1 to 3 weeks, the usual regimen being 200 mg of either ester intramuscularly every 2 weeks. Because the esters are hydrolyzed before the hormones act, therapy can be monitored by assaying the plasma testosterone level at various times after administration.

The oral effectiveness of 17α-alkylated androgens (such as meth-

FIGURE 335-7 Some of the androgen preparations available for pharmacologic use.

yltestosterone and methandrostenolone) is due to slower hepatic catabolism, which allows the alkylated derivatives to reach the systemic circulation. For this reason, 17α-methyl or -ethyl substitution is a feature of most orally active androgens. Unfortunately, all 17α-alkylated steroids can cause abnormal liver function, and for this reason they have a limited role in therapy.

Other alterations of the ring structure have been adopted empirically; some slow the rate of inactivation, others enhance the potency of a given molecule, and some alter the conversion to other active metabolites. For example, the potency of fluoxymesterone may be due to the fact that, unlike most androgens, it is a poor precursor for conversion to estrogens in peripheral tissues.

Three transdermal preparations are available in which a testosterone-loaded patch is applied to the skin each day. One is a scrotal patch (Testoderm) that contains no permeation enhancers, which may irritate the skin, but it has a low rate of acceptance. The other two systems (Androderm, Testosterone TTS) are applied to the trunk, arms, or thighs. Each patch provides physiologic testosterone levels that mimic the normal diurnal variation with higher levels in the morning hours. High rates of dermatologic problems have been reported with the Androderm transdermal system.

Side effects of androgens All androgens carry the risk of inducing virilization in women. Early manifestations include acne, coarsening of the voice, hirsutism, and menstrual irregularities. If treatment is discontinued as soon as these effects develop, the manifestations may slowly subside. Long-term side effects such as male-pattern baldness, marked hirsutism, voice changes, and hypertrophy of the clitoris are largely irreversible. At physiologic replacement doses, testosterone esters have few toxic effects in mature men. At supraphysiologic doses, however, gonadotropin secretion is inhibited, the testes shrink, and the sperm count falls (indeed, androgen abuse can be associated with low sperm counts that may persist for 9 months or longer after cessation of the steroid). In some older men, testosterone therapy may cause polycythemia (hematocrit >52%); in men predisposed to obstructive sleep apnea, androgen therapy may initiate or worsen symp-

toms. In older men, the presence of benign prostatic hyperplasia is not a contraindication for androgen therapy, but such men should be screened for prostate cancer before initiating androgen replacement (Chap. 95).

The so-called toxic side effects vary among the different agents and with the clinical setting in which they are used. Retention of a limited amount of sodium is an inevitable consequence of androgen therapy and may lead to edema in patients with underlying heart disease or renal failure, or when androgens are administered in enormous amounts. Although androgens do not cause malignancy, they may promote the growth of and intensify pain from carcinomas of the prostate and breast in men.

The feminizing side effects of androgen therapy in men are poorly understood. Testosterone (but not 5α-reduced androgens) can be converted (aromatized) in extraglandular tissues to estradiol. The most common manifestation of feminization is the development of gynecomastia. Such breast enlargement is common in children given androgens, possibly because of a greater capacity to convert androgens to estrogens in childhood. The administration of testosterone esters to men results in an increase in plasma estrogen levels, but in men with normal liver function gynecomastia usually develops only after use of high doses.

All 17α-alkylated androgens can produce liver function abnormalities such as elevated plasma levels of alkaline phosphatase and conjugated bilirubin. The incidence of clinical liver disease probably depends on the previous integrity of the liver, but jaundice may occur in the absence of preexisting liver disease. 17α-Alkylated drugs also increase the levels of a variety of plasma proteins that are synthesized in the liver. The most serious complications of 17α-alkylated androgens are peliosis hepatis (blood-filled cysts in the liver) and hepatoma. These disorders were initially described in patients with aplastic anemia, many of whom had Fanconi anemia, itself a predisposing factor for the development of malignancy. However, both lesions can occur after administration of substituted androgens for other indications, including use by athletes. These tumors may either follow a benign course after discontinuation of the drugs or be rapidly fatal.

One indication for 17α-alkylated androgens is in the treatment of hereditary angioedema in which the desired therapeutic benefit (increased level of the inhibitor of the first component of complement) may actually be an effect of the 17-alkylated side chain rather than of the parent androgen. As a consequence, weak androgens such as danazol are effective in this disorder (Fig. 335-7). Danazol is also used in the management of endometriosis (Chap. 52).

Replacement therapy The aim of androgen therapy in hypogonadal men is to restore or bring to normal male secondary sexual characteristics (beard, body hair, external genitalia) and male sexual behavior and to mimic the hormonal effects on somatic development (hemoglobin, muscle mass, nitrogen balance, and epiphyseal closure). Since an assay for plasma testosterone is available for monitoring therapy, the treatment of androgen deficiency is almost universally successful. The parenteral administration of a long-acting testosterone ester such as 100 to 200 mg testosterone enanthate at 1- to 2-week intervals results in a sustained increase in plasma testosterone to the normal male range. Alternatively, testosterone may be administered transdermally. Testosterone patches, which are available in different doses, are replaced daily. If hypogonadism is primary and of long duration (as in the Klinefelter syndrome), suppression of plasma LH to the normal range may not occur for many weeks, if at all. There is considerable variability in the relation between plasma testosterone and male sexual behavior, but in cases of postpubertal testicular failure (even of many years duration), normal sexual activity usually is resumed after adequate replacement. Androgen administration does not restore spermatogenesis in hypogonadal states, but the volume of the ejaculate (derived largely from the prostate and seminal vesicles) and other male secondary sex characteristics return to normal. The effects of endogenous androgen on hemoglobin, nitrogen retention, and skeletal development are also reproduced.

In men of all ages in whom hypogonadism developed before exit is appropriate to bring plasma testosterone into the adult range slowly. When therapy is commenced at the time of expected puberty in such men, the normal events of puberty proceed in the usual fashion. If therapy is delayed until after the time of usual puberty, the degree to which normal virilization will occur is variable, but many patients undergo a relatively complete anatomic and functional maturation. Intermittent low-dose androgen therapy is indicated in prepubertal hypogonadal boys with microphallus to bring the external genitalia into the normal range. If such patients are monitored closely and given androgens for only short periods, therapy usually has no adverse effects on somatic growth.

In boys of pubertal age with either isolated gonadotropin deficiency or primary testicular disease, the usual practice is to institute androgen therapy between the ages of 12 and 14 years, depending on the subjective need for sexual development. The initial administration of small doses of testosterone esters followed by a gradual increase to 100 to 150 mg/m² of body surface area every 1 to 3 weeks should result in a normal pubertal growth spurt. The time from the start of treatment to the appearance of secondary sex characteristics is variable. Penile development, deepening of the voice, and the appearance of other secondary sexual characteristics usually commence during the first year of treatment. In normal boys, puberty extends over several years, and treatment designed to replicate normal development does not shorten the process greatly.

Testosterone exerts its full action only in the presence of a balanced hormonal environment and, particularly, in the presence of adequate levels of growth hormone. Consequently, prepubertal boys with coexisting growth hormone and androgen deficiency respond poorly to androgens unless growth hormone is given simultaneously.

Pharmacologic uses   Androgens have been used for a variety of disorders unassociated with hypogonadism in the hope that potential benefits from the nonvirilizing actions of the agents (such as increases in nitrogen retention, muscle mass, and hemoglobin) would outweigh any deleterious actions of the drugs. The most common nonreplacement uses of androgen have been attempts to improve nitrogen balance in catabolic states (e.g., AIDS), self-administration by athletes to increase muscle mass and/or athletic performance, attempts to enhance erythropoiesis in refractory anemias (including the anemia of renal failure), treatment of hereditary angioedema and endometriosis, and management of growth retardation of various etiologies. Most of the expected benefits in these disorders have not been realized for two reasons. First, modest pharmacologic doses of androgens have little physiologic effect in men when superimposed on normal testicular androgen, and in women the virilizing side effects of androgens are formidable. Second, no androgen has been devised that exhibits only the nonvirilizing effects of the hormone. This conclusion is not surprising in view of the fact that the physiologic actions of androgens are mediated by a single, high-affinity receptor (Fig. 335-5).

The most pervasive form of androgen abuse is by male athletes in the expectation that muscle development and athletic performance will be improved. In controlled studies using modest pharmacologic doses (two to four times the usual replacement doses), these agents do not improve performance consistently. However, at the doses frequently taken by athletes (which sometimes exceed 10 times the replacement dose), androgens do enhance nitrogen balance and muscle mass; since the drugs have multiple side effects at high doses, these benefits do not outweigh the risks associated with androgen abuse in man, and the use of androgens by female athletes is associated with disfiguring virilization. Thus this practice cannot be condemned too harshly. The only established indications for androgen therapy outside of male hypogonadism are in selected patients with anemia due to bone marrow failure or hereditary angioedema and as an adjunct to growth hormone therapy.

Gonadotropins   Gonadotropin therapy is used to establish or restore fertility in patients with gonadotropin deficiency of any cause. Several gonadotropin preparations are available. Human menopausal gonadotropin (hMG) (purified from the urine of postmenopausal

women) contains 75 IU FSH and 75 IU LH per vial. hCG (purified from the urine of pregnant women) has little FSH activity and resembles LH in its ability to stimulate testosterone production by Leydig cells. Because of the expense of hMG, treatment is usually begun with hCG alone, and hMG is added later to promote the FSH-dependent stages of spermatid development. A high ratio of LH to FSH activity and treatment for 6 to 18 months may be necessary to bring about maturation of the prepubertal testes. Recombinant human FSH is also available and has been used mainly for ovulation induction in women. Trials are underway to examine its effects on spermatogenesis in men with hypogonadotropic hypogonadism. Once spermatogenesis is restored with combined FSH and LH therapy, hCG alone is often sufficient to maintain spermatogenesis.

The dose of hCG required to maintain a normal testosterone level varies from 1000 to 5000 IU weekly. A number of regimens have been used to induce maturation of spermatogenesis. Most involve starting with 2000 IU hCG three or more times a week until most of the clinical parameters, including plasma testosterone levels, are normal. hMG (usually one ampule) is then added three times a week to complete the development of spermatogenesis. The length of therapy required to restore spermatogenesis may be as long as 12 months.

GnRH and GnRH Analogues   GnRH (gonadorelin) is available for endocrine testing and is used by some physicians for chronic therapy of the infertility of hypogonadotropic hypogonadism. In the latter instance, it is necessary to administer GnRH in frequent boluses (25 to 200 ng/kg of body weight every 2 h) with the use of portable infusion pumps, analogous to those used for insulin administration. In general, pulsatile GnRH does not appear to be more efficacious than gonadotropin in returning sperm counts to normal. GnRH analogues (leuprolide, nafarelin, histrelin) are available for the suppression of gonadotropin secretion, leading to hypogonadism. In prostatic cancer, testicular androgen production can be blocked by monthly injection of 7.5 mg leuprolide in depot form.

BIBLIOGRAPHY

BAKER HWG: Male infertility, in *Endocrinology*, 3d ed, LLJ deGroot (ed). Philadelphia, Saunders, 1995, pp 2404–2433

BHASIN S, SALEHIAN B: Gonadotropin therapy of men with hypogonadotropic hypogonadism, in *Current Therapy in Endocrinology and Metabolism*, 6th ed, CW Bardin (ed). St. Louis, Mosby, 1997, pp 349–352

CARR BR, GRIFFIN JE: Fertility control and its complications, in *Williams Textbook of Endocrinology*, 9th ed, JD Wilson, DW Foster (eds). Philadelphia, Saunders, 1998, pp 901–926

CHILLON M et al: Mutations in the cystic fibrosis gene in patients with congenital absence of the vas deferens. N Engl J Med 332:1475, 1995

DE KRETSER DM: Declining sperm counts. BMJ 312:457, 1996

DRINKA PJ et al: Polycythemia as a complication of testosterone therapy in nursing home men with low testosterone levels. J Am Geriat Soc 43:899, 1995

FORESTA C et al: Y-chromosome deletions in idiopathic severe testiculopathies. J Clin Endocrinol Metab 82:1075, 1997

GNESSI L et al: Gonadal peptides as mediators of development and functional control of the testis. Endocrine Rev 18:541, 1997

GOLDZIEHER JW et al: Improving the diagnostic reliability of rapidly fluctuating plasma hormone levels by optimized multiple-sampling techniques. J Clin Endocrinol Metab 43:824, 1976

GRAY A et al: Age, disease and changing sex hormone levels in middle-aged men: Results of the Massachusetts male aging study. J Clin Endocrinol Metab 73:1016, 1991

GRIFFIN JE, WILSON JD: Disorders of the testes and male reproductive tract, in *Williams Textbook of Endocrinology*, 9th ed, JD Wilson et al (eds). Philadelphia, Saunders, 1998, pp 819–876

GRINSPOON S et al: Sustained anabolic effects of long-term androgen administration in men with AIDS wasting. Clin Infect Dis 28:634, 1999

GRUMBACH MM, STYNE DM: Puberty: Ontogeny, neuroendocrinology, physiology, and disorders, in *Williams Textbook of Endocrinology*, 9th ed, JD Wilson et al (eds). Philadelphia, Saunders, 1998, pp 1509–1626

HANDELSMAN DJ: Testicular dysfunction in systemic disease. Endocrinol Metab Clin North Am 23:839, 1994

HAYES FJ et al: Differential control of gonadotropin secretion in the human: endocrine role of inhibin. J Clin Endocrinol Metab 83:1835, 1998

——— et al: Hypogonadotropic hypogonadism. Endocrinol Metab Clin North Am 27: 739, 1998

LESCHEK EW et al: Six year results of spironolactone and testolactone treatment of familial male-limited precocious puberty with addition of deslorelin after central puberty onset. J Clin Endocrinol Metab 84:175, 1999

MACDONALD PC et al: Origin of estrogen in normal men and in women with testicular feminization. J Clin Endocrinol Metab 49:905, 1979

MARSHALL WA, TANNER JM: Variation in the pattern of pubertal changes in boys. Arch Dis Child 45:13, 1970

NAJMABADI H et al: Substantial prevalence of microdeletions of the Y-chromosome in infertile men with idiopathic azoospermia and oligospermia detected using a sequence-tagged site-based mapping strategy. J Clin Endocrinol Metab 81:1347, 1996

PALERMO GD et al: Intracytoplasmic sperm injection: A novel treatment for all forms of male factor infertility. Fertil Steril 63:1231, 1995

PARKER S, ARMITAGE M: Experience with transdermal testosterone replacement therapy for hypogonadal men. Clin Endocrinol 50:57, 1999

RUGARLI EI, BALLABIO A: Kallmann syndrome. From genetics to neurobiology. JAMA 270:2713, 1993

SALEHIAN B et al: Testicular pathologic changes and the pituitary-testicular axis during human immunodeficiency virus infection. Endocr Pract 5:1, 1999

SCHNEIDER BK et al: Influence of testosterone on breathing during sleep. J Appl Physiol 61:618, 1986

SNYDER PF, LAWRENCE DA: Treatment of male hypogonadism with testosterone enanthate. J Clin Endocrinol Metab 51:1335, 1980

WHITCOMB RW, CROWLEY WF JR: Hypogonadotropic hypogonadism: Gonadotropin-releasing hormone therapy, in *Current Therapy in Endocrinology and Metabolism*, 6th ed, CW Bardin (ed). St Louis, Mosby, 1997, pp 353–355

336   *Bruce R. Carr, Karen D. Bradshaw*

DISORDERS OF THE OVARY AND FEMALE REPRODUCTIVE TRACT

ACTH	adrenocorticotropic hormone	HPV	human papilloma virus
CT	computed tomography	LH	luteinizing hormone
ER	estrogen receptor	MRI	magnetic resonance imaging
FSH	follicle-stimulating hormone	PCOS	polycystic ovarian syndrome
GnRH	gonadotropin-releasing hormone	TGF	transforming growth factor
hCG	Human chorionic gonadotropin	TSH	thyroid-stimulating hormone
hMG	human menopausal gonadotropin		

The ovary is the source of ova for reproduction and of the hormones that regulate female sexual life. The anatomic structure, response to hormonal stimuli, and secretory capacity of the ovary vary at different periods of life. This chapter will review normal ovarian physiology as a background for understanding ovarian abnormalities and will consider other disorders of the female reproductive tract.

DEVELOPMENT, STRUCTURE, AND FUNCTION OF THE OVARY

EMBRYOLOGY   During the third week of gestation, the primordial germ cells differentiate from the endoderm lining the yolk sac at the caudal end of the embryo. The germ cells migrate to the genital ridge adjacent to the mesonephric kidney by the fifth week of gestation and undergo mitotic division. The gonads exist in an undifferentiated state until the seventh week of fetal life, at which time the primitive ovary can be distinguished from the testis (Chap. 338). Estrogen formation in the ovary commences between weeks 8 and 10, and by 10 to 11 weeks of gestation, oogonia in the ovarian cortex begin developing into primary oocytes. The ovary contains a finite number of germ cells, the number peaking at about 7 million oogonia by the fifth to sixth month of gestation. Subsequently, the germ cells decrease in number through a process of atresia so that only 1 million remain at birth, 400,000 are present at menarche, and only a few remain at meno-

pause. Two normal X chromosomes are required for development of the ovary; in individuals with a 45,X karyotype, ovarian development occurs, but the rate of atresia is accelerated so that only a fibrous streak remains at birth (Chap. 338).

After the oogonia cease to proliferate, meiosis commences, continues until the diplotene stage of the first meiotic division is completed, and then is arrested until the onset of ovulation at puberty. From the fifth month of fetal life, the primordial follicle consists of the primary oocyte arrested in meiosis, a single surrounding layer of granulosa cells, and a basement membrane that separates the primordial follicle from surrounding stromal (interstitial) tissues.

PUBERTAL MATURATION   The final maturation of ovarian follicles commences during puberty. The two major hormones that regulate follicular development are the pituitary gonadotropins—follicle-stimulating hormone (FSH) and luteinizing hormone (LH) (Fig. 336-1). During the second trimester of fetal development, the plasma gonadotropins rise to levels similar to those at menopause. This peak in gonadotropin levels may be responsible for the simultaneous peak in oocyte replication. After the second trimester, the hypothalamic-pituitary axis (the so-called gonadostat) becomes functional and is sensitive to negative feedback by steroid hormones, particularly estrogen and progesterone produced in the placenta. The levels of circulating gonadotropins consequently decrease, and gonadotropins are almost undetectable at the time of birth. In the neonate, concomitant with the decrease in estrogen and progesterone levels caused by separation from the placenta, there is a rebound increase in gonadotropin secretion for the first few months of life. With continued maturation of the hypothalamic-pituitary system, the gonadostat becomes exquisitely sensitive to negative feedback by low levels of circulating steroid hormones, and plasma gonadotropins again decrease.

As the time of puberty nears, a decrease in the sensitivity of the gonadostat allows for increased secretion of FSH and LH, possibly secondary to increased episodic or pulsatile secretion of gonadotropin-releasing hormone (GnRH) by the hypothalamus (Chap. 328). A sleep-induced, pulsatile pattern of LH secretion then ensues, the first step in the development of a cyclic pattern of gonadotropin secretion (Fig. 336-1). The increase in estrogen secretion exerts a positive feedback, which leads to an exaggeration of the pulsatile release of LH and eventually to menarche and ovulation, after which plasma gonadotropin concentrations reach adult values, which are similar during day and night. After the menopause, plasma gonadotropin levels rise, then plateau 5 to 10 years after menopause and remain fairly constant until the eighth to ninth decade of life, when the levels may fall. Although ovarian function is regulated primarily by LH and FSH, the ovary is a source of peptide and protein hormones and growth factors such as inhibin and activin that may play a role in ovarian function and regulation. The production of inhibin by the mature ovary accounts, in part, for the relative reduction in FSH that is seen during the reproductive years (Fig. 336-1).

With puberty the sensitivity of the hypothalamic-pituitary centers to circulating steroid hormones is decreased, GnRH release by the hypothalamus increases, gonadotropin secretion by the pituitary is enhanced, ovarian estrogen secretion increases, and the anatomic changes of puberty ensue. At age 10 to 11, the first secondary sexual characteristics begin to appear in girls, namely, development of the breast buds (thelarche), followed by the development of pubic hair (pubarche), and later by the development of axillary hair (adrenarche). The growth of pubic and axillary hair is believed to be initiated by adrenal androgens, the levels of which begin to rise at approximately 6 to 8 years of age. A growth spurt ensues, and peak growth rate is attained by age 12.

The culmination of puberty is the onset of predictable, cyclic menses. The average time between the beginning of breast development and the onset of menses (menarche) is 2 years. During the first few years after menarche, menstrual cycles are often irregular and unpredictable due to anovulation. The age of menarche is variable and is influenced by socioeconomic and genetic factors and by general health. In the United States, the mean age of menarche is believed to have

FIGURE 336-1 Pattern of gonadotropin secretion during different stages of life in women. FSH, follicle-stimulating hormone; LH, luteinizing hormone. The secretory patterns of LH during the waking hours (clear area) and night (stippled area) for each stage are indicated in the upper insets. (*After C Faiman et al: Clin Obstet Gynaecol 3:467, 1976.*)

decreased at a rate of 3 to 4 months per decade over the past 100 years and is now around 12 years, a change believed to be due to improved nutrition. A body weight of around 48 kg or some critical combination of weight, body water, and body fat is associated with development of hypothalamic insensitivity to feedback by steroids that leads to increased secretion of gonadotropins and finally to menarche. Obese girls have earlier menarche than girls with normal weights. In contrast, active participation in sports or ballet, malnutrition, and chronic debilitating disease can delay menarche.

MATURE OVARY   Morphology   The anatomic components and function of the adult ovary are illustrated schematically in Fig.

336-2. Under the influence of gonadotropins, a group of primary follicles are recruited, and by day 6 to 8 of the menstrual cycle, one follicle becomes mature or "dominant," a process characterized by accelerated growth of granulosa cells and enlargement of the fluid-filled antrum. The recruited follicles not destined to ovulate undergo degeneration, similar to the atresia that occurs in other follicles during embryogenesis. Just prior to ovulation, meiosis resumes in the ovum of the dominant follicle, and the first meiotic division results in formation of the first polar body. The antrum rapidly enlarges (up to 10 to 25 mm in size), follicular fluid increases in amount, and the follicular surface thins and forms a conical stigma. Ovulation from the dom-

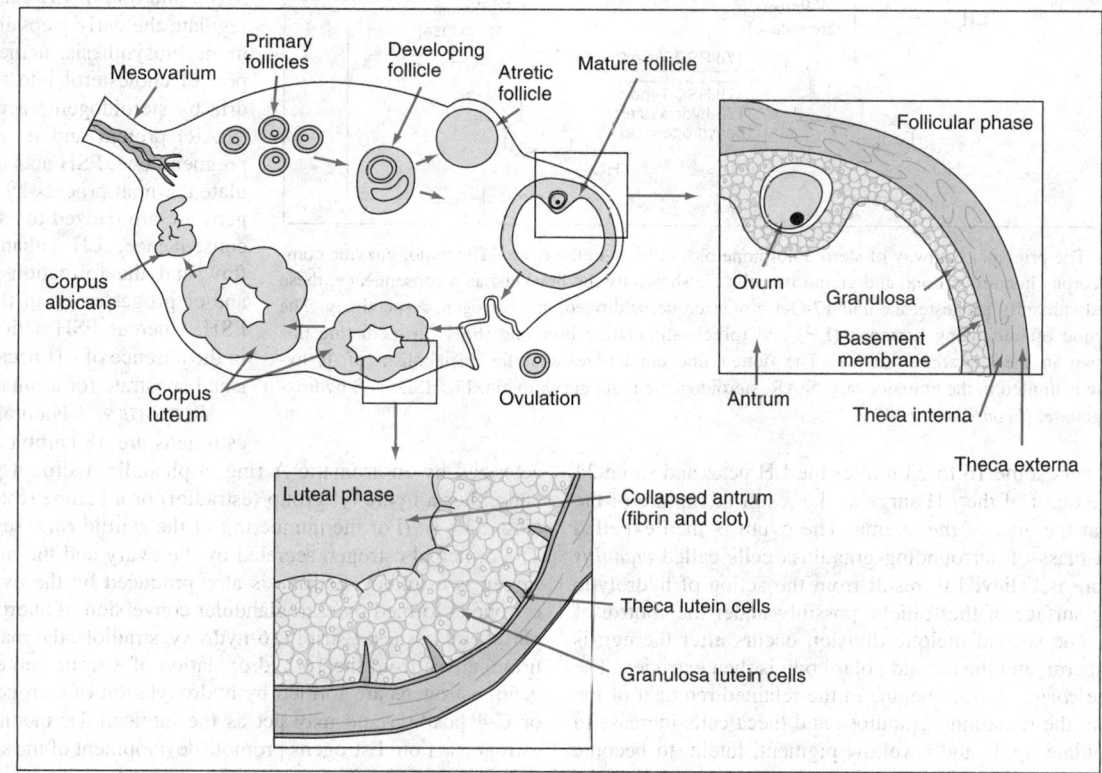

FIGURE 336-2   Developmental changes in the adult ovary during a complete 28-day cycle.

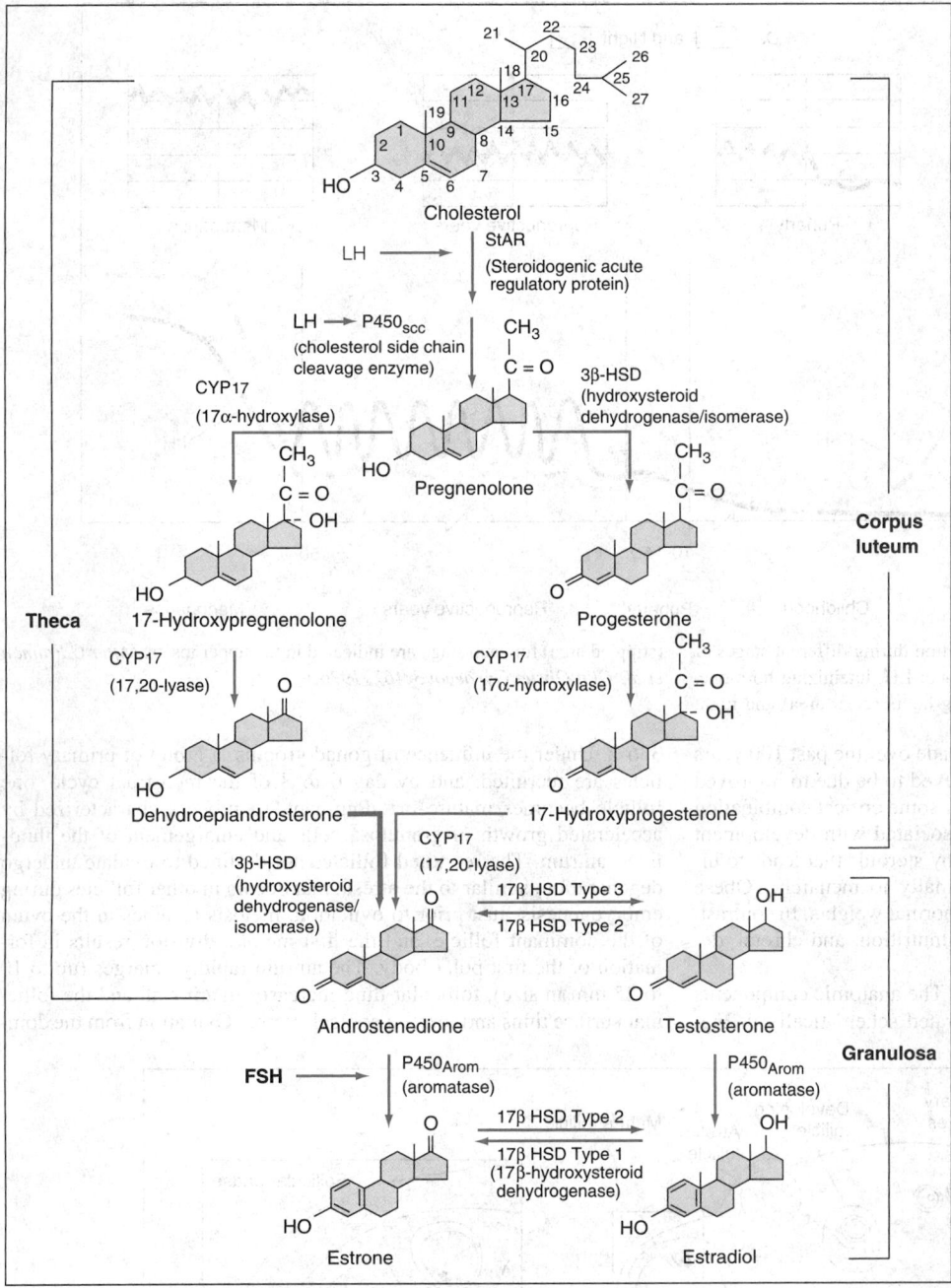

FIGURE 336-3 The principal pathway of steroid hormone biosynthesis in the ovary. The major enzyme complements for the corpus luteum, stroma, and granulosa cells are shown by the brackets; as a consequence, these cells produce predominantly progesterone and 17-OH progesterone, androgen, and estrogen, respectively. The major sites of action of luteinizing hormone (LH) and follicle-stimulating hormone (FSH) in mediating this pathway are shown in the horizontal arrows. The dotted line emphasizes that the metabolism of 17-hydroxyprogesterone is limited in the human ovary. StAR, steroidogenic regulatory protein. 17βHSD, 17-β-hydroxysteroid dehydrogenase. (*From Carr, 1998.*)

in time by a fibrous scar, the *corpus albicans*. The factors that limit the life span of the human corpus luteum are not known, but if pregnancy occurs, the corpus luteum persists under the influence of placental or chorionic gonadotropins, and progesterone is produced by the corpus luteum for the support of pregnancy.

Hormone Formation • *Steroid hormones* Like other steroid hormones, ovarian steroids are derived from cholesterol (Fig. 336-3). The ovary can synthesize cholesterol de novo and can also utilize cholesterol obtained from circulating lipoproteins as substrate for steroid hormone formation (Fig. 336-4). Virtually all ovarian cells are believed to possess the complete complement of enzymes required for the synthesis of estradiol from cholesterol (Fig. 336-3); however, different cell types in the ovary contain different amounts of these enzymes so that the main steroids produced differ in different compartments. For example, the corpus luteum forms mainly progesterone and 17-hydroxyprogesterone, whereas theca and stromal cells convert cholesterol to androstenedione and testosterone. Granulosa cells are particularly rich in the aromatase enzyme responsible for estrogen synthesis and utilize as substrates for this process androgens synthesized in the granulosa cells and the adjacent theca cells.

The principal sites of action of LH and FSH are also illustrated in Figs. 336-3 and 336-4. LH acts primarily to regulate the early steps in steroid hormone biosynthesis, namely, the transport of cholesterol into the mitochondria by steroidogenic acute regulatory (StAR) protein and its conversion to pregnenolone. FSH acts mainly to regulate the final process by which androgens are aromatized to estrogens. As a consequence, LH enhances substrate flow and the formation of androgens and/or progesterone in the absence of FSH, whereas FSH action is impeded in the absence of LH because of diminished substrate for aromatization.

ESTROGENS Naturally occurring estrogens are 18-carbon steroids characterized by an aromatic A ring, a phenolic hydroxyl group at C-3, and either a hydroxyl group (estradiol) or a ketone (estrone) at C-17 (Fig. 336-3). (For the numbering of the steroid ring, see Fig. 335-1.) The principal estrogen secreted by the ovary and the most potent estrogen is estradiol. Estrone is also produced by the ovary, but most estrone is formed by extraglandular conversion of androstenedione in peripheral tissues. Estriol (16-hydroxyestradiol), the main estrogen in urine, arises from the 16-hydroxylation of estrone and estradiol. Catechol estrogens are formed by hydroxylation of estrogens at the C-2 or C-4 position and may act as the intracellular mediators of some estrogen action. Estrogens promote development of the secondary sexual characteristics in women and cause uterine growth, thickening of the vaginal mucosa, thinning of the cervical mucus, and development

inant follicle occurs some 16 to 23 h after the LH peak and some 24 to 38 h after the onset of the LH surge as the result of rupture of the follicular wall at the area of the stigma. The ovum is then expelled together with a mass of surrounding granulosa cells called *cumulus cells*. The rupture is believed to result from the action of hydrolytic enzymes on the surface of the follicle, possibly under the control of prostaglandins. The second meiotic division occurs after the egg is fertilized by a sperm, and the second polar body is then extruded. The formation of the *corpus luteum* begins in the retained remnant of the ovulated follicle; the remaining granulosa and theca cells increase in size and accumulate lipids and a yellow pigment, lutein, to become "luteinized." After a period of 14 ± 2 days (the functional life of the corpus luteum), the corpus luteum begins to atrophy, to be replaced

Follicular phase

Theca

Granulosa

LDL-Cholesterol

Antrum

Cholesterol

LH

Androstenedione

FSH

Androstenedione

Estradiol

Basement membrane

Luteal phase

Theca lutein cells

Blood vessel invasion

Granulosa lutein cells

LDL-Cholesterol

Cholesterol

LH

Progesterone

FIGURE 336-4 Cellular interactions in the ovary during the follicular phase (*top*) and luteal phase (*bottom*). LDL, low-density lipoprotein; FSH, follicle-stimulating hormone; LH, luteinizing hormone. (*From BR Carr et al: Fertil Steril 38:303, 1982.*)

of the ductule system of the breasts. Estrogens also alter lipid profiles and exert vascular effects that help prevent cardiovascular disease. The mechanism of estrogen action in target tissues is similar to that for other steroid hormones and involves binding to a nuclear steroid receptor—either estrogen receptor (ER)α or ERβ—and enhancement of the transcription of messenger RNA, which in turn causes increased protein synthesis in the cell cytoplasm (Chap. 327). These receptors have specific tissue site expression and bind various estrogens with different affinities, thereby conferring selective actions.

PROGESTERONE Progesterone, a 21-carbon steroid (Fig. 336-3), is the principal hormone secreted by the corpus luteum and is responsible for progestational effects, i.e., induction of secretory activity in the endometrium of the estrogen-primed uterus in preparation for implantation of the fertilized egg. Progesterone also induces a decidual reaction in endometrium. Other effects include inhibition of uterine contractions, an increase in the viscosity of cervical mucus, glandular development of the breasts, and an increase in basal body temperature (thermogenic effect).

ANDROGENS The ovary synthesizes a variety of 19-carbon steroids, including dehydroepiandrosterone, androstenedione, testosterone, and dihydrotestosterone, principally in stromal and thecal cells. The major ovarian 19-carbon steroid is androstenedione (Fig. 336-3), part of which is secreted into the plasma and part of which is converted to estrogen in granulosa cells or to testosterone in the interstitium. Androstenedione can also be converted to testosterone and estrogens in peripheral tissues. Only testosterone and dihydrotestosterone are true androgens that interact with the androgen receptor and induce virilizing signs in women (Chaps. 53 and 335).

Other hormones *Inhibin* is secreted in two forms (A and B) by the follicle and inhibits the release of FSH by the hypothalamic-pituitary unit. *Activin* is also secreted by the follicle and may enhance FSH secretion as well as having local effects on ovarian steroidogenesis. *Follistatin* is an activin-binding protein that attenuates the actions of activin and other members of the transforming growth factor (TGF)β family.

Some ovarian hormones play an uncertain role in human physiology. *Relaxin*, a polypeptide hormone produced by the human corpus luteum and by the decidua, causes softening of the cervix and loosening of the symphysis pubis in preparation for parturition in animals. *Oxytocin, vasopressin*, and other hypothalamic and pituitary hormones are also present in granulosa and/or luteal cells, but their function in these cells is unknown. *Follicle regulatory protein* (FRP), found in human follicular fluid, inhibits granulosa secretion and growth. *Gonadocrinins*, peptides purified from rat follicular fluid, stimulate the release of both FSH and LH from the pituitary in vitro and in vivo. Granulosa cells secrete *oocyte maturation inhibitor* (OMI), a factor that prevents premature ovulation. In addition, in the gonads of both sexes a *meiosis-inducing substance* (MIS) triggers the onset of meiosis, an event that occurs earlier in ovarian than in testicular development. Local growth factors [including insulin-like growth factors (IGFs) 1 and 2 and TGFα and -β] may also influence steroid secretion by the ovary.

The Normal Menstrual Cycle The menstrual cycle is divided into a follicular or proliferative phase and a luteal or secretory phase (Fig. 336-5). The secretion of FSH and LH is fundamentally under negative feedback control by ovarian steroids (particularly estradiol) and by inhibin (which selectively suppresses FSH), but the response of gonadotropins to different levels of estradiol varies. FSH secretion is inhibited progressively as estrogen levels increase—typical negative feedback. In contrast, LH secretion is suppressed maximally by sustained low levels of estrogen and is enhanced by a rising level of estradiol—positive feedback. Feedback of estrogen involves both the hypothalamus and pituitary. Negative feedback suppresses GnRH and inhibits gonadotropin production. Positive feedback is associated with an increased frequency of GnRH secretion and enhanced pituitary sensitivity to GnRH.

The length of the menstrual cycle is defined as the time from the onset of one menstrual bleeding episode to onset of the next. In women of reproductive age, the cycle averages 28 $\pm$ 3 days and the mean duration of flow is 4 $\pm$ 2 days. Longer menstrual cycles (usually characterized by anovulation) occur at menarche and near the onset of menopause. At the end of a cycle plasma levels of estrogen and progesterone fall, and circulating levels of FSH increase. Under the influence of FSH, follicular recruitment results in development of the follicle that will be dominant during the next cycle.

After the onset of menses, follicular development continues, but FSH levels decrease. Approximately 8 to 10 days prior to the midcycle LH surge, plasma estradiol levels begin to rise as the result of estradiol formation by the granulosa cells of the dominant follicle. During the second half of the follicular phase, LH levels also begin to rise (owing to positive feedback). Just before ovulation, estradiol secretion reaches a peak and then falls. Immediately thereafter, a further rise in the plasma level of LH mediates the final maturation of the follicle, followed by follicular rupture and ovulation 16 to 23 h after the LH peak. The rise in LH is accompanied by a smaller increase in the level of plasma FSH, the physiologic significance of which is unclear. The plasma progesterone level also begins to rise just prior to midcycle and facilitates the positive feedback action of estradiol on LH secretion.

At the onset of the luteal phase, plasma gonadotropins decrease and plasma progesterone increases. A secondary rise in estrogens causes further gonadotropin suppression. Near the end of the luteal phase, progesterone and estrogen levels fall, and FSH levels begin to rise to initiate the development of the next follicle (usually in the

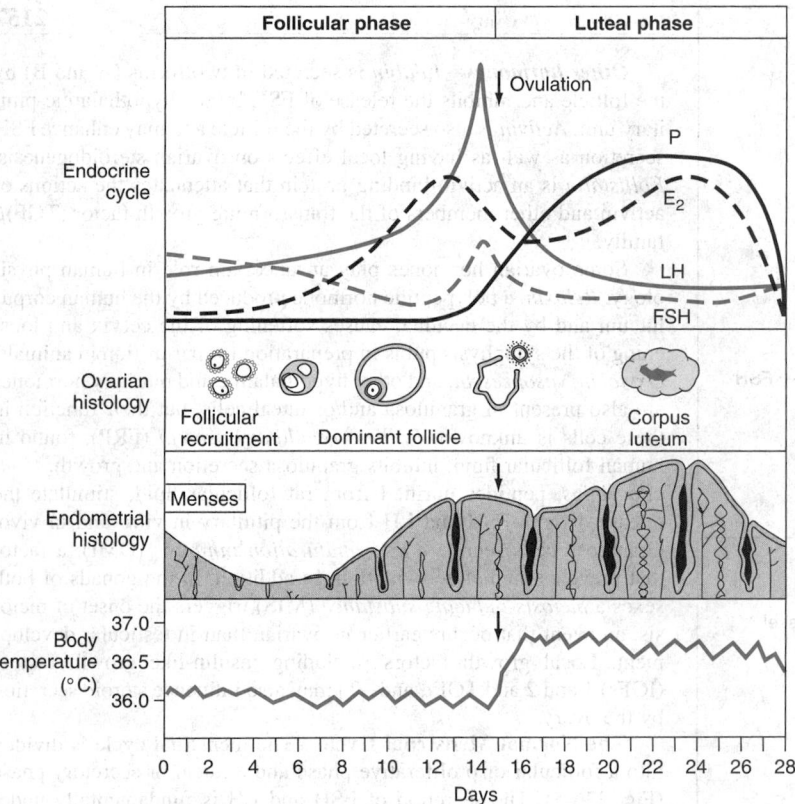

FIGURE 336-5 The hormonal, ovarian, endometrial, and basal body temperature changes and relationships throughout the normal menstrual cycle.

contralateral ovary) and the next menstrual cycle. Inhibin A levels are low in the follicular phase but reach a peak in the luteal phase. Inhibin B levels, in contrast, are increased in the follicular phase and low in the luteal phase.

The endometrium lining the uterine cavity undergoes marked alterations in response to the changing plasma levels of ovarian hormones (Fig. 336-5). Concurrent with the decrease in plasma estrogen and progesterone and the decline of corpus luteum function in the late luteal phase, intense vasospasm occurs in the spiral arterioles supplying blood to the endometrium, causing ischemic necrosis, endometrial desquamation, and bleeding. This vasospasm is caused by locally synthesized prostaglandins. The onset of bleeding marks the first day of the menstrual cycle. By the fourth to fifth day of the cycle, the endometrium is thin. During the proliferative phase, glandular growth of the endometrium is mediated by estrogen. After ovulation, increased progesterone levels lead to further thickening of the endometrium, but the rapid growth slows. The endometrium then enters the secretory phase, characterized by tortuosity of the glands, curling of the spiral arterioles, and glandular secretion. As corpus luteum function begins to wane in the absence of conception, the sequence of events leading to menstruation is again set into action.

Biphasic changes in basal body temperature are characteristic of the ovulatory cycle and are mediated by alterations in progesterone levels (Fig. 336-5). An increase in basal body temperature by 0.3 to 0.5°C begins after ovulation, persists during the luteal phase, and returns to the normal baseline (36.2 to 36.4°C) after the onset of the subsequent menses.

Cellular Interactions in the Ovary during the Normal Cycle LH stimulates thecal cells surrounding the follicle to form androgens, and androstenedione diffuses across the basement membrane of the follicle into granulosa cells, where it is aromatized to estrogen (Figs. 336-3 and 336-4).

The increase of FSH late in the preceding menstrual cycle stimulates growth and recruitment of the primary follicles by enhancing granulosa cell proliferation, resulting ultimately in the formation of the dominant follicle. This function of FSH is underscored by the fact that only primary follicles are seen in patients with mutations in FSH or the FSH receptor. In the granulosa cells, FSH also stimulates estrogen synthesis. Enhanced secretion of estradiol causes an increase in the number of estradiol receptors and further proliferation of granulosa cells. In the late follicular phase, FSH, in concert with estradiol, causes induction of LH receptors on the granulosa cells. LH acts via these receptors to increase progesterone secretion at midcycle. The amount of progesterone formed by the follicle is believed to be limited by the availability of cholesterol to serve as substrate for steroidogenesis and by the fact that most of the progesterone is converted to androstenedione by thecal cells. Prior to ovulation, the granulosa cells of the follicle are bathed in follicular fluid but have limited access to circulating blood and consequently to plasma low-density lipoprotein (LDL). As depicted in Fig. 336-4, the granulosa cells become vascularized after ovulation, and plasma cholesterol is made available to serve as the major substrate for progesterone synthesis by the corpus luteum. Thus, increased progesterone synthesis by the corpus luteum is the consequence of increased substrate availability. The peak in progesterone secretion by the corpus luteum occurs 8 days after ovulation at the time of maximal vascularization of the granulosa cells.

MENOPAUSE The *menopause* is defined as the final episode of menstrual bleeding in women. However, the term is used commonly to refer to the time interval that encompasses the transitional period between the reproductive years up to and after the last episode of menstrual bleeding. During this period, there is a progressive loss of ovarian function and a variety of endocrine, somatic, and psychological changes.

The median age of women at the time of cessation of menstrual bleeding is 50 to 51 years. Since the life expectancy of women is close to 80 years, approximately one-third of life occurs after cessation of reproductive function. Preceding the menopause, the pattern of menstrual cycles is variable, but the interval between menses usually becomes shorter, as follicular recruitment is hastened by increases in FSH. Day 3 FSH and E_2 levels are often elevated. Ovulatory cycles continue for some period of time, then anovulation becomes common.

The menopause is the consequence of the exhaustion of ovarian follicles. The decrease in the number of ova begins in intrauterine life; by the time of the menopause, few ova remain, and these appear to be nonfunctional. Only a small number of ova are lost as the result of ovulation during reproductive life; the majority are lost by atresia. The cessation of follicular development results in decreased production of estradiol, inhibin, and other hormones, which causes a loss of negative feedback on the hypothalamic-pituitary centers. In turn, the levels of plasma gonadotropins increase, with FSH levels rising earlier and higher than LH levels (Figs. 336-1 and 336-6). The higher concentration of FSH than LH in postmenopausal women may result from the decrease in inhibin secretion by the ovary, from the fact that FSH is cleared from plasma less rapidly than LH, and possibly from the loss of positive feedback on LH production by estradiol.

The ovaries of postmenopausal women are small and wrinkled, and the residual cells are predominantly stromal. Estrogen and androgen levels in plasma are reduced but not absent (Fig. 336-6). Before the menopause, plasma androstenedione is derived almost equally from the adrenals and the ovaries; after menopause the ovarian contribution ceases so that the plasma levels of androstenedione fall by 50% (Fig. 336-6). However, the menopausal ovary continues to secrete testosterone, presumably formed in stromal cells.

Circulating estrogens in the ovulating woman are derived from two sources. Some 60% of mean estrogen formation during the menstrual cycle is in the form of estradiol, formed primarily by ovaries, and the

FIGURE 336-6 Differences in hormone concentration in women during the reproductive years and in women during the menopause. FSH, follicle-stimulating hormone; LH, luteinizing hormone; E_2, estradiol-17β; E_1, estrone; Δ^4-A, androstenedione; T, testosterone. *From SSC Yen et al (eds), Reproductive Endocrinology. Philadelphia, Saunders, 1999; and from DR Mishell Jr, V Dajavan (eds), Reproductive Endocrinology, Infertility, and Contraception, 2d ed, Philadelphia, Davis, 1986.*

remainder is estrone, formed mainly in extraglandular tissues from androstenedione. After menopause, extraglandular estrogen formation is the major pathway for estrogen synthesis. Because adipose tissue is a major site of extraglandular estrogen production, peripheral estrogen formation may actually be enhanced in obese postmenopausal women, so that total estrogen production rates may be as great or greater than in premenopausal women. The predominant estrogen formed is estrone rather than estradiol.

The most common menopausal symptoms are vasomotor instability (hot flashes), atrophy of the urogenital epithelium and skin, decreased size of the breasts, and osteoporosis. Approximately 40% of menopausal women develop symptoms serious enough to seek medical assistance.

The pathogenesis of the hot flash is uncertain. There is a close temporal relationship between the onset of the hot flash and pulses of LH secretion, which reflect hypothalamic secretion of GnRH. Alterations in catecholamine, prostaglandin, endorphin, or neurotensin metabolism may play a role in conjunction with low estrogen production. Symptoms associated with the hot flash, including nervousness, anxiety, irritability, and depression, may or may not be caused entirely by estrogen deficiency.

The decrease in size of the tissues of the female reproductive tract and breasts in the menopause is due to estrogen deficiency. The vaginal mucosa and the endometrium usually become thin and atrophic (although endometrial hyperplasia occurs in one-fifth of postmenopausal women).

Osteoporosis is one of the dread afflictions of aging, and there is a close relationship between estrogen deprivation and its development. Approximately one-fourth of aging women and one-tenth of elderly men sustain a vertebral or hip fracture between the ages of 60 and 90, and the incidence is highest in elderly white women. Such fractures are a major cause of loss of independence, death and morbidity, and the fracture-related mortality increases from <10% in the 60- to 64-year age group to >30% in patients over 80 (Chap. 342). Many factors affect the development of osteoporosis, including ethnic origin, diet, activity, smoking, and general health, and estrogen deprivation is of particular importance. White and Asian postmenopausal women are more predisposed to osteoporosis and its consequences because bone mass in this group is lower prior to menopause, so loss in bone density has more severe consequences. Further evidence that osteoporosis is a disease of estrogen deprivation is suggested by the early development of osteoporosis in women with premature menopause due to either natural causes or surgical castration. After the menopause women ex-

perience an increase in the incidence of cardiovascular disease as the result of a decrease in the level of high-density lipoprotein (HDL) cholesterol as well as the effects of hypoestrogenism on vascular endothelium and reactivity.

LABORATORY AND CLINICAL ASSESSMENT OF HORMONAL STATUS

The hormonal status of women can usually be assessed by history and physical examination. In general, the presence of secondary sexual characteristics such as normal female breast development indicates adequate estrogen secretion in the past, and the presence of regular, predictable, cyclic menses implies that ovulation and the production of gonadotropins, estrogen, progesterone, and androgens are adequate and that the outflow tract is intact. Such a history may be more valuable than laboratory tests in evaluating ovarian hormone status. However, laboratory tests provide valuable ancillary information in the evaluation of women with endocrine dysfunction or infertility (Chap. 54).

PITUITARY GONADOTROPINS Plasma gonadotropins are assessed by radioimmunoassay (RIA), fluoroimmunoassay (FIA), or immunoradiometric assay (IRMA). Because both FSH and LH are secreted in a pulsatile manner, the results obtained from a single serum sample may be difficult to interpret. Consequently, multiple samples taken at 20-min intervals over 2 h may be pooled to obtain a mean value. Serum gonadotropin measurements are of the most use in evaluating women with suspected ovarian failure and in supporting the diagnosis of polycystic ovarian syndrome (PCOS) and hypogonadotropic hypogonadism. The normal ranges for serum LH and FSH in ovulating women are 0.8 to 57 and 1.4 to 21 IU/L, respectively. FSH levels that are persistently >40 IU/L are diagnostic of ovarian failure, and an LH value <0.8 IU/L suggests hypogonadotropic hypogonadism. In practice, however, gonadotropin values may be equivocal and must be interpreted in light of the remainder of the findings.

OVARIAN HORMONES The mean plasma levels and production rates of the principal ovarian hormones are presented in Table 336-1.

Estrogen The presence of normal secondary sexual characteristics implies that estrogen production was adequate in the past. The current estrogen status can be estimated by pelvic examination. The presence of a moist, rugated vagina with copious, clear, thin cervical mucus that can be stretched and that exhibits arborization or ferning when spread on a slide is strong evidence of adequate estrogen production. Cytologic demonstration of mature vaginal epithelial cells and abundant cornified squamous epithelial cells with pyknotic nuclei confirms the presence of adequate estrogen levels.

The progesterone-withdrawal test provides a functional assessment

Table 336-1   Concentrations of the Major Ovarian Steroid Hormones in Blood of Ovulatory Women

Steroid	Binding[a]	Phase of Menstrual Cycle	Plasma Concentration, nmol/L (ng/mL)
Estradiol	SHBG and albumin	Follicular	0.07–2.6 (0.02–0.7)
		Luteal	0.7 (0.2)
Estrone	Albumin	Follicular	0.2–1.1 (0.05–0.3)
		Luteal	0.4 (0.1)
Progesterone	CBG and albumin	Follicular	3 (1)
		Luteal	16–80 (5–25)
Androstenedione	Albumin	—	5.6 (1.6)
Testosterone	SHBG and albumin	—	1.4 (0.4)

[a] SHBG, sex hormone binding globulin; CBG, cortisol-binding globulin.
SOURCE: Modified from MB Lipsett, in *Reproductive Endocrinology*, SSC Yen et al (eds). Philadelphia, Saunders, 1999.

of the endometrium, outflow tract, and estrogen status. If menses appear within a week to 10 days after the end of a trial of medroxyprogesterone acetate (10 mg by mouth once or twice a day for 5 days) or after a single intramuscular injection of progesterone (100 mg), then prior estrogen priming was adequate to allow withdrawal bleeding.

Owing to its variable level in plasma during the normal cycle and the difficulty of estimating the day of the cycle in women with abnormal cycles, the measurement of estrogen levels in plasma or urine is of little use in the routine assessment of estrogen status. Measurement of plasma estradiol is useful during attempts to induce ovulation with gonadotropins to prevent the development of the ovarian hyperstimulation syndrome and is used along with ultrasound assessment to monitor follicular growth in women who are to undergo in vitro fertilization.

Progesterone Cyclic, predictable menses also imply that adequate progesterone is secreted during the luteal phase of the menstrual cycle. Assessment of progesterone is useful to detect ovulation and to evaluate the adequacy of the luteal phase in infertile women. Several functional assays of progesterone can be used. The least expensive and most useful is the daily measurement of basal body temperature throughout a cycle. Owing to the thermogenic properties of progesterone, a normal biphasic monthly curve showing a temperature elevation lasting for approximately 2 weeks after ovulation is a valid indication of progesterone secretion during the luteal phase (Fig. 336-5). The presence of viscous cervical mucus that does not stretch or fern and of predominantly intermediate cells on vaginal cytology or demonstration of a secretory epithelium in an endometrial biopsy during the luteal phase on days 20 to 22 of the cycle provides additional assessment of progesterone secretion. In addition, serum progesterone can be measured to assess the function of the corpus luteum.

Androgen Under normal conditions, the ovary secretes androstenedione, testosterone, and dehydroepiandrosterone. In conditions of androgen excess, hirsutism and/or virilization are common. The evaluation of androgen excess is discussed in Chap. 53.

DIAGNOSIS OF PREGNANCY Pregnancy is usually recognized on the basis of the history and physical examination. That is, a woman with previously cyclic, predictable menses develops amenorrhea accompanied by breast tenderness, malaise, lassitude, and nausea, and on physical examination the uterus is soft and enlarged.

Assays of placental products facilitate the diagnosis of pregnancy. Human chorionic gonadotropin (hCG) is secreted by the trophoblastic cells of the placenta into the maternal plasma and excreted in the urine. Assays of the hCG content of serum or urine use antibodies against hCG and make it possible to detect pregnancies 8 to 10 days after ovulation, before the first missed menstrual period and long before pregnancy can be diagnosed by clinical assessments. Assay of the β subunit of hCG in serum or urine makes it possible to differentiate between excess LH and hCG, an important distinction in evaluating women with trophoblastic disease such as hydatidiform mole or choriocarcinoma. Sensitive and specific hCG-based pregnancy tests are now available for testing by patients at home.

DISORDERS OF OVARIAN FUNCTION

PREPUBERTAL YEARS Puberty is said to be *precocious* if breast budding begins before age 8 or if menarche occurs before age 9. Those disorders in which the developing sexual characteristics are appropriate for the genetic and gonadal sex—i.e., feminization in girls or virilization in boys—are termed *isosexual precocity*, whereas *heterosexual precocity* occurs when sexual characteristics are not in accord with the genetic sex, namely, virilization in girls or feminization in boys. Pubertal disorders of boys are described in Chap. 335.

Isosexual Precocious Puberty Isosexual precocious puberty in girls can be divided into three major categories (Table 336-2).

True precocious puberty True precocious puberty is characterized by an early but otherwise normal sequence of pubertal develop-

Table 336-2 Differential Diagnosis of Sexual Precocity

I. Isosexual precocity
  A. True precocious puberty
    1. Constitutional
    2. Organic brain disease
    3. Congenital adrenal hyperplasia
  B. Precocious pseudopuberty
    1. Ovarian tumors
    2. Adrenal tumors
    3. McCune-Albright syndrome
    4. Hypothyroidism
    5. Russell-Silver syndrome
    6. Estrogen-containing medications
  C. Incomplete sexual precocity
    1. Premature thelarche
    2. Premature adrenarche
    3. Premature pubarche
II. Heterosexual precocity
  A. Ovarian tumors
  B. Adrenal tumors
  C. Congenital adrenal hyperplasia

ment, including increased secretion of gonadotropins and ovulatory menstrual cycles. Constitutional or idiopathic precocious puberty accounts for 90% of cases. In these individuals, no cause for the premature maturation of the central nervous system—hypothalamic-pituitary axis can be identified, and the diagnosis is confirmed by finding an adult pattern of LH and FSH release on a GnRH stimulation test. As many as half these individuals have abnormal findings on electroencephalograms. Premature appearance of secondary sexual characteristics and of ovulatory cycles with the accompanying risk of fertility may cause significant emotional disturbance. Therefore, prompt initiation of therapy is imperative. GnRH analogues suppress gonadotropins and inhibit estrogen synthesis, thereby blocking precocious puberty; they may also prevent premature closure of the epiphyses and the resulting short stature.

About 10% of cases are due to organic brain diseases, including brain tumors (hypothalamic gliomas, astrocytomas, ependymomas, germinomas, and hamartomas), encephalitis, meningitis, hydrocephalus, head injury, tuberous sclerosis, and neurofibromatosis. It is essential to distinguish this group of patients from those with the idiopathic disorder, and patients whose disorder is designated as idiopathic occasionally prove to have such tumors. Fortunately, most patients with organic lesions serious enough to cause precocious puberty have obvious neurologic signs and symptoms. Evaluation of all patients with precocious puberty should include, at a minimum, skull films and computed tomography (CT) or magnetic resonance imaging (MRI) of the brain. The success of treatment depends on the nature of the lesion, but surgical and radiation treatment of well-localized tumors is occasionally successful.

A rare cause of isosexual precocity is congenital adrenal hyperplasia due to 21-hydroxylase deficiency in girls in whom treatment is delayed until 4 to 8 years of age. After initiation of glucocorticoid replacement, such individuals may undergo isosexual precocious puberty (Chap. 331).

Precocious pseudopuberty Precocious pseudopuberty occurs when girls undergo feminization as a consequence of enhanced estrogen formation but do not ovulate or develop cyclic menses. Ovarian cysts or tumors that secrete estrogen (granulosa-theca cell tumors) are the most frequent cause of precocious pseudopuberty. Granulosa-theca cell tumors associated with intestinal polyps and pigmentation of the mucous membranes occur in the Peutz-Jeghers syndrome. Other ovarian tumors that secrete estrogens (or androgens that can be converted to estrogens at extraglandular sites) include dysgerminomas, teratomas, cystadenomas, and ovarian carcinomas (Chap. 97). Ovarian tumors can usually be detected by rectoabdominal examination or by sonography, CT, MRI, and/or laparoscopy. Ovarian teratomas and choriocarcinomas and other carcinomas that secrete hCG do not cause precocious puberty in girls unless they also secrete estrogen (hCG or

LH in the absence of FSH does not induce ovarian estrogen production). Rarely, feminizing tumors of the adrenal cause isosexual precocious puberty by direct formation of estrogens or by secretion of weak androgens, which are converted to estrogens in extraglandular tissues.

Other causes of precocious pseudopuberty include the following:

1. The McCune-Albright syndrome (polyostotic fibrous dysplasia) is due to an activating mutation in the G-protein, Gsα, that occurs during embryogenesis, leading to a mosaic pattern of expression in various tissues. It is characterized by café au lait spots, cystic fibrous dysplasia of bones, and sexual precocity. In the ovary, the Gsα mutation mimics the action of FSH, leading to autonomous follicle development and estrogen formation. Occasionally, this disorder leads to true precocious puberty (Chap. 343).
2. Primary hypothyroidism is occasionally associated with enhanced secretion of FSH, inducing ovarian estrogen secretion. High levels of thyroid-stimulating hormone (TSH) caused by hypothyroidism may also stimulate the FSH receptor.
3. The Russell-Silver syndrome, or congenital asymmetry, is associated with short stature and precocious feminization.
4. Estrogen-containing medications, including use of estrogen-containing creams for diaper rash or the ingestion of meat from estrogen-treated animals or poultry or of any estrogen by mouth, can cause this disorder.

Incomplete isosexual precocity This term is used to describe the premature development of a single pubertal event and encompasses several entities. Breast budding prior to age 7 (*premature thelarche*) without other evidence of estrogen secretion and without premature bone maturation is believed to be due to a transient increase in estrogen secretion or to a temporary increase in sensitivity to the small amounts of circulating estrogens formed prior to puberty. Usually, the disorder is self-limited and resolves spontaneously. Occasionally, axillary hair and/or pubic hair (*premature adrenarche* and *premature pubarche*) appear without any other secondary sexual development. The phenomenon is associated with adrenal androgen secretion in the range of normal puberty and can be distinguished from syndromes of virilization by the absence of clitoromegaly. It requires no treatment, and patients enter puberty at about the average time.

Heterosexual Precocity Virilization in a prepubertal female is usually due to congenital adrenal hyperplasia or to androgen secretion by an ovarian or adrenal tumor. The manifestations of virilization are described in Chaps. 53 and 331. Virilization in girls with congenital adrenal hyperplasia usually takes place in a background of variable sexual ambiguity (see Chap. 338).

Evaluation of Sexual Precocity The evaluation of sexual precocity involves a careful history and physical examination, including rectoabdominal examination, abdominal sonography, determination of bone age, and GnRH stimulation test, and measurement of thyroid hormones, TSH, and gonadotropins (and androgen or estrogen levels when appropriate). MRI and/or CT scans should be obtained if a neurologic disorder is suspected and no evidence of ovarian or adrenal tumor is found.

REPRODUCTIVE YEARS Disorders of the Menstrual Cycle • *Abnormal uterine bleeding* Between menarche and the menopause, almost every woman experiences one or more episodes of abnormal uterine bleeding, here defined as any bleeding pattern that differs in frequency, duration, or amount from the pattern observed during a normal menstrual cycle. A variety of descriptive terms (such as *menorrhagia*, *metrorrhagia*, and *menometrorrhagia*) have been used to characterize patterns of abnormal uterine bleeding. A more logical approach is to divide abnormal uterine bleeding into those patterns associated with ovulatory cycles and those associated with anovulatory cycles.

Ovulatory cycles Normal menstrual bleeding with ovulatory cycles is spontaneous, regular, cyclic, and predictable and is frequently associated with discomfort (*dysmenorrhea*). Deviations from this pattern associated with cycles that are still regular and predictable are most often due to organic disease of the outflow tract. For example, regular but prolonged and excessive bleeding episodes unassociated with bleeding dyscrasias (hypermenorrhea or menorrhagia) can result from abnormalities of the uterus such as submucous leiomyomas, adenomyosis, or endometrial polyps. Regular, cyclic, predictable menstruation characterized by spotting or light bleeding is termed *hypomenorrhea* and is due to obstruction of the outflow tract as from intrauterine synechiae or scarring of the cervix. Intermenstrual bleeding between episodes of regular, ovulatory menstruation is also often due to cervical or endometrial lesions. An exception to the association between organic disease and abnormal uterine bleeding is the occurrence of regular menstruation more frequently than 21 days apart (*polymenorrhea*). Such cycles may be a normal variant.

Anovulatory cycles Uterine bleeding that is unpredictable with respect to amount, onset, and duration and usually painless is described as *dysfunctional uterine bleeding*. This disorder is not due to abnormalities of the uterus but rather to chronic anovulation and occurs when there is interruption of the normal sequence of follicular and luteal phases under the influence of a dominant follicle and its resulting corpus luteum. As discussed above, uterine bleeding in ovulatory cycles is due to progesterone withdrawal and requires that the endometrium first be primed with estrogen. (When castrates or postmenopausal women are given progesterone, withdrawal bleeding usually does not occur.)

Dysfunctional uterine bleeding can occur in women who have a transient disruption of the synchronous hypothalamic-pituitary-ovarian patterns necessary for ovulatory cycles, most often at the extremes of the reproductive life—in the early menarche and in the perimenopausal period—but also after temporary stress or intercurrent illness.

Primary dysfunctional uterine bleeding can result from three disorders.

1. *Estrogen withdrawal bleeding* occurs when estrogen is given to a castrated or postmenopausal woman and then withdrawn. As in other types of dysfunctional uterine bleeding, this form of menstrual bleeding is usually painless.
2. *Estrogen breakthrough bleeding* occurs when there is continuous estrogen stimulation of the endometrium not interrupted by cyclic progesterone secretion and withdrawal. This is the most common type of dysfunctional uterine bleeding and is usually due to anovulation associated with chronic acyclic estrogen production, as in women with PCOS. Such women may have histories of irregular, unpredictable menses, oligomenorrhea, or amenorrhea (see below). Alternatively, estrogen breakthrough bleeding can occur in hypogonadal women given estrogens chronically rather than intermittently and in women with estrogen-secreting tumors of the ovary. Estrogen breakthrough bleeding may be profuse and is unpredictable with respect to duration, amount of flow, and time of occurrence. The endometrium is typically thin because its repair between episodes of bleeding is incomplete.
3. *Progesterone breakthrough bleeding* occurs in the presence of abnormally high ratios of progesterone to estrogen, e.g., in women using continuous low-dose oral contraceptives.

The approach to a patient with dysfunctional uterine bleeding begins with a careful history of menstrual patterns and prior hormonal therapy. Since not all urogenital tract bleeding is from the uterus, rectal, bladder, and vaginal or cervical sources must be excluded by physical examination. If the bleeding is from the uterus, a pregnancy-related disorder such as abortion or ectopic pregnancy must be ruled out.

℞ TREATMENT Once the diagnosis of dysfunctional uterine bleeding is established, a rational approach to management is as follows: During a first episode of dysfunctional bleeding the patient can simply be observed, provided the bleeding is not copious and no evidence of bleeding dyscrasia is present. If bleeding is moderately severe, control can be achieved with relatively high dose estrogen oral contraceptives for 3 weeks. Alternatively, a regimen of three or four low-dose oral contraceptive pills per day for 1 week followed by tapering to the usual dosage for up to 3 weeks is also effective. If uterine bleeding is more severe, hospitalization, bed rest, and intramuscular injections of estradiol valerate (10 mg) and hydroxyprogesterone caproate (500 mg) or intravenous or intramuscular conjugated estrogens (25 mg) usually control the bleeding. After initial treatment, iron replacement should be instituted, and recurrence can be prevented by cyclic oral contraceptives for 2 to 3 months (or more if pregnancy is not desired). Alternatively, menses can be induced every 2 to 3 months with medroxyprogesterone acetate, 10 mg by mouth once or twice a day for 10 days. If hormone therapy fails to control uterine bleeding, an endometrial biopsy, hysteroscopy, or dilatation and curettage may be required for diagnosis and therapy. Indeed, uterine sampling should be performed prior to hormone therapy in women at risk for endometrial cancer (i.e., in women who are approaching the age of menopause or are massively obese); endometrial cancer is rare in ovulatory women of reproductive age.

Amenorrhea An acceptable definition of amenorrhea is failure of menarche by age 15, irrespective of the presence or absence of secondary sexual characteristics, or the absence of menstruation for 6 months in a woman with previous periodic menses. However, women who do not fulfill these criteria should be evaluated if (1) the patient and/or her family are greatly concerned, (2) no breast development has occurred by age 13, or (3) any sexual ambiguity or virilization is present (Chap. 338). Amenorrhea is commonly categorized as either primary (the woman has never menstruated) or secondary (when menstruation has been present for a variable period of time in the past and has ceased). However, some disorders can cause either primary or secondary amenorrhea. For example, most women with gonadal dysgenesis have primary amenorrhea, but some have a few follicles and ovulate for short periods so that pregnancy occurs rarely. Furthermore, patients with chronic anovulation (PCOS) usually have secondary amenorrhea but on occasion have primary amenorrhea. For these reasons, categorization of amenorrhea into primary and secondary types is less helpful than a classification based on the underlying physiologic derangements: (1) anatomic defects, (2) ovarian failure, and (3) chronic anovulation with or without estrogen present.

ANATOMIC DEFECTS Anatomic or structural defects of the genital tract can preclude menstrual bleeding. Starting from the caudal end of the female genital tract, labial fusion is often associated with disorders of sexual development, particularly female pseudohermaphroditism (congenital adrenal hyperplasia or exposure to maternal androgens in utero; Chap. 338). Congenital defects of the vagina, imperforate hymen, and transverse vaginal septae can also cause amenorrhea. These women frequently have accumulation of menstrual blood behind the obstruction and may have cyclic, predictable episodes of abdominal pain.

More severe müllerian anomalies include müllerian agenesis (the Mayer-Rokitansky-Küster-Hauser syndrome; Chap. 338), second in frequency only to gonadal dysgenesis as a cause of primary amenorrhea. It can be caused by mutations in the genes encoding anti-müllerian hormone (AMH) or its receptor (AMHR). Women with this syndrome have a 46,XX karyotype, female secondary sex characteristics, and normal ovarian function, including cyclic ovulation, but have absence or hypoplasia of the vagina. The uterus usually consists of only rudimentary bicornuate cords, but if the uterus contains endometrium, cyclic abdominal pain and accumulation of blood may occur, as in other forms of outlet obstruction. One-third of women with this syndrome have abnormalities of the urogenital tract, and one-tenth have skeletal anomalies, usually involving the spine. The major diagnostic problem is distinguishing müllerian agenesis from complete testicular feminization, in which 46,XY genetic males with testes differentiate as phenotypic women but with a blind vaginal pouch and no uterus. Women with testicular feminization have feminized breasts but a paucity of pubic and axillary hair. The disorder is X-linked and is caused by mutations in the androgen receptor that result in profound resistance to the action of testosterone (Chap. 338). Testicular feminization can be diagnosed by demonstrating a male level of serum testosterone and a 46,XY karyotype, whereas demonstration of a 46,XX karyotype, the biphasic basal body temperature curve characteristic of ovulation, and elevated levels of progesterone during the luteal phase establish the diagnosis of müllerian agenesis.

A rare cause of absence of the uterus in 46,XY phenotypic women who are sexually infantile is the so-called testicular regression syndrome or testicular agenesis (Chap. 338).

Other abnormalities of the uterus that cause amenorrhea include obstruction due to scarring or stenosis of the cervix, often resulting from surgery, electrocautery, laser therapy, or cryosurgery. Such destruction of the endometrium (Asherman's syndrome) usually follows vigorous curettage for postpartum hemorrhage or after therapeutic abortion complicated by infection. This diagnosis is confirmed by hysterosalpingography or by direct visual examination of the endometrial scarring or synechiae using a hysteroscope.

Treatment of disorders of the outflow tract is surgical.

OVARIAN FAILURE Primary ovarian failure is associated with elevated plasma gonadotropin levels and can result from several causes. The most frequent cause is *gonadal dysgenesis*, in which the germ cells are absent and the ovary is replaced by a fibrous streak (Chaps. 65 and 338). Women with gonadal dysgenesis can be divided into two broad groups on the basis of chromosomal karyotype. The most common type is due to deletion of genetic material in the X chromosomes and accounts for about two-thirds of cases of gonadal dysgenesis. A 45,X karyotype is found in about half of women with this disorder, and most have somatic defects, including short stature, webbed neck, shield chest, and cardiovascular defects, collectively termed the *Turner phenotype*. The remainder of women with X chromosome abnormalities have chromosomal mosaicism with or without associated structural abnormalities of the X. The most common form of mosaicism is 45,X/46,XX. Gonadal tumors are rare in 45,X patients, but gonadal malignancies may occur in women with chromosomal mosaicism involving the Y chromosome. Therefore, chromosomal analysis should be performed in all cases of amenorrhea associated with ovarian failure, and the streak gonad should be removed if a Y chromosome is present. One means of identifying the presence of a Y chromosome is to amplify the sex-determining regions of the Y chromosome (SRY) by means of the polymerase chain reaction (Chap. 338). Approximately 90% of women with gonadal dysgenesis due to partial or complete deletion of the X never have menstrual bleeding, and the remaining 10% have sufficient follicles to experience menses and, rarely, fertility; the menstrual and reproductive lives of such individuals are invariably brief.

One-tenth of individuals identified as having bilateral streak gonads have a normal 46,XX or 46,XY karyotype and are said to have *pure gonadal dysgenesis*. These individuals have either normal or above-average stature, owing to failure of estrogen-mediated epiphyseal closure in the presence of a normal chromosomal constitution. Pure gonadal dysgenesis does not constitute a phenotypic or chromosomally homogeneous disorder (Chap. 338). Occasional women with a 46,XY karyotype develop signs of virilization, including clitoromegaly, and have an increased incidence of tumors in the gonadal streaks; as a consequence, gonadal streaks should be removed prophylactically, as discussed above, when a Y chromosome is present. Approximately two-thirds of women with 46,XX gonadal dysgenesis experience no menses, while the remainder have one or more menstrual episodes and are occasionally fertile.

Other causes of ovarian failure and amenorrhea include deficiency of the *CYP17* gene that encodes 17α-hydroxylase and 17,20-lyase activities, premature ovarian failure, the resistant-ovary syndrome, and ovarian failure secondary to chemotherapy or radiation therapy for malignancy. *17α-Hydroxylase deficiency* is characterized by primary amenorrhea, sexual infantilism, and hypertension, the latter due to increased production of desoxycorticosterone (DOC); whereas women with *17,20-lyase deficiency* have primary amenorrhea and sexual infantilism with normal blood pressure (Chaps. 331 and 338). The diagnosis of *premature ovarian failure* or *premature menopause* is applied to women who cease menstruating before age 40. The ovaries in such women are similar to the ovaries of postmenopausal women, containing few or no follicles as the result of accelerated follicular atresia. Premature ovarian failure due to ovarian antibodies may be one component of polyglandular failure, together with adrenal insufficiency, hypothyroidism, and other autoimmune disorders (Chap. 339). A rare form of ovarian failure is the *resistant-ovary syndrome*, in which the ovaries contain many follicles that are arrested in development prior to the antral stage, possibly because of resistance to the action of FSH in the ovary. A subset of these individuals have mutations in FSH or its receptor. To differentiate this disorder from the 46,XX variety of pure gonadal dysgenesis, which is also associated with sexual immaturity, it is necessary to perform ovarian biopsy. However, it is not clinically useful to make this distinction, since the conventional treatment of infertility in both conditions is usually unsuccessful. Women with ovarian failure who desire pregnancy have been treated with hormone replacement and transfer of donor embryos to the uterine cavity or fallopian tubes.

Chronic anovulation   At least 80% or more of gynecologic endocrine disorders result from chronic anovulation. Women with chronic anovulation fail to ovulate spontaneously but may ovulate with appropriate therapy. The ovaries of such women do not secrete estrogen in a normal cyclic pattern; it is clinically useful to differentiate those women who produce enough estrogen to have withdrawal bleeding after progestogen therapy from those who do not; the latter often have hypothalamic-pituitary dysfunction.

CHRONIC ANOVULATION WITH ESTROGEN PRESENT   Women with chronic anovulation who experience withdrawal bleeding after progestogen administration are said to be in a state of "estrus" due to the acyclic production of estrogen, largely estrone, by extraglandular aromatization of circulating androstenedione. This disorder is commonly termed *polycystic ovarian syndrome* (PCOS) and is characterized by infertility, hirsutism, obesity, and amenorrhea or oligomenorrhea. When spontaneous uterine bleeding occurs in women with PCOS, it is unpredictable as to time of onset, duration, and amount; on occasion the bleeding can be severe. The dysfunctional uterine bleeding is usually due to estrogen breakthrough (see above).

The disorder, as originally described by Stein and Leventhal, was characterized by enlarged, polycystic ovaries, but it is now known to be associated with a variety of pathologic findings in the ovaries, only some of which result in enlargement and none of which are pathognomonic. The most common finding is a white, smooth, sclerotic ovary with a thickened capsule, multiple follicular cysts in various stages of atresia, a hyperplastic theca and stroma, and rare or absent corpora albicans. Other ovaries have hyperthecosis in which the ovarian stroma is hyperplastic and may contain lipid-laden luteal cells. Thus, the diagnosis of PCOS is a clinical one, based on the coexistence of chronic anovulation and varying degrees of androgen excess. The fundamental defect that causes PCOS is unknown, and it is likely to have several distinct causes.

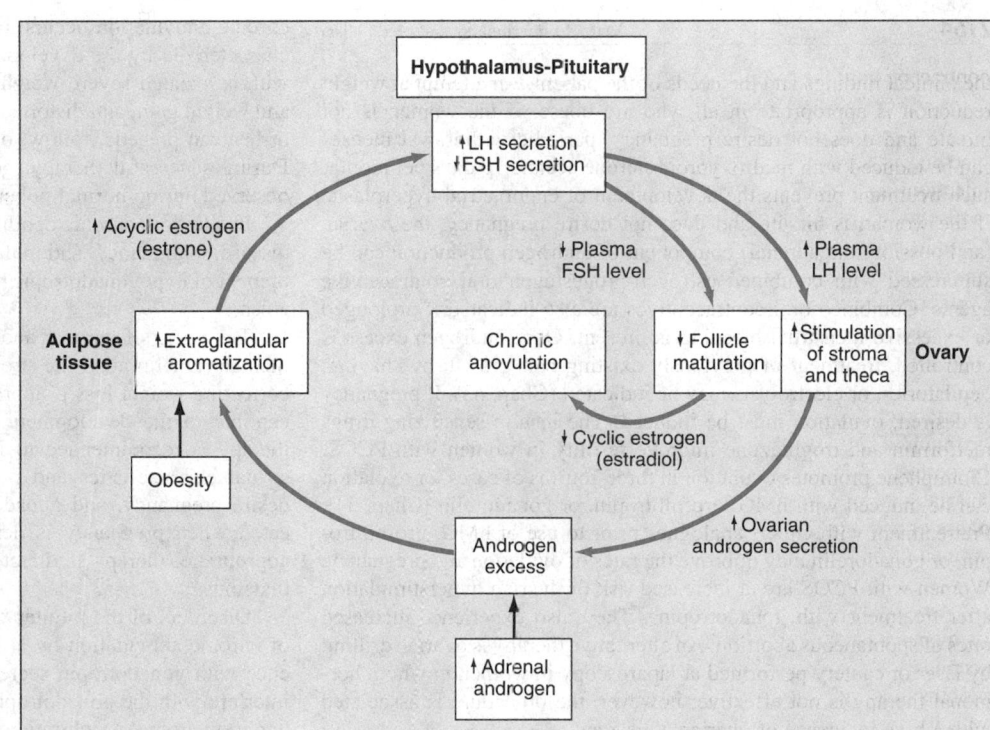

FIGURE 336-7   Proposed mechanism for the initiation and perpetuation of chronic anovulation in polycystic ovarian syndrome (PCOS). This cycle may be entered or initiated via adrenal androgen excess or obesity, both of which result in enhanced extraglandular formation of estrogens. The therapy of PCOS involves interruption of the cycle at any of several steps. *From SSC Yen et al (eds), Reproductive Endocrinology. Philadelphia, Saunders, 1999; and from U Goebelsmann, in Reproductive Endocrinology, Infertility, and Contraception, 2d ed, DR Mishell Jr, V Davajan (eds), Philadelphia, Davis, 1986.*

In most women with PCOS, menarche occurs at the expected time, but uterine bleeding is unpredictable in onset, duration, and amount. Amenorrhea ensues after a variable period, although primary amenorrhea occurs in some women. Signs of androgen excess (hirsutism) usually become evident around the time of menarche. One scenario suggests that this disorder originates as an exaggerated adrenarche in obese girls (Fig. 336-7). The combination of elevated levels of adrenal androgens and obesity leads to increased formation of extraglandular estrogen. This estrogen exerts a positive feedback on LH secretion and negative feedback on FSH secretion, resulting in a ratio of LH to FSH levels in plasma that is characteristically greater than 2. The increased LH levels can then lead to hyperplasia of the ovarian stroma and theca cells and increased androgen production, which in turn provides more substrate for peripheral aromatization and perpetuates the chronic anovulation. In the advanced stage of the disorder, the ovary is the major site of androgen production, but the adrenal may continue to secrete excess androgen as well. The greater the obesity, the more strongly this sequence would be perpetuated because more androgen is converted to estrogen by adipose tissue stromal cells, which in turn exaggerates inappropriate LH release by positive feedback. Ovarian follicles from women with PCOS have low aromatase activity, but normal aromatase can be induced by treatment with FSH. An association exists between PCOS/hyperthecosis, virilization, acanthosis nigricans, and insulin resistance; in the ovary, insulin may interact via the insulin-like growth factor receptors to enhance androgen synthesis in insulin-resistant states.

℞   **TREATMENT**   Treatment of PCOS is directed toward interrupting the self-perpetuating cycle and can be accomplished in several ways, such as by decreasing ovarian androgen secretion (by wedge resection or the use of oral contraceptive agents), decreasing peripheral estrogen formation (by weight reduction), or enhancing FSH secretion [by administration of clomiphene, human menopausal gonadotropin (hMG), GnRH (gonadorelin) by portable infusion pump, or purified FSH (urofollitropin)]. The choice of therapy depends on the clinical findings and the needs of the patient. An attempt at weight reduction is appropriate in all who are obese. If the woman is not hirsute and does not desire pregnancy, periodic withdrawal menses can be induced with medroxyprogesterone acetate 10 days per month; such treatment prevents the development of endometrial hyperplasia. If the woman is hirsute and does not desire pregnancy, the ovarian (and possibly the adrenal) component of androgen production can be suppressed with combined estrogen-progestogen oral contraceptive agents. Combined oral contraceptives are also indicated if prolonged or excessive menstrual bleeding is present. Once androgen excess is controlled, treatment of previously existing hair growth by shaving, depilatories, or electrolysis may be indicated (Chap. 53). If pregnancy is desired, ovulation must be induced. The insulin-sensitizing drugs metformin and troglitazone improve fertility in women with PCOS. Clomiphene promotes ovulation in three-fourths of cases, or ovulation can be induced with hMG, urofollitropin, or gonadorelin (Chap. 54). Pretreatment with GnRH analogues prior to use of hMG, urofollitropin, or gonadorelin may improve the rates of ovulation and pregnancy. Women with PCOS are at increased risk of ovarian hyperstimulation after treatment with gonadotropins. They also experience increased rates of spontaneous abortion. An alternative therapy is ovarian drilling by laser or cautery performed at laparoscopy in women in whom hormonal therapy is not effective; however, the procedure is associated with a high incidence of ovarian adhesions.

Chronic anovulation with estrogen present also may occur with tumors of the ovary. These include granulosa-theca cell tumors, Brenner tumors, cystic teratomas, mucous cystadenomas, and Krukenberg tumors (Chap. 97). Such tumors can either secrete excess estrogen themselves or produce androgens that are aromatized in extraglandular sites. Chronic anovulation and the clinical features of PCOS result. Occasionally, areas of the ovary not involved with tumors show the characteristic histologic changes of PCOS. Other causes of chronic anovulation with estrogen present include adrenal production of excess androgen (usually adult-onset adrenal hyperplasia due to partial 21-hydroxylase deficiency) and various thyroid disorders.

CHRONIC ANOVULATION WITH ESTROGEN ABSENT   Women with chronic anovulation who have low or absent estrogen production and do not experience withdrawal bleeding after progestogen treatment usually have hypogonadotropic hypogonadism due to disease of either the pituitary or the central nervous system.

Isolated hypogonadotropic hypogonadism associated with defects of smell (olfactory bulb defects) is known as the *Kallmann syndrome* (Chaps. 328 and 335). Affected women are sexually infantile and have a defect in the synthesis and/or release of GnRH. Hypothalamic lesions that impair GnRH production and cause hypogonadotropic hypogonadism include craniopharyngioma, germinoma (pinealoma), glioma, Hand-Schüller-Christian disease, teratomas, endodermal-sinus tumors, tuberculosis, sarcoidosis, and metastatic tumors that cause suppression or destruction of the hypothalamus. Central nervous system trauma and irradiation can also cause hypothalamic amenorrhea and deficiencies in secretion of growth hormone, adrenocorticotropic hormone (ACTH), vasopressin, and thyroid hormone.

More commonly, gonadotropin deficiency leading to chronic anovulation is believed to arise from functional disorders of the hypothalamus or higher centers. A history of a stressful event in a young woman is frequent. For example, chronic anovulation can begin suddenly in a woman who leaves home for the first time or experiences the death of a loved one. Gonadotropin and estrogen levels are in the low to low-normal range as compared with normal women in the early follicular phase of the cycle. In addition, rigorous exercise, such as jogging or ballet, and diets that result in excessive weight loss may lead to chronic anovulation, particularly in girls with a history of prior menstrual irregularity. The amenorrhea in these women does not appear to be due to weight loss alone but to a combination of a decrease in body fat and chronic stress. An extreme form of weight loss with chronic anovulation occurs in anorexia nervosa. Anorexia nervosa is characterized by the development in a young woman of amenorrhea with associated severe weight loss, distorted attitudes toward eating and weight gain, and distorted body image. In anorexia nervosa amenorrhea can precede, follow, or coincide with weight loss (Chap. 78). During successful therapy, gonadotropin changes recapitulate those observed during normal puberty (Fig. 336-1).

In addition, chronic debilitating diseases such as end-stage kidney disease, malignancy, and malabsorption are believed to lead to development of hypogonadotropic hypogonadism via a hypothalamic mechanism.

Treatment of chronic anovulation due to hypothalamic disorders includes ameliorating the stressful situation, decreasing exercise, and correcting weight loss if appropriate. These women appear to be susceptible to the development of osteoporosis; estrogen replacement therapy is recommended to induce and maintain normal secondary sexual characteristics and prevent bone loss in those who do not desire pregnancy, and gonadotropin or gonadorelin therapy is indicated when pregnancy is desired (see "Treatment," below). When appropriate, therapy is directed at the primary disease of the hypothalamus.

Disorders of the pituitary can lead to the estrogen-deficient form of chronic anovulation by at least two mechanisms—direct interference with gonadotropin secretion by lesions that either obliterate or interfere with the gonadotropic cells (chromophobe adenomas, Sheehan's syndrome) or inhibition of gonadotropin secretion in association with excess prolactin (prolactinoma). *Pituitary tumors* make up approximately 10% of all intracranial tumors and may secrete no hormone, one hormone, or more than one hormone (Chap. 328). Prolactin levels are elevated in 50 to 70% of patients with pituitary tumors, either because of prolactin secretion by the tumor itself (in the case of prolactinomas) or because the tumor mass interferes with the normal hypothalamic inhibition of prolactin secretion.

Prolactinomas can be divided into microadenomas (<10 mm in diameter) and macroadenomas (>10 mm). Prolactin excess associated with low levels of LH and FSH constitutes a specific subtype of hypogonadotropic hypogonadism. One-tenth or more of amenorrheic women have increased levels of serum prolactin, and more than half of women with both galactorrhea and amenorrhea have elevated prolactin levels. The amenorrhea is most often associated with decreased or absent estrogen production, but prolactin-secreting tumors on occasion are associated with normal ovulatory menses or chronic anovulation with estrogen present. The increased frequency of diagnosis of prolactin-secreting adenomas is probably due to several factors, including increased awareness, improved radiographic detection methods, and availability of radioimmunoassays for prolactin. Since in older autopsy series a 9 to 23% prevalence of pituitary adenomas was observed in asymptomatic women, the clinical and prognostic significance of small microadenomas in asymptomatic individuals is unclear. However, when tumors of any size are associated with symptoms of amenorrhea or galactorrhea, particularly when visual field defects or severe headaches are present, bromocriptine therapy or neurosurgical evaluation is indicated. In the latter half of pregnancy, prolactin-secreting pituitary tumors may expand, leading to headaches, compression of the optic chiasm, bitemporal hemianopsia, and blindness. Therefore, before inducing ovulation for the purposes of achieving pregnancy, it is mandatory to exclude the presence of a pituitary tumor. →*The evaluation, differential diagnosis, and management of hyperprolactinemia are described in Chap. 328.*

Large pituitary tumors such as null cell adenomas—whether or not hyperprolactinemia is present—are likely to be associated with deficiency of hormones in addition to gonadotropins (Chap. 328).

Craniopharyngiomas, which are thought to arise from remnants of Rathke's pouch, account for 3% of intracranial neoplasms, occur most frequently in the second decade of life, and may extend into the suprasellar region. Many of these tumors calcify and can be diagnosed by conventional skull films. Patients often present with sexual infantilism, delayed puberty, and amenorrhea due to gonadotropin deficiency; secretion of TSH, ACTH, growth hormone, and vasopressin may also be impaired.

Panhypopituitarism can occur spontaneously, be caused by mutations in transcription factors (Pit1; Prop1) involved in pituitary gland development, result from surgical or radiation treatment of pituitary adenomas, or develop after postpartum hemorrhage (Sheehan's syndrome). Patients with the latter disorder characteristically have failure to lactate or ovulate, loss of genital and axillary hair, hypothyroidism, and adrenal insufficiency (Chap. 328).

Evaluation of amenorrhea A general scheme for the evaluation of women with amenorrhea is given in Fig. 336-8. On physical examination, attention should be given to three features: (1) the degree of maturation of the breasts, pubic and axillary hair, and external genitalia; (2) the current estrogen status; and (3) the presence or absence of a uterus. Pregnancy should be excluded in all women with amenorrhea; it is prudent to perform a suitable pregnancy screening test even when the history and physical examination are not suggestive. Once that is done, the cause of amenorrhea can frequently be diagnosed clinically. For example, Asherman's syndrome is suggested by a history of curettage in a woman who previously menstruated; in women with primary amenorrhea and sexual infantilism, the essential differential diagnosis is between gonadal dysgenesis and hypopituitarism, and the diagnosis of gonadal dysgenesis (Turner's syndrome) or of anatomic defects of the outflow tract (müllerian agenesis, testicular feminization, and cervical stenosis) is frequently suggested on the basis of physical findings. When a specific cause is suspected, it is appropriate to proceed directly to confirm the diagnosis (obtaining a chromosomal karyotype or measurement of plasma gonadotropins). It is also useful to measure serum prolactin and FSH levels during the initial evaluation.

Estrogen status is evaluated by determining if the vaginal mucosa is moist and rugated and if the cervical mucus can be stretched and shown to fern upon drying. If these criteria are indeterminate, a progestational challenge is indicated, most often the administration of 10 mg medroxyprogesterone acetate by mouth once or twice daily for 5 days or 100 mg progesterone in oil intramuscularly. (It should be emphasized that progestogen should never be administered until pregnancy is excluded.) If estrogen levels are adequate (and the outflow tract is intact), menstrual bleeding should occur within 1 week of ending the progestogen treatment. If withdrawal bleeding occurs, the diagnosis is chronic anovulation with estrogen present, usually caused by PCOS.

If no withdrawal bleeding or only minimal vaginal spotting occurs, the nature of the subsequent workup depends on the results of the initial prolactin assay. If plasma prolactin is elevated, or if galactorrhea is present, radiography of the pituitary should be undertaken. When the plasma prolactin level is normal in an anovulatory woman with estrogen absent and with elevated FSH levels, the diagnosis is ovarian failure. If the gonadotropins are in the low or normal range, the diagnosis is either hypothalamic-pituitary disorder or an anatomic defect of the outflow tract. As indicated previously, the diagnosis of outflow tract disorder is usually suspected or established on the basis of the history and physical findings. When the physical findings are not clear-cut, it is useful to administer cyclic estrogen plus progestogen (1.25 mg oral conjugated estrogens per day for 3 weeks, with 10 mg medroxyprogesterone acetate added for the last 7 to 10 days of estrogen treat-

FIGURE 336-8 Flow diagram for the evaluation of women with amenorrhea. The most common diagnosis for each category is shown in parentheses. The dotted lines indicate that in some instances a correct diagnosis can be reached on the basis of history and physical examination alone.

ment), followed by 10 days of observation. If no bleeding occurs, the diagnosis of Asherman's syndrome or another anatomic defect of the outflow tract is confirmed by hysterosalpingography or hysteroscopy. If withdrawal bleeding occurs following the estrogen-progestogen combination, the diagnosis of chronic anovulation with estrogen absent (functional hypothalamic amenorrhea) is suggested. Radiologic evaluations of the pituitary-hypothalamic areas may be indicated in the latter cases—irrespective of the prolactin level—because of the danger of overlooking a pituitary-hypothalamic tumor and because the diagnosis of functional hypothalamic amenorrhea is one of exclusion (Chap. 328).

Infertility Infertility, the failure to become pregnant after 1 year of unprotected intercourse, affects approximately 10 to 15% of couples and is a common reason for seeking gynecologic assistance (Chap. 54). Male factors account for 40% of infertility problems (Chap. 335). In women, failure of ovulation accounts for 30% of cases; pelvic factors, such as tubal disease or endometriosis, account for half; and a cervical factor is implicated in about one-tenth. In 10 to 20% of infertile women no etiology is found.

Medical Aspects of Pregnancy (See also Chap. 7) The possibility of pregnancy should be considered in all women of reproductive age who are evaluated for medical illness or considered for surgery. Procedures such as x-ray exposure, drugs, and anesthetics may be harmful to the developing fetus, and a variety of medical problems may worsen during pregnancy, including hypertension; diseases of the heart, lungs, kidney, and liver; and metabolic and endocrine disorders. Abnormal vaginal bleeding or amenorrhea during the reproductive years should prompt consideration of a complication of pregnancy, such as incomplete abortion, ectopic pregnancy, or trophoblastic disease (hydatidiform mole or choriocarcinoma). Women who present with these complications of pregnancy often have histories of abdominal pain and vaginal bleeding and may have evidence of intraabdominal hemorrhage.

Choriocarcinoma is a particular problem because of its protean manifestations. Half these malignancies follow pregnancies complicated by hydatidiform mole, and the remainder occur after spontaneous abortion, ectopic pregnancy, or normal deliveries. Patients may present with intraabdominal bleeding due to rupture of the uterus, liver, or ovary, with pulmonary manifestations (cough, hemoptysis, pleuritic pain, dyspnea, and respiratory failure) or gastrointestinal symptoms, usually chronic blood loss or melena. In addition, patients can present with cerebral metastases or renal involvement. The diagnosis can be established by demonstrating an elevated level of the β subunit of hCG in plasma. Treatment and cure are possible with chemotherapeutic agents (dactinomycin and/or methotrexate). →*The manifestations of choriocarcinoma in men are discussed in Chap. 96.*

Ovarian Tumors   See Chap. 97

℞ **TREATMENT**   **Progestogens**   The major use of progestogens is in conjunction with estrogen to ensure the full maturation of the endometrium, both in combination birth control pills and in the therapy of hypogonadal states. In certain circumstances, however, progestogen therapy is appropriate by itself—to induce a progestational effect on the estrogen-primed endometrium (in diagnostic tests for the evaluation of amenorrhea), to inhibit pituitary gonadotropins for contraception (the progestogen-only birth control pill or progestogen-containing implants), for prophylaxis to prevent hyperplasia in PCOS, for palliation in cases of endometrial and breast carcinoma, and for treatment of endometriosis. Even when a direct progestational effect is desired, the available oral drugs substitute a synthetic derivative for the naturally occurring hormone. Oral progestogens include medroxyprogesterone acetate, megestrol acetate, norethindrone, norgestrel, and micronized progesterone. Parenteral agents include progesterone in oil, medroxyprogesterone acetate suspension, and 17-hydroxyprogesterone caproate. Vaginal progesterone suppositories are used for treatment of luteal-phase defects, and progestogen implants are available for long-term contraception.

The most common undesirable side effect is breakthrough bleeding, which occurs when progestogens are used continuously. Other complications include nausea, vomiting, and hirsutism. Abnormal liver function is a side effect of those derivatives with alkyl substitution in the 17α position. Synthetic progestogens are contraindicated if pregnancy is known or suspected, because of the risk of birth defects.

Estrogens   Estrogens are used for the treatment of gonadal failure, the control of fertility, and the management of dysfunctional uterine bleeding. However, none of the available oral or parenteral hormones replaces the pattern of circulating estradiol levels characteristic of the normally cycling, premenopausal woman (Fig. 336-5). Estrogens that can be given by mouth are either nonsteroidal agents (such as diethylstilbestrol) that mimic the action of estradiol, estrogen conjugates that must be hydrolyzed before they become active (usually estrone sulfate from pregnant mare's urine), or estrogen analogues that cannot be metabolized to estradiol (mestranol, quinestrol; Fig. 336-9). Even when micronized estradiol is given orally, it is rapidly converted in the body to estrone. Because oral therapy neither replaces nor mimics the daily secretory pattern of the deficient hormone, such therapy must be viewed as a pharmacologic substitution rather than a physiologic replacement. Likewise, the use of parenteral estrogens rarely mimics the physiologic situation. Parenteral preparations of conjugated estrogens, like the oral derivatives, are poor precursors of estradiol, and estradiol esters (estradiol benzoate and valerate) rarely result in plasma estradiol levels that mimic the normal monthly secretory cycle of the hormone. Transdermal estradiol results in constant levels of blood estradiol and is effective in the treatment of menopausal symptoms. Estrogen vaginal rings and creams can be used for local treatment of vaginal atrophy, but systemic absorption is variable. The side effects of estrogen substitution differ at various times of life.

Hypoestrogenism   In women with decreased estrogen production, whether due to disease of the ovaries (gonadal dysgenesis) or to hypogonadotropic hypogonadism, treatment with cyclic estrogens should be instituted at the time of expected puberty to induce the development and maintenance of female secondary sexual characteristics and to prevent osteoporosis. The most commonly used medications are conjugated estrogens (0.625 to 1.25 mg/d by mouth) together

FIGURE 336-9   The circulating forms of administered estrogenic drugs.

with medroxyprogesterone acetate (2.5 mg/d or 5 to 10 mg during the last several days of monthly estrogen treatment to prevent development of endometrial hyperplasia). Alternatively, oral contraceptives may be given (Chap. 54). Abnormal bleeding in women receiving estrogen replacement mandates histologic evaluation of the endometrium. Such substitution therapy or the use of oral contraceptives may also be used for the purpose of suppressing pituitary gonadotropins, as in women with PCOS, in whom the major therapeutic aim is suppression of ovarian androgen production.

Temporary administration of estrogens in larger quantities (up to two times the usual adult maintenance dose) may be necessary to induce the full development of secondary sexual characteristics in girls and for the control of menopausal symptoms. Even larger doses of parenteral estrogens (10 mg estradiol valerate or 25 mg conjugated estrogen) in conjunction with progestogen may be required in some instances of dysfunctional uterine bleeding. In addition to the potential long-term side effects of all estrogens (see below), high doses may cause nausea, vomiting, and edema.

Contraceptives   See Chap. 54

Estrogen Treatment of the Menopause   The use of estrogens in postmenopausal women is based on evidence that they may relieve some of the complications of the postmenopausal state, including osteoporosis, and some manifestations of aging itself. In some parts of the United States, as many as half of women in the menopausal age group used one or more forms of estrogen replacement for a median period of 5 years.

The menopause is not, however, a state of simple estrogen deprivation, as some estrogens continue to be produced. It is instead a state of altered estrogen metabolism; the predominant estrogen becomes estrone, which is formed by extraglandular conversion of prehormone, rather than estradiol secreted by the ovary. As is true for all estrogen therapy, the estrogen treatment of the menopause is actually a pharmacologic substitution of one or another estrogen analogue for estradiol rather than a physiologic replacement of the missing steroid. The estrogens available for replacement therapy include conjugated estrogens, estrogen substitutes (diethylstilbestrol), synthetic estrogen (ethinyl estradiol or derivatives), micronized estradiol, estrogen-containing vaginal creams, and estrogen-containing dermal patches. Selective ER modulators (e.g., raloxifene) have estrogenic activity in the bone and the cardiovascular system but are antiestrogenic in breast and uterus. Raloxifene binds to the ER, with a conformational change in the domain of the receptor involved in transcription. Regimens associated with a low risk of complications include the following: (1) cyclic estrogen therapy in the lowest effective dose for 25 days per month or continuous estrogens given each day of the month, (2) estrogens plus the addition of progestogen during the last 10 to 14 days of estrogen therapy, (3) low-dose continuous progestogen plus estrogen given daily, and (4) daily selective ER modulators (SERM).

The most clear-cut early benefit of estrogen therapy in the menopause is the relief of vasomotor instability (hot flashes) and of atrophy of the urogenital epithelium and skin. Estrogen therapy ameliorates these symptoms in most cases. When estrogen therapy is intended to treat hot flashes alone, it should be continued for only a few years, since hot flashes tend to diminish after 3 to 4 years in untreated women. Selective ER modulators have no effect on hot flashes.

Several lines of evidence indicate that routine estrogen therapy is beneficial in preventing the complications of menopausal osteoporosis, especially in high-risk women (i.e., thin white women; Chap. 342). First, in women undergoing premature menopause, the incidence and complication rates of osteoporosis are increased, and long-term estrogen replacement appears to be beneficial. Second, estrogen therapy has short-term positive effects on calcium balance and long-term beneficial effects on bone density. Third, in women given estrogen therapy, the incidence of fractures is decreased.

Of the potential side effects, the possibility of an increased risk of endometrial carcinoma is perhaps most worrisome. The relative risk of developing endometrial adenocarcinoma in estrogen users is between six and eight times the risk in nonusers. This risk increases with increasing duration and dosage of estrogen but is largely negated in women given combination estrogen-progestogen therapy. Despite the large body of evidence linking endometrial carcinoma and estrogen use, the increased incidence primarily involves low-grade malignancies that may be difficult to distinguish histologically from hyperplasia. These forms of malignancy have little effect on life expectancy.

Apprehension concerning worsening of hypertension and thromboembolic disease appears to be due to reports of the effects of estrogen-progestogen oral contraceptives during the reproductive years and not to estrogen use in postmenopausal women. There is no conclusive evidence that low-dose estrogen therapy after menopause increases the incidence or the severity of breast cancer or hypertension, but the risk for venous thromboembolism is slightly increased. Low-dose estrogen treatment after menopause does not appear to influence the development of atherosclerosis, myocardial infarction, or stroke. Strong evidence suggests that, in fact, estrogens may decrease the incidence of death from myocardial infarction. There is a slightly increased risk for the development of gallbladder disease with postmenopausal estrogen use.

A reasonable approach to the postmenopausal use of estrogens is as follows: (1) For long-term use, estrogens should be given in the minimal effective doses (0.625 mg conjugated estrogen orally or 1.0 mg micronized estradiol or transdermal estradiol 0.05 to 1.0 mg in a formulation that is changed every 3.5 days or every week). For women with an intact uterus, it is the practice in some clinics to give estrogens alone for 15 days and estrogen plus a daily progestogen dose for the remainder of the month. The most common regimens involve continuous estrogen plus low-dose continuous progestogen. (2) Such replacement therapy is indicated routinely in women undergoing premature menopause (surgically induced or spontaneous). (3) Estrogen therapy is also indicated routinely in women of all ages who have severe hot flashes or symptomatic atrophy of the urogenital epithelium. Hot flashes rarely persist for longer than 7 years, so, if therapy is given for this purpose, its duration can be limited. (4) In women who have had a hysterectomy, the potential benefits of treatment appear to outweigh the dangers, and in such women cyclic or continuous estrogen without progestogen is recommended. Whether estrogens should be given routinely to all women with intact uteri is an unsettled question, but the authors prescribe it in the absence of contraindications in hopes of ameliorating osteoporosis and reducing the risk of cardiovascular disease. (5) Raloxifene is given as a 60-mg tablet daily when the goal

is to provide protection against bone loss without incurring additional risk of estrogen-dependent breast cancer. Each woman receiving estrogens must be monitored indefinitely at yearly intervals.

Induction of Ovulation   See Chap. 54

OTHER DISORDERS OF THE FEMALE REPRODUCTIVE TRACT

VULVA   Most disorders of the vulva are due to venereal disease, most commonly syphilis (painless chancre), condylomata acuminata (venereal warts), and herpes vulvitis (painful ulcers; Chap. 132). All other lesions of the vulva, particularly in older women, must be biopsied. Early biopsy of cancer of the vulva is mandatory, because when it becomes symptomatic (pruritus and bleeding), it has often progressed to an advanced stage.

VAGINA   Infections of the vagina usually present as vaginal discharge and pruritus. The most frequent organisms are *Trichomonas*, *Candida albicans*, and *bacterial vaginalis* (Chap. 132). The diagnosis is made by microscopic examination of the discharge, and appropriate therapy can be instituted using vaginal or oral antibiotics.

Abnormalities of the vagina and cervix in female offspring of women given diethylstilbestrol during pregnancy include adenosis of the vagina and structural abnormalities of the vagina, cervix, and uterus; the risk of developing a rare vaginal cancer (adenocarcinoma, clear cell type) is increased (2 per 10,000 exposed women). Periodic examination of women at risk should begin at age 12 to 14, and reexamination should be done after any episode of abnormal bleeding.

CERVIX   Preinvasive lesions of the cervix (also known as *cervical intraepithelial neoplasia*) and invasive carcinoma of the cervix can be detected reliably by obtaining a Papanicolaou (Pap) smear.

Evaluation of the Pap Smear   The incidence of invasive cervical cancer has declined as a result of Pap smear screening. In the United States, approximately 2 to 3 million abnormal Pap smears are found each year. Most represent low-grade lesions but require appropriate follow-up. The follow-up of abnormal Pap smears requires an understanding of the Bethesda system for evaluating such smears (see below) and of the limitations of cytologic screening systems. Further evaluation may require repeat cytologic examination, colposcopy, or both.

Current Screening Recommendations   Risk factors for cervical neoplasia include a history of multiple sexual partners, coitus beginning at an early age, a history of infection with human papilloma virus (HPV), infection with HIV or another immunosuppressed state, and a history of cancer of the lower genital tract. Cervical cancer screening is recommended annually beginning at 18 years of age or when the woman becomes sexually active, if earlier than age 18. "Less frequent" screening is performed when three consecutive, negative, satisfactory annual Pap smears have been obtained or if the woman is in a low-risk category. There is no upper age limit for screening, because the prevalence of invasive cancer shows a linear increase with age, most of these cancers being diagnosed after age 50. Even after hysterectomy, annual screening should be performed if there is a history of abnormal Pap smears or other lower genital tract neoplasia.

The Bethesda System of Cytologic Examination   Pap smears are evaluated in regard to the adequacy of the specimen (satisfactory for evaluation, satisfactory but limited, or unsatisfactory for evaluation because of a stated reason), the general diagnosis (normal or abnormal), and a descriptive diagnosis if the smear is abnormal. The descriptive diagnoses include benign cellular changes, reactive cellular changes, and epithelial cell abnormalities, the latter including (1) atypical squamous cells of undetermined significance (ASCUS); (2) low-grade squamous intraepithelial lesion (LSIL), which is further categorized to include HPV infection, cervical intraepithelial neoplasia (CIN 1), and high-grade squamous intraepithelial lesion (HSIL, which is itself subdivided into CIN 2 and CIN 3); and (3) squamous cell carcinoma.

Guidelines for the Management of Women with Abnormal Pap Smears For ASCUS smears that are unqualified or suggest a reactive process, a repeat smear should be obtained every 4 to 6 months for 2 years until three consecutive negative smears have been obtained. For ASCUS smears that are unqualified but have severe inflammation, any specific cause should be treated, and the smear should be repeated in 2 to 3 months; because invasive carcinoma can be obscured by severe inflammation, clinical evaluation is mandatory. For postmenopausal women not using hormone replacement, a course of topical estrogen should be given before the test is repeated. For LSIL smears, the Pap test is repeated every 4 to 6 months for 2 years until three consecutive negative smears have been obtained; treatment of HPV is of no established benefit, and there is a high rate of regression of LSIL, so that in compliant, low-risk individuals, the outcome is usually favorable. If LSIL is persistent, colposcopy with directed biopsy is performed, and endocervical curettage is undertaken if a specific diagnosis is made by biopsy. Cervical cone biopsy or loop electrosurgical excision procedures are performed for higher-grade lesions such as HSIL. If cervical cancer is diagnosed by biopsy, clinical staging is performed, and the patient is treated with radiation therapy or surgery.

UTERUS Only 40% of cases of endometrial adenocarcinoma are detected by Pap smear. In women at high risk for endometrial carcinoma (because of obesity, a history of chronic anovulatory cycles, diabetes mellitus, hypertension, or estrogen treatment), yearly endometrial sampling should be performed. Measurement of endometrial thickness by sonography can indicate which patients are at risk for endometrial pathology. Endometrial thickness <5 mm is rarely associated with either hyperplasia or cancer. Low-dose oral estrogen therapy rarely causes breakthrough or withdrawal bleeding in postmenopausal women. Therefore, irrespective of whether the patient is using estrogen therapy, the occurrence of postmenopausal bleeding makes it mandatory to obtain a tissue diagnosis by either endometrial sampling or curettage to exclude endometrial cancer.

One of the most common disorders of the uterus and the most frequent tumor of women (one of four women affected) is the uterine leiomyoma, or fibroid tumor. Three-fourths of women with leiomyoma are asymptomatic, and the diagnosis is made on routine pelvic examination. When the tumor is associated with excessive menstrual blood loss, is large or fast-gowing, or causes significant pelvic pain (Chap. 52), the preferred treatment is hysterectomy if there is no desire for further childbearing. In young women, myomectomy is sometimes indicated when infertility or repeated fetal wastage is a manifestation or where future childbearing is desired.

FALLOPIAN TUBES AND OVARIES Infectious pelvic inflammatory disease is a common disorder of the fallopian tubes and usually becomes symptomatic after a menstrual period; the symptoms include fever, chills, abdominal pain, and vaginal discharge, and pelvic tenderness on physical examination is common. The initiating organism most often is *Chlamydia trachomatis* or *Neisseria gonorrhoeae*, but tuboovarian abscess and sterility are probably caused by mixed aerobic and anaerobic superinfections and require wide-spectrum antibiotic treatment (Chap. 133).

Endometriosis is a benign disorder characterized by the presence and proliferation of endometrial tissue (stroma and glands) outside the endometrial cavity. The clinical manifestations are variable. Endometriosis occurs most commonly between the ages of 30 and 40 and is found incidentally at the time of surgery in approximately one-fifth of all gynecologic operations. The fertility rate is reduced in affected women. The disorder usually involves the posterior cul-de-sac or the ovaries and can give rise to ovarian enlargement (endometriomas), although it may involve distant sites (lung, umbilicus). The major symptom is pelvic pain, characteristically dysmenorrhea (Chap. 52). However, the frequency and severity of symptoms correlate poorly with the extent of disease. Other manifestations include dyspareunia, pain with defecation, and infertility. The characteristic physical findings are multiple tender nodules palpable along the uterosacral ligament at the time of rectal-vaginal examination, a posteriorly fixed uterus, or enlarged, cystic ovaries. The diagnosis can only be confirmed by direct visualization, usually at diagnostic laparoscopy. Treatment depends on the degree of involvement and the desires of the patient and includes observation for mild disease with no associated infertility or pain, hormonal suppressive therapy, conservative surgery by laparoscopy or laparotomy if fertility is desired, or removal of the uterus, tubes, and ovaries in severe disease. Endometriosis is rare after the menopause.

Any adnexal mass that persists for more than 6 weeks or is larger than 6 cm must be evaluated. Although ovarian cysts and neoplasms are the most common pelvic adnexal masses (see above), tumors of the fallopian tubes, uterus, gastrointestinal tract, or urinary tract should also be considered. Sonography or radiographic evaluation is often helpful in identifying the nature of the adnexal mass prior to surgical exploration.

BIBLIOGRAPHY

ADASHI EV, LEUNG PCK: *The Ovary.* New York, Raven Press, 1993

BRZOSOWSKI AM et al: Molecular bases of agonist and antagonism in the oestrogen receptor. Nature 389:753, 1997

CARR BR: Disorders of the ovary and reproductive tract, in *Williams Textbook of Endocrinology*, 9th ed, JD Wilson et al (eds). Philadelphia, Saunders, 1998, pp 751–817

————, BLACKWELL RE (eds): *Textbook of Reproductive Medicine.* Stamford, CT, Appleton & Lange, 1998

CUNNINGHAM FG et al: *Williams' Obstetrics*, 20th ed. Stamford, CT, Appleton & Lange, 1993

DELMUS PD et al: Effects of raloxifene on bone mineral density, serum cholesterol concentrations, and uterine endometrium in postmenopausal women. N Engl J Med 337:1641, 1997

FUTTERWEIT W: *Polycystic Ovarian Disease.* New York, Springer-Verlag, 1984

GRAVE GD, CUTLER GB: *Sexual Precocity.* New York, Raven Press, 1993

GRUMBACH MM, CONTE FA: Disorders of sex differentiation, in *Williams Textbook of Endocrinology*, 9th ed, JD Wilson et al (eds). Philadelphia, Saunders, 1998, pp 1303–1425

————, STYNE DM: Puberty: Ontogeny, neuroendocrinology, physiology and disorders, in *Williams Textbook of Endocrinology*, 9th ed, JD Wilson et al (eds). Philadelphia, Saunders, 1998, pp 1509–1625

HERBST AL et al: *Comprehensive Gynecology*, 2d ed. St. Louis, Mosby, 1992

KAPLAN SA (ed): *Clinical Pediatric Endocrinology.* Philadelphia, Saunders, 1990

KNOBIL E, NEILL JD (eds): *The Physiology of Reproduction*, 2d ed. New York, Raven Press, 1994

LOBO RA: *Treatment of the Menopausal Woman.* New York, Raven Press, 1994

MILLER WL, STYNE DM: Disorders of puberty in the male and female, in *Reproductive Endocrinology*, SSC Yen et al (eds). Philadelphia, Saunders, 4th ed. 1999, pp 388–412

NESTLER JE et al: Effects of metformin on spontaneous and clomiphene-induced ovulation in the polycystic ovarian syndrome. N Engl J Med 338:1876, 1998

ROCK JA et al: *Female Reproductive Surgery.* Baltimore, Williams & Wilkins, 1992

SEIBEL MM: A new era in reproductive technology. N Engl J Med 318:828, 1988

SODERSTROM RM: *Operative Laparoscopy.* New York, Raven Press, 1993

SPEROFF L et al: *Clinical Gynecologic Endocrinology and Infertility*, 5th ed. Baltimore, Williams & Wilkins, 1994

STUDD JWW, WHITEHEAD MI (eds): *The Menopause.* Oxford, Blackwell, 1988

THOMPSON JD, ROCK JA: *Te Lindes Operative Gynecology.* 8th ed. Philadelphia, Lippincott, 1992

YEN SSC et al (eds): *Reproductive Endocrinology*, 4th ed. Philadelphia, Saunders, 1999

337 *Jean D. Wilson*

ENDOCRINE DISORDERS OF THE BREAST

The breasts are the site of fatal and preventable cancer in women and provide clues to underlying systemic illness in both men and women. Consequently, examination of the breasts is an important part of the physical examination. It is the duty of every physician to distinguish the abnormal from the normal at the earliest possible stage and to seek referral if there is any doubt. →*For discussion of cancer of the breast, see Chap. 89.*

ENDOCRINE CONTROL OF THE BREAST There is no histologic or functional difference in the breasts of prepubertal boys and girls, but a profound sexual dimorphism in breast development ensues at the time of puberty. The endocrine control of female breast development is illustrated in Fig. 337-1. Growth of the female breast at puberty is mediated primarily by estradiol, which induces the enlargement, division, and elongation of the tubular duct system and maturation of the nipples. Administration of estrogen to men is equally effective in this regard. To produce true alveolar development at the ends of the ducts, however, the synergistic action of progesterone is required. Within the gland a variety of mediators influence epithelial cell division and differentiation, including stimulatory factors such as the insulin-like growth factors, transforming growth factor α, and epidermal growth factor and inhibitory factors such as transforming growth factor β. Once the anatomic development of the ducts and alveoli is complete, the continued action of estrogen and progesterone is not required for lactation itself.

The endocrine control of milk formation is complex, requiring, in addition to appropriate priming by estrogen and progesterone, lactogenic hormones and the permissive action of glucocorticoid, insulin, thyroxine, and, in some species, growth hormone. There are two lactogenic hormones: (1) human placental lactogen (hPL, or chorionic somatomammotropin) and (2) prolactin. hPL is secreted in large amounts by the placenta during the latter part of gestation and prepares the breast for milk production. It disappears from the maternal (and fetal) circulation shortly after termination of pregnancy. The secretion of pituitary prolactin (Chap. 328) rises during pregnancy and plays the critical role in the initiation and maintenance of lactation in the puerperium. During late pregnancy and lactation, 60 to 80% of the anterior pituitary may consist of prolactin-secreting lactotrope cells, reflecting the stimulatory effects of estrogen on these cells.

Unlike most pituitary hormones, prolactin secretion is controlled predominantly by tonic inhibition. Under basal conditions inhibitory hypothalamic hormones, the most important being dopamine, are delivered from the central nervous system to the pituitary via the hypothalamic portal system and inhibit the release of prolactin into the blood (Chap. 328). Most factors that influence prolactin secretion do so by affecting the synthesis or release of dopamine. Basal prolactin levels in the mother fall after delivery, but prolactin secretion is enhanced by stimulation of the breasts, such as the act of nursing (the so-called sucking reflex), a phenomenon that is probably mediated by the reflex release of oxytocin, which acts as a prolactin-releasing factor. Prolactin binds to specific receptors on the cell surface of the breast acinar cells and activates the JAK-STAT signal transduction cascade to stimulate the synthesis of β-casein, whey acidic protein, and other milk constituents. In the postgestational state, the normal lactating woman forms about a liter of milk per day containing 38 g fat, 70 g lactose, and 12 g protein. Lactation can be suppressed by the administration of estrogens or diethylstilbestrol, which inhibit milk production by direct effects on the breast, or dopamine agonists such as bromocriptine, which inhibit prolactin secretion by the pituitary. Alternatively, if a woman does not nurse or use breast pumps postpartum, lactation usually ceases in 1 to 2 weeks.

GALACTORRHEA *Galactorrhea* refers to the nonpuerperal discharge of milk-containing fluid from the breast. The definition of exactly what constitutes galactorrhea is not always clearly defined in the literature. According to the studies of Friedman and Goldfein, breast secretions are absent in normal, regularly menstruating nulligravid women. However, breast secretions can be demonstrated in a fourth of normal women who have been pregnant in the past; thus breast secretions in small amounts may be of no clinical significance in these instances. Spontaneous leakage of milk from the breasts is usually of more significance than milk that must be expressed. When the secretion is milky or white, it is safe to assume that it contains fat, casein, and lactose and is in fact milk; the concentration of milk constituents may increase after repeated sampling. When the secretion is brown or greenish, it rarely contains normal milk constituents and consequently may not result from an underlying endocrinopathy. Bloody discharges may be due to neoplasms of the breast. With these issues in mind, galactorrhea can be defined as inappropriate production of milk that is persistent or worrisome to the patient, recognizing that in some instances no underlying pathology may be demonstrated.

Since the action of a lactogenic hormone is necessary for the initiation of milk production, it is logical to consider galactorrhea as a consequence of deranged prolactin physiology. However, as indicated above, a complex hormonal milieu is necessary for lactation. Milk production does not take place in many instances in which prolactin is elevated, both in men and in women who have not been exposed to the necessary hormonal environment. As a consequence, hyperprolactinemia is more common than galactorrhea. Furthermore, while enhanced prolactin secretion is necessary for the initiation of lactation, continued production can be maintained in the presence of minimally or intermittently elevated prolactin levels so that basal plasma prolactin levels are not always elevated in patients with galactorrhea. In some such women prolactin levels may be elevated during sleep or with stimulation of the nipple; in others, hyperprolactinemia may have been present transiently. Perhaps the strongest evidence for a critical role for prolactin in galactorrhea is the fact that administration of dopaminergic agents that suppress plasma prolactin levels corrects galactorrhea even when the basal plasma prolactin levels are normal.

Differential Diagnosis Galactorrhea can be due to failure of the normal hypothalamic inhibition of prolactin release, to increased prolactin-releasing factor(s), or to autonomous prolactin secretion by tumors (Table 337-1). Pituitary stalk section, whether traumatic or secondary to the mass effects of sellar tumors, results in increases in prolactin secretion due to interruption in the delivery of dopamine to the pituitary. Likewise, many drugs that influence the central nervous system (CNS) (including virtually all psychotropic agents, methyldopa, reserpine, and antiemetics) enhance prolactin release, presumably by inhibiting synthesis, release, or action of dopamine. Estrogens increase prolactin secretion, but estrogen withdrawal (as in the discontinuation of oral contraceptives) may also trigger the onset of galactorrhea. CNS diseases outside the pituitary can cause galactorrhea presumably by interfering with the production or delivery of dopamine to the pituitary (CNS sarcoidosis, craniopharyngioma, pinealoma, encephalitis, meningitis, hydrocephalus, hypothalamic tumors).

In primary hypothyroidism, galactorrhea results from the enhanced production of thyrotropin-releasing hormone (TRH), which also stimulates prolactin release; thyroid hormone replacement corrects the galactorrhea. A similar mechanism, involving enhanced secretion of ox-

Stage	Duct system	Major hormones	Permissive hormones
Prepubertal		None	Unknown
Adult		Estrogen (progesterone)	
Pregnancy		Estrogen Progesterone Prolactin Human placental lactogen	Insulin Thyroxine Glucocorticoids Growth hormone
Lactation		Prolactin Oxytocin	

FIGURE 337-1 Endocrine control of female breast development and function at various stages of life.

Table 337-1 Classification of Galactorrhea

I. Failure of normal hypothalamic inhibition of prolactin release
   A. Pituitary stalk section
   B. Drugs (phenothiazines, butyrophenones, methyldopa, tricyclic antide-
      pressants, opiates, reserpine, verapamil, paroxetine, rispiradone,
      metoclopramide, sertraline)
   C. Central nervous system disease, including extrapituitary tumors and
      null cell adenomas of the pituitary
II. Enhanced prolactin release
   A. Hypothyroidism
   B. Sucking reflex and breast trauma
III. Autonomous prolactin release
   A. Pituitary tumors
      1. Prolactin-secreting tumors
      2. Mixed growth hormone and prolactin-secreting tumors
      3. Null cell adenomas
   B. Ectopic production of human placental lactogen and/or prolactin
      1. Hydatidiform moles and choriocarcinomas
      2. Bronchogenic carcinoma and hypernephroma
IV. Idiopathic

ytocin, may cause the galactorrhea that follows breast surgery or breast
trauma.

Enhanced prolactin release can also occur from pituitary or nonpituitary tumors. Three types of pituitary tumors (Chap. 328) can cause
galactorrhea: (1) pure prolactin-secreting micro- or macroadenomas,
(2) mixed tumors that secrete both growth hormone and prolactin and
cause acromegaly with galactorrhea, and (3) large null cell adenomas.
The latter may interfere with the delivery of dopamine to the pituitary,
either by mass effects on the hypothalamus or by compressing the
pituitary stalk. Excess growth hormone secretion, in the absence of
hyperprolactinemia, on occasion causes galactorrhea. Rarely, prolactin
is secreted by bronchogenic carcinomas, and hydatidiform moles and
choriocarcinomas may secrete placental lactogen.

In series involving several hundred patients with galactorrhea, a
pituitary tumor was identified in about one-fourth, other known causes
were identified in another fourth or fifth, and the remaining half fell
into the idiopathic category. Many of the latter group ultimately developed prolactin-secreting pituitary tumors, some probably had subtle
disorders of hypothalamic function, and in others a drug-related cause
may have been missed. The fact remains that no satisfactory diagnosis
is reached in many patients. When menses are normal, the likelihood
of establishing a cause for galactorrhea is poor.

Galactorrhea is unusual in men, even in the presence of profound
elevations of plasma prolactin; when it does occur, it is usually upon
the background of a feminizing state (see below).

Diagnostic Evaluation If hyperprolactinemia is present, the
evaluation is fundamentally that of a pituitary tumor once drug causes
and hypothyroidism are excluded (Chap. 328). Even when a specific
cause cannot be identified and the diagnosis of idiopathic galactorrhea
is made by exclusion, it is necessary to remember that pituitary tumors
may subsequently become manifest. The higher the prolactin values
and the more persistent the galactorrhea, the greater is the likelihood
of such a development.

℞ **TREATMENT** Breast binders can be effective in patients with
mild galactorrhea of unknown etiology, presumably by preventing stimulation of the nipple and the consequent perpetuation of lactation. The aim of treatment in other instances is to correct the elevated
prolactin level, and treatment of a pituitary tumor, cessation of causative drugs, or correction of hypothyroidism is often followed by the
disappearance of galactorrhea. Dopamine agonists that suppress
plasma prolactin have been used to treat idiopathic hyperprolactinemia, prolactin-secreting tumors of the pituitary (Chap. 328), and even
normoprolactinemic galactorrhea. These drugs suppress lactation and
may cause resumption of menstrual cycles (and even fertility) in
women with amenorrhea and galactorrhea.

GYNECOMASTIA Enlargement of the male breast, or *gynecomastia*, can be a normal physiologic phenomenon at certain times
of life or the result of several pathologic states (Table 337-2). A central
issue in the evaluation of breast tissue in adult men is the separation
of the normal from the abnormal, as gynecomastia can be an important
indicator of underlying disease. It is sometimes difficult to distinguish
true breast tissue enlargement from adipose tissue (*lipomastia*). True
glandular tissue is often palpable, especially around the areolae, as it
is firmer and contains cordlike features that are distinct from the texture of adipose tissue. In difficult cases, true gynecomastia can be
identified by mammography or ultrasonography. In this discussion, we
shall assume that any palpable breast tissue in men (except for the
three physiologic states see below) can be due to an underlying endocrinopathy and deserves, at a minimum, a limited evaluation.

Early gynecomastia is characterized by proliferation in the breast
of both the fibroblastic stroma and the duct system, which elongates,
buds, and duplicates. As gynecomastia persists, progressive fibrosis
and hyalinization are associated with regression of epithelial proliferation and, eventually, a decrease in the number of ducts. When the
cause of the gynecomastia is corrected early in the course, resolution
occurs by reduction in size and epithelial content with gradual disappearance of the ducts, leaving hyaline bands that eventually disappear.

Growth of the breast in men, as in women, is mediated by estrogen
and results from an decrease in the ratio of active androgen to estrogen.
As described in Chap. 335, estradiol formation in normal men occurs
principally by the conversion of circulating androgen to estrogen in
extraglandular tissues; the normal ratio of the two hormones in plasma
is about 300:1. Growth of the breast ensues in men when the normal

Table 337-2 Differential Diagnosis of Gynecomastia

PHYSIOLOGIC GYNECOMASTIA

Newborn
Adolescence
Aging

PATHOLOGIC GYNECOMASTIA

I. Deficient production or action of testosterone
   A. Congenital anorchia
   B. Androgen resistance (testicular feminization and Reifenstein syn-
      drome)
   C. Defects of testosterone synthesis
   D. Klinefelter syndrome
   E. Viral orchitis
   F. Trauma
   G. Castration
   H. Neurologic and granulomatous diseases
   I. Renal failure
II. Increased estrogen production
   A. Increased estrogen secretion
      1. Testicular tumors
      2. True hermaphroditism
      3. Carcinoma of the lung and other tumors producing hCG
   B. Increased substrate for extraglandular aromatase
      1. Adrenal disease
      2. Liver disease
      3. Malnutrition
      4. Hyperthyroidism
   C. Increase in extraglandular aromatase
III. Drugs
   A. Estrogens (diethylstilbestrol, birth control pills, digitalis, estrogen-
      containing cosmetics, estrogen-contaminated foods, phytoestrogens)
   B. Drugs that enhance endogenous estrogen secretion (gonadotropins,
      clomiphene)
   C. Inhibitors of testosterone synthesis and/or action (ketoconazole,
      metronidazole, alkylating agents, cisplatin, spironolactone, cimeti-
      dine, flutamide, etomidate)
   D. Unknown mechanisms (busulfan, isoniazid, methyldopa, tricyclic an-
      tidepressants, penicillamine, diazepam, omeprazole, calcium channel
      blockers, angiotensin-converting enzyme inhibitors, marijuana,
      heroin, finasteride, growth hormone, antiretroviral agents)
IV. Idiopathic

Note: hCG, human chorionic gonadotropin.

ratio decreases as the result of diminished testosterone production or action, enhanced estrogen formation, or both processes occurring simultaneously.

337 Endocrine Disorders of the Breast **2171**

Physiologic Gynecomastia In the *newborn* transient enlargement of the breast is due to the action of maternal and/or placental estrogens. The enlargement usually disappears in a few weeks but may persist longer. *Adolescent* gynecomastia is common at some time during puberty. The median age of onset is 14; it is often asymmetric or transiently unilateral, frequently tender, and it regresses so that by age 20 only a small number of men have palpable vestiges of glandular tissue in one or both breasts. Although the origin of the excess estrogen has not been identified, the onset of gynecomastia correlates with the increase in adrenal androgens at adrenarche. In addition, the luteinizing hormone (LH) stimulation of androgen synthesis by the Leydig cell in early puberty may be associated with transient elevations of plasma estradiol so that the ratio of potent androgen to estrogen is low prior to the completion of puberty. *Gynecomastia of aging* also occurs in 40% or more of otherwise healthy elderly men. A likely explanation is the increase with age in the conversion of androgens to estrogens in extraglandular tissues. Abnormal liver function or drug therapy may be contributing causes in such men.

Pathologic Gynecomastia Pathologic gynecomastia can result from one of three basic mechanisms: deficiency in testosterone production or action (with or without a secondary increase in estrogen production), increase in estrogen production, or drugs (Table 337-2). Most of the disorders that cause primary and secondary testicular failure are discussed in Chap. 335. The fact that deficient testosterone production can cause gynecomastia is illustrated by the syndrome of congenital anorchia in which normal (or slightly low) estradiol levels, in the presence of profoundly decreased testosterone production, results in florid gynecomastia. Decreased testosterone production is also responsible for gynecomastia in some men with Klinefelter syndrome or testicular failure of other causes. In the disorders of androgen resistance, such as testicular feminization, deficient androgen action and increased testicular estrogen production are both present.

A primary increase in estrogen production can result from a variety of causes. Increased secretion of testicular estrogen may result from elevations in plasma gonadotropins, as in cases of aberrant production of chorionic gonadotropin by testicular tumors or by bronchogenic carcinomas, from the ovarian elements in the gonads of men with true hermaphroditism, or as the result of formation by testicular tumors (particularly Leydig and Sertoli cell tumors). Increased conversion of androgen to estrogens in extraglandular tissues can be due either to increased availability of substrate (androstenedione) for extraglandular estrogen formation (congenital adrenal hyperplasia, hyperthyroidism, and most feminizing adrenal tumors), or to diminished catabolism of androstenedione (liver disease) so that estrogen precursors are shunted to aromatase in peripheral sites. Extraglandular aromatase can be increased in tumors of the liver or adrenal gland and rarely as a result of an inherited disorder manifested by gynecomastia in affected males and macromastia in females.

Drugs can cause gynecomastia by several mechanisms. Many drugs either act directly as estrogens or cause an increase in plasma estrogen activity (e.g., in men receiving diethylstilbestrol for prostatic carcinoma and in transsexuals in preparation for sex-change operations). Boys and young men are particularly sensitive to estrogen and can develop gynecomastia after the use of dermal ointments containing estrogen or after the ingestion of milk or meat from estrogen-treated animals. The gynecomastia of digitalis ingestion is usually attributed to an estrogen-like side effect of the drug, but it occurs most commonly in men with abnormal liver function. A second mechanism of drug-induced gynecomastia is illustrated by clomiphene and human chorionic gonadotropin (hCG), which cause enhanced testicular secretion of estrogen. Other drugs cause gynecomastia by interfering with testosterone synthesis (ketoconazole and alkylating agents) and/or testosterone action, for instance, by blocking the binding of androgen to its receptor protein in target tissues (spironolactone and cimetidine). Finally, drugs that cause gynecomastia by mechanisms that have not

been defined include busulfan, ethionamide, isoniazid, methyldopa, tricyclic antidepressants, penicillamine, omeprazole, calcium channel blocking agents, angiotensin-converting enzyme inhibitors, metoclopramide, antiretroviral agents, diazepam, marijuana, and heroin. In some instances, the feminization is due to effects of drugs on liver function. Treatment with growth hormone can cause gynecomastia even in prepubertal boys, suggesting that growth hormone itself or one of the insulin-like growth factors has a direct effect on the breast.

Diagnostic Evaluation The evaluation of patients with gynecomastia should include: (1) a careful drug history; (2) measurement and examination of the testes (if both are small, a chromosomal karyotype should be obtained; if the testes are asymmetric, a workup for testicular tumor should be instituted); (3) evaluation of liver function; and (4) endocrine workup to include measurement of serum androstenedione or 24-h urinary 17-ketosteroids (usually elevated in feminizing adrenal states), measurement of plasma estradiol and hCG (helpful if elevated but usually normal), and measurement of plasma LH and testosterone. If LH is high and testosterone is low, the diagnosis is usually testicular failure; if LH and testosterone are both low, the diagnosis is most likely increased primary estrogen production (e.g., a Sertoli cell tumor of the testis), provided hypogonadotropic hypogonadism has been excluded; and if both LH and testosterone are elevated, the diagnosis is either an androgen-resistance state or a gonadotropin-secreting tumor.

A satisfactory diagnosis can be made in only half or fewer of patients referred for gynecomastia. This implies either that the diagnostic techniques are not sufficiently refined to recognize mild disturbances, that many causes of gynecomastia are as yet undefined, that the causes may be transient and difficult to diagnose, or that gynecomastia may in some instances be normal rather than due to a pathologic state. Because of the problem of separating the normal from the abnormal, gynecomastia should probably be worked up routinely only if the drug history is negative, the breast is tender (indicating rapid growth), or the breast mass is >4 cm in diameter. However, the decision to perform an endocrine evaluation depends on the clinical context. For example, gynecomastia associated with signs of underandrogenization should always be evaluated. A firm or hard breast mass should raise suspicion of male breast cancer (Chap. 89).

TREATMENT When the primary cause can be identified and corrected, the breast enlargement usually subsides promptly and eventually disappears. For example, androgen replacement therapy may produce dramatic improvement in men with testicular insufficiency. However, if the gynecomastia is of long duration (and fibrosis has replaced the original ductal hyperplasia), correction of the primary defect may not be followed by resolution. In such instances and when the primary cause cannot be corrected, surgery is the only effective therapy. Indications for surgery include several psychological and/or cosmetic problems, continued growth or tenderness, or suspected malignancy. Although the relative risk of carcinoma of the breast is increased in men with gynecomastia, it is rare nevertheless. Prophylactic radiation of the breasts prior to the institution of diethylstilbestrol or estrogen therapy is effective in preventing gynecomastia and has a low complication rate. In patients who have painful gynecomastia and who are not candidates for other therapy, treatment with antiestrogens such as tamoxifen may be indicated.

BIBLIOGRAPHY

GALACTORRHEA

ABDEL-GADIR A et al: The aetiology of galactorrhea in women with regular menstruation and normal prolactin levels. Human Reprod 7:912, 1992

BENJAMIN F: Normal lactation and galactorrhea. Clin Obstet Gynecol 37:887, 1994

EGBERTS AC et al: Non-puerperal lactation associated with antidepressant drug use. Br J Clin Pharmacol 44:277, 1997

FRANTZ AG, WILSON JD: Endocrine disorders of the breast, in *Williams Textbook of Endocrinology*, 9th ed, JD Wilson, DW Foster, HM Kronenberg, PR Larsen (eds). Philadelphia, Saunders, 1998, pp 877–900

FRIEDMAN S, GOLDFEIN A: Breast secretions in normal women. Am J Obstet Gynecol 104:846, 1969

HANEY AF: Galactorrhea, in *Current Therapy in Endocrinology and Metabolism*, 6th ed, CW Bardin (ed). St. Louis, Mosby, 1997, pp 393–396

JOHNSON DG et al: Prolactin secretion and biological activity in females with galactorrhoea and normal circulating prolactin concentrations at rest. Clin Endocrinol 22:661, 1985

KULSKI JK et al: Changes in the milk composition of nonpuerperal women. Am J Obstet Gynecol 139:597, 1981

LAURENCE DJ et al: The development of the normal human breast. Oxf Rev Reprod Biol 13:149, 1991

SAUER HJ: Physiology of lactation and factors affecting lactation. Obstet Gynecol Clin North Am 14:615, 1987

STRATAKIS CA et al: The aromatase excess syndrome is associated with feminization of both sexes and autosomal dominant transmission of aberrant P450 aromatase gene transcription. J Clin Endocrinol Metab 83:1348, 1998

TURKSOY RN et al: Diagnostic and therapeutic modalities in women with galactorrhea. Obstet Gynecol 56:323, 1980

YAZIGI RA et al: Prolactin disorders. Fertil Steril 67:215, 1997

GYNECOMASTIA

AGARWAL VR et al: Molecular basis of severe gynecomastia associated with aromatase expression in a fibrolamellar hepatocellular carcinoma. J Clin Endocrinol Metab. 83: 1797, 1998

APPELBAUM AH et al: Mammographic appearance of male breast disease. Radiographics 19:559, 1999

BLETHEN SL et al: Safety of recombinant deoxyribonucleic acid–derived growth hormone: The national cooperative growth study experience. J Clin Endocrinol Metab 81:1704, 1996

BRAUNSTEIN GD, GLASSMAN HA: Gynecomastia, in *Current Therapy in Endocrinology and Metabolism*, 6th ed, CW Bardin (ed). St Louis, Mosby, 1997, pp 401–404

CAVANAUGH J et al: Gynecomastia and cirrhosis of the liver. Arch Intern Med 150:563, 1990

DE GASPARO M et al: Antialdosterones: Incidence and prevention of sexual side effects. J Steroid Biochem 32:223, 1989

FELDMAN D: Ketoconazole and other imidazole derivatives as inhibitors of steroidogenesis. Endocr Rev 7:409, 1986

FRANTZ AG, WILSON JD: Endocrine disorders of the breast, in *Williams Textbook of Endocrinology*, 9th ed, JD Wilson, DW Foster, HM Kronenberg, PR Larsen (eds). Philadelphia, Saunders, 1998, pp 887–900

GEORGIADIS E et al: Incidence of gynaecomastia in 954 young males and its relationship to somatometric parameters. Ann Hum Biol 21:579, 1994

MABUCHI K et al: Risk factors for male breast cancer. J Natl Cancer Inst 74:371, 1985

MAHONEY CP: Adolescent gynecomastia: Differential diagnosis and management. Pediatr Clin North Am 37:1389, 1990

ROSE DP: Endocrine epidemiology of male breast cancer (review). Anticancer Res 8:845, 1988

SHER ES et al: Evaluation of boys with marked breast development at puberty. Clinic Pediatr (Phila) 37:367, 1998

STAIMAN VR, LOWE FC: Tamoxifen for flutamide/finasteride-induced gynecomastia. Urology 50:929, 1997

THOMPSON DF, CARTER R: Drug-induced gynecomastia. Pharmacotherapy 13:37, 1993

338   *Jean D. Wilson, James E. Griffin*

DISORDERS OF SEXUAL DIFFERENTIATION

Sexual differentiation is a sequential and ordered process. *Chromosomal sex*, established at the moment of fertilization, determines *gonadal sex*, and gonadal sex, in turn, causes the development of *phenotypic sex*, in which the male or female urogenital tract is formed (Fig. 338-1). A disturbance of any step in this process during embryogenesis may impair sexual differentiation (Table 338-1). Known causes of such disorders include environmental insults as in the ingestion of a virilizing drug during pregnancy, nonfamilial aberrations of the sex chromosomes as in 45,X gonadal dysgenesis, birth defects of multifactorial etiology as in most cases of hypospadias, and disorders due to single gene mutations as in the testicular feminization syndrome.

Limitations of knowledge make it necessary to make empirical assignments as to the type of derangement in some disorders, but specific diagnoses can usually be made as the result of genetic, endocrine, phenotypic, and chromosomal assessment. As a consequence, gender assignment in the newborn is usually appropriate, even in extreme instances of ambiguous genitalia.

NORMAL SEXUAL DIFFERENTIATION

The first event in sexual differentiation is the establishment of chromosomal sex, the heterogametic sex (XY) being male and the homogametic sex (XX) female. The embryos of both sexes then develop in an identical fashion until approximately 40 days of gestation.

The second phase of sexual differentiation is the conversion of the indifferent gonad into a testis or an ovary. No matter how many X chromosomes are present (as in 47,XXY, 48,XXXY, etc.), a testis will develop as long as a normal Y chromosome is present. Differentiation of the indifferent gonad into a testis is initiated by the actions of a single gene on the short arm of the Y chromosome (*SRY*); expression of an *SRY* transgene into female mice causes them to develop as males. The gene encodes a DNA-binding protein, but the mechanism by which *SRY* promotes testicular development remains poorly defined. At least four additional genes are also necessary for normal testicular development: (1) the Wilms' tumor–related gene (*WT1*), (2) steroidogenic factor 1 (*SF1*), (3) *SRY*-related HMG-box 9 (*SOX9*), and (4) *d*osage-sensitive sex reversal–*a*drenal hypoplasia congenita critical region on the *X* chromosome gene *1* (*DAX1*). These genes each encode putative transcription factors that regulate the expression of genes necessary for gonadal survival; mutations in *SRY* or any of the four downstream genes impair testicular development. It remains unclear if there are analogous "ovarian-determining genes," or if ovarian development is a default pathway in the absence of testicular determination genes. Mutations in some of the genes noted above (e.g., *SF1*) also prevent normal ovarian development.

The final process in sexual differentiation, the translation of gonadal sex into phenotypic sex (formation of the male or female urogenital tracts), is the consequence of the type of gonad formed and the endocrine secretions of the fetal gonads. The internal urogenital tract is derived from the wolffian and müllerian ducts that exist side by side in early embryos of both sexes (Fig. 338-1*A*). In the male the wolffian ducts give rise to the epididymides, vasa deferentia, and seminal vesicles, and the müllerian ducts disappear. In the female the müllerian ducts are converted into the fallopian tubes, uterus, and upper vagina, and the wolffian ducts regress. The external genitalia and urethra in the two sexes develop from common anlage—the urogenital sinus and the genital tubercle, folds, and swellings (Fig. 338-1*B*). The urogenital sinus gives rise to the prostate and prostatic urethra in the male and to the urethra and lower portion of the vagina in the female. The genital tubercle gives rise to the glans penis in the male and the clitoris in the female. The urogenital swellings become the scrotum or the labia majora, and the urethral folds form the labia minora or fuse to form the shaft of the penis and the male urethra.

In the absence of the testes, as in the normal female or in the male embryo castrated prior to the onset of gonadal differentiation, phenotypic sex develops along female lines. Thus, masculinization of the fetus is induced by hormones from the fetal testes, whereas female development does not require the presence of the ovary. Phenotypic sex normally conforms to chromosomal sex. That is, chromosomal sex determines gonadal sex, and gonadal sex, in turn, controls phenotypic sex.

Formation of the male phenotype is vested in the action of three hormones. Two—antimüllerian hormone (AMH) and testosterone—are secreted by the fetal testis. AMH [also termed *müllerian-inhibiting substance* (MIS)] is a protein that suppresses the müllerian ducts and prevents development of the uterus and fallopian tubes in the male. Testosterone acts directly to virilize the wolffian duct and is the precursor for the third embryonic male hormone, dihydrotestosterone (Chap. 335), which promotes development of the male urethra and prostate and formation of the penis and scrotum. Testosterone and dihydrotestosterone induce formation of the male urogenital tract during fetal life by acting through the same nuclear androgen receptor by which they act in postembryonic life (Chap. 335).

The secretion of testosterone by the fetal testes approaches a maximum by the tenth week of gestation, and formation of the sexual phenotypes is largely completed by the end of the first trimester. During the latter phases of gestation, the ovarian follicles develop and the vagina matures in the female, and testicular descent and phallic growth take place in the male.

DISORDERS OF CHROMOSOMAL SEX

Disorders of chromosomal sex (Table 338-2) occur when the number or structure of the X or Y chromosomes is abnormal (Chap. 66).

KLINEFELTER SYNDROME
Clinical Features Klinefelter syndrome is characterized by small, firm testes, azoospermia, gynecomastia, and elevated levels of plasma gonadotropins in men with two or more X chromosomes. The common karyotype is either a 47,XXY chromosomal pattern (the classic form) or 46,XY/ 47,XXY mosaicism. It is the most frequent major abnormality of sexual differentiation, the incidence being around 1 in 500 men.

Prepubertally, the testes are small but otherwise appear normal. After puberty, the disorder is manifest as infertility, gynecomastia, or occasionally underandrogenization (Table 338-3). Hyalinization of the seminiferous tubules and azoospermia are consistent features of the 47,XXY variety. The small, firm testes are usually <2 cm and always <3.5 cm in length (corresponding to 2- and 12-mL volume, respectively). Longer legs cause increased mean height. Gynecomastia is common and ordinarily develops during adolescence, is generally bilateral and painless, and may become disfiguring (Chap. 337). Obesity and varicose veins occur in one-third to one-half, and leg ulcers are associated with deficiency of plasminogen activator inhibitor-1. The diagnosis is made most frequently in boys with developmental delay and/or learning disabilities and social maladjustment; abnormalities of thyroid function, diabetes mellitus, and pulmonary disease are also common. The risk of breast cancer is 20 times that of normal men (but only about a fifth that in women). Most have male psychosexual orientation and function sexually as normal men.

About 10% of the patients have the mosaic form, as estimated by chromosomal karyotypes on peripheral blood leukocytes. The frequency of this variant may be underestimated, since chromosomal mosaicism can be present in the testes when the peripheral leukocyte karyotype is normal. The mosaic form is usually not as severe as the 47,XXY variety, and the testes may be normal (Table 338-3). The endocrine abnormalities are less severe, and gynecomastia and azoospermia are less common, and occasional mosaic individuals are fertile. In some the diagnosis may not be suspected because the manifestations are so mild.

Approximately 30 additional variants of Klinefelter syndrome have been described, including those with uniform cell lines (such as 48,XXYY, 48,XXXX, and 49,XXXXY) and a variety of mosaicisms

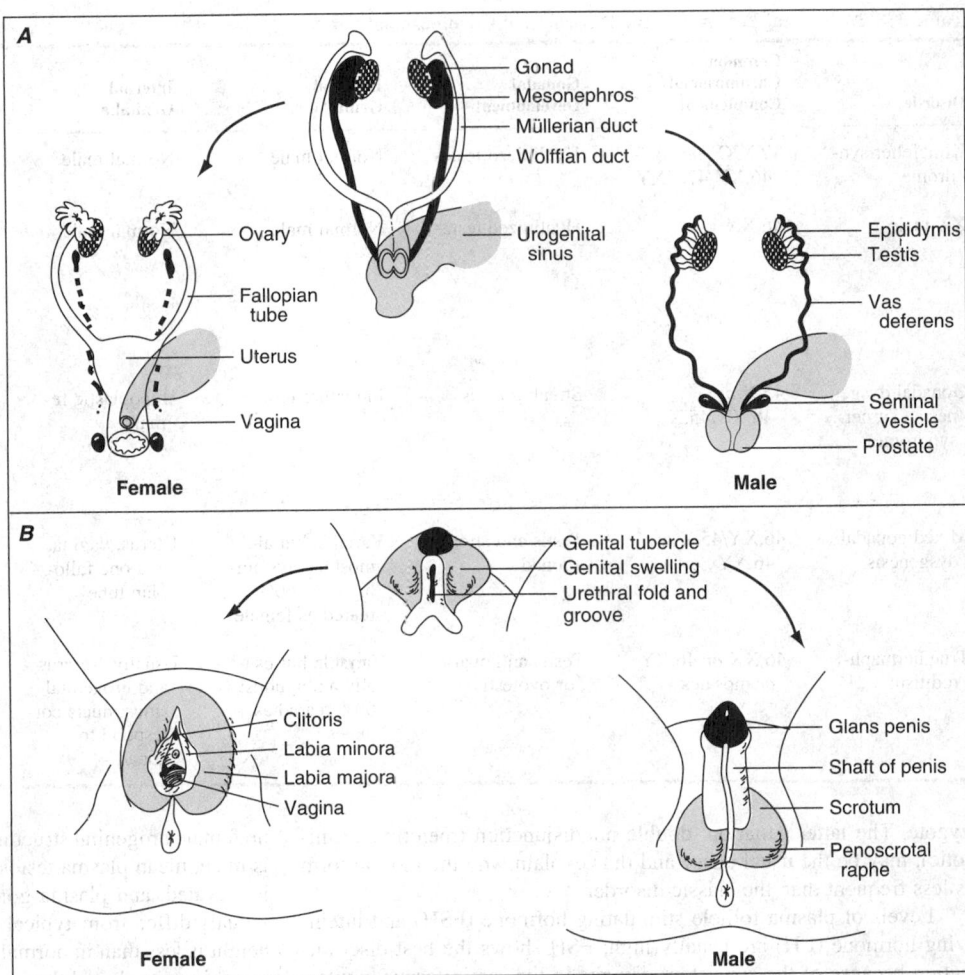

FIGURE 338-1 Normal sexual differentiation. *A.* Internal urogenital tract. *B.* External genitalia.

of the X chromosome with or without associated structural abnormalities of the X. In general, the greater the chromosomal abnormality the more severe the manifestations.

Pathophysiology The classic form is due to meiotic nondisjunction of the chromosomes during gametogenesis (Fig. 338-2). About 40% of the responsible meiotic nondisjunctions occur during spermatogenesis, and 60% occur during oogenesis. Advanced maternal age is a predisposing factor. The mosaic form is thought to result from chromosomal mitotic nondisjunction after fertilization of the zygote and can take place in either a 46,XY zygote (Fig. 338-2) or a 47,XXY

Table 338-1 Classification of Disorders of Sexual Development

Disorders of chromosomal sex
  Klinefelter syndrome
  XX male
  Gonadal dysgenesis
  Mixed gonadal dysgenesis
  True hermaphroditism
Disorders of gonadal sex
  Pure gonadal dysgenesis
  Dysgenetic testes
  Absent testis syndrome
Disorders of phenotypic sex
  Female pseudohermaphroditism
    Congenital adrenal hyperplasia
    Nonadrenal female pseudohermaphroditism
    Developmental disorders of müllerian ducts
  Male pseudohermaphroditism
    Abnormalities in androgen synthesis
    Abnormalities in androgen action
    Persistent müllerian duct syndrome
    Development defects of male genitalia

Table 338-2 Clinical Features of the Disorders of Chromosomal Sex

Disorder	Common Chromosomal Complement	Gonadal Development	External Genitalia	Internal Genitalia	Breast Development	Comment
Klinefelter syndrome	47,XXY *or* 46,XY/47,XXY	Hyalinized testes	Normal male	Normal male	Gynecomastia	Most common disorder of sexual differentiation; tall stature.
XX male	46,XX	Hyalinized testes	Normal male	Normal male	Gynecomastia	Shorter than normal men; increased incidence of hypospadias. Similar to Klinefelter syndrome. May be familial.
Gonadal dysgenesis (Turner syndrome)	45,X *or* 46,XX/45,X	Streak gonads	Immature female	Hypoplastic female	Immature female	Short stature and multiple somatic abnormalities. May be 46,XX with structurally abnormal X chromosome.
Mixed gonadal dysgenesis	46,XY/45,X *or* 46,XY	Testis and streak gonad	Variable but almost always ambiguous; 60% reared as female	Uterus, vagina, and one fallopian tube	Usually male	Second most common cause of ambiguous genitalia in the newborn; tumors common.
True hermaphroditism	46,XX *or* 46,XY *or* mosaics	Testis and ovary or ovotestis	Variable but usually ambiguous; 60% reared as males	Usually a uterus and urogenital sinus; ducts correspond to gonad	Gynecomastia in 75%	May be familial.

zygote. The latter situation, double nondisjunction (meiotic and mitotic), may be the usual cause and thus explain why the mosaic form is less frequent than the classic disorder.

Levels of plasma follicle stimulating hormone (FSH) and luteinizing hormone (LH) are usually high; FSH shows the best discrimination because of the consistent damage to the seminiferous tubules. The plasma testosterone level averages half normal but may overlap the normal range. Mean plasma estradiol levels are elevated; early, estradiol secretion by the testes may increase in response to the elevated plasma LH level, but the testicular secretion of estradiol and testosterone eventually declines. Elevated plasma estradiol late in the course is probably due both to decreased metabolic clearance and increased conversion of testosterone to estradiol in extragonadal tissues. The net result both early and late is a variable degree of feminization and virilization. Feminization, including gynecomastia, depends on the ratio of circulating estrogen to androgen (relative or absolute), and individuals with low plasma testosterone and high plasma estradiol levels are more likely to develop gynecomastia (Chap. 337). Men with untreated Klinefelter syndrome may have enlarged pituitary glands, presumably due to hyperplasia of the gonadotrophs due to inadequate testosterone feedback.

℞ TREATMENT In men with some sperm production, or in whom spermatids can be recovered from testicular biopsy, fertility is possible with in vitro fertilization (Chap. 335). Gynecomastia should be treated surgically. Some underandrogenized men benefit from supplemental androgen, particularly in those with decreased bone density, but such treatment may worsen the gynecomastia, presumably by providing increased substrate for estrogen formation in peripheral tissues. Testosterone should be injected in the form of testosterone cypionate or testosterone enanthate or administered via the transdermal route (Chap. 335). Following the administration of testosterone, the plasma LH level returns to normal only after several months, if at all.

XX MALE SYNDROME A 46,XX karyotype is found in approximately 1 in 20,000 phenotypic males. The findings resemble those in Klinefelter syndrome: the testes are small and firm (generally <2 cm), gynecomastia is frequent, the penis is normal to small in size, azoospermia and hyalinization of the seminiferous tubules are usual,

no female urogenital structures are present, psychosexual identification is male, mean plasma testosterone level is low, plasma estradiol level is elevated, and plasma gonadotropin levels are high. Affected individuals differ from typical Klinefelter patients only in that average height is less than in normal men, the incidence of cognitive problems is not increased, and the incidence of hypospadias is increased.

The majority of XX males have Y-related DNA (e.g., detected by polymerase chain reaction of the *SRY* gene); thus an X-Y or Y-autosome translocation appears to be the common cause. Some 46,XX males are negative for all Y-specific DNA, suggesting that their disorder is due to mutation in a downstream, autosomal or X-linked gene involved in development of the testes. The management is similar to that of Klinefelter syndrome.

GONADAL DYSGENESIS (TURNER SYNDROME) Clinical Features Gonadal dysgenesis is characterized by primary amenorrhea, sexual infantilism, short stature, multiple congenital anomalies, and bilateral streak gonads in phenotypic women with any of several defects of the X chromosome. This condition should be distinguished from (1) mixed gonadal dysgenesis in which a unilateral testis and a contralateral streak gonad may be present; (2) pure gonadal dysgenesis in which bilateral streak gonads are associated with a normal 46,XX or 46,XY karyotype, normal stature, and primary amenorrhea; and (3)

Table 338-3 Characteristics of Patients with Classic versus Mosaic Klinefelter Syndrome[a]

	47,XXY, %	46,XY/47,XXY, %
Abnormal testicular histology	100	94[b]
Decreased length of testis	99	73[b]
Azoospermia	93	50[b]
Decreased testosterone	79	33
Decreased facial hair	77	64
Increased gonadotropins	75	33[b]
Decreased sexual function	68	56
Gynecomastia	55	33[b]
Decreased axillary hair	49	46
Decreased length of penis	41	21

[a] Table based on 519 XXY patients and 51 XY/XXY patients.
[b] Significantly different at $p < .05$ or better.
SOURCE: After DL Gordon et al: Arch Intern Med 130:726, 1972.

the Noonan syndrome, an autosomal dominant disorder in both sexes characterized by webbed neck, short stature, congenital heart disease, cubitus valgus, and other congenital defects despite normal karyotypes and normal gonads.

The incidence is estimated at 1 in 3000 newborn females; the prenatal incidence may be as high as 2% of all human conceptuses, only a small fraction of whom survive to term. The diagnosis is made either at birth because of the associated anomalies or at puberty when amenorrhea and failure of sexual development are noted in conjunction with the associated anomalies. Gonadal dysgenesis is the most common cause of primary amenorrhea, accounting for a third of such patients. The external genitalia are unambiguously female but remain immature, and there is no breast development unless exogenous estrogen is given. The fallopian tubes and uterus are immature, and bilateral streak gonads are present in the broad ligaments. Primordial germ cells are present transiently during embryogenesis but disappear because of an accelerated rate of atresia (Chap. 336). After the age of expected puberty, these streaks lack identifiable follicles and ova and consist of fibrous tissue that is indistinguishable from normal ovarian stroma.

The somatic abnormalities primarily involve the skeleton and connective tissue. Lymphedema of the hands and feet, webbing of the neck, low hairline, redundant skin folds on the back of the neck, a shieldlike chest with widely spaced nipples, and growth retardation are features that suggest the diagnosis in infancy. Micrognathia, epicanthal folds, prominent low-set or deformed ears, a fishlike mouth, and ptosis may be present. Short fourth metacarpals are present in half, and 10 to 20% have coarctation of the aorta. In adults, the average height rarely exceeds 150 cm. Associated conditions include renal malformations, pigmented nevi, hypoplastic nails, tendency to keloid formation, perceptive hearing loss, unexplained hypertension, glucose intolerance, and autoimmune thyroid disease.

Pathophysiology About half have a 45,X karyotype, approximately one-fourth have mosaicism with no structural abnormality (46,XX/45,X), and the remainder have a structurally abnormal X chromosome with or without mosaicism (Chap. 66). The mechanism of chromosome loss is unknown and may occur during gametogenesis in either parent or as a mitotic error during one of the early cleavage divisions of the fertilized zygote (Fig. 338-2). Short stature and other somatic features result from haploinsufficiency of one or more genes encoded on the short arm of the X chromosome. Streak gonads result when genetic material is missing from either the long or short arm of the X. In individuals with mosaicism or structural abnormalities of the X, the phenotype on average is less severe than in the 45,X variety. In some patients with hypertrophy of the clitoris, an unidentified fragment of a chromosome is present and is assumed to be an abnormal Y; gonadoblastoma may develop in the streak gonads in this subset of patients. The Y-linked genes that predispose to gonadoblastoma are distinct from *SRY* because XY women with *SRY* deletions or mutations are also at risk for such tumors. Rarely, familial transmission of gonadal dysgenesis can be the result of a balanced X-autosome translocation (Chap. 66). Analysis of chromosomal karyotype is necessary to establish the diagnosis and to identify the group with Y chromosomal elements and hence a chance of developing malignancy in the streak gonads.

After the time of expected puberty, pubic and axillary hair remain sparse, the breasts are infantile, and no menses occur. Serum FSH is

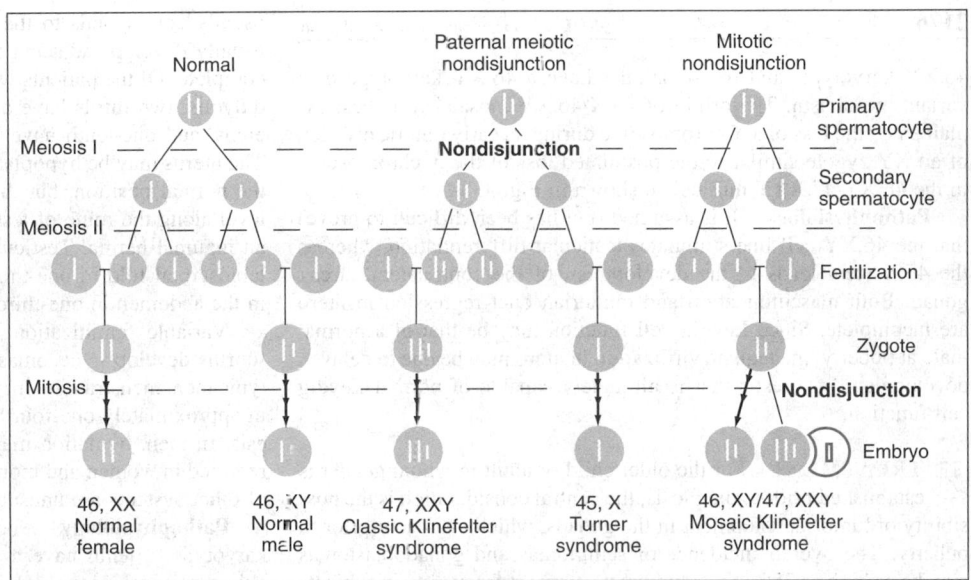

FIGURE 338-2 Schema for normal spermatogenesis and fertilization showing effects of meiotic and mitotic nondisjunction leading to classic Klinefelter syndrome, Turner syndrome, and mosaic Klinefelter. The schema would be similar if the abnormal events took place during oogenesis.

elevated in infancy, falls during midchildhood to the normal range, and increases to castrate levels at the age of 9 or 10. At this time, the serum LH level is also elevated, and plasma estradiol levels are low [<40 pmol/L (<10 pg/mL)]. Approximately 2% of 45,X and 12% of mosaic women have sufficient residual follicles to allow some menstruation, and occasionally minimally affected women become pregnant; the reproductive life in such individuals is brief.

TREATMENT At the anticipated time of puberty, replacement therapy with estrogen should be instituted to induce maturation of the breasts, labia, vagina, uterus, and fallopian tubes (Chap. 336). Linear growth and bone maturation rates usually double during the first year of treatment with estradiol, but the eventual height rarely approaches the predicted height. Combination therapy with oxandrolone and/or growth hormone accelerates growth and increases final height. Streak gonads should be removed in all women who are virilized or have Y-chromosome sequences.

MIXED GONADAL DYSGENESIS **Clinical Features** Mosaicism for a Y-bearing cell line, usually the 45,X/46,XY karyotype, is responsible for most instances of mixed gonadal dysgenesis. Affected individuals usually have a testis on one side and a streak gonad on the other, but bilateral dysgenetic testes or bilateral streak gonads may be present. The incidence is unknown, but in most hospitals the disorder is the second most common cause of ambiguous genitalia in the neonate after congenital adrenal hyperplasia.

The phenotype varies depending on the proportion of XY cells and their distribution. About two-thirds of such children are reared as females. Many have ambiguous genitalia, including phallic enlargement, a urogenital sinus, and some labioscrotal fusion. In most the testis is intraabdominal; individuals with a testis in the inguinal or scrotal position are usually reared as males. A uterus, vagina, and at least one fallopian tube are almost invariably present.

The prepubertal testis appears relatively normal. The postpubertal testis contains abundant Leydig cells, but the seminiferous tubules lack germinal elements and contain only Sertoli cells. The streak gonad, a thin, pale, elongated structure located either in the broad ligament or along the pelvic wall, is composed of ovarian stroma. At puberty the testis secretes androgen, causing virilization and phallic enlargement. Feminization is rare; when it occurs, estrogen secretion from a gonadal tumor should be suspected.

Approximately a third of these individuals exhibit somatic features of 45,X gonadal dysgenesis. Approximately two-thirds have the 45,X/

46,XY karyotype, and the remainder have a 46,XY karyotype or a variant mosaicism. The origin of 45,X/46,XY mosaicism is best explained by the loss of a Y chromosome during an early mitotic division of an XY zygote similar to the postulated loss of the X chromosome in the 46,XY/47,XXY mosaicism shown in Fig. 338-2.

Pathophysiology   It is assumed (but has been difficult to prove) that the 46,XY cell line stimulates testicular differentiation, whereas the 45,X stem leads to the development of the contralateral streak gonad. Both masculinization and müllerian duct regression in utero are incomplete. Since Leydig cell function may be that of a normal male at puberty, inadequate virilization in utero may be due to delayed development of a testis that is ultimately capable of normal Leydig cell function.

℞ TREATMENT   For the older child or adult in whom gender is established prior to diagnosis, the central consideration is the possibility of tumor development in the gonads, which can occur prior to puberty. The overall incidence of seminomas and gonadoblastomas may be as high as 25%. Such tumors occur most frequently in subjects with a female phenotype who lack the somatic features of 45,X gonadal dysgenesis and are more common in testes than in the streak gonad. When the diagnosis is established in phenotypic females, prophylactic gonadectomy should be performed because gonadal tumors may occur in childhood and because the testes secrete androgen at puberty and thus cause virilization. Such women, like those with gonadal dysgenesis, are then given estrogen to induce and maintain feminization.

When the diagnosis is established in phenotypic males during late childhood or in adults, the management is more complicated. Men with mixed gonadal dysgenesis are infertile (no germinal elements are present in the testes) and have a high risk of developing gonadal tumors. In deciding which testes can be safely conserved the following observations apply: (1) tumors develop in scrotal streak gonads but not in scrotal testes, (2) tumors that develop in intraabdominal testes are always associated with ipsilateral müllerian duct structures, and (3) tumors in streak gonads are always associated with tumors in the contralateral abdominal testis. Based on these observations, it is recommended that (1) all streak gonads should be removed, (2) scrotal testes should be preserved, and (3) intraabdominal testes should be excised unless they can be relocated in the scrotum and are not associated with ipsilateral müllerian duct structures. Reconstructive surgery of the phallus should be performed when appropriate.

When the diagnosis is established in early infancy and the genitalia are ambiguous, gender assignment is usually female, and resection of the phallus and gonadectomy can be performed in infancy, sometimes in one procedure. If the decision is for male gender assignment, the same criteria apply as to which testes should be removed as in older males.

TRUE HERMAPHRODITISM   Clinical Features   True hermaphroditism is a condition in which both an ovary and a testis or one or more gonads with features of both (ovotestis) are present. To justify the diagnosis, both types of gonadal epithelium must be documented histologically, the presence of ovarian stroma without oocytes not being sufficient. The incidence is unknown, but more than 400 cases have been reported. Three categories are recognized: (1) one-fifth are bilateral—testicular and ovarian tissue (ovotestes) on each side; (2) two-fifths are unilateral—an ovotestis on one side and an ovary or a testis on the other; and (3) the remainder are lateral—a testis on one side and an ovary on the other.

The external genitalia exhibit all gradations of the male-to-female spectrum. Two-thirds of affected individuals are sufficiently masculinized to be reared as males, but fewer than one-tenth have normal male external genitalia; most have hypospadias and incomplete labioscrotal fusion. Two-thirds of phenotypic females have an enlarged clitoris, and most have a urogenital sinus. Differentiation of the internal ducts

usually corresponds to the adjacent gonad. Although an epididymis usually develops adjacent to a testis, the vas deferens is usually incomplete. Of the patients with an ovotestis, three-fourths have an epididymis, two-thirds have a fallopian tube, one-tenth have a vas deferens, and one-tenth have both a vas deferens and a fallopian tube. The uterus may be hypoplastic or unicornuate. The ovary is usually in the normal position, but the testis or ovotestis may be found at any level along the route of testicular descent, frequently associated with an inguinal hernia. Testicular tissue is present in the scrotum or the labioscrotal fold in one-third, in the inguinal canal in one-third, and in the abdomen in one-third.

Variable feminization and virilization ensue at puberty; three-fourths develop gynecomastia, and about half menstruate. In phenotypic men, menstruation may cause cyclic hematuria. Ovulation occurs in approximately one-fourth and is more common than spermatogenesis. In men, ovulation may cause testicular pain. Fertility has been reported in women and more rarely in men. Congenital malformations of other systems are unusual.

Pathophysiology   About two-thirds of individuals have a 46,XX karyotype, a tenth have a 46,XY karyotype, and the remainder are chimeras or mosaics in whom a Y cell line is present. The mechanism responsible for the abnormal gonadal development is unknown. Only 10% of 46,XX true hermaphrodites are *SRY* positive, presumably the consequence of mosaicism or translocation of a portion of the Y chromosome; the remainder are believed to result from gain-of-function mutations in downstream genes involved in *SRY* action. On occasion, multiple sibs with a 46,XX karyotype are affected, possibly the result of an autosomal or X-linked mutation.

Because corpora lutea are frequently present in the ovaries, it is presumed that the female neuroendocrine axis functions normally in such individuals. Feminization (gynecomastia and menstruation) is the result of secretion of estradiol by ovarian tissue. In masculinized patients, secretion of androgen predominates, and some produce sperm.

℞ TREATMENT   When the diagnosis is made in early infancy, gender assignment depends on the anatomic features. In older children and adults, gonads and internal duct structures that are contradictory to the predominant phenotype (and the gender of rearing) should be removed, and the external genitalia should be modified when appropriate. Gonadal tumors are rare but have been reported in true hermaphrodites who carry Y chromosome sequences. Consequently, the possibility of future tumor development must be taken into account when the decision is made to preserve gonadal tissue.

DISORDERS OF GONADAL SEX

Disorders of gonadal sex result when chromosomal sex is normal but differentiation of the gonads is abnormal. Thus, gonadal sex does not correspond to chromosomal sex.

PURE GONADAL DYSGENESIS   Clinical Features   Pure gonadal dysgenesis is a disorder in which phenotypic females with gonads and genitalia characteristic of gonadal dysgenesis (bilateral streaks, infantile uterus and fallopian tubes, and sexual infantilism) have normal height, few if any somatic anomalies, and either a normal 46,XX or 46,XY karyotype. This disorder is about one-tenth as common as gonadal dysgenesis. It is genetically distinct but cannot be distinguished clinically from those instances of gonadal dysgenesis with minimal somatic abnormalities. The height is normal or greater than normal, some individuals being >170 cm. Estrogen levels vary from profound deficiency typical of 45,X gonadal dysgenesis to some breast development and menses that terminate in an early menopause. About 40% have some feminization. Axillary and pubic hair is scanty, and the internal genitalia consist of müllerian derivatives only. In both the 46,XX and the 46,XY forms the disorder prevents differentiation of ovary or testis, respectively; the development of the female phenotype and the elevation of gonadotropin secretion are due to failure of gonadal development.

Tumors may develop in the streak gonads, particularly dysgerminoma or gonadoblastoma in the 46,XY disorder. Such tumors may be heralded by the development of virilizing signs or a pelvic mass.

Pathophysiology Although chromosomal mosaicisms have been described under this nosology, the designation here is restricted to women with uniform 46,XX or 46,XY karyotypes. (Those with mosaicism are variants of gonadal dysgenesis or mixed gonadal dysgenesis, as described above.) The rationale for this restricted definition is based on the fact that both the XX and XY varieties can result from single gene mutations that are presumed to involve gene(s) essential for gonadal development. Several sibships have been reported in which more than one individual is affected with the 46,XX disorder, frequently the result of consanguineous matings, suggesting an autosomal recessive inheritance.

The 46,XY variety may occur in families; in some the disorder appears to be inherited as an X-linked trait, and in others the pattern suggests a male-limited autosomal recessive inheritance. About 15% of 46,XY women have either a deletion or a mutation in the *SRY* coding sequence. Other instances could be due to mutations in *SRY* outside the coding sequence, in other genes that influence *SRY* expression, or in the downstream genes that are controlled by *SRY*. Indeed, mutations in several genes that are downstream of *SRY* are now known to be a cause of the dysgenetic testes syndrome (also termed *dysgenetic male pseudohermaphroditism*; see below).

℞ **TREATMENT** The management of the estrogen deficiency is identical to that in gonadal dysgenesis; namely, appropriate estrogen replacement therapy is initiated at the time of expected puberty and maintained in adult life (Chap. 336). Because of the high frequency of gonadal tumors in the 46,XY variety, the streak gonads should be removed once the diagnosis is made; development of virilizing signs is indication for immediate surgery. The natural history of the gonadal tumors is uncertain, but the prognosis after surgical removal is usually good.

DYSGENETIC TESTES Individuals with these disorders are genetic males with disorders of testicular development that vary from streak gonads similar to those in gonadal dysgenesis to less severe defects. The disorders are frequently associated with systemic abnormalities, because many of the genes involved are also involved in the development of other tissues. The first of these genes to be identified was the Wilms' tumor gene *WT1*; mutations of this gene cause two disorders—the Denys-Drash and Frasier syndromes. *Denys-Drash syndrome* is an autosomal dominant disorder characterized by development of Wilms' tumors in males with a spectrum of gonadal defects ranging from streak gonads to less severely affected testes; urogenital defects include diffuse mesangial sclerosis of the kidneys. The underlying mutations in the zinc finger region of WT-1 are believed to inhibit the function of the wild-type protein and hence act as dominant negative mutations. Patients with *Frasier syndrome* have gonadal dysgenesis, impaired virilization, and focal sclerosis of the kidney but do not develop Wilms' tumors. Mutations in intron 9 of the *WT1* gene that cause Frasier syndrome interfere with the synthesis of specific splice variants of *WT1*.

A second downstream gene that is essential for differentiation of the testes is *SF1* (also known as *FTZF1*), a member of the nuclear hormone receptor superfamily. SF-1 regulates the expression of many genes involved in adrenal and gonadal development and steroidogenesis, as well as the *AMH* gene. Heterozygous mutation of this autosomal gene has been associated with 46,XY gonadal dysgenesis with adrenal insufficiency.

Another downstream gene is *SOX9*, a close relative of *SRY* that maps to chromosome 17q. This gene is expressed in high levels in the testes, where it is believed to be a key regulator of male differentiation. Heterozygous mutations of this gene cause 46,XY gonadal dysgenesis and skeletal abnormalities (*campomelic dysplasia*).

46,XY gonadal dysgenesis is also associated with duplication of the short arm of the X chromosome (Xp21), a phenomenon termed *dosage-sensitive sex reversal*. Loss-of-function mutations of the *DAX1*

gene in this region of the X chromosome are associated with adrenal hypoplasia congenita and hypogonadotrophic hypogonadism. The DAX-1 protein inhibits the expression of SF-1-regulated genes, providing a potential mechanism by which an excess of DAX-1 could cause gonadal dysgenesis in genetic males with Xp21 duplications.

THE ABSENT TESTES SYNDROME (ANORCHIA, TESTICULAR REGRESSION, GONADAL AGENESIS, AGONADISM) Clinical Features A spectrum of phenotypes occurs in 46,XY males with absent or rudimentary testes but in whom unequivocal evidence exists that endocrine function of the testis (e.g., consistent müllerian duct regression and variable testosterone synthesis) was present at some time during embryonic life. In pure gonadal dysgenesis, in contrast, no evidence can be inferred for gonadal function during embryonic development. The manifestations vary from complete failure of virilization to incomplete virilization of the external genitalia to otherwise normal men with bilateral anorchia.

The purest form is represented by 46,XY females with absent testes, sexual infantilism, and absence of both müllerian duct derivatives and accessory organs of male reproduction. Such individuals differ from those with 46,XY pure gonadal dysgenesis in that no gonadal remnant can be identified, including no streak gonad and no müllerian derivatives. Testicular failure must have occurred, therefore, between the onset of AMH synthesis and the onset of testosterone secretion (e.g., after development of Sertoli cells but before the onset of Leydig cell function).

In others, testicular failure occurred later in gestation, and these individuals may constitute problems in gender assignment. In some, failure of müllerian regression is more pronounced than failure of testosterone secretion, but none exhibit normal müllerian development. In those with more extensive virilization, the external genitalia are phenotypically male, but rudimentary oviducts and vasa deferentia may coexist internally.

At the final extreme is the syndrome of bilateral anorchia in which phenotypic men have absence of müllerian structures and gonads but male wolffian duct derivatives and external genitalia. Microphallus implies that failure of testosterone secretion occurred late in embryogenesis after anatomic development of the male urethra was complete. Gynecomastia may or may not be present.

Pathophysiology The pathogenesis is not understood. Testicular regression could be the result of mutant genes, teratogen, or trauma, and the disorder may well be heterogeneous in origin. Several instances of agonadism have occurred in the same family, some unilateral and others bilateral. Some individuals in whom no testes can be identified at laparotomy have blood testosterone values above the castrate range, presumably derived from remnant testes.

℞ **TREATMENT** The management of the two extremes is clearcut. Sexually infantile, phenotypic females should be given adequate estrogen to ensure appropriate feminization, and any coexisting vaginal agenesis should be treated by surgical or medical means. Likewise, phenotypic males with anorchia should be given androgen replacement to allow normal male secondary sexual development. Individuals with incomplete virilization or ambiguous external genitalia demonstrate a more complex problem and require careful assessment to determine appropriate gender assignment, hormonal therapy at the time of expected puberty, and surgical correction of the external genitalia when appropriate.

DISORDERS OF PHENOTYPIC SEX

Disorders of phenotypic sex occur in 46,XX or 46,XY individuals with appropriate gonadal sex but in whom development of the urogenital tract is inappropriate for the chromosomal/gonadal sex.

FEMALE PSEUDOHERMAPHRODITISM Female pseudohermaphroditism occurs in 46,XX women with bilateral ovaries but

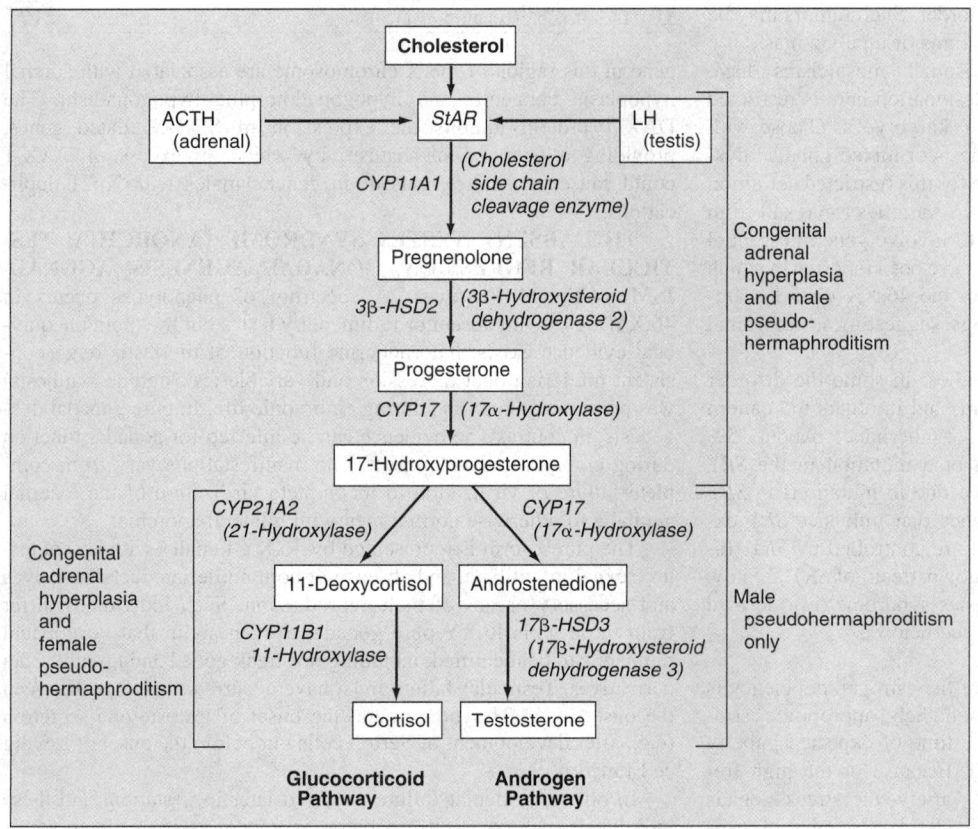

FIGURE 338-3 Pathways of glucocorticoid and androgen synthesis. Note abnormal conditions corresponding to impaired enzyme reactions.

with variable virilization of the urogenital tract because of androgen excess during fetal life.

Congenital Adrenal Hyperplasia · Clinical features The pathways by which glucocorticoids are synthesized in the adrenal gland and androgens are formed in the testis and adrenal are summarized in Fig. 338-3. Three reactions are common to both pathways (cholesterol side chain cleavage, 3β-hydroxysteroid dehydrogenase/isomerase, and 17α-hydroxylase); impairment of any of these reactions results in deficiency of glucocorticoid and androgen synthesis and consequently causes both congenital adrenal hyperplasia (due to enhanced ACTH levels) and defective virilization of the male embryo (male pseudohermaphroditism). Two reactions are involved exclusively in androgen synthesis (17,20-lyase and 17β-hydroxysteroid dehydrogenase); deficiency in either results in pure male pseudohermaphroditism with normal glucocorticoid synthesis. Deficiency of either of the terminal two enzymes of glucocorticoid synthesis (21-hydroxylase and 11β-hydroxylase) impairs formation of hydrocortisone; the compensatory increase in ACTH secretion causes adrenal hyperplasia and a secondary increase in androgen formation that virilizes the female and induces precocious masculinization in the male.

The major features of congenital adrenal hyperplasia are listed in Table 338-4. The *adrenal insufficiency* can be equally severe and life-threatening in both sexes and is described in Chap. 331. Some defects in steroidogenesis cause female pseudohermaphroditism, and some cause male pseudohermaphroditism. (3β-hydroxysteroid dehydrogenase/isomerase deficiency can cause either male or female pseudohermaphroditism, but since incomplete virilization of the male is more common, the disorder will be discussed under male pseudohermaphroditism.)

Congenital adrenal hyperplasia due to classic 21-hydroxylase deficiency is the most common cause of ambiguous genitalia in the newborn, with an incidence of between 1 in 5000 and 1 in 15,000 live births in Europe and the United States; it may or may not be associated with mineralocorticoid deficiency (salt loss) (Table 338-4). Virilization is usually apparent at birth in the female and within the first 2 to 3 years of life in the male. Manifestations in females include hypertrophy of the clitoris with ventral chordee, partial fusion of the labioscrotal folds, and variable virilization of the urethra. The uterus, fallopian tubes, and ovaries are normal, and the wolffian ducts do not virilize, probably because adrenal function begins relatively late in embryogenesis. The external appearance of an affected female newborn is similar to that of a male with bilateral cryptorchidism and hypospadias. The labioscrotal folds are bulbous and rugated and resemble a scrotum. Rarely, the virilization is so severe that development of a complete penile urethra and prostate results in errors in sex assignment at birth. Radiography following the injection of radiopaque dye into the external genital orifice is helpful in demonstrating the presence of vagina, uterus, and (sometimes) fallopian tubes. Occasionally, virilization of the female is slight or absent at birth and becomes evident in later infancy, adolescence, or adulthood (the so-called nonclassic or late-onset form of the disorder). In both sexes, rapid somatic maturation results in premature epiphyseal closure and a short adult height. The untreated female with the classic disorder grows rapidly during the first year of life and has progressive virilization. At the time of expected puberty

Table 338-4 Forms of Congenital Adrenal Hyperplasia

Deficiency	Cortisol	Aldosterone	Degree of Virilization of Females	Failure of Virilization in Males	Dominant Steroid Secreted	Comment
Classic 21-hydroxylase:						
Partial (simple virilizing or compensated)	Normal	↑	++++	none	17-Hydroxyprogesterone	Most common type (95% of total); from one- to two-thirds salt losers
Severe (salt-losing)	↓	↓	++++	none	17-Hydroxyprogesterone	
11β-Hydroxylase (hypertension)	↓	↓	++++	none	11-Deoxycortisol and 11-deoxycorticosterone	Hypertension
3β-Hydroxysteroid dehydrogenase/isomerase 2	↓	↓	+	++++	Δ⁵-3β-OH compounds (dehydroepiandrosterone)	Probably second most common, usually salt loss
17α-Hydroxylase	↓	↓	none	++++	Corticosterone and 11-deoxycorticosterone	No feminization of female, hypertension
StAR protein	absent	absent	none	++++	Cholesterol(?)	Rare, usually salt loss

there is a failure of normal female sexual development and absence of menstruation.

Since male phenotypic differentiation is normal, the condition is usually not recognized at birth in boys in the absence of adrenal insufficiency. However, early maturation of the external genitalia, development of secondary sex characteristics, coarsening of the voice, frequent erections, and excessive muscular development are noticeable during the first few years of life. Virilization in the male can follow two patterns. Excessive adrenal androgens can inhibit gonadotropin production so that the testes remain infantile in size despite the acceleration of masculinization. Such untreated adult men are capable of erection and ejaculation but have no spermatogenesis. Alternatively, adrenal androgen secretion can induce premature maturation of the hypothalamic-pituitary axis and initiate a true precocious puberty including early maturation of spermatogenesis (Chap. 335). The untreated male is also subject to the development of ACTH-dependent "tumors" of the adrenal rest cells of the testes.

In classic 21-hydroxylase deficiency, which accounts for about 95% of congenital adrenal hyperplasia, decreased production of hydrocortisone leads to increased release of ACTH, enlargement of the adrenal glands, and partial or complete compensation of the defect in the secretion of hydrocortisone. In about half, the enzyme defect appears to be partial, and cortisol secretion is normal. This form is termed *simple virilizing*. When deficiency of the enzyme is more complete, the so-called salt-losing form of 21-hydroxylase deficiency, production of cortisol and aldosterone is inadequate, leading to severe salt wastage with anorexia, vomiting, volume depletion, and vascular collapse within the first few weeks of life. In untreated patients, there is overproduction of the cortisol precursors prior to the 21-hydroxylase step, causing an increase in plasma progesterone and 17-hydroxyprogesterone. These steroids are weak aldosterone antagonists at the receptor level; in the compensated state aldosterone production increases to attempt to maintain normal sodium balance. Increased substrate availability is also responsible for the enhanced androgen synthesis and hence for the virilization.

Female pseudohermaphroditism also occurs in 11β-hydroxylase deficiency. In this disorder, a block in hydroxylation at the 11-carbon results in the accumulation of 11-deoxycortisol and deoxycorticosterone (DOC), a potent salt-retaining hormone that causes hypertension rather than salt loss. The clinical features that stem from glucocorticoid deficiency and androgen excess are similar to those in 21-hydroxylase deficiency.

Pathophysiology Both disorders are due to autosomal recessive mutations. The carrier frequency for CYP21A2 deficiency is about 1 in 50. Because the gene is located on the sixth chromosome close to the HLA-B locus, heterozygous carriers and homozygotes within a given family can be identified on the basis of the HLA haplotype. At the molecular level the mutations that give rise to 21-hydroxylase deficiency are highly polymorphic; indeed, partial gene deletions (10 to 30%), conversion of the gene from a functional state to a form that is not transcribed normally (10%), and point mutations (60 to 75%) have been characterized in the disorder. The classic disorder is due to mutations that severely impair enzyme activity, and less severe mutations cause the nonclassic, or late-onset, variety. 11β-hydroxylase activity is encoded by two genes on chromosome 8; mutations of the *CYP11B1* gene are responsible for this disorder. The *CYP11B2* gene encodes aldosterone synthase. A late-onset variant of 11β-hydroxylase deficiency exists but has not been characterized at the molecular level.

Urinary excretion of 17-ketosteroids and of the metabolites that accumulate proximal to the enzymatic blocks is increased. Plasma ACTH is elevated. In CYP21A2 deficiency, 17-hydroxyprogesterone accumulates in blood and is excreted predominantly as pregnanetriol. In CYP11B1 deficiency, 11-deoxycortisol accumulates in blood and is excreted predominantly as tetrahydrocortexolone. →*For additional discussion of the endocrine pathology, see Chap. 331.*

℞ **TREATMENT** Gender assignment should correspond to the chromosomal and gonadal sex, and appropriate surgical correc-

tion of the external genitalia should be undertaken as early as possible. This is of importance because appropriately treated men and women are capable of fertility. However, if the correct diagnosis is made late (after 3 years of age), gender assignment should be changed only after careful consideration of the psychosexual background.

Treatment with appropriate glucocorticoids prevents the consequences of hydrocortisone deficiency, arrests the rapid virilization, and prevents premature somatic and epiphyseal maturation. The suppression of the abnormal steroid secretion corrects the hypertension in CYP11B1 deficiency and in both disorders allows normal onset of menses and development of female secondary sex characteristics. In males, glucocorticoid therapy suppresses adrenal androgens and results in normal gonadotropin secretion, testicular development, and spermatogenesis. The usual maintenance dose of hydrocortisone is 10 to 20 mg/m^2 per day, given in three divided doses. However, the dose must be adjusted on an individual basis to optimize ACTH suppression while avoiding glucocorticoid side effects, which include growth retardation as well as Cushingoid features. Measurements of plasma 17-hydroxyprogesterone, androstenedione, ACTH, and renin levels have all been used to assess adequacy of replacement therapy. In severe CYP21A2 deficiency associated with salt loss or elevated plasma renin activity, treatment with mineralocorticoids is also indicated, and plasma renin levels should be monitored to assess the adequacy of mineralocorticoid replacement. Trials are underway to assess the potential use of antiandrogens (e.g., spironolactone, cyproterone acetate, flutamide) or aromatase inhibitors (e.g., latrazole, testolactone) as adjunctive therapy that may allow reductions in glucocorticoid dose. Treatment of affected fetuses in utero (beginning at 4 to 6 weeks) has been accomplished by administering dexamethasone (which crosses the placenta) to the mother. Though this treatment can reduce the extent of virilization in some girls, it is associated with maternal side effects, and the long-term consequences have not been established.

Other Causes of Female Pseudohermaphroditism Placental aromatase deficiency due to mutations in the gene encoding aromatase (*CYP19*) causes virilization of female embryos because of defective conversion of androgens to estrogens in the placenta and the secondary increase in testosterone levels in the fetus; in postnatal life CYP19 deficiency in women causes hirsutism and development of polycystic ovaries. Female pseudohermaphroditism can also occur in babies born to mothers with virilizing tumors of the ovary (e.g., arrhenoblastomas or luteomas of pregnancy) and, rarely, to mothers with virilizing adrenal tumors. In the past, the administration to pregnant women of progestogens with androgenic side effects (such as 17α-ethinyl-19-nor-testosterone) to prevent abortion resulted in masculinization of female fetuses.

Developmental Disorders of Müllerian Ducts (Congenital Absence of the Vagina, Müllerian Agenesis) • *Clinical features* Congenital hypoplasia or absence of the vagina in combination with abnormal or absent uterus (the Mayer-Rokitansky-Kuster-Hauser syndrome) is second to gonadal dysgenesis as a cause of primary amenorrhea. Most patients are ascertained after the time of expected puberty because of failure to menstruate. The height is normal, and the breasts, axillary and pubic hair, and habitus are feminine in character. The uterus can vary from almost normal, lacking only a conduit to the introitus, to the characteristic rudimentary bicornuate cords with or without a lumen. In some patients cyclic abdominal pain indicates that sufficient functional endometrium is present to result in retrograde menstruation and/or hematometra.

About one-third have abnormal kidneys, most commonly agenesis, ectopy, fused kidneys of the horseshoe type, or solitary ectopic kidneys in the pelvis. Skeletal abnormalities are present in one-tenth; most involve the spine, and limb and rib defects account for the rest. Specific abnormalities include wedge vertebrae, fused rudimentary or asymmetric vertebral bodies, supernumerary vertebrae, and the Klippel-Feil syndrome (congenital fusion of the cervical spine, short neck, low posterior hairline, and painless limitation of cervical movement).

Pathophysiology   The karyotype is 46,XX. Familial occurrence has been described, and the pattern of inheritance in most is consistent with a sex-limited autosomal dominant mutation. Sporadic cases may represent new mutations of the type responsible for the familial disorder or be multifactorial in etiology. In the familial cases, expressivity is variable; some have skeletal or renal abnormalities only, and some have other abnormalities of müllerian derivatives such as a double uterus. Bilateral renal aplasia in stillborn infants is commonly associated with absence of the uterus and vagina. Thus, the family history should be probed for isolated skeletal and renal abnormalities and for stillbirths that might result from congenital absence of both kidneys. Ovarian function is normal, and successful pregnancies have occurred after corrective vaginal surgery in patients with a normal uterus.

℞ **TREATMENT**   Vaginal agenesis can be treated by surgical or nonsurgical means. Surgical repair generally utilizes a split-thickness skin graft around a solid rubber mold to create an artificial vagina. Medical therapy involves the repeated application of pressure against the vaginal dimple with a simple dilator to force development of adequate vaginal depth. In view of complication rates of 5 to 10% in surgical series, surgery should be reserved for patients in whom a well-formed uterus is present and the possibility of fertility exists. Frequent coitus or instrumental dilatation is essential for maintaining patency of neovaginas formed by either technique.

MALE PSEUDOHERMAPHRODITISM   Defective virilization of the 46,XY embryo (male pseudohermaphroditism) can result from defects in androgen synthesis, defects in androgen action, defects in müllerian duct regression, and uncertain causes.

Abnormalities in Androgen Synthesis • *Clinical features*   Enzymatic defects that result in defective testosterone synthesis (Fig. 338-3) account for only about a fifth of cases of male pseudohermaphroditism (Tables 338-4 and 338-5). Each of the defects blocks a step in the conversion of cholesterol to testosterone. Three enzymatic reactions are common to the synthesis of other adrenal hormones as well: cholesterol side chain cleavage, 3β-hydroxysteroid dehydrogenase/isomerase, and 17α-hydroxylase (CYP17). Consequently, their deficiency results in congenital adrenal hyperplasia (Table 338-4) as well as male pseudohermaphroditism. Two others (17,20-lyase and 17β-hydroxysteroid dehydrogenase 3) are unique to the pathway of androgen synthesis, and their deficiency results only in male pseudohermaphroditism. Since androgens are obligatory precursors of estrogens, synthesis of estrogen is also low in all but the terminal defect (17β-hydroxysteroid dehydrogenase 3 deficiency).

Adrenal dysfunction is described in Chap. 331, and the present discussion concerns the abnormal sexual development. In genetic males with defective testosterone synthesis, absence of the uterus and fallopian tubes indicates that müllerian duct inhibition was normal during embryogenesis. Masculinization of the urogenital tract and external genitalia and virilization at puberty vary from almost normal to absent, and, therefore, the manifestations vary from men with mild hypospadias to phenotypic women who prior to puberty resemble women with complete testicular feminization. This heterogeneity is the consequence of varying severity of the enzymatic defects, varying effects of the steroids that accumulate proximal to the various metabolic blocks, and the presence of alternative enzymatic pathways in some disorders. In patients with partial defects in whom the plasma testosterone level is normal, the diagnosis can only be made by measuring the steroids that accumulate proximal to the metabolic block.

Congenital lipoid adrenal hyperplasia is an autosomal recessive disorder in which virtually no urinary steroids (either 17-ketosteroids or 17-hydroxycorticoids) can be detected. Since the defect blocks the conversion of cholesterol to pregnenolone, a step catalyzed by the cholesterol side chain cleavage enzyme (CYP11A1), it was originally assumed that the defect must involve this enzyme. However, the disorder is instead caused by mutations in the *st*eroidogenic *a*cute *r*egulatory (*StAR*) gene, which encodes the protein that transports cholesterol from the cytosol to the inner mitochondrial membrane in the adrenal and gonads. Manifestations of the disorder include salt wasting and profound adrenal insufficiency, and most affected individuals die during infancy. At autopsy, the adrenals and testes are enlarged and infiltrated with lipid. Affected males are incompletely masculinized, whereas affected female infants have normal genital development because lipid accumulation in the ovary does not occur until there is follicular development and active steroidogenesis.

3β-Hydroxysteroid dehydrogenase/isomerase 2 deficiency causes varying failure of masculinization and the development of a vagina in male infants. Female infants may be modestly virilized at birth due to the weak androgenic potency of dehydroepiandrosterone, the major steroid secreted. If the enzyme is absent in both the adrenal and testis, no urinary steroids contain a Δ^4-3-keto configuration, whereas in patients in whom the defect is partial or affects only the testis, the urine may contain normal or elevated levels of Δ^4-3-ketosteroids. Most patients have marked salt wasting and profound adrenal insufficiency, and long-term survival in untreated cases occurs only in states of partial deficiency. Minimally affected males may experience an otherwise normal male puberty except for profound gynecomastia. In these boys, a low-normal blood testosterone level is accompanied by elevated Δ^5 precursor steroids. 3β-Hydroxysteroid dehydrogenase activity is catalyzed by more than one isoenzyme. The type 2 isoenzyme is expressed in adrenals and gonads; the disorder described above is due to any of several mutations in this enzyme. The coding sequence of this gene is said to be normal in several individuals with the late-onset variant of the disease, the pathophysiology of which is unclear.

17α-Hydroxylase-17,20-lyase (CYP17) *deficiency* impairs the introduction of the 17-hydroxyl and the scission of the C-17,20 carbon bond that convert pregnenolone and progesterone to dehydroepiandrosterone and androstenedione, respectively. These reactions are mediated by a single enzyme CYP17, which is encoded on chromosome 10; it remains unclear why both reactions occur in the ovary and testis, whereas in the adrenal 17-hydroxyprogesterone is largely converted to glucocorticoids and mineralocorticoids rather than the 19-carbon steroids. Of note, some patients appear to have selective impairment of either 17α-hydroxylase or 17,20-lyase activity. These mutations have identified enzyme domains proposed to undergo posttranslational modification and selective interactions with cofactors that switch enzymatic activity. Whatever the mechanism, the consequences of 17α-hydroxylase and 17,20-lyase deficiencies are different.

17α-Hydroxylase deficiency is characterized by hypogonadism, absence of secondary sex characteristics, hypokalemic alkalosis, hypertension, and virtually undetectable hydrocortisone secretion in phenotypic women. Formation of both corticosterone and DOC by the adrenal is elevated, and urinary 17-ketosteroids are low. Aldosterone secretion is low due to high plasma DOC and depressed angiotensin levels and returns to normal after suppressive doses of glucocorticoids. In 46,XX individuals, amenorrhea, absent sexual hair, and hypertension are common, but the phenotype is that of a normal prepubertal woman. In males, the deficiency results in defective virilization that varies from complete male pseudohermaphroditism to ambiguous genitalia with perineoscrotal hypospadias and, in some, gynecomastia. Adrenal insufficiency does not develop, since the secretion of both corticosterone (a weak glucocorticoid) and DOC (a mineralocorticoid) is elevated. Hypertension and hypokalemia are prominent (even in the neonatal period) and remit after suppression of the DOC secretion by glucocorticoid replacement. A variety of point mutations, deletions, and insertions in the *CYP17* gene have been characterized in affected individuals.

17,20-Lyase deficiency in males is associated with normal function of the adrenal cortex and a variable pattern of male pseudohermaphroditism. In the majority there is genital ambiguity at birth, with some virilization at the time of expected puberty. Rare 46,XY patients

| Disorder | Inheritance | Phenotype | | | | | | Endocrine Profile Relative to Normal Male | | |
		Müllerian Ducts	Wolffian Ducts	Spermato-genesis	Urogenital Sinus	External Genitalia	Breast	Testosterone Production	Estrogen Production	LH
DEFECTS IN TESTOSTERONE SYNTHESIS										
Five enzymatic defects	Autosomal recessive	Absent	Variable development	Normal or decreased	Variable from male to female	Generally female	Usually male	Normal to decreased	Variable	High
DEFECTS IN ANDROGEN ACTION										
Steroid 5α-reductase 2 deficiency	Autosomal recessive	Absent	Male	Normal or decreased	Female	Clitoromegaly	Male	Normal	Normal	Normal or increased
Receptor disorders:										
Complete testicular feminization	X-linked recessive	Absent	Absent	Absent	Female	Female	Female	High	High	High
Incomplete testicular feminization	X-linked	Absent	Male	Absent	Female	Clitoromegaly and posterior fusion	Female	High	High	High
Reifenstein syndrome	X-linked recessive	Absent	Variable development	Absent	Variable from male to female	Incomplete male development	Female	High	High	High
Infertile or undervirilized fertile male	X-linked recessive	Absent	Male	Absent to normal	Male	Male	Usually male	Normal or high	Normal or high	Normal or high
DEFECTS IN MÜLLERIAN REGRESSION										
Persistent müllerian duct syndrome	Autosomal recessive	Rudimentary uterus and fallopian tubes	Male	Normal	Male	Male	Male	Normal	Normal	Normal

have had a female phenotype and no virilization at the time of expected puberty. The disorder has been recognized in one 46,XX woman with sexual infantilism. Mutations of *CYP17* that cause this disorder involve an area of the gene that is known to encode a binding site for the redox-partner of the enzyme.

17β-Hydroxysteroid dehydrogenase 3 (17β-HSD-3) *deficiency* involves the final step in testosterone biosynthesis, reduction of the 17-keto group of androstenedione. This is the most common enzymatic defect in testosterone synthesis. Affected 46,XY males usually have a female phenotype with a blind-ending vagina and absence of müllerian derivatives, but inguinal or abdominal testes and virilized wolffian duct structures are present. At the time of expected puberty, both virilization (with phallic enlargement and development of facial and body hair) and a variable degree of feminization take place. In some untreated patients, reversal of gender behavior from female to male occurs at puberty. Plasma testosterone level may be in the low-normal range, making it essential to document elevation in plasma androstenedione to make the diagnosis. Isoenzymes encoded by several different genes possess 17β-hydroxysteroid dehydrogenase activity, but the isoenzyme 3 is expressed in the testes. A variety of mutations have been characterized in the 17β-HSD-3 gene in affected individuals.

Pathophysiology These various disorders are inherited as autosomal recessive traits. The pattern of steroid secretion and excretion depends on the site of the various metabolic blocks (Fig. 338-3). In general, gonadotropin secretion is high, and many individuals with incomplete defects are able to compensate so that the steady-state levels of testosterone may be normal or almost normal.

In rare cases of male pseudohermaphroditism, testosterone formation is deficient for reasons other than a single enzyme defect in androgen synthesis. These include disorders in which Leydig cell agenesis is due to autosomal recessive loss-of-function mutations of

the LH receptor or to the secretion of a biologically inactive LH molecule. In addition, as described above, several disorders, including familial 46,XY pure gonadal dysgenesis, sporadic dysgenetic testes, and the absent testis syndrome, are characterized by deficient testosterone production due to abnormal gonadal development.

TREATMENT Therapy with glucocorticoids and in some instances mineralocorticoids is indicated in those disorders causing adrenal hyperplasia. The management of the genital abnormalities depends on the individual case. Fertility has not been reported, and its consideration does not enter into sex assignment. In genetic females there is no problem (except in diagnosis), in that affected individuals are raised appropriately as females and estrogen therapy is begun at the time of expected puberty to promote development of female secondary sex characteristics. Whether newborn males with ambiguous genitalia should be raised as males or females depends on the anatomic defect; in general, the more severely affected should be raised as females, and corrective surgery of the genitalia and removal of the testes should be undertaken as early as possible. In such women estrogen therapy is begun at the appropriate age to allow development of normal female secondary sex characteristics. In individuals raised as males, corrective surgery is indicated for any coexisting hypospadias, and plasma androgens should be monitored at the time of expected puberty to determine whether testosterone therapy is appropriate.

Abnormalities in Androgen Action Several disorders of male phenotypic development result from abnormalities of androgen action. The spectrum of phenotypes is described in Tables 338-4 and 338-5. In these disorders, testosterone formation and müllerian regression are normal, but male development is impaired because of resistance to androgen action in target tissues.

Steroid 5α-reductase 2 deficiency This autosomal recessive disorder is characterized by (1) severe perineoscrotal hypospadias; (2) a blind vaginal pouch of variable size opening either into the urogenital sinus or into the urethra; (3) testes with normal epididymides, vasa deferentia, and seminal vesicles, and termination of the ejaculatory ducts in the blind-ending vagina; (4) a female habitus with normal axillary and pubic hair but without female breast development; (5) the absence of uterus and fallopian tubes; (6) normal male plasma testosterone; and (7) masculinization to a variable degree at the time of puberty.

The realization that virilization during embryogenesis is defective only in the urogenital sinus and the external genitalia provided insight into the fundamental abnormality. Testosterone, the androgen secreted by the fetal testis, is responsible for conversion of the wolffian duct into the epididymis, vas deferens, and seminal vesicle, whereas dihydrotestosterone mediates virilization of the urogenital sinus and the external genitalia. Consequently, impairment of dihydrotestosterone formation in a male embryo would be expected to cause the phenotype in this disorder—normal male wolffian duct derivatives with defective masculinization of the external genitalia and urogenital sinus. Since testosterone itself regulates LH secretion (Chap. 335), plasma LH level is normal or minimally elevated. As a result, testosterone and estrogen production rates are those of normal men, and gynecomastia does not develop.

The fact that 5α-reductase 2 enzyme is deficient in this disorder was established by assay of biopsied tissues and cultured fibroblasts from affected individuals. Deletions or point mutations in the gene encoding steroid 5α-reductase 2 have been identified in most families studied. Approximately 40% are compound heterozygotes.

Receptor disorders The androgen receptor is a member of the steroid/thyroid family of receptors with steroid-binding, DNA-binding, and functional domains and is encoded by a gene on the long arm of the X chromosome. Mutations of this gene impair receptor function and hence impair male phenotypic differentiation and/or virilization.

CLINICAL FEATURES   *Complete testicular feminization* (also called *complete androgen insensitivity*) is a common form of male pseudohermaphroditism; estimates of frequency vary from 1 in 20,000 to 1 in 64,000 male births. It is the third most common cause of primary amenorrhea after gonadal dysgenesis and congenital absence of the vagina. The features are characteristic. Namely, a woman is ascertained either because of inguinal hernia (prepubertal) or primary amenorrhea (postpubertal). The development of the breasts, the habitus, and the distribution of body fat are female in character so that most have a truly feminine appearance. Axillary and pubic hair is absent or scanty, but some vulval hair is usually present. Scalp hair is that of a normal woman, and facial hair is absent. The external genitalia are unambiguously female, and the clitoris is normal. The vagina is short and blind-ending and may be absent or rudimentary. All internal genitalia are absent except for testes that contain normal Leydig cells and seminiferous tubules without spermatogenesis. The testes may be located in the abdomen, along the course of the inguinal canal, or in the labia majora. Occasionally, remnants of müllerian or wolffian duct origin are present in the paratesticular fascia or in fibrous bands extending from the testis. Patients tend to be rather tall, and bone age is normal. Psychosexual development is unmistakably female with regard to behavior, outlook, and maternal instincts.

The major complication of undescended testes in this disorder, as in all forms of cryptorchidism, is the development of tumors (Chap. 96). Since affected individuals undergo normal pubertal growth and feminize at the time of expected puberty and since testicular tumors rarely develop until after puberty, it is usual to delay gonadectomy until after the time of expected puberty. Prepubertal gonadectomy is indicated if the testes are present in the inguinal region or labia majora and result in discomfort or hernia formation. (If hernia repair is indicated prepubertally, most physicians prefer to remove the testes at the same time to limit the number of operative procedures.) If the testes are removed prepubertally, estrogen therapy is required at the appropriate age to ensure normal growth and breast development. Postpubertal gonadectomy causes menopausal symptoms and other evidence of estrogen withdrawal, and suitable estrogen replacement is indicated (Chap. 336).

Incomplete testicular feminization is about one-tenth as frequent as the complete form. In this disorder there is minor virilization of the external genitalia (partial fusion of the labioscrotal folds and/or some degree of clitoromegaly), normal pubic hair, and mixed virilization and feminization at the time of expected puberty. The vagina is short and blind-ending, but in contrast to the complete form, the wolffian duct derivatives are often partially developed. Since women with the incomplete disorder virilize at the time of expected puberty, gonadectomy should be performed before the expected time of puberty in all prepubertal patients with clitoromegaly or posterior labial fusion.

Reifenstein syndrome (also called *partial androgen insensitivity*) is the term applied to forms of incomplete male pseudohermaphroditism initially described by a number of eponyms (Reifenstein syndrome, Gilbert-Dreyfus syndrome, Lubs syndrome). These syndromes are mutations that partially impair the function of the androgen receptor. The most common phenotype is a man with perineoscrotal hypospadias and gynecomastia, but the spectrum of defective virilization in affected families ranges from men with azoospermia to phenotypic women with pseudovaginas. Axillary and pubic hair is normal, but chest and facial hair is scanty. Cryptorchidism is common, the testes are small, and azoospermia is present. Some have defects in wolffian duct derivatives such as absence or hypoplasia of the vas deferens. Since the psychological development in most is unequivocally male, the hypospadias and cryptorchidism should be corrected surgically. The treatment of the gynecomastia is surgical removal.

A disorder of the androgen receptor that is not actually a form of male pseudohermaphroditism is manifested as *infertility and/or undervirilization in phenotypic men*. Some such individuals are minimally affected members of families with Reifenstein syndrome in whom azoospermia is the only manifestation of the receptor defect. The *undervirilized fertile male* is an even more subtle manifestation of androgen receptor defect. In these families, affected men have gynecomastia and undervirilization, and some are fertile. More commonly, however, individuals with negative family histories present with male infertility with or without undervirilization.

PATHOPHYSIOLOGY   The karyotype is 46,XY, and the mutation is X-linked. The frequency of a positive family history varies from about two-thirds of patients with testicular feminization and Reifenstein syndrome to only occasional patients with the infertile male syndrome. The disorder in subjects with a negative family history is believed to be the result of new mutations.

Hormone dynamics are similar in all disorders of the androgen receptor. Plasma testosterone levels and rates of testosterone production by the testes are normal or high. Elevated testosterone production is caused by the high mean plasma level of LH, which, in turn, is due to defective feedback regulation caused by resistance to the action of androgen at the hypothalamic-pituitary level. Elevated LH concentration is responsible also for the increased estrogen production by the testes (Chap. 337). (In normal men, most estrogen is derived from peripheral formation from circulating androgens, but when the plasma LH level is elevated, the testes secrete increased amounts of estrogen into the circulation.) Thus resistance to the feedback regulation of LH secretion by circulating androgen results in elevated plasma LH levels, and this, in turn, results in the enhanced secretion of both testosterone and estradiol by the testes. Gonadotropin levels rise even higher (and menopausal symptoms may develop) when the testes are removed, indicating that gonadotropin secretion is under partial feedback control. Presumably, in the steady state and in the absence of an androgen effect, estrogen alone regulates LH secretion, a control purchased at the expense of an elevated plasma estrogen concentration for a male.

The hormonal changes in the infertile male syndrome are similar to those in the other receptor disorders but less marked. Some men with this syndrome do not have an elevation of plasma LH or plasma testosterone level.

Feminization in these disorders is the result of two interlocking phenomena. First, androgens and estrogens have antagonistic effects, and in the absence of androgen action, the cellular effect of estrogen is unopposed. Second, the testicular production of estradiol is greater than that of the normal male (although less than that of the normal female). Variable degrees of androgen resistance and enhanced estradiol production result in different degrees of defective virilization and enhanced feminization in the four clinical syndromes.

Each of these syndromes is the result of defects in the androgen receptor. In most families, the fundamental defect is due to point mutations in the coding sequence leading to premature termination codons or to amino acid substitutions in the hormone-binding domain. Such mutations impair receptor function to variable degrees. Some families with clinical syndromes typical of an androgen receptor disorder have normal androgen binding in fibroblasts; in most, point mutations in the DNA-binding domain of the androgen receptor are responsible for the androgen resistance.

℞ TREATMENT Individuals with 5α-reductase deficiency who are raised as females but elect at the time of expected puberty to change social sex to male or who are raised from the first as males should be monitored carefully and given supplemental androgens, preferably those such as nandrolone decanoate that do not require 5α-reduction for activation, when virilization is incomplete. Fertility has been reported in such an individual. Individuals with 5α-reductase deficiency who continue to function as females should be gonadectomized, given feminizing doses of estrogens indefinitely, and receive surgical correction of the introitus when appropriate. The management of subjects with androgen receptor defects depends on the phenotypic manifestations. Women with testicular feminization should be castrated (preferably after the completion of the pubertal growth spurt and the feminization of the breasts) to prevent tumor development in the testes and receive estrogen replacement to maintain feminization, prevent hot flashes, and protect the bones; shallow vaginal depth can usually be treated medically with the Frank technique. Men with the Reifenstein phenotype should have surgical correction of the hypospadias and may require surgery for gynecomastia; supplemental androgen therapy in these men rarely improves the incomplete virilization.

Persistent Müllerian Duct Syndrome Men with this uncommon disorder have testes and male phenotypic development and in addition have fallopian tubes and a uterus. In some, one or both testes are descended and the uterus and ipsilateral fallopian tube are in the inguinal canal or scrotum; both testes and fallopian tubes may be present in the hernia sac or can be drawn into it. In others, the testes are located high in the abdomen and hernias are not present. In both types, the vasa deferentia are embedded in the wall of the uterus, a feature that complicates surgical procedures designed to preserve potential fertility. Most individuals have uninformative family histories, but in some the condition is inherited as an autosomal recessive trait. Because the external genitalia are well developed and the subjects masculinize normally at puberty, it is assumed that during the critical stage of embryonic differentiation the fetal testes produce a normal amount of androgen. However, müllerian regression does not occur. Two types of mutations have been described in this disorder. In one the gene that encodes AMH is defective, and blood levels of AMH are usually low or undetectable; in the other the AMH receptor is defective, and blood levels of AMH are elevated. To minimize the chance of tumor development and to maintain virilization, orchiopexy should be performed. Malignancy in the uterus or vagina has not been described, and because the vasa deferentia are closely associated with the broad ligaments, the uterus and vagina should be left in place to

avoid disruption of the vasa deferentia during removal and consequently to preserve possible fertility.

Developmental Defects of the Male Genitalia • *Hypospadias* Hypospadias is a congenital anomaly in which the urethra terminates in an abnormal position along the ventral midline of the penis at some site between the normal urethral meatus and the perineum. This malformation occurs in 0.5 to 0.8% of male births in the United States and is often associated with ventral contraction and bowing of the penis (chordee). It is common to categorize hypospadias as glandular (involving the glans penis), penile, or perineoscrotal. Since androgens control penile development, hypospadias is generally assumed to result from some unidentified defect in androgen formation or action during embryogenesis. Indeed, hypospadias occurs in most disorders of male sexual differentiation, and a rare cause of hypospadias is maternal ingestion of progestational agents early in pregnancy. However, the known causes (single-gene defects, chromosomal abnormalities, and maternal drug ingestion) account for only about one-fourth of cases, and the etiology of most is unknown. The management is surgical.

Cryptorchidism The control of testicular descent is poorly understood, both in regard to the nature of the forces that cause the movement and to the hormonal factors that regulate the process. In anatomic terms, testicular descent can be divided into three phases: (1) transabdominal movement of the testis from its site of origin above the kidney to the inguinal ring, (2) formation of the opening in the inguinal canal (processus vaginalis) through which the testis exits the abdominal cavity, and (3) actual movement of the testis through the inguinal canal to its permanent site in the scrotum. This process occurs over a 6- to 7-month period during gestation, beginning at about the sixth week, and is not completed in some until after birth. Impairment at any stage in this process can impair descent of one or both testes. About 3% of full-term and 30% of premature male infants have at least one cryptorchid testis at birth, but descent is usually completed within the first few weeks of life, so that the incidence of failure of descent by 6 to 9 months of age is only 0.6 to 0.7%. It is this latter category of maldescent that requires intervention.

Permanent cryptorchidism can be classified as intraabdominal (10%), canalicular (in the inguinal canal) (20%), high scrotal (40%), or obstructed (30%), in which maldescent is due to a physical barrier between the inguinal pouch and the inlet of the scrotum. These disorders must be distinguished from the temporarily retracted normal testis.

The cryptorchid testis functions poorly after puberty, but the extent to which maldescent is the result of an abnormality of the testis or the cause of abnormal function is unknown. Two general theories have been advanced as to the etiology—inadequate intraabdominal pressure and deficient endocrine function of the testis either because of deficient testosterone synthesis or inadequate formation of AMH. Indeed, defects that result in inadequate development of intraabdominal pressure or inadequate development of the testes can cause cryptorchidism. As in hypospadias, however, the known causes of cryptorchidism constitute only a small fraction of the cases, and the etiology in most remains to be identified. Two complications of cryptorchidism are important; spermatogenesis cannot occur at the temperature of the abdominal cavity, and it is necessary to correct the process as early as possible to allow possible fertility. The fact that infertility is common in men who have been treated for unilateral as well as bilateral cryptorchidism suggests that maldescent is usually the consequence rather than the cause of the testicular malfunction. There is also a greater frequency of malignancy in undescended testes, which should be surgically corrected for this reason (Chap. 96).

BIBLIOGRAPHY

ACHERMANN JC et al: A mutation in the gene encoding steroidogenic factor-1 causes XY sex reversal and adrenal failure in humans. Nat Genet 22:125, 1999

AFFARA NA et al: Analysis of the *SRY* gene in 22 sex-reversed XY females identifies four new point mutations in the conserved DNA binding domain. Hum Mol Genet 2:785, 1993

ANDERSSON S et al: Molecular genetics and pathophysiology of 17β-hydroxysteroid dehydrogenase 3 deficiency. J Clin Endocrinol Metab 81:130, 1996

BEHRINGER RR: The in vivo roles of mullerian-inhibiting substance. Curr Top Dev Biol 29:171, 1994

BOUCEKKINE C et al: Clinical and anatomical spectrum in XX sex reversed patients. Relationship to the presence of Y-specific DNA sequences. Clin Endocrinol 40:733, 1994

BULUN SE: Aromatase deficiency in women and men: Would you have predicted the phenotype? J Clin Endocrinol Metab 81:867, 1996

CHAN WY: Molecular genetic, biochemical, and clinical implications of gonadotropin receptor mutations. Mol Genet Metab 63:75, 1998

DONAHOE PA et al: Mixed gonadal dysgenesis, pathogenesis and management. J Pediatr Surg 14:287, 1979

——— et al: Congenital adrenal hyperplasia, in *The Metabolic and Molecular Bases of Inherited Disease*, 8th ed, CR Scriver et al (eds). New York, McGraw-Hill, 2001, pp 4077–4115

EDMAN CD et al: Embryonic testicular regression: A clinical spectrum of XY agonadal individuals. Obstet Gynecol 49:208, 1977

FOSTER JW et al: Campomelic dysplasia and autosomal sex reversal caused by mutations in an *SRY*-related gene. Nature 372:525, 1994

GEORGE FW, WILSON JD: Sex determination and differentiation, in *The Physiology of Reproduction*, 2d ed, E Knobil, JD Neill (eds). New York, Raven Press, 1994, vol 1, pp 3–28

GRIFFIN JE et al: Congenital absence of the vagina: The Mayer-Rokitansky-Kuster-Hauser syndrome. Ann Intern Med 85:224, 1976

——— et al: The androgen resistance syndromes: 5α-Reductase deficiency, and related disorders, in *The Metabolic and Molecular Bases of Inherited Disease*, 8th ed, CR Scriver et al (eds). New York, McGraw-Hill, 2001, pp 4117–4146

GRUMBACH MM, CONTE FA: Disorders of sexual differentiation, in *Williams Textbook of Endocrinology*, 9th ed, JD Wilson, et al (eds). Philadelphia, Saunders, 1998, pp 1303–1425

HAWKINS JR et al: Mutational analysis of *SRY*: Nonsense and missense mutations in XY sex reversal. Hum Genet 88:471, 1992

IMBEAUD S et al: A 27-base pair deletion of the anti-mullerian type II receptor gene is the most common cause of the persistent mullerian duct syndrome. Hum Mol Genet 5:1269, 1996

JOSSO N et al: Clinical aspects and molecular genetics of the persistent mullerian duct syndrome. Clin Endocrinol 47:137, 1997

KROB G et al: True hermaphroditism: Geographical distribution, clinical findings, chromosomes and gonadal histology. Eur J Pediatr 153:2, 1994

MILLER WL, STRAUSS JF III: Molecular pathology and mechanism of action of the steroidogenic acute regulatory protein, StAR. J Steroid Biochem Mol Biol 69:131, 1999

——— et al: The molecular basis of isolated 17,20 lyase deficiency. Endocrine Res 24: 817, 1998

MISHINA Y et al: Genetic analysis of the mullerian-inhibitory substance signal transduction pathway in mammalian sexual differentiation. Genes Dev 10:2577, 1996

PARKER KL et al: Gene interactions in gonadal development. Ann Rev Physiol 61:417, 1999

ROSENFELD R, GRUMBACH MM (eds): *Turner Syndrome*. New York, Marcel Dekker, 1990

ROVET J et al: The psychoeducational profile of boys with Klinefelter syndrome. J Learn Disabil 29:180, 1996

SIMARD J et al: Molecular biology and genetics of the 3β-hydroxysteroid dehydrogenase/Δ5-Δ4 isomerase gene family. J Endocrinol 150 (Suppl):S189, 1996

SMYTH CM, BREMNER WJ: Klinefelter syndrome. Arch Intern Med 158:1309, 1998

STRUBBE EH et al: The Mayer-Rokitansky-Kuster-Hauser (MRKH) syndrome without and with associated features: Two separate entities? Clin Dysmorphol 3:192, 1994

SWAIN A, LOVELL-BADGE R: Mammalian sex determination: A molecular drama. Genes Dev 13:755, 1999

YANASE T et al: 17α-Hydroxylase/17,20-lyase defects. J Steroid Biochem Mol Biol 53: 153, 1995

ZINN AR, ROSS JL: Turner syndrome and haploinsufficiency. Curr Opin Genet Dev 8: 322, 1998

339   *Steven I. Sherman, Robert F. Gagel*

DISORDERS AFFECTING MULTIPLE ENDOCRINE SYSTEMS

ACTH adrenocorticotropin	MEN multiple endocrine neoplasia
CT computed tomography	MRI magnetic resonance imaging
CRH corticotropin-releasing hormone	MTC medullary thyroid carcinoma
FHH familial hypocalciuric hypercalcemia	PGA polyglandular autoimmune
FMTC familial medullary thyroid carcinoma	POEMS polyneuropathy, organomegaly, endocrinopathy, M-proteins, and skin changes
GH growth hormone	TSH thyroid stimulating hormone
GHRH growth hormone–releasing hormone	VIP vasoactive intestinal peptide
	ZES Zollinger-Ellison syndrome

NEOPLASTIC DISORDERS AFFECTING MULTIPLE ENDOCRINE ORGANS

Several distinct genetic disorders predispose to endocrine gland neoplasia and cause hormone excess syndromes (Table 339-1). DNA-based genetic testing is now available for these disorders, but effective management requires an understanding of endocrine neoplasia and the range of clinical features that may be manifest in an individual patient.

MULTIPLE ENDOCRINE NEOPLASIA (MEN) TYPE 1 Clinical Manifestations   MEN 1, or Wermer's syndrome, is characterized by neoplasia of parathyroid, pituitary, and pancreatic islet cells (Table 339-1). The syndrome is inherited as an autosomal dominant trait, so that each child of an affected parent has a 50% chance of inheriting the predisposing gene.

Several features of the pathogenesis of MEN 1 have important implications for its management. Though each tumor is derived from a single cell (clonal in origin), any endocrine cell within the affected organs can become transformed. Hyperplasia is the initiating lesion, followed later by adenomatous or carcinomatous changes. Consequently, the disease process within a single organ is multicentric. Neoplasia in one organ may affect the progression of disease in another organ. For example, the ectopic production of hypothalamic releasing hormones by a pancreatic tumor may stimulate the growth of a pituitary tumor. Because MEN 1 generally evolves over a 30- to 40-year period, the manifestations depend in part on when the disorder is identified.

Hyperparathyroidism is the most common manifestation of MEN 1. Hypercalcemia may be present during the teenage years, and most individuals are affected by age 40 (Fig. 339-1). Screening for hyperparathyroidism involves measurement of either an albumin-adjusted or ionized serum calcium level. The diagnosis is established by demonstrating elevated levels of serum calcium and intact parathyroid hormone. Manifestations of hyperparathyroidism in MEN 1 do not differ substantially from those in sporadic hyperparathyroidism and include calcium-containing kidney stones, bone abnormalities, and gastrointestinal and musculoskeletal complaints (Chap. 341).

Other familial disorders associated with hypercalcemia include familial parathyroid hyperplasia, familial adenomatous hyperparathyroidism, and familial hypocalciuric hypercalcemia (FHH). Calcium excretion is usually elevated in the patient with MEN 1 or other forms of primary hyperparathyroidism and low in FHH. Another distinguishing feature is that the serum calcium level is rarely elevated at birth in patients with MEN 1 but is frequently elevated in newborns with FHH. Differentiation of hyperparathyroidism of MEN 1 from other forms of familial primary hyperparathyroidism is usually based on family history, histologic features of resected parathyroid tissue, and, sometimes, long-term observation to determine whether other manifestations of MEN 1 develop. FHH is due to inactivating mutations of the calcium sensor, a transmembrane G protein–coupled receptor found in parathyroid tissue and kidney (Chap. 341).

Parathyroid hyperplasia is the common cause of hyperparathyroidism in MEN 1, although single and multiple adenomas have been described. Hyperplasia of one or more parathyroid glands is common in younger patients; adenomas are usually found in older patients or those with long-standing disease.

Neoplasia of the pancreatic islets is the second most common manifestation of MEN 1 and tends to occur in parallel with hyperparathyroidism (Fig. 339-1). Increased pancreatic islet cell hormones include pancreatic polypeptide (75 to 85%), gastrin [60%; Zollinger-Ellison syndrome (ZES)], insulin (25 to 35%), vasoactive intestinal peptide (VIP) (3 to 5%; Verner-Morrison or watery diarrhea syndrome), glucagon (5 to 10%), and somatostatin (1 to 5%). The tumors rarely produce adrenocorticotropin (ACTH), corticotropin-releasing hormone (CRH), growth hormone–releasing hormone (GHRH), calcitonin gene products, neurotensin, gastric inhibitory peptide, and others. Many of the tumors produce more than one peptide. The pancreatic neoplasms differ from the other components of MEN 1 in that approximately one-third of the tumors display malignant features, including hepatic metastases (Chap. 93).

Pancreatic islet cell tumors are diagnosed by identification of a characteristic clinical syndrome, hormonal assays with or without provocative stimuli, or radiographic techniques. One approach involves annual screening of people at risk with measurement of basal and meal-stimulated levels of pancreatic polypeptide to identify the tumors as early as possible; the rationale of this screening strategy is the concept that surgical removal of islet cell tumors at an early stage will be curative. Other approaches to screening include measurement of serum gastrin and pancreatic polypeptide levels every 2 to 3 years, with the rationale that pancreatic neoplasms will be detected at a later stage but can be managed medically, if possible, or by surgery. High-resolution, early-phase computed tomography (CT) scanning provides the best noninvasive technique for identification of these tumors, but intraoperative ultrasonography is the most sensitive method for detection of small tumors.

ZES is caused by excessive gastrin production and occurs in more than half of MEN 1 patients with pancreatic islet cell tumors (Fig. 339-1) (Chap. 93). Clinical features include increased gastric acid production, recurrent peptic ulcers, diarrhea, and esophagitis. The ulcer diathesis is refractory to conservative therapy such as antacids. The diagnosis is made by finding increased gastric acid secretion, elevated basal gastrin levels in serum [generally >115 pmol/L (200 pg/mL)], and an exaggerated response of serum gastrin to either secretin or calcium. Other causes of elevated serum gastrin levels, such as achlorhydria, treatment with H_2 receptor antagonists or omeprazole, retained gastric antrum, small-bowel resection, gastric outlet obstruction, and hypercalcemia, should be excluded. Gastrin-producing carcinoid-like tumors are frequently present in the duodenal wall.

Insulinoma causes hypoglycemia in about one-third of MEN 1 patients with pancreatic islet cell tumors (Fig. 339-1). The tumors may be benign or malignant (25%). The diagnosis can be established by documenting hypoglycemia during a short fast with simultaneous inappropriate elevation of serum insulin and C-peptide levels. More commonly, it is necessary to subject the patient to a supervised 72-h fast to provoke hypoglycemia (Chap. 334). Large insulinomas may be identified by CT scanning; small tumors not detected by radiographic techniques may be localized by selective arteriographic injection of calcium into each of the arteries that supply the pancreas and sampling the hepatic vein for insulin to determine the anatomic region containing the tumor. Intraoperative ultrasonography can also be used to lo-

calize these tumors, but preoperative calcium injection data are helpful in guiding the subtotal pancreatectomy if multiple or no abnormalities are detected by intraoperative ultrasonography.

Glucagonoma in occasional MEN 1 patients causes a syndrome of hyperglycemia, skin rash (necrolytic migratory erythema), anorexia, glossitis, anemia, depression, diarrhea, and venous thrombosis. In about half of these patients the plasma glucagon level is high, leading to its designation as the *glucagonoma syndrome*, although elevation of plasma glucagon level in MEN 1 patients is not necessarily associated with these symptoms. The glucagonoma syndrome may represent a complex interaction between glucagon overproduction and the nutritional status of the patient.

The *Verner-Morrison* or *watery diarrhea syndrome* consists of watery diarrhea, hypokalemia, hypochlorhydria, and metabolic acidosis. The diarrhea can be voluminous and is almost always found in association with an islet cell tumor, prompting use of the term *pancreatic cholera*. However, the syndrome is not restricted to pancreatic islet tumors and has been observed with carcinoids or other tumors. This syndrome is believed to be due to overproduction of VIP, although plasma VIP levels may not be elevated. Hypercalcemia may

Table 339-1   Disease Associations in the Multiple Endocrine Neoplasia (MEN) Syndromes

| | MEN 2 | | |
MEN 1	MEN 2A	MEN 2B	Mixed Syndromes
Parathyroid hyperplasia or adenoma	MTC	MTC	Familial pheochromocytoma and islet cell tumor
Islet cell hyperplasia, adenoma, or carcinoma	Pheochromocytoma	Pheochromocytoma	von Hippel–Lindau syndrome, pheochromocytoma, and islet cell tumor
Pituitary hyperplasia or adenoma	Parathyroid hyperplasia or adenoma	Mucosal and gastrointestinal neuromas	
Other less common manifestations: foregut carcinoid, pheochromocytoma, subcutaneous or visceral lipomas, dermal angiofibromas or collagenomas	Cutaneous lichen amyloidosis	Marfanoid features	Neurofibromatosis with features of MEN 1 or 2
	Hirschsprung disease		Myxomas, spotty pigmentation, and generalized endocrine overactivity in a single family
	FMTC		

NOTE: MTC, medullary thyroid carcinoma; FMTC, familial MTC.

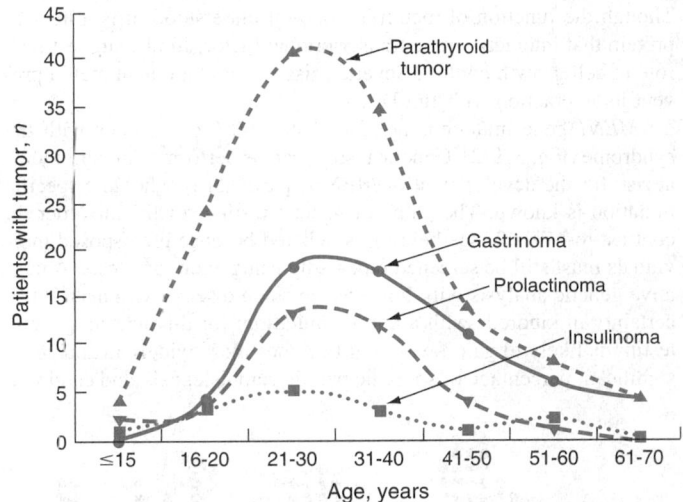

FIGURE 339-1 Age at onset of endocrine tumor expression in multiple endocrine neoplasia type 1 (MEN 1). Data derived from retrospective analysis for each endocrine organ hyperfunction in 130 cases of MEN 1. Age at onset is the age at first symptom or, with tumors not causing symptoms, age at the time of the first abnormal finding on a screening test. The rate of diagnosis of hyperparathyroidism increased sharply between ages 16 and 20 years. (*Reprinted with permission from Marx et al.*)

be induced by the effects of VIP on bone as well as by hyperparathyroidism.

Pituitary tumors occur in more than half of patients with MEN 1 and tend to be multicentric, making them difficult to resect (Chap. 328). Prolactinomas are most common (Fig. 339-1) and are diagnosed by finding serum prolactin levels >200 μg/L, with or without a pituitary mass evident by magnetic resonance imaging (MRI). Values <200 μg/L may be due to a prolactin-secreting neoplasm or to compression of the pituitary stalk by a different type of pituitary tumor. Acromegaly due to excessive growth hormone (GH) production is the second most common syndrome caused by pituitary tumors in MEN 1 (Chap. 328) but can rarely be due to production of GHRH by an islet cell tumor. Cushing's disease can be caused by ACTH-producing pituitary tumors or by ectopic production of ACTH or CRH by other tumors in the MEN 1 syndrome. Diagnosis of pituitary Cushing's disease is generally best accomplished by a high-dose dexamethasone suppression test or by petrosal venous sinus sampling for ACTH after intravenous injection of CRH (Chap. 328). Differentiation of a primary pituitary tumor from an ectopic CRH-producing tumor may be difficult because the pituitary is the source of ACTH in both disorders; documentation of CRH production by a pancreatic islet or carcinoid tumor may be the only method of proving ectopic CRH production. Adrenal cortical tumors are found in almost one-half of gene carriers but are rarely functional; malignancy in the cortical adenomas is uncommon.

Unusual manifestations of MEN 1   The rare carcinoid tumors in MEN 1 are of the foregut type and are derived from thymus, lung, stomach, or duodenum; they may metastasize or be locally invasive. These tumors usually produce serotonin, calcitonin, or CRH; the typical carcinoid syndrome with flushing, diarrhea, and bronchospasm is rare (Chap. 93). Subcutaneous or visceral lipomas and cutaneous leiomyomas may also be present but rarely undergo malignant transformation. Skin angiofibromas or collagenomas are seen in most patients with MEN 1 when carefully sought.

GENETIC CONSIDERATIONS   MEN 1 is transmitted as an autosomal dominant trait, reflecting the fact that the *MEN1* gene, located on chromosome 11q13, encodes a tumor suppressor protein termed *menin* (Fig. 339-2). Affected individuals typically harbor a germline mutation in *MEN1* and acquire a "second hit" in the normal gene as a result of another mutation or, more commonly, loss of the portion of chromosome 11 that contains the *MEN1* locus (Chap. 81). Though the function of menin is not well understood, it is a nuclear protein that interacts with a transcriptional factor, Jun D, suggesting a role in cell growth control. Several missense mutations in menin prevent its interaction with Jun D.

MEN1 gene mutations are found in >90% of families with the syndrome (Fig. 339-2). Genetic testing can be performed in individuals at risk for the development of MEN 1, particularly when the specific mutation is known. The value of genetic testing for this disorder, in contrast to MEN 2 (see below), is debated because predisposed individuals must still be screened repeatedly using endocrine tests. A negative genetic analysis will, however, exclude disease with near 100% certainty in kindreds with a known mutation; for this reason, genetic testing is likely to gain favor as it becomes more widely available. A significant percentage of sporadic parathyroid, islet cell, and carcinoid

tumors also have loss or mutation of *MEN1*. It is presumed that these mutations are somatic and occur in a single cell, leading to subsequent transformation. ■

TREATMENT   Almost everyone who inherits a mutant *MEN1* gene develops at least one clinical manifestation of the syndrome. Most develop hyperparathyroidism, 80% develop pancreatic islet cell tumors, and more than half develop pituitary tumors. For most of these tumors, initial surgery is not curative and patients frequently require multiple surgical procedures and surgery on two or more endocrine glands during a lifetime. For this reason, it is essential to establish clear goals for management of these patients rather than to recommend surgery casually each time a tumor is discovered. Ranges for acceptable management are discussed below.

Hyperparathyroidism   Individuals with serum calcium levels >3.0 mmol/L (12 mg/dL), evidence of calcium nephrolithiasis or renal dysfunction, neuropathic or muscular symptoms, or bone involvement (including osteopenia) should undergo parathyroid exploration. In MEN 1 an additional criterion for parathyroid surgery is hypercalcemia associated with elevated gastrin levels, because elevated serum calcium may stimulate gastrin production and ZES, a condition that may be improved by return of calcium levels to normal. There is less agreement regarding the necessity for parathyroid exploration in individuals who do not meet these criteria, and observation may be appropriate in the MEN 1 patient with asymptomatic hyperparathyroidism.

When parathyroid surgery is indicated in MEN 1, all parathyroid tissue should be identified and removed at the time of primary operation, and parathyroid tissue should be implanted in the nondominant forearm. Thymectomy should also be performed because of the potential for later development of malignant carcinoid tumors. If reoperation is necessary, transplanted tissue can be resected under local anesthesia with titration of tissue removal to return the serum calcium level to normal. A less desirable approach is to remove 3 to 3½ parathyroid glands from the neck, carefully marking the location of residual tissue so that the remaining tissue can be located easily during subsequent surgery.

Pancreatic Islet Tumors   (See Chap. 93 for discussion of pancreatic islet tumors not associated with MEN 1.) Two features of pancreatic islet cell tumors in MEN 1 complicate the management. First, the pancreatic islet cell tumors are multicentric, malignant about a third of the time, and cause death in 10 to 20% of patients. Second, removal of all pancreatic islets to prevent malignancy causes diabetes mellitus, a disease with severe long-term complications. These features make it difficult to formulate clear-cut guidelines, but some general concepts appear to be valid. First, islet cell tumors producing insulin, glucagon, VIP, GHRH, or CRH should be resected because medical therapy is generally ineffective. Second, gastrin-producing islet cell tumors that cause ZES are frequently multicentric. Recent experience suggests that a high percentage of ZES in MEN 1 is caused by duodenal wall tumors and that resection of these tumors improves the cure rate. Treatment with H_2 receptor antagonists (cimetidine or ranitidine) and the H^+,K^+-ATPase inhibitors (omeprazole or lansoprazole) provides an alternative to surgery for control of ulcer disease in patients with multicentric tumors or with hepatic metastases. Third, in families in which there is a high incidence of malignant islet cell tumors that cause death, total pancreatectomy at an early age may be justified to prevent malignancy.

Management of metastatic islet cell carcinoma is unsatisfactory.

FIGURE 339-2   Schematic depiction of the *MEN1* gene and the distribution of mutations. The shaded areas show coding sequence. The closed circles show the relative distribution of mutations, mostly inactivating, in each exon. Mutation data are derived from the Human Gene Mutation Database from which more detailed information can be obtained (www.uwcm.ac.uk/uwcm/mg/hgmd0.html) (*From M Krawczak, DN Cooper: Trends Genet 13:1321, 1998.*)

Hormonal abnormalities can sometimes be controlled. For example, ZES can be treated with H_2 receptor antagonists or H^+,K^+-ATPase inhibitors; the somatostatin analogue, octreotide, is useful in the management of carcinoid and the watery diarrhea syndrome. Bilateral adrenalectomy may be required for ectopic ACTH syndrome if medical therapy is ineffective (Chap. 331). Islet cell carcinomas frequently metastasize to the liver but may grow slowly. Hepatic artery embolization or chemotherapy (5-fluorouracil, streptozocin, chlorozotocin, doxorubicin, or dacarbazine) may reduce tumor mass, control symptoms of hormone excess, and prolong life; however, these treatments are never curative.

Pituitary Tumors Treatment of prolactinomas with dopamine agonists (bromocriptine, cabergoline, or quinagolide) usually returns the serum prolactin level to normal and prevents further tumor growth (Chap. 328). Surgical resection of a prolactinoma is rarely curative but may relieve mass effects. Transsphenoidal resection is appropriate for neoplasms that secrete ACTH, GH, or the α-subunit of the pituitary glycoprotein hormones. Octreotide reduces tumor mass in one-third of GH-secreting tumors and reduces GH and insulin-like growth factor I levels in 75% of patients. Radiation therapy may be useful for large or recurrent tumors.

Improvements in the management of MEN 1, particularly islet cell and pituitary tumors, have improved outcome in these patients substantially. As a result, other neoplastic manifestations, such as carcinoid syndrome, are now seen with increased frequency.

MULTIPLE ENDOCRINE NEOPLASIA TYPE 2 **Clinical Manifestations** Medullary thyroid carcinoma (MTC) and pheochromocytoma are associated in two major syndromes: MEN type 2A and MEN type 2B (Table 339-1). MEN 2A is the combination of MTC, hyperparathyroidism, and pheochromocytoma. Three subvariants of MEN 2A are familial medullary thyroid carcinoma (FMTC), MEN 2A with cutaneous lichen amyloidosis, and MEN 2A with Hirschsprung disease. MEN type 2B is the combination of MTC, pheochromocytoma, mucosal neuromas, intestinal ganglioneuromatosis, and marfanoid features.

Multiple endocrine neoplasia type 2A MTC is the most common manifestation. This tumor usually develops in childhood, beginning as hyperplasia of the calcitonin-producing cells (C cells) of the thyroid. MTC is typically located at the junction of the upper one-third and lower two-thirds of each lobe of the thyroid, reflecting the high density of C cells in this location; tumors >1 cm in size are frequently associated with local or distant metastases. Measurement of the serum calcitonin level after calcium or pentagastrin injection makes it possible to diagnose this disorder when the likelihood of metastasis is low (see below).

Pheochromocytoma occurs in approximately 50% of patients with MEN 2A and causes palpitations, nervousness, headaches, and sometimes sweating (Chap. 332). About half the tumors are bilateral, and >50% of patients who have had unilateral adrenalectomy develop a pheochromocytoma in the contralateral gland within a decade. A second feature of these tumors is a disproportionate increase in the secretion of epinephrine relative to norepinephrine. Capsular invasion is common, but malignant behavior is uncommon.

FIGURE 339-3 Schematic diagram of the *RET* proto-oncogene showing mutations found in MEN type 2 and sporadic medullary thyroid carcinoma (MTC). The *RET* proto-oncogene is located on the proximal arm of chromosome 10q (10q11.2). Activating mutations of two functional domains of RET tyrosine kinase receptor have been identified. The first affects a cysteine-rich (Cys-Rich) region in the extracellular portion of the receptor. Each germline mutation changes a cysteine at codons 609, 611, 618, 620, or 634 to another amino acid. The second region is the intracellular tyrosine kinase (TK) domain. Codon 634 mutations account for approximately 80% of all germline mutations. Mutations of codons 630, 768, 883, and 918 have been identified as somatic (nongermline) mutations that occur in a single parafollicular or C cell within the thyroid gland in sporadic MTC. A codon 918 mutation is the most common somatic mutation. Abbreviations: MEN 2, multiple endocrine neoplasia type 2; CLA cutaneous lichen amyloidosis; FMTC, familial medullary thyroid carcinoma; Signal, the signal peptide; Cadherin, a cadherin-like region in the extracellular domain; TM, transmembrane domain; TK, tyrosine kinase domain.

Hyperparathyroidism occurs in 15 to 20% of patients, with the peak incidence in the third or fourth decade. The manifestations of hyperparathyroidism do not differ from those in other forms of primary hyperparathyroidism (Chap. 341), with nephrolithiasis being common. Diagnosis is established by finding hypercalcemia, hypophosphatemia, hypercalciuria, and an inappropriately high serum level of intact parathyroid hormone. Multiglandular parathyroid hyperplasia is the most common histologic finding, although with long-standing disease adenomatous changes may be superimposed on hyperplasia.

Multiple endocrine neoplasia type 2B The association of MTC, pheochromocytoma, mucosal neuromas, and a marfanoid habitus is designated MEN 2B. MTC in MEN 2B develops earlier and is more aggressive than in MEN 2A. Metastatic disease has been described prior to 1 year of age, and death commonly occurs in the second or third decade of life. However, the prognosis is not invariably bad even in patients with metastatic disease, as evidenced by a number of multigenerational families with this disease.

Pheochromocytoma occurs in more than half of MEN 2B patients and does not differ from that in MEN 2A. Hypercalcemia is rare in MEN 2B, and there are no well-documented examples of hyperparathyroidism.

The mucosal neuromas and marfanoid body habitus are the most distinctive features and are recognizable in childhood. Neuromas are present on the tip of the tongue, under the eyelids, and throughout the gastrointestinal tract and are true neuromas, distinct from neurofibromas. Children may present with gastrointestinal symptoms, including increased gas, intermittent obstruction, and diarrhea caused by neuromas.

GENETIC CONSIDERATIONS Mutations of the *RET* protooncogene have been identified in 93 to 95% of patients with MEN 2 (Fig. 339-3). *RET* encodes a tyrosine kinase receptor that is normally activated by glial cell line–derived neurotropic factor. *RET* mutations induce constitutive activity of the receptor, explaining the autosomal dominant transmission of the disorder.

Naturally occurring mutations localize to two regions of the RET tyrosine kinase receptor. The first is a cysteine-rich extracellular domain; point mutations in the coding sequence for one of five cysteines (codons 609, 611, 618, 620, or 634) cause amino acid substitutions that induce receptor dimerization and activation in the absence of its ligand. Codon 634 mutations occur in 80% of MEN 2A kindreds and are most commonly associated with classic MEN 2A features (Figs. 339-3 and 339-2); an arginine substitution at this codon accounts for half of all MEN 2A mutations. All reported families with MEN 2A and cutaneous lichen amyloidosis are consistently associated with a codon 634 mutation. Mutations of codons 609, 611, 618, or 620 occur in 10 to 15% of MEN 2A kindreds and are more commonly associated with FMTC (Fig. 339-3). Mutations in codons 609, 618, and 620 have also been identified in MEN 2A and in the Hirschsprung variant (Fig. 339-3).

The second region of the RET tyrosine kinase that is mutated in MEN 2 is in the substrate recognition pocket at codon 918 (Fig. 339-3). This activating mutation is present in approximately 95% of patients with MEN 2B and accounts for 10 to 15% of all *RET* proto-oncogene mutations in MEN 2. Mutations of codon 883 and 22 have also been identified in a few patients with MEN 2B.

From 3 to 5% of kindreds with FMTC have no identifiable mutation of either of these regions. In a few such kindreds mutations of codons 768, 790, 791, 804, and 891 have been identified (Fig. 339-3).

Somatic mutations (found only in the tumor and not transmitted in the germline) of the *RET* proto-oncogene have been identified in sporadic MTC; 25 to 35% of sporadic tumors have codon 918 mutations, and somatic mutations in codons 630, 768, and 804 have also been identified (Fig. 339-3). Germline mutations of the *RET* proto-oncogene are present in about 6% of patients with apparent sporadic MTC, indicating that other family members may be at risk for the disease. ■

℞ **TREATMENT   Screening for Multiple Endocrine Neoplasia Type 2**   Death from MTC can be prevented by early thyroidectomy. The identification of *RET* proto-oncogene mutations and the application of DNA-based molecular diagnostic techniques to identify these mutations has simplified the screening process. During the initial evaluation of a kindred, a *RET* proto-oncogene analysis should be performed on an individual with proven MEN 2A. Establishment of the specific mutation in a kindred facilitates the subsequent analysis of other family members. Each family member at risk should be tested twice for the presence of the specific mutation; the second analysis should be performed on a new DNA sample and, ideally, in a second laboratory to exclude sample mix-up or technical error (see *endrcr06.mda.uth.tmc.edu* for a list of laboratory testing sites). Individuals in a kindred with a known mutation who have two normal analyses can be excluded from further screening.

There is general consensus that children with codon 883, 918, and 922 mutations, or those associated with MEN 2B, should have a total thyroidectomy and central lymph node dissection (level VI) performed during the first months of life or soon after identification of the syndrome. If local metastasis is discovered, a more extensive lymph node dissection (levels II to V) is generally indicated. In children with codon 611, 618, 620, 630, 634, and 891 mutations, thyroidectomy should be performed before the age of 6 years because of reports of local metastatic disease in children this age. Finally, there are kindreds with codon 609, 768, 790, 791, and 804 mutations where the phenotype of MTC appears to be less aggressive. In these kindreds, and in those with rare mutations, two management approaches have been suggested in association with genetic counseling: (1) perform a total thyroidectomy with or without central node dissection at some arbitrary age

(perhaps 6 to 12 years of age), or (2) continue annual or biannual provocative testing for calcitonin release with performance of total thyroidectomy with or without central neck dissection when the test becomes abnormal. The pentagastrin test involves measurement of serum calcitonin basally and 2, 5, 10, and 15 min after a bolus injection of 5 μg pentagastrin per kilogram body weight. Patients should be warned before injection of epigastric tightness, nausea, warmth, and tingling of extremities and reassured that the symptoms will last approximately 2 min. The recent unavailability of pentagastrin in the United States has led to use of a short calcium infusion, performed by obtaining a baseline serum calcitonin and then infusing 150 mg calcium salt intravenously over 10 min with measurement of serum calcitonin at 5, 10, 15, 30 min after initiation of the infusion.

The *RET* proto-oncogene analysis should be performed in patients with suspected MEN 2B to detect codon 883, 918, and 922 mutations, especially in newborn children where the diagnosis is suspected but the clinical phenotype is not fully developed. Other family members at risk for MEN 2B should also be tested because the mucosal neuromas can be subtle and not always identified. In the rare families with proven germline transmission of MTC but no identifiable *RET* proto-oncogene mutation, annual pentagastrin or calcium-pentagastrin testing should be performed on members at risk.

Annual screening for pheochromocytoma in subjects with germline *RET* mutations should be performed by measuring basal plasma or 24-h urine catecholamines and metanephrines. The goal is to identify a pheochromocytoma before it causes significant symptoms or is likely to cause sudden death, an event most commonly associated with large tumors. Although there are kindreds with FMTC and specific *RET* mutations in which no pheochromocytomas have been identified (Fig. 339-3), it is not clear that a large enough experience has been gained to exclude pheochromocytoma screening in these individuals. Radiographic studies, such as MRI or CT scans, are generally reserved for individuals with abnormal screening tests or with symptoms suggestive of pheochromocytoma (Chap. 332). Women should be tested during pregnancy because undetected pheochromocytoma can cause maternal death during childbirth.

Measurement of serum calcium and parathyroid hormone levels every 2 to 3 years provides an adequate screen for hyperparathyroidism, except in those families in which hyperparathyroidism is a prominent component, where measurements should be made annually.

Treatment of Medullary Thyroid Carcinoma   MTC is a multicentric disorder. Total thyroidectomy with a central lymph node dissection should be performed in children who carry the mutant genes. Incomplete thyroidectomy leaves the possibility of later transformation of residual long-term C cells. The goal of early therapy is cure, and a strategy that does not accomplish this goal is short-sighted. Long-term follow-up studies indicate an excellent outcome with approximately 90% of children free of disease 15 to 20 years after surgery. In contrast, 15 to 25% of patients in whom the diagnosis is made on the basis of a palpable thyroid nodule die from the disease within 15 to 20 years.

In adults with MTC >1 cm in size, metastases to regional lymph nodes are common. Total thyroidectomy with central lymph node dissection and selective dissection of other regional chains provide the best chance for cure. In patients with extensive local metastatic disease in the neck, external radiation may prevent local recurrence or reduce tumor mass but is not curative. Chemotherapy with combinations of adriamycin, vincristine, cyclophosphamide, and dacarbazine may provide palliation.

Treatment of Pheochromocytoma   The long-term goal for management of pheochromocytoma is to prevent death and cardiovascular complications. Improvements in radiographic imaging of the adrenals make direct examination of the apparently normal contralateral gland during surgery less important, and the rapid evolution of laparoscopic surgery has simplified management of early pheochromocytoma. The major question is whether to remove both adrenal glands or to remove only the affected adrenal at the time of primary surgery. Issues to be considered in making this decision include the possibility of malignancy (<15 reported cases), the likelihood of developing pheochromocytoma in the apparently unaffected gland over an 8- to 10-year period, and the risks of adrenal insufficiency caused by removal of both glands (at least two deaths related to adrenal insufficiency in MEN 2 patients). Most clinicians recommend removing only the affected gland. If both adrenals are removed, glucocorticoid and mineralocorticoid replacement is mandatory. An alternative approach is to remove the pheochromocytoma and adrenal medulla, leaving the adrenal cortex behind. This approach is usually successful and eliminates the necessity for steroid hormone replacement, although the pheochromocytoma recurs in some.

Treatment of Hyperparathyroidism Hyperparathyroidism has been managed by one of two approaches. Removal of 3½ glands with maintenance of the remaining half gland in the neck is the usual procedure. In families in whom hyperparathyroidism is a prominent manifestation (almost always associated with a codon 634 *RET* mutation) and recurrence is common, total parathyroidectomy with transplantation of parathyroid tissue into the nondominant forearm is preferred. This approach is discussed above in the context of hyperparathyroidism associated with MEN 1.

OTHER GENETIC TUMOR SYNDROMES

A number of mixed syndromes exist in which the neoplastic associations differ from those in MEN 1 or 2 (Table 339-1).

The cause of von Hippel–Lindau (VHL) syndrome, the association of central nervous system tumors, renal cell carcinoma, pheochromocytoma, and islet cell neoplasms, is mutations in the *VHL* tumor-suppressor gene. Germline-inactivating mutations of the *VHL* gene cause tumor formation when there is additional loss or somatic mutation of the normal *VHL* allele in brain, kidney, pancreatic islet, or adrenal medullary cells. A specific subset of mutations is more common in families with pheochromocytomas.

The molecular defect in type 1 neurofibromatosis inactivates neurofibromin, a cell membrane–associated protein that normally activates a GTPase. Inactivation of this protein impairs GTPase and causes continuous activation of p21 Ras and its downstream tyrosine kinase pathway. Endocrine tumors also form in less common neoplastic genetic syndromes. These include Cowden's disease, Carney complex, familial acromegaly, and familial carcinoid syndrome.

IMMUNOLOGIC SYNDROMES AFFECTING MULTIPLE ENDOCRINE ORGANS

When immune dysfunction affects two or more endocrine glands and other nonendocrine immune disorders are present, the *polyglandular autoimmune* (PGA) *syndromes* should be considered. The PGA syndromes are classified as two main types: the type I syndrome starts in childhood and is characterized by mucocutaneous candidiasis, hypoparathyroidism, and adrenal insufficiency; the type II, or *Schmidt syndrome*, is more likely to present in adults and most commonly comprises adrenal insufficiency, thyroiditis, and type 1 diabetes mellitus. However, the type II syndrome is heterogeneous and may consist of autoimmune thyroid disease along with a variety of other autoimmune endocrine disorders (Table 339-2).

POLYGLANDULAR AUTOIMMUNE SYNDROME TYPE I

PGA type I is usually recognized in the first decade of life and requires two of three components for diagnosis: mucocutaneous candidiasis, hypoparathyroidism, and adrenal insufficiency. Mineralocorticoids and glucocorticoids may be lost simultaneously or sequentially. This disorder is also called *autoimmune polyendocrinopathy-candidiasis-ectodermal dystrophy* (APECED). Other endocrine defects can include gonadal failure, hypothyroidism, anterior hypophysitis, and, less commonly, destruction of the β cells of the pancreatic islets and development of insulin-dependent (type 1) diabetes mellitus. Additional features include hypoplasia of the dental enamel, ungual dystrophy, tympanic membrane sclerosis, vitiligo, keratopathy, and gas-

Table 339-2 Features of Polyglandular Autoimmune (PGA) Syndromes

PGA I	PGA II
EPIDEMIOLOGY	
Autosomal recessive	Polygenic inheritance
Mutations in APECED gene	HLA-DR3 and HLA-DR4 associated
Childhood onset	Adult onset
Equal male:female ratio	Female predominance
DISEASE ASSOCIATIONS	
Mucocutaneous candidiasis	Adrenal insufficiency
Hypoparathyroidism	Hypothyroidism
Adrenal insufficiency	Graves' disease
Hypogonadism	Type 1 diabetes
Alopecia	Hypogonadism
Hypothyroidism	Hypophysitis
Dental enamel hypoplasia	Myasthenia gravis
Malabsorption	Vitiligo
Chronic active hepatitis	Alopecia
Vitiligo	Pernicious anemia
Pernicious anemia	Celiac disease

NOTE: APECED, autoimmune polyendocrinopathy-candidiasis-ectodermal dystrophy.

tric parietal cell dysfunction resulting in pernicious anemia. Some patients develop autoimmune hepatitis, malabsorption (variably attributed to intestinal lymphangiectasia, IgA deficiency, bacterial overgrowth, or hypoparathyroidism), asplenism, achalasia, and cholelithiasis (Table 339-2). At the outset, only one organ may be involved, but the number increases with time so that patients eventually manifest two to five components of the syndrome.

Most patients initially present with oral candidiasis in childhood; it is poorly responsive to treatment and relapses frequently. Chronic hypoparathyroidism usually occurs before adrenal insufficiency develops. More than 60% of postpubertal women develop premature hypogonadism. The endocrine components, including adrenal insufficiency and hypoparathyroidism, may not develop until the fourth decade, making continued surveillance necessary.

Type I PGA syndrome allows no HLA associations and is inherited as an autosomal recessive trait. The responsible gene, designated as either *APECED* or *AIRE*, encodes a transcription factor that is expressed in thymus and lymph nodes; a variety of different mutations have been reported.

POLYGLANDULAR AUTOIMMUNE SYNDROME TYPE II

PGA type II is characterized by two or more of the endocrinopathies listed in Table 339-2. Most often these include primary adrenal insufficiency, Graves' disease or autoimmune hypothyroidism, type 1 diabetes mellitus, and primary hypogonadism. Because adrenal insufficiency is relatively rare, it is frequently used to define the presence of the syndrome. Among patients with adrenal insufficiency, type 1 diabetes mellitus coexists in 52% and autoimmune thyroid disease occurs in 69%. However, many patients with antimicrosomal and antithyroglobulin antibodies never develop abnormalities of thyroid function. Thus, increased antibody titers alone are poor predictors of future disease. Other associated conditions include hypophysitis, celiac disease, atrophic gastritis, and pernicious anemia. Vitiligo, caused by antibodies against the melanocyte (see Plate IIA-11), and alopecia are less common than in the type I syndrome. Mucocutaneous candidiasis does not occur. A few patients develop a late-onset, usually transient hypoparathyroidism caused by antibodies that compete with parathyroid hormone for binding to the parathyroid hormone receptor. Up to 25% of patients with myasthenia gravis, and an even higher percentage who have myasthenia and a thymoma, have PGA type II (Chap. 380).

The type II syndrome is familial in nature but does not exhibit a characteristic Mendelian pattern of transmission. Like many of the individual autoimmune endocrinopathies, certain HL-DR3 and HLA-

DR4 alleles increase disease susceptibility; several different genes probably contribute to the expression of this syndrome.

A variety of autoantibodies are seen in PGA type II, including antibodies directed against: (1) thyroid antigens such as thyroid peroxidase, thyroglobulin, or the thyroid stimulating hormone (TSH) receptor; (2) adrenal side chain cleavage enzyme, steroid 21-hydroxylase, or ACTH receptor; and (3) pancreatic islet glutamic acid decarboxylase or the insulin receptor, among others. The roles of cytokines such as interferon and cell-mediated immunity are unclear.

DIAGNOSIS The clinical manifestations of adrenal insufficiency often develop slowly, may be difficult to detect, and can be fatal if not diagnosed and treated appropriately. Thus, prospective screening should be performed routinely in all patients and family members at risk for PGA types I and II. The most effective screening test for adrenal disease is a cosyntropin stimulation test (Chap. 331). A fasting blood glucose level can be obtained to screen for hyperglycemia. Additional screening tests should include measurements of TSH, luteinizing hormone, follicle-stimulating hormone, and, in men, testosterone levels. In families with suspected type I PGA syndrome, calcium and phosphorus levels should be measured. These screening studies should be performed every 1 to 2 years up to about age 50 in families with PGA type II syndrome and until about age 40 in patients with type I syndrome. Screening measurements of autoantibodies against potentially affected endocrine organs are of uncertain prognostic value. The differential diagnosis of PGA syndrome should include the DiGeorge syndrome (hypoparathyroidism due to glandular agenesis and mucocutaneous candidiasis), Kearns-Sayre syndrome (hypoparathyroidism, primary hypogonadism, type 1 diabetes mellitus, and panhypopituitarism), Wolfram's syndrome (congenital diabetes insipidus and diabetes mellitus), and congenital rubella (type 1 diabetes mellitus and hypothyroidism).

[Rx] **TREATMENT** With the exception of Graves' disease, the management of each of the endocrine components of the disease involves hormone replacement and is covered in detail in the chapters on adrenal, thyroid, gonadal, and parathyroid disease (Chaps. 330, 331, 335, 336, and 341). One aspect of therapy deserves special emphasis. Namely, primary hypothyroidism can mask adrenal insufficiency by prolonging the half-life of cortisol; consequently, administration of thyroid hormone to a patient with unsuspected adrenal insufficiency can precipitate adrenal crisis. Thus, all patients with hypothyroidism in the context of PGA syndrome should be screened for adrenal disease and, if it is present, be treated with glucocorticoids prior to or concurrently with thyroid hormone therapy.

OTHER AUTOIMMUNE ENDOCRINE SYNDROMES
Insulin Receptor Antibodies   Rare insulin-resistance syndromes occur in patients who develop antibodies that block the interaction of insulin with its receptor. Conversely, other classes of anti-insulin receptor antibodies can activate the receptor and can cause hypoglycemia; this disorder should be considered in the differential diagnosis of fasting hypoglycemia (Chap. 334).

Patients with insulin receptor antibodies and acanthosis nigricans are often middle-aged women who acquire insulin resistance in association with other autoimmune disorders such as systemic lupus erythematosus or Sjögren's syndrome. Vitiligo, alopecia, Raynaud's phenomenon, and arthritis may also be seen. Other autoimmune endocrine disorders, including thyrotoxicosis, hypothyroidism, and hypogonadism, occur rarely. Acanthosis nigricans, a velvety, hyperpigmented, thickened skin lesion, is prominent on the dorsum of the neck and other skin fold areas in the axillae or groin and often heralds the diagnosis in these patients. However, acanthosis nigricans also occurs in patients with obesity or polycystic ovarian syndrome, in which insulin resistance appears to be due to a postreceptor defect; thus acan-

thosis nigricans itself is not diagnostic of the immunologic form of insulin resistance.

Some patients with acanthosis nigricans have mild glucose intolerance, with a compensatory increase in insulin secretion that is only detected when insulin levels are measured. Others have severe diabetes mellitus requiring massive doses of insulin (several thousand units per day) to lower the blood glucose levels. The nature of the antibodies determines the manifestations; though insulin resistance is more common, fasting hypoglycemia can result from insulinomimetic antibodies.

Ataxia telangiectasia is an autosomal recessive disorder caused by mutations in *ATM*, a gene involved in cellular responses to ionizing radiation and oxidative damage (Chap. 364). This disorder is characterized by ataxia, telangiectasia, immune abnormalities, and an increased incidence of malignancies. Insulin-resistant diabetes mellitus occurs and is associated with anti-insulin antibodies.

Autoimmune Insulin Syndrome with Hypoglycemia   This disorder typically occurs in patients with other autoimmune disorders and is caused by polyclonal insulin-binding autoantibodies that bind to endogenously synthesized insulin. If the insulin dissociates from the antibodies several hours or more after a meal, hypoglycemia can result. Most cases of the syndrome have been described from Japan, and there may be a genetic component. In plasma cell dyscrasias such as multiple myeloma, the plasma cells may produce monoclonal antibodies against insulin and cause hypoglycemia by a similar mechanism.

Antithyroxine Antibodies and Hypothyroidism   Circulating autoantibodies against thyroid hormones in patients with both immune thyroid disease and plasma cell dyscrasias such as Waldenström's macroglobulinemia can bind thyroid hormones, decrease their biologic activity, and result in primary hypothyroidism. In other patients the antibodies simply interfere with thyroid hormone immunoassays and cause false elevations or decreases in measured hormone levels.

Crow-Fukase Syndrome   The features of this syndrome are highlighted by an acronym that emphasizes its important features: *p*olyneuropathy, *o*rganomegaly, *e*ndocrinopathy, *M*-proteins, and *s*kin changes (POEMS). The most important feature is a severe, progressive sensorimotor polyneuropathy associated with a plasma cell dyscrasia. Localized collections of plasma cells (plasmacytomas) can cause sclerotic bone lesions and produce monoclonal IgG or IgA proteins. Endocrine manifestations include amenorrhea in women and impotence and gynecomastia in men, hypogonadism, hyperprolactinemia, type 2 diabetes mellitus, primary hypothyroidism, and adrenal insufficiency. Skin changes include hyperpigmentation, thickening of the dermis, hirsutism, and hyperhidrosis. Hepatomegaly and lymphadenopathy occur in about two-thirds of patients, and splenomegaly is seen in about one-third. Other manifestations include increased cerebrospinal fluid pressure with papilledema, peripheral edema, ascites, pleural effusions, glomerulonephritis, and fever. Five-year survival is about 60%.

The systemic nature of the disorder may cause confusion with other connective tissue diseases. The endocrine manifestations suggest an autoimmune basis of the disorder, but circulating antibodies against endocrine cells have not been demonstrated. Increased serum and tissue levels of interleukin 6, interleukin 1β, vascular endothelial growth factor, and tumor necrosis factor α are present, but the pathophysiologic basis for the POEMS syndrome is uncertain. Therapy directed against the plasma cell dyscrasia such as local radiation of bony lesions, chemotherapy, plasmapheresis, and treatment with all-*trans* retinoic acid may result in endocrine improvement.

MISCELLANEOUS DISORDERS WITH ENDOCRINE MANIFESTATIONS

A variety of other clinical and genetic disorders are associated with multiple endocrine manifestations are summarized in Table 339-3.

Table 339-3 Other Disorders with Common Polyglandular Manifestations

Condition	Clinical Features	Type of Endocrine Involvement Hypothalamic-Pituitary	Thyroid	Parathyroid	Pancreas	Adrenal	Gonads	Inheritance/ Molecular Defect
Ataxia-telangiectasia	Early ataxia Oculocutaneous telangiectasia Immunologic deficiency	Occasional diminished pituitary reserve			Diabetes mellitus	Cortical hypoplasia	Dysgenetic gonads: gonadoblastomas later in females	Autosomal recessive Mutation of *ATM* gene
Pseudohypoparathyroidism	Short stature Short metacarpals and metatarsals Round facies Ectopic calcification	Variable deficiency of all pituitary hormones including prolactin	Hypo- or hyper-thyroidism	Elevated parathyroid hormone levels with normo- or hypocalcemia	Diabetes mellitus		Ovarian failure	Mutation of the $G_{\alpha s}$
Myotonic dystrophy	Muscular dystrophy Premature baldness Mental retardation	Gonadotropin and growth hormone abnormalities, ? related to central integrative defect	Hypothyroidism		Diabetes mellitus		Primary gonadal failure	Insertion of unstable CTG repeat in myotonic dystrophy gene on chromosome 19
Noonan syndrome	Short stature Ptosis Webbed neck Pulmonary stenosis	Gonadotropin deficiency	Thyroiditis				Primary gonadal failure	Autosomal dominant
Fanconi syndrome	Short stature Bone marrow hypoplasia Abnormal skin pigmentation Radius malformations	Panhypopituitarism			Diabetes mellitus	Adrenal atrophy	Gonadal atrophy	Autosomal recessive Mutation of *FAA* gene
Werner syndrome	Premature aging Atropic skin Cataracts Early osteopenia		Papillary thyroid carcinoma		Diabetes mellitus		Gonadal atrophy	Autosomal recessive Mutation of *WRN* gene

NOTE: ATM, ataxia telangiectasia mutated; FAA, Fanconi anemia A; WRN, Werner.

BIBLIOGRAPHY

AGARWAL SK et al: Menin interacts with the AP1 transcription factor JunD and represses JunD-activated transcription. Cell 84:730, 1999

BETTERLE C et al: Clinical review 93: Autoimmune polyglandular syndrome type I. J Clin Endocrinol Metab 83:1049, 1998

BONI R et al: Somatic mutations of the MEN1 tumor suppressor gene detected in sporadic angiofibromas. J Invest Dermatol 111:539, 1998

CHANDRASEKHARAPPA SC et al: Positional cloning of the gene for multiple endocrine neoplasia-type 1. Science 276:404, 1997

DRALLE H et al: Prophylactic thyroidectomy in 75 children and adolescents with hereditary medullary thyroid carcinoma: German and Austrian experience. World J Surg 22:744, 1998

EISENHOFER G et al: Plasma normetanephrine and metanephrine for detecting pheochromocytoma in von Hippel–Lindau disease and multiple endocrine neoplasia type 2. N Engl J Med 340:1872, 9, 1999

GAGEL RF: Multiple endocrine neoplasia, in *Williams Textbook of Endocrinology*, 9th ed, JD Wilson, et al (eds). Philadelphia, Saunders, 1998

HEINO M et al: Mutation analyses of North American APS-1 patients. Hum Mutat 13:69, 1999

MARX S et al: Multiple endocrine neoplasia type 1: Clinical and genetic topics. Ann Intern Med 129:484, 1998

NORTON JA et al: Surgery to cure the Zollinger-Ellison syndrome. N Engl J Med 341:635, 1999

SCOTT HS et al: Common mutations in autoimmune polyendocrinopathy-candidiasis-ectodermal dystrophy patients of different origins. Mol Endocrinol 12:1112, 1998

SOUBRIER MJ et al: POEMS syndrome: Study of 25 cases and a review of the literature. Am J Med 97:543, 1994

340 | *Michael F. Holick, Stephen M. Krane*

INTRODUCTION TO BONE AND MINERAL METABOLISM

BONE STRUCTURE AND METABOLIM
(See also Chap. 343)

Bone is a dynamic tissue that is remodeled constantly throughout life. The arrangement of compact and cancellous bone provides a strength and density suitable for mobility. In addition, bone provides a reservoir for calcium, magnesium, phosphorus, sodium, and other ions necessary for homeostatic functions. The skeleton is highly vascular and receives about 10% of the cardiac output.

The extracellular components of bone consist of a solid mineral phase in close association with an organic matrix, of which 90 to 95% is type I collagen (Chap. 351). The noncollagenous portion of the organic matrix contains proteins derived from serum (albumin and α_2-HS glycoproteins), proteins containing α-carboxyglutamic acid (GLA) [*bone GLA protein (BGP)*, *osteocalcin*, and a matrix GLA protein], the glycoprotein *osteonectin*, the phosphoprotein *osteopontin*, sialoproteins, *thrombospondin*, and other less well characterized proteins. Some of these proteins may function in initiating mineralization and in binding of the mineral phase to the matrix. The mineral phase is made up of calcium and phosphate and is best characterized as a poorly crystalline hydroxyapatite. The mineral phase of bone is deposited initially in intimate relation to the collagen fibrils and is found in specific locations in the "holes" between the collagen fibrils. This architectural arrangement of mineral and matrix results in a two-phase material well suited to withstand mechanical stresses.

Osteoblasts synthesize and secrete the organic matrix. Mineralization of the matrix, both in trabecular bone and in osteones of compact cortical bone (haversian systems), begins soon after the matrix is secreted (primary mineralization) but is not completed until after several weeks (secondary mineralization). Osteoblasts are derived from cells of mesenchymal origin (Fig. 340-1*A*). Although relatively little is known about the controls of osteoblast development, two genes have been shown to be important: core-binding factor A1 (*CBFA1*) and Indian hedgehog (*Ihh*). CBFA1 is a transcription factor and a homologue of the Drosophila factor, runt, and is expressed specifically in osteoblast progenitors and regulates the expression of several osteoblast-specific genes including osteopontin, bone sialoprotein, type I collagen, osteocalcin, and receptor-activator of NFκB (RANK) ligand. CBFA1 expression is regulated, in part, by bone morphogenic proteins (BMPs). *Cbfa1*-deficient mice are devoid of osteoblasts. Mice with a functional deletion of *Cbfa1* (*Cbfa1* $-/-$) have a cartilaginous skeleton but no osteoblasts and no bone, whereas mice with a deletion of only one allele (*Cbfa1* $+/-$) do have an osseous skeleton but have a delay in intramembranous bone formation of some cranial bones and the clavicles. The latter abnormalities are similar to those in the human disorder cleidocranial dysplasia, which maps to the locus that corresponds to *Cbfa1*.

The growth factor Ihh also plays a critical role in osteoblast development, as evidenced by the fact that Ihh-deficient mice lack osteoblasts in bone formed by endochondral ossification. Numerous other growth-regulatory factors affect osteoblast function, including transforming growth factor (TGF) β types I and II, acidic fibroblast growth factor (aFGF) and basic fibroblast growth factor (bFGF), platelet-derived growth factor (PDGF), and insulin-like growth factors (IGFs) I and II. Active osteoblasts are characterized by their location and morphology; the presence of a specific skeletal form of alkaline phosphatase; the presence of receptors for parathyroid hormone (PTH) and 1,25-dihydroxyvitamin D [1,25(OH)$_2$D]; and the ability to synthesize specific matrix proteins, such as type I collagen, osteocalcin, and osteopontin. As an osteoblast secretes matrix, which is then mineralized, the cell becomes an *osteocyte*, still connected with its blood supply through a series of canaliculi. Osteocytes are thought to be the mechanosensors in bone that communicate signals to surface osteoblasts and their progenitors through the canalicular network.

Resorption of bone is carried out mainly by *osteoclasts*, multinucleated cells that are formed by fusion of cells derived from hematopoietic stem cells related to the mononuclear phagocyte series. Multiple factors regulating osteoclast development have been identified (Fig. 340-1*B*). Macrophage colony stimulating factor (M-CSF) plays a critical role at several steps in the pathway that ultimately leads to fusion of osteoclast progenitor cells to form multinucleated, active osteoclasts. Discovery of the RANK signaling pathway provides new insight into the pathway that links osteoblast and osteoclast development (Fig. 343-2). RANK ligand is expressed on the surface of osteoblast progenitors and stromal fibroblasts. In a process involving cell-cell interactions, it binds to the RANK receptor on osteoclast progenitors, stimulating a signal transduction cascade that leads to osteoclast differentiation and activation. Al-

A

Mesenchymal osteoblast progenitor → Osteoblast precursor → Active osteoblast

BMPs

PTH, Vit D
IGFs, BMPs, others

CBFA1+

Collagen (I)
Alkaline phosphatase
Osteocalcin, osteopontin
Bone sialoprotein

B

Hematopoietic osteoclast progenitor → Osteoblast precursor → Mononuclear osteoclast → Quiescent osteoclast → Active osteoclast

M-CSF

Rank Ligand

M-CSF
Rank ligand
IL-1, IL-6

Rank Ligand
IL-1

Commitment

Differentiation

Fusion

PU-1+

c-fos+
NF-kB+
TRAP+

c-src+
β3 integrin+
PYK2 kinase+
Cathepsin K+
TRAF+
Carbonic anhydrase II+

FIGURE 340-1 Pathways regulating development of (*A*) osteoblasts and (*B*) osteoclasts. Hormones, cytokines, and growth factors that control cell proliferation and differentiation are shown above the arrows. Transcription factors and other markers specific for various stages of development are depicted below the arrows. BMPs, bone morphogenic proteins; PTH, parathyroid hormone; Vit D, vitamin D; IGFs, insulin-like growth factors; CBFA1, core binding factor A1; M-CSF, macrophage colony stimulating factor; PU-1, a monocyte- and B lymphocyte–specific ets family transcription factor; NFκB, nuclear factor κB; TRAF, tumor necrosis factor receptor–associated factors; RANK ligand, receptor activator of NFκB ligand; IL-1, interleukin-1; IL-6, interleukin-6. (*Modified from Suda et al.*)

ternatively, a soluble decoy receptor, referred to as *osteoprotegerin* (OPG), can bind RANK ligand and inhibit osteoclast differentiation. Several growth factors and cytokines, including interleukins (IL) 1, 6, and 11, tumor necrosis factor (TNF), interferon γ, and M-CSF, modulate the osteoclast differentiation and function. Osteoclasts are also regulated indirectly by osteoblasts and adjacent stromal fibroblasts in the marrow. For example, PTH receptors are not found on mature osteoclasts, and PTH increases osteoclastic bone resorption by first acting on osteoblasts or stromal fibroblasts. 1,25(OH)$_2$D receptors are found in precursor cells that can differentiate into monocytes or osteoclasts, and 1,25(OH)$_2$D also promotes differentiation along the osteoclast pathway.

In the embryo and in the growing child, bone develops by remodeling and replacing previously calcified cartilage (endochondral bone formation) or is formed without a cartilage matrix (intramembranous bone formation). The PTH/PTHrP receptor plays a central role in the control of chondrocyte differentiation at growth plates (Chap. 341). Ihh production by growth plate chondrocytes stimulates the production of PTH-related peptide (PTHrP), which slows the differentiation of chondrocytes. This pathway creates a local feedback system as Ihh is suppressed by the actions of PTHrP. Consistent with this mechanism, mice with null mutations of the PTH/PTHrP receptor or PTHrP exhibit growth plate chondrodysplasia that reflects accelerated differentiation of proliferating chondrocytes. In humans, homozygous inactivating mutations of the PTH/PTHrP receptor cause Blomstrand's chondrodysplasia.

New bone, whether formed in infants or in adults during repair, has a relatively high ratio of cells to matrix and is characterized by coarse fiber bundles of collagen that are interlaced and randomly dispersed (woven bone). In adults, the more mature bone is organized with fiber bundles regularly arranged in parallel or concentric sheets (lamellar bone). In long bones, deposition of lamellar bone in a concentric arrangement around blood vessels forms the haversian systems. Growth in length of bones is dependent on proliferation of cartilage cells and on the endochondral sequence at the growth plate. Growth in width and thickness is accomplished by formation of bone at the periosteal surface and by resorption at the endosteal surface, with the rate of formation exceeding that of resorption. In adults, after the epiphyses close, growth in length and endochondral bone formation cease, except for some activity in the cartilage cells beneath the articular surface. Even in adults, however, remodeling of bone (remodeling of haversian systems as well as trabecular bone) continues throughout life. In adults, ~4% of the surface of trabecular bone (such as iliac crest) is involved in active resorption, whereas 10 to 15% of trabecular surfaces is covered with osteoid. Radioisotope studies indicate that as much as 18% of the total skeletal calcium is deposited and removed each year. Thus, bone is an active metabolizing tissue that requires an intact blood supply.

The response of bone to fractures, infection, and interruption of blood supply and to expanding lesions is relatively limited. Dead bone must be resorbed, and new bone must be formed, a process carried out in association with growth of new blood vessels into the involved area. In injuries that disrupt the organization of the tissue, such as a fracture in which apposition of fragments is poor or when motion exists at the fracture site, the progenitor stromal cells differentiate into cells with functional capacities different from those of osteoblasts, and varying amounts of fibrous tissue and cartilage are formed. When there is good apposition with fixation and little motion at the fracture site, repair occurs predominantly by formation of new bone without other scar tissue.

FIGURE 340-2 Schematic representation of bone remodeling. The cycle of bone remodeling is carried out by the basic multicellular unit (BMU), comprising a group of osteoclasts and osteoblasts. In cortical bone, the BMUs tunnel through the tissue, whereas in cancellous bone, they move across the trabecular surface. The process of bone remodeling is initiated by contraction of the lining cells and the recruitment of osteoclast precursors. These precursors fuse to form multinucleated, active osteoclasts that mediate bone resorption. Osteoclasts adhere to bone and subsequently remove it by acidification and proteolytic digestion. As the BMU advances, osteoclasts leave the resorption site and osteoblasts move in to cover the excavated area and begin the process of new bone formation by secreting osteoid, which is eventually mineralized into new bone. After osteoid mineralization, osteoblasts flatten and form a layer of lining cells over new bone.

Remodeling of bone occurs along lines of force modulated by the mechanical stresses to which it is subjected. The signals from these mechanical stresses are sensed by osteocytes, which then transmit other signals to osteoclasts (or their precursors) or osteoblasts (or their precursors). A bowing deformity increases new bone formation at the concave surface and resorption at the convex surface, seemingly designed to produce the strongest mechanical structure. Expanding lesions in bone, such as tumors, induce resorption at the surface in contact with the tumor. Even in a disorder as architecturally disruptive as Paget's disease, remodeling is dictated by mechanical forces. Thus, the plasticity of bone is due to the interaction of cells with each other and with the environment.

The cycle of bone resorption and formation is a highly orchestrated process carried out by the basic multicellular unit (BMU), composed of a group of osteoclasts and osteoblasts (Fig. 340-2). Osteoclast-mediated resorption of bone takes place in scalloped spaces (*Howship's lacunae*) where the osteoclasts are attached through a specific αv,β3 integrin to components of the bone matrix such as osteopontin. This clear zone contains contractile proteins. The resorbing end of the cell forms a specialized ruffled border, which is in contact with the bone. Proteins, including a specialized proton-pump ATPase, are found in the ruffled border membrane and contribute to the acid environment, which solubilizes the mineral phase. In addition to the proton pump, carbonic anhydrase (type II isoenzyme) is required to maintain the acid pH. Other features of active osteoclasts include expression of the proto-oncogene c-*src*, tartrate-resistant acid phosphatase, cell-surface receptors for calcitonin, sodium pumps of the kidney type, a bicarbonate/chloride exchanger of the band 3 family, and an ability to resorb mineralized bone. The bone matrix is resorbed in the acid environment adjacent to the ruffled border by proteinases that act at low pH, such as cathepsin K, following solubilization of the mineral phase.

Bone formation involves deposition of an organic matrix by osteoblasts followed by mineralization. The mineral phase is composed of calcium and phosphorus, and the concentration of these ions in the plasma and extracellular fluid (ECF) influences the rate at which mineral is formed. In vitro, mineralization can proceed and crystals of hydroxyapatite can grow at concentrations of calcium and phosphorus similar to those in an ultrafiltrate of plasma. The calcium phosphate solid phase at the inception of mineralization is brushite (CaHPO$_4$ · 2H$_2$O). As mineralization progresses, the solid phase is a poorly crystalline hydroxyapatite with a relatively low (~1.2) calcium/phosphate molar ratio. With age and maturation, the perfection of the crystals and the calcium/phosphate ratio increase. Fluoride ions, when incorporated into the mineral phase, decrease the proportion of amorphous calcium phosphate and enhance the crystal structure.

There is a limit for the concentration of calcium and phosphorus ions in the ECF below which mineralization does not occur. A "solubility product" for bone mineral is difficult to calculate because (1) the mineral phase itself is of variable composition, and (2) the various components in ECF that regulate this solubility product are not known. Nevertheless, when the concentrations of calcium and phosphorus in ECF are excessive, a mineral phase may form in areas (e.g., soft tissues) that are not normally mineralized.

Collagens from a variety of sources can catalyze the nucleation of a mineral phase of calcium and phosphorus from solutions of these ions. The organization of collagen probably influences the amount and type of mineral phase formed in bone. The primary structures of type I collagen in skin and bone tissues are similar. There are differences, however, in posttranslational modifications of type I collagen, such as hydroxylations; glycosylations; and the type, number, and distribution of intermolecular cross-links (Chap. 351). In addition, the holes in the packing structure of the collagen are larger in mineralized collagen of bone and dentin than in unmineralized collagens such as tendon. Single amino-acid substitutions in the helical portion of either the α1 or α2 chain of type I collagen due to mutations in the *COL1A1* or *COL1A2* genes in osteogenesis imperfecta disrupt the organization of bone, and this indicates the importance of the fibrillar matrix in the structure of bone. At the time of their discovery, it was thought that some of the non-collagenous bone proteins—e.g., osteocalcin (bone-GLA protein), osteonectin, and osteopontin—played a role in mineralization, although such a role has not been established. Osteocalcin, a product exclusively of osteoblasts, is measurable by immunoassays in normal human serum, and its levels correlate with other measurements of bone formation. Matrix-GLA protein (MGP), a component of bone as well as non-osseous tissues, acts to inhibit mineralization in the non-osseous tissues. Thus, functional deletion of the MGP gene in mice results in massive soft tissue calcification, particularly in arterial walls.

Alkaline phosphatase is a marker for osteoblasts, and cellular levels of this enzyme correlate with rates of bone formation. Although mineralization defects occur in individuals with mutations that decrease alkaline phosphatase activity (hypophosphatasia), the function of alkaline phosphatase in mineralization is not completely understood. Other circulating markers of bone formation include osteocalcin and type I procollagen C-terminal peptides. Urinary markers for bone resorption are hydroxyproline, hydroxylysine and its glycosides, and the bone-specific hydroxypyridinium collagen cross-links (Chap. 342). Inorganic pyrophosphate is a potent inhibitor of mineralization at levels below those necessary to bind calcium ions.

CALCIUM METABOLISM

A total of 1 to 2 kg of calcium is present in the average adult, >98% of it in the skeleton. The calcium of the mineral phase at the surface of the crystals is in equilibrium with that in the ECF, but only a minor fraction of the total pool (~0.5%) is exchangeable. In normal adults plasma levels range from 2.2 to 2.6 mmol/L (8.8 to 10.4 mg/dL). The calcium in plasma is present as three forms: free ions, ions bound to plasma proteins, and, to a small extent, diffusible complexes. The concentration of free calcium ions, averaging 1.2 mmol/L (4.8 mg/dL), influences many cellular functions and is subjected to tight hormonal control, especially through PTH (Chap. 341). The concentration of serum proteins is an important determinant of calcium ion concentration; most calcium ion is bound to albumin. Ionized calcium can be measured directly with the use of calcium-specific electrodes. If ionized calcium cannot be measured, certain approximations can be used to estimate the protein-bound and ionized fractions. One formula that approximates the amount of calcium bound to protein is

$$\% \text{ protein-bound Ca} = 0.8 \times \text{albumin (g/L)} + 0.2 \times \text{globulin (g/L)} + 3$$

A simplified correction is sometimes used to assess whether the total serum calcium concentration is abnormal when serum proteins are low.

The correction is to add 1 mg/dL to the serum calcium level for every 1 g/dL by which the serum albumin level is below 4.0 g/dL. If the serum calcium level, for example, is 7.8 mg/dL (a subnormal value) and the serum albumin level is only 3.0 g/dL, then the stated serum calcium level is corrected by adding 1 mg/dL; the corrected value of 8.8 mg/dL is within the normal range.

The concentration of calcium ions in the ECF is kept constant by processes that constantly add and remove calcium. Calcium enters the plasma via absorption from the intestinal tract and resorption of ions from the bone mineral. Calcium leaves the ECF via secretion into the gastrointestinal tract (~100 to 200 mg/d), urinary excretion (~50 to 300 mg/d), deposition in bone mineral, and losses in sweat (up to 100 mg/d). Bone resorption and formation are tightly coupled, with approximately 12 mmol (500 mg) calcium entering and leaving the skeleton daily (Fig. 340-3). Calcium ions inside the cell mediate a variety of cellular functions. The level of free calcium in the cell is very low, approximately 0.1 μmol/L; thus, the gradient between plasma and intracellular free calcium is about 10,000 to 1. This gradient is tightly regulated by various channels and ion pumps.

The average dietary calcium intake for most adults in the United States is approximately 15 to 20 mmol/d (0.6 to 0.8 g/d). However, with heightened awareness of the role of adequate calcium intake for the prevention of osteoporosis, many adults on supplements have an intake of 20 to 37 mmol/d (0.8 to 1.5 g/d). Less than half of dietary calcium is absorbed in adults. Calcium absorption increases during periods of rapid growth in children, in pregnancy, and in lactation and decreases with advancing age. Most of the calcium is absorbed in the proximal small intestine, and the efficiency of absorption decreases in the more distal intestinal segments. Both active transport and diffusion-limited absorption are involved; the former is more important in the upper intestine and the latter in the lower intestine. Both processes are influenced by vitamin D (see below). All forms of calcium in the diet are not equally absorbed; calcium as the chloride is probably absorbed more efficiently than that in other preparations. Secretion of calcium into the intestinal lumen is constant and independent of absorption. If calcium availability in the diet is low [<12 mmol/d (500 mg/d)], a positive calcium balance requires an efficiency of absorption >30 to 40%.

The urinary calcium excretion of normal adults having an average calcium intake ranges between 2.5 and 10 mmol/d (100 and 400 mg/d). When the dietary calcium level is <5 mmol/d (200 mg/d), urinary calcium excretion is usually <5 mmol/d (200 mg/d). However, in most normal individuals, wide variations in dietary intake have little effect on urinary calcium. Hence, when the diet is low in calcium, the

FIGURE 340-3   Calcium homeostasis. Schematic illustration of calcium content of extracellular fluid (ECF) and bone as well as of diet and feces; magnitude of calcium flux per day as calculated by various methods is shown at sites of transport in intestine, kidney, and bone. Ranges of values shown are approximate and chosen to illustrate certain points discussed in text. In conditions of calcium balance, rates of calcium release from and uptake into bone are equal.

relative inefficiency of renal calcium conservation leads to a negative calcium balance unless calcium absorption is maximal (Fig. 340-3).

The amount of calcium in the urine is small compared with that filtered by the glomerulus [~150 to 250 mmol/d (6 to 10 g/d)] because the rates of reabsorption of the filtered calcium are high. Reabsorption takes place predominantly in the proximal tubule (~60%) and in Henle's loop (~25%) and to a small extent in the distal tubule. The calcium-sensing receptor also plays a role in renal calcium excretion, though the mechanisms that regulate its function have not been fully defined (Chap. 341). The excretion of other electrolytes affects the urinary excretion of calcium. For example, urinary calcium is usually proportional to urinary sodium; sulfate also increases calcium excretion.

A deficiency of PTH or vitamin D, intestinal disease, or severe dietary calcium deprivation may provide challenges to calcium homeostasis that cannot be compensated adequately by renal calcium conservation, resulting in a negative calcium balance. Increased bone resorption may protect against ECF calcium depletion even in states of chronic negative calcium balance but only at the expense of progressive bone loss.

PATHOPHYSIOLOGY A decrease in the concentration of free calcium ions in plasma results in increased neuromuscular irritability and tetany. This syndrome is characterized by peripheral and perioral paresthesia, carpal spasm, pedal spasm, anxiety, seizures, bronchospasm, laryngospasm, Chvostek's sign, Trousseau's sign, and Erb's sign, and lengthening of the QT interval of the electrocardiogram. In infants tetany may be manifested only by irritability and lethargy. The level of calcium ions that determines which features of tetany will be manifested varies among individuals. Tetany is also influenced by other components of the ECF; e.g., hypomagnesemia and alkalosis lower whereas hypokalemia and acidosis raise the threshold for tetany.

Increases in total serum calcium concentration are usually accompanied by increases in free calcium levels and may be associated with anorexia, nausea, vomiting, constipation, hypotonia, depression, and occasionally lethargy and coma. Persistent hypercalcemia, especially when accompanied by normal or elevated levels of serum phosphate, may cause ectopic deposition of a solid phase of calcium and phosphate in walls of blood vessels, connective tissue about the joints, gastric mucosa, cornea, and renal parenchyma. Hypercalcemia per se alters renal function in addition to the pathologic effects of calcium phosphate deposition.

PHOSPHORUS METABOLISM

Phosphorus is a major component of bone and of all other tissues and in some form is involved in almost all metabolic processes, including energy storage, membrane transport, membrane composition, and signal transduction. About 600 g of phosphorus is present in the normal adult, of which 85% is present in the crystalline structure of the skeleton.

In plasma from fasting subjects, most of the phosphorus is present as inorganic orthophosphate in concentrations of approximately 0.75 to 1.45 mmol/L (2.5 to 4.5 mg/dL). In contrast to calcium, of which ~50% is bound, only ~12% of the phosphorus in plasma is bound to proteins. Free HPO_4^{2-} and $NaHPO_4^-$ normally account for ~75% of the total phosphorus, and free $H_2PO_4^-$ accounts for ~10%. Since so many species are present, depending on pH and other factors, concentrations are usually expressed in terms of elemental phosphorus, in units of mmol/L or mg/dL. The serum phosphorus, however, can vary based on age; young children have almost twice the serum phosphorus as adults due to the need for rapid skeletal mineralization. Postmenopausal women also have higher circulating phosphorus levels. After ingesting a meal containing carbohydrate, there is a decrease in serum phosphorus levels [by 0.3 to 0.5 mmol/dL (1.0 to 1.5 mg/dL)] in response to the increase in insulin secretion, which enhances cellular phosphorus uptake and utilization. An increase in serum pH will decrease serum phosphorus, whereas a decrease in pH increases phos-

phorus concentration. There is a circadian variation in phosphorus concentration even during a 24-h fast: the nadir occurs between 9:00 A.M. and noon followed by an increase to a plateau in the afternoon and another small peak after midnight.

Phosphorus is plentiful in the diet. Common sources include dairy products, meats, eggs, and carbonated beverages that contain phosphoric acid. Approximately 60 to 70% of phosphorus is passively absorbed in the small intestine (Fig. 340-4). 1,25(OH)$_2$D enhances phosphorus absorption along the entire small intestine, with the highest efficiency in the jejunum and ileum. Chronic low phosphorus intake (<2 mg/kg of body weight per day) decreases serum phosphorus levels. Low serum phosphorus stimulates the renal production of 1,25(OH)$_2$D, which, in turn, increases the efficiency intestinal absorption up to 80 to 90%. 1,25(OH)$_2$D also decreases PTH secretion and, thereby reduces renal tubular loss of phosphorus.

The major control of phosphorus balance is exerted by the kidney. Approximately 90% of phosphorus in the circulation is filtered through the glomerulus and is largely absorbed by the proximal tubule such that only 10 to 15% of the filtered load is normally excreted. Urinary phosphorus excretion is reflective of dietary intake. Phosphorus absorption in the proximal tubule is coupled with sodium absorption. The primary regulation of phosphorus metabolism occurs in the distal convoluted tubule, and this mechanism is independent of sodium reabsorption. Volume expansion and decreased sodium reabsorption increase phosphorus clearance.

HYPOPHOSPHATEMIA **Causes** Although there are many potential causes for hypophosphatemia (Table 340-1), the most common etiologies include: (1) decreased intestinal phosphorus absorption, either due to vitamin D deficiency or the presence of a phosphorus-binding antacid; (2) urinary losses that are PTH- or alcohol-mediated; and (3) a shift of phosphorus from extracellular to intracellular compartments due to exogenous administration of insulin or consumption of nutrients that stimulate insulin release (e.g., carbohydrates). Increased renal clearance of phosphorus occurs in primary hyperparathyroidism, vitamin D deficiency, vitamin D–resistant and D–dependent rickets, hyperglycemic states, and oncogenic osteomalacia. In vitamin D deficiency, serum phosphorus is low because

FIGURE 340-4 Phosphate homeostasis. Schematic illustration of inorganic phosphorus content (termed here *phosphate*) in extracellular fluid (ECF) and bone as well as diet and feces; magnitude of phosphorus flux per day as estimated by various methods is shown at transport sites in intestine, kidney, and bone. Range of values shown illustrates special features of phosphorus metabolism discussed in text. The compartment labeled ICF refers to intracellular phosphorus, both organic and inorganic; rapid shifts of phosphorus into cells (and corresponding, possibly slower, efflux of phosphorus from cells) contribute to changes in ECF phosphorus. These shifts between ECF and ICF and phosphorus release from and uptake by bone are equal in conditions of phosphorus balance.

Table 340-1   Causes of Hypophosphatemia

Decreased intestinal phosphate absorption
  Vitamin D deficiency
  Vitamin D–dependent rickets types I and II
  Malabsorption
  Phosphate-binding antacids
  Extracellular shift of phosphorus to intracellular compartment
Increased renal phosphate excretion
  Hyperparathyroidism
  Vitamin D deficiency
  Vitamin D–dependent rickets types I and II
  X-linked hypophosphatemic rickets
  Fanconi syndromes
  Oncogenic osteomalacia
  Hyperglycemic states
  Alcoholism and alcohol withdrawal
  Ketoacidosis
Other
  Respiratory alkalosis
  Blast crisis in leukemia
  Starvation
  Insulin therapy
  Hungry bone syndrome after parathyroidectomy
  Recovery from hypothermia
  Sepsis

of decreased intestinal absorption as well as secondary hyperparathyroidism, which increases phosphorus losses in the urine. In X-linked hypophosphatemic rickets, there is a genetic defect in the *PHEX* gene, which encodes a neutral endopeptidase presumed to degrade the phosphaturia hormone known as *phosphatonin*. The disorder is associated with a severe renal leak of phosphorus into the urine. In addition, there is a defect in hypophosphatemia-mediated stimulation of 25(OH)D-1α-hydroxylase, resulting in decreased intestinal phosphorus absorption. Acidosis and hyperglycemic states associated with polyuria also cause excessive phosphorus loss in the urine. Ketoacidosis enhances intracellular and organic phosphorus degradation, thereby releasing large amounts of inorganic phosphorus into the circulation that is cleared into the urine. In ketosis, the serum phosphorus is often normal because of the continuous shift of phosphorus from intracellular to extracellular pools. However, when the ketosis is corrected, hypophosphatemia is apparent because of the return of phosphorus into the intracellular compartment (Chap. 333). A severe, acquired form of hypophosphatemia, *oncogenic osteomalacia*, is associated with vascular, mesenchymal tumors such as hemangiopericytomas but occasionally also with small cell lung cancer, prostate cancer, and other malignant tumors. It is likely that these tumors secrete a substance similar or identical to phosphatonin. The phosphorus levels in these patients are usually extremely low [0.4 to 0.5 mmol/L (1.2 to 1.5 mg/dL)], and the 1,25(OH)$_2$D levels are low or undetectable. The disorder is associated with severe fatigue, muscle weakness, and unrelenting bone discomfort.

Alcohol abuse is the most common cause of severe hypophosphatemia, which is caused by poor dietary intake of phosphorus, ethanol-enhanced urinary excretion of inorganic phosphorus, the use of calcium- or aluminum-containing antacids, and vomiting. Hypophosphatemia may transiently worsen with refeeding. Alcoholics may also have associated calcium and vitamin D deficiency and secondary hyperparathyroidism, which enhances phosphorus-wasting in the urine. Alcoholic ketoacidosis induces marked phosphaturia. Intense hyperventilation for prolonged periods may depress serum phosphorus levels due to associated alkalosis. Rapid correction of chronic respiratory acidosis has also been associated with hypophosphatemia and can lead to diaphragm weakness and an exacerbation of respiratory failure. Advanced leukemia with blast crisis (leukocyte counts usually >100,000) may cause severe hypophosphatemia; the likely cause is a rapid uptake of phosphorus into the rapidly dividing cells.

Laboratory and Clinical Findings   Serum phosphorus levels should be determined in a fasting state. Mild hypophosphatemia is not usually associated with clinical symptoms. In severe hypophosphatemia [≤0.3 mmol/L (≤1.0 mg/dL)], multiple organ systems are affected. Patients become irritable, apprehensive, and hyperventilate, resulting in complaints of muscle weakness, numbness, and paresthesia. In the most severe form, they are confused or obtunded and suffer from seizures and coma, which can ultimately lead to death. This metabolic encephalopathy is often associated with slowing of the electroencephalogram.

Phosphorus is essential for muscle function because of the need for large amounts of ATP and creatine phosphate. Patients with severe hypophosphatemia often complain of fatigue, muscle weakness, myalgia, and myopathy. Hypophosphatemia can cause rhabdomyolysis, which is particularly common in chronic alcoholics or during alcohol withdrawal. Rhabdomyolysis can be precipitated during treatment for diabetic ketoacidosis or by hyperalimentation or refeeding in a malnourished patient. Cardiomyopathy can also occur, resulting in reduced cardiac output, impaired pressor responsiveness to catecholamines, hypotension, and ventricular arrhythmias. Restoration of phosphorus deficits can result in prompt reversal. Severe muscle weakness can lead to respiratory insufficiency.

Erythrocytes and leukocytes are highly dependent on phosphorus for their function. Chronic hypophosphatemia decreases 2,3-bisphosphoglycerate and ATP, enhancing oxygen dissociation from hemoglobin and leading to tissue hypoxia. Hypophosphatemia causes impaired phagocytosis and opsonization and, therefore, increases susceptibility to bacterial and fungal infections.

Chronic hypophosphatemia causes a mineralization defect of the skeleton. In children, this causes rickets. In adults, chronic hypophosphatemia (often due to vitamin D deficiency) causes osteomalacia (see below). Patients with severe renal phosphorus-wasting and severe chronic hypophosphatemia may have marked fatigue, muscle weakness, and severe bone pain, especially of their long bones and ribcage.

TREATMENT   Mild hypophosphatemia usually resolves spontaneously when the underlying cause is corrected. Oral phosphorus replacement is sufficient if serum phosphorus is >0.3 mmol/L (1 mg/dL) and the patient is asymptomatic. Milk is an excellent source of phosphorus as it contains 1 g of inorganic phosphorus per liter. Carbonated beverages that contain phosphoric acid provide another source of phosphorus, especially for patients with lactase deficiency. Pharmaceutical preparations of phosphorus, such as Neutraphos or KPhos, contain sodium and potassium salts of phosphate. Depending on the degree of hypophosphatemia, up to 3 g/d can be given in four to six divided doses per 24 h. These doses usually do not cause diarrhea; >5 g/d will induce diarrhea.

For severe hypophosphatemia, with serum phosphorus levels <0.2 to 0.3 mmol/L (<0.5 to 1.0 mg/dL), ≥3 g/d of phosphorus may be required over several days to replete body stores. In patients with severe symptomatic hypophosphatemia who are unable to eat, intravenous phosphorus can be given, up to 1 g in 1 L of fluid over 8 to 12 h. Some caution is necessary when giving phosphorus intravenously because of the potential for precipitating soft tissue calcification. A serum calcium × serum phosphorus product >70 markedly increases the risk of soft tissue calcification and nephrocalcinosis. Patients with chronic hypophosphatemia caused by inherited or acquired renal phosphorus leak require vigilance when receiving high doses of oral phosphorus. Transiently elevated serum phosphorus levels can decrease ionized calcium levels, resulting in chronic stimulation of the parathyroid gland and leading to autonomous, persistent hyperplasia of the parathyroid glands. Thus, it is best to give frequent divided doses of phosphorus (four to six times a day), equaling a total of 2 to 3 g/d.

Phosphorus should not be given intramuscularly or subcutaneously because it can cause soft tissue necrosis and severe discomfort. Intravenous sodium or potassium phosphate, 15 mmol (0.465 g) of elemental phosphorus given in 100 mL of 0.9% saline over 60 min, el-

Decreased renal phosphate excretion	Other
Acute renal failure	Vitamin D intoxication
Chronic renal failure	Acidosis, respiratory or metabolic
Hypoparathyroidism	Crush injuries
Pseudohypoparathyroidism	Rhabdomyolysis
Tumoral calcinosis	Cytotoxic therapy and tumor lysis
Bisphosphonates	Fulminant hepatitis
Acromegaly	Extracellular shift from intracellular compartment
	Artifactual due to hemolysis

evates serum phosphorus levels by an average of 0.6 to 1.2 mmol/L (1.75 to 3.8 mg/dL).

HYPERPHOSPHATEMIA In adults, hyperphosphatemia is defined as a serum phosphorus level >1.6 mmol/L (5 mg/dL). In children, this level is much higher. The most common causes of hyperphosphatemia are acute and chronic renal failure (Table 340-2). In renal failure, the loss of tubular function impairs phosphorus excretion. This results in a cascade of events that can also affect calcium and phosphorus metabolism. The increase in serum phosphorus levels reduces serum calcium levels and the production of $1,25(OH)_2D$, leading to decreased intestinal calcium absorption and secondary hyperparathyroidism. Patients with pseudohypoparathyroidism and tumoral calcinosis also have decreased renal phosphorus clearance that results in hyperphosphatemia. Hypothyroidism reduces renal phosphorus excretion and may increase circulating concentrations of phosphorus. Vitamin D intoxication, due to excessive ingestion of either vitamin D or one of its analogues, can cause hyperphosphatemia along with hypercalcemia. Severe hypothermia, crush injuries, nontrauma rhabdomyolysis, tumoral calcinosis, and cytotoxic therapy of hematologic malignancies such as acute lymphoblastic leukemia can be associated with hyperphosphatemia. The serum phosphorus level can be artifactually elevated due to hemolysis of the blood sample. Thrombocytosis and multiple myeloma can cause spuriously elevated serum phosphorus levels due to thrombocytolysis.

Laboratory and Clinical Findings A rapid elevation of serum phosphorus can cause hypocalcemia and symptoms of neuromuscular irritability and tetany. Chronic hyperphosphatemia in association with normocalcemia can result in nephrocalcinosis and soft tissue calcification.

℞ **TREATMENT** In addition to treating the underlying disorder, dietary phosphorus intake should be limited by restricting carbonated beverages containing phosphoric acid and decreasing milk and dairy product consumption. The dietary intake of phosphorus should be between 600 and 1000 mg a day with modest protein restriction. For control of chronic hyperphosphatemia, usually in patients with chronic renal failure, oral aluminum hydroxide or aluminum carbonate gels are indicated. Prolonged use of aluminum-containing compounds is not recommended because of aluminum toxicity causing adynamic bone disease, proximal myopathy, encephalopathy, and anemia. When hyperphosphatemia is due to vitamin D intoxication, calcium salts are contraindicated because the high efficiency of calcium absorption can lead to severe hypercalcemia, soft tissue calcification, and nephrocalcinosis.

MAGNESIUM METABOLISM

Magnesium is the most abundant intracellular divalent cation. It is an essential cofactor for a multitude of enzymatic reactions that are important for the generation of energy from ATP. Approximately 30% of magnesium in the serum is protein-bound, 55% is ionized, and the remaining 15% is complexed. Like calcium, magnesium is bound to albumin, and it is the ionized fraction that is important for physiologic processes including neuromuscular function and maintenance of cardiovascular tone.

The serum concentration of magnesium is tightly regulated within a narrow range of approximately 0.7 to 1.1 mmol/L (1.4 to 2.2 meq/L)(1.7 to 2.6 mg/dl) as a result of the efficient absorption of dietary magnesium by the small intestine and conservation of magnesium in the kidney. About 30% of dietary magnesium is absorbed in the small intestine, but this fraction increases markedly when intake is substantially reduced. Approximately 96% of filtered magnesium is reabsorbed along the nephron, and only 4% is excreted into the urine. Because there is no regulation of magnesium absorption in the distal tubule and because magnesium reabsorption is very efficient, an increase in distal delivery increases magnesium loss in the urine.

HYPOMAGNESEMIA Although magnesium deficiency is a common clinical problem, serum magnesium levels are often overlooked or not measured in patients at risk for the disorder. Approximately 10% of patients admitted to city hospitals are hypomagnesemic, and up to 65% of patients in intensive care units may be magnesium-deficient. Hypomagnesemia is caused primarily by renal or gastrointestinal losses or decreased efficiency of intestinal magnesium absorption (Table 340-3). Reduced renal reabsorption due to loop diuretics and alcohol use is a common cause of hypomagnesemia. Because magnesium excretion is tightly coupled to sodium and calcium excretion, intravenous fluid therapy and volume-expanded states, such as primary hyperaldosteronism, may result in hypomagnesemia. Hypercalcemia and hypercalciuria decrease tubular reabsorption of magnesium. Osmotic diuresis in diabetes mellitus is one of the more common causes of hypomagnesemia.

Vomiting and nasogastric suctioning can cause severe magnesium depletion because intestinal tract fluids contain ~0.5 mmol/L (1.2 mg/dL)(1 meq/L). Fluid loss from diarrhea can contain as much as 7.4 mmol/L (18 mg/dL)(15 meq/L). Consequently, ulcerative colitis, Crohn's disease, and intestinal or biliary fistulas can result in magnesium depletion. Hypomagnesemia is prevalent in alcoholics. Ethanol causes a transient loss of magnesium in the urine. In most alcoholics, however, the magnesium deficit is modest. A more profound fall in serum magnesium levels may occur during alcohol withdrawal, where the decrease is associated with falls in levels of serum phosphate and potassium, probably due to shifts of these ions into intracellular compartments. The use of loop diuretics, as well as aminoglycosides, cisplatin, cyclosporine, and amphotericin B can increase renal loss of magnesium.

The clinical manifestations of hypomagnesemia are similar to those of severe hypocalcemia. The signs and symptoms of hypomagnesemia include muscle weakness, prolonged PR and QT intervals, and cardiac arrhythmias. Positive Chvostek's and Trousseau's signs indicative of hypocalcemia are often positive in hypomagnesemic patients as well; carpopedal spasm can also occur with hypomagnesemia. Magnesium is important for effective PTH secretion as well as the

Table 340-3 Causes of Hypomagnesemia

Increased renal excretion	Metabolic and endocrine
Volume expansion	Diabetes mellitus
Hypercalcemia	Primary hyperparathyroidism
Osmotic diuresis	Primary aldosteronism
Renal disease with magnesium wasting	Hypoparathyroidism
Metabolic acidosis	Hyperthyroidism
Gitelman's syndrome	Phosphate depletion
Bartter's syndrome	Ketoacidosis with treatment
Increased intestinal losses	Acute and chronic diarrhea
Vomiting	Intestinal resection or bypass
Nasal-gastric suctioning	Drugs
Malabsorption syndromes	Diuretics
Ileitis	Aminoglycosides
Colitis	Cisplatin
Intestinal and biliary fistulas	Cyclosporine
Alcoholism	Amphotericin B
	Ethanol
	Pentamidine

Table 340-4 Causes of Hypermagnesemia

Renal failure receiving magnesium-containing antacid, laxative, or infusion
Acute renal failure with rhabdomyolysis
Ketoacidosis without treatment
Familial hypocalciuric hypercalcemia
Volume depletion
Lithium
Accidental Epsom salt (magnesium sulfate) ingestion

renal and skeletal responsiveness to PTH; thus, hypomagnesemia is often associated with hypocalcemia due to impaired PTH secretion and function (Chap. 341).

Low serum magnesium levels <0.7 mmol/L (1.8 mg/dL)(1.5 meq/L) are indicative of magnesium deficiency. For mild deficiency, oral magnesium replacement is effective. The major side effect is diarrhea. Symptoms often occur when the serum magnesium is <0.5 mmol/L (1.2 mg/dL)(1.0 meq/L). This level is indicative of significantly depleted total-body magnesium stores. Because most magnesium resides in the intracellular space, the total-body magnesium deficit is often ~200 mmol (4800 mg) by the time serum levels fall to <0.5 mmol/L (1.2 mg/dL)(1.0 meq/L). Parenteral magnesium administration is usually needed under these circumstances. Two grams of magnesium sulfate [8.0 mmol (192 mg)(16.2 meq) of magnesium] can be given intravenously, with a cumulative dose up to 24 mmol (576 mg) (48 meq) over 24 h. Alternatively, a 50% solution of 2 g of magnesium sulfate can be given every 8 h intramuscularly although these injections can be painful. Patients with severe hypomagnesemia and associated seizures or acute arrhythmias can be given 4 to 8 mmol (96 to 192 mg)(8 to 16 meq) of magnesium as an intravenous injection over 5 to 10 min, followed by 24 mmol/d (576 mg/d)(48 meq/d).

A normal serum magnesium concentration attained after acute magnesium repletion is not necessarily indicative of repletion of the total-body magnesium stores. Restoration of urinary magnesium excretion is a better indicator of magnesium repletion. Once urinary magnesium excretion increases, the body stores are usually replenished. Patients who have chronic magnesium loss from intestinal or renal sources may require continued oral magnesium supplementation on a daily basis of up to 12.5 mmol/d (300 mg/d) in divided doses. Patients with renal failure need to be monitored carefully to prevent hypermagnesemia.

HYPERMAGNESEMIA Hypermagnesemia is rare but can be seen in renal failure when patients are taking magnesium-containing antacids, laxatives, enemas, or infusions (Table 340-4). It can also be seen in acute rhabdomyolysis.

The most readily detected clinical sign of hypermagnesemia is the disappearance of deep tendon reflexes. Neuromuscular symptoms include depressed respiration and apnea due to paralysis of the voluntary muscles, prolonged PR intervals, and increased QRS duration and QT interval; complete heart block and cardiac arrest can occur. Hypocalcemia may occur because hypermagnesemia depresses PTH secretion and induces an end-organ resistance to PTH similar to the effect seen in hypomagnesemia.

Treatment includes stopping the antacid or other preparations that contain large amounts of magnesium. The excess magnesium is quickly excreted by the kidney. Renal failure patients may require dialysis against a low magnesium bath. For severe hypermagnesemia with associated life-threatening complications, intravenous calcium in doses of 100 to 200 mg (elemental) over 5 to 10 min will antagonize the toxic effects of magnesium.

VITAMIN D

Vitamin D is a hormone rather than a classic vitamin, since with adequate exposure to sunlight, no dietary supplements are needed. Vitamin D exerts its physiologic effects on bone, intestine, kidney, and the parathyroid glands to modulate calcium and phosphorus metabolism. The active principle of vitamin D is synthesized under metabolic control via successive hydroxylations in the liver and kidney and is transported through the blood to its main target tissues (the small intestine and bone), where it regulates calcium homeostasis.

PHOTOBIOGENESIS Vitamin D_3 is a derivative of 7-dehydrocholesterol (provitamin D_3), the immediate precursor of cholesterol. When skin is exposed to sunlight or certain artificial light sources, the ultraviolet radiation enters the epidermis and causes transformation of 7-dehydrocholesterol to vitamin D_3. Wavelengths between 290 and 315 nm are absorbed by the conjugated double bonds at C_5 and C_7 of 7-dehydrocholesterol to produce previtamin D_3 (Fig. 340-5). Vitamin D_3 is made in the skin from the previtamin for many hours after a single sun exposure (Fig. 340-5). Once vitamin D_3 is synthesized, it is translocated from the epidermis into the circulation by the vitamin D–binding protein. Melanin in the skin competes with 7-dehydrocholesterol for ultraviolet photons and thus can limit the synthesis of previtamin D_3. The photochemical isomerization of previtamin D_3 and vitamin D_3 to biologically inert products appears to be more important in preventing excessive production of previtamin D_3 and vitamin D_3 during prolonged exposure to the sun.

Aging decreases the capacity of the skin to produce vitamin D_3; this capacity is reduced more than fourfold after age 70. Topical sunscreens can reduce or prevent cutaneous production of vitamin D_3 by absorbing the solar radiation responsible for previtamin D_3 synthesis in the skin. Other factors that affect the cutaneous synthesis of vitamin D_3 include altitude, geographic location, time of day, and area exposed. Latitude has profound effects on the cutaneous synthesis of vitamin D_3. As the zenith angle of the sun increases with approaching winter, more of the high-energy ultraviolet photons responsible for formation of the previtamin are absorbed by the ozone layer. In an area such as Boston (42°N), the absorption of these photons is so complete that essentially no vitamin D_3 is made in the skin between the months of November through February.

When the entire body is exposed to sufficient sunlight to cause mild erythema, the increase in the blood vitamin D is approximately equivalent to consuming oral doses of 10,000 to 25,000 international units (1 IU = 0.025 μg) of vitamin D. Only when skin irradiation is insufficient to produce the required quantities of vitamin D_3 is dietary supplementation needed to prevent skeletal mineralization defects. The fortification of milk and some cereals with either crystalline vitamin D_2 (Fig. 340-5) or vitamin D_3 should prevent rickets and osteomalacia. A survey of the vitamin D content in milk from the United States and western Canada revealed, however, that 71% did not contain 80 to 120% of the amount of vitamin D on the label and that ~15% of skim milk did not contain detectable vitamin D.

In 1997, the Food and Nutrition Board for the Institute of the Medicine recommended 200 IU/d as the adequate intake of vitamin D for neonates, children, and adults up to 50 years. For adults 51 to 70 and >71 years, the committee recommended 400 and 600 IU/d, respectively. In the absence of adequate sunlight exposure, all children and adults require at least 400 to 600 IU/d.

METABOLISM In the liver, vitamin D is metabolized to 25-hydroxyvitamin D [25(OH)D] by hepatic mitochondrial and/or microsomal enzyme(s) (Fig. 340-5). 25(OH)D is one of the major circulating metabolites, and its half-life is about 21 days. The concentrations of 25(OH)D and some of its metabolites in the serum are measured using competitive binding assays. The normal serum 25(OH)D concentration varies among different laboratories from 20 to 200 nmol/L (8 to 80 ng/mL). Individuals exposed to excessive sunlight may have concentrations of 25(OH)D up to 250 nmol/L (100 ng/mL) without adverse effects on calcium metabolism. The serum 25(OH)D levels usually reflect both 25-hydroxyvitamin D_2 [25(OH)D_2] and 25-hydroxyvitamin D_3 [25(OH)D_3]. The ratio of these two 25-hydroxylated derivatives depends on the relative amounts of vitamins D_2 or D_3 present in the diet and the amount of previtamin D_3 produced by exposure to sunlight.

The hepatic 25-hydroxylation of vitamin D is regulated by a product feedback mechanism. This regulation, however, is not tight; an increase in dietary intake or endogenous production of vitamin D_3 increases 25(OH)D levels in the serum. The levels can rise to >1200 nmol/L (500 ng/mL) when the intake of vitamin D is excessive. Serum 25(OH)D levels are reduced in severe chronic liver disease (Table 340-5). 25(OH)D is probably not biologically active at physiologic levels in vivo but is active in vitro at high concentrations.

After formation in the liver, 25(OH)D is bound by the vitamin D–binding protein and transported to the kidney for an additional stereospecific hydroxylation on either C_1 or C_{24} (Fig. 340-5). The kidney plays a pivotal role in the metabolism of 25(OH)D to the biologically active metabolite. The renal mitochondrial 25(OH)D-1-hydroxylase activity is enhanced by hypocalcemia to increase the rate of conversion of 25(OH)D to 1,25(OH)$_2$D. Hypocalcemia may not control this hydroxylation directly, however. Any decrease in the serum concentration of calcium below normal is a stimulus for increased secretion of PTH, which increases the synthesis of 1,25(OH)$_2$D in the renal proximal convoluted tubule. The renal production of 1,25(OH)$_2$D enhances the effects of PTH in lowering circulating concentrations (and presumably renal intracellular concentrations) of phosphate (Fig. 340-6). 1,25(OH)$_2$D also influences the renal metabolism of 25(OH)D by diminishing 25(OH)D-1α-hydroxylase activity and enhancing the metabolism of 25(OH)D to 24R,25-dihydroxyvitamin D [24,25(OH)$_2$D].

24,25(OH)$_2$D is normally present in serum at a concentration of 1 to 10 nmol/L (0.5 to 5.0 ng/mL). 24,25(OH)$_2$D is also a substrate for renal 25(OH)D-1α-hydroxylase and is converted to 1α,24R,25-trihydroxyvitamin D [1,24,25(OH)$_3$D], which, in turn, is metabolized to the biologically inactive substance calcitroic acid (Fig. 340-5). Cultured cells that possess nuclear receptors for 1,25(OH)$_2$D, such as chondrocytes, skin keratinocytes and fibroblasts, and intestinal and melanoma cells, also metabolize 25(OH)D to 24,25(OH)$_2$D. Studies of the vitamin D-24-hydroxylase null mice indicate that the major role of 24-hydroxylation is in the regulation of levels of 1,25(OH)$_2$D.

PHYSIOLOGY 1,25(OH)$_2$D, produced by the kidney and the placenta, is the only known important metabolite of vitamin D; the potential roles of other metabolites have not been clarified. 1,25(OH)$_2$D bound to a vitamin D–binding protein is delivered to various target organs, where the free form is taken up by cells and transported to a specific nuclear receptor protein. The vitamin D receptor (VDR) belongs to the nuclear receptor superfamily of steroid-retinoid-thyroid hormone-vitamin D transcription regulatory factors (Chap. 327). The VDR interacts with the retinoic acid X receptor (RXR) to form a heterodimeric (RXR-VDR) complex that binds to specific DNA sequences, termed the *vitamin D response elements* (VDREs). After 1,25(OH)$_2$D binds to the receptor, it induces conformational changes that result in the recruitment of a multitude of transcriptional coactivators that stimulate the transcription of target genes. In the intestine, the activated VDR stimulates calcium-binding protein

FIGURE 340-5 The photobiogenesis and metabolism of vitamin D. 7-Dehydrocholesterol can be either reduced by 7-dehydrocholesterol reductase (Δ^7ase) to cholesterol or photolyzed in the skin by solar ultraviolet B radiation (UVB) to previtamin D_3. Once formed, previtamin D_3 thermally isomerizes to vitamin D_3. Exposure of previtamin D_3 and vitamin D_3 to UVB radiation results in the generation of a variety of biologically inert photoproducts. Vitamin D_3 enters the circulation and is hydroxylated by the hepatic vitamin D-25-hydroxylase (step 25) to 25-hydroxyvitamin D_3, shown as 25(OH)D_3. 25-Hydroxyvitamin D_3 can be metabolized by a 25(OH)D-24-hydroxylase (step 24R) to 24,25-dihydroxyvitamin D_3, i.e., 24,25(OH)$_2$D$_3$. 25-Hydroxyvitamin D_3 is converted in the kidney by the 25-OH-D-1α-hydroxylase (step 1α) to its biologically active form, 1,25-dihydroxyvitamin D_3, i.e., 1,25(OH)$_2$D$_3$. As shown in the top two inserts, the vitamin D receptor (VDR), a member of the steroid superfamily of receptors, interacts with 1,25(OH)$_2$D$_3$ (identified as D_3), resulting in the phosphorylation of the 1,25(OH)$_2$D$_3$–VDR complex. This complex interacts with the retinoic acid X receptor (RXR) to form a heterodimer, which, in turn, interacts with the vitamin D–responsive element (VDRE) in the promoters of target genes. In the bone, this interaction increases the expression of mRNAs for osteocalcin (OC) and osteopontin (OP). 1,25-Dihydroxyvitamin D_3 can undergo multiple hydroxylations in its side chain that may ultimately result in the formation of the water-soluble biologically inactive calcitroic acid. The lower insert is the structure for vitamin D_2. It is structurally different from vitamin D_3 in having a double bond between C_{22} and C_{23} and a methyl group on C_{24}.

been clarified. 1,25(OH)$_2$D bound to a vitamin D–binding protein is delivered to various target organs, where the free form is taken up by cells and transported to a specific nuclear receptor protein. The vitamin D receptor (VDR) belongs to the nuclear receptor superfamily of steroid-retinoid-thyroid hormone-vitamin D transcription regulatory factors (Chap. 327). The VDR interacts with the retinoic acid X receptor (RXR) to form a heterodimeric (RXR-VDR) complex that binds to specific DNA sequences, termed the *vitamin D response elements* (VDREs). After 1,25(OH)$_2$D binds to the receptor, it induces conformational changes that result in the recruitment of a multitude of transcriptional coactivators that stimulate the transcription of target genes. In the intestine, the activated VDR stimulates calcium-binding protein

synthesis; in bone, it stimulates production of osteocalcin, osteopontin, and alkaline phosphatase. 1,25(OH)$_2$D also may have nonnuclear effects on its target tissues; 1,25(OH)$_2$D increases the transport of calcium from the extracellular to intracellular space, and it can mobilize calcium from intracellular calcium pools and enhance phosphatidylinositol metabolism. In the intestine, the net effect of 1,25(OH)$_2$D is to stimulate calcium and phosphate transport from the lumen of the small intestine into the circulation (Fig. 340-6). The effect of 1,25(OH)$_2$D on the enhancement of bone resorption is synergistic with that of PTH. Mature osteoclasts do not possess receptors for either PTH or 1,25(OH)$_2$D. Both PTH and 1,25(OH)$_2$D interact with their specific receptors on osteoblasts or stromal fibroblasts to induce the production

Table 340-5   Serum Concentrations of 25(OH)D in Disorders of Calcium, Phosphorus, and Bone Metabolism

Disease States	Serum 25(OH)D
Vitamin D deficiency	↓
Intestinal malabsorption syndromes	↓
Liver disorders (chronic and severe)	↓
Nephrotic syndrome	↓
Osteopenia in the aged	N or ↓
Vitamin D intoxication	↑

NOTE: ↓, decreased; N, normal; ↑, increased.

of RANK ligand on the osteoblast's cell surface. As described above, the RANK ligand interacts with the RANK receptor on immature osteoclasts, stimulating immature osteoclastic precursors to differentiate into mature osteoclasts. The role of $1,25(OH)_2D$ in the renal handling of calcium and phosphorus remains uncertain. Whatever the role of extraintestinal VDRs may be, the compelling evidence is that the phenotype of VDR null mice is corrected in the setting of normal mineral ion homeostasis. Thus the skeletal consequences of VDR ablation are the result of impaired intestinal calcium absorption and/or the accompanying secondary hyperparathyroidism and hypophosphatemia.

Receptors for $1,25(OH)_2D$ are also present in cells not classically considered target organs for this hormone, including skin, breast, pituitary, parathyroids, pancreatic beta cells, gonads, brain, skeletal muscle, circulating monocytes, and activated B and T lymphocytes. Although its physiologic role in these cells remains to be determined,

$1,25(OH)_2D$ inhibits proliferation of keratinocytes and fibroblasts, stimulates terminal differentiation of keratinocytes, induces monocytes to produce interleukin (IL)1 and to differentiate into macrophages and osteoclast-like cells, inhibits the production of PTH, and inhibits the production of IL-2 and immunoglobulin by activated T and B lymphocytes, respectively.

In addition, a variety of tumor cell lines, including lines derived from breast carcinomas, melanomas, and promyeloblasts, possess receptors for $1,25(OH)_2D$. Tumor cell lines that have $1,25(OH)_2D$ receptors respond to the hormone by decreasing the rate of proliferation and enhancing differentiation. For example, when malignant receptor-positive human promyelocytic cells (HL-60) are exposed to $1,25(OH)_2D$, the cells mature into functioning macrophages within 1 week. Although calcitriol [$1,25(OH)_2D$] is not useful for the treatment of leukemia, the antiproliferative effects of calcitriol and its analogue calcipotriene provide the rationale for their use in the treatment of psoriasis.

$1,25(OH)_2D$ regulates PTH synthesis by negative feedback (Fig. 340-6). This effect is the rationale for giving $1,25(OH)_2D_3$, and its less calcemic-inducing analogue 19-nor-$1,25$-dihydroxyvitamin D_3 (Fig. 340-7), to lower circulating levels of PTH in patients with chronic renal failure (Chap. 341).

The principal physiologic mechanism regulating the production of $1,25(OH)_2D$ appears to involve changes in serum extracellular calcium concentrations that result in reciprocal changes in secretion of PTH, the latter controlling, possibly through actions on serum or tissue phosphorus levels, the rate of $1,25(OH)_2D$ production. Other factors that enhance $1,25(OH)_2D$ production include estrogen, prolactin, and

FIGURE 340-6 Schematic representation of the hormonal control loop for vitamin D metabolism and function. A reduction in the serum calcium level below ~2.2 mmol/L (8.8 mg/dL) prompts a proportional increase in the secretion of parathyroid hormone (PTH) and so mobilizes additional calcium from the bone. PTH promotes the synthesis of $1,25(OH)_2D$ in the kidney, which, in turn, stimulates the mobilization of calcium from bone and intestine and regulates the synthesis of PTH by negative feedback.

FIGURE 340-7 Structure of 1,25-dihydroxyvitamin D_3, i.e., $1\alpha,25(OH)_2D_3$, and some of its clinically important analogues. When vitamin D_3 is hydrogenated, its A ring is rotated 180°, placing the 3β-OH in a pseudo 1α spatial orientation. This analogue, dihydrotachysterol (DHT$_3$) is metabolized by a liver 25-hydroxylase (step 25) to 25-hydroxydihydrotachysterol, i.e., 25(OH)DHT$_3$. It is believed that 25(OH)DHT$_3$ is the biologically active form that mimics $1,25(OH)_2D_3$ in its activity. Two clinically important analogues of $1\alpha,25(OH)_2D_3$ include its 25-deoxy derivative 1α-hydroxyvitamin D_3, i.e., $1\alpha(OH)D_3$, and calcipotriene. $1\alpha(OH)D_3$ is metabolized in the liver by 25-hydroxylase to $1\alpha,25(OH)D_3$. Calcipotriene is an analogue that is currently being used in Europe for the topical treatment of psoriasis.

growth hormone. Humans adapt to increased calcium requirements during growth, pregnancy, and lactation by increasing the efficiency of intestinal calcium absorption, possibly by enhancing 25(OH)D-1α-hydroxylase activity. During the first two trimesters of pregnancy, the levels of 1,25(OH)$_2$D increase in proportion to the concentration of the vitamin D–binding protein; levels of free 1,25(OH)$_2$D do not change. During the last trimester, the need for calcium for mineralization of the fetal skeleton is met by an increase in the concentrations of free 1,25(OH)$_2$D and enhanced maternal intestinal calcium absorption.

Most measurements of circulating 1,25(OH)$_2$D in various physiologic or pathologic states utilize a receptor/competitive binding assay. Serum levels of vitamin D and 25(OH)D vary with the season and with vitamin D intake, whereas levels of 1,25(OH)$_2$D appear to be unaltered by seasonal variation, by increases in dietary vitamin D, or by exposure to sunlight (Table 340-6); as long as vitamin D supplies and circulating concentrations of 25(OH)D are sufficient, metabolic influences control the renal 25(OH)D-1α-hydroxylase to ensure a closely regulated circulating concentration of 1,25(OH)$_2$D. The serum concentration of 1,25(OH)$_2$D ranges from 40 to 160 pmol/L (16 to 65 pg/mL), and its serum half-life is from 3 to 6 h.

PHARMACOLOGY Casual exposure to sunlight provides most people with adequate vitamin D. In elderly individuals, exposure of hands, face, and arms to a suberythemal dose of sunlight two to three times a week is usually adequate. A variety of over-the-counter vitamin preparations contain 400 IU of either vitamin D$_2$ (ergocalciferol) or vitamin D$_3$ (cholecalciferol). More potent preparations of vitamin D (calciferol) are available in capsule and tablet form (50,000 IU), as oil (500,000 IU/mL), and in oral solution (8000 IU/mL). A single oral dose of 50,000 IU of vitamin D$_2$ increases the circulating concentration of vitamin D from <25 nmol/L (10 ng/mL) to 130 to 260 nmol/L (50 to 100 ng/mL) within 12 to 24 h; the plasma half-life is about 2 days. Serum concentrations of 25(OH)D and 1,25(OH)$_2$D are not changed by these doses of vitamin D. For treatment of vitamin D deficiency, 50,000 IU of vitamin D once a week for 8 weeks raises the circulating concentration of 25(OH)D into the normal range; in the presence of secondary hyperparathyroidism, the circulating concentrations of 1,25(OH)$_2$D can increase to supranormal levels [up to 600 pmol/L (250 pg/mL)]. 25(OH)D$_3$ (calcifediol) available in capsules

Table 340-6 Serum Concentrations of 1,25(OH)$_2$D in Disorders of Calcium, Phosphorus, and Bone Metabolism

Disease States	Serum 1,25(OH)$_2$D
Vitamin D deficiency	↓ [a]
Renal failure:	
GFR > 30 (mL/min)/1.7 m^2	↓ or N
GFR < 30 (mL/min)/1.7 m^2	↓
Hypoparathyroidism	↓ or N
Pseudohypoparathyroidism	↓ or N
Vitamin D–dependent rickets:	
Type I	↓
Type II	↑
X-linked vitamin D–resistant rickets	↓ or N
Tumor-induced osteomalacia	↓
Oncogenic hypercalcemia	↓
Some lymphomas	↑
Hyperparathyroidism	↑
Sarcoidosis, tuberculosis, silicosis	↑
Idiopathic hypercalciuria	N or ↑
Williams' syndrome	↑
Vitamin D intoxication	N or ↑

[a] Serum 1,25(OH)$_2$D concentrations are normal or elevated in occasional patients with biopsy-proven osteomalacia and undetectable or low circulating concentrations of 25(OH)D. These patients also have secondary hyperparathyroidism and may represent a partially treated state; if a small amount of vitamin D is obtained from the diet or generated in the skin in these patients, the vitamin is efficiently converted to 1,25(OH)$_2$D. The net effect is low or undetectable circulating concentrations of 25(OH)D along with normal or elevated concentrations of 1,25(OH)$_2$D. However, in extreme vitamin D deficiency, circulating concentrations of 1,25(OH)$_2$D are low or undetectable.

NOTE: ↓ decreased; N, normal; ↑, increased; GFR, glomerular filtration rate.

containing either 20 or 50 μg may be useful in treating vitamin D deficiency [low 25(OH)D concentrations] in patients with severe liver dysfunction. Pharmacologic doses are used to treat disorders of 25(OH)D metabolism; in pharmacologic doses, 25(OH)D$_3$ is believed to act via interaction with the VDR. Calcitriol is available in capsules containing 0.25 or 0.5 μg and as a solution for intravenous use (1.0 and 2.0 μg/mL). Calcitriol is efficacious in a variety of disorders (Chap. 341), but even low doses can cause hypercalcemia, leading to attempts to develop analogues with less calcemic activity. Two such calcitriol analogues have been approved in the United States for the treatment of renal osteodystrophy; 19-nor-1,25-dihydroxyvitamin D$_2$, and 24-epi-1,25-dihydroxyvitamin D$_2$ (Fig. 340-7). 1α-Hydroxyvitamin D$_3$ [1(OH)D$_3$] is a potent 1,25(OH)$_2$D$_3$ agonist that is used in Europe and Japan. The structure of this analogue is identical to that of the natural renal hormone with the exception that it lacks a C$_{25}$ OH. In humans, this analogue is rapidly metabolized by the liver to 1,25(OH)$_2$D$_3$. Topical preparations of calcitriol (3 μg/g) in Europe and calcipotriene (50 μg/g) in Europe and the United States are used for the treatment of psoriasis. When applied over a large surface area, both can potentially cause hypercalcemia and hypercalciuria. Oral calcitriol is also effective for psoriasis and psoriatic arthritis.

When vitamin D is chemically manipulated to rotate the A ring through 180°, the C$_3$ β-OH assumes a geometric position that mimics the C$_1$ α-OH (Fig. 340-7). These compounds, called *pseudo-1α-hydroxyvitamin D analogues*, include the clinically useful dihydrotachysterol (DHT). This analogue is less effective in stimulating intestinal calcium transport on a weight basis than either vitamin D or 1,25(OH)$_2$D. Because it does not require 1α-hydroxylation to be active on intestinal calcium transport, it is 3 to 10 times more potent than vitamin D in disease states that impair renal 25(OH)D-1α-hydroxylase, such as hypoparathyroidism and chronic renal failure. Dihydrotachysterol is efficiently metabolized in the liver to 25-hydroxy-DHT, which is the biologically active form.

RICKETS AND OSTEOMALACIA

Rickets and osteomalacia are disorders in which mineralization of the organic matrix of the skeleton is defective. These disorders are caused by a number of different conditions associated with vitamin D deficiency or resistance (Table 340-7). In *rickets*, the growing skeleton is involved; defective mineralization occurs both in the bone and cartilaginous matrix of the growth plate. The term *osteomalacia* is usually used for this mineralization disorder in the adults in whom epiphyseal growth plates are closed.

For normal skeletal mineralization, sufficient calcium and phosphate must be present at the mineralization sites. In addition, intact metabolic and transport functions of osteoblasts and chondrocytes and adequate production of cross-linked collagen matrix are required. In cartilage, the initial mineral phase is enclosed in membrane-bound extracellular vesicles. If the osteoblast continues to produce matrix components that cannot be mineralized adequately, rickets or osteomalacia results. A characteristic feature of these disorders is therefore an increase in osteoid volume and thickness (the latter being normally <12 to 14 μm) and a decrease in calcification of the mineralization front. This can be detected in unmineralized sections by the fluorescence of previously ingested tetracyclines or by special stains. The inadequate mineralization of the matrix of cartilage in growing children leads to a widening of the epiphyseal plates of the long bones due to a disorganization of the otherwise highly ordered columns of hypertrophied cartilage cells. In addition, the poorly mineralized long bones are incapable of withstanding usual mechanical stresses and tend to undergo bowing deformities. Growth of the epiphyseal plates is diminished, stunting the growth of the long bones. Osteomalacia also compromises the architectural structure and strength of the skeleton in adults, causing an increase in fractures.

Table 340-7 Classification of Rickets and Osteomalacia

Vitamin D deficiency
  Dietary deficiency
  Deficient endogenous synthesis
Gastrointestinal disorders
  Small-intestinal diseases with malabsorption
  Partial or total gastrectomy
  Hepatobiliary disease
  Chronic pancreatic insufficiency
Disorders of vitamin D metabolism
  Hereditary: pseudovitamin D deficiency or vitamin
    D dependency types I and II
  Acquired: Anticonvulsants
        Chronic renal failure
        Tumor-associated (oncogenic) rickets and osteomalacia
Acidosis
  Distal renal tubular acidosis (classic or type I)
  Secondary forms of renal acidosis
  Ureterosigmoidostomy
  Drug-induced disease: Chronic acetazolamide ingestion
           Chronic ammonium chloride ingestion
Chronic renal failure
Phosphate depletion
  Dietary: low phosphate intake plus ingestion of nonabsorbable antacids
  Impaired renal tubular phosphate reabsorption
    Hereditary
      X-linked hypophosphatemic rickets (vitamin D–resistant rickets)
      Adult-onset vitamin D–resistant hypophosphatemic osteomalacia
    Acquired
      Sporadic hypophosphatemic osteomalacia (phosphate diabetes)
      Tumor-associated (oncogenic) rickets and osteomalacia
      Neurofibromatosis
      Fibrous dysplasia
Generalized renal tubular disorders (Fanconi's syndrome)
  Primary renal
  Associated with systemic metabolic abnormality
    Cystinosis
    Glycogenosis
    Lowe's syndrome
  Systemic disorder with associated renal disease
    Hereditary
      Inborn errors: Wilson's disease
              Tyrosinemia
      Neurofibromatosis
    Acquired: Multiple myeloma
          Nephrotic syndrome
          Transplanted kidney
    Intoxications: Cadmium
            Lead
            Outdated tetracycline
Primary mineralization defects
  Hereditary: hypophosphatasia
  Acquired: Disodium etidronate treatment (Note: Of the bis-
          phosphonates, only etidronate has this effect)
      Fluoride treatment
States of rapid bone formation with or without a relative
 defect in bone resorption
  Postoperative hyperparathyroidism with osteitis
   fibrosa cystica
  Osteopetrosis
Defective matrix synthesis: fibrogenesis imperfecta ossium
Miscellaneous: Magnesium-dependent conditions
          Axial osteomalacia
          Parenteral alimentation
          Aluminum intoxication

PATHOPHYSIOLOGY A large number of disorders are associated with rickets or osteomalacia, primarily through alterations of vitamin D nutrition or metabolism or because of phosphate wasting (Table 340-7). *Hypovitaminosis D* results from inadequate endogenous production of vitamin D$_3$ in the skin, from insufficient dietary supplementation, and/or from an inability of the small intestine to absorb adequate amounts of the vitamin from the diet. Resistance to the effects of vitamin D can result from (1) use of drugs that antagonize vitamin D action, (2) alterations in the metabolism of vitamin D, or (3) deficient or defective receptors for 1,25(OH)$_2$D. The consequences of hypovitaminosis D include (1) disturbances of mineral ion metabolism and secretion of PTH, and (2) mineralization defects in the skeleton (e.g., rickets in children, osteomalacia in adults). With an adequate glomerular filtration rate (GFR), the main changes are hypophosphatemia, normal or near-normal serum calcium levels, increased levels of PTH, and low levels of 25(OH)D (Table 340-5).

With regard to calcium metabolism, lack of vitamin D action leads to insufficient intestinal calcium absorption and hypocalcemia. The latter stimulates the secretion of PTH (secondary hyperparathyroidism), which enhances calcium release from bone, decreases calcium clearance by the kidney, and tends to blunt the hypocalcemia; as a consequence, most patients have a normal or low-normal serum calcium level. (Late in the course of untreated hypovitaminosis D, severe hypocalcemia develops.) Hypophosphatemia is more marked than hypocalcemia, especially in early stages of the deficiency. The efficiency of intestinal phosphate absorption is also decreased. The increased secretion of PTH, although partially effective in minimizing hypocalcemia, leads to urinary phosphate wasting because of decreased renal tubular reabsorption. This latter effect is the most significant factor in causing hypophosphatemia. Aging decreases the responsiveness of the renal 25(OH)D-1-hydroxylase to PTH, decreasing circulating levels of 1,25(OH)$_2$D and contributing to decreased calcium absorption in the elderly.

Although the conversion of vitamin D to 25(OH)D is impaired in severe chronic liver disease, there is not a strong correlation between low serum 25(OH)D levels and osteopenia. Patients with nephrotic syndrome with >4 g/d of proteinuria may have low 25(OH)D levels owing to loss in the urine of the vitamin D–binding protein with its associated tightly bound 25(OH)D. Circulating levels of 25(OH)D may also be decreased when the metabolism of 25(OH)D to 1,25(OH)$_2$D is increased, as in sarcoidosis and hyperparathyroidism. Chronic anticonvulsant therapy can also cause the development of osteomalacia or rickets; mineralization defects are worse in patients receiving multiple drug therapy and when vitamin D intake or exposure to sunlight is inadequate. Anticonvulsant drugs have multiple effects on calcium metabolism. Phenobarbital induces hepatic microsomal enzymes, alters the kinetics of the vitamin D-25-hydroxylase, and stimulates bile secretion, resulting in decreased serum concentrations of vitamin D and 25(OH)D. Phenytoin and phenobarbital inhibit intestinal calcium transport and bone mineral mobilization, independent of effects on vitamin D metabolism.

Glucocorticoids in high doses cause osteoporosis but do not induce osteomalacia and rickets (Chap. 342). Glucocorticoids directly inhibit vitamin D–mediated intestinal calcium absorption and bone mineral mobilization. Patients receiving glucocorticoids chronically may have depressed circulating levels of 1,25(OH)$_2$D; the mechanism(s) is unknown. Glucocorticoids also exert direct effects to induce apoptosis of osteoblasts and osteocytes.

A genetic defect in the hepatic 25-hydroxylation of vitamin D has not been described, but in one inherited disorder of calcium and bone metabolism, renal production of 1,25(OH)$_2$D is defective because of recessive mutations 25(OH)D-1α-hydroxylase activity. In this syndrome of pseudovitamin D–deficient rickets (also known as vitamin D–dependent rickets type I), renal production of 1,25(OH)$_2$D is impaired, circulating levels of 1,25(OH)$_2$D are low, but the therapeutic response to physiologic doses of calcitriol (0.25 to 1.0 μg/d) is normal. In patients with a similar phenotype, pseudovitamin D–resistant rickets (vitamin D–dependent rickets type II), mutations in the vitamin D receptor impair its function by altering the binding of the hormone to the receptor or by altering the binding of the receptor heterodimer complex to DNA. Individuals with this disorder have high circulating levels of 1,25(OH)$_2$D, but the hormone is ineffective because of the receptor defect. Alopecia is another feature of this disorder, suggesting a role for the VDR in hair follicle development.

Inherited forms of phosphate wasting disorders include X-linked hypophosphatemic rickets and autosomal dominant hypophosphatemic rickets. The gene responsible for the autosomal form is unknown but has been mapped to chromosome 12p13. The X-linked disorder is caused by mutations in the *PHEX* (phosphate-regulating gene with homology to endopeptidases on the X-chromosome) gene. The *PHEX* gene is postulated to encode an osteoblast protein that inactivates phosphatonin, a phosphaturic factor. Consequently, inactivating mutations result in phosphate wasting. The gene is expressed in heterozygotes, suggesting that the disorder is caused by haploinsufficiency. In patients with X-linked hypophosphatemic rickets, serum concentrations of $1,25(OH)_2D$ are normal or low. Since hypophosphatemia is a potent stimulator of the renal $25(OH)D-1\alpha$-hydroxylase, levels of $1,25(OH)_2D$ should be high, which suggests the existence of a functional defect in the $25(OH)D-1\alpha$-hydroxylase in this disorder. Therefore, the combination of calcitriol and phosphate supplements is more effective than therapy with phosphate supplements alone.

Patients with hypocalcemia due to hypoparathyroidism or pseudohypoparathyroidism have lower-than-normal mean serum concentrations of $1,25(OH)_2D$, although individual values may be in the normal range. In these patients, small replacement doses of calcitriol (0.25 to 1.0 μg/d) are effective even when the serum $25(OH)D$ concentrations are elevated. These observations indicate that absent or ineffective action of PTH decreases the activity of renal $25(OH)D-1\alpha$-hydroxylase. It is not known whether serum $1,25(OH)_2D$ levels would be restored if the hyperphosphatemia were controlled.

Patients with tumor-induced (oncogenic) osteomalacia have low levels of serum phosphorus and $1,25(OH)_2D$. Some of these tumors, especially malignant carcinomas, produce PTHrP (Chap. 341), leading to hypercalcemia as well as hypophosphatemia. Other tumors, particularly more benign neoplasms of vascular or mesenchymal origin, may be responsible for severe hypophosphatemia in the presence of normocalcemia. The mechanism for inhibition of $1,25(OH)_2D$ synthesis remains unknown; after removal of the tumor, however, the serum phosphorus and $1,25(OH)_2D$ levels return to normal.

It has been suggested that alteration of vitamin D receptor levels in target tissues (such as intestine) could affect calcium and bone metabolism, and bone mineral density appears to be associated with specific polymorphisms of the VDR gene. These polymorphisms affect the noncoding intervening DNA sequences (introns) or the coding sequence in a way that does not alter the amino acid sequence of the VDR. Some reports suggest that polymorphisms involving the endonucleases Bsm-I and Taq-I (bb, TT) are associated with higher bone mineral density; other studies have not confirmed these findings. The genetic contribution of VDR polymorphic variants to bone mineral density, as well as a number of other diseases with which they have been associated, require additional, larger-scale studies.

CLINICAL FEATURES The clinical manifestations of rickets are the result of skeletal deformities, susceptibility to fractures, weakness and hypotonia, and disturbances in growth. As the disorder progresses, particularly that associated with vitamin D deficiency, children are unable to walk without support due to the skeletal deformities in the lower limbs and severe muscle weakness (Fig. 340-8). Abnormal parietal flattening and frontal bossing develops in the skull. The calvariae are softened (*craniotabes*) and sutures may be widened. Prominence of the costochondral junctions is called the *rachitic rosary* and the indentation of the lower ribs at the site of attachment of the diaphragm is known as *Harrison's groove*. If untreated, deformities of the pelvis and extremities progress, with bowing being particularly common in the tibia, femur, radius, and ulna. For women, the flattening of the pelvis increases the risk of maternal and infant morbidity and mortality during childbirth. Fractures are frequent, dental eruption is often delayed, and enamel defects are common.

The presentation of osteomalacia in adults is usually more insidious. Bone pain and muscle weakness are common complaints and may be overlooked as indicators of vitamin D deficiency. It is estimated in the United States and Europe that >40% of the adult population over the age of 50 are vitamin D deficient. Although the standard lower

FIGURE 340-8 Typical clinical features of rickets. The child in the middle is normal; the children on either side have severe muscle weakness and bony deformities including bowed legs (right) or knock knees (left). *[Reproduced with permission from F Bicknell, F Prescott: in W Heineman (ed) The Vitamins in Medicine, 2ᵈ ed. London, Random House UK, 1948.]*

limit of the normal range for $25(OH)D$ is 10 ng/mL, several studies suggest that the cutoff for vitamin D deficiency should be increased to 20 ng/mL. This suggestion is based on PTH responses to various serum levels of $25(OH)D$. For example, elevated levels of PTH are frequently seen in individuals with $25(OH)D$ levels between 10 and 20 ng/mL, and administration of vitamin D (50,000 units of vitamin D once a week for 8 weeks) lowers PTH levels. Defects in skeletal mineralization may accompany these disturbances in vitamin D and mineral metabolism.

Pain in the hips may result in an antalgic gait. Muscle weakness is often associated with osteomalacia but is difficult to distinguish from hesitancy to move because of skeletal pain. Proximal weakness may mimic that of primary muscle disorders and contribute to the waddling gait. Many factors, including secondary hyperparathyroidism, hypophosphatemia, and vitamin D deficiency, contribute to the myopathy. Fractures of the involved bones may occur with minimal trauma. When the ribs are involved, severe deformities may develop in the thorax, and the collapse of the vertebral bodies may produce loss of height.

RADIOLOGIC FEATURES In rickets, the most prominent radiologic alteration is evident at the growth plate (physis) which is increased in thickness, cupped, and hazy at the metaphyseal border owing to decreased calcification of the hypertrophic zone and inadequate mineralization of the primary spongiosa. The trabecular pattern of the metaphysis is abnormal, the cortices of the diaphysis may be thinned, and the shafts may be bowed.

In osteomalacia, a decrease in bone density is usually associated with loss of trabeculae and thinning of the cortices. Radiologic and bone densitometric changes are indistinguishable from those in osteoporosis (Chap. 342). Trabecular patterns may be blurred, producing a homogeneous "ground glass" appearance. Radiolucent bands, ranging from a few millimeters to several centimeters in length and usually oriented perpendicular to the surface of the bones, suggest the presence of osteomalacia. They are particularly common at the inner aspects of the femur (especially near the femoral neck), in the pelvis, in the outer edge of the scapula, in the upper fibula, and in the metatarsals. These radiolucent bands, called *pseudofractures* or *Looser's zones*, occur most often where major arteries cross the bones and are thought to be due to the pulsation of these vessels in the undermineralized area (Fig. 340-9). Increased rather than decreased density of bones may be observed in patients who have renal tubular disorders rather than vitamin D deficiency and may produce a striking thickening of the cortices and a trabecular pattern of the spongy bone. Despite the increase in bone mass per unit volume, the trabeculae are covered with thickened osteoid seams typical of osteomalacia. Similar findings may occur in patients with chronic renal failure. The reason for the hyperostosis is unknown; the bone is architecturally abnormal and is subject to fracture with minimal trauma.

LABORATORY FINDINGS   Changes in serum concentration of calcium, inorganic phosphorus, 25(OH)D, and 1,25(OH)$_2$D vary with the different disorders. In vitamin D deficiency, whether due to dietary lack, inadequate sunlight exposure, or intestinal malabsorption, serum calcium levels are normal or low, whereas phosphorus and 25(OH)D levels are consistently low, the latter usually <15 nmol/L (<10 ng/mL) depending on the assay used. In contrast, levels of 1,25(OH)$_2$D may be normal or elevated owing to secondary hyperparathyroidism and the fact that circulating levels of 1,25(OH)$_2$D are 1000-fold less than those of 25(OH)D. Only when vitamin D deficiency is chronic and severe is hypocalcemia observed. It may be sufficiently severe to produce tetany. Mild acidosis and generalized aminoaciduria result from secondary hyperparathyroidism. Patients with renal tubular disorders have normal serum calcium levels and hypophosphatemia. Other laboratory findings such as glucosuria, aminoaciduria, acidosis, and hypouricemia reflect variable degrees of disturbance of proximal tubular function or are features of underlying disease (e.g., low plasma ceruloplasmin in Wilson's disease or abnormalities of immunoglobulins in multiple myeloma). In chronic renal failure, hyperphosphatemia and hypocalcemia are usually accompanied by normal 25(OH)D and low 1,25(OH)$_2$D levels. In nephrotic syndrome, serum 25(OH)D levels can be low owing primarily to urinary losses of vitamin D binding protein–bound 25(OH)D. Serum phosphorus levels are also normal or elevated in hypophosphatasia. Markers of bone resorption increase when secondary hyperparathyroidism and excessive bone resorption are associated with the defect in mineralization. Alkaline phosphatase levels in serum are usually elevated in rickets and osteomalacia.

TREATMENT   In rickets and osteomalacia due to dietary absence of vitamin D or inadequate exposure to sunlight, vitamin D$_2$ (ergocalciferol) or vitamin D$_3$ (cholecalciferol) is given orally in doses of 800 to 4000 IU (0.02 to 0.1 mg) daily for 6 to 12 weeks, followed by daily supplements of 200 to 600 IU, which are adequate to prevent the development of the disorder in otherwise normal persons. In elderly persons with vitamin D deficiency, the administration of 50,000 IU vitamin D by mouth once each week for 8 weeks raises the serum levels of 25(OH)D into the mid-normal range. In infants and children, such treatment causes improvement in muscle tone and strength, an increase in serum calcium and phosphorus levels, and a decrease in alkaline phosphatase levels after several weeks. Radiologic evidence of healing appears within weeks, and healing may be complete by a few months. Calcium supplements and larger initial doses of vitamin D may be necessary in infants and children with tetany. In adults with nutritional osteomalacia, healing of pseudofractures may be evident within 3 to 4 weeks after therapy with as little as 2000 IU (0.5 mg) vitamin D daily. Healing is usually complete by 6 months.

Patients with osteomalacia due to intestinal malabsorption do not respond to small doses of vitamin D. In the presence of active steatorrhea, daily oral doses of vitamin D of 50,000 to 100,000 IU (1.25 to 2.5 mg) and large doses of calcium (e.g., 15 g calcium lactate or 4 g calcium carbonate orally per day) may be required. In some instances, oral vitamin D is ineffective, and the parenteral route is required (e.g., 10,000 IU/d intramuscularly). Another approach is the use of artificial ultraviolet B radiation or exposure to sunlight in addition to supplemental calcium. Small doses of calcitriol (0.5 to 1.0 μg daily) are also usually effective in this form of osteomalacia. Inorganic phosphate therapy is not indicated either in deficiency or in intestinal malabsorption of the vitamin, since hypocalcemia will develop and intestinal calcium absorption will remain inadequate. In all patients in whom large doses of vitamin D are used, serum calcium and 25(OH)D levels should be monitored periodically. Semiquantitative urinary calcium measurements are inadequate.

In patients treated with multiple anticonvulsant agents, it is usually necessary to continue the drugs while adding 1000 IU/d of vitamin D and to monitor levels of serum calcium and serum 25(OH)D until a therapeutic response (evidence of radiologic healing, improvement in symptoms) is obtained.

Treatment of rickets and osteomalacia in the presence of renal tubular disorders is more difficult. Oral supplements of inorganic phosphate in divided doses of phosphorus (as elemental P), 1.0 to 3.6 g/d (50 mg/kg body weight per day for children), and calcitriol, 0.5 to 2.0 μg/d (30 ng/kg body weight per day for children), constitute the best regimen to restore skeletal growth and heal the bone disease. Patients with nephrotic syndrome and low serum 25(OH)D levels benefit from modest vitamin D supplementation (800 to 1000 IU/d). Small doses of calcitriol are equally effective in treating hypocalcemia and osteodystrophy resulting from chronic renal failure. The recommended initial dose of calcitriol is 0.25 μg/d. If after 2 to 4 weeks on this dose the biochemical parameters are unaltered, the dose is increased by 0.25 μg/d every 2 to 4 weeks until a satisfactory clinical biochemical response (including elevation of serum calcium levels and decrease in PTH levels) is obtained. The usual dose is 0.5 to 1.0 μg/d. Calcitriol may also be administered intravenously (1.0 to 2.5 μg three times weekly) to patients on dialysis, particularly to treat refractory osteitis fibrosa. Serum calcium levels should be monitored frequently during the first 1 to 2 months of therapy and less frequently once a stable dose has been established.

In patients who have had rickets in childhood, the abnormal mechanical stress of severe deformities may contribute to the develop-

FIGURE 340-9   Radiograph of the scapula of a 58-year-old woman with phosphate diabetes as a cause of osteomalacia. The presence of a pseudofracture or Looser's zone is indicated by an arrow.

ment of degenerative joint disease, particularly in the hips and knees. Osteotomies at the proper time after healing may prevent this complication and the requirement for more extensive arthroplasties later in life.

BIBLIOGRAPHY

Bone Structure and Metabolism

Avioli LV, Krane SM (eds): *Metabolic Bone Disease*, 3d ed. San Diego, Academic Press, 1998

Burger EH, Klein-Nulend J: Mechanotransduction in bone—role of the lacunocanalicular network. FASEB J 13:S101, 1999

Ducy P et al: Osf2/Cbfa1: A transcriptional activator of osteoblast differentiation. Cell 89:677, 1997

——— et al: Leptin inhibits bone formation through a hypothalamic relay: A central control of bone mass. Cell 100:197, 2000

Karsenty G: The genetic transformation of bone biology. Genes Dev 13:3037, 1999

Kronenberg HM et al: Functional analysis of the PTH/PTHrP network of ligands and receptors. Recent Prog Horm Res 53:283, 1998

Li J et al: RANK is the intrinsic hematopoietic cell surface receptor that controls osteoclastogenesis and regulation of bone mass and calcium metabolism. Proc Natl Acad Sci USA 97:1566, 2000

Manolagas SC: Birth and death of bone cells: Basic regulatory mechanisms and implications for the pathogenesis and treatment of osteoporosis. Endocrine Rev 21:115, 2000

Mundlos S et al: Mutations involving the transcription factor CBFA1 cause cleidocranial dysplasia. Cell 89:773, 1997

Russell RG et al: The pharmacology of bisphosphonates and the new insights into their mechanisms of action. J Bone Miner Res 14(Suppl 2):53, 1999

Soriano P et al: Targeted disruption of the c-*src* proto-oncogene leads to osteopetrosis in mice. Cell 64:693, 1991

Suda T et al: Modulation of osteoclast differentiation and function by the new members of the tumor necrosis factor receptor and ligand families. Endocrine Rev 20:345, 1999

Zhang P et al: A homozygous inactivating mutation in the parathyroid hormone/parathyroid hormone-related peptide receptor causing Blomstrand chondrodysplasia. J Clin Endocrinol Metab 83:3365, 1998

Calcium, Phosphorus, and Magnesium

Bringhurst FR: Regulation of calcium and phosphate homeostasis, in *Endocrinology*, 4th ed, LJ DeGroot, JL Jameson (eds). Philadelphia, Saunders, 2000

Bryant RJ et al: The new dietary reference intakes for calcium: Implications for osteoporosis. J Am Coll Nutr 18(5Suppl):406S, 1999

Dresner MK: *PHEX* gene and hypophosphatemia. Kidney Int 57:9, 2000

Econs MJ: New insights into the pathogenesis of inherited phosphate wasting disorders. Bone 25:131, 1999

Holick MF: Evaluation and treatment of disorders in calcium, phosphorus, and magnesium metabolism, in *Primary Care and General Medicine*, 2d ed, J Noble (ed). St. Louis, Mosby, 1996, pp 545–557

Hruska KA, Lederer ED: Hyperphosphatemia and hypophosphatemia, in *Primer on Metabolic Bone Diseases and Disorders of Mineral Metabolism*, 4th ed, MJ Favus (ed). Philadelphia, Lippincott-Raven, 1999, pp 245–253

Matkovic V: Calcium intake and peak bone mass. N Engl J Med 327:119, 1992

Rude RK: Magnesium depletion and hypermagnesemia, in *Primer on Metabolic Bone Diseases and Disorders of Mineral Metabolism*, 4th ed, MJ Favus (ed). Philadelphia, Lippincott-Raven, 1999, pp 241–245

Scheinman SJ et al: Isolated hypercalciuria with mutation in CLCN5: Relevance to idiopathic hypercalciuria. Kidney Int 57:232, 2000

Yamaguchi T et al: G protein–coupled extracellular Ca^{2+} (Ca^{2+})-sensing receptor (CaR) in cell signaling and control of diverse cellular functions. Adv Pharmacol 47:209, 2000

Vitamin D

Bouillon R: The many faces of rickets. N Engl J Med 338:681, 1998

———: Vitamin D: From photosynthesis, metabolism, and action, to clinical applications, in *Endocrinology*, 4th ed, LJ DeGroot, JL Jameson (eds). Philadelphia, Saunders, 2000

Darwin H, DeLuca H: Vitamin D-regulated gene expression. Crit Rev Eukaryotic Gene Expr 3:89, 1993

Holick MF (ed): *Vitamin D—Physiology, Molecular Biology and Clinical Applications*. Totowa, NJ, Humana Press, 1998

———, Adams JS: Vitamin D metabolism and biological function, in *Metabolic Bone Disease*, 3rd ed, LV Avioli, SM Krane (eds). San Diego, Academic Press, 1998, pp 123–163

Kitanaka S et al: Inactivating mutations in the 25-hydroxyvitamin D_3 1α-hydroxylase gene in patients with pseudovitamin D-deficiency rickets. N Engl J Med 338:653, 1998

341   *John T. Potts, Jr*

DISEASES OF THE PARATHYROID GLAND AND OTHER HYPER- AND HYPOCALCEMIC DISORDERS

AHO Albright's hereditary osteodystrophy	IP_3 inositol triphosphate
CGRP calcitonin gene–related peptide	MEN multiple endocrine neoplasia
CT computed tomography	PTH parathyroid hormone
DAG diacylglycerol	PTHrP parathyroid hormone–related peptide
ECF extracellular fluid	PHP pseudohypoparathyroidism
FHH familial hypocalciuric hypercalcemia	PPHP pseudopseudohypoparathyroidism
GPCR G protein–coupled receptor	SERMs selective estrogen receptor modulators

The four parathyroid glands are located posterior to the thyroid gland. They produce parathyroid hormone (PTH), which is the primary regulator of calcium physiology. PTH acts directly on bone, where it induces calcium resorption, and on the kidney, where it stimulates calcium reabsorption and synthesis of 1,25-dihydroxyvitamin D [$1,25(OH)_2D$], a hormone that stimulates gastrointestinal calcium absorption. Serum PTH levels are tightly regulated by a negative feedback loop. Calcium, acting through the calcium-sensing receptor, and vitamin D, acting through its nuclear receptor, inhibit PTH synthesis and release. Understanding the hormone pathways that regulate calcium levels and bone metabolism is essential for effective diagnosis and management of a wide array of hyper- and hypocalcemic disorders.

Hyperparathyroidism, characterized by excess production of PTH, is a common cause of hypercalcemia and is usually the result of autonomously functioning adenomas or hyperplasia. Surgery for this disorder is highly effective and has been shown recently to reverse some of the deleterious effects of long-standing PTH excess on bone density. Hypercalcemia of malignancy is also common and is usually due to the overproduction of parathyroid hormone–related peptide (PTHrP) by cancer cells. The similarities in the biochemical characteristics of hyperparathyroidism and hypercalcemia of malignancy, first noted by Albright in 1941, are now known to reflect the actions of PTH and PTHrP through the same G protein–coupled (GPC) PTH/PTHrP receptor.

Clarification over the past decade of genetic influences on parathyroid gland and bone cell function helps in constructing a logical approach to hyper- and hypocalcemic disorders. Advances that have occurred include elucidation of the genetic basis of multiple endocrine neoplasia (MEN) types 1 and 2, familial hypocalciuric hypercalcemia (FHH), the different forms of pseudohypoparathyroidism (PHP), Jansen's syndrome, disorders of vitamin D synthesis and action, and the molecular events associated with parathyroid gland neoplasia. The advent of new drugs, including bisphosphonates and selective estrogen receptor modulators (SERMs), offers new avenues for the treatment and prevention of metabolic bone disease. PTH analogues are promising therapeutic agents for the treatment of postmenopausal or senile osteoporosis, and calcimimetic agents, which act through the calcium-sensing receptor, may provide new approaches for PTH suppression.

PARATHYROID HORMONE

PHYSIOLOGY   The primary function of PTH is to maintain the extracellular fluid (ECF) calcium concentration within a narrow normal range. The hormone acts directly on bone and kidney and indirectly on intestine through its effects on synthesis of $1,25(OH)_2D$ to increase serum calcium concentrations; in turn, PTH production is closely regulated by the concentration of serum ionized calcium. This feedback system is the critical homeostatic mechanism for maintenance of ECF calcium. Any tendency toward hypocalcemia, as might be induced by calcium-deficient diets, is counteracted by an increased secretion of PTH. This in turn (1) acts to increase the rate of dissolution of bone mineral, thereby increasing the flow of calcium from bone into blood; (2) reduces the renal clearance of calcium, returning more of the calcium filtered at the glomerulus into ECF; and (3) increases the efficiency of calcium absorption in the intestine. Immediate control of blood calcium is probably due to effects of the hormone on bone and, to a lesser extent, on renal calcium clearance. Maintenance of steady-state calcium balance, on the other hand, probably results from the effects of $1,25(OH)_2D$ on calcium absorption (Chap. 340). The renal actions of the hormone are exerted at multiple sites and include inhibition of phosphate transport (proximal tubule), increased reabsorption of calcium (distal tubule), and stimulation of the renal $25(OH)D-1\alpha$-hydroxylase. As much as 12 mmol (500 mg) calcium is transferred between the ECF and bone each day (a large amount in relation to the total ECF calcium pool), and PTH has a major effect on this transfer. The homeostatic role of the hormone can preserve calcium concentration in blood acutely at the cost of bone destruction.

PTH has multiple actions on bone, some direct and some indirect. It increases the rate of calcium release from bone into blood acutely; PTH-mediated changes in bone calcium release can be seen within minutes. The chronic effects of PTH are to increase the number of bone cells, both osteoblasts and osteoclasts, and to increase the remodeling of bone; these effects are apparent within hours after the hormone is given and persist for hours after PTH is withdrawn. Continuous exposure to elevated levels of PTH for days (as in hyperparathyroidism or long-term infusions in animals) leads to increased osteoclast-mediated bone resorption. However, the administration of PTH intermittently over days in animals or osteoporotic patients leads to a net stimulation of bone formation rather than bone breakdown. Striking increases, especially in trabecular bone in the spine and hip, have been reported with the use of PTH in combination with estrogen. PTH as monotherapy caused a highly significant reduction in fracture incidence in a worldwide placebo-controlled trial.

Osteoblasts (or stromal cell precursors), which have PTH receptors, are crucial to this bone-forming effect of PTH; osteoclasts, which appear to lack PTH receptors, mediate bone breakdown. PTH-mediated stimulation of osteoclasts is believed to be indirect, acting in part through cytokines released from osteoblasts to activate osteoclasts; in experimental studies of bone resorption in vitro, osteoblasts must be present for PTH to activate osteoclasts to resorb bone. The nature of the cytokines that stimulate osteoclasts is a subject of major interest. Insulin-like growth factor 1, interleukin 6, granulocyte-macrophage colony stimulating factor, and possibly other agents are candidates, but the definitive messenger(s) has not been determined. Direct cell-to-cell contact between osteoblasts (stromal cells) and osteoclast precursors is also key to osteoclast function. Cell-associated ligands and receptors, as well as soluble decoy receptors, are involved in these interactions (Chap. 340).

STRUCTURE PTH is an 84-amino-acid single-chain peptide. The amino acid sequence of PTH has been characterized in multiple mammalian species, revealing marked conservation in the amino-terminal portion, which is critical for many biologic actions of the molecule. Synthetic fragments of the amino-terminal sequence as small as 1–14 residues are sufficient to activate the major receptor (see below). Biologic roles for the carboxyl-terminal region of PTH are under investigation; a separate receptor may exist for this region of the molecule. Fragments shortened or modified at the amino terminus still bind to the PTH receptor but lose the capacity to stimulate biologic responses. For example, the peptide composed of sequences 7–34 is a competitive inhibitor of active hormone binding to receptors in vitro but is a weak inhibitor in vivo.

BIOSYNTHESIS, SECRETION, AND METABOLISM

Synthesis Parathyroid cells have multiple methods of adapting to increased needs for PTH production. Most rapid (within minutes) is secretion of preformed hormone in response to hypocalcemia. Second, within hours, changes in gene activity and increased PTH mRNA are induced by sustained hypocalcemia. Finally, protracted challenge leads within days to cellular replication to increase gland mass.

PTH is initially synthesized as a larger molecule (preproparathyroid hormone, consisting of 115 amino acids), which is then reduced in size by a second cleavage (proparathyroid hormone, 90 amino acids) before secretion as the 84-amino-acid peptide. The hydrophobic regions of the preproparathyroid hormone serve a role in guiding transport of the polypeptide from sites of synthesis on polyribosomes through the endoplasmic reticulum to secretory granules. In one kindred with hypoparathyroidism, a mutation in the preprotein region of the gene disrupts this critical hydrophobic sequence and interferes with hormone secretion.

Studies with cloned and expressed PTH genes in vitro have demonstrated DNA regions involved in transcriptional control, including sites for interaction and regulation by the vitamin D receptor, as well as sites through which ambient calcium regulates transcription. Suppression of PTH gene activity at the transcriptional level by calcium is nearly maximal at physiologic concentrations; hypercalcemia results in no significant change. Hypocalcemia, however, increases transcriptional activity within hours. $1,25(OH)_2D_3$ strongly suppresses PTH gene transcription, though not when chronic hypocalcemia is induced experimentally in animals. In patients with renal failure, however, intravenous administration of supraphysiologic levels of $1,25(OH)_2D_3$ or analogues of the active metabolite can dramatically suppress PTH overproduction, which is sometimes difficult to control due to severe secondary hyperparathyroidism. Control over hormone stores is exerted by variation in the rates of proteolytic destruction of preformed hormone under the control of ECF calcium; high calcium increases and low calcium inhibits the proteolytic destruction of hormone stores. Regulation of hormone precursor processing and proteolytic destruction of preformed hormone (posttranslational regulation of hormone production) is an important mechanism for mediating rapid (minutes) changes in hormone availability.

Regulation of PTH Secretion PTH secretion increases steeply to a maximum value of five times the basal rate of secretion as calcium concentration falls from normal to the range of 1.9 to 2.0 mmol/L (7.5 to 8.0 mg/dL) (measured as total calcium). The ionized fraction of blood calcium is the important determinant of hormone secretion. Magnesium may influence hormone secretion in the same direction as calcium. It is unlikely, however, that physiologic variations in magnesium concentration affect PTH secretion. Severe intracellular magnesium deficiency impairs PTH secretion (see below).

The level of ECF calcium controls PTH secretion by interaction with a calcium sensor, a GPCR for which Ca^{2+} ions act as the ligand (see below). This receptor is a member of a distinctive subfamily of the GPCR superfamily that is characterized by a large extracellular domain suitable for "clamping" the small-molecule ligand. Stimulation of the receptor by high calcium levels leads to suppression of PTH secretion. The intracellular signals generated by the active receptor appear to be inositol triphosphate (IP_3) and diacylglycerol (DAG) formed by activation of phospholipase. The receptor is present in parathyroid glands and the calcitonin-secreting cells (C cells) of the thyroid, brain, and kidney. Genetic evidence has revealed a key biologic role for the calcium-sensing receptor in parathyroid gland responsiveness to calcium and, unexpectedly, in renal calcium clearance. Point mutations associated with loss of function cause a syndrome resembling hyperparathyroidism (FHH) but with hypocalciuria. On the other hand, gain-of-function mutations cause a form of hypocalcemia resembling hypoparathyroidism (see below).

Metabolism The secreted form of PTH is indistinguishable by immunologic criteria and by molecular size from the 84-amino-acid peptide (PTH 1–84) extracted from glands. However, much of the immunoreactive material found in the circulation is smaller than the extracted or secreted hormone. The principal circulating fragments of immunoreactive hormone lack a portion of the critical amino-terminal sequence required for biologic activity and, hence, are biologically inactive fragments (so-called middle- and carboxyl-terminal fragments). Much of the proteolysis of hormone occurs in the liver and kidney. However, fragments corresponding to the middle- and carboxyl-terminal portions have also been detected in effluent blood from the parathyroids and in the peripheral circulation; there is no convincing evidence, however, for circulating amino-terminal fragments. Peripheral metabolism of PTH does not appear to be regulated by physiologic states (high versus low calcium, etc.); hence peripheral metabolism of hormone, although responsible for rapid clearance of secreted hormone, appears to be a high-capacity, metabolically invariant catabolic process.

The rate of clearance of the secreted 84-amino-acid peptide from blood is more rapid than the rate of clearance of the biologically inactive fragment(s) corresponding to the middle- and carboxyl-terminal regions of PTH. Consequently, the interpretation of PTH immunoassays is influenced by the nature of the peptide fragments detected by the antibodies. Before the introduction of double-antibody assays designed to detect intact, biologically active hormone, most immunoassays also measured biologically inert long-lived fragments. Changes in the rate of production or clearance of fragments therefore alter the concentration of immunoreactive hormone.

Although the problems inherent in PTH measurements have been largely circumvented by use of double-antibody assays that detect only the intact molecule, new evidence has revealed the existence of a hitherto unappreciated larger PTH fragment that may affect the interpretation of most currently available double-antibody assays as well. A large amino-terminally truncated form of PTH, possibly PTH(7–84), is present in normal and uremic individuals in addition to PTH(1–84). The concentration of the putative 7–84 fragment relative to that of intact PTH(1–84) is higher with induced hypercalcemia (e.g., in uremic patients) than in eucalcemic or hypocalcemic conditions. The large fragment almost certainly cannot have (on the basis of structure-activity studies with PTH discussed above) much, if any, of the biologic potency of PTH. The suggestion that the PTH(7–84)-like fragment might act as an inhibitor of PTH action remains to be clarified. The identification of this fragment has clinical significance, particularly in renal failure, as efforts to prevent secondary hyperparathyroidism by a variety of measures (vitamin D analogues, higher calcium intake, and phosphate-lowering strategies) may have led to oversuppression of biologically active intact PTH when the presence of the amino-terminally truncated PTH was not appreciated. The role, if any, of excessive PTH suppression due to inaccurate measurement of PTH in adynamic bone disease in renal failure (see below) is unknown. Newer assays with extreme amino-terminal epitopes are being studied intensively.

PARATHYROID HORMONE–RELATED PROTEIN

The paracrine factor termed *PTHrP* is responsible for most instances of hypercalcemia of malignancy, a syndrome that resembles hyperparathyroidism. Many different cell types produce PTHrP, including brain, pancreas, heart, lung, mammary tissue, placenta, endothelial cells, and smooth muscle. In fetal animals, PTHrP directs transplacental calcium transfer, and high concentrations of PTHrP are produced in mammary tissue and secreted into milk. Human and bovine milk, for example, contain very high concentrations of the hormone; the biologic significance of the latter is unknown. PTHrP may also play a role in uterine contraction and other biologic functions, still being clarified in other tissue sites.

PTH and PTHrP, although distinctive products of different genes, exhibit considerable functional and structural homology (Fig. 341-1) and may have evolved from a shared ancestral gene. The structure of the gene for human PTHrP, however, is more complex than that of PTH, containing multiple exons and multiple sites for alternate splicing patterns during formation of the mRNA. Protein products of 141, 139, and 173 amino acids are produced, and other molecular forms may result from tissue-specific degradation at accessible internal cleavage sites. The biologic roles of these various molecular species and the nature of the circulating forms of PTHrP are unclear. It is uncertain whether PTHrP circulates at any significant level in normal human adults; as a paracrine factor, PTHrP may be produced, act, and be destroyed locally within tissues. In adults PTHrP appears to have little influence on calcium homeostasis, except in disease states, when large tumors, especially of the squamous cell type, lead to massive overproduction of the hormone (Fig. 341-1).

PTH AND PTHrP HORMONE ACTION Because PTHrP shares a significant homology with PTH in the critical amino terminus, it binds to and activates the PTH/PTHrP receptor, indistinguishably from effects seen with PTH. The 500-amino-acid PTH/PTHrP receptor (also known as the PTH1 receptor) belongs to a subfamily of GPCR that includes those for glucagon, secretin, and vasoactive intestinal peptide. The extracellular regions are involved in hormone binding, and the intracellular domains, after hormone activation, bind G protein subunits to transduce hormone signaling into cellular responses through stimulation of second messengers (Fig. 341-2). A second PTH receptor (PTH2 receptor) is expressed in brain, pancreas, and several other tissues. Its amino acid sequence and the pattern of its binding and stimulatory response to PTH and PTHrP differ from those of the PTH1 receptor. The PTH/PTHrP receptor responds equivalently to PTH and PTHrP, whereas the PTH2 receptor responds only to PTH. The endogenous ligand and the physiologic significance of this receptor are not completely defined.

FIGURE 341-1 Schematic diagram to illustrate similarities and differences in structure of human parathyroid hormone (PTH) and human PTH-related peptide (PTHrP). Close structural (and functional) homology exists between the first 30 amino acids of hPTH and hPTHrP. The PTHrP sequence may be 144 amino acid residues in length or longer. PTH is only 84 residues long; after residue 30, there is little structural homology between the two. Dashed lines in the PTHrP sequence indicate homology; underlined residues, although different from those of PTH, still represent conservative changes (charge or polarity preserved). Eleven amino acids are identical, and a total of 21 of 30 are homologues.

FIGURE 341-2 Schematic model of parathyroid hormone (PTH) action. Only one PTH receptor has been identified in bone and kidney. Different G proteins—G_s, G_q, etc.—activate a cellular second messenger pathway involving either an effect on adenyl cyclase (AC) to enhance cyclic AMP (cAMP) or phospholipase C (PL-C) activation of diacylglycerol (DAG) and inositol triphosphate (IP_3). These second messengers then activate protein kinase A (PK-A) or protein kinase C (PK-C). Phosphorylation of specific proteins, mostly still unidentified, leads to distal biologic responses. Cellular specificity or other factors (e.g., hormone levels, receptor expression levels) must determine which pathway is activated predominantly in a given cell type. Although only one form of receptor appears to be present in kidney and bone, another receptor (PTH2 receptor) has been described in brain, and others may exist.

The PTH1 and PTH2 receptors can be traced backward in evolutionary time to fish. The zebrafish PTH1 and PTH2 receptors exhibit the same selective responses to PTH and PTHrP as do the human PTH1 and PTH2 receptors. The evolutionary conservation of structure and function suggests unique biologic roles for these receptors. Recently, a 39-amino-acid hypothalamic peptide, tubular infundibular peptide (TIP-39), has been characterized and is a likely natural ligand of the PTH2 receptor.

G proteins of the G_s class link the PTH/PTHrP receptor to adenylate cyclase, an enzyme that generates cyclic AMP, leading to activation of protein kinase A. Coupling to G proteins of the G_q class links hormone action to phospholipase C, an enzyme that generates inositol phosphates (e.g., IP_3) and DAG, leading to activation of protein kinase C and intracellular calcium release (Fig. 341-2). Studies using the cloned PTH/PTHrP receptor confirm that it can be coupled to more than one G protein and second-messenger kinase pathway, apparently explaining the multiplicity of pathways stimulated by PTH. Incompletely characterized second-messenger responses may be independent of phospholipase C or adenylate cyclase stimulation (the latter, however, is the strongest and best characterized second messenger signaling pathway for PTH).

The details of the biochemical steps by which an increased intracellular concentration of cyclic AMP, IP_3, DAG, and intracellular Ca^{2+} lead to ultimate changes in ECF calcium and phosphate ion translocation or bone cell function are unknown. Stimulation of protein kinases (A and C) and calcium transport channels is associated with a variety of hormone-specific tissue responses. These responses include inhibition of phosphate and bicarbonate transport, stimulation of calcium transport, and activation of renal 1α-hydroxylase in the kidney. The responses in bone include effects on collagen synthesis; increased alkaline phosphatase, ornithine decarboxylase, citrate decarboxylase, and glucose-6-phosphate dehydrogenase activities; DNA, protein, and phospholipid synthesis; and calcium and phosphate transport. Ultimately, these biochemical events lead to an integrated hormonal response in bone turnover and calcium homeostasis.

PTH also activates Na^+/Ca^{2+} exchanges in renal distal tubular sites and stimulates translocation of preformed calcium transport channels, moving them from the interior to the apical surface to mediate in-

Paracrine Actions   **Calcium Homeostasis**

FIGURE 341-3 Dual role for the actions of the PTH/PTHrP receptor. Parathyroid hormone (PTH; endocrine-calcium homeostasis) and PTH-related peptide (PTHrP; paracrine–multiple tissue actions including growth plate cartilage in developing bone) use the single receptor for their disparate functions.

creased tubular uptake of calcium. PTH-dependent stimulation of phosphate excretion (blocking reabsorption—the opposite effect from actions on calcium in the kidney) involves the sodium-dependent phosphate cotransporter, NPT-2, lowering its apical membrane content (and therefore function). Similar shifts may be involved in other renal tubular transport effects of PTH.

PTHrP exerts important developmental influences on fetal bone development and in adult physiology. A homozygous knockout of the PTHrP gene (or the gene for the PTH receptor) in mice causes a lethal deformity in which animals are born with severe skeletal deformities resembling chondrodysplasia (Fig. 341-3).

CALCITONIN (See also Chap. 339)

Calcitonin is a hypocalcemic peptide hormone that in several mammalian species acts as the physiologic antagonist to PTH. Calcitonin seems to be of limited physiologic significance in humans, at least in calcium homeostasis, as contrasted with a clearly definable role in calcium metabolism in many other mammalian species. Calcitonin is of medical significance, however, because of its role as a tumor marker in sporadic and hereditary cases of medullary carcinoma and its medical use as an adjunctive treatment in severe hypercalcemia and in Paget's disease of bone.

The hypocalcemic activity of calcitonin is accounted for primarily by inhibition of osteoclast-mediated bone resorption and secondarily by stimulation of renal calcium clearance. These effects are mediated by receptors on osteoclasts and renal tubular cells. Calcitonin exerts additional effects through receptors present in brain, gastrointestinal tract, and the immune system. The hormone, for example, exerts analgesic effects directly on cells in the hypothalamus and related structures, possibly by interacting with receptors for related peptide hormones, such as calcitonin gene–related peptide (CGRP) or amylin. The latter ligands have specific high-affinity receptors and also can bind to and trigger calcitonin receptors. The calcitonin receptors are homologous in structure to the PTH/PTHrP receptor.

The thyroid is the major source of the hormone, and the cells involved in calcitonin synthesis arise from neural crest tissue. During embryogenesis, these cells migrate into the ultimobranchial body, derived from the last branchial pouch. In submammalian vertebrates, the ultimobranchial body constitutes a discrete organ, anatomically separate from the thyroid gland; in mammals, the ultimobranchial gland fuses with and is incorporated into the thyroid gland.

The naturally occurring calcitonins consist of a peptide chain of 32 amino acids. There is considerable sequence variability among species. Calcitonin from salmon is 10 to 100 times more potent than mammalian forms in lowering serum calcium in animals. Calcitonin is synthesized as a precursor molecule that is four times larger than calcitonin itself. Analysis of the sequence of the coding portions of the gene for rat calcitonin indicates that at least two peptides flank calcitonin. It is likely (by analogy with the common precursor for adrenocorticotropic hormone and endorphin) that these peptides, of still uncharacterized biologic function, are released along with calcitonin.

There are two calcitonin genes, α and β, located on chromosome 11 in the general region of the β-globulin and PTH genes; the transcriptional control of these genes is complex. Two different mRNA molecules are transcribed from the α gene; one is translated into the precursor for calcitonin, and the other message is translated into an alternative product, CGRP. CGRP is synthesized wherever the calcitonin mRNA is expressed, e.g., in medullary carcinoma of the thyroid. The β, or CGRP-2, gene is transcribed into the mRNA for CGRP in the central nervous system (CNS); this gene does not produce calcitonin, however. CGRP has cardiovascular actions and may serve as a neurotransmitter or play a developmental role in the CNS.

The secretion of calcitonin is under the direct control of blood calcium. The circulating level of calcitonin in humans is lower than that in many other species. In humans, changes in calcium and phosphate metabolism are not seen despite extreme variations in calcitonin production; no definite effects are attributable to calcitonin deficiency (totally thyroidectomized patients receiving only replacement thyroxine) or excess (patients with medullary carcinoma of the thyroid, a calcitonin-secreting tumor) (Chap. 339). Although there are no obvious abnormalities in calcium metabolism in patients with elevated calcitonin levels, bone remodeling is chronically suppressed. Calcitonin has been a useful pharmacologic agent to suppress bone resorption in Paget's disease (Chap. 343), has had limited use in the treatment of osteoporosis (Chap. 342), and is useful in early phases of treatment of severe hypercalcemia (see below).

HYPERCALCEMIA

Hypercalcemia can be a manifestation of a serious illness such as malignancy or can be detected coincidentally by laboratory testing in a patient with no obvious illness. The number of patients recognized with asymptomatic hypercalcemia, usually hyperparathyroidism, increased in the late twentieth century but is now declining somewhat, perhaps due to decreased use of routine blood calcium measurements or for other unknown reasons.

Whenever hypercalcemia is confirmed, a definitive diagnosis must be established. Although hyperparathyroidism, a frequent cause of asymptomatic hypercalcemia, is a chronic disorder in which manifestations, if any, may be expressed only after months or years, hypercalcemia can also be the earliest manifestation of malignancy, the second most common cause of hypercalcemia in the adult. The causes of hypercalcemia are numerous (Table 341-1), but hyperparathyroidism and cancer account for 90% of cases.

Before undertaking a workup, it is essential to be sure that true hypercalcemia, not a false-positive laboratory test, is present. A false-positive diagnosis of hypercalcemia is usually the result of inadvertent hemoconcentration during blood collection or elevation in serum proteins such as albumin. Hypercalcemia is a chronic problem, and it is cost-effective to obtain several serum calcium measurements; these tests need not be in the fasting state.

Clinical features are helpful in differential diagnosis. Hypercalcemia in an adult who is asymptomatic is usually due to primary hyperparathyroidism. In malignancy-associated hypercalcemia the disease is usually not occult; rather, symptoms of malignancy bring the patient to the physician, and hypercalcemia is discovered during the workup. In such patients the interval between detection of hypercalcemia and death is often <6 months. Accordingly, if an asymptomatic individual has had hypercalcemia or some manifestation of hypercalcemia, such as kidney stones, for >1 or 2 years, it is unlikely that malignancy is the cause. Nevertheless, differentiating primary hyperparathyroidism from *occult* malignancy can occasionally be difficult, and careful evaluation is required, particularly when the duration of the hypercalcemia is unknown. Hypercalcemia not due to hyperparathyroidism or malignancy can result from excessive vitamin D action,

high bone turnover from any of several causes, or from renal failure (Table 341-1). Dietary history and a history of ingestion of vitamins or drugs are often helpful in diagnosing some of the less frequent causes. PTH immunoassays based on double-antibody methods serve as the principal laboratory test in differential diagnosis.

Hypercalcemia from any cause can result in fatigue, depression, mental confusion, anorexia, nausea, vomiting, constipation, reversible renal tubular defects, increased urination, a short QT interval in the electrocardiogram, and, in some patients, cardiac arrhythmias. There is a variable relation from one patient to the next between the severity of hypercalcemia and the symptoms. Generally, symptoms are more common at calcium levels >2.9 to 3 mmol/L (11.5 to 12.0 mg/dL), but some patients, even at this level, are asymptomatic. When the calcium level is >3.2 mmol/L (13 mg/dL), calcification in kidneys, skin, vessels, lungs, heart, and stomach occurs and renal insufficiency may develop, particularly if blood phosphate levels are normal or elevated due to impaired renal function. Severe hypercalcemia, usually defined as ≥3.7 to 4.5 mmol/L (15 to 18 mg/dL) can be a medical emergency; coma and cardiac arrest can occur.

Except in malignancy-associated hypercalcemia, acute management of the hypercalcemia is usually successful prior to definitive therapy. The type of treatment is based on the severity of the hypercalcemia and the nature of associated symptoms.

PRIMARY HYPERPARATHYROIDISM Natural History and Incidence Primary hyperparathyroidism is a generalized disorder of calcium, phosphate, and bone metabolism due to an increased secretion of PTH. The elevation of circulating hormone usually leads to hypercalcemia and hypophosphatemia. There is great variation in the manifestations. Patients may present with multiple signs and symptoms, including recurrent nephrolithiasis, peptic ulcers, mental changes, and, less frequently, extensive bone resorption. However, with greater awareness of the disease and wider use of multiphasic screening tests, including blood calcium assays, the diagnosis is frequently made in patients who have no symptoms and minimal, if any, signs of the disease other than hypercalcemia and elevated levels of PTH. The manifestations may be subtle, and the disease may have a benign course for many years or a lifetime. Rarely, hyperparathyroidism develops or worsens abruptly and causes severe complications, such as marked dehydration and coma, so-called hypercalcemic parathyroid crisis.

The annual incidence of the disease is estimated to be as high as 0.2% in patients >60, with an estimated prevalence, including undis-

Table 341-1 Classification of Causes of Hypercalcemia

I. Parathyroid-related
   A. Primary hyperparathyroidism
      1. Solitary adenomas
      2. Multiple endocrine neoplasia
   B. Lithium therapy
   C. Familial hypocalciuric hypercalcemia
II. Malignancy-related
   A. Solid tumor with metastases (breast)
   B. Solid tumor with humoral mediation of hypercalcemia (lung, kidney)
   C. Hematologic malignancies (multiple myeloma, lymphoma, leukemia)
III. Vitamin D–related
   A. Vitamin D intoxication
   B. ↑ 1,25(OH)$_2$D; sarcoidosis and other granulomatous diseases
   C. Idiopathic hypercalcemia of infancy
IV. Associated with high bone turnover
   A. Hyperthyroidism
   B. Immobilization
   C. Thiazides
   D. Vitamin A intoxication
V. Associated with renal failure
   A. Severe secondary hyperparathyroidism
   B. Aluminum intoxication
   C. Milk-alkali syndrome

covered asymptomatic patients, of ≥1%. The disease has a peak incidence between the third and fifth decades but occurs in young children and in the elderly.

Etiology • *Solitary adenomas* The cause of hyperparathyroidism is one or more hyperfunctioning glands. The traditional view has been that a single abnormal gland is the cause in approximately 80% of patients; the abnormality in the gland is usually a benign neoplasm or adenoma and rarely a parathyroid carcinoma. Some surgeons and pathologists report that the enlargement of multiple glands is common; double adenomas are reported. In approximately 15% of patients, all glands are hyperfunctioning; *chief cell parathyroid hyperplasia* is usually hereditary and frequently associated with other endocrine abnormalities.

Multiple endocrine neoplasia Hereditary hyperparathyroidism can occur without other endocrine abnormalities but is usually part of a *multiple endocrine neoplasia* syndrome (Chap. 339). MEN 1 (Wermer's syndrome) consists of hyperparathyroidism and tumors of the pituitary and pancreas, often associated with gastric hypersecretion and peptic ulcer disease (Zollinger-Ellison syndrome). MEN 2A is characterized by pheochromocytoma and medullary carcinoma of the thyroid, as well as hyperparathyroidism; MEN 2B has additional associated features such as multiple neuromas but usually lacks hyperparathyroidism. Each of these MEN syndromes is transmitted in an autosomal dominant manner.

Pathology Adenomas are most often located in the inferior parathyroid glands, but in 6 to 10% of patients, parathyroid adenomas may be located in the thymus, the thyroid, the pericardium, or behind the esophagus. Adenomas are usually 0.5 to 5 g in size but may be as large as 10 to 20 g (normal glands weigh 25 mg on average). Chief cells are predominant in both hyperplasia and adenoma. The adenoma is sometimes encapsulated by a rim of normal tissue. With chief cell hyperplasia, the enlargement may be so asymmetric that some involved glands appear grossly normal. If generalized hyperplasia is present, however, histologic examination reveals a uniform pattern of chief cells and disappearance of fat even in the absence of an increase in gland weight. Thus, microscopic examination of biopsy specimens of several glands is essential to interpret findings at surgery. When an adenoma is present, the other glands are usually normal and contain a normal distribution of all cell types (rather than only chief cells) and normal amounts of fat.

Parathyroid carcinoma is usually not aggressive in character. Long-term survival without recurrence is common if at initial surgery the entire gland is removed without rupture of the capsule. Recurrent parathyroid carcinoma is usually slow-growing with local spread in the neck, and surgical correction of recurrent disease may be feasible. Occasionally, however, parathyroid carcinoma is more aggressive, with distant metastases (lung, liver, and bone) found at the time of initial operation. It may be difficult to appreciate initially that a primary tumor is carcinoma; increased numbers of mitotic figures and increased fibrosis of the gland stroma may precede invasion. The diagnosis of carcinoma is often made in retrospect. Hyperparathyroidism from a parathyroid carcinoma may be indistinguishable from other forms of primary hyperparathyroidism; a potential clue to the diagnosis, however, is provided by the degree of calcium elevation. Calcium values of 3.5 to 3.7 mmol/L (14 to 15 mg/dL) are frequent with carcinoma and may alert the surgeon to remove the abnormal gland with care to avoid capsular rupture.

GENETIC CONSIDERATIONS **Defects Associated with Hyperparathyroidism** As in many other types of neoplasia, two fundamental types of genetic defects have been identified in parathyroid gland tumors: (1) overactivity of protooncogenes, and (2) loss of function of tumor suppressor genes. The former, by definition, can lead to uncontrolled cellular growth and function by activation (gain-of-function mutation) of a single allele of the responsible gene, whereas the latter requires loss of function of both allelic copies.

Mutations in the *MENIN* gene locus on chromosome 11q13 are responsible for causing MEN 1; the normal allele of this gene fits the definition of a tumor suppressor gene. A mutation of one allele is inherited; loss of the other allele via somatic cell mutation leads to monoclonal expansion and tumor development in tissues such as the parathyroids. In approximately 20% of sporadic parathyroid adenomas, the *MENIN* locus on chromosome 11 appears to be deleted, implying that the same defect responsible for MEN 1 can also cause the sporadic disease (Fig. 341-4*A*). Consistent with the Knudson hypothesis for two-step neoplasia in certain inherited cancer syndromes (Chap. 81), the earlier onset of hyperparathyroidism in the hereditary syndromes reflects the statistical probability of only one mutational event triggering the monoclonal outgrowth. In sporadic adenomas, typically occurring later in life, two different somatic events must occur before the *MENIN* gene is silenced.

The *MENIN* gene codes for a novel protein consisting of 610 amino acids. The protein has a nuclear localization signal and appears to interact with the transcription factor Jun D. Most of the mutations are clearly of the inactivating type (nonsense, deletions); there is not, however, a good correlation between clinical features in different kindreds and the specific mutation detected (e.g., penetrance or age of onset of pituitary or pancreatic tumors). This is in contrast to the correlation between genotype and phenotype in MEN 2 (see below).

Other presumptive antioncogenes involved in hyperparathyroidism include a gene mapped to chromosome 1p seen in 40% of sporadic parathyroid adenomas and a gene mapped to chromosome Xp11 in patients with secondary hyperparathyroidism and renal failure, who progressed to "tertiary" hyperparathyroidism, now known to reflect monoclonal outgrowths within previously hyperplastic glands.

The *Rb* gene, a tumor suppressor gene located on chromosome 13q14, was initially associated with retinoblastomas but has since been implicated in many other forms of neoplasia including parathyroid carcinoma. Allelic deletion (with a presumed point mutation in the second allele) has been identified in all parathyroid carcinomas examined; there is also an abnormal staining pattern of the protein product of the gene. Allelic deletion is also seen in 10% of parathyroid adenomas, although the abnormal staining pattern of the Rb protein is not seen. Other gene loci on chromosome 13 may be involved in addition to the *Rb* locus.

There are two rare syndromes associated with hyperparathyroidism that involve one or more genes located on chromosome 1q. The hereditary hyperparathyroidism jaw tumor (HPT-JT) syndrome shows an autosomal dominant inheritance pattern; the jaw tumors are benign, but the parathyroid pathology may involve carcinoma as well as adenoma. Parathyroid carcinoma may also appear in the other syndrome, familial isolated primary hyperparathyroidism (FIPH). Both syndromes have been mapped through linkage studies to the chromosome 1q21-q31 region. Certain findings have led to speculation that this chromosome region might contain a protooncogene rather than an antioncogene.

In some parathyroid adenomas, activation of a protooncogene has been identified (Fig. 341-4*B*). A reciprocal translocation involving chromosome 11 has been identified that juxtaposes the PTH gene promoter upstream of a gene product termed *PRAD-1*, a cyclin D protein that plays a key role in normal cell division. This translocation is found in as many as 15% of parathyroid adenomas, usually in larger tumors. Targeted overexpression of cyclin D_1 in the parathyroid glands of transgenic mice causes the development of hyperparathyroidism, consistent with the role of this cell cycle control protein in parathyroid neoplasia.

A mutated protooncogene, *RET*, is involved in each of the clinical variants of MEN2 (Chap. 339). *RET* encodes a tyrosine kinase–type receptor; specific mutations lead to constitutive activity of the receptor, thereby explaining the autosomal dominant mode of transmission and the relatively early onset of neoplasia. ∎

Signs and Symptoms Half or more of patients with hyperparathyroidism are asymptomatic. In series in which patients are followed without operation, as many as 80% are classified as without symptoms.

A

B

FIGURE 341-4 *A.* Schematic diagram indicating concept of autosomal recessive rather than autosomal dominant inheritance of tumor susceptibility. The patient with the hereditary abnormality (multiple endocrine neoplasia, or MEN) is envisioned as having one defective gene (mutant receptor) inherited from the affected parent on chromosome 11, but one copy of the normal gene is present from the other parent. In the monoclonal tumor (benign tumor), a somatic event, here partial chromosomal deletion, removes the remaining normal gene from a cell. In nonhereditary tumors, two successive somatic mutations must occur, a process that takes a longer time. By either pathway, the cell, deprived of growth-regulating influence from this gene, has unregulated growth and becomes a tumor. A different genetic locus also involving loss of a tumor suppressor gene on chromosome 13 is involved in the pathogenesis of parathyroid carcinoma. *B.* Schematic illustration of the mechanism and consequences of gene rearrangement and overexpression of the PRAD 1 proto-oncogene (pericentromeric inversion of chromosome 11) in parathyroid adenomas. The excessive expression of PRAD 1 (a cell cycle control protein, cyclin D_1) by the highly active PTH gene promoter in the parathyroid cell contributes to excess cellular proliferation. *(From Habener et al, with permission.)*

Manifestations of hyperparathyroidism involve primarily the kidneys and the skeletal system. Kidney involvement, due either to deposition of calcium in the renal parenchyma or to recurrent nephrolithiasis, was present in 60 to 70% of patients prior to 1970. With earlier detection, renal complications occur in <20% of patients in many large series. Renal stones are usually composed of either calcium oxalate or calcium phosphate. In occasional patients, repeated episodes of nephrolithiasis or the formation of large calculi may lead to urinary tract obstruction, infection, and loss of renal function. Nephrocalcinosis may also cause decreased renal function and phosphate retention.

The distinctive bone manifestation of hyperparathyroidism is *osteitis fibrosa cystica*, which in series reported 50 years ago occurred in 10 to 25% of patients. In recent years, osteitis fibrosa cystica is very rare in primary hyperparathyroidism, probably due to the increased incidence of mild disease. Histologically, the pathognomonic features are an increase in the giant multinucleated osteoclasts in scalloped areas on the surface of the bone (Howship's lacunae) and a replacement of the normal cellular and marrow elements by fibrous tissue. X-ray changes include resorption of the phalangeal tufts and replacement of the usually sharp cortical outline of the bone in the digits by an irregular outline (subperiosteal resorption).

With the use of multiple markers of bone turnover, such as formation indices (bone-specific alkaline phosphatase, osteocalcin, and type I procollagen peptides) and bone resorption indices (including hydroxypyridinium collagen cross-links and telopeptides of type I collagen), increased skeletal turnover is detected in essentially all patients with established hyperparathyroidism.

Computed tomography (CT) scan and dual-energy x-ray absorptiometry (DEXA) of the spine provide reproducible quantitative estimates (within a few percent) of spinal bone density (Chap. 342). Similarly, cortical bone density in the extremities can be quantified by single-photon densitometry, usually of the distal radius at a site chosen to be primarily cortical. Studies reveal that cortical bone density is reduced while cancellous bone density, especially in the spine, is rel-

atively preserved. Serial studies in patients who choose to be followed without surgery have indicated that in the majority there is little further change over a number of years, consistent with laboratory data indicating relatively unchanged blood calcium and PTH levels. After an initial loss of bone mass in patients with mild asymptomatic hyperparathyroidism, a new equilibrium may be reached, with bone density and biochemical manifestations of the disease remaining relatively unchanged. This clinical course has led to the recommendations (discussed below) that asymptomatic patients may be safely followed with medical supervision. Certain recent findings have raised questions about the impact of asymptomatic hyperparathyroidism on the skeleton, however. In one careful, long-term study, parathyroidectomy led to improvements in bone density in the spine and hip in 10 to 15% of patients; the improved bone density has been maintained for a number of years of follow-up. Another group compared fracture incidence in a large cohort of hyperparathyroid patients followed for years without surgery versus those seen in an age- and sex-matched control population. The incidence of fractures of the spine, wrist, and ribs was significantly increased in the hyperparathyroid group (although there were no data available on bone density).

In symptomatic patients, dysfunctions of the central nervous system, peripheral nerve and muscle, gastrointestinal tract, and joints also occur. An awareness of the signs and symptoms of hyperparathyroidism may give the initial clue to the diagnosis. It has been reported that severe neuropsychiatric manifestations may be reversed by parathyroidectomy; it remains unclear, in the absence of controlled studies, whether this improvement has a defined cause-and-effect relationship. Generally, the fact that hyperparathyroidism is common in elderly patients, in whom there are often other problems, suggests the possibility that such coexisting problems as hypertension, renal deterioration, and depression may not be parathyroid-related and suggests caution in recommending parathyroid surgery as a cure for these conditions.

Neuromuscular manifestations may include proximal muscle weakness, easy fatigability, and atrophy of muscles and may be so striking as to suggest a primary neuromuscular disorder. The distinguishing feature is the complete regression of neuromuscular disease after surgical correction of the hyperparathyroidism.

Gastrointestinal manifestations are sometimes subtle and include vague abdominal complaints and disorders of the stomach and pancreas. Again, cause and effect are unclear. In MEN 1 patients with hyperparathyroidism, duodenal ulcer may be the result of associated pancreatic tumors that secrete excessive quantities of gastrin (Zollinger-Ellison syndrome). Pancreatitis has been reported in association with hyperparathyroidism, but the incidence and the mechanism are not established.

Chondrocalcinosis and pseudogout are said to be sufficiently frequent in hyperparathyroidism that screening of such patients is warranted. Occasionally, pseudogout is the initial manifestation.

Diagnosis   The diagnosis is typically made by detecting an elevated immunoreactive PTH level in a patient with asymptomatic hypercalcemia (see "Differential Diagnosis: Special Tests," below). Serum phosphate is usually low but may be normal, especially if renal failure has developed. Hypophosphatemia is a less specific diagnostic finding than hypercalcemia for two reasons: (1) phosphate levels are influenced by dietary intake, diurnal variations, and other factors; to be useful, samples must be obtained in the morning under fasting conditions; and (2) patients with severe hypercalcemia of any cause may have a low serum phosphate.

Many tests based on renal responses to excess PTH (renal calcium and phosphate clearance; blood phosphate, chloride, magnesium; urinary or nephrogenous cyclic AMP) were used in earlier decades. These tests have low specificity for hyperparathyroidism and are therefore not cost-effective; they have been replaced by PTH immunoassays.

℞ **TREATMENT   Medical Treatment**   Management of hyperparathyroidism involves two separate issues. The critical question is whether the disease should be treated surgically. If severe hypercalcemia [3.7 to 4.5 mmol/L (15 to 18 mg/dL)] is present, surgery is mandatory as soon as the diagnosis can be confirmed by a PTH immunoassay. However, in most patients with hyperparathyroidism, hypercalcemia is mild and does not require urgent surgical or medical treatment.

Several hundred patients have been closely followed without surgery in attempts to define the natural history of the disease and the benefits of surgery versus the risks of medical observation. Large-scale randomized, prospective clinical trials have not been undertaken, however. Rather, the long-term effects of hyperparathyroidism have been assessed in patients who do not have kidney stones, osteitis fibrosa cystica, or other clear-cut symptoms. Progressive loss of bone mass is a worrisome problem in women who face the problem of age-dependent and estrogen-deficient bone loss in the absence of hyperparathyroidism. The principal concern is that such patients, even though asymptomatic, will suffer sufficient bone loss due to PTH excess to make them more vulnerable to developing symptomatic osteoporosis.

The National Institutes of Health held a Consensus Conference on Management of Asymptomatic Hyperparathyroidism in 1991. *Asymptomatic hyperparathyroidism* was defined as documented (presumptive) hyperparathyroidism without signs or symptoms attributable to the disease. The consensus was that patients <50 should undergo surgery, given the long surveillance that would be required. Patients >50 are appropriate for medical monitoring if certain criteria are met and the patients wish to avoid surgery. Guidelines for recommending surgery in patients with asymptomatic hyperparathyroidism include the following:

1. Elevation of serum calcium, >0.25 to 0.40 mmol/L (1 to 1.6 mg/dL) above the upper limit of normal for the test laboratory.
2. History of life-threatening hypercalcemia, such as an episode induced by dehydration and recurring illness.

3. Reduction of age-matched creatinine clearance by >30% without a known cause. Presence of kidney stones detected by abdominal radiograph even if they are asymptomatic.
4. Elevation of 24-h urinary calcium excretion >400 mg.
5. Reduction of bone mass more than 2 standard deviations below normal using one of several noninvasive methods.

Other considerations that favor surgery include concern that consistent follow-up would be unlikely or that coexistent illness would complicate management. More recent data indicated that a subgroup of patients had selective vertebral osteopenia out of proportion to bone loss at other sites and responded to surgery with striking restoration of bone mass (average >20%), suggesting that such patients might also be recommended for surgery. Asymptomatic patients should be monitored regularly. Surgical correction of hyperparathyroidism can always be undertaken when indicated, since the success rate is high (>90%), mortality is low, and morbidity is minimal. The goals of monitoring are early detection of worsening hypercalcemia, deteriorating bone or renal status, or other complications of hyperparathyroidism.

The consensus panel did not make a recommendation as to estrogen use in patients for whom surgery was not elected because there was insufficient cumulative experience with such therapy to balance theoretical risks (breast and endometrial cancer) versus benefits. New medical therapies may change the approach to the disease in the future. Raloxifene (Evista), the first of the SERMS, has been shown to have many of the bone protective effects of estrogen in osteoporotic subjects yet at the same time lowers the incidence of breast cancer; use of this agent has not yet been reported in a series of hyperparathyroid patients, however. Early experience with calcimimetics, drugs that selectively stimulate the calcium sensor and suppress PTH secretion, indicates that these agents decrease PTH levels for several hours after a single dose.

European investigators have reported serious cardiovascular complications in patients with hyperparathyroidism that reverse, at least in part, after surgery. They also found an increased incidence of malignancy and an absolute increase in age-adjusted mortality due to hyperparathyroidism. These reports clearly describe experiences in a group of patients with more advanced disease, at least based on laboratory tests such as blood PTH levels, than the patients followed in the United States. In fact, a recent long-term epidemiologic study of a large cohort of patients in the United States, with a milder form of the disease (fitting the criteria for medical surveillance listed above), had an age-adjusted mortality no different than that of euparathyroid patients and no increased incidence of malignancy.

Surgical Treatment   Parathyroid exploration is challenging and is best undertaken by an experienced surgeon with the help of an experienced pathologist. Certain features help in predicting the pathology (e.g., multiple abnormal glands in familial cases). However, some critical decisions regarding management can be made only during the operation. The examination by frozen section of tissue removed at surgery helps direct the subsequent course of the operation.

As discussed above, there are many unresolved issues to consider in surgery for this disease. At the extreme of conservatism, the surgical approach is based on the view that typically only one gland (the adenoma) is abnormal. If an enlarged gland is found, a normal gland should be sought. In this view, if a biopsy of a normal-sized second gland confirms its histologic (and presumed functional) normality, no further exploration, biopsy, or excision is needed. At the other extreme is the minority viewpoint that all four glands be sought and that most of the total parathyroid tissue mass should be removed. The concern with the former approach is that the recurrence rate of hyperparathyroidism may be high if a second abnormal gland is missed; the latter approach could involve unnecessary surgery and an unacceptable rate of hypoparathyroidism. The majority viewpoint, judged by surgical reviews, is in favor of conservative surgery, i.e., removal of what is usually only one enlarged gland but only after four-gland exploration to eliminate the possibility that more than one gland is abnormal.

When normal glands are found in association with one enlarged gland, excision of the single adenoma usually leads to cure or symptom-free disease, although long-term follow-up studies are limited.

Surgical management has been enhanced recently by the use of preoperative ^{99m}Tc sestamibi scans to predict the location of an abnormal gland and intraoperative sampling of PTH before and at 5- to 15-min intervals after removal of a suspected adenoma to confirm a rapid fall (>50%) in PTH levels. In several centers, a combination of preoperative sestamibi imaging, cervical block anesthesia, minimal surgical incision, and intraoperative PTH measurements has allowed successful outpatient surgical management with a clear-cut cost benefit compared to general anesthesia and more extensive neck surgery. The use of these minimally invasive approaches requires clinical judgment to select patients unlikely to have multiple gland disease (e.g., MEN or secondary hyperparathyroidism).

Multiple gland hyperplasia, as predicted in familial cases, poses more difficult questions of surgical management. Once a diagnosis of hyperplasia is established, all the glands must be identified. Two schemes have been proposed for surgical management. One is that three glands be totally removed and the fourth gland be partially excised; care is taken to leave a good blood supply for the remaining gland. Other surgeons advocate total parathyroidectomy with immediate transplantation of a portion of a removed, minced parathyroid gland into the muscles of the forearm, with the view that surgical excision is easier from the ectopic site in the arm if there is recurrent hyperfunction. When parathyroid carcinoma is encountered, the tissue should be widely excised; care must be taken to avoid rupture of the capsule to prevent local seeding of tumor cells.

In a minority of cases, if no abnormal parathyroid glands are found in the neck, the issue of further exploration must be decided. There are documented cases of five or six parathyroid glands and of unusual locations for adenomas, such as in the mediastinum. A variety of techniques have been developed to aid in the preoperative localization of the abnormal parathyroid tissue. Usually these techniques are reserved for patients with initial unsuccessful neck explorations, since the combined success of the localization techniques is not better than that of an experienced parathyroid surgeon in finding the abnormal tissue at the first operation. Noninvasive or minimally invasive techniques include ultrasound, CT scan of the neck and mediastinum, and differential scanning after technetium-sestamibi administration.

When a second parathyroid exploration is indicated, the minimally invasive techniques such as ultrasound, CT scan, and isotope scanning should probably be combined with venous sampling and/or selective digital arteriography in one of the centers specializing in these techniques. Intraoperative monitoring of PTH levels by rapid PTH immunoassays may be useful in guiding the surgery, especially in patients who are reexplored after an initial unsuccessful operation. At one center, long-term cures have been achieved with selective embolization or injection of large amounts of contrast material into the endarterial circulation feeding the parathyroid tumor.

A decline in serum calcium occurs within 24 h after successful surgery; usually blood calcium falls to low-normal values for 3 to 5 days until the remaining parathyroid tissue resumes hormone secretion. Severe postoperative hypocalcemia is likely only if osteitis fibrosa cystica is present or if injury to all the normal parathyroid glands occurs during surgery.

In general, patients who do not have symptomatic bone disease or a large deficit in bone mineral and who have good renal and gastrointestinal function have few problems with postoperative hypocalcemia. The extent of postoperative hypocalcemia varies with the surgical approach. If all glands are biopsied, hypocalcemia may be transiently symptomatic and more prolonged. Hypocalcemia is more likely to be symptomatic after second parathyroid explorations, particularly when normal parathyroid tissue was removed at the initial operation and when the manipulation and/or biopsy of the remaining normal glands is more extensive in the search for the missing adenoma.

Patients with hyperparathyroidism have efficient intestinal calcium absorption due to the increased levels of 1,25(OH)$_2$D stimulated by PTH excess. Once hypocalcemia signifies successful surgery, patients can be put on a high-calcium intake or be given oral calcium supplements. Despite mild hypocalcemia, most patients do not require parenteral therapy. If the serum calcium falls to <2 mmol/L (8 mg/dL), *and if the phosphate level rises simultaneously*, the possibility that surgery has caused hypoparathyroidism must be considered. Coexistent hypomagnesemia should be checked for, as it interferes with PTH secretion and causes functional hypoparathyroidism (see below). Parenteral calcium replacement at a low level should be instituted when hypocalcemia is symptomatic. Such indications include a general sense of anxiety and positive Chvostek and Trousseau signs coupled with serum calcium consistently <2 mmol/L (8 mg/dL). For parenteral therapy, calcium (gluconate or chloride) solutions are prepared at a concentration of 1 mg/mL in 5% dextrose in water. The rate and duration of intravenous therapy are determined by the severity of the symptoms and the response of the serum calcium. An infusion of 0.5 to 2 (mg/kg)/h or 30 to 100 mL/h of a 1-mg/mL solution usually suffices to relieve symptoms. Usually, parenteral therapy is required for only a few days. If symptoms worsen or if parenteral calcium is needed for >2 to 3 days, therapy with a vitamin D analogue and/or oral calcium (2 to 4 g/d) should be started (see below). It is cost-effective to use calcitriol (doses of 0.5 to 1.0 μg/d) because of the rapidity of onset and rapidity of cessation of action, in comparison to other forms of vitamin D (see below). A rise in blood calcium after several months of vitamin D replacement may indicate restoration of parathyroid function to normal. It is also appropriate to monitor serum PTH serially to estimate gland function in such patients.

Magnesium deficiency may also complicate the postoperative course. Magnesium deficiency impairs the secretion of PTH, and so hypomagnesemia should be corrected whenever detected. Magnesium chloride is effective by mouth, but this compound is not widely available. Repletion is usually parenteral. Because the depressant effect of magnesium on central and peripheral nerve functions does not occur at levels <2 mmol/L (normal range 0.8 to 1.2 mmol/L), parenteral replacement can be given rapidly. A cumulative dose as great as 0.5 to 1 mmol/kg of body weight can be administered if severe hypomagnesemia is present; often, however, total doses of 20 to 40 mmol are sufficient. The magnesium is given either as an intravenous infusion over 8 to 12 h or in divided doses intramuscularly (magnesium sulfate, USP).

OTHER PARATHYROID-RELATED CAUSES OF HYPERCALCEMIA   Lithium Therapy   Lithium, used in the management of bipolar depression and other psychiatric disorders, causes hypercalcemia in approximately 10% of treated patients. The hypercalcemia is dependent on continued lithium treatment, remitting and recurring when lithium is stopped and restarted. The parathyroid adenomas reported in some hypercalcemic patients with lithium therapy may reflect the presence of an independently occurring parathyroid tumor; a permanent effect of lithium on parathyroid gland growth need not be implicated as most patients have complete reversal of hypercalcemia when lithium is stopped. However, long-standing stimulation of parathyroid cell replication by lithium may predispose to development of adenomas (as is documented in secondary hyperparathyroidism and renal failure).

The presence of hypercalcemia does not correlate with plasma lithium level, but the frequency with which hypercalcemia occurs is sufficiently high to support a causal relationship between lithium and the hypercalcemia, particularly the dependence of the hypercalcemia on the continuation of the lithium. At the levels achieved in blood in treated patients, lithium can be shown in vitro to shift the PTH secretion curve in response to calcium to the right; i.e., higher calcium levels are required to lower PTH secretion, probably acting at the calcium sensor (see below). It is logical to assume that this effect can cause elevated PTH levels and consequent hypercalcemia in otherwise normal individuals. If persistent hypercalcemia is detected during lithium therapy, it may be necessary to try alternative medication for the underlying psychiatric illness. Parathyroid surgery should not be recommended unless hypercalcemia and elevated PTH levels persist after lithium is discontinued.

GENETIC DISORDERS CAUSING HYPERPARATHYROID-LIKE SYNDROMES   Familial Hypocalciuric Hypercalcemia

FHH (also called *familial benign hypercalcemia*) is inherited as an autosomal dominant trait. Affected individuals are discovered because of asymptomatic hypercalcemia. This disorder and Jansen's disease (discussed below) are variants of hyperparathyroidism. FHH involves excessive secretion of PTH, whereas Jansen's disease is caused by excessive biologic activity of the PTH receptor in target tissues. Neither disorder, however, involves a primary growth disorder of the parathyroids.

The pathophysiology of FHH is now understood. The primary defect is abnormal sensing of the blood calcium by the parathyroid gland and renal tubule, causing inappropriate secretion of PTH and excessive renal reabsorption of calcium (Fig. 341-5). The calcium sensor is a member of the third family of GPCR (type C or III) and is located on chromosome 3. The receptor responds to the ECF calcium concentration, suppressing PTH secretion through second messenger signaling, thereby providing negative-feedback regulation of PTH secretion. More than 20 different mutations in the calcium-sensing receptor have been identified in patients with FHH (Fig. 341-6). These mutations lower the capacity of the sensor to bind calcium, and the mutant receptors function as though blood calcium levels are low; excessive secretion of PTH occurs from an otherwise normal gland. Approximately two-thirds of patients with FHH have mutations within the protein-coding region of the gene. The remaining one-third of kindreds may have mutations in the gene promoter or in other regions of the genome identified through mapping studies (e.g., chromosome 19).

Even before elucidation of the pathophysiology of FHH, abundant clinical evidence served to separate the disorder from primary hyperparathyroidism. Patients with primary hyperparathyroidism have <99% renal calcium reabsorption, whereas most patients with FHH have >99% reabsorption. The hypercalcemia in FHH is often detectable in affected members of the kindreds in the first decade of life, whereas hypercalcemia rarely occurs in patients with primary hyperparathyroidism or the MEN syndromes who are <10. PTH may be elevated in FHH, but the values are usually normal or lower for the same degree of calcium elevation than in patients with primary hyperparathyroidism. Parathyroid surgery in a few patients with FHH led

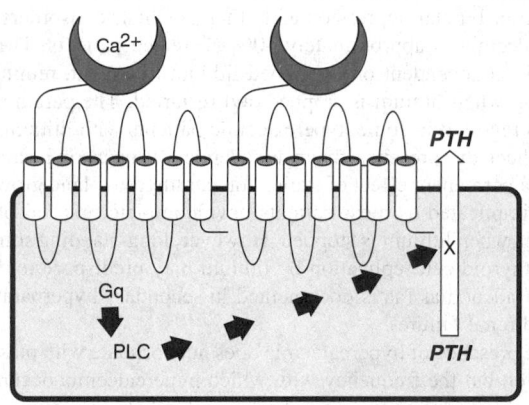

Parathyroid cell

FIGURE 341-5 The calcium sensor's role in parathyroid hormone (PTH) secretion and calcium homeostasis. The extracellular domain closes upon binding to calcium. PLC, phospholipase C; the G protein is shown as G_q (the subclass of G protein thought to activate PLC). When calcium in the blood is low, the sensor is less active and suppression of PTH secretion is lowered (i.e., more PTH is secreted). *(From BR Conklin, HR Bourne: Nature 367:22, 1994, with permission.)*

to permanent hypoparathyroidism, but hypocalciuria persisted nevertheless, establishing that hypocalciuria, therefore, is not PTH-dependent (now known to be due to the abnormal calcium sensor in the kidney).

Few clinical signs or symptoms are present in patients with FHH, and other endocrine abnormalities are not present. Most patients are detected as a result of family screening after hypercalcemia is detected in a proband. In those patients inadvertently operated upon, the parathyroids appeared normal or moderately hyperplastic. Parathyroid surgery is not appropriate, nor, in view of the lack of symptoms, does medical treatment seem needed to lower the calcium. Calcimimetic agents that bind to the calcium sensor and elevate the set point are under investigation.

One striking exception to the rule against parathyroid surgery in this syndrome is the occurrence, usually in consanguinous marriages (due to the rarity of gene), of a homozygous or compound heterozygote state, resulting in complete loss of the calcium sensor function. In this condition, neonatal severe hypercalcemia, total parathyroidectomy is mandatory.

Jansen's Disease   Mutations in the PTH/PTHrP receptor have been identified as responsible for this rare autosomal dominant syndrome. Because the mutations lead to constitutive receptor function, one abnormal copy of the mutant receptor is sufficient to cause the disease, thereby accounting for its dominant mode of transmission. The disorder leads to short-limbed dwarfism due to abnormal regulation of the bone growth plate. In adult life, there are numerous abnormalities in bone, including multiple cystic resorptive areas resembling those seen in severe hyperparathyroidism. Hypercalcemia and hypophosphatemia with undetectable or low PTH levels are typically seen. The pathogenesis of the disease has been confirmed by transgenic experiments in which targeted expression of the mutant receptor to the growth plate emulated several features of the disorder.

MALIGNANCY-RELATED HYPERCALCEMIA   Clinical Syndromes and Mechanisms of Hypercalcemia

Hypercalcemia due to malignancy is common (occurring with 10 to 15% of certain types of tumor, such as lung carcinoma), often severe and difficult to manage, confusing as to etiology, and sometimes difficult to distinguish from primary hyperparathyroidism. Although malignancy is often clinically obvious, hypercalcemia can occasionally be due to an occult tumor. Previously, hypercalcemia associated with malignancy was thought to be due to local invasion and destruction of bone by tumor cells; many cases are now known to result from the elaboration by the malignant cells of humoral mediators of hypercalcemia. PTHrP is the responsible humoral agent in most cases.

The histologic character of the tumor is more important than the extent of skeletal metastases in predicting hypercalcemia. Small cell carcinoma (oat cell) and adenocarcinoma of the lung, although the most common lung tumors associated with skeletal metastases, rarely cause hypercalcemia. By contrast, as many as 10% of patients with squamous cell carcinoma of the lung develop hypercalcemia. Histologic studies of bone in patients with squamous cell or epidermoid carcinoma of the lung, in sites invaded by tumor as well as areas remote from tumor invasion, reveal bone remodeling, including osteoclastic and osteoblastic activity. In contrast, minimal skeletal metabolic activation occurs even if there are extensive skeletal metastases of small cell (oat cell) carcinoma.

Two main mechanisms of hypercalcemia are operative in cancer hypercalcemia. Many solid tumors associated with hypercalcemia, particularly squamous cell and renal tumors, produce and secrete humoral factors that cause increased bone resorption and mediate the hypercalcemia through systemic actions on the skeleton. Alternatively, direct bone marrow invasion occurs with hematologic malignancies such as leukemia, lymphoma, and multiple myeloma. Lymphokines and cytokines produced by cells involved in the marrow response to the tumors promote resorption of bone through local destruction. Several hormones, hormone analogues, cytokines, and growth factors have been implicated as the result of clinical assays, in vitro tests, or chemical isolation. In some lymphomas, typically B cell lymphomas, there is an increased blood level of 1,25(OH)$_2$D, which is probably produced by lymphocytes. The etiologic factor produced by activated normal lymphocytes and by myeloma and lymphoma cells, termed *osteoclast activation factor*, now appears to represent the biologic action of several different cytokines, probably interleukin 1 and lymphotoxin or tumor necrosis factor.

The more common mechanism, humoral hypercalcemia of malignancy, occurs with cancers of the lung and kidney, in particular, in which bone metastases are absent, minimal, or not detectable clinically. The clinical picture resembles primary hyperparathyroidism (hypophosphatemia accompanies hypercalcemia), and elimination or regression of the primary tumor leads to disappearance of the hypercalcemia. The disorder is due to secretion by the tumors of the PTH-like factor, PTHrP, that activates the PTH/PTHrP receptor (see above).

As in hyperparathyroidism, patients with the humoral hypercalcemia of malignancy have elevated urinary nephrogenous cyclic AMP excretion, hypophosphatemia, and increased urinary phosphate clearance. However, in humoral hypercalcemia of malignancy, immunoreactive PTH is undetectable or suppressed, making the differential diagnosis easier. Other features of the disorder differ from those of true hyperparathyroidism. Patients may have high, rather than low, renal calcium clearance (relative to serum calcium when compared to true hyperparathyroidism, unlike the expected elevation) and low to normal levels of 1,25(OH)$_2$D. The reason that the humoral syndrome differs from hyperparathyroidism in these parameters is unclear since the biologic actions of PTH and PTHrP are presumably exerted through the same receptor. Other cytokines elaborated by the malignancy may be responsible for these variations from hyperparathyroidism. In some patients with the humoral hypercalcemia of malignancy, osteoclastic resorption is unaccompanied by an osteoblastic or bone-forming response, implying inhibition of the normal coupling of bone formation and resorption. Thus the interaction of more than one substance may determine whether hypercalcemia develops in a particular patient.

Several different assays (single- or double-antibody, different epitopes) have been developed to detect PTHrP. Most data indicate that circulating PTHrP levels are undetectable (or low) in normal individuals, elevated in most cancer patients with the humoral syndrome, and high in human milk. Despite the discovery of PTHrP, identifying the etiologic mechanisms in cancer hypercalcemia is often complex. For example, in breast carcinoma (metastatic to bone) and in a distinctive type of T cell lymphoma/leukemia initiated by human T cell lymphotropic virus I, hypercalcemia is caused by direct local lysis of bone as well as by a humoral mechanism involving excess production of PTHrP.

Diagnostic Issues Levels of PTH measured by the double-antibody technique are undetectable or extremely low in tumor hypercalcemia, as would be expected with the mediation of the hypercalcemia by a factor other than PTH (the hypercalcemia suppresses the normal parathyroid glands). In a patient with minimal symptoms referred for hypercalcemia, low or undetectable PTH and elevated PTHrP levels would focus attention on occult malignancy.

Ordinarily, the diagnosis of cancer hypercalcemia is not difficult because tumor symptoms are prominent when hypercalcemia is detected. Indeed, hypercalcemia may be noted incidentally during the workup of a patient with known or suspected malignancy. Clinical suspicion that malignancy is the cause of the hypercalcemia is heightened when there are other paraneoplastic signs or symptoms, such as weight loss, fatigue, muscle weakness, or unexplained skin rash, or when symptoms specific for a particular tumor are present. Squamous cell tumors are most frequently associated with hypercalcemia, partic-

FIGURE 341-6 Mutations in the calcium sensor receptor. The identified sequence alterations (X) cause loss of function and lead to inadequate suppression of parathyroid hormone release and, therefore, mild hypercalcemia (FHH); ♦, a gain-of-function mutation that causes hypocalcemia; S, a stop codon that is a loss of function mutation; •, conserved residues; ▲, acidic residues. *(From EM Brown et al: J Nutr 125:1965S, 1995, with permission.)*

ularly tumors of the lung, kidney, head and neck, and urogenital tract. Radiologic examinations can focus on these areas when clinical evidence is unclear. Bone scans with technetium-labeled bisphosphonate are useful for detection of osteolytic metastases; the sensitivity is high, but specificity is low; results must be confirmed by conventional x-rays to be certain that areas of increased uptake are due to osteolytic metastases per se. Bone marrow biopsies are helpful in patients with anemia or abnormal peripheral blood smears.

TREATMENT Treatment of the hypercalcemia of malignancy is first directed to control of the tumor; reduction of tumor mass usually corrects hypercalcemia. If a patient has severe hypercalcemia yet has a good chance for effective tumor therapy, treatment of the hypercalcemia should be vigorous while awaiting the results of definitive therapy. If hypercalcemia occurs in the late stages of a tumor that is resistant to therapy, the treatment of the hypercalcemia should be judicious as high calcium levels can have a mild sedating effect. Standard therapies for hypercalcemia (discussed below) are applicable to patients with malignancy.

VITAMIN D–RELATED HYPERCALCEMIA Hypercalcemia caused by vitamin D can be due to excessive ingestion or abnormal metabolism of the vitamin. Abnormal metabolism of the vitamin is usually acquired in association with a widespread granulomatous disorder. Vitamin D metabolism is carefully regulated, particularly the activity of renal 1α-hydroxylase, the enzyme responsible for the production of 1,25(OH)$_2$D (Chap. 340). The regulation of 1α-hydroxylase and the normal feedback suppression by 1,25(OH)$_2$D seem to work less well in infants than in adults and to operate poorly, if at all, in sites other than the renal tubule; these phenomena explain the occurrence of hypercalcemia secondary to excessive 1,25(OH)$_2$D$_3$ production in infants with Williams' syndrome (see below) and in adults with sarcoidosis or lymphoma.

Vitamin D Intoxication Chronic ingestion of 50 to 100 times the normal physiologic requirement of vitamin D (amounts >50,000 to 100,000 U/d) is usually required to produce significant hypercalcemia in normal individuals. An upper limit of dietary intake of 2000 U/d (50 μg/d) in adults is now recommended because of concerns about potential toxic effects of cumulative supraphysiologic doses. Vitamin D excess increases intestinal calcium absorption and, if severe, also increases bone resorption.

Hypercalcemia in vitamin D intoxication is due to an excessive biologic action of the vitamin, perhaps the consequence of increased levels of 25(OH)D rather than increased levels of the usual active metabolite 1,25(OH)$_2$D (the latter is frequently not elevated in vitamin D intoxication). 25(OH)D has definite, if low, biologic activity in intestine and bone. The production of 25(OH)D is less tightly regulated than is the production of 1,25(OH)$_2$D. Hence concentrations of 25(OH)D are elevated several-fold in patients with excess vitamin D intake.

The diagnosis is substantiated by documenting elevated levels of 25(OH)D >100 ng/mL. Hypercalcemia is usually controlled by restriction of dietary calcium intake and appropriate attention to hydration. These measures, plus discontinuation of vitamin D, usually lead to resolution of hypercalcemia. However, vitamin D stores in fat may be substantial, and vitamin D intoxication may persist for weeks after vitamin D ingestion is terminated. Such patients are responsive to glucocorticoids, which in doses of 100 mg/d of hydrocortisone or its equivalent, usually return serum calcium levels to normal over several days; severe intoxication may require intensive therapy.

Sarcoidosis and Other Granulomatous Diseases   In patients with sarcoidosis and other granulomatous diseases, such as tuberculosis and fungal infections, excess 1,25(OH)$_2$D is synthesized in macrophages or other cells in the granulomas. Indeed, increased 1,25(OH)$_2$D levels have been reported in anephric patients with sarcoidosis and hypercalcemia. Macrophages obtained from granulomatous tissue convert 25(OH)D to 1,25(OH)$_2$D at an increased rate. There is a positive correlation in patients with sarcoidosis between 25(OH)D levels (reflecting vitamin D intake) and the circulating concentrations of 1,25(OH)$_2$D, whereas normally there is no increase in 1,25(OH)$_2$D with increasing 25(OH)D levels due to multiple feedback controls on renal 1α-hydroxylase (Chap. 340). The usual regulation of active metabolite production by calcium or PTH does not operate in these patients; hypercalcemia does not lead to a reduction in the blood levels of 1,25(OH)$_2$D in patients with sarcoidosis. Clearance of 1,25(OH)$_2$D from blood may be decreased in sarcoidosis as well. PTH levels are usually low and 1,25(OH)$_2$D levels are elevated, but primary hyperparathyroidism and sarcoidosis may coexist in some patients.

Management of the hypercalcemia can often be accomplished by avoiding excessive sunlight exposure and limiting vitamin D and calcium intake. Presumably, however, the abnormal sensitivity to vitamin D and abnormal regulation of 1,25(OH)$_2$D synthesis will persist as long as the disease is active. Alternatively, glucocorticoids in the equivalent of ≤100 mg/d of hydrocortisone control hypercalcemia. Glucocorticoids appear to act by blocking excessive production of 1,25(OH)$_2$D as well as the response to it in target organs.

Idiopathic Hypercalcemia of Infancy   This rare disorder, usually referred to as *Williams' syndrome*, is an autosomal dominant disorder characterized by multiple congenital development defects, including supravalvular aortic stenosis, mental retardation, and an elfin facies, in association with hypercalcemia due to abnormal sensitivity to vitamin D. The syndrome was first recognized in England after the fortification of milk with vitamin D. Levels of 1,25(OH)$_2$D are elevated, ranging from 46 to 120 nmol/L (150 to 500 pg/mL). The mechanism of the abnormal sensitivity to vitamin D and of the increased circulating levels of 1,25(OH)$_2$D is still unclear. Studies suggest that mutations involving the elastin locus and perhaps other genes on chromosome 7 may play a role in the pathogenesis.

HYPERCALCEMIA ASSOCIATED WITH HIGH BONE TURNOVER   Hyperthyroidism   As many as 20% of hyperthyroid patients have high-normal or mildly elevated serum calcium concentrations; hypercalciuria is even more common. The hypercalcemia is due to increased bone turnover, with bone resorption exceeding bone formation. Severe calcium elevations are not typical, and the presence of such suggests a concomitant disease such as hyperparathyroidism. Usually, the diagnosis is obvious, but signs of hyperthyroidism may occasionally be occult, particularly in the elderly (Chap. 330). Hypercalcemia is managed by treatment of the hyperthyroidism.

Immobilization   Immobilization is a rare cause of hypercalcemia in adults in the absence of an associated disease but may cause hypercalcemia in children and adolescents, particularly after spinal cord injury and paraplegia or quadriplegia. With resumption of ambulation, the hypercalcemia in children usually returns to normal.

The mechanism appears to involve a disproportion between bone formation and bone resorption. Hypercalciuria and increased mobilization of skeletal calcium can develop in normal volunteers subjected to extensive bed rest, although hypercalcemia is unusual. Immobilization of an adult with a disease associated with high bone turnover, such as Paget's disease, may cause hypercalcemia.

Thiazides   Administration of benzothiadiazines (thiazides) can cause hypercalcemia in patients with high rates of bone turnover, such as patients with hypoparathyroidism treated with high doses of vitamin D. Traditionally, thiazides are associated with aggravation of hypercalcemia in primary hyperparathyroidism, but this effect can be seen in other high-bone-turnover states as well. The mechanism of thiazide action is complex. Chronic thiazide administration leads to reduction in urinary calcium; the hypocalciuric effect appears to reflect the enhancement of proximal tubular resorption of sodium and calcium in response to sodium depletion. Some of this renal effect is due to augmentation of PTH action and is more pronounced in individuals with intact PTH secretion. However, thiazides cause hypocalciuria in hypoparathyroid patients on high-dose vitamin D and oral calcium replacement if sodium intake is restricted. This finding is the rationale for the use of thiazides as an adjunct to therapy in hypoparathyroid patients, as discussed below. Thiazide administration to normal individuals causes a transient increase in blood calcium (usually within the high-normal range) that reverts to preexisting levels after a week or more of continued administration. If hormonal function and calcium and bone metabolism are normal, homeostatic controls are reset to counteract the calcium-elevating effect of the thiazides. In the presence of hyperparathyroidism or increased bone turnover from another cause, homeostatic mechanisms are ineffective. The abnormal effects of the thiazide on calcium metabolism disappear within days of cessation of the drug.

Vitamin A Intoxication   Vitamin A intoxication is a rare cause of hypercalcemia and is most commonly a side effect of dietary faddism (Chap. 75). Calcium levels can be elevated into the 3 to 3.5 mmol/L (12 to 14 mg/dL) range after the ingestion of 50,000 to 100,000 units of vitamin A daily (10 to 20 times the minimum daily requirement). Typical features of severe hypercalcemia include fatigue, anorexia, and, in some, severe muscle and bone pain. Excess Vitamin A intake is presumed to increase bone resorption.

The diagnosis can be established by history and by measurement of vitamin A levels in serum, which may be severalfold above normal. Occasionally, skeletal x-rays reveal periosteal calcifications, particularly in the hands. Withdrawal of the vitamin is usually associated with prompt disappearance of the hypercalcemia and reversal of the skeletal changes. As in vitamin D intoxication, administration of 100 mg/d hydrocortisone or its equivalent leads to a rapid return of the serum calcium to normal.

HYPERCALCEMIA ASSOCIATED WITH RENAL FAILURE   Severe Secondary Hyperparathyroidism   Secondary hyperparathyroidism occurs when partial resistance to the metabolic actions of PTH leads to excessive production of the hormone. Parathyroid gland hyperplasia occurs because resistance to the normal level of PTH leads to hypocalcemia, which, in turn, is a stimulus to parathyroid gland enlargement. This concept is supported by studies of the treatment of patients treated with bisphosphonates, which block the skeletal resorptive response. Because a portion of PTH secretion by each parathyroid cell is not suppressible by any degree of elevation of

Secondary hyperparathyroidism occurs not only in patients with renal failure but also in those with osteomalacia due to multiple causes (Chap. 340), including deficiency of vitamin D action, and PHP (deficient response to PTH at the level of the receptor). Hypocalcemia seems to be the common denominator in initiating secondary hyperparathyroidism. Only in patients with renal failure, however, is hypercalcemia sometimes encountered despite appropriate medical management regimens (see below). Primary and secondary hyperparathyroidism can be distinguished conceptually by the autonomous growth of the parathyroid glands in primary hyperparathyroidism (presumably irreversible) and the adaptive response of the parathyroids in secondary hyperparathyroidism (typically reversible). In fact, reversal over weeks from an abnormal pattern of secretion, presumably accompanied by involution of parathyroid gland mass to normal, occurs in patients who have been treated effectively to reverse the resistance to PTH (such as with calcium and vitamin D in osteomalacia).

Patients with secondary hyperparathyroidism may develop bone pain, ectopic calcification, and pruritus. The bone disease seen in patients with secondary hyperparathyroidism and renal failure is termed *renal osteodystrophy*. Osteomalacia (predominantly due to vitamin D and calcium deficiency) and/or osteitis fibrosa cystica (excessive PTH action on bone) may occur.

Two other skeletal disorders are associated with long-term dialysis in patients with renal failure. Aluminum deposition (see below) is associated with an osteomalacia-like picture. The other entity is a low-bone-turnover state termed "aplastic" or "adynamic" bone disease; PTH levels are lower than in typical secondary hyperparathyroidism. It is believed that the condition is caused, at least in part, by excessive PTH suppression, which may be even greater than previously appreciated in light of evidence that some of the immunoreactive PTH detected by most commercially available PTH assays is not the full-length biologically active molecule (as discussed above).

℞ **TREATMENT** Medical therapy to reverse secondary hyperparathyroidism includes reduction of excessive blood phosphate by restriction of dietary phosphate, the use of nonabsorbable antacids, and careful, selective addition of calcitriol (0.25 to 2.0 μg/d); calcium carbonate is preferred over aluminum-containing antacids to prevent aluminum toxicity. Intravenous calcitriol, administered as several pulses each week, helps control secondary hyperparathyroidism. Aggressive but carefully administered medical therapy can often, but not always, reverse hyperparathyroidism and its symptoms and manifestations.

Occasional patients develop severe manifestations of secondary hyperparathyroidism, including hypercalcemia, pruritus, extraskeletal calcifications, and painful bones, despite aggressive medical efforts to suppress the hyperparathyroidism. PTH hypersecretion no longer responsive to medical therapy, a state of severe hyperparathyroidism in patients with renal failure that requires surgery, has been referred to as *tertiary hyperparathyroidism*. Parathyroid surgery is necessary to control this condition. Based on genetic evidence from examination of tumor samples in these patients, the emergence of autonomous parathyroid function is due to a monoclonal outgrowth of one or more previously hyperplastic parathyroid glands.

Aluminum Intoxication Aluminum intoxication (and often hypercalcemia as a complication of medical treatment) may occur in patients on chronic dialysis; manifestations include acute dementia and unresponsive and severe osteomalacia. Bone pain, multiple nonhealing fractures, particularly of the ribs and pelvis, and a proximal myopathy may occur. Hypercalcemia develops when these patients are treated with vitamin D or calcitriol because of impaired skeletal responsiveness. Aluminum is present at the site of osteoid mineralization, osteoblastic activity is minimal, and calcium incorporation into the skeleton is impaired. Prevention is accomplished by avoidance of alu-

minum excess in the dialysis regimen; treatment of established disease involves mobilizing aluminum through the use of the chelating agent deferoxamine (Chap. 348).

Milk-Alkali Syndrome The milk-alkali syndrome is due to excessive ingestion of calcium and absorbable antacids such as milk or calcium carbonate. It is much less frequent since nonabsorbable antacids and other treatments became available for peptic ulcer disease. However, the increased use of calcium carbonate in the management of osteoporosis has led to reappearance of the syndrome. Several clinical presentations—acute, subacute, and chronic—have been described, all of which feature hypercalcemia, alkalosis, and renal failure. The chronic form of the disease, termed *Burnett's syndrome*, is associated with irreversible renal damage. The acute syndromes reverse if the excess calcium and absorbable alkali are stopped.

Individual susceptibility is important in the pathogenesis, as many patients are treated with calcium carbonate alkali regimens without developing the syndrome. One variable is the fractional calcium absorption as a function of calcium intake. Some individuals absorb a high fraction of calcium, even with intakes as high as 2 g or more of elemental calcium per day, instead of reducing calcium absorption with high intake, as occurs in most normal individuals. Resultant mild hypercalcemia after meals in such patients is postulated to contribute to the generation of alkalosis. Development of hypercalcemia causes increased sodium excretion and some depletion of total-body water. These phenomena and perhaps some suppression of endogenous PTH secretion due to mild hypercalcemia lead to increased bicarbonate resorption and to alkalosis in the face of continued calcium carbonate ingestion. Alkalosis per se selectively enhances calcium resorption in the distal nephron, thus aggravating the hypercalcemia. The cycle of mild hypercalcemia → bicarbonate retention → alkalosis → renal calcium retention → severe hypercalcemia perpetuates and aggravates hypercalcemia and alkalosis as long as calcium and absorbable alkali are ingested.

DIFFERENTIAL DIAGNOSIS: SPECIAL TESTS Differential diagnosis of hypercalcemia is best achieved by using clinical criteria, but the immunoassay for PTH is especially useful in distinguishing among major causes (Fig. 341-7). The clinical features that deserve emphasis are the presence or absence of symptoms or signs of disease and evidence of chronicity. If one discounts fatigue or depression, >90% of patients with primary hyperparathyroidism have *asymptomatic hypercalcemia*; symptoms of malignancy are usually present in cancer-associated hypercalcemia. Disorders other than hyperparathyroidism and malignancy cause <10% of cases of hypercalcemia, and some of the nonparathyroid causes are associated with clear-cut manifestations such as renal failure.

Hyperparathyroidism is the likely diagnosis in patients with *chronic hypercalcemia*. If hypercalcemia has been manifest for >1 year, malignancy can usually be excluded as the cause. A striking feature of malignancy-associated hypercalcemia is the rapidity of the course, whereby signs and symptoms of the underlying malignancy are evident within months of the detection of hypercalcemia. A careful history of dietary supplements and drug use may suggest intoxication with vitamins D or vitamin A or the use of thiazides.

Although clinical considerations are helpful in arriving at the correct diagnosis of the cause of hypercalcemia, appropriate laboratory testing is essential for definitive diagnosis. The immunoassay for PTH should separate hyperparathyroidism from all other causes of hypercalcemia. Patients with hyperparathyroidism have elevated PTH levels despite hypercalcemia, whereas patients with malignancy and the other causes of hypercalcemia (except for disorders mediated by PTH such as lithium-induced hypercalcemia) have levels of hormone below normal or undetectable. Assays based on the double-antibody method for PTH exhibit very high sensitivity (especially if serum calcium is simultaneously evaluated) and specificity for the diagnosis of primary hyperparathyroidism (Fig. 341-8).

In summary, PTH values are elevated in >90% of parathyroid-

FIGURE 341-7 Algorithm for the evaluation of patients with hypercalcemia. See text for details. FHH, familial hypocalciuric hypercalcemia; MEN, multiple endocrine neoplasia; PTH, parathyroid hormone; PTHrP, parathyroid hormone–related peptide.

related causes of hypercalcemia, undetectable or low in malignancy-related hypercalcemia, and undetectable or normal in vitamin D–related and high-bone-turnover causes of hypercalcemia. In view of the specificity of the PTH immunoassay and the high frequency of hyperparathyroidism in hypercalcemic patients, it is cost-effective to measure the PTH level in all hypercalcemic patients unless malignancy or a specific nonparathyroid disease is obvious. False-positive PTH assay results are rare. There are very rare reports of ectopic production of excess PTH by nonparathyroid tumors. Immunoassays for PTHrP are helpful in diagnosing certain types of malignancy-associated hypercalcemia. Although FHH is parathyroid-related, the disease should be managed distinctively from hyperparathyroidism. Clinical features and the low urinary calcium excretion can help make the distinction. Because the incidence of malignancy and hyperparathyroidism both increase with age, they can coexist as two independent causes of hypercalcemia.

1,25(OH)$_2$D levels are elevated in many (but not all) patients with primary hyperparathyroidism. In other disorders associated with hypercalcemia, concentrations of 1,25(OH)$_2$D are low or, at the most, normal. However, this test is of low specificity and is not cost-effective, as not all patients with hyperparathyroidism have elevated 1,25(OH)$_2$D levels, and not all nonparathyroid hypercalcemic patients have suppressed 1,25(OH)$_2$D. Measurement of 1,25(OH)$_2$D is, however, critically valuable in establishing the cause of hypercalcemia in sarcoidosis and certain B cell lymphomas.

A useful general approach is outlined in Fig. 341-7. If the patient is *asymptomatic* and there is evidence of *chronicity* to the hypercalcemia, hyperparathyroidism is almost certainly the cause. If PTH levels (usually measured at least twice) are elevated, the clinical impression is confirmed and little additional evaluation is necessary. If there is only a short history or no data as to the duration of the hypercalcemia, *occult malignancy* must be considered; if the PTH levels are not elevated, then a thorough workup must be undertaken for malignancy, including chest x-ray, CT of chest and abdomen, and bone scan. Immunoassays for PTHrP may be especially useful in such situations. Attention should also be paid to clues for underlying hematologic disorders such as anemia, increased plasma globulin, and abnormal serum immunoelectrophoresis; bone scans can be negative in some patients with metastases, such as in multiple myeloma. Finally, if a patient with chronic hypercalcemia is asymptomatic and malignancy therefore seems unlikely on clinical grounds, but PTH values are not elevated,

it is useful to search for other chronic causes of hypercalcemia, such as occult sarcoidosis.

℞ TREATMENT Hypercalcemic States The approach to medical treatment of hypercalcemia varies with its severity. Mild hypercalcemia, <3.0 mmol/L (12 mg/dL), can be managed by hydration. More severe hypercalcemia [levels of 3.2 to 3.7 mmol/L (13 to 15 mg/dL)] must be managed aggressively; above that level, hypercalcemia can be life-threatening and requires emergency measures. By using a combination of approaches, the serum calcium concentration can be decreased by 0.7 to 2.2 mmol/L (3 to 9 mg/dL) within 24 to 48 h in most patients, enough to relieve acute symptoms, prevent death from hypercalcemic crisis, and permit diagnostic evaluation. Therapy can then be directed at the underlying disorder—the second priority.

Hypercalcemia develops because of excessive skeletal calcium release, increased intestinal calcium absorption, or inadequate renal calcium excretion. Understanding the particular pathogenesis helps guide therapy. For example, hypercalcemia in patients with malignancy is primarily due to excessive skeletal calcium release and is, therefore, minimally improved by restriction of dietary calcium. On the other hand, patients with vitamin D hypersensitivity

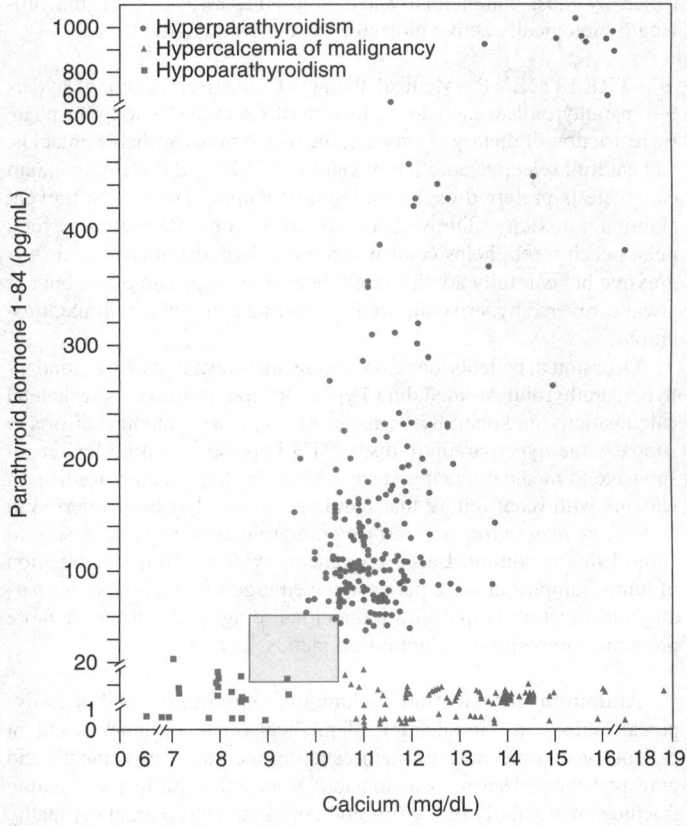

FIGURE 341-8 Levels of immunoreactive parathyroid hormone (PTH) detected in patients with primary hyperparathyroidism, hypercalcemia of malignancy, and hypoparathyroidism. Boxed area represents the upper and normal limits of blood calcium and/or immunoreactive PTH. (*From Nussbaum and Potts, with permission.*)

or vitamin D intoxication have excessive intestinal calcium absorption, and restriction of dietary calcium is beneficial. Decreased renal function or ECF depletion decreases urinary calcium excretion. In such situations, rehydration may rapidly reduce or reverse the hypercalcemia, even though increased bone resorption persists. As outlined below, the more severe the hypercalcemia, the greater the number of combined therapies that should be used. Rapid acting (hours) approaches—rehydration, forced diuresis, and calcitonin—can be used with the most effective antiresorptive agents, such as bisphosphonates (since severe hypercalcemia usually involves excessive bone resorption).

Hydration, increased salt intake, mild and forced diuresis The first principle of treatment is to restore normal hydration. Many hypercalcemic patients are dehydrated because of vomiting, inanition, and/or hypercalcemia-induced defects in urinary concentrating ability. The resultant drop in glomerular filtration rate is accompanied by an additional decrease in renal tubular sodium and calcium clearance. Restoring a normal ECF volume corrects these abnormalities and increases urine calcium excretion by 2.5 to 7.5 mmol/d (100 to 300 mg/d). Increasing urinary sodium excretion to 400 to 500 mmol/d increases urinary calcium excretion even further than simple rehydration. After rehydration has been achieved, saline can be administered or furosemide or ethacrynic acid can be given twice daily to depress the tubular reabsorptive mechanism for calcium (care must be taken to prevent dehydration). The combined use of these therapies can increase urinary calcium excretion to $\geq$12.5 mmol/d (500 mg/d) in most hypercalcemic patients. Since this is a substantial percentage of the exchangeable calcium pool, the serum calcium concentration usually falls 0.25 to 0.75 mmol/L (1 to 3 mg/dL) within 24 h. Precautions should be taken to prevent potassium and magnesium depletion; calcium-containing renal calculi are a potential complication.

Under life-threatening circumstances, the preceding approach can be pursued more aggressively, giving as much as 6 L isotonic saline (900 mmol sodium) daily plus furosemide or equivalent in doses up to 100 mg every 1 to 2 h or ethacrynic acid in doses to 40 mg every 1 to 2 h. Urinary calcium excretion may exceed 25 mmol/d (1000 mg/d), and the serum calcium may decrease by $\geq$1 mmol/L (4 mg/dL) within 24 h. Depletion of potassium and magnesium is inevitable unless replacements are given; pulmonary edema can be precipitated. The potential complications can be reduced by careful monitoring of central venous pressure and plasma or urine electrolytes; catheterization of the bladder may be necessary. This treatment approach should be supplemented with agents to block bone resorption. Though these agents do not become effective for several days, forced diuresis is difficult to sustain even in patients with good cardiopulmonary and renal function.

Bisphosphonates The bisphosphonates are analogues of pyrophosphate, with high affinity for bone, especially in areas of increased bone turnover, where they are powerful inhibitors of bone resorption. These bone-seeking compounds are stable in vivo because phosphatase enzymes cannot hydrolyze the central carbon-phosphorus-carbon bond. The bisphosphonates are concentrated in areas of high bone turnover and are taken up by and inhibit osteoclast action; the mechanism of action is complex. Bisphosphonates alter osteoclast proton pump function or impair the release of acid hydrolases into the extracellular lysosomes contiguous with mineralized bone. They may also inhibit the differentiation of monocyte-macrophage precursors into osteoclasts and possibly have effects on osteoblasts as well. The bisphosphonate molecules that contain amino groups in the side chain structure (see below) interfere with prenylation of proteins and can lead to cellular apoptosis. The highly active non-amino group–containing bisphosphonates are also metabolized to cytotoxic products.

The initial bisphosphonate widely used in clinical practice, etidronate, was effective but had several disadvantages, including the capacity to inhibit bone formation as well as blocking resorption. Subsequently, a number of second-generation compounds have become the mainstays of antiresorptive therapy for treatment of hypercalcemia. The most widely used, pamidronate, is a potent inhibitor of osteoclast-

mediated skeletal resorption yet does not cause mineralization defects at ordinary doses. Several additional bisphosphonates (alendronate, tiludronate, and risedronate) are potent and also have a highly favorable ratio of blocking resorption versus inhibiting bone formation. Though the bisphosphonates have similar structures, the routes of administration, efficacy, toxicity, and side effects vary. The potency of the compounds for inhibition of bone resorption varies a thousandfold in the order of etidronate, tiludronate, pamidronate, alendronate, and risedronate. Oral alendronate is approved for the therapy of osteoporosis in the United States, and in Europe oral preparations of these bisphosphonates are used in the chronic treatment of hypercalcemia. Only the intravenous use of pamidronate is approved for this purpose in the United States; between 30 and 90 mg pamidronate, given as a single intravenous dose over a few hours, returns serum calcium to normal within 24 to 48 h with an effect that lasts for weeks in 80 to 100% of patients.

Pamidronate causes low-grade fever in as many as 20% of patients, likely related to release of cytokines from osteoclasts, monocytes, and macrophages (Table 341-2). This effect is usually seen only with the initial doses. Etidronate causes hyperphosphatemia through a direct renal mechanism, whereas hypophosphatemia is seen after therapy with other bisphosphonates. Overall, second-generation bisphosphonates are now the agents of choice in severe hypercalcemia, particularly that associated with malignancy. Zoledronate, a third-generation bisphosphonate, is claimed to be 100 to 800 times more potent than pamidronate and to normalize calcium more quickly and for longer periods.

Calcitonin Calcitonin acts within a few hours of its administration, through receptors on osteoclasts, to block bone resorption and, in addition, to increase urinary calcium excretion by inhibition of renal tubular calcium reabsorption. However, calcitonin leads to variable and usually minimal lowering of calcium. Tachyphylaxis, a known phenomenon with this drug, may explain the variable results. However, in life-threatening hypercalcemia, calcitonin can be used effectively within the first 24 h in combination with rehydration and saline diuresis while waiting for more sustained effects from a simultaneously administered bisphosphonate such as pamidronate. Usual doses of calcitonin are 2 to 8 U/kg of body weight intravenously, subcutaneously, or intramuscularly every 6 to 12 h.

Other therapies *Plicamycin* (mithramycin), which inhibits bone resorption, has been a useful therapeutic agent but is now little used because of the effectiveness of bisphosphonates. Plicamycin must be given intravenously, either as a bolus injection or by slow infusion. The usual dose is 25 μg/kg body weight. Major side effects include thrombocytopenia, hepatocellular necrosis with increased lactic acid dehydrogenase (LDH) and aspartate aminotransferase (AST) levels, and decreased levels of clotting factors with resultant epistaxis, bruising, hemorrhage, and bleeding gums.

Gallium nitrate exerts a hypocalcemic action by inhibiting bone resorption and altering the structure of bone crystals. Major disadvantages include the 5-day duration of infusion and the potential for nephrotoxicity and relatively shorter duration of action than bisphosphonates. Accordingly it is not often used because of superior alternatives.

Glucocorticoids increase urinary calcium excretion and decrease intestinal calcium absorption when given in pharmacologic doses, but they also cause negative skeletal calcium balance. In normal individuals and in patients with primary hyperparathyroidism, glucocorticoids neither increase nor decrease the serum calcium concentration. In patients with hypercalcemia due to certain osteolytic malignancies, however, glucocorticoids may be effective as a result of antitumor effects. The malignancies in which hypercalcemia responds to glucocorticoids include multiple myeloma, leukemia, Hodgkin's disease, other lymphomas, and carcinoma of the breast, at least early in the course of the disease. Glucocorticoids are also effective in treating hypercalcemia due to vitamin D intoxication and sarcoidosis. In all the preceding situations, the hypocalcemic effect develops over several days,

Table 341-2 Therapies for Severe Hypercalcemia

Treatment	Onset of Action	Duration of Action	Advantages	Disadvantages
MOST USEFUL THERAPIES				
Hydration with saline	Hours	During infusion	Rehydration invariably needed	Volume overload, cardiac decompensation, intensive monitoring, electrolyte disturbance, inconvenience
Forced diuresis; saline plus loop diuretic	Hours	During treatment	Rapid action	
Bisphosphonates 1st generation: etidronate	1–2 days	5–7 days in doses used	First available bisphosphonate; intermediate onset of action	Less effective than other bisphosphonates
2d generation: pamidronate	1–2 days	10–14 days to weeks	High potency; intermediate onset of action	Fever in 20% hypophosphatemia, hypocalcemia, hypomagnesemia
Calcitonin	Hours	1–2 days	Rapid onset of action; useful as adjunct in severe hypercalcemia	Rapid tachyphylaxis
SPECIAL USE THERAPIES				
Phosphate Oral	24 h	During use	Chronic management (with hypophosphatemia); low toxicity if P < 4 mg/dL	Limited use except as adjuvant or chronic therapy
Intravenous	Hours	During use and 24–48 h afterward	Rapid action, highly potent but *rarely used* except with severe hypercalcemia and cardiac and renal decompensation present	Ectopic calcification; renal damage, fatal hypocalcemia
Glucocorticoids	Days	Days, weeks	Oral therapy, antitumor agent	Active only in certain malignancies; glucocorticoid side effects
Dialysis	Hours	During use and 24–48 h afterward	Useful in renal failure; onset of effect in hours; can immediately reverse life-threatening hypercalcemia	Complex procedure, reserved for extreme or special circumstances

and the usual glucocorticoid dosage is 40 to 100 mg prednisone (or its equivalent) daily in four divided doses. The side effects of chronic glucocorticoid therapy may be acceptable in some circumstances.

Dialysis is often the treatment of choice for hypercalcemia complicated by renal failure, which is difficult to manage. Peritoneal dialysis with calcium-free dialysis fluid can remove 5 to 12.5 mmol (200 to 500 mg) of calcium in 24 to 48 h and lower the serum calcium concentration by 0.7 to 3 mmol/L (3 to 12 mg/dL). Large quantities of phosphate are lost during dialysis, and serum inorganic phosphate concentrations usually fall, thus aggravating hypercalcemia. Therefore, the serum inorganic phosphate concentration should be measured after dialysis, and phosphate supplements should be added to the diet or to dialysis fluids if necessary.

Phosphate therapy, oral or intravenous, has a limited role in certain circumstances. Patients with primary hyperparathyroidism are frequently hypophosphatemic, and hypercalcemia of other causes also may be complicated by hypophosphatemia. Hypophosphatemia decreases the rate of calcium uptake into bone, increases intestinal calcium absorption, and directly and indirectly stimulates bone breakdown. These effects aggravate hypercalcemia, and correcting hypophosphatemia lowers the serum calcium concentration. The usual treatment is 1 to 1.5 g phosphorus per day for several days, given in four divided doses to minimize the chances of developing hyperphos-

phatemia. Such therapy has been administered for prolonged periods in selected patients. It is generally believed, but not established, that toxicity does not occur if therapy is limited to restoring serum inorganic phosphate concentrations to normal.

Raising the serum inorganic phosphate concentration above normal decreases serum calcium levels, sometimes strikingly. Intravenous phosphate is one of the most dramatically effective treatments available for severe hypercalcemia but is toxic and even dangerous (fatal hypocalcemia). For these reasons, it is used rarely and only in severely hypercalcemic patients with cardiac or renal failure. A phosphate phosphorus dose of ≥ 1500 mg intravenously over 6 to 8 h leads to a prompt decrease in serum calcium of as much as 1.2 to 2.5 mmol/L (5 to 10 mg/dL) in patients with initially normal serum inorganic phosphate concentrations. This therapy should be employed only in extreme emergencies. Inorganic phosphate is commercially available for oral use in liquid, powder, and capsule form and as a liquid for intravenous use. It is important to calculate doses in terms of phosphate phosphorus.

Summary The various therapies for hypercalcemia are listed in Table 341-2. The choice depends on the underlying disease, the severity of the hypercalcemia, the serum inorganic phosphate level, and the renal, hepatic, and bone marrow function. Mild hypercalcemia [≤ 3 mmol/L (12 mg/dL)] can usually be managed by hydration. Severe hypercalcemia [3.7 mmol/L (15 mg/dL)] requires rapid correction. Calcitonin should be given for its rapid, albeit short-lived, blockade of bone resorption, and intravenous pamidronate should be administered, although its onset of action is delayed for 1 to 2 days. In addition, for the first 24 to 48 h, aggressive sodium-calcium diuresis with intravenous saline and large doses of furosemide and ethacrynic acid following initial hydration should be initiated, but only if appropriate monitoring is available and cardiac and renal function are adequate. Otherwise, dialysis may be necessary. Intermediate degrees of hypercalcemia between 3.0 and 3.7 mmol/L (12 and 15 mg/dL) should be approached with vigorous hydration and then the most appropriate selection for the patient of the combinations used with severe hypercalcemia.

HYPOCALCEMIA

PATHOPHYSIOLOGY OF HYPOCALCEMIA: CLASSIFICATION BASED ON MECHANISM *Chronic hypocalcemia* is less common than hypercalcemia; causes include chronic renal failure, hereditary and acquired hypoparathyroidism, vitamin D deficiency, PHP, and hypomagnesemia.

Critically ill patients may have transient hypocalcemia with severe sepsis, burns, acute renal failure, and extensive transfusions with citrated blood. Acute hypocalcemia with certain medications is usually transient and may produce no symptoms. Although as many as half of patients in an intensive care setting are reported to have calcium concentrations <2.1 mmol/L (8.5 mg/dL), <10% have a reduction in ionized calcium. Patients with severe sepsis may have a decrease in ionized calcium (true hypocalcemia), but in other severely ill individuals, hypoalbuminemia is the primary cause of the reduced total calcium concentration. Alkalosis increases calcium binding to proteins, and in this setting direct measurements of ionized calcium should be made.

Medications such as protamine, heparin, and glucagon may cause transient hypocalcemia. These forms of hypocalcemia are usually not associated with tetany and resolve with improvement in the overall medical condition. The hypocalcemia after repeated transfusions of citrated blood usually resolves quickly.

Patients with *acute pancreatitis* have hypocalcemia that persists during the acute inflammation and varies in degree with the severity of the pancreatitis. The cause of hypocalcemia remains unclear. PTH values are reported to be low, normal, or elevated, and both resistance to PTH and impaired PTH secretion have been postulated. Occasionally, a chronic low total calcium and low ionized calcium concentration are detected in an elderly patient without obvious cause and with a paucity of symptoms; the pathogenesis is unclear.

Chronic hypocalcemia, however, is usually symptomatic and requires treatment. Neuromuscular and neurologic manifestations of chronic hypocalcemia include muscle spasms, carpopedal spasm, facial grimacing, and, in extreme cases, laryngeal spasm and convulsions. Respiratory arrest may occur. Increased intracranial pressure occurs in some patients with long-standing hypocalcemia, often in association with papilledema. Mental changes include irritability, depression, and psychosis. The QT interval on the electrocardiogram is prolonged, in contrast to its shortening with hypercalcemia. Arrhythmias occur, and digitalis effectiveness may be reduced. Intestinal cramps and chronic malabsorption may occur. Chvostek's or Trousseau's sign can be used to confirm latent tetany.

The classification of hypocalcemia shown in Table 341-3 is based on the premise that PTH is responsible for minute-to-minute regulation of plasma calcium concentration and, therefore, that the occurrence of hypocalcemia must mean a failure of the homeostatic action of PTH. Failure of the PTH response can occur due to hereditary or acquired parathyroid gland failure, if PTH is ineffective in target organs, or if the action of the hormone is overwhelmed by the loss of calcium from the ECF at a rate faster than it can be replaced.

PTH ABSENT Whether hereditary or acquired, hypoparathyroidism has a number of common components. Acute and chronic symptoms of untreated hypocalcemia are shared by both types of hypoparathyroidism, although the onset of hereditary hypoparathyroidism is more gradual and is often associated with other developmental defects. Basal ganglia calcification and extrapyramidal syndromes are more common and earlier in onset in hereditary hypoparathyroidism. In earlier decades, acquired hypoparathyroidism secondary to surgery in the neck was more common than hereditary hypoparathyroidism, but the frequency of surgically induced parathyroid failure has diminished as a result of improved surgical techniques that spare the parathyroid glands and increased use of nonsurgical therapy for hyperthyroidism. PHP, an example of ineffective PTH action rather than a failure of parathyroid gland production, may share several features with hypoparathyroidism, including extraosseous calcification and extrapyramidal manifestations such as choreoathetotic movements and dystonia.

Papilledema and raised intracranial pressure may occur in both hereditary or acquired hypoparathyroidism, as do chronic changes in fingernails and hair and lenticular cataracts, the latter usually reversible with treatment of hypocalcemia. Certain skin manifestations, including alopecia and candidiasis, are characteristic of hereditary hypoparathyroidism associated with autoimmune polyglandular failure (Chap. 339).

Hypocalcemia associated with hypomagnesemia is associated with both deficient PTH release and impaired responsiveness to the hormone. Patients with hypocalcemia secondary to hypomagnesemia have absent or low levels of circulating PTH, indicative of diminished hormone release despite maximum physiologic stimulus by hypocalcemia. Plasma PTH levels return to normal with correction of the hypomagnesemia. Thus hypoparathyroidism with low levels of PTH in blood can be due to hereditary gland failure, acquired gland failure, or acute but reversible gland dysfunction (hypomagnesemia).

Genetic Abnormalities and Hereditary Hypoparathyroidism Hereditary hypoparathyroidism can occur as an isolated entity without other endocrine or dermatologic manifestations (idiopathic hypoparathyroidism); more typically, it occurs in association with other abnormalities such as defective development of the thymus or failure of function of other endocrine organs such as the adrenal, thyroid, or ovary (Chap. 339). Idiopathic and hereditary hypoparathyroidism are often manifest within the first decade but may appear later.

A rare form of hypoparathyroidism associated with defective development of both the thymus and the parathyroid glands is termed the *DiGeorge syndrome* (DGS), or the *velocardiofacial syndrome* (VCFS). Congenital cardiovascular, facial, and other developmental defects are present, and most patients die in early childhood with severe infections, hypocalcemia and seizures, or cardiovascular complications. Some survive into adulthood, and milder, incomplete forms occur. Most cases are sporadic, but an autosomal dominant form involving microdeletions of chromosome 22q11.2 has been described. Smaller deletions in this region are seen in incomplete forms of the DGS syndrome, appearing in childhood or adolescence, that are manifest primarily by parathyroid gland failure.

Hypoparathyroidism can occur in association with a complex hereditary autoimmune syndrome involving failure of the adrenals, the ovaries, the immune system, and the parathyroids in association with recurrent mucocutaneous candidiasis, alopecia, vitiligo, and pernicious anemia (Chap. 339). The responsible gene on chromosome 21q22.3 has been identified. The protein product, which resembles a transcription factor, has been termed the *AIRE* (autoimmune regulator). A stop codon mutation occurs in many Finnish families with the disorder, commonly referred to as *polyglandular autoimmune type 1 deficiency*.

Gain-of-function mutations in the calcium-sensing receptor cause *autosomal dominant hypocalcemia* (ADH). These mutations induce constitutive receptor functions that lead to features that are the inverse of FHH. The activated receptor suppresses PTH, leading to hypocalcemia; receptor activation in the kidney results in excessive renal calcium excretion. Recognition of the syndrome is important because efforts to treat the hypocalcemia of these patients with vitamin D analogues and increased oral calcium exacerbate the already excessive urinary calcium secretion (several grams or more per 24 h), leading to irreversible renal damage from stones and ectopic calcification.

Table 341-3 Functional Classification of Hypocalcemia (Excluding Neonatal Conditions)

PTH ABSENT

Hereditary hypoparathyroidism	Hypomagnesemia
Acquired hypoparathyroidism	

PTH INEFFECTIVE

Chronic renal failure	Active vitamin D ineffective
Active vitamin D lacking	Intestinal malabsorption
↓ Dietary intake or sunlight	Vitamin D–dependent rickets type II
Defective metabolism:	Pseudohypoparathyroidism
Anticonvulsant therapy	
Vitamin D–dependent rickets type I	

PTH OVERWHELMED

Severe, acute hyperphosphatemia	Osteitis fibrosa after parathyroidectomy
Tumor lysis	
Acute renal failure	
Rhabdomyolysis	

NOTE: PTH, parathyroid hormone.

Hypoparathyroidism is seen in two disorders associated with mitochondrial dysfunction and myopathy, one termed the *Kearns-Sayre syndrome* (KSS), with ophthalmaplegia and pigmentary retinopathy, and the other termed the *MELAS syndrome*, *m*itochondrial *e*ncephalopathy, *l*actic *a*cidosis, and *s*troke-like episodes. Mutations or deletions in mitochondrial genes have been identified (Chap. 67).

The two other rare forms of hypoparathyroidism with other multisystem developmental abnormalities follow either an autosomal dominant pattern, with deafness and/or renal dysplasia, or an autosomal recessive pattern, with growth retardation and dysmorphic features.

Hereditary hypoparathyroidism occurs also as an isolated entity without any other defects. The pattern of inheritance varies and includes autosomal dominant, autosomal recessive, and X-linked inheritance patterns. In one family in which the disorder is transmitted as an autosomal dominant trait, a structural abnormality in the PTH gene has been identified. A defect in the signal sequence needed for processing of the hormone impairs PTH secretion. In another kindred with autosomal recessive inheritance, the mutant allele in the first intron of the PTH gene causes a splicing defect in mRNA production. An X-linked recessive form of hypoparathyroidism has been described in males from two kindreds that are probably related. The locus of the defect has been located to chromosome Xq26-q27.

Acquired Hypoparathyroidism *Acquired chronic hypoparathyroidism* is usually the result of inadvertent surgical removal of all the parathyroid glands; in some instances, not all the tissue is removed, but the remainder undergoes vascular supply compromise secondary to fibrotic changes in the neck after surgery. In the past, the most frequent cause of acquired hypoparathyroidism was surgery for hyperthyroidism. Hypoparathyroidism now usually occurs after surgery for hyperparathyroidism when the surgeon, facing the dilemma of removing too little tissue and thus not curing the hyperparathyroidism, removes too much. Parathyroid function may not be totally absent in all patients with postoperative hypoparathyroidism.

Even rarer causes of acquired chronic hypoparathyroidism include radiation-induced damage subsequent to radioiodine therapy of hyperthyroidism and glandular damage in patients with hemochromatosis or hemosiderosis after repeated blood transfusions. Infection may involve one or more of the parathyroids but usually does not cause hypoparathyroidism because all four glands are rarely involved.

Transient hypoparathyroidism is frequent following surgery for hyperparathyroidism. After a variable period of hypoparathyroidism, normal parathyroid function may return due to hyperplasia or recovery of remaining tissue. Occasionally, recovery occurs months after surgery.

℞ **TREATMENT** Treatment of acquired and hereditary hypoparathyroidism involves replacement with vitamin D or 1,25(OH)$_2$D$_3$ (calcitriol) combined with a high oral calcium intake. In most patients, blood calcium and phosphate levels are satisfactorily regulated, but some patients show resistance and a brittleness with a tendency to alternate between hypocalcemia and an overshoot hypercalcemia. For many patients, vitamin D in doses of 1 to 3 mg/d (40,000 to 120,000 U/d) combined with ≥1 g elemental calcium is satisfactory. The wide dosage range reflects the variation encountered from patient to patient; precise regulation of each patient is required. Compared to typical daily requirements in euparathyroid patients of 200 U/d, the high dose of vitamin D reflects the reduced conversion of vitamin D to 1,25(OH)$_2$D. Many physicians now use 0.5 to 1.0 μg of calcitriol in management of such patients, especially if they are difficult to control. When vitamin D (because of storage in fat) is withdrawn, weeks are required for the disappearance of the biologic effects, compared with a few days for calcitriol, which has a rapid turnover.

Oral calcium and vitamin D restore the overall calcium-phosphate balance but do not reverse the lowered urinary calcium reabsorption typical of hypoparathyroidism. Therefore, care must be taken to avoid excessive urinary calcium excretion after vitamin D and calcium replacement therapy; otherwise, kidney stones can develop. Thiazide diuretics lower urine calcium by as much as 100 mg/d in hypoparathyroid patients on vitamin D, provided they are maintained on a low-sodium diet. Use of thiazides seems to be of benefit in mitigating hypercalciuria and easing the daily management of these patients.

Hypomagnesemia Severe hypomagnesemia is associated with hypocalcemia (Chap. 340). Restoration of the total-body magnesium deficit leads to rapid reversal of hypocalcemia. There are at least two causes of the hypocalcemia—impaired PTH secretion and reduced responsiveness to PTH.

Hypomagnesemia is generally classified as primary or secondary; primary hypomagnesemia is due to hereditary defects in intestinal absorption or renal reabsorption of magnesium. Secondary hypomagnesemia, a more common condition, occurs on a nutritional basis or as a result of acquired intestinal or renal disorders. The most common causes of the secondary disorder are chronic alcoholism with poor nutritional intake, intestinal malabsorption syndromes, and parenteral nutrition when magnesium replacement is omitted.

The effects of magnesium on PTH secretion are similar to those of calcium; hypermagnesemia suppresses and hypomagnesemia stimulates PTH secretion. The effects of magnesium on PTH secretion are normally of little significance, however, because the calcium effects dominate. Greater change in magnesium than in calcium is needed to influence hormone secretion. Nonetheless, hypomagnesemia might be expected to increase hormone secretion. It is therefore surprising to find that severe hypomagnesemia is associated with blunted secretion of PTH. The explanation for the paradox is that severe, chronic hypomagnesemia leads to intracellular magnesium deficiency, which interferes with secretion and peripheral responses to PTH. The mechanism of the cellular abnormalities caused by hypomagnesemia is unknown, although effects on adenylate cyclase (for which magnesium is a cofactor) have been proposed.

Serum magnesium must usually fall below 0.4 mmol/L (1.0 mg/dL) to cause hypocalcemia. PTH levels are undetectable or inappropriately low despite the stimulus of severe hypocalcemia, and acute repletion of magnesium leads to a rapid increase in PTH level. Serum phosphate levels are often not elevated, in contrast to the situation with acquired or idiopathic hypoparathyroidism, probably because phosphate deficiency is a frequent accompaniment of hypomagnesemia.

Diminished peripheral responsiveness to PTH also occurs in some patients, as documented by subnormal response in urinary phosphorus and urinary cyclic AMP excretion after administration of exogenous PTH to patients who are hypocalcemic and hypomagnesemic. Both blunted PTH secretion and lack of renal response to administered PTH can occur in the same patient. When acute magnesium repletion is undertaken, the restoration of PTH levels to normal or supranormal may precede restoration of normal serum calcium by several days.

℞ **TREATMENT** Repletion of magnesium cures the condition, and attention must be given to restoring the intracellular deficiency, which may be considerable. Repletion should be parenteral. After intravenous magnesium administration, serum magnesium may return transiently to the normal range, but unless replacement therapy is adequate serum magnesium will again fall. If renal function is normal, urinary magnesium excretion is a useful indicator of magnesium repletion, as magnesium is retained by the kidney until the deficiency is corrected. Intracellular deficits can be ≥50 mmol. Parenteral administration of 10 to 14 mmol magnesium usually reverses the signs of magnesium deficiency, but greater amounts may occasionally be required if the deficit is large. If the cause of the hypomagnesemia is renal magnesium wasting, magnesium may have to be given chronically to prevent recurrence (Chap. 340).

PTH INEFFECTIVE PTH is ineffective when the hormone receptor–guanyl nucleotide–binding protein complex is defective (PHP,

Typically, hypophosphatemia is more severe than hypocalcemia in vitamin D deficiency states because of the increased secretion of PTH, which, although only partly effective in elevating blood calcium, is capable of promoting phosphaturia.

PHP, on the other hand, has a pathophysiology different from the other disorders of ineffective PTH action. PHP resembles hypoparathyroidism (in which PTH synthesis is deficient) and is manifested by hypocalcemia and hyperphosphatemia. The cause of the disorder is defective hormone activation of guanyl nucleotide–binding proteins, resulting in failure of PTH to increase intracellular cyclic AMP (see below).

Chronic Renal Failure Improved medical management of chronic renal failure and/or a more indolent course of the renal disease now allow many patients to survive long enough to develop features of renal osteodystrophy. Phosphate retention and impaired production of $1,25(OH)_2D$ are the principal factors that cause calcium deficiency, secondary hyperparathyroidism, and bone disease. The uremic state also causes impairment of intestinal absorption by mechanisms other than defects in vitamin D metabolism. Nonetheless, treatment with supraphysiologic amounts of vitamin D or calcitriol corrects the impaired calcium absorption.

Hyperphosphatemia in renal failure lowers blood calcium levels by several mechanisms, including extraosseous deposition of calcium and phosphate, impairment of the bone-resorbing action of PTH, and reduction in $1,25(OH)_2D$ production by remaining renal tissue. Low levels of $1,25(OH)_2D$ due to hyperphosphatemia and destruction of renal tissue and are critical in the development of hypocalcemia.

℞ TREATMENT Therapy of chronic renal failure (Chap. 270) involves appropriate management of patients prior to dialysis and adjustment of regimens once dialysis is initiated. Attention should be paid to restriction of phosphate in the diet; use of calcium-containing salts as phosphate-binding antacids is preferable, rather than aluminum, to avoid the problem of aluminum intoxication; provision of an adequate calcium intake by mouth, usually 1 to 2 g/d; and supplementation with 0.25 to 1.0 μg/d calcitriol. Each patient must be monitored closely. The aim of therapy is to restore normal calcium balance to prevent osteomalacia and secondary hyperparathyroidism. Reduction of hyperphosphatemia and restoration of normal intestinal calcium absorption by calcitriol can improve blood calcium levels and reduce the manifestations of secondary hyperparathyroidism. Since adynamic bone disease can occur in association with low PTH levels, it is important to avoid excessive suppression of the parathyroid glands while recognizing the beneficial effects of controlling the secondary hyperparathyroidism. These patients should probably be closely monitored with PTH assays that detect only the full-length PTH 1–84 to avoid interference by biologically inactive amino-terminally truncated PTH.

Vitamin D Deficiency due to Inadequate Diet and/or Sunlight
Vitamin D deficiency due to inadequate intake of dairy products enriched with vitamin D, lack of vitamin supplementation, and reduced sunlight exposure in the elderly, particularly during winter in northern latitudes, is more common in the United States than previously recognized. Biopsies of bone in elderly patients with hip fracture (documenting osteomalacia) and abnormal levels of vitamin D metabolites, PTH, calcium, and phosphate indicate that vitamin D deficiency may occur in as many as 25% of elderly patients, particularly in areas where there is little ambient sunlight. Concentrations of 25(OH)D are low or low-normal in these patients. Quantitative histomorphometry of bone biopsy specimens reveals widened osteoid seams consistent with osteomalacia. PTH hypersecretion compensates for the tendency for the blood calcium to fall but also induces renal phosphate wasting and results in osteomalacia.

Treatment involves adequate replacement with vitamin D and cal-

cium until the deficiencies are corrected. Severe hypocalcemia rarely occurs in moderately severe vitamin D deficiency of the elderly, but vitamin D deficiency must be considered in the differential diagnosis of mild hypocalcemia.

Defective Vitamin D Metabolism • *Anticonvulsant therapy*
Anticonvulsant therapy with any of several agents induces acquired vitamin D deficiency by increasing the conversion of vitamin D to inactive compounds. The more marginal the vitamin D intake in the diet, the more likely that anticonvulsant therapy will lead to abnormal mineral and bone metabolism (Chap. 340).

Although $1,25(OH)_2D$ levels are lower in patients treated with chronic anticonvulsants than in the normal population, there is a great deal of variation. The greater prevalence of the disorder in some European populations and in the mentally retarded may reflect the lower vitamin D intake of those groups. Restoration of bone mineral mass and reversal of hypocalcemia can be accomplished with vitamin D replacement plus oral calcium. Administration of 50,000 units of vitamin D monthly may be preventive if anticonvulsant therapy needs to be given chronically.

Vitamin D–dependent rickets type I Rickets can be due to *resistance to the action* of vitamin D as well as to vitamin D deficiency. Vitamin D–dependent rickets type I, previously termed *pseudo-vitamin D–resistant rickets*, differs from true vitamin D–resistant rickets (vitamin D-dependent rickets type II, see below) in that it is less severe and the biochemical and radiographic abnormalities can be reversed with appropriate doses of the vitamin or the active metabolite, $1,25(OH)_2D_3$.

Clinical features include hypocalcemia, often with tetany or convulsions, hypophosphatemia, secondary hyperparathyroidism, and osteomalacia, often associated with skeletal deformities and increased alkaline phosphatase. Physiologic amounts of calcitriol cure the disease (Chap. 340). This finding fits with the pathophysiology as the disorder, which is autosomal recessive, is now known to be caused by a series of mutations in the gene for the 25(OH)D-1α-hydroxylase. Over 20 different mutations have been identified. All patients have both alleles inactivated, but often the genetic pattern is that of a compound heterozygote. Response to high doses of vitamin D or calcifediol, as noted in prior years, is probably due to direct effects of 25(OH)D at high levels. Treatment begins with 1 to 2 μg/d calcitriol, but maintenance is satisfactory with physiologic doses of calcitriol (0.5 to 1.0 μg/d). Careful adjustment of calcitriol dose is required, particularly during growth periods.

Vitamin D Ineffective • *Intestinal malabsorption* Mild hypocalcemia, secondary hyperparathyroidism, severe hypophosphatemia, and a variety of nutritional deficiencies occur with gastrointestinal diseases. Hepatocellular dysfunction can lead to reduction in 25(OH)D levels, as in portal or biliary cirrhosis of the liver, and malabsorption of vitamin D and its metabolites, including $1,25(OH)_2D$, may occur in a variety of bowel diseases, hereditary or acquired. Hypocalcemia itself can lead to steatorrhea, due to deficient production of pancreatic enzymes and bile salts. Depending on the disorder, vitamin D or its metabolites can be given parenterally, guaranteeing adequate blood levels of active metabolites.

Vitamin D–dependent rickets type II Vitamin D–dependent rickets type II results from end-organ resistance to the active metabolite $1,25(OH)_2D_3$. The clinical features resemble those of the type I disorder and include hypocalcemia, hypophosphatemia, secondary hyperparathyroidism, and rickets. A clear distinction is partial or total alopecia in type II. Plasma levels of $1,25(OH)_2D$ are at least three times normal, in keeping with the refractoriness of the end organs. Some patients respond to very high doses of vitamin D or vitamin D metabolites (e.g., 17 to 20 μg/d calcitriol). Earlier suggestions that there were both receptor and postreceptor defects are incorrect. All of the genetically characterized phenotypes have mutations in the gene for the vitamin D receptor. Nineteen mutations have been identified that affect different regions of the receptor primarily in the DNA binding

Table 341-4 Classification of Pseudohypoparathyroidism (PHP) and Pseudopseudohypoparathyroidism (PPHP)

Type	Hypocalcemia, Hyperphosphatemia	Response of Urinary cAMP to PTH	Serum PTH	$G_{s\alpha}$ Subunit Deficiency	AHO	Resistance to Hormones in Addition to PTH
PHP-Ia	Yes	↓	↑	Yes	Yes	Yes
PHP-Ib	Yes	↓	↑	No	No	No
PHP-II	Yes	Normal	↑	No	No	No
PPHP	No	Normal	Normal	Yes	Yes	±

NOTE: ↓, decreased; ↑, increased; AHO, Albright's hereditary osteodystrophy; PTH, parathyroid hormone.

domain (with normal ligand binding: these were the so-called postreceptor defects detected by earlier indirect methods) or in the ligand-binding domain (classified previously as receptor negative).

Pseudohypoparathyroidism   PHP is a hereditary disorder characterized by symptoms and signs of hypoparathyroidism, typically in association with distinctive skeletal and developmental defects. The hypoparathyroidism is due to a deficient end-organ response to PTH. Hyperplasia of the parathyroids, a response to hormone resistance, causes elevation of PTH levels. Studies, both clinical and basic, have clarified some aspects of this syndrome, including the variable clinical spectrum, the pathophysiology, the genetic defects, and the inheritance.

A working classification of the various forms of PHP is given in Table 341-4. The classification scheme is based on the signs of ineffective PTH action (low calcium and high phosphate), urinary cyclic AMP response to exogenous PTH, the presence or absence of *Albright's hereditary osteodystrophy* (AHO), and assays of the concentration of the $G_{s\alpha}$ subunit of the adenylate cyclase enzyme. Using these criteria, there are four types: PHP type I, subdivided into a and b categories; PHP-II; and pseudopseudohypoparathyroidism (PPHP).

PHP-Ia and PHP-Ib   Individuals with PHP-I, the most common of the disorders, show a deficient urinary cyclic AMP response to administration of exogenous PTH. Patients with PHP-I are divided into type a, who have reduced amounts of $G_{s\alpha}$ in vitro assays with erythrocytes, and type b, with normal amounts of $G_{s\alpha}$ in erythrocytes. There is a third type (PHP-Ic, reported in a few patients) that differs from PHP-Ia only in having normal erythrocyte levels of $G_{s\alpha}$ despite having AHO, hypocalcemia, and decreased urinary cyclic AMP responses to PTH (presumably with a post-$G_{s\alpha}$ defect in adenyl cyclase stimulation).

Most patients show characteristic features of AHO, consisting of short stature, round face, skeletal anomalies (brachydactyly), and heterotopic calcification. Patients have low calcium and high phosphate levels, as with true hypoparathyroidism. PTH levels, however, are elevated, reflecting resistance to hormone action.

Amorphous deposits of calcium and phosphate are found in the basal ganglia in about half of patients. The defects in metacarpal and metatarsal bones are sometimes accompanied by short phalanges as well, possibly reflecting premature closing of the epiphyses. The typical findings are short fourth and fifth metacarpals and metatarsals. The defects are usually bilateral. Exostoses and radius curvus are frequent. Impairments in olfaction and taste and unusual dermatoglyphic abnormalities have been reported.

PPHP   The initial view that the defect responsible for PHP-Ia was simply the deficiency of $G_{s\alpha}$ subunits was temporarily confounded by the subsequent discovery that the same 50% reduction in $G_{s\alpha}$ subunits was seen in patients with PPHP, who have typical features of the hereditary osteodystrophy syndrome despite normal serum calcium levels and normal response of urinary cyclic AMP to exogenous PTH.

Multiple defects have now been identified in the *GNAS-1* gene in PHP-Ia and PPHP patients. This gene, which is located on chromosome 20q13, encodes the stimulatory G protein subunit $G_{s\alpha}$, among other products (see below). Mutations include abnormalities in splice junctions associated with deficient mRNA production and point mu-

tations that result in a protein with defective function as well as the 50% reduction in $G_{s\alpha}$ levels in erythrocytes.

Detailed analyses of disease transmission in affected kindreds have clarified many features of PHP-Ia, PPHP, and PHP-Ib (Fig. 341-9). The former two entities, traced through multiple kindreds, have an inheritance pattern consistent with gene imprinting—only females, not males, can transmit the full disease with hypocalcemia—and PHP and PPHP do not coexist in the same generation. The phenomenon of gene imprinting involves selective inactivation of either the maternal or the paternal allele (Chap. 65). In the case of the $G_{s\alpha}$ gene, it is paternally imprinted (silenced) so that the disease PHP-Ia is never inherited from the father carrying the defective allele but only from the mother. On the other hand, the defective allele is not imprinted or silenced in all tissues. It seems possible, therefore, that the AHO phenotype recognized in PPHP as well as PHP-Ia reflects haplotype insufficiency. In the renal cortex, however, it is postulated that only the maternal allele is normally active, such that lack of activity from a defective paternal allele is not of consequence. This explains the occurrence in PHP-Ia of hypocalcemia, hyperphosphatemia, and other stigmata such as variable resistance to other hormones (if similar tissue-specific imprinting occurs in other organs). Strong evidence favoring this overall hypothesis comes from gene knockout studies in the mouse (ablating exon 2 of the gene). Mice inheriting the mutant allele from the female had undetectable $G_{s\alpha}$ protein in renal cortex and were hypocalcemic and resistant to renal actions of PTH. Offspring inheriting the mutant allele from the male showed no evidence of PTH resistance or hypercalcemia.

The complex mechanisms that control the GNAS-1 gene also con-

FIGURE 341-9 Paternal imprinting of renal parathyroid hormone (PTH) resistance (*GNAS-1* gene for $G_{s\alpha}$ subunit) in pseudohypoparathyroidism (PHP). An impaired excretion of urinary cyclic AMP and phosphate is observed in patients with PHP. In the renal cortex, there is selective silencing of the paternal $G_{s\alpha}$ gene mRNA. The disease becomes manifest only in patients who inherit the defective gene from an obligate female carrier (*left*). If the genetic defect is inherited from an obligate male gene carrier, there is no biochemical abnormality; administration of PTH causes an appropriate increase in the urinary cyclic AMP and phosphate concentration [pseudo-PHP (PPHP); *right*]. Both patterns of inheritance lead to Albright's hereditary osteodystrophy (AHO), perhaps because of haplotype insufficiency—i.e., both copies of $G_{s\alpha}$ must be active in the fetus for normal bone development. If an abnormal allele is inherited from a father with AHO (PPHP), PTH resistance is not transmitted to offspring, but they have AHO (haplotype insufficiency); if the abnormal allele comes from the mother (with the normal paternal allele silenced in the kidney cortex), the full disease spectrum results.

tribute to challenges involved in unraveling the pathogenesis of these disorders. Alternative splicing patterns produce three different transcripts that encode distinct proteins. In addition to $G_s\alpha$, this gene encodes a second protein product with a unique NH_2-terminus (the XL exon); $XL_\alpha s$ includes exons 2–13. It is unknown whether this protein can function as a stimulatory G protein, but the mRNA encoding it is expressed in numerous endocrine tissues and is transcribed from only the paternal allele. A third transcript is transcribed from only the maternal allele and encodes the protein product, NESP55, which contains no homology with $XL_\alpha s$ or $G_s\alpha$.

PHP-Ib, lacking the AHO phenotype, shares with PHP-Ia the resistance to PTH action and a blunted urinary cyclic AMP response to administered PTH, a standard test for hormone resistance (Table 341-4). PHP-Ib patients, however, show normal levels of $G_s\alpha$ in erythrocytes. Bone responsiveness may be excessive rather than blunted in PHP-Ib compared to PHP-Ia patients, based on case reports that have emphasized an osteitis fibrosa–like pattern in some PHP patients who lack the AHO phenotype. The inheritance patterns in PHP-Ib kindreds are clearly consistent with paternal imprinting and lack male transmission of symptomatic disease; gene cloning studies have narrowed the responsible region to chromosome 20, close to—if not within—the *GNAS-1* gene locus. Elucidation of the responsible genetic and pathogenetic mechanisms in this disorder may further illuminate the function of the complex *GNAS-1* gene and the role of its products in hormonal signaling.

PHP-II refers to patients with hypocalcemia and hyperphosphatemia who have a normal urinary cyclic AMP response to PTH. These patients are assumed to have a defect in the response to PTH at a locus distal to cyclic AMP production, although at least some patients may instead have occult vitamin D deficiency.

The diagnosis of these hormone-resistant states can usually be made without difficulty when there is a positive family history for developmental defects and/or the presence of developmental anomalies, including brachydactyly, in association with the signs and symptoms of hypoparathyroidism. In all categories—PHP-Ia, -Ib, and -II—serum PTH levels are elevated, particularly when patients are hypocalcemic. However, patients with PHP-Ib or PHP-II do not have phenotypic abnormalities, only hypocalcemia with high PTH levels, confirming hormone resistance. In PHP-Ib, the response of urinary cyclic AMP to the administration of exogenous PTH is blunted. Levels of $G_s\alpha$ subunits in erythrocyte membranes are, however, normal in those with PHP-Ib. The diagnosis of PHP-II is more complex, in that cyclic AMP responses in urine are, by definition, normal. Since vitamin D deficiency itself can dissociate phosphaturic and urinary cyclic AMP responses to exogenous PTH, vitamin D deficiency must be excluded before the diagnosis of PHP-II can be entertained.

TREATMENT Treatment of PHP is similar to that of hypoparathyroidism, except that the doses of vitamin D and calcium are usually lower than those required in true hypoparathyroidism, presumably because the defect in PHP is only partial because of imprinting in specific tissues (renal cortex vs. renal medulla). Variability in response makes it necessary to establish the optimal regimen for each patient, based on maintaining the appropriate blood calcium level and urinary calcium excretion.

PTH Overwhelmed Occasionally, loss of calcium from the ECF is so severe that PTH cannot compensate. Such situations include acute pancreatitis and severe, acute hyperphosphatemia, often in association with renal failure, conditions in which there is rapid efflux of calcium from extracellular fluid. Severe hypocalcemia can occur quickly; PTH rises in response to hypocalcemia but does not return blood calcium to normal.

Severe, Acute Hyperphosphatemia Severe hyperphosphatemia is associated with extensive tissue damage or cell destruction (Chap. 340). The combination of increased release of phosphate from muscle and impaired ability to excrete phosphorus because of renal failure causes moderate to severe hyperphosphatemia, the latter causing cal-

cium loss from the blood and mild to moderate hypocalcemia. Hypocalcemia is usually reversed with tissue repair and restoration of renal function as phosphorus and creatinine values return to normal. There may even be a mild hypercalcemic period in the oliguric phase of renal function recovery. This sequence, severe hypocalcemia followed by mild hypercalcemia, reflects widespread deposition of calcium in muscle and subsequent redistribution of some of the calcium to the ECF after return of phosphate levels to normal.

Other causes of hyperphosphatemia include hypothermia, massive hepatic failure, and hematologic malignancies, either because of high cell turnover of malignancy or because of cell destruction by chemotherapy.

TREATMENT Treatment is directed toward lowering of blood phosphate by the administration of phosphate-binding antacids or dialysis, often needed for the management of renal failure. Although calcium replacement may be necessary if hypocalcemia is severe and symptomatic, calcium administration during the hyperphosphatemic period tends to increase extraosseous calcium deposition and aggravate tissue damage. The levels of $1,25(OH)_2D$ may be low during the hyperphosphatemic phase and return to normal during the oliguric phase of recovery.

Osteitis Fibrosis after Parathyroidectomy Severe hypocalcemia after parathyroid surgery is less common now that osteitis fibrosa cystica is an infrequent manifestation of hyperparathyroidism. When osteitis fibrosa cystica is severe, however, bone mineral deficits can be large. After parathyroidectomy, hypocalcemia can persist for days if calcium replacement is inadequate. Treatment may require parenteral administration of calcium; addition of calcitriol and oral calcium supplementation is sometimes needed for weeks to a month or two until bone defects are filled (which, of course, is of therapeutic benefit in the skeleton), making it possible to discontinue parenteral calcium and/or reduce the amount.

DIFFERENTIAL DIAGNOSIS OF HYPOCALCEMIA Care must be taken to ensure that true hypocalcemia is present; in addition, acute transient hypocalcemia can be a manifestation of a variety of severe, acute illnesses, as discussed above. *Chronic hypocalcemia*, however, can usually be ascribed to a few disorders associated with absent or ineffective PTH. Important clinical criteria include the duration of the illness, signs or symptoms of associated disorders, and the presence of features that suggest a hereditary abnormality. A nutritional history can be helpful in recognizing a low intake of vitamin D and calcium in the elderly, and a history of excessive alcohol intake may suggest magnesium deficiency.

Hypoparathyroidism and PHP are typically lifelong illnesses, usually (but not always) appearing by adolescence; hence a recent onset of hypocalcemia in an adult is more likely due to nutritional deficiencies, renal failure, or intestinal disorders that result in deficient or ineffective vitamin D. Neck surgery, even long past, however, can be associated with a delayed onset of postoperative hypoparathyroidism. A history of seizure disorder raises the issue of anticonvulsive medication. Developmental defects, particularly in childhood and adolescence, may point to the diagnosis of PHP. Rickets and a variety of neuromuscular syndromes and deformities may indicate ineffective vitamin D action, either due to defects in vitamin D metabolism or to vitamin D deficiency.

A pattern of *low calcium with high phosphorus* in the absence of renal failure or massive tissue destruction almost invariably means hypoparathyroidism or PHP. A *low calcium and low phosphorus* points to absent or ineffective vitamin D, thereby impairing the action of PTH on calcium metabolism (but not phosphate clearance). The relative ineffectiveness of PTH in vitamin D deficiency, anticonvulsant therapy, gastrointestinal disorders, and hereditary defects in vitamin D metabolism leads to secondary hyperparathyroidism as a compensation. The relatively unopposed action of the excess PTH on renal tubule phosphate transport, which is less dependent on vitamin D than calcium transport, accounts for renal phosphate wasting and hypophosphatemia.

Exceptions to these patterns may occur. Most forms of hypomagnesemia are due to long-standing nutritional deficiency as seen in chronic alcoholics. Despite the fact that the hypocalcemia is principally due to an acute absence of PTH, phosphate levels are usually low, rather than elevated as in hypoparathyroidism. Chronic renal failure is often associated with hypocalcemia and hyperphosphatemia, despite secondary hyperparathyroidism.

Diagnosis is usually established by application of the PTH immunoassay, tests for vitamin D metabolites, and measurements of the urinary cyclic AMP response to exogenous PTH. In hereditary and acquired hypoparathyroidism and in severe hypomagnesemia, PTH is either undetectable or in the normal range. This finding in a hypocalcemic patient is supportive of hypoparathyroidism, as distinct from ineffective PTH action, in which even mild hypocalcemia is associated with elevated PTH levels. Hence a failure to detect elevated PTH levels establishes the diagnosis of hypoparathyroidism; elevated levels suggest the presence of secondary hyperparathyroidism, as found in many of the situations in which the hormone is ineffective due to associated abnormalities in vitamin D action. Assays for 25(OH)D and 1,25(OH)$_2$D can be helpful. Low or low normal 25(OH)D indicates vitamin D deficiency due to lack of sunlight, inadequate vitamin D intake, or intestinal malabsorption. A low level of 1,25(OH)$_2$D in the presence of elevated concentrations of PTH suggests ineffective PTH action in disorders such as chronic renal failure, severe vitamin D deficiency, vitamin D–dependent rickets type I, and PHP. Recognition that mild hypocalcemia, rickets, and hypophosphatemia are due to anticonvulsant therapy is made by history.

℞ **TREATMENT** **Hypocalcemic States** The management of hypoparathyroidism, PHP, chronic renal failure, and hereditary defects in vitamin D metabolism involves the use of vitamin D or vitamin D metabolites and calcium supplementation. Vitamin D itself is the least expensive form of vitamin D replacement and is frequently used in the management of uncomplicated hypoparathyroidism and some disorders associated with ineffective vitamin D action. When vitamin D is used prophylactically, as in the elderly or in those with chronic anticonvulsant therapy, there is a wider margin of safety than with the more potent metabolites. However, most of the conditions in which vitamin D is administered chronically for hypocalcemia require amounts 50 to 100 times the daily replacement dose because the formation of 1,25(OH)$_2$D is deficient. In such situations, vitamin D is no safer than the active metabolite because intoxication can occur with high-dose therapy (because of storage in fat). Calcitriol is more rapid in onset of action and also has a short biologic half-life.

Vitamin D (5 μg/d) or calcifediol and lower doses of calcitriol (0.25 to 1.0 μg/d) are required to prevent rickets in normal individuals. In contrast, 1 to 3 mg (1000 to 3000 μg of vitamin D$_2$ or D$_3$ is typically required in hypoparathyroidism; doses of calcifediol are also high (several hundred micrograms per day). The dose of calcitriol is unchanged in hypoparathyroidism, since the defect is in hydroxylation by the 25(OH)D-1α-hydroxylase.

Patients with hypoparathyroidism should be given 2 to 3 g elemental calcium by mouth each day. The two agents, vitamin D or calcitriol and oral calcium, can be varied independently. If hypocalcemia alternates with episodes of hypercalcemia in more brittle patients with hypoparathyroidism, administration of calcitriol and use of thiazides, as discussed above, may make management easier.

BIBLIOGRAPHY

ARNOLD A et al: Monoclonality of parathyroid tumors in chronic renal failure and in primary parathyroid hyperplasia. J Clin Invest 95:2047, 1995

BASTEPE M, JÜPPNER H: Pseudohypoparathyroidism: New insights into an old disease. Endocrinol Metab Clin North Am, in press, 2000

BODY JJ et al: A dose-finding study of zoledronate in hypercalcemic cancer patients. J Bone Miner Res 14:1557, 1999

CHEN H et al: Outpatient minimally invasive parathyroidectomy: A combination of sestamibi-SPECT localization, cervical block anesthesia, and intraoperative parathyroid hormone assay. Surgery 126:1021, 1999

CHOU Y-H W et al: Mutations in the human Ca^{2+}-sensing-receptor gene that cause hypocalciuric hypercalcemia. Am J Hum Genet 56:1075, 1995

CRYNS VL et al: Frequent loss of chromosome arm 1p DNA in parathyroid adenomas. Genes Chromosomes Cancer 13:9, 1995

HABENER J et al: Hyperparathyroidism, in *Endocrinology*, 4th ed, L DeGroot et al (eds). Philadelphia, Saunders, 2000

HERBERT SC et al: Role of the Ca^{2+}-sensing receptor in divalent mineral ion homeostasis. J Exp Biol 200:295, 1997

JÜPPNER H et al: The gene responsible for pseudohypoparathyroidism type Ib is paternally imprinted and maps in four unrelated kindreds to chromosome 20q13.3 Proc Natl Acad Sci USA 95:11798, 1998

MALLETTE LE, EICHORN E: Effects of lithium carbonate on human calcium metabolism. Arch Intern Med 146:770, 1986

NEMETH EF et al: Calcimimetics with potent and selective activity on the parathyroid calcium receptor. Proc Natl Acad Sci USA 95:4040, 1998

NUSSBAUM SR, POTTS JT JR: Medical management of hyperparathyroidism and hypercalcemia, in *Endocrinology*, 4th ed, L DeGroot et al (eds). Philadelphia, Saunders, 2000

PIERCE SH et al: A familial syndrome of hypocalcemia with hypercalciuria due to mutations in the calcium-sensing receptor (see comments). N Engl J Med 335:1115, 1996

POLLAK MR et al: Familial hypocalciuric hypercalcemia and neonatal severe hyperparathyroidism. Effects of mutant gene dosage on phenotype. J Clin Invest 93:1108, 1994

POTTS JT JR et al (eds): Proceedings of the NIH Consensus Development Conference on Diagnosis and Management of Asymptomatic Primary Hyperparathyroidism. J Bone Miner Res 6 (Suppl 2):S1, 1991

——— et al: Parathyroid hormone and parathyroid hormone–related peptide in calcium homeostasis, bone metabolism, and bone development: The proteins, their genes, and receptors, in *Metabolic Bone Disease*, LV Avioli, SM Krane (eds.). New York, Academic, 1997, p 51

SALUSKY IB et al: The renal osteodystrophies, in *Endocrinology*, 4th ed, L DeGroot et al (eds). Philadelphia, Saunders, 2000

SCHWINDINGER WF et al: Targeted disruption of *Gnas* in embryonic stem cells. Endocrinology 138:4058, 1997

SEGRE GV, POTTS JT JR: Differential diagnosis of hypercalcemia, in *Endocrinology*, 4th ed., L DeGroot et al (eds). Philadelphia, Saunders, 2000

SILVERBERG SJ et al: Longitudinal measurements of bone density and biochemical indices in untreated primary hyperparathyroidism. J Clin Endocrinol Metab 80:723, 1995

——— et al: Primary hyperparathyroidism: 10-year course with or without parathyroid surgery. N Engl J Med 341:1249, 1999

STEWART AF et al: Malignancy-associated hypercalcemia, in *Endocrinology*, 4th ed, L DeGroot et al (eds). Philadelphia, Saunders, 2000

THAKKER RV: Molecular genetics of parathyroid disease. Curr Opin Endocrinol Diab 3:521, 1996

WERMERS RA et al: Survival after the diagnosis of hyperparathyroidism. Am J Med 104:115, 1998

YU S et al: Variable and tissue-specific hormone resistance in heterotrimeric Gs protein α-subunit (G$_s\alpha$) knockout mice is due to tissue-specific imprinting of the G$_s\alpha$ gene. Proc Natl Acad Sci USA 95:8715, 1998

ZHANG P et al: A homozygous inactivating mutation in the parathyroid hormone/parathyroid hormone–related peptide receptor causing Blomstrand chondrodysplasia. J Clin Endocrinol Metab 83:3365, 1998

342   *Robert Lindsay, Felicia Cosman*

OSTEOPOROSIS

Osteoporosis, characterized by decreased bone strength, is prevalent among postmenopausal women but also occurs in men and women with underlying conditions or major risk factors associated with bone demineralization. Its chief clinical manifestations are vertebral and hip fractures. Osteoporosis affects >10 million individuals in the United States, but only 10 to 20% are diagnosed and treated.

DEFINITION *Osteoporosis* is defined as a reduction of bone mass (or density) or the presence of a fragility fracture. This reduction in bone tissue is accompanied by deterioration in the architecture of the skeleton, leading to a markedly increased risk of fracture. Osteoporosis is defined operationally as a bone density that falls 2.5 standard deviations (SD) below the mean—also referred to as a *T-score* of −2.5. Those who fall at the lower end of the young normal range (a T-score of >1 SD below the mean) have low bone density and are considered to be at increased risk of osteoporosis.

EPIDEMIOLOGY In the United States, as many as 8 million women and 2 million men have osteoporosis (T-score < −2.5), and an additional 18 million individuals have bone mass levels that put them at increased risk of developing osteoporosis (e.g., bone mass T-score <−1.0). Osteoporosis occurs more frequently with increasing age as bone tissue is progressively lost. In women, the loss of ovarian function at menopause (typically after age 50) precipitates rapid bone loss such that most women meet the criteria for osteoporosis by age 70.

The epidemiology of fractures follows similar trends as the loss of bone density. Fractures of the distal radius increase in frequency before age 50 and plateau by age 60, with only a modest age-related increase thereafter. In contrast, incidence rates for hip fractures double every 5 years after age 70 (Fig. 342-1). This distinct epidemiology may be related to the way people fall as they age, with fewer falls on an outstretched hand. At least 1.5 million fractures occur each year in the United States as a consequence of osteoporosis. As the population continues to age, the total number of fractures will continue to escalate.

About 300,000 hip fractures occur each year in the United States, most of which require hospital admission and surgical intervention. The probability that a 50-year-old white individual will have a hip fracture during his or her lifetime is 14% for women and 5% for men; the risk for African Americans is much lower (about half these rates). Hip fractures are associated with a high incidence of deep vein thrombosis and pulmonary embolism (20 to 50%) and a mortality rate between 5 and 20% during the few months after surgery.

There are about 500,000 vertebral crush fractures per year in the United States. Only a fraction of these are recognized clinically, since many are relatively asymptomatic and are identified incidentally during radiography for other purposes (Fig. 342-2). Vertebral fractures rarely require hospitalization but are associated with long-term morbidity and a slight increase in mortality. Multiple fractures lead to height loss (often of several inches), kyphosis, and secondary pain and discomfort related to altered biomechanics of the back. Thoracic fractures can be associated with restrictive lung disease, whereas lumbar fractures are associated with abdominal symptoms including distention, early satiety, and constipation.

Approximately 200,000 wrist fractures occur in the United States each year. Fractures of other bones also occur with osteoporosis, which is not surprising given that bone loss is a systemic phenomenon. Frac-

FIGURE 342-2 Lateral spine x-ray showing severe osteopenia and a severe wedge-type deformity (severe anterior compression).

tures of the pelvis and proximal humerus are clearly associated with osteoporosis. Although some fractures are clearly the result of major trauma, the threshold for fracture is reduced for an osteoporotic bone (Fig. 342-3). A list of common risk factors for osteoporotic fractures is summarized in Table 342-1. Prior fractures, a family history of osteoporotic fractures, and low body weight are each independent predictors of fracture. Chronic diseases that increase the risk of falling or frailty, including dementias, Parkinson's disease, and multiple sclerosis, also increase fracture risk.

In the United States and Europe, osteoporosis-related fractures are more common among women than men, presumably due to a lower peak bone mass as well as postmenopausal bone loss in women. However, this gender difference in bone density and age-related increase in hip fractures is not as apparent in some other cultures, possibly due to genetics, physical activity level, or diet.

PATHOPHYSIOLOGY   Bone Remodeling Osteoporosis results from bone loss due to normal age-related changes in bone remodeling as well as extrinsic and intrinsic factors that exaggerate this process. These changes may be superimposed on a low peak bone mass. Consequently, the bone remodeling process is fundamental for understanding the pathophysiology of osteoporosis (Chap. 340). The skeleton increases in size by linear growth and by apposition of new bone tissue on the outer surfaces of the cortex (Fig. 342-4). This latter process is the phenomenon of modeling, which also allows the long

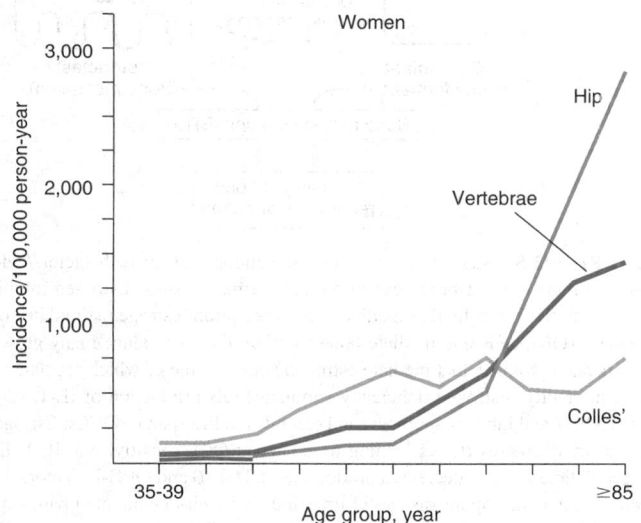

FIGURE 342-1 Epidemiology of vertebral, hip, and Colles' fractures with age. (*Adapted from LJ Melton III, in BL Riggs, LJ Melton II (eds): Osteoporosis: Etiology, Diagnosis and Management, 2d ed. Rochester, MN, Mayo Foundation, 1995.*)

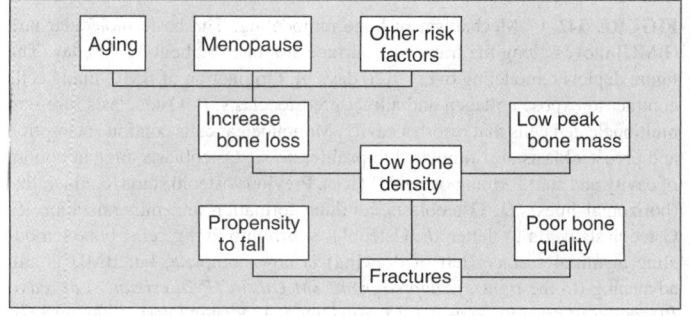

FIGURE 342-3 Factors leading to osteoporotic fractures.

Table 342-1 Risk Factors for Osteoporosis Fracture

Nonmodifiable	Estrogen deficiency
Personal history of fracture as an adult	Early menopause (<45 years) or bilateral ovariectomy
History of fracture in first-degree relative	Prolonged premenstrual amenorrhea (>1 year)
Female sex	Low calcium intake
Advanced age	Alcoholism
Caucasian race	Impaired eyesight despite adequate correction
Dementia	Recurrent falls
Potentially modifiable	Inadequate physical activity
Current cigarette smoking	Poor health/frailty
Low body weight [<58 kg (127 lb)]	

bones to adapt in shape to the stresses placed upon them. Increased sex hormone production at puberty is required for maximum skeletal maturation, which reaches maximum mass and density in early adulthood. Nutrition and lifestyle also play an important role in growth, though genetic factors are the major determinants of peak skeletal mass and density. Numerous genes control skeletal growth, peak bone mass, and body size, but it is likely that separate genes control skeletal structure and density. Heritability estimates of 50 to 80% for bone density and size have been derived based on twin studies. Though peak bone mass is often lower among individuals with a family history of osteoporosis, association studies of candidate genes [vitamin D receptor; Type I collagen, the estrogen receptor (ER), interleukin (IL) 6; and insulin-like growth factor (IGF) I] have not been consistently replicated. Linkage studies suggest that a genetic locus on chromosome 11 is associated with high bone mass.

Once peak skeletal mass has been attained, the process of remodeling becomes the principal metabolic activity of the skeleton. This process has three primary functions: (1) to repair microdamage within

the skeleton, (2) to maintain skeletal strength, and (3) to supply calcium from the skeleton to maintain serum calcium. Acute demands for calcium involve osteoclast-mediated resorption as well as calcium transport by osteocytes. The activation of remodeling may be induced by microdamage to bone due to excessive or accumulated stress.

Bone remodeling is also regulated by several circulating hormones, including estrogens, androgens, vitamin D, and parathyroid hormone (PTH), as well as locally produced growth factors such as IGF-I and -II, transforming growth factor (TGF) β, parathyroid hormone-related peptide (PTHrP), ILs, prostaglandins, tumor necrosis factor (TNF), and osteoprotegrin ligand (Fig. 342-5). Additional influences include include nutrition (particularly calcium intake) and physical activity level. The end result of this remodeling process is that the resorbed bone is replaced by an equal amount of new bone tissue. Thus, the mass of the skeleton remains constant after peak bone mass is achieved in adulthood. After age 30 to 45, however, the resorption and formation processes become imbalanced, and resorption exceeds formation. This imbalance may begin at different ages and varies at different skeletal sites; it becomes exaggerated in women after menopause. Excessive bone loss can be due to an increase in osteoclastic activity and/or a decrease in osteoblastic activity. In addition, an increase in remodeling activation frequency can magnify the small imbalance seen at each remodeling unit.

In trabecular bone, if the osteoclasts are sufficiently aggressive to penetrate trabeculae, they leave no template for new bone formation to occur and, consequently, may cause rapid bone loss. In cortical bone, increased activation of remodeling creates more porous bone. The effect of this increased porosity on cortical bone strength may be modest if the overall diameter of the bone is not changed. However, decreased apposition of new bone on the periosteal surface coupled

FIGURE 342-4 Mechanism of bone remodeling. The basic molecular unit (BMU) moves along the trabecular surface at a rate of about 10 μm/day. The figure depicts remodeling over ~120 days. *A.* Origination of BMU-lining cells contract to expose collagen and attract preosteoclasts. *B.* Osteoclasts fuse into multinucleated cells that resorb a cavity. Mononuclear cells continue resorption and preosteoblasts are stimulated to proliferate. *C.* Osteoblasts align at bottom of cavity and start forming osteoid (black). Previous osteoid starts to mineralize (horizontal lines). *D.* Osteoblasts continue formation and mineralization. *E.* Osteoblasts begin to flatten. *F.* Osteoblasts turn into lining cells; bone remodeling at initial surface (left of drawing) is now complete, but BMU is still advancing (to the right). *[Adapted from: SM Ott, in JP Bilezikian et al (eds): Principles of Bone Biology, vol. 18. San Diego, Academic Press, 1996, pp 231–241.]*

FIGURE 342-5 Steroid actions and interactions with growth factors/cytokines in bone cells at bone resorption and formation sites. Estrogen inhibits osteoclasts (OCL), cells that mediate bone resorption; estrogen stimulates osteoblasts (OB), cells that mediate bone formation. OBs produce many growth factors and cytokines that mediate estrogen action, some of which regulate the OCL indirectly. Estrogen deficiency stimulates OB production of IL-1, IL-6, and TNFα (and inhibits apoptosis and extends the life span of OCLs. Estrogen deficiency decreases IL-1ra leading to enhanced OCL sensitivity to IL-1. Estrogen deficiency also decreases production of TGF-β and OPG-L, factors that mediate osteoclast apoptosis. Solid lines indicate well-documented pathways. Dashed lines indicate less well defined pathways. ER, estrogen receptor; AR, androgen receptor; OPG, osteoprotegerin; OPG-L, osteoprotegerin-ligand; IL, interleukin; IL-1ra, interleukin 1 receptor antagonist; TGF-β, transforming growth factor β; TNFα, tumor necrosis factor α. *(Adapted from TC Spelsberg et al: Mol Endocrinol 13:819, 1999.)*

with increased endocortical resorption of bone decreases the biomechanical strength of long bones. Even a slight exaggeration in normal bone loss patterns increases the risk of osteoporotic fracture.

Calcium Nutrition Peak bone mass may be impaired by inadequate calcium intake during growth, thereby leading to increased risk of osteoporosis in later life. During the adult phase of life, calcium deprivation induces secondary hyperparathyroidism and an increase in the rate of remodeling. PTH stimulates the hydroxylation of vitamin D in the kidney, leading to increased levels of 1,25-dihydroxyvitamin D [$1,25(OH)_2D$] and enhanced gastrointestinal calcium absorption. PTH also reduces renal calcium loss. Though these are appropriate short-term homeostatic responses for improving calcium economy, the long-term effects are detrimental to the skeleton because of the ongoing imbalance at remodeling sites.

Total daily calcium intakes of <400 mg are likely to be detrimental to the skeleton, but there is more doubt about intakes in the 600- to 800-mg range, which is the average intake among adults in the United States. The recommended daily required intake of 1000 to 1200 mg for adults accomodates population heterogeneity in controlling calcium balance (Chap. 73).

Vitamin D (See also Chap. 340) Severe vitamin D deficiency causes rickets in children or osteomalacia in adults. There is accumulating evidence that vitamin D deficiency may be more prevalent than previously thought, particularly among individuals at increased risk, such as the elderly; those living in northern latitudes; and in individuals with poor nutrition, malabsorption, or chronic liver or renal disease. Modest vitamin D deficiency leads to compensatory secondary hyperparathyroidism and is an important risk factor for osteoporosis and fractures. Some studies have shown that >50% of inpatients on a general medical service exhibit biochemical features of vitamin D deficiency, including increased levels of PTH and alkaline phosphatase and lower levels of ionized calcium. In women living in northern latitudes, it has been shown that vitamin D levels decline during the winter months. This is associated with a striking seasonal bone loss, reflecting increased bone turnover. Treatment with vitamin D and calcium supplementation prevents this seasonal effect on bone metabolism. Reduced fracture rates have also been documented among individuals in northern latitudes who have greater vitamin D intake and have higher 25-hydroxyvitamin D [$25(OH)D$] levels (see below).

Estrogen Status Estrogen deficiency probably causes bone loss by two distinct but interrelated mechanisms: (1) activation of new bone remodeling sites, and (2) exaggeration of the imbalance between bone formation and resorption. The change in activation frequency causes a transient bone loss until a new steady state between resorption and formation is achieved. The remodeling imbalance, however, results in a permanent decrement in mass that can only be corrected by a remodeling event during which bone formation exceeds resorption. In addition, the very presence of more remodeling sites in the skeleton increases the probability that trabeculae will be penetrated, thereby eliminating the template upon which new bone can be formed and accelerating the loss of bony tissue.

The most frequent estrogen-deficient state is the cessation of ovarian function at the time of menopause, which occurs on average at the age of 51. Thus, with current life expectancy, an average woman will spend about 30 years without ovarian supply of estrogen. The mechanism by which estrogen deficiency causes bone loss is summarized in Fig. 342-5. Marrow cells (macrophages, monocytes, osteoclast precursors, mast cells) as well as bone cells (osteoblasts, osteocytes, osteoclasts) express ERs α and β. The net effect of estrogen deficiency is increased osteoclast recruitment and perhaps activity. Estrogen may also play an important role in determining the life span of bone cells by controlling the rate of apoptosis. Thus, in situations of estrogen deprivation, the life span of osteoblasts may be decreased whereas the longevity of osteoclasts is increased.

Since remodeling is initiated at the surface of bone, it follows that trabecular bone—which has a considerably larger surface area (80% of the total) than cortical bone—will be preferentially affected by estrogen deficiency. Fractures occur earliest at sites where trabecular

bone contributes most to bone strength; consequently, vertebral fractures are the most common early consequence of estrogen deficiency.

Physical Activity Inactivity, such as prolonged bed rest or paralysis, results in significant bone loss. Concordantly, athletes have higher bone mass than the general population. These changes in skeletal mass are most marked when the stimulus begins during growth and before the age of puberty. Adults are less capable than children of increasing bone mass following restoration of physical activity. Epidemiologic data support the beneficial effects on the skeleton of chronic high levels of physical activity. Fracture risk is lower in rural communities and in countries where physical activity is maintained into old age. However, when exercise is initiated during adult life, the effects of moderate exercise are modest, with a bone mass increase of 1 to 2%. It is argued that more active individuals are less likely to fall and are more capable of protecting themselves upon falling, thereby reducing fracture risk.

Chronic Disease Various genetic and acquired diseases are associated with an increase in the risk of osteoporosis (Table 342-2). Mechanisms that contribute to bone loss are unique for each disease and typically result from multiple factors including nutrition, reduced physical activity levels, and factors that affect bone-remodeling rates.

Medications A large number of medications used in clinical practice have potentially detrimental effects on the skeleton (Table 342-3). *Glucocorticoids* are a common cause of medication-induced osteoporosis. It is often not possible to determine the extent to which osteoporosis is related to the glucocorticoid or to other factors, as treatment is superimposed on the effects of the primary disease, which may itself be associated with bone loss (e.g., rheumatoid arthritis). Excessive doses of thyroid hormone can accelerate bone remodeling and result in bone loss.

Other medications have less detrimental effects upon the skeleton than pharmacologic doses of glucocorticoids. *Anticonvulsants* are thought to increase the risk of osteoporosis, although many affected individuals have concomitant vitamin D insufficiency, as anticonvulsants that induce the cytochrome P450 system alter vitamin D metabolism. Patients undergoing transplantation are at high risk for rapid bone loss and fracture not only from glucocorticoids but also from

Table 342-2 Diseases Associated with an Increased Risk of Generalized Osteoporosis in Adults

Hypogonadal states	Hematologic disorders/malignancy
Turner syndrome	Multiple myeloma
Klinefelter syndrome	Lymphoma and leukemia
Anorexia nervosa	Malignancy-associated parathyroid
Hypothalamic amenorrhea	hormone–related (PTHrP) production
Hyperprolactinemia	Mastocytosis
Other primary or secondary	Hemophilia
hypogonadal states	Thalassemia
Endocrine disorders	Selected inherited disorders
Cushing's syndrome	Osteogenesis imperfecta
Hyperparathyroidism	Marfan syndrome
Thyrotoxicosis	Hemochromatosis
Insulin-dependent diabetes	Hypophosphatasia
mellitus	Glycogen storage diseases
Acromegaly	Homocystinuria
Adrenal insufficiency	Ehlers-Danlos syndrome
Nutritional and gastrointestinal	Porphyria
disorders	Menkes' syndrome
Malnutrition	Epidermolysis bullosa
Parenteral nutrition	Other disorders
Malabsorption syndromes	Immobilization
Gastrectomy	Chronic obstructive pulmonary disease
Severe liver disease, especially biliary cirrhosis	Pregnancy and lactation
	Scoliosis
Pernicious anemia	Multiple sclerosis
Rheumatologic disorders	Sarcoidosis
Rheumatoid arthritis	Amyloidosis
Ankylosing spondylitis	

Table 342-3   Drugs Associated with an Increased Risk of Generalized Osteoporosis in Adults

Glucocorticoids	Excessive thyroxine
Cyclosporine	Aluminum
Cytotoxic drugs	Gonadotropin-releasing hormone agonists
Anticonvulsants	Heparin
Excessive alcohol	Lithium

treatment with other *immunosuppressants*, such as cyclosporine and tacrolimus (FK506). In addition, these patients often have underlying metabolic abnormalities, such as hepatic or renal failure, that predispose to osteopenia.

Cigarette Consumption   The use of cigarettes over a long period has detrimental effects on bone mass. These effects may be mediated directly, by toxic effects on osteoblasts, or indirectly by modifying estrogen metabolism. On average, cigarette smokers reach menopause 1 to 2 years earlier than the general population. Cigarette smoking also has secondary effects on bone growth, such as illness, frailty, decreased exercise, and the need for additional medications (e.g., glucocorticoids for lung disease).

MEASUREMENT OF BONE MASS   Several noninvasive techniques are now available for estimating skeletal mass or density. These include dual-energy x-ray absorptiometry (DXA), single-energy xray absorptiometry (SXA), quantitative computed tomography (CT), and ultrasound.

DXA is a highly accurate x-ray technique that has become the standard for measuring bone density in most centers. Though it can be used for measurements of any skeletal site, clinical determinations are usually made of the lumbar spine and hip. Portable DXA machines have been developed that measure the heel (calcaneus), forearm (radius and ulna), or finger (phalanges), and DXA can also be used to measure body composition. In the DXA technique, two x-ray energies are used to estimate the area of mineralized tissue, and the mineral content is divided by the area, which partially corrects for body size. However, this correction is only partial since DXA is a two-dimensional scanning technique and cannot estimate the depths or posteroanterior length of the bone. Thus, small people tend to have lower-than-average bone mineral density (BMD). Bone spurs, which are frequent in osteoarthritis, tend to falsely increase bone density of the spine. Because DXA instrumentation is provided by several different manufacturers, the output varies in absolute terms. Consequently, it has become standard practice to relate the results to "normal" values using T-scores, which compare individual results to those in a young population that is matched for race and gender. Alternatively, Z-scores compare individual results to those of an age-matched population that is also matched for race and gender. Thus, a 60-year-old woman with a Z-score of -1 (1 SD below mean for age) could have a T-score of -2.5 (2.5 SD below mean for a young control group) (Fig. 342-6).

CT is used primarily to measure the spine, and peripheral CT is used to measure bone in the forearm or tibia. Research into the use of CT for measurement of the hip is ongoing. The results obtained from CT are different from all others currently available since this technique specifically analyzes trabecular bone and can provide a true density (mass of bone per unit volume) measurement. However, CT remains expensive, involves greater radiation exposure, and is less reproducible.

Ultrasound is used to measure bone mass by calculating the attenuation of the signal as it passes through bone or the speed with which it traverses the bone. It is unclear whether ultrasound assesses bone quality, but this may be an advantage of the technique. Because of its relatively low cost and mobility, ultrasound is amenable for use as a screening procedure.

All of these techniques for measuring BMD have been approved by the U.S. Food and Drug Administration (FDA) based upon their capacity to predict fracture risk. The hip is the preferred site of meas-

FIGURE 342-6   Relationship between Z-scores and T-scores in a 60-year-old woman. (BMD, bone mineral density; SD, standard deviation.)

urement in most individuals, since it directly assesses bone mass at an important fracture site. When hip measurements are performed by DXA, the spine can be measured at the same time. In younger individuals, such as perimenopausal women, spine measurements may be the most sensitive indicator of bone loss.

When to Measure Bone Mass   Clinical guidelines developed by the National Osteoporosis Foundation recommend bone mass measurements in postmenopausal women, assuming they have risk factors for osteoporosis in addition to age, gender, and estrogen deficiency. The guidelines further recommend that bone mass measurement be considered in *all* women by age 60 to 65. Criteria approved for Medicare reimbursement of BMD are summarized in Table 342-4.

When to Treat Based Upon Bone Mass Results   The guidelines developed by the National Osteoporosis Foundation suggest that patients be considered for treatment when BMD > 2.5 SD below the mean value for young adults (T-score ≤ -2.5). Treatment should also be considered in women with risk factors in addition to menopause, if measurement of BMD of the hip gives a T score < -2.0. Because the fracture risk increases continuously as T-scores decline, there is no critical threshold and treatment decisions must be individualized. Cost-benefit analyses in this area are changing rapidly because of the availability of new drugs [e.g., bisphosphonates, selective estrogen receptor modulators (SERMs)] and the results of trials [e.g., the Heart and Estrogen-Progestin Replacement Study (HERS)] examining the long-term cardiovascular effects of hormone replacement therapy (HRT).

Approach to the Patient

The perimenopausal transition is a good opportunity to initiate discussion about risk factors for osteoporosis and to consider indications for a BMD test. A careful history and physical examination should be performed to identify risk factors for osteoporosis. As noted above, a low Z-score increases the suspicion of a secondary disease. Height loss >2.5 to 3.8 cm (1 to 1.5 in.) is an indication for radiography to rule out asymptomatic vertebral fractures, as is the presence of significant kyphosis or back pain, particularly if it began after menopause. For patients who present with fractures, it is important to ensure that the fractures are truly due to trauma or osteoporosis and not to secondary underlying malignancy. Usually this is clear on routine radi-

Table 342-4   FDA-Approved Indications for BMD Tests[a]

Estrogen deficient women at clinical risk of osteoporosis
Vertebral abnormalities on x-ray suggestive of osteoporosis (osteopenia, vertebral fracture)
Glucocorticoid treatment equivalent to $\geq$7.5 mg of prednisone, or duration of therapy >3 months
Primary hyperparathyroidism
Monitoring response to an FDA-approved medication for osteoporosis
Repeat BMD evaluations at >23-month intervals, or more frequently, if medically justified

[a] Criteria adapted from the 1998 Bone Mass Measurement Act.
NOTE: FDA, U.S. Food and Drug Administration; BMD, bone mineral density.

ography, but on occasion, CT, magnetic resonance imaging, or radionuclide scans may be helpful. Severe unremitting back pain also raises the suspicion of other causes such as malignancy (especially myeloma).

Routine Laboratory Evaluation There is no established algorithm for the evaluation of women presenting with osteoporosis. A general evaluation that includes complete blood count, serum calcium, and perhaps urine calcium is helpful for identifying selected secondary causes of low bone mass, particularly for women with fractures or very low Z-scores. An elevated serum calcium level suggests hyperparathyroidism or malignancy, whereas a reduced serum calcium level may reflect malnutrition and osteomalacia. In the presence of hypercalcemia, a serum PTH level differentiates between hyperparathyroidism (PTH ↑) and malignancy (PTH ↓), and a high PTHrP level can help document the presence of humoral hypercalcemia of malignancy (Chap. 341). A low urine calcium (<50 mg/24 h) suggests osteomalacia, malnutrition, or malabsorption; a high urine calcium (>300 mg/24 h) is indicative of hypercalciuria and must be investigated further. Hypercalciuria occurs primarily in three situations: (1) a renal calcium leak, which is more frequent in males with osteoporosis; (2) absorptive hypercalciuria, which can be idiopathic or associated with increased $1,25(OH)_2D$ in granulomatous disease; or (3) hematologic malignancies or conditions associated with excessive bone turnover such as Paget's disease, hyperparathyroidism, and hyperthyroidism.

When there is clinical suspicion of hyperthyroidism or Cushing's syndrome, thyroid stimulating hormone (TSH) or urinary free cortisol levels should be measured. When bowel disease, malabsorption, or malnutrition is suspected, serum albumin, cholesterol, and a complete blood count should be checked. Asymptomatic malabsorption might be suspected if there is anemia (macrocytic—vitamin B_{12} or folate deficiency; or microcytic—iron deficiency), or low serum cholesterol or urinary calcium levels. If these or other features suggest malabsorption, further evaluation is required. Asymptomatic celiac sprue with selective malabsorption is not uncommon; the diagnosis requires antigliadin and antiendomysial antibody tests and often a small-bowel biopsy. A trial of a gluten-free diet may be confirmatory (Chap. 286).

Myeloma can masquerade as generalized osteoporosis, although it more commonly presents with bone pain and characteristic "punched-out" lesions on radiography. Serum and urine electrophoresis and evaluation for light chains in urine are required to exclude this diagnosis. A bone marrow biopsy may be required to rule out myeloma (in patients with equivocal electrophoretic results) and can also be used to exclude mastocytosis, leukemia, and other marrow infiltrative disorders, such as Gaucher's disease.

Bone Biopsy Although the use of bone biopsy is rarely required today, it remains an important tool in clinical research. Tetracycline labeling of the skeleton allows determination of the rate of remodeling as well as evaluation for other metabolic bone diseases. The current use of BMD tests, in combination with hormonal evaluation and biochemical markers of bone remodeling, has largely replaced bone biopsy.

Biochemical Markers Several biochemical tests are now available that provide an index of the overall rate of bone remodeling (Table 342-5). Biochemical markers are usually characterized as those related primarily to *bone formation* or *bone resorption*. These tests measure the overall state of bone remodeling at a single point in time. Clinical use of these tests has been hampered by biologic variability (in part related to circadian rhythm) as well as to analytical variability.

For the most part, remodeling markers do not predict rates of bone loss well enough to use this information clinically. However, markers of bone resorption may help in the prediction of fracture risk, particularly in older individuals. In women ≥65 years, when bone density results are greater than the usual treatment thresholds noted above, a high level of bone resorption should prompt consideration of treatment. The primary use of biochemical markers is for monitoring the response to treatment. With the introduction of antiresorptive therapeutic agents, bone remodeling declines rapidly, with the fall in resorption occurring earlier than the fall in formation. Inhibition of bone

Table 342-5 Biochemical Markers of Bone Metabolism in Clinical Use

Bone formation
   Serum bone-specific alkaline phosphatase
   Serum osteocalcin
   Serum propeptide of type I procollagen
Bone resorption
   Urine and serum cross-linked N-telopeptide
   Urine and serum cross-linked C-telopeptide
   Urine total free deoxypyridinoline
   Urine hydroxyproline
   Serum tartrate-resistant acid phosphatase
   Serum bone sialoprotein
   Urine hydroxylysine glycosides

resorption is maximal within 3 to 6 months. Thus, measurement of bone resorption prior to initiating therapy and 4 to 6 months after starting therapy provides an earlier estimate of patient response than does bone densitometry. A decline in resorptive markers can be ascertained after treatment with bisphosphonates and HRT; this effect is less marked after treatment with either raloxifene or intranasal calcitonin. A biochemical marker response to therapy is particularly useful for asymptomatic patients and helps to ensure long-term compliance. When agents that stimulate bone formation become available, bone remodeling markers may be useful to help select therapy. However, since all current therapeutic approaches reduce bone turnover, this strategy currently has little value.

℞ TREATMENT Management of Osteoporotic Fractures
Treatment of the patient with osteoporosis frequently involves management of acute fractures as well as treatment of the underlying disease. Hip fractures almost always require surgical repair if the patient is to become ambulatory again. Depending on the location and severity of the fracture, condition of the neighboring joint, and general status of the patient, procedures may include open reduction and internal fixation with pins and plates, hemiarthroplasties, and total arthroplasties. These surgical procedures are followed by intense rehabilitation in an attempt to return patients to their prefracture functional level. Long bone fractures often require either external or internal fixation. Other fractures (e.g., vertebral, rib, and pelvic fractures) are usually managed with only supportive care, requiring no specific orthopedic treatment.

Only ~25 to 30% of vertebral compression fractures present with sudden-onset back pain. For acutely symptomatic fractures, treatment with analgesics is required, including nonsteroidal anti-inflammatory agents and/or acetaminophen, sometimes with the addition of a narcotic agent (codeine or oxycodone). A few small, randomized clinical trials have demonstrated that calcitonin may reduce pain related to acute vertebral compression fracture. A recently developed, but still experimental, technique involves percutaneous injection of artificial cement (polymethylmethacrylate) into the vertebral body (vertebroplasty or kyphoplasty); this has been reported to offer significant immediate pain relief in the majority of patients. Short periods of bed rest may be helpful for pain management, but, in general, early mobilization is recommended as it helps prevent further bone loss associated with immobilization. Occasionally, use of a soft elastic-style brace may facilitate earlier mobilization. Muscle spasms often occur with acute compression fractures and can be treated with muscle relaxants and heat treatments.

Severe pain usually resolves within 6 to 10 weeks. Chronic pain is probably not bony in origin; instead, it is related to abnormal strain on muscles, ligaments, and tendons and to secondary facet-joint arthritis associated with alterations in thoracic and/or abdominal shape. Chronic pain is difficult to treat effectively and may require analgesics, sometimes including narcotic analgesics. Frequent intermittent rest in a supine or semireclining position is often required to allow the soft tissues, which are under tension, to relax. Back-strengthening exercises (paraspinal) may be beneficial. Heat treatments help relax muscles and reduce the muscular component of discomfort. Various physical modalities, such as ultrasound and transcutaneous nerve stimulation, may be beneficial in some patients. Pain also occurs in the neck region, not as a result of compression fractures (which almost never occur in the cervical spine as a result of osteoporosis) but because of chronic strain associated from trying to elevate the head in a person with a severe thoracic kyphosis.

Multiple vertebral fractures are often associated with psychological symptoms, not always commonly appreciated. The changes in body configuration and back pain can lead to marked loss of self-image and a secondary depression. Altered balance, precipitated by the kyphosis and the anterior movement of the body's center of gravity, leads to a fear of falling, a consequent tendency to remain indoors, and the onset of social isolation. These symptoms can sometimes be alleviated by family support and/or psychotherapy. Medication may be necessary when depressive features are present.

Management of the Underlying Disease • *Risk factor reduction* Patients should be thoroughly educated to reduce the likelihood of any risk factors associated with bone loss and falling. Medications should be reviewed to ensure that any glucocorticoid medication is truly indicated and is being given in doses as low as possible. For those on thyroid hormone replacement, TSH testing should be performed to ensure that an adequate, but not excessive, dose is being used, as excess can be associated with increased bone loss. In patients who smoke, efforts should be made to facilitate smoking cessation. Reducing risk factors for falling also includes alcohol abuse treatment and a review of the medical regimen for any drugs that might be associated with orthostatic hypotension and/or sedation, including hypnotics and anxiolytics. If nocturia occurs, the frequency should be reduced, if possible (e.g., by decreasing or modifying diuretic use), as arising in the middle of sleep is a common precipitant of a fall. Patients should be instructed about environmental safety with regard to eliminating exposed wires, curtain strings, slippery rugs, and mobile tables. Avoiding stocking feet on wood floors, checking carpet condition (particularly on stairs), and providing good light in paths to bathrooms and outside the home are good preventive measures. Treatment for impaired vision is recommended, particularly a problem with depth perception, which is specifically associated with increased falling risk. Elderly patients with neurologic impairment (e.g., stroke, Parkinson's disease, Alzheimer's disease) are particularly at risk of falling and require specialized supervision and care.

Nutritional recommendations • CALCIUM A large body of data indicates that optimal calcium intake reduces bone loss and suppresses bone turnover. Recommended intakes from a recent report from the Institute of Medicine are shown in Table 342-6. The National Health and Nutritional Evaluation Studies (NHANES) have consistently documented that average calcium intakes fall considerably short of these recommendations. The preferred source of calcium is from dairy products and other foods, but many patients require additional calcium supplementation. Food sources of calcium are dairy products (milk,

yogurt, and cheese) and fortified foods such as certain cereals, waffles, snacks, juices, and crackers. Some of these fortified foods contain as much calcium per serving as milk.

If a calcium supplement is required, it should be taken in doses ≤600 mg at a time, as the calcium absorption fraction decreases at higher doses. Calcium supplements should be calculated based on the elemental calcium content of the supplement, not the weight of the calcium salt (Table 342-7). Calcium supplements containing carbonate are best taken with food since they require acid for solubility. Calcium citrate supplements can be taken at any time.

Several controlled clinical trials of calcium plus vitamin D have confirmed reductions in clinical fractures, including fractures of the hip (~20 to 30% risk reduction). All recent studies of pharmacologic agents have been conducted in the context of calcium replacement (± vitamin D). Thus, it is standard practice to ensure an adequate calcium and vitamin D intake in patients with osteoporosis, whether they are receiving additional pharmacologic therapy or not.

Although side effects from supplemental calcium are minimal, individuals with a history of kidney stones should have a 24-h urine calcium determination before starting increased calcium to avoid hypercalciuria. Furthermore, a thiazide-containing diuretic might be indicated in some patients to increase renal tubular calcium reabsorption and to reduce urine calcium levels.

VITAMIN D Vitamin D is synthesized in skin under the influence of heat and ultraviolet light (Chap. 340). However, large segments of the population do not obtain sufficient vitamin D to maintain what is now considered an adequate supply [serum 25(OH)D consistently >15 to 20 ng/mL]. Since vitamin D supplementation at doses that would achieve these serum levels is safe and inexpensive, it is now routine to recommend supplemental vitamin D. The Institute of Medicine recommends daily intakes of 200 IU for adults <50 years of age, 400 IU for those from 50 to 70 years, and 600 IU for those >70 years. Multivitamin tablets usually contain 400 IU, and many calcium supplements also contain vitamin D.

OTHER NUTRIENTS Other nutrients such as salt and caffeine may have modest effects on calcium excretion or absorption. Adequate vitamin K states is required for optimal carboxylation of osteocalcin. States in which vitamin K nutrition or metabolism is impaired, such as with long-term coumadin therapy, have been associated with reduced bone mass.

Magnesium is abundant in foods, and magnesium deficiency is quite rare in the absence of a serious chronic disease. Magnesium supplementation may be warranted in patients with inflammatory bowel disease, celiac sprue, chemotherapy, severe diarrhea, malnutrition, or alcoholism. Phytoestrogens may impact skeletal health, although the degree of this effect is unclear. Dietary phytoestrogens, which are derived primarily from soy products and legumes (e.g., garbanzo beans, chickpeas, and lentils), are insufficiently potent to justify their use in place of a pharmacologic agent in the treatment of osteoporosis.

Patients with hip fracture are often frail and relatively malnourished. Some data suggest an improved outcome in such patients when they are provided calorie and protein supplementation.

Exercise Exercise in young individuals increases the likelihood that they will attain the maximal genetically determined peak bone

Table 342-6 Adequate Calcium Intake

Life Stage Group	Estimated Adequate Daily Calcium Intake, mg/d
Young Children (1–3 years)	500
Older children (4–8 years)	800
Adolescents and young adults (9–18 years)	1300
Men and women (19–50 years)	1000
Men and women (51 and older)	1200

NOTE: Pregnancy and lactation needs are the same as for nonpregnant women (e.g., 1300 mg/d for adolescents/young adult and 1000 mg/d for ≥19 years.)
SOURCE: Adapted from the Standing Committee on the Scientific Evaluation of Dietary Reference Intakes. Food and Nutrition Board. Institute of Medicine. Washington, DC, 1997. National Academy Press.

Table 342-7 Elemental Calcium Content of Various Oral Calcium Preparations

Calcium Preparation	Elemental Calcium Content
Calcium citrate	40 mg/300 mg
Calcium lactate	80 mg/600 mg
Calcium gluconate	40 mg/500 mg
Calcium carbonate	400 mg/g
Calcium carbonate + 5 μg vitamin D₂ (OsCal 250)	250 mg/tablet
Calcium carbonate (Tums 500)	500 mg/tablet

SOURCE: SM Krane and MF Holick, Chap. 355 in HPIM, 14 ed, 1998.

mass. Meta-analyses of studies performed in postmenopausal women indicate that weight-bearing exercise prevents bone loss but does not appear to result in substantial bone gain. When the exercise is discontinued, any effects on bone mass wane. It is important to note, however, that exercise also has beneficial effects on neuromuscular function. Exercise can improve coordination, balance, and strength and thereby reduce the risk of falling, as well as the severity of injury upon a fall. Therefore, the beneficial effects of exercise on muscle mass and reduced risk of falling justify its recommendation for all age groups. A walking program is a practical way to start. Other activities such as dancing, racquet sports, cross-country skiing, and use of gym equipment are also recommended, depending on the patient's personal preference. Even women who cannot walk benefit from swimming or water exercises, not so much for the effects on bone, which are quite minimal, but because of effects on muscle. Exercise habits should be consistent, optimally at least three times a week.

FIGURE 342-7 Results of hormone-replacement therapy (HRT) regimens on bone mineral density (BMD) of the spine (*A*) and hip (*B*). Unadjusted mean percent change in BMD in the hip by treatment assignment and visit: adherent PEPI participants only. Results From the Postmenopausal Estrogen/ Progestin Interventions (PEPI) Trial. Estrogen, conjugated equine estrogen 0.625 mg/d; Progestin, medroxyprogesterone acetate 10 mg/d. (*Adapted from TL Bush et al: JAMA 276:1389, 1996.*)

Pharmacologic Therapies Until fairly recently, estrogen treatment, either by itself or in concert with a progestin, was the primary therapeutic agent for prevention or treatment of osteoporosis. Over the past 5 years, a number of new drugs have appeared, and more are expected in the near future. Some are agents that specifically treat osteoporosis (bisphosphonates, calcitonin); others, such as tissue-selective estrogens (or SERMs), have broader effects. The availability of these drugs allows therapy to be tailored to the needs of an individual patient. The evidence supporting the effectiveness of each remedy is variable, in part because these treatments are new.

Estrogens A large body of clinical trial data indicates that various types of estrogens (conjugated equine estrogens, estradiol, estrone, esterified estrogens, ethinyl estradiol, and mestranol) reduce bone turnover, prevent bone loss, and induce small increases in bone mass of the spine, hip, and total body. The effects of estrogen are seen in women with natural or surgical menopause and in late postmenopausal women with or without established osteoporosis. Estrogens are efficacious when administered orally, buccally, vaginally, percutaneously, subcutaneously, and transdermally. For both oral and transdermal routes of administration, combined estrogen/progestin preparations are now available in many countries, obviating the problem of taking two tablets or using a patch and oral progestin. One large study, referred to as PEPI (Postmenopausal Estrogen/ Progestin Intervention Trial), indicated that C-21 progestins alone do not augment the effect of estrogen on bone mass (Fig. 342-7).

DOSE OF ESTROGEN For oral estrogens, the recommended dose is 0.3 mg/d for esterified estrogens, 0.625 mg/d for conjugated equine estrogens, and 5 μg/d for ethinyl estradiol. For transdermal estrogen, the commonly used dose supplies 50 μg estradiol per day, but a lower dose may be appropriate for some individuals. Dose-response data are not available for other routes of administration.

FRACTURE DATA In contrast to the body of clinical trial data evaluating the effects of estrogen on bone mass, its effects on fracture occurrence have been less well studied. Epidemiologic databases indicate that women who take estrogen replacement have a 50% reduction, on average, of osteoporotic fractures, including hip fractures. The beneficial effect of estrogen is greatest among those who start replacement early and continue the treatment; the benefit wanes after discontinuation such that there is no residual protective effect against fracture by 10 years after discontinuation. There are no clinical trial data confirming that estrogen administration reduces the risk of hip fracture. In fact, the HERS trial of women with established coronary artery disease showed no reduction in the risk of hip or clinical fractures in the estrogen-progestin arm relative to the placebo group. These data

may not be definitive, however, since the women were not chosen for osteoporosis risk and were at unknown risk of osteoporotic fracture. Furthermore, radiographic vertebral fractures were not assessed in this study. One clinical study which looked at all nonvertebral fractures suggested a reduction in HRT-treated women.

A few clinical trials have evaluated spine fracture occurrence as an outcome with estrogen therapy. One that used high doses of estrogen (2.5 mg conjugated equine estrogen per day) indicated marked vertebral fracture reduction in estrogen-treated women. Several other small studies, using lower estrogen doses, have consistently shown that estrogen treatment reduces the incidence of vertebral compression fracture. The ongoing Women's Health Initiative will provide additional data about the effects of estrogen on the risk of other osteoporosis-related fractures.

Long-term estrogen use may be associated with an increase in the risk of venous thromboembolism and gallbladder, uterine, and breast cancer; in observational studies, estrogens have been associated with a significant reduction in myocardial infarction, although this was not so in HERS. The WHI will provide further information.

MODE OF ACTION Two subtypes of ERs, α and β, have been identified in bone and other tissues. Cells of monocyte lineage express both ERα and -β, as do osteoblasts. Estrogen-mediated effects vary depending on the receptor type. Using ER knockout mouse models, elimination of ERα produces a modest reduction in bone mass, whereas ERβ null animals had very little abnormality, except greater cortical bone mass. A male patient with a homozygous mutation of ERα had markedly decreased bone density as well as abnormalities in epiphyseal closure, confirming the important role of ERα in bone biology. The mechanism of estrogen action in bone is an area of active investigation (Fig. 342-5). Though data are conflicting, estrogens appear to inhibit osteoclasts directly. However, the majority of estrogen (and androgen) effects on bone resorption are mediated indirectly through paracrine factors produced by osteoblasts. These actions include: (1) increasing IGF-1 and TGF-β, and (2) suppressing IL-1 (α and β), IL-6, TNF-α, and osteocalcin synthesis. The consequence of these effects is primarily to decrease bone resorption.

Progestins In women with a uterus, daily progestin or cyclical progestins at least 12 days per month are prescribed in combination with estrogens to reduce the risk of uterine cancer. Medroxyprogesterone acetate and norethindrone acetate blunt the high-density lipoprotein response to estrogen, but micronized progesterone does not. Neither medroxyprogesterone acetate nor micronized progesterone appears to have an independent effect on bone; at lower doses, norethindrone acetate might have an additive benefit. On breast tissue, progestins may increase the risk of breast cancer, though this is by no means definite.

FIGURE 342-8 Alendronate treatment. Percentage change in bone mineral density in women receiving alendronate or placebo over 3 years. *(From UA Liberman et al: N Engl J Med 333:1437, 1995.)*

Legend: ●— Placebo   ◇— 5 mg   ■— 10 mg   △— 20, then 5 mg

Lumbar spine
Femoral neck
Trochanter
Total body

Y-axis: Mean change in bone mineral density, %
X-axis: Month

Tissue-selective estrogens, or SERMs Two SERMs are currently being used in postmenopausal women: raloxifene, which is approved for prevention and treatment of osteoporosis, and tamoxifen, which is approved for the prevention and treatment of breast cancer.

Tamoxifen reduces bone turnover and bone loss in postmenopausal women compared to placebo groups. These findings support the concept that tamoxifen acts as an estrogenic agent in bone. There are limited data on the effect of tamoxifen on fracture risk, but the Breast Cancer Prevention study indicated a possible reduction in clinical vertebral, hip, and Colles' fractures. The major benefit of tamoxifen is on breast cancer occurrence. The breast cancer prevention trial indicated that tamoxifen administration over 4 to 5 years reduced the incidence of new invasive and noninvasive breast cancer by approximately 45% in women at increased risk of breast cancer. The incidence of ER-positive breast cancers was reduced by 65%.

Raloxifene (60 mg/d) has effects on bone turnover and bone mass that are very similar to those of tamoxifen, indicating that this agent is also estrogenic on the skeleton. The effect of raloxifene on bone density (+1.4 to 2.8% versus placebo in the spine, hip, and total body) is somewhat less than that seen with standard doses of estrogens. Raloxifene reduces the occurrence of vertebral fracture by 30 to 50%, depending on the subpopulation.

Raloxifene, like tamoxifen and estrogen, has effects throughout other organ systems. The most positive effect appears to be a reduction in invasive breast cancer (mainly decreased ER-positive) occurrence of about 70% in women who take raloxifene compared to placebo. In contrast to tamoxifen, raloxifene is not associated with an increase in the risk of uterine cancer or benign uterine disease. Raloxifene increases the occurrence of hot flashes. Although raloxifene reduces serum total and low-density lipoprotein cholesterol, lipoprotein(a), and

fibrinogen, no studies including cardiovascular disease or cerebrovascular disease endpoints are available.

MODE OF ACTION OF SERMS All SERMs bind to the ER, but each agent produces a unique receptor conformation. As a result, specific coactivator or corepressor proteins are bound to the receptor (Chap. 327), resulting in differential effects on gene transcription that vary according to other transcription factors present in the cell. Another aspect of selectivity is the affinity of each SERM for the different ERα and β subtypes, which are expressed differentially in various tissues. These tissue-selective effects of SERMs offer the possibility of tailoring estrogen therapy to best meet the needs and risk factor profile of an individual patient.

Bisphosphonates Both alendronate and risendronate are approved for the prevention and treatment of postmenopausal osteoporosis and treatment of steroid-induced osteoporosis. Risedronate is also approved for the prevention of steroid-induced osteoporosis.

Alendronate has been shown to have dramatic effects in patients with osteoporosis, decreasing bone turnover and increasing bone mass in the spine by up to 8% versus placebo and by 6% versus placebo in the hip (Fig. 342-8). Multiple trials have evaluated the effect of alendronate on fracture occurrence. The Fracture Intervention Trial provided evidence in over 2000 women with prevalent vertebral fractures that daily alendronate treatment (5 mg/d for 2 years and 10 mg/d for 9 months afterwards) reduces vertebral fracture risk by about 50%, multiple vertebral fractures by up to 90%, and hip fractures by up to 50% (Fig. 342-9). Several subsequent trials have confirmed these findings. For example, in a study of >1900 women with low bone mass treated with alendronate (10 mg/d) versus placebo, the incidence of all nonvertebral fractures was reduced by ~47% after just 1 year.

Alendronate (5 to 10 mg/d) should be given with a full glass of water before breakfast, as bisphosphonates are poorly absorbed. Because of the potential for esophageal irritation, alendronate is contraindicated in patients who have stricture or inadequate emptying of the esophagus. It is recommended that patients remain upright for at least 30 min after taking the medication to avoid esophageal irritation. Cases of esophagitis, esophageal ulcer, and esophageal stricture have been described, but the incidence appears to be low. In clinical trials, overall gastrointestinal symptomatology was no different with alendronate compared to placebo.

Risedronate produces a dramatic reduction in bone turnover and an increase in bone mass. Controlled clinical trials have demonstrated >40% reduction in vertebral fracture risk over 3 years, accompanied by a 33% reduction in clinical nonspine fractures. Reports from several studies show a 40% reduction in hip fracture in patients with osteoporosis, with a somewhat greater effect in patients with prevalent vertebral fractures. Patients should take risedronate (5.0 mg orally) with a full glass of plain water [0.18 to 0.25 L (6 to 8 oz)], to facilitate delivery to the stomach, and should not lie down for 30 min after taking the drug. The incidence of gastrointestinal side effects in these trials with risedronate was similar to that of placebo.

Etidronate was the first bisphosphonate to be approved, initially for use in Paget's disease and hypercalcemia. This agent has also been used in osteoporosis trials of smaller magnitude than those performed for alendronate and risedronate. Etidronate probably has some efficacy against vertebral fracture when given as an intermittent cyclical regimen (2 weeks on, 2 1/2 months off).

MODE OF ACTION Bisphosphonates are structurally related to pyrophosphates, compounds that are incorporated into bone matrix. Through mechanisms that remain to be fully elucidated, bisphosphonates specifically impair osteoclast function and reduce osteoclast number, in part by the induction of apoptosis. Recent evidence suggests that the nitrogen-containing bisphosphonates also inhibit protein pren-

FIGURE 342-9 Cumulative proportions of women with osteoporosis who suffered clinical vertebral, hip, or wrist fracture during 3 years of treatment with alendronate or placebo (FIT 1). *(From DM Black et al: Lancet 348:1535, 1996.)*

ylation, one of the end products in the mevalonic acid pathway. This effect disrupts intracellular protein trafficking and may ultimately lead to apoptosis. Bisphosphonates have very long retention in the skeleton and may exert long-term effects.

Calcitonin Calcitonin is a polypeptide hormone produced by the thyroid gland (Chap. 341). Its physiologic role is unclear as no skeletal disease has been described in association with calcitonin deficiency or calcitonin excess. Calcitonins are approved by the FDA approved for Paget's disease, hypercalcemia, and osteoporosis in women >5 years past menopause.

Injectable calcitonin produces small increments in bone mass of the lumbar spine. However, difficulty of administration and frequent reactions, including nausea and facial flushing, make general use limited. In 1995, a nasal spray containing calcitonin (200 IU/d) was approved for treatment of osteoporosis in postmenopausal women. Several studies indicate that nasal calcitonin produces small increments in bone mass and a small reduction in new vertebral fractures in calcitonin-treated patients versus those on calcium alone.

Calcitonin is not indicated for prevention of osteoporosis and is not sufficiently potent to prevent bone loss in early postmenopausal women. As mentioned above, calcitonin might have an analgesic effect on bone pain, both in the subcutaneous and possibly the nasal form.

MODE OF ACTION Calcitonin suppresses osteoclast activity by direct action on the osteoclast calcitonin receptor. Osteoclasts exposed to calcitonin cannot maintain their active ruffled border, which normally maintains close contact with underlying bone. Calcitonin also affects osteoclast mobility and the movement of enzyme-containing cytoplasmic granules.

Experimental agents • *PARATHYROID HORMONE* Endogenous PTH is an 84-amino-acid peptide that is largely responsible for calcium

homeostasis (Chap. 341). Although chronic elevation of PTH, as occurs in hyperparathyroidism, is associated with bone loss (particularly cortical bone), PTH can also exert anabolic effects on bone. Consistent with this, some observational studies have indicated that mild elevations in PTH are associated with maintenance of trabecular bone mass. On the basis of these findings, preclinical and early clinical studies have been performed using an exogenous PTH analogue (1-34 PTH). The first randomized controlled trial in postmenopausal women showed that PTH, when superimposed on ongoing estrogen therapy, produced substantial increments in bone mass (13% over a 3-year period compared to estrogen alone). This increment in bone mass was also associated with a reduction in risk of vertebral compression deformity (Fig. 342-10). More recent studies have confirmed the ability of combined treatment with estrogen and PTH to induce striking increases in bone mass.

PTH use may be limited by its mode of administration, which currently requires subcutaneous injection. Alternative modes of delivery are being investigated, including transdermal and inhalation routes. The optimal frequency of administration also remains to be established, and it is possible that PTH might also be effective when used in high doses, 1 month out of every 3.

MODE OF ACTION Exogenously administered PTH appears to have direct actions on osteoblast activity, with biochemical and histomorphometric evidence of de novo bone formation early in response to PTH, prior to activation of bone resorption. Subsequently, PTH activates bone remodeling but still appears to favor bone formation over bone resorption. PTH stimulates IGF-I and collagen production and appears to increase osteoblast number by inhibiting apoptosis and stimulating replication.

FLUORIDE Fluoride has been available for many years and is a potent stimulator of osteoprogenitor cells when studied in vitro. It has been used in multiple osteoporosis studies with conflicting results, in part related to use of varying doses and preparations. Fluoride produces marked effects on bone mass, especially in the spine, where gains of around 10% per year have been observed. However, despite increments in bone mass, there is no consistent effect of fluoride on vertebral or nonvertebral fracture, which might actually increase when high doses of fluoride are used. Furthermore, animal data suggest that there is reduced biomechanical strength when fluoride is incorporated into bone as fluoroapatite, with excess osteoid accumulation and evidence of woven rather than lamellar bone formation, especially at high doses. For these reasons, fluoride remains an experimental agent, despite its long history and multiple studies.

OTHER POTENTIAL ANABOLIC AGENTS Several small studies of growth hormone (GH), alone or in combination with other agents, have not shown consistent or substantial positive effects on skeletal mass. Many of these studies are relatively short-term, and the effects of GH

FIGURE 342-10 Number of incident vertebral deformities (15% and 20% reductions) in women with osteoporosis on HRT, compared to HRT + PTH over 3 years. (HRT, hormone-replacement therapy; PTH, parathyroid hormone.) *(From Lindsay et al.)*

and the IGFs are still under investigation. Anabolic steroids, mostly derivatives of testosterone, act primarily as antiresorptive agents to reduce bone turnover but may also stimulate osteoblastic activity. Effects on bone mass remain unclear but appear weak, in general, and use is limited by masculinizing side effects. Several recent observational studies suggest that the statin drugs, currently used to treat hypercholesterolemia, may be associated with increased bone mass and reduced fractures, but there are not clinical trial data.

Nonpharmacologic Approaches   Protective pads worn around the outer thigh, which cover the trochanteric region of the hip can prevent hip fractures in elderly residents in nursing homes. The use of hip protectors is limited largely by compliance and comfort, but new devices are being developed that may circumvent these problems and provide adjunctive treatments.

Treatment Monitoring   There are currently no well-accepted guidelines for monitoring treatment of osteoporosis. Because most osteoporosis treatments produce small or moderate bone mass increments on average, it is reasonable to consider BMD as a monitoring tool. As with any biologic or assay determination, there is precision error with repeated measurements. Changes must exceed ~4% in the spine and 6% in the hip to be considered significant in any individual. The hip is the preferred site due to larger surface area and greater reproducibility. Medication-induced increments may require several years to produce changes of this magnitude (if they do at all). Consequently, it can be argued that BMD should not be repeated at intervals <2 years. Only significant BMD reductions should prompt a change in medical regimen, as it is expected that many individuals will not show responses greater than the detection limits of the current measurement techniques.

Biochemical markers of bone turnover may prove useful for treatment monitoring, but there is currently little hard evidence to support this concept; it remains unclear which endpoint is most useful. If bone turnover markers are used, a determination should be made before starting therapy and repeated ≥4 months after therapy is initiated. In general, a change in bone turnover markers must be 30 to 40% lower than the baseline to be significant because of the biologic and technical variability in these tests. A positive change in biochemical markers and/or bone density can be useful to help patients adhere to treatment regimens.

GLUCOCORTICOID-INDUCED OSTEOPOROSIS   Osteoporotic fractures are a well-characterized consequence of the hypercortisolism associated with Cushing's syndrome. However, the therapeutic use of glucocorticoids is by far the most common form of glucocorticoid-induced osteoporosis. Glucocorticoids are widely used in the treatment of a variety of disorders, including chronic lung disorders, rheumatoid arthritis and other connective tissue diseases, inflammatory bowel disease, and posttransplantation. Osteoporosis and related fractures are serious side effects of chronic glucocorticoid therapy. Because the effects of glucocorticoids on the skeleton are often superimposed upon the consequences of aging and menopause, it is not surprising that women and the elderly are most frequently affected. The skeletal response to steroids is remarkably heterogeneous, however, and even young, growing individuals treated with glucocorticoids can present with fractures.

The risk of fractures depends on the dose and duration of glucocorticoid therapy. Thus, cumulative dose is an important determinant of fracture risk. Bone loss is more rapid during the early months of treatment, and trabecular bone is more severely affected than cortical bone. Bone loss has been documented with the use of oral prednisone at doses that are generally considered to be less than replacement levels, and the lower threshold is not known. High-dose inhaled glucocorticoids can produce systemic effects on the skeleton, as can intra-articular injections. Alternate-day delivery does not appear to ameliorate the skeletal effects of glucocorticoids. The prevalence of vertebral fractures in asthmatic patients treated for 1 year with glucocorticoids is 11%, and increased risk of fractures has been demonstrated in most other disease states treated with glucocorticoids.

Pathophysiology   Glucocorticoids increase bone loss by multiple mechanisms including: (1) inhibition of osteoblast function and potential increase in osteoblast apoptosis, resulting in impaired synthesis of new bone; (2) stimulation of bone resorption, probably as a secondary effect; (3) impairment of the absorption of calcium across the intestine, probably by a vitamin D–independent effect; (4) increase of urinary calcium loss and induction of some degree of secondary hyperparathyroidism; (5) reduction of adrenal androgens and suppression of ovarian and testicular secretion of estrogens and androgens; and (6) potential induction of glucocorticoid myopathy, which may exacerbate effects on skeletal and calcium homeostasis, as well as increase the risk of falls.

Evaluation of the Patient   Because of the prevalence of glucocorticoid-induced osteopenia, it is important to evaluate the status of the skeleton in all patients being initiated on or already receiving long-term glucocorticoid therapy. Modifiable risk factors should be identified, including those for falls. Examination should include height and muscle strength testing. Laboratory evaluation should include an assessment of 24-h urinary calcium. A task force of the American College of Rheumatology recommends that all patients who are being initiated on glucocorticoids and patients already on long-term (>6 months) glucocorticoids have measurement of bone mass at both the spine and hip using DXA. If only one skeletal site can be measured, it is best to assess the spine in individuals <60 years and the hip for those >60 years.

Prevention   Bone loss caused by glucocorticoids can be prevented, and the risk of fractures significantly reduced. Strategies must include using the lowest dose of glucocorticoid for disease management. Topical and inhaled routes of administration are preferred, where appropriate. Risk factor reduction is important, including smoking cessation, limitation of alcohol consumption, and participation in weight-bearing exercise, where appropriate. All patients should receive an adequate calcium and vitamin D intake from the diet or from supplements.

℞   **TREATMENT**   Only bisphosphonates have been demonstrated in large clinical trials to reduce the risk of fractures in patients being treated with glucocorticoids. Risedronate has been shown to prevent bone loss and to reduce vertebral fracture risk by about 70%. Similar beneficial effects are observed in studies of alendronate and etidronate. Controlled trials of HRT have shown bone-sparing effects, and calcitonin also has some protective effect. Thiazides reduce urine calcium loss, but their role in prevention of fractures is unclear.

BIBLIOGRAPHY

BERARD A et al: Meta-analysis of the effectiveness of physical activity for the prevention of bone loss in postmenopausal women. Osteoporos Int 7:331, 1997

CAULEY JA et al: Estrogen replacement therapy and fractures in older women. Study of Osteoporotic Fractures Research Group. Ann Intern Med 122:9, 1995

CHAPUY MC et al: Effect of calcium and cholecalciferol treatment for three years on hip fractures in elderly women. BMJ 308:1081, 1994

COLLABORATIVE GROUP ON HORMONAL FACTORS IN BREAST CANCER: Breast cancer and hormone replacement therapy: Collaborative reanalysis of data from 51 epidemiological studies of 52705 women with breast cancer and 108411 women without breast cancer. Lancet 350:1047, 1997

COSMAN F, LINDSAY R Selective estrogen receptors modulators: Clinical spectrum. Endocr Rev 20: 418, 1999

CUMMINGS SR et al: The effect of raloxifene on risk of breast cancer in postmenopausal women: Results from the MORE randomized trial. Multiple Outcomes of Raloxifene Evaluation. JAMA 281:2189, 1999

EARLY BREAST CANCER TRIALISTS COLLABORATIVE GROUP: Tamoxifen for early breast cancer: An overview of the randomised trials. Lancet 351:1451, 1998

EASTELL RD: Treatment of postmenopausal osteoporosis. N Engl J Med 338:736, 1998

ETTINGER B et al: Reduction of vertebral fracture risk in postmenopausal women with osteoporosis treated with raloxifene: Results from a 3-year randomized clinical trial. Multiple Outcomes of Raloxifene Evaluation (MORE) Investigators. JAMA 282:637, 1999

GREGG EW et al: Physical activity and osteoporotic fracture risk in older women. Ann Intern Med 129:81, 1998

HARRIS ST et al: Effects of risedronate treatment on vertebral and nonvertebral fractures in women with postmenopausal osteoporosis: A randomized controlled trial. Vertebral Efficacy with Risedronate Therapy (VERT) Study Group. JAMA 282:1344, 1999

HOSKING D et al: Prevention of bone loss with alendronate in postmenopausal woman under 60 years of age. N Engl J Med 338: 485, 1998

HULLEY S et al: Randomized trial of estrogen plus progestin for secondary prevention of coronary heart disease in postmenopausal women. Heart and Estrogen/progestin Replacement Study (HERS) Research Group. JAMA 280:605, 1998

LINDSAY R: Clinical utility of biochemical markers. Osteoporos Int 9 (Suppl): S29, 1999

——— et al: Randomized controlled study of effect of parathyroid hormone on vertebral-bone mass and fracture incidence among postmenopausal women on estrogen with osteoporosis. Lancet 350:550, 1997

MARCUS R et al: *Osteoporosis*. San Diego, Academic, 1996, pp. 1–1373

OVERGAARD K et al: Effect of calcitonin given intranasally on bone mass and fracture rates in a dose response study. BJM 305:556, 1992

PAK CY et al: Treatment of postmenopausal osteoporosis with slow release sodium fluoride. Final report of a randomized controlled trial. Ann Intern Med 123:401, 1995

POLS HAP et al: Multinational, placebo-controlled, randomized trial of the effects of alendronate on bone density and fracture risk in postmenopausal women with low bone mass: Results of the FOSIT study. Fosamax International Trial Study Group. Osteoporosis Int 9: 461, 1999

SAAG KG et al: Alendronate for the prevention and treatment of glucocorticoid-induced osteoporosis. Glucocorticoid-Induced Osteoporosis Intervention Study Group. N Engl J Med 339:292, 1998

WASNICH RD et al: Antifracture efficacy of antiresorptive agents are related to changes in bone density. J Clin Endocrinol Metab 85: 231, 2000

343   *Stephen M. Krane, Alan L. Schiller*

PAGET'S DISEASE AND OTHER DYSPLASIAS OF BONE

PAGET'S DISEASE OF BONE

Paget's disease of bone (osteitis deformans) is characterized by excessive resorption of bone by osteoclasts, followed by the replacement of normal marrow by vascular, fibrous connective tissue. At some stage and to a variable degree, the resorbed bone is replaced by coarse-fibered, dense trabecular bone organized in haphazard fashion. The irregular and often rapid deposition of this new bone, to a great extent still lamellar, results in an increase in the number of prominent, irregular cement lines that give the bone its characteristic "mosaic" pattern. Most lesions show both excessive resorption and chaotic new bone formation. The disorder is usually focal but may be widespread.

INCIDENCE The prevalence is difficult to determine because the disease is often asymptomatic. It is frequently detected when roentgenograms are obtained for other reasons or because of a high level of alkaline phosphatase on routine blood screening. On the basis of autopsy examination, the incidence is estimated to be about 3% in individuals over age 40; the likelihood of occurrence increases with age. The incidence varies in different parts of the world. Radiologic surveys indicate that the frequency in adults is <1% in the United States, Great Britain, and Australia. In India, Japan, the Middle East, and Scandinavia, the disease is rare.

ETIOLOGY The cause is unknown. Some of the manifestations can be suppressed with glucocorticoids, salicylates, and cytotoxic drugs, but there is no convincing evidence that the fundamental lesion is inflammatory. Intranuclear inclusions have been found by electron microscopy in osteoclasts in pagetic bone. Some of the inclusions resemble nucleocapsids of viruses belonging to the measles group. Indirect immunofluorescence studies using antibodies to measles virus suggest that the inclusions are indeed measles virus nucleocapsids. The presence of mutations in specific regions of the viral genome is consistent with persistent infection. In some individuals with Paget's disease, osteoclasts and bone marrow mononuclear cells contain nucleocapsids of respiratory syncytial virus alone or in addition to nucleocapsids of measles virus; in some areas of Britain, canine distemper virus sequences have been identified in pagetic bone cells. Thus, different paramyxoviruses may have roles in the initiation or propagation of Paget's disease. Further evidence supporting the potential role of measles virus in the pathogenesis of the excessive bone resorption in Paget's disease has been obtained from studies of osteoclast precursors in vitro. Normal bone marrow–derived CD34+ cells transduced with a measles virus nucleocapsid gene differentiate into abnormal multinucleated osteoclasts that can resorb bone.

There is renewed interest in genetic factors that might be important in the predisposition to and pathogenesis of Paget's disease. Several large kindreds have been identified in which Paget's disease affects two or more generations with a pattern of inheritance consistent with autosomal dominant transmission. A rare Paget's disease–like disorder, familial expansile osteolysis, has been mapped to chromosome 18q21-22; Paget's disease was mapped to the same locus in several families. However, in other families with Paget's disease, there is no linkage to 18q21-22, indicating genetic heterogeneity. In some sporadic osteosarcomas, there is constitutional loss of heterozygosity mapped to the same region of chromosome 18, and the rare sarcomas associated with Paget's disease (see below) also exhibit loss of heterozygosity in this region. It is of great interest that the gene within the 18q21-22 locus (*TNFRS-F11A* gene) responsible for familial expansile osteolysis encodes the receptor activator of NfκB (RANK), a member of the tumor necrosis factor (TNF) superfamily crucial for osteoclast differentiation (see below). The mutation results in constitutive activation of RANK. It is unknown whether similar mutations occur in some individuals with Paget's disease.

PATHOPHYSIOLOGY The characteristic feature is increased resorption of bone accompanied by an increase in bone formation. In the early phase, bone resorption predominates (e.g., in the variant *osteoporosis circumscripta*) and the bones are very vascular. This has been termed the *osteoporotic, osteolytic*, or *destructive phase* of disease. Body calcium balance may be negative. Commonly, the excessive resorption is followed closely by formation of new pagetic bone. In this so-called mixed phase of the disease, the rate of bone formation is so geared to that of bone resorption that the magnitude of the increase in bone turnover is not reflected in the overall calcium balance. As the activity decreases, the resorptive rate may decline progressively relative to formation, eventually leading to development of hard, dense, less vascular bone (the so-called *osteoplastic* or *sclerotic phase*) and a positive calcium balance. The rates of bone turnover may be increased enormously in the early phases of the disease, occasionally more than 20 times normal.

Increased generation and overactivity of osteoclasts are considered the major abnormality. The osteoclasts are larger than normal and contain multiple pleomorphic nuclei. Increased numbers of osteoclast-like multinucleated cells are generated from hematopoietic precursors in long-term marrow cultures from individuals with Paget's disease. Production of interleukin (IL) 6 by the pagetic bone (marrow) cells is increased, and the cells are more sensitive than normal to the proresorptive effects of $1,25(OH)_2D_3$.

The calcification rate is characteristically increased in pagetic bone. Bone turnover correlates with the increased plasma level of bone alkaline phosphatase, which is higher in Paget's disease than in any other condition except for hereditary hyperphosphatasia. Although increased bone resorption enhances release of calcium and phosphate ions from bone, the plasma concentrations of these ions are usually normal, presumably because of mineral deposition in new bone and because of feedback control of parathyroid hormone secretion. The concentration of phosphate in the plasma is normal or slightly elevated. When the imbalance between bone formation and resorption favors resorption, as after prolonged immobilization or fractures, urinary calcium excretion may be increased and on occasion hypercalcemia may occur. If, on the other hand, bone formation exceeds resorption (relatively uncommon), circulating levels of parathyroid hormone may be increased. Significant increases in trabecular bone resorption and osteoid surfaces in normal bone from patients with Paget's disease may be due to compensatory, secondary hyperparathyroidism. Resorption involves both the organic and mineral phases of bone. While the inorganic ions of the mineral phase are reutilized for bone formation, amino acids such as hydroxyproline and hydroxylysine and the hydroxypyridinium cross-link compounds are released during resorption of the collagen matrix of bone and are not reutilized for collagen biosynthesis. The increased urinary excretion of small peptides containing hydroxyproline reflects increased bone resorption. The pyridinium cross-link compounds pyridinoline (Pyr) and deoxypyridinoline (D-Pyr) are released from bone collagen during osteoclastic bone resorption and can be measured in urine by several commercial assays. The C- and N-telopeptide measurements are also useful for monitoring therapy, but measurements of serum alkaline phosphatase activity alone are usually sufficient.

RADIOLOGIC CHANGES   The pelvic bones are most commonly involved, followed by the femur, skull, tibia, lumbosacral spine, dorsal spine, clavicles, and ribs; small bones are not as frequently diseased. The lytic phase of the disease may be overlooked except when it occurs in the skull as osteoporosis circumscripta, with areas of sharply demarcated radiolucency in the frontal, parietal, and occipital bones. In the long bones, the lytic areas are usually first seen at one end and progress toward the other end with a V-shaped advancing edge. The lesion may cause expansion of the cortex and exhibit features suggesting malignancy. Usually lysis is followed by a zone of increased density, representing the new bone formation of the mixed phase of the disease. In general, the bone enlarges with an irregularly widened cortex in a coarse, striated pattern and with increased density, occasionally focal in distribution. Perpendicular lines of radiolucency (cortical infractions) are frequent and occur on the convex side of bowed long bones, particularly the femur and tibia. The remodeling of the pagetic bone usually follows the lines of stress produced by muscle pull or gravity, accounting for the characteristic lateral bowing of the femur or anterior bowing of the tibia and the tendency for most of the dense bone to be deposited on the concave side of the bowed bone. In the mixed stage, there is enlargement and thickening of the skull, especially of the outer table, with irregular, spotty areas of increased density (Fig. 343-1). The changes in the pelvis reflect the varying degrees of bone resorption and new bone formation and are frequently accompanied by a characteristic thickening of the pelvic brim. In the sclerotic phase of the disease, the bone may show uniform increase in density, often in the absence of striations. This feature is common in the facial bones but occasionally occurs in the vertebrae, where a homogeneous, dense pattern gives an "ivory" appearance sim-

ilar to that typical of Hodgkin's disease, although the involved vertebrae in Hodgkin's disease are not enlarged. Computed tomography (CT) and magnetic resonance imaging (MRI) are useful in defining atypical lesions, particularly when neoplastic involvement is suspected. Technetium 99m diphosphonate bone scans are useful in documenting the extent of disease when therapy is contemplated or to confirm the diagnosis when radiologic findings are inconclusive.

CLINICAL MANIFESTATIONS   The clinical presentation is a function of the extent of the disease, the particular bones involved, and the presence of complications. Many patients are asymptomatic. In these individuals the disorder is discovered during radiologic examination of the pelvis or spine for another problem or because of the finding of an elevated level of plasma alkaline phosphatase. Other individuals may gradually become aware of a swelling or deformity of a long bone or develop a disturbance in gait due to unequal length of the lower extremities. Enlargement of the skull is often not noticed by the patients, except by awareness of increasing hat size. Facial pain and headache are initial complaints in some; backache and leg pain are common. The pain is usually dull but may be shooting or knifelike. Back pain is most common in the lumbar region and may radiate into the buttocks or lower extremities. This pain can be due to the pagetic process itself, to distortion of articular facets, or to secondary osteoarthritis. Pain in the lower extremities may be associated with the transverse cortical infractions along the convex lateral surface of the femur or the anterior surface of the tibia. New lytic lesions detected on bone scan may be the most painful. Pain may also be due to involvement of the hip joint resembling degenerative joint disease, which is characterized by narrowing of the joint space, bony lipping at the margin of the acetabulum, and deepening of the acetabulum. Angioid streaks may be present in the retina. Hearing loss can be due to direct involvement of the ossicles of the inner ear, involvement of bone in the region of the cochlea, or impingement on the eighth cranial nerve in the auditory foramen. More serious neurologic complications can result from overgrowth of bone at the base of the skull (platybasia) and compression of the brainstem. Compression of the spinal cord can cause paraplegia, particularly with involvement of the mid-dorsal spine. Pathologic fractures of vertebrae may also produce spinal cord lesions.

COMPLICATIONS   Blood flow may be markedly increased in extremities involved with Paget's disease. There is proliferation of blood vessels in pagetic bone, but anatomic and functional studies have not confirmed the presence of arteriovenous fistulas. Although blood flow is increased in bone, cutaneous vasodilatation in the pagetic extremities accounts for the increased warmth noted clinically. When the disease is widespread, involving one-third or more of the skeleton, the increased blood flow raises *cardiac output* and rarely leads to high-output heart failure. However, heart disease in individuals with Paget's disease is usually due to the same conditions that occur in other patients of similar age. *Pathologic fracture* may occur at any stage but is more common in the destructive phase of the disease. In the weight-bearing bones fractures are often incomplete, multiple, and on the convex side of the bone. They may occur spontaneously or after slight trauma. Though many lesions heal with no major disability, more serious fractures also occur. Complete fractures are often transverse as if the bone was snapped like a piece of chalk.

There is no characteristic level of urinary calcium excretion, but it tends to be higher when the resorptive phase predominates, possibly accounting for the somewhat higher incidence of *urinary stones* in these patients. *Hyperuricemia* and gout are common in men with Paget's disease, and calcific periarthritis may occur.

Sarcoma is the dread complication. The incidence is probably ≤1%, although higher incidence has been noted in series that include many patients with polyostotic involvement. The sarcomas most frequently arise in the femur, humerus, skull, facial bones, and pelvis and rarely in the vertebrae. Pagetic osteosarcomas are lytic in appearance on radiographs, in contrast to the sclerotic appearance of radiation-induced osteosarcomas. The tumors are multicentric in about 20% of patients. Fibrosarcomas and chondrosarcomas have also been found.

FIGURE 343-1   Lateral roentgenogram of the skull from a 58-year-old woman with Paget's disease of bone.

Pain and swelling are the common complaints that lead to recognition of the sarcomas. The extent and character of the neoplastic involvement are established by CT and/or MRI. In occasional patients, an "explosive rise" of the phosphatase level may accompany the growth of the sarcoma, whereas in patients with limited Paget's disease, phosphatase levels may be only slightly elevated and give no clue to the development of the malignant lesion. The prognosis is poor following the development of sarcomas, and ablative surgery is rarely successful. In contrast to the successful treatment of some osteosarcomas in children, chemotherapy has little effect on survival of patients with pagetic osteosarcomas. Reparative granulomas resembling giant cell tumors may cause local destruction, but they do not metastasize.

TREATMENT Most patients require no treatment, since the disease is localized and does not cause symptoms. Indications for therapy include persistent pain in involved bones, neural compression, rapidly progressive deformity resulting in disabling disturbance of posture and/or gait, high-output congestive heart failure, hypercalcemia, severe hypercalciuria with or without formation of renal stones, repeated fractures or nonunion, and preparation for major orthopedic surgery. Nonsteroidal anti-inflamatory drugs, such as one of the COX2 inhibitors or acetaminophen, may be useful to relieve pain, especially that involving the hip joints. Patients with severe hip or knee pain, unrelieved by analgesics and not responsive to therapy with agents that inhibit bone resorption, are candidates for total joint replacement. Results of joint replacement are often excellent, although patients with Paget's disease have an increased risk of ectopic bone formation around the operative site. Osteotomies are also useful in patients with bowing deformities of the tibia. In patients who have undergone surgical procedures, early ambulation and adequate fluid intake are important to prevent the development of hypercalciuria and hypercalcemia.

Potent bisphosphonates can inhibit bone resorption and are usually well tolerated. They appear to act by adsorbing to the surface of the calcium/phosphate mineral phase of bone and inhibiting osteoclast function. Bisphosphates are chemically stable analogues of inorganic pyrophosphate and are available in two classes: nitrogen-containing and non-nitrogen-containing. The non-nitrogen-containing bisphosphates (e.g., clodronate and etidronate) are metabolically incorporated into nonhydrolyzable analogues of ATP that may inhibit ATP-mediated reactions. The nitrogen-containing bisphosphates (e.g., pamidronate, alendronate, and risedronate) do not form ATP compounds, but they do inhibit enzymes in the mevalonate pathway, particularly enzymes involved in the synthesis of farnesyl pyrophosphate and geranylgeranyl pyrophosphate. The latter compounds are involved in protein prenylation reactions.

The first bisphosphate available for treatment of Paget's disease in the United States, editronate, was moderately effective in alleviating symptoms but did not decrease biochemical indices to the normal range. Editronate also inhibits mineralization of bone and produces osteomalacia. The newer bisphosphonates such as alendronate, pamidronate, risedronate, and tiludronate are more potent than etidronate and do not produce mineralization defects. Consequently, editronate is no longer indicated for treatment of Paget's disease. In the United States, pamidronate is approved for intravenous use, and alendronate and risedronate are approved for oral administration.

The bisphosphonates as a class are poorly absorbed from the gastrointestinal tract. Alendronate should be given orally with water after an overnight fast 30 to 60 min before breakfast; the dose is 40 mg/d for 6 months. Risedronate is administered at 30 mg/d for 2 to 3 months. Gastric irritability and rarely esophageal ulcerations may occur. Several regimens are advocated for the intravenous administration of pamidronate. For example, pamidronate is used intravenously as an infusion of 30 mg/d over 3 to 4 h in 5% glucose in water or normal saline on three or four successive days. Responses are usually rapid, with decreases in urinary excretion of hydroxyproline and pyridinium cross-link compounds within days to weeks, followed by a fall in levels of serum alkaline phosphatase. Flulike symptoms accompanied by fever may occur but usually subside rapidly.

Patients given bisphosphonates should also be given daily calcium supplements of 1 to 1.5 g and approximately 400 IU of vitamin D. Clinical and biochemical improvement often lasts for more than a year after bisphosphonate therapy. Clinical evaluation and assessment of alkaline phosphatase levels at 3-month intervals are useful for assessing the need for retreatment. Radiographs at 6-month intervals may be indicated for evaluation of lytic lesions, which usually heal with these agents.

Calcitonin therapy has largely been replaced by bisphosphonates for primary treatment of severe disease, but calcitonin may still be useful in patients who cannot tolerate alendronate or residronate because of gastrointestinal side effects or who prefer to avoid intravenous therapy with pamidronate. The administration of porcine, salmon, and human *calcitonins* for prolonged periods decreases plasma alkaline phosphatase and urinary hydroxyproline excretion. Treatment with calcitonin variably decreases bone pain due to suppression of the pagetic lesion as well as to an independent, centrally mediated analgesic effect. The calcitonins are probably most useful in patients with pain in areas of pagetic involvement not due to associated joint disease. The dose of salmon calcitonin is 50 to 100 MRC units daily given subcutaneously. In most cases, it is possible to reduce the dose to three times weekly. Some patients develop a sensation of warmth and/or nausea 30 min to several hours after injection. Nasal spray formulations of calcitonin can be administered at doses of 200 IU/d. Cytotoxic drugs such as plicamycin and dactinomycin no longer have a place in therapy.

Although the bisphosphonates and calcitonins act primarily to decrease bone resorption, the rate of new bone formation subsequently falls. As a result, the state of high bone turnover is shifted to a state of lower turnover, where rates of formation and resorption are still apparently geared to each other. In this lower turnover state, collagen fibers of the bone matrix are deposited in a more orderly fashion similar to normal bone.

HYPEROSTOSIS

A number of disease states have in common an increase in the mass of bone per unit volume (*hyperostosis*) (Table 343-1). This increase in bone mass is often associated with disturbance in the architecture of the tissue. The additional bone may be located at the periosteum, within the compact bone of the cortex, or in the trabeculae of the cancellous regions. In some diseases, the increase in bone mass may be spotty, as in osteopoikilosis, whereas in others, most of the skeleton may be involved, as in the malignant form of osteopetrosis in children. The increase in mass is usually not due to an excessive amount of mineral relative to matrix, except in disorders where islands of calcified cartilage may persist such as osteopetrosis. In some diseases, such as the osteosclerosis of untreated renal insufficiency, bone mass and radiodensity may be increased, even though the new bone formed is poorly mineralized and contains widened osteoid seams.

Although hyperostosis is usually due to decreased numbers of osteoclasts or altered osteoclast function, dysfunction of osteoblasts can also occur. For example, an engineered null mutation of the osteocalcin gene in mice results in a higher bone mass due to increased bone formation without change in bone resorption. Infection of newborn mice also produces an osteopetrosis-like phenotype in which osteoblast progenitors appear to induce increased bone formation. In human osteopetrosis of the relatively benign and sporadic type, viral nucleocapsid particles have been found in osteoclasts, and it is possible that viral infection accounts for the excessive bone mass.

OSTEOPETROSIS Also known as Albers-Schönberg or marble bone disease, osteopetrosis is clinically, biochemically, and genetically heterogeneous. Although osteopetrosis has many causes, a defect in bone resorption is always the underlying mechanism.

Table 343-1   Causes of Hyperostosis

Endocrine disorders
  Primary hyperparathyroidism
  Hypothyroidism
  Acromegaly
Radiation osteitis
Chemical poisoning
  Fluoride
  Elemental phosphorus
  Beryllium
  Arsenic
  Vitamin A intoxication
  Lead
  Bismuth
Osteomalacia
  Renal tubular osteomalacia (vitamin D resistance or phosphate diabetes)
  Chronic renal glomerular failure
Osteosclerosis (localized) associated with chronic infection
Osteosclerotic phase of Paget's disease
Osteosclerosis associated with carcinomatous metastases, malignant lymphoma, and hematologic disorders (myeloproliferative disorders, sickle cell disease, leukemia, multiple myeloma, systemic mastocytosis)
Osteosclerosis of erythroblastosis fetalis
Osteopetrosis
  Infantile (malignant, autosomal recessive form)
  Adult (benign, dominant form)
  Intermediate form with carbonic anhydrase II deficiency and renal tubular acidosis
Unclassified disorders
  Pyknodysostosis
  Osteomyelosclerosis
  Hyperostosis corticalis generalisata
  Hyperostosis generalisata with pachydermia
  Hereditary hyperphosphatasia
  Progressive diaphyseal dysplasia (osteopathia hyperostotica multiplex infantilis; Camurati-Engelmann disease)
  Melorheostosis
  Osteopoikilosis
  Hyperostosis frontalis interna

Several inherited forms of osteopetrosis occur in rodents, some of which can be cured by bone marrow transplantation from a normal littermate and are probably due to stem cell defects. The osteopetrosis in *op/op* mice and in *tl/tl* toothless rats is not cured by bone marrow transplantation, however. These animals have few osteoclasts, and those that are present appear to be defective. The *op/op* mice have a defect in the coding region of the gene for macrophage colony stimulating factor (M-CSF). The skeletal defects in these animals and in *tl/tl* rats can be reversed by treatment with M-CSF. Another form of osteopetrosis has been produced in mice by targeted disruption of the c-*src* gene, which is normally expressed at high levels in osteoclasts. These *src*−/− mice still have osteoclasts on bone surfaces, but they fail to form a ruffled border at the bone-resorbing surface. Disruption of the c-*fos* gene results in osteopetrosis in which osteoclasts are absent.

Important advances have also been made in understanding the interactions between osteoblasts/stromal cells and hemopoietic osteoclast precursor cells that lead to osteoclastogenesis (Fig. 343-2). A novel member of the TNF receptor superfamily, referred to as *osteoprotegerin* (OPG; also known as *osteoclastogenesis inhibitory factor*, OCIF) functions as a soluble decoy receptor that binds, and presumably neutralizes, RANK ligand, a transmembrane ligand expressed on osteoblasts/stromal cells. RANK ligand binds to RANK, a transmembrane receptor on hemopoietic osteoclast precursor cells, to activate osteoclast differentiation and function (Chap. 340). The RANK receptor binds to intracellular signaling molecules called *TNF receptor–associated factors* (TRAFs) that activate NFκB, a transcription factor known to be required for normal osteoclast function. Genetic models in mice are beginning to unravel this complex signaling pathway. Ex-

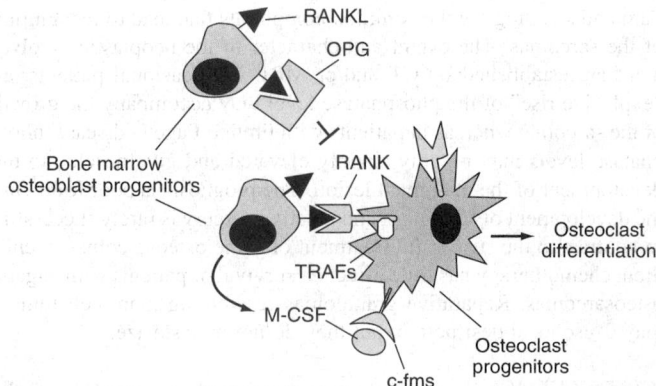

FIGURE 343-2   Role of the RANK pathway in osteoclast differentiation and function. Stromal bone marrow cells produce multiple growth factors and cytokines, including macrophage colony stimulating factor (M-CSF), to modulate osteoclastogenesis. RANKL (receptor activator of NFκB ligand) is produced by osteoblast progenitors. It can bind to a soluble decoy receptor known as OPG (osteoprotegerin) to inhibit action of the RANKL. Alternatively, a cell-cell interaction between osteoblast and osteoclast progenitors allows RANKL to bind to its membrane-bound receptor, RANK, thereby stimulating osteoclast differentiation and function. RANK binds intracellular proteins called TRAFs (tumor necrosis factor receptor–associated factors) that mediate receptor signaling through transcription factors such as NFκB. M-CSF binds to its receptor, c-fms, the cellular homologue of the *fms* oncogene. See text for the potential role of these pathways in disorders of osteoclast function such as osteopetrosis.

pression of a soluble version of RANK ligand stimulates osteoclast differentiation. Overexpression of OPG in transgenic mice leads to osteopetrosis, apparently by blocking RANK ligand. Mice deficient in RANK lack osteoclasts and develop severe osteopetrosis (as well as T cell immunologic defects). TRAF6-deficient mice also develop osteopetrotic features because of defective osteoclast function. It is clear, based on these and other lines of evidence, that the RANK ligand/OPG/RANK/TRAF/NFκB pathway plays a pivotal role in the control of osteoclast development and function.

In humans the infantile autosomal recessive form of osteopetrosis, until recently, has been of unknown cause. It is a severe bone disease that is usually fatal within the first decade of life. Osteoclasts are usually present in normal or increased numbers. In addition, since bone resorption is markedly suppressed, it has been assumed that the defect is not in genes responsible for osteoclast differentiation but in those responsible for osteoclast function. This form of osteopetrosis is manifested in utero and progresses after birth with anemia, hepatosplenomegaly, hydrocephalus, cranial nerve involvement, and death, often due to infections. Transplantation of bone marrow from allogeneic donors to provide normal osteoclast precursor cells has been successful in several patients, in whom osteopetrotic bone was repopulated with donor osteoclasts that produced radiologic and/or bone-biopsy evidence of bone resorption. Nearly 100 bone marrow transplantations have been reported over the past 15 years. If the transplants are successful, markers of donor cells can be found in bone resorbing areas and skeletal improvement persists for years. Although restoration of visual acuity usually does not occur with successful transplantation, this is the only means of approaching cure even in mild cases. The genetic defect in about half of the subjects studied has now been identified. The gene in the human disease was mapped to chromosome 11q13, a region that contains several potential candidate genes. In mice, introduction of a null mutation in one of the genes in this region, *Tcirg1*, that encodes the osteoclast-specific (*OC116*) subunit of the vacuolar proton pump ([V]-type H⁺-ATPase) responsible for acidification of the extracellular compartment adjacent to the brush border, results in osteopetrosis with abundant osteoclasts. Furthermore a deletion of the 5′ portion of the gene is the cause for the defect in *oc/oc* mice with spontaneous osteopetrosis. In approximately half of the human subjects with the autosomal recessive form of osteopetrosis so far examined, missense, frameshift, or potential splicing mutations have just been identified in the homologous gene, *TC1RG1*. Thus, mutations in *TG1RG1* are a frequent, although not the sole, cause of this form of osteopetrosis.

Less fulminant forms of osteopetrosis occur in older children and adults. In some the disorder appears to be sporadic, and in others the osteopetrosis is inherited as an autosomal dominant trait and progresses with age; anemia is not as severe, neurologic abnormalities are not as frequent, and recurrent pathologic fractures are the main feature. Although the disorder is most common in infants and children, the diagnosis may be made in adults when roentgenograms are obtained because of fractures or unrelated diseases.

An "intermediate" form of autosomal recessive osteopetrosis has been described in kindreds in which the skeletal abnormality is associated with renal tubular acidosis and cerebral calcification. This form is compatible with long survival and is associated with profound impairment of the activity of one of the isoenzymes of carbonic anhydrase (carbonic anhydrase II). Carbonic anhydrase II is a major component of the system that generates the acid environment adjacent to the ruffled border of the osteoclast. Deficiency of the enzyme impairs bone resorption. The defect in remodeling results in disorganization of bone structure, with thickened cortices and lack of funnelization of metaphyses. Despite increased density, the bone may be abnormal mechanically and can fracture readily. Osteomalacia or rickets is sometimes a component of osteopetrosis in children.

Roentgenograms reveal uniformly dense, sclerotic bone, often with no distinction between the cortical and cancellous regions (Fig. 343-3). In the severe infantile form, there is persistence of the primary spongiosa with central calcified cartilage cores surrounded by woven bone. Osteoclasts may be increased in number but do not function normally due to the acidification defect that results from the mutated vacuolar proton pump. In other forms of osteopetrosis, there may be different morphologic abnormalities such as loss of ruffled borders. The variability may reflect heterogeneity in this syndrome, as in the osteopetrosis in rodents. The long bones are usually involved, with increased density along the entire shaft. The metaphyses have a characteristic clubbed or splayed appearance. Alternating horizontal bands of increased and decreased density in the long bones and vertebrae suggest that the defect is intermittent during periods of growth. The skull, pelvis, ribs, and other bones may be involved. The phalanges and the distal humerus are usually spared.

Encroachment of bone on the marrow cavity, particularly in the severe infantile disorder, is associated with anemia of the myelophthisic type with extramedullary hematopoiesis in liver, spleen, and lymph nodes and enlargement of these organs. Neurologic abnormal-

FIGURE 343-3 Roentgenogram of the spine and pelvis of a 55-year-old man with the more benign, dominant form of osteopetrosis.

ities caused by encroachment on cranial nerves include optic atrophy, nystagmus, papilledema, exophthalmos, and impairment of extraocular muscles. Facial paralysis and deafness are frequent; trigeminal lesions and anosmia are less common. In infants, macrocephaly, hydrocephalus, and convulsions may occur, and infections such as osteomyelitis are frequent. Renal tubular acidosis is a feature of the osteopetrosis associated with carbonic anhydrase II deficiency.

In the less severe forms, about half of patients have no symptoms, and the disorder is discovered incidentally on roentgenograms. Others present with fractures, bone pain, osteomyelitis, and cranial nerve palsies.

Fractures may occur with trivial trauma. Healing of such fractures is usually slow but satisfactory. When the disease is manifested first in adult life, fractures may be the only clinical problem. Levels of calcium and alkaline phosphatase in the plasma are usually normal in adults, but hypophosphatemia and moderate hypocalcemia may occur in children. Serum acid phosphatase levels are usually increased.

As mentioned, in children with severe osteopetrosis, bone marrow transplantation from allogeneic donors or HLA-identical siblings has resulted in histologic and radiologic increases in bone resorption and variable improvement in anemia, vision, hearing, and growth and development. Unfortunately, it is not always possible to find appropriate donors, or patients may not be good candidates for bone marrow transplantation. In some patients with the lethal forms of the disorder, calcitriol therapy is associated with the appearance of osteoclasts with normal ruffled borders and other evidence of increased bone resorption.

PYKNODYSOSTOSIS Pyknodysostosis is an autosomal recessive form of osteosclerosis that superficially resembles osteopetrosis. It is a form of short-limbed dwarfism associated with bone fragility and a tendency to fracture with minimal trauma. Nevertheless, life span is usually normal. In addition to a generalized increase in bone density, features include short stature; separated cranial sutures; hypoplasia of the mandible; kyphoscoliosis and deformities of the trunk; persistence of deciduous teeth; progressive acroosteolysis of the terminal phalanges; high, arched palate; proptosis; blue sclerae; and a pointed, beaked nose. Patients usually present because of frequent fractures. The disorder is caused by mutations in a gene on chromosome 1q21 that encodes cathepsin K, a cysteine protease that is expressed in normal osteoclasts. Null mutations in the cathepsin K gene in mice result in a phenotype with many features of pyknodysostosis. Osteoclasts are present but do not function normally since there is no proteinase secreted into the area adjacent to the ruffled border where bone collagen resorption normally takes place.

OSTEOMYELOSCLEROSIS In osteomyelosclerosis, the marrow cells are replaced by diffuse fibroplasia, occasionally accompanied by osseous metaplasia and increased skeletal density on roentgenograms. In early stages woven bone may be found in intratrabecular locations, whereas in more advanced stages, woven bone is observed in the medulla. The disorder is probably a phase in the course of the myeloproliferative disorders and is characteristically accompanied by extramedullary hematopoiesis.

Hyperostosis corticalis generalisata (van Buchem's disease) is characterized by osteosclerosis of the skull (base and calvaria), lower jaw, clavicles, and ribs and thickening of the diaphyseal cortices of the long and short bones. Alkaline phosphatase levels in the serum are elevated, and the disorder may be due to increased formation of bone of normal structure. The major manifestations are due to neural compression and consist of optic atrophy, facial paralysis, and perception deafness. In *hyperostosis generalisata with pachydermia* (Uehlinger), the sclerosis is due to increased formation of subperiosteal spongy bone and involves the epiphyses, metaphyses, and diaphyses. Pain, swelling of joints, and thickening of the skin of the lower arms are common.

HEREDITARY HYPERPHOSPHATASIA This disorder is characterized by structural deformities of the skeleton, with increased thickness of the calvaria, increased density at the base of the skull, and widening and loss of normal architecture of the shafts and the epiphyses of the long and short bones. The failure to deposit normal bone and the haphazard orientation of lamellae suggest active remodeling that resembles that of Paget's disease. Osteoclasts with multiple nuclei characteristic of Paget's disease and the typical "mosaic" pattern of faceted units of lamellar bone are not found, however. Levels of plasma alkaline phosphatase and urinary excretion of hydroxyproline peptides and other collagen-degradation products are increased. The disorder is apparently inherited as an autosomal recessive trait. Treatment with bisphosphonates or calcitonin therapy may be of value.

PROGRESSIVE DIAPHYSEAL DYSPLASIA (CAMU-RATI-ENGELMANN DISEASE) This is an autosomal dominant disorder in which a symmetric thickening and increased diameter of the diaphyses of long bones occurs, particularly in the femur, tibia, fibula, radius, and ulna. Pain over affected areas, fatigue, abnormal gait, and muscle wasting are the major manifestations. Serum alkaline phosphatase levels may be elevated, and, on occasion, hypocalcemia and hyperphosphatemia may be found. Other abnormalities include anemia, leukopenia, and an elevated erythrocyte sedimentation rate. Linkage studies have localized a candidate gene (*DPD1*) to chromosome 19q13.2. Clinical and biochemical improvement may result from the use of glucocorticoids.

MELORHEOSTOSIS This rare, sporadic condition usually begins in childhood and is characterized by a slowly progressive linear hyperostosis in one or more bones of one limb, usually in a lower extremity. All segments of the bone may be involved, with sclerotic areas that have a "flowing" distribution. The involved limb is often extremely painful. Soft tissue masses, not connected to bone, are often mineralized and are composed of osseous or cartilaginous tissue. Other types of soft tissue masses are associated with joint contractures or consist of fibrofatty, lymphatic, or vascular tissue.

OSTEOPOIKILOSIS This is a benign autosomal dominant trait usually discovered by chance. In some families, the occurrence of melorheostosis suggests that these disorders may involve the same genetic locus. Osteopoikilosis is characterized by dense spots of trabecular bone <1 cm in diameter, usually of uniform density, located in the epiphyses and adjacent parts of the metaphyses. All bones may be involved except the skull, ribs, and vertebrae.

HYPEROSTOSIS FRONTALIS INTERNA This is an abnormality of the inner table of the frontal bones of the skull consisting of smooth, rounded enostoses covered by dura and projecting into the cranial cavity. These enostoses are usually <1 cm at their greatest diameter and do not extend posteriorly beyond the coronal suture. The abnormality is found almost exclusively in women who are frequently obese, hirsute, and may have a variety of neuropsychiatric complaints (Morgagni-Stewart-Morel syndrome). The disorder also occurs in women with no obvious illness or particular associated disease. The finding in the skull may be a manifestation of a generalized metabolic disorder.

FIBROUS DYSPLASIA (MCCUNE-ALBRIGHT SYNDROME)

The bony lesions of fibrous dysplasia are characterized by proliferation of fibroblast-like cells that in some areas have features of osteoblasts, with production of an extracellular matrix that may be calcified and have the appearance of woven bone. In other areas the cells have features of chondrocytes and produce a cartilage-like extracellular matrix. The lesions of fibrous dysplasia are usually focal and have a radiolucent appearance; they may be monostotic or polyostotic. The disorder occurs with equal frequency in both sexes. Some individuals have distinctive areas of skin pigmentation and precocious puberty (McCune-Albright syndrome) (Chap. 336). These diverse manifestations are the consequence of postzygotic mutations in the gene encoding the regulatory $G_{s\alpha}$ proteins.

INCIDENCE The monostotic form is the most common type of fibrous dysplasia. The lesions can be asymptomatic, can be associated with local pain, or predispose to pathologic fracture. Most of the lesions are in the ribs or in the craniofacial bones, especially the maxillae. Other bones that may be affected include metaphyseal or diaphyseal portions of the proximal femurs or tibias. Monostotic fibrous dysplasia is most often diagnosed in patients between 20 and 30 years of age. There are usually no associated skin lesions. Approximately one-quarter of the individuals with the polyostotic form have more than half the skeleton involved by disease. One side of the body may be affected, and the lesions may be distributed segmentally in a limb, particularly in the lower extremities. Craniofacial lesions are present in approximately half of patients with the polyostotic form. Whereas the monostotic form is usually detected in young adults, fractures and skeletal deformities occur in childhood in the polyostotic form; early-onset disease is generally more severe. Lesions, especially monostotic lesions, can become quiescent at puberty and worsen during pregnancy. McCune-Albright syndrome (polyostotic fibrous dysplasia, multiple café au lait spots, and sexual precocity) is more common (10:1) in females. Short stature is due to premature closure of the epiphyses.

PATHOPHYSIOLOGY Histologically, the lesions contain benign-appearing fibroblastic tissue arranged in a loose whorled pattern (Fig. 343-4). Malignant transformation of either monostotic or polyostotic fibrous dysplasia occurs with a frequency of <1%. The malignant change is usually detected in the third or fourth decade in individuals who have had lesions first identified in childhood. In about one-third of the cases the neoplasms arise in previously irradiated lesions. Ossifying fibroma of long bones is a peculiar fibroosseous cortical lesion that may be a variant of fibrous dysplasia. It is most common in the tibial shaft in teenagers. Although benign, the lesion has a tendency to recur if not adequately excised.

Fibrous dysplasia and McCune-Albright syndrome represent a phenotypic spectrum of disorders caused by activating mutations in the *GNAS1* gene, which encodes the $G_{s\alpha}$ protein. Because these postzygotic mutations occur at different stages in early development, the extent and type of tissues affected by the mutations are variable, explaining the mosaic pattern of skin and bone changes. The mutations occur in regions (e.g., Arg 201) of $G_{s\alpha}$ that selectively inhibit its GTPase activity. Because the GTP-bound form of the regulatory protein confers its active state (Chap. 341), the mutations confer constitutive stimulation of the cyclic AMP–protein kinase A signal transduction pathway. The mutations in *GNAS1* are also found in patients with fibrous dysplasia without manifestations of the McCune-Albright syndrome. Thus, in the boney lesions these mutations result in abnormalities in osteoblastic differentiation and the production of abnormal bone. In addition, there is an associated increase in osteoclastic bone resorption that provides a rationale for therapy with the bisphosphonate, pamidronate. Other tissues in which growth control and function are strongly regulated by $G_{s\alpha}$ protein–coupled receptors are particularly susceptible to the mutations. In addition to bone (parathyroid hormone receptor) and skin (melanocyte-stimulating hormone receptor), various endocrine glands, including the ovary (follicle-stimulating hormone receptor), thyroid (thyroid-stimulating hormone receptor), adrenal (ACTH-receptor), and pituitary (growth hormone–

FIGURE 343-4 Photomicrograph of the lesion of fibrous dysplasia. Note spicules of dark-staining woven bone (WB) surrounded by loose fibroblastic tissue.

releasing hormone receptor), are commonly affected by the $G_{s\alpha}$ mutations. It is of interest that the genetic abnormality in Albright's hereditary osteodystrophy (pseudohypoparathyroidism) is the opposite of that found in the McCune-Albright syndrome. In the former, alterations in $G_{s\alpha}$ function or expression result in *deficient* activity and decreased responsiveness to hormones that function through cyclic AMP–mediated signal transduction pathways (Chap. 341).

RADIOLOGIC CHANGES The roentgenographic appearance of the lesions is that of a radiolucent area with a well-delineated, smooth or scalloped border, typically associated with focal thinning of the cortex of the bone (Fig. 343-5). Fibrous dysplasia can cause bones to become larger than normal, a feature characteristic of Paget's disease as well. The "ground-glass" appearance is due to the thin spicules of calcified woven bone. Deformities can include coxa vara, shepherd's-crook deformity of the femur, bowing of the tibia, Harrison's grooves, and protrusio acetabuli. Involvement of facial bones, usually with lesions of increased radiodensity, may create a leonine appearance (*leontiasis ossea*). Fibrous dysplasia of the temporal bones can cause progressive loss of hearing and obliteration of the external ear canal. Advanced skeletal age in girls is correlated with sexual precocity but can occur in boys without sexual precocity. Occasionally, a focus of fibrous dysplasia may undergo cystic degeneration, with an enormous distortion of the shape of the bone, and mimic the so-called aneurysmal bone cyst.

CLINICAL MANIFESTATIONS The clinical course is variable. Skeletal lesions are usually detected because of localized pain, deformities, or fractures. Other symptoms ascribable to bone involvement are headache, seizures, cranial nerve abnormalities, hearing loss, narrowing of the external ear canal, or even spontaneous scalp hemorrhages if there is craniofacial bone disease. On rare occasions the onset of sexual precocity is the first clinical manifestation of the McCune-Albright syndrome. Serum calcium and phosphorus values are usually normal. In approximately one-third of patients with the polyostotic form, bone turnover is increased, as reflected by high levels of serum alkaline phosphatase and increased urinary excretion of collagen breakdown products. In some patients high cardiac output resembles that in extensive Paget's disease. Widespread disease does not usually develop when the disease is mild at the outset.

The cutaneous pigmentation in most patients with McCune-Albright syndrome consists of isolated dark-brown to light-brown macules that tend to be located on one side of the midline (Fig. 343-6). The border is usually, although not always, irregular or jagged ("coast of Maine"), in contrast to the smooth borders of the pigmented macules of neurofibromatosis ("coast of California"). As a rule, there are fewer than six of the lesions, which range in size from 1 cm to very large lesions, covering areas such as the back, buttocks, or sacral regions. When the lesions are in the scalp, the overlying hair may be more deeply pigmented. Localized alopecia is associated with osteomas of the skin, and such lesions tend to overly skeletal lesions. The pigmentation also tends to be on the same side as the skeletal lesions and actually to overlie them. Occasionally, neurofibromatosis and fibrous dysplasia coexist.

Sexual precocity occurs more commonly in girls than in boys. Premature vaginal bleeding, breast development, and growth of axillary and pubic hair are the usual features. Sexual precocity is due to autonomous end-organ activity, not to pituitary or hypothalamic dysfunction. Thus, girls have high estrogen levels and low or undetectable gonadotropins. The characteristic pigmented macules are usual but not invariable. Hyperthyroidism occurs with increased frequency, and rare associations include Cushing's syndrome, acromegaly, pulmonary lesions, and soft tissue myxomas. Hypophosphatemic osteomalacia may also accompany fibrous dysplasia and resembles the disorder associated with other skeletal and nonskeletal tumors.

Although the lytic lesions of fibrous dysplasia resemble the brown tumors of hyperparathyroidism, the age of the patient, normal calcium levels, increased density of bone in the skull, and areas of cutaneous pigmentation identify the former condition. Fibrous dysplasia and hyperparathyroidism may coexist, however. Neurofibromas may involve bone and produce cutaneous pigmentation as well as nodules in the skin. The pigmented macules of neurofibromatosis are more numerous and more widely distributed than in fibrous dysplasia, usually have smooth borders, and tend to involve areas such as the axillary folds. Other lesions that have roentgenographic features similar to those of isolated fibrous dysplasia are unicameral bone cysts, aneurysmal bone cysts, and nonossifying fibromas. Leontiasis ossea is most often due to fibrous dysplasia, although other disorders may also produce this appearance, such as craniometaphyseal dysplasia, hyperphosphatasia, and, in adults, Paget's disease.

℞ TREATMENT Fibrous dysplasia is not curable. The skeletal lesions, however, can be improved by orthopedic procedures such as casting, osteotomy with internal fixation, curettage, and bone grafting, depending on the lesion and the age of the patient. Indications for such procedures include progressive deformity, nonunion of fractures,

FIGURE 343-5 Roentgenogram of the upper extremity from a 33-year-old woman with fibrous dysplasia of bone. Typical lesions involve the entire humerus as well as the scapula and proximal ulna.

FIGURE 343-6 Typical pigmented café au lait lesion of the skin in an 11-year-old boy with polyostotic fibrous dysplasia. The border has the jagged "coast of Maine" appearance that is characteristic of McCune-Albright's syndrome. Note that the lesion is limited to one side (left) of the body.

and pain unresponsive to conservative treatment. Calcitonin may be effective in treatment of widespread disease associated with bone pain and high serum alkaline phosphatase levels. Pamidronate (0.5 to 1 mg/kg per day intravenously for 2 to 3 days) at 6-month or yearly intervals has been shown to reduce bone pain with refilling of osteolytic lesions in about half of patients and to decrease elevated levels of serum alkaline phosphatase and urinary hydroxyproline excretion. Precocious puberty does not respond to long-acting gonadotropin-releasing hormone (GnRH) analogues, consistent with the autonomous function of the gonads. Aromatase inhibitors, such as testolactone (22 mg/kg per day), have been used to block estrogen production, but with limited efficacy. Promising initial results have been seen with estrogen antagonists, such as tamoxifen. In addition to preventing pubertal progression, blockade of estrogen action is helpful to prevent early epiphyseal closure and short stature.

OTHER DYSPLASIAS OF BONE AND CARTILAGE

A variety of diseases of bone and cartilage have been called *dystrophies* or *dysplasias*. The *osteochondrodysplasias* are heritable disorders of connective tissue characterized by primary abnormalities of cartilage that lead to disturbances in cartilage and bone growth and development. They comprise several hundred distinct entities, which can be distinguished on the basis of clinical, genetic, and radiologic features. The molecular defects in a number of these disorders have been identified utilizing positional cloning and screening of candidate genes. Several of the disorders are due to mutations in collagen genes. →*For discussion of chondrodysplasias, see Chap. 351.*

SPONDYLOEPIPHYSEAL DYSPLASIA The *spondyloepiphyseal dysplasias* are disorders in which abnormalities of growth occur in various bones, including the vertebrae, pelvis, carpal and tarsal bones, and the epiphyses of tabular bones. On the basis of roentgenographic findings, this group can be divided into (1) those with generalized platyspondyly, (2) those with multiple epiphyseal dysplasias, and (3) those with epiphysometaphyseal dysplasias. *Morquio's syndrome*, in which there is a defect in degradation of glycosaminoglycans (therefore, a "mucopolysaccharidosis"), is inherited as an autosomal recessive trait and is associated with corneal opacities, dental defects, variable disturbances in intellect, and increased urinary excretion of keratosulfate; it belongs in the first group (Chap. 349). Other forms of spondyloepiphyseal dysplasia, some of which are accounted for by defects in type II collagen, may not be recognized until late in childhood or young adult life. Flat vertebral bodies are associated with other abnormalities in shape and alignment. The disordered development of the capital femoral epiphyses leads to irregularities in shape and flattening of the femoral heads and early onset of osteoarthritis of the hips.

ACHONDROPLASIA This disorder is among the more common types of dwarfism (1 in 15,000 to 1 in 40,000 live births). It is inherited as an autosomal dominant trait, although most cases are sporadic and due to new fibroblast growth factor receptor 3 (FGFR3) mutations (see below). The appearance of short limbs, particularly the proximal portions, with a normal trunk is characteristically accompanied by a large head, a saddle nose, and an exaggerated lumbar lordosis. The length of the spine is almost always normal. Features of the disorder are usually recognizable at birth. Those who survive infancy usually have normal mental and sexual development, and life span may be normal. Spinal deformity nevertheless may lead to a cord compression and nerve root encroachment, especially in those with kyphoscoliosis. Homozygous achondroplasia is a more serious disorder and a cause of neonatal death.

The most common mutation responsible for achondroplasia substitutes an arginine for glycine in the transmembrane domain of FGFR3 and causes a gain-of-function, implying that fibroblast growth factor normally acts via the FGFR3 to inhibit chondrocyte proliferation

in the growth plate. The abnormal proliferation at the growth plate, leaving other areas relatively unaffected in the tubular bones, causes production of short bones that are proportionately thick. Formation and maturation of the secondary ossification centers and articular cartilage are not disturbed. Appositional growth at the metaphysis continues, with resulting flare in this region of the bone; intramembranous bone formation at the periosteum is normal. Consistent with the inhibitory role of the FGFR3, a null mutation of the *Fgfr3* gene in mice causes increased growth in the physis. Mutations in other domains of the *FGFR3* gene have been described in thanatophoric dysplasia, the most severe and lethal dysplasia. In several types of the so-called craniosynostosis syndromes (Pfeiffer, Crouzon, Jackson-Weiss, and Apert syndromes), mutations have been identified in the *FGFR1* or *FGFR2* genes.

Pseudoachondroplasia clinically resembles achondroplasia with respect to the limb deformities but there are no skull abnormalities. Affected individuals have mutations in the gene encoding a non-collagenous component of cartilage called cartilate oligomeric matrix protein (COMP). Mutations in the *COMP* gene have also been described in one of the less severe forms of multiple epiphyseal dysplasia (EDM1).

ENCHONDROMATOSIS (DYSCHONDROPLASIA, OLLIER'S DISEASE) This is also a disorder of the growth plate in which the hypertrophic cartilage is not resorbed and ossified normally. It results in masses of cartilage with disorderly arrangement of the chondrocytes showing variable proliferative and hypertrophic changes. These masses are located in the metaphyses in close association with the growth plate in children but may be diaphyseal in teenagers and young adults. The disorder is usually recognized in childhood by the appearance of deformities or retardation in growth. The most common sites of involvement are the ends of long bones, usually in the region where rate of growth is most marked. The pelvis is often involved, but ribs, sternum, and skull are seldom affected. There is a tendency toward unilateral involvement. Chondrosarcoma develops occasionally in the enchondromata. The association of enchondromatosis and cavernous hemangiomata in the soft tissues including the skin is known as *Maffucci's syndrome*. Both Ollier's disease and Maffuci's syndrome have been associated with other primary malignancies as diverse as granulosa cell tumor of the ovary and cerebral gliomas.

MULTIPLE EXOSTOSES (DIAPHYSEAL ACLASIS OR OSTEOCHONDROMATOSIS) This is a disorder of the metaphysis, transmitted in an autosomal dominant manner, in which areas of the growth plate become displaced, presumably by growing through a defect in the perichondrium, or so-called ring of Ranvier. The spongiosa forms within the mass as vessels invade the cartilage. Therefore, the diagnostic radiographic finding is the direct continuity of the mass to the marrow cavity of the parent bone with absence of underlying cortex. Usually the growth of these exostoses ceases when growth of the adjacent plate ceases. The lesions may be solitary or multiple and are usually located in the metaphyseal areas of long bones, with the apex of the exostosis directed toward the diaphysis. Often the lesions produce no symptoms, but occasionally, interference with the function of a joint or tendon or compression of nerves may result. Dwarfism may occur. The metacarpals may be shortened, resembling those seen in Albright's hereditary osteodystrophy. Multiple exostoses are sometimes seen in patients with pseudohypoparathyroidism.

An exostosis may suddenly begin to enlarge long after growth should have ceased, and rarely, chondrosarcomas may develop from the cartilage cap of an exostosis. Although pregnancy may stimulate growth of an exostosis that clinically may mimic malignancy, the lesion merely undergoes exuberant endochondral ossification and cartilage hyperplasia without malignant changes.

Multiple inactivating mutations or deletions have been identified in the *EXT1* or *EXT2* genes in patients with hereditary multiple exostoses. The *EXT* genes probably function normally as a tumor suppressor, and mutations in *EXT* could contribute both to the development of the exostoses and to the malignant transformation to chondrosarcoma that sometimes occurs. Mutations in *EXT* genes apparently cause abnormal processing the cytoskeletal proteins in chondrocytes.

BIBLIOGRAPHY

BERNARD MA et al: Cytoskeletal abnormalities in chondrocytes with EXT1 and EXT2 mutations. J Bone Miner Res 15:442, 2000

BIANCO P et al: Mutations of the GNAS1 gene, stromal cell dysfunction, and osteomalacic changes in non-McCune-Albright fibrous dysplasia of bone. J Bone Miner Res 15: 120, 2000

CHAPURLAT RD, MEUNIER PJ: Fibrous dysplasia of bone. Baillieres Best Pract Res Clin Rheumatol 14:385, 2000

COOPER HA et al: SPONASTRIME dysplasia: Report of an 11-year-old boy and review of the literature. Am J Med Genet 92:33, 2000

DEERE M et al: Identification of nine novel mutations in cartilage oligomeric matrix protein in patients with pseudoachondroplasia and multiple epiphyseal dysplasia. Am J Hum Genet 85:486, 1999

DINI G et al: Long-term follow-up of two children with a variant of mild autosomal recessive osteopetrosis undergoing bone marrow transplantation. Bone Marrow Transplant 26:219, 2000

DREZNER MK: Proceeding of the third international symposium on Paget's disease. Napa, California, USA, November 29–30, 1998. J Bone Miner Res. 14(Suppl 2):1, 1999

EUGSTER EA et al: Tamoxifen treatment of progressive precocious puberty in a patient with McCune-Albright syndrome. J Pediatr Endocrinol Metab 12:681, 1999

FISHER JE et al: Alendronate mechanism of action: Geranylgeraniol, an intermediate in the mevalonate pathway, prevents inhibition of osteoclast formation, bone resorption, and kinase activation in vitro. Proc Natl Acad Sci USA 96:133, 1999

FRATTINI A et al: Defects in TCIRG1 subunit of the vacuolar proton pump are responsible for a subset of human autosomal recessive osteopetrosis. Nature Genet 25:343, 2000

GELB BD et al: Pycnodysostosis, a lysosomal disease caused by cathepsin K deficiency. Science 273:1236, 1996

GLASER RL et al: Paternal origin of FGFR2 mutations in sporadic cases of Crouzon syndrome and Pfeiffer syndrome. Am J Hum Genet 66:768, 2000

HOCKING L et al: Familial Paget's disease of bone: Patterns of inheritance and frequency of linkage to chromosome 18q. Bone 26:577, 2000

HUGHES AE et al: Mutations in TNFRS11A, affecting the signal peptide of RANK, cause familial expansile osteolysis. Nat Genet 24:45, 2000

JANSSENS K et al: Localisation of the gene causing diaphyseal dysplasia Camurati-Engelmann to chromosome 19q13. J Med Genet 37:245, 2000

KARSENTY G: The genetic transformation of bone biology. Genes Dev 13:3037, 1999

KORNAK U et al: Mutations in the α3 subunit of the vacuolar H⁺-ATPase cause infantile malignant osteopetrosis. Hum Mol Genet 9:2059, 2000

KURIHARA N et al: Osteoclasts expressing the measles virus nucleocapsid gene display a pagetic phenotype. J Clin Invest 105:607, 2000

LALA R et al: Pamidronate treatment of bone fibrous dysplasia in nine children with McCune-Albright syndrome. Acta Paediatr 89:188, 2000

LI J et al: RANK is the intrinsic hematopoietic cell surface receptor that controls osteoclastogenesis and regulation of bone mass and calcium metabolism. Proc Natl Acad Sci USA 97:1566, 2000

NELLISSERY MJ et al: Evidence for a novel osteosarcoma tumor-suppressor gene in the chromosome 18 region genetically linked with Paget disease of bone. Am J Hum Genet 63:817, 1998

NEVIN NC et al: Melorheostosis in a family with autosomal dominant osteopoikilosis. Am J Med Genet 82:409, 1999

RINGEL MD et al: Clinical implications of genetic defects in G proteins. The molecular basis of McCune-Albright syndrome and Albright hereditary osteodystrophy. Medicine 75:171, 1996

SAFTIG P et al: Functions of cathepsin K in bone resorption. Lessons from cathepsin K deficient mice. Adv Exp Biol 477:293, 2000

SILVE C: Hereditary hypophosphatasia and hyperphosphatasia. Curr Opin Rheumatol 6: 336, 1994

SINGER FR, KRANE SM: Paget's disease of bone, in Metabolic Bone Disease and Clinically Related Disorders, LV Avioli, SM Krane (eds). San Diego, Academic Press, 1998, pp 545–603

VAJO Z et al: The molecular and genetic basis of fibroblast growth factor receptor 3 disorders: The achondrodysplasia family of skeletal dysplasias, Muenke craniosyntosis, and Crouzon syndrome with acanthosis nigricans. Endocrine Rev 21:23, 2000

WHYTE MP, MURPHY WA: Osteopetrosis and other sclerosing bone disorders, in Metabolic Bone Disease and Clinically Related Disorders, LV Avioli, SM Krane (eds). San Diego, Academic Press, 1998

WUYTS W, VAN HUL W: Molecular basis of muliple exostoses: Mutations in the EXT1 and EXT2 genes. Hum Mutat 15:220, 2000

Section 3
DISORDERS OF INTERMEDIARY METABOLISM

344

Henry N. Ginsberg,, Ira J. Goldberg

DISORDERS OF LIPOPROTEIN METABOLISM

CETP cholesteryl ester transfer protein	LCAT lecithin:cholesterol acyltransferase
CHD coronary heart disease	LDL low-density lipoprotein
CPK creatine phosphokinase	LPL lipoprotein lipase
DM diabetes mellitus	LRP LDL receptor–related protein
FCHL familial combined hyperlipidemia	NCEP National Cholesterol Education Program
FH familial hypercholesterolemia	PLTP phospholipid transfer protein
HDL high-density lipoproteins	TSH thyroid-stimulating hormone
HTGL hepatic triglyceride lipase	VLDL very low density lipoproteins
IDL intermediate-density lipoproteins	

Lipoproteins are macromolecular complexes that carry hydrophobic plasma lipids, particularly cholesterol and triglyceride, in the plasma. More than half of the coronary heart disease (CHD) in the United States is attributable to abnormalities in the levels and metabolism of plasma lipids and lipoproteins. Some premature CHD is due to mutations in major genes involved in lipoprotein metabolism. However, elevated lipoprotein levels in most patients with CHD reflect the adverse impact of a sedentary lifestyle, excess body weight, and diets high in total and saturated fat superimposed on a genetic background that confers susceptibility to increased circulating lipids. A large body of evidence indicates that lifestyle changes and drug treatment strategies that correct hyperlipidemias reduce CHD risk (Chap 242). More than 70 clinical trials examining the effects of cholesterol reduction have been reported, including several large-scale studies using the potent cholesterol-lowering HMG-CoA reductase inhibitors (also known as statins). These studies unequivocally demonstrate that lowering low-density lipoprotein (LDL) cholesterol reduces fatal and nonfatal heart attacks (Table 344-1).

This chapter focuses on the major lipid disorders, including both the dyslipoproteinemias caused by single-gene defects and the disorders that are likely to be multifactorial in origin. A practical approach is provided to assist in the identification, evaluation, and treatment of patients with increased risk of CHD.

LIPID AND LIPOPROTEIN TRANSPORT

LIPOPROTEIN STRUCTURE Lipoproteins are spherical particles made up of hundreds of lipid and protein molecules. They are smaller than red blood cells and visible only by electron microscopy. However, when the larger, triglyceride-rich lipoproteins are present in high concentration, plasma can appear turbid or milky to the naked eye. The major lipids of the lipoproteins are cholesterol, triglycerides, and phospholipids. Triglycerides and the esterified form of cholesterol (cholesteryl esters) are nonpolar lipids that are insoluble in aqueous environments (hydrophobic) and comprise the core of the lipoproteins. Phospholipids and a small quantity of free (unesterified)

Table 344-1   Summary of Selected Major Lipid-Lowering Trials Investigating Effects on CHD

Trial [a]	Year Published	Treatment	Lipid Characteristics	1° or 2° [b]	Results
Los Angeles VA	1968	Unsaturated fat diet	—	1	↓ MI
Oslo	1981	Diet and smoking	—	1	↓ Reduced sudden death and MI
LRC Trial	1984	Cholestyramine	—	2	↓ Cardiac events [c]
Coronary Drug Project	1985	Niacin	—	2	↓ Cardiac death over 15 years
Helsinki	1987	Gemfibrozil	—	1	↓ Cardiac events
POSCH	1990	Ileal bypass	—	1	↓ Cardiac events
FATS	1990	Combination	—	2	↓ Cardiac events
4S	1994	Simvastatin	High cholesterol	2	↓ Death, cardiac events, and stroke
WOSCOPS	1995	Pravastatin	High cholesterol	1	↓ Cardiac events
CARE	1996	Pravastatin	Average LDL	2	↓ Cardiac events and stroke
LIPID	1998	Pravastatin	Variable LDL	2	↓ Cardiac events
AFCAPS/Tex-CAPS	1998	Mevacor	Average LDL Low HDL	1	↓ Cardiac events
VA HIT	1999	Gemfibrozil	Low-normal LDL Low HDL	2	↓ Cardiac events
AVERT	1999	Atorvastatin	—	2	↓ Time to new events compared to angioplasty

[a] LRC, Lipid Research Clinics; 4S, Scandanavian Simvastatin Survival Study; WOSCOPS, West of Scotland Coronary Prevention Study; CARE, Cholesterol and Recurrent Events Trial; AFCAPS/TexCAPS, Air Force/Texas Coronary Atherosclerosis Prevention Study; POSCH, Program on the Surgical Control of the Hyperlipidemias; FATS, Familial Atherosclerosis Treatment Study; LIPID, Long-Term Intervention with Pravastatin in Ischemic Disease; VA HIT, Veterans Administration-HDL Intervention Trial; AVERT, Atorvastatin versus Revascularization Treatments.
[b] 1°, Primary prevention trial in population without known CHD; 2°, secondary prevention trial in population with established (CHD) assessed for recurrent clinical episodes.
[c] Cardicac events, fatal and nonfatal CHD.
NOTE: CHD, coronary heart disease; MI, myocardial infarction; LDL, low-density lipoprotein; HDL, high-density lipoprotein.

cholesterol, which are soluble in both lipid and aqueous environments (amphipathic), cover the surface of the particles, where they act as the interface between the plasma and core components. A family of proteins, the apolipoproteins, also occupies the surface of the lipoproteins; the apolipoproteins play crucial roles in the regulation of lipid transport and lipoprotein metabolism.

Lipoproteins have been classified on the basis of their densities into five major classes:(1) chylomicrons, (2) very low density lipoproteins (VLDL), (3) intermediate-density lipoproteins (IDL), (4) LDL, and (5) high-density lipoproteins (HDL). The physical-chemical characteristics of the major lipoprotein classes are presented in Table 344-2.

APOLIPOPROTEINS The apolipoproteins (apos) provide structural stability to the lipoproteins and determine the metabolic fate of the particles upon which they reside. They were named in an arbitrary alphabetical order and, for the purposes of this discussion, will be described in relation to their association with lipoprotein classes (Table 344-3).

There are two forms of apo B—apo B100 and apo B48. Apo B100 is the major apolipoprotein of VLDL, IDL, and LDL, comprising approximately 30, 60, and 95% of the protein in these lipoproteins, respectively. Apo B100 has a molecular mass of about 545 kDa and is

synthesized in the liver. It is essential for the assembly and secretion of VLDL from the liver and is the ligand for the removal of LDL by the LDL receptor. The LDL receptor is a cell-surface protein that binds and internalizes lipoproteins that contain apo B100 or apo E. The LDL receptor binding domain of apo B100 is the sequence between amino acids 3200 and 3600, a region that is absent in apo B48.

Apo B48 is essential for the assembly and secretion of chylomicrons. Apo B48 is encoded by the same gene and messenger ribonucleic acid (mRNA) as Apo B100. However, the mRNA is edited in an unusual way: A cytidine deaminase in the intestine changes a cytidine to a uridine in base 6666 of the apo B100 mRNA to produce a stop codon so that apo B48 contains only the N-terminal 48% of the full-length apo B100. In contrast, the apo B100 mRNA in human liver is not edited. The role of apo B48 in the metabolism of chylomicrons in plasma is unclear. Individuals with mutations that interfere with the normal synthesis of apo B have absent or very low levels of chylomicrons, VLDL, IDL and LDL.

The apolipoproteins of the C series are synthesized in the liver and are present in all plasma lipoproteins (trace amounts in LDL). Individual apo Cs have different metabolic roles, but all inhibit the removal of plasma chylomicrons and VLDL remnants by the liver. Overexpression of apo CI in transgenic mice inhibits the uptake of chylomicron and VLDL remnants by the liver. Apo CI under- or overexpression has not been described in humans. Apo CII is an essential activator of the enzyme lipoprotein lipase (LPL), which hydrolyzes triglycerides in chylomicrons and VLDL; individuals lacking apo CII have severe hypertriglyceridemia. Apo CIII inhibits LPL, and apo CIII overexpression in transgenic mice causes severe hypertriglyceridemia. Humans who lack apo CIII have accelerated rates of VLDL triglyceride lipolysis.

Apo E is synthesized mainly in hepatocytes but is also made in other cells, including macrophages, neurons, and glial cells. It is found in chylomicrons, IDL, VLDL, and HDL and mediates the uptake of these lipoproteins in the liver by both the LDL receptor and the LDL receptor–related protein (LRP). Apo E also binds to heparin-like proteoglycan molecules on the surface of all cells. There are three major apo E alleles: E2, E3, and E4; these isoforms differ in sequence at two positions and have frequencies of about 0.12, 0.75, and 0.13, respectively, in the general population. Apo E2 binds to the LDL receptor with lower affinity than apo E3 or E4. Individuals who are homozygous for apo E2 may develop severe hyperlipidemia (type III dysbetalipoproteinemia); complete absence of apo E increases plasma levels of chylomicron and VLDL remnants and causes early atherosclerosis.

Apo AI, apo AII, and apo AIV are found primarily on HDL. Apo AI and apo AII are synthesized in the small intestine and the liver; apo AIV is made only in the intestine. Apo AI comprises about 70 to 80% of the protein of HDL and plays a critical structural role in HDL particles. Individuals with a profound deficiency of apo AI also lack HDL. Apo AI activates the enzyme lecithin:cholesterol acyl-

Table 344-2   Physical-Chemical Characteristics of the Major Lipoprotein Classes

Lipoprotein	Density, g/dL	Molecular Mass, kDa	Diameter, nm	Lipid, % [a]		
				TG	Chol	PL
Chylomicrons	0.95	400×10^3	75–1200	80–95	2–7	3–9
VLDL	0.95–1.006	$10–80 \times 10^3$	30–80	55–80	5–15	10–20
IDL	1.006–1.019	$5–10 \times 10^3$	25–35	20–50	20–40	15–25
LDL	1.019–1.063	2.3×10^3	18–25	5–15	40–50	20–25
HDL	1.063–1.210	$1.7–3.6 \times 10^2$	5–12	5–10	15–25	20–30

[a] The remaining percent composition is made up of the apoproteins.
NOTE: TG, triglyceride; Chol, the sum of free and esterified cholesterol; PL, phospholipid; VLDL, very low density lipoprotein; IDL, intermediate density lipoprotein; LDL, low-density lipoprotein; HDL, high-density lipoprotein.

transferase (LCAT), which esterifies free cholesterol in plasma. Plasma levels of HDL cholesterol and apo AI are inversely related to risk for CHD, and some patients with apo AI deficiency develop early, severe atherosclerosis. Transgenic mice that overexpress human apo AI are resistant to atherosclerosis. Apo AII is the second most abundant apoprotein in HDL, but its function has not been determined; transgenic mice that overexpress apo AII have high plasma levels of both HDL cholesterol and triglycerides but may be susceptible to atherosclerosis. Apo AII knockout mice have low levels of HDL, indicating that apo AII is also necessary for the integrity of HDL particles. Apo AIV, a minor component of HDL and chylomicrons may play a role in the activation of LCAT.

Apoprotein(a), a large glycoprotein that shares a high degree of sequence homology with plasminogen, is made by hepatocytes and is secreted into plasma where it forms a covalent linkage with the apo B100 of LDL to form lipoprotein(a). The physiologic role of lipoprotein(a) is not known, but elevated levels are associated with an increased risk for atherosclerosis.

ENZYMES INVOLVED IN LIPOPROTEIN METABOLISM
LPL is synthesized in fat and muscle, secreted into the interstitial space, transported across endothelial cells, and bound to proteoglycans on the luminal surfaces in the adjacent capillary beds. LPL mediates the hydrolysis of the triglycerides of chylomicrons and VLDL to generate free fatty acids and glycerol. The free fatty acids diffuse into adjacent tissues to be burned for energy or stored as fat. Most circulating LPL is associated with LDL. Insulin stimulates the synthesis and secretion of LPL; reduced LPL activity in diabetes mellitus can lead to impaired triglyceride clearance. Homozygotes for mutations that impair LPL have severe hypertriglyceridemia that usually manifests in childhood (type I hyperlipidemia). Heterozygotes for LPL defects have mild to moderate fasting hypertriglyceridemia but may have marked hypertriglyceridemia after consuming a high-fat meal. LPL is also expressed in macrophages, including cholesteryl ester–laden macrophages (foam cells) in atherosclerotic lesions. In this setting, secreted LPL may associate with LDL, causing retention of the lipoprotein in the subendothelial space.

Hepatic triglyceride lipase (HTGL), a member of a family of enzymes that includes LPL and pancreatic lipase, is synthesized in the liver and interacts with lipoproteins in hepatic sinusoids. HTGL removes triglycerides from VLDL remnants (IDL), thus promoting the conversion of VLDL to LDL. It may also play a role in the clearance of chylomicron remnants and in the conversion of HDL$_2$ to HDL$_3$ in the liver by hydrolyzing the triglyceride and phospholipid in HDL (see below). Severe hypertriglyceridemia in individuals with genetic deficiency of HTGL is due to the accumulation of chylomicron and VLDL remnants in plasma. In contrast to most patients with hypertriglyceridemia, however, individuals with HTGL deficiency have normal levels of HDL.

LCAT is synthesized in the liver and secreted into plasma where it is bound predominantly to HDL. LCAT mediates the transfer of linoleate from lecithin to free cholesterol on the surface of HDL to form cholesteryl esters that are then transferred to VLDL and eventually LDL. Apo AI is a cofactor for esterification of free cholesterol by LCAT. Deficiency of LCAT can be caused by mutations in the enzyme or in Apo A1. LCAT deficiency causes low levels of cholesteryl esters and HDL, and it can lead to corneal clouding and renal insufficiency.

Cholesteryl ester transfer protein (CETP) is synthesized primarily in the liver and circulates in plasma in association with HDL. CETP mediates the exchange of cholesteryl esters from HDL with triglyceride from chylomicrons or VLDL. This exchange can explain much of the inverse relationship between plasma levels of triglycerides and HDL cholesterol. LDL cholesteryl ester can also be exchanged with triglyceride from chylomicrons and VLDL, leading to the generation of small, dense LDL. Individuals who are homozygotes for mutations in the CETP gene have marked elevations of HDL cholesterol and apo AI. Heterozygotes for these mutations have slight elevations of HDL, indicating that CETP plays an important role in the removal of cholesteryl esters from HDL.

Phospholipid transfer protein (PLTP) is synthesized in the liver and lung. The production of mature HDL particles depends on PLTP, which provides phospholipid to the enlarging particles.

TRANSPORT OF EXOGENOUS (DIETARY) LIPIDS
Exogenous lipid transport in chylomicrons and chylomicron remnants is depicted in Fig. 344-1A. In western societies, where individuals ordinarily consume 50 to 100 g of fat and 0.5 g of cholesterol during three or four meals, transport of dietary fats is essentially continual. Normolipidemic individuals dispose of most dietary fat in the bloodstream within 8 h of the last meal, but some individuals with dyslipidemia, particularly those with elevated fasting levels of VLDL triglyceride, have measurable levels of intestinally derived lipoproteins in the circulation as long as 24 h after the last meal.

In the intestinal mucosa dietary triglyceride and cholesterol are incorporated into the core of nascent chylomicrons. The surface coat of the chylomicron is composed of phospholipid, free cholesterol, apo B48, apo AI, apo AII, and apo AIV. The chylomicron, essentially a fat droplet containing 80 to 95% triglycerides, is secreted into lacteals and transported to the circulation via the thoracic duct. In the plasma, apo C proteins are transferred to the chylomicron from HDL. Apo CII mediates hydrolysis of triglycerides by activating LPL on capillary endothelial cells in fat and muscle. After the triglyceride core has been hydrolyzed, apo CII and apo CIII recirculate back to HDL. The addition of apo E allows the chylomicron remnant to bind first to heparan sulfate proteoglycans within the space of Disse and then to hepatic LDL receptors and/or LDL receptor-related protein. As a consequence, dietary triglyceride is delivered to adipocytes and muscle cells as fatty acids, and dietary cholesterol is taken up by the liver where it can be used for bile acid formation, incorporated into membranes, resecreted as lipoprotein cholesterol back into the circulation, or excreted as cho-

Table 344-3 Characteristics of the Major Apolipoproteins

Apolipoprotein	Molecular Mass, Da	Lipoproteins	Metabolic Functions
Apo AI	28,016	HDL, chylomicrons	Structural component of HDL; LCAT activator
Apo AII	17,414	HDL, chylomicrons	Unknown
Apo AIV	46,465	HDL, chylomicrons	Unknown: possibly facilitates transfer of other apos between HDL and chylomicrons
Apo B48	264,000	Chylomicrons	Necessary for assembly and secretion of chylomicrons from the small intestine
Apo B100	540,000	VLDL, IDL, LDL	Necessary for assembly and secretion of VLDL from the liver; structural protein of VLDL, IDL, LDL; ligand for LDL receptor
Apo CI	6630	Chylomicrons, VLDL, IDL, HDL	May inhibit hepatic uptake of chylomicron and VLDL remnants
Apo CII	8900	Chylomicrons, VLDL, IDL, HDL	Activator of lipoprotein lipase
Apo CIII	8800	Chylomicrons, VLDL, IDL, HDL	Inhibitor of lipoprotein lipase; may inhibit hepatic uptake of chylomicron and VLDL remnants
Apo E	34,145	Chylomicrons, VLDL, IDL, HDL	Ligand for binding of several lipoproteins to the LDL receptor, to LRP, and possibly to a separate hepatic apo E receptor

NOTE: HDL, high-density lipoprotein; LCAT, lecithin:cholesterol acyltransferase; VLDL, very low density lipoprotein; IDL, intermediate-density lipoprotein; LDL, low-density lipoprotein; LRP, LDL receptor–related protein.

FIGURE 344-1   *A.* Transport of endogenous hepatic lipids via VLDL, IDL, and LDL. Note the relative and absolute changes in apoproteins, other than apo B100, as VLDL is converted to IDL and LDL. The sites of action of the two lipases, LPL and HTGL, are denoted as well, though the role of HTGL has not been completely defined. *B.* A schematic depiction of the transport of exogenously derived lipids from the intestine to peripheral tissues and liver via the chylomicron system. The cyclic movement of several apoproteins between HDL and chylomicrons is also represented. *C.* Simplified representation of HDL metabolism and the role of HDL in reverse cholesterol transport. Free cholesterol is accepted from peripheral tissues by HDL₃ and, after esterification, may be transferred to apo B100 lipoproteins. Cholesteryl ester may also be delivered to the liver by HDL itself. The significance of each of the three possible transport systems for cholesterol in overall reverse cholesterol transport is unknown. CETP, cholesteryl ester transfer protein; FFA, free fatty acids; HDL, high-density lipoprotein; HTGL, hepatic triglyceride lipase; IDL, intermediate-density lipoprotein; LDL, low-density lipoprotein; LPL, lipoprotein lipase; PL, phospholipase; TG, triglyceride; VLDL, very low density lipoprotein. *[From HN Ginsberg, Endocrinol Metab Clin North Am 19(2): 211, 1990.]*

lesterol into bile. Dietary cholesterol also regulates endogenous hepatic cholesterol synthesis.

Abnormal transport and metabolism of chylomicrons may predispose to atherosclerosis, and postprandial hyperlipidemia may be a risk factor for CHD. Chylomicrons and their remnants can be taken up by cells of the vessel wall, including monocyte-derived macrophages that migrate into the vessel wall from plasma. Cholesteryl ester accumulation by these macrophages transforms them into foam cells, the earliest cellular lesion of the atherosclerotic plaque (Chap. 241). If the postprandial levels of chylomicrons or their remnants are elevated, or if their removal from plasma is prolonged, cholesterol delivery to the artery wall may be increased.

TRANSPORT OF ENDOGENOUS LIPIDS   The endogenous lipid transport system, which conveys lipids from the liver to peripheral tissues and from peripheral tissues back to the liver, can be separated into two subsystems: the apo B100 lipoprotein system (VLDL, IDL, and LDL) and the apo AI lipoprotein system (HDL).

The Apo B100 Lipoprotein System (See Fig. 344-1*B*)   In the liver, triglycerides are made from fatty acids that are either taken up from plasma or synthesized de novo within the liver. Cholesterol can also be synthesized by the liver or delivered to the liver via lipoproteins, particularly chylomicron remnants. These core lipids are packaged together with apo B100 and phospholipids into VLDL and secreted into plasma where apos CI, CII, CIII, and E are added to the nascent VLDL particles. Triglycerides make up the bulk of the VLDL (55 to 80% by weight), and the size of the VLDL is determined by the amount of triglyceride available. Hence, very large triglyceride-rich VLDL are secreted in situations where excess triglycerides are synthesized, such as in states of caloric excess, in diabetes mellitus, and after alcohol consumption. Small VLDL are secreted when fewer triglycerides are available. Although VLDL are the principal hepatic lipoprotein secreted by most individuals, VLDL and cholesteryl ester–enriched IDL and/or LDL-like particles may be secreted by the liver in individuals with combined hyperlipidemia (see below).

In the plasma, triglycerides are hydrolyzed by LPL and VLDL particles are converted to VLDL remnants (IDL). In contrast to chylomicron remnants, VLDL remnants can either enter the liver or give rise to LDL. Larger VLDL particles carry more triglycerides and are likely to be removed directly from plasma without being converted to LDL; apo E in the VLDL remnants binds to the LDL receptor to mediate removal from the plasma. Smaller, more dense VLDL particles are more efficiently converted to LDL; apo E and HTGL play important roles in this process. Individuals with deficiency of either apo E2 or HTGL accumulate IDL in plasma. Apo B100 is the only protein that remains on the surface of the LDL particle.

The half-life of LDL in plasma is determined principally by the availability (or "activity") of LDL receptors. Most plasma LDL is taken up by the liver, and the remainder is delivered to peripheral tissues, including the adrenals and gonads, which utilize cholesterol as a precursor for steroid hormone synthesis. The adrenals have the highest concentration of LDL receptors per cell in the body. Overall, about 70 to 80% of LDL catabolism occurs via LDL receptors, and the remainder is removed by fluid endocytosis and possibly by other receptors.

The LDL receptor, a glycoprotein with a molecular mass of approximately 160 kDa, is present on the surfaces of nearly all cells in the body. Goldstein and Brown characterized the molecular genetics and cell biology of the LDL receptor and defined its role in cholesterol metabolism. They showed that cholesterol delivered to the cytoplasm by LDL regulates both the rate of cholesterol synthesis in the liver and the number of LDL receptors on the surface of hepatocytes. LDL receptor synthesis is mediated by sterol response element regulatory proteins (SREBPs). These transcription factors are activated in the absence of cholesterol, proteolytically cleaved, and transferred from the endoplasmic reticulum into the nucleus where they stimulate LDL receptor gene expression. Though the LDL receptor is a major factor in determining plasma LDL cholesterol levels, the rates of entry of VLDL into plasma and the efficiency with which VLDL is converted to LDL also influence steady-state LDL concentrations in plasma.

Increased levels of plasma LDL cholesterol and apo B100 are risk factors for atherosclerosis. Normal LDL does not cause foam cell formation when incubated with cultured macrophages or smooth-muscle cells. But, when LDL undergoes lipid peroxidation, it becomes a ligand for alternative, scavenger receptors that are present on endothelial cells and macrophages. Uptake of modified (oxidized) lipoproteins by these receptors in macrophages results in formation of cholesterol-laden foam cells. In addition to inducing foam cell formation, oxidized LDL acts in the vessel wall to stimulate the secretion of cytokines and growth factors by endothelial cells, smooth-muscle cells, and mono-cyte-derived macrophages (Chap. 242). The consequence is recruit-ment of more monocytes to the lesion and proliferation of smooth-muscle cells, which synthesize and secrete increased amounts of extracellular matrix, such as collagen. The critical role of LDL in ath-erosclerosis has been confirmed in genetically altered mice. Although mice are normally resistant to atherosclerosis, increased plasma levels of remnant lipoproteins or LDL lead to atherosclerosis in this species.

The role of VLDL in atherogenesis is less certain. The major rea-son for this uncertainty derives from the inverse relationship between elevated levels of triglyceride-rich lipoproteins and reduced levels of the antiatherogenic HDL cholesterol. It is possible, for example, that hypertriglyceridemia may not be directly atherogenic but rather the surrogate of other lipoprotein abnormalities. If postprandial hyperlip-idemia is a risk factor for CHD, individuals who have normal fasting plasma triglyceride levels but develop postprandial hypertriglyceri-demia after consumption of a fat load would be misclassified as "nor-mal" in studies in which only fasting blood samples are analyzed. It is clear that cholesteryl ester–enriched VLDL, isolated from choles-terol-fed animals, can be taken up by receptors on macrophages and smooth-muscle cells and cause foam cell formation. These cholesteryl ester–laden VLDLs are enriched in apo E and are probably repre-sentative of VLDL remnants. Thus, the risk of atherosclerosis from hypertriglyceridemia and elevated VLDL levels may be determined by the level of cholesteryl ester–enriched VLDL remnants. The athero-genic potential of IDL is probably similar to that of VLDL remnants.

Apo AI–Containing Lipoproteins (See Fig. 344-1*C*) In con-trast to atherogenic apo B lipoproteins, the apo AI–containing HDL appear to be antiatherogenic. In fact, in some studies, HDL cholesterol levels are as strong an indicator of protection from CHD as LDL cho-lesterol levels are an indicator of risk. Although a great deal is known about the HDL transport system, the mechanism by which these lipo-proteins protect against atherosclerosis is poorly defined.

HDL particles are formed in plasma from the coalescence of in-dividual phospholipid-apolipoprotein complexes. Apo AI appears to be the crucial, structural apoprotein for HDL, and apo AI/phospholipid complexes probably fuse with other phospholipid vesicles that contain apo AII and apo AIV to form the various types of HDL. The C apo-proteins can be added to HDL after their secretion as phospholipid complexes or by their transfer from triglyceride-rich lipoproteins. This may involve the action of PLTP. These small, cholesterol-poor HDL particles are heterogeneous in size and content and are referred to as HDL$_3$. Free cholesterol is transferred from cell membranes to HDL$_3$: a cholesterol transporter called ABC1 mediates this important first step in reverse cholesterol transport. Free cholesterol in HDL$_3$ is con-verted to cholesteryl ester by LCAT, and the cholesteryl ester moves into the core of the HDL. Formation of cholesteryl ester increases the capacity of the HDL$_3$ to accept more free cholesterol and enlarge to form the more buoyant class of HDL particles termed *HDL$_2$*. HDL$_2$ can be metabolized by two pathways: (1) cholesteryl esters can be transferred from HDL$_2$ to apo B lipoproteins or cells, or (2) the entire HDL$_2$ particle can be removed from plasma. The transfer of cholesteryl ester from HDL to triglyceride-rich apo B lipoproteins (chylomicrons and VLDL in the fed and fasted states, respectively) is mediated by CETP. Triglyceride is transferred to HDL in this process and is a substrate for lipolysis by LPL and/or HTGL. As a result, HDL$_2$ is converted back into HDL$_3$. When the apo B lipoproteins are removed

by the liver, reverse cholesterol transfer is complete. HDL cholesteryl ester may also be transferred selectively to cells via interaction of HDL with the scavenger receptor B-1, a receptor expressed by hepatocytes and steroid-producing cells. HDL-mediated reverse cholesterol trans-port (from peripheral tissues to the liver) is thought to be the primary mechanism by which HDL protects against atherosclerosis.

Rarely, low plasma HDL is due to a genetic deficiency of one of the structural components of HDL (such as apo AI). However, low HDL cholesterol levels are usually the secondary consequence of in-creased plasma levels of VLDL and IDL (or chylomicrons and their remnants). Mutations in the *ABC1* gene (see above) are associated with Tangier's disease, a rare form of low HDL. Low levels of HDL cho-lesterol and apo AI may increase atherosclerosis risk by any of several mechanisms. HDL could remove cholesterol from foam cells in athero-sclerotic lesions or protect LDL from oxidative modification. Alter-natively, the atherosclerotic risk of low HDL may be due to the com-monly associated elevations of apo B–containing lipoproteins, which accept HDL cholesteryl esters and deliver cholesteryl esters to the vessel wall.

THE HYPERLIPOPROTEINEMIAS (See Table 344-4)

HYPERCHOLESTEROLEMIA Elevated levels of fasting plasma total cholesterol in the presence of normal levels of triglycer-ides are almost always associated with increased concentrations of plasma LDL cholesterol (type IIa), as LDL carries about 65 to 75% of total plasma cholesterol. A rare individual with markedly elevated HDL cholesterol may also have increased plasma total cholesterol lev-els. Elevations of LDL cholesterol can result from single-gene defects, polygenic disorders, or from the secondary effects of other disease states.

Familial Hypercholesterolemia (FH) FH is a codominant ge-netic disorder that occurs in the heterozygous form in approximately 1 in 500 individuals. FH is due to mutations in the gene for the LDL receptor and is genetically heterogeneous, >200 different mutations in the gene having been described. Plasma levels of LDL cholesterol are elevated at birth and remain so throughout life. In untreated adults, total cholesterol levels range from 7 to 13 mmol/L (275 to 500 mg/dL). Plasma triglyceride levels are typically normal, and HDL choles-terol levels are normal or reduced. As would be expected of a disorder with decreased numbers of LDL receptors, the fractional clearance of LDL apo B is reduced. LDL production is increased because the liver secretes more VLDL and IDL and more IDL particles are converted to LDL rather than taken up by the hepatic LDL receptors. FH heter-ozygotes usually develop severe atherosclerosis in early or middle age. *Tendon xanthomas*, which are due to both intracellular and extracel-lular deposits of cholesterol, most commonly involve the Achilles ten-dons and the extensor tendons of the knuckles; they are found in about 75% of adults with FH. *Tuberous xanthomas*, which are softer, pain-less nodules on the elbows and buttocks, and *xanthelasmas*, which are barely elevated deposits of cholesterol on the eyelids, are common in heterozygous FH. CHD develops in men by the fourth decade of life or earlier.

The homozygous form of FH occurs in 1 out of 1 million individ-uals and is associated with a marked increase of plasma cholesterol levels (>13 mmol/L; >500 mg/dL), large xanthelasmas, and promi-nent tendon and planar xanthomas. These individuals have severe, pre-mature CHD that can be manifested in childhood.

Familial Defective Apo B100 This autosomal dominant disor-der is a phenocopy of FH and is due to a missense mutation at amino acid 3500 that reduces the affinity of LDL for the LDL receptor and, thus, impairs LDL catabolism. The prevalence and manifestations of both the heterozygous and homozygous forms are similar to those produced by mutations of the LDL receptor.

Polygenic Hypercholesterolemia Most moderate hypercholes-terolemia [plasma cholesterol levels between 6.5 and 9 mmol/L (240

Table 344-4 Characteristics of Common Hyperlipidemias

Lipid Phenotype	Plasma Lipid Levels, mmol/L (mg/dL)	Lipopoteins Elevated	Phenotype	Clinical Signs
ISOLATED HYPERCHOLESTEROLEMIA				
Familial hypercholesterolemia	Heterozygotes: total chol = 7–13 (275–500)	LDL	IIa	Usually develop xanthomas in adulthood and vascular disease at 30–50 years
	Homozygotes: total chol > 13 (>500)	LDL	IIa	Usually develop xanthomas and vascular disease in childhood
Familial defective apo B100	Heterozygotes: total chol = 7–13 (275–500)	LDL	IIa	
Polygenic hypercholesterolemia	Total chol = 6.5–9.0 (250–350)	LDL	IIa	Usually asymptomatic until vascular disease develops; no xanthomas
ISOLATED HYPERTRIGLYCERIDEMIA				
Familial hypertriglyceridemia	TG = 2.8–8.5 (250–750) (plasma may be cloudy)	VLDL	IV	Asymptomatic; may be associated with increased risk of vascular disease
Familial lipoprotein lipase deficiency	TG > 8.5 (>750) (plasma may be milky)	Chylomicrons	I, V	May be asymptomatic; may be associated with pancreatitis, abdominal pain, hepatosplenomegaly
Familial apo CII deficiency	TG > 8.5 (>750) (plasma may be milky)	Chylomicrons	I, V	As above
HYPERTRIGLYCERIDEMIA AND HYPERCHOLESTEROLEMIA				
Combined hyperlipidemia	TG = 2.8–8.5 (250–750) Total chol 6.5–13.0 (250–500)	VLDL, LDL	IIb	Usually asymptomatic until vascular disease develops; familial form may also present as isolated high TG or an isolated high LDL cholesterol
Dysbetalipoproteinemia	TG = 2.8–5.6 (250–500) Total chol 6.5–13.0 (250–500)	VLDL, IDL; LDL normal	III	Usually asymptomatic until vascular disease develops; may have palmar or tubo-eruptive xanthomas

NOTE: total chol, the sum of free and esterified cholesterol; LDL, low-density lipoprotein; TG, triglycerides; VLDL, very low density lipoproteins; IDL, intermediate-density lipoprotein.

and 350 mg/dL)] is polygenic in origin. Multiple genes interact with environmental factors to contribute to the hypercholesterolemia, and both overproduction and reduced catabolism of LDL are thought to play roles in the pathophysiology. The severity is probably affected by the consumption of saturated fat and cholesterol, age, and the level of physical activity. Plasma triglyceride and HDL cholesterol are usually normal. These individuals are at increased risk of atherosclerosis. Tendon xanthomas are not present. Genes involved in cholesterol and bile acid metabolism may be involved in the pathogenesis.

HYPERTRIGLYCERIDEMIA The diagnosis of hypertriglyceridemia is made by determining plasma lipids after an overnight fast. Because of the less certain association of triglycerides with CHD (compared to LDL cholesterol), plasma concentrations greater than the 90th or 95th percentile for age and sex have been used to define hypertriglyceridemia. Some studies show, however, that plasma triglyceride levels >130 to 150 mg/dL are associated with low HDL cho-

lesterol levels and small, dense LDL particles. Furthermore, a meta-analysis of several prospective population studies confirms that triglyceride concentrations are independent predictors of CHD risk. Isolated elevations of plasma triglycerides can be due to increased levels of VLDL (type IV) or combinations of VLDL and chylomicrons (type V). Rarely, only chylomicron levels are elevated (type I). Plasma is usually clear when triglyceride levels are <4.5 mmol/L (<400 mg/dL) and cloudy when levels are higher and VLDL (and/or chylomicron) particles become large enough to scatter light. When chylomicrons are present, a creamy layer floats to the top of plasma after refrigeration for several hours. Tendon xanthomas and xanthelasmas do not occur with isolated hypertriglyceridemia, but eruptive xanthomas (small orange-red papules) can appear on the trunk and extremities when triglyceride levels are >11.5 mmol/L (>1000 mg/dL) (i.e., when chylomicronemia is present). At these high levels of triglycerides, the retinal vessels can appear to be orange-yellow in color (lipemia retinalis). Pancreatitis is the major risk associated with plasma triglyceride concentrations >11 mmol/L (>1000 mg/dL).

Elevations in plasma triglycerides are usually associated with increased synthesis and secretion of VLDL triglycerides by the liver. Hepatic triglyceride synthesis is regulated by substrate flow (the availability of free fatty acids), energy balance (the level of glycogen stores in the liver), and hormonal status (the balance between insulin and glucagon). Obesity, excessive consumption of simple sugars and saturated fats, inactivity, alcohol consumption, and insulin resistance are commonly associated with hypertriglyceridemia. In most of these situations, increased free fatty acid flux from adipose tissue to the liver stimulates the assembly and secretion of VLDL. When VLDL triglyceride levels are markedly elevated [>11.5 mmol/L (>1000 mg/dL)], LPL may be saturated

so that an acquired LPL deficiency develops during the postprandial period even if there is no underlying genetic disorder. The addition of chylomicrons to the circulation may cause dramatic increases in plasma triglycerides.

Familial Hypertriglyceridemia Familial hypertriglyceridemia appears to be transmitted as an autosomal dominant disorder, though the underlying mutation(s) have not been identified. The pathophysiology is complex: both reduced catabolism of triglyceride-rich lipoproteins and overproduction of VLDL have been reported. Elevated levels of fasting plasma triglycerides in the range of 2.3 to 8.5 mmol/L (200 to 750 mg/dL) are usually associated with increased levels of VLDL triglycerides only. When VLDL triglyceride levels are markedly elevated (regardless of etiology), chylomicron triglycerides can also be present, even after a 14-h fast. A 20-year follow-up of individuals with familial hypertriglyceridemia demonstrated a moderate increase in CHD risk.

Familial Lipoprotein Lipase Deficiency This autosomal recessive disorder is due to the severe impairment or absence of LPL, leading to massive accumulation of chylomicrons in plasma. Manifestations begin in infancy and include pancreatitis, eruptive xanthomas, hepatomegaly, splenomegaly, foam cell infiltration of the bone marrow, and, when the level of triglycerides is >11 mmol/L (1000 mg/dL), lipemia retinalis. Atherosclerosis is not accelerated. The diagnosis is suspected by finding a creamy layer (chylomicrons) at the top of plasma that has incubated overnight at 4°C; it is confirmed by demonstrating that LPL levels in plasma do not increase after the administration of heparin (which normally releases LPL from endothelial surfaces). Manifestations recede dramatically when patients are placed on fat-free diets.

LPL levels are within the normal range in most patients with moderate hypertriglyceridemia [2.8 to 5.6 mmol/L (250 to 500 mg/dL)]. Heterozygous mutations in the LPL gene are present in 5 to 10% of hypertriglyceridemic individuals; LPL activity may be reduced by 20 to 50% in these individuals. Heterozygotes for LPL deficiency may also present with severe hypertriglyceridemia if they have poorly controlled diabetes, are pregnant, consume excessive quantities of alcohol, take exogenous estrogen, or are obese.

Familial Apoprotein CII Deficiency This rare autosomal recessive disorder causes a functional deficiency of LPL and clinical manifestations similar to those of familial LPL deficiency. Deficiency of apoprotein CII impairs hydrolysis of chylomicrons and VLDL so that either, or both, lipoproteins accumulate in blood. The diagnosis is suspected in children or adults with recurrent attacks of pancreatitis and confirmed by demonstrating the absence of apo CII on gel electrophoresis and that plasma transfusion (which contains abundant apo CII) causes a dramatic fall in plasma triglycerides. Heterozygotes have half-normal levels of apo CII, may have mild elevations of triglycerides, and are asymptomatic. Dietary fat restriction should be lifelong.

Hepatic Lipase Deficiency Total deficiency of HTGL is a rare autosomal recessive disorder that impairs the final catabolism and/or remodeling of small VLDL and IDL. Subjects with HTGL deficiency often have elevated levels of VLDL remnants; HDL$_2$ levels may be elevated because HTGL participates in the conversion of HDL$_2$ to HDL$_3$. HTGL activity is frequently increased in hypertriglyceridemic individuals, but the meaning of this association is unclear.

HYPERCHOLESTEROLEMIA WITH HYPERTRIGLYCERIDEMIA Concomitant hypercholesterolemia and hypertriglyceridemia occurs in two disorders—familial combined hyperlipidemia (FCHL) and dysbetalipoproteinemia.

Familial Combined Hyperlipidemia FCHL is transmitted as an autosomal dominant disorder. Probands (the initial case discovered within a family) typically have combined hyperlipidemia, isolated hypertriglyceridemia, or isolated elevated levels of LDL cholesterol. The diagnosis requires documentation at some time of combined hyperlipidemia in the proband or, if the proband has isolated hypercholesterolemia or hypertriglyceridemia, the various lipid phenotypes in first-degree relatives at risk. The lipoprotein phenotype in affected individuals may change over time. The underlying defect in this disorder is not known, though mutations or polymorphisms in the LPL gene and in the gene cluster for apo AI, apo CIII, and apo AIV may contribute to the disorder in some families. Insulin resistance is present in many individuals with FCHL; the link may result from increased free fatty acid flux driving assembly and secretion of apo B100 lipoproteins.

FCHL is associated with increased secretion of VLDL particles, as determined by the flux of VLDL apo B. The lipoprotein patterns associated with the disorder are most likely determined by genetic polymorphisms in genes that regulate the metabolism of VLDL. For example, if the affected individual also has a defect in LPL, hypertriglyceridemia will be present. Since the hydrolysis of VLDL triglycerides also regulates the generation of LDL in plasma, individuals with FCHL who have inefficient catabolism of VLDL may also have reduced levels of LDL cholesterol and high VLDL cholesterol. Finally, individuals with FCHL who synthesize normal quantities of triglycerides and secrete VLDL that carries normal amounts of triglyceride generate increased numbers of LDL particles and present with isolated elevations of plasma LDL cholesterol. These variations in VLDL catabolism, together with additional genetic heterogeneity and environmental variability, form the basis for the variable phenotype in this disorder. FCHL may occur in as many as 0.5 to 1.0% of Americans and is the most common familial lipid disorder in survivors of myocardial infarction. The increased risk for atherosclerosis is due to the presence of increased numbers of small, atherogenic VLDLs and the conversion of VLDL to the more atherogenic IDL and LDL. Persons with FCHL usually have clear plasma and do not have xanthomas or xanthelasma.

Dysbetalipoproteinemia This rare disorder affects 1 in 10,000 persons and is due to homozygosity for apo E2, the binding-defective form of apo E. Because apo E plays a crucial role in the catabolism of chylomicron and VLDL remnants, affected individuals have elevations in both VLDL triglyceride and VLDL cholesterol, and chylomicron remnants are present in fasting plasma. The ratio of total cholesterol to triglyceride approximates 1.0, and the ratio of VLDL cholesterol to triglyceride is greater than 0.25. LDL and HDL cholesterol levels are usually low. Although 1% of the population is homozygous for apo E2, most have normal plasma triglyceride and cholesterol levels. Thus, a second defect in lipid metabolism must be present in the 0.01% of individuals with dysbetalipoproteinemia. These individuals may have tuberous xanthomas and deposits of cholesterol in the palmar creases (striae palmaris); the latter, appearing as yellow-orange lines, are specific for dysbetalipoproteinemia. The risk for atherosclerosis and its complications is increased, with onset in the fourth and fifth decades. The incidence of peripheral vascular disease is higher than in FH.

REDUCED HDL CHOLESTEROL Low levels of HDL cholesterol can be defined as <0.9 mmol/L (<35 mg/dL) in men and <1 to 1.2 mmol/L (<40 to 45 mg/dL) in women. Low concentrations of HDL cholesterol are usually associated with coexistent hypertriglyceridemia, though "primary hypoalphalipoproteinemia" has been identified in both individuals and families. The relationship between hypertriglyceridemia and low HDL levels probably derives from: (1) CETP-mediated transfer of cholesteryl ester from the core of HDL to VLDL; (2) shift of surface components, particularly phospholipids apo CII, and apo CIII, from HDL to VLDL; and (3) increased fractional catabolism of the cholesteryl ester–poor apoAI that results from the first two processes. The complexity of the relationship between HDL and triglyceride levels is highlighted by the fact that HDL levels do not return to normal when fasting plasma triglycerides are reduced in most persons with hypertriglyceridemia and low HDL cholesterol levels. Low HDL is clinically silent, and the plasma is usually clear (it can be cloudy or creamy if there is concomitant hypertriglyceridemia).

Primary hypoalphalipoproteinemia refers to the state where HDL cholesterol concentrations are markedly reduced but plasma triglyceride concentrations are normal. Many individuals with this phenotype have had hypertriglyceridemia in the past or have an older (or more obese) first-degree relative who has both low HDL and increased triglyceride levels. Hence, both family studies and long-term follow-up may be required to identify individuals with primary reductions in HDL cholesterol. Rare mutations have been described in the apo AI gene that lead to reductions in apo AI synthesis or increases in catabolism. One mutation that is common in Italy, apo AI-Milano, is associated with a high fractional clearance rate of apo AI but is not associated with increased risk for atherosclerosis.

Some rare genetic disorders of lipid metabolism are summarized in Table 344-5.

SECONDARY CAUSES OF HYPERLIPOPROTEINEMIA (See Table 344-6) **Diabetes Mellitus** Diabetes can affect lipid and lipoprotein metabolism through several mechanisms (Chap. 333). In type 1 diabetes mellitus (DM) (formerly called insulin-dependent di-

Table 344-5 Rare Genetic Disorders of Lipid Metabolism

Disorder	Typical Age of Onset	Plasma Lipid Abnormality	Major Clinical Manifestations	Pathogenesis	Treatment
Hypobetalip-oproteinemia, abetalipopro-teinemia	Early childhood	Very low cholesterol and tri-glyceride levels	Malabsorption of fat, ataxia, neuropathy, reti-nitis pigmentosa, acan-thocytosis	Defective synthesis or secre-tion of apo B leads to low or absent chylomicrons, VLDL, and LDL in plasma	Vitamin E
Tangier disease	Childhood	Low cholesterol; triglycer-ides, normal to slightly ele-vated	Large orange tonsils, cor-neal opacities, relapsing polyneuropathy No premature atheroscle-rosis	Defect in ABC transporter 1; abnormal cholesterol uptake into and/or efflux from macrophages; increased apo AI clearance	None
Lecithin: choles-terol acyltrans-ferase (LCAT) deficiency (fish-eye disease)	Young adult	Total plasma cholesterol level variable with marked decrease in esterified cho-lesterol and increase in unesterified choles-terol; elevated VLDL level; structure of all lipoproteins is abnormal	Corneal opacities, hemo-lytic anemia, renal in-sufficiency, premature atherosclerosis	Decreased LCAT activity in plasma leads to accumula-tion of excess unesterified cholesterol in plasma and body tissues	Fat-restricted diet, kidney transplanta-tion
Cerebrotendinous xanthomatosis	Young adult	None	Progressive cerebellar ataxia, dementia and spinal cord paresis; sub-normal intelligence, ten-don xanthomas, cata-racts	Defect in sterol 27 hydroxy-lase; defective synthesis of primary bile acids in liver leads to increased hepatic synthesis of cholesterol and cholestanol, which accumu-late in brain, tendons, and other tissues	Chenodeoxy-cholic acid
Sitosterolemia	Childhood	Elevated levels of plant ster-ols in plasma, elevated or normal levels of choles-terol, normal triglyceride levels	Tendon xanthomas	Increased intestinal absorp-tion of dietary cholesterol, sitosterol, and other plant sterols with accumulation in plasma and tendons	Diet low in plant ster-ols and cholesterol

NOTE: VLDL, very low density lipoprotein; LDL, low-density lipoprotein.
SOURCE: Modified from MS Brown and JL Goldstein in *Harrison's Principles of Internal Medicine*, 13th ed, KJ Isselbacher et al (eds), New York, McGraw-Hill, 1994.

Table 344-6 Secondary Causes of Lipoprotein Abnormalities

HYPERCHOLESTEROLEMIA

Hypothyroidism	Acute intermittent porphyria
Obstructive liver disease	Drugs: progestogens, cyclosporine,
Nephrotic syndrome	thiazides
Anorexia nervosa	

HYPERTRIGLYCERIDEMIA

Obesity	Pregnancy
Diabetes mellitus	Drugs: estrogen, isotretinoin, beta
Chronic renal failure	blockers, glucocorticoids, bile
Lipodystrophy	acid–binding resins, thiazides
Glycogen storage disease	Acute hepatitis
Alcohol	Systemic lupus erythematosus
Ileal bypass surgery	Monoclonal gammopathy: multiple
Stress	myeloma, lymphomas
Sepsis	AIDS: protease inhibitors

HYPOCHOLESTEROLEMIA

Malnutrition	Monoclonal gammopathy
Malabsorption	Chronic liver disease
Hyperthyroidism	
Myeloproliferative diseases	
Chronic infectious diseases: AIDS, tuberculosis	

LOW HDL

Malnutrition	Beta blockers
Obesity	Anabolic steroids
Cigarette smoking	

NOTE: HDL, high-density lipoprotein.

abetes mellitus), plasma lipids are usually normal when control of diabetes with insulin is adequate. In diabetic ketoacidosis, hypertri-glyceridemia can be severe due to increases in both VLDL and chy-lomicrons. These abnormalities are associated with overproduction of VLDL and LPL deficiency secondary to insulinopenia. They usually improve with tight control of the diabetes. In type 2 DM (formerly called non-insulin-dependent diabetes mellitus), insulin resistance and obesity combine to cause mild to moderate hypertriglyceridemia and low HDL cholesterol levels. In general, this pattern of dyslipidemia is due to overproduction of VLDL. LDL cholesterol is usually normal in type 2 DM, though the LDLs are small, dense, and perhaps more atherogenic. Treatment of type 2 DM and weight reduction improve, but usually do not completely correct, the dyslipidemia (particularly the low HDL cholesterol levels). Therapy of hyperlipidemia should not be delayed in patients with type 2 DM, as they are at increased risk for CHD. It is recommended that patients with diabetes should be treated as if they already have CHD, i.e., the treatment goal is to reduce their LDL to <2.6 mmol/L (<100 mg/dL) (Fig. 344-2).

Hypothyroidism Hypothyroidism accounts for about 2% of all cases of hyperlipidemia and is second only to DM as a cause of sec-ondary hyperlipidemia. Levels of LDL cholesterol can be elevated, even in patients with subclinical disease in whom thyroid-stimulating hormone (TSH) levels are elevated but other thyroid function tests are normal. Hypertriglyceridemia can occur if obesity is present. Hypo-thyroidism is also associated with increased levels of HDL cholesterol, probably because of reduced HTGL activity. Correction of hypothy-roidism reverses the lipid abnormalities.

Renal Disease Renal disease causes a wide range of lipid ab-normalities. The nephrotic syndrome can be accompanied by eleva-tions in LDL, VLDL, or both. The severity of the hyperlipidemia cor-

A

B

FIGURE 344-2 Algorithms for the evaluation and treatment of hypercholesterolemia (*A*) and hypertriglyceridemia (*B*). Statin, HMG-CoA reductase inhibitor; Chol, cholesterol; HDL, high-density lipoprotein; LDL, low-density lipoprotein; TG, triglyceride; TSH, thyroid-stimulating hormone; CHD, coronary heart disease.

relates with the degree of hypoproteinemia. Renal failure is associated with hypertriglyceridemia and low HDL cholesterol concentrations.

Ethanol The metabolism of ethanol enhances the level of NADH in the liver which, in turn, stimulates the synthesis of fatty acids and their incorporation into triglycerides. Moderate ethanol consumption raises plasma VLDL levels, with the degree of elevation dependent on the baseline level. Severe hypertriglyceridemia and pancreatitis usually develop on the background of a genetic hyperlipidemia and heavy alcohol intake. Because ethanol also stimulates the synthesis of apo AI and inhibits CETP, ethanol-associated hypertriglyceridemia is usually accompanied by normal or elevated levels of HDL cholesterol.

Liver Disease Primary biliary cirrhosis and extrahepatic biliary obstruction can cause hypercholesterolemia and elevated levels of plasma phospholipids associated with increased levels of an abnormal lipoprotein (lipoprotein X; Chap. 299) and LDL. Severe liver injury often leads to a decrease in levels of both cholesterol and triglyceride. Acute hepatitis can cause elevated levels of VLDL and impairment of LCAT formation.

AIDS Use of protease inhibitor therapies has been associated with a generalized metabolic syndrome that includes hypertriglyceridemia, alterations in fat distribution, and occasionally type 2 DM (Chap. 309).

DIAGNOSIS Although the initial indication of an abnormality in lipoprotein metabolism is via blood measurements of triglyceride and cholesterol, the disorders are due to abnormalities of specific lipoproteins. Thus, lipoprotein analysis should assess VLDL, LDL, and HDL levels. Direct measurements of plasma LDL require laborious centrifugation techniques. However, LDL cholesterol concentrations can be estimated indirectly in individuals with triglyceride levels <4.5 mmol/L (<400 mg/dL) by subtracting the HDL and VLDL cholesterol from the total plasma cholesterol. HDL cholesterol is determined after chemical precipitation of VLDL and LDL. VLDL cholesterol is estimated to be the plasma triglyceride level divided by five. Therefore

$$\text{LDL cholesterol} = \text{total cholesterol} - (\text{HDL} + \text{triglycerides}/5)$$

where all values are measured in milligrams per deciliter.

In persons with triglyceride levels >4.5 mmol/L (>400 mg/dL), the ratio of triglyceride to cholesterol in VLDL is >5, and this equation cannot be used to calculate the plasma LDL cholesterol level. The other disorder that is not detected with this method is dysbetalipoproteinemia because the ratio of triglyceride to cholesterol in the VLDL is ≪5. In these two situations, direct measurement of LDL cholesterol must be performed in ultracentrifuged plasma. Commercial methods for the measurement of "direct LDL" are available. Although these methods appear to be precise and accurate, the measured values for LDL cholesterol are 0.06 to 0.17 mmol/L (5 to 15 mg/dL) less than estimated LDL because the estimated value is actually the combination of IDL and LDL. If a "direct LDL" measurement is used, the National Cholesterol Education Program (NCEP) guidelines (based on estimated LDL) must be adjusted before therapeutic decisions are made.

Because plasma triglyceride levels rise and both HDL and LDL cholesterol levels fall modestly after a fat-containing meal (due to the action of CETP), it is preferable to measure plasma lipids after a 12-h fast. Measuring cholesterol levels alone will not detect individuals with isolated low HDL; screening for CHD should therefore include measurement of HDL. Because serum lipid levels vary from day to day, at least two to three measurements should be made days or weeks apart before initiating therapy. Some experts advocate the use of total cholesterol/HDL ratios as a better assessment of individual risk. This is a reasonable approach provided both the patient and physician are aware that the treatment goal is to reduce LDL. In addition, rare patients with very high or very low levels of both LDL and HDL have ratios that are not interpretable on the basis of population studies. Although some laboratories offer measurements of individual apoproteins (e.g., apo B100 and apo AI), or size estimates of LDL, this information is not generally helpful in decision-making. Measurement of lipoprotein (a) levels can provide an indication of risk that cannot be gleaned from lipid measurements. Lipoprotein electrophoresis is not useful except for the diagnosis of dysbetalipoproteinemia, a diagnosis that otherwise requires ultracentrifugation methods. Apo E genotyping is also helpful in the diagnosis of dysbetalipoproteinemia (although rarely the disorder can be due to other defects in the apo E gene).

Both LDL and HDL cholesterol levels are temporarily decreased for several weeks after myocardial infarction or acute inflammatory states but can be accurately measured if blood is obtained within 8 h of the event.

Approach to the Patient

Elevated LDL Cholesterol   Treatment of elevated LDL cholesterol can have either of two aims—*primary prevention* of the complications of atherosclerosis or *secondary treatment* after complications have occurred. The rationale for primary prevention is based on the large body of data linking elevated levels of LDL cholesterol with increased CHD risk and an impressive body of clinical and experimental data demonstrating that reducing LDL cholesterol slows progression and may actually induce regression of atherosclerotic lesions (Chap. 242). Both primary and secondary intervention trials indicate that total mortality can be reduced when the LDL cholesterol is lowered (Table 344-1). A meta-analysis of four randomized trials (4S, CARE, AFCAPS/TexCAPS, LIPID) comparing HMG-CoA reductase inhibitors to control included 30,817 participants and found that HMG-CoA reductase inhibitor treatment was associated with: (1) a 20% decrease in total cholesterol, a 28% decrease in LDL cholesterol, a 13% decrease in triglycerides, and a 5% increase in HDL cholesterol; (2) a 31% decrease in major coronary events and a 21% decrease in all-cause mortality; (3) similar risk reduction in women and men; and (4) no effect on noncardiovascular mortality. Unexpectedly, the risk of stroke was also reduced 19 to 32% by HMG-CoA reductase inhibitor treatment, even though previous observational studies show a relatively weak association between cholesterol level and stroke risk.

Dietary Alterations   A fundamental starting point for both primary prevention and secondary treatment involves counseling to modify diet, exercise, smoking, and other life-style factors that increase the risk of CHD. The typical American diet derives about 35% of its calories from fat (14 to 15% from saturated fat) and contains 400 to 500 mg/d of cholesterol. Individuals with hyperlipidemia should be encouraged to eat a diet lower in cholesterol and saturated fat. The NCEP Step 1 diet, which is recommended for all Americans above age 2, provides 30% of calories from fat, <10% of calories from saturated fat, and <300 mg/d of cholesterol (Table 344-7). Carbohydrate is the typical nutrient used to replace fat in patients with isolated hypercholesterolemia. In general, whole-milk dairy products, egg yolks, meats, palm oil, and coconut oil should be replaced with fresh fruits and vegetables, complex carbohydrates (especially whole-grain products), and low-fat dairy products. Shellfish are low in fat content and, except for shrimp, also have low cholesterol levels; shrimp, in moderation, is acceptable. Portion size needs to be stressed; the protein and fat-rich portion of meat in a given meal should be <115 g (4 oz), the size of a deck of cards. Substitutions with any food low in saturated fat such as bran, nuts, and olive oil will have positive effects on LDL. Hydrogenation of vegetable oils increases the saturation of the fatty acids. In particular, trans-fatty acids, mainly found in commercially hydrogenated vegetable oils, raise LDL and can lower HDL cholesterol levels. Use of stanol-containing margarines has, by contrast, lowered LDL cholesterol about 5 to 10% by blocking cholesterol absorption in the small intestine. When further diet therapy is indicated, the NCEP Step 2 diet provides 30% of calories as fat but <7% of calories from saturated fat, and <200 mg/d of cholesterol. After changing from

Table 344-7   The Two-Step Approach to Treating Hypercholesterolemia

Nutrient	Step 1 Diet	Step 2 Diet
Total fat	<30% calories	<30% calories
Fatty acids		
Saturated	<10% calories	<7% calories
Polyunsaturated	≤10% calories	≤10% calories
Monounsaturated	10–15% calories	10–15% calories
Carbohydrates	50–60% calories	50–60% calories
Protein	10–20% calories	10–20% calories
Cholesterol	<300 mg/d	<200 mg/d

a Total calories: to achieve and maintain desirable body weight.

Table 344-8   Hypolipidemic Drugs

Drugs	Mode of Action	Lipoprotein Class Affected
HMG-CoA reductase inhibitors		
Lovastatin (Mevacor) 10–80 mg/d	↓ Cholesterol synthesis	↓ LDL 25–55%
Pravastatin (Pravachol) 10–40 mg/d	↑ LDL receptors	↓ VLDL, ↓ TG 10–20%
Simvastatin (Zocor) 5–40 mg/d		↑ HDL 5–10%
Fluvastatin (Lescol) 20–40 mg/d		
Atorvastatin (Lipitor) 10–80 mg/d		
Cerivastatin (Baycol) 0.3–0.4 mg/d		
Nicotinic acid		
Niacin 50–100 mg tid initially, then increase to 1.0–2.5 g tid	↓ Synthesis of VLDL and LDL; mechanism not defined	↓ TG 25–35%
Niaspan 1–2 g/d		↓ VLDL 25–35%
		↓ LDL 15–25%
		↑ HDL 15–30%
Bile acid–binding resins		
Cholestyramine (Questran) 8–12 g bid or tid	Interruption of the enterohepatic recycling of bile acids;	↓ LDL 20–30%
Cholestipol (Cholestid) 10–15 g bid or tid	↑ Synthesis of new bile acids from cholesterol	↑ HDL 5%
	↑ LDL receptors	↑ TG 10%
Fibric acid derivatives		
Clofibrate (Atromid) 1000 mg bid	↑ LPL and ↑ triglyceride hydrolysis;	↓ TG 25–40%
Gemfibrozil (Lopid) 600 mg bid	↓ VLDL synthesis	↑ or ↓ LDL
Fenofibrate (Tricor) 200 mg qd	↑ LDL catabolism	↑ HDL 5–15%
Probucol		
Probucol (Lorelco) 500 mg bid	↑ LDL clearance from plasma	↓ LDL 10–15%
	↓ Apo A I synthesis	↓ HDL 20–25%
	Antioxidant	

NOTE: LDL, low-density lipoprotein; VLDL, very low density lipoprotein; TG, triglycerides; HDL, high-density lipoprotein; LPL, lipoprotein lipase; CPK, creative phosphokinase.

the average American diet to the Step 1 diet, the LDL cholesterol usually drops 8 to 10%; an additional reduction of 5 to 7% can be achieved by advancing to the Step 2 diet. There is, however, great individual variability in diet responsiveness, and several values should be obtained before judging the efficacy of any diet treatment.

Primary Prevention The NCEP Adult Treatment Panel recommends measuring plasma cholesterol in all adults older than age 20 at least every 5 years. Ideally, this testing involves a lipoprotein profile to allow better risk stratification. Primary prevention goals include LDL cholesterol <3.36 mmol/L (<130 mg/dL), triglycerides <1.7 mmol/L (<150 mg/dL), and HDL cholesterol >1.03 mmol/L (>40 mg/dL) for men and >1.29 mmol/L (>50 mg/dL) for women. In individuals without DM or known CHD, treatment recommendations for primary prevention are outlined in Fig. 344-2. Assessment of risk factors in addition to LDL cholesterol is an essential part of this decision-making process. Risk factors include: (1) family history of premature CHD (<55 years in a male parent or sibling or <65 in female relatives), (2) hypertension (even if it is controlled with medications), (3) cigarette smoking (>10 cigarettes per day), (4) DM, and (5) low HDL [<0.9 mmol/L (<35 mg/dL)]. In addition, because CHD is more prevalent in older individuals, age (men >45 years, women >55 years, or younger women with premature menopause without estrogen replacement) is also an important risk factor. HDL cholesterol >1.6 mmol/L (>60 mg/dL) is a negative risk factor, i.e., one other risk factor can be negated by a high HDL cholesterol level.

In individuals with fewer than two risk factors, life-style modifications alone and follow-up testing may be used if LDL is <4.14 mmol/L (<160 mg/dL). For those with LDL >4.91 mmol/L (>190 mg/dL), drug treatment is indicated. If two or more risk factors are present, drug treatment in addition to life-style modifications should be instituted if LDL cholesterol is >3.36 mmol/L (>130 mg/dL). HMG-CoA reductase inhibitors are first-line medications for most patients; niacin and resins are second-line treatments (see below).

Secondary Prevention The NCEP guidelines are stringent for the secondary treatment of patients with CHD. Patients with CHD should be screened for lipid abnormalities during and after their initial diagnoses. A goal of lowering plasma LDL concentrations to <2.6 mmol/L (<100 mg/dL) is advocated for such individuals as well as for patients with DM (Fig. 344-2). As described below, this requires modifications of diet in addition to the use of one or more medications.

If a patient with CHD has only a modestly elevated LDL cholesterol level [e.g., <3.36 mol/L (<130 mg/dL)], a 4- to 6-week period of Step 1 diet therapy can precede the addition of drugs. In such a patient, moving to the Step 2 diet, which provides the same total fat but <7% of calories from saturated fat, can be useful. If, however, the LDL cholesterol is >3.36 mmol/L (>130 mg/dL), drug therapy should be instituted along with diet therapy (Fig. 344-2).

High Triglycerides and Low HDL The evidence that treatment to reduce plasma triglyceride levels or increase levels of HDL cholesterol leads to long-term health benefits is less compelling than that for treatment of high LDL levels. Two recent clinical trials have shown, however, that lowering triglycerides (using fibric acids) or lowering LDL (HMG-CoA reductase inhibitors) decreases CHD events in these patients. There have been no intervention trials in which only increases in HDL cholesterol concentrations have been achieved. Beneficial effects of niacin have been attributed, in part, to its HDL-raising effect and its action to reduce triglycerides and LDL. Even with drugs that primarily affect LDL cholesterol levels, such as bile acid–binding resins and HMG-CoA reductase inhibitors, some of the benefits achieved may be related to increases in HDL cholesterol levels.

In patients with isolated elevations of triglyceride levels or with hypertriglyceridemia and high LDL cholesterol, life-style modifications should be introduced as described above, and weight reduction

Common Side Effects	Contraindications	Drug Interactions	Combined Use
Hepatic dysfunction <2%, severe myositis <1%, ↑ CPK, len opacities may occur	Risk of myositis increased by impaired renal function and in combination with gemfibrozil or nicotinic acid	Fibric acid derivatives, niacin, ketoconazole, cyclosporine, erythromycin, coumadin	Bile acid resins; increased myositis risk when combined with gemfibrozil, niacin
Flushing (may be relieved by aspirin), hepatic dysfunction, tachycardia, atrial arrythmias, pruritus, dry skin, nausea, diarrhea, glucose intolerance, hyperuricemia	Peptic ulcer disease, cardiac arrhythmias, hepatic disease, gout, diabetes mellitus	Synergistic with ganglionic blocking agents used to treat hypertension	Bile acid resins, HMG-CoA reductase inhibitors, fibric acid derivatives
Constipation, gastric discomfort, nausea, hemorrhoidal bleeding, theoretical ↑ lithogenicity of bile	Biliary tract obstruction, gastric outlet obstruction	↓ Absorption of phenylbutazone, phenobarbital, thyroid hormone, digoxin, coumadin, thiazide diuretics, and some antibiotics; binds fat-soluble vitamins (A,D,E,K);	Nicotinic acid, HMG-CoA reductase inhibitors, fibric acid derivatives
↑ Lithogenicity of bile, gallstones, nausea, hepatic dysfunction, myositis <1%, cardiac arrythmias	Hepatic or biliary disease, renal insufficiency associated with ↑ risk of myositis	↑ Anticoagulant activity of coumadin	Bile acid resins
Diarrhea, nausea, abdominal pain, cardiac arrhythmias	Prolonged QT interval, primary biliary cirrhosis		Bile acid resins

should be strongly encouraged if obesity is present. Fat intake should be decreased, but the concomitant increase in carbohydrate intake may raise triglyceride and lower HDL cholesterol levels. If this occurs, replacing some of the saturated fat with monounsaturated fat, which will not raise LDL cholesterol, may be valuable. Severe hypertriglyceridemia and hyperchylomicronemia require very low fat diets, avoidance of free sugars, and decreased alcohol intake. Patients with genetic LPL deficiency are instructed to prepare their food using medium-chain triglycerides, which are not incorporated into chylomicrons. Fish oils decrease triglyceride synthesis, and high doses may be used for severe hypertriglyceridemia.

The management of hypertriglyceridemia focuses on the associated LDL and HDL concentrations as guidelines for therapy. Thus, the overall risk profile can be used to set goals for LDL cholesterol, using a low HDL level (commonly associated with hypertriglyceridemia) as a concomitant major risk factor for atherosclerosis. However, when triglyceride levels are >5.6 mmol/L (>500 mg/dL), the risk of developing pancreatitis increases, and a direct focus on lowering triglycerides is recommended. Thus, triglyceride levels >5.6 mmol/L (>500 mg/dL) are generally treated with drugs, whereas lower levels [2.2 to 5.6 mmol/L (200 to 500 mg/dL)] are not treated unless other CHD risk factors are present (Fig. 344-2).

℞ **TREATMENT** Three classes of lipid-lowering agents are recommended as first-line therapy against hypercholesterolemia: (1) the HMG-CoA reductase inhibitors; (2) niacin; and (3) the bile acid–binding resins (Table 344-8). Fibric acid derivatives are second-line agents for hypercholesterolemia and are most effective for lowering triglycerides.

HMG-CoA Reductase Inhibitors This class of drugs, which include lovastatin, simvastatin, pravastatin, fluvastatin, atorvastatin, and cerivastatin, inhibits the rate-limiting step in hepatic cholesterol biosynthesis (the conversion of HMG-CoA to mevalonate), causing an increase in LDL receptor levels in hepatocytes and enhanced receptor-mediated clearance of LDL cholesterol from the circulation. At usual doses, the HMG-CoA reductase inhibitors decrease total cholesterol by 20 to 30% and LDL cholesterol by 25 to 40%. Larger reductions may be achieved with higher doses. Treatment with reductase inhibitors often reduces triglycerides by 10 to 20%, possibly due to reduced secretion of VLDL by the liver. Higher doses of more potent reductase inhibitors, which can lower LDL cholesterol by 45 to 60%, can lower triglycerides by 30 to 45%. HDL cholesterol levels rise about 5 to 10%. In comparison with other lipid-lowering agents, HMG-CoA reductase inhibitors are relatively free of side effects. Mild, transient elevations in liver enzymes occur with all of the agents at the highest doses, but elevations in serum aminotransferases to more than three times the upper limits of normal occur in <2% of patients. Therapy should be discontinued when elevations of this magnitude occur. A rare but potentially serious adverse effect of HMG-CoA reductase inhibitors is myopathy, manifest by muscle pain with elevation of serum creatine phosphokinase (CPK). This occurs in <1% of patients treated with reductase inhibitors alone but is more common (about 2 to 3%) when used in combination with gemfibrozil, niacin, or cyclosporine.

Niacin The mechanism of action of niacin is not fully understood, but it appears to inhibit the secretion of lipoproteins containing apo B100 from the liver. Niacin decreases both total and LDL cholesterol approximately 15 to 25%, reduces VLDL levels by 25 to 35%, and raises HDL cholesterol levels by as much as 15 to 25%. Thus, niacin exerts favorable changes on the three major lipoproteins (VLDL, LDL, and HDL). Efficacy of monotherapy was confirmed in a long-term secondary prevention trial in which niacin significantly reduced the incidence of myocardial infarction. An even longer-term follow-up of that study (15 years total) showed an 11% decrease in all-cause mortality among patients randomized to niacin. Because of its ability to reduce VLDL synthesis, niacin is also a first-line drug for treatment of hypertriglyceridemia.

Niacin is safe, having been in use for almost 30 years, but unpleasant side effects, including cutaneous flushing with or without pruritus, may limit patient acceptability. The cutaneous symptoms tend to subside after several weeks and may be minimized by initiating therapy at low doses or by administering aspirin 30 min before the niacin dose. Less common adverse effects include elevations of liver enzymes, gastrointestinal distress, impaired glucose tolerance, and elevated serum uric acid levels with or without gouty arthritis. Liver enzymes may be elevated in 3 to 5% of patients on full doses of niacin (>2 g/d). Because of its propensity to worsen the control of blood sugar, niacin should be used with caution in patients with DM. Niaspan, an intermediate-release form of niacin, appears to exhibit lipid-altering activity similar to regular niacin.

Bile Acid–Binding Resins Cholestyramine and colestipol have been in use as lipid-lowering agents for almost three decades. These drugs interfere with reabsorption of bile acids in the intestine, resulting in a compensatory increase in bile acid synthesis and upregulation of LDL receptors in hepatocytes. The bile acid sequestrants are useful in the treatment of patients with elevated levels of LDL cholesterol and normal triglycerides. Sequestrants produce dose-dependent decreases on the order of 15 to 25% in total cholesterol and of 20 to 35% in LDL cholesterol. The agents cause modest increases in HDL cholesterol. A limitation of the sequestrants is their tendency to raise triglyceride levels through compensatory increases in hepatic synthesis of VLDL; they should not be given to hypertriglyceridemic individuals. Bile acid–binding resins are efficacious and safe and are recommended for young adult men and premenopausal women with moderate cholesterol elevations. Patient compliance is low, in part because of the need to dissolve these powdered agents in fluid; the availability of colestipol as a tablet may alleviate this problem. Gastrointestinal side effects include constipation, bloating, and gas.

Combination Therapy Combinations of bile acid–binding resins and reductase inhibitors are effective for the treatment of severe, isolated elevations of LDL cholesterol. Combinations of reductase inhibitors and niacin, or resins and niacin, are useful for the treatment of high LDL and low HDL cholesterol levels, though the former combination carries an increased risk of myositis (2 to 3%). If triglyceride and LDL levels are both elevated (HDL is usually reduced as well), resins and niacin are an excellent combination, with resins and gemfibrozil (see below) as an alternative. The combination of a reductase inhibitor and gemfibrozil can be useful when LDL cholesterol is very high in the face of concomitant hypertriglyceridemia, but the risk of myositis (about 2 to 3%) must be considered. Combinations of reductase inhibitors with either niacin or gemfibrozil might best be reserved for patients with CHD and combined hyperlipidemia.

LDL Apheresis In patients with homozygous FH and in ordinary FH patients who respond poorly to diet and drug therapy or who cannot tolerate drugs, apheresis at 7- to 14-day intervals can cause profound lowering of LDL cholesterol levels. Diet and drug regimens are continued during treatment. This approach should be considered for patients with few therapeutic options.

Fibric Acids Gemfibrozil and fenofibrate stimulate the activity of a liver transcription factor termed $PPAR\alpha$ that increases LPL activity and production of apo AI. Moreover, these drugs reduce VLDL triglyceride entry into plasma and reduce synthesis of apo CIII, which might improve LPL-induced lipolysis or reduce VLDL secretion. Stimulation of peroxisomal fatty acid oxidation by fibrates may also contribute to the triglyceride-lowering actions. Gemfibrozil and fenofibrate treatment is associated with 25 to 40% reductions in plasma triglyceride levels. Postprandial triglyceride levels, which are linked to fasting concentrations, are also reduced. HDL cholesterol levels increase 5 to 15% with fibrate treatment. Fibric acids and a low-fat diet are particularly useful in the treatment of dysbetalipoproteinemia and are first-line therapy for this disorder except in postmenopausal women, who should initially be given estrogen replacement (if not contraindicated).

Significant increases in LDL cholesterol can accompany otherwise potentially beneficial falls in triglycerides and increases in HDL cholesterol during fibrate therapy. Such rises may require a change to another drug or addition of a second agent.

In the short term, these drugs are well tolerated; mild gastrointestinal distress in the form of epigastric pain is the major side effect. Elevations of liver enzymes occur in 2 to 3% of patients but do not usually require cessation of treatment. Rarely, hepatitis can occur. Fibrates appear to make the bile more lithogenic, and long-term use is probably associated with a twofold increase in gallstone formation. Myopathy with myositis is a rare occurrence with the fibrates, either alone or in combination with HMG CoA reductase inhibitors.

Fish Oils Large doses of omega-3 fatty acids reduce triglyceride levels by diminishing their production. In the United States, omega-3 fatty acid capsules contain 40 to 60% omega-3 fatty acids; the rest of the fatty acids are omega-6. Therefore, to consume 2 to 4 g of omega-3 fatty acids, an individual must take 5 to 10 capsules per day.

HYPOCHOLESTEROLEMIA

A low total cholesterol concentration [<2.6 mmol/L (<100 mg/dL)] in an adult can be due to rare hereditary traits or secondary to a number of diseases. As described earlier, mutations in the gene for apo B100 that disrupt synthesis or produce truncated forms of apo B100 are associated with hypobetalipoproteinemia. These mutations are inherited as codominant traits; heterozygotes have plasma cholesterol levels in the range of 1.3 to 2.6 mmol/L (50 to 100 mg/dL), with reduced LDL cholesterol levels but normal plasma HDL cholesterol levels. Heterozygotes are asymptomatic, whereas hypolipoproteinemia homozygotes (or compound heterozygotes) have even lower total and LDL cholesterol concentrations and may have malabsorption of fats and fat-soluble vitamins similar to that in abetalipoproteinemia.

Abetalipoproteinemia (Table 344-5) is a rare, autosomal recessive disorder in which there are mutations in the microsomal triglyceride transfer protein (MTP) gene. Individuals who are homozygous for this disorder have total cholesterol levels <1.3 mmol/L (<50 mg/dL) and essentially no VLDL, IDL, LDL, or chylomicrons. Because dietary fat and vitamins A and E are transported from the intestine in chylomicrons, these patients may have malabsorption of fat and fat-soluble vitamins. Vitamin E deficiency in infancy and early childhood can result in neurologic problems (Chap. 75). If vitamin replacement is adequate, individuals with abetalipoproteinemia can live normal, healthy lives.

Moderately low levels of total cholesterol may also be associated with extreme reductions in HDL cholesterol. As noted above, these are almost always secondary to mutations in the gene for apo AI and a lack of apo AI in plasma.

A number of systemic diseases can cause low cholesterol concentrations. Malnutrition, often associated with alcoholism or gastrointestinal disease, can cause low levels of total and LDL cholesterol. Hyperthyroidism, particularly when severe, can reduce cholesterol levels. Patients with uncontrolled AIDS may have total cholesterol levels <2.1 mmol/L (<80 mg/dL), usually associated with severe wasting, diarrhea, and a poor prognosis. Several neoplasms, particularly those involving the hematopoietic system, are associated with hypocholesterolemia. Patients with acute and chronic myelogenous leukemia and myeloid metaplasia with splenomegaly can have severe reductions in both LDL and HDL levels. Other diseases with concomitant splenomegaly, including lipid storage diseases such as Gaucher's disease and Niemann-Pick disease, can cause very low LDL and HDL cholesterol concentrations due to increased lipoprotein catabolism.

BIBLIOGRAPHY

GOLDSTEIN JL et al: Familial hypercholesterolemia, in *The Metabolic and Molecular Bases of Inherited Disease*, 8th ed, CR Scriver et al (eds). New York, McGraw-Hill, 2001, pp 2863–2913

GOTTO AM Jr.: Triglyceride as a risk factor for coronary artery disease. Am J Cardiol 82: 22Q, 1998

GRUNDY SM: Primary prevention of coronary heart disease: Integrating risk assessment with intervention. Circulation 100:988, 1999

KNOPP RH: Drug treatment of lipid disorders. N Engl J Med 341:498, 1999

KRAUSS RM et al: Dietary guidelines for healthy American adults. A statement for health professionals from the Nutrition Committee, American Heart Association. Circulation 94:1795, 1996

LAROSA JC et al: Effect of statins on risk of coronary disease: A meta-analysis of randomized controlled trials. JAMA 282:2340, 1999

RIFKIND BM: Clinical trials of reducing low-density lipoprotein concentrations. Endocrinol Metab Clin North Am 27:585, 1998

STEINBERG D, GOTTO AM: Preventing coronary artery disease by lowering cholesterol levels: Fifty years from bench to bedside. JAMA 282:2043, 1999

Summary of the Second Report of the National Cholesterol Education Program expert panel on detection, evaluation, and treatment of high blood cholesterol in adults. JAMA 269:3015, 1993

345 *Lawrie W. Powell, Kurt J. Isselbacher*

HEMOCHROMATOSIS

DEFINITION Hemochromatosis is a common disorder of iron storage in which an appropriate increase in intestinal iron absorption results in deposition of excessive amounts of iron in parenchymal cells with eventual tissue damage and impaired function of organs, especially the liver, pancreas, heart, joints, and pituitary. The disease was termed *hemochromatosis* and the iron-storage pigment was called *hemosiderin* because it was believed that the pigment was derived from the blood. The terms *hemosiderosis* and *siderosis* are often used to describe the presence of stainable iron in tissues, but tissue iron must be quantified to assess body iron status (see below and Chap. 105). *Hemochromatosis* implies potentially severe progressive iron overload leading to fibrosis and organ failure. Cirrhosis of the liver, diabetes mellitus, arthritis, cardiomyopathy, and hypogonadotrophic hypogonadism are common manifestations.

Although there is debate about definitions, it seems logical to use the following terminology:

1. *Hereditary* or *genetic hemochromatosis*: This disorder is most often caused by inheritance of a mutant *HFE* gene, which is tightly linked to the HLA-A locus on chromosome 6p (see below). The genetic disease can be recognized during its early stages when iron overload and organ damage are minimal. At this stage the disease is best referred to as *early* or *precirrhotic hemochromatosis* (Fig. 345-1).

2. *Secondary iron overload*: Tissue injury usually occurs secondary to an iron-loading anemia such as thalassemia or sideroblastic anemia, in which increased erythropoiesis is ineffective. In the acquired iron-loading disorders, massive iron deposits in parenchymal tissues can lead to the same clinical and pathologic features as in hemochromatosis.

PREVALENCE Hemochromatosis is one of the most common genetic diseases, although its prevalence varies in different ethnic groups. It is most common in populations of northern European extraction in whom approximately 1 in 10 persons are heterozygous carriers and 0.3 to 0.5% are homozygotes. However, expression of the disease is modified by several factors, especially dietary iron intake, blood loss associated with menstruation and pregnancy, and blood donation. The clinical expression of the disease is 5 to 10 times more frequent in men than in women. Nearly 70% of affected patients develop the first symptoms between ages 40 and 60. The disease is rarely evident before age 20, although with family screening (see below) and periodic health examinations, asymptomatic subjects with iron overload can be identified, including young menstruating women. A recent study in a European non-blood bank population revealed that 30% of homozygous individuals did not have evidence of iron overload. Thus, the penetrance of the mutation is variable.

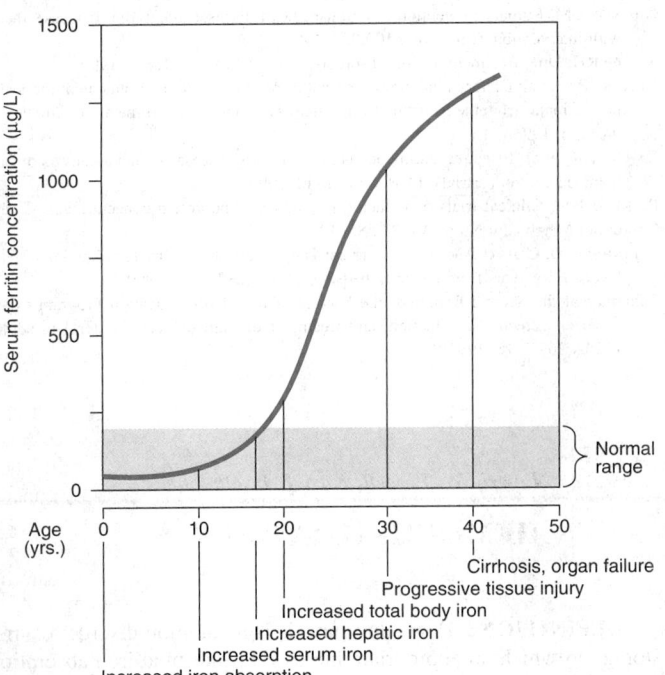

FIGURE 345-1 Sequence of events in genetic hemochromatosis and their correlation with the serum ferritin concentration. Increased iron absorption is present throughout life. Overt, symptomatic disease usually develops between ages 40 and 60, but latent disease can be detected long before this.

GENETIC BASIS AND MODE OF INHERITANCE The gene involved in the most common form of hemochromatosis was cloned in 1996 and is termed *HFE*. A homozygous G→A mutation resulting in a cysteine to tyrosine substitution at position 282 (C282Y) is the most common mutation. It was identified in 85 to 100% of patients with hereditary hemochromatosis in populations of northern European descent but was found in only 60% of cases from Mediterranean populations (e.g., southern Italy). A second, relatively common *HFE* mutation has also been identified. This results in an amino acid substitution of histidine to aspartic acid at position 63 (H63D). Some compound heterozygotes (e.g., one copy each of C282Y and H63D) have increased body iron stores. Thus, *HFE*-associated hemochromatosis is inherited as an autosomal recessive trait; heterozygotes have no, or minimal, increase in iron stores. However, in some cases this slight increase in hepatic iron acts as a cofactor that aggravates other diseases such as porphyria cutanea tarda (PCT) and nonalcoholic steatohepatitis.

Mutations in other genes, currently unidentified, are responsible for non-*HFE* associated hemochromatosis, including juvenile hemochromatosis, which affects subjects in the second and third decade of life (Table 345-1).

PATHOGENESIS Normally, the body iron content of 3 to 4 g is maintained such that intestinal mucosal absorption of iron is equal to iron loss. This amount is approximately 1 mg/d in men and 1.5 mg/d in menstruating women. In hemochromatosis, mucosal absorption is inappropriate to body needs and amounts to 4 mg/d or more. The progressive accumulation of iron causes an early elevation in plasma iron, an increased saturation of transferrin, and progressive elevation of plasma ferritin level (Fig. 345-1).

The *HFE* gene encodes a 343 amino acid protein that is structurally related to MHC class I proteins. The basic defect in hemochromatosis is a lack of cell surface expression of HFE (due to the C282Y mutation). The normal (wild type) HFE protein forms a complex with β_2-microglobulin and transferrin, and the C282Y mutation completely abrogates this interaction. As a result, the mutant HFE protein remains trapped intracellularly, reducing transferrin receptor-mediated iron up-

Table 345-1 Classification of Iron Overload States

Hereditary hemochromatosis
  Hemochromatosis, *HFE*-related
    C282Y homozygosity
    C282Y/H63D compound heterozygosity
  Hemochromatosis non-*HFE*-related
  Juvenile hemochromatosis
  Autosomal dominant hemochromatosis (Solomon Islands)
Acquired iron overload
  Iron-loading anemias
    Thalassemia major
    Sideroblastic anemia
    Chronic hemolytic anemias
    Transfusional and parenteral iron overload
  Dietary iron overload
  Chronic liver disease
    Hepatitis C
    Alcoholic cirrhosis, especially when advanced
    Nonalcoholic steatohepatitis
    Porphyria cutanea tarda
    Dysmetabolic iron overload syndrome
    Post portacaval shunting
Miscellaneous
  Iron overload in sub-Sahara Africa
  Neonatal iron overload
  Aceruloplasminemia
  Congenital atransferrinemia

take by the intestinal crypt-cell. This is postulated to upregulate the divalent metal transporter (DMT-1) on the brush border of the villous cells, leading to inappropriately increased intestinal iron absorption. In advanced disease, the body may contain 20 g or more of iron that is deposited mainly in parenchymal cells of the liver, pancreas, and heart. Iron may be increased 50- to 100-fold in the liver and pancreas and 5- to 25-fold in the heart. Iron deposition in the pituitary causes hypogonadotropic hypogonadism in both men and women. Tissue injury may result from disruption of iron-laden lysosomes, from lipid peroxidation of subcellular organelles by excess iron, or from stimulation of collagen synthesis by activated stellate cells.

Secondary iron overload with deposition in parenchymal cells occurs in chronic disorders of erythropoiesis, particularly in those due to defects in hemoglobin synthesis or ineffective erythropoiesis such as sideroblastic anemia and thalassemia (Chap. 106). In these disorders, the absorption of iron is increased. Moreover, these patients require blood transfusions and are also frequently treated inappropriately with iron. PCT, a disorder characterized by a defect in porphyrin biosynthesis (Chap. 346), is also sometimes associated with excessive parenchymal iron deposits. The magnitude of the iron load in PCT is usually insufficient to produce tissue damage. However, recent reports have found that many patients with PCT also have mutations in the *HFE* gene, and some have associated hepatitis C infection. Although the relationship among these disorders remains to be clarified, iron overload accentuates the inherited enzyme deficiency in PCT and should be avoided along with other agents (alcohol, estrogens, haloaromatic compounds) that may exacerbate PCT. Another cause of hepatic parenchymal iron overload is hereditary aceruloplasminemia. In this disorder, impairment of iron mobilization due to deficiency of ceruloplasmin (a ferroxidase) causes iron overload in hepatocytes.

Alcoholic subjects with end-stage chronic liver disease may have increased tissue iron stores of the degree seen in hemochromatosis. The increased iron may be caused by cell death and uptake of the released iron, as well as by hemolysis associated with spur-cell anemia (Chap. 108). Hemochromatosis in a heavy drinker can be distinguished from alcoholic liver disease by the presence of the C282Y mutation.

Excessive iron ingestion over many years rarely results in hemochromatosis. An important exception has been reported in South Africa among groups who brew fermented beverages in vessels made of iron. Hemochromatosis has on occasion been described in apparently normal subjects who have taken medicinal iron over many years, but such individuals probably have a genetic disorder.

The common denominator in all patients with hemochromatosis is *excessive amounts of iron in parenchymal tissues*. Parenteral administration of iron in the form of blood transfusions or iron preparations results predominantly in reticuloendothelial cell iron overload. This appears to lead to less tissue damage than iron loading of parenchymal cells.

PATHOLOGY At autopsy, the enlarged nodular liver and pancreas are rusty in color. Histologically, iron is increased in amount in many organs, particularly in the liver, heart, and pancreas, and to a lesser extent in the endocrine glands. The epidermis of the skin is thin, and melanin is increased in the cells of the basal layer. Deposits of iron are present around the synovial lining cells of the joints.

In the liver of patients with hemochromatosis, parenchymal iron is in the form of ferritin and hemosiderin. In the early stages these deposits are seen in the periportal parenchymal cells, especially within lysosomes in the pericanalicular cytoplasm of the hepatocytes. This stage progresses to perilobular fibrosis and eventually to deposition of iron in bile duct epithelium, Kupffer cells, and fibrous septa. In the advanced stage, a macronodular or mixed macro- and micronodular cirrhosis develops.

CLINICAL MANIFESTATIONS Initial symptoms include weakness, lassitude, weight loss, change in skin color, abdominal pain, loss of libido, and symptoms of diabetes mellitus. Hepatomegaly, increased pigmentation, spider angiomas, splenomegaly, arthropathy, ascites, cardiac arrhythmias, congestive heart failure, loss of body hair, testicular atrophy, and jaundice are prominent in advanced disease.

The *liver* is usually the first organ to be affected, and hepatomegaly is present in more than 95% of symptomatic patients. Hepatic enlargement may exist in the absence of symptoms or of abnormal liver function tests. Indeed, over half of patients with symptomatic hemochromatosis have little laboratory evidence of functional impairment of the liver, in spite of hepatomegaly and fibrosis. Loss of body hair, palmar erythema, testicular atrophy, and gynecomastia are common. Manifestations of portal hypertension and esophageal varices occur less commonly than in cirrhosis from other causes. Hepatocellular carcinoma develops in about 30% of patients with cirrhosis, and it is the most common cause of death in treated patients; hence the importance of early diagnosis and therapy. Its incidence increases with age, is more common in men, and occurs almost exclusively in cirrhotic patients. Splenomegaly occurs in approximately half of symptomatic cases.

Excessive skin pigmentation is present in over 90% of symptomatic patients at the time of diagnosis. The characteristic metallic or slate gray hue is sometimes referred to as bronzing and results from increased melanin and iron in the dermis. Pigmentation usually is diffuse and generalized, but it may be more pronounced on the face, neck, extensor aspects of the lower forearms, dorsa of the hands, lower legs, genital regions, and in scars.

Diabetes mellitus occurs in about 65% of patients and is more likely to develop in those with a family history of diabetes, suggesting that direct damage to the pancreatic islets by iron deposition occurs in combination with a genetic predisposition. The management is similar to that of other forms of diabetes, although pronounced insulin resistance is more common in association with hemochromatosis. Late complications are the same as seen in other causes of diabetes mellitus.

Arthropathy develops in 25 to 50% of patients. It usually occurs after age 50, but may occur as a first manifestation, or long after therapy. The joints of the hands, especially the second and third metacarpophalangeal joints, are usually the first joints involved, a feature that helps to distinguish the chondrocalcinosis associated with hemochromatosis from the idiopathic form (Chap. 322). A progressive polyarthritis involving wrists, hips, ankles, and knees also may ensue. Acute brief attacks of synovitis may be associated with deposition of calcium pyrophosphate (chondrocalcinosis or pseudogout), mainly in the knees. Radiologic manifestations include cystic changes of the subchondral bones, loss of articular cartilage with narrowing of the joint space, diffuse demineralization, hypertrophic bone proliferation, and calcification of the synovium. The arthropathy tends to progress despite removal of iron by phlebotomy. Although the relation of these abnormalities to iron metabolism is not known, the fact that similar changes occur in other forms of iron overload suggests that iron is directly involved.

Cardiac involvement is the presenting manifestation in about 15% of patients. The most common manifestation is congestive heart failure, which occurs in about 10% of young adults with the disease, especially those with juvenile hemochromatosis. Symptoms of congestive failure may develop suddenly, with rapid progression to death if untreated. The heart is diffusely enlarged and may be misdiagnosed as idiopathic cardiomyopathy if other overt manifestations are absent. Cardiac arrhythmias include premature supraventricular beats, paroxysmal tachyarrhythmias, atrial flutter, atrial fibrillation, and varying degrees of atrioventricular block.

Hypogonadism occurs in both sexes and may antedate other clinical features. Manifestations include loss of libido, impotence, amenorrhea, testicular atrophy, gynecomastia, and sparse body hair. These changes are primarily the result of decreased production of gonadotropins due to impairment of hypothalamic-pituitary function by iron deposition; however, primary testicular dysfunction may be seen in some cases. Adrenal insufficiency, hypothyroidism, and hypoparathyroidism may also occur.

DIAGNOSIS The association of (1) hepatomegaly, (2) skin pigmentation, (3) diabetes mellitus, (4) heart disease, (5) arthritis, and (6) hypogonadism should suggest the diagnosis. However, a parenchymal iron overload of comparatively short duration or modest degree may exist with none or only some of these manifestations [e.g., in young subjects (Fig. 345-1)]. Therefore, a high index of suspicion is needed to make the diagnosis early. This is particularly important because treatment before there is permanent organ damage can reverse the iron toxicity and restore life expectancy to normal (see below).

The history should be particularly detailed in regard to disease in other family members, alcohol ingestion, iron intake, and ingestion of large doses of ascorbic acid, which promotes iron absorption (Chap. 75). Appropriate tests should be performed to exclude iron deposition due to hematologic disease. The presence of liver, pancreatic, cardiac, and joint disease should be confirmed by physical examination, roentgenography, and standard function tests of these organs. The degree of increase in total-body iron stores should be assessed with particular attention to an increase in parenchymal iron concentration, with or without tissue damage.

The methods available for assessing parenchymal iron stores include (1) measurement of serum iron and the percent saturation of transferrin (or the unsaturated iron-binding capacity); (2) measurement of serum ferritin concentration; (3) liver biopsy with measurement of the iron concentration and calculation of the hepatic iron index (Table 345-2), (4) estimation of chelatable iron stores following the administration of deferoxamine; and (5) computed tomography (CT) and/or magnetic resonance imaging (MRI) of the liver. Each has its advantages and limitations. The serum iron level and percent saturation of transferrin are elevated early in the course, but their specificity is reduced by significant false-positive and false-negative rates. For example, serum iron concentration may be increased in patients with alcoholic liver disease without iron overload; in this situation, however, the hepatic iron index is usually not increased as in hemochromatosis (Table 345-1). In otherwise healthy persons, a fasting serum transferrin saturation greater than 50% is abnormal and suggests homozygosity for hemochromatosis.

The serum ferritin concentration is usually a good index of body iron stores, whether decreased or increased. In fact, an increase of 1 μg/L in serum ferritin level reflects an increase of about 65 mg in body stores. In most untreated patients with hemochromatosis, the serum ferritin level is greatly increased (Fig. 345-1 and Table 345-1). However, in patients with inflammation and hepatocellular necrosis, serum ferritin levels may be elevated out of proportion to body iron stores due to increased release from tissues. A repeat determination of serum

Table 345-2 Representative Iron Values in Normal Subjects, Patients with Hemochromatosis, and Patients with Alcoholic Liver Disease

Determination	Normal	Symptomatic Hemochromatosis	Homozygotes with Early, Asymptomatic Hemochromatosis	Heterozygotes	Alcoholic Liver Disease
Plasma iron, μmol/L (μg/dL)	9–27 (50–150)	32–54 (180–300)	Usually elevated 36–54 (200–300)	Elevated or normal	Often elevated 45–66 (250–370)
Total iron-binding capacity, μmol/L (μg/dL)	45–66 (250–370)	36–54 (200–300)	36–54 (200–300)	Elevated or normal	45–66 (250–370)
Transferrin saturation, percent	22–46	50–100	50–100	Normal or elevated	27–60
Serum ferritin, μg/L	10–200	900–6000	200–500	Usually <500	10–500
Urinary iron,[a] mg/24 h	0–2	9–23	2–5	2–5	Usually <5
Liver iron, μg/g dry wt	300–1400	6000–18,000	2000–4000	300–3000	300–2000
Hepatic iron index (μg/g dry wt) 56 × age	<1.0	>2	Usually >2	<2	<2

[a] After intramuscular administration of 0.5 g deferoxamine.

ferritin should therefore be carried out after acute hepatocellular damage has subsided, e.g., in alcoholic liver disease. Ordinarily, the combined measurements of the percent transferrin saturation and serum ferritin level provide a simple and reliable screening test for hemochromatosis, including the precirrhotic phase of the disease. If either of these tests is abnormal, genetic testing for hemochromatosis should be performed (Fig. 345-2).

The role of liver biopsy in the diagnosis and management of hemochromatosis is being reassessed as a result of the widespread availability of genetic testing for the C282Y mutation. The absence of severe fibrosis can be accurately predicted in most patients using clinical and biochemical variables. Thus, there is virtually no risk of severe fibrosis in a C282Y homozygous subject with: (1) serum ferritin level less than 1000 μg/L; (2) normal serum alanine amino transaminase values; (3) no hepatomegaly; and (4) no excess alcohol intake. However, it should be emphasized that liver biopsy is the only reliable method for establishing or excluding the presence of hepatic cirrhosis, which is the critical factor determining prognosis and the risk of developing hepatocellular carcinoma. Biopsy also permits histochemical estimation of tissue iron and measurement of hepatic iron concentration. Increased density of the liver due to iron deposition can be demonstrated by CT or MRI. A retrospective assessment of body iron storage is also provided by performing weekly phlebotomy and calculating the amount of iron removed before iron stores are exhausted (1 mL blood = approximately 0.5 mg iron).

SCREENING FOR HEMOCHROMATOSIS When the diagnosis of hemochromatosis is established, it is important to counsel and screen other family members (Chap. 68). Asymptomatic as well as symptomatic family members with the disease usually have an increased saturation of transferrin and an increased serum ferritin concentration. These changes occur even before the iron stores are greatly increased (Fig. 345-1). All first-degree relatives of patients with hemochromatosis should be tested for the C282Y and H63D mutations and advised appropriately. In affected individuals, it is important to confirm or exclude the presence of cirrhosis, and begin therapy as early as possible. When children of a proband are affected, a homozygote-heterozygote mating is most likely.

The role of population screening for hemochromatosis is controversial. Hemochromatosis fulfills the criteria established by the World Health Organization for population screening, and DNA testing could, in principle, be performed along with other neonatal tests. However, because iron overload does not develop until the second, third, or fourth decades, and the degree of penetrance is still uncertain, screening by phenotypic expression is more practical at present (Fig. 345-2).

TREATMENT The therapy of hemochromatosis involves removal of the excess body iron and supportive treatment of damaged organs. Iron removal is best begun by weekly or twice-weekly phlebotomy of 500 mL. Although there is an initial modest decline in the volume of packed red blood cells to about 35 mL/dL, the level stabilizes after several weeks. The plasma transferrin saturation remains increased until the available iron stores are depleted. In contrast, the plasma ferritin concentration falls progressively, reflecting the gradual decrease in body iron stores. Since one 500-mL unit of blood contains 200 to 250 mg iron and about 25 g iron should be removed, weekly phlebotomy may be required for 1 or 2 years. When the transferrin saturation and ferritin level become normal, phlebotomies are performed at appropriate intervals to maintain levels within the normal range. The measurements promptly become abnormal with iron reaccumulation. Usually one phlebotomy every 3 months will suffice.

Chelating agents such as deferoxamine, when given parenterally, remove 10 to 20 mg iron per day, which is much less than that mobilized by once-weekly phlebotomy. Phlebotomy is also less expensive, more convenient, and safer for most patients. However, chelating agents are indicated when anemia or hypoproteinemia is severe enough to preclude phlebotomy. Subcutaneous infusion of deferoxamine using a portable pump is the most effective means of administration.

The management of hepatic failure, cardiac failure, and diabetes mellitus is similar to conventional therapy for these conditions. Loss of libido and change in secondary sex characteristics are partially relieved by parenteral testosterone or gonadotropin therapy (Chap. 335).

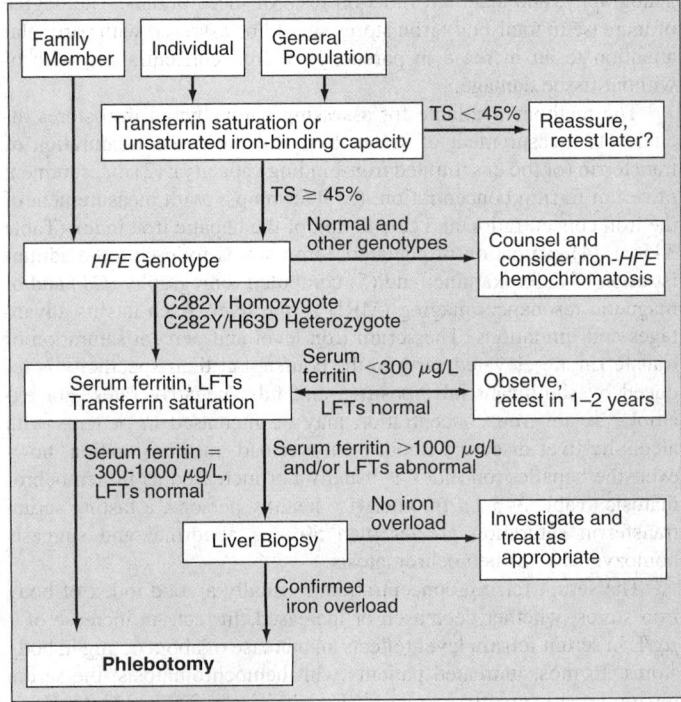

FIGURE 345-2 Algorithm for screening for *HFE*-associated hemochromatosis. LFT, liver function tests; TS, transferrin saturation. (*With permission from The Canadian Journal of Gastroenterology.*)

PROGNOSIS The principal causes of death in untreated patients are cardiac failure (30%), hepatocellular failure or portal hypertension (25%), and hepatocellular carcinoma (30%).

Life expectancy is improved by removal of the excessive stores of iron and maintenance of these stores at near-normal levels. The 5-year survival rate with therapy increases from 33 to 89%. With repeated phlebotomy, the liver and spleen decrease in size, liver function improves, pigmentation of skin decreases, and cardiac failure may be reversed. Diabetes improves in about 40%, but removal of excess iron has little effect on hypogonadism or arthropathy. Hepatic fibrosis may decrease, but cirrhosis is irreversible. End-stage liver disease can be treated with orthotopic liver transplantation, but the results are suboptimal unless excess iron stores are first corrected. Hepatocellular carcinoma usually occurs as a late sequela in patients who are cirrhotic at presentation. The apparent increase in its incidence in treated patients is probably related to their increased life span. Hepatocellular carcinoma does not appear to develop if the disease is treated in the precirrhotic stage. Indeed, the life expectancy of homozygotes treated before the development of cirrhosis is normal.

The importance of family screening and early therapy cannot be emphasized too strongly. Asymptomatic subjects detected by family studies should have phlebotomy therapy if iron stores are moderately to severely increased. Assessment of iron stores at appropriate intervals is also important. With this management approach, most manifestations of the disease can be prevented.

BIBLIOGRAPHY

ADAMS PC: Population screening for hemochromatosis. Hepatology 29:1324, 1999

BACON BR et al: Molecular medicine and hemochromatosis: At the crossroads. Gastroenterology 116:193, 1999

BONKOVSKY HL et al: Porphyria cutanea tarda, hepatitis C and HFE gene mutations in North America. Hepatology 27:1661, 1998

BROCK J et al: *Iron Metabolism in Health and Disease.* London, Saunders, 1994

CAMASCHELLA C et al: Juvenile and adult hemochromatosis are distinct genetic disorders. Eur J Hum Genet 5:371, 1997

EDWARDS CQ et al: Prevalence of hemochromatosis among 11,065 presumably healthy blood donors. N Engl J Med 318:1355, 1988

FEDER JN et al: A novel MHC class I-like gene is mutated in patients with hereditary hemochromatosis. Nat Genet 13:399, 1996

FEDER JN et al: The hemochromatosis founder mutation in HLA-H disrupts β_2 microglobulin interaction and cell surface expression. J Biol Chem 272:14025, 1997

GUYADER D et al: Noninvasive prediction of fibrosis in C282Y homozygous hemochromatosis. Gastroenterology 115:929, 1998

LUDWIG K et al: Hemosiderosis in cirrhosis: A study of 447 native livers. Gastroenterology 112:882, 1997

NEIDERAU C et al: Long-term survival in patients with hereditary hemochromatosis. Gastroenterology, 110:1107, 1996

OLYNYK JK et al: A population based study of the clinical expression of the hemochromatosis gene. N Engl J Med 341:718, 1999

346 Robert J. Desnick

THE PORPHYRIAS

AIP	acute intermittent porphyria	HMB	hydroxymethylbilane
ALA	δ-aminolevulinic acid	PBG	porphobilinogen
CEP	congenital erythropoietic porphyria	PCT	porphyria cutanea tarda
COPRO	coproporphyrinogen	PROTO	protoporphyrinogen
EPP	erythropoietic protoporphyria	URO	uroporphyrinogen
HCP	hereditary coproporphyria	VP	variegate porphyria
HEP	hepatoerythropoietic porphyria	XLSA	X-linked sideroblastic anemia

The porphyrias are inherited or acquired disorders of specific enzymes in the heme biosynthetic pathway (Fig. 346-1). These disorders are classified as either *hepatic* or *erythropoietic* depending on the primary site of overproduction and accumulation of the porphyrin precursor or porphyrin (Tables 346-1 and 346-2), although some have overlapping features. The major manifestations of the hepatic porphyrias are neurologic, including neuropathic abdominal pain, neuropathy, and mental disturbances, whereas the erythropoietic porphyrias characteristically cause cutaneous photosensitivity. The reason for neurologic involvement in the hepatic porphyrias is poorly understood. Cutaneous sensitivity to sunlight is due to the fact that excitation of excess porphyrins in the skin by long-wave ultraviolet light leads to cell damage, scarring, and deformation. Steroid hormones, drugs, and nutrition influence the production of porphyrin precursors and porphyrins, thereby precipitating or increasing the severity of some porphyrias. Thus, the porphyrias are multifactorial genetic disorders, in which environmental, physiologic, and genetic factors interact to cause disease (Chap. 68).

Because many symptoms of the porphyrias are nonspecific, diagnosis is often delayed. Laboratory testing is required to confirm or exclude the various types of porphyria (Table 346-2). Urinary δ-aminolevulinic acid (ALA) and porphobilinogen (PBG) are easily quantitated by chemical methods; the urinary porphyrin isomers can be separated and quantitated by high-performance liquid chromatography. The diagnostic profile of accumulated precursors and/or porphyrins in each disorder can also be defined by extraction and thin-layer chromatography of fecal porphyrins. However, a definite diagnosis requires demonstration of the specific enzyme deficiency or gene defect. The isolation and characterization of the cDNAs encoding the heme biosynthetic enzymes have permitted identification of the genetic basis of each porphyria. Molecular genetic analyses now make it possible to provide precise heterozygote identification and prenatal diagnoses in families with known mutations or with informative polymorphisms.

HEME BIOSYNTHESIS The first and last three enzymes in the heme biosynthetic pathway are located in the mitochondrion, whereas the other four are in the cytosol (Fig. 346-1). The first enzyme, δ-aminolevulinate synthase (ALA synthase), catalyzes the condensation of glycine, activated by pyridoxal phosphate and succinyl coenzyme A, to form ALA. In the liver, this rate-limiting enzyme can be induced by a variety of drugs, steroids, and other chemicals. Distinct erythroid-specific and nonerythroid (e.g., housekeeping) forms of ALA synthase are encoded by separate genes; defects in the erythroid form cause X-linked sideroblastic anemia (XLSA).

The second enzyme, δ-aminolevulinate dehydratase (ALA dehydratase), catalyzes the condensation of two molecules of ALA to form PBG. Four molecules of PBG condense to form the tetrapyrrole uroporphyrinogen (URO) III by a two-step process catalyzed by hydroxymethylbilane (HMB) synthase (also known as PBG deaminase or URO I synthase) and URO III synthase. HMB synthase catalyzes the head-to-tail condensation of four PBG molecules by a series of deaminations to form the linear tetrapyrrole HMB. URO synthase catalyzes the rearrangement and rapid cyclization of HMB to form the asymmetric, physiologic, octacarboxylate porphyrinogen URO III isomer.

The fifth enzyme in the pathway, URO decarboxylase, catalyzes the sequential removal of the four carboxyl groups from the acetic acid side chains of URO III to form coproporphyrinogen (COPRO) III, a tetracarboxylate porphyrinogen. This compound then enters the mitochondrion, where COPRO oxidase, the sixth enzyme, catalyzes the decarboxylation of two of the four propionic acid groups to form the two vinyl groups of protoporphyrinogen (PROTO) IX, a dicarboxylate porphyrinogen. Next, PROTO oxidase oxidizes PROTO IX to protoporphyrin IX by the removal of six hydrogen atoms. The product of the reaction is a porphyrin (oxidized form), in contrast to the preceding tetrapyrrole intermediates, which are porphyrinogens (reduced forms). Finally, ferrous iron is inserted into protoporphyrin IX to form heme, a reaction catalyzed by the eighth enzyme in the pathway, ferrochelatase (also known as heme synthetase or protoheme ferrolyase).

MITOCHONDRIA

Succinyl COA

Glycine

ALA-SYNTHASE

B_6 CoASH CO_2

δ-Aminolevulinic acid

FEEDBACK REPRESSION

Heme

$2 H^+$
Fe^{++}

FERROCHELATASE

Protoporphyrin IX

6H

PROTO-OXIDASE

COPRO-OXIDASE

$2CO_2$ $2 H$

Protoporphyrinogen IX

CYTOPLASM

ALA-DEHYDRATASE

H_2O

Porphobilinogen

HMB-SYNTHASE

$4 NH_3$

Hydroxymethylbilane

URO-SYNTHASE

H_2O

Uroporphyrinogen III

URO-DECARBOXYLASE

$4 H$
$4 CO_2$

Coproporphyrinogen III

FIGURE 346-1 The human heme biosynthetic pathway.

Each of the heme biosynthetic enzymes is encoded by a separate gene. Full-length human cDNAs for each of the enzymes, including those for both forms of ALA synthase, have been isolated and sequenced, and the chromosomal locations of the genes have been identified (Table 346-3).

REGULATION OF HEME BIOSYNTHESIS About 85% of the heme produced in the body is synthesized in erythroid cells to provide heme for hemoglobin; most of the remainder is produced in the liver, where the biosynthetic pathway is under negative feedback control (Chap. 104). "Free" heme in the liver regulates the synthesis and mitochondrial translocation of the housekeeping form of ALA synthase. Heme represses the synthesis of the ALA synthase mRNA and interferes with the transport of the enzyme from the cysotol into

mitochondria. ALA synthase is increased by many of the same chemicals that induce the cytochrome P450 enzymes in the endoplasmic reticulum of the liver. Because most of the heme in the liver is used for the synthesis of cytochrome P450 enzymes, hepatic ALA synthase and the cytochrome P450s are regulated in a coordinated fashion.

Different regulatory mechanisms control production of heme for hemoglobin. The erythroid-specific ALA synthase encoded on the X chromosome is expressed at higher levels than the hepatic enzyme, and an erythroid-specific control mechanism regulates iron transport into erythroid cells. During erythroid differentiation, the activities of the heme biosynthetic enzymes are increased.

THE HEPATIC PORPHYRIAS

The acute hepatic porphyrias are characterized by the rapid onset of neurologic manifestations. During the acute attack, individuals have markedly elevated plasma and urinary concentrations of the porphyrin precursors ALA and PBG, which originate from the liver.

ALA DEHYDRATASE–DEFICIENT PORPHYRIA This is a rare autosomal recessive disorder that has been described in only a few patients. Onset and severity of the disease are variable, presumably depending on the amount of residual ALA dehydratase activity. Treatment and prevention of the neurologic complications are the same as for other acute porphyrias (see below).

Clinical Features The clinical presentation is variable. The first reported cases were in two unrelated German men who had clinical onset during adolescence of abdominal pain and neuropathy, resembling acute intermittent porphyria (AIP; see below). A Swedish infant presented with failure to thrive and required transfusions and parenteral nutrition. Presumably, the earlier age of onset and more severe manifestations reflect a more complete enzyme deficiency. A Belgian man developed an acute motor polyneuropathy and polycythemia at age 63. Recently a Japanese woman was described who had her first acute attack and the syndrome of inappropriate secretion of antidiuretic hormone at age 69.

Diagnosis Patients have increased urinary levels of ALA and coproporphyrin. ALA dehydratase activity in erythrocytes is <5% of normal. Because either succinylacetone (which accumulates in hereditary tyrosinemia and is structurally similar to ALA) or lead can inhibit ALA dehydratase, increase urinary excretion of ALA, and cause manifestations that resemble those of the acute porphyrias, lead intoxication and hereditary tyrosinemia (fumarylacetoacetase deficiency) should be considered in the differential diagnosis of ALA dehydratase–deficient porphyria. Immunologic studies in the reported cases demonstrated the presence of nonfunctional enzyme proteins that cross-reacted with anti-ALA dehydratase antibodies. DNA analysis revealed different missense mutations that resulted in the amino acid substitutions G133R and V275M in the infantile-onset patient, and R240W and A274T in a juvenile-onset patient.

Heterozygotes are clinically asymptomatic and do not excrete increased levels of ALA, but they can be detected by demonstration of intermediate levels of erythrocyte ALA dehydratase activity or by demonstrating a specific mutation in the *ALA dehydratase* gene. Prenatal diagnosis of this disorder has not been achieved but should be possible by determination of the ALA dehydratase activity in cultured chorionic villi or amniocytes.

℞ TREATMENT Treatment is similar to that of AIP (see below). The severely affected infant was supported by hyperalimentation and periodic blood transfusions. Continued failure to thrive led to liver transplantation, which did not improve the hematologic manifestations.

ACUTE INTERMITTENT PORPHYRIA This hepatic porphyria is an autosomal dominant condition resulting from the half-normal level of HMB synthase (also termed PBG deaminase) activity. The disease is widespread but is especially common in Scandinavia and perhaps Great Britain. The enzyme deficiency can be demonstrated in most heterozygous individuals, but clinical expression is highly variable. Activation of the disease is related to environmental or hormonal factors, such as drugs, diet, and steroid hormones, which can precipitate the manifestations. Attacks can be prevented by avoiding known precipitating factors.

Clinical Features Most heterozygotes remain clinically asymptomatic (latent) unless exposed to factors that increase the production of porphyrins. Endogenous and exogenous gonadal steroids, porphyrinogenic drugs, alcohol ingestion, and low-calorie diets, usually instituted for weight loss, are common precipitating factors. Table 346-4 lists the major drugs that are harmful in AIP [and also in hereditary coproporphyria (HCP) and variegate porphyria (VP)] and some drugs and anesthetic agents known to be safe. More extensive lists of drugs considered harmful or safe are available (see the bibliography), but information is incomplete for many of them. Attacks also can be provoked by infections and by surgery.

Because the neurovisceral symptoms rarely occur before puberty and are often nonspecific, a high index of suspicion is required to make the diagnosis. The disease can be disabling but is rarely fatal. Abdominal pain, the most common symptom, is usually steady and poorly localized but may be cramping. Ileus, abdominal distention, and decreased bowel sounds are common. However, increased bowel sounds and diarrhea may occur. Abdominal tenderness, fever, and leukocytosis are usually absent or mild because the

symptoms are neurologic rather than inflammatory. Nausea, vomiting, constipation, tachycardia, hypertension, mental symptoms, pain in the limbs, head, neck, or chest, muscle weakness, sensory loss, dysuria, and urinary retention are characteristic. Tachycardia, hypertension, restlessness, tremors, and excess sweating are due to sympathetic overactivity.

The peripheral neuropathy is due to axonal degeneration (rather than demyelination) and primarily affects motor neurons. Significant neuropathy does not occur with all acute attacks; abdominal symptoms are usually more prominent. Motor neuropathy affects the proximal muscles initially, more often in the shoulders and arms. The course and degree of involvement are variable. Deep tendon reflexes may be normal or hyperactive but are usually decreased or absent with advanced neuropathy. Motor weakness can be asymmetric and focal and may involve cranial nerves. Sensory changes such as paresthesia and loss of sensation are less prominent. Progressive muscle weakness can lead to respiratory and bulbar paralysis and death when diagnosis and

Table 346-1 Classification of the Human Porphyrias

Type/Porphyria	Deficient Enzyme	Inheritance[a]	Photosensitivity	Neurovisceral Symptoms
HEPATIC PORPHYRIAS				
ALA dehydratase deficiency (ADP)	ALA dehydratase	AR	−	+
Acute intermittent porphyria (AIP)	HMB synthase	AD	−	+
Porphyria cutanea tarda (PCT)	URO decarboxylase	AD	+++	−
Hereditary coproporphyria (HCP)	COPRO oxidase	AD	+	+
Variegate porphyria (VP)	PROTO oxidase	AD	+	+
ERYTHROPOIETIC PORPHYRIAS				
X-linked sideroblastic anemia (XLSA)	ALA synthase	XLR	−	−
Congenital erythropoietic porphyria (CEP)	URO synthase	AR	+++	−
Erythropoietic protoporphyria (EPP)	Ferrochelatase	AD	+	−

[a] AR, autosomal recessive; AD, autosomal dominant; XLR, X-linked recessive.
NOTE: ALA, δ-aminolevulinic acid; HMB, hydroxymethylbilane; URO, uroporphyrinogen; COPRO, copoporphyrinogen; PROTO, protoporphyrinogen.

Table 346-2 The Major Metabolites Accumulated in the Human Porphyrias

Type/Porphyria	Increased Erythrocyte Porphyrins	Porphyrin Excretion	
		Urine	Stool
HEPATIC PORPHYRIAS			
ALA dehydratase deficiency (ADP)	PROTO	ALA, COPRO III	—
Acute intermittent porphyria (AIP)	—	ALA, PBG	—
Porphyria cutanea tarda (PCT)	—	URO I, 7-carboxylate porphyrin	ISOCOPRO
Hereditary coproporphyria (HCP)	—	ALA, PBG, COPRO III	COPRO III
Variegate porphyria (VP)	—	ALA, PBG COPRO III	PROTO IX, 5-carboxylate porphyrin
ERYTHROPOIETIC PORPHYRIAS			
X-linked sideroblastic anemia (XLSA)	—	—	—
Congenital erythropoietic porphyria (CEP)	URO I	URO I	COPRO I, URO I
Erythropoietic protoporphyria (EPP)	PROTO IX	—	PROTO IX

NOTE: ALA, δ-aminolevulinic acid; PBG, porphobilinogen; COPRO I, coproporphyrinogen; ISOCOPRO, isocoproporphyrin; URO, uroporphyrinogen; PROTO, protoporphyrinogen.

Gene	Chromosome Location	cDNA/ Protein	Genomic Organization Length/# Exons
δ-Aminolevulinate synthase			
Housekeeping	3p21.1	2,199 bp/640 aa	17 kb/11 exons
Erythroid-specific	Xp11.21	1,937 bp/587 aa	22 kb/11 exons
δ-Aminolevulinate dehydratase	9q34		
Housekeeping		1,149 bp/330 aa	15.9 kb/exons 1A, 2–12
Erythroid-specific		1,154 bp/330 aa	15.9 kb/exons 1B, 2–12
Hydroxymethylbilane synthase	11q23.3		
Housekeeping		1,086 bp/361 aa	11 kb/exons 1, 3–15
Erythroid-specific		1,035 bp/344 aa	11 kb/exons 2–15
Uroporphyrinogen III synthase	10q25.2→q26.3		
Housekeeping		1,296 bp/265 aa	34 kb/exons 1, 2B–10
Erythroid-specific		1,216 bp/265 aa	34 kb/exons 2A, 2B–10
Uroporphyrinogen decarboxylase	1p34	1,104 bp/367 aa	3 kb/10 exons
Coproporphyrinogen oxidase	3q12	1,062 bp/354 aa	14 kb/7 exons
Protoporphyrinogen oxidase	1q23	1,431 bp/477 aa	5.5 kb/13 exons
Ferrochelatase	18q21.3	1,269 bp/423 aa	45 kb/11 exons

[a] cDNA basepairs (bp), number of encoded amino acids (aa), genomic length in kilobases (kb), and number of exons are indicated.

treatment are delayed. Sudden death may result from sympathetic overactivity and cardiac arrhythmia.

Mental symptoms such as anxiety, insomnia, depression, disorientation, hallucinations, and paranoia can occur in acute attacks. Seizures can be due to neurologic effects or to hyponatremia. Treatment of seizures is difficult because virtually all antiseizure drugs (except bromides) may exacerbate AIP (clonazepam may be safer than phenytoin or barbiturates). Hyponatremia results from hypothalamic involvement and inappropriate vasopressin secretion or from electrolyte depletion due to vomiting, diarrhea, poor intake, or excess renal sodium loss. Persistent hypertension and impaired renal function may occur. When an attack resolves, abdominal pain may disappear within hours, and paresis begins to improve within days and may continue to improve over several years.

Diagnosis ALA and PBG levels are increased in plasma and urine during acute attacks. Urinary PBG excretion is usually 220 to 880 μmol/d (50 to 200 mg/d) [normal, 0 to 18 μmol/d (0 to 4 mg/d)], and urinary ALA excretion is 150 to 760 μmol/d (20 to 100 mg/d) [normal, 8 to 53 μmol/d (1 to 7 mg/d)]. The excretion of these compounds generally decreases with clinical improvement, particularly after hematin infusions (see below). A normal urinary PBG level effectively excludes AIP as a cause for current symptoms. Fecal porphyrins are usually normal or minimally increased in AIP, in contrast to HCP and VP. Most asymptomatic ("latent") heterozygotes with HMB syn-

Table 346-4 Categories of Unsafe and Safe Drugs in AIP, HCP, and VP

Unsafe	Safe
Barbiturates	Narcotic analgesics
Sulfonamide antibiotics	Aspirin
Meprobamate	Acetaminophen
Glutethimide	Phenothiazines
Methyprylon	Penicillin and derivatives
Ethchlorvynol	Streptomycin
Mephenytoin	Glucocorticoids
Succinimides	Bromides
Carbamazepine	Insulin
Valproic acid	Atropine
Pyrazolones	
Griseofulvin	
Ergots	
Synthetic estrogens and progestogens	
Danazol	
Alcohol	

NOTE: AIP, acute intermittent porphyria; HCP, hereditary coproporphyria; VP, variegate porphyria.

thase deficiency have normal urinary excretion of ALA and PBG. Therefore, measurement of HMB synthase in erythrocytes is useful to confirm the diagnosis and to screen asymptomatic family members.

The enzyme deficiency is detectable in erythrocytes from most AIP heterozygotes (*classic AIP*). Note that the activity is higher in young erythrocytes and may increase into the normal range in AIP when erythropoiesis is increased due to a concurrent condition. However, patients with the rare erythroid form of AIP (*erythroid, or variant, AIP*) have normal enzyme levels in erythrocytes and deficient activity in nonerythroid tissues (see below). The erythroid and housekeeping forms of HMB synthase are encoded by a single gene, which has two promoters: one promoter generates the ubiquitously expressed housekeeping mRNA; the other promoter transcribes the erythroid-specific mRNA. Several deletions and over 150 different point mutations have been found in the coding region of the gene in unrelated AIP families (Fig. 346-2). These mutations alter the kinetic properties and/or stability of the mutant enzymes or create premature termination codons. Mutations that cause erythroid AIP variants with half-normal enzyme in nonerythroid tissues, but normal activity in erythrocytes, include point mutations in the initiation methionine codon (which prevent translation) or in the 5' donor splice site of intron 1 (which cause abnormal splicing of the HMB synthase transcript).

Heterozygotes can be identified using various polymorphic sites in the *HMB synthase* gene. Efforts are now under way to identify the specific mutations in the *HMB synthase* gene in all AIP families; this information will make it possible to identify all heterozygotes in affected families and to advise them to avoid the factors that cause acute attacks. The prenatal diagnosis of a fetus at risk can be made with cultured amniotic cells or chorionic villi.

TREATMENT During acute attacks, narcotic analgesics may be required for abdominal pain, and phenothiazines are useful for nausea, vomiting, anxiety, and restlessness. Chloral hydrate can be given for insomnia, and benzodiazepines are probably safe in low doses, if a minor tranquilizer is required. Although intravenous glucose (at least 300 g/d) can be effective in acute attacks of porphyria, a more complete parenteral nutritional regimen may be beneficial if oral feeding is not possible for a prolonged period. However, intravenous heme is more effective than glucose in reducing porphyrin precursor excretion and probably leads to more rapid recovery. The response to heme therapy is reduced if therapy is delayed. Therefore, 3 to 4 mg of heme, in the form of hematin (Abbott Laboratories), heme albumin, or heme arginate (Leiras Oy, Turku, Finland), may be infused daily for 4 days beginning as soon as possible after onset of an attack. Heme arginate and heme albumin are chemically stable and are less likely than hematin to produce phlebitis or an anticoagulant effect. The rate of recovery from an acute attack depends on the degree of neuronal damage and may be rapid (1 to 2 days) with prompt therapy. Recovery from severe motor neuropathy may require months or years. Identification and avoidance of inciting factors can hasten recovery from an attack and prevent future attacks. Multiple inciting factors may contribute to a symptomatic episode. Frequent clear-cut cyclical attacks occur in some women and can be prevented with a long-acting gonadotropin-releasing hormone analogue (this indication is not approved by the U.S. Food and Drug Administration) (Chap. 336).

PORPHYRIA CUTANEA TARDA Porphyria cutanea tarda (PCT), the most common of the porphyrias, can be sporadic (type I) or familial (types II and III) and can also develop after exposure to halogenated aromatic hydrocarbons. Hepatic URO decarboxylase is deficient in all types of PCT. In type I PCT, URO decarboxylase activity is normal in erythrocytes. In type II PCT, an autosomal dominant disorder, the enzyme is deficient in erythrocytes and other tissues. In type III PCT, deficiency of the enzyme is limited to the liver. Deficient hepatic URO decarboxylase and a porphyrin pattern resembling PCT can be produced by exposure of normal individuals to a number of halogenated aromatic hydrocarbons. Hepatoerythropoietic porphyria (HEP) is an autosomal recessive form of porphyria that results from marked systemic deficiency of URO decarboxylase activity.

Clinical Features Cutaneous photosensitivity is the major clinical feature. Neurologic manifestations are not observed. Fluid-filled vesicles and bullae develop on sun-exposed areas such as the face, the dorsa of the hands and feet, the forearms, and the legs. The skin in these areas is friable, and minor trauma may lead to the formation of bullae. The appearance of small white plaques, termed *milia*, may precede or follow vesicle formation. Bullae and denuded skin heal slowly and are subject to infection. Other features include hypertrichosis and hyperpigmentation, especially of the face, and thickening, scarring, and calcification resembling the cutaneous changes of systemic sclerosis.

FIGURE 346-2 Mutations in the *HMB synthase* gene causing acute intermittent porphyria. Mutation nomenclature: letters, one-letter code for amino acids; numbers, codon positions.

A number of factors contribute to the development of hepatic URO decarboxylase deficiency, including excess alcohol, iron, and estrogens. The importance of excess hepatic iron as a precipitating factor is underscored by the finding that the incidence of the common hemochromatosis-causing mutations, *HFE* C282Y and H63D, are increased in patients with types I and II PCT (Chap. 345). Various chemicals can also induce PCT; an epidemic of PCT occurred in eastern Turkey in the 1950s as a consequence of wheat contaminated with the fungicide hexachlorobenzene. PCT also occurs after exposure to other chemicals, including di- and trichlorophenols and 2,3,7,8-tetrachlorodibenzo-(*p*)-dioxin (TCDD, dioxin). Patients with PCT characteristically have liver damage and are at risk for hepatocellular carcinoma. These carcinomas do not produce porphyrins.

HEP resembles congenital erythropoietic porphyria (CEP) and usually presents with blistering skin lesions, hypertrichosis, scarring, and red urine in infancy or childhood.

Diagnosis Porphyrins are increased in the liver, plasma, urine, and stool. The urinary ALA level may be slightly increased, but the PBG level is normal. Urinary porphyrins consist mostly of uroporphyrin and 7-carboxylate porphyrin, with lesser amounts of coproporphyrin and 5- and 6-carboxylate porphyrins. Plasma porphyrins are also increased in a pattern that resembles that in urine. Isocoproporphyrins are increased in feces and sometimes in plasma and urine. The finding of increased isocoproporphyrins is diagnostic for a deficiency of hepatic URO decarboxylase.

Type II PCT and HEP can be distinguished by finding decreased URO decarboxylase in erythrocytes. URO decarboxylase activity in liver, erythrocytes, and cultured skin fibroblasts in type II PCT is approximately 50% of normal in affected individuals and in family members with latent disease. In HEP, the URO decarboxylase activity is markedly deficient, with typical levels of 3 to 10% of normal. Several point mutations have been identified in the coding region of the *URO decarboxylase* gene from unrelated type II PCT and HEP patients (Fig. 346-3). Excess hepatic iron contributes to development of sporadic and familial forms of PCT. As noted above, coinheritance of *HFE* mutations that cause hemochromatosis increases susceptibility to PCT-precipitating factor. In the familial forms (types II and III), iron inhibits the residual normal enzyme, so that enzymatic activity in liver is <50% of normal. In type I PCT the decreased hepatic URO decarboxylase activity is not accompanied by a decrease in the amount of enzyme protein, suggesting that the enzyme is present in an inactive form; hepatic URO decarboxylase activity gradually increases after a remission is induced by phlebotomy.

TREATMENT Alcohol, estrogens, iron supplements, and, if possible, any drugs that may exacerbate the disease should be discontinued, but this step does not always lead to improvement. A complete response can almost always be achieved by repeated phlebotomy to reduce hepatic iron. A unit (450 mL) of blood can be removed every 1 to 2 weeks. Because iron overload is not marked in most cases, remission may occur after only five or six phlebotomies. Hemoglobin levels or hematocrits and serum ferritin should be followed closely to prevent development of iron deficiency and anemia. After remission, continued phlebotomy may not be needed even if ferritin levels return to normal. Relapses are treated by additional phlebotomy.

PCT can also be treated with chloroquine or hydroxychloroquine, both of which complex with the excess porphyrins and promote their excretion. Small doses (e.g., 125 mg chloroquine phosphate twice weekly) should be given, because standard doses can induce transient,

FIGURE 346-3 Mutations in the *URO synthase* gene causing familial porphyria cutanea tarda (*bottom*) and hepatoerythropoietic porphyria. (*top*) Mutation nomenclature as in Fig. 346-2.

sometimes marked increases in photosensitivity and hepatocellular damage. Hepatic imaging can diagnose or exclude complicating hepatocellular carcinoma. Treatment of PCT in patients with end-stage renal disease is facilitated by administration of erythropoietin.

HEREDITARY COPROPORPHYRIA HCP is an autosomal dominant form of hepatic porphyria that results from half-normal levels of COPRO oxidase activity. Photosensitivity may occur. A few cases of homozygous HCP have been reported.

Clinical Features HCP is influenced by the same factors that cause attacks in AIP. The disease is latent before puberty, and symptoms are more common in women. Neurovisceral symptoms and other manifestations are virtually identical to those of AIP. Photosensitivity may resemble that in PCT and VP. Cutaneous lesions may begin in childhood in rare homozygous cases.

Diagnosis Coproporphyrin is markedly increased in the urine and feces in symptomatic disease and sometimes when there are no symptoms. Urinary ALA and PBG levels are increased during acute attacks but may return to normal when symptoms resolve. Although the diagnosis can be confirmed by measuring COPRO oxidase activity, these assays are not widely available and require cells other than erythrocytes.

TREATMENT Neurologic symptoms are treated as in AIP (see above). Phlebotomy and chloroquine are ineffective when cutaneous lesions are present.

VARIEGATE PORPHYRIA VP, a hepatic porphyria that results from the deficient activity of PROTO oxidase, is transmitted in an autosomal dominant manner and can present with neurologic symptoms, photosensitivity, or both.

Clinical Features Neurovisceral signs and symptoms develop after puberty and are similar to those of AIP or HCP (see above). Attacks are provoked by the same drugs, steroids, and nutritional factors that are detrimental in AIP. Skin manifestations are more common than in HCP but usually occur apart from the neurovisceral symptoms. Because the skin lesions in VP, HCP, and PCT are not distinguishable by clinical examination or biopsy, these conditions must be diagnosed by assay of porphyrins and porphyrin precursors in blood, urine, and feces.

VP is particularly common in South Africa, where 3 of every 1000 whites have the disorder. Most are descendants of a couple who emigrated from Holland to South Africa in 1688. Homozygous VP is

associated with photosensitivity, neurologic symptoms, and developmental disturbances, including growth retardation, in infancy or childhood; all cases had increased erythrocyte levels of zinc protoporphyrin, a characteristic finding in all homozygous porphyrias so far described.

Dual porphyria, the simultaneous occurrence of VP and familial PCT, has been documented in several kindreds. *Chester porphyria* was described in a large British family in which individuals had acute porphyric attacks and deficiency of both PROTO oxidase and HMB synthase. Photosensitivity was not observed. It is unclear whether Chester porphyria is a variant of VP or AIP.

Diagnosis When VP is symptomatic, levels of fecal protoporphyrin and coproporphyrin and of urinary coproporphyrin are increased. Urinary ALA and PBG levels are increased during acute attacks. Plasma levels of porphyrins are increased, particularly when there are cutaneous lesions. VP can be distinguished rapidly from all other porphyrias by examining the fluorescence emission spectrum of porphyrins in plasma at neutral pH. This test is particularly useful for differentiating VP from PCT.

Assays of PROTO oxidase activity in cultured fibroblasts or lymphocytes are not widely available. Some latent cases of VP can be diagnosed by measurement of fecal porphyrins in relatives of VP patients.

TREATMENT Acute attacks are treated with hematin as in AIP. Other than avoiding sun exposure, there are few effective measures for treating the skin lesions. β-Carotene, phlebotomy, and chloroquine are not helpful.

THE ERYTHROPOIETIC PORPHYRIAS

In the erythropoietic porphyrias, porphyrins from bone marrow erythrocytes and plasma are deposited in the skin and lead to cutaneous photosensitivity.

X-LINKED SIDEROBLASTIC ANEMIA XLSA results from the deficient activity of the erythroid form of ALA synthase and is associated with ineffective erythropoiesis, weakness, and pallor.

Clinical Features Typically, males with XLSA develop refractory hemolytic anemia, pallor, and weakness during infancy. They have secondary hypersplenism, become iron overloaded, and can develop hemosiderosis. The severity depends on the level of residual erythroid ALA synthase activity and on the responsiveness of the specific mutation to pyridoxal 5'-phosphate supplementation (see below). Peripheral blood smears reveal a hypochromic, microcytic anemia with striking anisocytosis, poikilocytosis, and polychromasia; the leukocytes and platelets appear normal. Hemoglobin content is reduced, and the mean corpuscular volume and mean corpuscular hemoglobin concentration are decreased. Patients with milder, late-onset disease have been reported recently.

Diagnosis Bone marrow examination reveals hypercellularity with a left shift and megaloblastic erythropoiesis with an abnormal maturation. A variety of Prussian blue–staining sideroblasts are observed. Levels of urinary porphyrin precursors and of both urinary and fecal porphyrins are normal. The level of erythroid ALA synthase is decreased in bone marrow, but this enzyme is difficult to measure in the presence of the normal ALA synthase housekeeping enzyme. Definitive diagnosis requires the demonstration of mutations in the *erythroid ALA synthase* gene.

℞ **TREATMENT** The severe anemia may respond to pyridoxine supplementation. This cofactor is essential for ALA synthase activity, and mutations in the pyridoxine binding site of the enzyme have been found in several responsive patients. Cofactor supplementation may make it possible to eliminate or reduce the frequency of transfusion. Unresponsive patients may be transfusion-dependent and require chelation therapy.

CONGENITAL ERYTHROPOIETIC PORPHYRIA

CEP is an autosomal recessive disorder, also known as *Gunther's disease*, that is due to the markedly deficient activity of URO synthase; it is associated with hemolytic anemia and cutaneous lesions. CEP is characterized by accumulation of uroporphyrin I and coproporphyrin I isomers.

Clinical Features Severe cutaneous photosensitivity begins in early infancy. The skin over sun-exposed areas is friable, and bullae and vesicles are prone to rupture and infection. Skin thickening, focal hypo- and hyperpigmentation, and hypertrichosis of the face and extremities are characteristic. Secondary infection of the cutaneous lesions can lead to disfigurement of the face and hands. Porphyrins are deposited in teeth and in bones. As a result, the teeth are reddish brown and fluoresce on exposure to long-wave ultraviolet light. Hemolysis is probably due to the marked increase in erythrocyte porphyrins and leads to splenomegaly. Adults with a milder form of the disease have been described.

Diagnosis Uroporphyrin and coproporphyrin (mostly type I isomers) accumulate in the bone marrow, erythrocytes, plasma, urine, and feces. The diagnosis should be confirmed by demonstration of markedly deficient URO synthase activity. The disease can be detected in utero by measuring porphyrins in amniotic fluid and URO synthase activity in cultured amniotic cells or chorionic villi. Molecular analyses of the mutant alleles from over 20 unrelated patients have revealed the presence of gene rearrangements, an mRNA processing defect, and several point mutations that cause amino acid substitutions.

℞ **TREATMENT** The transfusion of sufficient blood to suppress erythropoiesis is effective but results in iron overload. Splenectomy may reduce hemolysis and decrease transfusion requirements. Protection from sunlight and from minor skin trauma is important. β-Carotene may be of some value. Complicating bacterial infections should be treated promptly. Recently, bone marrow transplantation has proven effective in several transfusion-dependent children, providing the rationale for stem-cell gene therapy.

ERYTHROPOIETIC PROTOPORPHYRIA

Erythropoietic protoporphyria (EPP) is an autosomal dominant disorder due to the partial deficiency of ferrochelatase activity. Protoporphyrin accumulates in erythroid cells and plasma and is excreted in bile and feces. EPP is the most common erythropoietic porphyria and, after PCT, the second most common porphyria.

Clinical Features Skin photosensitivity usually begins in childhood. The skin manifestations differ from those of other porphyrias. Vesicular lesions are uncommon. Redness, swelling, burning, and itching can develop within minutes of sun exposure and resemble angioedema. Symptoms may seem out of proportion to the visible skin lesions. Sparse vesicles and bullae occur in 10% of cases. Chronic skin changes may include lichenification, leathery pseudovesicles, labial grooving, and nail changes. Severe scarring is rare, as are pigment changes, friability, and hirsutism.

The primary source of excess protoporphyrin is the bone marrow reticulocyte. Erythrocyte protoporphyrin is free (not complexed with zinc) and is mostly bound to hemoglobin. In plasma, protoporphyrin is bound to albumin. Hemolysis and anemia are usually absent or mild.

Liver function is usually normal, but in some patients accumulation of protoporphyrin causes chronic liver disease that can progress to liver failure and death. The hepatic complications are often preceded by increasing levels of erythrocyte and plasma protoporphyrin and probably result, in part, from protoporphyrin accumulation in the liver. Protoporphyrin is insoluble, forms crystalline structures in liver cells, and can decrease hepatic bile flow. Gallstones composed at least in part of protoporphyrin occur in some patients.

Some obligate heterozygotes are asymptomatic and have little or no increase in erythrocyte protoporphyrin. Thus there is phenotypic variation in this disease.

Diagnosis Protoporphyrin levels are increased in bone marrow, circulating erythrocytes, plasma, bile, and feces. Urinary levels of porphyrin and porphyrin precursors are normal. Ferrochelatase activity in cultured lymphocytes or fibroblasts is decreased.

℞ **TREATMENT** Oral β-carotene (120 to 180 mg/d) improves tolerance to sunlight in many patients. The dosage may need to be adjusted to maintain serum carotene levels in the recommended range of 10 to 15 μmol/L (600 to 800 μg/dL). Mild skin discoloration due to carotenemia is the only significant side effect. The beneficial effects of β-carotene may involve quenching of singlet oxygen or free radicals. Unfortunately, this drug is less effective in other forms of porphyria associated with photosensitivity.

Treatment of hepatic complications is difficult. However, cholestyramine and other porphyrin absorbents such as activated charcoal may interrupt the enterohepatic circulation of protoporphyrin and promote its fecal excretion, leading to some improvement. Splenectomy may be helpful when the disease is accompanied by hemolysis and significant splenomegaly. Caloric restriction and drugs or hormones that may induce the heme pathway or impair hepatic excretory function should be avoided. Iron deficiency should be prevented or treated. Transfusions or intravenous heme therapy may suppress erythroid and hepatic protoporphyrin production and are sometimes beneficial. Liver transplantation has been carried out in some patients with severe liver complications.

BIBLIOGRAPHY

ANDERSON KE et al: Disorders of heme biosynthesis: X-linked sideroblastic anemia and the porphyrias, in *The Metabolic and Molecular Bases of Inherited Disease*, 8th ed, CR Scriver et al (eds). New York, McGraw-Hill, 2001, pp 2991–3062

BONKOVSKY HL et al: Porphyria cutanea tarda, hepatitis C and HFE gene mutations in North America. Hepatology 27:1661, 1998

DE SIERVI A et al: Identification and characterization of hydroxymethylbilane synthase mutations causing acute intermittent porphyria: Evidence for an ancestral founder of the common G111R mutation. Am J Med Genet 86:366, 1999

DESNICK RJ, ANDERSON KE: Heme biosynthesis and its disorders: Porphyrias and sideroblastic anemias, in *Hematology: Basic Principles and Practices*, 2d ed, R Hoffman et al (eds). New York, Churchill Livingstone, 1995, pp 523–545

——— et al: Molecular genetics of congenital erythropoietic porphyria. Semin Liver Dis 18:77, 1998

LINDBERG RL et al: Motor neuropathy in porphobilinogen deaminase–deficient mice imitates the peripheral neuropathy of human acute porphyria. J Clin Invest 103:1127, 1999

MAY A, BISHOP DF: The molecular biology and pyridoxine responsiveness of X-linked sideroblastic anaemia. Haematologica 83:56, 1998

MENDEZ M et al: Familial prophyria cutanea tarda: Characterization of seven novel uroporphyrinogen decarboxylase mutations and frequency of common hemochromatosis alleles. Am J Hum Genet 63:1363, 1998

MOORE MR et al: *Disorders of Porphyrin Metabolism*. New York, Plenum, 1987

TEZCAN I et al: Congenital erythropoietic porphyria successfully treated by allogeneic bone marrow transplantation. Blood 92:4053, 1998

XU W et al: Congenital erythropoietic porphyria: Identification and expression of 10 mutations in the uroporphyrinogen III synthase gene. J Clin Invest 95:905, 1995

347 **Robert L. Wortmann**

DISORDERS OF PURINE AND PYRIMIDINE METABOLISM

amidoPRT amidophosphoribosyl-transferase	5-FU 5-fluorouracil
AMP adenosine monophosphate	GMP guanosine monophosphate
APRT adenine phosphoribosyltransferase	HPRT hypoxanthine phosphoribosyltransferase
DPD dihydropyrimidine dehydrogenase	IMP inosine monophosphate
	PRPP phosphoribosylpyrophosphate
	UMP uridine-5′-monophosphate

Purines and pyrimidines are the bases that, when linked to sugars (ribose or deoxyribose) and phosphate groups, create the nucleic acids that comprise the building blocks of RNA and DNA. The main purine bases are adenine and guanine; the pyrimidine bases include cytosine, thymine, and uracil. In addition, purines participate in diverse cellular functions, including intracellular energy metabolism (e.g., ATP), cell signaling pathways (e.g., GTP), and intercellular communication (e.g., adenosine). The nucleotides therefore serve fundamental roles in the replication of genetic material, gene transcription, protein synthesis, and cellular metabolism. Disorders that involve abnormalities of nucleotide metabolism range from relatively common diseases such as hyperuricemia and gout, in which there is increased production or impaired excretion of a metabolic end product of purine metabolism (uric acid), to rare enzyme deficiencies that affect purine and pyrimidine synthesis or degradation. Understanding these biochemical pathways has led, in some instances, to the development of specific forms of treatment, such as the use of allopurinol to reduce uric acid production.

URIC ACID METABOLISM

Uric acid is the final breakdown product of purine degradation in humans. It is a weak acid with pK_as of 5.75 and 10.3. Urates, the ionized forms of uric acid, predominate in plasma extracellular fluid and synovial fluid, with approximately 98% existing as monosodium urate at pH 7.4. Monosodium urate is easily dialyzed from plasma. Binding of urate to plasma proteins has little physiologic significance.

Plasma is saturated with monosodium urate at a concentration of 415 μmol/L (6.8 mg/dL) at 37°C. At higher concentrations, plasma is therefore supersaturated, creating the potential for urate crystal precipitation. However, precipitation sometimes does not occur even at plasma urate concentrations as high as 4800 μmol/L (80 mg/dL), perhaps because of the presence of solubilizing substances in plasma.

Uric acid is more soluble in urine than in water, possibly because of the presence of urea, proteins, and mucopolysaccharides. The pH of urine greatly influences its solubility. At pH 5.0, urine is saturated with uric acid at concentrations ranging from 360 to 900 μmol/L (6 to 15 mg/dL). At pH 7.0, saturation is reached at concentrations between 9480 and 12,000 μmol/L (158 and 200 mg/dL). Ionized forms of uric acid in urine include mono- and disodium, potassium, ammonium, and calcium urates.

Although purine nucleotides are synthesized and degraded in all tissues, urate is produced only in tissues that contain xanthine oxidase, primarily the liver and small intestine. The amount of urate in the body is the net result of the amount produced and the amount excreted (Fig. 347-1). Urate production varies with the purine content of the diet and the rates of purine biosynthesis, degradation, and salvage. Normally, two-thirds to three-fourths of urate is excreted by the kidneys, and most of the remainder is eliminated through the intestines. A four-component model describes the renal handling of uric acid in humans and includes: (1) glomerular filtration, (2) tubular reabsorption, (3) secretion, and (4) postsecretory reabsorption (Fig. 347-2). Approxi-

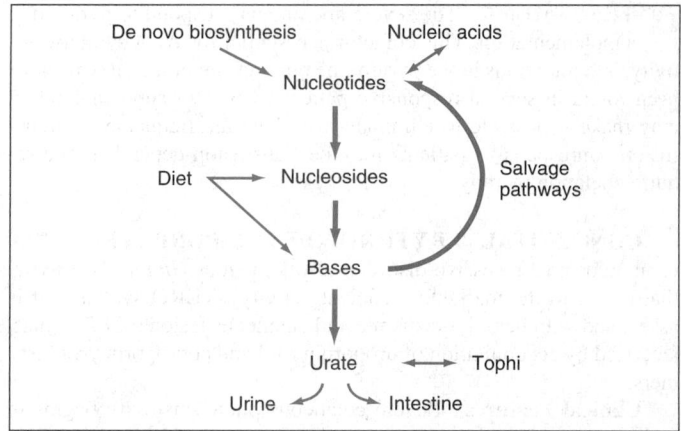

FIGURE 347-1 The total-body urate pool is the net result between urate production and excretion. Urate production is influenced by dietary intake of purines and the rates of de novo biosynthesis of purines from nonpurine precursors, nucleic acid turnover, and salvage by phosphoribosyltransferase activities. The formed urate is normally excreted by urinary and intestinal routes. Hyperuricemia can result from increased production, decreased excretion, or a combination of both mechanisms. When hyperuricemia exists, urate can precipitate and deposit in tissues as tophi.

mately 8 to 12% of urate filtered by the glomeruli is excreted in the urine as uric acid. After filtration, 98 to 100% of the urate is reabsorbed; about half the reabsorbed urate is secreted back into the proximal tubule, and about 40% of that is again reabsorbed.

Serum urate levels vary with age and sex. Most children have serum urate concentrations of 180 to 240 μmol/L (3.0 to 4.0 mg/dL). Levels begin to rise during puberty in males but remain low in females until menopause. Although the cause of this gender variation is not completely understood, it is due in part to a higher excretion of urate in females. Mean serum urate values of adult men and premenopausal women are 415 and 360 μmol/L (6.8 and 6.0 mg/dL), respectively. After menopause, values for women increase to approximate those of men. In adulthood, concentrations rise steadily over time and vary with height, body weight, blood pressure, renal function, and alcohol intake.

HYPERURICEMIA

Hyperuricemia can result from increased production or decreased excretion of uric acid or from a combination of the two processes. When sustained hyperuricemia exists, plasma and extracellular fluids are supersaturated with respect to urate, and total body urate is increased. Sustained hyperuricemia predisposes some individuals to develop clinical manifestations including gouty arthritis (Chap. 322) and renal dysfunction (see below).

Hyperuricemia may be defined as a plasma (or serum) urate concentration >420 μmol/L (7.0 mg/dL). This definition is based on physicochemical, epidemiologic, and disease-related criteria. Physicochemically, hyperuricemia is the concentration of urate in the blood that exceeds the solubility limits of monosodium urate in plasma, 415 μmol/L (6.8 mg/dL). In epidemiologic studies, hyperuricemia is defined as the mean plus 2 standard deviations of values determined from

FIGURE 347-2 Schematic for handling of uric acid by the kidney. Components are illustrated with the percentage of filtered urate.

a randomly selected healthy population. When measured in unselected individuals, 95% have serum urate concentrations <420 μmol/L (7.0 mg/dL). Finally, hyperuricemia can be defined in relation to the risk of disease. The risk of developing gouty arthritis or urolithiasis increases with urate levels >420 μmol/L (7.0 mg/dL) and escalates in proportion to the degree of elevation. Hyperuricemia is present in between 2.0 and 13.2% of ambulatory adults and somewhat more frequently in hospitalized individuals.

CAUSES OF HYPERURICEMIA Hyperuricemia may be classified as primary or secondary depending on whether the cause is innate or is the result of an acquired disorder (Table 347-1). However, it is more useful to classify hyperuricemia in relation to the underlying pathophysiology, i.e., whether it results from increased production, decreased excretion, or a combination of the two (Fig. 347-1, Table 347-2).

Increased Urate Production Diet provides an exogenous source of purines and, accordingly, contributes to the serum urate in proportion to its purine content. Strict restriction of purine intake reduces the mean serum urate level by about 60 μmol/L (1.0 mg/dL) and urinary uric acid excretion by approximately 1.2 mmol/d (200 mg/d). Because about 50% of ingested RNA purine and 25% of ingested DNA purine appear in the urine as uric acid, foods high in nucleic acid content have a significant effect on the serum urate level. Such foods include liver, "sweetbreads" (i.e., thymus and pancreas), kidney, and anchovy.

Endogenous sources of purine production also influence the serum urate level (Fig. 347-3). De novo purine biosynthesis, the formation of a purine ring from nonring structures, is an 11-step process that results in formation of inosine monophosphate (IMP). The first step combines phosphoribosylpyrophosphate (PRPP) and glutamine and is catalyzed by amidophosphoribosyltransferase (amidoPRT). The rates of purine biosynthesis and urate production are determined, for the most part, by this enzyme. AmidoPRT is regulated by the substrate PRPP, which drives the reaction forward, and by the end products of biosynthesis (IMP and other ribonucleotides), which provide feedback inhibition. A secondary regulatory pathway is the salvage of purine bases by hypoxanthine phosphoribosyltransferase (HPRT). HPRT catalyzes the combination of the purine bases hypoxanthine and guanine with PRPP to form the respective ribonucleotides IMP and guanosine monophosphate (GMP). Increased salvage activity thus retards de novo synthesis by reducing PRPP levels and increasing concentrations of inhibitory ribonucleotides.

Serum urate levels are closely coupled to the rates of de novo purine biosynthesis, which is driven in part by the level of PRPP, as evidenced by two inborn errors of purine metabolism. Both increased

Table 347-1 Classification of Hyperuricemia by Cause

Primary
  No recognized cause
  Hypoxanthine phosphoribosyltransferase deficiency
  Increased phosphoribosyl pyrophosphatase activity
Secondary
  Hereditary fructose intolerance
  Glycogen storage disease
  Myeloproliferative disease
  Lymphoproliferative disease
  Hemolytic anemia
  Psoriasis
  Obesity
  Renal insufficiency
  Lead intoxication
  Chronic beryllium disease
  Sarcoidosis
  Drugs
    Low-dose salicylates
    Diuretics
    Pyrazinamide
    Ethambutol
    Nicotinamide
    Ethanol

Table 347-2 Classification of Hyperuricemia by Pathophysiology

URATE OVERPRODUCTION

Primary idiopathic	Myeloproliferative diseases	Rhabdomyolysis
HPRT deficiency	eases	Exercise
PRPP synthetase over-activity	Polycythemia vera	Alcohol
	Psoriasis	Obesity
Hemolytic processes	Paget's disease	Purine-rich diet
Lymphoproliferative diseases	Glycogenosis III, V, and VII	

DECREASED URIC ACID EXCRETION

Primary idiopathic	Starvation ketosis	Drug ingestion
Renal insufficiency	Berylliosis	Salicylates (>2 g/d)
Polycystic kidney disease	Sarcoidosis	Diuretics
	Lead intoxication	Alcohol
Diabetes insipidus	Hyperparathyroidism	Levodopa
Hypertension	Hypothyroidism	Ethambutol
Acidosis	Toxemia of pregnancy	Pyrazinamide
Lactic acidosis	Bartter's syndrome	Nicotinic acid
Diabetic keto-acidosis	Down syndrome	Cyclosporine

COMBINED MECHANISM

Glucose-6-phosphatase deficiency	Fructose-1-phosphate aldolase deficiency	Alcohol
		Shock

NOTE: HPRT, hypoxanthine phosphoribosyltransferase; PRPP, phosphoribosylpyrophosphate.

PRPP synthetase activity and HPRT deficiency are associated with overproduction of purines, hyperuricemia, and hyperuricaciduria (see below for clinical descriptions). An X-linked disorder that causes an increase in activity of the enzyme PRPP synthetase leads to increased

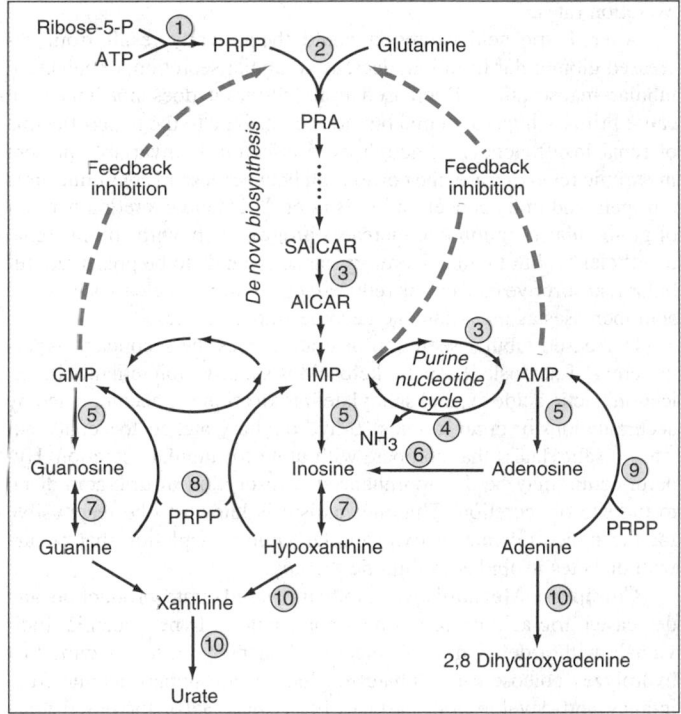

FIGURE 347-3 Abbreviated scheme of purine metabolism. (1) Phosphoribosylpyrophosphate (PRPP) synthetase, (2) amidophosphoribosyltransferase (amidoPRT), (3) adenylosuccinate lyase, (4) adenylate (AMP) deaminase, (5) 5'-nucleotidase, (6) adenosine deaminase, (7) purine nucleoside phosphorylase, (8) hypoxanthine phosphoribosyltransferase (HPRT), (9) adenine phosphoribosyltransferase (APRT), and (10) xanthine oxidase. PRA, phosphoribosylamine; SAICAR, succinylaminoimidazole carboxamide ribotide; AICAR, aminoimidazole carboxamide ribotide; GMP, guanylate; IMP, inosinate.

PRPP production and accelerated de novo biosynthesis. PRPP is a substrate and allosteric activator of amidoPRT, the first enzyme in the de novo pathway. HPRT deficiency is also X-linked and enhances urate biosynthesis in two ways. PRPP is accumulated as a result of decreased utilization in the salvage pathway and, in turn, provides increased substrate for amidoPRT and de novo biosynthesis. In addition, decreased formation of the nucleoside monophosphates, IMP and GMP, via the salvage pathway impairs feedback inhibition on amidoPRT, further enhancing de novo biosynthesis.

Accelerated purine nucleotide degradation can also cause hyperuricemia, i.e., with conditions of rapid cell turnover, proliferation, or cell death, as in leukemic blast crises, cytotoxic therapy for malignancy, hemolysis, or rhabdomyolysis. Nucleic acids released from cells are hydrolyzed by the sequential activities of nucleases and phosphodiesterases, forming nucleoside monophosphates, which in turn are degraded to nucleosides, bases, and urate. Hyperuricemia can result from excessive degradation of skeletal muscle ATP after strenuous physical exercise or status epilepticus and in glycogen storage diseases types III, V, and VII (Chap. 350). The hyperuricemia of myocardial infarction, smoke inhalation, and acute respiratory failure may also be related to accelerated breakdown of ATP.

Decreased Uric Acid Excretion Over 90% of individuals with sustained hyperuricemia have a defect in the renal handling of uric acid. In hyperuricemia with gout the renal defect is evidenced by a lower than normal ratio of urate clearance to glomerular filtration rate (or urate to insulin clearance rate) over a wide range of filtered loads. As a result, gouty individuals excrete approximately 40% less uric acid than nongouty individuals for any given plasma urate concentration. Uric acid excretion increases in gouty and nongouty individuals when plasma urate levels are raised by purine ingestion or infusion, but in those with gout, plasma urate concentrations must be 60 to 120 μmol/L (1 to 2 mg/dL) higher than normal to achieve equivalent uric acid excretion rates.

Altered uric acid excretion could theoretically result from decreased glomerular filtration, decreased tubular secretion, or enhanced tubular reabsorption. Decreased urate filtration does not appear to cause primary hyperuricemia but does contribute to the hyperuricemia of renal insufficiency. Although hyperuricemia is invariably present in chronic renal disease, the correlation between serum creatinine, urea nitrogen, and urate concentration is poor. Uric acid excretion per unit of glomerular filtration rate increases progressively with chronic renal insufficiency, but tubular secretory capacity tends to be preserved, tubular reabsorptive capacity is reduced, and extrarenal clearance of uric acid increases as renal damage becomes more severe.

Decreased tubular secretion of urate causes the secondary hyperuricemia of acidosis. Diabetic ketoacidosis, starvation, ethanol intoxication, lactic acidosis, and salicylate intoxication are accompanied by accumulations of organic acids (β-hydroxybutyrate, acetoacetate, lactate, or salicylates) that compete with urate for tubular secretion. Hyperuricemia may be due to enhanced reabsorption of uric acid distal to the site of secretion. This mechanism is known to be responsible for the hyperuricemia of extracellular volume depletion that occurs with diabetes insipidus or diuretic therapy.

Combined Mechanisms Both increased urate production and decreased uric acid excretion may contribute to hyperuricemia. Individuals with a deficiency of glucose-6-phosphatase, the enzyme that hydrolyzes glucose-6-phosphate to glucose, are hyperuricemic from infancy and develop gout early in life (Chap. 350). Increased urate production results from accelerated ATP degradation during fasting or hypoglycemia. In addition, the lower levels of nucleoside monophosphates decrease feedback inhibition of amidoPRT, thereby accelerating de novo biosynthesis. Glucose-6-phosphatase–deficient individuals may also develop hyperlacticacidemia, which blocks uric acid excretion by decreasing tubular secretion.

Patients with hereditary fructose intolerance caused by fructose-1-phosphate aldolase deficiency also develop hyperuricemia by both

mechanisms. In homozygotes, vomiting and hypoglycemia after fructose ingestion can lead to hepatic failure and proximal renal tubular dysfunction. Ingestion of fructose, the substrate for the enzyme, causes accumulation of fructose-1-phosphate. This action results in ATP depletion, accelerated purine nucleotide catabolism, and hyperuricemia. Both lactic acidosis and renal tubular acidosis contribute to urate retention. Heterozygous carriers develop hyperuricemia, and perhaps one-third develop gout. The heterozygous state has a prevalence of 0.5 to 1.5%, suggesting that fructose-1-phosphate aldolase deficiency may be a relatively common cause of familial gout.

Alcohol also promotes hyperuricemia by both mechanisms. Excessive alcohol consumption accelerates hepatic breakdown of ATP and increases urate production. Alcohol consumption can also induce hyperlacticacidemia, which blocks uric acid secretion. The higher purine content in some alcoholic beverages such as beer may also be a factor.

EVALUATION OF HYPERURICEMIA Hyperuricemia does not necessarily represent a disease, nor is it a specific indication for therapy. Rather, the finding of hyperuricemia is an indication to determine its cause. The decision to treat depends on the cause and the potential consequences of the hyperuricemia in each individual.

Quantification of uric acid excretion can be used to determine whether hyperuricemia is caused by overproduction or decreased excretion. On a purine-free diet, men with normal renal function excrete <3.6 mmol/d (600 mg/d). Thus, the hyperuricemia of individuals who excrete uric acid above this level while on a purine-free diet is due to purine overproduction, whereas it is due to decreased excretion in those who excrete lower amounts on the purine-free diet. If the assessment is performed while the patient is on a regular diet, the level of 4.2 mmol/d (800 mg/d) can be used as the discriminating value. With renal insufficiency, less urate is filtered in the glomeruli and less uric acid appears in the urine. Consequently, a lower 24-h urinary uric acid value in the presence of renal insufficiency does not necessarily rule out urate overproduction, but an elevated value provides strong evidence of urate overproduction. Spuriously high values can occur if a uricosuric agent is being taken at the time of urine collection. Glucocorticoids, ascorbic acid, salicylates in doses >2 g/d, and other agents that promote urate excretion interfere with the interpretation of results.

Assessment of the ratio of uric acid to creatinine (or the ratio of uric acid clearance to creatinine clearance) in spot or random urine samples is not a reliable method to screen for urate overproduction. However, this is a useful tool for evaluating individuals with acute renal failure suspected of having acute uric acid nephropathy (see below).

Pyrazinamide, which has a suppressive action on tubular secretion, can be used to investigate presecretory reabsorption of uric acid. Probenecid, an agent that inhibits postsecretory reabsorption, can be used to evaluate tubular secretion and postsecretory reabsorption.

COMPLICATIONS OF HYPERURICEMIA The most recognized complication of hyperuricemia is *gouty arthritis*. In the general population the prevalence of hyperuricemia ranges between 2.0 and 13.2%, and the prevalence of gout is between 1.3 and 3.7%. The higher the serum urate level, the more likely an individual is to develop gout. In one study, the incidence of gout was 4.9% for individuals with serum urate concentrations >540 μmol/L (9.0 mg/dL) compared with 0.5% for those with values between 415 and 535 μmol/L (7.0 and 8.9 mg/dL). The complications of gout correlate with both the duration and severity of hyperuricemia. →*For further discussion of gout, see Chap. 322.*

Hyperuricemia also causes several renal problems: (1) nephrolithiasis; (2) urate nephropathy, a rare cause of renal insufficiency attributed to monosodium urate crystal deposition in the renal interstitium; and (3) uric acid nephropathy, a reversible cause of acute renal failure resulting from deposition of large amounts of uric acid crystals in the renal collecting ducts, pelvis, and ureters.

Nephrolithiasis Uric acid nephrolithiasis occurs most commonly, but not exclusively, in individuals with gout. In gout, the prevalence of nephrolithiasis correlates with the serum and urinary uric acid levels, reaching approximately 50% with serum urate levels of 770 μmol/L (13 mg/dL) or urinary uric acid excretion >6.5 mmol/d (1100 mg/d).

Uric acid stones can develop in individuals with no evidence of arthritis, only 20% of whom are hyperuricemic. Uric acid can also play a role in other types of kidney stones. Some nongouty individuals with calcium oxalate or calcium phosphate stones have hyperuricemia or hyperuricaciduria. Uric acid may act as a nidus on which calcium oxalate can precipitate or lower the formation product for calcium oxalate crystallization.

Urate Nephropathy Urate nephropathy, sometimes referred to as *urate nephrosis*, is a late manifestation of severe gout and is characterized histologically by deposits of monosodium urate crystals surrounded by a giant cell inflammatory reaction in the medullary interstitium and pyramids. The disorder is now rare and cannot be diagnosed in the absence of gouty arthritis. The lesions may be clinically silent or cause proteinuria, hypertension, and renal insufficiency.

Uric Acid Nephropathy This reversible cause of acute renal failure is due to precipitation of uric acid in renal tubules and collecting ducts that causes obstruction to urine flow. Uric acid nephropathy develops following sudden urate overproduction and marked hyperuricaciduria. Factors that favor uric acid crystal formation include dehydration and acidosis. This form of acute renal failure occurs most often during an aggressive "blastic" phase of leukemia or lymphoma prior to or coincident with cytolytic therapy but has also been observed in individuals with other neoplasms, following epileptic seizures, and after vigorous exercise with heat stress. Autopsy studies have demonstrated intraluminal precipitates of uric acid, dilated proximal tubules, and normal glomeruli. The initial pathogenic events are believed to include obstruction of collecting ducts with uric acid and obstruction of distal renal vasculature.

If recognized, uric acid nephropathy is potentially reversible. Appropriate therapy has reduced the mortality from about 50% to practically nil. Serum levels cannot be relied on for diagnosis because this condition has developed in the presence of urate concentrations varying from 720 to 4800 μmol/L (12 to 80 mg/dL). The distinctive feature is the urinary uric acid concentration. In most forms of acute renal failure with decreased urine output, urinary uric acid content is either normal or reduced, and the ratio of uric acid to creatinine is <1. In acute uric acid nephropathy the ratio of uric acid to creatinine in a random urine sample or 24-h specimen is >1, and a value that high is essentially diagnostic.

℞ **TREATMENT Asymptomatic Hyperuricemia** Hyperuricemia is present in approximately 5% of the population and in up to 25% of hospitalized individuals. The vast majority are asymptomatic with regard to their hyperuricemia and are at no clinical risk because of it. Elevated serum urate concentrations have been associated with insulin resistance, obesity, hypertension, dyslipidemia (sometimes referred to as syndrome X), and atherosclerotic disease. However, urate does not appear to have a causal role in the development of coronary heart disease or death from cardiovascular disease. In the past, the association of hyperuricemia with cardiovascular disease and renal failure led to the use of urate-lowering agents for people with asymptomatic hyperuricemia. This practice is no longer recommended with the exception of individuals receiving cytolytic therapy for neoplastic disease, in which treatment is given in an effort to prevent uric acid nephropathy.

Hyperuricemic individuals are at risk to develop gouty arthritis, especially those with higher serum urate levels. However, treatment of asymptomatic hyperuricemia to prevent the first attack of gouty arthritis is not indicated because most hyperuricemic people never develop gout. Furthermore, neither structural kidney damage nor tophi are identifiable before the first attack. Reduced renal function cannot be attributed to asymptomatic hyperuricemia, and treatment of asymptomatic hyperuricemia does not alter the progression of renal dysfunction in patients with renal disease. Although nephrolithiasis is common in gouty patients, and a number of individuals with nephrolithiasis are hyperuricemic, increased risk of stone formation in people with asymptomatic hyperuricemia is not established.

Thus, because treatment with antihyperuricemic agents entails inconvenience, cost, and potential toxicity, routine treatment of asymptomatic hyperuricemia cannot be justified other than for prevention of acute uric acid nephropathy. In addition, routine screening for asymptomatic hyperuricemia is not recommended. If hyperuricemia is diagnosed, however, the cause should be determined. Causal factors should be corrected if the condition is secondary, and associated problems such as hypertension, hypercholesterolemia, diabetes mellitus, and obesity should be treated.

Symptomatic Hyperuricemia (See Chap. 322 for treatment of gout) • *Nephrolithiasis* Antihyperuricemic therapy is recommended for the individual who has both gouty arthritis and either uric acid– or calcium-containing stones, both of which may occur in association with hyperuricaciduria. Regardless of the nature of the calculi, fluid ingestion should be sufficient to produce a daily urine volume >2 L. Alkalinization of the urine with sodium bicarbonate or acetazolamide may be justified to increase the solubility of uric acid. Specific treatment of uric acid calculi requires reducing the urine uric acid concentration with allopurinol. Allopurinol administration decreases the serum urate concentration and the urinary excretion of uric acid in the first 24 h, with a maximum reduction occurring within 2 weeks. The average effective dose of allopurinol is 300 mg/d. Allopurinol can be given once a day because of the long half-life (18 h) of its active metabolite oxypurinol. The drug is effective in patients with renal insufficiency, but the dose should be reduced. Allopurinol is also useful in reducing the recurrence of calcium oxalate stones in gouty patients and in nongouty individuals with hyperuricemia or hyperuricaciduria. Potassium citrate (30 to 80 mmol/d orally in divided doses) is an alternative therapy for patients with uric acid stones alone or mixed calcium/uric acid stones. Allopurinol is also indicated for the treatment of 2,8-dihydroxyadenine kidney stones.

Uric acid nephropathy Uric acid nephropathy is often preventable, and immediate, appropriate therapy has greatly reduced the mortality rate. Vigorous intravenous hydration and diuresis with furosemide dilute the uric acid in the tubules and promote urine flow to ≥100 mL/h. The administration of acetazolamide, 240 to 500 mg every 6 to 8 h, and sodium bicarbonate, 89 mmol/L, intravenously enhances urine alkalinity and thereby solubilizes more uric acid. It is important to ensure that the urine pH remains >7.0 and to watch for circulatory overload. In addition, antihyperuricemic therapy in the form of allopurinol in a single dose of 8 mg/kg is administered to reduce the amount of urate that reaches the kidney. If renal insufficiency persists, subsequent daily doses should be reduced to 100 to 200 mg because oxypurinol, the active metabolite of allopurinol, accumulates in renal failure. Despite these measures, hemodialysis may be required.

HYPOURICEMIA

Hypouricemia, defined as a serum urate concentration <120 μmol/L (2.0 mg/dL) can result from decreased production of urate, increased excretion of uric acid, or a combination of both mechanisms. It occurs in <0.2% of the general population and <0.8% of hospitalized individuals. Hypouricemia causes no symptoms or pathology and therefore requires no therapy. It is, however, a sign of potential pathology, and its cause should be determined.

Most hypouricemia results from increased renal uric acid excretion. The finding of normal amounts of uric acid in a 24-h urine collection in an individual with hypouricemia is evidence for a renal cause. Medications with uricosuric properties (Table 347-3) include aspirin (at doses >2.0 g/d), x-ray contrast materials, and glyceryl-guaiacholate. Total parenteral hyperalimentation can also cause hypouricemia, possibly a result of the high glycine content of the infusion formula. Other causes of increased urate clearance include conditions

Table 347-3 Medications with Uricosuric Activity

Acetohexamide	Glyceryl guaiacolate
ACTH	Glycopyrrolate
Ascorbic acid	Halofenate
Azauridine	Meclofenamate
Benzbromarone	Phenolsulfonphthalein
Calcitonin	Phenylbutazone
Chlorprothixene	Probenecid
Citrate	Radiographic contrast agents
Dicumarol	Salicylates (>2 g/2d)
Diflunisal	Sulfinpyrazone
Estrogens	Tetracycline that is outdated
Glucocorticoids	Zoxazolamine

such as neoplastic disease, hepatic cirrhosis, diabetes mellitus, and inappropriate secretion of vasopressin; defects in renal tubular transport such as primary Fanconi syndrome and Fanconi syndromes caused by Wilson's disease, cystinosis, multiple myeloma, and heavy metal toxicity; and isolated congenital defects in the bidirectional transport of uric acid.

Hypouricemia from decreased production of urate is accompanied by very low urinary uric acid levels. Accumulation of other purine nucleosides and bases may occur depending on the specific defect. Individuals treated with allopurinol and some patients with neoplastic disease or severe hepatic dysfunction are hypouricemic and excrete increased quantities of hypoxanthine and xanthine in the urine. Xanthine oxidase deficiency can be inherited or acquired. Inherited forms include isolated xanthine oxidase deficiency and combined xanthine oxidase and sulfite oxidase deficiencies. Both cause hypouricemia and xanthinuria. Affected individuals excrete essentially no uric acid and may develop xanthine nephrolithiasis. Individuals with purine nucleoside phosphorylase deficiency, an inborn error of metabolism causing T cell–deficient immune dysfunction, are hypouricemic and excrete increased quantities of guanosine, deoxyguanosine, inosine, and deoxyinosine in the urine.

INBORN ERRORS OF PURINE METABOLISM
(See also Table 347-4, Fig. 347-3)

HPRT DEFICIENCY A complete deficiency of HPRT, the Lesch-Nyhan syndrome, is characterized by hyperuricemia, self-mutilative behavior, choreoathetosis, spasticity, and mental retardation.

Table 347-4 Inborn Errors of Purine Metabolism

Enzyme	Activity	Inheritance	Clinical Features
Hypoxanthine phosphoribosyltransferase	Complete deficiency	X-linked	Self-mutilation, choreoathetosis, hyperuricemia, gout, and uric acid lithiasis
	Partial deficiency	X-linked	Hyperuricemia, gout, and uric acid lithiasis
Phosphoribosylpyrophosphate synthetase	Overactivity	X-linked	Hyperuricemia, gout, uric acid lithiasis, and deafness
Adenine phosphoribosyltransferase	Deficiency	Autosomal recessive	2,8-Dihydroxyadenine lithiasis
Xanthine oxidase	Deficiency	Autosomal recessive	Xanthinuria and xanthine lithiasis
Adenylosuccinate lyase	Deficiency	Autosomal recessive	Autism and psychomotor retardation
Myoadenylate deaminase	Deficiency	Autosomal recessive	Myopathy with exercise intolerance or asymptomatic
Adenosine deaminase	Deficiency	Autosomal recessive	Severe combined immunodeficiency disease and chondro-osseous dysplasia
Purine nucleoside phosphorylase	Deficiency	Autosomal recessive	T cell–mediated immunodeficiency

A partial deficiency of HPRT, the Kelley-Seegmiller syndrome, is associated with hyperuricemia but no central nervous system manifestations. In both disorders, the hyperuricemia results from urate overproduction and can cause uric acid crystalluria, nephrolithiasis, obstructive uropathy, and gouty arthritis. Early diagnosis and appropriate therapy with allopurinol can prevent or eliminate all the problems attributable to hyperuricemia but have no effect on the behavioral or neurologic abnormalities.

HPRT catalyzes the reaction that combines PRPP and the purine bases hypoxanthine and guanine to form the respective nucleoside monophosphate IMP or GMP and pyrophosphate. The enzyme is encoded by a single gene located on the X chromosome in region q26-q27. Consequently, affected males are hemizygous for the trait and inherit the mutant allele from their asymptomatic mother, who is a carrier, or are the result of spontaneous gene mutations. The deficiency state is generally the result of point mutations, small deletions or insertions, or endoduplication of exons rather than major gene alterations.

INCREASED PRPP SYNTHETASE ACTIVITY Cells from individuals with increased PRPP synthetase activity contain elevated levels of PRPP. The high substrate content drives de novo purine synthesis, causing overproduction of uric acid. Like the HPRT deficiency states, PRPP synthetase overactivity is X-linked and results in gouty arthritis and uric acid nephrolithiasis. Nerve deafness occurs in some families.

ADENINE PHOSPHORIBOSYLTRANSFERASE (APRT) DEFICIENCY Individuals with a deficiency of APRT develop kidney stones composed of 2,8-dihydroxyadenine. APRT catalyzes the conversion of adenine to adenosine monophosphate (AMP). In the absence of APRT, adenine is converted by xanthine oxidase to 2,8-dihydroxyadenine, which is insoluble in urine. Reports of 2,8-dihydroxyadenine stones are rare, most likely because of its chemical similarity to uric acid. Analysis by x-ray powder diffraction is necessary for correct identification. Because this technique is rarely employed, many 2,8-dihydroxyadenine stones are incorrectly called uric acid. The consequence of this misidentification is not deleterious, as allopurinol therapy is the correct treatment for each type of stone.

APRT deficiency is inherited as an autosomal recessive trait. Caucasians with the disorder have a complete deficiency (type I), whereas Japanese subjects have some measurable enzyme activity (type II). Expression of the defect is similar in the two populations, as is the frequency of the heterozygous state (0.4 to 1.1 per 100).

HEREDITARY XANTHINURIA A deficiency of xanthine oxidase causes all purine in the urine to occur in the form of hypoxanthine and xanthine. About two-thirds of deficient individuals are asymptomatic. The remainder develop kidney stones composed of xanthine. A very small number of symptomatic individuals also have myopathy or recurrent polyarteritis. Xanthinuria appears to be inherited in an autosomal recessive pattern.

In a second form of inherited xanthinuria, the deficiency of xanthine oxidase is associated with a deficiency of sulfite oxidase. Neurologic symptoms attributable to the sulfite oxidase deficiency predominate over those of xanthinuria in individuals with the combined deficiency.

MYOADENYLATE DEAMINASE DEFICIENCY Adenylate deaminase (AMP deaminase) catalyzes the conversion of AMP to IMP with the release of ammonia and is an integral component of the purine nucleotide cycle, which plays an important role in skeletal muscle energy metabolism. Both primary (inherited) and secondary (acquired) forms of myoadenylate deaminase deficiency have been described. Myoadenylate deaminase is the only activity affected in the inherited form, whereas other muscle enzymes (creatine kinase and myokinase) are also decreased in the acquired deficiencies. In contrast, mRNA abundance is low in muscle from patients with acquired deficiencies, suggesting a different molecular basis for this form.

The primary form is inherited as an autosomal recessive trait. Clinically, this form does not appear to cause disease, and most individuals with this defect may be asymptomatic. Another explanation for the myopathy should be sought in symptomatic patients with this deficiency. The acquired deficiency occurs in association with a wide variety of neuromuscular disease, including muscular dystrophies, neuropathies, inflammatory myopathies, and collagen vascular diseases.

ADENYLOSUCCINATE LYASE DEFICIENCY Adenylosuccinate lyase participates in the synthesis of purine nucleotides in two ways. It catalyzes the conversion of succinylaminoimidazole carboxamide ribotide (SAICAR) to aminoimidazole carboxamide ribotide (AICAR) in the de novo pathway and in the conversion of AMP succinate to AMP in the purine nucleotide cycle. Deficiency of this enzyme is due to an autosomal recessive trait and causes profound psychomotor retardation, seizures, and other movement disorders. All individuals with this deficiency are mentally retarded, and most are autistic.

ADENOSINE DEAMINASE DEFICIENCY AND PURINE NUCLEOSIDE PHOSPHORYLASE DEFICIENCY See Chap. 308.

PYRIMIDINE DISORDERS

The pyrimidine, cytidine, is found in both DNA and RNA; it is a complementary base pair for guanine. Thymidine is found only in DNA where it is paired with adenine. Uridine is found only in RNA and can pair with either adenine or guanine in RNA secondary structures. Pyrimidines can be synthesized by a de novo pathway (Fig. 347-4) or reused in a salvage pathway. More than 25 different enzymes are involved in pyrimidine synthesis, salvage, and degradation pathways. Nonetheless, disorders of pyrimidine metabolism are rare. They are more difficult to recognize than purine disorders because of het-

erogeneous phenotypes and the absence of readily detected biochemical markers. Three disorders of pyrimidine metabolism are discussed below.

OROTIC ACIDURIA Hereditary orotic aciduria is an autosomal recessive disorder caused by mutations in a bifunctional enzyme, uridine-5′-monophosphate (UMP) synthase, which converts orotic acid to UMP in the de novo synthesis pathway (Fig. 347-4). The same protein encodes two distinct enzymatic activities. The disorder is characterized by hypochromic megaloblastic anemia that is unresponsive to vitamin B$_{12}$ and folic acid, growth retardation, and neurologic abnormalities. Increased excretion of orotic acid causes crystalluria and obstructive uropathy. Replacement of uridine (100 to 200 mg/kg per day) corrects the anemia, reduces orotic acid excretion, and improves the other sequelae of the disorder.

PYRIMIDINE 5′-NUCLEOTIDASE DEFICIENCY Pyrimidine 5′-nucleotidase catalyzes the removal of the phosphate group from pyrimidine ribonucleoside monophosphates (cytidine-5′-monophosphate or UMP) (Fig. 347-4). Deficiency of this enzyme is transmitted as a recessive trait and causes hemolytic anemia with prominent basophilic stippling of erythrocytes. The accumulation of pyrimidines or cytidine diphosphate choline (CDPC) is thought to induce hemolysis. The enzyme deficiency alters nucleoside composition and thereby generates a characteristic ultraviolet spectrum in deproteinized erythrocytes. There is no specific treatment.

DIHYDROPYRIMIDINE DEHYDROGENASE DEFICIENCY Dihydropyrimidine dehydrogenase (DPD) is the rate-limiting enzyme in the pathway of uracil and thymine degradation (Fig. 347-4). Deficiency of this enzyme causes excessive urinary excretion of uracil and thymine. DPD deficiency is transmitted in a recessive manner and causes nonspecific cerebral dysfunction with convulsive disorders, motor retardation, and mental retardation. A splice donor site mutation, which causes deletion of exon 14, accounts for 52% of mutant alleles. No specific treatment is available. DPD is also involved in the degradation of 5-fluorouracil (5-FU), a chemotherapeutic agent that inhibits thymidylate synthase. Consequently, deficiency of this enzyme is associated with 5-FU neurotoxicity.

MEDICATION EFFECTS ON PYRIMIDINE METABOLISM In addition to the role of DPD in 5-FU degradation (see above), other medications can influence pyrimidine metabolism. Leflunomide, which is used to treat rheumatoid arthritis, inhibits de novo pyrimidine synthesis by inhibiting dihydroorotate dehydrogenase, resulting in an antiproliferative effect on T cells. Allopurinol, an inhibitor of xanthine oxidase and purine synthesis, also inhibits orotidine-5′-phosphate decarboxylase, a step in UMP synthesis. Consequently, allopurinol use is associated with increased excretion of orotidine and orotic acid; there are no known clinical effects of this inhibition.

BIBLIOGRAPHY

BECKER MA et al: Purines and pyrimidines, in *The Metabolic and Molecular Bases of Inherited Disease*, 7th ed, CR Scriver et al (eds). New York, McGraw-Hill, 1995, pp 1655–1841

CULLETON BF et al: Serum uric acid risk for cardiovascular disease and death: The Framingham heart study. Ann Intern Med 131:7, 1999

SEEGMILLER JE et al: Metabolism of purines and genetic defects leading to hyperuricemia and gout, in *Gout, Hyperuricemia, and Other Crystal-Associated Arthropathies*, CJ Smyth, VM Holers (eds). New York, Marcel Dekker, 1999, p 127

SUCHI M et al: Molecular cloning of the human UMP synthase gene and characterization of point mutations in two hereditary orotic aciduria families. Am J Hum Genet 60: 525, 1997

VAN KUILENBURG ABP et al: Genotype and phenotype in patients with dihydropyrimidine dehydrogenase deficiency. Hum Genet 104:1, 1999

WEBSTER DR et al: Hereditary orotic aciduria and other disorders of pyrimidine metabolism, in *The Metabolic and Molecular Bases of Inherited Disease*, 8th ed, CR Scriver et al (eds). New York, McGraw-Hill, 2001, pp 2663–2702

WORTMANN RL: Gout and hyperuricemia, in *Kelly's Textbook of Rheumatology*, 6th ed, ED Harris, Jr, S Ruddy, CB Sledge (eds). Philadelphia, Saunders, 2000, in press

———, BENTZEL CJ: Renal handling of uric acid, in *Textbook of Nephrology*, 4th ed, SG Massary, RJ Glassrock (eds). Philadelphia, Lippincott Williams & Wilkins, in press

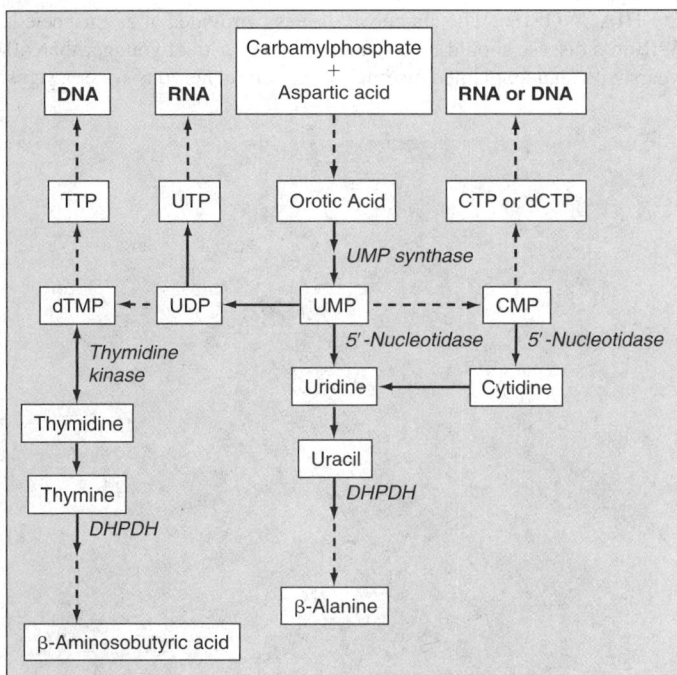

FIGURE 347-4 Abbreviated scheme of pyrimidine metabolism. Deficiency of uridine-5′-monophosphate (UMP) synthase causes orotic aciduria. Deficiency of pyrimidine-5′-nucleotidase causes a form of hemolytic anemia. Dihydropyrimidine dehydrogenase (DHPDH) deficiency impairs degradation of thymine and uracil, leading to seizure disorders and cerebral dysfunction. This enzyme is also required for metabolism of 5-fluorouracil. DTMP, deoxythymidine-5′-monophosphate; CMP, cytidine-5′-monophosphate.

348   *I. Herbert Scheinberg*

WILSON'S DISEASE

Wilson's disease is an inherited disorder of copper metabolism in individuals with two mutant *ATP7B* genes. Impairment of the normal excretion of hepatic copper results in toxic accumulation of the metal in liver, brain, and other organs. The disease occurs in every ethnic and geographic population, with a worldwide prevalence of ~1 in 30,000, and a heterozygous carrier frequency of ~1 in 90.

NATURAL HISTORY   The average concentrations of ceruloplasmin and hepatic copper are indistinguishable in normal neonates and in patients with Wilson's disease. In normal infants, however, the ceruloplasmin concentration increases and the hepatic copper concentration falls to adult levels during the first 3 months of life. In infants with Wilson's disease, the neonatal deficiency of ceruloplasmin and excess of hepatic copper persist indefinitely. Clinical manifestations are rare before age 6, occur most frequently in mid-adolescence, and eventually develop in all untreated patients.

In about half of patients any of four types of hepatic disturbances may herald the clinical onset. *Acute hepatitis* is usually self-limited, is often mistaken for viral hepatitis or infectious mononucleosis, and may be forgotten later in life. *Parenchymal liver disease* may persist after acute hepatitis or may develop insidiously without prior acute disease into a histologic and clinical picture indistinguishable from chronic active hepatitis and cirrhosis. In other patients *cirrhosis* may develop insidiously after a lapse of decades with no prior sign or symptom of liver disease. *Fulminant hepatitis*, generally fatal, is characterized by progressive jaundice, ascites, encephalopathy, hypoalbuminemia, hypoprothrombinemia, moderately elevated plasma levels of liver enzymes, and Coombs-negative hemolytic anemia.

In most other patients neurologic or psychiatric disturbances are the first clinical signs and are always accompanied by Kayser-Fleischer rings (**Plate III-16**). These golden deposits of copper in Descemet's membrane of the cornea do not interfere with vision but indicate that copper has been released from the liver and has probably caused brain damage. If a patient with frank neurologic or psychiatric disease does not have Kayser-Fleischer rings when examined by a trained observer using a slit lamp, the diagnosis of Wilson's disease can be excluded. Rarely, Kayser-Fleischer rings may be accompanied by sunflower cataracts.

The neurologic manifestations include resting and intention tremors, spasticity, rigidity, chorea, drooling, dysphagia, and dysarthria. Babinski responses may be present, and abdominal reflexes are often absent. Inexplicably—in view of the ubiquity of copper excess in the brain—sensory changes never occur, except for headache.

Psychiatric disturbances are present in most patients with neurologic symptoms. Schizophrenia, manic-depressive psychoses, and classic neuroses may occur, but the commonest disturbances are bizarre behavioral patterns that defy classification. Improvement in the psychiatric state can occur with pharmacologic reduction of the copper excess, but psychotherapy and additional pharmacotherapy may be required.

In about 5% of patients the clinical onset reflects neither a hepatic nor a central nervous system disturbance. The first manifestation may be primary or secondary amenorrhea or repeated and unexplained spontaneous abortions, perhaps due to excess free copper in intrauterine secretions. Kayser-Fleischer rings may occasionally first be discovered during routine ophthalmologic examination.

PATHOGENESIS   The metabolic defect in Wilson's disease is an inability to maintain a near-zero balance of copper. Dietary copper is generally in excess of the small amount that is essential to life. Normally, any excess absorbed copper is excreted by the liver; in patients with Wilson's disease, copper accumulates in the liver, reaching a mean level of about 1000 μg/g dry weight—40 times normal.

Fatty infiltration of the hepatic parenchyma and nuclear glycogen deposits are the earliest findings by light microscopy (Fig. 348-1). With electron microscopy, characteristic mitochondrial abnormalities appear to be specific for Wilson's disease. Later, necrosis, inflammation, fibrosis, bile duct proliferation, and cirrhosis ensue. Abnormalities in liver chemistries, particularly elevations in aminotransferases, may be seen at any stage. The capacity of hepatocytes to store copper is eventually exceeded, and copper is released into blood and taken up into extrahepatic tissues with disastrous effects in the brain (Table 348-1).

With magnetic resonance imaging, the effects of copper toxicity in the brain are seen most frequently in the lenticular nuclei and less commonly in the pons, medulla, thalamus, cerebellum, and cerebral cortex. Opalski and Alzheimer type II cells are present early in the course, although neither is specific for Wilson's disease, and neuronal necrosis and cavitation develop later.

An increased copper concentration in the kidney produces little, if any, structural change and usually does not alter renal function. Microscopic hematuria and/or minimal proteinuria occur occasionally; and nephrocalcinosis, renal calculi, and renal tubular acidosis are rare. Pathologic effects in other organs and tissues are minor.

GENETIC CONSIDERATIONS   The autosomal recessive Wilson disease gene, *ATP7B*, and the X-linked Menkes disease gene, *ATP7A*, are membrane-bound, P-type, copper-transporting ATPases containing 6 copper-binding sites (Chap. 353). The amino acid sequences of these genes are 54% identical. In liver the Wilson protein incorporates copper ions into apoceruloplasmin to form ceruloplasmin whose catabolism is accompanied by biliary excretion of its copper ions. In fetal liver the Menkes protein incorporates copper ions into apoceruloplasmin to form fetal ceruloplasmin whose catabolism is accompanied by hepatic retention of its copper ions. In Wilson's disease, ceruloplasmin that is synthesized in the presence of the *ATP7B* mutant is catabolized like fetal ceruloplasmin, leading to hepatic retention of its copper ions. ∎

DIAGNOSIS   The diagnosis is easy provided it is suspected. Wilson's disease should be considered in any patient younger than 40 years with an unexplained disorder of the central nervous system, signs

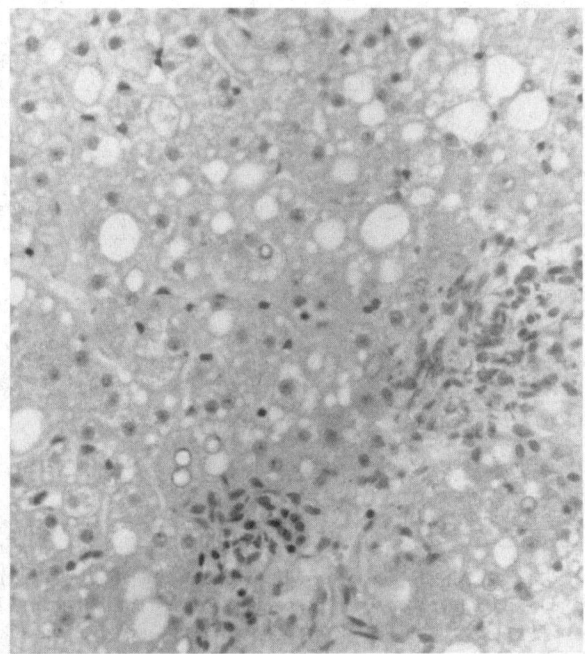

FIGURE 348-1   Macro- and microvesicular fatty changes, glycogen deposits in nuclei, and cellular infiltrates in a hematoxylin- and eosin-stained section of liver from an asymptomatic boy with Wilson's disease.

Group	Serum Ceruloplasmin		Hepatic Copper Concentration	
	No. of Patients	Mean ± SD, mg/dL	No. of Patients	Mean ± SD, μg/g Dry Weight
Wilson's disease				
Asymptomatic	31	3.6 ± 5.3	36	983.5 ± 368
Symptomatic	84	5.9 ± 7.1	33	588.3 ± 304
Heterozygous carriers	95[a]	28.4 ± 8.5	14	117.0 ± 51
Control subjects	180	30.7 ± 3.5	16	31.5 ± 6.8

[a] 71 parents of patients with Wilson's disease and 24 children, each of whom had one parent with Wilson's disease.

SOURCE: Sternlieb and Scheinberg, 1968.

or symptoms of hepatitis, chronic active hepatitis, unexplained persistent elevations of serum aminotransferase, hemolytic anemia in the presence of hepatitis, or unexplained cirrhosis and in any patient who has a relative with Wilson's disease.

The diagnosis is confirmed by the demonstration of either (1) a serum ceruloplasmin level <20 mg/dL *and* Kayser-Fleischer rings or (2) a serum ceruloplasmin level <20 mg/dL *and* a concentration of copper in a liver biopsy sample >250 μg/g dry weight. Most symptomatic patients excrete >100 μg copper per day in urine and have histologic abnormalities on liver biopsy.

℞ **TREATMENT** Treatment consists of removing and detoxifying the deposits of copper as rapidly as possible and must be instituted once the diagnosis is secure whether the patient is ill or asymptomatic. Penicillamine is administered orally in an initial dose of 1 g daily in a single or divided doses at least 30 min before and 2 h after eating. Because penicillamine has an antipyridoxine effect, 25 mg/d of pyridoxine is also given. In ~10% of patients sensitivity to penicillamine develops early, making it necessary to monitor the body temperature and skin daily. White blood cell and platelet counts should be assessed and urinalysis performed several times during the first month of treatment. Penicillamine should be discontinued and replaced by trientine, if rash, fever, leukopenia, thrombocytopenia, lymphadenopathy, or proteinuria develops, or if neurologic worsening accompanies the institution of penicillamine and persists for a week or more.

After therapy with penicillamine has been successfully instituted, the patient should be seen at 1- to 3-month intervals to assess the effectiveness of therapy and monitor for late drug toxicity. The history and the physical examination should focus on hepatic, neurologic, and psychiatric signs and symptoms. Slit-lamp examination of the corneas should be performed by an ophthalmologist if neurologic or psychiatric disturbances appear or worsen. White blood cell and platelet counts, transaminase levels, albumin, bilirubin, and free serum copper (total serum copper minus ceruloplasmin-bound copper) should be measured, the aim being a concentration of free copper less than ~0.2 μmol/dL (10 μg/dL). A persistent concentration >0.4 μmol/dL (20 μg/dL) indicates that the dose of penicillamine is too low or that the patient is noncompliant. For patients who are asymptomatic or who have improved maximally after several years on 1 g/d of penicillamine, the usual effective maintenance dose is 0.75 g/d taken 45 min before breakfast.

At any time, even after years of uneventful penicillamine administration, granulocytopenia, thrombocytopenia, the nephrotic syndrome, Goodpasture's syndrome, systemic lupus erythematosus, severe arthralgias, myasthenia, mammary gigantism, or elastosis perforans serpiginosa may supervene. Except for transient thrombocytopenia or granulocytopenia, these reactions mandate the replacement of penicillamine with trientine.

The dose of trientine is 1g/d on an empty stomach. Most patients find it convenient to take four 250-mg capsules, delaying breakfast for about an hour. Pyridoxine need not be given. Although the only reported toxic reaction to trientine is sideroblastic anemia, the same clinical procedures and laboratory determinations should be performed during its administration as are used during penicillamine therapy. Except for systemic lupus erythematosus and, occasionally, elastosis perforans serpiginosa, the other late penicillamine-induced toxic reactions disappear or improve with trientine therapy. Moreover, trientine is as effective therapeutically as penicillamine.

Zinc acetate or gluconate are effective as maintenance therapy, at doses of 150 mg/d of elemental zinc, for patients who are asymptomatic or have improved maximally on penicillamine or trientine. Zinc must *not*, however, be given together with penicillamine or trientine, both of which can chelate zinc and form complexes that are therapeutically ineffective.

Treatment must be continued for life. Inadequate treatment or interruption of therapy can be fatal or cause irreversible relapse. Indeed, of 11 patients who voluntarily discontinued penicillamine after years of successful treatment, 8 died after an average of 2.6 years of noncompliance. In contrast, of 13 patients in whom trientine was substituted because of an adverse reaction to penicillamine, 1 died accidentally, 5 were lost to follow-up, and 7 are alive and well 11 to 23 years later.

Prophylactic treatment of more than 100 asymptomatic patients with a documented diagnosis of Wilson's disease has shown that continual therapy with penicillamine or trientine can maintain the asymptomatic state indefinitely. Several such patients have been treated with penicillamine for >30 years.

Patients with severe neurologic disease who do not improve with penicillamine or trientine therapy that has reduced serum free copper to <0.3 μmol/dL (15 μg/dL) may benefit significantly from treatment with dimercaprol. Intramuscular injections of 3 mL (containing 300 mg of dimercaprol) are given on five successive weekdays for 4 weeks. Treatment is interrupted for 1 week, and a second 4-week course is given. If there is neurologic improvement, additional courses are given as long as improvement continues. If no improvement is seen after two courses, it is unlikely that additional courses will be effective.

The simultaneous occurrence of fulminant hepatitis and Coombs-negative hemolytic anemia may be the initial clinical manifestation of Wilson's disease or may occur in a noncompliant patient. The syndrome is almost always fatal, usually within a week or two, unless liver transplantation is performed. Transplantation is also indicated if progressive hepatic insufficiency occurs despite adequate treatment with penicillamine or trientine.

More than 150 women with Wilson's disease treated with penicillamine and more than 20 women treated with trientine have had successful and uneventful pregnancies.

BIBLIOGRAPHY

BREWER GJ et al: Treatment of Wilson's disease with zinc: XI. Interaction with other anticopper agents. J Am Coll Nutr 12:26, 1993

KRESSNER MS et al: Origins of biliary copper. Hepatology 4:867, 1984

PETRUKHIN K et al: Mapping, cloning and genetic characterization of the region containing the Wilson disease gene. Nat Genet 5:338, 1993

SCHEINBERG IH, STERNLIEB I: Wilson's and Menkes' Diseases. Cambridge, Harvard University Press (in preparation)

———, ———: Treatment of the neurological manifestations of Wilson's disease. Arch Neurol 52:339, 1995

———, ———: The use of trientine in preventing the effects of interrupting penicillamine therapy in Wilson's disease. N Engl J Med 317:209, 1987

SCHILSKY ML et al: Liver transplantation for Wilson's disease: Indications and outcome. Hepatology 19:583, 1994

STERNLIEB I, SCHEINBERG IH: Prevention of Wilson's disease in asymptomatic patients. N Engl J Med 278:352, 1968

VULPE C et al: Isolation of a candidate gene for Menkes disease and evidence that it encodes a copper-transporting ATPase. Nat Genet 3:7, 1993

349 *Gregory A. Grabowski*

LYSOSOMAL STORAGE DISEASES

GENERAL FEATURES

Lysosomes are heterogeneous subcellular organelles containing specific hydrolyases that allow targeted processing or degradation of proteins, nucleic acids, carbohydrates, and lipids. There are >30 different lysosomal storage diseases, and they vary greatly in the types of metabolic abnormalities that occur as well as in their clinical manifestations. Nonetheless, these disorders are considered together because they share a related pathophysiology that involves the accumulation of specific macromolecules within cells that normally process large amounts of these substrates. The disorders are classified based on the nature of the stored material and include mucopolysaccharidoses (MPS), gangliosidoses, glycosphingolipidoses, glycoproteinoses, mucolipidoses, leukodystrophies, and lipid storage disorders (Table 349-1). The most prevalent lysosomal storage diseases in adults are Fabry disease, Gaucher disease, and Niemann Pick disease (NPD).

Lysosomal storage diseases should be considered in the differential diagnosis of patients with neurologic or muscular degeneration, unexplained hepatomegaly or splenomegaly, or skeletal dysplasias and deformations. Physical findings are disease-specific, and definitive diagnosis is made by enzyme assays.

PHYSIOLOGY OF LYSOSOMES Lysosomal biogenesis is a continuous process that involves ongoing synthesis of lysosomal hydrolases, membrane constitutive proteins, and new membranes. Lysosomes originate from the fusion of *trans*-golgi network (TGN) vesicles with late endosomes. Progressive vesicular acidification accompanies the maturation of TGN vesicles, which contain various hydrolases, into lysosomes. Early endosomes have an internal pH of ~6.0 to 6.2; late endosomes and lysosomes have a pH of ~5.5 to 6.0 and ≤5, respectively. This gradient facilitates the pH-dependent dissociation of receptors and ligands [e.g., the mannose-6-phosphate (M6P) receptor and M6P-containing oligosaccharides] as well as activating lysosomal hydrolase function. This dynamic system, which has supplanted the static view of the lysosome, is consistent with the presence of heterogeneous populations of similar organelles whose contents differ significantly in time and location within the cell.

The accurate sorting, targeting, and activation of lysosomal enzymes is essential for maintaining normal cellular function. Abnormalities at several steps along the biosynthetic pathway can impair enzyme activation and lead to a lysosomal storage disorder. After cleavage of the hydrophobic signal peptide in the endoplasmic reticulum (ER) membrane, *N*-glycosylation occurs cotranslationally in the lumen of the ER. Complex oligosaccharide modifications occur during transit through the Golgi. The M6P modification of high-mannose oligosaccharide chains of many soluble lysosomal hydrolases occurs early in this process. Defects of this modification result in inappropriate extracellular secretion of most soluble lysosomal hydrolases, leading to severe phenotypes (I-cell disease). Lysosomal integral or associated membrane proteins (LIMPS or LAMPS) are sorted to the membrane or interior of the lysosome by several different signals. Phosphorylation, sulfation, additional proteolytic processing, and macromolecular assembly of heteromers occur concurrently and are critical to enzyme function. Defects in the latter can result in multiple enzyme/protein deficiencies.

PATHOGENESIS OF LYSOSOMAL STORAGE DISEASES The final common pathway for lysosomal storage diseases is the accumulation of specific macromolecules within tissues and cells that normally have a high flux of these substrates. The majority of lysosomal enzyme deficiencies result from point mutations or genetic rearrangements at a locus that encodes a single lysosomal hydrolase.

However, some mutations cause deficiencies of several different lysosomal hydrolases by altering the enzymes/proteins involved in targeting, active site modifications, or macromolecular association or trafficking. All are inherited as autosomal recessive disorders, except Hunter (MPS II) and Fabry diseases, which are X-linked. Lysosomal distortion, which is caused by substrate accumulation, probably has significant pathologic consequences. However, abnormal amounts of metabolites may also have pharmacologic effects important to disease pathophysiology.

For many lysosomal diseases, the accumulated substrates are endogenously synthesized within particular tissue sites of pathology. Other diseases have greater exogenous substrate supplies; that is, they are delivered by low-density lipoprotein receptor–mediated uptake in Fabry and cholesteryl ester storage diseases or by phagocytosis in Gaucher disease type 1.

The concept of the *threshold hypothesis* has important implications for disease classification, pathophysiology, and treatment. It implies a threshold of enzyme activity below which disease develops. Consequently, small changes in enzyme activity near the threshold can lead to or prevent disease. A critical element of this model is that enzymatic activity can be challenged by changes in substrate flux based on genetic background, cell turnover, recycling, or metabolic demands. Thus, a set level of residual enzyme may be adequate for substrate in some tissues or cells, but not in others. For some lysosomal storage diseases [e.g., metachromatic leukodystrophy (MLD), Tay-Sachs disease, Gaucher disease], genotype-phenotype correlations may help to predict the severity of clinical consequences associated with certain levels of enzyme activity. Defining enzyme activity thresholds may also be useful for predicting dose-response relationships for treatment and for the evaluation of exogenous enzyme replacement therapy.

SPECIFIC DISORDERS

MUCOPOLYSACCHARIDOSES (MPS) The various forms of MPS result from deficiencies of lysosomal enzymes needed for glycosaminoglycan (GAG) catabolism. GAGs are long-chain, complex carbohydrates that are linked to proteins in connective tissue. They are components of proteoglycans and include: chondroitin-4-sulfate, chondroitin-6-sulfate, heparan sulfate, dermatan sulfate, keratan sulfate, and hyaluronic acid. The particular accumulated GAG is determined by the specific enzyme deficiency. GAG accumulation in various tissues produces a spectrum of clinical features that can include skeletal abnormalities, corneal clouding, organomegaly, joint stiffness, hernias, short stature, and, in some disorders, mental retardation. Vacuolated lymphocytes in the peripheral smear and excessive urinary GAGs are typical findings. Clinical and laboratory features overlap among the MPS diseases and are not diagnostic. The MPS diseases occur with individual frequencies of about 1/50,000 to 1/100,000 in most populations.

The diagnosis is established by specific enzyme assays or, when known, DNA mutation analysis. Prenatal diagnosis is conducted most frequently with cultured amniotic cells. Mutation studies for carriers can be performed, if the mutation is known.

Treatment of the MPS diseases requires comprehensive, multisystem evaluations. Symptomatic therapies currently include corneal transplantation, correction of nerve entrapment, and heart valve replacement. Physical therapy for joint contractures is needed in all but MPS IV. In MPS III variants, psychotropic drugs are used to control behavior. For patients with MPS IH and IV, cervical myelopathy can be prevented by prospective cervical spinal fusion. The efficacy of bone marrow transplantation and enzyme replacement is under investigation.

MPS IH (Hurler Disease) This a severe autosomal recessive disorder that results from numerous different mutations of α-L-iduronidase. Progressive mental retardation, hepatosplenomegaly, skeletal malformations, and cardiopulmonary compromise typically lead to death during the first decade. Affected individuals appear normal at birth but exhibit accelerated growth and mild coarsening of facial features in the first year. Subsequently, there is slowing of growth, leading to short stature. In the first 2 years, clinical diagnosis is suggested by hepatosplenomegaly, corneal clouding, coarse features, large tongue, joint stiffness, and characteristic dysostosis multiplex on skeletal x-rays. Instability of the cervical vertebral bodies can lead to paralysis, particularly with subluxation on hyperextension. Developmental delay is apparent by 12 to 28 months, with subsequent slow mental regression. Additional features of this multisystem disease include hearing loss, chronic respiratory infections, valvular heart disease, and brain ventricular enlargement. The latter occurs from involvement of the arachnoid granulations.

MPS (Scheie Disease) and MPS I H/S (Hurler-Scheie Disease) These MPS variants are less severe than MPS IH (Hurler disease). They result from allelic mutations in the α-L-iduronidase gene, presumably with a less severe effect on enzyme function. Patients with MPS IS can survive into late adulthood with normal intelligence, though with severe progressive skeletal disease that resembles osteoarthritis. Bone marrow transplantation in MPS IH, if instituted before substantial central nervous system CNS involvement, has shown therapeutic promise. Preliminary intravenous enzyme administration has led to improvement in hepatosplenomegaly and connective tissue involvement.

MPS II (Hunter Syndrome) This is an X-linked recessive disorder that results from deletions and point mutations in the gene encoding iduronate sulfatase. Clinically, MPS IH and II are similar, though corneal clouding is absent in MPS II. Clinical manifestations range from severe CNS and visceral involvement with death in late childhood to milder forms with normal CNS function and survival into adulthood. Bone marrow transplantation has not been successful for treating the severe variants, and experience in the less severe variants is too limited to permit conclusions. Enzyme therapy trials are imminent.

MPS IIIA, IIIB, IIIC, and IIID (the Sanfilippo Syndromes) These autosomal recessive disorders are caused by various enzymatic deficiencies as summarized in Table 349-1. Skeletal defects and hepatosplenomegaly are less pronounced in this group of MPS variants, though progressive behavioral problems, mental retardation, and seizures are present. Affected patients can survive into the third or fourth decade with progressive CNS disease.

MPS IV (Morquio Syndrome) These MPS variants are autosomal recessive disorders characterized by severe skeletal diseases that resemble the spondyloepiphyseal dysplasias. There is extreme shortening of the trunk due to multiple vertebral collapses. The long bones are relatively spared. Joint laxity can lead to osteoarthritis-like destruction of the joints. Upper cervical spinal cord compression due to atlantoaxial instability predisposes to subluxation and paralysis. Many patients have mitral valve insufficiency that can be functionally significant. The A and B variants are distinguished clinically by more severe skeletal disease, N-acetylgalactosamine-6-sulfate sulfatase deficiency in A, than in β-galactosidase defects in B. Enzyme therapy trials will begin in the near future.

MPS VI (Maroteaux-Lamy Disease) Mutations in the arylsulfatase B gene cause this autosomal recessive disorder. Although clinically variable, the general phenotype resembles Hurler disease. Intelligence is normal, and the life span can extend beyond three decades. Cardiac valvular disease and progressive pulmonary hypertension are frequent causes of death. Bone marrow transplantation may be useful in diminishing these manifestations.

GM₂ GANGLIOSIDOSES The Tay-Sachs and Sandhoff disease variants are caused by defects in β-hexosaminidase (Hex) A and/or B. Hex A is a heteromeric protein with α and β chains, whereas Hex B contains only β chains. The α and β chains are encoded by different genes. Infantile, juvenile, and adult-onset variants are distinguished by age at onset and rate of progression.

In addition to other clinical manifestations described below, specific neurologic features, such as the retinal cherry red spot, suggest the diagnosis of Tay-Sachs and Sandhoff diseases. Diagnosis is confirmed by Hex A and/or B levels in blood plasma or nucleated cells. Screening for Tay-Sachs disease carriers in the Ashkenazi Jewish population is recommended.

Tay-Sachs Disease About 1 in 30 Ashkenazi Jews is a carrier for Tay-Sachs disease, which is caused by total Hex A deficiency. The infantile form is a fatal neurodegenerative disease that is characterized by macrocephaly, loss of motor skills, increased startle reaction, and macular pallor with cherry red spot on retinal examination. The juvenile-onset form presents with ataxia and dementia, with death by age 10 to 15 years. The adult-onset disorder is characterized by clumsiness in childhood; progressive motor weakness in adolescence; and additional spinocerebellar, lower motor neuron symptoms, and dysarthria in adulthood. Intelligence declines slowly, and psychosis is also common.

Sandhoff Disease Sandhoff disease is nearly identical to Tay-Sachs disease, though hepatosplenomegaly and bony dysplasias are present in the former. The later onset variants are characterized by progressive visceral and CNS disease. Treatment is supportive.

NEUTRAL GLYCOSPHINGOLIPID LIPID STORAGE DISORDERS **Fabry Disease** This is an X-linked disorder that results from a variety of mutations in the α-galactosidase gene. This enzyme cleaves the terminal α-galactosyl moiety from globotriaosylceramide (trihexosylceramide, THC), a key step in glycosphingolipid metabolism. Clinically, the disease manifests with angiokeratomas (telangiectatic skin lesions); hypohidrosis; corneal and lenticular opacities; acroparesthesia; and small-vessel disease of the kidney, heart, and brain. The estimated prevalence of hemizygous males with Fabry disease is 1/40,000.

The angiokeratomas and acroparesthesia may appear in childhood and lead to early diagnosis, if suspected. Angiokeratomas are punctate, dark red to blue-black, flat or slightly raised, usually symmetric, and do not blanch with pressure. They range from barely visible to several millimeters in diameter and have a tendency to increase in size and number with age. Characteristically, they are most dense between the umbilicus and knees—"the bathing suit area"—but may occur anywhere, including the mucosal surfaces. Corneal and lenticular lesions, detectable on slit-lamp examination, are present in affected men and ~70% of heterozygous women. Tortuosity of the conjunctival and retinal vessels is common. The acroparesthesia can be debilitating in childhood and adolescence, with a tendency to decrease after the third decade. Episodic agonizing, burning pain of the hands, feet, and proximal extremities can last from minutes to days and can be precipitated by exercise, fatigue, or fever. Abdominal pain can resemble that from appendicitis or renal colic.

Casts and microscopic hematuria can occur early, whereas proteinuria, isosthenuria, and progressive renal dysfunction occur in the second to fourth decades. Progressive renal failure occurs and requires transplantation. Hypertension, left ventricular hypertrophy, anginal chest pain with or without myocardial ischemia or infarction, and congestive heart failure can occur in the third to fourth decades. Leg lymphedema without hypoproteinemia and episodic diarrhea also occur. Death is due to renal failure or cardiovascular or cerebrovascular disease in untreated patients. Variants with residual α-galactosidase activity may have late-onset manifestations limited to the cardiovascular system that resemble hypertrophic myocardiopathies. Heterozygous females may exhibit some of these clinical manifestations but usually not the severe organ involvement.

Acroparesthesia, hypohidrosis or anhidrosis, angiokeratomas, and the typical corneal and lenticular lesions provide a presumptive diagnosis in males. Angiokeratomas are not diagnostic, however, and also occur in Fordyce scrotal angiokeratoma and several other lysosomal storage diseases.

Phenytoin and carbamazepine diminish the chronic and episodic acroparesthesia. Chronic hemodialysis or kidney transplantation can be lifesaving in patients with renal failure. Initial enzyme therapy results are promising.

Table 349-1   Selected Lysosomal Storage Diseases

Disorder[a]	Enzyme Deficiency	Stored Material	Clinical Types (Onset)	Inheritance	Neurologic
MUCOPOLYSACCHARIDOSES (MPS)					
MPS I H, Hurler (136)	α-L-Iduronidase	Dermatan sulfate Heparan sulfate	Infantile	AR	Mental retardation
MPS I H/S, Hurler/Scheie			Intermediate		Mental retardation
MPS I S, Scheie			Adult		None
MPS II, Hunter (136)	Iduronate sulfatase	Dermatan sulfate Heparan sulfate	Severe infantile Mild juvenile	X-linked	Mental retardation, less in mild form
MPS III A, Sanfilippo A (136)	Heparan-N-sulfatase	Heparan sulfate	Late infantile	AR	Severe mental retardation
MPS III B, Sanfilippo B	N-Acetyl-α-glucosaminidase	Heparan sulfate	Late infantile	AR	Severe mental retardation
MPS III C, Sanfilippo C	Acetyl-CoA: α-glucosaminide N-acetyltransferase	Heparan sulfate	Late infantile	AR	Severe mental retardation
MPS III D, Sanfilippo D	N-Acetylglucosamine-6-sulfate sulfatase	Heparan sulfate	Late infantile	AR	Severe mental retardation
MPS IV A, Morquio (136)	N-Acetylgalactosamine-6-sulfate sulfatase	Keratan sulfate Chondroitin-6 sulfate	Childhood	AR	None
MPS VI B, Morquio (136)	β-Galactosidase		Childhood	AR	None
MPS VI, Maroteaux-Lamy (136)	Arylsulfatase B	Dermatan sulfate	Late infantile	AR	None
MPS VII (136)	β-Glucuronidase	Dermatan sulfate Heparan sulfate	Neonatal Infantile Adult	AR	Mental retardation, absent in some adults
GM₂ GANGLIOSIDOSES					
Tay-Sachs' disease (153)	β-Hexosaminidase A	GM₂ gangliosides	Infantile Juvenile	AR	Mental retardation, seizures, later juvenile form
Sandhoff's disease (153)	β-Hexosaminidases A and B	GM₂ gangliosides	Infantile	AR	Mental retardation, seizures
NEUTRAL GLYCOSPHINGOLIPIDOSES					
Fabry disease (150)	α-Galactosidase A	Globotriaosylceramide	Childhood	X-linked	Painful acroparesthesias
Gaucher disease (146)	Acid β-Glucosidase	Glucosylceramide	Type 1 Type 2 Type 3	AR	None ++++ ++
Niemann-Pick disease (144) A and B	Sphingomyelinase	Sphingomyelin	Neuronopathic, type A Nonneuronopathic, type B	AR	Mental retardation and seizures
GLYCOPROTEINOSES					
Fucosidosis (140)	α-Fucosidase	Glycopeptides, oligosaccharides	Infantile Juvenile	AR	Mental retardation
α-Mannosidosis (140)	α-Mannosidase	Oligosaccharides	Infantile Milder variant	AR	Mental retardation
β-Mannosidosis (140)	β-Mannosidase	Oligosaccharides		AR	Seizures, mental retardation
Aspartylglucosaminuria (140)	Aspartylglucosaminidase	Aspartylglucosamine, glycopeptides	Young adult onset	AR	Mental retardation
Sialidosis (140)	Neuraminidase	Sialyloligosaccharides	Type I, congenital Type II, infantile and juvenile forms	AR	Myoclonus, mental retardation
MUCOLIPIDOSES (ML)					
ML-II, I-cell disease (138)	UDP-N-Acetylglucosamine-1-phosphotransferase	Glycoprotein, glycolipids	Infantile	AR	Mental retardation
ML-III, pseudo-Hurler polydystrophy (138)	UDP-N-Acetylglucosamine-1-phosphotransferase	Glycoprotein, glycolipids	Late infantile	AR	Mild mental retardation
LEUKODYSTROPHIES					
Krabbe's disease (147)	Galactosylceramidase	Galactosylceramide, Galactosyl sphingosine	Infantile	AR	Mental retardation
Metachromatic leukodystrophy (148)	Arylsulfatase A	Cerebroside sulfate	Infantile Juvenile Adult	AR	Mental retardation, dementia, and psychosis in adult
Multiple sulfatase deficiency (149)	Active site cysteine to C$_\alpha$-formylglycine-converting enzyme	Sulfatides, mucopolysaccharides	Late infantile	AR	Mental retardation
DISORDERS OF NEUTRAL LIPIDS					
Wolman disease (142)	Acid lysosomal lipase	Cholesterol esters, triglycerides	Infantile	AR	Mild mental retardation
Cholesteryl ester storage disease (142)	Acid lysosomal lipase	Cholesteryl esters	Childhood	AR	None
Farber disease (142)	Acid ceramidase	Ceramide	Infantile Juvenile	AR	Occasional mental retardation

[a] Numbers in parentheses refer to the chapters in Scriver et al, 8th edition, for detailed reviews.
NOTE: AR, autosomal recessive.

Liver and/or Spleen Enlargement	Skeletal Disease	Ophthalmologic	Hematologic	Unique Features
+++	++++	Corneal clouding	Vacuolated lymphocytes	Coarse facies, cardiovascular involvement, joint stiffness
+++	++++	Retinal degeneration, no corneal clouding	Granulated lymphocytes	Coarse facies, cardiovascular, joint stiffness, distinctive pebbly skin lesions
+	+	None	Granulated lymphocytes	Mild coarse facies
+	+	None	Granulated lymphocytes	Mild coarse facies
+	+	None	Granulated lymphocytes	Mild coarse facies
+	+	None	Granulated lymphocytes	Mild coarse facies
+	++++	Corneal clouding	Granulated neutrophils	Distinctive skeletal deformity, odontoid hypoplasia, aortic valve disease
±	++++			
++	++++	Corneal clouding	Granulated neutrophils and lymphocytes	Coarse facies, valvular heart disease
+++	+++	Corneal clouding	Granulated neutrophils	Coarse facies, vascular involvement, hydrops fetalis in neonatal form
None	None	Cherry red spot in infantile form	None	Macrocephaly, hyperacusis in infantile form
++	±	Cherry red spot	None	Macrocephaly, hyperacusis
None	None	Corneal dystrophy, vascular lesions	None	Cutaneous angiokeratomas, hypohydrosis
++++	++++	None	Gaucher cells in bone marrow, cytopenias	Adult form highly variable
+++	+	Eye movements		
++++	++++	Eye movements		
++++	None	Macular degeneration	Foam cells in bone marrow	Pulmonary infiltrates
	Osteo-Porosis			Lung failure
++	++	None	Vacuolated lymphocytes, foam cells	Coarse facies, angiokeratomas in juvenile form
+++	++	Cataracts, corneal clouding	Vacuolated lymphocytes, granulated neutrophils	Coarse facies, enlarged tongue
	++	None	Vacuolated lymphocytes, foam cells	Angiokeratomas
±	++	None	Vacuolated lymphocytes, foam cells	Coarse facies
++, less in type I	++ less in type I	Cherry red spot	Vacuolated lymphocytes	MPS phenotype in type II
±	++++	Corneal clouding	Vacuolated and granulated neutrophils	Coarse facies, absence of mucopolysacchariduria, gingival hypoplasia
None	+++	Corneal clouding, mild retinopathy, hyperopic astigmatism		Coarse facies, stiffness of hands and shoulders
None	None	None	None	White matter globoid cells
None	None	Optic atrophy	None	Gait abnormalities in late infantile form
+	++	Retinal degeneration	Vacuolated and granulated cells	Absent activity of all known cellular sulfatases
+++	None	None	None	Adrenal calcification
Hepatomegaly	None	None	None	Cirrhosis
+/−	None	Macular degeneration	None	Arthropathy, subcutaneous nodules

Gaucher Disease This is an autosomal recessive disorder that results from defective activity of acid β-glucosidase; >175 mutations have been described. This enzyme cleaves glucosylceramide, the parent compound of many glycosphingolipids and related glucolipids. Disease variants are classified based on the absence or presence and severity of neuronopathic involvement.

Type 2 Gaucher disease is a rare, severe CNS disease that leads to death by 2 years of age; it will not be addressed here.

Type 3 Gaucher disease has highly variable manifestations in the CNS and viscera. It can present in early childhood with rapidly progressive, massive visceral disease and slowly progressive to static CNS involvement; in adolescence with dementia; or in early adulthood with rapidly progressive, uncontrollable myoclonic seizures and mild visceral disease. Variants that span this spectrum also occur. Visceral disease in type 3 is nearly identical to that in type 1 but is generally more severe (see below). Early CNS findings may be limited to defects in lateral gaze tracking, which may remain static for decades. Mental retardation can be slowly progressive or static. This variant is most frequent among individuals of Swedish descent.

Type 1 Gaucher disease is a highly variable nonneuronopathic disease that can present in childhood to adulthood with slowly to rapidly progressive visceral disease. There is marked variability in age at onset and degree and progression of visceral involvement. In general, earlier diagnoses are associated with worse prognosis. The average age at diagnosis is ~20 years in Caucasian populations and somewhat younger in other groups. This pattern of presentation is distinctly bimodal, however, with peaks at <10 to 15 years and at ~25 years. Younger patients tend to have a greater degree of hepatosplenomegaly and accompanying blood cytopenias. In contrast, the older group has a greater tendency for chronic bone disease. Hepatosplenomegaly occurs in virtually all symptomatic patients and can be minor or massive. Accompanying anemia and thrombocytopenia are variable and are not linearly related to liver or spleen volume. Severe liver dysfunction is unusual, though minor liver function abnormalities are common. Splenic infarctions can resemble an acute abdomen. Pulmonary hypertension and alveolar Gaucher cell accumulation are uncommon, but life-threatening, and can occur at any age.

Though it is more common in adult patients, clinically evident skeletal disease in children can be devastating, resulting in massive destruction of the axial and peripheral skeleton. All patients with Gaucher disease have nonuniform infiltration of bone marrow by lipid-laden macrophages, termed *Gaucher cells*. This can lead to marrow packing with subsequent infarction, ischemia, necrosis, and cortical bone destruction. Bone marrow involvement spreads from proximal to distal in the limbs and can involve the axial skeleton extensively, causing vertebral collapse. In addition to bone marrow involvement, bone remodeling is defective, with loss of total bone calcium leading to osteopenia, osteonecrosis, avascular infarction, and vertebral compression fractures and spinal cord involvement. Aseptic necrosis of the femoral head is common, as is fracture of the femoral neck. The mechanism by which diseased bone marrow macrophages interact with osteoclasts and/or osteoblasts to lead to this complex bone disease is not well understood.

Affected patients experience chronic, ill-defined bone pain that can be debilitating and poorly correlated with radiographic findings. These are treated symptomatically. Some patients have one or more "bone crises" in their lifetimes that are associated with localized, excruciating pain, and, on occasion, local erythema, fever, and leukocytosis. Some patients have frequent crises, whereas other patients experience only one. Any bone can be involved, though the femurs and vertebral bodies are affected most often. These crises represent acute infarctions of bone, as evidenced in nuclear scans by localized absent uptake of pyrophosphate agents. X-rays are usually negative initially but may show lytic lesions 4 to 6 months after the acute phase. Osteomyelitis should be excluded by appropriate cultures. Bone cultures should be obtained only under sterile operating room conditions to minimize the chance of seeding an infection.

The diagnosis of Gaucher disease is established by demonstrating decreased acid β-glucosidase activity (0 to 20% of normal) in nucleated cells. The enzyme is not present in bodily fluids. The sensitivity of enzyme testing is poor for detecting heterozygous carriers; molecular testing is preferred when the mutations are known. The disease frequency varies from about 1 in 1000 in Ashkenazi Jews to <1 in 100,000 in some other populations. About 1 in 12 to 15 Ashkenazi Jews carries a Gaucher disease allele. Four common mutations account for ~90 to 95% of the mutations in affected patients: N370S (1226G), 84GG (a G insertion at cDNA position 84), L444P (1448C), and IVS-2 (an intron 2 splice junction mutation).

Genotype/phenotype studies indicate a significant correlation, though not absolute, between disease type and severity and the acid β-glucosidase genotype. For example, the most common mutation in the Ashkenazi Jewish population (N370S) shares a 100% association (to date) with nonneuronopathic, type 1 Gaucher disease, possibly because the N370S enzyme retains significant activity. The N370S/N370S and N370S/other mutant allele genotypes are associated with later onset/less severe and earlier onset/severe disease, respectively. The other alleles are L444P (very low activity), 84GG (null), or IVS-2 (null), and rare/private or uncharacterized alleles. As many as 50 to 60% of N370S/N370S patients are discovered as asymptomatic family members. The N370S/other mutant allele genotypes have disease onset about 2 decades earlier than those with N370S/N370S. The L444P/L444P patients almost always have life-threatening to very severe/early-onset disease, and many, though not all, develop CNS involvement in the first 2 decades of life. Some patients with this genotype have lethal neuronopathic disease at <1 year (type 2). Thus, this genotype is prognostic of very severe disease, with or without obvious CNS involvement.

Symptomatic management of the blood cytopenias and joint replacement surgeries continue to have important roles in the treatment of affected patients. However, enzyme therapy is currently the treatment of choice in significantly affected patients. Cerezyme, a recombinantly produced mannose-terminated (macrophage-targeted) acid β-glucosidase, has proved highly efficacious and safe in diminishing the hepatosplenomegaly and improving bone marrow involvement and hematologic findings.

Niemann-Pick Disease NPD is an autosomal recessive trait that occurs as several variants. Types A and B result from defects in acid sphingomyelinase; various mutations have been detected at this locus. Other variants, including NPD C, result from defective transport of cholesterol across the lysosomal membrane. Only NPD variants A and B will be considered here.

NPD A and B are distinguished primarily by an early age of onset and progressive CNS disease in A. NPD A typically has onset in the first 6 months, with rapidly progressive CNS deterioration, spasticity, failure to thrive, and massive hepatosplenomegaly. In contrast, NPD B has a later, more variable onset and progression of hepatosplenomegaly, with eventual development of cirrhosis and hepatic replacement by foam cells. Affected patients develop progressive pulmonary disease with dyspnea, hypoxemia, and a reticular infiltrative pattern on chest x-ray. Foam cells are present in alveoli, lymphatic vessels, and pulmonary arteries. Progressive hepatic or lung disease with associated bronchopneumonia, pulmonary hypertension, cor pulmonale, and decreased diffusion capacities lead to demise in adolescence to early adulthood.

The diagnosis is established by markedly decreased (1 to 10% of normal) sphingomyelinase activity in nucleated cells. Enzyme assays to detect NPD A or B carriers are unreliable. In families with known mutations, the molecular defect in heterozygotes can be identified by DNA analysis.

There is no specific treatment for NPD. The efficacy of hepatic or bone marrow transplantation has not been proven. Clinical trials using enzyme therapy are anticipated to begin soon.

THE LEUKODYSTROPHIES Globoid cell leukodystrophy and metachromatic leukodystrophy variants are autosomal recessive disorders that primarily involve CNS white matter and myelinated peripheral nervous system tracts.

Globoid Cell Leukodystrophy (GCL) The GCL variants are due to mutations in the galactosylceramidase gene. The term *globoid cell* is derived from the presence of characteristic multinucleated cells filled with galactosylceramide in the brains of affected patients. Infantile GCL (Krabbe disease) is a rapidly progressive, fatal disorder; patients succumb in the first 2 years. Juvenile and adult variants present with more slowly progressive dementia. For all variants, manifestations are confined to the CNS and peripheral nervous system. Diagnosis is confirmed by demonstrating defective galactosylceramidase activity in nucleated cells. Treatment is supportive, but bone marrow transplantation has shown some promise in the later onset variants.

Metachromatic Leukodystrophy MLD is due to defects in arylsulfatase A and accumulation of its substrate, galactosylceramide sulfate or sulfatide. The late-infantile form presents in the second year with progressive regression of developmental milestones and intellectual development. The disease is fatal in the first decade. The juvenile and adult forms have variable manifestations and present with gait disturbances, ataxia, mental regression, peripheral neuropathy, and/or seizures. In adults, behavioral disturbances, psychosis, and dementia tend to predominate. These later onset diseases may respond to bone marrow transplantation.

The diagnosis is established by demonstrating a deficiency of arylsulfatase A in nucleated cells. Homozygosity for a null allele (splicing defect in intron 2) produces severe infantile disease, whereas P426L homozygotes develop adult-onset disease. Compound heterozygotes, such as null and P426L alleles, have juvenile-onset variants. The diagnosis of MLD is complicated by the presence of a very frequent (10 to 15%) "pseudodeficiency allele" for arylsulfatase A. Although in vitro activity with synthetic substrates is deficient, cleavage of sulfatide is low-normal in vivo. Compound heterozygotes for the pseudodeficiency allele and true MLD alleles therefore appear to have deficient arylsulfatase A activity, diagnostic of MLD, but these individuals are not affected by the disease. MLD-causing mutations also occur on the background of the pseudodeficient allele, emphasizing the importance of careful genetic testing.

GLYCOGEN STORAGE DISEASE TYPE II (See also Chap. 350) Glycogen storage disease type II is an autosomal recessive disorder due to defects in acid α-glucosidase that lead to lysosomal glycogen accumulation. Numerous mutations have been found at this locus in affected patients. Skeletal and cardiac muscles are primarily involved. The infantile form (Pompe disease) is a fatal disorder characterized by hypertrophic cardiomegaly, macroglossia, and hypotonia due to glycogen accumulation in muscle. The juvenile form has progressive proximal muscle weakness, including impairment of respiratory function. Adult patients have phenotypes resembling slowly progressive muscular dystrophies. Prenatal diagnosis can be performed. Treatment is supportive, and enzyme trials are underway.

MUCOLIPIDOSES Mucolipidoses II (I-cell) and III (pseudo-Hurler polydystrophy) are rare autosomal recessive diseases. Both are caused by defective targeting of lysosomal hydrolases that require the M6P signal for sorting to the lysosome. As a result, >20 enzymes are secreted out of the cell and their substrates accumulated in specific cell types. N-acetylglucosamine-1-phosphotransferase activity, which is necessary for developing the M6P signal, is defective in these diseases. I-cell disease has a phenotype similar to MPS IH, whereas mucolipidosis-III is more similar to MPS IH/S; mental retardation is a feature of both. Diagnosis is suspected based on the characteristic phenotype and is established by demonstrating greatly elevated serum levels of lysosomal enzymes, as well as their deficiency in cells. Specific enzyme assays can also be performed. Carrier detection is possible but is not straightforward. Prenatal diagnosis can be performed using amniotic fluid and cells in at-risk families. Treatment is supportive.

BIBLIOGRAPHY

BEIGHTON P (ed): *McKusick's Heritable Disorders of Connective Tissue*, 5th ed. St. Louis, Mosby, 1993

SCRIVER CR et al (eds): *The Metabolic and Molecular Bases of Inherited Diseases*, 8th ed. New York, McGraw-Hill, 2000

WATTS RWE, GIBBS DA (eds): *Lysosomal Storage Diseases: Biochemical and Clinical Aspects.* Philadelphia, Taylor and Francis, 1986

350 *Yuan-Tsong Chen*

GLYCOGEN STORAGE DISEASES AND OTHER INHERITED DISORDERS OF CARBOHYDRATE METABOLISM

Carbohydrate synthesis and degradation play a vital role in cellular function by providing the energy required for most metabolic processes. The carbohydrates to be discussed include three monosaccharides: glucose, galactose, and fructose, and a polysaccharide, glycogen; the relevant biochemical pathways involved in the metabolism of these carbohydrates are shown in Fig. 350-1. Glucose is the principle substrate of energy metabolism in humans. Metabolism of glucose generates ATP via glycolysis and mitochondrial oxidative phosphorylation. A continuous source of glucose from dietary intake, gluconeogenesis, and degradation of glycogen maintain normal blood glucose levels. Sources of glucose in our diet are obtained by ingesting polysaccharides, primarily starch, and disaccharides including lactose, maltose, and sucrose. Galactose and fructose are two other monosaccharides that provide fuel for cellular metabolism; however, their role as fuel sources is much less significant than that of glucose. Galactose is derived from lactose (galactose + glucose), which is found in milk and milk products. If necessary, galactose can be incorporated into glycogen and thus becomes a source of glucose. Galactose is also an important component for certain glycolipids, glycoproteins, and glycosaminoglycans. The two dietary sources of fructose are sucrose (fructose + glucose), a commonly used sweetener, and fructose itself, which is found in fruits, vegetables, and honey.

This chapter is devoted to the inherited disorders of carbohydrate metabolism caused by defects in enzymes or transport proteins involved in glycogen metabolism, gluconeogenesis, and glycolysis (Table 350-1). Defects in glycogen metabolism typically cause an accumulation of glycogen in the tissues; hence, the name *glycogen storage diseases*. The defects in gluconeogenesis or glycolytic pathways including galactose and fructose metabolism do not usually result in glycogen accumulation.

Clinical manifestations of the various disorders of carbohydrate metabolism differ markedly. The symptoms range from harmless to lethal. Unlike disorders of lipid metabolism, mucopolysaccharidoses, or other storage diseases, dietary therapy has been effective in many of the carbohydrate disorders. Almost all the genes responsible for the inherited defects of carbohydrate metabolism have been cloned, and mutations have been identified. Advances in our understanding of the molecular basis of these diseases are being used to improve diagnosis and management, and some of these disorders are candidates for early trials of gene therapy.

Glycogen, the storage form of glucose in animal cells, is composed of glucose residues joined in straight chains by α1-4 linkages and branched at intervals of 4 to 10 residues with α1-6 linkages. The tree-like molecule can have a molecular weight of many millions and may aggregate to form structures recognizable by electron microscopy. In muscle, glycogen forms β particles, which are spherical and contain

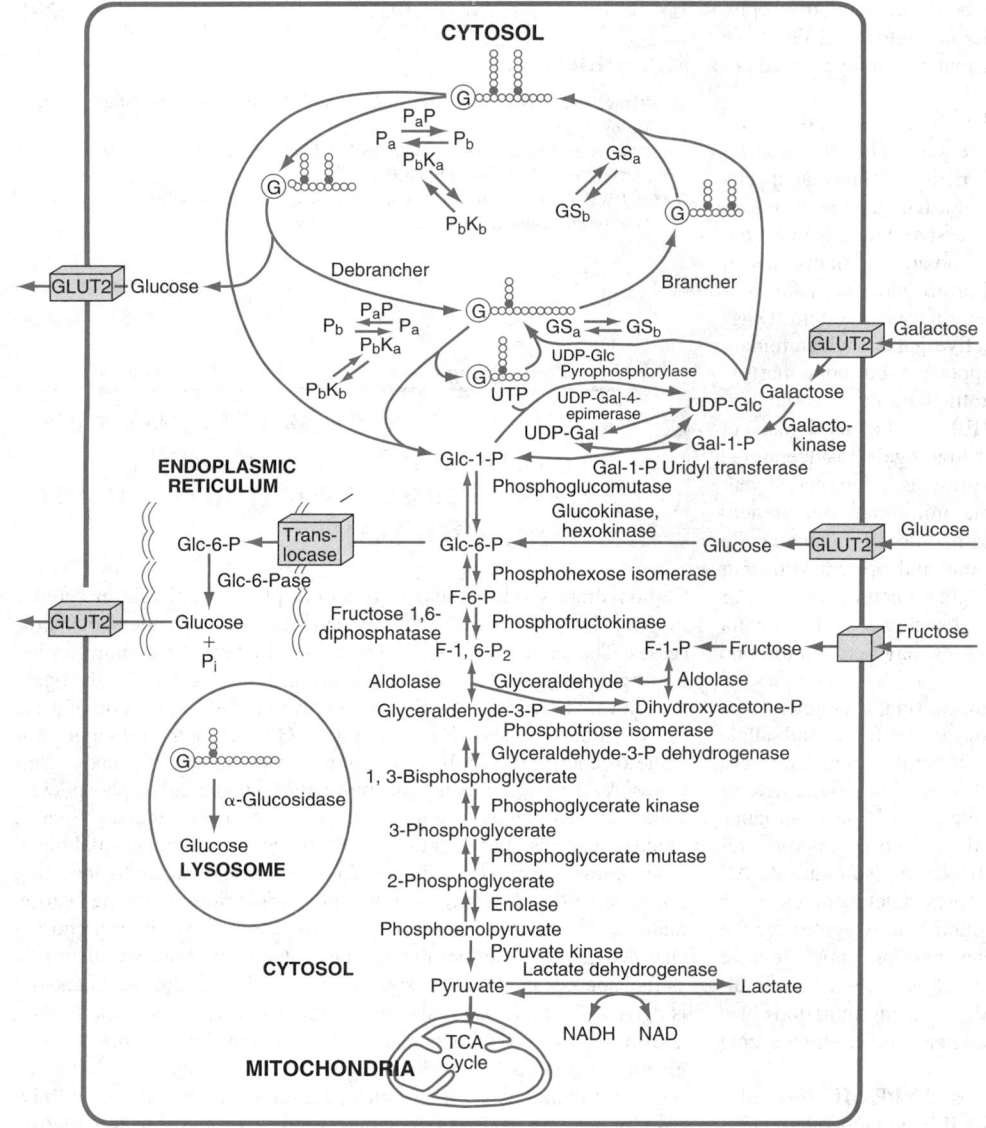

FIGURE 350-1 Metabolic pathways related to glycogen storage diseases and galactose and fructose disorders. Nonstandard abbreviations are as follows: GS_a, active glycogen synthase; GS_b, inactive glycogen synthase; P_a, active phosphorylase; P_b, inactive phosphorylase; P_aP, phosphorylase *a* phosphatase; P_bK_a, active phosphorylase *b* kinase; P_bK_b, inactive phosphorylase *b* kinase; G, glycogenin, the primer protein for glycogen synthesis. *[Modified from AR Beaudet: Glycogen storage disease, in KJ Isselbacher et al. (ed): Harrison's Principles of Internal Medicine, 13th ed., New York, McGraw-Hill, 1994, p 1855.]*

such as overtreatment of diabetes mellitus with insulin or administration of pharmacologic amounts of glucocorticoids.

Historically, the glycogen storage diseases were categorized numerically in the order in which the enzymatic defects were identified. They can also be classified by the organs involved and clinical manifestations, the system followed in this chapter (Table 350-1).

Because liver and muscle have abundant glycogen, they are the most commonly and seriously affected tissues. The hepatic glycogen storage diseases can be divided into two groups, with some overlap. The first is characterized by hepatomegaly and hypoglycemia. Because carbohydrate metabolism in the liver controls plasma glucose levels, the disorders of hepatic glycogen degradation and glucose release cause fasting hypoglycemia. Diseases in this group include glucose-6-phosphatase deficiency (type I), debranching enzyme deficiency (type III), liver phosphorylase deficiency (type VI), phosphorylase kinase deficiency (type IX), glycogen synthase deficiency (type 0), and glucose transporter-2 defects (type XI). The second group, characterized by cirrhosis of the liver and hepatomegaly, is associated with accumulation of abnormal forms of glycogen, which may be the cause of the hepatocellular injury. This group is represented by branching enzyme deficiency (type IV).

The role of glycogen in muscle is to provide substrates for the generation of sufficient ATP for muscle contraction. The muscle glycogen storage diseases can also be divided into two groups. The first is a muscle-energy disorder characterized by muscle pain, exercise intolerance, myoglobinuria, and susceptibility to fatigue. This group includes type V (McArdle disease), a muscle phosphorylase deficiency, and deficiencies of phosphofructokinase (type VII), phosphoglycerate kinase, phosphoglycerate mutase, lactase dehydrogenase, fructose 1,6-biphosphate aldolase A, and pyruvate kinase. Some of these latter enzyme deficiencies are associated with a compensated hemolysis, suggesting a more generalized defect in glucose metabolism. The second group of muscle disorders is characterized by progressive skeletal muscle weakness and atrophy and/or cardiomyopathy; it includes a lysosomal enzyme deficiency (acid α-glucosidase, type II) and deficiency of cardiac-specific phosphorylase kinase. Some glycogen storage diseases such as debranching enzyme deficiency (type IIIa) and branching enzyme deficiency (type IV) involve both muscle and liver.

The overall frequency of all forms of glycogen storage disease is approximately 1 in 20,000 live births; most are inherited as autosomal recessive traits, but phosphoglycerate kinase deficiency and one form of phosphorylase kinase deficiency are X-linked disorders. The most common childhood disorders are glucose-6-phosphatase deficiency (type I), lysosomal acid α-glucosidase deficiency (type II), debrancher deficiency (type III), and liver phosphorylase kinase deficiency (type IX). The most common adult disorder is myophosphorylase deficiency

up to 60,000 glucose residues. Each β particle contains a covalently linked protein called *glycogenin*. Liver contains β particles and rosettes of glycogen called α particles, which appear to be aggregated β particles.

The primary function of glycogen varies in different tissues. In skeletal muscle, stored glycogen is a source of fuel that is used for short-term, high-energy consumption during muscle activity; in the brain, the small amount of stored glycogen is used during brief periods of hypoglycemia or hypoxia as an emergency supply of energy. In contrast, the liver takes up glucose from the bloodstream after a meal and stores it as glycogen. When blood glucose levels start to fall, the liver converts glycogen back into glucose and releases it into the blood for use by tissues such as brain and erythrocytes that cannot store significant amounts of glycogen.

Glycogen storage diseases are inherited disorders that affect glycogen metabolism. Disorders in virtually every enzyme involved in the synthesis or degradation of glycogen and its regulation cause some type of glycogen storage disease (Fig. 350-1) in which glycogen is abnormal in quantity, quality, or both. Excluded from this chapter are those conditions in which tissue glycogen accumulation is secondary,

Table 350-1   Features of Glycogen Storage Diseases and Galactose and Fructose Disorders

Type/Common Name	Basic Defect	Clinical Features	Comments
LIVER GLYCOGENOSES			
Disorders with hepatomegaly and hypoglycemia			
Ia/von Gierke	Glucose-6-phosphatase	Growth retardation, enlarged liver and kidney, hypoglycemia, elevated blood lactate, cholesterol, triglycerides, and uric acid	Common, severe hypoglycemia
Ib	Glucose-6-phosphate translocase	As for Ia, with additional findings of neutropenia and neutrophil dysfunction	~10% of type I
IIIa/Cori or Forbes	Liver and muscle debranching enzyme	Childhood: Hepatomegaly, growth retardation, muscle weakness, hypoglycemia, hyperlipidemia, elevated liver transaminases; liver symptoms improve with age. Adulthood: muscle atrophy and weakness; onset: third to fourth decades; variable cardiomyopathy	Common, intermediate severity of hypoglycemia. Liver cirrhosis can occur in adulthood
IIIb	Liver debranching enzyme (normal muscle debrancher activity)	Liver symptoms same as in type IIIa; no muscle symptoms	~15% of type III
VI/Hers	Liver phosphorylase	Hepatomegaly, mild hypoglycemia, hyperlipidemia and ketosis; symptoms improve with age	Rare, "benign" glycogenosis
IX/phosphorylase kinase deficiency	Liver phosphorylase kinase α subunit	As for VI	Common, "benign glycogenosis," X-linked
0/glycogen synthase deficiency	Glycogen synthase	Fasting hypoglycemia and ketosis, elevated lactic acid and hyperglycemia after glucose load	Decreased glycogen stores
XI/Fanconi-Bickel	Glucose transporter-2	Failure to thrive, rickets, hepatomegaly, proximal renal tubular dysfunction, impaired glucose and galactose utilization	Rare, consanguinity in 70%
Disorders associated with liver cirrhosis			
IV/Andersen	Branching enzyme	Failure to thrive, hypotonia, hepatomegaly, splenomegaly, progressive liver cirrhosis and failure (death usually before fifth year); some without progression	One of the rarer glycogenoses; other neuromuscular variants exist
MUSCLE GLYCOGENOSES			
Disorders with muscle-energy impairment			
V/McArdle	Muscle phosphorylase	Exercise intolerance, muscle cramps, myoglobinuria on strenuous exercise, increased CK	Common, male predominance
VII/Tarui	Phosphofructokinase—M subunit	As for type V, with additional findings of a compensated hemolysis	Prevalent in Ashkenazi Jews and Japanese
Phosphoglycerate kinase deficiency	Phosphoglycerate kinase	As for type V, with additional findings of a hemolytic anemia and CNS dysfunction	Rare, X-linked
Phosphoglycerate mutase deficiency	Phosphoglycerate mutase—M subunit	As for type V	Rare; most patients are African American
Lactate dehydrogenase deficiency	Lactic acid dehydrogenase—M subunit	As for type V, with additional findings of erythematous skin eruption and uterine stiffness resulting in childbirth difficulty in female	Rare
Fructose 1,6-bisphosphate aldolase A deficiency	Fructose 1,6-bisphosphate aldolase A	As for type V, with additional finding of hemolytic anemia	Rare
Pyruvate kinase deficiency	Pyruvate kinase—muscle isozyme	Muscle cramps and/or fixed muscle weakness	Rare
Muscle phosphorylase kinase deficiency	Muscle-specific phosphorylase kinase	As for type V, some patients may have muscle weakness and atrophy	Rare, autosomal recessive
Disorders with progressive skeletal myopathy and/or cardiomyopathy			
II/Pompe	Lysosomal acid α-glucosidase	Infantile: hypotonia, muscle weakness, cardiac enlargement and failure, fatal early. Juvenile and adult: progressive skeletal muscle weakness and atrophy, proximal muscle and respiratory muscle are seriously affected	Common, undetectable, or very low level of enzyme activity in infantile form; residual enzyme activity in late-onset
Cardiac phosphorylase kinase deficiency	Cardiac-specific phosphorylase kinase	Severe cardiomyopathy and early heart failure	Very rare
GALACTOSE DISORDERS			
Galactosemia with uridyl transferase deficiency	Galactose 1-phosphate uridyl transferase	Vomiting, hepatomegaly, jaundice, cataracts, amino aciduria, failure to thrive	Long-term complications exist despite early diagnosis and treatment
Galactokinase deficiency	Galactokinase	Cataracts	Benign
Uridine diphosphate galactose 4-epimerase deficiency	Uridine diphosphate galactose 4-epimerase	Similar to transferase deficiency with additional findings of hypotonia and nerve deafness	Benign variant exists

(continued)

2283

Type/Common Name	Basic Defect	Clinical Features	Comments
FRUCTOSE DISORDERS			
Essential fructosuria	Fructokinase	Asymptomatic, positive urine reducing substance	Benign
Hereditary fructose intolerance	Fructose 1-phosphate aldolase B	Vomiting, lethargy, failure to thrive, hepatic failure	Prognosis good with early diagnosis and fructose restriction
Fructose 1,6-diphosphatase deficiency	Fructose 1,6-diphosphatase	Episodic hypoglycemia and lactic acidosis	Avoid fasting, good prognosis

NOTE: CK, creatine kinase; M, muscle; CNS, central nervous system.

(type V, or McArdle disease). In the past, the prognosis for many glycogen storage diseases was guarded. However, early diagnosis and better management have improved the survival rates, and many affected children are now adults.

GLYCOGEN STORAGE DISEASES: LIVER GLYCOGENOSES

DISORDERS WITH HEPATOMEGALY AND HYPO-GLYCEMIA   Type I Glycogen Storage Disease (Glucose-6-Phosphatase or Translocase Deficiency, von Gierke Disease)   Type I glycogen storage disease is due to a defect in glucose-6-phosphatase in liver, kidney, and intestinal mucosa. It can be divided into two subtypes: type Ia, in which the glucose-6-phosphatase enzyme is defective, and type Ib, which is due to a defect in the translocase that transports glucose-6-phosphate across the microsomal membrane. The defects in both subtypes lead to inadequate conversion in the liver of glucose-6-phosphate to glucose and thus make affected individuals susceptible to fasting hypoglycemia.

GENETIC CONSIDERATIONS   Type I glycogen storage disease is an autosomal recessive disorder. Both types Ia and Ib disease have been reported in many ethnic groups, but type Ia is rarely seen in blacks. The structural gene for glucose-6-phosphatase is located on chromosome 17q21; three common mutations (R83C, 130X, Q347X) are responsible for 70% of the known disease alleles. The structural gene for glucose 6-phosphate translocase is located on chromosome 11q23; two mutations, G339C and 1211delCT, appear to be prevalent in Caucasian patients, while W118R appears to be most common in Japanese patients. Carrier detection and prenatal diagnosis are possible with the use of molecular techniques. ■

Clinical and laboratory findings   Persons with type I disease may develop hypoglycemia and lactic acidosis during the neonatal period, but, more commonly, they present at 3 to 4 months of age with hepatomegaly and/or hypoglycemia. These children often have doll-like faces with fat cheeks, relatively thin extremities, short stature, and a protuberant abdomen that is due to massive hepatomegaly; the kidneys are enlarged, but the spleen and heart are of normal size.

The hallmarks of the disease are hypoglycemia, lactic acidosis, hyperuricemia, and hyperlipidemia. Hypoglycemia and lactic acidosis can develop after a short fast. Hyperuricemia is present in young children, but gout rarely develops before puberty. Despite hepatomegaly, liver enzymes are usually normal or near normal. Intermittent diarrhea may occur (the mechanism is not known). Easy bruising and epistaxis are associated with a prolonged bleeding time as a result of impaired platelet aggregation/adhesion.

Hypertriglyceridemia may cause the plasma to appear "milky," and cholesterol and phospholipids are also elevated. The lipid abnormality resembles type IV hyperlipidemia and is characterized by increased levels of very low-density lipoprotein (VLDL); low-density lipoprotein (LDL); increased levels of apoliproteins B, C, and E; and normal or reduced levels of apoliproteins A and D. The hepatocytes are distended by glycogen and fat with large and prominent lipid vacuoles. There is little associated fibrosis.

All these findings apply to both types Ia and Ib disease, but type Ib has the additional feature of recurrent bacterial infections due to neutropenia and impaired neutrophil function. Oral and intestinal mucosa ulcerations are common, and inflammatory bowel disease may occur.

Long-term complications   Although type I glycogen storage disease mainly affects the liver, multiple organ systems are also involved. Gout usually becomes symptomatic around puberty as a result of the long-term hyperuricemia. Puberty is often delayed, but fertility appears to be normal. Hypertriglyceridemia causes an increased risk of pancreatitis, but premature atherosclerosis has not been documented. Impaired platelet aggregation may reduce the risk of atherosclerosis.

By the second or third decade of life, most patients with type I glycogen storage disease develop hepatic adenomas that can hemorrhage and, in rare cases, may become malignant. Other complications include pulmonary hypertension and osteoporosis.

Renal disease is a late complication, and almost all patients older than 20 years have proteinuria. Many have hypertension, kidney stones, nephrocalcinosis, and altered creatinine clearance. Glomerular hyperfiltration, increased renal plasma flow, and microalbuminuria can occur before the onset of gross proteinuria. In young patients, hyperfiltration and hyperperfusion may be the only signs of renal abnormalities. With advanced renal disease, focal segmental glomerulosclerosis and interstitial fibrosis are evident on biopsy. In some patients, renal function deteriorates and progresses to failure, requiring dialysis or transplantation. Other abnormalities in renal function include amyloidosis, Fanconi-like syndrome, and distal renal tubular acidification defect. The increases in renal perfusion and maternal blood volume that normally occur in pregnancy can exacerbate renal problems. In addition, hypoglycemia may also become more difficult to control.

Diagnosis   The diagnosis of type I disease can be suspected on the basis of clinical presentation and abnormal plasma lactate and lipid values. In addition, administration of glucagon or epinephrine causes little or no rise in blood glucose but increases lactate levels significantly. Before the glucose 6-phosphatase and glucose 6-phosphate translocase genes were cloned, a definitive diagnosis required a liver biopsy to demonstrate a deficiency. Gene-based mutation analysis now provides a noninvasive way of diagnosis for most patients with types Ia and Ib disease.

TREATMENT   Treatment is designed to maintain normal blood glucose levels and is achieved by continuous nasogastric infusion of glucose or oral administration of uncooked cornstarch. Nasogastric drip feeding in early infancy may consist of an elemental enteral formula or may contain only glucose to maintain normoglycemia during the night; frequent feedings with a high-carbohydrate content are given during the day.

Uncooked cornstarch acts as a slow-release form of glucose and can be given at a dose of 1.6 g/kg every 4 h for infants younger than 2 years. As the child grows older, the cornstarch regimen can be changed to every 6 h, and it can be given by mouth as a liquid (1:2, weight:volume) at a dose of 1.75 to 2.5 g/kg of body weight. Because fructose and galactose cannot be converted to free glucose, their dietary intake should be restricted, and dietary supplements of multivitamins and calcium are required. Allopurinol is given to lower the levels of uric acid. In patients with type Ib disease, granulocyte and granulocyte-macrophage colony stimulating factors have been used successfully to correct the neutropenia, decrease the severity of bacterial infection, and improve the chronic inflammatory bowel disease.

Before surgery, the bleeding status of the patient should be evaluated, and good metabolic control should be established. Prolonged bleeding time can be corrected by the administration of a constant intravenous glucose infusion for 24 to 48 h before surgery. Vasopressin can be given during surgery to reduce bleeding complications, and normal glucose levels should be maintained throughout surgery.

Prognosis In the past, many patients with type I glycogen storage disease died, and the prognosis was guarded for those who survived. The long-term complications discussed above occur mostly in adults whose disease was not adequately treated during childhood. Early diagnosis and initiation of effective treatment have improved the outcome, but it is not known if all long-term complications can be avoided through good metabolic control.

Type III Glycogen Storage Disease (Debrancher Deficiency, Limit Dextrinosis) Type III glycogen storage disease is caused by a deficiency of glycogen debranching enzyme. Debranching enzyme and phosphorylase are responsible for complete degradation of glycogen; when debranching enzyme is defective, glycogen breakdown is incomplete, and an abnormal glycogen accumulates that has short outer chains and resembles limit dextrin.

GENETIC CONSIDERATIONS The type III glycogenoses are inherited as autosomal recessive traits. The disease has been reported in many different ethnic groups, and the frequency is relatively high in non-Ashkenazi Jews of North African descent. The gene for debranching enzyme is located on chromosome 1p21. At least 20 different mutations that cause type III disease have been identified. Two mutations (17delAG and Q6X), both located in exon 3 at amino acid codon 6, are exclusively found in the subtype IIIb. Carrier detection and prenatal diagnosis are possible with DNA-based linkage or mutation analysis. ■

Clinical and laboratory findings Deficiency of glycogen debranching enzyme causes hepatomegaly, hypoglycemia, short stature, variable skeletal myopathy, and cardiomyopathy. The disorder usually involves both liver and muscle and is termed *type IIIa glycogen storage disease*. However, in about 15% of patients, the disease appears to involve only the liver and is classified as *type IIIb*.

During infancy and childhood, the disease may be almost indistinguishable from type I disease because hepatomegaly, hypoglycemia, hyperlipidemia, and growth retardation are common features of both. Splenomegaly may be present, but the kidneys are not enlarged in type III disease. Remarkably, hepatomegaly and hepatic symptoms in most patients with type III disease improve with age and usually disappear after puberty. However, progressive liver cirrhosis with failure may occur and seems especially common in Japanese patients.

In patients with muscle involvement (type IIIa), muscle weakness is usually minimal during childhood but can become severe during the third or fourth decade of life, as evidenced by slowly progressive weakness and muscle wasting. Electromyographic (EMG) changes are consistent with a widespread myopathy, and nerve conduction may be abnormal. Ventricular hypertrophy is frequent, but overt cardiac dysfunction is rare. Hepatic symptoms may be so mild that the diagnosis is not made until adulthood, when neuromuscular disease becomes manifest. Polycystic ovaries appear to be a common finding in female patients; fertility, however, does not seem to be affected.

Hypoglycemia, hyperlipidemia, and elevated liver transaminases occur in children. In contrast to type I disease, fasting ketosis is prominent, and blood lactate and uric acid concentrations are usually normal. The administration of glucagon 2 h after a carbohydrate meal causes a normal rise of blood glucose, but after an overnight fast glucagon may provoke no change in blood glucose. Serum creatine kinase levels can sometimes be used to identify patients with muscle involvement, but normal levels do not rule out muscle enzyme deficiency.

The histology of the liver is characterized by a universal distention

of hepatocytes by glycogen and by the presence of fibrous septa. The fibrosis and the paucity of fat distinguish type III from type I glycogenosis. The fibrosis can range from minimal periportal fibrosis to micronodular cirrhosis.

Diagnosis In type IIIa glycogen storage disease, deficient debranching enzyme activity can be demonstrated in liver, skeletal muscle, and heart. In contrast, patients with type IIIb have debranching enzyme deficiency in the liver but not in muscle. In the past, definitive assignment of subtype required enzyme assays in both liver and muscle. DNA-based analyses now provide a noninvasive way of subtyping these disorders in most patients.

TREATMENT Dietary management of type III disease is less demanding than that of type I. If hypoglycemia is present, frequent high-carbohydrate meals with cornstarch supplements or nocturnal gastric drip feedings are usually effective. A high-protein diet during the day plus overnight protein enteral infusion may be tried in patients with myopathy, but it is not established whether such a regimen is effective. Patients do not need to restrict dietary intake of fructose and galactose, as do those with type I disease.

Prognosis Liver symptoms improve with age and usually disappear after puberty. Cirrhosis of the liver may occur later in life. In type IIIa disease, muscle weakness and atrophy worsen during adulthood.

Type VI Glycogen Storage Disease [Liver Phosphorylase Deficiency (Hers Disease)] The number of patients with enzymatically documented liver phosphorylase deficiency is small. It appears that patients with liver phosphorylase deficiency have a benign course. These patients present with hepatomegaly and growth retardation early in childhood. Hypoglycemia, hyperlipidemia, and hyperketosis are usually mild if present. Plasma lactic acid and uric acid levels are normal. The heart and skeletal muscles are not involved. The hepatomegaly and growth retardation improve with age and usually disappear at puberty. Treatment is symptomatic. A high-carbohydrate diet and frequent feeding are effective in preventing hypoglycemia, but most patients require no specific treatment. The liver phosphorylase gene is located on chromosome 14q21. A splicing site mutation in intron 13 has been identified in a large Mennonite kindred, and four other mutations have been found in patients with different ethnic backgrounds.

Type IX Glycogen Storage Disease (Liver Phosphorylase Kinase Deficiency) Defects of phosphorylase kinase cause a heterogeneous group of glycogenoses. The heterogeneity is due to the complexity of the phosphorylase kinase enzyme complex. It consists of four subunits (α, β, γ, and δ), each encoded by different genes (X chromosome as well as autosomes) that are differentially expressed in various tissues. Phosphorylase kinase deficiency can be divided into several subtypes on the basis of the gene/subunit involved, the tissues that are primarily affected, and the mode of inheritance.

Subtypes of phosphorylase kinase deficiency • *X-LINKED LIVER PHOSPHORYLASE KINASE DEFICIENCY* X-linked liver phosphorylase kinase deficiency is one of the most common liver glycogenoses. Phosphorylase kinase activity may also be deficient in erythrocytes and leukocytes but is normal in muscle. Typically, a child between the ages of 1 and 5 years presents with growth retardation and hepatomegaly. Levels of cholesterol, triglycerides, and liver enzymes are mildly elevated. Ketosis may occur after fasting. Lactic and uric acid levels are normal. Hypoglycemia is mild, if present. The rise in the blood glucose level after the administration of glucagon is normal. Hepatomegaly and abnormal blood chemistries gradually return to normal with age. Most adults achieve a normal final height and are practically asymptomatic, despite a persistent phosphorylase kinase deficiency.

Liver histology shows glycogen-distended hepatocytes. The accumulated glycogen (α particles, rosette form) has a frayed or burst appearance and is less compact than in type I or type III disease. Fibrous septa and low-grade inflammatory changes may be present.

The structural gene for the liver isoform of the phosphorylase kinase α-subunit is located on chromosome Xp22, and mutations of this gene have been found in the disorder. Subtle mutations tend to retain the phosphorylase kinase activity in blood cells, whereas nonsense mutations cause enzyme deficiency in both liver and blood cells.

AUTOSOMAL LIVER AND MUSCLE PHOSPHORYLASE KINASE DEFICIENCY An autosomal recessive form of liver and muscle phosphorylase kinase deficiency has been reported in several patients. As in the X-linked form of the disorder, hepatomegaly and growth retardation are the predominant symptoms in early childhood. Some patients also exhibit muscle hypotonia and have reduced activity of phosphorylase kinase in muscle. This form of the phosphorylase kinase deficiency is caused by mutations in the β-subunit of the gene located on chromosome 16q12-13.

AUTOSOMAL LIVER PHOSPHORYLASE KINASE DEFICIENCY In contrast to the benign course of X-linked phosphorylase kinase deficiency, patients with the autosomal recessive form of liver phosphorylase kinase deficiency have more severe phenotypes and often develop liver cirrhosis. This form of phosphorylase kinase deficiency is due to mutations in the testis/liver isoform of the γ-subunit gene located on chromosome 16p.

MUSCLE-SPECIFIC PHOSPHORYLASE KINASE DEFICIENCY Muscle-specific phosphorylase kinase deficiency causes cramps and myoglobinuria on exercise or progressive muscle weakness and atrophy. The activity of the enzyme is decreased in muscle but normal (when determined) in liver and blood cells. There is no hepatomegaly or cardiomegaly. The disorder may be due to mutation in the muscle isoform of the α-subunit located on the X chromosome.

CARDIAC-SPECIFIC PHOSPHORYLASE KINASE DEFICIENCY Several sporadic cases of cardiac-specific phosphorylase kinase deficiency have been reported. All patients died during infancy from cardiac failure due to massive glycogen deposition in the myocardium. The molecular basis has not been defined.

Diagnosis Definitive diagnosis of phosphorylase kinase deficiency requires demonstration of the enzymatic defect in affected tissues. Although phosphorylase kinase can be measured in leukocytes and erythrocytes, the enzyme has many tissue-specific isozymes, and the diagnosis can be missed without studies of the liver, muscle, or heart.

TREATMENT The treatment for liver phosphorylase or phosphorylase kinase deficiency is based on symptoms. A high-carbohydrate diet and frequent feedings are effective in preventing hypoglycemia, but most patients require no specific treatment. Prognosis is usually good; adult patients have normal stature and minimal hepatomegaly. There is no treatment for the fatal form of isolated cardiac phosphorylase kinase deficiency.

Type 0 Glycogen Storage Disease (Glycogen Synthase Deficiency) Strictly speaking, type 0 is not a glycogen storage disease, as the deficiency of the enzyme leads to decreased glycogen stores. The patients present in early infancy with morning drowsiness and fatigue and sometimes convulsions associated with hypoglycemia and hyperketonemia. There is no hepatomegaly or hyperlipidemia. Prolonged hyperglycemia and elevated lactate levels with normal insulin levels after administration of glucose suggest a possible diagnosis of glycogen synthase deficiency. Definitive diagnosis requires a liver biopsy to measure the enzyme activity. Treatment is symptomatic and involves frequent feedings rich in protein and nighttime supplements of uncooked cornstarch to alleviate hypoglycemia. Prognosis is good as patients survive to adulthood with a resolution of hypoglycemia except during pregnancy. Mutations in the liver glycogen synthase gene (located on chromosome 12p12.2) that cause glycogen synthase deficiency have been identified.

Type XI Glycogen Storage Disease (Hepatic Glycogenosis with Renal Fanconi Syndrome, Fanconi-Bickel Syndrome) This rare autosomal recessive disease is caused by defects in the facilitative glucose transporter 2 (GLUT-2) which transports glucose in and out of hepatocytes, pancreatic cells, and the baso-lateral membranes of intestinal and renal epithelial cells. The disease is characterized by proximal renal tubular dysfunction, impaired glucose and galactose utilization, and accumulation of glycogen in liver and kidney.

GENETIC CONSIDERATIONS The low prevalence of Fanconi-Beckel syndrome (fewer than 100 cases reported worldwide) is underscored by the fact that consanguinity is found in 70% of the patients with a detectable GLUT-2 mutation. The gene for GLUT-2 is located on chromosome 3q26 and most mutations detected so far cause premature termination of translation. ∎

Clinical and laboratory findings The affected child presents in the first year of life with failure to thrive, rickets, and a protuberant abdomen due to liver and kidney enlargement. Laboratory findings include glucosuria, phosphaturia, generalized aminoaciduria, bicarbonate wasting, hypophosphatemia, increased serum alkaline phosphatase levels, and radiologic findings of rickets. Mild fasting hypoglycemia and hyperlipidemia may be present. Liver transaminases, plasma lactate, and uric acid levels are usually normal. Oral galactose or glucose tolerance tests show intolerance to these sugars, which may be caused by the functional loss of GLUT-2, which prevents liver uptake of these sugars. Tissue biopsies show marked accumulation of glycogen in hepatocytes and proximal renal tubular cells, presumably due to the altered transport of glucose out of these organs.

TREATMENT There is no specific therapy. Growth retardation persists through adulthood. Symptomatic replacement of water, electrolytes, and vitamin D, restriction of galactose intake, and a diabetes mellitus-like diet, presented in frequent and small meals with a cornstarch supplement, may improve growth.

DISORDERS ASSOCIATED WITH LIVER CIRRHOSIS
Type IV Glycogen Storage Disease (Branching Enzyme Deficiency, Amylopectinosis, or Andersen Disease) Deficiency of branching enzyme activity results in accumulation of an abnormal glycogen with poor solubility. The disease is referred to as *type IV glycogen storage disease or amylopectinosis*, because the abnormal glycogen has fewer branch points, more 1-4 linked glucose units, and longer outer chains, resulting in a structure resembling amylopectin.

GENETIC CONSIDERATIONS Type IV glycogen storage disease is a rare autosomal recessive disease. Prenatal diagnosis is available with use of cultured amniocytes or chorionic villi to measure the level of enzymatic activity. The glycogen branching enzyme gene is located on chromosome 3p12. Both hepatic and neuromuscular forms of the disease are caused by mutations in the same branching enzyme gene; its characterization in individual patients may be useful in predicting the clinical course. ∎

Clinical and laboratory findings This disorder is clinically variable. The most common form is characterized by progressive cirrhosis of the liver and is manifest in the first 18 months of life as hepatosplenomegaly and failure to thrive. The cirrhosis progresses to cause portal hypertension, ascites, esophageal varices, and liver failure that leads to death by age 5. Less frequently, patients survive without progression of liver disease.

Tissue deposition of amylopectin-like materials can be demonstrated in liver, heart, muscle, skin, intestine, brain, spinal cord, and peripheral nerve. The histologic findings in the liver are characterized by both micronodular cirrhosis and faintly stained basophilic inclusions in the hepatocytes. The inclusions consist of coarsely clumped, stored material that is periodic acid Schiff-positive and partially resistant to diastase digestion. Electron microscopy shows, in addition to the conventional χ and β glycogen particles, an accumulation of fibrillar aggregations typical of amylopectin. Definitive diagnosis re-

A neuromuscular form of type IV glycogen storage disease has also been reported. Patients with this disease may present (1) at birth with severe hypotonia, muscle atrophy, and neuronal involvement and die during the neonatal period; (2) in late childhood with myopathy or cardiomyopathy; or (3) as adults with diffuse central and peripheral nervous system dysfunction accompanied by accumulation of polyglucosan bodies in the nervous system (so-called adult polyglucosan body disease). Definitive diagnosis of the adult disease requires assay of the branching enzyme in leukocytes or nerve biopsy, as the deficiency is limited to those tissues.

TREATMENT There is no specific treatment for type IV glycogen storage disease. For progressive hepatic failure, liver transplantation has been performed. However, caution should be taken in selecting patients for liver transplantation because a nonprogressive hepatic form of the disease exists, and extra hepatic manifestations of the disease may occur after transplantation.

GLYCOGEN STORAGE DISEASES: MUSCLE GLYCOGENOSES

DISORDERS WITH MUSCLE-ENERGY IMPAIRMENT

Type V Glycogen Storage Disease (Muscle Phosphorylase Deficiency, McArdle Disease) Deficiency of muscle phosphorylase is the prototype muscle-energy disorder. Deficiency of this enzyme in muscle limits ATP generation by glycogenolysis and results in glycogen accumulation.

GENETIC CONSIDERATIONS Type V glycogen storage disease is an autosomal recessive disorder that does not appear to have ethnic predilection. The gene for muscle phosphorylase is located on chromosome 11q13. The most common mutation in patients in the United States is a nonsense mutation that changes an arginine to a stop codon (R49X), and the most common mutation in the Japanese is deletion of a single codon (F708). These features allow DNA-based diagnosis and carrier detection in these two populations. ∎

Clinical and laboratory findings Symptoms usually develop first in adulthood and are characterized by exercise intolerance with muscle cramps. Two types of activity tend to cause symptoms: (1) brief exercise of great intensity, such as sprinting or carrying heavy loads; and (2) less intense but sustained activity, such as climbing stairs or walking uphill. Moderate exercise, such as walking on level ground, can be performed by most patients for long periods. Many patients experience a characteristic "second wind" phenomenon; if they rest briefly at the first appearance of muscle pain, they can resume exercise with more ease. About half of patients report burgundy-colored urine after exercise, the consequence of myoglobinuria secondary to rhabdomyolysis. Intense myoglobinuria after vigorous exercise may cause renal failure. Although most patients are diagnosed in the second or third decade, many report weakness and lack of endurance since childhood. In rare cases, EMG findings may suggest an inflammatory myopathy, and the diagnosis can be confused with polymyositis.

The level of serum creatine kinase is usually elevated at rest and increases more after exercise. Exercise also increases the levels of blood ammonia, inosine, hypoxanthine, and uric acid. The latter abnormalities are attributed to accelerated recycling of muscle purine nucleotides in the face of insufficient ATP production.

Diagnosis Lack of an increase in blood lactate and exaggerated blood ammonia elevations after an ischemic exercise test are indicative of muscle glycogenosis and suggest a defect in the conversion of glycogen or glucose to lactate. The abnormal exercise response, however, is not limited to type V disease and can occur with other defects in glycogenolysis or glycolysis, such as deficiencies of muscle phosphofructokinase or debranching enzyme (when the test is done after fasting). Definitive diagnosis is made by enzymatic assay in muscle tissue or by mutation analysis of the myophosphorylase gene.

TREATMENT In general, avoidance of strenuous exercise can prevent major episodes of rhabdomyolysis. Exercise tolerance can be augmented by aerobic training or by ingestion of glucose or fructose. A high-protein diet may increase exercise endurance in some patients. Longevity does not appear to be affected.

Type VII Glycogen Storage Disease (Muscle Phosphofructokinase Deficiency, Tarui Disease) Type VII disease is caused by a deficiency of muscle phosphofructokinase, which catalyzes the conversion of fructose-6-phosphate to fructose-1,6-diphosphate and is a key regulatory enzyme of glycolysis.

Phosphofructokinase is composed of three isozyme subunits (M, muscle; L, liver; and P, platelet), which are encoded by different genes and are differentially expressed in tissues. Skeletal muscle contains only M isozyme, and red blood cells contain a hybrid of L and M forms. Type VII disease is due to defective M isoenzyme, which causes complete enzyme deficiency in muscle and partial deficiency in red blood cells.

GENETIC CONSIDERATIONS Type VII glycogen storage disease is inherited as an autosomal recessive trait. The disease appears to be rare, and most reported patients are either Ashkenazi Jews or Japanese. The gene for the M isoenzyme is located on chromosome 12q13.3. In Ashkenazi Jews, 95% of mutant alleles are either a splicing defect or a nucleotide deletion. ∎

Clinical and laboratory findings The features are similar to those in type V disease, namely, early onset of fatigue and pain with exercise. Vigorous exercise causes severe muscle cramps and myoglobinuria. However, several features of type VII disease are distinctive. (1) Exercise intolerance is usually evident in childhood, is more severe than in type V disease, and may be associated with nausea and vomiting. (2) A compensated hemolysis occurs as evidenced by an increased level of serum bilirubin and reticulocyte count. (3) Hyperuricemia is common and becomes more marked after exercise. (4) An abnormal glycogen resembling amylopectin is present in muscle fibers; it is periodic acid Schiff-positive and resistant to diastase digestion. (5) Exercise intolerance is particularly acute after meals rich in carbohydrate because glucose cannot be utilized in muscle and because the ingested glucose inhibits lipolysis and thus deprives muscle of fatty acid and ketone substrates. In contrast, patients with type V disease can metabolize glucose derived from either liver glycogenolysis or exogenous glucose. Indeed, glucose infusion improves exercise tolerance in patients with type V disease.

Two rare type VII variants have been reported. One begins in infancy with hypotonia and limb weakness, and a rapidly progressive myopathy leads to death by age 4. The other occurs in adults and is characterized by a slowly progressive, fixed muscle weakness rather than by cramps and myoglobinuria.

Diagnosis The M isoenzyme defect must be demonstrated in muscle, red blood cells, or cultured skin fibroblasts by biochemical or histochemical techniques.

TREATMENT There is no specific treatment. Avoidance of strenuous exercise prevents acute attacks of muscle cramps and myoglobinuria.

Other Muscle Glycogenoses with Muscle-Energy Impairment Five additional enzyme defects produce muscle glycogenoses, namely, deficiencies in phosphoglycerate kinase, phosphoglycerate mutase, lactate dehydrogenase, fructose 1,6-bisphosphate aldolase A, and pyruvate kinase. All five enzymes affect terminal glycolysis, and deficiency causes muscle-energy impairment similar to that in type V and type VII disease. The failure of blood lactate to increase in response to exercise can be used to separate muscle glycogenoses from disorders of lipid metabolism, such as carnitine palmitoyl transferase II deficiency and very long chain acyl-coenzyme A dehydrogenase deficiency, which also cause muscle cramps and myoglobinuria. Muscle glycogen levels may be normal in the disorders affecting terminal glycolysis, and definitive diagnosis is made by assaying the enzymatic activity in muscle.

DISORDERS WITH PROGRESSIVE SKELETAL MUSCLE MYOPATHY AND/OR CARDIOMYOPATHY **Type II Glycogen Storage Disease (Acid α-1,4 Glucosidase Deficiency, Pompe Disease)** (See also Chap. 349) Type II disease is caused by a deficiency of lysosomal acid α-1,4 glucosidase (acid maltase), an enzyme responsible for the degradation of glycogen in lysosomal vacuoles. It is characterized by the accumulation of glycogen in lysosomes as opposed to its accumulation in cytoplasm in the other glycogenoses.

GENETIC CONSIDERATIONS Pompe disease is an autosomal recessive disorder and does not appear to have an ethnic predilection. The gene for acid α-glucosidase is on chromosome 17q25. A splice site mutation (IVS1-13TG) is common in patients with adult-onset disease. Prenatal diagnosis with amniocytes or chorionic villi is available. ∎

Clinical and laboratory findings The disorder encompasses a range of phenotypes, each including myopathy but differing in age of onset, organ involvement, and clinical severity. The most severe is the infantile-onset disease with cardiomegaly, hypotonia, and death before 1 year of age. Infants appear normal at birth but soon develop generalized muscle weakness with feeding difficulties, macroglossia, hepatomegaly, and congestive heart failure due to a hypertrophic cardiomyopathy. Electrocardiographic findings include a high-voltage QRS complex and a shortened PR interval. Death usually occurs from cardiorespiratory failure.

The juvenile or late-childhood form is characterized by skeletal muscle manifestations, usually without cardiac involvement, and a slowly progressive course. The juvenile form typically presents as delayed motor milestones (if age of onset is early enough) and difficulty in walking; these manifestations are followed by swallowing difficulties, proximal muscle weakness, and respiratory muscle involvement. This form can cause death before the end of the second decade.

An adult form of type II disease presents as a slowly progressive myopathy without cardiac involvement and has its onset between the second and seventh decades. The clinical picture is dominated by slowly progressive proximal muscle weakness with truncal involvement. The pelvic girdle, paraspinal muscles, and the diaphragm are most seriously affected. The initial symptoms may be respiratory insufficiency manifested by somnolence, morning headache, orthopnea, and exertional dyspnea.

Laboratory findings include elevated levels of serum creatine kinase, aspartate transaminase, and lactate dehydrogenase, particularly in infants. Muscle biopsy shows the presence of vacuoles that stain positively for glycogen, and muscle acid phosphatase is increased, presumably from a compensatory increase of lysosomal enzymes. Electron microscopy reveals the glycogen accumulation. EMG reveals myopathic features with irritability of muscle fibers and pseudomyotonic discharges. Serum creatine kinase is not always elevated in adults and, depending on the muscle biopsied or tested, muscle histology or EMG may not be abnormal. It is prudent to examine affected muscle.

Diagnosis Diagnosis can be established by demonstration of the absence or reduced levels of acid α-glucosidase activity in muscle or cultured skin fibroblasts. Deficiency is usually more severe in the infantile form than in the juvenile and adult disorders.

TREATMENT No effective treatment for the infantile form is currently available. Enzyme replacement is a promising therapy for this fatal lysosomal storage disease, and clinical trials are ongoing to test its safety and efficacy. A high-protein diet may be useful for the juvenile and adult forms. Nocturnal ventilatory support can improve the quality of life.

DISORDERS OF GALACTOSE METABOLISM

GALACTOSE 1-PHOSPHATE URIDYL TRANSFERASE DEFICIENCY GALACTOSEMIA "Classic" galactosemia is a serious disease with an early onset of symptoms; the incidence is 1 in 60,000. The newborn infant normally receives up to 20% of caloric intake as lactose, which consists of glucose and galactose. Without the transferase, the infant is unable to metabolize galactose 1-phosphate (Fig. 350-1), the accumulation of which results in injury to parenchymal cells of the kidney, liver, and brain.

GENETIC CONSIDERATIONS Galactosemia caused by transferase deficiency is inherited as an autosomal recessive trait; there are several enzymatic variants. The Duarte variant exhibits diminished red cell enzyme activity that is usually of no clinical significance. Some African-American patients have milder symptoms despite the absence of measurable transferase activity in erythrocytes; these patients retain 10% of the enzyme activity in liver and intestinal mucosa. Most Caucasian patients have no detectable enzyme activity in any of these tissues. The gene for galactose-1 phosphate uridyl transferase is located on chromosome 9p13. In African Americans, 48% of the mutant alleles are represented by the S135L substitution, perhaps accounting for the milder phenotype. In the Caucasian population, 70% of mutant alleles are represented by the Q188R substitution. Carrier testing and prenatal diagnosis can be carried out by direct enzyme analysis of amniocytes or chorionic villi. DNA-based testing can also be performed. ∎

Clinical and laboratory findings The clinical manifestations of uridyl transferase deficiency are myriad, necessitating a high index of suspicion if the diagnosis is to be made. Clinical features may include: jaundice, hepatomegaly, vomiting, hypoglycemia, convulsions, lethargy, irritability, feeding difficulties, poor weight gain, aminoaciduria, cataracts, vitreous hemorrhage, hepatic cirrhosis, ascites, splenomegaly, or mental retardation. Patients with galactosemia are at increased risk for *Escherichia coli* neonatal sepsis; the onset of sepsis often precedes the diagnosis of galactosemia. When the diagnosis is not made at birth, damage to the liver (cirrhosis) and brain (mental retardation) becomes increasingly severe and irreversible. For this reason, routine neonatal screening tests for galactosemia have been instituted in many parts of the world.

Diagnosis The preliminary diagnosis of galactosemia is made by demonstrating a reducing substance (by Clinitest) in urine specimens collected while the patient is receiving human or cow's milk or another formula containing lactose. The reducing substance found in urine, which is negative in a glucose oxidase test, can be identified as galactose with chromatography or an enzymatic test specific for galactose. Definitive diagnosis requires the demonstration of deficient activity of galactose-1-phosphate uridyl transferase in erythrocytes or other tissues, which also exhibit increased concentrations of galactose-1-phosphate.

TREATMENT Because of widespread newborn screening for galactosemia, patients are now being identified and treated early. Elimination of galactose from the diet reverses growth failure, renal, and hepatic dysfunction. Cataracts regress and most patients have no impairment of eyesight. Early diagnosis and treatment have improved the prognosis of galactosemia; on long-term follow-up, however, patients still have ovarian failure manifest as primary or secondary amenorrhea, as well as developmental delay and learning disabilities, which increase in severity with age. In addition, most patients have speech disorders and a smaller number demonstrate poor growth and impaired motor function and balance (with or without overt ataxia). The relative control of galactose-1-phosphate levels does not always correlate with long-term outcome, suggesting that other factors, such as uridine diphosphate (UDP)-galactose deficiency (a donor for galacto-lipids and proteins), may be responsible for some of the metabolic consequences of the disease.

GALACTOKINASE DEFICIENCY In contrast to the multiple systems that are affected in uridyl transferase deficiency, cataracts are usually the sole manifestation of galactokinase deficiency. The affected infant is otherwise asymptomatic. This disorder is characterized by elevated blood galactose levels with normal uridyl transferase activity and an absence of galactokinase activity in erythrocytes. Treatment is dietary restriction of galactose intake. Mutations leading to galactokinase deficiency have been identified in the gene coding for galactokinase (located on chromosome 17q24).

URIDINE DIPHOSPHATE GALACTOSE 4-EPIMERASE (UDP GAL 4-EPIMERASE) DEFICIENCY The abnormally accumulated metabolites in this disorder are very much like those seen in uridyl transferase deficiency; however, there is also an increase in cellular UDP galactose. There are two distinct forms of epimerase deficiency. A benign form was discovered incidentally as a result of the neonatal screening program. Affected persons in this case are healthy; the enzyme deficiency is limited to leukocytes and erythrocytes, without deranged metabolism in other tissues, and no treatment is required. The second form of epimerase deficiency is severe with clinical manifestations resembling uridyl transferase deficiency. Additional features include hypotonia and nerve deafness. The enzyme deficiency is generalized, and clinical symptoms respond to restriction of dietary galactose. Although this form of galactosemia is very rare, it must be considered in a symptomatic patient who has normal transferase activity. The gene for epimerase is located on chromosome 1p35-36; mutations responsible for both forms of the epimerase deficiency have been identified.

DISORDERS OF FRUCTOSE METABOLISM

DEFICIENCY OF FRUCTOKINASE (BENIGN FRUCTOSURIA) This condition is not associated with any clinical manifestations. It is an incidental finding, usually made through the detection of fructose as a reducing substance in the urine. No treatment is necessary.

DEFICIENCY OF FRUCTOSE 1,6-BISPHOSPHATE ALDOLASE (ALDOLASE B) (HEREDITARY FRUCTOSE INTOLERANCE) This is a severe disease of infants that appears with the ingestion of fructose-containing food. It is caused by deficiency of fructose 1,6-bisphosphate aldolase B activity in the liver, kidney, and intestine. The enzyme catalyzes the hydrolysis of fructose 1-phosphate and fructose 1,6-bisphosphate into the 3-carbon sugars, dihydroxyacetone phosphate, glyceraldehyde-3-phosphate, and glyceraldehyde (Fig. 350-1). Deficiency of this enzyme activity causes rapid accumulation of fructose 1-phosphate and initiates severe toxic symptoms when exposed to fructose.

GENETIC CONSIDERATIONS The true incidence of hereditary fructose intolerance is not known but may be as high as 1 in 23,000. The gene for aldolase B is on chromosome 9q22.3. Several mutations causing heredity fructose intolerance have been identified. A single missense mutation, which results in substitution of proline for alanine at position 149, is the most common mutation identified in northern Europeans. This mutation plus two other point mutations account for approximately 80 to 85% of hereditary fructose intolerance in Europe and the United States. The diagnosis of hereditary fructose intolerance can thus be made in most cases by direct DNA analysis. Prenatal diagnosis should be possible from either amniocentesis or chorionic villi with the use of DNA for mutational or linkage analysis. ■

Clinical and laboratory findings Patients with fructose intolerance are healthy and asymptomatic until fructose or sucrose (table sugar) is ingested (usually from fruit, fruit juice, or sweetened cereal). Clinical manifestations may resemble those of galactosemia and include jaundice, hepatomegaly, vomiting, lethargy, irritability, and convulsions. Laboratory findings include prolonged clotting time, hypoalbuminemia, elevation of bilirubin and transaminases, and proximal renal tubular dysfunction. If the disease is not diagnosed and intake of the noxious sugar persists, hypoglycemic episodes recur, and liver and kidney failure progress, eventually leading to death.

Diagnosis Suspicion of the enzyme deficiency is suggested by the presence of a reducing substance in the urine during an attack. The diagnosis is supported by an intravenous fructose tolerance test, which will cause a rapid decline of serum phosphate, followed by blood glucose, and a subsequent rise of uric acid and magnesium. An oral tolerance test should not be performed as patients may become acutely ill. Definitive diagnosis is made by assay of fructaldoase B activity in the liver.

TREATMENT Treatment consists of the complete elimination of all sources of sucrose, fructose and sorbitol from the diet. With this treatment, liver and kidney dysfunction improve, and catch-up growth is common. Intellectual development is usually unimpaired. As the patient matures, symptoms become milder, even after fructose ingestion, and the long-term prognosis is good. Owing to dietary avoidance of sucrose, affected patients have few dental caries.

FRUCTOSE 1,6-DIPHOSPHATASE DEFICIENCY Fructose 1,6-diphosphatase deficiency is a defect in gluconeogenesis. The disease is characterized by life-threatening episodes of acidosis, hypoglycemia, hyperventilation, convulsions, and coma. These episodes are triggered by febrile infections and gastroenteritis when oral food intake decreases. Laboratory findings include low blood glucose, high lactate and uric acid levels, and a blood gas picture of metabolic acidosis. In contrast to hereditary fructose intolerance, there is usually no aversion to sweets, and renal tubular and liver functions are normal. Treatment of acute attacks consists of correction of hypoglycemia and acidosis by intravenous infusion; the response is usually rapid. Later, avoidance of fasting and elimination of fructose and sucrose from the diet prevent further episodes. For long-term prevention of hypoglycemia, a slowly released carbohydrate such as cornstarch is useful. Patients who survive childhood seem to develop normally.

Diagnosis The diagnosis is established by demonstrating enzyme deficiency in either the liver or an intestinal biopsy specimen. The enzyme defect may also be demonstrated in leukocytes in some cases. The gene coding for fructose 1,6-diphosphatase is located on chromosome 9q22. In patients with known mutations, carrier detection and prenatal diagnosis are possible by DNA-based testing.

BIBLIOGRAPHY

ALI M et al: Hereditary fructose intolerance. J Med Genet 35:353, 1998

CHEN Y-T: Glycogen storage diseases, in *The Metabolic and Molecular Bases of Inherited Disease*, 8th ed, CR Scriver et al (eds). New York, McGraw-Hill, 2001, pp 1521–1551

DIMAURO S, BRUNO C: Glycogen storage disease of muscle. Curr Opin Neurol 11:477, 1998

ELPELEG ON: The molecular background of glycogen metabolism disorders. J Ped Endocrinol Metab 12:363, 1999

FERNANDEZ J, CHEN Y-T: The glycogen storage diseases, in *Inborn Metabolic Disease: Diagnosis and Treatment*, J Fernandez et al (eds). Berlin, New York, Springer-Verlag, 1995, p 71–87

HIRSCHHORN R, REUSER AJ: Glycogen storage disease type II: Acid α-glucosidase (acid maltase) deficiency, in *The Metabolic and Molecular Bases of Inherited Disease*, 8th ed, CR Scriver et al (eds). New York, McGraw-Hill, 2001, pp 1389–1420

KIKUCHI T et al: Clinical and metabolic correction of Pompe disease by enzyme therapy in acid maltase deficient quail. J Clin Invest 101:827, 1998

SEGAL S, BERRY GT: Disorders of galactose metabolism, *The Metabolic and Molecular Bases of Inherited Disease*, 7th ed, CR Scriver et al (eds). New York, McGraw-Hill, 1995, pp 967–1000

SANTER R et al: Mutations in *GLUT2*, the gene for the liver-type glucose transporter, in patients with Fanconi-Bickel syndrome. Nat Genet 17:324, 1997

SHEN J-J et al: Mutations in exon 3 of the glycogen debranching enzyme gene are associated with glycogen storage disease type III that is differentially expressed in liver and muscle. J Clin Invest 98:352, 1996

VEIGA DA CUNHA M et al: A gene on chromosome 11q23 coding for a putative glucose 6-phosphate translocase is mutated in glycogen storage disease type Ib and type Ic. Am J Hum Genet 63:976, 1998

WALTER JH et al: Recommendations for the management of galactosemia. UK Galactosemia Steering Group. Arch Dis Child 80:93, 1999

351   *Darwin J. Prockop, Helena Kuivaniemi,
Gerard Tromp, Leena Ala-Kokko*

INHERITED DISORDERS OF CONNECTIVE TISSUE

Heritable disorders that involve the major connective tissues of the body such as bone, skin, cartilage, blood vessels, and basement membranes are among the most common genetic diseases in human beings. Here we will focus primarily on those disorders that can have severe manifestations, are relatively common, and are sufficiently understood at the molecular level to provide useful paradigms: osteogenesis imperfecta (OI), the Ehlers-Danlos syndrome (EDS), chondrodysplasias (CDs), the Marfan syndrome (MFS), epidermolysis bullosa (EB), and the Alport syndrome (AS).

THE CHALLENGE OF CLASSIFYING THE DISEASES

The original classification of connective tissue diseases was based on the pattern of inheritance, the cluster of signs and symptoms, the histologic changes in tissues, and limited information about the molecular defects involved. This classification included about a dozen types and subtypes for OI, about the same number for the EDS, and over 150 for the CDs. Several limitations in these original classifications are now apparent. One is that the same mutation does not always produce the same disease phenotype in terms of severity of the condition or its clinical course. Such phenotypic variation occurs in many genetic diseases, including the connective tissue disorders, in which some members of a family are severely affected, whereas others with the same mutation have a mild disorder.

Most patients with classic features of a severe connective tissue disease have a mutation in a gene or genes coding for a single protein.

For example, the majority of patients with OI have a mutation in one of the two genes coding for type I procollagen. Similarly, most patients with MFS have mutations in a gene for fibrillin. For other disease categories, the situation is more complex. In EDS, for example, the type IV variant is usually caused by mutations in the gene for type III procollagen, the type VI variant by defects in the gene for lysyl hydroxylase, and the type VII variant by defects that impair the processing of type I procollagen to type I collagen.

Classifications of these disorders also tend to overemphasize the etiologic differences between severe genetic diseases that are apparent in infants and the more common diseases that appear much later in life. Single-gene defects can cause subsets of late-onset diseases such as osteoporosis, aneurysms, and osteoarthritis. For example, a small subset of patients with postmenopausal osteoporosis have mutations in the genes for procollagen I similar to the mutations in the same genes that produce lethal variants of OI. Likewise, a subset of patients with familial aortic aneurysms have mutations in the gene for procollagen III similar to the mutations in the same gene that cause lethal variants of type IV EDS, and occasional patients with osteoarthritis have mutations in the gene for procollagen II similar to the mutations in the same gene that cause lethal CDs. There is disagreement as to the best diagnosis for such patients in that some investigators feel that after a mutation similar to those seen in the early-onset diseases is identified, the patients should be reclassified as having mild forms of OI, EDS, or CD, even though they do not have definitive evidence of the early-onset diseases or seek medical attention until adulthood. Therefore, the category of diseases referred to as *inherited disorders of connective tissue* may have to be expanded as we obtain additional information about more common diseases.

DEFINITION AND COMPOSITION OF CONNECTIVE TISSUES

Connective tissues are composed of specific macromolecules, many of which are also constituents of the lung, the kidney, the walls of blood vessels, the vitreous gel of the eye, and the synovial fluid. Indeed, most organs and tissues contain small amounts of the same macromolecules assembled into membranes and septa. Therefore, virtually all structures contain some connective tissue.

The distinguishing feature of connective tissues is that the component macromolecules are assembled into an insoluble extracellular matrix (Table 351-1). The macromolecules include at least 19 different types of collagens, the related fibrous proteins known as *elastin* and *fibrillin*, a series of proteoglycans, and components whose structure and function are only partially defined.

Differences in the connective tissues of bone, skin, and cartilage are in part explained by differences in the content of specific components (Table 351-1). For example, tendons and ligaments consist primarily of type I collagen fibrils and small amounts of other components that help organize the type I fibrils into fibers and fiber bundles. Cartilage consists primarily of fibrils of type II collagen in the form of arcades that are distended by highly charged proteoglycans. The extracellular matrix of the aorta contains collagens that provide tensile strength and elastin that provides elasticity. Differences among the connective tissues also depend on the three-dimensional organization of the molecular components. The type I collagen fibrils in tendon are packed into thick, parallel bundles of fibers, whereas type I collagen fibrils in skin are randomly oriented. In cortical bone, helical arrays of type I collagen fibrils are deposited around haversian canals.

Table 351-1   Constituents of Connective Tissues in Various Tissues

Connective Tissue	Major Constituents	Approximate Amounts, % dry wt	Characteristics or Functions
Dermis, ligaments, tendons	Type I collagen	80	Bundles of fibrils
	Type III collagen	5–15	Thin fibrils
	Type IV collagen, laminin, nidogen	<5	In basal laminae under epithelium and endothelium
	Types V, VI, and VII collagens	<5	VII forms anchoring fibrils; others unknown
	Elastin, fibrillin	<5	Provides elasticity
	Fibronectin	<5	Associated with collagen fibers and cell surfaces
	Proteoglycans,[a] hyaluronate	0.5	Provide resiliency
Bone (demineralized)	Type I collagen	90	Complex fibril network
	Type VI collagen	1–2	Function unclear
	Proteoglycans[a]	1	Function unclear
	Osteonectin, osteopontin, osteocalcin, α2-glycoprotein, sialoproteins	1–5	May regulate mineralization
Aorta	Type I collagen	20–40	Fibril network
	Type III collagen	20–40	Thin fibrils
	Elastin, fibrillin	20–40	Provide elasticity
	Type IV collagen, laminin, nidogen	<5	Form basal lamina
	Types V and VI collagens	<2	Functions unclear
	Proteoglycans[a]	<3	Provide resiliency
Cartilage	Type II collagen	40–50	Arcades of thin fibrils
	Type IX collagen	5–10	Links type II fibrils
	Type X collagen	5–10	Surrounds hypertrophic cells
	Type XI collagen	<10	Function unclear
	Proteoglycans,[a] hyaluronate	15–50	Provides resiliency

[a] As discussed in text, >30 proteoglycans have now been identified. They differ in the structures of their core proteins and their contents of glycosaminoglycans side chains of chondroitin-4-sulfate, chondroitin-6-sulfate, dermatan sulfate, and keratin sulfate. Basal lamina contain a proteoglycan with a side chain of heparan sulfate that resembles heparin.

BIOSYNTHESIS OF CONNECTIVE TISSUE

Connective tissues form primarily by a process of self-assembly, in which a molecule of the correct size, shape, and surface properties binds to other molecules with the same or similar structure in a spontaneous but ordered manner. The molecular mechanisms and driving forces are similar to those involved in crystal formation.

Collagen Synthesis The self-assembly of connective tissue is illustrated by the assembly of collagen into fibrils. The collagen molecule that forms fibrils is a long, thin rod consisting of three polypeptide α chains wrapped into a rigid, ropelike triple helix (Fig. 351-1). The molecule has a triple-helical conformation, because each of the three α chains has a simple, repetitive amino acid sequence of about 1000 amino acids in which glycine (Gly) appears as every third amino acid. Therefore, the sequence of each α chain can be designated as $(-Gly-X-Y-)_{333}$, where X and Y represent amino acids other than glycine. To fold into a triple helix, every third amino acid in an α chain must be glycine, the smallest amino acid, since this residue must fit in a sterically restricted space where the three chains of the triple helix come together. Many of the X- and Y-position amino acids are proline and hydroxyproline, which provide rigidity to the triple helix. The remaining amino acids form clusters of hydrophobic and charged regions on the surface of the molecule that direct how one molecule spontaneously binds to other collagen molecules and thereby self-assembles into the large collagen fibrils in tissues (see Fig. 351-1).

More than 19 different collagens have been identified. Most are minor constituents that probably have highly specialized functions. The fibrillar collagens are found in tissues as long, highly ordered fibrils with a characteristic banding pattern by electron microscopy. Type I collagen, the most abundant, is found as cross-striated fibrils in a large number of tissues (Table 351-1). It is composed of two identical α chains called $\alpha1(I)$ and a third called $\alpha2(I)$. Type II collagen, another fibrillar collagen of cartilage, is composed of three identical α chains called $\alpha1(II)$. Type III collagen is found in small amounts in many tissues that contain type I collagen and in large amounts in large blood vessels; it is composed of three identical chains called $\alpha1(III)$. The nonfibrillar collagens are similar to the fibrillar collagens in that they contain -Gly-X-Y- sequences of amino acids that form triple-helical domains, but they also contain large globular domains. Self-assembly of most of the nonfibrillar collagens usually involves binding between the globular domains to form networks. For example, the type IV collagen in basement membranes self-assembles into a complex three-dimensional network that provides a diffusion barrier in the renal glomerulus and pulmonary alveolus. The network also provides support for epithelial and endothelial cells in these tissues and in skin, the gastrointestinal tract, and blood vessels. Some nonfibrillar collagens bind to the surface of fibrils formed by the more abundant collagens and alter the lateral growth of the fibrillar collagens or prevent the fibrils from coalescing into fiber bundles.

Because the molecules or monomers fibrillar collagens spontaneously self-assemble into fibrils, they are first synthesized as larger and more soluble precursors called *procollagens* and composed of proα chains. As the proα chains of procollagen are synthesized on ribosomes, the free ends move into the cisternae of the rough endoplasmic reticulum (Fig. 351-1). Hydrophobic signal peptides at the N termini are cleaved, and additional posttranslational reactions begin. Proline residues in the Y position of the repeating -Gly-X-Y- sequences are

FIGURE 351-1 Schematic representation of synthesis of a type I collagen fibril by a fibroblast. *A.* Intracellular steps in the assembly of the procollagen molecule. Hydroxylations and glycosylations of the proα chains begin soon after the amino termini pass into the cisternae of the rough endoplasmic reticulum and continue after the three chains associate through their carboxy-terminal propeptides and become disulfide linked. *B.* Cleavage of procollagen to collagen, self-assembly of the collagen molecule into quarter-staggered fibrils, and cross-linking of the molecules in the fibrils. Cleavage of the propeptides may occur within crypts of the fibroblast, as shown here, or some distance from the cell. Mutations (depicted by X) cause the synthesis of structurally abnormal pro$\alpha1(I)$ or pro$\alpha2(I)$ chains of type I procollagen by interfering either with protein assembly (procollagen suicide) (*A*) or with processing to normal collagen fibrils (*B*). (*From DJ Prockop et al, Am J Med Genet 34:60, 1989, with permission.*)

converted to hydroxyproline by prolyl hydroxylase in a reaction requiring ascorbic acid. Lysine residues in the Y position are similarly hydroxylated to hydroxylysine by lysyl hydroxylase. Many of the hydroxylysine residues are glycosylated with galactose or with galactose and glucose. A large mannose-rich oligosaccharide is assembled on the C-terminal propeptide of each chain. The association of the proα chains is directed by the structure and the surface properties of the globular C-propeptides. After the C-propeptides assemble correctly, the structure is locked in place by the formation of interchain disulfide bonds. Posttranslational modifications of the proα chains continue until each chain acquires about 100 hydroxyproline residues. Then a few of the hydroxyproline-rich -Gly-X-Y- sequences at the C terminus of the protein fold into a triple helix. The short region of triple helix becomes a nucleus for self-assembly of the triple helix of the whole protein, much like a nucleus for crystallization, in that the triple-helical conformation in one -Gly-X-Y- sequence induces the next -Gly-X-Y- sequence to fold into the same conformation. As a result, the conformation is propagated in a zipper-like fashion from the C terminus to the N terminus of the molecule, and the entire α-chain domain becomes a continuous triple helix. The protein then passes from the rough endoplasmic reticulum to other compartments and is secreted. The requirement for ascorbic acid in the hydroxylation of prolyl residues explains why wounds fail to heal in scurvy (Chap. 75). If sufficient proline residues are not converted to hydroxyproline, collagen cannot fold into a triple helix that is stable at body temperature. The abnormal protein accumulates in the cisternae of the rough endoplasmic reticulum and is slowly degraded.

After secretion, procollagen is processed to collagen by cleavage of the N-propeptides by procollagen N-proteinase and of the C-propeptides by procollagen C-proteinase. The processing of type I procollagen by the two proteinases converts the precursor to type I collagen and thereby decreases the solubility of the protein about 1000-fold. The 1000-fold decrease in solubility provides the entropic energy that drives the spontaneous self-assembly of the collagen into fibrils. Collagen monomers first assemble into a nucleus that grows by addition of monomers as determined by the structure of the nucleus. The nucleus and the final fibril can be assembled spontaneously from a single kind of collagen such as type I or type II. Fibrils can also be assembled as copolymers in which two or more collagens are incorporated into the same fibril simultaneously. Alternatively, a second collagen or a proteoglycan can bind to the surface of a growing fibril or to a fully formed fibril and thereby influence the final structure and the functional properties of the fibrils. The final structure of the fibrils in tissues is also influenced by the pressure and tensions on the fibrils, particularly after their tips are inserted into muscle and bone. The tension on tendons, for example, probably makes the initial thin fibrils coalesce into large fiber bundles.

Self-assembled collagen fibers have considerable tensile strength, which is increased by cross-linking reactions that form covalent bonds between α chains in one molecule and α chains in adjacent molecules. The first step in cross-linking is oxidation by lysyl oxidase of amino groups on a few lysine or hydroxylysine residues to form aldehydes that interact to form stable covalent bonds.

During growth and development, the collagen fibrils in all tissues undergo repeated synthesis, degradation, and resynthesis. The degradation of collagen fibers in tissues is initiated by specific collagenases found in leukocytes, fibroblasts, synovial cells, or related cell types. The collagenases cleave the collagen molecule at a point about three-quarters of the distance from its N terminus. The cleavage apparently triggers unfolding of the molecules on the surface of a fibril and further degradation by other proteinases.

Collagen fibers in most tissues of normal adults undergo very little metabolic turnover. One exception to this is the collagen fibrils that are degraded and resynthesized as part of the continual remodeling of bone. Although the collagen in many adult tissues is metabolically stable, the rate of turnover changes under some circumstances. In starvation, a large fraction of the collagen in skin and other connective tissues is degraded, thus providing amino acids for gluconeogenesis. Large losses of collagen also occur in most connective tissues during immobilization or prolonged periods of low-gravitational stress. In rheumatoid arthritis, pannus invasion causes a rapid degradation of collagen in the articular cartilage. Glucocorticoids decrease the collagen content of most connective tissues, including bone, by decreasing the rate of collagen synthesis. Decreases in collagen weaken tissues. In many pathologic states, however, collagen is deposited in excess. With injury to tissue, inflammation is usually followed by increased deposition primarily of type I collagen fibrils in the form of fibrotic tissue and scars. The deposition of collagen fibrils during the repair process is largely irreversible and is a major feature of the pathologic changes in hepatic cirrhosis, pulmonary fibrosis, atherosclerosis, and nephrosclerosis and in the scarring in skin and ligaments after surgery or trauma.

Elastin Synthesis Elastin assembly appears to be closely related to that of collagen, since a few of the prolines in the protein are hydroxylated to hydroxyproline by prolyl hydroxylase. The elastin monomer, however, is a single polypeptide that does not fold into a defined three-dimensional structure and is not synthesized as a larger precursor molecule. Instead, it is slowly secreted from cells into extracellular compartments, where it forms amorphous deposits around previously deposited microfibrils. The elastin deposits then become covalently cross-linked through oxidation of lysine residues to aldehydes by the same lysyl oxidase that initiates the cross-linking of collagen. The microfibrils in elastin deposits are largely composed of fibrillin, a large protein that forms beadlike strands.

Proteoglycan Synthesis The synthesis of proteoglycans begins in the cisternae of the rough endoplasmic reticulum with assembly of a core protein that then undergoes modification by sugar and sulfate transferases that generate large side chains of glycosaminoglycans. At least 30 proteoglycans have been identified by differences in the structures of their core proteins. The major proteoglycan of cartilage, called *aggrecan*, has a core protein of about 2000 amino acids to which are bound multiple side chains of chondroitin sulfate and keratin sulfate, polysaccharides consisting of highly charged and repetitive disaccharide sequences. After secretion from cells, the aggrecan monomer binds to a smaller protein called a *link protein*. The complex of core protein and link protein then spontaneously binds to a long chain of hyaluronic acid to form a huge copolymer called a *proteoglycan aggregate*. The highly charged proteoglycan aggregate binds water and small ions and thereby provides a large swelling pressure and resiliency to cartilage. Smaller proteoglycans such as decorin, biglycan, and fibromodulin have smaller core proteins with fewer and different polysaccharide side chains. They do not form large aggregates with hyaluronate but bind to fibrils of collagen or fibronectin and may thereby help regulate the assembly or spatial orientation of fibrils. One group of small proteoglycans known as *syndecans* binds to the plasma membranes of cells and may have a role in cell migration along fibrils or in signal transduction.

The assembly of bone follows much the same principles as the assembly of other connective tissues (Chap. 340). The first step is deposition of osteoid tissue that consists largely of type I collagen fibrils. Mineralization of osteoid occurs by steps that are still incompletely defined; proteins such as osteopontin and osteocalcin probably bind to the collagen fibrils and chelate calcium to initiate mineralization. Small proteoglycans such as decorin or fibromodulin may also play a role.

MUTATIONS THAT PRODUCE DISEASES OF CONNECTIVE TISSUES Because of the large number of tissue-specific macromolecules present in connective tissues, a large number of gene-protein systems are candidates for mutations that might cause disease of the tissues.

The most complete data on mutations causing heritable disorders of connective tissue are available on OI. Most patients with severe OI (types II and III) have mutations in either the gene for the proα1(I) chain or the gene for the proα2(I) chain of type I procollagen (the COL1A1 and COL1A2 genes). In patients with mild disease, many of the mutations decrease expression of protein from one allele of the genes. Most of the mutations in patients with severe OI cause synthesis of a structurally abnormal but partially functional proα chain. Mutations that cause synthesis of structurally abnormal proα chains include partial gene deletions, partial gene duplications, and RNA splicing mutations. The most common mutations, however, cause the substitution of single amino acids with bulky side chains for the glycine residues that appear as every third amino acid in the triple helix of a proα chain (Fig. 351-2). The structurally abnormal proα chains exert their effects primarily through one of three mechanisms (Fig. 351-1). First, the presence of an abnormal proα chain in a procollagen molecule containing two normal proα chains can prevent folding of the protein into a triple-helical conformation and lead to degradation of the whole molecule in a process called *procollagen suicide*. Similar dominant negative mutations are seen with other multisubunit proteins. The net result of procollagen suicide is accumulation of the unfolded protein in the rough endoplasmic reticulum of cells and a reduction in the amount of collagen available for fibril assembly. Second, the presence of one abnormal proα chain in a procollagen molecule can interfere with cleavage of the N-propeptide from the protein. The persistence of the N-propeptide on a fraction of the molecules interferes with the self-assembly of normal collagen so that thin and irregular collagen fibrils are formed. Third, the substitution of a bulkier amino acid for glycine can produce a change in the conformation of the molecule and result in the assembly of collagen fibrils that are abnormally branched or abnormally thick and short. Also, copolymerization of the mutated collagen with normal collagen can slow fibril assembly and decrease the total amount of collagen incorporated into fibrils.

Over 300 mutations in the two genes for type I procollagen have been found in patients with OI (Fig. 351-2). Initially, there was concern that many of the mutations might be neutral variations in the structure of the genes and not the cause of the disease phenotypes. However, the causal relationship between most of the mutations and the disease has been established by several kinds of evidence: (1) DNA linkage studies in families with mild variants of OI showed that specific mutated alleles were coinherited with the disease phenotypes. (2) Probands with lethal variants of OI were shown to have new mutations not found in the normal parents or in only a few cells from a mosaic parent (see below). (3) Studies with cultured skin fibroblasts from patients demonstrated that the mutations either produced specific disruptions in the biosynthesis of type I procollagen or caused synthesis of a type I procollagen that formed abnormal collagen fibrils (Fig. 351-1). (4) The mutations in probands with OI were not found in normal alleles for the genes. (5) Expression of several of the mutated genes for type I procollagen in transgenic mice generated disease phenotypes similar to those seen in patients who inherited the mutated genes (Fig. 351-3).

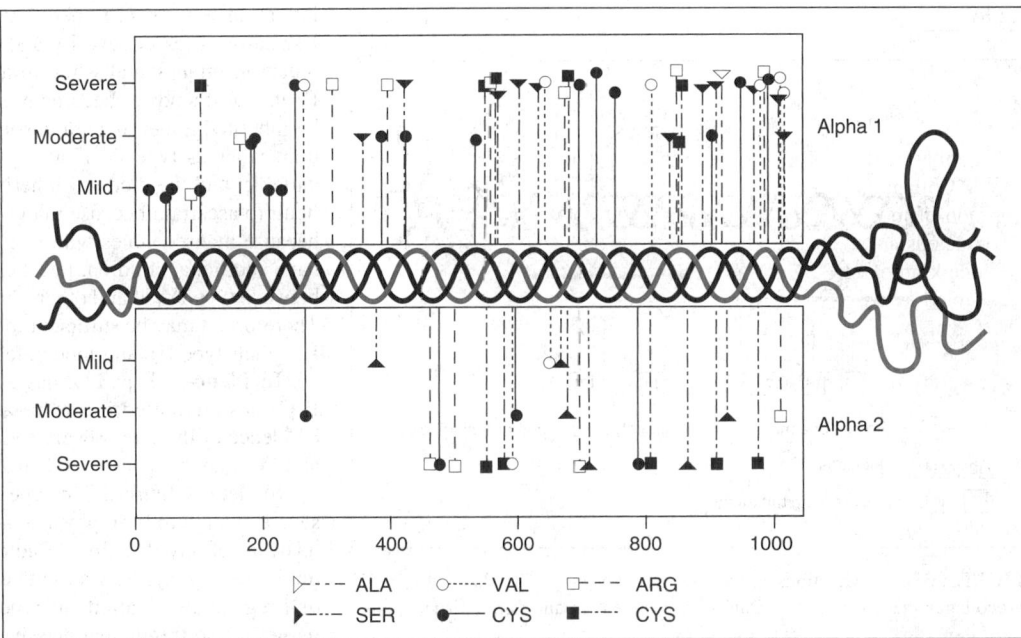

FIGURE 351-2 Examples of single-base mutations found in type I procollagen in patients with osteogenesis imperfecta (OI) and osteoporosis. Mild refers to type I OI, severe to type II OI, and moderate to type III or type IV OI.

The data on mutations in type I procollagen that cause OI have been used as a paradigm for defining other mutations in other collagen and procollagen genes that cause other disorders of connective tissue. For example, similar mutations in the gene for type III procollagen occur in patients with the type IV variant of EDS, which causes early death because of rupture of the aorta or other hollow organs (Fig. 351-4). Also, similar mutations in the gene for type II procollagen (COL2A1) are found in a number of patients with CDs (Fig. 351-5). In addition, transgenic mice expressing mutated genes for type II procollagen develop phenotypes resembling the CDs. Similar mutations in the gene for type VII collagen (COL7A1) are found in patients with the dystrophic form of EB, and mutations in the genes for type IV collagen are found in many patients with AS. As discussed below, the paradigm for defining the consequences of mutations in procollagen genes also helps explain findings on mutations in a fibrillin gene that cause MFS and mutations in keratin genes that cause the simplex variant of EB.

Several generalizations can be made about mutations in collagen genes. One is that unrelated patients rarely have the same mutation in the same gene. Another is that mutations that cause the most severe disease are usually new mutations in one allele that occur either during the generation of the germline in one of the parents or during meiosis in the fertilized egg (Chap. 65). Still another generalization is that most mild variants are caused by mutations that are specific or "private" to a given family. Indeed, the number of recurrent mutations in structural genes are so infrequent that there are, in effect, no common mutations responsible for the disorders in unrelated patients and no "hot spots" that contain most of the mutations.

Another general trend is that similar mutations in the same gene can produce different disease syndromes in terms of both severity and the major tissues involved. One reason for heterogeneity in pathologic manifestations is that different regions of a large molecule may be more important for its function in some connective tissues than in others. For example, some regions of the type I collagen molecule may be essential for the binding of mineralizing proteins in bone so that mutations in these regions cause fragile bones but do not impair func-

tion in skin and other nonmineralizing tissues. It is more difficult, however, to explain how the same mutation can produce a severe phenotype in some and a mild phenotype in other members of the same family. Such phenotypic variation appears to be characteristic of OI, where some subjects are short and have multiple fractures from minor trauma, whereas others in the same family can be of normal stature and free of fractures. In the past, such phenotypic variation was explained by undefined variations in the genetic background of different family members. Studies in transgenic mice, however, demonstrated similar phenotypic variation with expression of a mutated collagen gene in an inbred strain of mice in whom the genetic background is uniform. Therefore, the phenotypic variation is probably caused by undefined stochastic or chance events during embryonic and fetal development. Although dramatic phenotypic variations are relatively rare in OI and related disorders, it is important to consider in counseling families about the consequences of inherited mutations.

OSTEOGENESIS IMPERFECTA OI is an inherited disorder that causes a generalized decrease in bone mass (osteopenia) and makes the bones brittle. The disorder is frequently associated with blue sclerae, dental abnormalities (dentinogenesis imperfecta), progressive hearing loss, and a positive family history. The most severe forms cause death in utero, at birth, or shortly thereafter. The course of mild and moderate forms is more variable. Some patients appear normal at

FIGURE 351-3 Similarities of the phenotypes in transgenic mice with mutated type I procollagen and in a child with osteogenesis imperfecta. Note in both pictures the waviness of the ribs due to fractures in utero.

FIGURE 351-4 Mutations in the gene for the proα1(III) chain of type III procollagen that cause Ehlers-Danlos syndrome type and familial aneurysms.

birth and become progressively worse. Some have multiple fractures in infancy and childhood, improve after puberty, and fracture more frequently later in life. Women are particularly prone to fracture during pregnancy and after menopause. A few women from families with mild variants of OI do not develop fractures until after menopause, and their disease may be difficult to distinguish from postmenopausal osteoporosis.

Classification　The most common classification for OI was developed by Sillence (Table 351-2). Type I, the mildest form, is inherited as an autosomal dominant trait. Most patients have distinctly blue sclerae. Type I is subdivided into types IA and IB depending on whether or not dentinogenesis imperfecta is present. Type II is lethal in utero or shortly after birth. Radiographic criteria can be used to subdivide type II into five groups, with subgroup 1 showing the most severe changes and subgroup 5 the least. Types III and IV OI are

FIGURE 351-5　Mutations in the gene for the proα1(II) chain of type II procollagen that cause chondrodysplasia and related disorders.

intermediate in severity between types I and II. They differ from type I because of lesser severity and because the sclerae are only slightly bluish in infancy and white in adulthood. Type III differs from type IV in that it tends to become more severe with age. Also, type III can be inherited either as an autosomal recessive or autosomal dominant trait, whereas type IV is always dominant. The clinical courses are variable, and the mode of inheritance in types III and IV may be difficult to ascertain because many patients have sporadic mutations and because many couples with one child severely affected by OI do not have additional children. For these and related reasons, the distinction between type IV OI and other severe variants of OI may not be helpful. Therefore, it may be sufficient to classify patients simply as mild (type I), lethal (type II), and moderately severe (type III).

Incidence　Type I OI has a frequency of about 1 in 30,000. Type II OI has a reported incidence at birth of about 1 in 60,000, but the incidence of the three severe forms recognizable at birth (types II, III, and IV) may be as high as 1 in 20,000.

Skeletal Changes　In type I OI, the fragility of bones may be severe enough to limit physical activity or so mild that individuals are unaware of any disability. Radiographs of the skull of patients with mild disease may show a mottled appearance because of small islands of irregular ossification. In type II OI, bones and other connective tissues are so fragile that massive injuries can occur in utero or during delivery (Fig. 351-3). Ossification of many bones is frequently incomplete. Continuously beaded or broken ribs and crumpled long bones (accordina femora) may be present. For unclear reasons, the long bones may be either thick or thin. In types III and IV, multiple fractures from minor physical stress can produce severe deformities. Kyphoscoliosis can impair respiration, cause cor pulmonale, and predispose to pulmonary infections. The appearance on radiographs of "popcorn-like" deposits of mineral on the ends of long bones is an ominous sign. Progressive neurologic symptoms may result from basilar compression and communicating hydrocephalus.

In all forms of OI, bone mineral density in unfractured bone is decreased. However, the degree of osteopenia may be difficult to evaluate because recurrent fractures limit exercise and thereby worsen the decrease in bone mass. Surprisingly, fractures appear to heal normally.

Ocular Changes　The sclerae can be normal, slightly bluish, or bright blue. The color is probably caused by a thinness of the collagen layers of the sclerae that allows the choroid layers to be seen. Blue sclerae, however, are an inherited trait in some families who do not have increased bone fragility.

Dentinogenesis Imperfecta　The teeth may be normal, moderately discolored, or grossly abnormal. The enamel generally appears normal, but the teeth may have a characteristic amber, yellowish brown, or translucent bluish gray color because of improper deposition or deficiency of dentin. The deciduous teeth are usually smaller than normal, whereas permanent teeth are frequently bell-shaped and restricted at the base. In some patients, the teeth readily fracture and need to be extracted. The defect in dentin is directly attributable to the fact that normal dentin is rich in type I collagen. Similar tooth defects, however, can be inherited without any evidence of OI.

Hearing Loss　Hearing loss usually begins during the second decade of life and occurs in over 50% of subjects over age 30. The loss can be conductive, sensorineural, or mixed and varies in severity. The middle ear usually exhibits maldevelopment, deficient ossification, persistence of cartilage in areas that are normally ossified, and abnormal calcium deposits.

Associated Features　Other connective tissue involvement can include thin skin that scars extensively, joint laxity with permanent dislocations indistinguishable from those of EDS, and, occasionally, cardiovascular manifestations such as aortic regurgitation, floppy mitral valves, mitral incompetence, and fragility of large blood vessels. For unknown reasons, some patients develop a hypermetabolic state with elevated serum thyroxine levels, hyperthermia, and excessive sweating.

Molecular Defects　Most patients with OI have mutations in one of the two genes that encode type I procollagen. Over 90% of patients with type I OI and blue sclerae have mutations in the proα1(I) gene that decrease the steady-state levels of the mRNA for proα1(I) chains and decrease the rates of synthesis of proα1(I) chains relative to those for proα2(I) chains. In more severe forms (types II, III, and IV), the effects of mutations that cause synthesis of abnormal proα chains are amplified by the three mechanisms discussed above (Fig. 351-1). Mutations that change the structure of the protein near the N-proteinase cleavage site cause accumulation of a partially processed procollagen and produce lax joints similar to those in type VII EDS that is caused by mutations in the gene for the N-proteinase. Mutations that change the structure in the middle or near the C terminus of the molecule tend to cause severe or lethal variants of OI. It is difficult, however, to correlate the site or nature of the mutation and the clinical phenotype (Fig. 351-2). Most patients are heterozygotes with mutations in a single allele, but rare patients are homozygotes with two mutated alleles for proα1(I) or proα2(I) chains.

Mosaicism in Germ-Line Cells and in Somatic Cells Most lethal OI is the result of new autosomal dominant mutations. The frequency of a second child with lethal OI in the same family, however, is about 7% because of germ-line mosaicism in one of the parents. The presence of germ-line mosaicism has been demonstrated in several fathers of patients with type II OI by demonstrating the mutated gene in a fraction of their sperm. Apparently normal parents of children with severe OI may also have somatic cell mosaicism in which the mutated allele is present in a fraction of somatic cells such as fibroblasts, leukocytes, and hair root cells. Because of the possibility of germ-line mosaicism, asymptomatic parents of a child with severe OI should be counseled that recurrence can occur.

Diagnosis The diagnosis is usually made on the basis of clinical criteria. The presence of fractures together with blue sclerae, dentinogenesis imperfecta, or family history of the disease is usually sufficient to make the diagnosis. Other causes of pathologic fractures must be excluded, including the battered child syndrome, nutritional deficiencies, malignancies, and other inherited disorders such as CDs and hypophosphatasia (Table 351-3). X-rays usually reveal a decrease in bone density that can be verified by photon or x-ray absorptiometry. There is no consensus, however, as to whether the diagnosis can be made by microscopy of bone. A molecular defect in type I procollagen can be demonstrated in half or more of patients by incubating skin fibroblasts with radioactive amino acids and then analyzing the proα chains by polyacrylamide gel electrophoresis. The analysis detects decreases in the rate of synthesis of proα1(I) chains relative to proα2(I) chains, abnormally long proα chains, abnormally short proα chains, and proα chains with abnormal posttranslational modification because of an amino acid substitution that impairs folding of the triple helix. The mutations themselves can be defined in most patients by sequencing of genomic DNA. Because each proband and family usually has a "private" mutation, extensive analysis of about 10,000 bases in each of the two genes is required to identify the exact mutation. After a mutation in a type I procollagen gene is identified, a test based on the polymerase chain reaction can be used to screen family members at risk and for prenatal diagnosis.

℞ **TREATMENT** Many patients with OI have successful careers despite severe deformities. Those with mild disorder may need little treatment when fractures decrease after puberty, but women require special attention during pregnancy and after menopause, when fractures again increase. More severely affected children require a comprehensive program of physical therapy, surgical management of fractures and skeletal deformities, and vocational education.

Many of the fractures are only slightly displaced and have little soft tissue swelling. Therefore, they can be treated with minimal support or traction for a week or two followed by a light cast. If fractures are relatively painless, physical therapy can be initiated early. A judicious amount of exercise prevents loss of bone mass secondary to physical inactivity. Some physicians advocate insertion of steel rods into long bones to correct limb deformities; the risk/benefits and cost/benefits of such procedures are difficult to evaluate. Aggressive conventional intervention is usually warranted for pneumonia and cor pulmonale. For severe hearing loss, stapedectomy or replacement of the stapes with a prosthesis may be successful. Moderately to severely affected patients should be evaluated periodically to anticipate possible neurologic problems. About half of children have a substantial increase in growth when given growth hormone. Treatment with bisphosphonates to decrease bone loss has been introduced on an experimental basis. Initial results are promising, but the long-term effects of decreasing bone resorption are unknown. Also, a clinical trial has been initiated to use stromal cells from bone marrow that can differentiate into osteoblasts after systemic infusion. In the first phase of the trial, three children with severe OI (type III) showed clinical improvement after marrow ablation and transplantation of whole bone marrow from an HLA-compatible sibling.

A program for careful orthotic management developed by Bleck and a program for compressive management developed by Marini are useful. Counseling and emotional support are important for patients and parents, and lay organizations in some countries provide help in these areas. Prenatal ultrasonography will detect severely affected fetuses at about 16 weeks of pregnancy. Diagnosis by demonstrating synthesis of abnormal proα chains or by DNA sequencing can be carried out in chorionic villa biopsies at 8 to 12 weeks of pregnancy.

EHLERS-DANLOS SYNDROME EDS is characterized by hyperelasticity of the skin and hypermobile joints.

Classification Five types of EDS were initially defined based primarily on the extent to which the skin, joints, and other tissues are

Table 351-2 Classification of Osteogenesis Imperfecta (OI)

Type	Bone Fragility	Blue Sclerae	Abnormal Dentition	Hearing Loss	Inheritance[a]
I	Mild	Present	Absent in IA, present in IB	Present in most	AD
II	Extreme	Present	Present in some	Unknown	S, rarely AR
III	Severe	Bluish at birth	Present in some	High incidence	AR or AD
IV	Variable	Absent	Absent in IVA, present in IVB	High incidence	AD

[a] AD, autosomal dominant; AR, autosomal recessive; S, sporadic.

Table 351-3 Differential Diagnosis of Osteogenesis Imperfecta

Age	Diagnosis	Distinguishing Features
At birth	Hypophosphatasia	Unmineralized skull
	Achondrogenesis	Unmineralized vertebrae
	Thanatophoric dwarfism	H-shaped vertebrae
	Asphyxiating thoracic dystrophy	Cylindrical thorax
	Achondroplasia	Large head, short, tubular bones
Infancy	Battered child syndrome	Skull and rib fractures more common; soft tissue bruises
	Immobilization osteogenesis	
	Scurvy	
	Congenital syphilis	
	Infantile cortical hyperostosis (Coffey's disease)	
	Pyknodystosis	
	Osteopetrosis	
Childhood	Homocystinuria	Marfanoid appearance and mental deficiency
	Celiac disease	Steatorrhea, anemia
	Adrenal cortical tumor	
	Glucocorticoid therapy	
	Juvenile osteoporosis	
	Fibrous dysplasia	
	Sarcoma	

SOURCE: After R Smith et al: *The Brittle Bone Syndrome: Osteogenesis Imperfecta.* London, Butterworth, 1983.

Table 351-4 Clinical Features, Mode of Inheritance, and Biochemical Defects in Ehlers-Danlos Syndrome

Type	Clinical Features	Inheritance[a]	Biochemical Defects
I, gravis	Soft, velvety, hyperextensible skin; easy bruising; "cigarette paper" scars; hypermobile joints; varicose veins; prematurity	AD	Some in $\alpha1(V)$ and $\alpha2(V)$ chains of type V collagen
II, mitis	Similar to type I but less severe	AD	Some in $\alpha1(V)$ chain of type V collagen
III, familial hypermobility	Soft skin, no scarring, marked hypermobility	AD	Not known
IV, acrogeric, ecchymotic, vascular	Thin, translucent skin with visible veins; increased bruisability, skin and joints have normal extensibility; arterial, bowel, and uterine rupture	AD	Mutations in type III procollagen (see Fig. 351-4)
V, X-linked	Similar to type II	XLR	Not known
VI, ocular-scoliotic	Soft, velvety, hyperextensible skin; hypermobile joints; scoliosis; ocular fragility and keratoconus	AR	Lysyl hydroxylase deficiency
VII, arthrochalasis multiplex congenita	Marked joint hypermobility, soft skin with normal scarring	AD	A. Structural defect in the pro$\alpha1$(I) chain
		AD	B. Structural defect in the pro$\alpha2$(I) chain
		AR	C. Procollagen N-proteinase deficiency
VIII, periodontal	Generalized periodontitis, skin similar to type II but fragile and scars	AD	Not known
IX, cutis laxa occipital horn syndrome	Vacant, now recategorized as a disorder of copper transport		
X	Similar to type II	AR	Possible defect in fibronectin
XI, familial joint instability	Vacant, now recategorized with familial articular hypermobility syndromes		Not known

[a] AD, autosomal dominant; AR, autosomal recessive; XLR, X-linked recessive.
SOURCE: Adapted from Steinmann et al; A De Paepe et al: Am J Hum Genet 60, 547, 1997; and K. Michalickova et al: Hum Mol Genet 7:249, 1998.

involved, but the classification has now been extended (Table 351-4). Type I is the classic, severe form of the disease, with both severe joint hypermobility and skin that is velvety in texture, hyperextensible, and easily scarred. Type II is similar to type I but milder. In type III joint hypermobility is more prominent than skin changes. In type IV the skin changes are more prominent than joint changes. However, type IV patients are predisposed to sudden death from rupture of large blood vessels or other hollow organs. Type V is similar to type II but is inherited as an X-linked trait. Type VI is characterized by scoliosis, ocular fragility, and a cone-shaped deformity of the cornea (keratoconus). Type VII is characterized by marked joint hypermobility that is difficult to distinguish from type III except by the specific molecular defects in the processing of type I procollagen to collagen. Type VIII is distinguished by periodontal changes. Types IX, X, and XI were defined on the basis of preliminary biochemical and clinical data, but these classifications have not proven useful. Because of overlapping signs and symptoms, many patients and families with some of the features of EDS cannot be assigned to any of the defined types.

Incidence The incidence of EDS is difficult to establish, largely because patients with mild skin or joint symptoms rarely seek medical attention. It is also difficult to define the normal range of variation for joint mobility or skin elasticity. The incidence may be about 1 in 5000 births, although a higher value has been reported for blacks. Types I, II, and III account for most diagnoses.

Skin The changes vary from thin and velvety skin to skin that is either dramatically hyperextensible ("rubber man" syndrome) or easily torn or scarred. Type I patients develop characteristic "cigarette-paper" scars. In type IV extensive scars and hyperpigmentation develop over bony prominences, and the skin may be so thin that sub-cutaneous blood vessels are visible. In type VIII the skin is more fragile than hyperextensible, and it heals with atrophic, pigmented scars. Easy bruisability occurs in several types of EDS.

Ligament and Joint Changes Laxity and hypermobility of joints vary from mild to unreducible dislocations of hips and other large joints. In mild forms patients learn to reduce dislocations themselves and to avoid them by limiting physical activity. In more severe forms, surgical repair may be required. Some patients have progressive difficulty with age, but severe joint laxity is compatible with a normal life span.

Associated Changes Mitral valve prolapse and hernias occur, particularly in type I. Pes planus and mild to moderate scoliosis are common. Extreme joint laxity and repeated dislocations may lead to degenerative arthritis. In type VI the eye may rupture with minimal trauma, and kyphoscoliosis can cause respiratory impairment. Sclerae may be blue in type VI.

Molecular Defects Mutations in two of the three genes for type V collagen have been found in patients with types I and II EDS. The mutations include glycine substitutions in the triple-helical domain, RNA splicing mutations, exon skipping mutations, a small deletion of 7 bp, and a substitution of serine for cysteine in the C-propeptide. Mutations in both the $\alpha1(V)$ and $\alpha2(V)$ chain are found in patients with type I EDS, but to date only mutations in the $\alpha1(V)$ chain have been found in patients with type II EDS. Electron microscopy of skin from some patients with types I, II, or III EDS are consistent with mutations in a low-abundance collagen such as types III or V that either copolymerize with or bind to the surface of type I fibrils. However, irregular fibrils are not seen in all patients, and similar irregular fibrils can be seen in normal skin.

Most patients with type IV EDS have a defect either in the synthesis or structure of type III procollagen, a finding consistent with the fact that these patients are prone to spontaneous rupture of the aorta and intestines, tissues rich in type III collagen. The thinness and scarring of skin are more difficult to explain, since type III constitutes a small fraction of the collagen in skin (Table 351-1). The >50 mutations identified in the type III procollagen gene include partial gene deletions, RNA splicing mutations, and single-base mutations that cause substitution of glycine by amino acids with bulkier side chains (Fig. 351-4). In effect, most of the mutations lead to synthesis of abnormal but partially functional pro$\alpha1$(III) chains that produce procollagen suicide or alter fibril formation by the same mechanisms that amplify the effects of mutations in the genes for type I procollagen. Similar mutations in type III procollagen can cause aortic aneurysms in some individuals without other evidence of EDS type IV, MFS, or other inherited disorders of connective tissue.

Type VI EDS is caused by mutations in the gene that encodes lysyl hydrolase. In one series, all the patients were homozygous or compound heterozygotes for the mutated genes, and all the mutations caused profound deficiency of lysyl hydroxylase, a decrease in the hydroxylysine content of collagen, and a decrease in the cross-links in collagen fibers. The decrease in cross-links is explained by the observation that some cross-links are less stable if formed from lysine instead of hydroxylysine.

Type VII EDS is due to a defect in the conversion of procollagen to collagen caused either by mutations that make type I procollagen resistant to cleavage by procollagen N-proteinase or by mutations that decrease the activity of the enzyme. The type VIIA mutations alter the cleavage site in the proα1(I) chain, and the type VIIB mutations alter the cleavage site in the proα2(I) chain. Both types are dominantly inherited. Type VIIC is caused by mutations that decrease the activity of procollagen N-proteinase and is inherited as an autosomal recessive trait. In all three forms of type VII EDS, the persistence of the N-propeptide causes the formation of collagen fibrils that are thin and irregular. Since most patients do not have clinical osteopenia, the thin and irregular fibrils apparently suffice for the mineralization of bone but do not provide the necessary tensile strength for ligaments and joint capsules. However, some patients fracture easily and are difficult to distinguish from variants of OI.

The cause of type VIII EDS is unknown. Type IX is a disorder of copper transport. The syndrome, also referred to as *Menkes' syndrome*, is due to an X-linked defect and is associated with cutis laxa, hypopigmentation, unusual hair ("kinky"), vascular aneurysms, neurologic degeneration, and mental retardation. Mutations in a gene coding for a copper-transporting ATPase cause the disease (Chaps. 348 and 353). Type X EDS may be caused by defects in fibronectin, but no specific mutations have been defined.

Diagnosis The diagnosis is based on clinical criteria. Biochemical assays and gene analyses for known molecular defects in EDS are difficult and time-consuming, but specific diagnostic tests should be available in the future for families in which the genes at fault have been defined.

TREATMENT There is no specific therapy. Surgical repair and tightening of joint ligaments require careful evaluation of individual patients, as the ligaments frequently do not hold sutures. Patients with easy bruisability should be evaluated for other bleeding disorders. Patients with type IV EDS and members of their families should probably be evaluated at regular intervals by sonography and related techniques for early detection of aneurysms. Surgical repair of aneurysms may be difficult because of increased friability of tissues, and there is limited experience with elective surgery in such patients. Also, women with type IV EDS should be counseled about the increased risk of uterine rupture, bleeding, and other complications of pregnancy.

CHONDRODYSPLASIAS (See also Chap. 343) The CDs are inherited skeletal disorders that cause dwarfism and abnormal body proportions. The category also includes some individuals with normal stature and body proportions who have features such as ocular changes or cleft palate that are common in more severe CDs. Many patients develop degenerative joint changes, and mild CD in adults may be difficult to differentiate from primary generalized osteoarthritis. Some authors refer to the disorders as "skeletal dysplasias," but CD is a more widely used term.

Classification Over 150 distinct types and subtypes have been defined (Table 351-5) based on criteria such as "bringing death" (thanatophoric), causing "twisted" bones (diastrophic), affecting metaphyses (metaphyseal), affecting epiphyses (epiphyseal), and producing histologic changes such as an apparent increase in the fibrous material in the epiphyses (fibrochondrogenesis). Also, a number of eponyms

Table 351-5 Some Gene Mutations in Chondrodysplasias (CD)

Disease	Major Findings	Gene	Protein
SED congenita	Short-trunk dwarfism, hearing loss, cleft palate	COL2A1	Type II collagen
Achondrogenesis II/hypochondrogenesis	Short-limb dwarfism, large head, lethal	COL2A1	Type II collagen
Stickler syndrome			
Classic	Myopia, vitreoretinal degeneration, hearing loss, cleft palate, arthropathy	COL2A1/COL11A1	Type II or type XI collagen
Nonocular	Same as above, but no eye findings	COL11A2	Type XI collagen
Marshall syndrome	Similar to classic Stickler but less severe eye changes and more severe hearing loss	COL11A1	Type XI collagen
Kniest dysplasia	Short limbs and trunks, enlarged joints, myopia, hearing loss, cleft palate	COL2A1	Type II collagen
Metaphyseal CD, Schmidt type	Short limb dwarfism, flaring of metaphyses	COL10A1	Type X collagen
Pseudochondrodysplasia	Short stature, early OA	COMP	Cartilage oligomeric matrix protein
Multiple epiphyseal dysplasia	Short stature (variable), early OA	COMP COL9A2 COL9A3	Cartilage oligomeric matrix protein/type IX collagen
OA with mild CD	Early onset OA with mild epiphyseal changes	COL2A1	Type II collagen

NOTE: OA, osteoarthritis; SED, spondyloepiphyseal dysplasia: spondylo-, spinal changes including irregular endplates, flattened or wedge-shaped vertebrae; -epiphyseal, widening or irregularities of epiphyses; -metaphyseal, flared, cupped, irregularly mineralized or fragmented metaphyses.

are based on the first or most comprehensive case reports. Severe forms of the diseases produce gross distortions of most cartilaginous structures and of the eye. Mild forms are more difficult to classify. Among the features are cataracts, degeneration of the vitreous and retinal detachment, high forehead, hypoplastic facies, cleft palate, short extremities, and gross distortions of the epiphyses, metaphyses, and joint surfaces.

Incidence Data on the frequency of most CDs are not available, but the incidence of the Stickler syndrome may be as high as 1 in 10,000. Therefore, the diseases are probably among the more common heritable disorders of connective tissue.

Molecular Defects The first mutations shown to cause CDs were in the COL2A1 gene for type II collagen, the most abundant protein in cartilage. A number of mutations in this gene have now been reported in variants of CD ranging from mild to lethal (Fig. 351-5). A large fraction of patients with lethal CDs, a smaller number of patients with moderately severe CDs, and about 2% of families with early-onset generalized osteoarthritis have mutations in the same gene. However, similar phenotypes can also be caused by mutations in other genes, including genes for three other collagens, additional components of the cartilage matrix, growth factors, growth factor receptors, and transcription factors (see Table 351-6 for selected examples). The number of mutated genes reported does not necessarily reflect the incidence of such mutations in the diseases themselves but rather the complexity of the genes and the technical difficulties in searching the complete gene for mutations. Also, it reflects the availability of large families for DNA linkage analysis and the vigor with which investigators have pursued their interest in a given gene. It is likely that mutations in additional genes will be found.

Mutations in the COL2A1 gene were first found in patients with severe CDs characterized by gross deformities of bones and cartilage such as spondyloepiphyseal dysplasia congenita, hypochondrogenesis/achondrogenesis II, and the Kniest syndrome. However, mutations in the COL2A1 gene have been found in a few families in which few if any symptoms are present in childhood but in which joint stiffness, joint pain, and degenerative changes of osteoarthritis develop in midlife. The mutations in the COL2A1 gene are similar to the mutations in the genes for types I and III procollagens (Fig. 351-5), and the

Table 351-6 Examples of Genetic Mutations in Signaling Pathways and Developmental Genes

Category	Mutated Gene	Consequences	Clinical Phenotype
Transcription factor/extracellular signaling	Deficiency of GLI-3 transcription factor	Upregulation of sonic hedgehog pathway	Polysyndactyly and bifid phalanges with craniofacial defects (Greig syndrome)
	Truncation of GLI-3 transcription factor	Downregulation of sonic hedgehog pathway	Polydactyly, short limbs, imperforate anus, laryngeal cleft, and hypothalamic hamartoblastoma (Pallister-Hall syndrome)
Receptors	Missense in FGF-3 receptor	Increased FGF signaling	Short-trunk dwarfism (achondrodysplasia; hypochondrodysplasia; thanatrophoric dysplasia)
Developmental genes	HOXD-13	Inactivation of homeobox gene	Polysyndactyly
	PAX-3	Inactivation of paired-box gene	Hearing loss, abnormal pigmentation, craniofacial changes (Waardenburg syndrome)
Transcription factor	SOX-9	Slowed chondrocyte differentiation, decreased expression of type II collagen	Sex reversal, abnormal skeletal development (campomelic dysplasia)

correlations between genotype and the severity of the phenotype are equally difficult. In addition, mutations that change a codon for a Y-position amino acid in the -Gly-X-Y- repeat sequence from an arginine to cystine were found in families with early-onset osteoarthritis and minimal evidence of CDs. Stickler syndrome and related syndromes are caused by mutations in three different genes: the COL2AI gene for type II collagen and the COL11A1 and COL11A2 genes for type XI collagen. A series of mutations that introduce premature terminal signals in the COL2A1 gene lead to classic Stickler syndrome. However, some patients with classic Stickler syndrome have glycine substitutions in COL11A1. RNA splicing mutations in the COL11A1 gene are found in patients with the Marshall syndrome, which is similar to classic Stickler syndrome but with milder eye changes and more severe hearing loss. Patients classified as having nonocular Stickler syndrome have RNA splicing mutations in the COL11A2 gene.

Many individuals with the Schmid metaphyseal CD, characterized by short stature, *coxa vara*, flaring metaphyses, and waddling gait, have mutations in the gene for the type X collagen, a short, network-forming collagen found primarily in the hypertrophic zone of endochondral cartilage.

Mutations in the receptor for fibroblast growth factor 3 (FGFR-3) are present in most patients with achondroplasia, the most common cause of short-limbed dwarfism accompanied by macrocephaly and dysplasias of the metaphyses of long bones (Table 351-6). The same single-base mutation in the gene that converts glycine to arginine at position 380 is present in >90% of patients. Most patients represent sporadic new mutations, and this nucleotide change must be one of the most common recurring mutations in the human genome. The mutation causes unregulated signal transduction through the receptor and inappropriate development of cartilage. Mutations that alter other domains of FGFR-3 have been found in patients with the more severe disorders hypochondroplasia and thanatophoric dysplasia and in a few families with a variant of craniosynostosis. However, most patients with craniosynostosis appear to have mutations in the related gene FGFR-2 gene.

Mutations in the gene for the cartilage oligomeric matrix protein (COMP) have been found in patients with multiple epiphyseal dysplasia or pseudoachondroplasia, and in related syndromes characterized by short limbs and degenerative arthritis. However, some families with multiple epiphyseal dysplasia had a mutation in the gene for the α2(IX) or α3(IX) chain of type IX collagen (COL9A2 and COL9A3). All the known mutations in these two type IX collagen genes in patients with multiple epiphyseal dysplasia cause splicing out of the codons of exon 3. A mutation in the COL9A2 gene was also found in patients with the common condition of sciatica and herniations of vertebral discs. About 4% of Finnish probands with the phenotype had a single base substitution that converted a codon for glutamate to tryptophan in the α2(IX) chain of type IX collagen.

Diagnosis The diagnosis of severe forms of CD is made on the basis of the physical appearance, x-ray findings, histologic changes, and clinical course (Table 351-5).

℞ TREATMENT No definitive therapy is available. Symptomatic treatment is directed to secondary features such as degenerative arthritis. Many patients require joint replacement surgery and corrective surgery for cleft palate. The eyes should be monitored carefully for the development of cataracts and for the need for laser therapy to prevent retinal detachment. Patients should probably be advised to avoid obesity and contact sports. Counseling for the psychological problems of short stature is critical, and support groups have formed in many countries. Ultrasonography is sometimes successful for prenatal diagnosis but less frequently than with OI. Specific DNA tests are available for the CDs caused by mutations in the genes for types II, X, and XI collagens.

MARFAN SYNDROME Severe MFS is characterized by a triad of features: (1) long, thin extremities frequently associated with other skeletal changes, such as loose joints and arachnodactyly; (2) reduced vision as the result of dislocations of the lenses (ectopia lentis); and (3) aortic aneurysms that typically begin at the base of the aorta.

Classification The clinical diagnosis is frequently problematic because some affected members of families with MFS present with only one or two features of the typical clinical trial. Also, many patients present with one or two of the features of MFS without a family history, apparently because they represent sporadic mutations. Therefore, it is frequently difficult to determine on the basis of clinical data alone whether a patient with ectopia lentis or the characteristic body habitus of MFS is at risk for developing a life-threatening aortic aneurysm. The new DNA diagnostic tests for mutations in the fibrillin-1 and fibrillin-2 genes can probably resolve most, but not all, of these problems. Most patients who are prone to develop an aortic aneurysm as a component of MFS can be identified by detection of mutations in the fibrillin-1 gene. Some of these patients develop aortic aneurysms because of a mutation in the fibrillin-1 gene without the skeletal or ocular changes characteristic of MFS. Patients with the rarer form of MFS that is characterized by contractural arachnodactyly instead of loose joints can usually be identified by detection of a mutation in the fibrillin-2 gene that is similar in structure to the gene for fibrillin-1. Preliminary data suggest that patients with mutations in the fibrillin-2 gene are not prone to develop aneurysms. However, affected members of some rare families with a mutation in the fibrillin-1 gene also do not develop aortic aneurysms, even though they may show the skeletal or ocular changes. Therefore, the DNA tests are most helpful if: (1) a mutation is detected in either of the two genes, and (2) informative data are available on the clinical symptoms that the same mutation produces in the patient's family or in other families with similar clinical features.

Incidence and Inheritance   MFS has an incidence of about 1 in 10,000 in most racial and ethnic groups. The disorder is inherited as an autosomal dominant trait; at least one-fourth of patients do not have an affected parent, and their cases are probably due to new mutations.

Skeletal Changes   Patients are usually tall compared with other members of the same family and have long limbs. The ratio of the upper segment (top of the head to top of the pubic ramus) to the lower segment (top of the pubic ramus to the floor) is usually 2 SDs below mean for age, race, and sex. The fingers and hands are long and slender and have a spider-like appearance (arachnodactyly). Many patients have severe chest deformities, including depression (pectus excavatum), protrusion (pectus carinatum), or asymmetry. Scoliosis is frequent and usually accompanied by kyphosis. High-arched palate and high pedal arches or pes planus are common. A few patients have severe joint hypermobility similar to EDS.

Cardiovascular Changes   Cardiovascular abnormalities are the major source of morbidity and mortality (Chap. 247). Mitral valve prolapse develops early in life and in about one-quarter progresses to mitral valve regurgitation of increasing severity because of redundancy of the leaflets, stretching of the chordae tendineae, and dilatation of the valvulae annulus. Dilatation of the root of the aorta and the sinuses of Valsalva are characteristic and ominous features of the disease that can develop at any age and in rare instances may be detected by echocardiography in utero. The rate of dilatation is unpredictable, but it can lead to aortic regurgitation, dissection of the aorta, and rupture. Dilatation is probably accelerated by physical and emotional stress, as well as by pregnancy.

Ocular Changes   Dislocations of the lens may be readily apparent, but diagnosis usually requires pupillary dilatation and slit-lamp examination. The displacement is usually not progressive but may contribute to the formation of cataracts. The ocular globe is frequently elongated, most patients are myopic, and some develop retinal detachment. A few patients have lattice degeneration and retinal tears; most have adequate vision.

Associated Changes   Striae may occur over the shoulders and buttocks. Otherwise the skin is normal. A number of patients develop spontaneous pneumothorax. Inguinal and incisional hernias are common. Marked dilatation of the dural sac is seen frequently in computed tomography scans, but the condition is usually asymptomatic. Patients are typically thin with little subcutaneous fat, but adults may develop centripetal obesity.

Molecular Defects   Most patients with the classic features of MFS are heterozygotes for mutations in a gene on chromosome 15 that encodes fibrillin-1, a glycoprotein of 350 kDa that is a major component of elastin-associated microfibrils. These microfibrils are abundant in large blood vessels and the suspensory ligaments of the lens. Mutations in the fibrillin-1 gene include missense, nonsense, inframe deletions, and RNA splicing mutations. Many of the mutations are single amino acid substitutions in the epidemal growth factor-like domains of the molecule that may be involved with calcium binding. Mutations in the fibrillin-2 gene that cause the MFS variant characterized by contractures appear to follow a similar pattern. As with most genetic diseases, the nature and location of mutations in the genes are only an approximate guide to the severity of the phenotype unless the same mutation has been seen in other members of the same family or in similar unrelated patients. However, there is a clustering of mutations in the middle portion of the molecule of fibrillin-1 encoded by exons 23 to 32 that causes the most severe phenotype, referred to as *neonatal lethal MFS*. The function of fibrillin has not been defined, but the data suggest that fibrillin self-assembles into a fibrillar structure and that the conformation and surface properties of the entire molecule are critical for normal assembly. Therefore, the functional consequences of mutations that change the amino acid sequence of fibrillin may be similar to the effects of mutations that change the conformation of a fibrillar collagen.

Diagnosis   The diagnosis is easily established if the patient and other members of the family have dislocated lenses, aortic dilatation, and long and thin extremities together with kyphoscoliosis or other chest deformities. The diagnosis is frequently made if ectopia lentis and an aneurysm of the ascending aorta occur in the absence of a Marfan habitus or a positive family history. All patients in whom the diagnosis is suspected should have a slit-lamp examination and an echocardiogram. Also, homocystinuria (Table 351-3) should be ruled out by a negative cyanide-nitroprusside test for disulfides in the urine (Chap. 352). A few patients with types I, II, and III EDS have ectopia lentis but lack the Marfan habitus and instead have characteristic skin changes not present in MFS. Patients with familial aortic aneurysms tend to develop aneurysms at the base of the abdominal aorta. The location of the aneurysms, however, is somewhat variable, and the high incidence of aortic aneurysms in the general population (1 in 100) makes the differential diagnosis difficult unless other features of MFS are clearly present. A few families with familial aortic aneurysms have mutations in the gene for type III procollagen (Fig. 351-4).

TREATMENT   There is no established treatment, but several investigators have recommended use of propranolol or other β-adrenergic blocking agents to lower blood pressure and thereby delay or prevent aortic dilatation. Surgical replacement of the aorta, aortic valve, and mitral valve has been successful in some patients, and all patients should be followed carefully with echocardiography and other techniques for evaluation of cardiovascular changes (Chap. 247). Patients should probably be advised of the risks of severe physical and emotional stress and of pregnancy.

The scoliosis tends to be progressive and should be treated by mechanical bracing and physical therapy if >20° or by surgery if it progresses to >45°. Estrogen has been tried in girls with scoliosis, but the results are inconclusive. Dislocated lenses rarely require surgical removal, but patients should be followed closely for retinal detachment.

Diagnostic tests based on detection of fibrillin defects in cultured skin fibroblasts or DNA analysis of the gene are now available from several laboratories.

DISEASES RELATED TO ELASTIN   As may be expected from the role of elastin in maintaining the elasticity of skin, mutations in the elastin gene cause *cutis laxa*, a rare and heterogeneous group of disorders characterized by skin that is both lax and inelastic. Three different frame-shift mutations were found in three unrelated families with dominant forms of the disease. Surprisingly, other mutations in the elastin gene produce phenotypes that primarily involve the aorta, whose elasticity also depends on the presence of elastin. A large deletion that includes the elastin gene and probably several adjacent genes causes the *Williams syndrome*, characterized by supravalvular aortic stenosis, growth retardation, characteristic facies, and an unusual mental phenotype of low intelligence quotient together with a high degree of sociability.

EPIDERMOLYSIS BULLOSA   EB consists of a group of similar disorders in which the skin and related epithelial tissues break and blister as the result of minor trauma. As with most heritable disorders of connective tissues, the clinical manifestations range from lethal to mild.

Classification   Four types of EB are defined on the basis of the level at which blistering occurs: EB simplex for blistering in the epidermis, EB hemidesmosomal for fissures between kerotinocytes and between kerotinocytes and the basal lamina, EB junctional for blistering in the dermal-epidermal junction, and EB dystrophica for blistering in the dermis (Table 351-7).

Incidence   The incidence of EB in the United States is estimated to be 1 in 50,000.

Molecular Defects   The molecular basis of several specific variants of EB has been defined. A series of patients with EB simplex were found to have mutations in either keratin 14 or keratin 5, two of the major keratins in basal epithelial cells. Patients with the related

Table 351-7   Clinical Variants of Epidermolysis-Bullosa (EB)

EB Variant	Level of Tissue Separation	Mutated Gene
Simplex	Intraepidermal	KRT5
		KRT14
Hemidesmosomal[a]	Basal keratinocyte/ lamina lucida interface	
GABEB		COL17A1
EB-PA		ITGA6
		ITGB4
EB-MD		PLEC1
Junctional	Lamina lucida	LAMA3
		LAMB3
		LAMC2
Dystrophic	Sub-lamina densa	COL7A1

[a] GABEB, generalized atrophic benign EB; EB-PA, EB with pyloric artresia; EB-MD, EB with late-onset muscular dystrophy.
SOURCE: Modified from Pulkkinen and Uitto.

syndrome, epidermolytic icthyosis, have mutations in keratin 1 and keratin 10. The new disease phenotype of hemidesmosomal EB has three clinical variants that are caused by mutations in one of four genes (Table 351-7): (1) A generalized atrophic and benign form of EB is caused by mutations in the COL17A1 gene for type XVII collagen; (2) a variant with EB associated with pyloric atresia and other intestinal abnormalities is caused by mutations in either the gene for the $\alpha6$ integrin (ITG A6) or the gene for the $\beta4$ integrin (ITG B4); and (3) another variant characterized by relatively mild blistering at birth but associated with late-onset muscular dystrophy is caused by mutations in the gene for plectin (PLEC-1). Junctional EB is caused by mutations in any one of three genes for laminin (LAMA-3, LAMB-3, LAMC-2). The most severe dystrophic form of EB is caused by mutations in the gene for type VII collagen (COL7A1).

Diagnosis   The diagnosis is based on skin that readily breaks and forms blisters. EB simplex and EB hemidesmosomal are generally milder than EB junctional or EB dystrophica. EB dystrophica variants usually cause large and prominent scars. Precise classification within subtypes usually requires electron microscopy. The treatment is symptomatic.

ALPORT SYNDROME   (See also Chap. 275)   AS is an inherited disorder characterized by hematuria. Four forms of the disease are now recognized: (1) classic AS, which is inherited as an X-linked disorder with hematuria, sensorineural deafness, and conical deformation of the anterior surface of the lens (lenticonus); (2) a subtype of the X-linked form associated with diffuse leiomyomatosis; (3) an autosomal recessive form; and (4) an autosomal dominant form. The two autosomal forms can cause renal disease without deafness or lenticonus.

Incidence   The incidence of AS is about 1 in 10,000 in the general population and as high as 1 in 5000 in some ethnic groups. About 80% of AS patients have the X-linked variant.

Molecular Defects   Electron microscopy of kidneys from patients with classic AS demonstrates that the glomerular basement membrane is up to five times thicker than normal and that the lamina densa is distorted and split. The X-linked and autosomal recessive forms are caused primarily by mutations in genes for the $\alpha3(IV)$, $\alpha4(IV)$, $\alpha5(IV)$, or $\alpha6(IV)$ chains of type IV collagen, a major component of basement membranes. The type IV collagen in most membranes consists primarily of $\alpha1(IV)$ and $\alpha2(IV)$ chains folded into a large, rodlike molecule with globular ends and a long triple-helical domain that is interrupted by short sequences that do not form triple helices. The molecules self-assemble through both the globular ends and the long triple-helical domain to form a complex three-dimen-

sional network. The four additional α chains of type IV collagen are minor components of basement membranes, similar in structure, and are probably incorporated into the same or similar molecules. The six genes for the proteins are arranged in tandem pairs on different chromosomes in a head-to-head orientation and with overlapping promoters, i.e., the $\alpha1(IV)$ and $\alpha2(IV)$ genes are head-to-head on chromosome 13q34, the $\alpha3(IV)$ and $\alpha4(IV)$ genes are on chromosome 2q35-37, and the $\alpha5(IV)$ and $\alpha6(IV)$ genes are on chromosome Xq22. An X-linked variant is caused by mutations in the COL4A5 gene, and the X-linked variant associated with leiomyomatosis is caused by deletions that involve both the COL4A5 gene and the nearby COL4A6 gene. The autosomal recessive variants are caused by mutations in either the COL4A3 or COL4A4 genes. The mutations responsible for the autosomal dominant variants are still unknown, but they have been mapped to the same locus as the COL4A3 and COL4A4 genes.

Diagnosis   The diagnosis of classic AS is based on X-linked inheritance of hematuria, sensorineural deafness, and lenticonus. Because of the X-linked transmission, women are usually less severely affected than men and are generally underdiagnosed. The hematuria progresses to nephritis and may cause renal failure in late adolescence in affected males and at older ages in some women. The sensorineural deafness is primarily in the high-tone range. It can frequently be detected only by an audiogram and is usually not progressive. The lenticonus can occur without nephritis but is generally considered to be pathognomonic of classic AS.

 TREATMENT   There is no known treatment, but renal transplantation is usually successful.

BIBLIOGRAPHY

BYERS PH: Osteogenesis imperfecta, in *Connective Tissue and Its Heritable Disorders*, PM Royce, B Steinmann (eds). New York, Wiley-Liss, 1993, p 317

DE PAEPE A et al: Revised diagnostic criteria for the Marfan syndrome. Am J Med Genet 62:417, 1996

GLORIEUX FH et al: Cyclic administration of pamidronate in children with severe osteogenesis imperfecta. N Engl J Med 339:947, 1998

HORTON WA, HECHT JT: The chondrodysplasias, in *Connective Tissue and Its Heritable Disorders*, PM Royce, B Steinmann (eds). New York, Wiley-Liss, 1993, p 641

INTERNATIONAL WORKING GROUP ON CONSTITUTIONAL DISEASES OF BONE: International nomenclature and classification of the osteochondrodysplasias (1997). Am J Med Genet 79:376, 1998

KASHTAN CE: Alport syndrome: An inherited disorder of renal, ocular, and cochlear basement membranes. Medicine 78:838, 1999

KUIVANIEMI H et al: Mutations in the fibrillar collagens (types I, II, III, IX and XI), and fibril-associated collagen, and the network-forming collagen (type X) cause a spectrum of diseases of bone, cartilage and blood vessels. Hum Mutat, 9:300, 1997

MANOUVRIER-HANU S et al: Genetics of limb anomalies in humans. Trends Genet 15: 409, 1999

MARINI JC: Osteogenesis imperfecta. Comprehensive management. Adv Pediatr 35:391, 1988

MUNDLOS S, OLSEN BR: Heritable diseases of the skeleton. Part II: Molecular insights into skeletal development-matrix components and their homeostasis. FASEB J 11: 227, 1997

PEPIN M et al: Clinical and genetic features of Ehlers-Danlos syndrome type IV, the vascular type. N Engl J Med 342:673, 2000

PROCKOP DJ: Mutations in collagen genes as a cause of connective-tissue diseases. N Engl J Med 326:540, 1992

———, KIVIRIKKO KI: Collagen: Molecular biology, diseases and potentials for therapy. Annu Rev Biochem 64:403, 1996

PULKKINEN L, UITTO J: Mutations analysis and molecular genetics of epidermolysis bullosa. Matrix Biol 18:29, 1999

RAMIREZ F et al: Marfan syndrome: New clues to genotype-phenotype correlations. Ann Med 31:202, 1999

STEINMANN B et al: The Ehlers-Danlos syndrome, in *Connective Tissue and Its Heritable Disorders*, PM Royce, B Steinmann (eds). New York, Wiley-Liss, 1993, p 351

TASSABEHJI M et al: An elastin gene mutation producing abnormal tropoelastin and abnormal elastic fibres in a patient with autosomal dominant cutis laxa. Hum Mol Genet 7:1021, 1998

INHERITED DISORDERS OF AMINO ACID METABOLISM AND STORAGE

All polypeptides and proteins are polymers of amino acids. Eight amino acids, referred to as *essential*, cannot be synthesized by humans and must be obtained from dietary sources. The others are formed endogenously. Although most of the body's amino acids are "tied up" in proteins, small intracellular pools of *free* amino acids are in equilibrium with extracellular reservoirs in plasma, cerebrospinal fluid, and the lumina of the gut and kidney. Physiologically, amino acids are more than mere "building blocks" of proteins. Some (glycine, glutamate, γ-aminobutyric acid) are neurotransmitters. Others (phenylalanine, tyrosine, tryptophan, glycine) are precursors of hormones, coenzymes, pigments, purines, or pyrimidines. Each has a unique degradative pathway by which its nitrogen and carbon components are used for the synthesis of other amino acids, carbohydrates, and lipids.

More than 70 disorders of amino acid metabolism are now known. The catabolic and storage defects (approximately 60) discussed in this chapter far outnumber the transport abnormalities (approximately 10) considered in Chap. 353. Each of these disorders is rare—the incidences range from 1 in 10,000 for cystinuria or phenylketonuria to 1 in 200,000 for homocystinuria or alkaptonuria. Collectively, however, they occur in perhaps 1 in 500 to 1 in 1000 live births. Almost all are transmitted as autosomal recessive traits.

The features of inherited disorders of amino acid catabolism are summarized in Table 352-1. In general, these disorders are named for the compound that accumulates to highest concentration in blood (-*emias*) or urine (-*urias*). For many conditions (often called *aminoacidopathies*), the parent amino acid is found in excess; for others, generally referred to as *organic acidemias*, products in the catabolic pathway accumulate. Which compound(s) accumulates depends, of course, on the site of the enzymatic block, the reversibility of the reactions proximal to the lesion, and the availability of alternative pathways of metabolic "runoff." For some amino acids, such as the sulfur-containing or branched-chain molecules, defects have been described at nearly each step in the catabolic pathway. For others, only small numbers of defective reactions have been described. Biochemical and genetic heterogeneity is common. Four distinct forms of hyperphenylalaninemia, seven forms of homocystinuria, and seven types of methylmalonic acidemia are recognized. Such heterogeneity reflects the presence of an even larger array of molecular defects.

The manifestations of these conditions differ widely (Table 352-1). Some, such as sarcosinemia or hyperprolinemia, produce no clinical consequences. At the other extreme, complete deficiency of ornithine transcarbamylase or of branched-chain keto acid dehydrogenase is lethal in the untreated neonate. Central nervous system (CNS) dysfunction, in the form of developmental retardation, seizures, alterations in sensorium, or behavioral disturbances, is present in more than half the disorders. Protein-induced vomiting, neurologic dysfunction, and hyperammonemia occur in many disorders of urea cycle intermediates. Metabolic ketoacidosis, often accompanied by hyperammonemia, is a frequent presenting finding in the disorders of branched-chain amino acid metabolism. Occasional disorders produce focal tissue or organ involvement such as liver disease, renal failure, cutaneous abnormalities, or ocular lesions.

The clinical manifestations in many of these conditions can be prevented or mitigated if diagnosis is achieved early and appropriate treatment (i.e., dietary protein or amino acid restriction or vitamin supplementation) is instituted promptly. For this reason, several aminoacidopathies and organic acidemias are routinely screened in newborns using an array of chemical and microbiologic techniques. Once a presumptive diagnosis is made, confirmation can be provided by direct enzyme assay on extracts of leukocytes, erythrocytes, or cultured fibroblasts. DNA-based testing is possible for several disorders including phenylketonuria, ornithine transcarbamylase deficiency, citrullinemia, gyrate atrophy of the retina, propionic acidemia, and methylmalonic acidemia. As additional mutations are defined, DNA-based analysis may allow better predictions of outcome and improved therapeutic plans.

Several of these disorders (including branched-chain ketoaciduria, isovaleric acidemia, propionic acidemia, methylmalonic acidemia, homocystinuria, cystinosis, phenylketonuria, ornithine transcarbamylase deficiency, citrullinemia, argininosuccinic aciduria) can be diagnosed prenatally by chemical analysis of amniotic fluid or by chemical, enzymatic, or DNA-based studies of fresh or cultured amniotic fluid cells. In addition to predicting genotype and alleviating parental anxiety, prenatal diagnosis has led to improved treatment of affected newborns.

The focus of this chapter is on selected disorders that illustrate the principles, properties, and problems presented by the disorders of amino acid metabolism.

THE HYPERPHENYLALANINEMIAS

DEFINITION The hyperphenylalaninemias (Table 352-1) result from impaired conversion of phenylalanine to tyrosine. The most common and clinically important is *phenylketonuria*, which is characterized by an increased concentration of phenylalanine in blood, increased concentrations of phenylalanine and its by-products (notably phenylpyruvate, phenylacetate, phenyllactate, and phenylacetylglutamine) in urine, and severe mental retardation if untreated in infancy.

GENETIC CONSIDERATIONS Each of the hyperphenylalaninemias results from reduced activity of phenylalanine hydroxylase. In humans, this complete enzyme system is expressed only in liver. Phenylalanine and molecular oxygen are substrates, and a reduced pteridine, tetrahydrobiopterin, is a cofactor (Fig. 352-1). Tyrosine and dihydrobiopterin are the products of this catalytic system, the latter being reconverted to tetrahydrobiopterin by two enzymes, pterin-4α-carbinolamine dehydratase and dihydropteridine reductase.

Abnormalities in phenylalanine metabolism are autosomal recessive traits that occur in about 1 in 10,000 births. Phenylketonuria type I is widely distributed among whites and Orientals. It is rare in blacks. Phenylalanine hydroxylase activity in obligate heterozygotes is low but higher than in affected homozygotes. Adult heterozygous carriers are clinically well but can be identified by an increased ratio of phenylalanine/tyrosine in plasma in the semifasting state. They may have transient cognitive impairment after phenylalanine loads. Hyperphenylalaninemias are caused by mutations in the gene encoding phenylalanine hydroxylase (*PAH*) or in genes encoding enzymes involved in tetrahydrobiopterin synthesis or recycling. In the vast majority of patients, mutations occur in the *PAH* gene (causing phenylketonuria type I), and >300 mutations have been identified. Mutations causing a complete impairment of enzyme activity, such as the R408W, are associated with a more severe outcome requiring stringent dietary restriction of phenylalanine. Mutations causing a less complete deficiency of the enzyme, such as the I65T, are associated with milder forms of phenylketonuria.

In fewer than 2% of patients with phenylketonuria, mutations occur in other genes, including dihydrobiopterin reductase (*DHPR*) (30%), 6-pyruvoyl-tetrahydropterin synthase (*6-PTS*) (60%), GTP cyclohydrolase I (*GTP-CH*) (5%), and pterin-4α-carbinolamine dehydratase (*PCD*) (5%). In these cases, the impairment in phenylalanine hydroxylation results from tetrahydrobiopterin deficiency due to blocks in the pathway by which tetrahydrobiopterin is synthesized from GTP (phenylketonuria type III and malignant hyperphenylalaninemia) or deficiency of dihydropterine reductase (phenylketonuria type II), the enzyme that regenerates tetrahydrobiopterin from dihydrobiopterin (Fig. 352-1). Tyrosine hydroxylase and tryptophan hy-

Table 352-1   Inherited Disorders of Amino Acid Catabolism

Amino Acid(s) Affected	Disorder or Condition	Enzyme Defect	Clinical Manifestations[a]						Inheritance Pattern[b]
			Mental Retardation	Neuro-psychiatric Dysfunction	Protein Intolerance	Metabolic Ketoacidosis	Ammonia Intoxication	Other	
AROMATIC—HETEROCYCLIC									
Phenylala-nine	Phenylketo-nuria type I (severe to mild)	Phenylalanine hydroxylase	+	+	−	−	−	Hypopig-mented skin and hair, eczema	AR
	Phenylketo-nuria type II	Dihydropteridine reductase	+	+	−	−	−		AR
	Phenylketo-nuria type III	6-Pyruvoyl-tetra-hydropterin synthase	+	+	−	−	−		AR
	Malignant hy-perphenylalan-inemia	GTP cyclohydro-lase	+	+	−	−	−		AR
	Hyperphenyla-laninemia with primap-terinuria	Pterin-4α-carbinol-amine dehydra-tase	−	±	−	−	−	Transient hy-perphenyl-alaninemia	AR
Tyrosine	Tyrosinemia type I (hepa-torenal)	Fumarylacetoace-tate hydrolase	−	−	±	−	−	Cirrhosis, he-patic failure, renal tubular defects, rickets	AR
	Tyrosinemia type II (oculo-cutaneous)	Tyrosine transami-nase	±	−	−	−	−	Palmoplantar keratosis, painful cor-neal erosions with photo-phobia	AR
	Tyrosinemia type III	4-Hydroxyphe-nylpyruvate di-oxygenase	−	−	−	−	−		AR
	Hawkinsinuria	4-Hydroxyphe-nylpyruvate di-oxygenase	−	−	−	−	−	Failure to thrive, meta-bolic acidosis in infancy, fine hairs	AD
	Alkaptonuria	Homogentisic acid oxidase	−	−	−	−	−	Ochronosis, arthritis	AR
	Albinism (ocu-locutaneous)	Tyrosinase	−	−	−	−	−	Hypopigmen-tation of hair, skin, and optic fundus	AR
	Albinism (ocular)	Unknown	−	−	−	−	−	Hypopigmen-tation of optic fundus	XL, AR
Trypto-phan	Tryptophanuria	Unknown	+	+	−	−	−	Photosensi-tive skin rash	AR
	Xanthurenic aciduria	Kynureninase	?	−	−	−	−		?
Histidine	Histidinemia	Histidine-ammonia lyase	±	±	−	−	−	Hearing and speech deficit	AR
	Urocanic aciduria	Urocanase	+	+	−	−	−		?
	Formiminoglu-tamic aciduria	Formiminotrans-ferase	?	+	−	−	−		(AR)
GLYCINE-IMINO ACIDS									
Glycine	Hyperglycine-mia	Glycine cleavage	+	+	−	−	−		AR
	Sarcosinemia	Sarcosine dehy-drogenase	−	−	−	−	−		AR
	Hyperoxaluria (type I)	Alanine: glyoxy-late amino-trans-ferase	−	−	−	−	−	Calcium oxa-late nephroli-thiasis, renal failure	AR
	Hyperoxaluria (type II)	D-Glyceric acid dehydrogenase/ glyoxylate reduc-tase	−	−	±	−	−	Calcium oxa-late nephroli-thiasis, renal failure	AR

(continued)

Table 352-1—(continued)

Amino Acid(s) Affected	Disorder or Condition	Enzyme Defect	Clinical Manifestations[a]					Other	Inheritance Pattern[b]
			Mental Retardation	Neuro-psychiatric Dysfunction	Protein Intolerance	Metabolic Ketoacidosis	Ammonia Intoxication		
Imino acids	Hyperprolinemia (type I)	Proline oxidase	−	−	−	−	−		AR
	Hyperprolinemia (type II)	Δ′-Pyrroline dehydrogenase	−	−	−	−	−		AR
	Hyperhydroxyprolinemia	Hydroxyproline reductase	−	−	−	−	−		AR
	Iminopeptiduria	Prolidase	+					Crusting erythematous, ecchymotic dermatitis, recurrent infections	AR
SULFUR-CONTAINING									
Methionine	Hypermethioninemia	Methionine adenosyltransferase	−	−	−	−	−		?
Homocystine	Homocystinuria	Cystathionine β-synthase	±	±	−	−	−	Dislocated lenses, osteoporosis, thrombotic vascular disease	AR
	Homocystinuria	5,10-Methylene-tetrahydrofolate reductase	+	+	−	−	−		AR
	Homocystinuria and methylmalonic acidemia (cblC, -D)[c]	Cobalamin (vitamin B$_{12}$) reductase (cytosol)	+	+	−	−	−	Megaloblastic anemia	AR
	Homocystinuria and methylmalonic acidemia (cblF)	Lysosomal efflux	+	+	−	−	−		(?)
	Homocystinuria (cblE, -G)	Methionine synthase (MS) and MS reductase	+	+	−	−	−	Megaloblastic anemia	AR
Cystathionine	Cystathioninuria	Cystathionase	−	−	−	−	−		AR
Cystine	Cystinosis	Lysosomal efflux	−	−	−	−	−	Fanconi syndrome, renal failure, photophobia	AR
S-Sulfo-L-cysteine	S-Sulfo-L-cysteine, sulfite, thiosulfaturia	Sulfite oxidase	+	+	−	−	−	Dislocated lenses	AR
CATIONIC									
Lysine	Hyperlysinemia	α-Aminoadipic semialdehyde synthase			−	−	−		AR
	Saccharopinuria	δ-Aminoadipic semialdehyde synthase	−	−	−	−	−		?
	α-Ketoadipic aciduria	α-Ketoadipic acid dehydrogenase			−	−	−		?
	Glutaric aciduria (type I)	Glutaryl CoA dehydrogenase	−	+	−	−	−	Progressive dystonia and athetosis	AR
	Glutaric aciduria (type II)	Electron transfer flavoprotein; or ETF-ubiquinone oxidoreductase	−	+	−	+	−	Hypoglycemia, acidosis, "sweaty feet" odor, hypotonia, fatty degeneration of liver and kidney	AR

(continued)

Table 352-1   Inherited Disorders of Amino Acid Catabolism—*(continued)*

Amino Acid(s) Affected	Disorder or Condition	Enzyme Defect	Clinical Manifestations[a]						Inheritance Pattern[b]
			Mental Retardation	Neuro-psychiatric Dysfunction	Protein Intolerance	Metabolic Ketoacidosis	Ammonia Intoxication	Other	
Ornithine	Hyperornithinemia, hyperammonemia, homocitrullinuria	Mitochondrial ornithine transporter-1	+	+	+	−	+		AR
	Hyperornithinemia	Ornithine-D-aminotransferase	−	−	−		−	Gyrate atrophy of choroid and retina	AR
UREA CYCLE									
Carbamylphosphate	Hyperammonemia (type I)	Carbamylphosphate synthetase I	+	+	+	−	+		AR
N-acetylglutamate	Hyperammonemia (type IA)	N-acetylglutamate synthetase	±	+	+		+		AR
Ornithine	Hyperammonemia (type II)	Ornithine transcarbamylase	+	+	+	−	+		XL
Citrulline	Citrullinemia-1	Argininosuccinate synthetase	+	+	+		+		AR
	Citrullinemia-2	Activating protein (?)	±	+	−	−	+		AR
Argininosuccinic acid	Argininosuccinic aciduria	Argininosuccinase	+	+	+	−	+		AR
Arginine	Argininemia	Arginase	+	+	+	−	+		AR
BRANCHED-CHAIN									
Valine	Hypervalinemia	Valine aminotransferase	+	+	+	−	−		AR
Leucine, isoleucine	Hyperleucine-isoleucinemia	Leucine-isoleucine aminotransferase	+	+	+	−	−		?
Valine, leucine, isoleucine	Classic branched-chain ketoaciduria[c]	Branched-chain ketoacid dehydrogenase	+	+	+	±	−	"Maple syrup" odor	AR
	Intermittent branched-chain ketoaciduria	Branched-chain ketoacid dehydrogenase	±	−	+	+	−		AR
Leucine	Isovaleric acidemia	Isovaleryl CoA dehydrogenase	±	±	+	+	±	"Sweaty feet" odor	AR
	β-Methylcrotonyl glycinuria	β-Methylcrotonyl CoA carboxylase	+	+	−	+	−	"Cat's urine" odor	AR
	β-Hydroxy-β-methylglutaric aciduria	β-Hydroxy-β-methylglutaryl CoA lyase	−	+	+	+	−		AR
Isoleucine, valine	α-Methylacetoacetic aciduria	β-Ketothiolase	±	±	+	+	+		AR
	Propionic acidemia (pcc A, B, C)[c]	Propionyl CoA carboxylase	±	±	+	+	+		AR
	Propionic acidemia (bio)[c]	Holocarboxylase synthetase; biotinidase	+	±	+	+	−		AR
	Methylmalonic acidemia (mut)[c]	Methylmalonyl CoA mutase	±	±	+	+	+		AR
	Methylmalonic acidemia (cbl A)[c]	Cobalamin (vitamin B$_{12}$) reductase (mitochondrial) (?)	±	±	+	+	+		AR
	Methylmalonic acidemia (cbl B)[c]	Cobalamin (vitamin B$_{12}$): ATP adenosyltransferase	±	±	+	+	+		AR

[a] +, Regularly present; ±, sometimes present; −, absent; ?, uncertain; all designations refer to manifestations in untreated disorder.

[b] AR, autosomal recessive; XL, X-linked; (AR), probably autosomal recessive.

[c] Designations in parentheses refer to complementation groups assigned by genetic analysis with cultured cells.

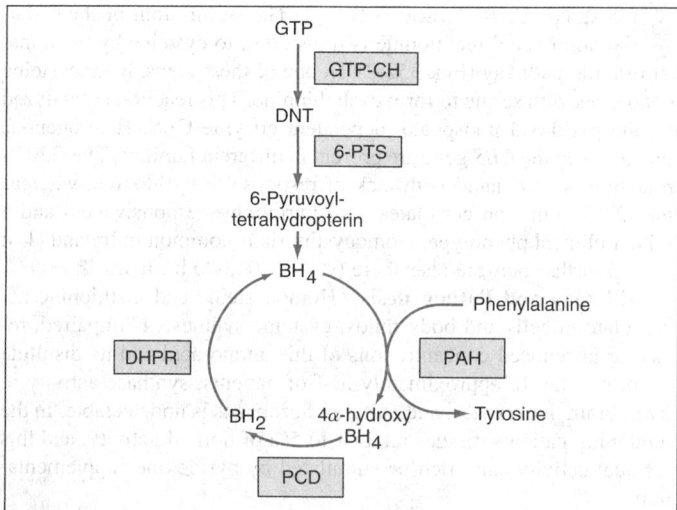

FIGURE 352-1 Pathways, enzymes, and coenzymes involved in the hyperphenylalaninemias. Blocked-in symbols highlight points of etiologic or therapeutic significance to the various genetic defects underlying these disorders. Abbreviations: GTP, guanosine triphosphate; GTP-CH, guanosine triphosphate cyclohydrolase; DNT, dihydroneopterin triphosphate; 6-PTS, 6-pyruvoyltetrahydropterin synthase; BH4, tetrahydrobiopterin; BH2, dihydrobiopterin; DHPR, dihydropteridine reductase; PAH, phenylalanine hydroxylase; PCD, pterin-4α−carbinolamine dehydratase.

droxylase also require tetrahydrobiopterin. Their products (L-dopa and 5-hydroxytryptophan) are essential for the synthesis of neurotransmitters. Heterozygotes for these conditions do not have hyperphenylalaninemia, but carriers of mutations in GTP cyclohydrolase have a peculiar form of dystonia, transmitted as a dominant trait with variable expressivity and higher penetrance in females; it is exquisitely responsive to levodopa. Neurotransmitter levels are not altered in transient hyperphenylalaninemia (sometimes called *transient phenylketonuria*), which has been described in some patients with pterin-4α-carbinolamine dehydratase deficiency. ■

Etiology and Pathogenesis Phenylalanine accumulation in blood and urine and reduced tyrosine formation are direct consequences of the impaired hydroxylation. In untreated phenylketonuria and in its tetrahydrobiopterin-deficient variants, plasma concentrations of phenylalanine become sufficiently high [1 mmol/L (16 mg/dL)] to activate alternative pathways of metabolism and lead to formation of phenylpyruvate, phenylacetate, phenyllactate, and other derivatives that are rapidly cleared by the kidney and excreted in urine. The severe brain damage is due to several consequences of phenylalanine accumulation: competitive inhibition of transport of other amino acids required for protein synthesis, impaired polyribosome formation or stabilization, reduced synthesis and increased degradation of myelin, and inadequate formation of norepinephrine and serotonin. Phenylalanine is a competitive inhibitor of tyrosinase, a key enzyme in the pathway of melanin synthesis. This block, plus reduced availability of the melanin precursor tyrosine, accounts for the hypopigmentation of hair and skin.

Clinical Manifestations No abnormalities are apparent at birth, but untreated children with classic phenylketonuria fail to attain early developmental milestones, develop microcephaly, and demonstrate progressive impairment of cerebral function. Hyperactivity, seizures, and severe mental retardation are major clinical problems later in life. Electroencephalographic abnormalities; "mousy" odor of skin, hair, and urine (due to phenylacetate accumulation); and a tendency to hypopigmentation and eczema complete the devastating clinical picture. In contrast, affected children who are detected at birth and treated promptly show none of these abnormalities. Children with tetrahydrobiopterin deficiency, however, suffer a worse clinical course. Seizures appear early, followed by progressive cerebral and basal ganglia dysfunction (rigidity, chorea, spasms, hypotonia). Most succumb

to secondary infection within a few years despite early diagnosis and vigorous treatment.

A number of women with phenylketonuria who have been treated since infancy have reached adulthood and become pregnant. If maternal phenylalanine levels are not strictly controlled before and during pregnancy, their offspring are at risk, even if they are heterozygous, for *maternal phenylketonuria*. Affected children have microcephaly and an increased risk of congenital defects. After birth, these children have severe neurodevelopmental delay and growth retardation.

Diagnosis Plasma phenylalanine concentrations are usually normal at birth in the hyperphenylalaninemias but rise rapidly after institution of protein feedings. To prevent mental retardation, diagnosis and initiation of dietary treatment of classic phenylketonuria must occur before the child is 3 weeks of age. For this reason, most newborns in North America and Europe are screened by determinations of blood phenylalanine concentration using the Guthrie bacterial inhibition assay. Abnormal values are confirmed using quantitative analysis of plasma amino acids. Prenatal diagnosis of type I phenylketonuria is now feasible using DNA-based tests that detect specific mutations or polymorphic markers that are linked to the *PAH* gene.

In newborns with type I phenylketonuria, plasma levels depend on the amount of phenylalanine in the diet and the degree of impairment of phenylalanine hydroxylase. Dietary phenylalanine restriction is usually instituted if blood phenylalanine levels are >250 μmol/L (4 mg/dL). Careful monitoring of these infants reveals the degree of phenylalanine hydroxylase impairment and dictates the degree of dietary phenylalanine restriction.

Deficiency of tetrahydrobiopterin, which occurs in 1 to 2% of newborns with increased blood phenylalanine, is excluded by screening the urinary pteridine profile and by assay of dihydropteridine reductase activity on dried blood specimens. Dihydropteridine reductase deficiency and the blocks in tetrahydrobiopterin synthesis can be detected in utero using assays on cultured amniocytes. Tetrahydrobiopterin deficiency manifests with hyperphenylalaninemia and progressive neurologic impairment despite prompt dietary restriction of phenylalanine.

TREATMENT Phenylketonuria is the first inherited metabolic disease in which a strategy of reducing the accumulation of the offending metabolite prevented the dire clinical consequences. This was accomplished by a special diet low in phenylalanine and supplemented with tyrosine. Tyrosine becomes an essential amino acid in phenylalanine hydroxylase deficiency. Sufficient phenylalanine is provided for new protein synthesis and normal growth. This amount varies with age and requires frequent adjustments, especially early in life. Ordinarily, plasma phenylalanine concentrations are maintained between 120 and 360 μmol/L (2 and 6 mg/dL). Such diet therapy must be instituted during the first 3 weeks of life. Even then, modest CNS dysfunction may occur with more deleterious mutations or after excess protein intake. Because uncontrolled hyperphenylalaninemia results in brain damage, dietary restriction should be continued and monitored indefinitely, recognizing that transient phenylketonuria may not require lifelong therapy. An enteric-coated formulation of phenylalanine ammonia lyase, which degrades phenylalanine in the gut, is under investigation for its potential to reduce the strain imposed by the special diet.

Children with tetrahydrobiopterin deficiency deteriorate despite dietary phenylalanine restriction. Such patients may be helped, however, by a regimen in which dietary phenylalanine restriction is combined with tetrahydrobiopterin supplements, levodopa, 5-hydroxytryptophan, and carbidopa. Finally, the deleterious consequences of maternal phenylketonuria can be minimized by continuing lifelong phenylalanine-restricted diets in females with phenylketonuria and assuring strict phenylalanine restriction prior to conception and throughout gestation.

THE HOMOCYSTINURIAS
(HYPERHOMOCYSTEINEMIAS)

The homocystinurias are seven biochemically and clinically distinct disorders (Table 352-1), each characterized by increased concentration of the sulfur-containing amino acid homocystine in blood and urine. The most common form results from reduced activity of cystathionine β-synthase (CBS), an enzyme in the transsulfuration pathway that converts methionine to cysteine (Fig. 352-2). The other forms are the result of impaired conversion of homocysteine to methionine, a reaction catalyzed by homocysteine:methyltetrahydrofolate methyltransferase (also known as *methionine synthase*) and two essential cofactors, methyltetrahydrofolate and methylcobalamin (methyl-vitamin B_{12}). Depending on the underlying disorder, some patients show chemical and, in some instances, clinical improvement following administration of specific vitamin supplements (pyridoxine, folate, or cobalamin) (Chap. 75). In classic homocystinuria, the levels of free homocystine in plasma increase and result in homocystinuria. *Hyperhomocysteinemia* refers to increased total plasma concentration of homocysteine in the sulfhydryl and disulfide form, free and protein-bound. Hyperhomocysteinemia, in the absence of significant homocystinuria, is found in individuals who are heterozygous or homozygous for certain genetic defects that impair folate or vitamin B_{12} metabolism or cause cystathionine synthase deficiency. Changes of homocysteine levels are also observed with increasing age; in postmenopausal women; in patients with renal failure, hypothyroidism, leukemias, or psoriasis; and during therapy with drugs such as methotrexate, nitrous oxide, isoniazid, and some antiepileptic agents.

Homocysteine acts as an atherogenic and thrombophilic agent. An increase in total plasma homocysteine represents an independent risk factor for coronary, cerebrovascular, and peripheral arterial disease as well as for deep-vein thrombosis (Chap. 241). Homocysteine is synergistic with hypertension and smoking, and it is additive with other risk factors that predispose to peripheral arterial disease. In addition, hyperhomocysteinemia and folate and vitamin B_{12} deficiency have been associated with an increased risk of neural tube defects in pregnant women.

CYSTATHIONINE β-SYNTHASE DEFICIENCY   Definition
Deficiency of this enzyme leads to increased concentrations of methionine and homocystine in body fluids and to decreased concentrations of cysteine and cystine. Clinical hallmarks include dislocation of optic lenses (usually downward and medially), mental retardation, marfanoid habitus, osteoporosis, and thrombotic vascular disease.

GENETIC CONSIDERATIONS   The sulfur atom of the essential amino acid methionine is transferred to cysteine by the transsulfuration pathway (Fig. 352-2). In one of these steps, homocysteine condenses with serine to form cystathionine. This reaction is catalyzed by the pyridoxal phosphate–dependent enzyme CBS. Heterogenous mutations in the *CBS* gene are present in different families. The G307S mutation is associated with lack of response to pyridoxine, whereas the I278T mutation correlates with pyridoxine-responsiveness and a milder clinical phenotype. Homocystinuria is common in Ireland (1 in 60,000 births) but rare elsewhere (<1 in 200,000 births). ■

Etiology and Pathogenesis   Homocysteine and methionine accumulate in cells and body fluids; cysteine synthesis is impaired, resulting in reduced concentrations of this amino acid and its disulfide form, cystine. In approximately half of patients, synthase activity in liver, brain, leukocytes, and cultured fibroblasts is undetectable. In the remaining patients, tissues retain 1 to 5% of normal activity, and this residual activity can often be stimulated by pyridoxine supplementation.

Homocysteine interferes with the normal cross-linking of collagen, an effect that likely plays an important role in the ocular, skeletal, and vascular complications. Altered collagen in the suspensory ligament of the optic lens and in bone matrix may account for the dislocated lenses and osteoporosis. Similarly, interference with normal ground substance metabolism in vascular walls may predispose to the arterial and venous thrombotic diathesis. Increased platelet adhesiveness may result from homocysteine accumulation, thereby contributing to the thrombotic occlusive disease so often observed. Recurrent cerebrovascular accidents secondary to thrombotic disease may account for the mental retardation, but direct chemical effects on cerebral cell metabolism have not been excluded.

Clinical Manifestations   More than 80% of homozygotes for complete CBS deficiency develop dislocated optic lenses. This abnormality usually appears by 3 to 4 years of age and often results in glaucoma and impaired visual acuity. Mental retardation occurs in about half of such patients, often accompanied by ill-defined behavioral disturbances. Osteoporosis is a common radiologic finding (seen in two-thirds of patients by age 15) but rarely causes clinical disease. Life-threatening vascular complications, probably initiated by damage to vascular endothelium, are the major cause of morbidity and mortality. Occlusion of coronary, renal, and cerebral arteries with attendant tissue infarction can occur during the first decade of life. Nearly a fourth of patients die of vascular disease before age 30. These vascular complications seem to be exacerbated by angiographic procedures. Importantly, pyridoxine-responsive patients have milder clinical manifestations in all regards and may escape newborn screening and present with ectopia lentis or premature vascular occlusion. Hetero-

FIGURE 352-2   Pathways, enzymes, and coenzymes involved in the homocystinurias. Blocked-in symbols highlight specific moieties of particular etiologic or therapeutic significance to the various genetic defects underlying these disorders. Abbreviations: B_{12}, hydroxocobalamin; MeCbl, methylcobalamin; MTFR, methylenetetrahydrofolate reductase; PLP, pyridoxal phosphate; CBS, cystathionine β-synthase; BHMT, betaine:homocysteine methyl transferase; MS, methionine synthase (5-methyltetrahydrofolate:homocysteine transferase).

zygous carriers for *CBS* deficiency (about 1 in 70 in the population) may have hyperhomocysteinemia, with an increased risk for premature coronary, peripheral, and cerebral occlusive vascular disease.

Diagnosis The cyanide-nitroprusside test is a simple way of demonstrating increased excretion of sulfhydryl-containing compounds in urine. This is confirmed by measurement of free plasma methionine and homocystine. Plasma methionine tends to be increased in synthase-deficient patients and normal or low in those with other causes of homocystinuria and impaired methionine formation (see below). Diagnostic confirmation depends on measurements of CBS activity in tissue extracts or cells cultured from patients. Heterozygotes can be identified by measurement of peak serum homocystine after an oral methionine load (100 mg/kg) and by measurement of tissue synthase activity.

℞ TREATMENT As with classic phenylketonuria, effective treatment depends on early diagnosis. A number of infants diagnosed in the newborn period have been treated successfully with methionine-restricted, cystine-supplemented diets. In approximately half of patients, oral pyridoxine (25 to 500 mg/d) produces a fall in plasma and urinary methionine and homocystine and an increase in cystine concentration in body fluids. This effect probably reflects a modest increase in CBS activity in cells of patients in whom the defect is characterized either by reduced affinity for cofactor or by accelerated degradation of mutant enzyme. Vitamin supplementation at these doses is apparently harmless and should be tried in all patients. Folate deficiency should be prevented by adequate supplementation. Betaine has also been effective in reducing homocystine levels in pyridoxine-unresponsive patients.

5,10-METHYLENETETRAHYDROFOLATE REDUCTASE (MTFR) DEFICIENCY

Definition Hyperhomocysteinemia with normal or decreased methionine levels is caused by deficiency of MTFR, the enzyme involved in the synthesis of 5-methyltetrahydrofolate, a cofactor in the enzymatic formation of methionine from homocysteine (Fig. 352-2). CNS dysfunction and premature vascular occlusion may occur.

Genetic Basis and Pathogenesis 5-Methyltetrahydrofolate:homocysteine methyltransferase (methionine synthase) catalyzes the conversion of homocysteine to methionine. A primary defect in MTFR activity results, secondarily, in deficient methyltransferase activity and impaired conversion of homocysteine to methionine. This series of reactions is critical to normal DNA and RNA synthesis. Methionine deficiency and impaired nucleic acid synthesis may contribute to CNS dysfunction, while homocystine accumulation may predispose to thrombosis.

Hyperhomocysteinemia is inherited as an autosomal recessive trait and is caused by mutations in the MTFR (*MTHFR*) gene, which is located on chromosome 1p36.3. A thermolabile variant form of this enzyme, which has reduced activity, may be a common cause of hyperhomocysteinemia associated with increased risk of vascular disease in young adults.

Clinical Manifestations More than 30 patients with homocystinuria due to MTFR deficiency have been reported. The most severely affected have developmental retardation and cerebral atrophy early in life. Others have behavioral disturbances (catatonia) during the second decade or mild retardation. The severity of the clinical manifestations reflects the severity of the reductase deficiency.

Diagnosis Increased concentrations of free homocystine in body fluids with normal or decreased concentrations of methionine suggest severe MTFR deficiency. Total plasma homocysteine levels slightly above the normal range suggest milder dysfunction of this enzyme. Serum folate concentration is low in some patients. Confirmation requires direct MTFR assays in cultured fibroblasts.

℞ TREATMENT Therapeutic experience is limited. Folate, vitamin B_{12}, methionine, or betaine supplementation decrease

homocystine urinary excretion and improve the clinical manifestations in some patients.

DEFICIENCY OF COBALAMIN (VITAMIN B_{12}) COENZYME SYNTHESIS **Definition** Five other forms of homocystinuria also reflect impaired conversion of homocysteine to methionine. The primary defects in these entities, however, are in the synthesis of methylcobalamin, a cobalamin (vitamin B_{12}) coenzyme required by methionine synthase (MS) (Fig. 352-2). In some, methylmalonic acid accumulates in body fluids because of impaired synthesis of a second coenzyme, adenosylcobalamin, required for isomerization of methylmalonyl coenzyme A (CoA) to succinyl CoA. These disorders are designated cblC, -D, -E, -F, and -G.

Etiology and Pathogenesis As with MTFR deficiency, each disorder impairs remethylation of homocysteine. Since methylcobalamin is required for methyl-group transfer from methyltetrahydrofolate to homocysteine, impaired cobalamin metabolism leads to deficient methyltransferase activity. The defects responsible for impaired synthesis of methylcobalamin involve one of several steps in lysosomal or cytosolic activation of the vitamin precursor (Fig. 352-2). Somatic cell genetic studies indicate that each of the five abnormalities (cblC to -G) is distinct and imply that all are inherited as autosomal recessive traits.

Clinical Manifestations More than 45 patients—mostly children—with these defects in cobalamin metabolism have been described. Although clinical manifestations vary, abnormalities include developmental delay, dementia, spasticity, megaloblastic anemia, and pancytopenia. It is not possible to define a specific clinical syndrome for each of the defects in cobalamin metabolism.

Diagnosis Homocystinuria, homocysteinemia, and hypomethioninemia are the chemical hallmarks. Methylmalonic acidemia, too, has been noted in those defects resulting from defective synthesis of both cobalamin coenzymes. These findings may also be present in juvenile- or adult-onset pernicious anemia in which intestinal cobalamin absorption is impaired. Measurement of serum cobalamin concentrations, low in pernicious anemia and normal in patients with defective conversion of cobalamin vitamin to coenzymes, helps in the differential diagnosis. Definitive diagnosis depends on demonstrating impaired coenzyme synthesis in cultured cells.

℞ TREATMENT Treatment of affected children with hydroxycobalamin injections (1 to 2 mg/QD) and betaine supplements decreases homocystine and methylmalonate excretion; the hematologic and neurologic deficits have also been diminished to variable degrees in some patients. Intervention early in life seems to offer the best long-term prognosis.

ALKAPTONURIA

Definition Alkaptonuria is a rare disorder of tyrosine catabolism in which deficiency of homogentisate 1,2-dioxygenase (also known as *homogentisic acid oxidase*) leads to excretion of large amounts of homogentisic acid in urine and accumulation of oxidized homogentisic acid pigment in connective tissues (*ochronosis*). After many years, ochronosis produces a distinctive form of degenerative arthritis.

Genetic Basis and Pathogenesis Alkaptonuria was the first human disease shown to be inherited as an autosomal recessive trait. Affected homozygotes occur with a frequency of about 1 in 200,000. Heterozygous carriers are clinically well and excrete no homogentisic acid in urine, even after loading doses of tyrosine. The gene for homogentisate 1,2-dioxygenase (*HGD*) maps to chromosome 3q21-q23 and encodes a 445 amino acid protein expressed not only in liver and kidney but also in small intestine, colon, and prostate. Expression in this latter organ is consistent with accumulation of black calculi of homogentisic acid in the prostate of patients with alkaptonuria, sometimes requiring prostatectomy.

Patients have minimally increased concentrations of homogentisic acid in blood because it is rapidly cleared by the kidney. However, homogentisic acid accumulates in cells and body fluids. Its oxidized polymers bind to collagen, leading to the progressive deposition of a gray to bluish-black pigment. The mechanism(s) by which this deposition causes degenerative changes in cartilage, intervertebral disk, and other connective tissues is unknown but may involve direct chemical irritation, impaired collagen cross-linking, disturbed articular chondrocyte metabolism, or some combination of factors.

Clinical Manifestations   Alkaptonuria may go unrecognized until middle life when degenerative joint disease develops. Prior to this time, the tendency of the patient's urine to darken on standing may go unnoticed, as may slight pigmentation of the sclerae and ears. The latter manifestations are generally the earliest external evidence of the disorder and develop after age 20 to 30. Foci of gray-brown scleral pigment and generalized darkening of the concha, anthelix, and finally, helix of the ear are typical. Ear cartilages may be irregular and thickened. *Ochronotic arthritis* is heralded by pain, stiffness, and some limitation of motion of the hips, knees, and shoulders. Acute arthritis may resemble rheumatoid arthritis, but small joints are usually spared. Limitation of motion and ankylosis of the lumbosacral spine are common late manifestations. Pigmentation of heart valves, larynx, tympanic membranes, and skin occurs, and occasional patients develop pigmented renal or prostatic calculi. Degenerative cardiovascular disease may be increased in older patients.

Diagnosis   A patient whose urine darkens to blackness on standing must be suspected of having alkaptonuria, but this may not be observed with the use of modern plumbing conditions. The diagnosis is usually made from the triad of degenerative arthritis, ochronotic pigmentation, and urine that turns black upon alkalinization. Homogentisic acid in urine may be identified presumptively by other tests: after addition of ferric chloride, a purple-black color is observed; treatment with Benedict's reagent yields a brown color; addition of a saturated silver nitrate solution produces an intermediate black color. These screening tests can be confirmed by chromatographic, enzymatic, or spectrophotometric determinations of homogentisic acid. X-rays of the lumbar spine show degeneration and dense calcification of the intervertebral disks and narrowing of the intervertebral spaces (bamboo-like appearance).

℞ **TREATMENT**   There is no specific treatment for ochronotic arthritis. Joint manifestations might be mitigated if homogentisic acid accumulation and deposition could be curbed by dietary restriction of phenylalanine and tyrosine, but the long-term nature of the disease discourages such therapeutic attempts. Ascorbic acid impedes oxidation and polymerization of homogentisic acid in vitro, but the efficacy of this form of treatment has not been established. Symptomatic treatment is similar to that for osteoarthritis (Chap. 321).

CYSTINOSIS

Definition   Cystinosis is a rare disorder characterized by the intralysosomal accumulation of free cystine in body tissues. This results in the appearance of cystine crystals in the cornea, conjunctiva, bone marrow, lymph nodes, leukocytes, and internal organs. Three variants have been identified: an infantile (nephropathic) form leading to the Fanconi syndrome and renal insufficiency in the first decade, a juvenile (intermediate) form in which renal disease is manifest during the second decade, and an adult (benign) form characterized by deposition of cystine in the cornea but not in the kidney.

§ **GENETIC CONSIDERATIONS**   All types are inherited as autosomal recessive traits. The gene for the infantile form of nephropathic cystinosis encodes an integral membrane protein, which is a putative lysosomal cystine transporter. The gene is located on chromosome 17p13 and is designated *CTNS*. It is highly expressed in the pancreas, kidney, skeletal muscle, placenta, and heart. A common 65-kb deletion accounts for the majority of patients of European ancestry with infantile cystinosis. The juvenile- and adult-onset forms of nephropathic cystinosis are allelic with the infantile form. Obligate heterozygotes have intracellular cystine concentrations intermediate between those of normal persons and affected patients, but they are free of clinical abnormalities.

The basic defect involves impaired efflux of cystine from lysosomes rather than an abnormality in cystine catabolism. Lysosomal cystine efflux is an active, ATP-dependent process. The cystine content of tissues may be more than 100 times normal in the infantile form and more than 30 times normal in the adult form. Intracellular cystine in lysosomes does not exchange with other intra- or extracellular pools of this amino acid. Neither plasma nor urinary concentrations of cystine are particularly elevated. Cystine accumulation in the kidney causes renal insufficiency in the infantile and juvenile forms. Patchy depigmentation and degeneration of the peripheral retina occur in the infantile and juvenile forms. Cystine crystals may also be deposited in the cornea, ocular conjunctiva, or uvea. ■

Clinical Manifestations   In the infantile form, abnormalities are usually apparent by 6 to 10 months of age. Growth retardation, vomiting, fever, vitamin D–resistant rickets, polyuria, dehydration, and metabolic acidosis are prominent. Generalized proximal tubular dysfunction (the Fanconi syndrome) leads to hyperphosphaturia and hypophosphatemia, renal glycosuria, generalized amino aciduria, low plasma carnitine, hypouricemia, and often hypokalemia. Death due to uremia or intercurrent infection usually occurs before age 10. Ocular manifestations are prominent. Photophobia is usually demonstrable within the first years of life due to cystine deposits in the cornea, and retinal degeneration may appear even earlier. Hypothyroidism, insulin-dependent diabetes mellitus, and delayed puberty are often observed in older patients.

In contrast, patients with the adult form have only ocular abnormalities. Photophobia, headache, and burning or itching of the eyes are major complaints. Glomerular and tubular function and the integrity of the retina are preserved. The findings in the juvenile variant fall between these extremes. Ocular and renal manifestations do not become significant until the second decade. The renal lesion, albeit milder than that in the infantile form, eventually leads to renal insufficiency.

Diagnosis   Cystinosis must be considered in any child with vitamin D–resistant rickets, the Fanconi syndrome, or glomerular insufficiency. Hexagonal or rectangular cystine crystals can be detected in the cornea (by slit-lamp examination), in leukocytes from peripheral blood or bone marrow, or in biopsies of rectal mucosa. Diagnosis is confirmed by measurement of cystine in leukocytes. The infantile form has been diagnosed prenatally by the demonstration of increased cystine content in cultured amniotic fluid cells.

℞ **TREATMENT**   The adult form is benign and requires no treatment. Symptomatic treatment of renal disease in the infantile or juvenile form includes maintenance of adequate fluid intake to prevent dehydration; correction of the metabolic acidosis; administration of supplementary calcium, phosphate, and vitamin D to heal the rickets; and carnitine supplements (100 mg/kg per day) to correct the increased urinary losses. Specific therapy with the free thiol cysteamine slows the progression of renal dysfunction and improves growth. This compound acts in lysosomes by forming a mixed disulfide with cysteine, allowing it to be transported out of the organelle by an unrelated transporter not affected by the disease. Treatment is more effective if initiated before the patient is 2 years of age. Eye drops containing cysteamine can remove corneal crystals but requires frequent applications (10 to 14 times a day).

Children with nephropathic cystinosis and end-stage renal disease benefit from kidney transplantation. Patients who tolerate the procedure and do not develop immunologic problems have return of kidney function toward normal. The transplanted kidneys have not developed the functional abnormalities typical of cystinosis (i.e., the Fanconi syndrome or glomerular insufficiency). Patients may, however, continue to accumulate cystine in the cornea and other organs (thyroid, brain, and muscle).

PRIMARY HYPEROXALURIA

Definition Primary hyperoxaluria is the designation for two rare autosomal recessive disorders characterized by chronic excessive urinary excretion of oxalic acid and by calcium oxalate nephrolithiasis and nephrocalcinosis. Typically, patients with both forms develop renal insufficiency early in life and die of uremia. Calcium oxalate deposits are widespread in renal and extrarenal tissues, causing a condition referred to as *oxalosis*.

GENETIC CONSIDERATIONS The metabolic basis for the primary hyperoxalurias involves pathways of glyoxylate metabolism. In type I hyperoxaluria, urinary excretion of oxalate and of the oxidized and reduced forms of glyoxylate is increased. The excessive synthesis of these substances results from a block in glyoxylate metabolism. The primary defect in most patients is deficiency of the hepatic peroxisomal enzyme alanine:glyoxylate amino transferase. The gene (*AGXT*) for this enzyme maps to 2q36-37, and several distinct mutations have been defined in patients with type I hyperoxaluria. Some of these mutations misdirect the enzyme to mitochondria and render it nonfunctional.

In type II hyperoxaluria, L-glyceric acid is excreted in excess along with oxalate. In this condition, activity of D-glyceric acid dehydrogenase, which catalyzes the reduction of hydroxypyruvate to D-glyceric acid in the catabolic pathway of serine metabolism, is absent in leukocytes (and presumably other tissues). The accumulated hydroxypyruvate is instead reduced by lactic dehydrogenase to the L-isomer of glycerate, which is excreted in the urine. The same enzyme possesses glyoxylate reductase activity, and its deficiency promotes the oxidation of glyoxylate to oxalate, thus causing the formation of increased oxalate.

Stone formation, nephrocalcinosis, and oxalosis are due to insolubility of calcium oxalate. Extrarenal deposits of oxalate are prominent in the heart, walls of arteries and veins, male urogenital tract, and bone, particularly in type I hyperoxaluria. ■

Clinical Manifestations Nephrolithiasis and oxalosis may be manifest during the first year of life. Most patients experience renal colic or hematuria between ages 2 and 10 and succumb to uremia before age 20. With the onset of uremia, patients may develop severe peripheral arterial spasm and necrosis with resulting vascular insufficiency. Oxalate excretion falls as renal failure worsens. In patients with delayed onset of symptoms, survival to age 50 or 60 has been reported, despite recurrent nephrolithiasis. Type II hyperoxaluria is a milder disease with less involvement of extrarenal organs and delayed impairment of kidney function.

Diagnosis Oxalate excretion in normal children or adults is <0.5 mmol (60 mg) per 1.73 m^2 surface area per day. Patients with type I or type II hyperoxaluria excrete two to four times this amount. Distinction between the two types depends on the identification of the other organic acids that identify them: glycolic acid in type I and L-glyceric acid in type II. Since patients with pyridoxine deficiency or chronic ileal disease may excrete excessive amounts of oxalate, these conditions must be excluded.

TREATMENT There is no satisfactory treatment. Increasing the volume of urine can transiently reduce urinary oxalate concentration. Large doses of pyridoxine (100 mg/d) may reduce urinary oxalate in some patients, but long-term effects are not dramatic. A diet high in phosphate content seems to reduce the frequency of attacks of renal colic, but oxalate excretion is unaffected. Combined liver-kidney transplantation can correct the enzyme deficiency and replace the damaged organs. Liver transplantation seems promising in patients diagnosed before the onset of kidney failure.

ACKNOWLEDGMENT
This chapter includes the contributions of Dr. Leon E. Rosenberg and Dr. Louis J. Elsas from previous editions.

BIBLIOGRAPHY

DANPURE CJ: Primary hyperoxaluria, in *The Molecular and Metabolic Bases of Inherited Disease*, 8th ed, CR Scriver et al (eds). New York, McGraw-Hill, 2001, pp 3323–3367

ELSAS LJ, ACOSTA PB: Nutritional support of inherited metabolic diseases, in *Modern Nutrition in Health and Disease*, 9th ed, ME Shils et al (eds). Baltimore, Williams & Wilkins, 1998, Chap 61

GAHL WA: Cystinosis: A disorder of lysosomal membrane transport, in *The Molecular and Metabolic Bases of Inherited Disease*, 8th ed, CR Scriver et al (eds). New York, McGraw-Hill, 2001, pp 5085–5108

LA DU BN: Alkaptonuria, in *The Molecular and Metabolic Bases of Inherited Disease*, 8th ed, CR Scriver et al (eds). New York, McGraw-Hill, 2001, pp 2109–2123

MUDD SH et al: Disorders of transsulfuration, in *The Molecular and Metabolic Bases of Inherited Disease*, 8th ed, CR Scriver et al (eds). New York, McGraw-Hill, 2001, pp 2007–2056

NYHAN WL, OZAND PT: *Atlas of Metabolic Diseases*. London, Chapman & Hall Medical, 1998

ROSENBERG LE, SCRIVER CR: Disorders of amino acid metabolism, in *Metabolic Control and Disease*, 8th ed, PK Bondy, LE Rosenberg (eds). Philadelphia, Saunders, 1980, pp 583–776

ROSENBLATT DS, FENTON WA: Inherited disorders of folate and cobalamin transport and metabolism, in *The Molecular and Metabolic Bases of Inherited Disease*, 8th ed, CR Scriver et al (eds). New York, McGraw-Hill, 2001, pp 3897–3933

SCRIVER CR, KAUFMAN S: Hyperphenylalaninemia: Phenylalanine hydroxylase deficiency, in *The Molecular and Metabolic Bases of Inherited Disease*, 8th ed, CR Scriver et al (eds). New York, McGraw-Hill, 2001, pp 1667–1724

353 *Nicola Longo*

INHERITED DEFECTS OF MEMBRANE TRANSPORT

Specific membrane transporters mediate the passage of a wide variety of substances across plasma cell membranes. Classes of substrates represented include amino acids, sugars, cations, anions, vitamins, and water. The disorders considered in this chapter have three features in common: each is characterized by a specific defect in the transport of one or more compounds; each is inherited as a dominant or recessive trait, implying that variation in a single genetic locus is involved; and each is presumed to reflect a primary alteration in a specific membrane protein. Many of these defects have been well characterized physiologically and genetically. Inherited defects impairing the transport of amino acids, hexoses, and chloride are discussed here as examples of the abnormalities encountered; others are considered elsewhere in this text.

The number of inherited disorders of membrane transport continues to increase with the identification of new transporters and the clarification of the molecular basis of diseases with previously unknown pathophysiology. The first transport disorders identified affected the gut or the kidney, but transport processes are now proving essential for the normal function of every organ. Mutations in transporter molecules have been demonstrated in disorders of the heart, muscle, brain, and endocrine and sensory organs (see examples in Table 353-1). In some cases, the same phenotype can be caused by mutations in different genes (*nonallelic heterogeneity*), often because they encode interacting proteins. In other cases, distinct mutations in the same gene (*allelic heterogeneity*) can cause different diseases depending on the degree of functional inactivation caused by the mutation, the presence of dominant-negative effects, or paradoxical activation of function.

Table 353-1 Genetic Disorders of Membrane Transport

Class of Substance and Disorder	Individual Substrates	Tissues Manifesting Transport Defect	Proposed Molecular Basis of Defect	Major Clinical Manifestations	Mode of Inheritance	Location of Discussion
AMINO ACIDS						
Classic cystinuria	Cystine, lysine, arginine, ornithine	Proximal renal tubule, jejunal mucosa	Shared dibasic-cystine transport protein	Cystine nephrolithiasis	Autosomal recessive	Chap. 353
Dibasic amino-aciduria	Lysine, arginine, ornithine	Proximal renal tubule, jejunal mucosa	Dibasic transport protein	Type I: Benign; Type II: Protein intolerance, hyperammonemia, retardation	Autosomal recessive	Chap. 353
Hypercystinuria	Cystine	Proximal renal tubule	Cystine transport protein	Some risk of cystine nephrolithiasis	Autosomal recessive	Chap. 353
Lysinuria	Lysine	Proximal renal tubule, jejunal mucosa	Lysine transport protein	Seizures, physical and mental retardation	Possible autosomal recessive	Chap. 353
Hartnup disease	Neutral amino acids	Proximal renal tubule, jejunal mucosa	Shared neutral amino acid transport protein	Constant neutral aminoaciduria, intermittent symptoms of pellagra	Autosomal recessive	Chap. 353
Tryptophan malabsorption	Tryptophan	Jejunal mucosa	Tryptophan transport protein	Indoluria, ?hypercalcemia, ?nephrocalcinosis	Probable autosomal recessive	Chap. 353
Methionine malabsorption	Methionine	Jejunal mucosa	Methionine transport protein	α-Hydroxybutyricaciduria, white hair, mental retardation, convulsions, hyperpneic attacks, edema	Probable autosomal recessive	Chap. 353
Histidinuria	Histidine	Proximal renal tubule, jejunal mucosa	Histidine transport protein	Mental retardation	Autosomal recessive	Chap. 353
Iminoglycinuria	Glycine, proline, hydroxyproline	Proximal renal tubule, jejunal mucosa	Shared glycine–imino acid transport protein	None	Autosomal recessive	Chap. 353
Dicarboxylicaminoaciduria	Glutamic acid, aspartic acid	Proximal renal tubule, jejunal mucosa	Shared dicarboxylic amino acid transport protein	None	Probable autosomal recessive	Chap. 353
Cystinosis	Cystine	Lysosomal membranes	Cystine transport protein	Renal failure, hypothyroidism, blindness	Autosomal recessive	Chap. 352
HEXOSES						
Renal glycosuria	D-Glucose	Proximal renal tubule	D-glucose transport protein (Na$^+$-dependent)	Glycosuria with normal blood glucose	Autosomal recessive	Chap. 353
Glucose-galactose malabsorption	D-Glucose, D-Galactose	Jejunal mucosa, proximal renal tubule	Shared Na$^+$-dependent glucose-galactose transport protein	Watery diarrhea on feeding glucose, lactose, sucrose, or galactose	Autosomal recessive	Chaps. 286, 352
Glucose-transporter protein syndrome	D-Glucose	Ubiquitous	Facilitative glucose transporter GLUT1	Seizures, mental retardation	Autosomal recessive	Chap. 353
Fanconi-Bickel syndrome	D-Glucose	Liver, kidney, pancreas, intestine	Facilitative glucose transporter GLUT2	Growth retardation rickets, hepatorenal glycogenosis, hypo- and hyperglycemia	Autosomal recessive	Chap. 353
Glycogen storage disease type ID (?)	D-Glucose	Liver microsomes	Facilitative glucose transporter GLUT7	Hypoglycemia, neutropenia, glycogen storage disease	Autosomal recessive	Chap. 350
LIPIDS						
Familial hypercholesterolemia	Cholesterol	Fibroblasts, lymphoid lines, leukocytes	Membrane LDL–cholesterol receptor protein	Hypercholesterolemia, tendon xanthomas, arcus corneae, coronary artery atherosclerosis	Autosomal dominant	Chap. 344

(continued)

Table 353-1—(continued)

Class of Substance and Disorder	Individual Substrates	Tissues Manifesting Transport Defect	Proposed Molecular Basis of Defect	Major Clinical Manifestations	Mode of Inheritance	Location of Discussion
Defect in transport of long-chain fatty acids	Long-chain fatty acids	Liver	Fatty acid transporter	Nonketotic hypoglycemia, acute liver failure	Autosomal recessive	
URATE						
Hypouricemia	Uric acid	Proximal renal tubule	Urate transport protein	Hypouricemia, hyperuricosuria, ?hypercalciuria	Autosomal recessive	Chap. 278
ANIONS						
Familial hypophosphatemic rickets	Inorganic phosphate	Proximal renal tubule, jejunal mucosa	Phosphate-regulator homologue to endopeptidases PHEX	Hypophosphatemia, phosphaturia, phosphopenic rickets/osteomalacia	X-linked dominant	Chap. 342
Congenital chloridorrhea	Chloride, sulfate	Ileal and colonic mucosa	Cl^-/HCO_3^- exchange pump carrier protein (DRA)	Hydramnios, watery diarrhea, elevated fecal chloride, achloriduria, metabolic alkalosis with volume depletion, hyperaldosteronism	Autosomal recessive	Chaps. 286, 353
Dent's syndrome, X-linked recessive hypophosphatemic rickets and nephrocalcinosis	Chloride, phosphate	Proximal renal tubule	Voltage-gated Cl^- channel CLCN5	Proteinuria, hypercalciuria, nephrocalcinosis, nephrolithiasis, rickets	X-linked recessive	Chap. 342
Hypophosphatemic rickets with hypercalciuria	Phosphate	Renal tubule	Phosphate transporter	Hypophosphatemic rickets, hypercalciuria	Autosomal recessive	Chap. 342
Bartter's syndrome	Sodium, chloride	Renal tubule	Na,K,2·Cl cotransporter, apical ATP-regulated K^+ channel, basolateral Cl^- channel	Hypochloremic metabolic alkalosis, hypercalciuria, hyperaldosteronism	Autosomal recessive	Chaps. 49, 276
Gitelman's syndrome	Sodium, chloride	Distal convoluted tubule	Na^+/Cl^- cotransporter SLC12A3	Hypokalemic metabolic alkalosis, hypomagnesemia, hypocalciuria	Autosomal recessive	Chaps. 49, 276
Congenital myotonia	Chloride	Muscle	Cl^- channel CLCN1	Myotonia, muscle cramps	Autosomal dominant and recessive	Chap. 383
Pendred syndrome	Iodide, chloride	Thyroid, cochlea	Na^+-independent I^- and Cl^- transporter	Deafness, ± goiter	Autosomal recessive	Chap. 330
Cystic fibrosis	Chloride	Lung, pancreas, sweat gland	Ion channel protein	Pulmonary, pancreatic destruction	Autosomal recessive	Chap. 257
Distal renal tubular acidosis (type I—gradient)	Chloride, bicarbonate	Distal renal tubule, erythrocytes	Anion exchanger SLC4A1	Hyperchloremic acidosis, hypokalemia, acquired nephrocalcinosis, hypercalciuria, elliptocytosis	Autosomal dominant	Chap. 276
Familial goiter	Inorganic iodide	Thyroid gland, salivary gland, gastric mucosa	Iodide transport protein	Congenital hypothyroidism (cretinism), goiter	Probable autosomal recessive	Chap. 330
Achondrogenesis type 1B, astelosteogenesis type 2, diatrophic dysplasia	Sulfate	Osteoblasts, chondrocytes	Sulfate transporter	Skeletal dysplasia, dwarfism, deformities	Autosomal recessive	Chap. 343
Dubin-Johnson syndrome	Bile acids	Liver	Biliary organic anion transporter ABCC2	Jaundice, hepatomegaly, conjugated hyperbilirubinemia	Autosomal recessive	Chap. 294

(continued)

Table 353-1 Genetic Disorders of Membrane Transport—(*continued*)

Class of Substance and Disorder	Individual Substrates	Tissues Manifesting Transport Defect	Proposed Molecular Basis of Defect	Major Clinical Manifestations	Mode of Inheritance	Location of Discussion
CATIONS						
Proximal renal tubular acidosis (type II—HCO₃⁻ wasting)	Hydrogen ion	Proximal renal tubule	Proximal tubule H^+ pump carrier protein	Hyperchloremic acidosis, bicarbonate wasting	Probable autosomal recessive	Chap. 276
Menkes' disease	Copper	Most tissues except liver	Copper-transporting ATPase (ATP7A)	Severe mental retardation, pili torti (kinky hair), typical facies, arterial tortuosity, excess Wormian bones, thermal instability	X-Linked recessive	Chap. 355
Distal renal tubular acidosis	Hydrogen ion	Distal nephron, cochlea	H^+ ATPase ATP6B1	Hyperchloremic acidosis, growth retardation, sensineural deafness	Autosomal recessive	Chaps. 49, 276
Liddle's syndrome	Sodium	Collecting tubule	Epithelial Na^+ channel SCNN1 (activation)	Hypertension, hypokalemia, metabolic alkalosis	Autosomal dominant	Chaps. 49, 276
Type I pseudohypoaldosteronism	Sodium	Collecting tubule	Epithelial Na^+ channel SCNN1 (inactivation)	Hyponatremia, growth retardation, hyperkalemia	Autosomal recessive	Chaps. 49, 331
Hyperkalemic periodic paralysis, paramyotonia congenita	Sodium	Muscle	Muscle Na^+ channel α subunit SCN4A	Periodic paralysis, muscle wasting, variable myotonia	Autosomal dominant	Chap. 383
Nesidioblastosis of pancreas	Potassium	Pancreatic β cell	Sulfonylurea receptor SUR1, K^+ channel KCNJ11	Neonatal hypoglycemia, hyperinsulinemia	Autosomal recessive	Chap. 334
Wilson's disease	Copper	Liver and kidney	Copper-transporting ATPase (ATP7B)	Motor and psychiatric disturbances, hepatolenticular degeneration	Autosomal recessive	Chap. 348
Darier disease	Calcium	Keratinocytes, muscle, brain	Sarcoplasmic Ca^{2+}-ATPase ATP2A2	Keratotic skin papules, bullous lesions, psychosis	Autosomal dominant	Chap. 57
Long QT syndrome	Potassium, sodium	Heart	Voltage-gated K^+ channels KCNQ1, KCNH2, KCNE2, Na^+ channel SCN5A	Syncope, arrhythmia, sudden death	Autosomal dominant	Chap. 230
Jervell and Lange-Nielsen syndrome	Potassium	Heart, inner ear	Voltage-gated K^+ channels KCNQ1, KCNE1	Syncope, arrhythmia, sudden death, deafness	Autosomal recessive	Chap. 234
Benign familial neonatal epilepsy	Potassium	Brain	Voltage-gated K^+ channels KCNQ2, KCNQ3	Neonatal convulsions normal development	Autosomal dominant	Chap. 360
WATER						
Nephrogenic diabetes insipidus (AVP-resistant)	Water	Distal renal tubule	AVP receptor	Polyuria, polydipsia, hyposthenuria	X-linked recessive	Chap. 276, 329
Nephrogenic diabetes insipidus	Water	Collecting tubule	Aquaporin 2 (water channel)	Polyuria, dehydration, hyposthenuria	Autosomal recessive and dominant	Chap. 329
VITAMINS						
Juvenile pernicious anemia	Cobalamin (vitamin B_{12})	Ileal mucosa	Receptor for intrinsic factor–cobalamin complex	Megaloblastic anemia	Autosomal recessive	Chap. 107
Folate malabsorption	Folic acid	Small bowel	Folate transport protein	Megaloblastic anemia	Autosomal recessive	Chap. 107

(continued)

Table 353-1—(continued)

Class of Substance and Disorder	Individual Substrates	Tissues Manifesting Transport Defect	Proposed Molecular Basis of Defect	Major Clinical Manifestations	Mode of Inheritance	Location of Discussion
Rogers' syndrome	Thiamine	Ubiquitous	Thiamine transporter SLC19A2	Megaloblastic anemia, diabetes, deafness	Autosomal recessive	Chap. 75
OTHER						
Sialic acid storage	Sialic acid (monosaccharide)	Lysosomes	Sialic acid transport protein AST	Retardation	Autosomal recessive	Chap. 349
Carnitine transport	Carnitine	Muscle, kidney, fibroblasts	High-affinity carnitine transporter OCTN2	Hypoketotic hypoglycemia, cardiomyopathy, hypotonia	Autosomal recessive	Chap. 334
Benign recurrent and progressive familial intrahepatic cholestasis	Bile salts	Liver	Phosphatidylcholine transporter MDR3, phospholipid transporter FIC1, bile salt export pump	Cholestasis, hepatomegaly, cirrhosis, liver failure	Autosomal recessive	Chap. 294
Primary bile acid malabsorption	Bile salts	Gut	Na⁺-dependent bile acid transporter	Congenital diarrhea, steatorrhea	Autosomal recessive	Chap. 294
Glycogen storage disease type Ib	D-Glucose	Liver microsomes	Glucose-6-phosphate transporter	Hypoglycemia, neutropenia, glycogen storage disease	Autosomal recessive	Chap. 350

DISORDERS OF AMINO ACID TRANSPORT

As listed in Table 353-1, 10 disorders of amino acid transport have been described. Five (cystinuria, dibasic aminoaciduria, Hartnup disease, iminoglycinuria, and dicarboxylic aminoaciduria) show transport abnormalities for structurally related amino acids, thereby implying the existence of group-specific membrane receptors or carriers. With the exception of iminoglycinuria and dicarboxylic aminoaciduria, the defects have important clinical consequences. The remaining five disorders affect the transport of only one amino acid, implying the existence of substrate-specific transport systems. Each of these conditions affects transport in the kidney, gut, or both; none has been shown to alter transport in other tissues.

CYSTINURIA **Definition** Cystinuria, the most common inborn error of amino acid transport, is characterized by impaired renal tubular reabsorption and excessive urinary excretion of the dibasic amino acids lysine, arginine, ornithine, and cystine. A similar transport defect exists in the intestinal mucosa. Because cystine is the least soluble of the naturally occurring amino acids, its overexcretion predisposes to the formation of renal, ureteral, and bladder stones. Such stones are responsible for the signs and symptoms of the disorder.

GENETIC CONSIDERATIONS Cystinuria is among the most common inborn errors, with a frequency of 1 in 10,000 to 1 in 15,000 in many ethnic groups. The disorder is transmitted as an autosomal recessive trait and results from impaired function of membrane carrier proteins in the apical brush border of proximal renal tubule and small intestinal cells.

There are three genetic variants of cystinuria. The urinary excretion patterns and renal clearance abnormalities in each type are similar in homozygotes, but the three variants are distinguished by studies of intestinal transport in homozygotes and urinary excretion patterns in heterozygotes. Type I homozygotes lack mediated intestinal transport of cystine, lysine, arginine, and ornithine; heterozygotes have normal urinary amino acid excretion patterns. Type II homozygotes lack mediated lysine transport in the gut but retain some capacity for cystine transport; heterozygotes have moderately increased urinary excretion of each of the four amino acids. Type III homozygotes retain some capacity for mediated intestinal transport of the four involved substrates; heterozygotes have modestly increased urinary lysine and cystine. The gene for type I cystinuria (*SLC3A1*) encodes solute carrier family 3 and maps to chromosome 2p16.3. The other two types of

cystinuria (types II and III) are caused by mutations in *SLC7A9*, which maps to chromosome 19q13 and encodes the light subunit needed for the correct processing of SLC3A1. ■

Clinical Manifestations Massive excretion of cystine and the other dibasic amino acids occurs in homozygotes with classic cystinuria. Cystine stones account for 1 to 2% of all urinary tract calculi but are the most common cause of stones in children. The maximum solubility of cystine in the physiologic urinary pH range of 4.5 to 7.0 is about 1200 μmol/L (300 mg/L). Since affected homozygotes regularly excrete 2400 to 7200 μmol (600 to 1800 mg) daily, crystalluria and stone formation are a constant threat. Stone formation usually becomes manifest in the second or third decade but may occur in the first year of life or as bladder calculi at birth. Symptoms and signs are those typical of urolithiasis: hematuria, flank pain, renal colic, obstructive uropathy, and infection (Chap. 279). Recurrent urolithiasis may lead to progressive renal insufficiency.

Diagnosis The presence of cystine in a urinary tract stone is pathognomonic of cystinuria. However, because half the stones in cystinuric individuals are of mixed composition, and because the cystine core in as many as 10% may not be detected, a urinary nitroprusside test should be performed on all patients with urolithiasis to exclude this diagnosis. The nitroprusside test is also positive (appearance of a cherry red color) in some heterozygotes for cystinuria and in patients with hypercystinuria, homocystinuria, and mercaptolactate-cysteine disulfiduria. When cystine content exceeds 1000 μmol/L (250 mg/L), cystine crystals may be seen in the sediment of acidified, concentrated, chilled urine. These hexagonal crystals are pathognomonic of cystine overexcretion in patients not taking sulfonamides.

Diagnostic confirmation of cystinuria depends on demonstration of the characteristic amino acid excretion pattern in the urine. Selective overexcretion of cystine, lysine, arginine, and ornithine can be demonstrated by qualitative and quantitative chromatography. Quantitation is important for differentiating heterozygotes from homozygotes and for following free cystine excretion during therapy.

TREATMENT Management is aimed at preventing cystine crystal formation by reducing the concentration of cystine in urine. This aim is accomplished by increasing urinary volume and by maintaining an alkaline urine pH. Fluid ingestion in excess of 4 L/d is essential, and 5 to 7 L/d is optimal. Urinary cystine concentration should be <1000 to 1200 μmol/L (250 to 300 mg/L). The daily fluid ingestion necessary to maintain this dilution of excreted cystine should be spaced over 24 h, with one-third of the total volume ingested between bedtime and 2 to 3 A.M. Stones can be prevented and even dissolved by such hydration. It must be made clear to individuals with cystinuria that water is a necessary drug for them. Solubility of cystine in urine rises sharply above pH 7.5, and urinary alkalinization can be therapeutic in some situations. Vigorous administration of sodium bicarbonate, acetazolamide, and polycitrates is required to maintain a persistently alkaline pH, but this measure introduces the danger of inducing formation of calcium oxalate, calcium phosphate, and magnesium ammonium phosphate stones and of producing nephrocalcinosis.

Another treatment involves administration of penicillamine, which undergoes sulfhydryl-disulfide exchange with cystine to form the mixed disulfide of penicillamine and cysteine. Since this disulfide is more than 50 times as soluble as cystine, penicillamine (1 to 3 g/d) reduces free cystine excretion markedly, thereby preventing new stone formation and promoting dissolution of existing calculi. Unfortunately, side effects include acute serum sickness, agranulocytosis, pancytopenia, immune glomerulitis, and the Goodpasture syndrome. Thus its use should be reserved for patients who fail to respond to hydration alone or who are in a high-risk category (one remaining kidney, renal insufficiency). Tiopronin (α-mercaptopropionylglycine, 800 to 1200 mg/d in four divided doses) has a mechanism of action similar to that of penicillamine, has lower toxicity, and is a suitable alternative. Captopril, a sulfhydryl-containing antihypertensive agent, has limited efficacy to reduce cystine excretion. When medical management fails, urologic surgery is required, but it should be a last resort as cystine stones reform more easily in scarred epithelium. Small (<1.5 cm) cystine stones can be treated with extracorporeal shock wave lithotripsy. Ureteroscopic removal is effective for ureteral stones, while larger or branched cystine stones require percutaneous nephrostolithotomy, sometimes associated with other procedures. All these procedures may produce smaller fragments, which can cause severe renal colic. Occasional patients progress to renal failure and require kidney transplantation.

DIBASIC AMINOACIDURIA   This disorder is characterized by a defect in renal tubular reabsorption of the three dibasic amino acids lysine, arginine, and ornithine but *not* cystine. There are two variants, transmitted as autosomal recessive traits. In the common form of dibasic aminoaciduria (type II), also known as *lysinuric protein intolerance*, homozygotes show defective intestinal transport of dibasic amino acids as well as exaggerated renal losses. It is most common in Finland (1 in 60,000) and is rare elsewhere. The transport defect affects basolateral rather than luminal membrane transport and is associated with impairment of the urea cycle. The defective gene (*SLC7A7*) in this condition maps to chromosome 14q11.2 and encodes a unique membrane transporter, y$^+$LAT, that associates with the cell-surface glycoprotein 4F2 heavy chain to form the complete sodium-independent transporter y$^+$L. The requirement for multiple gene products in the formation of this dimeric transporter probably explains part of the intrafamilial variability observed in lysinuric protein intolerance.

Manifestations are related to the losses of ornithine, arginine, and lysine. Affected patients present in childhood with hepatosplenomegaly, protein intolerance, and episodic ammonia intoxication. Older patients may present with severe osteoporosis, impairment of kidney function, or interstitial changes in the lungs. Plasma concentrations of lysine, arginine, and ornithine are reduced, whereas urinary excretion of lysine and orotic acid are increased. Hyperammonemia may develop after the ingestion of protein loads or with infections, probably due to insufficient amounts of arginine and ornithine to maintain proper function of the urea cycle. The clinical features have been attributed to the hyperammonemia and to insufficient amounts of lysine to support protein synthesis during growth.

Type I dibasic aminoaciduria has been described in a large French-Canadian kindred. Type I patients have profound mental retardation without hyperammonemia and protein intolerance. The condition also differs from type II by the presence of a modest excess of dibasic amino acids in the urine of asymptomatic heterozygotes. Type I disease may involve the same transport system as that impaired in the more common type II dibasic aminoaciduria.

℞ **TREATMENT**   Dietary protein should be restricted in conjunction with supplementation of citrulline (2 to 8 g/d), a neutral amino acid that fuels the urea cycle when metabolized to arginine and ornithine. Carnitine supplements may improve growth by sparing lysine and by enhancing fatty acid oxidation. Pulmonary disease responds to glycocorticoids in some patients.

HARTNUP DISEASE   Pellagra-like skin lesions, variable neurologic manifestations, and neutral or aromatic aminoaciduria characterize this disease. Alanine, serine, threonine, valine, leucine, isoleucine, phenylalanine, tyrosine, tryptophan, glutamine, asparagine, and histidine are excreted in urine in quantities 5 to 10 times normal, and intestinal transport of these same amino acids is defective. The clinical manifestations result from nutritional deficiency of the essential amino acid tryptophan, caused by its intestinal and renal malabsorption. Manifestations are episodic, related in part to metabolic demands for tryptophan. Only a small fraction of patients with the chemical findings of this disorder develop a pellagra-like syndrome, implying that manifestations depend on other factors in addition to the transport defect.

Hartnup disease is inherited as an autosomal recessive trait, and the gene has been mapped to chromosome 11q13. Homozygotes occur with a frequency of about 1 in 24,000 births. Heterozygotes exhibit no clinical or chemical abnormalities. In patients with Hartnup disease, the renal and intestinal transport defect for tryptophan leads to niacin deficiency. Tryptophan metabolism leads to the synthesis of niacin and nicotinamide-adenine dinucleotide and supplies about half the daily niacin needs. The transport defect likely reflects abnormalities of a group-specific system for neutral amino acids. Some residual reabsorptive capacity persists for each involved amino acid. This suggests that they are transported by other carrier systems as well, a conclusion supported by the identification of patients with substrate-specific transport defects for tryptophan, methionine, and histidine.

The diagnosis of Hartnup disease should be suspected in any patient with clinical features of pellagra without a history of dietary niacin deficiency (Chap. 75). The neurologic and psychiatric manifestations range from attacks of cerebellar ataxia to mild emotional lability to frank delirium and are usually accompanied by exacerbations of the erythematous, eczematoid skin rash. Fever, sunlight, stress, and sulfonamide therapy provoke clinical relapses. Diagnosis is made by detection of the neutral aminoaciduria, which does not occur in dietary niacin deficiency. Treatment is directed at niacin repletion and includes a high-protein diet and daily nicotinamide supplementation (50 to 250 mg). Tryptophan ethyl esters can also bypass the absorption defect.

IMINOGLYCINURIA   This benign autosomal recessive trait is characterized by excessive urinary excretion of glycine and the imino acids proline and hydroxyproline. Homozygotes occur with a frequency of about 1 in 16,000. The enhanced excretion of glycine, proline, and hydroxyproline reflects a defect in the tubular transport system shared by these three compounds. An intestinal transport defect may also be present. This suggests that more than one mutation may lead to iminoglycinuria, a thesis corroborated by the demonstration that obligate heterozygotes from some, but not all, families have glycinuria. No consistent clinical abnormalities have been reported in homozygotes that are usually detected by urinary amino acid screening programs.

DICARBOXYLIC AMINOACIDURIA   Selective urinary loss and exaggerated endogenous renal clearance of glutamic and aspartic acids have been described in two unrelated children. Intestinal absorption of these dicarboxylic amino acids was impaired in one. This patient suffered from recurrent hypoglycemia; the other was asymptomatic.

SUBSTRATE-SPECIFIC DEFECTS IN AMINO ACID TRANSPORT Rare pedigrees exist in which individuals have defective renal tubular reabsorption and/or impaired intestinal absorption of a single free amino acid (Table 353-1). These disorders, each apparently inherited as an autosomal recessive trait, suggest that transport of amino acids is catalyzed by substrate-specific as well as group-specific transport mechanisms. Examples include hypercystinuria, lysinuria, histidinuria, and selective malabsorption of methionine or tryptophan.

DISORDERS OF HEXOSE TRANSPORT

D-Glucose is the major carbohydrate used by the cell for energy production and many other anabolic purposes. A number of transporter proteins work together to maintain glucose homeostasis in the intact organism by coordinating absorption and utilization of D-glucose by all cells in the body. Two main classes of glucose transporters have been identified in humans: active Na^+-glucose cotransporters (SGLT) and the facilitative glucose transporters (GLUT). Na^+-glucose cotransporters actively concentrate glucose inside intestinal and renal cells using the electrochemical potential of Na^+ as their energy source. Defects in this class of transporters cause renal glycosuria (SGLT2) and intestinal glucose-galactose malabsorption (SGLT1). Facilitative glucose transporters allow glucose to enter cells using its own concentration gradient. This process is essential for the delivery of glucose to the cell for energy production. Defects in facilitative transporters cause the glucose-transporter protein syndrome (GLUT1) and the Fanconi-Bickel syndrome (GLUT2) and may be involved in one subtype of glycogen storage disorder (GLUT7).

DISORDERS OF CONCENTRATIVE GLUCOSE TRANSPORTERS *Renal glycosuria* is characterized by the urinary excretion of glucose at normal concentrations of blood glucose. The renal tubular malabsorption is specific for glucose. Unlike generalized tubular dysfunction, other compounds such as phosphate and amino acids are transported normally. The genetic basis for this condition is not known at present. The condition is benign, but occasionally glycosuria may be severe enough to cause polyuria and polydipsia. Even more rarely, dehydration or ketosis may develop under conditions of stress such as pregnancy or starvation.

In normal persons, glucose is present in the glomerular filtrate at a concentration equal to that in plasma water and is reabsorbed throughout the proximal renal tubule by a sodium-dependent, phlorizin-inhibitable transport process. Reabsorptive capacity exceeds normal plasma glucose concentration. The plasma concentration at which filtered glucose begins to escape proximal tubular reabsorption is usually around 10 mmol/L (200 mg/dL). Maximal renal absorptive capacity is exceeded at a filtered load of around 2 mmol (325 mg)/min per 1.73 m² body surface area, and this value is defined as the tubular maximum for glucose (TmG).

Two patterns of glycosuria are recognized: type A, characterized by a reduced tubular maximum reabsorptive capacity, and type B, showing a reduced threshold for glycosuria, an increased "splay" in the titration curve, and a normal TmG. Renal glycosuria occurs in homozygotes with either of these recessively inherited mutations and in compound heterozygotes with these presumably allelic mutations. Modest reduction in renal threshold or TmG is present in heterozygotes in some families; modest glycosuria occurs in such family members when plasma glucose is elevated. In the few patients studied, renal glycosuria was not associated with impaired intestinal transport.

Glucose-galactose malabsorption is characterized by profuse, watery diarrhea in infants fed milk or foods containing lactose, sucrose, glucose, or galactose. The primary defect involves the sodium-hexose cotransporter in the intestinal and renal brush border. A specific defect in intestinal absorption of glucose and galactose can be demonstrated by oral tolerance tests that produce little or no increase in plasma glucose or galactose. Active D-glucose and D-galactose transport is absent in affected children, and intermediate transport capacity is present in their parents. Fructose-containing or carbohydrate-free formulas are well tolerated. Treatment with a glucose- and galactose-free diet leads to resolution of symptoms in childhood. Although the basic transport defect is present throughout life, most patients show an improved tolerance for glucose and galactose with age.

A number of these patients have renal glycosuria at normal plasma glucose concentrations. Renal titration studies generally demonstrate a reduced threshold for glucose reabsorption (type B renal glycosuria) and a normal TmG. Urinary glucose loss is not as severe as in isolated renal glycosuria. This finding suggests the presence of multiple glucose transport proteins in the kidney. One, whose gene remains to be identified, is responsible for the bulk of glucose reabsorption in the proximal convoluted tubule and is believed to be abnormal in renal glycosuria. Another transporter, SGLT1, is shared by glucose and galactose and is responsible for the reabsorption of the least traces of glucose in the late proximal straight tubule. Its function is abnormal in glucose-galactose malabsorption, and heterogeneous mutations have been found in the *SGLT1* gene on chromosome 22q. In glucose-galactose malabsorption, as in renal glycosuria, transport of sugars in other tissues is normal, reflecting the multiplicity and tissue specificity of hexose transporters.

DISORDERS OF FACILITATIVE GLUCOSE TRANSPORTERS At least five different facilitative glucose transporters (GLUT1, -2, -3, -4, and -7) mediate the influx and efflux of glucose in mammalian cells. Disease-causing mutations have been identified in two of these transporters (GLUT1 and GLUT2). The tissue specificity and redundancy of facilitative glucose transporters in different tissues helps to explain the clinical manifestations that result from their defective function. De novo mutations in the gene encoding the ubiquitous GLUT1 transporter cause the glucose-transporter protein syndrome. Patients present with seizures, developmental delay, and acquired microcephaly. These patients have normal blood glucose concentration but markedly decreased concentration of glucose in their cerebrospinal fluid. GLUT1 is the predominant glucose transporter in the blood-brain barrier. Haploinsufficiency reduces the transfer of glucose through the blood-brain barrier, restricting the energy supply to the brain. This defect is expressed in other cells, such as erythrocytes and fibroblasts, that have less stringent energy requirements or express additional glucose transporters, preventing cellular damage and clinical sequelae. Therapy in the glucose-transporter protein syndrome consists of using a ketogenic diet to deliver alternative fuels to the brain.

The GLUT2 transporter is expressed mainly in liver, pancreatic β cells, and in the basolateral membrane of gut and renal tubular cells. Truncating mutations in the *GLUT2* transporter gene have been identified in the autosomal recessive disorder Fanconi-Bickel syndrome. Patients present early in life with failure to thrive and polydipsia, with prominent glycosuria and aminoaciduria, rickets, fasting hypoglycemia with ketonuria, and prolonged postprandial hyperglycemia. Glycogen is accumulated in the liver and kidney, reflecting the inability to release glucose through the GLUT2 transporter. This results in fasting hypoglycemia and ketonuria and in generalized renal tubular dysfunction. The prolonged postprandial hyperglycemia is due to decreased sugar uptake by the liver and by the pancreatic β cell, the latter resulting in defective insulin synthesis and release. Affected patients do not develop diabetes because human pancreatic β cells have alternative glucose transporters (GLUT1 and GLUT3) that can partially compensate for the absence of GLUT2 transporters. Therapy consists of symptomatic replacement of the renal losses of water and electrolytes, vitamin D replacement, and a diet plan consisting of frequent meals rich in complex carbohydrates to prevent hypoglycemia, analogous to the treatment of patients with glycogen storage diseases (Chap. 350).

DEFECTIVE ANION TRANSPORT: CHLORIDORRHEA

This rare, autosomal recessive disease results from impairment of active transport of chloride in the ileum and colon. Absence of chloride-bicarbonate ion exchange causes profound symptoms even before birth (polyhydramnios and absence of meconium). Massive watery diarrhea is apparent from the first days of life. This fluid loss, with its attendant impairment of electrolyte homeostasis, is life-threatening. A hypokalemic, hypochloremic, hyponatremic metabolic alkalosis develops with dehydration and secondary hyperaldosteronism. Fecal fluid contains an excess of chloride ion over the sum of the accompanying cations sodium and potassium. Fecal chloride concentration always exceeds 90 mmol/L when volume and serum electrolyte disturbances are corrected, and this chloridorrhea is diagnostic. Renal chloride transport is normal. Decreased urine chloride results from the kidney's attempts to conserve salt and water. The defective gene in this condition, called *DRA* (for downregulated in adenoma), maps to chromosome 7q and encodes an anion transporter, which is expressed only in the gastrointestinal tract. A deletion of the Val 317 codon in the *DRA* gene is responsible for the Finnish form of congenital chloride diarrhea.

Treatment requires adequate, lifelong repletion of electrolyte and fluid losses. Exact replacement of water, sodium chloride, and potassium chloride can prevent the growth and psychomotor retardation and the development of progressive renal damage. The renal lesion, with hyalinized glomeruli, juxtaglomerular hyperplasia, calcifications, and arteriolar changes, is probably a result of chronic volume depletion. Treatment of hyperreninemia and hypokalemia with prostaglandin inhibitors may reduce renal damage but does not alter intestinal symptoms or the need for chronic sodium chloride repletion. Omeprazole, while not decreasing the need for adequate oral replacement of electrolytes, may decrease stool output and improve the social life of patients.

ACKNOWLEDGMENT
This chapter includes the contributions of Dr. Leon E. Rosenberg and Dr. Louis J. Elsas from previous editions.

BIBLIOGRAPHY

BORSANI G et al: SLC7A7, encoding a putative permease-related protein, is mutated in patients with lysinuric protein intolerance. Nat Genet 21:297, 1999

DESJEUX J-F et al: Congenital selective Na⁺ D-glucose cotransport defects leading to renal glycosuria and congenital selective intestinal malabsorption of glucose and galactose, in *The Molecular and Metabolic Bases of Inherited Disease*, 7th ed, CR Scriver et al (eds). New York, McGraw-Hill, 1995, pp 3563–3580

ELSAS LJ, ROSENBERG LE: Renal glycosuria, in *Strauss and Welt's Diseases of the Kidney*, 3d ed, LE Earley, CW Gottschalk (eds). Boston, Little, Brown, 1979, pp 1021–1028

LEVY HL: Hartnup disorder, in *The Molecular and Metabolic Bases of Inherited Disease*, 8th ed, CR Scriver et al (eds). New York, McGraw-Hill, 2001, pp 4957–4969

LONGO N, ELSAS LJ: Human glucose transporters. Adv Pediatr 45:293, 1998

PALACIN M et al: Cystinuria, in *The Molecular and Metabolic Bases of Inherited Disease*, 8th ed, CR Scriver et al (eds). New York, McGraw-Hill, 2001, pp 4909–4932

SHORT EM, ROSENBERG LE: Renal aminoaciduria, in *Strauss and Welt's Diseases of the Kidney*, 3d ed, LE Earley, CW Gottschalk (eds). Boston, Little, Brown, 1979, pp 975–1020

TORRENTS D et al: Identification of SLC7A7, encoding y+LAT-1, as the lysinuric protein intolerance gene. Nat Genet 21:293, 1999

354

Abhimanyu Garg

THE LIPODYSTROPHIES AND OTHER PRIMARY DISORDERS OF ADIPOSE TISSUE

The distribution and quantity of adipose tissue are controlled by multiple factors, including genetic background, diet, hormones, and exercise. The lipodystrophies are a heterogeneous group of adipose tissue disorders characterized by a selective loss of body fat (Tables 354-1 and 354-2). Patients with lipodystrophies have a propensity to develop insulin resistance, hypertriglyceridemia, diabetes mellitus, and fatty liver.

FAMILIAL OR GENETIC LIPODYSTROPHIES

CONGENITAL GENERALIZED LIPODYSTROPHY (BERARDINELLI-SEIP SYNDROME) *Clinical features* The primary diagnostic features of congenital generalized lipodystrophy (CGL) include a near-total lack of body fat and a marked muscular appearance from birth (Fig. 354-1A). On careful physical examination, however, fat can be detected in the palms and soles; with magnetic resonance imaging (MRI), normal amounts of fat can also be visualized in the orbits, scalp, perineum, and juxtaarticular and epidural regions (where the cushioning or protective functions of adipose tissue are critical). MRI studies also reveal a near-complete absence of metabolically active adipose tissue from most subcutaneous areas, intra-abdominal and intrathoracic regions, and bone marrow.

Children exhibit accelerated linear growth and advanced bone age, but plasma levels of growth hormone or insulin-like growth factor I (IGF-I) are normal. Their basal metabolic rate is relatively high. It is unclear, however, whether hypermetabolism results from a primary increase in sympathetic nervous system activity or whether it is a compensatory response to protect against excessive heat loss due to extreme lack of body fat. Other features include acanthosis nigricans, prominent umbilicus or hernia, and an acromegalic appearance with coarse facial features and large hands and feet. Occasionally, excess body hair and hyperhidrosis have been noted. Fatty liver has been noted during infancy and can lead to cirrhosis and its complications. Liver, spleen, and kidney enlargement can cause abdominal protuberance. A few patients develop hypertrophic cardiomyopathy, but it rarely leads to heart failure.

Postpubertal women may have clitoromegaly, mild hirsutism, polycystic ovaries, and oligomenorrhea. Successful pregnancy in affected women is rare, whereas affected males have normal reproductive potential. Penile enlargement may be noted in childhood. After puberty, the skeleton appears sclerotic and focal lytic lesions develop in the appendicular bones. Some patients develop goiter.

Metabolic abnormalities Patients with CGL have markedly elevated fasting serum insulin and C-peptide concentrations, as well as extreme insulin resistance. Diabetes mellitus appears during the pubertal years, and pancreatic pathology reveals severe amyloidosis of

Table 354-1 Classification of Lipodystrophies

FAMILIAL OR GENETIC FORMS

Congenital generalized lipodystrophy (CGL; Berardinelli-Seip Syndrome)
Familial partial lipodystrophy
   Dunnigan variety (FPLD)
   Köbberling variety
   Mandibuloacral dysplasia variety
Other types

ACQUIRED FORMS

Acquired generalized lipodystrophy (Lawrence syndrome)
Acquired partial lipodystrophy (Barraquer-Simons syndrome)
HIV-1 protease inhibitor–induced lipodystrophy
Localized lipodystrophies

Table 354-2 Distinguishing Features of Various Lipodystrophies

Feature	Congenital Generalized	Familial Partial (Dunnigan)	Acquired Generalized	Acquired Partial	HIV-1 Protease Inhibitor–induced
Pathogenesis	Genetic, autosomal recessive	Genetic, autosomal dominant	Autoimmune or post-viral infection	Autoimmune or post-viral infection	Drug-induced
Age of onset	Birth	Puberty	Childhood	Childhood	All ages
Sex incidence	Equal	Equal	Female preponderance	Female preponderance	Male preponderance
Areas with fat loss	Face, neck, trunk, limbs, intraabdominal, intrathoracic, bone marrow	Trunk, limbs	Face, neck, trunk, limbs, palms, soles	Face, neck, upper trunk, and upper limbs	Face, trunk, limbs
Areas with excess fat	None	Face, neck, intraabdominal	None	Lower abdomen, hips, lower limbs	Neck, upper back, intraabdominal
Insulin resistance	Severe	Mild to moderate	Severe	Usually absent	Mild to moderate
Diabetes mellitus	During teenage	After 2nd decade	During teenage	Rare	Occasional
Hypertriglyceridemia	Moderate to severe	Moderate to severe	Moderate to severe	Rare	Moderate to severe
Fatty liver, hepatomegaly	Severe	Mild to moderate	Severe	Usually absent	Mild
Acanthosis nigricans	Severe	Absent or mild	Absent or mild	Absent	Absent
Polycystic ovaries, menstrual abnormalities	Frequent	In one-fifth	None	None	None
Umbilical hernia	Present	Absent	Absent	Absent	Absent
Kidney pathology	Nephromegaly; diabetic nephropathy later	Diabetic nephropathy later	Diabetic nephropathy later	Membranocapillary glomerulonephritis	None
Autoimmune diseases	None	None	Relatively common	Relatively common	None

the pancreatic islets with loss of β cells. Plasma leptin concentrations are low, as expected in view of the reduced adipose tissue. Fasting plasma free fatty acid concentrations are normal. Hypertriglyceridemia may be observed during childhood, and patients can develop chylomicronemia, eruptive xanthomas, and acute pancreatitis. Low concentrations of high-density lipoprotein (HDL) cholesterol are also common.

Course Patients with CGL are at risk of early mortality from cirrhosis and its complications, acute pancreatitis, or diabetic nephropathy. They also may develop diabetic retinopathy. Despite long-standing hypertriglyceridemia and hyperglycemia, atherosclerotic vascular complications are rare.

GENETIC CONSIDERATIONS Approximately 120 patients of various ethnic backgrounds have been reported with this autosomal recessive form of lipodystrophy. The absence of fat could result from agenesis, failure of differentiation of preadipocytes, or an inability of mature adipocytes to synthesize and/or store triglycerides. Numerous candidate genes have been excluded, including the insulin receptor, β_3-adrenergic receptor, fatty acid binding protein 2, IGF-I receptor, insulin receptor substrate-1, hormone-sensitive lipase, leptin, and peroxisome proliferator–activated receptor γ. Genome-wide linkage analysis of 17 families revealed genetic heterogeneity, but a candidate *CGL1* gene was localized to chromosome 9q34; the defective *CGL* gene(s) have yet to be identified. ■

FAMILIAL PARTIAL LIPODYSTROPHY Dunnigan Variety • Clinical features Patients with familial partial lipodystrophy, Dunnigan variety (FPLD) appear normal during childhood. During puberty, however, these patients begin to lose subcutaneous fat from the limbs and trunk, while exhibiting "increased muscularity" (Fig. 354-1*B*). Many patients accumulate excess fat in the face and neck, often resulting in a double chin, supraclavicular humps, and round face. Occasionally, fat accumulates in the axillae. Labia majora appear prominent in women. MRI demonstrates excess fat inside the abdomen and in the intermuscular fasciae. Bone marrow and fat in certain mechanical locations, such as the orbits and joints, are normal. Acanthosis nigricans, hirsutism, menstrual abnormalities, and polycystic ovaries are infrequent. Hepatomegaly due to fatty liver is common, but progression to cirrhosis has not been reported.

Metabolic abnormalities Patients with FPLD have mild to moderate insulin resistance, and diabetes mellitus develops, usually after

the second decade. Patients have low serum HDL cholesterol and can develop severe hypertriglyceridemia. Fasting plasma free fatty acid concentrations may be elevated.

Course Major causes of morbidity and mortality in patients with FPLD include coronary heart disease, other atherosclerotic vascular complications, and acute pancreatitis.

GENETIC CONSIDERATIONS This rare autosomal dominant disorder has been reported in 35 Caucasian families and one Indian family comprising approximately 200 affected individuals. The *FPLD* locus has been mapped to chromosome 1q21-22. Recently, several missense mutations in the gene encoding the nuclear envelope protein lamin A/C (*LMNA*) have been found to be responsible for FPLD. Alternative splicing of *LMNA* produces Lamins A and C, members of the intermediate filament multigene family. All mutations causing typical FPLD cluster in exon 8 of *LMNA*, affecting the globular C-terminal tail of the Lamin A/C protein except one in exon 11 that only affects Lamin A and causes an atypical mild FPLD. The loss of subcutaneous adipose tissue in the limbs and trunk in FPLD may be due to adipocyte apoptosis and degeneration. Fat accumulation in the face and neck may be a secondary phenomenon, since it is not always present. ■

Köbberling Variety Characteristic features include loss of fat from the limbs with preservation of facial fat; truncal subcutaneous fat may be excessive. Most patients have hypertriglyceridemia and diabetes mellitus. Still unknown are the pattern of inheritance, age of onset, and whether this disorder is a distinct entity or a variant of the Dunnigan variety. Only a few women from two small pedigrees and four sporadic cases have been reported; it is not yet clear whether men can also be affected.

Mandibuloacral Dysplasia Variety This autosomal recessive disorder is characterized by short stature, high-pitched voice, mandibular and clavicular hypoplasia, dental abnormalities, acroosteolysis, stiff joints, and ectodermal defects. A few patients have also exhibited loss of limb fat. Insulin resistance and diabetes mellitus are rare.

OTHER TYPES An autosomal dominant type of generalized lipodystrophy with acromegaloid features has been reported in a pedigree from Brazil. The onset of lipodystrophy occurred after 18 years of age. In another form of lipodystrophy, marked loss of subcutaneous fat from the limbs, face, palms, and soles, but excess subcutaneous fat in the neck and trunk has been noted.

FIGURE 354-1 Anterior view of patients with different forms of lipodystrophy. *A.* Congenital generalized lipodystrophy: a 16-year-old girl with generalized loss of fat, acromegaloid features, severe acanthosis nigricans affecting axillae and abdomen, umbilical hernia. *B.* Familial partial lipodystrophy, Dunnigan variety: a 43-year-old woman with marked loss of subcutaneous fat from both the limbs and trunk and excess fat deposition in the face, chin, supraclavicular area, and labia majora. *C.* Acquired generalized lipodystrophy: a 10-year-old boy who developed generalized loss of fat that also affected the palms and soles after panniculitis at the age of 3 months. *D.* Acquired partial lipodystrophy: a 30-year-old woman with onset of lipodystrophy at age 14 years shows loss of fat from the face, neck, upper limbs, trunk, and anterior thighs. There is accumulation of excess fat in the hips and other regions of lower limbs. *(Parts A and B are reproduced with permission from the Endocrine Society and Nature Genetics.)*

ACQUIRED LIPODYSTROPHIES

ACQUIRED GENERALIZED LIPODYSTROPHY (LAW-RENCE SYNDROME) This form of lipodystrophy has been reported in approximately 50 patients and is characterized by a generalized disappearance of fat, mostly during childhood or adolescence. It is three times more common in females than males.

Clinical features Fat loss affects the face, neck, trunk, and extremities and usually occurs over several months or years; superficial veins and muscles become prominent (Fig. 354-1*C*). Fat loss can include the palms and soles. In some, the onset of the disorder was reported after infections such as varicella, measles, pertussis, diphtheria, pneumonia, osteomyelitis, parotitis, infectious mononucleosis, or hepatitis. In others, lipodystrophy starts with painful, purple-brown subcutaneous nodules that leave depressed areas with loss of subcutaneous fat. Adipose tissue may show infiltration with lymphocytes, mononuclear macrophages, fat-cell necrosis, and fat-filled macrophages; this infiltration is consistent with a type of acute panniculitis. Almost one-third of these patients develop acanthosis nigricans, and some have mild hirsutism. Hepatomegaly due to fatty infiltration is a consistent finding and can lead to cirrhosis. Splenomegaly has also been reported.

Metabolic abnormalities Ketosis-resistant diabetes mellitus usually occurs after the onset of lipodystrophy, and metabolic abnormalities are similar to those in CGL. Severely hyperglycemic patients may have elevated plasma free fatty acids.

Pathogenesis It is not yet known whether preceding infections play a causal role in this disorder. Some patients reportedly develop autoimmune diseases, including childhood dermatomyositis, juvenile rheumatoid arthritis, Hashimoto's thyroiditis, vitiligo, hemolytic anemia, or chronic active hepatitis. Autoantibodies against adipocyte membranes have been reported; it seems likely that antibody- and/or cell-mediated adipocyte lysis causes fat loss in these patients.

ACQUIRED PARTIAL LIPO-DYSTROPHY (BARRAQUER-SIMONS SYNDROME) This form of lipodystrophy affects females three times more often than males and has been reported in about 200 patients. The onset usually occurs during childhood or adolescence. Fat loss typically affects the face, neck, upper limbs, thorax, and upper abdomen, and there is increased fat deposition in the hips and lower extremities (Fig. 354-1*D*).

Clinical features Fat loss occurs gradually over 1 to 2 years and initially affects the face; other areas are affected later. In most cases, the lower abdomen, hips, and lower extremities are spared. In general, patients do not develop insulin resistance and other metabolic abnormalities, acanthosis nigricans, hirsutism, or menstrual problems. Approximately one-third of patients develop mesangiocapillary glomerulonephritis, usually 10 years after disease onset. Systemic lupus erythematosus and other autoimmune diseases have also been reported, including childhood dermatomyositis, thyroiditis, pernicious anemia, celiac disease, dermatitis herpetiformis, rheumatoid arthritis, Sjögren's syndrome, temporal arteritis, and leukocytoclastic vasculitis. In addition, many patients have serum antinuclear and anti-double-stranded DNA antibodies.

Pathogenesis C3 nephritic factor (C3NeF), a polyclonal IgG immunoglobulin, can be detected in the serum of up to 90% of these patients. Serum C3 is universally low, but C1q, C4, C5, C6, factor B, and properdin concentrations are usually normal (which suggests activation of the alternative complement pathway). Loss of fat may be due to C3NeF-induced lysis of adipocytes that express factor D. C3NeF also binds and inactivates factor H, which can induce glomerulonephritis by mechanisms similar to those seen in genetic factor H deficiency.

HIV-1 PROTEASE INHIBITOR–INDUCED LIPODYSTROPHY Highly active antiretroviral therapy (HAART) therapy for HIV, a combination which includes HIV-1 protease inhibitors, is associated with the development of lipodystrophy in the majority of patients after 18 months to 2 years of treatment (Chap. 309). It is characterized by marked reduction in subcutaneous fat from the face, trunk, and limbs, resulting in an appearance of "increased muscularity." Excess fat may also accumulate around the neck (double chin and buffalo hump) and inside the abdomen. Patients are prone to develop insulin resistance, diabetes mellitus, and hypertriglyceridemia. It is unclear whether this disorder is caused by a side effect of one or more of the drugs (most likely a protease inhibitor) or by a metabolic response to dramatic reduction of viral load. Hormonal causes, such as hypercortisolism, have been excluded.

LOCALIZED LIPODYSTROPHIES These disorders are characterized by a loss of subcutaneous adipose tissue from small areas or parts of a limb. Fat loss may occur secondary to injections of insulin, glucocorticoids, antibiotics, iron dextrans, or diphtheria/pertussis/tetanus vaccine. Repeated pressure against any body part, such as the thigh or chin, can cause lipodystrophy. In some patients, acute panniculitis causes localized lipodystrophy without progressing further. *Centrifugal lipodystrophy* begins in the abdomen, groin, and axillae of children under the age of 3, and eventually spreads to involve the entire abdomen. The surrounding areas show slightly erythematous and scaly changes with an accumulation of lymphocytes and histiocytes on histology. Complete or partial improvement occurs spontaneously after 8 to 10 years.

℞ **TREATMENT** Patients with lipodystrophies have cosmetic problems that warrant judicious treatment. Facial reconstruction can be accomplished with free flaps, transposition of facial muscle, and silicone or other implants. In acquired partial lipodystrophy, adipose tissue transplantation from the thigh to face lasts for only 2 to 5 years. In FPLD, excess fat in the face and neck may require liposuction or lipectomy. Etretinate and fish oil have improved acanthosis nigricans in some patients with generalized lipodystrophy.

Dietary fat should be restricted for patients with severe hypertriglyceridemia. Reduced energy intake and increased physical activity can mitigate insulin resistance. In children, however, enough energy should be provided to allow for normal growth and development. Medium chain triglycerides have been reported to benefit some patients with acquired generalized lipodystrophy.

In patients with CGL, diabetes control may require extremely high doses of insulin. Oral hypoglycemic agents may also be used (Chap. 333). Glycemic control can mitigate dyslipidemia and prevent diabetic complications. Severe hypertriglyceridemia should be treated with fibrates and/or omega-3 polyunsaturated fatty acids. Niacin worsens glycemic control and should not be used. Estrogens should be avoided because they may accentuate hypertriglyceridemia and can cause acute pancreatitis.

LIPOMATOSIS

MULTIPLE SYMMETRIC LIPOMATOSIS (MADELUNG DISEASE) This type of lipomatosis affects men 4 to 15 times more frequently than women. It is characterized by a symmetric, progressive growth of nonencapsulated subcutaneous adipose tissue, primarily in the neck (bull neck with buffalo hump and double chin) and supraclavicular and shoulder regions. Fat may also accumulate in the trunk and proximal limbs, though the distal arms and legs are spared. Rarely, laryngeal, tracheal, or vena caval compression may occur from deep lipomatous infiltration in the neck and mediastinum. Many patients also have peripheral neuropathy; hypertriglyceridemia and hyperuricemia are uncommon. Serum HDL cholesterol levels are usually elevated, and diabetes mellitus has not been reported.

Most of these patients have a preceding history of heavy ethanol intake. The underlying mechanisms and predisposing factors for the disorder, however, remain unknown. The lipomatous tissue contains small adipocytes (but not brown fat) with increased lipoprotein lipase activity and reduced catecholamine-stimulated lipolysis. In several families and in some sporadic cases, mitochondrial DNA mutations A-to-G and G-to-A transitions at nucleotides 8344 and 8363, respectively, or deletions in the tRNA^{Lys} gene have been reported. Most of these patients had multiple, discrete, and encapsulated lipomas in the neck and trunk, which is distinct from the features of typical patients with multiple symmetric lipomatosis. These patients also have associated peripheral neuropathy, myopathy, cerebellar ataxia, myoclonus, or hearing loss. Mitochondrial DNA mutations have not been found in many patients with typical multiple symmetric lipomatosis.

Surgical resection may be required to relieve compression or for cosmetic reasons. Cessation of alcohol intake does not result in regression but may slow growth rate.

OTHER FORMS OF LIPOMATOSIS *Mediastinal lipomatosis* is characterized by local overgrowth of adipose tissue in the mediastinum. It occurs in patients with Cushing's syndrome and can occasionally cause tracheal compression.

Pelvic lipomatosis is characterized by overgrowth of pelvic fat, causing bladder dysfunction (frequency, dysuria, and nocturia), constipation, and lower abdominal pain. Bilateral ureteral obstruction may also occur. The male:female ratio is 18:1. The etiology is not known, but the condition may result from a localized manifestation of obesity. Surgery may be needed to relieve urinary tract obstruction.

Epidural lipomatosis occurs in obese patients or in those receiving exogenous steroid therapy. Fat deposition most often occurs in the thoracic or lumbar spine, causing back pain, radicular pain, or spinal cord compression. Laminectomy may be indicated for cord compression. Weight loss or discontinuation of steroid therapy may also be helpful.

ADIPOSIS DOLOROSA (DERCUM DISEASE)

This is a rare disease of unknown etiology that mainly affects obese postmenopausal women (female:male ratio, 30:1). It is characterized by the presence of multiple circumscribed or diffuse painful subcutaneous fat deposits on the trunk and limbs, particularly near the knees. Patients also report weakness, fatigue, and emotional lability. Relief of pain is difficult; intravenous lidocaine, glucocorticoids, surgical excision, and liposuction are sometimes helpful.

ACUTE PANNICULITIS

A variety of systemic diseases including collagen vascular diseases such as systemic lupus erythematosus and scleroderma are associated with *acute panniculitis*, or *nodular fat necrosis* (Chap. 311). Panniculitis may also occur as a manifestation of lymphoproliferative disorders (Chap. 112).

Disseminated fat necrosis is usually associated with acute pancreatitis or pancreatic carcinoma. It may be caused by the release of pancreatic enzymes into the circulation (Chap. 304).

HORMONAL EFFECTS ON ADIPOSE DISTRIBUTION

A variety of hormones influence the distribution of adipose tissue. Growth hormone, for example, reduces truncal fat but can increase fat in the palms and soles. Insulin enhances lipogenesis and fat storage. Thyroid hormones increase metabolic rate, including energy expenditure by fat tissue. Estrogens induce fat accumulation in the hips, legs, breasts and other subcutaneous regions. Glucocorticoids redistribute adipose tissue from peripheral to central locations. In Cushing's syndrome, characteristic features include buffalo hump, increased supraclavicular and truncal fat.

BIBLIOGRAPHY

BRODOVSKY J et al: Adiposis dolorsa (Dercum's disease): 10 year follow-up. Ann Plast Surg 33:664, 1994

CARR A et al: A syndrome of peripheral lipodystrophy, hyperlipidaemia and insulin resistance in patients receiving HIV protease inhibitors. AIDS 2:F51, 1998

GAMEZ J et al: Familial multiple symmetric lipomatosis associated with the A8344G mutation of mitochondrial DNA. Neurology 51:258, 1998

GARG A: Lipodystrophies. Am J Med 108:143, 2000

GARG A et al: Adipose tissue distribution pattern in patients with familial partial lipodystrophy (Dunnigan variety). J Clin Endocrinol Metab 84:170, 1999

——— et al: A gene for congenital generalized lipodystrophy maps to human chromosome 9q34. J Clin Endocrinol Metab 84:3390, 1999

KOBBERLING J et al: Lipodystrophy of the extremities. A dominantly inherited syndrome associated with lipoatrophic diabetes. Humangenetik 29:111, 1975

PETERS JM et al: Localization of the gene for familial partial lipodystrophy (Dunnigan variety) to chromosome 1q21-22. Nat Genet 18:292, 1998

SEIP M, TRYGSTAD O: Generalized lipodystrophy, congenital and acquired (lipoatrophy). Acta Paediatr Suppl 413:2, 1996

SPECKMAN RA et al: Mutational and haplotype analyses of families with familial partial lipodystrophy (Dunnigan variety) reveal recurrent missense mutations in the globular C-terminal domain of lamin A/C. Am J Hum Genet 66:1192, 2000

Frederick G. Banting was born on November 14, 1891, in Alliston, Ontario, Canada. He was the youngest of five children born to Margaret and William Banting, hard-working farmers. After high school Banting was accepted to the University of Toronto to study for the Methodist ministry; however, at the end of the first year he switched to medicine. In 1917, after completion of medical school, he saw service in World War I in France, where he was wounded and received the Military Cross. After the war he sought a permanent position in surgery at the University of Toronto based on his wartime experiences but was unsuccessful; he therefore entered private practice. He obtained, however, an appointment as a demonstrator at the University of Western Ontario, where he became interested in medical research. Banting's private practice did not flourish, and he became quite frustrated. On the background of a faltering practice, Banting had two other possibilities—accompany an oil exploration to Northwest Canada as a doctor or find a laboratory in which to pursue his ideas about diabetes.

It is said that his interest in diabetes occurred at an early age when he lost a childhood friend to the disease. Banting had read an article about the pancreas and diabetes in which two areas of the pancreas were discussed: one produced exocrine substances for food digestion in the intestine, and the other, the islets of Langerhans, appeared to be degenerated in diabetic patients. However, multiple researchers had failed to treat diabetic patients successfully with various pancreatic extracts. Banting reasoned that if the pancreatic ducts were ligated, the exocrine portion of the pancreas would atrophy, thereby facilitating the isolation of the endocrine extract that was lacking in the diabetic patient. Banting contacted John J.R. Macleod, Professor of Physiology at the University of Toronto, with his idea. The senior Macleod was quite skeptical, in part because of Banting's lack of research experience. Nevertheless, Macleod thought it was worth a try and appointed Charles Best, who was in his final undergraduate year in physiology and biochemistry, as Banting's assistant.

After many dogs had died, Banting and Best finally had an animal whose pancreatic ducts had been tied and the exocrine portion of the pancreas had degenerated. The extract of the remaining portion of the pancreas rapidly lowered the blood and urine sugar in a pancreatectomized diabetic dog. A second diabetic dog was near coma and actually awakened and walked on administration of the pancreatic extract (figure). Both dogs, however, died one day later. James Collip, a biochemist with expertise in processing tissue extracts, was then enlisted to provide a purer pancreatic extract for administration to humans with diabetes. In January, 1922, a 14-year-old diabetic boy received the first purified extract; he improved immediately. Similar results were obtained with six other diabetic patients. In 1923 Banting shared the Nobel Prize in Physiology or Medicine with John Macleod for his discovery of insulin. He shared the monetary award of the prize with Charles Best.

John J. R. Macleod was born on September 6, 1876, in Cluny, Perthshire, Scotland to Jane and Robert Macleod, a minister. Macleod received his early schooling at Aberdeen Gramar School and then matriculated into the University of Aberdeen to study medicine. He graduated with honors, then studied biochemistry at the University of Leipzig in Germany. Macleod then was a demonstrator in physiology and later a lecturer in biochemistry. In 1903 he was appointed Professor of Physiology at Western Reserve University in the United States where he commenced his studies in diabetes mellitus. In 1918 he was appointed Professor and Head of the Physiology Department at the University of Toronto in Canada where Frederick G. Banting contacted him about conducting research in diabetes. Prior to this time, Macleod had focused his research predominantly on non-pancreatic aspects of glucose regulation, particularly the role of the liver and the central nervous system. With the discovery of insulin and the award of the Nobel Prize to Banting and Macleod, there was substantial debate about what role Macleod had played in the discovery. He certainly had lent the facilities of his department for Best's and Banting's research. As Banting shared his prize money with Best, Macleod shared his prize money with James Collip who had purified the pancreatic extract.

REFERENCES

1. Aaseng N: *The Disease Fighters*. Minneapolis, Lerner Publications, 1987
2. Magill FN (ed): *Nobel Prize Winners: Physiology and Medicine*, vol 1. Pasadena, Salem Press, 1993
3. Schrier RW: *A Salute to Nobel Laureates in Physiology and Medicine*
4. Sourkes TL: *Nobel Prize Winners in Medicine and Physiology 1901–1965*. London, Abelard-Schuman, 1967

Robert W. Schrier, MD

Best and Banting with pancreatectomized dog, Marjorie, whose diabetic coma was treated with insulin. (Reprinted with permission from Ref. 1.)

Section 1
DIAGNOSIS OF NEUROLOGIC DISORDERS

355 *Stephen L. Hauser, M. Flint Beal*

NEUROBIOLOGY OF DISEASE

The human nervous system is the organ of consciousness, cognition, ethics, and behavior; as such, it is the most intricate structure known to exist. One-third of the 100,000 genes encoded in the human genome is expressed in the nervous system. Each mature brain is composed of 100 billion neurons, several million miles of axons and dendrites, and more than 10^{15} synapses. Neurons exist within a dense parenchyma of multifunctional glial cells that synthesize myelin, preserve homeostasis, and regulate immune responses. Measured against this background of complexity, the achievements of molecular neuroscience have been extraordinary. Advances in cell biology and genetics have provided new tools to explore the pathophysiology of nervous system diseases, clarifying their underlying causes, revealing new unanticipated groupings, and raising realistic hope that novel therapies and prevention strategies will be possible. This chapter reviews selected themes in neurobiology that provide a context for understanding fundamental mechanisms underlying neurologic disorders. →*The reader is also referred to related discussions of neurogenetic disorders (Chap. 359) and the neurobiology of addiction (Chap. 386), and to the individual chapters on specific disorders.*

ION CHANNELS AND CHANNELOPATHIES The resting potential of neurons and the action potentials responsible for impulse conduction are generated by ion currents and ion channels. Most ion channels are gated, meaning that they can transition between conformations that are open or closed to ion conductance. Individual ion channels are distinguished by the specific ions they conduct; by their kinetics; and by whether they directly sense voltage, are linked to receptors for neurotransmitters or other ligands such as neurotrophins, or are activated by second messengers. The diverse characteristics of different ion channels provide a means by which neuronal excitability can be exquisitely modulated at both the cellular and the subcellular levels. Mutations in ion channels—channelopathies—are responsible for a growing list of human neurologic disorders (Table 355-1). One example is epilepsy, a syndrome of diverse causes characterized by repetitive, synchronous firing of neuronal action potentials. Action potentials are normally generated by the opening of sodium channels and the inward movement of sodium ions down the intracellular concentration gradient. Depolarization of the neuronal membrane opens potassium channels, resulting in outward movement of potassium ions, repolarization, closure of the sodium channel, and hyperpolarization. Sodium or potassium channel subunit genes have long been considered candidate disease genes in inherited epilepsy syndromes, and recently such mutations have been identified (Chap. 360). These mutations appear to alter the normal gating function of these channels, increasing the inherent excitability of neuronal membranes in regions where the abnormal channels are expressed.

Whereas the specific clinical manifestations of channelopathies are quite variable, one common feature is that manifestations tend to be intermittent or paroxysmal, such as occurs in epilepsy, migraine, ataxia, myotonia, or periodic paralysis. Exceptions are clinically progressive channel disorders such as spinocerebellar ataxia type 6 (SCA6) and autosomal dominant hearing impairment. The neurologic channelopathies identified to date are all uncommon disorders caused by obvious mutations in channel genes. As the full repertoire of human ion channels and related proteins are identified, it is likely that additional channelopathies will be discovered. In addition to rare disorders that result from obvious mutations, it is possible that subtle allelic variations in channel genes or in their pattern of expression might underlie susceptibility to some common forms of epilepsy, migraine, or other disorders.

NEUROTRANSMITTERS AND NEUROTRANSMITTER RECEPTORS Synaptic neurotransmission is the predominant means by which neurons communicate with each other. Classic neurotransmitters are synthesized in the presynaptic region of the nerve terminal; stored in vesicles; and released into the synaptic cleft, where they bind to receptors on the postsynaptic cell. Secreted neurotransmitters are eliminated by reuptake into the presynaptic neuron (or glia), by diffusion away from the synaptic cleft, and/or by specific inactivation. In addition to the classic neurotransmitters, many neuropeptides have been identified as definite or probable neurotransmitters; these include substance P, neurotensin, enkephalins, β-endorphin, histamine, vasoactive intestinal polypeptide, cholecystokinin, neuropeptide Y, and somatostatin. Peptide neurotransmitters are synthesized in the cell body rather than the nerve terminal and may colocalize with classic neurotransmitters in single neurons. Nitric oxide and carbon monoxide are gases that appear also to function as neurotransmitters, in part by signaling in a retrograde fashion from the postsynaptic to the presynaptic cell.

Neurotransmitters modulate the function of postsynaptic cells by binding to specific neurotransmitter receptors, of which there are two major types. *Ionotropic receptors* are direct ion channels that open after engagement by the neurotransmitter. *Metabotropic receptors* interact with G proteins, stimulating production of second messengers and activating protein kinases, which modulate a variety of cellular events. Ionotropic receptors are multiple subunit structures, whereas

Table 355-1 **Examples of Neurologic Channelopathies**

Category	Disorder	Channel Type	Gene	Chap. Ref.
Ataxias	Episodic ataxia-1	K	*KCNAI*	364
	Episodic ataxia-2	Ca	*CACNLIAd*	
	Spinocerebellar ataxia-6	Ca	*CACNLIAd*	
Migraine	Familial hemiplegic migraine	Ca	*CACNLIAd*	15
Epilepsy	Benign neonatal familial convulsions	K	*KCNQ2, KCNQ3*	360
	Generalized epilepsy with febrile convulsions plus	Na	*SCNIβ*	
Periodic paralysis	Hyperkalemic periodic paralysis	Na	*SCN4A*	383
	Hypokalemic periodic paralysis	Ca	*CACNLIA3*	
Myotonia	Myotonia congenita	C1	*CLCN1*	383
	Paramyotonia congenita	Na	*SCN4A*	
Deafness	Jorvell and Lange-Nielsen syndrome (deafness, prolonged QT interval, and arrythmia)	K	*KCNQ1, KCNE1*	29
	Autosomal dominant progressive deafness	K	*KCNQ4*	

metabotropic receptors are composed of single subunits only. One important difference between ionotropic and metabotropic receptors is that the kinetics of ionotropic receptor effects are fast (generally less than a millisecond) because neurotransmitter binding directly alters the electrical properties of the postsynaptic cell, whereas metabotropic receptors function over longer time periods. These different properties contribute to the potential for selective and finely modulated signaling by neurotransmitters.

Individual neurotransmitter systems are perturbed in a large number of clinical disorders, examples of which are highlighted in Table 355-2. One example is the involvement of dopaminergic neurons originating in the substantia nigra of the midbrain and projecting to the striatum (nigrostriatal pathway) in Parkinson's disease and in heroin addicts after the ingestion of the toxin MPTP (1-methyl-4-phenyl-

1,2,5,6-tetrahydropyridine) (Chap. 363). A second important dopaminergic system arising in the subtantia nigra is the mesolimbic pathway, which influences behavior and appears to be important in the pathogenesis of addiction. Addictive drugs share the property of increasing dopamine release, and blockade of dopamine in the nucleus accumbens (a part of the mesolimbic pathway) terminates the rewarding effects of addictive drugs (Chap. 386).

CELL TO CELL COMMUNICATION THROUGH GAP JUNCTIONS Not all cell-to-cell communication in the nervous system occurs via neurotransmission. Gap junctions provide for direct neuron-neuron electrical conduction and also create openings for the diffusion of ions and metabolites between cells. In addition to neurons, gap junctions are also widespread in glia, creating a syncytium that protects neurons by removing glutamate and potassium from the extracellular environment. Gap junctions consist of membrane-spanning proteins termed connexins that pair across adjacent cells. Mechanisms

Table 355-2   Principal Classic Neurotransmitters

Neurotransmitter	Anatomy	Clinical Aspects
Acetylcholine (Ach) $CH_3-\overset{\overset{O}{\|\|}}{C}-O-CH_2-CH_2-N-(CH_3)_3$	Motor neurons in spinal cord → neuromuscular junction	Acetylcholinesterases (nerve gases) Myasthenia gravis (antibodies to Ach receptor) Congenital myasthenic syndromes (mutations in Ach receptor subunits) Lambert-Eaton syndrome (Antibodies to Ca channels impair Ach release) Botulism (toxin disrupts Ach release by exocytosis)
	Basal forebrain → widespread cortex	Alzheimer's disease (selective cell death) Autosomal dominant frontal lobe epilepsy (mutations in CNS Ach receptor)
	Interneurons in striatum Autonomic nervous system (preganglionic and postganglionic sympathetic)	Parkinson's disease (tremor)
Dopamine (structure) $CH_2-CH_2-NH_3$ with HO, HO on ring	Substantia nigra → striatum (nigrostriatal pathway)	Parkinson's disease (selective cell death) MPTP parkinsonism (toxin transported into neurons)
	Substantia nigra → limbic system and widespread cortex	Addiction, behavioral disorders
	Arcuate nucleus of hypthalamus → anterior pituitary (via portal veins)	Inhibits prolactin secretion
Norepinephrine (NE) (structure) $CH-CH_2-NH_2$ with OH, HO, HO	Locus ceruleus (pons) → limbic system, hypothalamus, cortex	Mood disorders (MAO-A inhibitors and tricyclics increase NE and improve depression)
	Medulla → locus ceruleus, spinal cord	Anxiety
	Postganglionic neurons of sympathetic nervous system	Orthostatic tachycardia syndrome (mutations in NE transporter)
Serotonin (indole structure) HO, $CH_2-CH_2-NH_2$	Pontine raphe nuclei → widespread projections	Mood disorders (SSRIs improve depression) Migraine pain pathway
	Medulla/pons → dorsal horn of spinal cord	Pain pathway
γ-aminobutyric acid (GABA) $H_2N-CH_2-CH_2-CH_2-COOH$	Major inhibitory neurotransmitter in brain; widespread cortical interneurons and long projection pathways	Stiff person syndrome (antibodies to glutamic acid decarboxylase, the biosynthetic enzyme for GABA) Epilepsy (Gabapentin and valproic acid increase GABA)
Glycine H_2N-CH_2-COOH	Major inhibitory neurotransmitter in spinal cord	Spasticity Hyperekplexia (myoclonic startle syndrome) due to mutations in glycine receptor
Glutamate $H_2N-\underset{\underset{COOH}{\|}}{CH}-CH_2-CH_2-COOH$	Major excitatory neurotransmitter; located throughout CNS, including cortical pyramidal cells	Seizures due to ingestion of domoic acid (a glutamate analogue) Rasmussen's encephalitis (antibody against glutamate receptor 3) Excitotoxic cell death

that involve gap junctions have been related to a variety of neurologic disorders. Mutations in connexin 32, a gap junction protein expressed by Schwann cells, are responsible for the X-linked form of Charcot-Marie-Tooth disease (Chap. 379). Mutations in either of two gap junction proteins expressed in the inner ear—connexin 26 and connexin 31—result in autosomal dominant progressive hearing loss (Chap. 29). Glial calcium waves mediated through gap junctions also appear to explain the phenomenon of spreading depression associated with migraine auras and the march of epileptic discharges. Spreading depression is a neural response that follows a variety of different stimuli and is characterized by a circumferentially expanding negative potential that propagates at a characteristic speed of 20 μm/s and is associated with an increase in extracellular potassium.

SIGNALING PATHWAYS AND GENE TRANSCRIPTION The fundamental issue of how memory, learning, and thinking are encoded in the nervous system is likely to be clarified by identifying the signaling pathways involved in neuronal differentiation, axon guidance, and synapse formation, and by understanding how these pathways are modulated by experience. Many families of transcription factors, each comprising multiple individual components, are expressed in the nervous system. Elucidation of these signaling pathways has already begun to provide insights into the cause of a variety of neurologic disorders, including inherited disorders of cognition such as X-linked mental retardation. This syndrome affects approximately 1 in 500 males, and linkage studies in different families suggest that as many as 60 different X-chromosome encoded genes may be responsible. A number of disease genes have now been identified. Three encode proteins that regulate members of the ras family of GTP-binding proteins thought to have roles in regulation of the actin cytoskeleton and in neurite outgrowth (*OPHN1*, *PAK3*) or synaptic vesicle transport and neurotransmitter release (*GDI1*); one (*IL1RAPL*) has homology to an interleukin (IL)1 receptor accessory protein involved in IL-1 signaling; and one (*FMR2*) functions as a nuclear transcriptional regulatory protein. Rett syndrome, a common cause of (dominant) X-linked progressive mental retardation in females, is also due to a mutation in a gene (*MECP2*) encoding a DNA-binding protein involved in transcriptional repression. As the X chromosome comprises only approximately 3% of germline DNA, then by extrapolation the number of genes that potentially contribute to clinical disorders affecting intelligence in humans must be potentially very large.

MYELIN Myelin is the multilayered insulating substance that surrounds axons and speeds impulse conduction by permitting action potentials to jump between naked regions of axons (nodes of Ranvier) and across myelinated segments. A single oligodendrocyte usually ensheaths multiple axons in the central nervous system (CNS), whereas in the peripheral nervous system (PNS) each Schwann cell typically myelinates a single axon. Myelin is a lipid-rich material formed by a spiraling process of the membrane of the myelinating cell around the axon, creating multiple membrane bilayers that are tightly apposed (compact myelin) by charged protein interactions. A number of clinically important neurologic disorders are caused by inherited mutations in myelin proteins of the CNS or PNS. Constituents of myelin also

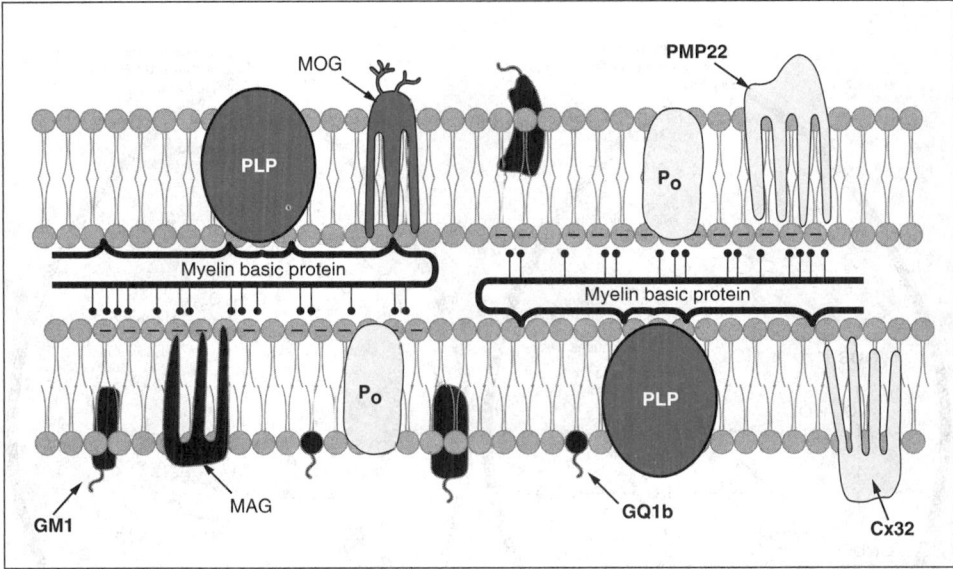

FIGURE 355-1 The molecular architecture of the myelin sheath illustrating the most important disease-related proteins. The illustration represents a composite of CNS and PNS myelin. Proteins restricted to CNS myelin are shown in dark blue, proteins of PNS myelin are light blue, and proteins present in both CNS and PNS are black.

In the CNS, the X-linked allelic disorders, Pelizaeus Merzbacher disease and one variant of familial spastic paraplegia, are caused by mutations in the gene for proteolipid protein (PLP) that normally promotes extracellular compaction between adjacent myelin lamellae. The homologue of PLP in the PNS is the P_0 protein, mutations in which cause the neuropathy Charcot-Marie-Tooth disease (CMT) type 1B. The most common form of CMT is the 1A subtype caused by a duplication of the *PMP22* gene; deletions in *PMP22* are responsible for another inherited neuropathy termed hereditary liability to pressure palsies (Chap. 379).

In multiple sclerosis (MS), myelin basic protein (MBP) and the quantitatively minor CNS protein, myelin oligodendrocyte glycoprotein (MOG), are likely T cell and B cell antigens, respectively (Chap. 371). The location of MOG at the outermost lamella of the CNS myelin membrane may facilitate its targeting by autoantibodies. In the PNS, autoantibodies against myelin gangliosides are implicated in a variety of disorders, including GQ1b in the Fisher variant of Guillain-Barré syndrome, GM1 in multifocal motor neuropathy, and sulfatide constituents of myelin-associated glycoprotein (MAG) in peripheral neuropathies associated with monoclonal gammopathies (Chap. 378).

have a propensity to be targeted as autoantigens in autoimmune demyelinating disorders (Fig. 355-1).

NEUROTROPHIC FACTORS Neurotrophic factors (Table 355-3) are secreted proteins that modulate neuronal growth, differentiation, repair, and survival; some have additional functions, including roles in neurotransmission and in the synaptic reorganization involved in learning and memory. Because of their survival promoting and antiapoptotic effects, neurotrophic factors are in theory outstanding candidates for therapy of disorders characterized by premature death of neurons such as occurs in amyotrophic lateral sclerosis (ALS) and other degenerative motor neuron disorders. Knockout mice lacking receptors for ciliary neurotrophic factor (CNTF) receptor or brain-derived neurotrophic factor (BDNF) show loss of motor neurons, and experimental motor neuron death can be rescued by treatment with various neurotrophic factors including CNTF and BDNF. However, in phase 3 clinical trials both CNTF and BDNF were ineffective in human ALS, and two other trials of insulin-like growth factor 1 yielded con-

Table 355-3 Neurotrophic Factors

Neurotrophin family	Transforming growth factor β family
Nerve growth factor	
Brain-derived neurotrophic factor	Glial-derived neurotrophic family
Neurotrophin-3	Neurturin
Neurotrophin-4	Persephin
Neurotrophin-6	Fibroblast growth factor family
Cytokine family	Hepatocyte growth factor
Ciliary neurotrophic factor	Insulin-like growth factor (IGF) family
Leukemia inhibitory factor	
Interleukin-6	IGF-1
Cardiotrophin-1	IGF-2

FIGURE 355-2 Involvement of mitochondria in cell death. A severe excitotoxic insult (*A*) results in cell death by necrosis, whereas a mild excitotoxic insult (*B*) results in apoptosis. After a severe insult (such as ischemia), there is a large increase in glutamate activation of NMDA receptors, an increase in intracellular Ca^{2+} concentrations, activation of nitric oxide synthase (NOS), and increased mitochondrial Ca^{2+} and superoxide generation followed by the formation of $ONOO^-$. This sequence results in damage to cellular macromolecules including DNA, leading to activation of poly-ADP-ribose polymerase (PARS). Both mitochondrial accumulation of Ca^{2+} and oxidative damage lead to activation of the permeability transition pore (PTP) that is linked to excitotoxic cell death.

A mild excitotoxic insult can occur due either to an abnormality in an excitotoxicity amino acid receptor, allowing more Ca^{2+} flux, or to impaired functioning of other ionic channels or of energy production, which may allow the voltage-dependent NMDA receptor to be activated by ambient concentrations of glutamate. This event can then lead to increased mitochondrial Ca^{2+} and free radical production, yet relatively preserved ATP generation. The mitochondria may then release cytochrome c (Cyt c), caspase 9, apoptosis-inducing factor (Aif), and perhaps other mediators that lead to apoptosis. The precise role of the PTP in this mode of cell death is still being clarified, but there does appear to be involvement of the adenine nucleotide transporter that is a key component of the PTP.

flicting results with little evidence of clinically significant efficacy. Current understanding of the redundancy and diversity of neurotrophic factor activities at different stages in the life and health of individual neurons is extremely limited, and data obtained in rodent systems are not always applicable to humans. For example, CNTF knockout mice show a partial loss of motoneurons, yet humans who have homozygous mutations that inactivate the gene for CNTF gene are asymptomatic.

STEM CELLS AND TRANSPLANTATION The nervous system is traditionally considered to be a nonmitotic organ, in particular with respect to neurons. These concepts have been challenged by the finding that neural progenitor or stem cells exist in the adult CNS that are capable of differentiation, migration over long distances, and extensive axonal arborization and synapse formation with appropriate targets. These capabilities also indicate that the repertoire of factors required for growth, survival, differentiation, and migration of these cells exist in the mature nervous system. The poor outcome associated with many neurologic disorders, however, clearly indicates that any potential for functional neuronal reconstitution after injury must be extremely limited in most clinical contexts. In rodents, neural stem cells, defined as progenitor cells capable of differentiating into mature cells of neural or glial lineage, have been experimentally propagated from fetal CNS and neuroectodermal tissues, and also from adult ger-

minal matrix and ependyma regions. Human fetal CNS tissue is also capable of differentiation into cells with neuronal, astrocyte, and oligodendrocyte morphology when cultured in the presence of particular growth factors. Impressively, such cells could be stably engrafted into mouse CNS tissue, creating neural chimeras. Once the repertoire of signals required for cell type specification are better understood, differentiation into specific neural or glial subpopulations can be directed in vitro; such cells could also be engineered to express therapeutic molecules.

Experimental transplantation of human fetal dopaminergic neurons in patients with Parkinson's disease has shown that these transplanted cells can survive within the host striatum. Studies of transplantation for patients with Huntington's disease have also reported encouraging, although very preliminary, results. Oligodendrocyte precurser cells transplanted into mice with a dysmyelinating disorder effectively migrated in the new environment, interacted with axons, and mediated myelination; such experiments raise hope that similar transplantation strategies may be feasible in human disorders of myelin such as multiple sclerosis. Enthusiasm for transplantation therapy must be tempered by unresolved concerns over safety (including the theoretical risk of malignant transformation of transplanted cells), ethics (particularly with respect to use of fetal tissue), and efficacy.

CELL DEATH—EXCITOTOXICITY AND APOPTOSIS Excitotoxicity refers to neuronal cell death caused by activation of excitatory amino acid receptors (Fig. 355-2). Compelling evidence for a role of excitotoxicity, especially in ischemic neuronal injury, is derived from experiments in animal models. Experimental models of stroke are associated with increased extracellular concentrations of the excitatory amino acid neurotransmitter glutamate, and neuronal damage is attenuated by denervation of glutamine-containing neurons or the administration of glutamate receptor antagonists. The distribution of cells sensitive to ischemia corresponds closely with that of *N*-methyl-D-aspartate (NMDA) receptors (except for cerebellar Purkinje cells, which are vulnerable to hypoxia-ischemia but lack NMDA receptors); and competitive and noncompetitive NMDA antagonists are effective in preventing focal ischemia. In global cerebral ischemia, non-NMDA receptors (kainic acid and AMPA) are activated, and antagonists to these receptors are protective. Experimental brain damage induced by hypoglycemia is also attenuated by NMDA antagonists.

Excitotoxicity is not a single event but rather a cascade of cell injury. Excitotoxicity causes influx of calcium into cells and much of the calcium is sequestered in mitochondria rather than in the cytoplasm. Increased mitochondrial calcium causes metabolic dysfunction and free radical generation; activates protein kinases, phospholipases, nitric oxide synthase, proteases, and endonucleases; and inhibits protein synthesis. Activation of nitric oxide synthase generates nitric oxide ($NO^{\bullet}$), which can react with superoxide ($O_2^{\bullet-}$) to generate peroxynitrite ($ONOO^-$), which may play a direct role in neuronal injury. Another critical pathway is activation of poly-ADP-ribose polymerase, which occurs in response to free radical-mediated DNA damage. Ex-

2324

perimentally, mice with knockout mutations of neuronal nitric oxide synthase or poly-ADP-ribose polymerase, or those that overexpress superoxide dismutase, are resistant to focal ischemia.

Apoptosis, or programmed cell death, plays an important role in both physiologic and pathologic conditions. During embryogenesis, apoptotic pathways operate to destroy neurons that fail to differentiate appropriately or reach their intended targets. There is mounting evidence for an increased rate of apoptotic cell death in a variety of acute and chronic neurologic diseases. Apoptosis is characterized by neuronal shrinkage, chromatin condensation, and DNA fragmentation, whereas necrotic cell death is associated with cytoplasmic and mitochondrial swelling followed by dissolution of the cell membrane. Apoptotic and necrotic cell death can coexist or be sequential events depending on the severity of the initiating insult. Cellular energy reserves appear to have an important role in these two forms of cell death, with apoptosis favored under conditions in which ATP levels are preserved. Evidence of DNA fragmentation has been found in a number of degenerative neurologic disorders, including Alzheimer's disease, Huntington's disease, and ALS. The best characterized genetic neurologic disorder related to apoptosis is infantile spinal muscular atrophy (Werdnig-Hoffmann disease), in which two genes thought to be involved in the apoptosis pathways are causative.

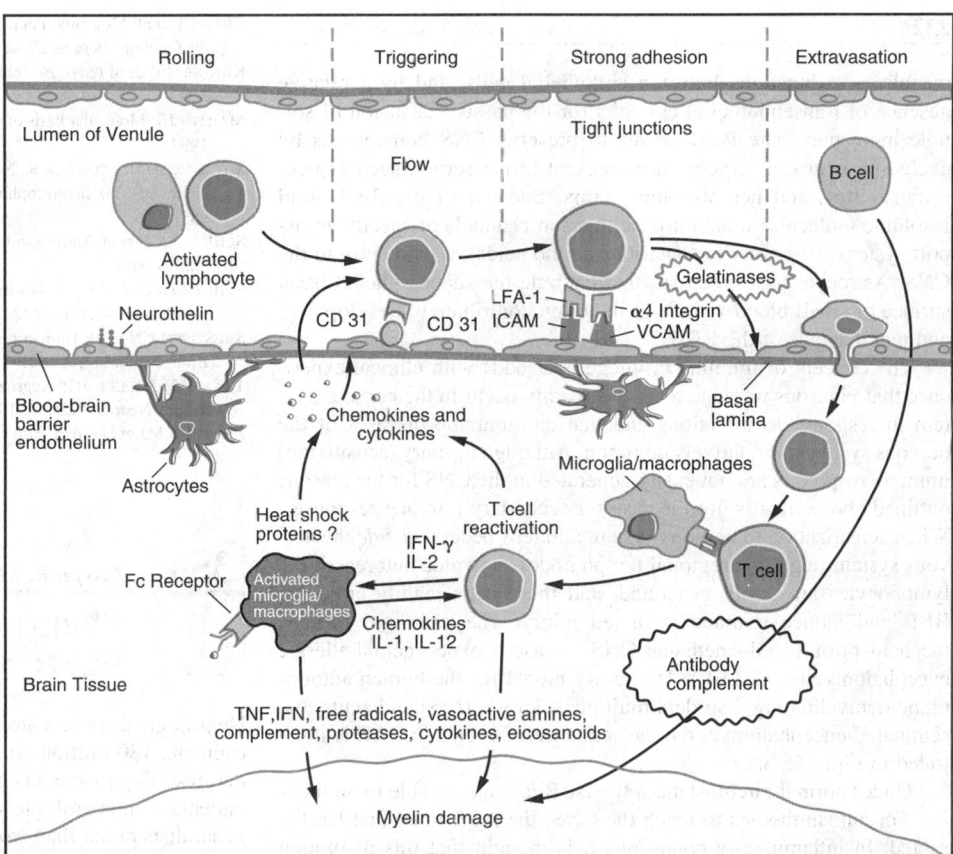

FIGURE 355-3 A model for experimental allergic encephalomyelitis (EAE). Crucial steps for disease initiation and progression include peripheral activation of preexisting autoreactive T cells; homing to the CNS and extravasation across the blood-brain barrier; reactivation of T cells by exposed autoantigens; secretion of cytokines; activation of microglia and astrocytes and recruitment of a secondary inflammatory wave; and immune-mediated myelin destruction. ICAM, intercellular adhesion molecule; LFA-1, leukocyte function-associated antigen-1; VCAM, vascular cell adhesion molecule; IFN, interferon; IL, interleukin; TNF, tumor necrosis factor.

Mitochondria are essential in controlling specific apoptosis pathways. The redistribution of cytochrome c from mitochondria during apoptosis leads to the activation of a cascade of intracellular proteases known as caspases. Redistribution of cytochrome c is prevented by overproduction of the apoptotic protein BCL2 and is promoted by the proapoptotic protein BAX. These pathways may be triggered by activation of a large pore in the mitochondrial inner membrane known as the permeability transition pore. Recent studies suggest that blocking this pore reduces both hypoglycemic and ischemic cell death.

PROTEIN AGGREGATION AND NEURODEGENERATION The possibility that protein aggregation plays a role in the pathogenesis of neurodegenerative diseases is a major focus of current research. Protein aggregation is a major histopathologic hallmark of neurodegenerative diseases. Deposition of β-amyloid is strongly implicated in the pathogenesis of Alzheimer's disease. Genetic mutations in familial Alzheimer's disease produce increased amounts of β-amyloid with 42 amino acids, which has an increased propensity to aggregate, as compared to β-amyloid with 40 amino acids. Mutations in genes encoding the microtubule associated protein tau lead to altered splicing of tau and the production of neurofibrillary tangles in frontotemporal dementia and progressive supranuclear palsy. Familial Parkinson's disease is associated with mutations in α-synuclein and the ubiquitin carboxy-terminal hydrolase. The characteristic histopathologic feature of Parkinson's disease is the Lewy body, an eosinophilic cytoplasmic inclusion that contains both neurofilaments and α-synuclein. Huntington's disease and cerebellar degenerations are associated with expansions of polyglutamine repeats in proteins, which aggregate to produce neuronal intranuclear inclusions. Familial ALS is associated with superoxide dismutase mutations and cytoplasmic inclusions containing superoxide dismutase. In autosomal dominant neurohypo-

physeal diabetes insipidus, mutations in vasopressin result in abnormal protein processing, accumulation in the endoplasmic reticulum, and cell death (Chap. 329).

The major scientific question presently is whether protein aggregates contribute to neuronal death or whether they are merely a secondary bystander. Protein aggregates are usually ubiquinated, which targets them for degradation by the 26S component of the proteosome. An inability to degrade protein aggregates could lead to cellular dysfunction, impaired axonal transport, and cell death by apoptotic mechanisms.

In experimental models of Huntington's disease and cerebellar degeneration, protein aggregates are not well correlated with neuronal death. A number of compounds have been developed to block β-amyloid production and/or aggregation, and these agents are being studied in early clinical trials in humans.

NEUROIMMUNOLOGY The nervous system is traditionally considered to be an immunologically privileged organ, a concept originally derived from observations that tissue grafts implanted in the brain were not rejected efficiently. In this context, immune privilege of the CNS may be maintained by a variety of mechanisms including: the lack of an efficient surveillance function by T cells; the absence of a traditional lymphoid system; limited expression of major histocompatibility complex (MHC) molecules required for T cell recognition of antigen; effects of regulatory cytokines secreted spontaneously or in response to mediators such as nerve growth factor (NGF), creating an immunosuppressive milieu; and also from expression of fas ligand that can induce apoptosis of fas-expressing immune cells that enter the brain. The blood-brain barrier (BBB) partially isolates the brain from the peripheral environment and contributes to immune privilege. Anatomically, the barrier is created by the presence of imper-

2325

meable tight junctions between endothelial cells, and by a relative absence of transendothelial conduits for the passive diffusion of soluble molecules. The BBB serves to preserve CNS homeostasis by excluding neuroactive substances present in the serum, such as neurotransmitters and neurotrophic factors. Because of the BBB, lipid insoluble molecules must utilize either ion channels or specific transport systems (for glucose or various amino acids) to gain entry to the CNS. Astrocyte foot processes that encircle the subendothelial basal surface of small blood vessels in the brain contribute to development and maintenance of the BBB.

The concept of immune privilege is at odds with clinical experience that vigorous immune reactions readily occur in the nervous system in response to infections and that autoimmune diseases of the nervous system are relatively common. Although primary (sensitizing) immune responses are not easily generated in the CNS for the reasons outlined above, this is not the case for secondary immune responses. When sensitization to nervous system antigens occurs *outside* the nervous system (e.g., in a regional lymph node), activated autoreactive T lymphocytes are easily generated, and these cells readily cross the BBB and induce immune mediated injury. The paradigm for this mechanism of T cell–mediated CNS disease is experimental allergic encephalomyelitis (EAE), a laboratory model for the human autoimmune demyelinating disorders multiple sclerosis (MS) and acute disseminated encephalomyelitis; the sequence of events in EAE is illustrated in Fig. 355-3.

Under normal circumstances the BBB is impermeable to antibodies. For autoantibodies to reach the CNS, the BBB must first be disrupted. In inflammatory conditions it is thought that this disruption most often occurs via actions of proinflammatory cytokines elaborated within the brain consequent to interactions between pathogenic T cells and antigen-presenting cells (APCs). In contrast to the BBB, in the PNS the blood-nerve barrier is incomplete. Endothelial tight junctions are lacking, and the capacity of charged molecules, including antibodies, to cross the barrier appears to be greatest in two regions of the PNS: proximally in the spinal roots and distally at neuromuscular junctions. This anatomic feature is likely to contribute to the propensity of antibody-mediated autoimmune disorders of the PNS to target proximal nerves (Guillain-Barré syndrome) or the neuromuscular junction (myasthenia gravis, Eaton-Lambert syndrome).

The major APCs in the CNS are microglial cells and macrophages; both cell types express MHC class 2 molecules as well as costimulatory molecules required for antigen presentation. Neurons do not express MHC class 2 molecules; however, some neurons express MHC class 1 proteins, which may be further increased in response to neuronal activity. Neuronal MHC class 1 molecules may function as retrograde postsynaptic signaling molecules that interact with presynaptic CD3ζ molecules to stabilize active synapses and transynaptically modulate neuronal function. Studies in mice also indicate that MHC class 1 molecules influence the mating behavior of females; a hierarchichal pattern of preference is determined by the specific class 1 alleles expressed by potential male suitors. This behavior appears to be mediated by distinctive odors imparted either by the class 1 molecules themselves or by other families of molecules controlled by class 1 alleles. Thus, it appears likely that MHC molecules subserve a variety of signaling and adhesion functions that influence nervous system function far beyond their well-established roles as mediators of APC-T lymphocyte interactions.

BIBLIOGRAPHY

ALBRIGHT TD et al: Neural science: A century of progress and the mysteries that remain. Cell 25:S1, 2000

BERKE JD, HYMAN SE: Addiction, dopamine, and the molecular mechanisms of memory. Neuron 25:515, 2000

COOPER EC, JAN LY: Ion channel genes and human neurological disease: Recent progress, prospects, and challenges. Proc Natl Acad Sci USA 96:4759, 1999

DARNELL RB: Immunologic complexity in neurons. Neuron 21:947, 1998

GREEN T et al: Molecular neurobiology and genetics: Investigation of neural function and dysfunction. Neuron 20:427, 1998.

KANDEL ER et al (eds): *Principles of Neural Science*, 4th ed. New York, McGraw-Hill, 2000

MARTIN JB: Molecular basis of the neurodegenerative disorders. N Engl J Med 340:1970, 1999

MITSUMOTO H, TSUZAKA K: Neurotrophic factors and neuromuscular disease: 1. General comments, the neurotrophin family, and neuropoietic cytokines. Muscle/Nerve 22: 983, 1999

SCHEFFLER B et al: Marrow-mindedness: A perspective on neuropoiesis. Trends Neurosci 22:348, 1999

SCHULZ JB et al: Caspases as treatment targets in stroke and neurodegenerative diseases. Ann Neurol 45:421, 1999

SVENDSEN CN et al: Human neural stem cells: Isolation, expansion and transplantation. Brain Pathol 9:499, 1999

TRAN PB, MILLER RJ: Aggregates in neurodegenerative disease: Crowds and power? Trends Neurosci 22:194, 1999

ZIGMOND MJ et al (eds): *Molecular neuroscience*. London, Academic Press, 1999

356

Joseph B. Martin, Stephen L. Hauser

APPROACH TO THE PATIENT WITH NEUROLOGIC DISEASE

Neurologic disorders are common and costly. According to one recent estimate, 180 million Americans suffer from a nervous system disorder, resulting in annual cost of 634 billion dollars (Table 356-1). Most patients with neurologic symptoms seek care from internists and other generalists rather than from neurologists, and this situation is likely to continue as primary care–based health care systems become increasingly prevalent and access to specialists is reduced. Because useful therapies now exist for many neurologic disorders, a skillfull approach to their diagnosis is important. Many errors result from an over-reliance on neuroimaging and other laboratory tests at the expense of a primary focus on the history and examination. These errors can be avoided by adherence to an approach in which the patient's illness is defined first in *anatomic* and then in *pathophysiologic* terms; only then should a specific diagnosis be entertained. Arrival at a diagnosis permits the physician to institute therapy and to inform and counsel patients and their families about the expected disease course.

THE NEUROLOGIC METHOD OF CLINICAL EVALUATION

LOCATE THE LESION(S) The first priority is to define the anatomic substrate responsible for the patient's illness by seeking to determine what part of the neural axis is likely to be involved in causing the neurologic symptoms. Can the disorder be mapped to one specific site in the nervous system, is it multifocal, or is there evidence of a more diffuse neurologic disease? Is the disorder restricted to the nervous system, or does it arise in the context of a systemic illness? Is it in the central nervous system (CNS), the peripheral nervous system (PNS), or both? If in the CNS, is the process restricted to the cerebral cortex, or is there evidence of basal ganglia, brainstem, cerebellum, and/or spinal cord involvement? Are the pain-sensitive meninges involved? If in the PNS, could the disorder be located in peripheral nerves and, if so, are motor or sensory nerves primarily affected, or is a lesion in the neuromuscular junction or muscle more likely?

The first clues to defining the anatomic area of involvement appear in the history, and the examination is then directed to confirm or rule out these impressions and to clarify uncertainties suggested by the history. A more detailed examination of a particular region of the CNS or PNS is often indicated. For example, the examination of a patient who presents with a history of ascending paresthesias and weakness should be directed toward deciding, among other things, if the location of the lesion is in the spinal cord or peripheral nerves. Focal back pain,

Table 356-1 Impact of Neurologic and Psychiatric Diseases in the United States

Disorder	Patients in Millions	Cost in $ Billions
Addiction	17.5	160
Alzheimer's disease	4	100
Blindness/vision loss	13	38.4
Deafness/hearing loss	28	56
Depression/manic depressive illness	17.5	47.3
Developmental disorders	8.6	30
Epilepsy	2.5	3.5
Head injury	2	25
Huntington's disease	0.03	—
Multiple sclerosis	0.3	2.5
Pain	80	100
Parkinson's disease	1	6
Schizophrenia	2	30
Spinal cord injury	0.25	5
Stroke	3	30
Total	**180**	**634**

SOURCE: Modified from Dana Alliance for Brain Initiatives.

a spinal cord sensory level, and incontinence suggest a spinal cord origin, whereas a stocking-glove pattern of sensory loss suggests peripheral nerve disease; areflexia usually indicates peripheral neuropathy but may also be present with spinal shock in acute spinal cord disorders.

Deciding "where the lesion is" accomplishes the task of limiting the possible etiologies to a manageable, finite number. In addition, this strategy safeguards against making tragic errors. Symptoms of recurrent vertigo, diplopia, and nystagmus should not trigger "multiple sclerosis" as an answer (etiology) but "brainstem" or "pons" (location); then a diagnosis of brainstem arteriovenous malformation will not be missed for lack of consideration. Similarly, the combination of optic neuritis and spastic ataxic paraparesis should initially suggest optic nerve and spinal cord disease; multiple sclerosis, CNS syphilis, and vitamin B_{12} deficiency are treatable disorders that can produce this syndrome. Once the question, "Where is the lesion?" is answered, then the question, "What is the lesion?" can be addressed.

DEFINE THE PATHOPHYSIOLOGY Clues to the pathophysiology of the disease process may also be present in the history. Primary neuronal (gray matter) disorders may present as early cognitive disturbances, movement disorders, or seizures, whereas white matter involvement produces predominantly "long tract" disorders of motor, sensory, visual and cerebellar pathways. Progressive and symmetric symptoms often have a metabolic or degenerative origin; in such cases lesions are usually not sharply circumscribed. Thus, a patient with paraparesis and a clear spinal cord sensory level is unlikely to have vitamin B_{12} deficiency as the explanation. A Lhermitte symptom (electric shock–like sensations evoked by neck flexion) is due to ectopic impulse generation in white matter pathways and occurs with demyelination in the cervical spinal cord. Symptoms that worsen after exposure to heat or exercise may indicate conduction block in demyelinated axons and suggest a diagnosis of multiple sclerosis. Slowly advancing visual scotoma with luminous edges, termed fortification spectra, are diagnostic of spreading cortical depression, such as occurs in migraine.

ESTABLISH AN ETIOLOGIC DIAGNOSIS The clinical data obtained from the history and the examination are assembled into one of the known syndromes and are interpreted and translated in terms of neuroanatomy and neurophysiology. From the syndrome the physician should be able to determine the anatomic localization(s) that best explains the clinical findings. The proper selection of laboratory tests is important to arrive at an anatomic, but more particularly an etiologic, diagnosis. The laboratory assessment of a patient with positive neurologic findings may include (1) serum electrolytes, complete blood count, and renal, liver, and endocrine studies; (2) cerebrospinal fluid (CSF) examination (see below); (3) neuroimaging studies (Chap.

358); or (4) electrophysiologic studies (Chap. 357). The anatomic localization, mode of onset and course of illness, other medical data, and laboratory findings are then integrated to establish an etiologic diagnosis.

THE NEUROLOGIC HISTORY

Attention to the description of the symptoms as experienced by the patient and substantiated by family members or friends often permits an accurate localization and determination of the probable cause of the complaints even before the neurologic examination is undertaken. Two principles should be followed. First, each complaint should be pursued as far as possible in an effort to delineate where the lesion might be or, more importantly, to formulate a set of questions to be answered by the examination. A patient complains of weakness of the right arm. What are the associated features? Is this weakness for brushing the hair (proximal) or opening a twist-top bottle (distal)? Second, negative associations may also be crucial. A patient with a right hemiparesis without a language deficit likely has a lesion (and likely an etiology) different from that of a patient with a right hemiparesis and aphasia. Additional features of the history include the following:

1. *Temporal course of the illness.* It is important to ascertain the precise time of appearance and rate of progression of the symptoms experienced by the patient. The rapid onset of a neurologic complaint, occurring within seconds or minutes, usually indicates a cerebrovascular event, a seizure, or rarely migraine. The onset of sensory symptoms located in one extremity that spread over a few seconds to adjacent portions of that extremity and then to the other limb or to the face suggests a seizure. A more gradual onset and less well localized sensory symptoms point to the possibility of a transient ischemic attack (TIA). A similar but slower temporal march of a sensory change occurring with headache, nausea, or visual disturbance suggests migraine. In general, the march of migraine is slower than that of seizure, and a TIA tends to be more generalized in location on the side of the body or extremities. The presence of "positive" sensory symptoms (e.g., tingling) or involuntary motor movements suggests a seizure; in contrast, transient loss of function (negative symptoms) suggests a TIA. A stuttering onset where symptoms appear, stabilize, and then progress over hours or days also suggests cerebrovascular disease; an additional history of transient remission or regression indicates that the process is due to ischemia and not hemorrhage. On occasion, a demyelinating process may also produce new symptoms that evolve rapidly over the course of a few hours. Progressing symptoms associated with the systemic manifestations of fever, stiff neck, and altered level of consciousness raise the possibility of an infectious process. Relapsing and remitting symptoms involving different levels of the neuraxis suggest multiple sclerosis. Slowly progressive symptoms without remissions are characteristic of neurodegenerative disorders.

2. *Subjective descriptions of the complaint.* The same words often mean different things to different patients. "Dizziness" may imply impending syncope, a sense of giddiness, or true spinning vertigo. "Numbness" may mean a complete loss of feeling, a positive sensation of tingling, or paralysis. "Blurred vision" may be used to describe unilateral visual loss, as in transient monocular blindness, or diplopia. It is important to define the contextual meaning of the patient's complaint to understand its true significance.

3. *Corroboration of the history by others.* It is often useful to obtain additional information from family, friends, or observers to corroborate or expand the patient's description. Memory loss, aphasia, loss of insight, drug or alcohol abuse, and other factors may impair the patient's capacity to communicate normally with the examiner or prevent openness about factors that have contributed to the illness. Episodes of loss of consciousness that may be due to syncope or seizures necessitate that details be sought from observers to ascertain the exact circumstances.

4. *Family history.* Many neurologic disorders have an underlying genetic component. The presence of a Mendelian disorder, such as Huntington's disease or Charcot-Marie-Tooth neuropathy, is often obvious if appropriate family data are available. In polygenic disorders such as multiple sclerosis or migraine, a positive family history, when present, may be helpful. It is important to elicit family history about all illnesses, in addition to neurologic and psychiatric disorders. A familial propensity to hypertension or heart disease may be relevant to a patient who presents with a stroke. Many inherited neurologic illnesses are associated with multisystem manifestations that may provide clues to the correct diagnosis (e.g., the phakomatoses, hepatocerebral disorders, neuro-ophthalmic syndromes).

5. *Medical illnesses.* Many neurologic illnesses occur in the context of systemic disorders. Disorders such as diabetes mellitus, hypertension, and abnormalities of blood lipids predispose to cerebrovascular disease. Marfan's syndrome and related collagen disorders predispose to dissection of the cranial arteries and also to aneurysmal subarachnoid hemorrhage; the latter may also occur with polycystic kidney disease. A recent onset of asthma suggests the possibility of polyarteritis nodosa. Various neurologic disorders occur with dysthyroid states. A solitary mass lesion may be a brain abscess in a patient with valvular heart disease, a primary hemorrhage in a patient with a coagulopathy, a metastasis in a patient with underlying cancer, or a lymphoma or toxoplasmosis in a patient with AIDS. The presence of systemic diseases that are associated with peripheral neuropathy should be explored. Most patients with coma in a hospital setting can be shown to have a metabolic, toxic, or infectious process.

6. *The patient's perception of the disease.* It is frequently helpful to ask patients what they perceive to be wrong. Patients who complain of failing memory are often concerned that they have early symptoms of Alzheimer's disease; more often they are found to suffer from depression. Patients with headaches may fear that a tumor or an impending stroke is a possibility. Patients with sensory symptoms frequently are concerned about the possibility of multiple sclerosis. The patient may seek medical attention because a relative or friend has been diagnosed with a serious neurologic illness.

7. *Drug use and abuse and toxin exposure.* It is essential to inquire about the history of drug use, both prescribed and illicit. Digitalis use may provoke complaints of yellow vision. Excessive vitamin ingestion may lead to disease; for example, vitamin A and pseudotumor cerebri, or pyridoxine and peripheral neuropathy. Aminoglycoside antibiotics may exacerbate symptoms of weakness in patients with disorders of neuromuscular transmission, such as myasthenia gravis. Dizziness may be secondary to ototoxicity caused by aminoglycosides. Many patients are unaware that over-the-counter sleeping pills, cold preparations, and diet pills are actually drugs. Alcohol, the most prevalent neurotoxin, is often not recognized as such by patients. A history of environmental or industrial exposure to neurotoxins may provide an essential clue; consultation with the patient's family or employer may be required.

8. *History of malignancy.* Patients with malignancy may present with nervous system metastases, a paraneoplastic syndrome (Chap. 101), or complications from chemotherapy or radiotherapy.

9. *Formulating an impression of the patient.* Use the opportunity while taking the history to form an impression of the patient. Is there evidence of anxiety, depression, hypochondriasis? Are there any clues to defects of language, memory, inappropriate behavior, or secondary gain? The neurologic assessment begins as soon as the patient walks into the room and the first introduction is made.

THE NEUROLOGIC EXAMINATION

A systematic neurologic examination should encompass a survey of all functions from the cerebrum to the peripheral nerve and muscle, i.e., from the mental status examination to the simplest reflexes. Phy-

sicians should acquire skills that come only from the repeated use of the same techniques and instruments on a large number of individuals with and without neurologic disease. Errors and serious omissions are avoided if the examination procedure is orderly and systematic, beginning with mental (cerebral) functions and continuing with cranial nerves; then with motor, reflex, and sensory functions of the arms, trunk, and legs; and finishing with an analysis of posture and gait (Table 356-2).

This detailed examination is undertaken only if there are symptoms of disturbed nervous system functioning. If none are present, it suffices to do an abbreviated examination that includes evaluation only of pupils, ocular movements, optic fundi, facial movements, speech, strength of arm and leg muscles, tendon and plantar reflexes, pain and vibratory sensation in hands and feet, and gait. All this can be completed in 3 to 5 min.

Several additional points about the examination are worth noting. First, in recording observations, it is important to describe what is found rather than to apply a poorly defined medical term (i.e., "patient groans to sternal rub" rather than "obtunded"). Second, if the patient's complaint is brought out by some activity, reproduce the activity in the office. If the complaint is of dizziness when raising the right arm and turning the head to the left, have the patient do it. If pain occurs after walking two blocks, have the patient demonstrate it, and repeat the examination. Finally, the use of tests that are individually tailored to the patient's problem can be of value in assessing changes over time. Tests of walking a 25-ft distance (normal, 5 to 6 s; note assistance, if any), repetitive finger or toe tapping (normal, 20 to 25 taps in 5 s), or handwriting are examples.

The neurologic examination may be normal even in patients with a serious neurologic disease, such as one that causes seizures or syncope. A comatose patient may arrive with no available history; the examination proceeds along the lines described in Chap. 24. An inadequate history may be compensated for to some extent by a succession of examinations from which the course of the illness may be plotted.

LUMBAR PUNCTURE

The clinical indications for lumbar puncture (LP) are listed in Table 356-3. In experienced hands, LP is a safe procedure. The patient is asked to lie on his or her side facing away from the examiner. The back is positioned at the edge of the bed or table near the examiner. The patient is asked to "roll up into a ball"—the neck is gently flexed and the knees drawn up to the abdomen. Proper positioning is essential for success; the examiner should ensure that the shoulders and pelvis are vertically aligned without forward or backward tilt. A pillow is placed under the neck for comfort and a blanket offered for warmth. Because the spinal cord terminates at approximately the L1 vertebral level, the LP is performed below this level; i.e., at or below the L2–L3 interspace. A useful anatomic guidepost is the iliac crest which corresponds to the L3–L4 interspace. The interspace is chosen after gentle palpation to identify the spinous processes at each lumbar level. The skin is cleansed with an antibacterial liquid and alcohol, and the area is draped with sterile cloths. Local anesthetic, typically 1% lidocaine, is injected into the subcutaneous tissue; a topical anesthetic cream (lidocaine 2.5%/prilocaine 2.5%) applied 90 min before the procedure can eliminate pain associated with injection. Approximately 5 min after the lidocaine injection, the LP needle (typically 22 gauge) is inserted in the midline between two spinous processes and slowly advanced at a slightly cephalic angle aiming at the umbilicus. The bevel of the needle should be maintained in a horizontal position, parallel to the direction of the dural fibers; this minimizes injury to the fibers as the dura is penetrated. In most adults, the needle is advanced 4 to 5 cm (1½ to 2 in.) before the subarachnoid space is reached, and the examiner usually recognizes entry as a sudden release of resistance. Some examiners prefer to remove the stylet periodically as the needle is advanced to look for CSF flow. If the needle cannot be advanced because bone is hit, if the patient experiences sharp radiating pain

Table 356-2   The Neurologic Examination

Mental Status Examination (See also Chaps. 24 to 26)

These tests are designed to evaluate attention, orientation, memory, insight, judgment, and grasp of general information. A series of numbers can be recited and the patient asked to respond every time a specific item recurs (attention). The patient can be asked his or her name, the place, the day, and the date. Retentive memory and immediate recall can be tested by determining the number of digits that can be repeated in sequence. Recent memory is evaluated by testing recall of a series of objects after defined times (e.g., 5 and 15 min). More remote memory is evaluated by assessment of the patient's ability to provide a coherent chronologic history of his or her illness or personal life events. Recall of major historical or current events can be used to assess the fund of general knowledge. If answers suggest that there may be a problem with insight, the patient should be asked whether anything is wrong with his or her health. Interpretation of proverbs (e.g., "People who live in glass houses..."; "A bird in the hand....") can provide information relative to judgment and capacity to reason in an abstract manner. Specific higher cortical functions can be tested when clinical circumstances suggest that deficits may be present. Evaluation of language function should include assessment of spontaneous speech, naming, repetition, reading, writing, and comprehension. Calculations, identification of right from left, identification of fingers, praxis (whistling, brushing teeth, combing hair, saluting), and ability to draw and copy figures may also be assessed.

Cranial Nerve (CN) Examination (See also Chaps. 28, 29, and 367)

CN I   Occlude each nostril sequentially. Use a mild test stimulus such as soap, toothpaste, coffee, or lemon oil. With the eyes closed, the patient sniffs and tries to identify the stimulus.

CN II   Check visual acuity (with eyeglasses or pinhole correction) using a Snellen chart (distance) or Jaeger's test type (near). Map visual fields by confrontation testing in each quadrant of the visual field for each eye individually. The best method is to sit facing the patient [0.6 to 1.0 m (2 to 3 ft) apart] and ask him or her to gently cover one eye and fix the uncovered eye on the examiner's nose. A small object (e.g., a white hatpin or cotton-tipped applicator) is then moved from the periphery of the field toward the center until appreciated by the patient. The patient's visual field should be mapped against the examiner's for comparison. The size of the blind spot can also be estimated in this manner; for central vision, use of a red pin will improve sensitivity of the study. Formal perimetry and tangent screen examinations may be required to identify and delineate small defects. Optic fundi should be examined with an ophthalmoscope, and the color, size, and degree of swelling or elevation of the optic disc recorded. The retinal vessels should be checked for size, regularity, arterial-venous nicking at crossing points, hemorrhage, exudates, aneurysms, etc. Normally, 8 to 12 vessels course over the disc margin, and the darker arterioles are approximately two-thirds the size of the lighter colored venules.

CN III, IV, VI   Describe the size and shape of pupils and direct and consensual pupillary reactions to light. Check for pupillary accommodation with convergence (ask the patient to follow a small object as it moves towards the bridge of the nose). Check for lid droop, lag, or retraction. Ask the patient to follow a small object (e.g., a hatpin) at a distance of 0.6 m (2 ft). Move the target slowly in both horizontal and vertical planes; observe any paresis, nystagmus, or abnormality of smooth pursuit (saccades, oculomotor ataxia, etc.). Horizontal nystagmus is best assessed at 45° and not at extreme lateral gaze. Incomplete eye movements may result from a nuclear or supranuclear cause; a supranuclear cause is present if full eye movements are present with doll's-head maneuver (gentle, rapid side-to-side or up-and-down movements of the neck).

CN V   Feel the masseter and temporalis muscles as the patient bites down. Test jaw opening, protrusion, and lateral motion against resistance. Examine sensation over the entire face and corneas using a light wisp of cotton.

CN VII   Look for facial asymmetry at rest and with spontaneous movements. Test eyebrow elevation, forehead wrinkling, eye closure, smiling, frowning, cheek puff, whistle, lip pursing, and chin muscle contraction. Look in particular for differences in strength of the lower versus upper facial muscles. Taste on the anterior two-thirds of the tongue may be impaired by lesions of the nerve proximal to the chordi tympani. Test taste for sweet (sugar), salt, sour (lemon), and bitter (quinine) using cotton-tipped applicators moistened in the appropriate solution and placed on the lateral margin of the protruded tongue halfway back from the tip.

CN VIII   Check the ability to hear a tuning fork, finger rub, watch tick, and whispered voice with each ear. Check for air versus mastoid bone conduction (Rinne) and lateralization of a tuning fork placed on the center of the forehead (Weber). Examine the tympanic membranes. Quantitative testing of hearing requires formal audiometry.

CN IX, X   Check for symmetric elevation of the palate-uvula with phonation ("aah") as well as the position of the uvula and palatal arch at rest. Sensation in the region of the tonsils, posterior pharynx, and tongue may also require testing in some patients. Pharyngeal ("gag") reflex is evaluated by stimulating the posterior pharyngeal wall on each side with a blunt object (e.g., tongue blade). Direct examination of vocal cords by laryngoscopy may be necessary.

CN XI   Check shoulder shrug (trapezius muscle) and head rotation to each side (sternocleidomastoid muscle) against resistance.

CN XII   Examine the bulk and power of the tongue. Look for atrophy, deviation from midline with protrusion, tremor, and small flickering or twitching movements (fibrillations, fasciculations).

Motor Examination (See also Chap. 22)

Inspection   Muscles are examined for atrophy or hypertrophy. Fasciculations may be observed as fine twitching that occurs spontaneously or is induced by light percussion. Involuntary movements may be present at rest (e.g., tics, myoclonus, choreoathetosis, ballismus), during maintained posture (pill-rolling tremor of Parkinson's disease), or with voluntary action (intention tremor of cerebellar disease or familial tremor).

Tone   Muscle tone is tested by resistance to passive motion of a relaxed limb. During testing, it is useful to distract the patient from the examination to minimize active movements. In the upper limbs, tone is assessed by repetitive pronation and supination of the forearm and by rolling the hand at the wrist. In the lower limbs, the examiner's hands are placed behind the thighs and rapidly raised; with normal tone the ankles drag along the table surface for a variable distance before rising, whereas increased tone results in an immediate lift of the heel off the surface. Decreased tone is most commonly due to lower motor neuron, peripheral nerve, or cerebellar pathway disorders. Increased tone may be evident as spasticity (resistance determined by the angle and direction of motion; corticospinal tract disease), rigidity (similar resistance at all angles of motion; extrapyramidal disease), or paratonia/Gegenhalten (fluctuating changes in resistance to repetitive passive movements; frontal lobe pathways). One frequently observed type of rigidity is the cogwheel rigidity of Parkinson's disease, in which passive motion elicits jerky interruptions in resistance.

Strength   Muscle strength is tested by evaluating flexion, extension, adduction, and abduction at each joint, and recorded using the following scale:

0 = no movement	4− = movement against a mild degree of resistance
1 = flicker or trace of contraction but no associated movement at a joint	4 = movement against moderate resistance
2 = movement with gravity eliminated	4+ = movement against strong resistance
3 = movement against gravity but not against resistance	5 = full power

Reflexes

Muscle Stretch Reflexes   Commonly tested are the biceps (**C5, C6**), brachioradialis (**C5, C6**), triceps (**C7, C8**), and finger flexor (**C8**) reflexes in the upper limbs and the patellar or quadriceps (**L3, L4**) and Achilles (**S1, S2**) reflexes in the lower limbs. Stretch reflexes are best elicited in a relaxed limb. It is sometimes useful to use conversation to distract the patient during reflex testing. Reflexes may be enhanced by asking the patient to voluntarily contract other, distant muscle groups (Jendrassik maneuver). For example, upper limb reflexes may be reinforced by voluntary teeth-clenching, and the Achilles reflex by hooking the flexed fingers of the two hands together and by attempting to pull them apart. For each reflex tested, left and right limbs should be similarly positioned and the two sides tested sequentially. It is more useful to determine the smallest stimulus required to elicit a reflex rather than the maximum response that can be obtained.

(continued)

Table 356-2   The Neurologic Examination—*(continued)*

Reflexes are graded according to the following scale:

0 = absent
1 = present but diminished
2 = normoactive
3 = exaggerated
4 = clonus

Clonus refers to repetitive rhythmic contractions evoked by a stretch stimulus; it is most commonly noted at the Achilles tendon. Occasional normal individuals will have two or three beats of physiologic ankle clonus, but sustained ankle clonus is an abnormal finding that signifies hyperactivity of the motor unit resulting from an upper motor neuron lesion.

Cutaneous Reflexes   The plantar reflex is elicited by stroking, with a noxious stimulus (i.e., a key or tongue blade), the lateral surface of the sole beginning near the heel and moving across the ball of the foot to the great toe. The normal reflex consists of plantar flexion of the toes. With upper motor neuron lesions above the S1 level of the spinal cord, a paradoxical extension of the great toe is noted, associated with fanning and extension of the other toes (extensor plantar response or Babinski sign); a prominent extensor plantar response may be accompanied by triple flexion at the ankle, knee, and hip. In some patients with corticospinal tract lesions, the great toe on the involved side may assume an extensor posture at rest or after movement of the foot. Some patients may voluntarily withdraw from the plantar stroke, simulating an extensor response. In these situations, the true direction of the plantar response may be determined by pressure applied to the anterior tibia, stroking towards the ankle (Oppenheim sign), pressure applied to the calf (Gordon sign) or ankle (Schaefer sign), or pricking of the dorsum of the great toe (Bing sign).

Superficial abdominal reflexes are elicited by lightly stroking the abdominal wall with a sharp object (e.g., a pin) and observing movement of the umbilicus. The upper abdominal reflex (spinal cord level T9) is elicited by stroking the upper lateral corner of the abdomen towards the umbilicus, whereas the lower abdominal reflex (T12) is elicited by a stimulus beginning at the lower lateral abdomen. The normal response consists of diagonal movement of the umbilicus toward the origin of the stimulus. With upper motor neuron lesions, these reflexes are absent. They are most helpful when there is preservation of upper but not lower abdominal reflexes, indicating a spinal lesion between T9 and T12, or when the response is asymmetric. Obese individuals or multiparous women may lack visible superficial abdominal reflexes. Other useful cutaneous reflexes include the cremasteric (ipsilateral elevation of the testicle following stroking of the medial thigh), anal (contraction of the anal sphincter following pinprick stimulation of the perianal region), and bulbocavernosus (contraction of urethra and anal sphincter after a stimulus to the glans penis) reflexes.

Primitive Reflexes   In disease of the frontal lobe pathways, several primitive reflexes not normally present in the adult may appear. The suck response is elicited by lightly touching the center of the lips, and the root response the corner of the lips, with a tongue blade; the patient will move the lips to suck or root in the direction of the stimulus. The grasp reflex is elicited by touching the palm, and in particular the area between the thumb and index finger, with the examiner's fingers; a positive (abnormal) response consists of a forced grasp of the stimulated hand. The palmomental response consists of contraction of the mentalis muscle ipsilateral to a scratch stimulus diagonally applied to the palm.

Sensory Examination (See also Chap. 23)

Five primary sensory modalities—vibration, joint position, light touch, pinprick, and temperature—are routinely tested in each limb. Vibration testing generally utilizes a 128-Hz weighted tuning fork applied to the terminal phalynx of the great toe or middle finger just below the nail bed. The examiner compares the patient's threshold of vibration perception with his or her own or compares distal and proximal thresholds in the patient. For joint position testing, the examiner grasps the limb laterally and distal to the joint to be assessed; small 1–2 mm excursions are normally appreciated. Light touch is best assessed with a wisp of cotton, pinprick with a new pin (compare sharp versus blunt end), and temperature initially with a tuning fork immersed in cold and warm water. Patients with lesions above the level of the thalamus may have disorders of "discriminative sensation," resulting in an inability to perceive double simultaneous stimuli, to localize stimuli accurately, to identify closely approximated stimuli as separate (two-point discrimination), to identify objects by touch alone (stereognosis), or identify letters or numbers written on the skin surface (graphesthesia).

Coordination (See also Chap. 22)

The patient is asked to touch his or her index finger repetitively to the nose and then to the examiner's outstretched finger; the examiner's finger can be moved with each repetition. Another useful test is to ask the patient to alternate tapping the palm then the back of one hand on the thigh. To test coordination in the legs, in the supine position the patient is asked to slide the heel (not the arch!) of each foot from the knee down the shin of the other leg, and to raise the leg and touch with the great toe the examiner's index finger. For all these movements, the accuracy, speed, and rhythm are noted.

Gait (See also Chap. 22)

Gait testing is essential; unexpected abnormalities may be detected that prompt the examiner to return, in more detail, to other aspects of the examination. Normal gait requires that multiple systems—including power, sensation, coordination, and praxis—function in a coordinated fashion. The ability to rise from the sitting or lying position, to walk, turn, and heel-toe walk along a straight line should be noted. A positive Romberg test consists of an ability to stand with feet together and eyes open but not with eyes closed, and usually signifies a proprioceptive sensory deficit. The examination may reveal decreased arm swing on one side (corticospinal tract disease), a stooped posture and short-stepped gait (parkinsonism), a broad-based unstable gait (ataxia), scissoring (spasticity), or a high-stepped, slapping gait (posterior column or peripheral nerve disease), or the patient may appear to be stuck in place (apraxia).

---

down one leg, or if the tap is "dry," the needle is removed completely and repositioned.

Once the subarachnoid space is reached, a manometer is attached to the needle and the CSF pressure is measured. The examiner should look for normal oscillations in CSF pressure associated with pulse and respirations. Depending on the clinical indication, fluid is then obtained for studies that include the following: (1) cell count, differential, and presence of microorganisms—it is often useful to repeat the cell count in the first and last tube; (2) protein, glucose, and other chemical measurements; (3) cytology; (4) bacteriologic cultures and virus isolation; (5) VDRL, cryptococcal antigen, and serologic and genetic tests for other microorganisms as appropriate; (6) immunoelectrophoresis for determination of gamma globulin level (paired serum sample essential), oligoclonal banding, and other special biochemical tests (NH_3, pH, CO_2, enzymes). Normal values of CSF constituents are shown in

Appendix A. Under most conditions, the physician should not be concerned about removing too large a quantity of CSF. A sufficient volume to obtain all the data required is essential. In particular, adequate volumes for cytology, when indicated, should be removed.

Failure to enter the lumbar subarachnoid space after two or three trials can usually be corrected by repositioning the patient in the sitting position and then assisting them to lie on their side. The "dry tap" is more often due to an improperly placed needle than to a pathologic obliteration of subarachnoid space by a compressive lesion of the spinal cord or by chronic adhesive arachnoiditis. A bloody tap due to penetration of a meningeal vessel may be confused with subarachnoid hemorrhage. In these situations a specimen of CSF should be centrifuged immediately after it is obtained; clear supernatant CSF after centrifugation supports the diagnosis of a bloody tap, whereas xanthochromic supernatant suggests subarachnoid hemorrhage. In

Table 356-3 Indications for Diagnostic Lumbar Puncture

Absolute Indications
Meningitis
Encephalitis
Meningeal cancer
Guillain-Barré syndrome
Acute demyelinating disorders
Acute disseminated encephalomyelitis
Transverse myelitis
Brainstem encephalomyelitis
Benign intracranial hypertension (pseudotumor cerebri)
Unexplained neurologic disorders
Seizure
Stroke
Polyneuropathy
Dementia
Altered level of consciousness
Possible indications (Depending on the clinical situation)
Multiple sclerosis
Subarachnoid hemorrhage (if CT negative)

general, bloody CSF due to a meningeal vessel puncture clears gradually in successive tubes, whereas blood due to a subarachnoid hemorrhage does not. In addition to subarachnoid hemorrage, xanthochromic CSF may also be present in patients with liver disease or when the level of CSF protein is elevated [>1.5 to 2.0 g/L (150 to 200 mg/dL)].

There are several absolute or relative contraindications to LP. The procedure should be undertaken with particular care in patients with thrombocytopenia or disorders of blood coagulation because serious hemorrhage into the extradural or intradural space may occur. In these situations, it is prudent whenever possible to transfuse platelets, administer fresh frozen plasma, or reverse therapeutic anticoagulation before the procedure. Patients receiving low-molecular-weight heparin may be at risk of hemorrhage unless doses are held for 24 h. An LP through areas of cutaneous or soft tissue infection may spread infection to the meninges; thus LP at these sites should be avoided.

In patients with elevated CSF pressure, potentially fatal cerebellar or tentorial herniation may follow LP. This possibility should be considered in all patients with focal neurologic findings, altered mental status, or papilledema. If CSF examination is required in such cases, it is wise to first obtain a neuroimaging scan to exclude a mass lesion. An exception to this rule is suspected meningitis, where immediate CSF examination is indicated. In this situation, the LP may be performed with a fine-bore (24-gauge) needle. If the pressure is >400 mmHg, the minimum required sample of fluid should be obtained, the needle removed, and, according to the suspected clinical disease and the patient's condition, intravenous mannitol administered in a dose of 0.75 to 1.0 mg/kg; unless contraindicated, dexamethasone may also be started in a dose of 4 to 6 mg every 6 h.

After LP, the patient is normally positioned in a comfortable, recumbant position for 1 h before rising. The principal complication of LP is headache, occurring in 10 to 30% of patients, caused by a drop in CSF pressure related to persistent leakage of CSF. Such headaches typically begin 12 to 48 h after the procedure and may last from several days to 2 weeks, rarely longer. These headaches are strikingly positional in character; they are worsened by an upright posture and are relieved by lying flat. →*Therapy is discussed in Chap. 15.*

BIBLIOGRAPHY

ADAMS RD et al: *Principles of Neurology*, 6th ed. New York, McGraw-Hill, 1997
AMERICAN ACADEMY OF NEUROLOGY: Practice parameter: Lumbar puncture (summary statement). Report of the Quality Standards Subcommittee. Neurology 43:625, 1993
DANA ALLIANCE FOR BRAIN INITIATIVES: *Delivery Results: A Progress Report on Brain Research.* New York, Dana Press, 1996
FISHMAN RA: *Cerebrospinal Fluid in Diseases of the Nervous System*, 2d ed. Philadelphia, Saunders, 1992
FULLER G: Neurological examination made easy. New York. Churchill Livingstone, 1999
GOPAL AK et al: Cranial computed tomography before lumbar puncture: a prospective clinical evaluation. Arch Int Med 159:2681, 1999
HAERER AF: *DeJong's The Neurologic Examination*. Philadelphia, Lippincott, 1992
QUINT DJ: Indications for emergent MRI of the central nervous system. JAMA 283:853, 2000

357 Michael J. Aminoff

ELECTROPHYSIOLOGIC STUDIES OF THE CENTRAL AND PERIPHERAL NERVOUS SYSTEMS

ELECTROENCEPHALOGRAPHY

The electrical activity of the brain [the *electroencephalogram* (EEG)] is easily recorded from electrodes placed on the scalp. The potential difference between pairs of electrodes on the scalp (bipolar derivation) or between individual scalp electrodes and a relatively inactive common reference point (referential derivation) is amplified and displayed on paper or the screen of an oscilloscope. The findings depend on the patient's age and level of arousal. The rhythmic activity normally recorded represents the postsynaptic potentials of vertically oriented pyramidal cells of the cerebral cortex and is characterized by its frequency. In normal awake adults lying quietly with the eyes closed, an 8- to 13-Hz alpha rhythm is seen posteriorly in the EEG, intermixed with a variable amount of generalized faster (beta) activity, and it is attenuated when the eyes are opened (Fig. 357-1). During drowsiness, the alpha rhythm is also attenuated; with light sleep, slower activity in the theta (4 to 7 Hz) and delta (<4 Hz) ranges becomes more conspicuous.

The EEG is best recorded from several different electrode arrangements (montages) in turn, and activating procedures are generally undertaken in an attempt to provoke abnormalities. Such procedures commonly include hyperventilation (for 3 or 4 min), photic stimulation, sleep, and the deprivation of sleep on the night prior to the recording.

Electroencephalography is relatively inexpensive and may aid clinical management in several different contexts.

THE EEG AND EPILEPSY The EEG is most useful in evaluating patients with suspected epilepsy. The presence of *electrographic seizure activity*, i.e., of abnormal, repetitive, rhythmic activity having an abrupt onset and termination, clearly establishes the diagnosis. The absence of such electrocerebral accompaniment does not exclude a seizure disorder, however, because there may be no change in the scalp-recorded EEG during simple or complex partial seizures. With generalized tonic-clonic seizures, however, the EEG is always abnormal during the episode. It is often not possible to obtain an EEG during clinical events that may represent seizures, especially when such events occur unpredictably or infrequently. The development of portable equipment to record the EEG continuously on cassettes for 24 h or longer in ambulatory patients has made it easier to capture the electrocerebral accompaniments of such clinical episodes, and monitoring by this means is sometimes helpful in confirming that seizures are occurring, characterizing the nature of clinically equivocal episodes, and determining the frequency of epileptic events.

The EEG findings may also be helpful in the interictal period by showing certain abnormalities that are strongly supportive of a diagnosis of epilepsy. Such *epileptiform activity* consists of bursts of abnormal discharges containing spikes or sharp waves. The presence of epileptiform activity is not specific for epilepsy, but it has a much greater prevalence in epileptic patients than in normal individuals. When epileptiform activity is found in the EEG of a patient with ep-

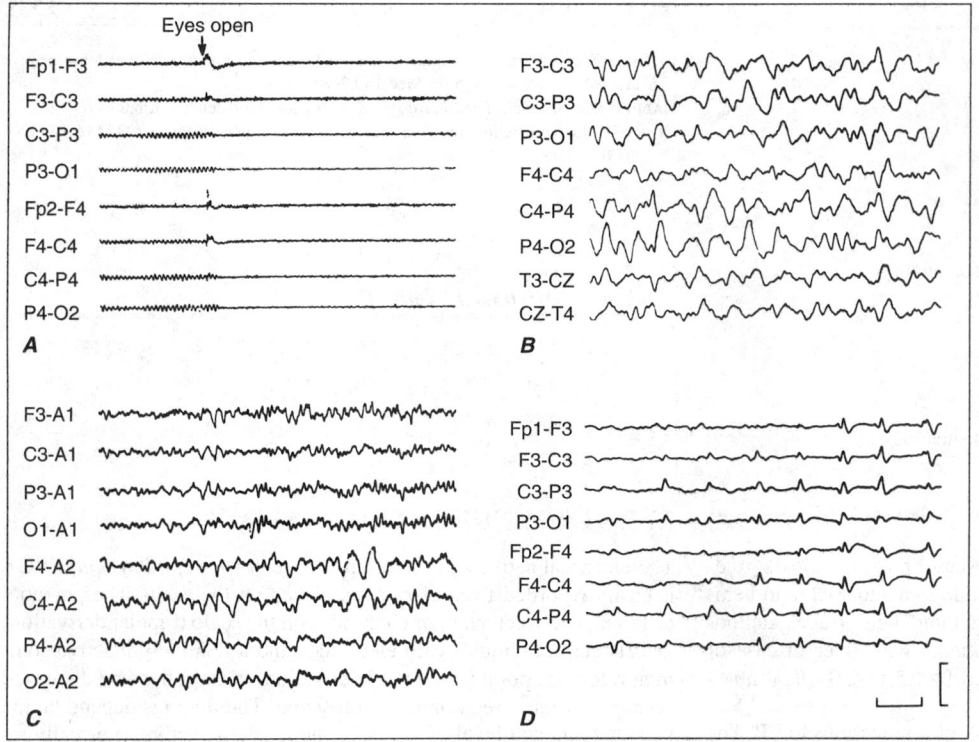

FIGURE 357-1 *A.* Normal EEG showing a posteriorly situated 9-Hz alpha rhythm that attenuates with eye opening. *B.* Abnormal EEG showing irregular diffuse slow activity in an obtunded patient with encephalitis. *C.* Irregular slow activity in the right central region, on a diffusely slowed background, in a patient with a right parietal glioma. *D.* Periodic complexes occurring once every second in a patient with Creutzfeldt-Jakob disease. Horizontal calibration: 1 s; vertical calibration: 200 μV in A, 300 μV in other panels. *(From Aminoff, 1999.)* In this and the following figure, electrode placements are indicated at the left of each panel and accord with the international 10:20 system. A, earlobe; C, central; F, frontal; Fp, frontal polar; P, parietal; T, temporal; O, occipital. Right-sided placements are indicated by even numbers, left-sided placements by odd numbers, and midline placements by Z.

isodic behavioral disturbances that clinically might be epileptic in nature, the likelihood that epilepsy is the correct diagnosis is markedly increased.

The EEG findings have also been used in classifying seizure disorders and selecting appropriate anticonvulsant medication for individual patients (Fig. 357-2). The episodic generalized spike-wave activity that occurs during and between seizures in patients with typical absences (petit mal epilepsy) contrasts with the normal findings, focal interictal epileptiform discharges, or ictal patterns found in patients with complex partial seizures. These latter seizures may have no correlates in the scalp-recorded EEG or may be associated with abnormal rhythmic activity of variable frequency, a localized or generalized distribution, and a stereotyped pattern that varies with the patient. Focal or lateralized epileptogenic lesions are important to recognize, especially if surgical treatment is contemplated. Intensive long-term monitoring of clinical behavior and the EEG is required for operative candidates, however, and this generally also involves recording from intracranially placed electrodes (which may be subdural, extradural, or intracerebral in location).

The findings in the routine scalp-recorded EEG may indicate the prognosis of seizure disorders: in general, a normal EEG implies a better prognosis than otherwise, whereas an abnormal background or profuse epileptiform activity suggests a poor outlook. The EEG findings are not helpful in determining which patients with head injuries, stroke, or brain tumors will go on to develop seizures, because in such circumstances epileptiform activity is commonly encountered regardless of whether seizures occur. The EEG findings are sometimes used to determine whether anticonvulsant medication can be discontinued in epileptic patients who have been seizure-free for several years, but the findings provide only a general guide to prognosis: further seizures may occur after withdrawal of anticonvulsant medication despite a

normal EEG or, conversely, may not occur despite a continuing EEG abnormality. The decision to discontinue anticonvulsant medication is made on clinical grounds, and the EEG does not have a useful role in this context except for providing guidance when there is clinical ambiguity or the patient requires reassurance about a particular course of action.

The EEG has no role in the management of tonic-clonic status epilepticus except when there is clinical uncertainty whether seizures are continuing in a comatose patient. In patients treated by pentobarbital-induced coma for refractory status epilepticus, the EEG findings are useful in indicating the level of anesthesia and whether seizures are occurring. During status epilepticus, the EEG shows repeated electrographic seizures or continuous spike-wave discharges. In nonconvulsive status epilepticus, a disorder that may not be recognized unless an EEG is performed, the EEG may also show continuous spike-wave activity ("spike-wave stupor") or, less commonly, repetitive electrographic seizures (complex partial status epilepticus).

THE EEG AND COMA In patients with an altered mental state or some degree of obtundation, the EEG tends to become slower as consciousness is depressed, regardless of the underlying cause (Fig. 357-1). Other findings may also be present and may suggest diagnostic possibilities, as when electrographic seizures are found or there is a focal abnormality indicating a structural lesion. The EEG generally slows in metabolic encephalopathies, and triphasic waves may be present. The findings do not permit differentiation of the underlying metabolic disturbance but help to exclude other encephalopathic processes by indicating the diffuse extent of cerebral dysfunction. The response of the EEG to external stimulation is helpful prognostically because electrocerebral responsiveness implies a lighter level of coma than a nonreactive EEG. Serial records provide a better guide to prognosis than a single record and supplement the clinical examination in following the course of events. As the depth of coma increases, the EEG becomes nonreactive and may show a burst-suppression pattern, with bursts of mixed-frequency activity separated by intervals of relative cerebral inactivity. In other instances there is a reduction in amplitude of the EEG until eventually electrocerebral activity cannot be detected. Such electrocerebral silence does not necessarily reflect irreversible brain damage, because it may occur in hypothermic patients or with drug overdose. The prognosis of electrocerebral silence, when recorded using an adequate technique, depends upon the clinical context in which it is found. In patients with severe cerebral anoxia, for example, electrocerebral silence in a technically satisfactory record implies that useful cognitive recovery will not occur.

In patients with clinically suspected brain death, an EEG, when recorded using appropriate technical standards, may be confirmatory by showing electrocerebral silence. However, complicating disorders that may produce a similar but reversible EEG appearance (e.g., hypothermia or drug intoxication) must be excluded. The presence of residual EEG activity in suspected brain death fails to confirm the diagnosis but does not exclude it. The EEG is usually normal in patients with locked-in syndrome and helps in distinguishing this dis-

FIGURE 357-2 Electrographic seizures. *A*. Onset of a tonic seizure showing generalized repetitive sharp activity with synchronous onset over both hemispheres. *B*. Burst of repetitive spikes occurring with sudden onset in the right temporal region during a clinical spell characterized by transient impairment of external awareness. *C*. Generalized 3-Hz spike-wave activity occurring synchronously over both hemispheres during an absence (petit mal) attack. Horizontal calibration: 1 s; vertical calibration: 400 μV in A, 200 μV in B, and 750 μV in C. *(From Aminoff, 1999.)*

order from the comatose state with which it is sometimes confused clinically.

THE EEG IN OTHER NEUROLOGIC DISORDERS In the developed countries, computed tomography (CT) scanning and magnetic resonance imaging (MRI) have taken the place of EEG as a noninvasive means of screening for focal structural abnormalities of the brain, such as tumors, infarcts, or hematomas (Fig. 357-1). Nonetheless, the EEG is still used for this purpose in many parts of the world, although infratentorial or slowly expanding lesions may fail to cause any abnormalities. Focal slow-wave disturbances, a localized loss of electrocerebral activity, or more generalized electrocerebral disturbances are common findings but provide no reliable indication about the nature of the underlying pathology.

In patients with an acute encephalopathy, focal or lateralized periodic slow-wave complexes, sometimes with a sharpened outline, sug-

gest a diagnosis of herpes simplex encephalitis, and periodic lateralized epileptiform discharges (PLEDs) are commonly found with acute hemispheric pathology such as a hematoma, abscess, or rapidly expanding tumor. The EEG findings in dementia are usually nonspecific and do not distinguish between the different causes of cognitive decline except in rare instances when the presence of complexes occurring with a regular repetition rate (so-called periodic complexes) in dementing disorders, for example, supports a diagnosis of Creutzfeldt-Jakob disease (Fig. 357-1) or subacute sclerosing panencephalitis. In most patients with dementias, the EEG is normal or diffusely slowed, and the EEG findings alone cannot indicate whether a patient is demented or distinguish between dementia and pseudodementia.

EVOKED POTENTIALS

SENSORY EVOKED POTENTIALS The noninvasive recording of spinal or cerebral potentials elicited by stimulation of specific afferent pathways is an important means of monitoring the functional integrity of these pathways but does not indicate the pathologic basis of lesions involving them. Such evoked potentials (EPs) are so small compared to the background EEG activity that the responses to a number of stimuli have to be recorded and averaged with a computer in order to permit their recognition and definition. The background EEG activity, which has no fixed temporal relationship to the stimulus, is averaged out by this procedure.

Visual evoked potentials (VEPs) are elicited by monocular stimulation with a reversing checkerboard pattern and are recorded from the occipital region in the midline and on either side of the scalp. The component of major clinical importance is the so-called P100 response, a positive peak having a latency of approximately 100 ms. Its presence, latency, and symmetry over the two sides of the scalp are noted. Amplitude may also be measured, but changes in size are much less helpful for the recognition of pathology. VEPs are most useful in detecting dysfunction of the visual pathways anterior to the optic chiasm. In patients with acute severe optic neuritis, the P100 is frequently lost or grossly attenuated; as clinical recovery occurs and visual acuity improves, the P100 is restored but with an increased latency that generally remains abnormally prolonged indefinitely. The VEP findings are therefore helpful in indicating previous or subclinical optic neuritis. They may also be abnormal with ocular abnormalities and with other causes of optic nerve disease, such as ischemia or compression by a tumor. Normal VEPs may be elicited by flash stimuli in patients with cortical blindness.

Brainstem auditory evoked potentials (BAEPs) are elicited by monaural stimulation with repetitive clicks and are recorded between the vertex of the scalp and the mastoid process or earlobe. A series of potentials, designated by roman numerals, occurs in the first 10 ms after the stimulus and represents in part the sequential activation of different structures in the pathway between the auditory nerve (wave I) and the inferior colliculus (wave V) in the midbrain. The presence, latency, and interpeak latency of the first five positive potentials recorded at the vertex are evaluated. The findings are helpful in screening for acoustic neuromas, detecting brainstem pathology, and evaluating comatose patients. The BAEPs are normal in coma due to metabolic/toxic disorders or bihemispheric disease but abnormal in the presence of brainstem pathology.

Somatosensory evoked potentials (SEPs) are recorded over the scalp and spine in response to electrical stimulation of a peripheral (mixed or cutaneous) nerve. The configuration, polarity, and latency of the responses depend on the nerve that is stimulated and on the recording arrangements. SEPs are used to evaluate proximal (otherwise inaccessible) portions of the peripheral nervous system and the integrity of the central somatosensory pathways.

Clinical Utility of Sensory Evoked Potentials EP studies may detect and localize lesions in afferent pathways in the central nervous system (CNS). They have been used particularly to investigate patients with suspected multiple sclerosis (MS), the diagnosis of which requires the recognition of lesions involving several different regions of the central white matter. In patients with clinical evidence of only one lesion, the electrophysiologic recognition of abnormalities in other sites helps to suggest or support the diagnosis but does not establish it unequivocally. Multimodality EP abnormalities are not specific for MS; they may occur in AIDS, Lyme disease, systemic lupus erythematosus, neurosyphilis, spinocerebellar degenerations, familial spastic paraplegia, and deficiency of vitamin E or B_{12}, among other disorders. The diagnostic utility of the electrophysiologic findings therefore depends upon the circumstances in which they are found. Abnormalities may aid in the localization of lesions to broad areas of the CNS, but attempts at precise localization on electrophysiologic grounds are misleading because the generators of many components of the EP are unknown.

The EP findings are sometimes of prognostic relevance. Bilateral loss of SEP components that are generated in the cerebral cortex implies that cognition may not be regained in posttraumatic or postanoxic coma, and EP studies may also be useful in evaluating patients with suspected brain death. In patients who are comatose for uncertain reasons, preserved BAEPs suggest either a metabolic-toxic etiology or bihemispheric disease. In patients with spinal cord injuries, SEPs have been used to indicate the completeness of the lesion—the presence or early return of a cortically generated response to stimulation of a nerve below the injured segment of the cord indicates an incomplete lesion and thus a better prognosis for functional recovery than otherwise. In surgery, intraoperative EP monitoring of neural structures placed at risk by the procedure may permit the early recognition of dysfunction and thereby permit a neurologic complication to be averted or minimized.

Visual and auditory acuity may be determined using EP techniques in patients whose age or mental state precludes traditional ophthalmologic or audiologic examinations.

COGNITIVE EVOKED POTENTIALS Certain EP components depend upon the mental attention of the subject and the setting in which the stimulus occurs, rather than simply on the physical characteristics of the stimulus. Such "event-related" potentials (ERPs) or "endogenous" potentials are related in some manner to the cognitive aspects of distinguishing an infrequently occurring target stimulus from other stimuli occurring more frequently. For clinical purposes, attention has been directed particularly at the so-called P3 component of the ERP, which is also designated the P300 component because of its positive polarity and latency of approximately 300 to 400 ms after onset of an auditory target stimulus. The P3 component is prolonged in latency in many patients with dementia, whereas it is generally normal in patients with depression or other psychiatric disorders that might be mistaken for dementia. ERPs are therefore sometimes helpful in making this distinction when there is clinical uncertainty, although a response of normal latency does not exclude a dementing disorder.

MOTOR EVOKED POTENTIALS The electrical potentials recorded from muscle or the spinal cord following stimulation of the motor cortex or central motor pathways are referred to as *motor evoked potentials*. For clinical purposes such responses are recorded most often as the compound muscle action potentials elicited by transcutaneous magnetic stimulation of the motor cortex. A strong but brief magnetic field is produced by passing a current through a coil, and this induces stimulating currents in the subjacent neural tissue. The procedure is painless and apparently safe. Abnormalities have been described in several neurologic disorders with clinical or subclinical involvement of central motor pathways, including MS and motor neuron disease. In addition to a possible role in the diagnosis of neurologic disorders or in evaluating the extent of pathologic involvement, the technique provides information of prognostic relevance (e.g., in suggesting the likelihood of recovery of motor function after stroke) and

is useful as a means of monitoring intraoperatively the functional integrity of central motor tracts.

ELECTROPHYSIOLOGIC STUDIES OF MUSCLE AND NERVE

The motor unit is the basic element subserving motor function. It is defined as an anterior horn cell, its axon and neuromuscular junctions, and all the muscle fibers innervated by the axon. The number of motor units in a muscle ranges from approximately 10 in the extraocular muscles to several thousand in the large muscles of the legs. There is considerable variation in the average number of muscle fibers within the motor units of an individual muscle, i.e., in the innervation ratio of different muscles. Thus the innervation ratio is less than 25 in the human external rectus or platysma muscle and between 1600 and 1700 in the medial head of the gastrocnemius muscle. The muscle fibers of individual motor units are divided into two general types by distinctive contractile properties, histochemical stains, and characteristic responses to fatigue. Within each motor unit, all of the muscle fibers are of the same type.

ELECTROMYOGRAPHY The pattern of electrical activity in muscle [i.e., the *electromyogram* (EMG)], both at rest and during activity, may be recorded from a needle electrode inserted into the muscle. The nature and pattern of abnormalities relate to disorders at different levels of the motor unit.

Relaxed muscle normally is electrically silent except in the endplate region, but abnormal spontaneous activity (Fig. 357-3) occurs in various neuromuscular disorders, especially those associated with denervation or inflammatory changes in affected muscle. Fibrillation potentials and positive sharp waves (which reflect muscle fiber irritability) and complex repetitive discharges are most often—but not always—found in denervated muscle and may also occur after muscle injury and in certain myopathic disorders, especially inflammatory disorders such as polymyositis. After an acute neuropathic lesion they are found earlier in proximal rather than distal muscles and sometimes do not develop distally in the extremities for 4 to 6 weeks; once present, they may persist indefinitely unless reinnervation occurs or the muscle degenerates so completely that no viable tissue remains. Fasciculation potentials (which reflect the spontaneous activity of individual motor units) are characteristic of slowly progressive neuropathic disorders, especially those with degeneration of anterior horn cells (such as amyotrophic lateral sclerosis). Myotonic discharges—high-frequency discharges of potentials derived from single muscle

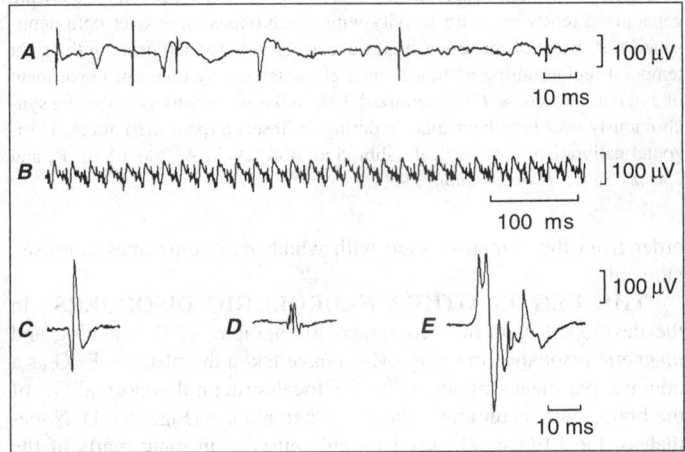

FIGURE 357-3 Activity recorded during EMG. *A.* Spontaneous fibrillation potentials and positive sharp waves. *B.* Complex repetitive discharges recorded in partially denervated muscle at rest. *C.* Normal triphasic motor unit action potential. *D.* Small, short-duration, polyphasic motor unit action potential such as is commonly encountered in myopathic disorders. *E.* Long-duration polyphasic motor unit action potential such as may be seen in neuropathic disorders.

fibers that wax and wane in amplitude and frequency—are the signature of myotonic disorders such as myotonic dystrophy or myotonia congenita but occur occasionally in polymyositis or other, rarer, disorders.

Slight voluntary contraction of a muscle leads to activation of a small number of motor units. The potentials generated by any muscle fibers of these units that are within the pick-up range of the needle electrode will be recorded (Fig. 357-3). The parameters of normal motor unit action potentials depend on the muscle under study and age of the patient, but their duration is normally between 5 and 15 ms, amplitude is between 200 μV and 2 mV, and most are bi- or triphasic. The number of units activated depends on the degree of voluntary activity. An increase in muscle contraction is associated with an increase in the number of motor units that are activated (recruited) and in the frequency with which they discharge. With a full contraction, so many motor units are normally activated that individual motor unit action potentials can no longer be distinguished, and a complete interference pattern is said to have been produced.

The incidence of small, short-duration, polyphasic motor unit action potentials (i.e., having more than four phases) is usually increased in myopathic muscle, and an excessive number of units is activated for a specified degree of voluntary activity. By contrast, the loss of motor units that occurs in neuropathic disorders leads to a reduction in number of units activated during a maximal contraction and an increase in their firing rate, i.e., there is an incomplete or reduced interference pattern; the configuration and dimensions of the potentials may also be abnormal, depending on the duration of the neuropathic process and on whether reinnervation has occurred. The surviving motor units are initially normal in configuration but, as reinnervation occurs, they increase in amplitude and duration and become polyphasic (Fig. 357-3).

Action potentials from the same motor unit sometimes fire with a consistent temporal relationship to each other, so that double, triple, or multiple discharges are recorded, especially in tetany, hemifacial spasm, or myokymia.

Electrical silence characterizes the involuntary, sustained muscle contraction that occurs in phosphorylase deficiency, which is designated a *contracture*.

EMG enables disorders of the motor units to be detected and characterized as either neurogenic or myopathic. In neurogenic disorders, the pattern of affected muscles may localize the lesion to the anterior horn cells or to a specific site as the axons traverse a nerve root, limb plexus, and peripheral nerve to their terminal arborizations. The findings do not enable a specific etiologic diagnosis to be made, however, except in conjunction with the clinical findings and results of other laboratory studies.

The findings may provide a guide to the severity of an acute disorder of a peripheral or cranial nerve (by indicating whether denervation has occurred and the completeness of the lesion), and whether the pathologic process is active or progressive in chronic or degenerative disorders such as amyotrophic lateral sclerosis. Such information is important for prognostic purposes.

Various quantitative EMG approaches have been developed. The most common is to determine the mean duration and amplitude of 20 motor unit action potentials using a standardized technique. The technique of macro-EMG provides information about the number and size of muscle fibers in a larger volume of the motor unit territory and has also been used to estimate the number of motor units in a muscle. Scanning EMG is a computer-based technique that has been used to study the topography of motor unit action potentials and, in particular, the spatial and temporal distribution of activity in individual units. The technique of single-fiber EMG is discussed separately below.

NERVE CONDUCTION STUDIES Recording of the electrical response of a muscle to stimulation of its motor nerve at two or more points along its course (Fig. 357-4) permits conduction velocity to be determined in the fastest-conducting motor fibers between the points of stimulation. The latency and amplitude of the electrical re-

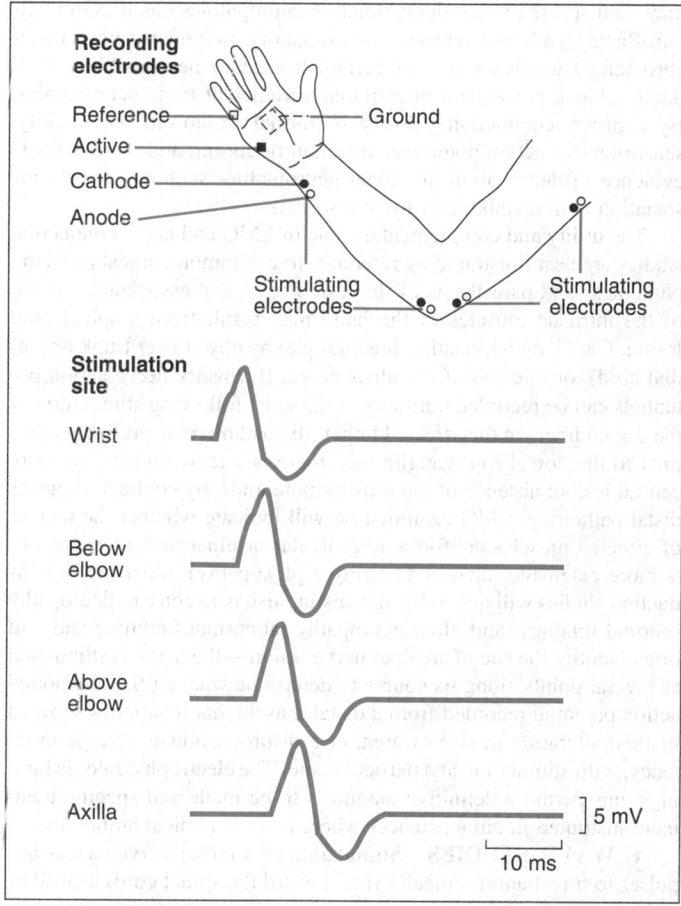

FIGURE 357-4 Arrangement for motor conduction studies of the ulnar nerve. Responses are recorded with a surface electrode from the abductor digiti minimi muscle to supramaximal stimulation of the nerve at different sites, and are shown in the lower panel. *(From Aminoff, 1998.)*

sponse of muscle (i.e., of the compound muscle action potential) to stimulation of its motor nerve at a distal site are also compared with values defined in normal subjects. Sensory nerve conduction studies are performed by determining the conduction velocity and amplitude of action potentials in sensory fibers when these fibers are stimulated at one point and the responses are recorded at another point along the course of the nerve. In adults, conduction velocity in the arms is normally between 50 and 70 m/s, and in the legs is between 40 and 60 m/s.

Nerve conduction studies complement the EMG examination, enabling the presence and extent of peripheral nerve pathology to be determined. They are particularly helpful in determining whether sensory symptoms are arising from pathology proximal or distal to the dorsal root ganglia (in the former instance, peripheral sensory conduction studies will be normal) and whether neuromuscular dysfunction relates to peripheral nerve disease. In patients with a mononeuropathy, they are invaluable as a means of localizing a focal lesion, determining the extent and severity of the underlying pathology, providing a guide to prognosis, and detecting subclinical involvement of other peripheral nerves. They enable a polyneuropathy to be distinguished from a mononeuropathy multiplex when this is not possible clinically, an important distinction because of the etiologic implications. Nerve conduction studies provide a means of following the progression and therapeutic response of peripheral nerve disorders and are being used increasingly for this purpose in clinical trials. They may suggest the underlying pathologic basis in individual cases. Conduction velocity is often markedly slowed, terminal motor latencies are prolonged, and compound motor and sensory nerve action potentials may be dispersed in the demyelinative neuropathies (such as in Guillain-Barré syndrome, chronic inflammatory polyneuropathy, metachromatic leukodystrophy, or certain hereditary neuropathies); conduction block is frequent in acquired varieties of these neuropathies. By contrast, conduction velocity is normal or slowed only mildly, sensory nerve action potentials are small or absent, and there is EMG evidence of denervation in axonal neuropathies such as occur in association with metabolic or toxic disorders.

The utility and complementary role of EMG and nerve conduction studies are best illustrated by reference to a common clinical problem. Numbness and paresthesia of the little finger, and associated wasting of the intrinsic muscles of the hand may result from a spinal cord lesion, C8/T1 radiculopathy, brachial plexopathy (lower trunk or medial cord), or a lesion of the ulnar nerve. If sensory nerve action potentials can be recorded normally at the wrist following stimulation of the digital fibers in the affected finger, the pathology is probably proximal to the dorsal root ganglia, i.e., there is a radiculopathy or more central lesion; absence of the sensory potentials, by contrast, suggests distal pathology. EMG examination will indicate whether the pattern of affected muscles conforms to radicular or ulnar nerve territory, or is more extensive (thereby favoring a plexopathy); ulnar motor conduction studies will generally also distinguish between a radiculopathy (normal findings) and ulnar neuropathy (abnormal findings) and will often identify the site of an ulnar nerve lesion—the nerve is stimulated at several points along its course to determine whether the compound action potential recorded from a distal muscle that it supplies shows a marked alteration in size or area, or a disproportionate change in latency, with stimulation at a particular site. The electrophysiologic findings thus permit a definitive diagnosis to be made and specific treatment instituted in circumstances where there is clinical ambiguity.

F WAVE STUDIES   Stimulation of a motor nerve causes impulses to travel antidromically (i.e., toward the spinal cord) as well as orthodromically (to the nerve terminals). Such antidromic impulses cause a few of the anterior horn cells to discharge, producing a small motor response that occurs considerably later than the direct response elicited by nerve stimulation. The F wave so elicited is sometimes abnormal (absent or delayed) with proximal pathology of the peripheral nervous system, such as a radiculopathy, and may therefore be helpful in detecting abnormalities when conventional nerve conduction studies are normal. In general, however, the clinical utility of F wave studies has been disappointing, except perhaps in Guillain-Barré syndrome, where they are often absent or delayed.

H REFLEX STUDIES   The H reflex is easily recorded only from the soleus muscle (S1) in normal adults. It is elicited by low-intensity stimulation of the tibial nerve and represents a monosynaptic reflex in which spindle (Ia) afferent fibers constitute the afferent arc and alpha motor axons the efferent pathway. The H reflexes are often absent bilaterally in elderly patients or with polyneuropathies and may be lost unilaterally in S1 radiculopathies.

MUSCLE RESPONSE TO REPETITIVE NERVE STIMULATION   The size of the electrical response of a muscle to supramaximal electrical stimulation of its motor nerve relates to the number of muscle fibers that are activated. Neuromuscular transmission can be tested by several different protocols, but the most helpful is to record with surface electrodes the electrical response of a muscle to supramaximal stimulation of its motor nerve by repetitive (2 to 3 Hz) shocks delivered before and at selected intervals after a maximal voluntary contraction.

There is normally little or no change in size of the compound muscle action potential following repetitive stimulation of a motor nerve at 2 to 3 Hz with stimuli delivered at intervals after voluntary contraction of the muscle for about 20 to 30 s, even though preceding activity in the junctional region influences the release of acetylcholine and thus the size of the endplate potentials elicited by a test stimulus. This is because more acetylcholine is normally released than is required to bring the motor endplate potentials to the threshold for generating muscle fiber action potentials. In disorders of neuromuscular transmission this safety factor is reduced. Thus, in myasthenia gravis repetitive stimulation, particularly at a rate of between 2 and 5 Hz, may lead to a depression of neuromuscular transmission, with a decrement in size of the response recorded from affected muscles. Similarly, immediately after a period of maximal voluntary activity, single or repetitive stimuli of the motor nerve may elicit larger muscle responses than before, indicating that more muscle fibers are responding. This postactivation facilitation of neuromuscular transmission is followed by a longer-lasting period of depression, maximal between 2 and 4 min after the conditioning period and lasting for as long as 10 min or so, during which responses are reduced in size.

Decrementing responses to repetitive stimulation at 2 to 5 Hz are common in myasthenia gravis but may also occur in the congenital myasthenic syndromes. In Lambert-Eaton myasthenic syndrome, in which there is defective release of acetylcholine at the neuromuscular junction, the compound muscle action potential elicited by a single stimulus is generally very small. With repetitive stimulation at rates of up to 10 Hz, the first few responses may decline in size, but subsequent responses increase. If faster rates of stimulation are used (20 to 50 Hz), the increment may be dramatic so that the amplitude of compound muscle action potentials eventually reaches a size that is several times larger than the initial response. In patients with botulism, the response to repetitive stimulation is similar to that in Lambert-Eaton syndrome, although the findings are somewhat more variable and not all muscles are affected.

SINGLE-FIBER ELECTROMYOGRAPHY   The technique is particularly helpful in detecting disorders of neuromuscular transmission. A special needle electrode is placed within a muscle and positioned to record action potentials from two muscle fibers belonging to the same motor unit. The time interval between the two potentials will vary in consecutive discharges, and this is called the *neuromuscular jitter*. The jitter can be quantified as the mean difference between consecutive interpotential intervals and is normally between 10 and 50 μs. This value is increased when neuromuscular transmission is disturbed for any reason, and in some instances impulses in individual muscle fibers may fail to occur because of impulse blocking at the neuromuscular junction. Single-fiber EMG is more sensitive than repetitive nerve stimulation or determination of acetylcholine receptor antibody levels in diagnosing myasthenia gravis.

Single-fiber EMG can also be used to determine the mean fiber density of motor units (i.e., mean number of muscle fibers per motor unit within the recording area) and to estimate the number of motor units in a muscle, but this is of less immediate clinical relevance.

BLINK REFLEXES   Electrical or mechanical stimulation of the supraorbital nerve on one side leads to two separate reflex responses of the orbicularis oculi—an ipsilateral R1 response having a latency of approximately 10 ms and a bilateral R2 response with a latency in the order of 30 ms. The trigeminal and facial nerves constitute the afferent and efferent arcs of the reflex, respectively. Abnormalities of either nerve or intrinsic lesions of the medulla or pons may lead to uni- or bilateral loss of the response, and the findings may therefore be helpful in identifying or localizing such pathology.

BIBLIOGRAPHY

AMINOFF MJ: *Electromyography in Clinical Practice: Electrodiagnostic Aspects of Neuromuscular Disease*, 3d ed. New York, Churchill Livingstone, 1998

———— (ed): *Electrodiagnosis in Clinical Neurology*, 4th ed. New York, Churchill Livingstone, 1999

BRIL V et al: Electrophysiological monitoring in clinical trials. Muscle Nerve 11:1368, 1998

DALY DD, PEDLEY TA (eds): *Current Practice of Clinical Electroencephalography*, 2d ed. New York, Raven Press, 1990

DUMITRU D: *Electrodiagnostic Medicine*. Philadelphia, Hanley and Belfus, 1995

EBERSOLE JS (ed): *Ambulatory EEG Monitoring*. New York, Raven Press, 1988

KIMURA J: *Electrodiagnosis in Diseases of Nerve and Muscle*, 2d ed. Philadelphia, Davis, 1989

NIEDERMEYER E, LOPES DA SILVA F (eds): *Electroencephalography*, 3d ed. Baltimore, Urban & Schwarzenberg, 1993

NEUROIMAGING IN NEUROLOGIC DISORDERS

A dramatic increase in the role of imaging in diagnosis of neurologic diseases occurred with the development of computed tomography (CT) in the early 1970s and of magnetic resonance imaging (MRI) in the 1980s. MRI has gradually replaced CT for many indications and has also reduced the indications for invasive neuroimaging techniques, such as myelography and angiography. In general, MRI is more sensitive than CT for the evaluation of most lesions affecting the central nervous system, particularly those in the spinal cord, cranial nerves, and posterior fossa. CT is more sensitive than MRI for visualizing fine osseous detail, such as temporal bone anatomy and fractures. Recent developments, such as helical CT, CT angiography (CTA), MR angiography (MRA), positron emission tomography (PET), Doppler ultrasound, and interventional angiography have continued to advance diagnosis and guide therapy. Conventional angiography is reserved for cases in which small-vessel detail is essential for diagnosis (Table 358-1).

COMPUTED TOMOGRAPHY **Technique** The CT image is a computer-generated cross-sectional representation of anatomy cre-

Table 358-1 Guidelines for the Use of CT , Ultrasound, and MRI

Condition	Recommended Technique
Hemorrhage	
Acute parenchymal	CT > MRI
Subacute/chronic	MRI
Subarachnoid hemorrhage	CT, lumbar puncture → angiography
Aneurysm	Angiography > ?MRA
Ischemic infarction	
Hemorrhagic infarction	CT or MRI
Bland infarction	MRI > CT
Carotid or vertebral dissection	MRI/MRA
Vertebral basilar insufficiency	MRI/MRA
Carotid stenosis	Doppler ultrasound, MRA, CTA
Suspected mass lesions	
Neoplasm, primary or metastatic	MRI + contrast
Infection/abscess	MRI + contrast
Immunosuppression with focal findings	MRI + contrast
Vascular malformations	MRI ± angiography
White matter disorders	MRI
Demyelinating disease	MRI ± contrast
Dementia	MRI or CT
Trauma	
Acute trauma	CT (noncontrast)
Shear injury/chronic hemorrhage	MRI
Headache/migraine	CT (noncontrast) or MRI
Seizure	
First time, no focal neurologic deficits	MRI > CT as screen
Partial complex/refractory	MRI + coronal T2W imaging
Cranial neuropathy	MRI + contrast
Meningeal disease	MRI + contrast
SPINE	
Low back pain	
No neurologic deficits	Conservative therapy, consider MRI or CT after 4 weeks
With focal deficits	MRI > CT
Spinal stenosis	MRI or CT
Cervical spondylosis	MRI or CT myelography
Infection	MRI + contrast > CT
Myelopathy	MRI + contrast, consider myelography if MRI negative
Arteriovenous malformations	MRI, myelography/angiography

NOTE: CT, computed tomography; MRI, magnetic resonance imaging; MRA, MR angiography; CTA, CT angiography; T2W, T2-weighted.

ated by an analysis of the attenuation of x-ray beams passed through various points around a section of the body. As the x-ray source, collimated to the desired slice thickness, rotates around the patient, sensitive x-ray detectors aligned 180° from the source detect x-rays attenuated by the patient's anatomy. A computer calculates a "back projection" image from the 360° x-ray attenuation profile. Greater x-ray attenuation, as caused by bone, results in areas of high "density," while soft tissue structures, which attenuate x-rays less, are lower in density. The resolution of an image depends on the radiation dose, the collimation (slice thickness), the field of view, and the matrix size of the display. A typical modern CT scanner is capable of obtaining sections 1 to 2, 5, and 10 mm thick at a speed of 1 to 3 s per section; complete studies of the brain can be completed in <2 to 3 min.

Intravenous contrast is often administered prior to or during a CT study to identify vascular structures and to detect defects in the blood-brain barrier (BBB) associated with disorders such as tumors, infarcts, and infections. An intact BBB prevents contrast molecules, which are large, from exiting the intravascular compartment. In the normal central nervous system, only vessels and those structures not having a BBB (e.g., the pituitary gland, choroid plexus, and dura) enhance. The use of contrast agents carries a risk of allergic reaction, increases the dose of radiation when both noncontrast and contrast CT scans are to be obtained, adds expense, and may mask hemorrhage; thus, before contrast is administered, the indication for its use should always be considered carefully.

Helical CT is a new technique in which continuous three-dimensional CT information is obtained. In the helical scan mode, the table moves continuously through the rotating x-ray beam, generating a "helix" of information that can be reformatted into various slice thicknesses. Advantages include shorter scan times, reduced patient and organ motion, and the ability to acquire images during the infusion of intravenous contrast. The contrast images can be used to construct CT angiograms of vascular structures. CTA images require a workstation to threshold and segment CT images for display (Fig. 358-1). CTA has proven useful in assessing the carotid bifurcation and intracranial arterial anatomy in selected instances in which a contraindication to MRA exists. Newer "multidetector" scanners allow multiple sections to be obtained with each revolution of the gantry. These scanners have further decreased the time per examination and permit rapid assessment of vascular anatomy (Fig. 358-2).

Indications The indications for CT have decreased since the development of MRI. While MRI gives greater soft tissue contrast and is more sensitive than CT in detecting early brain damage, CT is useful in imaging osseous structures of the spine, skull base, and temporal bones. CT is also more sensitive and specific than MRI for acute subarachnoid hemorrhage. In the spine, CT is useful in evaluating patients

FIGURE 358-1 CT angiography (CTA) of middle cerebral aneurysm. A right middle cerebral aneurysm (*arrow*) is shown on CTA (*left image*) and confirmed by conventional internal carotid angiography (*right image*). CTA image is produced by helical scans or 1-mm CT scans performed during a rapid bolus infusion of intravenous contrast medium. Subtraction of background nonenhancing brain results in the CTA image. (*From RA Alberico et al: Am J Neuroradiol 16:1571, 1995.*)

FIGURE 358-2 A 65-year-old man with aphasia of 5 h duration. Prior right lacunar infarctions were noted by history. *A.* Noncontrast CT scan through the lateral ventricles demonstrates two low-density foci representing old cerebral infarctions on the right. No pathology is seen in the left hemisphere, the site of his acute symptoms. B. Single axial CT image from a CT angiography (CTA) examination obtained in 45 s through the entire supraortic vasculature, cervical carotids, and circle of Willis. Normal right common carotid artery is homogeneously opacified (*arrows*). Left internal carotid artery lumen is narrowed by eccentric low-density atherosclerotic plaque (*arrowheads*), which narrows the lumen to approximately 40%. (C, common carotid artery; V, internal jugular vein; I, internal carotid artery; E, external carotid artery.) *C.* Sagittal reformation through the cervical carotid vasculature from the CTA data set demonstrates the plaque at the origin of the internal carotid artery (*arrow*). *D.* Axial T2-weighted FLAIR (fluid-attenuated inversion recovery) MR image 7 h following onset of aphasia demonstrates a focal cortical high signal intensity (*arrows*) consistent with a small infarction in the posterior temporal lobe. Following anticoagulation, patient improved to his baseline status.

with osseous spinal stenosis and spondylosis, but MRI is often preferred in those with neurologic deficits. CT can also be obtained following intrathecal contrast injection to evaluate the intracranial cisterns for cerebrospinal fluid (CSF) fistula, as well as the spinal subarachnoid space.

Complications CT is safe and reliable. Radiation exposure is between 3 and 5 cGy per examination. The most frequent complications are associated with use of intravenous contrast agents. Two broad categories of contrast media, ionic and nonionic, are in use. Ionic agents are relatively safe and inexpensive but cause a higher incidence of toxicity reactions than nonionic agents.

Nephrotoxicity caused by contrast administration (*contrast nephropathy*) may result from hemodynamic changes, tubular obstruction and cell damage, or immunologic reactions to contrast agents. A rise in serum creatinine of at least 85 μmol/L (1 mg/dL) within 48 h of contrast administration is often used as a definition of contrast nephropathy, although other causes of acute renal failure must be excluded. The prognosis is usually favorable, with serum creatinine levels returning to baseline within 1 to 2 weeks. Risk factors for contrast nephropathy include advanced age, preexisting renal disease, diabetes, dehydration, and high contrast dose. Patients with diabetes and those with mild renal failure should be well hydrated prior to the administration of nonionic agents. Nonionic, low-osmolar media produce fewer abnormalities in renal blood flow and less endothelial cell damage than ionic agents (see guidelines on p. 2339).

A *sensation of heat*, *pain*, *nausea*, and *vomiting* are well-known side effects following intravenous administration of ionic contrast media, and they become more important as studies require longer imaging times and repeated contrast injections. Pain and the sensation of heat are probably due to the osmolality of the agent and vasodilation. These side effects are less intense or nonexistent with nonionic contrast media.

Anaphylactoid reactions to intravenous contrast media range from mild hives to bronchospasm to acute anaphylaxis and death. The pathogenesis of these allergic reactions is not fully understood, but it is thought to include the release of mediators such as histamine, antibody-antigen reactions, and complement activation. Severe allergic reactions occur in approximately 0.04% of patients receiving nonionic media, sixfold fewer than with ionic media. Risk factors include a history of prior contrast reaction, allergy (asthma and hay fever), and cardiac disease. In these patients, a noncontrast CT or MRI procedure should be considered as an alternative to contrast administration. If contrast is absolutely required, a nonionic agent should be used in conjunction with pretreatment with glucocorticoids and antihistamines (Table 358-2 and guidelines on p. 2339). Patients with allergic reactions to iodinated contrast material do not usually react against gadolinium-based magnetic resonance (MR) contrast material, although it would be wise to pretreat in a similar fashion prior to MR contrast administration.

MAGNETIC RESONANCE IMAGING Technique The phenomenon of magnetic resonance is a complex interaction between protons in biologic tissues, a static and alternating magnetic field (the magnet), and energy in the form of radiofrequency waves of a specific frequency (Rf), introduced by coils placed next to the body part of interest. The energy state of the hydrogen protons is transiently excited. The subsequent return to equilibrium (*relaxation*) of the protons results in a release of Rf energy (the *echo*), which can be measured by the same surface coils that delivered the Rf pulses. The complex Rf signal, or echo, is transformed by Fourier analysis into the information used to form an MR image.

T1 and T2 relaxation times The rate of return to equilibrium of perturbed protons is called the *relaxation rate*. The relaxation rate is different for different normal and pathologic tissues. The relaxation rate of a hydrogen proton in a tissue is influenced by surrounding

Guidelines for Use of Intravenous Contrast in Patients with Impaired Renal Function

Serum Creatinine Level, μmol/L (mg/dL)[a]	Recommendations
<133 (<1.5)	Use either ionic or nonionic contrast at 2 mL/kg to 150 mL total
133–177 (1.5–2.0)	Use nonionic contrast; hydrate diabetics
>177 (>2.0)	Consider noncontrast CT or MRI; use nonionic contrast if required
177–221 (2.0–2.5)	Use nonionic contrast only if required (as above); contraindicated in diabetics
>265 (>3.0)	Nonionic contrast given only to patients undergoing dialysis within 24 h

[a] Risk is greatest in patients with rising creatinine levels.
NOTE: CT, computed tomography; MRI, magnetic resonance imaging.

molecular environment and atomic neighbors. Two relaxation rates, the T1 and T2 relaxation times, are measurable. The T1 relaxation rate is the time for 63% of the protons to return to their normal equilibrium state, while the T2 relaxation rate is the time for 63% of the protons to become dephased owing to interactions among adjacent protons. The intensity of the signal, and thus the image contrast, can be modulated by altering certain parameters, such as the interval between Rf pulses (TR) and the time between the Rf pulse and the signal reception (TE). So-called T1-weighted (T1W) images are produced by keeping the TR and TE relatively short. Under these conditions, contrast between structures is based primarily on their T1 relaxation differences. T2-weighted (T2W) images are produced by using longer TR and TE times. Fat and subacute hemorrhage have short T1 relaxation rates and a high signal intensity on T1W images. Watery media, such as CSF and edematous tissue, have long T1 and T2 relaxation rates, a low signal intensity on T1W images, and a high signal intensity on T2W images. As white matter contains more lipid (due to myelin), it contains 10 to 15% less water than gray matter. These two chemical differences account for much of the contrast difference between gray and white matter on MRI (Fig. 358-3). T2W images are more sensitive than T1W images to edema or myelin destruction (Fig. 371-2).

MR images can be generated in sagittal, coronal, axial, and oblique planes without changing the patient's position. Each plane obtained requires a separate sequence lasting 5 to 10 min. Unlike CT, movement of the patient during a sequence will distort *all* the images; therefore, patient cooperation is important. Approximately 5% of the population experience claustrophobia in the MR environment. This can be reduced by mild sedation. Three-dimensional volumetric imaging is also possible with MR, resulting in data that can be reformatted in any plane and manipulated in a real-time fashion to highlight certain disease processes. Fluid-attenuated inversion recovery, or FLAIR, is a pulse sequence that produces T2W images in which the CSF signal is suppressed. FLAIR images are more sensitive than standard spine echo images for cortical lesions and meningeal processes (Fig. 358-2D).

Table 358-2   Indications for the Use of Nonionic Contrast Media

- Prior adverse reaction to contrast media, with the exception of heat, flushing, or an episode of nausea or vomiting
- Asthma or other serious lung disease
- History of atopic allergies (pretreatment with glucocorticoids and antihistamines recommended)
- Age under 2 years old
- Renal failure or a creatinine level >177 μmol/L (>2.0 mg/dL)
- Cardiac dysfunction, including cardiac failure, severe arrhythmias, unstable angina pectoris, recent myocardial infarction, or pulmonary hypertension
- Diabetes
- Severe debilitation

Guidelines for the Premedication of Patients with Prior Allergic Reaction to Contrast Agents

12 h before examination:
  Prednisone, 40 mg PO *or* methylprednisolone, 32 mg PO
2 h before examination:
  Prednisone, 40 mg PO *or* methylprednisolone, 32 mg PO
    and
  Cimetidine, 300 mg PO *or* ranitidine, 150 mg PO
Immediately before examination:
  Benadryl, 50 mg IV (alternatively, can be given PO 2 h before exam)

Contrast material   The heavy-metal element *gadolinium* forms the basis of all current intravenous MR contrast agents. Gadolinium is a paramagnetic substance, which means that it reduces the T1 and T2 relaxation times of nearby water protons, resulting in a high signal on T1W images. The metal is chelated to an agent such as DTPA, which allows renal excretion without toxicity. Approximately 0.2 mL/kg body weight is administered intravenously (10 to 15 mL for the average-sized adult); the cost is approximately $60 per 20 mL. Gadolinium contrast does not cross a normal BBB, and thus it causes enhancement of brain tissue only at sites of abnormalities in the BBB (Fig. 371-2D) and in areas of the brain that normally have no BBB, such as the pituitary gland. Allergic reactions are extremely rare; renal failure does not occur. These agents can be administered safely to children as well as adults.

MAGNETIC RESONANCE ANGIOGRAPHY Flowing blood exhibits complex MR signals that range from bright to dark relative to background stationary tissue (Fig. 358-3). Fast-flowing blood, such as arterial blood, shows no signal on routine MR images. Slower flow, as in veins or distal to arterial stenoses, may appear high in signal. It is possible, by varying the MR image parameters, to assess blood flow either qualitatively or quantitatively. This is the basis of MRA, which capitalizes on the differences in signal between moving blood and stationary tissue on gradient echo images (Fig. 358-4). *Gradient echo images* differ from standard spin echo images in being more sensitive to blood products, calcification, and other susceptibility artifacts. The suppression of background signal achieved in short-flip-angle gradient echo images provides the contrast needed for flowing blood to appear bright in signal on MRA images.

It is important to understand that MRA provides a *vascular flow map* rather than the anatomic map given by conventional angiography. Two MRA techniques, time-of-flight (TOF) and phase-contrast, are used. TOF, currently the technique used most frequently, relies on the suppression of nonmoving tissue to provide a background for the high signal intensity of flowing blood. A typical TOF angiography sequence results in a series of contiguous thin MR sections (0.9 mm thick), which can be viewed as a stack to create an angiographic image data set that can be reformatted or viewed in various planes and angles to reveal the vascular relationships (Fig. 358-4). Either arterial (MRA) or venous (MRV) structures may be highlighted.

Phase-contrast MRA has a longer acquisition time than TOF MRA but reveals the velocity and direction of blood flow in addition to providing anatomic information similar to that of TOF imaging. Through the selection of different imaging parameters, differing blood velocities can be highlighted; selective venous and arterial MRA images thus can be obtained. One advantage of phase-contrast MRA is the excellent suppression of background signal.

MRA has lower resolution than conventional angiography and therefore cannot detect small-vessel detail, such as is needed in the workup of vasculitis. It is also less sensitive to slow flow and thus may not differentiate occlusive disease from near-occlusive disease. Motion, either by the patient or by anatomic structures, may distort the images, creating artifacts that may be misinterpreted as stenoses

FIGURE 358-3 MRI scans of the normal brain. *A, B*. Axial T2-weighted images through (*A*) the lateral ventricles and (*B*) the circle of Willis. Note that gray matter is slightly higher in signal intensity than white matter. Cerebrospinal fluid (CSF) has a bright signal intensity owing to its free mobile water content. Moving protons in arterial structures demonstrate a signal void (*ar-* *rows*). *C*. T1-weighted image. Less contrast is visible between gray and white matter structures; however, white matter appears slightly higher in signal intensity than gray matter owing to a shorter T1 relaxation time. Signal flow voids are seen in arterial structures and CSF spaces.

or occlusions. These limitations notwithstanding, MRA has proved useful in evaluation of the cervical carotid artery and larger-caliber intracranial arterial and venous structures. It has also proved useful in the noninvasive detection of intracranial aneurysms (Fig. 361-13) and vascular malformations.

ECHO-PLANAR MR IMAGING Recent improvements in gradients, software, and high-speed computer processors now permit MR imaging of the brain on the order of milliseconds. With echo-planar MRI (EPI), fast gradients are switched on and off at high speeds to create the information used to form an image. In routine spin echo imaging, images of the brain can be obtained in 5 to 10 min. With EPI, all of the information required for processing an image is accumulated in 50 to 150 ms, and the information for the entire brain is obtained in 5 to 10 s. EPI allows motion-free imaging, as well as perfusion imaging, diffusion imaging (Fig. 358-4*A*), functional MRI, and kinematic motion studies.

EPI techniques are making their way into clinical practice. The hope for these techniques is that they will provide useful functional data in addition to exquisite anatomic images. EPI *perfusion imaging* and *diffusion imaging* are useful in early detection of ischemic injury of the brain, and may be useful in demonstrating "tissue at risk" of further infarction (Fig. 358-4*A*). Diffusion imaging may also be useful in the characterization of white matter tracts. *Functional MRI* of the brain is a technique that localizes regions of activity in the brain following task activation. Tasks alter the balance of oxyhemoglobin and deoxyhemoglobin within specific regions of the activated cortex. Repetitive actions such as finger tapping elicit an increase in the amount of blood flow delivered to a specific region of the brain, resulting in a slight increase in oxyhemoglobin and a 2 to 3% change in signal intensity. Further work will determine whether these techniques are cost-effective or clinically useful, but currently somatosensory and auditory cortex localization are possible.

Complications of MRI and Patient Safety MRI is considered safe for patients, even at very high field strengths. Serious injuries have been caused, however, by the high magnetic fields used. Ferromagnetic (metal) objects are attracted to the magnet and may act as missiles if brought too close to the magnet. Likewise, ferromagnetic aneurysm clips may torque within the magnet, causing hemorrhage and even death. Metallic foreign bodies in the eye have moved and caused hemorrhage, so screening for ocular metallic fragments is indicated in those with a history of ocular metallic foreign bodies. Implanted cardiac pacemakers are a contraindication to MRI owing

to the risk of induced arrhythmias. All personnel and patients must be screened and educated thoroughly to prevent such disasters. Table 358-3 lists several of the more common contraindications for MRI.

POSITRON EMISSION TOMOGRAPHY PET relies on the detection of positrons emitted during the decay of a radionuclide that has been injected into a patient. The most frequently used moiety is 2-[^{18}F]fluoro-2-deoxy-D-glucose (FDG), which is an analogue of glucose and is taken up by cells competitively with 2-deoxyglucose. Multiple images of glucose uptake activity are formed after 45 to 60 min. Images reveal differences in regional glucose activity among normal and pathologic brain structures. FDG PET scanning has been used to assist in differentiating radiation necrosis from active neoplasm following therapy, in localizing temporal lobe epileptic foci, and in detecting metastatic disease and determining cardiac viability. A lower activity of FDG in the parietal lobes has been associated with Alzheimer's disease (Fig. 362-1).

MYELOGRAPHY **Technique** Myelography involves the intrathecal instillation of 8 to 15 mL of water-soluble iodinated contrast medium (180 to 300 mg/mL) into the lumbar or cervical subarachnoid space via a percutaneously placed spinal needle (22 gauge or smaller). Contrast is maneuvered into the area of interest by fluoroscopic guidance and patient rotation. *Conventional myelography* involves a relatively high concentration and volume of contrast material and visualization by x-ray "spot films" and formal "overhead" plain films. The radiation exposure during conventional myelography is 4 to 8 cGy, making it one of the more radiation-intense procedures. The gonads should be shielded if possible, although doing so is sometimes difficult. CT scanning is often performed after myelography (*CT myelography*), to better demonstrate the spinal cord and roots as filling defects in the opacified subarachnoid space. CT myelography alone, in which CT is performed after the subarachnoid injection of a small amount of relatively dilute contrast material, has replaced conventional myelography for many indications, thereby reducing exposure to radiation and contrast media. CT slices 3 mm thick are routinely obtained through the area of interest.

Indications For diagnosis of diseases of the spinal canal and cord, myelography has been largely replaced by CT, CT myelography, and MRI (Table 358-1). The remaining indications for conventional plain film myelography include the evaluation of suspected meningeal or arachnoid cysts and the localization of spinal dural arteriovenous fistulas and CSF fistulas. Conventional myelography and CT myelog-

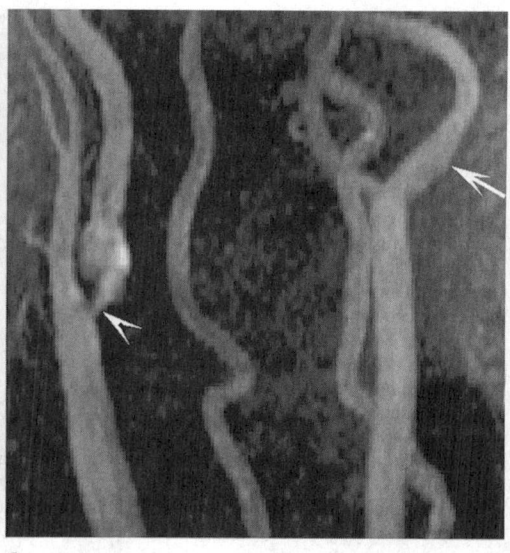

A   B   C

FIGURE 358-4 *A.* Axial echo-planar diffusion-weighted MR image demonstrates three foci of reduced diffusion consistent with acute cerebral ischemia (*arrowheads*) located in the subcortical white matter of the frontal lobe. Reduced diffusion is consistent with cytotoxic edema and is most commonly associated with acute cerebral infarction. *B.* Axial postcontrast T2-weighted image demonstrates two foci of subcortical enhancement consistent with sub-

acute cerebral ischemia. *C.* A 15° projection from a three-dimensional time-of-flight magnetic resonance angiogram through the cervical carotid arteries. Note the normal internal carotid artery on the left (*arrow*). The right internal carotid artery demonstrates a high-grade stenosis at the carotid bifurcation and origin of the internal carotid artery (*arrowhead*).

raphy provide the most precise information in patients with prior spinal fusion and spinal fixation hardware.

Contraindications Myelography is relatively safe. However, it should be performed with caution in any patient with suspected herniation, elevated intracranial pressure, or a history of allergic reaction to intrathecal contrast media. In patients with a suspected spinal block, only a small amount of contrast medium should be instilled below the level of the block to minimize the risk of deterioration. Lumbar puncture is to be avoided in patients with bleeding disorders, including patients receiving anticoagulant therapy (Chap. 356).

Complications Complications resulting from myelography are related to the needle puncture and to reactions to intrathecal contrast material.

Vasovagal syncope may occur during lumbar puncture; it is accentuated by the upright position used during lumbar myelography. Adequate hydration before and after myelography will reduce the incidence of this complication.

Headache, nausea, and *vomiting* are the most frequent complications of dural puncture and myelography, occurring in up to 38% of patients. These symptoms are thought to result from neurotoxic effects of the contrast agent, persistent leakage of CSF at the puncture site, or psychological reactions to the procedure. The incidence of headache has been reduced with the use of smaller-gauge spinal needles and nonionic, water-soluble contrast agents.

Postural headache (post–lumbar puncture headache) is generally due to prolonged leakage of CSF from the puncture site, resulting in CSF hypotension. Intravenous hydration may be helpful, and an autologous epidural blood patch is indicated in patients with persistent headache 48 h after myelography (Chap. 15).

Hearing loss is a rare complication. It may result from a direct toxic effect of the contrast medium or from an alteration of the pressure equilibrium between CSF and perilymph in the inner ear.

Puncture of the spinal cord is a rare but serious complication of cervical (C1-2) and high lumbar puncture. The cervical approach requires proper alignment of the patient and is best performed in the prone position using fluoroscopic guidance. Direct puncture of the spinal cord, laceration of epidural and vertebral venous and arterial structures, and hyperextension of the neck are reported complications.

Injection of contrast material into the spinal cord can precipitate acute neurologic decline or subacute hemorrhagic necrosis of the gray matter. The risk of cord puncture is greatest in patients with spinal stenosis or conditions that reduce CSF volume. In these settings, a low-dose lumbar injection followed by thin-section CT is a safer alternative to cervical puncture.

Intrathecal contrast reactions are rare, but aseptic meningitis and encephalopathy may occur. The latter is usually dose-related and associated with contrast entering the intracranial subarachnoid space. *Seizures* occur following myelography in 0.1 to 0.3% of patients. Risk factors include a preexisting seizure disorder and the use of a total iodine dose of >4500 mg. Other reported symptoms include headache, hyperthermia, hallucinations, depression, and anxiety states. These neurotoxic side effects have been reduced by the development of nonionic, water-soluble contrast agents, as well as by head elevation and generous hydration following myelography.

Arachnoiditis, or inflammation of the leptomeninges, has also been ascribed to the use of contrast agents for myelography. Pantopaque, an oil-soluble contrast agent no longer used, was first noted to cause arachnoiditis, especially in cases where myelography resulted in subarachnoid bleeding (i.e., traumatic tap). The incidence of arachnoiditis with new water-soluble, nonionic contrast agents is much lower than with Pantopaque and with ionic, water-soluble agents (metrizamide). Other variables that increase the likelihood of arachnoiditis include trauma, infection, and subarachnoid hemorrhage.

ANGIOGRAPHY **Technique** Angiography is essential in the diagnostic evaluation of many patients with vascular pathology. However, it carries the greatest risk of morbidity of all diagnostic imaging procedures, owing to the necessity of inserting a catheter into a blood vessel, directing the catheter to the required location, injecting contrast material to visualize the vessel, and removing the catheter while maintaining hemostasis. Therapeutic transcatheter procedures (see below) have become important options for the treatment of some cerebrovascular diseases. The decision to undertake a diagnostic or therapeutic angiographic procedure requires careful assessment of the goals of the investigation and its attendant risks.

Patients undergoing angiography should be well hydrated before and after the procedure to better tolerate the contrast agents. Since the

Table 358-3 Common Contraindications for MRI[a]

Cardiac pacemaker or permanent pacemaker leads
Internal defibrillatory devices
Cochlear prostheses
Bone growth stimulators
Implanted spinal cord stimulators
Electronic infusion devices
Intracranial aneurysm clips (some but not all)
Ocular implants (some) or ocular metallic foreign body
McGee stapedectomy piston prosthesis
Omniphase penile implant
Swan-Ganz catheter
Magnetic stoma plugs
Magnetic dental implants
Magnetic sphincters
Ferromagnetic IVC filters, coils, stents—considered safe at 6 weeks after implantation
Tattooed eyeliner (contains ferromagnetic material and may result in eye irritation)

[a] For a complete list, see Shellock and Kanal.

femoral route is used most commonly, the femoral artery must be compressed after the procedure to prevent a hematoma from developing. The puncture site and distal pulses should be evaluated carefully after the procedure; complications can include thigh hematoma or distal emboli.

Indications   Table 358-1 lists some of the indications for conventional angiography. Over the past 20 years, angiography has been replaced for many indications by CT or MRI. However, it is still used today for evaluating intracranial small-vessel pathology (such as vasculitis), for assessing vascular malformations and aneurysms, and in intravascular therapeutic procedures.

Complications   The vast majority of aortic arch, carotid, and vertebral arteriograms are carried out via transfemoral arterial access. A common femoral arterial puncture provides retrograde access via the aorta to the aortic arch and great vessels. The most feared complication of cerebral angiography is stroke. Thrombus can form on or inside the tip of the catheter, and atherosclerotic thrombus or plaque can be dislodged by the catheter or guidewire or by the force of injection and can embolize distally in the cerebral circulation. The duration and extent of the resulting ischemic neurologic deficit depends on the size and length of the embolus, its composition (fresh thrombus is thought to fragment more readily), its location, and the available collateral circulation. Risk factors for ischemic complications include limited experience on the part of the angiographer, atherosclerosis, vasospasm, low cardiac output, decreased oxygen-carrying capacity, advanced age, and possibly migraine. The risk of a neurologic complication varies but is approximately 4% for transient ischemic attack and stroke, 1% for permanent deficit, and <0.1% for death.

Ionic contrast material injected into the cerebral vasculature can be neurotoxic if the BBB is breached, either by an underlying disease or by the injection of hyperosmolar contrast agent. Ionic contrast media are less well tolerated than nonionic media, probably because they can induce changes in cell membrane electrical potentials. Patients with dolichoectasia of the basilar artery can suffer reversible brainstem dysfunction and acute short-term memory loss during angiography owing to the slow percolation of the contrast material and the consequent prolonged exposure of the brain. Rarely, an intracranial aneurysm ruptures during an angiographic contrast injection, causing subarachnoid hemorrhage, perhaps as a result of injection under high pressure.

Spinal Angiography   Spinal angiography may be indicated to evaluate vascular malformations and tumors and to identify the artery of Adamkiewicz prior to aortic aneurysm repair. The procedure is lengthy and requires the use of relatively large volumes of contrast; the incidence of serious complications, including paraparesis, subjective visual blurring, and altered speech, is approximately 2%.

Interventional Neuroradiology   This rapidly developing field is providing new therapeutic options for patients with difficult neurovascular problems. Available procedures include detachable coil therapy for aneurysms, particulate or liquid adhesive embolization of arteriovenous malformations, balloon angioplasty and stenting of stenosis or vasospasm, transarterial or transvenous embolization of dural arteriovenous fistulas, balloon occlusion of carotid-cavernous and vertebral fistulas, endovascular treatment of vein-of-Galen malformations, preoperative embolization of tumors, and thrombolysis of acute arterial or venous thrombosis. Many of these disorders place the patient at high risk of cerebral hemorrhage, stroke, or death. The therapeutic risks are comparable to those of neurosurgery rather than routine diagnostic radiographic procedures.

The highest complication rates are found with the therapies designed to treat the highest-risk diseases. In a large series of surgically difficult intracranial aneurysms treated with detachable balloons, Higashida and colleagues reported a 7.4% incidence of stroke and a 9.8% death rate. These figures must be considered in light of the high morbidity and mortality associated with untreated and surgically unapproachable aneurysms (Chap. 361). The advent of the electrolytically detachable coil has reduced these rates and ushered in a new era in the treatment of cerebral aneurysms. It remains to be determined what the role of coils will be relative to surgical options, but in many centers, coiling of aneurysms has become standard therapy for many aneurysms.

BIBLIOGRAPHY

GONZÁLEZ RG et al: Diffusion-weighted MR imaging: Diagnostic accuracy in patients imaged within 6 hours of stroke symptom onset. Radiology 210:155, 1999

HIGASHIDA RT et al: Intracranial aneurysms: Interventional neurovascular treatment with detachable balloons—results in 215 cases. Radiology 178:663, 1991

MULLER M et al: Ischemia after carotid endarterectomy: Comparison between transcranial Doppler sonography and diffusion-weighted MR imaging (see comments). AJNR Am J Neuroradiol 21:47, 2000

PROVENZALE JM, SORENSON AG: Diffusion-weighted MR imaging in acute stroke: Theoretic considerations and clinical applications. AJR Am J Roentgenol 173:1459, 1999

SORENSEN AG et al: Hyperacute stroke: Evaluation with combined multisection diffusion-weighted and hemodynamically weighted echo-planar MR imaging. Radiology 199(2):391, 1996

YOSHIURA T et al: Advanced MR techniques: Diffusion MR imaging, perfusion MR imaging, and spectroscopy. Neuroimaging Clin North Am 9:439, 1999

359   Joseph B. Martin, Frank M. Longo

MOLECULAR DIAGNOSIS OF NEUROLOGIC DISORDERS

AD	Alzheimer's disease	HD	Huntington's disease
ALS	amyotrophic lateral sclerosis	HYPP	hyperkalemic periodic paralysis
BMD	Becker muscular dystrophy	OMIM	Online Mendelian Inheritance
CMT1A	Charcot-Marie-Tooth	in Man	
DM	dystrophia myotonica	PCR	polymerase chain reaction
DMD	Duchenne muscular	SCA	spinocerebellar ataxia
	dystrophy	UTR	untranslated region
FA	Friedreich's ataxia		

Completion of the Human Genome Project, along with evolving strategies for linking disease phenotypes with gene loci, will increase the rate at which genes responsible for neurologic disorders are discovered. The widespread availability of DNA testing has already changed traditional diagnostic approaches and raised novel ethical issues. For example, the discovery of "susceptibility" genes that do not directly cause disease but modify the age of disease onset or rate of disease progression creates complexity in the application of molecular diagnosis, particularly in guiding the use of preventative therapies. In this chapter we review molecular diagnostic approaches relevant to neurologic disease and illustrate how they contribute to patient care.

359 Molecular Diagnosis of Neurologic Disorders **2343**

DNA-BASED DIAGNOSIS OF NEUROLOGIC DISORDERS Appropriate use of DNA testing in the clinical setting requires that the clinician have a general understanding of the available molecular diagnostic approaches and the limitations in their application and interpretation. For many of the disorders listed in Table 359-1, the identification of specific disease-causing mutations has made direct DNA diagnosis possible. Most disease-causing mutations consist of single base substitutions leading to amino acid substitutions (missense mutations), premature translation stop signals (nonsense mutations), or abnormal RNA transcript splicing. Other mutations result from DNA deletions, DNA duplications, or instability of trinucleotide repeats. The ability to detect a mutation eliminates the need for additional diagnostic studies. For disorders that have been linked to specific gene loci but for which specific mutations have not been identified, DNA diagnosis may be possible by family linkage analysis. Linkage analysis requires that family relationships (such as paternity) are correctly established, that informative markers are available, and that an adequate number of family members are genotyped and clinically evaluated. For many patients, lack of this information makes DNA diagnosis impossible.

Approaches for Detection of DNA Mutations • *Direct sequencing of patient DNA* These methods generally require amplification of DNA by the polymerase chain reaction (PCR). With most current sequencing methods, only 300 to 400 DNA bases are determined in each sequencing reaction; therefore, sequencing-based strategies are best applied when a limited region contains the majority of potential mutation sites. Direct DNA sequencing allows novel mutations to be detected and decreases the chances of a false-negative result. In some cases, the significance of previously uncharacterized missense mutations will be difficult to interpret. While they may code for harmless amino acid polymorphisms, in other cases they may be the cause of the disease. The segregation of the same mutation with the disease phenotype within a family or the substitution of nonconserved amino acids, especially in critical protein regions, suggests the latter.

Allele-specific oligonucleotide hybridization This technique, in which sequence-specific oligonucleotides differentially recognize DNA segments with normal or mutated sequence, is best suited for detecting known mutations and can be applied to a large number of samples.

Differential restriction endonuclease patterns of PCR-amplified DNA DNA is digested with restriction enzymes that recognize either normal or mutated DNA sequence; the size pattern of resulting DNA fragments indicates whether the DNA sample contains normal or variant sequence (Chap. 65). This method is directed toward detecting known mutations.

Analysis of unstable repeats The number of trinucleotide (or other sized) repeats at a specific DNA locus can be counted by amplifying the DNA segment using PCR and then applying electrophoresis to determine the repeat number present in the amplified DNA. Large repeat expansions such as occur in myotonic dystrophy often prevent reliable application of PCR and require Southern blot analysis for detection.

Analysis of single-stranded conformation polymorphisms Gene segments of several hundred bases are PCR-amplified and electrophoresed under denaturing conditions. Mutation-induced alterations of DNA structure lead to altered electrophoretic patterns. This approach can detect novel mutations directly. Large numbers of samples, either covering many exons of a large gene or from many patients, can be analyzed using this method.

Detection of DNA deletions by fluorescence in situ hybridization DNA deletions are detected by hybridizing chromosomes with a fluorescent probe corresponding to the gene of interest. Fluorescence in situ hybridization (FISH) can detect deletions smaller than the 2000- to 3000-kb minimum detected by banding techniques.

Detection of DNA deletions or duplications by pulsed-field electrophoresis with Southern blot analysis DNA deletions and duplications can also be detected using an electrophoresis technique (pulsed-field) optimized for separation of large DNA segments. This method is used for the detection of chromosome 17p11.2-12 duplications or deletions in the diagnosis of Charcot-Marie-Tooth disease type 1A (CMT1A) and hereditary neuropathy with liability to pressure palsies (HNPP), respectively.

Cytogenetic testing Chromosomes isolated from peripheral blood lymphocytes or tissue are stained, allowing identification of insertions, deletions, other chromosome imbalances, and assessment of chromosomal number (Chap. 66).

Some disorders such as Duchenne muscular dystrophy (DMD), Becker muscular dystrophy (BMD), neurofibromatosis (type 1 and 2), and familial amyotrophic lateral sclerosis (ALS) can be caused by dozens of different mutations within one gene. Heterogeneity over a wide region of a given gene is common for many genes involved in metabolic diseases. Many methods of DNA analysis focus on recurring point mutations or relatively short segments of DNA. Using such focused DNA analysis, mutations are found in only about two-thirds of DMD, BMD, and neurofibromatosis type 2 patients and in fewer than half of those with neurofibromatosis type 1. Advances in multiplex PCR and single-strand chain polymorphism analysis have increased this yield, but the clinician should be aware of the sensitivity of each DNA analysis.

Detection of Protein Abnormalities For some applications, diagnostic methods based on protein properties or function are more effective and efficient than DNA-based tests. Traditional enzyme activity–based assays continue to be useful for diagnosis of many metabolic diseases, and additional protein functions can be used to detect other disorders. For example, immunostaining or western blot analysis using dystrophin antibodies may reveal decreased protein levels or aberrant distribution of dystrophin in a muscle biopsy of a patient in whom no DNA mutations are detected.

COMPLICATIONS AND LIMITATIONS OF GENETIC TESTING The limitations of DNA testing must be considered. If the presumed diagnosis is in error or if the phenotype overlaps with other disorders, the failure to detect a given mutation does not rule out other phenotype-causing mutations in the same gene or other genes. Different mutations in the same gene can result in different phenotypes (*allelic heterogeneity*), and mutations in different genes can result in the same phenotype (*nonallelic genetic heterogeneity*). Other phenomena such as phenocopies, incomplete penetrance, age-dependent onset of phenotype, polygenic inheritance, imprinting, mitochondrial inheritance, and dynamic mutations (trinucleotide repeats) may also make interpretation of genetic testing difficult.

Nonallelic Genetic Heterogeneity Nonallelic genetic heterogeneity (also known simply as genetic heterogeneity) exists when individuals or families have similar pathologic and/or clinical syndromes caused by mutations in different genes, as in the multiple demyelinating forms of CMT disease (Table 359-1). For CMT type 1A the locus is 17p11.2, and mutations are present in the *PMP-22* gene encoding the peripheral myelin protein. CMT type 1B, which is clinically similar to CMT 1A but less common, is caused by a mutation on chromosome 1q22 in the *PMZ* gene encoding the P_o protein, a component of compact myelin. Familial Alzheimer's disease (AD) is caused by mutations in genes located on chromosome 14 (*presenilin 1*, causing 70 to 80% of early-onset AD), 1 (*presenilin 2*), and 21 (*amyloid precursor protein*). Type I autosomal dominant spinocerebellar ataxias (SCAs) are caused by mutations in at least 10 different genes. The phenotypically similar limb-girdle muscular dystrophies (LGMD) are also caused by mutations in a large number of distinct genes, several of which encode products in distinct protein families. As disease-causing mutations continue to be identified, genetic heterogeneity is emerging as a common theme.

An intriguing basis of genetic heterogeneity consists of mutations in distinct genes encoding proteins that function via direct interaction in common mechanistic pathways. The phenotypically similar X-

Table 359-1 Selected Neurogenetic Diseases

Disorder	Chromosomal Localization	Principal Clinical Findings—Phenotype	Mode of Inheritance	Gene Product/Function	Chapter or Reference (OMIN)
DEMENTIAS					
Alzheimer's disease, early onset, familial (AD1)	21q21.3-22.05	Rare cause of early-onset AD	AD	Point mutations in gene encoding the APP protein alter APP metabolism	362, Selkoe (104760)
Alzheimer's disease, late onset, familial and sporadic (AD2)	19q13.2	Memory loss, dementia	Co-Dom	ε4 allele of the ApoE gene associated with increased risk and earlier onset	362 (107741)
Alzheimer's disease, early onset, familial (AD3)	14q24.3	Dementia, memory loss, typical AD	AD	Mutations in gene encoding presenilin-1 lead to elevated Aβ42 production	362 (104311)
Alzheimer's disease, early onset, familial (AD4)	1q31-42	Dementia, memory loss, typical AD	AD	Mutations in gene encoding presenilin-2 lead to elevated Aβ42 production	362 (600759)
Familial Creutzfeldt-Jakob disease	20pter-p12	Spongiform encephalopathy with dementia, myoclonus	AD	Mutations in gene encoding the prion protein	375 (123400)
Fatal familial insomnia	20pter-p12	Adult-onset insomnia	AD	Mutations in gene encoding the prion protein	27, 375 (600072)
Gerstmann-Sträussler-Scheinker	20pter-p12	Spongiform encephalopathy with dementia, myoclonus	AD	Mutations in gene encoding the prion protein	375 (137440)
Hereditary frontotemporal dementia (FTD)	17q21.2	Insidious mood and behavioral changes beginning prior to dementia; some cases with ALS/parkinsonism	AD	Mutations in the gene encoding the tau protein; changes in protein structure alter tau-microtubule interactions	362, Wilhelmsen et al. Lee and Trojanowski (601630)
MOVEMENT DISORDERS					
Dystonia DYT1	9q34	Early onset, generalized dystonia, starts in a limb	AD	A 3-bp (GAG) deletion in the gene encoding torsin A; homology to heat-shock/chaperone proteins	363, Ozelius et al. Klein et al. (128100)
Dystonia DYT2	Unknown	Early onset, generalized or segmental	AR	Unknown	(224500)
Dystonia DYT3	Xq13.1	~50% of cases with parkinsonism	XL-R	Unknown	(314250)
Dystonia DYT4	Unknown	Whispering dysphonia	AD	Unknown	(128101)
Dystonia DYT5a	14q22.1-22.2	Onset in first decade; starts in distal lower extremity and spreads; diurnal fluctuation; responds to levodopa	AD	Mutations in gene encoding GTP cyclohydrolase I	(128230)
Dystonia DYT5b	11p15.5	Dopa-responsive dystonia	AR	Mutations in gene encoding tyrosine hydroxylase	(191290)
Dystonia DYT6	8p21-22	Onset in adolescence, segmental	AD	Unknown	(602629)
Dystonia DYT7	18p	Adult onset, focal (writer's cramp, toricollis, dysphonia, blepharospasm)	AD	Unknown	(602124)
Dystonia DYT8	2q33-25	Paroxysmal dystonia-choreoathetosis precipitated by stress, fatigue, alcohol	AD	Unknown	(118800)
Dystonia DYT9	1p21-13.8	Paroxysmal dystonia; paresthesias, diplopia; spastic paraplegia between attacks	AD	Unknown	(118800)
Dystonia DYT10	Unknown	Paroxysmal dystonia-choreoathetosis precipitated by sudden movements	AD	Unknown	(128200)
Dystonia DYT11	11q23	Myoclonus combined with dystonia	AD	Unknown	(159900)
Dystonia DYT12	19q	Rapid-onset dystonia and parkinsonism		Mutations in gene encoding D₂ dopamine receptor	(128235)
Familial Parkinson's disease (PD), Park 1	4q21-23	Family of Italian descent; very rare familial cause of PD	AD	Point mutation in gene encoding α-synuclein	363, Spacy and Wood (601508)
Familial Parkinson's disease, Park 2	6q25.2-27	Juvenile-onset parkinsonism and a marked response to levodopa	AR	Point mutations or deletions in *parkin* gene	363 (602544)
Huntington's disease	4p16.3	Chorea, depression, dementia; rigidity and epilepsy in juvenile patients	AD	Expansion of CAG repeat in ORF of gene encoding huntingtin	362 (143100)
Wilson's disease	13q14.3	Extrapyramidal signs, psychiatric disorder	AR	Mutations in gene encoding a P-type ATPase regulating copper transport	348 (277900)

(continued)

Table 359-1—*(continued)*

Disorder	Chromosomal Localization	Principal Clinical Findings— Phenotype	Mode of Inheritance	Gene Product/Function	Chapter or Reference (OMIN)
ATAXIAS					
Ataxia telangiectasia	11q22.3	Cerebellar degeneration, choreoathetosis, ocular apraxia, oculocutaneous tenalgiectasia, immunodeficiency, endocrinopathy	AR	Mutations in *ATM* gene which encodes P1-3 kinase signaling protein; regulates cell cycle and differentiation	364 (208900)
Ataxia with vitamin E deficiency (AVED)	8q13	Same as Friedreich's ataxia but with severe vitamin E deficiency	AR	Mutations in gene encoding α-tocopherol transfer protein	364 (600415)
Dentatorubral-pallidoluysian atrophy (DRPLA)	12p12.3-13.1	Ataxia, choreoathetosis, myoclonus, dementia, seizures	AD	Expansion of CAG repeat in ORF of gene encoding DRPLA (atrophin) protein	364 (125370)
Episodic ataxia type 1 (EA-1)	12p13	Ataxic episodes, seconds to minutes, myokymia, paroxysmal kinesogenic choreoathetosis, acetazolamide and phenytoin responsive	AD	Mutations in gene encoding the KCNA1 potassium channel	364 (160120)
Episodic ataxia type 2 (EA-2)	19p13	Ataxic episodes lasting hours to days, downgaze nystagmus, headache, progressive cerebellar signs and atrophy, acetazolamide responsive	AD	Mutations in gene encoding α1A voltage-gated calcium channel; allelic with familial hemiplegic migraine and spinocerebellar ataxia type 6	364 (108500)
Friedreich's ataxia	9q13-21.1	Onset during puberty, ataxia, dysarthria, absent reflexes, decreased vibration, joint position sense, cardiomyopathy, diabetes mellitus	AR	Expansion of trinucleotide repeat (GAA) in intron of *frataxin* gene	364 (229300)
Spinocerebellar ataxia-1 (SCA1)	6p22-23	Ataxia, ophthalmoparesis, spasticity, onset 3rd or 4th decade	AD	Expansion of CAG repeat in ORF of gene encoding ataxin-1	364 (164400)
Spinocerebellar ataxia-2 (SCA2)	12q23-24.1	Features similar to SCA1, can include hypotonia and ophthalmoplegia	AD	Expansion of CAG repeat in ORF of gene encoding ataxin-2	364 (183090)
Spinocerebellar ataxia-3 (SCA3), Machado-Joseph disease (MJD)	14q32-24.3	Ataxia, ophthalmoparesis, bulging eyes, corticospinal signs, dystonia-rigidity, amyotrophy	AD	Expansion of CAG repeat in ORF of *MJD1* gene	364 (109150)
Spinocerebellar ataxia-4 (SCA4)	16q22.1	Ataxia, sensory axonal neuropathy, normal eye movements, corticospinal signs	AD	Unknown	364 (600223)
Spinocerebellar ataxia-5 (SCA5)	11p11-q11 (centromeric)	Ataxia, dysarthria; mild	AD	Unknown	364 (600224)
Spinocerebellar ataxia-6 (SCA6)	19p13	Slowly progressive ataxia; predominant cerebellar signs, gaze-evoked and vertical nystagmus	AD	Expansion of CAG repeat in ORF of gene encoding α1A calcium channel; allelic with familial hemiplegic migraine and episodic ataxia type 2	364 (184086)
Spinocerebellar ataxia-7 (SCA7)	3p13-12	Ataxia, retinal degeneration	AD	Expansion of CAG repeat in ORF of gene encoding ataxin-7	364 (164500)
Spinocerebellar ataxia-8 (SCA8)	13q21	Ataxia, bulbar findings, sensory neuropathy	AD	Expansion of CTG repeat in 3′ UTR of antisense *SCA8* transcripts; CTG repeat not found in sense *SCA8* transcripts; whether expansions are causative or polymorphic remains to be established.	364, Koob et al. (603680)
Spinocerebellar ataxia-10 (SCA10)	22q13	Ataxia, epilepsy	AD	Unknown	364, Zu et al. (603516)
Spinocerebellar ataxia-11 (SCA11)	15q15-21.3	Slowly progressive ataxia; predominant cerebellar signs; similar to SCA6	AD	Unknown	364 (604432)

(continued)

Table 359-1   Selected Neurogenetic Diseases—*(continued)*

Disorder	Chromosomal Localization	Principal Clinical Findings—Phenotype	Mode of Inheritance	Gene Product/Function	Chapter or Reference (OMIN)
Spinocerebellar ataxia-12 (SCA12)	5q31-33	Ataxia, corticospinal signs, abnormal eye movements	AD	Expansion of CAG repeat in 5'UTR region of *PPP2R2B* gene encoding a brain-specific regulator subunit of the protein phosphatase PP2A	364, Holmes et al. (604326)
SPASTIC PARAPLEGIAS					
Autosomal dominant hereditary spastic paraplegias (AD-HSP)	SPG3:14q11-22 SPG4:2p21-22 SPG6:15q11.1 SPG8: 8q23-24	"Uncomplicated" spastic paraplegia primarily involving corticospinal tracts; SPG4 locus accounts for 40–50% of AD-HSP families	AD	In 2p21-22-linked forms, mutations present in gene coding spastin, a ubiquitously expressed ATPase	365, Fink and Hedera Hazan et al. (182600; 182601; 600363; 603563)
Autosomal recessive hereditary spastic paraplegias (AR-HSP)	SPG5:8q11-13 SPG7: 16q24.3 SPG9:15q13-15	Either pure spastic paraplegia or including involvement of other CNS systems	AR	In 16q-linked forms, mutations present in the gene encoding paraplegin, a mitochondrial metalloprotease	365, Pearce (270800; 602783; 601162)
X-linked hereditary spastic paraplegias	SPG1: Xq28 SPG2: Xq21-22	Initial pure spastic paraplegia; involvement of entire CNS over years;	X-LR	SPG1: mutations in L1CAM gene; allelic with X-linked hydrocephalus and MASA syndrome; SPG2: mutations in proteolipid protein (PLP) gene; allelic with Pelizaeus-Merzbacher disease	365, Fransen et al. (312900; 312920)
VASCULAR DISEASES					
Cerebral autosomal dominant arteriopathy with subcortical infarcts and leukoencephalopathy (CADASIL)	19p13.1	Multiple subcortical infarcts, leukoencephalopathy, vascular dementia	AD	Mutations in gene encoding the Notch3 protein, a transmembrane signal transduction protein	361, Dichgans et al. Joutel et al. (125310)
Cerebral cavernous malformation (CCM1)	7q11.2-21	Headache, intracerebral hemorrhage, seizures, neurologic deficits	AD	Unknown	Craig et al. (116860)
Cerebral cavernous malformation (CCM2)	7p13-15	Headache, intracerebral hemorrhage, seizures, neurologic deficits	AD	Unknown	(603284)
Cerebral cavernous malformation (CCM3)	3q25.2-27	Headache, intracerebral hemorrhage, seizures, neurologic deficits	AD	Unknown	(603285)
Familial cerebral amyloid angiopathy (Dutch type)	21q21.3-22.05	Cerebral hemorrhage	AD	Mutation in gene encoding APP	Watson et al. (104760)
Familial hemiplegic migraine	19p13	Onset 5–30 years, aura with unilateral paresis and other focal symptoms lasting 30–60 min; headache, ± cerebellar signs	AD	Mutations in gene encoding α1A voltage-gated calcium channel; allelic with EA-2 and SCA6	15, Lehmann-Horn and Jurkat-Rott Davies and Hanna (141500)
EPILEPSY SYNDROMES					
Autosomal dominant nocturnal frontal lobe epilepsy (ADNFLE)	20q13.2	Seizures begin in childhood, occur at night; predominantly motor and occasionally violent	AD	Mutations in gene encoding the α_4 subunit of the neuronal nicotinic acetylcholine receptor (CHRNA4)	360, McNamara (600513)
Benign neonatal epilepsy-1 (EBN1)	20q13.3	Generalized seizures, neonatal onset, benign course, usually resolving at 6–12 months, 10–15% have seizures later in life	AD	Mutations in gene encoding the KCNQ2 potassium channel	360, McNamara (121200)
Benign neonatal epilepsy-2 (EBN2)	8q24	Clinically indistinguishable from EBN1	AD	Mutations in gene encoding the KCNQ3 potassium channel	360, McNamara (121201)
Epilepsy, progressive myoclonic (Unverricht-Lundborg type) (EPM1)	21q22.3	Generalized seizures, stimulus-reactive myoclonus, onset age 6–15, progressive	AD	Most common mutation is expansion of a dodecamer repeat in the 5' UTR of the gene encoding cystatin B, an inhibitor of cystein protease	360, Serratosa et al. (254800)
Epilepsy, progressive myoclonic (Lafora disease) (EPM2A)	6q24	Onset of seizures and myoclonus at age 15 followed by myoclonus; intracellular Lafora bodies	AR	Mutations in *EPM2A* gene which encodes a protein tyrosine phosphatase	(254780)

(continued)

Table 359-1—(continued)

Disorder	Chromosomal Localization	Principal Clinical Findings—Phenotype	Mode of Inheritance	Gene Product/Function	Chapter or Reference (OMIN)
Generalized epilepsy with febrile seizures plus (GEFS+)	19q13.1	Febrile seizures before 3 months of age or after 3 years of age	AD	Mutations in gene encoding the β_1 subunit of the voltage-gated sodium channel (SCN1B)	360, McNamara (604236)
Progressive epilepsy with mental retardation (EPMR)	8pter-p22	Normal at birth, generalized seizures onset age 5–10 years, severe mental retardation after seizure onset	AR	Mutations in *CLN8* gene, encoding a putative transmembrane protein	360, Ranta et al. (600143)
MOTOR NEURON DISEASES					
Familial amyotrophic lateral sclerosis, adult, dominant (ALS1)	21q22.1	Weakness, muscle atrophy, spasticity, increased TRDs; about 10% of cases are familial, indistinguishable clinically from sporadic form	AD	Point mutations in gene encoding Cu, Zn-superoxide dismutase (SOD1) in some families (20%); altered SOD1 protein structure may lead to aberrant and toxic copper-mediated catalysis	365, Cleveland (105400)
Familial amyotrophic lateral sclerosis, juvenile, recessive (ALS2)	2q33-34	Earlier onset and slower progression than ALS1	AR	Unknown; mapped to a 8-Mb region	365 (205100)
Familial amyotrophic lateral sclerosis, adult, dominant (ALS3)	22q12.2	Similar to ALS1	AD	Mutations in neurofilament protein heavy chain gene in ~1% of "sporadic" cases; disruption of neurofilament cross-linking; mutations might be either causative or constitute risk factors	365 (162230)
Spinobulbar muscular atrophy (SBMA; Kennedy syndrome)	Xq12	Muscular weakness and atrophy	X-LR	Expansion of CAG repeat in ORF of gene encoding androgen receptor	365 (313200)
Spinal muscular atrophy I–III (SMA)	5q13	SMA I: infantile, Werdnig-Hoffman disease—present by 3 mos., hypotonia, proximal weakness, areflexia. SMA II: childhood onset, limb-girdle weakness, areflexia, 70% never ambulate independently. SMA III: juvenile, Kugelberg-Welander disease—onset after age 2, slowly progressive symmetric proximal muscle weakness sparing bulbar muscles	AR	All three types of SMA are caused by mutations in the survival motor neuron (SMN1) gene; most cases show homozygous absence of specific SMN1 exons; severity of phenotype may be related to SMH1 protein levels	365, Wirth (253300; 253550; 253400)
NEUROPATHIES					
Charcot-Marie-Tooth disease, type 1A (CMT1A)	17p11.2	HMSN I: Variable onset, motor > sensory neuropathy, distal muscle atrophy, absent reflexes, high arches in feet, decreased nerve conduction velocities, +/− nerve enlargement; (~50% of hereditary neuropathy)	AD	Majority with 1.5 Mb duplication in gene encoding peripheral myelin protein (PMP-22), a component of compact myelin; point mutations also found.	379, Chance Warner et al (118220)
Charcot-Marie-Tooth disease, type 1B (CMT1B)	1q22-23	Similar to HMSN I (~40 families identified)	AD	Mutations in *MPZ* gene encoding P_o protein, a component of compact myelin	379 (118200)
Charcot-Marie-Tooth disease, types 1,2,3 X-linked (CMTX1,2,3)	CMTX1: Xq13.1 CMTX2: Xp22.2 CMTX3:Xq26	HMSN I (~10–15% of hereditary neuropathy)	X-linked dominant	CMTX1: mutations in gene encoding connexin32, a gap junction protein localized to uncompacted peripheral myelin at the nodes of Ranvier and Schmidt-Lanterman clefts; CMTX2,3: genes unknown	379 (302800) (302801) (302802)
Charcot-Marie-Tooth disease, type 2A (CMT2A)	1p35-36	HMSNII: Later onset, sensorimotor axonal neuropathy, near-normal nerve conduction velocities (20–50% of hereditary neuropathy)	AD	Unknown	379 (118210)

(continued)

Table 359-1 Selected Neurogenetic Diseases—*(continued)*

Disorder	Chromosomal Localization	Principal Clinical Findings—Phenotype	Mode of Inheritance	Gene Product/Function	Chapter or Reference (OMIN)
Charcot-Marie-Tooth disease, type 2B (CMT2B)	3q13-22	HSMNII (several families)	AD	Unknown	379 (600882)
Charcot-Marie-Tooth disease, type 4A (CMT4A)	8q13-21.1	HMSN I (few families; Tunisia)	AR	Unknown	379 (214400)
Congenital hypomyelinating neuropathy (CH)	10q21.1-22.1 1q22-23	Neonatal hypomyelinating neuropathy with extremely slow nerve conduction velocities	AD and AR	Cases mapped to 10q21.1-22.1 demonstrate mutations in the *EGR2* gene encoding a zinc finger DNA binding protein; cases mapped to 1q22-23 show mutations in the *MPZ* gene coding P$_o$ protein, a component of compact myelin	379 (129010; 159440)
Déjerine-Sottas disease (DSDA)	17p11.2-12 1q22-23	HSMNIII: Onset birth/infancy, slowly progressive sensorimotor deficits, high arches, scoliosis, ataxia, enlarged nerves, markedly decreased conduction velocities	AD	17p-linked: mutations in gene encoding PMP22 (see above) 1q-linked: mutations in *MPZ* gene encoding P$_o$ (see above)	379 (145900)
Familial amyloidotic polyneuropathy (FAP)	18q11.2-12.1 and other loci	Sensory/autonomic peripheral neuropathy, cardiomyopathy	AD	Mutations in gene encoding transthyretin; amyloid formation	379 (176300)
Hereditary neuropathy with pressure palsies (HNPP)	17p11.2	Recurrent entrapment/pressure neuropathies, segmental demyelination (relatively frequent, 1:10,000; underrecognized)	AD	Deletions or point mutations in gene encoding PMP-22; HNPP and CMT1A may result from reciprocal products of unequal crossover	379 Stogbauer et al. (162500)
NEUROMUSCULAR JUNCTION DISORDERS					
Congenital myasthenic syndrome type Ia (familial infantile myasthenia)	17p12-11	Onset at birth to early childhood, myasthenic weakness and possible respiratory distress	AR	Loss-of-function mutations in gene encoding the ε subunit of the acetylcholine receptor (AChR) cause decreased response to ACh or decreased levels of the AChR	380, Engel et al. (254210)
Congenital myasthenic syndrome type II ("slow-channel" syndrome)	2q24-32 17p12-11	Onset at birth to early childhood, myasthenic weakness and possible respiratory distress	AD	Gain-of-function mutations in genes encoding the α, β, or ε subunits of the AChR cause increased response to ACh	380, Engel et al. (601462)
MYOPATHIES					
Central core disease (CCD)	19q13.1	Nonprogressive primarily proximal myopathy, onset in infancy	AD	Mutation in ryanodine receptor gene (RYR1); allelic with malignant hyperthermia syndrome (MHS1)	383 (117000)
Congenital muscular dystrophy (merosin deficient) (CMD)	6q22-23	Weakness and hypotonia at birth, limb contractures at birth or later	AR	Mutations in *LAMA2* gene encoding merosin	383 (156225)
Duchenne/Becker muscular dystrophy (DMD/BMD)	Xp21.2	DMD: onset of muscular weakness early in life, progressive; BMD: later onset, less severe	X-LR	Mutations in dystrophin gene resulting in complete absence or major deletions of dystrophin (DMD), or less severe derangement of dystrophin structure (BMD)	383, Hoffman (310200)
Emery-Dreifuss muscular dystrophy	Xq28 1q21.2	Childhood onset, benign course with early contractures; progressive muscle wasting with humeral/peroneal predominance, cardiac conduction defects; X-linked and AD forms have similar phenotype	X-LR AD	Xq28: mutations in gene encoding emerin, an inner nuclear membrane protein; 1q11-q23: mutations in gene encoding the lamin A/C protein; main A/C interaction with emerin may be involved in targeting emerin to the nuclear envelope	383, Bonne et al. (310300; 181350)

(continued)

Table 359-1—(continued)

Disorder	Chromosomal Localization	Principal Clinical Findings—Phenotype	Mode of Inheritance	Gene Product/Function	Chapter or Reference (OMIN)
Facioscapulohumeral dystrophy	4q35	Weakness, atrophy; face and shoulder muscles	AD	Associated with deletion of variable number of 3.3 kb repeat units; more severe phenotype with larger deletions; nature of gene products affected by deletion are unknown	383, Fitzsimons (158900)
Fukuyama-type congenital muscular dystrophy (FCMD)	9q31	Weakness and hypotonia at birth, cerebral and cerebellar polymicrogyria and cerebellar cysts, ocular anomalies; overlaps with Walker-Warberg syndrome	AR	3 kb retrotransposal insertion in the 3′UTR of the gene encoding fukutin, a putative secreted protein of unknown function; severe phenotypes including Walker-Warburg syndrome associated with compound heterozygotes	383, Kondo-Iida et al. Toda (253800)
Hyperkalemic periodic paralysis (HYPP)	17q23.1-25.3	Myotonia, periodic areflexic paralysis	AD	Mutations in gene encoding α subunit, sodium channel (SCN4A); allelic with paramyotonia congenita (PC)	383 (170500)
Hypokalemic periodic paralysis (HOKPP)	1q32	Similar to HYPP, but attacks accompanied by hypokalemia, triggered by insulin or glucose	AD	Loss-of-function mutations in α_1 subunit of the dihydropyridine (DHP)–sensitive calcium channel	383 (170400)
Limb-girdle muscular dystrophy, autosomal dominant forms	LGMD1A: 5q31 LGMD1B: 1q11-21 LGMD1C: 3p25	Late (third decade) onset muscular dystrophy, sparing the face; slow progression	AD	LGMD1C: mutations in gene encoding caveolin-3; genes unknown for LGMD1A and LGMD1B	383 (601253)
Limb-girdle muscular dystrophy, autosomal recessive forms (clinical and genetic overlap with severe childhood autosomal recessive muscular dystrophy, SCARMD)	LGMD2A: 15q LGMD2B: 2p16-13 LGMD2C: 13q LGMD2D: 17q LGMD2E: 4q LGMD2F: 5q LGMD2G: 17q LGMD2H: 9q	Heterogeneous group of myopathies with progressive weakness of shoulder and pelvic muscles; severe forms with onset in first decade and milder forms with later onset; disorders caused by mutations in genes encoding sarcoglycan are also known as "sarcoglycanopathies"	AR	Mutations in genes encoding: calpain 3 (LGMD2A); dysferlin (LGMD2B); telethonin (LGMD2G). Sarcoglycanopathies: γ-sarcoglycan (LGMD2C); α-sarcoglycan (adhalin) (LGMD2D); β-sarcoglycan (LGMD2E); δ-sarcoglycan (LGMD2F)	383, Bushby Moreira et al. Vainzof et al. (253600)
Malignant hyperthermia (MHS1) and central core disease (CCD)	19q13.1 Other candidate loci: 1q, 3q, 5p, 7q, 17q	Sensitivity to volatile anesthetics, muscle contraction	AD	In 19q-linked forms (~50% of cases) mutations in gene encoding ryanodine receptor (RYR1) cause disturbances in calcium flux	383, Jurkat-Rott et al. (145600)
Desmin-related myopathy (myofibrillar myopathy; hereditary distal myopathy)	2q35 11q22.3-23.1 and other loci	Proximal and distal weakness, cardiomyopathy, neuropathy	AR and AD	2q35-linked forms: mutations in gene encoding desmin 11q21-linked forms: mutations in gene encoding αB-crystallin, a chaperone for desmin	383, Engel (601419)
Myotonia congenita (dominant myotonia congenita, Thomsen's disease)	7q35	Onset in first decade, muscle stiffness/myotonia, muscle hypertophy without weakness	AD	Mutations in gene encoding the ClC-1 chloride channel lead to a dominant loss of function within the homomultimeric channel	383 (160800)
Myotonia congenita (recessive myotonia congenita, Becker)	7q35	Similar to dominant myotonia congenita	AR	Loss-of-function mutations in gene encoding the ClC-1 chloride channel	383 (160800)
Myotonic dystrophy	19q13.3	Multisystem disorder; cataracts, myotonia, weakness, frontal baldness, mental retardation	AD	CTG repeats 3′ UTR of gene encoding myotonin protein kinase, localized to membranes of neuromuscular and myotendinous junctions; expression of adjacent genes may also be affected	383 (160900)

(continued)

Table 359-1   Selected Neurogenetic Diseases—*(continued)*

Disorder	Chromosomal Localization	Principal Clinical Findings—Phenotype	Mode of Inheritance	Gene Product/Function	Chapter or Reference (OMIN)
Nemaline myopathy	1q22-23 2q21.2-22 1q42.1	Most commonly congenital nonprogressive or slowly progressive myopathy; forms range from severe congenital to mild adult	AD and AR	Dominant 1p22-linked form: mutations in α-tropomyosin gene (*TPM3*) leading to increased tropomyosin-actin affinity; 2q21-linked form: mutations in gene encoding nebulin; 1q42 linked form: mutations in gene coding α-actin (*ACTA1*)	383, Nowak et al. Wallgren-Pettersson et al. (161800)
Oculopharyngeal muscular dystrophy (OPMD)	14q11.2-13	Onset usually after age 50, ptosis, dysphagia, and proximal limb weakness	AD	Mutation in gene encoding the poly(A) binding protein 2 (PABP2); a GCG repeat encoding a polyalanine tract expands from 6 to 8–13 repeats	383, Brais et al. (164300)
Paramyotonia congenita (PC)	17q23.1-25.3	Cold-induced muscle stiffness (myotonia) and weakness, occasional periodic paralysis	AD	Mutations in gene encoding α subunit, sodium channel (SCN4A); allelic with HYPP	383 (168300)
Startle disease (hyperexplexia)	5q21-31	Exaggerated startle, neonatal hypertonia, nocturnal myoclonus	AD, AR	Mutations in gene coding the $α_1$ subunit of the inhibitory glycine receptor	22 (149400)
Walker-Warburg syndrome (WWS)	9q33-31	Congenital muscular dystrophy, lissencephaly, ocular anomalies, hydrocephalus, callosal hypoplasia, septal agenesis	AR	Mutation in gene encoding fukutin; often compound heterozygote mutations; allelic with Fukuyama-type congenital muscular dystrophy (FCMD)	(236670)

NEUROCUTANEOUS SYNDROMES

Disorder	Chromosomal Localization	Principal Clinical Findings—Phenotype	Mode of Inheritance	Gene Product/Function	Chapter or Reference (OMIN)
Neurofibromatosis, type 1 (NF1) (Von Recklinghausen's disease)	17q11.2	Café au lait spots, neurofibromas, axillary or inguinal freckling, Lisch nodules in iris; affects 1 in 4000 individuals	AD	Mutations in the gene encoding neurofibromin, a member of the Ras-GTPase activating protein (GAP) family	370 (162200)
Neurofibromatosis, type 2 (NF2)	22q12.2	Acoustic neuromas, bilateral meningiomas; affects 1 in 50,000 individuals	AD	Deletions in the gene that encodes merlin, a membrane-cytoskeletal linkage protein	370 (101000)
Tuberous sclerosis, type 1 (TSC1)	9q34	Epilepsy, facial angiofibromas, mental retardation; ~50% of TSC families linked to TSCI and ~50% to TSC2; two-thirds of TCS cases arise from spontaneous mutations, with the majority TSC2-linked	AD	Mutations in gene encoding hamartin, a putative membrane-associated protein that forms cytosolic complexes with tuberin	370, Crino and Henske Nellist et al. (191100)
Tuberous sclerosis, type 2 (TSC2)	16p13.3	Epilepsy, facial angiofibromas, mental retardation	AD	Mutations in gene encoding tuberin, which has homology to GTPase activating proteins; tuberin binds to hamartin, possibly acting as a chaperon	370 (191092)

NOTE: OMIN web site www3.ncbi.nlm.nih.gov/omin/ AD, autosomal dominant; ALS, amyotrophic lateral sclerosis; APP, amyloid precursor protein; AR, autosomal recessive; CNS, central nervous system; Co-Dom, codominant; TRDs, trinucleotide repeat disorders; HMSN, hereditary motor and sensory neuropathy; MASA, mental retardation, aphasia, shuffling gait, adducted thumbs; ORF, open reading frame; X-LR, X-linked recessive; UTR, untranslated region.

linked and autosomal dominant Emery-Dreifuss muscular dystrophies are caused by mutations in genes encoding emerin and lamin A/C, respectively. Emerin and lamin A/C interaction is likely to be important for targeting emerin to the nuclear envelope. Tuberous sclerosis types 1 and 2 are caused by mutations in the genes encoding tuberin and hamartin, respectively. Evidence suggests that tuberin binds to hamartin, possibly acting as a chaperon.

Allelic Heterogeneity   Different mutations in the same gene (allelic mutations) can cause markedly distinct clinical phenotypes. Mutations in the α1A voltage-gated calcium channel subunit can cause either familial hemiplegic migraine, SCA type 6, or episodic ataxia type 2 (EA-2). Familial Creutzfeldt-Jakob disease, fatal familial insomnia, and Gerstmann-Sträussler-Scheinker disease are all caused by allelic mutations in the prion protein gene (20pter-p12), each of which results in distinct aberrant protein isoforms or alterations in expression. Mutations in the gene encoding the L1 cell adhesion molecule (L1CAM) can cause either isolated hydrocephalus or MASA syndrome (mental retardation, aphasia, shuffling gait, and adducted thumbs). Mutations in the sodium channel α subunit (SCN4A) can cause either hyperkalemic periodic paralysis (HYPP) or paramyotonia congenita (PC). In cases of allelic heterogeneity, different mutations cause distinct alterations in protein structure and function, resulting in separate phenotypes.

Phenocopies   Patients may have a clinical presentation that resembles the phenotype of a genetic disorder but that has a nongenetic cause. Examples include vascular dementia appearing as familial AD,

Variable Expressivity Variable expressivity occurs when the severity of a trait resulting from a mutant allele varies from mild to severe. Expression of the disease phenotype can be modified by other factors such as predisposing alleles of other genes, environmental agents, sex, and age. Variation in expression can also occur following somatic variations in trinucleotide repeats, as occurs in myotonic dystrophy (dystrophia myotonica, or DM).

Incomplete Penetrance Penetrance refers to the all-or-none expression of a mutant genotype. If a disease is expressed in <100% of individuals carrying the abnormal allele, it is said to have incomplete penetrance.

Polygenic Inheritance and Complex Traits The majority of diseases listed in Table 359-1 are caused by mutations in single genes. In disorders such as "sporadic" AD, Parkinson's disease, and multiple sclerosis, it is likely that disease onset is determined by concomitant mutations or polymorphisms in large numbers of genes. Genetic testing for susceptibility or diagnosis will require assessment of multigene "panels."

INFLUENCE OF GENETIC BACKGROUND Machado-Joseph disease (MJD) and SCA type 3 are autosomal dominant ataxias originally described in different ethnic backgrounds with distinct features. MJD occurs in families, often of Portuguese-Azorean origin, and is manifest as hereditary ataxia with dystonia, rigidity, faciolingual fasciculation, and bulging eyes. In French families with a syndrome of progressive ataxia and dysarthria recognizably distinct from that found in Portuguese-Azorean families, the SCA3 gene was mapped to a site on chromosome 14q near the MJD locus. It is now clear that MJD and SCA3 are both caused by expansion of the same tract of CAG repeats in the same gene (*MJD1*) at 14q32.1. Although expansions in *MJD1* are the most common mutations in German SCA patients, the diagnosis of MJD had not previously been considered in this population. The extent to which different genetic background causes phenotypic heterogeneity will require further studies.

SUSCEPTIBILITY GENES Allelic variations or mutations can cause increased susceptibility to specific diseases. Detection of such DNA polymorphisms can influence differential diagnosis, as in the genotyping of *APOE* alleles in the diagnosis of AD. Apolipoprotein E (apoE) is a 299-amino-acid protein involved in mobilization and reutilization of lipoprotein cholesterol. ApoE secreted by astrocytes appears to be internalized by neurons via low-density lipoprotein-related receptors where it contributes to neuronal function. The three isoforms of apoE (apoE2, apoE3, and apoE4) are derived from three corresponding alleles of the *APOE* gene located at 19q13.2; the apoE4 allele is overrepresented in sporadic and familial AD and is a significant risk factor for the disease. In contrast, the apoE2 allele is underrepresented and thus may have a "protective" effect (Chap. 362).

The increased incidence of the *APOE4/4* genotype in AD patients has raised the possibility that ascertainment of *APOE* genotype might be useful in the diagnostic assessment of patients with dementia. For example, since AD accounts for some two-thirds of late-onset dementia, the prior probability of an elderly patient with dementia having AD is approximately 0.66. In many populations the probability of a demented patient with the *APOE4/4* genotype having AD increases to >0.90. However, since the relationship between *APOE4* genotype and probability of AD changes with age, gender, and ethnic background, application of population-based probabilities to specific individuals is limited. If a 25-year-old presents with dementia and has the *APOE4/4* genotype, it is very unlikely that this patient has AD. Since individuals with all *APOE* genotypes can have AD, genotypes cannot absolutely rule in or rule out this diagnosis. Even if genotyping increases the odds that a given patient has AD, it does not rule out the possibility that a treatable cause of dementia is present. Current diagnostic studies for demented patients are focused on detecting reversible causes of dementia (Chap. 26) *APOE* genotype results would not change the diagnostic evaluation and should not be ordered on a routine basis. Nevertheless, *APOE* genotyping might eventually be combined with yet-to-be developed diagnostic tests to form a "panel" of data with acceptable sensitivity and specificity for diagnosis (Chap. 362).

The availability of *APOE* genotyping raises questions about the use of predictive testing in asymptomatic individuals. Until preventive therapy is available, many clinicians would consider such predictive testing unethical. Moreover, useful predictions of age of onset based solely on *APOE* genotyping are not possible. For the 2% of the population with the high-risk *E4/E4* genotype, the period of risk extends from the fifties to beyond the nineties.

APPROACHES TO GENETIC TESTING One indication for DNA analysis is to confirm the diagnosis of a specific disease already suggested by clinical assessment. DNA testing can also be used to narrow the differential diagnosis in cases with multiple diagnostic possibilities. DNA testing for HD allows patients to avoid neuroimaging and other diagnostic studies. When a patient presents with a well-established and relatively specific clinical phenotype, such as that of HD, initial genetic testing can focus on a single gene. In other disorders, such as the SCAs, the high degree of phenotypic overlap calls for concomitant testing of a panel of genes (*SCA1*, *SCA2*, *SCA3*, *SCA6*, and *SCA7*). Another application of genetic analysis is presymptomatic testing in members of families known or suspected to have a specific disorder. In these cases the most common reasons for testing are life management issues, reproductive planning decisions, and eliminating the stress of unknown carrier status. Development of new therapies that delay onset or progression of neurodegenerative diseases will provide additional indications for presymptomatic testing.

Genetic testing should be conducted only in the context of comprehensive genetic counseling, in which the implications of potential test results are fully explained and adequate support services are available. Clinicians ordering genetic studies should be familiar with issues regarding informed consent, suicide risk, ongoing patient support, insurance, employment discrimination, testing of minors, and testing of fetal tissue.

A directory of diseases for which DNA diagnostic testing is available, along with a listing of testing sites, on the www.genetests.org, web site. This site was developed at the University of Washington, Seattle, and is supported by the U.S. National Library of Medicine and Maternal and Child Health Bureau.

CLINICAL AND GENETIC CLASSIFICATION OF GENE DISORDERS Neurogenetic disorders have traditionally been classified and subtyped on the basis of clinical and pathophysiologic concepts. Their complexity, phenotypic variability, and overlapping features limit the resolution of phenotype-based classification and confound nosology. Identification of tightly linked disease markers and discovery of disease-causing mutations have provided a basis for refining such classifications. For example, the clinical distinction between neurofibromatosis type 1 and type 2 has been upheld by the discovery that they are caused by mutations in different genes, encoding the GTPase-activating protein and the merlin (schwannomin) cytoskeletal protein, respectively. In contrast, the finding that DMD and BMD are caused by mutations in the same gene points to shared pathophysiologic mechanisms and blurs the distinctions between these disorders. Mutations in different genes can lead to overlapping clinical syndromes as in the inherited ataxias. In other instances, phenotypically dissimilar disorders are caused by mutations in the same gene, as described above for the α1A voltage-gated calcium channel subunit gene.

Neurogenetic disorders with known chromosomal gene localization are organized primarily by clinical phenotype in Table 359-1. As in any clinical classification, there is frequent overlap in specific phenotypic features. Reference numbers from the Online Mendelian Inheritance in Man (OMIM) database (described below) are included to facilitate access to continuously updated disease information.

Different modes of inheritance occur in each of these categories. Neurologic genetic disorders inherited in Mendelian autosomal dominant mutations include HD, familial AD, ALS, DM, CMT, familial HYPP, SCA, and tuberous sclerosis. Autosomal recessive disorders include FA, Wilson's disease, and ataxia telangiectasia. X-linked recessive traits include DMD, spinobulbar muscular atrophy (Kennedy syndrome), and fragile X syndrome. Non-Mendelian patterns of transmission such as maternal inheritance can result from mitochondrial mutations (Chap. 383) and unstable trinucleotide repeats (see below).

The types of mutations causing neurologic genetic disorders include gene deletions (the most common finding in DMD), insertions (e.g., Fukuyama-type congenital muscular dystrophy), duplications (e.g., CMT1A), translocations that interrupt the gene (neurofibromatosis type 1), and point mutations (e.g., in the superoxide dismutase gene in ALS). Point mutations, either missense or nonsense, are considered "static" mutations because they generally remain stable during meiosis and provide the basis for classic Mendelian inheritance. Unstable trinucleotide repeats cause "dynamic" mutations and account for the clinical phenomenon of anticipation.

GENETICALLY INDUCED MECHANISMS OF CELL DEATH Three general mechanisms of cell death in genetic disorders have been proposed: loss of function, dominant-negative effects, and gain of function.

In *loss-of-function disorders*, the mutation causes a deficiency in an enzyme or protein resulting in cellular dysfunction. The best defined examples are the lysosomal storage disorders in which enzymatic deficiencies in complex lipid metabolism lead to accumulation of normal or abnormal cellular constituents. The mode of inheritance in these disorders is most often autosomal recessive, but it can also be X-linked or the combined result of an inherited germline mutation and an acquired somatic mutation ("second hit") that knocks out both alleles (such as the loss of a growth-suppressor gene in tumors such as retinoblastoma). It is less common for loss-of-function disorders to result from autosomal dominant mutations.

In the case of a *dominant-negative effect*, the abnormal mutation competes with or abolishes the normal allelic function at either the DNA, RNA, or protein level. A dominant-negative mechanism in DM has been suggested by observations that RNA transcripts with expanded CTG repeats precipitate normal RNA transcripts. In myotonia congenita, abnormal protein isoforms combined with normal isoforms of the CLC-1 chloride channel disrupt overall homomultimeric channel function.

In *gain-of-function effects*, the abnormal cellular function exerted by the mutation at one allele in some way renders the cell susceptible to toxic effects, whether or not the normal allele is expressed.

True dominant disorders such as HD and SCA1, in which the heterozygote genotype elicits the full disease phenotype, could be the result of (1) dominant-negative effects, in which proteins with expanded polyglutamine tracts would form oligomers with normal protein isoforms and thereby interfere with their function; or (2) toxic gain-of-function effects.

DISORDERS ASSOCIATED WITH TRINUCLEOTIDE REPEATS An important group of neurologic disorders is caused by abnormal expansions of trinucleotide repeats (Table 359-2). A useful way of organizing repeat diseases and understanding their mechanisms is based on the location of the repeat expansions within the gene. Expansions can occur in the 5′ untranslated region (UTR), within the open reading frame (translated portion of the gene), within the 3′ UTR, or within introns.

The first category of trinucleotide repeat disorders in which repeats are located in the 5′ UTR includes fragile X syndrome and SCA12. Expansions in this region lead to impaired transcription with subsequent loss of protein expression.

The second category of trinucleotide diseases consists of neurodegenerative disorders in which expansion of a CAG repeat in the open reading frame encodes an aberrant protein with an expanded polyglutamine tract. The stretches of CAG repeats, which vary between 5 and 37 in the normal alleles of each gene, are increased two- to fourfold in the mutation. There is a striking correlation between larger numbers of repeats and both increased severity of the neurologic disorder and earlier age of onset. HD patients homozygous for the disease allele have phenotypes similar to heterozygous patients.

These observations suggest a model in which a gain of function is toxic to neurons. One possibility is that expanded polyglutamine tracts provide a substrate for aberrant protein–protein interactions. Such interactions might lead to a loss of function of a critical protein or toxic accumulations of protein aggregates. Several lines of evidence support such a protein-based hypothesis. Open reading frame CAG repeats are indeed translated into protein. Transgenic mice expressing a human *SCA1* gene with an expanded CAG repeat develop the characteristic phenotype only when the transgene is expressed. One study has suggested that polyglutamine tracts of the proteins that cause HD and dentatorubral-pallidoluysian atrophy (DRPLA) interact with glyceraldehyde-3-phosphate dehydrogenase and thereby might have a deleterious effect on neuronal energy metabolism.

Table 359-2 Neurologic Diseases Caused by Expansion of Trinucleotide Repeats

Disorder	Site of Repeat/*Gene*	Effect on Gene Expression or Protein Structure
Fragile X	CGG repeat in 5′ UTR/*FMR1*	Decreased transcript expression and loss of FMRP protein
Spinocerebellar ataxia SCA-12	CAG repeat in 5′UTR/*PPP2R2B*	Likely decreased transcript expression and loss of regulator subunit of the protein phosphatase PP2A
Huntington's disease	CAG repeat in ORF/*ITI5 (HD)*	Expanded polyglutamine tract in huntingtin protein
Dentatorubropallidoluysian atrophy (DRPLA)	CAG repeat in ORF/*atrophin-1*	Expanded polyglutamine tract in atrophin-1 protein
Spinal and bulbar muscular atrophy (SBMA)	CAG repeat in ORF/*AR*	Expanded polyglutamine tract in androgen receptor
Spinocerebellar ataxia (SCA)		
SCA-1	CAG repeat in ORF/*SCA-1*	Expanded polyglutamine tract in ataxin-1 protein
SCA-2	CAG repeat in ORF/*SCA-2*	Expanded polyglutamine tract in ataxin-2 protein
SCA-3 (MJD)	CAG repeat in ORF/*MJD*	Expanded polyglutamine tract in MJD protein
SCA-6	CAG repeat in ORF/*CACNL1A4*	Expanded polyglutamine tract in α1A calcium channel
SCA-7	CAG repeat in ORF/*SCA-7*	Expanded polyglutamine tract in ataxin-7 protein
Oculopharyngeal muscular dystrophy (OPMD)	GCG repeat in ORF/*PABP2*	Expanded polyalanine tract in poly(A) binding protein 2
SCA-8	CTG repeat in 3′UTR/*SCA-8*	CTG repeat found in antisense but not sense transcripts; may lead to decreased levels of sense transcripts
Myotonic dystrophy	CTG repeat in 3′UTR/*DMPK*	Possible alterations in DMPK transcript processing, functions of 3′UTR-binding proteins, and expression of adjacent *DMR-N9* and *DMAHP* genes
Friedreich's ataxia	GAA repeat in intron/*X25*	Altered gene structure interferes with transcription leading to loss of frataxin protein

NOTE: MJD, Machado-Joseph disease; ORF, open reading frame; UTR, untranslated region.

Gain-of-function models of polyglutamine tract diseases must also reconcile the observations that each neurodegenerative disease affects only regionally specific populations of neurons, yet proteins associated with these disorders are widely expressed. One possibility is that each of these polyglutamine tract proteins interacts with yet-to-be discovered proteins that are indeed cell-type specific. The huntingtin-associated protein (HAP1) is one such candidate. HAP1 is selectively expressed in brain tissue and demonstrates enhanced association with forms of huntingtin protein with increased lengths of glutamine repeats. Another potential mechanism of cell-type specificity is that somatic instability of CAG repeats leads to greater expansions in specific cell populations. However, the relatively small variations of three to five in the number of triplet repeats in the HD gene in different regions of the brain makes this explanation less likely.

In the third category of trinucleotide repeat disorders, repeat expansion occurs in the 3′ UTR. In DM, a GTC (CAG in the antisense) repeat in the 3′ UTR of the DM kinase gene expands manyfold, from 5 to 40 repeats in normal alleles to up to 2700 in severe cases. The repeat expansion is variable in different tissues, indicating that errors in DNA replication can occur during meiosis and during somatic cell mitosis. Since DNA sequence motifs in the 3′ UTR of RNA transcripts regulate transcript stability and processing, expansions in this region might affect transcript levels and alter DM kinase protein levels. Quantitative analysis of messenger RNA in muscle biopsies has demonstrated marked disease-specific decreases in DM kinase mRNA in adult-onset DM patients. Levels of normal as well as mutant DM transcripts were decreased, suggesting a novel mechanism of a dominant-negative mutation occurring at the RNA level.

A second potential mechanism in DM is that expansion of the GTC repeat could inhibit expression of the adjacent *DMR-N9* (telomeric) and *DMAHP* (centromeric) genes. Disruption of adjacent chromatin structure by repeat expansion is one mechanism by which expression of adjacent genes could be inhibited. Alternatively, repeat expansions at one locus might affect expression of more than one gene by a *cis*-acting effect, and expansion-containing transcripts may alter levels of transcripts derived from a separate allele by a *trans*-acting effect.

A fourth category of trinucleotide repeat disease occurs with repeat expansion in an intron. FA is caused by the expansion of a GAA triplet in intron 1 of the *X25* gene. Repeat expansions with associated alterations in DNA structure are likely to impair *X25* transcription. Consistent with an autosomal recessive pattern of inheritance and a loss-of-function disease mechanism, the majority of FA patients tested to date demonstrate homozygosity for expanded alleles, while a smaller number are heterozygous with a combination of one expanded allele and point mutations in the other allele. FA is not associated with anticipation (see below) and manifests more often during adolescence rather than middle age, distinguishing it from other trinucleotide repeat diseases.

The discovery of triplet repeats has given molecular precision to old concepts such as *anticipation* (earlier onset of the disease in successive generations, which is associated with further expansion of the abnormal repeats in more severely affected individuals) and has helped to account for variations in gene expression. Variations in trinucleotide repeats in HD, and particularly in DM have given a molecular explanation for *variable expression*, where variations in repeats occurring among individual members of the family can lead to earlier onset or more severe symptoms and signs, as occurs in juvenile HD. Studies suggesting that other neurologic and psychiatric disorders involve anticipation raise the possibility that additional trinucleotide repeat diseases will be discovered.

ONLINE MENDELIAN INHERITANCE IN MAN The OMIM catalogue contains a frequently updated listing of all known genetic traits. For each disease it includes information on clinical manifestations, mapping studies and identity (if available) of the relevant gene, and status of genetic testing. OMIM is administered by the National Center for Biotechnologic Information and is on the Internet at www3.ncbi.nlm.nih.gov/omim/.

BIBLIOGRAPHY

BIRD TD: Apolipoprotein E genotyping in the diagnosis of Alzheimer's disease: A cautionary view. Ann Neurol 38:2, 1995

———: Risks and benefits of DNA testing for neurogenetic disorders. Semin Neurol 19: 253, 1999

BONNE G et al: Mutations in the gene encoding lamin A/C cause autosomal dominant Emery-Dreifuss muscular dystrophy. Nat Genet 21:285, 1999

BRAIS B et al: Short GCG expansions in the PABP2 gene cause oculopharyngeal muscular dystrophy. Nat Genet 18:164, 1998

BUSHBY KMD: Making sense of the limb-girdle muscular dystrophies. Brain 122:1403, 1999

CHANCE PF: Molecular genetics of hereditary neuropathies. J Child Neurol 14:43, 1999

CLEVELAND DW: From Charcot to SOD1: Mechanisms of selective motor neuron death in ALS. Neuron 24:515, 1999

CRAIG HD et al: Multilocus linkage identifies two new loci for a Mendelian form of stroke, cerebral cavernous malformation, at 7p15-13 and 3q25.2-27. Hum Mol Genet 7:1851, 1998

CRINO PB, HENSKE EP: New developments in the neurobiology of the tuberous sclerosis complex. Neurology 53:1384, 1999

DAVIES NP, HANNA MG: Neurological channelopathies: Diagnosis and therapy in the new millennium. Ann Med 31:406, 1999

DICHGANS M et al: The phenotypic spectrum of CADASIL: Clinical findings in 102 cases. Ann Neurol 44:731, 1998

ENGEL AG: Myofibrillar myopathy. Ann Neurol 46:681, 1999

——— et al: Congenital myasthenic syndromes. Arch Neurol 56:163, 1999

FIGLEWICZ DA, BIRD TD: "Pure" hereditary spastic paraplegias. The story becomes complicated. Neurology 53:5, 1999

FINK JK: Approach to patients with inherited neurological disorders. Semin Neurol 18: 211, 1998

———, HEDERA P: Hereditary spastic paraplegia: Genetic heterogeneity and genotype-phenotype correlation. Semin Neurol 19:301, 1999

FITZSIMONS RB: Facioscapulohumeral muscular dystrophy. Curr Opin Neurol 12:501, 1999

FRANSEN E et al: Genotype-phenotype correlation in L1 associated diseases. J Med Genet 35:399, 1998

HAZAN J et al: Spastin, a new AAA protein, is altered in the most frequent form of autosomal dominant spastic paraplegia. Nat Genet 23:296, 1999

HOFFMAN EP: Muscular dystrophy: Identification and use of genes for diagnostics and therapeutics. Arch Pathol Lab Med 123:1050, 1999

HOH HH, OTT J: Complex inheritance and localizing disease genes. Hum Hered 50:85, 2000

HOLMES SE et al: Expansion of a novel CAG trinucleotide repeat in the 5′ region of *PPP2R2B* is associated with SCA12. Nat Genet 23:391, 1999

JOUTEL A et al: *Notch3* mutations in CADASIL, a hereditary adult-onset condition causing stroke and dementia. Nature 383:707, 1996

JURKAT-ROTT K et al: Genetics and pathogenesis of malignant hyperthermia. Muscle Nerve 23:4, 2000

KLEIN C et al: Genetics of primary dystonia. Semin Neurol 19:271, 1999

KONDO-IIDA E et al: Novel mutations and genotype-phenotype relationships in 107 families with Fukuyama-type congenital muscular dystrophy (FCMD). Hum Mol Genet 8:2303, 1999

KOOB MD et al: An untranslated CTG expansion causes a novel form of spinocerebellar ataxia (SCA8). Nat Genet 21:379, 1999

LEE VM-Y, TROJANOWSKI JQ: Neurodegenerative tauopathies: Human disease and transgenic mouse models. Neuron 24:507, 1999

LEHMANN-HORN F, JURKAT-ROTT K: Voltage-gated ion channels and hereditary disease. Physiol Rev 79:1317, 1999

LIN X et al: Expanding our understanding of polyglutamine diseases through mouse models. Neuron 24:499, 1999

MARTIN JB: Molecular basis of the neurodegenerative disorders. N Engl J Med 340:1970, 1999

McNAMARA JO: Emerging insights into the genesis of epilepsy. Nature 399:A15, 1999

MOREIRA ES et al: Limb-girdle muscular dystrophy type 2G is caused by mutations in the gene encoding the sarcomeric protein telethonin. Nat Genet 24:163, 2000

NELLIST M et al: Characterization of the cytosolic tuberin-hamartin complex. J Biol Chem 274:35647, 1999

NOWAK KJ et al: Mutations in the skeletal muscle a-actin gene in patients with actin myopathy and nemaline myopathy. Nat Genet 23:208, 1999

OZELIUS LJ et al: The TOR1A (DYT1) gene family and its role in early onset torsion dystonia. Genomics 62:377, 1999

PANDOLFO M: Friedreich's ataxia: Clinical aspects and pathogenesis. Semin Neurol 19: 311, 1999

PEARCE DA: Hereditary spastic paraplegia: Mitochondrial metalloproteases of yeast. Hum Genet 104:443, 1999

RANTA S et al: The neuronal ceroid lipfuscinoses in human EPMR and mnd mutant mice are associated with mutations in CLN8. Nat Genet 23:233, 1999

REDDY PH et al: Recent advances in understanding the pathogenesis of Huntington's disease. Trends Neurosci 22:248, 1999

SELKOE DJ: Translating cell biology into therapeutic advances in Alzheimer's disease. Nature 399:A23, 1999

SERRATOSA JM et al: The molecular genetic bases of the progressive myoclonus epilepsies. Adv Neurol 79:383, 1999

SPACY SD, WOOD NW: The genetics of Parkinson's disease. Curr Opin Neurol 12:427, 1999

STEVANIN G et al: Are (CTG)n expansions at the SCA8 locus rare polymorphisms? Nat Genet 24:213, 2000

STOGBAUER F et al: Hereditary recurrent focal neuropathies. Neurology 54:546, 2000

THOMSON G, ESPOSITO MS: The genetics of complex diseases. Trends Cell Biol 9:M17, 1999

TIMCHENKO LT, CASKEY CT: Triplet repeat disorders: Discussion of molecular mechanisms. Cell Mol Life Sci 55:1432, 1999

TODA T et al: Fukuyama-type congenital muscular dystrophy: The first human disease to be caused by an ancient retrotransposal integration. J Mol Med 77:816, 1999

TOURNIER-LASSERVE E: CACNA1A mutations. Hemiplegic migraine, episodic ataxia type 2 and the others. Neurology 53:3, 1999

VAINZOF M et al: Sarcoglycanopathies are responsible for 68% of severe autosomal recessive limb-girdle muscular dystrophy in the Brazilian population. J Neurol Sci 164: 44, 1999

VNENCAK-JONES CL: Molecular testing for inherited diseases. Am J Clin Pathol 112:S19, 1999

WALLGREN-PETTERSSON C et al: Clinical and genetic heterogeneity in autosomal recessive nemaline myopathy. Neuromuscul Disord 9:564, 1999

WARNER LE et al: Hereditary peripheral neuropathies: Clinical forms, genetics, and molecular mechanisms. Annu Rev Med 50:263, 1999

WATSON DJ et al: Effects of the amyloid precursor protein Glu693Gln 'Dutch' mutation on the production and stability of amyloid beta-protein. Biochem J 340:703, 1999

WILHELMSEN KC et al: Tau mutations in frontotemporal dementia. Dement Geriatr Cogn Disord 10:S88, 1999

WIRTH B: An update of the mutation spectrum of the survival motor neuron gene (SMN1) in autosomal recessive spinal muscular atrophy (SMA). Hum Mutat 15:228, 2000

WORTH PF et al: Large, expanded repeats in SCA8 are not confined to patients with cerebellar ataxia. Nat Genet 34:214, 2000

ZU L et al: Mapping of a new autosomal dominant spinocerebellar ataxia to chromosome 22. Am J Hum Genet 64:594, 1999

Section 2
DISEASES OF THE CENTRAL NERVOUS SYSTEM

360 Daniel H. Lowenstein

SEIZURES AND EPILEPSY

CT computed tomography	MRI magnetic resonance imaging
CNS central nervous system	MTLE mesial temporal lobe epilepsy
EEG electroencephalogram	PET positron emission tomography
GABA γ-aminobutyric acid	SPECT single photon emission
ILAE International League Against	computed tomography
Epilepsy	VNS vagus nerve stimulation
JME juvenile myoclonic epilepsy	

A *seizure* (from the Latin *sacire*, "to take possession of") is a paroxysmal event due to abnormal, excessive, hypersynchronous discharges from an aggregate of central nervous system (CNS) neurons. Depending on the distribution of discharges, this abnormal CNS activity can have various manifestations, ranging from dramatic convulsive activity to experiential phenomena not readily discernible by an observer. Although a variety of factors influence the incidence and prevalence of seizures, approximately 5 to 10% of the population will have at least one seizure during their lifetime, with the highest incidence occurring in early childhood and late adulthood. Because seizures are common, this clinical problem is encountered frequently during medical practice in a variety of settings.

The meaning of the term seizure needs to be carefully distinguished from that of epilepsy. *Epilepsy* describes a condition in which a person has *recurrent* seizures due to a chronic, underlying process. This definition implies that a person with a single seizure, or recurrent seizures due to correctable or avoidable circumstances, does not necessarily have epilepsy. Epilepsy refers to a clinical phenomenon rather than a single disease entity, since there are many forms and causes of epilepsy. However, among the many causes of epilepsy there are various *epilepsy syndromes* in which the clinical and pathologic characteristics are distinctive and suggest a specific underlying etiology.

Using the definition of epilepsy as two or more unprovoked seizures, the incidence of epilepsy is approximately 0.3 to 0.5% in different populations throughout the world, and the prevalence of epilepsy has been estimated at 5 to 10 persons per 1000.

CLASSIFICATION OF SEIZURES

An essential step in the evaluation and management of a patient with a seizure is to determine the type of seizure that has occurred. The importance of this cannot be overemphasized—classifying the seizure is essential for focusing the diagnostic approach on particular etiologies, selecting the appropriate therapy, and providing potentially vital information regarding prognosis. In 1981, the International League Against Epilepsy (ILAE) published a modified version of the International Classification of Epileptic Seizures that has continued to be a useful classification system (Table 360-1). This system is based on the clinical features of seizures and associated electroencephalographic findings. Other potentially distinctive features such as etiology or cellular substrate are not considered in this classification system, although this will undoubtedly change in the future as more is learned about the pathophysiologic mechanisms that underlie specific seizure types.

The main characteristic that distinguishes the different categories of seizures is whether the seizure activity is partial (synonymous with focal) or generalized. *Partial seizures* are those in which the seizure activity is restricted to discrete areas of the cerebral cortex. *General-*

Table 360-1 Classification of Seizures

1. Partial seizures
   a. Simple partial seizures (with motor, sensory, autonomic, or psychic signs)
   b. Complex partial seizures
   c. Partial seizures with secondary generalization
2. Primarily generalized seizures
   a. Absence (petit mal)
   b. Tonic-clonic (grand mal)
   c. Tonic
   d. Atonic
   e. Myoclonic
3. Unclassified seizures
   a. Neonatal seizures
   b. Infantile spasms

ized seizures involve diffuse regions of the brain simultaneously in a bilaterally symmetric fashion. Partial seizures are often associated with structural abnormalities of the brain. In contrast, generalized seizures may result from cellular, biochemical, or structural abnormalities that have a more widespread distribution.

PARTIAL SEIZURES Partial seizures occur within discrete regions of the brain. If consciousness is fully preserved during the seizure, the clinical manifestations are considered relatively simple and the seizure is termed a *simple partial seizure*. If consciousness is impaired, the symptomatology is more complex and the seizure is termed a *complex partial seizure*. An important additional subgroup comprises those seizures that begin as partial seizures and then spread diffusely throughout the cortex, i.e., *partial seizures with secondary generalization*.

Simple Partial Seizures Simple partial seizures cause motor, sensory, autonomic, or psychic symptoms without an obvious alteration in consciousness. For example, a patient having a partial motor seizure arising from the right primary motor cortex in the vicinity controlling hand movement will note the onset of involuntary movements of the contralateral, left hand. These movements are typically clonic (i.e., repetitive, flexion/extension movements) at a frequency of approximately 2 to 3 Hz; pure tonic posturing may be seen as well. Since the cortical region controlling hand movement is immediately adjacent to the region for facial expression, the seizure may also cause abnormal movements of the face synchronous with the movements of the hand. The electroencephalogram (EEG) recorded with scalp electrodes during the seizure (i.e., an ictal EEG) may show abnormal discharges in a very limited region over the appropriate area of cerebral cortex if the seizure focus involves the cerebral convexity (Chap. 357). Seizure activity occurring within deeper brain structures is often not recorded by the standard EEG, however, and may require intracranial electrodes for its detection.

Three additional features of partial motor seizures are worth noting. First, in some patients the abnormal motor movements may begin in a very restricted region such as the fingers and gradually progress (over seconds to minutes) to include a larger portion of the extremity. This phenomenon was originally described by Hughlings Jackson and is known as a "Jacksonian march," representing the spread of seizure activity over a progressively larger region of motor cortex. Second, patients may experience a localized paresis (Todd's paralysis) for minutes to many hours in the involved region following the seizure. Third, in rare instances the seizure may continue for hours or days. This condition, termed *epilepsia partialis continua*, is often quite refractory to medical therapy.

Other forms of simple partial seizures include those that cause changes in somatic sensation (e.g., paresthesias), vision (flashing lights or formed hallucinations), equilibrium (sensation of falling or vertigo), or autonomic function (flushing, sweating, piloerection). Simple partial seizures arising from the temporal or frontal cortex may also cause alterations in hearing, olfaction, or higher cortical function (psychic symptoms). This includes the sensation of unusual, intense odors (e.g., burning rubber or kerosene) or sounds (crude or highly complex sounds), or an epigastric sensation that rises from the stomach or chest to the head. Some patients describe odd, internal feelings such as fear, a sense of impending change, detachment, depersonalization, déjà vu, or illusions that objects are growing smaller (micropsia) or larger (macropsia). When such symptoms precede a complex partial or secondarily generalized seizure, these simple partial seizures serve as a warning, or *aura*.

Complex Partial Seizures Complex partial seizures are characterized by focal seizure activity accompanied by a transient impairment of the patient's ability to maintain normal contact with the environment. Operationally this means that the patient is unable to respond appropriately to visual or verbal commands during the seizure and has impaired recollection or awareness of the ictal phase. The seizures frequently begin with an aura (i.e., a simple partial seizure) that is stereotypic for the patient. The start of the ictal phase is often a sudden behavioral arrest or motionless stare, and this marks the onset

of the event for which the patient will be amnestic. The behavioral arrest is usually accompanied by automatisms, which are involuntary, automatic behaviors that have a wide range of manifestations. Automatisms may consist of very basic behaviors such as chewing, lip smacking, swallowing, or "picking" movements of the hands, or more elaborate behaviors such as a display of emotion or running. The patient is typically confused following the seizure, and the transition to full recovery of consciousness may range from seconds up to an hour. Careful examination of the patient immediately following the seizure may show an anterograde amnesia or, in cases involving the dominant hemisphere, a postictal aphasia.

The routine, interictal (i.e., between seizures) EEG in patients with complex partial seizures is often normal, or may show brief discharges termed *epileptiform spikes*, or *sharp waves*. Since complex partial seizures can arise from the medial temporal lobe or inferior frontal lobe, i.e., regions distant from the scalp, the EEG recorded during the seizure may be nonlocalizing. However, the seizure focus is often detected using special electrodes such as sphenoidal or surgically placed intracranial electrodes.

The range of potential clinical behaviors linked to complex partial seizures is so broad that extreme caution is advised before concluding that stereotypic episodes of bizarre or atypical behavior are not due to seizure activity. In such cases it is imperative to consider more detailed EEG studies to determine whether the behaviors are caused by a seizure disorder.

Partial Seizures with Secondary Generalization Partial seizures can spread to involve both cerebral hemispheres and produce a generalized seizure, usually of the tonic-clonic variety (discussed below). Secondary generalization is observed frequently following simple partial seizures, especially those with a focus in the frontal lobe, but may also be associated with partial seizures occurring elsewhere in the brain. A partial seizure with secondary generalization is often difficult to distinguish from a primarily generalized tonic-clonic seizure, since bystanders tend to emphasize the more dramatic, generalized convulsive phase of the seizure and overlook the more subtle, focal symptoms present at onset. In some cases, the focal onset of the seizure becomes apparent only when a careful history identifies a preceding aura (i.e., simple partial seizure). Often, however, the focal onset is not clinically evident and may be established only through careful EEG analysis. Nonetheless, distinguishing between these two entities is extremely important, as there may be substantial differences in the evaluation and treatment of partial versus generalized seizure disorders.

GENERALIZED SEIZURES By definition, generalized seizures arise from both cerebral hemispheres simultaneously. However, it is currently impossible to exclude entirely the existence of a focal region of abnormal activity that initiates the seizure prior to rapid secondary generalization. For this reason, generalized seizures may be practically defined as bilateral clinical and electrographic events without any detectable focal onset. Fortunately, a number of the subtypes of generalized seizures have distinctive features that facilitate clinical diagnosis.

Absence Seizures (Petit Mal) Absence seizures are characterized by sudden, brief lapses of consciousness without loss of postural control. The seizure typically lasts for only seconds, consciousness returns as suddenly as it was lost, and there is no postictal confusion. Although the brief loss of consciousness may be clinically inapparent or the sole manifestation of the seizure discharge, absence seizures are usually accompanied by subtle, bilateral motor signs such as rapid blinking of the eyelids, chewing movements, or small-amplitude, clonic movements of the hands.

Absence seizures usually begin in childhood (ages 4 to 8) or early adolescence and are the main seizure type in 15 to 20% of children with epilepsy. The seizures can occur hundreds of times per day, but the child may be unaware of or unable to convey their existence. This can lead to a situation in which the patient is constantly struggling to piece together experiences that have been interrupted by the seizures. Since the clinical signs of the seizures are subtle, especially to new parents, it is not surprising that the first clue to absence epilepsy is often unexplained "daydreaming" and a decline in school performance recognized by a teacher.

The electrophysiologic hallmark of typical absence seizures is a generalized, symmetric, 3-Hz spike-and-wave discharge that begins and ends suddenly on a normal EEG background (Chap. 357). Periods of spike-and-wave discharges lasting more than a few seconds usually correlate with the clinical signs, but the EEG often shows many more periods of abnormal cortical activity than were suspected clinically. Hyperventilation tends to provoke these electrographic discharges and even the seizures themselves and is routinely used when recording the EEG.

Typical absence seizures are often associated with generalized, tonic-clonic seizures, but patients usually have no other neurologic problems and respond well to treatment with specific anticonvulsants. Although estimates vary, approximately 60 to 70% of such patients will have a spontaneous remission during adolescence.

Atypical Absence Seizures Atypical absence seizures have features that deviate from both the clinical and EEG features of typical absence seizures. For example, the lapse of consciousness is usually of longer duration and less abrupt in onset and cessation, and the seizure is accompanied by more obvious motor signs that may include focal or lateralizing features. The EEG shows a generalized, slow spike-and-wave pattern with a frequency of ≤2.5/s, as well as other abnormal activity. Atypical absence seizures are usually associated with diffuse or multifocal structural abnormalities of the brain and therefore may accompany other signs of neurologic dysfunction such as mental retardation. Furthermore, the seizures are less responsive to anticonvulsants compared to typical absence seizures.

Generalized, Tonic-Clonic Seizures (Grand Mal) Primarily generalized, tonic-clonic seizures are the main seizure type in approximately 10% of all persons with epilepsy. They are also the most common seizure type resulting from metabolic derangements and are therefore frequently encountered in many different clinical settings. The seizure usually begins abruptly without warning, although some patients describe vague premonitory symptoms in the hours leading up to the seizure. This prodrome should be distinguished from the stereotypic auras associated with focal seizures that secondarily generalize. The initial phase of the seizure is usually tonic contraction of muscles throughout the body, accounting for a number of the classic features of the event. Tonic contraction of the muscles of expiration and the larynx at the onset will produce a loud moan or cry. Respirations are impaired, secretions pool in the oropharynx, and the patient becomes cyanotic. Contraction of the jaw muscles may cause biting of the tongue. A marked enhancement of sympathetic tone leads to increases in heart rate, blood pressure, and pupillary size. After 10 to 20 s, the tonic phase of the seizure typically evolves into the clonic phase, produced by the superimposition of periods of muscle relaxation on the tonic muscle contraction. The periods of relaxation progressively increase until the end of the ictal phase, which usually lasts no more than 1 min. The postictal phase is characterized by unresponsiveness, muscular flaccidity, and excessive salivation that can cause stridorous breathing and partial airway obstruction. Bladder or bowel incontinence may occur at this point as well. Patients gradually regain consciousness over minutes to hours, and during this transition there is typically a period of postictal confusion. Patients will subsequently complain of headache, fatigue, and muscle ache that can last for many hours. The duration of impaired consciousness in the postictal phase can be extremely long, i.e., many hours, in patients with prolonged seizures or underlying CNS diseases such as alcoholic cerebral atrophy.

The EEG during the tonic phase of the seizure shows a progressive increase in generalized low-voltage fast activity, followed by generalized high-amplitude, polyspike discharges. In the clonic phase, the high-amplitude activity is typically interrupted by slow waves to create a spike-and-wave pattern. The postictal EEG shows diffuse slowing that gradually recovers as the patient awakens.

There are many variants of the generalized tonic-clonic seizure, including pure tonic and pure clonic seizures. Brief tonic seizures lasting only a few seconds are especially noteworthy since they are usually associated with known epileptic syndromes having mixed seizure phenotypes, such as the Lennox-Gastaut syndrome (discussed below).

Atonic Seizures Atonic seizures are characterized by sudden loss of postural muscle tone lasting 1 to 2 s. Consciousness is briefly impaired, but there is usually no postictal confusion. A very brief seizure may cause only a quick head drop or nodding movement, while a longer seizure will cause the patient to collapse. This can be quite dramatic and extremely dangerous, since there is a substantial risk of direct head injury with the fall. The EEG shows brief, generalized spike-and-wave discharges followed immediately by diffuse slow waves that correlate with the loss of muscle tone. Similar to pure tonic seizures, atonic seizures are usually seen in association with known epileptic syndromes.

Myoclonic Seizures Myoclonus is a sudden and brief muscle contraction that may involve one part of the body or the entire body. A normal, common physiologic form of myoclonus is the sudden jerking movement observed while falling asleep. Pathologic myoclonus is most commonly seen in association with metabolic disorders, degenerative CNS diseases, or anoxic brain injury (Chap. 22). Although the distinction from other forms of myoclonus is imprecise, myoclonic seizures are considered to be true epileptic events since they are caused by cortical (versus subcortical or spinal) dysfunction. The EEG shows bilaterally synchronous spike-and-wave discharges. Myoclonic seizures usually coexist with other forms of generalized seizure disorders but are the predominant feature of juvenile myoclonic epilepsy (discussed below).

UNCLASSIFIED SEIZURES Not all seizure types can be classified as partial or generalized. This appears to be especially true of seizures that occur in neonates and infants. The distinctive phenotypes of seizures at these early ages likely result, in part, from differences in neuronal function and connectivity in the immature versus mature CNS.

EPILEPSY SYNDROMES

In addition to recognizing the patterns of different types of seizures, it is also useful to be familiar with some of the more common epilepsy syndromes, since this often helps in the determination of therapy and prognosis. Epilepsy syndromes are disorders in which epilepsy is a predominant feature, and there is sufficient evidence (e.g., through clinical, EEG, radiologic, or genetic observations) to suggest a common underlying mechanism. Three important epilepsy syndromes are listed below; additional examples with a known genetic basis are shown in Table 360-2.

JUVENILE MYOCLONIC EPILEPSY Juvenile myoclonic epilepsy (JME) is a generalized seizure disorder of unknown cause that appears in early adolescence and is usually characterized by bilateral myoclonic jerks that may be single or repetitive. The myoclonic seizures are most frequent in the morning after awakening and can be provoked by sleep deprivation. Consciousness is preserved unless the myoclonus is especially severe. Many patients also experience generalized tonic-clonic seizures, and up to one-third have absence seizures. The condition is otherwise benign, and although complete remission is uncommon, the seizures respond well to appropriate anticonvulsant medication. There is often a family history of epilepsy, and genetic linkage studies suggest a polygenic cause.

LENNOX-GASTAUT SYNDROME Lennox-Gastaut syndrome occurs in children and is defined by the following triad: (1) multiple seizure types (usually including generalized tonic-clonic, atonic, and atypical absence seizures); (2) an EEG showing slow (<3 Hz) spike-and-wave discharges and a variety of other abnormalities; and (3) impaired cognitive function in most but not all cases. Lennox-Gastaut syndrome is associated with CNS disease or dysfunc-

Table 360-2 Examples of Genes Associated with Epilepsy Syndromes[a]

Gene (Locus)	Function of Gene	Clinical Syndrome	Comments
CHRNA4 (20q13.2)	Nicotinic acetylcholine receptor subunit; mutations cause a decrease in Ca^{2+} flux through the receptor; this may reduce amount of GABA release in presynaptic terminals	Autosomal dominant nocturnal frontal lobe epilepsy (ADNFLE); childhood onset; brief, nighttime seizures with prominent motor movements; often misdiagnosed as primary sleep disorder	Rare; first identified in a large Australian family; additional CHRNA4 mutation found in a Norweigan family with similar phenotype; second ADNFLE locus found on 15q24
KCNQ2 (20q13.3) KCNQ3 (8q24)	Voltage-gated potassium channel subunits; mutation in pore regions may cause a 20–40% reduction of potassium currents, which will lead to impaired repolarization	Benign familial neonatal convulsions (BFNC); autosomal dominant inheritance; onset in 1st week of life in infants who are otherwise normal; remission usually within weeks to months; long-term epilepsy in 10–15%	Rare; sequence and functional homology to KCNQ1, mutations of which cause long QT syndrome and a cardiac-auditory syndrome
SCN1B (19q12.1)	β-subunit of a voltage-gated sodium channel; mutation disrupts disulfide bridge that is crucial for structure of extracellular domain; mutated β-subunit leads to slower sodium channel inactivation	Generalized epilepsy with febrile seizures plus (GEFS+); autosomal dominant inheritance; presents with febrile seizures at either <3 months or >3 years, then variable seizure types not associated with fever	Incidence uncertain; GEFS+ identified in other families without SCN1B mutations; significant phenotypic heterogeneity within same family, including members with febrile seizures only
CSTB (21q22.3)	Cystatin B, a noncaspase cysteine protease inhibitor; normal protein may block neuronal apoptosis by inhibiting caspases directly or indirectly (via cathepsins), or controlling proteolysis	Progressive myoclonus epilepsy (PME) (Unverricht-Lundborg disease); autosomal recessive inheritance; age of onset between 6–15 years, myoclonic seizures, ataxia, and progressive cognitive decline; brain shows neuronal degeneration	Overall rare, but relatively common in Finland and Western Mediterranean (>1 in 20,000); precise role of cystatin B in human disease unknown, although mice with null mutations of cystatin B have similar syndrome
EPM2A (6q24)	Laforin, a protein tyrosine phosphatase (PTP); may influence glycogen metabolism, which is known to be regulated by phosphatases	Progressive myoclonus epilepsy (Lafora's disease); autosomal recessive inheritance; onset age 6–19 years, death within 10 years; brain degeneration associated with polyglucosan intracellular inclusion bodies in numerous organs	Most common PME in Southern Europe, Middle East, Northern Africa, and Indian subcontinent; genetic heterogeneity; unknown whether seizure phenotype due to degeneration or direct effects of abnormal laforin expression.
Doublecortin (Xq21-24)	Doublecortin, expressed primarily in frontal lobes; function unknown; potentially an intracellular signalling molecule	Classic lissencephaly associated with severe mental retardation and seizures in males; subcortical band heterotopia with more subtle findings in females (presumably due to random X-inactivation); X-linked dominant	Relatively rare but of uncertain incidence, recent increased ascertainment due to improved imaging techniques; relationship between migration defect and seizure phenotype unknown

[a] The first three syndromes listed in the table (ADNFLE, BFNC, and GEFS+) are all the currently known idiopathic generalized epilepsies associated with identified gene mutations. The last three syndromes are examples of the numerous Mendelian disorders in which seizures are one part of the phenotype.

NOTE: GABA, γ-aminobutyric acid.

tion from a variety of causes, including developmental abnormalities, perinatal hypoxia/ischemia, trauma, infection, and other acquired lesions. The multifactorial nature of this syndrome suggests that it is a nonspecific response of the brain to diffuse neural injury. Unfortunately, many patients have a poor prognosis due to the underlying CNS disease and the physical and psychosocial consequences of severe, poorly controlled epilepsy.

MESIAL TEMPORAL LOBE EPILEPSY SYNDROME
Mesial temporal lobe epilepsy (MTLE) is the most common syndrome associated with complex partial seizures and is an example of a symptomatic, partial epilepsy. Distinctive clinical, electroencephalographic, and pathologic features define this syndrome (Table 360-3). High-resolution magnetic resonance imaging (MRI) can detect the characteristic hippocampal sclerosis that appears to be an essential element in the pathophysiology of MTLE for many patients (Fig. 360-1). Recognition of this syndrome is especially important because it tends to be refractory to treatment with anticonvulsants but responds extremely well to surgical intervention. Major advances in the understanding of basic mechanisms of epilepsy have come through studies of experimental models of MTLE, discussed below.

THE CAUSES OF SEIZURES AND EPILEPSY

Seizures are a result of a shift in the normal balance of excitation and inhibition within the CNS. Given the numerous properties that control

Table 360-3 Characteristics of the Mesial Temporal Lobe Epilepsy (MTLE) Syndrome

History	
History of febrile seizures	Seizures may remit and reappear
Positive family history of epilepsy	Seizures often intractable
Early onset	
Rare secondarily generalized seizures	
Clinical Observations	
Aura common	Postictal disorientation, memory
Behavioral arrest/stare	loss, dysphasia (with focus in
Complex automatisms	dominant hemisphere)
Unilateral posturing	
Laboratory Studies	
Unilateral or bilateral anterior temporal spikes on EEG	
Hypometabolism on interictal PET	
Hypoperfusion on interictal SPECT	
Material-specific memory deficits on intracranial amobarbital (Wada) test	
MRI findings	
Small hippocampus with increased signal on T2-weighted sequences	
Small temporal lobe	
Enlarged temporal horn	
Pathologic findings	
Highly selective loss of specific cell populations within hippocampus in most cases	

NOTE: EEG, electroencephalogram; PET, positron emission tomography; SPECT, single photon emission computed tomography.

FIGURE 360-1   Mesial temporal lobe epilepsy. The EEG suggested a right temporal lobe focus. Coronal high-resolution T2-weighted fast spin echo magnetic resonance image obtained through the body of the hippocampus demonstrates abnormal high signal intensity in the right hippocampus (white arrows; compare with the normal hippocampus on the left, black arrows) consistent with mesial temporal sclerosis.

neuronal excitability, it is not surprising that there are many different ways to perturb this normal balance, and therefore many different causes of both seizures and epilepsy. Our understanding of the basic mechanisms involved remains very limited, and consequently there is not a rigorous, mechanistic-based framework for organizing all the etiologies. Conceptually, however, three important clinical observations emphasize how a variety of factors determine why certain conditions may cause seizures or epilepsy in a given patient.

1. *The normal brain is capable of having a seizure under the appropriate circumstances, and there are differences between individuals in the susceptibility or threshold for seizures.* For example, seizures may be induced by high fevers in children who are otherwise normal and who never develop other neurologic problems, including epilepsy. However, febrile seizures occur only in a relatively small proportion of children. This implies there are various underlying, *endogenous factors* that influence the threshold for having a seizure. Some of these factors are clearly genetic, as it has been shown that a family history of epilepsy will influence the likelihood of seizures occurring in otherwise normal individuals. Normal development also plays an important role, since the brain appears to have different seizure thresholds at different maturational stages.

2. *There are a variety of conditions that have an extremely high likelihood of resulting in a chronic seizure disorder.* One of the best examples of this is severe, penetrating head trauma, which is associated with up to a 50% risk of subsequent epilepsy. The high propensity for severe traumatic brain injury to lead to epilepsy suggests that the injury results in a long-lasting, pathologic change in the CNS that transforms a presumably normal neural network into one that is abnormally hyperexcitable. This process is known as *epileptogenesis*, and the specific changes that result in a lowered seizure threshold can be considered *epileptogenic factors*. Other processes associated with epileptogenesis include stroke, infections, and abnormalities of CNS development. Likewise, the genetic abnormalities associated with epilepsy likely involve processes that trigger the appearance of specific sets of epileptogenic factors.

3. *Seizures are episodic.* Patients with epilepsy have seizures intermittently and, depending on the underlying cause, many patients are completely normal for months or even years between seizures. This implies there are important provocative or *precipitating factors* that

induce seizures in patients with epilepsy. Similarly, precipitating factors are responsible for causing the single seizure in someone without epilepsy. Precipitants include those due to intrinsic physiologic processes, such as psychological or physical stress, sleep deprivation, or hormonal changes associated with the menstrual cycle. They also include exogenous factors such as exposure to toxic substances and certain medications.

These observations emphasize the concept that the many causes of seizures and epilepsy result from a dynamic interplay between endogenous factors, epileptogenic factors, and precipitating factors. The potential role of each needs to be carefully considered when determining the appropriate management of a patient with seizures. For example, the identification of predisposing factors (e.g., family history of epilepsy) in a patient with febrile seizures may increase the necessity for closer follow-up and a more aggressive diagnostic evaluation. Finding an epileptogenic lesion may help in the estimation of seizure recurrence and duration of therapy. Finally, removal or modification of a precipitating factor may be an effective and safer method for preventing further seizures than the prophylactic use of anticonvulsant drugs.

CAUSES ACCORDING TO AGE   In practice, it is useful to consider the etiologies of seizures based on the age of the patient, as age is one of the most important factors determining both the incidence and likely causes of seizures or epilepsy (Table 360-4). During the *neonatal period and early infancy*, potential causes include hypoxic-ischemic encephalopathy, trauma, CNS infection, congenital CNS abnormalities, and metabolic disorders. Babies born to mothers using neurotoxic drugs such as cocaine, heroin, or ethanol are susceptible to drug-withdrawal seizures in the first few days after delivery. Hypoglycemia and hypocalcemia, which can occur as secondary complications of perinatal injury, are also causes of seizures early after delivery. Seizures due to inborn errors of metabolism usually present once regular feeding begins, typically 2 to 3 days after birth. Pyridox-

Table 360-4   The Causes of Seizures

Neonates (<1 month)	Perinatal hypoxia and ischemia
	Intracranial hemorrhage and trauma
	Acute CNS infection
	Metabolic disturbances (hypoglycemia, hypocalcemia, hypomagnesemia, pyridoxine deficiency)
	Drug withdrawal
	Developmental disorders
	Genetic disorders
Infants and children (>1 mo and <12 years)	Febrile seizures
	Genetic disorders (metabolic, degenerative, primary epilepsy syndromes)
	CNS infection
	Developmental disorders
	Trauma
	Idiopathic
Adolescents (12–18 years)	Trauma
	Genetic disorders
	Infection
	Brain tumor
	Illicit drug use
	Idiopathic
Young adults (18–35 years)	Trauma
	Alcohol withdrawal
	Illicit drug use
	Brain tumor
	Idiopathic
Older adults (>35 years)	Cerebrovascular disease
	Brain tumor
	Alcohol withdrawal
	Metabolic disorders (uremia, hepatic failure, electrolyte abnormalities, hypoglycemia)
	Alzheimer's disease and other degenerative CNS diseases
	Idiopathic

NOTE: CNS, central nervous system.

ine (vitamin B₆) deficiency, an important cause of neonatal seizures, can be effectively treated with pyridoxine replacement. The idiopathic or inherited forms of benign neonatal convulsions are also seen during this time period.

The most common seizures arising in *late infancy and early childhood* are febrile seizures, which are seizures associated with fevers but without evidence of CNS infection or other defined causes. The overall prevalence is 3 to 5% and even higher in some parts of the world, such as Asia. Patients often have a family history of febrile seizures or epilepsy. Febrile seizures usually occur between 3 months and 5 years of age and have a peak incidence between 18 and 24 months. The typical scenario is a child who has a generalized, tonic-clonic seizure during a febrile illness in the setting of a common childhood infection such as otitis media, respiratory infection, or gastroenteritis. The seizure is likely to occur during the rising phase of the temperature curve (i.e., during the first day) rather than well into the course of the illness. A *simple* febrile seizure is a single, isolated event, brief, and symmetric in appearance. *Complex* febrile seizures have repeated seizure activity, last >15 min, or have focal features. Approximately one-third of patients with febrile seizures will have a recurrence, but <10% have three or more episodes. Recurrences are much more likely when the febrile seizure occurs in the first year of life. Simple febrile seizures are not associated with an increase in the risk of developing epilepsy, while complex febrile seizures have a risk of 2 to 5%; other risk factors include the presence of preexisting neurologic deficits and a family history of nonfebrile seizures.

Childhood marks the age at which many of the well-defined epilepsy syndromes present. Some children who are otherwise normal develop idiopathic, generalized tonic-clonic seizures without other features that fit into specific syndromes. Temporal lobe epilepsy usually presents in childhood and may be related to mesial temporal lobe sclerosis (as part of the MTLE syndrome) or other focal abnormalities such as cortical dysgenesis. Other types of partial seizures, including those with secondary generalization, may be the relatively late manifestation of a developmental disorder, an acquired lesion such as head trauma, CNS infection (especially viral encephalitis), or very rarely a CNS tumor.

The period of *adolescence and early adulthood* is one of transition during which the idiopathic or genetically based epilepsy syndromes, including JME and juvenile absence epilepsy, become less common, while epilepsies secondary to acquired CNS lesions begin to predominate. Seizures that begin in patients in this age range may be associated with head trauma, CNS infections (including parasitic infections such as cysticercosis), brain tumors, congenital CNS abnormalities, illicit drug use, or alcohol withdrawal.

Head trauma is a common cause of epilepsy in adolescents and adults. The head injury can be caused by a variety of mechanisms, and the likelihood of developing epilepsy is strongly correlated with the severity of the injury. A patient with a penetrating head wound, depressed skull fracture, intracranial hemorrhage, or prolonged posttraumatic coma or amnesia has a 40 to 50% risk of developing epilepsy, while a patient with a closed head injury and cerebral contusion has a 5 to 25% risk. Recurrent seizures usually develop within 1 year after head trauma, although intervals of 10 years or longer are well known. In controlled studies, mild head injury, defined as a concussion with amnesia or loss of consciousness of <30 min, was not found to be associated with an increased likelihood of epilepsy. Nonetheless, most epileptologists know of patients who have partial seizures within hours or days of a mild head injury and subsequently develop chronic seizures of the same type; such cases may represent rare examples of chronic epilepsy resulting from mild head injury.

The causes of seizures in *older adults* include cerebrovascular disease, trauma (including subdural hematoma), CNS tumors, and degenerative diseases. Cerebrovascular disease may account for approximately 50% of new cases of epilepsy in patients older than 65. Acute seizures (i.e., occurring at the time of the stroke) are seen more often with embolic rather than hemorrhagic or thrombotic stroke. Chronic seizures typically appear months to years after the initial event and are associated with all forms of stroke.

Table 360-5 Drugs and Other Substances that Can Cause Seizures

Antimicrobials/antivirals	Psychotropics
β-lactam and related compounds	Antidepressants
Quinolones	Antipsychotics
Acyclovir	Lithium
Isoniazid	Radiographic contrast agents
Ganciclovir	Theophylline
Anesthetics and Analgesics	Sedative-hypnotic drug with-
Meperidine	drawal
Tramadol	Alcohol
Local anesthetics	Barbiturates
Class 1B agents	Benzodiazepines
Immunomodulatory drugs	Drugs of abuse
Cyclosporine	Amphetamine
OKT3 (monoclonal antibodies to T cells)	Cocaine
	Phencyclidine
Tacrolimus (FK-506)	Methylphenidate
Interferons	Flumazenil[a]

[a] In benzodiazepine-dependent patients.

Metabolic disturbances such as electrolyte imbalance, hypo- or hyperglycemia, renal failure, and hepatic failure may cause seizures at any age. Similarly, endocrine disorders, hematologic disorders, vasculitides, and many other systemic diseases may cause seizures over a broad age range. A wide variety of medications and abused substances are known to precipitate seizures as well (Table 360-5).

BASIC MECHANISMS

MECHANISMS OF SEIZURE INITIATION AND PROPAGATION Partial seizure activity can begin in a very discrete region of cortex and then spread to neighboring regions, i.e., there is a *seizure initiation* phase and a *seizure propagation* phase. Studies of experimental models of these phases suggest that the initiation phase is characterized by two concurrent events in an aggregate of neurons: (1) high-frequency bursts of action potentials, and (2) hypersynchronization. The bursting activity is caused by a relatively long-lasting depolarization of the neuronal membrane due to influx of extracellular calcium (Ca²⁺), which leads to the opening of voltage-dependent sodium (Na⁺) channels, influx of Na⁺, and generation of repetitive action potentials. This is followed by a hyperpolarizing afterpotential mediated by γ-aminobutyric acid (GABA) receptors or potassium (K⁺) channels, depending on the cell type. The synchronized bursts from a sufficient number of neurons result in a so-called spike discharge on the EEG.

Normally, the spread of bursting activity is prevented by intact hyperpolarization and a region of surrounding inhibition created by inhibitory neurons. With sufficient activation there is a recruitment of surrounding neurons via a number of mechanisms. Repetitive discharges lead to the following: (1) an increase in extracellular K⁺, which blunts the extent of hyperpolarization and depolarizes neighboring neurons; (2) accumulation of Ca²⁺ in presynaptic terminals, leading to enhanced neurotransmitter release; and (3) depolarization-induced activation of the *N*-methyl-D-aspartate (NMDA) subtype of the excitatory amino acid receptor, which causes more Ca²⁺ influx and neuronal activation. The recruitment of a sufficient number of neurons leads to a loss of the surrounding inhibition and propagation of seizure activity into contiguous areas via local cortical connections, and to more distant areas via long commissural pathways such as the corpus callosum.

Many factors control neuronal excitability, and thus there are many potential mechanisms for altering a neuron's propensity to have bursting activity. Examples of mechanisms *intrinsic* to the neuron include changes in the conductance of ion channels, response characteristics of membrane receptors, cytoplasmic buffering, second-messenger systems, and protein expression as determined by gene transcription, translation, and posttranslational modification. Mechanisms *extrinsic* to the neuron include changes in the amount or type of neurotransmitters present at the synapse, modulation of receptors by extracellular ions and other molecules, and temporal and spatial properties of both synaptic and nonsynaptic input. Nonneural cells, such as astrocytes and oligodendrocytes, have an important role in many of these mechanisms as well.

Certain known causes of seizures are explained by these mechanisms. For example, accidental ingestion of domoic acid, which is an analogue of glutamate (the principal excitatory neurotransmitter in the brain), causes profound seizures via direct activation of excitatory amino acid receptors throughout the CNS. Penicillin, which can lower the seizure threshold in humans and is a potent convulsant in experimental models, reduces inhibition by antagonizing the effects of GABA at its receptor. The basic mechanisms of other precipitating factors of seizures, such as sleep deprivation, fever, alcohol withdrawal, hypoxia, and infection, are not as well understood but presumably involve analogous perturbations in neuronal excitability. Similarly, the endogenous factors that determine an individual's seizure threshold may relate to these properties as well.

Knowledge of the mechanisms responsible for the initiation and propagation of most generalized seizures (including tonic-clonic, myoclonic, and atonic types) remains rudimentary and reflects the limited understanding of the connectivity of the brain at a systems level. Much more is understood about the origin of generalized spike-and-wave discharges in absence seizures. These appear to be related to oscillatory rhythms that are normally generated during sleep by circuits connecting the thalamus and cortex. This oscillatory behavior involves an interaction between $GABA_B$ receptors, T-type Ca^{2+} channels, and K^+ channels located within the thalamus. Pharmacologic studies indicate that modulation of these receptors and channels can induce absence seizures, and there is speculation that the genetic forms of absence epilepsy may be associated with mutations of components of this system.

MECHANISMS OF EPILEPTOGENESIS Epileptogenesis refers to the transformation of a normal neuronal network into one that is chronically hyperexcitable. For example, there is often a delay of months to years between an initial CNS injury such as trauma, stroke, or infection and the first seizure. The injury appears to initiate a process that gradually lowers the seizure threshold in the affected region until a spontaneous seizure occurs. In many genetic and idiopathic forms of epilepsy, epileptogenesis is presumably determined by developmentally regulated events.

Pathologic studies of the hippocampus from patients with temporal lobe epilepsy have led to the suggestion that some forms of epileptogenesis are related to *structural changes in neuronal networks*. For example, many patients with MTLE syndrome have a highly selective loss of neurons that has been proposed to contribute to inhibition of the main excitatory neurons within the dentate gyrus. There is also evidence that, in response to the loss of neurons, there is reorganization or "sprouting" of surviving neurons in a way that affects the excitability of the network. Some of these changes can be seen in experimental models of prolonged electrical seizures or traumatic brain injury. Thus, an initial injury such as head injury may lead to a very focal, confined region of structural change that causes local hyperexcitability. The local hyperexcitability leads to further structural changes that evolve over time until the focal lesion produces clinically evident seizures. Similar models have also provided strong evidence for long-term alterations in *intrinsic, biochemical properties of cells* within the network, such as chronic changes in glutamate receptor function.

GENETIC CAUSES OF EPILEPSY The most important recent progress in epilepsy research has been the identification of genetic mutations associated with a variety of epilepsy syndromes. Table 360-2 describes some of these in further detail. Although all of the mutations identified to date cause rare forms of epilepsy, they have led to extremely important conceptual advances. For example, it appears that many of the inherited, idiopathic epilepsies (i.e., the relatively "pure"

forms of epilepsy in which seizures are the phenotypic abnormality and brain structure and function are otherwise normal) are due to mutations affecting ion channel function. These syndromes are therefore part of the larger group of "channelopathies" causing paroxysmal disorders such as cardiac arrhythmias, episodic ataxia, periodic weakness, and familial hemiplegic migraine (Chap. 15). In contrast, gene mutations observed in symptomatic epilepsies (i.e., disorders in which other neurologic abnormalities, such as cognitive impairment, coexist with seizures) are proving to be associated with pathways influencing CNS development or neuronal homeostasis. A current challenge is to identify the multiple susceptibility genes that underlie the more common forms of idiopathic epilepsies.

MECHANISMS OF ACTION OF ANTIEPILEPTIC DRUGS Currently available antiepileptic drugs appear to act primarily by blocking the initiation or spread of seizures. This occurs through a variety of mechanisms, and in most cases the drugs have pleiotropic effects. The mechanisms include inhibition of Na^+-dependent action potentials in a frequency-dependent manner (e.g., phenytoin, carbamazepine, topiramate, zonisamide), inhibition of voltage-gated Ca^{2+} channels (phenytoin), decrease of glutamate release (lamotrigine), potentiation of GABA receptor function (benzodiazepines and barbiturates), and increase in the availability of GABA (valproic acid, gabapentin, tiagabine). The two most effective drugs for absence seizures, ethosuximide and valproic acid, probably act by inhibiting T-type Ca^{2+} channels in thalamic neurons.

In contrast to the relatively large number of antiepileptic drugs that can attenuate seizure activity, there are currently no drugs known to prevent the formation of a seizure focus following CNS injury in humans. The eventual development of such "antiepileptogenic" drugs will provide an important means of preventing the emergence of epilepsy following injuries such as head trauma, stroke, and CNS infection.

EVALUATION OF THE PATIENT WITH A SEIZURE

When a patient presents shortly after a seizure, the first priorities are attention to vital signs, respiratory and cardiovascular support, and treatment of seizures if they resume (see "Treatment"). Life-threatening conditions such as CNS infection, metabolic derangement or drug toxicity must be recognized and managed appropriately.

When the patient is not acutely ill, the evaluation will initially focus on whether or not there is a history of earlier seizures (Fig. 360-2). If this is the patient's first seizure, then the emphasis will be to (1) establish whether the reported episode was a seizure rather than another paroxysmal event, (2) determine the cause of the seizure by identifying risk factors and precipitating events, and (3) decide whether anticonvulsant therapy is required in addition to treatment for any underlying illness.

In the patient with prior seizures or a known history of epilepsy, the evaluation is directed toward (1) identification of the underlying cause and precipitating factors, and (2) determination of the adequacy of the patient's current therapy.

HISTORY AND EXAMINATION The history should first determine whether the event was truly a seizure. It is essential to take the time to gather an in-depth history, for *in many cases the diagnosis of a seizure is based solely on clinical grounds—the examination and laboratory studies are often normal*. Keeping in mind the characteristics of different seizure types, questions need to focus precisely on the symptoms before, during, and after the episode in order to discriminate a seizure from other paroxysmal events (see "Differential Diagnosis of Seizures"). Seizures frequently occur out-of-hospital, and the patient may be unaware of the ictal and immediate postictal phases; thus witnesses to the event should be interviewed carefully.

The history should also focus on risk factors and predisposing events. Clues for a predisposition to seizures include a history of febrile seizures, earlier auras or brief seizures not recognized as such, and a family history of seizures. Epileptogenic factors such as prior head trauma, stroke, tumor, or vascular malformation should be identified. In children, a careful assessment of developmental milestones may provide evidence for underlying CNS disease. Precipitating factors such as sleep deprivation, systemic diseases, electrolyte or metabolic derangements, acute infection, drugs that lower the seizure threshold (Table 360-5), or alcohol or illicit drug use should also be identified.

The general physical examination includes a search for signs of infection or systemic illness. Careful examination of the skin may reveal signs of neurocutaneous disorders, such as tuberous sclerosis or neurofibromatosis, or chronic liver or renal disease. A finding of organomegaly may indicate a metabolic storage disease, and limb asymmetry may provide a clue for brain injury early in development. Signs of head trauma and use of alcohol or illicit drugs should be sought. Auscultation of the heart and carotid arteries may identify an abnormality that predisposes to cerebrovascular disease.

All patients require a complete neurologic examination, with particular emphasis on eliciting signs of cerebral hemispheric disease (Chap. 356). Careful assessment of mental status (including memory, language function, and abstract thinking) may suggest lesions in the anterior frontal, parietal, or temporal lobes. Testing of visual fields will help screen for lesions in the optic pathways and occipital lobes. Screening tests of motor function such as pronator drift, deep tendon reflexes, gait, and coordination may suggest lesions in motor (frontal) cortex, and cortical sensory testing (e.g., double simultaneous stimulation) may detect lesions in the parietal cortex.

LABORATORY STUDIES

Routine blood studies are indicated to identify the more common metabolic causes of seizures, such as abnormalities in electrolytes, glucose, calcium, or magnesium, and hepatic or renal disease. A screen for toxins in blood and urine should also be obtained from all patients in the appropriate risk groups, especially when no clear precipitating factor has been identified. A lumbar puncture is indicated if there is any suspicion of meningitis or encephalitis and is mandatory in all patients infected with HIV, even in the absence of symptoms or signs suggesting infection.

All patients who have a possible seizure disorder should be evaluated with an EEG (Chap. 357) as soon as possible. The EEG may help to establish the diagnosis of epilepsy, classify the seizure type, and provide evidence for the existence of a particular epilepsy syndrome. If the patient is having frequent seizures, such as a child with absence epilepsy, the EEG may confirm the pres-

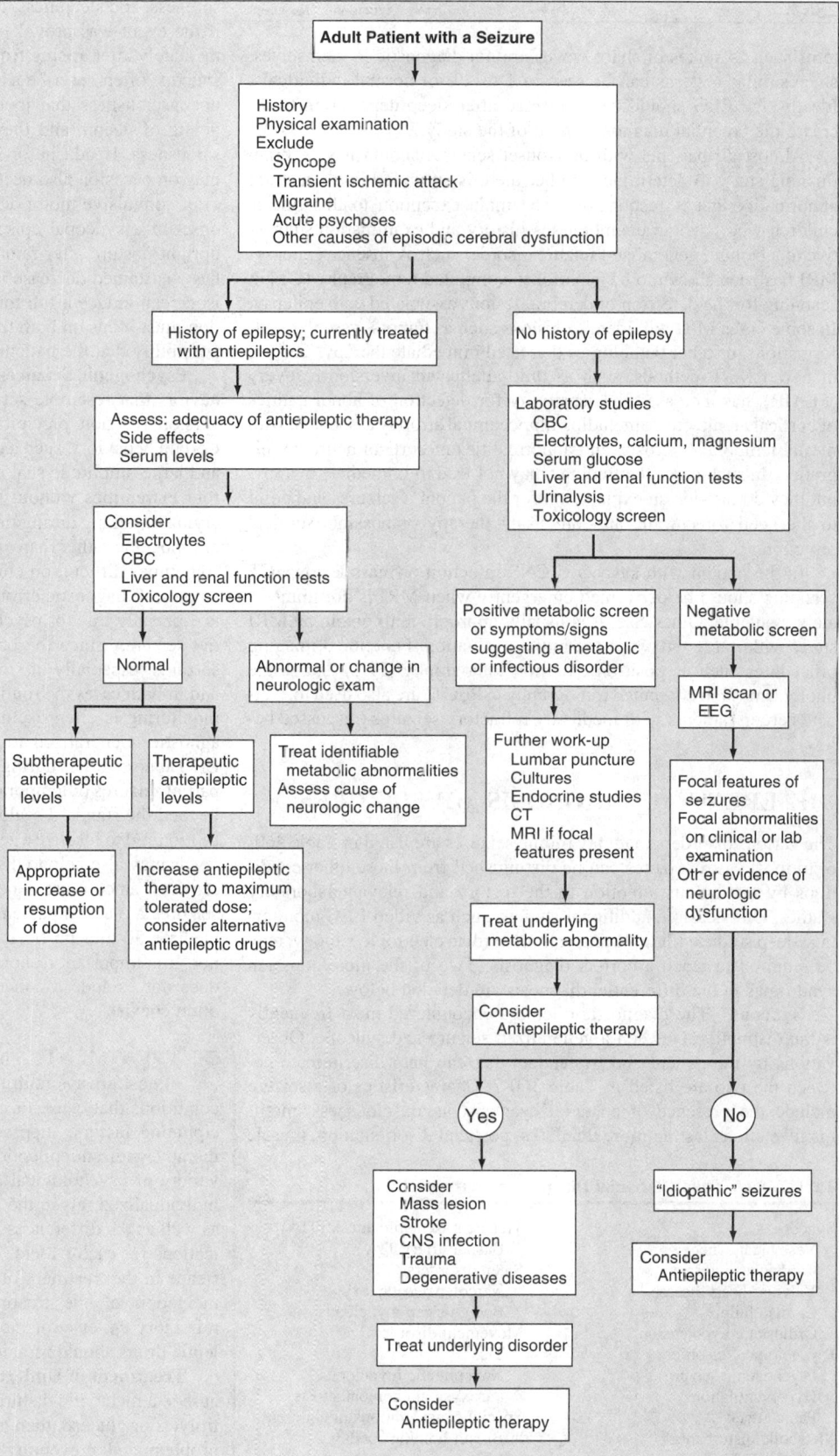

FIGURE 360-2 Evaluation of the adult patient with a seizure. CBC, complete blood count; CT, computed tomography; MRI, magnetic resonance imaging; EEG, electroencephalogram; CNS, central nervous system.

ence of seizures and help to identify the seizure type. In patients with infrequent seizures, the EEG may reveal potentially abnormal interictal activity that, when combined with clinical or radiologic data, aids in establishing the diagnosis. However, the existence of epileptiform patterns such as spikes or sharp waves are not diagnostic in themselves, since similar patterns can be seen in 1 to 2% of normal individuals. Ideally, the EEG should be performed after sleep deprivation to increase the potential diagnostic yield of the study.

Almost all patients with new-onset seizures should have a brain imaging study to determine whether there is an underlying structural abnormality that is responsible. The main exception to this rule is children who have an unambiguous history and examination suggestive of a benign, generalized seizure disorder such as absence epilepsy. MRI has been shown to be superior to computed tomography (CT) in scanning for the detection of cerebral lesions associated with epilepsy. In some cases MRI will identify lesions such as tumors, vascular malformations, or other pathologies that need immediate therapy. The use of newer MRI methods, such as fluid-attenuated inversion recovery (FLAIR), has increased the sensitivity for detection of abnormalities of cortical architecture, including hippocampal atrophy associated with mesial temporal sclerosis, and abnormalities of cortical neuronal migration. In such cases the findings may not lead to immediate therapy, but they do provide an explanation for the patient's seizures and point to the need for chronic anticonvulsant therapy or possible surgical resection.

In the patient with suspected CNS infection or mass lesions, CT scanning should be performed emergently when MRI is not immediately available. Otherwise, it is usually appropriate to obtain an MRI study within a few days of the initial evaluation. Functional imaging procedures such as positron emission tomography (PET) and single photon emission computed tomography (SPECT) are also used to evaluate certain patients with medically refractory seizures (discussed below).

DIFFERENTIAL DIAGNOSIS OF SEIZURES

The various disorders that may mimic seizures are listed in Table 360-6. In most cases seizures can be distinguished from these other conditions by meticulous attention to the history and relevant laboratory studies. On occasion, additional studies, such as video-EEG monitoring, sleep studies, tilt table analysis, or cardiac electrophysiology, may be required to reach a correct diagnosis. Two of the more common syndromes in the differential diagnosis are detailed below.

Syncope   The diagnostic dilemma encountered most frequently is the distinction between a generalized seizure and syncope. Observations by the patient and bystanders that can help discriminate between the two are listed in Table 360-7. Characteristics of a seizure include the presence of an aura, cyanosis, unconsciousness, motor manifestations lasting more than 30 s, postictal disorientation, muscle

Table 360-6 The Differential Diagnosis of Seizures

Syncope	Transient ischemic attack (TIA)
Vasovagal syncope	Basilar artery TIA
Cardiac arrhythmia	Sleep disorders
Valvular heart disease	Narcolepsy/cataplexy
Cardiac failure	Benign sleep myoclonus
Orthostatic hypotension	Movement disorders
Psychological disorders	Tics
Psychogenic seizure	Nonepileptic myoclonus
Hyperventilation	Paroxysmal choreoathetosis
Panic attack	Special considerations in children
Metabolic disturbances	Breath-holding spells
Alcoholic blackouts	Migraine with recurrent abdominal pain and cyclic vomiting
Delirium tremens	Benign paroxysmal vertigo
Hypoglycemia	Apnea
Hypoxia	Night terrors
Psychoactive drugs (e.g., hallucinogens)	Sleepwalking
Migraine	
Confusional migraine	
Basilar migraine	

soreness, and sleepiness. In contrast, a syncopal episode is more likely if the event was provoked by acute pain or anxiety or occurred immediately after arising from the lying or sitting position. Patients with syncope often describe a stereotyped transition from consciousness to unconsciousness that includes tiredness, sweating, nausea, and tunneling of vision, and they experience a relatively brief loss of consciousness. Headache or incontinence usually suggests a seizure but may on occasion also occur with syncope. A brief period (i.e., 1 to 10 s) of convulsive motor activity is frequently seen immediately at the onset of a syncopal episode, especially if the patient remains in an upright posture after fainting (e.g., in a dentist's chair) and therefore has a sustained decrease in cerebral perfusion. Rarely, a syncopal episode can induce a full tonic-clonic seizure. In such cases the evaluation must focus on both the cause of the syncopal event as well as the possibility that the patient has a propensity for recurrent seizures.

Psychogenic Seizures   Psychogenic seizures are nonepileptic behaviors that resemble seizures. The behavior is often part of a conversion reaction precipitated by underlying psychological distress. Certain behaviors, such as side-to-side turning of the head, asymmetric and large-amplitude shaking movements of the limbs, twitching of all four extremities without loss of consciousness, pelvic thrusting, and crying or talking during the event, are more commonly associated with psychogenic rather than epileptic seizures. However, the distinction is sometimes difficult on clinical grounds alone, and there are many examples of diagnostic errors made by experienced epileptologists. This is especially true for psychogenic seizures that resemble complex partial seizures, since the behavioral manifestations of complex partial seizures (especially of frontal lobe origin) can be extremely unusual, and in both cases the routine surface EEG may be normal. Video-EEG monitoring is often useful when the clinical observations are nondiagnostic. Generalized tonic-clonic seizures always produce marked EEG abnormalities during and after the seizure. For suspected complex partial seizures of temporal lobe origin, the use of additional electrodes beyond the standard scalp locations (e.g., sphenoidal electrodes) may be required to localize a seizure focus. Measurement of serum prolactin levels may also help to discriminate between organic and psychogenic seizures, since most generalized seizures and many complex partial seizures are accompanied by rises in serum prolactin (during the immediate 30-min postictal period), whereas psychogenic seizures are not. It is important to note that the diagnosis of psychogenic seizures does not exclude a concurrent diagnosis of epilepsy, since the two often coexist.

℞ **TREATMENT**   Therapy for a patient with a seizure disorder is almost always multimodal and includes treatment of underlying conditions that cause or contribute to the seizures, avoidance of precipitating factors, suppression of recurrent seizures by prophylactic therapy with antiepileptic medications or surgery, and addressing a variety of psychological and social issues. Treatment plans must be individualized, given the many different types and causes of seizures as well as the differences in efficacy and toxicity of antiepileptic medications for each patient. In almost all cases a neurologist with experience in the treatment of epilepsy should design and oversee implementation of the treatment strategy. Furthermore, patients with refractory epilepsy or those who require polypharmacy with antiepileptic drugs should remain under the regular care of a neurologist.

Treatment of Underlying Conditions   If the sole cause of a seizure is a metabolic disturbance such as an abnormality of serum electrolytes or glucose, then treatment is aimed at reversing the metabolic problem and preventing its recurrence. Therapy with antiepileptic drugs is usually unnecessary unless the metabolic disorder cannot be corrected promptly and the patient is at risk of having further seizures. If the apparent cause of a seizure was a medication (e.g., theophylline) or illicit drug use (e.g., cocaine), then appropriate therapy is avoidance of the drug and there is usually no need for antiepileptic medications unless subsequent seizures occur in the absence of these precipitants.

Seizures caused by a structural CNS lesion such as a brain tumor, vascular malformation, or brain abscess may not recur after appropriate treatment of the underlying lesion. However, despite removal of the structural lesion, there is a risk that the seizure focus will remain in the surrounding tissue or develop de novo as a result of gliosis and other processes induced by surgery, radiation, or other therapies. Most patients are therefore maintained on an antiepileptic medication for at least 1 year, and an attempt is made to withdraw medications only if the patient has been completely seizure-free. If the seizures are refractory to medication, the patient may benefit from surgical removal of the epileptic brain region (see "Surgical Treatment of Refractory Epilepsy").

Avoidance of Precipitating Factors Unfortunately, little is known about the specific factors that determine precisely when a seizure will occur in a patient with epilepsy. Some patients can identify particular situations that appear to lower their seizure threshold; these situations should be avoided. For example, a patient who has seizures in the setting of sleep deprivation should obviously be advised to maintain a normal sleep schedule. Many patients note an association between alcohol intake and seizures, and they should be encouraged to modify their drinking habits accordingly. There are also relatively rare cases of patients with seizures that are induced by highly specific stimuli such as a video game monitor, music, or an individual's voice ("reflex epilepsy"). If there is an association between stress and seizures, stress reduction techniques such as physical exercise, meditation, or counseling may be helpful.

Antiepileptic Drug Therapy Antiepileptic drug therapy is the mainstay of treatment for most patients with epilepsy. The overall goal is to completely prevent seizures without causing any untoward side effects, preferably with a single medication and a dosing schedule that is easy for the patient to follow. Seizure classification is an important element in designing the treatment plan, since some antiepileptic drugs have different activities against various seizure types. However, there is considerable overlap between many antiepileptic drugs, such that the choice of therapy is often determined more by specific needs of the patient, especially the patient's assessment of side effects.

When to initiate antiepileptic drug therapy Antiepileptic drug therapy should be started in any patient with recurrent seizures of unknown etiology or a known cause that cannot be reversed. Whether to initiate therapy in a patient with a single seizure is controversial. Patients with a single seizure due to an identified lesion such as a CNS tumor, infection, or trauma, in which there is strong evidence that the lesion is epileptogenic, should be treated. The risk of seizure recurrence in a patient with an apparently unprovoked or idiopathic seizure is uncertain, with estimates ranging from 31 to 71% in the first 12 months after the initial seizure. This uncertainty arises from differences in the underlying seizure types and etiologies in various published epidemiologic studies. Generally accepted risk factors associated with recurrent seizures include the following: (1) an abnormal neurologic examination, (2) seizures presenting as status epilepticus, (3) postictal Todd's paralysis, (4) a strong family history of seizures, or (5) an abnormal EEG. Most patients with one or more of these risk factors should be treated. Issues such as employment or driving may influence the decision whether or not to start medications as well. For example, a patient with a single, idiopathic seizure and whose job depends on driving may prefer taking antiepileptic drugs rather than risking a seizure recurrence and the potential loss of driving privileges.

Selection of antiepileptic drugs The choices of antiepileptic drugs in the United States for different seizure types are shown in Table 360-8, and the main pharmacologic characteristics of commonly used drugs are listed in Table 360-9. Older medications such as phenytoin, valproic acid, carbamazepine, and ethosuximide are generally used as first-line therapy for most seizure disorders since, overall, they are as effective as recently marketed drugs and significantly less expensive. Of the new drugs that have become available in the United States in the past decade, most are currently being used as add-on or alternative therapy.

In addition to efficacy, other factors influencing the specific choice of an initial medication for a patient include the relative convenience of dosing schedule (e.g., once daily versus three or four times daily) and potential side effects. Almost all of the commonly used antiepileptic drugs can cause similar, dose-related side effects such as sedation, ataxia, and diplopia. Close follow-up is required to ensure these are promptly recognized and reversed. Most of the drugs may also cause idiosyncratic toxicity such as rash, bone marrow suppression, or hepatotoxicity. Although rare, these side effects need to be carefully considered during drug selection, and patients require laboratory tests (e.g., complete blood count and liver function tests) prior to the institution of a drug (to establish baseline values) and during initial dosing and titration of the agent.

ANTIEPILEPTIC DRUG SELECTION FOR PARTIAL SEIZURES Carbamazepine or phenytoin is currently the initial drug of choice for the treatment of partial seizures, including those that secondarily generalize. Overall they have very similar efficacy, but differences in phar-

Table 360-7 Clinical Features of a Generalized Tonic-Clonic Seizure Versus Syncope

Features	Seizure	Syncope
Immediate precipitating factors	Usually none	Emotional stress, valsalva, orthostatic hypotension, cardiac etiologies
Premonitory symptoms	None or aura (e.g., odd odor)	Tiredness, nausea, diaphoresis, tunneling of vision
Posture at onset	Variable	Usually erect
Transition to unconsciousness	Often immediate	Gradual over seconds[a]
Duration of unconsciousness	Minutes	Seconds
Duration of tonic or clonic movements	30–60 s	Never more than 15 s
Facial appearance during event	Cyanosis, frothing at mouth	Pallor
Disorientation and sleepiness after event	Many minutes to hours	<5 min
Aching of muscles after event	Often	Sometimes
Biting of tongue	Sometimes	Rarely
Incontinence	Sometimes	Unusual
Headache	Sometimes	Rarely

[a] May be sudden with certain cardiac arrhythmias.

Table 360-8 Antiepileptic Drugs of Choice

	Primary Generalized Tonic-Clonic	Partial[a]	Absence	Atypical Absence, Myoclonic, Atonic
First-Line	Valproic acid Lamotrigine	Carbamazepine Phenytoin Valproic acid Lamotrigine	Ethosuximide Valproic acid	Valproic acid
Alternatives	Phenytoin Carbamazepine Topiramate Primidone Phenobarbital Felbamate	Gabapentin[b] Topiramate[b] Tiagabine[b] Primidone Phenobarbital	Lamotrigine Clonazepam	Lamotrigine Topiramate[b] Clonazepam Felbamate

[a] Includes simple partial, complex partial, and secondarily generalized seizures.
[b] As adjunctive therapy.

Table 360-9 Commonly Used Antiepileptic Drugs

Generic Name	Trade Name	Principal Uses	Typical Dosage and Dosing Intervals	Half-Life	Therapeutic Range	Adverse Effects Neurologic	Adverse Effects Systemic	Drug Interactions
Phenytoin (diphenyl-hydantoin)	Dilantin	Tonic-clonic (grand mal) Focal-onset	300–400 mg/d (3–6 mg/kg, adult; 4–8 mg/kg, child) qd-bid	24 h (wide variation, dose-dependent)	10–20 μg/mL	Dizziness Diplopia Ataxia Incoordination Confusion	Gum hyperplasia Lymphadenopathy Hirsutism Osteomalacia Facial coarsening Skin rash	Level increased by isoniazid, sulfonamides Level decreased by enzyme-inducing drugs[a] Altered folate metabolism
Carbamazepine	Tegretol Carbatrol	Tonic-clonic Focal-onset	600–1800 mg/d (15–35 mg/kg, child) bid-qid	10–17 h	6–12 μg/mL	Ataxia Dizziness Diplopia Vertigo	Aplastic anemia Leukopenia Gastrointestinal irritation Hepatotoxicity Hyponatremia	Level decreased by enzyme-inducing drugs[a] Level increased by erythromycin, propoxyphene, isoniazid, cimetidine
Valproic acid	Depakene Depakote	Tonic-clonic Absence Atypical absence Myoclonic Focal-onset	750–2000 mg/d (20–60 mg/kg) bid-qid	15 h	50–150 μg/mL	Ataxia Sedation Tremor	Hepatotoxicity Thrombocytopenia Gastrointestinal irritation Weight gain Transient alopecia Hyperammonemia	Level decreased by enzyme-inducing drugs[a]
Lamotrigine	Lamictal	Focal-onset Tonic-clonic Atypical absence Myoclonic Lennox-Gastaut syndrome	150–500 mg/d bid	25 h 14 h (with enzyme-inducers) 59 h (with valproic acid)	Not established	Dizziness Diplopia Sedation Ataxia Headache	Skin rash Stevens-Johnson syndrome	Level decreased by enzyme-inducing drugs[a] Level increased by valproic acid
Ethosuximide	Zarontin	Absence (petit mal)	750–1250 mg/d (20-40 mg/kg) qd-bid	60 h, adult 30 h, child	40–100 μg/mL	Ataxia Lethargy Headache	Gastrointestinal irritation Skin rash Bone marrow suppression	
Gabapentin	Neurontin	Focal-onset	900–2400 mg/d tid-qid	5–9 h	Not established	Sedation Dizziness Ataxia Fatigue	Gastrointestinal irritation	No known significant interactions
Topiramate	Topamax	Focal-onset Tonic-clonic	400 mg/d bid	20–30 h	Not established	Psychomotor slowing Sedation Speech or language problems Fatigue Paresthesias	Renal stones (avoid use with other carbonic anhydrase inhibitors)	Level decreased by enzyme-inducing drugs[a]

(continued)

Table 360-9—(continued)

Generic Name	Trade Name	Principal Uses	Typical Dosage and Dosing Intervals	Half-Life	Therapeutic Range	Adverse Effects		Drug Interactions
						Neurologic	Systemic	
Tiagabine	Gabatril	Focal-onset Tonic-clonic Lennox-Gastaut syndrome	32–56 mg/d bid-qid	7–9 h	Not established	Confusion Sedation Depression Dizziness Speech or language problems Paresthesias Psychosis	Gastrointestinal irritation	Level decreased by enzyme-inducing drugs[a]
Phenobarbital	Luminol	Tonic-clonic Focal-onset	60–180 mg/d (1–4 mg/kg, adult); (3–6 mg/kg, child) qd	90 h (70 h in children)	10–40 μg/mL	Sedation Ataxia Confusion Dizziness Decreased libido Depression	Skin rash	Level increased by valproic acid, phenytoin Enhances metabolism of other drugs via liver enzyme induction
Primidone	Mysoline	Tonic-clonic Focal-onset	750–1000 mg/d (10–25 mg/kg) bid-tid	Primidone, 8–15 h Phenobarbital, 90 h	Primidone, 4–12 μg/mL Phenobarbital, 10–40 μg/mL	Same as phenobarbital		
Clonazepam	Klonopin	Absence Atypical absence Myoclonic	1–12 mg/d (0.1–0.2 mg/kg) qd-tid	24–48 h	10–70 ng/mL	Ataxia Sedation Lethargy	Anorexia	Level decreased by enzyme-inducing drugs[a]
Felbamate	Felbatol	Focal-onset Lennox-Gastaut syndrome	2400–3600 mg/d, (45 mg/kg, child) tid-qid	16–22 h	Not established	Insomnia Dizziness Sedation Headache	Aplastic anemia Hepatic failure Weight loss Gastrointestinal irritation	Increases phenytoin, valproic acid, active carbamazepine metabolite
Levetiracetam	Keppra	Focal-onset	1000–3000 mg/d bid	6–8 h	Not established	Sedation Fatigue Incoordination Psychosis	Anemia Leukocytopenia	None known
Zonisamide	Zonegran	Focal-onset	200–800 mg/d	50–68 h	Not established	Sedation Dizziness Confusion Headache	Anorexia Renal stones	Level decreased by enzyme-inducing drugs[a]
Oxcarbazepine	Trileptal	Focal-onset	900–2400 mg/d bid	10–17 h (for active metabolite)	6–12 μg/mL	Fatigue Ataxia Dizziness Diplopia Vertigo Headache	See carbamazepine	Level decreased by enzyme-inducing drugs[a] May increase phenytoin

[a] Phenytoin, carbamazepine, phenobarbital

macokinetics and toxicity are the main determinants for use in a given patient. Phenytoin has a relatively long half-life and offers the advantage of once or twice daily dosing compared to two or three times daily dosing for carbamazepine (although a more expensive, extended-release form of carbamazepine is now available). An advantage of carbamazepine is that its metabolism follows first-order pharmacokinetics, and the relationship between drug dose, serum levels, and toxicity is linear. By contrast, phenytoin shows properties of saturation kinetics, such that small increases in phenytoin doses above a standard maintenance dose can precipitate marked side effects. This is one of the main causes of acute phenytoin toxicity. Long-term use of phenytoin is associated with untoward cosmetic effects (e.g., hirsutism, coarsening of facial features, and gingival hypertrophy), so it is often avoided in young patients who are likely to require the drug for many years. Carbamazepine can cause leukopenia, aplastic anemia, or hepatotoxicity and would therefore be contraindicated in patients with predispositions to these problems.

Valproic acid is an effective alternative for some patients with partial seizures, especially when the seizures secondarily generalize. Gastrointestinal side effects are fewer when using the valproate semisodium formulation (Depakote). Valproic acid also rarely causes reversible bone marrow suppression and hepatotoxicity, and laboratory testing is required to monitor toxicity. This drug should generally be avoided in patients with preexisting bone marrow or liver disease. Irreversible, fatal hepatic failure appearing as an idiosyncratic rather than dose-related side effect is a relatively rare complication; its risk is highest in children <2 years old, especially those taking other antiepileptic drugs or with inborn errors of metabolism. Valproic acid therapy should therefore only be used in infants and young children when the benefits clearly exceed this risk.

Lamotrigine, gabapentin, topiramate, tiagabine, and phenobarbital are additional drugs currently used for the treatment of partial seizures with or without secondary generalization. Lamotrigine appears to have an overall efficacy profile similar to the more standard drugs and is now being used as monotherapy. All patients, particularly children, need to be monitored closely for a lamotrigine-induced rash during the initiation of therapy. Also, lamotrigine must be started very slowly when used as add-on therapy with valproic acid, since valproic acid can inhibit its metabolism, thereby substantially prolonging its half-life. Gabapentin is unique in not having any significant drug interactions. This makes it potentially useful as add-on therapy, especially in patients who are particularly susceptible to side effects of other medications. Until recently, phenobarbital and other barbiturate compounds were commonly used as first-line therapy for many forms of epilepsy. However, the barbiturates frequently cause sedation in adults, hyperactivity in children, and other more subtle cognitive changes; thus, their use should be limited to situations in which no other suitable treatment alternatives exist.

ANTIEPILEPTIC DRUG SELECTION FOR GENERALIZED SEIZURES Valproic acid is currently considered the best initial choice for the treatment of primarily generalized, tonic-clonic seizures and lamotrigine, followed by carbamazepine and phenytoin, are suitable alternatives. Valproic acid is also particularly effective in absence, myoclonic, and atonic seizures and is therefore the drug of choice in patients with generalized epilepsy syndromes having mixed seizure types. Ethosuximide remains the preferred drug for the treatment of uncomplicated absence seizures, but it is not effective against tonic-clonic or partial seizures. Ethosuximide rarely causes bone marrow suppression, so that periodic monitoring of blood cell counts is required. Although approved for use in partial seizure disorders, lamotrigine appears to be effective in epilepsy syndromes with mixed, generalized seizure types such as JME and Lennox-Gastaut syndrome.

Initiation and monitoring of therapy   Because the response to any antiepileptic drug is unpredictable, patients should be carefully educated about the approach to therapy. Patients need to understand that the goal is to prevent seizures and minimize the side effects of therapy; determination of the optimal dose is often a matter of trial and error. This process may take months or longer if the baseline seizure frequency is low. Most anticonvulsant drugs need to be introduced relatively slowly to minimize side effects, and patients should expect that minor side effects such as mild sedation, slight changes in cognition, or imbalance will typically resolve within a few days. Starting doses are usually the lowest value listed under the dosage column

in Table 360-9. Subsequent increases should be made only after achieving a steady state with the previous dose (i.e., after an interval of five or more half-lives).

Monitoring of serum antiepileptic drug levels can be very useful for establishing the initial dosing schedule. However, the published therapeutic ranges of serum drug concentrations are only an approximate guide for determining the proper dose for a given patient. The key determinants are the clinical measures of seizure frequency and presence of side effects, not the laboratory values. Conventional assays of serum drug levels measure the total drug (i.e., both free and protein-bound), yet it is the concentration of free drug that reflects extracellular levels in the brain and correlates best with efficacy. Thus, patients with decreased levels of serum proteins (e.g., decreased serum albumin due to impaired liver or renal function) may have an increased ratio of free to bound drug, yet the concentration of free drug may be adequate for seizure control. These patients may have a "subtherapeutic" drug level, but the dose should be changed only if seizures remain uncontrolled, not just to achieve a "therapeutic" level. It is also useful to monitor free drug levels in such patients. In practice, other than during the initiation or modification of therapy, monitoring of antiepileptic drug levels is most useful for documenting compliance.

If seizures continue despite gradual increases to the maximum tolerated dose and documented compliance, then it becomes necessary to switch to another antiepileptic drug. This is usually done by maintaining the patient on the first drug while a second drug is added. The dose of the second drug should be adjusted to decrease seizure frequency without causing toxicity. Once this is achieved, the first drug can be gradually withdrawn (usually over weeks unless there is significant toxicity). The dose of the second drug is then further optimized based on seizure response and side effects.

When to discontinue therapy   Overall, about 70% of children and 60% of adults who have their seizures completely controlled with antiepileptic drugs can eventually discontinue therapy. Clinical studies suggest that the following patient profile yields the greatest chance of remaining seizure-free after drug withdrawal: (1) complete medical control of seizures for 1 to 5 years; (2) single seizure type, either partial or generalized; (3) normal neurologic examination, including intelligence; and (4) normal EEG. The appropriate seizure-free interval is unknown and undoubtedly varies for different forms of epilepsy. However, it seems reasonable to attempt withdrawal of therapy after 2 years in a patient who meets all of the above criteria, is motivated to discontinue the medication, and clearly understands the potential risks and benefits. In most cases it is preferable to reduce the dose of the drug gradually over 2 to 3 months. Most recurrences occur in the first 3 months after discontinuing therapy, and patients should be advised to avoid potentially dangerous situations such as driving or swimming during this period.

Treatment of refractory epilepsy   Approximately one-third of patients with epilepsy do not respond to treatment with a single antiepileptic drug, and it becomes necessary to try a combination of drugs to control seizures. Patients who have focal epilepsy related to an underlying structural lesion or those with multiple seizure types and developmental delay are particularly likely to require multiple drugs. There are currently no clear guidelines for rational polypharmacy, but in most cases the initial combination therapy combines first-line drugs, i.e., carbamazepine, phenytoin, valproic acid, and lamotrigine. If these drugs are unsuccessful, then the addition of a newer drug such as topiramate or gabapentin is indicated. Patients with myoclonic seizures resistant to valproic acid may benefit from the addition of clonazepam, and those with absence seizures may respond to a combination of valproic acid and ethosuximide. The same principles concerning the monitoring of therapeutic response, toxicity, and serum levels for monotherapy apply to polypharmacy, and potential drug interactions need to be recognized. If there is no improvement, a third drug can be added while the first two are maintained. If there is a response, the least effective of the first two drugs should be gradually withdrawn.

Surgical Treatment of Refractory Epilepsy   Approximately 20% of patients with epilepsy are resistant to medical therapy despite efforts to find an effective combination of antiepileptic drugs. For some, surgery can be extremely effective in substantially reducing seizure frequency and even providing complete seizure control. Understanding the potential value of surgery is especially important when, at the time of diagnosis, a patient has an epilepsy syndrome that is considered likely to be drug-resistant. Rather than submitting the patient to years of unsuccessful medical therapy and the associated psychosocial trauma of ongoing seizures, the patient should have an efficient but relatively brief attempt at medical therapy and then be referred for surgical evaluation.

The most common surgical procedure for patients with temporal lobe epilepsy involves resection of the anteromedial temporal lobe (temporal lobectomy) or a more limited removal of the underlying hippocampus and amygdala. Focal seizures arising from extratemporal regions may be suppressed by a focal neocortical resection or precise removal of an identified lesion (lesionectomy). When the cortical region cannot be removed, multiple subpial transection, which disrupts intracortical connections, is sometimes used to prevent seizure spread. Hemispherectomy or multilobar resection is useful for some patients with severe seizures due to hemispheric abnormalities such as hemimegaloencephaly or other dysplastic abnormalities, and corpus callosotomy has been shown to be effective for disabling tonic or atonic seizures, usually when they are part of a mixed-seizure syndrome (e.g., Lennox-Gastaut syndrome).

Presurgical evaluation is designed to identify the functional and structural basis of the patient's seizure disorder. Inpatient video-EEG monitoring is used to define the anatomic location of the seizure focus and to correlate the abnormal electrophysiologic activity with behavioral manifestations of the seizure. Routine scalp or scalp-sphenoidal recordings are usually sufficient for localization, and advances in neuroimaging have made the use of invasive electrophysiologic monitoring such as implanted depth electrodes or subdural electrodes much less common. A high-resolution MRI scan is routinely used to identify structural lesions. Functional imaging studies such as SPECT and PET are adjunctive tests that may help verify the localization of an apparent epileptogenic region with an anatomic abnormality. Once the presumed location of the seizure onset is identified, additional studies, including neuropsychological testing and the intracarotid amobarbital test (Wada test) may be used to assess language and memory localization and to determine the possible functional consequences of surgical removal of the epileptogenic region. In some cases, the exact extent of the resection to be undertaken is determined by performing cortical mapping at the time of the surgical procedure. This involves electrophysiologic recordings and cortical stimulation in the awake patient to identify the extent of epileptiform disturbances and the function of cortical regions in question.

Advances in presurgical evaluation and microsurgical techniques have led to a steady increase in the success of epilepsy surgery. Clinically significant complications of surgery are <5%, and the use of functional mapping procedures has markedly reduced the neurologic sequelae due to removal or sectioning of brain tissue. For example, about 70% of patients treated with temporal lobectomy will become seizure-free, and another 15 to 25% will have at least a 90% reduction in seizure frequency. Marked improvement is also usually seen in patients treated with hemispherectomy for catastrophic seizure disorders due to large hemispheric abnormalities. Postoperatively, patients generally need to remain on antiepileptic drug therapy, but the marked reduction of seizures following surgery can have a very beneficial effect on their quality of life.

Vagus Nerve Stimulation (VNS) VNS is a new treatment option for patients with medically refractory epilepsy who are not candidates for resective brain surgery. The procedure involves placement of a bipolar electrode on the midcervical portion of the left vagus nerve. The electrode is connected to a small, subcutaneous generator located in the infraclavicular region, and the generator is programmed to deliver intermittent electrical pulses to the vagus nerve. The precise mechanism of action of VNS is unknown, although experimental studies have shown that stimulation of vagal nuclei leads to widespread activation of cortical and subcortical pathways and an associated increased seizure threshold. In practice, the efficacy of VNS appears to be no greater than recently introduced anticonvulsant medications. Adverse effects of the surgery are rare, and stimulation-induced side effects, including transient hoarseness, cough, and dyspnea, are usually mild and well tolerated.

STATUS EPILEPTICUS Status epilepticus refers to continuous seizures or repetitive, discrete seizures with impaired consciousness in the interictal period. The duration of seizure activity sufficient to meet the definition of status epilepticus has traditionally been specified as 15 to 30 min. However, a more practical definition is to consider status epilepticus as a situation in which the duration of seizures prompts the acute use of anticonvulsant therapy, typically when seizures last beyond 5 min.

Status epilepticus is an emergency and must be treated immediately, since cardiorespiratory dysfunction, hyperthermia, and metabolic derangements can develop as a consequence of prolonged seizures, and these can lead to irreversible neuronal injury. Furthermore, CNS injury can occur even when the patient is paralyzed with neuromuscular blockade but continues to have electrographic seizures. The most common causes of status epilepticus are anticonvulsant withdrawal or noncompliance, metabolic disturbances, drug toxicity, CNS infection, CNS tumors, refractory epilepsy, and head trauma.

Generalized status epilepticus is obvious when the patient is having overt convulsions. However, after 30 to 45 min of uninterrupted seizures, the signs may become increasingly subtle. Patients may have mild clonic movements of only the fingers, or fine, rapid movements of the eyes. There may be paroxysmal episodes of tachycardia, hypertension, and pupillary dilation. In such cases, the EEG may be the only method of establishing the diagnosis. Thus, if the patient stops having overt seizures, yet remains comatose, an EEG should be performed to rule out ongoing status epilepticus.

The first step in the management of a patient in status epilepticus is to attend to any acute cardiorespiratory problems or hyperthermia, perform a brief medical and neurologic examination, establish venous access, and send samples for laboratory studies to identify metabolic abnormalities. Anticonvulsant therapy should then begin without delay; a treatment approach is shown in Fig. 360-3.

BEYOND SEIZURES: OTHER MANAGEMENT ISSUES

Interictal Behavior The adverse effects of epilepsy often go beyond the occurrence of clinical seizures, and the extent of these effects depends largely upon the etiology of the seizure disorder, the degree to which the seizures are controlled, and the presence of side effects from antiepileptic therapy. Many patients with epilepsy are completely normal between seizures and able to live highly successful and productive lives. In contrast, patients with seizures secondary to developmental abnormalities or acquired brain injury may have impaired cognitive function and other neurologic deficits. Frequent interictal EEG abnormalities have been shown to be associated with subtle dysfunction of memory and attention. Patients with many seizures, especially those emanating from the temporal lobe, often note an impairment of short-term memory that may progress over time.

Patients with epilepsy are at risk of developing a variety of psychiatric problems including depression, anxiety, and psychosis. This risk varies considerably depending on many factors, including the etiology, frequency, and severity of seizures and the patient's age and previous history. Depression occurs in approximately 20% of patients, and the incidence of suicide is higher in epileptic patients than in the general population. Depression should be treated through counseling or medication. The selective serotonin reuptake inhibitors typically

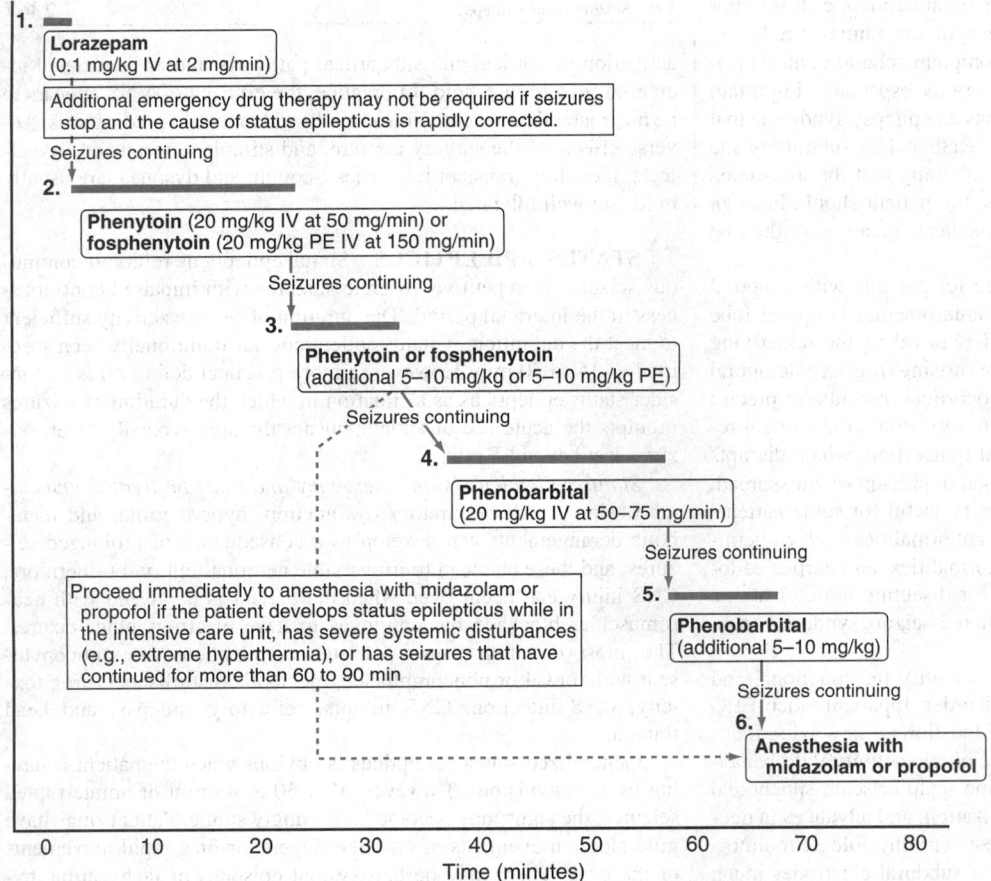

1.
Lorazepam
(0.1 mg/kg IV at 2 mg/min)

Additional emergency drug therapy may not be required if seizures stop and the cause of status epilepticus is rapidly corrected.

Seizures continuing

2.
Phenytoin (20 mg/kg IV at 50 mg/min) or **fosphenytoin** (20 mg/kg PE IV at 150 mg/min)

Seizures continuing

3.
Phenytoin or fosphenytoin
(additional 5–10 mg/kg or 5–10 mg/kg PE)

Seizures continuing

4.
Phenobarbital
(20 mg/kg IV at 50–75 mg/min)

Seizures continuing

Proceed immediately to anesthesia with midazolam or propofol if the patient develops status epilepticus while in the intensive care unit, has severe systemic disturbances (e.g., extreme hyperthermia), or has seizures that have continued for more than 60 to 90 min

5.
Phenobarbital
(additional 5–10 mg/kg)

Seizures continuing

6.
Anesthesia with midazolam or propofol

Time (minutes)
0 10 20 30 40 50 60 70 80

FIGURE 360-3 Pharmacologic treatment of generalized tonic-clonic status epilepticus in adults. IV, intravenous; PE, phenytoin equivalents. The horizontal bars indicate the approximate duration of drug infusions.

have no effect on seizures, while the tricyclic antidepressants may lower the seizure threshold. Anxiety can appear as a manifestation of a seizure, and anxious or psychotic behavior can sometimes be observed as part of a postictal delirium. Interictal psychosis is a rare phenomenon that typically occurs after a period of increased seizure frequency. There is usually a brief lucid interval lasting up to a week, followed by days to weeks of agitated, psychotic behavior. The psychosis will usually resolve spontaneously but may require treatment with antipsychotic or anxiolytic medications.

There is ongoing controversy as to whether some patients with epilepsy (especially temporal lobe epilepsy) have a stereotypical "interictal personality." The predominant view is that the unusual or abnormal personality traits observed in such patients are, in most cases, not due to epilepsy but result from an underlying structural brain lesion, the effects of antiepileptic drugs, or psychosocial factors.

Mortality of Epilepsy Patients with epilepsy have an increased risk of death that is roughly two to three times greater than what would be expected in a matched population without epilepsy. Most of the increased mortality is due to the underlying etiology of epilepsy, i.e., more widespread neurologic or systemic diseases in children and tumors or strokes in older adults. However, a small number of patients die from a syndrome known as *sudden unexpected death in epileptic patients* (SUDEP), which usually affects young people with convulsive seizures and tends to occur at night. The cause(s) remain unknown, although the leading theories propose brainstem-mediated effects of seizures on cardiac rhythms or pulmonary function.

Psychosocial Issues There continues to be a cultural stigma about epilepsy, although it is slowly declining in societies with effective health education programs. Because of this stigma, many patients with epilepsy harbor fears, such as the fear of becoming mentally retarded or dying during a seizure. These issues need to be carefully addressed by educating the patient about epilepsy and by ensuring that family members, teachers, fellow employees, and other associates are equally well informed. The Epilepsy Foundation of America (1-800-EFA-1000) is a patient advocacy organization and a useful source of educational material.

Employment and Driving
Many patients with epilepsy face difficulty in obtaining or maintaining employment, even when their seizures are well controlled. Federal and state legislation is designed to prevent employers from discriminating against patients with epilepsy, and patients should be encouraged to understand and claim their legal rights. Patients in these circumstances also benefit greatly from the assistance of health providers who act as strong patient advocates.

Loss of driving privileges is one of the most disruptive social consequences of epilepsy. Physicians should be very clear about local regulations concerning driving and epilepsy, since the laws vary considerably among states and countries. In all cases, it is the physician's responsibility to warn patients of the danger imposed on themselves and others while driving if their seizures are uncontrolled (unless the seizures are not associated with impairment of consciousness or motor control). In general, most states allow patients to drive after a seizure-free interval (on or off medications) between 3 months and 2 years.

SPECIAL ISSUES RELATED TO WOMEN AND EPILEPSY

Catamenial Epilepsy Some women experience a marked increase in seizure frequency around the time of menses. This is thought to reflect either the effects of estrogen and progesterone on neuronal excitability or changes in antiepileptic drug levels due to altered protein binding. Acetazolamide (250 to 500 mg/d) may be effective as adjunctive therapy in some cases when started 7 to 10 days prior to the onset of menses and continued until bleeding stops. Some patients may benefit from increases in antiepileptic drug dosages during this time or from control of the menstrual cycle through the use of oral contraceptives.

Pregnancy Most women with epilepsy who become pregnant will have an uncomplicated gestation and deliver a normal baby. However, epilepsy poses some important risks to a pregnancy. Seizure frequency during pregnancy will remain unchanged in approximately 50% of women, increase in 30%, and decrease in 20%. Changes in seizure frequency are attributed to endocrine effects on the CNS, variations in antiepileptic drug pharmacokinetics (such as acceleration of hepatic drug metabolism or effects on plasma protein binding), and changes in medication compliance. It is therefore useful to see patients at more frequent intervals during pregnancy and monitor serum antiepileptic drug levels. Measurement of the unbound drug concentrations may be useful if there is an increase in seizure frequency or worsening of side effects of antiepileptic drugs.

The overall incidence of fetal abnormalities in children born to mothers with epilepsy is 5 to 6%, compared to 2 to 3% in healthy women. Part of the higher incidence is due to teratogenic effects of antiepileptic drugs, and the risk increases with the number of medications used (e.g., 10% risk of malformations with three drugs). A syndrome comprising facial dysmorphism, cleft lip, cleft palate, cardiac defects, digital hypoplasia, and nail dysplasia was originally ascribed to phenytoin therapy, but it is now known to occur with other first-line antiepileptic drugs (i.e., valproic acid and carbamazepine) as well. Also, valproic acid and carbamazepine are associated with a 1 to 2% incidence of neural tube defects compared with a baseline of 0.5 to 1%. Little is currently known about the safety of newer drugs.

Since the potential harm of uncontrolled seizures on the mother and fetus is considered greater than the teratogenic effects of antiepileptic drugs, it is currently recommended that pregnant women be maintained on effective drug therapy. When possible, it seems prudent to have the patient on monotherapy at the lowest effective dose, especially during the first trimester. Patients should also take folate (1 to 4 mg/d), since the antifolate effects of anticonvulsants are thought to play a role in the development of neural tube defects, although the benefits of this treatment remain unproved in this setting.

Enzyme-inducing drugs such as phenytoin, phenobarbital, and primidone cause a transient and reversible deficiency of vitamin K–dependent clotting factors in approximately 50% of newborn infants. Although neonatal hemorrhage is uncommon, the mother should be treated with oral vitamin K (20 mg daily) in the last 2 weeks of pregnancy, and the infant should receive an intramuscular injection of vitamin K (1 mg) at birth.

Contraception Special care should be taken when prescribing antiepileptic medications for women who are taking oral contraceptive agents. Drugs such as carbamazepine, phenytoin, phenobarbital, and topiramate can significantly antagonize the effects of oral contraceptives via enzyme induction and other mechanisms. Patients should be advised to consider alternative forms of contraception, or their contraceptive medications should be modified to offset the effects of the antiepileptic medications.

Breast Feeding Antiepileptic medications are excreted into breast milk to a variable degree. The ratio of drug concentration in breast milk relative to serum is approximately 80% for ethosuximide, 40 to 60% for phenobarbital, 40% for carbamazepine, 15% for phenytoin, and 5% for valproic acid. Given the overall benefits of breast feeding and the lack of evidence for long-term harm to the infant by being exposed to antiepileptic drugs, mothers with epilepsy should be encouraged to breast feed. This should be reconsidered, however, if there is any evidence of drug effects on the infant, such as lethargy or poor feeding.

BIBLIOGRAPHY

BATE L, GARDINER M: Genetics of inherited epilepsies. Epileptic Disorders 1:7, 1999

BRODIE MJ, DICHTER MA: Antiepileptic drugs. N Engl J Med 334:168, 1996

CHADWICK D: Seizures and epilepsy after traumatic brain injury. Lancet 355:334, 2000

DEVINSKY O: Patients with refractory seizures. N Engl J Med 340:1565, 1999

ENGEL J JR: Surgery for seizures. N Engl J Med 334:647, 1996

KOTAGAL P, LUDERS HO (eds): *The Epilepsies: Etiologies and Prevention.* San Diego, Academic Press, 1999

LOWENSTEIN DH, ALLDREDGE BK: Status epilepticus. N Engl J Med 338:970, 1998

MCNAMARA JO: Emerging insights into the genesis of epilepsy. Nature 339(6738 Suppl): A15, 1999

SACKELLARES JC, BERENT S (eds): *Psychological Disturbances in Epilepsy.* Boston, Butterworth-Heinemann, 1997

SCHILLER Y et al: Discontinuation of antiepileptic drugs after successful epilepsy surgery. Neurology 54:346, 2000

WYLLIE E (ed): *The Treatment of Epilepsy: Principles and Practice*, 2d ed. Baltimore, Williams & Wilkins, 1997

361

Wade S. Smith, Stephen L. Hauser, J. Donald Easton

CEREBROVASCULAR DISEASES

Cerebrovascular diseases occur predominately in the middle and late years of life. They cause approximately 200,000 deaths in the United States each year, as well as considerable neurologic disability. The incidence of stroke increases with age; thus the disability affects many people in their "golden years," a segment of the population that is growing rapidly in Western countries. Categories of cerebrovascular diseases include ischemia-infarction and intracranial hemorrhage (Table 361-1). Many of the arterial and cardiac disorders underlying these diseases are preventable; the morbidity and mortality from cerebrovascular diseases has been diminishing in recent years, apparently because of better recognition and treatment of hypertension.

Most cerebrovascular diseases are manifest by the abrupt onset of a focal neurologic deficit. The deficit may remain fixed or may rapidly improve or progressively worsen. It is this abrupt onset of a nonconvulsive and focal neurologic deficit that defines a *stroke*, or cerebrovascular accident (CVA).

Cerebral ischemia is caused by a reduction in blood flow that lasts for several seconds to a few minutes. Neurologic symptoms are manifest within 10 s because neurons lack glycogen and suffer rapid energy failure. When blood flow is rapidly restored brain tissue can recover fully, and the patient's symptoms are only transient: a transient ischemic attack (TIA) is said to have occurred. Typically the neurologic signs and symptoms of TIA last for 5 to 15 min but, by definition, must last <24 h. If the cessation of flow lasts for more than a few minutes, *infarction* or death of brain tissue results. Stroke has occurred if the neurologic signs and symptoms last for >24 h. A *generalized* reduction in cerebral blood flow due to systemic hypotension (e.g., cardiac arrhythmia, myocardial infarction, or hemorrhagic shock) usually produces syncope (Chap. 21). If low cerebral blood flow is maintained for a longer duration, then infarction in the border zones between the major cerebral artery distributions or widespread brain necrosis develops. This process is termed *global hypoxia-ischemia* and a patient with cognitive sequelae is said to have *hypoxic-ischemic encephalopathy* (Chap. 376). *Focal* ischemia or infarction, on the other hand, is usually caused by thrombosis of the cerebral vessels themselves or by emboli from a proximal arterial source or the heart. A comprehensive list of causes of ischemia-infarction is shown in Table 361-2.

Cerebral hemorrhage produces neurologic symptoms by producing a mass effect on neural structures or from the toxic effects of blood itself; debate exists as to how much injury occurs from tamponade of surrounding blood vessels. As with ischemia-infarction, the causes are numerous (Tables 361-1 and 361-7).

When faced with an acute stroke, the clinician must rapidly differentiate between ischemia-infarction and hemorrhage, because the method of emergency treatment depends on cause. The clinician should focus on two goals: (1) to prevent or reverse acute brain injury, and (2) to prevent future neurologic injury. The first goal involves identifying those patients who may benefit from thrombolysis and attending to acute medical issues of airway, blood pressure, and concomitant organ failure; the second goal is achieved once the mechanism of stroke is elucidated and the proper secondary prevention strategy prescribed.

ISCHEMIC STROKE

MECHANISMS AND DEFINITIONS Several pathophysiologic processes may produce cerebral ischemia and infarction. A common form is atherosclerotic damage to the aortic arch, carotid bifurcation, or intracranial vessels that produces local thrombosis and distal

Table 361-1 Pathophysiologic Classification of Cerebrovascular Diseases

Stroke Subtype	Frequency, %	CT Findings	Causes
Ischemic	85		
Thrombotic	25		
Lacunar stroke	20–25	Hypodensity usually <1 cm³	Lipohyalinosis of small vessels
Large vessel	1–5	Varies	Atherosclerosis of intracranial arteries
Embolic	75		
Cardioembolic	20	Wedge-shaped cortical/sub-cortical hypodensity	See Table 361-2
Artery-artery	15	Wedge-shaped cortical/sub-cortical hypodensity	Aortic, carotid or intracranial atherosclerosis
Cryptogenic	30	Wedge-shaped cortical/sub-cortical hypodensity	Extensive workup reveals no cause
Other	10	Varies	
Hemorrhagic	15		
Intraparenchymal	10	Hyperdensity within brain substance	Hypertension, AVM, amyloid angiopathy
Subdural	<1	Hyperdensity within sub-dural space	Trauma
Epidural	<1	Hyperdensity within epidural space	Trauma
Subarachnoid	1–2	Hyperdensity within sub-arachnoid space	Ruptured aneurysm, trauma

NOTE: AVM, arteriovenous malformation; CT, computed tomography.

embolism of the clot. The released clot travels until it occludes a distal vessel and prevents distal cerebral blood flow. Such strokes are called *atherothromboembloic strokes*, or simply *embolic strokes*, and are a subset of *artery-artery embolic strokes*. Stroke produced by thrombosis of large (~0.5 to 3 mm) intracranial vessels in situ from atherosclerosis is termed *atherothrombotic stroke*. Unlike coronary arteries in which vascular occlusion may be sudden and complete, sudden thrombosis of intracranial vessels occurs less frequently. It may be more likely that atherosclerosis of an intracranial vessel will produce stroke by distal embolism rather than by occlusion. Stenosis of an extra- or intracranial vessel may produce a *low-flow stroke* or TIA if cardiac output or systemic blood pressure is reduced below some threshold. This mechanism was thought to be the cause of stroke from carotid atherosclerosis, but it is now clear that carotid disease produces stroke primarily by an embolic mechanism. True flow-related TIAs and stroke are rare, but it is important to identify them since they will respond to revascularization procedures rather than standard antithrombotic treatment. Thrombotic occlusion of smaller intracranial vessels (~30 to 100 μm), in contrast to larger vessel thrombosis, is a frequent cause of stroke. These end-arteries typically supply a small volume of brain tissue, and their occlusion may result in a *lacunar syndrome*, of which there are >30 types. A patient who has a stroke from this event is said to have *lacunar stroke*. The underlying pathology of this form of stroke is usually lipohyalinosis or microatheromata with thrombosis of the vascular lumen.

Clinically, thrombotic strokes are more gradual in onset or may stutter. It is common for a person to experience several TIAs of the lacunar type prior to eventual stroke. *Crescendo TIAs*—the occurrence of increasing number and frequency of TIAs—have a particularly high likelihood of evolving to stroke. *Stroke in progression* is said to be present if a patient suffers progressive neurologic deficits over a few hours or days that are not accounted for by cerebral edema. This may happen as a small vessel slowly thromboses or, more ominously, as a larger intracranial vessel such as the basilar artery progressively thromboses, producing an ever enlarging region of cerebral ischemia. Heparin and thrombolytic treatment may arrest progression, but it has been difficult to demonstrate in clinical trials whether or not such treatments improve outcome.

Embolism from a cardiac source is most commonly from red atrial thrombi but can arise from numerous sources. In most cases the clinician does not observe clot within the heart and makes the diagnosis by associating a known cardiac cause (e.g., atrial fibrillation, recent myocardial infarction) with a sudden large-vessel occlusion in the brain. Such strokes are called *cardioembolic strokes*. Some patients, however, may develop sudden occlusion of a large intracranial vessel, and despite extensive evaluation, no cause is apparent. These strokes are called *cryptogenic strokes*.

Clinically, embolic events usually produce a sudden onset of neurologic dysfunction that is maximum at onset. The extent of neuronal ischemia is determined by the location of the occlusion and the degree to which collateral flow is offered to the ischemic tissue bed, the blood pressure and body temperature, and other factors. Embolic strokes have a higher risk of transforming into hemorrhagic stroke in which petechial bleeding or frank hemorrhage occurs into the infarcted tissue hours or days following the initial embolic occlusion. This natural history risk of spontaneous hemorrhage must be taken into account in acute stroke trials testing the safety of thrombolytic treatment.

RISK FACTORS FOR ISCHEMIC STROKE Older age, family history of thrombotic stroke, diabetes mellitus, hypertension, tobacco smoking, elevated blood cholesterol levels, and other factors are risk factors for atherosclerosis and

Table 361-2 Causes of Stroke

Common Causes	Uncommon Causes
Thrombosis	Hypercoagulable disorders
Lacunar stroke (small vessel)	Protein C deficiency
Large vessel thrombosis	Protein S deficiency
Dehydration	Antithrombin III deficiency
Embolic occlusion	Antiphospholipid syndrome
Artery-to-artery	Factor V Leiden mutation[a]
Carotid bifurcation	Prothrombin G20210 mutation[a]
Aortic arch	Systemic malignancy
Arterial dissection	Sickle cell anemia
Cardioembolic	β-Thalassemia
Atrial fibrillation	Polycythemia vera
Mural thrombus	Systemic lupus erythematosus
Myocardial infarction	Homocysteinemia
Dilated cardiomyopathy	Thrombotic thrombocytopenic purpura
Valvular lesions	Disseminated intravascular coagulation
Mitral stenosis	Dysproteinemias
Mechanical valve	Nephrotic syndrome
Bacterial endocarditis	Inflammatory bowel disease
Paradoxical embolus	Oral contraceptives
Atrial septal defect	Venous sinus thrombosis[b]
Patent foramen ovale	Fibromuscular dysplasia
Atrial septal aneurysm	Vasculitis
Spontaneous echo contrast	Systemic vasculitis (PAN, Wegner's, Takayasu's, giant cell arteritis)
	Primary CNS vasculitis
	Meningitis (syphilis, tuberculosis, fungal, bacterial, zoster)
	Cardiogenic
	Mitral valve calcification
	Atrial myoxoma
	Intracardiac tumor
	Marantic endocarditis
	Libman-Sacks endocarditis
	Subarachnoid hemorrhage vasospasm
	Drugs: cocaine, amphetamine
	Moyamoya disease
	Eclampsia

[a] Chiefly cause venous sinus thrombosis.
[b] May be associated with any hypercoagulable disorder.
NOTE: CNS, central nervous system; PAN, polyarteritis nodosa.

hence either proven or probable risk factors for ischemic stroke. Risk of second stroke is strongly influenced by prior stroke or TIA (Table 361-3). Many cardiac conditions predispose to stroke, including atrial fibrillation and recent myocardial infarction. Oral contraceptives may increase stroke risk slightly, and certain inherited and acquired hypercoagulable states predispose to stroke. Identification of modifiable risk factors and prophylactic interventions to lower risk is probably the best treatment for stroke overall, as the total number of strokes could be reduced substantially by these means. (See below for recommendations for risk factor modification.)

ACUTE STROKE Clinical Encounter Patients with acute stroke often do not seek medical assistance on their own, perhaps because it is rarely painful but also because they may lose the appreciation that something is wrong with them (*anosognosia*). It is often a family member or a bystander who calls for help, and many gain entry into the medical system through emergency medical services, such as the 911 system in the United States. Use of such a system allows rapid evaluation of patients for consideration for time-sensitive treatments such as thrombolysis. Patients at risk for stroke should be counseled to call emergency medical services if they experience the sudden onset of any of the following: loss of sensory and/or motor function on one half of the body; change in vision, gait, or ability to speak or understand; or a sudden, severe headache.

The differential diagnosis of neurologic symptoms of sudden onset includes stroke (ischemic or hemorrhagic), TIA, seizure with postictal Todd's paralysis, intracranial tumor, migraine, and metabolic encephalopathy (Table 361-4). An adequate history from an observer that no convulsive activity occurred at the onset reasonably excludes seizure. Tumors may present with acute neurologic symptoms due to hemorrhage, seizure, or hydrocephalus. Surprisingly, migraine can mimic cerebral ischemia, even in patients without a significant migraine history. When it develops without head pain (*acephalgic migraine*), the diagnosis may remain elusive. Elderly patients without any prior history of complicated migraine may develop acephalgic migraine after age 65. The sensory disturbance is often prominent, and the sensory deficit, as well as any motor deficits, tends to migrate slowly across a limb over minutes. The diagnosis of migraine becomes more likely as the cortical disturbance begins to cross vascular boundaries. At times it may be difficult to make the diagnosis until multiple episodes have occurred leaving behind no residual stroke or brain imaging abnormality. Classically, metabolic encephalopathies produce a fluctuating mental status without focal neurologic findings. However, in the setting of prior stroke or brain injury, a patient with fever or sepsis will manifest hemiparesis, which clears rapidly when the infection is remedied. The metabolic process serves to "unmask" a prior deficit.

STROKE SYNDROMES A careful history and neurologic examination can often localize the region of brain dysfunction; if this region corresponds to a particular arterial distribution, the possible causes responsible for the syndrome can be narrowed. This is of particular importance when the patient presents with a TIA and a normal examination. For example, if a patient develops language loss and a

Table 361-3 Annual Vascular Event Rates for Patients with Atherosclerotic Cerebral Vascular Disease

Cerebrovascular Features	Annual Probability, %, of		
	Stroke	Vascular Death	All Death
General elderly male population	0.6		
Asymptomatic carotid disease	1.3	3.4	6.0
Transient monocular blindness	2.2	3.5	4.3
Transient ischemic attack	3.7	2.3	4.0
Minor stroke	6.1	3.2	4.9
Major stroke	9.0	3.5	7.6
Symptomatic carotid stenosis, >70%	15.0	2.0	

SOURCE: Modified with permission from JL Wilterdink, JD Easton: Outcome rates for vascular events in patients with atherosclerotic cerebral vascular disease. Arch Neurol 49: 857, 1992.

Table 361-4 Clinical Management of Acute Stroke

New onset of neurologic deficit: Stroke or TIA?	Differential diagnosis of new focal deficit 　Stroke or TIA 　Seizure with postictal Todd's paresis 　Tumor 　Migraine 　Metabolic encephalopathy 　　Fever/infection and old stroke 　　Hyperglycemia 　　Hypercalcemia 　　Hepatic encephalopathy
Initial assessment and management	ABCs, serum glucose Noncontrast head CT 　Hemorrhage 　　Medical and surgical management 　Tumor or other CNS process 　　Treat accordingly 　Normal or hypodense area consistent with acute ischemic stroke 　　Consider thrombolysis, heparin, aspirin 　　Maintain blood pressure and hydrate 　　Admit patient to appropriate level of care depending on concomitant medical problems and airway
Subsequent hospital management	Establish cause of stroke and risk factors Plan for secondary prophylaxis (drugs, risk factor modifications) Obtain physical, occupational, and speech therapy consultation and social work as appropriate Establish nutrition Discharge planning should include prescriptions for risk factor reduction, including when to institute antihypertensive treatment, and antithrombotic medication prophylaxis

NOTE: ABCs, airway management, breathing, cardiac status; CNS, central nervous system; CT, computed tomography; TIA, transient ischemic attack.

right homonymous hemianopia, a search for causes of left middle cerebral emboli should be performed. A finding of an isolated stenosis of the right internal carotid artery in that patient suggests an asymptomatic carotid stenosis, which carries a significantly lower risk than symptomatic stenosis (i.e., stenosis of the left internal carotid artery). The following sections describe the clinical findings of arterial ischemia associated with cerebral vascular territories depicted in Figs. 361-1 through 361-9. Stroke syndromes are divided into: (1) large vessel stroke within the anterior circulation, (2) large vessel stroke within the posterior circulation, and (3) small vessel disease of either vascular bed.

Large Vessel Stroke within the Anterior Circulation • *Pathophysiology* The internal carotid artery and its branches comprise the anterior circulation of the brain. These vessels can be occluded by intrinsic disease of the vessel (e.g., atherosclerosis or dissection) or by embolic occlusion from a proximal source. The causes of occlusion are enumerated here, and the clinical manifestations are listed in the next section.

EXTRACRANIAL INTERNAL CAROTID ARTERY The origin of the internal carotid artery is probably the most common site of atherosclerosis that leads to TIA or stroke. Atherosclerosis is usually most severe in the first 2 cm and arises from the posterior wall, often extending downward into the common carotid artery. Atherosclerosis at this site is often manifested by a TIA or minor stroke, presumably caused by embolism or, less frequently, low flow.

Dissection of the carotid artery produces cerebral ischemia by distal embolization and/or low flow to the anterior circulation. When low flow is the mechanism, there is presumably inadequate collateral flow through the circle of Willis. Fibromuscular dysplasia of the carotids may produce distal emboli or dissection.

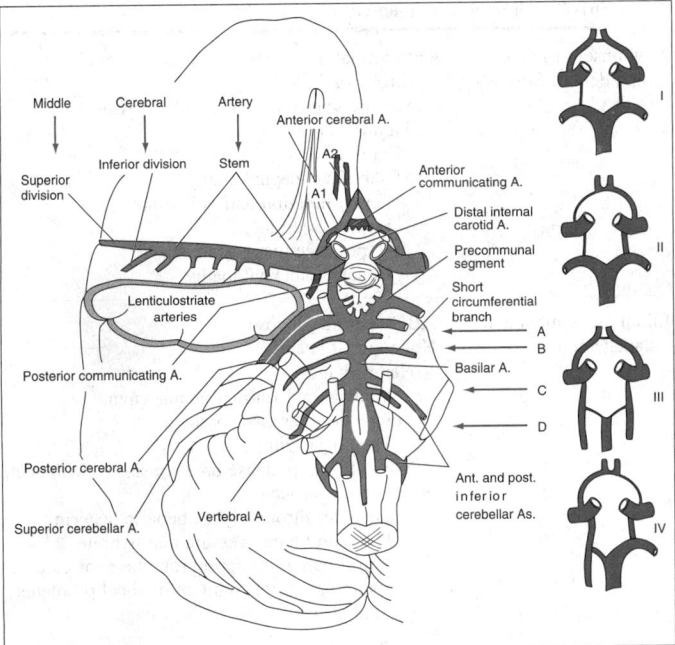

FIGURE 361-1 Diagram of the brainstem, cerebellum, inferior right frontal lobe, and transected temporal lobe. Principal branches of the vertebral basilar arterial system are pictured. The stem of the middle cerebral artery with its small, deep penetrating lenticulostriate arteries and the circle of Willis with its small, deep penetrating branches are shown. Roman numerals I, II, III, and IV represent some of the possible variations of the circle of Willis due to atresia of one or more of its arterial components. *A, B, C,* and *D* arrows indicate the four levels of the brainstem diagrammed below (*D,* Fig. 361-6; *A,* Fig. 361-7; *B,* Fig. 361-8; *C,* Fig. 361-9). Although typical vascular syndromes of the pons and medulla have been designated by the shaded areas in Figs. 361-6 to 361-9, the shading is approximate only. Great variability in infarct size and location occurs when the basilar or vertebral arteries or one of their penetrating branches becomes occluded. This variability is because of variation in arterial anatomic location and available collateral circulation. Thus the stroke syndromes produced are often atypical, incomplete, or merge with one another. *(Courtesy of CM Fisher, MD.)*

Rarely a large embolus will lodge in the common or internal carotid artery. Emboli of a size sufficient to block the internal carotid most often originate from pulmonary veins or extensive atrial or myocardial thrombi. *Takayasu's arteritis* (Chap. 317) is the most common form of vasculitis that affects the carotid artery.

INTRACRANIAL INTERNAL CAROTID ARTERY Atheromatous disease at the petrous inlet, the siphon (S-shaped portion of the internal carotid artery in the cavernous sinus), or the proximal segment of the middle or anterior cerebral arteries may produce distal embolization. These intracranial sites predominate in African Americans, Hispanics, and Asians. *Moyamoya syndrome* results from progressive stenosis and occlusion of the distal internal carotid artery and/or proximal middle and anterior cerebral arteries. It is idiopathic in children and acquired secondary to atherosclerosis in adults. Ischemia is produced by breakdown in lenticulostriate collaterals that form to reconstitute flow in the middle cerebral artery (MCA) or by progressive sclerosis of cortical vessels. Capsular hemorrhage may occur from rupture of the enlarged lenticulostriate vessels.

MIDDLE CEREBRAL ARTERY In contrast to the internal carotid artery, occlusion of the proximal MCA or one of its major branches is most often due to an embolus (artery-to-artery, cardiac, or of unknown source) rather than intracranial atherothrombosis. Atherosclerosis of the proximal MCA may cause distal emboli to the middle cerebral territory or, less commonly, may produce low-flow TIAs. Collateral formation via leptomeningeal vessels often prevents MCA stenosis from becoming symptomatic.

ANTERIOR CEREBRAL ARTERY Atheromatous deposits in the proximal segment of the anterior cerebral artery rarely cause symptoms because the effects of occlusion are usually circumvented by collateral circulation through the anterior communicating artery. If the anterior communicating artery is congenitally atretic or the atheromatous lesion occurs distally in the anterior cerebral artery, TIAs and stroke may occur. The anterior cerebral artery is rarely the recipient of emboli.

Clinical manifestations • MIDDLE CEREBRAL ARTERY The cortical branches of the MCA supply the lateral surface of the hemisphere except for (1) the frontal pole and a strip along the superomedial border of the frontal and parietal lobes supplied by the anterior cerebral artery and (2) the lower temporal and occipital pole convolutions supplied by the posterior cerebral artery (Figs. 361-2, 361-4, and 361-5).

The proximal MCA (M1 segment) gives rise to penetrating branches (termed *lenticulostriate arteries*) that supply the putamen, outer globus pallidus, posterior limb of the internal capsule above the plane of the upper border of the globus pallidus, the adjacent corona radiata, and the body and upper and lateral head of the caudate nucleus. In the sylvian fissure, the middle cerebral artery in most patients divides into *superior* and *inferior* divisions (M2 branches). Branches of the inferior division supply the inferior parietal and temporal cortex, and those from the superior division supply the frontal and superior parietal cortex (Fig. 361-3). There is considerable variability in the parietal lobe supply between the two divisions, with about two-thirds of individuals having an inferior division that supplies regions above the angular gyrus.

If the entire MCA is occluded at its origin (blocking both its penetrating and cortical branches) and the distal collaterals are limited, the clinical findings are contralateral hemiplegia, hemianesthesia, homonymous hemianopia, and a day or two of gaze preference to the ipsilateral side. When the dominant hemisphere is involved, global aphasia is present also, and when the nondominant hemisphere is affected, anosognosia, constructional apraxia, and neglect are found (Fig. 361-3). Dysarthria may also occur.

Complete MCA syndromes occur most often when an embolus occludes the stem of the artery. Cortical collateral blood flow and differing arterial configurations are probably responsible for the development of many partial syndromes. Partial syndromes also may be due to emboli that enter the proximal MCA without complete occlusion, occlude distal MCA branches, or fragment and move distally.

Partial syndromes due to embolic occlusion of a single branch include hand, or arm and hand, weakness alone (brachial syndrome) or facial weakness with nonfluent (expressive, Broca) aphasia (Chap 25), with or without arm weakness (frontal opercular syndrome). A

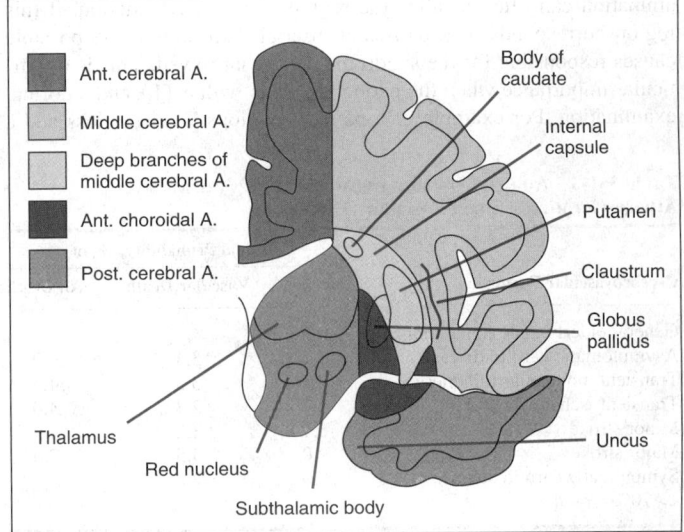

FIGURE 361-2 Diagram of a cerebral hemisphere in coronal section showing the territories of the major cerebral vessels. *(Courtesy of C M Fisher, MD.)*

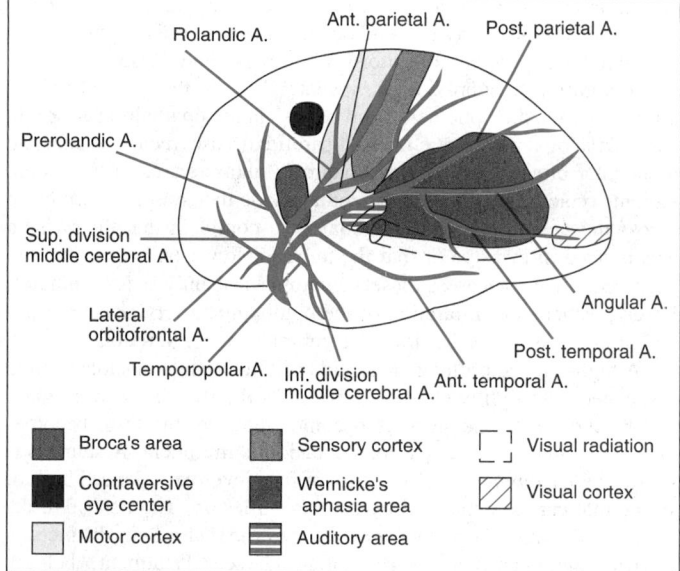

FIGURE 361-3 Diagram of a cerebral hemisphere, lateral aspect, showing the branches and distribution of the middle cerebral artery and the principal regions of cerebral localization. Note the bifurcation of the middle cerebral artery into a superior and inferior division. *(Courtesy of CM Fisher, MD.)*

Signs and symptoms: *Structures involved*

Paralysis of the contralateral face, arm, and leg; sensory impairment over the same area (pinprick, cotton touch, vibration, position, two-point discrimination, stereognosis, tactile localization, barognosis, cutaneographia): *Somatic motor area for face and arm and the fibers descending from the leg area to enter the corona radiata and corresponding somatic sensory system*

Motor aphasia: *Motor speech area of the dominant hemisphere*

Central aphasia, word deafness, anomia, jargon speech, sensory agraphia, acalculia, alexia, finger agnosia, right-left confusion (the last four comprise the Gerstmann syndrome): *Central, suprasylvian speech area and parietooccipital cortex of the dominant hemisphere*

Conduction aphasia: *Central speech area (parietal operculum)*

Apractognosia of the minor hemisphere (amorphosynthesis), anosognosia, hemiasomatognosia, unilateral neglect, agnosia for the left half of external space, dressing "apraxia," constructional "apraxia," distortion of visual coordinates, inaccurate localization in the half field, impaired ability to judge distance, upside-down reading, visual illusions (e.g., it may appear that another person walks through a table): *Nondominant parietal lobe (area corresponding to speech area in dominant hemisphere); loss of topographic memory is usually due to a nondominant lesion, occasionally to a dominant one*

Homonymous hemianopia (often homonymous inferior quadrantanopia): *Optic radiation deep to second temporal convolution*

Paralysis of conjugate gaze to the opposite side: *Frontal contraversive field or projecting fibers*

combination of sensory disturbance, motor weakness, and nonfluent aphasia suggests that an embolus has occluded the proximal superior division and infarcted large portions of the frontal and parietal cortices (Fig. 361-3). If a fluent (Wernicke's) aphasia occurs without weakness, the inferior division of the MCA supplying the posterior part (temporal cortex) of the dominant hemisphere is probably involved (Fig. 361-3). Jargon speech and an inability to comprehend written and spoken language are prominent features, often accompanied by a contralateral, homonymous superior quadrantanopia. Hemineglect or spatial agnosia without weakness indicates that the inferior division of the MCA in the nondominant hemisphere is involved.

ANTERIOR CEREBRAL ARTERY The anterior cerebral artery is divided into two segments: the precommunal (A1) circle of Willis, or stem, which connects the internal carotid artery to the anterior communicating artery, and the postcommunal (A2) segment distal to the anterior communicating artery (Figs. 361-1 and 361-4). The A1 segment gives rise to several deep penetrating branches that supply the anterior limb of the internal capsule, the anterior perforate substance,

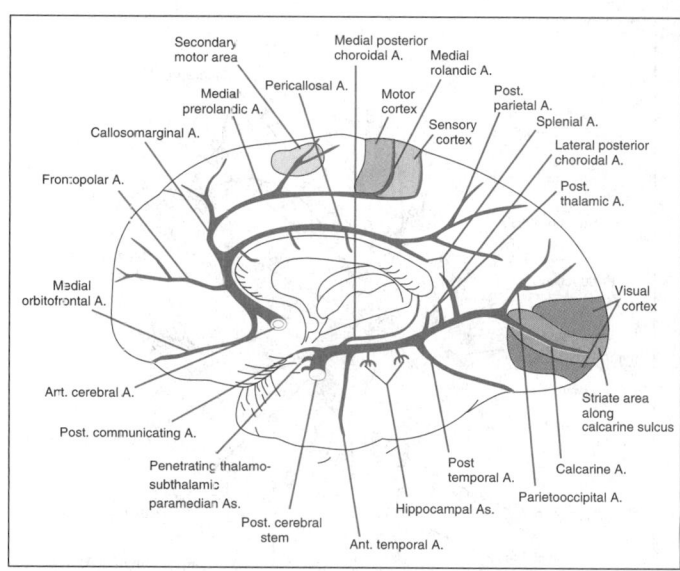

FIGURE 361-4 Diagram of a cerebral hemisphere, medial aspect, showing the branches and distribution of the anterior cerebral artery and the principal regions of cerebral localization. *(Courtesy of CM Fisher, MD.)*

Signs and symptoms: *Structures involved*

Paralysis of opposite foot and leg: *Motor leg area*

A lesser degree of paresis of opposite arm: *Arm area of cortex or fibers descending to corona radiata*

Cortical sensory loss over toes, foot, and leg: *Sensory area for foot and leg*

Urinary incontinence: *Sensorimotor area in paracentral lobule*

Contralateral grasp reflex, sucking reflex, gegenhalten (paratonic rigidity): *Medial surface of the posterior frontal lobe (?) supplemental motor area*

Abulia (akinetic mutism), slowness, delay, intermittent interruption, lack of spontaneity, whispering, reflex distraction to sights and sounds: *Uncertain localization—probably cingulate gyrus and medial inferior portion of frontal, parietal, and temporal lobes*

Impairment of gait and stance (gait apraxia): *Frontal cortex near leg motor area*

Dyspraxia of left limbs, tactile aphasia in left limbs: *Corpus callosum*

amygdala, anterior hypothalamus, and the inferior part of the head of the caudate nucleus (Fig. 361-2).

Occlusion of the proximal anterior cerebral artery is usually well tolerated because of collateral flow. Occlusion of a single A2 segment results in the contralateral symptoms noted in the legend of Fig. 361-4. If both A2 segments arise from a single anterior cerebral stem (contralateral A1 segment atresia), the occlusion affects both hemispheres. Profound abulia (a delay in verbal and motor response) and bilateral pyramidal signs with paraparesis and urinary incontinence result.

ANTERIOR CHOROIDAL ARTERY This artery arises from the internal carotid artery and supplies the posterior limb of the internal capsule and the white matter posterolateral to it, through which pass some of the geniculocalcarine fibers (Figs. 361-2 and 361-5). The complete syndrome of anterior choroidal artery occlusion consists of contralateral hemiplegia, hemianesthesia (hypesthesia), and homonymous hemianopia. However, because this territory is also supplied by penetrating vessels of the proximal MCA and the posterior communicating and posterior choroidal arteries, minimal deficits may occur, and patients frequently recover substantially.

INTERNAL CAROTID ARTERY The clinical picture of internal carotid occlusion varies depending on whether the cause of ischemia is propagated thrombus, embolism, or low flow. The cortex supplied by the middle cerebral territory is affected most often. With a competent circle of Willis, occlusion may go unnoticed. If the thrombus propagates up the internal carotid artery into the MCA, or embolizes it, symptoms are identical to proximal MCA occlusion (see above).

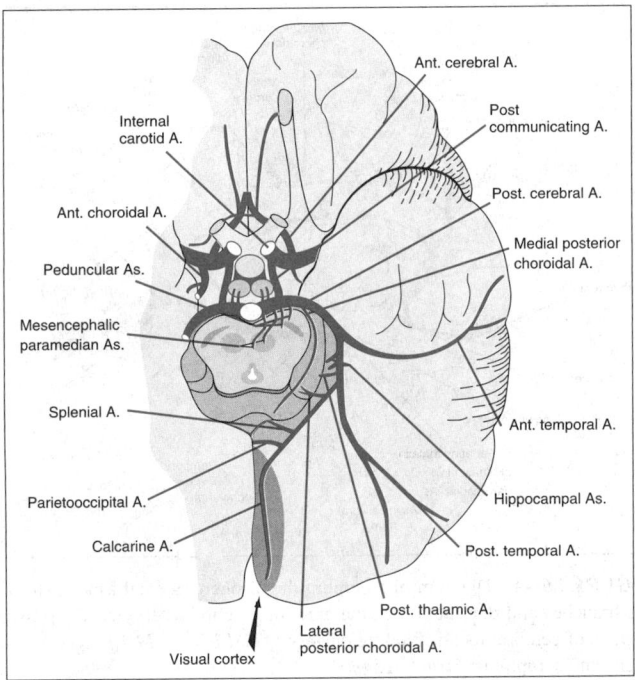

FIGURE 361-5 Inferior aspect of the brain with the branches and distribution of the posterior cerebral artery and the principal anatomic structures shown. *(Courtesy of CM Fisher, MD.)*

Signs and Symptoms: *Structures involved*

1. Peripheral territory (see also Fig. 361-4). Homonymous hemianopia (often upper quadrantic): *Calcarine cortex or optic radiation nearby.* Bilateral homonymous hemianopia, cortical blindness, awareness or denial of blindness; tactile naming, achromatopia (color blindness), failure to see to-and-fro movements, inability to perceive objects not centrally located, apraxia of ocular movements, inability to count or enumerate objects, tendency to run into things that the patient sees and tries to avoid: *Bilateral occipital lobe with possibly the parietal lobe involved.* Verbal dyslexia without agraphia, color anomia: *Dominant calcarine lesion and posterior part of corpus callosum.* Memory defect: *Hippocampal lesion bilaterally or on the dominant side only.* Topographic disorientation and prosopagnosia: *Usually with lesions of nondominant, calcarine, and lingual gyrus.* Simultagnosia, hemivisual neglect: *Dominant visual cortex, contralateral hemisphere.* Unformed visual hallucinations, peduncular hallucinosis, metamorphopsia, teleopsia, illusory visual spread, palinopsia, distortion of outlines, central photophobia: *Calcarine cortex.* Complex hallucinations: *Usually nondominant hemisphere.*

2. Central territory. Thalamic syndrome: sensory loss (all modalities), spontaneous pain and dysesthesias, choreoathetosis, intention tremor, spasms of hand, mild hemiparesis: *Posteroventral nucleus of thalamus; involvement of the adjacent subthalamus body or its afferent tracts.* Thalamoperforate syndrome: crossed cerebellar ataxia with ipsilateral third nerve palsy (Claude's syndrome): *Dentatothalamic tract and issuing third nerve.* Weber's syndrome: third nerve palsy and contralateral hemiplegia: *Third nerve and cerebral peduncle.* Contralateral hemiplegia: *Cerebral peduncle.* Paralysis or paresis of vertical eye movement, skew deviation, sluggish pupillary responses to light, slight miosis and ptosis (retraction nystagmus and "tucking" of the eyelids may be associated): *Supranuclear fibers to third nerve, interstitial nucleus of Cajal, nucleus of Darkschewitsch, and posterior commissure.* Contralateral rhythmic, ataxic action tremor; rhythmic postural or "holding" tremor (rubral tremor): *Dentatothalamic tract (?).*

Sometimes there is massive infarction of the entire deep white matter and cortical surface. When the origins of both the anterior and middle cerebral arteries are occluded at the top of the carotid artery, abulia or stupor occurs with hemiplegia, hemianesthesia, and aphasia or anosognosia. When the posterior cerebral artery arises from the internal

carotid artery (an unusual configuration called a *fetal posterior cerebral artery*), it also may become occluded and give rise to symptoms referable to its peripheral territory (Figs. 361-4 and 361-5).

In addition to supplying the ipsilateral brain, the internal carotid artery perfuses the optic nerve and retina via the ophthalmic artery. In about 25% of symptomatic internal carotid disease, recurrent transient monocular blindness (TMB or amaurosis fugax) warns of the lesion. Patients typically describe a horizontal shade that sweeps down or up across the field of vision. They may also complain that their vision was blurred in that eye or that the upper or lower half of vision disappeared. In most cases, these symptoms last only a few minutes. Rarely, ischemia or infarction of the ophthalmic artery or central retinal arteries occurs at the time of cerebral TIA or infarction.

A high-pitched prolonged carotid bruit fading into diastole is often associated with tightly stenotic lesions. As the stenosis grows tighter and flow distal to the stenosis becomes reduced, the bruit becomes fainter and may disappear when occlusion is imminent. A stenosis is said to be *asymptomatic* if the patient has never experienced TIA or stroke that can be explained by the carotid lesion. The risk of stroke with this finding is low. *Symptomatic carotid stenosis*, in distinction, carries a significantly higher risk for stroke (see "Treatment," below).

COMMON CAROTID ARTERY   All symptoms and signs of internal carotid occlusion may also be present with occlusion of the common carotid artery. Bilateral common carotid artery occlusions at their origin may occur in Takayasu's arteritis (Chap. 317).

Large Vessel Stroke within the Posterior Circulation   The posterior circulation is composed of the paired vertebral arteries, the basilar artery, and the paired posterior cerebral arteries. The vertebral arteries join to form the basilar artery at the pontomedullary junction. The basilar artery divides into two posterior cerebral arteries in the interpeduncular fossa (Fig. 361-1). These major arteries gives rise to long and short circumferential branches and to smaller deep penetrating branches that supply the cerebellum, medulla, pons, midbrain, subthalamus, thalamus, hippocampus, and medial temporal and occipital lobes. Occlusion of each vessel produces its own distinctive syndrome.

Pathophysiology • POSTERIOR CEREBRAL ARTERY   In 75% of cases, both posterior cerebral arteries arise from the bifurcation of the basilar artery; in 20%, one has its origin from the ipsilateral internal carotid artery via the posterior communicating artery; in 5%, both originate from the respective ipsilateral internal carotid arteries (Fig. 361-1). The precommunal, or P1, segment of the true posterior cerebral artery is atretic in such cases.

Atheroma formation or emboli that lodge at the top of the basilar artery or along the P1 segment may cause symptoms by occluding one or more of the small brainstem-penetrating branches (Figs. 361-1 and 361-5) that supply the middle cerebral peduncles, the substantia nigra, red nucleus, oculomotor nuclei, midbrain reticular formation, subthalamic nucleus, decussation of the superior cerebellar peduncles, the medial longitudinal fasciculus, and the medial lemniscus. The *artery of Percheron* arises from either the right or the left precommunal segment of the posterior cerebral artery; it divides in the subthalamus to supply the inferomedial and anterior portions of the thalamus and subthalamus bilaterally. The *thalamogeniculate branches*, which also originate from the precommunal portion of the posterior cerebral artery, supply the dorsal, dorsomedial, anterior and inferior thalamus, and the medial geniculate body. The *medial posterior choroidal artery* supplies the superior dorsomedial and dorsoanterior thalamus and the medial geniculate body in addition to the tela choroidea of the third ventricle. The *lateral posterior choroidal artery* supplies the choroid plexus of the lateral ventricle.

Occlusions in the posterior cerebral artery distal to the junction with the posterior communicating artery (P2 segment) (Fig. 361-5) may disrupt small circumferential branches that course around the midbrain to supply the lateral part of the cerebral peduncles, medial lemniscus, tegmentum of the midbrain, superior colliculi, lateral geniculate body, and posterolateral nucleus of the thalamus, choroid plexus, and hippocampus. On the rare occasions when atheroma occur more distally in the posterior cerebral artery (Fig. 361-5), occlusion may produce ischemia in the inferomedial temporal lobe, parahippocampal and hippocampal gyri, and occipital lobe—including the primary visual cortex and the visual association areas.

In addition to atherothrombosis and embolism, posterior circulation disease may also be caused by dissection of either vertebral artery and fibromuscular dysplasia.

VERTEBRAL AND POSTERIOR INFERIOR CEREBELLAR ARTERIES The vertebral artery, which arises from the innominate artery on the right and the subclavian artery on the left, divides into four anatomic segments. The first (V1) extends from its origin to its entrance into the sixth or fifth transverse vertebral foramen. The second segment (V2) transverses the vertebral foramina from C6 to C2. The third (V3) passes through the transverse foramen and circles around the arch of the atlas to pierce the dura at the foramen magnum. The fourth (V4) segment courses upward to join the other vertebral artery to form the basilar artery; only the fourth segment gives rises to branches that supply the brainstem and cerebellum. The *posterior inferior cerebellar artery* (PICA) in its proximal segment supplies the lateral medulla and, in its distal branches, the inferior surface of the cerebellum. Anastomotic channels exist among the ascending cervical arteries, the thyrocervical arteries, the occipital artery (branch of the external carotid artery), and the second segment of the vertebral artery.

Atherothrombotic lesions have a predilection for V1 and V4 segments of the vertebral artery. The first segment may become diseased at the origin of the vessel and may produce posterior circulation emboli; collateral flow from the contralateral vertebral artery or the ascending cervical, thyrocervical, or occipital arteries is usually sufficient to prevent low-flow TIAs or stroke. When one vertebral artery is atretic and an atherothrombotic lesion threatens the origin of the other, the collateral circulation, which may also include retrograde flow down the basilar artery, is often insufficient (Figs. 361-1 and 361-5). In this setting, low-flow TIAs may occur, consisting of syncope, vertigo, and alternating hemiplegia; this state also sets the stage for thrombosis. Disease of the distal fourth segment of the vertebral artery can promote thrombus formation manifest as embolism or with propagation as basilar artery thrombosis. Stenosis proximal to the origin of the posterior inferior cerebellar artery can threaten the lateral medulla and posterior inferior surface of the cerebellum.

If the subclavian artery is occluded proximal to the origin of the vertebral artery, there is a reversal in the direction of blood flow in the ipsilateral vertebral artery. Exercise of the ipsilateral arm may increase demand on vertebral flow, producing posterior circulation TIAs, or "subclavian steal."

Although atheromatous disease rarely narrows the second and third segments of the vertebral artery, this region is subject to dissection, fibromuscular dysplasia, and, rarely, encroachment by osteophytic spurs within the vertebral foramina.

BASILAR ARTERY Branches of the basilar artery supply the base of the pons and superior cerebellum and fall into three groups: (1) paramedian, 7 to 10 in number, which supply a wedge of pons on either side of the midline; (2) short circumferential, 5 to 7 in number, which supply the lateral two-thirds of the pons and middle and superior cerebellar peduncles; and (3) bilateral long circumferential (superior cerebellar and anterior inferior cerebellar arteries), which course around the pons to supply the cerebellar hemispheres.

Atheromatous lesions can occur anywhere along the basilar trunk but are most frequent in the proximal basilar and distal vertebral segments. Typically, lesions occlude either the proximal basilar and one or both vertebral arteries. The clinical picture varies depending on the availability of retrograde collateral flow from the posterior communicating arteries. Rarely, dissection of a vertebral artery may involve the basilar artery and, depending on the location of true and false lumen, may produce multiple penetrating artery strokes.

Although atherothrombosis occasionally occludes the distal portion of the basilar artery, emboli from the heart or proximal vertebral or basilar segments are more commonly responsible for "top of the basilar" syndromes.

Clinical manifestations • *POSTERIOR CEREBRAL ARTERY* Embolic occlusion is the usual cause of stroke in this vascular territory. Two syndromes are commonly observed: (1) midbrain, subthalamic, and thalamic signs, which are due to disease of the P1 segment or of its penetrating branches; and (2) cortical temporal and occipital lobe signs, due to occlusion of the P2 segment.

1. *P1 syndromes.* If the P1 segment is occluded, infarction usually occurs in the ipsilateral subthalamus and medial thalamus and in the ipsilateral cerebral peduncle and midbrain (Fig. 361-5). A third nerve palsy with contralateral ataxia (Claude's syndrome) or with contralateral hemiplegia (Weber's syndrome) may result. The ataxia indicates involvement of the red nucleus or dentatorubrothalamic tract; the hemiplegia is localized to the cerebral peduncle. If the subthalamic nucleus is involved, contralateral hemiballismus may occur. Occlusion of the artery of Percheron produces paresis of upward gaze and drowsiness, and often abulia. Extensive infarction in the midbrain and subthalamus occurring with bilateral proximal posterior cerebral artery occlusion presents as coma, unreactive pupils, bilateral pyramidal signs, and decerebrate rigidity.

Atheromatous occlusion of the penetrating branches of thalamic and thalamogeniculate arteries produces less extensive thalamic and thalamocapsular lacunar syndromes. The *thalamic Déjerine-Roussy syndrome* is the best known. Its main feature is contralateral hemisensory loss followed later by an agonizing, searing or burning pain in the affected areas. It is persistent and responds poorly to analgesics. Anticonvulsants (carbamazepine or gabapentin) or tricyclic antidepressants may be beneficial. Associated motor signs include hemiparesis, hemiballismus, choreoathetosis, intention tremor, incoordination, and posturing of the hand and arm, particularly while walking.

2. *P2 syndromes* (see also Fig. 361-5). Occlusion of the distal posterior cerebral artery causes infarction of the medial temporal and occipital lobes. Contralateral homonymous hemianopia with macula sparing is the usual manifestation. Occasionally, only the upper quadrant of visual field is involved. If the visual association areas are spared and only the calcarine cortex is involved, the patient may be aware of visual defects. Medial temporal lobe and hippocampal involvement may cause an acute disturbance in memory, particularly if it occurs in the dominant hemisphere. The defect usually clears because memory has bilateral representation. If the dominant hemisphere is affected and the infarct extends to involve the splenium of the corpus callosum, the patient may demonstrate alexia without agraphia. Visual agnosia for faces, objects, mathematical symbols, and colors and anomia with paraphasic errors (amnestic aphasia) may also occur in this setting, even without callosal involvement. Occlusion of the posterior cerebral artery can produce *peduncular hallucinosis* (visual hallucinations of brightly colored scenes and objects).

Bilateral infarction in the distal posterior cerebral arteries produces cortical blindness (blindness with preserved pupillary light reaction). The patient is often unaware of the blindness or may even deny it (*Anton's syndrome*). Tiny islands of vision may persist, and the patient may report that vision fluctuates as images are captured in the preserved portions. Rarely, only peripheral vision is lost and central vision is spared, resulting in "gun-barrel" vision. A constellation of symptoms termed *Balint's syndrome* can occur, usually with bilateral visual association area lesions. It includes optic ataxia (inability to visually guide limb movements), ocular ataxia (inability to direct eyes to a precise point in the visual field), inability to enumerate objects in a picture (simultagnosia) or extract meaning from a picture, and inability to avoid objects in one's path. Balint's syndrome occurs most often with infarctions secondary to low flow in the "watershed" between the distal posterior and middle cerebral artery territories, as occurs after cardiac arrest. Patients may even experience persistence of a visual image for several minutes despite gazing at another scene (*palinopia*). Embolic occlusion of the top of the basilar artery can produce any or all of the central or peripheral territory symptoms. The hallmark is the sudden onset of bilateral signs, including ptosis, pupillary asymmetry or lack of reaction to light, and somnolence.

VERTEBRAL AND POSTERIOR INFERIOR CEREBELLAR ARTERIES Embolic occlusion or thrombosis of a V4 segment causes ischemia of the lateral medulla. The constellation of vertigo, numbness of the ipsilateral face and contralateral limbs, diplopia, hoarseness, dysarthria, dysphagia, and ipsilateral Horner's syndrome is called the lateral medullary (or Wallenberg's) syndrome (Fig. 361-6). Most cases result from ipsilateral vertebral artery occlusion; in the remainder, PICA occlusion is responsible. Occlusion of the medullary penetrating branches of the vertebral artery or PICA results in partial syndromes. *Hemiparesis is not a feature of vertebral artery occlusion.*

Rarely, a *medial medullary syndrome* occurs with infarction of the pyramid and contralateral hemiparesis of the arm and leg, sparing the face. If the medial lemniscus and emerging hypoglossal nerve fibers are involved, contralateral loss of joint position sense and ipsilateral tongue weakness occur.

Cerebellar infarction with edema can lead to *sudden respiratory arrest* due to raised intracranial pressure (ICP) in the posterior fossa. Drowsiness, Babinski signs, dysarthria, and bifacial weakness may be absent, or present only briefly, before respiratory arrest ensues. Gait unsteadiness, dizziness, nausea, and vomiting may be the only early symptoms and signs and should arouse suspicion of this impending complication, which may require neurosurgical decompression, often with an excellent outcome.

BASILAR ARTERY Because the brainstem contains many structures in close apposition, a diversity of clinical syndromes may emerge with ischemia, reflecting involvement of the corticospinal and corticobulbar tracts, ascending sensory tracts, and cranial nerve nuclei (Figs. 361-7, 361-8, and 361-9).

The symptoms of transient ischemia or infarction in the territory of the basilar artery often do not indicate whether the basilar artery itself or one of its branches is diseased, yet this distinction has important implications for therapy. *The picture of complete basilar occlusion, however, is easy to recognize as a constellation of bilateral long tract signs (sensory and motor) with signs of cranial nerve and cerebellar dysfunction.* A "locked-in" state of preserved consciousness with quadriplegia and cranial nerve signs suggest complete pontine and lower midbrain infarction. The therapeutic goal is to identify *impending* basilar occlusion before devastating infarction occurs. A series of TIAs and a slowly progressive, fluctuating stroke are extremely significant as they often herald an atherothrombotic occlusion of the distal vertebral or proximal basilar artery.

TIAs in the proximal basilar distribution may produce dizziness (often described by patients as "swimming," "swaying," "moving," "unsteadiness" or "light-headedness"). Other symptoms that warn of basilar thrombosis include diplopia, dysarthria, facial or circumoral numbness, and hemisensory symptoms. In general, symptoms of basilar branch TIAs affect one side of the brainstem, whereas symptoms of basilar artery TIAs usually affect both sides, though a "herald" hemiparesis has been emphasized as an initial symptom of basilar occlusion. Most often TIAs, whether due to impending occlusion of the basilar artery or a basilar branch, are short-lived (5 to 30 min) and repetitive, occurring several times a day. The pattern suggests intermittent reduction of flow. Many neurologists treat with heparin to prevent clot propagation.

Atherothrombotic occlusion of the basilar artery with infarction usually causes *bilateral* brainstem signs. A gaze paresis or internuclear ophthalmoplegia associated with ipsilateral hemiparesis may be the only manifestations of bilateral brainstem ischemia. More often, unequivocal signs of bilateral pontine disease are present. Complete basilar thrombosis carries a high mortality.

Occlusion of a branch of the basilar artery usually causes *unilateral* symptoms and signs involving motor, sensory, and cranial nerves. As long as symptoms remain unilateral, concern over pending basilar occlusion should be reduced.

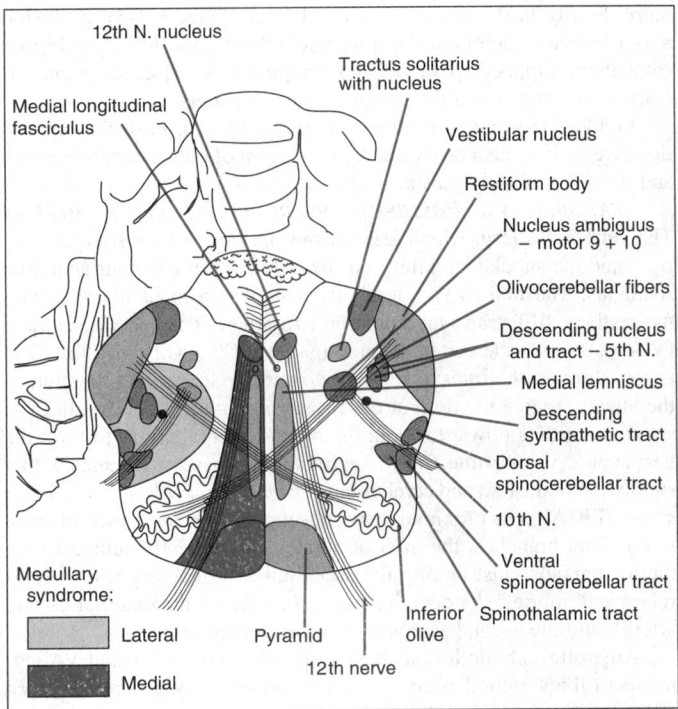

FIGURE 361-6 *(Courtesy of CM Fisher, MD.)*
Signs and Symptoms: *Structures involved*

1. Medial medullary syndrome (occlusion of vertebral artery or of branch of vertebral or lower basilar artery)
   On side of lesion
     Paralysis with atrophy of half the tongue: *Ipsilateral twelfth nerve*
   On side opposite lesion
     Paralysis of arm and leg sparing face; impaired tactile and proprioceptive sense over half the body: *Contralateral pyramidal tract and medial lemniscus*

2. Lateral medullary syndrome (occlusion of any of five vessels may be responsible—vertebral, posterior inferior cerebellar, superior, middle, or inferior lateral medullary arteries)
   On side of lesion
     Pain, numbness, impaired sensation over half the face: *Descending tract and nucleus fifth nerve*
     Ataxia of limbs, falling to side of lesion: *Uncertain—restiform body, cerebellar hemisphere, cerebellar fibers, spinocerebellar tract (?)*
     Nystagmus, diplopia, oscillopsia, vertigo, nausea, vomiting: *Vestibular nucleus*
     Horner's syndrome (miosis, ptosis, decreased sweating): *Descending sympathetic tract*
     Dysphagia, hoarseness, paralysis of palate, paralysis of vocal cord, diminished gag reflex: *Issuing fibers ninth and tenth nerves*
     Loss of taste: *Nucleus and tractus solitarius*
     Numbness of ipsilateral arm, trunk, or leg: *Cuneate and gracile nuclei*
   On side opposite lesion
     Impaired pain and thermal sense over half the body, sometimes face: *Spinothalamic tract*

3. Total unilateral medullary syndrome (occlusion of vertebral artery): Combination of medial and lateral syndromes

4. Lateral pontomedullary syndrome (occlusion of vertebral artery): Combination of lateral medullary and lateral inferior pontine syndromes

5. Basilar artery syndrome (the syndrome of the lone vertebral artery is equivalent): A combination of the various brainstem syndromes plus those arising in the posterior cerebral artery distribution
   Bilateral long tract signs (sensory and motor; cerebellar and peripheral cranial nerve abnormalities): *Bilateral long tract; cerebellar and peripheral cranial nerves*
   Paralysis or weakness of all extremities, plus all bulbar musculature: *Corticobulbar and corticospinal tracts bilaterally;*

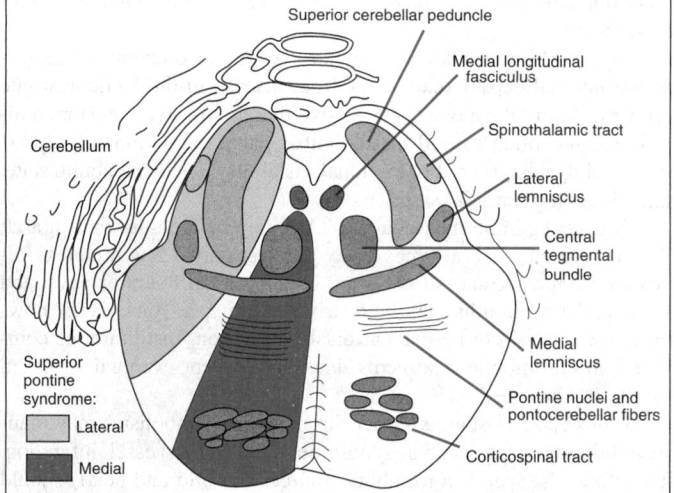

FIGURE 361-7 *(Courtesy of CM Fisher, MD.)*

Signs and Symptoms: *Structures involved*

1. Medial superior pontine syndrome (paramedian branches of upper basilar artery)

   On side of lesion

   Cerebellar ataxia (probably): *Superior and/or middle cerebellar peduncle*

   Internuclear ophthalmoplegia: *Medial longitudinal fasciculus*

   Myoclonic syndrome, palate, pharynx, vocal cords, respiratory apparatus, face, oculomotor apparatus, etc.: *Localization uncertain—central tegmental bundle (?), dentate projection (?), inferior olivary nucleus (?)*

   On side opposite lesion

   Paralysis of face, arm, and leg: *Corticobulbar and corticospinal tract*

   Rarely touch, vibration, and position are affected: *Medial lemniscus*

2. Lateral superior pontine syndrome (syndrome of superior cerebellar artery)

   On side of lesion

   Ataxia of limbs and gait, falling to side of lesion: *Middle and superior cerebellar peduncles, superior surface of cerebellum, dentate nucleus*

   Dizziness, nausea, vomiting; horizontal nystagmus: *Vestibular nucleus;*

   Paresis of conjugate gaze (ipsilateral): *Pontine contralateral gaze*

   Skew deviation: *Uncertain*

   Miosis, ptosis, decreased sweating over face (Horner's syndrome): *Descending sympathetic fibers*

   Tremor: *Dentate nucleus (?), superior cerebellar peduncle (?)*

   On side opposite lesion

   Impaired pain and thermal sense on face, limbs, and trunk: *Spinothalamic tract*

   Impaired touch, vibration, and position sense, more in leg than arm (there is a tendency to incongruity of pain and touch deficits): *Medial lemniscus (lateral portion)*

Superior Cerebellar Artery   Occlusion results in severe ipsilateral cerebellar ataxia, nausea and vomiting, dysarthria, and contralateral loss of pain and temperature sensation over the extremities, body, and face (spino- and trigeminothalamic tract). Partial deafness, ataxic tremor of the ipsilateral upper extremity, Horner's syndrome, and palatal myoclonus may occur rarely. Partial syndromes occur frequently (Fig. 361-7). With large strokes, swelling and mass effects may compress the midbrain or produce hydrocephalus; these symptoms may evolve rapidly. Neurosurgical intervention may be lifesaving in such cases.

Anterior Inferior Cerebellar Artery   Occlusion produces variable degrees of infarction because the size of this artery and the territory it supplies vary inversely with those of the PICA. The principal symptoms include: (1) ipsilateral deafness, facial weakness, vertigo, nausea and vomiting, nystagmus, tinnitus, cerebellar ataxia, Horner's syndrome, and paresis of conjugate lateral gaze; and (2) contralateral loss of pain and temperature sensation. An occlusion close to the origin of the artery may cause corticospinal tract signs (Fig. 361-9).

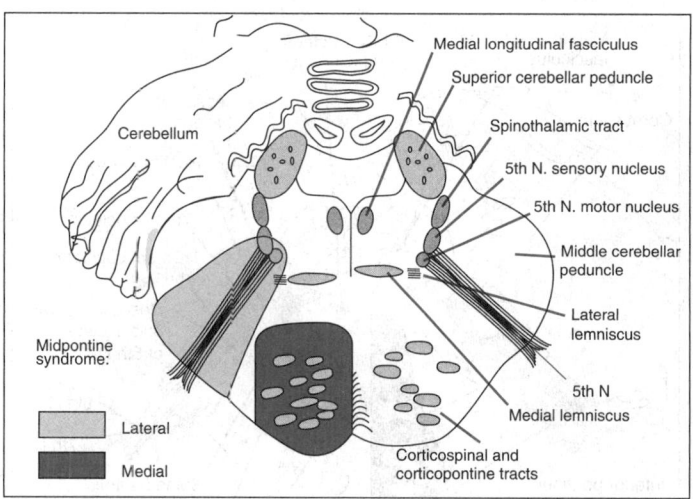

FIGURE 361-8 *(Courtesy of CM Fisher, MD.)*

Signs and Symptoms: *Structures involved*

1. Medial midpontine syndrome (paramedian branch of midbasilar artery)

   On side of lesion

   Ataxia of limbs and gait (more prominent in bilateral involvement): *Pontine nuclei*

   On side opposite lesion

   Paralysis of face, arm, and leg: *Corticobulbar and corticospinal tract*

   Variable impaired touch and proprioception when lesion extends posteriorly: *Medial lemniscus*

2. Lateral midpontine syndrome (short circumferential artery)

   On side of lesion

   Ataxia of limbs: *Middle cerebellar peduncle*

   Paralysis of muscles of mastication: *Motor fibers or nucleus of fifth nerve*

   Impaired sensation over side of face: *Sensory fibers or nucleus of fifth nerve*

   On side opposite lesion

   Impaired pain and thermal sense on limbs and trunk: *Spinothalamic tract*

Occlusion of one of the short circumferential branches of the basilar artery affects the lateral two-thirds of the pons and middle or superior cerebellar peduncle, whereas occlusion of one of the paramedian branches affects a wedge-shaped area on either side of the medial pons (Figs. 361-7 to 361-9).

Small Vessel "Lacunar" Stroke   The term *lacunar infarction* refers to infarction following atherothrombotic or lipohyalinotic occlusion of one of the small, penetrating branches of the circle of Willis, middle cerebral artery stem, or vertebral and basilar arteries. The term *small vessel stroke* denotes occlusion of a small penetrating artery, regardless of mechanism.

Pathophysiology   The middle cerebral artery stem, the arteries comprising the circle of Willis (A1 segment, anterior and posterior communicating arteries, and P1 segment), and the basilar and vertebral arteries all give rise to 100- to 300-μm branches that penetrate the deep gray and white matter of the cerebrum or brainstem (Fig. 361-1). Each of these small branches can occlude either by atherothrombotic disease at its origin or by the development of lipohyalinotic thickening. Thrombosis of these vessels causes small infarcts that are referred to as *lacunes* (Latin for "lake" of fluid noted at autopsy). They range in size from 3 or 4 mm to 1 or 2 cm. Hypertension and age are the principal risk factors. Lacunar infarcts cause approximately 20% of all strokes.

Clinical manifestations   The most common *lacunar syndromes* are the following: (1) Pure motor hemiparesis from an infarct in the posterior limb of the internal capsule or basis pontis; the face, arm and leg are almost always involved. (2) Pure sensory stroke from an infarct in the ventrolateral thalamus. (3) Ataxic hemiparesis from an infarct

FIGURE 361-9 *(Courtesy of CM Fisher, MD.)*
Signs and symptoms: *Structures involved*

1. Medial inferior pontine syndrome (occlusion of paramedian branch of basilar artery)
    On side of lesion
    Paralysis of conjugate gaze to side of lesion (preservation of convergence): *"Center" for conjugate lateral gaze*
    Nystagmus: *Vestibular nucleus*
    Ataxia of limbs and gait: *Middle cerebellar peduncle (?)*
    Diplopia on lateral gaze: *Abducens nerve*;
    On side opposite lesion
    Paralysis of face, arm, and leg: *Corticobulbar and corticospinal tract in lower pons*
    Impaired tactile and proprioceptive sense over half of the body: *Medial lemniscus*

2. Lateral inferior pontine syndrome (occlusion of anterior inferior cerebellar artery)
    On side of lesion
    Horizontal and vertical nystagmus, vertigo, nausea, vomiting, oscillopia: *Vestibular nerve or nucleus*
    Facial paralysis: *Seventh nerve*
    Paralysis of conjugate gaze to side of lesion: *"Center" for conjugate lateral gaze*
    Deafness, tinnitus: *Auditory nerve or cochlear nucleus*
    Ataxia: *Middle cerebellar peduncle and cerebellar hemisphere*
    Impaired sensation over face: *Descending tract and nucleus fifth nerve*
    On side opposite lesion
    Impaired pain and thermal sense over half the body (may include face): *Spinothalamic tract*

in the base of the pons. (4) Dysarthria and a clumsy hand or arm due to infarction in the base of the pons or in the genu of the internal capsule. (5) Pure motor hemiparesis with "motor (Broca's) aphasia" due to thrombotic occlusion of a lenticulostrate branch supplying the genu and anterior limb of the internal capsule and adjacent white matter of the corona radiata.

Syndromes 1 and 2 often overlap. Syndromes resulting from occlusion of the penetrating arteries of the proximal posterior cerebral artery were discussed above. Syndromes resulting from occlusion of the penetrating arteries of the basilar artery (Figs. 361-7 to 361-9) include ipsilateral ataxia and contralateral crural (leg) paresis, hemiparesis with horizontal gaze palsy, and hemiparesis with a crossed sixth nerve palsy. Lower basilar branch syndromes include internu-

clear ophthalmoplegia, horizontal gaze palsy, and appendicular cerebellar ataxia.

An anarthric pseudobulbar syndrome due to bilateral infarctions in the internal capsule can occur from disease in the lenticulostrate arteries. Before the advent of effective therapy for hypertension, multiple lacunes often caused pseudobulbar palsy (predominantly dysarthria and dysphagia) with emotional instability, a slowed abulic state, and bilateral pyramidal signs.

Transient symptoms (lacunar TIAs) may herald a lacunar infarct; they may occur several times a day and last only a few minutes. Recovery from a lacunar stroke often begins within hours or days, and over weeks or months may be nearly complete; in some cases, however, there is severe permanent disability. Often, institution of combined antithrombotic treatments does not prevent eventual stroke in "stuttering lacunes."

A large vessel source (either thrombosis or embolism) may manifest initially as a lacunar syndrome with small vessel infarction. Therefore, the search for embolic sources (carotid and heart) should not be abandoned in the evaluation of these patients.

FINDING THE CAUSE OF STROKE   The clinical presentation, temporal profile, and signs found on examination often establish the cause or narrow the possibilities to a few. Judicious use of laboratory testing and imaging studies complete the initial evaluation. For stroke without an identified cause (cryptogenic stroke), the exact diagnosis may be made months or years later as new symptoms develop. Unfortunately, nearly 30% of strokes remains unexplained despite extensive evaluation; nevertheless, they occur in patients with the same clinical profiles as those whose strokes are due to atherothrombosis.

Clinical examination should be focused on the peripheral vascular system (carotid auscultation for bruits, blood pressure, and pressure comparison between arms), the heart (dysrhythmia, murmurs), extremities (peripheral emboli), and retina [effects of hypertension and cholesterol emboli (Hollenhorst plaques)]; with a complete neurologic examination to localize the site of stroke. A chest x-ray, electrocardiogram (ECG), urinalysis, complete blood count, erythrocyte sedimentation rate, serum electrolytes, blood urea nitrogen, creatinine, blood sugar, serologic test for syphilis, serum lipid profile, prothrombin time, and partial thromboplastin time should be evaluated in all patients. An ECG may demonstrate conduction abnormalities and arrhythmias or reveal evidence of recent myocardial infarction. A lumbar puncture (LP) will generally confirm or exclude subarachnoid hemorrhage (SAH) and can reveal meningitis as a cause for stroke. However, an LP should not be performed on patients with a possible intracranial mass lesion and therefore should generally be avoided in patients with a suspected stroke who are comatose or who have lateralizing neurologic signs with indications of increased ICP. Finally, an imaging study of the brain is nearly always performed and is required for patients being considered for thrombolysis.

BRAIN IMAGING (See also Chap. 358)   **Computed Tomographic Scans**   Computed tomography (CT) images identify or exclude hemorrhage as the cause of stroke, and they identify extraparenchymal hemorrhages, neoplasms, abscesses, and other conditions masquerading as stroke. Scans obtained in the first several hours after an infarction generally show no abnormality, and the infarct may not be seen reliably for 24 to 48 h. Even later, CT may fail to show small ischemic strokes in the posterior fossa because of bone artifact and may also miss small infarcts on the cortical surface. The CT scan documents most supratentorial lacunar infarcts. Lacunar infarction is diagnosed when the infarct size is <2 cm and its location is consistent with occlusion of a small penetrating branch of a major artery at the base of the brain. Larger deep white matter infarcts in the territory of the MCA may present as a lacunar syndrome but are caused by occlusions of large vessels and compensatory collateral perfusion.

Contrast-enhanced CT scans add specificity by showing contrast enhancement of subacute infarcts and allow visualization of venous structures. Coupled with newer generation scanners, administration of intravenous contrast allows visualization of large cerebral arteries.

Such "CT angiograms" may be useful in acute stroke management to reveal the presence or absence of large vessel pathology.

Magnetic Resonance Imaging (MRI) MRI reliably documents the extent and location of infarction in all areas of the brain, including the posterior fossa and cortical surface, if appropriate imaging sequences are obtained. It also identifies intracranial hemorrhage and other abnormalities. The higher the field strength, the more reliable and precise the image. Diffusion-weighted imaging is more sensitive for early brain infarction than standard magnetic resonance (MR) sequences (Fig. 361-10) as is FLAIR (fluid-attenuated inversion recovery) imaging (Chap. 358). MR angiography is highly sensitive for extracranial internal carotid plaque as well as intracranial stenosis of large vessels. With higher degrees of stenosis, MR angiography tends to overestimate the degree of stenosis when compared to conventional x-ray angiography. MRI with fat saturation is an imaging sequence used to visualize extra- or intracranial arterial dissection. This sensitive technique images clotted blood within the dissected vessel wall and has revealed carotid or vertebral dissection as the cause of stroke in a sizable fraction of young patients (age <45). Stroke with neck, jaw, or retroauriclar pain, with or without Horner's syndrome, should prompt this imaging modality or conventional x-ray angiography.

MRI is less sensitive for acute blood products than CT and is more expensive and less readily available. Claustrophobia also limits its application. Most acute stroke protocols use CT because of these limitations. However, outside this setting, MRI provides superior information compared with CT in nearly every case of stroke.

Cerebral Angiography Conventional x-ray cerebral angiography is the "gold standard" for identifying and quantifying atherosclerotic stenoses of the cerebral arteries and other pathologies, including aneurysm, vasospasm, intraluminal thrombi, fibromuscular dysplasia, arteriovenous fistula, vasculitis, and collateral channels of blood flow. Endovascular techniques, which are evolving rapidly, can be used to deploy stents within delicate intracranial vessels and perform balloon angioplasty of stenotic lesions. Recent studies have documented that intraarterial delivery of thrombolytic agents to patients with acute MCA stroke can effectively recanalize vessels and improve clinical outcomes. Although investigational in many centers, use of cerebral angiography coupled with endovascular techniques for cerebral revascularization may become routine in the near future.

Ultrasound Techniques Stenosis at the origin of the internal carotid artery can be identified and quantified reliably by ultrasonography that combines a B-mode ultrasound image with a Doppler ultrasound assessment of flow velocity ("Duplex" ultrasound). Transcranial Doppler (TCD) assessment of middle, anterior, and posterior cerebral artery flow and of vertebrobasilar flow is also useful. This latter technique can detect stenotic lesions in the middle cerebral stem, the distal vertebral arteries, and the basilar artery because such lesions increase systolic flow velocity. When there is an occlusion or hemodynamically significant stenosis at the origin of the internal carotid artery or in the carotid siphon, TCD assesses collateral flow across the anterior or posterior circle of Willis. In many cases, MR angiography combined with carotid and transcranial ultrasound studies eliminates the need for conventional x-ray angiography in evaluating carotid artery lesions for surgery. The combination of the two studies is less expensive than x-ray angiography and reduces the risk of stroke secondary to the procedure.

Ultrasound cannot distinguish reliably between complete and near-complete carotid occlusion; this distinction can be made reliably only by x-ray angiography.

Other Techniques Both xenon techniques (principally xenon-CT) and positron emission tomography (PET) can quantify cerebral blood flow. These tools are generally used for research (Chap. 358) but can be useful for determining the significance of arterial stenosis

FIGURE 361-10 Magnetic resonance imaging of acute stroke. *A.* Diffusion-weighted image of the posterior fossa in a woman with sudden-onset left palate and tongue weakness, showing restricted diffusion in the left basis pontis. T2-weighted MRI at the same time as image *A* showed no evidence of infarction (not shown). *B.* T2-weighted image 2 days later clearly defines the area of infarct.

and planning for revascularization surgery. Single photon emission tomography (SPECT), CT-perfusion, and MR-perfusion techniques report relative cerebral blood flow and currently are research tools.

FINDING EMBOLIC SOURCES If the clinical syndrome of stroke suggests large vessel ischemia or is sudden in onset or if imaging studies reveal infarction consistent with embolism, a search for the cause of embolism is warranted. Documentation of the exact embolic source can direct therapy that can lessen mortality and morbidity. Embolic stroke is classified by the artery involved (e.g., embolic MCA stroke, as discussed above) or by the source of embolism, either from another artery (artery-to-artery embolic stroke) or cardioembolic. Both causes of embolic stroke are discussed below.

Cardioembolic Stroke • *Pathophysiology* Cardioembolism causes approximately 20% of all ischemic strokes. Stroke caused by heart disease is primarily due to embolism of thrombotic material forming on the atrial or ventricular wall or the left heart valves. These thrombi then detach and embolize the arterial circulation. The thrombus may fragment or lyse quickly, producing only TIA. Alternatively, the arterial occlusion may last longer, producing stroke. Subsequent thrombosis distal to the obstruction may occur, producing stroke in progression.

Emboli from the heart most often lodge in the MCA or one of its branches; infrequently, the anterior cerebral artery territory is involved. Emboli large enough to occlude the stem of the MCA (3 to 4 mm) lead to large infarcts that involve both deep gray and white matter and some portions of the cortical surface and its underlying white matter. A smaller embolus may occlude a small cortical or penetrating arterial branch. The location and size of an infarct within a vascular territory often depend on the extent of the collateral circulation.

Vascular congestion of varying degree is common to all ischemic strokes, but extravasation of blood is often associated with embolic infarcts. Because emboli migrate and lyse, recirculation into the infarcted brain may cause petechial hemorrhages. Sometimes there is enough seepage of blood into the infarct to cause visible hemorrhagic infarction on a CT scan. This *hemorrhagic transformation* of a pale infarct typically occurs from 12 to 36 h after embolization and is often asymptomatic. Frank hemorrhage into the infarct sometimes occurs and almost always causes clinical worsening. This is more likely to occur when the stem of the MCA is occluded and a large infarct develops in the territory of the lenticulostriate arteries before recirculation occurs. Edema invariably accompanies the tissue necrosis. In large infarcts, massive edema may compress adjacent tissue, adding to the ischemic process; it also increases ICP and may cause herniation of the brain from one intracranial compartment to another.

The most frequent causes of cardioembolic stroke in most of the world are nonrheumatic (often called nonvalvular) atrial fibrillation, myocardial infarction, prosthetic valves, rheumatic heart disease, and ischemic cardiomyopathy (Table 361-2). Cardiac disorders causing brain embolism are discussed in the respective chapters on heart diseases. A few pertinent aspects are highlighted here.

Nonrheumatic atrial fibrillation is the most common cause of cerebral embolism. Patients with atrial fibrillation have an average annual risk of stroke of ~5%. The risk varies according to the presence of certain risk factors, including older age, hypertension, poor left ventricular function, prior cardioembolism, diabetes, and thyrotoxicosis. Patients younger than 60 with none of these risk factors have an annual risk for stroke of about 0.5%, while those with most of the factors have a rate of about 15%. Guidelines for the use of warfarin are based on risk factors (Table 361-5). The presumed stroke mechanism is thrombus formation in the fibrillating atrium or atrial appendage with subsequent embolization. Left atrial enlargement and congestive heart failure are additional risk factors for formation of atrial thrombi. Rheumatic heart disease usually causes ischemic stroke when there is prominent mitral stenosis or atrial fibrillation.

The cardioembolic causes of stroke are enumerated in Table 361-2. A recent myocardial infarction may be a source of emboli, especially when transmural and involving the anteroapical ventricular wall. Mitral valve prolapse is not usually a source of emboli unless the prolapse is severe.

Paradoxical embolization occurs when venous thrombi migrate to the arterial circulation, usually via a patent foramen ovale or atrial septal defect, which may be occult. Bubble-contrast echocardiography (intravenous injection of agitated saline coupled with either transthoracic or transesophageal echocardiography) can demonstrate a right-to-left shunt, revealing the conduit for paradoxical embolization. Alternatively, a right-to-left shunt is implied if immediately following intravenous injection of agitated saline, high-intensity transients (HITs) can be observed during TCD insonation of the MCA. Both techniques are highly sensitive for detection of right-to-left shunts. Fat and tumor emboli, bacterial endocarditis, and air and amniotic fluid emboli associated with delivery may occasionally be responsible.

Bacterial endocarditis causes valvular vegetations that can give rise to multiple septic emboli (Chap. 126). The appearance of multifocal or diffuse symptoms and signs in a patient with stroke makes bacterial endocarditis a more likely consideration. Infarcts of microscopic size occur, and large septic infarcts may evolve into brain abscesses. Large septic emboli may cause hemorrhage into the infarct, which usually precludes use of anticoagulation or thrombolytics. Mycotic aneurysms caused by septic emboli give rise to SAH or intracerebral hemorrhage.

Clinical manifestations   The stroke is nearly always sudden and maximal at onset. Certain neurologic syndromes suggest embolism, often cardioembolism, as their cause. In the MCA territory these include (1) the frontal opercular syndrome, with facial weakness and severe aphasia or dysarthria; (2) the brachial or hand plegia syndrome, in which the arm or hand is paralyzed with or without cortical sensory abnormalities; (3) Broca's or Wernicke's aphasia alone; or (4) left visual neglect, when the nondominant parietal lobe is involved. Sudden hemianopia suggests a posterior cerebral artery embolus, and sudden foot and shoulder weakness suggests an anterior cerebral embolus.

Table 361-5   **Consensus Recommendation for Antithrombotic Prophylaxis in Atrial Fibrillation**

Age	Risk Factors[a]	Recommendation
Age ≤65	≥1	Warfarin INR 2–3
	0	Aspirin or no treatment
Age 65–75	≥1	Warfarin INR 2–3
	0	Warfarin INR 2–3 or aspirin
Age >75		Warfarin INR 2–3

[a] Risk factors include previous transient ischemic attack or stroke, hypertension, heart failure, diabetes, clinical coronary artery disease, mitral stenosis, prosthetic heart valves, or thyrotoxicosis.
SOURCE: Modified from Laupacis et al.

Sudden sleepiness and inability to look up associated with bilateral ptosis suggest an embolus to the top of the basilar artery, specifically to the artery of Percheron (see above).

Seizures at the time of stroke occur in 3 to 5% of infarctions, are more often associated with embolic stroke rather than thrombosis, and are usually associated with supratentorial cortical surface infarctions. Another 3 to 5% of patients develop epilepsy 6 to 18 months after stroke. Many cases of idiopathic epilepsy in the elderly are probably the result of silent cortical infarction.

Artery-to-Artery Stroke   Thrombus formation on atherosclerotic plaques may embolize to distant arteries. The most common source is the carotid bifurcation, but any diseased vessel may be a source, including the aortic arch and common carotid, internal carotid, and vertebral-basilar arteries.

Dissection of the internal carotid or vertebral arteries or even vessels beyond the circle of Willis is a common source of embolic stroke in young patients. The dissection is usually painful and precedes stroke by several hours or days. Extracranial dissections rarely cause hemorrhage because of the tough adventitia of these vessels. Intracranial dissections, on the other hand, may produce SAH because the adventitia of intracranial vessels is thin, and pseudoaneurysms may form, requiring treatment to prevent rerupture. The cause of dissection is usually unknown and recurrence is rare. Ehlers-Danlos type IV, Marfan's disease, cystic medial necrosis, and fibromuscular dysplasia are associated with dissections. Trauma (usually a motor vehicle accident or a sports injury) can cause carotid and vertebral artery dissections. Chiropractic neck manipulation is also associated with dissection and stroke.

Laboratory and Imaging Evaluation for Embolic Stroke   A thorough cardiac evaluation should be undertaken in patients in whom the suspicion of cardioembolism is high. This includes the young, those with a history of heart disease, those with multifocal or hemorrhagic infarcts, and those with seizures at onset. Continuous ECG monitoring may reveal intermittent atrial fibrillation. An echocardiogram may disclose mitral valve disease, an intracardiac thrombus or tumor, or a dyskinetic area of myocardium. Spontaneous echo contrast within the atrial appendage is associated with stroke and may represent a tendency for spontaneous clotting of blood within the atrium. Transesophageal echocardiography is superior to the transthoracic technique for visualization of valves, left atrium, and aortic arch. Intravenous bubble contrast should be administered to all patients undergoing echocardiography in search of an embolic source. The presence of atrial fibrillation alone is sufficient to establish cause, even in the absence of a left atrial clot.

Embolic infarction may appear as a single low-density area compatible with pale infarction on CT imaging. Petechial hemorrhages within the area may be seen as well and are more likely a day or two after the infarction. MRI scanning better documents infarction both supra- and infratentorially; when coupled with MR angiography, it can help identify arterial sources of emboli from either the extra- or intracranial vessels. MRI with fat saturation should be performed on patients with neck pain preceding stroke, as this technique is highly sensitive for detecting arterial dissection. Carotid ultrasonography and TCD techniques may reveal carotid atherosclerosis or intracranial stenosis, respectively. Conventional x-ray angiography is rarely indicated.

Arterial imaging (CT or MR angiography or TCD) performed in the early hours of stroke often shows occlusion of one or more vessels. Complete lysis of emboli often occurs, and angiography performed after several days may be normal.

LESS COMMON CAUSES OF STROKE   (Table 361-2) *Hypercoagulable disorders* (Chap. 62) primarily cause increased venous thrombotic risk and therefore may cause venous sinus thrombosis. Protein S deficiency and homocysteinemia may cause arterial thromboses as well. Systemic lupus erythematosus with Libman-Sacks endocarditis can be a cause of embolic stroke. These conditions overlap with the antiphospholipid syndrome, which probably requires long-term anticoagulation to prevent further stroke.

Venous sinus thrombosis of the lateral or sagittal sinus or of small cortical veins (cortical vein thrombosis) occurs as a complication of pregnancy and the postpartum period, sepsis, and intracranial infections (meningitis). It is seen with increased incidence in patients with laboratory-confirmed thrombophilia (Table 361-2) including polycythemia, sickle cell anemia, proteins C and S deficiency, factor V Leiden mutation (resistance to activated protein C), antithrombin III deficiency, homocysteinemia, and the prothrombin G20210 mutation. Women who take oral contraceptives and have the prothrombin G20210 mutation may be at high risk for sinus thrombosis. Patients present with headache, focal neurologic signs (especially paraparesis), and seizures. Often, CT imaging is normal unless an intracranial venous hemorrhage has occurred, but the venous sinus occlusion is readily visualized using MR venography or conventional x-ray angiography. With greater degrees of sinus thrombosis, the patient may develop signs of increased ICP and coma. Intravenous heparin, regardless of the presence of intracranial hemorrhage, has been shown to reduce morbidity and mortality, and the long-term outcome is generally good. Heparin prevents further thrombosis and reduces venous hypertension and ischemia. If an underlying hypercoagulable state is not found, many physicians treat with warfarin for 3 to 6 months then convert to aspirin, depending on the degree of resolution of the venous sinus clot, and continue indefinite anticoagulation if thrombophilia is diagnosed.

Fibromuscular dysplasia affects the cervical arteries and occurs mainly in women. The carotid or vertebral arteries show multiple rings of segmental narrowing alternating with dilatation. Occlusion is usually incomplete. The process is often asymptomatic but occasionally is associated with an audible bruit, TIAs, or stroke. The cause and natural history of fibromuscular dysplasia is unknown (Chap. 248). TIA or stroke generally occurs only when the artery is severely narrowed or dissects. Anticoagulation or antiplatelet therapy may be helpful.

Temporal (giant cell) arteritis (Chap. 317) is a relatively common affliction of elderly persons in which the external carotid system, particularly the temporal arteries, becomes the site of a subacute granulomatous inflammation with giant cells. Occlusion of posterior ciliary arteries derived from the ophthalmic artery results in blindness in one or both eyes and can be prevented with glucocorticoids. It rarely causes stroke as the internal carotid artery is usually not inflamed. Idiopathic giant cell arteritis involving the great vessels arising from the aortic arch (Takayasu's arteritis) may cause carotid or vertebral thrombosis; it is rare in the western hemisphere.

Necrotizing (or granulomatous) arteritis, occurring alone or in association with generalized polyarteritis nodosa or Wegener's granulomatosis, involves the distal small branches (<2 mm diameter) of the main intracranial arteries and produces small ischemic infarcts in the brain, optic nerve, and spinal cord. The cerebrospinal fluid often shows pleocytosis, and the protein level is elevated. *Primary central nervous system vasculitis* is rare; small or medium-sized vessels are usually affected. Brain biopsy or high-resolution conventional x-ray angiography is usually required to make the diagnosis. Patients with any form of vasculitis may present with insidious progression of combined white and gray matter infarctions, prominent headache, and cognitive decline. Aggressive immunosuppression with glucocorticoids, and often cyclophosphamide, is usually necessary to reverse the ischemia. Depending upon the duration of the disease, many patients can make an excellent recovery.

Drugs, in particular amphetamines and perhaps cocaine, may cause stroke on the basis of acute hypertension and drug-induced vasculitis. Abstinence appears to be the best treatment, as no data exist on use of any treatment.

Arteritis can also occur as a consequence of bacterial, tuberculous, and syphilitic meningitis.

Moyamoya disease is a poorly understood occlusive disease involving large intracranial arteries, especially the distal internal carotid artery and the stem of the middle and anterior cerebral arteries. Vascular inflammation is absent. The lenticulostriate arteries develop a rich collateral circulation around the occlusive lesion, which gives the impression of a "puff of smoke" ("moyamoya" in Japanese) on conventional x-ray angiography. Other collaterals include transdural anastomoses between the cortical surface branches of the meningeal and the scalp arteries. The disease occurs mainly in Asian children or young adults but can occur in adults who have atherosclerosis. The etiology of the childhood form is unknown. Because of the occurrence of SAH from rupture of the transdural anastomotic channels, anticoagulation is risky. Breakdown of dilated lenticulostriate arteries may produce parenchymal hemorrhage, and progressive occlusion of large surface arteries can occur, producing large artery distribution strokes. Bypass of extracranial carotid arteries to the dura or MCAs may prevent stroke and hemorrhage.

Reversible widespread cerebral segmental vasoconstriction is hypothesized to occur in certain patients with headache and fluctuating neurologic symptoms and signs. Sometimes cerebral infarction ensues. The cause is unknown. Head injury, migraine, sympathomimetic drug use, eclampsia, and the postpartum period have all been associated with this entity. Conventional x-ray angiography is the only means of establishing the diagnosis, but because angiography itself can cause spasm of vessels, even the existence of this vascular entity is debated.

Binswanger's disease (chronic progressive subcortical encephalopathy) is a rare condition in which infarction of the subcortical white matter occurs subacutely. CT or MRI scans detect periventricular white matter infarcts and gliosis. There is lipohyalinosis in the small arteries of the deep white matter, as in hypertension. There are usually associated lacunar infarcts. Binswanger's disease may represent a type of border zone ischemic infarction in the deep white matter between the penetrating arteries of the circle of Willis and of the cortex. The pathophysiologic basis of the disease is unclear, but it typically occurs in older patients with severe long-standing hypertension.

CADASIL (cerebral autosomal dominant arteriopathy with subcortical infarcts and leukoencephalopathy) is an inherited disorder that presents as small vessel strokes, progressive dementia, and extensive symmetric white matter changes visualized by MRI. Approximately 40% of patients have migraine with aura, often manifest as transient motor or sensory deficits. Onset is usually in the fourth or fifth decade of life. This autosomal dominant condition is caused by a missense mutation in Notch-3, a member of a highly conserved gene family characterized by epidermal growth factor repeats in its extracellular domain. Definitive diagnosis is made by brain biopsy revealing typical osmophilic inclusions within smooth-muscle cells of blood vessels; these inclusions may also be present in skin biopsy sections. CADASIL is the only monogenic ischemic stroke syndrome so far described. Genetic testing is not currently available except on a research basis.

℞ **TREATMENT** **Acute Stroke Management** After the clinical diagnosis of stroke is made, an orderly process of evaluation and treatment should follow (Table 361-4). The first goal is to prevent or reverse brain injury. After initial stabilization, an emergency noncontrast head CT scan should be performed to differentiate ischemic from hemorrhagic stroke; there are no reliable clinical findings that conclusively separate ischemia from hemorrhage, although a more depressed level of consciousness and higher initial blood pressure favor hemorrhage, and a deficit that remits suggests ischemia. The second goal is to obtain an accurate understanding of the stroke mechanism so one can halt progression of brain injury or begin to prevent a second stroke. Often this is done during an acute hospitalization, but depending on stroke severity, it may be performed in the outpatient setting. There exists no consensus on the rate with which this evaluation should proceed, primarily because there are few data on the daily risks of recurrence following an initial stroke.

General principles During focal brain ischemia, a gradation in brain perfusion exists such that a core of tissue is infarcted within minutes but a shell of surrounding tissue is only marginally ischemic.

This *ischemic penumbra* may progress to infarction within minutes to hours depending on a number of factors (Chap. 376). Salvage of this "at risk" tissue is the goal of emergency stroke therapy. The penumbral tissue will infarct with only minor drops in systemic blood pressure because cerebral autoregulation within this zone is impaired. *Therefore, a patient's blood pressure at presentation should not be lowered unless it is* >185/110 and thrombolytic therapy will be given (see below). Revascularization of the parent vessel occlusion can restore blood flow to the penumbra and prevent infarction. This concept fuels research into intravenous and intraarterial thrombolysis as well as mechanical means of arterial thrombectomy.

Treatments designed to reverse or lessen the amount of tissue infarction fall within five categories: (1) medical support, (2) thrombolysis, (3) anticoagulation, (4) antiplatelet agents, and (5) neuroprotection.

Medical support When cerebral infarction occurs, the immediate goal is to optimize cerebral perfusion in the surrounding ischemic area. Attention is also directed toward preventing the common complications of bedridden patients—infections (pneumonia, urinary tract, and skin) and deep venous thrombosis with pulmonary embolism.

Elevated blood pressure should not be lowered unless there is malignant hypertension (Chap. 246) or concomitant myocardial ischemia. When faced with the competing demands of myocardium and brain, heart rate lowering with the β_1-adrenergic blocker esmolol can be a first step to decrease cardiac work and maintain blood pressure. If the blood pressure is low, raising it is advisable, using intravenous fluids or vasopressor drugs to enhance perfusion within the ischemic penumbra. Fever is detrimental and should be treated with antipyretics.

Between 5 and 10% of patients develop enough cerebral edema to cause obtundation or brain herniation. Edema peaks on the second or third day but causes mass effect for 10 days. The larger the infarct, the greater the likelihood that clinically significant edema will develop. Even small amounts of cerebellar edema can acutely increase ICP in the posterior fossa. The resulting brainstem compression may result in coma and respiratory arrest and require emergency surgical decompression. Water restriction and intravenous mannitol may be used to raise the serum osmolarity, but hypovolemia should be avoided as this may contribute to hypotension and worsening infarction. Trials are under way to test the clinical benefits of craniotomy and elevation of the skull (hemicraniectomy) for large hemispheric infarcts with marked cerebral edema.

Thrombolysis The use of thrombolytic agents in acute cerebral infarction has been studied extensively. Angiography performed within a few hours of infarction frequently demonstrates arterial occlusions corresponding to patients' presenting signs and symptoms. It is this association of arterial occlusion with acute neurologic symptoms that prompted the study of thrombolytic agents in stroke patients.

Three early intravenous streptokinase trials were stopped because of a higher death rate in the streptokinase-treated patients, mainly due to symptomatic intracranial bleedings. These trials enrolled patients several hours into the stroke process, which may account for the high hemorrhage rates.

The European Cooperative Acute Stroke Study (ECASS) tested intravenous recombinant tissue plasminogen activator (rtPA; 1.1 mg/kg to a 100 mg max.; 10% as a bolus, then the remainder over 60 min) vs. placebo in patients with ischemic stroke within 6 h of onset of symptoms. The median time to treatment was 4 h. Overall, thrombolysis was not beneficial because of an excess of cerebral hemorrhage. However, in those patients who had no signs of major infarction on the initial CT scan, the functional outcome was improved.

The National Institute of Neurological Disorders and Stroke (NINDS) rtPA Stroke Study showed a clear benefit for rtPA in selected patients with acute stroke. The NINDS study used intravenous rtPA (0.9 mg/kg to a 90 mg max.; 10% as a bolus, then the remainder over 60 min) vs. placebo in patients with ischemic stroke within 3 h of onset. Half of the patients were treated within 90 min. Symptomatic

intracerebral hemorrhage occurred in 6.4% of patients on rtPA and 0.6% on placebo. There was a nonsignificant 4% reduction in mortality on rtPA, (21% on placebo and 17% on rtPA) and a significant 12% absolute increase in the number of patients with only minimal disability (32% on placebo and 44% on rtPA.) Thus, despite an increased incidence of symptomatic intracerebral hemorrhage, treatment with intravenous rtPA within 3 h of the onset of ischemic stroke improved clinical outcome. A lower dose of rtPA was used than in the ECASS, and half of the patients were treated within 90 min of stroke onset. These two features may account for much of the increase in benefit and decrease in bleeding hazard compared to the results seen in ECASS.

Finally, ECASS-II tested the NINDS dose of rtPA (0.9 mg/kg, maximum dose 90 mg) but allowed patients to receive drug up to the sixth hour, as in ECASS-I. No significant benefit was found, but improvement was found in post hoc analyses.

Because of the marked differences in trial design, including drug and dose used, time to thrombolysis, and severity of stroke, the precise efficacy of intravenous thrombolytics for acute ischemic stroke remains unclear. The risk of intracranial hemorrhage appears to rise with larger strokes, longer times from onset of symptoms, and higher doses of rtPA administered. The established dose of 0.9 mg/kg administered intravenously within 3 h of stroke onset appears safe. Many hospitals have developed expert stroke teams to facilitate this treatment. The drug is now approved in the United States and Canada for acute stroke when given within 3 h from the time the stroke symptoms began, and efforts should be made to give it as early in this 3-h window as possible. The time of stroke onset is defined as the time the patient's symptoms began or the time the patient was last seen as normal. A patient who awakens with stroke has the onset defined as when they went to bed. Table 361-6 summarizes eligibility criteria and instructions for administration of rtPA.

A recent trial of the fibrinolytic agent ancrod provides further evidence that this approach is effective in acute ischemic stroke.

There is growing interest in using thrombolytics via an intraarterial

Table 361-6 Administration of Intravenous Recombinant Tissue Plasminogen Activator (rtPA) for Acute Ischemic Stroke[a]

Indication	Contraindication
Clinical diagnosis of stroke	Sustained BP > 185/110
Onset of symptoms to time of drug administration ≤3 h	Platelets < 100,000; HCT < 25%; glucose < 50 or > 400
CT scan showing no hemorrhage or significant edema	Use of heparin within 48 h and prolonged PTT, or elevated INR
Age ≥18 years	Rapidly improving symptoms
Consent by patient or surrogate	Prior stroke or head injury within 3 months; prior intracranial hemorrhage
	Major surgery in preceding 14 days
	Minor stroke symptoms
	Gastrointestinal bleeding in preceding 21 days
	Recent myocardial infarction
	Coma or stupor

Administration of rtPA
  Intravenous access with two peripheral IV lines (avoid arterial or central line placement)
  Review eligibility for rtPA
  Administer 0.9 mg/kg intravenously (maximum 90 mg) IV as 10% of total dose by bolus, followed by remainder of total dose over 1 h
  Continous cuff blood pressure monitoring
  No other antithrombotic treatment for 24 h
  For decline in neurologic status or uncontrolled blood pressure, stop infusion, give cryoprecipitate, and reimage brain emergently
  Avoid urethral catheterization for ≥2 h

[a] See Activase (tissue plasminogen activator) package insert for complete list of contraindications and dosing.
NOTE: BP, blood pressure; CT, computed tomography; HCT, hematocrit; INR, international normalized ratio; PTT, partial thromboplastin time.

route to increase the concentration of drug at the clot and minimize systemic bleeding complications. Two recent trials [PROACT and PROACT II (prolyse in acute cerebral thromboembolism)] using intraarterial thrombolysis for acute MCA occlusions up to the sixth hour following onset of stroke showed benefit. Nevertheless, intraarterial use in ischemic stroke is not approved by the FDA. Intraarterial treatment of basilar artery occlusions may also be beneficial for selected patients, but all intraarterial therapy remains experimental.

Anticoagulation   The role of anticoagulation in atherothrombotic cerebral ischemia is uncertain. Several recent trials have investigated antiplatelet versus anticoagulant medications given within 12 to 24 h of the initial event. The U.S. Trial of Organon 10172 in Acute Stroke Treatment (TOAST), an investigational low-molecular-weight heparin, failed to show any benefit over aspirin. Use of subcutaneous unfractionated heparin versus aspirin was tested in two trials, the International Stroke Trial (IST) and the Chinese Acute Stroke Trial (CAST). Taken together, the trials, which studied an aggregate of 40,541 patients, showed a reduction in stroke and death by 1% within 2 to 4 weeks in patients treated with aspirin rather than placebo. Heparin given subcutaneously [without monitoring the partial thromboplastin time (PTT)] afforded no additional benefit over aspirin and increased bleeding rates. Therefore, trials do not support the use of heparin for patients with atherothrombotic stroke of $\geq$12 h duration.

The use of antiplatelet or anticoagulant medication in acute stroke (i.e., <6 h) is less well studied. Heparin is widely used for crescendo TIAs, despite the absence of data from controlled studies regarding this indication. In approximately 20% of patients with acute stroke, deficits will progress over several hours to 1–2 days. Many physicians heparinize all patients with recent mild ischemic stroke in order to prevent some of this worsening. Theoretically, heparin may prevent propagation of clot within a thrombosed vessel or may prevent more emboli from occurring. Some neurologists use heparin until carotid and intracranial vessel patency can be assessed then convert to aspirin if the large vessels are patent. The bleeding complication rate for 7 days of heparin is about 10% with a serious bleed rate of ~2%. Clearly the value of this approach must be clarified.

Heparinization is generally accomplished by beginning an infusion without bolus and is monitored to maintain the activated PTT at approximately twice normal. This regimen is maintained for 2 to 5 days. During this time the patient is monitored for hemorrhagic complications, the evaluation is completed, and a decision is made regarding the need for carotid endarterectomy, long-term anticoagulation, or an antiplatelet therapy. If long-term anticoagulation is chosen, warfarin is administered and heparin discontinued when the international normalized ratio (INR) is in the range of 2 to 3.

Antiplatelet agents   Aspirin is the only antiplatelet agent that has been prospectively studied for the treatment of acute ischemic stroke. The recent large trials, IST and CAST, found that the use of aspirin within 48 h of stroke onset reduced both stroke recurrence risk and mortality minimally. Among 19,435 patients in IST, those allocated to aspirin had slightly fewer deaths within 14 days (9.0 vs. 9.4%), significantly fewer recurrent ischemic strokes (2.8 vs. 3.9%), no excess of hemorrhagic strokes (0.9 vs. 0.8%), and a trend towards a reduction in death or dependence at 6 months (61.2 vs. 63.5%). In CAST, 21,106 patients with ischemic stroke received 160 mg/d of aspirin or a placebo for up to 4 weeks. There were very small reductions in the aspirin group in early mortality (3.3 vs. 3.9%), recurrent ischemic strokes (1.6 vs. 2.1%), and dependency at discharge or death (30.5 vs. 31.6%). These trials demonstrate that the use of aspirin in the treatment of acute ischemic stroke is safe and produces a small but definite net benefit. For every 1000 acute strokes treated with aspirin, about 9 deaths or nonfatal stroke recurrences will be prevented in the first few weeks and approximately 13 fewer patients will be dead or dependent at 6 months.

Agents that act at the glycoprotein IIb/IIIa receptor are undergoing clinical trials in acute stroke treatment.

Neuroprotection   Neuroprotection is the concept of providing a treatment that prolongs the brain's tolerance to ischemia long enough to allow other measures to be employed to mitigate ischemia. Hypothermia is probably the most powerful neuroprotectant but is only now the subject of clinical trials. Drugs that block the excitatory amino acid pathways have been shown to protect neurons and glia in animals, but despite multiple clinical trials they have not yet been proven to be beneficial in humans.

Primary and Secondary Prevention • *General principles*
A number of medical and surgical interventions, as well as life-style modifications, are available for preventing stroke. Some of these can be widely applied because of their low cost and minimal risk; others are expensive and carry substantial risk, but may be valuable for selected high-risk patients.

Evaluation of a patient's *clinical risk profile* can help determine which preventive treatments to offer. In addition to known risk factors for ischemic stroke (above), certain clinical characteristics also contribute to an increased risk of stroke (Table 361-3). The North American Symptomatic Carotid Endarterectomy Trial (NASCET; see below) found that even in patients with the same degree of carotid artery stenosis, specifically 70 to 99%, nine prospectively selected risk factors predicted the risk of vascular outcomes in the medically treated patients. The overall risk of stroke was much greater in a high-risk group (those with more than six risk factors) than in a low-risk group (those with fewer than six risk factors). Fully 39% of patients in the high-risk group treated medically experienced an ipsilateral stroke within 2 years. The rate for the low-risk group was less than half that but was still 17%.

Atherosclerosis risk factors   The relationship of various factors to the risk of atherosclerosis is described in Chap. 241. Older age, family history of thrombotic stroke, diabetes mellitus, hypertension, tobacco smoking, elevated blood cholesterol, and other factors are either proven or probable risk factors for ischemic stroke, largely by their link to atherosclerosis. Hypertension is the most significant of the risk factors; in general, all hypertension should be treated. The presence of known cerebrovascular disease is not a contraindication to treatment aimed at achieving normotension. Also, the value of treating systolic hypertension in older patients has been clearly established. Care must be taken to avoid overtreatment of hypertension, however; the treatment goal is to achieve normotension gradually.

Treatment of hypercholesterolemia has been well established for coronary artery disease but has been studied little in the prevention of stroke. In several recent studies, statin drugs were found to lower stroke risk. Since coronary artery disease is the most common cause of death in patients with cerebrovascular disease, treatment of hypercholesterolemia seems prudent for both the heart and brain. Tobacco smoking should be discouraged in all patients (Chap. 390). Whether or not tight control of blood sugar in patients with diabetes lowers stroke risk is uncertain.

Antiplatelet agents • ATHEROTHROMBOTIC STROKE Platelet *antiaggregation agents* can prevent atherothrombotic events, including TIA and stroke, by inhibiting the formation of intraarterial platelet aggregates. These can form on diseased arteries, induce thrombus formation, and occlude the artery or embolize into the distal circulation. Aspirin, clopidogrel, and the combination of aspirin plus extended-release dipyridamole are the antiplatelet agents used most for this purpose. Ticlopidine has been largely abandoned because of its adverse effects.

Aspirin is the most widely studied antiplatelet agent. Its antiplatelet effect is accomplished by acetylating the cyclooxygenase enzyme in platelets. This irreversibly inhibits the formation in platelets of thromboxane A_2, a platelet aggregating and vasoconstricting prostaglandin. This effect is permanent and lasts for the usual 8-day life of the platelet. Paradoxically, aspirin also inhibits the formation in endothelial cells of prostacyclin, an antiaggregating and vasodilating prostaglandin. This effect is transient. As soon as the aspirin is cleared from the blood, the nucleated endothelial cells again produce prostacyclin. Aspirin in low doses given once daily inhibits the production of thromboxane A_2 in platelets without substantially inhibiting prostacyclin formation. The FDA recommends 50 to 325 mg of aspirin daily for stroke prevention.

Ticlopidine blocks the ADP receptor on platelets and thus prevents the cascade resulting in activation of the glycoprotein IIb/IIIa receptor that leads to fibrinogen binding to the platelet and consequent platelet aggregation. Ticlopidine is more effective than aspirin; however, it has the disadvantage of causing diarrhea, skin rash, a low incidence of neutropenia, and thrombotic thrombocytopenic purpura. Clopidogrel works by the same mechanism as ticlopidine and is not associated with these important side effects. Although many physicians have accepted clopidogrel as equivalent to ticlopidine in stroke prevention, the CAPRIE (Clopidogrel versus Aspirin in Patients at Risk of Ischemic Events) trial, which led to FDA approval, showed less robust efficacy. Studies of clopidogrel in combination with aspirin are in progress in both cerebrovascular and cardiovascular patients.

Dipyridamole is an antiplatelet agent that inhibits the uptake of adenosine by a variety of cells, including those of the vascular endothelium. The accumulated adenosine is an inhibitor of aggregation. At least in part through its effects on platelet and vessel wall phosphodiesterases, dipyridamole also potentiates the antiaggregatory effects of prostacyclin and nitric oxide produced by the endothelium and acts by inhibiting platelet phosphodiesterase, which is responsible for the breakdown of cyclic AMP. The resulting elevation in cyclic AMP inhibits aggregation of platelets. Dipyridamole has a controversial history in stroke prevention. The European Stroke Prevention Study-2 showed efficacy of both 50 mg daily of aspirin and extended-release dipyridamole in preventing stroke, and a significantly better risk reduction when the two agents were combined. A combination capsule of extended-release dipyridamole and aspirin is approved for prevention of stroke.

Many large clinical trials have demonstrated clearly that most antiplatelet agents reduce the risk of all important vascular atherothrombotic events (i.e., ischemic stroke, myocardial infarction, and death due to all vascular causes) in patients at risk for these events. The overall *relative* reduction in risk of nonfatal stroke is about 25 to 30% and of all vascular events is about 25%. The *absolute* reduction varies considerably depending on the particular patient's risk. Individuals at very low risk for stroke seem to experience the same relative reduction, but their risk may be so low that the "benefit" is meaningless. On the other hand, individuals with a 10 to 15% risk of vascular events per year experience a reduction to about 7.5 to 11%.

Aspirin is inexpensive, can be given in low doses, and could be recommended for all adults to prevent both stroke and myocardial infarction. However, it causes epigastric discomfort, gastric ulceration, and gastrointestinal hemorrhage, which may be asymptomatic or life-threatening. Consequently, not every 40- or 50-year old should be advised to take aspirin regularly because the risk of atherothrombotic stroke is extremely low and is outweighed by the risk of adverse side effects. Conversely, every patient who has experienced an atherothrombotic stroke and has no contraindication should be taking an antiplatelet agent regularly because the average annual risk of another stroke is 8 to 10%; another few percent will experience a myocardial infarction or vascular death. Clearly, the likelihood of benefit far outweighs the risks of treatment.

The choice of antiplatelet agent, and dose, similarly must balance the risk of stroke against the risks and cost of the treatments against the expected benefits. But these data are less definitive, and opinions therefore vary. Many authorities believe low-dose (30 to 75 mg daily) and high-dose (650 to 1300 mg daily) aspirin are about equally effective. Some advocate very low doses to avoid adverse effects, and still others advocate very high doses to be sure the benefit is maximal. Most physicians in North America recommend 325 mg daily, while most Europeans recommend 50 to 100 mg. Similarly, the choice of aspirin, clopidogrel, or dipyridamole plus aspirin must balance the fact that the latter are more effective than aspirin but the cost is higher.

EMBOLIC STROKE Although warfarin is more effective than aspirin in preventing ischemic stroke associated with atrial fibrillation, some patients with atrial fibrillation have a low rate of ischemic stroke, and others have a high risk of hemorrhage and lose all of the expected benefit of anticoagulation by this complication. Still others are at such high risk for ischemic stroke that the benefits of warfarin override even the high hemorrhage rate. Preventive treatment depends on knowing the relative risks and benefits for the particular patient.

The Stroke Prevention in Atrial Fibrillation II trial showed that in "low-risk" patients (those without hypertension, recent heart failure, or prior thromboembolism) younger than 75 years given aspirin, the thromboembolism rate was only 0.5% per year. Consequently, one could reasonably recommend that patients <75 years with no risk factors be treated with aspirin only (Table 361-5).

Anticoagulation therapy • *ATHEROTHROMBOTIC STROKE* There are few data to support the use of long-term warfarin for preventing atherothrombotic stroke, either intracranially or extracranially. Several large trials are in progress.

EMBOLIC STROKE Several recent trials demonstrated that anticoagulation (INR range 2 to 3) in patients with chronic nonvalvular (nonrheumatic) atrial fibrillation prevents cerebral embolism and is safe. For primary prevention and for patients who have experienced stroke or TIA, anticoagulation with warfarin reduces the risk by about 65% and clearly outweighs the 1% per year rate of major bleeding complication.

The decision to use anticoagulation for primary prevention is based primarily on risk factors (Table 361-5). The presence of any risk factor tips the balance in favor of anticoagulation.

Because of the high annual stroke risk in untreated rheumatic heart disease, primary prophylaxis against stroke has not been studied in a double-blind fashion. These patients generally receive long-term anticoagulation.

Anticoagulation also reduces the risk of embolism in acute myocardial infarction. Most clinicians recommend a 3-month course of anticoagulation when there is anterior Q-wave infarction, substantial left ventricular dysfunction, congestive heart failure, mural thrombosis, or atrial fibrillation. Warfarin is recommended long-term if atrial fibrillation persists.

Thromboembolism is one of the most serious complications of prosthetic heart valve implantation. Anticoagulation has been proven effective for preventing strokes in this situation, while antiplatelet therapy alone has not. However, coupled with warfarin anticoagulation, aspirin adds substantial benefit. A greater degree of anticoagulation (INR of 3 to 4, depending on valve type) is recommended for prosthetic heart valve patients.

If the embolic source cannot be eliminated, anticoagulation should in most cases be continued indefinitely. Many neurologists recommend combining antiplatelet agents with anticoagulants for patients who "fail" one form of therapy (i.e., have another stroke of TIA). This empirical approach subjects the patient to an increased bleeding risk.

Secondary prophylaxis for ischemic stroke of unknown origin is controversial. Some physicians prescribe anticoagulation for 3 to 6 months followed by antiplatelet treatment. The results of ongoing stroke trials may help to clarify the best treatment.

SURGICAL THERAPY Surgery for atherosclerotic occlusive disease is largely limited to *carotid endarterectomy* for plaques located at the origin of the internal carotid artery in the neck (see below).

Balloon angioplasty coupled with stenting is being used with increasing frequency to open stenotic carotid arteries and maintain their patency. This method has not been compared prospectively with endarterectomy. Concern exists about distal embolization of plaque during vessel dilation. Some neurointerventional centers are treating *intracranial* atherosclerotic disease with angioplasty and stenting. Surgery in the proximal common carotid, the subclavian, and the vertebral arteries is uncommon and is being replaced by endovascular stenting and angioplasty. Extracranial to intracranial bypass surgery has been proven ineffective for atherosclerotic stenoses that are inaccessible to conventional carotid endarterectomy. Although experimental, bypass surgery may have a role in patients with moyamoya disease or the unusual patient with intracranial stenosis and flow-related TIA.

Carotid disease Carotid endarterectomy is a proven effective prophylaxis against stroke and TIA. Approximately 100,000 of these procedures are performed annually in the United States to remove obstructing atherosclerotic plaques. The most important clinical distinction is between symptomatic and asymptomatic carotid stenosis. Symptomatic stenosis is defined as carotid stenosis ipsilateral to the vascular distribution of a stroke or TIA; e.g., a left carotid stenosis in a patient with transient expressive aphasia. Asymptomatic carotid stenosis is defined by the absence of clinical signs or symptoms of stroke or TIA relevant to the carotid lesion. The distinction is important because the natural history of these conditions is markedly different.

Symptomatic carotid stenosis was studied in the NASCET and the European Carotid Surgery Trial (ECST). Both showed a substantial benefit for surgery in patients with a stenosis of >70%. In NASCET, the average cumulative ipsilateral stroke rate at 2 years was 26% for patients treated medically and 9% for those receiving the same medical treatment plus a carotid endarterectomy. This 17% *absolute* reduction in the surgical group is a 65% *relative* risk reduction favoring surgery. NASCET also showed a significant benefit for patients with 50 to 70% stenosis, although less robust. ECST found harm for patients with stenosis in the 0 to 30% range treated surgically.

A patient's risk of stroke and possible benefit from surgery is related to the presence of retinal versus hemispheric symptoms, degree of arterial stenosis, extent of associated medical conditions, institutional surgical morbidity and mortality, and other factors. A patient with multiple atherosclerosis risk factors, symptomatic hemispheric ischemia, very high grade stenosis in the appropriate internal carotid artery, and an institutional perioperative morbidity and mortality rate of ≤6% generally should undergo carotid endarterectomy. If the perioperative stroke rate is >6% for any particular surgeon, however, the benefits of carotid endarterectomy are lost.

The indications for surgical treatment of *asymptomatic carotid disease* have been clarified by the results of the Asymptomatic Carotid Atherosclerosis Study (ACAS), which randomized patients with ≥60% stenosis to medical treatment with aspirin or the same medical treatment plus carotid endarterectomy. The surgical group had a risk over 5 years for ipsilateral stroke (and any perioperative stroke or death) of 5.1%, compared to a risk in the medical group of 11%. While this demonstrates a 53% *relative* risk reduction, the *absolute* risk reduction is only 5.9% over 5 years, or 1.2% annually. The perioperative complication rate was higher in women, so they received only a 17% relative risk reduction over 5 years. Nearly half of the strokes in the surgery group were caused by preoperative angiograms.

The natural history of asymptomatic stenosis is an approximate 2% per year stroke rate, while symptomatic patients experience a 13% per year risk of stroke. Whether to recommend carotid revascularization for an asymptomatic patient remains controversial and depends on many factors including patient preference, age, and comorbidities. Medical therapy for reduction of atherosclerosis risk factors and aspirin, 325 mg/d, are generally recommended for patients with asymptomatic carotid stenosis. As with atrial fibrillation, it is imperative to counsel the patient about TIAs so their therapy can be revised if they become symptomatic.

Stroke Centers and Rehabilitation Comprehensive stroke units that care for the acute patient followed by rehabilitation services

Table 361-7 Causes of Intracranial Hemorrhage

Cause	Location	Comments
Head trauma	Intraparenchymal: frontal lobes, anterior temporal lobes; subarachnoid	Coup and contracoup injury during brain deceleration
Hypertensive hemorrhage	Putamen, globus pallidus, thalamus, cerebellar hemisphere, pons	Chronic hypertension produces hemorrhage from small (~100 μm) vessels in these regions
Transformation of prior ischemic infarction	Basal ganglion, subcortical regions, lobar	Occurs in 1–6% of ischemic strokes with predilection for large hemispheric infarctions
Metastatic brain tumor	Lobar	Lung, choriocarcinoma, melanoma, renal cell carcinoma, thyroid, atrial myxoma
Coagulopathy	Any	Uncommon cause; often associated with prior stroke or underlying vascular anomaly
Drug	Lobar, subarachnoid	Cocaine, amphetamine
Arteriovenous malformation	Lobar, intraventricular, subarachnoid	Risk is approximately 2–4% per year for bleeding
Aneurysm	Subarachnoid, intraparenchymal, rarely subdural	Mycotic and nonmycotic forms of aneurysms
Amyloid angiopathy	Lobar	Degenerative disease of intracranial vessels; linkage to Alzheimer's disease, rare in patients <60
Cavernous angioma	Intraparenchymal	Multiple cavernous angiomas linked to chromosome 7q
Dural arteriovenous fistula	Lobar, rarely subarachnoid	Produces bleeding by venous hypertension
Capillary telangiectasias	Usually brainstem	Rare cause of hemorrhage

have been shown to improve neurologic outcomes and reduce mortality. Use of clinical pathways and dedicating staff to the stroke patient can improve the efficacy of care. Stroke teams that provide emergency 24-h evaluation of acute stroke patients for consideration of thrombolysis and acute medical management are essential components of the care process.

Proper rehabilitation of the stroke patient includes early physical, occupational, and speech therapy. It is directed toward educating the patient and family about the patient's neurologic deficit, preventing the complications of immobility (e.g., pneumonia, deep vein thrombosis and pulmonary embolism, pressure sores of the skin, muscle contractures), and providing encouragement and instruction in overcoming the deficit. The goal of rehabilitation is to return the patient to home and to maximize recovery by providing a safe, progressive regimen suited to the individual patient.

INTRACRANIAL HEMORRHAGE

Blood can extravasate anywhere within the cranial vault or spinal column. Hemorrhages are classified by their location and the underlying vascular pathology. Bleeding into subdural and epidural spaces is principally produced by trauma (Chap. 369). Intraparenchymal, intraventricular, and subarachnoid hemorrhage will be considered here.

DIAGNOSIS Intracranial hemorrhage is often discovered on noncontrast CT imaging of the brain during the acute evaluation of stroke. CT is more sensitive than routine MRI for acute blood. The location of hemorrhage narrows the differential diagnosis to a few entities. Table 361-7 lists the causes and anatomic spaces involved in hemorrhages.

EMERGENCY MANAGEMENT Close attention should be paid to airway management since a reduction in the level of consciousness is common. The initial blood pressure should be maintained until the results of the CT scan are reviewed. Patients with acute SAH should have blood pressure lowered to a normal range with nonvasodilating agents such as labetalol or esmolol. Patients with cerebellar hemorrhages or with depressed mental status and radiographic evidence of hydrocephalus should undergo urgent neurosurgical evaluation. Based on the clinical examination and CT findings, further imaging studies may be necessary, including MRI or conventional x-ray angiography. Stuporous or comatose patients generally are treated presumptively for elevated ICP, with tracheal intubation and hyperventilation, mannitol administration, and elevation of the head of the bed while surgical consultation is obtained (Chap. 376).

INTRAPARENCHYMAL HEMORRHAGE Intraparenchymal hemorrhage is the most common type of intracranial hemorrhage. It is an important cause of stroke, especially in Asians and blacks. Hypertension, trauma, and cerebral amyloid angiopathy cause the majority of these hemorrhages. Advanced age and heavy alcohol consumption increase the risk, and cocaine use is one of the most important causes in the young.

Hypertensive Intraparenchymal Hemorrhage • *Pathophysiology* Hypertensive parenchymal hemorrhage (hypertensive hemorrhage or hypertensive intracerebral hemorrhage) usually results from spontaneous rupture of a small penetrating artery deep in the brain. The most common sites are the basal ganglia (putamen, thalamus, and adjacent deep white matter), deep cerebellum, and pons. When hemorrhages occur in other brain areas or in nonhypertensive patients, greater consideration should be given to hemorrhagic disorders, neoplasms, vascular malformations, and other causes. The small arteries in these areas seem most prone to hypertension-induced vascular injury. The hemorrhage may be small or a large clot may form and compress adjacent tissue, causing herniation and death. Blood may dissect into the ventricular space, which substantially increases morbidity and may cause hydrocephalus. If the patient survives, the clot liquefies, is absorbed, and leaves only a small residual cleft.

Most hypertensive intraparenchymal hemorrhages develop over 30 to 90 min, whereas those associated with anticoagulant therapy may evolve for as long as 24 to 48 h. Within 48 h macrophages begin to phagocytize the hemorrhage at its outer surface. After 1 to 6 months, the hemorrhage is generally resolved to a slitlike orange cavity lined with glial scar and hemosiderin-laden macrophages.

Clinical manifestations Although not particularly associated with exertion, intracerebral hemorrhages almost always occur while the patient is awake and sometimes when stressed. The hemorrhage generally presents as the abrupt onset of focal neurologic deficit. Seizures are uncommon. The focal deficit typically worsens steadily over 30 to 90 min and is associated with a diminishing level of consciousness and signs of increased ICP, such as headache and vomiting.

The putamen is the most common site for hypertensive hemorrhage, and the adjacent internal capsule is invariably damaged (Fig. 361-11). Contralateral hemiparesis is therefore the sentinel sign. When

FIGURE 361-11 Acute onset of right hemiparesis. Transaxial noncontrast CT scan through the region of the basal ganglia reveals a hematoma involving the left putamen. This is a typical hypertensive hemorrhage.

mild, the face sags on one side over 5 to 30 min, speech becomes slurred, the arm and leg gradually weaken, and the eyes deviate away from the side of the hemiparesis. The paralysis may worsen until the affected limbs become flaccid or extend rigidly with a Babinski sign on the same side. When hemorrhages are large, drowsiness gives way to stupor as signs of upper brainstem compression appear. Coma ensues, accompanied by deep, irregular, or intermittent respiration; a dilated and fixed ipsilateral pupil; bilateral Babinski signs; and decerebrate rigidity. In milder cases, edema in adjacent brain tissue may cause progressive deterioration over 12 to 72 h.

Thalamic hemorrhages also produce a contralateral hemiplegia or hemiparesis from pressure on, or dissection into, the adjacent internal capsule. A prominent sensory deficit involving all modalities is usually present. Aphasia, often with preserved verbal repetition, may occur after hemorrhage into the dominant thalamus, and apractognosia or mutism occurs in some cases of nondominant hemorrhage. There may also be a homonymous visual field defect. Thalamic hemorrhages cause several typical ocular disturbances by virtue of extension medially into the upper midbrain. These include deviation of the eyes downward and inward so that they appear to be looking at the nose, unequal pupils with absence of light reaction, skew deviation with the eye opposite the hemorrhage displaced downward and medially, ipsilateral Horner's syndrome, absence of convergence, paralysis of vertical gaze, and retraction nystagmus. Patients may later develop a chronic, contralateral pain syndrome (see Déjerine-Roussy syndrome, above).

In pontine hemorrhages, deep coma with quadriplegia usually occurs over a few minutes. There is often prominent decerebrate rigidity and "pin-point" (1 mm) pupils that react to light. There is impairment of reflex horizontal eye movements evoked by head turning (doll's-head or oculocephalic maneuver) or by irrigation of the ears with ice water (Chap. 24). Hyperpnea, severe hypertension, and hyperhidrosis are common. Death usually occurs within a few hours, but there are occasional survivors.

Cerebellar hemorrhages usually develop over several hours and are characterized by occipital headache, repeated vomiting, and ataxia of gait. In mild cases there may be no other neurologic signs other than gait ataxia. Dizziness or vertigo may be prominent. There is often paresis of conjugate lateral gaze toward the side of the hemorrhage, forced deviation of the eyes to the opposite side, or an ipsilateral sixth nerve palsy. Less frequent ocular signs include blepharospasm, involuntary closure of one eye, ocular bobbing, and skew deviation. Dysarthria and dysphagia may occur. There are no Babinski signs until late in the evolution of the hemorrhage as it compresses or dissects into the ventral brainstem. As the hours pass, the patient often becomes stuporous and then comatose from brainstem compression or obstructive hydrocephalus; immediate surgical evacuation may be life-saving.

Laboratory and Imaging Evaluation The CT scan reliably detects acute focal hemorrhages in the supratentorial space. Small pontine hemorrhages may not be identified because of motion and bone-induced artifact that obscure structures in the posterior fossa. After the first 2 weeks, x-ray attenuation values of clotted blood diminish until they become isodense with surrounding brain. Mass effect and edema may remain. In some cases, a surrounding rim of contrast enhancement appears after 2 to 4 weeks and may persist for months. MRI, though more sensitive for delineating posterior fossa lesions, is generally not necessary in most instances. Images of flowing blood on MRI scan may identify arteriovenous malformations (AVMs) as the cause of the hemorrhage. MRI and conventional x-ray angiography are used when the cause of intracranial hemorrhage is uncertain, particularly if the patient is young or not hypertensive and the hematoma is not in one of the four usual sites for hypertensive hemorrhage. For example, hemorrhage into the temporal lobe suggests rupture of a MCA saccular aneurysm.

Since these patients typically have focal neurologic signs and obtundation, and often show signs of increased ICP, an LP should be avoided as it may induce cerebral herniation.

TREATMENT **Acute Management**   Nearly 50% of patients with a hypertensive intracerebral hemorrhage die. The volume and location of the hematoma determine the prognosis. In general, supratentorial hematomas with volumes <30 mL have a good prognosis, 30 to 60 mL an intermediate prognosis, and >60 mL a poor prognosis during initial hospitalization. Infratentorial pontine hematomas >3 cm are usually fatal. Extension into the ventricular system, especially the fourth ventricle, worsens the prognosis. Except in patients who are on therapeutic anticoagulation or who have a bleeding disorder, little can be done about the hemorrhage itself. Hematomas may expand for several hours following the initial hemorrhage, so treating severe hypertension seems reasonable to prevent hematoma progression. As with ischemic stroke, lowering blood pressure too much or too quickly might cause cerebral ischemia around the hemorrhage cavity.

Evacuation of the hematoma is usually not helpful, except in cerebellar hemorrhages. For cerebellar hemorrhages, a neurosurgeon should be consulted immediately to assist with the evaluation; most cerebellar hematomas >3 cm in diameter will require surgical evacuation. If the patient is alert without focal brainstem signs and if the hematoma is <1 cm in diameter, surgical removal is usually unnecessary. Patients with hematomas between 1 and 3 cm require careful observation for signs of impaired consciousness, which usually means surgery is required.

Tissue surrounding hematomas is displaced and compressed but not necessarily infarcted. Hence, in survivors, major improvement commonly results as the hematoma is reabsorbed and the adjacent tissue regains its function. Careful management of the patient during the acute phase of the hemorrhage can lead to considerable recovery.

Surprisingly, despite large intraparenchymal hemorrhages, ICP is often not elevated. However, if the hematoma causes marked midline shift of structures with consequent obtundation or coma or hydrocephalus, osmotic agents coupled with induced hyperventilation can be instituted to lower ICP (Chap. 376). These maneuvers will provide enough time to place a ventriculostomy or ICP monitor. Once ICP is recorded, further hyperventilation and osmotic therapy can be tailored to the individual patient. For example, if ICP is found to be high, cerebrospinal fluid (CSF) can be drained from the ventricular space and osmotic therapy continued; persistent or progressive elevation in ICP may prompt surgical evacuation of the clot or withdrawal of support. Alternately, if ICP is normal or only mildly elevated, induced hyperventilation can be reversed and osmotic therapy tapered. Since hyperventilation may actually produce ischemia by cerebral vasoconstriction, as a general management principal induced hyperventilation should be limited to acute resuscitation of the patient with presumptive high ICP and eliminated once other treatments (osmotic therapy or surgical treatments) have been instituted. Glucocorticoids are not helpful for the edema from intracerebral hematoma.

Prevention   Hypertension is the leading cause of primary intracerebral hemorrhage. Prevention is aimed at reducing hypertension, excessive alcohol use, and use of illicit drugs such as cocaine and amphetamines.

OTHER CAUSES OF INTRACEREBRAL HEMORRHAGE

Cerebral amyloid angiopathy is a disease of the elderly in which arteriolar degeneration occurs and amyloid is deposited in the walls of the cerebral arteries but not elsewhere. Amyloid angiopathy causes both single and recurrent lobar hemorrhages and is probably the most common cause of lobar hemorrhage in the elderly. It accounts for some intracranial hemorrhages associated with intravenous thrombolysis given for myocardial infarction. This disorder can be suspected in patients who present with multiple hemorrhages (and infarcts) over several months or years, but it is definitively diagnosed by demonstration of Congo red staining of amyloid in cerebral vessels.

Cocaine-induced stroke is an important cause of stroke, particularly in patients <40. Intracerebral hemorrhage, ischemic stroke, and SAH are all associated with cocaine use. Angiographic findings vary from completely normal arteries to large vessel occlusion or stenosis, vasospasm, or changes consistent with vasculitis. The mechanism of cocaine-related stroke is not known, but cocaine enhances sympathetic activity causing acute, sometimes severe, hypertension, and this may lead to hemorrhage. Slightly more than half of cocaine-related intracranial hemorrhages are intracerebral, and the rest are subarachnoid. In cases of SAH, a saccular aneurysm is usually identified. Presumably, acute hypertension causes aneurysmal rupture.

Head injury often causes intracranial bleeding. The common sites are intracerebral (especially temporal and inferior frontal lobes) and into the subarachnoid, subdural, and epidural spaces. Trauma must be considered in any patient with an unexplained acute neurologic deficit (hemiparesis, stupor, or confusion), particularly if the deficit occurred in the context of a fall (Chap. 369).

Intracranial hemorrhages associated with *anticoagulant therapy* can occur at any location; they are often lobar or subdural. Anticoagulant-related intracerebral hemorrhages may evolve slowly, over 24 to 48 h. Coagulopathy should be reversed with fresh-frozen plasma and vitamin K to limit the volume of hemorrhage. When intracerebral hemorrhage is associated with thrombocytopenia (platelet count <50,000/μl), transfusion of fresh platelets is indicated. Intracerebral hemorrhage associated with *hematologic disorders* (leukemia, aplastic anemia, thrombocytopenic purpura) can occur at any site and may present as multiple intracerebral hemorrhages. Skin and mucous membrane bleeding is usually evident and offers a diagnostic clue.

Hemorrhage into a *brain tumor* may be the first manifestation of neoplasm. Choriocarcinoma, malignant melanoma, renal cell carcinoma, and bronchogenic carcinoma are among the most common metastatic tumors associated with intracerebral hemorrhage. Glioblastoma multiforme in adults and medulloblastoma in children may also have areas of intracerebral hemorrhage.

Hypertensive encephalopathy is a complication of malignant hypertension. In this acute syndrome, severe hypertension is associated with headache, nausea, vomiting, convulsions, confusion, stupor, and coma. Focal or lateralizing neurologic signs, either transitory or permanent, may occur but are infrequent and therefore suggest some other vascular disease (hemorrhage, embolism, or atherosclerotic thrombosis). There are retinal hemorrhages, exudates, papilledema (hypertensive retinopathy grade IV), and evidence of renal and cardiac disease. In most cases ICP and CSF protein levels are elevated. The hypertension may be essential or due to chronic renal disease, acute glomerulonephritis, acute toxemia of pregnancy, pheochromocytoma, or other causes. Lowering the blood pressure reverses the process, but stroke can occur. Neuropathologic examination reveals multifocal to diffuse cerebral edema and hemorrhages of various sizes from petechial to massive. Microscopically, there are necrosis of arterioles, minute cerebral infarcts, and hemorrhages. The term *hypertensive encephalopathy* should be reserved for this syndrome and not for chronic recurrent headaches, dizziness, recurrent TIAs, or small strokes that often occur in association with high blood pressure.

Primary intraventricular hemorrhage is rare. It usually begins within the substance of the brain and dissects into the ventricular system without leaving signs of intraparenchymal hemorrhage. Vasculitis, usually polyarteritis nodosa or lupus erythematosus, can produce hemorrhage into any region of the central nervous system; most hemorrhages are associated with hypertension, but the arteritis itself may cause bleeding by disrupting the vessel wall. *Sepsis* can cause small petechial hemorrhages throughout the cerebral white matter. *Moyamoya disease*, mainly an occlusive arterial disease that causes ischemic symptoms, may on occasion produce multiple small aneurysms that rupture. Hemorrhages into the spinal cord are usually the result of an AVM or metastatic tumor. *Epidural spinal hemorrhage* produces a rapidly evolving syndrome of spinal cord or nerve root compression (Chap. 368).

Clinical Manifestations   Symptoms and signs appear over several minutes. Most lobar hemorrhages are small and cause a restricted clinical syndrome that simulates an embolus to an artery supplying one lobe. For example, the major neurologic deficit with an occipital hemorrhage is hemianopia; with a left temporal hemorrhage, aphasia and delirium; with a parietal hemorrhage, hemisensory loss; and with frontal hemorrhage, arm weakness. Large hemorrhages may be associated with stupor or coma if they compress the thalamus or midbrain. Most patients with lobar hemorrhages have focal headaches, and more than half vomit or are drowsy. Stiff neck and seizures are uncommon. Spinal hemorrhages usually present with sudden back pain and some manifestation of myelopathy.

Laboratory and Imaging Evaluation CT scanning reliably detects even very small supratentorial hemorrhages. MRI is more sensitive for delineating associated abnormalities, such as aneurysm, vascular malformation, and neoplasm, and is superior for imaging the posterior fossa and spinal column. MRI with gadolinium contrast enhancement is useful for revealing tumors and AVMs. Using special sequences sensitive for hemosiderin, MRI may show evidence of multiple prior hemorrhages, suggesting amyloid angiopathy and vascular anomalies. Repeating an MRI scan at 4 to 8 weeks may be necessary to reveal the underlying cause of hemorrhage, as the acute hematoma may obscure an underlying vascular anomaly or tumor. Conventional x-ray angiography is used when the cause of hemorrhage is uncertain, especially in the young and the middle-aged, or when better delineation of vascular anomalies is necessary.

Treatment The recommendations for management of hypertensive intracerebral hemorrhage generally apply. If a causative lesion is found, it is treated appropriately.

SUBARACHNOID HEMORRHAGE Excluding head trauma, the most common cause of SAH is rupture of a saccular aneurysm. Other causes include bleeding from a vascular anomaly and extension into the subarachnoid space from a primary intracerebral hemorrhage. Many idiopathic SAHs are localized to the perimesencephalic cisterns and are benign; they probably have a venous or capillary source, and angiography is unrevealing.

Saccular Aneurysm Autopsy studies have found that 3 to 4% of the population harbor aneurysms, for a prevalence of 8 to 10 million people in the United States. The incidence of bleeding is only 25,000 to 30,000 cases per year. The mortality rate for patients who arrive alive at hospital is about 50% during the first month. Of those who survive, more than half are left with major neurologic deficits as a result of the initial hemorrhage, cerebral vasospasm with infarction, or hydrocephalus. If the patient survives but the aneurysm is not obliterated, the annual rebleed rate is about 3%. Given these alarming figures, the major therapeutic emphasis is on preventing the predictable early complications of the rupture.

Unruptured, asymptomatic aneurysms are much less dangerous than a recently ruptured aneurysm. The annual risk of rupture for aneurysms <10 mm in size is approximately 0.1%, and for aneurysms ≥10 mm in size is approximately 0.5%; the surgical morbidity far exceeds these percentages. As more data become available, a true risk-benefit analysis for treating these aneurysms will result.

Giant aneurysms, those >2.5 cm in diameter, occur at the same sites (see below) as small aneurysms and account for 5% of cases. The three most common locations are the terminal internal carotid artery, MCA bifurcation, and top of the basilar artery. Their risk of rupture is about 6% in the first year after identification and may remain high indefinitely. They often cause symptoms by compressing the adjacent brain or cranial nerves.

Mycotic aneurysms are usually located distal to the first bifurcation of major arteries of the circle of Willis. Most result from infected emboli due to bacterial endocarditis causing septic degeneration of arteries and subsequent dilatation and rupture. Whether these lesions should be sought and repaired prior to rupture, or left to heal spontaneously, is controversial.

Pathophysiology Saccular aneurysms occur at the bifurcations of the large arteries at the base of the brain; rupture is into the subarachnoid space in the basal cisterns and often into the parenchyma of the adjacent brain. Approximately 85% of aneurysms occur in the

anterior circulation, mostly on the circle of Willis. Common sites include the junction of the anterior communicating artery with the anterior cerebral artery, the junction of the posterior communicating artery with the internal carotid artery, the bifurcation of the MCA, the top of the basilar artery, the junction of the basilar artery and the superior cerebellar artery or the anterior inferior cerebellar artery, and the junction of the vertebral artery and the posterior inferior cerebellar artery. About 20% of patients have multiple aneurysms, many at mirror sites bilaterally. As an aneurysm develops, it typically forms a neck with a dome. The length of the neck and the size of the dome vary greatly and are factors that are important in planning both neurosurgical obliteration or endovascular embolization. The arterial internal elastic lamina disappears at the base of the neck. The media thins, and connective tissue replaces smooth-muscle cells. At the site of rupture (most often the dome) the wall thins, and the tear that allows bleeding is often no more than 0.5 mm long. It is not currently possible to predict which aneurysms are likely to rupture, but limited data suggest that most ruptured aneurysms are >7 mm in diameter.

Clinical manifestations Most aneurysms present as a sudden SAH. At the moment of aneurysmal rupture with major SAH, the ICP suddenly rises. Abrupt, severe, and generalized vasospasm may occur transiently. These events may account for the sudden transient loss of consciousness that occurs in nearly half of patients. Sudden loss of consciousness may be preceded by a brief moment of excruciating headache, but most patients first complain of headache upon regaining consciousness. In 10% of cases, aneurysmal bleeding is severe enough to cause loss on consciousness for several days. In about 45% of cases, severe headache associated with exertion is the presenting complaint. The patient often calls the headache "the worst headache of my life." However, the clinician should be sensitive to the less dramatic features of sudden onset of headache or to a new or different headache than what the patient has ever experienced. The headache is usually generalized, and vomiting is common.

Although sudden headache in the absence of focal neurologic symptoms is the hallmark of aneurysmal rupture, focal neurologic deficits may occur. Anterior communicating artery or middle cerebral bifurcation aneurysms may rupture into the adjacent brain or subdural space and form a hematoma large enough to produce mass effect. The common deficits that result include hemiparesis, aphasia, and abulia.

Occasionally, prodromal symptoms suggest the location of a progressively enlarging unruptured aneurysm. A third cranial nerve palsy, particularly when associated with pupillary dilatation, loss of light reflex, and focal pain above or behind the eye, may occur with an expanding aneurysm at the junction of the posterior communicating artery and the internal carotid artery. A sixth nerve palsy may indicate an aneurysm in the cavernous sinus, and visual field defects can occur with an expanding supraclinoid carotid or anterior cerebral artery aneurysm. Occipital and posterior cervical pain may signal a posterior inferior cerebellar artery or anterior inferior cerebellar artery aneurysm. Pain in or behind the eye and in the low temple can occur with an expanding MCA aneurysm. Growing aneurysms rarely cause head pain in the absence of neurologic symptoms and signs.

Aneurysms can undergo small ruptures and leaks of blood into the subarachnoid space, so-called sentinel bleeds. Sudden unexplained headache at any location should raise suspicion of SAH and be investigated because a major hemorrhage may be imminent.

DELAYED NEUROLOGIC DEFICITS There are four major causes of delayed neurologic deficits; reapture, hydrocephalus, vasospasm, and hyponatremia.

1. *Rerupture* The incidence of rerupture of an untreated aneurysm in the first month following SAH is about 30% with the peak at 7 days. It is associated with a 60% mortality and poor outcome. Early treatment eliminates this risk.

2. *Hydrocephalus* Acute hydrocephalus can cause stupor and coma. More often, subacute hydrocephalus develops over a few days or weeks and causes progressive drowsiness or slowed mentation (abulia) with incontinence. Differentiating hydrocephalus from cerebral vasospasm is accomplished with a CT scan, TCD ultrasound, or con-

ventional x-ray angiography. Hydrocephalus may clear spontaneously or require temporary ventricular drainage. Chronic hydrocephalus may develop weeks to months after SAH and manifest as gait difficulty, incontinence, or impaired mentation. Subtle signs may be a lack of initiative in conversation or a failure to recover independence.

3. *Vasospasm* Narrowing of the arteries at the base of the brain following SAH occurs regularly. This vasospasm causes symptomatic ischemia and infarction in approximately 30% of patients and is the major cause of delayed morbidity or death. Signs of ischemia appear 4 to 14 days after the hemorrhage, most frequently at about 7 days. The severity and distribution of vasospasm determine whether infarction will occur.

The mechanism of delayed vasospasm is likely to be related to direct effects of clotted blood and its breakdown products on the artery. In general, the more blood that surrounds the arteries, the greater the chance of symptomatic vasospasm. Spasm of the MCA typically causes contralateral hemiparesis and dysphasia (dominant hemisphere). Proximal anterior cerebral artery vasospasm causes abulia and incontinence, while severe vasospasm of the posterior cerebral artery causes hemianopia. Severe spasm of the basilar or vertebral arteries occasionally produces focal brainstem ischemia. All of these focal symptoms may present abruptly, fluctuate, or develop over a few days.

Vasospasm can be detected reliably with conventional x-ray angiography, but this invasive procedure is expensive and carries risk of stroke and other complications. TCD ultrasound is based on the principle that the velocity of blood flow within an artery will rise as the lumen diameter is narrowed. By directing the probe along the MCA and proximal anterior cerebral, carotid terminus, vertebral, and basilar arteries on a daily or every-other-day basis, vasospasm can be reliably detected noninvasively and treatments initiated to prevent cerebral ischemia (see below).

Severe cerebral edema in patients with infarction from vasospasm may increase the ICP enough to reduce cerebral perfusion pressure. Treatment is with mannitol and hyperventilation (Chap. 376).

4. *Hyponatremia* Hyponatremia may be profound and develop quickly in the first 2 weeks following SAH. It usually results from inappropriate secretion of vasopressin (Chap. 329) and secretion of atrial and brain natriuretic factors, which produce a natriuresis. This "cerebral salt-wasting syndrome" clears over the course of 1 to 2 weeks and, in the setting of SAH, arguably should not be treated with free-water restriction (see below).

Laboratory evaluation and imaging (Fig. 361-12) The hallmark of aneurysmal rupture is blood in the CSF. More than 95% of cases have enough blood to be visualized on a high-quality noncontrast CT scan obtained within 72 h. If the scan fails to establish the diagnosis of SAH and no mass lesion or obstructive hydrocephalus is found, an LP should be performed to establish the presence of subarachnoid blood. Lysis of the red blood cells and subsequent conversion of hemoglobin to bilirubin stains the spinal fluid yellow within 6 to 12 h of SAH. This xanthochromic spinal fluid peaks in intensity at 48 h and lasts for 1 to 4 weeks, depending on the amount of subarachnoid blood.

The extent and location of subarachnoid blood on noncontrast CT scan help locate the underlying aneurysm, identify the cause of any neurologic deficit, and predict delayed vasospasm. A high incidence of symptomatic vasospasm in the middle and anterior cerebral arteries has been found when early CT scans show subarachnoid clots >5 × 3 mm in the basal cisterns or layers of blood >1 mm thick in the cerebral fissures. CT scans less reliably predict vasospasm in the vertebral, basilar, or posterior cerebral arteries.

LP prior to scanning is indicated only if a CT scan is not available at the time of the suspected SAH. Once the diagnosis of hemorrhage from a ruptured saccular aneurysm is suspected, four-vessel conventional x-ray angiography (both carotids and both vertebrals) is generally performed to localize and define the anatomic details of the aneurysm and to determine if other unruptured aneurysms exist. At certain centers, the ruptured aneurysm can be treated using endovascular techniques at the time of the initial angiogram (see following treatment).

FIGURE 361-12 Subarachnoid hemorrhage. Sudden onset of headache and altered mental status. Noncontrast CT scan at the level of the suprasellar cistern revealed subarachnoid hemorrhage. Communicating hydrocephalus is present, indicated by dilation of the temporal horns of the lateral ventricle. Angiography demonstrated an aneurysm of the anterior communicating artery, which had ruptured.

The ECG frequently shows ST-segment and T-wave changes similar to those associated with cardiac ischemia. Prolonged QRS complex, increased QT interval, and prominent "peaked" or deeply inverted symmetric T waves are usually secondary to the intracranial hemorrhage. The cause of these changes is debated, but there is evidence that structural myocardial lesions produced by circulating catecholamines may occur after SAH.

Serum electrolytes are obtained because hyponatremia may develop. Close monitoring (daily or twice daily) of serum sodium is important since hyponatremia can occur precipitously during the first 2 weeks following SAH (see above).

TCD ultrasound assessment of proximal middle, anterior, and posterior cerebral and basilar artery flow is helpful in detecting the onset of vasospasm and in following its course and response to therapy.

TREATMENT Aneurysm rerupture is common in the early days after SAH and is associated with a 60% incidence of death or poor outcome. Early aneurysm repair prevents future hemorrhage and allows the safe application of techniques to improve blood flow (e.g., induced hypertension and hypervolemia) should symptomatic vasospasm develop. An aneurysm can be "clipped" by a neurosurgeon or "coiled" by a neurointerventional radiologist. Surgical repair involves placing a metal clip across the aneurysm neck, with the advantage that rebleeding risk is eliminated immediately. This approach requires craniotomy and brain retraction, which is associated with neurologic deficits. The newer endovascular technique involves placing platinum coils within the aneurysm via a catheter from the femoral artery. The aneurysm is packed tightly to enhance thrombosis and over time is walled-off from the circulation. The safety and efficacy of these two techniques are being compared in an ongoing European trial.

The medical management of SAH centers on airway protection, blood pressure management before and after aneurysm treatment, preventing rebleeding prior to treatment, managing vasospasm, treating hydrocephalus, and treating hyponatremia.

Intracranial hypertension following aneurysmal rupture occurs secondary to subarachnoid blood, parenchymal hematoma, acute hydrocephalus, or loss of vascular autoregulation. Patients who are stuporous should undergo emergent ventriculostomy to prevent cerebral ischemia from high ICP. Medical therapies designed to combat raised ICP (e.g., mild hyperventilation, mannitol, and sedation) can also be used as needed (Chap. 376). High ICP refractory to treatment carries a poor prognostic sign.

Prior to definitive treatment of the ruptured aneurysm, care is required to maintain adequate cerebral perfusion pressure while avoiding excessive elevation of arterial pressure. Occasionally an intracranial hematoma causing neurologic deterioration requires removal.

Because rebleeding is common, all patients who are not candidates for early surgical treatment are put on bed rest in a quiet, preferably darkened, room and are given stool softeners to prevent constipation. If headache or neck pain is severe, mild sedation and analgesia are prescribed. Extreme sedation is avoided because it can obscure changes in neurologic status. Adequate hydration is necessary to avoid a decrease in blood volume predisposing to brain ischemia.

Seizures are uncommon at the onset of aneurysmal rupture. The quivering, jerking, and extensor posturing that often accompany loss of consciousness are probably related to the sharp rise in ICP or, perhaps, acute generalized vasospasm. However, phenytoin is often given as prophylactic therapy since a seizure may promote rebleeding.

Glucocorticoids may help reduce the head and neck ache caused by the irritative effect of the subarachnoid blood. There is no good evidence they reduce cerebral edema, are neuroprotective, or reduce vascular injury, and their routine use therefore is controversial.

Antifibrinolytic agents are not routinely prescribed but may be considered in patients in whom aneurysm treatment cannot proceed immediately. They are associated with a reduced incidence of aneurysmal rerupture but are also associated with an increased incidence of delayed cerebral infarction and deep venous thrombosis.

Vasospasm remains the leading cause of morbidity and mortality following aneurysmal SAH and treatment of the aneurysm. Treatment with the calcium channel antagonist nimodipine (60 mg orally q6h) has been reported to be beneficial, but the effects seem to be modest. Nimodipine can cause significant hypotension in some patients, which may worsen cerebral ischemia in patients with vasospasm. The most widely accepted therapy for symptomatic cerebral vasospasm is to increase the cerebral perfusion pressure by raising mean arterial pressure through plasma volume expansion and the judicious use of vasopressor agents, usually phenylephrine or dopamine. Raised perfusion pressure has been associated with clinical improvement in many patients, but high arterial pressure may promote rebleeding in unprotected aneurysms. Treatment with induced hypertension and hypervolemia generally requires monitoring of arterial and central venous pressures and in severe cases, the pulmonary artery wedge pressure. Volume expansion helps prevent hypotension, augments cardiac output, and reduces blood viscosity by reducing hematocrit. This method is called "triple-H" (hypertension, hemodilution, and hypervolemic) therapy.

If symptomatic vasospasm persists despite optimal medical therapy, intraarterial papaverine and percutaneous transluminal angioplasty are considered. Vasodilatation following angioplasty appears to be permanent, allowing triple-H therapy to be tapered sooner. The vasodilating effects of papaverine do not last more than 12 to 24 h.

Acute hydrocephalus can cause stupor or coma. It may clear spontaneously or require temporary ventricular drainage. When chronic hydrocephalus develops, ventricular shunting is the treatment of choice.

Free-water restriction is contraindicated in patients with SAH at risk for vasospasm because hypovolemia and hypotension may occur and precipitate cerebral ischemia. Many patients continue to experience a decline in serum sodium despite normal saline parenteral fluids. Frequently, supplemental oral salt coupled with normal saline will mitigate hyponatremia, but often patients will need hypertonic saline in addition. Care must be taken to not correct serum sodium too quickly in patients with marked hyponatremia of several days' duration, as central pontine myelinolysis (Chap. 376) may occur. All patients should have pneumatic compression stockings applied to prevent pulmonary embolism. Systemic heparin is contraindicated in patients with ruptured and untreated aneurysms; it is a relative contraindication following craniotomy, and it may delay thrombosis of a coiled aneurysm.

Vascular Anomalies   Vascular anomalies can be divided into congenital vascular malformations and acquired vascular lesions.

Congenital vascular malformations   True AVMs, venous anomalies, and capillary telangiectasias are congenital lesions that usually remain clinically silent through life.

True *arteriovenous malformations* are congenital shunts between the arterial and venous systems that may present as headache, focal seizures, and intracranial hemorrhage. AVMs consist of a tangle of abnormal vessels across the cortical surface or deep within the brain substance. AVMs vary in size from a small blemish a few millimeters in diameter to a huge mass of tortuous channels composing an arteriovenous shunt of sufficient magnitude to raise cardiac output. The blood vessels forming the tangle interposed between arteries and veins are usually abnormally thin and do not have a normal structure. AVMs occur in all parts of the cerebral hemispheres, brainstem, and spinal cord, but the largest ones are most frequently in the posterior half of the hemispheres, commonly forming a wedge-shaped lesion extending from the cortex to the ventricle.

Although the lesion is present from birth, bleeding or other symptoms are most common between the ages of 10 and 30, occasionally as late as the fifties. AVMs are more frequent in men, and rare familial cases have been described.

Headache (without bleeding) may be hemicranial and throbbing, like migraine, or diffuse. Focal seizures, with or without generalization, occur in about 30% of cases. Half of AVMs become evident as intracerebral hemorrhages. In most, the hemorrhage is mainly intraparenchymal with a small amount of spillage into the subarachnoid space. Blood is usually not deposited in the basal cisterns, and symptomatic cerebral vasospasm is rare. The threat of rerupture in the early weeks is low. Hemorrhages may be massive, leading to death, or may be as small as 1 cm in diameter, leading to minor focal symptoms or no deficit. The AVM may be large enough to steal blood away from adjacent normal brain tissue or to increase venous pressure significantly to produce venous ischemia locally and in remote areas of the brain. This is seen most often with large AVMs in the territory of the MCA.

Large AVMs of the anterior circulation may be associated with a systolic and diastolic bruit (sometimes self-audible) over the eye, forehead, or neck and a bounding carotid pulse. Headache at the onset of AVM rupture is not generally as explosive as with aneurysmal rupture. MRI is better than CT for diagnosis, although contrast CT scanning sometimes detects calcification of the AVM.

Surgical treatment of symptomatic AVMs, often with preoperative embolization to reduce operative bleeding, is generally indicated for accessible lesions. Sterotaxic radiation, an alternative to surgery, can produce a slow sclerosis of arterial channels over 1 to 2 years.

Most data suggest that patients with asymptomatic AVMs have a low risk for hemorrhage; the risk increases after a first hemorrhage to about 2 to 3% annually. Several angiographic features of the AVM can be used to help predict future bleeding risk. Paradoxically, smaller lesions seem to have a higher hemorrhage rate. The mortality rate with each bleed is about 15%.

Venous anomalies are the result of development of anomalous cerebral, cerebellar, or brainstem drainage. These structures, unlike AVMs, are functional venous channels. They are of little clinical significance and should be ignored if found incidentally on brain imaging studies. Surgical resection of these anomalies may result in venous infarction and hemorrhage. Venous anomalies may be associated with cavernous malformations (see below), which do carry some bleeding risk. If resection of a cavernous malformation is attempted, the venous anomaly should not be disturbed.

Capillary telangiectasias are true capillary malformations that often form extensive vascular networks through an otherwise normal brain structure. The pons and deep cerebral white matter are typical locations, and these capillary malformations can be seen in patients with hereditary hemorrhagic telangiectasia (Osler-Rendu-Weber) syndrome. If bleeding does occur, it rarely produces mass effect or significant symptoms. No treatment options exist.

Acquired vascular lesions Cavernous angiomas are tufts of capillary sinusoids that form within the deep hemispheric white matter and brainstem with no normal intervening neural structures. The pathogenesis is unclear. Familial cavernous angiomas have been mapped to several different chromosomal loci; the gene responsible for 7q-linked form encodes a protein that interacts with a member of the RAS family of GTPases. Cavernous angiomas are typically <1 cm in diameter and are often associated with a venous anomaly. Bleeding is usually of small volume, causing slight mass effect only. The bleeding risk for single cavernous malformations is 0.7 to 1.5% per year and may be higher for patients with prior clinical hemorrhage or multiple malformations. Seizures may occur if the malformation is located near the cerebral cortex. Surgical resection eliminates bleeding risk and may reduce seizure risk, but it is reserved for those malformations that form near the brain surface. Radiation treatment has not been shown to be of benefit.

Dural arteriovenous fistulas are acquired connections usually from a dural artery to a dural sinus. Patients may complain of a pulse-synchronous cephalic bruit ("pulsatile tinnitus") and headache. Depending on the magnitude of the shunt, venous pressures may rise high enough to cause cortical ischemia or venous hypertension and hemorrhage. Surgical and endovascular techniques are usually curative. These fistulas may form because of trauma, but most are idiopathic. There is an association between fistulas and dural sinus thrombosis. Fistulas have been observed to appear months to years following venous sinus thrombosis, suggesting that angiogenesis factors elaborated from the thrombotic process may cause these anomalous connections to form. Alternatively, dural arteriovenous fistulas can produce venous sinus occlusion over time, perhaps from the high pressure and high flow through a venous structure.

BIBLIOGRAPHY

ALBERS GW et al: Antithrombotic and thrombolytic therapy for ischemic stroke. Fifth ACCP Consensus Conference on Antithrombotic Therapy. Chest 114:683S, 1998

BARNETT HJ et al: Benefit of carotid endarterectomy in patients with symptomatic moderate or severe stenosis. North American Symptomatic Carotid Endarterectomy Trial Collaborators. N Engl J Med 339:1415, 1998

BILLER J et al: *Guidelines for Carotid Endarterectomy*. A statement for healthcare professionals from a Special Writing Group of the Stroke Council, American Heart Association. Circulation 97:501, 1998

CAPRIE STEERING COMMITTEE: A randomised, blinded, trial of clopidogrel versus aspirin in patients at risk of ischaemic events (CAPRIE). Lancet 348:1329, 1996

CAST: Randomised placebo-controlled trial of early aspirin use in 20,000 patients with acute ischaemic stroke. CAST (Chinese Acute Stroke Trial) Collaborative Group. Lancet 349:1641, 1997

EUROPEAN CAROTID SURGERY TRIALISTS' COLLABORATIVE GROUP: MRC European Carotid Surgery Trial: Interim results for symptomatic patients with severe (70–99%) or with mild (0–29%) carotid stenosis. Lancet 337:1235, 1991

EXECUTIVE COMMITTEE FOR THE ASYMPTOMATIC CAROTID ATHEROSCLEROSIS STUDY: Endarterectomy for asymptomatic carotid artery stenosis. JAMA 273:1421, 1995

GORTER JW: Major bleeding during anticoagulation after cerebral ischemia: Patterns and risk factors. Stroke Prevention In Reversible Ischemia Trial (SPIRIT). European Atrial Fibrillation Trial (EAFT) study groups. Neurology 53:1319, 1999

HACKE W et al: Randomised double-blind placebo-controlled trial of thrombolytic therapy with intravenous alteplase in acute ischaemic stroke (ECASS II). Second European-Australasian Acute Stroke Study Investigators. Lancet 352:1245, 1998

INTERNATIONAL STUDY OF UNRUPTURED INTRACRANIAL ANEURYSMS INVESTIGATORS: Unruptured intracranial aneurysms—risk of rupture and risks of surgical intervention. N Engl J Med 339:1725, 1998

INZITARI D et al: The causes and risk of stroke in patients with asymptomatic internal-carotid-artery stenosis. N Engl J Med 342:169, 2000

LABERGE-LE COUTEULX CS et al: Truncating mutations in CCM1, encoding KRIT1, cause hereditary cavernous angiomas. Nat Genet 23:189, 1999

LAUPACIS A et al: Antithrombotic therapy for atrial fibrillation. Chest 114:579S, 1998

PLEHN JF et al: Reduction of stroke incidence after myocardial infarction with pravastatin: The Cholesterol and Recurrent Events (CARE) study. The Care Investigators. Circulation 99:216, 1999

SHERMAN DG et al: Intravenous ancrod for treatment of acute ischemic stroke. The STAT study: A randomized controlled trial. JAMA 283:2395, 2000

THE INTERNATIONAL STROKE TRIAL (IST): A randomised trial of aspirin, subcutaneous heparin, both, or neither among 19,435 patients with acute ischaemic stroke. International Stroke Trial Collaborative Group. Lancet 349:1569, 1997

THE NATIONAL INSTITUTE OF NEUROLOGICAL DISORDERS AND STROKE RT-PA STROKE STUDY GROUP: Tissue plasminogen activator for acute ischemic stroke. N Engl J Med 333:1581, 1995

THE PUBLICATIONS COMMITTEE FOR THE TRIAL OF ORG 10172 IN ACUTE STROKE TREATMENT (TOAST) INVESTIGATORS: Low molecular weight heparinoid, ORG 10172 (danaparoid), and outcome after acute ischemic stroke: A randomized controlled trial. JAMA 279:1265, 1998

THE STROKE PREVENTION IN REVERSIBLE ISCHEMIA TRIAL (SPIRIT) STUDY GROUP: A randomized trial of anticoagulants versus aspirin after cerebral ischemia of presumed arterial origin. Ann Neurol 42:857, 1997

TURPIE AGG et al: A comparison of aspirin with placebo in patients treated with warfarin after heart-valve replacement. N Engl J Med 329:534, 1993

WILTERDINK JL, EASTON JD: Dipyridamole plus aspirin in cerebrovascular disease. Arch Neurol 56:1087, 1999

| 362 | *Thomas D. Bird* |

ALZHEIMER'S DISEASE AND OTHER PRIMARY DEMENTIAS

AD	Alzheimer's disease	FTD	frontotemporal dementia
ALS	amyotrophic lateral sclerosis	HD	Huntington's disease
APP	amyloid precursor protein	MRI	magnetic resonance imaging
CAT	choline acetyltransferase	NFTs	neurofibrillary tangles
CJD	Creutzfeldt-Jakob disease	NPH	normal-pressure hydrocephalus
CSF	cerebrospinal fluid	PET	positron emission tomography
CT	computed tomography	SSRIs	selective serotonin reuptake
EEG	electroencephalogram		inhibitors
FAD	familial AD		

ALZHEIMER'S DISEASE   Alzheimer's disease (AD) is the most common cause of dementia in western countries. Approximately 10% of all persons over the age of 70 have significant memory loss; in more than half the cause is AD. This translates into approximately 3 to 4 million persons with AD in the United States, with a total health care cost of more than $80 billion per year. It is estimated that the annual total cost of caring for a single AD patient in an advanced stage of the disease is $47,000. The disease also exacts a heavy emotional toll on family members and caregivers. AD was first described in 1907 in a 55-year-old woman by Professor Alois Alzheimer in Germany. The condition was initially thought to represent a relatively uncommon form of presenile dementia. However, it has become clear that AD can occur in any decade of adulthood and is the most common cause of dementia in the elderly. The disease is defined as a clinical-pathologic entity. Clinically, AD most often presents with subtle onset of memory loss followed by a slowly progressive dementia that has a course of several years. Pathologically there is gross, diffuse atrophy of the cerebral cortex with secondary enlargement of the ventricular system. Microscopically there are extracellular neuritic plaques containing $A\beta$ amyloid, silver-staining neurofibrillary tangles in neuronal cytoplasm, and accumulation of $A\beta$ amyloid in arterial walls of cerebral blood vessels (see "Pathogenesis," below). The recent identification of four different susceptibility genes for AD has provided a foundation for rapid progress in understanding the biologic basis of the disease.

Clinical Manifestations   In the early stages of the disease, the memory loss may go unrecognized or may be ascribed to benign forgetfulness. Slowly the cognitive problems begin to interfere with daily activities, such as keeping track of finances, following instructions on the job, driving, shopping, and housekeeping. Some patients are unstages of the disease, some persons remain ambulatory but wander aimlessly and may have complete loss of judgment, reason, and cognitive abilities. Hallucinations and delusions are common; they are usually concrete and not too complex or bizarre. For example, patients may falsely accuse a spouse of infidelity, not recognize an old friend, think a visitor is a burglar, or become frightened of their own image in a mirror. Loss of inhibitions and belligerence may occur and may even alternate with passivity and social withdrawal. Sleep-wake patterns may be disturbed, and nighttime wandering may be very disruptive to the household. Some patients develop a shuffling gait with generalized muscle rigidity associated with slowness and awkwardness of movement. The patients often look parkinsonian but rarely have a rapid, rhythmic, resting tremor. In end-stage AD, patients frequently, but not always, become rigid, mute, incontinent, and bedridden. Help may be needed with the simplest tasks, such as eating, dressing, and toilet function. They may show hyperactive tendon reflexes and primitive sucking and snouting reflexes. Myoclonic jerks (sudden brief contractions of various muscles or the whole body) may occur spontaneously or in response to physical or auditory stimulation. This phenomenon raises the possibility of Creutzfeldt-Jakob disease (CJD) (Chap. 375), but the course of AD is much more prolonged. Generalized seizures may also occur. Death usually results from malnutrition, secondary infections, or heart disease. The typical duration of AD is 8 to 10 years, but the course can range from 1 to 25 years. For unknown reasons, some AD patients show a steady downhill decline in function, while others have prolonged plateaus without major deterioration.

Differential Diagnosis Early in the disease course, other etiologies of dementia should be excluded. These include treatable entities such as thyroid disease, vitamin deficiencies, brain tumor, drug and medication intoxication, chronic infection, and severe depression (pseudodementia) (see Chap. 26). Neuroimaging studies [computed tomography (CT) and magnetic resonance imaging (MRI)] are not specific for AD and may be normal early in the course of the disease. However, neuroimaging helps to exclude other disorders, such as primary and secondary neoplasms, multiinfarct dementia, diffuse white matter disease, and normal-pressure hydrocephalus. As AD progresses, diffuse cortical atrophy becomes apparent, and detailed MRI scans show atrophy of the hippocampus (Fig. 362-1A). The electroencephalogram (EEG) in AD may be normal or show nonspecific slowing. Routine spinal fluid examination gives normal results. Research studies have indicated a general decrease in cerebrospinal fluid (CSF) Aβ amyloid levels with an increase in tau protein. There is considerable overlap of these levels with those of the normal aged population, and the usefulness of these measurements in diagnosis remains unclear. Combining the results of both measurements may prove to be most helpful. The use of blood apolipoprotein (Apo) E genotyping is discussed under "Pathogenesis," below. Slowly progressive decline in memory and orientation, normal results on laboratory tests, and an MRI or CT scan showing only diffuse cortical atrophy including the hippocampus is highly suggestive of AD. A clinical diagnosis of AD reached after careful evaluation is confirmed at autopsy 80 to 90% of the time. The misdiagnosed cases usually represent one of the other dementing disorders described later in this chapter. Relatively simple clinical clues are useful in the differential diagnosis. Early prominent gait disturbance with only mild memory loss suggests normal-pressure hydrocephalus (see below). Resting tremor with stooped posture, bradykinesia, and masked face suggests

FIGURE 362-1 Alzheimer's disease. Axial T1-weighted MR images through the midbrain of a normal 86-year-old athletic individual (*A*) and a 77-year-old male (*B*) with Alzheimer's disease. Note that both individuals have prominent sulci and slight dilatation of the lateral ventricles. However, there is a reduction in the volume of the hippocampus of the patient with Alzheimer's disease (*arrows*) compared with the normal-for-age hippocampus of the older individual. Below, fluorodeoxyglucose positron emission tomographic scans of a normal control (*C*) and a patient with Alzheimer's disease (*D*). Note that the patient has decreased activity in the parietal lobes bilaterally (*arrows*), a typical finding in this condition. (*Images courtesy of TF Budinger, University of California.*)

aware of these difficulties (agnosognosia), and others have considerable insight, resulting in frustration and anxiety. These major differences in insight have no clear explanation. Change of environment may be bewildering, and the patient may become lost on walks or while driving an automobile. In the middle stages of the disease, the patient is unable to work, is easily lost and confused, and requires daily supervision. Social graces, routine behavior, and superficial conversation may be surprisingly retained. Language may be impaired, especially comprehension and naming of objects. In some patients, aphasia is an early and prominent feature. Word-finding difficulties and circumlocution may be a problem even when formal testing demonstrates intact naming and fluency. Although confrontation naming is frequently deficient, there are often other language deficits as well, including impairments in fluency, comprehension, and repetition. Various apraxias are also common, i.e., deficits in performing sequential motor tasks such as dressing, eating, solving simple puzzles, and copying geometric figures. Patients may be unable to do simple calculations or tell time. Rarely, AD patients may have a form of cortical blindness in which they deny their inability to see. This correlates at autopsy with severe neuropathologic changes in the visual cortex. In the late

Parkinson's disease (Chap. 363). Chronic alcoholism suggests vitamin deficiency. Loss of sensibility to position and vibration stimuli accompanied by Babinski responses suggests vitamin B_{12} deficiency (Chap. 368). Early onset of a seizure suggests a metastatic or primary brain neoplasm (Chap. 370). A past history of long-term depression suggests pseudodementia (see below). A history of treatment for insomnia, anxiety, psychiatric disturbance, or epilepsy suggests chronic drug intoxication. Rapid progression over a few weeks or months associated with ataxia, rigidity, and myoclonus suggests CJD (Chap. 375). Prominent behavioral changes with intact memory and lobar atrophy on brain imaging suggests frontotemporal dementia (FTD). A positive family history of dementia suggests either one of the familial forms of AD or one of the other genetic disorders associated with dementia, such as Huntington's disease (see below), familial FTD (see below), familial forms of prion diseases, or rare forms of hereditary ataxias (Chap. 364).

Pathogenesis The most important risk factors for AD are old age and a positive family history. The frequency of AD increases with each decade of adult life to reach 20 to 40% of the population over the age of 85. A positive family history of dementia suggests a genetic cause of AD, as discussed below. Female gender may also be a risk factor independent of the greater longevity of women. Unconfirmed studies have suggested that postmenopausal estrogen use is associated with a decreased frequency of AD. Some AD patients have a past history of head trauma with concussion, but this appears to be a relatively minor risk factor. There is some suggestion that AD is more common in groups with lower educational attainment, but education influences test-taking ability, and it is clear that AD can affect persons of all intellectual levels. One unconfirmed study found that the capacity to express complex written language in early adulthood correlated with a decreased risk for AD. Numerous environmental factors, including aluminum, mercury, viruses, and prions, have been proposed as causes of AD, but none has been proved to play a role. Preliminary studies have suggested that inflammation may play some role in the pathogenesis of AD, as the use of nonsteroidal anti-inflammatory agents is associated with decreased risk. Vascular disease does not seem to be a direct cause of AD, even though there is an associated amyloid angiopathy.

Positron emission tomography (PET) has indicated that the earliest metabolic changes in AD occur in parietal cortex (Fig. 362-1C, D). At autopsy, the most severe pathology is usually seen in the hippocampus, temporal cortex, and nucleus basalis. The most important microscopic findings are neuritic "senile" plaques and cytoplasmic neurofibrillary tangles (NFTs). These two lesions accumulate in small numbers during normal aging of the brain but occur in quantitative excess in the dementia of AD. The neuritic plaques contain a central core that includes $A\beta$ amyloid, proteoglycans, Apo E, α_1 antichymotrypsin, and other proteins. $A\beta$ amyloid is a 4.2-kDa protein of 39 to 42 amino acids that is derived proteolytically from a larger transmembrane protein (amyloid precursor protein, APP) through cleavage by two enzymes termed β and γ secretase. The normal function of $A\beta$ amyloid is unknown. APP has been shown to have neurotrophic and neuroprotective activities. The plaque core is surrounded by the debris of degenerating neurons, microglia, and macrophages. The accumulation of $A\beta$ amyloid in cerebral arterioles is termed *amyloid angiopathy*. The NFTs were first noted by Alzheimer. They are silver-staining, twisted neurofilaments in neuronal cytoplasm that represent abnormally phosphorylated tau (τ) protein and appear as paired helical filaments by electron microscopy. Tau is a microtubule-associated protein that may function to assemble and stabilize the microtubules that convey cell organelles, glycoproteins, and other important materials through the neuron. The ability of tau protein to bind to microtubule segments is determined partly by the number of phosphate groups attached to it. Increased phosphorylation of tau protein may disturb this normal process. Biochemically, AD is associated with a decrease in the cerebral cortical levels of several proteins and neurotransmitters, especially acetylcholine, its synthetic enzyme choline acetyltransferase (CAT), and nicotinic cholinergic receptors. Reduction of acetylcholine may be related

in part to degeneration of cholinergic neurons in the nucleus basalis of Meynert that project to many areas of cortex. There is also reduction in norepinephrine levels in brainstem nuclei such as the locus coeruleus.

Several genetic factors are known to play important roles in the pathogenesis of at least some cases of AD. One is the *APP* gene on chromosome 21. Adults with trisomy 21 (Down's syndrome) consistently develop the typical neuropathologic hallmarks of AD if they survive beyond age 40. Many also develop a progressive dementia superimposed on their baseline mental retardation. APP is a membrane-spanning protein that is subsequently processed into smaller units, including the $A\beta$ amyloid that is deposited in the neuritic plaques of AD. Presumably the extra dose of the *APP* gene on chromosome 21 is the initiating cause of AD in adult Down's syndrome and eventually results in an excess of cerebral $A\beta$ amyloid. Furthermore, a few families with early-onset familial AD (FAD) have been discovered to have point mutations in the *APP* gene. Although very rare, these families were the first indication of a single-gene autosomal dominant transmission of AD. The most frequent of these *APP* mutations is substitution of valine for isoleucine at position 717. Elevated plasma $A\beta$ peptide may be a risk factor for developing AD in the general population.

Investigation of large families with multigenerational FAD led subsequently to the discovery of two additional AD genes, termed the *presenilins*. Presenilin-1 (*PS-1*) is on chromosome 14 and encodes a protein called S182. Mutations in this gene cause an early-onset AD (onset before age 60 and often before age 50) that is transmitted in an autosomal dominant, highly penetrant fashion. More than 40 different mutations have been found in the *PS-1* gene in families from a wide range of ethnic backgrounds. Presenilin-2 (*PS-2*) is on chromosome 1 and encodes a protein called STM2. A mutation in the *PS-2* gene was first found in a group of American families with Volga German ethnic background. The two genes (*PS-1* and *PS-2*) are highly homologous and encode similar proteins that at first appeared to have seven transmembrane domains (hence the designation *STM*), but subsequent studies have suggested eight such domains with a ninth submembrane region. The normal function of these proteins and the means by which mutations affecting them result in AD is unknown. Both S182 and STM2 are cytoplasmic neuronal proteins that are widely expressed throughout the nervous system. They are homologous to a cell-trafficking protein, sel 12, that is found in the nematode *Coenorhabditis elegans*. Knockout of the *PS-1* gene in mice causes embryonic death, but PS-2 knockout mice have only mild pulmonary pathology, suggesting very different primary functions of the two proteins. The AD pathology in transgenic mice carrying both APP and PS-1 mutations is worse than that in mice with only a single mutation. Also, the mutant human *PS-1* gene protects PS-1 knockout mice from embryonic lethality, and this observation fits with the idea that *PS-1* mutations cause disease by a toxic gain of function. Patients with mutations in these genes have elevated plasma levels of $A\beta$ amyloid, suggesting a possible link between the presenilins and APP. There is evidence that presenilin-1 may normally cleave APP at the γ secretase site, and mutations in either gene (*PS-1* or *APP*) may disturb this function. Mutations in *PS-1* have thus far proved to be the most common cause of early-onset FAD, representing 40 to 70% of this relatively rare syndrome. Mutations in *PS-1* tend to produce AD with an earlier age of onset (mean, 45 years) and a shorter, more rapidly progressive course (mean duration, 6 to 7 years) than the disease caused by mutations in *PS-2* (onset, 53 years; duration, 11 years). Some carriers of uncommon *PS-2* mutations have had onset of dementia after the age of 70. Mutations in the presenilins are rarely involved in the more common sporadic cases of late-onset AD occurring in the general population. Molecular DNA blood testing for these uncommon mutations is now possible on a research basis, and mutation analysis of *PS-1* is commercially available. Such testing is likely to be positive only in early-onset cases of FAD. Any testing of asymptomatic persons at risk must be done in the context of formal, thoughtful genetic counseling (Chap. 359).

A discovery of great importance has implicated the *Apo E* gene on chromosome 19 in the pathogenesis of late-onset familial and sporadic forms of AD. Apo E is involved in cholesterol transport (Chap. 344) and has three alleles: ε2, ε3, and ε4. The ε4 allele of *Apo E* shows a strong association with AD in the general population, including sporadic and late-onset familial cases. Approximately 24 to 30% of the normal white population has at least one ε4 allele (12 to 15% allele frequency), and about 2% are ε4/4 homozygotes. In a group of AD patients, approximately 40 to 65% have at least one ε4 allele, a highly significant difference compared with controls. On the other hand, many AD patients have no ε4 allele, and individuals with ε4 may never develop AD. Therefore, ε4 is neither necessary nor sufficient as a cause of AD. Nevertheless, it is clear that the Apo E ε4 allele, especially in the homozygous 4/4 state, is an important risk factor for AD. It appears to act as a dose-dependent modifier of age of onset, with the earliest onset associated with the ε4/4 homozygous state. One study found a 45% risk for developing AD by age 73 in females who were 4/4 homozygotes. It is unknown how Apo E functions as a risk factor modifying age of onset. Apo E is present in the neuritic amyloid plaques of AD, and may also be involved in NFT formation, because it binds to tau protein. Apo E4 decreases neurite outgrowth in cultures of dorsal root ganglion neurons. There is suggestive evidence that the ε2 allele may be "protective." Interesting but unconfirmed reports suggest that AD patients with an ε4 allele may be less responsive cholinesterase inhibitor drugs. The use of Apo E testing in the diagnosis of AD is controversial. It is not indicated as a predictive test in normal persons, because its precise predictive value is unclear, and many individuals with the ε4 allele never develop dementia. However, some cognitively normal ε4/4 homozygotes have been found by PET to have decreased cerebral cortical metabolic rates, suggesting possible presymptomatic abnormalities compatible with the earliest stage of AD. Studies show that in demented persons who meet clinical criteria for AD, the finding of an ε4 allele increases the reliability of diagnosis. However, the absence of an ε4 allele does not eliminate the diagnosis of AD. Furthermore, all patients with dementia, including those with an ε4 allele, require a search for reversible causes of their cognitive impairment. Nevertheless, Apo E remains the single most important biologic marker associated with risk for AD, and studies of its functional role and diagnostic usefulness are progressing rapidly. Its association (or lack thereof) with other dementing illnesses needs to be fully evaluated. The ε4 allele is not associated with the dementia of Parkinson's disease, FTD, or CJD.

Additional genes are also likely to be involved in AD, including a potential candidate on chromosome 12 (α_2-macroglobulin).

TREATMENT The management of Alzheimer's disease is difficult and frustrating, because there is no specific treatment and the primary focus is on long-term amelioration of associated behavioral and neurologic problems. Building rapport with the patient, family members, and other caregivers is essential to successful management.

Tacrine (tetrahydroaminoacridine) and donepezil (Aricept) are the only drugs presently approved by the U.S. Food and Drug Administration (FDA) for treatment of AD. Their pharmacologic action is presumed to be inhibition of cholinesterase, with a resulting increase in cerebral levels of acetylcholine. Double-blind, placebo-controlled, crossover studies with cholinesterase inhibitors have shown them to be associated with improved caregiver ratings of patients' functioning and with an apparent decreased rate of decline in cognitive test scores over periods of up to 2 years. Such studies are difficult to perform because of the subjective nature of many of the observations and the lack of a uniform rate of decline among patients. Nevertheless, a small but important minority of AD patients (approximately 10 to 20%)

appear to show a modest response to these agents and tolerate their side effects (which include dose-related nausea, vomiting, diarrhea, bradycardia, and dizziness). Even without actual improvement these agents may provide stabilization of the patient's condition for a period of months. There is no evidence that these drugs are beneficial in the late stages of AD. Tacrine may be hepatotoxic, necessitating frequent testing of liver function and adjustment of the dose. Donepezil is not hepatotoxic and can be administered once daily (5 to 10 mg). Contraindications for cholinesterase inhibitor treatment include liver disease, alcoholism, peptic ulcer disease, chronic obstructive pulmonary disease; and bradycardia. Clinical trials of other anticholinesterase drugs are in progress.

In a recent prospective observational study, the use of estrogen replacement therapy appeared to protect—by about 50%—against development of AD in women. This study appeared to confirm the results of two earlier case-controlled studies. On the other hand, a prospective treatment study of women with AD found no difference between estrogen and placebo. The mechanism of possible estrogen effects on Alzheimer's disease is unknown but may result from direct effects on cholinergic neurons, antioxidant properties, or a lowering of levels of Apo E. A prospective randomized clinical trial of estrogen replacement therapy in women is underway.

In patients with moderately advanced AD, a prospective trial of the antioxidants selegiline, α tocopherol (vitamin E), or both demonstrated no significant benefit on primary outcomes of progression. However, a modest beneficial effect of each treatment compared to placebo was present in secondary analyses that controlled for intergroup difference in baseline dementia scores. These possible beneficial effects are small in magnitude and require confirmation.

A randomized, double-blind, placebo-controlled trial of an extract of *Ginkgo biloba* found modest improvement in cognitive function in subjects with AD and vascular dementia. This study requires confirmation before *G. biloba* is considered an effective treatment for dementia, because there was a high subject dropout rate and no improvement on a clinician's judgment scale.

As noted above, several retrospective studies have also suggested a protective effect on dementia of nonsteroidal anti-inflammatory agents. Controlled prospective studies are in progress.

In an APP mutation mouse model of AD, weekly immunization with Aβ peptide both prevented the occurrence and reversed the accumulation of amyloid plaques in the brain. The possible benefit of this treatment strategy in humans is unknown and is under evaluation. In addition, the identification of a protease that acts as the APP β secretase has raised the possibility that inhibiting this enzyme might decrease amyloid accumulation in brain, another potential therapeutic strategy for AD.

Mild to moderate depression is common in the early stages of AD and may respond to antidepressant medication. Selective serotonin reuptake inhibitors (SSRIs) are commonly used, as are tricyclic antidepressants with low anticholinergic side effects (desipramine and nortriptyline). Generalized seizures should be treated with an appropriate anticonvulsant, such as phenytoin or carbamazepine. Agitation, insomnia, hallucinations, and belligerence are especially troublesome characteristics of some AD patients and often are responsible for nursing home placement. Mild sedation with benadryl may help insomnia, and agitation has been variously treated with phenothiazines (such as thioridazine), haloperidol, risperidone, and benzodiazepines (such as lorazepam). These medications frequently have untoward side effects, including sedation, confusion, increased muscle tone, and adventitious movements. Low-dose haloperidol (0.5 to 2 mg), trazodone, buspirone, propranolol, and olanzapine may be the most helpful and have the fewest side effects. The few controlled studies comparing drugs with behavioral intervention in the treatment of agitation suggest that both approaches are equally effective. However, careful, daily, nondrug behavior management is often not available, rendering medication necessary. In the early stages of AD, memory aids such as notebooks and posted daily reminders are helpful. Common sense and clinical studies have shown that family members should emphasize activities that are pleasant and deemphasize those that are unpleasant. Kitchens, bathrooms, and bedrooms need to be made safe, and patients eventually must stop driving. Loss of independence and change of environment may worsen confusion, agitation, and anger. Communication and repeated calm reassurance are necessary. Caregiver "burnout" is common, often resulting in nursing home placement of the patient and respite breaks for the caregiver help to maintain successful long-term management of the patient. Use of adult daycare centers can be most helpful. Local and national support groups, such as the Alzheimer's Disease and Related Disorders Association, are valuable resources.

VASCULAR DEMENTIA Dementia associated with cerebral vascular disease can be divided into two general categories: multi-infarct dementia and diffuse white matter dementia (also called subcortical arteriosclerotic encephalopathy or Binswanger's disease). Cerebral vascular disease appears to be a more common cause of dementia in Asia than in Europe and North America. Individuals who have had several strokes may develop chronic cognitive deficits, commonly called *multi-infarct dementia*. The strokes may be large or small (sometimes lacunar) and usually involve several different brain regions. In fact, one study has shown that lacunar stroke is the most common stroke subtype associated with dementia. The occurrence of dementia seems to depend partly on the total volume of damaged cortex, but it is also more common in individuals with left-hemisphere lesions, independent of any language disturbance, and when the stroke involves the hippocampus. Subcortical infarction has been associated with both frontal and global cerebral hypometabolism, which may in turn lead to dementia. The patients give a history of episodes of sudden neurologic deterioration. Multi-infarct dementia patients usually also have a history of hypertension, diabetes, coronary artery disease, or other manifestations of diffuse atherosclerosis. Physical examination usually reveals focal neurologic deficits such as hemiparesis, unilateral Babinski reflex, a visual field defect, or pseudobulbar palsy. The recurrent strokes result in a stepwise progression of disease. Neuroimaging studies clearly show the multiple areas of infarction. Thus, the history and neuroimaging findings differentiate this condition from AD. However, AD and multiple infarctions are both common and sometimes occur together. With normal aging, there is also an accumulation of amyloid in cerebral blood vessels, leading to a condition called *cerebral amyloid angiopathy of aging* (not associated with dementia), which predisposes older persons to hemorrhagic lobar stroke. AD patients with amyloid angiopathy and hypertension also appear to be at increased risk of cerebral infarction. Apo E ε4 has been reported to be a risk factor for amyloid angiopathy independent of AD.

Some persons with dementia are discovered on MRI studies to have bilateral abnormalities of subcortical white matter, termed *diffuse white matter disease* (or leukoaraiosis) (Fig. 362-2). The dementia may be of subtle onset and slow progression, features that distinguish it from multi-infarct dementia. (A few such patients have been described with apparently sudden onset of cognitive impairment.) Early symptoms are mild confusion, apathy, change in personality, and memory deficit. Marked difficulties in judgment and orientation and dependence on others for daily activities develop later. Euphoria, elation, or aggressive behavior are common. A mixed picture of pyramidal and cerebellar signs may be present in the same patient. Lateralizing motor signs are uncommon. A gait disorder appears in at least half the patients. In advanced cases, urinary incontinence and dysarthria with or without pseudobulbar features are frequent. Seizures and myoclonic jerks appear in a minority of patients. This disorder appears to be the result of chronic ischemia due to occlusive disease of small penetrating cerebral arteries and arterioles (microangiopathy). The patients usually, but not always, have a history of hypertension, but any disease causing stenosis of small cerebral vessels may be the critical underlying factor. An association with abnormalities of the coagulation-fibrinolysis pathway has been reported. Binswanger described several

FIGURE 362-2 Diffuse white matter disease (Binswanger's disease). Axial T2-weighted MR image through the lateral ventricles reveals multiple areas of abnormal high signal intensity involving the periventricular white matter as well as the corona radiata and lentiform nuclei (*arrows*). While seen in some individuals with normal cognition, this appearance is more pronounced in patients with dementia of a vascular etiology.

patients with this condition, but the term *Binswanger's disease* should be used with caution, because it does not really identify a single entity. Other rare causes of white matter disease may also present with dementia, such as adult metachromatic leukodystrophy and progressive multifocal leukoencephalopathy (papovavirus infection). The term *CADASIL* refers to an inherited form of diffuse white matter disease described as *c*erebral *a*utosomal *d*ominant *a*rteriopathy with *s*ubcortical *i*nfarcts and *l*eukoencephalopathy. Clinically there is a progressive dementia developing in the fifth to seventh decades in multiple family members who may also have a history of migraine and recurrent stroke without hypertension. Skin biopsy may show characteristic dense bodies in the media of arterioles. The disease is caused by mutations in the notch 3 gene, but there is no commercially available genetic test. The frequency of this disorder is unknown.

Treatment of vascular dementia must be focused on the underlying causes, such as hypertension, atherosclerosis, and diabetes. Recovery of lost cognitive function is not likely to occur.

FRONTOTEMPORAL DEMENTIA AND PICK'S DISEASE FTD may be the cause of as many as 10% of all cases of dementia and an even greater proportion of presenile onset (<65 years) cases. The patients are often irritable; have loss of inhibitions; and do better on construction, copying, and calculation tasks than patients with AD. Memory is often intact early in the disease. Patients may be socially inappropriate or remote and withdrawn. Hoarding, overeating, and weight gain are common. Rigidity and mutism often occur late in the disease. Imaging studies reveal atrophy confined to the frontal or frontal and temporal lobes. The condition is heterogeneous, and the broad designation FTD usually includes Pick's disease (discussed below) as a subcategory. An autosomal dominant genetic form of FTD has been linked to DNA markers on chromosome 17. Some of these families have disinhibition dementia associated with motor neuron disease, whereas others display parkinsonian features. Cytoplasmic aggregations of tau protein are found in many neurons of cortex, striatum, and substantia nigra. These aggregates sometimes resemble those found in progressive supranuclear palsy (Chap. 363) or AD. This con-

A   **B**

FIGURE 362-3 Normal pressure hydrocephalus. *A.* Sagittal T1-weighted MR image demonstrates dilatation of the lateral ventricle and stretching of the corpus callosum (*arrows*), depression of the floor of the third ventricle (*single arrowhead*), and enlargement of the aqueduct (*double arrowheads*). Note the diffuse dilatation of the lateral, third, and fourth ventricles with a patent aqueduct, typical of communicating hydrocephalus. *B.* Axial T2-weighted MR images demonstrate dilatation of the lateral ventricles without cortical atrophy. This patient underwent successful ventriculoperitoneal shunting.

dition is referred to as *frontotemporal dementia with parkinsonism linked to chromosome 17* (FTDP-17). Many FTDP-17 families have been found to inherit missense mutations in the tau gene that disturb the microtubule-binding function of tau or alter the carefully regulated alternative splicing of the gene. Recent studies show that only a small portion of sporadic FTD patients have tau mutations, which are more commonly found in familial FTD cases with known tau neuropathology at autopsy.

Pick's disease is a commonly discussed disorder that is difficult to differentiate clinically from AD and is less well defined as a distinct entity. The major distinguishing hallmark is marked symmetric lobar atrophy of temporal and/or frontal lobes, which can be visualized by neuroimaging studies (CT, MRI, or single photon emission CT) and is readily apparent at autopsy. The atrophy is sometimes asymmetric and may involve the basal ganglia. Microscopic findings include gliosis, neuronal loss, and swollen or ballooned neurons, which frequently contain silver-staining cytoplasmic inclusions referred to as *Pick bodies*. Pick bodies consist of straight and constricted fibrils that share antigenic determinants with the NFTs of AD, including the microtubule-associated protein tau, suggesting that Pick bodies derive from altered components of the neuronal cytoskeleton. Onset is usually in the fifth through seventh decades. Clinically, there is a slowly progressive dementia often associated with hyper-oral behavior, bulimia, language disturbance, emotional disinhibition, irritability, and persistent aimless wandering. In the early stages the behavioral changes are more prominent than memory loss. The language disturbance may be aphasia or forced repetitive speech patterns, sometimes progressing to echolalia, language impoverishment, and mutism. These clinical characteristics may sometimes occur in AD, so that the clinical diagnosis of Pick's disease often requires confirmation at autopsy. Some brains containing Pick bodies may also have varying quantities of amyloid plaques and NFTs, blurring the distinction from AD. Examples of familial Pick's disease that display an autosomal dominant-like pattern of inheritance have been reported. There is no specific treatment.

DIFFUSE LEWY BODY DISEASE Lewy bodies are intraneuronal cytoplasmic inclusions that stain with periodic acid–Schiff and ubiquitin. They are composed of straight neurofilaments 7 to 20 nm long with surrounding amorphous material. They contain epitopes recognized by antibodies against phosphorylated and nonphosphorylated neurofilament proteins, ubiquitin, and a presynaptic protein called α-synuclein. Lewy bodies are traditionally found in the substantia nigra of patients with idiopathic Parkinson's disease (Chap. 363). Large numbers of such inclusions have also been discovered in cortical neurons in patients with dementia. In patients without other pathologic features, the condition is referred to as *diffuse Lewy body disease*. In patients whose brains also contain amyloid plaques and NFTs, the condition is called the *diffuse Lewy body variant of Alzheimer's disease*. The quantity of Lewy bodies required to establish the diagnosis is uncertain. The diagnosis is primarily a neuropathologic entity; however, there is some evidence that there is a characteristic clinical syndrome. In addition to chronic progressive dementia, these patients often also have parkinsonian features, in particular rigidity, which may be combined with an intention tremor. Frequent fluctuations of behavior, cognitive ability, and level of alertness may occur. These fluctuations can be marked, with the occurrence of episodic confusion and lucid intervals suggesting delirium. However, despite the fluctuating pattern, the clinical features persist over a long period, unlike a typical transient delirium. Delusions and visual hallucinations are common, and auditory hallucinations may also occur. Repeated unexplained falls are often noted. Frequently there is an unusual sensitivity to neuroleptic medications and benzodiazepines, with exaggerated adverse responses to standard doses. In most patients, this condition is difficult to distinguish from AD or Parkinson's disease with dementia. The population prevalence of diffuse Lewy body disease is not known, but it is now more commonly diagnosed than in the past because of the use of ubiquitin staining during neuropathologic studies. At autopsy, 10 to 30% of demented patients may show cortical Lewy bodies. It is not yet clear what role Apo E may play in Lewy body disease without AD changes. There is no specific treatment.

NORMAL-PRESSURE HYDROCEPHALUS Normal-pressure hydrocephalus (NPH) is a syndrome with distinct clinical, physiologic, and neuroimaging characteristics. The clinical triad includes an abnormal gait (ataxic or apractic), dementia (usually mild to moderate), and urinary incontinence. Neuroimaging studies of the brain reveal enlarged lateral ventricles (hydrocephalus) with little or no cortical atrophy. This is a communicating hydrocephalus with a patent aqueduct of Sylvius and upward stretching of the corpus callosum (Fig. 362-3). Lumbar puncture opening pressure is in the high normal range, and the CSF protein and sugar concentrations and cell count are normal. NPH is presumed to be caused by obstruction to normal flow of CSF over the cerebral convexity and delayed absorption into the venous system. The indolent nature of the process results in enlarged lateral ventricles but relatively little increase in CSF pressure. There is presumably stretching and distortion of white matter tracts in the corona radiata, but the exact physiologic cause of the clinical syndrome is unclear. Some patients with NPH have a history of conditions producing scarring of the basilar meninges (blocking upward flow of CSF) such as previous meningitis, subarachnoid hemorrhage, or head trauma. Most patients seem to have no pertinent past history. In contrast to patients with AD, the patient with NPH has an early and prominent gait disturbance and no evidence of cortical atrophy on CT or MRI. A number of attempts have been made to use various special studies to improve the diagnosis of NPH and predict the success of ventricular shunting. These include radionuclide cisternography (showing a delay in CSF absorption over the convexity) and various attempts to monitor and alter CSF flow dynamics, including a constant-pressure infusion test. None of these studies has proven to be specific or consistently useful. There is sometimes a transient improvement in gait or cognition following lumbar puncture (or serial punctures) with removal of 30 to 50 mL of CSF, but this finding also has not proved to be consistently predictive of post-shunt improvement. One study determined that no more than 1 to 2% of a large group of demented patients had NPH. AD often masquerades as NPH, because the gait may be abnormal in AD and cortical atrophy is sometimes difficult to determine by CT or MRI early in the disease. Hippocampal atrophy on MRI may be a clue suggesting AD (Fig. 362-1). Approximately 30 to 50% of pa-

A   *B*

FIGURE 362-4   Huntington's disease *A*. Sagittal T1-weighted MRI shows enlargement of the lateral ventricles reflecting typical caudate atrophy (*arrows*). *B*. Axial T2-weighted image demonstrates abnormal high signal intensity in the putamen (*arrows*).

tients identified by careful diagnosis as having NPH will show improvement with a ventricular shunting procedure. Gait may improve more than memory. Transient, short-lasting improvement is common. Patients should be carefully selected for this operation, because subdural hematoma and infection are known complications. A recent study limited to four patients showed benefit from aggressive siphoning of CSF to reduce ventricular size, but there were frequent perioperative complications.

HUNTINGTON'S DISEASE   Huntington's disease (HD) is a genetic, autosomal dominant, degenerative brain disorder. It has a population frequency of about 10/100,000. The two clinical hallmarks of the disease are chorea and behavioral disturbance. The illness may begin with either or both of these symptoms predominating. Onset is usually in the fourth or fifth decade, but there is a wide range in age of onset, from childhood to >75 years. The chorea begins as subtle fidgeting that may be unrecognized by the patient and family. However, the movement disorder is usually slowly progressive and eventually may become disabling. There are frequent, irregular, sudden jerks and movements of any of the limbs or trunk. Grimacing, grunting, and poor articulation of speech may be prominent. The gait is disjointed and poorly coordinated and has a so-called dancing (choreic) quality. Memory is frequently not impaired until late in the disease, but attention, judgment, awareness, and executive functions may be seriously deficient at an early stage. Depression, apathy, social withdrawal, irritability, and intermittent disinhibition are common. Delusions and obsessive-compulsive behavior may occur. Schizophrenia is occasionally the initial diagnosis. The disease duration is typically about 15 years but also shows a wide range. Early onset before the age of 20 (juvenile HD) is associated with rigidity, ataxia, cognitive decline, and more rapid progression, with a typical duration of about 8 years. Seizures are rare with adult-onset HD but more common with juvenile-onset disease. There is no specific treatment, but the adventitious movements and behavioral changes may partially respond to phenothiazines, haloperidol, benzodiazepines, or olanzepine. SSRIs may help with the frequently associated depression.

Neuropathologically, the disease predominantly strikes the striatum. Atrophy of the caudate nuclei, which form the lateral margins of the lateral ventricles, can be visualized on neuroimaging studies in the middle and late stages of the disease (Fig. 362-4). More diffuse cortical atrophy can be seen late in the disease. Microscopically there are no dramatic pathologic characteristics, such as the plaques and tangles seen with AD. However, there is gliosis and neuronal loss, especially of medium-sized spiny neurons in the caudate and putamen. Some neurons contain intranuclear inclusions that stain with antibodies to polyglutamine. There is relative sparing of large cholinergic aspiny neurons. (Treatment with 3-nitroproprionic acid, a succinate dehydrogenase inhibitor, has produced HD-like pathologic changes in experimental animals). Neurochemically there is a marked decrease of γ-aminobutyric acid (GABA) and its synthetic enzyme glutamic acid decarboxylase throughout the basal ganglia. The levels of other neurotransmitters, including substance P and enkephalins, are also reduced. Magnetic resonance spectroscopy (MRS) in living subjects with HD has shown elevated levels of lactate in the basal ganglia.

The HD gene, called *IT15*, is located on chromosome 4p, contains a CAG trinucleotide repeat expansion, and codes for a protein called *huntingtin*. The protein is found in neurons throughout the brain; its normal function is unknown. Inactivation of the homologous gene in mice causes embryonic death in homozygotes, but heterozygotes are phenotypically normal. Transgenic mice with an expanded CAG repeat in the HD gene develop a progressive movement disorder. The CAG repeat codes for a long polyglutamine domain in the expressed protein. The disease process may result from a toxic gain of function (Chap. 359). One hypothesis is that these polyglutamine tracts cause abnormal protein-binding reactions, which then interfere with other cell processes such as mitochondrial activity. The HD mutation may lead to abnormal cleavage of the huntingtin protein, passage of protein fragments from cytoplasm to nucleus, and interference of nuclear mechanisms leading to apoptosis and neuronal death.

The DNA repeat expansion forms the basis of a diagnostic blood test for the disease gene. Persons having 38 or more CAG repeats in the HD gene have inherited the disease mutation and will eventually develop symptoms if they live to an advanced age. Each of their children has a 50% risk of also inheriting the abnormal gene. There is a rough correlation between a larger number of repeats and an earlier age of onset, but most patients fall into a range of intermediate repeat numbers (40 to 49 repeats) in which this correlation is not clinically useful. For unclear reasons, juvenile onset with a large repeat expansion most often occurs when the father is the affected parent (a form of genetic anticipation). There is a CAG repeat range (about 26 to 37) in the HD gene that is rarely associated with clinical symptoms, but it is unstable and may expand to a symptomatic range when passed to a child. Asymptomatic adult children at risk for HD should receive careful genetic counseling prior to DNA testing, because a positive result may have serious emotional and social consequences. Detailed testing and counseling protocols have been published. In addition to use in genetic counseling of persons at risk for HD, the DNA test can also be used in differential diagnosis. For example, some persons with late-onset, apparently sporadic "senile" chorea have been found to carry the HD mutation. Also, disorders that may mimic HD, such as schizophrenia, benign familial chorea, inherited ataxias, neural acanthocytosis, and FAD, will not show the CAG expansion in the HD gene.

OTHER DEGENERATIVE DEMENTIAS Several other primary neurologic disorders have been associated with dementia and are the result of various poorly understood degenerative neuronal processes. These conditions include progressive supranuclear palsy, cortical basal degeneration, primary progressive aphasia, and the amyotrophic lateral sclerosis (ALS)/parkinsonian/dementia complex of Guam. These are progressive dementing illnesses of unknown cause whose names are descriptive of the typical clinical signs or the anatomic brain areas that are involved with nonspecific atrophy and neuronal degeneration.

Progressive supranuclear palsy (Chap. 363) is a degenerative disease that involves both the brainstem and neocortex with diffuse NFTs. Clinically, this disorder begins with vertical supranuclear gaze paresis and progresses slowly to include symmetric rigidity and dementia. Stiff, unstable posture with hyperextension of the neck and slow gait with frequent falls are common. Early in the disease, the patients have difficulty with downgaze and lose vertical opticokinetic nystagmus on downward movement of the target. Although the patients have very limited voluntary eye movements, their eyes still retain oculocephalic reflexes (doll's head maneuver). The dementia is considered to be of the subcortical type, with slowed thought processes, impaired verbal fluency, and difficulty with sequential actions and with shifting from one task to another. Seizures and sleep apnea may occur. There is only a limited response to L-dopa, and there is no other effective treatment. Death occurs within 5 to 10 years. At autopsy, the NFTs are found in multiple subcortical structures (including the subthalamus, globus pallidus, substantia nigra, locus coeruleus, periaqueductal gray matter, superior colliculi, and oculomotor nuclei) as well as in the neocortex. The NFTs have similar staining characteristics to those of AD, but on electron microscopy they generally are seen to consist of straight tubules rather than the paired helical filaments found in AD.

Progressive supranuclear palsy is often confused with idiopathic *Parkinson's disease* (Chap. 363). Although elderly Parkinson's patients may have some difficulty with upgaze, they do not develop significant downgaze paresis or progressive supranuclear palsy, and neurologic findings in Parkinson's disease are more likely to be asymmetric. However, dementia does occur in approximately 20% of Parkinson's disease patients. The occurrence of dementia in Parkinson's disease is more likely with increasing age, increasing severity of extrapyramidal signs, and the presence of depression. These patients may also show cortical atrophy on brain imaging. Neuropathologically, there may be Alzheimer changes in the cortex (amyloid plaques and NFTs), neuronal Lewy body inclusions in both the substantia nigra and the cortex, or no specific microscopic changes other than gliosis and neuronal loss.

Cortical basal ganglionic degeneration is a slowly progressive dementing illness associated with severe gliosis and neuronal loss in both the neocortex and basal ganglia (substantia nigra and striatum). There is often a unilateral onset with rigidity, dystonia, and apraxia of one arm and hand ("alien hand" syndrome). Eventually the condition becomes bilateral and includes dysarthria, slow gait, action tremor, and dementia. The microscopic features include enlarged, achromatic neurons in the cortex, and there may also be NFTs and amyloid plaques. The condition is rarely familial; the cause is unknown; and there is no specific treatment.

Another entity is *primary progressive aphasia* (Chap. 25). Patients with this disorder have aphasia associated with asymmetric atrophy of the left hemisphere and occasionally go on to develop dementia. Neuroimaging studies show the left hemisphere atrophy. Some patients are nonfluent, with hesitant, telegraphic speech associated with impaired comprehension and naming. Neuropathologic studies have shown a heterogeneous group of abnormalities, including Pick's disease, AD, CJD, and nonspecific gliosis.

The *ALS/parkinsonian/dementia complex of Guam* is a rare degenerative disease that occurs in the Chamorro natives on the island of Guam. Individual patients may have any combination of parkinsonian features, dementia, and motor neuron disease. The most characteristic pathologic features are the presence of NFTs in degenerating neurons of the cortex and substantia nigra and loss of motor neurons in the spinal cord. Epidemiologic evidence supports a probable environmental cause, such as exposure to a neurotoxin with a long latency period. One interesting but unproven candidate neurotoxin occurs in the seed of the false palm tree (cycad), which Guamanians traditionally used to make flour. The possibility of a contributing genetic factor has not been excluded. The ALS syndrome is decreasing in frequency on Guam, but a dementing illness with rigidity continues to be seen.

Finally, rare forms of degenerative dementia continue to be reported, such as dementia lacking specific histologic features and an early-onset hereditary dementia caused by mutations in neuroserpin, a type of serine protease inhibitor.

BIBLIOGRAPHY

BIRD TD, BENNETT RL: Why do DNA testing? Practical and ethical implications of new neurogenetic tests. Ann Neurol 38:141, 1995

BOWEN J et al: Progression to dementia in patients with isolated memory loss. Lancet 349:763, 1998

BREITNER JCS et al: Apo E-ε4 count predicts age when prevalence of AD increases, then declines. Neurology 53:321, 1999

CAPLAN LR: Binswanger's disease—revisited. Neurology 45:626, 1995

DANIEL SE et al: The clinical and pathological spectrum of Steele-Richardson-Olszewski syndrome (progressive supranuclear palsy): A reappraisal. Brain 118:759, 1995

DUBINSKY RM et al: Practice parameter: Risk of driving and Alzheimer's disease (an evidence-based review). Report of the Quality Standards Subcommittee of the American Academy of Neurology. Neurology 54:2205, 2000

LENDON C et al: Exploring the etiology of Alzheimer disease using molecular genetics. JAMA 277:825, 1997

LIM A et al: Clinico-neuropathological correlation of Alzheimer's disease in a community-based case series. J Am Geriatr Soc 47:564, 1999

MALM J et al: The predictive value of cerebrospinal fluid dynamic tests in patients with the idiopathic adult hydrocephalus syndrome. Arch Neurol 52:783, 1995

MARTIN JB: Molecular basis of the neurodegenerative disorders. N Engl J Med 340:1970, 1999

MAYEUX R et al: Utility of the apolipoprotein E genotype in the diagnosis of Alzheimer's disease. N Engl J Med 338:506, 1998

MAYEUX R, SANO M: Treatment of Alzheimer's Disease. N Engl J Med 341:1670, 1999

MCKEITH IG et al: An evaluation of the predictive validity and inter-rater reliability of clinical diagnostic criteria for senile dementia of Lewy body type. Neurology 44:872, 1994

MENDEZ MF et al: Pick's disease versus Alzheimer's disease: A comparison of clinical characteristics. Neurology 43:289, 1993

RABER J et al: Apolipoprotein E and cognitive performance. Nature 404:352, 2000

RAFTOPOULOS C et al: Cognitive recovery in idiopathic normal pressure hydrocephalus: A prospective study. Neurosurgery 35:397, 1994

REIMAN EM et al: Preclinical evidence of Alzheimer's disease in persons homozygous for the ε4 allele for apolipoprotein E. N Engl J Med 334:752, 1996

SCHENK D et al: Immunization with amyloid-β attenuates Alzheimer disease-like pathology in the PDAPP mouse. Nature 400:173, 1999

SHERRINGTON R et al: Cloning of a gene bearing missense mutations in early-onset familial Alzheimer's disease. Nature 375:754, 1995

TATEMICHI TK et al: Dementia after stroke: Baseline frequency, risks, and clinical features in a hospitalized cohort. Neurology 42:1185, 1992

TERRY RD et al: *Alzheimer Disease*, 2d ed. New York, Lippincott Williams & Wilkins, 1999

TISON F et al: Dementia in Parkinson's disease: A population-based study in ambulatory and institutionalized individuals. Neurology 45:705, 1995

VANNESTE JAL: Three decades of normal pressure hydrocephalus: Are we wiser now? J Neurol Neurosurg Psychiatry 57:1021, 1994

VASSAR R et al: β-Secretase cleavage of Alzheimer's amyloid precursor protein by the transmembrane aspartic protease BACE. Science 286:735, 1999

WILHELMSEN KC: Frontotemporal dementia genetics. J Geriatr Psychiatry Neurol 11:55, 1998

PARKINSON'S DISEASE AND OTHER EXTRAPYRAMIDAL DISORDERS

PARKINSON'S DISEASE Parkinsonism is a syndrome consisting of a variable combination of tremor, rigidity, bradykinesia, and a characteristic disturbance of gait and posture. Parkinson's disease is a chronic, progressive disorder in which idiopathic parkinsonism occurs without evidence of more widespread neurologic involvement.

Parkinson's disease generally commences in middle or late life and leads to progressive disability with time. The disease occurs in all ethnic groups, has an equal sex distribution, and is common, with a prevalence of 1 to 2 per 1000 of the general population and 2 per 100 among people older than 65 years. Signs of parkinsonism are extremely common in the elderly; one survey indicated that 15% of individuals between 65 and 74 years of age, and more than half of all individuals after age 85, have abnormalities on examination consistent with the presence of an extrapyramidal disorder.

Neuroanatomy Symptoms of Parkinson's disease are caused by loss of nerve cells in the pigmented substantia nigra pars compacta and the locus coeruleus in the midbrain. Cell loss also occurs in the globus pallidus and putamen. Eosinophilic intraneural inclusion granules (Lewy bodies) are present in the basal ganglia, brainstem, spinal cord, and sympathetic ganglia.

Pars compacta neurons of the substantia nigra provide dopaminergic input to the striatum, which is part of the basal ganglia (Fig. 22-4*A*). In Parkinson's disease, loss of pars compacta neurons leads to striatal dopamine depletion and ultimately to reduced thalamic excitation of the motor cortex (Fig. 22-4*B*). Other neurotransmitters, such as norepinephrine, are also depleted, with clinical consequences that are uncertain but perhaps contribute to depression, dysautonomia, and "freezing" episodes of marked akinesia. →*The neural pathways that modulate motor activity are considered in detail in Chap. 22.*

Pathogenesis Parkinsonism can be induced in primates by exposure to 1-methyl-4-phenyl-1,2,3,6-tetrahydropyridine (MPTP), which is converted by monoamine oxidase B to *N*-methyl-4-phenylpyridinium (MPP+), an active toxin. MPP+ is taken up by dopaminergic nigral neurons through an active transport system that is normally involved in dopamine reuptake, and then inhibits oxidative phosphorylation, possibly at the level of complex I in the respiratory chain. This results in the death of nigrostriatal neurons, dopamine depletion in the basal ganglia, and parkinsonism. In addition to energy failure, MPP+ may also generate free radicals and oxidative stress.

The cause of Parkinson's disease is unknown. One suggested cause is exposure to an unrecognized environmental toxin, perhaps structurally similar to MPTP. Such exposure may have occurred years before the onset of any clinical disturbance, because symptoms will not develop until the cumulative cell loss from toxin exposure and natural aging approximates 80% of the original cell population. Alternatively or additionally, endogenous toxins may be responsible. In particular, the normal neurotransmitter dopamine readily oxidizes to produce free radicals, which can cause cell death. Although the precise role of dopamine itself remains unclear, the evidence relating Parkinson's disease to damage by free radicals is compelling.

Oxidative stress is likely when dopamine turnover is increased, glutathione is reduced (leaving neurons more vulnerable to oxidant stress), and reactive iron is increased (promoting the generation of potentially toxic hydroxyl radicals). A mitochondrial complex 1 defect occurs in Parkinson's disease and may contribute to neuronal vulnerability and loss through free radical generation.

Accumulating evidence suggests a genetic susceptibility to the disease. An increased incidence of parkinsonism has been noted in the monozygotic twins of patients developing Parkinson's disease prior to

the age of 50. First-degree relatives of patients are twice as likely to develop the disease as controls. Approximately 5% of parkinsonian patients have a familial form of the disorder. Three genes for the parkinsonian phenotype have recently been identified. Two different mutations of the α synuclein gene (in the q21-23 region of chromosome 4) have been identified in dominantly inherited parkinsonism; the α synuclein protein is of uncertain function but is abundant in neurons, especially at synaptic terminals, and in Lewy bodies. Homozygous deletions of the parkin gene (6q25.2-q27) have been associated with autosomal recessive parkinsonism; parkin is a protein expressed in the substantia nigra. Finally, a heterozygous missense mutation of the gene for ubiquitin carboxy-terminal hydrolase L1 has been identified in a parkinsonian family. The mechanism by which these mutations leads to parkinsonism remains to be determined, but the phenotype clearly has genetic heterogeneity.

Clinical Manifestations The 4- to 6-Hz *tremor* is typically most conspicuous at rest and worsens with emotional stress. It often begins with rhythmic flexion-extension of the fingers, hand, or foot, or with rhythmic pronation-supination of the forearm, and may be confined initially to one limb or to the two limbs on one side before becoming more generalized. It may also involve the mouth and chin. In 10 to 15% of patients, however, the tremor is faster (7 to 8 Hz) and postural, resembling essential tremor (see below) both clinically and in its response to pharmacotherapy.

Rigidity, defined as an increase in resistance to passive movement (Chap. 22), is a common clinical feature that accounts for the flexed posture of many patients. The most disabling feature, however, is *bradykinesia* (or, in its most severe form, akinesia), a slowness of voluntary movement and an associated reduction in automatic movements, such as swinging of the arms when walking. There is a fixity of facial expression, with widened palpebral fissures and infrequent blinking. There may be blepharoclonus (fluttering of the closed eyelids), blepharospasm (involuntary closure of the eyelids), and drooling of saliva from the mouth. The voice is hypophonic and poorly modulated. Power is preserved, but fine or rapidly alternating movements are impaired. The combination of tremor, rigidity, and bradykinesia results in small, tremulous, and often illegible handwriting. Patients have difficulty in rising from bed or an easy chair and tend to assume a flexed posture when erect. Walking is often difficult to initiate, and patients may have to lean forward increasingly until they can advance. They walk with small, shuffling steps, have no arm swing, are unsteady (especially on turning), and may have difficulty in stopping. Some patients walk with a *festinating gait*, i.e., at an increasing speed to prevent themselves from falling because of their abnormal center of gravity.

The tendon reflexes are unaltered, and the plantar responses are flexor. Repetitive tapping (at about 2 Hz) over the glabella produces a sustained blink response (Myerson's sign), in contrast to the response of normal subjects. A depressed mood is common, and an impairment of cognitive function—sometimes amounting to a frank dementia—is frequently evident in advanced cases.

Differential Diagnosis Parkinsonism is simulated by certain disorders. *Depression* is associated with changes in the voice and facial appearance and a poverty of spontaneous activity, such as occur in Parkinson's disease. A trial of treatment with antidepressant drugs helps to clarify the diagnosis if uncertainty persists and other signs of parkinsonism are absent. *Essential (benign, familial) tremor* may be mistaken for parkinsonian tremor, but a family history of tremor is common; alcohol in small quantities may ameliorate the tremor, and other neurologic signs are lacking. Moreover, essential tremor commonly involves the head (with a nodding or no-no tremor), whereas parkinsonism spares the head but affects the face and lips. *Normal-pressure hydrocephalus* (Chap. 362) causes an apraxic gait disturbance (sometimes resembling the gait of parkinsonism), urinary incontinence, and dementia. Imaging studies reveal dilation of the ventricular system without cortical atrophy, and surgical shunting procedures to

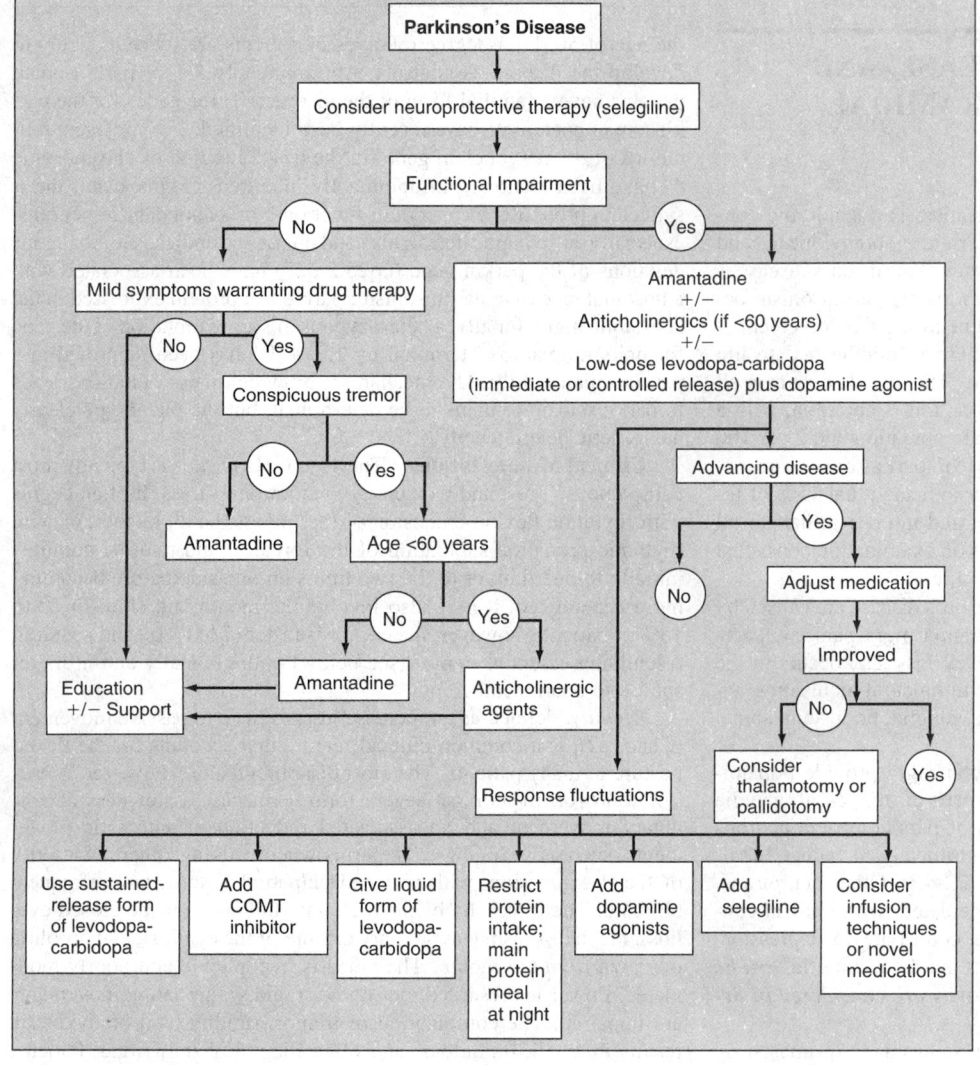

FIGURE 363-1 Algorithm for the management of patients with Parkinson's disease.

bypass any obstruction to the flow of cerebrospinal fluid (CSF) may be helpful.

Parkinsonism may occur as part of various neurologic diseases that are important to distinguish from Parkinson's disease for prognostic and therapeutic purposes. In *Wilson's disease* (Chap. 348), other abnormal movements are also usually present. The family history, early age of onset, associated Kayser-Fleischer rings, and low serum copper and ceruloplasmin levels distinguish it from Parkinson's disease. *Huntington's disease* (Chap. 362) sometimes presents with rigidity and akinesia, but the family history and any accompanying dementia point to the correct diagnosis, which can be confirmed by genetic studies. The *Shy-Drager syndrome* (Chap. 366) is a degenerative disorder characterized by parkinsonism, impaired autonomic function (resulting in postural hypotension, abnormal thermoregulatory sweating, disturbances of bladder and bowel control, impotence, and gastroparesis) and by signs of more widespread neurologic involvement (pyramidal, cerebellar, or lower motor neuron signs). There is generally no treatment except for the postural hypotension, which may respond to the measures discussed in Chap. 366. The response to antiparkinsonian agents is usually disappointing. *Striatonigral degeneration* (see below) leads to bradykinesia and rigidity, but tremor is usually inconspicuous. Cerebellar deficits sometimes occur (multisystem atrophy), and there may be autonomic insufficiency (Shy-Drager syndrome). Antiparkinsonian drugs are generally ineffective. *Progressive supranuclear palsy* (discussed separately, below) causes bradykinesia and rigidity, but conspicuous abnormalities of voluntary eye movements (especially vertical gaze), dementia, pseudobulbar palsy, and axial dystonia dis-

tinguish it from Parkinson's disease. There is little or no response to antiparkinsonian drugs. *Cortical-basal ganglionic degeneration* may be mistaken for Parkinson's disease, but intellectual decline, aphasia, apraxia, sensory neglect, and other evidence of cortical dysfunction should suggest the correct diagnosis. In *diffuse Lewy body disease*, parkinsonism is joined with a conspicuous dementia and with evidence of more widespread neurologic involvement. In *Creutzfeldt-Jakob disease*, any parkinsonian features are overshadowed by the rapidly progressive dementia; myoclonus is common, ataxia or pyramidal signs may occur, visual disturbances are sometimes conspicuous, and the electroencephalographic findings are often characteristic. Similarly, in *Alzheimer's disease* there may be minor extrapyramidal deficits, but these are generally inconsequential compared with the marked cognitive impairment that characterizes the disorder. →*Alzheimer's disease and diffuse Lewy body disease are considered in Chap. 362, and Creutzfeldt-Jakob disease is discussed in Chap. 375.*

Parkinsonism sometimes occurs as a consequence of a systemic disorder. Drug-induced *secondary parkinsonism* is especially common (discussed below). MPTP-induced parkinsonism has occurred in several humans who inadvertently took this meperidine analogue for recreational purposes. The mechanisms involved are discussed above, and the history of exposure, unusually early age of onset, and rapid progression should suggest the correct diagnosis. Exposure to various toxins, such as manganese dust or carbon disulfide, also causes parkinsonism, and the diagnosis is suggested by an accurate occupational history. Parkinsonism sometimes occurs as a result of severe carbon monoxide poisoning or develops after an encephalitic illness. Postencephalitic parkinsonism was especially common after the outbreak of encephalitis lethargica that occurred in an early part of the twentieth century.

TREATMENT Approaches to treatment are summarized in Fig. 363-1.

Symptomatic Pharmacologic Treatment Nonselective muscarinic antagonists (*anticholinergic drugs*) are sometimes helpful, especially in relieving tremor. Various preparations are available, including trihexyphenidyl, benztropine, procyclidine, and orphenadrine. The usual maintenance doses are shown in Table 363-1. Common side effects include dryness of the mouth, constipation, urinary retention, and blurred vision. Narrow-angle glaucoma may be aggravated. Con-

Table 363-1 Commonly Used Muscarinic Antagonists (Anticholinergic Drugs) for the Treatment of Parkinson's Disease

Generic Name	Proprietary Name	Tablet Strength	Usual Dose, mg
Benztropine	Cogentin	0.5, 1, 2	0.5–2 tid
Biperiden	Akineton	2	1–3 qid
Orphenadrine	Disipal	100	100 tid
Procyclidine	Kemadrin	5	2.5–10 tid
Trihexyphenidyl	Artane	2, 5	2–5 tid

fusion and hallucinations are especially troublesome in the elderly. Treatment is started with the preparation of choice in a small initial dose that is gradually increased, depending on response and tolerance. If the drug is unhelpful, another anticholinergic preparation is substituted.

Amantadine, either alone or combined with an anticholinergic agent, is sometimes helpful for mild parkinsonism; it acts by potentiating the release of endogenous dopamine. It may improve all major clinical features of the disorder, has relatively uncommon side effects (restlessness, confusion, skin rashes, edema, disturbances of cardiac rhythm), and is given in a standard dose (100 mg twice daily). However, many patients derive only transient, if any, benefit from it.

Levodopa, the metabolic precursor of dopamine (Fig. 363-2), provides symptomatic benefit in most patients with parkinsonism and is often particularly helpful in relieving bradykinesia. The presence in the intestinal mucosa of dopa decarboxylase, which converts levodopa to dopamine, means that most of an ingested dose of levodopa is lost before it even enters the general circulation. Administration of levodopa in combination with an extracerebral dopa-decarboxylase inhibitor reduces the extracerebral metabolism of levodopa and also reduces the incidence of peripheral side effects. Levodopa is therefore administered routinely in combination with a peripheral dopa-decarboxylase inhibitor (carbidopa in the United States; benserazide in Europe). In the United States, the combination of carbidopa and levodopa (in 1:10 and 1:4 ratios) is available commercially as Sinemet. Standard formulations are Sinemet 25/100, 10/100, and 25/250 mg. A common starting dose is 25/100 mg three times daily, which is increased gradually to 25/250 mg three or four times daily, taken 1 h before or 2 h after meals to maximize absorption and transport across the blood-brain barrier.

There was initially concern that the early introduction of levodopa might accelerate the death of nigrostriatal neurons because of a hypothetical increase in dopamine-mediated neurotoxicity. It is now clear that levodopa should be introduced as soon as is warranted by the patient's clinical state, rather than postponed out of concern for this theoretical possibility. However, initial treatment with a dopamine agonist may provide similar benefit to levodopa and thus allow introduction of the latter to be postponed; in consequence, emergence of late side effects may be delayed. The most common initial side effects of levodopa are nausea, vomiting, postural hypotension, and, occasionally, cardiac arrhythmias. Abnormal movements (dyskinesias), restlessness (akathisia), and confusion tend to occur somewhat later and are dose-related. Dyskinesias may be present during most of the day, occur only when plasma levodopa levels peak, or develop when the plasma levodopa concentration reaches a certain submaximal level. Management depends on distinguishing these possibilities by the temporal profile of the dyskinesia. When dyskinesias occur only at a certain submaximal blood level of levodopa, adjustment of the daily dose to produce higher or lower blood levels may alleviate them; dyskinesias related to peak blood levels of levodopa are helped by a reduction in dose.

Important late complications of levodopa therapy are the wearing-off effect (transient deterioration shortly before the next dose is due) and the "on-off" phenomenon—abrupt but transient fluctuations in

FIGURE 363-2 Diagrammatic representation of a dopaminergic nerve terminal and the associated postsynaptic dopamine receptors. The metabolic pathways for the synthesis and breakdown of dopamine are shown. The circled numbers indicate the site of action of several drugs used in the treatment of Parkinson's disease: ①, the site of action of levodopa (L-dopa); ②, that of dopamine agonist drugs; and ③, that of selegiline. DA, dopamine.

clinical state that occur frequently during the day, without warning or an obvious relationship to dosing schedule, resulting in alternating periods of marked akinesia or greater mobility accompanied by iatrogenic dyskinesias. Response fluctuations can be controlled in part by reducing dosing intervals, administering levodopa 1 h before meals and restricting dietary protein intake (to reduce any competition by various amino acids with levodopa for the active carrier system that transports it into the blood and from the blood into the brain), or treatment with dopamine agonists. The addition of selegiline (5 mg at breakfast and lunch), a monoamine oxidase B inhibitor, reduces the metabolic breakdown of dopamine and may also be helpful (see "Neuroprotective Treatment," below).

Response fluctuations to oral levodopa may also be reduced or eliminated by catechol-*O*-methyltransferase (COMT) inhibitor agents or by frequent or continuous administration of levodopa intravenously, intraduodenally, or by intragastric infusion. A commercially available controlled-release formulation of Sinemet (Sinemet CR 25/100 or 50/200 mg) sometimes helps in reducing the dosing frequency and maintaining steady blood levels of levodopa, but it is of only limited benefit in reducing response fluctuations. Surgical treatment is also effective (see later). The pathogenesis of the on-off phenomenon is obscure, but proposed mechanisms relate to the pharmacokinetics of levodopa, degeneration of presynaptic dopaminergic nerve terminals, altered sensitivity of dopamine receptors, and abnormalities of nondopaminergic neurotransmitter systems.

Dopamine agonist drugs may produce symptomatic benefit by direct stimulation of dopamine receptors (Fig. 363-2). There are five major dopamine-receptor subtypes classified into two groups. The D_1 group is made of the D_1 and D_5 subtypes, and the D_2 group consists of D_2, D_3, and D_4 subtypes. Drug efficacy and toxicity may relate to receptor specificity of dopamine agonists. The absorption and cerebral distribution of dopamine agonist drugs are less erratic than with levodopa, and they do not require enzymatic conversion to an active metabolite. Their early introduction either prior to Sinemet or in conjunction with low-dose Sinemet therapy (25/100 mg three times daily) yields sustained benefit and a lower incidence of late complications (such as response fluctuations and dyskinesias) than when levodopa is used alone and in a higher dose.

The agonists initially available were bromocriptine and pergolide, which are ergot derivatives. Bromocriptine, which stimulates dopamine D_2 receptors (Fig. 22-4), is introduced in a dose of 1.25 mg/d for 1 week and 2.5 mg/d for the next week, after which the daily dose is increased by 2.5-mg increments every 2 weeks, depending on response and tolerance. Maintenance doses range between 2.5 and 10 mg three times daily when the drug is taken with Sinemet. Pergolide activates both D_1 and D_2 dopamine receptors. It is introduced in a dose of 0.05 mg daily for 2 days; the dose is then increased by 0.1 to 0.15 mg/ d every 3 days for 12 days and by 0.25 mg/d every 3 days thereafter. The usual maintenance dose is 1 mg three times daily. Side effects are similar to those of levodopa, but psychiatric effects such as delusions or hallucinations are more common, and dyskinesias are less common, than with levodopa. Other adverse effects include headache, nasal congestion, erythromelalgia, pleural and retroperitoneal fibrosis, pulmonary infiltrates, and vasopasm. These agonists are contraindicated in patients with psychotic disorders and are best avoided in those with recent myocardial infarction, severe peripheral vascular disease, or active peptic ulceration.

Pramipexole and ropinirole are new dopamine agonists. Their selective nature suggested that they might be more effective and have fewer side effects that the first-generation agonists, but this remains uncertain from the few studies comparing them to bromocriptine or pergolide. Because of their non-ergoline structure, adverse effects such as erythromelalgia, vasospasm, and pleural or retroperitoneal fibrosis are unlikely. Both agents, however, may cause postural hypotension, lassitude, sleep disturbances, peripheral edema, constipation, nausea, dyskinesias, and confusion. Excessive or uncontrollable somnolence may require withdrawal of the medication.

Pramipexole, an aminobenzthiazol-derived selective D_3 agonist, provides worthwhile benefit when used alone for mild parkinsonism or when taken together with Sinemet for advanced disease. It permits a reduction in Sinemet dosage and smooths response fluctuations. It may also benefit associated affective symptoms. Pramipexole is absorbed rapidly from the gastrointestinal tract, reaches peak plasma concentrations in about 2 h, and is excreted by the kidneys; renal failure may therefore necessitate reduction in daily dose. The starting dose is 0.125 mg three times daily, with doubling of the dose after 1 week, and again after another week. The daily dose is then increased by 0.75 mg at weekly intervals depending on need and tolerance. The usual maintenance dose is 0.5 to 1.5 mg three times daily. Ropinirole, a selective D_2 agonist, is also effective for mild or advanced disease. It is started at 0.25 mg three times daily; total daily dose is increased by 0.75 mg at weekly intervals until the fourth week and then by 1.5 mg as needed. The usual maintenance dose is between 2 and 8 mg three times daily. It is metabolized by CYP1A2, and its clearance may be reduced by drugs undergoing hepatic metabolism.

Various new dopamine agonists are being evaluated, and new means of administering them (e.g., by subcutaneous infusion pump or transdermally) may lead to a steadier clinical response.

Selective COMT inhibitors such as tolcapone and entacapone enhance the benefits of levodopa therapy by reducing the conversion of levodopa to 3-O-methyldopa (which competes with levodopa for an active carrier mechanism) and by increasing the availability in the brain of levodopa. They are helpful in patients with response fluctuations to Sinemet, leading to a smoother response, greater "on" time, and reduction in daily levodopa requirement. Both agents are absorbed rapidly, bound to plasma proteins, and metabolized before being excreted. Both have peripheral effects, but tolcapone is also active centrally. Tolcapone is slightly more potent, has a longer duration of action, and is usually taken in a dose of 100 mg (rarely, 200 mg) three times daily, whereas entacapone (200 mg) is taken with each dose of Sinemet and may thus be taken four to six times daily. When COMT inhibitors are introduced, the daily dose of Sinemet may have to be

reduced by up to 30% in the first 48 h to prevent or minimize such complications as dyskinesias, nausea, and confusion. Other adverse effects include diarrhea, abdominal pain, postural hypotension, sleep disturbances, and discolored urine. Acute hepatic failure has occurred in rare patients receiving tolcapone, and a transient increase in liver enzymes is not uncommon. Accordingly, when tolcapone is prescribed, a consent form should be signed by the patient and liver function monitored every 2 weeks for the first year and less frequently thereafter, as recommended by the manufacturer.

Experimental studies suggest that glutamate antagonists may benefit patients with Parkinson's disease, and clinical studies of such agents are planned. G_{M1} ganglioside and various neurotrophic factors influence dopaminergic nigrostriatal cells, and work is continuing to develop delivery systems that will permit their use in the treatment of Parkinson's disease.

Surgical Treatment Destructive neurosurgical procedures were used for some years to treat parkinsonism, but their use declined with the advent of levodopa. Unilateral posteroventral pallidotomy or thalamotomy was resurrected in the 1990s as a therapeutic approach for relieving rigidity, bradykinesia, and tremor in patients with advanced disease in whom antiparkinsonian medication was ineffective or poorly tolerated. A positive (but incomplete) response to surgery is reported in >90% of patients; the beneficial effect predominates on the side contralateral to the procedure. Complications include cerebral infarction or hemorrhage, dysarthria or hypophonia, cognitive disturbances, and—after pallidotomy—visual field defects. Bilateral procedures have a higher morbidity and are generally discouraged. Such surgery is being replaced in some centers by high-frequency stimulation of selected locations in the brain, using an implanted electrode and stimulator, to induce a functional but reversible lesion. Thalamic stimulation is very effective in relieving tremor, and preliminary studies suggest that stimulation of the globus pallidus internus or subthalamic nucleus increases "on" time and improves clinical status in those with advanced parkinsonism and response fluctuations. Brain stimulation surgery has a lower morbidity than ablative surgery, but neither approach is warranted in patients with secondary or atypical parkinsonism or dementia.

There is ongoing interest in transplantation of fetal midbrain dopaminergic (nigral) cells into the putamen of patients with Parkinson's disease. Survival of engrafted cells has been documented by enhancement of fluorodopa uptake as visualized by positron emission tomography (PET), and in one autopsy study there was extensive striatal reinnervation by the transplanted cells. Fetal nigral transplantation remains an experimental procedure, and the nature of any long-term benefit is uncertain. Transplantation of autologous adrenal medullary tissue has also been attempted for Parkinson's disease, with mixed results; benefit seems most likely to occur in individuals younger than 50 years of age.

Neuroprotective Treatment Selective inhibitors of monoamine oxidase B such as selegiline (Eldepryl; Deprenyl) may reduce oxidative damage and thus slow disease progression, but the evidence for this effect is incomplete. In a large multicenter study, treatment with selegiline delayed the need for symptomatic therapy in patients with untreated parkinsonism, suggesting that progression of the disease had been retarded, but it was subsequently found that selegiline itself has a mild effect on symptoms. Thus, the basis of the observed effect is uncertain. The use of selegiline for protective purposes should probably be discussed with all patients unless they have end-stage disease or are very elderly, but the uncertainty of any benefit should be indicated. Selegiline in a standard dose (5 mg with breakfast and 5 mg with lunch) is not associated with the hypertensive ("cheese") effect of nonselective monoamine oxidase inhibitors. Acute toxic interactions may, however, occur with meperidine, tricyclic drugs, or serotonin reuptake inhibitors, and selegiline should not be prescribed to patients receiving those medications. Selegiline is metabolized to amphetamine and methamphetamine, so some patients may experience anxiety or insomnia. Moreover, an increased mortality rate has recently been found among patients receiving selegiline, raising concerns about its long-term safety. Patients must understand that selegiline is not intended to relieve symptoms and that there is no means of determining whether it is affecting disease progression in individual cases. Other inhibitors of monamine oxidase B are currently being evaluated for their effect on the natural history of Parkinson's disease and may clarify the issue.

Tocopherol (vitamin E) is an important scavenger of free radicals, but in a large study it failed to provide any protective benefit when taken in a dose of 2000 units daily. The extent to which it penetrates the brain, however, is not clear.

General Measures Physical therapy and speech therapy may help patients with moderately severe parkinsonism. In advanced cases, the quality of life can be improved by certain aids to daily living, such as extra rails or banisters placed in the home, table cutlery with large handles, nonslip table mats, voice amplifiers, and chairs that can gently eject the occupant.

FAMILIAL OR BENIGN ESSENTIAL TREMOR

A postural tremor (Chap. 22) may develop in otherwise normal individuals, sometimes on a familial basis with autosomal dominant inheritance. The pathophysiologic basis of the disorder is unknown.

Symptoms can develop at any age but often do not appear until middle or later life. Typically one or both hands, the head, and the voice are affected in any combination; the legs are generally spared. Apart from the tremor, no other abnormalities are present on neurologic examination. The tremor may worsen with time and ultimately become an embarrassment, but it generally causes no disability except when it disturbs handwriting or performance of fine tasks with the hands. A small quantity of alcohol sometimes relieves the tremor for a short period.

Rx **TREATMENT** Treatment is often unnecessary and is best delayed for as long as possible because, once initiated, it generally needs to be continued indefinitely. Propranolol, 40 to 120 mg orally twice daily, may reduce the amplitude of the tremor. A single oral dose (40 to 120 mg) may be taken in anticipation of known precipitating circumstances. Primidone is also effective but has to be introduced gradually. Other agents that may be helpful include alprazolam and mirtazapine. Thalamic stimulation (discussed earlier) may be helpful for severe tremor unresponsive to medical treatment.

PROGRESSIVE SUPRANUCLEAR PALSY

Progressive supranuclear palsy (also referred to as *Steele-Richardson-Olszewski syndrome*) is a sporadic degenerative disorder characterized pathologically by neuronal loss, gliosis, and neurofibrillary tangles in the midbrain, pons, basal ganglia, and dentate nuclei of the cerebellum. The neurofibrillary tangles of this disorder are distinct from those of Alzheimer's disease in that they are composed of straight filaments rather than paired helical filaments. The microtubule-associated protein tau is a constituent of the tangles, and a genetic association between an intrinsic polymorphism of tau and progressive supranuclear palsy has recently been reported. Thus, progressive supranuclear palsy may represent a tau pathologic process. There are also decreased concentrations of dopamine and homovanillic acid in the caudate nucleus and putamen.

Clinical Manifestations This uncommon disorder generally begins between the ages of 45 and 75 years; it affects men twice as frequently as women. Supranuclear ophthalmoplegia is characteristic. There is conspicuous failure of voluntary saccadic gaze (and of the fast phase of optokinetic nystagmus) in a vertical plane, especially downward, with later involvement of horizontal gaze. Eventually, smooth pursuit movements are also affected. Oculocephalic (e.g., doll's-head) and oculovestibular (caloric) reflexes are intact. Axial dystonia in extension, especially of the neck, is common and is frequently accompanied by limb rigidity and bradykinesia that may mimic Parkinson's disease. Tremor, however, is unusual. The combination of supranuclear ophthalmoplegia and axial rigidity accounts for the common presenting complaint of frequent falls. There may be

facial weakness, dysarthria, dysphagia, and exaggerated jaw jerk and gag reflexes (pseudobulbar palsy) as well as exaggerated and inappropriate emotional responses (pseudobulbar affect). Brisk tendon reflexes, extensor plantar responses, and cerebellar signs are sometimes encountered. A global impairment of intellectual function is frequent, but focal cortical dysfunction is rare.

Progressive supranuclear palsy should be considered whenever a middle-aged or elderly person with repeated falls has an extrapyramidal syndrome accompanied by nuchal dystonia and paralysis of voluntary downgaze. The marked impairment of voluntary downward and horizontal gaze distinguishes this disorder from Parkinson's disease, as does the extended rather than flexed dystonic posturing of the axial musculature, the absence of tremor, and the poor response to antiparkinsonian medications.

Rx **TREATMENT** The course is generally progressive, with aspiration or inanition leading to a fatal outcome within 10 years. Dopaminergic preparations sometimes reduce rigidity and bradykinesia, and anticholinergic (trihexyphenidyl, 6 to 15 mg/d) or tricyclic drugs (amitriptyline, 50 to 75 mg at bedtime) may benefit speech, gait, and pseudobulbar affect, but any benefit is limited and not sustained.

CORTICAL-BASAL GANGLIONIC DEGENERATION

This rare sporadic disorder typically begins in middle or later life with functional impairment of one or more limbs. Examination reveals signs of parkinsonism, but the extrapyramidal abnormalities are generally insufficient to account for the clinical deficit, which results from apraxia. As the disorder progresses, other evidence of cortical dysfunction also appears, such as aphasia, agnosia, sensory inattention, and mild dementia. Pathologically there is cell loss and gliosis in the cerebral cortex as well as the substantia nigra. The response to antiparkinsonian medication is disappointing, and the course is generally progressive, with increasing disability and dependence leading ultimately to death.

STRIATONIGRAL DEGENERATION

In a few patients with seemingly classic Parkinson's disease, there is little or no response to dopaminergic medication, and pathologic study at autopsy reveals neuronal loss and gliosis in the putamen, globus pallidus, caudate and subthalamic nuclei, and substantia nigra. This disorder has therefore been called *striatonigral degeneration*. It has an age and gender distribution similar to those of Parkinson's disease. Clinical examination reveals the findings of parkinsonism, but tremor is usually relatively inconspicuous. Cognitive function is preserved.

There may be an accompanying impairment of autonomic function (Shy-Drager syndrome; Chap. 366), and examination in such cases often reveals that a combination of pyramidal and cerebellar signs is also present. Indeed, in some cases the cerebellar findings are so conspicuous that the disorder is more properly called *spinocerebellar ataxia type 1* (olivopontocerebellar atrophy; Chap. 364).

The management of patients with striatonigral degeneration is difficult. Antiparkinsonian medications generally are prescribed but are usually ineffective.

MACHADO-JOSEPH DISEASE (SPINOCEREBELLAR ATAXIA TYPE 3)

Machado-Joseph disease is an autosomal dominant form of striatonigral degeneration that generally begins in the third or fourth decade. Most affected individuals are of Portuguese ancestry. There may be only mild parkinsonian signs, whereas spasticity, hyperreflexia, extensor plantar responses, cerebellar findings, external ophthalmoplegia and, sometimes, peripheral neuropathy are conspicuous. Cognitive function is preserved. Pathologically the findings are similar to those of striatonigral degeneration, but the dentate nucleus of the cerebellum is also involved. There is no specific treatment. →*The different clinical subtypes of the disease, their genetic basis, and related autosomal dominant ataxias with some extrapyramidal features are discussed in Chap. 364.*

IDIOPATHIC TORSION DYSTONIA

The occurrence of dystonic movements and postures without other neurologic signs in patients with a normal birth and developmental history is designated *idiopathic torsion dystonia.* The pathophysiologic and biochemical basis of this entity is unknown. Pathologic examination reveals no specific abnormalities, but the disorder is attributed to basal ganglia dysfunction partly because of observations made in cases of secondary dystonia. Other possible causes of dystonia (Chap. 22) should be excluded before this diagnosis is made. The disorder may occur on a sporadic or hereditary basis. In cases with onset in childhood or adolescence, inheritance is commonly autosomal dominant, with the gene, designated DYT1, localized to 9q32-34 and involving a GAG deletion. The gene codes for the protein Torsin A, the function of which is unclear. Onset is typically in a limb (commonly the leg), with subsequent spread to the other limbs and trunk, but sparing of the cranial muscles. Other autosomal dominant forms present in children or adults and begin in limb, axial, or cranial muscles; cranial involvement (facial, laryngeal, cervical) is common. This gene (DYT6) has been mapped to chromosome 8 in certain families. In a few families with autosomal dominant, adult-onset cranial, cervical, or upper limb dystonia, the responsible gene (DYT7) has been mapped to chromosome 18p. In other families, other unmapped genetic loci appear to be involved. Autosomal recessive and X-linked recessive (Xq21.3) forms are also described. Onset in childhood is associated with a positive family history, symptoms that begin in the legs, and greater disability than with later onset. About one-third of patients eventually become chair- or bedbound.→*A summary of the genetic loci responsible for the various dystonic disorders is provided in Table 359-1.*

Examination reveals the abnormal movements and sustained postures that characterize the disorder. There may be involvement of the neck, trunk, limbs, and face (blepharospasm or oromandibular dystonia). A description of these various motor abnormalities is provided in Chap. 22. Initially they may be brought out by voluntary activity, but eventually they are present constantly, leading to deformity and disability.

Occasional patients have *dopa-responsive dystonia,* which is inherited in an autosomal dominant manner with incomplete penetrance. The responsible gene (DYT5) maps to chromosome 14q. Onset is usually in childhood, and examination typically reveals associated bradykinesia and rigidity. The response to low-dose levodopa therapy is dramatic.

℞ **TREATMENT**   Treatment is symptomatic and is often unsatisfactory. Anticholinergic drugs in high doses (e.g., trihexyphenidyl, 30 to 50 mg/d) are probably the most effective means of providing some relief of the abnormal movements and postures. They are introduced in a low dose and built up gradually, depending on response and tolerance. Phenothiazines or haloperidol are sometimes helpful but usually cause mild parkinsonism. Diazepam, baclofen, and carbamazepine are helpful occasionally. Stereotactic thalamotomy may be beneficial when dystonia is predominantly unilateral and involves the limbs.

FOCAL TORSION DYSTONIA   Dystonia may occur as an isolated phenomenon affecting a discrete part of the body, rather than having the more generalized distribution described above. Such focal or segmental dystonias probably represent variants of idiopathic torsion dystonia; its genetic basis was discussed earlier. Both *blepharospasm* (spontaneous, involuntary forced closure of the eyelids) and *oromandibular dystonia* can occur as isolated focal dystonias. Oromandibular dystonia consists of involuntary contractions of the masticatory, lingual, and perioral muscles, leading to opening or closure of the mouth; pouting, pursing, or retraction of the lips; and roving or protruding movements of the tongue. The combination of blepharospasm and oromandibular dystonia is called *Meige syndrome.*

Spasmodic torticollis is characterized by a tendency for the head to turn to one side. The designation *anterocollis* indicates that the head is flexed forward, and *retrocollis* that it is pulled backward. These cervical dystonias are often intermittent initially, but eventually the head is held continuously in the abnormal position. Spontaneous remission occurs occasionally, especially in the first few months after onset, but thereafter the disorder is likely to be permanent and may worsen with time.

℞ **TREATMENT**   Pharmacotherapy is usually unrewarding, but the drugs used in treating idiopathic torsion dystonia are helpful in some patients. Local injection of botulinum toxin into the overactive muscles often produces a benefit lasting several weeks or months by producing a temporary presynaptic block of neuromuscular transmission, and injections can be repeated as needed. This is the most effective treatment available for most focal dystonias. Selective section of the spinal accessory nerve (cranial nerve XI) and the upper cervical nerve roots is sometimes helpful for patients with cervical dystonia unresponsive to other measures.

TASK-SPECIFIC FOCAL DYSTONIA   Writer's cramp is a task-specific dystonia in which abnormal posturing of the hand and forearm occurs when the hand is used for writing. As the disorder worsens, abnormal posturing may also occur with other tasks, such as applying cosmetics, shaving, or using table cutlery. Drug treatment is usually unrewarding, and it is often necessary for patients to learn to use the other hand for these tasks. Injections of botulinum toxin into the involved muscles are sometimes helpful, but function usually remains impaired. Other task-specific dystonias include violinist's cramp, barber's cramp, and telegrapher's cramp, in each of which dystonic posturing occurs when the hand is used for a skilled, occupationally related function. The pathophysiologic basis of these disorders is uncertain, but recent work relates it to abnormal processing of sensory input from the affected extremity during the activity.

DRUG-INDUCED MOVEMENT DISORDERS   Parkinsonism   Parkinsonism is a frequent complication of treatment with dopamine-depleting agents such as reserpine or antipsychotic dopamine antagonists such as the phenothiazines or butyrophenones. The antipsychotic drugs most likely to cause parkinsonism are those that are potent D_2 receptor antagonists having little anticholinergic effect, such as piperazine phenothiazines, haloperidol, and thiothixene. Women and the elderly have an increased risk of this complication. In comparison with Parkinson's disease, tremor is less common and bradykinesia is typically symmetric, but the two disorders are sometimes impossible to distinguish except by the history of drug ingestion. Signs usually develop within 3 months of starting the causal agent and may persist for several months (or longer) after its withdrawal. Drug-induced parkinsonism is best managed by discontinuing the antipsychotic drug when possible, substituting an antipsychotic with greater anticholinergic potency, or adding an anticholinergic drug such as trihexyphenidyl. Levodopa should not be prescribed—it is of no help if the offending neuroleptic agent is continued, and it may worsen the underlying psychotic disorder.

Acute Dystonia or Dyskinesia   Acute dystonia (such as blepharospasm or torticollis) or dyskinesia (such as chorea or facial grimacing) may complicate treatment with a dopamine receptor antagonist. It typically commences within 1 week of the introduction of such medication, usually in the first 48 h, and is more common in young patients. Its pathophysiologic basis is uncertain. Treatment with an anticholinergic drug (e.g., benztropine, 2 mg, or diphenhydramine, 50 mg intravenously) is usually helpful.

Tardive Akathisia   *Akathisia* denotes a motor restlessness. Patients are unable to sit still and feel obliged to move about. It is commonly induced by chronic antipsychotic drug treatment, especially in women, and is treated like drug-induced parkinsonism.

Tardive Dyskinesia or Dystonia   Tardive dyskinesia or dystonia is a common complication of long-term antipsychotic drug treatment (with dopamine receptor antagonists). The risk of its development increases with advancing age, but its pathogenesis is unclear. One suggestion is that it is related to drug-induced supersensitivity of striatal dopamine receptors. However, although supersensitivity is an inevitable accompaniment of chronic antipsychotic drug treatment, tardive dyskinesia does not always occur. Moreover, the time courses of the two phenomena are different. Supersensitivity occurs relatively early during treatment and reverses when medication is withdrawn, whereas tardive dyskinesia usually requires exposure for at least 6 months before it develops and may persist indefinitely. Another suggestion is that it involves an abnormality of γ-aminobutyric acid (GABA)-ergic neurons. This is supported by observations that GABA and glutamic acid decarboxylase (its synthesizing enzyme) are depleted in the basal ganglia by long-term administration of antipsychotic drugs to animals and that CSF levels of GABA are reduced in patients with tardive dyskinesia.

The clinical features of tardive dyskinesia include abnormal choreoathetoid movements, especially involving the face and mouth in adults and the limbs in children. Tardive dystonia may be focal, producing, for example, blepharospasm, torticollis, or oromandibular dystonia, or it may affect contiguous body parts (e.g., the face and neck or arm and trunk). Generalized dystonia is uncommon, especially in older patients. It may be impossible to distinguish these disturbances from those of Huntington's disease (Chap. 362), Sydenham's chorea (Chap. 235), or idiopathic torsion dystonia except by the history of drug exposure. The iatrogenic disorder often resolves spontaneously in children or young adults but frequently persists in middle-aged or older individuals.

℞ **TREATMENT** Treatment of the established disorder is often unsatisfactory. It is therefore important that antipsychotic drugs be prescribed only when necessary and that their long-term use be accompanied by periodic drug holidays to determine whether treatment is still required. Drug holidays may actually unmask incipient dyskinesias, which often worsen on withdrawal of the causal agent. In such circumstances, permanent withdrawal of the antipsychotic medication, if this is possible, may lead to remission of the dyskinesia. Treatment with antidopaminergic agents such as haloperidol or phenothiazines (which cause the disorder) often suppresses the dyskinesias at least for a period, but these agents are best avoided, because they may exacerbate the underlying problem. Treatment with dopamine-depleting agents, such as reserpine, 0.25 mg gradually increased to 2 to 4 mg/d, or tetrabenazine (in countries where it is available), 12.5 mg gradually increased to as much as 200 mg/d, is sometimes worthwhile in reducing the severity of the dyskinesia. Other pharmacologic approaches are unrewarding in most instances. Tardive dystonia may respond to tetrabenazine (if available) or to anticholinergic drugs used as for idiopathic torsion dystonia.

Tardive tic resembles Gilles de la Tourette's syndrome (see below) and is best treated with clonidine or clonazepam.

Neuroleptic Malignant Syndrome Rigidity, hyperthermia, altered mental status resembling catatonia, labile blood pressure, and autonomic dysfunction characterize this serious complication of treatment with antipsychotic (neuroleptic) agents, especially haloperidol. Associated clinical features include tachycardia, tachypnea, metabolic acidosis, and myoglobinuria that may be fatal. The cause is unknown, but antagonism of dopamine is a likely contributor. The prevalence of this syndrome among patients receiving neuroleptics is <2%, with the disorder occurring most commonly in young adults. Symptoms evolve over 1 to 2 days. The syndrome can develop at any time during exposure to the medication, but it usually occurs within the first 30 days of use.

The differential diagnosis includes infection, malignant hyperthermia, and alcohol- or drug-withdrawal states. Drug-induced parkinsonism may be similar but is not associated with fever or the autonomic features described above.

℞ **TREATMENT** Treatment includes immediate withdrawal of antipsychotic drugs and also of lithium and anticholinergic agents, which may increase the risk of developing the disorder. Symptomatic treatment is also necessary and includes antipyretics and artificial cooling, rehydration, and measures to maintain the blood pressure. Serum potassium should be monitored. Dantrolene, bromocriptine or another dopamine agonist, levodopa, amantadine, or benzodiazepines are sometimes helpful, but the mortality rate is on the order of 5 to 20%. Subcutaneous heparin administration reduces the risk of venous thrombosis. Most survivors recover completely, but potential complications include renal failure, pulmonary embolism, and a chronic cerebellar syndrome (related to the hyperthermia). Recovery generally occurs over 2 to 3 weeks.

Other Drug-Induced Movement Disorders Dyskinesia or dystonia may complicate therapy with levodopa or dopamine agonists as a dose-related phenomenon that is reversed by withdrawal of the medication or reduction of the dose. Reversible chorea may also complicate treatment with anticholinergic drugs, phenytoin, carbamazepine, amphetamines, lithium, and oral contraceptives; dystonia may follow treatment with lithium, carbamazepine, and metoclopramide; and postural tremor from theophylline, caffeine, lithium, thyroid hormone, tricyclic antidepressants, valproic acid, and isoproterenol.

GILLES DE LA TOURETTE'S SYNDROME Gilles de la Tourette's syndrome, which has a prevalence in the United States of approximately 0.05%, consists of chronic multiple motor and phonic tics that have no known cause. The disorder is not related to social or ethnic background or to perinatal abnormalities. Symptoms typically begin between 5 and 15 years of age and follow a relapsing and remitting course. A family history is sometimes obtained, and partial expression of the trait may occur in siblings or offspring of patients. In most families with chronic tic disorders, there is an autosomal dominant mode of inheritance with variable penetrance that is gender related. Boys are affected much more commonly than girls.

The pathophysiology is obscure, and no structural pathology has been recognized. A dopaminergic excess has been suggested by the clinical observation that the tics may respond to treatment with dopamine-blocking drugs.

Clinical Manifestations The first signs consist of single or multiple motor tics in 80% of cases and of phonic tics in 20%. Motor tics commonly affect the face and may consist of repetitive sniffing, winking, blinking, elevation of the eyelids, eye closure, pursing of the lips, or facial twitching. Patients eventually develop several different motor and phonic tics, the latter frequently taking the form of grunts, barks, hisses, sighs, throat-clearing, coughing, and verbal utterances that may involve coprolalia (involuntary and inappropriate swearing or obscene speech), echolalia (involuntary repetition of the phrases of others), and palilalia (repetition of words or phrases). The tics may change in location, severity, complexity, and character with time; are worsened by emotional stress; and can be suppressed voluntarily for short periods. In some cases, tics are complex (such as jumping up in the air) or involve repetitive self-mutilating activities (such as nail-biting, hair-pulling, or lip-biting). Tics that involve repetitive sensory phenomena, such as pressure, tickle, or thermal sensations, also occur. Many patients have associated behavioral abnormalities, especially obsessive-compulsive disorder and attention deficit hyperactivity disorder.

Apart from the presence of tics, physical examination typically reveals no other abnormalities, but the incidence of left-handedness or ambidexterity is greater than among normal persons, and many patients have nonspecific electroencephalographic abnormalities of no diagnostic significance.

The diagnosis is often delayed for years, the symptoms sometimes being attributed to psychiatric illness. Patients may be subjected to unnecessary and expensive treatment before the correct diagnosis is made. Depression, sometimes leading to suicide, may result from social embarrassment caused by the tics.

Differential Diagnosis Many children develop transient or chronic simple tics, and these have a benign prognosis and require no treatment. In some instances, simple or multiple tics persist for several years but resolve in late adolescence. Wilson's disease, a treatable cause of dyskinesias and tics, is generally associated with hepatic and renal involvement, Kayser-Fleischer corneal rings, low serum copper and ceruloplasmin levels, and increased 24-h urinary copper excretion (Chap. 348). The associated dementia, the character of the abnormal movements, and genetic studies distinguish Huntington's disease (Chap. 362). Sydenham's chorea (Chap. 235) may be confused with Gilles de la Tourette's syndrome when a history of rheumatic fever or polyarthritis is lacking and there is no cardiac involvement, but it usually resolves over 3 to 6 months. Tics may also occur in postencephalitic syndromes and as a side effect of stimulant or neuroleptic medication.

℞ **TREATMENT**   Treatment is symptomatic and may need to be continued indefinitely.

Clonidine alleviates motor and phonic tics in some children, possibly by reducing activity in noradrenergic neurons of the locus coeruleus. The initial dose is 2 to 3 μg/kg per day, increased after 2 weeks to 4 μg/kg per day and then, if required, to 5 μg/kg per day. There may be a transient fall in blood pressure when this agent is introduced. Other side effects are sedation, reduced or excessive salivation, and diarrhea.

Haloperidol has been used widely for many years. It is introduced in a low daily dose (0.25 mg), which is gradually increased by 0.25 mg every 5 days, depending on response and tolerance. The optimal dose is usually 2 to 8 mg/d. Side effects include extrapyramidal movement disorders, sedation, xerostomia, blurred vision, and gastrointestinal disturbances. Pimozide, another dopaminergic-receptor antagonist, may be of benefit when haloperidol is unhelpful or poorly tolerated. It may produce widening of the QT interval and sudden death at high doses, so the electrocardiogram should be monitored routinely. Its long-term safety is unknown. It is introduced in a dose of 1 mg/d, and the dose is then increased by 2 mg every 10 days; most patients require 7 to 16 mg/d. The total dose should not exceed 0.3 mg/kg per day. Phenothiazines such as fluphenazine sometimes help, but patients unresponsive to haloperidol do not usually benefit from these drugs. Clonazepam or carbamazepine can also be tried. Family counseling and psychotherapy are sometimes helpful.

RESTLESS LEGS SYNDROME   The restless legs syndrome is a common, chronic disorder that often has a familial basis, with evidence of autosomal dominant inheritance. It is characterized by a need to move because of unpleasant creeping sensations that arise deep within the legs and occasionally also in the arms, especially when patients are relaxed. For this reason, there is often difficulty in settling down to sleep at night. Periodic leg movements may also occur during sleep and can be documented by polysomnography. The cause is unknown, although the disorder is common during pregnancy and is sometimes associated with uremic or diabetic neuropathy, primary amyloidosis, or malignancy. Clinical examination may reveal evidence of underlying systemic disease or mild peripheral neuropathy but is more often normal. Symptoms may respond to correction of coexisting iron-deficiency anemia or to treatment with dopaminergic medication (such as levodopa, bromocriptine, or pergolide), benzodiazepines (diazepam or clonazepam), or opiates (codeine, propoxyphene, or oxycodone).

BIBLIOGRAPHY

BENNETT DA et al: Prevalence of parkinsonian signs and associated mortality in a community population of older people. N Engl J Med 334:771, 1996

DUNNETT SB, BJORKLUND A: Prospects for new restorative and neuroprotective treatments in Parkinson's disease. Nature 399:A32, 1999

FINE J et al: Long-term follow-up of unilateral pallidotomy in advanced Parkinson's disease. N Engl J Med 342:1708, 2000

GRATZ SS, SIMPSON GM: Neuroleptic malignant syndrome. Diagnosis, epidemiology and treatment. CNS Drugs 2:429, 1994

HYDE TM, WEINBERGER DR: Tourette's syndrome: A model neuropsychiatric disorder. JAMA 273:498, 1995

IANNACCONE S et al: Evidence of peripheral axonal neuropathy in primary restless legs syndrome. Mov Disord 10:2, 1995

JANKOVIC J: New and emerging therapies for Parkinson disease. Arch Neurol 56:785, 1999

KOLLER W et al: High-frequency unilateral thalamic stimulation in the treatment of essential and parkinsonian tremor. Ann Neurol 42:292, 1997

KORDOWER JH et al: Neuropathological evidence of graft survival and striatal reinnervation after the transplantation of fetal mesencephalic tissue in a patient with Parkinson's disease. N Engl J Med 332:1118, 1995

KURTH MC et al: Tolcapone improves motor function and reduces levodopa requirement in patients with Parkinson's disease experiencing motor fluctuations: A multicenter, double-blind, randomized, placebo-controlled trial. Neurology 48:81, 1997

LANG AE, LOZANO AM: Parkinson's disease. N Engl J Med 339:1044, 1130, 1998

——— et al: Posteroventral medial pallidotomy in advanced Parkinson's disease. N Engl J Med 337:1036, 1997

LIMOUSIN P et al: Electrical stimulation of the subthalamic nucleus in advanced Parkinson's disease. N Engl J Med 339:1105, 1998

MARTIN JB: Molecular basis of the neurodegenerative disorders. N Engl J Med 340:1970, 1999

NYGAARD TG et al: Linkage mapping of dopa-responsive dystonia (DRD) to chromosome 14q. Nat Genet 5:386, 1993

OLANOW CW, TATTON WG: Etiology and pathogenesis of Parkinson's disease. Annu Rev Neurosci 22:123, 1999

OZELIUS LJ et al: The early-onset torsion dystonia gene (DYT1) encodes an ATP-binding protein. Nat Genet 17:40, 1997

PARKINSON STUDY GROUP: Effects of tocopherol and deprenyl on the progression of disability in early Parkinson's disease. N Engl J Med 328:176, 1993

———: Impact of deprenyl and tocopherol treatment on Parkinson's disease in DATATOP subjects not requiring levodopa. Ann Neurol 39:29, 1996

POLYMEROPOULOS MH et al: Mapping of a gene for Parkinson's disease to chromosome 4q21-q23. Science 274:1197, 1996

QUINN N: Drug treatment of Parkinson's disease. BMJ 310:575, 1995

SCHUURMAN PR et al: A comparison of continuous thalamic stimulation and thalamotomy for suppression of severe tremor. N Engl J Med 342:461, 2000

STARR PA et al: Ablative surgery and deep brain stimulation for Parkinson's disease. Neurosurgery 43:989, 1998

TANNER CM et al: Parkinson disease in twins: An etiologic study. JAMA 281:341, 1999

UITTI RJ et al: Unilateral pallidotomy for Parkinson's disease: Comparison of outcome in younger versus older patients. Neurology 49:1072, 1997

364   *Roger N. Rosenberg*

ATAXIC DISORDERS

AT	ataxia telangiectasia	MJD	Machado-Joseph disease
AVED	Ataxia of the Friedreich's phenotype with vitamin E deficiency	MRI	magnetic resonance imaging
CNS	central nervous system	mtDNA	mitochondrial DNA
CT	computed tomography	MTP	microsomal triglyceride transfer protein
DRPLA	dentatorubropallidoluysian atrophy	SCAs	spinocerebellar ataxias
EA	episodic ataxia	VLDL	very-low-density lipoprotein

Approach to the Patient

Ataxia is a common and important neurologic finding. Symptoms and signs of ataxia consist of gait impairment, unclear ("scanning") speech, visual blurring due to nystagmus, hand incoordination, and tremor with movement (Chap. 22). These result from the involvement of the cerebellum and its afferent and efferent pathways including the spinocerebellar pathways, and the frontopontocerebellar pathway originating in the rostral frontal lobe (Brodmann's area 10). True cerebellar ataxia must be distinguished from ataxia associated with vestibular nerve or labyrinthine disease, as the latter results in a disorder of gait associated with a significant degree of dizziness, light-headedness, or the perception of movement (Chap. 21). True cerebellar ataxia is devoid of these vertiginous complaints and is clearly an unsteady gait due to imbalance. Weakness of proximal leg muscles and a variant of acute idiopathic polyneuritis (Miller-Fisher syndrome) can on occasion simulate the imbalance of cerebellar disease. In the patient who presents with ataxia, the rate and pattern of the development of cerebellar symptoms are important in determining the diagnostic possibilities (Table 364-1). A gradual and progressive increase in symptoms with bilateral and symmetric involvement suggests a biochemical, metabolic, immune, or toxic etiology. Conversely, focal, unilateral symptoms with headache and impaired level of consciousness accompanied by ipsilateral cranial nerve palsies and contralateral weakness imply a space-occupying cerebellar lesion.

Symmetric Ataxia Progressive and symmetric ataxia can be classified with respect to onset as acute (over hours or days), subacute (weeks or months), or chronic (months to years). Acute and reversible ataxias include those caused by intoxication with alcohol, phenytoin, lithium, barbiturates, and other drugs. Intoxication caused by toluene exposure, gasoline sniffing, glue sniffing, spray painting, or exposure to methyl mercury or bismuth are additional causes of acute or subacute ataxia, as is treatment with cytotoxic chemotherapeutic drugs such as flourouracil and paclitaxel. Children with a postinfectious syndrome (especially after varicella) may develop gait ataxia and mild dysathria, which are both reversible (Chap. 371). Rare infectious causes of acquired ataxia include poliovirus, coxsackievirus, echovirus, Epstein-Barr virus, toxoplasmosis, *Legionella*, and the prion protein responsible for Creutzfeldt-Jakob disease. The subacute development of ataxia of gait over weeks to months (acute cerebellar degeneration of the vermis) may be due to the combined effects of alcoholism and malnutrition, particularly with deficiencies of vitamins B_1 and B_{12}. Hyponatremia has also been associated with ataxia. A paraneoplastic syndrome, which may be associated with myoclonus and opsoclonus, may present as incapacitating gait ataxia. Specific autoantibodies (Yo, Ri, and PCD) have been identified that are responsible for cerebellar degeneration involving principally the midline or vermis (Chap. 101). Female patients may present with cerebellar ataxia before the identification of a breast or ovarian carcinoma. Removal of the tumor may prevent further progression of symptoms and in some patients result in gait improvement. Chronic symmetric gait ataxia of months' to years' duration suggests an inherited ataxia (discussed below), a metabolic disorder, or a chronic infection. Hypothyroidism must always be considered as a readily treatable and reversible form of gait ataxia. Infectious diseases that can present with ataxia are meningovascular syphilis and tabes dorsalis due to degeneration of the posterior columns and spinocerebellar pathways in the spinal cord. Lyme disease may cause ataxic symptoms.

Focal Ataxia Acute focal ataxia commonly results from cerebrovascular disease, usually ischemic infarction, hemorrhagic infarction, or cerebellar hemorrhage. These lesions typically produce cerebellar symptoms ipsilateral to the injured cerebellum and may be associated with an impaired level of consciousness due to brainstem compression and increased intracranial pressure; ipsilateral pontine signs, including sixth and seventh nerve palsies, may be present. Focal and worsening signs of acute ataxia should also prompt consideration of a posterior fossa subdural hematoma, bacterial abscess, primary or metastatic cerebellar tumor, or acute demyelinating lesion of multiple sclerosis. Computed tomography (CT) or magnetic resonance imaging (MRI) studies will reveal clinically significant processes of this type, which may require surgical decompression. Many of these lesions represent true neurologic emergencies, as sudden herniation, either rostrally through the tentorium or caudal herniation of cerebellar tonsils

Table 364-1 Etiology of Cerebellar Ataxia

Symmetrical and Progressive Signs			Focal and Ipsilateral Cerebellar Signs		
Acute (Hours to Days)	Subacute (Days to Weeks)	Chronic (Months to Years)	Acute (Hours to Days)	Subacute (Days to Weeks)	Chronic (Months to Years)
Intoxication: alcohol, lithium, diphenylhydantoin, barbiturates (positive history and toxicology screen) Acute viral cerebellitis (CSF supportive of acute viral infection) Postinfection syndrome	Intoxication: mercury, solvents, gasoline, glue; cytotoxic chemotherapeutic drugs Alcoholic-nutritional (vitamin B_1 and B_{12} deficiency) Lyme disease	Paraneoplastic syndrome Hypothyroidism Inherited diseases Tabes dorsalis (tertiary syphilis)	Vascular: Cerebellar infarction, hemorrhage, or subdural hematoma Infectious: cerebellar abscess (positive mass lesion on MRI/CT, positive history in support of lesion)	Neoplastic: cerebellar glioma or metastatic tumor (positive for neoplasm on MRI/CT) Demyelinating: Multiple sclerosis (history, CSF and MRI are consistent) AIDS-related multifocal leukoencephalopathy (positive HIV test and CD4+ cell count for AIDS)	Stable gliosis secondary to vascular lesion or demyelinating plaque (stable lesion on MRI/CT older than several months) Congenital lesion: Chiari or Dandy-Walker malformations (malformation noted on MRI/CT)

ABBREVIATIONS: CSF, cerebrospinal fluid; CT, computed tomography; MRI, magnetic resonance imaging.

through the foramen magnum can occur and is usually devastating (Chap. 376). Lymphoma or progressive multifocal leukoencephalopathy (PML) in a patient with AIDS may present with an acute or subacute focal cerebellar syndrome. Chronic etiologies of ataxia include multiple sclerosis and congenital lesions such as the Chiari type I malformation, and congenital cysts of the posterior fossa (Dandy-Walker syndrome).

THE INHERITED ATAXIAS

Of the syndromes that constitute the inherited ataxias, some show autosomal dominant or autosomal recessive modes of inheritance, and some are caused by mitochondrial mutations and thus show a maternal mode of inheritance. Substantial progress has been made in recent years in identifying the molecular basis of these syndromes (Table 364-2), so that a genomic classification is superseding previous ones based on clinical expression alone.

Although the clinical manifestations and neuropathologic findings of cerebellar disease dominate the clinical picture, there may also be characteristic changes in the basal ganglia, brainstem, spinal cord, optic nerves, retina, and peripheral nerves. In large families with dominantly inherited disease, there are many gradations from purely cerebellar manifestations to mixed cerebellar and brainstem disorders, cerebellar and basal ganglia syndromes, and spinal cord or peripheral nerve disease. Rarely, dementia is present as well. The clinical picture may be consistent within a family with dominantly inherited ataxia, but sometimes most affected family members show one characteristic syndrome, while one or several members have an entirely different phenotype.

The autosomal spinocerebellar ataxias (SCAs) are caused by CAG triplet repeat expansions in different genes including SCA1, SCA2, MJD, SCA6, SCA7, and SCA13. SCA8 is due to a CTG repeat expansion (Table 364-2). The clinical phenotypes of these SCAs overlap. A single phenotype can result from several different genotypes, and conversely a single genotype can be associated with more than one different phenotype. The genotype has become the gold standard for diagnosis and classification. CAG encodes glutamine, and these expanded CAG triplet repeat expansions result in expanded polyglutamine proteins, termed *ataxins*, that produce a toxic gain of function with

Table 364-2 Genotype Classification of the Spinocerebellar Ataxias

Name	Locus	Phenotype
SCA1 (autosomal dominant type 1)	6p22-p23 with CAG repeats (exonic) Ataxin-1	Ataxia with ophthalmoparesis, pyramidal and extrapyramidal findings
SCA2 (autosomal dominant type 2)	12q23-q24.1 with CAG repeats (exonic) Ataxin-2	Ataxia with slow saccades and minimal pyramidal and extrapyramidal findings
Machado-Joseph disease/SCA3 (autosomal dominant type 3)	14q24.3-q32 with CAG repeats (exonic) MJD–ataxin-3	Ataxia with ophthalmoparesis and variable pyramidal, extrapyramidal, and amyotrophic signs
SCA4 (autosomal dominant type 4)	16q24-ter	Ataxia with normal eye movements, sensory axonal neuropathy, and pyramidal signs
SCA5 (autosomal dominant type 5)	Centromeric region of chromosome 11	Ataxia and dysarthria; family descended from paternal grandparents of President Lincoln
SCA6 (autosomal dominant type 6)	19p13 with CAG repeats in α_{1A}-voltage–dependent calcium channel gene (exonic)	Ataxia and dysarthria, nystagmus, mild proprioceptive sensory loss
SCA7 (autosomal dominant type 7)	3p14.1-p21.1 with CAG repeats (exonic) Ataxin-7	Ophthalmoparesis, visual loss, ataxia, dysarthria, extensor plantar response, pigmentary retinal degeneration; severity varies from asymptomatic to late onset/mild to early onset/aggressive
SCA8 (autosomal dominant type 8)	13q21 with CTG repeats (untranslated)	Gait ataxia, dysarthria, nystagmus; leg spasticity and reduced vibratory sensation
SCA10 (autosomal dominant type 10)	22q	Gait ataxia, dysarthria, nystagmus; partial complex and generalized motor seizures
SCA11 (autosomal dominant type 11)	15q14-q21.3 by linkage	Slowly progressive gait and extremity ataxia, dysarthria, vertical nystagmus, hyperreflexia
SCA12 (autosomal dominant type 12)	5q31-q33 by linkage	Tremor, decreased movement, increased reflexes, dystonia, ataxia, dysautonomia, dementia
SCA13 (single case)	6q27 with CAG repeats in the TATA binding-protein gene	Gait and extremity ataxia, hyperreflexia, extensor plantar responses, dysarthria, dysphagia, severe mental retardation
Dentatorubropallidoluysian atrophy (autosomal dominant)	12p12-ter with CAG repeats (exonic) Atrophin	Ataxia, choreoathetosis, dystonia, seizures, myoclonus, dementia
Friedreich's ataxia (autosomal recessive)	9q13-q21.1 with intronic GAA repeats Frataxin	Ataxia, areflexia, extensor plantar responses, position sense deficits, cardiomyopathy, diabetes mellitus, scoliosis, foot deformities; defective iron transport from mitochondria
Friedreich's ataxia (autosomal recessive)	8q13.1-q13.3; α-TTP deficiency	Same as phenotype that maps to 9q but associated with vitamin E deficiency
Kearns-Sayre syndrome (sporadic)	mtDNA deletion and duplication mutations	Ptosis, ophthalmoplegia, pigmentary retinal degeneration, cardiomyopathy, diabetes mellitus, deafness, heart block, increased CSF protein, ataxia
Myoclonus epilepsy and ragged red fiber syndrome (MERRF) (maternal inheritance)	Mutation in mtDNA of the tRNA^{lys} at 8344; also mutation at 8356	Myoclonic epilepsy, ragged red fiber myopathy, ataxia
Mitochondrial encephalopathy, lactic acidosis, and stroke syndrome (MELAS) (maternal inheritance)	tRNA^{leu} mutation at 3243; also at 3271 and 3252	Headache, stroke, lactic acidosis, ataxia
Leigh's disease; subacute necrotizing encephalopathy (maternal inheritance or autosomal recessive)	mtDNA complex V defect (ATPase gene at 8993) or mitochondrial protein synthesis defect (both maternally inherited); or complex IV defect (autosomal recessive)	Obtundation, hypotonia, cranial nerve defects, respiratory failure, hyperintense signals on T2-weighted magnetic resonance images in basal ganglia, cerebellum, or brainstem; ataxia
Episodic ataxia, type 1 (EA-1) (autosomal dominant)	12p; potassium channel gene, KCNA1	Episodic ataxia for minutes; provoked by startle or exercise; with facial and hand myokymia; cerebellar signs are not progressive; responds to phenytoin
Episodic ataxia, type 2 (EA-2) (autosomal dominant)	19p13(CACNA1A) (allelic with SCA6) (α_{1a}-voltage–dependent calcium channel subunit)	Episodic ataxia for days; provoked by stress, fatigue; with down-gaze nystagmus; cerebellar atrophy results; progressive cerebellar signs; responds to acetazolamide
Ataxia telangiectasia (autosomal recessive)	11q22-q23; ATM gene for regulation of cell cycle; mitogenic signal transduction and meiotic recombination	Telangiectasia, ataxia, dysarthria, pulmonary infections, neoplasms of lymphatic system; IgA and IgG deficiencies; diabetes mellitus, breast cancer
Infantile-onset spinocerebellar ataxia of Nikali et al. (autosomal recessive)	10q23.3-q24.1	Infantile ataxia, sensory neuropathy; athetosis, hearing deficit, ophthalmoplegia, optic atrophy; primary hypogonadism in females

autosomal dominant inheritance. Although the phenotype is variable for any given disease gene, a pattern of neuronal loss with gliosis is produced that is relatively unique for each ataxia. Immunohistochemical and biochemical studies have shown cytoplasmic (SCA2), neuronal (SCA1, MJD, SCA7), and nucleolar (SCA7) accumulation of the specific mutant polyglutamine containing ataxin proteins. Expanded polyglutamine ataxins with more than approximately 40 glutamines are potentially toxic to neurons for a variety of reasons including the following: high levels of gene expression for the mutant polyglutamine ataxin in affected neurons; conformational change of the aggregated protein to a β-pleated structure; abnormal transport of the ataxin into the nucleus (SCA1, MJD, SCA7); binding to other polyglutamine proteins, including the TATA-binding transcription protein and the CREB-binding protein, impairing their functions; altering the efficiency of the ubiquitin-proteosome system of protein turnover; and inducing neuronal apoptosis. An earlier age of onset (anticipation) and more aggressive disease in subsequent generations are due to further expansion of the CAG triplet repeat and increased polyglutamine number in the mutant ataxin. A new classification based on the genotype and its specific mutant ataxin is presented in Table 364-2, and the salient features of the most common disorders are discussed below.

AUTOSOMAL DOMINANT ATAXIAS The new genomic classification of the dominantly inherited ataxias includes SCA type 1 through SCA13, dentatorubropallidoluysian atrophy (DRPLA), and episodic ataxia (EA) types 1 and 2 (Table 364-2).

SCA1 SCA1 was previously referred to as *olivopontocerebellar atrophy*, but genomic data have shown that that entity represents several different genotypes with overlapping clinical features.

Symptoms and signs SCA1 is characterized by the development in early or middle adult life of progressive cerebellar ataxia of the trunk and limbs, impairment of equilibrium and gait, slowness of voluntary movements, scanning speech, nystagmoid eye movements, and oscillatory tremor of the head and trunk. Dysarthria, dysphagia, and oculomotor and facial palsies may also occur. Extrapyramidal symptoms include rigidity, an immobile face, and parkinsonian tremor. The reflexes are usually normal, but knee and ankle jerks may be lost, and extensor plantar responses may occur. Dementia may be noted but is usually mild. Impairment of sphincter function is common, with urinary and sometimes fecal incontinence. Cerebellar and brainstem atrophy are evident on MRI (Fig. 364-1).

Marked shrinkage of the ventral half of the pons, disappearance of the olivary eminence on the ventral surface of the medulla, and atrophy of the cerebellum are evident on gross postmortem inspection of the brain. Variable loss of Purkinje cells, reduced numbers of cells in the molecular and granular layer, demyelination of the middle cerebellar peduncle and the cerebellar hemispheres, and severe loss of cells in the pontine nuclei and olives are found on histologic examination. Degenerative changes in the striatum, especially the putamen, and loss of the pigmented cells of the substantia nigra may be found in cases with extrapyramidal features. More widespread degeneration in the central nervous system (CNS), including involvement of the posterior columns and the spinocerebellar fibers, is often present, especially in the cases with autosomal dominant inheritance.

GENETIC CONSIDERATIONS SCA1 was mapped positionally to chromosome 6 (6p22-p23), and the causal gene was found to contain CAG expanded DNA repeats (Chap. 359). The mutant allele

FIGURE 364-1 Sagittal MRI of the brain of a 60-year-old man with gait ataxia and dysarthria due to SCA1, illustrating cerebellar atrophy.

has >40 CAG repeats, whereas alleles from unaffected individuals have ≤36 repeats. A few patients with 38 to 40 CAG repeats have been described. There is a direct correlation between a larger number of repeats and a younger age of onset for SCA1. Juvenile patients have higher numbers of repeats, and anticipation is present in subsequent generations. The SCA1 gene is 450 kilobases (kb) long and has nine exons, with the first seven exons located in a 5' untranslated region and the last two exons containing the coding region. The SCA1 transcript contains 10,660 bases and is transcribed from both the wild-type allele and SCA1 alleles. The CAG repeat, which codes for a polyglutamine tract, lies within the coding region. The SCA1 gene product, called ataxin-1, is a novel protein of unknown function. Recently, polyglutamine aggregates bound to ubiquitin have been described in neuronal nuclei that are undergoing degeneration. Similar neuronal nuclear inclusions have been seen in cerebellar Purkinje cells of transgenic mice overexpressing an expanded variant of the ataxin-1 gene that causes human SCA1. Other transgenic mice carrying the SCA1 gene but with the self-association region deleted, so that polyglutamine aggregation did not occur, still developed ataxia and Purkinje cell pathology. Thus, although nuclear localization of ataxin-1 is necessary, nuclear aggregation of ataxin-1 is not required to initiate pathogenesis in transgenic mice. ■

SCA2 • Symptoms and signs Another clinical phenotype, SCA2, has been described in Cubans. These patients probably are descendants of a common ancestor, and the population may be the largest homogeneous group of patients with ataxia yet described. The age of onset ranges from 2 to 65 years, and there is considerable clinical variability within families. Although neuropathologic and clinical findings are compatible with a diagnosis of SCA1, including parkinsonian rigidity, optic disk pallor, mild spasticity, and retinal degeneration, it appears that SCA2 is a unique form of cerebellar degenerative disease.

GENETIC CONSIDERATIONS The gene in SCA2 families has been mapped to 12q23-q24.1. Thus, the similar clinical phenotypes of SCA1 and SCA2, mapped respectively to 6p and 12q, represent different genotypes. The gene has recently been identified, and it also contains CAG repeat expansions coding for a polyglutamine-containing protein, ataxin-2. Normal alleles contain 15 to 24 repeats; mutant alleles have 35 to 59 repeats. ■

Machado-Joseph Disease/SCA3 Machado-Joseph disease (MJD) is an autosomal dominant spinocerebellar degenerative disease first described among the Portuguese and their descendants in New England and California. Subsequently, MJD has been found in families from Portugal, Australia, Brazil, Canada, China, England, France, India, Israel, Italy, Japan, Spain, Taiwan, and the United States. In most populations, it is the most common inherited autosomal dominant ataxia.

Symptoms and signs MJD has been classified into three clinical types. In type I MJD (amyotrophic lateral sclerosis–parkinsonism–dystonia type), neurologic deficits appear in the first two decades and involve weakness and spasticity of extremities, especially the legs, often with dystonia of the face, neck, trunk, and extremities. Patellar and ankle clonus are common, as are extensor plantar responses. The gait is slow and stiff, with a slightly broadened base and lurching from side to side; this gait results from spasticity, not true ataxia. There is no truncal titubation. Pharyngeal weakness and spasticity cause difficulty with speech and swallowing. Of note is the prominence of horizontal and vertical nystagmus, loss of fast saccadic eye movements, hypermetric and hypometric saccades, and impairment of upward vertical gaze. Facial fasciculations, facial myokymia, lingual fasciculations without atrophy, ophthalmoparesis, and ocular prominence are common and early manifestations.

In type II MJD (ataxic type), true cerebellar deficits appear, including dysarthria and gait and extremity ataxia, beginning in the second to fourth decades, along with corticospinal and extrapyramidal deficits of spasticity, rigidity, and dystonia. Type II is the most common form of MJD. Ophthalmoparesis, upward vertical gaze deficits, and facial and lingual fasciculations are also present. Type II MJD must be distinguished from the clinically similar disorders SCA1 and SCA2.

Type III MJD (ataxic-amyotrophic type) presents in the fifth to the seventh decades with a pancerebellar disorder that includes dysarthria and gait and extremity ataxia. Distal sensory loss involving pain, touch, vibration, and position senses and distal atrophy are prominent, indicating the presence of peripheral neuropathy. The deep tendon reflexes are depressed to absent, and there are no corticospinal or extrapyramidal findings.

The mean age of onset of symptoms in MJD is 25 years. Neurologic deficits invariably progress and lead to death from debilitation within 15 years of onset, especially in patients with types I and II disease. Usually, patients retain full intellectual function.

The major pathologic findings are variable loss of neurons and glial replacement in the corpus striatum and severe loss of neurons in the pars compacta of the substantia nigra. A moderate loss of neurons occurs in the dentate nucleus of the cerebellum and in the red nucleus. Purkinje cell loss and granule cell loss occur in the cerebellar cortex. Cell loss also occurs in the dentate nucleus and in the cranial nerve motor nuclei. Sparing of the inferior olives distinguishes MJD from other dominantly inherited ataxias.

GENETIC CONSIDERATIONS   The gene locus for MJD has been mapped to 14q24.3-q32. The genes from families with MJD in Japan and North and South America all map to the same locus. Unstable CAG repeat expansions are present in the MJD gene coding for a polyglutamine-containing protein named ataxin-3 or MJD-ataxin. An earlier age of onset is associated with longer repeats. Alleles from normal individuals have between 12 and 37 CAG repeats, and MJD alleles have 60 to 84 CAG repeats. A patient with autonomic dysfunction and ataxia has been described with 56 CAG repeats. Polyglutamine-containing aggregates of ataxin-3 (MJD-ataxin) have been described in neuronal nuclei undergoing degeneration. ■

SCA6   Genomic screening for CAG repeats in other families with autosomal dominant ataxia and vibratory and proprioceptive sensory loss have yielded another locus. Of interest is that different mutations in the same gene for the α_{1A} voltage-dependent calcium channel subunit (CACNLIA4) (also referred to as the CACNA1A gene) at 19p13 result in different clinical disorders. CAG repeat expansions (21 to 27 in patients; 4 to 16 triplets in normal individuals) result in late onset progressive ataxia with cerebellar degeneration. Missense mutations in this gene result in familial hemiplegic migraine. Non-sense mutations resulting in termination of protein synthesis of the gene product yield hereditary paroxysmal cerebellar ataxia or episodic ataxia. Some patients with familial hemiplegic migraine develop progressive ataxia and also have cerebellar atrophy.

Dentatorubropallidoluysian Atrophy   DRPLA is a disorder of variable clinical presentation that is characterized by progressive ataxia, choreoathetosis, dystonia, seizures, myoclonus, and dementia. DRPLA is due to unstable CAG triplet repeats in the open reading frame of a gene named atrophin located on chromosome 12p12-ter. Larger expansions are found in patients with earlier onset. The number of repeats is ≥49 in patients with DRPLA; it is ≤26 in normal individuals. Anticipation occurs; successive generations in individual families show progressively earlier onset of disease in association with an increasing CAG repeat number. Larger expansions occur in children who inherit the disease from their father.

Episodic Ataxia   Types 1 and 2 are two rare dominantly inherited disorders that have been mapped to chromosomes 12p (a potassium channel gene) for type 1 and 19p for type 2. Patients with EA-1 have brief episodes of ataxia with myokymia and nystagmus that last only minutes. Startle, sudden change in posture, and exercise can induce episodes. Acetazolamide or anticonvulsants may be therapeutic. Patients with EA-2 have episodes of ataxia with nystagmus that can

last for hours or days. Stress, exercise, or excessive fatigue may be precipitants. Acetazolamide may be therapeutic and can reverse the relative intracellular alkalosis detected by MR spectroscopy. Stop codon, non-sense mutations causing EA-2 have been found in the CACNA1A gene, encoding the α_{1A} voltage-dependent calcium channel subunit (see SCA6 above). See Table 364-2 for details.

AUTOSOMAL RECESSIVE ATAXIAS   Friedreich's Ataxia   This is the most common form of inherited ataxia, comprising one-half of all hereditary ataxias. It can occur in a classic form or in association with a genetically determined vitamin E deficiency syndrome; the two forms are clinically indistinguishable.

Symptoms and signs   Friedreich's ataxia presents before 25 years of age with progressive staggering gait, frequent falling, and titubation. The lower extremities are more severely involved than the upper ones. Dysarthria occasionally is the presenting symptom; and rarely progressive scoliosis, foot deformity, nystagmus, or cardiopathy are initial signs.

The neurologic examination reveals nystagmus, loss of fast saccadic eye movements, truncal titubation, dysarthria, dysmetria, and ataxia of extremity and truncal movements. Extensor plantar responses (with normal tone in trunk and extremities), absence of deep tendon reflexes, and weakness (greater distally than proximally) are usually found. Loss of vibratory and proprioceptive sensation occurs. The median age of death is 35 years. Women have a significantly better prognosis than men; the 20-year survival rate is 100% in women and 63% in men.

Cardiac involvement occurs in 90% of patients. Cardiomegaly, symmetric hypertrophy, murmurs, and conduction defects are reported. Idebenone, a free-radical scavenger, has been shown in preliminary studies to protect heart muscle from iron-induced injury and to decrease myocardial hypertrophy. Iron chelators and antioxidant drugs are potentially harmful. Moderate mental retardation or psychiatric syndromes are present in a small percentage of patients. A high incidence of diabetes mellitus (20%) is found and is associated with insulin resistance and pancreatic β-cell dysfunction. However, no linkage is reported between the Friedreich's ataxia gene and loci predisposing to diabetes mellitus. Musculoskeletal deformities are common and include pes cavus, pes equinovarus, and scoliosis. MRI of the spinal cord shows significant cord atrophy in affected patients (Fig. 364-2).

The primary sites of pathology are the spinal cord, dorsal root ganglion cells, and the peripheral nerves. Slight atrophy of the cerebellum and cerebral gyri may occur. Sclerosis and degeneration occur

FIGURE 364-2 Sagittal MRI of the brain and spinal cord of a patient with Friedreich's ataxia, demonstrating spinal cord atrophy

predominantly in the spinocerebellar tracts, lateral corticospinal tracts, and posterior columns. Degeneration of the glossopharyngeal, vagus, hypoglossal, and deep cerebellar nuclei is described. The cerebral cortex is histologically normal except for loss of Betz cells in the precentral gyri. The peripheral nerves are extensively involved, with a loss of large myelinated fibers. The density of small myelinated fibers is normal, but axonal size and myelin thickness are diminished. Cardiac pathology consists of myocytic hypertrophy and fibrosis, focal vascular fibromuscular dysplasia with subintimal or medial deposition of periodic acid–Schiff (PAS)-positive material, myocytopathy with unusual pleomorphic nuclei, and focal degeneration of myelinated and unmyelinated nerves and cardiac ganglia.

§ **GENETIC CONSIDERATIONS** The classic form of Friedreich's ataxia has been mapped to 9q13-q21.1, and the mutant gene, frataxin, contains expanded GAA triplet repeats in the first intron. There is homozygosity for expanded GAA repeats in most patients. Normal persons have 7 to 22 GAA repeats, and patients have 200 to 900 GAA repeats. Patients with Friedreich's ataxia have undetectable or extremely low levels of frataxin mRNA, as compared with carriers and unrelated individuals; thus, disease appears to be caused by a loss of expression of the frataxin protein. Frataxin is a mitochondrial protein involved in iron homeostasis. Mitochondrial iron accumulation due to loss of the iron transporter coded by the mutant frataxin gene results in oxidized intramitochondrial iron. Excess oxidized iron results in turn in the oxidation of cellular components and irreversible cell injury.

Two forms of hereditary ataxia associated with abnormalities in the interactions of vitamin E (α-tocopherol) with very-low-density lipoprotein (VLDL) have been delineated. Ataxia of the Friedreich's phenotype with vitamin E deficiency (AVED) and abetalipoproteinemia (Bassen-Kornzweig syndrome) have both been clarified at the molecular genetic level. Abetalipoproteinemia is caused by mutations in the gene coding for the larger subunit of the microsomal triglyceride transfer protein (MTP). Defects in MTP result in impairment of formation and secretion of VLDL in liver. This defect results in a deficiency of delivery of vitamin E to tissues, including the central and peripheral nervous system, as VLDL is the transport molecule for vitamin E and other fat-soluble substitutes. AVED is due to mutations in the gene for α-tocopherol transfer protein (α-TTP) on chromosome 8 (8q13). These patients have an impaired ability to bind vitamin E into the VLDL produced and secreted by the liver, resulting in a deficiency of vitamin E in peripheral tissues. Hence, either absence of VLDL (abetalipoproteinemia) or impaired binding of vitamin E to VLDL (AVED) causes an ataxic syndrome. Once again, a genotype classification has proved to be essential in sorting out the various clinical forms of the Friedreich's disease syndrome. ■

Ataxia Telangiectasia • *Symptoms and signs* Patients present in the first decade of life with progressive telangiectatic lesions associated with deficits in cerebellar function and nystagmus. The neurologic manifestations correspond to those in Friedreich's disease, which should be included in the differential diagnosis. Truncal ataxia, extremity ataxia, dysarthria, extensor plantar responses, myoclonic jerks, areflexia, and distal sensory deficits may develop. There is a high incidence of recurrent pulmonary infections and neoplasms of the lymphatic and reticuloendothelial system in patients with ataxia telangiectasia (AT) as well as an increased incidence of cancer. Thymic hypoplasia with cellular and humoral (IgA and IgG2) immunodeficiencies, premature aging, and endocrine disorders such as insulin-dependent diabetes mellitus are described. There is an increased incidence of lymphomas, Hodgkin's disease, and acute leukemias of the T cell type. There is also an increased incidence of breast cancer in women who are heterozygous for AT. The immunologic defects and increased susceptibility to cancer have been causally linked to cellular disorders in AT. Exposure of cultured cells to ionizing radiation slows the rate of DNA replication and increases the frequency of chromosomal aberrations.

The most striking neuropathologic changes include loss of Pur-

kinje, granule, and basket cells in the cerebellar cortex as well as of neurons in the deep cerebellar nuclei. The inferior olives of the medulla also may have neuronal loss. There is a loss of anterior horn neurons in the spinal cord and of dorsal root ganglion cells associated with posterior column spinal cord demyelination. A poorly developed or absent thymus gland is the most consistent defect of the lymphoid system.

§ **GENETIC CONSIDERATIONS** The gene for AT (the *ATM* gene) has been positionally mapped to chromosome 11q22-q23. *ATM*, which has a 12-kb transcript, was mutated in AT patients from all complementation groups described previously. A partial *ATM* cDNA clone of 5.9 kb encodes a protein that is similar to several yeast and mammalian phosphatidylinositol-3'-kinases involved in mitogenic signal transduction, meiotic recombination, and cell cycle control. Defective DNA repair in AT fibroblasts exposed to ultraviolet light has been demonstrated. The discovery of *ATM* will make possible the identification of heterozygotes who are at risk for cancer (e.g., breast cancer) and permit early diagnosis. ■

Mitochondrial Ataxias Spinocerebellar syndromes have been identified with mutations in mitochondrial DNA (mtDNA). Thirty pathogenic mtDNA point mutations and >60 different types of mtDNA deletions are known, several of which cause or are associated with ataxia (Chap. 383).

Xeroderma Pigmentosum Xeroderma pigmentosum is a rare autosomal recessive neurocutaneous disorder caused by the inability to repair damage to DNA, such as that produced by ultraviolet radiation. In addition to skin lesions, patients may show progressive mental deterioration, microcephaly, ataxia, spasticity, choreoathetosis, and hypogonadism. Nerve deafness, peripheral neuropathy (predominantly axonal), electroencephalographic abnormalities, and seizures are reported. Neuronal death occurs in pyramidal cells, cerebellar Purkinje cells, the deep nuclei of the cerebellum, the brainstem, the spinal cord, and peripheral nerves.

Cockayne Syndrome This is a rare autosomal recessive disorder first described by Cockayne in 1936. Clinical features are mental retardation, optic atrophy, dwarfism, neural deafness, hypersensitivity of skin to sunlight, cataracts, and retinal pigmentary degeneration. Cerebellar, pyramidal, and extrapyramidal deficits and peripheral neuropathy may occur, with a "bird-headed" facial appearance and normal-pressure hydrocephalus. Skin fibroblasts exposed to ultraviolet light demonstrate defective DNA repair.

Marinesco-Sjögren Syndrome This rare syndrome, in which progressive cerebellar deficits begin early in childhood, is another example in which a Friedreich's syndrome is associated with additional specific features. In this case, cataracts, mental retardation, multiple skeletal abnormalities, hypogonadotropic hypogonadism, and severe cerebellar atrophy are associated. The syndrome is likely a lysosomal storage disorder caused by an enzymatic defect, but the pathophysiology is unknown.

℞ **TREATMENT** The physician's most important task in the management of patients with ataxia is to identify treatable disease entities. Malignancies may present with chronic progressive ataxia either directly with a mass effect in the posterior fossa or indirectly by paraneoplastic degeneration. Other mass lesions can be treated appropriately. Malabsorption syndromes leading to vitamin E deficiency may lead to ataxia. The vitamin E deficiency form of Friedreich's ataxia must be considered, and serum vitamin E levels measured. Vitamin E therapy is indicated for these rare patients. There is preliminary evidence that idebenone, a free-radical scavenger, is therapeutic for patients with classic Friedreich ataxia by reducing myocardial hypertrophy. There is no current evidence that it improves neurologic function. Iron chelators and antioxidant drugs are potentially harmful as they may increase heart muscle injury. Vitamin B_1 and B_{12} levels in serum must be measured, and the vitamins should be administered to patients having deficient levels. The deleterious effects of diphenylhydantoin and alcohol on the cerebellum are well known. Hypothyroidism is easily treated. Aminoacidopathies, leukodystrophies, urea-cycle abnormalities, and mitochondrial encephalomyopathies may produce ataxia, and some dietary or metabolic therapies are available. The cerebrospinal fluid should be tested for a syphilitic infection in patients with progressive ataxia and other features of tabes dorsalis. Similarly, antibody titers for Lyme disease and *Legionella* should be measured, and appropriate antibiotic therapy should be instituted in antibody-positive patients. There is no proven therapy for the dominant ataxias (SCA1 to 13). The identification of gene defects will, it is hoped, lead to specific pharmacologic therapy. At present, identification of an at-risk person's genotype, together with appropriate family and genetic counseling, can reduce the incidence of these cerebellar syndromes (Chaps. 68, 359).

BIBLIOGRAPHY

BRADLEY JL et al: Clinical, biochemical and molecular genetic correlations in Friedreich's ataxia. Hum Mol Genetics 9(2):275, 2000

CONNER KE, ROSENBERG RN: The hereditary ataxias, in *The Molecular and Genetic Basis of Neurological Disease*, 2d ed, RN Rosenberg et al (eds). Boston, Butterworth-Heinemann, 1997, pp 503–544

HOLMES SE et al: A novel CAG trinucleotide repeat expansion adjacent to a gene encoding a subunit of protein phosphatase 2A is associated with a progressive neurological disorder. Soc Neurosci 25:1096, 1999

MATSUURA T et al: Mapping of the gene for a novel spinocerebellar ataxia with pure cerebellar signs and epilepsy. Ann Neurol 45:407, 1999

PANDOLFO M, MONTERMINI L: Molecular genetics of the hereditary ataxias. Adv Genet 38:31, 1998

PAULSON HL: Human Genetics '99: Trinucleotide repeats: Protein fate in neurodegenerative proteinopathies: Polyglutamine diseases join the (Mis)fold. Am J Hum Genet 64:339, 1999

ROSENBERG RN: Autosomal dominant cerebellar phenotypes: The genotype has settled the issue. Neurology 45:1, 1995

TERRY JB, ROSENBERG RN: Frontal lobe ataxia. Surg Neurol 44:583, 1995

365   Robert H. Brown, Jr.

AMYOTROPHIC LATERAL SCLEROSIS AND OTHER MOTOR NEURON DISEASES

AMYOTROPHIC LATERAL SCLEROSIS Amyotrophic lateral sclerosis (ALS) is the most common form of progressive motor neuron disease. It is a prime example of a neuronal system disease and is arguably the most devastating of the neurodegenerative disorders.

Pathology The pathology of motor neuron degenerative disorders involves lower motor neurons (consisting of anterior horn cells in spinal cord and their brainstem homologues innervating bulbar muscles) and upper, or corticospinal, motor neurons (emanating from layer five of motor cortex to descend via the pyramidal tract to synapse with lower motor neurons, either directly or indirectly via interneurons; (Chap. 22). Although at its onset ALS may involve selective loss of function of only upper or lower motor neurons, it ultimately causes progressive loss of both categories of motor neurons. Indeed, in the absence of clear involvement of both motor neuron types, the diagnosis of ALS is questionable.

Other motor neuron diseases involve only particular subsets of motor neurons (Tables 365-1 and 365-2). Thus, in bulbar palsy and spinal muscular atrophy (SMA, also called progressive muscular atrophy), the lower motor neurons of brainstem and spinal cord, respectively, are most severely involved. By contrast, pseudobulbar palsy, primary lateral sclerosis (PLS), and familial spastic paraplegia (FSP) affect only upper motor neurons innervating the brainstem and spinal cord.

Table 365-1 Sporadic Motor Neuron Diseases

CHRONIC

Upper and lower motor neurons
    Amyotrophic lateral sclerosis
Predominantly upper motor neurons
    Primary lateral sclerosis
Predominantly lower motor neurons
    Multifocal motor neuropathy with conduction block
    Motor neuropathy with paraproteinemia or cancer
    Motor-predominant peripheral neuropathies
Other
    Associated with other degenerative disorders
    Secondary motor neuron disorders (see Table 365-3)

ACUTE

Poliomyelitis
Herpes zoster
Coxsackie virus

In each of these diseases, the affected motor neurons undergo shrinkage, often with accumulation of the pigmented lipid (lipofuscin) that normally develops in these cells with advancing age. In ALS, the motor neuron cytoskeleton is typically affected early in the illness. Focal enlargements are frequent in proximal motor axons; ultrastructurally, these "spheroids" are composed of accumulations of neurofil-

Table 365-2 Genetic Motor Neuron Diseases

Disease	Locus	Gene
I. Upper and lower motor neurons (familial ALS)		
A. Autosomal dominant	21q	Superoxide dismutase
	22q	Neurofilament heavy subunit
	X_{cent}	Unknown
B. Autosomal recessive (juvenile)	2q	Unknown
	15q	Unknown
C. Mitochondrial	mtDNA	Cytochrome c oxidase
II. Upper motor neurons		
A. Familial spastic paraplegia (FSP)		
1. Autosomal dominant	2p	Spastin
	14q	Unknown
2. Autosomal recessive	8p	Unknown
	16q	Paraplegin
3. X-linked	Xq21	Proteolipid protein
	Xq28	L1 CAM
B. Adrenomyeloneuropathy	Xq21	Adrenoleukodystrophy protein
III. Lower motor neurons		
A. Spinal muscular atrophies	5q	Survival motor neuron protein
1. Infantile: Werdnig-Hoffmann disease		Survival motor neuron protein
2. Childhood		Survival motor neuron protein
3. Adolescent: Kugelberg-Welander disease		Survival motor neuron protein
B. X-linked spinobulbar muscular atrophy	Xq	Androgen receptor
C. G_{M2} gangliosidosis		
1. Adult Tay-Sach's disease	15q	Hexosaminidase A
2. Sandhoff disease	5q	Hexosaminidase B
3. AB variant	5q	GM2 activator protein
IV. ALS-plus syndromes		
A. ALS with frontotemporal dementia	9q	Unknown
B. Amyotrophy with behavioral disorder and parkinsonian features	17q	Tau protein

aments. Beyond some astroglial proliferation, which is the inevitable accompaniment of all degenerative processes in the central nervous system (CNS), the interstitial and supportive tissues and the macrophage system remain largely inactive, and there is no inflammation.

The death of the peripheral motor neurons in the brainstem and spinal cord leads to denervation and consequent atrophy of the corresponding muscle fibers. Histochemical and electrophysiologic evidence indicates that in the early phases of the illness denervated muscle can be reinnervated by sprouting of nearby distal motor nerve terminals, although reinnervation in this disease is considerably less extensive than in most other disorders affecting motor neurons (e.g., poliomyelitis, peripheral neuropathy). As denervation progresses, muscle atrophy is readily recognized in muscle biopsies and on clinical examination. This is the basis for the term *amyotrophy* in the name for the disease. The loss of cortical motor neurons results in thinning of the corticospinal tracts that travel via the internal capsule and brainstem to the lateral and anterior white matter columns of the spinal cord. The loss of fibers in the lateral columns and resulting fibrillary gliosis impart a particular firmness (*lateral sclerosis*) (Fig. 365-1). A remarkable feature of the disease is the selectivity of neuronal cell death. By light microscopy, the entire sensory apparatus, the regulatory mechanisms for the control and coordination of movement, and the components of the brain that are needed for cognitive processes remain intact. However, immunostaining indicates that neurons bearing ubiquitin, a marker for degeneration, are also detected in nonmotor systems. Moreover, studies of glucose metabolism in the illness also indicate that there is neuronal dysfunction outside of the motor system. Within the motor system, there is some selectivity of involvement. Thus, motor neurons required for ocular motility remain unaffected, as do the parasympathetic neurons in the sacral spinal cord (the nucleus of Onufrowicz, or Onuf) that innervate the sphincters of the bowel and bladder.

Clinical Manifestations The manifestations of ALS are somewhat variable depending on whether corticospinal or lower motor neu-

rons in the brainstem and spinal cord are more prominently involved. Typically, with lower motor neuron dysfunction and early denervation, the initial sign of the disease is insidiously developing asymmetric weakness, usually first evident distally in one of the limbs. A detailed history often discloses recent development of cramping with volitional movements, typically in the early hours of the morning (e.g., while stretching in bed). Weakness caused by denervation is associated with progressive wasting and atrophy of muscles and, particularly early in the illness, spontaneous twitching of motor units, or fasciculations. In the hands, a preponderance of extensor over flexor weakness is common. When the initial denervation involves bulbar rather than limb muscles, the problem at onset is difficulty with chewing, swallowing, and movements of the face and tongue. Early involvement of the muscles of respiration may lead to death before the disease is far advanced elsewhere.

With prominent corticospinal involvement, there is hyperactivity of the muscle-stretch reflexes (tendon jerks) and, often, spastic resistance to passive movements of the affected limbs. Patients with significant reflex hyperactivity complain of muscle stiffness often out of proportion to weakness. Degeneration of the corticobulbar projections innervating the brainstem results in dysarthria and exaggeration of the motor expressions of emotion. The latter leads to involuntary excess in weeping or laughing (so-called pseudobulbar affect).

Virtually any muscle group may be the first to show signs of the disease, but, as time passes, more and more muscles become involved until ultimately the disorder takes on a symmetric distribution in all regions. It is characteristic of ALS that, regardless of whether the initial disease involves upper or lower motor neurons, both will eventually be implicated. Even in the late stages of the illness, sensory, bowel and bladder, and cognitive functions are preserved. Even when there is severe brainstem disease, ocular motility is spared until the very late stages of the illness. Dementia is not a component of sporadic ALS. In some families, ALS is co-inherited with frontotemporal dementia, characterized by early behavioral abnormalities with prominent behavioral features indicative of frontal lobe dysfunction.

A committee of the World Federation of Neurology has established diagnostic guidelines for ALS. Essential for the diagnosis is the presence of simultaneous upper and lower motor neuron involvement with progressive weakness, and the exclusion of all alternative diagnoses. The disorder is classified as "definite" ALS when three or four of the following sites are involved: bulbar, cervical, thoracic, and lumbosacral motor neurons. When two sites are involved, the diagnosis is "probable"; when only one site is implicated, the diagnosis is "possible." An exception is made for those who have progressive upper and lower motor neuron signs at only one site and a mutation in the gene encoding superoxide dismutase (below).

Epidemiology The illness is relentlessly progressive, leading to death from respiratory paralysis; the median survival is from 3 to 5 years. There are very rare reports of stabilization or even regression of ALS. In most societies there is an incidence of 1 to 3 per 100,000 and a prevalence of 3 to 5 per 100,000. Several endemic foci of higher prevalence exist in the western Pacific (e.g., in specific regions of Guam or Papua New Guinea). In the United States and Europe, males are somewhat more frequently affected than females. While ALS is overwhelmingly a sporadic disorder, some 5 to 10% of cases are inherited as an autosomal dominant trait.

Familial ALS Several forms of selective motor neuron disease are heritable (Table 365-2). Two involve both corticospinal and lower motor neurons. The most common is familial ALS (FALS). Apart from its inheritance as an autosomal dominant trait, it is clinically indistinguishable from sporadic ALS. Genetic studies have identified mutations in the gene encoding the cytosolic enzyme superoxide dismutase (SOD1) as the cause of one form of FALS. However, this accounts for only 20% of inherited cases of ALS; there clearly are other ALS genes to be identified. There is a juvenile-onset, dominantly inherited form of ALS that is genetically mapped to the long-arm of chromo-

FIGURE 365-1 Amyotrophic lateral sclerosis. Axial T2-weighted MRI scan through the lateral ventricles of the brain reveals abnormal high signal intensity within the corticospinal tracts (*arrows*). This MRI feature represents an increase in water content in myelin tracts undergoing Wallerian degeneration secondary to cortical motor neuronal loss. This finding is commonly present in ALS, but can also be seen in AIDS-related encephalopathy, infarction, or other disease processes that produce corticospinal neuronal loss in a symmetric fashion.

some 9. Two recessively inherited forms of juvenile-onset ALS with long survival map to chromsomes 2 and 15. Another familial, adult-onset disorder that may mimic aspects of ALS is Kennedy's syndrome, described below.

Differential Diagnosis Because ALS is currently untreatable, it is imperative that potentially remediable causes of motor neuron dysfunction be excluded (Table 365-3). This is particularly true in cases that are atypical by virtue of (1) restriction to either upper or lower motor neurons, (2) involvement of neurons other than motor neurons, and (3) evidence of motor neuronal conduction block on electrophysiologic testing. Compression of the cervical spinal cord or cervicomedullary junction from tumors in the cervical regions or at the foramen magnum or from cervical spondylosis with osteophytes projecting into the vertebral canal can produce weakness, wasting, and fasciculations in the upper limbs and spasticity in the legs, closely resembling ALS. The absence of cranial nerve involvement may be helpful in differentiation, although some foramen magnum lesions may compress the twelfth cranial (hypoglossal) nerve, with resulting paralysis of the tongue. Absence of pain or of sensory changes, normal

Table 365-3 Etiology and Investigation of Motor Neuron Disorders

Diagnostic Categories	Investigations
Structural lesions	MRI scan of head (including foramen magnum), cervical spine[a]
Parasagittal or foramen magnum tumors	
Cervical spondylosis	
Chiari malformation or syrinx	
Spinal cord arteriovenous malformation	
Infections	CSF exam, culture[a]
Bacterial—tetanus, Lyme	Lyme antibody titer[a]
Viral—poliomyelitis, herpes zoster	Antiviral antibody titers (e.g., enteroviruses)
Retroviral myelopathy	HTLV-1, HTLV-2 titers
Intoxications, physical agents	
Toxins—lead, aluminum, other metals	24-h urine for heavy metals[a] Serum and urine for lead, aluminum
Drugs—strychnine, phenytoin	
Electric shock, x-irradiation	
Immunologic mechanisms	Complete blood count[a]
Plasma cell dyscrasias	Sedimentation rate[a]
Autoimmune polyradiculoneuropathy	Immunoprotein electrophoresis[a] Anti-G_{M1} antibodies[a]
Motor neuropathy with conduction block	
Paraneoplastic	Anti-Hu antibody
Paracarcinomatous/lymphoma	MRI scan, bone marrow biopsy
Metabolic	
Hypoglycemia	Fasting blood sugar (FBS), routine chemistries including calcium[a]
Hyperparathyroidism	PTH, calcium, phosphate
Hyperthyroidism	Thyroid functions[a]
Deficiency of folate, vitamins B_{12}, E, and folate	Vitamin B_{12}, vitamin E, folate levels[a]
Malabsorption	24-h stool fat, carotene, prothrombin time
Mitochondrial dysfunction	Fasting lactate, pyruvate, ammonia Consider mtDNA analysis
Hereditary biochemical disorders	
Superoxide dismutase 1 mutation	White blood cell DNA analysis
Androgen receptor defect (Kennedy's disease)	Abnormal CAG insert in androgen receptor gene
Hexosaminidase deficiency	Lysosomal enzyme screen
Infantile (α-glucosidase deficiency) (Pompe's disease)	
Hyperlipidemia	Lipid electrophoresis
Hyperglycinuria	Urine and serum amino acids
Methylcrotonylglycinuria	CSF amino acids

[a] Denotes studies that should be obtained in all cases.
NOTE: CSF, cerebrospinal fluid; HTLV, human T cell leukemia virus; MRI, magnetic resonance imaging.

bowel and bladder function, normal roentgenographic studies of the spine, and normal cerebrospinal fluid (CSF) all favor ALS. Where doubt exists, magnetic resonance imaging (MRI) scans should be performed to visualize the cervical spinal cord.

Another important entity in the differential diagnosis of ALS is multifocal motor neuropathy (MMN) with conduction block, discussed below and in Chap. 378. A diffuse, lower motor axonal neuropathy mimicking ALS sometimes evolves in association with hematopoietic disorders such as lymphoma (Chap. 101). The underlying marrow pathology is often signaled by the presence of an M-component in serum which, in this clinical setting, should prompt consideration of a bone marrow biopsy. Lyme infection may also cause an axonal, lower motor neuropathy.

Other treatable disorders that occasionally mimic ALS are chronic lead poisoning and thyrotoxicosis. These disorders may be suggested by the patient's social or occupational history or by unusual clinical features. When the family history is positive, disorders involving the genes encoding SOD1, hexosaminidase A, or α-glucosidase deficiency must be excluded (Chap. 349). These are readily identified by appropriate laboratory tests. Benign fasciculations are occasionally a source of concern because on inspection they resemble the fascicular twitchings that accompany motor neuron degeneration. The absence of weakness, atrophy, or denervation phenomena on electrophysiologic examination usually excludes ALS or other serious neurologic disease. Patients who have recovered from poliomyelitis may experience a delayed deterioration of motor neurons that presents clinically with progressive weakness, atrophy, and fasciculations. Its cause is unknown but is thought to reflect sublethal prior injury to motor neurons by poliovirus (Chap. 193).

Rarely, ALS develops concurrently with features indicative of more widespread neurodegeneration. Thus, one infrequently encounters otherwise typical ALS patients with a Parkinsonian movement disorder or dementia. It remains unclear whether this reflects the unlikely simultaneous occurrence of two disorders or a primary defect triggering two forms of neurodegeneration. The latter is suggested by the observation that multisystem neurodegenerative diseases may be inherited. For example, prominent amyotrophy has been described as a dominantly inherited disorder in individuals with bizarre behavior and a movement disorder suggestive of parkinsonism; many such cases have now been ascribed to mutations that alter the expression of isoforms of tau protein in brain (Chap. 362). In other cases, ALS develops simultaneously with a striking frontotemporal dementia. These disorders may be dominantly co-inherited; in some families, this trait is linked to a locus on chromosome 9q, although the underlying genetic defect is not established.

Pathogenesis The cause of sporadic ALS is not well defined. Some data suggest that excitotoxic neurotransmitters such as glutamate may participate in the death of motor neurons in ALS. This may be a consequence of diminished uptake of synaptic glutamate by an astroglial glutamate transporter, EAAT2. In one study of sporadic ALS brains, this loss of transport function was attributed to abnormal splicing of the mRNA transcript for the EAAT2 transporter selectively in motor cortex. It is striking that one cellular defense against such excitotoxicity is the enzyme SOD1, which detoxifies the free radical superoxide anion. Because SOD1 is mutated in some familial cases of ALS, it may be that glutamate excitotoxicity and ALS result from free radical accumulations in motor neurons. Precisely why the SOD1 mutations are toxic to motor nerves is not established, although it is clear that the effect is not simply loss of normal scavenging of the superoxide anion.

TREATMENT There is no treatment capable of arresting the underlying pathologic process in ALS. The drug riluzole was approved for use in ALS because it produces a modest lengthening of survival. In one trial, the survival rate at 18 months with riluzole (100 mg/d) was similar to placebo at 15 months. The mechanism of this effect is not known with certainty; it may reduce excitotoxicity by diminishing glutamate release. Side effects of riluzole may include nausea, dizziness, weight loss, and elevated liver enzymes. In a single study, insulin-like growth factor (IGF-1) was found to slow the progression of ALS modestly; because this effect was not confirmed in a second trial, IGF-1 is not routinely available as an ALS treatment at this time. Clinical trials of several other agents are in progress, including brain-derived neurotrophic factor, glial-derived neurotrophic factor, the anti-glutamate compound topiramate, and creatine. Creatine has proven to be beneficial in SOD-1 transgenic ALS mice, perhaps by augmenting intracellular ATP stores. In a single study in France, vitamin E was beneficial in sporadic ALS. It is also modestly beneficial in the ALS mice and thus is now used empirically by many individuals with ALS. On the basis of successful animal experiments, trials of neural stem therapy of the spinal cord are also being developed in ALS.

In the absence of a primary therapy for ALS, a variety of rehabilitative aids may substantially assist ALS patients. Foot-drop splints facilitate ambulation by avoiding tripping on a floppy foot and obviating excessive hip flexion. Finger-extension splints can potentiate grip. Respiratory support may be life-sustaining. For patients electing against long-term ventilation by tracheostomy, positive-pressure ventilation by mouth or nose provides transient (several weeks) relief from hypercarbia and hypoxia. Also extremely beneficial for some patients is a respiratory device (In-exsufflator, Emerson) that produces an artificial cough. This is highly effective in clearing airways and preventing aspiration pneumonia. When bulbar disease prevents normal chewing and swallowing, gastrostomy is uniformly helpful, restoring normal nutrition and hydration. Fortunately, an increasing variety of speech synthesizers are now available to augment speech when there is advanced bulbar palsy. Because they facilitate oral communication and may be effective for telephone use, such devices are helpful in preserving patient autonomy.

In contrast to ALS, several of the disorders (Table 365-2) that bear some clinical resemblance to ALS are treatable; for this reason, a careful search for such forms of secondary motor neuron disease is warranted.

SELECTED DISORDERS OF THE LOWER MOTOR NEURON In the varieties of motor neuron disease grouped under this heading, the peripheral motor neurons are affected without evidence of involvement of the corticospinal motor system (Table 365-1).

X-Linked Spinobulbar Muscular Atrophy (Kennedy's Disease) This is an X-linked lower motor neuron disorder in which progressive weakness and wasting of limb and bulbar muscles begins in males in midadult life and is conjoined with androgen insensitivity manifested by gynecomastia and reduced fertility (Chap. 335). In addition to gynecomastia, which may be subtle, two findings distinguishing this disorder from ALS are the absence of signs of pyramidal tract disease (spasticity) and the presence of a subtle sensory neuropathy in some patients. The underlying molecular defect is an expanded trinucleotide repeat (-CAG-) in the first exon of the androgen receptor gene on the X chromosome; this may be readily screened from DNA from blood. An inverse correlation appears to exist between the number of -CAG- repeats and the age of onset of the disease (Chap. 359).

Adult Tay-Sach's Disease Several reports have described adult-onset, predominantly lower motor neuropathies arising from deficiency of the enzyme β-hexosaminidase (hex A). These tend to be distinguishable from ALS because they are very slowly progressive; dysarthria and radiographically evident cerebellar atrophy may be prominent. In rare cases, spasticity may also be present, although it is generally absent (Chap. 349).

Spinal Muscular Atrophy The SMAs are a family of selective lower motor neuron diseases of early onset. Despite some phenotypic variability (largely in age of onset), the defect in the majority of families with SMA is genetically linked to a locus on the proximal long arm of chromosome 5. The affected gene at this locus is a putative motor neuron survival protein (SMN, for survival motor neuron) that is important in the formation and trafficking of RNA complexes across

the nuclear membrane. All types of SMA are transmitted as traits. Neuropathologically these disorders are characterized by extensive loss of large motor neurons; muscle biopsy reveals evidence of denervation atrophy. Several clinical forms are described.

Infantile SMA (SMA I, Werdnig-Hoffmann Disease) has the earliest onset and most rapidly fatal course. In some instances it is apparent even before birth, as indicated by decreased fetal movements late in the third trimester. Though alert, afflicted infants are weak and floppy (hypotonic) and lack muscle stretch reflexes. Death generally ensues within the first year of life. When the family history is unclear, it is difficult in the early weeks and months to distinguish SMA I from benign congenital hypotonia. An electromyogram is often particularly helpful as SMA I usually demonstrates fulminant denervation; in congenital hypotonia the electromyogram is often myopathic or normal.

Chronic childhood SMA (SMA II) begins later in childhood and evolves with a more slowly progressive course. *Juvenile SMA* (SMA III, Kugelberg-Welander disease) manifests during late childhood and runs a slow, indolent course. Unlike most denervating diseases, in this chronic disorder weakness is greatest in the proximal muscles; indeed, the pattern of clinical weakness can suggest a primary myopathy such as limb-girdle dystrophy. Electrophysiologic and muscle biopsy evidence of denervation distinguish SMA III from the myopathic syndromes.

Multifocal Motor Neuropathy with Conduction Block In this disorder lower motor neuron function is regionally and chronically disrupted by remarkably focal blocks in conduction. Many patients have elevated serum titers of mono- and polyclonal antibodies to ganglioside G_{M1}; it is hypothesized that the antibodies produce selective, focal, paranodal demyelination of motor neurons. MMN is not typically associated with corticospinal signs. In contrast to ALS, MMN may respond dramatically to therapy such as intravenous immunoglobulin or chemotherapy; it is thus imperative that MMN be excluded when considering a diagnosis of ALS. →*A detailed discussion of this condition can be found in Chap. 378.*

Other Forms of Lower Motor Neuron Disease In individual families, other syndromes characterized by selective lower motor neuron dysfunction in an SMA-like pattern have been described. There are rare X-linked and autosomal dominant forms of apparent SMA. There is an ALS variant of juvenile onset, the Fazio-Londe syndrome, which involves mainly the musculature innervated by the brainstem. A component of lower motor neuron dysfunction is also found in degenerative disorders such as Machado-Joseph disease and the related olivopontocerebellar degenerations (Chap. 364).

SELECTED DISORDERS OF THE UPPER MOTOR NEURON **Primary Lateral Sclerosis** This exceedingly rare disorder arises sporadically in adults in mid- to late life. Clinically PLS is characterized by progressive spastic weakness of the limbs, preceded or followed by spastic dysarthria and dysphagia, indicating combined involvement of the corticospinal and corticobulbar tracts. Fasciculations, amyotrophy, and sensory changes are absent; neither electromyography nor muscle biopsy shows denervation. On neuropathologic examination there is selective loss of the large pyramidal cells in the precentral gyrus and degeneration of the corticospinal and corticobulbar projections. The peripheral motor neurons and other neuronal systems are spared. The course of PLS is variable; while long-term survival is documented, the course may be as aggressive as in ALS, with approximately 3-year survival from onset to death. Early in its course, PLS raises the question of multiple sclerosis or other demyelinating diseases such as adrenoleukodystrophy as diagnostic considerations. A myelopathy suggestive of PLS is infrequently seen with infection with the human T cell leukemia virus (HTLV-I) (Chap. 368). The clinical course and laboratory testing will distinguish these possibilities.

Familial Spastic Paraplegia In its pure form, FSP is usually transmitted in families as an autosomal dominant trait; most adult-onset cases are dominantly inherited. It arises in the third or fourth decade and is characterized by progressive spastic weakness beginning in the distal lower extremities. Patients with FSP typically have long survival, presumably because respiratory function is spared. Late in the illness there may be urinary urgency and incontinence and sometimes fecal incontinence; sexual function tends to be preserved. In pure forms of FSP, ataxia, posterior column sensory loss, and amyotrophy are absent or minimal; however, in some patients, minor sensory changes (impaired vibration and position sense) may be observed in late stages. Some family members may show isolated spasticity without other clinical symptoms. Neuropathologically, in FSP there is degeneration of the corticospinal tracts, which appear nearly normal in the brainstem but show increasing atrophy at more caudal levels in the spinal cord. It is now apparent that defects at several different loci underlie both dominantly and recessively inherited forms of FSP (Table 365-2). An infantile-onset form of X-linked, recessive FSP arises from mutations in the gene for proteolipid protein. This is an example of rather striking allelic variation, as most other mutations in the same gene cause not FSP but Pelizaeus-Merzbacher disease, a disorder of CNS myelin. Defects in two other genes encoding the proteins "spastin" and "paraplegin" have recently been associated, respectively, with dominantly and recessively inherited FSP. The latter gene is of particular interest as it has homology to metalloproteases that are important in mitochondrial function in yeast.

Rarely, FSP may arise concomitantly with significant involvement of other regions of the nervous system. Thus, it has been described concurrently with amyotrophy, mental retardation, mental retardation with skin thickening, optic atrophy, and sensory neuropathy. In some cases there is loss of fibers in the ascending posterior columns and the spinocerebellar tracts, features reminiscent of Friedreich's ataxia. These complicated forms of FSP emphasize the challenge inherent in classifying the neurodegenerative disorders; there may be considerable overlap of the clinical phenotypes in diseases otherwise classified as distinct. Fortunately, it is likely that increasingly available genetic testing will clarify these nosologic difficulties.

WEB SITES Several web sites provide valuable information on ALS including those offered by the Muscular Dystrophy Association (www.mdausa.org), the Amyotrophic Lateral Sclerosis Association (www.alsa.org), and the World Federation of Neurology (www.wfnals.org).

BIBLIOGRAPHY

BROWN RH et al: *Amyotrophic Lateral Sclerosis.* London, Martin Dunitz, 1999

CASARI G: Spastic paraplegia and OXPHOS impairment caused by mutations in paraplegin, a nuclear-encoded mitochondrial metalloprotease. Cell 93:973, 1998

CLEVELAND DW: From Charcot to SOD1: Mechanisms of selective motor neuron death in ALS. Neuron 24:515, 1999

COMI GP et al: Cytochrome c oxidase subunit I microdeletion in a patient with motor neuron disease. Ann Neurol 43:110, 1998

LACOMBLEZ L et al: Dose-ranging study of riluzole in amyotrophic lateral sclerosis. Lancet 347:1425, 1997

LAI EC et al: Effect of recombinant human insulin-like growth factor-1 on progression of ALS. A placebo-controlled study. Neurol 49:1621, 1997

MARTIN JB: Molecular basis of the neurodegenerative disorders. N Engl J Med 340:1970, 1999

MILLER RG et al: The ALS patient care database: Goals, design and early results. Neurology 54:53, 2000

PELLIZZONI L et al: A novel function of SMN, the spinal muscular atrophy disease gene product, in pre-mRNA splicing. Cell 95:615, 1998

ROSEN DR et al: Mutations in Cu/Zn superoxide dismutase gene are associated with familial amyotrophic lateral sclerosis. Nature 362:59, 1993

TRAYNOR BJ et al: Amyotrophic lateral sclerosis mimic syndromes: A population based study. Arch Neurol 54:109, 2000

366

John W. Engstrom, Joseph B. Martin

DISORDERS OF THE AUTONOMIC NERVOUS SYSTEM

Rapid adjustments in vital physiologic mechanisms critical to survival are accomplished by the autonomic nervous system (ANS). The importance of this regulation is emphasized by the extent and severity of disability resulting from compromised ANS function. This chapter describes the clinical manifestations, diagnosis, and treatment of ANS disorders. →*The functional anatomy and relevant pharmacology of the sympathetic and parasympathetic components of the ANS are discussed in Chap. 72. Hypothalamic disorders that cause disturbances in homeostasis are discussed in Chaps. 17 and 328.*

CLINICAL MANIFESTATIONS Classification Disorders of the ANS may result from central nervous system (CNS) or peripheral nervous system (PNS) causes (Table 366-1). In many instances, the clinical signs and symptoms are due to interruption of a reflex arc controlling autonomic responses. The interruption can occur in the afferent limb, CNS processing centers, or efferent limb of the reflex arc. For example, a lesion of the medulla produced by a posterior fossa tumor can impair blood pressure (BP) responses to postural changes and result in orthostatic hypotension. Hypotension can also be caused by lesions of the spinal cord or peripheral vasomotor nerve fibers (diabetes mellitus). Diagnosis of the site of reflex interruption is dependent on the clinical context, ANS tests, and neuroimaging. Important elements of the clinical context include the presence or absence of CNS signs (pathophysiology and prognosis differ), association with sensory or motor polyneuropathy, family history, and pathologic findings. Some syndromes do not fit easily into any classification scheme because little is known about etiology, pathology, or treatment.

Table 366-1   Classification of ANS Disorders

I. With CNS signs
    Multiple system atrophy
    Spinal cord disorders (multiple sclerosis, tabes dorsalis, trauma, syrinx, hereditary degenerations)
    Parkinson's disease
    Huntington's disease
    Tumors, multiple cerebral infarcts
    Hypothalamic disorders
    Wernicke's encephalopathy
II. Without CNS signs
    Diabetes mellitus
    Other peripheral neuropathies (alcoholism, amyloidosis, porphyria, uremia, collagen vascular disease, leprosy, Chagas disease, vitamin B_{12} deficiency, HIV)
    Pure autonomic failure
    Acute pandysautonomia
    Chronic idiopathic anhidrosis
    Familial dysautonomia—Riley-Day syndrome
    Guillain-Barré syndrome
    Toxic neuropathies (vincristine, heavy metals, propafenone, uremia)
    Paraneoplastic (sensory neuropathy, enteric neuropathy)
    Tangier's and Fabry's diseases
    Neuromuscular junction (botulism, Lambert-Eaton syndrome)
III. Miscellaneous
    Postural orthostatic tachycardia syndrome (POTS)
    Prolonged bed rest or space flight
    Raynaud's syndrome
    Advanced age
    Dopamine β-hydroxylase deficiency
    Monamine oxidase deficiency
IV. Focal ANS disorders
    Complex regional pain syndrome type I (reflex sympathetic dystrophy, shoulder–hand syndrome)
    Complex regional pain syndrome type II (causalgia)
    Radiculopathy
    Horner's syndrome
    Adie's syndrome
    Reinnervation anomalies ("crocodile" tears)

Symptoms of Autonomic Dysfunction The clinical manifestations of autonomic lesions are influenced by the organ involved, the normal balance of sympathetic–parasympathetic innervation, the nature of the underlying illness, and the severity and stage of progression. *Impotence* often heralds autonomic failure in men and may precede other symptoms by more than a decade (Chap. 51). A decrease in the frequency of spontaneous early morning erections may occur months before loss of nocturnal penile tumescence and development of total impotence. *Bladder dysfunction* may appear early in men and women, particularly in those with CNS involvement. Brain and spinal cord disease above the level of the lumbar spine results first in urinary frequency and small bladder volumes, and eventually in incontinence (*upper motor neuron* or *spastic bladder*). Disease of PNS autonomic nerve fibers to and from the bladder results in large bladder volumes, urinary frequency, and overflow incontinence (*lower motor neuron bladder* or *flaccid bladder*). Measurement of bladder volume (postvoid residual) is a useful bedside test for distinguishing between upper and lower motor neuron bladder dysfunction. *Gastrointestinal autonomic dysfunction* typically presents as severe constipation. Diarrhea occurs occasionally (as in diabetes mellitus) due to rapid transit of contents or uncoordinated small bowel motor activity, or on an osmotic basis from bacterial overgrowth associated with small bowel stasis. Impaired glandular secretory function may cause difficulty with food intake due to decreased salivation or eye irritation due to decreased lacrimation. Occasionally, temperature elevation and vasodilation can result from *anhidrosis* because sweating is normally important for heat dissipation (Chap. 17).

Orthostatic hypotension (OH) (also called "postural hypotension") is the most disabling feature of autonomic dysfunction. OH can cause a variety of symptoms, including dimming or loss of vision, lightheadedness, diaphoresis, diminished hearing, pallor, and weakness. Syncope results when the drop in BP impairs cerebral perfusion. Other manifestations of impaired cardiovascular control from baroreflex dysfunction include supine hypertension, a heart rate that is fixed regardless of posture, and postprandial hypotension. The most common causes of OH are not neurologic in origin (Table 366-2) and must be distinguished from neurogenic etiologies (Table 366-1). →*Neurocardiogenic and cardiac syncope are considered in Chap. 20.*

Approach to the Patient

The most common, clinically significant autonomic disorders present with symptoms of OH. The first step in the evaluation of symptomatic orthostasis is the exclusion of treatable causes. The history should include a review of current medications which may cause OH (e.g., diuretics, antihypertensives, antidepressants, phenothiazines, ethanol, narcotics, insulin, barbiturates, and β-adrenergic and calcium channel blockers). Exaggerated responses to medications may be the first sign of an underlying autonomic disorder. The history may reveal a potential underlying cause for symptoms (e.g., diabetes, Parkinson's disease) or may reveal specific underlying mechanisms (e.g., cardiac pump failure, reduced intravascular volume). Inappropriate or extreme venous pooling may contribute to symptomatic OH. The relationship of symptoms to meals (splanchnic shunting of blood), or standing on awakening in the morning (due to relative intravascular volume depletion) should be sought.

Physical examination includes measurement of supine and standing pulse and BP, with a period of at least 2 min between positions. Sustained drops in systolic (>20 mmHg) or diastolic (>10 mmHg) BP after standing for at least 2 min that are not associated with an increase in pulse rate of >15 beats per minute suggest an autonomic deficit. In nonneurogenic causes of OH, the BP drop is accompanied by a compensatory increase in heart rate of >15 beats per minute. The requirement that the hypotension is sustained differentiates autonomic failure from sluggish baroreceptor responses that are common in the elderly. Other common signs of ANS dysfunction include supine hypertension or postprandial hypotension. Neurologic evaluation should include a mental status examination (to exclude neurodegenerative dis-

Table 366-2   Nonneurogenic Causes of Orthostatic Hypotension

Cardiac pump failure	Venous pooling
Myocardial infarction	Alcohol
Myocarditis	Postprandial dilation of
Constrictive pericarditis	splanchnic vessel beds
Aortic stenosis	Vigorous exercise with dila-
Tachyarrhythmias	tion of skeletal vessel beds
Bradyarrhythmias	Heat: hot environment, hot
Salt-losing nephropathy	showers and baths, fever
Adrenal insufficiency	Prolonged recumbancy or
Diabetes insipidus	standing
Venous obstruction	Sepsis
Reduced intravascular volume	Medications
Straining of heavy lifting, urination,	Antihypertensives
defecation	Diuretics
Dehydration	Vasodilators: nitrates, hydrala-
Diarrhea, emesis	zine
Hemorrhage	Alpha- and beta-blocking
Burns	agents
Metabolic	CNS sedatives: barbiturates,
Adrenocortical insufficiency	opiates
Hypoaldosteronism	Tricylic antidepressants
Pheochromocytoma	Phenothiazines
Severe potassium depletion	

orders), cranial nerve examination (to detect the impaired downgaze found with progressive supranuclear palsy), motor examination (for Parkinson's disease and parkinsonian syndromes), and sensory examination (for polyneuropathies). In patients without a clear initial diagnosis, follow-up neurologic evaluations performed over years may reveal an evolution of neurologic findings that makes it possible to reach a specific diagnosis.

Disorders of autonomic function should be considered in the differential diagnosis of patients with symptoms of altered sweating (hyperhidrosis or hypohidrosis), constipation, impotence, or bladder dysfunction (urinary frequency, hesitancy, or incontinence). An initial practical approach to the patient with OH or autonomic symptoms is summarized in Table 366-3.

Autonomic Testing (See also Chap. 357)   Autonomic function tests are helpful when the history and physical examination findings are inconclusive, when detection of subclinical involvement is important to evaluate the extent and severity of abnormalities, or to monitor the effects of therapy. Both physiologic and pharmacologic tests are available to assess the functional characteristics of the ANS. Commonly used physiologic tests assess autonomic aspects of cardiovascular function. These tests are noninvasive and provide quantitative and regional data about autonomic function. Pharmacologic tests can elucidate pathophysiologic abnormalities and guide the development of rational therapy.

Heart rate variation with deep breathing This is a test of parasympathetic influence on cardiovascular function. Results are influenced by the subject's posture, rate and depth of respiration [5 to 6 breaths per minute and a forced vital capacity (FVC) >1.5 L are optimal], age, medications, and hypocapnea. Interpretation of results requires comparison of test data with results from normal individuals collected under the same test conditions. For example, the lower limit of normal heart rate variation with deep breathing in persons younger than 20 years is >15 to 20 beats/min, but for persons over age 60 it is 5 to 8 beats/min. Heart rate variation with deep

Table 366-3   Initial Evaluation of OH or ANS Symptoms

Review medication use
Review coexisting medical disorders
Determine the relationship of OH to meals, exercise, straining, and standing
  up from bed in the morning
Record supine and standing BP and pulse
Complete neurologic examination

Table 366-4 Normal Blood Pressure and Heart Rate Changes during the Valsalva Maneuver

Phase	Maneuver	Blood Pressure	Heart Rate	Comments
I	Onset of expiration against a partially closed glottis	Rises due to aortic compression	Decreases	
II *early*	Continued expiration	Falls due to decreased venous return	Increases	
II *late*	Continued expiration	Total peripheral vascular resistance increases (increased sympathetic discharge and plasma epinephrine)	Increases at slower rate	Requires efferent sympathetic response
III	End of expiration	Falls due to increased capacitance of pulmonary bed	Increases further	
IV	Recovery	Increases ("overshoot") due to vasoconstriction and increased cardiac output	Compensatory bradycardia	Requires efferent sympathetic response

breathing (respiratory sinus arrhythmia) is abolished by the administration of atropine.

Valsalva response This response assesses integrity of the afferent limb, central processing, and efferent limb of the baroreceptor reflex (Table 366-4). The response is obtained with the subject sitting or supine. A constant expiratory pressure of 40 mmHg is maintained for 15 s while changes in heart rate and beat-to-beat BP are measured. There are four phases of BP and heart rate response to the Valsalva maneuver. Phases I and III are mechanical and related to changes in intrathoracic and intraabdominal pressure. In early phase II, reduced stroke volume and venous return results in a fall in BP, reflex tachycardia, and increased total peripheral resistance. Increased total peripheral resistance arrests the BP drop approximately 5 to 8 s after the onset of the maneuver. Late phase II begins with a progressive rise in BP toward baseline. Venous return and cardiac output return to normal in phase IV. Persistent peripheral arteriolar vasoconstriction results in a temporary BP overshoot and phase IV bradycardia (mediated by the baroreceptor reflex).

Autonomic function during the Valsalva maneuver can be measured in several ways. The *Valsalva ratio* is calculated from heart rate changes during the maneuver and is defined as the maximum phase II tachycardia divided by the minimum phase IV bradycardia. The ratio reflects the integrity of the entire baroreceptor reflex arc and of sympathetic efferents to blood vessels; sympathetic efferent function is assessed in the phase II BP response and the BP overshoot. Test results depend on the age and posture of the subject, the expiratory pressure, the duration of expiration, the FVC, and medications. Noninvasive recording of beat-to-beat BP changes provides a direct measure of sympathetic efferent input to blood vessels during phases II and IV that does not depend on the presence of a normal baroreceptor reflex arc.

Sudomotor function The capacity to produce sweat can be assessed quantitatively or qualitatively. Sweating is induced by release of acetylcholine from sympathetic postganglionic fibers. The *quantitative sudomotor axon reflex test* (QSART) is a measure of regional autonomic function mediated by acetylcholine-induced sweating. A reduced or absent response indicates a lesion of the postganglionic sudomotor axon. For example, sweating may be reduced in the legs as a result of peripheral neuropathy (e.g., in diabetes) before other signs of autonomic dysfunction emerge. The *thermoregulatory sweat test* (TST) is a *qualitative* measure of regional sweat production in response to an elevation of body temperature. An indicator powder placed on the anterior body surface changes color with sweat production during temperature elevation. The pattern of color changes is a measure of regional sweat secretion. The pattern of sweat abnormality may suggest a peripheral or central cause for the deficit. For example, a unilateral decrease over half the body suggests a central lesion. Measurement of galvanic skin responses in the limbs after an induced electrical potential is another qualitative test for detecting the presence or absence of sweating. The response is simple to measure, but habituation occurs.

Orthostatic blood pressure recordings Beat-to-beat BP measurements determined in supine, 80° tilt, and tilt-back positions are useful to quantitate orthostatic failure of BP control. It is important to allow a 20-min period of supine rest before assessing changes in BP during tilting. The test can be useful for the evaluation of patients with unexplained syncope and to detect vagally mediated syncope.

Cold pressor test The cold pressor test assesses sympathetic function. The individual immerses one hand in ice water (1° to 4°C) and BP is measured at 30 s and 1 min. The systolic and diastolic pressures normally rise by 10 to 20 mmHg. The afferent pathway is spinothalamic and thus is distinct from the afferent limb of the baroreceptor reflex arc. When spinothalamic pathways are intact, an abnormal response indicates an abnormality of autonomic central processing or sympathetic efferent function. When the response to the cold pressor test is normal and the Valsalva response is abnormal, the lesion is located in the afferent limb of the baroreceptor reflex arc.

Pharmacologic tests Pharmacologic assessments can help localize an autonomic defect to the CNS or the PNS. The test is controlled for time of day, position of the patient, level of patient activity, and food intake. Measures should be taken to minimize patient stress. Measurement of plasma levels of neurotransmitter metabolites and BP responses to infused drugs helps to distinguish between central and peripheral causes of autonomic dysfunction (Table 366-5); however, these studies are not routine clinical tools.

SPECIFIC SYNDROMES OF ANS DYSFUNCTION Multiple System Atrophy Multiple system atrophy (MSA) is an uncommon entity that comprises several overlapping clinical syndromes, including striatonigral degeneration (Shy-Drager syndrome), progressive supranuclear palsy (Chap. 363), and olivopontocerebellar atrophy (Chap. 364). The clinical syndrome can include various combinations of symptoms of autonomic dysfunction (OH, impotence, bladder and bowel dysfunction, and defective sweating), as well as additional symptoms of CNS disease such as rigidity, tremor, loss of associative movements, or abnormal eye movements. Most patients present with autonomic dysfunction alone, and other neurologic manifestations usually develop within 5 years. Patients with the striatonigral variant exhibit a form of parkinsonism in which bradykinesia and rigidity are more prominent than tremor. Patients with either a pure cerebellar

Table 366-5 Pharmacology Testing of Central and Peripheral Causes of Autonomic Failure

	Central	Peripheral	Intact
Supine plasma NE level	Normal	Low	Normal
Standing plasma NE level	No change	Low	Doubles
Blood pressure response to infused NE	Normal/increased	Exaggerated response	Normal/increased

syndrome or striatonigral degeneration may also develop pyramidal tract involvement. Some patients have features of both subtypes.

These disorders progress relentlessly to death 7 to 10 years after onset. Pharmacologic differences distinguish MSA from peripheral causes of autonomic failure (Table 366-4). Neuropathologic changes include primary neuronal degeneration with loss of neurons and gliosis in many CNS regions, including the brainstem, the cerebellum, the striatum, and the intermediolateral cell column of the thoracolumbar spinal cord. ANS abnormalities are also associated with Parkinson's disease and Huntington's disease.

Spinal Cord Lesions Spinal cord lesions from any cause may result in focal autonomic deficits or autonomic hyperreflexia. Descending pathways from the brain normally modulate organized patterns of sympathetic activity and modulate segmental autonomic reflexes. Spinal cord transection or hemisection may be attended by autonomic hyperreflexia affecting bowel, bladder, sexual, temperature-regulation, or cardiovascular functions. Dangerous increases or decreases in body temperature may result from inability to experience the sensory accompaniments of heat or cold exposure below the level of the injury. Quadriparetic patients exhibit both supine hypertension and OH after upward tilting. Markedly increased autonomic discharge can be elicited by bladder pressure or stimulation of the skin or muscles; suprapubic palpation of the bladder, catheter insertion, catheter obstruction, or urinary infection are common and correctable precipitants. This phenomenon, termed autonomic dysreflexia, affects 85% of patients with a traumatic spinal cord lesion above the C6 level. In patients with supine hypertension, BP can be lowered by tilting the head upward. Vasodilator drugs may be used to treat acute elevations in BP. Clonidine is used prophylactically to reduce the hypertension resulting from bladder stimulation. Sudden, dramatic increases in BP can lead to intracranial hemorrhage and death.

Peripheral Nerve and Neuromuscular Junction Disorders Peripheral neuropathies (Chap. 377) are the most common cause of chronic autonomic insufficiency. Neuropathies that affect small myelinated and unmyelinated fibers of the sympathetic and parasympathetic nerves occur in diabetes mellitus, amyloidosis, chronic alcoholism, porphyria, and Guillain-Barré syndrome. Neuromuscular junction disorders include botulism and Lambert-Eaton syndrome.

Diabetes mellitus Autonomic involvement in diabetes may begin at any stage in the disease (Chap. 333) and often presents with asymptomatic abnormalities in vagal function that can be detected as reduced heart rate variation with deep breathing. Loss of small myelinated and unmyelinated nerve fibers in the splanchnic distribution, carotid sinus, and vagus nerves is characteristic. Widespread enteric neuropathy can cause profound disturbances in gut motility (gastroparesis), nausea and vomiting, malnutrition, achlorhydria, and bowel incontinence. Other symptoms may include impotence, urinary incontinence, pupillary abnormalities, and OH. Typical symptoms and signs of hypoglycemia may fail to appear because damage to the sympathetic innervation of the adrenal gland can result in a lack of epinephrine release. Insulin excess may also cause profound hypotension. Autonomic dysfunction may lengthen the QT interval and enhance the risk of sudden death. Hyperglycemia appears to be one risk factor for autonomic involvement. Biochemical and pharmacologic studies in diabetic neuropathy are compatible with autonomic failure localized to the PNS [low supine plasma norepinephrine (NE) levels and exaggerated pressor responsiveness].

Amyloidosis Autonomic neuropathy occurs in both sporadic and familial forms of amyloidosis (Chap. 319). Although patients usually present with a distal painful neuropathy accompanied by sensory loss, autonomic insufficiency can precede the development of the polyneuropathy. Death is usually due to cardiac or renal impairment. Postmortem studies reveal amyloid deposition in many organs, including two sites that contribute to autonomic failure: intraneural blood vessels and autonomic ganglia. Pathologic examination reveals a loss of unmyelinated and myelinated nerve fibers.

Alcoholic neuropathy Abnormal parasympathetic vagal and efferent sympathetic function occurs in individuals with chronic alco-

holism. Pathologic changes can be demonstrated in the parasympathetic (vagus) and sympathetic fibers and in ganglia. Impotence is a major problem, but concurrent gonadal hormone abnormalities may obscure the parasympathetic component to this symptom. Clinical symptoms of autonomic failure generally appear when the polyneuropathy is severe. OH may also be prominent in Wernicke's encephalopathy (Chap. 376). Autonomic involvement may contribute to the high mortality rates associated with alcoholism (Chap. 387).

Porphyria Although each of the porphyrias can cause autonomic dysfunction, the condition is most extensively documented in the acute intermittent type (Chap. 346). Autonomic symptoms include tachycardia, sweating, urinary retention, and hypertension or, less commonly, hypotension. Other prominent symptoms include anxiety, abdominal pain, nausea, and vomiting. Abnormal autonomic function can occur both during acute attacks and during remissions. Elevated catecholamine levels during acute attacks correlate with the degree of tachycardia and hypertension.

Guillain-Barré syndrome BP fluctuations and arrhythmias can be severe (Chap. 378). It is estimated that 2 to 10% of seriously ill patients with Guillain-Barré syndrome suffer fatal cardiovascular collapse. Abnormal sweating, sphincter disturbance, and pupillary dysfunction also occur. Demyelination has been described in the vagus and glossopharyngeal nerves, the sympathetic chain, and the white rami communicantes. The presence of autonomic involvement is not clearly related to the severity of motor or sensory involvement.

Botulism The toxin binds presynaptically to cholinergic nerve terminals and, after uptake into the cytosol, blocks acetycholine release by digesting key proteins involved in neurotransmitter release. Manifestations of this blockade consist of motor paralysis and autonomic disturbances, including blurred vision, dry mouth, nausea, unreactive or sluggishly reactive pupils, constipation, and urinary retention (Chap. 144).

Pure Autonomic Failure (PAF) This sporadic syndrome consists of postural hypotension, impotence, bladder dysfunction, and defective sweating. The disorder begins in the middle decades and occurs in women more than in men. The symptoms can be disabling, but the disease does not shorten life span. The clinical and pharmacologic characteristics suggest a primary involvement of postganglionic sympathetic neurons. There is a severe reduction in the density of neurons within sympathetic ganglia, resulting in low supine plasma NE levels and noradrenergic supersensitivity (Table 366-5). The clinical diagnosis may be difficult in early stages because patients may present with isolated OH, raising a question of PAF, but they later develop signs of multiple system atrophy (discussed above).

Postural Orthostatic Tachycardia Syndrome (POTS) This syndrome is characterized by symptomatic orthostatic intolerance (*not* OH) and an increase in heart rate to >120 beats per minute or by 30 beats per minute with standing. The condition affects young adult women most commonly, but it can occur over a wide age range. Associated symptoms include light-headedness, shortness of breath, and exercise intolerance. The pathogenesis is unclear in most cases; hypovolemia, venous pooling, impaired brainstem regulation, or β-receptor supersensitivity may play a role. In one affected individual, a mutation in the NE transporter resulting in impaired NE clearance from synapses was responsible. Only one-fourth of patients eventually resume their usual daily activities. Expansion of fluid volume and postural training are initial approaches to treatment. If the response to treatment is inadequate, then fludrocortisone, phenobarbital, beta blockers, and clonidine have been used with some success.

Postprandial Hypotension The importance of postprandial hypotension (PPH) among healthy elderly persons, hypertensive patients, and elderly patients in nursing homes has probably been underestimated. Abnormally reduced peripheral vasoconstriction in response to shunting of blood to the splanchnic circulation after a meal contributes to PPH. The wisdom of administering cardiovascular medications that have hypotensive effects at mealtimes to healthy and hypertensive elderly patients is questionable. PPH is also associated with diabetes, Parkinson's disease, renal failure treated with hemodialysis, cardiovascular disease, paraplegia, and autonomic failure.

Inherited Disorders   Riley-Day syndrome (familial dysautonomia) is an autosomal recessive disorder of infants and children that occurs among Ashkenazi Jews. The defective gene, located on the long arm of chromosome 9, has not been identified. Decreased tearing, hyperhidrosis, reduced sensitivity to pain, areflexia, absent fungiform papillae on the tongue, and labile BP may be present. Episodic abdominal crises and fever are common. Increased sensitivity to intraocular methacholine and absent axon flare response to intradermal histamine injection are useful diagnostic markers. Normal resting plasma NE levels that do not increase on standing are consistent with an afferent lesion. Pathologic examination of nerves reveals a loss of small myelinated and unmyelinated nerve fibers.

Primary Hyperhidrosis   This syndrome presents with excess sweating of the palms of the hands and soles of the feet. The disorder affects 0.6 to 1.0% of the population; the etiology is unclear (there may be a genetic component). While not dangerous, the condition can be socially embarrassing (e.g., shaking hands) or disabling (e.g., inability to write without soiling the paper). Onset of symptoms is usually in adolescence; the condition tends to improve with age. Topical antiperspirants (e.g., Drysol) are occasionally helpful. T2 ganglionectomy or sympathectomy is successful in >90% of patients with palmar hyperhidrosis. The advent of endoscopic transaxillary T2 sympathectomy has lowered the complication rate of the procedure. The most common complication is compensatory hyperhidrosis, which improves spontaneously over months; other potential complications include recurrent hyperhidrosis (16%), Horner's syndrome (<2%), gustatory sweating, wound infection, hemothorax, and intercostal neuralgia. Local injection of botulinum toxin has been used to block cholinergic, post-ganglionic sympathetic fibers to sweat glands in patients with palmar hyperhidrosis; however, the technique is limited by the need for repetitive injections (the effect usually lasts 4 months before waning), pain with injection, the high cost of botulinum toxin, and the possibility of temporary intrinsic hand muscle weakness. Tap water iontophoresis has been successful for some patients.

Miscellaneous   The importance of autoimmunity in the pathogenesis of autonomic failure has been underestimated; autoantibodies against acetylcholine receptors in autonomic ganglia have been found in some patients with acute pandysautonomia and paraneoplastic autonomic neuropathy. Other conditions associated with autonomic failure include infections, poisoning (organophosphates), malignancy, and aging. Disorders of the hypothalamus can affect autonomic function and produce abnormalities in temperature control, satiety, sexual function, and circadian rhythms (Chap. 328).

Reflex Sympathetic Dystrophy and Causalgia   The failure to identify a primary role of the ANS in the pathogenesis of these disorders has resulted in a change of nomenclature. *Complex regional pain syndrome* (CRPS) *types I* and *II* are now used in place of reflex sympathetic dystrophy (RSD) and causalgia, respectively.

CRPS type I is a regional pain syndrome that usually develops after tissue trauma. Examples of associated trauma include myocardial infarction, minor shoulder or limb injury, and stroke. *Allodynia* (the perception of a nonpainful stimulus as painful), *hyperpathia* (an exaggerated pain response to a mildly painful stimulus), and spontaneous pain occur; these symptoms are unrelated to the severity of the initial trauma and are not confined to the distribution of a single peripheral nerve. CRPS type II is a regional pain syndrome that develops after injury to a peripheral nerve. Spontaneous pain initially develops within the territory of the affected nerve but eventually may spread outside the nerve distribution.

Pain is the primary clinical feature of CRPS. Vasomotor abnormalities, sudomotor abnormalities, or focal edema may occur alone or in combination, but must be present for diagnosis. Limb pain syndromes that do not meet these criteria are best classified as "limb pain—not otherwise specified (NOS)". In CRPS, localized sweating (increased resting sweat output) and changes in blood flow may produce temperature differences between affected and unaffected limbs.

CRPS type I (RSD) has classically been divided into three clinical phases but is now considered to be more variable than previously thought. Phase I consists of pain and swelling in the distal extremity occurring within weeks to 3 months after the precipitating event. The pain is diffuse, spontaneous, and either burning, throbbing, or aching in quality. The involved extremity is warm and edematous, and the joints are tender. Increased sweating and hair growth are present. In phase II (3 to 6 months after onset), thin, shiny, cool skin appears. After an additional 3 to 6 months (phase III), atrophy of the skin and subcutaneous tissue plus flexion contractures complete the clinical picture.

Therapy for both types of CRPS is unsatisfactory. The desire to provide relief for these severely disabling pain syndromes has produced a variety of surgical and medical treatments with conflicting reports of efficacy. Clinical trials suggest that early mobilization with physical therapy or a brief course of steroids may be helpful for CRPS type I. The long-term results of this treatment are unclear. Other medical treatments have included the use of adrenergic blockers, nonsteroidal anti-inflammatory drugs (NSAIDs), calcium channel blockers, phenytoin, opioids, and calcitonin. Stellate ganglion blockade is a commonly used invasive therapeutic technique. Although stellate ganglion blocks often provide temporary pain relief, the efficacy of repetitive blocks is uncertain.

℞ TREATMENT   Management of autonomic failure is usually limited to alleviating the disability caused by symptoms. Treatment of the primary disorder does not generally improve autonomic function. The history and examination are key to the identification of easily reversible conditions (Table 366-3).

OH is often severely disabling but may be mild. Neurogenic OH should be treated only if symptoms are present that limit activities of daily living. Nonpharmacologic interventions can be helpful. Patients should avoid sodium depletion or dehydration by maximizing salt intake (eating salty foods) and deliberately drinking at least 2 to 2.5 L/d of water. Sleeping in a head-up tilt position reduces nocturnal diuresis, morning postural hypotension and hypovolemia, and minimizes supine hypertension. Patients are often advised to sit with legs dangling over the edge of the bed for several minutes before attempting to stand in the morning. Isotonic exercise is desirable, but vigorous exercise or prolonged recumbency should be avoided. Circumstances that accentuate vasodilation (alcohol intake, high ambient temperature) may precipitate severe hypotension. Nonprescription medicines containing sympathomimetics must be used carefully because they may cause severe hypertension in the setting of autonomic failure accompanied by denervation supersensitivity. Compressive garments are of questionable value.

Most patients require pharmacologic therapy for the management of OH. Fludrocortisone is the initial drug of choice; at doses between 0.1 mg/d and 0.3 mg bid orally, it enhances renal sodium conservation and increases the sensitivity of arterioles to norepinephrine. Susceptible patients may develop fluid overload, congestive heart failure, supine hypertension, or hypokalemia; with chronic administration, potassium supplements are often necessary. Sustained elevations of supine BP above 200/110 should be avoided.

OH of moderate severity can be treated with a combination of fludrocortisone and the α_1-receptor agonist midodrine. Midodrine is well absorbed when given orally and causes arteriolar and venous constriction without CNS or cardiac stimulation. It is administered orally 30 to 45 min before meals at an initial dose of 5 mg tid, increasing to a maximum of 10 mg q4h. Side effects include pruritus, uncomfortable piloerection, and supine hypertension.

OH with a postprandial component may respond to several measures. Frequent, small, low-carbohydrate meals may diminish splanchnic shunting of blood after meals and reduce PPH. Prostaglandin inhibitors (ibuprofen or indomethacin) taken with meals can prevent

PPH. Caffeine (250 mg or two cups of coffee) can be given once per day, usually in the morning. The somatostatin analogue octreotide can be useful in the treatment of postprandial syncope by inhibiting the release of gastrointestinal peptides that have vasodilator and hypotensive effects. The dose ranges from 25 μg subcutaneously bid to 100 to 200 μg subcutaneously tid. Despite the lack of a pressor effect, octreatide may also be useful for preventing the PPH that occurs in normal elderly patients.

OH accompanied by diarrhea may respond to the α_2 agonist clonidine; coincident causes of nonneurogenic OH must be excluded before this treatment is begun because the risk of associated hypotension is significant. Initial doses are 0.1 to 0.2 mg orally every morning; the dose is gradually increased if drowsiness, dry mouth, constipation, supine hypertension, or hypotension are not dose-limiting. Octreotide may also be useful for some patients with this condition.

OH associated with anemia may respond to erythropoietin. One study found that systolic BP increased by 20 mmHg and orthostatic symptoms improved with normalization of the hematocrit. Erythropoietin is administered subcutaneously at doses of 25 to 75 U/kg three times per week. The hematocrit increases after 2 to 6 weeks. A weekly maintenance dose is usually necessary. The increased intravascular volume that accompanies the rise in hematocrit can exacerbate supine hypertension.

Many patients with ANS failure exhibit exaggerated sensitivity to various drugs. Compounds with hypotensive actions should generally be avoided. For example, anticholinergic agents are a better initial choice than dopaminergic compounds for parkinsonism. Anesthetic management poses unique problems since these patients may have abnormal baroreceptor reflexes, impaired sympathetic innervation of peripheral arterioles, exaggerated pharmacologic responses, abnormal fluid balance, or adrenal medullary insufficiency. More important than the choice of anesthetic is awareness by the physician of the implications that autonomic failure may have for peri- and postoperative monitoring and management.

BIBLIOGRAPHY

BRAUS DF et al: The shoulder-hand syndrome after stroke: A prospective clinical trial. Ann Neurol 36:728, 1994

JANSEN RW, LIPSITZ LA: Postprandial hypotension: Epidemiology, pathophysiology, and clinical management. Ann Intern Med 122:286, 1995

LOW PA (ed): *Clinical Autonomic Disorders*, 2d ed. New York, Lippincott-Raven, 1997

―――― et al: Efficacy of midodrine vs. placebo in neurogenic orthostatic hypotension. JAMA 277:1046, 1997

MATHIAS CJ: Orthostatic hypotension: Causes, mechanisms, and influencing factors. Neurology 45(Suppl 5):S6, 1995

MCLEOD JG: Autonomic dysfunction in peripheral nerve disease. Invited review. Muscle Nerve 15:3, 1992

POLINSKY RJ: Clinical autonomic neuropharmacology. Neurol Clin 8:77, 1990

ROBERTSON D, DAVIS TL: Recent advances in the treatment of orthostatic hypotension. Neurology 45(Suppl 5):S26, 1995

SHANNON JR et al: Orthostatic intolerance and tachycardia associated with norepinephrine-transporter deficiency. N Engl J Med 342:541, 2000

STOLMAN LP: Treatment of hyperhidrosis. Dermatol Clin 16:863–67, 1998

VELDMAN PHJM et al: Signs and symptoms of reflex sympathetic dystrophy: Prospective study of 829 patients. Lancet 342:1012, 1993

VERNINO S et al: Autoantibodies to ganglionic acetylcholine receptors in autoimmune autonomic neuropathies. N Engl J Med 343:847, 2000

367 M. Flint Beal, Stephen L. Hauser

COMMON DISORDERS OF THE CRANIAL NERVES

Symptoms and signs of cranial nerve pathology are common in internal medicine. They often develop in the context of a widespread neurologic disturbance, and in such situations cranial nerve involvement may represent the initial manifestation of the illness. In other disorders, involvement is largely restricted to one or several cranial nerves; these distinctive disorders are reviewed in this chapter. Disorders of ocular movement are discussed in Chap 28; disorders of smell, taste, and hearing in Chap 29; and vertigo and disorders of vestibular function in Chap 21.

DISORDERS OF FACIAL SENSATION

The trigeminal (fifth cranial) nerve supplies sensation to the skin of the face and anterior half of the head (Fig. 367-1). Its motor part innervates the masseter and pterygoid masticatory muscles.

TRIGEMINAL NEURALGIA (TIC DOULOUREUX) The most striking disorder of trigeminal nerve function is tic douloureux, a condition characterized by excruciating paroxysms of pain in the lips, gums, cheek, or chin and, very rarely, in the distribution of the ophthalmic division of the fifth nerve. The disorder occurs almost exclusively in middle-aged and elderly persons. The pain seldom lasts more than a few seconds or a minute or two but may be so intense that the patient winces, hence the term *tic*. The paroxysms recur frequently, both day and night, for several weeks at a time. Another characteristic feature is the initiation of pain by stimuli applied to certain areas on the face, lips, or tongue ("trigger zones") or by movement of these parts. *Objective signs of sensory loss cannot be demonstrated.* The adequate stimulus to a trigger zone for precipitating an attack is a tactile one and possibly tickle, rather than a noxious or thermal stimulus. Usually a spatial and temporal summation of impulses is necessary to trigger an attack, which is followed by a refractory period of up to 2 or 3 min.

The *diagnosis* of this disorder rests on these strict clinical criteria, and the condition must be distinguished from other forms of facial and cephalic neuralgia and pain arising from diseases of the jaw, teeth, or sinuses (Chap. 15). Tic douloureux is usually without assignable cause; in typical cases, neuroimaging studies are not necessary. On occasion, when trigeminal neuralgia develops in a younger adult, it may be due to a plaque of multiple sclerosis at the root entry zone of the fifth nerve in the pons. Very rarely it occurs with herpes zoster or a tumor. To a degree that remains uncertain, pain of tic douloureux may be caused by a redundant or tortuous blood vessel in the posterior fossa, causing an irritative lesion of the nerve or its root. Usually, however, lesions such as aneurysms, neurofibromas, or meningiomas affecting the nerve produce a loss of sensation (trigeminal neuropathy, see below).

FIGURE 367-1 The three major sensory divisions of the trigeminal nerve consist of the ophthalmic, maxillary, and mandibular nerves.

℞ **TREATMENT** Drug therapy with carbamazepine is the initial treatment of choice and is effective in approximately 50 to 75% of patients. Carbamazepine should be started as a single daily dose of 100 mg taken with food, and increased gradually (by 100 mg daily every 1 to 2 days) until substantial (>50%) pain relief is achieved. Most patients require a maintenance dose of 200 mg qid. Doses >1200 mg daily provide no additional benefit. Dizziness, imbalance, sedation, and rare cases of agranulocytosis are the most important side effects of carbamazepine. If treatment is effective, it is usually continued for approximately 1 month and then tapered as tolerated. If carbamazepine is not well tolerated or is ineffective, phenytoin, 300 to 400 mg daily, can be tried. Baclofen may also be administered, either alone or in combination with carbamazepine or phenytoin. The initial dose is 5 to 10 mg tid, gradually increasing as needed to 20 mg qid.

If drug treatment fails, surgical therapy should be offered. The most widely applied procedure creates a heat lesion of the trigeminal (gasserian) ganglion or nerve, a method termed *radiofrequency thermal rhizotomy*. Injection of glycerol in Meckel's cave is a method preferred by some surgeons. Either procedure produces short-term relief in >95% of patients; however, long-term studies indicate that pain recurs in a substantial percentage of treated patients in some series. Complications and morbidity are infrequent in experienced hands. These procedures result in partial numbness of the face and carry a risk of corneal denervation with secondary keratitis when used for the rare instances of first-division trigeminal neuralgia.

A third treatment, microvascular decompression, requires a suboccipital craniectomy, a major procedure requiring several days of hospitalization. It has an 80% efficacy rate, but the pain may recur, and, in a small number of cases, there is damage to the eighth or seventh nerve.

TRIGEMINAL NEUROPATHY A variety of diseases in addition to tic douloureux may affect the trigeminal nerve (Table 367-1). Most present with sensory loss on the face or with weakness of the jaw muscles. Deviation of the jaw on opening indicates weakness of the pterygoids on the side to which the jaw deviates. Tumors of the middle cranial fossa (meningiomas), of the trigeminal nerve (schwannomas), or of the base of the skull (metastatic tumors) may cause a combination of motor and sensory signs. Lesions in the cavernous sinus can affect the first and second divisions of the trigeminal nerve, and lesions of the superior orbital fissure can affect the first (ophthalmic) division. The accompanying corneal anesthesia increases the risk of ulceration (neurokeratitis).

Loss of sensation over the chin (mental neuropathy) can be the only manifestation of systemic malignancy. Rarely, an idiopathic form of trigeminal neuropathy is observed. It is characterized by feelings of numbness and paresthesias, sometimes bilaterally, with loss of sensation in the territory of the trigeminal nerve but without weakness of

Table 367-1 Trigeminal Nerve Disorders

Nuclear (brainstem) lesions	Peripheral nerve lesions
Multiple sclerosis	Nasopharyngeal carcinoma
Stroke	Trauma
Syringobulbia	Guillain-Barré syndrome
Glioma	Sjögren's syndrome
Lymphoma	Collagen-vascular diseases
Preganglionic lesions	Sarcoidosis
Acoustic neuroma	Leprosy
Meningioma	Drugs (stilbamidine, trichloroethylene)
Metastasis	Idiopathic trigeminal neuropathy
Chronic meningitis	
Cavernous carotid aneurysm	
Gasserian ganglion lesions	
Trigeminal neuroma	
Herpes zoster	
Infection (spread from otitis media or mastoiditis)	

the jaw. Recovery is the rule, but the symptoms may be troublesome for many months, or even years. Leprosy may involve the trigeminal nerves.

Tonic spasm of the masticatory muscles, known as *trismus*, is symptomatic of tetanus (Chap. 143). It may also occur as an idiosyncratic reaction in patients treated with phenothiazine drugs; lesser degrees may be associated with disease of the pharynx, temporomandibular joint, teeth, and gums.

DISORDERS OF THE FACIAL NERVE

The seventh cranial nerve supplies all the muscles concerned with facial expression. The sensory component is small (the nervus intermedius); it conveys taste sensation from the anterior two-thirds of the tongue and probably cutaneous impulses from the anterior wall of the external auditory canal. The motor nucleus of the seventh nerve lies anterior and lateral to the abducens nucleus. After leaving the pons, the seventh nerve enters the internal auditory meatus with the acoustic nerve. The nerve continues its course in its own bony channel, the facial canal, and exits from the skull via the stylomastoid foramen. It then passes through the parotid gland and subdivides to supply the facial muscles.

A complete interruption of the facial nerve at the stylomastoid foramen paralyzes all muscles of facial expression. The corner of the mouth droops, the creases and skin folds are effaced, the forehead is unfurrowed, and the eyelids will not close. Upon attempted closure of the lids, the eye on the paralyzed side rolls upward (Bell's phenomenon). The lower lid sags also, and the punctum falls away from the conjunctiva, permitting tears to spill over the cheek. Food collects between the teeth and lips, and saliva may dribble from the corner of the mouth. The patient complains of a heaviness or numbness in the face, but sensory loss is rarely demonstrable and taste is intact.

If the lesion is in the middle ear portion, taste is lost over the anterior two-thirds of the tongue on the same side. If the nerve to the stapedius is interrupted, there is hyperacusis (painful sensitivity to loud sounds). Lesions in the internal auditory meatus may also affect the adjacent auditory and vestibular nerves, causing deafness, tinnitus, or dizziness. Intrapontine lesions that paralyze the face usually affect the abducens nucleus as well, and often the corticospinal and sensory tracts.

If the peripheral facial paralysis has existed for some time and recovery of motor function is incomplete, a continuous diffuse contraction of facial muscles may appear. The palpebral fissure becomes narrowed, and the nasolabial fold deepens. Attempts to move one group of facial muscles may result in contraction of all of them (associated movements, or *synkinesis*). Facial spasms may develop and persist indefinitely, being initiated by every facial movement (*hemifacial spasm*). This condition may represent a transient or permanent sequela to a Bell's palsy but may also be due to an irritative lesion of the facial nerve (e.g., an acoustic neuroma, an aberrant artery that compresses the nerve and is relieved by surgery, or a basilar artery aneurysm). However, in the most common form of hemifacial spasm, the cause and pathology are unknown. Anomalous regeneration of the seventh nerve fibers may result in other troublesome phenomena. If fibers originally connected with the orbicularis oculi come to innervate the orbicularis oris, closure of the lids may cause a retraction of the mouth, or if fibers originally connected with muscles of the face later innervate the lacrimal gland, anomalous tearing ("crocodile tears") may occur with any activity of the facial muscles, such as eating. Yet another unusual facial synkinesia is one in which jaw opening causes a closure of the eyelids on the side of the facial palsy (jaw-winking).

BELL'S PALSY The most common form of facial paralysis is idiopathic, i.e., *Bell's palsy*. The incidence rate of this disorder is about 23 per 100,000 annually, or about 1 in 60 or 70 persons in a lifetime. The pathogenesis of the paralysis is unproven, but an association with herpes simplex virus type 1 DNA in endoneurial fluid and posterior auricular muscle has been documented.

Clinical Manifestations   The onset of Bell's palsy is fairly abrupt, maximal weakness being attained by 48 h as a general rule. Pain behind the ear may precede the paralysis for a day or two. Taste sensation may be lost unilaterally, and hyperacusis may be present. In some cases there is mild cerebrospinal fluid (CSF) lymphocytosis. Magnetic resonance imaging (MRI) may reveal swelling and uniform enhancement of the geniculate ganglion and facial nerve, and, in some cases, entrapment of the swollen nerve in the temporal bone is noted. Fully 80% of patients recover within a few weeks or months. Electromyography may be of some prognostic value; evidence of denervation after 10 days indicates that there has been axonal degeneration and that there will be a long delay (3 months, as a rule) before regeneration occurs and that it may be incomplete. The presence of incomplete paralysis in the first week is the most favorable prognostic sign.

Differential Diagnosis   There are many other causes of facial palsy that must be considered in the differential diagnosis of idiopathic Bell's palsy. Tumors that invade the temporal bone (carotid body, cholesteatoma, dermoid) may produce a facial palsy, but the onset is insidious and the course progressive. The *Ramsay Hunt syndrome*, presumably due to herpes zoster of the geniculate ganglion, consists of a severe facial palsy associated with a vesicular eruption in the pharynx, external auditory canal, and other parts of the cranial integument; often the eighth cranial nerve is affected as well. *Acoustic neuromas* frequently involve the facial nerve by local compression. Infarcts, demyelinating lesions of multiple sclerosis, and tumors are the common pontine lesions that interrupt the facial nerve fibers; other signs of brainstem involvement are usually present. Bilateral facial paralysis (facial diplegia) occurs in *Guillain-Barré syndrome* (Chap. 378) and also in a form of sarcoidosis known as *uveoparotid fever* (*Heerfordt syndrome*). Lyme disease is a frequent cause of facial palsies in endemic areas. The *Melkersson-Rosenthal syndrome* consists of a rarely encountered triad of recurrent facial paralysis, recurrent—and eventually permanent—facial (particularly labial) edema, and less constantly, plication of the tongue; its cause is unknown. Leprosy frequently involves the facial nerve, and facial neuropathy may also occur in diabetes mellitus.

All these forms of nuclear or peripheral facial palsy must be distinguished from the supranuclear type. In the latter, the frontalis and orbicularis oculi muscles are involved less than those of the lower part of the face, since the upper facial muscles are innervated by corticobulbar pathways from both motor cortices, whereas the lower facial muscles are innervated only by the opposite hemisphere. In supranuclear lesions there may be a dissociation of emotional and voluntary facial movements, and often some degree of paralysis of the arm and leg or an aphasia (in dominant hemisphere lesions) is conjoined.

Laboratory Evaluation   The diagnosis of Bell's palsy can usually be made clinically in patients with (1) a typical presentation, (2) no risk factors or preexisting symptoms for other causes of facial paralysis, (3) absence of cutaneous lesions of herpes zoster in the external ear canal, and (4) a normal neurologic examination with the exception of the facial nerve. Particular attention to the eighth cranial nerve, which courses near to the facial nerve in the pontomedullary junction and in the temporal bone, and to other cranial nerves is essential. In atypical or uncertain cases, an erythrocyte sedimentation rate, testing for diabetes mellitus, a Lyme titer, chest x-ray for possible sarcoidosis, or MRI scanning may be indicated.

℞   **TREATMENT**   Symptomatic measures include (1) the use of paper tape to depress the upper eyelid during sleep and prevent corneal drying, and (2) massage of the weakened muscles. A course of glucocorticoids, given as prednisone 60 to 80 mg daily during the first 5 days and then tapered over the next 5 days, appears to shorten the recovery period and modestly improve the functional outcome. In one double-blind study, patients treated within 3 days of onset with both prednisone and acyclovir (400 mg five times daily for 10 days) had a better outcome than patients treated with prednisone alone.

OTHER FACIAL DISORDERS   *Facial hemiatrophy* occurs mainly in females and is characterized by a disappearance of fat in the dermal and subcutaneous tissues on one side of the face. It usually begins in adolescence or early adult years and is slowly progressive. In its advanced form, the affected side of the face is gaunt, and the skin is thin, wrinkled, and rather brown. The facial hair may turn white and fall out, and the sebaceous glands become atrophic. The muscles and bones are not involved as a rule. Sometimes the atrophy becomes bilateral. The condition is a form of lipodystrophy. Treatment is cosmetic, consisting of transplantation of skin and subcutaneous fat.

Facial myokymia refers to a fine rippling activity of the facial muscles; it may be caused by a plaque of multiple sclerosis. *Blepharospasm* is an involuntary recurrent spasm of both eyelids that occurs in elderly persons as an isolated phenomenon or with varying degrees of spasm of other facial muscles. Severe, persistent cases of blepharospasm or hemifacial spasm can be treated by local injection of botulinus toxin into the orbicularis oculi; the spasms are relieved for 3 to 4 months, and the injections can be repeated.

GLOSSOPHARYNGEAL NERVE DISORDERS

GLOSSOPHARYNGEAL NEURALGIA   This form of neuralgia resembles trigeminal neuralgia in many respects but is much less common. The pain is intense and paroxysmal; it originates in the throat, approximately in the tonsillar fossa. In some cases the pain is localized in the ear or may radiate from the throat to the ear because of involvement of the tympanic branch of the glossopharyngeal nerve. Spasms of pain may be initiated by swallowing. There is no demonstrable sensory or motor deficit. Cardiac symptoms—bradycardia, hypotension, and fainting—have been reported. A trial of carbamazepine or phenytoin is the recommended therapy, but if that is unsuccessful, division of the glossopharyngeal nerve near the medulla is the definitive treatment. Percutaneous rhizotomy of glossopharyngeal and vagal fibers in the jugular foramen alleviates pain in some patients.

Very rarely, herpes zoster involves the glossopharyngeal nerve. Glossopharyngeal neuropathy in conjunction with vagus and accessory nerve palsies may also occur with a tumor or aneurysm in the posterior fossa or in the jugular foramen. Hoarseness due to vocal cord paralysis, some difficulty in swallowing, deviation of the soft palate to the intact side, anesthesia of the posterior wall of the pharynx, and weakness of the upper part of the trapezius and sternocleidomastoid muscles make up the syndrome (Table 367-2, jugular foramen syndrome).

DISORDERS OF THE VAGUS NERVE

DYSPHAGIA AND DYSPHONIA   Complete interruption of the intracranial portion of one vagus nerve results in a characteristic paralysis. The soft palate droops ipsilaterally and does not rise in phonation. There is loss of the gag reflex on the affected side, as well as of the "curtain movement" of the lateral wall of the pharynx, whereby the faucial pillars move medially as the palate rises in saying "ah." The voice is hoarse and slightly nasal, and the vocal cord lies immobile midway between abduction and adduction. There may also be a loss of sensibility at the external auditory meatus and the posterior pinna.

The pharyngeal branches of both vagi may be affected in diphtheria; the voice has a nasal quality, and regurgitation of liquids through the nose occurs during the act of swallowing.

The vagus nerve may be involved at the meningeal level by neoplastic and infectious processes and within the medulla by tumors, vascular lesions (e.g., the lateral medullary syndrome of Wallenberg), and motor neuron disease. This nerve may be involved by the inflammatory lesion of herpes zoster. Polymyositis and dermatomyositis, which cause hoarseness and dysphagia by direct involvement of laryngeal and pharyngeal muscles, may be confused with diseases of the vagus nerves. Also, dysphagia is a symptom in some patients with

Table 367-2 Cranial Nerve Syndromes

Site	Cranial Nerves Involved	Usual Cause
Sphenoid fissure (superior orbital)	III, IV, first division V, VI	Invasive tumors of sphenoid bone; aneurysms
Lateral wall of cavernous sinus	III, IV, first division V, VI, often with proptosis	Infection, thrombosis, aneurysm, or fistula of cavernous sinus; invasive tumors from sinuses and sella turcica; benign granuloma responsive to glucocorticoids
Retrosphenoid space	II, III, IV, V, VI	Large tumors of middle cranial fossa
Apex of petrous bone	V, VI	Petrositis; tumors of petrous bone
Internal auditory meatus	VII, VIII	Tumors of petrous bone (dermoids, etc.); infectious processes; acoustic neuroma
Pontocerebellar angle	V, VII, VIII, and sometimes IX	Acoustic neuroma; meningioma
Jugular foramen	IX, X, XI	Tumors and aneurysms
Posterior laterocondylar space	IX, X, XI, XII	Tumors of parotid gland and carotid body and metastatic tumors
Posterior retroparotid space	IX, X, XI, XII and Horner syndrome	Tumors of parotid gland, carotid body, lymph nodes; metastatic tumor; tuberculous adenitis

myotonic dystrophy. →See Chap. 40 for discussion of nonneurologic forms of dysphagia.

The recurrent laryngeal nerves, especially the left, are most often damaged as a result of intrathoracic disease. Aneurysm of the aortic arch, an enlarged left atrium, and tumors of the mediastinum and bronchi are much more frequent causes of an isolated vocal cord palsy than are intracranial disorders.

When confronted with a case of laryngeal palsy, the physician must attempt to determine the site of the lesion. If it is intramedullary, there are usually other signs, such as ipsilateral cerebellar dysfunction, loss of pain and temperature sensation over the ipsilateral face and contralateral arm and leg, and an ipsilateral Horner syndrome. If the lesion is extramedullary, the glossopharyngeal and spinal accessory nerves are frequently involved (see jugular foramen syndrome, Table 367-2). If it is extracranial in the posterior laterocondylar or retroparotid space, there may be a combination of ninth, tenth, eleventh, and twelfth cranial nerve palsies and a Horner syndrome (Table 367-2). If there is no sensory loss over the palate and pharynx and no palatal weakness or dysphagia, the lesion is below the origin of the pharyngeal branches, which leave the vagus nerve high in the cervical region; the usual site of disease is then the mediastinum.

DISORDERS OF THE ACCESSORY NERVE

Isolated involvement of the accessory, or eleventh cranial, nerve can occur anywhere along its route, resulting in partial or complete paralysis of the sternocleidomastoid and trapezius muscles. More commonly, involvement occurs in combination with deficits of the ninth and tenth cranial nerves in the jugular foramen or after exit from the skull (Table 367-2). An idiopathic form of accessory neuropathy, akin to Bell's palsy, has been described, and it may be recurrent in some cases. Most but not all patients recover.

DISORDERS OF THE HYPOGLOSSAL NERVE

The twelfth cranial nerve supplies the ipsilateral muscles of the tongue. The nucleus of the nerve or its fibers of exit may be involved by intramedullary lesions such as tumor, poliomyelitis, or most often motor neuron disease. Lesions of the basal meninges and the occipital bones (platybasia, invagination of occipital condyles, Paget's disease)

may compress the nerve in its extramedullary course or in the hypoglossal canal. Isolated lesions of unknown cause can occur. Atrophy and fasciculation of the tongue develop weeks to months after interruption of the nerve.

MULTIPLE CRANIAL NERVE PALSIES

Several cranial nerves may be affected by the same disease process. In this situation, the main clinical problem is to determine whether the lesion lies within the brainstem or outside it. Lesions that lie on the surface of the brainstem are characterized by involvement of adjacent cranial nerves (often occurring in succession) and late and rather slight involvement of the long sensory and motor pathways and segmental structures lying within the brainstem. The opposite is true of intramedullary, intrapontine, and intramesencephalic lesions. The extramedullary lesion is more likely to cause bone erosion or enlargement of the foramens of exit of cranial nerves. The intramedullary lesion involving cranial nerves often produces a crossed sensory or motor paralysis (cranial nerve signs on one side of the body and tract signs on the opposite side).

Involvement of multiple cranial nerves outside the brainstem is frequently the result of diabetes or trauma (sudden onset), localized infections such as herpes zoster (acute onset), infectious and noninfectious causes of meningitis (Chap. 374) or granulomatous diseases such as Wegener's granulomatosis (subacute onset), Behçet's disease, or tumors and enlarging saccular aneurysms (chronic development). Of the tumors, lymphomas, neurofibromas, meningiomas, chordomas, cholesteatomas, carcinomas, and sarcomas have all been observed to involve a succession of lower cranial nerves. Owing to their anatomic relationships, the multiple cranial nerve palsies form a number of distinctive syndromes, listed in Table 367-2. Sarcoidosis is the cause of some cases of multiple cranial neuropathy, and chronic glandular tuberculosis (scrofula) the cause of a few others. Midline granuloma of the nasopharynx may also affect multiple cranial nerves, as do nasopharyngeal tumors, platybasia, basilar invagination of the skull, and the adult Chiari malformation. A purely motor disorder without atrophy always raises the question of myasthenia gravis (Chap. 380). Guillain-Barré syndrome commonly affects the facial nerves bilaterally (facial diplegia). In the Fisher variant of the Guillain-Barré syndrome, oculomotor paresis occurs with ataxia and areflexia in the limbs (Chap. 378). Wernicke encephalopathy can cause a severe ophthalmoplegia combined with other brainstem signs.

The cavernous sinus syndrome is a distinctive and frequently life-threatening disorder. It often presents as orbital or facial pain; orbital swelling and chemosis due to occlusion of the ophthalmic veins; fever; oculomotor neuropathy affecting the third, fourth, and sixth cranial nerves; and trigeminal neuropathy affecting the ophthalmic (V_1) and occasionally the maxillary (V_2) divisions of the trigeminal nerve. Cavernous sinus thrombosis, often secondary to infection from orbital cellulitis (frequently Staphylococcus aureus), a cutaneous source on the face, or sinusitis (especially with mucormycosis in diabetic patients), is the most frequent cause; other etiologies include aneurysm of the carotid artery, a carotid-cavernous fistula (orbital bruit may be present), meningioma, nasopharyngeal carcinoma or other tumor, or an idiopathic granulomatous disorder (Tolosa-Hunt syndrome). Due to the anatomy of the cavernous sinus (Fig. 367-2) the syndrome may extend to become bilateral. Early diagnosis is essential, especially in cases due to infection, and treatment depends upon the underlying etiology. In infectious cases, prompt administration of broad-spectrum antibiotics, drainage of any abcess cavities, and identification of the offending organism is essential. Anticoagulant therapy may benefit cases of primary thrombosis. Repair or occlusion of the carotid artery may be required for treatment of fistulas or aneurysms. The Tolosa-Hunt syndrome generally responds to glucocorticoids.

An idiopathic form of multiple cranial nerve involvement on one or both sides of the face is occasionally seen (see Juncos and Beal). The syndrome consists of a subacute onset of boring facial pain, followed by paralysis of motor cranial nerves. The clinical features over-

Ant. cerebral a.
Int. carotid a.
Ant. clinoid process
Subarachnoid space
Optic chiasma
Oculomotor (III) n.
Trochlear (IV) n.
Hypophysis
Ophthalmic (V_I) n.
Maxillary (V_2) n.
Sphenoid sinus
Pia
Arachnoid
Dura
Abducens (VI) n.

FIGURE 367-2 Anatomy of the cavernous sinus in coronal section, illustrating the location of the cranial nerves in relation to the vascular sinus, internal carotid artery (which loops anteriorly to the section), and surrounding structures.

lap those of the Tolosa-Hunt syndrome and appear to be due to idiopathic inflammation of the dura mater, which may be visualized by MRI. The syndrome is frequently responsive to glucocorticoids.

ACKNOWLEDGMENT
The authors acknowledge the contributions of Dr. Joseph B. Martin and Dr. Maurice Victor to this chapter in previous editions.

BIBLIOGRAPHY

ADAMS RD, VICTOR M: *Principles of Neurology*, 6th ed. New York, McGraw-Hill, 1997, chap 47, pp 1370–1385

ADOUR KK et al: Bell's palsy treatment with acyclovir and prednisone compared with prednisone alone: A double-blind, randomized, controlled trial. Ann Otol Rhinol Laryngol 105:371, 1996

BARKER FG et al: The long-term outcome of microvascular decompression for trigeminal neuralgia. N Engl J Med 334:1077, 1996

CHALK C, ISAACS H: Recurrent spontaneous accessory neuropathy. J Neurol Neurosurg Psychiatry 53:621, 1990

DELZELL JE, GRELLE AR: Trigeminal neuralgia: New treatment options for a well-known cause of facial pain. Arch Fam Med 8:264, 1999

FURUTA Y et al: Reactivation of herpes simplex virus type 1 in patients with Bell's palsy. J Med Virol 54:162, 1998

JACKSON CG, VON DOERSTEN PG: The facial nerve. Current trends in diagnosis, treatment, and rehabilitation. Med Clin North Am 83:179, 1999

JANKOVIC J, BRIN MF: Therapeutic uses of botulinum toxin. N Engl J Med 324:1186, 1991

JUNCOS JL, BEAL MF: Idiopathic cranial polyneuropathy. Brain 110:197, 1987

KEANE JR: Bilateral seventh nerve palsy: Analysis of 43 cases and review of the literature. Neurology 44:1198, 1994

KEANE JR: Fourth nerve palsy: Historical review and study of 215 inpatients. Neurology 43:2439, 1993

———: Twelfth-nerve palsy. Arch Neurol 53:561, 1996

LECKY BRF et al: Trigeminal sensory neuropathy. Brain 110:1463, 1987

LOSSOS A, SIEGAL T: Numb chin syndrome in cancer patients: Etiology, response to treatment, and prognostic significance. Neurology 42:1181, 1992

MIWA H et al: Recurrent cranial neuropathy as a clinical presentation of idiopathic inflammation of the dura mater: A possible relationship to Tolosa-Hunt syndrome and cranial pachymeningitis. J Neurol Sci 154:101, 1998

PHATOUROS CC et al: Carotid artery cavernous fistulas. Neurosurg Clin N Am 11:67, 2000

STEINER I, MATTAN Y: Bell's palsy and herpes viruses: to (acyclo)vir or not to (acyclo)vir? J Neurol Sci 170:19, 1999

WANG A, JANKOVIC J: Hemifacial spasm: Clinical findings and treatment. Muscle Nerve 21:1740, 1998

YOON KB et al: Long-term outcome of thermocoagulation for trigeminal neuralgia. Anaesthesia 54:803, 1999

368 *Stephen L. Hauser*

DISEASES OF THE SPINAL CORD

Diseases of the spinal cord are frequently devastating. They can produce quadriplegia, paraplegia, and sensory deficits far beyond the damage they would inflict elsewhere in the nervous system because the spinal cord contains, in a small cross-sectional area, almost the entire motor output and sensory input systems of the trunk and limbs. Many spinal cord diseases are reversible if recognized and treated at an early stage (Table 368-1); thus, they are among the most critical of neurologic emergencies. The efficient use of diagnostic procedures, guided by a working knowledge of the relevant anatomy and clinical features of common spinal cord diseases, is often the key to a successful outcome.

Approach to the Patient

Spinal Cord Anatomy Relevant to Clinical Signs The spinal cord is a thin, tubular extension of the central nervous system contained within the bony spinal canal. It originates at the medulla and continues caudally to terminate at the filum terminale, a fibrous extension of the conus medullaris that terminates at the coccyx. The adult spinal cord is approximately 18 inches long, oval or round in shape, and enlarged in the cervical and lumbar regions, where neurons that innervate the upper and lower extremities, respectively, are located. The white matter tracts containing ascending sensory and descending motor pathways are located peripherally, whereas nerve cell bodies are clustered in an inner region shaped like a four-leaf clover that surrounds the central canal (anatomically an extension of the fourth ventricle). The membranes that cover the spinal cord—the pia, arachnoid, and dura—are continuous with those of the brainstem and cerebral hemispheres.

The spinal cord is somatotopically organized, consisting of 31 segments, each containing an exiting ventral motor root and entering dorsal sensory root (Fig. 368-1). During embryologic development, growth of the cord lags behind that of the vertebral column, and in the adult the spinal cord ends at approximately the first lumbar vertebral body. The lower spinal nerves take an increasingly downward course to exit via the appropriate intervertebral foramina. The first seven pairs of cervical spinal nerves exit above the same-numbered vertebral bodies, whereas all the subsequent nerves exit below the same-numbered vertebral bodies; this situation is due to the presence of eight cervical spinal cord segments but only seven cervical vertebrae. The approxi-

Table 368-1 Some Treatable Spinal Cord Disorders

Compressive
  Epidural, intradural, or intramedullary neoplasm
  Epidural abscess
  Epidural hemorrhage
  Cervical spondylosis
  Herniated disc
  Posttraumatic compression by fractured or displaced vertebra or hemorrhage
Vascular
  Arteriovenous malformation
Inflammatory
  Transverse myelitis
  Multiple sclerosis
Infectious
  Viral: Herpes simplex type 2
  Bacterial: Syphilis, tuberculosis, listeria, other
  Parasitic: Schistosomiasis, toxoplasmosis
Developmental
  Syringomyelia
Metabolic
  Subacute combined degeneration

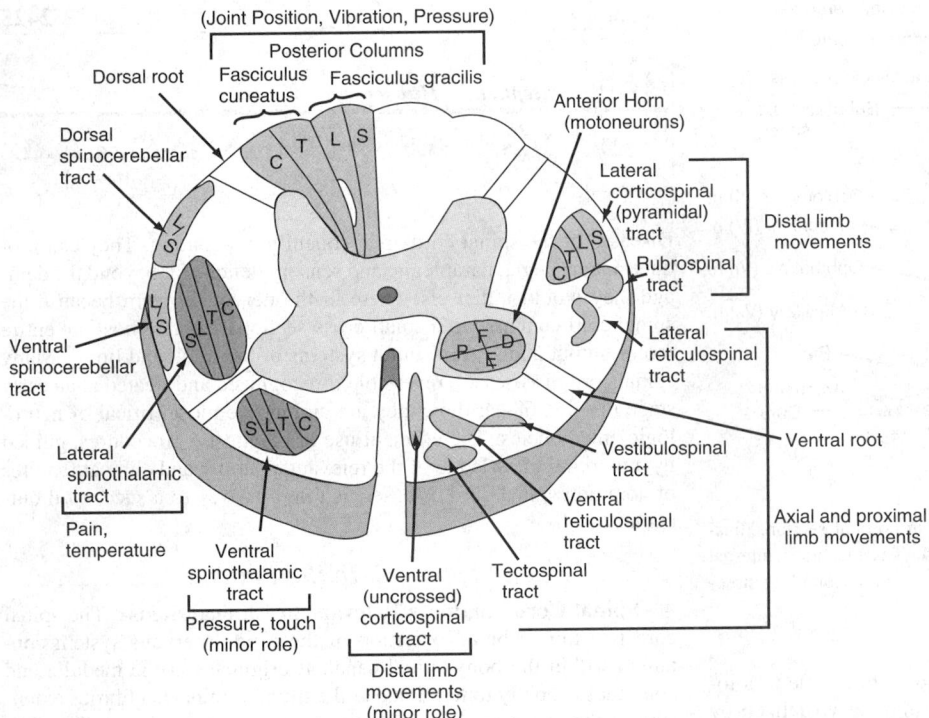

(Joint Position, Vibration, Pressure)

Posterior Columns

Fasciculus cuneatus · Fasciculus gracilis

Dorsal root

Dorsal spinocerebellar tract

Anterior Horn (motoneurons)

Lateral corticospinal (pyramidal) tract

Distal limb movements

Rubrospinal tract

Ventral spinocerebellar tract

Lateral reticulospinal tract

Lateral spinothalamic tract

Ventral root

Pain, temperature

Vestibulospinal tract

Ventral spinothalamic tract

Ventral reticulospinal tract

Axial and proximal limb movements

Pressure, touch (minor role)

Ventral (uncrossed) corticospinal tract

Tectospinal tract

Distal limb movements (minor role)

FIGURE 368-1 Transverse section through the spinal cord, composite representation, illustrating the principal ascending (*left*) and descending (*right*) pathways. The lateral and ventral spinothalamic tracts (*dark-blue*) ascend contralateral to the side of the body that is innervated. C, cervical; T, thoracic; L, lumbar; S, sacral; P, proximal; D, distal; F, flexors; E, extensors.

mate relationship between spinal cord segments and the corresponding vertebral bodies is shown in Table 368-2. These relationships assume importance for localization of lesions that cause spinal cord compression; a T10 spinal cord level, for example, indicates involvement of the cord adjacent to the seventh or eighth thoracic vertebral body.

Level of the lesion The presence of a *level* below which sensory, motor, and/or autonomic function is disturbed is a hallmark of spinal cord disease. A sensory level is sought by asking the patient to identify as sharp a pinprick stimulus or as cool a cold stimulus (a dry tuning fork after immersion in cold water) applied to the low back and sequentially moved up toward the neck on each side. In general, a sensory level to pinprick or temperature, indicating damage to the spinothalamic tract, is located one to two segments below the actual level of a unilateral spinal cord lesion, but it may be at the level of the lesion when bilateral. That is because sensory fibers enter the cord at the dorsal root, synapse in the dorsal horn, and then ascend ipsilaterally for several segments before crossing just anterior to the central canal to join the opposite spinothalamic tract. Lesions that disrupt descending corticospinal and bulbospinal tracts cause paraplegia or quadriplegia, with increased muscle tone, exaggerated deep tendon reflexes, and extensor plantar signs. Such lesions also typically produce autonomic disturbances, with disturbed sweating and bladder, bowel, and sexual dysfunction. A sweat level may be determined by drawing a spoon up the torso. There will be little resistance to movement of the spoon along the dry, nonsweating skin; at the level at which sweating begins, resistance will suddenly increase.

Table 368-2 Spinal Cord Levels Relative to the Vertebral Bodies

Spinal Cord Level	Corresponding Vertebral Body
Upper cervical	Same as cord level
Lower cervical	1 level higher
Upper thoracic	2 levels higher
Lower thoracic	2 to 3 levels higher
Lumbar	T10–T12
Sacral	T12–L1
Coccygeal	L1

The uppermost level of a spinal cord lesion is often localized by attention to *segmental signs* corresponding to disturbed motor or sensory innervation by an individual cord segment. A band of altered sensation (hyperalgesia or hyperpathia) at the upper end of the sensory disturbance, fasciculations or atrophy in muscles innervated by one or several segments, or a single diminished or absent deep tendon reflex may be noted. These signs may also occur with focal root or peripheral nerve disorders; thus, segmental signs are most useful when they occur with other signs of cord disease. With severe and acute transverse lesions, the limbs may be flaccid rather than spastic (so-called spinal shock). This state may last for several days, rarely for weeks, and may be initially mistaken for extensive damage to many segments of the cord (as in ascending necrotic myelopathy associated with cancer) or as polyneuropathy. Brief clonic or myoclonic movements of the limbs often precede paralysis in acute transverse lesions, particularly those due to cord infarction.

Patterns of spinal cord disease The location of the major ascending and descending pathways of the spinal cord are shown in Fig. 368-1. Most fiber tracts—including the posterior columns and the spinocerebellar and pyramidal tracts—travel ipsilateral to the side of the body they innervate. As noted above, afferent fibers mediating pain and temperature sensation are unusual in that they ascend contralaterally as the spinothalamic tract. The anatomic relationships of these various fiber tracts and nuclei produce distinctive clinical syndromes that are pathognomonic of spinal cord disease and that often provide clues to the underlying disease process.

BROWN-SEQUARD HEMICORD SYNDROME This syndrome consists of ipsilateral weakness (pyramidal tract) and loss of joint position and vibratory sense (posterior column), with contralateral loss of pain and temperature sense (spinothalamic tract) below the lesion. The sensory level for pain and temperature is one or two levels below the lesion. Segmental signs, such as radicular pain, muscle atrophy, or loss of a deep tendon reflex, when they occur, are unilateral. Pure examples of hemicord syndromes are rare; partial or bilateral forms are more common. Partial syndromes may involve the dorsal (posterior) quadrant, producing ipsilateral loss of vibration and position sense, or ventral (anterior) quadrant with ipsilateral paralysis and contralateral loss of pain and temperature sense.

CENTRAL CORD SYNDROME The central cord syndrome results from disorders of gray matter nerve cells and crossing spinothalamic tracts near the central canal. In the cervical cord, the central cord syndrome produces arm weakness out of proportion to leg weakness and a "dissociated" sensory loss consisting of loss of pain and temperature sense in a cape distribution over the shoulders, lower neck, and upper trunk with intact light touch, joint position, and vibration sense. Trauma, syringomyelia, tumors, and anterior spinal artery ischemia are common causes of the central cord syndrome.

ANTERIOR TWO-THIRDS SYNDROME This syndrome results from extensive bilateral disease of the spinal cord that spares the posterior columns. All spinal cord functions—motor, sensory and autonomic—are lost below the level of the lesion, with the striking exception of intact vibration and position sensation. The etiology is vascular, either thromboembolism of the anterior spinal artery or compression of this vessel by mass lesions within the spinal canal.

INTRAMEDULLARY AND EXTRAMEDULLARY SYNDROMES The diagnosis of spinal cord disorders frequently requires that intramedullary processes, which arise within the substance of the cord, be distinguished from extramedullary processes that compress the spinal cord or its vascular supply. Distinguishing features are relative and serve only as rough guides to clinical decision making. With extramedullary lesions, radicular pain is often prominent, and there is early sacral sensory loss (lateral spinothalamic tract) and spastic weakness in the legs (corticospinal tract) due to the superficial location of these fibers in the lateral spinal cord, which renders them susceptible to external compression. Intramedullary lesions tend to produce poorly localized burning pain rather than radicular pain and spare sensation in the perineal and sacral areas; corticospinal tract signs may appear late. With extramedullary lesions, the distinction between extradural and intradural masses is important, as the former are generally malignant and the latter benign; a long duration of symptoms favors an intradural origin.

Specific localizing signs • CERVICAL CORD High cervical cord lesions are frequently life-threatening, producing quadriplegia and weakness of respiratory muscles innervated by the phrenic nerve (C3-C5). There is diaphragmatic paralysis, and breathing is possible only by use of accessory muscles of respiration. Extensive lesions near the junction of the cervical cord and medulla are usually fatal owing to involvement of adjacent medullary centers, which results in vasomotor and respiratory collapse. Partial lesions in this area, generally due to trauma, may interrupt decussating pyramidal tract fibers destined for the legs, which cross below those of the arms, resulting in a "crural paresis" of the lower limbs. Compressive lesions near the foramen magnum may produce weakness of the ipsilateral shoulder and arm followed by weakness of the ipsilateral leg, then the contralateral leg, and finally the contralateral arm; the patient may complain of suboccipital pain spreading to the neck and shoulders. Lesions at C4-C5 produce quadriplegia with preserved respiratory function. At the mid-cervical (C5-C6) level, there is relative sparing of shoulder muscles and loss of biceps and brachioradialis reflexes. Lesions at C7 spare the biceps but produce weakness of finger and wrist extensors and loss of the triceps reflex. Lesions at C8 paralyze finger and wrist flexion, and the finger flexor reflex is lost. In general, cervical cord disorders are best localized by the pattern of weakness that ensues, whereas sensory deficits have less localizing value. A Horner's syndrome (miosis, ptosis, and facial hypohidrosis) may also occur ipsilateral to cervical cord lesions at any level.

THORACIC CORD Lesions of the thoracic cord are best localized by identification of a sensory level on the trunk. Sensory dermatomes of the body are shown in Fig. 23-2; useful markers are at the nipples (T4) and umbilicus (T10). Weakness of the legs and disturbances of bladder, bowel, or sexual function may also accompany damage to the thoracic cord. The abdominal wall musculature, supplied by the lower thoracic cord, is observed during movements of respiration or coughing or by asking the patient to interlock the fingers behind the head in the supine position and attempt to sit up. Lesions at T9-T10 paralyze the lower, but spare the upper, abdominal muscles, resulting in upward movement of the umbilicus when the abdominal wall contracts (Beevor's sign) and in loss of lower, but not upper, superficial abdominal reflexes (Chap. 356). With unilateral lesions, attempts to contract the abdominal wall produce movement of the umbilicus to the normal side; superficial abdominal reflexes are absent on the involved side. Midline back pain is a useful localizing sign in the thoracic region.

LUMBAR CORD The lumbar and sacral cord segments progressively decrease in size, and focal lesions of these segments are less easily localized than in cervical and thoracic regions. Lesions at L2-L4 paralyze flexion and adduction of the thigh, weaken leg extension at the knee, and abolish the patellar reflex. Lesions at L5-S1 paralyze movements of the foot and ankle, flexion at the knee, and extension of the thigh, and abolish the ankle jerk (S1). A cutaneous reflex useful in localization of lumbar cord disease is the cremasteric reflex (Chap. 356), which is segmentally innervated at L1-L2.

SACRAL CORD/CONUS MEDULLARIS The conus medullaris is the tapered caudal termination of the spinal cord, comprising the lower sacral and single coccygeal segments. Isolated lesions of the conus medullaris spare motor and reflex functions in the legs. The conus syndrome is distinctive, consisting of bilateral saddle anesthesia (S3-S5), prominent bladder and bowel dysfunction (urinary retention and incontinence with lax anal tone), and impotence. The bulbocavernosus (S2-S4) and anal (S4-S5) reflexes are absent (Chap. 356). Muscle strength is largely preserved. Lesions of the conus medullaris must be distinguished from those of the cauda equina, the cluster of nerve roots derived from the lower cord as they descend to their exits in the intervertebral foramina. Cauda equina lesions are characterized by severe low back or radicular pain, asymmetric leg weakness or sensory loss, variable areflexia in the lower extremities, and relative sparing of bowel and bladder function. Mass lesions in the lower spinal canal may produce a mixed clinical picture in which elements of both cauda equina and conus medullaris syndromes coexist. →*Cauda equina syndromes are discussed in Chap. 16.*

ACUTE AND SUBACUTE SPINAL CORD DISEASES

Acute and subacute spinal cord disorders are commonly due to extramedullary compression (tumor, infection, spondylosis, or trauma), infarction or hemorrhage, or inflammation. In this category are some of the most dangerous—and treatable—disorders in clinical practice. Early recognition is the key to successful management. Epidural compression due to malignancy often presents with warning signs, generally neck or back pain, bladder disturbances, or sensory symptoms, that precede the development of paralysis. Infarction, hemorrhage, or spinal subluxation is more likely to produce sudden "strokelike" myelopathy without antecedent symptoms.

NEOPLASTIC SPINAL CORD COMPRESSION Neoplasms of the spinal canal may be extramedullary (epidural or intradural) or intramedullary. In adults, most neoplasms are epidural in origin, resulting from metastases to the adjacent vertebral body, spinous or transverse process, or pedicle. Vertebral metastases are essentially bone-marrow metastases, and the propensity of solid tumors to metastasize to the vertebral column probably reflects the high percentage of bone marrow located in the axial skeleton of older individuals. Retroperitoneal neoplasms (especially lymphomas or sarcomas) may enter the spinal canal through the intervertebral foramina; typically they produce radicular pain and other signs of root involvement prior to cord compression. Almost any malignant tumor can metastasize to the spinal canal, although breast, lung, prostate, kidney, lymphoma, and plasma cell dyscrasia are particularly frequent. The thoracic cord is most commonly involved; exceptions are metastases from prostate and ovarian cancer, which occur disproportionately in the sacral and lumbar vertebrae, perhaps resulting from spread through Batson's plexus, a network of veins along the anterior surface of the spinal cord in the epidural space.

Pain is the initial symptom; it may be either aching and localized or sharp and radiating in quality. Pain indicates displacement of pain-sensitive structures, especially periosteum and meninges. The pain worsens with movement, coughing, or sneezing and may awaken patients at night. The recent onset of back pain, particularly if in the thoracic spine (which is uncommonly involved by spondylosis), should prompt consideration of vertebral metastasis. Rarely, pain is mild or absent. Pain typically precedes signs of cord compression by weeks or even months, but once cord compression occurs, it is always progressive and may advance rapidly. Therapy is effective only if administered early, when signs of cord dysfunction are mild or absent; therapy will not reverse a complete paralysis that has been present for >48 h. These realities highlight the importance of prompt recognition and efficient management of these lesions.

Plain radiographs of the spine and radionuclide bone scans have only a limited role in diagnosis because they fail to identify 15 to 20% of metastatic vertebral lesions and may miss paravertebral masses that reach the epidural space by growth through the intervertebral foramina.

Magnetic resonance imaging (MRI) provides excellent anatomic resolution of the site and extent of the tumor (Fig. 368-2); at most centers, MRI has largely replaced computed tomography (CT) and myelography in the diagnosis of epidural masses. MRI can often distinguish between malignant lesions and other masses—epidural abscess, tuberculoma, or epidural hemorrhage, among others—that present in a similar fashion. Vertebral metastases are usually hypointense relative to a normal bone marrow signal on T1-weighted MRI scans; after the administration of gadolinium, contrast enhancement may "normalize" the appearance of the tumor by increasing its intensity to that of normal bone marrow. In contrast to infection, vertebral metastases typically do not cross the disk space. Nonetheless, it can be difficult to distinguish between infection and malignancy by MRI.

Because imaging resources are scarce, and both cancer and back pain are common, it is important to convey to the radiologist an estimate of the urgency of the imaging procedure requested. If signs of spinal cord involvement are present, imaging should be obtained on an emergency basis. If there are radicular symptoms but no evidence of myelopathy, it is usually safe to defer imaging for 24 to 48 h. With back or neck pain only, imaging studies should be obtained within a few days. Finally, up to 40% of patients who present with symptomatic disease at one level are found to have asymptomatic epidural disease elsewhere; thus, the entire spine should be imaged in all patients with epidural malignancy.

R_x TREATMENT Management includes glucocorticoids to reduce interstitial edema, local radiotherapy (initiated as early as possible) to the symptomatic lesion, and specific therapy for the underlying tumor type. Glucocorticoids (dexamethasone, 40 mg daily) can be administered before the imaging study if the clinical suspicion is strong and continued at a lower dose (20 mg daily in divided doses) until radiotherapy (a total of 3000 cGy administered in 15 daily fractions) is completed. Radiotherapy appears to be as effective as surgery, even for classically radioresistant metastases. Biopsy of the epidural mass is usually unnecessary in patients with known preexisting cancer, but biopsy is indicated if a history of underlying cancer is lacking. Surgery, either decompression or vertebral body resection, should be considered when signs of cord compression worsen despite radiotherapy, when the maximum tolerated dose of radiotherapy has been delivered previously to the site, or when a vertebral compression fracture contributes to cord compression. A good response to radiotherapy can

be expected in individuals who are ambulatory at presentation; new weakness is prevented, and some recovery of motor function occurs in approximately half of treated patients. Fixed motor deficits—paraplegia or quadriplegia—do not usually respond to either radiotherapy or surgery.

In contrast to tumors of the epidural space, most intradural mass lesions are slow-growing and benign. Meningiomas and neurofibromas account for most of these lesions, with occasional cases representing chordoma, lipoma, dermoid, or sarcoma. Meningiomas (Fig. 368-3) are often located posterior to the thoracic cord or near the foramen magnum, although they can arise from the meninges anywhere along the spinal canal. Neurofibromas are benign tumors of the nerve sheath that typically arise near the posterior root; when multiple, neurofibromatosis (Chap. 370) is the likely etiology. Symptoms usually begin with radicular sensory symptoms followed by an asymmetric, progressive spinal cord syndrome. Therapy is surgical resection.

Primary intramedullary tumors of the spinal cord are uncommon. They typically present as central cord or hemicord syndromes, often in the cervical region; there may be poorly localized burning pain in the extremities and sparing of sacral sensation. In adults, most of these lesions are either ependymomas, hemangioblastomas, or low-grade astrocytomas (Fig. 368-4). Complete resection of an intramedullary ependymoma is often possible with microsurgical techniques. Debulking of an intramedullary astrocytoma can also be helpful, as these are often slowly growing lesions; the value of adjunctive radiotherapy is uncertain. Secondary (metastatic) intramedullary tumors are rare.

SPINAL CORD INFARCTION The spinal cord is supplied by three arteries that course vertically over its surface, a single anterior spinal artery, and paired posterior spinal arteries. At each segment, paired penetrators branching from the anterior spinal artery supply the anterior two-thirds of the spinal cord; the posterior spinal arteries, which often become less distinct below the midthoracic level, supply the posterior columns. Rostrally, the spinal arteries arise from the vertebral arteries. During embryogenesis, arterial feeders arise at each segmental level, but most involute before birth; generally, between

FIGURE 368-2 Epidural spinal cord compression due to breast carcinoma. Sagittal T1-weighted (*A*) and T2-weighted (*B*) MRI scans through the cervicothoracic junction reveal a compression fracture of the second thoracic vertebral body with posterior displacement and compression of the upper thoracic spinal cord. The low-intensity bone marrow signal in *A* signifies replacement by tumor.

FIGURE 368-3 MRI of a thoracic meningioma. Coronal T1-weighted postcontrast image through the thoracic spinal cord demonstrates intense enhancement of a well-circumscribed extramedullary mass (*arrows*) which displaces the spinal cord to the left, widening the cistern adjacent to the mass.

FIGURE 368-4 MRI of an intramedullary astrocytoma. Sagittal T1-weighted postcontrast image through the cervical spine demonstrates expansion of the upper cervical spine by a mass lesion emanating from within the spinal cord at the cervicomedullary junction. Irregular peripheral enhancement occurs within the mass (*arrows*).

three and eight major feeders remain, arising from the vertebral, sub-clavian, intercostal (off the aorta), iliac, and sacral arteries. In addition to the vertebral arteries, in adults, anterior spinal artery feeders often occur at C6, at an upper thoracic level, and at T11-L2 (artery of Adam-kiewicz). Feeders from the aorta are more likely to arise from the left side.

Spinal cord ischemia can occur at any level. The signs are deter-mined by the level of the lesion and by the individual vascular anat-omy, including areas of watershed flow and potential for anastomosis. The anterior spinal artery is discontinuous in some individuals, in-creasing the importance of feeders to the lower cord. With systemic hypotension, cord infarction occurs at the level of greatest ischemic risk, often T3-T4, and also at boundary zones between the anterior and posterior spinal artery territories. The latter may result in an acute—or more commonly progressive—syndrome of weakness and spastic-ity with little sensory change resembling amyotrophic lateral sclerosis (ALS).

Acute infarction in the territory of the anterior spinal artery pro-duces paraplegia or quadriplegia, dissociated sensory loss affecting pain and temperature sense but sparing vibration and position sense, and loss of sphincter control. Onset may be sudden and dramatic or progressive over minutes or hours. Sharp midline or radiating back pain localized to the area of ischemia is frequently noted. Partial in-farction of one anterior hemicord (hemiplegia or monoplegia and crossed pain and temperature loss) may also occur. Areflexia due to spinal shock is often present initially; with time, hyperreflexia and spasticity appear.

The acute onset of pain, sparing of posterior column function, and sharply demarcated spinal cord level distinguish anterior spinal artery infarction from epidural spinal cord compression, in which pain is often chronic, posterior column sense is impaired, and a cord level is indistinct. An exception to this rule is when epidural tumors compress or invade vascular structures, resulting in an anterior spinal artery syn-drome. Infarction in the territory of the posterior spinal arteries, re-sulting in loss of posterior column function, also occurs and may be underrecognized as a cause of loss of position and vibration sense.

Spinal cord infarction is associated with aortic atherosclerosis, dis-secting aortic aneurysm (chest or back pain with diminished pulses in legs), or hypotension from any cause. Cardiogenic emboli, vasculitis related to collagen vascular disease, and surgical clipping of aortic aneurysms are other predisposing conditions. Occasional cases de-velop either during pregnancy or after acute back trauma or exercise that by an unknown mechanism leads to embolism of nucleus pulposus material into spinal vessels. In a substantial number of cases, no cause can be found, and thromboembolism in arterial feeders is suspected.

MRI is often normal but is useful to exclude other causes of acute myelopathy, in particular epidural compression, spinal cord hemor-rhage (hematomyelia), infectious myelitis, or transverse myelitis. Lumbar puncture is indicated whenever the underlying cause has not been clarified by MRI. Other useful laboratory studies include a sed-imentation rate to search for an underlying vasculitis, Venereal Disease Research Laboratories test, and evaluation for aortic or cardiac disease or for a hypercoagulable state.

Therapy is directed at treatment of any predisposing condition. In cord infarction due to presumed thromboembolism, anticoagulation is probably not indicated, with the exception of the unusual transient ischemic attack or incomplete infarction with a stuttering or progres-sive course.

EPIDURAL HEMATOMA Hemorrhage into the epidural (or subdural) space can compress the spinal cord or roots. Presenting symptoms are the acute onset of focal or radicular pain followed by variable signs of a spinal cord or conus medullaris disorder. Trauma, tumor, or blood dyscrasias are predisposing conditions. Rare cases complicate lumbar puncture or epidural anesthesia, sometimes in as-sociation with use of low-molecular-weight heparin. Epidural hema-toma can also occur on an idiopathic basis. MRI confirms the clinical suspicion and can delineate the extent of the bleed. Extrinsic spinal cord compression from any cause is a medical emergency, and appro-priate treatment consists of prompt recognition, reversal of any un-derlying clotting disorder, and emergency surgical decompression. Surgery may be followed by substantial recovery, especially in patients with some preservation of motor function preoperatively. Because of the risk of hemorrhage, lumbar puncture should be avoided whenever possible in patients with thrombocytopenia or other coagulopathies (including those due to therapeutic anticoagulation) until the under-lying bleeding disorder is reversed.

HEMATOMYELIA Hemorrhage into the substance of the spi-nal cord is rare. It may result from trauma, an intraparenchymal vas-cular malformation (see below), vasculitis due to polyarteritis nodosa or lupus erythematosus, bleeding disorders, or spinal cord infection or neoplasm. Hematomyelia presents as an acute painful transverse my-elopathy. With large lesions, extension into the subarachnoid space may occur, resulting in subarachnoid hemorrhage (Chap. 361). Diag-nosis is best made by MRI. Therapy is supportive, and surgical inter-vention is generally not useful. An exception is hematomyelia due to an underlying vascular malformation; in such cases, selective spinal angiography may be indicated, followed by acute surgical intervention to evacuate the clot and remove the underlying vascular lesion.

EPIDURAL ABSCESS Spinal epidural abscess presents as a clinical triad of pain, fever, and rapidly progressive weakness. Prompt recognition of this distinctive and treatable medical emergency will in most cases prevent severe and permanent sequelae. Epidural abscesses can form anywhere along the spinal canal. Pain is almost always present, either midline along the spine or radicular in type. The du-ration of pain prior to presentation is generally two weeks or less, but in some chronic cases it may be several months or longer. Fever is common, often accompanied by an elevated white blood cell count or sedimentation rate. As the abscess expands, spinal cord injury results from venous congestion and thrombosis, thrombophlebitis of the ep-idural space, spinal artery disease, or cord compression. Once weak-ness and other signs of myelopathy appear, progression is often rapid, although it may be gradual.

Risk factors include impaired immune status (diabetes mellitus, renal failure, alcoholism, malignancy), intravenous drug abuse, and infections of the skin or other tissues. Two-thirds of epidural infections result from hematogenous spread from the skin (furunculosis), soft tissue (pharyngeal or dental abscesses), or deep viscera (bacterial endocarditis). One-third result from direct extension of a local infection to the subdural space; examples of local predisposing conditions are vertebral osteomyelitis, decubitus ulcers, or iatrogenic complications of lumbar puncture, epidural anesthesia, or spinal surgery.

Most cases are due to *Staphylococcus aureus*; gram-negative bacilli, *Streptococcus*, anaerobes, and fungi can also cause epidural abscesses. Tuberculosis from an adjacent vertebral source remains an important cause in the underdeveloped world. As the population ages and the number of immunosuppressed individuals increases, an increase in the incidence of spinal epidural abscess (currently 2 per 1000 hospital admissions) has been noted.

MRI scans (Fig. 368-5) localize the abscess and exclude a primary intraparenchymal lesion, for example, transverse myelitis or hematomyelia. Lumbar puncture is often not required but may be indicated if encephalopathy or other clinical signs raise the question of associated meningitis, which is present in fewer than 25% of cases. In such situations, the level of the tap should be planned carefully to minimize the risk of inducing either meningitis by passage of the needle through infected tissue or herniation from decompression below an area of obstruction to the flow of cerebrospinal fluid (CSF). A high cervical tap is often the safest approach. CSF abnormalities in subdural abscess consist of pleocytosis with a preponderance of polymorphonuclear cells, an elevated protein level, and a reduced glucose level. Blood cultures are positive in <25% of cases.

℞ TREATMENT   Treatment is emergency decompressive laminectomy with debridement combined with long-term antibiotic treatment. Surgical evacuation prevents development of paralysis and may improve or reverse paralysis in evolution, but it is unlikely to improve deficits of more than several days duration. Antibiotics should be started empirically before surgery, modified on the basis of culture results, and usually continued for at least 4 weeks. If surgery is contraindicated or if there is a fixed paraplegia or quadriplegia that is unlikely to improve following surgery, long-term administration of systemic and oral antibiotics can be used; in such cases, coverage may be guided by results of positive blood cultures. However, paralysis may develop or progress during antibiotic therapy; thus, initial surgical management remains the treatment of choice.

FIGURE 368-5   MRI of a spinal epidural abscess due to tuberculosis. *A*. Sagittal T2-weighted free spin-echo MR sequence. A hypointense mass replaces the posterior elements of C3 and extends epidurally to compress the spinal cord (*arrows*). *B*. Sagittal T1-weighted image after contrast administration reveals a diffuse enhancement of the epidural process (*arrows*) with extension into the epidural space.

TRANSVERSE MYELITIS   Transverse myelitis is an acute or subacute, generally monophasic, inflammatory disorder of the spinal cord. The initial symptom is focal neck or back pain, followed by various combinations of paresthesias, sensory loss, motor weakness, and sphincter disturbance evolving within hours to several days. There may be mild sensory symptoms only, or a devastating functional transection of the cord. Partial forms may selectively involve posterior columns, anterior spinothalamic tracts, or one hemicord. Dysesthesias may begin in the feet and ascend either symmetrically or asymmetrically, earlier in one leg than in the other; these symptoms may initially raise a question of Guillain-Barré syndrome, but involvement of the trunk with a sharply demarcated spinal cord level indicates the myelopathic nature of the process. In severe cases, areflexia indicating spinal shock may be present, but hyperreflexia soon supervenes; persistent areflexic paralysis indicates necrosis over multiple segments of the spinal cord.

Up to 40% of cases are associated with an antecedent infection or recent vaccination. Many infectious agents have been implicated, including influenza, measles, varicella, rubeola, mumps, and Epstein-Barr virus and cytomegalovirus, as well as *Mycoplasma*. As in the related disorder acute disseminated encephalomyelitis (Chap. 371), transverse myelitis often begins as the patient appears to be recovering from the infection, and infectious agents have not been isolated from the nervous system of affected individuals. These features suggest that transverse myelitis results from an autoimmune response triggered by infection and not from direct infection of the spinal cord.

Multiple sclerosis (MS) (see below) may present initially as transverse myelitis. MS-associated transverse myelitis usually is not associated with an antecedent infection or vaccination. Devic's disease (Chap. 371) is a demyelinating disorder that presents as transverse myelitis associated with optic neuritis that is typically bilateral. Transverse myelitis, at times recurrent, has also been associated with systemic lupus erythematosus and other collagen-vascular diseases, Sjögren's syndrome, and Behçet's disease; sarcoidosis may produce a subacute transverse myelopathy with severe cord swelling.

MRI findings consist of variable swelling of the cord and diffuse or multifocal areas of abnormal bright signal on T2-weighted sequences, often extending over several cord segments. Contrast enhancement, indicating disruption in the blood-brain barrier associated with perivenous inflammation, is present in acute cases. MRI is also useful to exclude cord compression. A brain MRI should be obtained in all cases to assess the likelihood that the transverse myelitis represents an initial attack of MS. A normal scan indicates that the risk of evolution to MS is low—approximately 5% over 3 to 5 years; by contrast, the finding of multiple periventricular T2-bright lesions indicates a risk of 50% or greater over the same time period. CSF may be normal, but more often there is pleocytosis, with up to several hundred mononuclear cells per microliter; in severe or rapidly evolving cases, polymorphonuclear cells may be present. CSF protein levels are normal or at most mildly elevated; oligoclonal banding is a variable finding but, when present, is associated with future evolution to MS.

There are no prospective trials of therapy. Intravenous methylprednisolone (500 mg qd for 3 days) followed by oral prednisone (1 mg/kg per day for several weeks, then gradual taper) is used for treatment of moderate to severe symptoms.

ACUTE INFECTIOUS MYELOPATHIES   These inflammatory disorders result from direct invasion of the spinal cord by infectious agents. Bacterial etiologies are rare; almost any pathogenic species may be responsible and in one recent review *Listeria monocytogenes* was most frequently identified. Poliomyelitis is the prototypic virus that produces acute infection of the spinal cord. Herpes zoster is currently the most common viral cause of acute myelitis; cytomegalovirus, herpes simplex virus type 1, Epstein-Barr virus, and rabies virus have been identified in occasional cases. Herpes simplex virus 2 may produce a recurrent sacral myelitis, which could be mistaken for MS, in association with outbreaks of genital herpes. →*Viral infections of the spinal cord are discussed in Chap. 373.*

Schistosomiasis (Chap. 222) is an important cause of parasitic myelitis worldwide. The myelitis is intensely inflammatory and granulomatous in nature, caused by a local response to tissue-digesting enzymes produced by ova from the parasite. Toxoplasmosis (Chap. 217) can cause a focal myelopathy, and this diagnosis should be considered in patients with AIDS owing to the high frequency of nervous system toxoplasmosis in this population.

CHRONIC MYELOPATHIES

SPONDYLITIC MYELOPATHY Neck and shoulder pain with stiffness are early symptoms; pressure on nerve roots results in radicular arm pain, most often in a C5 or C6 distribution. Compression of the cervical cord produces a slowly progressive spastic paraparesis, at times asymmetric, and often accompanied by paresthesias in the feet and hands. Vibratory sense is frequently diminished in the legs, and occasionally there is a sensory level for vibration on the upper thorax. Coughing or straining often produces leg weakness or radiating arm or shoulder pain. Dermatomal sensory loss in the arms, atrophy of intrinsic hand muscles, increased deep tendon reflexes in the legs, and extensor plantar responses are common. Urinary urgency or incontinence occurs in advanced cases. Reflexes in the arms are often diminished at some level, often the biceps (C5-C6). In individual cases, radicular, myelopathic, or combined signs may predominate. The diagnosis should be considered in cases of progressive cervical myelopathy, paresthesias of the feet and hands, or wasting of the hands. Spondylitic myelopathy is also one of the most common causes of gait difficulty in the elderly.

Diagnosis is best made by MRI. Extrinsic compression is appreciated on axial views, and T2-weighted sequences may reveal abnormal areas of high signal intensity within the cord adjacent to the site of compression. Definitive therapy consists of surgical relief of the compression, generally by posterior laminectomy. When that is not feasible, an anterior approach with resection of the protruded disc material may be required.→*Cervical spondylosis and related degenerative diseases of the spine are discussed in Chap. 16.*

VASCULAR MALFORMATIONS Although uncommon, vascular malformations are important lesions because they represent a treatable cause of progressive myelopathy. Arteriovenous malformations (AVMs) are most often located posteriorly, within the dura or along the surface of the cord, at or below the midthoracic level. The typical presentation is a middle-aged man with a progressive myelopathy. The myelopathy may worsen slowly or rapidly or may have periods of apparent remission with superimposed worsenings resembling MS. Acute deterioration due to hemorrhage into the spinal cord or subarachnoid space may also occur. At presentation, most patients have sensory, motor, and bladder disturbances. The motor disorder may predominate and produce a mixture of upper and lower motoneuron signs, simulating ALS. Pain, either dysesthesias or radicular pain, is also common. Other symptoms suggestive of AVM include intermittent claudication (symptoms that appear with exercise and are relieved by rest), or an effect of posture, menses, or fever on symptoms. A rare AVM syndrome presents as a progressive thoracic myelopathy with paraparesis developing over weeks or several months, associated with abnormally thick, hyalinized vessels (Foix-Alajouanine syndrome).

AVMs located at cervical or upper thoracic levels are distinctive; they occur equally in males and females, tend to be located anterior rather than posterior to the cord, often have an intramedullary component to the malformation, and may bleed (see "Hematomyelia," above).

Examination of the skin overlying the spine may reveal a vascular lesion, lipoma, or area of altered pigmentation, all clues to a spinal cord AVM. Bruits are rare but should be sought at rest or after exercise. High-resolution MRI with contrast administration detects most AVMs (Fig. 368-6). A small number of AVMs not detected by MRI may be visualized by CT myelography as enlarged vessels along the surface of the cord. Definitive diagnosis requires selective spinal angiography, which will also define the vascular feeders and extent of the malfor-

FIGURE 368-6 Arteriovenous malformation. Sagittal MR scans of the thoracic spinal cord: T2 fast spin-echo technique (*left*) and T1 post-contrast image (*right*). On the T2-weighted image (*left*), abnormally high signal intensity is noted in the central aspect of the spinal cord (*arrowheads*). Numerous punctate flow voids indent the dorsal and ventral spinal cord (*arrow*). These represent the abnormally dilated venous plexus supplied by a dural arteriovenous fistula. After contrast administration (*right*), multiple, serpentine, enhancing veins (*arrows*) on the ventral and dorsal aspect of the thoracic spinal cord are visualized, diagnostic of arteriovenous fistula. This patient was a 54-year-old man with a 4-year history of progressive paraparesis.

mation. Embolization with occlusion of the major feeding vessels may stabilize a progressive neurologic deficit or produce a gradual recovery.

RETROVIRUS-ASSOCIATED MYELOPATHIES The myelopathy associated with the human T cell lymphotropic virus type I (HTLV-I) presents as a slowly progressive spastic paraparesis with variable sensory and bladder disturbance. The myelopathy is typically thoracic. Approximately half of patients have back or leg pain. Signs may be asymmetric, may lack a well-defined sensory level, and may spare upper extremity function, although hyperreflexia in the arms is common. Onset is generally insidious, and the tempo of progression is variable, but most patients are nonambulatory within 10 years of onset. This presentation may resemble primary progressive MS or a thoracic AVM. Diagnosis is made by demonstration of HTLV-I–specific antibody in serum by enzyme-linked immunosorbent assay (ELISA), confirmed by radioimmunoprecipitation or Western blot analysis of specific antibody directed against protein products of the viral *gag* and *env* genes. There is no effective treatment; symptomatic therapy for spasticity and bladder symptoms may be helpful. →*HTLV-I infections of the nervous system are discussed in Chap. 373.*

A progressive myelopathy may also occur in AIDS, characterized by vacuolar degeneration of the posterior and lateral tracts resembling subacute combined degeneration (see below).

SYRINGOMYELIA Syringomyelia is a cavitary expansion of the spinal cord that may produce a progressive myelopathy. Syrinxes commonly occur in the lower cervical/high thoracic region or in the high cervical region, where they may extend rostrally to the medulla or pons (syringobulbia); any region of the spinal cord may be involved. More than half of all cases are associated with Chiari malformations. In the Chiari type 1 malformation, the cerebellar tonsils protrude through the foramen magnum and into the cervical spinal canal; when this abnormality is associated with protrusion of meninges (meningocele) or meninges and cord (meningomyelocele) through a spinal canal that has incompletely closed, it is designated a Chiari type 2 (or Arnold-Chiari) malformation. Acquired cases are often associated with trauma, inflammatory spinal cord disorders such as transverse myelitis, chronic arachnoiditis due to tuberculosis or other etiologies, or spinal cord tumors. Occasional cases are idiopathic.

Syringomyelia has been proposed to result from interference with the normal outflow of CSF from the fourth ventricle to the subarachnoid space due to obstruction of the foramina of Luschka and Magendie. This blockage leads to downward pressure on the cervical spinal cord and progressive syrinx formation. However, syringomyelia may occur without foraminal obstruction, indicating that other factors, for example interference with normal upward CSF flow in the spinal canal, may also be important. Syrinxes associated with Chiari type 1 malformations generally communicate freely with the subarachnoid space, and the syrinx fluid resembles normal CSF; by contrast, in many acquired cases the syrinx cavities do not communicate, and the fluid is proteinaceous.

The classic presentation is a central cord syndrome with dissociated sensory loss and areflexic weakness in the upper limbs. The sensory deficit consists of loss of pain and temperature sensation which is "suspended" over the nape of the neck, shoulders, and upper arms in a cape distribution or is in the hands; vibration and position sensation is largely preserved. Most cases begin asymmetrically with unilateral sensory loss. Muscle wasting in the lower neck, shoulders, arms, and hands with asymmetric or absent reflexes reflects extension of the cavity to the anterior horns. As the lesion enlarges, spasticity and weakness of the legs, bladder and bowel dysfunction, and, in some cases, a Horner's syndrome appear. Thoracic kyphoscoliosis is a frequent additional finding. Some patients develop numbness and sensory loss on the face from damage to the descending tract of the trigeminal nerve (C2 level or above). With Chiari malformations, cough headache, and neck, arm, or facial pain are common. Syringobulbia may present as palatal or vocal cord paralysis, dysarthria, horizontal or vertical nystagmus, episodic dizziness, and/or tongue weakness.

Symptoms typically begin insidiously in adolescence or early adulthood, progress irregularly, and may undergo spontaneous arrest for several years. Onset or sudden deterioration may follow trauma, neck manipulation or extension, or severe cough. Symptoms of syringobulbia may progress rapidly.

MRI scans accurately identify syrinx cavities and associated spinal cord enlargement (Fig. 368-7). In all cases, MRI scans of the brain and the entire spinal cord should be obtained to delineate the full extent of the syrinx, assess posterior fossa structures, and determine whether hydrocephalus is present. If a Chiari malformation is not found, a contrast-enhanced MRI scan should be obtained to search for abnormal enhancement from an associated spinal cord tumor.

℞ TREATMENT   Treatment is surgical. Syringomyelia associated with tonsillar herniation is treated with posterior fossa decompression, generally consisting of suboccipital craniectomy, upper cervical laminectomy, and placement of a dural graft. If obstruction of fourth ventricular outflow is present, flow is reestablished by enlargement of the opening. If the syrinx cavity is large, some surgeons recommend direct decompression of the fluid cavity, but the added benefit of this procedure is uncertain, and morbidity may occur. With Chiari malformations, shunting of hydrocephalus should generally precede any attempt to correct the syrinx. Surgical results are often excellent, with stabilization of the neurologic deficit in most cases; some patients have improvement postoperatively. Syringomyelia secondary to trauma or infection is treated with a decompression and drainage procedure in which a small shunt is inserted between the syrinx cavity and the subarachnoid space. Finally, syringomyelia due to an intramedullary spinal cord tumor is managed by resection of the tumor if

FIGURE 368-7   MRI of a syringomyelia associated with a Chiari malformation. Sagittal T1-weighted image through the cervical and upper thoracic spine demonstrates descent of the cerebellar tonsils and vermis below the level of the foramen magnum (*black arrows*). Within the substance of the cervical and thoracic spinal cord, a CSF collection dilates the central canal (*white arrows*).

feasible; decompression of the cyst cavity may produce temporary relief, but recurrence is common.

MULTIPLE SCLEROSIS   Spinal cord involvement is common in MS. It may develop acutely as an exacerbation in a patient with known MS or appear as the presenting manifestation of the disease (see "Transverse Myelitis," above). Chronic progressive myelopathy is the most frequent cause of disability in both primary progressive and secondary progressive forms of MS. Involvement is typically asymmetric, producing motor, sensory, and bladder/bowel disturbances. Diagnosis is facilitated by identification of earlier attacks that may not be initially recalled by the patient; by MRI, CSF and evoked response testing; and by exclusion of other conditions. The diagnosis may be particularly difficult to establish in patients with primary progressive MS. Therapy with interferon β or glatiramer acetate is indicated for many patients with MS-related myelopathy that is not due to primary progressive MS. →*MS is discussed in Chap. 371.*

SUBACUTE COMBINED DEGENERATION (VITAMIN B$_{12}$ DEFICIENCY)   This treatable myelopathy presents with parasthesias in the hands and feet, early loss of vibration and position sensation, and a progressive spastic and ataxic weakness. Loss of reflexes due to a superimposed peripheral neuropathy, present in many patients, is an important diagnostic clue. Optic atrophy and irritability and other mental changes may be prominent in advanced cases and on occasion are the presenting symptoms (megaloblastic madness). The myelopathy of subacute combined degeneration tends to be diffuse rather than focal; signs are generally symmetric and reflect predominant involvement of the posterior and lateral tracts. The diagnosis is confirmed by the finding of a low serum B$_{12}$ concentration, elevated levels of homocysteine and methylmalonic acid in uncertain cases, and a positive Schilling test (Chap. 75).

TABES DORSALIS   Tabes dorsalis and meningovascular syphilis of the spinal cord are presently rare but must be considered in the differential diagnosis of spinal cord syndromes, in particular those that arise in individuals infected with HIV. The most common symptoms of tabes are characteristic fleeting and repetitive, lancinating pains, which occur mostly in the legs and less commonly in the back, thorax, abdomen, arms, and face. Ataxia of the legs and gait due to loss of position sense occurs in half of patients. Paresthesias, bladder disturbances, and acute abdominal pain with vomiting (visceral crisis) occur in 15 to 30% of patients. The cardinal signs of tabes are loss of reflexes in the legs, impaired position and vibratory sense, Romberg's sign, and bilateral Argyll Robertson pupils, which fail to constrict to light but react with accommodation.

FAMILIAL SPASTIC PARAPLEGIA
Occasional cases of progressive myelopathy occur on a familial basis. Most present with progressive spasticity and weakness in the legs. Sphincter disturbances and mild degrees of sensory loss may also be present. On examination, a sharply defined spinal cord level is not detected, in contrast to many focal spinal cord disorders. In some families, whose condition is referred to as "complicated" familial spastic paraplegia, additional neurologic signs, for example, nystagmus, ataxia, or optic atrophy, occur. Onset may be as early as the first year of life or as late as middle adulthood. The genetic basis of several forms of familial spastic paraplegia is now known (Table 368-3). No disease-modifying therapy exists.

ADRENOMYELONEUROPATHY
This X-linked disorder, a variant of adrenoleukodystrophy, most commonly presents as a progressive spastic paraparesis beginning in early adulthood; some patients also have a mild peripheral neuropathy. Affected males usually have a history of adrenal insufficiency beginning in childhood. Rare heterozygous females may also present with adult-onset myelopathy. Diagnosis is usually made by demonstration of elevated levels of very long chain fatty acids in plasma and in cultured fibroblasts. The responsible gene, located at Xq17-28, encodes a protein involved in peroxysomal transport. Steroid replacement is indicated if hypoadrenalism is present, and bone marrow transplantation has been attempted for this condition without clear evidence of efficacy.

OTHER CHRONIC MYELOPATHIES
Primary lateral sclerosis (Chap. 365) is characterized by progressive spasticity with weakness, often accompanied by dysarthria and dysphonia. Sensory function is spared. The disorder resembles ALS, but there is no evidence of a lower motor neuron disturbance. Toxic causes include (1) lathyrism due to ingestion of chick peas containing the excitotoxin β-N-oxalylaminoalanine (BOAA) and seen primarily in the undeveloped world, and (2) nitrous oxide inhalation producing a myelopathy identical to subacute combined degeneration. Systemic lupus erythematosus (Chap. 311) and Sjögren's syndrome (Chap. 314) have both been associated with progressive myelopathy. Cancer-related causes include chronic paraneoplastic myelopathy (Chap. 101) or radiation injury (Chap. 370). Finally, in some patients the etiology of a chronic myelopathy may not be determined initially. A cause can ultimately be identified in most idiopathic cases and thus periodic reassessment is essential.

→ *Traumatic spinal cord lesions are discussed in Chap. 369.*

MEDICAL REHABILITATION OF SPINAL CORD DISORDERS

The prospects for significant recovery from an acute spinal cord lesion fade after approximately 4 months. There are currently no effective means to promote repair of injured spinal cord tissue; promising experimental approaches include the use of factors that influence reinnervation by axons of the corticospinal tract or nerve graft bridges that promote reinnervation across spinal cord lesions. The disability associated with irreversible spinal cord damage is determined primarily by the level of the lesion and by whether the disturbance in function is complete or incomplete (Table 368-4). Even a complete high cervical cord lesion may be compatible with a productive life. Development of a rehabilitation plan framed by realistic expectations, and attention to the neurologic, medical, and psychological complications that commonly arise, are primary goals of treatment.

The usual symptoms associated with medical illnesses may be lacking, because of the destruction of afferent pain pathways in the cord. Unexplained fever, worsening of spasticity, or deterioration in neurologic function should prompt search for an underlying cause such as infection, thrombophlebitis, or an intraabdominal pathology; these etiologies are far more likely to be responsible than primary neurologic events such as meningitis, secondary syringomyelia, or chronic arachnoiditis. The loss of normal thermoregulation and inability to maintain normal body temperature can produce recurrent fever (*quadriplegic fever*), although most episodes of fever are due to infection of the urinary tract, lung, skin, or bone.

Bladder dysfunction generally results from loss of supraspinal innervation of the detrusor muscle of the bladder wall and the sphincter musculature. Detrusor spasticity is treated with anticholinergic drugs (oxybutinin, 2.5 to 5 mg qid) or tricyclic antidepressants with anticholinergic properties (imipramine, 25 to 200 mg/d). Failure of the sphincter muscle to relax during bladder emptying (urinary dyssynergia) may be managed with the α-adrenergic blocking agent terazosin

Table 368-3 Inherited (Monogenic) Myelopathies[a]

Designation	Clinical Presentation	Genetics
Autosomal recessive	Early onset (age 1–20), progressive spasticity of legs, mild loss of vibration and position sense, bladder symptoms	Linkage to chromosome 16q; encodes paraplegin, a mitochondrial ATPase involved in diverse cellular functions. Additional loci exist at 8q and 15q.
Autosomal dominant	Most common form; families have either early or late onset (before or after age 35)	Linkage to chromosome 2p for both early and late onset; encodes spastin, an ATPase that may be involved in function of nuclear protein complexes. Other loci exist at 14q, 15q, and 8q.
X-linked	Early childhood onset as pure spastic paraplegia or "complicated" with nystagmus, ataxia, or other neurologic signs	"Complicated" form due to mutation of proteolipid protein gene; differs from the dysmyelinating disorder Pelizaeus-Merzbacher disease in that the allelic protein DM20, essential for oligodendrocyte development, is normal
X-linked	Pure or "complicated"	Mutations in neural cell adhesion molecule L1CAM. Allelic disorders X-linked hydrocephalus and MASA syndrome (mental retardation, aphasia, shuffling gait, adducted thumbs).

[a] See also Chap. 359.

Table 368-4 Expected Neurologic Function Following Complete Cord Lesions

Level	Self-Care	Transfers	Maximum Mobility
High quadriplegia (C1-C4)	Dependent on others; requires respiratory support	Dependent on others	Motorized wheelchair
Low quadriplegia (C5-C8)	Partially independent with adaptive equipment	May be dependent or independent	May use manual wheelchair, drive an automobile with adaptive equipment
Paraplegia (below T1)	Independent	Independent	Ambulates short distances with aids

SOURCE: Adapted from Ditunno and Formal.

hydrochloride (1 to 2 mg tid or qid), with intermittent catheterization, or, if that is not feasible, by use of a condom catheter in men or a permanent indwelling catheter. Surgical options include the creation of an artificial bladder by isolating a segment of intestine that can be catheterized intermittently (enterocystoplasty) or can drain continuously to an external appliance (urinary conduit). Bladder areflexia due to acute spinal shock or conus lesions is best treated by catheterization.

Bladder dysfunction predisposes the patient to urinary tract infection. Bacteriuria due to asymptomatic colonization is extremely common and is generally not treated. Prophylaxis with antiseptics or antibiotics is of little value. Urinary tract infections may present only as foul-smelling urine or a change in voiding pattern; the development of high fever or other systemic signs often indicates pyelonephritis. Bowel regimens and disimpaction are necessary in most patients to ensure at least biweekly evacuation and avoid colonic distention or obstruction.

High cervical cord lesions cause various degrees of mechanical respiratory failure requiring artificial ventilation. In cases of incomplete respiratory failure, chest physical therapy is useful, and a negative-pressure cuirass may alleviate atelectasis, particularly if the major lesion is below C4. With severe respiratory failure, tracheal intubation, followed by tracheotomy, provides tracheal access for ventilation and suctioning. Phrenic nerve pacing may be useful in some patients with lesions at C5 or above.

Patients with acute cord injury are at high risk for venous thrombosis and pulmonary embolism. During the first two weeks, use of calf-compression devices and anticoagulation with heparin (5000 U subcutaneously every 12 h) or warfarin (INR, 2 to 3) are recommended. In cases of persistent paralysis, anticoagulation should probably be continued for 3 months.

Prophylaxis against decubitus ulcers should involve frequent changes in position in a chair or bed, the use of special mattresses, and cushioning of areas where pressure sores often develop, such as the sacral prominence and heels. Early treatment of ulcers with careful cleansing, surgical or enzyme debridement of necrotic tissue, and appropriate dressing and drainage may prevent infection of adjacent soft tissue or bone.

Spasticity (Chap. 22) is often a late manifestation of spinal cord disease, occurring weeks or even months after the initial insult. Stretching exercises are useful to maintain mobility of joints. Drug treatment is effective but may result in reduced function, as some patients use their spasticity as an aid to stand, transfer, or walk. Baclofen (15 to 240 mg/d in divided doses) is the most effective drug available; it acts by facilitating GABA-mediated inhibition of motor reflex arcs. Diazepam acts by a similar mechanism and is useful for leg spasms that interrupt sleep (2 to 4 mg at bedtime). For nonambulatory patients, the direct muscle inhibitor dantrolene (25 to 100 mg qid) may be used, but it is potentially hepatotoxic. In severe cases, intrathecal baclofen administered via an implanted pump, botulinum toxin injections, or dorsal rhizotomy may be required to control spasticity.

Paroxysmal autonomic hyperreflexia may occur following lesions above the major splanchnic sympathetic outflow at T6. Headache, flushing, and diaphoresis above the level of the lesion, and hypertension with bradycardia or tachycardia, are the major symptoms. The trigger is typically a noxious stimulus—for example, bladder or bowel distention, a urinary tract infection, or a decubitus ulcer—below the level of the cord lesion. Ascending sensory fibers are thought to activate, via interneurons, sympathetic neurons of the intermediolateral nuclei in the thoracic spinal cord, producing vasoconstriction, tachycardia, and systemic hypertension. Reflex pathways, activated by carotid and aortic baroreceptors and projecting to the central nervous system via the vagus and glossopharyngeal nerves, then inhibit sympathetic activity above the cord lesion, producing vasodilation, but below the lesion descending pathways are blocked and sympathetic hyperactivity continues. Treatment consists of removal of offending

stimuli; ganglionic blocking agents (mecamylamine, 2.5 to 5 mg) or other short-acting antihypertensive drugs are useful in some patients (see review by Colachis).

BIBLIOGRAPHY

BLAIVAS JG: Bladder function in the SCI patient. J Neurol Rehab 8:47, 1994

CHAN CT, GOLD WL: Intramedullary abcess of the spinal cord in the antibiotic era: Clinical features, microbial etiologies, trends in pathogenesis, and outcomes. Clin Infect Dis 27:619, 1998

COLACHIS SC: Autonomic hyperreflexia with spinal cord injury. J Am Paraplegia Soc 15(3):172, 1992

CRISTANTE L, HERRMANN H-D: Surgical management of intramedullary spinal cord tumors: Functional outcome and sources of morbidity. Neurosurgery 35:69, 1994

DAROUICHE RO et al: Bacterial spinal epidural abscess: Review of 43 cases and literature survey. Medicine 71:369, 1992

DITUNNO JF, FORMAL CS: Chronic spinal cord injury. N Engl J Med 330:550, 1994

HAZAN J et al: Spastin, a new AAA protein, is altered in the most frequent form of autosomal dominant spastic paraplegia. Nat Genet 23:296, 1999

KATZ JD, ROPPER AH: Progressive necrotic myelopathy: Clinical course in 9 patients. Arch Neurol 57:355, 2000

MILHORAT TH et al: Chiari1 malformation redefined: Clinical and radiologic findings for 364 symptomatic patients. Neurosurgery 44:1005, 1999

SCOTT TF et al: Transverse myelitis: Comparison with spinal cord presentations of multiple sclerosis. Neurology 50:429, 1998

SMALL JA, SHERIDAN PH: Research priorities for syringomyelia: A National Institute of Neurologic Disorders and Stroke workshop summary. Neurology 46:577, 1996

SMYTH MD, PEACOCK WH: The surgical treatment of spasticity. Muscle Nerve 23:153, 2000

369　　*Allan H. Ropper*

TRAUMATIC INJURIES OF THE HEAD AND SPINE

Head injuries are frequent in industrialized countries and affect many individuals in the prime of life. Almost 10 million head injuries occur annually in the United States alone, about 20% of which are serious enough to cause brain damage. Among men under 35 years, accidents, usually motor vehicle collisions, are the chief cause of death, and >70% of these involve head injury. Minor head injuries are so common that almost all physicians encounter patients requiring immediate care or suffering from various sequelae. Traumatic spinal cord injuries often occur in conjunction with head injury. The two are best considered together in the context of trauma to the nervous system.

A recent decline in mortality from head and spinal cord injuries can be attributed mainly to the use of seat belts and motorcycle helmets and the development of ambulance systems with trained personnel. In addition, a systematic approach to the evaluation of patients with head and spine trauma, beginning at the scene of the accident, has contributed to the improvement in outcome. Also, the wide availability of computed tomography (CT) and magnetic resonance imaging (MRI) has contributed to advances in diagnosis and intensive care treatment and an understanding of the pathologic lesions that are produced by trauma.

TYPES OF HEAD INJURIES

SKULL FRACTURES A blow to the skull causes a fracture if the elastic tolerance of the bone is exceeded. Intracranial lesions accompany two-thirds of skull fractures, and the presence of a skull fracture increases manyfold the chances of an underlying subdural or epidural hematoma. Consequently, fractures are important primarily as markers of the site and severity of injury. They are also the cause of cranial nerve injuries and the source of entry pathways to the cerebrospinal fluid (CSF) for bacteria (meningitis), air (pneumocephalus), and leakage of CSF.

Fractures are classified as *linear, basilar, compound,* or *depressed.*

Linear fractures, which are most often associated with subdural or epidural hematomas, account for 80% of all skull fractures. They are usually oriented from the point of impact toward the base of the skull. Basilar skull fractures are often extensions of adjacent fractures over the convexity of the skull but may occur independently owing to stresses on the floor of the middle cranial fossa or occiput. They are usually located parallel to the petrous bone or along the sphenoid bone toward the sella turcica and ethmoidal groove. Although most are uncomplicated, basilar skull fractures can cause CSF leakage, pneumocephalus, and cavernous-carotid fistulas. Hemotympanum (blood behind the tympanic membrane), delayed ecchymosis over the mastoid process (Battle's sign), or periorbital ecchymosis ("racoon sign") all signify fracture of the basilar skull. Because routine x-ray examination may fail to disclose basilar fractures, they should be suspected if these clinical signs are present. CSF may leak through the cribriform plate or the adjacent sinus and manifest as a watery discharge from the nose (CSF rhinorrhea). Persistent rhinorrhea and recurrent meningitis are indications for surgical repair of torn dura underlying the fracture. The precise site of the leak is often difficult to determine, but useful diagnostic tests include the instillation of water-soluble contrast into the CSF followed by CT with the patient in various positions, and injection of radionuclide compounds or fluorescein into the CSF with an assessment of uptake of these compounds by absorptive nasal pledgets. The site of an intermittent leak is rarely delineated, and most resolve spontaneously. Sellar fractures, even ones associated with serious neuroendocrine dysfunction, are sometimes radiologically occult. Fractures of the dorsum sella may cause sixth or seventh nerve palsies or optic nerve damage. An air-fluid level in the sphenoid sinus suggests a fracture of the sellar floor.

Petrous bone fractures, especially those oriented along the long axis of the bone, may be associated with facial palsy, disruption of ear ossicles, and CSF otorrhea. Transverse petrous fractures are less common; they almost always damage the cochlea or labyrinths and often the facial nerve. External bleeding from the ear is usually from local abrasion of the external canal but can also result from petrous fracture.

Fractures of the frontal bone are often depressed, involving the frontal and paranasal sinuses and the orbits; permanent anosmia results if the olfactory filaments in the cribriform plate are disrupted. Depressed skull fractures are typically compound, but they are often neurologically asymptomatic because the impact energy is dissipated in breaking the bone; however, some are associated with brain contusions and focal neurologic signs caused by damage to the underlying cortical area. Prompt debridement and exploration of compound fractures are required in order to avoid infection.

CRANIAL NERVE INJURIES The cranial nerves likely to be injured with head trauma include the olfactory, optic, oculomotor, and trochlear nerves; the first and second branches of the trigeminal nerve; and the facial and auditory nerves. Anosmia and an apparent loss of taste (actually a loss of perception of aromatic flavors, with elementary tastes retained) occur in ~10% of persons with serious head injuries, particularly with falls on the back of the head. This sequela results from displacement of the brain and shearing of the olfactory nerve filaments and may occur in the absence of a fracture. Recovery is the rule, leaving residual hyposmia, but if bilateral anosmia persists for several months, the prognosis is poor. Fractures of the sphenoid bone may rarely bruise or transect the optic nerve, resulting in unilateral partial or complete blindness and an unreactive pupil, usually equal in size to that of the other side and with a preserved consensual light response. Partial optic nerve injuries from closed trauma result in blurring of vision, central or paracentral scotomas, or sector defects. Direct orbital injury may cause short-lived blurred vision for close objects and pupillary paralysis because of reversible iridoplegia. Diplopia limited to downward gaze, which suggests trochlear nerve damage, occurs as an isolated problem after minor injury and can develop after a delay of several days; it may also result from fracture of the lesser wing of the sphenoid bone. The diplopia is corrected if the head is tilted away from the affected eye. Direct facial nerve injury by a basal fracture is present immediately in 3% of severe

injuries; it may also be delayed 5 to 7 days. Fractures through the petrous bone, particularly the less common transverse type, are liable to produce this injury. Delayed facial palsy, the mechanism of which is unknown, has a good prognosis. Injury to the eighth cranial nerve from a fracture of the petrous bone causes loss of hearing, vertigo, and nystagmus immediately after injury. Deafness from nerve injury must be distinguished from that due to rupture of the eardrum, blood in the middle ear, or disruption of the ossicles from fracture through the middle ear. A high-tone hearing loss occurs with direct cochlear concussion.

SEIZURES *Convulsions* are surprisingly uncommon immediately after a head injury, but a brief period of tonic extensor posturing or a few clonic movements of the limbs just after the moment of impact may occur. However, the superficial cortical scars that evolve from contusions are highly epileptogenic and may later manifest as seizures, even after many years (Chap. 360). The severity of injury determines the risk of future seizures. It has been estimated that 17% of individuals with brain contusion, subdural hematoma, or prolonged loss of consciousness will develop a seizure disorder and that this risk extends for an indefinite period of time, whereas the risk is only 2% after mild injury; the majority of convulsions in the latter group occur within 5 years of injury.

CONCUSSION *Concussion* refers to an immediate but transient loss of consciousness that is associated with a short period of amnesia and described as the experience or appearance of being dazed or "star struck." It typically occurs after a blunt impact that creates a sudden deceleration of the cranium and a movement of the brain within the skull. Severe concussion may precipitate a brief convulsion or autonomic signs such as facial pallor, bradycardia, faintness with mild hypotension, or sluggish pupillary reaction, but most patients are neurologically normal. Higher primates are particularly susceptible to concussion; in contrast, billy goats, rams, and woodpeckers can tolerate impact velocity and deceleration 100-fold greater than that experienced by humans. The mechanism of loss of consciousness in concussion is believed to be a transient electrophysiologic dysfunction of the reticular activating system in the upper midbrain caused by rotation of the cerebral hemispheres on the relatively fixed brainstem (Chap. 24).

Gross and light-microscopic changes in the brain are usually absent following concussion, but biochemical and ultrastructural changes, such as mitochondrial ATP depletion and local disruption of the blood-brain barrier, suggest that complex abnormalities occur. CT and MRI scans are usually normal; however, approximately 3% of patients will be found to have an intracranial hemorrhage of some type.

The amnesia of concussion typically follows at least a few moments of unresponsiveness, but rarely there is no loss of consciousness. The memory loss spans the time of, and moments before, mild impact injuries but may encompass previous weeks (rarely months) in cases of more severe trauma. The extent of retrograde amnesia has been suggested as a rough measure of the severity of injury. Any anterograde amnesia is usually brief and disappears rapidly in alert patients. Memory is regained in an orderly way from the most distant to recent memories, with islands of amnesia occasionally remaining in severe cases. The mechanism of peritraumatic amnesia is not known. Hysterical posttraumatic amnesia is not uncommon and should be suspected when inexplicable abnormalities of behavior occur, such as recounting events that cannot be recalled on later testing, a bizarre affect that emulates the lay notion of amnesia or psychosis (Ganser syndrome), forgetting one's own name, or a persistent anterograde deficit that is excessive in comparison with the degree of injury.

A single, uncomplicated head injury only infrequently produces permanent neurobehavioral changes in patients who are free of preexisting psychiatric problems and substance abuse. However, there has been increasing attention to minor problems in memory and concentration that may have an anatomic correlate in small shearing or other microscopic lesions (see below).

FIGURE 369-1 *A.* Traumatic cerebral contusion. Noncontrast CT scan demonstrating a hyperdense hemorrhagic region in the anterior temporal lobe. *B.* Cerebral contusions adjacent to the bony prominences of the skull. Hemorrhagic areas are seen in the basal frontal and temporal regions where the brain is impelled against the sphenoid and petrous bones.

CONTUSION, BRAIN HEMORRHAGE, AND SHEARING LESIONS A surface bruise of the brain, or *contusion*, consists of varying degrees of petechial hemorrhage, edema, and tissue destruction. Contusions and deeper hemorrhages result from mechanical forces that displace the hemispheres forcefully relative to the skull by deceleration of the brain against the inner skull, either under a point of impact (coup lesion) or, as the brain swings back, in the antipolar area (contrecoup lesion). Trauma sufficient to cause prolonged unconsciousness usually produces some degree of contusion. Because the motion of the hemispheres brings them into contact with the prominences of the sphenoid and other frontal basal bones, blunt impact, as from an automobile dashboard or from falling forward while drunk, typically causes contusions on the orbital surfaces of the frontal lobes and the anterior and basal portions of the temporal lobes. With lateral forces, as from the doorframe of a car, the contusions are situated on the lateral convexity of the hemispheres. In both instances there may be obverse contrecoup contusions.

Contusions are visible on CT and MRI scans, appearing early as inhomogeneous hyperdensities on CT and as hyperintensities on MRI; the signal changes reflect small scattered areas of cortical and subcortical blood and localized brain edema (Fig. 369-1); there is also some degree of subarachnoid bleeding, which may be detected by scans or lumbar puncture. Confluent, roughly spherical contusions can be distinguished from cerebral hemorrhages by their involvement of the cortical surface. Contusions may acquire a surrounding ringlike contrast enhancement after a week that may be mistaken for tumor or abscess. Glial and macrophage reactions begin within 2 days and result years later in scarred, hemosiderin-stained depressions on the surface (*plaques jaunes*) that are one source of posttraumatic epilepsy.

The clinical signs produced by contusions vary with their location and size; a hemiparesis or gaze preference, similar to the signs of a middle cerebral artery stroke, is fairly typical. Large bilateral contusions produce coma with extensor posturing. Contusions limited to the frontal lobes produce an abulic-taciturn state and those in the temporal lobe may cause an aggressive, combative, or delirous syndrome, described below. The secondary effects of progressive edema are the most threatening aspect of contusion injury and lead to coma and signs of secondary brainstem compression (pupillary enlargement).

Deep hemorrhages in the central white matter may result from confluent contusions in the depths of a sulcus. However, ganglionic, diencephalic, and other deep hematomas due to torsion or shearing forces in the brain occur independently of surface damage. Large single hemorrhages after minor trauma may bring to attention a bleeding diathesis or cerebrovascular amyloidosis in the elderly. For unexplained reasons, deep cerebral hemorrhages may not develop until several days after severe injury. Sudden neurologic deterioration in a comatose patient or an unexplained rise in intracranial pressure (ICP) should therefore prompt investigation with a CT scan.

Another type of deep white matter lesion consists of widespread acute disruption, or "shearing," of axons at the time of impact. Characteristically there are small areas of tissue disruption in the corpus callosum and dorsolateral pons, but these areas may not be appreciated in scans. The presence of widespread axonal damage of both hemispheres, a state called *diffuse axonal injury*, has been proposed as the explanation of persistent coma or vegetative state, but small ischemic-hemorrhagic lesions in the midbrain and low diencephalon are as often the cause. Only severe shearing lesions that contain blood are visualized by CT, usually in the corpus callosum and centrum semiovale (Fig. 369-2); however, within days of the injury, MRI scan demonstrates such lesions throughout the white matter, especially with the use of gradient echo MRI sequences.

On occasion, especially in children, cranial trauma causes diffuse brain swelling within a few hours after injury, even though CT may not reveal focal contusions or hemorrhages. The swelling creates a mass effect with disastrous consequences. Swelling is likely due to microvascular disruption and greatly increased cerebral blood flow. Episodes of moderate hypotension after the injury may play a role in this complication.

Residual symptoms and signs of primary or secondary compressive brainstem hemorrhages or ischemic lesions include cerebellar tremor, pupillary enlargement, eye movement abnormalities, and the "locked-in" syndrome (Chap. 24).

SUBDURAL AND EPIDURAL HEMATOMAS Hemorrhages beneath the dura (subdural) or between the dura and skull (epidural) may be associated with contusions and other injuries, making it difficult to determine their relative contribution to the clinical state. However, subdural and epidural hematomas more often occur as the sole manifestation of injury, and each has characteristic clinical and radiologic features. Because the mass effect and the rise in ICP caused by these hemorrhages may be life threatening, it is imperative that they be identified immediately by CT or MRI scan and evacuated when appropriate.

Acute Subdural Hematoma These lesions become symptomatic minutes or hours after injury. Up to one-third of patients have a lucid interval before coma supervenes, but most are drowsy or comatose from the moment of injury. Direct cranial trauma is not required for acute subdural hemorrhage to occur; acceleration forces alone, as from whiplash, are adequate, especially in the elderly and those taking anticoagulant medications. A unilateral headache and slightly enlarged pupil on the same side are frequently but not invar-

FIGURE 369-2 Multiple small areas of hemorrhage and tissue disruption in the white matter of the frontal lobes on noncontrast CT scan. These appear to reflect an extreme type of the "diffuse axonal shearing" lesions that occur with closed head injury.

FIGURE 369-3 Acute subdural hematoma in a noncontrast CT scan. The hyperdense clot has an irregular border with the brain and typically causes more horizontal displacement (mass effect) than might be expected from its thickness. The disproportionate mass effect is the result of the large rostral-caudal extent of these hematomas. Compare to Fig. 369-4.

iably found. Stupor or coma, a hemiparesis, and unilateral pupillary enlargement are the typical signs of larger hematomas; pupillary dilation is contralateral to the hematoma in 5 to 10%. In an acutely deteriorating patient with diminished alertness and with pupillary enlargement, burr (drainage) holes or an emergency craniotomy are appropriate, at times even without prior radiographic confirmation of subdural hematoma. Small subdural hematomas may be asymptomatic and usually do not require therapy. A more subacute syndrome from subdural hematoma occurs days to weeks after injury with drowsiness, headache, confusion, or mild hemiparesis; it is seen in alcoholics and in the elderly. Chronic subdural hematoma is described below.

Most subdural hematomas appear as crescentic collections over the convexity of the hemisphere and are located over the frontotemporal region, less often in the inferior middle fossa or over the occipital poles (Fig. 369-3). The degree of midline shift is disproportionately greater than the apparent size of the clot in any one axial CT scan, but the guidelines relating shift to the level of consciousness outlined in Chap. 24 remain useful. Less common instances of interhemispheric, posterior fossa, or bilateral convexity clots are difficult to diagnose clinically, although drowsiness and the signs expected for each region can be detected (Chap 25). Larger clots are thought to be primarily venous in origin, though additional arterial bleeding sites are often found; some large clots, when explored surgically, appear to be exclusively arterial.

Acute Epidural Hematoma Epidural hematomas evolve more rapidly than subdural hematomas and are therefore more treacherous. They occur in up to 10% of severe trauma cases and are less often associated with underlying cortical damage than are subdural hematomas. Most patients are unconscious when first seen. A "lucid interval" of several minutes to hours before coma supervenes is said to be most characteristic of epidural hemorrhage, although it is not common, and epidural hemorrhage by no means is the only cause of this temporal profile.

An epidural hematoma located over the convexity of either lateral temporal lobe is explained by its origin from a torn dural vessel, most commonly the middle meningeal artery, which is transected by a fracture of the squamous portion of the temporal bone. Frontal, inferior temporal, or occipitoparietal epidural hematomas are less frequent, occurring when fractures disrupt branches of the middle meningeal

artery. The hematoma strips the tightly attached dura from the inner table of the skull, producing a characteristic lenticular shaped clot on CT (Fig. 369-4). Epidural hematomas may be less frequent in the elderly because of the tighter attachment of dura to skull that occurs with aging. Posterior fossa epidural hematomas are rare and difficult to detect clinically; most result from surgery in that region, such as resection of an acoustic schwannoma.

Chronic Subdural Hematoma A history of trauma may or may not be elicited; 20 to 30% of patients recall no head injury, particularly the elderly and those with a bleeding diathesis. The causative injury may be trivial (striking the head against the branch of a tree, a sudden stop in a car, or minor head contact during a fall or faint) and is often

FIGURE 369-4 Acute epidural hematoma. The typical lenticular shape is due to the dura, which is tightly adherent to the skull. Epidural hematomas are usually caused by disruption of the middle meningeal artery following fracture of the temporal bone.

forgotten because it was remote. Headaches (common but not invariable), slowed thinking, change in personality, a seizure, or a mild hemiparesis emerges weeks or months afterwards. The headache may fluctuate in severity, sometimes with positional changes. Many chronic subdural hematomas are bilateral and produce perplexing clinical syndromes. The initial clinical impression is of a stroke, brain tumor, drug intoxication, depression, or a dementing illness because drowsiness, inattentiveness, and incoherence of thought are more prominent than focal signs such as hemiparesis. Patients with undetected small bilateral subdural hematomas seem to have a low tolerance for surgery, anesthesia, and drugs that depress the nervous system, remaining drowsy or confused for long periods postoperatively. Occasionally a chronic hematoma causes brief episodes of hemiparesis or aphasia that are indistinguishable from transient ischemic attacks.

Skull x-rays are usually normal except for a shift of the calcified pineal body to one side or an occasional unexpected fracture. In very long-standing cases the irregular calcification of membranes that surround the collection may be appreciated. CT performed without contrast infusion shows a low-density mass over the convexity of the hemisphere (Fig. 369-5), but between 2 to 6 weeks after the initial bleeding the clot appears isodense compared to adjacent brain. Bilateral chronic hematomas may fail to be detected because of the absence of lateral tissue shifts; this circumstance is suggested by a "hypernormal" CT scan with fullness of the cortical sulci and small ventricles in an older patient. CT with contrast demonstrates the vascular fibrous capsule surrounding the clot; MRI can reliably identify either a subacute or chronic clot. Lumbar puncture is not recommended for diagnosis because of the risk of worsening tissue shifts but, if performed, shows xanthochromia of the spinal fluid and a variable number of red blood cells. Chronic subdural hematomas can expand gradually and clinically resemble tumors of the brain.

Clinical observation and serial imaging are reasonable in patients with few symptoms and small subdural collections. Treatment with glucocorticoids alone is sufficient in some cases, but surgical evacuation is more often successful. The fibrous membranes that grow from the dura and encapsulate the region require surgical resection to prevent recurrent fluid accumulation. Small hematomas are largely resorbed, leaving only the organizing membranes, which become calcified after many years.

PENETRATING INJURIES, COMPRESSIONS, AND LACERATIONS Tangential scalp wounds from bullets are capable of producing neurologic signs or delayed seizures because small hemorrhages or contusions arise even in the absence of missile penetration. Bullets entering the brain cause considerable damage because of their tremendous kinetic energy. A cylindrical area of necrosis surrounds the bullet track, but the nature of injury differs for different projectiles. Soft civilian bullets typically shatter on impact and leave a track of metallic fragments with moderate parenchymal damage, whereas military bullets, because of their high velocity and energy, disrupt tissue at great distances from the track and produce massive brain destruction. All of these penetrating injuries cause a rapid increase in ICP for several minutes, followed by a drop depending on the volume of secondary hemorrhage and the degree of developing edema. Infection is a risk mainly from shell fragments, shrapnel, grenades, and mines, because such small projectiles carry surface bacteria and dirt into the brain. Most neurosurgeons administer systemic antibiotics prophylactically and perform local debridement for all types of penetrating injuries. Aneurysms may form as a result of disruption of vessel walls from the shock wave of the passing projectile; facial-orbital entrance wounds have the highest incidence of this complication. The aneurysms have an unpredictable course, but most that rupture do so in the first month. The prognosis for survival after missile injuries is good if consciousness is preserved and poor if coma is present from the outset.

In civilian practice, intracranial foreign bodies such as knives, picks, studgun staples, or high-speed tool bits may be missed unless skull x-rays are taken after what are seemingly minor penetrating injuries. Surgical removal of the object, debridement, and extensive exploration for hemorrhage and necrotic tissue are required.

TRAUMATIC VASCULAR DISSECTION AND OCCLUSION The kinetic energy of minor or more severe head or neck trauma can produce dissection of the internal carotid or vertebral arteries by stripping the intima or the media. Chiropractic neck manipulation accounts for some cases. Severe blunt impacts to the neck can initiate a dissection several centimeters above the origins of the internal carotid or vertebral arteries. There is usually local neck pain over the affected carotid artery, a Horner's syndrome, and headache over the ipsilateral anterior cranium. Some patients with carotid dissection subsequently have large middle cerebral artery strokes with hemiplegia after a period of fluctuating hemiparesis. In drowsy or comatose patients, evidence of dissection or subsequent stroke is difficult to determine, but its presence is suggested by unexplained hemiplegia, unilateral miosis, or appearance of cerebral infarction on CT scan.

Traumatic vertebral artery dissection causes vertigo, vomiting, suboccipital or supraorbital headache, and other signs of lateral medullary or cerebellar ischemia. These symptoms may be attributed erroneously to vestibular concussion. In comatose patients, the only indication may be inferior cerebellar infarction on imaging studies. Vasospasm from traumatic subarachnoid blood may also be involved in the development of infarction after head injury.

Cavernous sinus arteriovenous fistulas are rare but serious complications in patients who survive severe head injury. The problem is first evident as a self-audible bruit (many are also audible to the examiner), proptosis, conjunctival injection, or visual impairment. Angiography shows early filling of the cavernous sinus and its draining tributaries. The fistula enlarges, causing increasingly severe local changes around the eye and orbit and decreased chances of visual recovery. About 10%, mostly small fistulas, resolve spontaneously. Many surgical approaches have been tried, including ligation of the carotid artery and direct obliteration of the fistula or cavernous sinus, but a detachable balloon that is delivered by an intravascular catheter has proved most successful.

FIGURE 369-5 CT scan of chronic bilateral subdural hematomas of different ages. The collections began as acute hematomas and have become hypodense (called *hygromas*) in comparison to the adjacent brain after a period during which they were isodense and difficult to appreciate. Some areas of resolving blood are contained on the more recently formed collection on the left.

Raised ICP arising from contusion, hematoma, and subsequent progressive edema accounts for at least 50% of deaths after head injury; outcome is inversely related to the level of ICP. Aggressive treatment of raised ICP in modern intensive care units is believed to contribute to improved survival after severe head injury, but many other factors pertain, and the role of direct monitoring of ICP to guide therapy, while favored in many centers, is still uncertain.

For several minutes to an hour after acute head injury, cerebral blood flow increases in most patients, although metabolic demands and oxygen consumption of the cerebrum are diminished. Autoregulation—the ability of the cerebral vasculature to maintain a constant blood flow in response to decreased or increased perfusion pressure—is impaired globally and even more so in damaged regions. The rise in cerebral blood volume caused by the failure of autoregulation is thought to account for approximately two-thirds of the rise in ICP after severe head injury. The blood-brain barrier also becomes more permeable in contused regions, promoting edema formation. Resting ICP is spontaneously interrupted by rises in ICP, termed *plateau waves*, which arise as a result of a loss of cerebrovascular tone and a resultant increase in cerebral blood volume. Plateau waves may be precipitated by iatrogenic maneuvers such as suctioning, physical therapy, excess fluid administration, or pain but also by mild, often unnoticed hypotension that causes cerebrovascular dilation. Signs of clinical deterioration, such as pupillary enlargement, may occur after plateau waves; occasionally, brain death ensues. Other secondary systemic phenomena after severe head injury, particularly hypotension and hypoxia, cause brain damage and greatly alter outcome. →*The regulation of ICP and its relationship to cerebral blood flow (CBF) are discussed in Chap. 376.*

CLINICAL SYNDROMES AND TREATMENT OF HEAD INJURY

MINOR INJURY The patient who is fully alert and attentive after head injury but who has one or more symptoms of headache, faintness, nausea, a single episode of emesis, difficulty with concentration, or slight blurring of vision has a good prognosis with little risk of subsequent deterioration. Such patients have usually sustained a concussion and are expected to have a brief amnestic epoch. Children and young adults are particularly prone to drowsiness, vomiting, and irritability, which is sometimes delayed for several hours after apparently minor injuries. Occasionally, vasovagal syncope occurs several minutes to an hour after the injury and may cause undue concern. Constant generalized or frontal headache is common in the days following trauma; it may be migrainous (throbbing and hemicranial) in nature. After several hours of observation, patients with this category of injury may be accompanied home and observed by a family member or friend. Most patients with a minor syndrome do not have a skull fracture on skull x-ray or hemorrhage on CT. The decision to perform these tests depends largely on clinical signs suggesting that the impact was severe (e.g., prolonged concussion, periorbital or mastoid hematoma, repeated vomiting), on the seriousness of other bodily injuries, and on the degree of surveillance that can be expected at home. Persistent severe headache and repeated vomiting in the context of normal alertness and no focal neurologic signs are usually benign, but radiologic studies should be obtained and observation in the hospital is justified.

INJURY OF INTERMEDIATE SEVERITY Patients who are not comatose but who have persistent confusion, behavioral changes, subnormal alertness, extreme dizziness, or focal neurologic signs such as hemiparesis should be admitted to the hospital and soon thereafter have a CT scan. Usually a contusion or hematoma is found. The clinical syndromes most common in this group, in addition to

postconcussive headache, dizziness, and vomiting, include (1) delirium with a disinclination to be examined or moved, expletive speech, and resistance if disturbed (anterior temporal lobe contusions); (2) a quiet, disinterested, slowed mental state (abulia) with dull facial appearance and irascibility (inferior frontal and frontopolar contusions); (3) a focal deficit such as aphasia or mild hemiparesis (due to subdural hematoma or convexity contusion, or, less often, carotid artery dissection); (4) confusion with inattention, poor performance on simple mental tasks, and fluctuating or slightly erroneous orientation (associated with several types of injuries, including the first two described above as well as medial frontal contusions and interhemispheric subdural hematoma); (5) repetitive vomiting, nystagmus, drowsiness, and unsteadiness (usually labyrinthine concussion, but occasionally due to a posterior fossa subdural hematoma or vertebral artery dissection); and (6) diabetes insipidus (damage to the median eminence or pituitary stalk). It needs to be emphasized that intermediate-grade injuries are often complicated by drug or alcohol intoxication.

Clinical observation is necessary to detect increasing drowsiness, change in respiratory pattern, or pupillary enlargement and to ensure restriction of free water (unless there is diabetes insipidus). Asymmetry in limb posture, limb movement, or gaze preference suggests a subdural or epidural hematoma or large contusion. Most patients in this category improve over several days. During the first week, the state of alertness, memory, and other cognitive performance often fluctuate, and irascibility or agitation is common. Behavioral changes are worst at night, as with most other encephalopathies, and may be treated with small doses of antipsychotic medications. Subtle abnormalities of attention, intellect, spontaneity, and memory tend to return to normal weeks or months after the injury, sometimes surprisingly abruptly; persistent losses in cognition are discussed below.

SEVERE INJURY Patients who are comatose from the onset require immediate neurologic attention and often resuscitation. After intubation, with care taken to avoid deforming the cervical spine, the depth of coma, pupillary size and reactivity, limb movements, and Babinski responses are assessed. As soon as vital functions permit and cervical spine x-rays and a CT scan have been obtained, the patient should be transported to a critical care unit. The finding of an epidural or subdural hematoma or large intracerebral hemorrhage is an indication for prompt surgery and intracranial decompression in otherwise salvageable patients. Subsequent treatment is probably best guided by direct measurement of ICP but may proceed on a presumptive basis using clinical status and CT scan as guides. All potential exacerbating factors must be eliminated. Hypoxia, hyperthermia, hypercarbia, awkward head positions, and high mean airway pressures from mechanical ventilation all increase cerebral blood volume and ICP. Many, but not all, patients will have lower ICP when the head and trunk are elevated. Active management of raised ICP includes hyperosmolar dehydration with 20% mannitol (0.25 to 1 g/kg every 3 to 6 h), preferably using directly measured ICP as a guide. Otherwise, a serum osmolality of ~300 mosmol/L is desirable. It is customary to restrict free water administration in order to maintain high serum osmolarity, but there is no rationale for a reduction in the total volume of fluids administered if they are iso- or hyperosmolar, e.g., normal saline. Induced hypocarbia to an initial level of 28 to 33 mmHg P_{CO_2} is rapidly effective in reducing ICP, but its duration of effect is limited and its use has fallen out of favor, perhaps excessively so.

Persistently raised ICP after inception of this conservative therapy generally indicates a poor outcome. Although the addition of high-dose barbiturates may further lower ICP, there is no beneficial effect on overall outcome. In many instances, barbiturates cause a parallel reduction in ICP and BP without a net improvement in cerebral perfusion. Systolic BP should be maintained >100 mmHg by vasopressor agents, if necessary. Mean BP levels >110 to 120 mmHg may exaggerate brain edema, but some neurosurgeons allow the BP to rise above normal on the basis that this may abort plateau waves. A conventional approach to extreme hypertension utilizes diuretics and β-adrenergic blocking agents, angiotensin-converting enzyme inhibitors, or intermittent doses of barbiturates. A number of other antihypertensive drugs, including some calcium channel blockers and nitrates, are said to be relatively contraindicated because they may raise ICP. Antacids administered by nasogastric tube or direct-acting drugs are utilized to keep gastric pH >3.5 and prevent gastrointestinal bleeding as described below. The use of large doses of glucocorticoids in severe head injury does not improve outcome. Several studies suggest that early nutritional support results in faster neurologic recovery from head injury. If the patient remains comatose, it is worthwhile to repeat the CT or MRI scan to exclude a delayed surface or intracerebral hemorrhage. Intensive care salvages some critically ill head-injured patients by concentrating efforts on simple treatments that avoid medical complications, particularly pneumonia and sepsis and preventable increases in ICP.

SYSTEMIC DERANGEMENTS RESULTING FROM SEVERE HEAD TRAUMA   Injuries outside the cranium should be searched for at the outset, because they are likely to be forgotten if not initially noted. In particular, associated spinal, long bone, and abdominal injuries may cause delayed difficulties in management. Over half of patients who persist in coma for 24 h after head injury develop *abnormalities of electrolytes or fluid balance*. Diabetes insipidus should be suspected if urine output increases and urine specific gravity is low (Chap. 329). Replacement of water losses suffices for mild cases, but vasopressin may be required. Secretion of aldosterone and antidiuretic hormone (vasopressin, AVP) in response to stress favor the retention of sodium and free water, respectively. The latter usually predominates, leading to mild hypervolemic hyponatremia, but this is obscured if osmotic dehydrating agents have been used.

Some patients with head injuries suffer *hypoxia* acutely after injury without obvious pulmonary infiltrates. Aspiration pneumonia presents a great risk; lung injury from aspirated gastric contents, infection, and atelectasis may combine to produce the adult respiratory distress syndrome (ARDS) and severe arteriovenous shunting (Chap. 265). ARDS also occurs owing to disseminated intravascular coagulopathy, fat embolism, or, rarely, "neurogenic" pulmonary edema (see below). The effect of positive end-expiratory pressure (PEEP) on ICP is complex, but PEEP should not be withheld if necessary for oxygenation. *Atelectasis* is common in all poorly responsive patients and is treated with chest physical therapy and adequate ventilator tidal volumes. *Pulmonary embolism* is also a major threat to bedridden patients, and intermittent pneumatic calf compression or modest doses of subcutaneous heparin may be useful prophylaxis. The latter has not predisposed to intracerebral or gastrointestinal bleeding. Early recognition of deep leg vein thrombosis and aggressive treatment by occlusion of the inferior vena cava may prevent later emboli.

Patients with severe long bone injuries are subject to widespread *cerebral fat embolism*. For uncertain reasons, this complication is seen less often than previously, perhaps because of better fluid replacement. In the typical case, head injury is a minor part of the overall trauma; nonetheless, severe cranial injury masks the syndrome. Several days after the bone fractures occur, restlessness, delirium or drowsiness progressing to coma in severe cases, seizures, generalized brain edema, and hypoxia develop. About half the patients have retinal and punctate conjunctival hemorrhages or fat that is visible in retinal vessels. A petechial rash (prominent in the anterior axillary folds and supraclavicular fossae), diffuse interstitial infiltrates on the chest x-ray, fat in the urine, and/or renal failure occur in some patients. Severe reduction in arterial oxygen content is common from widespread lung injury (ARDS). Cerebral fat embolism causes a cerebral purpura, mainly in the white matter, due to capillary occlusion by fat globules. There is evidence that patients in whom this complication is recognized and treated early have a better prognosis. Massive doses of glucocorticoids and administration of positive-pressure ventilation with high end-expiratory pressures have been claimed to be useful.

Most patients with severe head injuries develop gastric erosions, but only a few have clinically significant hemorrhages. *Gastrointestinal bleeding* usually occurs in the first days to 1 week after injury. Unlike the majority of patients in shock or with stress ulceration, head-trauma patients often have elevated gastric acidity. Prophylactic treatment with gastric coating agents as discussed above, with H_2 receptor blockers, or with frequent antacid administration probably reduces gastric hemorrhage in other stress states and is commonly used in head trauma.

Acute head trauma may cause transient apnea and cardiac arrest. In the absence of overwhelming brain damage, recovery from the arrest is the rule. Subsequently, a sympathoadrenal discharge or raised ICP causes *systemic hypertension*, either with the classically associated bradycardia of the Cushing response or, almost as frequently, with tachycardia. Cardiac arrhythmias are common, most notably sinus bradycardia, supraventricular tachycardias, nodal rhythm, and heart block. T-wave inversion and alterations in the ST segment may simulate subendocardial ischemia. In some instances these changes are due to cardiac muscle contusion.

Neurogenic pulmonary edema is a form of respiratory failure in which the alveoli fill with fluid, as in congestive heart failure, but left ventricular end-diastolic pressure is normal after the infiltrates are established. The nature of this pulmonary vascular leak is not settled, but it may be the result of a sudden shift of intravascular volume from the systemic to the pulmonary circulation or there may be a direct cerebral neurogenic influence on the pulmonary microvasculature. The alveolar capillary leak may continue despite a return of pulmonary vascular pressure to normal.

Many patients demonstrate a mild *coagulopathy*, and 5 to 10% have various degrees of disseminated intravascular coagulation, a harbinger of poor outcome. There is a correlation between the severity of injury and the level of increased fibrin degradation products in blood, and one cause of the coagulopathy may be the release of highly thromboplastic material from damaged brain tissue.

PROGNOSIS   Extensive work by Jennet's group in Glasgow and by the Traumatic Coma Data Bank has provided data on the outcome in severe head injury. Verbal output, eye opening, and the best motor response of the limbs have been found to be predictive of outcome and are summarized using the "Glasgow Coma Scale" (Table 369-1). Over 85% of patients with aggregate scores of 3 or 4 die within 24 h. However, a number of patients with slightly higher scores but a poor initial prognosis, including absent pupillary light responses, survive, suggesting that an initially aggressive approach is justified in most patients. Patients <20 years, particularly children, may make remarkable recoveries after having grave early neurologic signs. In

Table 369-1   Glasgow Coma Scale for Head Injury

Eye opening (E)	
Spontaneous	4
To loud voice	3
To pain	2
Nil	1
Best motor response (M)	
Obeys	6
Localizes	5
Withdraws (flexion)	4
Abnormal flexion posturing	3
Extension posturing	2
Nil	1
Verbal response (V)	
Oriented	5
Confused, disoriented	4
Inappropriate words	3
Incomprehensible sounds	2
Nil	1

NOTE: Coma score = E + M + V. Patients scoring 3 or 4 have an 85 percent chance of dying or remaining vegetative, while scores above 11 indicate only a 5 to 10 percent likelihood of death or vegetative state and 85 percent chance of moderate disability or good recovery. Intermediate scores correlate with proportional chances of recovery.

one large study of severe head injury, 55% of children had a good outcome at 1 year, compared with 21% of adults. Older age, increased ICP, hypoxia and hypotension, and CT scan evidence of compression of the cisterns surrounding the brainstem and shift of midline structures are all poor prognostic signs. Delayed evacuation of large intracerebral clots is also associated with a poor prognosis.

Evoked potentials have prognostic value in head injury, similar to their use in ischemic-hypoxic brain injury, and their accuracy in predicting a poor outcome probably exceeds that of purely clinical methods. The results obtained from somatosensory evoked potentials are clearest, with the bilateral absence of cortical potentials (more caudal potentials present) predicting death or a vegetative state in over 90% of patients. A normal or mildly abnormal test, however, does not reliably predict a good functional outcome.

NEUROPSYCHOLOGICAL OUTCOME AFTER HEAD INJURY

A structural basis has been sought for the posttraumatic nervous instability termed the *postconcussion syndrome*, which consists of fatigue, dizziness, headache, and difficulty in concentration after mild or moderate injury. Most instances are difficult to distinguish from asthenia and depression. However, with intermediate-grade injury there is probably a substantial incidence of difficulty with attention and memory as well as other subtle cognitive deficits. Based on experimental models, some investigators believe that subtle axonal shearing lesions or biochemical alterations account for these symptoms despite normal findings on brain imaging, evoked potentials, and electroencephalogram. In moderate and severe trauma, neuropsychological changes are found routinely, but some of these deficits identified in formal testing are not important in daily functioning. Test scores tend to improve rapidly during the first 6 months after injury, then more slowly for years.

SPINAL CORD TRAUMA

Approximately 10,000 patients a year in the United States, mostly young and otherwise healthy, become paraplegic or quadriplegic because of spinal cord injuries; there are an estimated 200,000 quadriplegics in the nation. Most spinal cord injuries in civilian life result from fracture or dislocation of the surrounding vertebral column. Vertical compression with flexion is the main mechanism of injury in the thoracic cord, and hyperextension or flexion is the main cause of injury in the cervical cord. Preexisting spondylosis, a congenitally narrowed spinal canal, hypertrophied ligamentum flavum (Chap. 16), and instability of the apophyseal joints from diseases such as rheumatoid arthritis predispose to severe spinal cord damage even after minor degrees of injury.

PATHOPHYSIOLOGY AND PATHOLOGY OF SPINAL CORD INJURY Considerable spinal cord damage results from secondary phenomena that arise in the minutes and hours following injury. Even when a complete transverse myelopathy is evident immediately after impact, some secondary changes and the resultant damage may be reversible. The immediate compression of the cord causes pericapillary hemorrhages that coalesce and enlarge, particularly in the gray matter. Infarction of gray matter and early white matter edema are evident within 4 hours of experimental blunt injury. Eight hours after injury, there is global infarction at the traumatized level, and only at this point does necrosis of white matter and paralysis below the level of the lesion become irreversible. The necrosis and central hemorrhages enlarge to occupy one or two levels above and below the point of primary impact. Gliosis progresses over several months, and the affected regions may cavitate, causing a syringomyelic syndrome.

A large number of interventions for acute spinal compression injury have been of uncertain benefit, but high doses of methylprednisolone (typically 30 mg/kg followed by 5.4 mg/kg hourly for 23 h) administered within 8 hours of injury is associated with a slightly improved outcome. The critical factor for recoverable function is the time from injury to the institution of any therapy.

MANAGEMENT OF SPINAL CORD INJURY SYNDROMES Any patient with an injury that involves the spine or head potentially has an associated instability of the spinal column. The care of such patients begins at the scene of the accident: the neck should be immobilized, and care should be taken during transport and during the physical and radiologic examinations to prevent extension or rotation of the neck and torsion-rotation of the thoracic spine. Intubation, if necessary, can be accomplished by a blind nasotracheal technique or over an endoscope in order to avoid neck extension. High thoracic or cervical cord transection causes hypotension and bradycardia because of a functional sympathectomy (sometimes corroborated by bilateral ptosis and miosis—Horner's syndrome), which responds to infusion of crystalloid or colloid.

The neurologic assessment in the awake patient with possible spinal injury focuses on neck or back pain, diminished limb power, a sensory level on the trunk, and on deep tendon reflexes, which are usually absent below the level of acute cord injury. The level of injury can be approximated from the upper dermatome of sensory loss. Injuries above C5 cause quadriplegia and respiratory failure. At C5 and C6 the biceps are weak, whereas the deltoid and the supra- and infraspinatus are spared. C7 injuries cause weakness of the triceps, wrist extensors, and forearm pronators. Injuries at T1 and below cause paraplegia. Compression in the lower thoracic and lumbar spine causes a conus medullaris or cauda equina syndrome. Cauda equina injuries are usually incomplete, involving peripheral nerves rather than spinal cord, and therefore are surgically remediable for longer periods after injury than spinal cord compression. In a comatose patient, absent reflexes, especially with small pupils or paradoxical breathing and hypotension, signify a high cervical cord injury. →*The principles of spinal cord localization are considered in detail in Chap. 368.*

Reversible and preventable causes of spinal cord compression must be detected and surgically remedied. These include dislocation of a vertebral body, or an unstable vertebral fracture that can lead to misalignment and cord compression in the future. Treatment of fractures through the pedicles, facets, or vertebral bodies varies; some fractures heal with immobilization and time, usually 2 to 3 months, while others require surgical fusion to ensure stability. Many traumatic myelopathies have no clearly associated fracture or dislocation, but there is generally rupture of the supporting ligaments that has produced transient cord compression during the impact. If x-rays suggest any aberration in the position of vertebrae, then realignment should generally be undertaken quickly. CT or MRI exam is the most useful for demonstrating spinal misalignment and fractures. The role of myelography is not as compelling as it was in the past, but many neurosurgeons choose to instill a few drops of water-soluble contrast medium into the spinal subarachnoid space to demonstrate a block to the flow of CSF by CT or conventional myelography. Decompression within 2 hours of severe injury may lead to some recovery of spinal cord function. With incomplete myelopathies, especially if the limbs are becoming progressively weaker, early realignment is performed even many hours after injury. The surgical approaches to decompressing the spinal column depend on the specific nature of the injury. In complete transverse myelopathies beyond 6 to 12 hours after injury, decompressive laminectomies are usually unsuccessful in restoring function.

Atlantoaxial dislocation can cause immediate death from respiratory failure, an event that may occur unexpectedly even without other neurologic signs. Rheumatoid arthritis predisposes to this injury. Atlantooccipital dislocations occur predominantly in children and are almost always fatal. "Jefferson's fractures" are burst fractures of the ring of the atlas resulting from a force descending on the vertex of the skull, as in diving accidents; they are usually asymptomatic. "Hangman's fractures" are produced by hyperextension and longitudinal distraction of the upper cervical spine, as occurs with penal hanging or striking the chin on a steering wheel in a head-on collision. These are usually fractures through the pedicles of C2 with subluxation anteriorly of C2 on C3. Traction reduction and prolonged immobilization usually allow proper healing.

Hyperflexion dislocation of the cervical vertebrae commonly causes quadriplegia. Occasionally, a markedly displaced injury is unassociated with neurologic dysfunction, presenting only with neck pain. Any degree of subluxation must be considered as potentially unstable.

Compression fracture of the cervical spine can cause neurologic damage if a bone fragment is driven backward (burst fracture) into the spinal cord. "Teardrop fractures" with crushing of a vertebral body, leaving a fragment of bone anteriorly, are usually associated with ligamentous disruption and spinal instability. Single compression fractures of the thoracic spine are usually stable because the thoracic cage provides support, but they may be associated with anterior spinal cord compression and require decompression and stabilization with the insertion of metal rods.

Mild *cervical hyperextension* injuries may cause only disruption of supporting ligamentous structures and can be well tolerated. More severe injuries cause vertebral displacement and cord compression. The "central cord syndrome" is produced by brief compression of the cervical cord and disruption of the central gray matter. It usually occurs in patients with an already narrow spinal canal, either congenitally or from cervical spondylosis. There is weakness of the arms with pinprick loss over the arms and shoulders, and relative sparing of leg power and sensation on the trunk and legs. Abnormality of bladder function is variable. The prognosis for recovery is good.

Thoracolumbar fracture is produced by impact in the high or middle back, usually while the patient is bent over. Impingement on the spinal canal results in a complex combination of cauda equina and conus medullaris dysfunction. Purely lumbar fractures with displacement of a vertebral body produce cauda equina compression. Surgical decompression is usually recommended, even with severe neurologic deficits, because there is considerable potential for recovery of the nerve roots of the cauda.

The subsequent care of patients with spinal cord injury is best undertaken in specialized centers. →*General principles of medical and urologic management are discussed in Chap. 368.*

BIBLIOGRAPHY

ANNEGERS JF et al: A population-based study of seizures after traumatic brain injury. N Engl J Med 338:20, 1998

COLLINS MW et al: Current issues in managing sports-related concussion. JAMA 282: 2283, 1999

DACEY RG et al: Neurosurgical complications after apparently minor head injury. J Neurosurg 65:203, 1986

EISENBERG HM et al: Report of the Traumatic Coma Data Bank. J Neurosurg 75(Suppl): S1, 1991

GOLDSTEIN M: Traumatic brain injury: A silent epidemic. Ann Neurol 27:327, 1990

LANGFITT TW, GENARELLI TA: Can the outcome from head injury be improved? J Neurosurg 56:19, 1982

LEVIN HS et al: Neurobehavioral outcome following minor head injury: A three center study. J Neurosurg 66:234, 1987

MCCRORY PR, BERKOVIC SF: Video analysis of acute motor and convulsive manifestations in sport-related concussion. Neurology 54:1488, 2000

ROPPER AH (ed): *Neurological and Neurosurgical Intensive Care*, 3d ed. New York, Raven, 1993

ROSNER MJ et al: Cerebral perfusion pressure: Management protocol and clinical results. J Neurosurg 83:949, 1995

RUFF RM et al: Predictors of outcome following severe head trauma: Follow-up data from the Traumatic Coma Data Bank. Brain Inj 7:101, 1993

STEIN SC et al: Delayed and progressive brain injury in closed-head trauma: Radiological demonstration. Neurosurgery 32:25, 1993

370

Stephen M. Sagar, Mark A. Israel

PRIMARY AND METASTATIC TUMORS OF THE NERVOUS SYSTEM

CEA	carcinoembryonic antigen	PET	positron emission tomography
CNS	central nervous system	PNET	primitive neuroectodermal
CSF	cerebrospinal fluid		tumors
CT	computed tomography	SPECT	single-photon emission
EEG	electroencephalography		computed tomography
MRI	magnetic resonance imaging	VHL	von Hippel–Lindau

Malignant primary tumors of the central nervous system (CNS) occur in approximately 18,000 individuals and account for an estimated 13,300 deaths in the United States annually, a mortality rate of 5 per 100,000. An almost equal number of benign tumors of the CNS were diagnosed, with a much lower mortality rate. Glial tumors account for 50 to 60% of primary brain tumors, meningiomas account for about 25%, schwannomas for about 10%, and all other CNS tumors for the remainder. An increase in the frequency of diagnosis of malignant gliomas in the elderly has been reported in recent years. It is unclear if this change represents a true increased incidence or is the result of more frequent use of modern neuroimaging techniques.

Brain and vertebral metastases from systemic tumors are more prevalent than primary CNS tumors. About 15% of patients who die of cancer (80,000 individuals each year in the United States) have symptomatic brain metastases; an additional 5% suffer spinal cord involvement. These tumors, therefore, pose a major problem in the management of systemic cancer.

BRAIN TUMORS

Approach to the Patient

Clinical Features Brain tumors usually present with one of three syndromes: (1) subacute progression of a focal neurologic deficit; (2) seizure; or (3) nonfocal neurologic disorder such as headache, dementia, personality change, or gait disorder. The presence of systemic symptoms such as malaise, weight loss, anorexia, or fever suggests a metastatic rather than a primary brain tumor.

Progressive focal neurologic deficits result from compression of neurons and white matter tracts by expanding tumor and surrounding edema. Less commonly, a brain tumor may present with a stroke-like onset of focal neurologic deficit. Although this presentation may be caused by hemorrhage into the tumor, often no hemorrhage can be demonstrated and the mechanism is obscure. Tumors frequently associated with hemorrhage include high-grade astrocytomas and metastatic melanoma and choriocarcinoma.

Seizures may result from disruption of cortical circuits. Tumors that invade or compress the cerebral cortex, even small meningiomas, are more likely to be associated with seizures than subcortical neoplasms. Nonfocal neurologic dysfunction usually reflects increased intracranial pressure, hydrocephalus, or diffuse tumor spread. Tumors in some areas of the brain may produce subtle deficits; for example, frontal lobe tumors may present with personality change, dementia, or depression.

Headache may result from focal irritation or displacement of pain-sensitive structures (Chap. 15) or from a generalized increase in intracranial pressure. A headache that worsens rather than abates with recumbency is suggestive of a mass lesion. The headache of increased intracranial pressure has a characteristic pattern. Early on, these headaches are usually holocephalic and episodic, occurring more than once a day. They typically develop rapidly over several minutes, persist for 20 to 40 min, and subside quickly. They may awaken the patient from a sound sleep, generally 60 to 90 min after retiring, or may be precipitated by coughing, sneezing, or straining. Vomiting may occur with severe headaches. As elevated intracranial pressure becomes sustained, the headache becomes continuous but varying in intensity. Elevated intracranial pressure may cause papilledema (Chap. 28), although it is often not present in patients over 55 years old.

Infrequent but characteristic brain tumor presentations include anosmia from a meningioma arising along the cribiform plates and olfactory tracts and unilateral hearing loss from schwannomas of the eighth cranial nerve. Asymptomatic brain tumors, most often meningiomas, are commonly discovered incidentally on imaging studies obtained for unrelated purposes.

The Karnofsky performance scale is useful in assessing and following patients with brain tumors (Chap. 79). A score ≥70 indicates that the patient is ambulatory and independent in self-care activities; it has often been taken as a level of function justifying aggressive therapy.

Table 370-1 Hereditary Syndromes Associated with Brain Tumors

Syndrome	Gene (Locus)	Gene Product (Function)	Nervous System Neoplasms
Neurofibromatosis type 1 (von Recklinghausen's Disease)[a]	NF1 (17q)	Neurofibromin (GTPase activating protein)	Neuroma, schwannoma, meningioma, optic glioma
Neurofibromatosis type 2[a]	NF2 (22q)	Merlin (cytoskeletal protein)	Schwannoma, glioma, ependymoma, meningioma
Tuberous sclerosis	TSC1 (9q) TSC2 (16p)	Hamartin (unknown function) Tuberin (GTPase activating protein)	Astrocytoma
von Hippel-Lindau[a]	VHL (3p)	pVHL (modulator of mRNA elongation)	Hemangioblastoma of retina, cerebellum and spinal cord; pheochromocytoma
Li-Fraumeni[a]	p53 (17p)	TP53 (cell cycle and transcriptional regulator)	Malignant glioma
Retinoblastoma[a]	RB1 (13q)	RB (cell cycle regulator)	Retinoblastoma, pineoblastoma, malignant glioma
Turcot	APC (5q) (adenomatous polyposis coli)	APC (cell adhesion)	Medulloblastoma, malignant glioma
Gorlin (basal cell nevus syndrome)	PTCH (9q) (patched)	PTH (developmental regulator)	Medulloblastoma
Multiple endocrine neoplasia 1 (Werner syndrome)[a]	MEN1 (11q13)	Menin (cofactor for transcription)	Pituitary adenoma, malignant schwannoma

[a] Genetic testing possible.

Laboratory Examination Primary brain tumors typically do not produce serologic abnormalities such as an elevated sedimentation rate or tumor-specific antigens associated with systemic cancers. In contrast, metastases to the nervous system, depending on the type and extent of the primary tumor, may be associated with systemic signs of malignancy (Chap. 83). Lumbar puncture may precipitate brain herniation in patients with mass lesions, and should be performed only in patients with suspected CNS infection or meningeal metastasis. Findings in the cerebrospinal fluid (CSF) of patients with primary and metastatic nervous system tumors may include raised opening pressure, elevated protein level, and a mild lymphocytic pleocytosis. Astrocytomas that extend to the ventricular surface, or the rupture of an epidermoid cyst, can occasionally produce an intense CSF inflammatory reaction simulating infectious meningitis. The CSF rarely contains malignant cells, with the important exceptions of leptomeningeal metastases, primary CNS lymphoma and primitive neuroectodermal tumors, including medulloblastoma.

Neuroimaging Computed tomography (CT) and magnetic resonance imaging (MRI) reveal mass effect and contrast enhancement. Mass effect reflects the volume of neoplastic tissue as well as surrounding edema. Brain tumors typically produce a vasogenic pattern of edema, with accumulation of excess water in white matter. The normal blood-brain barrier results from tight junctions between endothelial cells that prevent entry of most charged molecules into the nervous system. Contrast enhancement reflects a breakdown of the blood-brain barrier within the tumor, permitting leakage of contrast agent. Low-grade gliomas typically do not exhibit contrast enhancement.

Positron emission tomography (PET) and single-photon emission tomography (SPECT) have ancillary roles in the imaging of brain tumors, primarily in distinguishing tumor recurrence from tissue necrosis that can occur after irradiation (see below). Electroencephalography (EEG) has a role in the evaluation of patients with possible seizures. Functional imaging with PET, MRI, or magnetoencephalography may be of use in surgical or radiosurgical planning to define the anatomic relationship of the tumor to critical brain regions such as the primary motor cortex.

TREATMENT Symptomatic Glucocorticoids decrease the volume of edema surrounding brain tumors and improve neurologic function; dexamethasone (12 to 20 mg/d in divided doses orally or intravenously) is used because it has relatively little mineralocorticoid activity.

Tumors that involve the cerebral cortex or hippocampus may produce epilepsy. Anticonvulsants are therefore used therapeutically and prophylactically; phenytoin, carbamazepine, and valproic acid are equally effective (Chap. 360). If the tumor is subcortical in location, prophylactic anticonvulsants are unnecessary.

Gliomas are associated with an increased risk for deep vein thrombosis and pulmonary embolism, probably because these tumors secrete procoagulant factors into the systemic circulation. Whether this risk extends to other brain tumors is unknown. Even though hemorrhage within gliomas is a frequent histopathologic finding, patients with gliomas appear to be at no increased risk for symptomatic intracranial bleeding following treatment with an anticoagulant. Prophylaxis with low-dose subcutaneous heparin should be considered for patients with gliomas who have lower limb immobility, which places them at risk for deep venous thrombosis.

PRIMARY BRAIN TUMORS

ETIOLOGY Exposure to ionizing radiation is the only well-documented environmental risk factor for the development of brain tumors. A number of hereditary syndromes are associated with an increased risk of brain tumors (Table 370-1). Genes that contribute to the development of brain tumors, as well as other malignancies, fall into two general classes, *tumor-suppressor genes* and *proto-oncogenes* (Chap. 81). Whereas germ line mutations of tumor suppressor genes are rare, somatic mutations are almost invariably found in malignant tumors, including brain tumors. Likewise, the over-expression of proto-oncogenes is frequent in brain tumors as well as systemic malignancies. Moreover, cytogenetic analysis often reveals characteristic changes. In astrocytic tumors, DNA is commonly lost on chromosomes 10p, 17p, 13q, and 9. Oligodendrogliomas frequently have deletions of 1p and 19q. In meningiomas portions of 22q, which contains the gene for neurofibromatosis type 2, are often lost. Less frequently there is evidence of amplification of specific genes, for example *EGFR* in some astrocytomas.

The particular constellation of genetic alterations varies among individual gliomas, even those that are histologically indistinguishable. Moreover, gliomas are genetically unstable, genetic abnormalities tend to accumulate with time, and these changes correspond with increasingly aggressive malignant behavior. There appear to be at least two genetic routes for the development of malignant glioma (Fig. 370-1). One route involves the progression, generally over years, from a low grade astrocytoma with early deletions of chromosome 17 and inactivation of the p53 gene to a malignant glioma with additional chromosomal deletions. The second route is characterized by the de novo appearance of a malignant glioma with amplification of the *EGFR* gene and an intact p53 gene. In both pathways, inactivation of the *PTEN* gene as a result of the loss of chromosome 10 occurs frequently.

ASTROCYTOMAS   Tumors derived from astrocytes are the most common primary intracranial neoplasms (Fig. 370-2). Their neuropathologic appearance is highly variable. The most widely used histologic grading system is the World Health Organization (WHO) four-tiered grading system. Grade I is reserved for special histologic variants of astrocytoma that have an excellent prognosis after surgical excision. These include *juvenile pilocytic astrocytoma*, *subependymal giant cell astrocytoma* (which occurs in patients with tuberous sclerosis), and *pleiomorphic xanthoastrocytoma*. At the other extreme is

FIGURE 370-2   Malignant astrocytoma (glioblastoma). Coronal proton density-weighted MR scan through the temporal lobes demonstrates a heterogeneous right temporal lobe mass (*arrows*) compressing the third and lateral ventricles. The area of hypointense signal (*double arrows*) indicates either hemorrhage or calcification. Heterogeneous MR signal intensity is typical of glioblastoma.

grade IV, *glioblastoma multiforme*, a clinically aggressive tumor. *Astrocytoma* (grade II) and *anaplastic astrocytoma* (grade III) are intermediate. The histologic features associated with higher grade are hypercellularity, nuclear and cytoplasmic atypia, endothelial proliferation, mitotic activity, and necrosis. Endothelial proliferation and necrosis are especially robust predictors of aggressive behavior.

A limitation of all grading schemes, especially when applied to a single biopsy, is that astrocytic tumors are histologically variable from region to region, and their histopathology may change with time. It is common for low-grade astrocytomas to progress over time to a higher histopathologic grade and a more aggressive clinical course.

Quantitative measures of mitotic activity also correlate with prognosis. The proliferation index can be determined by immunohistochemical staining with antibodies to the proliferating cell nuclear antigen (PCNA) or with a monoclonal antibody termed *Ki-67*, which recognizes a histone protein expressed in proliferating but not quiescent cells. These measures provide estimates of DNA synthesis and correlate with malignant clinical behavior of the tumor.

The overall prognosis is poor. In a representative Finnish population, the median survival was 93.5 months for patients with grade I or II astrocytomas, 12.4 months for patients with grade III (anaplastic astrocytoma), and 5.1 months for patients with grade IV (glioblastoma) tumors. In the United States, the median survival of patients with high-grade brain tumors is approximately 12 months. In addition to histopathology, features that correlate with poor prognosis include age over 65 and a poor functional status, as defined by the Karnofsky performance scale (see Table 79-2).

Low-Grade Astrocytoma   Low-grade astrocytomas are more common in children than adults. Pilocytic astrocytoma, named for its characteristic spindle-shaped cells, is the most common childhood brain tumor. It frequently occurs in the cerebellum. Typically, this tumor is cystic and well demarcated from adjacent brain. Complete surgical excision usually produces long-term, disease-free survival.

The optimal management of other low-grade astrocytomas, termed fibrillary astrocytomas, is controversial. For patients who are symptomatic from mass effect or poorly controlled epilepsy, surgical excision can relieve symptoms. For patients who are asymptomatic or minimally symptomatic at presentation, a diagnostic biopsy should be performed and, when surgically feasible, the tumor may be resected. The indications for postoperative radiation therapy are uncertain. In

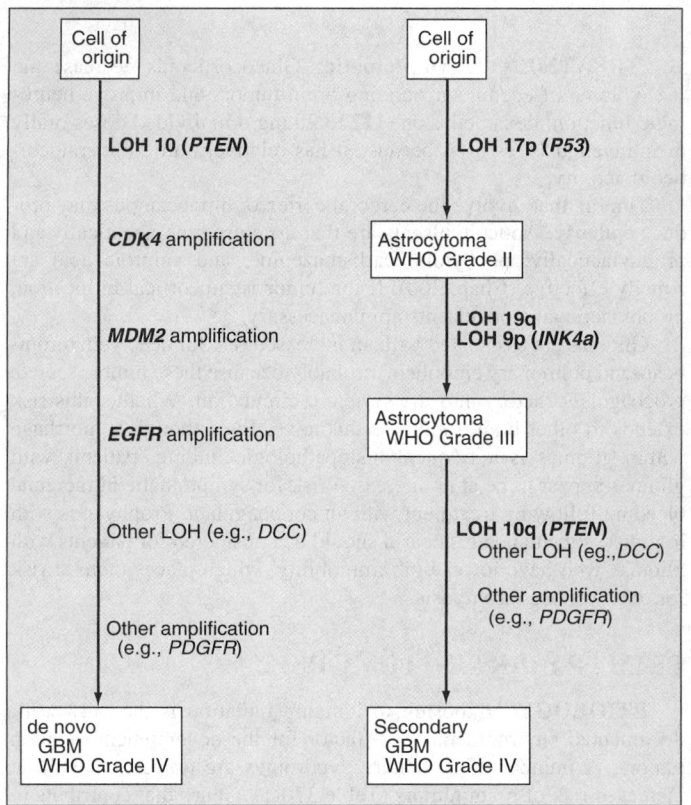

FIGURE 370-1   Proposed model for the pathogenesis of human astrocytoma. The highest grade of astrocytoma, glioblastoma multiforme (GBM), typically presents without evidence of a precursor lesion, although it is associated with multiple genetic alterations. The most diagnostic of these is amplification of the epidermal growth factor receptor (*EGFR*). Tumors with such a presentation are referred to as de novo GBM. Less commonly, GBM arises in association with progressive genetic alterations after the diagnosis of a lower grade astrocytoma. These tumors are referred to as secondary GBM. The most widely described alterations are mutations of *P53* and *INK4a*. Other genes implicated in the development of these primary brain tumors include *CDK4, MDM2, DDC,* and *PDGFR*. LOH, loss of heterozygosity.

many centers, when only a biopsy or partial resection is possible, postoperative external beam radiation therapy is administered, whereas it is not used if a gross total tumor resection can be achieved. Other centers reserve radiation therapy for tumor recurrence or progression, at which time the tumor may display a more malignant phenotype. No role for chemotherapy in the management of low-grade astrocytoma has been defined.

High-Grade Astrocytoma The large majority of astrocytomas arising in adults are high grade, supratentorial, and do not have a clearly defined margin. Neoplastic cells migrate away from the main tumor mass and infiltrate adjacent brain, often tracking along white matter pathways. Imaging studies do not indicate the full extent of the tumor. These tumors are eventually fatal, although prolonged survival occurs in a few patients. Longer survival correlates with younger age, better performance status, and greater extent of surgical resection. Late in their course, gliomas, especially those

FIGURE 370-3 Oligodendroglioma. *A*. Noncontrast CT scan reveals a calcified mass involving the left temporal lobe (*arrows*) associated with mild mass effect but little edema. *B*. An MR T2-weighted image demonstrates a heterogeneous mass with hypointense signal (*black arrows*) surrounded by a zone of higher signal intensity (*white arrows*), consistent with a calcified temporal lobe mass. The tumor extends into the left medial temporal lobe and compresses the midbrain.

located in the posterior fossa, can metastasize along CSF pathways to the spine. Metastases outside the CNS are rare.

High-grade astrocytomas are managed with glucocorticoids, surgery, radiation therapy, and chemotherapy. Dexamethasone is generally administered at the time of diagnosis and continued for the duration of radiation therapy. After completion of radiotherapy, the dose of dexamethasone is tapered to the lowest tolerated dose.

Because astrocytomas infiltrate adjacent normal brain, total surgical excision is not possible. Surgery is indicated to obtain tissue for pathologic diagnosis and to control mass effect. Moreover, retrospective studies indicate that the extent of tumor resection correlates with survival, at least in younger patients. Therefore, accessible astrocytomas are resected aggressively in patients younger than 65 years old who are in good general medical condition.

Postoperative radiation therapy prolongs survival and improves quality of life, although the duration of benefit is only a few months. Treated with dexamethasone alone following surgery, the mean survival of patients under 65 years of age with glioblastoma is 7 to 9 months. Survival is prolonged to 11 to 13 months with radiation therapy. Focal brain irradiation is less toxic and is as effective as whole-brain radiation for the treatment of primary glial tumors. Radiation is generally administered to the tumor mass, as defined by contrast enhancement on a CT or MRI scan, plus a 3- to 4-cm margin. A total dose of 5000 to 7000 cGy is administered in 25 to 35 equal fractions, 5 days per week.

The roles of stereotaxic radiosurgery and interstitial brachytherapy in glioma treatment are uncertain. *Stereotaxic radiosurgery* is the administration of a focused high dose of radiation to a precisely defined volume of tissue in a single treatment, usually using the gamma knife. Stereotaxic radiosurgery can potentially achieve tumor ablation without surgery. A major limitation of stereotaxic radiosurgery is that it can be used for only relatively small tumors, generally less than 3 cm in maximum diameter. *Interstitial brachytherapy*, the implantation of radioactive beads into the tumor mass, is generally reserved for tumor recurrence because of its associated toxicity—in particular, necrosis of adjacent brain tissue.

Chemotherapy is marginally effective and is often used as an adjuvant following surgery and radiation therapy. Nitrosoureas, including carmustine (BCNU) and lomustine (CCNU), are the most effective available agents. Since a typical glioma infiltrates normal brain where

the blood-brain barrier is relatively intact, lipid-soluble agents such as the nitrosoureas, which cross the blood-brain barrier, may reach more malignant cells than water-soluble agents. Experimental approaches include intraarterial infusion of chemotherapy, the implantation of chemotherapy-releasing wafers or injection of chemotherapeutic agents into the tumor resection cavity, administration of chemotherapy after disruption of the blood-brain barrier, and intensive chemotherapy regimens supported by autologous bone marrow transplantation.

Gliomatosis cerebri is a rare form of astrocytoma in which there is diffuse infiltration of the brain by malignant astrocytes without a focal enhancing mass. It generally presents as a multifocal CNS syndrome or a more generalized disorder including dementia, personality change, or seizures. Neuroimaging studies are often nonspecific, and biopsy is required to establish the diagnosis. Gliomatosis is treated with whole-brain radiation therapy and, in selected patients, with systemic chemotherapy.

OLIGODENDROGLIOMAS Oligodendrogliomas have a more benign course and are more responsive to cytotoxic treatment than astrocytomas. Five-year survival is greater than 50%, and 10-year survival is 25 to 34%.

Oligodendrogliomas occur chiefly in supratentorial locations; in adults about 30% contain areas of calcification (Fig. 370-3). Many gliomas contain mixtures of cells with astrocytic and oligodendroglial features. If this mixed histology is prominent, the tumor is termed a *mixed glioma* or an *oligoastrocytoma*. The greater the oligodendroglial component, the more benign the clinical course. As a rule, oligodendrogliomas are less infiltrative than astrocytomas, permitting more complete surgical excision. The histologic features of mitoses, necrosis, and nuclear atypia are associated with a more aggressive clinical course. If these features are prominent, the tumor is termed an *anaplastic oligodendroglioma*.

The optimal management of oligodendrogliomas has not been defined. Surgery, at minimum a stereotaxic biopsy, is necessary to establish a diagnosis. Many oligodendrogliomas are amenable to gross total surgical resection. In addition, oligodendrogliomas may respond dramatically to systemic combination chemotherapy with procarbazine, lomustine and vincristine (PCV). Oligodendrogliomas with deletions of chromosomes 1p and 19q typically respond to PCV, but only about 25% of oligodendrogliomas lacking these genetic markers respond to chemotherapy. Chemotherapy may be used as the initial treatment, and residual tumor can be surgically excised or treated with stereotaxic radiosurgery. An alternative approach is to first excise the accessible tumor mass, then administer systemic chemotherapy and finally, employ stereotaxic radiosurgery or external beam radiation for residual tumor.

EPENDYMOMAS   In adults ependymomas are typically located in the spinal canal, especially in the lumbosacral region, arising from the filum terminale of the spinal cord. These tumors often have a myxopapillary histology, with a papillary arrangement of cells and mucin production. In children, ependymomas occur within the ventricles, most often the fourth ventricle, and may exhibit diagnostic ependymal rosettes. Ependymomas with histologic signs of malignancy, including cellular atypia, frequent mitotic figures, or a high labeling index, virtually always recur after surgical resection. Imaging with CT or MRI scans reveals ependymomas as uniformly enhancing masses that are relatively well demarcated from adjacent neural tissue. Ependymomas may metastasize via CSF pathways: brain tumor metastases that spread to the spinal cord by this means are termed *drop metastases*.

Following the gross total excision of an ependymoma, the prognosis is excellent. The 5-year disease-free survival is >80%. However, many ependymomas cannot be totally excised, and postoperative focal external beam radiation or stereotaxic radiosurgery is used. Whether focal radiation is adequate or whether the entire neuraxis needs to be irradiated is not resolved.

GERMINOMAS   These tumors most commonly present during the second decade of life, generally at sites within or adjacent to the third ventricle including the pineal region. Germinomas are the most frequent variety of *germ cell tumor*, a tumor type arising in midline structures and including *teratoma*, yolk sac tumor (*endodermal sinus tumor*), *embryonal carcinoma*, and *choriocarcinoma*. Germinomas of the CNS may be benign but are more often aggressive and invasive. Due to their location, patients frequently present with hypothalamic-pituitary dysfunction including diabetes insipidus, visual field deficits, disturbances of memory or mood, or hydrocephalus (Chap. 328). Neuroimaging demonstrates germinomas to be uniformly enhancing masses with or without well-defined borders. The treatment of choice is complete surgical resection. For unresectable tumors, a stereotaxic biopsy is performed for diagnosis, and focal radiation is the primary therapy. When the extent of disease or very young age precludes radiotherapy as primary treatment, platinum-based chemotherapy may decrease tumor size and facilitate subsequent radiation therapy of residual disease or recurrent tumor. Prognosis depends on the histology and surgical resectability of the tumor. Germinomas are generally radiosensitive and chemosensitive, and 5-year survival is >85%.

MEDULLOBLASTOMAS AND PRIMITIVE NEUROECTODERMAL TUMORS (PNET)   These highly cellular malignant tumors are thought to arise from neural precursor cells. Medulloblastomas of the posterior fossa are the most frequent malignant brain tumor of children. If the tumor is not disseminated at presentation, the prognosis is generally favorable; subsets of pediatric patients have >70% survival rates at 5 years, although <50% of all children with medulloblastoma survive to adulthood. PNET is a term applied to tumors histologically indistinguishable from medulloblastoma but occurring either in adults or supratentorially in children. In adults, >50% present in the posterior fossa, but these tumors frequently disseminate along CSF pathways.

If possible, these tumors should be surgically excised, although outcome is not related to the extent of surgery. In adults, surgical excision of a PNET should be followed by chemotherapy and irradiation of the entire neuraxis, with a boost in radiation dose to the primary tumor. Aggressive treatment can result in prolonged survival, although half of adult patients relapse within 5 years of treatment.

CNS LYMPHOMA   Primary CNS Lymphoma   These are B cell malignancies of intermediate to high grade that present within the neuraxis without evidence of systemic lymphoma. They occur most frequently in immunocompromised individuals, specifically organ transplant recipients or patients with AIDS (Chap. 309), but the incidence of primary CNS lymphoma is increasing in both immunocompetent and immunocompromised patients. In immunocompromised patients, CNS lymphomas are invariably associated with Epstein-Barr virus (EBV) infection of the tumor cells. Chromosomal translocations involving the c-*myc* gene occur in EBV-associated lymphomas outside the CNS (Chap. 112) but not in primary CNS lymphoma.

In immunocompetent patients, neuroimaging studies most often reveal a uniformly enhancing mass lesion. In immunocompromised patients, primary CNS lymphoma is likely to be multicentric and exhibit ring enhancement or to arise in the meninges (Fig. 370-4). Stereotaxic needle biopsy can be used to establish the diagnosis. Leptomeningeal involvement is present in approximately 15% of patients

FIGURE 370-4   CNS lymphoma. *A.* Proton density–weighted MR image through the temporal lobe demonstrates a low signal intensity nodule (*small arrows*) surrounded by a ring of high signal intensity edema (*larger arrows*). *B.* T1-weighted contrast-enhanced axial MRI demonstrates ring enhancement surrounded by a nonenhanced rim of edema. In this patient with AIDS, a solitary lesion of this type is consistent with either lymphoma or toxoplasmosis; the presence of multiple lesions favors toxoplasmosis. *C.* In a different patient with lymphomatous meningitis, an axial postcontrast T1-weighted MRI through the midbrain demonstrates multiple areas of abnormal enhancement in periventricular and subependymal regions (*arrows*). Lymphoma tends to spread subependymally at interfaces of CSF and brain parenchyma.

at presentation and in 50% at some time during the course of the illness. Moreover, the disease extends to the eyes in up to 15% of patients. Therefore, a slit-lamp examination and, if indicated, anterior chamber paracentesis or vitreous biopsy is necessary before radiation therapy to define radiation ports.

The prognosis of primary CNS lymphoma is poor compared to histologically similar lymphoma occurring outside the CNS. Many patients experience a favorable clinical and radiographic response to glucocorticoids that may be dramatic; however, it is invariably transient and relapse occurs within weeks. Radiotherapy has been the mainstay of treatment, but systemic combination chemotherapy including high-dose methotrexate is also effective. Intrathecal chemotherapy with methotrexate should also be used if leptomeningeal disease is present. Despite aggressive therapy, >90% of patients develop recurrent CNS disease. Historically, the survival of immunocompetent patients with CNS lymphoma has been approximately 18 months, and may now be longer with the use of systemic chemotherapy. In organ transplant recipients, reversal of the immunosuppressed state can improve outcome. Survival with AIDS-related primary CNS lymphoma is very poor, generally ≤3 months; pretreatment performance status, the degree of immunosuppression, and the extent of CNS dissemination at diagnosis all appear to influence outcome.

Secondary CNS Lymphoma Secondary CNS lymphoma almost always occurs in association with progressive systemic disease in adults with B cell lymphoma or B cell leukemia who have tumor involvement of bone, bone marrow, testes, or the cranial sinuses. Leptomeningeal lymphoma is usually detectable with contrast-enhanced CT or gadolinium-enhanced MRI of the brain and spine or by CSF examination. Treatment consists of systemic chemotherapy, intrathecal chemotherapy, and CNS irradiation. It is usually possible to effectively suppress the leptomeningeal disease, although the overall prognosis is determined by the course of the systemic lymphoma.

PITUITARY ADENOMAS See Chap. 328.

MENINGIOMAS Meningiomas are derived from mesoderm, probably from cells giving rise to the arachnoid granulations. These tumors are usually benign and attached to the dura. They may invade the skull but only infrequently invade the brain. Meningiomas most often occur along the sagittal sinus, over the cerebral convexities, in the cerebellar-pontine angle, and along the dorsum of the spinal cord. They are more frequent in women than men, with a peak incidence in middle age.

Meningiomas may be found incidentally on a CT or MRI scan or may present with a focal seizure, a slowly progressive focal deficit, or symptoms of raised intracranial pressure. The radiologic image of a dural-based, extra-axial mass with dense, uniform contrast enhancement is essentially diagnostic, although a dural metastasis must also be considered (Fig. 370-5). A meningioma may have a "dural tail," a streak of dural enhancement flanking the main tumor mass; however, this finding may be present with other dural tumors.

Total surgical resection of benign meningiomas is curative. If a total resection cannot be achieved, local external beam radiotherapy reduces the recurrence rate to <10%. For meningiomas that are not surgically accessible, targeted radiosurgery with the gamma knife or heavy particle radiation should be considered. Small asymptomatic meningiomas incidentally discovered in older patients can safely be followed radiologically; these tumors grow at an average rate of approximately 0.24 cm in diameter per year and only rarely become symptomatic.

Rare meningiomas invade the brain or have histologic evidence of malignancy such as nuclear pleomorphism and cellular atypia. A high mitotic index is also predictive of aggressive behavior. *Hemangiopericytoma*, although not strictly a meningioma, is a meningeal tumor with an especially aggressive behavior. Meningiomas with features of aggressiveness and hemangiopericytomas, even if totally excised by gross inspection, frequently recur and should receive postoperative radiotherapy. Chemotherapy has no proven benefit.

SCHWANNOMAS These tumors are also called *neuromas*, *neurinomas*, or *neurolemmomas*. They arise from Schwann cells of

FIGURE 370-5 Meningioma. Coronal postcontrast T1-weighted MR image demonstrates an enhancing extraaxial mass arising from the falx cerebri (*arrows*).

nerve roots, most frequently in the eighth cranial nerve (vestibular schwannoma, formerly termed acoustic schwannoma). The fifth cranial nerve is the second most frequent site; however, schwannomas may arise from any cranial or spinal root except the optic and olfactory nerves, which are myelinated by oligodendroglia rather than Schwann cells. Neurofibromatosis (NF) type 2 (see below) strongly predisposes to vestibular schwannoma. Schwannomas of spinal nerve roots are also seen in these patients as well as patients with NF type 1.

Eighth nerve schwannomas typically arise from the vestibular division of the nerve. Because the vestibular system adapts to slow destruction of the eighth nerve, vestibular schwannomas characteristically present as progressive unilateral hearing loss rather than with dizziness or other vestibular symptoms. Unexplained unilateral hearing loss always merits evaluation, including audiometry and either brainstem auditory evoked potentials or an MRI scan (Chap. 29). As a vestibular schwannoma grows, it can compress the cerebellum, pons, or facial nerve, producing associated symptoms. With rare exceptions schwannomas are histologically and clinically benign. They appear as dense and uniformly enhancing neoplasms on MRI (Fig. 370-6). Vestibular schwannomas enlarge the internal auditory canal, an imaging feature that helps distinguish them from other cerebellopontine angle masses.

Whenever possible, schwannomas should be surgically excised. When the tumors are small, it is usually possible to preserve hearing in the involved ear. In the case of large tumors, the patient is usually deaf at presentation; nonetheless, surgery is indicated to prevent further compression of posterior fossa structures. Gamma knife treatment is also effective for schwannoma but is equivalent in cost and complication rate to surgery. Moreover, the long-term consequences of stereotaxic radiosurgery, including the possibility of secondary radiation-induced neoplasms, are unknown.

OTHER BENIGN BRAIN TUMORS *Epidermoid tumors* are cystic tumors with proliferative epidermal cells at the periphery and more mature epidermal cells towards the center of the cyst. The mature cells desquamate into the liquid center of the cyst. Epidermoid tumors are thought to arise from embryonic epidermal rests within the cranium. They occur extraaxially near the midline, in the middle cranial fossa, the suprasellar region, or the cerebellopontine angle. Epidermoid cysts are well-demarcated lesions that are amenable

FIGURE 370-6 Vestibular schwannoma. *A.* Axial noncontrast MR scan through the cerebellopontine angle demonstrates an extraaxial mass that extends into a widened internal auditory canal, displacing the pons (*arrows*). *B.* Postcontrast T1-weighted image demonstrates intense enhancement of the vestibular schwannoma (*white arrow*). Abnormal enhancement of the left fifth nerve (*black arrow*) most likely represents another schwannoma in this patient with neurofibromatosis type 2.

to complete surgical excision. Postoperative radiation therapy is unnecessary.

Dermoid cysts are thought to arise from embryonic rests of skin tissue trapped within the CNS during closure of the neural tube. The most frequent locations are in the midline supratentorially or at the cerebellopontine angle. Histologically, they are composed of all elements of the dermis, including epidermis, hair follicles, and sweat glands; they frequently calcify. Treatment is surgical excision.

Craniopharyngiomas are thought to arise from remnants of Rathke's pouch, the mesodermal structure from which the anterior pituitary gland is derived (Chap. 328). Craniopharyngiomas typically present as suprasellar masses. Histologically, craniopharyngiomas resemble epidermoid tumors; they are usually cystic, and in adults 80% are calcified. Because of their location, they may present as growth failure in children, endocrine dysfunction in adults, or visual loss in either age group. Treatment is surgical excision; postoperative external beam radiation or stereotaxic radiosurgery is added if total surgical removal cannot be achieved.

Colloid cysts are benign tumors of unknown cellular origin that occur within the third ventricle and can obstruct CSF flow. *Rare benign primary brain tumors* include neurocytomas, subependymomas, and pleomorphic xanthoastrocytomas. Surgical excision of these neoplasms is the primary treatment and can be curative.

NEUROCUTANEOUS SYNDROMES

This group of genetic disorders, also known as the *phakomatoses*, produces a variety of developmental abnormalities of skin along with an increased risk of nervous system tumors (Table 370-1). These disorders are inherited as autosomal dominant conditions with variable penetrance.

NEUROFIBROMATOSIS TYPE 1 (VON RECKLINGHAUSEN'S DISEASE) NF1 is characterized by cutaneous *neurofibromas*, pigmented lesions of the skin called *café au lait spots*, freckling in non-sun exposed areas such as the axilla, hamartomas of the iris termed Lisch nodules, and pseudoarthrosis of the tibia. Neurofibromas are benign peripheral nerve tumors composed of proliferating Schwann cells and fibroblasts. They present as multiple, palpable, rubbery, cutaneous tumors. They are generally asymptomatic; however, if they grow in an enclosed space, e.g., the intervertebral foramen, they may produce a compressive radiculopathy or neuropathy. Aqueductal stenosis with hydrocephalus, scoliosis, short stature, hypertension, epilepsy, and mental retardation may also occur.

Mutation of the *NF1* gene on chromosome 17 causes von Recklinghausen's disease. The *NF1* gene is a tumor suppressor gene; it encodes a protein, *neurofibromin*, which modulates signal transduction through the *ras* GTPase pathway. Patients with NF1 are at increased risk of developing nervous system neoplasms, including plexiform neurofibromas, optic gliomas, ependymomas, meningiomas, astrocytomas, and pheochromocytomas. Neurofibromas may undergo secondary malignant degeneration and become sarcomas.

NEUROFIBROMATOSIS TYPE 2 NF2 is characterized by the development of bilateral vestibular schwannomas in >90% of individuals who inherit the gene. Patients with NF2 also have a predisposition for the development of meningiomas, gliomas, and schwannomas of cranial and spinal nerves. In addition, a characteristic type of cataract, juvenile posterior subcapsular lenticular opacity, occurs in NF2. Multiple café au lait spots and peripheral neurofibromas occur rarely.

In patients with NF2, vestibular schwannomas usually present with progressive unilateral deafness early in the third decade of life. Bilateral vestibular schwannomas are generally detectable by MRI at that time (Fig. 370-6). Surgical management, designed to treat the underlying tumor and preserve hearing as long as possible, is difficult.

The *NF2* gene on chromosome 22q codes for a protein called *neurofibromin 2*, *schwannomin*, or *merlin*, with homology to a family of cytoskeletal proteins that includes moesin, ezrin, and radixin.

TUBEROUS SCLEROSIS (BOURNEVILLE'S DISEASE) Tuberous sclerosis is characterized by cutaneous lesions, seizures, and mental retardation. The cutaneous lesions include adenoma sebaceum (facial angiofibromas), ash leaf–shaped hypopigmented macules (best seen under ultraviolet illumination with a Wood's lamp), shagreen patches (yellowish thickenings of the skin over the lumbosacral region of the back), and depigmented nevi. On neuroimaging studies, the presence of subependymal nodules, which may be calcified, is characteristic. Patients inheriting the tuberous sclerosis gene are at increased risk of developing ependymomas and childhood astrocytomas, of which >90% are *subependymal giant cell astrocytomas*. These are benign neoplasms that may develop in the retina or along the border of the lateral ventricles. They may obstruct the foramen of Monro and produce hydrocephalus. Rhabdomyomas of the myocardium and angiomyomas of the kidney, liver, adrenals, and pancreas may also occur.

Treatment is symptomatic. Anticonvulsants for seizures, shunting for hydrocephalus, and behavioral and educational strategies for mental retardation are the mainstays of management. Severely affected individuals generally die before age 30.

Mutations at both 9q(TSC-1) and 16p(TSC-2) are associated with tuberous sclerosis. The mutated genes code for *tuberins*, proteins that modulate the GTPase activity of other cellular proteins.

VON HIPPEL–LINDAU SYNDROME This syndrome consists of retinal, cerebellar, and spinal hemangioblastomas, which are slowly growing cystic tumors. Hypernephroma, renal cell carcinoma, pheochromocytoma, and cysts of the kidneys, pancreas, epididymis, or liver may also occur. Erythropoietin production by hemangioblastomas may result in polycythemia. The von Hippel–Lindau (VHL) tumor suppressor gene on chromosome 3p encodes a protein that appears to suppress transcription elongation by RNA polymerase II.

TUMORS METASTATIC TO BRAIN

MECHANISMS OF BRAIN METASTASES The large majority of brain metastases disseminate by hematogenous spread. The anatomic distribution of brain metastases generally parallels regional cerebral blood flow, with a predilection for the gray matter–white matter junction and for the border zone between middle cerebral and posterior cerebral artery distributions. The lung is the most common origin of brain metastases; both primary lung cancer and cancers metastatic to the lung can metastasize to the brain. Breast cancer has a propensity to metastasize to the cerebellum and the posterior pituitary gland. This propensity could be explained by patterns of retrograde venous flow from the thorax into the skull or by an especially hospitable environment for breast cancer cells provided by the cerebellum and pituitary (the "seed and soil" hypothesis).

Lung cancer (adenocarcinoma and small cell lung cancer), breast cancer (especially ductal carcinoma), gastrointestinal malignancies, and melanoma are common tumors that metastasize to brain (Table 370-2). Certain less common tumors have a special propensity to metastasize to brain, including germ cell tumors and thyroid cancer. By contrast, prostate cancer, ovarian cancer, and Hodgkin's disease rarely metastasize to the brain. Moreover, breast cancer that metastasizes to bone tends not to metastasize to the brain. Therefore, the cellular environment of the brain is hospitable to only a subset of systemic cancers. Parenchymal spinal cord metastases are rare.

EVALUATION OF METASTASES FROM KNOWN CANCER On MRI scans brain metastases typically appear as well-demarcated, approximately spherical lesions that are hypointense or isointense relative to brain on T1-weighted images and bright on T2-weighted images. They invariably enhance with gadolinium, reflecting extravasation of gadolinium through tumor vessels that lack a blood-tumor barrier (Fig. 370-7). Small metastases often enhance uniformly. Larger metastases typically produce ring enhancement surrounding a central mass of nonenhancing necrotic tissue that develops as the metastasis outgrows its blood supply. Metastases are surrounded by variable amounts of edema. Blood products may also be seen, reflecting hemorrhage of abnormal tumor vessels.

The radiologic appearance of a brain metastasis is not specific. The differential diagnosis of ring-enhancement lesions includes brain abscess, radiation necrosis, toxoplasmosis, granulomas (tuberculosis, sarcoidosis), demyelinating lesions, primary brain tumors, primary CNS lymphoma, stroke, hemorrhage, and trauma. Contrast-enhanced CT scanning is less sensitive than MRI for the detection of brain metastases. Cytologic examination of the CSF is not indicated, since intraparenchymal brain metastases almost never shed cells into CSF. Measuring CSF levels of tumor markers such as carcinoembryonic antigen (CEA) is rarely helpful in management.

BRAIN METASTASES WITHOUT A KNOWN PRIMARY TUMOR In general hospital populations, up to one-third of patients presenting with brain metastases do not have a known underlying cancer. These patients generally present with either a seizure or a progressive neurologic deficit. Neuroimaging studies demonstrate one or multiple ring-enhancement lesions. In individuals who are not immunocompromised and not at risk for brain abscesses, this radiologic pattern is most likely due to brain metastasis.

Diagnostic evaluation begins with a search for the primary tumor. Blood tests should include CEA and liver function tests. A careful examination of the skin for melanoma and the thyroid gland for masses should be carried out. A CT scan of the chest, abdomen, and pelvis should be obtained. If these are all negative, further imaging studies, including bone scan, other radionuclide scans, and upper and lower gastrointestinal barium studies, are unlikely to be productive. The search for a primary cancer most often discloses lung cancer, particularly small cell lung cancer, or melanoma. In 30% of patients no primary tumor can be identified even after extensive evaluation.

A tissue diagnosis is essential. If a primary tumor is found, it will usually be more

Table 370-2 Frequency of Primary Tumors that Metastasize to the Nervous System

Site of Primary Tumor	Brain Metastases, %	Leptomeningeal Metastases, %	Spinal Cord Compression, %
Lung	40	24	18
Breast	19	41	24
Melanoma	10	12	4
Gastrointestinal tract	7	13	6
Genitourinary tract	7		18
Other	17	10	30

accessible to biopsy than a brain lesion. If a single brain lesion is found in a surgically accessible location, if a primary tumor is not found, or if the primary tumor is in a location difficult to biopsy, the brain metastasis should be biopsied or resected.

TREATMENT Once a systemic cancer metastasizes to the brain it is, with rare exception, incurable. Therapy is therefore palliative, designed to prevent disability and suffering and, if possible, to prolong life. Published outcome studies have focused on survival as the primary end point, leaving questions regarding quality of life unanswered. There is, however, widespread agreement that glucocorticoids, anticonvulsants, and radiation therapy improve the quality of life for many patients. The roles of surgery and chemotherapy are less well established.

General Measures High-dose glucocorticoids frequently ameliorate symptoms of brain metastases. Improvement is often dramatic, occurs within 6 to 24 h, and is sustained with continued administration, although the toxicity of glucocorticoids is cumulative. Therefore, if possible, a more definitive therapy for metastases should be instituted to permit withdrawal of glucocorticoid therapy. One-third of patients with brain metastases have one or more seizures. Anticonvulsants are empirically used for seizure prophylaxis when supratentorial metastases are present.

Specific Measures • *Radiation therapy* Radiation is the primary treatment for brain metastases. Since multiple microscopic deposits of tumor cells throughout the brain are likely to be present in addition to metastases visualized by neuroimaging studies, whole-brain irradiation is usually used. Its benefit has been established in controlled studies, but no clear dose response has been shown. Usually, 30–37.5 Gy is administered in 10 to 15 fractions; an additional dose

FIGURE 370-7 Brain metastasis. *A.* Axial T2-weighted MRI through the lateral ventricles reveals two isodense masses, one in the subependymal region and one near the cortex (*arrows*). *B.* T1-weighted postcontrast image at the same level as *A* reveals enhancement of the two masses seen on the T2-weighted image as well as a third mass in the left frontal lobe (*arrows*).

("boost") of focal irradiation to a single or large metastasis may also be administered.

Surgery Up to 40% of patients with brain metastases have only a single tumor mass identified by CT. Accessible single metastases are usually surgically excised as a palliative measure. If the systemic disease is under control, total resection of a single brain lesion has been demonstrated to improve survival and minimize disability. Survival appears to be improved if surgery is followed by whole-brain irradiation.

Chemotherapy Brain metastases of certain tumors, including breast cancer, small cell lung cancer, and germ cell tumors, are often responsive to systemic chemotherapy. Although metastases frequently do not respond as well as the primary tumor, dramatic responses to systemic chemotherapy or hormonal therapy may occur in some cases. In patients who are neurologically stable, two to four cycles of systemic chemotherapy may be administered initially to reduce tumor mass and render the residual tumor more amenable to radiation therapy. Even if a complete radiologic remission is achieved from chemotherapy, whole-brain irradiation should then be administered.

Experimental therapies These include stereotaxic radiosurgery, gene therapy, immunotherapy, intraarterial chemotherapy, and chemotherapy administered following osmotic disruption of the blood-brain barrier.

LEPTOMENINGEAL METASTASES

Leptomeningeal metastases are also called *carcinomatous meningitis*, *meningeal carcinomatosis*, and, in the cases of specific tumors, *leukemic meningitis* or *lymphomatous meningitis*. Clinical evidence of leptomeningeal metastases is present in 8% of patients with metastatic solid tumors; at necropsy, the prevalence is as high as 19%. Among solid tumors, adenocarcinomas of the breast and lung and melanoma are most often responsible (Table 370-2). In one-quarter of patients the systemic cancer is under control; thus effective control of leptomeningeal disease can improve the quality and duration of life.

Pathologically, three patterns of tumor involvement may be seen: (1) a diffuse coating of the leptomeninges by a thin layer of tumor cells, (2) nodular growth of macroscopic tumor metastases in meninges and on nerve roots, or (3) plaque-like metastases in the leptomeninges with many cells shed into the subarachnoid space and extension of tumor into Virchow-Robin spaces. Leptomeningeal metastases may coexist with parenchymal CNS metastases.

Cancer usually metastasizes to the meninges via the bloodstream. Alternatively, a superficially located parenchymal metastasis may shed cells directly into the subarachnoid space. Some tumors, including squamous cell carcinoma of the skin and some non-Hodgkin's lymphomas, have a propensity to grow along peripheral nerves and may seed the meninges by that route.

CLINICAL FEATURES Leptomeningeal metastases present with signs and symptoms at multiple levels of the nervous system, most often in a setting of known systemic malignancy. Encephalopathy is frequent, and cranial neuropathy or spinal radiculopathy from nodular nerve root compression is characteristic. Hydrocephalus results from obstruction of CSF outflow in the posterior fossa. Focal neurologic deficits from coexisting intraparenchymal metastases may occur.

LABORATORY EVALUATION Leptomeningeal metastases are diagnosed by cytologic demonstration of malignant cells in the CSF, by MRI demonstration of nodular tumor deposits in the meninges or diffuse meningeal enhancement (Fig. 370-8), or by meningeal biopsy. CSF findings are usually those of an inflammatory meningitis, consisting of lymphocytic pleocytosis, elevated protein levels, and normal or low CSF glucose. A complete MRI examination of the neuraxis may demonstrate hydrocephalus due to obstruction of CSF pathways and identify nodular meningeal metastases.

FIGURE 370-8 Carcinomatous meningitis. Sagittal postcontrast MRI through the lower thoracic region demonstrates diffuse pial enhancement along the surface of the spinal cord (*arrows*), typical of CSF spread of neoplasm.

℞ **TREATMENT** In selected patients, intrathecal chemotherapy and focal external beam radiotherapy to sites of leptomeningeal disease are the mainstays of management. Although the prognosis of leptomeningeal metastases is poor, approximately 20% of patients aggressively treated for leptomeningeal metastases can expect a sustained response of approximately 6 months. Intrathecal therapy exposes meningeal tumor to high concentrations of chemotherapy with minimal systemic toxicity. Methotrexate can be safely administered intrathecally and is effective against leptomeningeal metastases from a variety of solid tumors and lymphoma; ara-C and thio-TEPA are alternative agents. Intrathecal chemotherapy may be administered either by repeated lumbar puncture or through an indwelling Ommaya reservoir, which consists of a catheter in one lateral ventricle attached to a reservoir implanted under the scalp. If there is a question of patency of CSF pathways, a radionuclide flow study may be performed.

Large deposits of tumor on the meninges or along nerve roots are unlikely to respond to intrathecal chemotherapy, as the barrier to diffusion is too great. Therefore, external beam radiation is employed. Hydrocephalus is treated with a ventriculoperitoneal shunt, although seeding of the peritoneum by tumor is a risk.

MALIGNANT SPINAL CORD COMPRESSION

Spinal cord compression from solid tumor metastases usually results from expansion of a vertebral metastasis into the epidural space. Primary tumors that frequently metastasize to bone include lung, breast, and prostate cancer. Back pain is usually the first symptom and is prominent at presentation in 90% of patients. The pain is typically dull, aching, and may be associated with localized tenderness. If a nerve root is compressed, radicular pain is also present. The neurologic signs that accompany spinal cord compression are determined by the spinal level of the lesion; the thoracic cord is most often affected. Weakness, sensory loss, and autonomic dysfunction (urinary urgency and incontinence, fecal incontinence, and sexual impotence in men) are the hallmarks of spinal cord compression. Once signs of spinal cord compression appear, they tend to progress rapidly. It is thus essential to recognize and treat this devastating complication of malignancy at the earliest possible time in order to prevent irreversible neurologic deficits. →*Diagnosis and management are discussed in Chap. 368.*

Systemic cancer may compress or invade peripheral nerves. Compression of the brachial plexus may occur by direct extension of Pancoast's tumors (cancer of the apex of the lung) or by extension of local lymph node metastases of breast or lung cancer or lymphoma. The lumbosacral plexus may be compressed by the retroperitoneal spread of prostate or ovarian cancer or lymphoma. Skull metastases may compress cranial nerve branches as they pass through the skull, and pituitary metastases may extend into the cavernous sinus. The epineurium generally provides an effective barrier to invasion of the peripheral nerves by solid tumors, but certain tumors characteristically invade and spread along peripheral nerves. Squamous cell carcinoma of the skin may spread along branches of the trigeminal nerve and extend intracranially. Non-Hodgkin's lymphoma may be neurotrophic and cause a syndrome resembling mononeuropathy multiplex. Focal external beam radiation may reduce pain, prevent irreversible loss of peripheral nerve function, and possibly restore function.

In patients with cancer who have brachial or lumbosacral plexopathy, it may be difficult to distinguish tumor invasion from radiation injury. High radiation dose or the presence of myokymia (rippling contractions of muscle) suggests radiation injury, whereas pain suggests tumor. Radiographic imaging studies may be equivocal, and surgical exploration is sometimes required.

COMPLICATIONS OF THERAPY

RADIATION TOXICITY The nervous system is vulnerable to delayed injury by therapeutic radiation. The mechanism of injury is unknown, but radiation-induced free radical production is probably contributory. Histologically, there is demyelination, hyaline degeneration of small arterioles, and eventually brain infarction and necrosis. However, radiation injury can occur without vasculopathy, suggesting that ischemia is a late manifestation and does not account entirely for the tissue damage.

Radiation injury to the brain is classified by the time of its occurrence. *Acute radiation injury* occurs during or immediately after therapy. It is rarely seen with current protocols of external beam radiation but may occur after stereotaxic radiosurgery. Manifestations include headache, sleepiness, and worsening of preexisting neurologic deficits. *Early delayed radiation injury* occurs within 4 months of therapy. It is associated with an increased white matter T2 signal on MRI scans.

In children, the *somnolence syndrome* is a common form of early delayed radiation injury in which somnolence and ataxia develop after whole-brain irradiation. Irradiation of the cervical spine may cause Lhermitte's phenomenon, an electricity-like sensation evoked by neck flexion (Chap. 368). Acute and early delayed radiation injury are steroid-responsive and self-limited disorders and do not appear to increase the risk of late radiation injury.

Late delayed radiation injury produces permanent damage to the nervous system. It occurs more than 4 months (generally 8 to 24 months) after completion of therapy; onset 15 years after therapy has been described. After whole-brain irradiation, progressive dementia can occur, sometimes accompanied by gait apraxia. White matter signal abnormalities are present on MRI studies (Fig. 370-9). Following focal brain irradiation, radiation necrosis occurs within the radiation field, producing a contrast-enhanced mass, frequently with ring enhancement. MRI or CT scans are often unable to distinguish radiation necrosis from recurrent tumor, but PET or SPECT scans may demonstrate that glucose metabolism is increased in tumor tissue but decreased in radiation necrosis. Biopsy is frequently required to establish the correct diagnosis. Peripheral nerves, including the brachial and lumbosacral plexuses, may also develop late delayed radiation injury over a time span similar to that observed in the CNS.

If untreated, radiation necrosis of the CNS may act as an expanding mass lesion, although it may resolve spontaneously or after steroid treatment. Progressive radiation necrosis is best treated with surgical resection if the patient has a life expectancy of at least 6 months and a good Karnofsky performance score. There are anecdotal reports that anticoagulation with heparin or coumadin may be beneficial. Radiation injury also accelerates the development of atherosclerosis in large arteries, but an increase in the risk of stroke becomes significant only years after radiation treatment.

Endocrine dysfunction frequently follows exposure of the hypothalamus or pituitary gland to therapeutic radiation. Growth hormone is the pituitary hormone most sensitive to radiation therapy, and thyroid-stimulating hormone is the least sensitive; ACTH, prolactin, and the gonadotropins have an intermediate sensitivity.

Development of a second neoplasm is another risk of therapeutic radiation that generally occurs many years after radiation exposure. Depending on the irradiated field, the risk of gliomas, meningiomas, sarcomas, and thyroid cancer is increased.

FIGURE 370-9 Radiation injury. *A.* Late-delayed radiation injury 1 year after whole-brain radiation (5500 cGy). T2-weighted MR image at the level of the temporal lobes reveals high signal intensity abnormality in periventricular white matter (*arrows*). *B* and *C.* Focal radiation necrosis 3 years after radiotherapy (7000 cGy) for carcinoma of the nasopharynx. Axial T2-weighted MRI (*B*) demonstrates a mass in the right frontal lobe with surrounding vasogenic edema. Abnormal signal changes are also present on the left. T1-weighted postcontrast MRI (*C*) reveals a heterogeneously enhancing mass in the right cingulate gyrus.

COMPLICATIONS OF CHEMOTHERAPY   Chemotherapy regimens used to treat primary brain tumors have generally included a nitrosourea and are well tolerated. Infrequently, nitrosoureas and other drugs used to treat CNS neoplasms cause altered mental states (e.g., confusion, depression), ataxia, and seizures. Chemotherapy for systemic malignancy is a more frequent cause of nervous system toxicity. Cisplatin commonly produces tinnitus and high-frequency bilateral hearing loss, especially in younger patients. At cumulative doses >450 mg/m^2, cisplatin can produce a symmetric, large fiber axonal predominantly sensory neuropathy; paclitaxel (Taxol) produces a similar picture. Fluorouracil and high-dose cytosine arabinoside can cause cerebellar dysfunction that resolves after discontinuation of therapy. Vincristine, which is commonly used to treat lymphoma, may cause an acute ileus and is frequently associated with development of a progressive distal, symmetric sensory-motor neuropathy with foot drop and paresthesias.

BIBLIOGRAPHY

BIGNER DD, MCLENDON RE, BRUNER JM (eds): *Russell and Rubinstein's Pathology of Tumors of the Nervous System.* New York, Oxford Univ Press, 1998

BIGNER SH: Cerebrospinal fluid cytology: Current status and diagnostic applications. J Neuropath Exp Neurol 51:235, 1992

BYRNE TN: Spinal cord compression from epidural metastases. N Engl J Med 327:614, 1992

CAIRNCROSS JG et al: Specific genetic predictors of chemotherapeutic response and survival in patients with anaplastic oligodendrogliomas. J Natl Cancer Inst 90:1473, 1998

GUTMANN DH et al: The diagnostic evaluation and multidisciplinary management of neurofibromatosis 1 and neurofibromatosis 2. JAMA 278:51, 1997

KORI SH et al: Brachial plexus lesions in patients with cancer: 100 cases. Neurology 31:45, 1981

MAHER ER, KAELIN WG: von Hippel-Lindau disease. Medicine 76:381, 1997

MCKUSICK VA (ed): *Online Mendelian Inheritance in Man.* URL: www.ncbi.nlm.nih.gov/Omim/. Washington, DC, National Library of Medicine, 1999

MECKLING S et al: Malignant supratentorial glioma in the elderly: Is radiotherapy useful? Neurology 47:901, 1996

NG H-K, LAM PYP: The molecular genetics of central nervous system tumors. Pathology 30:196, 1998

OLSON JD et al: Long-term outcome of low-grade oligodendroglioma and mixed glioma. Neurology 54:1442, 2000

PATCHELL RA et al: A randomized trial of surgery in the treatment of single metastases to the brain. N Engl J Med 322:494, 1990

POSNER JB: *Neurologic Complications of Cancer.* Philadelphia, FA Davis, 1995

SKLAR CA, CONSTINE LS: Chronic neuroendocrinological sequelae of radiation therapy. Int J Radiation Oncol Biol Phys 31:1113, 1995

VON DEIMLING A et al: Molecular pathways in the formation of gliomas. Glia 15:328, 1995

WILSON CB: Meningiomas: Genetics, malignancy, and the role of radiation in induction and treatment. J Neurosurg 81:666, 1994

371	*Stephen L. Hauser, Donald E. Goodkin*

MULTIPLE SCLEROSIS AND OTHER DEMYELINATING DISEASES

ADEM acute disseminated encephalomyelitis	MOG myelin oligodendrocyte glycoprotein
CNS central nervous system	MRI magnetic resonance imaging
CSF cerebrospinal fluid	MS multiple sclerosis
EAE experimental allergic encephalomyelitis	PNS peripheral nervous system
IFN interferon	PPMS primary progressive MS
IL interleukin	RRMS relapsing-remitting MS
MBP myelin basic protein	SPMS secondary progressive MS
MHC major histocompatibility complex	TNF tumor necrosis factor

The demyelinating diseases occupy a unique place in neurology owing to their frequency; tendency to strike young adults; diversity of manifestations; and range of fundamental questions in neurobiology, immunology, virology, and genetics that arise regarding their pathogenesis. These disorders share features of inflammation and selective destruction of central nervous system (CNS) myelin; the peripheral nervous system (PNS) is spared. No specific tests for the demyelinating diseases exist, and diagnosis is based on recognition of the distinctive clinical patterns of CNS injury they produce.

MULTIPLE SCLEROSIS

Multiple sclerosis (MS) is characterized by (1) a relapsing-remitting or progressive course and (2) a pathologic triad of CNS inflammation, demyelination, and gliosis (scarring). Lesions of MS are classically said to be *disseminated* in time and space. MS affects approximately 350,000 Americans and 1.1 million individuals worldwide. In Western societies, MS is second only to trauma as a cause of neurologic disability arising in early to middle adulthood. Current evidence indicates that MS is an autoimmune disease that develops in genetically susceptible individuals who have resided in certain permissive environments. Manifestations of MS vary from a benign illness to a rapidly evolving and incapacitating disease requiring profound adjustments in life-style and goals for patients and their families. Complications from MS affect multiple body systems; hence, a multidisciplinary approach is recommended to optimize clinical care.

PATHOGENESIS   Anatomy   MS derives its name from the multiple scarred areas visible on macroscopic examination of the brain. These lesions, termed *plaques*, are sharply demarcated gray or pink areas easily distinguished from surrounding white matter. Plaques vary in size from 1 or 2 mm to several centimeters. The acute MS lesion, rarely found at autopsy, consists of perivenular cuffing by inflammatory mononuclear cells, predominantly T lymphocytes and macrophages, which also infiltrate white matter tissue and appear to orchestrate demyelination. At sites of inflammation, the blood-brain barrier is disrupted but the vessel wall itself is preserved, distinguishing the MS lesion from vasculitis. In some inflammatory lesions, a distinctive pattern of myelin damage, termed *vesicular demyelination*, can be appreciated. This change consists of dissolution of the multilamellated compact myelin sheaths that surround axon cylinders and their reconstitution as a lattice-like network of myelin membrane fragments. Myelin-specific autoantibodies (see "Immunology," below) are bound to the vesiculated myelin membranes, at least in some patients; these autoantibodies are thought to promote demyelination and stimulate macrophages and microglial cells (specialized CNS phagocytes of bone marrow origin) that scavenge the myelin debris. As lesions evolve, astrocytes proliferate extensively (gliosis). Oligodendrocytes, the myelin-producing cells, also proliferate initially in most MS lesions, but these cells are often destroyed as the infiltration and gliosis progress. Surviving oligodendrocytes or those that newly differentiate from a precursor pool may partially remyelinate naked axons, resulting in *shadow plaques*. MS lesions may enlarge by gradual concentric outward growth; some chronic plaques display histologic gradations of increasing acuity from the center to the lesion edge.

The correspondence between number and size of plaques ("plaque burden") and the severity of clinical symptoms is imprecise. Hence, an extensive plaque burden may be associated with mild symptoms; or, conversely, seemingly minor pathologic changes may be present in some severely disabled individuals. Occasional cases either are clinically silent or produce "nonspecific" isolated symptoms such as facial pain, and evidence of MS is found unexpectedly at autopsy.

Recent ultrastructural studies of MS lesions suggest that different underlying pathologies may be present in different patients. Heterogeneity has been identified both in terms of the fate (i.e., death or survival) of oligodendrocytes in plaques and by the presence or absence of antibody and complement deposition. In primary progressive MS (PPMS; see below), a distinctive oligodendroglial cytopathy has been reported based on examination of a limited number of cases; if confirmed, this finding would suggest that PPMS is a unique disorder. Finally, although selective demyelination with sparing of axon cylinders is the hallmark of MS, partial or total axonal destruction, and in extreme cases cavitation, may also occur. The extent of axonal loss appears to correlate with irreversible neurologic disability. Axonal loss and cavitation are particularly prominent in the subtype of MS known as neuromyelitis optica or Devic's syndrome (see below).

Physiology Demyelination may have either negative or positive effects on axonal conduction. *Negative conduction abnormalities* consist of slowed axonal conduction, variable conduction block that occurs in the presence of high- but not low-frequency volleys of impulses, or complete conduction block. Conduction block in demyelinated fibers may also occur in response to raised temperature or metabolic derangements. The mechanism of conduction block appears to involve a hyperpolarization of the resting axon potential due to the exposure of voltage-dependent potassium channels that are normally buried underneath the myelin sheath. *Positive conduction abnormalities* include generation of ectopic impulses, spontaneously or after mechanical deformation, and abnormal "crosstalk" between demyelinated axons. Variable conduction block may explain the fluctuations in function that vary from hour to hour and from day to day in many patients and the characteristic worsening that is associated with fever or exercise. Ectopic impulse generation or "crosstalk" might give rise to Lhermitte's symptom, paroxysmal symptoms, or paresthesias (see below). Experimental therapies designed to alleviate conduction abnormalities in MS have included the use of calcium channel blockers to reduce the threshold for impulse generation and pharmacologic blockade (with 4-aminopyridine) of potassium channels.

Epidemiology MS is approximately twice as common in females as in males. In both sexes, the incidence rises steadily from adolescence to age 35 and declines gradually thereafter. The mean age of onset is slightly later in men than in women, due in part to a relative overrepresentation of males in PPMS, which has a later mean age of onset. MS beginning as early as age two years or as late as the eighth decade of life is rare but well documented. Various epidemiologic observations, summarized below, support of the role of an environmental exposure of some type in MS.

Location and risk MS is primarily a disease of individuals living in temperate climates. The prevalence increases with increasing distance from the equator; this finding appears to be true in both the northern and southern hemispheres. Prevalence rates and north-south gradients are generally similar in North America and Europe. The highest known prevalence (250 per 100,000) occurs in the Orkney islands, located north of the mainland of Scotland, and MS is also common throughout Scandinavia and northern Europe. Numerous studies also suggest that location influences MS risk. For example, the prevalence of MS is low in Japan (2 per 100,000) but moderate (15 per 100,000) in Japanese Americans.

Changes in prevalence Studies from the United States, Europe, and Australia suggest that the prevalence of MS may have increased during the twentieth century, however these findings could represent an artifact due to improved detection of cases in the modern era.

Reported clusters Several possible point epidemics of MS have been described, the most convincing of which occurred in the Faeroe Islands off the coast of Denmark after the British occupation during World War II.

GENETIC CONSIDERATIONS An inherent genetic susceptibility to MS exists, as summarized by the following observations:

Risk in Different Ethnic Groups The prevalence of MS differs among ethnic groups that reside in the same environment. In the United States, the prevalence of MS is higher in Caucasians than in other racial groups, consistent with observations in other parts of the world.

Familial Aggregation First-, second-, and third-degree relatives of patients with MS are at increased risk for the disease. Siblings of affected individuals have a lifetime risk of ~5%, whereas the risk to parents or children of affected individuals is somewhat lower. Studies

of adoptees, half-siblings, and spouses of patients with MS strongly indicate that familial aggregation is primarily determined by shared genetic, and not environmental, factors.

Twin Studies The most compelling evidence for a genetic effect on MS is derived from twin studies, which demonstrate concordance rates of ~30% in monozygotic twins and 5% in dizygotic twins (similar to the risk in nontwin siblings).

The inheritance of MS cannot be explained with a simple genetic model. A single-gene hypothesis is at odds with concordance estimates in twin and family studies and with the observed nonlinear decrease in disease risk as the genetic distance from the MS proband is increased. It is likely that susceptibility is determined by multiple independent genetic loci (polygenic inheritance), each with a relatively small contribution to the overall risk. It is also possible that different genetic causes of susceptibility to MS (genetic heterogeneity) may exist. Linkage and association studies have identified the major histocompatibility complex (MHC) on chromosome 6 as one genetic determinant for MS. This complex encodes the histocompatibility antigens (the HLA system) that present peptide antigens to T cells. The class II (HLA-D) region of the MHC is most strongly associated with MS, and susceptibility appears to result from the presence of the DR2 allele and its corresponding haplotype, defined by molecular criteria as DRB1*1501, DQA1*0102, DQB1*0602. Other genetic regions implicated in MS susceptibility include loci on chromosomes 3, 5, 16, and 19. ■

Immunology MS appears to be an autoimmune disease mediated, at least in part, by T lymphocytes. Evidence in support of this concept is derived from analogy to the laboratory model experimental allergic encephalomyelitis (EAE) and from direct studies of the immune system of MS patients.

Autoreactive T lymphocytes Myelin basic protein (MBP) is an important T cell antigen in EAE and probably also in human MS. In patients with MS but not in unaffected individuals activated MBP-reactive T cells can be identified in the peripheral blood. In cerebrospinal fluid (CSF), the frequency of T cells reactive against MBP (and other myelin proteins) is also higher in patients with MS than in unaffected individuals. Direct evidence that MBP-reactive T cells are present in MS lesions has also been suggested by sequence analysis of the antigen-binding domain of T cell receptor molecules cloned from plaque tissue. The susceptibility gene DR2 may influence the immune response to MBP because it binds with high affinity to a fragment of MBP spanning amino acids 89 to 101; this region of MBP appears to be immunodominant for T cell responses in DR2-positive individuals.

Autoantibodies Increasing evidence suggests that autoantibodies play some role in MS, probably acting in concert with a pathogenic T cell response. In EAE, autoantibodies directed against myelin oligodendrocyte glycoprotein (MOG), a quantitatively minor myelin protein, were found to mediate MS-like demyelinating lesions; and recently anti-MOG antibodies were also detected in actively demyelinating MS lesions. MOG is thus a good candidate as a humoral autoantigen in MS. Evidence of an abnormal humoral immune response is present in the CSF of patients with MS. Membrane attack complexes can be detected in the CSF, suggesting a role for complement-mediated antibody damage. Elevated levels of immunoglobulin are easily measured and are characteristic of CSF in MS. Oligoclonal antibody—derived from expansion of a small number of different molecules—is also present in most cases. Oligoclonal immunoglobulin is also detected in other chronic inflammatory responses, including infections, and thus is not specific to MS. It is synthesized locally, and the specific pattern is unique to each patient. Attempts to identify an antigen against which most oligoclonal immunoglobulin is directed have been unsuccessful.

Cytokines Numerous cytokines and chemokines have been detected in brain, CSF, and peripheral blood of patients with MS, and it is probable that these molecules regulate many of the cellular interactions that operate in this disease (Chap. 305). By analogy to EAE T_H1 cytokines that regulate cellular immunity, including interleukin (IL) 2, tumor necrosis factor (TNF) α, and interferon (IFN) γ have traditionally been thought to be central to MS pathogenesis. TNF-α or IFN-γ may contribute directly to tissue damage by injuring oligodendrocytes or the myelin membrane. Unfortunately, treatment strategies designed to blunt the T_H1 response have thus far not been successful in treating MS. Furthermore, a recent clinical trial with a humanized antibody to TNF-α appeared to worsen MS. The identification of autoantibodies in MS suggests that T_H2 cytokines (including IL-4, IL-5, and IL-10) may play a pathogenic role in MS, and may explain why the results of T_H1-based approaches have been disappointing.

Triggers Magnetic resonance imaging (MRI) scans indicate that many patients with relapsing forms of MS have bursts of multifocal inflammation that occur approximately monthly, or 7 to 10 times more frequently than clinical attacks. This finding suggests the presence of a large reservoir of subclinical disease in MS. Bursts appear to be associated with the migration of activated T cells from the peripheral blood across the blood-brain barrier and into brain; the triggers responsible for these bursts are not known. Patients may experience relapses after nonspecific upper respiratory infections, suggesting that molecular mimicry between viruses and myelin antigens may trigger attacks, or that some viruses may function as superantigens capable of activating disease-inducing T cells in MS (Chap. 305).

Microbiology As noted above, epidemiologic evidence supports the role of an environmental exposure in MS. MS risk also correlates with high socioeconomic status, which may reflect improved sanitation and delayed initial exposures to infectious agents. Some viruses, e.g., poliomyelitis and measles viruses, produce neurologic sequelae more frequently when the age of initial infection is delayed. The most widely studied experimental model of virus-induced demyelinating disease is infection with Theiler virus, a murine coronavirus similar to measles virus and canine distemper virus. Infection with some Theiler strains produces a chronic infection of oligodendrocytes with multifocal perivascular lymphocytic infiltration and demyelination, closely resembling lesions of MS.

In patients with MS, high antibody titers have been reported in serum and CSF against many viruses, including measles, herpes simplex, varicella, rubella, Epstein-Barr, and influenza C and some parainfluenza strains. Furthermore, numerous viruses and bacteria (or their genomic sequences) have been recovered from MS tissues and fluids. The most recent claims have involved human herpes virus type 6 (HHV-6) and chlamydia pneumoniae. A causal role for any infectious agent in MS remains unproven.

CLINICAL MANIFESTATIONS The onset of MS may be abrupt or insidious. Symptoms may be severe or seem so trivial that a patient may not seek medical attention for months or years. Initial symptoms are commonly one or more of the following: weakness or diminished dexterity in one or more limbs, a disturbance of gait, optic neuritis, sensory disturbance, diplopia, and ataxia (Table 371-1).

Weakness of the limbs may manifest as fatigue, disturbance of gait,

or loss of dexterity. Initially, weakness may be detected only after physical exertion. Weakness is frequently accompanied by pyramidal signs including increased motor tone (spasticity), hyperreflexia, an extensor plantar response, and an absent superficial abdominal reflex. Occasionally, a tendon reflex may be lost (simulating a peripheral nerve lesion) if afferent fibers of the motor reflex arc are disrupted by a lesion in the dorsal root entry zone.

Optic neuritis generally presents as diminished acuity, dimness, or color desaturation in the central field of vision. These symptoms may be mild or progress over hours or days to severe visual loss, or rarely to complete loss of light perception. Visual symptoms are generally monocular but may occur bilaterally. Periorbital pain frequently precedes or accompanies diminished visual acuity and may be aggravated by eye movement. An afferent pupillary response (Fig. 28-2) may be detected by a swinging flashlight test. Funduscopic examination may be normal or reveal swelling of the optic disc (papillitis). Venous sheathing of retinal vessels, due to the transendothelial migration of lymphocytes, is occasionally present. Pallor of the optic disc (optic atrophy) commonly follows an episode of optic neuritis. Uveitis occurs rarely.

Visual blurring in MS may result from optic neuritis or diplopia. These two causes are distinguished by asking the patient to cover each eye sequentially and observing whether the visual difficulty clears. *Diplopia* may result from an internuclear ophthalmoplegia (INO) or extraocular muscle weakness of the sixth (or rarely the third or fourth) cranial nerves. An INO consists of impaired or slowed adduction of one eye from a lesion in the ipsilateral medial longitudinal fasciculus. This tract connects the sixth cranial nerve nucleus with the contralateral third nerve nucleus. Prominent nystagmus is often observed in the abducting eye, along with a small skew deviation. An INO can resemble an isolated medial rectus palsy. Convergence is often preserved in INO, helping to differentiate between these two entities. The finding of bilateral INO is highly suggestive of MS. Other common gaze disturbances in MS include a horizontal gaze palsy due to an ipsilateral lesion in the abducens nucleus or the paramediam pontine reticular formation, a "one and a half" syndrome from a horizontal gaze palsy plus an INO, and acquired pendular nystagmus.

Sensory symptoms commonly include paresthesias (tingling, "pins and needles," or painful burning) or hypesthesia (numbness or a "dead" feeling). Complaints of unpleasant feelings of "swollen," "wet,", "raw", or "tightly wrapped" body parts are common. Sensory symptoms often begin in a focal area of a limb, the torso, or the head and spread over hours or days to adjacent ipsilateral or contralateral areas of the body. Involvement of the trunk with a "cord level" is diagnostically helpful because it identifies the spinal cord and not the PNS as the origin of the sensory symptoms.

Ataxia of gait and limbs reflects demyelination in the cerebellum or cerebellar pathways. In advanced MS cerebellar dysarthria (scanning speech) is common. The true extent of cerebellar involvement may be uncertain when motor and sensory deficits coexist.

Bladder dysfunction manifests as urgency or hesitancy in voiding, incomplete emptying, or incontinence. Constipation is also common. One or more of these symptoms occurs at some time in most patients with MS and may be present at onset. Fecal urgency or bowel incontinence occur less commonly.

Cognitive dysfunction may be recognized early or late in the course of MS. Cognitive deficits most commonly include memory loss, impaired attention, problem-solving difficulties, slowed information processing, and difficulties in shifting between cognitive tasks. Impaired judgment and emotional liability may be evident. These symptoms impair activities of daily living in as many as 20% of patients.

Depression is experienced by ~60% of patients during the course of the illness. Suicide is 7.5-fold more common than in age-matched controls.

Fatigue occurs in most patients with MS. It may be maximum during mid-afternoon or continuous throughout the day. Symptoms of fatigue include generalized motor weakness, limited ability to concentrate or read, lassitude, and sleepiness.

Table 371-1 Initial Symptoms of MS

Symptom	Percent of Cases	Symptom	Percent of Cases
Weakness	35	Lhermitte	3
Sensory loss	37	Pain	3
Paresthesias	24	Dementia	2
Optic neuritis	36	Visual loss	2
Diplopia	15	Facial palsy	1
Ataxia	11	Impotence	1
Vertigo	6	Myokymia	1
Paroxysmal attacks	4	Epilepsy	1
Bladder	4	Falling	1

SOURCE: After WB Matthews et al, *McAlpine's Multiple Sclerosis,* New York, Churchill Livingstone, 1991.

Heat sensitivity is experienced as the appearance of new symptoms or the worsening of preexisting symptoms on exposure to heat. For example, transient visual blurring may become apparent during a hot shower or with physical exercise. It is a common phenomenon for symptoms of MS to worsen transiently, sometimes in a dramatic fashion, during the course of a febrile illness (see pseudoexacerbation, below).

Ancillary Symptoms *Lhermitte's symptom* is the sensation of a momentary electric current or shock evoked by neck flexion, other neck movements, or cough. The symptom typically radiates down the spine into the legs, but it may radiate into the arms or be provoked by movements of the lumbar spine. Lhermitte's symptom is not specific to MS; it also occurs with other spinal cord disorders, including cervical spondylosis.

Paroxysmal symptoms are brief and stereotypic. Tonic spasms consist of an unpleasant tingling or other sensation association with tonic contraction of a limb, face, or trunk. Other paroxysmal symptoms include dysarthria and ataxia, diplopia, transient unilateral paralysis, hemifacial spasm, paresthesias, and pain. Attacks may be momentary or persist for ≥30 s. They generally begin in clusters, occurring many times throughout the day, and the patient may identify precipitating factors such as hyperventilation or particular movements.

Trigeminal neuralgia, a lancinating facial pain, may also occur; features that suggest MS rather than an idiopathic etiology (Chap. 367) include onset before 50 years of age, bilateral occurrence, objective facial sensory loss, and constant rather than paroxysmal pain.

Facial weakness may resemble idiopathic Bell's palsy; however, facial weakness due to MS is generally not associated with ipsilateral loss of taste sensation or retroauricular pain (Chap. 367).

Facial myokymia, or chronic flickering contractions of the facial musculature, are also common. The movements commonly involve the orbicularis oculus muscle and appear under the eye. Facial myokymia may arise from lesions of the corticobulbar tracts or brainstem course of the facial nerve.

Vertigo may appear suddenly and in dramatic fashion with gait unsteadiness and vomiting, resembling acute labyrinthitis. A brainstem rather than end-organ origin of vertigo is suggested by the presence of coexisting trigeminal or facial nerve involvement, vertical nystagmus, or nystagmus that is unaccompanied by latency of onset, direction reversal, or fatigue (Chap. 21). Hearing loss may also occur but is uncommon.

DISEASE COURSE Approximately 85% of patients with MS experience an abrupt onset of symptoms and signs at disease onset. Thereafter, the clinical course may be characterized by acute episodes of worsening (exacerbations or relapses), gradual progression of disability, or combinations of both. Four clinical patterns are recognized by international consensus. Patients with *relapsing-remitting MS* (RRMS) experience relapses with or without complete recovery and are clinically stable between these episodes (Fig. 371-1, A and B). Approximately 50% of patients with RRMS convert to *secondary progressive MS* (SPMS) within 10 years of disease onset. The secondary progressive phase is characterized by gradual progression of disability with or without superimposed relapses (Fig. 371-1, C and D). In contrast, patients with *primary progressive MS* (PPMS) experience gradual progression of disability from onset without superimposed relapses (Fig. 371-1, E and F). Approximately 10% of patients with MS experience this clinical pattern. Patients with *progressive relapsing MS* experience gradual progression of disability from disease onset later accompanied by one or more relapses; this clinical pattern affects ~5% of patients (Fig. 376-1G).

DIAGNOSIS There is no definitive diagnostic test. Diagnostic criteria for clinically definite MS require documentation of two or more episodes of symptoms and two or more signs that reflect pathology in anatomically noncontiguous white matter tracts of the CNS (Table 371-2). Symptoms must last more than one day and occur as distinct episodes that are separated by 28 or more days. At least one of the two required signs must be present on neurological examination. The second may be documented as an abnormal paraclinical test, either

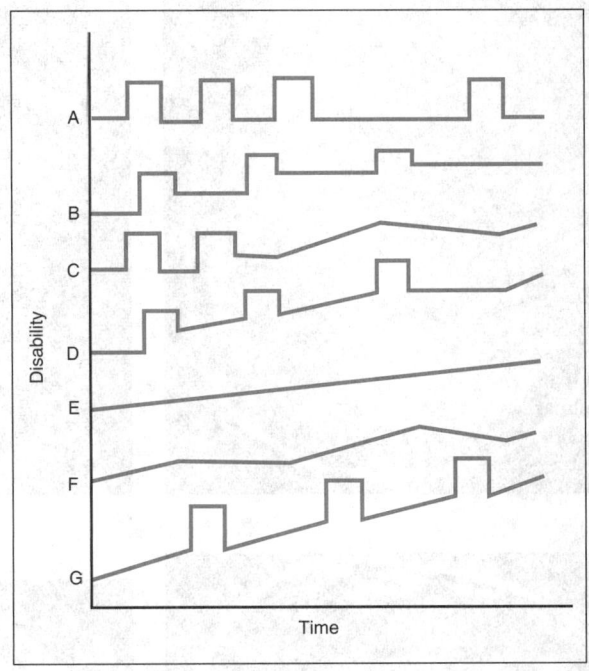

FIGURE 371-1 Clinical patterns of MS. A, B, relapsing-remitting; C, D, secondary progressive; E, F, primary progressive; G, progressive relapsing.

Table 371-2 Diagnostic Criteria for MS

1. Examination must reveal *objective* abnormalities of the CNS.
2. Involvement must reflect predominantly disease of white matter long tracts, usually including (a) pyramidal pathways, (b) cerebellar pathways, (c) medial longitudinal fasciculus, (d) optic nerve, and (e) posterior columns.
3. Examination or history must implicate involvement of two or more areas of the CNS.
   a. MRI may be used to document a *second* lesion when only one site of abnormality has been demonstrable on examination. A confirmatory MRI must have either four lesions involving the white matter or three lesions if one is periventricular in location. Acceptable lesions must be >3 mm in diameter. For patients older than 50 years, two of the following criteria must also be met: (a) lesion size >5 mm, (b) lesions adjacent to the bodies of the lateral ventricles, and (c) lesion(s) present in the posterior fossa.
   b. Evoked response testing may be used to document a *second* lesion not evident on clinical examination.
4. The clinical pattern must consist of (a) two or more separate *episodes* of worsening involving different sites of the CNS, each lasting at least 24 h and occurring at least 1 month apart, or (b) gradual or stepwise *progression* over at least 6 months if accompanied by increased CSF IgG synthesis or two or more oligoclonal bands.
5. Age of onset between 15 and 60 years.
6. The patient's neurologic condition could not be better attributed to another disease. Laboratory testing that may be advisable in certain cases includes (a) CSF analysis, (b) MRI of the head or spine, (c) serum vitamin B_{12} level, (d) human T cell lymphotropic virus type I (HTLV-I) titer, (e) erythrocyte sedimentation rate, (f) rheumatoid factor, antinuclear, anti-DNA antibodies (SLE), (g) serum VDRL, (h) angiotensin-converting enzyme (sarcoidosis), (i) *Borrelia* serology (Lyme disease), (j) very-long-chain fatty acids (adrenoleukodystrophy), and (k) serum or CSF lactate, muscle biopsy, or mitochondrial DNA analysis (mitochondrial disorders).

DIAGNOSTIC CATEGORIES

1. *Definite MS:* All six criteria fulfilled.
2. *Probable MS:* All six criteria fulfilled except (a) only one objective abnormality despite two symptomatic episodes or (b) only one symptomatic episode despite two or more objective abnormalities.
3. *At risk for MS:* All six criteria fulfilled except only one symptomatic episode and one objective abnormality.

FIGURE 371-2 MRI findings in MS. *A.* Axial first-echo image from T2-weighted sequence demonstrates multiple bright signal abnormalities in white matter, typical for MS. *B.* Sagittal T2-weighted FLAIR (fluid attenuated inversion recovery) image in which the high signal of CSF has been suppressed. CSF appears dark, while areas of brain edema or demyelination appear high in signal as shown here in the corpus callosum (*arrows*). Lesions in the anterior corpus callosum are frequent in MS and rare in vascular disease. *C.* Sagittal T2-weighted fast spin echo image of the thoracic spine demonstrates a fusiform high signal intensity lesion in the mid thoracic spinal cord. *D.* Sagittal T1-weighted image obtained afer the intravenous administration of gadolinium DTPA reveals focal areas of blood-brain barrier disruption, identified as high-signal-intensity regions (*arrows*).

served pathologically in MS (Dawson's fingers). Lesions are also commonly found within the brainstem, corpus callosum, cerebellum, and spinal cord. Lesions of the anterior corpus callosum are particularly useful diagnostically because this site is usually spared in cerebrovascular disease. Specific criteria for the use of MRI in support of a diagnosis of MS have been proposed (Table 371-2).

The correlation between the total volume of T2-weighted signal abnormality—the "lesion burden"—and clinical measures of disability is poor. Approximately one-third of hyperintense T2-weighted lesions appear hypointense on T1-weighted imaging sequences. These "black holes" provide more specific imaging markers of irreversible demyelination and axonal loss that correlate more robustly with clinical measures of disability. The correlation between MRI measures and clinical status is even stronger with emerging imaging techniques, including magnetization transfer imaging and proton-magnetic resonance spectroscopic imaging, which can distinguish irreversible demyelination and axonal loss from reversible edema and inflammation.

Evoked Responses Evoked response testing may detect slowed or absent conduction in visual, auditory, somatosensory, or motor pathways (Chap. 357). These tests use computer averaging techniques to record the electrical response evoked in the nervous system after repetitive sensory stimuli. One or several evoked responses are abnormal in 80 to 90% of patients with MS. Abnormalities in evoked responses occur with a variety of neurologic disorders that disrupt pathways being measured; thus, they are not specific to MS. Testing is of diagnostic value when it provides evidence of a subclinical second lesion in a patient who manifests only one abnormality on neurologic examination (Table 371-2).

brain or spinal cord MRI, or visual, auditory, or somatosensory evoked electrical response. In patients who experience gradual progression of disability for 6 or more months without superimposed relapses, documentation of intrathecal IgG may be used to support the diagnosis.

DIAGNOSTIC TESTS **Magnetic Resonance Imaging** Widespread availability of brain and spinal cord MRI has revolutionized the diagnosis and management of MS. Disease-related changes are detected by MRI (Fig. 371-2) in >95% of patients who otherwise meet diagnostic criteria for definite MS (Table 371-2). An increase in vascular permeability, detected by leakage of the intravenous contrast agent gadolinium DPTA into the brain, appears to be a very early event in the formation of new MS lesions and perhaps is a marker of inflammation. Gadolinium enhancement persists for 2 to 8 weeks; and the residual mixture of edema, inflammation, demyelination, axonal loss, and gliosis in the MS plaque remains visible as a focal area of hyperintensity on spin-echo (T2-weighted) and proton-density images. Lesions often appear to extend outward from the ventricular surface, corresponding to a pattern of perivenous demyelination that is ob-

Cerebrospinal Fluid (CSF) CSF abnormalities consist of abnormally increased levels of intrathecally synthesized IgG, oligoclinal banding, and mononuclear cell pleocytosis. Various formulas are used to distinguish intrathecally synthesized IgG from serum IgG that may have entered the CNS passively across a disrupted blood-brain barrier. One formula expresses the ratio of IgG to albumin in the CSF divided by the ratio in the serum ("the CSF IgG index"). Oligoclonal banding of CSF IgG is detected by agarose gel electrophoresis techniques. Two or more oligoclonal bands are found in 75 to 90% of patients with MS. Oligoclonal banding may be absent at the onset of MS, and in individual patients the number of bands present may increase with time. It is important that paired serum samples be studied to exclude a systemic origin of the oligoclonal bands.

Other CSF abnormalities also occur but are less specific for MS. In one large series, CSF mononuclear pleocytosis (>5 cells/μL) was present in 25% of patients with MS. CSF cell counts are generally <20/μL in patients with MS, and counts >50/μL are unusual but may

of polymorphonuclear leukocytes in CSF makes the diagnosis of MS
unlikely. Pleocytosis is more common in young patients with relapsing-remitting MS than in older patients with progressive forms
of MS. The total CSF protein content is usually normal or only
slightly increased. A protein elevation >100 mg/dL is rare and should
prompt consideration of alternative diagnosis such as an infection or
tumor.

DIFFERENTIAL DIAGNOSIS Numerous diagnostic formulas have been proposed for MS (Table 371-2); although useful, they
cannot replace sound clinical judgment. No single clinical sign or test
is diagnostic of MS. The diagnosis is usually easily made in a young
adult with relapsing and remitting symptoms referable to different areas of CNS white matter. The possibility of an alternate diagnosis
should be considered when (1) symptoms are localized exclusively to
the posterior fossa, craniocervical junction, or spinal cord; (2) the patient is younger than 15 or older than 60 years; (3) the clinical course
is progressive from onset; and (4) the patient has never experienced
visual, sensory or bladder symptoms. Diagnosis may also be difficult
in patients with a rapid or even explosive onset suggesting a cerebrovascular accident, or mild symptoms only and a normal neurologic
examination. In such situations, the patient should be questioned
carefully for a history of prior attacks that may not be recalled
initially. Rarely, a mass lesion resulting from intense inflammation and
swelling may occur in MS and may mimic a primary or metastatic
tumor.

Examination reveals evidence of neurologic disease in most patients. Abnormal signs are often more widespread than expected from
the interview. For example, a patient with MS may present with symptoms in one leg and signs in both. This type of finding is helpful when
it permits exclusion of a single focal lesion as the source of a patient's
symptoms. Conversely, the presence of features that are uncommon
or rare in MS should call the diagnosis into question. These include
aphasia, extrapyramidal syndromes suggesting parkinsonism, chorea,
isolated dementia, amyotrophy with fasciculations, peripheral neuropathy, fever, headache, seizures, or coma.

Systemic lupus erythematosus (SLE) rarely produces a relapsing
or progressive disorder that mimics MS; other manifestations of SLE
are usually present (Chap. 311). Behçet's syndrome may produce a
chronic illness with optic neuropathy and myelopathy but more often
presents as an acute or subacute multifocal CNS disorder; characteristic oral and genital lesions, uveitis, and an elevated ESR are distinguishing features (Chap. 316). Relapsing-remitting CNS syndromes
have also been described in Sjögren's syndrome. Sarcoidosis may produce cranial nerve palsies (especially of the seventh cranial nerve),
progressive optic atrophy, or myelopathy (Chap. 318). Systemic involvement helps to distinguish these conditions from MS. Lyme borreliosis may involve the optic nerve, brainstem, or spinal cord in the
absence of characteristic rash, fever, or meningoradiculitis (Chap.
176). Other chronic infections, including meningovascular syphilis
and infection with HIV, may need to be considered. HTLV type I–
associated myelopathy (HAM; tropical spastic paraparesis) is characterized by back pain, progressive spasticity affecting predominantly
the lower limbs, and bladder symptoms (Chap. 373). Diagnosis is
based on identification of specific antibody to HTLV-I in serum and
CSF and by direct virus isolation. Infection with the HTLV-II retrovirus may cause a progressive myelopathy similar to that caused by
HTLV-I.

As noted above, the acute onset of a focal CNS disturbance in a
previously healthy individual may suggest a stroke or migraine. Progressive focal deficits should always prompt consideration of a compressive lesion. Primary CNS lymphoma may produce single or multiple lesions that contrast-enhance on MRI and may resemble acute
lesions of MS. A progressive or relapsing brainstem disturbance may
be due to a vascular malformation in the posterior fossa. Pontine
glioma is distinguished from MS by its tendency to produce progressive deficits that involve contiguous structures. Chiari malformations

presenting in adulthood may cause cerebellar ataxia, nystagmus, and
spastic weakness of the limbs; headache, lower cranial nerve palsies,
and a syringomyelic syndrome are useful distinguishing features. Progressive myelopathies may result from cervical spondylosis, spinal
cord tumor, or arteriovenous malformation (Chap. 368).

A positive family history, neurologic signs suggesting diffuse
symmetric demyelination, and lack of characteristic CSF changes raise
the possibility of a metabolic or genetic condition that may mimic MS.
Subacute combined degeneration due to vitamin B$_{12}$ deficiency may
produce an MS-like syndrome in the absence of megaloblastic anemia
(Chap. 368). Uncommon genetic disorders that may mimic MS include
Krabbe's disease, metachromatic leukodystrophy, methylenetetrahydrofolate reductase deficiency, biotinidase deficiency, adrenomyelo-
neuropathy, familial spastic paraparesis, spinocerebellar ataxia, mitochondrial encephalopathy with lactic acidosis and stroke (MELAS),
Leber's disease, and subacute necrotizing encephalomyelopathy
(Leigh's disease).

PROGNOSIS Most patients with MS experience progressive
disability. Fifteen years after diagnosis, fewer than 20% of patients
with MS have no functional limitation, 50 to 60% require assistance
when ambulating, 70% are limited or unable to perform major activities of daily living, and 75% are not employed. In 1998, it was estimated that the total annual economic burden of MS in the United States
exceeded 6.8 billion. The following clinical and brain MRI features
may confer a more favorable prognosis: presentation with isolated optic neuritis or sensory symptoms, complete recovery from a first attack,
age of onset younger than 40 years, female sex, relapsing-remitting
clinical course, and fewer than two relapses in the first year of illness.
In general, patients who experience minimal neurologic impairment 5
years after the first symptoms are least likely to be severely disabled
10 to 15 years later. By comparison, patients with persistent truncal
ataxia, severe action tremor, or a disease course that is progressive
from the onset are more likely to experience progression of disability.

In patients who experience an initial attack of monosymptomatic
optic neuritis, brainstem signs, or myelopathy, brain MRI provides
useful prognostic information. If the brain MRI reveals multiple T2-
weighted lesions, the risk of developing definite MS within a 10-year
period of follow-up is 70 to 80%. Conversely, if the brain MRI is
normal, <10% of patients will experience a second episode of symptoms consistent with MS within 10 years.

TREATMENT The treatment of MS may be divided into two
categories: (1) treatments designed to modify the disease process
and (2) symptomatic management. Longitudinal scoring of the functional consequences of MS is essential for treatment decisions. The
Kurtzke Expanded Disability Status Score (EDSS) is the most widely
used measure of neurologic impairment in MS (Table 371-3).

Disease Modifying Therapies for RRMS (Fig. 371-3)
Three treatment options for patients with RRMS are approved for use
in the United States: (1) IFN-β1b (Betaseron), (2) IFN-β1a (Avonex),
and (3) glatiramer acetate (Copaxone). Each of these treatments is also
prescribed for patients with SPMS who experience frequent exacerbations because this clinical pattern cannot be distinguished reliably
from RRMS with incomplete recovery from exacerbations. In Phase
III clinical trials, recipients of IFN-β1b, IFN-β1a, and glatiramer acetate experienced ~30% fewer clinical exacerbations and significantly
fewer new MRI lesions compared to placebo recipients. IFN-β1b and
IFN-β1a also convincingly delayed time to onset of sustained progression of disability. Furthermore, IFN-β1a was found to delay the
development of clinically definite MS in patients who experience a
single episode of demyelination and have MRI findings indicating
prior subclinical disease.

Treatment effects with IFN-β1b and IFN-β1a may be mediated by
down regulating (1) expression of MHC molecules on the surface of
antigen-presenting cells, (2) actions of proinflammatory cytokines, and

Table 371-3 Scoring Systems for MS

KURTZKE EXPANDED DISABILITY STATUS SCORE (EDSS)

0.0 = Normal neurologic exam [all grade 0 in functional status (FS)]
1.0 = No disability, minimal signs in one FS (i.e., grade 1)
1.5 = No disability, minimal signs in more than one FS (more than one grade 1)
2.0 = Minimal disability in one FS (one FS grade 2, others 0 or 1)
2.5 = Minimal disability in two FS (two FS grade 2, others 0 or 1)
3.0 = Moderate disability in one FS (one FS grade 3, others 0 or 1) or mild disability in three or four FS (three/four FS grade 2, others 0 or 1) though fully ambulatory
3.5 = Fully ambulatory but with moderate disability in one FS (one grade 3) and one or two FS grade 2; or two FS grade 3; or five FS grade 2 (others 0 or 1)
4.0 = Ambulatory without aid or rest for ≥ 500 m
4.5 = Ambulatory without aid or rest for ≥ 300 m
5.0 = Ambulatory without aid or rest for ≥ 200 m
5.5 = Ambulatory without aid or rest for ≥ 100 m

6.0 = Unilateral assistance required to walk about 100 m with or without resting
6.5 = Constant bilateral assistance required to walk about 20 m without resting
7.0 = Unable to walk beyond about 5 m even with aid; essentially restricted to wheelchair; wheels self and transfers alone
7.5 = Unable to take more than a few steps; restricted to wheelchair; may need aid to transfer
8.0 = Essentially restricted to bed or chair or perambulated in wheelchair, but out of bed most of day; retains many self-care functions; generally has effective use of arms
8.5 = Essentially restricted to bed much of the day; has some effective use of arm(s); retains some self-care functions
9.0 = Helpless bed patient; can communicate and eat
9.5 = Totally helpless bed patient; unable to communicate or eat
10.0 = Death due to MS

FUNCTIONAL STATUS (FS) SCORE

A. Pyramidal functions
0 = Normal
1 = Abnormal signs without disability
2 = Minimal disability
3 = Mild or moderate paraparesis or hemiparesis, or severe monoparesis
4 = Marked paraparesis or hemiparesis, moderate quadriparesis, or monoplegia
5 = Paraplegia, hemiplegia, or marked quadriparesis
6 = Quadriplegia

B. Cerebellar functions
0 = Normal
1 = Abnormal signs without disability
2 = Mild ataxia
3 = Moderate truncal or limb ataxia
4 = Severe ataxia all limbs
5 = Unable to perform coordinated movements due to ataxia

C. Brainstem functions
0 = Normal
1 = Signs only
2 = Moderate nystagmus or other mild disability
3 = Severe nystagmus, marked extraocular weakness, or moderate disability of other cranial nerves
4 = Marked dysarthria or other marked disability
5 = Inability to swallow or speak

D. Sensory functions
0 = Normal
1 = Vibration or figure-writing decrease only, in 1 or 2 limbs
2 = Mild decrease in touch or pain or position sense, and/or moderate decrease in vibration in 1 or 2 limbs, or vibratory decrease alone in 3 or 4 limbs
3 = Moderate decrease in touch or pain or position sense, and/or essentially lost vibration in 1 or 2 limbs, or mild decrease in touch or pain, and/or moderate decrease in all proprioceptive tests in 3 or 4 limbs
4 = Marked decrease in touch or pain or loss of proprioception, alone or combined, in 1 or 2 limbs or moderate decrease in touch or pain and/or severe proprioceptive decrease in more than 2 limbs

5 = Loss (essentially) of sensation in 1 or 2 limbs or moderate decrease in touch or pain and/or loss of proprioception for most of the body below the head
6 = Sensation essentially lost below the head

E. Bowel and bladder functions
0 = Normal
1 = Mild urinary hesitancy, urgency, or retention
2 = Moderate hesitancy, urgency, retention of bowel or bladder, or rare urinary incontinence
3 = Frequent urinary incontinence
4 = In need of almost constant catheterization
5 = Loss of bladder function
6 = Loss of bowel and bladder function

F. Visual (or optic) functions
0 = Normal
1 = Scotoma with visual acuity (corrected) better than 20/30
2 = Worse eye with scotoma with maximal visual acuity (corrected) of 20/30 to 20/59
3 = Worse eye with large scotoma, or moderate decrease in fields, but with maximal visual acuity (corrected) of 20/60 to 20/99
4 = Worse eye with marked decrease of fields and maximal acuity (corrected) of 20/100 to 20/200; grade 3 plus maximal acuity of better eye of 20/60 or less
5 = Worse eye with maximal visual acuity (corrected) less than 20/200; grade 4 plus maximal acuity of better eye of 20/60 or less
6 = Grade 5 plus maximal visual acuity of better eye of 20/60 or less

G. Cerebral (or mental) functions
0 = Normal
1 = Mood alteration only (does not affect EDSS score)
2 = Mild decrease in mentation
3 = Moderate decrease in mentation
4 = Marked decrease in mentation
5 = Chronic brain syndrome—severe or incompetent

SOURCE: After JF Kurtzke, Neurology 33:1444, 1983.

---

(3) expression of vascular endothelial adhesion molecules and matrix metalloproteinases that mediate trafficking of activated lymphocytes and macrophages into the CNS. Glatiramer acetate, a synthetic polypeptide designed to resemble MBP, may act by (1) inducing antigen-specific suppressor T cells as a result of shared determinants between copolymer 1 and MBP and (2) binding to MHC molecules on the surface of antigen-presenting cells.

IFN-β1b, 8.0 million international units (MIU), is administered by subcutaneous injection every other day. IFN-β1a, 6.0 MIU, is administered by intramuscular injection once every week. Glatiramer acetate, 20 mg, is administered by subcutaneous injection every day. IFN-β1b, IFN-β1a and glatiramer acetate are generally well tolerated. Erythematous reactions at the injection site are common with IFN-β1b and glatiramer acetate. Transient flu-like symptoms frequently occur at the

beginning of IFN-β treatment; these symptoms, which usually resolve within several months, can be managed with ibuprofen, acetaminophen or other analgesic medications. Approximately 15% of glatiramer acetate recipients experience one or more episodes of flushing, chest tightness, dyspnea, palpitations, and anxiety after injection. This systemic reaction is unpredictable, self-limited, and generally lasts <1 h. Approximately 40% of IFN-β1b recipients and 5 to 25% of IFN-β1a recipients develop neutralizing antibodies within 12 months of initiating therapy. Data suggest that neutralizing antibodies may degrade clinical efficacy, but this relationship is not apparent in all patients. The clinical usefulness of commercially available tests for neutralizing antibodies is unclear.

In the United States, ~90% of treated patients with RRMS receive one of the interferons as first-line therapy, and the remaining 10%

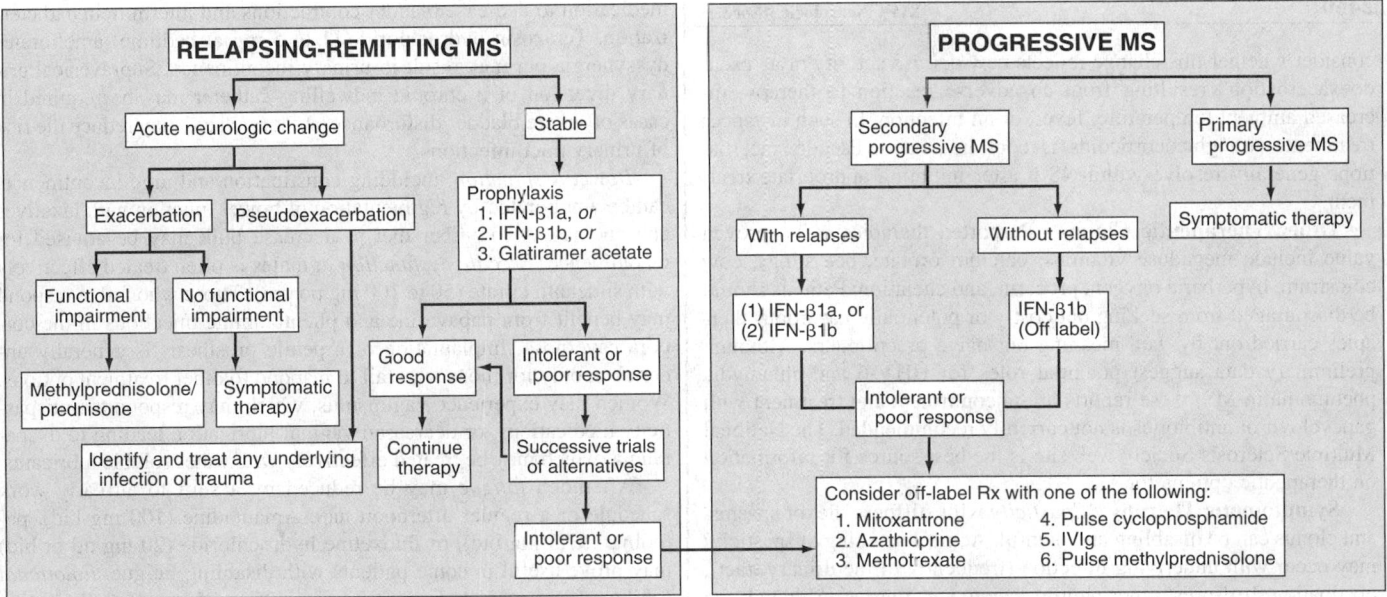

FIGURE 371-3 Therapeutic decision making for MS.

receive glatiramer acetate. Irrespective of the agent chosen, treatment should probably be discontinued in patients who continue to experience frequent clinical exacerbations or gradual progression of disability for ≥6 months. It is unknown whether patients who fail to respond adequately to treatment with any one of these interventions will respond more favorably to another; thus, it is reasonable to try a second agent (Fig. 371-3). The value of combination therapy is also unknown at this time.

Disease Modifying Therapies for SPMS IFN-β1b (Betaferon) and mitoxantrone (novantrone) were each shown to reduce annual exacerbation rates and MRI activity and delay time to onset of sustained progression of disability in patients with SPMS. Applications for approval of use of these drugs are filed in the United States. IFN-β1b is currently approved for treatment of SPMS in Canada and Europe. IFN-β1b, 8.0 MIU, is administered subcutaneously every other day. Mitoxantrone, 12 mg/m², is administered by intravenous infusion every third month. It may act as a T and B cell immunosuppressant and an enhancer of suppressor cell function. Mitoxantrone may cause mild nausea, slight hair thinning, leukopenia, thrombocytopenia and irreversible amennorhea. Dose-related cardiac toxicity is of concern, and treatment with mitoxantrone should be considered only in patients with normal ventricular ejection fractions; periodic echocardiograms are advised if cumulative doses of mitoxantrone exceed 100 mg/m².

Other Off-Label Treatment Options for RRMS and SPMS *Azathioprine*, 2 to 3 mg/kg body weight, is administered orally each day. This drug modestly reduces annual exacerbation rates in patients with RRMS and SPMS. Its effect on sustained progression of disability is less convincing

Methotrexate, 7.5 mg, is administered orally once each week. This drug, when administered for up to 2 years, modestly reduces disease activity in patients with SPMS as assessed by MRI and standardized tests of manual dexterity. An important practical advantage of methotrexate is the simplicity of a weekly oral dosing schedule.

Cyclophosphamide (CTX) reduces progression of disability in patients with SPMS when compared to ACTH. However, this observation has not been convincingly demonstrated in a placebo-controlled trial. Some investigators advocate pulse CTX therapy for young adults with aggressive forms of MS who fail to respond to approved treatment options.

Intravenous immunoglobulin (IVIg), 0.15 to 0.20 g/kg body weight, administered monthly for up to 2 years convincingly reduced annual exacerbation rates, but its effects on disability and MRI activity

were not investigated. At higher doses, 1g/kg body weight daily for 2 days every 6 months, IVIg significantly reduced new MRI activity. Use of this treatment will probably be limited because of its high cost, questions about optimal dose, and uncertainty about the effect of long-term treatment on disability.

Methylprednisolone administered in bimonthly cycles at high doses modestly delays time to onset of sustained progression of disability.

2-Chlorodeoxyadenosine (2-CDA, cladribine) significantly reduces MRI activity in patients with SPMS. However, significant clinical benefits were not observed during 12 months of therapy in a Phase III clinical trial. In the absence of convincing clinical benefit, it is unlikely that 2-CDA will be commonly prescribed.

Disease-Modifying Therapies for PPMS No approved therapies for PPMS exist at this time. The results of ongoing trials of IFN-β1a, glatiramer acetate, and mitoxantrone in PPMS are awaited.

Therapy for Exacerbations The severity and duration of acute exacerbations of MS are reduced by treatment with glucocorticoids. Although methylprednisolone (MePDN) is most commonly prescribed, there is no consensus for the optimal dose and route of administration. Clinical exacerbations that impair activities of daily living can be treated with MePDN, 1000 mg, administered intravenously each day for 3 days followed by oral prednisone, 60 mg daily for 5 days, then tapering by 10 mg each day thereafter. A similar approach is employed for treatment of initial attacks of demyelinating disease. With the exception of severe attacks that jeopardize patient safety, treatment can generally be administered in an outpatient setting. Physical and occupational therapy should be prescribed when impaired mobility or decreased manual dexterity impair activities of daily living.

Common side effects of short-term glucocorticoid therapy include fluid retention, potassium loss, weight gain, gastric disturbances, acne, and emotional lability. Salt and fluid retention are managed with a low-salt, potassium-rich diet and avoidance of potassium-wasting diuretics. In patients who have heart disease or require concurrent diuretic therapy, oral potassium supplementation is advised. Lithium carbonate (300 mg orally bid) may provide effective prophylaxis for patients who experience emotional lability and insomnia associated with glucocorticoid therapy. For patients with a history of peptic ulcer disease, cimetidine (400 mg bid) or ranitidine (150 mg bid) is advised.

In one small controlled trial, plasma exchange (7 treatments given over 2 weeks) was effective in some patients with unusually fulminant attacks of demyelination unresponsive to glucocorticoids.

When patients experience an acute deterioration, it is important to consider whether this change reflects new disease activity or a "pseudoexacerbation" resulting from an adverse reaction to therapy, increased ambient temperature, fever, or an infection. In such instances treatment with glucocorticoids is contraindicated. Pseudoexacerbations generally resolve within 48 h after initiating appropriate treatment.

Other Therapeutic Claims Purported therapies of no proven value include megadose vitamins, calcium orotate, bee stings, cow colostrum, hyperbaric oxygen, procarin, and chelation. Patients should be discouraged from seeking out costly or potentially hazardous therapies carried out by well-meaning but naive practitioners. Although preliminary data suggest potential roles for HHV-6 and chlamydia pneumonia in MS, these reports are unconfirmed, and treatment with gancyclovir or antibiotics is not currently recommended. The National Multiple Sclerosis Society web site is the best source for information on therapeutic options for MS.

Symptomatic Therapy *Spasticity* with stiffness, flexor spasms, and clonus can be disabling and painful. Acute worsening of spasticity may occur with underlying infection (frequently of the urinary tract), obstipation, bedsores, other painful lesions, or injuries. Although the mechanisms are poorly understood, spasticity may also worsen following IFN-β therapy. These potential precipitants should be considered and treated specifically. All medications for spasticity have limited efficacy and may produce symptomatic worsening in patients who rely upon spasticity to provide leg strength necessary for effective ambulation. Baclofen (15 to 80 mg/d in divided doses) is the most useful drug available. In refractory cases, baclofen administered orally in higher doses (up to 240 mg/d) or intrathecally via an indwelling catheter may be effective. Tizanidine (2 to 8 mg tid) and diazepam (1 to 2 mg bid or tid) are particularly effective for painful nocturnal spasms, but daytime use is often limited by excessive somnolence. Cyclobenzaprine hydrochloride (5 to 10 mg bid or tid), clonazepam (0.5 to 1.0 mg tid, including a bedtime dose), and clonidine hydrochloride (0.1 to 0.2 mg tid, including a bedtime dose) may be useful for patients who otherwise fail to respond. Dantrolene may produce unacceptable weakness, and its use is usually reserved for nonambulatory patients. A course of glucocorticoids may be given in exceptional cases where other agents have failed, but benefits seldom last more than 2 to 3 weeks.

Pain, including trigeminal neuralgia and painful dysesthesias, may respond to carbamazepine (100 to 1200 mg/d in divided, escalating doses), gabapentin (300–3600 mg/d), dilantin (300–400 mg/d), amitriptyline (25–150 mg/d), or baclofen (10–80 mg/d). In patients with unilateral leg pain, it may be difficult to distinguish dysesthesias due to MS from radiculopathy due to lumbar disk disease; nonsurgical therapy is justified in the absence of convincing signs of nerve root compression.

Paroxysmal symptoms respond to carbamazepine (up to 1200 mg in divided doses), gabapentin (100 to 600 mg tid), or acetazolamide (125 to 250 mg tid). Although no treatment for tremor is satisfactory, slight improvement is occasionally seen with clonazepam (0.5 to 1.0 mg bid or tid), primidone (125 to 250 mg bid or tid), ondansetron (4 to 8 mg bid or tid), and isoniazid (up to 1200 mg in divided doses). Stereotaxic thalamotomy may be considered in cases of disabling tremor in which a unilateral reduction in symptoms is required, but the general experience with this procedure has been disappointing.

Because specific symptoms of *bladder dysfunction* correlate poorly with physiologic findings, urodynamic evaluation is often required. The pathophysiology of abnormal micturition also may change over time in MS. Bladder hyperreflexia is treated with anticholinergics: oxybutynin (5 mg bid or tid), tolterodine (1 to 2 mg bid), or propantheline (7.5 to 15 mg qid). Urinary retention due to bladder hyporeflexia may respond to the cholinergic drug bethanecol (10 to 50 mg tid or qid). Dyssynergia between detrusor and external sphincter muscles may be treated effectively with a combination of anticholinergic medication to decrease bladder contractions and intermittent catheterization. Terazosin hydrochloride (1 to 5 mg at bedtime) ameliorates dyssynergia but may result in urinary incontinence. Supravesical urinary diversion or a chronic indwelling catheter may be required in cases of severe bladder disturbance. Ascorbic acid may reduce the risk of urinary tract infections.

Bowel dysfunction, including constipation and urge incontinence, can be ameliorated by regimentation of bowel function with laxatives and enemas. A low-fiber diet to decrease bulk may be advised for incontinence. *Erectile dysfunction* in males is often treated effectively with sildenafil citrate (50 to 100 mg po prn). Those who fail to respond may benefit from papaverine and phentolamine injections in the corpora cavernosa. Implantation of a penile prosthesis is generally undertaken only for those who fail to respond to other treatment options. Women may experience vaginismus, which may respond to antispasticity medications, or decreased vaginal lubrication leading to dyspareunia, which may be treated effectively with water soluble lubricants.

Afternoon *fatigue* may be reduced by a shift to an early work schedule or a regular afternoon nap. Amantadine (100 mg bid), pemoline (37.5 mg bid), or fluoxetine hydrochloride (20 mg qd or bid) may prove useful in some patients with disabling fatigue. *Emotional lability* often responds to amitriptyline (25 to 75 mg/d) or fluoxetine (20 mg/d). It is essential to be vigilant for clinical evidence of *depression*, since the risk of suicide is increased in patients with MS. Occupational counseling and other support services may assist patients and their families in coping with the effects of the disease. Health maintenance should be emphasized, including stress reduction, a balanced diet, avoidance of rapid change in weight, and adequate rest. Although there is little evidence linking vaccination with relapses of MS, it is prudent to avoid unnecessary immunizations. Swimming is an ideal form of exercise for many patients because of the buoyant support and hypothermia that is achieved.

Pregnancy may affect the course of MS. Compared with nonpregnant MS patients, pregnant patients experience fewer attacks during gestation but more attacks in the first 3 months after parturition. The two effects appear to be roughly similar in magnitude; thus, no effect of pregnancy on disability or on the overall disease course has been identified. Although it has been hypothesized that high levels of prolactin induced in the postpartum period and maintained by breast feeding result in immune stimulation that predisposes to relapses of MS, studies indicate no effect of breast feeding on attack frequency in the postpartum period. The advisability of childbearing should be determined primarily by the patient's physical state and available social support.

CLINICAL VARIANTS OF MS *Neuromyelitis optica (Devic's syndrome)* is characterized by separate attacks of acute optic neuritis and myelitis. Optic neuritis may be unilateral or bilateral and precede or follow an attack of myelitis by days, months, or years. Respiratory failure may result from cervical cord lesions. CSF neutrophil counts $>50/\mu L$ are reported to occur in as many as 20% of patients. In contrast to patients with MS, patients with Devic's syndrome do not experience brainstem, cerebellar, and cognitive involvement, and the brain MRI is normal. Characteristically, MRI demonstrates a transiently enhancing focal region of swelling and cavitation that extends over three or more spinal cord segments. In contrast to MS, histopathology of these lesions may reveal areas of necrosis and thickening of blood vessel walls. Thus, it remains uncertain whether Devic's syndrome is a variant of MS or a separate entity. The role of disease-modifying therapies for MS has not been rigorously studied in patients with Devic's syndrome. This syndrome is unusual in Caucasians but appears to be more common in Asians. The 5-year survival rate in the Mayo Clinic series was ~70%.

Acute MS (Marburg's variant) is a rare acute fulminant process that generally ends in death from brainstem involvement within one year. There are no remissions. Diagnosis can be established only at postmortem examination; widespread demyelination, axonal loss, edema, and macrophage infiltration are characteristic, and discrete plaques may also be seen. In contrast to postinfectious encephalomyelitis (see below), this disorder does not follow exanthematous infection or vaccination. It has been suggested that acute MS may be associated with an immature form of myelin that is more susceptible to breakdown. As with Devic's syndrome, it is unclear whether this syndrome represents an extreme form of MS or another disease altogether.

ACUTE DISSEMINATED ENCEPHALOMYELITIS

In contrast to MS, acute disseminated encephalomyelitis (ADEM) is distinguished by a monophasic course and a frequent association with antecedent immunization (postvaccinal encephalomyelitis) or infection (postinfectious encephalomyelitis). The pathologic hallmark of ADEM is the presence of widely scattered small foci of perivenular inflammation and demyelination. In its most explosive form, acute hemorrhagic leukoencephalitis, lesions are vasculitic and hemorrhagic, and the clinical course is devastating.

Postvaccinal encephalomyelitis may follow the administration of smallpox and certain rabies vaccines. Postinfectious encephalomyelitis is most frequently associated with the viral exanthems of childhood. Natural infection with measles virus is the most common antecedent (1 in 1000 cases). Worldwide, measles encephalomyelitis remains a common illness, but in developed countries use of the live measles vaccine has dramatically reduced its incidence. An ADEM-like illness rarely follows vaccination with live measles vaccine (1 to 2 in 10^6 immunizations). ADEM is now most frequently associated with varicella (chickenpox) infections (1 in 4000 to 10,000 cases). It also may follow infection with rubella, mumps, influenza, parainfluenza, and infectious mononucleosis viruses and with *Mycoplasma*. Some patients may have a nonspecific upper respiratory infection or no known antecedent illness.

An autoimmune response to MBP can be detected in the CSF from many patients with ADEM. This response has been most clearly established after rabies vaccination and infection with measles virus. With measles infection, the induction of immune responses to a variety of CNS antigens may occur, but only the response to MBP correlates with the development of ADEM. Many cases of postvaccinal encephalomyelitis may result from sensitization with brain material that contaminates the viral vaccines. Attempts to demonstrate direct viral invasion of the CNS have been unsuccessful. The molecular mechanism responsible for virus-induced triggering of an autoimmune response to MBP is not known but may include molecular mimicry due to antigens shared between the virus and host determinants or to virus-mediated CNS injury with secondary sensitization to MBP.

CLINICAL MANIFESTATIONS The severity of ADEM varies. In severe cases, the onset is abrupt, and progression is rapid (hours to days). In postinfectious ADEM, the neurologic syndrome generally begins late in the course of the viral illness as the exanthem is fading. Fever reappears, and headache, meningismus, and lethargy progressing to coma may develop. Seizures are common. Signs of disseminated neurologic disease are consistently present. Motor findings may include hemiparesis or quadriparesis and extensor plantar responses. Tendon reflexes may be lost initially, later to become hyperactive. Variable degrees of sensory loss and of brainstem involvement may occur. In ADEM due to complications from chickenpox, cerebellar involvement is often prominent. CSF protein is modestly elevated (50 to 150 mg/dL). Lymphocytic pleocytosis, generally ≤200 cells per microliter, occurs in 80% of patients. Occasional patients have higher counts or a mixed polymorphonuclear-lymphocytic pattern during the initial days of the illness. Transient CSF oligoclonal banding has been reported. MRI may reveal extensive gadolinium enhancement of white matter in brain and spinal cord.

DIAGNOSIS The diagnosis is easily established when there is a history of recent vaccination or exanthematous illness. In severe cases with predominantly cerebral involvement, acute encephalitis due to infection with herpes simplex or other viruses may be difficult to exclude. In the absence of a specific viral prodrome or of immunization, it may not be possible to distinguish ADEM from acute MS. The simultaneous onset of disseminated symptoms and signs indicating optic nerve, brain, and spinal cord involvement is common in ADEM and rare in MS. Similarly, meningismus, drowsiness or coma, or seizures suggest ADEM. Optic nerve involvement is generally bilateral in ADEM and unilateral in MS, and transverse myelopathy is usually complete in the former and partial in the latter. The CSF protein level is normal in most patients with MS; lymphocyte counts are rarely >50 cells/μL, and polymorphonuclear leukocytes are not present. MRI findings that may support a diagnosis of ADEM include extensive and relatively symmetric white matter abnormalities and diffuse gadolinium enhancement of all abnormal areas, indicating active disease and a monophasic course.

TREATMENT Therapy consists of intravenous methylprednisolone as employed for exacerbations of MS. Uncontrolled studies have found ACTH and plasmapheresis also to be of benefit. Occasional patients show evidence of relapse shortly after termination of therapy, and for them, reinstitution of therapy may be useful. The prognosis reflects the severity of the underlying acute illness. Measles encephalomyelitis is associated with a mortality rate of 5 to 20%, and most survivors have permanent neurologic sequelae. Children who recover may have persistent seizures and behavioral and learning disorders.

BIBLIOGRAPHY

ARCHELOS JJ et al: The role of B cells and autoantibodies in multiple-sclerosis. Ann Neurol 47:694, 2000

CONFAVREUX C et al: Rate of pregnancy-related relapse in multiple sclerosis. N Engl J Med 339:285, 1998

EUROPEAN STUDY GROUP ON INTERFERON β-1B IN SECONDARY PROGRESSIVE MS. Placebo-controlled multicentre randomised trial of interferon β-1b in treatment of secondary progressive multiple sclerosis. Lancet 352:1491, 1998

FAZEKAS F et al: Randomized placebo-controlled trial of monthly intravenous immunoglobin therapy in relapsing-remitting multiple sclerosis. Lancet 349:589, 1997

GENAIN C et al: Identification of autoantibodies associated with myelin damage in multiple sclerosis. Nat Med 5:2, 1999

JACOBS LD et al: Intramuscular interferon beta 1a initiated during a first demyelinating event in multiple sclerosis. N Engl J Med 343:898, 2000

JOHNSON KP et al: Extended use of glatiramer acetate (copaxone) is well tolerated and maintains its clinical effect on multiple sclerosis relapse rate and degree of disability. Neurology 50:701, 1998

LUCCHINETTI C et al: Heterogeneity of multiple sclerosis lesions: Implications for the pathogenesis of demyelination. Ann Neurol 47:707, 2000

THE MULTIPLE SCLEROSIS GENETICS GROUP: Linkage of the MHC to familial multiple sclerosis suggests genetic heterogeneity. Hum Mol Gen 7:8, 1998

NOSEWORTHY JH et al: Medical progress: multiple sclerosis. N Engl J Med 343:938, 2000

THE OWIMS STUDY GROUP: Evidence of interferon β-1a dose response in relapsing-remitting MS. Neurology 53:679, 1999

OKSENBERG JR, HAUSER SL: The molecular pathogenesis of multiple sclerosis, in Molecular Neurology, JB Martin (ed). New York, Scientific American Medicine, 1998

PRISMS STUDY GROUP: Randomised double-blind placebo-controlled study of interferon β-1a in relapsing-remitting multiple sclerosis. Lancet 352:1498, 1998

RUDICK RA, GOODKIN DE (eds): Multiple Sclerosis Therapeutics. London, Martin Dunitz, 1999

STUVE O, ZAMVIL S: Pathogenesis, diagnosis, and treatment of acute disseminated encephalomyelitis (ADEM). Curr Opin Neurol 12:395, 1999

WEINSHENKER BG et al: A randomized trial of plasma exchange in acute central nervous system inflammatory disease. Ann Neurol 46:878, 1999

ZHAO GJ et al: Effect of interferon beta-1b in MS: Assessment of annual accumulation of PD/T2 activity on MRI. UBC MS/MRI Analysis Group and the MS Study Group. Neurology 54:200, 2000

372

Karen L. Roos, Kenneth L. Tyler

BACTERIAL MENINGITIS AND OTHER SUPPURATIVE INFECTIONS

CNS	central nervous system	LPS	lipopolysaccharide
CPP	cerebral perfusion pressure	MAP	mean arterial pressure
CSF	cerebrospinal fluid	MIC	minimal inhibitory concentration
CT	computed tomography	MRI	magnetic resonance imaging
EEG	electroencephalogram	PCR	polymerase chain reaction
Hib	*H. influenzae* type b	PMNs	polymorphonuclear neutrophils
HSV	herpes simplex virus	SAH	subarachnoid hemorrhage
ICP	intracranial pressure	SDE	subdural empyema
IL	interleukin	TNF	tumor necrosis factor
LA	latex particle agglutination		

ACUTE BACTERIAL MENINGITIS

DEFINITION Bacterial meningitis is an acute purulent infection within the subarachnoid space. It is associated with a central nervous system (CNS) inflammatory reaction that may result in decreased consciousness, seizures, raised intracranial pressure, and stroke. The meninges, the subarachnoid space, and the brain parenchyma are all involved in the inflammatory reaction; as such, *meningoencephalitis* is the more accurate descriptive term.

EPIDEMIOLOGY Bacterial meningitis is the most common form of suppurative intracranial infection, with an annual incidence >2.5 cases/100,000 population. The epidemiology of bacterial meningitis has changed in recent years. Currently, the organisms most commonly responsible for community-acquired bacterial meningitis are *Streptococcus pneumoniae* (~50%), *Neisseria meningitidis* (~25%), group B streptococci (~10%), and *Listeria monocytogenes* (~10%). *Haemophilus influenzae* was once the most common cause of bacterial meningitis in the United States. The incidence of *H. influenzae* meningitis declined precipitously following the introduction of the *H. influenzae* type b (Hib) vaccine in 1987, and *H. influenzae* now accounts for <10% of bacterial meningitis cases. There have also been major changes in the epidemiology of pneumococcal disease, with the global emergence and increasing prevalence of penicillin- and cephalosporin-resistant strains of *S. pneumoniae*. As of 1998, ~44% of clinical isolates of *S. pneumoniae* in the United States had intermediate or high levels of resistance to penicillin. In the past several years, there has been an increase in the incidence of meningococcal infections on college campuses and an increase in the incidence of meningococcal disease in North America and Europe due to the emergence of a virulent strain of serogroup C, serotype 2a *N. meningitidis*. An increasing incidence of *N. meningitidis* strains with moderate or relative resistance to penicillin and a decreased susceptibility to ampicillin has been reported worldwide, but the clinical significance of these strains is still unknown. Annual meningitis epidemics, caused primarily by the serogroup A meningococcus, continue to occur in the meningitis belt of sub-Saharan Africa. Epidemics due to the serogroup B meningococcus continue to occur in Europe, Latin America, and New Zealand. Group B streptococcus or *S. agalactiae* was previously responsible for meningitis predominantly in neonates, but it has been reported with increasing frequency in individuals >50 years, particularly those with underlying diseases. *L. monocytogenes* has emerged as an important cause of bacterial meningitis in the elderly and in individuals with impaired cell-mediated immunity.

ETIOLOGY *S. pneumoniae* (Chap. 140) is the most common cause of meningitis in adults >20 years. There are a number of predisposing conditions that increase the risk of pneumococcal meningitis, the most important of which is pneumococcal pneumonia. Additional risk factors include coexisting acute or chronic otitis media, alcoholism, diabetes, splenectomy, hypogammaglobulinemia, complement deficiency, and head trauma with basilar skull fracture and cerebrospinal fluid (CSF) rhinorrhea.

N. meningitidis (Chap. 146) accounts for nearly 60% of bacterial meningitis cases in children and young adults between the ages of 2 and 20. The nasopharynx is initially colonized by this organism, resulting in either an asymptomatic carrier state or invasive meningococcal disease. The risk of invasive disease following nasopharyngeal colonization depends on both bacterial virulence factors and host immune defense mechanisms, including the host's capacity to produce antimeningococcal antibodies and to lyse meningococci by both the classic and alternative complement pathways. Individuals with deficiencies of any of the complement components, including properdin, are highly susceptible to meningococcal infections.

Enteric gram-negative bacilli are the causative organisms of meningitis that is associated with chronic and debilitating diseases such as diabetes, cirrhosis or alcoholism, and chronic urinary tract infections and following neurosurgical procedures, particularly craniotomy or craniectomy.

Resistance to infection with *L. monocytogenes* requires effective cell-mediated immunity. As a result, elderly individuals and those with impaired cell-mediated immunity due to organ transplantation, pregnancy, malignancy, chronic illness, or immunosuppressive therapy are all at increased risk for listerial meningitis. Infection is acquired by ingesting foods contaminated by this organism. Foodborne human listerial infection has been reported from contaminated coleslaw, milk, deli meat, and soft cheeses.

The frequency of *H. influenzae* type b meningitis in children has declined dramatically since the introduction of the Hib conjugate vaccine, although rare cases of Hib meningitis in vaccinated children have been reported. More frequently, *H. influenzae* causes meningitis in unvaccinated children and adults.

Staphylococcus aureus and coagulase-negative staphylococci are predominant organisms causing meningitis that follows invasive neurosurgical procedures, particularly shunting procedures for hydrocephalus, or occurs as a complication of the use of subcutaneous Ommaya reservoirs for the administration of intrathecal chemotherapy.

PATHOPHYSIOLOGY The most common bacteria that cause meningitis, *S. pneumoniae* and *N. meningitidis*, initially colonize the nasopharynx by attaching to nasopharyngeal epithelial cells. Bacteria are transported across epithelial cells in membrane-bound vacuoles to the intravascular space or invade the intravascular space by creating separations in the apical tight junctions of columnar epithelial cells. Once the bacteria gain access to the bloodstream, they are able to avoid phagocytosis by neutrophils and classic complement–mediated bactericidal activity because of the presence of a polysaccharide capsule. Once in the bloodstream, bacteria can reach the intraventricular choroid plexus. Infection of choroid plexus epithelial cells allows bacteria direct access to the CSF. Some bacteria, such as *S. pneumoniae*, can adhere directly to cerebral capillary endothelial cells and subsequently migrate through or between these cells to reach the CSF. Bacteria are able to multiply rapidly within CSF because of the absence of effective host immune defenses. Normal CSF contains few white blood cells (WBCs) and relatively small amounts of complement proteins and immunoglobulins. The paucity of the latter two prevents effective opsonization of bacteria, an essential prerequisite for bacterial phagocytosis by neutrophils. Phagocytosis of bacteria is further impaired by the fluid nature of CSF, which is less conducive to phagocytosis than a solid tissue substrate.

A critical event in the pathogenesis of bacterial meningitis is the inflammatory reaction induced by the invading bacteria. Many of the neurologic manifestations and complications of bacterial meningitis result from the immune response to the invading pathogen rather than from direct bacteria-induced tissue injury. As a result, neurologic injury can progress even after the CSF has been sterilized by antibiotic therapy.

The lysis of bacteria with the subsequent release of cell-wall components into the subarachnoid space is the initial step in the induction of the inflammatory response and the formation of a purulent exudate in the subarachnoid space (Fig. 372-1). Bacterial cell-wall components, such as the lipopolysaccharide (LPS) molecules of gram-negative bacteria and teichoic acid and peptidoglycans of *S. pneumoniae*, induce meningeal inflammation by stimulating the production of inflammatory cytokines and chemokines by microglia, astrocytes, monocytes, microvascular endothelial cells, and CSF leukocytes. In experimental models of meningitis, cytokines including tumor necrosis factor (TNF) and interleukin (IL) 1 are present in CSF within 1 to 2 h of intracisternal inoculation of LPS. This cytokine response is quickly followed by an increase in CSF protein concentration and leukocytosis. Chemokines (cytokines that induce chemotactic migration in leukocytes) and a variety of other proinflammatory cytokines are also produced and secreted by leukocytes and tissue cells that are stimulated by IL-1 and TNF. In addition, bacteremia and the inflammatory cytokines induce the production of excitatory amino acids, reactive oxygen and nitrogen species (free oxygen radicals, nitric oxide, and peroxynitrite), and other mediators that can induce death of brain cells.

Much of the pathophysiology of bacterial meningitis is a direct consequence of elevated levels of CSF cytokines and chemokines. TNF and IL-1 act synergistically to increase the permeability of the blood-brain barrier, resulting in induction of vasogenic edema and the leakage of serum proteins into

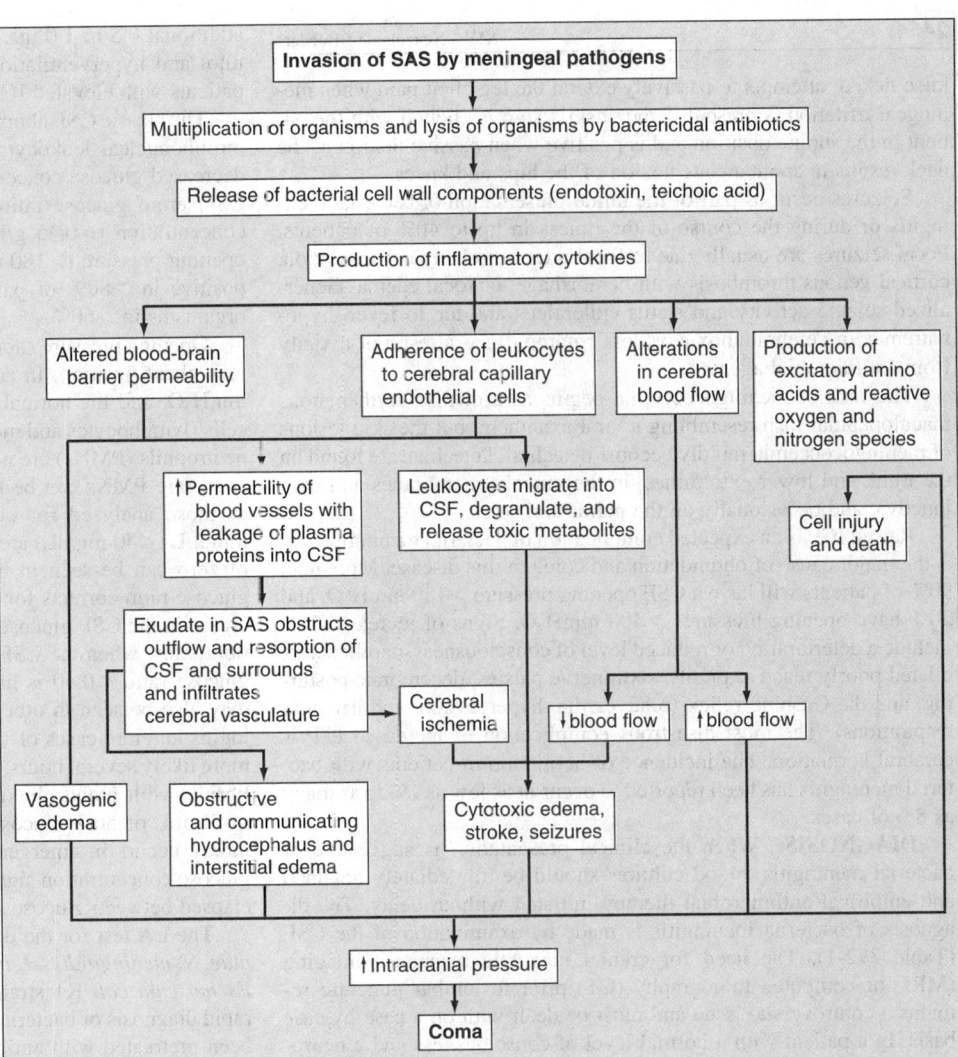

FIGURE 372-1 The pathophysiology of the neurologic complications of bacterial meningitis. SAS, subarachnoid space; CSF, cerebrospinal fluid (©Kroos).

the subarachnoid space (Fig. 372-1). The subarachnoid exudate of proteinaceous material and leukocytes obstructs the flow of CSF through the ventricular system and diminishes the resorptive capacity of the arachnoid granulations in the dural sinuses, leading to obstructive and communicating hydrocephalus and concomitant interstitial edema.

Inflammatory cytokines upregulate the expression of selectins on cerebral capillary endothelial cells and leukocytes, which allows for leukocytes to adhere to vascular endothelial cells and to subsequently migrate into the CSF. The adherence of leukocytes to capillary endothelial cells increases the permeability of blood vessels, allowing for the leakage of plasma proteins into the CSF, which adds to the inflammatory exudate. Neutrophil degranulation results in the release of toxic metabolites that contribute to cytotoxic edema, cell injury, and death. Contrary to previous beliefs, CSF leukocytes probably do little to contribute to the clearance of CSF bacterial infection.

During the very early stages of meningitis there is an increase in cerebral blood flow, soon followed by a decrease in cerebral blood flow and a loss of cerebrovascular autoregulation. Cerebral perfusion pressure (CPP) is defined as the difference between the mean arterial pressure (MAP) and the intracranial pressure (ICP), i.e., CPP = MAP − ICP. CPP is protected by cerebrovascular autoregulation, which dilates or constricts cerebral resistance vessels in response to alterations in CPP, due to changes in either the MAP or the ICP. Loss of cerebrovascular autoregulation means that any increase in systemic blood pressure leads to an increase in cerebral blood flow and ICP. Conversely, a decrease in mean systemic arterial pressure, for example, associated with septic shock, results in a decrease in cerebral blood

flow and subsequent cerebral ischemia and infarction. The cerebrovascular complications of bacterial meningitis include not only a loss of autoregulation but also narrowing of the large arteries at the base of the brain due to encroachment on the vessel by the purulent exudate in the subarachnoid space and infiltration of the arterial wall by inflammatory cells with intimal thickening (vasculitis); this may result in ischemia and infarction, obstruction of branches of the middle cerebral artery by thrombosis, thrombosis of the major cerebral venous sinuses, and thrombophlebitis of the cerebral cortical veins. The combination of interstitial, vasogenic, and cytotoxic edema leads to raised ICP and coma. Cerebral edema, either focal or generalized, can lead to cerebral herniation (see below). Focal or diffuse cerebral edema is the most likely cause of meningitis-associated brain herniation; however, hydrocephalus and dural sinus or cortical vein thrombosis may also play a role.

CLINICAL PRESENTATION Meningitis can present as either an acute fulminant illness that progresses rapidly in a few hours or as a subacute infection that progressively worsens over several days. The classic clinical triad of meningitis is fever, headache, and nuchal rigidity ("stiff neck"). Each of these signs and symptoms occurs in >90% of cases. Alteration in mental status occurs in 75% of patients and can vary from lethargy to coma. Nausea, vomiting, and photophobia are also common complaints. Nuchal rigidity is the pathognomonic sign of meningeal irritation and is present when the neck resists passive flexion. Kernig's and Brudzinski's signs are also classic signs of meningeal irritation. Kernig's sign is elicited with the patient in the supine position. The thigh is flexed on the abdomen, with the knee flexed; attempts to passively extend the leg elicit pain when meningeal irritation is present. Brudzinski's sign is elicited with the patient in the supine position and is positive when passive flexion of the neck results in spontaneous flexion of the hips and knees.

Seizures occur as part of the initial presentation of bacterial meningitis or during the course of the illness in up to 40% of patients. Focal seizures are usually due to focal arterial ischemia or infarction, cortical venous thrombosis with hemorrhage, or focal edema. Generalized seizure activity and status epilepticus are due to fever, hyponatremia, or cerebral anoxia or, less commonly, as a result of toxicity from antimicrobial agents.

The rash of meningococcemia begins as a diffuse erythematous maculopapular rash resembling a viral exanthem, but the skin lesions of meningococcemia rapidly become petechial. Petechiae are found on the trunk and lower extremities, in the mucous membranes and conjunctiva, and occasionally on the palms and soles.

Raised ICP is an expected complication of bacterial meningitis and is the major cause of obtundation and coma in this disease. More than 90% of patients will have a CSF opening pressure >180 mmH$_2$O, and 20% have opening pressures >400 mmH$_2$O. Signs of increased ICP include a deteriorating or reduced level of consciousness, papilledema, dilated poorly reactive pupils, sixth nerve palsies, decerebrate posturing, and the Cushing reflex (bradycardia, hypertension, and irregular respirations). The most disastrous complication of increased ICP is cerebral herniation. The incidence of herniation in patients with bacterial meningitis has been reported to occur in as few as 1% to as many as 8% of cases.

DIAGNOSIS When the clinical presentation is suggestive of bacterial meningitis, blood cultures should be immediately obtained and empirical antimicrobial therapy initiated without delay. The diagnosis of bacterial meningitis is made by examination of the CSF (Table 372-1). The need for cranial magnetic resonance imaging (MRI) or computed tomography (CT) prior to lumbar puncture remains a controversial issue and must be dealt with on a case-by-case basis. In a patient with a normal level of consciousness and a neurologic examination with no evidence of papilledema or focal deficits, it is safe to perform lumbar puncture without prior neuroimaging studies. If lumbar puncture is delayed in order to obtain neuroimaging studies, empirical antibiotic therapy should be initiated after blood cultures are obtained. Antibiotic therapy for several hours prior to lumbar puncture will not significantly alter the CSF white blood cell count or glucose concentration, nor is it likely to sterilize the CSF so that the organism cannot be identified on Gram's stain. Increased ICP should be treated in patients with clinical signs of increased pressure, and lumbar puncture performed with a 22- or 25-gauge needle. Only a minimum amount of CSF need be removed for analysis; ~3.5 mL of CSF is sufficient to obtain a cell count (1.0 mL), glucose and protein concentrations (1.0 mL), latex particle agglutination (LA) tests (0.5 mL), and Gram's stain and bacterial cultures (1.0 mL). If possible, an additional 0.5 to 1.0 mL should be saved. Preadministration of mannitol and hyperventilation further decrease the risk of herniation in patients with elevated ICP.

The classic CSF abnormalities in bacterial meningitis are: (1) polymorphonuclear leukocytosis (>100 cells per microliter in 90%), (2) decreased glucose concentration [<2.2 mmol/L (<40 mg/dL) and/or CSF/serum glucose ratio of <0.4 in ~60%], (3) increased protein concentration [>0.45 g/L (>45 mg/dL) in 90%], and (4) increased opening pressure (>180 mmH$_2$O in 90%). CSF bacterial cultures are positive in >80% of patients, and CSF Gram's stain demonstrates organisms in >60%.

Opening pressure should be measured with the patient in the lateral recumbent position. In adults, the normal opening pressure is <180 mmH$_2$O, and the normal white blood cell count is <5 mononuclear cells (lymphocytes and monocytes) per microliter. Polymorphonuclear neutrophils (PMNs) are not found in cell counts of normal CSF; however, rare PMNs can be found in concentrated CSF specimens, such as those analyzed for cytology. CSF glucose concentrations <2.2 mmol/L (<40 mg/dL) are abnormal, and a CSF glucose concentration of zero can be seen in bacterial meningitis. Use of the CSF/serum glucose ratio corrects for hyperglycemia that may mask a relative decrease in the CSF glucose concentration. The CSF glucose concentration is low when the CSF/serum glucose ratio is <0.6. A CSF/serum glucose ratio <0.40 is highly suggestive of bacterial meningitis but may also be seen in other conditions, including carcinomatous meningitis and rare cases of viral meningitis. It takes at least 30 min, and more likely several hours, for CSF glucose concentration to reach equilibrium with blood glucose concentrations; therefore, administration of 50 mL of 50% glucose (D50) prior to lumbar puncture, as commonly occurs in emergency room settings, is unlikely to alter CSF glucose concentration significantly unless more than a few hours have elapsed between glucose administration and lumbar puncture.

The LA test for the detection of bacterial antigens of *S. pneumoniae*, *N. meningitidis*, *H. influenzae* type b, group B streptococcus, and *Escherichia coli* K1 strains in the CSF is very useful for making a rapid diagnosis of bacterial meningitis, especially in patients who have been pretreated with antibiotics and in whom CSF Gram's stain and culture are negative. The CSF LA test has a *specificity* of 95 to 100% for *S. pneumoniae* and *N. meningitidis*, so a positive test is virtually diagnostic of bacterial meningitis by these organisms. However, the *sensitivity* of the CSF LA test is only 70 to 100% for detection of *S. pneumoniae* and 33 to 70% for detection of *N. meningitidis* antigens, so a negative test does not exclude infection by these organisms. The Limulus amebocyte lysate assay is a rapid diagnostic test for the detection of gram-negative endotoxin in CSF, and thus for making a diagnosis of gram-negative bacterial meningitis. The test has a specificity of 85 to 100% and a sensitivity approaching 100%. Thus, a positive Limulus amebocyte lysate assay occurs in virtually all patients with gram-negative bacterial meningitis, but false-positives may occur. CSF polymerase chain reaction (PCR) tests are not as useful in the diagnosis of bacterial meningitis as they are in the diagnosis of viral CNS infections. A CSF PCR test has been developed for detecting DNA from bacteria in CSF, but its sensitivity and specificity need to be better characterized before its role in diagnosis can be defined.

Almost all patients with bacterial meningitis will ultimately have neuroimaging studies performed. MRI is preferred over CT because of its superiority in demonstrating areas of cerebral edema and ischemia. In patients with bacterial meningitis, diffuse meningeal enhancement is often seen after the administration of gadolinium. Meningeal enhancement is not diagnostic of meningitis but occurs in any CNS disease associated with increased blood-brain barrier permeability.

Petechial skin lesions, if present, should be biopsied. The rash of meningococcemia results from the dermal seeding of organisms with vascular endothelial damage, and biopsy may reveal the organism on Gram's stain.

DIFFERENTIAL DIAGNOSIS Foremost in the differential diagnosis of bacterial meningitis is viral meningoencephalitis, specifically herpes simplex virus (HSV) encephalitis (Chaps. 182, 373). The

Table 372-1 Cerebrospinal Fluid Abnormalities in Bacterial Meningitis

Opening pressure	>180 mmH$_2$O
White blood cells	>10/μL to <10,000/μL; neutrophils predominate
Red blood cells	Absent, unless traumatic tap
Glucose	<2.2 mmol/L (<40 mg/dL)
CSF serum:glucose ratio	<0.40
Protein	>0.45 g/L (>45 mg/dL)
Gram's stain	Positive in 70–90% of untreated cases
Culture	Positive in 80% of cases
Latex agglutination	Specific for antigens of *S. pneumoniae*, *N. meningitidis*, *E. coli*, *H. influenzae*, type b, and group B streptococcus
Limulus amebocyte lysate assay	Positive in gram-negative meningitis
PCR for bacterial DNA	Specificity and sensitivity unknown

NOTE: PCR, polymerase chain reaction.

clinical presentation of HSV encephalitis includes headache, fever, altered consciousness, focal neurologic deficits (e.g., dysphasia, hemiparesis), and focal or generalized seizures. Features that distinguish herpes encephalitis from bacterial meningitis include the findings on CSF studies, neuroimaging, and electroencephalogram (EEG). The classic CSF profile in patients with viral CNS infections is a lymphocytic pleocytosis with a normal glucose concentration, as contrasted with the PMN pleocytosis and hypoglycorrhachia characteristic of bacterial meningitis. MRI abnormalities other than meningeal enhancement are not seen in uncomplicated bacterial meningitis. Patients with HSV encephalitis frequently have MRI abnormalities, including increased signal within the orbitofrontal and medial temporal lobes and insular cortex on T2-weighted and FLAIR images. There is a distinctive EEG pattern in HSV encephalitis consisting of periodic, stereotyped, sharp-and-slow wave complexes originating in one or both temporal lobes and repeating at regular intervals of 2 to 3 s. The periodic complexes are typically noted between the second and the fifteenth day of the illness and are present in two-thirds of pathologically proven cases of HSV encephalitis.

The clinical presentation of encephalitis caused by arthropod-borne viruses (Chap. 198) can also resemble that of bacterial meningitis. Another consideration is rickettsial disease (Chap. 177). Rocky Mountain spotted fever (RMSF) is transmitted by a tick bite and caused by the bacteria *Rickettsia rickettsii*. The disease may resemble bacterial meningitis because of its common presentation with high fever, prostration, myalgia, headache, and nausea and vomiting. Most patients develop a characteristic rash within 96 h of the onset of symptoms. The rash is initially a diffuse erythematous maculopapular rash that may be difficult to distinguish from that of meningococcemia. It progresses to a petechial rash, then to a purpuric rash, and, if untreated, to skin necrosis or gangrene. The color of the lesions changes from bright red to very dark red, then yellowish-green to black. The rash typically begins in the wrist and ankles, and then spreads distally and proximally within a matter of a few hours and involves the palms and soles. Diagnosis is made by immunofluorescent staining of skin biopsy specimens.

Focal suppurative CNS infections (see below), including subdural and epidural empyema and brain abscess, should also be considered. The presence of focal features in a patient with suspected bacterial meningitis should prompt immediate neuroimaging studies; MRI is preferable to CT and is extremely sensitive and specific for diagnosis.

Among noninfectious CNS processes, subarachnoid hemorrhage (SAH; Chap. 361) is generally the major consideration. A classic presentation of SAH is the explosive onset of a severe headache or a sudden transient loss of consciousness followed by a severe headache. Nuchal rigidity and vomiting are frequently present and contribute to the resemblance between SAH and meningitis. CT scan is a sensitive indicator of the presence of SAH and usually allows for prompt diagnosis, although occasional patients with suspected SAH have a normal CT scan. In these patients a lumbar puncture is indicated, and the presence of grossly bloody CSF allows SAH to be immediately distinguished from bacterial meningitis.

℞ **TREATMENT Empirical antimicrobial therapy** (Table 372-2) Bacterial meningitis is a medical emergency. The goal is to begin antibiotic therapy within 60 min of a patient's arrival in the emergency room. Empirical antimicrobial therapy is initiated in patients with suspected bacterial meningitis before the results of CSF Gram's stain and culture are known. *S. pneumoniae* (Chap. 140) and *N. meningitidis* (Chap. 146) are the most common etiologic organisms of community-acquired bacterial meningitis. Due to the emergence of penicillin- and cephalosporin-resistant *S. pneumoniae*, empirical therapy of community-acquired bacterial meningitis in children and adults should include a third-generation cephalosporin (e.g., ceftriaxone or cefotaxime) and vancomycin. Ceftriaxone or cefotaxime provide good coverage for susceptible *S. pneumoniae*, group B streptococci, and *H. influenzae* and adequate coverage for *N. meningitidis*. Ampicillin should be added to the empirical regimen for coverage of *L. mono-*

Table 372-2 Antibiotics Used in Empirical Therapy of Bacterial Meningitis and Focal CNS Infections

Indication	Antibiotic
Preterm infants to infants <1 month	Ampicillin + cefotaxime
Infants 1–3 months	Ampicillin + (cefotaxime or ceftriaxone) (consider adjunctive dexamethasone)
Immunocompetent children >3 months, adults <50	(Cefotaxime or ceftriaxone) + vancomycin
Adults >50, individuals with alcoholism or other debilitating illnesses	Ampicillin + vancomycin + (cefotaxime or ceftriaxone)
Hospital-acquired meningitis, meningitis after head trauma or neurosurgery, neutropenic patients	Ceftazidime + vancomycin
Impaired cell-mediated immunity (at any age)	Ceftazidime (in place of cefotaxime or ceftriaxone) + ampicillin

Antimicrobial Agent	Total Daily Dose and Dosing Interval	
	Child (> 1 month)	Adult
Ampicillin	200–300 (mg/kg)/d, q4h	12 g/d, q4h
Cefotaxime	300 (mg/kg)/d, q6h	12 g/d, q4h
Ceftriaxone	100–200 (mg/kg)/d, q12h	4 g/d, q12h
Ceftazidime	150 (mg/kg)/d, q8h	6 g/d, q8h
Metronidazole	30 (mg/kg)/d, q6h	2000 mg/d, q6h
Nafcillin	100–200 (mg/kg)/d, q6h	9–12 g/day, q4h
Vancomycin	60 (mg/kg)/d, q6h	2 g/d, q6h

cytogenes in individuals under three months of age, those over age 55, or those with suspected impaired cell-mediated immunity because of chronic illness, organ transplantation, pregnancy, malignancies, or immunosuppressive therapy. In hospital-acquired meningitis, and particularly meningitis following neurosurgical procedures, staphylococci and gram-negative organisms including *Pseudomonas aeruginosa* are the most common etiologic organisms. In these patients, empirical therapy should include a combination of vancomycin and ceftazidime. Ceftazidime should be substituted for ceftriaxone or cefotaxime in neurosurgical patients and in neutropenic patients, as *P. aeruginosa* may be the meningeal pathogen, and ceftazidime is the only cephalosporin with adequate activity against *P. aeruginosa* in the CNS.

Specific antimicrobial therapy (Table 372-3) • *Meningococcal meningitis* Although ceftriaxone and cefotaxime provide adequate empirical coverage for *N. meningitidis*, penicillin G remains the antibiotic of choice for meningococcal meningitis caused by susceptible strains. Isolates of *N. meningitidis* with moderate resistance to penicillin have been identified, but patients infected with these strains have still been successfully treated with penicillin. CSF isolates of *N. meningitidis* should be tested for penicillin and ampicillin susceptibility, and if resistance is found, cefotaxime or ceftriaxone should be substituted for penicillin. A 7-day course of intravenous antibiotic therapy is adequate for uncomplicated meningococcal meningitis. The index case and all close contacts should receive chemoprophylaxis with a 2-day regimen of rifampin (600 mg every 12 h for 2 days in adults and 10 mg/kg every 12 h for 2 days in children >1 year). Rifampin is not recommended in pregnant women. Alternatively, adults can be treated with one dose of ciprofloxacin (750 mg), one dose of azithromycin (500 mg), or one IM dose of ceftriaxone (250 mg). Close contacts are defined as those individuals who have had contact with oropharyngeal secretions either through kissing or by sharing toys, beverages, or cigarettes.

Pneumococcal meningitis Antimicrobial therapy of pneumococcal meningitis is initiated with a third-generation cephalosporin (ceftriaxone or cefotaxime) and vancomycin (Tables 372-2 and 372-3). All CSF isolates of *S. pneumoniae* should be tested for sensitivity to penicillin and the third-generation cephalosporins. Once the results

Table 372-3 Antimicrobial Therapy of CNS Bacterial Infections Based on Pathogen[a]

Organism	Antibiotic	Total Daily Adult Dose and Dosing Interval
Neisseria meningitidis		
Penicillin-sensitive	Penicillin G	20–24 million U/d, q4h
	or	
	Ampicillin	12 g/d, q4h
Penicillin-resistant	Ceftriaxone	4 g/d, q12h
	or	
	Cefotaxime	12 g/d, q4h
Streptococcus pneumoniae		
Penicillin-sensitive	Penicillin G	20–24 million U/d, q4h
Relatively penicillin-resistant	Ceftriaxone	4 g/d, q12h
	or	
	Cefotaxime	12 g/d, q4h
Penicillin-resistant	Vancomycin	2 g/d, q6h
	plus	
	Ceftriaxone	4 g/d, q12h
	or	
	Cefotaxime	12 g/d, q4h
	±	
	Intraventricular vancomycin	20 mg/d
Gram-negative bacilli (except *P. aeruginosa*)	Ceftriaxone	4 g/d, q12h
	or	
	Cefotaxime	12 g/d, q4h
Pseudomonas aeruginosa	Ceftazidime	6 g/d, q8h
Staphylococci		
Methicillin-sensitive	Nafcillin	9–12 g/d, q4h
Methicillin-resistant	Vancomycin	2 g/d, q6h
Listeria monocytogenes	Ampicillin	12 g/d, q4h
Haemophilus influenzae	Ceftriaxone	4 g/d, q12h
	or	
	Cefotaxime	12 g/d, q4h
Streptococcus agalactiae	Ampicillin	12 g/d, q4h
	or	
	Penicillin G	20–24 million U/d, q4h
Bacteroides fragilis	Metronidazole	2000 mg/d, q6h
Fusobacterium spp.	Metronidazole	2000 mg/d, q6h

[a] All antibiotics are administered intravenously; doses indicated are for patients with normal renal function.

of antimicrobial susceptibility tests are known, therapy can be modified accordingly. For *S. pneumoniae* meningitis, an isolate of *S. pneumoniae* is considered to be susceptible to penicillin with a minimal inhibitory concentration (MIC) < 0.06 μg/mL, to have intermediate resistance when the MIC is 0.1 to 1.0 μg/mL, and to be highly resistant when the MIC > 1.0 μg/mL. Isolates of *S. pneumoniae* that have cephalosporin MICs ≤ 0.5 μg/mL are considered sensitive to the cephalosporins (cefotaxime, ceftriaxone, cefepime). Those with MICs of 1 μg/mL are considered to have intermediate resistance, and those with MICs ≥ 2 μg/mL are considered resistant. Penicillin-resistant strains of *S. pneumoniae* are more common than cephalosporin-resistant strains of *S. pneumoniae*. For meningitis due to pneumococci with cefotaxime or ceftriaxone MICs ≤ 0.5 μg/mL, treatment with cefotaxime or ceftriaxone is usually adequate. If the MIC is ≥ 1 μg/mL, vancomycin is the antibiotic of choice. Rifampin can be added to vancomycin for its synergistic effect but is inadequate as monotherapy because resistance develops rapidly when it is used alone.

Patients with *S. pneumoniae* meningitis should have a repeat lumbar puncture performed 24 to 36 h after the initiation of antimicrobial therapy to document sterilization of the CSF. Failure to sterilize the CSF after 24 to 36 h of antibiotic therapy should be considered presumptive evidence of antibiotic resistance. Patients with penicillin- and cephalosporin-resistant strains of *S. pneumoniae* who do not respond to intravenous vancomycin alone may benefit from the addition of intraventricular vancomycin. The intraventricular route of administration is preferred over the intrathecal route because adequate con-

centrations of vancomycin in the cerebral ventricles are not always achieved with intrathecal administration. A 2-week course of intravenous antimicrobial therapy is recommended for pneumococcal meningitis.

L. monocytogenes meningitis Meningitis due to this organism is treated with ampicillin for at least 3 weeks (Table 372-3). Gentamicin is often added (2 mg/kg loading dose then 5.1 mg/kg per day given every 8 h and adjusted for serum levels and renal function). The combination of trimethoprim [10 to 20 (mg/kg)/d] and sulfamethoxazole [50 to 100 (mg/kg)/d] given every 6 h may provide an alternative in penicillin-allergic patients.

Staphylococcal meningitis Meningitis due to susceptible strains of *S. aureus* or coagulase-negative staphylococci is treated with nafcillin (Table 372-3). Vancomycin is the drug of choice for methicillin-resistant staphylococci and for patients allergic to penicillin. In these patients, the CSF should be monitored during therapy. If the CSF is not sterilized after 48 h of intravenous vancomycin therapy, then either intrathecal or intraventricular vancomycin, 20 mg once daily, can be added.

Gram-negative bacillary meningitis The third-generation cephalosporins, cefotaxime, ceftriaxone, and ceftazidime, are equally efficacious for the treatment of gram-negative bacillary meningitis, with the exception of meningitis due to *P. aeruginosa*, which should be treated with ceftazidime (Table 372-3). A 3-week course of intravenous antibiotic therapy is recommended for meningitis due to gram-negative bacilli.

Newer antibiotics Cefepime is a broad-spectrum fourth-generation cephalosporin with in vitro activity similar to that of cefotaxime or ceftriaxone against *S. pneumoniae* and *N. meningitidis* and greater activity against *Enterobacter* spp. and *P. aeruginosa*. The dose of cefepime is 2 g intravenously every 12 h in adults. In clinical trials, cefepime has been demonstrated to be equivalent to cefotaxime in the treatment of pneumococcal and meningococcal meningitis, but its efficacy in bacterial meningitis caused by penicillin- and cephalosporin-resistant pneumococcal organisms, *Enterobacter* spp., and *P. aeruginosa* has not been established. Meropenem is a carbapenem antibiotic structurally related to imipenem, but reportedly with less seizure proclivity than imipenem. Meropenem is highly active in vitro against *L. monocytogenes*, has been demonstrated to be effective in cases of meningitis caused by *P. aeruginosa*, and shows good activity against penicillin-resistant pneumococci. In experimental pneumococcal meningitis, meropenem was comparable to ceftriaxone and inferior to vancomycin in sterilizing CSF cultures. The dose of meropenem is 1 to 2 g intravenously every 8 h for adults. The number of patients with bacterial meningitis enrolled in clinical trials of meropenem has not been sufficient to definitively assess the epileptogenic potential of this antibiotic. Firm recommendations regarding the use of cefepime and meropenem in bacterial meningitis await more clinical experience.

Adjunctive therapy The release of bacterial cell-wall components by bactericidal antibiotics leads to the production of the inflammatory cytokines IL-1 and TNF in the subarachnoid space (Fig. 372-1). Dexamethasone exerts its beneficial effect by inhibiting the synthesis of IL-1 and TNF at the level of mRNA, decreasing CSF outflow resistance, and stabilizing the blood-brain barrier. The rationale for giving dexamethasone 20 min before antibiotic therapy is that dexamethasone inhibits the production of TNF by macrophages and microglia only if it is administered before these cells are activated by endotoxin. Dexamethasone does not alter TNF production once it has been induced. The results of clinical trials of dexamethasone therapy in children, predominantly with meningitis due to *H. influenzae* and *S. pneumoniae*, have demonstrated its efficacy in decreasing meningeal inflammation and neurologic sequelae such as the incidence of sensorineural hearing loss. Evidence for efficacy of dexamethasone in other types of bacterial meningitis remains much more limited. The American Academy of Pediatrics recommends the consideration of dexamethasone for bacterial meningitis in infants and children ≥2 months. The recommended dose is 0.6 mg/kg per day in four divided doses given intravenously for the first 2 days of antibiotic therapy or

0.8 mg/kg per day in two divided doses given for 2 days. The first dose of dexamethasone should be administered before or at least with the first dose of antibiotic.

The role of dexamethasone in the treatment of bacterial meningitis in adults remains uncertain. In a single clinical trial, dexamethasone was demonstrated to reduce the incidence of mortality in adults from pneumococcal meningitis. Other clinical trials of dexamethasone therapy in adults with bacterial meningitis are in progress. The suggested dose of dexamethasone is 0.6 mg/kg per day in four divided doses for the first 2 to 4 days of antimicrobial therapy. For the reasons cited earlier, dexamethasone should ideally be given 20 min before, or not later than simultaneous with, the first dose of antibiotics. It is unlikely to be of significant benefit if started ≥6h after antimicrobial therapy has been initiated. Dexamethasone may decrease the penetration of vancomycin into CSF, and it delays the sterilization of CSF in experimental models of *S. pneumoniae* meningitis. As a result, its potential benefit should be carefully weighed when vancomycin is the antibiotic of choice. The third-generation cephalosporins and rifampin penetrate the CSF extremely well, even in the presence of dexamethasone, and may provide an alternative when adjunctive dexamethasone is being used to treat *S. pneumoniae* meningitis.

Increased Intracranial Pressure Emergency treatment of increased ICP includes elevation of the patient's head to 30 to 45°, intubation and hyperventilation (Pa$_{CO_2}$ 25 to 30 mmHg), and mannitol. Patients with increased ICP should be managed in an intensive care unit. In these patients, accurate ICP measurements are best obtained with an ICP monitoring device. →*Increased intracranial pressure is discussed in detail in Chap. 376.*

PROGNOSIS Mortality is 3 to 7% for meningitis caused by *H. influenzae*, *N. meningitidis*, or group B streptococci; 15% for that due to *L. monocytogenes*; and 20% for *S. pneumoniae*. In general, the risk of death from bacterial meningitis is significantly associated with (1) decreased level of consciousness on admission, (2) onset of seizures within 24 h of admission, (3) signs of increased ICP, (4) young age (infancy) and age >50, (5) the presence of comorbid conditions including shock and/or the need for mechanical ventilation, and (6) delay in the initiation of treatment. Decreased CSF glucose concentration [<2.2 mmol/L (<40 mg/dL)] and markedly increased CSF protein concentration [>3 g/L (>300 mg/dL)] have been predictive of increased mortality and poorer outcomes in some series. Moderate or severe sequelae occur in ~25% of survivors of bacterial meningitis, although the exact incidence varies with the infecting organism. Common sequelae include decreased intellectual function, memory impairment, seizures, hearing loss and dizziness, and gait disturbances.

BRAIN ABSCESS

DEFINITION A brain abscess is a focal, suppurative process within the brain parenchyma; it begins in an area of devitalized brain tissue as a localized area of cerebritis and develops into a collection of pus surrounded by a well-vascularized capsule.

EPIDEMIOLOGY A bacterial brain abscess is a relatively uncommon intracranial infection, with an incidence of approximately 1 in 100,000 persons per year. Predisposing conditions include paranasal sinusitis, otitis media, and dental infections. Brain abscess is an extremely uncommon complication of these common infections, reflecting the efficiency with which they are treated with oral antimicrobial therapy, thereby minimizing the risk of subsequent intracranial spread of infection. In most modern series, a significant percentage of brain abscesses are not caused by classic pyogenic bacteria, but rather by *Toxoplasmi gondii*, *Aspergillus* spp., *Nocardia* spp., *Mycobacteria* spp., and fungi such as *Cryptococcus neoformans*. This distribution reflects the importance of brain abscesses in hosts whose immune systems are compromised, whether from HIV infection, organ transplantation, cancer, or immunosuppressive therapy. In Latin America and in immigrants from Latin America, the most common cause of brain abscess is *Taenia solium* (neurocysticercosis). The discussion that follows is limited to bacterial brain abscess; the other etiologies are discussed elsewhere.

ETIOLOGY A brain abscess may develop (1) by direct spread from a contiguous cranial site of infection, such as paranasal sinusitis, otitis media, mastoiditis, or dental infection; (2) following head trauma or a neurosurgical procedure; or (3) as a result of hematogenous spread from a remote site of infection. In 20 to 30% of cases no obvious primary source of infection is apparent (cryptogenic brain abscess).

Abscesses that develop as a result of direct spread of infection from the frontal, ethmoidal, or sphenoidal sinuses and those that occur due to dental infections are usually located in the frontal lobes. The most common pathogens in brain abscesses associated with paranasal sinusitis are microaerophilic and anaerobic streptococci, *Haemophilus* spp., *Bacteroides* spp. (non-*fragilis*), and *Fusobacterium* spp. The most common pathogens in brain abscess from dental infections are streptococci and *Prevotella* and *Porphyromonas* (formerly *Bacteroides*) spp.

The majority of brain abscesses associated with otititts media and mastoiditis occur in the temporal lobe and cerebellum and are caused by streptococci, *Bacteroides* spp. (including *B. fragilis*), *P. aeruginosa*, and Enterobacteriaceae. A brain abscess that is the result of hematogenous spread of infection from a site elsewhere in the body can occur anywhere in the brain but tends to form primarily in areas supplied by the middle cerebral artery (i.e., posterior frontal or parietal lobes). Metastatic abscesses are usually located at the interface of the gray-white matter and are often multiple. The microbiology of these brain abscesses is dependent on the primary source of infection. For example, brain abscesses that develop as a complication of infective endocarditis are often due to viridans streptococci or *S. aureus*; those that follow pyogenic lung infection are often due to *Streptococcus*, *Actinomyces*, or *Fusobacterium* species; those resulting from urinary sepsis are often caused by Enterobacteriaceae or *Pseudomonas aeruginosa*; and those associated with an intraabdominal source are frequently caused by *Streptococcus* spp., Enterobacteriaceae, or anaerobes. Abscesses that follow penetrating head trauma are frequently due to *S. aureus*, *Clostridium* spp., or Enterobacteriaceae, and those following a neurosurgical procedure are usually due to staphylococci, Enterobacteriaceae, or *P. aeruginosa*. Congenital cardiac malformations that produce a right-to-left shunt, such as tetralogy of Fallot, and atrial and ventricular septal defects allow bloodborne bacteria to bypass the pulmonary capillary bed and reach the brain. The decreased arterial oxygenation and saturation from the right-to-left shunt and polycythemia may cause focal areas of cerebral ischemia, thus providing a nidus for microorganisms that bypassed the pulmonary circulation to multiply and form an abscess. Streptococci are the most common pathogens in this setting.

PATHOGENESIS AND HISTOPATHOLOGY Results of experimental models of brain abscess formation suggest that for bacterial invasion of brain parenchyma to occur, there must be preexisting or concomitant areas of ischemia, necrosis, or hypoxia in brain tissue. The intact brain parenchyma is relatively resistant to infection. Once bacteria have established infection, brain abscess formation evolves through four stages, regardless of the infecting organism. The early cerebritis stage (days 1 to 3) is characterized by a perivascular infiltration of inflammatory cells, which surround a central core of coagulative necrosis. Marked edema surrounds the lesion at this stage. In the late cerebritis stage (days 4 to 9), pus formation leads to enlargement of the necrotic center, which is surrounded at its border by an inflammatory infiltrate of macrophages and fibroblasts. A thin capsule of fibroblasts and reticular fibers gradually develops, and the surrounding area of cerebral edema becomes more distinct than in the previous stage. The third stage, early capsule formation (days 10 to 13), is characterized by the formation of a capsule that is better developed on the cortical than on the ventricular side of the lesion. This stage correlates with the appearance of a ring-enhancing capsule on neuroimaging studies. The final stage, late capsule formation (day 14 and be-

FIGURE 372-2 Pneumococcal brain abscess. Note that the abscess wall has hyperintense signal on the axial T1-weighted image (*A*, black arrow), hypointense signal on the axial proton density images (*B*, black arrow), and enhances prominently after gadolinium administration on the coronal T1-weighted image (*C*). The abscess is surrounded by a large amount of vasogenic edema and has a small "daughter" abscess (*C*, white arrow). (*Courtesy of Joseph Lurito, MD.*)

yond), is defined by a well-formed necrotic center surrounded by a dense collagenous capsule. The surrounding area of cerebral edema has regressed, but marked gliosis with large numbers of reactive astrocytes has developed outside the capsule. This gliotic process may contribute to the development of seizures as a sequelae of brain abscess.

CLINICAL PRESENTATION A brain abscess presents as an expanding intracranial mass lesion, rather than as an infectious process. The most common symptom is headache, occurring in >75% of patients. The headache is often characterized as a constant, dull, aching sensation, either hemicranial or generalized, and it becomes progressively more severe and refractory to therapy. Fever is present in only 50% of patients at the time of diagnosis and is typically low-grade. Thus the absence of fever should not exclude the diagnosis. The new onset of focal or generalized seizure activity is a presenting sign in 25 to 30% of patients. In most large series, a focal neurologic deficit is part of the initial presentation in >60% of patients.

The clinical presentation of a brain abscess depends on its location and on the presence of raised ICP, which develops as edema surrounds the evolving abscess. Hemiparesis is the most common localizing sign of a frontal lobe abscess. A temporal lobe abscess may present with a disturbance of language (dysphasia) or an upper homonymous quadrantanopia. Nystagmus and ataxia are signs of a cerebellar abscess. The earliest signs of increased ICP in a patient with a brain abscess are papilledema, nausea and vomiting, and drowsiness or confusion. Meningismus is not present unless the abscess has ruptured into the ventricle or the infection has spread to the subarachnoid space.

DIAGNOSIS The diagnosis of a brain abscess is made by neuroimaging studies. CT has the advantage of greater feasibility in acutely ill patients, but MRI is better for demonstrating abscesses in the early (cerebritis) stages and is superior to CT for identifying abscesses in the posterior fossa. Cerebritis appears on MRI as an area of low-signal intensity on T1-weighted images with irregular postgadolinium enhancement and as an area of increased signal intensity on T2-weighted images. Cerebritis is often not visualized by CT scan. As the abscess matures, the appearance of the lesion changes. On a contrast-enhanced CT scan, a mature brain abscess appears as a focal area of hypodensity surrounded by ring enhancement. On T1-weighted MRI, a mature brain abscess has the characteristics demonstrated in Fig. 372-2. On T2-weighted MRI, there is a hyperintense central area of pus surrounded by a well-defined hypointense capsule and a hyperintense area of edema.

The microbiologic diagnosis is made by Gram's stain and culture of abscess material obtained by stereotactic needle aspiration. Lumbar puncture should not be performed in patients with known or suspected focal intracranial infections such as abscess or empyema; CSF analysis contributes nothing to diagnosis or therapy, and lumbar puncture increases the risk of herniation.

Additional laboratory studies that may provide clues to the diagnosis of brain abscess in patients with a CNS mass lesion include the peripheral white blood cell count and erythrocyte sedimentation rate; the latter will be elevated in about 60% of patients, and about 50% will have a peripheral leukocytosis.

DIFFERENTIAL DIAGNOSIS Conditions that can cause headache, fever, focal neurologic signs, and seizure activity include brain abscess, subdural empyema, bacterial meningitis, viral meningoencephalitis, superior sagittal sinus thrombosis, and acute disseminated encephalomyelitis. In unusual cases, tumors and, more rarely, cerebral infarction or hematoma can have an MRI or CT appearance resembling brain abscess.

TREATMENT Empirical therapy of a brain abscess depends on the source of infection (Table 372-4) and typically includes a third-generation cephalosporin (e.g., cefotaxime) and metronidazole (Table 372-3 for antibiotic dosages). Patients with multiple abscesses, which suggest the possibility of hematogenous spread, or those who develop abscesses following head trauma should have nafcillin added to this regimen for coverage of staphylococci. Patients who develop abscesses following neurosurgical procedures should be treated with vancomycin plus ceftazidime (in place of cefotaxime) for coverage of both staphylococci and *P. aeruginosa*.

Aspiration and drainage of the abscess under stereotactic guidance are beneficial for both diagnosis and therapy. Empirical antibiotic coverage can be modified based on the results of Gram's stain and culture of the abscess contents (Table 372-4). Complete excision of a bacterial abscess via craniotomy or craniectomy is generally reserved for multiloculated abscesses or those in which stereotactic aspiration is unsuccessful. Antibiotic therapy alone is generally not optimal for treatment of brain abscess and should be reserved for patients whose abscesses cannot be surgically aspirated or otherwise drained, for selected patients with multiple abscesses, and in patients whose condition is too tenuous to allow performance of a neurosurgical procedure. All patients should receive a minimum of 6 to 8 weeks of parenteral antibiotic therapy. The role, if any, of supplemental oral antibiotic therapy following completion of a standard course of parenteral therapy has never been adequately studied.

In addition to surgical drainage and antibiotic therapy, patients

Table 372-4 Empirical Therapy of Brain Abscess Based on Source of Infection

Source	Antimicrobial Therapy
Paranasal sinusitis	Penicillin or a third-generation cephalosporin (cefotaxime or ceftriaxone) + metronidazole
Otitis media	Penicillin + metronidazole + ceftazidime
Dental infection	Penicillin + metronidazole
Endocarditis	Nafcillin or vancomycin + metronidazole + third-generation cephalosporin
Lung abscess, urinary sepsis, intra-abdominal source	Ceftazidime + metronidazole + penicillin
Head trauma	Nafcillin or vancomycin + third-generation cephalosporin
Neurosurgical procedure	Vancomycin + ceftazidime
Cyanotic congenital heart disease	Penicillin or third-generation cephalosporin + metronidazole

should receive prophylactic anticonvulsant therapy because of the high risk of focal or generalized seizures. Anticonvulsant therapy is continued for at least 3 months after resolution of the abscess, and decisions regarding withdrawal are then based on the EEG. If the EEG is abnormal, anticonvulsant therapy should be continued. If the EEG is normal, anticonvulsant therapy can be slowly withdrawn, with close follow-up and repeat EEG after the medication has been discontinued.

Glucocorticoids should not be given routinely to patients with brain abscesses. Intravenous dexamethasone therapy (10 mg every 6 h) is usually reserved for patients with substantial periabscess edema and associated mass effect and increased ICP. Dexamethasone should be tapered as rapidly as possible to avoid delaying the natural process of encapsulation of the abscess.

Serial CT or MRI scans should be obtained on a monthly or twice-monthly basis to document resolution of the abscess. More frequent studies (e.g., weekly) are probably warranted in the subset of patients who are receiving antibiotic therapy alone. A small amount of enhancement may remain for months after the abscess has been successfully treated.

PROGNOSIS Bacterial abscess can be successfully treated in the majority of patients. Seizures, however, are a common complication and occur in as many as 70% of patients.

SUBDURAL EMPYEMA

DEFINITION A subdural empyema (SDE) is a collection of pus between the dura and arachnoid membranes (Fig. 372-3).

EPIDEMIOLOGY SDE is a rare intracranial infection. Sinusitis is the most common predisposing condition and typically involves the frontal sinuses, either alone or in combination with the ethmoid and maxillary sinuses. Sinusitis-associated empyema has a striking predilection for young males, possibly reflecting sex-related differences in sinus anatomy and development. SDE may also develop as a complication of head trauma or following neurosurgical drainage of a subdural hematoma. Secondary infection of a subdural effusion may also result in empyema, although secondary infection of hematomas, in the absence of a prior neurosurgical procedure, is rare.

ETIOLOGY Aerobic and microaerophilic streptococci and anaerobic bacteria are the most common causative organisms of sinusitis-associated SDE. Staphylococci and gram-negative bacilli are often the etiologic organisms when SDE follows neurosurgical procedures or head trauma. SDE should be distinguished from subdural effusions that, especially in infants and children, may complicate bacterial meningitis. Subdural effusions are sterile collections of protein-rich fluid that result from increased permeability of the thin-walled capillaries and veins in the inner layer of the dura.

PATHOPHYSIOLOGY Sinusitis-associated SDE develops as a result of either retrograde spread of infection from septic thrombophlebitis of the mucosal veins draining the sinuses or contiguous spread of infection to the brain from osteomyelitis in the posterior wall of the frontal or other sinuses. SDE may also develop from direct introduction of bacteria into the subdural space as a complication of a neurosurgical procedure. The evolution of SDE can be extremely rapid because the subdural space is a large compartment that offers few mechanical barriers to the spread of infection. In patients with sinusitis-associated SDE, suppuration typically begins in the upper and anterior portions of one cerebral hemisphere and then extends posteriorly. SDE is often associated with other intracranial infections including epidural empyema (40%), cortical thrombo-

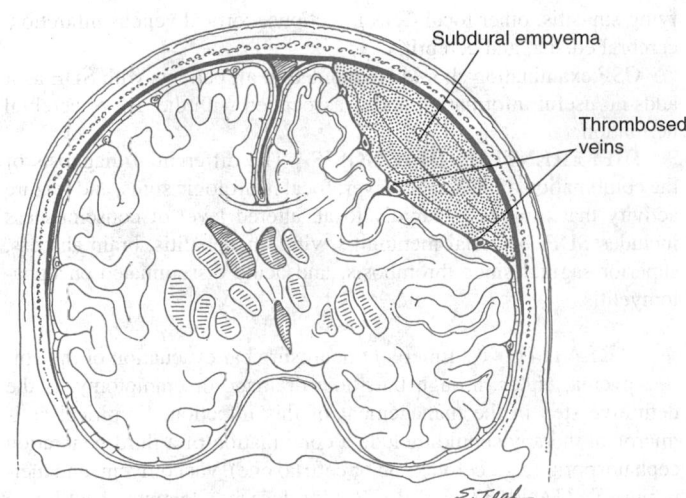

FIGURE 372-3 Subdural empyema is a collection of pus between the dura and arachnoid membranes.

phlebitis (35%), and intracranial abscess or cerebritis (>25%). Cortical venous infarction produces necrosis of underlying cerebral cortex and subcortical white matter, with focal neurological deficits and seizures (see below).

CLINICAL PRESENTATION A patient with SDE typically presents with fever and a progressively worsening headache. Patients may also have signs and symptoms related to sinusitis or other primary sites of intracranial infection. As the infection progresses, focal neurologic deficits, seizures, and signs of increased ICP commonly occur. Headache is the most common complaint at the time of presentation; initially it is localized to the side of the subdural infection but then becomes more severe and generalized. Contralateral hemiparesis or hemiplegia is the most common focal neurologic deficit and can occur from the direct effects of the SDE on the cortex or as a consequence of venous infarction. Seizures begin as partial motor seizures that then become secondarily generalized. Seizures may be due to the direct irritative effect of the SDE on the underlying cortex or result from cortical venous infarction (see above). In untreated SDE, the increasing mass effect and increase in ICP cause progressive deterioration in consciousness, leading ultimately to coma.

DIAGNOSIS Neuroimaging has greatly facilitated the diagnosis of SDE. MRI (Fig. 372-4) is superior to CT in identifying SDE and any associated intracranial infections. The administration of gadolinium greatly improves diagnosis by enhancing the rim of the empyema and allowing the empyema to be clearly delineated from the underlying brain parenchyma. Cranial MRI is also extremely valuable in identi-

FIGURE 372-4 Subdural empyema. There is marked enhancement of the dura and leptomeninges (*A, B*, straight arrows) along the left medial hemisphere. The pus is hypointense on T1-weighted images (*A, B*), but markedly hyperintense on the proton density–weighted (*C*, curved arrow) image. (*Courtesy of Joseph Lurito, MD.*)

fying sinusitis, other focal CNS infections, cortical venous infarction, cerebral edema, and cerebritis.

CSF examination should be avoided in all patients with SDE as it adds no useful information and is associated with the risk of cerebral herniation.

DIFFERENTIAL DIAGNOSIS   The differential diagnosis of the combination of headache, fever, focal neurologic signs, and seizure activity that progresses rapidly to an altered level of consciousness includes SDE, bacterial meningitis, viral encephalitis, brain abscess, superior sagittal sinus thrombosis, and acute disseminated encephalomyelitis.

℞ TREATMENT   Emergent neurosurgical evacuation of the empyema, either through burr-hole drainage or craniotomy, is the definitive step in the management of this infection. Empirical antimicrobial therapy should include a combination of a third-generation cephalosporin (e.g., cefotaxime or ceftriaxone), vancomycin, and metronidazole (Tables 372-3 and 372-4 for dosages). Parenteral antibiotic therapy should be continued for a minimum of 4 weeks. Specific diagnosis of the etiologic organisms is made based on Gram's stain and culture of fluid obtained via either burr holes or craniotomy; the initial empirical antibiotic coverage should be modified accordingly.

PROGNOSIS   Prognosis is influenced by the level of consciousness of the patient at the time of hospital presentation, the size of the empyema, and the speed with which therapy is instituted. Long-term neurologic sequelae, which include seizures and hemiparesis, occur in up to 50% of cases.

EPIDURAL ABSCESS

DEFINITION   Cranial epidural abscess is a suppurative infection occurring in the potential space between the inner skull table and the dura (Fig. 372-5).

ETIOLOGY AND PATHOPHYSIOLOGY   A cranial epidural abscess develops as a complication of a craniotomy or compound skull fracture or as a result of spread of infection from the frontal sinuses, middle ear, mastoid, or orbit. An epidural abscess may develop contiguous to an area of osteomyelitis, when craniotomy is complicated by infection of the wound or bone flap, or as a result of direct infection of the epidural space. Infection in the frontal sinus, middle ear, mastoid, or orbit can reach the epidural space through retrograde spread of infection from septic thrombophlebitis in the emissary veins that drain these areas or by way of direct spread of infection through areas of osteomyelitis. Unlike the subdural space, the epidural space is really a potential rather than an actual compartment. The dura is normally tightly adherent to the inner skull table, and infection must dissect the dura away from the skull table as it spreads. As a result,

FIGURE 372-5   Cranial epidural abscess is a collection of pus between the dura and the inner table of the skull.

epidural abscesses are often smaller than SDEs. Cranial epidural abscesses, unlike brain abscesses, only rarely result from hematogenous spread of infection from extracranial primary sites. The bacteriology of a cranial epidural abscess is similar to that of SDE (see above). The etiologic organisms of an epidural abscess that arises from frontal sinusitis, middle ear infections, or mastoiditis are usually streptococci or anaerobic organisms. Staphylococci or gram-negative organisms are the usual cause of an epidural abscess that develops as a complication of craniotomy or compound skull fracture.

CLINICAL PRESENTATION   Patients typically present with severe hemicranial headache and persistent fever. The diagnosis should always be suspected when these symptoms occur following recent head trauma or neurosurgery or in the setting of frontal sinusitis, mastoiditis, or otitis media.

DIAGNOSIS   Cranial MRI is the procedure of choice to demonstrate a cranial epidural abscess. The sensitivity of CT is limited by the presence of signal artifacts arising from the bone of the inner skull table. On MRI, an epidural abscess appears as a lentiform or crescent-shaped fluid collection that is hyperintense compared to CSF on T2-weighted images. On T1-weighted images, the fluid collection has a signal intensity that is intermediate between that of brain tissue and CSF. Following the administration of gadolinium, a significant enhancement of the dura is seen on T1-weighted images.

℞ TREATMENT   Immediate neurosurgical drainage is indicated. Empirical antimicrobial therapy, pending the results of Gram's stain and culture of the purulent material obtained at surgery, should include a combination of penicillin, a third-generation cephalosporin, nafcillin or vancomycin, and metronidazole (Tables 372-2 and 372-3). When the organism has been identified, antimicrobial therapy can be modified accordingly. Antibiotics should be continued for at least 3 weeks after surgical drainage.

SUPPURATIVE THROMBOPHLEBITIS

DEFINITION   Suppurative intracranial thrombophlebitis is septic venous thrombosis of cortical veins and sinuses. This may occur as a complication of bacterial meningitis, SDE, epidural abscess, or infection in the skin of the face, paranasal sinuses, middle ear, or mastoid.

ANATOMY AND PATHOPHYSIOLOGY   The cerebral veins and venous sinuses have no valves; therefore, blood within them can flow in either direction. The superior sagittal sinus is the largest of the venous sinuses (Fig. 372-6). It receives blood from the frontal, parietal, and occipital superior cerebral veins and the diploic veins, which communicate with the meningeal veins. Bacterial meningitis is a common predisposing condition for septic thrombosis of the superior sagittal sinus. The diploic veins, which drain into the superior sagittal sinus, provide a route for the spread of infection from the meninges, especially in cases where there is purulent exudate near areas of the superior sagittal sinus. Infection can also spread to the superior sagittal sinus from nearby SDE or epidural abscess. Dehydration from vomiting, hypercoagulable states, and immunologic abnormalities, including the presence of circulating antiphospholipid antibodies, also contribute to cerebral venous sinus thrombosis. Thrombosis may extend from one sinus to another, and often at autopsy thrombi of different histologic ages can be detected in several sinuses. Thrombosis of the superior sagittal sinus is often associated with thrombosis of superior cortical veins and small parenchymal hemorrhages.

The superior sagittal sinus drains into the transverse sinuses (Fig. 372-6). The transverse sinuses also receive venous drainage from small veins from both the middle ear and mastoid cells. The transverse sinus becomes the sigmoid sinus before draining into the internal jugular vein. Septic transverse/sigmoid sinus thrombosis can be a complication of acute and chronic otitis media or mastoiditis. Infection spreads from the mastoid air cells to the transverse sinus via the emissary veins or by direct invasion. The cavernous sinuses are inferior to the superior sagittal sinus at the base of the skull. The cavernous sinuses receive blood from the facial veins via the superior and inferior ophthalmic veins. Bacteria in the facial veins enter the cavernous sinus via these veins. Bacteria in the sphenoid and ethmoid sinuses can spread to the cavernous sinuses via the small emissary veins. The sphenoid and ethmoid sinuses are the most common sites of primary infection resulting in septic cavernous sinus thrombosis.

CLINICAL MANIFESTATIONS *Septic thrombosis of the superior sagittal sinus* presents as headache, nausea and vomiting, confusion, and focal or generalized seizures. There may be a rapid development of stupor and coma. Weakness of the lower extremities with bilateral Babinski signs or hemiparesis is often present. When superior sagittal sinus thrombosis occurs as a complication of bacterial meningitis, nuchal rigidity and Kernig's and Brudzinski's signs may be present.

The oculomotor nerve, the trochlear nerve, the abducens nerve, the ophthalmic and maxillary branches of the trigeminal nerve, and the internal carotid artery all pass through the cavernous sinus. The symptoms of *septic cavernous sinus thrombosis* are fever, headache, frontal and retroorbital pain, and diplopia. The classic signs are ptosis, proptosis, chemosis, and extraocular dysmotility due to deficits of cranial nerves III, IV, and VI. Hypo- or hyperesthesia of the ophthalmic and maxillary divisions of the fifth cranial nerve and a decreased corneal reflex may be detected. There may be evidence of dilated, tortuous retinal veins and papilledema.

Headache and earache are the most frequent symptoms of *transverse sinus thrombosis*. A transverse sinus thrombosis may also present with Gradinego's syndrome characterized by otitis media, sixth nerve palsy, and retroorbital or facial pain. Sigmoid sinus and internal jugular vein thrombosis may present with neck pain.

DIAGNOSIS The diagnosis of septic venous sinus thrombosis is suggested by an absent flow void within the affected venous sinus on MRI and confirmed by magnetic resonance venography or the venous phase of cerebral angiography. The diagnosis of thrombophlebitis of intracerebral and meningeal veins is suggested by the presence of intracerebral hemorrhage but requires cerebral angiography for definitive diagnosis.

℞ TREATMENT Septic venous sinus thrombosis is usually treated with antibiotics and hydration. The choice of antimicrobial therapy is based on the bacteria responsible for the predisposing or associated condition. Anticoagulation with dose-adjusted heparin has been reported to be beneficial in patients with aseptic venous sinus thrombosis; it is also used in the treatment of septic venous sinus thrombosis complicating bacterial meningitis in patients who are worsening despite antimicrobial therapy and intravenous fluids. The presence of a small intracerebral hemorrhage from septic thrombophlebitis is not an absolute contraindication to heparin therapy. Successful management of aseptic venous sinus thrombosis has been reported with urokinase therapy and with a combination of intrathrombus recombinant tissue plasminogen activator (rtPA) and intravenous heparin, but there is yet no reported experience with these therapies in septic venous sinus thrombosis.

BIBLIOGRAPHY

ACUTE BACTERIAL MENINGITIS

COYLE PK: Glucocorticoids in central nervous system bacterial infection. Arch Neurol 56:796, 1999

DURAND ML et al: Acute bacterial meningitis in adults: A review of 493 episodes. N Engl J Med 328:21, 1993

FANG CT et al: Klebsiella pneumoniae meningitis: Timing of antimicrobial therapy and prognosis. QJM 93:45, 2000

PELTOLA H: Prophylaxis of bacterial meningitis. Infect Dis Clin North Am 685, 13 1999

QUAGLIARELLO VJ, SCHELD WM: Treatment of bacterial meningitis. N Engl J Med 336: 708, 1997

FIGURE 372-6 Anatomy of the cerebral venous sinuses.

ROOS KL: *Meningitis: 100 Maxims in Neurology.* London, Arnold, and New York, Oxford University Press, 1996, 1–208

——— et al: Acute bacterial meningitis in children and adults, in *Infections of the Central Nervous System,* 2d ed, WM Scheld, RJ Whitley, DT Durack (eds). Philadelphia, Lippincott-Raven, 1997, 335–401

SCHUCHAT A et al: Bacterial meningitis in the United States in 1995. N Engl J Med 337: 970, 1997

TAUBER MG, MOSSER B: Cytokines and chemokines in meningeal inflammation: Biology and clinical implications. Clin Infect Dis 28:1, 1999

BRAIN ABSCESS

MAMELAK AN et al: Improved management of multiple brain abscesses: A combined surgical and medical approach. Neurosurg 36:76, 1995

MATHISEN GE, JOHNSON JP: Brain abscess. Clin Infect Dis 25:763, 1997

SUBDURAL EMPYEMA

DILL SR et al: Subdural empyema: Analysis of 32 cases and review. Clin Infect Dis 20: 372, 1995

NATHOO N et al: Intracranial subdural empyema in the era of computed tomography: A review of 699 cases. Neurosurgery 44:529, 1999

CRANIAL EPIDURAL ABSCESS

GELLIN BG et al: Epidural abscess, in *Infections of the Central Nervous System,* 2d ed, WM Scheld, RJ Whitley, DT Durack (eds). Lippincott-Raven, Philadelphia, 1997, 507–522

SILVERBERG AL, DINUBILE MJ: Subdural empyema and cranial epidural abscess. Med Clin North Am 69:361, 1985

SUPPURATIVE THROMBOPHLEBITIS

SOUTHWICK FS et al: Septic thrombosis of the dural venous sinuses. Medicine 65:82, 1986

373   *Kenneth L. Tyler*

VIRAL MENINGITIS AND ENCEPHALITIS

Hundreds of viruses have been reported to produce acute infection and injury to the central or peripheral nervous systems. Many aspects of the clinical characteristics of these diseases are determined by whether the infection is limited primarily to the meninges (*meningitis*) or extends to involve the parenchyma of the brain (*encephalitis*), spinal cord (*myelitis*), or nerve roots (*radiculitis*). In some cases more than one of these areas can be involved simultaneously (meningoencephalitis, myeloradiculitis, etc.). Viruses can also produce chronic or persistent infections of the central nervous system (CNS). →*Infections caused by HIV are discussed in Chap. 309, human T cell leukemia virus (HTLV) types I and II in Chap. 368, and prions in Chap. 375.*

ACUTE VIRAL INFECTIONS

VIRAL MENINGITIS Clinical Manifestations The syndrome of viral meningitis consists of fever, headache, and meningeal irritation coupled with an inflammatory cerebrospinal fluid (CSF) profile (see below). Fever may be accompanied by malaise, myalgia, anorexia, nausea and vomiting, abdominal pain, and/or diarrhea. It is not uncommon to see a mild degree of lethargy or drowsiness. The presence of more profound alterations in consciousness, such as stupor, coma, or marked confusion, should prompt consideration of alternative diagnoses. Similarly, seizures, cranial nerve palsies, or other focal neurologic signs or symptoms suggests parenchymal involvement and is not typical of uncomplicated viral meningitis. The headache associated with viral meningitis is usually frontal or retroorbital and often associated with photophobia and pain on moving the eyes. Nuchal rigidity is present in most cases but may be mild and present only near the limit of neck anteflexion. Evidence of severe meningeal irritation, such as Kernig's and Brudzinski's signs (Chap. 372), is generally absent.

Etiology Enteroviruses account for 75 to 90% of aseptic meningitis cases in most series (Table 373-1). Viruses belonging to the *Enterovirus* genus are members of the family Picornaviridae and include the coxsackieviruses, echoviruses, polioviruses, and human enteroviruses 68 to 71. Using a variety of diagnostic techniques including CSF polymerase chain reaction (PCR) tests, culture, and serology, a specific viral cause can be found in 75 to 90% of cases of viral meningitis. CSF cultures are positive in 30 to 70% of patients, the frequency of isolation depending on the specific viral agent. Approximately two-thirds of culture-negative cases of aseptic meningitis have a specific viral etiology identified by CSF PCR testing (see below).

Epidemiology The exact incidence of viral meningitis in the United States is impossible to determine since most cases go unreported to public health authorities. In temperate climates, there is a substantial increase in cases during the summer and early fall months, reflecting the seasonal predominance of enterovirus and arthropod-borne encephalitis virus ("arbovirus") infections, with a peak monthly incidence of about 1 reported case per 100,000 population. The dramatic seasonal predilections of some viruses causing meningitis provide a valuable but not always infallible clue to diagnosis (Table 373-2).

Laboratory Diagnosis • *CSF examination* The most important laboratory test in the diagnosis of meningitis is examination of the CSF. The typical profile in cases of viral meningitis is a lymphocytic pleocytosis (25 to 500 cells per microliter), a normal or slightly elevated protein level [0.2 to 0.8 g/L (20 to 80 mg/dL)], a normal glucose level, and a normal or mildly elevated opening pressure (100 to 350 mm H$_2$O). Organisms *are not* seen on Gram's or acid-fast stained smears or india ink wet mounts of CSF. Rarely, polymorphonuclear neutrophils (PMNs) may predominate in the first 48 h of illness, especially in patients with infections due to echovirus 9 or Eastern equine virus. However, the presence of a persisting PMN pleocytosis should always prompt consideration of bacterial meningitis or parameningeal infections. The total CSF cell count in viral meningitis is typically 25 to 500/μL, although cell counts of several thousand per microliter are occasionally seen, especially with infec-

Table 373-1 Viruses Causing Acute Meningitis

Common	Less Common	Rare
Enteroviruses	HSV-1	Adenoviruses
Arboviruses	LCMV	CMV
HIV	Mumps virus	EBV
HSV-2		Influenza A, B; measles; parainfluenza; rubella; VZV

NOTE: CMV, cytomegalovirus; EBV, Epstein-Barr virus; HIV, human immunodeficiency virus; HSV, herpes simplex virus; LCMV, lymphocytic choriomeningitis virus; VZV, varicella-zoster virus.

Table 373-2 Seasonal Prevalence of Viruses Commonly Causing Meningitis

Summer and Early Fall	Fall and Winter	Winter and Spring	Nonseasonal
Arboviruses	LCMV	Mumps	HIV
Enteroviruses			HSV

NOTE: As in Table 373-1.

tions due to lymphocytic choriomeningitis virus (LCMV) and mumps virus. The CSF glucose level is typically normal in viral infections, although it may be decreased in 10 to 30% of cases due to mumps as well as in cases due to LCMV. Rare instances of decreased CSF glucose concentration occur in cases of meningitis due to echoviruses and other enteroviruses, herpes simplex virus (HSV) type 2, and varicella-zoster virus (VZV). As a rule, a lymphocytic pleocytosis with a low glucose level should suggest fungal, listerial, or tuberculous meningitis or noninfectious disorders (e.g., sarcoid, neoplastic meningitis).

A number of tests measuring levels of various CSF proteins, enzymes, and mediators, including C-reactive protein, lactic acid, lactate dehydrogenase, neopterin, quinolinate, interleukin (IL) 1β, IL-6, soluble IL-2 receptor, β_2-microglobulin, and tumor necrosis factor (TNF), have been proposed as potential discriminators between viral and bacterial meningitis or as markers of specific types of viral infection (e.g., infection with HIV), but are of limited general use.

Polymerase chain reaction amplification of viral nucleic acid Amplification of viral-specific DNA or RNA from CSF using PCR amplification has become the single most important method for diagnosing CNS viral infections. HSV DNA is frequently amplified from the CSF of patients with herpes simplex encephalitis (HSV-1) and recurrent lymphocytic meningitis (HSV-2), even when standard culture techniques are negative. PCR is also used routinely to diagnose CNS viral infections caused by enteroviruses, cytomegalovirus (CMV), Epstein-Barr virus (EBV), and VZV. Genomic amplification and detection of enteroviral (coxsackie-, polio-, echo-, enterovirus) RNA in the CSF of patients with meningitis is now the diagnostic procedure of choice for this group of viruses.

CSF culture The overall results of CSF culture for the diagnosis of viral infection are disappointing (Table 373-3), presumably because of the generally low concentration of infectious virus present and the need to customize isolation procedures for individual viruses. For viral isolation, 2 mL of CSF should be brought promptly to the microbiology laboratory, where it should be refrigerated and processed as speedily as possible. CSF specimens for viral isolation should never be stored in a −20°C freezer since viruses are often unstable at this temperature, and most freezers have "frostfree" warm-up cycles that are detrimental to viral stability. Storage for >24 h is probably best done in a −70°C freezer.

Other sources for viral isolation Viruses may also be isolated from sites and body fluids other than CSF, including throat swabs, stool, blood, and urine. Enteroviruses and adenoviruses may be found in feces; arboviruses, some enteroviruses, and LCMV, in blood; mumps and CMV, in urine; and enteroviruses, mumps, and adenoviruses, in throat washings. During enteroviral infections, viral shedding in stool may persist for several weeks. The presence of enterovirus in stool is not diagnostic and may result from residual shedding from a

Table 373-3 Possibility of Culturing Specific Viruses from Cerebrospinal Fluid

Excellent	Fair	Poor or None
Coxsackievirus, echovirus, LCMV, mumps virus	HIV, adenovirus, arboviruses (most), HSV-2, VZV, rabies virus	Poliovirus, HSV-1, EBV, CMV

NOTE: As in Table 373-1.

previous enteroviral infection; it also occurs in some asymptomatic individuals during enteroviral epidemics.

Serologic studies For some viruses, such as the arboviruses, serologic studies remain an important diagnostic tool but are less useful for viruses such as HSV, VZV, CMV, and EBV for which the prevalence of antibody seropositivity in the general population is high. Diagnosis of viral infection can be made by documenting seroconversion between acute-phase and convalescent sera (typically obtained after 2 to 4 weeks), or by demonstrating the presence of virus-specific IgM antibodies. Antiviral antibodies may be measured in CSF (see below). The timing of the antibody response often means that serologic data are useful mainly for the retrospective establishment of a specific diagnosis, and their value in initial diagnosis and management is limited. Most viral infections of the CNS are associated with intrathecal synthesis of antiviral antibody. This results in an elevation in the ratio of antibody in CSF compared to serum (CSF/serum antibody index).

Agarose electrophoresis or isoelectric focusing of CSF γ-globulins may reveal the presence of oligoclonal bands. These bands have been found in association with a number of viral infections, including infections with HIV, HTLV type I, VZV, mumps, subacute sclerosing panencephalitis (SSPE), and progressive rubella panencephalitis. The associated antibodies are often directed against viral proteins. The finding of oligoclonal bands may be of some diagnostic utility, since typically they are not seen with arbovirus, enterovirus, or HSV infections. Oligoclonal bands are also encountered in certain noninfectious neurologic diseases (e.g., multiple sclerosis) and may be found in nonviral infections (e.g., syphilis, Lyme borreliosis).

Other laboratory studies All patients with suspected viral meningitis should have a complete blood count and differential; liver function tests; and measurement of the erythrocyte sedimentation rate (ESR), blood urea nitrogen (BUN), and plasma levels of electrolytes, glucose, creatinine, creatine kinase, aldolase, amylase, and lipase. Abnormalities in specific test results may suggest particular etiologic diagnoses. Magnetic resonance imaging (MRI), computed tomography (CT), electroencephalography (EEG), evoked response studies, electromyography (EMG), and nerve conduction studies are not necessary in most cases. They are best used selectively when atypical presentations or unusual features present diagnostic problems.

Differential Diagnosis The most important issue in the differential diagnosis is the exclusion of nonviral causes that can mimic viral meningitis. The major categories of disease that should always be considered and excluded are (1) bacterial meningitis and other infectious meningidities (e.g., *Mycoplasma, Listeria, Brucella, Coxiella,* and *Rickettsia*); (2) parameningeal infections or partially treated bacterial meningitis; (3) nonviral infectious meningitides where cultures may be negative (e.g., fungal, tuberculous, parasitic, or syphilitic disease); (4) neoplastic meningitis; and (5) meningitis secondary to noninfectious inflammatory diseases such as sarcoid, Behçet's disease, and the uveomeningitic syndromes.

Specific viral etiologies Enteroviruses (Chap. 193) are the most common cause of viral meningitis (>75% of cases with etiology identified) and should be considered the leading candidates when a typical case occurs in the summer months, especially in a child (<15 years) (Table 373-4). However,

Table 373-4   Serotypes of Enteroviruses Causing CNS Infections

Frequency as Cause of CNS Infections	Poliovirus	Coxsackievirus	Echovirus	Enterovirus
Frequent	—	B5	7, 9, 11, 30	70, 71
Common	—	A9, B3, B4	4, 6, 18	—
Rare	1–3	B1, B6	2, 3, 12, 22	—

NOTE: CNS, central nervous system.
SOURCE: After Rotbart.

despite their summer prevalence, sporadic cases of enteroviral CNS infection are seen year-round. The physical examination should include a careful search for exanthemata, hand-foot-mouth disease, herpangina, pleurodynia, myopericarditis, and hemorrhagic conjunctivitis, which may be stigmata of enterovirus infections. PCR amplification of enteroviral RNA from CSF has become the diagnostic procedure of choice for these infections.

Arbovirus infections typically occur in the summer months, have clear geographic localization, and occur in epidemics, all factors reflecting the ecology of their transmission through infected insect vectors (Fig. 373-1); Table 373-6; Chap. 198). Arboviral meningitis should be considered when clusters of meningitis cases occur in a restricted geographic region during the summer or early fall. A history of tick exposure or travel or residence in the appropriate geographic area should suggest the possibility of Colorado tick fever virus or Powassan virus infection, although nonviral diseases producing meningitis (e.g., Lyme disease) or headache with meningismus (e.g., Rocky Mountain spotted fever) may also present this way.

HSV-2 meningitis (Chap. 182) occurs in approximately 25% of women and 11% of men at the time of an initial (primary) episode of genital herpes. Of these patients, 20% go on to have recurrent attacks of meningitis. In some series, HSV-2 has been the most important cause of aseptic meningitis in adults, especially women, and overall it

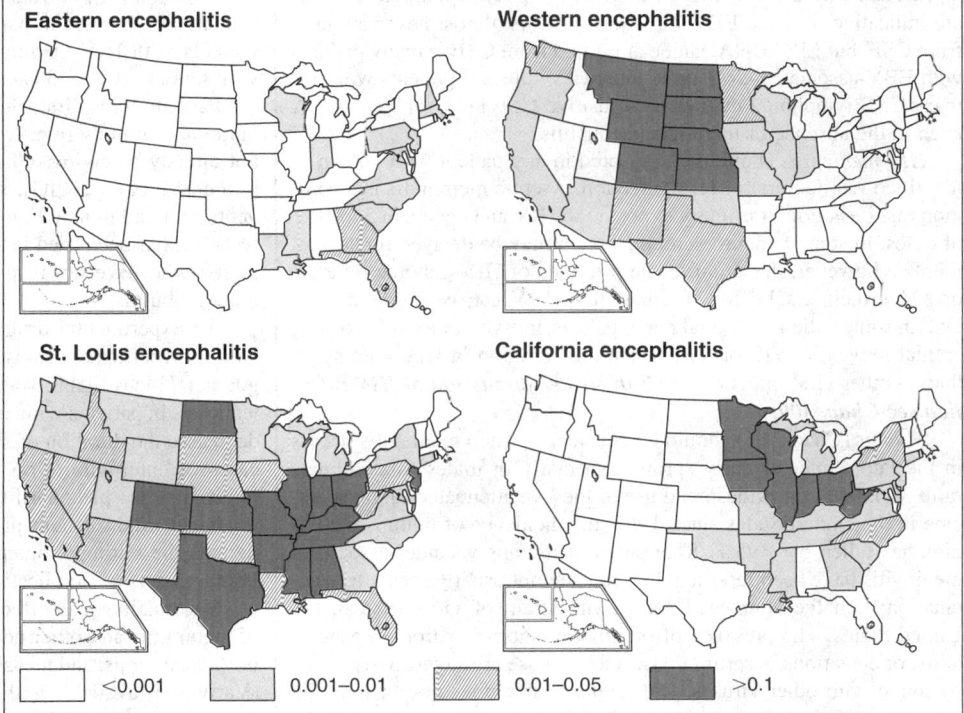

FIGURE 373-1 Incidence of selected forms of arboviral encephalitis in the United States; cases per 10,000 population per year for St. Louis and California encephalitis (bottom maps) and per 100,000 per year for eastern and western encephalitis (top maps). *(Modified from TF Tsai et al.)*

is probably second only to enteroviruses as a cause of viral meningitis. Although HSV-2 can be cultured from CSF during a first episode of meningitis, cultures are invariably negative during recurrent episodes of HSV-2 meningitis. Diagnosis depends on amplification of HSV-2 DNA from CSF by PCR. Almost all cases of recurrent HSV meningitis are due to HSV-2, although rare cases due to HSV-1 have been reported. Most cases of benign recurrent lymphocytic meningitis, including those meeting accepted diagnostic criteria for Mollaret's meningitis, appear to be due to HSV. Genital lesions may not be present, and most patients give no history of genital herpes. CSF cultures are negative, although HSV DNA can be amplified from CSF by PCR during attacks of meningitis but not during symptom-free intervals.

VZV meningitis should be suspected in the presence of concurrent chickenpox or shingles. However, it is important to recognize that in some series up to 40% of VZV meningitis cases have been reported to occur in the absence of rash. The frequency of VZV as a cause of meningitis is extremely variable, ranging from as low as 3% to as high as 20% in different series. The frequency would be expected to decline with the increasing utilization of the live attenuated varicella vaccine (Varivax) in children. In addition to meningitis, encephalitis (see below), and shingles (see below), VZV can also produce acute cerebellar ataxia. This typically occurs in children and presents with the abrupt onset of limb and truncal ataxia. A similar syndrome occurs less commonly in association with EBV and enteroviral infection. PCR has rapidly become a major tool in the diagnosis of VZV CNS infections. In patients with negative CSF PCR results, the diagnosis of VZV CNS infection can be made by the demonstration of VZV-specific intrathecal antibody synthesis and/or the presence of VZV CSF IgM antibodies, or by positive CSF cultures.

EBV infections may also produce aseptic meningitis, with or without accompanying evidence of the infectious mononucleosis syndrome. The diagnosis may be suggested by the finding of atypical lymphocytes in the CSF or an atypical lymphocytosis in peripheral blood. The demonstration of IgM antibody to viral capsid antigen (VCA), antibody to the diffuse (D) component of early antigen (EA), or subsequently a rising titer of antibody to nuclear antigen (EBNA) are indicative of acute EBV infection. EBV is almost never cultured from CSF, but EBV DNA can be amplified from CSF in many patients with EBV-associated CNS infections. HIV-infected patients with primary CNS lymphoma may have a positive CSF PCR for EBV DNA even in the absence of meningoencephalitis.

HIV meningitis should be suspected in any patient with known or identified risk factors for HIV infection. Aseptic meningitis is a common manifestation of primary exposure to HIV and occurs in 5 to 10% of cases. In some patients, seroconversion may be delayed for several months; however, detection of the presence of HIV genome by PCR or p24 protein establishes the diagnosis. HIV can be cultured from CSF in some patients. Cranial nerve palsies, most commonly involving cranial nerves V, VII, or VIII, are more common in HIV meningitis than in other viral infections. →*For further discussion of HIV infection see Chap. 309.*

Mumps (Chap. 196) should be considered when meningitis occurs in the late winter or early spring, especially in males (male/female ratio 3:1). With the widespread use of the live attenuated mumps vaccine in the United States since 1967, the incidence of mumps meningitis has fallen by >95%. Rare cases of mumps vaccine–associated meningitis have been reported, but they are not usually seen after vaccination with the attenuated Jeryl-Lynn strain of virus used in the United States. The presence of orchitis, oophoritis, parotitis, pancreatitis, or elevations in serum lipase and amylase are suggestive but can be found with other viruses, and their absence does not exclude the diagnosis. Clinical meningitis occurs in 5% of patients with parotitis, but only 50% of patients with meningitis have associated parotitis. Mumps infection confers lifelong immunity, so a documented history of previous infection excludes this diagnosis. The presence of hypo-

glycorrhachia (10 to 30%) may be an additional diagnostic clue, once other causes have been excluded (see above). Up to 25% of patients may have a PMN-predominant CSF pleocytosis, and CSF abnormalities may persist for months. Diagnosis is typically made by isolation of virus from CSF and/or demonstration of seroconversion between acute-phase and convalescent sera.

LCMV infection (Chap. 198) should be considered when aseptic meningitis occurs in the late fall or winter, and in individuals with a history of exposure to house mice (*Mus musculus*), pet or laboratory rodents (e.g., hamsters), or their excreta. Some patients have an associated rash, pulmonary infiltrates, alopecia, parotitis, orchitis, or myopericarditis. Laboratory clues to the diagnosis of LCMV, in addition to the clinical findings noted above, may include the presence of leukopenia, thrombocytopenia, or abnormal liver function tests. Some cases present with a marked CSF pleocytosis (>1000 cells per microliter) and hypoglycorrhachia (<30%).

℞ TREATMENT   In the usual case of viral meningitis, treatment is symptomatic, and hospitalization is not required. Exceptions include patients with deficient humoral immunity, neonates with overwhelming infection, and patients in whom the clinical or CSF profile suggests the possibility of a bacterial or other nonviral cause of infection. Patients with suspected bacterial meningitis should receive appropriate empirical therapy pending culture results (Chap. 372). Patients usually prefer to rest undisturbed in a quiet, darkened room. Analgesics can be used to relieve headache, which is often reduced by the initial diagnostic lumbar puncture. Antipyretics may help to reduce fever, which rarely exceeds 40°C. Hyponatremia may develop as a result of inappropriate vasopressin secretion (SIADH), so fluid and electrolyte status should be monitored. Repeat lumbar puncture is indicated only in patients whose fever and symptoms fail to resolve after a few days or if there is doubt about the initial diagnosis.

Oral or intravenous acyclovir may be of benefit in patients with meningitis caused by HSV-1 or -2 and in cases of severe EBV or VZV infection. Data concerning treatment of HSV, EBV, and VZV meningitis are extremely limited. Seriously ill patients should probably receive intravenous acyclovir (30 mg/kg per day in three divided doses) for 7 days. Oral acyclovir (800 mg, five times daily), famciclovir (500 mg, tid), or valacyclovir (1000 mg, tid) for a week may be tried in less severely ill patients, although data on efficacy are lacking. Patients with HIV meningitis should receive highly active antiretroviral therapy (Chap. 309).

Patients with viral meningitis who are known to have deficient humoral immunity (e.g. X-linked agammaglobulinemia), and who are not already receiving either intramuscular γ-globulin or intravenous immunoglobulin (IVIG), should be treated with these agents. Intraventricular administration of immunoglobulin through an Ommaya reservoir has been tried in some patients with chronic enteroviral meningitis who have not responded to intramuscular or intravenous immunoglobulin.

An experimental drug, pleconaril (Viropharma Inc., VP 63843), has shown efficacy against a variety of enteroviral infections and has good oral bioavailability and excellent CNS penetration. Ongoing clinical trials in patients with enteroviral meningitis suggest that pleconaril decreases the duration of symptoms compared to placebo. Since most cases of enteroviral CNS infection are benign and self-limited, the indications for pleconaril therapy need to be better defined. Antiviral treatment might benefit patients with chronic CNS enteroviral infections in the setting of agammaglobulinemia or those who develop poliomyelitis as a complication of polio vaccine administration.

Vaccination is an effective method of preventing the development of meningitis and other neurologic complications associated with poliovirus, mumps, and measles infection. A live attenuated VZV vaccine (Varivax) is available in the United States. Clinical studies indicate an effectiveness rate of 70 to 90% for this vaccine. Reduction in primary VZV infection would be expected to reduce the frequency and/or severity both of primary neurologic complications of varicella and of the consequences of later reactivation (e.g., shingles).

Prognosis In adults, the prognosis for full recovery from viral meningitis is excellent. Rare patients complain of persisting headache, mild mental impairment, incoordination, or generalized asthenia for weeks to months. The outcome in infants and neonates (<1 year) is less certain; intellectual impairment, learning disabilities, hearing loss, and other lasting sequelae have been reported in some studies.

VIRAL ENCEPHALITIS **Definition** In distinction to meningitis, where the infectious process and associated inflammatory response is limited largely to the meninges, in encephalitis the brain parenchyma is also involved. Many patients with encephalitis also have evidence of associated meningitis (meningoencephalitis) and, in some cases, involvement of the spinal cord or nerve roots (encephalomyelitis, encephalomyeloradiculitis).

Clinical Manifestations In addition to the acute febrile illness with evidence of meningeal involvement characteristic of meningitis, the patient with encephalitis commonly has an altered level of consciousness, an abnormal mental state, and evidence of either focal or diffuse neurologic signs and symptoms. Any degree of altered consciousness may occur, ranging from mild lethargy to deep coma. Patients with encephalitis are frequently confused, delirious, and disoriented. Mental aberrations may include hallucinations, agitation, personality change, behavioral disorders, and, at times, a frankly psychotic state. Focal or generalized seizures occur in >50% of patients with severe encephalitis. Virtually every possible type of focal neurologic disturbance has been reported in viral encephalitis; the signs and symptoms reflect the sites of infection and inflammation. The most commonly encountered focal findings are aphasia, ataxia, hemiparesis (with hyperactive tendon reflexes and extensor plantar responses), involuntary movements (e.g., myoclonic jerks), and cranial nerve deficits (e.g., ocular palsies, facial weakness). Involvement of the hypothalamic-pituitary axis may result in temperature dysregulation, diabetes insipidus, or the development of SIADH. Despite the clear neuropathologic evidence that viruses differ in the regions of the CNS they injure, it is often impossible to distinguish reliably on clinical grounds alone one type of viral encephalitis (e.g., that caused by HSV) from others (see "Differential Diagnosis," below).

Etiology The number of viruses reported to cause encephalitis is legion. In the United States, there are approximately 20,000 reported cases per year. The same organisms responsible for aseptic meningitis are also responsible for encephalitis, although their relative frequencies differ (Table 373-5; Fig. 373-1). The most important viruses causing sporadic cases of encephalitis in immunocompetent adults are HSV-1, VZV, and, less commonly, enteroviruses. Epidemics of encephalitis are caused by arboviruses, which belong to several different viral taxonomic groups including *Alphavirus* of the family Togaviridae (e.g. Eastern equine encephalitis virus, Western equine encephalitis virus), *Flavivirus* of the family Flaviviridae (e.g., St. Louis encephalitis virus, Powassan virus), and *Bunyavirus* of the family Bunyaviridae (e.g., California encephalitis virus serogroup, LaCrosse virus). In most years, the largest number of cases of arbovirus encephalitis are generally due to St. Louis encephalitis virus and the California encephalitis virus serogroup. New causes of viral encephalitis are constantly appearing, as evidenced by the recent outbreak of ~300 cases of encephalitis with a 40% mortality rate in Malaysia caused by Nipah virus, a new member of the Paramyxovirus family. Similarly, well-known viruses may suddenly appear in unexpected locations, as illustrated by a recent outbreak of encephalitis in New York City due to West Nile virus.

Table 373-5 Viruses Causing Encephalitis

Common	Less Common	Rare
Arboviruses, enteroviruses, HSV-1, mumps	CMV, EBV, HIV, measles, VZV	Adenoviruses, CTFV, influenza A, LCMV, parainfluenza, rabies, rubella

NOTE: As in Table 373-1; also, CTFV, Colorado tick fever virus.

Laboratory Diagnosis • *CSF examination* CSF examination should be performed in all patients with suspected viral encephalitis unless contraindicated by the presence of severely increased intracranial pressure (ICP). The characteristic CSF profile is indistinguishable from that of viral meningitis and consists of a lymphocytic pleocytosis, a mildly elevated protein level, and a normal glucose level. A CSF pleocytosis (>5 cells per microliter) occurs in >95% of patients with documented viral encephalitis, and its absence should prompt a careful search for other causes of an encephalopathy. In rare cases, a pleocytosis may be absent on the initial lumbar puncture but present subsequently. Patients who are severely immunocompromised by HIV infection, steroid or other immunosupressant drugs, chemotherapy, or certain lymphoreticular malignancies may fail to mount a CSF inflammatory response. CSF cell counts exceed 500/μL in only about 10% of patients with encephalitis. Infections with certain arboviruses (e.g., Eastern equine encephalitis or California encephalitis viruses), mumps, and LCMV may occasionally result in cell counts >1000/μL, but this degree of pleocytosis should suggest the possibility of nonviral infections or other inflammatory processes. Atypical lymphocytes in the CSF may be seen in EBV infection and less commonly with other viruses, including CMV, HSV, and enteroviruses. The presence of substantial numbers of PMNs after the first 48 h should prompt consideration of bacterial infection, leptospirosis, amebic infection, and noninfectious processes such as acute hemorrhagic leukoencephalitis. Large numbers of CSF PMNs may be present in patients with viral encephalitis due to Eastern equine encephalitis virus, echovirus 9, and, more rarely, other enteroviruses. About 20% of patients with encephalitis will have a significant number of red blood cells (>500/μL) in the CSF in a nontraumatic tap. The pathologic correlate of this may be the presence of a hemorrhagic encephalitis of the type seen with HSV, Colorado tick fever virus, and occasionally California encephalitis virus. A decreased CSF glucose level is distinctly unusual in viral encephalitis and should suggest the possibility of fungal, tuberculous, parasitic, leptospiral, syphilitic, sarcoid, or neoplastic meningitis. Rare patients with mumps, LCMV, or advanced HSV encephalitis may have low CSF glucose concentrations.

CSF PCR PCR amplification of viral nucleic acid has become the diagnostic procedure of choice for many types of viral encephalitis. Recent studies with HSV encephalitis indicate that the sensitivity (~98%) and specificity (~94%) of CSF PCR equal or exceed those of brain biopsy. Although less detailed specificity and sensitivity data are available for most other viruses, PCR has become the primary diagnostic test for CNS infections caused by CMV, EBV, VZV, and enteroviruses (see "Viral Meningitis," above). Studies of HSV encephalitis indicate that the incidence of positive CSF PCR gradually declines after the second week of illness. PCR results are generally not affected by ≤1 week of antiviral therapy. In one study 98% of CSF specimens remained PCR-positive during the first week of initiation of antiviral therapy, but the numbers fell to ~50% 8 to 14 days, and to ~21% by ≥15 days after initiation of therapy.

Patients suspected of having HSV encephalitis should be started on acyclovir (see below), and their CSF should be assayed for the presence of HSV DNA by PCR. A positive CSF PCR in the appropriate clinical setting is diagnostic of HSV encephalitis. A negative PCR test effectively excludes the diagnosis, unless the test is performed late in the course of illness or following prolonged antiviral therapy (see above). Blood or blood breakdown products may inhibit PCR reactions and generate false-negative results. Nonetheless the negative predictive value of a negative CSF PCR is ~98% and provides sufficient basis to discontinue acyclovir therapy unless mitigating circumstances likely to generate a false-negative PCR are present.

CSF culture Attempts to culture viruses from the CSF in cases of encephalitis are often disappointing (Table 373-3). Cultures are invariably negative in cases of HSV-1 encephalitis.

Serologic studies and antigen detection The basic approach to the serodiagnosis of viral encephalitis is identical to that discussed earlier for viral meningitis. In patients with HSV encephalitis, both antibodies to HSV-1 glycoproteins and glycoprotein antigens have been detected in the CSF. Optimal detection of both HSV antibodies and antigen typically occurs after the first week of illness, limiting the utility of these tests in acute diagnosis. Nonetheless, CSF HSV antibody testing may be of value in selected patients whose illness is >1 week's duration and who are CSF PCR-negative for HSV.

MRI, CT, EEG Patients with suspected encephalitis almost invariably undergo neuroimaging studies and often EEG. These tests help identify or exclude alternative diagnoses and assist in the differentiation between a focal, as opposed to diffuse, encephalitic process. Focal findings in a patient with encephalitis should always raise the possibility of HSV encephalitis. Examples of focal findings include: (1) areas of increased signal intensity in the frontotemporal, cingulate, or insular regions of the brain on T2-weighted spin-echo MRI images (Fig. 373-2); (2) temporoparietal areas of low absorption, mass effect, and contrast enhancement on CT; or (3) periodic focal temporal lobe spikes on a background of slow or low-amplitude ("flattened") activity on EEG. Approximately 10% of patients with PCR-documented HSV encephalitis will have a normal MRI, although nearly 90% will have abnormalities in the temporal lobe. CT is less sensitive than MRI and is normal in up to 33% of patients. EEG abnormalities occur in >90% of PCR-documented cases of HSV encephalitis; they typically involve the temporal lobes but are often nonspecific.

Brain biopsy Brain biopsy is now generally reserved for patients in whom CSF PCR studies fail to lead to a specific diagnosis, who have focal abnormalities on MRI, and who continue to show progressive clinical deterioration despite treatment with acyclovir and supportive therapy. The isolation of HSV from brain tissue obtained at biopsy was once considered the "gold standard" for the diagnosis of HSV encephalitis, although with the advent of CSF PCR tests for HSV it is no longer necessary to perform brain biopsy for this purpose. The need for brain biopsy to diagnose other forms of viral encephalitis has also declined greatly with the widespread availability of CSF PCR diagnostic tests for EBV, CMV, VZV, and enteroviruses. When biopsy is performed, the tissue is cultured for virus and examined histopathologically and ultrastructurally. The biopsy is typically carried out under general anesthesia through a craniectomy. Tissue should be taken from a site that appears to be significantly involved on the basis of clinical and laboratory criteria. Although brain biopsy is not an innocuous procedure, the mortality rate is low (<0.2%). Potential morbidity, in addition to that related to general anesthesia, includes local bleeding and edema, the development of a seizure focus, and wound dehiscence or infection. From a practical viewpoint, the incidence of serious morbidity appears to be between 0.5 and 2%.

Differential Diagnosis The differential diagnosis includes both infectious and noninfectious causes of encephalitis. Some of the most common illnesses masquerading as viral encephalitis, as identified in multicenter clinical trials using brain biopsy as a diagnostic standard, were vascular diseases; abscess and empyema; fungal, parasitic, rickettsial, and tuberculous infections; tumors; Reye's syndrome; toxic encephalopathy; subdural hematoma; and systemic lupus erythematosus. Of the nonviral infections, particular attention should be paid to *Listeria, Mycoplasma, Leptospira, Cryptococcus,* and *Mucor* infections, as well as to toxoplasmosis and tuberculosis.

Once nonviral causes of encephalitis have been excluded, the major diagnostic impetus is to distinguish HSV from other viruses that cause encephalitis. This distinction is particularly important because in virtually every other instance the therapy is supportive, whereas specific and effective antiviral therapy is available for HSV, and its efficacy is enhanced when it is instituted early in the course of infection. HSV encephalitis should be considered when clinical features suggesting involvement of the inferomedial frontotemporal regions of the brain are present, including prominent olfactory or gustatory hallucinations, anosmia, unusual or bizarre behavior or personality alterations, or memory disturbance. HSV encephalitis should always be suspected in patients with focal findings on clinical examination, neuroimaging studies, or EEG. The diagnostic procedure of choice in these patients is CSF PCR analysis for HSV. A positive CSF PCR establishes the diagnosis, and a negative test dramatically reduces the likelihood of HSV encephalitis (see above).

Epidemiologic factors may provide important clues. Particular attention should be paid to the season of the year (Table 373-2), the age of the patient (Table 373-6), the geographic location and travel history (Fig. 373-1; Table 373-6), and possible exposure to animal bites, rodents, and ticks. *Morbidity and Mortality Weekly Reports* provides regular information about the prevalence of particular viruses causing encephalitis by season and region of the country. State public health authorities provide another valuable resource concerning isolation of particular agents in individual regions.

℞ **TREATMENT** Specific antiviral therapy should be initiated when appropriate. Vital functions, including respiration and blood pressure, should be monitored continuously and supported as required. In the initial stages of encephalitis, many patients will require care in an intensive care unit. Basic management and supportive therapy should include careful monitoring of ICP, fluid restriction and avoidance of hypotonic intravenous solutions, and suppression of fever. Seizures should be treated with standard anticonvulsant regimens, and prophylactic therapy should be considered in view of the high frequency of seizures in severe cases of encephalitis (>50%). As with all seriously ill, immobilized patients with altered levels of consciousness, encephalitis patients are at risk for aspiration pneumonia, stasis ulcers and decubiti, contractures, deep venous thrombosis and its complications, and infections of indwelling lines and catheters.

Acyclovir is of benefit in the treatment of HSV and should be started empirically in all patients with suspected viral encephalitis. Treatment should be discontinued in patients found not to have HSV encephalitis, with the possible exception of patients with severe encephalitis due to VZV or EBV. HSV, VZV, and EBV all encode an enzyme, deoxypyrimidine (thymidine) kinase, that phosphorylates acyclovir to produce acyclovir-5'-monophosphate. Host cell enzymes then phosphorylate this compound to form a triphosphate derivative. It is the triphosphate that acts as an antiviral agent by inhibiting viral DNA polymerase and by causing premature termination of nascent viral DNA chains. The specificity of action depends on the fact that uninfected cells do not phosphorylate significant amounts of acyclovir

FIGURE 373-2 Coronal FLAIR magnetic resonance image from a patient with herpes simplex encephalitis. Note the area of increased signal in the temporal lobe (left) confined predominantly to the gray matter. This patient had predominantly unilateral disease; bilateral lesions are more common but may be quite asymmetric in their intensity.

to acyclovir-5′-monophosphate. A second level of specificity is provided by the fact that the acyclovir triphosphate is a more potent inhibitor of viral DNA polymerase than of the analogous host cell enzymes.

Adults should receive a dose of 10 mg/kg of acyclovir intravenously every 8 h (30 mg/kg per day total dose) for a minimum of 14 days. Although no studies directly addressing this issue are yet available, we suggest repeating the CSF PCR after completion of 14 days of acyclovir therapy, and discontinuing the acyclovir in PCR-negative patients. Patients with a persisting positive CSF PCR for HSV should be treated for an additional 7 days, and the PCR repeated. Neonatal HSV CNS infection is less responsive to acyclovir therapy than HSV encephalitis in adults; it is recommended that neonates with HSV encephalitis receive 20 mg/kg of acyclovir every 8 h (60 mg/kg per day total dose) for a minimum of 21 days.

Prior to intravenous administration, acyclovir should be diluted to a concentration ≤7 mg/mL. (A 70-kg person would receive a dose of 700 mg, which would be diluted in a volume of 100 mL.) Each dose should be infused slowly over 1 h rather than by rapid or bolus infusion, to minimize the risk of renal dysfunction. Care should be taken to avoid extravasation or intramuscular or subcutaneous administration. The alkaline pH of acyclovir can cause local inflammation and phlebitis (9%). Dose adjustment is required in patients with impaired renal glomerular filtration. Penetration into CSF is excellent, with average drug levels approximately 50% of serum levels. Complications of therapy include elevations in BUN and creatinine levels (5%), thrombocytopenia (6%), gastrointestinal toxicity (nausea, vomiting, diarrhea) (7%), and neurotoxicity (lethargy or obtundation, disorientation, confusion, agitation, hallucinations, tremors, seizures) (1%). Acyclovir resistance may be mediated by changes in either the viral deoxypyrimidine kinase or DNA polymerase. To date, acyclovir-resistant isolates have not been a significant clinical problem in immunocompetent individuals. However, there have been reports of clinically virulent acyclovir-resistant HSV isolates from sites outside the CNS in immunocompromised individuals, including those with AIDS.

Oral antiviral drugs with efficacy against HSV, VZV, and EBV, including acyclovir, famciclovir, and valacyclovir, have not been evaluated in the treatment of encephalitis either as primary therapy or as supplemental therapy following completion of a course of parenteral acyclovir. An NIAID/NINDS-sponsored phase III trial of supplemental oral valacyclovir therapy (2 g, tid for 3 months) following the initial 14- to 21-day course of therapy with parenteral acyclovir has recently been initiated in patients with HSV encephalitis; it may help clarify the role of extended oral antiviral therapy.

Both ganciclovir and foscarnet have been shown to be effective in the treatment of CMV-related CNS infections. These drugs are often used in combination. Cidofovir (see below) may provide an alternative in patients who fail to respond to ganciclovir and foscarnet, although data concerning its use in CMV CNS infections are extremely limited.

Ganciclovir is a synthetic nucleoside analogue of 2′-deoxyguanosine. The drug is preferentially phosphorylated by virus-induced cellular kinases. Ganciclovir triphosphate acts as a competitive inhibitor of the CMV DNA polymerase, and its incorporation into nascent viral DNA results in premature chain termination. Following intravenous administration, CSF concentrations of ganciclovir are 25 to 70% of coincident plasma levels. The usual dose for treatment of severe neurologic illnesses is 5 mg/kg every 12 h given intravenously at a constant rate over 1 h. Induction therapy is followed by maintenance therapy of 5 mg/kg every day for an indefinite period. Induction therapy should be continued until patients show a decline in CSF pleocytosis and a reduction in CSF CMV DNA copy number on quantitative PCR testing (where available). Doses should be adjusted in patients with renal insufficiency. Treatment is often limited by the development of granulocytopenia and thrombocytopenia (20 to 25%), which may require reduction in or discontinuation of therapy. Gastrointestinal side effects including nausea, vomiting, diarrhea, and abdominal pain occur in ~20% of patients. Some patients treated with ganciclovir for CMV retinitis have developed retinal detachment, but the causal relationship to ganciclovir treatment is unclear.

Foscarnet is a pyrophosphate analogue that inhibits viral DNA polymerases by binding to the pyrophosphate-binding site. Following intravenous infusion, CSF concentrations range from 15 to 100% of coincident plasma levels. The usual dose for serious CMV-related neurologic illness is 60 mg/kg every 8 h administered by constant infusion over 1 h. Induction therapy for 14 to 21 days is followed by maintenance therapy (60 to 120 mg/kg per day). Induction therapy may need to be extended in patients who fail to show a decline in CSF pleocytosis and a reduction in CSF CMV DNA copy number on quantitative PCR tests (where available). Approximately one-third of patients develop renal impairment during treatment, which is reversible following discontinuation of therapy in most, but not all, cases. This is often associated with elevations in serum creatinine and proteinuria and is less frequent in patients who are adequately hydrated. Many patients experience fatigue and nausea. Reduction in serum calcium, magnesium, and potassium occur in approximately 15% of patients and may be associated with tetany, cardiac rhythm disturbances, or seizures.

Cidofovir is a nucleotide analogue that is effective in treating CMV retinitis and equivalent or better than ganciclovir in some experimental models of murine CMV encephalitis, although data concerning its efficacy in human CMV CNS disease are limited. The usual dose is 5 mg/kg intravenously once weekly for 2 weeks, then biweekly for 2 or more additional doses, depending on clinical response. Patients must be prehydrated with normal saline (e.g., 1 L over 1 to 2 h) prior to each dose, and treated with probenecid (e.g., 1 g 3 h before cidofovir and 1 g 2 and 8 h after cidofovir). Nephrotoxicity is common; the dose should be reduced if renal function deteriorates.

Intravenous ribavarin (15 to 25 mg/kg per day in divided doses given every 8 h) has been reported to be of benefit in isolated cases of severe encephalitis due to California encephalitis (LaCrosse) virus. Ribavarin might be of benefit for the rare patients, typically infants or young children, with severe adenovirus or rotavirus encephalitis, and in patients with encephalitis due to LCMV or other arenaviruses. However, clinical trials are lacking. Hemolysis, with resulting anemia, has been the major side effect limiting therapy.

Sequelae There is considerable variation in the incidence and severity of sequelae in patients surviving viral encephalitis. In the case of Eastern equine encephalitis virus infection, nearly 80% of survivors have severe neurologic sequelae. At the other extreme are infections due to EBV, California encephalitis virus, and Venezuelan equine encephalitis virus, where severe sequelae are unusual. For example, approximately 5 to 15% of children infected with LaCrosse virus have a residual seizure disorder, and 1% have persistent hemiparesis. Detailed information about sequelae in patients with HSV encephalitis

Table 373-6 Features of Selected Arbovirus Encephalitides

Feature	WEE	EEE	VEE	SLE	CE
Region	West, midwest	Atlantic and Gulf	South	All	East and north-central
Age	Infants, adults >50 years	Children	Adults	Adults >50 years	Children
Deaths	5–15%	50–75%	1%	2–20%	<1%
Sequelae	Low to moderate	80%	Rare	20%	Rare
Vector	Mosquito	Mosquito	Mosquito	Mosquito	Mosquito
Animal host	Birds	Birds	Horses, small mammals	Birds	Rodents

NOTE: CE, California encephalitis virus; EEE, Eastern equine encephalitis virus; SLE, St. Louis encephalitis virus; VEE, Venezuelan equine encephalitis virus; WEE, Western equine encephalitis virus.
SOURCE: After Whitley.

treated with acyclovir are available from the NIAID-CASG trials. Of 32 acyclovir-treated patients, 26 survived (81%). Of the 26 survivors, 12 (46%) had no or only minor sequelae, 3 (12%) were moderately impaired (gainfully employed but not functioning at their previous level), and 11 (42%) were severely impaired (requiring continuous supportive care). The incidence and severity of sequelae were directly related to the age of the patient and the level of consciousness at the time of initiation of therapy. Patients with severe neurologic impairment (Glasgow coma score 6) at initiation of therapy either died or survived with severe sequelae. Young patients (<30 years) with good neurologic function at initiation of therapy did substantially better (100% survival, 62% with no or mild sequelae) compared with their older counterparts (>30 years); (64% survival, 57% no or mild sequelae). Recent studies using quantitative CSF PCR tests for HSV indicate that clinical outcome following treatment also correlates with the amount of HSV DNA present in CSF at the time of presentation.

ACUTE MYELITIS AND RADICULITIS

Myelitis is a viral infection of the spinal cord, which may occur as an isolated syndrome or in association with encephalitis (encephalomyelitis) or infection involving the nerve roots (myeloradiculitis). Viral infection involving sensory ganglia and nerve roots may also occur as an isolated syndrome, most commonly in the form of shingles.

MYELITIS   Clinical Features and Epidemiology   The prototypical viral myelitis is the syndrome of acute anterior poliomyelitis caused by polioviruses. Paralytic polio (Chap. 193) is a rarity in the United States (four to eight cases per year), although it remains a major problem in some regions of the world. Most cases of paralytic polio in the United States occur as a result of the exceedingly rare reversion of vaccine strains to virulence. The cases are divided among those recently vaccinated and unvaccinated nonimmune adults exposed to recently vaccinated children. Occasional outbreaks have occurred in nonimmunized populations such as the Amish in Pennsylvania. Illness typically begins with prodromal symptoms, including fever, headache, myalgia, pharyngitis, nausea and vomiting, and meningeal signs. These are associated with the typical CSF profile of aseptic meningitis. In some patients these symptoms are followed by the development of muscle weakness resulting from viral injury to the motor neurons in the anterior horn of the spinal cord or in brainstem motor nuclei. The incidence, severity, and pattern of weakness are age-dependent, with more severe disease being seen with increasing age. Young children often develop weakness of one leg, older children weakness of both legs, and adults asymmetric quadriparesis, often with associated urinary retention. Weakness is associated with fasciculations, loss of deep and superficial reflexes, and the development of atrophy. Involvement of the brainstem (bulbar polio) can result in dysphagia, dysarthria, respiratory impairment, and vasomotor disturbances. Although some patients complain of paresthesia, objective sensory loss is not present.

A distinctive polio-like syndrome is produced by enterovirus 70. Patients develop acute hemorrhagic conjunctivitis, followed days to weeks later by a poliomyelitis-like weakness.

Viruses may also affect both the anterior and posterior portions of the spinal cord over a considerable longitudinal extent, producing "transverse" myelitis. The clinical syndrome is one of acute muscle weakness, which may be of the flaccid hyporeflexic type initially but usually develops into spastic paralysis with hyperreflexia and extensor plantar responses. Sensory loss is almost invariably present and typically involves both pain-temperature and position-vibration modalities, producing a sensory level. Urinary symptoms (retention, overflow incontinence, or, in milder cases, hesitancy or decreased voiding sensation) and constipation or even fecal incontinence are present in virtually all patients. Although this syndrome can be caused by a variety of viruses, most cases in immunocompetent patients are due to HSV-2, VZV, or EBV. CMV is an important cause of myelitis in immunocompromised patients, notably those with HIV infection.

A mild form of myelitis predominantly affecting the sacral spinal cord occurs in association with genital HSV-2 infection. At the time of the first episode of genital herpes, about 25% of women, and a smaller percentage of men, develop an aseptic meningitis syndrome. In some individuals this may be associated with urinary retention, dysesthesia, paresthesia, or neuralgia in the legs, buttocks, or genital area, and weakness in one or both legs.

Chronic viral myelitis is associated with advanced HIV infection (vacuolar myelopathy) and with infection due to HTLV-1 (tropical spastic paraparesis and HTLV-I−associated myelopathy). →*For further discussion of these infections see Chap. 309.*

Diagnosis   Almost all patients with viral myelitis will have inflammatory changes in the CSF including a lymphocytic pleocytosis and elevated protein; glucose is normal. An exception to this pattern occurs in HIV-associated CMV myeloradiculopathy in which a polymorphonuclear pleocytosis and low CSF glucose are characteristic. For myelitis caused by HSV, EBV, CMV, and VZV, CSF PCR studies may be diagnostic. Some patients show evidence of intrathecal synthesis of antibody or the presence of CSF IgM antibodies, and these studies may be helpful in PCR-negative patients. Viral cultures are frequently positive in patients with CMV myelitis and may be positive in some cases of myelitis due to HSV-2. Neuroimaging studies may be helpful in identifying the site and extent of the myelitis. The usual findings are areas of increased T2 signal within the spinal cord parenchyma. Patients with HIV-associated CMV radiculomyelopathy may show increased signal and enhancement of the nerve roots. Perhaps the most important role of MRI is to exclude compressive lesions and other causes of acute myelopathy.

TREATMENT   Reports of treatment of viral myelitis are usually isolated case reports or small series. Patients with myelitis due to HSV, EBV, or VZV should be treated with intravenous acyclovir (10 mg/kg, tid) for 10 to 14 days. Patients with HIV-associated CMV radiculomyelopathy should receive ganciclovir plus foscarnet (see above under CMV encephalitis for dose), although the results of treatment are frequently disappointing.

GANGLIONITIS AND RADICULITIS   Herpes Zoster (See also Chap. 183) • *Clinical features*   Reactivation of VZV latent in neurons within the trigeminal or spinal sensory ganglia produces zoster (*shingles*). Zoster is a distinctive clinical syndrome consisting of paresthesia or dysesthesia in a dermatomal distribution followed by a localized cutaneous eruption. Zoster occurs in patients previously infected with chickenpox (varicella). During the initial varicella infection, virus in the skin travels up the sensory nerves to become latent within neurons in the trigeminal and spinal sensory ganglia. Reactivation results in active viral replication in sensory ganglia followed by spread of virus through nerves to the skin, where a dermatomal vesicular eruption occurs. The incidence of zoster increases with age and is higher in patients with compromised cellular immunity. The typical history is one of several days of itching, tingling, burning, or pain in a dermatomal distribution that is followed by a vesicular eruption consisting of clear vesicles on an erythematous base. The vesicles become cloudy, dry, and crust over after 1 to 2 weeks. The lesions are most commonly found in the thoracic dermatomes, with T5-T10 accounting for approximately two-thirds of cases. Most patients will have hypalgesia and hypesthesia in the affected dermatome. About 5% of patients develop motor weakness and atrophy (zoster paresis) in the associated myotome. Rare patients can have zoster-like neuralgic pain in the absence of a cutaneous eruption (*zoster sine herpete*). Diagnosis in these patients depends on serologic studies in serum or CSF or the identification of VZV DNA in CSF by PCR.

Characteristic syndromes result from zoster eruptions involving the trigeminal and geniculate distribution. In 10 to 15% of cases, reactivation of virus in the trigeminal ganglia results in a rash in the distribution of the ophthalmic division of the trigeminal nerve (*ophthalmic zoster*). Vesicular eruption may be conjoined with conjunctivitis, keratitis, ocular muscle palsies, ptosis, and mydriasis. In rare cases, an attack is followed by the development of cerebral angiitis involving the ipsilateral carotid and/or middle cerebral arteries. Vascular compromise may lead to hemiplegia, aphasia, or other focal deficits contralateral to the side of the facial eruption. Reactivation of virus from the geniculate ganglion produces the *Ramsay Hunt syndrome*, consisting of facial palsy often associated with loss of taste in the anterior tongue, tinnitus, hearing loss, and vertigo. Zoster eruptions are found in the external auditory meatus.

Some 45% of patients over age 50 who develop shingles will experience pain persisting for >6 weeks after disappearance of the rash (*postherpetic neuralgia*). Postherpetic neuralgia is almost never seen in children who develop zoster and is rare (6%) in adults younger than 50. (See "Treatment" below, and Chap. 183).

Diagnosis The diagnosis of shingles is generally made on clinical grounds. Recurrent HSV infection may produce a similar syndrome of a cutaneous eruption in a dermatomal distribution associated with paresthesia. Unlike shingles, in which more than two or three recurrences in a lifetime would be virtually unknown, multiple recurrences are characteristic of HSV infection. The presence of VZV can be confirmed by culture or PCR of material obtained from the vesicular lesions. Direct detection of varicella zoster virus antigens in vesicle scrapings by immunocytochemistry or fluorescent microscopy is more sensitive and specific than the traditional Tzanck preparation and more sensitive than culture. A Tzanck preparation is made by smearing material obtained from the base of a vesicle onto a slide, which is then stained with Wright or Giemsa stain. The presence of syncytial giant cells with intranuclear inclusions is typical of a herpesvirus infection but does not distinguish between VZV and HSV.

℞ **TREATMENT**   **Shingles in Immunocompetent Adults**
    Three antiviral drugs, acyclovir, famciclovir, and valacyclovir, are available for treatment of herpes zoster (shingles). Famciclovir is the diacetyl prodrug form of the nucleoside penciclovir. Following oral administration famciclovir is enzymatically converted to penciclovir (which is not absorbed well orally). Penciclovir acts intracellularly like acyclovir, but its active triphosphate metabolite has an extended half-life compared to acyclovir triphosphate in infected cells. Valacyclovir is the 6-valine ester of acyclovir and is enzymatically converted to acyclovir in the liver. Valacyclovir is better absorbed than acyclovir and allows for significantly (~fourfold) higher serum and CSF acyclovir levels than can be achieved with equimolar doses of oral acyclovir.

Acyclovir, valacyclovir, and famciclovir all produce more rapid resolution of cutaneous lesions and decreased duration of viral shedding compared to placebo if therapy is started within 72 h of rash onset, and decrease the duration of pain. These effects are generally modest, and supportive therapy alone is probably sufficient in immunocompetent patients <50 years who do not have significant pain and whose lesions do not involve the trigeminal dermatome. Immunocompetent patients with trigeminal zoster should be treated with antiviral drugs to reduce the risk of developing keratitis or other ophthalmologic complications of zoster. Patients >50 years should be treated with antiviral drugs in an effort to reduce the risk or duration of postherpetic neuralgia (see below). Typical doses in immunocompetent adults are acyclovir, 800 mg five times per day for 7 to 10 days; famciclovir, 500 mg tid for 7 days; and valacyclovir 1000 mg tid for 7 days.

The role of adjunctive glucocorticoid therapy has not been definitively established. Its use is not recommended in patients <50 or in immunocompromised individuals. In immunocompetent individuals >50, glucocorticoids do not appear to increase complications when used in conjunction with antiviral agents and may reduce the incidence of postherpetic neuralgia. A typical regimen, which should only be used in patients also receiving antiviral therapy, is prednisone, 30 mg bid for 1 week, then 15 mg bid for a second week, and 7.5 mg bid for a final week.

Shingles in Immunocompromised Patients   Immunocompromised patients, including those with HIV infection, who have evidence of disease involving more than one dermatome or in the trigeminal distribution should be treated with intravenous acyclovir (10 mg/kg tid for 10 to 14 days). Immunocompromised patients with mild disease limited to a single dermatome (other than the trigeminal) can be treated initially with oral agents. These patients should be closely monitored and switched to intravenous acyclovir if they show any signs of disease progression while receiving oral therapy. Adverse effects of famciclovir, valacyclovir, and acyclovir are generally minor, with headache and nausea being reported in about 8 to 20% of recipients. Patients with renal insufficiency require reduction in dosing.

Postherpetic Neuralgia   Controlled trials of both amitriptyline and desipramine have shown these drugs to be of benefit in the treatment of postherpetic neuralgia. Amitriptyline should be started at low dose (12.5 to 25 mg/d) and gradually increased until pain is controlled or side effects prevent further dose increases; the optimal dose is usually in the range of 75 to 150 mg/d. Desipramine is probably equally efficacious; however, selective serotonin reuptake inhibitors appear to be of limited utility. In a controlled study, carbamazepine was shown to be effective in reducing neuropathic lancinating pain but not continuous aching or burning pain. Treatment should be started at 200 mg/d and gradually increased until pain is controlled or side effects limit further therapy. The usual effective dose is ~600 mg/d, but some patients may require up to 1200 mg/d. Gabapentin has also been shown to be effective in a randomized controlled trial. Patients should be started on 300 mg tid, with a gradual increase to a maximum of 1200 mg tid. Phenytoin and valproate sodium may also be effective for neuropathic zoster pain. Topical agents such as 2.5% lidocaine–2.5% prilocaine cream or 5% lidocaine gel may benefit some patients with milder symptoms.

VIRAL INFECTION OF THE PERIPHERAL NERVOUS SYSTEM   The distinction between ganglionitis, radiculitis, and neuritis are somewhat arbitrary and depend largely on the whether the brunt of injury involves the ganglia, nerve roots (radiculitis), or peripheral nerves (neuritis). Direct viral infection of peripheral nerves is unusual and should be distinguished from postviral immune-mediated injury to nerves. Many viruses, including CMV, HSV, EBV, VZV, mumps virus, and hepatitis B virus (HBV) have been associated, based predominantly on seroepidemiologic studies, with Guillain-Barré syndrome. It is presumed that the antecedent viral infection triggers an immunologic reaction that subsequently results in damage to peripheral nerve myelin (Chap. 378). A Guillain-Barré–like syndrome can also be seen in association with HIV infection, although these patients typically have a CSF pleocytosis rather than the classic albuminocytologic dissociation (elevated protein, zero or few cells).

Patients with HIV infection may develop CMV infection of peripheral nerves, either alone or in combination with involvement of nerve roots and spinal cord. Patients present with back and leg pain, flaccid paraparesis with areflexia, multimodal sensory loss, and impairment of bowel and bladder function. The CSF shows a polymorphonuclear pleocytosis with an elevated protein and, in some patients, a decreased glucose. As noted earlier, this CSF profile is extremely unusual in viral infections and should suggest the diagnosis of CMV polyradiculopathy in the appropriate clinical setting. CMV inclusions and antigen can be detected in Schwann cells of affected nerves, and CSF cultures or PCR are frequently positive for CMV. Rare cases of CMV-associated multiple mononeuropathy have also been reported. Patients present with radial, peroneal, or sural neuropathies alone or in combination. CMV antigen can be detected in Schwann cells of involved nerves, indicating that the neuropathies are caused by direct viral infection. Evidence of demyelination may be present, and immune mechanisms may contribute to the pathogenesis of the nerve injury.

Viral spread from the site of initial inoculation to the CNS through nerves is integral to the pathogenesis of rabies virus infection (Chap. 197). Rabies virus particles have been detected by electron microscopy and rabies virus antigen by immunocytochemistry in nerves innervating the site of initial viral inoculation. Neural spread of virus is also a central feature of the pathogenesis of shingles (see above) and of recurrent herpes labialis and genitalis (Chap. 182).

Isolated cranial nerve palsies, especially of the facial nerve (Bell's palsy), have been attributed to HSV, VZV (Ramsay Hunt syndrome), HIV, EBV, enteroviruses, and mumps virus, although in many cases the etiologic relationship appears rather tenuous. Pathologic specimens are almost never available from acute cases of Bell's palsy because of the generally benign and self-limited nature of the illness. Virus has never been cultured from the facial nerve, nor have viral antigens or nucleic acid been detected. However, in a study of patients with peripheral facial palsy undergoing decompressive facial nerve surgery, HSV DNA was found by PCR in endoneurial fluid from the facial nerve in ~80% of 14 patients with Bell's palsy, and VZV DNA was found in ~90% of those with Ramsay Hunt syndrome. This represents the strongest evidence to date for the direct role of these viruses in facial palsy.

Auditory and/or vestibular syndromes may also result from viral injury to the eighth cranial nerve. Mumps, measles, and VZV have been associated with cases of unilateral or bilateral nerve deafness. Seroepidemiologic studies also suggest a possible role for parainfluenza viruses, adenoviruses, and HSV in acute hearing loss. HSV has also been suggested to have a role in the pathogenesis of some cases of vestibular neuritis, based on detection of HSV DNA by PCR in vestibular ganglia.

CHRONIC AND PERSISTENT VIRAL CNS DISEASE

PROGRESSIVE MULTIFOCAL LEUKOENCEPHALOPATHY   Clinical Features and Pathology   Progressive multifocal leukoencephalopathy (PML) is a progressive disorder characterized pathologically by multifocal areas of demyelination of varying size distributed throughout the CNS. In addition to demyelination, there are characteristic cytologic alterations in both astrocytes and oligodendrocytes. Astrocytes are tremendously enlarged and contain hyperchromatic, deformed, and bizarre nuclei and frequent mitotic figures. Oligodendrocytes have enlarged, densely staining nuclei that contain viral inclusions formed by crystalline arrays of JC virus particles. Patients often present with visual deficits (45%), typically a homonymous hemianopia, and mental impairment (38%) (dementia, confusion, personality change). Motor weakness may not be present early but eventually occurs in 75% of cases.

Almost all patients (>95%) have an underlying immunosuppressive disorder. Prior to the HIV epidemic, common associated diseases included lymphoproliferative disorders, immune deficiency states, myeloproliferative disease, and chronic infectious or granulomatous diseases. Since 1984, the importance of these associated disorders in PML has been dwarfed by that of AIDS; >60% of currently diagnosed PML cases occur in patients with AIDS. Conversely, it has been estimated that nearly 1% of AIDS patients will develop PML. Early indications suggest that the basic features of AIDS-associated PML do not differ significantly from those of non-AIDS-associated PML.

Diagnostic Studies   The diagnosis of PML is frequently suggested by MRI or less commonly CT. MRI is more sensitive than CT and reveals multifocal asymmetric, coalescing white matter lesions located periventricularly, in the centrum semiovale, in the parietal-occipital region, and in the cerebellum. These lesions have increased T2 and decreased T1 signal. The lesions of PML are generally nonenhancing or show only minimal peripheral enhancement and are not associated with edema or mass effect. CT shows hypodense nonenhancing white matter lesions without edema or mass effect.

The CSF is typically normal, although mild elevation in protein and/or IgG may be found. Pleocytosis occurs in <25% of cases, is predominantly mononuclear, and rarely exceeds 25 cells/μL. PCR amplification of JC virus DNA from CSF has become an important di-

agnostic tool. CSF PCR for JC virus DNA has high specificity, but sensitivity has varied among studies. Rare cases of positive CSF PCR for JC virus DNA in the absence of clinical or radiographic evidence of PML have been described in HIV-infected patients. It remains to be established whether these results are false positives or are indicative of preclinical PML.

The presence of a positive CSF PCR for JC virus DNA in association with typical MRI lesions in the appropriate clinical setting is diagnostic of PML. Patients with negative CSF PCR studies may require brain biopsy for definitive diagnosis. In biopsy or necropsy specimens of brain, JC virus antigen and nucleic acid can be detected by immunocytochemistry, in situ hybridization, or PCR amplification. Detection of JC virus antigen or genomic material should only be considered diagnostic of PML if accompanied by characteristic pathologic changes, since both antigen and genomic material have been found in the brains of normal patients.

TREATMENT   No effective therapy for PML is available. Intravenous and/or intrathecal cytarabine were not shown to be of benefit in a recent randomized controlled trial. Based on isolated case reports of benefit in some patients, a randomized controlled trial of cidofovir is currently under way. Some patients with HIV-associated PML have shown dramatic clinical improvement associated with improvement in their immune status following institution of highly active antiretroviral therapy.

SUBACUTE SCLEROSING PANENCEPHALITIS   Clinical Features and Epidemiology   SSPE is a rare chronic progressive demyelinating disease of the CNS associated with a chronic nonpermissive infection of brain tissue with measles virus. Fewer than 10 cases per year are reported in the United States. The incidence has declined substantially since the introduction of a measles vaccine. Most patients give a history of primary measles infection at an early age (2 years), which is followed after a latent interval of 6 to 8 years by the development of a progressive neurologic disorder. Some 85% of patients are between 5 and 15 years old at diagnosis. Initial manifestations include poor school performance and mood and personality changes. Typical signs of a CNS viral infection, including fever and headache, do not occur. As the disease progresses, patients develop progressive intellectual deterioration, focal and/or generalized seizures, myoclonus, ataxia, and visual disturbances. In the late stage of the illness, patients are unresponsive, quadriparetic, and spastic, with hyperactive tendon reflexes and extensor plantar responses.

Diagnostic Studies   The EEG shows a characteristic periodic pattern with bursts every 3 to 8 s of high-voltage, sharp slow waves, followed by periods of attenuated ("flat") background. The CSF is acellular with a normal or mildly elevated protein level and a markedly elevated γ-globulin level (>20% of total CSF protein). CSF antimeasles antibody levels are invariably elevated, and oligoclonal antimeasles antibodies are often present. CT and MRI show evidence of multifocal white matter lesions, cortical atrophy, and ex vacuo ventricular enlargement. Measles virus can be cultured from brain tissue using special cocultivation techniques. Viral antigen can be identified immunocytochemically, and viral genome can be detected by in situ hybridization or PCR amplification.

TREATMENT   No definitive therapy for SSPE is available. Treatment with Inosiplex (isoprinosine) (100 mg/kg per day), alone or in combination with intrathecal or intraventricular interferon, has been reported to prolong survival and produce clinical improvement in some patients but has never been subjected to a controlled clinical trial.

PROGRESSIVE RUBELLA PANENCEPHALITIS   Clinical Features and Epidemiology   This is an extremely rare disorder that primarily affects children with congenital rubella syndrome, although isolated cases have been reported following childhood rubella. All the approximately 20 cases reported to date have been in male children. After a latent period of 8 to 19 years, patients develop progressive neurologic deterioration. The initial manifestations are similar to those seen in SSPE and include decline in school performance, behavioral alterations, and seizures, followed by severe progressive dementia, prominent ataxia, pyramidal signs (spasticity, hyperreflexia, extensor plantar responses), and visual deterioration. In the terminal stages of the illness, patients are globally demented, mute, and quadriparetic, often with associated ophthalmoplegia.

Diagnostic Studies   CSF shows a mild lymphocytic pleocytosis, slightly elevated protein level, markedly increased γ-globulin, and rubella virus–specific oligoclonal bands. CT scan may show enlarged ventricles, cortical and cerebellar atrophy, and hypodensity in the white matter. Rubella virus has been isolated from explant and cocultivation cultures of brain biopsy material in one reported case.

℞ **TREATMENT**   No therapy is currently available. Isoprinosine and amantadine are of no benefit. Universal prevention of both congenital and childhood rubella through the use of the available live attenuated rubella vaccine would be expected to eliminate the disease.

BIBLIOGRAPHY

BALE JF: Viral encephalitis. Med Clin North Am 77:25, 1993

BERGER JR, CONCHA M: Progressive multifocal leukoencephalopathy: The evolution of a disease once considered rare. J Neurovirol 1:5, 1995

CINQUE P et al: The role of laboratory investigation in the diagnosis and management of patients with suspected herpes simplex encephalitis: A consensus report. J Neurol Neurosurg Psychiat 61:339, 1996

COHEN JI et al: Recent advances in varicella-zoster virus infection. Ann Intern Med 130: 922, 1999

CONNOLLY KJ, HAMMER SM: The acute aseptic meningitis syndrome. Infect Dis Clin North Am 4:599, 1990

DEBIASI R, TYLER KL: Polymerase chain reaction in the diagnosis and management of central nervous system infections. Arch Neurol 56:1215 , 1999

FONG IW, TOMA E: The natural history of progressive multifocal leukoencephalopathy in patients with AIDS. Clin Infect Dis 20:1305, 1995

GILDEN DH et al: Neurologic complications of the reactivation of varicella-zoster virus. N Engl J Med 342:635, 2000

GOH KJ et al: Clinical features of Nipah virus encephalitis among pig farmers in Malaysia. N Engl J Med 342:1229, 2000

JOHNSON RT: Acute encephalitis. Clin Infect Dis 20:971, 1995

———: *Viral Infections of the Nervous System*, 2d ed. Philadelphia, Lippincott Raven, 1998

LANCIOTTI RS et al: Origin of the West Nile virus responsible for an outbreak of encephalitis in the northeastern United States. Science 286:2333, 1999

ROOS KL (ed): Central nervous system infections. Semin Neurol 12:155, 1992

ROTBART HA: Enteroviral infections of the central nervous system. Clin Infect Dis 20: 971, 1995

RUST RS et al: La Crosse and other forms of California encephalitis. J Child Neurol 14: 1, 1999

SCHELD WM et al: *Infections of the Central Nervous System*, 2d ed. New York, Lippincott-Raven, 1997

TSAI TF: Arboviral infections in the United States. Infect Dis Clin North Am 5:73, 1991

TYLER KL, MARTIN JB (eds): Contemporary Neurology Series, vol 41: *Infectious Diseases of the Central Nervous System*. Philadelphia, FA Davis, 1993

374   *Walter J. Koroshetz, Morton N. Swartz*

CHRONIC AND RECURRENT MENINGITIS

Chronic inflammation of the meninges (pia, arachnoid, and dura) can produce profound neurologic disability and may be fatal if not successfully treated. The condition is most commonly diagnosed when a characteristic neurologic syndrome exists for >4 weeks and is associated with a persistent inflammatory response in the cerebrospinal fluid (CSF) (white blood cell count >5/μL). The causes are varied, and appropriate treatment depends on identification of the etiology. Five categories of disease account for most cases of chronic meningitis: (1) meningeal infections, (2) malignancy, (3) noninfectious in-

flammatory disorders, (4) chemical meningitis, and (5) parameningeal infections.

CLINICAL PATHOPHYSIOLOGY   Neurologic manifestations of chronic meningitis (Table 374-1) are determined by the anatomic location of the inflammation and its consequences. Persistent headache with or without stiff neck and hydrocephalus, cranial neuropathies, radiculopathies, and cognitive or personality changes are the cardinal features. These can occur alone or in combination. When they appear in combination, widespread dissemination of the inflammatory process along CSF pathways has occurred. In some cases, the presence of an underlying systemic illness points to a specific agent or class of agents as the probable cause. The diagnosis of chronic meningitis is usually made when the clinical presentation prompts the astute physician to examine the CSF for signs of inflammation.

CSF is produced by the choroid plexus of the cerebral ventricles, exits through narrow foramina into the subarachnoid space surrounding the brain and spinal cord, circulates around the base of the brain and over the cerebral hemispheres, and is resorbed by arachnoid villi projecting into the superior sagittal sinus. CSF flow provides a pathway for rapid spread of infectious and malignant processes over the brain, spinal cord, and cranial and spinal nerve roots. Spread from the subarachnoid space into brain parenchyma may occur via the arachnoid cuffs that surround blood vessels that penetrate brain tissue (Virchow-Robin spaces).

Intracranial Meningitis   Nociceptive fibers of the meninges (Chap. 15) are stimulated by the inflammatory process, resulting in headache or neck or back pain. Obstruction of CSF pathways at foramina or arachnoid villi may produce *hydrocephalus* and symptoms of raised intracranial pressure, including headache, vomiting, apathy or drowsiness, gait instability, papilledema, visual loss, impaired upgaze, or palsy of the seventh cranial nerve (CN) (Chap. 376). Cognitive and behavioral changes during the course of chronic meningitis may also result from vascular damage, which may similarly produce seizures, stroke, or myelopathy.

Inflammatory deposits seeded via the CSF circulation are often prominent around the brainstem and cranial nerves and along the undersurface of the frontal and temporal lobes. Such cases, termed *basal meningitis*, often present as multiple cranial neuropathies, with visual loss (CN II), facial weakness (CN VII), hearing loss (CN VIII), diplopia (CNs III, IV, and VI), sensory or motor abnormalities of the oropharynx (CNs IX, X, and XII), decreased olfaction (CN I), or facial sensory loss and masseter weakness (CN V).

Spinal Meningitis   Injury may occur to motor and sensory roots as they traverse the subarachnoid space and penetrate the meninges. These cases present as multiple radiculopathies with combinations of radicular pain, sensory loss, motor weakness, and sphincter dysfunc-

Table 374-1   Symptoms and Signs of Chronic Meningitis

Symptoms	Signs
Chronic headache	+/– Papilledema
Neck or back pain	Brudzinski's or Kernig's sign of meningeal irritation
Change in personality	Altered mental status—drowsiness, inattention, disorientation, memory loss, frontal release signs (grasp, suck, snout), perseveration
Facial weakness	Peripheral seventh CN palsy
Double vision	Palsy of CNs III, IV, VI
Visual loss	Papilledema, optic atrophy
Hearing loss	Eighth CN palsy
Arm or leg weakness	Myelopathy or radiculopathy
Numbness in arms or legs	Myelopathy or radiculopathy
Sphincter dysfunction	Myelopathy or radiculopathy Frontal lobe dysfunction
Clumsiness	Ataxia

NOTE: CN, cranial nerve.

tion. Meningeal inflammation can encircle the cord, resulting in myelopathy. Patients with slowly progressive involvement of multiple cranial nerves and/or spinal nerve roots are likely to have chronic meningitis. Electrophysiologic testing (electromyography, nerve conduction studies, and evoked response testing) may be helpful in determining whether there is involvement of cranial and spinal nerve roots.

Systemic Manifestations In some patients, evidence of systemic disease provides clues to the underlying cause of chronic meningitis. A careful history and physical examination are essential before embarking on a diagnostic workup, which may be costly, prolonged, and associated with risk from invasive procedures. A complete history of travel, sexual practice, and exposure to infectious agents should be sought. Infectious causes are often associated with fever, malaise, anorexia, and signs of localized or disseminated infection outside the nervous system. Infectious causes are of major concern in the immunosuppressed patient, especially in patients with AIDS, in whom chronic meningitis may present without headache or fever. Noninfectious inflammatory disorders often produce systemic manifestations, but meningitis may be the initial manifestation. Carcinomatous meningitis may or may not be accompanied by clinical evidence of the primary neoplasm.

Approach to the Patient

The occurrence of chronic headache, hydrocephalus, cranial neuropathy, radiculopathy, and/or cognitive decline in a patient should prompt consideration of a lumbar puncture for evidence of meningeal inflammation. On occasion the diagnosis is made when an imaging study [computed tomography (CT) or magnetic resonance imaging (MRI)] shows contrast enhancement of the meninges, always an abnormal finding except after a recent neurosurgical procedure. Once chronic meningitis is confirmed by CSF examination, effort is focused on identifying the cause (Tables 374-2 and 374-3) by (1) further analysis of the CSF, (2) diagnosis of an underlying systemic infection or noninfectious inflammatory condition, or (3) pathologic examination of meningeal biopsy specimens.

Two clinical forms of chronic meningitis exist. In the first, the symptoms are chronic and persistent, whereas in the second there are recurrent, discrete episodes of illness. In the latter group, all symptoms, signs, and CSF parameters of meningeal inflammation resolve completely between episodes without specific therapy. In such patients, the likely etiologies include infection with herpes simplex virus (HSV) type 2; chemical meningitis due to leakage into CSF of contents from an epidermoid tumor, craniopharyngioma, or cholesteatoma; primary inflammatory conditions, including Vogt-Koyanagi-Harada syndrome, Behçet's syndrome (Chap. 316), Mollaret's meningitis, and systemic lupus erythematosus (SLE; Chap. 311); and drug hypersensitivity with repeated administration of the offending agent. The duration of chronic meningitis may also be of value in diagnosis; for example, an untreated patient with tuberculous meningitis is unlikely to survive beyond 4 to 6 weeks.

The epidemiologic history is of considerable importance and may provide direction for selection of laboratory studies. Pertinent features include a history of tuberculosis or exposure to a likely case; past travel to areas endemic for fungal infections (the San Joaquin Valley in California and southwestern states for coccidioidomycosis; midwestern states for histoplasmosis, southeastern states for blastomycosis); travel to the Mediterranean region or ingestion of imported unpasteurized dairy products (*Brucella*); time spent in areas endemic for Lyme disease (e.g., Connecticut, New York, Massachusetts); exposure to sexually transmitted disease (syphilis); exposure of an immunocompromised host to pigeons and their droppings (*Cryptococcus*); gardening (*Sporothrix schenkii*); ingestion of poorly cooked meat or contact with a household cat (*Toxoplasma gondii*); residence in Thailand or Japan (*Gnathostoma spinigerum*) or the South Pacific (*Angiostrongylus can-*

tonensis); rural residence and raccoon exposure (*Baylisascaris procyonis*); and residence in Latin America, the Philippines, or Southeast Asia when eosinophilic meningitis is present (*Taenia solium*).

The presence of focal cerebral signs in a patient with chronic meningitis suggests the possibility of a brain abscess or other parameningeal infection; identification of a potential source of infection (chronic draining ear, sinusitis, right-to-left cardiac or pulmonary shunt, chronic pleuropulmonary infection) supports this diagnosis. In some cases, diagnosis may be established by recognition and biopsy of unusual skin lesions (Behçet's syndrome, cryptococcosis, blastomycosis, SLE, Lyme disease, intravenous drug use, sporotrichosis, trypanosomiasis) or enlarged lymph nodes (lymphoma, tuberculosis, sarcoid, infection with HIV, secondary syphilis, or Whipple's disease). A careful ophthalmologic examination may reveal uveitis [Vogt-Koyanagi-Harada syndrome, sarcoid, or central nervous system (CNS) lymphoma], keratoconjunctivitis sicca (Sjögren's syndrome), or iridocyclitis (Behçet's syndrome) and is essential to assess visual loss from hydrocephalus. Aphthous oral lesions, genital ulcers, and hypopyon suggest Behçet's syndrome. Hepatosplenomegaly suggests lymphoma, sarcoid, tuberculosis, or brucellosis. Herpetic lesions in the genital area or on the thighs suggests HSV-2 infection. A breast nodule, a suspicious pigmented skin lesion, or an abdominal mass directs attention to possible carcinomatous meningitis.

Imaging Once the clinical syndrome is recognized as a potential manifestation of chronic meningitis, proper analysis of the CSF is essential. However, if the possibility of raised intracranial pressure exists, a brain imaging study should be performed before lumbar puncture. In patients with communicating hydrocephalus caused by impaired resorption of CSF, lumbar puncture is safe and may lead to temporary improvement. However, if intracranial pressure is elevated because of a mass lesion, brain swelling, or a block in ventricular CSF outflow (obstructive hydrocephalus), then lumbar puncture carries the potential risk of brain herniation (Fig. 374-1). Obstructive hydrocephalus usually requires direct ventricular drainage of CSF.

Contrast-enhanced MRI or CT studies of the brain and spinal cord can identify meningeal enhancement, parameningeal infections (including brain abscess), encasement of the spinal cord (malignancy or inflammation and infection), or nodular deposits on the meninges or nerve roots (malignancy or sarcoidosis). Imaging studies are also useful to localize areas of meningeal disease prior to meningeal biopsy.

Cerebral angiography may be indicated in patients with chronic meningitis and stroke to identify cerebral arteritis (granulomatous angiitis, infectious arteritis).

Cerebrospinal Fluid Analysis The CSF pressure should be measured and samples sent for bacterial culture, cell count and differential, Gram's stain, and measurement of glucose and protein. In cases without a known cause, CSF should be sent for the Venereal Disease Research Laboratories (VDRL) test, acid-fast bacillus (AFB) stain and culture, fungal wet mount and India ink preparation and culture, culture for fastidious bacteria and fungi, assays for cryptococcal antigen and oligoclonal immunoglobulin bands, and cytology. Other specific CSF tests (Tables 374-2 and 374-3) or blood tests and cultures should be ordered as indicated on the basis of the history, physical examination, or preliminary CSF results (i.e., eosinophilic, mononuclear, or polymorphonuclear meningitis). Rapid diagnosis may be facilitated by polymerase chain reaction (PCR) testing to identify DNA sequences in the CSF that are specific for the suspected pathogenic organism.

In most categories of chronic (not recurrent) meningitis, mononuclear cells predominate in the CSF. When neutrophils predominate after 3 weeks of illness, the principal etiologic considerations are *Nocardia asteroides*, *Actinomyces israelii*, *Brucella*, *Mycobacterium tuberculosis* (5 to 10% of early cases only), various fungi (*Blastomyces dermatitidis*, *Candida albicans*, *Histoplasma capsulatum*, *Aspergillus* species, *Pseudallescheria boydii*, *Cladophialophora bantiana*) and noninfectious causes (SLE, exogenous chemical meningitis). When eosinophils predominate or are present in limited numbers in a primarily mononuclear cell response in the CSF, the differential diagnosis

Table 374-2   Infectious Causes of Chronic Meningitis

Causative Agent	CSF Formula	Helpful Diagnostic Tests	Risk Factors and Systemic Manifestations
COMMON BACTERIAL CAUSES			
Partially treated suppurative meningitis	Mononuclear or mixed mononuclear-polymorphonuclear cells	CSF culture and Gram's stain	History consistent with acute bacterial meningitis and incomplete treatment
Parameningeal infection	Mononuclear or mixed mononuclear-polymorphonuclear cells	Contrast-enhanced MRI or CT to detect parenchymal, subdural, epidural, or sinus infection	Otitis media, pleuropulmonary infection, right-to-left cardiopulmonary shunt for brain abscess, focal neurologic signs; neck, back, ear, or sinus tenderness
Mycobacterium tuberculosis	Mononuclear cells except polymorphonuclear cells in early infection (leukocytes commonly $<500/\mu L$); low CSF glucose, elevated protein	Tuberculin skin test may be negative; AFB culture of CSF (sputum, urine, gastric contents if indicated); tuberculostearic acid detection in CSF; identify tubercle bacillus on acid-fast stain of CSF or protein pellicle; PCR	Exposure history; previous tuberculous illness; immunosuppressed or AIDS; young children; fever, meningismus, night sweats, miliary TB on x-ray or liver biopsy; stroke due to arteritis
Lyme disease (Bannwarth's syndrome): *Borrelia burgdorferi*	Mononuclear cells; elevated protein	Serum Lyme antibody titer; western blot confirmation; (patients with syphilis may have false-positive Lyme titer)	History of tick bite or appropriate exposure history; erythema chronicum migrans rash; arthritis, radiculopathy, Bell's palsy, meningoencephalitis–multiple sclerosis-like syndrome
Syphilis (secondary, tertiary): *Treponema pallidum*	Mononuclear cells; elevated protein	CSF VDRL; serum VDRL (or RPR); FTA or MHA-TP; serum VDRL may be negative in tertiary syphilis	Appropriate exposure history; HIV seropositive individuals at increased risk of aggressive infection; "dementia"; cerebral infarction due to endarteritis
UNCOMMON BACTERIAL CAUSES			
Actinomyces	Polymorphonuclear cells	Anaerobic culture	Parameningeal abscess or sinus tract (oral or dental focus); pneumonitis
Nocardia	Polymorphonuclear cells; occasionally mononuclear cells; often low glucose	Isolation may require weeks; weakly acid fast	Associated brain abscess may be present
Brucella	Mononuclear cells (rarely polymorphonuclear); elevated protein; often low glucose	CSF antibody detection; serum antibody detection	Intake of unpasteurized dairy products; exposure to goats, sheep, cows; fever, arthralgia, myalgia, vertebral osteomyelitis
Whipple's disease: *Tropherema whippelii*	Mononuclear cells	Biopsy of small bowel or lymph node; CSF PCR for *T. whippelii*; brain and meningeal biopsy (with PAS stain and EM examination)	Diarrhea, weight loss, arthralgias, fever; dementia, ataxia, paresis, ophthalmoplegia, oculomasticatory myoclonus
RARE BACTERIAL CAUSES			
Leptospirosis (occasionally if left untreated may last 3–4 weeks); *Pseudoallescheria boydii* (neutrophilic pleocytosis)			
FUNGAL CAUSES			
Cryptococcus neoformans	Mononuclear cells; count not elevated in some patients with AIDS	India ink or fungal wet mount of CSF (budding yeast); blood and urine cultures; antigen detection in CSF	AIDS and immunosuppression; pigeon exposure; skin and other organ involvement due to disseminated infection
Coccidioides immitis	Mononuclear cells (sometimes 10–20% eosinophils); often low glucose	Antibody detection in CSF and serum	Exposure history—southwestern US; increased virulence in dark-skinned races
Candida sp.	Polymorphonuclear or mononuclear cells	Fungal stain and culture of CSF	IV drug abuse; recent surgery; prolonged intravenous therapy; disseminated candidiasis
Histoplasma capsulatum	Mononuclear cells; low glucose	Fungal stain and culture of large volumes of CSF; antigen detection in CSF, serum, and urine; antibody detection in serum, CSF	Exposure history—Ohio and central Mississippi River Valley; AIDS; mucosal lesions
Blastomyces dermatitidis	Mononuclear cells	Fungal stain and culture of CSF; biopsy and culture of skin, lung lesions; antibody detection in serum	Midwestern and southeastern US; usually systemic infection; abscesses, draining sinus, ulcers
Aspergillus sp.	Mononuclear or polymorphonuclear cells	CSF culture	Sinusitis; granulocytopenia or immunosuppression
Sporothrix schenckii	Mononuclear cells	Antibody detection in CSF and serum; CSF culture	Traumatic inoculation; IV drug use; ulcerated skin lesion
RARE FUNGAL CAUSES			
Cladophialophora bantiana (formerly *Cladosporium trichoides*) and other dark-walled (dematiaceous) fungi such as *Curvularia* and *Drechslera*; *Mucor*			

(continued)

Table 374-2   Infectious Causes of Chronic Meningitis—*(continued)*

Causative Agent	CSF Formula	Helpful Diagnostic Tests	Risk Factors and Systemic Manifestations
PROTOZOAL CAUSES			
Toxoplasma gondii	Mononuclear cells	Biopsy or response to empirical therapy in clinically appropriate context (including presence of antibody in serum)	Usually with intracerebral abscesses; common in HIV-seropositive patients
Trypanosomiasis *Trypanosoma gambiense*, *Trypanosoma rhodesiense*	Mononuclear cells, elevated protein level	Elevated CSF IgM; identification of trypanosomes in CSF and blood smear	Endemic in Africa; chancre, lymphadenopathy; prominent sleep disorder
RARE PROTOZOAL CAUSES			
Acanthamoeba sp. causing granulomatous amebic encephalitis and meningoencephalitis in immunocompromised and debilitated individuals			
HELMINTHIC CAUSES			
Cysticercosis (infection with cysts of *Taenia solium*)	Mononuclear cells; may have eosinophils; glucose level may be low	Indirect hemagglutination assay in CSF; ELISA immunoblotting in serum	Usually with multiple cysts in basal meninges and hydrocephalus; cerebral cysts, muscle calcification
Gnathostoma spinigerum	Eosinophils, mononuclear cells	Peripheral eosinophilia	History of eating raw fish; common in Thailand and Japan; subarachnoid hemorrhage; painful radiculopathy
Angiostrongylus cantonensis	Eosinophils, mononuclear cells	Recovery of worms from CSF	History of eating raw shellfish; common in tropical Pacific regions; often benign
Baylisascaris procyonis (raccoon ascarid)	Eosinophils, mononuclear cells		Infection follows accidental ingestion of *B. procyonis* eggs from raccoon feces; fatal meningoencephalitis
RARE HELMINTHIC CAUSES			
Trichinella spiralis (trichinosis); *Echinococcus* cysts; *Schistosoma* sp. The first may produce a lymphocytic pleocytosis, whereas the latter two may produce an eosinophilic response in CSF associated with cerebral cysts (*Echinococcus*) or granulomatous lesions of brain or spinal cord			
VIRAL CAUSES			
Mumps	Mononuclear cells	Antibody in serum	No prior mumps or immunization; may produce meningoencephalitis; may persist for 3–4 weeks
Lymphocytic choriomeningitis	Mononuclear cells	Antibody in serum	Contact with rodents or their excreta; may persist for 3–4 weeks
Echovirus	Mononuclear cells; may have low glucose	Virus isolation from CSF	Congenital hypogammaglobulinemia; history of recurrent meningitis
HIV (acute retroviral syndrome)	Mononuclear cells	p24 antigen in serum and CSF; high level of HIV viremia	HIV risk factors; rash, fever, lymphadenopathy; lymphopenia in peripheral blood; syndrome may persist long enough to be considered chronic meningitis; or chronic meningitis may develop in later stages (AIDS) due to HIV
Herpes simplex (HSV)	Mononuclear cells	PCR for HSV DNA; CSF antibody	Recurrent meningitis due to HSV-2 (rarely HSV-1) often associated with genital recurrences

ABBREVIATIONS: AFB, acid-fast bacillus stain; CSF, cerebrospinal fluid; ELISA, enzyme-linked immunosorbent assay; EM, electron microscopy; FTA, fluorescent treponemal antibody absorption test; IV, intravenous; MHA-TP, microhemagglutination assay-*Trepo-* *nema pallidum*; PAS, periodic acid–Schiff; PCR, polymerase chain reaction; RPR, rapid plasma reagin test; TB, tuberculosis; VDRL, Venereal Disease Research Laboratories test.

includes parasitic diseases (*A. cantonensis, G. spinigerum, B. procyonis,* or *Toxocara canis* infection, cysticercosis, schistosomiasis, echinococcal disease, *T. gondii* infection), fungal infections (6 to 20% eosinophils along with a predominantly lymphocyte pleocytosis, particularly with coccidioidal meningitis), neoplastic disease (lymphoma, leukemia, metastatic carcinoma), or other inflammatory processes (sarcoidosis, hypereosinophilic syndrome).

It is often necessary to broaden the number of diagnostic tests if the initial workup does not reveal the cause. In addition, repeated samples of large volumes of CSF may be required to diagnose certain infectious and malignant causes of chronic meningitis. For instance, lymphomatous or carcinomatous meningitis may be diagnosed by examination of sections cut from a cell block formed by spinning down the sediment from a large volume of CSF. The diagnosis of fungal meningitis may require large volumes of CSF for culture of sediment.

If standard lumbar puncture is unrewarding, a cervical cisternal tap to sample CSF near to the basal meninges may be fruitful.

Laboratory Investigation   In addition to the CSF examination, an attempt should be made to uncover pertinent underlying illnesses. Tuberculin skin test, chest radiograph, urine analysis and culture, blood count and differential, renal and liver function tests, and measurement of electrolytes (including calcium and phosphate), sedimentation rate, antinuclear antibody, and serum angiotensin-converting enzyme level are often indicated. Liver or bone marrow biopsy may be diagnostic in some cases of miliary tuberculosis, disseminated fungal infection, sarcoidosis, or metastatic malignancy. Abnormalities discovered on chest radiograph or chest CT can be pursued by bronchoscopy or transthoracic needle biopsy.

Meningeal Biopsy   A diagnostic meningeal biopsy should be strongly considered in patients who are severely disabled, who need

Table 374-3 Noninfectious Causes of Chronic Meningitis

Causative Agents	CSF Formula	Helpful Diagnostic Tests	Risk Factors and Systemic Manifestations
Malignancy	Mononuclear cells, elevated protein, low glucose	Repeated cytologic examination of large volumes of CSF; CSF exam by polarizing microscopy; clonal lymphocyte markers; deposits on nerve roots or meninges seen on myelogram or contrast-enhanced MRI; meningeal biopsy	Metastatic cancer of breast, lung, stomach, or pancreas; melanoma, lymphoma, leukemia; meningeal gliomatosis; meningeal sarcoma; cerebral dysgerminoma; meningeal melanoma or B cell lymphoma
Chemical compounds (may cause recurrent meningitis)	Mononuclear cells or PMNs, low glucose, elevated protein; xanthochromia from subarachnoid hemorrhage in week prior to presentation with ''meningitis''	Contrast-enhanced CT scan or MRI; cerebral angiogram to detect aneurysm	History of recent injection into the subarachnoid space; history of sudden onset of headache; recent resection of acoustic neuroma or craniopharyngioma; epidermoid tumor of brain or spine, sometimes with dermoid sinus tract; pituitary apoplexy
Primary inflammation CNS sarcoidosis	Mononuclear cells; elevated protein; often low glucose	Serum and CSF angiotensin-converting enzyme levels; biopsy of extraneural affected tissues or brain lesion/meningeal biopsy	CN palsy, especially of CN VII; hypothalamic dysfunction, especially diabetes insipidus; abnormal chest radiograph; peripheral neuropathy or myopathy
Vogt-Koyanagi-Harada syndrome (recurrent meningitis)	Mononuclear cells		Recurrent meningoencephalitis with uveitis, retinal detachment, alopecia, lightening of eyebrows and lashes, dysacusis, cataracts, glaucoma
Isolated granulomatous angiitis of the nervous system	Mononuclear cells, elevated protein	Angiography or meningeal biopsy	Subacute dementia; multiple cerebral infarctions; recent zoster ophthalmicus
Systemic lupus erythematosus	Mononuclear or polymorphonuclear cells	Anti-DNA antibody, antinuclear antibodies	Encephalopathy; seizures; stroke; transverse myelopathy; rash; arthritis
Behçet's syndrome (recurrent meningitis)	Mononuclear or polymorphonuclear cells, elevated protein		Oral and genital aphthous ulcers; iridocyclitis; retinal hemorrhages; pathergic lesions at site of skin puncture
Chronic benign lymphocytic meningitis	Mononuclear cells		Recovery in 2–6 months, diagnosis by exclusion
Mollaret's recurrent meningitis	Large endothelial cells and polymorphonuclear cells in first hours, followed by mononuclear cells	PCR for herpes; MRI/CT to rule out epidermoid tumor or dural cyst	Recurrent meningitis; exclude HSV-2; rare cases due to HSV-1; occasional case associated with dural cyst
Drug hypersensitivity	Polymorphonuclear cells; occasionally mononuclear cells or eosinophils		Exposure to ibuprofen, sulfonamides, isoniazid, tolmetin, ciprofloxacin, pyridium; improvement after discontinuation of drug; recurrent episodes with recurrent exposure
Wegener's granulomatosis	Mononuclear cells	Chest and sinus radiographs; urinalysis; ANCA antibodies in serum	Associated sinus, pulmonary, or renal lesions; CN palsies; skin lesions; peripheral neuropathy
Other: multiple sclerosis, Sjögren's syndrome, and rarer forms of vasculitis (e.g., Cogan's syndrome)			

ABBREVIATIONS: ANCA, anti-neutrophil cytoplasmic antibodies; PMN, polymorphonuclear neutrophil; PCR, polymerase chain reaction.

chronic ventricular decompression, or whose illness is progressing rapidly. The activities of the surgeon, pathologist, microbiologist, and cytologist should be coordinated so that a large enough sample is obtained and the appropriate cultures and histologic and molecular studies, including electron microscopic and PCR studies, are performed. The diagnostic yield of meningeal biopsy can be increased by targeting regions that enhance with contrast on MRI or CT. With current microsurgical techniques, most areas of the basal meninges can be accessed for biopsy via a limited craniotomy. In a series from the Mayo Clinic reported by Cheng et al., MRI demonstrated meningeal enhancement in 47% of patients undergoing meningeal biopsy. Biopsy of an enhancing region was diagnostic in 80% of cases; biopsy of nonenhancing regions was diagnostic in only 9%; sarcoid (31%) and metastatic adenocarcinoma (25%) were the most common conditions identified.

Approach to the Enigmatic Case In approximately one-third of cases, the diagnosis is not known despite careful evaluation of CSF and potential extraneural sites of disease. A number of the organisms that cause chronic meningitis may take weeks to be identified by cultures. In enigmatic cases several options are available, determined by the extent of the clinical deficits and rate of progression. It is prudent to wait until cultures are finalized if the patient is asymptomatic or symptoms are mild and not progressive. Unfortunately, in many cases progressive neurologic deterioration occurs, and rapid treatment is required. Ventricular-peritoneal shunts may be placed to relieve hydrocephalus, but the risk of disseminating the undiagnosed inflammatory process into the abdomen must be considered.

Empirical Treatment Diagnosis of the causative agent is essential because effective therapies exist for many etiologies of chronic meningitis, but if the condition is left untreated, progressive damage

FIGURE 374-1 Tuberculosis. A 38-year-old man presented with a 2-year history of episodic left-sided numbness, transient speech arrest, and a 3-month history of headache with nausea. Axial (*A*) and coronal (*B, C*) T_1-weighted gadolinium-enhanced MRI scans showed pial- and dural-based enhancing mass lesions consistent with multiple cerebral tuberculomas; right-to-left horizontal displacement is seen in *C*. The meningeal enhancement indicates complicating tuberculous meningitis due to rupture of a tuberculoma into the subarachnoid space.

to the CNS and cranial nerves and roots is likely to occur. Occasionally, empirical therapy must be initiated when all attempts at diagnosis fail. In general, empirical therapy in the United States consists of antimycobacterial agents, amphotericin for fungal infection, or glucocorticoids for noninfectious inflammatory causes. It is important to direct empirical therapy of lymphocytic meningitis at tuberculosis, particularly if the condition is associated with hypoglycorrhachia and sixth and other CN palsies, since untreated disease is fatal in 4 to 8 weeks. In the Mayo Clinic series, the most useful empirical therapy was administration of glucocorticoids rather than antituberculous therapy. Carcinomatous or lymphomatous meningitis may be difficult to diagnose initially, but the diagnosis becomes evident with time.

THE IMMUNOSUPPRESSED PATIENT Chronic meningitis is not uncommon in the course of HIV infection. Pleocytosis and mild meningeal signs often occur at the onset of HIV infection, and occasionally low-grade meningitis persists. Toxoplasmosis commonly presents as intracranial abscesses and may also be associated with meningitis. Other important causes of chronic meningitis in AIDS include infection with *Cryptococcus, Nocardia, Candida,* or other fungi; syphilis; and lymphoma. Toxoplasmosis, cryptococcosis, nocardiosis, and other fungal infections are important etiologic considerations in individuals with immunodeficiency states other than AIDS, including those due to immunosuppressive medications. Because of the increased risk of chronic meningitis and the attenuation of clinical signs of meningeal irritation in immunosuppressed individuals, CSF examination should be performed for any persistent headache or unexplained change in mental state.

BIBLIOGRAPHY

ANDERSON NE, WILLOUGHBY EW: Chronic meningitis without predisposing illness. A review of 83 cases. Q J Med 63:283, 1987

BOUZA E et al: Coccidioidal meningitis. Medicine 60:139, 1981

——— et al: Brucellar meningitis. Rev Infect Dis 9:810, 1987

BROSS JE, GORDON G: Nocardial meningitis. Rev Infect Dis 13:160, 1991

CHARLESTON AJ et al: Idiopathic steroid-responsive chronic lymphocytic meningitis—clinical features and long-term outcome in 17 patients. Aust N Z J Med 28:784, 1998

CHENG TM et al: Chronic meningitis: The role of meningeal or cortical biopsy. Neurosurgery 34:590, 1994

JINNAH HA et al: Chronic meningitis with cranial neuropathies in Wegener's granulomatosis: Case report and review of the literature. Arthritis Rheum 40:573, 1997

MAYER SA et al: Biopsy-proven isolated sarcoid meningitis. J Neurosurgery 78:994, 1993

PEACOCK JE et al: Persistent neutrophilic meningitis. Medicine 63:379, 1984

PHILLIPS ME et al: Neoplastic versus inflammatory meningeal enhancement with Gd-DTPA. J Comput Assisted Tomogr 14:536, 1990

REIK L et al: Granulomatous angiitis presenting as chronic meningitis and ventriculitis. Neurology 33:1609, 1983

SCHELD WM et al: *Infections of the Central Nervous System,* 2nd ed. New York, Raven Press, 1997

SMITH JE, AKSAMIT AJ: Outcome of chronic idiopathic meningitis. Mayo Clinic Proc 69:548, 1994

SWARTZ MN: "Chronic meningitis"—many causes to consider. N Engl J Med 317:957, 1987

THWAITS G et al: Tuberculous meningitis. J Neurol Neurosurg Psychiatry 68:289, 2000

WHEAT LJ et al: Histoplasma capsulatum infections of the central nervous system. Medicine 69:244, 1990

| 375 | *Stanley B. Prusiner, Patrick Bosque* |

PRION DISEASES

Creutzfeldt-Jakob disease (CJD) is a degenerative disease of the central nervous system (CNS) that is caused by infectious proteins called *prions.* CJD typically presents with dementia and myoclonus, is relentlessly progressive, and usually results in death within a year of onset. Most patients with CJD are between 50 and 75 years of age; however, patients as young as 17 years and as old as 83 years have been recorded.

In mammals, prions reproduce by binding to the normal, *c*ellular isoform of the *prion p*rotein (PrP^C) and stimulating its conversion into the di*sease-c*ausing isoform (PrP^Sc). PrP^C is rich in α-helix and has little β-sheet, while PrP^Sc has less α-helix and a high β-sheet content (Fig. 375-1). This α to β transition in prion protein (PrP) structure is the fundamental event underlying prion diseases, which are disorders of protein conformation (Table 375-1).

Four new concepts have emerged from studies of prions. First, prions are the only known infectious pathogens that are devoid of nucleic acid. All other infectious agents possess genomes composed of either RNA or DNA that direct the synthesis of their progeny. Second, prion diseases may be manifest as infectious, genetic, and sporadic disorders. No other group of illnesses with a single etiology presents with such a wide spectrum of clinical manifestations. Third, prion diseases result from the accumulation of PrP^Sc, the conformation of which differs substantially from that of its precursor PrP^C. Fourth, PrP^Sc can exist in a variety of different conformations, each of which seems to specify a specific disease phenotype. How a specific conformation of a PrP^Sc molecule is imparted to PrP^C during prion replication to produce nascent PrP^Sc with the same conformation is unknown. Additionally, it is unclear what factors determine where in the CNS a particular PrP^Sc molecule will be deposited.

SPECTRUM OF PRION DISEASES The sporadic form of CJD is the most common prion disorder in humans. Sporadic CJD (sCJD) accounts for ~85% of all cases of human prion disease, while inherited prion diseases account for 10 to 15% of all cases (Table 375-2). Familial CJD (fCJD), Gerstmann-Sträussler-Scheinker disease (GSS), and fatal familial insomnia (FFI) are all dominantly inherited prion diseases that are caused by mutations in the PrP gene.

Although infectious prion diseases account for <1% of all cases and infection does not seem to play an important role in the natural history of these illnesses, the transmissibility of prions is an important biologic feature. Kuru of the Fore people of New Guinea is thought to have resulted from the consumption of brains from dead relatives during ritualistic cannibalism. With the cessation of ritualistic cannibalism in the late 1950s, kuru has nearly disappeared with the exception of a few recent patients exhibiting incubation periods of almost 40 years. Iatrogenic CJD (iCJD) seems to be the result of the accidental inoculation of patients with prions. New variant CJD (nvCJD) in teenagers and young adults in Europe is the result of exposure to tainted beef from cattle with bovine spongiform encepalopathy (BSE).

Six diseases of animals are caused by prions (Table 375-2). Scrapie of sheep and goats is the prototypic prion disease. Mink encephalopathy, BSE, feline spongiform encephalopathy, and exotic ungulate encephalopathy are all thought to occur after the consumption of prion-infected foodstuffs. The origin of chronic wasting disease, a prion disease endemic in deer and elk in regions of North America, is uncertain.

EPIDEMIOLOGY CJD is found throughout the world. The incidence of sCJD is approximately one case per million population. Although many geographic clusters of CJD have been reported, each has been shown to segregate with a PrP gene mutation that results in a nonconservative substitution. Attempts to identify common exposure to some etiologic agent have been unsuccessful for both the sporadic and familial cases. Ingestion of scrapie-infected sheep or goat meat as a cause of CJD in humans has not been demonstrated by epidemiologic studies although speculation about this potential route of inoculation continues. Studies with Syrian hamsters demonstrate that oral infection with prions can occur, but the process is inefficient compared to intracerebral inoculation.

PATHOGENESIS The human prion diseases were initially classified as neurodegenerative disorders of unknown etiology on the basis of pathologic changes being confined to the CNS. With the transmission of kuru and CJD to apes, investigators began to view these diseases as CNS infectious illnesses caused by slow viruses. Even though the familial nature of a subset of CJD cases was well described, the significance of this observation became more obscure with the transmission of CJD to animals. Eventually, the meaning of heritable CJD became clear with the discovery of mutations in the PrP gene of these patients. The prion concept explains how a disease can manifest as a heritable as well as an infectious illness. Moreover, the hallmark common to all of the prion diseases, whether sporadic, dominantly inherited, or acquired by infection, is that they involve the aberrant metabolism of the prion protein.

A major feature that distinguishes prions from viruses is the finding that both PrP isoforms are encoded by a chromosomal gene. In humans, the PrP gene is designated PRNP and is located on the short arm of chromosome 20. Limited proteolysis of PrP^Sc produces a smaller, protease-resistant molecule of ~142 amino acids designated PrP 27-30; under the same conditions, PrP^C is completely hydrolyzed (Fig. 375-2). In the presence of detergent, PrP 27-30 polymerizes into amyloid. Prion amyloid formed by limited proteolysis and detergent extraction is indistinguishable from the filaments that aggregate to form PrP amyloid plaques in the CNS. Both the rods and the PrP amyloid filaments found in brain tissue exhibit similar ultrastructural morphology and green-gold birefringence after staining with Congo red dye.

FIGURE 375-1 Structures of prion proteins. *A.* NMR structure of Syrian hamster recombinant (rec) PrP(90–231). Presumably, the structure of the α-helical form of recPrP(90–231) resembles that of PrP^C. recPrP(90–231) is viewed from the interface where PrP^Sc is thought to bind to PrP^C. Shown are: α-helices A (residues 144–157), B (172–193), and C (200–227). Flat ribbons depict B-strands S1 (129–131) and S2 (161–163). *(Reprinted with permission from H Lui et al: Biochemistry 38:5362, 1999.)* *B.* Plausible model for the tertiary structure of human PrP^Sc. Shown are α-helices B (residues 178–191) and C (202–218). β-strands are 108–113, 116–122, 128–135 and 138–144. *[Reprinted from Les Prix Nobel T. Frängsmyr (ed), Stockholm, Norstedts Tryckeri, 1998, pp 268–323, with permission.]*

Species Barrier Studies on the role of the primary and tertiary structures of PrP in the transmission of prion disease have given new insights into the pathogenesis of these maladies. The amino acid sequence of PrP encodes the species of the prion, and the prion derives its PrP^Sc sequence from the last mammal in which it was passaged. While the primary structure of PrP is likely to be the most important or even sole determinant of the tertiary structure of PrP^C, PrP^Sc seems to function as a template in determining the tertiary structure of nascent PrP^Sc molecules as they are formed from PrP^C. In turn, prion diversity appears to be enciphered in the conformation of PrP^Sc, and thus, prion strains seem to represent different conformers of PrP^Sc.

In general, transmission of prion disease from one species to another is inefficient, in that not all intracerebrally inoculated animals develop disease, and those that fall ill do so only after long incubation times that can approach the natural lifespan of the animal. This "species barrier" to transmission is correlated with the degree of homology between the amino acid sequence of PrP^C in the inoculated host and of PrP^Sc in the prion inoculum. The importance of sequence homology

Table 375-1 Glossary of Prion Terminology

Prion	**Pro**teinaceous **in**fectious particle that lacks nucleic acid. Prions are composed largely, if not entirely, of PrP^Sc molecules. They can cause scrapie in animals and related neurodegenerative diseases of humans such as Creutzfeldt-Jakob disease (CJD). "Scrapie agent" is a synonym.
PrP^Sc	Scrapie isoform of the prion protein. This protein is the only identifiable macromolecule in purified preparations of scrapie prions.
PrP^C	Cellular isoform of the prion protein. PrP^C is the precursor of PrP^Sc.
PrP 27-30	Limited digestion of PrP^Sc with proteinase K generates PrP 27-30 by truncation of the N terminus.
PRNP	PrP gene located on human chromosome 20.
Prion rod	An aggregate of prions composed largely of PrP 27-30 molecules. Created by detergent extraction and limited proteolysis of PrP^Sc. Morphologically and histochemically indistinguishable from many amyloids.
PrP amyloid	Amyloid containing PrP in the brain of animals or humans with prion disease; often accumulates as plaques.

Table 375-2   The Prion Diseases

Disease	Host	Mechanism of Pathogenesis
Human		
Kuru	Fore people	Infection through ritualistic canni-balism
iCJD	Humans	Infection from prion-contaminated hGH, dura mater grafts, etc.
nvCJD	Humans	Infection from bovine prions?
fCJD	Humans	Germline mutations in PrP gene
GSS	Humans	Germline mutations in PrP gene
FFI	Humans	Germline mutation in PrP gene (D178N, M129)
sCJD	Humans	Somatic mutation or spontaneous conversion of PrP^C into PrP^{Sc}?
sFI	Humans	Somatic mutation or spontaneous conversion of PrP^C into PrP^{Sc}?
Animal		
Scrapie	Sheep	Infection in genetically suscepti-ble sheep
BSE	Cattle	Infection with prion-contaminated MBM
TME	Mink	Infection with prions from sheep or cattle
CWD	Mule deer, elk	Unknown
FSE	Cats	Infection with prion-contaminated beef
Exotic ungulate encephalopathy	Greater kudu, nyala, or oryx	Infection with prion-contaminated MBM

ABBREVIATIONS: BSE, bovine spongiform encephalopathy; CJD, Creutzfeldt-Jakob disease; sCJD, sporadic CJD; fCJD, familial CJD; iCJD, iatrogenic CJD; nvCJD, new variant CJD; CWD, chronic wasting disease; FFI, fatal familial insomnia; sFI, sporadic fatal insomnia; FSE, feline spongiform encephalopathy; GSS, Gerstmann-Sträussler-Scheinker disease; hGH, human growth hormone; MBM, meat and bone meal; TME, transmissible mink encephalopathy.

between the host and donor PrP argues that PrP^C directly interacts with PrP^{Sc} in the prion conversion process.

Prion Strains   The existence of prion strains raised the question of how heritable biologic information can be enciphered in a molecule other than nucleic acid. Strains or varieties of prions have been defined by incubation times and the distribution of neuronal vacuolation. Subsequently, the patterns of PrP^{Sc} deposition were found to correlate with vacuolation profiles, and these patterns were also used to characterize strains of prions.

Persuasive evidence that strain-specific information is enciphered in the tertiary structure of PrP^{Sc} comes from transmission of two different inherited human prion diseases to mice expressing a chimeric human-mouse PrP transgene. In FFI, the protease-resistant fragment of PrP^{Sc} after deglycosylation has a molecular mass of 19 kDa, whereas in fCJD and most sporadic prion diseases, it is 21 kDa (Table 375-3). This difference in molecular mass was shown to be due to different sites of proteolytic cleavage at the NH$_2$ termini of the two human PrP^{Sc} molecules, reflecting different tertiary structures. These distinct conformations were not unexpected because the amino acid sequences of the PrPs differ.

Extracts from the brains of patients with FFI transmitted disease into mice expressing a chimeric human-mouse PrP transgene and induced formation of the 19-kDa PrP^{Sc}, whereas fCJD and sCJD produced the 21-kDa PrP^{Sc} in mice expressing the same transgene. On second passage, these differences were maintained, demonstrating that chimeric PrP^{Sc} can exist in two different conformations based on the sizes of the protease-resistant fragments even though the amino acid sequence of PrP^{Sc} is invariant.

This analysis was extended when patients with sporadic fatal insomnia (sFI) were identified. Although they did not carry a *PrP* gene mutation, the clinical and pathologic phenotype was indistinguishable from that of patients with FFI. Furthermore, 19-kDa PrP^{Sc} was found in their brains, and on passage of prion disease to mice expressing a

FIGURE 375-2   Prion protein isoforms. *A.* Western immunoblot of brain homogenates from uninfected (lanes 1 and 2) and prion-infected (lanes 3 and 4) Syrian hamsters. Samples in lanes 2 and 4 were digested with proteinase K. PrP^C in lanes 2 and 4 was completely hydrolyzed under these conditions, whereas in PrP^{Sc} (lane 4), approximately 67 amino acids were digested from the NH$_2$-terminus to generate PrP 27–30. The blot was developed with anti-PrP polyclonal rabbit antiserum. Molecular size markers (*left*) are in kilodaltons. *B.* Bar diagram of Syrian hamster PrP, which consists of 254 amino acids. After processing of the NH$_2$ and COOH termini, both PrP^C and PrP^{Sc} consist of 209 residues. After limited proteolysis, the NH$_2$ terminus of PrP^{Sc} is truncated to form PrP 27–30 composed of approximately 142 amino acids. *[Reprinted from Les Prix Nobel T. Frängsmyr (ed), Stockholm, Norstedts Tryckeri, 1998, pp 268–323, with permission.]*

chimeric human-mouse PrP transgene, PrP^{Sc} was also found. These findings indicate that the disease phenotype is dictated by the conformation of PrP^{Sc} and not the amino acid sequence. PrP^{Sc} acts as a template for the conversion of PrP^C into nascent PrP^{Sc}.

SPORADIC AND INHERITED PRION DISEASES

Initiation of sporadic disease may hypothetically follow from a somatic mutation and thus follow a path similar to that for germline mutations in inherited disease. In this situation, the mutant PrP^{Sc} must be capable of targeting wild type PrP^C, a process known to be possible for some mutations but less likely for others. Alternatively, the activation barrier separating wild type PrP^C from PrP^{Sc} could be crossed on rare occasions when viewed in the context of a population. Most individuals would be spared, while presentations in the elderly with an incidence of ~1 per million would be seen.

Twenty different mutations resulting in nonconservative substitutions in the human *PrP* gene have, to date, been found to segregate with inherited human prion diseases. Missense mutations and expansions in the octapeptide repeat region of the gene are responsible for familial forms of prion disease. Five different mutations of the *PrP* gene have been linked genetically to heritable prion disease.

Although phenotypes may vary dramatically within families, specific phenotypes tend to associate with certain mutations. A clinical phenotype indistinguishable from typical sporadic CJD is usually seen with substitutions at codons 180, 183, 200, 208, 210, and 232. Substitutions at codons 102, 105, 117, 198, and 217 are associated with the GSS variant of prion disease. The normal human PrP sequence contains five repeats of an eight or nine peptide sequence. Insertions from two to nine extra octapeptide repeats are frequently associated with variable phenotypes ranging from a condition indistinguishable from sporadic CJD to a slowly progressive dementing illness of many years duration. A mutation at codon 178 resulting in substitution of asparagine for aspartate produces FFI if a methionine is encoded at the polymorphic 129 residue on the same allele. Typical CJD is seen if a valine is encoded at position 129 of the same allele.

Human *PrP* Gene Polymorphisms Polymorphisms influence the susceptibility to sporadic, inherited, and infectious forms of prion disease. The methionine/valine polymorphism at position 129 not only modulates the age of onset of some inherited prion diseases but also determines the clinical phenotype. The influence of the codon 129 polymorphism iatrogenic and sporadic forms of prion disease has also been documented. The finding that homozygosity at codon 129 predisposes to sCJD supports a model of prion production that favors PrP interactions between homologous proteins.

Substitution of the basic residue lysine at position 219 produced dominant negative inhibition of prion replication in neuroblastoma cells. A lysine at 219 has been found in 12% of the Japanese population, and this group seems to be resistant to prion disease. Dominant negative inhibition of prion replication was also found with substitution of the basic residue arginine at position 171; sheep with arginine are resistant to scrapie.

INFECTIOUS PRION DISEASES

IATROGENIC CJD Accidental transmission of CJD to humans appears to have occurred with corneal transplantation, contaminated electroencephalogram (EEG) electrode implantation, and surgical procedures. Corneas from donors with inapparent CJD have been transplanted to apparently healthy recipients who developed CJD after prolonged incubation periods. The same improperly decontaminated EEG electrodes that caused CJD in two young patients with intractable epilepsy caused CJD in a chimpanzee 18 months after their experimental implantation.

Surgical procedures may have resulted in accidental inoculation of patients with prions during their operations, presumably because some instrument or apparatus in the operating theater became contaminated when a CJD patient underwent surgery. Although the epidemiology of these studies is highly suggestive, no proof for such episodes exists.

Dura Mater Grafts More than 70 cases of CJD after implantation of dura mater grafts have been recorded. All of the grafts were thought to have been acquired from a single manufacturer whose preparative procedures were inadequate to inactivate human prions. One case of CJD occurred after repair of an eardrum perforation with a pericardium graft.

Table 375-3 Distinct Prion Strains Generated in Humans with Inherited Prion Diseases and Transmitted to Transgenic Mice[a]

Inoculum	Host Species	Host PrP Genotype	Incubation Time [days ± SEM] (n/n$_0$)	PrP^{Sc}(kDa)
None	Human	FFI(D178N, M129)		19
FFI	Mouse	Tg(MHu2M)	206 ± 7 (7/7)	19
FFI → Tg(MHu2M)	Mouse	Tg(MHu2M)	136 ± 1 (6/6)	19
None	Human	fCJD(E200K)		21
fCJD	Mouse	Tg(MHu2M)	170 ± 2 (10/10)	21
fCJD → Tg(MHu2M)	Mouse	Tg(MHu2M)	167 ± 3 (15/15)	21

[a] Tg(MHu2M) mice express a chimeric human-mouse PrP gene.
NOTE: Clinicopathologic phenotype is determined by the conformation of PrP^{Sc} in accord with the results of the transmission of human prions from patients with FFI to transgenic mice.

Human Growth Hormone and Pituitary Gonadotropin Therapy The possibility of transmission of CJD from contaminated human growth hormone (hGH) preparations derived from human pituitaries has been raised by the occurrence of fatal cerebellar disorders with dementia in >100 patients ranging in age from 10 to 41 years. These patients received injections of hGH every 2 to 4 days for 4 to 12 years. If it is assumed that these patients developed CJD from injections of prion-contaminated hGH preparations, the possible incubation periods range from 4 to 30 years. Even though several investigations argue for the efficacy of inactivating prions in hGH fractions prepared from human pituitaries with 6 *M* urea, it seems doubtful that such protocols will be used for purifying hGH because recombinant hGH is available. Four cases of CJD have occurred in women receiving human pituitary gonadotropin.

NEW VARIANT CJD The restricted geographic occurrence and chronology of nvCJD have raised the possibility that BSE prions have been transmitted to humans. Approximately 70 cases of nvCJD have been recorded, and the fact that the incidence has remained relatively constant has made establishing the origin of nvCJD difficult. No set of dietary habits distinguishes patients with nvCJD from apparently healthy individuals. Moreover, there is no explanation for the predilection of nvCJD for teenagers and young adults. Epidemiologic studies over the past three decades have failed to find evidence for transmission of sheep prions to humans. Attempts to predict the future number of cases of nvCJD on the basis of possible exposure to bovine prions before the offal ban in 1998 that prevented further feeding of meat and bone meal (MBM) to cattle have been uninformative because so few cases of nvCJD have occurred. Are we at the beginning of a human prion disease epidemic in Great Britain similar to those seen for BSE and kuru, or will the number of nvCJD cases remain small as seen with iCJD caused by cadaveric hGH?

It is possible that a particular conformation of bovine PrP^{Sc} was selected for heat resistance during the rendering process and was then reselected multiple times as cattle infected by ingesting prion-contaminated MBM were slaughtered and their offal rendered into more MBM. Recent studies of PrP^{Sc} from brains of patients who died of nvCJD show a pattern of PrP glycoforms different from those found for sCJD or iCJD. But the usefulness of measuring PrP glycoforms is questionable when trying to relate BSE to nvCJD because PrP^{Sc} is formed after the protein is glycosylated and enzymatic deglycosylation of PrP^{Sc} requires denaturation.

The most compelling evidence that nvCJD comes from BSE prions was obtained from experiments in mice expressing the bovine PrP transgene. Both BSE and nvCJD prions were efficiently transmitted to these transgenic mice. In contrast to sporadic CJD prions, nvCJD did not transmit disease efficiently to mice expressing a chimeric human-mouse PrP transgene. Earlier studies with nontransgenic mice suggested that nvCJD and BSE might be derived from the same source because both sources of inocula transmitted disease with similar but very long incubation periods.

NEUROPATHOLOGY Frequently, the brains of patients with CJD have no recognizable abnormalities on gross examination. Patients who survive for several years have variable degrees of cerebral atrophy.

On light microscopy, the pathologic hallmarks of CJD are spongiform degeneration and astrogliosis. The lack of an inflammatory response in CJD and other prion diseases is an important pathologic feature of these degenerative disorders. Spongiform degeneration is characterized by many 1- to 5-μm vacuoles in the neuropil between nerve cell bodies. Generally, the spongiform changes occur in the cerebral cortex, putamen, caudate nucleus, thalamus, and molecular layer of the cerebellum. Astrocytic gliosis is a constant but nonspecific feature of prion diseases. Widespread proliferation of fibrous astrocytes is found throughout the gray matter of brains infected with CJD prions. Astrocytic processes filled with glial filaments form extensive networks.

Amyloid plaques have been found in ~10% of CJD cases. Purified CJD prions from humans and animals exhibit the ultrastructural and histochemical characteristics of amyloid when treated with detergents during limited proteolysis. In first passage from some human Japanese CJD cases, amyloid plaques have been found in mouse brains. These plaques stain with antisera raised against PrP.

The amyloid plaques of GSS are morphologically distinct from those seen in kuru or scrapie. GSS plaques consist of a central dense core of amyloid surrounded by smaller globules of amyloid. Ultrastructurally, they consist of a radiating fibrillar network of amyloid fibrils with scant or no neuritic degeneration. The plaques can be distributed throughout the brain but are most frequently found in the cerebellum. They are often located adjacent to blood vessels. Congophilic angiopathy has been noted in some cases of GSS.

In nvCJD, a characteristic feature is the presence of "florid plaques." These are composed of a central core of PrP amyloid surrounded by vacuoles in a pattern suggesting petals on a flower.

CLINICAL FEATURES   Nonspecific prodromal symptoms occur in about a third of patients with CJD and may include fatigue, sleep disturbance, weight loss, headache, malaise, and ill-defined pain. Most patients with CJD present with deficits in higher cortical function. These deficits virtually always progress over weeks or months to a state of profound dementia characterized by memory loss, impaired judgment, and a decline in virtually all aspects of intellectual function. A few patients present with either visual impairment or cerebellar gait and coordination deficits. Frequently, the cerebellar deficits are rapidly followed by progressive dementia. Visual problems often begin with blurred vision and diminished acuity, rapidly followed by dementia.

Other symptoms and signs include extrapyramidal dysfunction manifested as rigidity, masklike facies, or choreoathetoid movements; pyramidal signs (usually mild); seizures (usually major motor) and, less commonly, hypesthesia; supranuclear gaze palsy; optic atrophy; and vegetative signs such as changes in weight, temperature, sweating, or menstruation.

Myoclonus   Most patients (~90%) with CJD exhibit myoclonus that appears at various times throughout the illness. Unlike other involuntary movements, myoclonus persists during sleep. Startle myoclonus elicited by loud sounds or bright lights is frequent. It is important to stress that myoclonus is neither specific nor confined to CJD. Dementia with myoclonus can also be due to Alzheimer's disease (AD) (Chap. 362), to cryptococcal encephalitis (Chap. 204), or to the myoclonic epilepsy disorder Unverricht-Lundborg disease (Chap. 360).

Clinical Course   In documented cases of accidental transmission of CJD to humans, an incubation period of 1.5 to 2.0 years preceded the development of clinical disease. In other cases, incubation periods of up to 30 years have been suggested. Most patients with CJD live 6 to 12 months after the onset of clinical signs and symptoms, whereas some live for up to 5 years.

DIAGNOSIS   The constellation of dementia, myoclonus, and periodic electrical bursts in an afebrile 60-year-old patient generally indicates CJD. Clinical abnormalities in CJD are confined to the CNS. Fever, elevated sedimentation rate, leukocytosis in blood, or a pleocytosis in cerebrospinal fluid (CSF) should alert the physician to another etiology to explain the patient's CNS dysfunction.

Important variations in the typical course of CJD appear in certain inherited and transmitted forms of the disease. fCJD has an earlier mean age of onset than sCJD. In GSS, ataxia is usually a prominent and presenting feature, with dementia occurring late in the disease course. GSS may present earlier than CJD (mean age, 43 years; range, 24 to 66 years) and is typically more slowly progressive than CJD; death usually occurs within 5 years of onset. FFI is characterized by insomnia and dysautonomia; dementia occurs only in the terminal phase of the illness. Rare sporadic cases have been identified. nvCJD has an unusual clinical course, with a prominent psychiatric prodrome that may include visual hallucinations and early ataxia, while frank dementia usually is a late sign of nvCJD (see below).

DIFFERENTIAL DIAGNOSIS   Many conditions may mimic CJD superficially. AD is occasionally accompanied by myoclonus but is usually distinguished by its protracted course and lack of motor and visual dysfunction.

Intracranial vasculitides (Chap. 317) may produce nearly all of the symptoms and signs associated with CJD, sometimes without systemic abnormalities. Myoclonus is exceptional with cerebral vasculitis, but focal seizures may confuse the picture; furthermore, myoclonus is often absent in the early stages of CJD. Stepwise change in deficits, prominent headache, abnormal cerebrospinal fluid, and focal magnetic resonance imaging (MRI) or angiographic abnormalities all favor vasculitis.

Neurosyphilis (Chap. 172) may present with dementia and myoclonus that progresses in a relatively rapid fashion but is easily distinguished from CJD by CSF findings, as is cryptococcal meningoencephalitis. A diffuse intracranial tumor (gliomatosis cerebri; Chap. 370) may occasionally be confused with CJD. In rare cases of CNS neoplasia, neuroimaging studies are normal and there are no signs of increased intracranial pressure; however, CSF protein is usually elevated. Adult onset leukodystrophies (ceroid lipofuscinosis or Kuf's disease) and myoclonic epilepsy with Lafora bodies (Chap. 360) may be responsible for dementia, myoclonus, and ataxia; but the less acute courses and prominent seizures distinguish them from CJD. A number of diseases that may simulate CJD are easily distinguished by noting the clinical setting in which they occur. These diseases include anoxic encephalopathy, subacute sclerosing panencephalitis, progressive rubella panencephalitis, herpes simplex encephalitis (in immunoincompetent hosts), dialysis dementia, uremia, and portasystemic shunt encephalopathy.

When CJD begins atypically, it may for a short time resemble other disorders such as Parkinson's disease, progressive supranuclear palsy (Chap. 363), or progressive multifocal leukoencephalopathy (Chap. 373). However, this resemblance usually fades early in the course of CJD.

Certain drug intoxications, particularly lithium and bismuth, may produce a syndrome with encephalopathy and myoclonus. The rare condition known as Hashimoto's encephalopathy, which presents with a subacutely progressive encephalopathy and myoclonus with periodic triphasic complexes on the EEG should be excluded in every case of suspected CJD. It is diagnosed by the finding of high titers of antithyroglobulin or antithyroid perioxidase (antimicrosomal) antibodies in the blood, and improves with glucocorticoid therapy. Unlike CJD, fluctuations in severity typically occur in Hashimoto's encephalopathy.

The AIDS dementia complex (Chap. 309) may occasionally imitate CJD in onset, early course, physical signs, computed tomography (CT) findings, and lack of abnormalities on routine CSF studies. The few such patients without manifestations of systemic immunodeficiency (<10%) should be questioned about risk factors and should have serum antibodies to HIV determined. Additionally, more specific CSF tests are likely to be abnormal; in one study, CSF oligoclonal bands were present in six of nine patients, and intra-blood-brain barrier synthesis of IgG specific for HIV was elevated in eight of nine.

LABORATORY TESTS   With the exception of brain biopsy, there are no specific tests for CJD. If the constellation of pathologic changes frequently found in CJD is seen in a brain biopsy, then the diagnosis is reasonably secure (see Neuropathology, above). The rapid and reliable diagnosis of CJD postmortem can be accomplished with antisera to PrP. Numerous western blotting studies have consistently demonstrated PrP immunoreactive proteins that are proteinase K–resistant in the brains of patients with CJD. Because PrP^{Sc} is not uniformly distributed throughout the CNS, the apparent absence of PrP^{Sc} in a limited sample such as a biopsy does not rule out prion disease. A highly sensitive and quantitative immunoassay was developed based on epitopes that are exposed in PrP^C but buried in PrP^{Sc}. Unlike all other immunoassays for PrP^{Sc}, this conformation-dependent immunoassay (CDI) does not require limited proteolysis to hydrolyze PrP^C before measurement of the protease-resistant core of PrP^{Sc} (PrP 27-30).

If the patient has a family history suggestive of inherited CJD, sequencing the *PrP* gene may facilitate the diagnosis. Sometimes, the PrP sequence is helpful for even seemingly nonfamilial cases.

CT may be normal or show cortical atrophy. The MRI scan may show a subtle increased intensity in the basal ganglia with T2 or diffusion weighted imaging, but this finding is neither sensitive nor specific enough to make a diagnosis. CSF is nearly always normal but may show a minimal protein elevation. Although the stress protein 14-3-3 is elevated in the CSF of most patients with CJD, similar elevations of 14-3-3 are found in herpes simplex virus encephalitis, multi-infarct dementia, and stroke. In AD, 14-3-3 is generally not elevated. In the serum of some patients with CJD, the S-100 protein is elevated; but like 14-3-3, this elevation is not specific.

The EEG is often useful in the diagnosis of CJD. During the early phase of CJD, the EEG is usually normal or shows only scattered theta activity. In most advanced cases, repetitive, high voltage, triphasic, and polyphasic sharp discharges are seen, but in many cases their presence is transient. The presence of these stereotyped periodic bursts of <200 ms duration, occurring every 1 to 2 s, makes the diagnosis of CJD very likely. These discharges are frequently but not always symmetric; there may be a one-sided predominance in amplitude. As CJD progresses, normal background rhythms become fragmentary and slower.

CARE OF CJD PATIENTS It is important to stress that CJD is neither a contagious nor a communicable disease, but it is transmissible. Although the risk of accidental inoculation by aerosols is very small, procedures producing aerosols should be performed in certified biosafety cabinets. Biosafety level 2 practices, containment equipment, and facilities are recommended by the Centers for Disease Control and Prevention and the National Institutes of Health. The primary problem in caring for patients with CJD is the inadvertent infection of healthcare workers by needle and stab wounds, whereas the possible transmission of a contagion through the air has never been documented. Electroencephalographic and electromyographic needles should not be reused after studies on patients with CJD have been performed.

There is no reason for pathologists or morgue dieners to resist performing autopsies on patients whose clinical diagnosis was CJD. Standard microbiologic practices outlined here, along with specific recommendations for decontamination, seem to be adequate precautions for the care of patients with CJD and the handling of infected specimens.

DECONTAMINATION OF CJD PRIONS Prions are extremely resistant to common inactivation procedures, and there is some disagreement about the optimal conditions for sterilization. Some investigators recommend treating CJD-contaminated materials once with 1 N NaOH at room temperature, but we believe this procedure may be inadequate for sterilization. Autoclaving at 132°C for 5 h or treatment with 2 N NaOH for several hours is recommended for sterilization of prions. The term "sterilization" implies complete destruction of prions; any residual infectivity can be hazardous.

PREVENTION AND THERAPEUTICS There is no known effective therapy for treating or preventing CJD. With one possible exception, there are no well-documented cases of patients with CJD showing recovery either spontaneously or after therapy.

Several compounds have been demonstrated to eliminate prions from prion-infected cultured cells. A class of compounds known as "dendrimers" seems particularly efficacious in this regard. Several drugs delay the onset of disease in animals inoculated with prions if the drugs are given around the time of the inoculation. The most common scenarios in which one would want to treat humans are either patients showing signs of disease or presymptomatic patients carrying mutations predisposing them to develop prion disease. No treatment has shown any efficacy in animal models of these two scenarios.

Structure-based drug design predicated on dominant negative inhibition of prion formation has produced several promising compounds. Whether this approach or that of enhanced clearance of misfolded proteins will provide general methods for developing novel therapeutics for Alzheimer's disease and Parkinson's disease, as well as amyotrophic lateral sclerosis (ALS), remains to be established.

BIBLIOGRAPHY

GAJDUSEK DC: Unconventional viruses and the origin and disappearance of kuru. Science 197:943, 1977

HARRIS DA: *Prions: Molecular and Cellular Biology.* Wymondham, Norfolk, Horizon Scientific Press, 1999

JOHNSON RT, GIBBS CJ JR.: Creutzfeldt-Jakob disease and related transmissible spongiform encephalopathies. N Engl J Med 339:1994, 1998

KIRSCHBAUM WR: *Jakob-Creutzfeldt Disease.* Amsterdam, Elsevier, 1968

PRUSINER SB: Prions. Proc Natl Acad Sci USA 95:13363, 1998

——— (ed): *Prion Biology and Diseases.* Cold Spring Harbor, New York, Cold Spring Harbor Laboratory Press, 1999

SEIPELT M et al: Hashimoto's encephalitis as a differential diagnosis of Creutzfeldt-Jakob disease. J Neurol Neurosurg Psychiatry 66:172, 1999

WILL RG et al: Diagnosis of new variant Creutzfeldt-Jacob disease. Ann Neurol 47:575, 2000

376 *J. Claude Hemphill, M. Flint Beal, Daryl R. Gress*

CRITICAL CARE NEUROLOGY

Advances in the understanding of the pathophysiology of acute nervous system injury and the development of treatments that target these injury mechanisms have led to the growth of critical care neurology as a discipline. Life-threatening neurologic illness may be caused by a primary disorder affecting any region of the neuroaxis or may occur as a consequence of a systemic disorder such as hepatic failure, multisystem organ failure (MSOF), or cardiac arrest (Table 376-1). Critical care neurology focuses on preservation of neurologic tissue and prevention of secondary brain injury caused by ischemia, edema, and elevated intracranial pressure (ICP).

PATHOPHYSIOLOGY **Brain Edema** Swelling, or edema, of brain tissue occurs with many types of brain injury. The two principal types of edema are vasogenic and cytotoxic. *Vasogenic edema* refers to the influx of fluid and solutes into the brain through an incompetent blood-brain barrier (BBB). In the normal cerebral vasculature, endothelial tight junctions associated with astrocytes create an impermeable barrier (the BBB), through which access into the brain interstitium is dependent upon specific transport mechanisms (Chap. 355). The BBB may be compromised in ischemia, trauma, infection, and metabolic derangements. Typically, vasogenic edema develops rapidly following injury. *Cytotoxic edema* refers to cellular swelling. Originally described as a response to exogenous toxins, cellular swelling occurs in a variety of settings including brain ischemia and trauma. Early astrocytic swelling is a hallmark of ischemia.

Brain edema that is clinically significant usually represents a combination of vasogenic and cellular components. Edema can lead to increased ICP as well as tissue shifts and brain displacement from focal

Table 376-1 Neurologic Disorders in Critical Illness

Localization Along Neuroaxis	Syndrome
Central Nervous System	
Brain: Cerebral hemispheres	Global encephalopathy
	Septic
	Organ failure—hepatic, renal
	Medication related
	Sedative/hypnotics/analgesics
	H₂ blockers, antihypertensives
	Drug overdose
	Electrolyte disturbance—hyponatremia; hypoglycemia
	Hypotension/hypoperfusion
	Hypoxia
	Meningitis
	Subarachnoid hemorrhage
	Wernicke's disease
	Seizure—postictal or nonconvulsive status
	Hypertensive encephalopathy
	Hypothyroidism—myxedema
	Focal deficits
	Ischemic stroke
	Tumor
	Abscess, subdural empyema
	Subdural/epidural hematoma
Brainstem	Mass effect and compression
	Ischemic stroke, intraparenchymal hemorrhage
	Hypoxia
Spinal cord	Mass effect and compression
	Disc herniation
	Epidural hematoma
	Ischemia—hypotension/embolic
	Subdural empyema
	Trauma, central cord syndrome
Peripheral nervous system	
Peripheral nerve	
Axonal	Critical illness polyneuropathy
	Possible neuromuscular blocking agent complication
	Metabolic disturbances, uremia—hyperglycemia
	Medication effects—chemotherapeutic, antiretroviral
Demyelinating	Guillian-Barré syndrome
	Chronic inflammatory demyelinating polyneuropathy
Neuromuscular junction	Prolonged effect of neuromuscular blockade
	Medication effects—aminoglycosides
	Myasthenia-gravis, Lambert-Eaton syndrome
Muscle	Septic myopathy
	Cachectic myopathy—with or without disuse atrophy
	Electrolyte disturbances—hypokalemia/hyperkalemia; hypophosphatemia
	Acute quadriplegic myopathy

processes. These tissue shifts can cause injury by mechanical distraction and compression in addition to the ischemia of impaired perfusion consequent to the elevated ICP.

Cerebral Perfusion and Autoregulation Brain tissue requires constant perfusion in order to ensure adequate delivery of substrate, principally oxygen and glucose. The hemodynamic response of the brain has the capacity to preserve perfusion across a wide range of systemic blood pressures. Cerebral perfusion pressure (CPP), defined as the mean systemic arterial pressure (MAP) minus the ICP, provides the driving force for circulation across the capillary beds of the brain. *Autoregulation* refers to the physiologic response whereby cerebral blood flow (CBF) remains relatively constant over a wide range of

blood pressures as a consequence of alterations of cerebrovascular resistance (Fig. 376-1). If systemic blood pressure drops, cerebral perfusion is preserved through vasodilatation of arterioles in the brain; likewise, arteriolar vasoconstriction occurs at high systemic pressures to prevent hyperperfusion. At the extreme limits of MAP or CPP (high or low), flow becomes directly related to perfusion pressure. These autoregulatory changes occur in the microcirculation and are mediated by vessels below the resolution of those seen on angiography. CBF is also strongly influenced by pH and P_{CO_2}. CBF increases with hypercapnia and acidosis and decreases with hypocapnia and alkalosis. This forms the basis for the use of hyperventilation to lower ICP, and this effect on ICP is mediated through a decrease in intracranial blood volume. Cerebral autoregulation is critical to the normal homeostatic functioning of the brain, and this process may be disordered focally and unpredictably in disease states such as traumatic brain injury and severe focal cerebral ischemia.

Cerebrospinal Fluid and Intracranial Pressure The cranial contents consist essentially of brain, cerebrospinal fluid (CSF), and blood. CSF is produced principally in the choroid plexus of each lateral ventricle, exits the brain via the foramina of Luschka and Magendi, and flows over the cortex to be absorbed into the venous system along the superior sagittal sinus. Approximately 150 mL of CSF are contained within the ventricles and surrounding the brain and spinal cord; the cerebral blood volume is also ~150 mL. The bony skull offers excellent protection for the brain but allows little tolerance for additional volume. Significant increases in volume eventually result in increased ICP. Obstruction of CSF outflow, edema of cerebral tissue, or increases in volume from tumor or hematoma may increase ICP. Elevated ICP diminishes cerebral perfusion and can lead to tissue ischemia. Ischemia in turn may lead to vasodilatation via autoregulatory mechanisms designed to restore cerebral perfusion. However, vasodilatation also increases cerebral blood volume, which in turn then increases ICP, lowers CPP, and provokes further ischemia (Fig. 376-2). This vicious cycle is commonly seen in traumatic brain injury, massive intracerebral hemorrhage, and large hemispheric infarcts with significant tissue shift.➔*Excitotoxicity and mechanisms of cell death are discussed in Chap. 355.*

Approach to the Patient

Critically ill patients with severe central nervous system dysfunction require rapid evaluation and intervention in order to limit primary and secondary brain injury. Initial neurologic evaluation should be performed concurrent with stabilization of basic respiratory, cardiac, and hemodynamic parameters. Significant barriers may exist to neurologic assessment in the critical care unit. Endotracheal intubation and the

FIGURE 376-1 Cerebral autoregulation curve (solid line). Cerebral perfusion is constant over a wide range of systemic blood pressure. Perfusion is increased in the setting of hypoxia or hypercarbia. BP, blood pressure; CBF, cerebral blood flow. (*Reprinted with permission from Anesthesiology 43:447, 1975. Copyright 1975, Lippincott Company.*)

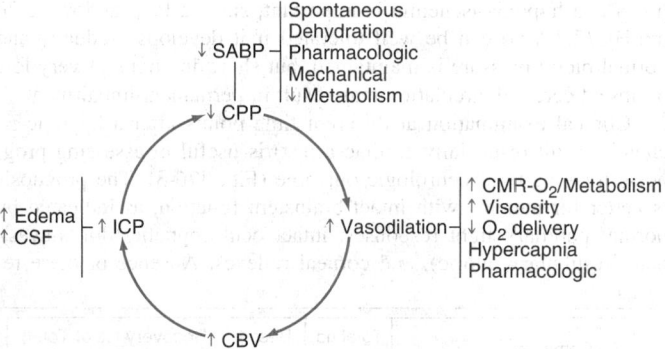

FIGURE 376-2 Ischemia and vasodilatation. Reduced cerebral perfusion pressure (CPP) leads to increased ischemia, vasodilatation, increased intracranial pressure, (ICP) and further reductions in CPP, a cycle leading to further neurologic injury. CBV, cerebral blood volume; CMR, cerebral metabolic rate; CSF, cerebrospinal fluid; SABP, systolic arterial blood pressure. *(From Rosner et al.)*

use of sedative or paralytic agents to facilitate critical care procedures can make clinical assessment challenging.

An impaired level of consciousness is frequent in critically ill patients. The essential first task in assessment is to determine whether the cause of dysfunction is related to a diffuse, usually metabolic, process or whether a focal, usually structural, process is implicated. Examples of diffuse processes include metabolic encephalopathies related to organ failure, drug overdose, or hypoxia-ischemia. Focal processes include ischemic and hemorrhagic stroke and traumatic brain injury, especially with intracranial hematomas. Since these two categories of disorders have fundamentally different causes, treatments, and prognoses, the initial focus is on making this distinction rapidly and accurately. →*The approach to the confused or comatose patient is discussed in Chap. 24; etiologies are listed in Table 24-1.*

Minor focal deficits may be present on the neurologic examination in patients with metabolic encephalopathies. However, the finding of prominent focal signs such as pupillary asymmetry, hemiparesis, gaze palsy, or paraplegia should alert the examiner to the possibility of a structural lesion. All patients with a decreased level of consciousness associated with focal findings should undergo an urgent neuroimaging procedure, as should all patients with coma of unknown etiology. Computed tomographic (CT) scanning is usually the most appropriate initial study because it can be performed quickly in critically ill patients and demonstrates hemorrhage, hydrocephalus, and intracranial tissue shifts well. Magnetic resonance imaging (MRI) may provide more specific information in some situations, such as acute ischemic stroke (diffusion-weighted imaging, DWI) and cerebral venous sinus thrombosis (magnetic resonance venography, MRV). Any suggestion of trauma from the history or examination should alert the examiner to the possibility of cervical spine injury and prompt an imaging evaluation using plain x-rays, MRI, or CT.

Other diagnostic studies are best utilized in specific circumstances, usually when neuroimaging studies fail to reveal a structural lesion and the etiology of the altered mental state remains uncertain. Electroencephalography (EEG) can be important in the evaluation of critically ill patients with severe brain dysfunction. The EEG of encephalopathy typically reveals generalized slowing. One of the most important uses of EEG is to help exclude inapparent seizures, especially nonconvulsive status epilepticus. Untreated continuous or frequently recurrent seizures may cause neuronal injury, making the diagnosis and treatment of seizure crucial in this patient group. Lumbar puncture (LP) may be necessary to exclude infectious processes, and an elevated opening pressure may be an important clue to cerebral venous sinus thrombosis. In patients with coma or profound encephalopathy, it is preferable to perform a neuroimaging study prior to LP. If bacterial meningitis is suspected, an LP may be performed first or antibiotics may be empirically administered before the diagnostic studies are completed. Standard laboratory evaluation of critically ill pa-

tients should include assessment of serum electrolytes (especially sodium and calcium), glucose, renal and hepatic function, complete blood counts, and coagulation. Serum or urine toxicology screens should be performed in patients with encephalopathy of unknown cause. EEG, LP, and other specific laboratory tests are most useful when the mechanism of the altered level of consciousness is uncertain; they are not routinely performed in clear-cut cases of stroke or traumatic brain injury.

Monitoring of ICP can be an important tool in selected patients. Indications for ICP monitoring, as well as specific types of monitors, vary. In general, patients who should be considered for ICP monitoring are those with primary neurologic disorders, such as stroke or traumatic brain injury, who are not moribund and who are at significant risk for secondary brain injury due to elevated ICP and decreased CPP. Such patients include those with severe traumatic brain injury resulting in coma [Glasgow Coma Scale (GCS) score of ≤8 (Table 369-1)]; those with large tissue shifts from supratentorial ischemic or hemorrhagic stroke resulting in decreased consciousness; and those with (or at risk for) hydrocephalus from subarachnoid hemorrhage, intraventricular hemorrhage, or posterior fossa stroke. An additional disorder in which ICP monitoring can add important information is fulminant hepatic failure, in which elevated ICP may be treated with barbiturates or, eventually, liver transplantation. In general, ventriculostomy is preferable to ICP monitoring devices that are placed in brain parenchyma, because ventriculostomy allows CSF drainage as a method of treating elevated ICP. However, parenchymal ICP monitoring is most appropriate for patients with diffuse edema and small ventricles (which may make ventriculostomy placement more difficult) or any degree of coagulopathy (in which ventriculostomy carries a higher risk of hemorrhagic complications).

Treatment of Elevated ICP Elevated ICP may occur in a wide range of disorders including head trauma, intracerebral hemorrhage, subarachnoid hemorrhage with hydrocephalus, and fulminant hepatic failure. Because CSF and blood volume can be redistributed initially, by the time elevated ICP occurs intracranial compliance is severely impaired. At this point, small changes in the volume of CSF, intravascular blood, edema, or a mass lesion may result in significant changes in ICP. Elevated ICP then diminishes cerebral perfusion. This is a fundamental mechanism of secondary ischemic brain injury and constitutes an emergency that requires immediate attention. Specific thresholds of ICP vary, but in general, ICP should be maintained at <20 mmHg and CPP should be maintained at ≥70 mmHg.

A number of different interventions may lower ICP, and ideally the selection of treatment will be based on the underlying mechanism responsible for the elevated ICP (Table 376-2). For example, in hydrocephalus from subarachnoid hemorrhage, the principal cause of elevated ICP is impairment of CSF drainage. In this setting, ventricular drainage of CSF is likely to be sufficient and most appropriate. In head trauma and stroke, cytotoxic edema may be most responsible, and the use of osmotic diuretics such as mannitol becomes an appropriate early step. As described above, elevated ICP may cause tissue ischemia, and, if cerebral autoregulation is intact, the resulting vasodilatation can lead to a cycle of worsening ischemia. Paradoxically, administration of vasopressor agents to increase mean arterial pressure may actually lower ICP by improving perfusion, thereby allowing autoregulatory vasoconstriction as ischemia is relieved and ultimately decreasing intracranial blood volume.

Early signs of elevated ICP include drowsiness and a diminished level of consciousness. Neuroimaging studies may reveal evidence of edema and mass effect. Hypotonic intravenous fluids should be avoided, and elevation of the head of the bed is recommended. Patients must be carefully observed for risk of aspiration and compromise of the airway as the level of alertness declines. Coma and unilateral pupillary changes are late signs and require immediate intervention. Emergent treatment of elevated ICP is most quickly achieved by intubation and hyperventilation, which causes vasoconstriction and re-

Table 376-2   Stepwise Approach to Treatment
of Elevated Intracranial Pressure (ICP)ᵃ

Insert ICP monitor—ventriculostomy versus parenchymal device
General goals: maintain ICP < 20 mmHg and CPP > 70 mmHg

For ICP > 20–25 mmHg for >5 min:
1. Drain CSF via ventriculostomy (if in place)
2. Elevate head of the bed
3. Osmotherapy—mannitol 25–100 g q4h as needed
   (maintain serum osmolality <320 mOsm/L)
4. Glucocorticoids—dexamethasone 4 mg q6h for vasogenic edema from
   tumor, abscess
   (avoid glucocorticoids in head trauma, ischemic and hemorrhagic
   stroke)
5. Sedation (e.g., morphine, propofol, or midazolam); add neuromuscular
   paralysis if necessary
   (patient will require endotracheal intubation and mechanical ventilation
   at this point, if not before)
6. Hyperventilation—to Pa_{CO_2} 30–35 mmHg
7. Pressor therapy—phenylephrine, dopamine, or norepinephrine to maintain adequate MAP to ensure CPP > 70 mmHg,
   (maintain euvolemia to minimize deleterious systemic effects of pressors)
8. Consider second-tier therapies for refractory elevated ICP
   a. High-dose barbiturate therapy ("pentobarb coma")
   b. Aggressive hyperventilation to Pa_{CO_2} < 30 mmHg
   c. Hemicraniectomy

ᵃ Throughout ICP treatment algorithm, consider repeat head CT to identify mass lesions
amenable to surgical evacuation.
NOTE: CPP, cerebral perfusion pressure; MAP, mean arterial pressure; Pa_{CO_2}, arterial partial pressure of carbon dioxide.

duces cerebral blood volume. Because of the concern of provoking or
worsening cerebral ischemia, hyperventilation is best used for short
periods of time until a more definitive treatment can be instituted.
Furthermore, the effects of continued hyperventilation on ICP are
short-lived, often only for several hours because of the buffering capacity of the cerebral interstitium, and rebound elevated ICP may accompany abrupt discontinuation of hyperventilation. As the level of
consciousness declines to coma, the ability to follow the neurologic
status of the patient by examination deteriorates and measurement of
ICP must be considered. If a ventriculostomy device is in place, direct
drainage of CSF to reduce ICP is possible. Finally, high-dose barbiturates or hypothermia are sometimes used for refractory elevated ICP,
although these have significant side effects and have not been shown
to improve outcome.

CRITICAL CARE DISORDERS OF THE CENTRAL NERVOUS SYSTEM ASSOCIATED WITH SYSTEMIC DISEASE

HYPOXIC-ISCHEMIC ENCEPHALOPATHY   Hypoxic-
ischemic encephalopathy occurs from lack of delivery of oxygen to
the brain because of hypotension or respiratory failure. The most common causes are myocardial infarction, cardiac arrest, shock, asphyxiation, paralysis of respiration, and carbon monoxide or cyanide poisoning. In some circumstances, hypoxia may predominate. Carbon
monoxide and cyanide poisoning are termed *histotoxic hypoxia* since
they cause a direct impairment of the respiratory chain.

Clinical Manifestations   Mild degrees of pure hypoxia, such as
occur at high altitudes, cause impaired judgment, inattentiveness, motor incoordination, and, at times, euphoria. However, with hypoxia-
ischemia, such as occurs with circulatory arrest, consciousness is lost
within seconds. If circulation is restored within 3 to 5 min, full recovery may occur, but if hypoxia-ischemia lasts beyond 3 to 5 min, some
degree of permanent cerebral damage is the rule. Except in extreme
cases, it may be difficult to judge the precise degree of hypoxia-ischemia, and some patients make a relatively full recovery after even 8 to
10 min of global cerebral ischemia. The distinction between pure hy-

poxia and hypoxia-ischemia is important, since a Pa_{O_2} as low as 20
mmHg (2.7 kPa) can be well tolerated if it develops gradually and
normal blood pressure is maintained, but short durations of very low
or absent cerebral circulation may result in permanent impairment.

Clinical examination at different time points after a hypoxic-ischemic insult (especially cardiac arrest) is useful in assessing prognosis for long-term neurologic outcome (Fig. 376-3). The prognosis
is better for patients with intact brainstem function, as indicated by
normal pupillary light responses, intact oculocephalic (doll's-eyes),
oculovestibular (caloric), and corneal reflexes. Absence of these re-

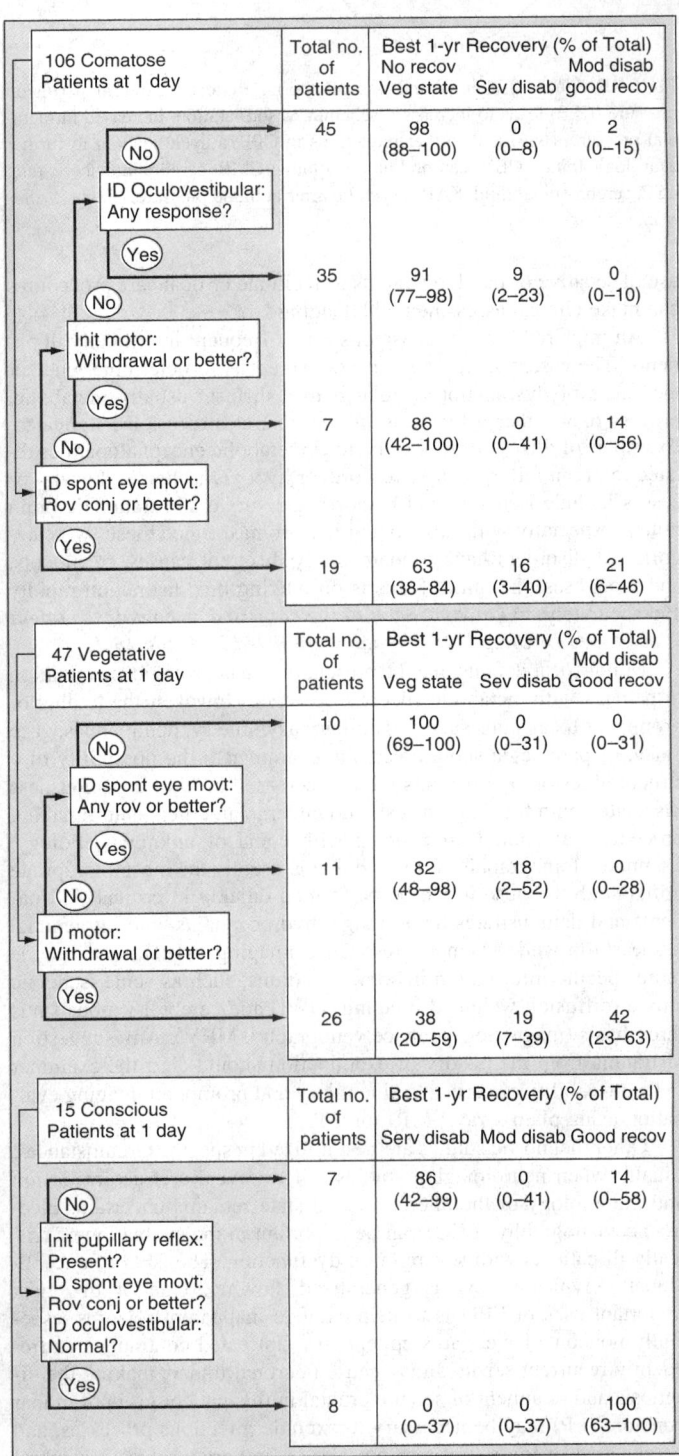

FIGURE 376-3   Clinical examination at day 1 provides useful prognostic
information in hypoxic-ischemic encephalopathy. Numbers in parentheses represent 95% confidence intervals. Recov, recovery; veg, vegetative; sev, severe;
mod, moderate; spont eye movt, spontaneous eye movement; rov conj, roving
conjugate. (*From Levy et al.*)

flexes and the presence of persistently dilated pupils that do not react
to light are grave prognostic signs. A uniformly dismal prognosis from
hypoxic-ischemic coma is conveyed by the clinical findings of absence
of pupillary light reflex or absence of a motor response to pain on day
3 following the injury. Electrophysiologically, the finding of bilateral
absence of the early cortical somatosensory evoked response (SSEPs)
in the first week also conveys a poor prognosis. Long-term consequences of hypoxic-ischemic encephalopathy include persistent coma
or vegetative state (Chap. 24), dementia, visual agnosia (Chap. 25),
parkinsonism, choreoathetosis, cerebellar ataxia, myoclonus, seizures,
and an amnestic state, which may be a consequence of selective damage to the hippocampus (Chap. 26).

Pathologic Findings   Principal histologic findings are extensive
multifocal or diffuse laminar cortical necrosis (Fig. 376-4), with almost invariable involvement of the hippocampus. The hippocampal
CA1 neurons are vulnerable to even brief episodes of hypoxia-ischemia, perhaps explaining why selective persistent memory deficits may
occur after brief cardiac arrest. Scattered small areas of infarction or
neuronal loss may be present in the basal ganglia, hypothalamus, or
brainstem. In some cases, extensive bilateral thalamic scarring may
affect thalamic and extrathalamic pathways that mediate arousal, and
this has been suggested as one pathologic explanation for the persistent
vegetative state. A specific form of hypoxic-ischemic encephalopathy,
so-called watershed infarcts, occurs at the distal territories between the
major cerebral arteries and can cause cognitive deficits, including visual agnosia, and weakness that is greater in proximal than in distal
muscle groups.

Diagnosis   Diagnosis is based upon the history of a hypoxic-
ischemic event such as cardiac arrest. Blood pressure <70 mmHg
systolic or Pa_{O_2} < 40 mmHg is usually necessary, although both absolute levels as well as duration of exposure are important determinants of cellular injury. Occasionally the clinical and radiographic features of a hypoxic-ischemic syndrome are seen without documented
profound hypotension or hypoxia. Carbon monoxide intoxication can
be confirmed by measurement of carboxyhemoglobin and is suggested
by a cherry red color of the skin.

| R_X | **TREATMENT**   Treatment should be directed at restoration of |

TREATMENT   Treatment should be directed at restoration of
normal cardiorespiratory function. This includes securing a clear
airway, ensuring adequate oxygenation and ventilation, and restoring
cerebral perfusion, whether by cardiopulmonary resuscitation, fluid,
pressors, or cardiac pacing. Hypothermia and neuroprotective agents
that target different aspects of the cell injury cascade are experimental
approaches that have not yet been shown to have clinical value.

FIGURE 376-4   Cortical laminar necrosis in hypoxic-ischemic encephalopathy. T1-weighted postcontrast magnetic resonance image shows cortical enhancement in a watershed distribution consistent with laminar necrosis.

Severe carbon monoxide intoxication may be treated with hyperbaric oxygen. Anticonvulsants may be needed to control seizures, although these are not usually given prophylactically. Posthypoxic
myoclonus may respond to oral administration of clonazepam at doses
of 1.5 to 10 mg daily or valproate at doses of 300 mg to 1200 mg
daily in divided doses. Myoclonic status epilepticus after a severe hypoxic-ischemic insult portends a universally poor prognosis, even if
seizures are controlled.

DELAYED POSTANOXIC ENCEPHALOPATHY   De-
layed postanoxic encephalopathy is an uncommon phenomenon in
which patients appear to make an initial recovery from hypoxic-ischemic insult but then develop a relapse characterized by apathy, confusion, and agitation. Progressive neurologic deficits may include shuffling gait, diffuse rigidity and spasticity, persistent parkinsonism or
myoclonus, and, on occasion, coma and death after 1 to 2 weeks.
Widespread cerebral demyelination may be present.

Carbon monoxide and cyanide intoxication can also cause a delayed encephalopathy. Little clinical impairment is evident when the
patient first regains consciousness, but a parkinsonian syndrome characterized by akinesia and rigidity without tremor may develop. Symptoms can worsen over months, accompanied by increasing evidence
of damage in the basal ganglia as seen on both CT and MRI.

METABOLIC ENCEPHALOPATHIES   Altered mental
states, variously described as confusion, delirium, disorientation, and
encephalopathy, are present in many patients with severe illness in an
intensive care unit (ICU). Older patients are particularly vulnerable to
delirium, a confusional state characterized by disordered perception,
frequent hallucinations, delusions, and sleep disturbance. This is often
attributed to medication effects, sleep deprivation, pain, and anxiety.
The term *ICU psychosis* has been used to describe a mental state
with profound agitation occurring in this setting. The presence of
family members in the ICU may help to calm and orient agitated patients, and in severe cases, low doses of neuroleptics (e.g., haloperidol
0.5 to 1 mg) can be useful. Ultimately, the psychosis resolves with
improvement in the underlying illness and a return to familiar
surroundings.

In the ICU setting, several metabolic causes of an altered level of
consciousness predominate. Hypercarbic encephalopathy can present
with headache, confusion, stupor, or coma. Hypoventilation syndrome
occurs most frequently in patients with a history of chronic CO_2 retention who are receiving oxygen therapy for emphysema or chronic
pulmonary disease (Chap. 263). The elevated Pa_{CO_2} leading to CO_2
narcosis may have a direct anesthetic effect, and cerebral vasodilatation from increased Pa_{CO_2} can lead to increased ICP. Hepatic encephalopathy is suggested by asterixis and can occur in chronic liver failure
or acute fulminant hepatic failure. Both hyperglycemia and hypoglycemia can cause encephalopathy, as can hypernatremia and hyponatremia. Confusion, impairment of eye movements, and gait ataxia are
the hallmarks of acute Wernicke's disease (see below).

SEPTIC ENCEPHALOPATHY   Pathogenesis   In patients
with sepsis, the systemic response to infectious agents leads to the
release of circulating inflammatory mediators that appear to contribute
to encephalopathy. Critical illness, in association with the systemic
inflammatory response syndrome (SIRS), can lead to MSOF. This syndrome can occur in the setting of apparent sepsis, severe burns, or
trauma, even without clear identification of an infectious agent. Many
patients with critical illness, sepsis, or SIRS develop encephalopathy
without obvious explanation. This condition is broadly termed *septic
encephalopathy*. While the specific mediators leading to neurologic
dysfunction remain uncertain, it is clear that the encephalopathy is not
simply the result of metabolic derangements of multiorgan failure. The
cytokines tumor necrosis factor α, interleukin (IL) 1, IL-2, and IL-6
are thought to play a role in this syndrome.

Diagnosis   Septic encephalopathy presents clinically as a diffuse
dysfunction of the brain without prominent focal findings. Confusion,

disorientation, agitation, and fluctuations in level of alertness are typical. In more profound cases, especially with hemodynamic compromise, the decrease in level of alertness can be more prominent, at times resulting in coma. Hyperreflexia and frontal release signs such as a grasp or snout reflex (Chap. 356) can be seen. Abnormal movements such as myoclonus, tremor, or asterixis can occur. Septic encephalopathy is quite common, occurring in the majority of patients with sepsis and MSOF. Diagnosis is often difficult because of the multiple potential causes of neurologic dysfunction in critically ill patients, and requires exclusion of structural, metabolic, toxic, and infectious (e.g., meningitis or encephalitis) causes. Although the mortality of patients with septic encephalopathy severe enough to produce coma approaches 50%, this reflects the severity of the underlying critical illness and is not a direct result of the septic encephalopathy. Neurologically, successful treatment of the underlying critical illness almost always results in complete resolution of the encephalopathy, without significant residua.

CENTRAL PONTINE MYELINOLYSIS This disorder typically presents in a devastating fashion as quadriplegia and pseudobulbar palsy. Predisposing factors include severe underlying medical illness or nutritional deficiency; most cases are associated with rapid correction of hyponatremia or with hyperosmolar states. The pathology consists of demyelination without inflammation in the base of the pons, with relative sparing of axons and nerve cells. MRI is useful in establishing the diagnosis (Fig. 376-5) and may also identify partial forms that present as confusion, dysarthria, and/or disturbances of conjugate gaze without quadriplegia. Therapeutic guidelines for the restoration of severe hyponatremia should aim for gradual correction, i.e., by ≤10 mmol/L (10 meq/L) within 24 h and 20 mmol/L (20 meq/L) within 48 h.

WERNICKE'S DISEASE Wernicke's disease is a common and preventable disorder due to a deficiency of thiamine (Chap. 75). In the United States, alcoholics account for most cases, but patients with malnutrition due to hyperemesis, starvation, renal dialysis, cancer, or AIDS are also at risk. The characteristic clinical triad is that of ophthalmoplegia, ataxia, and global confusion. However, only one-third of patients with acute Wernicke's disease present with the classic clinical triad. Most patients are profoundly disoriented, indifferent, and inattentive, although rarely they have an agitated delirium related to ethanol withdrawal. If the disease is not treated, stupor, coma, and death may ensue. Ocular motor abnormalities include horizontal nystagmus on lateral gaze, lateral rectus palsy (usually bilateral), conjugate gaze palsies, and rarely ptosis. Gait ataxia probably results from a combination of polyneuropathy, cerebellar involvement, and vestibular paresis. The pupils are usually spared, but they may become miotic with advanced disease.

Wernicke's disease is usually associated with other manifestations of nutritional disease, such as polyneuropathy. Rarely, amblyopia or

FIGURE 376-5 Central pontine myelinolysis. Axial T2-weighted magnetic resonance scan through the pons reveals a symmetric area of abnormal high signal intensity within the basis pontis (*arrows*).

FIGURE 376-6 Wernicke's disease. Coronal T1-weighted postcontrast magnetic resonance image reveals abnormal enhancement of the mammillary bodies (*arrows*), typical of acute Wernicke's encephalopathy.

spinal spastic ataxia occurs. Tachycardia and postural hypotension may be related to impaired function of the autonomic nervous system or to the coexistence of cardiovascular beriberi. Patients who recover show improvement in ocular palsies within hours after the administration of thiamine, but horizontal nystagmus may persist. Ataxia improves more slowly than the ocular motor abnormalities. Approximately half recover incompletely and are left with a slow, shuffling, wide-based gait and an inability to tandem walk. Apathy, drowsiness, and confusion improve more gradually. As these symptoms recede, an amnestic state with impairment in recent memory and learning may become more apparent (*Korsakoff's psychosis*). Korsakoff's psychosis is frequently persistent; the residual mental state is characterized by gaps in memory, confabulation, and disordered temporal sequencing.

Pathology Lesions in the periventricular regions of the diencephalon, midbrain, and brainstem as well as the superior vermis of the cerebellum consist of symmetric discoloration of structures surrounding the third ventricle, aqueduct, and fourth ventricle, with petechial hemorrhages in occasional acute cases and atrophy of the mamillary bodies in most chronic cases. There is frequently endothelial proliferation, demyelination, and some neuronal loss. These changes may be detected by MRI scanning (Fig. 376-6). The amnestic defect is related to lesions in the dorsal medial nuclei of the thalamus.

Pathogenesis Thiamine is a cofactor of several enzymes, including transketolase, pyruvate dehydrogenase, and α-ketoglutarate dehydrogenase. Thiamine deficiency produces a diffuse decrease in cerebral glucose utilization and results in mitochondrial damage. Glutamate accumulates owing to impairment of α-ketoglutarate dehydrogenase activity and, in combination with the energy deficiency, may result in excitotoxic cell damage.

℞ TREATMENT Wernicke's disease is a medical emergency and requires immediate administration of thiamine, in a dose of 50 mg either intravenously or intramuscularly. The dose should be given daily until the patient resumes a normal diet and should be begun prior to treatment with intravenous glucose solutions. Glucose infusions may precipitate Wernicke's disease in a previously unaffected patient or cause a rapid worsening of an early form of the disease. For this reason, thiamine should be administered to all alcoholic patients requiring parenteral glucose.

CRITICAL CARE DISORDERS OF THE PERIPHERAL NERVOUS SYSTEM ASSOCIATED WITH SYSTEMIC DISEASE

Critical illness with disorders of the peripheral nervous system (PNS) arises in two contexts: (1) primary neurologic diseases that require critical care interventions such as intubation and mechanical ventilation, and (2) secondary PNS manifestations of systemic critical illness, often involving MSOF. The former include acute polyneuropathies such as Guillain-Barré syndrome (Chap. 378), neuromuscular junction disorders including myasthenia gravis (Chap. 380) and botulism (Chap. 144), and primary muscle disorders such as polymyositis (Chap. 382). The latter result either from the systemic disease itself or as a consequence of interventions.

General principles of respiratory evaluation in patients with PNS involvement, regardless of cause, include assessment of pulmonary mechanics, such as maximal inspiratory force (MIF) and vital capacity (VC), and evaluation of strength of bulbar muscles. Regardless of the cause of weakness, endotracheal intubation should be considered when the MIF falls to <-25 cmH$_2$O or the VC is <1 L. Also, patients with severe palatal weakness may require endotracheal intubation in order to prevent acute upper airway obstruction or recurrent aspiration. Arterial blood gases and percutaneous oxygen saturation are used to follow patients with potential respiratory compromise from PNS dysfunction; however, intubation and mechanical ventilation should be undertaken long before oxygen saturation drops or CO$_2$ retention develops from hypoventilation. →*Principles of mechanical ventilation are discussed in Chap. 266.*

NEUROPATHY   While encephalopathy may be the most obvious neurologic dysfunction in critically ill patients, dysfunction of the PNS is also quite common. It is typically present in patients with prolonged critical illnesses lasting several weeks and involving sepsis; clinical suspicion is aroused when there is failure to wean from mechanical ventilation despite improvement of the underlying sepsis and critical illness. *Critical illness polyneuropathy* refers to the most common PNS complication related to critical illness; it is seen in the setting of prolonged critical illness, sepsis, and MSOF. Neurologic findings include diffuse weakness, decreased reflexes, and distal sensory loss. Electrophysiologic studies demonstrate a diffuse, symmetric, distal axonal sensorimotor neuropathy, and pathologic studies have confirmed axonal degeneration. The precise mechanism of critical illness polyneuropathy remains unclear, but circulating factors such as cytokines, which are associated with sepsis and SIRS, are thought to play a role. It has been reported that up to 70% of patients with the sepsis syndrome have some degree of neuropathy, although far fewer have a clinical syndrome profound enough to cause severe respiratory muscle weakness requiring prolonged mechanical ventilation or resulting in failure to wean. Treatment is supportive, with specific intervention directed at treating the underlying illness. While spontaneous recovery is usually seen, the time course may extend over weeks to months and necessitate long-term ventilatory support and care even after the underlying critical illness has resolved.

DISORDERS OF NEUROMUSCULAR TRANSMISSION

A defect in neuromuscular transmission may be a source of weakness in critically ill patients. Myasthenia gravis (Chap. 380) may be a consideration; however, persistent weakness secondary to impaired neuromuscular junction transmission is almost always due to administration of drugs. A number of medications impair neuromuscular transmission; these include antibiotics, especially aminoglycosides, and beta-blocking agents. In the ICU, the nondepolarizing neuromuscular blocking agents (nd-NMBAs), also known as muscle relaxants, are most commonly responsible. Included in this group of drugs are such agents as pancuronium, vecuronium, rocuronium, and atracurium. They are often used to facilitate mechanical ventilation or other critical care procedures, but with prolonged use persistent neuromuscular blockade may result in weakness even after discontinuation of these agents hours or days earlier. Risk factors for this prolonged action of neuromuscular blocking agents include female sex, metabolic acidosis, and renal failure.

Prolonged neuromuscular blockade does not appear to produce permanent damage to the PNS. Once the offending medications are discontinued, full strength is restored, although this may take days. In general, the lowest dose of neuromuscular blocking agent should be used to achieve the desired result, and, when these agents are used in the ICU, a peripheral nerve stimulator should be used to monitor neuromuscular junction function.

MYOPATHY   Critically ill patients, especially those with sepsis, frequently develop muscle wasting, often in the face of seemingly adequate nutritional support. The assumption has been that this represents a catabolic myopathy brought about as a result of multiple factors, including elevated cortisol and catecholamine release and other circulating factors induced by the SIRS. In this syndrome, known as *cachectic myopathy*, serum creatine kinase levels and electromyography (EMG) are normal. Muscle biopsy shows type II fiber atrophy. Panfascicular muscle fiber necrosis may also occur in the setting of profound sepsis. This so-called *septic myopathy* is characterized clinically by weakness progressing to a profound level over just a few days. There may be associated elevations in serum creatine kinase and urine myoglobin. Both EMG and muscle biopsy may be normal initially but eventually show abnormal spontaneous activity and panfascicular necrosis with an accompanying inflammatory reaction.

Acute quadriplegic myopathy describes a clinical syndrome of severe weakness seen in the setting of glucocorticoid and nd-NMBA use. The most frequent scenario in which this is encountered is the asthmatic patient who requires high-dose glucocorticoids and nd-NMBA to facilitate mechanical ventilation. This muscle disorder is not due to prolonged action of nd-NMBAs at the neuromuscular junction but, rather, is an actual myopathy with muscle damage; it has occasionally been described with high-dose glucocorticoid use alone. Clinically this syndrome is most often recognized when a patient fails to wean from mechanical ventilation despite resolution of the primary pulmonary process. Pathologically, there may be vacuolar changes in both type I and type II muscle fibers with evidence of regeneration. Acute quadriplegic myopathy has a good prognosis. If patients survive their underlying critical illness, the myopathy invariably improves and patients usually return to normal. However, because this syndrome is a result of true muscle damage, not just prolonged blockade at the neuromuscular junction, this process may take weeks or months, and tracheostomy with prolonged ventilatory support may be necessary. At present, it is unclear how to prevent this myopathic complication, except by avoiding use of nd-NMBAs, a strategy not always possible. Monitoring with a peripheral nerve stimulator can help to avoid the overuse of these agents. However, this is more likely to prevent the complication of prolonged neuromuscular junction blockade than it is to prevent this myopathy.

BIBLIOGRAPHY

BEAL AL, CERRA FB: Multiple organ failure syndrome in the 1990s. Systemic inflammatory response and organ dysfunction. JAMA 271:226, 1994

BOLTON CF et al: The neurological complications of sepsis. Ann Neurol 33:94, 1993

HIRANO M et al: Acute quadriplegic myopathy: A complication of treatment with steroids, nondepolarizing blocking agents, or both. Neurology 42:2082, 1992

KIMELBERG HK: Current concepts of brain edema. Review of laboratory investigations. J Neurosurg 83:1051, 1995

LARSSON L et al: Acute quadriplegia and loss of muscle myosin in patients treated with nondepolarizing neuromuscular blocking agents and corticosteroids: Mechanisms at the cellular and molecular levels. Crit Care Med 28:34, 2000

LAURENO R: Central pontine myelinolysis following rapid correction of hyponatremia. Ann Neurol 13:232, 1983

LEE JM et al: The changing landscape of ischemic brain injury mechanisms. Nature 399:A7, 1999

LEVY DE et al: Predicting outcome from hypoxic-ischemic coma. JAMA 253:1420, 1985

ROPPER AH: Neurological intensive care. Ann Neurol 32:564, 1992

ROSNER MJ et al: Cerebral perfusion pressure: Management protocol and clinical results. J Neurosurg 83:949, 1995

SEGREDO V et al: Persistent paralysis in critically ill patients after long-term administration of vecuronium. N Engl J Med 327:524, 1992

THE MULTI-SOCIETY TASK FORCE ON PVS: Medical aspects of the persistent vegetative state (2). N Engl J Med 330:1572, 1994

VICTOR M et al: *The Wernicke-Korsakoff Syndrome and Related Disorders Due to Alcoholism and Malnutrition.* Philadelphia, Davis, 1989

ZANDBERGEN EG et al: Systematic review of early prediction of poor outcome in anoxic-ischemic coma. Lancet 352:1808, 1998

ZOCHODNE DW et al: Critical illness polyneuropathy. A complication of sepsis and multiple organ failure. Brain 110:819, 1987

377 *Arthur K. Asbury*

APPROACH TO THE PATIENT WITH PERIPHERAL NEUROPATHY

Peripheral neuropathy is a general term indicating peripheral nerve disorders of any cause; the manifestations of neuropathy may be so diverse that it is difficult for the physician to know where to begin and how to proceed.

The clinical and electrodiagnostic (EDX) approach to evaluation and management of a neuropathic disorder is summarized in Fig. 377-1. The EDX approach consists of electrophysiologic examination of nerve and muscle, including nerve conduction studies and electromyography. It is part of the evaluation of any neuropathy and is considered to be an extension of the neurologic examination. Using this scheme, the examiner determines for each patient the tempo, distribution, and severity of the neuropathy and makes a judgment as to whether the problem represents a mononeuropathy, a mononeuropathy multiplex, or a polyneuropathy. Often this distinction is obvious. With the sum of clinical and EDX information in hand, the differential diagnostic possibilities and treatment options are usually narrowed to a manageable number.

MONONEUROPATHY *Mononeuropathy* refers to focal involvement of a single nerve trunk and therefore implies a local cause. Direct trauma, compression, and entrapment are the usual ones. Ulnar

neuropathies, due to lesions either at the ulnar groove or in the cubital tunnel, and median neuropathy due to compression in the carpal tunnel constitute the great majority of mononeuropathies encountered in clinical practice. These are described below, and other common mononeuropathies are listed in Table 377-1. EDX examination is part of the evaluation of mononeuropathies, mainly to judge the nature of the focal lesion (demyelinating or axonal degeneration) and, in severe mononeuropathies, to determine whether any nerve fibers remain in continuity.

In the absence of a history of trauma to the nerve trunk, factors favoring conservative management of a mononeuropathy include sudden onset, no motor deficit, few or no sensory findings (even though pain and sensory symptoms may be present), and no evidence of axonal degeneration by EDX criteria. Factors favoring active measures including surgical intervention are chronicity and worsening neurologic deficit on examination, particularly if motor and EDX evidence suggests that the lesion has produced a degree of wallerian degeneration.

Ulnar Neuropathy Complete ulnar paralysis results in a characteristic claw-hand deformity owing to wasting and weakness of many of the small hand muscles and hyperextension of the fingers at the metacarpophalangeal joints and flexion at the interphalangeal joints. The flexion deformity is most pronounced in the fourth and fifth fingers. Sensory loss occurs over the fifth finger, the ulnar aspect of the fourth finger, and the ulnar border of the palm. The superficial location of the nerve at the elbow makes it a common site of pressure palsy. The ulnar nerve may also become entrapped just distal to the

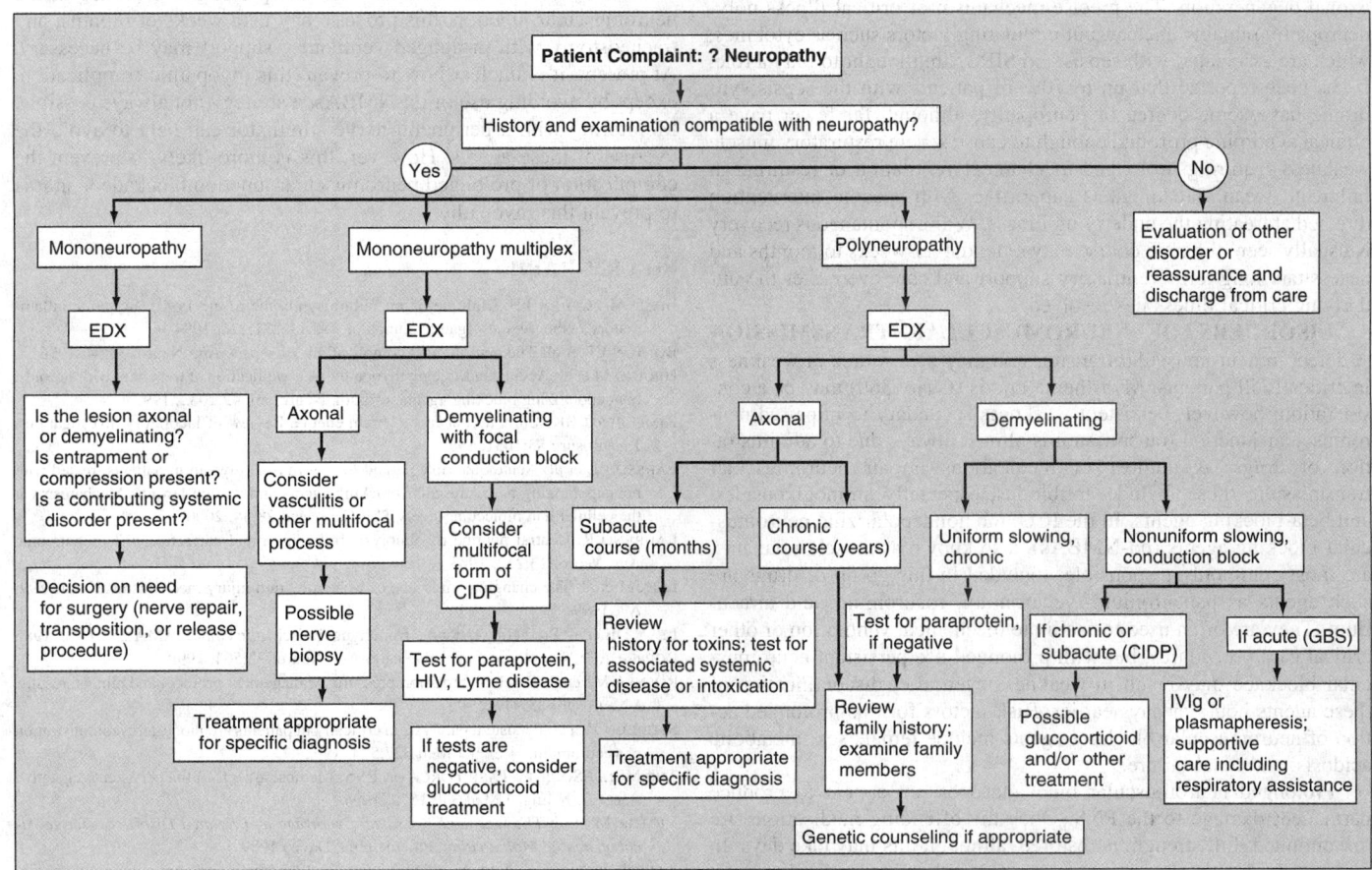

FIGURE 377-1 Approach to the evaluation of peripheral neuropathies. CIDP, chronic inflammatory demyelinating polyradiculoneuropathy; EDX, electrodiagnostic studies; GBS, Guillain-Barré syndrome; IVIg, intravenous immunoglobulin. *(After AK Asbury, in Harrison's Textbook of Internal Medicine, Update IV. New York, McGraw-Hill, 1983.)*

Table 377-1 Common Mononeuropathies

Nerve	Origin (Spinal Segments)	Muscles Innervated	Usual Site of Lesion	Clinical Features	Comments
UPPER EXTREMITY					
Suprascapular	C5, C6	Supraspinatus Infraspinatus	Suprascapular notch of scapula	Weakness of lateral rotation of the humerus	No sensory deficit
Long thoracic	C5–C7	Serratus anterior	Variable	Winging of scapula	No sensory deficit
Axillary	C5, C6	Deltoid, teres minor	Near shoulder joint	Weakness of shoulder abduction; atrophy of shoulder	Sensory deficit similar to C5 dorsal root lesion (See Figs. 23-2 and 23-3)
Radial	C5–T1	Triceps, brachioradialis, wrist, finger, and thumb extensors	Spiral groove of humerus	Wrist drop most obvious, also finger and thumb extensors paralyzed	Saturday night palsy (acute compression) is frequent cause
Posterior interosseous branch	C7, C8	Finger and thumb extensors	Edge of supinator muscle below elbow	Finger drop; wrist relatively spared	No sensory deficit
Ulnar	C8, T1	Ulnar flexor of the wrist, long flexors of 4th and 5th digits, and most intrinsic hand muscles	Ulnar groove at the elbow	Weakness of finger adduction and abduction and thumb adduction (see text); interosseous atrophy, claw-hand	May be acute or insidious; sensory symptoms/signs are distinctive (Figs. 23-2 and 23-3); see also text
			Cubital tunnel	Same as above	Often pain over medial proximal forearm (cubital tunnel)
			Medial base of palm	Intrinsic hand muscles only, interosseous atrophy	No sensory deficit
Median	C6–T1	Abductor pollicis brevis; more proximal muscles include forearm pronator, long finger and thumb flexors	Carpal tunnel	Characteristic sensory symptoms and deficit and inability to make a circle with thumb and index finger	Sensory deficit as per Figs. 23-2 and 23-3 (see text); known as carpal tunnel syndrome
Anterior interosseous branch	C7–T1	Long flexors of thumb and index and middle fingers	Anterior interosseus branch below the elbow	Weakness of pinch; pain in volar forearm	No sensory deficit
LOWER EXTREMITY					
Femoral	L2–L4	Iliopsoas (hip flexor) and quadriceps femoris (knee extensor)	Proximal to inguinal ligament	Knee buckling; absent knee jerk; weak anterior thigh muscles with atrophy	Association with diabetes mellitus; sensory disturbance as per Fig. 23-2
Lateral femoral cutaneous branch	L2, L3	None	Inguinal ligament	Dysesthetic hyperpathia of lateral thigh	Known as meralgia paresthetica
Obturator	L3, L4	Thigh adductors	Intrapelvic or at pubis	Weakness of hip adduction	Sensory deficit on medial thigh
Sciatic	L4–S3	Hamstring muscles, hip abductor, and all muscles below the knee	Near sciatic notch	Severe lower leg and hamstring weakness; flail foot; severe disability	Uncommon except from war wounds
Posterior tibial	L5–S2	Calf muscles (proximally), toe flexors and other intrinsic foot muscles	Tarsal tunnel, near medial malleolus	Pain and numbness of sole, weak toe flexors	Known as tarsal tunnel syndrome (see text)
Peroneal	L4–S1	Dorsiflexors of toes and foot, evertors of foot	At neck of fibula	Foot drop and weakness of foot eversion	Sensory deficit is similar in distribution to L5, S1 sensory roots

elbow in the cubital tunnel formed by the aponeurotic arch linking the two heads of the flexor carpi ulnaris. Also, prolonged pressure on the base of the palm, as occurs with use of hand tools or bicycle riding, may result in damage to the deep palmar branch of the ulnar nerve, causing weakness of the small hand muscles but no sensory loss (Table 377-1).

Carpal Tunnel Syndrome The median nerve in the carpal tunnel lies in close quarters with nine tendons. Entrapment of the nerve at the wrist (*carpal tunnel syndrome*) may be secondary to excessive use of the wrist, tenosynovitis with arthritis, or local infiltration, e.g., by a thickening of connective tissue as in acromegaly or by deposit of amyloid or by one of the mucopolysaccharidoses. Other systemic diseases associated with an increased incidence of carpal tunnel syndrome are hypothyroidism, rheumatoid arthritis, and diabetes mellitus, but underlying diseases account for only a small fraction of all cases. The main symptoms of carpal tunnel syndrome are nocturnal paresthesias of thumb, index, and middle fingers. With worsening, numbness occurs in that distribution, and is demonstrable by pin examination. Eventually weakness and atrophy of the abductor pollicis brevis (thenar eminence) becomes evident. The principal treatment of carpal tunnel syndrome is surgical section of the carpal ligament to relieve entrapment. Incomplete lesions of the median nerve between the axilla and wrist may result in *causalgia* (a particularly severe type of burning pain; Chap. 12; Table 377-1).

Tarsal Tunnel Syndrome The distal tibial nerve, along with several tendons and the posterior tibial artery, lies in the tarsal tunnel just posterior to the medial malleolus. Because of its superficial site, the distal tibial nerve is subject to compression or to direct trauma. Causes include sprain or fracture of the ankle, ill-fitting footwear, posttraumatic fibrosis, cysts, or ganglia adjacent to the nerve, arthritis, and tenosynovitis. Characteristic symptoms are pain in the ankle and the sole of the foot with paresthesias, particularly upon walking. On examination, the tibial nerve trunk in the tarsal tunnel is usually tender to palpation, sensory deficit should be demonstrable on the sole of the foot, and weakness of the toe plantar-flexor muscles may be noted. EDX examination and also nerve block using local anesthetic are useful in establishing the diagnosis. Definitive treatment is extensive surgical decompression of the tibial nerve in the tarsal tunnel. Tarsal tunnel syndrome, in terms of its pathophysiology and management, is similar to carpal tunnel syndrome but is much less common (Table 377-1).

POLYNEUROPATHY   The prototypical picture of polyneuropathy occurs with acquired toxic or metabolic neuropathic states. The first symptoms tend to be sensory and consist of tingling, prickling, burning, or bandlike dysesthesias in the balls of the feet or tips of the toes, or in a general distribution over the soles (Chap. 23). Symptoms and findings are usually symmetric and graded distally. If the polyneuropathy remains mild, objective motor or sensory signs may not be detectable.

With progression, dysesthesias spread up the lower legs. Pansensory loss is usually found over both feet, ankle jerks are lost, and weakness of dorsiflexion of the toes, best demonstrated in the great toe, is present. In some instances, the process begins with weakness in the feet, without preceding sensory symptoms. As worsening occurs, sensory loss moves centripetally in a graded "stocking" fashion, and the patient may complain that the feet have a numb or "wooden" feeling or may say "I feel as though I'm walking on stumps." Patients have difficulty walking on their heels during examination, and their feet may slap while walking. Later, the knee jerk reflex disappears and foot drop becomes more apparent. By the time sensory disturbance has reached the upper shin, dysesthesias are usually noticed in the tips of the fingers. The degree of spontaneous pain varies but is often considerable. Light stimuli to hypesthetic areas, once perceived, may be experienced as extremely uncomfortable (*hyperpathia*). Unsteadiness of gait may be out of proportion to muscle weakness because of proprioceptive loss.

Worsening is more severe in the legs than in the arms and proceeds in a centripetal, symmetrically graded manner with pansensory loss, areflexia, and muscle atrophy; motor weakness is usually greater in the extensor muscles than in corresponding flexor groups. When the sensory disturbance reaches the elbows and mid-thighs, a tent-shaped area of hypesthesia may often be demonstrated on the lower abdomen. This area will grow broader, and its apex will extend rostrally toward the sternum as the neuropathy worsens. By this time, patients generally cannot stand or walk or hold objects in their hands.

Overall, nerve fibers are affected according to axon length, without regard to root or nerve trunk distribution—hence the aptness of the term *stocking-glove* to describe the pattern of sensory deficit. In general, the motor deficit is also graded, distal, and symmetric.

Although *polyneuropathy* connotes a widespread symmetric process, usually distal and graded, polyneuropathies are quite diverse because of the variability of tempo, severity, mix of sensory and motor features, and presence or absence of positive symptoms. For instance, a patient with a subacute, severely dysesthetic sensory polyneuropathy and alopecia who is in the early phases of thallium intoxication bears little similarity to the patient with a 40-year history of insidiously progressive clumsiness of gait whose findings are foot drop, lower leg atrophy, pes cavus, and minimal asymptomatic distal sensory deficit due to a hereditary polyneuropathy (Chap. 379). These two patients fall at opposite ends of the spectrum of polyneuropathy.

The classification of peripheral neuropathies has become increasingly complex as the capacity to discriminate new subgroups and identify new associations with toxins and systemic disorders improves. Further, our grasp of the pathophysiologic basis of the clinical phenomena observed in neuropathy has increased rapidly. But these advances are primarily descriptive; little progress has been made in understanding the fundamental pathogenic events in nervous tissue that eventuate in any of the polyneuropathies.

The important features of each major grouping of polyneuropathies are summarized in Table 377-2, and key aspects of specific polyneuropathies are given in Tables 377-3 to 377-6.

MONONEUROPATHY   MULTIPLEX   (MULTIFOCAL NEUROPATHY)   *Mononeuropathy multiplex* refers to simultaneous or sequential involvement of individual noncontiguous nerve trunks, either partially or completely, evolving over days to years. Since the disease process underlying mononeuropathy multiplex involves peripheral nerves in a multifocal and random fashion, progression of the disease involves a tendency for the neurologic deficit to become less patchy and multifocal and more confluent and symmetric. As a result, some patients present with a distal symmetric neuropathy. Attention to the pattern of early symptoms is therefore important in making the judgment that a particular neuropathy is indeed a mononeuropathy multiplex.

ASSESSMENT AND DIAGNOSIS OF POLYNEUROPATHY AND MONONEUROPATHY MULTIPLEX   Clues to the diagnosis of these neuropathies often lie in unnoticed or forgotten events occurring weeks or months prior to the onset of symptoms. Inquiry should be made about recent viral illnesses; other systemic symptoms; institution of new medications; exposures to solvents, pesticides, or heavy metals; the occurrence of similar symptoms in family members or coworkers; habits concerning alcohol; and the presence of preexisting medical disorders. Patients should be asked if they would feel well if free of their neuropathic symptoms; answers will suggest the presence or absence of an underlying systemic illness.

Table 377-2   Major Types of Polyneuropathy

Type of Polyneuropathy	Evolution	Causes	Comments
Axonal			
Acute	Days to weeks	Porphyria	See Table 377-3; also Chap. 346
		Massive intoxications (arsenic; inhalants)	See Table 377-4
		Guillain-Barré syndrome—axonal form	See Chapter 378
Subacute	Weeks to months	Mostly toxic or metabolic polyneuropathies; see Tables 377-3 and 377-4	Treatment involves eliminating the toxins or treating the associated systemic disorder
Chronic	Months to years	<5 years, consider toxic/metabolic causes; >5 years, consider hereditary basis, also diabetic and dysproteinemic causes	See Tables 377-3 and 377-4; also Chap. 379 on hereditary neuropathy
Demyelinating			
Acute	Days to weeks	Almost all are the common form of Guillain-Barré syndrome; see Chap. 378	Rare possibilities include diphtheritic polyneuritis or buckthorn berry intoxication
Subacute	Weeks to months	Mostly relapsing form of CIDP (see Chap. 378)	Rarely, toxins mentioned above plus aurothioglucose and taxol (see Table 377-3)
Chronic	Months to years	Many possibilities including hereditary; inflammatory-autoimmune; dysproteinemias, other metabolic and toxic neuropathies	See Chaps. 378 and 379; also Tables 377-3 and 377-4

Table 377-3 Polyneuropathy Associated with Systemic Diseases

Systemic Disease (Occurrence)	Axonal[a]			Demyelinating[a]			Sensory vs. Motor[b]	Autonomic[a]	Comment
	Acute	Subacute	Chronic	Acute	Subacute	Chronic			
Diabetes mellitus (common)	−	±	+	−	±	+	S, SM, rarely M	± to +	See Table 377-5
Uremia (sometimes)	±	+	+	−	−	−	SM	±	Controllable with proper dialysis; curable with successful renal transplant
Porphyria (3 types) (rare)	+	±	−	−	−	−	M or SM	± to +	May be proximal > distal and may have atypical proximal sensory deficits
Hypoglycemia (rare)	±	+	±	−	−	−	M	−	Usually with insulinoma; arms often > legs
Vitamin deficiency, excluding B$_{12}$ (sometimes)	−	+	+	−	−	−	SM	±	Involves thiamine, pyridoxine, folate, pantothenic acid, and probably others
Vitamin B$_{12}$ deficiency (sometimes)	−	±	+	−	−	−	S	−	Neuropathy overshadowed by myelopathy
Critical illness (sepsis) (common)	−	+	±	−	−	−	M > S	−	Sepsis patients severely ill
Chronic liver disease (sometimes)	−	−	−	−	−	+	S or SM	−	Usually mild or subclinical
Primary biliary cirrhosis (rare)	−	±	+	−	−	−	S	−	Intraneural xanthomas; dysesthesia
Primary systemic amyloidosis (rare)	−	±	+	−	−	−	SM	+	Also in amyloidosis with myeloma or macroglobulinemia
Hypothyroidism (rare)	−	−	−	−	±	+	S	−	May respond to thyroid replacement
Chronic obstructive lung disease (rare)	−	±	+	−	−	−	S or SM	−	Severe pulmonary insufficiency
Acromegaly (rare)	−	−	+	−	−	−	S	−	Carpal tunnel syndrome also frequent
Malabsorption (sprue, celiac disease) (sometimes)	−	±	+	−	−	−	S or SM	±	Basis for neuropathy unclear; deficiency?
Carcinoma (sensory) (rare)	−	+	+	−	−	−	Pure S	−	Due to ganglionitis mostly small cell lung or breast carcinoma; paraneoplastic
Carcinoma (sensorimotor) (sometimes)	−	+	+	−	−	−	SM	±	Sensorimotor axonal neuropathy; mostly with lung cancer
Carcinoma (late) (common)	−	+	+	−	−	−	S > M	±	Mild, probably related to weight loss and wasting
Carcinoma (demyelinating) (sometimes)	−	−	−	+	+	±	SM	−	Acute or relapsing demyelinating neuropathy
HIV infection (sometimes)	−	±	+	−	−	−	S ≫ M	−	Late stages of AIDS; other neuropathies occur; see text
Lyme disease (sometimes)	−	±	+	−	−	−	S > M	−	Variable picture; see text
Lymphoma, including Hodgkin's (sometimes)	−	+	+	+	+	±	See above	±	Same as with carcinomatous types
Polycythemia vera (rare)	−	±	+	−	−	−	S	−	Also CNS manifestations; often shooting pains in limbs
Multiple myeloma, lytic type (sometimes)	−	±	+	−	−	−	S, M, or SM	±	Symptomatic neuropathy uncommon; subclinical neuropathy frequent
Multiple myeloma, osteosclerotic[c] (sometimes)	−	−	±	−	±	+	SM	−	May show severe slowing of nerve conduction velocity

(continued)

Table 377-3 Polyneuropathy Associated with Systemic Diseases—*(continued)*

Systemic Disease (Occurrence)	Axonal[a]			Demyelinating[a]			Sensory vs. Motor[b]	Autonomic[a]	Comment
	Acute	Subacute	Chronic	Acute	Subacute	Chronic			
Monoclonal gammopathy of undetermined significance (sometimes):									
IgA	−	±	+	−	−	−	SM	−	IgM$_\kappa$ mainly; may bind to myelin-associated glycoprotein (MAG) or other glycoconjugates
IgG	−	±	+	−	−	−	SM	−	
IgM	−	−	±	−	±	+	SM or S	−	
Cryoglobulinemia (rare)	−	±	+	−	−	−	SM	−	May be mononeuropathy multiplex in presentation

[a] +, Usually; ±, sometimes; −, rare, if ever.
[b] S, sensory; M, motor; SM, sensorimotor.
[c] Some cases associated with POEMS syndrome (*p*olyneuropathy, *o*rganomegaly, *e*ndocrinopathy, *M* proteins, and *s*kin changes; see Chap. 339).

How did symptoms first appear? Even with distal polyneuropathies, symptoms may appear in the sole of one foot a few days or a week before the other, but usually the patient will describe a distal graded disturbance that moves evenly and symmetrically in centripetal fashion. Symptoms that first appear in the distribution of individual digital nerves, involving only half of a digit at a time, and then gradually spread and coalesce suggest a multifocal process (mononeuropathy multiplex), as might occur with a systemic vasculitis or cryoglobulinemia.

The evolution of neuropathy ranges from rapid worsening over a few days to an indolent process lasting many years. Polyneuropathies that progress slowly, over more than 5 years, are most likely to be genetically determined, particularly if the major manifestations are distal atrophy and weakness with few or no positive sensory symptoms. Diabetic polyneuropathy and paraproteinemic neuropathies also progress insidiously over 5 to 10 years. Axonal degenerations of toxic or metabolic origin tend to evolve over several weeks to a year or more, and the rate of progression of demyelinating neuropathies is highly variable, ranging from a few days in Guillain-Barré syndrome (GBS; Chap. 378) to many years in others.

Major fluctuations in the course of neuropathy raise two possibilities: (1) relapsing forms of neuropathy and (2) repeated toxic exposures. Slow fluctuation in symptoms taking place over weeks or months (reflecting changes in the activity of neuropathy) should not be confused with day-to-day variation or diurnal undulation of symptoms. The latter are common to all neuropathic disorders. An example is carpal tunnel syndrome, in which dysesthesias may be prominent at night but absent during the day.

Palpation of the nerve trunk to detect enlargement is a frequently forgotten part of the neurologic examination. In mononeuropathy or mononeuropathy multiplex, the entire course of the nerve trunk in question should be explored manually for focal thickening, for the presence of neurofibroma, point tenderness, or Tinel's phenomenon (generation of a tingling sensation in the sensory territory of the nerve by tapping along the course of the nerve trunk); and for pain elicited by stretching of the nerve trunk. In leprous neuritis, fusiform thickening of nerve trunks is frequent, and beading of nerve trunks may be encountered in amyloid polyneuropathy. In genetically determined hypertrophic neuropathies, uniform thickening of all nerve trunks may occur, often to the caliber of a clothesline or larger.

Most neuropathies involve nerve fibers of all sizes, but damage is sometimes restricted to either large or small fibers. In a polyneuropathy affecting mainly small fibers, diminished pinprick and temperature sensation, often with painful, burning dysesthesias, will predominate, along with autonomic dysfunction but with relative sparing of motor power, balance, and tendon jerks. Some cases of amyloid and distal diabetic polyneuropathies fall into this category. In contrast, large-fiber polyneuropathy is characterized by areflexia, sensory ataxia, relatively minor cutaneous sensory deficit, and variable degrees of motor dysfunction, sometimes severe.

For patients with polyneuropathy or mononeuropathy multiplex, standard tests should include a complete blood count and measurement of erythrocyte sedimentation rate, urinalysis, chest x-ray, postprandial blood glucose determination, and serum protein electrophoresis. Further tests are dictated by the combined results of the history and the physical and EDX examination (Fig. 377-1).

Electrodiagnosis EDX examination is a key procedure in all patients with suspected neuropathy. It is generally not possible to make the distinction between axonal and demyelinating disorders by clinical examination alone; here EDX analysis is particularly useful. EDX features of demyelination are slowing of nerve conduction velocity (NCV), dispersion of evoked compound action potentials, conduction block (major decrease in amplitude of muscle compound action potentials on proximal stimulation of the nerve, as compared to distal stimulation), and marked prolongation of distal latencies (Chap. 357). In contrast, axonal neuropathies are characterized by a reduction in amplitude of evoked compound action potentials with relative preservation of NCV. The distinction between a primarily demyelinating neuropathy and an axonal neuropathy is crucial because of the differing approaches to diagnosis and management.

EDX studies also help to determine the presence or absence of a sensory involvement when that is not clear by clinical examination alone. It provides information about the distribution of subclinical findings, thus sharpening the diagnostic focus. Other issues that may be clarified by the electrodiagnostician include:

1. The distinction between disorders primary to nerve and to muscle (neuropathy versus myopathy)
2. The distinction between root or plexus involvement and more distal nerve trunk involvement
3. The distinction between generalized polyneuropathic processes and widespread multifocal nerve trunk involvement
4. The distinction between upper and lower motor neuron weakness
5. The distinction, in a given generalized polyneuropathic process, between primary demyelinating neuropathy and axonal degeneration
6. The assessment, in both primary axonal and demyelinating neuropathies, of features bearing on the nature, activity, and likely prognosis of the neuropathy
7. The assessment, in mononeuropathies, of the site of the lesion and its major effect on nerve fibers, especially the distinction between demyelinating conduction block and wallerian degeneration
8. The characterization of disorders of the neuromuscular junction
9. The identification, often in muscle of normal bulk and strength, of important features such as chronic partial denervation, fasciculations, and myotonia
10. The analysis of cramp, and its distinction from physiologic contracture

Table 377-4 Polyneuropathy Associated with Drugs and Environmental Toxins

	Axonal[a]			Demyelinating[a]			Sensory vs. Motor[b]	Autonomic[a]	CNS[a]	Comment
	Acute	Subacute	Chronic	Acute	Subacute	Chronic				
DRUGS[c]										
Amiodarone (antiarrhythmic)	−	−	+	−	−	+	SM	−	−	Dose-dependent neuropathy, reversible by decreasing dose
Aurothioglucose (antirheumatic)	±	±	−	+	+	−	SM	−	−	Idiosyncratic reaction; ? immune-mediated
Cisplatin (antineoplastic)	−	+	+	−	−	−	S			Severe sensory neuropathy, also ototoxicity; dose-related
Dapsone (dermatologic agent; used, e.g., for leprosy)	−	±	+	−	−	−	M	−	−	Dose-related pure motor neuropathy
Disulfiram (antialcoholism agent)	±	+	+	−	−	−	SM	−	±	Usually occurs after months of treatment
Hydralazine (antihypertensive)	−	±	+	−	−	−	S > M	−	−	A pyridoxine antagonist
Isoniazid	−	±	+	−	−	−	SM	±	−	A pyridoxine antagonist; neurotoxic in slow acetylators
Metronidazole (antiprotozoal)	−	−	±	−	−	−	S or SM	−	+	Dose-related central-peripheral distal axonopathy
Misonidazole (radiosensitizer)	−	±	+	−	−	−	S or SM	−	+	Neurotoxicity is the limiting factor
Nitrofurantoin (urinary antiseptic)	−	±	+	−	−	−	SM	−	−	Generally total dose-related; renal failure enhances toxicity
Nucleoside analogues (ddC, ddI, d4T) (antiretroviral agents)	±	+	+	−	−	−	S ≫ M	−	?	Dose-related; painful
Phenytoin (anticonvulsant)	−	−	+	−	−	−	S > M	−	−	After 20–30 years of phenytoin use
Pyridoxine (vitamin)	−	±	+	−	−	−	S	−	−	Occurs with large intake (>300 mg/d)
Suramin (antineoplastic)	+	+	−	+	+	−	M > S	−	−	Related to serum levels 350 μg/mL or above
Taxol (antineoplastic)	±	+	±	±	+	±	S > M	−	−	Dose-related
Vincristine (antineoplastic)	−	+	+	−	−	−	S > M	−	−	Sensory symptoms common, hands > feet; motor signs ominous; should stop treatment
TOXINS[c]										
Acrylamide (flocculant; grouting agent)	−	±	+	−	−	−	S > M	±	+	Large-fiber neuropathy; sensory ataxia
Arsenic (herbicide; insecticide)	±	+	−	−	−	−	SM	±	±	Skin changes, Mees' lines in nails; painful; systemic effects
Diphtheria toxin	−	−	−	+	+	−	SM	−	−	Clinically very rare; can be confused with GBS

(continued)

Table 377-4 Polyneuropathy Associated with Drugs and Environmental Toxins—*(continued)*

	Axonal[a]			Demyelinating[a]			Sensory vs. Motor[b]	Autonomic[a]	CNS[a]	Comment
	Acute	Subacute	Chronic	Acute	Subacute	Chronic				
γ-Diketone hexa-carbons (solvents)	−	±	+	−	−	+	SM	±	+	Neurofilamentous swelling of axons; these solvents now in restricted use
Inorganic lead	−	−	+	−	−	−	M > S or M	−	±	Selective motor neuropathy with prominent wrist drop
Organophosphates	−	±	+	−	−	−	SM	−	+	Brain and spinal cord also affected, the latter irreversibly
Thallium (rat poison)	−	+	+	−	−	−	SM	−	+	Also alopecia, Mees' lines in nails; painful

[a] +, Usually; ±, sometimes; −, rare, if ever.
[b] S, sensory; M, motor; SM, sensorimotor.
[c] The following drugs and environmental toxins are also neurotoxic, mainly to the peripheral nervous system:

Drugs: Amitriptyline, chloramphenicol, colchicine, ethambutol, nitrous oxide, perhexi-line maleate, sodium cyanate, thalidomide, L-tryptophan.
Environmental toxins: Allyl chloride, buckthorn berry, carbon disulfide, dimethylamino-proprionitrile (DMAPN), ethylene oxide, metallic mercury, methyl bromide, polychlorinated biphenyls, styrene, trichlorethylene, vacor.
NOTE: CNS, central nervous system; GBS, Guillain-Barré syndrome.

If in a particular instance of progressive polyneuropathy of subacute or chronic evolution the EDX findings are those of an axonopathy, a long list of metabolic states and exogenous toxins comes under consideration (Tables 377-3 and 377-4). If the course is protracted over several years, it raises the likelihood of a hereditary neuropathy (Chap. 379); family members must be examined and additional attention given to the family history. If the EDX findings indicate primary demyelination of nerve, the approach is entirely different. The possibilities then include acquired demyelinating neuropathy, thought to be immunologically mediated (Chap. 378), and genetically determined neuropathies, some of which are marked by uniform and drastic slowing of nerve conduction velocities (Chap. 379).

If the clinical features indicate mononeuropathy multiplex, the EDX question is whether the process is primarily axonal or demyelinating. Almost one-third of all adults with the clinical syndrome of mononeuropathy multiplex have a clear-cut picture of a demyelinating disorder, often with foci of persistent conduction block on EDX examination. Multifocal demyelinating neuropathy may represent part of the spectrum of chronic inflammatory demyelinating neuropathy (CIDP), or, if multifocal and only motor, would fit into the related category of multifocal motor neuropathy. →*For further discussion of the management of multifocal motor neuropathy, see Chap. 378.*

The remaining two-thirds of patients with mononeuropathy multiplex have a picture of patchy axonal involvement by EDX examination. Although ischemia should be suspected as the basis of neuropathy in these patients, only about one-half can be shown to have disease of the vasa nervorum, usually vasculitis. Management of those with proven vasculitis of vasa nervorum is often the same as treatment for systemic vasculitis (Chaps. 317 and 378). If the cause of mononeuropathy multiplex remains undiagnosed even on follow-up, management should be conservative. In many patients the disease will stabilize or reverse, at least partially.

Mononeuropathy multiplex syndrome may also be seen as a manifestation of leprosy, sarcoidosis, certain types of amyloidosis, hypereosinophilia syndrome, cryoglobulinemia, neuroAIDs, and multifocal types of diabetic neuropathy.

Nerve Biopsy The sural nerve at the ankle is the preferred site for cutaneous nerve biopsy. There are few indications to employ this invasive technique. The main one is in asymmetric and multifocal neuropathic disorders producing a clinical picture of mononeuropathy multiplex, the basis of which is still unclear after other laboratory investigations are complete. Diagnostic considerations include vasculitis, multifocal demyelinating neuropathies, amyloidosis, leprosy, and occasionally sarcoidosis. Nerve biopsy is also helpful when one or more cutaneous nerves are palpably enlarged. Another clinical application is in establishing the diagnosis in some genetically determined childhood disorders such as metachromatic leukodystrophy, Krabbe's disease, giant axonal neuropathy, and infantile neuroaxonal dystrophy. In all of these recessively inherited diseases, both the central nervous system and the peripheral nervous system are affected.

There is a tendency to carry out sural nerve biopsy in distal symmetric polyneuropathies of subacute or chronic evolution. This practice is discouraged because its yield is low. Nerve biopsy in this situation may be useful as part of an approved research protocol when the biopsy will provide crucial information not otherwise obtainable.

SPECIAL CATEGORIES OF NEUROPATHY Some neuropathies require individual description because of their importance or distinctiveness.

Diabetic Neuropathies The neuropathies of diabetes mellitus are classified in Table 377-5. A limitation of this classification is that most patients do not fit neatly into any single category but instead have overlapping clinical features of several. For instance, many diabetic patients with distal, primarily sensory polyneuropathy can also be shown to have autonomic dysfunction, usually in the form of vasomotor disturbance in the limbs and abnormalities of sweating. Similarly, patients who develop a proximal motor syndrome often have dysautonomic features (including sexual impotence in males) and some degree of distal sensory polyneuropathy. To compound matters, such patients appear at risk of developing a cranial mononeuropathy. Pain is a frequent feature of diabetic neuropathies (Table 377-5) but is variable in incidence and degree.

Table 377-5 Classification of Diabetic Neuropathies

Symmetric
1. Distal, primarily sensory polyneuropathy
   a. Mainly large fibers affected
   b. Mixed[a]
   c. Mainly small fibers affected[a]
2. Autonomic neuropathy
3. Chronically evolving proximal motor neuropathy[a,b]

Asymmetric
1. Acute or subacute proximal motor neuropathy[a,b]
2. Cranial mononeuropathy[b]
3. Truncal neuropathy[a,b]
4. Entrapment neuropathy in the limbs

[a] Often painful.
[b] Recovery, partial or complete, is likely.

Table 377-6 Sensory Neuropathies

| Cause or Association | Course | Nerve Fiber Size Affected | | | Comment |
		Small	Large	Neuronopathy	
TOXINS/DRUGS					
Cisplatin (antineoplastic)	Sub/Chr	+	++	+	Dose-related
Pyridoxine (vitamin, in megadose amounts)	Sub/Chr	+	++	+/−	Dose-related
Taxol (antineoplastic)	Acu/Sub	++	+	−	NGF may be protective
SYSTEMIC DISEASES					
Paraneoplastic	Sub	+	++	++	Most SCLC and breast
Sjögren's syndrome	Sub/Chr	+/−	+	++	Variable presentation
Dysproteinemia (mainly IgM$_\kappa$)	Chr	+	++	−	Demyelinating; may bind to MAG and other myelin glycoproteins
IDIOPATHIC					
Acute sensory neuronopathy	Acu	+/−	++	++	Poor recovery; persistent deficit
Chronic ataxic neuropathy	Chr	+/−	++	Prob.	Gradual progression
HEREDITARY					
Many varieties (see Chap. 379)	Chr	Variable		Some	Progressive

ABBREVIATIONS: ++, most; +, some; ±, occasionally; Prob, probable; Acu, acute; Sub, subacute; Chr, chronic; NGF, nerve growth factor;; MAG, myelin-associated glycoprotein; SCLC, small cell lung carcinoma.

Diabetic neuropathies occur in the setting of long-standing hyperglycemia (decades), whether the diabetes is insulin-dependent or not. By far the most common neuropathies related to diabetes mellitus are the diffuse sensory and autonomic types (categories 1 and 2 under "Symmetric" in Table 377-5). Sensory and autonomic polyneuropathy, chronic and indolent in evolution, may first be noticed in the third to fifth decades in patients with juvenile-onset diabetes but tends to occur after age 50 in patients with adult-onset diabetes. Focal and multifocal types of neuropathy are less common but quite dramatic (categories 1, 2, and 3 under "Asymmetric" in Table 377-5). They rarely occur before the age of 45 and are usually subacute or acute in onset. Cranial mononeuropathies are isolated sixth or third nerve palsies. The latter spares the pupil in three-fourths of cases, and some local pain or headache occurs in one-half. Truncal (thoracoabdominal) neuropathy is painful, involves one or more intercostal or lumbar nerves unilaterally, and frequently coexists with the asymmetric proximal motor neuropathy. In asymmetric proximal motor neuropathy, the most evident features are weakened muscles innervated by the femoral and obturator nerves (quadriceps femoris, iliopsoas, adductor magnus) and ipsilateral loss of the knee jerk reflex. Sensory deficit is minor, but pain in the hip and anterior thigh may be prominent. In all these multifocal and focal neuropathies, the pain usually subsides within weeks to a year, and function is usually partly or completely recovered. The same is true for symmetric proximal motor neuropathy (category 3 under "Symmetric" in Table 377-5).

Focal and multifocal diabetic neuropathies are considered to be ischemic in origin, and ischemia may also underlie symmetric polyneuropathies, which are also thought to involve abnormality of nerve metabolism.

Management of diabetic neuropathies is directed toward optimal glycemic control and symptomatic pain suppression. In the long-term Diabetes Control and Complications Trial, patients who controlled their diabetes meticulously showed significantly less neuropathy. The role of aldose reductase inhibitors in preventing or reversing diabetic complications, including neuropathy, remains unclear. Entrapment neuropathies are frequently amenable to surgical decompression.

Neuropathies with HIV Infection Neuropathies are common in infection with HIV, but different types of neuropathy are seen according to the stage of the disease. GBS or CIDP (Chap. 378) are the neuropathies likely to occur following conversion to seropositivity and during the asymptomatic phase of HIV infection. Treatment is the same as for HIV-negative patients. In later, symptomatic stages, mononeuritis multiplex, axonal in nature, can occur; the course is typically subacute or chronic. In some cases, vasculitis of the vasa nervorum has been demonstrated.

The most common neuropathy is a distal, symmetric, mainly sensory polyneuropathy, which evolves slowly in the late symptomatic stages of HIV infection and frequently coexists with symptomatic encephalopathy and myelopathy (Table 377-3; Chap. 309). Improvement of this polyneuropathy with zidovudine treatment has been claimed. Sensory polyneuropathy of late-stage HIV infection must be distinguished from toxic polyneuropathy that may result from the use of nucleoside analogue treatment (Table 377-4). Also in the late stages, a severe, destructive, subacute, asymmetric polyradiculopathy involving the cauda equina may be seen; it is caused by an opportunistic infection of the nerve roots with cytomegalovirus. Ganciclovir, started early, can arrest the disorder.

Neuropathies with Lyme Disease A focal or multifocal radiculoneuropathy may occur weeks, months, or even years after primary infection by the tick-borne spirochete *Borrelia burgdorferi*. Although usually sensory and either dysesthetic or painful, the neuropathy is variable in distribution, affecting cranial nerves and spinal roots or nerves in a patchy, asymmetric fashion. Neuropathy is often chronic and persistent; cerebrospinal fluid pleocytosis is the rule. In many, improvement occurs spontaneously, but the course is shortened by treatment with antibiotics, usually intravenous ceftriaxone (Chap. 176).

Herpes Zoster This is a sensory neuritis due to infection with varicella-zoster virus and is characterized by acute inflammation of one or more dorsal root ganglia. Lancinating pain and hyperalgesia over the skin surface supplied by the affected roots occur for 3 to 4 days, followed by the appearance in the same segment of a herpetic eruption characterized by painful raised blisters on reddened bases. Pain usually subsides in a few weeks. If the inflammatory process spreads to involve related motor roots, segmental motor weakness and wasting appear. Paralysis of the oculomotor nerves may occur in conjunction with involvement of the ophthalmic division of the trigeminal ganglion (ophthalmoplegic zoster). Facial paralysis may occur with involvement of the geniculate ganglion and herpetic eruption on the ipsilateral tympanic membrane or external ear canal (Ramsay Hunt syndrome).

In fewer than 5% of patients, neuropathic pain persists in the dermatomal distribution of the affected ganglia. This pain, known as *postherpetic neuralgia*, is intense, burning, hyperpathic, and unrelenting; it often dominates the lives of those affected. Advancing age is a risk factor for this outcome. In some patients, blunting of the pain to tolerable levels is achieved by use of carbamazepine or a tricyclic antidepressant such as desipramine (Chap. 12).

Leprous Neuritis   This is a major worldwide cause of neuropathy. *Mycobacterium leprae* organisms readily invade Schwann cells in cutaneous nerve twigs, particularly those associated with unmyelinated nerve fibers. *M. leprae* thrives best in the coolest tissues in the body. Two major forms of leprous neuritis are recognized, tuberculoid and lepromatous, which actually represent the ends of a spectrum of disease, the middle of which is called borderline (dimorphous) leprosy (patchy and multifocal involvement of skin and nerve). The treatment of a given case depends on where it falls in this spectrum (Chap. 170). Tuberculoid (high-resistance) leprosy consists of a single patch of hypesthetic or anesthetic skin in any location. The skin patch is frequently thickened, reddened, or hypopigmented. Few or no *M. leprae* bacilli may be demonstrated. If a superficially placed nerve trunk, typically a cutaneous nerve, courses just beneath the area of affected skin, it may be engulfed in the inflammatory reaction, resulting in an associated mononeuropathy. Such a nerve may be palpably enlarged and beaded. Lepromatous (low-resistance) leprosy is marked by immunologic tolerance, numerous bacilli, and widespread skin thickening, cutaneous anesthesia, and anhidrosis, which spare only the warmest parts of the body, notably the axilla, the groin, and beneath the scalp hair. Motor signs (focal weakness and atrophy) result from damage to mixed nerves lying close to the skin, particularly the median, ulnar, peroneal, and facial nerves.

Bell's Palsy   This seventh nerve palsy is due to inflammation of the facial nerve in the facial canal, the basis for which remains obscure. Edema may play a part in causing compression of nerve fibers, with resulting acute unilateral paralysis of facial muscles (Chap. 367).

Sarcoidosis   This may involve single or multiple peripheral nerves, producing asymmetric mononeuritis or polyneuritis. Unilateral or bilateral facial paralysis is described in association with parotitis and uveitis (Heerfordt's syndrome).

Polyneuritis Cranialis   This is a relapsing and remitting mononeuropathy multiplex restricted to cranial nerves (Chap. 367). It is usually associated with indolent tuberculous cervical adenitis (scrofula) or sarcoidosis. Treatment of the underlying condition will halt the cranial nerve palsies.

SPECIAL NEUROPATHIC PRESENTATIONS   Some disorders selectively affect the peripheral nervous system, limiting dysfunction to specific systems or sites, such as motor nerves, brachial plexus, or the autonomic nervous system.

Autonomic Neuropathy   The autonomic nervous system regulates the visceral organs and vegetative functions (Chap. 366). Many pharmacologic agents modify specific autonomic functions, but autonomic neuropathy (dysautonomia) with structural changes in pre- and postganglionic neurons can also occur. Usually autonomic neuropathy is a manifestation of a more generalized polyneuropathy also affecting somatic peripheral nervous function, as in diabetic neuropathy, GBS, and alcoholic polyneuropathy, but occasionally syndromes of pure pandysautonomia are encountered. Symptoms of dysautonomia are mainly negative (i.e., loss of function) and include postural hypotension with faintness or syncope, anhidrosis, hypothermia, bladder atony, obstipation, dry mouth and dry eyes from failure of salivary and lacrimal glands to secrete, blurring of vision from lack of pupillary and ciliary regulation, and sexual impotence in males. Positive phenomena (hyperfunction) may also occur and include episodic hypertension, diarrhea, hyperhidrosis, and either tachycardia or bradycardia. Management is symptomatic and also directed at the underlying cause, if it can be identified.

Pure Motor Neuropathy   Disorder affecting any level of the motor unit—anterior horn cell, motor axon, or neuromuscular junction—can result in a purely lower motor syndrome without sensory disturbance. Distinguishing anterior horn cell disorders (motor neuronopathies) from motor axonopathies may be difficult clinically because they share manifestations (weakness, muscle denervation atrophy, hypo- or areflexia, fasciculations). EDX examination may also fail to localize the primary site of the lesion (neuropathic versus neuronopathic) unless the lesion is demyelinating in nature, in which case it is by definition neuropathic.

Examples of motor neuronopathies include the lower-motor form of amyotrophic lateral sclerosis, poliomyelitis, hereditary spinal muscular atrophies, and adult variant of hexosaminidase A deficiency. Motor neuropathies may be seen with lead or dapsone intoxication, occasionally with porphyria, and also with multifocal motor neuropathy. The latter is a chronic asymmetric disorder of mid-life associated with persistent conduction block on EDX examination, and often high titers of antiganglioside antibodies (particularly anti-GM_1). Neuromuscular junction disorders (e.g., Lambert-Eaton myasthenic syndrome, tick bite paralysis, other types of toxic neuromuscular blockade) are purely motor and can be recognized and localized electrodiagnostically. Some motor-sensory polyneuropathies have predominant motor symptoms and signs, such as hereditary motor-sensory neuropathies, GBS, and CIDP, but the subclinical sensory component is readily demonstrated electrodiagnostically or by quantitative sensory testing.

Pure Sensory Neuropathy   Clinical presentations involving primary sensation only (Table 377-6; Chap. 23) are not uncommon. Manifestations may (1) reflect mainly large afferent fiber involvement with deficits of vibratory and proprioceptive sense, areflexia, and sensory ataxia with or without tingling dysesthesias; (2) reflect mainly small afferent fiber involvement with numbness and cutaneous hypesthesia to pin-prick and temperature stimuli, often with painful, burning dysesthesias; or (3) be pansensory, with both large and small fiber manifestations. The pattern of distribution, although variable, is often distal and symmetric, particularly for large-fiber neuropathies.

The most severe and widespread of these pure sensory syndromes exhibit poor or no recovery, suggesting irreversible lesions of nerve cell bodies in dorsal root and trigeminal ganglia. These are referred to as *sensory neuronopathies*. With sensory neurotoxins, moderate doses lead to potentially reversible neuropathy, but high doses appear to cause irreversible neuronopathy (Table 377-6).

Plexopathy   This term refers to disorders of either the brachial or the lumbosacral plexus. Lesions of the brachial plexus are characterized by motor and sensory signs different from those expected in either mononeuropathies of the upper limb or polyneuropathies. The usual causes are direct trauma to the plexus, idiopathic brachial neuritis (also called *neuralgic amyotrophy*), cervical rib or band, infiltration by malignant tumor, or prior radiation therapy. When the upper parts of the brachial plexus, arising from cervical roots 5 through 7, are affected, weakness and atrophy of shoulder girdle and upper arm muscles occur. Injuries to the lower brachial plexus, arising from the eighth cervical and first thoracic roots, produce distal arm weakness, atrophy, and focal sensory deficit in the forearm and hand. In general, idiopathic brachial neuritis, irradiation with >60 Gy (6000 rad), and particular types of trauma (arm jerked downward) result in damage to the upper portions of the brachial plexus. In contrast, infiltration by malignant tumor, cervical rib or band, and certain other types of trauma (arm jerked upward) cause damage to the lower brachial plexus. Lumbosacral plexopathies are less common; they may be due to idiopathic lumbosacral plexitis, retroperitoneal hemorrhage, or malignant tumor infiltration or may occur in association with long-standing diabetes mellitus.

Cold Effects   Cold exerts direct deleterious effects on peripheral nerve, independent of ischemia. Cold injury to nerve occurs after prolonged exposure, usually of a limb, to moderately low temperatures, as with immersion of the feet in seawater; actual freezing of tissue is not required. Axonal degeneration of myelinated fibers is the pathologic expression of cold injury. Frequently, limbs affected by cold injury to nerve show sensory deficit and dysesthesias, cutaneous vasomotor instability, pain, and marked sensitivity to minimal cold exposure, which persist for many years. The pathophysiology of these phenomena is uncertain.

Trophic Changes   The array of observable changes in completely denervated muscle, bone, and skin, including hair and nails, is well known, if incompletely understood. It is unclear what portion of the changes is due purely to denervation versus that caused by disuse, immobility, lack of weight bearing, and particularly recurrent, unnoticed, painless trauma. Considerable evidence favors the view that ulceration of skin, poor healing, tissue resorption, neurogenic arthropathy, and mutilation are the result of repeated unheeded injury to insensitive parts. This sequence of events is avoidable with proper attention to and care of the insensitive parts by both patient and physician.

RECOVERY FROM NEUROPATHY In contrast to axons in the central nervous system, peripheral nerve fibers have an excellent ability to regenerate under proper circumstances. The process of regeneration following axonal degeneration may take from 2 months to more than a year, depending on the severity of the neuropathy and the length of regeneration required. Regeneration can take place when the cause of the neuropathy has been eliminated, such as removal from contact with a neurotoxic substance or correction of an abnormal metabolic state. A deficit secondary to demyelination may recover rapidly, since intact axons may remyelinate in just a few weeks. For example, a patient with GBS, in whom demyelination but no secondary axonal degeneration has occurred, may recover to normal strength from bedfastness and paralysis of arms and legs in as little as 3 to 4 weeks.

PERIPHERAL NERVE TUMORS These tumors are mostly benign and can arise on any nerve trunk or twig. Although peripheral nerve tumors can occur anywhere in the body, including the spinal roots and cauda equina, many are subcutaneous in location and present as a soft swelling, sometimes with a purplish discoloration of the skin. Two major categories of peripheral nerve tumors are recognized: neurilemmoma (schwannoma) and neurofibroma. Neurilemmomas are usually solitary and grow in the nerve sheath, rendering the tumor relatively easy to dissect free. In contrast, neurofibromas tend to be multiple, grow in the endoneurial substance, which renders them difficult to dissect, may undergo malignant changes, and are the hallmark of von Recklinghausen's neurofibromatosis (NF1) (Chap. 370).

BIBLIOGRAPHY

ASBURY AK, THOMAS PK: *Peripheral Nerve Disorders*, 2d ed. Oxford, Butterworth-Heinemann, 1995

BOLTON CF, BREUER AC: Critical illness polyneuropathy. Muscle Nerve 22:419, 1999

CHALK CH: Acquired peripheral neuropathy. Neurol Clin 15:501, 1997

DAWSON DM et al: *Entrapment Neuropathies*, 3d ed. Philadelphia, Lippincott-Raven, 1999

DIABETES CONTROL AND COMPLICATIONS TRIAL RESEARCH GROUP: The effect of intensive diabetes therapy on the development and progression of neuropathy. Ann Intern Med 122:561, 1995

DYCK PJ, THOMAS PK (eds): *Diabetic Neuropathy*, 2d ed, Philadelphia, Saunders, 1999

——— et al (eds): *Peripheral Neuropathy*, 3d ed. Philadelphia, Saunders, 1992

HOLLAND NR et al: Small-fiber sensory neuropathies: Clinical course and neuropathology of idiopathic cases. Ann Neurol 44:47, 1998

MOORE RD et al: Incidence of neuropathy in HIV-infected patients on monotherapy vs those on combination therapy with didanosine, stavudine, and hydroxyurea. AIDS 14:273, 2000

STEWART JD: *Focal Peripheral Neuropathies*, 3d ed. Philadelphia, Lippincott Williams Wilkins, 1999

WARD JD: Improving prognosis in type 2 diabetes. Diabetes Care 22 (Suppl 2): B84, 1999

WOOLF CJ, MANNION RJ: Neuropathic pain: Aetiology, symptoms, mechanisms and management. Lancet 353:1954, 1999

ZOCHODNE DW: Diabetic neuropathies: Features and mechanisms. Brain Pathol 9:369, 1999

378 *Arthur K. Asbury, Stephen L. Hauser*

GUILLAIN-BARRÉ SYNDROME AND OTHER IMMUNE-MEDIATED NEUROPATHIES

AIDP acute inflammatory demyelinating polyneuropathy	MAG myelin-associated glycoprotein
CIDP chronic inflammatory demyelinating polyneuropathy	MFS M. Fisher syndrome
	MGUS monoclonal gammopathy of undetermined significance
CSF cerebrospinal fluid	MMN multifocal motor neuropathy
EAN experimental allergic neuritis	PAN polyarteritis nodosa
GBS Guillain-Barré syndrome	PE plasma exchange
IVIg intravenous immune globulin	SCLC small cell lung cancer

GUILLAIN-BARRÉ SYNDROME

Guillain-Barré syndrome (GBS) is an acute, frequently severe, and fulminant polyradiculoneuropathy that is autoimmune in nature. It occurs year-round at a rate of about one case per million per month, or approximately 3500 cases per year in the United States and Canada. Males and females are equally at risk, and in western countries adults are more frequently affected than children.

CLINICAL MANIFESTATIONS GBS manifests as rapidly evolving areflexic motor paralysis with or without sensory disturbance. The usual pattern is an ascending paralysis that may be first noticed as rubbery legs. Weakness typically evolves over hours to a few days and is frequently accompanied by tingling dysesthesias in the extremities. The legs are usually more affected than the arms, and facial diparesis is present in 50% of affected individuals. The lower cranial nerves are also frequently involved, causing bulbar weakness and difficulty with handling secretions and maintaining an airway. Most patients require hospitalization, and almost 30% require ventilatory assistance at some time during the illness. Fever and constitutional symptoms are absent at the onset, and, if present, cast doubt on the diagnosis. Deep tendon reflexes usually disappear within the first few days of onset. Cutaneous sensory deficits, e.g., loss of pain and temperature sensation, are usually relatively mild; but functions subserved by large sensory fibers, such as deep tendon reflexes and proprioception, are more severely affected. Bladder dysfunction may occur in severe cases but is usually transient. If bladder dysfunction is a prominent feature and comes early in the course, possibilities other than GBS should be considered, particularly spinal cord disease. Once clinical worsening stops and the patient reaches a plateau, the crisis is usually past. Improvement may begin within days of the plateau.

Several subtypes of GBS are now recognized, as determined primarily by electrodiagnostic and pathologic distinctions (Table 378-1). In severe cases of GBS requiring critical care management, autonomic involvement is common. Usual features are loss of vasomotor control with wide fluctuation in blood pressure, postural hypotension, and cardiac dysrhythmias. These features require close monitoring and management and can be fatal. Pain is another common feature of GBS; several types are encountered. Most common is deep aching pain in weakened muscles, which patients liken to having over-exercised the previous day. Other pains in GBS include back pain involving the entire spine and sometimes dysesthetic pain in the extremities as a manifestation of sensory nerve fiber involvement. These pains are self-limited and should be treated with standard analgesics.

A range of limited or regional GBS syndromes may be encountered, although uncommonly. These include (1) the M. Fisher syndrome (Table 378-1 and see "Immunopathogenesis," below); (2) pure sensory forms; (3) ophthalmoplegia with anti-GQ1b antibodies (see "Immunopathogenesis," below), as part of severe motor-sensory GBS; (4) GBS with severe bulbar and facial paralysis, sometimes associated

Table 378-1 Subtypes of Guillain-Barré Syndrome (GBS)

Subtype	Features	Electrodiagnosis	Pathology
Acute inflammatory demyelinating poly-neuropathy (AIDP)	Adults affected more than children; 90% of cases in western world; recovery rapid; anti-GM1 antibodies (<50%)	Demyelinating	First attack on Schwann cell surface; widespread myelin damage, macrophage activation, and lymphocytic infiltration; variable secondary axonal damage
Acute motor axonal neuropathy (AMAN)	Children and young adults; Prevalent in China and Mexico; May be seasonal; recovery rapid; anti-GD1a antibodies	Axonal	First attack at motor nodes of Ranvier; macrophage activation, few lymphocytes, frequent periaxonal macrophages; extent of axonal damage highly variable
Acute motor sensory axonal neuropathy (AMSAN)	Mostly adults; uncommon; recovery slow, often incomplete; closely related to AMAN	Axonal	Same as AMAN, but also affects sensory nerves and roots; axonal damage usually severe
M. Fisher syndrome (MFS)	Adults and children; uncommon; ophthalmoplegia, ataxia, and areflexia; Anti-GQ1b antibodies (90%)	Demyelinating	Few cases examined; resembles AIDP

with antecedent cytomegalovirus infection and anti-GM2 antibodies; and (5) acute pandysautonomia.

ANTECEDENT EVENTS Seventy-five percent of cases of GBS are preceded 1 to 3 weeks by an acute infectious process, usually respiratory or gastrointestinal. Culture and seroepidemiologic techniques show that 20 to 30% of all cases occurring in North America, Europe, and Australia are preceded by infection or reinfection with *Campylobacter jejuni*. A similar proportion is preceded by a human herpes virus infection, often cytomegalovirus or Epstein-Barr virus. Other viruses and also Mycoplasma pneumoniae have been identified as agents involved in antecedent infections. Recent immunization has also been associated with GBS. The swine influenza vaccine, administered widely in the United States in 1976, is the most notable example; influenza vaccines in use from 1992 to 1994, however, resulted in only one additional case of GBS per million persons vaccinated. Older type rabies vaccine, prepared in nervous system tissue, is implicated as a trigger of GBS in developing countries where it is still used; the mechanism is presumably immunization against neural antigens. GBS also occurs more frequently than can be attributed to chance alone in patients with lymphoma, including Hodgkin's disease (Chap. 112), in HIV-seropositive individuals (Chap. 309), and in patients with systemic lupus erythematosus (Chap. 311).

IMMUNOPATHOGENESIS Several lines of evidence support an autoimmune basis for acute inflammatory demyelinating polyneuropathy (AIDP), the most common and best studied type of GBS; by analogy the concept extends to all of the subtypes of GBS (Table 378-1).

It is likely that both cellular and humoral immune mechanisms contribute to tissue damage in AIDP. T cell activation is suggested by the finding that elevated levels of cytokines and cytokine receptors are present in serum [interleukin (IL)2, soluble IL-2 receptor] and in cerebrospinal fluid (CSF) [IL-6, tumor necrosis factor α, interferon-γ]. AIDP is also closely analogous to an experimental T cell–mediated immunopathy designated experimental allergic neuritis (EAN); EAN is induced in laboratory animals by immune sensitization against protein fragments derived from peripheral nerve proteins, and in particular against the P2 protein. Based on analogy to EAN, it was initially thought that AIDP was likely to be primarily a T cell–mediated dis-

order, however, abundant data now suggest that autoantibodies directed against nonprotein determinants may be central to many cases.

Circumstantial evidence suggests that all GBS results from immune responses to nonself antigens (infectious agents, vaccines) that misdirect to host nerve tissue through a resemblance-of-epitope (molecular mimicry) mechanism (Fig. 378-1) (Chap. 307). The neural targets are likely to be glycoconjugates, specifically gangliosides (Fig. 378-2). Gangliosides are complex glycosphingolipids that contain one or more sialic acid residues; various gangliosides participate in cell–cell interactions (including those between axons and glia), modulation of receptors, and regulation of growth. They are typically exposed on the plasma membrane of cells, rendering them susceptible to an antibody-mediated attack. Gangliosides and other glycoconjugates are present in large quantity in human nervous tissues and in key sites, such as nodes of Ranvier. Antiganglioside antibodies, most frequently to GM1, are common in GBS (20 to 50% of cases), particularly in those preceded by *C. jejuni* infection. Furthermore, isolates of *C. jejuni* from stool cultures of patients with GBS have surface glycolipid structures that antigenically cross react with gangliosides, including GM1, concentrated in human nerves. Another line of evidence is derived from experience in Europe with parenteral use of purified bovine brain gangliosides for treatment of various neuropathic disorders. Five to 15 days after injection some recipients developed acute motor axonal GBS with high titers of anti-GM1 antibodies that recognized epitopes at nodes of Ranvier and motor endplates.

Particularly noteworthy is the M. Fisher syndrome (MFS), which presents as rapidly evolving ataxia and areflexia of limbs without weakness, and ophthalmoplegia often with pupillary paralysis. The MFS variant accounts for ~5% of all GBS cases. Anti-GQ1b antibodies are found in >90% of patients with MFS (Table 378-1; Fig. 378-2), and titers of IgM and IgG are highest early in the course. Anti-GQ1b antibodies are not found in other forms of GBS unless there is extraocular motor nerve involvement. Of note, extraocular motor nerves are enriched in GQ1b gangliosides in comparison to limb nerves. Further, a monoclonal anti-GQ1b antibody raised against *C. jejuni* isolated from a patient with MFS blocked neuromuscular transmission experimentally.

Taken together, these observations provide strong but still inconclusive evidence that anti-ganglioside antibodies play an important pathogenic role in GBS. Definitive proof requires the passive transfer of GBS with specific antibodies; this procedure has not yet been accomplished, although a single case of apparent maternal-fetal transplacental transfer of GBS has been described.

PATHOPHYSIOLOGY In the demyelinating forms of GBS, the basis for flaccid paralysis and sensory disturbance is conduction block. This finding, demonstrable electrophysiologically, implies that the axonal connections remain intact. Hence, recovery can take place rapidly as remyelination occurs. In severe cases of demyelinating GBS, secondary axonal degeneration usually occurs; its extent can be estimated electrophysiologically. More secondary axonal degeneration correlates with a slower rate of recovery and a greater degree of residual disability. When a primary axonal pattern is encountered electrophysiologically, the implication is that axons have degenerated and become disconnected from their targets, specifically the neuromuscular junctions, and must therefore regenerate for recovery to take place. In motor axonal cases in which recovery is rapid, the lesion is thought to be localized to preterminal motor branches, allowing regeneration and reinnervation to take place quickly.

LABORATORY FEATURES CSF findings are distinctive, consisting of an elevated CSF protein level (100 to 1000 mg/dL) without accompanying pleocytosis. The CSF is often normal when symptoms have been present for ≤48 h; by the end of the first week the level of protein is usually elevated. An increased white cell count in the CSF (10 to 100/μL) in otherwise typical GBS raises the possibility of unrecognized HIV infection (Chap. 309). Electrodiagnostic features are mild or absent in the early stages and lag behind the clinical evolution. In cases with demyelination (Table 378-1) prolonged distal latencies, conduction velocity slowing, evidence of conduction block, and temporal dispersion of compound action potential are the usual features. In cases with primary axonal pathology, the principal electrodiagnostic finding is reduced amplitude of compound action potentials without conduction slowing or prolongation of distal latencies.

DIAGNOSIS GBS is a descriptive entity. The diagnosis is made by recognizing the pattern of rapidly evolving paralysis with areflexia, absence of fever or other systemic symptoms, and characteristic antecedent events (Table 378-2). In the early phases, laboratory tests are helpful only to exclude other disorders that can resemble GBS. Electrodiagnostic features may be minimal, and the CSF protein level may not rise until the end of the first week. If the diagnosis is strongly suspected, treatment should be initiated without waiting for evolution of the characteristic electrodiagnostic and CSF findings to occur. GBS patients with risk factors for HIV or with CSF pleocytosis should have a serologic test for HIV.

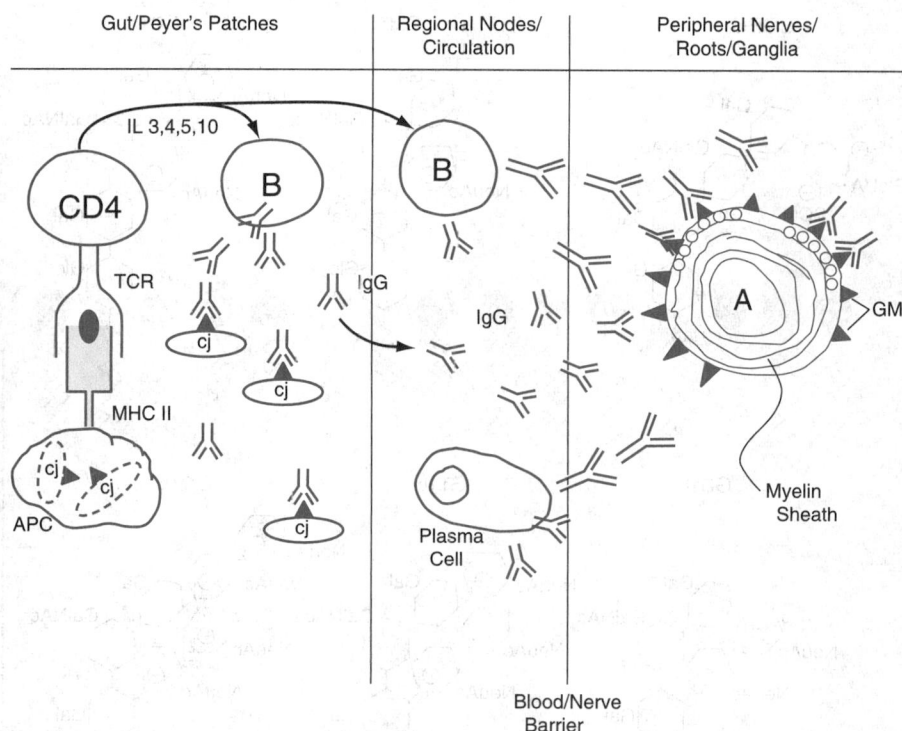

FIGURE 378-1 Postulated immunopathogenesis of GBS associated with *C. jejuni* infection. B cells recognize glycoconjugates on *C. jejuni* (Cj) (triangles) that cross-react with GM1 ganglioside present on peripheral nerve myelin. Some B cells, activated via a T cell–independent mechanism, secrete primarily IgM (not shown). Other B cells (upper left side) are activated via a partially T cell–dependent route and secrete primarily IgG; T cell help is provided by CD4 cells activated locally by fragments of Cj proteins that are presented on the surface of antigen-presenting cells (APC). A critical event in the development of GBS is the escape of activated B cells from Peyers patches into regional lymph nodes. Activated T cells probably also function to assist in opening of the blood-nerve barrier, facilitating penetration of pathogenic autoantibodies. The earliest changes in myelin (right) consist of edema between myelin lamellae and vesicular disruption (shown as circular blebs) of the outermost myelin layers. These effects are associated with activation of the C5b-C9 membrane attack complex and probably mediated by calcium entry; it is possible that the macrophage cytokine tumor necrosis factor (TNF) also participates in myelin damage. B, B cell; MHC II, class II major histocompatibility complex molecule; TCR, T cell receptor; A, axon.

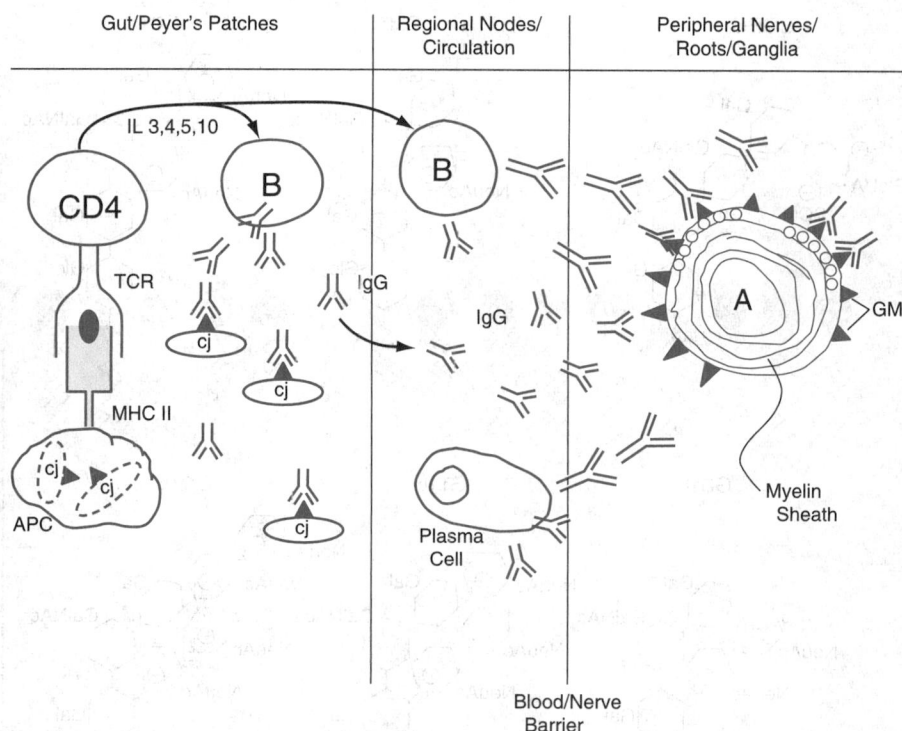

TREATMENT Treatment should be initiated as soon after diagnosis as possible. Each day counts; ~2 weeks after the first motor symptoms, immunotherapy is no longer effective. Either high-dose intravenous immune globulin (IVIg) or plasmapheresis can be initiated, as they are equally effective (Table 378-3). A combination of the two therapies is not significantly better than either alone. IVIg is usually administered as five daily infusions for a total dose of 2 g/kg body weight. A course of plasmapheresis, consisting of ~40 to 50 mL/kg plasma exchange (PE) daily for 4 to 5 days, is usually employed. In patients who are treated early in the course of GBS and improve, relapse may occur in the second or third week. Brief treatment with the original therapy is usually effective. Glucocorticoids have not been found to be effective in GBS.

In the worsening phase of GBS, most patients require monitoring in a critical care setting, with particular attention to vital capacity, cardiovascular status, and chest physiotherapy. As noted, ~30% of patients with GBS require ventilatory assistance, sometimes for prolonged periods of time (several weeks or longer). Frequent turning and assiduous skin care are important, as are daily range-of-motion exercises to avoid joint contractures.

PROGNOSIS AND RECOVERY Approximately 85% of patients with GBS achieve a full functional recovery within several months to a year, although minor findings on examination (such as areflexia) may persist. The mortality rate is <5% in optimal settings; death usually results from secondary pulmonary complications. The outlook is worst in patients with severe proximal motor and sensory axonal damage. Such axonal damage may be either primary or secondary in nature (see "Pathophysiology," above), but in either case successful regeneration cannot occur. Other factors that worsen the outlook for recovery are advanced age, a fulminant or severe attack, and a delay in the onset of treatment.

CHRONIC INFLAMMATORY DEMYELINATING POLYNEUROPATHY

Chronic inflammatory demyelinating polyneuropathy (CIDP) is distinguished from GBS by its chronic course. In other respects, this neuropathy shares many features with GBS, including elevated CSF protein levels and the electrodiagnostic findings of acquired demyelination. Most cases occur in adults, and males are affected slightly more often than females. The incidence of CIDP is lower than that of GBS, but due to the protracted course the prevalence is greater.

CLINICAL MANIFESTATIONS Onset is usually gradual, sometimes subacute; and, in a few, the initial attack is indistinguishable from that of GBS. Symptoms are both motor and sensory in most cases. Weakness of the limbs is usually symmetric but can be strikingly asymmetric. There is considerable variability from case to case. Some patients have a chronic progressive course, whereas others, usually younger patients, have a relapsing and remitting course. Some have only motor findings, and a small proportion present with a relatively pure syndrome of sensory ataxia. Tremor occurs in ~10% and may become more prominent during periods of subacute worsening or improvement. A small proportion have cranial nerve findings, including external ophthalmoplegia. CIDP tends to ameliorate over time with

FIGURE 378-2 Glycolipids implicated as antigens in immune-mediated neuropathies. Sulfate-3-glu-curonyl paragloboside (SGPG) is the glycolipid sharing a carbohydrate epitope with MAG, and the terminal sulfated glucuronic acid (shaded) is a key part of the epitope. GM1 is the ganglioside implicated in motor nerve disorders, and in most cases the terminal Gal (β1-3) GalNAc epitope (shaded), which is shared with GD1b, is involved. The disialosyl moiety implicated in sensory neuropathies consists of NeuAcα2–8NeuAc- (shaded) and is present in GD1b and GT1b gangliosides, as well as the simpler GD2 and GD3 gangliosides (not shown). GQ1b ganglioside that is an antigen in MFS has two disialosyl moieties. Although GD1a ganglioside has two sialic acid residues, they are not linked to each other, so it usually does not cross-react with the anti-GD1b antibodies. The shaded sugar moieties represent key aspects of the various epitopes, but carbohydrate sequences recognized by the antibodies may include additional sugar residues. GlcUA, glucuronic acid; Gal, galactose; GlcNAc, *N*-acetylglucosamine; Glc, glucose; GalNAc, *N*-acetylgalactosamine; NeuAc, *N*-acetylneuraminic acid (sialic acid). *(From MC Dalakis and RH Quarles: Ann Neurol 39:419, 1996, with permission.)*

treatment; the result is that many years after onset nearly 75% of patients have a reasonable functional recovery with only modest degrees of disability. Death from CIDP is uncommon.

DIAGNOSIS The diagnosis rests on characteristic clinical, CSF, and electrophysiologic findings. The CSF is usually acellular with an elevated protein level, sometimes several times normal. Electrodiagnostically, variable degrees of conduction slowing, prolonged distal latencies, temporal dispersion of compound action potentials, and conduction block are the principal features. In particular, the presence of conduction block is a certain sign of an acquired demyelinating process. Evidence of axonal loss, presumably secondary to demyelination, is present in >50% of patients. In all patients with CIDP, serum protein electrophoresis with immunofixation is indicated to screen for monoclonal gammopathy and associated conditions (see "Monoclonal Gammopathy of Undetermined Significance," below).

PATHOGENESIS Although there is evidence of immune activation in CIDP, the precise mechanisms of pathogenesis are unknown. Biopsy typically reveals little inflammation and onion-bulb thickening of nerves resulting from recurrent demyelination and remyelination. The response to therapy suggests that CIDP is immune-mediated; interestingly, CIDP responds to glucocorticoids (see below),

whereas GBS does not. Approximately 25% of patients with clinical features of CIDP also have a monoclonal gammopathy of undetermined significance (MGUS). Cases associated with monoclonal IgA or IgG usually respond to treatment as favorably as cases without a monoclonal gammopathy. Patients with IgM monoclonal gammopathy tend to have more sensory findings, a more protracted course and may have a less satisfactory response to treatment, although this is an area of controversy.

℞ TREATMENT Most authorities initiate treatment for CIDP when progression is rapid or walking is compromised. If the disorder is mild, management can be expectant, awaiting spontaneous remission. Controlled studies have shown that high dose IVIg, PE, and glucocorticoids are all more effective than placebo. Initial therapy is usually either IVIg or PE, which appear to be equally effective. IVIg is administered as 0.4 g/kg body weight daily for 5 days; most patients require periodic retreatment at approximately 6-week intervals. PE is initiated at 2 to 3 treatments per week for 6 weeks; periodic retreatment may also be required. Treatment with oral glucocorticoids is another option (60 to 80 mg prednisone daily for 1 to 2 months, followed by a gradual dose reduction of 10 mg per month as tolerated), but long-term adverse effects including bone demineralization, gastrointestinal bleeding, and cushingoid changes are problematic. Approximately one-half of patients with CIDP fail to adequately respond to the initial therapy chosen; a different treatment should then be tried. Patients who fail therapy with IVIg, PE, and glucocorticoids may benefit from treatment with immunosuppressive agents such as azathiaprine, methotrexate, cyclosporine, and cyclophosphamide, either alone or as adjunctive therapy. Use of these therapies requires periodic reassessment of their risks and benefits.

MULTIFOCAL MOTOR NEUROPATHY

Multifocal motor neuropathy (MMN) is a distinctive but uncommon neuropathy that presents as a slowly progres-

Table 378-2 Diagnostic Criteria for Guillain-Barré Syndrome

REQUIRED

1. Progressive weakness of 2 or more limbs due to neuropathy[a]
2. Areflexia
3. Disease course <4 weeks
4. Exclusion of other causes [e.g., vasculitis (polyarteritis nodosa, systemic lupus erythematosus, Churg-Strauss syndrome), toxins (organophosphates, lead), botulism, diphtheria, porphyria, localized spinal cord or cauda equina syndrome]

SUPPORTIVE

1. Relatively symmetric weakness
2. Mild sensory involvement
3. Facial nerve or other cranial nerve involvement
4. Absence of fever
5. Typical CSF profile (acellular, increase in protein level)
6. Electrophysiologic evidence of demyelination

---

[a] Excluding M. Fisher and other variant syndromes.
SOURCE: Modified from AK Asbury, DR Cornblath: Ann Neurol 27:S21, 1990

Trial/Site	Reference	No. Patients (N)/ Follow up (FU)/ Trial Arms	End Points	Results/p value	Comment
GBS Study Group; USA/Canada (18 centers)	Neurology 35:1096, 1985	N = 245 FU 6 months PE vs. none	1. % improved 1 grade at 4 weeks 2. days to improve 1 grade 3. days to reach grade 2	1. 59% (PE) vs. 39% (none) <0.001 2. 19 days (PE) vs. 40 days (none) <0.001 3. 53 days (PE) vs. 85 days (none) <0.001	First major trial showing efficacy—prior smaller trials showed conflicting results
French Coop. Group on PE in GBS; France/Switzerland (28 centers)	Ann Neurol 22:753, 1987; Ann Neurol 32:94, 1992	N = 220 FU = 1 year PE vs. none; Albumin vs. FFP in PE arm	1. days to walk w/ assistance 2. days to positive Δ score 3. Albumin vs. FFP	1. 30 days (PE) vs. 44 days (none) < 0.01 2. 4 days (PE) vs. 12 days (none) <0.001 3. No significant difference	At 1 year, full strength recovery in 71% (PE) vs. 52% (none); p = 0.007
Dutch GB Study Group; The Netherlands (15 centers)	N Engl J Med 326: 1123, 1992	N = 150 FU = 6 months IVIg vs. PE	1. % improved 1 grade at 4 weeks 2. days to reach grade 2	1. 53% (IVIg) vs. 34% (PE) p = 0.024 2. 55 days (IVIg) vs. 70 days (PE) p = 0.07	Patient assignment inadvertently favored IVIg group
Plasma Exchange/ Sandoglobulin GBS Trial (38 centers in 11 countries)	Lancet 349:225, 1997	N = 329 FU = 48 weeks IVIg vs. PE vs. both (3 arms)	1. % improved 1 grade at 4 weeks 2. Secondary end points: days to reach grade 2; days to off-respirator; disability at 48 weeks	No significant difference between the 3 groups for any end points	Nonsignificant trends favoring combined therapy

ABBREVIATIONS: PE, plasma exchange; IVIg, high dose intravenous immunoglobulin; FFP, fresh frozen plasma
NOTE: All studies except the French Coop. Group used the London grade scale: 0, healthy; 1, minor symptoms/signs; 2, walk 5 m unassisted; 3, walk 5 m with assistance; 4, bed/chairbound; 5, requiring assisted respiration; 6, dead.

sive motor weakness and atrophy evolving over years in the distribution of selected nerve trunks, associated with sites of persistent focal motor conduction block in the same nerve trunks. Sensory fibers are relatively spared. The arms are affected more frequently than the legs, and >75% of all patients are male. Some cases have been confused with lower motor neuron forms of amyotrophic lateral sclerosis (Chap. 365). Approximately 50% of patients present with high titers of polyclonal IgM antibody to the ganglioside GM1. It is uncertain how this finding relates to the discrete foci of persistent motor conduction block, but high concentrations of GM1 gangliosides are normal constituents of nodes of Ranvier in peripheral nerve fibers. Pathology reveals demyelination and mild inflammatory changes at the sites of conduction block.

Most patients with MMN respond to high-dose IVIg (dosages as for CIDP, above) and some refractory patients have responded to cyclophosphamide. Glucocorticoids and PE are not effective.

NEUROPATHIES WITH MONOCLONAL GAMMOPATHY

MULTIPLE MYELOMA   Clinically overt polyneuropathy occurs in ~5% of patients with the commonly encountered type of multiple myeloma, which exhibits either lytic or diffuse osteoporotic bone lesions. These neuropathies are sensorimotor, are usually mild but may be severe, and generally do not reverse with successful suppression of the myeloma. In most cases, electrodiagnostic and pathologic features are consistent with a process of axonal degeneration.

In contrast, myeloma with osteosclerotic features, although representing only 3% of all myelomas, is associated with polyneuropathy in one-half of cases. These neuropathies, which may also occur with solitary plasmacytoma, are distinct because they (1) are usually demyelinating in nature, (2) often respond to radiation therapy or removal of the primary lesion, (3) are associated with different monoclonal proteins and light chains (almost always lambda as opposed to primarily kappa in the lytic type of multiple myeloma), and (4) may occur in association with other systemic findings including thickening of the skin, hyperpigmentation, hypertrichosis, organomegaly, endocrinopathy, anasarca and clubbing of fingers. These are features of the POEMS syndrome (polyneuropathy, organomegaly, endocrinopathy, M protein, and skin changes). The pathogenesis of this uncommon syndrome and the explanation for its association with lambda light chains are unknown.

Neuropathies are also encountered in other systemic conditions with gammopathy including Waldenström's macroglobulinemia, primary systemic amyloidosis, and cryoglobulinemic states (mixed essential cryoglobulinemia, some cases of hepatitis C).

MONOCLONAL GAMMOPATHY OF UNDETERMINED SIGNIFICANCE   Chronic polyneuropathies occurring in association with MGUS are usually associated with the immunoglobulin isotypes IgG, IgA, and IgM. From a clinical standpoint, many of these patients are indistinguishable from patients with CIDP without monoclonal gammopathy (see Chronic Inflammatory Demyelinating Polyneuropathy, above), and their response to immunosuppressive agents is also similar. An exception is the syndrome of IgM kappa monoclonal gammopathy associated with an indolent, longstanding, sometimes static sensory neuropathy, frequently with tremor and sensory ataxia. Most patients are male and over age 50. In the majority, the monoclonal IgM immunoglobulin binds to a normal peripheral nerve constituent, myelin-associated glycoprotein (MAG), found in the paranodal regions of Schwann cells. Binding appears to be specific for a polysaccharide epitope that is also found in other normal peripheral nerve myelin glycoproteins, P0 and PMP22, and also in other normal nerve-related glycosphingolipids (Fig. 378-1). In the MAG-positive cases, IgM paraprotein is incorporated into the myelin sheaths of affected patients and widens the spacing of the myelin lamellae, thus producing a distinctive ultrastructural pattern. Demyelination and remyelination are the hallmarks of the lesions. The chronic demyelinating neuropathy appears to result from a destabilization of myelin metabolism rather than activation of an immune response. Therapy with chlorambucil or cyclophosphamide often results in improvement of the neuropathy associated with a prolonged reduction in the levels in the circulating paraprotein; chronic use of these alkylating agents is associated with significant risks (Chap. 84). In a small proportion of patients, MGUS will in time evolve into frankly malignant conditions, such as multiple myeloma (Chap. 113) or lymphoma (Chap. 112).

VASCULITIC NEUROPATHY

Peripheral nerve involvement is common in polyarteritis nodosa (PAN), appearing in half of all cases clinically and in 100% of cases at postmortem studies (Chap. 317). The most common pattern is multifocal (asymmetric) motor-sensory neuropathy (mononeuropathy multiplex) due to ischemic lesions of nerve trunks and roots; however, some cases of vasculitic neuropathy present as a distal, symmetric motor-sensory neuropathy. Symptoms of neuropathy are a common presenting complaint in patients with PAN. The electrodiagnostic findings are those of an axonal process. Small- to medium-sized arteries of the vasa nervorum, particularly the epineural vessels, are affected in PAN, resulting in a widespread ischemic neuropathy. A high frequency of neuropathy is also present in allergic angiitis and granulomatosis (Churg-Strauss syndrome).

Systemic vasculitis should always be considered when a subacute or chronically evolving mononeuropathy multiplex occurs in conjunction with constitutional symptoms (fever, anorexia, weight loss, loss of energy, malaise and nonspecific pains). Diagnosis of suspected vasculitic neuropathy is made by a combined nerve and muscle biopsy, with serial section or skip-serial techniques (Chap. 377).

Approximately one-third of biopsy-proven cases of vasculitic neuropathy are "nonsystemic" in that the vasculitis appears to affect only peripheral nerve. Constitutional symptoms are absent, and the course is more indolent than that of PAN. The erythrocyte sedimentation rate may be elevated, but other tests for systemic disease are negative. Nevertheless, clinically silent involvement of other organs is likely, and vasculitis is frequently found in muscle biopsied at the same time as nerve.

Vasculitic neuropathy may also be seen as part of the vasculitis syndrome occurring in the course of other connective tissue disorders. The most frequent is rheumatoid arthritis, but ischemic neuropathy due to involvement of vasa nervorum may also occur in mixed cryoglobulinemia, Sjögren's syndrome, Wegener's granulomatosis, hypersensitivity angiitis (Chap. 317), and progressive systemic sclerosis (Chap. 313). Management of these neuropathies including the "nonsystemic" vasculitic neuropathy consists of treatment of the underlying condition as well as the aggressive use of glucocorticoids and other immunosuppressant drugs, usually cyclophosphamide.

ANTI-HU PARANEOPLASTIC NEUROPATHY

This uncommon immune-mediated disorder manifests as a sensory neuronopathy, i.e., selective damage to dorsal root ganglia. The onset is often asymmetric with dysesthesias and sensory loss in the limbs that soon progress to affect all limbs, the torso, and face. Marked sensory ataxia, pseudoathetosis, and inability to walk, stand, or even sit unsupported are frequent features and are secondary to the extensive deafferentation. Subacute sensory neuronopathy is often idiopathic, but ~25% of cases are paraneoplastic, primarily related to lung cancer, and most of those are small cell lung cancer (SCLC) (Chap. 101). The gene *HuD*, ordinarily expressed only in neurons, is expressed in SCLC cells; the gene product functions as an RNA binding protein. Host anti-Hu antibodies to this tumor gene product cross-react with the same epitope expressed in dorsal root ganglion neurons, which results in immune-mediated neuronal destruction. An encephalomyelitis may accompany the sensory neuronopathy and presumably has the same pathogenesis. Neurologic symptoms usually precede, by 1 year on average, the identification of SCLC. The sensory neuronopathy runs its course in a few weeks or months and stabilizes, leaving the patient disabled. Most cases are unresponsive to treatment with glucocorticoids, IVIg, PE, or immunosuppressant drugs.

BIBLIOGRAPHY

GENERAL

BENATAR M et al: Immune-mediated peripheral neuropathies and voltage-gated sodium channels. Muscle Nerve 22:108, 1999

GOLD R et al: Mechanisms of immune regulation in the peripheral nervous system. Brain Pathol 9:343, 1999

QUARLES RH, WEISS D: Autoantibodies associated with peripheral neuropathy. Muscle Nerve 22:800, 1999

GUILLAIN-BARRÉ SYNDROME

HO TW et al: Anti-GD1a antibody is associated with axonal but not demyelinating forms of Guillain-Barré syndrome. Ann Neurol 45:168, 1999

JACOBS BC et al: The spectrum of antecedent infections in Guillain-Barré syndrome: A case control study. Neurology 51:1110, 1998

VAN KONINGSVELD R et al: Mild forms of Guillain-Barré syndrome in an epidemiologic survey in the Netherlands. Neurology 54:620, 2000

YUKI N et al: Clinical features and response to treatment in Guillain-Barré syndrome associated with antibodies to GM1b ganglioside. Ann Neurol 47:314, 2000

CHRONIC INFLAMMATORY DEMYELINATING POLYNEUROPATHY

BOUCHARD C et al: Clinicopathologic findings and prognosis of chronic inflammatory demyelinating polyneuropathy. Neurology 52:498, 1999

GORSON K et al: Chronic inflammatory demyelinating polyneuropathy: Clinical features and response to treatment in 67 consecutive patients with and without a monoclonal gammopathy. Neurology 48:321, 1997

MULTIFOCAL MOTOR NEUROPATHY

VAN DEN BERG L et al: The long-term effect of intravenous immunoglobulin treatment in multifocal motor neuropathy. Brain 121:421, 1998

NEUROPATHIES WITH MONOCLONAL GAMMOPATHY

PONSFORD S et al: Long-term clinical and neurophysiological follow-up of patients with peripheral neuropathy associated with benign monoclonal gammopathy. Muscle Nerve 23:164, 2000

ROPPER AH, GORSON KC: Neuropathies associated with paraproteinemia N Engl J Med 338:1601, 1999

VASCULITIC NEUROPATHY

SAID G: Necrotizing peripheral nerve vasculitis. Neurol Clin 15:835, 1997

ANTI-HU PARANEOPLASTIC NEUROPATHY

DALMAU J et al: Anti-Hu-associated paraneoplastic encephalomyelitis/sensory neuronopathy. A clinical study of 71 patients. Medicine 71:59, 1992

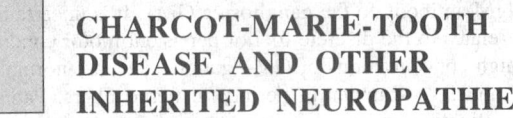

379 *Phillip F. Chance, Thomas D. Bird*

CHARCOT-MARIE-TOOTH DISEASE AND OTHER INHERITED NEUROPATHIES

CHARCOT-MARIE-TOOTH DISEASE

GENERAL CLINICAL FEATURES Charcot-Marie-Tooth (CMT) neuropathy comprises a heterogeneous group of inherited peripheral nerve diseases (Table 379-1). Transmission is most frequently autosomal dominant but may also be autosomal recessive or X-linked. An estimated 1 in 2500 persons has a form of CMT, making it one of the most frequently encountered inherited neurologic syndromes.

The neuropathy of CMT affects both motor and sensory nerves. Typical features consist of distal muscle weakness and atrophy, impaired sensation, and absent or hypoactive deep tendon reflexes. Common signs and symptoms are related to muscle loss and weakness, initially involving the feet and legs and later progressing to the hands and forearms. A history of an abnormal high-stepped (steppage) gait with frequent tripping and falling is frequently elicited. Complaints related to foot deformity (pes cavus, or high-arched feet) result from loss of intrinsic muscles of the feet. Despite the involvement of sensory nerves in CMT, complaints of limb pain or sensory disturbances are unusual.

Onset is most often during the first or second decade of life, although presentation in mid-adult life is not unusual. The variation in clinical presentation is exceptionally wide, ranging from individuals whose only clinical finding is pes cavus and minimal or no distal muscle weakness to those with severe distal atrophy and marked hand and foot deformity. However, it is unusual for patients with CMT to lose ambulation. There are no therapies that can prevent the onset or

Table 379-1 Genetic Spectrum of Inherited Neuropathies: Forms of Charcot-Marie-Tooth (CMT) Neuropathy/Hereditary Motor and Sensory Neuropathy (HMSN) and Related Disorders

	Locus	Gene	Mechanism
CHARCOT-MARIE-TOOTH TYPE 1			
(HMSNI)			
CMT1A	17p11.2-12	PMP22	Duplication/point mutation
CMT1B	1q22-23	P0	Point mutation
CMT1C	Unknown	Unknown	Unknown
CMT1?	10q21-22	EGR2	Point mutation
CMT4A	8q13-21	Unknown	Unknown
	5q23-33	Unknown	Unknown
CMT4B	11q13	MTMR2	Point mutation
CMTX	Xq13.1	CX32	Point mutation
CHARCOT-MARIE-TOOTH TYPE 2			
(HMSNII)			
CMT2A	1p35-36	Unknown	Unknown
CMT2B	3q13-22	Unknown	Unknown
CMT2C	Unknown	Unknown	Unknown
CMT2D	7p14	Unknown	Unknown
CMT2E	8p21	NF-L	Point mutation
DÉJERINE-SOTTAS			
(HMSNIII)			
DSD (CMT3)	17p11.2-12	PMP22	Point mutation
	1q22-23	P0	Point mutation
	10q21-22	EGR2	Point mutation
CONGENITAL HYPOMYELINATION			
CH	1q22-23	P0	Point mutation
	10q21-22	EGR2	Point mutation
HEREDITARY NEUROPATHY WITH PRESSURE PALSIES			
HNPP	17p11.2-12	PMP22	Deletion/point mutation

NOTE: PMP22, peripheral myelin protein 22; P_0, myelin protein zero; Cx32, connexin32; EGR2 (Krox-20) early growth response 2 gene; MTMR2, myotubularin-related protein-2; NF-L, neurofilament-light chain; CH, congenital hypomyelination.

delay progression of disability associated with CMT. Patients frequently benefit from physical therapy, use of ankle-foot orthroses (AFOs) to alleviate foot drop, and, in some cases, surgical procedures to the foot. Surgery should be undertaken only when pain or difficulty walking due to severe foot deformity cannot be managed by more conservative means.

CLASSIFICATION BY PHENOTYPE A widely accepted classification system distinguishes demyelinating forms of CMT (also designated as CMT type 1, or CMT1) from those due to axonal degeneration (CMT type 2, or CMT2). Individuals with CMT1 have electrophysiologic findings of reduced motor and sensory nerve conduction velocities (NCVs; typically <38 to 40 m/s) and pathologic findings of hypertrophic demyelinating neuropathy ("onion bulbs"). By contrast, in CMT2 there is relative preservation of the myelin sheath and these individuals have normal or near-normal NCVs. CMT3 refers to Déjerine-Sottas disease (DSD; see below), CMT4 to autosomal recessive forms of CMT, and CMTX to X-linked varieties.

An alternative classification system designates these disorders as hereditary motor and sensory neuropathies (HMSN); HMSNI refers to CMT1, HMSNII to CMT2, HMSNIII to DSD, and HMSNIV to Refsum disease (see below).

Approach to the Patient

A clinical diagnosis of an inherited peripheral neuropathy consistent with a form of CMT (CMT1 or CMT2) should be established prior to undertaking specific genetic tests. Other causes of peripheral neuropathy (e.g., diabetes mellitus, alcoholism, heavy metal poisoning, immune neuropathies) should also be considered and, if necessary, ruled out. An environmental exposure may affect multiple family members, thereby potentially mimicking a hereditary illness. CMT is usually a chronic, slowly progressive condition. One should be sus-

picious of cases that seem to have a rapid course of deterioration. As noted above, the neurologic findings show great variability in patients with CMT; mild pes cavus and depressed deep tendon reflexes may be the only signs of disease.

Although symptoms related to sensory disturbances are uncommon in CMT, a careful sensory examination is nonetheless essential. In patients who have no objective signs of sensory impairment and no evidence of sensory nerve dysfunction on electrophysiologic studies, alternative diagnoses including primary motor system disorders (e.g., distal spinal muscle atrophy, juvenile amyotrophic lateral sclerosis) should be considered.

The pedigree is of paramount importance in the diagnosis of CMT. Examination of multiple family members, particularly parents, for subtle signs of neuropathy may help to establish a diagnosis. If possible, it is also important to obtain NCVs and an electromyogram (EMG) from all at-risk family members.

GENETIC CONSIDERATIONS   CMT Neuropathy Type 1A (CMT1A) The overwhelming majority of autosomal dominant CMT1 pedigrees demonstrate linkage to chromosome 17p11.2-12 (CMT1A) and are most frequently associated with a tandem 1.5-megabase (Mb) DNA duplication in this chromosomal region. The DNA duplication is usually inherited as a stable Mendelian trait; however, it may also arise as a de novo event. The de novo duplication is responsible for most sporadic cases of CMT1 and may also account for some cases of CMT1 previously thought to occur on the basis of an autosomal recessive mode of inheritance. When present as a de novo event, the duplication results more commonly from an error in spermatogenesis; however, ~10% of de novo cases have been found to result from an error in oogenesis.

The critical gene for CMT1A is peripheral myelin protein-22 (PMP22), which is expressed in Schwann cells. The *PMP22* gene encodes a 160-amino-acid protein localized to the compact portion of peripheral nerve myelin; it contains four putative transmembrane domains and is highly conserved in evolution. The level of expression of PMP22 is crucial for proper myelination of peripheral nerves. The neuropathy in patients with the 17p11.2-12 duplication results from the presence of three copies of PMP22 leading to increased expression at this locus. In rare cases, patients homozygous for the CMT1A duplication have been identified, and in some cases these individuals exhibit a more severe phenotype than their heterozygous siblings or parents. As discussed below, monosomic underexpression of PMP22 results in hereditary neuropathy with liability to pressure palsies (HNPP).

Rare CMT1 pedigrees that are linked to chromosome 17p11.2-12 yet lack the DNA duplication may harbor missense mutations within the *PMP22* gene.

Approximately three-quarters of patients with a clinical diagnosis of CMT1 carry the 17p11.2-12 duplication. DNA testing for CMT1A (including the associated chromosome 17 duplication and sequencing to detect point mutations in PMP22) has become available and is now an accepted part of the evaluation of many patients with suspected hereditary neuropathies (see below).

CMT Neuropathy Type 1B (CMT1B) CMT1B is much less common than CMT1A; it results from mutations in the human myelin protein zero gene (*MPZ*, or P_0), which maps to chromosome 1q22-q23. P_0 is the major structural protein component of peripheral nervous system myelin (quantitatively 50% by weight) and represents ~10% of total Schwann cell mRNA. P_0 is a member of the immunoglobulin gene superfamily of cell adhesive molecules and localizes to the compact portion of peripheral nerve myelin. P_0 protein consists of 248 amino acids and contains an intracellular and a glycosylated extracellular domain with a single transmembrane segment. Many different point mutations in the P_0 gene have been found in patients with CMT1B, and these mutations predominately map to the extracellular domain of its gene product.

At the clinical level it is not possible to differentiate patients with CMT1A from those with CMT1B. Molecular genetic testing is available.

Déjerine-Sottas Disease   DSD (also called *HMSNIII*) is a severe, infantile or childhood onset, hypertrophic demyelinating polyneuropathy. NCVs are greatly prolonged (typically <10 m/s), and elevations in the cerebrospinal fluid (CSF) protein level are typically present. The clinical features of DSD overlap those of severe CMT1, and for this reason, the continued clinical separation of CMT1 and DSD is perhaps unwarranted. Many cases of DSD appear to be sporadic, occuring in the absence of a family history of neuropathy.

Molecular genetic studies indicate that DSD may be associated with point mutations in the P_0 or the *PMP22* genes, although pedigrees have been described that lack mutations in either the P_0, *PMP22*, or *Cx32* gene (see below). All DSD mutations identified to date appear to function as dominant genetic traits. Recently, a point mutation in the P_0 gene has been proposed as a mechanism for congenital hypomyelinating neuropathy (CHN), likely an even more severe form of DSD.

Hereditary Neuropathy with Liability to Pressure Palsies   HNPP (also called *tomaculous neuropathy*) is an autosomal dominant disorder that produces an episodic, recurrent demyelinating neuropathy. HNPP typically develops during adolescence and may cause attacks of numbness, muscular weakness, and atrophy. Peroneal palsies, carpal tunnel syndrome, and other entrapment neuropathies are manifestations of HNPP. Motor and sensory NCVs are mildly reduced in affected patients as well as in asymptomatic gene carriers. Pathologic changes observed in HNPP include segmental demyelination and tomaculous, or sausage-like, formations in peripheral nerves. Because of mild overlap of clinical features with CMT1, HNPP patients may on occasion be misdiagnosed as having CMT1.

The HNPP locus maps to chromosome 17p11.2-12 and is associated with a 1.5-Mb deletion. The duplicated CMT1A chromosome (described earlier) and the deleted HNPP chromosome are the reciprocal products of unequal crossing-over during meiosis. In the case of HNPP, loss of a copy of the *PMP22* gene and underexpression of this critical myelin gene lead to demyelination. Most HNPP patients have the associated chromosome 17 deletion; however, rare patients with HNPP have been found to have point mutations in the *PMP22* gene. Molecular genetic testing is clinically available.

Treatment for HNPP is largely supportive. Surgical decompression of nerves has been proposed but is controversial. There is some evidence that surgical repair of carpal tunnel syndrome in HNPP is of little benefit and that transposition of the ulnar nerve at the elbow may produce poor results because the nerves are especially sensitive to manipulation and minor trauma.

CMT Neuropathy Type 2   CMT2 is less common than CMT1, and less progress has been made towards its molecular understanding. In general, CMT2 has a later age of onset, produces less involvement of the intrinsic muscles of the hands, and lacks palpably enlarged nerves. Extensive demyelination with "onion bulb" formation is not present in CMT2. Motor NCVs are normal or only slightly reduced in affected persons. A CMT2 locus was assigned by linkage studies to the short arm of chromosome 1 (1p35-36) and designated as CMT2A. One CMT2 pedigree was found to demonstrate linkage to markers from chromosome 3q13-q22 and has been designated CMT2B. Further genetic heterogeneity within CMT2 is likely as kindreds with the features of axonal neuropathy, weakness of the diaphragm, and vocal cord paralysis have been described and are designated as having CMT2C. Another form of CMT2, designated CMT2D, has been mapped to chromosome 7p14. More recently, in a large Russian pedigree a CMT2 gene was mapped to chromosome 8p21 (designated CMT2E) and a mutation was found in the neurofilament-light gene. Additionally, certain P_0 or connexin32 (Cx32, see below) mutations have been found to be the underlying genetic defect in a subset of patients with CMT1 or CMTX who were initially thought to have CMT2 because of only mild slowing of NCVs. DNA testing is not available for CMT2.

X-linked CMT Neuropathy   The clinical features of X-linked CMT disease (CMTX) include demyelinating neuropathy, absence of male-to-male transmission, and an earlier age of onset and faster rate of progression in males. NCVs vary widely in CMTX from nearly normal to moderately slowed. CMTX accounts for ~10% of all patients thought to have a form of demyelinating CMT (i.e., CMT1). CMTX should be suspected when the commonly associated chromosome 17 duplication is not present and there is no history of father-to-son transmission of the neuropathy.

The gene for CMTX maps to chromosome Xq13-21 and results from point mutations in the connexin32 (*Cx32*) gene. Connexin32 encodes a major component of gap junctions and is expressed in peripheral nerves. Cx32 is structurally similar to PMP22, as both of these proteins contain four putative transmembrane domains in similar orientation. Over 200 different mutations in the *Cx32* gene have been described in patients with CMTX, and the distribution pattern of these mutations suggests that all parts of the connexin32 protein are functionally important. DNA testing is clinically available for Cx32 mutations causing CMTX.

Cx32 has a pattern of expression in peripheral nerve similar to that of other myelin protein genes; however, immunohistochemical studies show a different localization. Unlike PMP22 and P_0, which are present in compact myelin, Cx32 is located at uncompacted folds of Schwann cell cytoplasm around the nodes of Ranvier and at Schmidt-Lanterman incisures. This localization suggests a role for gap junctions composed of Cx32 in providing a pathway for the transfer of ions and nutrients around and across the myelin sheath. Mutations in the Cx32 protein have been suggested to alter its cellular localization and its trafficking and interfere with cell-to-cell communication.

CMT Variants   Mutations in the putative zinc finger domain of the early growth response 2 gene (*EGR2*, or *Krox-20*) have been implicated as the underlying defect in CMT1 families that were found to be negative for the CMT1A duplication, as well as for mutations in either PMP22, P_0, or Cx32. Studies have shown that EGR2 acts as a direct transactivator of myelination genes in differentiating Schwann cells. EGR2 mutations have also been reported in a family with CHN.

Rare families with autosomal recessive motor and sensory neuropathy have been reported, particularly Tunisian families with parental consanguinity. Both demyelinating and axonal types of neuropathy have been described and given the designation CMT4. One form of autosomal recessive demyelinating neuropathy has been mapped to chromosome 8q13-q21 (CMT4A). Another form of CMT, characterized by focally folded myelin sheaths (CMT4B), has been mapped to chromosome 11q23 and recently shown to be caused by mutations in MTMR2, a gene encoding myotubularin-related protein-2, which is thought to be a transcriptional regulator. An additional pedigree with phenotypic features of CMT4B did not show linkage to chromosome 11 or to any other known CMT loci, implicating further genetic heterogeneity. Currently, DNA testing is not clinically available for any form of CMT4 or for mutations in EGR2.

Genetic Evaluation of CMT and HNPP   An approach for evaluating an individual patient suspected of having an inherited peripheral neuropathy is presented in Fig. 379-1. If a proband has evidence for CMT1, determination of NCVs is a useful screening tool for parents and other at-risk family members. The *CMT1* gene is penetrant in early life, and correct disease status can probably be determined with nerve conduction screening by age 5. However, if a proband's nerve conduction is normal or only mildly prolonged, the diagnosis may be CMT2. In this case the screening examination will need to focus on determination of motor unit amplitudes and other electrical signs of denervation. Rare patients have been found to have point mutations in either P_0 or Cx32 resulting in very mild demyelination and misclassification as CMT2.

The overwhelming proportion of CMT1 and CMT2 pedigrees have autosomal dominant inheritance. In pedigrees lacking male-to-male inheritance and/or those in which males are more severely affected

FIGURE 379-1 Evaluation of patients suspected of having an inherited peripheral neuropathy. CMT, Charcot-Marie-Tooth; HNPP, hereditary neuropathy with liability to pressure palsies. *(Modified from Lynch and Chance.)*

than females and have an earlier onset, CMTX should be suspected. Determination of autosomal dominant versus X-linked CMT is important as the genetic counseling for these two modes of inheritance is different. For any form of autosomal dominant CMT, the likelihood of an affected parent (of either sex) having an affected child is 50% for each pregnancy, regardless of the sex of the child. For CMTX, all daughters of an affected father will inherit the gene, and none of the sons will be affected. For a woman with CMTX, there is a 50% likelihood that her children will be affected regardless of their sex.

Sporadic cases in males can be especially difficult to evaluate, as the neuropathy could be nongenetic or the pattern of inheritance could be autosomal dominant, X-linked, or even autosomal recessive. Sporadic cases may also represent de novo duplications (CMT1A) or de novo deletions (HNPP). False paternity is another explanation for apparent sporadic CMT or HNPP.

Molecular genetic testing is currently available for the DNA duplication (or deletion) associated with CMT1A or HNPP and for point mutations in the *PMP22*, P_0 or *Cx32* genes associated with other forms of CMT1 and CMTX. ■

CHEMOTHERAPY IN PATIENTS WITH CMT Chemotherapeutic agents known to affect peripheral nerves should be used with great caution in patients with inherited neuropathies, and in the case of vincristine, total avoidance is strongly advised. A number of reports have documented the serious consequences of vincristine treatment administered in standard oncologic dosages in patients with CMT, including well-documented CMT1A and CMT2. The complications ranged from the precipitation of severe neuropathies in clinically asymptomatic at-risk individuals, through degrees of marked clinical worsening, and even death due to respiratory collapse.

OTHER INHERITED NEUROPATHIES

HEREDITARY SENSORY NEUROPATHIES Hereditary sensory neuropathies (HSN) are a heterogeneous group of disorders affecting sensory neurons. The most common form of HSN, HSN type

I, is an autosomal degenerative disorder of sensory and motor neurons. Phenotypically, distal sensory loss, distal muscle wasting and weakness, and variable neural deafness are observed. The disease involves progressive loss of dorsal root ganglion cells and axons in peripheral nerves. Age of onset is the second decade of life or later. The HSN-I locus maps to chromosome 9q22.1-q22.3. Because of the presence of muscular weakness in some patients with HSN, this disorder may be clinically confused with CMT.

FAMILIAL AMYLOID NEUROPATHY Familial amyloid polyneuropathy (FAP) is an autosomal dominant disorder that classically presents as progressive sensory peripheral neuropathy, with early involvement of the autonomic nervous system and an associated cardiomyopathy. Postmortem studies have shown extensive amyloid deposition in multiple organs throughout the body. Transthyretin (TTR) is the most common constituent amyloid fibril protein deposited in FAP. Several different point mutations in the TTR gene have been described in TTR-related FAP, and DNA testing for these mutations is clinically available. →*Amyloidosis is discussed in Chap. 319.*

REFSUM DISEASE This autosomal recessive disorder is characterized by a progressive sensorimotor demyelinating polyneuropathy, associated with cerebellar ataxia and retinitis pigmentosa. Neural deafness, cardiomyopathy, cataracts, and icthyosis are additional features. Onset is in late childhood or early adulthood. Patients often complain of night blindness as the earliest symptom. The CSF protein is typically elevated. Diagnosis is made by demonstration of elevated levels of phytanic acid (a 20-carbon branched-chain fatty acid) in the serum and urine. The disorder appears to be due to a deficiency of a peroxysomal enzyme, phytanic acid oxidase, responsible for alpha oxidation of phytanic acid. Therapy, consisting of avoidance of dietary sources of phytanic acid, and plasmapheresis in some cases, is partially effective.

BIBLIOGRAPHY

BOERKOEL CF et al: Molecular mechanisms for CMT1A duplication and HNPP deletion. Ann NY Acad Sci. 883:22, 1999

CHANCE PF: Overview of hereditary neuropathy with liability to pressure palsies in Charcot-Marie-Tooth Disorders. Ann NY Acad Sci 883:14, 1999

DYCK PJ et al: Hereditary motor and sensory neuropathies, in PJ Dyck et al (eds): *Peripheral Neuropathy*. Philadelphia, Saunders, 1993, pp 1094–1136

KAMHOLZ J et al: Charcot-Marie-Tooth disease type 1: Molecular pathogenesis to gene therapy. Brain 123:222, 2000

KELLER MP, CHANCE PF: Inherited neuropathies: From gene to disease. Brain Pathol 9: 327, 1999

LYNCH D, CHANCE PF: Inherited peripheral neuropathies. *Neurologist* 3:277, 1997

MENSIYANOVA IV et al: A new variant of Charcot-Marie-Tooth disease type 2 is probably the result of a mutation in the neurofilament-light gene. Am J Hum Genet 67:37, 2000

PAREYSON D: Charcot-Marie-Tooth disease and related neuropathies: Molecular basis for distinction and diagnosis. Muscle Nerve 22:1498, 1999

WARNER LE et al: Hereditary peripheral neuropathies: Clinical forms, genetics, and molecular mechanisms. (Review). Annu Rev Med 50:263, 1999

380   *Daniel B. Drachman*

MYASTHENIA GRAVIS AND OTHER DISEASES OF THE NEUROMUSCULAR JUNCTION

Myasthenia gravis (MG) is a neuromuscular disorder characterized by weakness and fatigability of skeletal muscles. The underlying defect is a decrease in the number of available acetylcholine receptors (AChRs) at neuromuscular junctions due to an antibody-mediated autoimmune attack. Treatment now available for MG is highly effective, although a specific cure has remained elusive.

PATHOPHYSIOLOGY In the neuromuscular junction (Fig. 380-1), acetylcholine (ACh) is synthesized in the motor nerve terminal

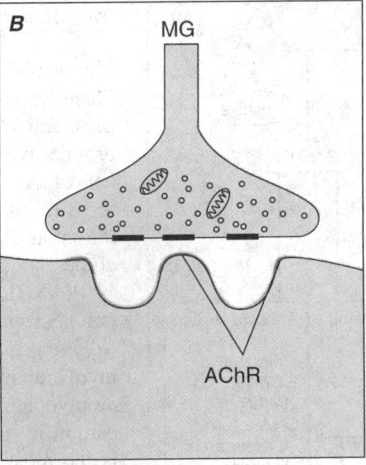

FIGURE 380-1 Diagrams of (*A*) normal and (*B*) myasthenic neuromuscular junctions. V, vesicles; M, mitochondria. See text for description of normal neuromuscular transmission. The MG junction shows a normal nerve terminal; a reduced number of AChRs (stippling); flattened, simplified postsynaptic folds, and a widened synaptic space.

and stored in vesicles (quanta). When an action potential travels down a motor nerve and reaches the nerve terminal, ACh from 150 to 200 vesicles is released and combines with AChRs that are densely packed at the peaks of postsynaptic folds. The structure of the AChR has been fully elucidated; it consists of five subunits (2α, β, δ, and γ or ϵ) arranged around a central pore. When ACh combines with the binding sites on the AChR, the channels in the AChRs open, permitting the rapid entry of cations, chiefly sodium, which produces depolarization at the end-plate region of the muscle fiber. If the depolarization is sufficiently large, it initiates an action potential that is propagated along the muscle fiber, triggering muscle contraction. This process is rapidly terminated by hydrolysis of ACh by acetylcholinesterase (AChE) and by diffusion of ACh away from the receptor.

In MG, the fundamental defect is a decrease in the number of available AChRs at the postsynaptic muscle membrane. In addition, the postsynaptic folds are flattened, or "simplified." These changes result in decreased efficiency of neuromuscular transmission. Therefore, although ACh is released normally, it produces small end-plate potentials that may fail to trigger muscle action potentials. Failure of transmission at many neuromuscular junctions results in weakness of muscle contraction.

The amount of ACh released per impulse *normally* declines on repeated activity (termed *presynaptic rundown*). In the myasthenic patient, the decreased efficiency of neuromuscular transmission combined with the normal rundown results in the activation of fewer and fewer muscle fibers by successive nerve impulses and hence increasing weakness, or *myasthenic fatigue*. This mechanism also accounts for the decremental response to repetitive nerve stimulation seen on electrodiagnostic testing.

The neuromuscular abnormalities in MG are brought about by an autoimmune response mediated by specific anti-AChR antibodies. The anti-AChR antibodies reduce the number of available AChRs at neuromuscular junctions by three distinct mechanisms: (1) accelerated turnover of AChRs by a mechanism involving cross-linking and rapid endocytosis of the receptors; (2) blockade of the active site of the AChR, i.e., the site that normally binds ACh; and (3) damage to the postsynaptic muscle membrane by the antibody in collaboration with complement. The pathogenic antibodies are IgG and are T cell dependent. Thus, immunotherapeutic strategies directed against T cells are effective in this antibody-mediated disease.

How the autoimmune response is initiated and maintained in MG is not completely understood. However, the thymus appears to play a role in this process. The thymus is abnormal in ~75% of patients with MG; in about 65% the thymus is "hyperplastic," with the presence of active germinal centers, while 10% of patients have thymic tumors (thymomas). Muscle-like cells within the thymus (myoid cells), which

bear AChRs on their surface, may serve as a source of autoantigen and trigger the autoimmune reaction within the thymus gland.

CLINICAL FEATURES MG is not rare, having a prevalence of at least 1 in 7500. It affects individuals in all age groups, but peaks of incidence occur in women in their twenties and thirties and in men in their fifties and sixties. Overall, women are affected more frequently than men, in a ratio of approximately 3:2. The cardinal features are *weakness* and *fatigability* of muscles. The weakness increases during repeated use (fatigue) and may improve following rest or sleep. The course of MG is often variable. Exacerbations and remissions may occur, particularly during the first few years after the onset of the disease. Remissions are rarely complete or permanent. Unrelated infections or systemic disorders often lead to increased myasthenic weakness and may precipitate "crisis" (see below).

The distribution of muscle weakness has a characteristic pattern. The cranial muscles, particularly the lids and extraocular muscles, are often involved early, and diplopia and ptosis are common initial complaints. Facial weakness produces a "snarling" expression when the patient attempts to smile. Weakness in chewing is most noticeable after prolonged effort, as in chewing meat. Speech may have a nasal timbre caused by weakness of the palate or a dysarthric "mushy" quality due to tongue weakness. Difficulty in swallowing may occur as a result of weakness of the palate, tongue, or pharynx, giving rise to nasal regurgitation or aspiration of liquids or food. In approximately 85% of patients, the weakness becomes generalized, affecting the limb muscles as well. The limb weakness in MG is often proximal and may be asymmetric. Despite the muscle weakness, deep tendon reflexes are preserved. If weakness of respiration becomes so severe as to require respiratory assistance, the patient is said to be in *crisis*.

DIAGNOSIS AND EVALUATION (Table 380-1) The diagnosis is suspected on the basis of weakness and fatigability in the typical distribution described above, without loss of reflexes or impairment of sensation or other neurologic function. The suspected diagnosis should always be confirmed definitively before treatment is undertaken; this is essential because (1) other treatable conditions may

Table 380-1 Diagnosis of Myasthenia Gravis (MG)

History
  Diplopia, ptosis, weakness
  Weakness in characteristic distribution
  Fluctuation and fatigue: worse with repeated activity, improved by rest
  Effects of previous treatments
Physical examination
  Ptosis, diplopia
  Motor power survey: quantitative testing of muscle strength
  Forward arm abduction time (5 min)
  Vital capacity
  Absence of other neurologic signs
Laboratory testing
  Anti-AChR radioimmunoassay: ~90% positive in generalized MG; 50% in ocular MG; definite diagnosis if positive; negative result does not exclude MG
  Edrophonium chloride (Tensilon) 2 mg + 8 mg IV; highly probable diagnosis if *unequivocally* positive
  Repetitive nerve stimulation; decrement of >15% at 3 Hz: highly probable
  Single-fiber electromyography: blocking and jitter, with normal fiber density; confirmatory, but not specific
  For ocular or cranial MG: exclude intracranial lesions by CT or MRI

NOTE: AChR, acetylcholine receptor; CT, computed tomography; MRI, magnetic resonance imaging.
SOURCE: From Drachman, 1994.

closely resemble MG, and (2) the treatment of MG may involve surgery and the prolonged use of drugs with adverse side effects.

Anticholinesterase Test Drugs that inhibit the enzyme AChE allow ACh to interact repeatedly with the limited number of AChRs, producing improvement in the strength of myasthenic muscles. Edrophonium is used most commonly, because of the rapid onset (30 s) and short duration (about 5 min) of its effect. An objective end-point must be selected to evaluate the effect of edrophonium. The examiner should focus on one or more unequivocally weak muscle groups and evaluate their strength objectively. For example, weakness of extraocular muscles, impairment of speech, or the length of time that the patient can maintain the arms in forward abduction may be useful measures. An initial dose of 2 mg of edrophonium is given intravenously. If definite improvement occurs, the test is considered positive and is terminated. If there is no change, the patient is given an additional 8 mg intravenously. The dose is administered in two parts because some patients react to edrophonium with unpleasant side effects such as nausea, diarrhea, salivation, fasciculations, and rarely syncope or bradycardia. Atropine (0.6 mg) should be drawn up in a syringe, ready for intravenous administration if these symptoms become troublesome.

False-positive tests occur in occasional patients with other neurologic disorders, such as amyotrophic lateral sclerosis, and in placebo-reactors. False-negative or equivocal tests also may occur. In some cases it is helpful to use a longer-acting drug such as neostigmine (15 mg given orally), since this permits more time for detailed evaluation of strength. In virtually all instances, it is desirable to carry out further testing to establish the diagnosis of MG definitively.

Electrodiagnostic Testing *Repetitive nerve stimulation* often provides helpful diagnostic evidence of MG. Anti-AChE medication is stopped 6 to 24 h before testing. It is best to test weak muscles or proximal muscle groups. Electric shocks are delivered at a rate of two or three per second to the appropriate nerves, and action potentials are recorded from the muscles. In normal individuals, the amplitude of the evoked muscle action potentials does not change at these rates of stimulation. However, in myasthenic patients there is a rapid reduction in the amplitude of the evoked responses of more than 10 to 15%. As a further test, a single dose of edrophonium may be given to prevent or diminish this decremental reaction.

Antiacetylcholine Receptor Antibody As noted above, anti-AChR antibodies are detectable in the serum of approximately 80% of all myasthenic patients, but in only about 50% of patients with weakness confined to the ocular muscles. The presence of anti-AChR antibodies is virtually diagnostic of MG, but a negative test does not exclude the disease. The measured level of anti-AChR antibody does not correspond well with the severity of MG in different patients. However, in an individual patient, a treatment-induced fall in the antibody level often correlates with clinical improvement.

Inherited Myasthenic Syndromes The *congenital myasthenic syndromes* (CMS) comprise a heterogeneous group of disorders of the neuromuscular junction that are not autoimmune, but rather are due to genetic mutations in which virtually any component of the neuromuscular junction may be affected. Alterations in function of the presynaptic nerve terminal, the various subunits of the AChR or AChE have

Table 380-2 The Congenital Myasthenic Syndromes

Type	Clinical Features	Electrophysiology	Genetics	Endplate Effects	Treatment
Slow channel	Most common; weak forearm extensors; onset 2d to 3d decade; variable severity	Repetitive muscle response on nerve stimulation; prolonged channel opening and MEPP	Autosomal dominant; α, β, ϵ AChR mutations	Excitotoxic end-plate myopathy; decreased AChRs; postsynaptic damage	Quinidine: decreases end-plate damage; made worse by Anti-AChE
Low-affinity fast channel	Onset early; moderately severe; ptosis, EOM involvement; weakness and fatigue	Brief and infrequent channel openings; opposite of slow channel syndrome	Autosomal recessive; may be heteroallelic	Normal end-plate structure	3,4-DAP; Anti-AChE
Severe AChR deficiencies	Early onset; variable severity; fatigue; typical MG features	Decremental response to repetitive nerve stimulation; decreased MEPP amplitudes	Autosomal recessive; ϵ mutations most common; many different	Increased span of end-plates; variable synaptic folds	Anti-AChE; ?3,4-DAP
AChE deficiency	Early onset; variable severity; scoliosis; may have normal EOM, absent pupillary responses	Decremental response to repetitive nerve stimulation	Mutant gene for AChE's collagen anchor	Small nerve terminals; degenerated junctional folds	Worse with Anti-AChE drugs

ABBREVIATIONS: AChR, acetylcholine receptor; AChE, acetylcholinesterase; EOM, extraocular muscles; MEPP, miniature endplate potentials; 3,4-DAP, 3-4-Diaminopyridine.

been identified in the various forms of CMS. These disorders share many of the clinical features of autoimmune MG, including weakness and fatigability of skeletal muscles, in some cases involving extraocular muscles (EOMs), lids, and proximal muscles, similar to the distribution in autoimmune MG. CMS should be suspected when symptoms of myasthenia have begun in infancy or childhood, and AChR antibody tests are consistently negative. Features of four of the most common forms of CMS are summarized in Table 380-2. Although clinical electrodiagnostic and pharmacologic tests may suggest the correct diagnosis, sophisticated electrophysiologic and molecular analysis are required for precise elucidation of the defect; this may lead to helpful treatment as well as genetic counseling. In the forms that involve the AChR, a wide variety of mutations have been identified in each of the subunits, but the ϵ subunit is affected in about 75% of these cases. In most of the recessively inherited forms of CMS, the mutations are heteroallelic; that is, *different* mutations affecting each of the two alleles are present.

Differential Diagnosis Other conditions that cause weakness of the cranial and/or somatic musculature include the nonautoimmune CMS discussed above, drug-induced myasthenia, Lambert-Eaton myasthenic syndrome (LEMS), neurasthenia, hyperthyroidism, botulism, intracranial mass lesions, and progressive external ophthalmoplegia. Treatment with *penicillamine* (used for scleroderma or rheumatoid arthritis) may result in true MG, but the weakness is usually mild, and recovery occurs within weeks or months after discontinuing its use. *Aminoglycoside antibiotics* in very large doses and *procainamide* can cause neuromuscular weakness in normal individuals or exacerbation of weakness in myasthenic patients.

LEMS is a presynaptic disorder of the neuromuscular junction that can cause weakness similar to that of MG. The proximal muscles of the lower limbs are most commonly affected, but other muscles may be involved as well. Cranial nerve findings, including ptosis of the eyelids and diplopia, occur in up to 70% of patients and resemble features of MG. However, the two conditions are readily distinguished, since patients with LEMS have depressed or absent reflexes, show autonomic changes such as dry mouth and impotence, and show incremental responses on repetitive nerve stimulation. It is now known that LEMS is caused by autoantibodies directed against P/Q type calcium channels at the motor nerve terminals, which can be detected in approximately 85% of LEMS patients. These autoantibodies result in impaired release of ACh from nerve terminals. A majority of patients with this syndrome have an associated malignancy, most commonly small cell carcinoma of the lung, which is thought to trigger the autoimmune response. The diagnosis of LEMS may signal the presence of the tumor long before it would otherwise be detected, permitting early removal. Treatment of the neuromuscular disorder involves plasmapheresis and immunosuppression, as for MG.

Neurasthenia may present with weakness and fatigue, but muscle testing usually reveals the "jerky release" or "give-away weakness" characteristic of nonorganic disorders, and the complaint of fatigue in these patients means tiredness or apathy rather than decreasing muscle power on repeated effort. *Hyperthyroidism* is readily diagnosed or excluded by tests of thyroid function, which should be carried out routinely in patients with suspected MG. Abnormalities of thyroid function (hyper- or hypothyroidism) may increase myasthenic weakness. *Botulism* can cause myasthenic-like weakness, but the pupils are often dilated, and repetitive nerve stimulation gives an *incremental* rather than decremental response. Diplopia that mimics the symptoms of MG may occasionally be due to an *intracranial mass lesion* that compresses nerves to the EOMs (e.g., sphenoid ridge meningioma), but magnetic resonance imaging (MRI) of the head and orbits usually reveals the lesion.

Progressive external ophthalmoplegia is a rare condition resulting in weakness of the EOMs, which may be accompanied by weakness of the proximal muscles of the limbs and other systemic features. Most patients with this condition have mitochondrial disorders that can be detected on muscle biopsy (Chaps. 67 and 383).

Search for Associated Conditions (Table 380-3) Myasthenic patients have an increased incidence of several associated disorders. *Thymic abnormalities* occur in ~75% of patients, as noted above. Neoplastic change (thymoma) may produce enlargement of the thymus, which is detected by computed tomography (CT) or MRI scanning of the anterior mediastinum. A thymic shadow on CT scan may normally be present through young adulthood, but enlargement of the thymus in a patient >40 years is highly suspicious of thymoma. *Hyperthyroidism* occurs in 3 to 8% of patients and may aggravate the myasthenic weakness. Tests of thyroid function should be obtained.

Table 380-3 Disorders Associated with Myasthenia Gravis and Recommended Laboratory Tests

Associated disorders
  Disorders of the thymus: thymoma, hyperplasia
  Other autoimmune disorders: thyroiditis, Graves' disease, rheumatoid arthritis, lupus erythematosus, skin disorders, family history of autoimmune disorder
  Disorders or circumstances that may exacerbate myasthenia gravis: hyperthyroidism or hypothyroidism, occult infection, medical treatment for other conditions (aminoglycoside antibiotics, quinine, antiarrhythmic agents)
  Disorders that may interfere with therapy: tuberculosis, diabetes, peptic ulcer, gastrointestinal bleeding, renal disease, hypertension, asthma, osteoporosis
Recommended laboratory tests or procedures
  CT or MRI of mediastinum
  Tests for lupus erythematosus, antinuclear antibody, rheumatoid factor, antithyroid antibodies
  Thyroid-function tests
  Tuberculin test
  Chest radiography
  Fasting blood glucose measurement
  Pulmonary-function tests
  Bone densitometry in older patients

SOURCE: From RT Johnson, JW Griffin (eds): *Current Therapy in Neurologic Disease,* 4th ed. St. Louis, Mosby Year Book, 1993, p 379.

Because of the *association of MG with other autoimmune disorders,* blood tests for rheumatoid factor and antinuclear antibodies should be carried out in all patients. Chronic infection of any kind can exacerbate MG and should be sought carefully. Finally, measurements of *ventilatory function* are valuable because of the frequency and seriousness of respiratory impairment in myasthenic patients.

Because of the side effects of glucocorticoids and other immunosuppressive agents used in the treatment of MG, a thorough medical investigation should be undertaken, searching specifically for evidence of chronic or latent infection (such as tuberculosis or hepatitis), hypertension, diabetes, renal impairment, and glaucoma.

℞ TREATMENT (Fig. 380-2) The prognosis has improved strikingly as a result of advances in treatment; virtually all myasthenic patients can be returned to full productive lives with proper therapy. The most useful treatments for MG include anticholinesterase medications, immunosuppressive agents, thymectomy, and plasmapheresis or intravenous immunoglobulin (IVIg).

Anticholinesterase Medications Anticholinesterase medication produces at least partial improvement in most myasthenic patients, although improvement is complete in only a few. There is no substantial difference in efficacy among the various anticholinesterase drugs;

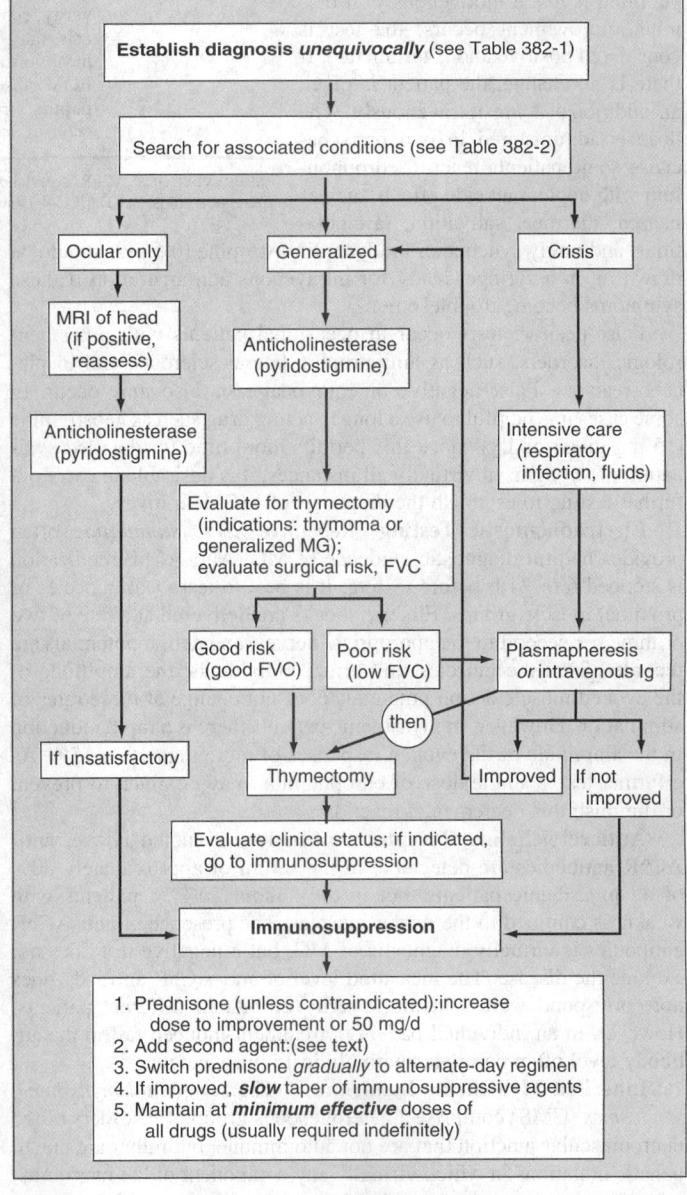

FIGURE 380-2 Algorithm for the management of myasthenia gravis. FVC, forced vital capacity.

oral pyridostigmine is the one most widely used in the United States. As a rule, the beneficial action of oral pyridostigmine begins within 15 to 30 min and lasts for 3 to 4 h, but individual responses vary. Treatment is begun with a moderate dose, e.g., 60 mg three to five times daily. The frequency and amount of the dose should be tailored to the patient's individual requirements throughout the day. For example, patients with weakness in chewing and swallowing may benefit by taking the medication before meals so that peak strength coincides with mealtime. Long-acting pyridostigmine tablets may help to get the patient through the night but should never be used for daytime medication because of their variable absorption. The maximum useful dose of pyridostigmine rarely exceeds 120 mg every 3 h during daytime. Overdosage with anticholinesterase medication may cause increased weakness and other side effects. In some patients, muscarinic side effects of the anticholinesterase medication (diarrhea, abdominal cramps, salivation, nausea) may limit the dose tolerated. In these cases, propantheline bromide may be used to block the autonomic side effects without altering the beneficial effects on skeletal muscle. Loperamide is useful for the treatment of diarrhea.

Thymectomy Two separate issues should be distinguished: (1) surgical removal of thymoma, and (2) thymectomy as a treatment for MG. Surgical removal of a thymoma is necessary because of the possibility of local tumor spread, although most thymomas are benign. In the absence of a tumor, the available evidence suggests that up to 85% of patients experience improvement after thymectomy; of these, ~35% achieve drug-free remission. However, the improvement is typically delayed for months to years. The advantage of thymectomy is that it offers the possibility of long-term benefit, in some cases diminishing or eliminating the need for continuing medical treatment. In view of these potential benefits and of the negligible risk in skilled hands, thymectomy has gained widespread acceptance in the treatment of MG. It is the consensus that thymectomy should be carried out in all patients with generalized MG who are between the ages of puberty and at least 55 years. Whether thymectomy should be recommended in children, in adults >55 years of age, and in patients with weakness limited to the ocular muscles is still a matter of debate. Thymectomy must be carried out in a hospital where it is performed regularly and where the staff is experienced in the pre- and postoperative management, anesthesia, and surgical techniques of total thymectomy.

Immunosuppression Immunosuppression using glucocorticoids, azathioprine, and other drugs is effective in nearly all patients with MG. The choice of drugs or other immunomodulatory treatments should be guided by the relative benefits and risks for the individual patient and the urgency of treatment. *It is helpful to develop a treatment plan based on short-term, intermediate-term, and long-term objectives. For example, if immediate improvement is essential either because of the severity of weakness or because of the patient's need to return to activity as soon as possible, plasmapheresis should be undertaken or intravenous immunoglobulin (IVIg) administered. For the intermediate term, glucocorticoids and cyclosporine generally produce clinical improvement within a period of 1 to 3 months. The beneficial effects of azathioprine and mycophenolate mofetil usually begin after many months (up to a year), but these drugs have advantages for the long-term treatment of patients with MG.* The side effects of each drug may preclude its use in some patients, as indicated below.

Assessment of patient's status In order to evaluate the effectiveness of treatment as well as drug-induced side effects, it is important to assess the patient's clinical status at baseline and on repeated interval examinations in a systematic manner. Because of the variability of symptoms of MG, the interval history as well as findings on examination must be taken into account. The most useful clinical tests

Myasthenia Gravis Worksheet

History

General	Normal	Good	Fair	Poor
Diplopia	None	Rare	Occasional	Constant
Ptosis	None	Rare	Occasional	Constant
Arms	Normal	Slightly limited	Some ADL impairment	Definitely limited
Legs	Normal	Walks/runs fatigues	Can walk limited distances	Minimal walking
Speech	Normal	Dysarthric	Severely dysarthric	Unintelligible
Voice	Normal	Fades	Impaired	Severely impaired
Chew	Normal	Fatigue on normal foods	Fatigue on soft foods	N-G tube
Swallow	Normal	Normal foods	Soft foods only	N-G tube
Respiration	Normal	Dyspnea on unusual effort	Dyspnea on any effort	Dyspnea at rest

Examination

BP_____ Pulse_____ Wt_____
Vital capacity_____
EOMS_____
Ptosis time_____
Edema_____
Face_____
Cataracts?   R_____   L_____

Arm abduction R_____ L_____
Deltoids   R_____ L_____
Biceps   R_____ L_____
Triceps   R_____ L_____
Grip   R_____ L_____
Iliopsoas   R_____ L_____
Quadriceps   R_____ L_____
Hamstrings   R_____ L_____

FIGURE 380-3 Abbreviated interval assessment form for use in evaluating treatment for myasthenia gravis.

include forward arm abduction time (up to a full 5 min), forced vital capacity, range of eye movements, and time to development of ptosis on upward gaze. Manual muscle testing or, preferably, quantitative dynamometry of limb muscles, especially proximal muscles, is also important. An interval form can provide a succinct summary of the patient's status and a guide to treatment results; an abbreviated form is shown in Fig. 380-3. A progressive reduction in the patient's AChR antibody level also provides clinically valuable confirmation of the effectiveness of treatment; conversely, a rise in AChR antibody levels warns that tapering of immunosuppressive medication may lead to clinical exacerbation. Reliable quantitative measurement of AChR antibody levels provides important information about the results of treatment. It is best to compare antibody levels from prior frozen serum samples with current serum in simultaneously run assays.

Glucocorticoid therapy Glucocorticoids, when used properly, produce improvement in myasthenic weakness in the great majority of patients. The initial dose of prednisone should be relatively low (15 to 25 mg/d) to avoid the early weakening that occurs in about one-third of patients treated initially with a high-dose regimen. The dose is increased stepwise, as tolerated by the patient (usually by 5 mg/d at 2- to 3-day intervals), until there is marked clinical improvement or a dose of 50 mg/d is reached. This dose is maintained for 1 to 3 months and then is gradually modified to an alternate-day regimen over the course of an additional 1 to 3 months; the goal is to reduce the dose to zero or to a minimal level on the "off day." Generally, patients begin to improve within a few weeks after reaching the maximum dose, and improvement continues to progress for months or years. The prednisone dosage may gradually be reduced, but usually months or years may be needed to determine the minimum effective dose, and close monitoring is required by patient and doctor. *Few patients are able to do without prednisone entirely.* Patients on long-term gluco-corticoid therapy must be followed carefully to prevent or treat adverse side effects. The most common errors in the steroid treatment of myasthenic patients include (1) insufficient persistence—improvement may be delayed and gradual; (2) too early, too rapid, or excessive tapering of steroid dosage; and (3) lack of attention to prevention and treatment of side effects. →*The management of patients treated with glucocorticoids is discussed in Chap. 331.*

Other immunosuppressive drugs Azathioprine, cyclosporine, mycophenolate mofetil, or occasionally cyclophosphamide is effective in many patients, either alone or in combination with glucocorticoid therapy. Azathioprine has been the most widely used of these drugs because of its relative safety in most patients and long track record. Its therapeutic effect may add to that of glucocorticoids and/or allow the steroid dose to be reduced. However, up to 10% of patients are unable to tolerate azathioprine because of idiosyncratic reactions consisting of flulike symptoms of fever and malaise, bone marrow depression, or abnormalities of liver function. An initial dose of 50 mg/d should be used to test for adverse side effects. If this dose is tolerated, it is increased gradually until the white blood count falls to approximately 3000 to 4000/μL. In patients who are receiving glucocorticoids concurrently, leukocytosis precludes the use of this measure. A reduction of the lymphocyte count to <1000/μL and/or an increase of the mean corpuscular volume of red blood cells may be used as indications of adequacy of azathioprine dosage. The typical dosage range is 2 to 3 mg/kg total body weight (including fat in obese patients). The beneficial effect of azathioprine takes at least 3 to 6 months to begin and even longer to peak.

Cyclosporine is approximately as effective as azathioprine and is being used increasingly in the management of MG. Its beneficial effect appears more rapidly than that of azathioprine. It may be used alone but is usually used as an adjunct to glucocorticoids to permit reduction of the steroid dose. The usual dose of cyclosporine is 4 to 5 mg/kg per day, given in two divided doses (to minimize side effects). Side effects of cyclosporine include hypertension and nephrotoxicity, which must be closely monitored. "Trough" blood levels of cyclosporine are measured 12 h after the evening dose. The therapeutic range, as measured by radioimmunoassay, is 150 to 200 ng/L.

Mycophenolate mofetil, which has been used for immunosuppression in transplant patients, is now proving useful in the treatment of MG. A dose of 1 g bid is recommended. Its mechanism of action involves inhibition of purine synthesis by the "de novo" pathway. Since lymphocytes lack the alternative "salvage" pathway that is present in all other cells, mycophenolate inhibits proliferation of lymphocytes but not proliferation of other cells. It does not kill or eliminate preexisting autoreactive lymphocytes, and therefore clinical improvement in autoimmune diseases such as MG may be delayed for many months to a year, until the preexisting autoreactive lymphocytes die spontaneously. The advantage of mycophenolate lies in its relative lack of adverse side effects, with only occasional production of diarrhea and rare development of leukopenia. This drug may become the choice for long-term treatment of myasthenic patients. Unfortunately, the present cost of mycophenolate may be prohibitively high.

Cyclophosphamide is reserved for occasional patients refractory to the other drugs, because of its relatively high risk of adverse side effects, including late development of malignancies.

Plasmapheresis and Intravenous Immunoglobulin Plasmapheresis has been used therapeutically in MG. Plasma, which contains the pathogenic antibodies, is mechanically separated from the blood cells, which are returned to the patient. A course of five exchanges (3 to 4 L per exchange) is generally administered over a 2-week period. Plasmapheresis produces a short-term reduction in anti-AChR antibodies, with clinical improvement in many patients. It is useful as a temporary expedient in seriously affected patients or to improve the patient's condition prior to surgery (e.g., thymectomy).

The indications for the use of IVIg are the same as those for plasma

exchange: to produce rapid improvement to help the patient through a difficult period of myasthenic weakness or prior to surgery. This treatment has the advantages of not requiring special equipment or large-bore venous access. The usual dose is 2 g/kg, which is typically administered over 5 days (400 mg/kg/per day). If tolerated, the course of IVIg can be shortened to administer the entire dose over a 3-day period. Improvement occurs in about 70% of patients, beginning during treatment, or within 4 to 5 days thereafter, and continuing for weeks to months. The mechanism of action of IVIg is not known; the treatment has no consistent effect on the measurable amount of circulating AChR antibody. Adverse reactions are uncommon, but include headache, fluid overload, and rarely renal shutdown.

The intermediate and long-term treatment of myasthenic patients requires other methods of therapy outlined earlier in this chapter.

Management of Myasthenic Crisis Myasthenic crisis is defined as an exacerbation of weakness sufficient to endanger life; it usually consists of respiratory failure caused by diaphragmatic and intercostal muscle weakness. Treatment should be carried out in an intensive care unit staffed with physicians experienced in the management of myasthenia gravis, respiratory insufficiency, infectious disease, and fluid and electrolyte therapy. The possibility that the deterioration could be due to excessive anticholinesterase medication ("cholinergic crisis") is best excluded by temporarily stopping anticholinesterase drugs. The most common cause of crisis is intercurrent infection. This should be treated *immediately*, because the mechanical and immunologic defenses of the patient can be assumed to be compromised. The myasthenic patient with fever and early infection should be treated like other immunocompromised patients. Early and effective antibiotic therapy, respiratory assistance, and pulmonary physiotherapy are essentials of the treatment program. As discussed above, plasmapheresis or IVIg is frequently helpful in hastening recovery.

BIBLIOGRAPHY

DRACHMAN DB: Myasthenia gravis: Medical progress. N Engl J Med 330:1797, 1994

——: Myasthenia gravis, in *The Autoimmune Diseases*, 3d ed, N Rose, I Mackay (eds). Orlando, FL, Academic, 1998, pp 637–662

——: The ten most frequently asked questions about myasthenia gravis. Neurologist 5: 350, 1999

ENGEL AG, et al: Congenital myasthenic syndromes: New insights from molecular genetic and patch-clamp studies. Ann N Y Acad Sci, 841:140, 1998

GAJDOS P: Intravenous immune globulin in myasthenia gravis. Clin Exp Immunol 197: 49, 1994

LENNON V: Serologic diagnosis of myasthenia gravis and the Lambert-Eaton myasthenic syndrome, in *Handbook of Myasthenia Gravis and Myasthenic Syndromes*, RP Lisak (ed). New York, Marcel Dekker, 1994, p 149

LINDSTROM JM: Acetylcholine receptors and myasthenia. Muscle Nerve 23:453, 2000

SANDERS DB: *Myasthenia Gravis and Myasthenic Syndromes.* Philadelphia, Saunders, 1994

381   *Jerry R. Mendell*

APPROACH TO THE PATIENT WITH MUSCLE DISEASE

Skeletal muscle diseases, or myopathies, are defined as disorders with structural changes or functional impairment of muscle. These conditions can be differentiated from other diseases of the motor unit by characteristic clinical and laboratory findings. →*Myasthenia gravis and related disorders are discussed in Chap. 380; inflammatory muscle diseases and inclusion body myositis in Chap. 382; muscular dystrophies and inherited, metabolic, and toxic myopathies in Chap. 383.*

CLINICAL FEATURES   **Muscle Weakness** Symptoms of muscle weakness can be either intermittent or persistent. Some patients complain of weakness that physicians more accurately classify as fatigue. Disorders causing intermittent weakness (Fig. 381-1) include myasthenia gravis, periodic paralyses (hypokalemic, hyperkalemic, and paramyotonia congenita), and metabolic energy deficiencies of glycolysis (especially myophosphorylase deficiency) and fatty acid utilization (carnitine palmitoyltransferase deficiency). The states of energy deficiency cause activity-related muscle breakdown accompanied by myoglobinuria, appearing as light-brown- to dark-brown-colored urine. Most muscle disorders cause persistent weakness (Fig. 381-2). In the majority of these, including most types of muscular dystrophy, polymyositis, and dermatomyositis, the proximal muscles are weaker than the distal, and the facial muscles are spared, a pattern referred to as *limb-girdle*. For other patterns of weakness the differential diagnosis is more restricted. Cranial innervated muscle weakness causing ptosis and extraocular muscle weakness without diplopia points to oculopharyngeal muscular dystrophy, mitochondrial myopathies, or myotubular myopathy. Facial weakness (difficulty with eye closure and impaired smile) and scapular winging (Fig. 381-3) are characteristic of facioscapulohumeral dystrophy. Facial and distal limb weakness associated with hand grip myotonia is virtually diagnostic of myotonic dystrophy. A pathognomonic pattern exclusive to inclusion body myositis includes loss of strength in both proximal and distal muscles, handgrip weakness, and wasting of quadriceps muscles. Less frequently, but important diagnostically, is the presence of a dropped head syndrome indicative of selective neck extensor muscle weakness. The most common neuromuscular diseases causing this pattern of weakness include myasthenia gravis, polymyositis, and amyotrophic lateral sclerosis. A final pattern, recognized because of preferential distal extremity weakness, is typical of a unique category of muscular dystrophy, the distal myopathies (Chap. 383).

It is important to examine functional capabilities to help disclose certain patterns of weakness (Table 381-1). The Gowers' sign (Fig. 381-4) is particularly useful. Observing the gait of an individual may disclose a lordotic posture caused by combined trunk and hip weakness, frequently exaggerated by toe walking (Fig. 381-5). A waddling gait is caused by the inability of weak hip muscles to prevent hip drop or hip dip. Hyperextension of the knee (genu recurvatum or backkneeing) is characteristic of quadriceps muscle weakness; and a steppage gait, due to footdrop, accompanies distal weakness.

Any disorder causing muscle weakness may be accompanied by fatigue, referring to an inability to maintain or sustain a force (pathologic fatigability). This condition must be differentiated from asthenia, a type of fatigue caused by excess tiredness or lack of energy (Fig.

381-2). Associated symptoms may help differentiate asthenia and pathologic fatigability. Asthenia is often accompanied by a tendency to avoid physical activities, complaints of daytime sleepiness, necessity for frequent naps, and difficulty concentrating on activities, such as reading. There may be feelings of overwhelming stress and depression. Thus, asthenia is not a myopathy. In contrast, pathologic fatigability occurs in disorders of neuromuscular transmission and in disorders altering energy production, including defects in glycolysis, lipid metabolism, or mitochondrial energy production. Pathologic fatigability also occurs in chronic myopathies because of difficulty accomplishing a task with less muscle. Pathologic fatigability is accompanied by abnormal clinical or laboratory findings. Fatigue without those supportive features almost never indicates a primary muscle disease.

Muscle Pain, Cramps, and Stiffness Muscle pain can be associated with involuntary muscle activity producing cramps, contractures, and stiff or rigid muscles (Chap. 22). In distinction, true myalgia (muscle aching), which can be localized or generalized, has no involuntary activity but may be accompanied by weakness, tenderness to palpation, or swelling. Certain drugs cause true myalgia (Table 381-2).

There are two painful muscle conditions of particular importance, neither of which is associated with muscle weakness. Fibromyalgia is a common, yet poorly understood type of myofascial pain syndrome. Patients complain of severe muscle pain and tenderness and have specific painful trigger points, sleep disturbances, and easy fatigability (Chap. 325). Polymyalgia rheumatica occurs in patients older than 50 years and is characterized by stiffness (without involuntary activity) and pain in the shoulders, lower back, hips, and thighs (Chap. 317). The erythrocyte sedimentation rate is elevated, and temporal arteritis may be present. Polymyalgia rheumatica is important to recognize because treatment with glucocorticoids can relieve discomfort and prevent the associated ischemic arteritis, which threatens vision.

Muscle cramps are painful, involuntary, localized, muscle contractions with a visible or palpable hardening of the muscle. They are abrupt in onset and short in duration, and they may cause abnormal posturing of the joint. The electromyogram (EMG) shows firing of motor units, reflecting an origin from spontaneous neurogenic activity. Muscle cramps are not a feature of most primary muscle diseases, although they occur commonly in Duchenne and related forms of mus-

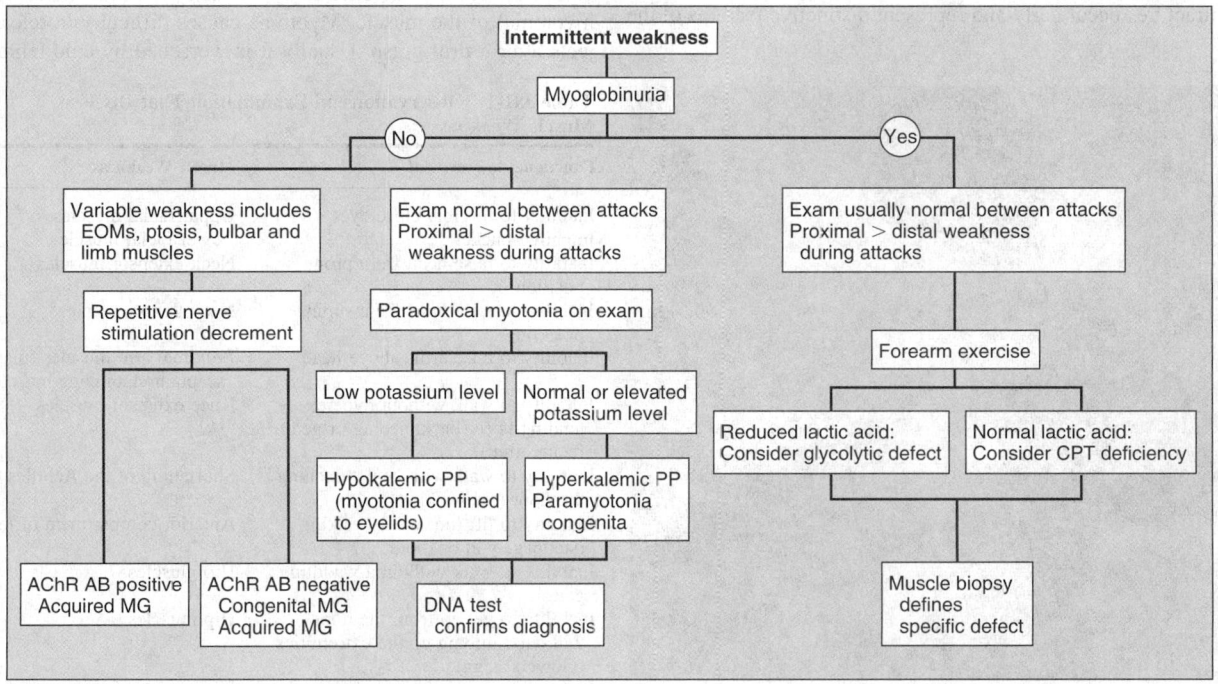

FIGURE 381-1 Diagnostic evaluation for intermittent weakness. EOMs, extraocular muscles; AChR AB, acetylcholine receptor antibody; PP, periodic paralysis; CPT, carnitine palmitoyltransferase; MG, myasthenia gravis.

FIGURE 381-2 Diagnostic evaluation for persistent weakness. EOM, extraocular muscle; OPMD, oculopharyngeal muscular dystrophy; FSHD, facioscapulohumeral muscular dystrophy; IBM, inclusion body myositis; DM, dermatomyositis; PM, polymyositis; MG, myasthenia gravis, ALS, amyotrophic lateral sclerosis; CK, creatine kinase.

cular dystrophy (Chap. 383). Muscle cramps more often accompany neurogenic disorders, especially motor neuron disease (Chap. 365), radiculopathies, and polyneuropathies (Chap. 377).

A muscle contracture is different from a muscle cramp. In both conditions, the muscle becomes hard, but a contracture is associated with energy failure in glycolytic disorders. The muscle is unable to relax after an active muscle contraction. The EMG shows electrical silence. Confusion is created because contracture also refers to a muscle that cannot be passively stretched to its proper length (fixed contracture) because of fibrosis. In some muscle disorders, especially Emery-Dreifuss muscular dystrophy and Bethlem myopathy (Chap. 383), fixed contractures occur early and represent distinctive features of the disease.

Muscle stiffness can refer to different phenomena. Some patients with inflammation of joints and periarticular surfaces feel stiff. This condition is different from the disorders of hyperexcitable motor nerves causing stiff or rigid muscles (Chap. 22). In *stiff-man syndrome* spontaneous discharges of the motor neuron of the spinal cord cause involuntary muscle contractions mainly involving the axial and proximal lower extremity muscles. Neuromyotonia (Isaac's syndrome) is another cause of motor nerve hyperexcitability.

Myotonia is a condition of prolonged muscle contraction followed by slow muscle relaxation. It always follows muscle activation, usually voluntary, but may be elicited by mechanical stimulation (percussion myotonia) of the muscle. Myotonia causes difficulty in releasing objects after a firm grasp. Usually it is worsened by cold temperatures

FIGURE 381-3 Facioscapulohumeral dystrophy with prominent scapular winging.

Table 381-1   Observations on Examination That Disclose Muscle Weakness

Functional Impairment	Muscle Weakness
Inability to forcibly close eyes	Upper facial muscles
Impaired pucker	Lower facial muscles
Inability to raise head from prone position	Neck extensor muscles
Inability to raise head from supine position	Neck flexor muscles
Inability to raise arms above head	Proximal arm muscles (may be only scapular stabilizing muscles)
Inability to walk without hyperextending knee (backkneeing or genu recurvatum)	Knee extensor muscles
Inability to walk with heels touching the floor (toe walking)	Shortening of the Achilles tendon
Inability to lift foot while walking (steppage gait or footdrop)	Anterior compartment of leg
Inability to walk without a waddling gait	Hip muscles
Inability to get up from the floor without climbing up the extremities (Gowers' sign)	Hip muscles
Inability to get up from a chair without using arms	Hip muscles

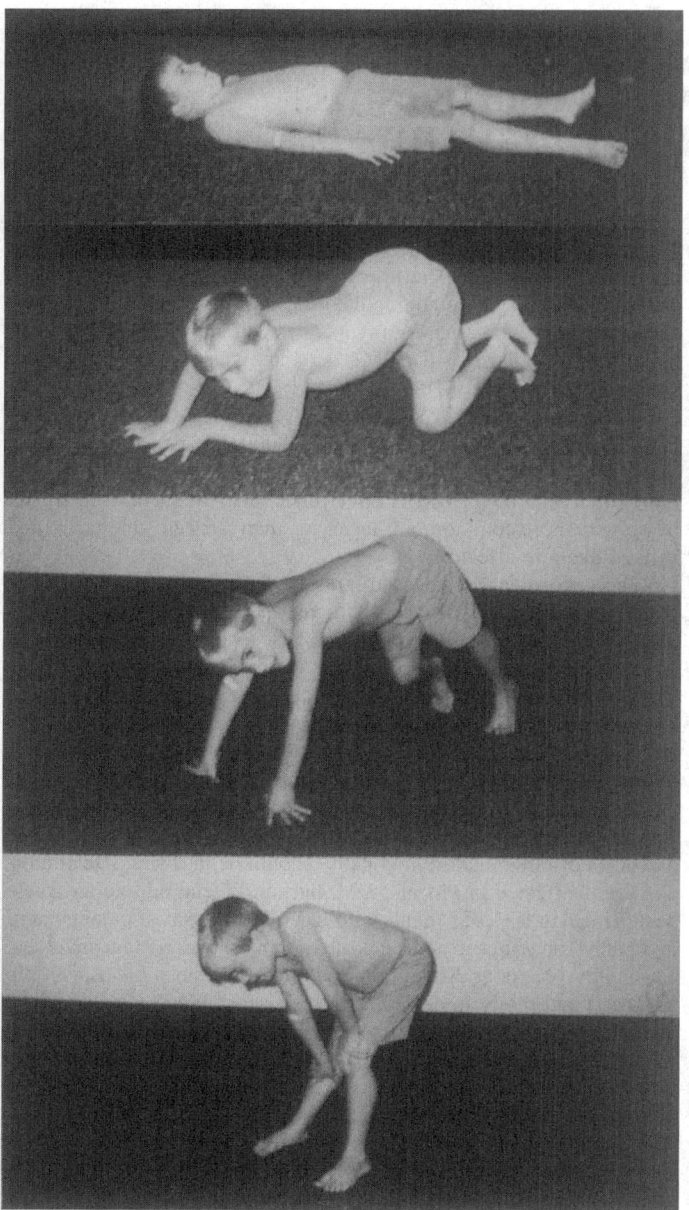

FIGURE 381-4   Gowers' sign showing a patient using arms to climb up the legs in attempting to get up from the floor.

FIGURE 381-5   Lordotic posture, exaggerated by standing on toes, associated with trunk and hip weakness.

and eases with continued activity. The sodium channelopathies (paramyotonia congenita and hyperkalaemic periodic paralysis) are accompanied by a unique phenomenon, paradoxical myotonia, in which repeated muscle contraction exacerbates the myotonia (Chap. 383). In hypokalemic periodic paralysis, myotonia of the eyelids may be present but limb muscles are usually spared.

Muscle Enlargement and Atrophy   In most myopathies muscle tissue is replaced by fat and connective tissue, but the size of the muscle is usually not affected. However, in Duchenne and Becker muscular dystrophies enlarged calf muscles are typical. In the patients with these forms of dystrophy, the enlargement represents true muscle hypertrophy. The calf muscles remain very strong even late in the course of the disease. The term "pseudohypertrophy" should be avoided when referring to these patients. Muscle enlargement can also result from infiltration by sarcoid granulomas, amyloid deposits, bacterial and parasitic infections, and focal myositis. A tendon rupture, especially a biceps brachii tendon, is a common cause of focal muscle enlargement.

LABORATORY EVALUATION   A limited battery of tests can be used to evaluate a suspected myopathy. Nearly all patients require serum enzyme level measurements and electrodiagnostic stud-

ies as screening tools to differentiate muscle disorders from other motor unit diseases. The other tests described—DNA studies, the forearm exercise test, and muscle biopsy—are used to diagnose specific types of myopathies.

Serum Enzymes   Creatine kinase (CK) is the preferred muscle enzyme to measure in the evaluation of myopathies. Damage to muscle causes the CK to leak from the muscle fiber to the serum. The MM isoenzyme predominates in skeletal muscle, while CK-MB is the marker for cardiac muscle. Serum CK can be elevated in normal individuals without provocation, presumably on a genetic basis or after strenuous activity, minor trauma (including the EMG needle), a prolonged muscle cramp, or a generalized seizure. Aspartate aminotransferase (AST), alanine aminotransferase (ALT), and lactic dehydrogenase (LDH) are enzymes sharing an origin in both muscle and liver. Problems arise when the levels of these enzymes are found to be elevated in a routine screening battery, leading to the erroneous assumption that liver disease is present when in fact muscle could be the cause. An elevated gamma-glutamyl transferase (GGT) helps to establish a liver origin since this enzyme is not found in muscle. Aldolase is often thought to be a muscle-specific enzyme but is also present in liver.

Electrodiagnostic Studies   EMG, repetitive nerve stimulation, and nerve conduction studies (Chap. 357) are essential methods for evaluation of the patient with suspected muscle disease. In combina-

Table 381-2   **Drugs That Cause True Myalgia**

Clofibrate	Emetine
Lovastatin	Labetalol
Gemfibrozil	Nifedipine
Vincristine	D-Penicillamine
Zidovudine	L-Tryptophan
Cyclosporine	Epsilon aminocaproic acid
Gold	Heroin
Danazol	Cocaine
Cimetidine	Methadone

tion they provide the information necessary to differentiate myopathies from neuropathies and neuromuscular junction diseases. Certain features of the EMG will point to an acquired, inflammatory muscle disorder (e.g., irritability on needle placement) versus a long-standing myopathic disorder that is more suggestive of a dystrophic process. The EMG can also be invaluable in helping to choose an appropriately affected muscle to sample for biopsy. The EMG can be used to fully characterize suspected involuntary activity seen during the examination, such as myokymia and myotonia.

DNA Analysis　Advances in molecular diagnosis have evolved over the past decade and now serve as important tools for diagnosis. Certain muscle disorders can be definitively diagnosed by DNA analysis; these are fully discussed in Chap. 383. Nevertheless, important limitations need to be mentioned in seeking a molecular diagnosis. For example, in some disorders, such as Duchenne and Becker dystrophies, two-thirds of patients have deletion- or duplication-mutations that are easy to detect, while the remainder have point mutations that are much more difficult to find. For patients without identifiable gene defects, the muscle biopsy remains the main diagnostic tool.

Forearm Exercise Test　In myopathies with intermittent symptoms, and especially those associated with myoglobinuria, there may be a defect in glycolysis. Many variations of the forearm exercise test exist. For safety, the test should not be performed under ischemic conditions to avoid an unnecessary insult to the muscle causing rhabdomyolysis. The test is performed by placing a small indwelling catheter into an antecubital vein. A baseline blood sample is obtained for lactic acid and ammonia. The forearm muscles are exercised by asking the patient to vigorously squeeze a sphygmomanometer bulb for 1 min. Blood is then obtained at intervals of 1, 2, 4, 6, and 10 min for comparison with the baseline sample. Normal controls must be established for each laboratory. A three- to fourfold rise of lactic acid is typical. The simultaneous measurement of ammonia serves as a control, since it should also rise with exercise. In patients with myophosphorylase deficiency or other glycolytic defects (Chap. 383), the lactic acid rise will be absent or below normal, while the rise in ammonia will reach control values. If there is lack of effort, neither lactic acid nor ammonia will rise. Patients with selective failure to increase ammonia may have myoadenylate deaminase deficiency. This condition has been reported to be a cause of myoglobinuria, but deficiency of this enzyme in asymptomatic individuals makes interpretation controversial.

Muscle Biopsy　Muscle biopsy analysis is an important step in establishing the final diagnosis of suspected myopathy. The microscopic evaluation uses a combination of techniques—histochemistry, immunocytochemistry with a battery of antibodies, and electron microscopy. Not all techniques need to be used on every case. A specific diagnosis can be established in many disorders. A combination of stains to identify mononuclear cells (polymyositis), complement (dermatomyositis), and amyloid (inclusion body myositis) help to distinguish the inflammatory myopathies. Mitochondrial and metabolic (e.g., myophosphorylase and acid maltase deficiencies) myopathies demonstrate distinctive histochemical and electron microscopic profiles. A battery of antibodies is available for the identification of missing components of the dystrophin-glycoprotein complex and related proteins to help diagnose specific types of muscular dystrophies. In addition, the congenital myopathies have distinctive histologic features essential for diagnosis.

BIBLIOGRAPHY

GRIGGS RC et al: Evaluation of the patient with myopathy, in *Evaluation and Treatment of Myopathies*, RC Griggs et al (eds). Philadelphia, FA Davis, 1995, pp 17–77

KINCAID JC: Muscle pain, fatigue, and fasiculations. Neurol Clin 15:697, 1997

WASIELEWSKI PG et al: Inherited neurologic disorders: Relevant considerations and new aspects, in Clinical Neurology, RJ Joynt, RC Griggs (eds). Philadelphia, Lippincott-Raven, 1996, pp 1–48

ZISMAN DA et al: Sarcoidosis presenting as a tumorlike muscular lesion. Medicine 78: 112, 1983

382

Marinos C. Dalakas, Jr.

POLYMYOSITIS, DERMATOMYOSITIS, AND INCLUSION BODY MYOSITIS

The inflammatory myopathies represent the largest group of acquired and potentially treatable causes of skeletal weakness. On the basis of well defined clinical, demographic, histologic and immunopathological criteria, the inflammatory myopathies can be classified into three major groups: polymyositis (PM), dermatomyositis (DM), and inclusion body myositis (IBM).

GENERAL CLINICAL FEATURES　The incidence of PM, DM, and IBM is approximately 1 in 100,000. PM is predominantly a disease of adults. DM affects both children and adults, and women more often than men. IBM is three times more frequent in men than in women, more common in Caucasians than African Americans, and is most likely to affect persons >50.

These disorders present as progressive and often symmetric muscle weakness. Patients usually report increasing difficulty with everyday tasks requiring the use of proximal muscles, such as getting up from a chair, climbing steps, stepping onto a curb, lifting objects, or combing hair. Fine-motor movements that depend on the strength of distal muscles, such as buttoning a shirt, sewing, knitting, or writing, are affected only late in the course of PM and DM, but fairly early in IBM. Falling is common in IBM because of early involvement of the quadriceps muscle with buckling of the knees. Ocular muscles are spared, even in advanced, untreated cases; if these muscles are affected, the diagnosis of inflammatory myopathy should be in doubt. Facial muscles are unaffected in PM and DM, but mild facial muscle weakness occurs in up to 60% of patients with IBM. In all forms of inflammatory myopathy, pharyngeal and neck-flexor muscles are often involved, causing dysphagia or difficulty in holding up the head (*neck drop*). In advanced and rarely in acute cases, respiratory muscles may also be affected. Severe weakness, if untreated, is almost always associated with muscle wasting. Sensation remains normal. The tendon reflexes are preserved but may be absent in severely weakened or atrophied muscles, especially in IBM where atrophy of the quadriceps and the distal muscles is common. Myalgia and muscle tenderness may occur in a small number of patients, usually early in the diseaese and more often in DM than in PM. Weakness in PM and DM progresses subacutely over a period of weeks or months and rarely acutely; by contrast, IBM progresses very slowly, over years, and its course may simulate late-life muscular dystrophies (Chap. 383) or slowly progressive motor neuron disorders (Chap. 365).

SPECIFIC FEATURES (Table 382-1)　**Polymyositis**　In most patients, the actual onset of PM is not easily determined, and patients typically delay seeking medical advice for several months. This is in contrast to DM, in which the rash facilitates early recognition (see below). PM is a subacute inflammatory myopathy affecting adults, and rarely children, who *do not have* any of the following: rash, involvement of the extraocular and facial muscles, family history of a neuromuscular disease, history of exposure to myotoxic drugs or toxins, endocrinopathy, neurogenic disease, muscular dystrophy, biochemical muscle disorder (deficiency of a muscle enzyme), or IBM as excluded by muscle biopsy analysis (see below). PM may occur either in isolation, in association with a systemic autoimmune or connective tissue disease, or with known viral or bacterial infection. D-Penicillamine and, on occasion, zidovudine (AZT) may also produce an inflammatory myopathy similar to PM.

Dermatomyositis　DM is a distinctive entity identified by a characteristic rash accompanying, or more often preceding, muscle weakness. The rash may consist of a heliotrope rash (blue-purple discoloration) on the upper eyelids with edema, a flat red rash on the face and upper trunk, and erythema of the knuckles with a raised violaceous scaly eruption (*Gottron rash*) that later results in scaling of the skin

Characteristic	Polymyositis	Dermatomyositis	Inclusion Body Myositis
Age at onset	>18 yr	Adulthood and childhood	>50 yr
Familial association	No	No	Yes, in some cases
Associated conditions			
Connective tissue diseases	Yes[a]	Scleroderma and mixed connective tissue disease (overlap syndromes)	Yes, in up to 20% of cases[a]
Other autoimmune diseases[b]	Frequent	Infrequent	Rare, but more frequently recognized
Malignancy	No	Yes, in up to 15% of cases	No
Viruses	Yes, with HIV, HTLV-I;[c] other viruses are uncertain	Unproven	Unproven (rare cases with HIV, HTLV-1)
Drugs[d]	Yes	Yes, rarely	No

[a] Systemic lupus erythematosus, rheumatoid arthritis, Sjögren's syndrome, systemic sclerosis, mixed connective tissue disease.

[b] Crohn's disease, vasculitis, sarcoidosis, primary biliary cirrhosis, adult celiac disease, chronic graft-versus-host disease, discoid lupus, ankylosing spondylitis, Behçet's syndrome, myasthenia gravis, acne fulminans, dermatitis herpetiformis, psoriasis, Hashimoto's disease, granulomatous diseases, agammaglobulinemia, monoclonal gammopathy, hypereosinophilic syndrome, Lyme disease, Kawasaki disease, autoimmune thrombocytopenia, hypergammaglobulinemic purpura, hereditary complement deficiency, IgA deficiency.

[c] HTLV-I, human T cell lymphotropic virus type I.

[d] Drugs include penicillamine (dermatomyositis and polymyositis), zidovudine (polymyositis), and contaminated tryptophan (dermatomyositis-like illness). Other myotoxic drugs may cause myopathy but not an inflammatory myopathy (see text for details).

(see Plates IIE-63 and IIE-65). The erythematous rash can also occur on other body surfaces, including the knees, elbows, malleoli, neck and anterior chest (often in a *V sign*), or back and shoulders (*shawl sign*), and may worsen after sun exposure. In some patients the rash is pruritic, especially on the scalp, chest, and back. Dilated capillary loops at the base of the fingernails are also characteristic. The cuticles may be irregular, thickened, and distorted, and the lateral and palmar areas of the fingers may become rough and cracked, with irregular, "dirty" horizontal lines, resembling *mechanic's hands*. The weakness can be mild, moderate, or severe enough to lead to quadraparesis. At times, the muscle strength appears normal, hence the term *dermatomyositis sine myositis*. When muscle biopsy is performed in such cases, however, significant perivascular and perimysial inflammation is seen. In children, DM resembles the adult disease, except for more frequent extramuscular manifestations, as discussed later. A common early abnormality in children is "misery," defined as an irritable child who appears uncomfortable, has a red flush on the face, is fatigued, does not wish to socialize, and has a varying degree of proximal muscle weakness. A tiptoe gait due to flexion contracture of the ankles is also common.

DM usually occurs alone but may overlap with scleroderma and mixed connective tissue disease. Fasciitis and thickening of the skin similar to that seen in chronic cases of DM have occurred in patients with the *eosinophilia–myalgia syndrome* associated with the ingestion of contaminated L-tryptophan.

Inclusion Body Myositis In patients ≥50, IBM is the most common of the inflammatory myopathies. It is often misdiagnosed as PM and suspected only retrospectively when a patient with presumed PM does not respond to therapy. Weakness and atrophy of distal muscles, especially foot extensors and deep finger flexors, occur in almost all cases of IBM and may be a clue to early diagnosis. Some patients present with falls because their knees collapse due to early quadriceps weakness. Others present with weakness in the small muscles of the

hands, especially finger flexors, and complain of inability to hold certain objects, such as golf clubs, or perform certain tasks, such as turning keys or tying knots. On occasion, the weakness and accompanying atrophy can be asymmetric and selectively involve the quadriceps, iliopsoas, triceps, biceps, and finger flexors, resembling a lower motor neuron disease. Dysphagia is common, occurring in up to 60% of IBM patients, and may lead to episodes of choking. Sensory examination is generally normal; some patients have mildly diminished vibratory sensation at the ankles that presumably is age-related. The distal weakness does not represent motor neuron or peripheral nerve involvement but results from the myopathic process affecting distal muscles. The diagnosis is always made by the characteristic findings on the muscle biopsy, as discussed below. Disease progression is slow but steady, and most patients require an assistive device such as cane, walker, or wheelchair within several years of onset.

In at least 20% of cases, IBM is associated with systemic autoimmune or connective tissue diseases. Familial aggregation has also been noted in coaffected siblings with typical IBM; such cases have been designated as *familial inflammatory IBM*. This disorder is distinct from *hereditary inclusion body myopathy* (h-IBM), which describes a heterogeneous group of recessive and less frequently dominant, inherited syndromes. The h-IBMs are noninflammatory myopathies with clinical profiles distinct from sporadic IBM. A subset of h-IBM that spares the quadriceps muscle has emerged as a distinct entity. This disorder, originally described in Iranian Jews and now seen in many ethnic groups, is linked to chromosome 9p1.

ASSOCIATED CLINICAL FINDINGS **Extramuscular Manifestations** In addition to the primary myopathy, a number of extramuscular manifestations may be present to a varying degree in patients with PM or DM:

1. *Systemic symptoms*, such as fever, malaise, weight loss, arthralgia, and Raynaud's phenomenon especially when inflammatory myopathy is associated with a connective tissue disorder.
2. *Joint contractures*, mostly in DM and especially in children.
3. *Dysphagia and gastrointestinal symptoms* due to involvement of the oropharyngeal striated muscles and upper esophagus. Dysphagia may be prominent in the active stages of DM and is frequent in IBM. Gastrointestinal ulcerations due to vasculitis and infection were common in children with DM before the use of immunosuppressive drugs.
4. *Cardiac disturbances*, including atrioventricular conduction defects, tachyarrhythmias, dilated cardiomyopathy, and low ejection fraction. Congestive heart failure and myocarditis may also occur, either from the disease itself or from hypertension associated with long-term use of glucocorticoids.
5. *Pulmonary dysfunction*, due to primary weakness of the thoracic muscles, drug-induced pneumonitis (e.g., from methotrexate), or interstitial lung disease may cause dyspnea, nonproductive cough, and aspiration pneumonia. Interstitial lung disease may precede myopathy or occur early in the disease, and develops in up to 10% of patients with PM or DM.
6. *Subcutaneous calcifications*, sometimes extruding on the skin and causing ulcerations and infections, are seen in DM, primarily in children.

Malignancies Although all the inflammatory myopathies can have a chance association with malignant lesions, especially in older age groups, the incidence of malignant conditions appears to be specifically increased only in patients with DM but not PM or IBM. The most common tumors associated with DM are ovarian cancer, breast cancer, melanoma, and colon cancer. The extent of the search that should be conducted for an occult malignant neoplasm in adults with DM depends on the clinical circumstances. Tumors in these patients are usually uncovered by abnormal findings in the medical history and physical examination and not through an extensive radiologic blind search. Thus the weight of evidence argues against performing expensive, invasive, and nondirected tumor searches. When a suspected malignancy is not apparent, a complete annual physical examination with pelvic, breast, and rectal examinations; urinalysis; complete blood count; blood chemistry tests; and a chest film should suffice.

Overlap The term *overlap syndrome* has been used loosely to describe the frequent association of inflammatory myopathies with connective tissue diseases. A well-characterized overlap syndrome occurs in patients with DM who also have manifestations of systemic sclerosis or mixed connective tissue disease, such as sclerotic thickening of the dermis, contractures, esophageal hypomotility, microangiopathy, and calcium deposits (Table 382-1). By contrast, signs of rheumatoid arthritis, systemic lupus erythematosus, or Sjögren's syndrome are very rare in patients with DM. Patients with the overlap syndrome of DM and systemic sclerosis may have a specific antinuclear autoantibody, the anti-PM/Scl, directed against a nucleolar-protein complex.

PATHOGENESIS An autoimmune origin of these disorders is supported by their association with other systemic autoimmune, viral, or connective tissue diseases; the presence of various autoantibodies; their association with histocompatibility genes; the evidence of T cell–mediated myocytotoxicity or complement-mediated microangiopathy; and their response to immunotherapies. However, the specific muscle or capillary target antigens have not been identified, and the agents initiating self-sensitization are still unknown.

Autoantibodies and Immunogenetics Various autoantibodies against nuclear antigens (antinuclear antibodies) and cytoplasmic antigens are found in up to 20% of patients with inflammatory myopathies. The antibodies to cytoplasmic antigens, present in <10% of PM and DM patients, are directed against cytoplasmic ribonucleoproteins, which are involved in translation and protein synthesis. They include antibodies against various synthetases, translation factors, and proteins of the signal-recognition particles. The antibody directed against the histidyl-transfer RNA synthetase, called *anti-Jo-1*, accounts for 75% of all the anti-synthetases and is clinically useful because up to 80% of patients with anti-Jo-1 antibodies have interstitial lung disease. Some patients with the anti-Jo-1 antibody may also have Raynaud's phenomenon, nonerosive arthritis, and the HLA antigens DR3 and DRw52. In both PM and IBM, there is an increased frequency (up to 75%) of haplotypes of DR3 (molecular designation DRB1*0301, DQB1*0201), suggesting that these alleles may be risk factors for the development of these disorders (Chap. 306).

Immunopathologic Mechanisms In DM, the endomysial infiltrates have a higher than normal percentage of B cells, a higher ratio of CD4+ cells (helper cells) to CD8+ cells (suppressor-cytotoxic T cells), proximity of CD4+ cells to B cells and macrophages, and a relative absence of lymphocytic invasion of nonnecrotic muscle fibers, all of which suggest a mechanism mediated primarily by humoral processes. The immune process is directed against microvascular antigens and is mediated by the complement C5b-9 membranolytic attack complex, resulting in necrosis of the endothelial cells, reduced numbers of endomysial capillaries, ischemia, muscle-fiber destruction often resembling microinfarcts, and inflammation. Larger intramuscular blood vessels may also be affected in the same pattern, leading to actual muscle infarction. Residual perifascicular atrophy reflects the endofascicular hypoperfusion that is prominent in the periphery of the fascicles. Complement activation is thought to trigger release of proinflammatory cytokines, induce expression of vascular cell adhesion molecule (VCAM)-1 and intracellular adhesion molecule (ICAM)-1 on endothelial cells, and facilitate migration of activated lymphoid cells to the perimysial and endomysial spaces.

In PM and IBM there is evidence not of microangiopathy and muscle ischemia, as in DM, but of an antigen-directed cytotoxicity mediated by CD8+ cytotoxic T cells. This conclusion is supported by the presence of CD8+ cells, which, along with macrophages, initially surround and eventually invade and destroy healthy, nonnecrotic muscle fibers that aberrantly express class I MHC molecules. MHC-I ex-pression, absent from the sarcolemma of normal muscle fibers, is probably induced by cytokines secreted by activated T cells and macrophages. The cytotoxic autoinvasive CD8+ T cells contain perforin and granzyme granules directed towards the surface of the muscle fibers and capable of inducing cell death. The infiltrating endomysial T cells appear to be clonally restricted, suggesting an antigen-driven T cell response. The putative antigens are more likely to be endogenous sarcolemmal or cytoplasmic self-proteins synthesized within the muscle, rather than endogenous viral peptides, because viruses have not been identified within the muscle fibers.

T cell–derived cytokines (interleukins 2, 4, and 5 and interferon γ), the macrophage-derived cytokines (interleukins 1 and 6 and tumor necrosis factor α), and adhesion molecules on leukocytes (L-selectin and integrins LFA-1, VLA-4) and their respective ligands on endothelial cells (GlyCAM-1, ICAM-1, VCAM-1) in patients with PM, DM, and IBM; these may facilitate the adhesion and transmigration of activated T cells through the endothelial cell wall. T cell metalloproteinases (MMP-2 and MMP-9) are also upregulated and may facilitate adhesion of T cells to muscle, enhancing cytotoxicity.

The Role of Nonimmune Factors in IBM In IBM, the presence of vacuoles, the amyloid-positive deposits within some vacuolated muscle fibers, the abnormal muscle mitochondria with mitochondrial DNA deletions, and the relative resistance of the disease to immunosuppressive therapies suggest that, in addition to the autoimmune component, there is also a degenerative process. Similar to Alzheimer's disease, the amyloid deposits in IBM are immunoreactive against amyloid precurser protein (APP), chymotrypsin, apolipoprotein E, and phosphorylated tau, but it is unclear whether these deposits directly contribute to disease pathogenesis or are secondary phenomena. The same can be said for the mitochondrial abnormalities, which may also be secondary caused by the effects of aging and upregulated cytokines.

Association with Viral Infections and the Role of Retroviruses Several viruses, including coxsackieviruses, influenza, paramyxoviruses, mumps, cytomegalovirus, and Epstein-Barr virus have been indirectly associated with chronic and acute myositis. For the coxsackieviruses, an autoimmune myositis triggered by molecular mimicry has been proposed because of structural homology between histidyl-transfer RNA synthetase that is the target of the Jo-1 antibody (see above) and genomic RNA of an animal picornavirus, the encephalomyocarditis virus. Very sensitive polymerase chain reaction (PCR) studies, however, have repeatedly failed to confirm the presence of such viruses in muscle biopsies from these patients.

The best evidence of a viral connection in PM and IBM is with the retroviruses. Monkeys infected with the simian immunodeficiency virus and humans infected with HIV and human T cell lymphotropic virus (HTLV) develop PM or, rarely, IBM. In humans infected with HIV or HTLV-1, an isolated inflammatory myopathy may occur as the initial manifestation of the retroviral infection or myositis may develop later in the disease course. Retroviral antigens have been detected only in occasional endomysial macrophages and not within the muscle fibers themselves, suggesting that persistent infection and viral replication within the muscle do not occur. Histologic findings in PM and IBM associated with HIV-1 and HTLV-1 infection are identical to retroviral-negative myositis, specifically CD8+ T cells and macrophages that invade or surround MHC-I antigen–expressing nonnecrotic muscle fibers. The development of PM or IBM in HIV-positive patients should be distinguished from a toxic myopathy related to long-term therapy with zidovudine, which is characterized by fatigue, myalgia, mild muscle weakness, and mild elevation of creatine kinase (CK). Zidovudine-induced myopathy, which generally improves when the drug is discontinued, is a mitochondrial disorder characterized histologically by the presence of numerous "ragged-red" fibers. Abnormal muscle mitochondria and depletion of the muscle mitochondrial DNA by zidovudine results from inhibition of γ-DNA polymerase, an enzyme found solely in the mitochondrial matrix.

DIFFERENTIAL DIAGNOSIS The clinical picture of skin rash and proximal or diffuse muscle weakness has few causes other than DM. However, proximal muscle weakness without skin involvement can be due to many conditions other than PM.

Subacute or Chronic Progressive Muscle Weakness This may be due to denervating conditions such as the spinal muscular atrophies or amyotrophic lateral sclerosis (Chap. 365). In addition to the muscle weakness, upper motor neuron signs in the latter aid in the diagnosis. The muscular dystrophies, such as those of Duchenne and Becker and the limb-girdle and facioscapulohumeral types, may be additional considerations (Chap. 383). However, the muscular dystrophies usually develop more slowly (over years rather than weeks or months) and rarely present after the age of 30. In rare patients it may be difficult, even with a muscle biopsy, to distinguish chronic PM from a rapidly advancing muscular dystrophy. This is particularly true of facioscapulohumeral muscular dystrophy, where interstitial inflammatory cell infiltration is commonly found early in the disease. Such doubtful cases should always be given an adequate trial of glucocorticoid therapy. Some metabolic myopathies, including glycogen storage disease due to myophosphorylase or acid maltase deficiency, lipid storage myopathies due to carnitine deficiency, and mitochondrial diseases produce muscle weakness, which is often associated with other characteristic clinical signs (Chap. 383); diagnosis rests upon histochemical and biochemical studies of the muscle biopsy. The endocrine myopathies such as those due to hypercorticosteroidism, hyper- and hypothyroidism, and hyper- and hypoparathyroidism require the appropriate laboratory investigations for diagnosis. Muscle wasting in patients with an underlying neoplasm may be due to disuse, cachexia, or rarely to a paraneoplastic neuromyopathy (Chap. 101).

Diseases of the neuromuscular junction, including myasthenia gravis or the Lambert-Eaton myasthenic syndrome, cause fatiguing weakness that also affects the eye and cranial muscles (Chap. 380). Repetitive nerve stimulation and single-fiber electromyography (EMG) studies aid in diagnosis.

Acute Muscle Weakness This may be caused by an acute neuropathy such as Guillain-Barré syndrome (Chap. 378) or a neurotoxin. When combined with painful muscle cramps, rhabdomyolysis, and myoglobinuria, it may be due to metabolic disorders including some of the glycogen storage diseases, such as myophosphorylase deficiency (McArdle's disease), carnitine palmityltransferase deficiency, and myoadenylate deaminase deficiency (Chap. 383). Acute viral infections may cause a similar syndrome. Several animal parasites, such as protozoa (*toxoplasma, trypanosoma*), cestodes (cysticerci), and nematodes (trichinae), may produce a focal or diffuse inflammatory myopathy known as *parasitic polymyositis. Staphylococcus aureus, Yersinia, Streptococcus,* or other anaerobic bacteria may produce a suppurative myositis, known as *tropical polymyositis,* or *pyomyositis.* Pyomyositis, previously rare in the west, is now seen in occasional AIDS patients. Other bacteria, such as *Borrelia burgdorferi* (Lyme disease) and *Legionella pneumophila* (Legionnaire's disease) may infrequently cause myositis.

Chronic alcoholics may develop a painful myopathy with myoglobinuria after a bout of heavy drinking; present with a painless acute hypokalemic myopathy, which is completely reversible; or show an asymptomatic elevation of serum CK and myoglobin. Acute muscle weakness with myoglobinuria may occur with prolonged severe hypokalemia or with hypophosphatemia and hypomagnesemia, often seen in chronic alcoholics and in patients on nasogastric suction receiving parenteral hyperalimentation.

Macrophagic Myofasciitis This distinctive inflammatory muscle disorder, recently described in France, presents as diffuse myalgias, fatigue, and mild muscle weakness. Muscle biopsy reveals pronounced infiltration of the connective tissue around the muscle (epimysium, perimysium, and perifascicular endomysium) by sheets of periodic acid–Schiff-positive macrophages and occasional CD8+ T cells. The CK or erythrocyte sedimentation rate is variably elevated. Most patients respond to glucocorticoid therapy, and the overall prognosis is favorable. Histologic involvement is focal and limited to sites of previous vaccinations, which may have been administered months or years earlier. This disorder, which to date has not been observed out-

side of France, has been linked to an aluminum-containing substrate used in vaccine preparation.

Drug-Induced Myopathies Penicillamine and procainamide may produce a true myositis resembling PM, and a DM-like illness has been associated with contaminated preparations of L-tryptophan. As noted above, zidovudine causes a mitochondrial myopathy. Other drugs may elicit a toxic noninflammatory myopathy that is histologically different from DM, PM, or IBM. The most common drugs are the cholesterol-lowering agents such as clofibrate, lovastatin, simvastatin, or provastatin, especially when combined with cyclosporine or gemfibrozil. Rhabdomyolysis and myoglobinuria have been associated with amphotericin B, ε-aminocaproic acid, fenfluramine, heroin, and phencyclidine. The use of amiodarone, chloroquine, colchicine, carbimazole, emetine, etretinate, ipecac syrup, chronic laxative use resulting in hypocalcemia, licorice, glucocorticoids, and growth hormone has also been associated with myopathy. Some neuromuscular blocking agents such as pancuronium, in combination with glucocorticoids, may cause the acute critical illness myopathy. A careful drug history is essential for diagnosis of these drug-induced myopathies, which do not require immunosuppressive therapy.

Pain on Movement and Muscle Tenderness A number of conditions including *polymyalgia rheumatica* and arthritic disorders of adjacent joints may enter into the differential diagnosis of inflammatory myopathy, even though they do not cause myositis (Chap. 317). The muscle biopsy is either normal or discloses type II fiber atrophy. Patients with *fibrositis* and *fibromyalgia* complain of focal or diffuse muscle tenderness, fatigue, and aching, which is sometimes poorly differentiated from joint pain. In other patients there may be minor signs of a collagen vascular disorder, such as an increased erythrocyte sedimentation rate, antinuclear antibody, or rheumatoid factor. Occasionally there is slight but transient elevation of the serum CK. The muscle biopsy is usually normal and the prognosis favorable. Many such patients show some response to nonsteroidal anti-inflammatory agents, though most continue to have indolent complaints. *Chronic fatigue syndrome,* which may follow a viral infection, can present with debilitating fatigue, fever, sore throat, painful lymphadenopathy, myalgia, arthralgia, sleep disorder, and headache (Chap. 384). These patients do not have muscle weakness, and the muscle biopsy is usually normal.

DIAGNOSIS The clinically suspected diagnosis of PM, DM, or IBM is confirmed by examining the serum muscle enzymes, EMG findings, and muscle biopsy (Table 382-2).

The most sensitive enzyme is CK, which in active disease can be elevated as much as 50-fold. Although the CK level usually parallels disease activity, it can be normal in some patients with active DM and is frequently normal or only slightly above normal in IBM, even from disease onset. CK may also be normal in patients with untreated, even active, childhood DM and in some patients with DM associated with a connective tissue disease, reflecting the concentration of the pathologic process in the intramuscular vessels and the perimysium. Along with the CK, the serum glutamic-oxaloacetic and glutamate pyruvate transaminases, lactate dehydrogenase, and aldolase may be elevated.

Needle EMG shows myopathic potentials characterized by short-duration, low-amplitude polyphasic units on voluntary activation and increased spontaneous activity with fibrillations, complex repetitive discharges, and positive sharp waves. Mixed potentials (polyphasic units of short and long duration) indicating a chronic process and muscle fiber regeneration are often present in IBM. These EMG findings are not diagnostic of an inflammatory myopathy but are useful to identify the presence of active or chronic myopathy and to exclude neurogenic disorders.

Magnetic resonance imaging is not routinely used for the diagnosis of PM, DM, or IBM. However, it may guide the location of the muscle biopsy in certain clinical settings.

Muscle biopsy is the definitive test for establishing the diagnosis of inflammatory myopathy and for excluding other neuromuscular dis-

Table 382-2 Criteria for Definite Diagnosis of Inflammatory Myopathies

Criterion	Polymyositis	Dermatomyositis	Inclusion Body Myositis
Muscle strength	Myopathic muscle weakness[a]	Myopathic muscle weakness[a,b]	Myopathic muscle weakness with early involvement of distal muscles[a]
Electromyographic findings	Myopathic	Myopathic	Myopathic with mixed potentials
Muscle enzymes	Elevated (up to 50-fold)	Elevated (up to 50-fold) or normal	Elevated (up to 10-fold) or normal
Muscle biopsy findings[c]	Diagnostic[d,e]	Diagnostic or nonspecific	Diagnostic[d,f]
Rash or calcinosis	Absent	Present and diagnostic[d,g]	Absent

[a] Myopathic muscle weakness, affecting proximal muscles more than distal ones and sparing eye and facial muscles, is characterized by a subacute onset (weeks to months) and rapid progression in patients who have no family history of neuromuscular disease, no endocrinopathy, no exposure to myotoxic drugs or toxins, and no biochemical muscle disease (excluded on the basis of muscle-biopsy findings).

[b] In some cases with the typical rash, the muscle strength is seemingly normal (*dermatomyositis sine myositis*); these patients often have new onset of easy fatigue and reduced endurance. Careful muscle testing may reveal mild muscle weakness.

[c] See text for details.

[d] An adequate trial of prednisone or other immunosuppressive drugs is warranted in probable cases. If, in retrospect, the disease is unresponsive to therapy, another muscle biopsy should be considered to exclude other diseases or possible evolution in inclusion body myositis.

[e] Probable polymyositis is present if muscle biopsy shows nonspecific myopathy without inflammation.

[f] Probable inclusion body myositis is present if muscle biopsy shows chronic nonspecific myopathy with inflammation but no vacuoles.

[g] If rash is absent but muscle biopsy findings are characteristic of dermatomyositis, diagnosis is definite.

eases. Inflammation is the histologic hallmark for these diseases; however, additional features are characteristic of each subtype.

In PM there are T cell infiltrates located primarily within the muscle fascicles (endomysially) and surrounding individual, healthy muscle fibers resulting in phagocytosis and necrosis. When the disease is chronic, connective tissue is increased and often reacts positively with alkaline phosphatase.

In DM the endomysial inflammation is predominantly perivascular or in the interfascicular septae and around, rather than within, the muscle fascicles. The intramuscular blood vessels show endothelial hyperplasia with tuboreticular profiles, fibrin thrombi (especially in children), and obliteration of capillaries. The muscle fibers undergo necrosis, degeneration, and phagocytosis, often in groups involving a portion of a muscle fasiculus in a wedgelike shape or at the periphery of the fascicle, due to microinfarcts within the muscle. This results in perifascicular atrophy, characterized by 2 to 10 layers of atrophic fibers at the periphery of the fascicles. The presence of perifascicular atrophy is diagnostic of DM, *even in the absence of inflammation.*

In IBM, the following occur: (1) intense endomysial inflammation with T cells invading muscle fibers in a pattern identical to (but often more severe) from that seen in PM; (2) basophilic granular deposits distributed around the edge of slitlike vacuoles (rimmed vacuoles); (3) loss of fibers, replaced by fat and connective tissue, and angulated or round fibers, scattered or in small groups; (4) eosinophilic cytoplasmic inclusions; (5) abnormal mitochondria characterized by the presence of ragged-red fibers and cytochrome-oxidase (COX)-negative fibers and supported by the presence of mitochondrial DNA deletions in up to 75% of patients; (6) tiny congophilic amyloid deposits within or next to the vacuoles, best visualized by Texas-red fluorescent optics; and (7) characteristic filamentous inclusions seen by electron microscopy in the vicinity of the rimmed vacuoles. Such filaments can be

seen in other vacuolar myopathies; thus they are not unique to IBM. Although demonstration of the filaments by electron microscopy was previously essential for the diagnosis of IBM, currently this is not absolutely necessary if all the other characteristic light-microscopic features, including amyloid deposits, are present.

In some patients with an acquired myopathy that fulfills the clinical criteria for PM or IBM, the muscle biopsy specimen may fail to confirm the suspected diagnosis; in such cases, a diagnosis of probable PM or probable IBM is assigned. An intramuscular inflammatory response around nonnecrotic muscle fibers is an invariable feature of both PM and IBM, and the absence of inflammation raises a critical question about the diagnosis. It is not unreasonable in such cases to obtain another muscle biopsy specimen from a different site. When the patient has the typical clinical phenotype of IBM but the muscle biopsy shows only features of chronic inflammatory myopathy without the typical vacuoles, the diagnosis of probable IBM is also appropriate.

Diagnostic criteria are summarized in Table 382-2. The diagnosis of PM is *definite* if a patient has an acquired, subacute myopathy fulfilling the exclusion criteria noted above, elevated CK levels, and a confirmatory muscle biopsy. The diagnosis of DM is *definite* if the characteristic rash is present, even if there is no inflammation in the muscle biopsy specimen. The diagnosis of IBM is *definite* when the characteristic histologic features are present in the muscle biopsy specimen from a patient with the appropriate clinical characteristics.

TREATMENT The goal of therapy is to improve muscle strength, thereby improving function in activities of daily living. When strength improves the serum CK falls concurrently; however, the reverse is not always true. Unfortunately, there is a common tendency to "chase" or treat the CK level instead of the muscle weakness, a practice that has led to prolonged and unnecessary use of immunosuppressive drugs and erroneous assessment of their efficacy. It is prudent to discontinue these drugs if, after an adequate trial, there is no objective improvement in muscle strength whether or not CK levels are reduced. Agents used in the treatment of PM and DM include:

1. *Glucocorticoids.* Oral prednisone is the initial treatment of choice; the effectiveness and side effects of this therapy determine the future need for stronger immunosuppressive drugs. High-dose prednisone, at least 1 mg/kg per day, is initiated as early in the disease as possible. After an initial period of 3 to 4 weeks, prednisone is tapered slowly over a period of 10 weeks to 1 mg/kg every other day. Then, if there is evidence of efficacy and no serious side effects, the dosage is further reduced by 5 or 10 mg every 3 to 4 weeks until the lowest possible dose that controls the disease is reached. The efficacy of prednisone is determined by an objective increase in muscle strength and activities of daily living, which almost always occurs by the third month of therapy. A feeling of increased energy or a reduction of the CK level without a concomitant increase in muscle strength is not a reliable sign of improvement. If prednisone provides no objective benefit after ~3 months of high-dose therapy, the disease is probably unresponsive to the drug and tapering should be accelerated while the next-in-line immunosuppressive drug is started. Although controlled trials have not been performed, almost all patients with true PM or DM respond to glucocorticoids to *some degree and for some period of time*; in general, DM responds better than PM.

The long-term use of prednisone may cause increased weakness associated with a normal or unchanged CK level; this effect is referred to as *steroid myopathy.* In a patient who previously responded to high doses of prednisone, the development of increased weakness may be related to steroid myopathy or to disease activity that either will respond to a higher dose of glucocorticoids or has become glucocorticoid-resistant. In these circumstances, the decision to raise or lower the prednisone dosage may be influenced by reviewing the patient's history of muscle strength (especially with respect to mobility), serum CK levels, and changes in medications during the preceding 2 months. In uncertain cases, the prednisone dosage can be adjusted arbitrarily;

2. *Immunosuppressive drugs*. Approximately 75% of patients ultimately require treatment with immunosuppressive drugs. Treatment is generally initiated when a patient fails to respond adequately to glucocorticoids after a 3-month trial, the patient becomes glucocorticoid-resistant, glucocorticoid-related side effects appear, attempts to lower the prednisone dose repeatedly result in a new relapse, or rapidly progressive disease with evolving severe weakness and respiratory failure develops.

Drug selection is largely empirical, with choices based on personal experience, relative efficacy, and safety. The following agents are commonly used: (1) *Azathioprine* is well tolerated, has few side effects, and appears to be as effective for long-term therapy as other drugs. The dose is up to 3 mg/kg daily. (2) *Methotrexate* has a faster onset of action than azathioprine. It is given orally starting at 7.5 mg weekly for the first 3 weeks (2.5 mg every 12 h for 3 doses), with gradual dose escalation by 2.5 mg per week to a total of 25 mg weekly. An important side effect is methotrexate pneumonitis, which can be difficult to distinguish from the interstitial lung disease of the primary myopathy associated with Jo-1 antibodies (described above). (3) *Cyclophosphamide* (0.5 to 1 g/m^2 intravenously monthly for 6 months) has limited success and significant toxicity. (4) *Chlorambucil* has variable results. (5) *Cyclosporine* has inconsistent and mild benefit. (6) *Mycophenolate mofetil* has recently shown some effectiveness.

3. *Immunomodulating procedures*. In a double-blind study of patients with refractory DM, intravenous immunoglobulin (IVIg) improved not only the strength and rash but also the underlying immunopathology. The benefit can be impressive but is short-lived ($\leq$8 weeks); repeated infusions every 6 to 8 weeks are required to maintain improvement. A dose of 2 g/kg divided over 2 to 5 days per course is recommended. A controlled double-blind study in PM is not yet completed, but uncontrolled observations suggest that IVIg is beneficial for some patients. Neither plasmapheresis or leukapheresis appears to be effective in PM and DM.

The following sequential empirical approach to the treatment of PM and DM is suggested: *Step 1*: High-dose prednisone; *step 2*: azathioprine or methotrexate; *step 3*: IVIg; *step 4*: a trial, with guarded optimism, of one of the following agents, chosen according to the patient's age, degree of disability, tolerance, experience with the drug, and the patient's general health: cyclosporine, chlorambucil, cyclophosphamide, mycophenolate. Patients with interstitial lung disease may benefit from aggressive treatment with cyclophosphamide.

Common pitfalls leading to failure of steroid or immunosuppressive treatment are inadequate initial dose of prednisone or cytotoxic drugs, short duration of therapy or quick tapering, early development of preventable side effects necessitating early discontinuation of prednisone, and wrong diagnosis. A patient with presumed PM who has not responded to any form of immunotherapy most likely has IBM or another disease. In these cases, a repeat muscle biopsy and a more vigorous search for the putative "other disease" are recommended. In addition to IBM, the most often misdiagnosed disorders are metabolic myopathy such as phosphorylase deficiency, a dystrophic process with endomysial inflammation resembling polymyositis, drug-induced myopathy, or an endocrinopathy.

Calcinosis, a manifestation of DM, is difficult to treat; however, new calcium deposits may be prevented if the primary disease responds to the available therapies. Diphosphonates, aluminum hydroxide, probenecid, colchicine, low doses of warfarin, calcium blockers, and surgical excision have all been tried without success.

IBM is resistant to immunosuppressive therapies. Prednisone together with azathioprine or methotrexate have been disappointing, but most experts try these agents for a few months in newly diagnosed patients. Because occasional patients may feel subjectively weaker after these drugs are discontinued, some clinicians prefer to maintain some patients on low-dose, every-other-day prednisone or weekly methotrexate in an effort to halt disease progression, even though there

is no objective evidence or controlled study to support this practice. In one double-blind study of IVIg in IBM, minimal benefit in up to 30% of the patients was found; the strength gains, however, were not of sufficient magnitude to justify the routine use of this drug. A second controlled trial combining IVIg with prednisone was ineffective in 36 IBM patients. Despite these disappointing results, many experts believe that a 2- to 3-month trial with IVIg may be reasonable for selected patients with IBM who experience rapid progression of muscle weakness or choking episodes due to worsening dysphagia.

PROGNOSIS Although accurate data from large series is not available, it is believed that the 5-year survival rate for treated patients with PM and DM is approximately 80%; death is usually due to pulmonary, cardiac, or other systemic complications. Patients severely affected at presentation or treated after long delays, those with severe dysphagia or respiratory difficulties, older patients, and those with associated cancer have a worse prognosis. DM responds more favorably to therapy than PM and thus has a better prognosis. Most patients improve with therapy, and many make a full functional recovery, which is often sustained with maintenance therapy. Up to 30% may be left with some residual muscle weakness. Relapses may occur at any time.

IBM has the least favorable prognosis of the inflammatory myopathies. Most patients will require the use of an assistive device such as a cane, walker, or wheelchair within 5 to 10 years of onset. In general, the older the age of onset in IBM, the more rapidly progressive is the course.

BIBLIOGRAPHY

ARGOV Z et al: Various types of hereditary inclusion body myopathies map to chromosome 9p1-q1. Ann Neurol 41:548, 1997

CALLEN JP: Dermatomyositis. Lancet 355:53, 2000

DALAKAS MC: Polymyositis, dermatomyositis, and inclusion-body myositis. N Engl J Med 325:1487, 1991

———: Molecular immunology and genetics of inflammatory muscle diseases. Arch Neurol 55:1509, 1998

———: Intravenous immunoglobulin in the treatment of autoimmune neuromuscular diseases: Present status and practical therapeutic guidelines. Muscle Nerve 22:1479, 1999

ENGEL AG et al: The polymyositis and dermatomyositis syndromes, in *Myology*, AG Engel, C Franzini-Armstrong (eds). New York, McGraw-Hill, 1994, pp 1335–1383

GHERARDI RK et al: Macrophagic myofasciitis: An emerging entity. Lancet 352:347, 1998

ILLA I et al: Immunocytochemical and virological characteristics of HIV-associated inflammatory myopathies: Similarities with seronegative polymyositis. Ann Neurol 39: 474, 1991

IOANNOU Y et al: Myositis overlap syndromes. Curr Opin Rheumatol 11:468, 1999

LEON-MONZON DM et al: Polymyositis in patients with HTLV-I: The role of the virus in the cause of the disease. Ann Neurol 36:643, 1994

MILLER FW et al: A randomized double-blind controlled trial of plasma exchange and leukapheresis in patients with polymyositis and dermatomyositis. N Engl J Med 326: 1380, 1992

OLDFORS A, LINDBERG G: Inclusion body myositis. Curr Opin Neurol 12:527, 1999

SIVAKUMAR K et al: An inflammatory, familial, inclusion body myositis with autoimmune features and a phenotype identical to sporadic inclusion body myositis: Studies in three families. Brain 120:653, 1997

383

Robert H. Brown, Jr., Jerry R. Mendell

MUSCULAR DYSTROPHIES AND OTHER MUSCLE DISEASES

The muscle disorders discussed in this chapter include diseases that cause acute, subacute, and chronic muscle weakness. Some cause pain in addition to or instead of weakness. →*Dermatomyositis and polymyositis are discussed in Chap. 382.*

HEREDITARY MYOPATHIES

Muscular dystrophy refers to a group of hereditary progressive diseases. Each type of muscular dystrophy has unique phenotypic and genetic features (Table 383-1).

DUCHENNE MUSCULAR DYSTROPHY   This X-linked recessive disorder, sometimes also called *pseudohypertrophic muscular dystrophy*, has an incidence of ~30 per 100,000 live-born males.

Clinical Features   Duchenne dystrophy is present at birth, but the disorder usually becomes apparent between ages 3 and 5. The boys fall frequently and have difficulty keeping up with their friends when playing. Running, jumping, and hopping are invariably abnormal. By age 5, muscle weakness is obvious by muscle testing. On getting up from the floor, the patient uses his hands to climb up himself (Gowers' maneuver). Contractures of the heel cords and iliotibial bands become apparent by age 6, when toe walking is associated with a lordotic posture. Loss of muscle strength is progressive, with predilection for proximal limb muscles and the neck flexors; leg involvement is more severe than arm involvement. Between ages 8 and 10 walking may require the use of braces; joint contractures and limitations of hip flexion, knee, elbow, and wrist extension are made worse by prolonged sitting. By age 12, most patients are wheelchair dependent. Contractures become fixed, and a progressive scoliosis often develops that may be associated with pain. The chest deformity with scoliosis impairs pulmonary function, which is already diminished by muscle weakness. By age 16 to 18, patients are predisposed to serious, sometimes fatal pulmonary infections. Other causes of death include aspiration of food and acute gastric dilation.

A cardiac cause of death is uncommon despite the presence of a cardiomyopathy in almost all patients. Congestive heart failure seldom occurs except with severe stress such as pneumonia. Cardiac arrhythmias are rare. The typical electrocardiogram (ECG) shows an increase net RS in lead V_1; deep, narrow Q waves in the precordial leads; and tall right precordial R waves in V_1. Intellectual impairment in Duchenne dystrophy is common; the average intelligence quotient (IQ) is approximately one standard deviation below the mean. Impairment of intellectual function appears to be nonprogressive and affects verbal ability more than performance.

Laboratory Features   Serum creatine kinase (CK) levels are invariably elevated to between 20 and 100 times normal. The levels are abnormal at birth but decline late in the disease because of inactivity and loss of muscle mass. Electromyography (EMG) demonstrates features typical of myopathy. The muscle biopsy shows muscle fibers of varying size as well as small groups of necrotic and regenerating fibers. Connective tissue and fat replace lost muscle fibers. A definitive diagnosis of Duchenne dystrophy can be established on the basis of dystrophin deficiency in a biopsy of muscle tissue or mutation analysis on peripheral blood leukocytes as discussed below.

GENETIC CONSIDERATIONS   Duchenne dystrophy is caused by a mutation of the gene that encodes dystrophin, a 427-kDa protein localized to the inner surface of the sarcolemma of the muscle fiber. The dystrophin gene is more than 2000 kb in size and thus is one of the largest identified human genes. It is localized to the short arm of the X chromosome at Xp21. At present, mutations of the gene can be identified (in approximately two-thirds of Duchenne patients) with a battery of cDNA probes. Deletions are not uniformly distributed over the gene, but rather are most common near the beginning (5' end) and middle of the gene. Deletion size does not correlate with severity of disease. Less often, Duchenne dystrophy is caused by a gene duplication or point mutation. Identification of a specific mutation allows for an unequivocal diagnosis, makes possible accurate testing of potential carriers, and is useful for prenatal diagnosis.

A diagnosis of Duchenne dystrophy can also be made by western

Table 383-1   Progressive Muscular Dystrophies

Type	Inheritance	Defective Gene/Protein	Onset Age (years)	Clinical Features	Other Organ Systems Involved
Duchenne	XR	Dystrophin	Before 5	Progressive weakness of girdle muscles Unable to walk after age 12 Progressive kyphoscoliosis Respiratory failure in 2d or 3d decade	Cardiomyopathy Mental impairment
Becker	XR	Dystrophin	Early childhood to adult	Progressive weakness of girdle muscles Able to walk after age 15 Respiratory failure may develop by 4th decade	Cardiomyopathy
Emery-Dreifuss	XR/AD	Emerin/Lamins A/C	Childhood to adult	Elbow contractures, humeral and peroneal weakness	Cardiomyopathy
Limb-girdle	AD/AR	Several (Table 383-2)	Early childhood to early adult	Slow progressive weakness of shoulder and hip girdle muscles	± Cardiomyopathy
Congenital	AR	Several (Table 383-3)	At birth or within first few months	Hypotonia, contractures, delayed milestones Progression to respiratory failure in some; static course in others	CNS abnormalities (hypomyelination, malformation) Eye abnormalities
Myotonic	AD	Expanded noncoding CTG repeat	Usually 2d decade May be infancy if mother affected	Slowly progressive weakness of face, shoulder girdle, and foot dorsiflexion	Cardiac conduction defects Mental impairment Cataracts Frontal baldness Gonadal atrophy
Facioscapulohumeral	AD	Deletion, distal 4q	Before age 20	Slowly progressive weakness of face, shoulder girdle, and foot dorsiflexion	Deafness Coats' (eye) disease
Oculopharyngeal	AD	Expansion, poly-A RNA binding protein	5th to 6th decade	Slowly progressive weakness of extraocular, pharyngeal, and limb muscles	—

ABBREVIATIONS: XR, X-linked recessive; AD, autosomal dominant; AR, autosomal recessive.

blot analysis of muscle biopsy specimens, revealing abnormalities on the quantity and molecular weight of dystrophin protein. In addition, immunocytochemical staining of muscle with dystrophin antibodies can be used to demonstrate absence or deficiency of dystrophin localizing to the sarcolemmal membrane. Carriers of the disease may demonstrate a mosaic pattern, but dystrophin analysis of muscle biopsy specimens for carrier detection is not reliable. ■

Pathogenesis Dystrophin is part of a large complex of sarcolemmal proteins and glycoproteins (Fig. 383-1). Dystrophin binds to F-actin at its amino terminus and to β-dystroglycan at the carboxyl terminus. β-Dystroglycan complexes to α-dystroglycan, which binds to laminin in the extracellular matrix (ECM). Laminin has a heterotrimeric molecular structure arranged in the shape of a cross with one heavy chain and two light chains, β1 and γ1. The laminin heavy chain of skeletal muscle is designated laminin α2. Peripheral to laminin in the ECM are collagen proteins IV and VI. Like β-dystroglycan, the

FIGURE 383-1 Dystrophin-associated protein complex. Dystrophin localizes to the cytoplasmic face of the membrane in a subsarcolemmal location. Dystrophin complexes with two transmembrane protein complexes, the dystroglycans and the sarcoglycans. The dystroglycans bind to the extracellular matrix protein laminin. The syntrophin complex and an isoform of nitric oxide synthase (nNOS) are shown in their presumed places in relation to the dystrophin-glycoprotein complex. Also shown are the transmembrane proteins caveolin-3 and α7 integrin that may respectively interact with nNOS and laminin. See text for further explanation.

transmembrane sarcoglycan proteins also bind to dystrophin; these five proteins (designated α- through ε-sarcoglycan) complex tightly with each other. More recently, other membrane proteins implicated in muscular dystrophy have been found to be loosely affiliated with constituents of the dystrophin complex. These include caveolin-3 and α7 integrin (Fig. 383-1).

The dystrophin-glycoprotein complex appears to confer stability to the sarcolemma, although the function of each individual component of the complex is incompletely understood. Deficiency of one member of the complex may cause abnormalities in other components. For example, a primary deficiency of dystrophin (Duchenne dystrophy) may lead to secondary loss of the sarcoglycans and dystroglycan. The primary loss of a single sarcoglycan (see "Limb-Girdle Muscular Dystrophy," below) results in a secondary loss of other sarcoglycans in the membrane without uniformly affecting dystrophin. In either instance, disruption of the dystrophin-glycoprotein complexes weakens the sarcolemma, causing membrane tears and a cascade of events leading to muscle fiber necrosis. This sequence of events occurs repeatedly during the life of a patient with muscular dystrophy.

℞ **TREATMENT** Glucocorticoids, administered as prednisone in a dose of 0.75 mg/kg per day, significantly slow progression of Duchenne dystrophy for up to 3 years. Some patients cannot tolerate glucocorticoid therapy; weight gain in particular represents a significant deterrent for some boys.

BECKER MUSCULAR DYSTROPHY This less severe form of X-linked recessive muscular dystrophy results from allelic defects of the same gene responsible for Duchenne dystrophy. Becker muscular dystrophy is approximately 10 times less frequent than Duchenne, with an incidence of about 3 per 100,000 live-born males.

Clinical Features The pattern of muscle wasting in Becker muscular dystrophy closely resembles that seen in Duchenne. Proximal muscles, especially of the lower extremities, are prominently involved. As the disease progresses, weakness becomes more generalized. Significant facial muscle weakness is not a feature. Hypertrophy of muscles, particularly in the calves, is an early and prominent finding.

Most patients with Becker dystrophy first experience difficulties between ages 5 and 15 years, although onset in the third or fourth decade or even later can occur. By definition, patients with Becker dystrophy walk beyond age 15, while patients with Duchenne dystrophy are typically in a wheelchair by the age of 12. Patients with Becker

dystrophy have a reduced life expectancy, but most survive into the fourth or fifth decade.

Mental retardation may occur in Becker dystrophy, but it is not as common as in Duchenne. Cardiac involvement occurs in Becker dystrophy and may result in heart failure.

Laboratory Features Serum CK levels, results of EMG, and muscle biopsy findings closely resemble those in Duchenne dystrophy. The diagnosis of Becker muscular dystrophy requires western blot analysis of muscle biopsy samples demonstrating dystrophin of reduced amount or abnormal size. Mutation analysis of DNA from peripheral blood leukocytes recognizes deletions and duplications of the dystrophin gene in 65% of patients with Becker dystrophy, approximately the same percentage as in Duchenne dystrophy. In both Becker and Duchenne dystrophies, the size of the DNA deletion does not predict clinical severity; however, in ~95% of patients with Becker dystrophy, the DNA deletion does not alter the translational reading frame of messenger RNA. These "in-frame" mutations allow for production of some dystrophin, which accounts for the presence of altered rather than absent dystrophin on western blot analysis.

℞ **TREATMENT** The use of glucocorticoids has not been adequately studied in Becker dystrophy.

LIMB-GIRDLE MUSCULAR DYSTROPHY The syndrome of limb-girdle muscular dystrophy (LGMD) represents more than one disorder.

Clinical Features Muscle weakness affects both males and females, with onset ranging from late in the first decade to the fourth decade. Most LGMDs are progressive and affect primarily the pelvic and shoulder girdle muscles. Respiratory insufficiency from weakness of the diaphragm may occur. The distribution of weakness and rate of progression vary from family to family. Similar to the dystrophinopathies, cardiac involvement may result in congestive heart failure or arrhythmias; occasional patients present with a cardiomyopathy. Intellectual function remains normal.

Laboratory Features An elevated serum CK level, myopathic EMG findings, and muscle biopsy features indicative of myopathy are characteristic. Careful attention is required to exclude phenotypically similar disorders, such as spinal muscular atrophy (Chap. 365), inflammatory myopathies (Chap. 382), and metabolic myopathies (see below). The availability of western blot analysis for dystrophin allows LGMD to be distinguished unequivocally from Becker and Duchenne muscular dystrophies.

§ **GENETIC CONSIDERATIONS**   LGMD may be transmitted by autosomal dominant or autosomal recessive inheritance. In a new genetic classification, *LGMD1* refers to the dominantly inherited form and *LGMD2* to the recessively inherited form. Genetic linkage has identified three dominantly inherited disorders, LGMD1A–C. The recessively inherited forms of LGMD now number eight. In each case genetic linkage has been established; the specific protein deficiency is known for most forms (Table 383-2 and Fig. 383-1). In LGMD2A the defect lies in a muscle-specific, calcium-activated neutral protease, calpain 3. LGMD2B arises from defects in dysferlin, a novel, membrane-associated muscle protein. Four sarcoglycans (α-δ) are deficient in LGMD2C–F. ■

℞ **TREATMENT**   At present, only supportive care can be offered. Long leg braces are useful for affected children but seldom helpful for adults. Wheelchairs may be essential or may be used to help preserve energy for work or recreational activities. Cardiac or respiratory muscle involvement may require individualized treatment. Studies of primary genetic therapy in LGMD are currently in progress.

EMERY-DREIFUSS MUSCULAR DYSTROPHY   This disorder is characterized by childhood onset of contractures at the elbows, weakness in the humeral and peroneal muscles, and cardiomyopathy. The contractures may precede the weakness. As the disease progresses, the weakness may spread to involve the proximal limb-girdle muscles. Perhaps the most critical clinical aspect of Emery-Dreifuss muscular dystrophy (EDMD) is the cardiomyopathy, which may appear as conduction defects of abrupt onset. Sudden death is not uncommon in EDMD, even in otherwise unaffected female carriers; early use of pacemakers may be lifesaving.

Most cases of EDMD are X-linked, arising because of defects in a gene encoding emerin, a nuclear membrane protein. Another group is inherited as autosomal dominant traits. In these instances the molecular defects are in the gene located on chromosome 1, encoding the proteins lamin A and lamin C. These proteins are splice variants that localize to the nuclear envelope where, in some cells, they co-localize with emerin.

CONGENITAL MUSCULAR DYSTROPHY   This rare autosomal recessive disorder includes at least six subgroups with overlapping clinical features. Variable involvement of the brain and eyes can help differentiate these conditions; three have been mapped to specific chromosomes, with a specific defect identified in each (Table 383-3). All the forms of congenital muscular dystrophy present at birth or in the first few months of life with hypotonia and proximal limb weakness. Varying degrees of joint contractures at the elbows, hips, knees, and ankles are seen in most patients. Contractures present at birth are referred to as *arthrogryposis*. Weakness of facial muscles may occur, but other cranial nerve musculature is spared. Severity varies greatly, but about half of affected individuals never achieve the

Table 383-2   Limb-Girdle Muscular Dystrophies

Disease	Chromosomal Location	Defective Gene/Protein	Protein Size (kDa)
Autosomal Dominant			
LGMD1A	5q	Unknown	Unknown
LGMD1B	1q11–21	Lamins A and C	70
LGMD1C	3p25	Caveolin-3	24
Autosomal Recessive			
LGMD2A	15q15	Calpain-3	95
LGMD2B	2p13	Dysferlin	200
LGMD2C	13q12	γ-Sarcoglycan	35
LGMD2D	17q21	α-Sarcoglycan	50
LGMD2E	4q12	β-Sarcoglycan	43
LGMD2F	5q33	δ-Sarcoglycan	35
LGMD2G	17q11–12	Telethonin	19
LGMD2H	9q31–33	Unknown	Unknown

Table 383-3   Congenital Muscular Dystrophies

Type	Inheritance	Chromosome	Defective Gene/Protein
Laminin α2 chain deficiency	AR	6q22–23	Laminin α2 chain
α7 integrin deficiency	AR	12q13	α7 integrin
Fukuyama CMD	AR	9q31–33	Fukutin
Walker-Warburg syndrome	AR	Unknown	Unknown
Muscle-eye-brain disease	AR	Unknown	Unknown
Unlinked CMD	AR	Unknown	Unknown

ABBREVIATIONS: AR, autosomal recessive; CMD, congenital muscular dystrophy.

ability to stand independently. Death may ensue because of respiratory insufficiency early in life. Some patients learn to walk, although difficulty in motor activities (e.g., running) persists.

In patients with a deficiency of laminin α2 (formerly called merosin), diffuse white matter changes typical of hypomyelination are seen by magnetic resonance imaging. The clinical manifestations of the cerebral hypomyelination are mild, with learning disability as the most severe problem. In *Fukuyama congenital muscular dystrophy*, found mainly in Japan, patients are severely disabled and mentally retarded; most have seizures and die by age 20. Microcephaly and enlarged ventricles occur. Micropolygyria is common. The primary defect in this dystrophy is in the gene encoding fukutin, a secreted protein whose function remains ill-defined. In some patients, the fukutin gene is disrupted by insertion of a transposon, a novel pathogenetic mechanism. Recently, it has been reported that a form of congenital muscular dystrophy arises from the absence of α7 integrin, a muscle membrane protein.

MYOTONIC DYSTROPHY   This disorder, the most common adult muscular dystrophy, has an incidence of 13.5 per 100,000 live births and affects males and females equally.

Clinical Features   The clinical expression of myotonic dystrophy varies widely and involves many systems other than muscle. Affected patients have a typical "hatchet-faced" appearance due to temporalis, masseter, and facial muscle atrophy and weakness. Neck muscles, including flexors and sternocleidomastoids, and distal limb muscles are involved early. Weakness of wrist extensors, finger extensors, and intrinsic hand muscles impairs function. Ankle dorsiflexor weakness may cause footdrop. Proximal muscles remain stronger throughout the course, although preferential atrophy and weakness of quadriceps muscles occur in many patients. Palatal, pharyngeal, and tongue involvement produce a dysarthric speech, nasal voice, and swallowing problems. Some patients have diaphragm and intercostal muscle weakness, resulting in respiratory insufficiency.

Myotonia, which usually appears by age 5, is demonstrable by percussion of the thenar eminence, the tongue, and wrist extensor muscles. Myotonia causes a slow relaxation of hand grip after a forced voluntary closure. Advanced muscle wasting makes myotonia more difficult to detect.

Congenital myotonic dystrophy is a more severe form of the disease and occurs in ~25% of infants of affected mothers. It is characterized by severe facial and bulbar weakness and transient neonatal respiratory insufficiency.

Cardiac disturbances occur in most patients with myotonic dystrophy. ECG abnormalities are common, including first-degree heart block and more extensive conduction system involvement. Complete heart block and sudden death can occur. Congestive heart failure occurs infrequently but may result from cor pulmonale secondary to respiratory failure. Mitral valve prolapse also occurs commonly.

Other features associated with myotonic dystrophy include intellectual impairment, hypersomnia, posterior subcapsular cataracts, frontal baldness, gonadal atrophy, insulin resistance, and decreased esophageal and colonic motility.

Laboratory Features The diagnosis of myotonic dystrophy can usually be made on the basis of clinical findings. Serum CK levels may be normal or mildly elevated. EMG evidence of myotonia is present in most cases. Muscle biopsy shows muscle atrophy, which selectively involves type 1 fibers in 50% of cases. Typically, increased numbers of central nuclei can be seen. Necrosis of muscle fibers and increased connective tissue, common in other muscular dystrophies, do not usually occur in myotonic dystrophy.

GENETIC CONSIDERATIONS Myotonic dystrophy is an autosomal dominant disorder. New mutations do not appear to contribute to the pool of affected individuals. The disorder is transmitted by an intronic mutation consisting of an unstable expansion of a CTG trinucleotide repeat sequence at 19q13.3. An increase in the severity of the disease phenotype in successive generations (genetic anticipation) is accompanied by an increase in the number of trinucleotide repeats. A similar type of mutation has been identified in fragile X syndrome (Chap. 359). The unstable triplet repeat in myotonic dystrophy can be used for prenatal diagnosis. Congenital disease occurs almost exclusively in infants born to affected mothers; it is possible that sperm with greatly expanded triplet repeats do not function well.

How the CTG expansions impair function of muscle and other cells is not understood. They may alter expression of an adjacent protein kinase gene or of other neighboring genes. Alternatively, the expanded CTG might act as a sink that binds and inactivates important RNA binding proteins.

A subset of patients with multisystemic disease features similar to myotonic dystrophy do not have the diagnostic CTG expansion. Their weakness tends to be proximal rather than distal. This condition, termed proximal myotonic myopathy (PROMM), is genetically distinct from myotonic dystrophy. ■

TREATMENT The myotonia in myotonic dystrophy rarely warrants treatment. Phenytoin is the preferred agent for the occasional patient who requires an antimyotonia drug; other agents, particularly quinine and procainamide, may worsen cardiac conduction. Cardiac pacemaker insertion should be considered for patients with unexplained syncope or advanced conduction system abnormalities with evidence of second-degree heart block, or trifascicular conduction disturbances with marked prolongation of the PR interval. Molded ankle-foot orthoses help prevent footdrop in patients with distal lower extremity weakness.

FACIOSCAPULOHUMERAL MUSCULAR DYSTROPHY

This form of muscular dystrophy has an incidence of approximately 1 in 20,000. It is distinct from a similar disorder known as scapuloperoneal dystrophy.

Clinical Features The condition typically has an onset in childhood and young adulthood. In most cases, facial weakness is the initial manifestation, appearing as an inability to smile, whistle, or fully close the eyes. Weakness of the shoulder girdles, rather than the facial muscles, usually brings the patient to medical attention. Loss of scapular stabilizer muscles makes arm elevation difficult. Scapular winging becomes apparent with attempts at abduction and forward movement of the arms. Biceps and triceps muscles may be severely affected, with relative sparing of the deltoid muscles. Weakness is invariably worse for wrist extension than for wrist flexion, and weakness of the anterior compartment muscles of the legs may lead to footdrop.

In most patients, the weakness remains restricted to facial, upper extremity, and distal lower extremity muscles. In 20% of patients, weakness progresses to involve the pelvic girdle muscles, and severe functional impairment and possible wheelchair dependency result.

Characteristically, patients with facioscapulohumeral (FSH) dystrophy do not have involvement of other organ systems, although labile hypertension is common, and there is an increased incidence of nerve deafness. Coats' disease, a disorder consisting of telangiectasia, exudation, and retinal detachment, also occurs.

Laboratory Features The serum CK level may be normal or mildly elevated. EMG usually indicates a myopathic pattern. The muscle biopsy shows nonspecific features of a myopathy. A prominent inflammatory infiltrate, which is often multifocal in distribution, is present in some biopsy samples. The cause or significance of this finding is unknown.

GENETIC CONSIDERATIONS An autosomal dominant inheritance pattern with almost complete penetrance has been established, but each family member should be examined for the presence of the disease, since ~30% of those affected are unaware of involvement. FSH dystrophy is caused by deletions of telomeric heterochromatin at chromosome 4q35. There is a significant correlation between disease severity and the size of the 4q35-associated deletion. Although a specific FSH gene and protein have not been identified, carrier detection and prenatal diagnosis are possible. Most sporadic cases represent new mutations. Genetic heterogeneity has been documented for FSH dystrophy; in occasional families, the disease is linked to chromosome 10. ■

TREATMENT No specific treatment is available; ankle-foot orthoses are helpful for patients with footdrop. Scapular stabilization procedures improve scapular winging but may not improve function.

OCULOPHARYNGEAL DYSTROPHY

This form of muscular dystrophy represents one of several disorders characterized by *progressive external ophthalmoplegia*, which consists of slowly progressive ptosis and limitation of eye movements with sparing of pupillary reactions for light and accommodation. Patients usually do not complain of diplopia, in contrast to patients having conditions with a more acute onset of ocular muscle weakness (e.g., myasthenia gravis).

Clinical Features Oculopharyngeal muscular dystrophy has a late onset; it usually presents with ptosis and/or dysphagia in the fourth to sixth decade. The extraocular muscle impairment is less prominent in the early phase but may be severe later. The swallowing problem may become debilitating and result in pooling of secretions and repeated episodes of aspiration. Mild weakness of the neck and extremities also occurs.

Laboratory Features The serum CK level may be two to three times normal. Myopathic EMG findings are typical. On biopsy, muscle fibers are found to contain vacuoles, which by electron microscopy are shown to contain membranous whorls, accumulation of glycogen, and other nonspecific debris related to lysosomes. A distinct feature of oculopharyngeal dystrophy is the presence of tubular filaments, 8.5 nm in diameter, in muscle cell nuclei.

GENETIC CONSIDERATIONS Oculopharyngeal dystrophy has an autosomal dominant inheritance pattern with complete penetrance. The incidence is high in French-Canadians and in Spanish-American families of the southwestern United States. Large kindreds of Italian and of eastern European Jewish descent have been reported. The molecular defect in oculopharyngeal muscular dystrophy is a subtle expansion of a modest polyanine repeat tract in a poly-RNA binding protein (PABP2) in muscle; this disorder maps to chromosome 14q. ■

TREATMENT Dysphagia can cause inanition, making oculopharyngeal muscular dystrophy a potentially life-threatening disease. Cricopharyngeal myotomy may improve swallowing, although it does not prevent aspiration. Eyelid crutches can improve vision in patients in whom ptosis obstructs vision; candidates for ptosis surgery must be carefully selected—those with severe facial weakness are not suitable.

DISTAL MYOPATHIES

Patients with predominantly distal weakness usually have a disease of peripheral nerve or anterior horn cells rather than of muscle. There is, however, a heterogeneous group of uncommon disorders of this type with histopathologic and electrophysiologic evidence of myopathy. These distal myopathies can be separated into two types with onset in late adulthood and two types with onset in early adulthood.

The most common late adult–onset form, described by Welander, is inherited as an autosomal dominant condition with onset in the fifth decade. Weakness begins in the hands, and distal anterior-compartment leg muscle involvement occurs later in the course. The serum CK level is either normal or mildly increased. Muscle biopsy shows vacuolated muscle fibers. This disorder genetically maps to chromosome 2p13.

Another late adult–onset form of distal myopathy, also inherited as an autosomal dominant trait, was first recognized in non-Scandinavian patients and also occurs in Finland. Weakness begins in the anterior compartment of the distal lower extremities. The serum CK level is normal or mildly elevated. Muscle fibers often have vacuoles. This disease, sometimes designated "Udd myopathy," maps to the locus for the skeletal muscle protein titin on chromosome 2q31–33.

Both of the distal myopathies with onset in early adulthood have autosomal recessive inheritance. In one type, the weakness usually begins in the anterior compartment of the distal lower extremities, although in some cases it begins in the hands. The serum CK level is moderately elevated (<10 times normal), and muscle biopsies reveal a myopathy with many fibers showing vacuoles. Many of these cases are genetically linked to the centromere on chromosome 9. The other form of early adult–onset distal myopathy (Miyoshi myopathy) is distinguished by weakness beginning in the posterior compartment, i.e., the gastrocnemius muscle. The serum CK level is markedly elevated (>10-fold), and biopsy shows a myopathy without vacuolated fibers. Like LGMB2B, Miyoshi myopathy is caused by defects in the gene encoding the protein dysferlin on chromosome 2p13.

CONGENITAL MYOPATHIES

These rare disorders are distinguished from muscular dystrophies by the presence of specific histochemical and structural abnormalities in muscle. Three major types are described: *central core disease, nemaline (rod) myopathy,* and *centronuclear (myotubular) myopathy.* Other rare types, such as multicore disease, fingerprint body myopathy, and sarcotubular myopathy, are not discussed here.

CENTRAL CORE DISEASE   Patients with central core disease may have decreased fetal movements and breech presentation. Hypotonia and delay in motor milestones, particularly in walking, are common. Later in childhood, patients develop problems with stair climbing, running, and getting up from the floor. On examination, there is mild facial, neck-flexor, and proximal-extremity muscle weakness. Legs are more affected than arms. Skeletal abnormalities include congenital hip dislocation, scoliosis, and pes cavus; clubbed feet also occur. Most cases are nonprogressive, but exceptions are well documented.

The serum CK level is usually normal. Needle EMG demonstrates a myopathic pattern. Muscle biopsy shows fibers with single or multiple central or eccentric discrete zones (cores) devoid of oxidative enzymes. Cores occur preferentially in type 1 fibers and represent poorly aligned sarcomeres associated with Z disk streaming.

GENETIC CONSIDERATIONS   Autosomal dominant inheritance is characteristic; sporadic cases also occur. The disease is caused by point mutations of the ryanodine receptor gene on chromosome 19q, encoding the calcium-release channel of the sarcoplasmic reticulum of skeletal muscle; mutations of this gene also account for some cases of inherited malignant hyperthermia (Chap. 17).

Specific treatment is not required, but establishing a diagnosis of central core disease is extremely important, because these patients have a known predisposition to malignant hyperthermia during anesthesia. ∎

NEMALINE MYOPATHY   The term *nemaline* refers to the distinctive presence in muscle fibers of rods or threadlike structures (Greek *nema,* "thread"). Nemaline myopathy is clinically heterogeneous. A severe neonatal form presents with hypotonia and feeding difficulties leading to early death. Most commonly, nemaline myopathy presents in infancy or childhood with delayed motor milestones. The course is nonprogressive or slowly progressive. The physical appearance may be striking because of the long, narrow facies, high-arched palate, and open-mouthed appearance due to a prognathous jaw. Other skeletal abnormalities include pectus excavatum, kyphoscoliosis, pes cavus, and clubfoot deformities. Facial and generalized muscle weakness are common. These two early childhood forms of nemaline myopathy are referred to as *congenital nemaline myopathy,* in contrast to an adult-onset disorder with progressive proximal weakness. Myocardial involvement is occasionally present in both the congenital and adult-onset forms of the disease.

The serum CK level is usually normal or slightly elevated. The EMG in weak muscles demonstrates a myopathic pattern with occasional fibrillation potentials. Muscle biopsy demonstrates clusters of small rods (nemaline bodies), which occur preferentially, but not exclusively, in type 1 muscle fibers. The muscle often shows type 1 muscle fiber predominance. Rods originate from the Z disk material of the muscle fiber. In the severe neonatal variant, rods are commonly observed in the nucleus of muscle fibers.

GENETIC CONSIDERATIONS   Nemaline myopathy shows at least two patterns of inheritance: autosomal recessive and autosomal dominant with incomplete penetrance. Sporadic cases also occur. Nemaline myopathy is associated with mutations of three genes: TPM3 (α-tropomyosin slow) in both dominant and recessive forms, NEB (encoding nebulin) in the slowly progressive autosomal dominant variant, and ACTA1 (α-actin) in the severe neonatal form. ∎

CENTRONUCLEAR MYOPATHY   Three distinct variants of centronuclear myopathy occur. A *neonatal form,* also known as myotubular myopathy, presents with severe hypotonia and weakness at birth. The *late infancy–early childhood form* presents with delayed motor milestones. Later, difficulty with running and stair climbing becomes apparent. A marfanoid, slender body habitus, long narrow face, and high-arched palate are typical. Scoliosis and clubbed feet may be present. Most patients exhibit progressive weakness, some requiring wheelchairs. Progressive external ophthalmoplegia with ptosis and varying degrees of extraocular muscle impairment are characteristic of both the neonatal and the late-infantile forms. A third variant, the *late childhood-adult form,* has an onset in the second or third decade. Patients have full extraocular muscle movements and rarely exhibit ptosis. There is mild, nonprogressive limb weakness and no associated skeletal abnormalities.

Normal or slightly elevated CK levels occur in each of the forms. EMG studies often give distinctive results, showing positive sharp waves and fibrillation potentials, complex and repetitive discharges, and rarely myotonic discharges. Muscle biopsy specimens in longitudinal section demonstrate rows of central nuclei, often surrounded by a halo. In transverse sections, central nuclei are found in 25 to 80% of muscle fibers.

GENETIC CONSIDERATIONS   A gene for the neonatal form of centronuclear myopathy has been localized to Xq28; this gene encodes myotubularin, a protein tyrosine phosphatase. Missense, frameshift and splice-site mutations predict loss of myotubularin function in affected individuals. Carrier identification and prenatal diagnosis are possible. The inheritance pattern for the late infancy–early childhood disorder is probably autosomal recessive, and for the late childhood–adult form is probably autosomal dominant. ∎

DISORDERS OF MUSCLE ENERGY METABOLISM

There are two principal sources of energy for skeletal muscle—fatty acids and glucose. Abnormalities in either glucose or lipid utilization can be associated with distinct clinical presentations that can range from an acute, painful syndrome with rhabdomyolysis and myoglobinuria to a chronic, progressive muscle weakness simulating muscular dystrophy.

GLYCOGEN STORAGE AND GYCOLYTIC DEFECTS These disorders can be divided into those that can cause exercise intolerance, particularly intermittent muscle pain and myoglobinuria, and those in which fixed muscle weakness is the predominant clinical feature. The latter can mimic LGMD or inflammatory myopathies.

Disorders of Glycogen Storage Causing Fixed Muscle Weakness Three clinical forms of acid maltase deficiency (*type II glycogenosis*) can be distinguished, all of which have autosomal recessive inheritance. The gene for acid maltase is found on the long arm of chromosome 17. The *infantile form* is the most common, with onset of symptoms in the first 3 months of life. Infants develop severe muscle weakness, cardiomegaly, hepatomegaly, and respiratory insufficiency. Glycogen accumulation in motor neurons of the spinal cord and brainstem contributes to muscle weakness. Death usually occurs by 1 year of age. In the *childhood form*, the picture resembles muscular dystrophy. Delayed motor milestones result from proximal limb muscle weakness and involvement of respiratory muscles. The heart may be involved, but the liver and brain are unaffected. The *adult form* begins in the third or fourth decade. Respiratory failure and diaphragmatic weakness are often initial manifestations heralding progressive proximal muscle weakness. The heart and liver are not involved.

In all forms of acid maltase deficiency, the serum CK level is 2 to 10 times normal. EMG examination demonstrates a myopathic pattern, but other features are especially distinctive, including myotonic discharges, trains of fibrillation and positive waves, and complex repetitive discharges. EMG discharges are very prominent in the lumbosacral paraspinal muscles. The muscle biopsy shows vacuoles containing glycogen and the lysosomal enzyme acid phosphatase. Electron microscopy reveals membrane-bound and free tissue glycogen. Definitive diagnosis is established by enzyme determination in muscle.

No satisfactory treatment exists for acid maltase deficiency. A high-protein diet has been advocated, but efficacy has not been documented. Intravenous enzyme replacement has not shown benefit.

In *debranching enzyme deficiency (type III glycogenosis)*, a slowly progressive form of muscle weakness can develop after puberty. Rarely, myoglobinuria may be seen. Patients are usually diagnosed in infancy, however, because of hypotonia and delayed motor milestones, hepatomegaly, growth retardation, and hypoglycemia. *Branching enzyme deficiency (type IV glycogenosis)* is a rare and fatal glycogen storage disease characterized by failure to thrive and hepatomegaly. Hypotonia and muscle wasting may be present, but the skeletal muscle manifestations are minor compared to liver failure.

Disorders of Glycolysis Causing Exercise Intolerance Five glycolytic defects are associated with recurrent myoglobinuria: *myophosphorylase deficiency (type V glycogenosis)*, *phosphofructokinase deficiency (type VII glycogenosis)*, *phosphoglycerate kinase deficiency (type IX glycogenosis)*, *phosphoglycerate mutase deficiency (type X glycogenosis)*, and *lactate dehydrogenase deficiency (glycogensosis type XI)*. Myophosphorylase deficiency, also known as McArdle's disease, is by far the most common of the glycolytic defects associated with exercise intolerance. All are inherited as autosomal recessive traits, except for phosphoglycerate kinase deficiency, which is X-linked recessive. These five glycolytic defects result in a common failure to support energy production at the initiation of exercise, although the exact site of energy failure remains controversial.

Clinical muscle manifestations in these five conditions usually begin in adolescence. Symptoms are precipitated by brief bursts of high-intensity exercise, such as running or lifting heavy objects. A history of myalgia and muscle stiffness usually precedes the intensely painful muscle contractures, which may be followed by myoglobinuria. Acute renal failure accompanies significant pigmenturia. Exercise tolerance can be enhanced by a slow induction phase (warm-up) or brief periods of rest, allowing for the start of the "second-wind" phenomenon (switching to utilization of fatty acids).

Certain features help distinguish some enzyme defects. Varying degrees of hemolytic anemia accompany deficiencies of both phosphofructokinase (mild) and phosphoglycerate kinase (severe). In phosphoglycerate kinase deficiency, the usual clinical presentation is a seizure disorder associated with mental retardation; exercise intolerance is an infrequent manifestation.

In all of these conditions, the serum CK levels fluctuate widely and may be elevated even during symptom-free periods. CK levels >100 times normal are expected, accompanying myoglobinuria. All patients with suspected glycolytic defects leading to exercise intolerance should undergo a forearm exercise test (Chap. 381). An impaired rise in venous lactate is highly indicative of a glycolytic defect. In lactate dehydrogenase deficiency, venous levels of lactate do not increase, but pyruvate rises to normal, after forearm exercise. In all glycolytic defects, a definitive diagnosis is made by muscle biopsy.

Training may enhance the second-wind phenomenon, but attempts to raise blood glucose or to modify these disorders through diet have not proved beneficial.

DISORDERS OF LIPID METABOLISM

Lipid is an important muscle energy source during rest and during prolonged, submaximal exercise. Fatty acids are derived from circulating very low–density lipoprotein (VLDL) in the blood or from triglycerides stored in muscle fibers. Oxidation of fatty acids occurs in the mitochondria. To enter the mitochondria, a fatty acid must first be converted to an "activated fatty acid," acyl-CoA. The acyl-CoA must be linked with carnitine by the enzyme carnitine palmitoyltransferase (CPT) I for transport into the mitochondria. CPT I is present on the inner side of the outer mitochondrial membrane. Carnitine is removed by CPT II, an enzyme attached to the inside of the inner mitochondrial membrane, allowing transport of acyl-CoA into the mitochondrial matrix for β-oxidation.

CARNITINE DEFICIENCY Deficiency of this important substrate results in a myopathic and a systemic disorder.

Myopathic carnitine deficiency is associated with generalized muscle weakness, usually beginning in childhood. The clinical features overlap with those of muscular dystrophy and polymyositis. Patients develop progressive, painless proximal weakness. A severe cardiomyopathy may be present. Serum CK levels may be mildly to markedly (>10-fold) elevated. The muscle biopsy shows striking lipid accumulation. The serum carnitine level is normal. The cause for decreased muscle carnitine is not understood. Most cases are sporadic, but the inheritance pattern is thought to be autosomal recessive. Some patients respond to oral carnitine supplementation; this treatment should be tried in all cases. Other patients have responded to prednisone, riboflavin, or propranolol. A diet substituting medium-chain for long-chain triglycerides has been helpful for some patients.

Systemic carnitine deficiency usually presents in infancy and early childhood and is characterized by progressive weakness and episodes of hepatic encephalopathy with nausea, vomiting, confusion, coma, and early death. Carnitine levels are reduced in muscle, liver, kidney, and heart; but the low serum carnitine levels are especially useful in distinguishing this condition from the myopathic form. No single cause has been identified to explain the low serum carnitine levels. Decreased hepatic synthesis explains some cases, while increased urinary excretion occurs in others. Serum CK levels may be slightly elevated. The muscle biopsy may show lipid storage. In some cases, the liver, heart, and kidney show increased lipid. Treatment with oral carnitine supplementation or glucocorticoids has helped some, but not all, patients.

Secondary carnitine deficiency accompanies a variety of disorders in which carnitine deficiency is caused by decreased synthesis (cirrhosis), insufficient intake (parenteral nutrition), or excessive loss (renal dialysis, Fanconi's syndrome, or organic acidemia). Carnitine deficiency may also be seen in the muscular dystrophies, where it is thought to be a nonspecific result of loss of muscle tissue. Oral carnitine supplementation has not been shown to clearly benefit patients with these secondary syndromes.

CARNITINE PALMITOYLTRANSFERASE DEFICIENCY
CPT II deficiency is the most common recognizable cause of recurrent myoglobinuria, more common than the glycolytic defects.

Clinical Features   Onset is usually in the teenage years or early twenties. Muscle pain and myoglobinuria occur after prolonged exercise. Fasting predisposes to the development of symptoms. In contrast to disorders caused by defects in glycolysis, in which muscle cramps follow short, intense bursts of exercise, the muscle pain in CPT II deficiency does not occur until the limits of utilization have been exceeded and muscle breakdown has already begun. Episodes of rhabdomyolysis may produce severe weakness. In contrast to carnitine deficiency, strength is normal between attacks.

Laboratory Findings   Serum CK levels and EMG findings are both usually normal between episodes. A normal rise of venous lactate during forearm exercise distinguishes this condition from glycolytic defects, especially myophosphorylase deficiency. Muscle biopsy does not show lipid accumulation and is usually normal between attacks. The diagnosis requires direct measurement of muscle CPT.

GENETIC CONSIDERATIONS   CPT II deficiency is much more common in men than women (5:1); nevertheless, all evidence indicates autosomal recessive inheritance. A mutation in the gene for CPT II causes the disease in some individuals. ∎

TREATMENT   It has been suggested that frequent meals and a low-fat, high-carbohydrate diet can prolong exercise tolerance. Others suggest substituting medium-chain triglycerides in the diet. Neither approach has proven beneficial.

MYOADENYLATE DEAMINASE DEFICIENCY
The muscle enzyme myoadenylate deaminase converts adenosine 5′-monophosphate (5′-AMP) to inosine monophosphate (IMP) with liberation of ammonia. Myoadenylate deaminase may play a role in regulating adenosine triphosphate (ATP) levels in muscles. Most individuals with myoadenylate deaminase deficiency have no symptoms. Many questions have been raised about the clinical effects of myoadenylate deaminase deficiency, and, specifically, its relationship to exertional myalgia and fatigability; but there is no consensus. There have been a few reports of patients with this disorder who have exercise-exacerbated myalgia and myoglobinuria. The full clinical significance of myoadenylate deaminase deficiency has not been established.

MITOCHONDRIAL MYOPATHIES

In 1972, Olson and colleagues recognized that muscle fibers with significant numbers of abnormal mitochondria could be highlighted with the modified trichrome stain; the term "ragged red fibers" was coined. By electron microscopy, the mitochondria in ragged red fibers are enlarged and often bizarrely shaped and have crystalline inclusions. Since that seminal observation, the understanding of these disorders of muscle and other tissues has expanded (Chap. 67).

Mitochondria play a key role in energy production. Oxidation of the major nutrients derived from carbohydrate, fat, and protein leads to the generation of reducing equivalents. The latter are transported through the respiratory chain in the process known as oxidative phosphorylation. The energy generated by the oxidation-reduction reactions of the respiratory chain is stored in an electrochemical gradient coupled to ATP synthesis.

A novel feature of mitochondria is their genetic composition. Each mitochondrion possesses a DNA genome that is distinct from that of the nuclear DNA. Human mitochondrial DNA (mtDNA) consists of a double-stranded, circular molecule comprising 16,569 base pairs. It codes for 22 transfer RNAs, 2 ribosomal RNAs, and 13 polypeptides of the respiratory chain enzymes. The genetics of mitochondrial diseases differ from the genetics of chromosomal disorders. The DNA of mitochondria is directly inherited from the cytoplasm of the gametes, mainly from the oocyte. The sperm contributes very little of its mitochondria to the offspring at the time of fertilization. Thus, mitochondrial genes are derived almost exclusively from the mother, accounting for maternal inheritance of some mitochondrial disorders.

mtDNA DISORDERS OF MUSCLE   Many different classifications of mitochondrial myopathies are possible. A convenient scheme allows for disorders to be grouped by the type of mtDNA mutation: deletions or point mutations.

Disorders Associated with mtDNA Deletions   The *Kearns-Sayre syndrome* (KSS) is a sporadic, noninherited disorder with onset before age 20. The characteristic findings include a triad of clinical features: progressive external ophthalmoplegia, pigmentary degeneration of the retina, and heart block. Some patients have only extraocular manifestations. Patients with KSS may also have short stature, ataxia, dementia, sensorineural hearing loss, diabetes, and hypothyroidism. Cerebrospinal fluid (CSF) lactate and pyruvate levels are elevated. The course is progressively downhill, and most patients die in their third or fourth decade. In KSS, two populations of mtDNA, wild type and mutant, are present in the same cell; the mutations in the latter consist of single mtDNA deletions. Heteroplasmy can be recognized on Southern blot analysis. The highest percentage of deleted mtDNA can be detected in postmitotic tissues, especially skeletal muscle. Other tissues can harbor the mutation (e.g., peripheral blood leukocytes, brain, liver, and fibroblasts). The absence of mutant mtDNA reflects both mitotic segregation early in embryogenesis and selection against a mutant cell line in a rapidly dividing tissue. KSS is not inherited, since mutations leading to an affected individual take place in the fertilized ovum.

An *autosomal dominant disorder with progressive external ophthalmoplegia and proximal weakness* shares clinical features with KSS: hearing loss, ataxia, peripheral neuropathy, mental retardation, and hypoparathyroidism. Some of these patients also have weakness of respiratory muscles, exercise intolerance, cataracts, and early death. The patients have ragged red fibers on muscle biopsy and multiple mtDNA deletions, rather than single deletions as in KSS. The mutation accounting for the autosomal dominant inheritance occurs in a nuclear gene that encodes a protein involved in the control of mtDNA replication. A failure or disruption of binding of this nuclear-encoded protein during mtDNA replication results in multiple deletions.

Disorders Associated with mtDNA Point Mutations   *Myoclonic epilepsy and ragged red fibers*, called the *MERRF syndrome*, consists of mitochondrial myopathy, myoclonus, generalized seizures, intellectual deterioration, ataxia, and hearing loss. Extraocular movements are normal in MERRF. Onset is often in childhood or early adult life. As with other mitochondrial disorders, individuals display varying manifestations of the disease. Serum and CSF lactate and pyruvate levels are increased. The course is progressively downhill, and most patients die with severe encephalopathy. MERRF syndrome is maternally inherited. Most often, point mutations in the lysine transfer RNA gene of mtDNA can be found. This abnormality can be detected in mtDNA isolated from peripheral blood leukocytes or skeletal muscle and is useful for clinical diagnosis and genetic counseling. These mutations alter the normal conformation of the transfer RNA, impairing translation probably at the ribosomal level.

Mitochondrial myopathy, encephalopathy, lactic acidosis, and stroke-like episodes are referred to by the acronym *MELAS*. This disorder is a multisystem mitochondrial encephalomyopathy that begins in childhood after normal birth and early development. Patients have stunted growth and recurrent stroke-like episodes manifesting as hemiparesis, hemianopia, or cortical blindness. Episodic vomiting may occur, and some patients have hearing loss. Focal or generalized seizures and myoclonic epilepsy may be present. Full expression of the disease leads to dementia, a bedridden state, and death often before age 20. Lactic acidosis may be present. MELAS can be maternally inherited, but sporadic cases are common. No large pedigrees have been reported. In 80 to 90% of patients, a point mutation of the leucine transfer RNA gene of mtDNA has been identified at nucleotide 3243. Some patients with this same mutation have only diabetes mellitus and hearing loss. Rarely, a mtDNA mutation of subunit 4 of complex I (ND4) of the respiratory chain causes MELAS. Mutation analysis provides a specific diagnostic test that can be performed on peripheral blood leukocytes or skeletal muscle.

A clinical syndrome with combined features of *skeletal and cardiac myopathies associated with lactic acidosis* that is distinct from MELAS has been described with a point mutation at nucleotide 3260 of the leucine transfer RNA gene of mtDNA.

ENDOCRINE AND METABOLIC MYOPATHIES

Many endocrine disorders cause weakness. Muscle fatigue is more common than true weakness. The cause of weakness in these disorders is not well defined. It is not even clear that weakness results from disease of muscle as opposed to another part of the motor unit since the serum CK level is often normal (except in hypothyroidism), and the muscle histology is characterized by atrophy rather than destruction of muscle fibers. Nearly all endocrine myopathies respond to treatment.

THYROID DISORDERS (See also Chap. 330) Abnormalities of thyroid function can cause a wide array of muscle disorders. These conditions relate to the important role of thyroid hormones in regulating the metabolism of carbohydrates and lipids as well as the rate of protein synthesis and enzyme production. Thyroid hormones also stimulate calorigenesis in muscle, increase muscle demand for vitamins, and enhance muscle sensitivity to circulating catecholamines.

Hypothyroidism Patients with hypothyroidism have frequent muscle complaints, and proximal muscle weakness occurs in about one-third of them. Muscle cramps, pain, and stiffness are common. Features of slow muscle contraction and relaxation occur in 25% of patients, and the relaxation phase of muscle stretch reflexes is characteristically prolonged. The serum CK level is often elevated (up to 10 times normal), even when there is minimal clinical evidence of muscle disease. In both children and adults, a distinct syndrome has been described. Severely hypothyroid children, especially boys, may have the Debré-Kocher-Sémélaigne syndrome, characterized by weakness, slowness of movement, and striking muscle hypertrophy, causing an "infant Hercules appearance." In adult hypothyroidism, Hoffman's syndrome results in prominent muscle enlargement and weakness with muscle stiffness. The cause of muscle enlargement in these two syndromes has not been determined. The muscle biopsy shows no distinctive morphologic abnormalities.

Hyperthyroidism Patients who are thyrotoxic commonly have proximal muscle weakness and atrophy on examination, but they rarely complain of the deficit. Muscle stretch reflexes are preserved and often brisk. Bulbar, respiratory, and even esophageal muscles may occasionally be affected, causing dysphagia, dysphonia, and aspiration. When bulbar involvement occurs, it is usually accompanied by chronic proximal limb weakness, but occasionally it presents in the absence of generalized thyrotoxic myopathy. Other neuromuscular disorders occur in association with hyperthyroidism, including periodic paralysis, myasthenia gravis, and a progressive ocular myopathy associated with proptosis (Graves' ophthalmopathy). Serum CK levels are not elevated in thyrotoxic myopathy. The muscle histology usually shows only atrophy of muscle fibers.

PARATHYROID DISORDERS (See also Chap. 341) **Hyperparathyroidism** Muscle weakness is an integral part of primary and secondary hyperparathyroidism. Proximal muscle weakness, muscle wasting, and brisk muscle stretch reflexes are the main features of this endocrinopathy. Serum CK levels are usually normal or slightly elevated. Serum calcium and phosphorus levels show no correlation with the clinical neuromuscular manifestations. Muscle biopsies show only varying degrees of atrophy without muscle fiber degeneration.

Hypoparathyroidism An overt myopathy due to hypocalcemia rarely occurs. Neuromuscular symptoms are usually related to localized or generalized tetany. Serum CK levels may be increased secondary to muscle damage after tetany. Hyporeflexia or areflexia is usually present and contrasts with the hyperreflexia in hyperparathyroidism.

ADRENAL DISORDERS (See also Chap. 331) Conditions associated with glucocorticoid excess cause a myopathy; in fact, steroid myopathy is the most commonly diagnosed endocrine muscle disease. Steroid excess, either endogenous or exogenous (see "Toxic Myopathies," below), produces various degrees of proximal limb weakness. Muscle wasting may be striking. A cushingoid appearance invariably precedes or accompanies clinical signs of myopathy. Histologic sections demonstrate muscle fiber atrophy rather than degeneration or necrosis of muscle fibers. Adrenal insufficiency commonly causes muscle fatigue. Objective weakness occurs less often and is typically mild.

In primary hyperaldosteronism, or Conn's syndrome, neuromuscular complications are due to potassium depletion. The clinical picture is one of persistent muscle weakness. Long-standing hyperaldosteronism may lead to proximal limb weakness and wasting. Serum CK levels may be elevated, and a muscle biopsy may demonstrate degenerating fibers, some with vacuoles. These changes relate to hypokalemia and are not a direct effect of aldosterone on skeletal muscle.

PITUITARY DISORDERS (See also Chap. 328) Patients with acromegaly usually have mild proximal weakness without muscle atrophy. Muscles often appear enlarged, but they have decreased force generation. The duration of acromegaly, rather than the serum growth hormone levels, correlates with the degree of myopathy.

DIABETES MELLITUS (See also Chap. 333) Neuromuscular complications of diabetes mellitus are most often related to neuropathy with cranial and peripheral nerve palsies or distal sensorimotor polyneuropathy. "Diabetic amyotrophy" is now known to be a neuropathy affecting the proximal major nerve trunks and lumbosacral plexus. More appropriate terms for this disorder include *diabetic proximal neuropathy* and *lumbosacral radiculoplexopathy*.

The only notable myopathy of diabetes mellitus is ischemic infarction of thigh muscles. This condition occurs in patients with poorly controlled diabetes and presents with acute onset of pain, tenderness, and edema of one thigh with a palpable mass. The muscles most often affected include the vastus lateralis, thigh adductors, and biceps femoris. Computed tomography or magnetic resonance imaging can demonstrate focal abnormalities in the affected muscle. Imaging of the muscle renders muscle biopsy unnecessary.

VITAMIN DEFICIENCY Vitamin D deficiency is the most important cause of myopathy occurring as an integral part of a vitamin deficiency. Vitamin D deficiency (Chaps. 75 and 340) due to either decreased intake, decreased absorption, or impaired vitamin D metabolism (as occurs in renal disease) may lead to chronic muscle weakness. Pain reflects the underlying bone disease (osteomalacia). Vitamin E deficiency has been associated with a vacuolar myopathy. It has not been established that deficiency of other vitamins causes a myopathy.

MYOPATHIES OF SYSTEMIC ILLNESS Systemic illnesses such as chronic respiratory, cardiac, or hepatic failure are frequently associated with severe muscle wasting and complaints of weakness. Strength testing often demonstrates mild weakness in such patients. Fatigue is a more significant problem.

Myopathy may be a manifestation of chronic renal failure, independent of the better known uremic polyneuropathy. Abnormalities of calcium and phosphorus homeostasis and bone metabolism in chronic renal failure result from a reduction in 1,25-dihydroxyvitamin D, leading to decreased intestinal absorption of calcium. Hypocalcemia, further accentuated by hyperphosphatemia due to decreased renal phosphate clearance, leads to secondary hyperparathyroidism. Renal osteodystrophy results from the compensatory hyperparathyroidism, which leads to osteomalacia from reduced calcium availability and to osteitis fibrosa from the parathyroid hormone excess. The clinical picture of the myopathy of chronic renal failure is identical to that of primary hyperparathyroidism and osteomalacia. There is proximal limb weakness with bone pain.

Gangrenous calcification represents a separate, rare, and sometimes fatal complication of chronic renal failure. In this condition, widespread arterial calcification occurs and results in ischemia. Extensive skin necrosis may occur along with painful myopathy and even myoglobinuria.

TOXIC MYOPATHIES

The classification of toxic myopathies is shown in Table 383-4. Drugs and chemicals may produce focal or generalized damage to skeletal muscle.

The most common cause of focal damage is the injection of narcotic analgesics. Three agents in particular—pentazocine, meperidine, and heroin—may cause a severe fibrotic reaction in muscle. Common injection sites include deltoid, triceps, gluteus maximus, and quadriceps muscles. The muscles become indurated and may have local abscess formation. Cutaneous ulcerations and depressions may occur. Severe joint contractures may develop.

Other drugs may induce generalized muscle weakness, particularly affecting the proximal muscles. In most cases the exact mechanism of drug toxicity is poorly understood. D-Penicillamine induces a condition simulating the clinical and pathologic picture of polymyositis. A similar condition has been reported with cimetidine. Procainamide may cause myositis as part of a systemic lupus erythematosus–like reaction. Chloroquine administration may cause a vacuolar myopathy.

Zidovudine, used in the treatment of AIDS, produces proximal weakness and pain. On muscle biopsy, zidovudine myopathy demonstrates a distinctive pathologic alteration of skeletal muscle, affecting mitochondria and resembling ragged red fibers. Some patients may tolerate the reintroduction of zidovudine in lower doses.

The cholesterol-lowering agents, including fibric acid derivatives (clofibrate, gemfibrozil), 3-hydroxy-methyl-glutaryl-coenzyme A reductase inhibitors (lovastatin, simivastatin, pravastatin), and niacin have all been implicated in myopathies, occasionally causing myoglobinuria. Emetine hydrochloride (used for treatment of amebiasis), ε-aminocaproic acid (an antifibrinolytic agent), and perhexiline (used for angina pectoris) have all been observed to cause muscle weakness and muscle fiber necrosis after several weeks of therapy.

Drug-induced myopathy accompanied by proximal weakness occurs with glucocorticoid therapy. Glucocorticoid drugs fluorinated in the 9α-position, such as triamcinolone, dexamethasone, and betamethasone, are most likely to cause weakness, but chronic administration of any glucocorticoid, including prednisone, causes weakness. Divided-dose, as opposed to single-morning-dose, regimens produce more severe weakness. A single-dose, alternate-day regimen is yet less toxic. The clinical diagnosis of steroid-induced muscle weakness can be difficult if the medication is being used to treat an underlying inflammatory myopathy. The presence of a normal serum CK level, minimal or no changes of myopathy on EMG, and type 2 muscle fiber atrophy on biopsy are helpful in suggesting steroid-induced weakness.

Excess alcohol intake causes acute muscle weakness with rhabdomyolysis and myoglobinuria by several different mechanisms, including prolonged obtundation, seizures, hypokalemia, and hypophosphatemia. The existence of a chronic myopathy causing slowly progressive weakness in this setting is controversial. Alcoholics often have chronic weakness resulting from neuropathy and poor nutrition.

A very serious drug-induced condition, *malignant hyperthermia*, occurs in susceptible individuals after exposure to certain general anesthetic and depolarizing muscle relaxants (Table 383-4). The local anesthetic amides, including lidocaine and mepivacaine, have also been implicated as precipitating agents.

DISORDERS OF MUSCLE MEMBRANE EXCITABILITY

Elucidation of the molecular defects in the primary periodic paralyses provides insight into their pathogenesis and forms the basis for their classification (Table 383-5). These diseases are all characterized by muscle stiffness due to electrical irritability of the muscle membrane (myotonia), usually without significant permanent muscle weakness until late in the course. These clinical features (myotonia without dystrophy) distinguish these disorders from myotonic dystrophy in which there is significant distal weakness. In the nondystrophic myotonias, onset is usually in childhood or at adolescence; episodic weakness beginning after age 25 is almost never due to periodic paralysis. Attacks typically occur after rest or sleep and almost never in the midst of vigorous activity, although antecedent exercise often provokes weakness. Patients remain alert during the attacks. Early in the course of these disorders, interattack strength is normal. After many years of attacks, interictal weakness develops and may be progressive. These disorders are amenable to treatment, and progressive weakness can be prevented and even reversed. Diagnosis is based on the clinical history and confirmed by appropriate evaluation of serum electrolytes during attacks, by evaluation of the response of strength to provocative testing with glucose, insulin, potassium, and cold, or by DNA analysis of the appropriate gene.

CALCIUM CHANNEL DISORDERS OF MUSCLE Hypokalemic Periodic Paralysis Hypokalemic periodic paralysis (hypoKPP) causes episodic weakness, which usually affects proximal limb muscles more than distal ones; rarely, ocular, bulbar, or respiratory muscles are affected. Respiratory muscle weakness may prove fatal. Meals high in carbohydrate or sodium can provoke attacks. Reflexes become hypoactive, and cardiac arrhythmias may occur during attacks owing to low serum potassium. Onset is at adolescence. Men are more often affected because of decreased penetrance in women. Some women have only infrequent attacks.

Diagnosis is established by demonstrating a low serum potassium level during a paralytic attack and by excluding secondary causes of

Table 383-4 Toxic Myopathies

Distribution	Clinical Features	Compound
Generalized		
	Myotonia	Propranolol, cyclosporine, iodides, clofibrate
	Inflamation	Cimetidine, penicillamine, procainamide
	Weakness, myalgias, rhabdomyolysis, myoglobinuria, high serum CK	Chloroquine, clofibrate, gemfibrozil, lovastatin, simivastatin, pravastatin, niacin, colchicine, cyclosporine, emetine, ε-aminocaproic acid, glucocorticoids, labetalol, perhexilline, propranolol, vincristine, zidovudine, alcohol, amphetamine, barbiturates, cocaine, heroin, phencyclidine
	Malignant hyperthermia	Ethyl chloride, ethylene, diethyl ether, gallamine, halothane, lidocaine, mepivacaine, methoxylflurane, trichloroethylene, succinylcholine
Focal	Possible focal weakness, myalgia	Pentazocine, meperidine, heroin

| Feature | Calcium Channel | | Sodium Channel | | Chloride Channel |
	Hypokalemic PP	Hyperkalemic PP	Paramyotonia Congenita	Sodium Channel Myotonia	Congenital Myotonia
Mode of inheritance	AD	AD	AD	AD	AD or AR
Age of onset	Adolescence	Early childhood	Early childhood	Early childhood	Early childhood
Myotonia[a]	No	Yes	Yes	Yes	Yes
Episodic weakness	Yes	Yes	Yes	No	No
Frequency of attacks of weakness	Daily to yearly	May be 2–3/d	With cold, usually rare	Never	Never
Duration of attacks of weakness	2–12 h	From 1–2 h to >1 day	2–24 h	None	None
Serum K+ level during attacks of weakness	Decreased	Increased or normal	Usually normal	(No attacks)	(No attacks)
Effect of K+ loading	No change	Increased myotonia, then weakness	Increased myotonia	Increased myotonia	No change
Effect of muscle cooling	No change	Increased myotonia	Increased myotonia, then weakness	Mild increase in myotonia	Increased myotonia
Fixed weakness	Yes	Yes	Yes	No	No

[a] May be paradoxical.

ABBREVIATIONS: AD, autosomal dominant; AR, autosomal recessive; PP, periodic paralysis.

hypokalemia. The molecular defect in the calcium channel can be defined in many patients. Muscle biopsy often shows the presence of single or multiple centrally placed vacuoles. Patients whose attacks are too infrequent for study of a spontaneous attack to be feasible require provocative testing with glucose and insulin administration. Provocative tests are potentially hazardous and require careful monitoring.

HypoKPP is caused by mutations in a voltage-sensitive, skeletal muscular calcium channel, although details of the pathogenesis are incompletely understood (Fig. 383-2).

The acute paralysis improves after the administration of potassium salts. Oral KCl (0.2 to 0.4 mmol/kg) should be given to patients with severe weakness and repeated at 15- to 30-min intervals depending on the response of the ECG, serum potassium level, and muscle strength. Milder attacks usually resolve spontaneously. When patients are unable to swallow or are vomiting, intravenous therapy may be necessary. Small, repeated boluses of KCl (0.1 mmol/kg) may be administered over 5 to 10 min with careful monitoring of the ECG and serum potassium level. If potassium is administered as a dilute solution (20 to 40 mmol/L) in 5% glucose or in physiologic saline solution, the serum potassium level may decline, and weakness may worsen. Mannitol is the preferred vehicle for administered intravenous potassium in such situations, since it facilitates rapid return of the serum potassium level to normal and does not cause the lowering of the serum potassium level that may be caused by glucose or saline solutions.

The goal of therapy is to eliminate attacks, which also prevents interattack weakness. Before effective means of attack prevention became available, chronic progressive interattack weakness frequently caused serious disability. Prophylactic administration of potassium salts, even in large doses, does not prevent attacks, but acetazolamide (125 to 1000 mg/d in divided doses) or dichlorphenamide (50 to 200 mg/d) abolishes attacks in most cases. The metabolic acidosis induced by acetazolamide may underlie the beneficial effect. Paradoxically, acetazolamide lowers the serum potassium level; to achieve an adequate response in some patients, it may be necessary to give supplementary potassium along with acetazolamide and to avoid high-carbohydrate meals. Chronic acetazolamide treatment may be associated with renal calculi, and patients should be monitored for this complication. In occasional patients, attacks may not respond to or may even be worsened by acetazolamide. In such patients, triamterene (25 to 100 mg/d) or spironolactone (25 to 100 mg/d) may prevent attacks.

SODIUM CHANNEL DISORDERS OF MUSCLE   Hyperkalemic Periodic Paralysis   Hyperkalemic periodic paralysis (hyperKPP) causes episodic weakness of limb muscles; cranial and respiratory muscles are rarely involved. The term "hyperkalemic" is misleading, since patients are often normokalemic during attacks. It is the fact that attacks are precipitated by potassium administration that best defines the disorder. Paresthesias and muscle pain are present during many attacks.

Diagnosis is suggested by a modest elevation of the serum potassium level during attacks in nearly half of patients; at times, however, the serum potassium level is normal or even low. The so-called hyperkalemic and normokalemic forms of this disorder are not separate entities. Intravenous glucose-insulin loading does not precipitate weakness, but potassium-loading tests (0.05 to 0.15 g/kg) do induce weakness in such patients. Potassium-loading tests are potentially hazardous and are contraindicated in patients with renal disease and diabetes. Random serum potassium measurements may suggest the diagnosis, since potassium level elevations are frequent during attack-free intervals. EMG evidence of myotonia and the finding of vacuoles on muscle biopsy provide supporting data.

Like hypoKPP, hyperKPP may also respond to chronic administration of acetazolamide or dichlorphenamide.

Paramyotonia Congenita   Paramyotonia congenita (PC) causes attacks of paralysis either spontaneously or with cold provocation. PC with periodic paralysis is similar to hyperKPP, except that paradoxical myotonia (i.e., myotonia worsening with activity) and objective cold sensitivity are more prominent in PC.

In PC, attacks of weakness are seldom severe enough to require emergency treatment and are never fatal. Oral administration of glucose or other carbohydrate hastens recovery. Since interattack weakness may develop after repeated attacks, prophylactic treatment is usually indicated in PC. Thiazide diuretics (e.g., chlorothiazide, 250 to 1000 mg/d) are reported to be effective.

Potassium-Aggravated Myotonia   Some patients with muscle sodium channel defects have severe muscle stiffness but no paralytic episodes. The stiffness is accentuated by elevations in serum potassium levels. Mutations in the skeletal muscle voltage-gated sodium channel SCN4A cause hyperKPP, PC and potassium-aggravated myotonia (PAM) (Fig. 383-2). In vitro study of these mutations demonstrates increased conductance through the sodium channels, often because of subnormal, slowed inactivation of the channel after action potential firing.

CHLORIDE CHANNEL DISORDERS OF MUSCLE   Myotonia Congenita   In some families, severe, cold-aggravated muscle stiffness with muscle hypertrophy is transmitted as an inherited trait (dominant or recessive). This problem is usually evident in childhood; symptoms may become less severe in the adult years. This problem is caused by mutations in a skeletal muscle chloride channel resulting in impaired membrane repolarization. Myotonia congenita due to chloride channel defects can be distinguished from sodium channel myo-

Sodium channel α subunit

○ HyperKPP   △ PC   ■ PAM

Calcium channel α subunit

Chloride channel

○ Myotonia Congenita   ▲ Myotonia Congenita   ☆ ADR (murine)
  Dominant   Recessive   insertion

                                                  ▽ adr^mto (murine)
                                                    stop

                                                  ▢ Myotonic goat
                                                    Ala → Pro

FIGURE 383-2 The sodium and calcium channels are depicted here as containing four homologous domains, each with six membrane-spanning segments. The fourth segment of each domain bears positive charges and acts as the "voltage sensor" for the channel. The association of the four domains is thought to form a pore through which ions pass. Sodium channel mutations are shown along with the phenotype that they confer. HyperKPP, hyperkalemic periodic paralysis; PC, paramyotonia congenita; PAM, potassium-aggravated myotonia. See text for details.

The chloride channel is envisioned to have ten membrane-spanning domains. The positions of mutations causing dominantly and recessively inherited myotonia congenita are indicated, along with mutations that cause this disease in mice and goats.

tonia by the rather striking muscle hypertrophy and by DNA mutational screening.

DISORDERS OF UNKNOWN PATHOGENETIC MECHANISM   Thyrotoxic Periodic Paralysis   This disorder is clinically indistinguishable from hypoKPP. It is common in young Latin American and Asian men, among whom up to 10% of thyrotoxic patients may have this condition. The thyrotoxicosis may be overlooked for many months. Occasionally, the only indication of thyrotoxicosis is a depressed level of thyroid-stimulating hormone. Acute attacks respond to potassium administration. Treatment of the underlying thyrotoxicosis abolishes attacks. β-Adrenergic blocking agents are useful for reducing the frequency and severity of attacks while measures to control thyrotoxicosis are instituted. Acetazolamide is not helpful in preventing attacks. The pathogenesis of thyrotoxic periodic paralysis is uncertain, but there is evidence for a decrease in the activity of the calcium pump.

Andersen's Syndrome   In this rare disorder patients manifest periodic paralysis (hyperkalemic or hypokalemic), cardiac dysrhythmias (even when normokalemic), and dysmorphic features (hypertelorism, low set ears, broad nose). Treatment of the episodic weakness is the same as for the other periodic paralyses, although cardiac status must be considered as well.

BIBLIOGRAPHY

ANDERSON LV et al: Dysferlin is a plasma membrane protein and is expressed early in human development. Hum Mol Genet 8:855, 1999

BAROHN RJ: Distal myopathies and dystrophies. Semin Neurol 13:247, 1993

BLAKE DJ, KRÖGER S: The neurobiology of Duchenne muscular dystrophy: Learning lessons from muscle? Trends Neurosci 23:92, 2000

BONNE G et al: Mutations in the gene encoding lamin A/C cause autosomal dominant Emery-Dreifuss muscular dystrophy. Nat Genet 21:285, 1999

CAMPBELL KP: Adhalin gene mutations and autosomal recessive limb-girdle muscular dystrophy. Ann Neurol 38:353, 1995

CANNON SC: Ion-channel defects and aberrant excitability in myotonia and periodic paralysis. Trends Neurosci 19:3, 1996

DIMAURO S et al: Mitochondrial encephalomyopathies, in *The Molecular and Genetic Basis of Neurologic Disease*, RN Rosenberg et al (eds). Boston, Butterworth-Heinemann, 1997

EMERY AEH (ed): *Neuromuscular Disorders: Clinical and Molecular Genetics*. Wiley, Chichester, 1999

GRIGGS RC et al: The muscular dystrophies, in *Evaluation and Treatment of Myopathies*, RC Griggs et al (eds). Philadelphia, FA Davis, 1995

INTERNATIONAL MUSCULAR DYSTROPHY CONSORTIUM (IDMC): The new nomenclature and DNA testing guidelines for myotonic dystrophy type 1 (DM1). Neurology 54:1218, 2000

KISSEL JT et al: Endocrine myopathies, in *Handbook of Clinical Neurology*, vol 19, LP Rowland, S DiMauro (eds). New York, Elsevier, 1992

LIU J et al: Dysferlin, a novel skeletal muscle gene, is mutated in Miyoshi myopathy and limb girdle muscular dystrophy. Nat Genet 20:31, 1998

MINETTI C et al: Mutations in the caveolin-3 gene cause autosomal dominant limb-girdle muscular dystrophy. Nat Genet 18:365, 1998

MOREIRA ES et al: Limb-girdle muscular dystrophy type 2G is caused by mutations in the gene encoding the sarcomeric protein telethonin. Nat Genet 24:163, 2000

TSAO C-Y et al: The childhood muscular dystrophies: Making order out of chaos. Semin Neurol 19:9, 1999

VARDERIO E et al: Carnitine palmitoyltransferase II deficiency: Structure of the gene and characterization of two novel disease-causing mutations. Hum Mol Genet 4:19, 1995

Stephen E. Straus

CHRONIC FATIGUE SYNDROME

DEFINITION *Chronic fatigue syndrome* (CFS) is the current name for a disorder characterized by debilitating fatigue and several associated physical, constitutional, and neuropsychological complaints (Table 384-1). This syndrome is not new; in the past, patients diagnosed with conditions such as the vapors, neurasthenia, effort syndrome, hyperventilation syndrome, chronic brucellosis, epidemic neuromyasthenia, myalgic encephalomyelitis, hypoglycemia, multiple chemical sensitivity syndrome, chronic candidiasis, chronic mononucleosis, chronic Epstein-Barr virus infection, and postviral fatigue syndrome may have had what is now called chronic fatigue syndrome. The U.S. Centers for Disease Control and Prevention (CDC) has developed diagnostic criteria for CFS based upon symptoms and the exclusion of other illnesses (Table 384-2).

EPIDEMIOLOGY Patients with CFS are twice as likely to be women as men and are generally 25 to 45 years old, although cases in childhood and in later life have been described.

Cases are recognized in many developed countries. Most arise sporadically, but many clusters have also been reported. The most famous outbreaks of CFS occurred in Los Angeles County Hospital in 1934; in Akureyri, Iceland, in 1948; in the Royal Free Hospital, London, in 1955; in Punta Gorda, Florida, in 1956; and in Incline Village, Nevada, in 1985. While these clustered cases suggest a common environmental or infectious cause, none has been identified.

Estimates of the prevalence of CFS have depended on the case definition used and the method of study. Chronic fatigue itself is a common symptom, occurring in as many as 20% of patients attending general medical clinics; CFS is far less common. Community-based studies find that 100 to 300 individuals per 100,000 population in the United States meet the current CDC case definition.

PATHOGENESIS The diverse names for the syndrome reflect the equally numerous and controversial hypotheses about its etiology. Several common themes underlie attempts to understand the disorder: It is often postinfectious, it is associated with immunologic disturbances, and it is commonly accompanied by neuropsychological complaints and depression.

Table 384-1 Specific Symptoms Reported by Patients with Chronic Fatigue Syndrome

Symptom	Percentage
Fatigue	100
Difficulty concentrating	90
Headache	90
Sore throat	85
Tender lymph nodes	80
Muscle aches	80
Joint aches	75
Feverishness	75
Difficulty sleeping	70
Psychiatric problems	65
Allergies	55
Abdominal cramps	40
Weight loss	20
Rash	10
Rapid pulse	10
Weight gain	5
Chest pain	5
Night sweats	5

SOURCE: From SE Straus: J Infect Diseases 157:405, 1988.

Table 384-2 CDC Criteria for Chronic Fatigue Syndrome

A case of chronic fatigue syndrome is defined by the presence of:
1. Clinically evaluated, unexplained, persistent or relapsing fatigue that is of new or definite onset; is not the result of ongoing exertion; is not alleviated by rest; and results in substantial reduction of previous levels of occupational, educational, social, or personal activities; and
2. Four or more of the following symptoms that persist or recur during six or more consecutive months of illness and that do not predate the fatigue:
   * Self-reported impairment in short-term memory or concentration
   * Sore throat
   * Tender cervical or axillary nodes
   * Muscle pain
   * Multijoint pain without redness or swelling
   * Headaches of a new pattern or severity
   * Unrefreshing sleep
   * Postexertional malaise lasting $\geq$24 h

SOURCE: Adapted from Fukuda et al.

Many studies in the 1980s and 1990s attempted to link CFS to infection with a persistent virus such as a lymphotropic herpesvirus, retrovirus, or enterovirus. In many patients with chronic fatigue, titers of antibodies to herpesviruses, measles virus, rubella virus, and coxsackievirus B are elevated. Reports that viral antigens and nucleic acids could be specifically identified in patients with CFS have not been confirmed. One study from the United Kingdom failed to detect any association between acute infections and subsequent prolonged fatigue. Another study found that chronic fatigue did not develop after typical upper respiratory infections but did in some individuals after infectious mononucleosis. Thus, while cumulative experience suggests that antecedent viral infections are associated with CFS, a direct viral pathogenesis is unproven.

Changes in immune parameters of uncertain functional significance have been reported in CFS. Modest and nonspecific elevations in titers of antinuclear antibodies, reductions in immunoglobulin subclasses, deficiencies in mitogen-driven lymphocyte proliferation, reductions in natural killer cell activity, disturbances in cytokine production, and shifts in lymphocyte subsets with increases in cells expressing activation markers have been described. None of the immune findings appears in all patients, nor do any correlate with the severity of CFS. None are specific; thus they remain nondiagnostic. In theory, symptoms of CFS could result from excessive production of a cytokine, such as interleukin 1, that induces asthenia and other flulike symptoms; however, conclusive data in support of this long-held hypothesis are lacking.

Disturbances in endocrine function, consistent with reduced production of corticotropin-releasing hormone in the hypothalamus, have been reported in controlled studies of CFS. Mean serum cortisol concentrations were lower in patients than in controls; levels of adrenocorticotropic hormone were correspondingly high. Hypothetically, these neuroendocrine abnormalities could contribute to the impaired energy and depressed mood of patients.

Mild to moderate depression is present in half to two-thirds of patients. Much of this depression may be reactive, but its prevalence exceeds that seen in other chronic medical illnesses. Some propose that CFS is fundamentally a psychiatric disorder and that the various neuroendocrine and immune disturbances arise secondarily.

MANIFESTATIONS Typically, CFS arises suddenly in a previously active individual. An otherwise unremarkable flulike illness or some other acute stress leaves unbearable exhaustion in its wake. Other symptoms, such as headache, sore throat, tender lymph nodes, muscle and joint aches, and frequent feverishness, lead to the belief that an infection persists, and medical attention is sought. Over several weeks, despite reassurances that nothing serious is wrong, the symptoms persist and other features of the syndrome become evident—disturbed sleep, difficulty in concentration, and depression (Table 384-1).

Depending on the dominant symptoms and the beliefs of the patient, additional consultations may be sought from allergists, rheumatologists, infectious disease specialists, psychiatrists, ecologic therapists, homeopaths, or other professionals, frequently with unsatisfactory results. Once the pattern of illness is established, the symptoms may fluctuate somewhat. Many patients report that diverse complaints are linked—that during periods of greatest fatigue they perceive the most pain and difficulty with concentration. Patients also commonly assert that excessive physical or emotional stress may exacerbate their symptoms.

Most patients remain capable of continuing to meet the obligations of family, work, or community despite their symptoms. The discretionary activities are abandoned first. Some feel unable to engage in any gainful employment. A minority of individuals require help with the activities of daily living.

Ultimately, isolation, frustration, and pathetic resignation can mark the protracted course of illness. Patients may become angry at physicians for failing to acknowledge or resolve their plight. Fortunately, CFS does not appear to progress. On the contrary, many patients experience gradual improvement, and a minority recover fully.

DIAGNOSIS   Physical examination and routine laboratory tests are required to rule out other causes of the patient's symptoms. Prominent abnormalities argue strongly in favor of alternative diagnoses. No laboratory test, however, can diagnose this condition or measure its severity. In most cases, elaborate, expensive workups are not helpful. Magnetic resonance imaging of the brain may identify small T2 hyperintense signals in a minority of patients, but these findings do not aid diagnosis nor are they prognostic. The dilemma for patient and clinician alike is that CFS has no pathognomonic features and remains a constellation of symptoms and a diagnosis of exclusion. Often the patient presents with features that also meet criteria for other subjective disorders such as fibromyalgia and irritable bowel syndrome.

℞ **TREATMENT**   The primary responsibility of a physician confronted with a chronically fatigued patient is to address the cause by taking a thorough history, conducting a complete physical examination, judiciously using the laboratory, and, throughout this process, considering the differential diagnosis. After other illnesses have been excluded, there are several points to address in the long-term care of a patient with chronic fatigue.

The patient should be informed about the illness and what is known of its pathogenesis; its potential impact on the physical, psychological, and social dimensions of life; and its prognosis. Patients are relieved when their complaints are taken seriously. Periodic reassessment is appropriate to identify a possible underlying process that is late in declaring itself and to address intercurrent symptoms that should not be simply dismissed as yet another subjective complaint.

Many symptoms of CFS respond to treatment. Nonsteroidal antiinflammatory drugs alleviate headache, diffuse pain, and feverishness. Allergic rhinitis and sinusitis are common; antihistamines or decongestants may be helpful. Although the patient may be averse to psychiatric diagnoses, depression is often a prominent symptom and, when present, should be treated. Expert psychiatric assessment is sometimes advisable. Nonsedating antidepressants improve mood and disordered sleep and thereby attenuate the fatigue somewhat. Even modest improvements in symptoms can make an important difference in the patient's degree of self-sufficiency and ability to appreciate life's pleasures.

Practical advice should be given regarding lifestyle. Sleep disturbances are common; consumption of heavy meals with alcohol and caffeine at night can make sleep even more elusive, compounding fatigue. Total rest leads to further deconditioning and the self-image of being an invalid, whereas overexertion may worsen exhaustion and lead to total avoidance of exercise. A moderate, carefully graded regimen should be encouraged and has been proven to relieve symptoms and enhance exercise tolerance.

Controlled therapeutic trials have established that acyclovir, intramuscular liver extract–folic acid–cyanocobalamin injections, and intravenous immunoglobulin, among others, are of no value. Two studies showed that low doses of hydrocortisone provide modest benefit, but they may lead to adrenal suppression. Countless anecdotes circulate regarding other traditional and nontraditional therapies. It is important to guide patients away from those therapeutic modalities that are toxic, expensive, or unreasonable.

The physician should promote the patient's efforts toward improvement. Three clinical trials in England showed behavioral therapy to be helpful. This approach aims to dispel misguided beliefs and fears about the illness that can contribute to inactivity and despair. For CFS, as for many other conditions, a comprehensive approach to physical, psychological, and social aspects of well-being is in order.

BIBLIOGRAPHY

FUKUDA K et al: The chronic fatigue syndrome: A comprehensive approach to its definition and study. Ann Intern Med 121:953, 1994

FULCHER KY, WHITE PD: Randomised controlled trial of graded exercise in patients with the chronic fatigue syndrome. BMJ 314:1647, 1997

SHARPE MC et al: Cognitive behaviour therapy for the chronic fatigue syndrome: A randomised controlled trial. BMJ 312:22, 1996

STEELE L et al: The epidemiology of chronic fatigue in San Francisco. Am J Med 105: 83S, 1998

STRAUS SE et al: *Chronic Fatigue Syndrome.* New York: Marcel Dekker, 1994

Section 5

PSYCHIATRIC DISORDERS

385	*Victor I. Reus*

MENTAL DISORDERS

The term "mental disorders," as defined in the 4th edition of the standard psychiatric *Diagnostic and Statistical Manual* (DSM-IV), encompasses a broad range of conditions characterized by patterns of abnormal behavioral and psychological signs and symptoms that result in dysfunction. The implication that mental disorders lack a physical cause is unfortunate and incorrect, and the term survives only for want of a better substitute. Mental disorders are highly prevalent in medical practice and may present either as a primary disorder or as a comorbid condition. The total direct and indirect costs of all mental disorders in the United States has been estimated to be $148 billion dollars, only slightly less than costs incurred by cardiovascular diseases.

The DSM-IV-PC (Primary Care) manual provides a useful synopsis of mental disorders most likely to be seen in primary care practice. The current system of classification is multiaxial and includes the presence or absence of a major mental disorder (axis I), any underlying personality disorder (axis II), general medical condition (axis III), psychosocial and environmental problems (axis IV), and overall rating of general psychosocial functioning (axis V).

Changes in health care delivery underscore the need for primary care physicians to assume responsibility for the initial diagnosis and treatment of the most common mental disorders. Prompt diagnosis is essential to ensure that patients have access to appropriate medical services and to maximize the clinical outcome. Validated patient-based questionnaires have been developed that systematically probe for signs and symptoms associated with the most prevalent psychiatric diagnoses and guide the clinician into a more targeted historic assessment. Prime MD and the Symptom-Driven Diagnostic System for Primary Care (SDDS-PC) are inventories that require only 10 min to complete and link patient responses to the formal diagnostic criteria of anxiety, mood, somatoform, and eating disorders and to alcohol abuse or dependence.

A physician who refers patients to a psychiatrist should know not only when doing so is appropriate but also how to do it, since societal misconceptions and the stigma of mental illness impede the process. Primary care physicians should base referrals to a psychiatrist on the presence of the signs and symptoms of a mental disorder and not simply on the absence of a physical explanation for a patient's complaint. The physician should discuss with the patient the reasons for requesting the referral or consultation and provide reassurance that he or she will continue to provide medical care and work collaboratively with the mental health professional. Consultation with a psychiatrist or transfer of care is appropriate when physicians encounter evidence of psychotic symptoms, mania, severe depression, or anxiety; symptoms of posttraumatic stress disorder (PTSD); suicidal or homicidal preoccupation; or a failure to respond to first-order treatment.→*Eating disorders are discussed in Chap. 78.*

ANXIETY DISORDERS

Anxiety disorders, the most prevalent psychiatric illnesses in the general community, are present in 15 to 20% of medical clinic patients. Anxiety, defined as a subjective sense of unease, dread, or foreboding, can indicate a primary psychiatric condition or can be a component of, or reaction to, a primary medical disease. The primary anxiety disorders are classified according to their duration and course and the existence and nature of precipitants.

When evaluating the anxious patient, the clinician must first determine whether the anxiety antedates or postdates a medical illness or is due to a medication side effect. Approximately one-third of patients presenting with anxiety have a medical etiology for their psychiatric symptoms, but an anxiety disorder can also present with somatic symptoms in the absence of a diagnosable medical condition.

PANIC DISORDER Clinical Manifestations Panic disorder is defined by the presence of recurrent and unpredictable panic attacks, which are distinct episodes of intense fear and discomfort associated with a variety of physical symptoms, including palpitations, sweating, trembling, shortness of breath, chest pain, dizziness, and a fear of impending doom or death (Table 385-1). Paresthesias, gastrointestinal distress, and feelings of unreality are also common. Panic attacks have a sudden onset, developing within 10 min and usually resolving over the course of an hour, and they occur in an unexpected fashion. The frequency and severity of panic attacks varies, ranging from once a week to clusters of attacks separated by months of well-being. The first attack is usually outside the home. Onset is usually in late adolescence to early adulthood. In some individuals, anticipatory anxiety develops over time and results in a generalized fear and a progressive avoidance of places or situations in which a panic attack might recur. *Agoraphobia*, which occurs commonly in patients with panic disorder, is an acquired irrational fear of being in places where one might feel trapped or unable to escape (Table 385-2). Typically, it leads the patient into a progressive restriction in life-style and, in a literal sense, in geography. Frequently, patients are embarrassed that they are housebound and dependent on the company of others to go out into the

Table 385-1 Diagnostic Criteria for Panic Attack

A discrete period of intense fear or discomfort, in which four or more of the following symptoms developed abruptly and reached a peak within 10 min:
1. Palpitations, pounding heart, or accelerated heart rate
2. Sweating
3. Trembling or shaking
4. Sensations of shortness of breath or smothering
5. Feeling of choking
6. Chest pain or discomfort
7. Nausea or abdominal distress
8. Feeling dizzy, unsteady, lightheaded, or faint
9. Derealization (feelings of unreality) or depersonalization (being detached from oneself)
10. Fear of losing control or going crazy
11. Fear of dying
12. Paresthesias (numbness or tingling sensations)
13. Chills or hot flushes

SOURCE: *Diagnostic and Statistical Manual of Mental Disorders*, 4th ed.

world and do not volunteer this information; thus physicians will fail to recognize the syndrome if direct questioning is not pursued.

Differential Diagnosis A diagnosis of panic disorder is made after a medical etiology for the panic attacks has been ruled out. A variety of cardiovascular, respiratory, endocrine, and neurologic conditions can present with anxiety as the chief complaint. Patients with true panic disorder will often focus on one specific feature to the exclusion of others. For example, 20% of patients who present with syncope as a primary medical complaint have a primary diagnosis of a mood, anxiety, or substance-abuse disorder, the most common being panic disorder. The differential diagnosis of panic disorder is complicated by a high rate of comorbidity with other psychiatric conditions, especially alcohol and benzodiazepine abuse, which patients initially use in an attempt at self-medication. Some 75% of panic disorder patients will also satisfy criteria for major depression at some point in their illness.

When the history is nonspecific, physical examination and focused laboratory testing must be used to rule out medical anxiety states, such as those resulting from pheochromocytoma, thyrotoxicosis, or hypoglycemia. Electrocardiogram (ECG) and echocardiogram may detect some cardiovascular conditions associated with panic, such as paroxysmal atrial tachycardia and mitral valve prolapse. In two studies, panic disorder was the primary diagnosis in 43% of patients with chest pain who had normal coronary angiograms and was present in 9% of all outpatients referred for cardiac evaluation. Panic disorder has also been diagnosed in many patients referred for pulmonary function testing or with symptoms of irritable bowel syndrome.

Etiology and Pathophysiology The etiology of panic disorder is unknown but appears to involve a genetic predisposition, altered

Table 385-2 Diagnostic Criteria for Agoraphobia

1. Anxiety about being in places or situations from which escape might be difficult (or embarrassing) or in which help may not be available in the event of having an unexpected or situationally predisposed panic attack or panic-like symptoms. Agoraphobic fears typically involve characteristic clusters of situations that include being outside the home alone; being in a crowd or standing in a line; being on a bridge; and traveling in a bus, train, or automobile.
2. The situations are avoided (e.g., travel is restricted) or else are endured with marked distress or with anxiety about having a panic attack or panic-like symptoms, or require the presence of a companion.
3. The anxiety or phobic avoidance is not better accounted for by another mental disorder, such as social phobia (e.g., avoidance limited to social situations because of fear of embarrassment), specific phobia (e.g., avoidance limited to a single situation like elevators), obsessive-compulsive disorder (e.g., avoidance of dirt in someone with an obsession about contamination), posttraumatic stress disorder (e.g., avoidance of stimuli associated with a severe stressor), or separation anxiety disorder (e.g., avoidance of leaving home or relatives).

SOURCE: *Diagnostic and Statistical Manual of Mental Disorders*, 4th ed.

Table 385-3 Antidepressants

Name	Usual Daily Dose, mg	Side Effects	Comments
SSRIs			
Fluoxetine (Prozac)	10–80	Headache; nausea and	Once daily dosing, usu-
Sertraline (Zoloft)	50–200	other GI effects; jitteri-	ally in A.M.; fluoxetine
Paroxetine (Paxil)	20–60	ness; insomnia; sexual	has very long half-life;
Fluvoxamine (Luvox)	100–300	dysfunction; can affect	must not be combined
Citalopram (Celexa)	20–60	plasma levels of other	with MAOIs
		meds (except sertraline);	
		akathisia rare	
TCAs			
Amitriptyline (Elavil)	150–300	Anticholinergic (dry	Once daily dosing, usu-
Nortriptyline (Pamelor)	50–200	mouth, tachycardia,	ally qhs; blood levels of
Imipramine (Tofranil)	150–300	constipation, urinary re-	most TCAs available;
Desipramine	150–300	tention, blurred vision);	can be lethal in O.D.
(Norpramin)		sweating; tremor; pos-	(lethal dose = 2 g); nor-
Doxepin (Sinequan)	150–300	tural hypotension; car-	triptyline best tolerated,
Clomipramine	150–300	diac conduction delay;	especially by elderly
(Anafranil)		sedation; weight gain	
Mixed norepinephrine/se-			
rotonin reuptake inhibi-			
tors			
Venlafaxine (Effexor)	75–375	Nausea; dizziness; dry	Bid-tid dosing; lower po-
		mouth; headaches; in-	tential for drug-drug in-
		creased blood pressure;	teractions than SSRIs;
		anxiety and insomnia	contraindicated with
Mirtazapine (Remeron)	15–45	Somnolence; weight	MAOIs.
		gain; neutropenia rare	Once daily dosing
Mixed-action drugs			
Bupropion	250–450	Jitteriness; flushing; sei-	Tid dosing, but sustained
(Wellbutrin)		zures in at-risk patients;	release also available;
		anorexia; tachycardia;	fewer sexual side effects
		psychosis	than SSRIs or TCAs;
			may be useful for adult
			ADD
Trazodone (Desyrel)	200–600	Sedation; dry mouth;	Useful in low doses for
		ventricular irritability;	sleep because of sedat-
		postural hypotension;	ing effects with no anti-
		priapism rare	cholinergic side effects
Nefazodone (Serzone)	300–600	Sedation; headache; dry	Once daily dosing; no ef-
		mouth; nausea; consti-	fect on REM sleep un-
		pation	like other antidepres-
			sants
MAOIs			
Phenelzine (Nardil)	45–90	Insomnia; hypotension;	May be more effective in
Tranylcypromine	20–50	anorgasmia; weight	patients with atypical
(Parnate)		gain; hypertensive cri-	features or treatment-
Isocarboxazid (Mar-	20–60	sis; tyramine cheese re-	refractory depressions
plan)		action; lethal reactions	
		with SSRIs; serious re-	
		actions with narcotics	

NOTE: ADD, attention deficit disorder; MAOI, monoamine oxidase inhibitor; REM, rapid eye movement; SSRI, selective serotonin reuptake inhibitor; TCA, tricyclic antidepressant.

autonomic responsivity, and social learning. Panic disorder shows familial aggregation, although concordance in monozygotic twins is only 30%. Acute panic attacks appear to be associated with increased noradrenergic discharge in the locus coeruleus. Intravenous infusion of sodium lactate evokes an attack in two-thirds of panic disorder patients, as do the α_2-adrenergic antagonist yohimbine and carbon dioxide inhalation. It is hypothesized that each of these stimuli activates a neural circuit involving noradrenergic neurons in the locus coeruleus and serotonergic neurons in the dorsal raphe. Agents that block serotonin reuptake are therapeutic in preventing attacks. It is theorized that panic-disorder patients have a heightened sensitivity to somatic symptoms, which triggers increasing arousal, setting off the "panic attack" mechanism. Accordingly, successful therapeutic intervention involves altering the patient's cognitive interpretation of anxiety-producing experiences as well as preventing the attack itself.

℞ TREATMENT Achievable goals of treatment are to decrease the frequency of panic attacks and to reduce their intensity. The cornerstone of drug therapy is antidepressant medications (Tables 385-3, 385-4, and 385-5). The tricyclic antidepressant (TCA) agents imipramine and clomipramine can benefit 75 to 90% of panic disorder patients. Low doses (e.g., 10 to 25 mg/d) are given initially to avoid any increased anxiety associated with heightened monoamine levels in the initial stages of treatment. Selective serotonin reuptake inhibitors (SSRIs) are equally effective and do not have the adverse effects of TCAs. SSRIs should be started at one-third to one-half of their usual antidepressant dose (e.g., 5 to 10 mg fluoxetine, 25 to 50 mg sertraline, 10 mg paroxetine). Monoamine oxidase inhibitors (MAOIs) are at least as effective as TCAs and may specifically benefit patients who have comorbid features of atypical depression (i.e., hypersomnia and weight gain). Insomnia, orthostatic hypotension, and the need to maintain a low-tyramine diet (avoidance of cheese and wine) have limited their use, however. Antidepressants typically take 2 to 6 weeks to become effective, and doses may need to be adjusted according to clinical response.

Because of anticipatory anxiety and the need for immediate relief of panic symptoms, benzodiazepines are useful early in the course of treatment and sporadically thereafter (Table 385-6). For example, alprazolam, starting at 0.5 mg qid and increasing to 4 mg/d in divided doses, is effective, but patients must be monitored closely, as some develop dependence and begin to escalate the dose of this medication. Clonazepam, at a final maintenance dose of 2 to 4 mg/d, is also helpful; its longer half-life permits twice-daily scheduling, and patients appear less likely to develop dependence on this agent.

Early psychotherapeutic intervention and psychoeducation aimed at symptom control enhances the effectiveness of drug treatment. Patients can be taught breathing techniques, can be educated about physiologic changes that occur with panic, and can learn to expose themselves voluntarily to precipitating events. Homework assignments and monitored compliance are important components of successful treatment. Once patients have achieved a satisfactory response, drug treatment should be maintained for 1 to 2 years to prevent relapse.

GENERALIZED ANXIETY DISORDER Clinical Manifestations Patients with generalized anxiety disorder (GAD) have persistent, excessive, and/or unrealistic worry associated with other signs and symptoms, which commonly include muscle tension, impaired concentration, autonomic arousal, feeling "on edge" or restless, and insomnia (Table 385-7). Onset is usually before age 20, and a history of childhood fears and social inhibition may be present. The incidence of GAD is increased in first-degree relatives of patients with the diagnosis; family studies also indicate that GAD and panic disorder segregate independently. Over 80% of patients with GAD also suffer from major depression, dysthymia, or social phobia. Comorbid substance abuse is common in these patients, particularly alcohol and/or sedative/hypnotic abuse. Patients with GAD readily admit to worrying excessively over minor matters, with life-disrupting effects; unlike in panic disorder, complaints of symptoms such as shortness of breath, palpitations, and tachycardia are relatively rare.

Table 385-4 Management of Antidepressant Side Effects

Symptoms	Comments and Management Strategies
Gastrointestinal	
Nausea, loss of appetite	Usually short-lived and dose-related; consider temporary dose reduction or administration with food and antacids
Diarrhea	Famotidine, 20–40 mg/d
Constipation	Wait for tolerance; try diet change, stool softener; avoid laxatives
Sexual dysfunction	Consider dose reduction; drug holiday
Anorgasmia/impotence; impaired ejaculation	Bethanechol, 10–20 mg, 2 h before activity, or cyproheptadine, 4–8 mg 2 h before activity, or bupropion, 100 mg bid or amantadine, 100 mg bid/tid
Orthostasis	Tolerance unlikely; increase fluid intake, use calf exercises/support hose; fludrocortisone, 0.025 mg/d
Anticholinergic	Wait for tolerance
Dry mouth, eyes	Maintain good oral hygiene; use artificial tears, sugar-free gum
Tremor/jitteriness	Antiparkinsonian drugs not effective; use dose reduction/slow increase; lorazepam, 0.5 mg bid, or propranolol, 10–20 mg bid
Insomnia	Schedule all doses for the morning; trazodone, 50–100 mg qhs
Sedation	Caffeine; schedule all dosing for bedtime; buproprion, 75–100 mg in afternoon
Headache	Evaluate diet, stress, other drugs; try dose reduction; amitriptyline, 50 mg/d
Weight gain	Decrease carbohydrates; exercise; consider fluoxetine
Loss of therapeutic benefit over time	Related to tolerance? Increase dose or drug holiday; add amantadine, 100 mg bid, buspirone, 10 mg tid, or pindolol, 2.5 mg bid

Etiology and Pathophysiology In experimental models of anxiety, anxiogenic agents share in common the property of altering the binding of benzodiazepines to the γ-aminobutyric acid (GABA) A receptor/chloride ion channel complex. Benzodiazepines are thought to bind two separate $GABA_A$ receptor sites: type I, which has a broad neuroanatomic distribution, and type II, which is concentrated in the hippocampus, striatum, and neocortex. The antianxiety effects of the various benzodiazepines and side effects such as sedation and memory impairment are influenced by their relative binding to type I and type II receptor sites. Serotonin [5-hydroxytriptamine (5HT)] also appears to have a role in anxiety. Buspirone, a partial $5HT_{1A}$ receptor agonist, and certain $5HT_{2A}$ and $5HT_{2C}$ receptor antagonists (e.g., nefazodone) may also have beneficial effects.

 TREATMENT A combination of pharmacologic and psychotherapeutic interventions is most effective in GAD, but complete

Table 385-5 Possible Drug Interactions with Selective Serotonin Reuptake Inhibitors

Agent	Effect
Monoamine oxidase inhibitors	Serotonin syndrome—absolute contraindication
Serotonergic agonists, e.g., tryptophan, fenfluramine	Potential serotonin syndrome
Drugs that are metabolized by P450 isoenzymes: tricyclics, other SSRIs, antipsychotics, beta blockers, codeine, terfenadine, astemizole, triazolobenzodiazepines, calcium channel blockers	Delayed metabolism resulting in increased blood levels and potential toxicity—possible fatality secondary to QT prolongation with terfenadine or astemizole
Drugs that are bound tightly to plasma proteins, e.g., warfarin, coumadin	Increased bleeding secondary to displacement
Drugs that inhibit the metabolism of SSRIs by P450 isoenzymes, e.g., quinidine	Increased SSRI side effects

NOTE: SSRI, selective serotonin reuptake inhibitor.

symptomatic relief is rare. A short course of a benzodiazepine is usually indicated, preferably lorazepam, oxazepam, or temazepam. (The first two of these agents are metabolized via conjugation rather than oxidation and thus do not accumulate if hepatic function is altered.) Administration should be initiated at the lowest dose possible and prescribed on an as-needed basis as symptoms warrant. Benzodiazepines differ in their milligram per kilogram potency, half-life, lipid solubility, metabolic pathways, and presence of active metabolites. Agents that are absorbed rapidly and are lipid soluble, such as diazepam, have a rapid onset of action and a higher abuse potential. Benzodiazepines should generally not be prescribed for >4 to 6 weeks because of the development of tolerance and the risk of abuse and dependence. It is important to warn patients that concomitant usage of alcohol or other sedating drugs may result in neurotoxicity and impair their ability to function. An optimistic approach that encourages the patient to clarify environmental precipitants, anticipate his or her reactions, and plan effective response strategies are essential elements of therapy.

Adverse effects of benzodiazepines generally parallel their relative half-lives. Longer-acting agents, such as diazepam, chlordiazepoxide, flurazepam, and clonazepam, tend to accumulate active metabolites, with resultant sedation, impairment of cognition, and poor psychomotor performance. Shorter-acting compounds, such as alprazolam and oxazepam, can result in daytime anxiety, early morning insomnia, and with discontinuation, rebound anxiety and insomnia. Although patients develop tolerance to the sedative effects of benzodiazepines, they are less likely to habituate to the adverse psychomotor effects. Withdrawal from the longer half-life benzodiazepines can be accomplished through gradual, stepwise dose reduction (by ~10% every 1 to 2 weeks) over 6 to 12 weeks. It is usually more difficult to taper patients off shorter-acting benzodiazepines. Physicians may need to switch the patient to a benzodiazepine with a longer half-life or use an adjunctive medication, such as a beta blocker or carbamazepine, before attempting to discontinue the benzodiazepine. Withdrawal reactions vary in severity and duration; they can include depression, anxiety, delirium, lethargy, diaphoresis, tinnitus, autonomic arousal, unusual neuromuscular movements, and, rarely, seizures.

Buspirone, an azaspirone, is a nonbenzodiazepine anxiolytic agent. It is nonsedating, does not lead to tolerance or dependence, does not interact with benzodiazepine receptors or alcohol, and has no abuse or disinhibition potential. However, it requires several weeks to take effect and requires thrice-daily dosing. Patients who were previously responsive to a benzodiazepine are unlikely to rate buspirone as equally effective, but patients with head injury or dementia who have symptoms of anxiety and/or agitation may do well with this agent.

Administration of benzodiazepines to geriatric patients requires special care. Such patients have increased drug absorption; decreased hepatic metabolism, protein binding, and renal excretion; and an increased volume of distribution. These factors, together with the likely presence of comorbid medical illnesses and medication, dramatically increase the likelihood of toxicity. Iatrogenic psychomotor impairment can result in falls and fractures, confusional states, or motor vehicle accidents. If used, agents in this class should be started at the lowest possible dose, and results should be monitored closely. Benzodiazepines are contraindicated during pregnancy and breast-feeding.

PHOBIC DISORDERS Clinical Manifestations The cardinal feature of phobic disorders is a marked and persistent fear of objects or situations, exposure to which results in an immediate anxiety reaction. The patient avoids the phobic stimulus, and this avoidance usually impairs occupational or social functioning. Panic attacks may be triggered by the phobic stimulus or may emerge spontaneously during the course of the illness. Unlike patients with other anxiety disorders, individuals with phobias experience anxiety only in specific situations. Common phobias include fear of closed spaces (claustrophobia), fear of blood, and fear of flying. Social phobia is distinguished

Table 385-6 Anxiolytics

Name	Equivalent PO dose, mg	Onset of Action	Half-life, h	Comments
Benzodiazepines:				
Diazepam (Valium)	5	Fast	20–70	Active metabolites; quite sedating
Flurazepam (Dalmane)	15	Fast	30–100	Flurazepam is a pro-drug; metabolites are active; quite sedating
Triazolam (Halcion)	0.25	Intermediate	1.5–5	No active metabolites; can induce confusion and delirium, especially in elderly
Lorazepam (Ativan)	1	Intermediate	10–20	No active metabolites; direct hepatic glucuronide conjugation; quite sedating
Alprazolam (Xanax)	0.5	Intermediate	12–15	Active metabolites; not too sedating; may have specific antidepressant and antipanic activity; tolerance and dependence develop easily
Chlordiazepoxide (Librium)	10	Intermediate	5–30	Active metabolites; moderately sedating
Oxazepam (Serax)	15	Slow	5–15	No active metabolites; direct glucuronide conjugation; not too sedating
Temazepam (Restoril)	15	Slow	9–12	No active metabolites; moderately sedating
Clonazepam (Klonopin)	0.5	Slow	18–50	No active metabolites; moderately sedating
Non-benzodiazepines				
Buspirone (BuSpar)	7.5	2 weeks	2–3	Active metabolites; tid dosing—usual daily dose 10–20 mg tid; nonsedating; no additive effects with alcohol; useful for agitation in demented or brain-injured patients

by a specific fear of social or performance situations in which the individual is exposed to unfamiliar individuals or to possible examination and evaluation by others. Examples include having to converse at a party, use public restrooms, and meet strangers. In each case, the affected individual is aware that the experienced fear is excessive and unreasonable given the circumstance. The specific content of a phobia may vary across gender, ethnic, and cultural boundaries.

Phobic disorders are common, with a 1-year prevalence rate of 9% and a lifetime rate of 10 to 11%. Onset is typically in childhood to

Table 385-7 Diagnostic Criteria for Generalized Anxiety Disorder

A. Excessive anxiety and worry (apprehensive expectation), occurring more days than not for at least 6 months, about a number of events or activities (such as work or school performance).

B. The person finds it difficult to control the worry.

C. The anxiety and worry are associated with three (or more) of the following six symptoms (with at least some symptoms present for more days than not for the past 6 months): (1) restlessness or feeling keyed up or on edge; (2) being easily fatigued; (3) difficulty concentrating or mind going blank; (4) irritability; (5) muscle tension; (6) sleep disturbance (difficulty falling or staying asleep, or restless unsatisfying sleep).

D. The focus of the anxiety and worry is not confined to features of an Axis I disorder, e.g., the anxiety or worry is not about having a panic attack (as in panic disorder), being embarrassed in public (as in social phobia), being contaminated (as in obsessive-compulsive disorder), being away from home or close relatives (as in separation anxiety disorder), gaining weight (as in anorexia nervosa), having multiple physical complaints (as in somatization disorder), or having a serious illness (as in hypochondriasis), and the anxiety and worry do not occur exclusively during posttraumatic stress disorder.

E. The anxiety, worry, or physical symptoms cause clinically significant distress or impairment in social, occupational, or other important areas of functioning.

F. The disturbance is not due to the direct physiologic effects of a substance (e.g., a drug of abuse, a medication) or a general medical condition (e.g., hyperthyroidism) and does not occur exclusively during a mood disorder, a psychotic disorder, or a pervasive developmental disorder.

SOURCE: *Diagnostic and Statistical Manual of Mental Disorders*, 4th ed.

early adulthood. Familial aggregation may occur. In one study of female twins, concordance rates for agoraphobia, social phobia, and animal phobia was found to be 23% for monozygotic twins and 15% for dizygotic twins. Full criteria for diagnosis are usually satisfied first in adulthood, but behavioral avoidance of unfamiliar people, situations, or objects dating from early childhood is common.

TREATMENT Recent controlled trials have documented the efficacy of several pharmacologic agents in the treatment of phobic disorders. Beta blockers (e.g., propranolol, 20 to 40 mg orally 2 h before the event) are particularly effective in the treatment of "performance anxiety" (but not general social phobia) and appear to achieve their benefit by preventing the occurrence of peripheral manifestations of anxiety, such as perspiration, tachycardia, palpitations, and tremor. MAOIs alleviate social phobia independently of their antidepressant activity, and SSRIs appear to be effective also. Benzodiazepines can be helpful in reducing fearful avoidance, but the chronic nature of phobic disorders limits their usefulness.

Behaviorally focused psychotherapy is an important component of treatment, as relapse rates are high when medication is used as the sole treatment. Cognitive-behavioral strategies are the cornerstone of treatment; these are based upon the finding that distorted perceptions and interpretations of fear-producing stimuli play a major role in perpetuation of phobias. Individual and group therapy sessions teach the patient to identify specific negative thoughts associated with the anxiety-producing situation and help to reduce the patient's fear of loss of control. In desensitization therapy, hierarchies of feared situations are constructed and the patient is encouraged to pursue and master gradual exposure to the anxiety-producing stimuli.

Patients with social phobia, in particular, have a high rate of comorbid alcohol abuse, as well as of other psychiatric conditions (e.g., eating disorders), necessitating the need for parallel management of each disorder if anxiety reduction is to be achieved.

STRESS DISORDERS **Clinical Manifestations** Patients may develop anxiety after exposure to extreme traumatic events such as the threat of personal death or injury or the death of a loved one. The reaction may occur shortly after the trauma (*acute stress disorder*) or be delayed and subject to recurrence (PTSD) (Table 385-8). In both syndromes, individuals experience associated symptoms of detachment and loss of emotional responsivity. The patient may feel depersonalized and unable to recall specific aspects of the trauma, though typically it is reexperienced through intrusions in thought, dreams, or flashbacks, particularly when cues of the original event are present. Patients often actively avoid stimuli that precipitate recollections of the trauma and demonstrate a resulting increase in vigilance, arousal, and startle response. Patients with stress disorders are at risk for the development of other anxiety, mood, and substance-related disorders. Between 5 and 10% of Americans will at some time in their life satisfy criteria for PTSD, with women more likely to be affected than men.

Risk factors for the development of PTSD include a past psychi-

Table 385-8 Diagnostic Criteria for Posttraumatic Stress Disorder

A. The person has been exposed to a traumatic event in which both of the following were present:
  1. The person experienced, witnessed, or was confronted with an event or events that involved actual or threatened death or serious injury, or a threat to the physical integrity of self or others.
  2. The person's response involved intense fear, helplessness, or horror.
B. The traumatic event is persistently reexperienced in one (or more) of the following ways:
  1. Recurrent and intrusive distressing recollections of the event, including images, thoughts, or perceptions.
  2. Recurrent distressing dreams of the event.
  3. Acting or feeling as if the traumatic event were recurring (includes a sense of reliving the experience, illusions, hallucinations, and dissociative flashback episodes, including those that occur on awakening or when intoxicated).
  4. Intense psychological distress at exposure to internal or external cues that symbolize or resemble an aspect of the traumatic event.
  5. Physiologic reactivity on exposure to internal or external cues that symbolize or resemble an aspect of the traumatic event.
C. Persistent avoidance of stimuli associated with the trauma and numbing of general responsiveness (not present before the trauma), as indicated by three or more of the following:
  1. Efforts to avoid thoughts, feelings, or conversations associated with the trauma
  2. Efforts to avoid activities, places, or people that arouse recollections of the trauma
  3. Inability to recall an important aspect of the trauma
  4. Markedly diminished interest or participation in significant activities
  5. Feeling of detachment or estrangement from others
  6. Restricted range of affect (e.g., unable to have loving feelings)
  7. Sense of a foreshortened future (e.g., does not expect to have a career, marriage, children, or a normal life span)
D. Persistent symptoms of increased arousal (not present before the trauma), as indicated by two (or more) of the following:
  1. Difficulty falling or staying asleep
  2. Irritability or outbursts of anger
  3. Difficulty concentrating
  4. Hypervigilance
  5. Exaggerated startle response
E. Duration of the disturbance (symptoms in criteria B, C, and D) is more than 1 month
F. The disturbance causes clinically significant distress or impairment in social, occupational, or other important areas of functioning.

SOURCE: *Diagnostic and Statistical Manual of Mental Disorders*, 4th ed.

atric history and personality characteristics of high neuroticism and extroversion. Studies of monozygotic and dizygotic twins showed a substantial influence of genetics on all symptoms associated with PTSD, with no evidence for an environment effect.

Etiology and Pathophysiology   It is hypothesized that in PTSD there is excessive release of norepinephrine from the locus coeruleus in response to stress. Increased noradrenergic activity at locus coeruleus projection sites in hippocampus and amygdala theoretically facilitates encoding of fear-based memories. Greater sympathetic responses to cues associated with the traumatic event occurs in PTSD.

℞ **TREATMENT** Acute stress reactions are usually self-limited, and treatment typically involves the short-term use of benzodiazepines and supportive/expressive psychotherapy. The chronic and recurrent nature of PTSD, however, requires a more complex approach employing drug and behavioral treatments. TCAs such as imipramine and amitriptyline, the MAOI phenelzine, and the SSRIs (fluoxetine, sertraline, citalopram, paroxetine) can all reduce anxiety, symptoms of intrusion, and avoidance behaviors. Trazodone, a sedating antidepressant, is frequently used at night to help with insomnia (50 to 150 mg qhs). Carbamazepine, valproic acid, or alprazolam have also independently produced improvement in uncontrolled trials. There is frequent comorbidity with substance abuse, especially alcohol.

Psychotherapeutic strategies are used in treatment of PTSD to help the patient overcome avoidance behaviors and demoralization and master fear of recurrence of the trauma; therapies that encourage the patient to dismantle avoidance behaviors through stepwise focusing on the experience of the traumatic event are the most effective.

OBSESSIVE-COMPULSIVE DISORDER   Clinical Manifestations Obsessive-compulsive disorder (OCD) was previously considered a relatively rare condition, but recent epidemiologic data indicate a lifetime prevalence of 2 to 3% worldwide. OCD is characterized by obsessive thoughts and compulsive behaviors that impair everyday functioning. Fears of contamination and germs are common, as are handwashing, counting behaviors, and having to check and recheck such actions as whether a door is locked. The degree to which the disorder is disruptive for the individual varies, but in all cases obsessive-compulsive activities take up >1 h per day and are undertaken to relieve the anxiety triggered by the core fear. Patients often conceal their symptoms, usually because they are embarrassed by the content of their thoughts or the nature of their actions. Physicians must ask specific questions regarding recurrent thoughts and behaviors, particularly if physical clues such as chafed and reddened hands or patchy hair loss (from repetitive hair pulling, or trichotillomania) are present. Tics are sometimes associated with OCD. OCD usually has a gradual onset, beginning in early adulthood, but childhood onset is not rare. The disorder usually has a waxing and waning course, but some cases may show a steady deterioration in psychosocial functioning.

Etiology and Pathophysiology A genetic contribution to OCD is suggested by a higher monozygotic than dizygotic concordance rate and the fact that familial studies show an aggregation with Tourette's disorder. OCD is more common in males and in first-born children.

The anatomy of obsessive-compulsive behavior is thought to involve a frontal-subcortical neural circuit involving the orbital frontal cortex, caudate nucleus, and globus pallidus. Neuroimaging studies have demonstrated a decrease in caudate nucleus volume, abnormalities in frontal lobe white matter, and increases in glucose metabolism in the orbital cortex of the frontal lobes and the head of the caudate nucleus. The caudate nucleus seems particularly involved in the acquisition and maintenance of habit and skill learning, and interventions that are successful in reducing obsessive-compulsive behaviors are paralleled by a comparable decrease in caudate glucose metabolic rate.

℞ **TREATMENT** Clomipramine, fluoxetine, and fluvoxamine are approved for the treatment of OCD. Clomipramine is a TCA that is often tolerated poorly owing to significant anticholinergic and sedative side effects at the doses required to treat the illness (150 to 250 mg/d). Its efficacy in OCD is unrelated to its antidepressant activity. Fluoxetine (40 to 60 mg/d) and fluvoxamine (100 to 300 mg/d) are as effective as clomipramine and show a more benign side-effect profile. Fluvoxamine, a structurally unique SSRI, is metabolized through the hepatic P450 microsomal system (as is fluoxetine); it appears to inhibit the III A4 isoenzyme specifically and should not be given with other drugs that act on III A4, such as terfenadine and astemizole, because life-threatening cardiac arrhythmias may result. Only 50 to 60% of patients with OCD show an acceptable degree of improvement with pharmacotherapy alone. In treatment-resistant cases, augmentation with other serotonergic agents, such as buspirone, or with a neuroleptic or benzodiazepine may be beneficial. When a therapeutic response is achieved, long-duration maintenance therapy is usually indicated.

For many individuals, particularly those with time-consuming compulsions, behavior therapy will result in as much improvement as that afforded by medication. Effective techniques include the gradual increase in exposure to stressful situations, maintenance of a diary to clarify stressors, and homework assignments that substitute new activities for their compulsive behavior.

MOOD DISORDERS

Mood disorders are characterized by a disturbance in the regulation of mood, behavior, and affect. Mood disorders are subdivided into (1) depressive disorders, (2) bipolar disorders, and (3) depression in association with medical illness or alcohol and substance abuse (Chaps. 387 through 389). Depressive disorders are differentiated from bipolar disorders by the absence of a manic or hypomanic episode. The relationship between pure depressive syndromes and bipolar disorders is not well understood; depression occurs at increased frequency in families of bipolar individuals, but the reverse is not true. Depression in general is associated with high disability and societal cost; in the Global Burden of Disease Study conducted by the World Health Organization, unipolar major depression ranked fourth in percentage of disability-adjusted life years and was projected to rank second in the year 2020.

DEPRESSION IN ASSOCIATION WITH MEDICAL ILLNESS Depression occurring in the context of medical illness is difficult to evaluate. Depressive symptomatology may reflect the psychological stress of coping with the disease, may be caused by the disease process itself or by the medications used to treat it, or may simply coexist in time with the medical diagnosis.

Virtually every class of *medication* includes some agent that can induce depression. Antihypertensive drugs, anticholesterolemic agents, and antiarrhythmic agents are commonly used classes of medications that can trigger depressive symptoms. Among the antihypertensive agents, β-adrenergic blockers and, to a lesser extent, calcium channel blockers are the most likely to cause depressed mood. Iatrogenic depression should also be considered in patients receiving glucocorticoids, antimicrobials, systemic analgesics, antiparkinsonian medications, and anticonvulsants. To decide whether a causal relationship exists between pharmacologic therapy and a patient's change in mood, it is necessary to chart the chronology of symptoms and sometimes to undertake an empirical trial of an alternative medication.

Between 20 and 30% of cardiac patients manifest a depressive disorder; an even higher percentage experience depressive symptomatology when self-reporting scales are used. Depressive symptoms following myocardial infarction impair rehabilitation and are associated with higher rates of mortality and medical morbidity. Depressed patients often show decreased variability in heart rate (an index of reduced parasympathetic nervous system activity), and this has been proposed as one mechanism by which depression may predispose individuals to ventricular arrhythmia and increased morbidity. Although TCAs have been used to treat depression in individuals with cardiac disease for a number of years, and although the quinidine-like effect of tricyclics may be useful in patients with preexisting arrhythmias, TCAs are contraindicated in patients with preexisting bundle branch block. They may also paradoxically precipitate arrhythmias. Tricyclic-induced tachycardia is an additional concern in patients with congestive heart failure. Experience with the SSRIs is more limited, but thus far they appear not to induce ECG changes or adverse cardiac events. SSRIs may interfere with hepatic metabolism of anticoagulants, however, causing increased anticoagulation.

Epidemiologic surveys of depression in patients with cancer show a wide variability in prevalence, as might be predicted by differences in tumor site, severity of illness, and type of medical or surgical intervention. There is an overall mean prevalence of 25%, but depression occurs in 40 to 50% of patients with cancers of the pancreas or oropharynx. Assessment of the validity of prevalence rates is complicated by the fact that extreme cachexia may be misinterpreted as part of the symptom complex of depression. The higher prevalence of depression in patients with pancreatic cancer nevertheless persists when patients are compared to those with advanced gastric cancer. Initiation of antidepressant medication in cancer patients has been shown to improve quality of life as well as mood. Psychotherapeutic approaches, particularly group therapy, may have some effect on short-term depression, anxiety, and pain symptoms and on recurrence rates and long-term survival. In a study of female patients with metastatic breast cancer, patients in group therapy had longer survival than control patients.

Depression occurs frequently in patients with *neurologic disorders*, particularly cerebrovascular disorders, Parkinson's disease, multiple sclerosis, and traumatic brain injury. Left-hemisphere strokes, particularly those involving the dorsal lateral frontal cortex, are most likely to cause depression. Both tricyclic and SSRI antidepressants are effective in the treatment of depression secondary to stroke, as are stimulant compounds and, in some patients, MAOIs.

The reported prevalence of depression in patients with *diabetes mellitus* varies from 8 to 27%, with the severity of the mood state correlating with the physical symptoms of illness and the degree of hyperglycemia. Pharmacologic treatment of depression is complicated by antidepressant effects on the blood glucose level. MAOIs can induce hypoglycemia and weight gain. TCAs can lead to hyperglycemia and carbohydrate craving. SSRIs, like MAOIs, may cause a reduction in fasting plasma glucose, but they are easier to use and may also improve dietary and medication compliance.

Hypothyroidism is frequently associated with features of depression, most commonly depressed mood and memory impairment. Hyperthyroid states may also present in a similar fashion, usually in geriatric populations. Improvement in mood usually follows normalization of thyroid function, but adjunctive antidepressant medication is sometimes required. Patients with subclinical hypothyroidism can also experience symptoms of depression and cognitive difficulty that respond to thyroid replacement.

DEPRESSIVE DISORDERS   Clinical Manifestations   *Major depression* is defined as depressed mood on a daily basis for a minimum duration of 2 weeks (Table 385-9). An episode may be characterized by sadness, indifference or apathy, or irritability and is usually associated with change in neurovegetative functions, including sleep patterns, appetite and weight, motor agitation or retardation, fatigue, impairment in concentration and decision making, feelings of

Table 385-9   Criteria for Major Depressive Episode

A. Five (or more) of the following symptoms have been present during the same 2-week period and represent a change from previous functioning; at least one of the symptoms is either (1) depressed mood or (2) loss of interest or pleasure. **Note:** Do not include symptoms that are clearly due to a general medical condition, or mood-incongruent delusions or hallucinations.

1. Depressed mood most of the day, nearly every day, as indicated by either subjective report (e.g., feels sad or empty) or observation made by others (e.g., appears tearful)
2. Markedly diminished interest or pleasure in all, or almost all, activities most of the day, nearly every day (as indicated by either subjective account or observation made by others)
3. Significant weight loss when not dieting or weight gain (e.g., a change of >5% of body weight in a month), or decrease or increase in appetite nearly every day
4. Insomnia or hypersomnia nearly every day
5. Psychomotor agitation or retardation nearly every day (observable by others, not merely subjective feelings of restlessness or being slowed down)
6. Fatigue or loss of energy nearly every day
7. Feelings of worthlessness or excessive or inappropriate guilt (which may be delusional) nearly every day (not merely self-reproach or guilt about being sick)
8. Diminished ability to think or concentrate, or indecisiveness, nearly every day (either by subjective account or as observed by others)
9. Recurrent thoughts of death (not just fear of dying), recurrent suicidal ideation without a specific plan, or a suicide attempt or a specific plan for committing suicide

B. The symptoms do not meet criteria for a mixed episode
C. The symptoms cause clinically significant distress or impairment in social, occupational, or other important areas of functioning
D. The symptoms are not due to the direct physiologic effects of a substance (e.g., a drug of abuse, a medication) or a general medical condition (e.g., hypothyroidism)
E. The symptoms are not better accounted for by bereavement; i.e., after the loss of a loved one, the symptoms persist for >2 months or are characterized by marked functional impairment, morbid preoccupation with worthlessness, suicidal ideation, psychotic symptoms, or psychomotor retardation

SOURCE: *Diagnostic and Statistical Manual of Mental Disorders*, 4th ed.

shame or guilt, and thoughts of death or dying. Patients with depression have a profound loss of pleasure in all enjoyable activities, exhibit early morning awakening, feel that the dysphoric mood state is qualitatively different from sadness, and often notice a diurnal variation in mood (worse in morning hours). Paradoxically, these more severe features predict a good response to antidepressant treatment.

Approximately 15% of the population experiences a major depressive episode at some point in life, and 6 to 8% of all outpatients in primary care settings satisfy diagnostic criteria for the disorder. Depression is often undiagnosed, and, even more frequently, it is treated inadequately. If a physician suspects the presence of a major depressive episode, the initial task is to determine whether it represents unipolar or bipolar depression or is one of the 10 to 15% of cases that are secondary to general medical illness or substance abuse. Physicians should also assess the risk of suicide by direct questioning, as patients are often reluctant to verbalize such thoughts without prompting. If specific plans are uncovered or if significant risk factors exist (e.g., a past history of suicide attempts, profound hopelessness, concurrent medical illness, substance abuse, or social isolation), the patient must be referred to a mental health specialist for immediate care. In evaluating suicidal risk the physician should specifically probe each of these areas in an empathic and hopeful manner, being sensitive to denial and possible minimization of distress. The presence of anxiety, panic, or agitation significantly increases near-term suicidal risk. Nearly 15% of patients whose depressive illness goes untreated will commit suicide; most will have sought help from a physician within 1 month of their death.

In some depressed patients, the mood disorder does not appear to be episodic and is not clearly associated with either psychosocial dysfunction or change from the individual's usual experience in life. *Dysthymic disorder* consists of a pattern of chronic (at least 2 years), ongoing, mild depressive symptoms that are less severe and less disabling than those found in major depression; the two conditions are sometimes difficult to separate, however, and can occur together ("double depression"). Many patients who exhibit a profile of pessimism, disinterest, and low self-esteem respond to antidepressant treatment. Dysthymic disorder exists in ~5% of primary care patients.

Studies of various cultures have shown that external manifestations of depression differ but the core symptoms remain the same. The incidence of depression increases with age; the disorder is approximately twice as prevalent in women as in men, regardless of age. These gender differences were previously believed to reflect sociocultural factors, but recent longitudinal twin studies indicate that the liability to major depression in adult women is largely genetic in origin, and that the effect of environmental factors is transitory and does not affect lifetime prevalence. The relationship between psychological stress, negative life events, and the onset of depressive episodes is complex. Negative life events can precipitate and contribute to depression, but recent data indicate that genetic factors influence the sensitivity of individuals to these stressful events. In most cases, both biologic and psychosocial factors are involved in the precipitation and unfolding of depressive episodes. The most potent stressors appear to involve death of a relative, assault, or severe marital or relationship problems.

Unipolar depressive disorders usually have their onset in early adulthood, and recurrences over the course of a lifetime are likely. The best predictor of future risk is the number of past episodes; 50 to 60% of patients who have a first episode have at least one or two more episodes. Some patients experience multiple episodes that become more severe and frequent over time. The duration of an untreated episode varies greatly, ranging from a few months to ≥1 year. The pattern of recurrence and clinical progression in a developing episode is also variable. Within an individual, there is often long-term stability in phenotype (presenting symptoms, frequency and duration of episodes). In a minority of patients, the severity of the depressive episode may progress to psychotic symptomatology; in elderly patients, depressive symptoms may be associated with confusion and mistaken for dementia (i.e., "pseudodementia"). A seasonal pattern of depression, called *seasonal affective disorder*, may manifest with onset and remission of episodes at predictable times of the year. This disorder is more common in women, whose symptoms are anergy, fatigue, weight gain, hypersomnia, and episodic carbohydrate craving. The prevalence increases with distance from the equator, and mood improvement may occur by altering light exposure.

Etiology and Pathophysiology The neurobiology of unipolar depression is poorly understood. Although evidence for genetic transmission is not as strong as in bipolar disorder, monozygotic twins have a higher concordance rate (46%) than dizygotic siblings (20%), with little evidence for any effect of a shared family environment. Parallels between the affective, motor, and cognitive dysfunctions seen in unipolar depression and those observed in diseases of the basal ganglia have suggested that neural networks involving prefrontal cortex and the basal ganglia may be involved. This hypothesis is supported by positron emission tomography (PET) studies of brain glucose metabolism that show a decrease in metabolic rate in the caudate nuclei and frontal lobes in depressed patients that returns to normal with recovery. Single-photon emission computed tomography (SPECT) studies show comparable changes in blood flow. Magnetic resonance imaging (MRI) findings in some patients include an increased frequency of subcortical white matter lesions. However, because these findings are more prevalent in patients with late onset of depressive illness, their significance remains unproven. A number of studies document increased ventricle-to-brain ratios in some patients with recurrent depression, but whether this finding is state-dependent or represents true cerebral atrophy is controversial.

Postmortem examination of brains of suicide victims suggest altered noradrenergic activity, including increased binding to α_1-, α_2-, and β-adrenergic receptors in the cerebral cortex and a decreased total number and density of noradrenergic neurons in the locus coeruleus. Involvement of the serotonin system is suggested by findings of reduced plasma tryptophan levels, a decreased cerebrospinal fluid level of 5-hydroxyindolacetic acid (the principal metabolite of serotonin in brain), and decreased platelet serotonergic transporter binding. An increase in brain serotonin receptors in suicide victims is also reported. Depletion of blood tryptophan, the amino acid precursor of serotonin, rapidly reverses the antidepressant benefit in depressed patients who have been successfully treated. However, a decrement in mood after tryptophan reduction is considerably less robust in untreated patients, indicating that, if presynaptic serotonergic dysfunction occurs in depression, it likely plays a contributing rather than a causal role.

Neuroendocrine abnormalities that reflect the neurovegetative signs and symptoms of depression include (1) increased cortisol and corticotropin-releasing hormone (CRH) secretion, (2) an increase in adrenal size, (3) a decreased inhibitory response of glucocorticoids to dexamethasone, and (4) a blunted response of thyroid-stimulating hormone (TSH) level to infusion of thyroid-releasing hormone (TRH). Antidepressant treatment leads to normalization of these pituitary-adrenal abnormalities.

Diurnal variations in symptom severity and alterations in circadian rhythmicity of a number of neurochemical and neurohumoral factors suggest that biologic differences may be secondary to a primary defect in regulation of biologic rhythms. Patients with major depression show consistent findings of a decrease in rapid eye movement (REM) sleep onset (REM latency), an increase in REM density, and, in some subjects, a decrease in stage IV delta slow-wave sleep.

Although antidepressant drugs result in a blockade of neurotransmitter uptake within hours, their therapeutic effects typically emerge over several weeks, implicating neuroadaptive changes in second messenger systems and transcription factors as possible mechanisms of action.

TREATMENT Treatment planning requires coordination of short-term symptom remission with longer term maintenance strategies designed to prevent recurrence. The most effective intervention for achieving remission and preventing relapse is medication, but combined treatment, incorporating psychotherapy to help the patient cope with decreased self-esteem and demoralization, improves outcome (Fig. 385-1). About 40% of primary care patients with depression drop out of treatment and discontinue medication if symptomatic improvement is not noted within a month, unless additional support is provided. Outcome improves with (1) increased intensity and frequency of visits during the first 4 to 6 weeks of treatment, (2) supplemental educational materials, and (3) psychiatric consultation as indicated. Despite the widespread use of SSRIs, there is no convincing evidence that this class of antidepressant is more efficacious than TCAs. Between 60 and 70% of all depressed patients respond to any drug chosen, if it is given in a sufficient dose for 6 to 8 weeks. There is no ideal antidepressant; no current compound combines rapid onset of action, moderate half-life, a meaningful relationship between dose and blood level, a low side effect profile, minimal interaction with other drugs, and safety in overdose. A rational approach to selecting which antidepressant to use involves matching the patient's preference and medical history with the metabolic and side effect profile of the drug (Tables 385-4 and 385-5). A previous response, or a family history of a positive response, to a specific antidepressant would suggest that that drug be tried first. Before initiating antidepressant therapy, the physician should evaluate the possible contribution of comorbid illnesses and consider their specific treatment. In individuals with suicidal ideation, particular attention should be paid to choosing a drug with a low toxicity if taken in overdose. The SSRIs and other newer antidepressant drugs are distinctly safer in this regard; nevertheless, the advantages of TCAs have not been completely superseded. The existence of generic equivalents make TCAs relatively cheap, and for several tricyclics, particularly nortriptyline, imipramine, and desipramine, well-defined relationships between dose, plasma level, and therapeutic response exist. The steady-state plasma level achieved for a given drug dose can vary more than tenfold between individuals. Plasma levels may help in understanding resistance to treatment and/or unexpected drug toxicity. The principal disadvantages of TCAs are antihistamine side effects (sedation) and anticholinergic side effects (constipation, dry mouth, urinary hesitancy, and blurred vision). Severe cardiac toxicity due to conduction block or arrhythmias can also occur but is uncommon at therapeutic levels. TCAs are probably contraindicated in patients with cardiovascular risk factors. Tricyclic agents are lethal in overdose, with desipramine carrying the greatest risk. Prescribing only a 10-day supply may be judicious. Most patients require a daily dose of 150 to 200 mg of imipramine or amitriptyline or its equivalent to achieve a therapeutic blood level of 150 to 300 ng/mL and a satisfactory remission; some patients show a partial effect at lower doses. Geriatric patients in particular may require a low starting dose and slow escalation. Ethnic differences in drug metabolism are significant; Hispanic, Asian, and African American patients generally require lower doses than Caucasians to achieve a comparable blood level.

Second-generation antidepressants include amoxapine, maprotiline, trazodone, and bupropion. Amoxapine is a dibenzoxazepine derivative that blocks norepinephrine and serotonin reuptake and has a metabolite that shows a degree of dopamine blockade. Long-term use of this drug carries a risk of tardive dyskinesia. Maprotiline is a potent noradrenergic reuptake blocker that has little anticholinergic effect but may produce seizures. Bupropion is a novel antidepressant whose mechanism of action is thought to involve enhancement of noradrenergic function. It has no anticholinergic, sedating, or orthostatic side effects and has a low incidence of sexual side effects. It may, however, be associated with aversive stimulant-like side effects, may lower seizure threshold, and has an exceptionally short half-life, requiring multiple dosing. An extended-release preparation is available.

SSRIs such as fluoxetine, sertraline, paroxetine, and citalopram cause a lower frequency of anticholinergic, sedating, and cardiovascular side effects but a possibly greater incidence of gastrointestinal complaints, sleep impairment, and sexual dysfunction than do TCAs. Akathisia, involving an inner sense of restlessness and anxiety, may also be more common, particularly during the first week of treatment. A serious concern, aside from drug interaction, is the risk of "serotonin syndrome," thought to result from hyperstimulation of brainstem $5HT_{1A}$ receptors and characterized by myoclonus, agitation, abdominal cramping, hyperpyrexia, hypertension, and potentially death. Combinations of serotonergic agonists should be monitored closely for this reason. Considerations such as half-life, compliance, toxicity, and drug-drug interactions may guide the choice of a particular SSRI. Fluoxetine and its principal active metabolite, norfluoxetine, for example, have a combined half-life of almost 7 days, resulting in a delay of 5 weeks before steady-state levels are achieved and a similar delay for complete drug excretion once its use is discontinued. All the SSRIs may impair sexual function, resulting in diminished libido, impotence, or difficulty in achieving orgasm. Sexual dysfunction frequently results in noncompliance and should be asked about specifically in patients using SSRIs. Sexual dysfunction can sometimes be ameliorated by lowering the dose, by instituting drug holidays over the weekend (two or three times a month), or by treatment with amantadine (100 mg tid), bethanechol (25 mg tid), or buspirone (10 mg tid). Paroxetine appears to be more anticholinergic than either fluoxetine or sertraline, and sertraline carries a lower risk of producing an adverse drug interaction than the other two. Rare side effects of SSRIs include vasospastic angina and alterations of prothrombin time. Citalopram is the most specific of currently available SSRIs and appears to have no specific inhibitory effects on the P450 system.

Venlafaxine, like imipramine, blocks the reuptake of both norepinephrine and serotonin, but it produces relatively little in the way of traditional tricyclic side effects. Unlike the SSRIs, it has a relatively linear dose-response curve. Patients should be monitored for a possible increase in diastolic blood pressure, and multiple daily dosing is required because of the drug's short half-life. An extended-release form is available and has a somewhat lower incidence of gastrointestinal

FIGURE 385-1 A guideline for the medical management of major depressive disorder. SSRI, selective serotonin reuptake inhibitor; TCA, tricyclic antidepressant.

side effects. Nefazadone is a selective $5HT_2$ receptor antagonist that also inhibits the presynaptic reuptake of serotonin and norepinephrine. Its side effects are similar to those of the SSRIs, and twice-daily dosing produces a steady state within 4 to 5 days. The drug is related structurally to trazodone, which is currently used more for its sedative than its antidepressant properties. Nefazadone appears to produce a lower incidence of sexual side effects than do the SSRIs. Mirtazapine is a tetracyclic antidepressant that has a comparatively unique spectrum of activity. It increases noradrenergic and serotonergic neurotransmission through a blockade of central α_2-adrenergic auto- and heteroreceptors and postsynaptic $5HT_2$ and $5HT_3$ receptors. It is also strongly antihistaminic and, as such, may produce sedation at lower doses.

With the exception of citalopram, each of the SSRIs, as well as nefazadone, may inhibit one or more cytochrome P450 enzymes (Table 385-5). Depending on the specific isoenzyme involved, the metabolism of a number of concomitantly administered medications can be dramatically affected. Fluoxetine and paroxetine, for example, by inhibiting 2D6, can cause dramatic increases in the blood level of type 1C antiarrhythmics, while sertraline and nefazadone, by acting on 3A4, may alter blood levels of terfenadine, carbamazepine, and astemizole. Because many of these compounds have a narrow therapeutic window and can cause iatrogenic ventricular arrhythmias at toxic levels, the possibility of an adverse drug interaction should be considered.

Other treatment options include the MAOIs and electroconvulsive therapy. The MAOIs are highly effective, particularly in atypical depression, but the risk of hypertensive crisis following intake of tyramine-containing food or sympathomimetic drugs makes them inappropriate as first-line agents. Common side effects include orthostatic hypotension, weight gain, insomnia, and sexual dysfunction. MAOIs should not be used concomitantly with SSRIs, because of the risk of serotonin syndrome, or with TCAs, because of possible hyperadrenergic effects. Electroconvulsive therapy is at least as effective as medication, but its use is reserved for treatment-resistant cases and delusional depressions.

Regardless of the medication chosen, the treatment response should be evaluated after approximately 2 months of therapy. Three-quarters of patients show an adequate response by this time, but if remission is inadequate, the patient should be questioned about medication compliance, and an increase in dose should be considered if side effects are not troublesome. If there is no improvement, consultation with or referral to a mental health specialist is advised. Strategies for treatment then include selection of an alternative drug, combinations of antidepressants, and/or adjunctive treatment with other classes of drugs, including lithium, thyroid hormone, and dopamine agonists. Patients whose response to an SSRI disappears over time may benefit from the addition of buspirone (10 mg tid) or pindolol (2.5 mg tid) or small amounts of a tricyclic antidepressant such as desipramine (25 mg bid or tid). Once significant remission is achieved, drug treatment should be continued for at least 6 to 9 months to prevent relapse. In patients who have had two or more episodes of depression, indefinite maintenance treatment should be considered.

It is essential to counsel patients about depression and the medications they are receiving. An educational approach is best, describing what is known about the depressive syndrome and how the medications may help. Advice about stress reduction, side effects, and expected length of treatment and cautions that alcohol may exacerbate depressive symptoms and impede drug response are helpful. Patients should be given time to describe their experience and the impact it has had on them, their family, and their outlook. Occasional empathic silence may be as helpful for the treatment alliance as verbal reassurance.

BIPOLAR DISORDER **Clinical Manifestations** Bipolar disorder is common, affecting approximately 3 million persons in the United States, but often difficult to diagnose. It is characterized by unpredictable swings in mood from mania (or hypomania) to depression. Some patients suffer only from recurrent attacks of *mania*, which in its pure form is associated with increased psychomotor activity;

excessive social extroversion; decreased need for sleep; impulsivity and impairment in judgment; and expansive, grandiose, and sometimes irritable mood (Table 385-10). In severe mania, patients may experience delusions and paranoid thinking indistinguishable from schizophrenia. Half of patients with bipolar disorder present with a mixture of psychomotor agitation and activation with dysphoria, anxiety, and irritability. It may be difficult to distinguish *mixed mania* from *agitated depression*. In some bipolar patients (*bipolar II disorder*), the full criteria for mania are lacking, and the requisite recurrent depressions are separated by periods of mild activation and increased energy (hypomania). In *cyclothymic disorder*, there are numerous hypomanic periods, usually of relatively short duration, alternating with clusters of depressive symptoms that fail, either in severity or duration, to meet the criteria of major depression. The mood fluctuations are chronic and should be present for at least 2 years before the diagnosis is made.

Manic episodes typically emerge over a period of days to weeks, but onset within hours is possible, usually in the early morning hours. An untreated episode of either depression or mania can be as short as several weeks or last as long as 8 to 12 months, and rare patients have an unremitting chronic course. The term *rapid cycling* is used for patients who have four or more episodes of either depression or mania in a given year. This pattern occurs in 15% of all patients, almost all of whom are women. In some cases, rapid cycling is linked to an underlying thyroid dysfunction and, in others, is iatrogenically triggered by prolonged antidepressant treatment.

Although bipolar illness is associated with frequent episodic recurrence, it was once thought to have a favorable prognosis and outcome. More recent data, however, show that approximately half of patients with the disorder have sustained difficulties in work performance and psychosocial functioning. The most frequent age of onset for bipolar disorder is between 20 and 30 years of age, but many individuals report premorbid symptoms in late childhood or early adolescence. The prevalence is similar for men and women; women are likely to have more depressive and men more manic episodes over a lifetime.

Differential Diagnosis The differential diagnosis of mania includes toxic effects of stimulant or sympathomimetic drugs as well as secondary mania induced by hyperthyroidism, AIDS, or neurologic

Table 385-10   Criteria for a Manic Episode

A. A distinct period of abnormally and persistently elevated, expansive, or irritable mood, lasting at least 1 week (or any duration if hospitalization is necessary)
B. During the period of mood disturbance, three (or more) of the following symptoms have persisted (four if the mood is only irritable) and have been present to a significant degree:
   1. Inflated self-esteem or grandiosity
   2. Decreased need for sleep (e.g., feels rested after only 3 hours of sleep)
   3. More talkative than usual or pressure to keep talking
   4. Flight of ideas or subjective experience that thoughts are racing
   5. Distractibility (i.e., attention too easily drawn to unimportant or irrelevant external stimuli)
   6. Increase in goal-directed activity (either socially, at work or school, or sexually) or psychomotor agitation
   7. Excessive involvement in pleasurable activities that have a high potential for painful consequences (e.g., engaging in unrestrained buying sprees, sexual indiscretions, or foolish business investments)
C. The symptoms do not meet criteria for a mixed episode.
D. The mood disturbance is sufficiently severe to cause marked impairment in occupational functioning or in usual social activities or relationships with others, or to necessitate hospitalization to prevent harm to self or others, or there are psychotic features.
E. The symptoms are not due to the direct physiologic effects of a substance (e.g., a drug of abuse, a medication, or other treatment) or a general medical condition (e.g., hyperthyroidism).

Note: Manic-like episodes that are clearly caused by somatic antidepressant treatment (e.g., medication, electroconvulsive therapy, light therapy) should not count toward a diagnosis of bipolar I disorder.

SOURCE: *Diagnostic and Statistical Manual of Mental Disorders*, 4th ed.

disorders, such as Huntington's or Wilson's disease, or cerebrovascular accidents. Comorbidity with alcohol and substance abuse is common, either because of poor judgment and increased impulsivity or because of an attempt at self-medication.

Etiology and Pathophysiology Evidence for a genetic predisposition to bipolar disorder is significant. The concordance rate for monozygotic twin pairs approaches 80%, and segregation analyses are consistent with autosomal dominant transmission. Several chromosomal locations for the gene have been proposed in the past decade on the basis of linkage analysis in affected families. None, however, has yet received convincing confirmation.

The pathophysiologic mechanisms underlying the profound and recurrent mood swings of bipolar disorder remain unknown. Cellular models of changes in membrane Na^+- and K^+-activated ATPase and proposals of disordered signal transduction mechanisms involving the phosphoinositol system and GTP-binding proteins have received the most attention. Alterations in glutamate regulation and in neuroprotective transcription factors are also being investigated as possible explanations for the therapeutic effects of lithium.

Neurophysiologic studies suggest that patients with bipolar disorder have altered circadian rhythmicity. Lithium may exert its therapeutic benefit through a resynchronization of intrinsic rhythms keyed to the light/dark cycle (Chap. 27). Neuroimaging techniques have also identified a higher rate of subcortical white matter abnormalities in patients than in age-matched controls.

℞ **TREATMENT** (Table 385-11) Lithium carbonate is the mainstay of treatment in bipolar disorder, although sodium valproate is equally effective in acute mania. Carbamazepine is also efficacious. The response rate to lithium carbonate is 70 to 80% in acute mania, with beneficial effects appearing in 1 to 2 weeks. Lithium also has a prophylactic effect in prevention of recurrent mania, and, to a lesser extent, in the prevention of recurrent depression. A simple cation, lithium is rapidly absorbed from the gastrointestinal tract and remains unbound to plasma or tissue proteins. Some 95% of a given dose is excreted unchanged through the kidneys within 24 h.

Serious side effects from lithium administration are rare, but minor complaints such as gastrointestinal discomfort, nausea, diarrhea, polyuria, weight gain, skin eruptions, alopecia, and edema are common. Over time, urine-concentrating ability may be decreased, but signifi-

cant nephrotoxicity does not occur. In a small subset of patients in whom excessive polyuria occurs (>3000 mL/24 h), dose or schedule adjustments or the adjunctive use of diuretics should be considered. Lithium exerts an antithyroid effect by interfering with the synthesis and release of thyroid hormones. Approximately 5% of patients taking lithium for ≥18 months develop hypothyroidism, with women more likely to be affected than men. Iatrogenic hypothyroidism should be ruled out in any patient who experiences a recurrence of depressive symptomatology during lithium treatment. More serious side effects include tremor, interference with concentration and memory, ataxia, dysarthria, and incoordination. ECG changes of T wave flattening and conduction delays may occur. There is suggestive, but not conclusive, evidence that lithium is teratogenic, inducing cardiac malformations in the first trimester.

In the treatment of acute mania, lithium is initiated at 300 mg bid or tid, and the dose is then increased by 300 mg every 2 to 3 days to achieve blood levels of 0.8 to 1.2 meq/L. Before initiating treatment the physician should obtain baseline measures of electrolytes, creatinine, thyroid function, and a complete blood count (CBC). Because the therapeutic effect of lithium may not appear until 7 to 10 days of treatment, adjunctive usage of lorazepam (1 to 2 mg every 4 h) or clonazepam (0.5 to 1 mg every 4 h) may be beneficial to control agitation. Antipsychotics are indicated in patients with severe agitation who respond only partially to benzodiazepines. These agents should be discontinued in the transition to maintenance lithium therapy. Patients using lithium should be monitored closely, since the blood levels required to achieve a therapeutic benefit are close to those associated with neurotoxicity. Risk factors for neurotoxicity include concomitant medical illness, decrease in salt intake, or concurrent use of medications that may increase the serum level of lithium (neuroleptics, diuretics, and calcium channel blockers). Once stabilization is achieved, the lithium level can be monitored on a bimonthly basis, and thyroid and renal functions on a biannual basis, or more frequently if clinical change occurs.

Valproic acid is an alternative in patients who cannot tolerate lithium or respond poorly to it. Valproic acid may be better than lithium for patients who have a rapid-cycling course (i.e., more than four episodes a year) or who present with a mixed or dysphoric mania. Valproic acid is usually started at 500 to 750 mg/d in divided doses. The dose is increased every several days to achieve blood levels in the range of 50 to 100 μg/mL, which typically are achieved at a dose of 1000 to 2500 mg/d. The most serious adverse effects of valproic acid are hepatoxicity, which may be fatal, and hyponatremia. Such cases are fortunately rare, but periodic monitoring of liver enzymes, particularly during the first 90 days of treatment, is indicated.

Carbamazepine, although not formally approved by the U.S. Food and Drug Administration (FDA) for bipolar disorder, has clinical efficacy in the treatment of acute mania. Carbamazepine is initiated at 400 to 600 mg/d in divided doses, and the dose is increased to achieve a blood level of 4 to 12 mg/L. Carbamazepine may induce a benign leukopenia, but the risk of aplastic anemia is minimal. Nevertheless, it is wise to obtain a CBC periodically.

Preliminary evidence also suggests that other anticonvulsant agents such as gabapentin, lamotrigine, and topiramate may possess some therapeutic benefit.

The recurrent nature of bipolar mood disorder necessitates maintenance treatment. Maintenance of blood lithium levels of at least 0.8 mg/L is important to achieve optimal prophylaxis. Compliance is frequently an issue and often requires enlistment and education of concerned family members to avoid relapse. Efforts to identify and limit psychosocial factors that may trigger episodes are important, as is an emphasis on life-style regularity. Antidepressant medications are sometimes required for the treatment of severe breakthrough depressions, but their use should generally be avoided during maintenance treatment because of the risk of precipitating mania or accelerating the cycle frequency. Loss of efficacy over time may be observed with any of the mood-stabilizing agents. In such situations, an alternative agent or combination therapy is usually helpful.

Table 385-11　Clinical Pharmacology of Mood Stabilizers

Agent and Dosing	Side Effects and Other Effects
Lithium 　Starting dose: 300 mg 　　bid or tid 　Therapeutic blood 　　level: 0.8–1.2 meq/L	*Common side effects:* nausea/anorexia/diarrhea, fine tremor, thirst, polyuria, fatigue, weight gain, acne, folliculitis, neutrophilia, hypothyroidism Blood level is increased by thiazides, tetracyclines, and NSAIDs Blood level is decreased by bronchodilators, verapamil, and carbonic anhydrase inhibitors *Rare side effects:* Neurotoxicity, renal toxicity, hypercalcemia, ECG changes
Valproic acid 　Starting dose: 250 mg 　　tid 　Therapeutic blood 　　level: 50–125 μg/mL	*Common side effects:* Nausea/anorexia, weight gain, sedation, tremor, rash, alopecia Inhibits hepatic metabolism of other medications *Rare side effects:* Pancreatitis, hepatoxicity, Stevens-Johnson syndrome
Carbamazepine 　Starting dose: 200 mg 　　bid 　Therapeutic blood 　　level: 4–12 μg/mL	*Common side effects:* Nausea/anorexia, sedation, rash, dizziness/ataxia Induces hepatic metabolism of other medications *Rare side effects:* Hyponatremia, agranulocytosis, Stevens-Johnson syndrome

NOTE: NSAID, nonsteroidal anti-inflammatory drug; ECG, electrocardiogram.

Table 385-12 Expert Consensus Guidelines on the Drug Treatment of Acute Mania and Bipolar Depression

Condition	Preferred Agents
Euphoric mania	Lithium
Mixed/dysphoric mania	Valproic acid
Mania with psychosis	Valproic acid with olanzapine
	Conventional antipsychotic or risperidone
Hypomania	Lithium or valproic acid alone
Severe depression with psychosis	Venlafaxine, bupropion, *or* paroxetine *plus* lithium *plus* olanzapine, *or* risperidone; consider ECT
Severe depression without psychosis	Bupropion, paroxetine, sertraline, venlafaxine, *or* citalopram *plus* lithium
Mild to moderate depression	Lithium alone; add bupropion if needed

NOTE: ECT, electroconvulsive therapy.
SOURCE: From GS Sachs et al: Postgrad Med April, 2000.

Consensus guidelines for the treatment of acute mania and bipolar depression are described in Table 385-12.

SOMATOFORM DISORDERS

CLINICAL MANIFESTATIONS Patients with multiple somatic complaints that cannot be explained by a known medical condition or by the effects of alcohol or of recreational or prescription drugs are seen commonly in primary care practice; one survey indicates a prevalence of 5%. The somatoform disorders include a variety of conditions that differ in terms of the specific symptoms that are present and in whether or not the symptoms are intentionally produced. In *somatization disorder*, the patient presents with multiple physical complaints referable to different organ systems (Table 385-13). Onset is usually before age 30, and the disorder is persistent. Formal diagnostic criteria require the recording of at least four pain, two gastro-intestinal, one sexual, and one pseudoneurologic symptom. Patients with somatization disorder often present with dramatic complaints, but the complaints are inconsistent. Symptoms of comorbid anxiety and mood disorder are common and may be the result of drug interactions due to regimens initiated independently by different physicians. Patients with somatization disorder may be impulsive and demanding and frequently qualify for a formal comorbid psychiatric diagnosis. In *conversion disorder*, the symptoms focus on deficits that involve voluntary motor or sensory function and on psychological factors that initiate or exacerbate the medical presentation. Like somatization disorder, the deficit is not intentionally produced or simulated, as is the case in factitious disorder (malingering). In *hypochondriasis*, the essential feature is a belief of serious medical illness that persists despite reassurance and appropriate medical evaluation. As with somatization disorder, patients with hypochondriasis have a history of poor relationships with physicians stemming from their sense that they have been evaluated and treated inappropriately or inadequately. Hypochondriasis can be disabling in intensity and is persistent, with waxing and waning symptomatology.

In *factitious illnesses*, the patient consciously and voluntarily produces physical symptoms of illness. The term *Munchausen's syndrome* is reserved for individuals with particularly dramatic, chronic, or severe factitious illness. In true factitious illness, the sick role itself is gratifying. A variety of signs, symptoms, and diseases have been either simulated or caused by factitious behavior, the most common including chronic diarrhea, fever of unknown origin, intestinal bleeding or hematuria, seizures, and hypoglycemia. Factitious disorder is usually not diagnosed until 5 to 10 years after its onset, and it can produce significant social and medical costs. In *malingering*, the fabrication derives from a desire for some external reward, such as a narcotic medication or disability reimbursement.

Table 385-13 Diagnostic Criteria for Somatization Disorder

A. A history of many physical complaints beginning before age 30 years that occur over a period of several years and result in treatment being sought or significant impairment in social, occupational, or other important areas of functioning.
B. Each of the following criteria must have been met, with individual symptoms occurring at any time during the course of the disturbance:
  1. *Four pain symptoms:* a history of pain related to at least four different sites or functions (e.g., head, abdomen, back, joints, extremities, chest, rectum, during menstruation, during sexual intercourse, or during urination)
  2. *Two gastrointestinal symptoms:* a history of at least two gastrointestinal symptoms other than pain (e.g., nausea, bloating, vomiting other than during pregnancy, diarrhea, or intolerance of several different foods)
  3. *One sexual symptom:* a history of at least one sexual or reproductive symptom other than pain (e.g., sexual indifference, erectile or ejaculatory dysfunction, irregular menses, excessive menstrual bleeding, vomiting throughout pregnancy)
  4. *One pseudoneurologic symptom:* a history of at least one symptom or deficit suggesting a neurologic condition not limited to pain (conversion symptoms such as impaired coordination or balance, paralysis or localized weakness, difficulty swallowing or lump in throat, aphonia, urinary retention, hallucinations, loss of touch or pain sensation, double vision, blindness, deafness, seizures; dissociative symptoms such as amnesia; or loss of consciousness other than fainting)
C. Either of the following:
  1. After appropriate investigation, each of the symptoms in criterion B cannot be fully explained by a known general medical condition or the direct effects of a substance (e.g., a drug of abuse, a medication)
  2. When there is a related general medical condition, the physical complaints or resulting social or occupational impairment are in excess of what would be expected from the history, physical examination, or laboratory findings
D. The symptoms are not intentionally produced or feigned (as in factitious disorder or malingering).

SOURCE: *Diagnostic and Statistical Manual of Mental Disorders,* 4th ed.

TREATMENT Patients with somatization disorders are frequently subjected to multiple diagnostic testing and exploratory surgeries in an attempt to find their "real" illness. Such an approach is doomed to failure and does not address the core issue. Successful treatment is best achieved through behavior modification, in which access to the physician is tightly regulated and adjusted to provide a sustained and predictable level of support that is less clearly contingent on the patient's level of presenting distress. Visits can be brief and should not be associated with a need for a diagnostic or treatment action. Although the literature is limited, some patients with somatization disorder may benefit from antidepressant treatment. Fluoxetine and MAOIs have both been found to be useful in reducing obsessive ruminations, dysphoria, and anxious preoccupation in patients with multiple somatic complaints.

The treatment of factitious disorder is complicated in that any attempt to confront the patient usually only creates a sense of humiliation and causes the patient to abandon treatment from that caregiver. A better strategy is to introduce psychological causation as one of a number of possible explanations and to include factitious illness as an option in the differential diagnoses that are discussed. Without directly linking psychotherapeutic intervention to the diagnosis, the patient can be offered a face-saving means by which the pathologic relationship with the health care system can be examined and alternative approaches to life stressors developed.

PERSONALITY DISORDERS

CLINICAL MANIFESTATIONS Personality disorders are characteristic patterns of thinking, feeling, and interpersonal behavior that are relatively inflexible and cause significant functional impairment or subjective distress for the individual. The observed behaviors are not secondary to another mental disorder, nor are they precipitated by substance abuse or a general medical condition. This distinction is often difficult to make in clinical practice, as personality change may be the first sign of serious neurologic, endocrine, or other medical illness. Patients with frontal lobe tumors, for example, can present with changes in motivation and personality while the results of the neurologic examination remain within normal limits. Personality traits are stable over time and environmental situation and are recognizable in adolescence or early adult life. Although DSM-IV portrays personality disorders as qualitatively distinct categories, there is an alternative perspective that personality characteristics vary as a continuum between normal functioning and formal mental disorder.

Personality disorders have been grouped into three clusters that share similar attributes. *Cluster A* includes paranoid, schizoid, and schizotypal personality disorders. It includes individuals who are odd and eccentric and who maintain an emotional distance from others. Individuals have a restricted emotional range and remain socially isolated. Patients with schizotypal personality disorder frequently have unusual perceptual experiences and express magical beliefs about the external world. The essential feature of paranoid personality disorder is a pervasive mistrust and suspiciousness of others to an extent that is unjustified by available evidence. *Cluster B* disorders include antisocial, borderline, histrionic, and narcissistic types and describe individuals whose behavior is impulsive, excessively emotional, and erratic. *Cluster C* incorporates avoidant, dependent, and obsessive-compulsive personality types; enduring traits are anxiety and fear. The boundaries between cluster types are to some extent artificial, and many patients who meet criteria for one personality disorder also meet criteria for aspects of another. The risk of a comorbid major mental disorder is increased in patients who qualify for a diagnosis of personality disorder.

℞ **TREATMENT** Historically, recommended treatment for personality disorders was long-term psychotherapy, in which the pathologic patterns of interaction with the world at large could be relived and examined through the corrective emotional experience of the controlled therapeutic relationship. More recently, the recognition that personality derives in part from biologically determined components of temperament has given rise to the empirical use of drugs to treat specific symptom clusters as well as any coexisting major mental disorder. Antidepressant medications and low-dose antipsychotic drugs have some efficacy in cluster A personality disorders, while anticonvulsant mood-stabilizing agents and MAOIs may be considered for patients with cluster B diagnoses who show marked mood reactivity, behavioral dyscontrol, and/or rejection hypersensitivity. Anxious or fearful cluster C patients often have a response to medication that parallels that for patients with axis I anxiety disorders. In all cases, it is important for both the physician and the patient to have reasonable expectations as to the possible effect of the medication and any associated side effects. Beneficial responses may be subtle and observable only over time.

SCHIZOPHRENIA

CLINICAL MANIFESTATIONS Schizophrenia is a heterogeneous syndrome characterized by perturbations of language, perception, thinking, social activity, affect, and volition. There are no pathognomonic features. The syndrome commonly begins in late adolescence, has an insidious onset, and, classically, a poor outcome, progressing from social withdrawal and perceptual distortions to a state of chronic delusions and hallucinations. Patients may present with positive symptoms (such as conceptual disorganization, delusions, or hallucinations) or negative symptoms (loss of function, anhedonia, decreased emotional expression, impaired concentration, and diminished social engagement) and must have at least two of these for a 1-month period and continuous signs for at least 6 months to meet formal diagnostic criteria. "Negative" symptoms predominate in one-third of the schizophrenic population and are associated with a poor long-term outcome and a poor response to drug treatment. However,

marked variability in the course and individual character of symptoms is typical.

Schizophrenia can be classified according to the specific symptomatology present, although such distinctions do not correlate well with either course of illness or response to treatment, and many individuals have symptoms of more than one type. The four main symptom subtypes are catatonic, paranoid, disorganized, and residual. *Catatonic-type* describes patients whose clinical presentation is dominated by profound changes in motor activity, negativism, and echolalia or echopraxia. *Paranoid-type* describes patients who have a prominent preoccupation with a specific delusional system and who otherwise do not qualify as having *disorganized-type* disease, in which disorganized speech and behavior are accompanied by a superficial or silly affect. In *residual-type* disease, negative symptomatology exists in the absence of delusions, hallucinations, or motor disturbance. The diagnosis of *schizophreniform disorder* is reserved for patients who meet the symptom requirements but not the duration requirements for schizophrenia, and that of *schizoaffective disorder* is used for those whose symptoms of schizophrenia are independent of associated periods of mood disturbance. Prognosis depends not on symptom severity but on the response to antipsychotic medication. Patients may present with acute rather than insidious onset of symptoms, and remission without recurrence does occur. About 10% of schizophrenic patients commit suicide. As currently defined, schizophrenia is present in 0.85% of individuals worldwide. Overall, lifetime prevalence is approximately 1 to 1.5%.

The societal costs of schizophrenia are substantial. An estimated 300,000 episodes of acute schizophrenia occur annually, resulting in direct and indirect costs that have been estimated at >$33 billion.

DIFFERENTIAL DIAGNOSIS For a diagnosis of schizophrenia to be made, the symptom complex must cause significant dysfunction in social or occupational domains and last for at least 6 months. The diagnosis is principally one of exclusion, requiring the absence of significant associated mood symptoms, any relevant medical condition, and substance abuse. Drug reactions that cause hallucinations, paranoia, confusion, or bizarre behavior may be dose-related or idiosyncratic; β-adrenergic blockers, clonidine, cycloserine, quinacrine, and procaine derivatives are most commonly associated with these symptoms. Drug causes should be ruled out in any case of newly emergent psychosis. The general neurologic examination in patients with schizophrenia is usually normal, but motor rigidity, tremor, and dyskinesias are noted in one-quarter of untreated patients.

EPIDEMIOLOGY AND PATHOPHYSIOLOGY Epidemiologic surveys identify three principal risk factors for schizophrenia: (1) genetic susceptibility, (2) early developmental insults, and (3) winter birth. Family, twin, and adoption studies show that genetic factors are involved in at least a subset of individuals who develop schizophrenia. Using conservative diagnostic definitions, schizophrenia is observed in approximately 6.6% of all first-degree relatives of an affected proband. If both parents are affected, the risk for offspring is 40%. The concordance rate for monozygotic twins is 50%, compared to 10% for dizygotic twins. Examination of families in which aggregation of schizophrenia occurs has revealed an increased incidence of other psychotic and nonpsychotic psychiatric disorders as well, including schizoaffective disorder and *schizotypal* and *schizoid personality disorders*, the latter terms designating individuals who show a lifetime pattern of social and interpersonal deficits characterized by an inability to form close interpersonal relationships, eccentric behavior, and mild perceptual distortions. Some relatives and individuals with schizophrenia have been found to have distinctive patterns in expressing emotion, most often involving increased criticism, hostility, and emotional overinvolvement.

There is evidence that environmental influences modulate genetic factors in the expression of schizophrenia, and, in sporadic cases, may serve as a sufficient cause. Gestational and birth complications, including Rh factor incompatibility, prenatal exposure to influenza during the second trimester, and prenatal nutritional deficiency have been implicated. Studies of monozygotic twins discordant for schizophrenia have reported neuroanatomic differences between affected and unaffected siblings, supporting a "two-strike" etiology involving both genetic susceptibility and an environmental insult. The latter might involve localized hypoxia during critical stages of brain development.

Neuroimaging and postmortem studies have identified a number of structural and functional abnormalities, including (1) enlargement of the lateral and third ventricles with associated cortical atrophy and sulcal enlargement; (2) volumetric reductions in the amygdala, hippocampus, right prefrontal cortex, and thalamus; (3) altered asymmetry of the planum temporale; and (4) decreases in neuronal metabolism in the thalamus and prefrontal cortex. Some, but not all, prospective studies record progressive reduction in hemispheric volume over years. Neuropathologic studies have reported changes in the size, orientation, and density of cells in the hippocampus and, in the prefrontal cerebral cortex, decreases in neuronal number and the density of interneurons in layer II as well as an increased density of pyramidal cells in layer V. These observations suggest that schizophrenia results from a disturbance in a cortical striatal–thalamic circuit resulting in deficits in sensory filtering and attentional behavior. Although the formal diagnostic requirements for schizophrenia are not usually met until early adult life, children who eventually develop the disorder may exhibit subtle deficits in motor function, cognition, and emotional expression from an early age.

The hypothesized alterations in cortical neuronal circuitry are paralleled clinically by impairments in attention and cortical information processing, autonomic nervous system activation, and habituation. Schizophrenic individuals are highly distractible and demonstrate deficits in perceptual-motor speed, ability to shift attention, and filtering out of background stimuli. Event-related evoked potential studies of schizophrenia have defined a specific reduction in P300 amplitude to a novel stimulus, which implicates an impairment in cognitive processing. Impaired information processing is found in unaffected family members.

Despite evidence for a genetic causation, the results of molecular genetic linkage studies in schizophrenia are inconclusive. Reports of linkage of schizophrenia to loci on chromosomes 1, 5, 6, 8, 11, and 22 and other regions have not been formally replicated and have led to larger scale association studies currently underway.

The *dopamine hypothesis* of schizophrenia is based on the serendipitous discovery that agents that diminish dopaminergic activity have beneficial effects in reducing the acute symptoms and signs of psychosis, specifically agitation, anxiety, and hallucinations. Amelioration of delusions and social withdrawal is less dramatic. Thus far, however, evidence for increased dopaminergic activity is indirect. An increase in the activity of nigrostriatal and mesolimbic systems and a decrease in mesocortical tracts innervating the prefrontal cortex is hypothesized, although it is likely that other neurotransmitters, including serotonin, acetylcholine, glutamate, and GABA also contribute to the pathophysiology of the illness. Involvement of excitatory amino acids is postulated, based on the finding that NMDA receptor antagonists and channel blockers, such as phencyclidine (PCP) and ketamine, produce characteristic signs of schizophrenia in normal individuals.

℞ **TREATMENT** Antipsychotic agents (Table 385-14) remain the cornerstone of acute and maintenance treatment of schizophrenia and are effective in the treatment of hallucinations, delusions, and thought disorders, regardless of etiology. The exact mechanism of action remains incompletely understood, but dopaminergic receptor blockade in the limbic system and basal ganglia appears to be an essential element, since the clinical potencies of traditional antipsychotic drugs parallel their affinities for the D_2 receptor, and even the newer "atypical" agents exert some degree of D_2 receptor blockade. All neuroleptics induce expression of the immediate-early gene c-*fos* in the nucleus accumbens, a dopaminergic site connecting prefrontal and limbic cortices. The clinical efficacy of newer atypical neuroleptics, however, may involve D_1, D_3, and D_4 receptor blockade, α_1- and α_2-noradrenergic activity and/or altering the relationship between $5HT_2$ and D_2 receptor activity.

Conventional neuroleptics differ in their potency and side-effect profile. Older agents, such as chlorpromazine and thioridazine, are more sedating and anticholinergic and more likely to cause orthostatic hypotension, while higher potency antipsychotics, such as haloperidol, perphenazine, and thiothixene, carry a higher risk of inducing extrapyramidal side effects. The model atypical antipsychotic agent is clozapine, a dibenzodiazepine that has a greater potency in blocking the $5HT_2$ than the D_2 receptor and a much higher affinity for the D_4 than the D_2 receptor. Its principal disadvantage is risk of blood dyscrasia, requiring regular monitoring of the CBC. Unlike other antipsychotics, clozapine does not cause a rise in prolactin level. Approximately 30% of patients have a better antipsychotic response to these agents than to traditional neuroleptics, suggesting that they will increasingly displace the older-generation drugs. Clozapine appears to be the most effective member of this class; however, its side-effect profile makes it most appropriate for treatment-resistant cases. *Clozapine* increases the activity of the immediate-early gene c-*fos* in the prefrontal cortex, the neuroanatomic region having the highest concentration of D_4 receptors and an area thought to mediate the specific executive functions that are prominently impaired in schizophrenia. *Risperidone*, a benzisoxazole derivative, is more potent at $5HT_2$ than D_2 receptor sites, like clozapine, but it also exerts significant α_2 antagonism, a property that may contribute to its perceived ability to improve mood and increase

Table 385-14 Antipsychotic Agents

Name	Usual PO Daily Dose, mg	Side Effects	Sedation	Comments
TYPICAL ANTIPSYCHOTICS				
Low-potency				
Chlorpromazine (Thorazine)	100–1000	Anticholinergic effects; orthostasis; photosensitivity; cholestasis	+ + +	EPSEs usually not prominent; can cause anticholinergic delirium in elderly patients
Thioridazine (Mellaril)	100–800		+ + +	
Mid-potency				
Trifluoperazine (Stelazine)	2–15	Fewer anticholinergic side effects; fewer EPSEs than with higher potency agents	+ +	Well tolerated by most patients
Perphenazine (Trilafon)	4–32		+ +	
High potency				
Haloperidol (Haldol)	0.5–10	No anticholinergic side effects; EPSEs often prominent	0/+	Often prescribed in doses that are too high; long-acting injectable forms of haloperidol and fluphenazine available
Fluphenazine (Prolixin)	1–10		0/+	
Thiothixene (Navane)	2–20		0/+	
NOVEL ANTIPSYCHOTICS				
Clozapine (Clozaril)	200–600	Agranulocytosis (1%); weight gain seizures; drooling; hyperthermia	+ +	Requires weekly WBC
Risperidone (Risperdal)	2–6	Orthostasis	+	Requires slow titration; EPSEs observed with doses >6 mg qd
Olanzapine (Zyprexa)	10–20	Weight gain	+ +	Generally well tolerated
Seroquel (Quetiapine)	300–400	Sedation; weight gain; anxiety	+ + +	Bid dosing

NOTE: EPSEs, extrapyramidal side effects; WBC, white blood count.

motor activity. Risperidone is not as effective as clozapine in treatment-resistant cases but does not carry a risk of blood dyscrasia. *Olanzapine* is more similar neurochemically to clozapine but has a significant risk of inducing weight gain. *Quetiapine* is distinct in having a weak D_2 effect but potent α_1 and histamine blockade.

Conventional antipsychotic agents are effective in ~70% of patients presenting with a first episode. Improvement may be observed within hours or days, but full remission usually requires 6 to 8 weeks. The choice of agent depends principally on the side-effect profile and cost of treatment or on a past personal or family history of a favorable response to the drug in question. Atypical agents appear to be more effective in treating negative symptoms and improving cognitive function. Equivalent treatment response can usually be achieved with relatively low doses of any drug selected, i.e., 4 to 6 mg/d of haloperidol, 10 to 15 mg of olanzapine, or 4 to 6 mg/d of risperidone. Doses in this range result in >80% D_2 receptor blockade, and there is little evidence that higher doses increase either the rapidity or degree of response. Maintenance treatment requires careful attention to the possibility of relapse and monitoring for the development of a movement disorder. Intermittent drug treatment is less effective than regular dosing, but gradual dose reduction is likely to improve social functioning in many schizophrenic patients who have been maintained at high doses. If medications are completely discontinued, however, the relapse rate is ~60% within 6 months. Long-acting injectable preparations (haloperidol decanoate and fluphenazine decanoate) are considered when noncompliance with oral therapy leads to relapses. In treatment-resistant patients, a transition to clozapine usually results in rapid improvement, but a prolonged delay in response in some cases necessitates a 6- to 9-month trial for maximal benefit to occur.

Antipsychotic medications can cause a broad range of side effects, including lethargy, weight gain, postural hypotension, constipation, and dry mouth. Extrapyramidal symptoms such as dystonia, akathisia, and akinesia are also frequent with traditional agents and may contribute to poor compliance if not specifically addressed. Anticholinergic and parkinsonian symptoms respond well to trihexyphenidyl, 2 mg bid, or benztropine mesylate, 1 to 2 mg bid. Akathisia may respond to beta blockers. In rare cases, more serious and occasionally life-threatening side effects may emerge, including ventricular arrhythmias, gastrointestinal obstruction, retinal pigmentation, obstructive jaundice, and neuroleptic malignant syndrome (characterized by hyperthermia, autonomic dysfunction, muscular rigidity, and elevated creatine phosphokinase levels). The most serious adverse effects of clozapine are agranulocytosis, which has an incidence of 1%, and induction of seizures, which has an incidence of 10%. Weekly white blood cell counts are required, particularly during the first 3 months of treatment.

A serious side effect of long-term use of the classic antipsychotic agents is *tardive dyskinesia*, characterized by repetitive, involuntary, and potentially irreversible movements of the tongue and lips (buccolinguo-masticatory triad), and, in approximately half of cases, choreoathetoid movements of the limbs (Chap. 22). Tardive dyskinesia has an incidence of ~4% per year of exposure, and a maximal prevalence of ~20% in chronic patients treated with high-dose neuroleptics. The risk associated with the newer atypical agents is unknown but expected to be much less. The prevalence increases with age and with total dose and duration of drug administration, but unknown individual factors play the greatest part in determining risk. The cause of tardive dyskinesia is unknown, but evidence suggests that chronic neuroleptic treatment increases the formation of free radicals and perhaps damages mitochondrial energy metabolism. Vitamin E may reduce abnormal involuntary movements if given early in the syndrome.

Drug treatment of schizophrenia is by itself insufficient. Psychoeducational efforts directed towards families and relevant community resources have proven to be necessary to maintain stability and optimize prognosis. A treatment model involving a multidisciplinary case-management team that seeks out and closely follows the patient in the community has proven particularly effective, not only in maintaining pharmacologic adherence but also in facilitating occupational achievement and interactions with welfare, legal, and primary medical care systems.

ASSESSMENT AND EVALUATION OF VIOLENCE

Primary care physicians may encounter situations in which familial, domestic, or societal violence is discovered or suspected. Such an awareness can carry legal and moral obligations; many state laws mandate reporting of child, spousal, and elder abuse. Physicians are frequently the first point of contact for both victim and abuser. Between 1 and 2 million older Americans and 1.5 million U.S. children are thought to experience some form of physical maltreatment each year. Spousal abuse is thought to be even more prevalent. A recent survey of internal medicine practices found that 5.5% of all female patients had experienced domestic violence in the previous year, and that these individuals were more likely to suffer from depression, anxiety, somatization disorder, and substance abuse and to have attempted suicide. When domestic violence is suspected, direct but nonjudgmental questioning should be pursued with each party separately—"Do you feel safe at home?" and "If there's a disagreement or a conflict between the two of you, how is it worked out?" In addition to obvious and suggestive physical injury, individuals who are abused frequently express low self-esteem, vague somatic symptomatology, social isolation, and a passive feeling of loss of control. Although it is essential to treat these elements in the victim, the first obligation is to ensure that the perpetrator has taken responsibility for preventing any further violence. Substance abuse and/or dependence and serious mental illness in the abuser may contribute to the risk of harm and require direct intervention. Depending on the situation, law enforcement agencies, community resources such as support groups and shelters, and individual and family counseling can be appropriate components of a treatment plan. A safety plan should be formulated with the victim, in addition to the provision of information about abuse, its likelihood of recurrence, and its tendency to increase in severity and frequency. Antianxiety and antidepressant medications may sometimes be useful in treating the acute symptoms, but only if independent evidence for an appropriate psychiatric diagnosis exists. Antidepressants are generally not indicated when the diagnosis is linked to the social situation, such as an adjustment disorder with depressed mood. The most important element in treatment is the development of a supportive doctor-patient relationship that avoids further blame of the victim.

In certain circumstances, a significant potential for societal violence may be discovered. Sympathetic, but direct, questioning about potential violent impulses, access to weapons, recreational drug use, and specific homicidal ideation is necessary and is sometimes therapeutic in its own right. The existence and possible contribution of such medical conditions as delirium and/or intoxication should be evaluated. Available disposition options for potentially violent patients include police custody, psychiatric hospitalization, and referral to home care, with involvement of family, friends, and caregivers. In deciding which treatment option is most appropriate, clinicians should endeavor to establish an empathic interaction with the patient, while avoiding interventions or stimuli that might precipitate or increase the risk of violent behavior. Formal verbal limit setting may be necessary if the patient reveals the existence of a weapon or becomes increasingly agitated or verbally abusive. Use of the least restrictive intervention is generally the best approach during the initial evaluation.

MENTAL HEALTH PROBLEMS IN THE HOMELESS

There is a high prevalence of mental disorders and substance abuse among homeless and impoverished people. The total number of homeless individuals in the United States is estimated at 2 to 3 million, one-third of whom qualify as having a serious mental disorder. Poor hygiene and nutrition, substance abuse, psychiatric illness, physical trauma, and exposure to the elements combine to make the provision of medical care a challenging enterprise. Only a minority of individuals receive formal mental health care; the main points of contact are outpatient medical clinics and emergency departments. Primary care settings represent a critical site in which housing needs, treatment of substance dependence, and evaluation and treatment of psychiatric illness can most efficiently take place. Successful intervention is dependent on breaking down traditional administrative barriers to health care and recognizing the physical constraints and emotional costs imposed by homelessness. Simplifying health care instructions and follow-up, allowing frequent visits, and dispensing medications in limited amounts that require ongoing contact are possible techniques for establishing a successful therapeutic relationship. Child neglect, resulting in developmental delay and emotional difficulty in addition to other health problems, is unfortunately common and necessitates an effort to evaluate the well being of any offspring independently.

BIBLIOGRAPHY

GENERAL

AMERICAN PSYCHIATRIC ASSOCIATION: *Diagnostic and Statistical Manual of Mental Disorders*, 4th ed. Washington DC, American Psychiatric Association, 1994

BERRETTINI WH: Genetics of psychiatric disease. Annu Rev Med 51:465, 2000

BROADHEAD WE et al: Development and validation of the SDDS-PC screen for multiple mental disorders in primary care. Arch Fam Med 4:211, 1995

EISENSTAT SA, BANCROFT L: Domestic violence. N Engl J Med 341:886, 1999

FUGH-BERMAN A, COTT JM: Dietary supplements and natural products as psychotherapeutic agents. Psychosom Med 61:712, 1999

PROCTOR R et al: Behavioural management in nursing and residential homes: A randomised controlled trial. Lancet 354:26, 1999

SPITZER RL et al: Utility of a new procedure for diagnosing mental disorders in primary care: The Prime-MD study. JAMA 272:1749, 1994

PSYCHOLOGICAL FACTORS IN MEDICAL ILLNESS

ALI A et al: Emotional abuse, self-blame and self-silencing in women with irritable bowel syndrome. Psychosom Med 62:76, 2000

BLOCK SD: Assessing and managing depression in the terminally ill patient. Ann Intern Med 132:209, 2000

BROERS S et al: Psychological functioning and quality of life following bone marrow transplantation: A 3-year follow-up study. J Psychosom Res 48:11, 2000

CARNEY RM et al: Can treating depression reduce mortality after an acute myocardial infarction? Psychosom Med 61:666, 1999

DROSSMAN DA: Presidential address: Gastrointestinal illness and the biopsychosocial model. Psychosom Med 60:258, 1998

MCDANIEL JS et al: Cancer and depression: Theory and treatment. Psychiat Ann 27:360, 1997

ROBINSON RG, YATES WR (eds): *Psychiatric Treatment of the Medically Ill*. New York, Marcel Dekker, 1999

SELNES OA et al: Neurobehavioural sequelae of cardiopulmonary bypass. Lancet 353:1601, 1999

ANXIETY DISORDERS

BARTOW DH et al: Cognitive-behavioral therapy, imipramine, or their combination for panic disorder. A randomized controlled trial. JAMA 283:2529, 2000

STOUDEMIRE A: Epidemiology and psychopharmacology of anxiety in medical patients. J Clin Psychiatry 57:64, 1996

MOOD DISORDERS

BALDESSARINI RJ, TONDO L: Does lithium treatment still work? Arch Gen Psychiatry 57:187, 2000

BALLENGER JC, et al: Consensus statement on the primary care management of depression from the International Consensus Group on Depression and Anxiety. J Clin Psychiatry 60:54, 1999

CASE DB, SLABY AE: The suicidal patient in family practice. Primary Psychiatry 3:30, 1996

DORIS A et al: Depressive illness. Lancet 354:1369, 1999

FRANK E, THASE ME: Natural history and preventative treatment of recurrent mood disorders. Annu Rev Med 50:453, 1999

IRWIN M et al: Screening for depression in the older adult. Arch Intern Med 159:1701, 1999

KELLER MB et al: A comparison of nefazodone, the cognitive behavioral-analysis system of psychotherapy, and their combination for the treatment of chronic depression. N Engl J Med 342:1462, 2000

KENT JM: SNaRIs, NaSSAs, and NaRIs: New agents for the treatment of depression. Lancet 355:911, 2000

LEIBENLUFT E, SUPPES T: Treating bipolar illness: Focus on treatment algorithms and management of the sleep-wake cycle. Am J Psychiatry 156:1976, 1999

PERSONS JB et al: The role of psychotherapy in the treatment of depression. Arch Gen Psychiatry 53:283, 1996

SOMATOFORM DISORDERS, PERSONALITY AND BEHAVIORAL DISORDERS

KEELEY R et al: Somatoform symptoms and treatment nonadherence in depressed family medicine outpatients. Arch Fam Med 9:46, 2000

SIMON GE et al: An international study of the relation between somatic symptoms and depression. N Engl J Med 341:1329, 1999

SCHIZOPHRENIA

BRZUSTOWICZ LM et al: Location of a major susceptibility locus for familial schizophrenia on chromosome 1q21-22. Science 288:678, 2000

LAURIELLO J et al: A critical review of research on psychosocial treatment of schizophrenia. Biol Psychiatry 46:1409, 1999

MCEVOY JP et al (eds): The expert consensus guideline series: Treatment of schizophrenia 1999. J Clin Psychiatry (Suppl) 60:1, 1999

PULVER AE: Search for schizophrenia susceptibility genes. Biol Psychiatry 47:221, 2000

SCHULTZ SK, ANDREASEN NC: Schizophrenia. Lancet 353:1425, 1999

Section 6
ALCOHOLISM AND DRUG DEPENDENCY

386

Robert O. Messing

BIOLOGY OF ADDICTION

Drug addiction is a chronic, relapsing disorder characterized by compulsion to take a drug and loss of self-control in limiting drug intake. The American Psychiatric Association (*DSM-IV*) uses the term *substance dependence* instead of drug addiction and requires at least three of the following symptoms to be present for diagnosis: (1) tolerance; (2) withdrawal; (3) persistent desire or unsuccessful attempts to reduce use; (4) use in larger amounts than intended; (5) reduction in important social, occupational, or recreational activities because of drug use; (6) considerable time spent obtaining the substance; and (7) continued use despite health, social, or economic problems resulting from substance use. *Substance abuse* is a milder disorder characterized by repetitive drug use that results in social or economic distress. Experimental studies in humans and in animal models (rodents and also simpler organisms such as flies and worms) have begun to elucidate the cellular and molecular mechanisms that mediate the loss of control in drug taking that is the hallmark of addiction. This chapter will review current understanding of the neurobiology of drug abuse relevant to the specific substances discussed in subsequent chapters, namely alcohol (Chap. 387), opioids (Chap. 388), cocaine and marijuana (Chap. 389), and nicotine (Chap. 390).

BEHAVIORAL RESPONSES TO DRUGS OF ABUSE

Drugs of abuse produce *euphoria*, which is an emotional state characterized by intensely pleasant feelings. A major reason why users are motivated to seek and take more of a drug is because they perceive

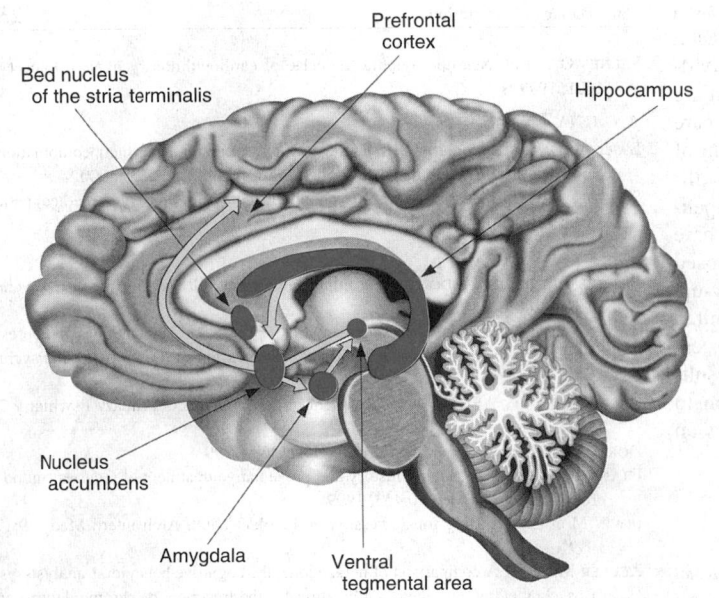

FIGURE 386-1 Mid-sagittal section of the human brain demonstrating limbic structures involved in brain reward pathways.

the experience as *rewarding*. *Reinforcement* refers to the ability of a drug to produce a pleasurable response that motivates the user to take the drug repeatedly. The powerful reinforcing and rewarding properties of abusable drugs can be measured by the tremendous effort experimental animals will expend, e.g., by pressing a lever multiple times, to obtain an oral or intravenous dose of a drug.

Tolerance is a reduction in response to a drug after repeated use and is a normal, adaptive, physiologic response. *Pharmacokinetic tolerance* may arise through an increase in the rate of metabolism. For example, barbiturates induce hepatic microsomal enzymes resulting in more rapid metabolism. *Pharmacodynamic tolerance* results from drug-induced changes in cell signaling and gene expression. Behavioral *sensitization* is a process whereby repeated administration of a drug leads to a progressively stronger behavioral response. Sometimes called "reverse tolerance," it is often measured by examining drug-induced locomotor activation. It generally requires longer intervals between doses to develop than does tolerance. Both tolerance and sensitization can promote repeated drug use. Tolerance develops to the rewarding properties of most abusable drugs, requiring the user to employ higher doses to achieve a euphoric effect. Sensitization also promotes drug self-administration, since rodents will expend greater effort in lever-pressing for drugs to which they are sensitized.

Physical dependence is an adaptive state that develops through resetting of homeostatic mechanisms to permit normal function despite the continued presence of a drug. When drug intake is abruptly terminated in a physically dependent individual, a withdrawal syndrome emerges. The symptoms of withdrawal tend to be opposite to those seen during acute drug exposure. Thus, abstinence from alcohol and other sedative-hypnotics causes nervous system hyperactivity, whereas withdrawal from cocaine and other stimulants is characterized by fatigue, sedation, and depression. Withdrawal symptoms are the principal evidence for physical dependence. Like tolerance, physical dependence is a normal physiologic response to repeated drug exposure and does not necessarily indicate drug abuse or addiction. However, withdrawal can cause intensely negative, unpleasant emotions such as dysphoria, anxiety, and irritability. In animal studies employing intracranial self-stimulation, withdrawal is also associated with reduced brain reward function. Thus, it appears that drug withdrawal can act as a negative reinforcer that contributes to repeated drug use.

Human patients prescribed opioids for treatment of pain may develop tolerance and physical dependence but rarely become addicted. Likewise, in experimental animals, establishing physical dependence

is not sufficient to induce voluntary drug self-administration. Instead, it appears that animals and humans seek abusable drugs mainly for their positive reinforcing properties. In susceptible persons, repeated use of abusable drugs induces drug *craving*, a powerful motivational state in which the addict seeks the drug to the exclusion of other activities. Craving is a manifestation of *psychological dependence* on a drug and is most severe during acute abstinence. It is a long-lasting, conditioned response that may be evoked by environmental cues such as sights, smells, or situations associated with previous drug use, even after long periods of drug abstinence. Understanding the mechanisms that underlie susceptibility to drug craving is a critical task in addiction research.

GENETIC FACTORS IN ADDICTION Genetic factors have been studied most extensively in alcoholism (Chap. 387). Patterns of inheritance in humans are most consistent with alcoholism being a polygenic disorder. Some genes confer a reduced risk for alcoholism. Approximately half of all individuals in Asian populations carry an allele of aldehyde dehydrogenase that encodes an isozyme with reduced enzymatic activity. After ingesting alcohol, they have increased blood levels of acetaldehyde and experience vasodilatation, tachycardia, hot sensations, and hypotension. They also report feeling intoxicated at very low doses of alcohol. Individuals expressing this isoenzyme rarely abuse alcohol. Other genetic factors predispose individuals to increased risk for alcoholism. A recent multicenter study of 105 families of alcoholics revealed evidence for susceptibility loci for alcohol dependence on chromosomes 1, 7, and possibly 2. An additional study of a Southwestern Native American population found evidence for genetic linkage to alcohol dependence on chromosomes 4 and 11. The identity of the genes associated with increased risk is not yet known.

NEUROANATOMY OF DRUG REWARD Early studies of intracranial electrical self-stimulation in rodents identified key structures involved in drug reward and motivational aspects of drug dependence (Fig. 386-1). These include the midbrain ventral tegmental area (VTA), median forebrain bundle (MFB), nucleus accumbens, medial frontal cortex, amygdala, and lateral hypothalamus. Many of these structures are key components of a *mesocorticolimbic dopamine system* that is now a principal focus of addiction research. Dopaminergic neurons in the VTA project axons via the MFB to the nucleus accumbens, amygdala, and frontal cortex. Reciprocal projections from γ-aminobutyric acid (GABA)-containing neurons in the nucleus accumbens project back through the MFB onto VTA neurons. Other brain regions modulate this system through opioid peptide, GABA, serotonin, and glutamate inputs that interact with the VTA, nucleus accumbens, and other structures within the system.

Certain nuclei within the mesocorticolimbic dopamine system share similarities in architecture, receptor expression, and connectivity with other brain regions. These related structures reside in the basal forebrain and include the central medial amygdala, bed nucleus of the stria terminalis, and shell of the nucleus accumbens. They appear to constitute a functional entity that has been called the "extended amygdala." The extended amygdala receives inputs from the hippocampus, basolateral amygdala, midbrain, and lateral hypothalamus and sends efferents to the ventral pallidum, VTA, and lateral hypothalamus.

MOLECULAR TARGETS OF ABUSED DRUGS Dopamine released from presynaptic terminals of VTA neurons in the nucleus accumbens is a major mediator of drug reward and reinforcement (Fig. 386-2A). Acute administration of all abusable drugs increases extracellular levels of dopamine in the shell of the nucleus accumbens. In addition, dopamine receptor antagonists injected into this region reduce drug self-administration in animals. Dopamine binds to a family of five G protein–coupled, seven-transmembrane receptors that can be grouped into two major classes, D_1-like (D_1 and D_5 receptors) and D_2-like (D_2, D_3, and D_4 receptors). D_1-like receptors activate adenylyl cyclase by coupling to the stimulatory G protein G_s, whereas D_2-like

FIGURE 386-2 Schematic representation of molecular targets for drugs of abuse. *A*. Dopaminergic synapse showing a presynaptic axon terminal of a ventral tegmental area dopaminergic neuron (*left*). Dopamine (DA) released from synaptic vesicles in the terminal bind to dopamine D_1-like and D_2-like receptors that regulate the activity of adenylyl cyclase (AC) in the dendritic terminal of a medium spiny GABA-ergic neuron (*right*) in the nucleus accumbens shell. *B*. Neurotransmitter receptor–gated ion channels (ionotropic receptors) regulated by ethanol, benzodiazepines, barbiturates, and nicotine. Stimulatory (+) and inhibitory (−) effects of these drugs on these channels are indicated. *C*. Seven-transmembrane receptors coupled to $G_{i/o}$ proteins (metabotropic receptors) that mediate actions of opioids and cannabinoids.

receptors inhibit adenylyl cyclase by coupling to inhibitory G_i proteins. Despite opposing actions on adenylyl cyclase, both classes of dopamine receptors appear to mediate drug reinforcement. Experimental animals will self-administer D_1-like and D_2-like receptor agonists, and antagonists of D_1, D_2, and D_3 receptors decrease the reinforcing properties of cocaine. These receptor-specific responses most likely result from dopamine actions on different subpopulations of cells in the nucleus accumbens.

Opioids, nicotine, psychostimulants, barbiturates, benzodiazepines, and cannabinoids elicit their acute behavioral effects by binding to specific seven-transmembrane neurotransmitter receptors (opioids and cannabinoids), neurotransmitter receptor–gated ion channels (nicotine, barbiturates, and benzodiazepines), or transporters (cocaine and amphetamines) on the plasma membrane of neuronal cells (Fig. 386-2). Ethanol interacts with several signaling proteins including serotonin 5HT-3 receptors, nicotinic receptors, voltage-gated calcium channels, and sodium-independent purine transporters, but GABA$_A$ receptors and the *N*-methyl-D-aspartate (NMDA) subtype of glutamate receptors appear to be most sensitive to intoxicating concentrations of

ethanol. As discussed below, drug actions at these targets lead to elevation of extracellular dopamine levels in the nucleus accumbens. This appears to be extremely important for the reinforcing properties of psychostimulants. For several other drugs of abuse, dopamine-independent pathways also contribute.

Dopamine Transporter Much evidence indicates that the rewarding properties of cocaine and amphetamine are due primarily to their ability to elevate extracellular dopamine levels in the nucleus accumbens. Specific populations of neurons within the nucleus accumbens are activated during cocaine self-administration in rodents. In addition, selective destruction of dopaminergic terminals within the nucleus accumbens or administration of dopamine receptor antagonists into that region eliminates cocaine self-administration. Cocaine and amphetamines act by altering transport of dopamine through plasma membrane dopamine transporters (DATs) in presynaptic nerve terminals (Fig. 386-2A). Reuptake of dopamine through DATs is the major mechanism for termination of dopaminergic neurotransmission. DAT is a 12-transmembrane glycoprotein and a member of the large sodium- and chloride-dependent transporter family, which also includes carriers for GABA, glycine, serotonin, norepinephrine, and other organic molecules. Cocaine binds to DATs and inhibits dopamine reuptake. Amphetamine causes intracellular release of dopamine from vesicles and reverse transport of dopamine through DATs. These actions serve to elevate levels of extracellular dopamine at dopaminergic synapses.

Recent studies of mice lacking the DAT gene have revealed redundancy in systems mediating cocaine reinforcement. Psychostimulants fail to alter extracellular dopamine levels or induce locomotor activity in these mice. However, DAT-null mice can still be trained to press a lever to receive intravenous cocaine, suggesting that other genes can also mediate the reinforcing properties of cocaine. In addition to inhibiting DAT function, cocaine blocks reuptake of serotonin and norepinephrine. In DAT-null mice, residual binding of a cocaine analogue can be displaced by serotonin reuptake inhibitors, and cocaine stimulates neurons in brain regions with a high density of serotonergic fibers. Therefore, inhibition of serotonin uptake through plasma membrane serotonin transporters may also contribute to psychostimulant reward.

GABA$_A$ Receptors The major inhibitory neurotransmitter in the nervous system is GABA. Binding of GABA to GABA$_A$ receptors activates a Cl^- current that is enhanced by benzodiazepines, barbiturates, and ethanol (Fig. 386-2B). Activation of this current maintains the neuronal plasma membrane close to its resting potential and thereby inhibits the generation of action potentials. GABA$_A$ receptors appear to be pentameric membrane glycoproteins composed of α, β, γ, and possibly δ peptide subunits. Fifteen subunits are known to be expressed in the mammalian central nervous system (six α, three β, three γ, one δ, one ϵ, one θ) and RNA splice variants have been identified. In rodents, the GABA$_A$ receptor agonist muscimol substitutes for ethanol in tests of drug discrimination; when injected into the nucleus accumbens, muscimol terminates ethanol self-administration. These results suggest that the reinforcing properties of ethanol are mediated in part by ethanol's actions at GABA$_A$ receptors in the nucleus accumbens.

NMDA Receptors In the nervous system, excitatory synaptic activity evoked by glutamate and aspartate is mediated by neurotransmitter receptor–gated ion channels (ionotropic receptors) that regulate cation conductances and by G protein–coupled receptors (metabotropic receptors) that stimulate phosphoinositide hydrolysis. Ionotropic glutamate receptors have been subclassified based on activation by selective agonists into three groups: NMDA receptors, high-affinity kainate receptors, and α-amino-3-hydroxy-5-methyl-4-isoxazole propionic acid (AMPA) receptors. There is a rich glutamatergic projection from neurons in the frontal cortex to the nucleus accumbens where fibers terminate mainly on medium spiny GABA-ergic neurons. NMDA receptors in the nucleus accumbens appear to play a role in the rewarding properties of several drugs. Thus, phencyclidine and other NMDA antagonists have rewarding actions when administered in the nucleus accumbens. The rewarding properties of ethanol may also be partly due to inhibition of NMDA-activated calcium currents. In addition, NMDA receptors modulate responses to psychostimulants since administration of the NMDA receptor antagonist MK-801 prior to cocaine or amphetamine prevents sensitization to these drugs.

Nicotinic Receptors Like other drugs of abuse, nicotine elicits dopamine release in the nucleus accumbens, and intravenous self-administration of nicotine is blocked by dopamine antagonists and by neurochemical lesions that destroy dopaminergic fibers in the nucleus accumbens. Nicotine increases dopamine release by activating nicotinic acetylcholine receptors (nAChRs) on cell bodies and nerve terminals of dopaminergic VTA neurons. Neuronal nAChRs are receptor-gated ion channels that allow entry of sodium into cells when acetylcholine is present. They appear to be pentameric complexes composed of different combinations of at least 10 different subunits. Targeted disruption of the β_2 subunit gene eliminates most high-affinity nicotine binding in the brain and prevents nicotine-induced dopamine release in the nucleus accumbens. In addition, mice that lack the β_2 subunit show attenuated nicotine self-administration, indicating that β_2-containing nAChRs mediate the reinforcing properties of nicotine.

Opioid Receptors Morphine and other opioids activate opioid receptors, which are a family of seven-transmembrane, G protein–coupled receptors (Figs. 386-2C and 386-3). Three classes, μ, δ, and κ, have been identified. The rewarding action of opioids appears to be mediated by activation of μ receptors since opioid reinforcement is blocked by selective μ receptor antagonists and by targeted disruption of the μ receptor gene. Binding of opioid agonists to μ receptors activates the G proteins G_i and G_o. This results in inhibition of adenylyl cyclase, thereby decreasing levels of the intracellular second messenger cyclic AMP and reducing activity of cyclic AMP–dependent protein kinase A (PKA). In addition, these G proteins activate voltage-gated potassium channels and inhibit voltage-gated calcium channels. The net result is suppression of electrical excitability in neurons expressing μ receptors.

GABA-containing interneurons in the VTA suppress firing of dopaminergic VTA neurons that project to the nucleus accumbens. Opioids disinhibit these dopaminergic neurons by binding to μ receptors expressed by the GABA-containing interneurons. This increases the firing rate of dopaminergic VTA neurons and promotes dopamine release in the nucleus accumbens. Rodents will self-administer opioids into both the VTA and the nucleus accumbens. Opioid self-administration into the nucleus accumbens occurs even after dopaminergic projections to that region are destroyed. Thus, dopamine-dependent mechanisms involving the VTA and dopamine-independent mechanisms in the nucleus accumbens both contribute to opioid reward.

Opioid receptors also regulate ethanol consumption. Ethanol acutely inhibits opioid binding to δ-opioid receptors, and chronic ethanol exposure increases the density of μ- and δ-opioid receptors. Nonselective opioid antagonists reduce ethanol self-administration in animals. Several regions of the extended amygdala appear to mediate this response, although the central nucleus of the amygdala appears most important. In two independent clinical trials, the opioid receptor antagonist naltrexone, in combination with counseling, reduced craving and relapse in abstinent alcoholics. Thus, opioid systems appear to modulate ethanol craving in addicted individuals.

Cannabinoid Receptors The active ingredient of cannabis, Δ^9-tetrahydrocannabinol (Δ-9-THC), and the endogenous cannabinoid anandamide bind two subtypes of G protein–coupled cannabinoid receptors. Studies with mutant mice lacking the CB_1 receptor gene have revealed that the CB_1 receptor is responsible for the reinforcing properties of cannabinoids. When administered intravenously, Δ-9-THC increases dopamine levels in the nucleus accumbens. This is blocked by cannabinoid receptor antagonists and by μ-opioid receptor antagonists administered into the VTA. Conversely, morphine reinforcement and the severity of opioid withdrawal are reduced in mice that lack CB_1 receptors. These results suggest that opioids and cannabinoids share common signaling pathways in the brain and can interact to promote each other's reinforcing properties.

ADAPTATION TO CHRONIC DRUG USE Repeated drug exposure elicits changes in neural function that lead to drug dependence and craving. Several mechanisms are being elucidated, including drug-induced alterations in receptor and ion channel function, intracellular signal transduction, gene expression, and synaptic connectivity.

Chronic exposure to drugs of abuse can change the function of receptors and ion channels by altering their density, subunit composition, or coupling to signal transduction cascades. For example, chronic exposure to ethanol increases the density of NMDA receptors and L-type voltage-gated calcium channels in the brain. These changes contribute to neuronal hyperactivity observed during alcohol withdrawal since NMDA and L-type channel antagonists reduce signs of withdrawal in alcohol-dependent rodents deprived of ethanol. In addition, chronic exposure to ethanol decreases GABA$_A$ receptor function and abolishes potentiation by ethanol. Downregulation of GABA$_A$ receptor function contributes to manifestations of alcohol withdrawal since benzodiazepines and barbiturates, which activate GABA$_A$ receptors, are very helpful in reducing alcohol withdrawal symptoms.

Chronic exposure to many drugs of abuse induces adaptive changes in neuronal signal transduction pathways. This has been most clearly demonstrated for opioids, which increase cyclic AMP signaling in the locus coeruleus after chronic administration (Fig. 386-3). The locus coeruleus is the principal adrenergic nucleus in the brain and

FIGURE 386-3 Schematic representation of opioid signaling in the locus coeruleus. Brief exposure to opioids activates μ-opioid receptors leading to G protein dissociation and $G\alpha_i$-mediated inhibition of adenylyl cyclase (AC), cyclic AMP formation, and protein kinase A (PKA). In addition, the $\beta\gamma$ subunits of the dissociated G proteins inhibit presynaptic voltage-gated Ca^{2+} channels and enhance the function of G protein–gated, inwardly rectifying K^+ channels, leading to a decrease in cell excitability. Bold arrows indicate compensatory increases in AC, PKA, and cyclic AMP response element binding protein (CREB) levels, and increased function of Na^+ channels following chronic exposure to opioids. This leads to increased neuronal activity, thereby contributing to opioid tolerance and to hyperexcitability during acute opioid withdrawal. Increases in CREB-mediated gene expression may also lead to long-term changes in neuronal function that contribute to addiction.

regulates attention states and the autonomic nervous system. Hyperactivity of this nucleus has been implicated in opioid withdrawal. Chronic opioid exposure increases expression of adenylyl cyclase, PKA, and the cyclic AMP response element binding protein, CREB, which mediates cyclic AMP–dependent gene expression. These changes increase the intrinsic firing rate of neurons in the locus coeruleus, in part through activation of an inward sodium current. Thus, upregulation of cyclic AMP signaling opposes the acute inhibitory action of opioids on this pathway.

Chronic exposure to cocaine, opioids, or ethanol upregulates cyclic AMP–mediated signaling in other brain regions, including the VTA and the nucleus accumbens. Upregulation of cyclic AMP signaling in the nucleus accumbens contributes to psychostimulant tolerance since pharmacologic inhibition of PKA or overexpression of CREB in the nucleus accumbens decreases the rewarding properties of cocaine. Upregulation of cyclic AMP signaling may also account for supersensitivity of neurons in the nucleus accumbens to D_1 receptor agonists following chronic cocaine administration. Additional neuroadaptive changes in dopamine signaling can modify drug-seeking behavior in rodents. Rats can be readily trained to voluntarily self-administer intravenous cocaine for several hours. If during a course of self-administration, saline is substituted for cocaine, the rate of self-administration declines dramatically. However, exposure to a single intraperitoneal priming injection of cocaine or a D_2-like receptor agonist causes the animal to resume lever pressing. In contrast, treatment with a D_1-like receptor agonist blocks the ability of cocaine to reinstate drug-seeking behavior. It appears that D_1-like agonists inhibit relapse in drug seeking. Therefore, they may prove to be useful in treatment of cocaine addiction.

A current hypothesis views addiction as a form of learning mediated by maladaptive recruitment of memory systems involving limbic structures. Mechanisms that could contribute to such learned, long-term adaptation include drug-induced gene expression and synaptic reorganization. For example, the transcription factor CREB, which is activated by chronic drug use, has been implicated in models of learning. Repeated exposure to many drugs of abuse also causes prolonged activation of another transcription factor, *Fos*-related antigen, in the nucleus accumbens. Ethanol increases the number of dendritic spines on hippocampal pyramidal cells and somatosensory cortical neurons, whereas amphetamine increases dendritic length and the density of dendritic spines on neurons in the nucleus accumbens and prefrontal cortex. Such drug-induced changes in gene expression and neuronal connectivity could lead to long-term alterations in brain reward pathways that may underlie drug addiction in humans.

BIBLIOGRAPHY

AMARA SG, SONDERS MS: Neurotransmitter transporters as molecular targets for addictive drugs. Drug Alcohol Depend 51:87, 1998

BERKE JD, HYMAN SE: Addiction, dopamine, and the molecular mechanisms of memory. Neuron 25:515, 2000

CRABBE JC et al: Identifying genes for alcohol and drug sensitivity: Recent progress and future directions. Trends Neurosci 22:173, 1999

KANDEL ER et al (eds): *Principles of Neural Science*. 4th ed, New York, McGraw-Hill, 2000

KOOB GF et al: Neuroscience of addiction. Neuron 21:467, 1998

LEDENT C et al: Unresponsiveness to cannabinoids and reduced addictive effects of opiates in CB1 receptor knockout mice. Science 283:401, 1999

MESSING RO, DIAMOND I: Molecular biology of alcohol dependence, in *The Molecular and Genetic Basis of Neurological Disease*, 2d ed, R Rosenberg et al (eds). Boston, Butterworth-Heinemann, 1997, pp 1109–1126

NESTLER EJ: Molecular mechanisms of opiate and cocaine addiction. Curr Opin Neurobiol 7:713, 1997

ROBINSON TE, KOLB B: Persistent structural modifications in nucleus accumbens and prefrontal cortex neurons produced by previous experience with amphetamine. J Neurosci 17:8491, 1997

ROCHA BA et al: Cocaine self-administration in dopamine-transporter knockout mice [see comments]. Nat Neurosci 1:132, 1998

SELF DW et al: Opposite modulation of cocaine-seeking behavior by D1- and D2-like dopamine receptor agonists. Science 271:1586, 1996

387   *Marc A. Schuckit*

ALCOHOL AND ALCOHOLISM

The yearly cost of alcohol-related problems in the United States is as much as $300 billion, including accidents, health problems, lost productivity, crime, and treatment. There are more than 22,000 deaths from alcohol-related auto accidents per year, as well as almost 2 million nonfatal injuries and damage to almost 5 million vehicles. In addition, alcohol is responsible for almost 5% of missed work time, with a 25% decrease in work performance among heavy drinkers. Men and women who fulfill criteria for alcohol use disorders decrease their life span by approximately 15 years, with abuse and dependence responsible for almost 25% of premature deaths in men and 15% in women, figures that represent a three- to sixfold odds ratio of early death even among people with higher levels of education and socioeconomic functioning.

PHARMACOLOGY AND NUTRITIONAL IMPACT OF ETHANOL   Ethanol is a weakly charged molecule that moves easily through cell membranes, rapidly equilibrating between blood and tissues. The effects of drinking depend in part on the amount of ethanol consumed per unit of body weight; the level of alcohol in the blood is expressed as milligrams or grams of ethanol per deciliter (e.g., 100 mg/dL or 0.10 g/dL). A level of 0.02 to 0.03 results from the ingestion of one to two typical drinks. In round figures, 340 mL (12 oz) of beer, 115 mL (4 oz) of nonfortified wine, and 43 mL (1.5 oz) (a shot) of 80-proof beverage each contain approximately 10 g of ethanol; 0.5 L (1 pint) of 86-proof beverage contains approximately 160 g, and 1 L of wine contains approximately 80 g of ethanol. Congeners found in alcoholic beverages may contribute to body damage with heavy drinking; these include low-molecular-weight alcohols (e.g., methanol and butanol), aldehydes, esters, histamine, phenols, tannins, iron, lead, and cobalt.

Ethanol is a central nervous system (CNS) depressant that decreases activity of neurons, although some behavioral stimulation is observed at low blood levels. This drug has cross-tolerance and shares a similar pattern of behavioral problems with other brain depressants, including the benzodiazepines and barbiturates. Alcohol is absorbed from mucous membranes of the mouth and esophagus (in small amounts), from the stomach and large bowel (in modest amounts), and from the proximal portion of the small intestine (the major site). The rate of absorption is *increased* by rapid gastric emptying; by the absence of proteins, fats, or carbohydrates (which interfere with absorption); by the absence of congeners; by dilution to a modest percentage of ethanol (maximum at about 20% by volume); and by carbonation (e.g., champagne).

Between 2% (at low blood alcohol concentrations) and about 10% (at high blood alcohol concentrations) of ethanol is excreted directly through the lungs, urine, or sweat, but the greater part is metabolized to acetaldehyde, primarily in the liver. At least two metabolic routes, each with different optimal concentrations of ethanol (K_m), result in the metabolism of approximately one drink per hour. The most important pathway occurs in the cell cytosol where alcohol dehydrogenase (ADH) produces acetaldehyde, which is then rapidly destroyed by aldehyde dehydrogenase (ALDH) in the cytosol and mitochondria. Each of these steps requires nicotinamide adenine dinucleotide (NAD) as a cofactor, and it is the increased ratio of the reduced cofactor (NADH) to NAD (NADH:NAD) that is responsible for many of the metabolic derangements observed after drinking. A second pathway occurs in the microsomes of the smooth endoplasmic reticulum (the microsomal ethanol-oxidizing system, or MEOS), which is responsible for 10% or more of ethanol oxidation at high blood alcohol concentrations.

One gram of ethanol has approximately 29.7 kJ (7.1 kcal) of energy, and a drink contains between 293.0 and 418.6 kJ (70 and 100 kcal) from ethanol and other carbohydrates. However, these are "empty" of nutrients such as minerals, proteins, and vitamins. In addition, alcohol interferes with absorption of vitamins in the small intestine and decreases their storage in the liver. These actions affect folate (folacin or folic acid), pyridoxine (B_6), thiamine (B_1), nicotinic acid (niacin, B_3), and vitamin A. Heavy drinking can also produce low blood levels of potassium, magnesium, calcium, zinc, and phosphorus as a consequence of dietary deficiency and acid-base imbalances during excess alcohol ingestion or withdrawal.

An ethanol load in a fasting, healthy individual is likely to produce transient hypoglycemia within 6 to 36 h, secondary to the acute actions of ethanol on gluconeogenesis. This can result in glucose intolerance until the alcoholic has abstained for 2 to 4 weeks. Alcohol ketoacidosis, probably reflecting a decrease in fatty acid oxidation coupled with poor diet or recurrent vomiting, should not be misdiagnosed as diabetic ketosis. With the former, patients show an increase in serum ketones along with a mild increase in glucose but a large anion gap, a mild to moderate increase in serum lactate, and a β-hydroxybutyrate/lactate ratio of between 2:1 and 9:1 (with normal being 1:1).

BEHAVIORAL EFFECTS, TOLERANCE, AND DEPENDENCE The effects of any drug depend on the dose, the rate of increase in plasma, the concomitant presence of other drugs, and the past experience with the agent. With alcohol, an additional factor is whether blood alcohol levels are rising or falling; the effects are more intense during the former period.

Even though "legal intoxication" requires a blood alcohol concentration of at least 80 to 100 mg/dL, behavioral, psychomotor, and cognitive changes are seen at levels as low as 20 to 30 mg/dL (i.e., after one to two drinks). Deep but disturbed sleep can be seen at twice the legal intoxication level, and death can occur with levels between 300 and 400 mg/dL. Beverage alcohol is probably responsible for more overdose deaths than any other drug.

The intoxicating effects of alcohol appear to be due to actions at specific neurotransmitter receptors and transporters. Alcohol enhances γ-aminobutyric acid A ($GABA_A$) receptors, and inhibits N-methyl-D-asparate (NMDA) receptors (Chap. 386). In vitro studies suggest that additional effects involve inhibition of adenosine uptake and a translocation of the cyclic AMP–dependent protein kinase catalytic subunit from the cytoplasm to the nucleus. Neurons adapt quickly to these actions, and thus different effects may be present during chronic administration and withdrawal.

At least three types of compensation develop after repeated exposure to the drug, producing tolerance of higher ethanol levels. First, after 1 to 2 weeks of daily drinking, *metabolic or pharmacokinetic tolerance* develops, with a 30% increase in the rate of hepatic ethanol metabolism. This alteration disappears almost as rapidly as it develops. Second, *cellular or pharmacodynamic tolerance* develops through neurochemical changes that may also contribute to physical dependence. Third, individuals can learn to adapt their behavior so that they can function better than expected under drug influence (*behavioral tolerance*).

The cellular changes caused by chronic ethanol exposure may not resolve for several weeks or longer following cessation of drinking. In the interim, the neurons require ethanol to function optimally, and the individual can be said to be physically dependent. This physical condition is distinct from psychological dependence, a concept indicating that the person is psychologically uncomfortable without the drug.

THE EFFECTS OF ETHANOL ON BODY SYSTEMS

While one to two drinks per day in an otherwise healthy and nonpregnant individual can have some beneficial effects, at higher doses alcohol is toxic to most body systems. Knowledge about the deleterious effects of alcohol helps the practicing physician to identify alcoholic patients. Signs and symptoms of ethanol abuse can be used to help motivate the patient to abstain. It is important to remember that the typical white- or blue-collar alcoholic functions at a fairly high level for years, and that not everyone develops each problem.

CENTRAL NERVOUS SYSTEM Approximately 35% of drinkers may experience a *blackout*, an episode of temporary anterograde amnesia, in which the person forgets all or part of what occurred during a drinking evening. Another common problem, one seen after as few as one or two drinks, is that while alcohol can help someone to fall asleep, it also "fragments" the sleep pattern causing alterations between sleep stages and a deficiency in deep sleep. At the same time, alcohol diminishes rapid eye movement (REM) or dream sleep early in the evening, with resulting prominent and sometimes disturbing dreams later in the night. Finally, alcohol relaxes muscles in the pharynx, which can cause snoring and exacerbate sleep apnea, with symptoms of the latter in 75% of alcoholic men over age 60.

An additional problem related to the acute effects of alcohol on most drinkers is the impairment in judgment, balance, and motor coordination that contributes to the high incidence and severity of accidents. At least half of individuals who experience severe physical trauma in an accident have evidence of substance-related impairment, a finding that is consistent with the fact that 40% of drinkers in the United States have at some time driven while intoxicated with alcohol and that 15% of flight crews have evidence of repeated heavy drinking. Regarding the latter, at least one study noted that pilot performance is still impaired 14 h after a blood alcohol concentration of 100 mg/dL, despite subsequent abstinence.

The effect of alcohol on the nervous system is even more pronounced among alcohol-dependent individuals. Chronic intake of high doses of ethanol causes *peripheral neuropathy* in 5 to 15% of alcoholics, which is possibly related to thiamine deficiency. Patients complain of bilateral limb numbness, tingling, and paresthesias; symptoms are more pronounced distally than proximally. The treatment is abstinence and thiamine supplementation.

Wernicke's syndrome (ophthalmoparesis, ataxia, and encephalopathy) and *Korsakoff's syndrome* (alcohol-induced persisting amnestic disorder), are seen in the United States at a rate of approximately 50 per million people per year. These disorders are the result of thiamine deficiency in vulnerable individuals, possibly owing to interaction with a genetic transketolase deficiency. Korsakoff's syndrome presents as profound and persistent anterograde amnesia (inability to learn new material) and a milder retrograde amnesia. Additional symptoms can include impairment in visuospatial, abstract, and conceptual reasoning but with a normal intelligence quotient (IQ). Some patients demonstrate an acute onset of Korsakoff's syndrome in association with the neurologic stigmata seen with Wernicke's syndrome (e.g., sixth nerve palsy and ataxia), whereas others have a more gradual onset. With oral thiamine replacement (50 to 100 mg/d), only one-quarter of Korsakoff's patients achieve full recovery, one-half experience partial improvement, and one-quarter show no improvement, even after many months of supplementation. →*Wernicke's syndrome is discussed in detail in Chap. 376.*

About 1% of alcoholics develop *cerebellar degeneration*, a syndrome of progressive unsteady stance and gait often accompanied by mild nystagmus. Atrophy of the cerebellar vermis is seen on brain computed tomography and magnetic resonance imaging scans, but the cerebrospinal fluid is usually normal. Treatment consists of abstinence and multiple vitamin supplementation, although improvement is often minimal.

Alcoholics can show severe *cognitive* problems and impairment in recent and remote memory for weeks to months after an alcoholic binge. Increased size of the brain ventricles and cerebral sulci are seen in 50% or more of chronic alcoholics, but these changes are often reversible, returning toward normal after a year or more of abstinence. Permanent CNS impairment (alcohol-induced persisting dementia) can develop and accounts for up to 20% of chronically demented patients. There is no single alcoholic dementia syndrome; rather, this label is used to describe patients who have apparently irreversible cognitive changes (possibly from diverse causes) in the midst of chronic alcoholism.

Finally, almost every psychiatric syndrome can be seen temporarily during heavy drinking or subsequent withdrawal. These include intense *sadness* lasting for days to weeks in the midst of heavy drinking in 40% of alcoholics, which is classified as an alcohol-induced mood disorder in the *Fourth Diagnostic and Statistical Manual* of the American Psychiatric Association (DSM-IV); severe *anxiety* in 10 to 30% of alcoholics, often beginning during alcohol withdrawal and which can persist for many months after cessation of drinking (alcohol-induced anxiety disorder); and auditory *hallucinations* and/or *paranoid delusions* in the absence of any obvious signs of withdrawal—a state now called *alcohol-induced psychotic disorder*—and reported at sometime in 1 to 10% of alcoholics. Treatment of all forms of alcohol-induced psychopathology includes abstinence and supportive care, with the likelihood of full recovery within several days to 6 weeks. A history of alcohol intake is an important consideration in *any* patient with one of these psychiatric symptoms.

THE GASTROINTESTINAL SYSTEM   Esophagus and Stomach Acute alcohol intake can result in inflammation of the esophagus (possibly secondary to reflux of gastric contents) and stomach (resulting from both an increase in acid production and damage to the gastric mucosal barrier). Esophagitis can cause epigastric distress, and gastritis, the most frequent cause of gastrointestinal bleeding in heavy drinkers, can present as anorexia and/or abdominal pain. Chronic heavy drinking, if associated with violent vomiting, can produce a longitudinal tear in the mucosa at the gastroesophageal junction—a Mallory-Weiss lesion. Although many gastrointestinal problems are reversible, two complications of chronic alcoholism, esophageal varices secondary to cirrhosis-induced portal hypertension and atrophy of the gastric mucosa, may be irreversible.

Pancreas The incidence of acute pancreatitis in alcoholics (about 25 per 1000 per year) is almost threefold higher than in the general population, accounting for an estimated 10% or more of the cases of this disorder (Chap. 304).

Liver Ethanol absorbed from the small bowel is carried directly to the liver, where it becomes the preferred fuel; NADH accumulates and oxygen utilization escalates; gluconeogenesis is impaired (with a resulting fall in the amount of glucose produced from glycogen); lactate production increases; and there is a decreased oxidation of fatty acids in the citric acid cycle with an increase in fat accumulation within liver cells. In the healthy individual taking no medications, these changes are reversible, but with repeated exposure to ethanol, more severe changes in liver functioning are likely to occur. These include, in overlapping stages, fatty accumulation, alcohol-induced hepatitis, perivenular sclerosis, and cirrhosis, with the latter observed in an estimated 15 to 20% of alcoholics (Chap. 298).

CANCER As discussed briefly below, the leading cause of death in alcoholics is cardiovascular disease, but cancer occupies a solid second place. Women drinking as few as 1.5 drinks per day increase their risk of breast cancer 1.4-fold. For both genders, four drinks per day increases the risk for oral and esophageal cancers by approximately threefold and rectal cancers by a factor of 1.5, whereas seven to eight or more drinks per day enhances the risks for many of these cancers by a factor of five. Overall, it has been estimated that alcoholics have a rate of carcinoma 10 times higher than the general population.

HEMATOPOIETIC SYSTEM Ethanol exerts multiple reversible acute and chronic effects on all blood cells. The impact on red blood cells (RBC) is an increase in size (mean corpuscular volume, MCV), usually without anemia. This change appears to reflect the effect of alcohol on stem cells. If heavy drinking is accompanied by folic acid deficiency, there can also be hypersegmented neutrophils, reticulocytopenia, and hyperplastic bone marrow; if malnutrition is present, sideroblastic changes can also be observed. Chronic heavy drinking can also decrease production of most white blood cells (WBCs), decrease granulocyte mobility and adherence, and impair the

delayed-hypersensitivity response to new antigens (with a possible false-negative tuberculin skin test). Finally, many alcoholics present with mild thrombocytopenia. When due to repeated intoxication, the low platelet count usually resolves within a week of abstinence. Thrombocytopenia can also occur secondary to hepatic cirrhosis and congestive splenomegaly (increased destruction) or to folic acid deficiency (decreased production). Ethanol itself might not have a major effect on platelet function, but polyphenols and other constituents of some alcoholic beverages, particularly wine, may interfere with platelet aggregation.

CARDIOVASCULAR SYSTEM Acutely, ethanol decreases myocardial contractility and causes peripheral vasodilation, with a resulting mild decrease in blood pressure and a compensatory increase in cardiac output. Exercise-induced increases in cardiac oxygen consumption are higher after alcohol intake. These acute effects have little clinical importance for the average healthy drinker but can produce problems in men and women with cardiac disease.

Chronic intake of even modest doses of alcohol can have both deleterious and beneficial effects. Regarding the latter, a maximum of one to two drinks per day over long periods may decrease the risk for cardiovascular death, perhaps through an increase in high-density lipoprotein (HDL) cholesterol or changes in clotting mechanisms. In one large national study, cardiovascular mortality was reduced by 30 to 40% among individuals reporting one or more drinks daily compared to nondrinkers, with overall mortality lowest among those consuming approximately one drink per day. Recent data have also corroborated the decreased risk for ischemic, but not hemorrhagic, stroke associated with regular light drinking.

The consumption of three or more drinks per day results in a dose-dependent increase in blood pressure, which returns to normal within weeks of abstinence. As a result, heavy drinking is an important contributor to mild to moderate hypertension. Chronic heavy drinking can cause cardiomyopathy, with symptoms ranging from unexplained arrhythmias in the presence of left ventricular impairment to heart failure with dilation of all four heart chambers and hypocontractility of heart muscle. Perhaps one-third of cases of cardiomyopathy are alcohol-induced. Mural thrombi can form in the left atrium or ventricle, while heart enlargement exceeding 25% can cause mitral regurgitation. Atrial or ventricular arrhythmias, especially paroxysmal tachycardia, can also occur after a drinking binge in individuals showing no other evidence of heart disease—a syndrome known as the "holiday heart."

GENITOURINARY SYSTEM CHANGES, SEXUAL FUNCTIONING, AND FETAL DEVELOPMENT Acutely, modest ethanol doses (e.g., blood alcohol concentrations of 100 mg/dL or even less) can both increase sexual drive and decrease erectile capacity in men. Even in the absence of liver impairment, a significant minority of chronic alcoholic men may show irreversible testicular atrophy with concomitant shrinkage of the seminiferous tubules, decreases in ejaculate volume, and a lower sperm count (Chap. 335).

The repeated ingestion of high doses of ethanol by women can result in amenorrhea, a decrease in ovarian size, absence of corpora lutea with associated infertility, and spontaneous abortions. Heavy drinking during pregnancy results in the rapid placental transfer of both ethanol and acetaldehyde, which may have serious consequences for fetal development. The *fetal alcohol syndrome* can include any of the following: facial changes with epicanthal eye folds, poorly formed concha, and small teeth with faulty enamel; cardiac atrial or ventricular septal defects; an aberrant palmar crease and limitation in joint movement; and microcephaly with mental retardation. The specific amount of ethanol and/or specific time of vulnerability during pregnancy have not been defined, making it advisable for pregnant women to abstain completely.

OTHER EFFECTS OF ETHANOL Between one-half and two-thirds of alcoholics have evidence of decreased skeletal muscle strength caused by acute *alcoholic myopathy*, a condition that improves but which might not disappear with abstinence. Effects of repeated heavy drinking on the *skeletal system* include alterations in calcium metabolism, lower bone density, and less growth in the epiphyses, with an increased risk for fractures and osteonecrosis of the femoral head. *Hormonal changes* include an increase in cortisol levels, which can remain elevated during heavy drinking; inhibition of vasopressin secretion at rising blood alcohol concentrations and the opposite effect at falling blood alcohol concentrations (with the final result that most alcoholics are likely to be slightly overhydrated); a modest and reversible decrease in serum thyroxine (T_4); and a more marked decrease in serum triiodothyronine (T_3).

ALCOHOLISM (ALCOHOL ABUSE OR DEPENDENCE)

Because many drinkers occasionally imbibe to excess, temporary alcohol-related pathology is common in nonalcoholics. The period of heaviest drinking is usually the late teens to the late twenties. This is also a time of high risk for temporary alcohol-related social, occupational, or driving difficulties. These phenomena are often isolated events or self-limited, but when repeated problems in multiple life areas develop, the person is likely to meet criteria for alcohol abuse or dependence.

DEFINITIONS AND EPIDEMIOLOGY DSM-IV defines alcohol dependence as repeated alcohol-related difficulties in at least three of seven areas of functioning that cluster together over any 12-month period. These problems include any combination of tolerance, withdrawal, taking larger amounts of alcohol over longer periods than intended, an inability to control use, spending a great deal of time associated with alcohol use, giving up important activities to drink, and continued use of alcohol despite physical or psychological consequences. In this diagnosis a special emphasis is placed on evidence of tolerance and/or withdrawal, a condition referred to as "dependence with a physiological component" and which is associated wtih a more severe clinical course. Dependence occurs in both men and women, in individuals from all socioeconomic strata, and in people of all racial backgrounds. The diagnosis predicts a course of recurrent problems with the use of alcohol and the consequent shortening of the life span by a decade or more. In the absence of alcohol dependence, an individual can be given a diagnosis of *alcohol abuse* if he or she demonstrates *repetitive* problems with alcohol in any one of four life areas: an inability to fulfill major obligations, use in hazardous situations such as driving, legal problems, or use despite social or interpersonal difficulties.

The clinical diagnosis of alcohol abuse or dependence rests on the documentation of a pattern of *difficulties associated with alcohol use*; the definition is *not* based on the quantity and frequency of alcohol consumption. Thus, in screening for alcohol abuse or dependence, it is important to probe for life problems and then attempt to tie in use of alcohol or another substance. Information regarding marital or job problems, legal difficulties, histories of accidents, medical problems, evidence of tolerance, etc., is an important component of all evaluations and yields data that are of use even for nonalcoholic individuals.

The lifetime risk for alcohol dependence in most western countries is about 10 to 15% for men and 5% for women. When alcohol abuse is also considered, the rates are even higher. The typical alcoholic is a blue- or white-collar worker or homemaker and thus does not fit the common stereotype.

GENETICS OF ALCOHOLISM Alcoholism is a multifactorial disorder in which both environmental and biologic factors contribute. The importance of genetic influences in alcoholism is supported by the higher risk for this disorder in the identical versus fraternal twin of an alcoholic and the fourfold increased risk for children of alcoholics even if adopted at birth and raised without knowledge of the problems of their biologic parents.

The evidence supporting genetic influences in alcoholism has stimulated a search for trait markers of a vulnerability toward the disorder.

A 15-year follow-up of 453 men originally studied at age 20 has shown that subjects with alcoholic fathers demonstrated relatively lower levels of response to alcohol, including less intense subjective feelings of intoxication, less alcohol-related impairment in cognitive and psychomotor tests, and less intense alcohol-related changes in prolactin and cortisol secretion. This low level of response to alcohol at around age 20 was a powerful predictor of later alcoholism, explaining most of the relationship between a family history of this disorder and later alcohol problems. Additional genetically influenced characteristics that contribute to the risk of alcoholism appear to include some personality traits such as higher levels of impulsivity and sensation seeking, and several electrophysiologic measures such as the P300 wave of the event-related potential (Chap. 357), which might relate to cognitive styles or evidence of CNS disinhibition. All the genetic factors combined appear to explain up to 60% of the risk, with environmental influences contributing at least 40%.

NATURAL HISTORY For the "average" alcoholic, the age of first drink and first minor problems (e.g., an argument with a friend while drunk or an alcoholic blackout) are similar to those in the general population. However, by the early to mid-twenties, most men and women moderate their drinking (perhaps learning from minor problems), whereas difficulties for alcoholics are likely to escalate, with the first major life problem from alcohol appearing in the mid-twenties to early forties. Once established, the course of alcoholism is likely to be one of exacerbations and remissions. As a rule, there is remarkably little difficulty in stopping alcohol use when problems develop, and this step is often followed by days to months of carefully controlled drinking. Unfortunately, these periods are almost inevitably followed by escalations in alcohol intake and subsequent problems. The course is not hopeless, because between half and two-thirds of alcoholics maintain abstinence for extended periods after treatment. Even without formal treatment or self-help groups there is at least a 20% chance of long-term abstinence. However, should the alcoholic continue to drink, the life span is shortened by an average of 15 years, with the leading causes of death, in decreasing order, being heart disease, cancer, accidents, and suicide.

IDENTIFICATION OF THE ALCOHOLIC AND INTERVENTION Physicians even in affluent areas should recognize that approximately 20% of patients have alcoholism. Therefore, it is important to pay attention to the alcohol-related symptoms and signs described above as well as laboratory tests that are likely to be abnormal in the context of regular consumption of 6 to 8 or more drinks per day. These include a high-normal or slightly elevated MCV (e.g., ≥ 91 fL), γ-glutamyl transferase (GGT) (≥ 30 units), serum uric acid [>416 μmol/L (7 mg/dL)], carbohydrate-deficient transferrin (CDT) (≥ 20 g/L), and triglycerides [≥ 2.0 mmol/L (180 mg/dL)]. Mild and fluctuating hypertension (e.g., 140/95), repeated infections such as pneumonia, and otherwise unexplained cardiac arrhythmias should also raise the possibility that the patient is an alcoholic. Other disorders suggestive of alcoholism include cancer of the head and neck, esophagus, or stomach as well as cirrhosis, unexplained hepatitis, pancreatitis, bilateral parotid gland swelling, and peripheral neuropathy.

Once the likelihood of alcoholism is established, only a few moments are needed to gather the history of alcohol-related life problems. The patient and the spouse or another close family member should be asked about patterns of accidents, relationship difficulties, problems on the job, and driving-related difficulties, after which the role played by alcohol should be identified. All physicians should be able to take the time needed to gather such information. In addition, a simple 25-item form to be answered by the patient, the Michigan Alcohol Screening Test (MAST), is available to aid in identifying alcoholics. However, this is only a screening tool, and a careful face-to-face interview is still required for a meaningful diagnosis. The CAGE, which consists of asking about alcohol-related trouble *c*utting down on intake, being *a*nnoyed by criticisms, *g*uilt, or use of an "*e*ye-opener," can also be helpful as an initial screen.

After alcoholism is identified, the diagnosis must be shared with the patient. The presenting complaint can be used as an entrée to the hypertension could be told that these are clinically important symptoms and that physical findings and laboratory tests indicate that alcohol appears to have contributed to the complaints and is increasing the risk for further medical and psychological problems. The physician should share information about the course of alcoholism and explore possible avenues of attacking the problem. Some patients and family members will benefit from the opportunity to read additional material (see "Bibliography").

The process of intervention is rarely accomplished in one session. For the person who refuses to stop drinking at the first intervention, a logical step is to "keep the door open," establishing future meetings so that help is available as problems escalate. In the meantime the family may benefit from counseling or referral to self-help groups such as Al-Anon (the Alcoholics Anonymous group for family members) and Alateen (for teenage children of alcoholics). The patient should be reminded that driving while intoxicated is dangerous and illegal.

THE ALCOHOL WITHDRAWAL SYNDROME   Once the brain has been repeatedly exposed to high doses of alcohol, any sudden decrease in intake can produce symptoms of withdrawal. As with all CNS depressants, the symptoms are generally the opposite of those produced by intoxication. Features include tremor of the hands (shakes or jitters); agitation and anxiety; autonomic nervous system overactivity such as an increase in pulse, respiratory rate, and body temperature; insomnia, possibly accompanied by bad dreams; and gastrointestinal upset. These withdrawal symptoms generally begin within 5 to 10 h of decreasing ethanol intake, peak in intensity on day 2 or 3, and improve by day 4 or 5. Anxiety, insomnia, and mild levels of autonomic dysfunction may persist at decreasing levels for 6 months or more as a protracted abstinence syndrome, which may contribute to the tendency to return to drinking.

At some point in their lives, between 2 and 5% of alcoholics experience withdrawal seizures ("rum fits"), usually within 48 h of stopping drinking. These are usually generalized (unless there is an underlying focal lesion), and any electroencephalographic abnormalities are mild and generally return to normal within several days.

The term *delirium tremens* (DTs) refers to delirium (mental confusion with fluctuating levels of consciousness) along with a tremor, severe agitation, and autonomic overactivity (e.g., marked increases in pulse, blood pressure, and respirations). Fortunately, this serious and potentially life-threatening complication of alcohol withdrawal is rare. Only 5 to 10% of alcohol-dependent individuals ever experience DTs; the chance of DTs during any single withdrawal is less than 1% but is higher if there has been a withdrawal seizure. DTs are most likely to develop in patients with concomitant severe medical disorders or evidence of underlying brain damage, and thus can usually be avoided if the underlying medical problems can be identified and treated.

℞ **TREATMENT**   **Acute Intoxication**   The first priority is to be certain that the vital signs are relatively stable without evidence of respiratory depression, cardiac arrhythmia, or potentially dangerous changes in blood pressure. Life-threatening problems require appropriate emergency care and hospitalization. The clinician must recognize that a variety of causes may produce obtundation or coma in the alcoholic patient. The possibility of intoxication with other drugs should be considered, and a blood or urine sample is indicated to screen for opioids or other CNS depressants such as benzodiazepines or barbiturates. A coexisting seizure disorder, head injury, meningitis, brain abscess, or other potentially life-threatening neurologic disorder may be present. Other medical conditions that must be considered include hypoglycemia, hepatic failure, or diabetic ketoacidosis.

Patients who are medically stable should be placed in a quiet environment and asked to lie on their side if fatigued in order to minimize the risk of aspiration. When the behavior indicates an increased likelihood of violence, hospital procedures should be followed, including planning for the possibility of a show of force with an intervention team. In the context of aggressiveness, patients should be clearly reminded in a nonthreatening way that it is the goal of the staff to help

them to feel better and to avoid problems. If the aggressive behavior continues, relatively low doses of a short-acting benzodiazepine such as lorazepam (e.g., 1 mg by mouth) may be used and can be repeated as needed, but care must be taken so that the addition of this second CNS depressant does not destabilize vital signs or worsen confusion. An alternative approach is to use an antipsychotic medication (e.g., 5 mg of haloperidol liquid), but this has the potential danger of lowering the seizure threshold. If aggression escalates, the patient might require a short-term admission to a locked ward, where medications can be used more safely and vital signs more closely monitored.

Withdrawal   The first, and most important, step is to perform a *thorough* physical examination in all alcoholics who are considering stopping drinking. It is necessary to evaluate organ systems likely to be impaired, including a search for evidence of liver failure, gastrointestinal bleeding, cardiac arrhythmia, and glucose or electrolyte imbalance.

The second step in treating withdrawal for even the typical well-nourished alcoholic is to give patients adequate nutrition and rest. All patients should be given oral multiple B vitamins, including 50 to 100 mg of thiamine daily for a week or more. Most patients enter withdrawal with normal levels of body water or mild overhydration, and intravenous fluids should be avoided unless there is evidence of significant recent bleeding, vomiting, or diarrhea. Medications can usually be administered orally.

The third step in treatment is to recognize that most withdrawal symptoms are caused by the rapid removal of a CNS depressant. Therefore, patients can be weaned by administering any drug of this class and gradually decreasing the levels over 3 to 5 days. While many CNS depressants are effective, the *benzodiazepines* have the highest margin of safety and are, therefore, the preferred class of drugs in the treatment of alcohol withdrawal. Benzodiazepines with short half-lives (Chap. 385) are especially useful for patients with serious liver impairment or evidence of preexisting encephalopathy or brain damage. On the other hand, short-half-life benzodiazepines, e.g., oxazepam or lorazepam, result in rapidly changing drug blood levels and must be given every 4 h to avoid abrupt fluctuations in blood levels that may increase the risk for seizures. Therefore, most clinicians use drugs with longer half-lives, such as diazepam or chlordiazepoxide. The goal is to administer enough drug on day 1 to alleviate most of the symptoms of withdrawal (e.g., the tremor and elevated pulse), and then to decrease the dose by 20% on successive days over a period of 3 to 5 days. The approach is flexible; the dose is increased if signs of withdrawal escalate, and the medication is withheld if the patient is sleeping or shows signs of increasing orthostatic hypotension. The average patient requires 25 to 50 mg of chlordiazepoxide or 10 mg of diazepam given orally every 4 to 6 h on the first day.

For the patient with DTs, treatment can be difficult and the condition is likely to run a course of 3 to 5 days regardless of the therapy employed. The focus of care is to identify medical problems and correct them and to control behavior and prevent injuries. Many clinicians recommend the use of high doses of benzodiazepine (doses as high as 800 mg/day of chlordiazepoxide have been reported), a treatment that will decrease the agitation and raise the seizure threshold but probably does little to improve the confusion. Other clinicians recommend the use of antipsychotic medications, such as 20 mg or more per day of haloperidol, an approach less likely to exacerbate confusion but which may increase the risk of seizures. Antipsychotic drugs have no place in the treatment of mild withdrawal symptoms.

Generalized withdrawal seizures rarely require aggressive pharmacologic intervention beyond that given to the usual patient undergoing withdrawal, i.e., adequate doses of benzodiazepines. There is little evidence that anticonvulsants such as phenytoin are effective in drug-withdrawal seizures, and the risk of seizures has usually passed by the time effective drug levels are reached. →*The rare patient with status epilepticus must be treated aggressively, as outlined in Chap. 361, initially with intravenous lorazepam.*

While alcohol withdrawal is often treated in a hospital, efforts at reducing costs have resulted in the development of outpatient detoxification for relatively mild abstinence syndromes. This is appropriate for patients in good physical condition who demonstrate mild signs of withdrawal despite low blood alcohol concentrations and for those without prior history of DTs or withdrawal seizures. Such individuals still require a careful physical examination, evaluation of blood tests, and vitamin supplementation. Benzodiazepines can be given *in a 1- to 2-day supply* to be administered to the patient by a spouse or other family member four times a day. Patients are asked to *return daily* for evaluation of vital signs and to come to the emergency room if signs and symptoms of withdrawal escalate.

Rehabilitation of Alcoholics   After completing alcoholic rehabilitation, 60% or more of middle-class alcoholics maintain abstinence for at least a year, and many for a lifetime. As is true for any long-term disorder for which treatment requires changes in life-style (e.g., diabetes or hypertension), therapeutic approaches include general supports that meet commonsense guidelines. Considering the lack of evidence for the superiority of any specific treatment type, it is best to keep interventions simple.

Maneuvers in rehabilitation fall into two general categories. First are attempts to help the alcoholic achieve and maintain a high level of motivation toward abstinence. These include education about alcoholism and instructing family and/or friends to stop protecting the person from the problems caused by alcohol. The second step is to help the patient to readjust to life without alcohol and to reestablish a functional lifestyle through counseling, vocational rehabilitation, and self-help groups such as Alcoholics Anonymous. The third component, called *relapse prevention*, helps the person to identify situations in which a return to drinking is likely, formulate ways of managing these risks, and develop coping strategies that increase the chances of a return to abstinence if a slip occurs.

There is no convincing evidence that inpatient rehabilitation is always more effective for the average alcoholic than is outpatient care. However, more intense interventions work better than those that are less intensive, and some alcoholics do not respond to outpatient care. The decision to hospitalize can be made if (1) the patient has medical problems that are difficult to treat outside a hospital; (2) depression, confusion, or psychosis interferes with outpatient care; (3) the patient has such a severe life crisis that it is difficult to get his or her attention as an outpatient; (4) outpatient treatment has failed; or (5) the patient lives far from the treatment center. In any setting, the best predictors of continued abstinence include evidence of higher levels of life stability (e.g., supportive family and friends) and higher levels of functioning (e.g., job skills, higher levels of education, and absence of crimes unrelated to alcohol).

Whether the treatment begins in an inpatient or an outpatient setting, subsequent outpatient contact should be maintained for a minimum of 6 months and preferably a full year after abstinence is achieved. Counseling with an individual physician or through groups focuses on day-to-day living—emphasizing areas of improved functioning in the absence of alcohol (i.e., why it is a good idea to continue to abstain) and helping the patient to manage free time without alcohol, develop a nondrinking peer group, and handle stresses on the job without alcohol.

The physician serves an important role in identifying the alcoholic, treating associated medical or psychiatric syndromes, overseeing detoxification, referring the patient to rehabilitation programs, and providing counseling. The physician is also responsible for selecting which (if any) medication might be appropriate during alcoholism rehabilitation. Patients often complain of continuing sleep problems or anxiety when acute withdrawal treatment is over, problems that may be a component of protracted withdrawal. Unfortunately, there is no place for hypnotics or antianxiety drugs in the treatment of most alcoholics after acute withdrawal has been completed. Regarding insomnia, patients should be reassured that the trouble in sleeping is normal after alcohol withdrawal and will improve over the subsequent weeks and months. They should then follow a rigid bedtime and awakening schedule and avoid any naps or the use of caffeine in the evenings. The sleep pattern will improve rapidly. Anxiety can be approached by helping the person to gain insight into the temporary nature of the symptoms and to develop strategies to achieve relaxation as well as using forms of cognitive therapy.

In addition, while the mainstay of alcoholic rehabilitation involves counseling, education, and cognitive techniques, several interesting medications are under active evaluation and might prove to be useful. The first is the opioid-antagonist drug naltrexone, which has been reported in several small-scale, short-term studies to decrease the probability of a return to drinking and to shorten periods of relapse. While this medication looks promising, longer-term large-scale trials in more diverse clinical settings will be required before the cost-effectiveness of naltrexone can be established. A second medication, acamprosate, has been tested in over 5000 patients in Europe, with results that appear similar to those reported for naltrexone. Currently, acamprosate is not available in the United States, although a long-term, trial of naltrexone, acamprosate, and their combination is in progress. A third medication, which has historically been used in the treatment of alcoholism, is the ALDH inhibitor disulfiram. Taken in doses of 250 mg/day, this drug produces an unpleasant (and potentially dangerous) reaction in the presence of alcohol, a phenomenon related to rapidly rising blood levels of the first metabolite of alcohol, acetaldehyde. However, few adequate double-blind controlled trials have demonstrated the superiority of disulfiram over placebo. Disulfiram has many side effects, and the reaction with alcohol can be dangerous, especially for patients with heart disease, stroke, diabetes mellitus, and hypertension. Thus, most clinicians reserve this medication for patients who have a clear history of longer-term abstinence associated with prior use of disulfiram and for those who might take the drug under the supervision of another individual (such as a spouse), especially during discrete periods that they have identified as representing high-risk drinking situations for them (such as the Christmas holiday).

More data are required before any medication can be recommended for routine use in alcohol rehabilitation. However, additional support for alcoholics is available through Alcoholics Anonymous in almost every community. Alcoholics Anonymous is a self-help group of recovering alcoholics (men and women who have stopped drinking, perhaps many years ago) that offers an effective model of abstinence, provides a sober peer group, and makes crisis intervention available when the urge to drink escalates. No matter what type of rehabilitation program is planned, the alcoholic should be offered the option of joining Alcoholics Anonymous.

BIBLIOGRAPHY

LIEBER C: Medical disorders of alcoholism. N Engl J Med 333:1058, 1995

PRESCOTT CA, KENDLER KS: Genetic and environmental contributions to alcohol abuse and dependence in a population-based sample of male twins. Am J Psychiatry 156:34, 1999

PROJECT MATCH RESEARCH GROUP: Matching alcoholism treatments to client heterogeneity. J Stud Alcohol 58:7, 1997

SACCO RL et al: The protective effect of moderate alcohol consumption on ischemic stroke. JAMA 281:53, 1999

SCHUCKIT MA: Biological, psychological, and environmental predictors of the alcoholism risk: A longitudinal study. J Stud Alcohol 59:485, 1998

———: *Educating Yourself About Alcohol and Drugs: A People's Primer*. New York, Plenum, 1995

——— et al: Clinical implications for four drugs of the DSM-IV distinction between substance dependence with and without a physiological component. Am J Psychiatry 156:41, 1999

———: *Drug and Alcohol Abuse: A Clinical Guide to Diagnosis and Treatment*, 5th ed. New York, Plenum, 2000

——— et al: The clinical course of alcohol-related problems in alcohol dependent and nonalcohol dependent drinking women and men. J Stud Alcohol 59:581, 1998

THUN MJ et al: Alcohol consumption and mortality among middle aged and elderly U.S. adults. N Engl J Med 337:1705, 1997

WIESE JG et al: The alcohol hangover Ann Int Med 132:897, 2000

388

OPIOID DRUG ABUSE AND DEPENDENCE

The principal effects of the opioids (opiate-like drugs) are a damping of pain perception along with modest levels of sedation and euphoria. Drugs in this category include heroin, morphine, and codeine as well as many prescription analgesics and antitussive agents. Opioid drugs are widely used in medical practice, and, thus, dependence and abuse are not limited to the classic opiod-dependent person on the street.

Tolerance to any one opioid is likely to extend to the others (i.e., cross-tolerance is likely), and all opioids are associated with a similar pattern of drug-related problems. Each is capable of producing dependence as defined in the *Fourth Diagnostic and Statistical Manual* of the American Psychiatric Association (DSM-IV), including evidence of physical dependence, a diagnosis made in the context of a history of tolerance and/or withdrawal. The abstinence syndrome from any of the substances can be treated with administration of any of the others.

PHARMACOLOGY The prototypic opiates, morphine and codeine (3-methoxymorphine), are taken directly from the milky juice of the poppy *Papaver somniferum*. The semisynthetic drugs produced from the morphine or thebane molecules include hydromorphone, diacetylmorphine (heroin), and oxycodone. The purely synthetic opioids, sharing many of the basic properties of opium and morphine, include meperidine, propoxyphene, diphenoxylate, fentanyl, buprenorphine, methadone, and pentazocine. Despite claims to the contrary, all these substances (including almost all prescription analgesics) are capable of producing euphoria as well as psychological and physical dependence when taken in high enough doses over prolonged periods.

The opioids produce their effects by binding to different types of opioid receptors throughout the body, including the central nervous system (CNS). Endogenous opioid peptides (i.e., enkephalins, endorphins, dynorphins, and others) have been identified that appear to be natural ligands for opioid receptors. These peptides have a distinct distribution in the CNS. The receptors with which opioid peptides interact are differentially engaged in production of the various opiate effects, such as analgesia, respiratory depression, constipation, and euphoria. Substances capable of antagonizing one or more of these actions include nalorphine, levallorphan, cyclazocine, butorphanol, buprenorphine, and pentazocine, each of which has mixed agonist and antagonist properties, as well as naloxone, nalmefene, and naltrexone, which are pure opiate antagonists. All antagonist drugs (including those with mixed agonist properties), can precipitate withdrawal symptoms if administered to a patient who is physically dependent on other opioids. The availability of relatively specific antagonists has helped identify different receptor subtypes, including μ receptors, which influence some of the more classic opioid actions such as pain control, reinforcement, constipation, hormone levels, and respiration; κ receptors, with possible similar functions along with sedation and effects on hormones; and δ receptors, thought to relate mostly to analgesia, mood, reinforcement, and breathing. The major features of tolerance, dependence, and withdrawal are thought to be mediated primarily by μ receptors. All opioid receptors are coupled to inhibitory G proteins, which mediate their actions within cells (Chap. 386).

Opioid drugs are absorbed from the gastrointestinal system, the lungs, and/or the muscles. The most rapid and pronounced effects occur following intravenous administration, with only slightly less efficient absorption after smoking or inhaling the vapor ("chasing the dragon"), and the least intense actions are seen after absorption from the digestive tract. Most of the metabolism of opioids occurs in the liver, primarily through conjugation with glucuronic acid, and only small amounts are excreted directly in the urine or feces. The plasma half-lives of these drugs range from 2.5 to 3 h for morphine to more than 22 h for methadone and even longer for levomethadyl acetate (LAAM).

Street heroin is typically only 5 to 10% pure. The remainder consists of materials such as lactose and fruit sugars, quinine, powdered milk, phenacetin, caffeine, antipyrine, and strychnine, which are used to "cut" the drug and increase the profit margin. Any marked, unexpected increase in the purity of street drugs is likely to cause unintentional lethal overdoses in users expecting less effect from a "hit."

THE ACUTE AND CHRONIC EFFECTS OF OPIOID DRUGS With the exception of overdose and physical dependence, most opioid effects are relatively benign and rapidly reversible. A major danger, however, comes through the use of contaminated needles by intravenous users, which increases the risk of hepatitis B and C, bacterial endocarditis, and infection with HIV (Chap. 309).

Effects on Body Systems Acute changes in the *gastrointestinal system* are the result of decreased motility with resulting constipation and anorexia. Chronic gastrointestinal problems in opioid-dependent individuals typically occur as a consequence of hepatitis in injection drug users.

Effects of opiods in the CNS include intoxication-induced nausea and vomiting (medulla), decreased pain perception (spinal cord, thalamus, and periaqueductal gray region), euphoria (limbic system), and sedation (reticular activating system). The adulterants added to street drugs may contribute to some of the more permanent nervous system damage, including peripheral neuropathy, amblyopia, myelopathy, and leukoencephalopathy. One study revealed abnormalities in cognitive function and brain computed tomography scans of opioid-dependent subjects; whether these abnormalities are due to the opioid itself, the adulterants, the consequences of dirty needles, or an unhealthy lifestyle is unknown. Acute opioid administration decreases levels of luteinizing hormone, with a subsequent reduction in testosterone, which might contribute to the decreased sex drive reported by most opioid-dependent people. Other hormonal changes include a decrease in the release of thyrotropin and increases in prolactin and possibly growth hormone (Chap. 328).

Acute changes in the *respiratory system* include respiratory depression, which results from a decreased response of the brainstem to carbon dioxide tension, a component of the drug overdose syndrome described below. At even low drug doses, this effect can be clinically significant in individuals with underlying pulmonary disease. *Cardiovascular* changes tend to be relatively mild, with no direct opiate effect on heart rhythm or myocardial contractility, but there is a potential problem from orthostatic hypotension, probably secondary to dilation of peripheral vessels. Bacterial infections of the lungs and heart valves can occur from contaminated needles; the latter can result in emboli and thus an increased risk for stroke.

The Toxic Reaction or Overdose Syndrome High doses of opioids can result in a potentially lethal toxic reaction or overdose syndrome. While toxic reactions are seen with all opioids, the more potent drugs such as fentanyl (80 to 100 times more powerful than morphine) are especially dangerous. The typical syndrome, which occurs immediately with intravenous overdose, includes shallow respirations at a rate of two to four per minute, pupillary miosis (with mydriasis once brain anoxia develops), bradycardia, a decrease in body temperature, and a general absence of responsiveness to external stimulation. If this medical emergency is not treated rapidly, respiratory depression, cyanosis, cardiorespiratory arrest, and death can ensue. Postmortem examination reveals few specific changes except for diffuse cerebral edema. An "allergic-like" reaction to intravenous heroin, perhaps in part related to adulterants, can also occur and is characterized by decreased alertness, a frothy pulmonary edema, and an elevation in the blood eosinophil count.

The first step in managing overdose is to provide any needed respiratory or cardiovascular support including intubation for airway protection if needed. Definitive treatment for the typical opioid overdose is the administration of a narcotic antagonist such as naloxone in an initial dose of 0.4 mg to 2 mg intravenously, expecting a response in 1 to 2 min. This dose can be repeated every 2 to 3 min up to a dose of 10 mg. With the exception of overdoses with buprenorphine, if no response is seen after 10 mg, it is unlikely that an opioid overdose is responsible for the respiratory depression or coma. If an intravenous line is not available, the drug can be given intramuscularly. It is important to titrate the dose relative to the patient's symptoms. The goal is to ameliorate the respiratory depression but not provoke a severe withdrawal state. Because the effects of this drug diminish within 2 to 3 h, the individual must be monitored for at least 24 h after a heroin overdose and 72 h after an overdose of a longer-acting drug such as methadone. If there is little response to naloxone alone, the possibility of a concomitant overdose with a benzodiazepine should be considered and a challenge with intravenous flumazenil, 0.2 mg/min up to a maximum of 3 mg in an hour, might be used. Patients who are physically dependent on an opioid may experience a precipitous onset of an abstinence syndrome after administration of the opioid antagonist, but aggressive treatment of this syndrome is not appropriate until all vital signs are relatively stable.

As with any drug overdose, treatment of either the typical or the "allergic" type of opioid toxic reaction often requires continued supportive care until the drug effect subsides. Patients may require respiratory support (often with oxygen supplementation and positive-pressure breathing for the "allergic" type of overdose), intravenous fluids perhaps accompanied by pressor agents to support blood pressure, and gastric lavage to remove any remaining drug with care taken to use a cuffed endotracheal tube to prevent aspiration if the patient is not alert. It is important to evaluate and treat any possible anaphylactic reactions. Cardiac arrhythmias and/or convulsions, especially likely to be seen with codeine, propoxyphene, or meperidine, also need to be treated.

OPIOID ABUSE AND DEPENDENCE   **Definition and Epidemiology**   Repeated opioid use to the point of developing multiple problems is a good indicator that future abuse and dependence are likely. DSM-IV criteria for opioid dependence are the same as those for alcohol dependence (Chap. 387). An individual is dependent if within a 12-month period repeated difficulties occur in any three areas of functioning, including tolerance, withdrawal, use of greater amounts of opiates than intended, and use despite consequences. Patients who do not have dependence but demonstrate repeated difficulties with the law, impaired ability to meet obligations, use in hazardous situations, or continued use despite problems can be labeled as having abuse.

The use of opioids for intoxication is less prevalent than the use of alcohol, marijuana, and several other drugs. A 1997 national survey reported that almost 5% of men and women age 12 or above in the United States had used an opioid for intoxication, including almost 2% in the prior year and slightly less than 1% in the prior month. Focusing specifically on heroin, the lifetime prevalence was approximately 1%, with 0.3% having taken the drug in the prior year. Use patterns of these drugs were almost twice as high in another 1997 survey sampling 12th graders in high school. In all studies, prevalence rates were higher in males than females. None of the national surveys offered data regarding the prevalence of dependence.

Genetics   While most data on the importance of genetic influences in substance use disorders apply to alcoholism, there are interesting findings regarding other drugs. One large study of over 3000 male twin pairs reported that there are genetic influences that relate uniquely to heroin dependence and also noted additional genetic factors related to an overall vulnerability toward substance-related problems. The genetic influences operate in the context of additional environmental factors that are likely to relate both to the family of upbringing and the general environment. Genetic factors might influence personality characteristics such as impulsivity and sensation-seeking or susceptibility to develop antisocial personality disorder. Genes relating to the actions of the drug on specific neurochemical systems such as dopamine are also potential candidates for an enhanced vulnerability toward developing opioid dependence.

Natural History   Dependence on or abuse of opioids can be seen in at least three types of patients. First, a minority of people with nonfatal *chronic pain syndromes* (e.g., back, joint, and muscle disorders) misuse their prescribed drugs. If physical dependence is established, abstinence syndromes can then intensify the pain, promoting continued drug intake. Physicians can avoid contributing to physical dependence by helping the patient to accept the goal of minimization rather than disappearance of the pain and to recognize that discomfort may not be completely eliminated (Chap. 12). Analgesic medication should be only one component of treatment and limited to the oral administration of the least potent analgesic that is able to "take the edge off" the pain (e.g., ibuprofen or, if needed, propoxyphene). Behavior modification techniques, such as muscle relaxation and meditation, and carefully selected exercises should be used as appropriate to help increase function and decrease pain. Finally, nonmedicinal approaches, including electrical transcutaneous neurostimulation for muscle and joint disease, may be useful.

The second group at high risk are *physicians, nurses,* and *pharmacists,* primarily because of their easy access to substances of abuse. Physicians may begin to use opioids to help them sleep or to reduce stress or physical aches and pains. This group appears to be at especially high risk for developing dependence on the highly potent drugs such as fentanyl. Because of the growing awareness of these problems, impaired-physician programs have been established in many hospitals and by most state medical societies. Such groups attempt to identify and aid substance-impaired physicians, giving them peer support and education to help them achieve abstinence before problems escalate to the point of licensure revocation. All doctors are advised never to prescribe opioids for themselves or for members of their family—physicians deserve the same level of care and protection from future problems as their patients.

The third and most obvious group are those who buy street drugs to get high. While some of these men and women have prior histories of severe antisocial problems, most have a relatively high level of premorbid functioning. The typical person begins using opioids occasionally, often after experimenting with tobacco, then alcohol, then marijuana, and then brain depressants or stimulants. Occasional opiate use, or "chipping," might continue for some time, and some individuals never escalate their intake to the point of developing dependence.

Of course, opiate-dependent individuals are likely to continue to have experience with many other drugs. At least three of these often remain as problems during the course of opioid dependence. First, alcohol is typically used to moderate withdrawal problems, to enhance the opioid high, and as a substitute when the preferred drug is not readily available, including during methadone and other treatments. This pattern of problematic drinking, often meeting criteria for alcohol dependence, is present at some time in approximately half of opioid-dependent persons. The second drug, cocaine, appears to be taken for many of the same reasons as alcohol, and is often administered intravenously with the opioid in a mixture known as a "speedball." The third class of drugs misused in combination with opioids consists of the benzodiazepines, especially among people in methadone maintenance.

Once persistent opioid use is established, severe problems are likely to develop. At least 25% die within 10 to 20 years from suicide, homicide, accidents, or infectious diseases such as tuberculosis, hepatitis, or AIDS. The mortality rate has escalated in recent years in response to the AIDS epidemic among injection drug users, with an estimated 60% of these men and women carrying HIV (Chap. 309). At the same time, while the majority of opioid-dependent persons show frequent exacerbations and remissions, it is important to remember that approximately 35% achieve long-term, often permanent, abstinence. This remission is probably most often seen after the age of 40 but can occur at any point in the clinical course. While this favorable outcome can be observed in any opioid-dependent person, as is true with most drugs of abuse a better prognosis is associated with prior histories of marital and employment stability and fewer criminal activities unrelated to drugs.

℞ **TREATMENT**   The key to diagnosis is to discard the erroneous stereotype that opioid-dependent men and women are always unemployed and homeless. Abuse or dependence is possible in any patient who demonstrates symptoms of what might be opioid withdrawal; anyone who has a chronic pain syndrome; physicians, nurses, and pharmacists or others with easy access to opioids; and all patients who repeatedly seek out prescription analgesics. Therefore, it is important to take the time with *every* patient, especially those with complaints of pain, to gather a history that includes the patterns of opioid use and the list of doctors and clinics from which they have received prescriptions. If the chronic use of opioids is suspected, gathering further data from an additional informant such as a relative or close friend can be essential. Another indicator of an enhanced risk for opioid dependence is a history of pervasive antisocial problems beginning in the preteen years. Blood and urine screens can be used to identify opioids in patients in whom misuse is suspected, and clinicians should search for physical stigmata of misuse (e.g., needle marks).

After identifying opioid dependence, the next step is intervention. The need for active treatment of the abstinence syndrome can be presented, and the availability of help in establishing a drug-free life-style can be emphasized. The final decision, of course, rests with the patient. This approach to intervention is presented in relation to alcoholism in Chap. 387.

The Symptoms of Withdrawal   Withdrawal symptoms, usually the opposite of the acute effects of the drug, include nausea and diarrhea, coughing, lacrimation, mydriasis, rhinorrhea, profuse sweating, twitching muscles, piloerection (or "goose bumps") as well as mild elevations in body temperature, respiratory rate, and blood pressure. In addition, diffuse body pain, insomnia, and yawning occur, along with intense drug craving. Drugs with a short half-life, such as morphine or heroin, cause symptoms typically within 8 to 16 h of the last dose (thus, many dependent individuals awake in mild withdrawal every morning); symptom intensity peaks within 36 to 72 h after discontinuation of the drug, and the acute syndrome disappears within 5 to 8 days. However, a protracted abstinence phase of mild symptoms (e.g., moodiness, slight changes in pupillary size, autonomic dysfunction, changes in sleep pattern) may persist for 6 or more months. These lingering symptoms, which can be relieved by administering an opioid, probably contribute to relapse.

Treatment of the Withdrawal Syndrome   A thorough physical examination, including an assessment of neurologic function and a search for local and systemic infections, especially abscesses, is mandatory. Laboratory testing generally includes assessment of liver function and, in intravenous users, HIV status. Proper nutrition and rest must be initiated as soon as possible.

Optimal treatment of withdrawal requires administration of sufficient opioid medication on day 1 to decrease symptoms, followed by a more gradual withdrawal of the drug, usually over 5 to 10 days. Any opioid will work (all have some level of cross-tolerance), but for ease of administration, many physicians prefer to use a long-acting drug such as methadone. To estimate the first day's dose from the patient's history, 1 to 2 mg of methadone can be considered approximately equivalent to 3 mg of morphine, 1 mg of heroin, or 20 mg of meperidine. Most patients require between 10 and 25 mg of methadone orally twice on day 1, with higher doses given if prominent symptoms of withdrawal are not dampened. After several days of a stabilized drug dose, the opioid is then decreased by 10 to 20% of the original day's dose each day.

However, most states restrict the prescription of opioids to dependent persons, and, in the absence of special permits, detoxification with opioids is often proscribed or limited. Thus, pharmacologic treatments often center on relief of symptoms of diarrhea with Imodium or a nonopioid drug, of "sniffles" with decongestants, and pain with nonopioid analgesics (e.g., ibuprofen). Comfort can be enhanced with the α_2-adrenergic agonist clonidine to decrease sympathetic nervous system overactivity. Given at doses of approximately 5 μg/kg (up to 0.3 mg given two to four times a day), clonidine decreases autonomic nervous system dysfunction and produces sedation. Blood pressure should be monitored closely. Some clinicians augment this regimen with low to moderate doses of benzodiazepines for 2 to 5 days to decrease agitation.

A special case of opioid withdrawal is seen in the newborn made passively dependent through the mother's drug abuse during pregnancy. Some level of withdrawal develops in 50 to 90% of children of heroin-dependent mothers. As few as 25% of infants of methadone-maintenance mothers show clinically relevant withdrawal symptoms, probably because of the longer half-life of this drug. The syndrome consists of irritability, crying, a tremor (in 80%), increased reflexes, increased respiratory rate, diarrhea, hyperactivity (in 60%), vomiting (40%), and sneezing/yawning/hiccuping (in 30%). The child usually has a low birth weight but may be otherwise unremarkable until the second day, when symptoms are likely to begin.

The treatment follows the same general steps used in the treatment of the physically dependent adult. The child must be carefully evaluated to rule out medical problems such as hypoglycemia, hypocalcemia, infections, and trauma; general support in a warm, quiet environment and regulation of electrolytes and glucose are also required. The infant with moderate to severe symptoms can be treated with any of the following: paregoric (0.2 mL orally every 3 to 4 h), methadone (0.1 to 0.5 mg/kg per day), phenobarbital (8 mg/kg per day), or diazepam (1 to 2 mg/kg every 8 h). Medication should be given in decreasing levels for 10 to 20 days. Dependent infants of mothers on methadone maintenance also benefit by breast feeding while the mother continues to take methadone.

Rehabilitation of Opioid-Dependent Persons   Despite some differences in demographics, the same general rules for rehabilitation apply to opioid-dependent persons as to alcoholics. The basic strategy includes detoxification and family support, and the process can benefit from the use of reading materials or referral to self-help groups. It is also important to establish realistic patient goals and a program of counseling and education to increase motivation toward abstinence. A long-term commitment to rebuilding a life-style without the substance is essential for preventing recidivism.

Most rehabilitation approaches have common elements, regardless of the drug involved. Patients are educated about their responsibility for improving their lives, and *motivation for abstinence* is increased by providing information about the medical and psychological problems that can be expected if dependence continues. Patients and families are encouraged to *establish an opioid-free life-style* by learning to cope with chronic pain and develop realistic vocational planning (e.g., for pharmacists, physicians, and nurses). The dependent person is also encouraged to establish a drug-free peer group and to participate in self-help groups such as Narcotics Anonymous. Another important treatment component is *relapse prevention* aimed at identifying triggers for a return to drugs and developing appropriate coping strategies.

Much of this advice and counseling can be given by the physician, but many clinicians refer patients to more formal drug programs, including methadone maintenance clinics, programs using narcotic antagonists, and therapeutic communities. Long-term follow-up of treated patients indicates that approximately one-third were completely drug free in the previous year; 60% were no longer using opioids, although some were misusing other substances. Individuals who stay in methadone maintenance or in therapeutic communities show significant improvement in antisocial behavior and employment status. In general, the best prognosis is for those individuals who are employed, who have higher levels of education, and who remain in treatment for at least 2 months. Dependence among health care providers, such as physicians, is treated similarly, but in addition a closely supervised "diversion" procedure is usually instituted and carried out for 1 to 2 years or more.

Methadone maintenance   Maintenance programs with methadone and the even longer-acting agent LAAM should only be used in combination with education and counseling. It is important to note that drug maintenance is not aimed at "curing" opioid dependence; rather, it provides a substitute drug that is legally accessible, safer, can be taken orally, and has a long half-life so that it can be taken once a day. The goal is to help persons who have repeatedly failed in drug-free programs to improve functioning within the family and job, to decrease legal problems, and to improve health.

Methadone is a long-acting opioid that possesses almost all the physiologic properties of heroin. The recipient, who has been carefully screened to rule out prior psychiatric disorders, may be maintained on a relatively low dose (e.g., 30 to 40 mg/d); a better approach is to use a higher dose (80 to 120 mg/d), because it may be more effective in blocking heroin-induced euphoria and decreasing craving. There is some evidence that the higher methadone doses result in greater retention in treatment and consequently in lower levels of arrest and relapse to street drugs. Three-quarters or more of patients, especially those receiving the higher doses, are likely to remain heroin-free for 6 months or longer. Methadone is administered as an oral liquid given once a day at the program, with weekend doses taken by the patient at home. The longer-acting analogues, such as LAAM, can be given two or three times a week, with the dose of LAAM increased to as high as 80 mg three times a week if needed. After a period of maintenance (usually 6 months to 1 year or longer), the clinician can work closely with the patient to regulate the rate of drug decrease (by about 5% per week) if possible.

In the past, the British have used heroin maintenance with goals and guidelines similar to those of current methadone programs. There is no evidence that heroin maintenance has any advantages over methadone maintenance, but the heroin approach does add the risk that the drug will be easily sold on the streets. Treatment with mixed agonists-antagonists such as buprenorphine also appears beneficial, although results are not as good as with methadone.

Opioid antagonists   The opiate antagonists (e.g., naloxone) compete with heroin and other opioids for receptors, reducing the effects of the opioid agonists. Administered over long periods with the intention of blocking the "high" produced if the patient takes opioids, these drugs can be useful as part of an overall treatment approach that includes counseling and support. The most widely used antagonist in rehabilitation is naltrexone; 50 mg per day antagonizes 15 mg of heroin for 24 h, and higher doses (125 to 150 mg) block the effects of 25 mg of intravenous heroin for up to 3 days. Naltrexone is free of agonist properties, produces no known withdrawal symptoms when stopped, and its side effects tend to be mild. To avoid precipitating a withdrawal syndrome, patients should be free of opioids for a minimum of 5 days before beginning treatment with this medication. In addition, they should first be challenged with 0.4 or 0.8 mg of the shorter-acting agent naloxone to be certain they are able to tolerate the long-acting antagonist. Following this procedure, a test dose of 10 mg of naltrexone can be given, with the expectation that any withdrawal symptoms will be seen in 0.5 to 2 h. Several variations of this approach can be used with detoxification from methadone maintenance, including a fairly rapid, medically supervised plan. Over a 10-day period, the daily dose should be increased to about 100 mg on Mondays and Wednesdays and 150 mg on Fridays. Unfortunately, despite the apparent advantages of this treatment approach, some patients are resistant to continuing care. In one study, only about 60% of the patients completed 6 days of naltrexone induction, and only 10% remained in the program at the end of 6 months. However, another study reported much higher rates of compliance, with almost a third achieving continuous abstinence for at least a year.

Drug-free programs   Most existing halfway houses and recovery centers for opioid-dependent persons use some variant of the therapeutic community approach. This is an exception to the general preference for short-term residential (as opposed to outpatient) rehabilitation, since care can last a year or more while the person is taken out of the street culture and given a new life within the group. In this structure, members, including leaders who are themselves in the process of recovery, help participants gain insights into more successful strategies for coping with problems.

As is true for treatments of all substance-use disorders, it is likely that counseling, behavioral treatments, and relatively simple approaches to psychotherapy add significantly to a positive outcome. Most approaches focus on teaching participants to cope with stress, enhancing their understanding of personality attributes, teaching better cognitive styles, and, through the process of relapse prevention, addressing issues that might contribute to increased craving, easy access to drugs, or periods of decreased motivation. A combination of these therapies with the approaches described above appears to give the best results.

Finally, it is important to discuss prevention. Except for the terminally ill, physicians should carefully monitor opioid drug use in their patients, keeping doses as low as is practical and administering them over as short a period as the level of pain would warrant in the average person. Physicians must be vigilant regarding their own risk for opioid abuse and dependence, *never* prescribing these drugs for themselves. For the nonmedical intravenous drug–dependent person, all possible efforts must be made to prevent AIDS, hepatitis, bacterial endocarditis, and other consequences of contaminated needles both through methadone maintenance and by considering needle-exchange programs.

BIBLIOGRAPHY

AHMED SH, KOOB GF: Transition from moderate to excessive drug intake: Change in hedonic set point. Science 282:298, 1998

AMERICAN PSYCHIATRIC ASSOCIATION: Practical guidelines for the treatment of substance use disorders. Am J Psychiatry 52(Suppl):1, 1995

BALL J, ROSS A: *The Effectiveness of Methadone Maintenance Treatments.* New York, Springer-Verlag, 1991

CORNISH JW et al: Naltrexone pharmacotherapy for opioid dependent federal probationers. J Subst Abuse Treat 14:529, 1997

GOLDMAN D, BERGEN A: General and specific inheritance of substance abuse and alcoholism. Arch Gen Psychiatry 55:964, 1998

JONES JE et al: Induction with levomethadyl acetate. Arch Gen Psychiatry 55:729, 1998

KLEE H, MORRIS J: The role of needle exchanges in modifying sharing behavior: Cross-study comparisons 1989–1993. Addiction 90:1635, 1995

MAGURA S et al: Pre- and in-treatment predictors of retention in methadone treatment using survival analysis. Addiction 93:51, 1998

MANFREDINI R et al: Emergency admissions of opioid drug abusers for overdose: A chronobiological study of enhanced risk. Ann Emerg Med 24:615, 1994

MORRISON J, WICKERSHAM P: Physicians disciplined by a state medical board. JAMA 279:1889, 1998

SCHOTTENFELD RS et al: Buprenorphine vs methadone maintenance treatment for concurrent opioid dependence and cocaine abuse. Arch Gen Psychiatry 54:713, 1997

SCHUCKIT MA: *Educating Yourself about Alcohol and Drugs: A People's Primer.* New York, Plenum, 1998

————: *Drug and Alcohol Abuse: A Clinical Guide to Diagnosis and Treatment,* 5th ed. New York, Plenum, 2000

———— et al: Clinical implications for four drugs of the DSM-IV distinction between substance dependence with and without a physiological component. Am J Psychiatry 156:41, 1999

SEES KL et al: Methadone maintenance vs 180-day psychosocially enriched detoxification for treatment of opioid dependence. A randomized controlled trial. JAMA 283:1303, 2000

TSUANG MT et al: Co-occurrence of abuse of different drugs in men: The role of drug-specific and shared vulnerabilities. Arch Gen Psychiatry 55:967, 1998

389   *Jack H. Mendelson, Nancy K. Mello*

COCAINE AND OTHER COMMONLY ABUSED DRUGS

The abuse of cocaine and other psychostimulant drugs appears to be increasing in many metropolitan and rural areas throughout the world, according to a year 2000 report by the National Institute on Drug Abuse (NIDA). The number of deaths associated with these drugs has also increased. In several urban areas of the United States, use of these drugs has increased more sharply among women than men. Although enhanced legal enforcement as well as educational prevention procedures have attenuated, in part, the increase in psychostimulant abuse among youths in the United States, there appears to be an enhanced worldwide risk for psychostimulant abuse and dependence.

The initiation and continuation of drug abuse are determined by a complex interaction of the pharmacologic properties and relative availability of each drug, the personality and expectations of the user, and the environmental context in which the drug is used. Polydrug abuse, the concurrent use of several drugs with different pharmacologic effects, is increasingly common among individuals from all socioeconomic strata. There has been an alarming increase in particularly dangerous forms of polydrug abuse, such as the combined use of heroin and cocaine intravenously. There is no simple explanation for this change in polydrug use patterns. Drug abusers may attempt to attenuate one drug effect with another, as when heroin or alcohol is used to modulate the cocaine high. Sometimes one drug is used to enhance the effects of another, as with benzodiazepines and methadone, or cocaine plus heroin in methadone-maintained patients.

Chronic cocaine and psychostimulant abuse may cause a number of adverse health consequences, ranging from pulmonary disease to reproductive dysfunction. Preexisting disorders such as hypertension and cardiac disease may be exacerbated by drug abuse, and the combined use of two or more drugs may accentuate medical complications associated with abuse of one of them. The adverse health consequences of drug abuse are further complicated by AIDS.

Drug abuse increases the risk of exposure to HIV. Cocaine and psychostimulant abuse contribute to the risk for HIV infection in part by the adverse immunomodulatory effects of these drugs. In addition, concurrent use of cocaine and opiates (the "speedball") is frequently associated with needle-sharing by intravenous drug users. These individuals continue to represent the largest single group of persons with HIV infection in several major metropolitan areas in the United States as well as in urban areas in Scotland, Italy, Spain, Thailand, and China.

COCAINE Cocaine is a stimulant and local anesthetic with potent vasoconstrictor properties. The leaves of the coca plant (*Erythroxylon coca*) contain approximately 0.5 to 1% cocaine. The drug produces physiologic and behavioral effects when administered orally, intranasally (snorting), intravenously, or via inhalation following pyrolysis (smoking). Cocaine increases synaptic concentrations of the monoamine neurotransmitters dopamine, norepinephrine, and serotonin by binding to transporter proteins in presynaptic neurons and blocking reuptake. The reinforcing effects of cocaine are related to effects on dopaminergic neurons in the mesolimbic system (Chap. 386).

Prevalence of Cocaine Use Cocaine has become widely available throughout the United States, and cocaine abuse occurs in virtually all social and economic strata of society. The prevalence of cocaine abuse in the general population has been accompanied by an increase in cocaine abuse by heroin-dependent persons, including those in methadone maintenance programs. Intravenous cocaine is often used concurrently with intravenous heroin—a combination that purportedly attenuates the postcocaine "crash" and substitutes a cocaine "high" for the heroin "high" blocked by methadone.

Acute and Chronic Cocaine Intoxication There has been an increase in both intravenous administration and inhalation of pyrolyzed cocaine via smoking. Following intranasal administration, changes in mood and sensation are perceived within 3 to 5 min, and peak effects occur at 10 to 20 min. The effects rarely last >1 h. Inhalation of pyrolyzed materials includes inhaling crack/cocaine or smoking coca paste, a product made by extracting cocaine preparations with flammable solvents, and cocaine free-base smoking. Free-base cocaine, including the free base prepared with sodium bicarbonate (crack), is becoming increasingly popular because of the relative high potency of the compound and its rapid onset of action (8 to 10 s following smoking).

Cocaine produces a brief, dose-related stimulation and enhancement of mood and an increase in cardiac rate and blood pressure. Body temperature usually increases, and high doses of cocaine may induce

lethal pyrexia or hypertension. Because cocaine inhibits reuptake of catecholamines at adrenergic nerve endings, the drug potentiates sympathetic nervous system activity. Cocaine has a short plasma half-life of approximately 45 to 60 min. Cocaine is metabolized primarily by plasma esterases, and cocaine metabolites are excreted in urine. The very short duration of euphorigenic effects of cocaine observed in chronic abusers is probably due to both acute and chronic tolerance. Frequent self-administration of the drug (two to three times per hour) is often reported by chronic cocaine abusers. Alcohol is used to modulate both the cocaine high and the dysphoria associated with the abrupt disappearance of cocaine's effects. A metabolite of cocaine, cocaethylene, has been detected in blood and urine of persons who concurrently abuse alcohol and cocaine. Cocaethylene induces changes in cardiovascular function similar to those of cocaine alone, and the pathophysiologic consequences of alcohol abuse plus cocaine abuse may be additive when both are used together.

The prevalent assumption that cocaine inhalation or intravenous administration is relatively safe is contradicted by reports of death from respiratory depression, cardiac arrhythmias, and convulsions associated with cocaine use. In addition to generalized seizures, neurologic complications may include headache, ischemic or hemorrhagic stroke, or subarachnoid hemorrhage. Disorders of cerebral blood flow and perfusion in cocaine-dependent persons have been detected with magnetic resonance spectroscopy (MRS) studies. Severe pulmonary disease may develop in individuals who inhale crack cocaine; this effect is attributed both to the direct effects of cocaine and to residual contaminants in the smoked material. Hepatic necrosis has been reported to occur following crack cocaine use.

Although men and women who abuse cocaine may report that the drug enhances libidinal drive, chronic cocaine use causes significant loss of libido and adversely affects reproductive function. Impotence and gynecomastia have been observed in male cocaine abusers, and these abnormalities often persist for long periods following cessation of drug use. Women who abuse cocaine have reported major derangements in menstrual cycle function including galactorrhea, amenorrhea, and infertility. Chronic cocaine abuse may cause persistent hyperprolactinemia as a consequence of disordered dopaminergic inhibition of prolactin secretion by the pituitary. Cocaine abuse by pregnant women, particularly the smoking of crack, has been associated with both an increased risk of congenital malformations in the fetus and perinatal cardiovascular and cerebrovascular disease in the mother. However, cocaine abuse per se is probably not the sole cause of these perinatal disorders, since many problems associated with maternal cocaine abuse, including poor nutrition and health care status as well as polydrug abuse, also contribute to risk for perinatal disease.

Protracted cocaine abuse may cause paranoid ideation and visual and auditory hallucinations, a state that resembles alcoholic hallucinosis. Psychological dependence on cocaine, as manifested by inability to abstain from frequent compulsive use, has also been reported. Although the occurrence of withdrawal syndromes involving psychomotor agitation and autonomic hyperactivity remains controversial, severe depression ("crashing") following cocaine intoxication may accompany drug withdrawal.

℞ TREATMENT Treatment of cocaine overdose is a medical emergency that is often best managed in an intensive care unit. Cocaine toxicity produces a hyperadrenergic state characterized by hypertension, tachycardia, tonic-clonic seizures, dyspnea, and ventricular arrhythmias. Intravenous diazepam in doses up to 0.5 mg/kg administered over an 8-h period has been shown to be effective for control of seizures. Ventricular arrhythmias have been managed successfully by administration of 0.5 to 1.0 mg of propranolol intravenously. Since many instances of cocaine-related mortality have been associated with concurrent use of other illicit drugs (particularly heroin), the physician must be prepared to institute effective emergency treatment for multiple drug toxicities.

Treatment of chronic cocaine abuse requires combined efforts by primary care physicians, psychiatrists, and psychosocial care providers. Early abstinence from cocaine use is often complicated by symptoms of depression and guilt, insomnia, and anorexia, which may be as severe as those observed in major affective disorders. Individual and group psychotherapy, family therapy, and peer group assistance programs are often useful for inducing prolonged remission from drug use. A number of medications used for the treatment of various psychiatric disorders have been administered to reduce the duration and severity of cocaine abuse and dependence. However, no available medication is both safe and highly effective for either cocaine detoxification or maintenance of abstinence. Some psychotherapeutic interventions are occasionally effective; however, no specific form of psychotherapy or behavioral modification is uniquely beneficial.

MARIJUANA AND CANNABIS COMPOUNDS

Cannabis sativa contains >400 compounds in addition to the psychoactive substance, delta-9-tetrahydrocannabinol (THC). Marijuana cigarettes are prepared from the leaves and flowering tops of the plant, and a typical marijuana cigarette contains 0.5 to 1 g of plant material. Although the usual THC concentration varies between 10 and 40 mg, concentrations >100 mg per cigarette have been detected. Hashish is prepared from concentrated resin of *C. sativa* and contains a THC concentration of between 8 to 12% by weight. "Hash oil," a lipid-soluble plant extract, may contain a THC concentration of 25 to 60% and may be added to marijuana or hashish to enhance its THC concentration. Smoking is the most common mode of marijuana or hashish use. During pyrolysis, >150 compounds in addition to THC are released in the smoke. Although most of these compounds do not have psychoactive properties, they do have potential physiologic effects.

THC is quickly absorbed from the lungs into blood and is then rapidly sequestered in tissues. It is metabolized primarily in the liver, where it is converted to 11-hydroxy-THC, a psychoactive compound, and >20 other metabolites. Many THC metabolites are excreted through the feces at a rate of clearance that is relatively slow in comparison to that of most other psychoactive drugs.

Specific cannabinoid receptors (CB_1 and CB_2) have been identified in the central nervous system, including the spinal cord, and in the peripheral nervous system. High densities of these receptors have been found in the cerebral cortex, basal ganglia, and hippocampus. B lymphocytes also appear to have cannabinoid receptors. A naturally occurring THC-like ligand has been identified in the nervous system, where it is widely distributed.

Prevalence of Marijuana Use Marijuana is the most commonly used illegal drug in the United States. Use is particularly prevalent among adolescents; studies suggest that ~40% of high school students in the United States have used marijuana. Marijuana is relatively inexpensive and is considered by many persons to be less hazardous than the use of other controlled drugs and substances. Very potent forms of marijuana (sinsemilla) are now available in many communities, and concurrent use of marijuana with crack/cocaine and phencyclidine is increasing. Marijuana abuse by individuals from all social strata has been increasing.

Acute and Chronic Marijuana Intoxication Acute intoxication from marijuana and cannabis compounds is related to both the dose of THC and the route of administration. THC is absorbed more rapidly from marijuana smoking than from orally ingested cannabis compounds. Acute marijuana intoxication usually consists of a subjective perception of relaxation and mild euphoria resembling mild to moderate alcohol intoxication. This condition is usually accompanied by some impairment in thinking, concentration, and perceptual and psychomotor function. Higher doses of cannabis may produce behavioral effects analogous to severe alcohol intoxication. Although the effects of acute marijuana intoxication are relatively benign in normal users, the drug can precipitate severe emotional disorders in individuals who have antecedent psychotic or neurotic problems. As with other psychoactive compounds, both set (user's expectations) and setting (environmental context) are important determinants of the type and severity of behavioral intoxication.

As is true of alcoholics, chronic marijuana abusers may lose interest in common socially desirable goals and steadily devote more time to drug acquisition and use. However, THC does not cause a specific and unique "amotivational syndrome." The range of symptoms sometimes attributed to marijuana use is difficult to distinguish from mild to moderate depression and the maturational dysfunctions often associated with protracted adolescence. Chronic marijuana use has also been reported to increase the risk of psychotic symptoms in individuals with a past history of schizophrenia.

Physical Effects of Marijuana Conjunctival injection and tachycardia are the most frequent immediate physical concomitants of smoking marijuana. Tolerance for marijuana-induced tachycardia develops rapidly among regular users; angina may be precipitated by marijuana smoking in persons with a history of coronary insufficiency. Exercise-induced angina may be increased after marijuana use to a greater extent than after tobacco cigarette smoking. Patients with cardiac disease should be strongly advised not to use cannabis compounds.

Significant decrements in pulmonary vital capacity have been found in regular daily marijuana smokers. Because marijuana smoking typically involves deep inhalation and prolonged retention of marijuana smoke, marijuana smokers may develop chronic bronchial irritation. Impairment of single-breath carbon monoxide diffusion capacity (DL_{co}) is greater in persons who smoke both marijuana and tobacco than in tobacco smokers. Despite the well-documented association between tobacco smoking and lung cancer, at present there is no direct evidence that marijuana smoking induces lung cancer. However, heavy marijuana use among Americans may be too recent to permit detection of this problem.

Although marijuana has also been associated with adverse effects on a number of other systems, many of these studies await replication and confirmation. A reported correlation between marijuana use and decreased testosterone levels in males has not been confirmed. Decreased sperm count and sperm motility and morphologic abnormalities of spermatozoa following marijuana use have also been reported. Administration of high doses of marijuana to female rhesus monkeys suppresses pituitary gonadotropins and gonadal steroids. Prospective studies demonstrated a correlation between impaired fetal growth and development and heavy marijuana use during pregnancy. Marijuana has also been implicated in derangements of the immune system; in chromosomal abnormalities; and in inhibition of DNA, RNA, and protein synthesis; however, these findings have not been confirmed or related to any specific physiologic effect in humans.

Tolerance and Physical Dependence Habitual marijuana users rapidly develop tolerance to the psychoactive effects of marijuana and often smoke more frequently and try to secure more potent cannabis compounds. Tolerance for the physiologic effects of marijuana develops at different rates; e.g., tolerance develops rapidly for marijuana-induced tachycardia but more slowly for marijuana-induced conjunctival injection. Tolerance to both behavioral and physiologic effects of marijuana decreases rapidly upon cessation of marijuana use.

Withdrawal signs and symptoms have been reported in chronic cannabis users, with the severity of symptoms related to dosage and duration of use. These include tremor, nystagmus, sweating, nausea, vomiting, diarrhea, irritability, anorexia, and sleep disturbances. Withdrawal signs and symptoms observed in chronic marijuana users are usually relatively mild in comparison to those observed in heavy opiate or alcohol users and rarely require medical or pharmacologic intervention. More severe and protracted abstinence syndromes may occur after sustained use of high potency cannabis compounds.

Therapeutic Use of Marijuana Marijuana, administered as cigarettes or as a synthetic oral cannabinoid (dronabinol), has been proposed to have a number of properties that may be clinically useful in some situations. These include antiemetic effects in chemotherapy recipients, appetite-promoting effects in AIDS, reduction of intraocular pressure in glaucoma, and reduction of spasticity in multiple sclerosis and other neurologic disorders. With the possible exception of AIDS-related cachexia, none of these attributes of marijuana compounds is clearly superior to other readily available therapies. Furthermore, any therapeutic benefit of marijuana must be balanced against the many unhealthy psychoactive effects associated with its use.

METHAMPHETAMINE The abuse of methamphetamine, also referred to as "meth," "speed," "crank," "chalk," "ice," "glass," or "crystal," has been declining in many metropolitan areas and communities throughout the United States. This decrease is attributed in part to drug seizures and the closures of clandestine laboratories that produce methamphetamine illegally. Prevention programs focusing upon methamphetamine abuse have also increased.

Most persons who abuse amphetamine self-administer the drug orally, although there have been reports of methamphetamine administration by inhalation and intravenous injection. Individuals who abuse or become dependent upon methamphetamine state that use of this drug induces feelings of euphoria and decreases fatigue associated with aversive life situations. Adverse physiologic effects observed as a consequence of methamphetamine abuse include headache, difficulty concentrating, diminished appetite, abdominal pain, vomiting or diarrhea, disordered sleep, paranoid or aggressive behavior, and psychosis. Severe, life-threatening toxicity may present as hypertension, cardiac arrythmia or failure, subarachnoid hemorrhage, ischemic stroke, intracerebral hemorrhage, convulsions, or coma. Amphetamines increase the release of monoamine neurotransmitters (dopamine, norepinephrine, and serotonin) from presynaptic neurons. It is thought that the euphoric and reinforcing effects of this class of drugs are mediated through dopamine and the mesolimbic system, whereas the cardiovascular effects are related to norepinephrine. Magnetic resonance spectroscopy studies suggest that chronic abuse may injure the frontal areas and basal ganglia of the brain.

Therapy of acute methamphetamine overdose is largely symptomatic. Ammonium chloride may be useful to acidify the urine and enhance clearance of the drug. Hypertension may respond to sodium nitroprusside or α-adrenergic antagonists. Sedatives may reduce agitation and other signs of central nervous system overactivity. Treatment of chronic methamphetamine dependence may be accomplished in either an inpatient or outpatient setting using strategies similar to those described above for cocaine abuse.

MDMA (3,4-methylenedioxymethamphetamine), or *Ecstasy*, is a derivative of methamphetamine. Ecstasy is usually taken orally but may be injected or inhaled. In addition to amphetamine-like effects, MDMA can induce vivid hallucinations and other perceptual distortions. These toxicities are similar to those of lysergic acid diethylamide (LSD) and may be mediated through the release of serotonin.

LYSERGIC ACID DIETHYLAMIDE The discovery of the psychedelic effects of LSD in 1947 led to an epidemic of LSD abuse during the 1960s. Imposition of stringent constraints on the manufacture and distribution of LSD (classified as a Schedule I substance by the U.S. Food and Drug Administration), as well as public recognition that psychedelic experiences induced by LSD were a health hazard, have resulted in a reduction in LSD abuse. The drug still retains some popularity among adolescents and young adults, however, and there are indications that LSD use among young persons has been increasing in some communities in the United States.

LSD is a very potent drug; oral doses as low as 20 μg may induce profound psychological and physiologic effects. Tachycardia, hypertension, pupillary dilation, tremor, and hyperpyrexia occur within minutes following oral administration of 0.5 to 2 μg/kg. A variety of bizarre and often conflicting perceptual and mood changes, including visual illusions, synesthesias, and extreme lability of mood, usually occur within 30 min after LSD intake. The action of LSD may persist for 12 to 18 h, even though the half-life of the drug is only 3 h.

Tolerance develops rapidly for LSD-induced changes in psychological function when the drug is used one or more times per day for 4 or more days. Abrupt abstinence following continued use does not produce withdrawal signs or symptoms. There have been no clinical reports of death caused by the direct effects of LSD.

The most frequent medical emergency associated with LSD use is panic episode (the "bad trip"), which may persist up to 24 h. Management of this problem is best accomplished by supportive reassurance ("talking down") and, if necessary, administration of small doses of anxiolytic drugs. Adverse consequences of chronic LSD use include risk for schizophreniform psychosis and derangements in memory function, problem solving, and abstract thinking. Treatment of these disorders is best carried out in specialized psychiatric facilities.

PHENCYCLIDINE Phencyclidine (PCP), a cyclohexylamine derivative, is widely used in veterinary medicine to briefly immobilize large animals and is sometimes described as a dissociative anesthetic. PCP binds to ionotropic *n*-methyl-*d*-aspartate (NMDA) receptors in the nervous system blocking ion current through these channels. PCP is easily synthesized; its abusers are primarily young people and polydrug users. It is used orally, by smoking, or by intravenous injection. It is also used as an adulterant in THC, LSD, amphetamine, or cocaine. The most common street preparation, *angel dust*, is a white granular powder that contains 50 to 100% of the drug. Low doses (5 mg) produce agitation, excitement, impaired motor coordination, dysarthria, and analgesia. Users may have horizontal or vertical nystagmus, flushing, diaphoresis, and hyperacusis. Behavioral changes include distortions of body image, disorganization of thinking, and feelings of estrangement. Higher doses of PCP (5 to 10 mg) may produce hypersalivation, vomiting, myoclonus, fever, stupor, or coma. PCP doses of $\geq$10 mg cause convulsions, opisthotonus, and decerebrate posturing, which may be followed by prolonged coma.

The diagnosis of PCP overdose is difficult because the patient's initial symptoms may suggest an acute schizophrenic reaction. Confirmation of PCP use is possible by determination of PCP levels in serum or urine; PCP assays are available at most toxicologic centers. PCP remains in urine for 1 to 5 days following high-dose intake.

PCP overdose requires life-support measures, including treatment of coma, convulsions, and respiratory depression in an intensive care unit. There is no specific antidote or antagonist for PCP. PCP excretion from the body can be enhanced by gastric lavage and acidification of urine. Death from PCP overdose may occur as a consequence of some combination of pharyngeal hypersecretion, hyperthermia, respiratory depression, severe hypertension, seizures, hypertensive encephalopathy, and intracerebral hemorrhage.

Acute psychosis associated with PCP use should be considered a psychiatric emergency since patients may be at high risk for suicide or extreme violence toward others. Phenothiazines should not be used for treatment because these drugs potentiate PCP's anticholinergic effects. Haloperidol (5 mg intramuscularly) has been administered on an hourly basis to induce suppression of psychotic behavior. PCP, like LSD and mescaline, produces vasospasm of cerebral arteries at relatively low doses. Chronic PCP use has been shown to induce insomnia, anorexia, severe social and behavioral changes, and, in some cases, chronic schizophrenia.

POLYDRUG ABUSE Although drug abusers often report a preference for a particular drug, such as alcohol or opiates, the concurrent use of other drugs is common. Multiple drug use often involves substances that may have different pharmacologic effects from the preferred drug. Concurrent use of dissimilar compounds such as stimulants and opiates or stimulants and alcohol is not unusual. The diversity of reported drug use combinations suggests that achieving some perceptible change in state, rather than any particular direction of change (stimulation or sedation), may be the primary reinforcer in polydrug use and abuse. There is also evidence that intoxication with alcohol or opiates is associated with increased tobacco smoking. There is relatively little systematic information available about multiple drug abuse interactions. However, the combined use of cocaine, heroin, and alcohol increases the risk for toxic effects and adverse medical consequences over risks associated with use of a single drug. One determinant of polydrug use patterns is the relative availability and cost of the drugs. There are many examples of situationally determined drug-use patterns. For example, alcohol abuse, with its attendant medical complications, is one of the most serious problems encountered in former heroin addicts participating in methadone maintenance programs.

The physician must recognize that perpetuation of polydrug abuse and drug dependence is not necessarily a symptom of an underlying emotional disorder. Neither alleviation of anxiety nor reduction of depression accounts for initiation and perpetuation of polydrug abuse. Severe depression and anxiety are as frequently the consequences of polydrug abuse as they are the antecedents. There is also evidence that some of the most adverse consequences of drug use may be reinforcing and contributing to the continuation of polydrug abuse.

℞ **TREATMENT** Adequate treatment of polydrug abuse, as well as other forms of drug abuse, requires innovative programs of intervention. The first step in successful treatment is detoxification, a process that may be difficult because of the abuse of several drugs with different pharmacologic actions (e.g., alcohol, opiates, and cocaine). Since patients may not recall or may deny simultaneous multiple drug use, diagnostic evaluation should always include urinalysis for qualitative detection of psychoactive substances and their metabolites. Treatment of polydrug abuse often requires hospitalization or inpatient residential care during detoxification and the initial phase of drug abstinence. When possible, specialized facilities for the care and treatment of chemically dependent persons should be used. Outpatient detoxification of polydrug abuse patients is likely to be ineffective and may be dangerous.

As in the treatment of alcohol abuse, no single therapeutic modality has been shown to be uniquely effective in inducing remission. Polydrug abuse is a chronic disorder with an unpredictable pattern of remission and recrudescence. Even temporary remissions with attendant physical, social, and psychological improvements are preferable to the continuation or progressive acceleration of polydrug abuse and its related adverse medical and interpersonal consequences. In polydrug abuse, as in many chronic disorders, definitive "cures" rarely occur. The concerned physician should continue to assist polydrug abuse patients throughout the cyclic oscillations of this complex behavior disorder, recognizing that resumption of drug use may be the rule rather than the exception.

BIBLIOGRAPHY

ERNST T et al: Evidence for long-term neurotoxicity associated with methamphetamine abuse: A 1H MRS study. Neurology 54:1344, 2000

KAUFMAN MJ et al: Cocaine-induced cerebral vasoconstriction detected in humans with magnetic resonance angiography. JAMA 279:376, 1998

MENDELSON JH, MELLO NK: Drug therapy: Management of cocaine abuse and dependence. N Engl J Med 334:965, 1996

———— et al: Cocaine pharmacokinetics in men and in women during the follicular and luteal phase of the menstrual cycle. Neuropsychopharmacology 21:294, 1999

NAHAS GG et al: *Marihuana and Medicine*. Totowa, NJ, Humana Press, 1999

NATIONAL INSTITUTE ON DRUG ABUSE: *Epidemiologic Trends in Drug Abuse, Advance Report*. NIH Publication No. 00-4738, 2000

SCHUCKIT MA: *Drug and Alcohol Abuse: A Clinical Guide to Diagnosis and Treatment*, 5th ed. New York, Kluwer Academic/Plenum, 2000

SIEGEL AJ et al: Cocaine-induced erythrocytosis and increase in Von Willebrand factor. Arch Intern Med 159:1925, 1999

390   *David M. Burns*

NICOTINE ADDICTION

The use of tobacco leaf to create and satisfy nicotine addiction was introduced to Columbus by Native Americans and spread rapidly to Europe. The use of tobacco as cigarettes, however, is predominantly a twentieth century phenomenon, as is the epidemic of disease caused by this form of tobacco.

Nicotine is the principal constituent of tobacco responsible for its addictive character. Addicted smokers regulate their nicotine intake and blood levels by adjusting the frequency and intensity of their tobacco use both to obtain the desired psychoactive effects and avoid withdrawal.

Unburned cured tobacco contains nicotine, carcinogens, and other toxins capable of causing gum disease and oral cancer. When tobacco is burned, the resultant smoke contains, in addition to nicotine, carbon monoxide and >4000 other compounds that result from volatilization, pyrolysis, and pyrosynthesis of tobacco and various chemical additives used in making different tobacco products. The smoke is composed of a fine aerosol, with a particle size distribution predominantly in the range to deposit in the airways and alveolar surfaces of the lungs, and a vapor phase. The bulk of the toxicity and carcinogenicity of the smoke resides in the aerosolized particulate phase, which contains a large number of toxic constituents and >40 carcinogenic compounds. The aggregate of particulate matter, after subtracting nicotine and moisture, is referred to as tar. The vapor phase contains carbon monoxide, respiratory irritants, and ciliotoxins as well as many of the volatile compounds responsible for the distinctive smell of cigarette smoke.

The alkaline pH of smoke from blends of tobacco utilized for pipes and cigars allows sufficient absorption of nicotine across the oral mucosa to satisfy the smoker's need for this drug. Therefore, smokers of pipes and cigars tend not to inhale the smoke into the lung, confining the toxic and carcinogenic exposure (and the increased rates of disease) largely to the upper airway for most users of these products. The acidic pH of smoke generated by the tobacco used in cigarettes dramatically reduces absorption of nicotine in the mouth, necessitating inhalation of the smoke into the larger surface of the lungs in order to absorb quantities of nicotine sufficient to satisfy the smoker's addiction. The shift to using tobacco as cigarettes, with resultant increased deposition of smoke in the lung, has created the epidemic of heart disease, lung disease, and lung cancer that dominates the current disease manifestations of tobacco use.

DISEASE MANIFESTATIONS OF CIGARETTE SMOKING Over 400,000 individuals die prematurely each year in the United States from cigarette use; this represents approximately one out of every five deaths in the United States. Approximately 40% of cigarette smokers will die prematurely due to cigarette smoking unless they are able to quit.

The major diseases caused by cigarette smoking are listed in Table 390-1, with the relative risks for each disease listed for male and female current smokers. The incidence of smoking-related diseases is proportionately greater in younger than in older smokers, particularly for coronary artery disease and stroke. At older ages, the background rate of disease in nonsmokers increases, diminishing the fractional contribution of smoking and the relative risk; however, absolute excess rates of disease mortality found in smokers compared to nonsmokers increase with increasing age. The organ damage caused by smoking and the number of smokers who die from smoking are both greater among the elderly, as one would expect from a process of cumulative injury.

Cardiovascular Diseases Cigarette smokers are more likely than nonsmokers to develop large vessel atherosclerosis as well as small vessel disease. Approximately 90% of peripheral vascular disease in the nondiabetic population can be attributed to cigarette smoking, as can approximately 50% of aortic aneurysms. In contrast, 20 to 30% of coronary artery disease and approximately 10% of occlusive cerebrovascular disease are caused by cigarette smoking. There is a

Disease or Condition	Relative Risk	
	Males	Females
All causes of death	2.3	1.9
Coronary heart disease		
Age 35–64	2.8	3
Age >64	1.6	1.6
Cerebrovascular lesions		
Age 35–64	3.7	4.8
Age ≥65	1.9	1.5
Aortic aneurysm	4.7	3.9
Peripheral vascular disease	13.5	2.2
Chronic obstructive pulmonary disease	9.7	10.4
Cancer		
Lip, oral cavity, pharynx	27.5	5.6
Esophagus	7.6	10.3
Pancreas	2.1	2.3
Larynx	10.5	17.8
Lung	22.4	11.9
Kidney	3.0	1.4
Bladder, other urinary organs	2.9	2.6
Complications of pregnancy		1.4
Perinatal complications		1.3
Low birth weight		2.1

multiplicative interaction between cigarette smoking and other cardiac risk factors such that the increment in risk produced by smoking among individuals with hypertension or elevated serum lipids is substantially greater than the increment in risk produced by smoking for individuals without these risk factors.

In addition to its role in promoting atherosclerosis, cigarette smoking also increases the likelihood of myocardial infarction and sudden cardiac death by promoting platelet aggregation and vascular occlusion. Reversal of these effects may explain the rapid benefit of smoking cessation for a new coronary event demonstrable among those who have survived a first myocardial infarction. This effect may also explain the substantially higher rates of graft occlusion among continuing smokers following vascular bypass surgery for cardiac or peripheral vascular disease, as well as the high failure rate of angioplasty procedures among continuing smokers.

Cessation of cigarette smoking reduces the risk of a second coronary event within 6 to 12 months after quitting, and rates of first myocardial infarction or death from coronary heart disease also decline within the first few years following cessation. After 15 years of cessation, the risk of a new myocardial infarction or death from coronary heart disease in former smokers is similar to that in those who have never smoked.

Cancer Cancers of the lung, larynx, oral cavity, esophagus, pancreas, kidney, and urinary bladder are caused by cigarette smoking. In addition, there is evidence suggesting that cigarette smoking may play a role in increasing the risk of cervical and stomach cancer. There is conflicting evidence on the relationship of cigarette smoking and cancer of the breast, but overall there does not appear to be a causal link. There is a lower risk of uterine cancer among postmenopausal women who smoke.

The risks of cancer increase with the increasing number of cigarettes smoked per day and the duration of smoking, and there are synergistic interactions between cigarette smoking and alcohol use for cancer of the oral cavity, esophagus, and possibly lung. Several occupational exposures also synergistically increase lung cancer risk among cigarette smokers, most notably occupational asbestos and radon exposure.

Cessation of cigarette smoking reduces the risk of developing cancer relative to continuing smoking, but even 20 years after cessation there is a modest persistent increased risk of developing lung cancer.

Respiratory Disease Cigarette smoking is responsible for >90% of chronic obstructive pulmonary disease. Within 1 to 2 years of beginning to smoke regularly, many young smokers will develop inflammatory changes in their small airways, although lung function measures of these changes do not predict development of chronic air-

flow obstruction. After ≥20 years of smoking, pathophysiologic changes in the lungs develop and progress proportional to smoking intensity and duration. Chronic mucous hyperplasia of the larger airways results in a chronic productive cough in as many as 80% of smokers over age 60. Chronic inflammation and narrowing of the small airways and/or enzymatic digestion of alveolar walls resulting in pulmonary emphysema can result in reduced expiratory airflow sufficient to produce clinical symptoms of respiratory limitation in approximately 15% of smokers.

Changes in the small airways of young smokers will reverse after 1 to 2 years of cessation. There may also be a small increase in measures of expiratory airflow following cessation among individuals who have developed chronic airflow obstruction, but the major change following cessation is a slowing of the rate of decline in lung function with advancing age rather than a return of lung function toward normal.

Pregnancy Cigarette smoking is associated with several maternal complications of pregnancy: premature rupture of membranes, abruptio placentae, and placenta previa; there is also a small increase in the risk of spontaneous abortion among smokers. Infants of smoking mothers are more likely to experience preterm delivery, have a higher perinatal mortality, are small for their gestational age, are more likely to die of sudden infant death syndrome, and appear to have a developmental lag for at least the first several years of life.

Other Conditions Smoking delays healing of peptic ulcers; increases the risk of osteoporosis, senile cataracts, and macular degeneration; and results in premature menopause, wrinkling of the skin, gallstones and cholecystitis in women, and male impotence.

Environmental tobacco smoke Long-term exposure to environmental tobacco smoke increases the risk of lung cancer and coronary artery disease among nonsmokers. It also increases the incidence of respiratory infections, chronic otitis media, and asthma in children as well as causing exacerbation of asthma in children.

PHARMACOLOGIC INTERACTIONS Cigarette smoking may interact with a variety of other drugs in ways that may have clinically significant implications (Table 390-2). Cigarette smoking induces the cytochrome P450 system, which may alter the metabolic clearance of drugs such as theophylline. This effect may result in more drug toxicity among nonsmokers on fixed drug dosage schedules and in inadequate serum levels in smokers as outpatients when the dosage is established in the hospital under nonsmoking conditions. Correspondingly, serum levels may rise when smokers are hospitalized and not allowed to smoke. Smokers may also have higher first-pass clearance for drugs such as lidocaine, and the stimulant effects of nicotine may reduce the effect of benzodiazepines or beta blockers.

Table 390-2 Interactions of Smoking and Prescription Drugs

Drug	Interaction
Benzodiazepines	Less sedation
Beta blockers	Reduced lowering of heart rate and blood pressure
Caffeine	Faster metabolic clearance
Chlorpromazine	Decreased serum concentrations of uncertain clinical implications
Dextropropoxyphene	Less analgesia
Flecainide	Increased first-pass clearance
Fluvoxamine	Decreased serum concentrations of uncertain clinical implications
Haloperidol	Decreased serum concentrations of uncertain clinical implications
Heparin	Faster clearance
Imiprimine	Decreased serum concentrations of uncertain clinical implications
Insulin	Delayed absorption due to skin vasoconstriction
Lidocaine	Increased first-pass clearance
Mexiletine	Increased first-pass clearance
Pentazocine	Less analgesia, possibly increased clearance
Propranolol	Increased first-pass clearance
Tacrine	Faster metabolic clearance
Theophylline	Faster metabolic clearance

OTHER FORMS OF TOBACCO USE   Other major forms of tobacco use are moist snuff deposited between the cheek and gum, chewing tobacco, pipes and cigars, and recently bidi (tobacco wrapped in tendu or temburni leaf and commonly used in India) and clove cigarettes. Oral tobacco use leads to gum disease and can result in oral cancer. All forms of burned tobacco generate toxic and carcinogenic smoke similar to that of cigarette smoke. The differences in disease consequences of use relate to frequency of use and depth of inhalation. The risk of upper airway cancers is similar among cigarette and cigar smokers, while those who have smoked only cigars have a much lower risk of lung cancer, heart disease, and chronic obstructive pulmonary disease. However, cigarette smokers who switch to pipes or cigars do tend to inhale the smoke, increasing their risk; and it is likely that comparable inhalation and frequency of exposure to tobacco smoke from any of these forms of tobacco use will lead to comparable disease outcomes.

Recent prevalence-of-use data have suggested a resurgence of cigar and bidi use among adolescents of both genders, raising concerns that these older forms of tobacco use are once again causing a public health concern.

LOWER TAR AND NICOTINE CIGARETTES   Since the bulk of the toxicity of cigarette smoke is contained in the tar, and since nicotine is the principal addictive agent in cigarettes, it has been suggested that cigarettes that deliver less tar and nicotine to the smoker might be safer. Studies of smokers of low-yield cigarettes suggest that there may be a 10 to 20% reduction in the risk of developing lung cancer among those who reduce the nominal tar yield of their cigarettes by ≥50%. However, this benefit is only evident if smokers do not compensate for the lower nicotine delivery with an increased intensity of smoking, and most studies show that smokers of low-yield cigarettes do compensate. Because of their addiction to nicotine, most smokers tend to preserve their intake of nicotine, and correspondingly their tar intake, when they shift to lower nicotine cigarettes.

Newer, very low yield cigarettes commonly use vents in the filters or other engineering designs to reduce the tar and nicotine when the cigarette is smoked by machine. However, the delivery of tar and nicotine is much higher when these cigarettes are smoked by actual smokers. Current evidence suggests that if there is any disease-reduction benefit for smokers of low-yield cigarettes, it is too small to be clinically meaningful, and individuals should be discouraged from thinking of low-yield cigarettes as a substitute for cessation.

CESSATION   The process of stopping smoking is often a cyclical one, with the smoker sometimes making multiple attempts to quit and failing before finally being successful. Approximately 70 to 80% of smokers would like to quit smoking, approximately one-third of current smokers attempt to quit each year, and ≥90% of these unassisted quit attempts fail. Smokers have been categorized into those who are not thinking about quitting (precontemplation), those who are thinking about quitting (contemplation), and those who are in the action phase of quitting. A useful conceptualization of the cessation process is one where smokers cycle through the stages of cessation; each time smokers go around the cycle, a few more smokers become successful in their cessation efforts. One goal of clinician-based smoking interventions then becomes moving smokers from one stage of the cessation cycle to another, and efforts can be focused on moving the smoker to the next stage rather than focusing exclusively on immediate cessation.

The move from thinking about quitting to making a quit attempt is often triggered by a variety of environmental stimuli independent of physician control. The cost of cigarettes can be a powerful trigger for cessation attempts. Media campaigns, particularly when coupled with cessation events, are also able to trigger cessation attempts in large numbers of smokers. Changes in workplace rules to restrict smoking in the workplace have been associated with quit attempts in substantial numbers of workers. However, physician advice to quit, particularly around an acute illness, is also a powerful trigger for cessation activity, with up to half of patients who are advised to quit making a cessation effort.

Telephone counseling and nicotine-replacement therapy are all useful enhancers of long-term cessation success. Clinic-based cessation programs have a substantial benefit for long-term cessation for those who can be recruited to participate, and physician recommendation can double the fraction of smokers who are willing to participate in these programs.

PREVENTION   Approximately 90% of individuals who will become cigarette smokers initiate the behavior during adolescence. Factors that promote adolescent initiation are parental or older generation cigarette smoking, tobacco advertising and promotional activities, the availability of cigarettes, and the social acceptability of smoking. The need for an enhanced self-image and to imitate adult behavior is greatest for those adolescents who have the least external validation of their self-worth, which may explain in part the enormous differences in adolescent smoking prevalence by socioeconomic and school performance strata.

Prevention of smoking initiation must begin early, preferably in the elementary school years. Physicians who deal with adolescents should be sensitive to the prevalence of this problem in their patient population. Effective physician-based interventions for adolescent smokers remain to be developed, but current clinical guidelines suggest that physicians should ask all adolescents whether they have experimented with tobacco or currently use tobacco, reinforce the facts that most adolescents and adults do not smoke, and explain that all forms of tobacco are both addictive and harmful.

GENETIC CONSIDERATIONS   Several genes have been associated with nicotine addiction. Some reduce the clearance of nicotine, and others have been associated with an increased likelihood of becoming dependent on tobacco and other drugs as well as a higher incidence of depression. Genetic alterations that involve the neurotransmitter dopamine, and possibly the serotoninergic and cholinergic neuroregulatory pathways, are being explored for their contribution to development of addiction to tobacco and other substances. The precise role these genetic differences play in development and maintenance of nicotine addiction remains to be determined, but it is unlikely that genetic factors are the principal determinants of addiction. Rates of smoking initiation among males, and corresponding rates of nicotine addiction, have dropped by almost 50% since the mid-1950s, suggesting that factors other than genetics are the principal determinants of whether individuals will become addicted. It is more likely that genetic polymorphism represents a range of biologic susceptibility conditioning the intensity of cigarette use and the probability that experimentation with tobacco as an adolescent leads to addiction as an adult. ■

PHYSICIAN INTERVENTION   Physicians can make a clear difference in promoting successful cessation among their smoking patients, and the Agency for Health Care Policy and Research (AHCPR) has developed clinical guidelines for health care system–based smoking cessation (Table 390-3). All patients should be asked whether they smoke, their past experience with quitting, and whether they are currently interested in quitting. Those who are not interested in quitting should be encouraged and motivated to quit; provided a clear, strong, and personalized physician message that smoking is an important health concern; and offered assistance if they become interested in quitting in the future. There is a relationship between the amount of assistance a patient is willing to accept, and the success of the cessation attempt. A quit date should be negotiated, usually not the day of the visit but within the next few weeks, and a follow-up contact by office staff around the time of the quit date should be provided.

There are a variety of nicotine-replacement products, including over the counter nicotine patch and gum, as well as nicotine nasal and oral inhalers available by prescription. Clonidine and, more recently, antidepressants such as bupropion have also been shown to be effective; some evidence supports the combined use of nicotine-replacement therapy and antidepressants. Nicotine-replacement therapy is provided in different dosages for use with smokers of different numbers of cigarettes per day. Antidepressants are more effective in those with a history of depression symptoms. At this time there are few clear

Table 390-3 Clinical Practice Guidelines

390 Nicotine Addiction

2577

Physician Actions	Effective Pharmacologic Interventions	Other Effective Interventions
Ask: systematically identify all tobacco users at every visit	Nicotine patch or gum	Physician or other medical personnel counseling (10 min)
Advise: strongly urge all smokers to quit	Nicotine nasal inhaler	Intensive smoking cessation programs[a]
Identify smokers willing to quit	Nicotine oral inhaler	Clinic-based smoking status identification system
Assist the patient in quitting	Clonidine	Counseling by nonclinicians and social support by family and friends
Arrange follow-up contact	Bupropion	Telephone counseling

[a] At least four to seven sessions of 20- to 30-min duration, lasting at least 2 weeks, preferably 8 weeks.

indications favoring the use of one agent over another as initial therapy. Current recommendations are to offer pharmacologic treatment to all who will accept it and to provide counseling and other support to the patient as a part of the cessation attempt. Cessation advice alone is likely to increase success by 50% compared with no intervention; a more comprehensive approach with advice, pharmacologic assistance, and counseling can increase cessation success by almost threefold.

In order for physicians to incorporate cessation assistance into their practice successfully, it is essential to change the infrastructure in which the physician practices. The following are simple changes: (1) including questions on smoking and interest in cessation on patient-intake questionnaires, (2) asking patients whether they smoke as part of the initial vital sign measurements made by office staff, (3) listing smoking as a problem in the medical record, and (4) automating follow-up contact with the patient on their quit date. These changes are essential to institutionalizing smoking intervention within the practice setting; without this institutionalization, the best intentions of physicians to intervene with their patients who smoke are often lost in the time crush of a busy practice.

BIBLIOGRAPHY

NATIONAL CANCER INSTITUTE: *Changes in Cigarette-Related Disease Risks and Their Implication for Prevention and Control.* Smoking and Tobacco Control Monograph No. 8, USDHHS NIH NCI, (NIH) Publication 97-4213, 1997

PROCHAZKA AV: New developments in smoking cessation. Chest 17:169S, 2000

US DEPARTMENT OF HEALTH AND HUMAN SERVICES: *The Health Benefits of Smoking Cessation: A Report of the Surgeon General.* DHHS (CDC) Publication 90-8416, 1990

———: *Women and Tobacco. A Report of the Surgeon General.* DHHS (CDC), National Center for Chronic Disease Prevention and Health Promotion, Office on Smoking and Health, in press

———: *Smoking Cessation and Prevention.* Clinical Practice Guideline Number 18, Agency for Health Care Policy and Research Publication, Public Health Service, DHHS, 2000

ZEVIN S, BENOWITZ NL: Drug interactions with tobacco smoking: An update. Clin Pharmacokinet 36:426, 1999

NOBEL PRIZE IN PHYSIOLOGY OR MEDICINE, 1924

Willem Einthoven was born on May 16, 1860, in Semarang, Java, in the Dutch East Indies (Indonesia) to Jacob Einthoven and Louise de Vogel. He was the third of six children and his father was a practicing physician who died when Willem was only 10 years old. After his father's death, the family returned to the Netherlands. Einthoven attended the University of Utrecht where he received his B.S. degree in 1878, and then studied medicine at the same institution. During his medical studies, he undertook a number of research projects with outstanding investigators at Utrecht University that culminated in scientific publications, particularly in the area of eye physiology. On receiving his medical degree in 1885 and based on his scientific contributions, at the age of 25 years he was appointed a Professor of Physiology at the University of Leiden. In addition to his work in the physiology of the eye, he also studied the nervous control of bronchial vessels. He then commenced his work on the electrophysiology of the heart. The first study of the electrical deflections of the heart was by Augustus Waller, a friend of Einthoven, who used the capillary ergometer to show the electrical changes associated with the heartbeat. Waller rejected any importance of these electrical changes and did not pursue the work further. Einthoven, however, was convinced of the importance of these electrical impulses, but the capillary electrometer was too sensitive to be reliable. To counter this problem, Einthoven made a hole some 3.0 to 4.5 m (10 to 15 ft) below his laboratory and lined it with rocks to insulate the capillary ergometer from the vibrations caused by horse-drawn trucks as they passed the wooden building of his laboratory. Nevertheless, Einthoven's efforts with the capillary ergometer were still unsuccessful, so he turned to another device.

He began working with the d'Arsonval galvanometer and replaced the silver-plated quartz coil with a wire, which was much lighter than the coil. This change allowed not only increased sensitivity but also more rapid response time for recording the electrical potentials from the heart.

Using this string galvanometer, Einthoven demonstrated that there was a characteristic electrocardiogram for each individual. He labeled the waves of this electrocardiogram P, Q, R, S, and T—the nomenclature still used in electrocardiography. Einthoven then connected his laboratory to the hospital a mile away using a transmission wire owned by the telephone company. With this approach he could study the electrocardiograms of patients in the hospital from his own laboratory. This was the first instance of the development and use of the telecardiogram. Einthoven showed that patients with different heart diseases had different electrocardiograms including cardiac enlargement secondary to valvular problems, premature contractions, and heart block. He also described the electrical axis of the heart that correlated with the anatomical axis, another observation that is still key in cardiogram interpretation a century later. Einthoven also recognized that electrical deflection varied based on the position of the electrodes and therefore proposed a standardized system for placing the electrodes and gave the leads their current names I, II, and III. Throughout his career, Einthoven combined his knowledge of physiology and physics as he laid the groundwork for modern electrocardiography. Einthoven clearly deserves to be the "Father of Electrocardiography." For his accomplishments, he was awarded the Nobel Prize in Physiology or Medicine in 1924. Einthoven, however, received little public recognition during his lifetime for his contributions in electrocardiography, awareness of the value of the electrocardiogram in clinical medicine came later.

REFERENCES

1. Magill FN (ed): *Nobel Prize Winners: Physiology or Medicine*, vol 1. Pasadena, Salem Press, 1993
2. Schrier RW: *A Salute to Nobel Laureates in Physiology and Medicine*, Proceedings of the Association of American Physicians 108(1): Jan 1996
3. Sourkes TL: *Nobel Prize Winners in Medicine and Physiology 1901–1965*. London, Abelard-Schuman, 1967

Robert W. Schrier, MD

NOBEL PRIZE IN PHYSIOLOGY OR MEDICINE, 1929

Christiaan Eijkman, Jr., was born in Nijerk, the Netherlands, on August 11, 1858, the seventh child of a school-teacher. His family moved to Amsterdam where he received his early schooling and then entered the University of Amsterdam. The government paid for his tuition in medical school in exchange for his agreement to be an army physician. Thus, after graduation from medical school in 1883 he was sent to the Dutch East Indies, where he spent 2 years in Java and Sumatra. Eijkman had become quite interested in bacteriology and went to study this field in Berlin with Robert Koch.

While in Berlin, Eijkman met the members of a two-man commission being sent by the Dutch government to the Dutch East Indies to discover the cause of beriberi, then epidemic in tropical and subtropical countries. They went to Koch's laboratory before departing for the East Indies because they thought that bacteria must be causing beriberi. Beriberi was characterized by a polyneuritis with resulting paralysis of the lower extremities (*dry beriberi*) as well as respiratory and cardiac failure with edema (*wet beriberi*). Eijkman volunteered to accompany the team to help in isolating the proposed causative bacteria and then to implement sterilization techniques. The team at first believed that they had identified a bacterium as the cause of beriberi, and the other members of the team then returned to The Netherlands. Applying Koch's principles for proving a bacterial cause of beriberi, however, frustrated Eijkman since he could not document the transmission of the disease in any manner.

The investigation appeared to be at a dead end when a coincidence put Eijkman "on the right track." A disease quite similar to beriberi broke out among chickens in the Djakarta laboratory of a military hospital. The chickens had muscular weakness, could not use their wings or raise their heads, and died of respiratory failure. Microscopic examination demonstrated degeneration of the chickens' peripheral nerves. Eijkman attempted to pass the disease from one chicken to another and was unsuccessful. Again, there seemed to be an impasse in Eijkman's research, but suddenly the affected chickens began to improve and there were no new cases. Eijkman then focused on the chickens' food and found that they had been receiving leftover polished rice from the officers' dining room from June 17th to November 27th. Then a new cook took over, and the chickens again were fed with unpolished rice. The chickens' beriberi had commenced on July 10th and subsided during the last part of November. Eijkman was able to reproduce the symptoms of beriberi by again feeding the chickens polished rice and to reverse the disease by feeding the chickens unpolished (whole-grain) rice. Eijkman was then able to extract an active substance from the inner hull (pericarp) of the rice grain that could be administered either by mouth or by injection.

The final proof came when Eijkman learned that some prison inmates on the island of Java were fed polished rice and others were fed unpolished rice. Epidemiologic studies demonstrated a 300 times greater incidence of beriberi in those prisons using polished rice. The essential substance in the rice husk was found to be an amine, and thus the term *vital amine* was coined, later shortened to *vitamin*. Eijkman's discovery of the water-soluble vitamin, thiamine saved thousands of lives and opened the era whereby vitamins were recognized as essential elements of the diet.

Frederick Gowland Hopkins was born on June 20, 1861, at Eastbourne, England. He became interested in science at an early age with the worlds revealed by a microscope given to him by his father. He later said that the observations that he made at home with his microscope, ". . .were something very important—the most important thing that I had come against; so much more important than anything I was being taught in school." Although he received a "first class" in chemistry at the City of London School, he left school at 17 and became a bank clerk. However, after 6 months at that job he became an assistant to an analytic chemist. This work led him ultimately to a university degree in chemistry and finally a medical degree at age 32—quite an old age to become a physician in that era.

Hopkins clearly made up for any "lost time." In 1898 he moved to Cambridge University to teach the chemical aspects of physiology, became a Reader, and ultimately, in 1914, Professor of a new Department of Biochemistry at Cambridge. His Department of Biochemistry attracted some of the brightest young minds. He was one of the first to teach the dynamics of biochemistry; he thus not only observed what chemical substances are in living cells but what they do in the life of the living cell. Hopkins discovered tryptophan and glutathione but rather than pursue their structure, he immediately sought what they were doing in the body. On the background of Eijkman's discovery of thiamine deficiency as the cause of beriberi, and the British Navy's cure of scurvy by dietary means, Hopkins studied the factors involved in animal growth. He found that adequate amounts of fat, carbohydrates, proteins, and minerals were not sufficient to sustain normal animal growth. It was not until he added a milk supplement to the diet that normal growth was restored. He concluded that the failure to grow was not due to a lack of food intake but rather to an inability to use the food optimally. In his classic paper published in 1912, Hopkins concluded that milk and other foods must contain important accessory food factors. While Hopkins did not identify these factors, his studies were important in future discoveries of the roles of vitamin C and vitamin B complex (see figure).

REFERENCES

1. Aaseng N: *The Disease Fighters*. Minneapolis, Lerner Publications, 1987
2. Magill FN (ed): *Nobel Prize Winners: Physiology or Medicine*, vol. 1. Pasadena, Salem Press, 1993
3. Schrier RW: *A Salute to Nobel Laureates in Physiology and Medicine*, Proceedings of the Association of American Physicians 108(1): 1996
4. Sourkes TL: *Nobel Prize Winners in Medicine and Physiology 1901-1965*. London, Abelard-Schuman, 1967

Robert W. Schrier, MD

The chicken on the left was fed a normal diet, whereas the chicken on the right was fed a diet lacking in vitamins B and C. (Reprinted with permission from Ref. 1.)

Section 1
SPECIFIC ENVIRONMENTAL AND OCCUPATIONAL HAZARDS

---

391 *Howard Hu, Frank E. Speizer*

SPECIFIC ENVIRONMENTAL AND OCCUPATIONAL HAZARDS

It cannot be overemphasized that an appropriate environmental/occupational history is an essential part of the medical workup of many chronic diseases. The general approach to the patient whose illness may have been caused or exacerbated by environmental or occupational hazards is detailed in Chap. 5.

The term *hazards* in this context is generally synonymous with *toxins* and *toxic exposures* and encompasses chemical factors as well as other risks posed by the physical environment and by selected natural phenomena. These hazards may exist in the general environment or in the workplace. Strictly speaking, smoking, alcohol ingestion, nutritional factors, and infectious agents can also be considered chemical or environmental hazards.

Once a specific hazard has been identified as a factor in the pathogenesis of an illness or as an imminent threat, the clinical approach must include the development of a strategy for preventing further exposure and for treating the specific manifestations of the illness, using antidotes and supportive measures. In the following chapters, specific hazards are considered, including acute poisoning and drug overdose; heavy metal poisoning; disorders caused by venoms, bites, and stings; drowning and near-drowning; electrical injuries; and radiation injury. The health effects of ambient air pollution, occupational respiratory exposures, passive smoking, and assorted toxic air pollutants are discussed briefly in Chap. 254. Space does not allow specific discussion in this text of many other important categories of hazards, such as organic solvents; chemicals used in the plastics, synthetic textiles, and rubber industries; and pesticides. The reader should consult other detailed texts or electronic information sources for clinical data on these topics. In this volume, however, brief attention is focused on several selected issues in light of recent developments in research that have enhanced our understanding of the way these hazards may interact with human behavior and consequently pose increased risks to both individuals and society.

HAZARDOUS WASTE AND GROUNDWATER CONTAMINATION The term *hazardous waste* embodies toxic chemicals, radioactive materials, and biologic or infectious wastes. In many communities, hazardous waste has emerged as a major public health concern. In the United States, some 50,000 sites (defined by specific criteria) have been estimated to contain hazardous chemicals; 1000 or so of these have been included as "Superfund sites" on a National Priority List drawn up by the Environmental Protection Agency (EPA). New or unrecognized sites are likely to exist as well. These sites may require long-term remedial action. The spectrum of substances contained at the sites is wide and theoretically may include any of some 30,000 chemicals that are commonly used in commerce. However, the EPA keeps fewer than 200 chemicals on a special hazardous substance list in light of their toxicity, the frequency with which they are encountered, and other factors. One difficulty in anticipating risks associated with hazardous waste sites is that the substances are usually present in mixtures whose composition is seldom fully known. In addition, with respect to toxicity, chemicals may interact with one another in an additive, protective, or synergistic fashion, and little knowl-

edge exists on which to base predictions regarding the interactions of these complex mixtures.

Waste-site employees and the surrounding community can incur hazardous exposures through the inhalation of toxic vapors or dusts emanating directly from a waste site or an on-site incinerator; the ingestion of water contaminated by surface runoff or by material leaching through soil into surface water or groundwater; the ingestion of contaminated plants, fish, or other wildlife; or direct contact. This last risk is particularly likely for children, who may enter a poorly secured site. Perhaps the exposure of greatest concern to community residents has been the contamination of groundwater by volatile organic compounds or solvents (VOCs); together, the widespread detection of low levels of VOCs in groundwater and the several studies suggesting an association between heavy VOC contamination of drinking water and cancer probably account for the high priority given in public opinion polls to avoiding cancer risks. A 1983 study found that 11 of the 20 chemicals most commonly detected at National Priority List waste sites were VOCs (Table 391-1).

Current regulatory policy rests on the assumption that there is no threshold below which a carcinogen exerts no effect or risk. Thus, once a substance is identified as a probable carcinogen (see below), it is regulated to a concentration that is believed to be accompanied by an acceptable level of risk. Clearly, great uncertainty exists regarding methods used to classify drinking-water carcinogens and to extrapolate the risks related to exposure to these substances. Regardless, VOC contamination in groundwater is likely to continue to be a high-priority issue in the public arena.

ENVIRONMENTAL CARCINOGENS Based on studies and reviews of the literature by the International Agency for Research on Cancer, enough evidence exists to classify around 60 substances and processes as probably or definitely carcinogenic in humans (Table 391-2). Some processes are deemed carcinogenic on the basis of epidemiologic evidence, even though the specific causative agent cannot always be clearly identified. Tumor promoters are not distinguished from tumor initiators in this listing, and the chemical structures and modes of action are diverse. Around 150 additional agents and processes have been designated as possibly carcinogenic on the basis of studies of bacteria and animals as well as human epidemiologic studies. The

Table 391-1 Volatile Organic Compounds Most Frequently Detected in 1983 at National Priority List Hazardous Waste Sites (in Order of Frequency and Detection) and (When Known) Associated Cancer Risks

Chemical	Risk Level[a]
Trichloroethylene	3.0
Toluene	
Benzene	1.0
Chloroform	0.43
Tetrachloroethylene	0.7
1,1,1-Trichloroethane	
Ethylbenzene	
Trans-1,2-dichloroethane	0.4
Xylene	
Dichloromethane	
Vinyl chloride	0.02

[a] Concentration in water (μg/L) equivalent to a lifetime cancer risk of 1×10^{-6}. Risk estimates used in these calculations were derived from the U.S. Environmental Protection Agency (1990).

Table 391-2 Substances and Processes Classified as Definitely or Probably Carcinogenic by the International Agency for Research on Cancer

AGENTS AND GROUPS OF AGENTS	MIXTURES
Aflatoxins, naturally occurring [1402-68-2][a]	Alcoholic beverages
4-Aminobiphenyl [92-67-1]	Analgesic mixtures containing phenacetin
Arsenic [7440-38-2] and arsenic compounds	Betel quid with tobacco
Asbestos [1332-21-4]	Coal-tar pitches [65996-93-2]
Azathioprine [446-86-6]	Coal tars [8007-45-2]
Benzene [71-43-2]	Mineral oils, untreated and mildly treated
Benzidine [92-87-5]	Salted fish (Chinese style)
Beryllium [7440-41-7] and beryllium compounds	Shale oils [68308-34-9]
N,N-Bis(2-chloroethyl)-2-naphthylamine (chlornaphazine) [494-03-1]	Soots
Bis(chloromethyl)ether [542-88-1] and chloromethyl methyl ether [107-30-2]	Tobacco products, smokeless
1,4-Butanediol dimethanesulfonate (busulfan; Myleran) [55-98-1]	Tobacco smoke
Cadmium [7440-43-9] and cadmium compounds	Wood dust

AGENTS AND GROUPS OF AGENTS (continued):

Aflatoxins, naturally occurring [1402-68-2][a]
4-Aminobiphenyl [92-67-1]
Arsenic [7440-38-2] and arsenic compounds
Asbestos [1332-21-4]
Azathioprine [446-86-6]
Benzene [71-43-2]
Benzidine [92-87-5]
Beryllium [7440-41-7] and beryllium compounds
N,N-Bis(2-chloroethyl)-2-naphthylamine (chlornaphazine) [494-03-1]
Bis(chloromethyl)ether [542-88-1] and chloromethyl methyl ether [107-30-2]
1,4-Butanediol dimethanesulfonate (busulfan; Myleran) [55-98-1]
Cadmium [7440-43-9] and cadmium compounds
Chlorambucil [305-03-3]
1-(2-Chloroethyl)-3-(4-methylcyclohexyl)-1-nitrosourea (methyl-CCNU; Semustine) [13909-09-6]
Chromium [VI] compounds
Cyclosporine [79217-60-0]
Cyclophosphamide [50-18-0] [6055-19-2]
Diethylstilbestrol [56-53-1]
Erionite [66733-21-9]
Ethylene oxide [75-21-8]
Melphalan [148-82-3]
δ-Methoxypsoralen (methoxsalen) [298-81-7] plus ultraviolet radiation
MOPP and other combined chemotherapy including alkylating agents
Mustard gas (sulfur mustard) [505-60-2]
2-Naphthylamine [91-59-8]
Nickel compounds
Estrogen therapy, postmenopausal
Radon [10043-92-2] and its decay products
Silica [14808-60-7], crystalline
Solar radiation
Talc-containing asbestiform fibers (tamoxifen) [10540-29-1][b]
2,3,7,8-Tetrachlorodibenzo-para-dioxin [1746-01-6]
Thiotepa [52-24-4]
Treosulfan [299-75-2]
Vinyl chloride [75-01-4]

MIXTURES

Alcoholic beverages
Analgesic mixtures containing phenacetin
Betel quid with tobacco
Coal-tar pitches [65996-93-2]
Coal tars [8007-45-2]
Mineral oils, untreated and mildly treated
Salted fish (Chinese style)
Shale oils [68308-34-9]
Soots
Tobacco products, smokeless
Tobacco smoke
Wood dust

EXPOSURE CIRCUMSTANCES

Aluminum production
Auramine manufacturing
Boot and shoe manufacture and repair
Coal gasification
Coke production
Furniture and cabinet making
Hematite mining (underground) with exposure to radon
Iron and steel founding
Isopropanol manufacturing (strong-acid process)
Magenta manufacturing
Painting (occupational exposure)
Rubber industry
Strong-inorganic-acid mists containing sulfuric acid (occupational exposure)

[a] Numbers in brackets are Chemical Abstract Service Registration Numbers.
[b] There is also conclusive evidence that tamoxifen reduces the risk of contralateral breast cancer.

extent to which inferences can be made from nonhuman studies is controversial but certainly depends on minimal standards in the execution of such studies. For example, the Interagency Regulatory Liaison Group recommends that for a carcinogen assay to be considered positive, the test must have been performed on at least 50 animals of each sex in two different species with at least three dose groups (control and two dose levels) over the lifetime of the animals.

BUILDING-RELATED ILLNESSES Reports of discomfort and symptoms in relation to office environments began in the United States in the 1970s. Research has led to the recognition that some building-related illnesses have a clear etiology; these illnesses include hypersensitivity diseases, infections, and exacerbations of asthma due to airborne irritants. However, the majority of such complaints, particularly those of mucous membrane irritation, fatigue, and headache, have no clear etiology. Terms such as *sick-building syndrome* (SBS; also called *tight-building syndrome*) and *nonspecific building-related illnesses* have been used to designate this constellation of symptoms, which have been found in most investigations to occur most often in sealed buildings with centrally controlled mechanical ventilation. Early characterizations of SBS as mass psychogenic illness have not been borne out in the majority of cases by subsequent epidemiologic investigations. Since indoor air-exchange rates were sharply reduced in the 1970s to conserve energy, current hypotheses focus on inadequate dilution of irritants arising from building materials (such as formaldehyde-containing particle board), office supplies (such as carbonless copy paper and photocopy developer solution), toxins from mold and bacterial endotoxin, and personal care products used by occupants as risk factors for SBS. Confirmation of these hypotheses and further characterization of SBS await additional research.

MULTIPLE-CHEMICAL SENSITIVITY The multiple-chemical sensitivity (MCS) syndrome is a diagnosis that has increasingly been given to patients with a wide variety of symptoms that they attribute to exposure at very low levels to a number of commonly encountered chemicals. The syndrome usually begins after a well-defined environmental event, such as a reaction to a more clearly toxic dose of an organic solvent, pesticide, or respiratory irritant. Some cases of MCS begin as SBS. Affected persons commonly report symptoms such as fatigue, malaise, headache, dizziness, lack of concentration, memory loss, and "spaciness"—symptoms that overlap somewhat with those of other diagnoses of uncertain etiology, such as chronic fatigue syndrome. The pathogenesis of MCS is obscure, and no proven methods exist for its diagnosis, evaluation, and treatment. Case series suggesting a high prevalence of affective disorders indicate that psychological factors may play a role in causing MCS and/or in determining its severity; however, evidence does not support MCS as a purely psychogenic illness. A few studies of MCS patients suggest that the biologic mechanism of MCS may involve neurogenic inflammation of the nasal mucosa (as indicated by abnormal rhinolaryngoscopic findings) linked to central nervous system dysfunction (as indicated by alterations seen on single photon emission computed tomography); however, well-controlled research remains sparse, and no firm conclusions can be drawn. Other than the ruling out of other treatable conditions and the avoidance of exacerbating exposures, no specific recommendations for the management of MCS patients can yet be made. A panel of European scientists convened by the World Health Organization recommended that the designation *MCS* be replaced by the term *idiopathic environmental illness* (IEI).

PERSISTENT ORGANIC POLLUTANTS Persistent organic pollutants (POPs) are a class of chemical compounds that tend to travel thousands of miles if released into the atmosphere, to accumulate in the food chain, and to persist in the environment as well as in human tissues (principally fat cells). Although the list of POPs is long, 12 have been identified as particularly important: nine pesticides (aldrin, chlordane, DDT, dieldrin, endrin, heptachlor, hexachlorobenzene, mirex, and toxaphene), dioxins and furans (byproducts of incineration), and polychlorinated biphenyls (PCBs, fluids used mainly as dielectrics in transformers). The persistence and lipid solubility of these compounds allow them to bioconcentrate several thousand-fold as they are passed up the food chain to humans. High levels of exposure to a number of POPs have been shown to contribute to birth defects, infertility, immunosuppression, impaired cognitive development, and some types of cancers. These effects have been linked to the potential of POPs to act as endocrine disruptors—i.e., hormonal mimics. The further production and use of most POPs have been banned, but concern remains over the possible low-level effects of POPs that persist in the environment and in human tissues. Concern has been raised, for example, that population exposures to POPs are contributing to worldwide declines in sperm density and increased rates of congenital hypospadias and testicular and breast cancer; epidemiologic studies testing these theories have yielded mixed results, however, and more research is needed.

GLOBAL CLIMATIC CHANGES An increasing body of evidence indicates that human activities are responsible for global climatic changes, which, in turn, may be directly or indirectly increasing human exposure to environmental hazards. The depletion of stratospheric ozone by chlorinated fluorocarbons, with a consequent increase in ultraviolet radiation exposure, has been firmly established. Increased risks of skin cancers and cataracts are accepted as results of this phenomenon. Less clear is whether the immunosuppressive effects of ultraviolet radiation detected in animals and in vitro have significant clinical impacts on human resistance to infection. Although uncertainties in climate modeling persist, an increasing if not overwhelming amount of evidence indicates that anthropogenic greenhouse gases are fostering global warming. A prominent concern is that global warming can abet the introduction and dissemination of serious infectious diseases, such as mosquito-borne infections (malaria, dengue, and viral encephalitis) and waterborne infectious and toxin-related illnesses (cholera, shellfish poisoning). The World Health Organization has identified global warming as one of the largest public health challenges facing the twenty-first century.

BIBLIOGRAPHY

BARTHA L et al: Multiple chemical sensitivity: A 1999 consensus. Arch Environ Health 54:147, 1999

DOLK H et al: Risk of congenital anomalies near hazardous-waste landfill sites in Europe: The EUROHAZCON Study. Lancet 352:423, 1998

FISHER BE: Most unwanted—persistent organic pollutants. Environ Health Perspect 107: A18, 1999

GRAVELING RA et al: A review of multiple chemical sensitivity. Occup Environ Med 56: 73, 1999

JOHNSON BL, DEROSA C: The toxicologic hazard of Superfund hazardous-waste sites. Rev Environ Health 12:235, 1997

MCMICHAEL AJ, HAINES A: Global climate change: The potential effects on health. BMJ 315:805, 1997

MENZIES D, BOURBEAU J: Building-related illness. N Engl J Med 337:1524, 1997

PATZ JA et al: Global climate change and emerging infectious diseases. JAMA 275:217, 1996

392   *Jerome H. Modell*

DROWNING AND NEAR-DROWNING

It is an unexpected tragedy when a previously healthy person dies or is exposed to severe cerebral hypoxia and suffers permanent brain damage. For many years, drowning was considered a "fight for survival": Arms flailing and screaming for help, a person who could not swim struggled to remain on the surface of the water to reach safety. This situation, however, is rarely reported by persons at the scene of aquatic emergencies. Furthermore, no single set of circumstances comprises drowning or near-drowning. It may be a secondary event following such precursors as head or spinal trauma; hypoxia-induced unconsciousness; or unconsciousness due to preexisting cardiovascular disease, sudden cardiac death, or myocardial infarction. The initiating event is usually unknown, so the drowned or near-drowned victim must be treated based on probable physiologic effects of the near-drowning itself. If survival with normal brain function is to occur, a thorough understanding of the pathophysiology of drowning and an organized approach to therapy are imperative.

PATHOPHYSIOLOGY OF DROWNING Approximately 90% of near-drowning victims aspirate fluid into their lungs. In those who do not aspirate fluid, hypoxemia results simply from breath holding, laryngospasm, or apnea. In those who do aspirate, the volume and the composition of the fluid determine the physiologic basis of the hypoxemia. Freshwater aspiration alters the surface tension properties of pulmonary surfactant and makes alveoli unstable, which causes a decreased ventilation/perfusion ratio. Some alveoli collapse and become atelectatic, which produces a true or absolute intrapulmonary shunt, while others are poorly ventilated and produce a relative shunt; in either case, significant pulmonary venous admixture occurs. Fresh water in the alveoli is hypotonic and is rapidly absorbed and redistributed throughout the body. While some have proposed that water continues to enter the lungs after death, at autopsy the lungs of victims who died in the water frequently contain little water. Also, it has been shown experimentally that if a dead body is submerged in tagged or colored water, water is not found in the lungs at autopsy. These findings support the premise that active respiration determines the volume of water aspirated

Hypertonic seawater pulls additional fluid from the plasma into the lungs, and thus the alveoli are fluid-filled but perfused, which causes substantial pulmonary venous admixture. With both types of water, pulmonary edema may occur secondary to events such as fluid shifts, a change in capillary permeability, or cerebral hypoxia, which causes neurogenic pulmonary edema. Regardless of the cause, pulmonary edema adds to the ventilation/perfusion abnormality.

Water that is grossly contaminated with bacteria or that contains particulate matter may complicate the picture. Particulate matter can obstruct the smaller bronchi and respiratory bronchioles. Grossly contaminated water increases the risk of severe pulmonary infection. Neither problem is sufficiently common, however, to justify recommending specific therapy routinely for all victims.

At least 85% of near-drowned victims are thought to aspirate 22 mL/kg of water or less, which does not result in a clinically significant alteration of blood volume or serum electrolyte concentrations. After resuscitation, by the time blood is analyzed, serum electrolyte concentrations are usually normal or close to normal. Significant changes are documented in only approximately 15% of those who cannot be resuscitated and only rarely in those who are resuscitated. These findings suggest that either a small amount of water was aspirated, fluid was rapidly redistributed, or both. Therefore, electrolyte disturbance rarely needs treatment. When a large quantity of water is aspirated, seawater causes hypovolemia, which concentrates extracellular electrolytes, and fresh water causes acute hypervolemia. If enough water is aspirated that plasma becomes severely hypotonic and the patient is hypoxemic, red cell membranes can rupture, and plasma hemoglobin and serum potassium concentrations increase significantly. However, this development has been reported only rarely. With rapid redistribution of fluid and development of pulmonary edema, even freshwater victims frequently demonstrate hypovolemia by the time they reach the hospital.

Hypercarbia, which is associated with apnea and/or hypoventilation, is less often documented by blood gas analysis than is hypoxemia. While hypoxemia due to pulmonary venous admixture persists in all near-drowned victims who aspirate water, hypercarbia is usually corrected sooner with artificial mechanical ventilation and improved minute ventilation and, thus, is reported in only a small percentage of victims evaluated at the hospital. Besides hypoxemia, metabolic acidosis also persists in most patients. Abnormal cardiovascular function, usually ascribed to hypoxemia, is brief with effective, timely therapy. Abnormality in renal function is uncommon, but when it does occur, it too is secondary to hypoxemia, altered renal perfusion, or, in extremely rare circumstances, significant hemoglobinuria.

℞ **TREATMENT** The first step is retrieving the victim from the water, and, if necessary, performing artificial ventilation and circulation. The American Heart Association recommends that an ab-

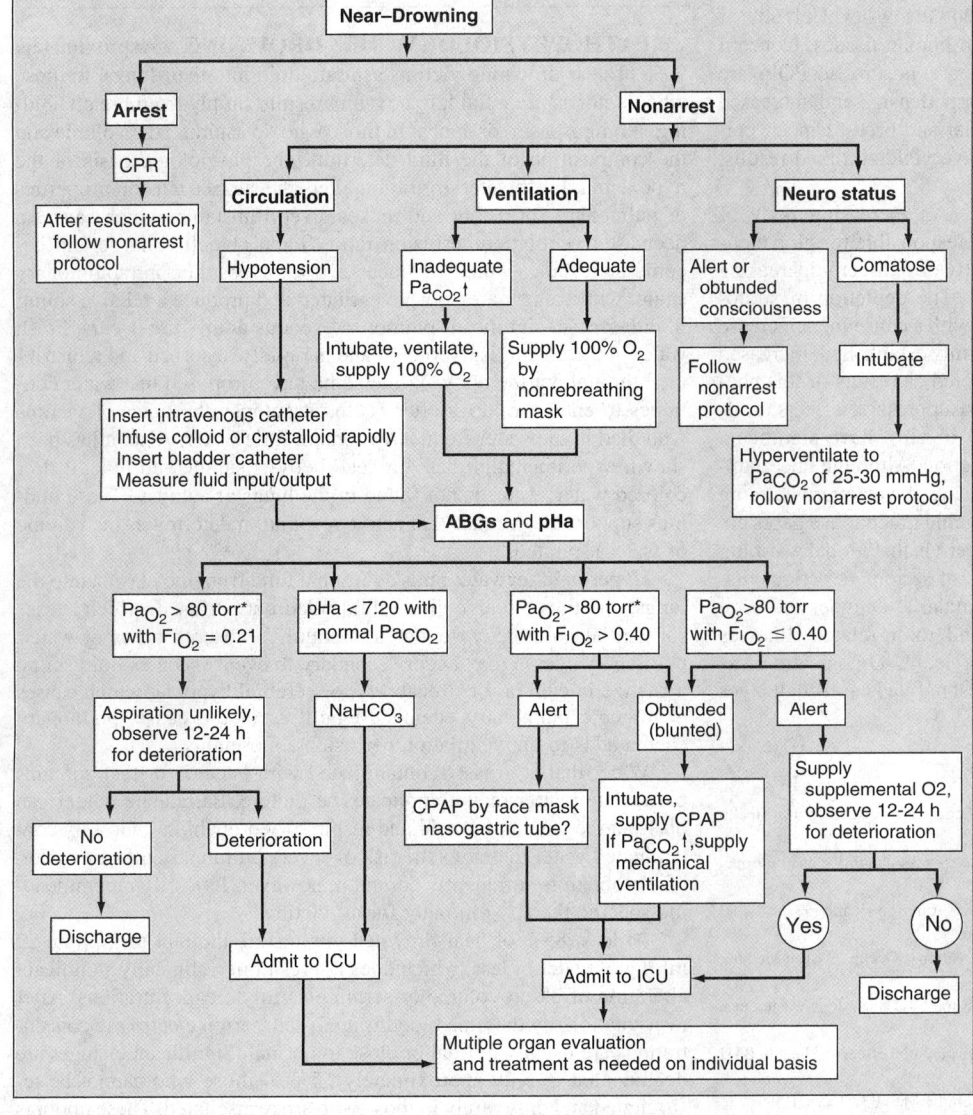

FIGURE 392-1 Treatment of a near-drowned victim should follow a sequence of priorities. *Guidelines only; assumes victim had normal arterial blood gas values (ABGs) before near-drowning. Abbreviations/definitions: CPAP, continuous positive airway pressure; CPR, cardiopulmonary resuscitation; $F_{I_{O_2}}$, fraction of inspired oxygen; intubate: endotracheal intubation; ICU, intensive care unit; $NaHCO_3$, bicarbonate; Pa_{O_2}/Pa_{CO_2}, arterial oxygen/carbon dioxide tension; pHa, arterial pH. *(Modified from Graves and Layon.)*

dominal thrust not be used routinely in victims of submersion. This recommendation was upheld by a special committee of the Institute of Medicine convened in 1994 specifically to evaluate the efficacy of an abdominal thrust in the treatment of near-drowned victims. In these patients, an abdominal thrust may lead to regurgitation of gastric contents and, thus, to aspiration of the vomitus. Further, an abdominal thrust may delay ventilatory or circulatory resuscitation. Therefore, an abdominal thrust should be used only when the airway is obstructed with a foreign body or when the victim fails to respond to mouth-to-mouth ventilation.

Because emergency services and intensive pulmonary and cardiovascular care have improved during the past 25 years, central nervous system depression now presents the major therapeutic challenge in near-drowning. The rate of survival with normal cerebral function varies considerably in retrospective studies. Some factors that adversely influence survival are prolonged submersion, delay in initiation of effective cardiopulmonary resuscitation, severe metabolic acidosis (pH < 7.1), asystole upon arrival at a medical facility, fixed dilated pupils, and a low Glasgow coma score (<5). None of these predictors is absolute, however, and, when maximally treated, normal survivors have been reported in all of the above categories. Absence of cortical

evoked potentials does indicate irreversibility of the cerebral hypoxic lesion; this test, however, cannot be done in the field to guide rescuers. A comparison of outcomes between one institution that added brain preservation techniques to intensive pulmonary and circulatory treatment and another institution that did not found no significant differences.

Hypothermia appears to be protective, but only if it occurs early, at the time of the accident, in which case it increases the victim's chance of cerebral salvage after relatively long periods of acute hypoxia and cardiac arrest. While hypothermia prolongs tolerance to hypoxia, it also can precipitate fatal cardiac arrhythmia; thus, its occurrence can be helpful on the one hand and harmful on the other. The diving reflex produces bradycardia, breath holding, and circulatory redistribution when the face is submerged in cold water. However, the effect of the diving reflex in explaining cerebral recovery after prolonged immersion has not been specifically documented.

Significant pulmonary venous admixture usually persists even after successful resuscitation; therefore, supplemental oxygen should be administered until arterial blood gas analysis confirms that oxygen is no longer needed. Intravenous access should be established as soon as possible. The trachea should be intubated if necessary for airway maintenance or to facilitate mechanical ventilatory support. Electrocardiographic monitoring will facilitate prompt treatment of cardiac arrhythmia.

Victims should be transported to a hospital for definitive testing of the adequacy of ventilation and blood gas exchange, cardiac activity, and effective circulating blood volume. Other variables, such as serum electrolyte concentrations, renal function, and cerebral status, should be analyzed as indicated.

The single most effective treatment for hypoxemia, regardless of cause, is mechanical ventilatory support including continuous positive airway pressure (CPAP). After freshwater aspiration, improvement in ventilation/perfusion matching is more consistent when CPAP is combined with mechanical inflation of the lung than with spontaneous respiration. The question of whether CPAP should be combined with spontaneous respiration or with mechanical ventilation should be decided by whether the specific patient can perform the necessary work of breathing, adequately eliminate carbon dioxide, and adequately match ventilation/perfusion ratios. Positive airway pressure should be withdrawn gradually as the lungs stabilize and ventilation/perfusion ratio returns toward normal.

The pH in near-drowned victims is commonly significantly acidotic, which, in turn, can depress cardiac function. The metabolic component of the acidosis, if it results in a pH < 7.20, should be corrected pharmacologically, although there is some disagreement on this point. With cardiovascular instability, cannulation of the pulmonary artery with a Swan-Ganz catheter or evaluation by transesophageal echocardiography is indicated. Many patients will be hypovolemic from loss of fluid into the lung as pulmonary edema or from decreased venous return secondary to increased intrathoracic pressure during mechanical ventilatory support.

Because recovery after long periods of submersion under frigid conditions has been reported, body temperature should be taken into account before a decision is made to terminate therapy. The body temperature of victims depends not only on the temperature of the water from which they are retrieved but also on how well they were insulated by clothing. The volume of water actually aspirated is also important, because a large volume, if distributed before cardiac arrest occurs, can produce rapid central cooling. Thus, cold water can be protective when it produces total-body hypothermia, which decreases metabolic oxygen requirement. On the other hand, cold water may also contribute to the accident if hypothermia occurs before total submersion, and severe, or even fatal, cardiac arrhythmia results. Several methods of rewarming hypothermic victims have been advocated, but any technique that increases oxygen utilization, such as shivering, should be avoided.

Regardless of the conditions surrounding a drowning or near-drowning, treatment should adhere to the following sequence of priorities (Fig. 392-1):

1. Remove the victim from the water as soon as possible and stabilize the patient's head and neck if trauma is suspected.
2. Immediately follow the ABCs of cardiopulmonary resuscitation—even in the water if this does not endanger the rescuer.
3. If the patient is unconscious, protect the airway as needed with endotracheal intubation.
4. Establish venous access as soon as possible.
5. Provide supplemental oxygen and ventilatory support until each is no longer needed. This can be judged from analysis of arterial blood for oxygen tension, carbon dioxide tension, and pH.
6. Monitor cardiac rhythm with an electrocardioscope as soon as possible.
7. Monitor body temperature and restore it to normal.
8. If the patient has persistent respiratory insufficiency, provide intensive pulmonary support with CPAP and mechanical ventilation therapy as necessary.
9. If the patient has cardiovascular instability, evaluate cardiac output and effective circulatory volume by invasive monitoring, and measure serum electrolyte concentrations. Intravenous fluid replacement should be provided as necessary.
10. Evaluate and treat renal function and cerebral status as indicated.

Glucocorticoid therapy, prophylactic antibiotic therapy, and monitoring of intracranial pressure are no longer recommended.

ACCIDENT PREVENTION Because drowning begins as an accident that results in a medical problem, the definitive strategy is to prevent the accident. For those victims in whom the accident is secondary to a medical condition, as in persons susceptible to syncope or seizure, the only way to prevent the accident is to identify those who ought to avoid the water or to encourage them to use the buddy system. For young children, early swimming lessons, vigilant caretakers, and stringent laws governing pool enclosures are needed. Those who teach parenting classes should routinely warn parents about the risk of toddlers' drowning in such household fixtures as toilets, buckets of water, and even washing machines. Preventing accidents during boating, athletics, and other water-related recreational activities requires public education. Rules associated with these activities to maximize safety and judicious, responsible behavior should be portrayed as life-saving measures. Similarly, drinking alcohol, a "ubiquitous catalyst" to drowning, should be portrayed as life-threatening whenever water is nearby.

BIBLIOGRAPHY

AMERICAN HEART ASSOCIATION: Guidelines for cardiopulmonary resuscitation and emergency cardiac care. JAMA 268:2171, 1992

BOHN DJ et al: Influence of hypothermia, barbiturate therapy, and intracranial pressure monitoring on morbidity and mortality after near-drowning. Crit Care Med 14:529, 1986

GRAVES SA, LAYON AJ: Drowning and near-drowning, in *Emergency Medicine: A Comprehensive Review*. 3d ed, TC Kravis et al (eds). New York, Raven, 1993, pp 689–700

LAYON AJ, MODELL JH: Drowning and near drowning, in *The Lung at Depth*, C Lundgren, JH Miller (eds). New York, Marcel Dekker, 1999, pp 395–415

MODELL JH: Drowning. N Engl J Med 328:253, 1993

———, GOODWIN SR: Drowning and near-drowning, in *Kendig's Disorders of the Respiratory Tract in Children*, 6th ed, V Chernick, TF Boat (eds). Philadelphia, Saunders, 1998, pp 572–584

——— et al: Drowning without aspiration: Is this an appropriate diagnosis. J Foren Sci. 44:1119, 1999

——— et al: Clinical course of 91 consecutive near-drowning victims. Chest 70:231, 1976

ROSEN P et al (eds): *The Use of the Heimlich Maneuver in Near-Drowning*. Committee on the Treatment of Near-Drowning Victims, Institute of Medicine, Washington, DC, 1994

SWANN HG et al: Freshwater and seawater drowning: A study of the terminal cardiac and biochemical events. Texas Rep Biol Med 5:423, 1947

393 *Raphael C. Lee*

ELECTRICAL INJURIES

EPIDEMIOLOGY Electrical injury occurs when the body experiences levels of current that alter electrophysiologic function or cause tissue damage. Most commonly, such injuries result from contact with commercial electrical power sources in the home and workplace. Microwave, radiofrequency, light irradiation, and other injuries are less common. Ionizing electromagnetic fields (radiation) involve atomic absorption and free radical production, leading to biochemical alterations.

Electrical shock is one of the leading causes of work related injury, comprising 7% of all workplace fatalities. The exact incidence is unknown because many victims don't report minor injuries. The economic impact of industrial electrical injury in the United States is estimated to be in excess of $1 billion annually. Approximately one-third of high-power electrical injuries occur in the construction industry, one-third occur in the utility and petrochemical industries, and one-third are non-work related. More than 90% of the injuries occur in males, most commonly between the ages of 20 and 34. The extremities are nearly always involved, and limb amputation may be required.

Most injuries are due to low-voltage (<1000 V) electrical shock. Low-voltage power-frequency electrical shocks usually occur in and around the home. The household electric power in the United States is 120 V, AC 60-cycle current. In Europe it is 220 V. Low-voltage shocks carry a significant risk of electrocution due to cardiac arrest because they may cause muscle spasm that results in prolonged contact. Roughly 3 to 4% of all United States hospital burn unit admissions are for electrical injury, mostly a result of high-voltage (>1000 V) shocks. Extensive tissue damage, rather than electrocution, is characteristic of high-voltage shocks.

PATHOPHYSIOLOGY The term *direct current* (DC) is used to indicate a field frequency of zero (i.e., constant voltage gradient), and *alternating current* (AC) indicates that the field is changing direction (i.e., alternating polarity) with time. DC electrical power passes through the body on direct electrical contact. AC current can be carried by direct contact, capacitive coupling, and magnetic induction.

Tissue damage can result from exposure to harmful levels of current at any frequency in the electromagnetic spectrum that ranges from DC to ζ-hertz (ionizing irradiation). The tissue effects of electricity depend as much on the frequency as on the magnitude of current. Table 393-1 presents a classification of electrical injury according to fre-

Table 393-1   Electrical Injuries by Frequency Range

Frequency Range	General Applications	Harmful Tissue Effects
Low (DC–10 KHz)	Commercial electrical power, batteries	Joule heating, cell membrane electro-poration
Radiofrequency (10 KHz–10 MHz)	Radiocommunication, diatherm, electro-cautery	Joule heating, dielec-tric heating of pro-teins
Microwave (10 MHz–10 GHz)	Microwave heating	Dielectric heating of water
Light and ionizing ($\geq 10^{15}$ Hz)	Photooptical and ion-izing irradiation (ul-traviolet, x-ray, gamma)	Reactive oxygen in-termediates produc-tion

quency range. Commercial electrical power operates in the narrow frequency range of DC to 150 Hz in the low frequency regime. An electrical shock in this frequency range is most common.

When the voltage is <1000 V, direct mechanical contact is usually required for electrical contact. For high voltages (>1000 V), arcing usually initiates the electrical contact. On direct electrical contact, the electron flow in the metal conductor or arc is converted at the skin surface into electrolyte ions that carry the current through the body. This electrochemical process generates heat and toxic chemical by-products that contribute to contact area injury. In high-voltage con-tacts, exposure to the expanding arc, an excellent conductor, brings the victim into the electrical circuit. The arc can reach very high tem-peratures, leading to skin burns or clothing ignition. At higher fre-quencies (>10 MHz) electrical power can couple electrical energy across an air gap into the body without charge transport across the skin surface (capacitive coupling).

Low-frequency electricity causes tissue injury primarily by per-meabilizing cell membranes, electroconformational denaturation of cell membrane proteins, and thermal denaturation of tissue proteins. Factors that determine the anatomic pattern, the extent of tissue injury, and the relative contribution of heat versus direct electrical damage include the amount of current, anatomic location, and the contact du-ration. The type of clothing, the use of protective gear, and the power capability of the electrical source also contribute to the wide range of clinical manifestations in victims of electrical shock. In addition, a very high-energy electrical arc can produce a strong thermoacoustic blast force leading to barotrauma. Associated falls and skin burns are frequent, exacerbating the injury. Cataracts characteristically occur af-ter rapid and brief exposure of the eyes to hot gases and arc-mediated electrical current. The latency period for development of cataracts av-erages approximately 6 months.

Peripheral nerve and skeletal muscle tissues are most vulnerable to membrane damage by applied electrical currents. The "no-let-go" phenomenon results from the passage of more than 14 to 16 mA lon-gitudinally through the forearm that induces tetanic contractions of muscles controlling handgrip. The resulting involuntary muscle spasm may lead to joint dislocations and spine fractures. When current of >50 mA is passed hand-to-hand or hand-to-foot, there is enough in-duced depolarization of myocardial membranes to cause cardiac ar-rhythmias, particularly if the induced depolarization occurs during early myocardial repolarization. Disruption of extremity skeletal mus-cle and nerve cell membranes by the process of electroporation results when more than 0.5 to 1 A is passed through the extremity. Electro-poration damage accumulates on the time scale of milliseconds, lead-ing to lethal cellular injury. With more prolonged contacts in the range of seconds, thermal damage in the subcutaneous tissues becomes sub-stantial. Because the vulnerability to supraphysiologic temperature ex-posure is similar regardless of tissue type, all tissues in the current path are burned when pathologic levels of heating occur. Extensive disruption of cell membranes leads to release of myoglobin and he-

moglobin, which enter the circulation. Acute renal failure can result from intrarenal crystalization of these molecules. Acute renal failure superimposed on extensive tissue injury has a very high mortality rate.

DIAGNOSIS   For the more common low-frequency electrical injuries, at least two skin contact wounds are present. Differences in wound size and topography are largely determined by the surface con-tact area, the shape of the objects that conducted the current through the victim, and the duration of contact.

Cardiac arrhythmias and most respiratory disturbances must be rapidly detected by examination of the pulse, chest, and electrocardi-ogram. The next priority is to determine the location and extent of tissue damage. Injured skeletal muscle and nerves are often found beneath undamaged skin. Lateral spine x-rays or computed tomogra-phy (CT) are needed to rule out unstable spine fracture patterns. X-ray images of the extremities involved are also important to rule out skeletal fractures or joint dislocations. Blood chemistries should be immediately evaluated and monitored. Metabolic acidosis and elevated serum potassium levels may exist as consequences of extensive skel-etal muscle injury. Serum CPK levels will rise over several hours if there is significant rhabdomyolysis.

Tissue edema begins to form because of increased vascular per-meability and the release of intracellular contents into the extravascular space. Muscle compartment syndrome and compression neuropathies are common manifestations. If available, magnetic resonance imaging (MRI) scans can rapidly localize tissue edema. Where severe heating has coagulated the blood vessels, tissue injury may exist in the absence of edema. Muscle compartment fluid pressures should be measured where edema is present. If MRI is not available, then the muscle com-partments in the current path between contact points should be mon-itored for elevated interstitial fluid pressure. Elevated compartment pressures may evolve during resuscitation. Muscle compartment fluid pressures >30 cmH₂0 are indications for fasciotomy. It may be nec-essary to check the pressures every 8 h for 24 h. Radionucleotide scanning with ^{99m}Tc-pyrophosphate can also be useful to detect tissue damage. These scans, however, take 4 to 6 h to complete and are mostly useful in the less severe injuries. If there is a history of loss of consciousness, CT of the head is indicated.

TREATMENT   The first priority is to disconnect the patient from the electrical power source. When high-capacity circuits are involved, disconnection must not be attempted before the circuit is deenergized. Cervical spine fracture should be assumed until proven otherwise. Critical initial considerations are evaluation and support of vital organ function and, secondarily, assessment of the extent of in-jury. After very-high voltage trauma, prolonged cardiopulmonary re-suscitation (CPR) may be necessary before the stunned myocardium regains the ability to sustain a coordinated rhythm.

Patients with significant wounds and tissue injury as well as those with vital organ injury require hospital admission. It is unlikely for cardiac arrhythmias to develop if cardiac injury is not detectable on initial presentation. Peripheral nerve injury invariably occurs even in minor shocks and usually resolves over several days. If symptoms persist, however, they may be controlled with cyclooxygenase inhib-itors alone or with antioxidants. Small wounds can be managed by cleaning and applying topical antibiotics. Major neuropsychological and stress disorders often follow a terrifying "no-let-go" experience. Management often involves psychiatric consultation.

For more substantial trauma, a Foley catheter and large bore pe-ripheral intravenous lines delivering normal saline at a rate sufficient to generate a 30 to 50 mL/h urine output are essential. If the urine is visibly pigmented with myoglobin or hemoglobin, the output should be doubled and alkalinized to a pH >6 by adding bicarbonate to the intravenous solutions until the urine has cleared. In the most severe injuries, hyperpermeability of peripheral capillaries may result in rapid interstitial (third space) fluid accumulation. In such cases, it may be necessary to increase blood oxygen levels and add dextran to resus-citation fluids.

Cardiac arrhythmias must be immediately controlled by antiarrhythmic drugs simultaneously with the correction of serum pH and electrolyte abnormalities. Brain injury–related seizures must be controlled with antiepileptic agents. Patients who have lost central nervous system (CNS) control of respiration or airways should be intubated and mechanically ventilated. A paralyzed ventilated patient may need monitoring by electroencephalogram (EEG) to assess seizure control. Appropriate management of corneal burns or abrasions, tympanic membrane rupture, and closed head injury should be instituted.

Large skin burn wounds are often present because of arc-mediated contacts and clothing ignition. Care should be taken to prevent rapid loss of body heat through open wounds. Tetanus prophylaxis should be administered.

Perfusion of devascularized tissue must be quickly restored. Diminished pulses or decreased tissue oxygen by transcutaneous pulse oximetry are indications for escharotomy releases. Fasciotomy is often required. The classic clinical signs of pain in acute compartment syndrome cannot be relied on because of associated nerve injury. In addition to decompression of extremity muscle compartments, decompression of nerve within edematous fibrous and osseous conduits (e.g., carpal tunnel, Guyon's canal, and tarsal tunnel) should be carried out to help prevent compression neuropathy. Care to avoid tissue drying or desiccation is important. Debridement of nonviable subcutaneous tissue should be performed as soon as a general anesthetic can be safely administered.

Anaerobic bacterial infection of devascularized skeletal muscle is a common complication. Intravenous penicillin G and/or hyperbaric oxygen as prophylactic antibiotics are sometimes utilized but have unproven value. Radiographs taken to rule out fractures may reveal air bubbles in the subcutaneous tissues. This gas results from tissue boiling when prolonged Joule heating has occurred.

Rehabilitation into society and gainful employment are the ultimate objectives. For severely injured victims these goals require functional muscle and nerve reconstruction as well as correction of scar contractures. Psychological and neurocognitive problems are expected and require treatment by experts. Persistent peripheral neurologic problems are also common and often require detailed evaluation and therapeutic intervention.

LIGHTNING INJURIES

Lightning injury is a powerful manifestation of arc-mediated electrical contact. Arcing occurs when the voltage gradient in air exceeds 2 million V/m. The arc consists of a hot ionized gas of subatomic particles that is highly conductive. Peak lightning currents reach into the range of 30,000 to 50,000 A for a duration of 5 to 10 μs. Lightning arc temperatures reach up to 30,000°K, which generates thermoacoustic blast waves, commonly called thunder. Peak blast pressures reach 4 or 5 atm in the immediate vicinity of a lightning strike, and up to 1 or 2 atm 1 m away. Substantial barotrauma can result.

Like radiofrequency current, lightning current flows along the surfaces of conducting objects. Initially, the flow of an enormous current through the lightning strike generates a very large surrounding magnetic field pulse. This magnetic field pulse can induce current flow in the body, enough to disrupt cardiac and CNS function. When lightning current enters the ground, it spreads out radially, which sets a large current traveling along the surfaces of the ground. A substantial voltage drop can occur between the feet of a nearby individual. The voltage drops between widely separated feet can reach 1500 to 2000 V and can induce a 2 to 3 A current flow in the legs for a 10-μs period.

Victims of direct lightning strikes experience a multimodal injury. Superficial burns on the skin represent the current path along the skin surface. The intense brief shock pulse seems to arrest all electrophysiologic processes. The victim appears lifeless. Prolonged CPR may be necessary. Muscle and nerve necrosis is rare in survivors. Deeper injury results when the victim is in contact with a large conducting object such as a truck or fence that has been struck by lightning, which then discharges over several milliseconds through the victim.

Delay in resuscitation is the most common cause of death. By-standers are usually afraid to touch the victim while precious minutes pass. However, unless the victim is on an insulating platform, there is no residual electric charge on the body after several milliseconds. When needed, CPR should be given without hesitation. Victims should be cared for in an intensive care unit until life-threatening CNS and cardiac injuries are ruled out. Late neurologic and ophthalmologic sequelae often develop.

BIBLIOGRAPHY

DeBono R: A histological analysis of a high voltage electric current injury to an upper limb. Burns 25:541, 1999

Lederer W et al: Electricity-associated injuries II: Outdoor management of lightning-induced casualties. Resuscitation 43:89, 2000

Lee RC: Injury by electrical forces: Pathophysiology, manifestations, and therapy. Curr Probl Surgery 34(9):677–764, 1997

Lee RC, Capelli-Schellpfeffer M, Kelley KM (eds): *Electrical Injury: A Multidisciplinary Approach to Therapy, Prevention and Rehabilitation.* Ann NY Acad Sci vol. 720, 1994

Luce EA: Electrical burns. Clin Plast Surg 27:133, 2000

394 *Stephen M. Hahn, Eli Glatstein*

RADIATION INJURY

All human beings are constantly exposed to ionizing radiation. Environmental sources include the cosmic radiation from space and radiation from the ground and from inhaled and ingested materials. Airline travel and mining both increase exposure to the background radiation. For example, air travel at 30,000 ft exposes individuals to a dose equivalent of 0.5 mrem/h. Radiation originating in the body comes mainly from radioactive potassium, which emits beta and gamma rays. Lungs are exposed to irradiation from inhaled air, which contains small amounts of radioactive radon. The cosmic exposure contributes approximately 28 mrem per year. The ground and internal sources contribute approximately 26 and 27 mrem per year, respectively. The most prominent man-made sources of radiation include x-ray equipment, nuclear weapons, and radioactive medications.

TERMINOLOGY AND DEFINITIONS

The first major unit of radiation exposure was the roentgen (R), defined as an amount of x-rays or gamma rays that produces a specific amount of ionization in a unit of air under standard temperature and pressure (Table 394-1); this quantity can be measured directly in an ionization chamber. The rad, or *r*adiation *a*bsorbed *d*ose, is defined as 100 ergs/g of tissue. Thus, the rad represents a net deposition of energy in a three-dimensional volume, because x-rays attenuate as they traverse tissue. The rad has been replaced by the Système Internationale (SI)

Table 394-1 Units and Definitions

Unit	Quantity Measured	Definition
Roentgen (R)	Exposure	Amount of x-rays or gamma rays that produces a specific amount of ionization in a given volume of air
Rad	Dose	100 ergs deposited per gram of tissue
Gray (Gy)	Dose	SI unit of dose; equals 100 rad
Rem	Dose equivalence	Unit that reflects the biologic response. It is used to compare various types of radiation
Sievert (Sv)	Dose equivalence	SI unit of dose equivalence; equals 100 rem

unit of the gray (Gy), which represents 100 rad. Roentgens and rads can be converted by means of various tables; the relation between them depends on photon energy.

The above definitions reflect physical variables. The unit that reflects the biologic response and that can be used to compare the effects of various types of radiation is the unit of *dose equivalence*, the rem (*roentgen equivalent in man*). The rem has been replaced by the SI unit, the sievert (Sv), which equals 100 rem. These units reflect the exposure or absorption dose multiplied by a biologic factor that represents the biologic effectiveness of the specific type of radiation (see below).

TYPES OF IONIZING RADIATION

The absorption of energy from radiation in tissue often leads to excitation or ionization. Excitation involves elevation of an electron in an atom or molecule to a higher energy state without actual ejection of the electron. Ionization involves actual ejection of one or more electrons from the atom. Ionizing radiation is subclassified as electromagnetic (photon) or particulate radiation (Table 394-2). X-rays and gamma rays are examples of electromagnetic photon radiation. They differ only in their source: X-rays are produced mechanically, by making electrons strike a target, which causes the electrons to give up their kinetic energy as x-rays, while gamma rays are produced by nuclear disintegration of radioactive isotopes.

X-rays can be thought of as packets of energy, or photons. X-rays have no mass or charge, travel in straight lines, and attenuate continuously as they traverse tissue. Gamma rays have similar properties. Each photon contains an amount of energy equal to $h\nu$, where h is Planck's constant. The critical difference between nonionizing and ionizing radiation is the energy of individual photons, not the energy of the total dose.

Types of *particulate radiation* include electrons, protons, alpha particles, neutrons, negative pi-mesons, and heavy charged ions; these have discrete mass and charge (except for neutrons, which lack charge; Table 394-2). *Electrons*, or *beta particles*, are small and negatively charged and can be accelerated to close to the speed of light. They decelerate fairly rapidly in tissue and penetrate it to only a limited depth. Thus, electron beams are often used to treat superficial problems. *Protons* are positively charged and have a mass about 2000 times that of an electron. Protons stop abruptly, depending on their energy; in the process of sudden deceleration, most of their energy is given up, which tends to cause ionization just before the proton stops. This region of enhanced ionization, sometimes called the Bragg peak, means that proton beams exert their effects in a relatively compact region. *Alpha particles* are helium nuclei, consisting of two protons

and two neutrons. The mass and charge are great enough that these particles do not penetrate far through matter unless they have tremendous energy; even a piece of paper is enough to protect against most alpha particles. Because these particles are charged, they can be accelerated in electrical fields.

Neutrons are similar in mass to protons (having an atomic mass of 1), but they are not charged and therefore cannot be accelerated in an electrical field. Neutron beams are produced by colliding charged particles into a suitable target or are emitted as a fission product of heavy radioactive atoms. *Heavy charged ions* are nuclei of heavier elements that have a positive charge owing to the stripping away of some or all of the orbiting electrons.

Equal doses of different types of radiation do not necessarily produce equal biologic effects; thus 1 Gy of neutrons produces a greater biologic effect than 1 Gy of x-rays. The biologic effects produced by a given dose of radiation can be quantified by the relative biologic effectiveness (RBE) value, which relates them to the effects produced by 250-kV photon radiation as a standard. In general, the greater the RBE value for a given type of radiation, the greater the biologic effect. The RBE value will be greater for more densely ionizing radiation, such as neutrons. The RBE value depends on the linear energy transfer (see below), the dose, the dose rate, and the nature of the biologic system.

The linear energy transfer (LET) is the amount of ionization occurring per unit length of the radiation track. It is usually expressed as kilovolts per micron and increases with the square of the charge of the incident particle. High-LET radiation is biologically different from low-LET (i.e., conventional) radiation: Hypoxic and oxygenated cells respond similarly to high-LET irradiation, whereas it takes about three times as much low-LET radiation to produce a given killing effect in hypoxic cells as in oxygenated cells. It is thought that low-LET radiation must produce multiple hits on DNA to destroy a cell, whereas high-LET radiation need produce only a single hit on DNA to kill a cell. Representative values of LET and RBE are given in Table 394-3.

Radiation, especially x-rays, is absorbed and causes ionization in three major ways: the *photoelectric effect*, the *Compton effect*, and *pair production*. At low energies (30 to 100 keV), as in diagnostic radiology, the photoelectric effect is important. In this process, the incident photon interacts with an electron in one of the outer shells of an atom (typically K, L, or M). If the energy of the photon is greater than the binding energy of the electron, then the electron is expelled from the orbit with a kinetic energy that is equal to the energy of the incident photon minus the binding energy of the electron. The photoelectric effect varies as a function of the cube of the atomic number of the material exposed (Z^3); this fact explains why bone is visualized much better than soft tissue on radiographs.

At higher energies, as used in therapeutic radiology, the Compton effect dominates. In this process, the incident photon interacts with an electron in an orbital shell. Part of the incident photon energy appears as kinetic energy of electrons, and the residual energy continues as a less energetic deflected photon.

At energy levels above 1.02 MeV, the photons may be absorbed

Table 394-2   Common Types of Ionizing Radiation

Type	Mass	Charge	Comment
Electromagnetic			
X-ray	0	0	X-rays and gamma rays do not differ except in the source. Gamma rays are produced intranuclearly, and x-rays are produced extranuclearly (i.e., mechanically).
Gamma ray	0	0	
Particulate			
Electron (e)	9.1×10^{-31} kg	-1	—
Proton (p)	$2000 \times e$	$+1$	Exhibits a Bragg peak
Neutron (n)	$2000 \times e$	0	Cannot be accelerated by an electrical field
Alpha particle	2p + 2n $\sim 8000 \times e$	$+2$	Helium nucleus

Table 394-3   Linear Energy Transfer (LET) and Relative Biologic Effectiveness (RBE) Values

Type of Radiation	LET Values, keV/μm
Cobalt-60 gamma rays	0.2
250-keV x-rays	2.0
10 MeV protons	4.7

Type of Radiation	RBE Values (Quality Factors)
X-rays, gamma rays, and electrons	1
Neutrons	3–20
Heavy particles	1–20

through pair production. In this process, both a positron and an electron are produced in the absorbing material. A positron has the same mass as an electron but has a positive instead of a negative charge. The positron travels a very short distance in the absorbing medium before it interacts with another electron. When that happens, the entire mass of both particles is converted to energy, with the emission of two photons in exactly opposite directions.

BIOLOGIC EFFECTS OF RADIATION

Radiation must produce double-strand breaks in DNA to kill a cell, owing partly to the high capacity of mammalian cells for repairing single-strand damage. Radiation can also produce effects indirectly by interacting with water (which makes up approximately 80% of a cell's volume) to generate free radicals, which can damage the cell. Free radicals are highly reactive chemical entities that lack a stable number of outer-shell electrons. A free radical is not stable and has a life span of a fraction of a second. It is estimated that most x-ray-induced cell damage is due to the formation of hydroxyl radicals, as follows:

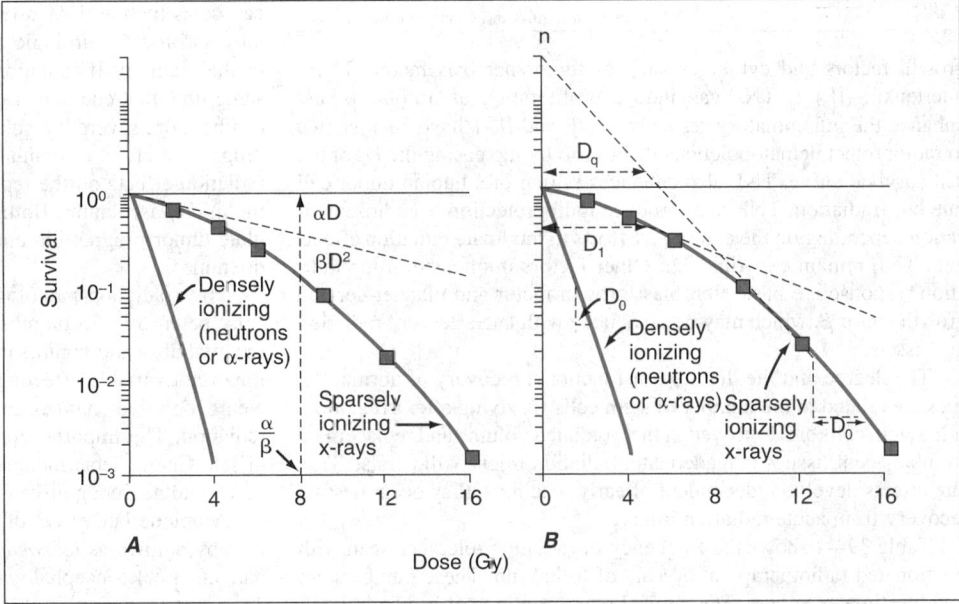

FIGURE 394-1 Shape of survival curve for mammalian cells exposed to radiation. The fraction of cells surviving is plotted on a logarithmic scale against dose on a linear scale. For alpha particles or low-energy neutrons (said to be densely ionizing) the dose-response curve is a straight line from the origin (i.e., survival is an exponential function of dose). The survival curve can be described by just one parameter, the slope. For x-rays or gamma rays (said to be sparsely ionizing), the dose-response curve has an initial linear slope, followed by a shoulder; at higher doses the curve tends to become straight again. A. The experimental data are fitted to a linear-quadratic function. There are two components of cell killing: one is proportional to dose (αD), while the other is proportional to the square of the dose (βD^2). The dose at which the linear and quadratic components are equal is the ratio α/β. The linear-quadratic curve bends continuously but is a good fit to experimental data for the first few decades of survival. B. The curve is described by the initial slope (D_1), the final slope (D_0), and a parameter that represents the width of the shoulder, either n or D_q. (From Hall, with permission.)

$$\text{Ionizing radiation} + H_2O \rightarrow H_2O^+ + e^-$$
$$H_2O^+ + H_2O \rightarrow H_3O^+ + OH\bullet$$
$$OH\bullet \rightarrow \text{Cell damage}$$

The result of radiation damage is cell death. The biologic effects on epithelial cell reproduction are typically expressed only when the damaged cells attempt to divide. Another biologic effect is the induction of cancerous growth by mutation many years after radiation exposure. Patients who receive radiation have a significant risk of neoplasm two to three decades after their exposure; this risk is significantly higher than that of the population as a whole.

RADIATION-INDUCED CHROMOSOME ABERRATIONS Chromosome breaks can occur when cells are irradiated. The broken ends of chromosomes can combine with broken ends of different chromosomes. These abnormal combinations are most readily seen during mitosis. Chromosome abnormalities typically occur in cells irradiated in the G1 phase of the cell cycle, before the doubling of genetic material. If cells are irradiated in the G2 phase, chromatid aberrations may result. The frequency of chromosomal aberrations in peripheral circulating lymphocytes correlates with the dose received. The dose can be estimated by comparing the chromosomal changes to in vitro cultures exposed to controlled doses of irradiation. The minimum dose that can be detected by peripheral lymphocyte analysis is about 0.1 to 0.2 Sv (10 to 20 rem). Lymphocyte analysis may provide evidence of recent total-body exposure.

CELL SURVIVAL CURVE The dose-response curve for all mammalian cells appears to have a linear-quadratic relationship. In simple terms, the mathematical model that explains the relationship between the dose and the fraction of surviving cells has both linear and exponential components. The linear component results from double-stranded chromosomal breaks produced by single hits. The exponential component represents breaks produced by multiple hits. Figure 394-1 shows the shape of a typical survival curve for mammalian cells exposed to radiation. The fraction of cells surviving is plotted on a semilogarithmic scale. For x-rays or gamma rays, the dose-response curve has a shoulder that is followed by a straight line curve as the dose is increased. The shoulder represents the cell's ability to repair sublethal injury. For alpha particles or lower energy neutrons, the dose-response curve is a straight line from the origin. Thus, the survival rate is an exponential function of the dose.

In all mammalian cell lines studied, increases in the radiation dose decrease the survival rate of cells. However, a number of factors may contribute to a relative resistance to radiation in human tumors in vivo, including hypoxia and expression of particular oncogenes, such as *ras*. The biologic basis for radiation resistance has not been fully defined.

Four important processes that occur after radiation exposure can be summarized as the "four R's" of radiobiology. The first is *repair*. Repair is temperature dependent and is thought to represent the enzymatic mechanisms for healing intracellular injury. The second R is *reoxygenation*, a process whereby oxygen (and other nutrients) are actually better distributed to viable cells following radiation injury and cell killing. The third R is *repopulation*, the ability of the cell population to continue to divide and to replace dying and dead cells. The fourth R is *redistribution*, which reflects the variability of a cell's radiosensitivity over the cell cycle. Radiosensitivity can vary through the cell cycle by as much as a factor of 3. The G1 phase has the most variable length of all the phases of the cell cycle. For most cell lines, cells that have a short G1 period are most sensitive at the G2/mitosis interface, less sensitive in G1, and most resistant toward the end of the synthesis (S) period.

Radiation therapy is effective in cancer treatment when it exerts greater cytotoxic effects on tumor cells than on normal tissues. A major determinant of the therapeutic index is exploiting differences in the four R's between tumor cells and normal tissues by delivering the radiation in dose fractions.

CLINICAL FINDINGS ON FRACTIONATION The clinical radiation response may be related to the interactions of various growth factors and cytokines. For example, radiation can induce growth factors and cytokines such as tumor necrosis factor (TNF), interleukin (IL) 1. TNF can induce proliferation of fibroblasts and enhance the inflammatory response. TNF and IL-1 have been shown to radioprotect hematopoietic cells in vitro by increasing the D_0 of the cell survival curve. TNF also enhances killing of a human tumor cell line by irradiation. TNF may produce radioprotection or radiosensitization depending on the cell type. Efforts to modulate radiation effects with TNF remain experimental. Other factors implicated in the radiation response are basic fibroblast growth factor and platelet-derived growth factor β, which may be associated with late effects of radiation on vessels.

The degree and the duration of functional recovery of normal tissues are related to the number of stem cells surviving after irradiation. If the stem cells are destroyed in the irradiated volume and replacement from adjacent tissues is inadequate, radiation injury will persist. True late effects develop independent of early reactions; they occur despite recovery from acute radiation injury.

Table 394-4 shows the frequency of radiation tolerance seen with fractionated radiotherapy at 5 years of follow-up. These numbers are rough estimates at best. The clinical manifestations of irradiation will depend on the volume of the organ irradiated, the total dose, the dose per fraction, and the length of time taken to deliver the dose. Dose per fraction is the most important factor determining normal tissue effects. In addition, the cellular consequences of treatment can be progressive over time. Thus, length of follow-up is also crucial in judging clinical sequelae.

Central Nervous System Traditionally, the central nervous system (CNS) has been described as relatively resistant to radiation-induced changes. When the human brain is treated with standard fractionation (1.8 to 2.0 Gy/d), acute reactions are seldom observed.

Subacute CNS reactions to radiation treatment are more common. The clinical manifestations may include *Lhermitte's sign*, which is a self-limited paresthesia occurring with flexion of the neck. It is believed to be due to transient demyelination of the spinal cord following significant radiation exposure. It can be seen 1 to 3 months after completion of radiation treatment to the spinal cord. The frequency of Lhermitte's sign varies according to the type of radiation therapy and

can be as high as 15% after mantle-field radiation. Mild encephalopathy and focal neurologic changes can occur after irradiation limited to the cranium. If radiation treatments to the brain are given at the same time that chemotherapeutic agents are administered, the effects can be more severe, presumably reflecting altered permeability to the drugs. The effect of cranial irradiation is believed to be secondary to radiation effects on the replicating oligodendrocytes and possibly on the microvasculature. Both clinical and radiologic changes may simulate tumor progression and can often pose diagnostic and treatment dilemmas.

Postirradiation pathology and associated clinical symptoms typically begin 6 to 36 months after radiation therapy and are related to the total dose and volume treated. Fraction size appears to be the most important variable affecting the rate of postirradiation brain necrosis. Neurocognitive changes can also be seen in children after cranial irradiation. The important pretreatment factors that predict the degree of late CNS effects include the age at which cranial irradiation was given and neurocognitive functional level at the time of treatment.

A unique late effect of cranial irradiation combined with chemotherapy, known as *leukoencephalopathy*, has been described in some patients. Leukoencephalopathy is a necrotizing reaction usually noted 4 to 12 months after combined treatment with methotrexate and cranial irradiation. Dementia and dysarthria may progress to seizures, ataxia, or death.

Transverse myelitis after radiation treatment is a spinal cord reaction similar to cerebral necrosis. This syndrome consists of progressive and irreversible leg weakness and loss of bladder function and sensation referrable to a single spinal cord level. Flaccid paralysis eventually occurs. Symptoms can occur as early as 6 months after radiation treatment, but the usual time to onset is 12 to 24 months. Lhermitte's sign does not correlate with transverse myelitis.

Skin Skin reaction can be seen within 2 weeks of fractionated radiotherapy, a delay that correlates with the time required for cells to move from the basal to the keratinized layer of skin. The severity of the reaction depends on the skin dose per fraction and the total dose delivered to an area of skin. Erythema is observed, soon followed by dry desquamation. The skin at this time can be erythematous, warm, and sometimes edematous. The vessels in the upper dermis are dilated, and inflammatory infiltration with granulocytes, macrophages, eosinophils, plasma cells, and lymphocytes is noted.

When a severe skin reaction occurs, it is usually located where the beam strikes the skin tangentially. *Moist desquamation* consists of eruption of the epidermal layer. Healing is through reepithelialization from cells of less affected basal layers. When skin reactions are severe, treatment interruptions are needed to permit healing.

Dry desquamation is treated conservatively. Symptoms of dryness can be alleviated by advising the patient to wear only cotton fabric next to the affected skin and to refrain from the use of irritants of any kind. If treatment becomes necessary, hydrophilic agents that do not contain heavy metals are recommended. Petroleum jellies should not be used, as they may trap bacteria and increase the chance of infection. Moist desquamation is best managed by leaving the affected area dry and open to air.

A chronic reaction to radiation can be seen starting 6 to 12 months after irradiation. The epidermis is usually atrophic and may be more easily injured than normal skin. Interstitial fibrosis may also be increased. Hyperpigmentation of irradiated skin outlining the treatment field can be seen within a couple of months after completion of irradiation. This will fade gradually. The skin becomes thin, and hair loss may be permanent. Radiation therapy can induce second malignancies, which tend to be more aggressive than cancers arising in patients without significant radiation exposure.

Heart and Blood Vessels When cardiac disease appears after radiation treatment, it is often difficult to tell to what extent the radiation treatment was causative. The pathogenesis of atherosclerotic heart disease is multifactorial. Exposure of a large heart volume to high-dose radiation therapy accelerates the development of coronary artery disease. Acute "pericarditis" may result from cardiac irradiation.

Table 394-4 Class 1 Organs: Fatal or Severe Morbidity Following Cumulative Doses of Radiation Delivered with Standard Fractionation

Organ	Injury	TD$_{5/5}$[a]	TD$_{50/5}$[b]	Whole or Partial Organ (Field Size or Length)
Bone marrow	Aplasia, pancytopenia	250	450	Whole
		3000	4000	Segmental
Liver	Acute and chronic hepatitis	2500	4000	Whole
		1500	2000	Whole (strip)
Stomach	Perforation, ulcer, hemorrhage	4500	5500	100 cm
Intestine	Ulcer, perforation, hemorrhage	4500	5500	400 cm
		5000	6500	100 cm
Brain	Infarction, necrosis	5000	6000	Whole
Spinal cord	Infarction, necrosis	4500	5500	10 cm
Heart	Pericarditis, pancarditis	4500	5500	60%
		7000	8000	25%
Lung	Acute and chronic pneumonitis	3000	3500	100 cm
		1500	2500	Whole
Kidney	Acute and chronic nephrosclerosis	1500	2000	Whole (strip)
		2000	2500	Whole
Fetus	Death	200	400	Whole

[a] TD$_{5/5}$ is the minimal tolerance dose—the dose that, when administered to a given patient population under a standard set of treatment conditions, results in a rate of severe complications of 5% or less within 5 years of treatment.

[b] TD$_{50/5}$ is the maximal tolerance dose—the dose that, when administered to a given population of patients under a standard set of treatment conditions, results in a rate of severe complications of 50% within 5 years of treatment.

SOURCE: From P Rubin et al (eds): *Radiation Biology and Radiation Pathology Syllabus*, set RT 1: *Radiation Oncology*. Chicago, American College of Radiology, 1975.

The symptoms may include chest pain and fever, with or without pericardial effusion. This syndrome is usually self-limited and typically manifests itself a few months after treatment. Asymptomatic pericardial effusion may be the most common manifestation of radiation-induced heart disease. It is usually detected by chest x-ray and confirmed by an echocardiogram.

Most patients with symptomatic radiation-induced constrictive pericarditis will have received more than 40 Gy to a large portion of the heart. The risk increases significantly with cardiac doses greater than 50 Gy.

Chronic cardiac changes may have their onset from 6 months to several years after irradiation. The clinical symptoms may indicate chronic constrictive disease due to pericardial, myocardial, and endocardial fibrosis—a pancarditis. The clinical signs may include dyspnea, chest pain, venous distention, pleural effusion, and paradoxical pulse.

Lung The clinical symptoms of radiation pneumonitis can be separated into early and late phases. During the early phase, clinical manifestations may include dyspnea, cough, and fever. Shortness of breath is relatively infrequent. It is more common to observe only the radiologic changes on a chest x-ray, without clinical symptoms. The clinical signs and symptoms of radiation pneumonitis may appear in 3 to 6 weeks if a large region of lung is irradiated to a dose above 25 Gy. An infiltrate outlining the treatment field may become evident on the chest x-ray. Radiation changes should not occur outside the treated field. Computed tomography can often help in distinguishing radiation pneumonitis from other causes of the infiltrate. The incidence of radiation pneumonitis can be reduced with careful treatment planning designed to lower the total dose given to the treated lung volume. Permanent scarring that results in respiratory compromise may develop if the dose and the volume of lung irradiated are excessive. Dyspnea and cough may be severe and debilitating.

Patients with symptoms of radiation pneumonitis may respond rapidly to glucocorticoids, but the medication has little effect on fibrotic changes. Glucocorticoids must be tapered very slowly to avoid rebound exacerbation of symptoms, which can prove lethal for some patients. Prophylactic administration of glucocorticoids is of no proven merit. Supportive care includes bronchodilators and oxygen at the lowest possible FI_{O_2}.

Digestive Tract Pathologic changes of the epithelial layer occur early during radiation treatments. The underlying submucosa may become edematous, with dilation of capillaries. Recovery from radiation damage can be expected within a few weeks after completion of radiation therapy, provided that sufficient numbers of stem cells are left. The radioresponsiveness of the aerodigestive tract, like that of other structures, is not uniform but varies according to the location.

Patients often have symptoms from radiation exposure that are similar to other forms of acute gastritis. The clinical signs include epigastric pain, loss of appetite, nausea, and vomiting. Decreased gastric acidity is observed after 15 to 20 Gy of fractionated radiation therapy. The tolerance of the stomach to radiation is also aggravated by addition of systemic chemotherapy, such as 5-fluorouracil.

The germinal centers of the bowel mucosa are in the crypts of Lieberkühn. Newly formed cells move upward along the walls of the crypts as transitional cells, undergoing maturation. The epithelial lining of the small bowel is the most rapidly renewed system in the human body and is completely renewed in 3 to 6 days. Within 12 to 24 h after the first dose of radiation therapy, pathologic evidence of dead cells are seen in the mucosal lining. Complete denudation of the mucosal surface rarely occurs during a regular course of radiation treatment because of the high capacity of the mucosa for regeneration. However, a focal area of erosion may be seen. The histologic appearance may be nearly normal within 2 to 3 weeks after radiation therapy.

Clinical manifestations of acute radiation enteropathy are nausea and vomiting, diarrhea, and cramping pain. Relevant factors contributing to the pathogenesis of diarrhea include malabsorption and alterations in the intestinal bacterial flora. The severity of symptoms, as in other anatomic areas, is proportional to the irradiated volume and the total dose.

Symptoms of chronic radiation enteropathy include diarrhea, abdominal cramping, nausea, malabsorption, vomiting, and obstruction. Progressive fibrosis, perforation, fistula formation, and stenosis of the irradiated portion of the bowel can occur during the chronic phase of radiation enteropathy. Most clinical manifestations of chronic changes occur between 6 months and 5 years after radiation therapy.

Conservative noninvasive treatment can frequently control gastrointestinal symptoms. A low-residue or elemental diet may be beneficial. When nonsurgical treatment fails to relieve severe symptoms, surgical intervention is often indicated.

Bladder Radiation injury to the bladder generally becomes symptomatic 3 to 6 weeks after the start of treatment, and symptoms usually subside 3 to 4 weeks after completion of radiation therapy. Patients often complain of increased frequency and dysuria. Cystoscopy often shows diffuse mucosal changes similar to those of acute cystitis. Sometimes desquamation and ulceration can be seen. Without infection, urinary symptoms are managed symptomatically. Concurrent chemotherapy with cytotoxic agents such as cyclophosphamide increases the severity of the acute bladder reaction.

The late effects of high radiation doses to the bladder may include interstitial fibrosis, telangiectasia, and ulceration. The blood vessels may be dilated and prone to rupture, resulting in painless hematuria. These changes are often difficult to distinguish from tumor recurrence and progression. A contracted bladder may result from doses in excess of 60 Gy.

Testes and Ovaries In general, type B spermatogonia are exquisitely sensitive to the effects of radiation. The type A spermatogonia are thought to be more resistant because their longer cell cycle time allows considerable variation in radiosensitivity among different phases of the cell cycle. Sertoli cells and Leydig cells are less radiosensitive than the spermatogonia. Elevated levels of follicle-stimulating hormone (FSH) and luteinizing hormone (LH) have been observed after as little as 75 cGy. Doses as low as 10 cGy to the testicles may result in injury to the type B spermatogonia. The single dose required for permanent sterilization on normal human males is believed to be between 6 and 10 Gy. In normal human males, sperm count recovery requires 9 to 18 months after a fractionated dose of 8 to 100 cGy.

The radiation dose necessary to induce ovarian failure is age-dependent. A single dose of 3 to 4 Gy can induce amenorrhea in almost all women over 40 years of age. In young women, oogenesis is much less sensitive to radiation than is spermatogenesis in men.

ACUTE TOTAL-BODY IRRADIATION The data regarding the acute effects of total-body irradiation on humans come primarily from Japanese survivors of the atomic bomb, Marshallese exposed to radioactive fall-out in 1954, and persons exposed to radiation from the Chernobyl nuclear accident. Early symptoms of acute total-body irradiation, known as the *prodromal radiation syndrome*, last for a limited time. Clinical manifestations depend on the total-body dose. At doses >100 Gy, death usually occurs 24 to 48 h later from neurologic and cardiovascular failure. This is known as the *cerebrovascular syndrome*. Because cerebrovascular damage causes death very quickly, the failures of other systems do not have time to develop.

At doses between 5 and 12 Gy, death may occur in a matter of days as a result of the *gastrointestinal syndrome*. The symptoms during this period may include nausea, vomiting, and prolonged diarrhea for several days leading to dehydration, sepsis, and death. A total-body dose >10 Gy is uniformly fatal unless supportive therapy (fluid, electrolytes, blood products, and antibiotics) is given. The process of intestinal denudation depends on the dose and may take between 3 and 120 days. Death from intestinal denudation usually occurs before the full effects of radiation on the blood-forming elements are seen.

At total-body doses between 2 and 8 Gy, death may occur 2 to 4 weeks after exposure from bone marrow failure, the *hematopoietic syndrome*. The full effect of radiation is not apparent until the mature

Table 394-5   Examples of Radiation-Induced Cancers

Types of Exposure	Types of Cancer Observed
Neck irradiation during infancy for benign conditions	Thyroid carcinoma
Radiation therapy for other malignant tumors	Thyroid carcinoma
	Breast cancer
	Gastric cancer
	Melanoma
	Lung cancer
	Sarcomas in the field
Cranial irradiation	Central nervous system tumors
Breast irradiation for postpartum mastitis	Breast cancer
Brush-licking by radium dial painters	Bone sarcomas
Uranium mining	Lung cancer
In utero exposure	Leukemia

hematopoietic cells are depleted. Clinical symptoms during this period may include chills, fatigue, and petechial hemorrhage. Peripheral blood lymphopenia develops during the first 12 to 48 h after any significant exposure. Beyond 5 to 6 Gy, the rate and magnitude of the drop are not well correlated to radiation exposure. Some stem cells may survive acute exposure to ≥ 10 Gy. Death is from infection or bleeding and usually occurs before anemia can develop (red blood cell half-life is 100 to 120 days).

The $LD_{50/60}$ (the dose at which 50% of the population is dead by 60 days) is around 3.25 Gy if support is not given. There is considerable variability in the total-body dose tolerated. The very young and the old are more radiosensitive than middle-aged and young adult individuals. Females in general appear to be more tolerant of radiation than males. Persons exposed to <2 Gy will require little or no therapy but should probably be observed closely with daily blood counts for a few days.

The role of bone marrow transplantation for patients exposed to acute total-body irradiation is debated. At doses <8 Gy, the patient is likely to survive with supportive care. Most people exposed to doses higher than 10 Gy will die from the gastrointestinal syndrome. Therefore, 8 to 10 Gy may be the dose range in which bone marrow transplantation could have a role, although the Chernobyl experience did not confirm this prediction. Estimating the dose received by a given patient after radiation exposure is difficult. However, exposure estimation must be done quickly because bone marrow transplantation is most effective if it is performed within the first 3 to 5 days after exposure.

RADIATION AND CANCER INDUCTION Some nonlethal changes in DNA sequences caused by irradiation may cause malignant transformations. Thus, it is not surprising that second neoplasms can be caused by exposure to ionizing radiation. However, paradoxically, this risk is actually less with doses above a certain level. Whether there is a "safe" dose that will not have any adverse biologic effect is unclear. Estimates of the risk of developing cancer after low-level exposure to ionizing radiation are often derived by extrapolation from the risks for higher doses and acute exposures. Predicted risks of cancer are, therefore, prone to modification depending on the assumptions made about the data available for analysis.

Throughout the history of human exposure to ionizing radiation, increased rates of cancer have been noted after exposure to radiation. The populations studied include survivors of the atomic bomb during World War II; radium watch-dial painters who shaped their brush tips with their tongues; and patients who underwent multiple fluoroscopic examinations for tuberculosis, received spinal irradiation for ankylosing spondylitis, and received breast irradiation for postpartum mastitis; and others. Exposure to ionizing radiation at an earlier age appears to increase the chance of developing radiation-induced carcinomas. However, the radiation-induced cancers have an age of onset similar to that of the native cancers, and the available data argue against radiation as

the only cause of the increased incidence of cancers seen after exposure to radiation. Table 394-5 shows examples of cancer observed in specific situations.

Because a safe dose of radiation is unknown at present, it is prudent to avoid routine exposures to ionizing irradiation.

ACKNOWLEDGMENT

The authors wish to acknowledge Dr. L. Chinsoo Cho for his contribution to this chapter in the 14th edition.

BIBLIOGRAPHY

HALL EJ: *Radiobiology for the Radiologist*, 4th ed. Philadelphia, Lippincott, 1994

METTLER FA JR, UPTON AC: *Medical Effects of Ionizing Radiation*, 2d ed, Philadelphia, Saunders, 1995

MOSS WT, COX JD: *Moss' Radiation Oncology: Rationale, Technique, Results*, 7th ed. St. Louis, Mosby, 1994

PEREZ CP, BRADY LW: *Principles and Practice of Radiation Oncology*, 3d ed. Philadelphia, Lippincott-Raven, 1998

RUBIN P: Late effects of normal tissues consensus conference. Int J Radiat Oncol Biol Phys 31:5, 1995

RUIFROK ACC, MCBRIDE WH: Growth factors: Biological and clinical aspects. Int J Radiat Oncol Biol Phys 43:877, 1999

395   *Howard Hu*

HEAVY METAL POISONING

Metals constitute a major category of toxins that pose a significant threat to health through occupational as well as environmental exposures. One indication of their importance relative to other potential hazards is their ranking by the U.S. Agency for Toxic Substances and Disease Registry, which lists all hazards present in toxic waste sites according to their prevalence and the severity of their toxicity. The first, second, third, and sixth hazards on the list are heavy metals: lead, mercury, arsenic, and cadmium, respectively. This chapter offers specific information on the sources and metabolism of each of these metals as well as on the toxic effects produced by each and the appropriate treatment for poisoning by each.

The intrinsic atomic stability of metals allows their relatively easy tracing and measurement in biologic material, although the clinical significance of the levels measured is not always clear. Metals are inhaled primarily as dusts and fumes (the latter defined as tiny particles generated by combustion). Metal poisoning can also result from exposure to vapors (e.g., mercury vapor in the manufacture of fluorescent lamps). When metals are ingested in contaminated food or drink or through hand-to-mouth activity (implicated especially often in children), their gastrointestinal absorption varies greatly with the specific chemical form of the metal and the nutritional status of the host. Once a metal is absorbed, blood is the main medium for its transport, with the precise kinetics dependent on diffusibility, binding forms, rates of biotransformation, availability of intracellular ligands, and other factors. Some organs (such as bone, liver, and kidney) sequester metals in relatively high concentrations for years. Most metals are excreted through renal clearance and gastrointestinal excretion; some proportion is also excreted through salivation, perspiration, exhalation, lactation, skin exfoliation, and loss of hair and nails.

Some metals, such as copper and selenium, are essential to normal metabolic function as trace elements (Chap. 75) but are toxic at high levels of exposure. Others, such as lead and mercury, are xenobiotic and theoretically are capable of exerting toxic effects at any level of exposure. Indeed, much research is currently focused on the contribution of low-level xenobiotic metal exposure to chronic diseases and to subtle changes in health that may have significant public health consequences.

The most important component of treatment for metal toxicity is the termination of exposure. Another component is the use of *chelating agents*, which are used to bind metals into stable cyclic compounds with relatively low toxicity and to enhance their excretion. The principal chelating agents are dimercaprol (British Anti-Lewisite, BAL), edetate (EDTA), succimer (DMSA, dimercaptosuccinic acid), and penicillamine; their specific use depends on the metal involved and the clinical picture. Activated charcoal does not bind metals and thus is of limited usefulness in cases of acute metal ingestion.

Besides the four metals discussed in detail in this chapter, several others deserve mention. *Aluminum* contributes to the encephalopathy occurring in patients with severe renal disease who are undergoing dialysis (Chap. 341). High levels of aluminum are found in the neurofibrillary tangles in the cerebral cortex and hippocampus of patients with Alzheimer's disease as well as in the drinking water and soil of areas with an unusually high incidence of Alzheimer's disease. The experimental and epidemiologic evidence for the aluminum–Alzheimer's disease link is so far relatively weak, however, and it cannot be concluded that aluminum is a causal agent or a contributing factor in neurodegenerative disease. Hexavalent *chromium* is corrosive and sensitizing. Workers in the chromate and chrome pigment production industries have consistently had an excess risk of lung cancer. The introduction of *cobalt* chloride as a fortifier in beer led to outbreaks of fatal cardiomyopathy among heavy consumers. Occupational exposure (e.g., of some miners, dry-battery manufacturers, and arc welders) to *manganese* can cause a Parkinsonian syndrome within 1 to 2 years, including gait disorders; postural instability; a masked, expressionless face; tremor; and psychiatric symptoms. With the introduction of methylcyclopentadienyl manganese tricarbonyl (MMT) as a gasoline additive, concern has arisen over the toxic potential of environmental manganese exposure. *Nickel* exposure induces an allergic response, and inhalation of nickel compounds with low aqueous solubility (such as nickel subsulfide and nickel oxide) in occupational settings is associated with an increased risk of cancer of the lung. Overexposure to *selenium* may cause local irritation of the respiratory system and eyes, gastrointestinal irritation, liver inflammation, loss of hair, depigmentation, and peripheral nerve damage. Workers exposed to certain organic forms of *tin* (particularly trimethyl and triethyl derivatives) have developed psychomotor disturbances, including tremor, convulsions, hallucinations, and psychotic behavior.

Finally, *thallium*, which is a component of some insecticides, metal alloys, and fireworks, is absorbed through the skin as well as through ingestion and inhalation. Severe poisoning follows a single ingested dose of >1 g or >8 mg/kg. Nausea and vomiting, abdominal pain, and hematemesis precede confusion, psychosis, organic brain syndrome, and coma. Thallium is radiopaque. Induced emesis or gastric lavage is indicated within 4 to 6 h of acute ingestion; Prussian blue prevents absorption and is given orally at 250 mg/kg in divided doses. Unlike other types of metal poisoning, thallium poisoning may be less severe when activated charcoal is used to interrupt its enterohepatic circulation. Other measures include forced diuresis, treatment with potassium chloride (which promotes renal excretion of thallium), and peritoneal dialysis.

LEAD

SOURCE Lead has been mined and used in industry and in household products for centuries. The dangers of lead toxicity, the clinical manifestations of which are termed *plumbism*, have been known since ancient times. The twentieth century saw both the greatest-ever exposure of the general population to lead and an extraordinary amount of new research on lead toxicity.

Populations are exposed to lead chiefly via paints, cans, plumbing fixtures, and leaded gasoline. The intensity of these exposures, while decreased by regulatory actions, remains high in some segments of the population because of the deterioration of lead paint used in the past and the entrainment of lead from paint and vehicle exhaust into soil and house dust. Many other environmental sources of exposure exist, such as leafy vegetables grown in lead-contaminated soil, improperly

glazed ceramics, lead crystal, and certain herbal folk remedies. Many industries, such as battery manufacturing, demolition, painting and paint removal, and ceramics, continue to pose a significant risk of lead exposure to workers and surrounding communities.

New research on lead toxicity has been stimulated by advances in toxicology and epidemiology as well as by a shift of emphasis in toxicology away from binary outcomes (life/death; 50% lethal dose) to grades of function, such as neuropsychological performance, indices of behavior, blood pressure, and kidney function.

Tests for levels of lead in blood have facilitated both research on lead and surveillance of individuals at risk. Blood lead is now measured with stringent quality controls in commercial laboratories throughout the United States. Measurement of the blood lead levels of children 6 months to 5 years of age is mandated by some states, and the U.S. Occupational Safety and Health Administration (OSHA) requires the testing of workers who may be exposed to lead in the course of their jobs.

METABOLISM Elemental lead and inorganic lead compounds are absorbed through ingestion or inhalation. Organic lead (e.g., tetraethyl lead, the lead additive to gasoline) is absorbed to a significant degree through the skin as well. Pulmonary absorption is efficient, particularly if particle diameters are $<1\ \mu m$ (as in fumes from burning lead paint). Children absorb up to 50% of the amount of lead ingested, whereas adults absorb only ~ 10 to 20%. Gastrointestinal absorption of lead is enhanced by fasting and by dietary deficiencies in calcium, iron, and zinc; such absorption is minimal, however, for lead in the form of lead sulfide, a common constituent of mining waste. Lead is absorbed into blood plasma, where it equilibrates rapidly with extracellular fluid, crosses membranes (such as the blood-brain barrier and the placenta), and accumulates in soft and hard tissues. In the blood, ~ 95 to 99% of lead is sequestered in red cells, where it is bound to hemoglobin and other components. As a consequence, lead is usually measured in whole blood rather than in serum. The largest proportion of absorbed lead is incorporated into the skeleton, which contains >90% of the body's total lead burden. Lead is excreted mainly in the urine (in a process that depends on glomerular filtration and tubular secretion) and in the feces. Lead also appears in hair, nails, sweat, saliva, and breast milk. The half-life of lead in blood is ~ 25 days; in soft tissue, ~ 40 days; and in the nonlabile portion of bone, >25 years. Thus, blood lead levels may decline significantly while the body's total burden of lead remains heavy.

The toxicity of lead is probably related to its affinity for cell membranes and mitochondria, as a result of which it interferes with mitochondrial oxidative phosphorylation and sodium, potassium, and calcium ATPases. Lead impairs the activity of calcium-dependent intracellular messengers and of brain protein kinase C. In addition, lead stimulates the formation of inclusion bodies that may translocate the metal into cell nuclei and alter gene expression.

CLINICAL TOXICOLOGY Symptomatic lead poisoning in childhood generally develops at blood lead levels $>3.9\ \mu mol/L$ (80 $\mu g/dL$) and is characterized by abdominal pain and irritability followed by lethargy, anorexia, pallor (resulting from anemia), ataxia, and slurred speech. Convulsions, coma, and death due to generalized cerebral edema and renal failure occur in the most severe cases. Subclinical lead poisoning [blood lead level $>1.4\ \mu mol/L$ ($> 30\ \mu g/dL$)] can cause mental retardation and selective deficits in language, cognitive function, balance, behavior, and school performance despite the lack of discernible symptoms. Epidemiologic studies and meta-analyses of studies regarding lead's effect on the intellectual function of children indicate that cognition is probably impaired in a dose-related fashion at blood lead levels well below $1.4\ \mu mol/L$ (30 $\mu g/dL$) and that no threshold for this effect is likely to exist above the lowest measurable blood lead level of $0.05\ \mu mol/L$ (1 $\mu g/dL$). The impact is greatest when the exposure is of long duration and has been most apparent when it takes place around the age of 2 years; however, the impact of fetal lead exposure remains to be clarified, particularly in view of the observation that maternal bone lead stores can be mobilized to a significant degree during pregnancy, with consequent exposure of the fetus.

In adults, symptomatic lead poisoning, which usually develops when blood lead levels exceed 3.9 μmol/L (80 μg/dL) for a period of weeks, is characterized by abdominal pain, headache, irritability, joint pain, fatigue, anemia, peripheral motor neuropathy, and deficits in short-term memory and the ability to concentrate. Encephalopathy is rare. A "lead line" sometimes appears at the gingiva-tooth border after prolonged high-level exposure. Some individuals develop these symptoms and signs at lower blood lead levels [1.9 to 3.9 μmol/L (40 to 80 μg/dL)] and/or with briefer periods of exposure. Chronic subclinical lead exposure is associated with interstitial nephritis, tubular damage (with tubular inclusion bodies), hyperuricemia (with an increased risk of gout), and a decline in glomerular filtration rate and chronic renal failure. Epidemiologic evidence also suggests that blood lead levels in the range of 0.34 to 1.7 μmol/L (7 to 35 μg/dL) are associated with increases in blood pressure, decreases in creatinine clearance, and decrements in cognitive performance that are too small to be detected as a lead effect in individual cases but nevertheless may contribute significantly to the causation of chronic disease.

An additional issue for both children and adults is whether lead that has accumulated in bone and lain dormant for years can pose a threat later in life, particularly at times of increased bone resorption such as pregnancy, lactation, and senile osteoporosis. Elevation of the bone lead level appears to be a risk factor for anemia, hypertension, cardiac conduction delays, and impairment of cognitive function. Hyperthyroidism has been reported to cause lead toxicity in adults by mobilizing stores of bone lead acquired during childhood.

Genetic polymorphisms, such as variants of the gene that codes for aminolevulinic acid dehydratase (a critical enzyme in the production of heme) or the C282Y hemochromatosis gene, may confer differences in susceptibility to lead retention and toxicity; ~15% of Caucasians have a variant form of one of these genes. This issue is the focus of continued research.

LABORATORY FINDINGS In 1991, the Centers for Disease Control and Prevention designated 0.48 μmol/L (10 μg/dL) as the blood lead level of concern in children. A specific set of interventions is recommended when the level exceeds this value. OSHA requires the regular measurement of blood lead in lead-exposed workers and the maintenance of blood lead levels <1.9 μmol/L (40 μg/dL). Concentrations of heme precursors (such as δ-aminolevulinic acid) in plasma and urine are sometimes increased at blood lead levels as low as 0.73 μmol/L (15 μg/dL). Levels of protoporphyrin (free erythrocyte or zinc) rise—although not consistently—once blood lead levels have exceeded 1.2 μmol/L (25 μg/dL) for several months. Lead-associated anemia is usually normocytic and normochromic and may be accompanied by basophilic stippling. Lead-induced peripheral demyelination is reflected by prolonged nerve conduction time and subsequent paralysis, usually of the extensor muscles of the hands and feet (wristdrop and footdrop). An increased density at the metaphyseal plate of growing long bones (lead lines) can develop in children and resemble those seen in rickets. Children with high-level lead exposure sometimes develop Fanconi's syndrome, pyuria, and azotemia. Adults chronically exposed to lead can develop elevated serum creatinine levels, decreased creatinine clearance rates, and chronic changes and intranuclear inclusion bodies (detected at renal biopsy). Deficits may be apparent in neuropsychometric tests of both children and adults; these abnormalities by themselves are not pathognomonic. Bone lead levels measured in vivo by K-x-ray fluorescence, a technique adapted for this purpose, are more sensitive than blood lead levels as a predictor of hypertension, cognitive impairments, and reproductive toxicity in epidemiologic studies; however, measurement of bone lead levels has not yet been shown to be of clinical value and is not widely available.

TREATMENT It is absolutely essential to prevent further exposure of affected individuals to lead. Cases of lead poisoning should be reported to OSHA (if the exposure is occupational) and to local boards of health so that home evaluations can be performed. Pharmacologic treatment for lead toxicity entails the use of chelating agents, principally edetate calcium disodium (CaEDTA), dimercaprol, penicillamine, and succimer, which is given orally and has relatively few side effects. Chelation is recommended for the treatment of all children whose blood lead levels are >2.7 μmol/L (55 μg/dL), with the addition of dimercaprol if lead encephalopathy is found. Chelation is also recommended for children if blood lead levels are between 1.2 and 2.7 μmol/L (25 and 55 μg/dL) and the total amount of lead excreted in urine during the 8 h after a single dose of edetate calcium disodium exceeds 9.7 μmol/L (200 μg/dL). Chelation is recommended for adults if blood lead levels exceed 3.9 μmol/L (80 μg/dL) or if these levels exceed 2.9 μmol/L (60 μg/dL) and symptoms have developed. The ability of chelation to improve subclinical outcomes (such as performance on psychometric testing) at lower levels of blood lead in both children and adults is the subject of current research.

MERCURY

SOURCE Metallic mercury (Hg⁰) is used in thermometers, dental amalgams, and some batteries. Mercurous mercury (Hg⁺) and mercuric mercury (Hg²⁺) can be combined with other chemicals, such as carbon, chlorine, or oxygen, to form inorganic or organic mercury compounds. All three forms of mercury are toxic to various degrees. Organic mercury compounds are slowly broken down into inorganic compounds; conversely, inorganic mercury can be converted by microorganisms in soil and water into the organic compound methyl mercury. Fish, particularly tuna and swordfish, can concentrate methyl mercury at high levels; such contamination of fish by industrial runoff and their subsequent ingestion was responsible for the Minamata Bay epidemic of mercury poisoning in Japan in 1955. Occupational exposure to inorganic mercury compounds continues in some chemical, metal-processing, electrical-equipment, automotive, and building industries and in medical and dental services. Environmental exposure probably takes place most commonly through ingestion of contaminated fish and through inhalation of the vapor generated by ordinary dental amalgam, which typically contains ~50% metallic mercury. There is also concern about exposure to drinking water contaminated by toxic waste sites included on the National Priority List, almost half of which contain mercury, and about the inhalation of fumes from incinerators burning mercury-contaminated waste products. Such incineration can also lead to environmental mercury contamination, methylation of the contaminating mercury by environmental bacteria, concentration of the resultant organic mercury compounds up the food chain, and consequent human exposure (particularly to contaminated fish). Ironically, the medical/hospital industry has been identified as a major incinerator of mercury-contaminated waste.

METABOLISM Elemental mercury is not well absorbed by the gastrointestinal tract and is excreted almost entirely in the feces after being ingested; however, when left standing, mercury is volatilized at room temperature into a vapor that is well absorbed by the lungs. Once absorbed, mercury in this form is lipid soluble, crosses the blood-brain barrier and the placenta, and can be oxidized by catalase and hydrogen peroxide into mercuric chloride, which is retained by the kidney and brain for years. Elemental mercury in blood has a half-life of ~60 days and is excreted mainly in the urine and feces.

The gastrointestinal and dermal absorption of inorganic mercury is significant. Large overdoses disrupt gastrointestinal barriers, further enhancing absorption. Once absorbed, inorganic mercury breaks down into metallic and mercuric mercury. Relatively little of this mercury crosses the blood-brain barrier; most is excreted in the urine or feces, with a half-life of 40 days, or is retained by the kidneys as mercuric mercury.

Organic mercury, particularly methyl mercury, can evaporate and undergo pulmonary absorption. Forms that are ingested (e.g., in contaminated fish) are well absorbed. Only small amounts are absorbed through the skin. Absorbed organic mercury is lipid soluble, readily crosses the blood-brain barrier and the placenta, appears in breast milk, and concentrates in the kidneys and central nervous system. Methyl mercury is acetylated in the liver, excreted in bile, reabsorbed, and then excreted in urine. Methyl mercury can also be conjugated with cysteine or glutathione. Only 1% of organic mercury is excreted unchanged into urine. The half-life of organic mercury compounds is in the range of 70 days. Exposure to mercury in any form stimulates the kidney to produce metallothionein, a metal-binding protein that affords partial protection against mercury toxicity.

CLINICAL TOXICOLOGY Inhalation of metallic mercury vapor is the form of mercury exposure that has been best studied in terms of toxicity. High levels of exposure are most likely in an occupational setting in which mercury vapors are generated by heat-induced volatilization of metallic mercury. Cough, dyspnea, and tightness or burning pain in the chest are common symptoms that may be accompanied by diffuse infiltrates or a pneumonitis-like appearance on chest x-ray. Respiratory distress, pulmonary edema, lobar pneumonia, fibrosis, and desquamation of the bronchiolar epithelium can occur in relatively severe cases and have sometimes led to death. Acute inhalation of mercury vapor can also cause neurologic toxicity manifested by tremors (beginning in the hands), emotional lability, headaches, and polyneuropathy. Chronic exposure to metallic mercury produces a characteristic intention tremor and mercurial *erethism*, a constellation of findings including excitability, memory loss, insomnia, timidity, and sometimes delirium that was described in workers with occupational exposure in the felt-hat industry—hence the expression "mad as a hatter." Dentists with occupational exposure to mercury score below normal on neurobehavioral tests of motor speed, visual scanning, verbal and visual memory, and visuomotor coordination. Low-level exposure from dental amalgams may also be associated with adverse immunologic reactions in individuals with certain major human leukocyte antigen genotypes; further research is needed in this area.

Acute high-dose ingestion of inorganic mercury causes severe gastrointestinal corrosion with nausea, vomiting, hematemesis, and abdominal pain; acute renal failure, cardiovascular collapse, and shock may ensue. The lethal dose of inorganic mercury is estimated to be in the range of 10 to 42 mg/kg. Lower levels of exposure cause milder forms of gastrointestinal inflammation, gingivitis and loosening of the teeth, increased blood pressure and tachycardia, and the nephrotic syndrome. Symptoms similar to erethism may develop. Skin exposure to mercuric salts can cause exfoliative dermatitis.

Ingestion of organic mercury compounds is followed by diarrhea, tenesmus, and blisters of the upper gastrointestinal tract. The fatal dose of organic mercury is estimated at 10 to 60 mg/kg. People who ingested flour contaminated with *N*-(ethylmercuri)-*p*-toluenesulfonanilide developed bradycardia, QT prolongation, ST-segment depression, and T-wave inversions. The neurotoxicity resulting from organic mercury exposure is characterized by paresthesia; impaired peripheral vision, hearing, taste, and smell; slurred speech; unsteadiness of gait and limbs; muscle weakness; irritability; memory loss; and depression. In general, such symptoms begin at doses >1.7 mg/kg. Autopsy findings suggest that lesions in the basal ganglia and gray matter of the cortex and cerebellum are chiefly responsible for these symptoms. Organic mercury exposure, primarily through the ingestion of grain treated with mercuric fungicides or of contaminated fish, is also associated with an increased risk of fetal toxicity. After the 1955 mercury poisoning outbreak in Minamata, Japan, exposed mothers gave birth to infants with mental retardation; retention of primitive reflexes; cerebellar symptoms; dysarthria; hyperkinesia; hypersalivation; atrophy of the cerebral cortex, corpus callosum, and cerebellum; and abnormal neuronal cytoarchitecture. This last change may reflect derangement of neuronal migration during fetal development.

Worthy of special note is dimethylmercury, a "supertoxic" compound encountered exclusively in laboratory settings. The physical properties of dimethylmercury permit transdermal absorption (against which latex gloves do not afford protection) as well as volatilization with inhalation. Exposure to ~400 mg (an amount equivalent to a few drops) is lethal, with cerebellar degeneration as a prominent feature.

Exposure of children to mercury in any of its forms can cause a particular syndrome known as *acrodynia*, or pink disease. This condition is characterized by flushing, itching, swelling, tachycardia, elevated blood pressure, excessive salivation or perspiration, irritability, weakness, morbilliform rashes, and desquamation of the palms and soles.

LABORATORY FINDINGS Levels of mercury in blood and urine should not exceed 180 nmol/L (3.6 μg/dL) and 0.7 μmol/L (15 μg/L), respectively. Symptoms may develop when blood and urine mercury levels exceed 1 μmol/L (20 μg/dL) and 3 μmol/L (60 μg/L), respectively. If a baseline 24-h urinary mercury value is low, repetition of the measurement after a single 2-g oral dose of succimer may be useful in documenting elevated renal mercury burdens in retired mercury-exposed workers; an increase of >20 μg in a 24-h urine sample suggests previous exposure. Levels in hair may be used as a dosimeter for chronic organic mercury exposure; neurobehavioral dysfunction in children may occur if the maternal mercury concentration in hair exceeds 30 nmol/g (6 μg/g).

TREATMENT Acute ingestion of mercuric salts can be treated by induced emesis or gastric lavage. Polythiol resins can be administered orally to bind mercury in the gastrointestinal tract. The most effective chelating agents are dimercaprol, succimer, and penicillamine, which have active mono- or dithiol groups. Acute inorganic mercury poisoning can be treated with dimercaprol at a dose not exceeding 24 mg/kg per day and given intramuscularly in divided doses. Therapy is usually given in 5-day courses separated by several days of rest. The *N*-acetyl form of penicillamine is also useful at a dose of 30 mg/kg per day in divided doses. Peritoneal dialysis, hemodialysis, and extracorporeal regional complexing hemodialysis with succimer have all been used with some success in the treatment of patients with renal failure.

Chronic inorganic mercury poisoning is best treated with *N*-acetyl penicillamine.

ARSENIC

SOURCE Significant exposure to arsenic occurs through both anthropogenic and natural sources. Arsenic is released into the air by volcanoes and is a natural contaminant of some deep-water wells. Occupational exposure to arsenic is common in the smelting industry (in which arsenic is a byproduct of ores containing lead, gold, zinc, cobalt, and nickel) and is increasing in the microelectronics industry (in which gallium arsenide is responsible). Low-level arsenic exposure continues to take place in the general population (as do some cases of high-dose poisoning) through the commercial use of inorganic arsenic compounds in common products such as wood preservatives, pesticides, herbicides, fungicides, and paints; through the consumption of foods and the smoking of tobacco treated with arsenic-containing pesticides; and through the burning of fossil fuels in which arsenic is a contaminant. Arsenic was also a major ingredient of Fowler's solution and continues to be found in some folk remedies.

METABOLISM The toxicity of an arsenic-containing compound depends on its valence state (zero-valent, trivalent, or pentavalent), its form (inorganic or organic), and the physical aspects governing its absorption and elimination. In general, inorganic arsenic is more toxic than organic arsenic, and trivalent arsenite is more toxic than pentavalent and zero-valent arsenic. The normal intake of arsenic by adults occurs primarily through ingestion and averages ~50 μg/d (range, 8 to 104 μg/d). Most (~64%) of this amount is accounted for by organic arsenic from fish, seafood, and algae; the specific arsenic compounds obtained from these sources are arsenobentaine and arsenocholine, which are relatively nontoxic and are rapidly excreted in unchanged form in the urine. After absorption, inorganic arsenic accumulates in the liver, spleen, kidneys, lungs, and gastrointestinal tract. It is then rapidly cleared from these sites but leaves a residue in keratin-rich tissues such as skin, hair, and nails. Arsenite (+5) undergoes biomethylation in the liver to the less toxic metabolites methylarsenic acid and dimethylarsenic acid; biomethylation can quickly become saturated, however, and the result is the deposition of increasing doses of inorganic arsenic in soft tissues. Arsenic, particularly in its trivalent form, inhibits critical sulfhydryl-containing enzymes. In the pentavalent form, the competitive substitution of arsenic for phosphate can lead to rapid hydrolysis of the high-energy bonds in compounds such as ATP.

CLINICAL TOXICOLOGY Acute arsenic poisoning from ingestion results in increased permeability of small blood vessels and inflammation and necrosis of the intestinal mucosa; these changes manifest as hemorrhagic gastroenteritis, fluid loss, and hypotension. Delayed cardiomyopathy accompanied by electrocardiographic abnormalities may develop. Symptoms include nausea, vomiting, diarrhea, abdominal pain, delirium, coma, and seizures. A garlicky odor may be detectable on the breath. Acute tubular necrosis and hemolysis may develop. The reported lethal dose of arsenic ranges from 120 to 200 mg in adults and is 2 mg/kg in children. Arsine gas causes severe hemolysis within 3 to 4 h of exposure and can lead to acute tubular necrosis and renal failure.

In chronic arsenic poisoning, the onset of symptoms comes at 2 to 8 weeks. Typical findings are skin and nail changes, such as hyperkeratosis, hyperpigmentation, exfoliative dermatitis, and Mees' lines (transverse white striae of the fingernails); sensory and motor polyneuritis manifesting as numbness and tingling in a "stocking-glove" distribution, distal weakness, and quadriplegia; and inflammation of the respiratory mucosa. Epidemiologic evidence has linked chronic consumption of water containing arsenic at concentrations in the range of 10 to 1820 ppb with diabetes, vasospasm, and peripheral vascular insufficiency culminating in "blackfoot disease," a gangrenous condition affecting the extremities. Chronic arsenic exposure has also been associated with a greatly elevated risk of skin cancer and possibly of cancers of the lung, liver (angiosarcoma), bladder, kidney, and colon.

LABORATORY FINDINGS When acute arsenic poisoning is suspected, an x-ray of the abdomen may reveal ingested arsenic, which is radiopaque. The serum arsenic level may exceed 0.9 μmol/L (7 μg/dL); however, arsenic is rapidly cleared from the blood. Electrocardiographic findings may include QRS complex broadening, QT prolongation, ST-segment depression, T-wave flattening, and multifocal ventricular tachycardia. Urinary arsenic should be measured in 24-h specimens collected after 48 h of abstinence from seafood ingestion; normally, levels of total urinary arsenic excretion are <0.67 μmol/d (50 μg/d). Arsenic may be detected in the hair and nails for months after exposure. Abnormal liver function, anemia, leukocytosis or leukopenia, proteinuria, and hematuria may be detected. Electromyography may reveal features similar to those of Guillain-Barré syndrome.

℞ **TREATMENT** Vomiting should be induced with ipecac in the alert patient with acute arsenic ingestion. Gastric lavage may be useful; activated charcoal with a cathartic (such as sorbitol) may be tried, although its efficacy is not clear. Aggressive therapy with intravenous fluid and electrolyte replacement in an intensive-care setting may be life-saving. Dimercaprol is the chelating agent of choice and is administered intramuscularly at an initial dose of 3 to 5 mg/kg on the following schedule: every 4 h for 2 days, every 6 h on the third day, and every 12 h thereafter for 10 days. (An oral chelating agent may be substituted.) Succimer is sometimes an effective alternative, particularly if adverse reactions to dimercaprol develop (such as nausea, vomiting, headache, increased blood pressure, and convulsions). In cases of renal failure, doses should be adjusted carefully, and hemodialysis may be needed to remove the chelating agent–arsenic complex. Arsine gas poisoning should be treated supportively with the goals of maintaining renal function and circulating red-cell mass. Other than the avoidance of additional exposure, specific treatment is not of proven benefit in chronic arsenic toxicity. Recovery, particularly from the resulting peripheral neuropathy, may take months and may never be complete.

CADMIUM

SOURCE Environmental exposure to cadmium can result from the ingestion of basic foodstuffs, especially grains, cereals, and leafy vegetables, which readily absorb cadmium occurring naturally or in soil contaminated by sewage sludge, fertilizers, and polluted groundwater. Serious cadmium poisoning can follow the contamination of food and water by mining effluents, as took place in the 1946 outbreak of *itai-itai* ("ouch-ouch") disease (so named because cadmium-induced bone toxicity caused painful bone fractures) in the Jintzu River basin in Japan. Airborne cadmium can be released during smelting or during the incineration of municipal waste containing plastics and nickel-cadmium batteries. Cigarette smoke contains cadmium. Occupational exposure takes place in the metal-plating, pigment, battery, and plastics industries.

METABOLISM The normal daily intake of cadmium through ingestion or inhalation is from 20 to 40 μg, although only 5 to 10% of this amount is absorbed. Most absorbed cadmium is concentrated in the liver and kidneys. In erythrocytes and soft tissues, cadmium is bound to metallothionein, a low-molecular-weight protein that mitigates the toxicity of the unbound ion. This complex is filtered at the glomerulus but is then reabsorbed by the proximal tubules. The lack of an effective elimination pathway is responsible for cadmium's biologic half-life of 10 to 30 years. The toxicity of cadmium may involve its binding to key cellular sulfhydryl groups, its competition with other metals (zinc and selenium) for inclusion in metalloenzymes, and its competition with calcium for binding sites on regulatory proteins such as calmodulin.

CLINICAL TOXICOLOGY Acute high-dose cadmium inhalation can cause severe respiratory irritation with pleuritic chest pain, dyspnea, cyanosis, fever, tachycardia, nausea, and life-threatening noncardiogenic pulmonary edema. The onset of symptoms may be delayed from 4 to 24 h. Acute exposure through ingestion can cause severe nausea, vomiting, salivation, abdominal cramps, and diarrhea. Single lethal oral doses have reportedly ranged from 350 to 8900 mg. Chronic effects of cadmium exposure are dose-dependent and include anosmia, yellowing of the teeth, emphysema, minor changes in liver function, microcytic hypochromic anemia unresponsive to iron therapy, renal tubular dysfunction characterized by proteinuria and increased urinary excretion of β_2-microglobulin, and (with prolonged poisoning) osteomalacia leading to bone lesions and pseudofractures. In follow-up studies of occupationally exposed workers, β_2-microglobulinuria was found to be irreversible. Associations with hypertension, prostate cancer, and lung cancer have been suggested by some studies but await confirmation. In one study of men and women living in an area moderately contaminated with cadmium, higher body cadmium burdens were found to be a significant risk factor for lower bone density, a higher incidence of fractures, and a faster decline in height. These changes may be related to cadmium's calciuric effect on the kidney.

LABORATORY FINDINGS The daily level of excretion of cadmium by persons without known cadmium exposures is usually <10 nmol/L (1 μg/L or 1 μg/g of creatinine). This level increases somewhat with age and smoking. Toxicity, including renal dysfunction, is considered unlikely until the urinary cadmium level exceeds 100 nmol/L (10 μg/g of creatinine). Serum cadmium levels reflect recent rather than chronic exposure and generally are <30 nmol/L (0.3 μg/dL) in unexposed persons. A blood level >500 nmol/L (5 μg/dL) is considered toxic. An increased urinary concentration of β_2-microglobulin is the most sensitive indicator of an elevated cadmium dose and of nephropathy but may also be detected in other renal diseases, such as chronic pyelonephritis.

R TREATMENT There is no effective treatment for cadmium poisoning. Chelation therapy is not useful, and dimercaprol is contraindicated as this agent may exacerbate nephrotoxicity. Avoidance of further exposure and supportive therapy (including vitamin D if osteomalacia exists) are the mainstays of management.

BIBLIOGRAPHY

GENERAL

APOSHIAN HV et al: Mobilization of heavy metals by newer, therapeutically useful chelating agents. Toxicology 97:23, 1995

GOYER RA: Nutrition and metal toxicity. Am J Clin Nutr 61:646S, 1995

LYZNICKI JM et al: Manganese in gasoline. J Occup Environ Med 41:140, 1999

ROELS HA et al: Usefulness of biomarkers of exposure to inorganic mercury, lead, or cadmium in controlling occupational and environmental risks of nephrotoxicity. Ren Fail 21:251, 1999

LEAD

GONZÁLEZ-COSSÍO T et al: Decrease in birth weight in relation to maternal bone lead burden. Pediatrics 100:856, 1997

HU H et al: The relationship of blood and bone lead to hypertension among middle-aged to elderly men. JAMA 275:1171, 1996

KIM R et al: A longitudinal study of low-level lead exposure and renal function in men from the Normative Aging Study. JAMA 275:1177, 1996

KORRICK SA et al: Lead and hypertension in a sample of middle-aged women. Am J Public Health 89:330, 1999

STEWART WF et al: Neurobehavioral function and tibial and chelatable lead levels in 543 former organolead workers. Neurology 52:1610, 1999

MERCURY

CLARKSON TW: Mercury: Major issues in environmental health. Environ Health Perspect 100:31, 1993

NIERENBERG DW et al: Delayed cerebellar disease and death after accidental exposure to dimethylmercury. N Engl J Med 338:1672, 1998

ROELS HA et al: Urinary excretion of mercury after occupational exposure to mercury vapour and influence of the chelating agent meso-w,e-dimercaptosuccinic acid (DMSA). Br J Ind Med 48:247, 1991

ARSENIC

ABERNATHY CO et al: Arsenic: Health effects, mechanisms of actions, and research issues. Environ Health Perspect 107:593, 1999

ÇÖL M et al: Arsenic-related Bowen's disease, palmar keratosis, and skin cancer. Environ Health Perspect 107:687, 1999

CADMIUM

LAUWERYS RR et al: Cadmium: Exposure markers as predictors of nephrotoxic effects. Clin Chem 40:1391, 1994

STAESSEN JA et al: Environmental exposure to cadmium, forearm bone density, and risk of fractures: Prospective population study. Lancet 353:1140, 1999

Section 2

ILLNESSES DUE TO POISONS, DRUG OVERDOSAGE, AND ENVENOMATION

396 *Christopher H. Linden, Michael J. Burns*

POISONING AND DRUG OVERDOSAGE

ARDS adult respiratory distress syndrome	G6PD glucose-6-phosphate dehydrogenase
AV atrioventricular	MAO monoamine oxidase
BUN blood urea nitrogen	NAC *N*-acetylcysteine
CNS central nervous system	NAPQI *n*-acetyl-*p*-benzoquinoneimine
COX cyclooxygenase	
ECG electrocardiogram	PEMA phenylethylmalonamide
EEG Electroencephalographic	SA sinoatrial
GABA γ-aminobutyric acid	SSRIs Selective serotonin reuptake inhibitors
GBL γ-butyrolactone	
GHB γ-hydroxybutyrate	TCAs Tricyclic antidepressants

Poisoning refers to the development of dose-related adverse effects following exposure to chemicals, drugs, or other xenobiotics. To paraphrase Paracelsus, the dose makes the poison. In excessive amounts, substances that are usually innocuous, such as oxygen and water, can cause poisoning. Conversely, in small doses, substances commonly regarded as poisons, such as arsenic and cyanide, can be consumed without ill effect. There is, however, substantial individual variability in the response to, and disposition of, a given dose (Chaps. 70 and 71). Some of this variability is genetic, and some is acquired on the basis of enzyme induction, inhibition, or because of tolerance. Poisoning may be local (e.g., skin, eyes, or lungs) or systemic depending on the chemical and physical properties of the xenobiotic, its mechanism of action, and the route of exposure. The severity and reversibility of poisoning also depend on the functional reserve of the individual or target organ, which is influenced by age and preexisting disease. All of these factors must be considered when attempting to predict the effects of a particular exposure.

EPIDEMIOLOGY

In the United States, exposure to xenobiotics results in over 5 million requests for medical advice or treatment each year. Most exposures are acute, accidental, involve a single agent, occur in the home, result in minor or no toxicity, and involve children under 6 years of age. Common routes of exposure are ingestion (74%), dermal (8.2%), inhalation (6.7%), ocular (6%), bites and stings (3.9%), and parenteral injections (0.3%). Exposures most frequently involve cleaning agents, analgesics, cosmetics, plants, cough and cold preparations, and bites and envenomations (Chaps. 397 and 398). Pharmaceuticals are involved in 41% of exposures and 75% of serious or fatal poisonings.

Accidental exposures can result from the improper use of chemicals at work or play; product mislabeling; label misreading; mistaken identification of unlabeled chemicals; uninformed self-medication; and dosing errors by nurses, parents, pharmacists, physicians, and the elderly. Excluding the recreational use of ethanol, attempted suicide is the most common reason for intentional exposure. Unintended poisonings may result from the intentional use of drugs for psychotropic effects (abuse) or excessive self-dosing (misuse).

About 5% of exposures require hospitalization. They account for 5 to 10% of all ambulance transports, emergency room visits, and intensive care unit admissions. Up to 30% of psychiatric admissions are prompted by attempted suicide via overdosage.

Overall, the mortality rate is low: 0.03% of all exposures. It is much higher (1 to 2%) in hospitalized patients with nonaccidental (suicidal) overdose, who account for the majority of serious poisonings. Carbon monoxide poisoning is the leading cause of death; patients with such poisoning are typically dead when discovered and are included in medical examiner but not hospital or poison center statistics. Drug-related fatalities are most commonly due to analgesics, antidepressants, sedative-hypnotics, neuroleptics, stimulants and street drugs, cardiovascular drugs, anticonvulsants, antihistamines, and asthma therapies. Nonpharmaceutical agents most often implicated in

Table 396-1 Differential Diagnosis of Poisoning Based on Physiologic Status as Determined by Vital Signs and CNS Activity

Excited	Depressed	Discordant	Normal

Sympathomimetic syndrome
  Amphetamines
  Bronchodilators (β_2-adrenergic agonists)
  Caffeine
  Cocaine
  Decongestants (α-adrenergic agonists)
  Ergot alkaloids
  MAO inhibitors
  Theophylline
  Thyroid hormones
	Sympatholytic syndrome
	  α-Adrenergic blockers
	  Angiotensin-converting enzyme inhibitors
	  Antiarrhythmics
	  Antidepressants (tricyclic)
	  β-Adrenergic blockers
	  Calcium channel blockers
	  Clonidine
	  Decongestants (imidazolines)
	  Digitalis
		Asphyxiants
		  Carbon monoxide
		  Cyanide
		  Hydrogen sulfide
		  Inert gases
		  Irritant fumes, gases, vapors
		  Methemoglobinemia
		  Nitrophenol herbicides
			Agents with slow absorption
			  Carbamazepine
			  Digitalis preparations
			  Dilantin Kapseals
			  Enteric-coated pills
			  Lomotil
			  Salicylates
			  Sustained-release preparations

Anticholinergic syndrome
  Antidepressants (tricyclic)
  Antihistamines
  Antiparkinsonian agents
  Antispasmodics (GI, GU)
  Belladonna alkaloids
  Cyclobenzaprine
  Mydriatics (topical)
  Orphenadrine
  Plants/mushrooms
  Phenothiazines
	Cholinergic syndrome
	  Bethanechol
	  Carbamate insecticides
	  Echothiophate
	  Myasthenia gravis drugs (e.g., pyridostigmine)
	  Organophosphate insecticides
	  Physostigmine
	  Pilocarpine
	  Urecholine
		CNS syndromes
		  Disulfiram
		  Dystonic/extrapyramidal reactions
		  Isoniazid
		  Neuroleptic malignant syndrome
		  Serotonin syndrome
		  Strychnine
		  Volatile hydrocarbon inhalation
			Agents with slow distribution
			  Digitalis preparations
			  Heavy metals
			  Lithium
			  Salicylates

Hallucinogenic syndrome
  LSD and its analogues
  Marijuana
  Mescaline and its analogues
  Phencyclidine
	Opioid syndrome
	  Analgesics
	  Antidiarrheal agents
	  Antispasmodics (GI)
	  Heroin
	  Opium
		Membrane-active agents
		  Amantadine
		  Antiarrhythmic agents
		  Antidepressants (cyclic)
		  β-Adrenergic blockers
		  Fluorides
		  Heavy metals
		  Lithium
		  Local anesthetics
		  Meperidine
		  Neuroleptic agents
		  Propoxyphene
		  Quinine and related antimalarial agents
			Agents that are activated metabolically
			  Acetaminophen
			  Chloramphenicol
			  Chlorinated hydrocarbons
			  Ethylene glycol
			  L-thyroxine
			  Methanol
			  Paraquat
			  Certain methemoglobin inducers

Withdrawal syndrome
  Antidepressants
  β-Adrenergic blockers
  Clonidine
  Ethanol
  Opioids
  Sedative-hypnotics
	Sedative-hypnotic syndrome
	  Alcohols
	  Anticonvulsants
	  Barbiturates
	  Benzodiazepines
	  Bromide
	  Ethchlorvynol
	  γ-Hydroxybutyrate
	  Hydrocarbons
	  Glutethimide
	  Methyprylon
	  Muscle relaxants
		Metabolic acidosis (low lactate; high anion gap)
		  Alcoholic ketoacidosis
		  Ethylene glycol
		  Methanol
		  Formaldehyde/paraldehyde
		  Salicylate
		  Sulfur/sulfate
		  Toluene
		  Valproic acid
			Inhibitors of metabolic pathways
			  Disulfiram
			  Inhibitors of thyroid hormone synthesis
			  MAO inhibitors
			  Salicylates
			
			Inhibitors of nucleic acid synthesis
			  Anticancer agents
			  Antiviral agents
			  Immunosuppressive drugs
			  Mushrooms (amatoxins)
			  Podophylline
			
			Nontoxic exposure
			
			Psychogenic illness

NOTE: CNS, central nervous system; MAO, monoamine oxidase; GI, gastrointestinal; GU, genitourinary; LSD, lysergic acid diethylamide.

fatal poisoning include alcohols and glycols, gases and fumes, chemicals, cleaning substances, pesticides, and automotive products.

DIAGNOSIS

Although poisoning can mimic other illnesses, the correct diagnosis can usually be established by the history, physical examination, routine and toxicologic laboratory evaluations, and characteristic clinical course. The *history* should include the time, route, duration, and circumstances (location, surrounding events, and intent) of exposure; the name and amount of each drug, chemical, or ingredient involved; the time of onset, nature, and severity of symptoms; the time and type of first aid measures provided; and the medical and psychiatric history.

In many cases the victim is confused, comatose, unaware of an exposure, or unable or unwilling to admit to one. Suspicious circumstances include unexplained illness in a previously healthy person; a history of psychiatric problems (particularly depression); recent changes in health, economic status, or social relationships; and onset of illness while working with chemicals or after ingesting food, drink (especially ethanol), or medications. Patients who become ill soon after arriving from a foreign country or being arrested for criminal activity should be suspected of "body packing" or "body stuffing" (ingesting or concealing illicit drugs in a body cavity). Relevant history may be available from family, friends, paramedics, police, pharmacists, physicians, and employers, who should be questioned regarding the patient's habits, hobbies, behavior changes, available medications, and antecedent events. A search of clothes, belongings, and place of discovery may reveal a suicide note or a container of drugs or chemicals. The imprint code on pills and the label on chemical products may be used to identify the ingredients and potential toxicity of a suspected poison by consulting a reference text, a computerized database, the manufacturer, or a regional poison information center.

In the absence of a history of exposure, the *clinical course* may suggest a diagnosis of poisoning. Poisoning typically evolves and resolves more rapidly than other disorders. Signs and symptoms characteristically develop within an hour of acute exposure, peak within several hours, and resolve over hours to days. However, the absence of signs and symptoms soon after an overdose does not rule out a poisoning.

The *physical examination* should focus initially on the vital signs, cardiopulmonary system, and neurologic status. On the basis of the pulse, blood pressure, respiratory rate, temperature, and mental status, the physiologic state can be characterized as excited, depressed, discordant, or normal. A differential diagnosis can then be formulated (Table 396-1). Examination of the eyes (for nystagmus, pupil size and reactivity), abdomen (for bowel activity and bladder size), and skin (for burns, bullae, color, warmth, moisture, pressure sores, and puncture marks) may narrow the diagnosis to a particular disorder. Grading the severity of poisoning (Table 396-2) is useful for assessing the clinical course and response to treatment.

The patient should also be examined for evidence of trauma and underlying illnesses. Except with carbon monoxide, theophylline, and drugs that cause hypoglycemia or hypoxia, seizures and neurologic manifestations of poisoning are nonfocal. Hence, focal findings should prompt evaluation for a structural central nervous system (CNS) lesion. When the history is unclear, all orifices should be examined for the presence of chemical burns and drug packets. The odor of breath or vomitus and the color of nails, skin, or urine may provide diagnostic clues.

Laboratory assessment may be helpful in the differential diagnosis

Table 396-2 Severity of Physiologic Stimulation and Depression in Poisoning and Drug Withdrawal

PHYSIOLOGIC STIMULATION

Grade 1 Anxious, irritable, tremulous; vital signs normal; diaphoresis, flushing or pallor, mydriasis, and hyperreflexia may be present

Grade 2 Agitated; may have confusion or hallucinations but is able to converse and follow commands; vital signs mildly to moderately increased

Grade 3 Delirious; unintelligible speech, uncontrollable motor hyperactivity; moderately to markedly increased vital signs; tachyarrhythmias possible

Grade 4 Coma, seizures, cardiovascular collapse

PHYSIOLOGIC DEPRESSION

Grade 1 Awake, lethargic, or sleeping but arousable by voice or tactile stimulation; able to converse and follow commands; may be confused

Grade 2 Responds to pain but not voice; can vocalize but not converse; spontaneous motor activity present; brainstem reflexes intact

Grade 3 Unresponsive to pain; spontaneous motor activity absent; brainstem reflexes depressed; motor tone, respirations, and temperature decreased

Grade 4 Unresponsive to pain; flaccid paralysis; brainstem reflexes and respirations absent; cardiovascular vital signs decreased

---

of poisoning (Fig. 396-1). An increased anion-gap metabolic acidosis is characteristic of advanced methanol, ethylene glycol, and salicylate intoxication but can occur with other agents (Table 396-1) and in any poisoning that results in hepatic, renal, or respiratory failure, seizures, or shock. The serum lactate concentration is low (less than the anion gap) in the former and high (nearly equal to the anion gap) in the latter. An abnormally low anion gap can be due to elevated blood levels of bromide, calcium, iodine, lithium, magnesium, or nitrate. An increased osmolal gap—the difference between the serum osmolality (measured by freezing point depression) and that calculated from the serum sodium, glucose, and blood urea nitrogen (BUN) of >10 mmol/L—suggests the presence of a low-molecular-weight solute such as an alcohol, glycol, or ketone or an unmeasured electrolyte or sugar. The osmolal gap can also provide an estimate of the amount of anion present (Table 396-3). Ketosis suggests acetone, isopropyl alcohol, or salicylate poisoning. Hypoglycemia may be due to poisoning with β-adrenergic blockers, ethanol, insulin, oral hypoglycemic agents, quinine, and salicylates, whereas hyperglycemia can occur in poisoning with acetone, β-adrenergic agonist, calcium channel blockers, iron, theophylline, or Vacor. Hypokalemia can be caused by barium, a β-adrenergic agonist, a diuretic, theophylline, or toluene; hyperkalemia suggests poisoning with an α-adrenergic agonist, a β-adrenergic blocker, cardiac glycosides, or fluoride.

Radiologic studies may also be useful for diagnostic purposes. Pulmonary edema (adult respiratory distress syndrome, or ARDS) can be caused by poisoning with carbon monoxide, cyanide, an opioid, paraquat, phencyclidine, a sedative-hypnotic, or salicylate; by inhalation of irritant gases, fumes, or vapors (ammonia, metal oxides, mercury); or by prolonged anoxia, hyperthermia, or shock. Aspiration pneumonia is common in patients with coma, seizures, and petroleum distillate ingestion. Ra-

diopaque densities may be visible on abdominal x-rays following the ingestion of calcium salts, chloral hydrate, chlorinated hydrocarbons, heavy metals, illicit drug packets, iodinated compounds, potassium salts, psychotherapeutic agents, lithium, phenothiazines, enteric-coated tablets, or salicylates.

The electrocardiogram (ECG) can be useful to assist with the differential diagnosis and to guide treatment. Bradycardia and atrioventricular (AV) block may occur in patients poisoned by α-adrenergic agonists, antiarrhythmic agents, beta blockers, calcium channel blockers, cholinergic agents (carbamate and organophosphate insecticides), cardiac glycosides, lithium, magnesium, or tricyclic antidepressants. QRS- and QT-interval prolongation may be caused by hyperkalemia and by membrane-active drugs (Table 396-1). Ventricular tachyarrhythmias may be seen in poisoning with cardiac glycosides, fluorides, membrane-active drugs, sympathomimetics, or agents that cause hyperkalemia or potentiate the effects of endogenous catecholamines (e.g., chloral hydrate, aliphatic and halogenated hydrocarbons).

Analysis of urine and blood (and occasionally of gastric contents and chemical samples) may be useful to confirm or rule out suspected poisoning. Interpretation of laboratory data requires knowledge of the tests used for screening and confirmation (thin-layer, gas-liquid, or high-performance liquid chromatography; colorimetric and fluorometric assays; enzyme-multiplied and radioimmunoassays; gas chromatography; mass spectrometry), their sensitivity (limit of detection) and specificity, the preferred biologic specimen for analysis, and the optimal time of specimen sampling. Personal communication with the laboratory is essential. A negative result on a screen may mean the substance is not detectable by the test used or that its concentration is too low for detection at the time of sampling. In the latter case, repeating the test at a later time may yield a positive result.

Although some rapid screening tests for a limited number of drugs of abuse are available, comprehensive screening tests require 2 to 6 h for completion, and immediate management must be based on the history, physical examination, and routine ancillary tests. In addition,

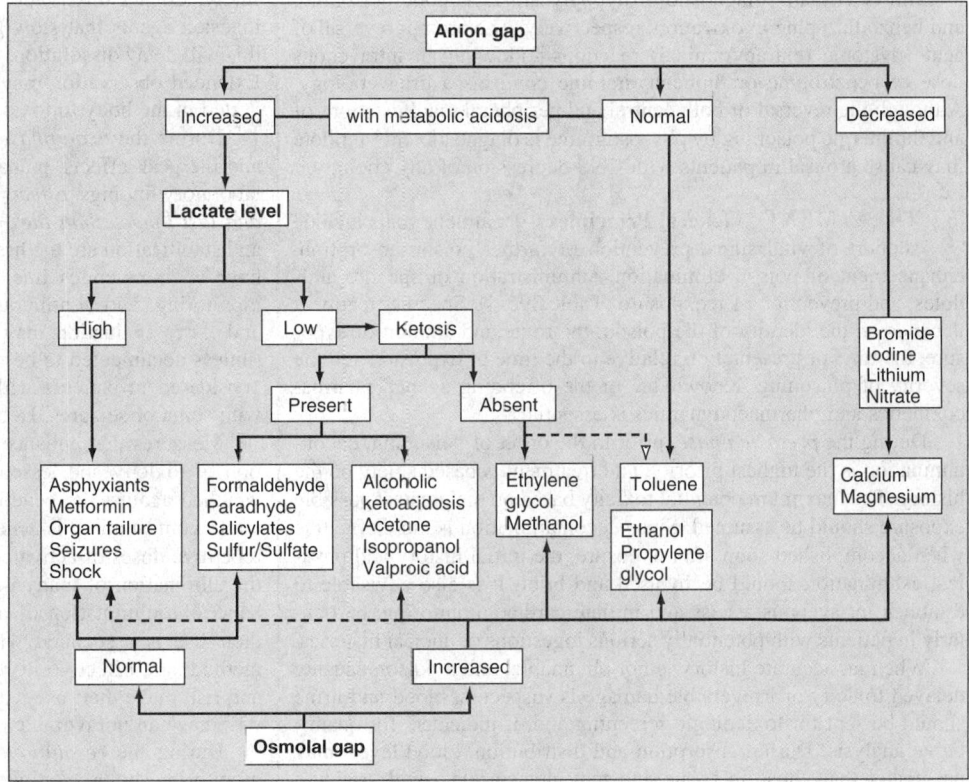

FIGURE 396-1 Differential diagnosis of poisoning based on the results of routine laboratory tests. Dashed lines indicate possible pathways.

Table 396-4   Fundamentals of Poisoning Management

Table 396-3   Solute Effects on Serum Osmolality

Agent	Approximate Serum Concentrations (mg/dL) of Solute That Will Increase the Serum Osmolality by 1 mmol/kg[a]
Alcohols	
Ethanol	4.6
Isopropanol	6.0
Methanol	2.6
Glycols	
Ethylene glycol	5.2
Propylene glycol	7.6
Ketones	
Acetone	5.8
Electrolytes	
Calcium	4
Magnesium	2.4
Sugars	
Mannitol	18
Sorbitol	18

[a] Equivalent to 2 mmol/L of calcium and magnesium and 1 mmol/L of all other compounds.

when the patient is asymptomatic, or when the clinical picture is consistent with the reported history, qualitative screening is neither clinically useful nor cost-effective. It is of greatest value in patients with severe or unexplained toxicity who have coma, seizures, cardiovascular instability, metabolic or respiratory acidosis, and nonsinus cardiac rhythms. Quantitative analysis is useful for poisoning with acetaminophen, acetone, alcohol (including ethylene glycol), antiarrhythmics, anticonvulsants, barbiturates, digoxin, heavy metals, lithium, paraquat, salicylate, and theophylline, as well as for carboxyhemoglobin and methemoglobin. Results can often be available within an hour.

The *response to antidotes* may be useful for diagnostic purposes. Resolution of altered mental status and abnormal vital signs within minutes of intravenous administration of dextrose, naloxone, or flumazenil is virtually diagnostic of hypoglycemia, narcotic poisoning, and benzodiazepine intoxication, respectively. The prompt reversal of acute dystonic (extrapyramidal) reactions following an intravenous dose of benztropine or diphenhydramine confirms a drug etiology. Although the reversal of both central and peripheral manifestations of anticholinergic poisoning by physostigmine is diagnostic, this antidote may cause arousal in patients with CNS depression of any etiology.

℞ **TREATMENT   General Principles**   Treatment goals include support of vital signs, prevention of further poison absorption, enhancement of poison elimination, administration of specific antidotes, and prevention of reexposure (Table 396-4). Specific treatment depends on the identity of the poison, the route and amount of exposure, the time of presentation relative to the time of exposure, and the severity of poisoning. Knowledge of the offending agents' pharmacokinetics and pharmacodynamics is essential.

During the *pretoxic phase*, prior to the onset of poisoning, decontamination is the highest priority, and treatment is based solely on the history. The maximum potential toxicity based on the greatest possible exposure should be assumed. Since decontamination is more effective when accomplished soon after exposure, the initial history and physical examination should be focused and brief. It is also advisable to establish intravenous access and initiate cardiac monitoring, particularly in patients with potentially serious ingestions or unclear histories.

When an accurate history is not obtainable, and a poison causing delayed toxicity or irreversible damage is suspected, blood and urine should be sent for toxicologic screening and, if indicated, for quantitative analysis. During absorption and distribution, blood levels may be greater than those in tissue and may not correlate with toxicity. However, high blood levels of agents whose metabolites are more toxic than the parent compound (acetaminophen, ethylene glycol, or

Table 396-4   Fundamentals of Poisoning Management

SUPPORTIVE CARE

Airway protection	Treatment of seizures
Oxygenation/ventilation	Correction of temperature abnormalities
Treatment of arrhythmias	Correction of metabolic derangements
Hemodynamic support	Prevention of secondary complications

PREVENTION OF FURTHER POISON ABSORPTION

Gastrointestinal decontamination	Decontamination of other sites
Syrup of ipecac–induced emesis	Eye decontamination
Gastric lavage	Skin decontamination
Activated charcoal	Body cavity evacuation
Whole-bowel irrigation	
Catharsis	
Dilution	
Endoscopic/surgical removal	

ENHANCEMENT OF POISON ELIMINATION

Multiple-dose activated charcoal	Extracorporeal removal
Forced diuresis	Peritoneal dialysis
Alteration of urinary pH	Hemodialysis
Chelation (Chap. 395)	Hemoperfusion
	Hemofiltration
	Plasmapheresis
	Exchange transfusion
	Hyperbaric oxygenation

ADMINISTRATION OF ANTIDOTES

Neutralization by antibodies	Metabolic antagonism
Neutralization by chemical binding	Physiologic antagonism

PREVENTION OF REEXPOSURE

Adult education	Notification of regulatory agencies
Child-proofing	Psychiatric referral

methanol) may indicate the need for additional interventions (antidotes, dialysis).

Most patients who remain or become asymptomatic 4 to 6 h after ingestion will not develop subsequent toxicity and can be discharged safely. Longer observation may be necessary for patients who have ingested agents that slow gastric emptying and intestinal motility as this will delay dissolution, absorption, and distribution characteristics. Extended observation may also be indicated for agents that are converted in the body to toxic metabolites (Table 396-1).

During the *toxic phase*, the time between the onset of poisoning and the peak effects, management is based primarily on clinical and laboratory findings. *Effects after an overdose begin sooner, peak later, and last longer than they do after a therapeutic dose.* Resuscitation and stabilization are the first priority. All symptomatic patients should have an intravenous line, oxygen saturation determination, cardiac monitoring, and continuous observation. Baseline laboratory, ECG, and x-ray evaluation may also be appropriate. Intravenous glucose (unless documented to be normal), naloxone, and thiamine should be considered in patients with altered mental status, particularly those with soma or seizures. Decontamiation may also be appropriate.

Measures that enhance poison elimination may shorten the duration of toxicity and lessen its severity. However, the risks must be weighed against the benefits. Diagnostic certainty (usually via laboratory confirmation) is generally a prerequisite. Intestinal dialysis with repetitive doses of activated charcoal is usually safe and can enhance the elimination of many poisons. Diuresis and chelation therapy enhance the elimination of a relatively small number of poisons, and their use is associated with potential complications. Extracorporal methods are effective in removing many poisons, but their expense and risk make their use reasonable only in patients who would otherwise have an unfavorable outcome.

During the *resolution phase* of poisoning, supportive care and monitoring should continue until clinical, laboratory, and ECG abnormalities have resolved. Since chemicals are eliminated from the blood before tissues, blood levels are usually lower than tissue levels during this phase and may not correlate with toxicity. This is particularly true when extracorporeal elimination procedures are used. Redistribution from tissues may cause a rebound increase in the blood level after termination of these procedures. When a metabolite is responsible for toxic effects, continued treatment of an asymptomatic patient might be necessary because of a potentially toxic blood level (acetaminophen, ethylene glycol, and methanol).

Supportive Care The goal of supportive therapy is to maintain physiologic homeostasis until detoxification is accomplished and to prevent and treat secondary complications such as aspiration, bedsores, cerebral and pulmonary edema, pneumonia, rhabdomyolysis, renal failure, sepsis, thromboembolic disease, and generalized organ dysfunction due to prolonged hypoxia or shock.

Admission to an intensive care unit is indicated for the following: patients with severe poisoning (coma, respiratory depression, hypotension, cardiac conduction abnormalities, cardiac arrhythmias, hypothermia or hyperthermia, seizures); those needing close monitoring, antidotes, or enhanced elimination therapy; those showing progressive clinical deterioration; and those with significant underlying medical problems. Patients with mild to moderate toxicity can be managed on a general medical service, intermediate care unit, or emergency department observation area, depending on the anticipated duration and level of monitoring needed (intermittent clinical observation versus continuous clinical, cardiac, and respiratory monitoring). Patients who have attempted suicide require continuous observation and measures to prevent self-injury until they are thought unlikely to make further attempts.

Respiratory care Endotracheal intubation for protection against the aspiration of gastrointestinal contents is of paramount importance in patients with CNS depression or seizures as this complication can increase morbidity and mortality. Mechanical ventilation may be necessary for patients with respiratory depression or hypoxia and to facilitate therapeutic sedation or paralysis in order to prevent hyperthermia, acidosis, and rhabdomyolysis associated with neuromuscular hyperactivity. Since clinical assessment of respiratory function is often inaccurate, the need for oxygenation and ventilation is best determined by oximetry or arterial blood gas analysis. The gag reflex is not a reliable indicator of the need for intubation. A patient may maintain airway patency while being stimulated but not if left unattended. Those who cannot respond to voice or who are unable to sit and drink fluids without assistance are best managed by prophylactic intubation.

Drug-induced pulmonary edema is usually noncardiac rather than cardiac in origin. Profound CNS depression and cardiac conduction abnormalities suggest the latter etiology. Measurement of pulmonary artery pressure may be necessary to establish etiology and direct appropriate therapy. Extracorporeal measures (membrane oxygenation, venoarterial perfusion, cardiopulmonary bypass), partial liquid (perfluorocarbon) ventilation, and hyperbaric oxygen therapy may be appropriate for severe but reversible respiratory failure.

Cardiovascular therapy Maintenance of normal tissue perfusion is critical to allow for complete recovery once the offending agent has been eliminated. If hypotension is unresponsive to volume expansion, treatment with norepinephrine, epinephrine, or high-dose dopamine may be necessary (Chap. 38). Intraaortic balloon pump counterpulsation and venoarterial or cardiopulmonary perfusion techniques should be considered for severe but reversible cardiac failure. Bardyarrhythmias associated with hypotension generally should be treated as described in Chap. 229. Glucagon and calcium may be effective in both beta blocker and calcium channel blocker poisoning. Antibody therapy may be indicated for cardiac glycoside poisoning.

Supraventricular tachycardia associated with hypertension and CNS excitation is almost always due to agents that cause generalized physiologic excitation (Table 396-1). Most cases are mild or moderate in severity and require only observation or nonspecific sedation with a benzodiazepine. For cases that are severe or associated with hemodynamic instability, chest pain, or ECG evidence of ischemia, specific therapy is indicated. For patients with sympathetic hyperactivity, treatment with a combined alpha and beta blocker (labetalol), a calcium

channel blocker (verapamil or diltiazem), or a combination of a beta blocker and a vasodilator (esmolol and nitroprusside) is preferred. For those with anticholinergic poisoning, physostigmine is the treatment of choice. Supraventricular tachycardia without hypertension is generally secondary to vasodilation or hypovolemia and responds to fluid administration.

Lidocaine and phenytoin are generally safe for ventricular tachyarrhythmias, but beta blockers can be hazardous unless the arrhythmia is clearly due to sympathetic hyperactivity. For ventricular tachyarrhythmias due to tricyclic antidepressants and probably other membrane-active agents (Table 396-1), class IA, IC, and III antiarrhythmic agents are contraindicated (because of similar electrophysiologic effects), but sodium bicarbonate may be helpful. Magnesium sulfate and overdrive pacing (by isoproterenol or a pacemaker) may be useful in patients with torsade de pointes and prolonged QT intervals. Magnesium and antidigoxin antibodies should be considered in patients with severe cardiac glycoside poisoning. Invasive (esophageal or intracardiac) ECG recording may be necessary to determine the origin (ventricular or supraventricular) of wide-complex tachycardias (Chap. 230). If the patient is hemodynamically stable, however, it may be prudent to observe rather than to treat with another potentially proarrhythmic agent. Arrhythmias may be resistant to drug therapy until underlying acid-base, electrolyte, oxygenation, and temperature derangements are corrected.

Central nervous system therapies Neuromuscular hyperactivity and seizures can lead to hyperthermia, lactic acidosis, and rhabdomyolysis, with their attendant complications, and should be treated aggressively. Seizures caused by excessive stimulation of catecholamine receptors (sympathomimetic or hallucinogen poisoning and drug withdrawal), or decreased activity of γ-aminobutyric acid (GABA) (isoniazid poisoning) or glycine (strychnine poisoning) receptors are best treated with enhancers of GABA effects such as benzodiazepines or barbiturates. Since benzodiazepines and barbiturates act by slightly different mechanisms (the former increases the frequency and the latter increases the duration of chloride channel opening in response to GABA), therapy with both may be effective when neither is effective alone. Seizures caused by isoniazid, which inhibits the synthesis of GABA, may require high doses of pyridoxine (which facilitates the synthesis of GABA). Seizures resulting from membrane destabilization (beta blocker or cyclic antidepressant poisoning) may require a membrane-active anticonvulsant such as phenytoin as well as GABA enhancers. For poisons with central dopaminergic effects (phencyclidine), an agent with opposing activity, such as haloperidol, may be useful. In anticholinergic and cyanide poisoning, specific antidotal therapy may be necessary. The treatment of seizures secondary to ischemia, edema, or metabolic abnormalities should include correction of the underlying cause. Neuromuscular paralysis is indicated in refractory cases. Electroencephalographic (EEG) monitoring and continuing treatment of seizures are necessary to prevent permanent neurologic damage.

Other measures Temperature extremes, metabolic abnormalities, hepatic and renal dysfunction, and secondary complications should be treated by standard therapies.

Prevention of Poison Absorption • *Gastrointestinal decontamination* Whether or not to perform gastrointestinal decontamination, and which procedure to use, depends on the time since ingestion; the existing and predicted toxicity of the ingestant; the availability, efficacy, and contraindications of the procedure; and the nature, severity, and risk of complications. In animal and human volunteer studies, the efficacy of activated charcoal, gastric lavage, and syrup of ipecac decreases with time, and there are insufficient data to support or exclude a beneficial effect when they are used more than 1 h after ingestion. Due to the lack of clinical studies using control groups without treatment, the efficacy of these procedures for improving the outcome of overdose patients has not been established.

The average time from ingestion to presentation for treatment is over 1 h for children and over 3 h for adults. Most patients will recover from poisoning uneventfully with good supportive care alone, but complications of gastrointestinal decontamination, particularly aspiration, can prolong this process. Hence, gastrointestinal contamination should be performed selectively, not routinely, in the management of overdose patients. It is clearly unnecessary when predicted toxicity is minimal or the time of expected maximal toxicity has passed without significant effect.

Activated charcoal has comparable or greater efficacy, fewer contraindications and complications, is less aversive and invasive than ipecac or gastric lavage, and is the preferred method of gastrointestinal decontamination in most situations.

Activated charcoal is prepared as a suspension in water, either alone or with a cathartic. It is given orally via a nippled bottle (for infants), or via a cup, straw, or small-bore nasogastric tube. The recommended dose is 1 g/kg body weight, using 8 mL of diluent per gram of charcoal if a premixed formulation is not available. Palatability may be increased by adding a sweetener (sorbitol) or a flavoring agent (cherry, chocolate, or cola syrup) to the suspension. Charcoal adsorbs ingested poisons within the gut lumen, allowing the charcoal-toxin complex to be evacuated with stool. The complex can also be removed from the stomach by induced emesis or lavage. In vitro, charcoal adsorbs ≥90% of most substances when given in an amount equal to 10 times the weight of the substance. Charged (ionized) chemicals such as mineral acids, alkalis, and highly dissociated salts of cyanide, fluoride, iron, lithium, and other inorganic compounds are not well adsorbed by charcoal. In animal and human volunteer studies, charcoal decreases the absorption of ingestants by an average of 73% when given within 5 min of ingestant administration, 51% when given at 30 min, and 36% at 60 min. Charcoal is at least equally as effective as ipecac syrup or gastric lavage. Experimentally, lavage followed by charcoal is more effective than charcoal alone, and charcoal before and after lavage is more effective than charcoal alone or charcoal after lavage. In the treatment of poisoned patients, however, charcoal alone generally results in a better clinical outcome than either treatment with ipecac followed by charcoal or lavage followed by charcoal. Side effects of charcoal include nausea, vomiting, and diarrhea or constipation. Charcoal may also prevent the absorption of orally administered therapeutic agents. Complications include mechanical obstruction of the airway, aspiration, vomiting, and bowel obstruction and infection caused by inspissated charcoal. Charcoal is not recommended for patients who have ingested corrosives because it obscures endoscopy.

Gastric lavage is performed by sequentially administering and aspirating about 5 mL fluid per kilogram of body weight through a no. 28 French orogastric tube in children and a no. 40 French tube in adults. Except for infants, tap water is acceptable. The patient should be placed in Trendelenburg and left lateral decubitus positions to prevent aspiration (even if an endotracheal tube is in place). Lavage decreases ingestant absorption by an average of 52% if performed within 5 min of ingestion administration, 26% if performed at 30 min, and 16% if performed at 60 min. Its efficacy is similar to that of ipecac. Significant amounts of ingested drug are recovered in one-tenth of patients. Aspiration is a common complication (occurring in up to 10% of patients), especially when lavage is perfomed improperly. Serious complications (tracheal lavage, esophageal and gastric perforation) occur in approximately 1% of patients. For this reason, the physician should personally insert the lavage tube and confirm its placement, and the patient must be cooperative or adequately restrained (with pharmacologic sedation if necessary) during the procedure. Gastric lavage is contraindicated in corrosive or petroleum distillate ingestions because of the respective risks of gastroesophageal perforation and aspiration-induced hydrocarbon pneumonitis.

Syrup of ipecac can be used for the home management of patients with accidental ingestions, reliable histories, and mild predicted toxicity. It may delay the administration and decrease the effectiveness of activated charcoal, oral antidotes, and whole-bowel irrigation and is very rarely appropriate for patients treated at a health care facility. It is administered orally in a dose of 30 mL for adults, 15 mL for children, and 10 mL for small infants. Clear liquids should also be given. Ipecac irritates the stomach and stimulates the central chemoreceptor trigger zone. Vomiting usually occurs about 20 min after administration. The dose may be repeated if vomiting does not occur. In animal and human volunteer studies, ipecac decreases ingestant absorption by an average of 60% if given within 5 min of ingestant administration, 32% if given at 30 min, and 30% if given at 60 min. Side effects include lethargy in children (12%) and protracted vomiting (8 to 17%). Chronic ipecac use (by patients with anorexia nervosa or bulimia) may cause electrolyte and fluid abnormalities, cardiac toxicity, and myopathy. Except for aspiration, serious complications are rare. Gastric or esophageal tears and perforations and stroke have been reported. Ipecac is contraindicated in patients with recent gastrointestinal surgery, CNS depression, or seizures, and in those who have ingested corrosives or rapidly acting CNS poisons (camphor, cyanide, tricyclic antidepressants, propoxyphene, strychnine).

Whole-bowel irrigation is performed by administering a bowel-cleansing solution containing electrolytes and polyethylene glycol (Golytely, Colyte) orally or by gastric tube at a rate of up 0.5 L/h in children and 2.0 L/h in adults until rectal effluent is clear. The patient must be in a sitting position. Although data are limited, whole-bowel irrigation may be at least equally as effective as other decontamination procedures. It may be appropriate for those who have ingested foreign bodies, packets of illicit drugs, slow-release or enteric-coated medications, and agents that are poorly adsorbed by charcoal (e.g., heavy metals). It is contraindicated in patients with bowel obstruction, ileus, hemodynamic instability, and compromised unprotected airways.

Cathartic salts (disodium phosphate, magnesium citrate and sulfate, sodium sulfate) or *saccharides* (mannitol, sorbitol) promote the rectal evacuation of gastrointestinal contents. The most effective cathartic is sorbitol in a dose of 1 to 2 g/kg of body weight. Alone, cathartics do not prevent ingestant absorption and should not be used as a method of gut decontamination. Their primary use is to prevent constipation following charcoal administration. Abdominal cramps, nausea, and occasional vomiting are side effects. Complications of repeated dosing include hypermagnesemia and excessive diarrhea. Cathartics are contraindicated in patients who have ingested corrosives and in those with preexisting diarrhea. Magnesium-containing cathartics should not be used in patients with renal failure.

Dilution (i.e., drinking 5 mL/kg of body weight of water or another clear liquid) should be accomplished as soon as possible after the ingestion of corrosives (acids, alkali). However, it may increase the dissolution rate (and hence absorption) of capsules, tablets, and other solid ingestants and should *not* be used in these circumstances.

Endoscopic or surgical removal of poisons may be useful in rare situations, such as ingestion of a potentially toxic foreign body that fails to transit the gastrointestinal tract, a potentially lethal amount of a heavy metal (arsenic, iron, mercury, thallium), or agents that have coalesced into gastric concretions or bezoars (barbiturates, glutethimide, heavy metals, lithium, meprobamate, sustained-release preparations). Patients who become toxic from cocaine due to its leakage from multiple ingested drug packets require immediate surgical intervention.

Decontamination of other sites   Immediate, copious flushing with water, saline, or another available clear, drinkable liquid is the initial treatment for topical exposures (exceptions include alkali metals, calcium oxide, phosphorus). Saline is preferred for eye irrigation. A triple wash (water, soap, water) may be best for dermal decontamination. Inhalational exposures should be treated initially with fresh air or oxygen. The removal of liquids from body cavities such as the vagina or rectum is best accomplished by irrigation. Solids (drug packets, pills) should be removed manually, preferably with visual guidance.

Enhancement of Poison Elimination   Although the elimination of most poisons can be accelerated by therapeutic interventions, the pharmacokinetic efficacy (removal of drug at a rate greater than that accomplished by intrinsic elimination) and clinical benefit (in terms of a shortened duration of toxicity or improved outcome) of such interventions are often more theoretical than proven. Hence, the decision to use such measures should be based on the actual or predicted toxicity and the potential efficacy, cost, and risks of therapy.

Multiple-dose activated charcoal Repetitive oral dosing with charcoal can enhance the elimination of previously absorbed substances by binding them within the gut as they are excreted in the bile, secreted by gastrointestinal cells, or passively diffuse into the gut lumen (reverse absorption or enterocapillary exsorption). Doses of 0.5 to 1 g/kg body weight every 2 to 4 h, adjusted downward to avoid regurgitation in patients with decreased gastrointestinal motility, are generally recommended. Experimentally, this treatment enhances the elimination of nearly all substances tested. Pharmacokinetic efficacy approaches that of hemodialysis for some agents (e.g., phenobarbital, theophylline). Multiple-dose therapy is not effective in accelerating elimination of chlorpropamide, tobramycin, or agents that adsorb poorly to charcoal. Complications include intestinal obstruction, pseudoobstruction, and nonocclusive intestinal infarction in patients with decreased gut motility.

Forced diuresis and alteration of urinary pH Diuresis and ion trapping via alteration of urine pH may prevent the renal reabsorption of poisons that undergo excretion by glomerular filtration and active tubular secretion. Since membranes are more permeable to nonionized molecules than to their ionized counterparts, acidic (low-pK_a) poisons are ionized and trapped in an alkaline urine, and basic poisons are ionized and trapped in an acid urine. Saline diuresis can enhance the renal excretion of alcohols, bromide, calcium, fluoride, lithium, meprobamate, potassium, and isoniazid. Alkaline diuresis (a urine pH $\geq$7.5 and a urine output of 3 to 6 mL/kg body weight per hour) enhances the elimination of chlorphenoxyacetic acid herbicides, chlorpropamide, diflunisal, fluoride, methotrexate, phenobarbital, sulfonamides, and salicylates. Contraindications include congestive heart failure, renal failure, and cerebral edema. Acid-base, fluid, and electrolyte parameters should be monitored carefully. Acid diuresis enhances the renal elimination of amphetamines, chloroquine, cocaine, local anesthetics, phencyclidine, quinidine, quinine, strychnine, sympathomimetics, tricyclic antidepressants, and tocainide. Its use, however, has been largely abandoned because of potential complications and lack of clinical efficacy.

Extracorporeal removal Peritoneal dialysis, hemodialysis, charcoal or resin hemoperfusion, hemofiltration, plasmapheresis, and exchange transfusion are capable of removing any toxin from the bloodstream. Agents most amenable to enhanced elimination by dialysis have low molecular mass (<500 Da), high water solubility, low protein binding, small volumes of distribution (<1 L/kg body weight), prolonged elimination (long half-life), and high dialysis clearance relative to total-body clearance. Molecular weight, water solubility, or protein binding do not limit the efficacy of the other forms of extracorporeal removal.

Dialysis should be considered in cases of severe poisoning due to barbiturates, bromide, chloral hydrate, ethanol, ethylene glycol, isopropyl alcohol, lithium, methanol, procainamide, theophylline, salicylates, and possibly heavy metals. Although hemoperfusion may be more effective in removing some of these poisons, it does not correct associated acid-base and electrolyte abnormalities. Hemoperfusion should be considered in cases of severe poisoning due to carbamazepine, chloramphenicol, disopyramide, and hypnotic-sedatives (barbiturates, ethchlorvynol, glutethimide, meprobamate, methaqualone), paraquat, phenytoin, procainamide, theophylline, and valproate. Both techniques require central venous access and systemic anticoagulation and often result in transient hypotension. Hemoperfusion may also cause hemolysis, hypocalcemia, and thrombocytopenia. Peritoneal dialysis and exchange transfusion are less effective but may be used when other procedures are either not available, contraindicated, or technically difficult (e.g., in infants). Exchange transfusion removes poisons affecting red blood cells (as in methemoglobinemia or arsine-

induced hemolysis). The roles of hemofiltration and plasmapheresis are not yet defined.

Candidates for these treatments include patients with severe toxicity who deteriorate despite aggressive supportive therapy; those with potentially prolonged, irreversible, or fatal toxicity; those with dangerous blood levels of toxins; those who lack the capacity for self-detoxification because of liver or renal failure; and those with a serious underlying illness or complication that will adversely affect recovery.

Other techniques The elimination of heavy metals can be enhanced by chelation, and the removal of carbon monoxide can be increased by hyperbaric oxygenation as discussed in sections on specific poisons.

Administration of Antidotes Antidotes counteract the effects of poisons by neutralizing them (e.g., antibody-antigen reactions, chelation, chemical binding) or by antagonizing their physiologic effects (e.g., activation of opposing nervous system activity, provision of competitive metabolic or receptor substrate). Poisons or conditions with specific antidotes include acetaminophen, anticholinergic agents, anticoagulants, benzodiazepines, beta blockers, calcium channel blockers, carbon monoxide, cardiac glycosides, cholinergic agents, cyanide, drug-induced dystonic reactions, ethylene glycol, fluoride, heavy metals, hydrogen sulfide, hypoglycemic agents, isoniazid, methemoglobinemia, narcotics, sympathomimetics, Vacor, and a variety of envenomations. Antidotes can significantly reduce morbidity and mortality, but most are potentially toxic. Since their safe use requires correct identification of a specific poisoning or syndrome, details of antidotal therapy are discussed with the conditions for which they are indicated.

Prevention of Reexposure Poisoning is a preventable illness. Unfortunately, some adults and children are poison-prone, and recurrences are common. Adults with accidental exposures should be instructed regarding the safe use of medications and chemicals (according to labeling instructions). Confused patients may need assistance with the administration of medications. Errors in dosing by health care providers may require educational efforts. Patients should be advised to avoid circumstances that result in chemical exposure or poisoning. Appropriate agencies and health departments should be notified in cases of environmental or workplace exposure. The best approach with young children and patients with intentional overdose is to limit access to poisons. In households where children live or visit, alcoholic beverages, medications, household products (automotive, cleaning, fuel, pet-care, toiletry products), nonedible plants, and vitamins should be kept out of reach or in locked or child-proof cabinets. Depressed or psychotic patients should receive psychiatric assessment, disposition, and follow-up. They should be given prescriptions for a limited supply of drugs and with a limited number of refills and be monitored for compliance and response to therapy.

SPECIFIC POISONS

The following discussion focuses on poisonings that are common, produce life-threatening toxicity, or require unique therapeutic interventions. Poisonings not covered here are described in the referenced texts. →*Alcohol, cocaine, hallucinogens, and opioids are discussed in Chaps. 386 to 389, and heavy metal poisoning is discussed in Chap. 395.*

ACETAMINOPHEN Acetaminophen is absorbed rapidly and has a volume of distribution of 1 L/kg body weight. Plasma concentrations range from 160 to 660 μmol/L (5 to 20 μg/mL) following therapeutic doses. Most acetaminophen is metabolized by hepatic conjugation with sulfate and glucuronide to form nontoxic metabolites, with minor amounts being excreted unchanged or oxidized by hepatic cytochrome P450 enzymes (primarily CYPIIE1) to form a highly reactive, electrophilic, and potentially toxic intermediary metabolite *n*-acetyl-*p*-benzoquinoneimine (NAPQI). After therapeutic doses, NAPQI is rapidly detoxified by conjugation with glutathione and excreted as cysteine and mercapturic acid conjugates. Following an acute ingestion of ≥140 mg/kg body weight, sulfate and glucuronide pathways become saturated, resulting in an increased fraction and amount of acetaminophen metabolized to NAPQI and eventual glutathione depletion. When this occurs, free NAPQI binds covalently to hepatocytes and causes their lysis (centrilobular necrosis). Less often, hepatotoxicity develops following the chronic ingestion of therapeutic or slightly greater amounts in conditions associated with decreased glutathione reserves (e.g., alcoholism, childhood, acute starvation, chronic malnutrition) and possibly in conditions with enhanced P450 enzyme activity (e.g., anticonvulsant and antituberculosis drug use). The plasma half-life is usually 2 to 4 h but may be prolonged if hepatotoxicity develops.

Clinical Toxicity Early manifestations of poisoning are nonspecific and not predictive of subsequent hepatotoxicity. Within 2 to 4 h of acute overdose, nausea, vomiting, diaphoresis, and pallor may develop. CNS depression is typically absent unless massive doses are ingested. Within 24 to 48 h, hepatotoxicity is evidenced by right upper quadrant tenderness and mild hepatomegaly. Renal function may also be impaired. Laboratory evidence of hepatic toxicity includes prolongation of the prothrombin time and elevation of serum bilirubin and transaminase activity (aspartate transaminase, alanine transaminase). Severe poisoning may cause hepatic failure. Greater than twofold prolongation of prothrombin time, a serum bilirubin level >68 μmol/L (4 mg/dL), pH <7.30, serum creatinine >3.3, and a high-grade encephalopathy indicate a poor prognosis. In patients who recover, liver function returns to normal within 1 week, and liver histology returns to normal within 3 months. Chronic poisoning is usually similar, but alcoholics may present with a syndrome of severe combined hepatic and renal insufficiency with dehydration, jaundice, coagulopathy, hypoglycemia, and acute tubular necrosis.

Diagnostic Evaluation A serum acetaminophen level should be obtained between 4 and 24 h after ingestion. A level above the lower line on the Rumack-Matthew nomogram (Fig. 396-2) indicates possible hepatotoxicity and the need for antidote therapy.

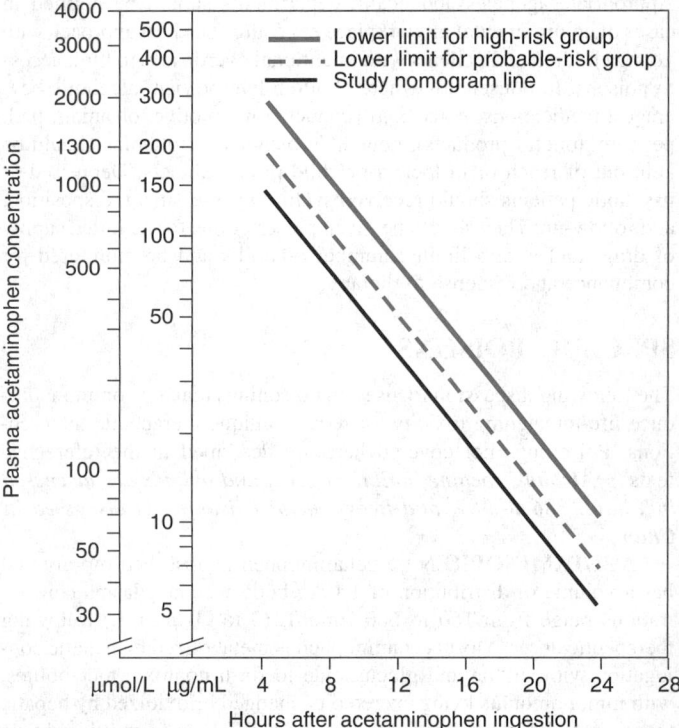

FIGURE 396-2 Nomogram to define risk according to initial plasma acetaminophen concentration. *(After BH Rumack, H Matthew: Pediatrics 55:871, 1975.)*

℞ TREATMENT Activated charcoal is recommended for patients who present within 4 h of ingestion. (Charcoal does not interfere significantly with acetylcysteine therapy.) Antidotal therapy consists of oral *N*-acetylcysteine (NAC), diluted 3:1 with a nonalcoholic, nondairy beverage. It is given at a loading dose of 140 mg/kg body weight, followed by a maintenance dose of 70 mg/kg body weight every 4 h for 17 additional doses. Treatment is most effective if started within 8 to 10 h of an overdose and should be administered before the serum level is known. If the level is subsequently shown to be nontoxic, therapy may be discontinued. Side effects of NAC include nausea, vomiting, and epigastric discomfort. The dose should be repeated if vomiting occurs within an hour of dosing. Antiemetics (metoclopramide, droperidol, odansetron) may be necessary. Liver and renal function should be monitored during therapy. Patients with severe hepatotoxicity should be considered for liver transplantation.

ACIDS AND ALKALI Common alkaline products include ammonia, bleach (sodium hypochlorite), drain cleaners (sodium hydroxide), surface cleaners (phosphates), laundry and dishwasher detergents (phosphates, carbonates), disk batteries, denture cleaners (borates, phosphates, carbonates), and Clinitest tablets (sodium hydroxides). Acids are used in toilet bowl cleaners (hydrofluoric, phosphoric, and sulfuric acids), soldering fluxes (hydrochloric acid), antirust compounds (hydrofluoric and oxalic acids), automobile battery fluid (sulfuric acid), and stone cleaners (hydrofluoric and nitric acids). Other corrosives include hydrogen peroxide, hydrazine, and phenol.

Alkalis produce liquefactive necrosis with rapidly penetrating tissue injury and a higher risk of perforation of the esophagus and stomach than do acids. Acids produce coagulative necrosis. Both may burn the mouth, esophagus, stomach, and proximal small bowel. Liquids tend to produce superficial, often circumferential burns over a larger surface area, while solids and tablets cause localized but deeper burns. The severity of the burn relates to the contact time, the amount ingested, and the pH (especially if <2 or >12) of the ingested product.

Clinical Toxicity Burns of the mouth result in excess salivation, pain, dysphonia, and dysphagia and are manifested by erythema, edema, ulceration, and necrosis. Deep burns may destroy mucosal nerve endings and produce anesthesia. Lack of oral findings does not rule out esophageal or gastric injury. Esophageal symptoms and signs include drooling, painful swallowing, retrosternal pain, and neck tenderness. Vomiting of blood and mucus may occur. Esophageal perforation is suggested by increased severity of chest pain, often with respiratory distress. Epigastric pain, vomiting, and tenderness may occur with burns to the stomach. Aspiration of acids and alkalis may cause fulminant tracheitis and bronchial pneumonia. In severe cases, hypotension, shock, metabolic acidosis, liver and renal dysfunction, hemolysis, and disseminated intravascular coagulation may be seen. Deep burns, particularly if extensive or circumferential, may be followed by fibrosis with stricture formation and obstruction of the esophagus (alkalis) or of the gastric outlet (acids).

Diagnosis Endoscopy, best performed 12 to 24 h after ingestion, is used to document the site of injury and its severity and should be performed in symptomatic patients. Chest and abdominal x-rays and routine laboratory testing should be obtained to evaluate for aspiration, perforation, and organ dysfunction. Residual effects of the ingestion can be assessed by barium swallow.

℞ TREATMENT Treatment includes immediate dilution with milk or water. Administration of a weak acid (carbonated beverage or citrus juice) or base (antacid) is also acceptable. Glucocorticoids and esophageal stents have traditionally been used for alkali burns to prevent esophageal stricture formation, but their efficacy is not proven. Animal studies suggest that glucocorticoids may be effective if begun immediately on presentation. If used, a dose of 1 to 2 mg of methylprednisolone per kilogram every 4 to 6 h for at least 2 weeks is suggested. Concomitant prophylactic broad-spectrum antibiotic use is also recommended. Glucocorticoids are not useful for acid burns. Antacids should be used for burns of the stomach. Esophageal stricture or gastric outlet obstruction may require subsequent dilatation and bouginage or surgical reconstruction.

ANTIARRHYTHMIC DRUGS Class IA (disopyramide, moricizine, procainamide, and quinidine), IB (lidocaine, mexiletine, phenytoin, and tocainide), and IC (encainide, flecainide, propafenone) antiarrhythmics block myocardial cell membrane fast sodium channels and slow cardiac conduction, whereas class III agents (amiodarone, bretylium, ibutilide, and sotalol) block potassium currents and prolong refractoriness. These agents are rapidly absorbed (except for disopyramide and sustained-release formulations), have volumes of distribution ranging from 1 to 10 L/kg, have half-lives of 3 to 16 h, and are eliminated mainly by hepatic metabolism.

Clinical Toxicity The acute ingestion of more than twice the usual daily dose is potentially toxic. Effects generally begin within 1 h and peak within several hours. Toxicity may also develop during chronic therapeutic use. Manifestations include nausea, vomiting, and diarrhea, followed by lethargy, confusion, ataxia, bradycardia, hypotension, and cardiovascular collapse. Anticholinergic effects (blurred vision, dry mucosae) may be seen in disopyramide poisoning. Quinidine and class IB agents may cause agitation, dysphoria, and seizures. ECG findings include bradycardia with AV block, ventricular tachycardia, ventricular fibrillation (including the polymorphous form, torsade de pointes), and QT-interval prolongation. More specifically, class IA agents prolong the PR, QRS, and JT intervals, class IC agents prolong the QRS interval, and class III agents prolong the JT interval. Class IB agents have little or no effects on conduction intervals. Depressed myocardial contractility and arrhythmias may lead to decreased cardiac output and pulmonary edema. Hypoglycemia and mild hypokalemia may be seen with disopyramide and quinidine intoxication, respectively.

Diagnosis Comprehensive toxicology screening will detect most of these agents. Measurement of serum levels are used for monitoring therapy and for confirmation of overdose.

℞ **TREATMENT** Activated charcoal is the procedure of choice for gastrointestinal decontamination. Hypotension, bradyarrhythmias, and seizures are treated with standard measures. Patients with persistent hypotension may benefit from pulmonary arterial pressure measurement. Cardiac pacing, intraaortic balloon pump counterpulsation, and cardiopulmonary bypass may be necessary. Ventricular tachyarrhythmias that cause hemodynamic instability should be treated with lidocaine. Bretylium is probably also safe. Sodium bicarbonate (0.5 to 1 mmol/kg by intravenous bolus) may be effective for tachyarrhythmias due to class IA or IC agents. Mild hypokalemia may be protective, and potassium levels as low as 3.0 mmol/L may be best treated by watchful waiting. Magnesium sulfate (4 g or 40 mL of a 10% solution given intravenously as an initial dose) and overdrive pacing (with isoproterenol or electricity) are used for torsade de pointes. Hemodialysis and hemoperfusion may enhance the elimination of disopyramide, the active procainamide metabolite *N*-acetylprocainamide, and possibly other agents.

ANTICHOLINERGIC AGENTS Agents that can competitively block the binding of acetylcholine to CNS and parasympathetic postganglionic muscarinic neuroreceptors include antihistamines (H_1 blockers), belladonna alkaloids and related agents (atropine, glycopyrrolate, homatropine, hyoscine, ipratropium, scopolamine), drugs for Parkinson's disease (benztropine, biperiden, trihexyphenidyl), topical mydriatics (cyclopentolate, tropicamide), neuroleptics (clozapine, olanzepine, phenothiazines), skeletal muscle relaxants (cyclobenzaprine, orphenadrine), smooth-muscle relaxants (clidinium, dicyclomine, isometheptene, oxybutynin), tricyclic antidepressants, and some plants (e.g., *Datura stramonium*, or jimson weed) and mushrooms. Their absorption can be delayed following an overdose. Most are weak bases, exhibit variable binding to plasma proteins (18 to 98%), and have moderate volumes of distribution (2 to 6 L/kg). They are elimi-

nated primarily by hepatic metabolism and have half-lives ranging from 2 to 24 h or more.

Clinical Toxicity Manifestations usually begin within an hour of acute overdosage and 1 to 3 days after beginning treatment in cases of chronic poisoning. Toxic doses are only slightly greater than therapeutic ones. CNS manifestations include agitation, ataxia, confusion, delirium, hallucinations, and movement disorders (choreoathetoid and picking movements). Lethargy, respiratory depression, and coma may occur. Peripheral nervous system findings include decreased or absent bowel sounds, dilated pupils, dry skin and mucosal surfaces, urinary retention, and increases in pulse rate, blood pressure, respiratory rate, and temperature. Neuromuscular hyperactivity may lead to rhabdomyolysis and hyperthermia. First-generation H_1 blockers (diphenhydramine and probably others) can sometimes cause tricyclic antidepressant–like cardiotoxicity and seizures. Because of class III antiarrhythmic activity, original nonsedating or second-generation antihistamines (astemizole, terfenadine) caused QT-interval prolongation with subsequent ventricular tachyarrhythmias, especially torsade de pointes, and were withdrawn from U.S. markets.

Diagnosis The diagnosis is supported by detecting these agents in the urine. It can be confirmed by demonstrating resolution of anticholinergic toxicity in response to physostigmine.

℞ **TREATMENT** Activated charcoal adsorbs these agents effectively and is the preferred method of gastrointestinal decontamination. Agitation may respond to benzodiazepines, and comatose patients may require intubation and mechanical ventilation. Cardiovascular toxicity and arrhythmias should be treated as described for antiarrhythmics and tricyclic antidepressants. Physostigmine, an acetylcholinesterase inhibitor, reverses anticholinergic toxicity. It is indicated primarily for uncontrolled agitation and delirium. The dose is 1 to 2 mg given intravenously over 2 to 5 min; the dose can be repeated if there is an incomplete response or recurrent toxicity. If signs of cholinergic poisoning occur (see "Organophosphate and Carbamate Insecticides," below), they can be reversed by atropine in half the amount of physostigmine given. Physostigmine should not be given for seizures or for coma; its arousal effects are nonspecific and cannot be used for diagnostic purposes. Physostigmine is contraindicated in the presence of cardiac conduction defects or ventricular arrhythmias because it can cause asystole in such patients.

ANTICONVULSANTS Carbamazepine, lamotrigine, phenytoin and other hydantoins, topiramate, and valproate act primarily to limit the spread of a seizure from its focus by inhibiting the passive influx of sodium through voltage-dependent sodium channels in neuronal membranes, an activity analogous to that of class I antiarrhythmics (see above). This action, and the resultant inhibition of the release of excitatory neurotransmitters (e.g., aspartate, glutamate), limits posttetanic potentiation of synaptic transmission. Like the barbiturates and benzodiazepines (see below), felbamate, gabapentin, and the investigational agents tiagabine and vigabatrin enhance synaptic transmission of the inhibitory neurotransmitter GABA. The succimides ethosuximide and methsuximide elevate the seizure threshold by reducing calcium conduction through T-type calcium channels. Valproate also inhibits GABA metabolism and calcium conductance. Valproate and its metabolites interfere with enzymes involved in fatty acid synthesis and oxidation, gluconeogenesis, and the urea cycle. Carbamazepine is structurally similar to the tricyclic antidepressants and can cause similar toxicity (see "Cyclic Antidepressant," below) in overdose.

Anticonvulsants are well absorbed after oral administration. Phenytoin is also available for intravenous use, both as phenytoin and the prodrug phosphenytoin. A prodrug formulation of valproate, divalproex, a molecule of which dissociates into two molecules of valproate, is also marketed. Gastrointestinal absorption is prolonged with regular and sustained-release formulations of carbamazepine, extended-release phenytoin, and enteric-coated divalproex, particularly following overdose. The volume of distribution is small for valproate (0.1 to 0.4 L/kg); moderate for phenytoin (0.5 to 0.8 L/kg); large for carbamazepine, felbamate, gabapentin, and lamotrigine (≥ 1 L/kg); and unknown for other agents. All are eliminated primarily by hepatic metabolism. Carbamazepine has an active (10,11-epoxide) metabolite. Half-lives, therapeutic doses, serum concentrations, adverse effects, and drug interactions are listed in Table 360-9. The half-life of phenytoin, valproate, and possibly carbamazepine and other agents is prolonged following overdose.

Clinical Toxicity   Anticonvulsants primarily cause CNS depression (Table 396-2). Cerebellar and vestibular function are affected first, with cerebral depression occurring later. Effects are the same and occur at similar blood levels, regardless of whether overdose is acute or chronic. Ataxia, blurred vision, diplopia, dizziness, nystagmus, slurred speech, tremors, and nausea and vomiting are common initial manifestations. Paradoxical excitation can occur, and membrane-active agents can sometimes cause de novo seizures and exacerbation of epilepsy. Coma with respiratory depression usually occurs at serum carbamazepine concentrations >20 $\mu g/mL$, serum phenytoin levels >60 $\mu g/mL$, and serum valproate levels >180 $\mu g/mL$. Anticholinergic effects (see above) may be present in carbamazepine poisoning, and tricyclic antidepressant–like cardiotoxicity (see below) can occur at drug levels >30 $\mu g/mL$.

Hypotension and arrhythmias (e.g., bradycardia, conduction disturbances, ventricular tachyarrhythmias) can occur during the rapid infusion of phenytoin. Although these effects have been attributed to its propylene glycol diluent, they have also been reported with rapid infusions of phosphenytoin, which does not contain this solvent. Cardiovascular toxicity after oral phenytoin overdose, however, is essentially nonexistent. Extravasation of phenytoin can result in local tissue necrosis due to the high pH of this formulation. Intravenous phenytoin may also cause the "purple glove syndrome" (limb edema, discoloration, and pain). This can occur hours after infusion and without signs of extravasation. A compartment syndrome with limb ischemia and muscle necrosis is a potential complication. Multiple metabolic abnormalities, including anion-gap metabolic acidosis, hyperosmolality, hypocalcemia, hypoglycemia, hypophosphatemia, hypernatremia, and hyperammonemia (with or without other evidence of hepatotoxicity), can occur in valproate poisoning. Three or more days may be required for resolution of toxicity in severe carbamazepine, phenytoin, and valproate poisoning.

Diagnosis   The diagnosis of carbamazepine, phenytoin, and valproate poisoning can be confirmed by measuring serum drug concentrations. Serial drug levels should be obtained until a peak is observed following acute overdose. Quantitative serum levels of other agents are not generally available. Most anticonvulsants can be detected by comprehensive urine screening tests.

℞ **TREATMENT**   Activated charcoal is the method of choice for gastrointestinal decontamination. Multiple-dose charcoal therapy can enhance the elimination of carbamazepine, phenytoin, valproate, and perhaps other agents. Airway protection and support of respiration with endotracheal intubation and mechanical ventilation, if necessary, are the mainstays of treatment. Seizures should be treated with benzodiazepines or barbiturates. Physostigmine (see "Anticholinergic Agents," above) should be considered for anticholinergic poisoning due to carbamazepine. The treatment of carbamazepine-induced hypotension, cardiac conduction disturbances, and ventricular tachyarrhythmias should include sodium bicarbonate (see "Antiarrhythmic Drugs," above). Phenytoin and phosphenytoin cardiotoxicity usually resolves promptly upon discontinuation of the infusion. Crystalloids and lidocaine can be given if necessary. Tissue injury secondary to phenytoin extravasation should be treated by standard wound care measures. Treatment of the purple glove syndrome includes elevation of the affected extremity. A vascular surgeon should evaluate this condition, if signs of ischemia are present. Occasionally, CNS depression

due to valproate will respond to naloxone (2 mg intravenously). Metabolic derangements should be corrected. Hemodialysis and hemoperfusion can enhance the elimination of valproate and its metabolites. Hemodialysis can also correct associated metabolic disturbances. Hemoperfusion only modestly increases carbamazepine elimination. These procedures should be reserved for patients with persistently high drug levels (e.g., carbamazepine ≥ 40 $\mu g/mL$ and valproate ≥ 1000 $\mu g/mL$) who do not respond to supportive care.

BARBITURATES   Barbiturates bind to the GABA receptor complex and prolong the opening of the chloride channels in response to GABA, thereby inhibiting excitable cells of the CNS and other tissues. They can be classified as long-acting (6 to 12 h; mephobarbital, barbital, phenobarbital, primidone), intermediate-acting (3 to 6 h; amobarbital, aprobarbital, butabarbital, butalbital), short-acting (1 to 3 h; hexobarbital, pentobarbital, and secobarbital), and ultrashort-acting ($<$30 min; methohexital, thiamylal, and thiopental).

Barbiturates are weak acids with pK_a values ranging from 7.2 to 8.5, volumes of distribution of 0.8 to 1.5 L/kg of body weight, and 45 to 70% protein binding in the plasma. With therapeutic doses, plasma concentrations generally peak in 1 to 4 h (earlier for short-acting agents than for long-acting ones). Most barbiturates are metabolized by the liver. Some are converted to active metabolites: mephobarbital to barbital, and primidone to phenobarbital and phenylethylmalonamide (PEMA). In contrast to short-acting agents, long-acting ones also undergo significant renal excretion: 95% for barbital, 25 to 33% for phenobarbital, 15 to 42% for primidone, and 95% for PEMA. Half-lives range from 1 h for ultrashort-acting agents to 6 d for long-acting ones.

Clinical Toxicity   Barbiturates cause CNS depression (Table 396-2). Hypothermia, hypotension, pulmonary edema, and cardiac arrest may occur in severe cases. Pressure sores, bullous skin lesions, and rhabdomyolysis can develop with prolonged coma. Maximal toxicity usually occurs within 4 to 6 h but may be delayed to 10 h or more after overdosage with long-acting barbiturates.

Diagnosis   Serum drug levels can confirm the diagnosis. Significant toxicity is usually apparent when serum concentrations of long-acting barbiturates exceed 170 $\mu mol/L$ (4 mg/dL) and those of short-acting barbiturates exceed 88 $\mu mol/L$ (2 mg/dL). Because of tolerance, the degree of CNS depression relative to dose and drug level is dependent on prior exposure to the drug.

℞ **TREATMENT**   Activated charcoal effectively adsorbs barbiturates and is the method of choice for gastrointestinal decontamination. Hemodynamic and respiratory support and correction of temperature and electrolyte derangements may be necessary. Renal elimination of phenobarbital (and probably other long-acting agents) is enhanced by alkalinization of urine to a pH of 8 (by giving intravenous sodium bicarbonate) and by saline diuresis. Elimination can also be enhanced by repeated doses of activated charcoal. Since short-acting barbiturates are predominantly metabolized by the liver, diuresis is ineffective. Hemodialysis and hemoperfusion are effective in removing both long- and short-acting barbiturates, but their use should be reserved for patients with refractory hypotension.

BENZODIAZEPINES   Benzodiazepines potentiate the inhibitory effect of GABA on CNS neurons by binding to the GABA receptor complex and increasing the frequency of opening of chloride channels in response to GABA stimulation. They can be classified as long-acting (chlordiazepoxide, clonazepam, clorazepate, diazepam, flurazepam, prazepam, quazepam), short-acting (alprazolam, flunitrazepam, lorazepam, and oxazepam), and ultrashort-acting (estazolam, midazolam, temazepam, and triazolam). Benzodiazepines are readily absorbed, exhibit 85 to 99% protein binding in the plasma, are lipid soluble, and have an apparent volume of distribution of 0.3 to 2 L/kg body weight. They are weak acids with pK_a values ranging from 1.3 to 6.2 and are eliminated mainly by hepatic metabolism. Some have active metabolites. Half-lives range from 2 h for short-acting agents to 8 days for long-acting ones.

Clinical Toxicity CNS depressant effects (Table 396-2) begin within 30 min of acute overdose. Coma and respiratory depression are rare but can occur with ultrashort-acting agents and when benzodiazepines are combined with other CNS depressants. Paradoxical excitation may occur early in the course of poisoning.

Diagnosis The diagnosis is supported by identification of benzodiazepine metabolites in urine. Since immunoassays do not detect all benzodiazepines, a negative result does not exclude the diagnosis. A response to flumazenil confirms the diagnosis.

℞ TREATMENT Activated charcoal adsorbs benzodiazepines and is the method of choice for gastrointestinal decontamination. Respiratory support should be provided as necessary. Flumazenil, a competitive benzodiazepine receptor antagonist, can reverse CNS and respiratory depression and obviate the need for endotracheal intubation. Doses of 0.1 mg should be given intravenously at 1-min intervals until the desired effect is achieved or a cumulative dose of 3 mg has been given. Since flumazenil has a relatively short duration of action, patients must be monitored carefully for relapse. Should relapse occur, treatment can be repeated (at intervals of 20 min with a maximum dose of 3 mg/h). Flumazenil can cause seizures in patients who have coingested stimulants and tricyclic antidepressants or who are physically dependent on benzodiazepines as a result of chronic use. It should not be used in patients with ECG evidence of tricyclic antidepressant cardiotoxicity.

β-ADRENERGIC BLOCKING AGENTS

β-Adrenergic blocking agents act by competitively inhibiting β-adrenergic neurohumoral receptors. This activity defines them as class II antiarrhythmics. At therapeutic doses, some beta blockers act at both β_1 and β_2 receptors and are "nonselective" (carvedilol, labetalol, nadolol, pindolol, propranolol, timolol); some act predominantly on β_1 receptors and are "cardioselective" (acebutolol, atenolol, betaxolol, bisoprolol, esmolol, metoprolol). Certain beta blockers have partial agonist or sympathomimetic activity (acebutolol, carteolol, pindolol, and possibly penbutolol), some have an α_1 blocking activity and the additional property of vasodilation (carvedilol, labetalol), and some have quinidine-like antiarrhythmic effects (acebutolol, metoprolol, pindolol, propranolol, sotalol, and possibly betaxolol). Antiarrhythmic effects are due to a reduction of sodium and calcium influx during membrane depolarization (phase 0) as a consequence of decreased production of cyclic AMP by adenylate cyclase. Decreased cardiac contractility results from inhibition of calcium influx into cells and the release of calcium from sarcoplasmic reticulum.

Beta blockers are readily absorbed and exhibit variable protein binding (5 to 93%), water solubility, and volumes of distribution (0.23 to 10.0 L/kg body weight). Most beta blockers are eliminated predominantly by hepatic metabolism. Atenolol, nadolol, and sotalol are eliminated primarily by renal excretion, and esmolol is metabolized by erythrocyte esterases.

Clinical Toxicity Effects usually begin within 1/2 h following an overdose and peak within 2 h. Onset may be delayed with the ingestion of sustained-release preparations. Findings include nausea and vomiting followed by bradycardia, hypotension, and CNS depression. However, agents with sympathomimetic activity can cause hypertension and tachycardia. CNS effects can include seizures and tend to be more pronounced with highly lipophilic agents (penbutolol, propranolol). The skin is often pale and cool. Bronchospasm and pulmonary edema are uncommon unless there is a history of asthma, chronic obstructive pulmonary disease, or congestive heart failure. Metabolic abnormalities include hyperkalemia and hypoglycemia (as a direct result of β-adrenergic receptor blockade) and metabolic acidosis (due to seizures, shock, or respiratory depression). ECG manifestations include all degrees of AV block, bundle branch block, prolonged QRS duration, and asystole. Sotalol may cause QT-interval prolongation with ventricular tachycardia, ventricular fibrillation, and torsade de pointes occurring up to 20 h after overdose. Patients with mild poisoning usually recover within 6 to 12 h, whereas those with

severe poisoning and ingestions of sustained-release preparations may be symptomatic for 24 to 48 h.

Diagnosis The diagnosis is primarily based on the clinical presentation. Urine toxicology screening may identify the presence of beta blockers, but blood levels are neither generally available nor helpful in guiding therapy.

℞ TREATMENT Activated charcoal adsorbs these agents effectively and is the preferred method of gastrointestinal decontamination. Gastric emptying procedures may produce vagal stimulation and exacerbate bradyarrhythmias. Bradycardia associated with hypotension will sometimes respond to atropine, isoproterenol, and vasopressors (amrinone, dopamine, dobutamine, epinephrine, and norepinephrine have been used with variable success, alone or in combination). With severe poisoning, these agents may be ineffective, and glucagon, calcium, cardiac pacing (external or internal), and intraaortic balloon pump support may be necessary. Glucagon, which stimulates adenylate cyclase by a nonadrenergic mechanism, is given at an initial dose of 5 to 10 mg. Patients who respond favorably can be treated with an infusion of 1 to 5 mg/h. Calcium and high-dose insulin can be given with glucose and potassium to reverse negative inotropic effects, as described for calcium channel blocker poisoning. Bronchospasm may be treated with an inhaled beta agonist, subcutaneous epinephrine, and intravenous aminophylline. Lidocaine, magnesium (as for antiarrhythmic poisoning), or overdrive pacing may be used for sotalol-induced ventricular tachyarrhythmias. Extracorporeal elimination procedures are probably not of benefit, except possibly for atenolol, metoprolol, nadolol, and sotalol.

CALCIUM CHANNEL BLOCKERS

Bepridil, diltiazem, verapamil, and the dihydropyridine derivatives amlodipine, felodipine, isradipine, nicardipine, nifedipine, nimodipine, and nisoldipine decrease the influx of calcium across slow (L-type) calcium channels in the membranes of myocardial and vascular smooth-muscle cells during phases 2 (plateau) and 4 (spontaneous depolarization) of the action potential. These actions define them as class IV antiarrhythmics. Bepridil also has class I antiarrhythmic activity. Electrophysiologic effects include decreased cardiac contractility, heart rate [sinoatrial (SA) node rate], and AV nodal conduction. At therapeutic doses, all calcium channel blockers cause vasodilation. Diltiazem and verapamil also have significant negative inotropic and chronotropic activity.

Calcium channel blockers are well absorbed and exhibit high (80 to 99%) plasma protein binding. Most have distribution volumes ranging from 1 to 8 L/kg body weight. They are eliminated mainly by hepatic metabolism, and the half-lives typically range from 1 to 24 h.

Clinical Toxicity Toxic effects begin within 2 h of ingestion of immediate-release preparations but may be delayed up to 18 h following overdoses of sustained-release preparations. Manifestations include nausea, vomiting, bradycardia, hypotension, and CNS depression (Table 396-2). Hypotension caused by diltiazem and verapamil is usually due to myocardial depression (decreased cardiac output), whereas that caused by the dihydropyridine derivatives is usually due to low peripheral vascular resistance. Reflexive tachycardia is sometimes seen in dihydropyridine poisoning. Seizures can occur and are the result of direct membrane effects as well as cerebral hypoperfusion. Hypotension may precipitate mesenteric or myocardial ischemia or infarction, and depression of cardiac function may lead to pulmonary edema. ECG findings include all degrees of AV block, prolonged QRS and QT intervals (mainly with verapamil), evidence of ischemia or infarction, and asystole. Metabolic acidosis (secondary to shock) and hyperglycemia (resulting from the inhibition of insulin release) may be present. Serum calcium levels, however, remain normal.

Diagnosis These agents can be detected by comprehensive urine screening tests. Serum levels are not generally available or helpful in guiding therapy.

℞ **TREATMENT**   Activated charcoal is preferred for gastrointestinal decontamination. Symptomatic bradycardia should be treated with atropine, calcium, isoproterenol, glucagon, and electrical (external or internal) pacing. Restoring perfusion is particularly important in patients with organ ischemia. The initial dose of calcium is 10 mL of 10% calcium chloride or 30 mL of the 10% gluconate solution intravenously over 2 min. This dose may be repeated up to four times in patients with a partial, transient, or absent response. High serum calcium levels may be required for a therapeutic effect. A continuous calcium infusion (0.2 mL/kg body weight per hour up to a maximum of 10 mL/h) may be appropriate when relapse occurs after an initial bolus. Although electrical pacing may be required, glucagon, in the same dose as for beta blocker poisoning, may also be effective. High-dose insulin (0.1–0.2 units/kg body weight of regular insulin as a bolus followed by 0.1–1 units/kg per hour) along with glucose (25-g bolus followed by 1 g/kg per hour of a 20% infusion) and potassium to maintain euglycemia and normokalemia should also be considered. This treatment enhances myocardial metabolism and improves myocardial contactility. It may be particularly effective in verapamil poisoning. Hypotension that persists despite resolution of bradycardia should initially be treated with fluids. Amrinone, dopamine, dobutamine, glucagon, and norepinephrine, alone or in combination, have also been used with success. Intraaortic balloon pump support should be used in patients with refractory shock. Patients with mild toxicity usually recover within a few hours, whereas those with severe toxicity or overdose with sustained-release preparations may remain symptomatic for 24 h or longer.

CARBON MONOXIDE   Carbon monoxide is produced in large amounts in industrial processes as well as by internal combustion engines, fossil-fueled home appliances (generators, heaters, stoves), and the incomplete combustion of nearly all natural materials and synthetic products. Methylene chloride, a solvent in paint removers, is metabolized to carbon monoxide.

Carbon monoxide is absorbed rapidly through the lungs and binds to hemoglobin (forming carboxyhemoglobin) with an affinity 210 times that of oxygen. Its binding reduces oxygen transport by hemoglobin and also decreases the release of oxygen in tissues (the oxygen dissociation curve shifts to the left). Carbon monoxide also binds to myoglobin, decreasing its oxygen-carrying capacity, and to mitochondrial cytochrome oxidase, inhibiting cellular respiration. The net effect is tissue hypoxia with anaerobic metabolism, lactic acidosis, lipid peroxidation, and free radical formation. Once carbon monoxide exposure is discontinued, dissociation of the hemoglobin–carbon monoxide complex occurs, and carbon monoxide is excreted through the lungs. At atmospheric pressure, the carboxyhemoglobin half-life is 4 to 6 h. It decreases to 40 to 80 min when breathing 100% oxygen and to 15 to 30 min with hyperbaric oxygen therapy. The apparent half-life after methylene chloride exposure is considerably longer.

Clinical Toxicity   Manifestations of carbon monoxide poisoning include shortness of breath, dyspnea, tachypnea, headache, emotional lability, confusion, impaired judgment, clumsiness, and syncope. Nausea, vomiting, and diarrhea may also occur. Cerebral edema, coma, respiratory depression, and pulmonary edema may be seen in severe poisoning. Cardiovascular manifestations include ischemic chest pain, arrhythmias, heart failure, and hypotension. In comatose patients, blisters and bullae may develop over pressure points. Serum creatine kinase and lactate dehydrogenase levels may be elevated. Myoglobinuria secondary to muscle necrosis may result in renal failure. Visual field defects, blindness, and venous engorgement with papilledema or optic atrophy may be noted. Arterial blood gas analysis may reveal metabolic acidosis, a normal P_{O_2}, decreased oxygen saturation (when measured by CO-oximetry, but not when calculated from the P_{O_2} or measured by pulse oximetry), and a variable P_{CO_2}. Oxygen saturation measured by pulse oximetry will be falsely elevated but less than normal. A cherry-red color of skin and mucous membranes is rare, and cyanosis is usual.

After brief exposure, carboxyhemoglobin fractions of 15 to 20% are associated with mild symptoms, 20 to 40% with moderate symptoms, and 40 to 50% with severe symptoms. Fractions >60% are often fatal. With prolonged exposure, toxicity occurs at lower fractions. Patients with loss of consciousness are at risk for developing neuropsychiatric sequelae 1 to 3 weeks after exposure. Manifestations vary from subtle personality changes and intellectual impairment to gross neurologic deficits such as blindness, deafness, incoordination, and parkinsonism.

Diagnosis   An elevated carboxyhemoglobin fraction confirms exposure, but the result must be interpreted with respect to the time elapsed from exposure to sampling. If the carboxyhemoglobin fraction cannot be measured directly, the difference between the oxygen saturation calculated from the P_{O_2} and that measured by CO-oximetry can be used to estimate the carboxyhemoglobin fraction.

℞ **TREATMENT**   In conscious patients, oxygen should be administered by a non-rebreather mask at 10 L/min until carboxyhemoglobin fraction is <10% and symptoms have resolved. Infants and pregnant women require treatment for several more hours, because fetal hemoglobin has a higher affinity for carbon monoxide than adult hemoglobin. Endotracheal intubation and mechanical ventilation with 100% oxygen are indicated in patients with coma, seizures, or cardiovascular instability. Arrhythmias and hypotension are treated by usual measures. Although hyperbaric oxygen therapy is often recommended for patients with coma, syncope, seizures, and cardiovascular instability, for those with less severe neurologic or cardiovascular dysfunction that does not resolve with oxygen and supportive measures, and for those who develop neurologic sequalae, recent data suggest that it is no more effective than prolonged high-flow normobaric oxygen in reversing acute toxicity and preventing sequelae.

CARDIAC GLYCOSIDES   Poisoning with digitalis and other cardiac glycosides occurs most often during therapeutic or suicidal use of digoxin. It can also occur when plants (foxglove, oleander, squill) or the skin (venom) of *Bufo* toads (Colorado River, Asian, Chinese, European) are ingested. Toad venom also contains hallucinogens and accounts for the practice of toad licking as a form of recreational drug abuse. At therapeutic doses, cardiac glycosides inhibit the enzyme Na^+, K^+-ATPase, leading to increased intracellular levels of Na^+ and Ca^{2+} and decreased intracellular K^+ levels. Increased cytosolic Ca^{2+} enhances the excitation-contraction coupling of actin and myosin during systole and improves myocardial contractility. Electrophysiologic effects are due to indirect sympatholytic and vagotonic effects and to direct effects on cardiac muscle, pacemaker, and conduction cells (reduced action potential duration and AV node resting potential, prolongation of the refractory period). ECG manifestations include prolongation of the PR interval, shortening of the QT interval, scooping and depression of the ST segment, and decreased T-wave amplitude. In toxic doses, SA node automaticity and AV nodal conduction are decreased. Sympathetic tone; automaticity in muscle, AV nodal, and conduction cells; and afterdepolarizations are increased. ECG manifestations include bradydysrhythmias as well as triggered tachydysrhythmias. Hypokalemia potentiates the electrophysiologic effects of cardiac glycosides, increases their tissue binding, and decreases their renal excretion. Magnesium blocks calcium channels and modulates their sympathetic effects, whereas calcium and hypoxia enhance their activity.

Digoxin is absorbed and distributed slowly. Serum levels may not correlate with clinical effect for up to 8 h following a dose. Digoxin is 25 to 30% protein bound in the plasma, has a large volume of distribution of 5 to 6 L/kg body weight, and is eliminated primarily by renal excretion. The half-life ranges between 36 and 45 h, is prolonged in hepatic failure and in renal failure, and may be shortened in overdose. Therapeutic serum concentrations range from 0.6 to 2.5 nmol/L (0.5 to 2.0 ng/mL).

Clinical Toxicity Symptoms include vomiting, confusion, delirium, and occasionally hallucinations, blurred vision, photophobia, scotomata, and chromotopsia (disturbed color perception). Cardiac manifestations include sinus arrhythmia, sinus bradycardia, and all degrees of AV block. Premature ventricular contractions, bigeminy, ventricular tachycardia, and fibrillation also occur. The combination of a supraventricular tachyarrhythmia and AV block (e.g., paroxysmal atrial tachycardia with second-degree AV block, atrial fibrillation with third-degree AV block) or the presence of bidirectional ventricular tachycardia is highly suggestive of cardiac glycoside poisoning. Bradyarrhythmias and hypokalemia are common with chronic intoxication, whereas tachyarrhythmias and hyperkalemia are generally seen with acute poisoning. Similarly, serum digoxin levels may be minimally elevated or even therapeutic in chronic toxicity, whereas they are usually markedly elevated following acute overdose. Since chronic poisoning occurs almost exclusively in patients with underlying heart disease, the incidence, variety, and severity of dysrhythmias tend to be greater than with acute poisoning. In patients taking digoxin, poisoning should be suspected when a normal or fast heart rate becomes slow or the rhythm becomes regularly irregular.

Diagnosis The diagnosis is confirmed by measuring the serum digoxin level. Levels must be interpreted with respect to the time of the last dose. Digoxin assays may cross-react with nondigoxin glycosides and produce a false-positive result. Toxicology screening tests do not detect cardiac glycosides.

℞ TREATMENT Activated charcoal is preferred for gastrointestinal decontamination. Emesis and gastric intubation may cause vagal stimulation and precipitate or worsen conduction disturbances. Repeated doses of charcoal can enhance the elimination of digoxin. Potassium, magnesium, and calcium abnormalities and hypoxia should be corrected. Sinus bradycardia and second- and third-degree heart block resulting in hypotension can be treated with atropine, dopamine, epinephrine, and possible phenytoin (100 mg intravenously every 5 min up to 15 mg/kg) and isoproterenol. Magnesium sulfate (as for antiarrhythmic poisoning), phenytoin, lidocaine, bretylium, and amiodarone may be given for ventricular tachyarrhythmias. Antidotal therapy with digoxin-specific Fab-fragment antibodies should be administered for potentially life-threatening dysrhythmias. A serum potassium level ≥5.5 meq/L following acute overdose is associated with severe poisoning and is an indication for antibody therapy in the absence of dysrhythmias. Electrical pacing may be necessary as a temporizing measure. Prophylactic pacing is not recommended, as the pacing wire may increase ventricular irritability and precipitate tachydysrhythmias. If defibrillation is necessary, a low energy level (e.g., 50 W·s) should be used initially as the electrical shock may precipitate arrhythmias, which are more malignant and refractory to treatment. Digoxin-specific Fab-fragment antibodies are given intravenously over 15 to 30 min, unless cardiac arrest has occurred, in which case the solution is given as a bolus. Effects are usually apparent within an hour. The drug-antibody complex is excreted in the urine with a half-life of 16 to 20 h. In patients with renal failure, the drug-antibody complex is metabolized over a period of days to weeks. Although free digoxin levels decrease rapidly to zero following antibody administration, routine methods used to measure digoxin do not differentiate between bound and unbound drug, so that drug levels do not correlate with toxicity after antibody therapy.

Each vial (40 mg) of digoxin antibody fragments can neutralize 0.6 mg of digoxin. Formulas and tables for calculating the dose of antibody are available in the package insert. Unfortunately, toxicity may occur before distribution is complete or before levels are available. In addition, the amount of an acute overdose may be unknown, and calculated doses often exceed the effective dose (leading to costly overtreatment). The following empirical dosing guidelines are therefore offered. With chronic intoxication, the total-body drug load and serum drug levels only slightly exceed therapeutic amounts, patients may be dependent on inotropic effects, and a dose of 1 to 4 vials is usually effective. In acute poisoning, drug load is generally quite high,

and 5 to 15 vials are usually required. Initial doses can be on the low side and repeated as necessary. Antibodies cross-react with other cardiac glycosides, but larger doses may be needed for toxicity not involving digoxin.

CYANIDE Cyanide salts are used in photography, metallurgy, electroplating, metal cleaning, and ore refining. Hydrogen cyanide gas, which is used as a fumigant rodenticide and in chemical syntheses, is liberated when they are combined with acids. Cyanide is also produced during the decomposition and metabolism of nitroprusside. Organic cyanides (nitriles) are used in making rubber, in artificial nail removers, and as rodenticides. Cyanogenic glycosides are present in the seeds of the chokeberry, cherry, plum, peach, apricot, pear, bean, apple, and crabapple.

Cyanide inhibits mitochondrial cytochrome oxidase, thereby blocking electron transport and preventing oxygen utilization and oxidative metabolism. Lactic acidosis occurs as a consequence of anaerobic metabolism. Cyanide is rapidly absorbed from the stomach, lungs, mucosal surfaces, and unbroken skin. Ingested salts react with gastric hydrochloric acid to form hydrocyanic acid, which is then absorbed. A dose of 200 mg of potassium or sodium cyanide, or 50 mg of hydrocyanic acid, is potentially lethal. Cyanide is 60% protein bound, concentrated in red cells, and has a volume of distribution of 1.5 L/kg body weight. Mitochondrial rhodanase mediates the transfer of sulfur from thiosulfate to the cyanide ion and converts it to less toxic thiocyanate, which is excreted in the urine. Cyanide poisoning during nitroprusside therapy can be prevented by the prophylactic administration of thiosulfate.

Clinical Toxicity Effects begin within seconds of inhalation and within 30 min of ingestion. Initial manifestations of cyanide poisoning include a burning sensation in the mouth and throat, agitation, anxiety, faintness, headache, nausea, vomiting, diaphoresis, dyspnea, tachycardia, and hypertension. A bitter almond odor may be detected on the breath. Later effects include coma, convulsions, opisthotonus, trismus, paralysis, respiratory depression, pulmonary edema, arrhythmias, bradycardia, and hypotension. A rough correlation exists between blood cyanide levels and symptoms: Levels<8 μmol/L (0.02 mg/L) are associated with no symptoms; 20 to 40 μmol/L (0.05 to 0.1 mg/dL) with flushing and tachycardia; 40 to 100 μmol/L (0.1 to 0.25 mg/dL) with obtundation; 100 to 200 μmol/L (0.25 to 0.3 mg/dL) with coma and respiratory depression; and levels >120 μmol/L (0.3 mg/dL) with death. With significant poisoning, lactic acidosis is invariably present. ECG abnormalities include both tachyarrhythmias and bradyarrhythmias.

Diagnosis The diagnosis is based on the history and physical examination. Although measurement of the whole-blood cyanide level will confirm the diagnosis, cyanide assays are not routinely available and treatment decisions must be based on clinical findings. Lactate levels have been used as a surrogate marker.

℞ TREATMENT Management involves supportive therapy, gastrointestinal decontamination, high-dose oxygen, and antidotal therapy with amyl nitrite, sodium nitrite, and sodium thiosulfate (the Lilly cyanide antidote kit). Nitrites convert hemoglobin to methemoglobin, which has a higher affinity for cyanide than does cytochrome oxidase and thus promotes its dissociation from this enzyme. Thiosulfate reacts with cyanide, which is slowly released from cyanomethemoglobin, to form thiocyanate. Oxygen reverses the binding of cyanide to cytochrome oxidase sites and enhances the efficacy of sodium nitrite and sodium thiosulfate, in addition to acting as a substrate for metabolism.

Indications for antidotal therapy include altered mental status, abnormal vital signs, and metabolic acidosis. Amyl nitrite, administered for 30 s of each minute and using a fresh ampule every 3 min, is a first-aid measure and is omitted when intravenous sodium nitrite is available or the patient has been intubated. The ampule is broken between two pads of gauze and placed over the airway while the patient breathes spontaneously or is ventilated by a bag-mask unit. Sodium nitrite is administered as a 3% solution at a dose of 10 to 15 mL (300 to 450 mg) over 1 to 2 min. Sodium thiosulfate is also administered intravenously, as a 25% solution at a dose of 50 mL (12.5 g) given over 1 to 2 min. With recurrent or persistent symptoms, doses of sodium nitrite and sodium thiosulfate can be repeated. Hyperbaric oxygen therapy should be considered in patients who fail to respond to antidotal therapy. Hydroxycobalamin, a vitamin B_{12} precursor that also binds cyanide ion, is an alternative antidote that is not yet widely available.

CYCLIC ANTIDEPRESSANTS   Tricyclic antidepressants (TCAs) such as amitriptyline, imipramine (and their respective active metabolites nortriptyline and desipramine), chlomipramine, doxepin, protriptyline, and trimipramine and polycyclic agents such as amoxapine, bupropion, maprotiline, mirtazepine, and trazodone (and its metabolite nefazodone) act primarily by blocking the presynaptic reuptake monoamine neurotransmitters in the CNS, most importantly norepinephrine and serotonin, but also dopamine. They also have anticholinergic, α-adrenergic receptor blocking, and quinidine-like (class IA antiarrhythmic) effects as well as variable and selective blocking activity at histamine and monoamine receptors. Bupropion, nefazodone, and trazodone have serotonin agonist activity. Selective serotonin reuptake inhibitors (SSRIs) such as fluoxetine, paroxetine, sertaline, citalopram, and fluvoxamine can enhance the presynaptic release of serotonin and block its receptors in addition to inhibiting its reuptake. The nonselective serotonin reuptake inhibitors such as venlafaxine also inhibit norepinephrine reuptake.

Cyclic antidepressants are well absorbed. Peak serum levels usually occur within 2 to 6 h of ingestion but can sometimes occur later. These agents exhibit high (about 95%) protein binding in the plasma, have large volumes of distribution (20 to 45 L/kg body weight), and are eliminated mainly by hepatic metabolism, with half-lives of 24 h or more.

Clinical Toxicity   Effects generally develop within 30 min of ingestion and peak within 6 h. Following low overdosage (about 10 mg/kg) of TCAs, anticholinergic effects predominate (see "Anticholinergic Agents," above). With larger doses, marked CNS depression (Table 396-2), cardiotoxicity, seizures, and hypotension occur. Ventricular tachyarrhythmias, atrioventricular and intraventricular conduction delays, terminal bradycardia, decreased cardiac output, and pulmonary edema may be seen. Death can occur within 6 h of ingestion from cardiovascular effects or much later from multiple organ failure or pulmonary complications. Terminal (last 40 ms) QRS right-axis deviation, an R wave greater than the S wave or >3 mm in lead aV_R, and prolongation of the QRS complex (>100 ms) of the ECG are sensitive indicators of TCA cardiotoxicity. Increasing duration of the QRS complex correlates with an increased risk of cardiac arrhythmias and seizures.

Although seizures can occur, CNS depression is typically mild with SSRIs and moderate with the polycyclic agents. Sinus tachycardia is common, but life-threatening cardiovascular effects are virtually nonexistent. An exception is trazodone, which can cause QT-interval prolongation and ventricular tachycardia. The serotonin syndrome (discussed separately) is also a potential complication of SSRI overdose.

Diagnosis   The diagnosis is supported by the presence of these drugs in the urine on comprehensive screening tests. TCA serum levels are diagnostic and generally correlate with severity. Serum levels of active metabolites should be summed with that of the parent compound when estimating the serum concentration. Levels ≤1000 nmol/L (300 ng/mL) are therapeutic. Levels >3300 nmol/L (1000 ng/mL) are associated with severe poisoning.

℞ **TREATMENT**   Activated charcoal is the preferred method of gastrointestinal decontamination. Repeated doses may enhance the elimination of some agents. Physostigmine (see "Anticholinergic

Agents," above) can reverse anticholinergic effects due to low-dose TCA poisoning and may be used if the ECG is normal and deterioration has been excluded by a suitable period of observation. For other toxicity, treatment includes support of respiration and volume expansion and norepinephrine or high-dose dopamine for hypotension. Seizures should be treated with benzodiazepines and barbiturates. Phenytoin is of uncertain benefit. Acidemia increases the likelihood of arrhythmias and should be corrected. Sodium bicarbonate should be given as a bolus following a seizure and as an infusion to maintain a serum pH of 7.45 to 7.50 in patients with QRS prolongation. Treatment of ventricular tachyarrhythmias is similar to that described for antiarrhythmic agents and should include sodium bicarbonate. Phenytoin is often recommended, but its efficacy is not established. β-Adrenergic blockers and class IA, IC, and III antiarrhythmics should be avoided. Cardiac pacing and invasive hemodynamic support may be necessary for severe cardiovascular depression.

ETHYLENE GLYCOL   Ethylene glycol is a colorless, odorless, sweet-tasting, water-soluble liquid used as a solvent for paints, plastics, and pharmaceuticals; in the manufacture of explosives, fire extinguishers, and foams; and as an ingredient in hydraulic fluids, windshield cleaners, radiator antifreeze, and de-icer solutions.

Ethylene glycol produces intoxication similar to that caused by ethanol but is more potent. Peak blood levels occur approximately 2 h after ingestion. The volume of distribution is 0.6 to 0.8 L/kg body weight. Ethylene glycol is oxidized by alcohol dehydrogenase to glycoaldehyde, which is metabolized successively to glycolic acid, glyoxylic acid, and oxalic acid. Pyridoxine and thiamine are cofactors in degradation pathways. As much as 20% is excreted unchanged in the urine. The half-life ranges from 3 to 8 h. Metabolites, primarily glycolic acid, cause CNS depression, metabolic acidosis with an increased anion gap, and interstitial and tubular damage to the kidney. Oxalic acid may precipitate as calcium oxalate in the brain, heart, kidney, lung, pancreas, and urine and cause hypocalcemia.

Ethanol and fomepizole bind to alcohol dehydrogenase with a higher affinity than ethylene glycol and hence block the production of toxic metabolites. Ethanol is metabolized by alcohol dehydrogenase, but fomepizole is not. Ethanol and fomepizole prolong the half-life of ethylene glycol to 15 to 20 h.

Clinical Toxicity   As little as 120 mg/kg body weight or 0.1 mL/kg body weight (one swallow) of pure ethylene glycol can result in a potentially toxic serum concentration of 3 mmol/L (20 mg/dL). Effects begin about 30 min after ingestion and include nausea, vomiting, slurred speech, ataxia, nystagmus, and lethargy. A faint, sweet aromatic odor may be detected on the breath, and the serum osmolality may be elevated. Effects caused by metabolites begin 3 to 12 h after ingestion (longer if ethanol has also been ingested) and include tachypnea, agitation, confusion, lethargy, back pain, hypotension, coma, and seizures. In severe cases, ARDS, cyanosis, pulmonary edema, and cardiomegaly may be seen. Laboratory findings include metabolic acidosis, an increased anion gap (low bicarbonate and chloride), hypocalcemia, leukocytosis, increased BUN and creatinine, calcium oxalate crystalluria, and proteinuria. Acute tubular necrosis with oliguria or anuria typically becomes evident 12 to 24 h following ingestion. Renal failure is usually reversible but may last days to weeks.

Diagnostic Evaluation   The diagnosis is established by measuring serum ethylene glycol and glycolate levels. The diagnosis is suggested by an elevated serum osmolality and ethanol-like effects soon after ingestion and by an increased anion-gap metabolic acidosis and crystalluria later on. If laboratory confirmation is not immediately available, the osmolal gap can also be used to estimate the serum ethylene glycol concentration (Table 396-3).

℞ **TREATMENT**   Gastric aspiration is the decontamination procedure of choice. Activated charcoal should also be administered. Supportive measures include protection of the airway, ventilatory and circulatory support, and anticonvulsants for seizures. Metabolic acidosis will not resolve spontaneously and should be corrected with sodium bicarbonate; large doses may be required. Sodium bicarbonate should also be given to alkalinize the urine as this will enhance the excretion of acid metabolites. Fluids and diuretics can be used to treat oliguria but they do not increase the excretion of ethylene glycol. Hypocalcemia is treated with intravenous calcium salts. Supplemental pyridoxine (50 mg qid) and thiamine (100 mg qid) may be beneficial.

Indications for ethanol or fomepizole therapy include an ethylene glycol concentration >3 mmol/L (20 mg/dL); an elevated osmolal gap, an increased anion-gap metabolic acidosis, back pain, laboratory evidence of renal toxicity, or ethanol-like intoxication in a patient with a history of ethylene glycol ingestion and a low or undetectable ethanol level; an elevated osmolal gap not accounted for by the presence of ethanol, isopropyl alcohol, acetone, or propylene glycol in a patient with ethanol-like intoxication; and an increased anion-gap metabolic acidosis with a low lactate level not explained by alcoholic or diabetic ketoacidosis, uremia, or salicylate, formaldehyde, paraldehyde, or toluene exposure. A serum ethanol level of ≥20 mmol/L (100 mg/dL) is required to inhibit the metabolism of ethylene glycol (higher levels may be needed with very high ethylene glycol concentrations). The loading dose of ethanol is 10 mL/kg of 10% ethanol intravenously or 1 mL/kg of 95% ethanol by mouth; the maintenance dose is 1.5 mL/kg per hour of 10% ethanol intravenously or 3 mL/kg per hour of 10% ethanol intravenously during hemodialysis. Maintaining a therapeutic concentration is often difficult; levels must be monitored frequently and the dose adjusted as necessary. Ethanol induces its own metabolism and progressively higher doses may be required as time passes. Fomepizole is diluted in 100 mL of intravenous fluid and administered over 30 min in a loading dose of 15 mg/kg followed by 10 mg/kg every 12 h for four doses and 15 mg/kg thereafter. Additional doses are required in patients undergoing dialysis. Although expensive (about $1000 U.S. per 1.5-g vial), fomepizole has a number of advantages over ethanol: it does not cause CNS depression, hypoglycemia, or fluid, electrolyte, and serum osmolality derangements; it has a longer duration of action; and does not require monitoring of serum drug levels. Although seizures have occurred after fomepizole, their etiology is unclear, and side effects have generally been limited to headache, nausea, dizziness, rash, eosinophilia, and mild self-limited hepatotoxicity. Serum ethylene glycol concentrations should be monitored frequently. Ethanol or fomepizole should be continued until the ethylene glycol level falls below 1.5 mmol/L (10 mg/dL).

Hemodialysis enhances the elimination of ethylene glycol and its toxic metabolites so that it is complete in about 3 h. Indications for hemodialysis include an ethylene glycol concentration >8 mmol/L (50 mg/dL) and metabolic acidosis not readily correctable with bicarbonate and antidotal therapy, lack of clinical improvement despite treatment, and laboratory evidence of renal toxicity (regardless of the ethylene glycol level). This therapy should be continued (repeated intermittently) until acidemia resolves and the ethylene glycol level is <3 mmol/L (20 mg/dL).

HYDROCARBONS Aromatic hydrocarbons, such as xylene and toluene, halogenated hydrocarbons, such as carbon tetrachloride and trichloroethane, and petroleum distillate hydrocarbons, such as gasoline, lacquer thinner, mineral seal oil, kerosene, and lighter fluid, are CNS depressants and gastrointestinal and respiratory tract irritants. They are absorbed rapidly following inhalation or pulmonary aspiration. Aromatic and halogenated hydrocarbons are also absorbed following ingestion and are toxic to the heart, liver, and kidneys. Aromatic hydrocarbons can cause bone marrow suppression and skeletal muscle damage. Petroleum distillate hydrocarbons are poorly absorbed following ingestion.

Clinical Toxicity Hydrocarbons produce CNS excitation in low doses and depression in high doses. Rarely, coma and seizures occur. Psychosis, cerebral and cerebellar atrophy, encephalopathy, and peripheral neuropathy can result from chronic inhalation. Other effects include nausea, vomiting, abdominal pain, hepatitis, renal tubular acidosis, acute hepatic or renal failure, and rhabdomyolysis. Sudden death due to myocardial irritability and ventricular fibrillation may

occur following hydrocarbon sniffing. After ingestion, hydrocarbons cause burning of the mouth and throat with subsequent nausea, vomiting, and diarrhea. Aspiration into the lungs may occur with ingestion or as a result of vomiting and cause pneumonia. Following aspiration, chest x-ray abnormalities include infiltrates, atelectasis, effusions, pneumothorax, and pneumatoceles. Renal tubular acidosis with decreased serum bicarbonate, calcium, phosphate, and potassium and increased serum chloride may result from chronic aromatic hydrocarbon inhalation.

Diagnosis The diagnosis is based on the clinical presentation. Assays for hydrocarbons are not routinely available.

TREATMENT The ingestion of aromatic and halogenated hydrocarbons requires prompt gastric lavage. More than one episode of ipecac-induced emesis is contraindicated, and the role of activated charcoal is controversial. Since the ingestion of other types of hydrocarbons is unlikely to result in systemic toxicity and since the risk of aspiration during gastric decontamination is greater than the potential benefit, decontamination is contraindicated for these ingestions. Supportive therapy includes oxygen, respiratory support, and monitoring of liver, renal, and myocardial function. Metabolic abnormalities should be corrected, and patients with aspiration pneumonitis should be monitored for superimposed bacterial infection. Glucocorticoids are ineffective.

HYDROGEN SULFIDE Hydrogen sulfide is a rapidly acting, malodorous ("rotten eggs"), colorless, irritating gas. It is encountered in the petroleum and mining industries, tanning of leather, vulcanization of rubber, the production of synthetic fabrics, metal refining, the production of heavy water for atomic reactors, and glue and felt manufacturing. It is also found in sewers, sulfur springs, and the holds of fishing vessels and as a byproduct of manure storage.

Sulfide anion inhibits electron transport in the cytochrome oxidase system, thereby inhibiting aerobic metabolism with resultant cellular anoxia and lactic acidosis. Hydrogen sulfide is rapidly detoxified by oxidation to sulfate products, which are excreted by the kidneys.

Clinical Toxicity Exposure to low concentrations of hydrogen sulfide results in rhinitis, conjunctivitis, and pharyngitis. Inhalation of large amounts causes headache, vertigo, nausea, vomiting, confusion, seizures, and coma. Hypoventilation, hypoxia, cyanosis, metabolic acidosis, pneumonia, and pulmonary edema can occur.

Diagnosis The diagnosis is based on the characteristic clinical features, including the characteristic odor, exposure setting, and rapidity of onset. Sulfide levels have been used to confirm the diagnosis but are not routinely available.

TREATMENT Treatment includes prompt removal of the victim from the site of exposure, assisted ventilation, and 100% oxygen. Although controversial, amyl and sodium nitrite, in the same dose as for cyanide poisoning, should be considered for patients with coma or cardiac arrest who fail to respond to oxygen therapy. Nitrites promote the dissociation of sulfide ions from cytochrome oxidase by providing an alternative binding site (methemoglobin). They also enhance detoxification by acting as a catalyst for sulfide oxidation. Hyperbaric oxygen should be considered in patients who do not respond to the preceding measures.

IRON Non-transferring-bound plasma iron catalyzes the formation of free radicals, which then cause mitochondrial injury, lipid peroxidation, increased capillary permeability, vasodilation, and intestinal, renal, hepatic, myocardial, and pulmonary toxicity. Ingestion of 20 mg/kg body weight of elemental iron typically produces gastrointestinal symptoms, and 60 mg/kg body weight may cause systemic toxicity. Ferrous sulfate, fumarate, gluconate, and succinate contains 20, 33, 12, and 35% elemental iron, respectively.

Ferrous iron is absorbed by duodenal and jejunal cells, oxidized to ferric iron, and bound to ferritin. It is then slowly released, binds to plasma transferrin (an iron-specific globulin) and other proteins, and is transported to tissues. Serum iron levels usually peak 4 to 6 h after overdosage (later for delayed-release formulations). Iron bound to transferrin is nontoxic.

Clinical Toxicity   Initial manifestations include vomiting and diarrhea (often bloody). X-rays may reveal iron tablets in the stomach or small bowel. Systemic effects include lethargy, hypotension, and metabolic acidosis. Seizures, coma, pulmonary edema, and vascular collapse may occur with severe poisoning. Jaundice, elevated hepatic enzyme levels, prolongation of prothrombin time, and hyperammonemia are indicative of liver injury. Proteinuria and cells in the urine indicate renal injury. In the recovering patient, gastric ulcerations and scars may cause outlet obstruction. Overgrowth of *Yersinia enterocolitica* with sepsis is a rare complication of iron overload.

Diagnosis   The diagnosis is primarily based on clinical findings. A serum iron concentration >50 μmol/L (300 μg/dL) is potentially toxic. A positive x-ray, fever >38.5°C, hyperglycemia >8.5 mmol/L (150 mg/dL), and leukocytosis (white blood cell count >15,000/μL) have also been associated with potential toxicity. Serious poisoning is generally associated with levels >80 μmol/L (500 μg/dL). A positive urine deferoxamine provocative challenge test (see below) is also diagnostic.

TREATMENT   Gastric lavage and whole-bowel irrigation are the preferred methods of gastrointestinal decontamination. When iron tablets are visible on x-ray, serial films can be used to assess their success. Endoscopic removal and gastrostomy may be necessary when these procedures are ineffective (e.g., large ingestions, concretions). Complexation of ingested iron with orally administered activated charcoal, bicarbonate, phosphate, deferoxamine, or magnesium hydroxide has not been shown to reduce toxicity.

Intravenous sodium bicarbonate should be used to correct metabolic acidosis. Nearly all patients are volume depleted and should be given intravenous crystalloid. Coagulation abnormalities should be treated with vitamin K or blood products.

Parenteral deferoxamine should be given to patients with elevated serum iron levels or clinical manifestations of poisoning. If the iron level is mildly elevated or not immediately available or if the patient has mild clinical toxicity, an intravenous challenge dose of 15 mg/kg per hour can be given. Urine becomes a vin rosé or rusty orange color in the presence of the iron-deferoxamine complex (ferrioxamine), indicating that free iron is present. Patients with a positive challenge test or significant clinical toxicity should be given intravenous deferoxamine at a rate of 10 to 15 mg/kg per hour. When iron levels exceed 180 μmol/L (1000 μg/dL), larger deferoxamine doses (up to 30 mg/kg per hour) can be given initially. Once the patient is asymptomatic or improved, deferoxamine therapy should be discontinued. Rapid infusion of deferoxamine can cause hypotension. Pulmonary edema is a complication of prolonged, high-dose therapy, and renal failure can occur if it is administered to hypovolemic patients. Exchange transfusion or plasmapheresis should be reserved for patients with renal failure or who fail to respond to the preceding therapy.

ISONIAZID   Toxic doses of isoniazid decrease the synthesis of the inhibitory CNS neurotransmitter GABA by interfering with the activation and supply of pyridoxal-5-phosphate, a cofactor for the enzyme glutamic acid decarboxylase, which converts glutamic acid to GABA. Isoniazid also causes pyridoxine depletion by complexing with pyridoxine to form hydrazides that are then excreted, and it forms hydrazones that inhibit the production and activity of pyridoxal phosphate enzymes. The resultant decrease in GABA can cause seizures with increased lactate production by muscle. Since isoniazid also inhibits the metabolism of lactate to pyruvate, profound and intractable lactic acid acidosis may ensue.

Isoniazid is rapidly absorbed, with peak serum concentrations

noted within 1 to 2 h. The volume of distribution is approximately 0.7 L/kg body weight. Serum protein binding is slight. Elimination is primarily by hepatic acetylation to acetylisoniazid followed by hydrolysis to isonicotinic acid. The rate of acetylation is genetically determined and characterized as either slow or fast with corresponding half-lives of 0.5 to 1.5 and 2 to 4 h.

Clinical Toxicity   Nausea, vomiting, dizziness, slurred speech, lethargy, and confusion begin within 30 min of ingestion of doses greater than 20 mg/kg body weight. Severe poisoning results in coma, respiratory depression, generalized seizures, and lactic acid acidosis. Seizures may be protracted and relatively unresponsive to standard anticonvulsant therapy. Acidosis does not occur when seizures are prevented.

Diagnosis   The diagnosis is primarily based on clinical findings. It can be confirmed by measuring isoniazid in blood, but isoniazid assays are not routinely available. Urine screening tests do not detect the drug.

TREATMENT   Activated charcoal adsorbs isoniazid quite well and is the preferred method of gastrointestinal decontamination. Ipecac-induced vomiting should be avoided because of the potential for rapid deterioration with coma and seizures. Seizures are sometimes responsive to benzodiazepines and barbiturates, but pyridoxine (vitamin B$_6$), which reverses isoniazid-induced enzyme inhibition, is often also necessary. Diazepam and pyridoxine are synergistic. Bicarbonate may be necessary to correct acidosis. Intravenous pyridoxine is given intravenously (over 5 min in patients with seizures and over 30 min in those without) in an amount equal to the ingested dose of isoniazid. When the ingested dose is not known, 5 g of pyridoxine should be administered. Seizures are usually promptly controlled, but the patient may not awake for several hours. The dose may be repeated if the response is partial or if symptoms recur. Saline diuresis enhances the excretion of isoniazid, and the drug is efficiently removed by hemodialysis. Because pyridoxine therapy is highly effective, these procedures are rarely necessary.

ISOPROPYL ALCOHOL AND ACETONE   Isopropyl alcohol is a component of rubbing alcohol, solvents, aftershave solutions, antifreeze, and window cleaners. Acetone is found in cleaners, solvents, and nail polish removers. Both are absorbed rapidly from the stomach and the lungs and distributed in body water with volumes of distribution of about 0.6 L/kg body weight. Isopropyl alcohol is metabolized to acetone in the liver by the enzyme alcohol dehydrogenase. Up to 20% is excreted unchanged in urine. Its half-life ranges from 3 to 6 h. Acetone is excreted by the kidneys and lungs with a half-life of 20 to 30 h. Isopropyl alcohol and acetone are CNS depressants and have about twice the potency of ethanol.

Clinical Toxicity   Effects begin within 30 min of ingestion and include vomiting, abdominal discomfort, and sometimes hematemesis as well as headache, dizziness, and ethanol-like intoxication. Obtundation, coma, respiratory depression, hypothermia, and hypotension may be seen with severe poisoning. Their characteristic odors may be detected on the breath or gastric contents. Both hypoglycemia and hyperglycemia can occur. Increased serum osmolality, mild ketoacidosis, and a falsely elevated serum creatinine with a normal BUN (due to the interference with creatinine assays by acetone) may be present.

Diagnosis   Characteristic clinical and laboratory findings suggest the diagnosis. Direct measurement of serum levels will confirm it. Routine urine screening tests do not detect these agents. If laboratory confirmation is not readily available, the osmolal gap can be used to estimate the serum concentration (Table 396-3).

TREATMENT   Gastric aspiration is the preferred method of gastrointestinal decontamination. Activated charcoal is ineffective. Intravenous fluids and possibly bicarbonate should be given for dehydration, hypotension, and acidosis. Ventilatory support may be necessary. Hemodialysis is effective for removing isopropyl alcohol and acetone and should be considered in patients with high serum levels who do not respond to conservative therapy.

LITHIUM   Lithium, an alkali metal like sodium and potassium, appears to act by substituting for endogenous cations, thereby intefering with cell membrane ion transport and excitability, adenylate cyclase activation, neurotransmitter (norepinephrine) release, and Na^+, K^+-ATPase activity. It is available as the carbonate salt in pill form and as the liquid citrate salt. These preparations contain 8 mmol (meq) of lithium per 300 mg and 5 mL, respectively.

Lithium is absorbed slowly, with peak serum levels occurring 2 to 4 h after ingestion (later with overdosage and with sustained-release preparations). Lithium is not bound to plasma proteins. It has an initial volume of distribution of 0.3 to 0.4 L/kg body weight and a final one of 0.7 to 1 L/kg. Therapeutic serum levels are 0.6 to 1.2 mmol/L. An increase in the postdistribution lithium level of 1 to 1.5 mmol/L for each mmol/kg ingested can be predicted following acute overdose. Levels obtained prior to complete distribution will be higher than those in tissue and not correlate with clinical effects. Elimination is primarily (95%) by renal excretion (glomerular filtration with significant reabsorption in the proximal tubule). Renal excretion is increased by diuresis and urinary alkalinization and decreased by hypovolemia and hyponatremia. The serum half-life ranges from 18 to 36 h and can be prolonged in patients with chronic intoxication.

Clinical Toxicity   Effects begin 1 to 4 h after acute ingestion. Onset can be delayed following overdose of sustained-release preparations. It typically occurs insidiously during chronic therapy, often resulting from an intercurrent illness that causes dehydration and decreased lithium elimination. Gastrointestinal effects include nausea, vomiting, and diarrhea; neuromuscular effects include weakness, confusion, ataxia, tremors, fasciculations, myoclonus, choreoathetosis, coma, and seizures; and cardiovascular effects include arrhythmias and hypotension. Hyperthermia can occur. Leukocytosis, hyperglycemia, albuminuria, glycosuria, nephrogenic diabetes insipidus, and a falsely elevated serum chloride level (due to interference by lithium with its assays) resulting in a low anion-gap may be present. ECG changes include sinus tachycardia or bradycardia, flattened or inverted T waves, AV block, and a prolonged QT interval. Prolonged or permanent encephalopathy and movement disorders can occur in patients with severe poisoning.

Diagnosis   Since lithium is not detected by routine screening tests, a serum level must be requested specifically. Because of slow absorption and distribution, serial drug levels should be obtained following acute overdosage. In chronic poisoning, severe toxicity may occur at serum levels of 3 to 4 mmol/L. Following acute overdose, only mild effects may be present despite serum levels that rise to ≥8 mmol/L. As distribution occurs and levels fall, progressive toxicity may ensue.

℞ **TREATMENT**   Gastric lavage and whole-bowel irrigation are the procedures of choice for gastrointestinal decontamination. Whole-bowel irrigation is preferred for sustained-release formulations because intact pills will not fit through a lavage tube. Endoscopy should be considered if a concretion is suspected (persistently high or rising drug levels 2 or more days following ingestion). Activated charcoal does not adsorb lithium. Experimentally, oral administration of the ion-exchange resin sodium polystyrene sulfonate (Kayexalate) can bind lithium, prevent its absorption, and enhance its elimination, but the clinical effectiveness of this therapy is unproven. Supportive therapy includes standard treatments for seizures, CNS depression, hypotension, and arrhythmias. Symptomatic patients should be given an intravenous saline bolus and infusion to correct dehydration, to achieve a normal urine output, and to replace fluid losses in those with diabetes insipidus. Although diuresis can enhance renal excretion of lithium, there is little evidence that this therapy is more effective than simply maintaining a normal urine output. Hemodialysis, however, is highly effective in enhancing lithium elimination. It is recommended for patients with coma, seizures, and severe, persistent or progressive con-

fusion, CNS depression, or movement disorders; lesser toxicity in the presence of renal failure; and when the peak lithium level exceeds 8 mmol/L following acute overdose (because of the likelihood of severe postdistribution toxicity). Because of slow redistribution, drug levels typically rise following dialysis. Dialysis should be repeated until the postredistribution level is <1 mmol/L. Despite dialysis, clinical recovery may take days to weeks. There is no conclusive evidence that dialysis decreases the incidence of permanent sequelae.

METHANOL   Methanol is a component of shellacs, varnishes, paint removers, canned fuel (Sterno), windshield-washer solutions, and copy machine fluid. It is also used to denature ethanol and render it unfit for consumption. It is a CNS depressant with a potency about half of that of ethanol. Methanol is initially metabolized by alcohol dehydrogenase to formaldehyde, with subsequent oxidation to formic acid, and then to carbon dioxide and water. Formic acid is responsible for metabolic acidosis and retinal toxicity. Its detoxification utilizes tetrahydrofolate as a cofactor.

Methanol is readily absorbed, with peak serum levels occurring 1 to 2 h after ingestion. It is distributed throughout body water, with a volume of distribution of 0.7 L/kg body weight. Protein binding is negligible. Elimination occurs mainly by hepatic metabolism, with up to 10% excreted unchanged by the lungs and kidneys. Elimination follows first-order kinetics, with a half-life of 2 to 4 h at low serum levels (≤9 mmol/L or 30 mg/dL). At higher levels, it changes to zero-order kinetics, with an elimination rate of about 3 mmol/L per hour (10 mg/dL per hour) and an apparent half-life of up to 30 h. As with ethylene glycol, ethanol and fomepizole block the production of methanol metabolites, by competitively inhibiting alcohol dehydrogenase, and increase its elimination half-life to 30 to 60 h.

Clinical Toxicity   As with ethylene glycol, as little as one swallow of pure methanol is potentially toxic. Effects begin within an hour of ingestion. Initial manifestations are caused by methanol itself and include nausea, vomiting (sometimes bloody), abdominal pain, headache, vertigo, and an ethanol-like intoxication. An increased osmolal gap may be present. Pancreatitis has been reported. Later effects are due to formic acid and include coma, seizures, an increased anion-gap metabolic acidosis, and retinal injury. Ophthalmologic manifestations occur 15 to 30 h after ingestion and include clouding and diminished vision, dancing and flashing spots, dilated or fixed pupils, hyperemia of optic disks, retinal edema, and blindness. These changes are potentially reversible with prompt institution of therapy. With severe poisoning, myocardial depression, bradycardia, and shock may occur.

Diagnosis   The diagnosis is confirmed by measurement of serum methanol and formate levels. Early in the course, the diagnosis is suggested by ethanol-like intoxication and an elevated serum osmolality. Later, the diagnosis is suggested by an increased-anion-gap metabolic acidosis and visual complaints. If laboratory confirmation is not immediately available, the osmolal gap can also be used to estimate the serum methanol concentration (Table 396-3).

℞ **TREATMENT**   Gastric aspiration is the treatment of choice for gastrointestinal decontamination. Supportive measures should include volume replacement, respiratory care, and treatment of seizures. Acidosis should be corrected with sodium bicarbonate; large amounts may be required. Sodium bicarbonate should also be given to alkalinize the urine as this will enhance the excretion of formic acid. Supplemental folate (50 mg qid) is recommended.

Indications for ethanol or fomepizole therapy include a methanol concentration >6 mmol/L (20 mg/dL); an elevated osmolal gap, an increased anion-gap metabolic acidosis, visual symptoms, or ethanol-like intoxication in a patient with a history of methanol ingestion and a low or undetectable ethanol level; an elevated osmolal gap not accounted for by the presence of ethanol, isopropyl alcohol, acetone, or propylene glycol in a patient with ethanol-like intoxication; and an increased anion-gap metabolic acidosis with a low lactate level not explained by alcoholic or diabetic ketoacidosis or uremia or by salicylate, formaldehyde, paraldehyde, or toluene exposure. Doses and treatment considerations are the same as for ethylene glycol. Serum methanol concentrations should be monitored frequently. Ethanol or fomepizole should be continued until the methanol level falls below 3 mmol/L (10 mg/dL).

Hemodialysis enhances the elimination of methanol and formic acid. Indications for hemodialysis include methanol levels >15 mmol/L (50 mg/dL) and metabolic acidosis not readily correctable with bicarbonate and antidotal therapy, lack of clinical improvement despite treatment, or visual symptoms (regardless of the methanol level). This therapy should be continued or repeated intermittently until acidemia resolves and the methanol level is <6 mmol/L (20 mg/dL).

METHEMOGLOBINEMIA   Methemoglobinemia results from exposure to chemicals that oxidize the ferrous (Fe^{2+}) iron in hemoglobin to the ferric (Fe^{3+}) state. Concomitant oxidation of hemoglobin protein may cause its precipitation in erythrocytes and consequent hemolytic anemia, manifest as Heinz bodies and "bite cells," respectively, on peripheral blood smear. Oxidizing agents include aniline and its derivatives, aminophenols, aminophenones, chlorates, dapsone, local anesthetics (particularly benzocaine), nitrites, nitrates, naphthalene, nitrobenzene and related chemicals, oxides of nitrogen, phenazopyridine, primaquine and related antimalarials, and sulfonamides.

Methemoglobin (ferric hemoglobin) cannot carry oxygen and causes a functional anemia. It also shifts the oxygen-dissociation curve to the left, limiting the release of oxygen to tissues. Symptoms are due to hypoxia and anaerobic metabolism.

Various systems normally operate to keep methemoglobin at physiologic levels (1% of the total hemoglobin concentration). Oxidizing agents are inactivated by enzymes that utilize ascorbic acid and sulfhydryl agents such as glutathione. Methemoglobin is reduced to hemoglobin by NADH-methemoglobin reductase (responsible for 95% of baseline reducing capacity), NADPH-methemoglobin reductase, and the ascorbic acid and glutathione enzyme systems. When supplied with the cofactor methylene blue, the activity of NADPH-methemoglobin reductase is greatly increased. Because this enzyme is dependent on NADPH, individuals with glucose-6-phosphate dehydrogenase (G6PD) deficiency have profound impairment in the ability to reduce methemoglobin after oxidant exposure.

Clinical Toxicity   Onset may be immediate or delayed depending on whether the parent compound or a metabolite is the oxidant. Cyanosis with a gray-brown hue that is unresponsive to oxygen occurs when the fraction of hemoglobin existing as methemoglobin exceeds 15% (about 15 g/L or 1.5 g/dL of absolute methemoglobin). Most patients are asymptomatic until the methemoglobin fraction is >20 to 30%, at which point fatigue, headache, tachycardia, dizziness, and weakness develop. At fractions >45%, dyspnea, bradycardia, hypoxia, metabolic (lactic) acidosis, seizures, coma, and cardiac arrhythmias may occur. Fractions >70% are rapidly fatal. Hemolytic anemia is typically delayed in onset and may cause hyperkalemia and renal failure.

Diagnosis   The diagnosis is confirmed by measuring the methemoglobin level by CO-oximetry. If CO-oximetry is not available, the methemoglobin fraction can be estimated by the difference between the oxygen saturation calculated from the P_{O_2} and that measured directly. Oxygen saturation measured by pulse oximetry will be subnormal but either falsely depressed or elevated with respect to the true value. Blood with high levels of methemoglobin is chocolate-colored when placed on filter paper and compared with normal blood. Urine toxicology testing may detect the oxidizing agent.

TREATMENT   Activated charcoal is the preferred method of gastrointestinal decontamination. Supplemental oxygen should be administered. Methylene blue is indicated for methemoglobin fractions

>30% and at lower fractions in patients with anemia or cardiovascular disease, particularly if manifestations of hypoxia or organ ischemia are present. Methylene blue is given at a dose of 1 to 2 mg/kg body weight as a 1% solution over 5 min. If a clinical response is not observed within 1 h, the dose may be repeated. As long as the oxidizing agent is present, methemoglobin will continue to be generated, and additional doses may be necessary. Side effects of methylene blue include anxiety, dysuria, precordial pain, and blue or green discoloration of the urine. It is contraindicated in patients with G6PD deficiency in whom it may induce hemolysis. In doses >7 mg/kg of body weight, methylene blue itself can cause methemoglobinemia. Exchange transfusion and hyperbaric oxygen therapy may be of benefit in patients with very high methemoglobin fractions or severe clinical toxicity that is refractory to the above and those with G6PD deficiency. Erythrocyte transfusion may be necessary if hemolysis is severe. Hemodialysis may be useful for removing the offending agent.

MONOAMINE OXIDASE INHIBITORS   The antidepressants isocarboxazid, phenelzine, and tranylcypromine and the chemotherapeutic agent procarbazine irreversibly and nonselectively block monoamine oxidase (MAO) isoenzymes in the brain, gut, and liver, thus inhibiting the catabolism of endogenous MAO substrates such as epinephrine, dopamine, norepinephrine, and serotonin and exogenous ones such as ingested tyramine. Clorgyline and moclobemide selectively inhibit MAO-A, which preferentially deaminates serotonin, and pargyline and selegiline selectively inhibit MAO-B. Toxicity results from the accumulation and effects of MAO substrates. A tyramine reaction can occur when foods with high tyramine content such as aged cheese, aged, pickled, or smoked meat and fish, and red wine are ingested by individuals taking MAO inhibitors. Interactions with sympathomimetics can result in exaggerated sympathetic effects, and interactions with serotonergic agents can cause the serotonin syndrome (discussed subsequently).

MAO inhibitors are absorbed and appear to have relatively large volumes of distribution (>1 L/kg body weight). They are eliminated primarily by hepatic metabolism and have half-lives ranging from several hours to >24 h.

Clinical Toxicity   Onset following overdose is typically delayed and insidious. Effects may not begin until 6 to 24 h after ingestion and progress slowly. Initial manifestations include dilated pupils, agitation, diaphoresis, tachycardia, hypertension, and tachypnea. Nausea and vomiting may also occur. Later, confusion, CNS depression, fasciculations, twitching, tremor, muscle rigidity, rhabdomyolysis, hyperthermia, and lactic acidosis may be noted. Terminal bradycardia and cardiovascular collapse may ensue.

Tyramine and sympathomimetic reactions occur within 30 to 90 min of food or drug ingestion and resolve within a few hours. Manifestations are similar to overdose. Reflex bradycardia, seizures, and intracranial hemorrhage have also been described.

Diagnosis   The diagnosis is based on the history and clinical presentation. Serum assays are not available, and urine screening tests do not usually detect these agents.

TREATMENT   Activated charcoal is the preferred method of gastrointestinal decontamination. Benzodiazepines should be given for neuromuscular hyperactivity. Therapeutic paralysis is recommended for refractory or progressive neuromuscular hyperactivity, particularly if concomitant rhabdomyolysis and hyperthermia are present. The treatment of hyperthermia should include external cooling measures. Replacement of insensible fluid losses is also important. Severe hypertension and tachycardia should be treated with labetalol or nitroprusside and esmolol. Hypotension should first be treated with intravenous fluids and then with pressors. Pressors should initially be given at lower than normal doses because of the possibility of an exaggerated response. In fact, before any drug is given, potential interaction with MAO inhibitors should be investigated. Because MAO inhibition may persist for up to 2 weeks after discontinuing therapy, drug and dietary precautions should be maintained during this period.

MUSCLE RELAXANTS AND MISCELLANEOUS SEDATIVE-HYPNOTICS

Muscle relaxants (baclofen, carisoprodol, chlorphenesin, chlorzoxazone, cyclobenzaprine, methocarbamol, and orphenadrine) and nonbarbiturate, nonbenzodiazepine sedative-hypnotics (buspirone, chloral hydrate, ethchlorvynol, glutethimide, meprobamate, methaqualone, methyprylon, zolpidem) including the street drugs γ-butyrolactone (GBL) and its metabolite γ-hydroxybutyrate (GHB) are primarily CNS depressants. Most interact with GABA receptor complexes, enhancing the effects of this inhibitory neurotransmitter. Some muscle relaxants also depress spinal synaptic reflexes. Cyclobenzaprine and orphenadrine have anticholinergic activity. Orphenadrine also has sodium channel blocking activity.

These agents are readily absorbed, with peak blood levels occurring 1 to 2 h after ingestion. They are eliminated primarily by hepatic metabolism. Baclofen, an exception, is largely excreted unchanged in the urine. Chloral hydrate is rapidly metabolized to trichloroethanol, an active compound with a much longer half-life than the parent drug. Carisoprodol is metabolized to meprobamate. Glutethimide also has an active metabolite. Half-lives are >20 h for cyclobenzaprine, ethchlorvynol, and methaqualone; 10 to 20 h for glutethimide, meprobamate, methyprylon, and orphenadrine; and <6 h for other agents.

Clinical Toxicity Effects begin within an hour of ingestion. All muscle relaxants cause CNS depression (Table 396-2). Nystagmus is usually present. Carisoprodol, chloral hydrate, chlorphenesin, chlorzoxazone, and methocarbamol also cause nausea and vomiting. Cyclobenzaprine and orphenadrine cause anticholinergic toxicity, and orphenadrine can cause ventricular tachyarrhythmias, including torsades de pointes. Baclofen can produce hypothermia, excitability, delirium myoclonus, seizures, cardiac conduction abnormalities, tachycardia bradycardia, and hypotension. Intrathecal baclofen overdose can lead to precipitous and profound effects. Supraventricular and ventricular tachycardia can occur in chloral hydrate poisoning. GBL and GHB can cause paradoxical agitation, seizures, miosis, and bradycardia in addition to CNS depression. The effects of GBL and GHB typically last only a few hours; the duration of toxicity from other agents is substantially longer. Coma from ethchlorvynol and glutethimide, which are highly lipophilic, and from meprobamate, which can form concretions, can last for several days. With glutethimide, erratic absorption can result in cyclic coma.

Diagnosis The clinical diagnosis is supported by detecting the drugs on comprehensive urine screening. Quantitative measurements of serum levels are not routinely available.

℞ **TREATMENT** Activated charcoal is preferred for gastrointestinal decontamination. Repetitive doses may enhance their elimination. The treatment of anticholinergic poisoning is discussed in the section pertaining to these agents. Although arrhythmias due to orphenadrine have responded to physostigmine, they are more likely due to sodium channel blockade than to anticholinergic effects and should probably be treated as described above for class I antiarrhythmics. Cerebrospinal fluid drainage may enhance the elimination of intrathecal baclofen. CNS depression from zolpidem may respond to flumazenil (see "Benzodiazepines," above). Treatment is otherwise supportive. Extracorporeal hemodynamic support and enhanced elimination procedures should be considered for patients with cardiovascular depression unresponsive to standard therapy.

NEUROLEPTIC AGENTS

Clozapine, chlorprothixene, droperidol, haloperidol, loxapine, molindone, olanzapine, pimozide, quetiapine, risperidone, sertindole, thiothixene, trimethobenzamide, ziprasidone, and the phenothiazines (chlorpromazine, fluphenazine, perphenazine, prochlorperazine, promazine, promethazine, thiethylperazine, thioridazine and its metabolite mesoridazine, trifluoperazine, triflupromazine, trimeperazine) primarily act by blocking type 2 dopamine receptors in the CNS. They also have variable inhibitory activity at α-adrenergic, histaminergic, muscarinic, serotonergic, and other dopamine receptor subtypes. Some phenothiazines have a quinidine-like activity. Acute extrapyramidal effects (dystonia, akathisia, Parkinsonism) result from an imbalance of cholinergic and dopaminergic activity in the basal ganglia. These effects are idiosyncratic rather than dose-related and can be delayed in onset. The neuroleptic malignant syndrome (Chaps. 17 and 363) rarely, if ever, occurs following acute overdose.

Neuroleptic agents are well absorbed, exhibit 90 to 95% protein binding in plasma, have large apparent volumes of distribution (10 to 40 L/kg body weight), and are eliminated slowly by hepatic metabolism with half-lives of 10 to 40 h.

Clinical Toxicity Toxic effects begin within 30 to 60 min of ingestion and include CNS depression (Table 396-2), respiratory depression, hypotension, pulmonary edema, and hypothermia. Pupils are often constricted, and the skin is usually warm and dry. Anticholinergic manifestations may be the predominant effect of low overdosage (see "Anticholinergic Agents," above). Cardiac effects include tachycardia, atrioventricular block, and atrial and ventricular arrhythmias. Torsade de pointes; prolonged PR, QRS, and QT intervals; and U- and T-wave abnormalities may be seen with pimozide, mesoridazine, risperidone, thioridazine ingestions and high-dose intravenous droperidol and haloperidol.

Acute dystonic reactions are characterized by sustained muscle contractions resulting in abnormal posturing of the eyes, face, tongue, jaw, neck, back, abdomen, and pelvis. Akathisia is the subjective sensation of motor restlessness, and Parkinsonism is manifest by akinesia and rigidity. Patients may be anxious but remain alert and oriented during these reactions.

Diagnosis The diagnosis is supported by detecting the presence of these agents on toxicologic screening of the urine. Quantitative measurement is not helpful.

℞ **TREATMENT** Activated charcoal is the preferred method of gastrointestinal decontamination. Supportive care includes airway protection and mechanical ventilation for CNS and respiratory depression, fluid resuscitation followed by pressors for hypotension, and anticonvulsants for seizures. Diuresis and dialysis are ineffective. Seizures should be treated with benzodiazepines, and hypotension should be managed with volume expanders and pressor agents. Physostigmine may be useful for anticholinergic toxicity (see "Anticholinergic Agents," above). Treatment of ventricular dysrhythmias is the same as described above for class I antiarrhythmics.

Acute extrapyramidal reactions usually respond rapidly to antimuscarinic therapy such as intravenous diphenhydramine (1 mg/kg body weight given over 2 min) or benztropine (1 to 2 mg). Doses may be repeated in 20 min if the response is incomplete. Treatment should be continued with an oral formulation for 2 to 3 days since these reactions can recur in the absence of additional exposure.

NONSTEROIDAL ANTI-INFLAMMATORY DRUGS

Diclofenac, diflunisal, etodolac, fenoprofen, flurbiprofen, ibuprofen, indomethacin, ketoprofen, ketorolac, meclofenamate, mefenamic acid, naproxen, oxaprozin, piroxicam, phenylbutazone, sulindac, and tolmetin inhibit prostaglandin and thromboxane synthesis by blocking cyclooxygenase (COX) isoenzymes: COX-1, the constitutive form in the gastrointestinal tract, kidney, and platelets, and COX-2, an inducible form that becomes expressed in response to bacterial toxins and cytokines (tissue inflammation). They are absorbed rapidly, and blood concentrations peak 1 to 2 h after ingestion. They are highly protein bound (>90%) and have volumes of distribution of less than 1.0 L/kg body weight. They are primarily eliminated by hepatic metabolism. Half-lives range from 1 to 16 h except for phenylbutazone, which has a half-life of 2 to 4 days.

Clinical Toxicity Effects are usually mild and include nausea, vomiting, abdominal pain, drowsiness, headache, glycosuria, hematuria, and proteinuria. Acute renal failure and hepatitis occur rarely. Diflunisal can cause hyperventilation, tachycardia, and sweating. Coma, respiratory depression, seizures, and cardiovascular collapse may occur with mefenamic acid and phenylbutazone. Ibuprofen can cause metabolic acidosis, coma, and seizures. Metabolic acidosis is relatively common in phenylbutazone poisoning and occurs rarely with naproxen. Seizures can also occur with ketoprofen and naproxen. Preliminary data indicates that selective COX-2 inhibitors, such as celecobix and rofecobix, do not share the toxicity of these nonselective inhibitors.

Diagnosis Comprehensive toxicology screening will identify these drugs in the urine, but quantitative analysis is not useful.

℞ **TREATMENT** Activated charcoal is the preferred method of gastrointestinal decontamination. Repeated doses may enhance the elimination of indomethacin, phenylbutazone, and piroxicam. Renal excretion is not increased by diuresis, and protein binding limits the efficacy of hemodialysis. Hemoperfusion might be useful in patients with hepatic or renal failure and severe clinical toxicity. Treatment is otherwise supportive.

ORGANOPHOSPHATE AND CARBAMATE INSECTI-CIDES

Organophosphorus compounds such as the insecticides chlorpyrifos, phosphorothioic acid (Diazinon), dichlorvos, fenthion, malathion, and parathion and the chemical warfare "nerve gases" such as sarin irreversibly inhibit acetylcholinesterase and cause accumulation of acetylcholine at muscarinic and nicotinic synapses and in the CNS. Carbamates such as the insecticides aldicarb, propoxur (Baygon), carbaryl (Sevin), and bendiocarb (Ficam) and the therapeutic agents ambenonium, neostigmine, physostigmine, and pyridostigmine reversibly inhibit this enzyme. Agents that directly stimulate cholinergic receptors such as arecholine (from betel nuts), bethanechol, pilocarpine, and urecholine have the same effect.

Organophosphates are absorbed through the skin, lungs, and gastrointestinal tract; are distributed widely in tissues; and are slowly eliminated by hepatic metabolism. Oxidative metabolites of parathion and malathion (paraoxon, malaoxon) are the active forms of these agents. Carbamates are eliminated rapidly by serum and liver enzymes.

Clinical Toxicity The time from exposure to the onset of toxicity varies from minutes to hours but is usually between 30 min and 2 h. Muscarinic effects include nausea, vomiting, abdominal cramps, urinary and fecal incontinence, increased bronchial secretions, cough, wheezing, dyspnea, sweating, salivation, miosis, blurred vision, lacrimation, and urinary frequency and incontinence. In severe poisoning, bradycardia, conduction block, hypotension, and pulmonary edema may occur. Nicotinic signs include twitching, fasciculations, weakness, hypertension, tachycardia, and in severe cases paralysis and respiratory failure. CNS effects include anxiety, restlessness, tremor, confusion, weakness, seizures, and coma. Toxicity due to carbamates is shorter in duration and usually less severe than that due to organophosphates. Most patients recover within 24 to 48 h, but fat-soluble organophosphates may cause effects for weeks to months. Death is most often due to pulmonary toxicity.

Diagnosis A reduction of cholinesterase activity in plasma and in red blood cells to <50% of normal confirms the diagnosis. A reduction in red blood cell cholinesterase activity is more specific; however, this test is less readily available, and some organophosphates inhibit only one type of cholinesterase. With carbamates, depression in plasma or red blood cell cholinesterase levels is transient because of the rapid reversibility of the inhibition. Since cholinesterase assays are not routinely or rapidly available, the initial diagnosis is clinical.

℞ **TREATMENT** Contaminated clothing should be removed, and the skin should be washed with soap and water. Gastrointestinal decontamination should include use of activated charcoal. Supportive measures include oxygen administration, ventilatory assistance, and treatment of seizures. Atropine, a muscarinic receptor antagonist, should be administered for muscarinic effects. A dose of 0.5 to 2 mg

is given intravenously every 5 to 15 min until bronchial and other secretions have dried. Repeated doses or a constant infusion may be necessary for recurrent toxicity. Pralidoxime (2-PAM) reactivates cholinesterases and is indicated for nicotinic symptoms due to organophosphate poisoning. The use of pralidoxime in carbamate poisoning is controversial. It is usually unnecessary, but its use is safe, particularly if it is administered in conjunction with atropine. A dose of 1 to 2 g is given intravenously over 5 to 30 min (depending on severity). It can be repeated in 30 min if the response is incomplete. Rapid injection can cause tachycardia, laryngospasm, muscle rigidity, and weakness. Repeated doses (every 4 to 6 h) or a continuous infusion (500 mg/h) are indicated for recurrent effects. Neither atropine nor pralidoxime is particularly effective at reversing CNS effects; seizures should be treated aggressively with benzodiazepines.

SALICYLATES Aspirin (acetylsalicyclic acid) and salicylate salts have activity similar to that of other nonsteroidal anti-inflammatory drugs described above. Aspirin, but not other salicylates, also inhibits platelet aggregation. Toxic doses increase the sensitivity of respiratory centers in the brain to changes in oxygen and carbon dioxide concentrations. They also uncouple oxidative phosphorylation, increase the rate of metabolism (oxygen consumption, glucose utilization, and carbon dioxide and heat production), and inhibit the Krebs cycle and carbohydrate and lipid metabolism. Metabolic effects lead to respiratory center stimulation and respiratory alkalosis early in the course of poisoning and lactic and ketoacidosis in later stages. Salicylates can also inhibit the hepatic synthesis of clotting factors.

With therapeutic doses, peak serum levels of 0.7 to 1.4 mmol/L (10 to 20 mg/dL) occur 1 to 2 h after ingestion, 50 to 80% is bound to albumin, the volume of distribution is small (0.2 L/kg body weight), and the half-life is 2 to 3 h. Being a weak acid, the unbound portion in the serum exists mainly in an ionized state. Elimination occurs primarily by hepatic metabolism, with about 10% being excreted unchanged.

Although salicylates are absorbed rapidly, absorption may continue for 24 h or longer after an overdose. Acidosis increases the nonionized (diffusable) fraction, and unbound salicylate promotes its tissue distribution (i.e., increases the volume of distribution). Saturation of metabolic pathways results in a prolonged half-life (20 to 36 h), and renal excretion becomes the most important route of elimination. Alkalinization of the urine enhances renal excretion by converting urinary salicylate to the ionized form, which cannot be reabsorbed.

Clinical Toxicity Initial manifestations occur 3 to 6 h after an overdose of ≥150 mg/kg and include vomiting, sweating, tachycardia, hyperpnea, fever, tinnitus, lethargy, confusion, respiratory alkalosis with compensatory bicarbonate excretion resulting in an alkaline urine (pH >6). Increases in the rate or depth of respirations may be subtle. Vomiting, diaphoresis, and hyperventilation may lead to dehydration and decreased renal function. As acid products of intermediary metabolism accumulate, increased anion-gap metabolic acidosis and ketosis develop, and their excretion results in the urine becoming acidic (pH <6). In moderate poisoning, both respiratory alkalosis and metabolic acidosis are present, usually with alkalemia and paradoxical aciduria, although the serum pH can be normal. Elevation of the hematocrit, white blood cell count, and platelet count; hypernatremia; hyperkalemia; hypoglycemia; and prolongation of the prothrombin time may be seen. Severe poisoning is manifest by coma, respiratory depression, seizures, cardiovascular collapse, and cerebral and pulmonary edema (both noncardiogenic and cardiogenic). At this stage, metabolic evaluation reveals acidemia (metabolic acidosis with respiratory alkalosis or acidosis) and aciduria.

Diagnosis The diagnosis should be suspected in anyone with an unexplained acid-base disorder. Salicylates are identified by a positive urine ferric chloride test (purple color), which is usually included in routine screening procedures, or quantitative serum analysis. Following acute overdose, a peak level of <2.2 mmol/L (30 mg/dL) is associated with little or no toxicity, one of 2.2 to 7 mmol/L (30 to 100 mg/dL) with mild to moderate effects, and one of >7 mmol/L (100 mg/dL) with severe poisoning. Because of delayed and prolonged absorption, serial levels should be obtained. In chronic poisoning, symptoms may occur at levels only slightly above the therapeutic range.

℞ **TREATMENT** Activated charcoal is the preferred method of gastrointestinal decontamination. Repeated doses may enhance elimination. Because of delayed absorption, decontamination may be helpful 12 to 24 h after ingestion. Gastric lavage and whole-bowel irrigation should be considered in patients with ingestions of >500 mg/kg, particularly when toxicity progresses and drug levels continue to rise following charcoal administration. Endoscopy may be useful for the diagnosis and removal of gastric bezoars. A bedside glucose level should be determined in patients with altered mental status. Intravenous saline should be given to replace fluid losses and to produce a brisk urine flow. The degree of dehydration is often underestimated; several liters or more may be necessary. Supplemental glucose and oxygen should also be given. Electrolyte and metabolic abnormalities should be corrected. Coagulopathy should be treated with intravenous vitamin K. Seizures and heart failure are treated with standard therapies. Saline diuresis and urinary alkalinization (to a pH of 8) enhance the elimination of salicylate and should be instituted in symptomatic patients and those with salicylate levels >2.2 mmol/L (30 mg/dL). Depending on severity, 50 to 150 mmol of bicarbonate (along with potassium) can be added to a liter of dextrose-containing saline solution (such that the final sodium concentration is nearly isotonic) and administered at a rate of 2 to 6 mL/kg per hour. Electrolytes, calcium, acid-base status, urine pH, and fluid balance must be monitored carefully during such therapy. When acidemia is present, bicarbonate should also be given to correct the serum pH, increase the ionization of serum salicylate, and limit its tissue distribution. Diuresis is contraindicated when cerebral or pulmonary edema and renal failure are present. Salicylates are effectively removed by hemodialysis. Indications for hemodialysis include severe clinical toxicity, levels that approach or exceed 7 mmol/L (100 mg/dL) following acute overdose, and contraindications or failure to respond to other treatment modalities.

SEROTONIN SYNDROME This syndrome is due to excessive CNS and peripheral serotonergic (5HT-1a and possibly 5HT-2) activity and results from the concomitant use of agents that promote the release of serotonin from presynaptic neurons (e.g., amphetamines, cocaine, codeine, methylenedioxy-methamphetamine or MDMA, reserpine, some MAO inhibitors), inhibit its reuptake (e.g., cyclic antidepressants, particularly the SSRIs, ergot derivatives, dextromethorphan, meperidine, pentazocine, sumatriptan and related agents, tramadol, some MAO inhibitors) or metabolism (e.g., cocaine, MAO inhibitors), or stimulate postsynaptic serotonin receptors (e.g., bromocriptine, bupropion, buspirone, levodopa, lithium, L-tryptophan, lysergic acid diethylamide or LSD, mescaline, trazodone). Less often, it results from the use or overdose of a single serotonergic agent or when one agent is taken soon after another has been discontinued (up to 2 weeks for some agents). Serotonergic effects also appear to have been responsible for pulmonary hypertension and valvulopathy associated with the anorexiants dexfenfluramine and fenfluramine (withdrawn from U.S. markets in 1997).

Clinical Toxicity Onset occurs as early as an hour after single or multiple drug overdose or the addition of another serotonergic agent to current therapy and as a long as several days after increasing the dose of one or more agents. Manifestations include altered mental status (agitation, confusion, delirium, mutism, coma, and seizures), neuromuscular hyperactivity (restlessness, incoordination, hyperreflexia, myoclonus, rigidity, and tremors), and autonomic dysfunction (abdominal pain, diarrhea, diaphoresis, fever, elevated and fluctuating blood pressure, flushed skin, mydriasis, tearing, salivation, shivering, and tachycardia). Complications include hyperthermia, lactic acidosis, rhabdomyolysis, kidney and liver failure, ARDS, and disseminated intravascular coagulation. Effects last from 6 to 48 h, depending on severity.

Diagnosis The diagnosis is based on clinical manifestations and the history of drug exposure. Toxicology testing is useful only for confirming an exposure or detecting an unsuspected one. In contrast to the neuroleptic malignant syndrome (Chap. 363), with which its shares many features, the serotonin syndrome becomes maximal and later resolves over a period of hours rather than days, and there is myclonus and hyperreflexia in contrast to "lead-pipe" rigidity.

℞ **TREATMENT** Gastrointestinal decontamination may be indicated for acute overdose. Supportive measures include hydration with intravenous fluids, airway protection and mechanical ventilation, benzodiazepines (and paralytics, if necessary) for neuromuscular hyperactivity, and mechanical cooling measures for hyperthermia.

The administration of serotonin-receptor antagonists may hasten the resolution of this syndrome. Cyproheptadine (Periactin), an antihistamine with 5HT-1a and 5HT2 receptor blocking activity, and chlorpromazine (Thorazine), a nonspecific serotonin receptor antagonist, have been used with success. Cyproheptadine is given orally or by gastric tube in an initial dose of 4 to 8 mg and repeated as necessary every 2 to 4 h up to a maximum of 32 mg in 24 h. A response is usually noted in 1 to 2 h but may be absent in severe cases. Chlorpromazine has the advantage that it can be given parenterally (intramuscularly or by slow intravenous injection in doses of 50 to 100 mg). Since it can cause hypotension, its use should be preceded by adequate fluid hydration. The use of chlorpromazine for the neuroleptic malignant syndrome misdiagnosed as the serotonin syndrome, and conversely, the use of bromocriptine for the serotonin syndrome misdiagnosed as the neuroleptic malignant syndrome may result in worsening of symptoms. Other medications with variable success in treating the serotonin syndrome include propranolol, methysergide, and dantrolene.

SYMPATHOMIMETICS Amphetamines (amphetamine itself, benzphetamine, dextroamphetamine, diethylpropion, methamphetamine, phendimetrazine, phentermine), cathinone (from khat, or the plant *Catha edulis*), ephedrine, mazindol, methylphenidate, and pemoline directly stimulate α- and β-adrenergic receptors. Some also induce the release of dopamine and norepinephrine. Phenylephrine, pseudoephedrine, and phenylpropanolamine primarily stimulate α receptors, whereas mephentermine and bronchodilators such as albuterol, bitoterol, isoetherine, etaproterenol, pirbuterol, and salmeterol primarily stimulate β receptors.

These agents are readily absorbed, with peak serum levels occurring 1 to 2 h after ingestion (sooner after nasal insufflation and with the "ice" or crystalline form of methamphetamine, which, like crack cocaine, can be smoked). They are weak bases with volumes of distribution of 2 to 6 L/kg body weight. Elimination occurs by a combination of hepatic metabolism and renal excretion of unchanged drug. Half-lives range from 2 to 34 h. Excretion is enhanced in an acid urine and slowed in an alkaline one.

Clinical Toxicity Effects are seen within 30 to 60 min after ingestion and include nausea, vomiting, abdominal cramps, and headache as well as manifestations of adrenergic and CNS stimulation (Table 396-2). Although hypertension and tachycardia occur with nonselective agents, hypertension with reflex bradycardia, and even AV block, may occur with agents that have predominantly alpha effects. Tachycardia with hypotension (as a result of vasodilation) can be seen with selective β agonists. Other findings may include combativeness, auditory and visual hallucinations, dilated pupils, dry mouth, pallor, and tachypnea. Complications include lactic acidosis, rhabdomyolysis, and intracranial hemorrhage. β-Adrenergic stimulation causes potassium to move into cells and may result in hypokalemia.

Diagnosis The diagnosis is supported by finding these agents in the urine by toxicology screening. Quantitative measurement is not useful.

℞ **TREATMENT** Activated charcoal is the preferred method of gastrointestinal decontamination. Benzodiazepines or barbiturates should be used to control neuromuscular hyperactivity and to treat seizures. A nonselective adrenergic blocker such as labetalol or the selective α-adrenergic antagonist phentolamine (1 to 5 mg intravenously every 5 min until the desired response is achieved) with or without a cardioselective beta blocker such as esmolol are recommended for severe or symptomatic hypertension; propranolol or a cardioselective beta blocker is recommended for severe or symptomatic tachycardia. Lidocaine and propranolol are preferred for the treatment of ventricular tachyarrhythmias. Hyperthermia should be treated with external cooling measures along with sedation and, if necessary, paralyzing agents. Although theoretically effective for enhancing drug elimination, acid diuresis is not recommended due to lack of documented clinical efficacy and risks of side effects such as worsening of acidosis and potential triggering of myoglobinuric renal failure.

THEOPHYLLINE Theophylline, caffeine, and other methylxanthines are phosphodiesterase inhibitors that reduce the degradation of intracellular cyclic AMP, thereby enhancing the actions of endogenous catecholamines and leading to β-adrenergic stimulation. Theophylline is absorbed rapidly from the stomach and upper small bowel. Following overdose, serum levels peak 1 to 2 h after ingestion of liquid preparations, 2 to 4 h after ingestion of tablets, and 6 to 24 h after ingestion of sustained-release preparations. Theophylline is approximately 60% bound to albumin and has a low volume of distribution (0.6 L/kg body weight). Therapeutic serum levels are 55 to 110 μmol/L (10 to 20 mg/L). Elimination occurs primarily by hepatic metabolism, which is saturable at levels in the high therapeutic range. The serum half-life, normally 4 to 6 h, is therefore prolonged in overdoses. Elimination is also decreased with impaired liver function, congestive heart failure, viral infections, and concomitantly administered drugs such as cimetidine, erythromycin, fluoroquinolones, and tetracycline.

Clinical Toxicity Effects begin 30 min to 2 h following overdose and include nausea, vomiting, psychomotor excitation, pallor, diaphoresis, tachypnea, tachycardia, and muscle tremors. Severe poisoning is characterized by coma, seizures, respiratory depression, cardiac arrhythmias, hypotension, and rhabdomyolysis. Seizures can be focal and are often protracted, repetitive, and resistant to therapy. Both atrial and ventricular tachyarrhythmias, including ventricular fibrillation, can occur. Hypotension develops only after acute overdose. Ketosis, metabolic acidosis, hyperamylasemia, hyperglycemia, hypokalemia, hypocalcemia, and hypophosphatemia may also be seen in acute poisoning.

Diagnosis The diagnosis is confirmed by measuring a serum drug level. Theophylline is not readily detected by routine urine screening. Wtih chronic exposure, arrhythmias and seizures occur at lower serum levels (200 to 300 μmol/L, or 40 to 60 mg/L) than the levels seen after acute overdose (400 to 500 μmol/L, 80 to 100 mg/L). Because of prolonged and delayed absorption after overdosage, particularly with sustained-release preparations, levels should be measured serially to determine the peak concentration.

℞ **TREATMENT** Activated charcoal is the preferred method of gastrointestinal decontamination. With sustained-release forms, whole-bowel irrigation should also be considered. Antiemetics are often required for vomiting. Seizures and neuromuscular hyperactivity should be treated with benzodiazepines and barbiturates and pharmacologic paralysis in refractory cases; phenytoin is ineffective. Intravenous propranolol is preferred for the treatment of tachyarrhythmias. It can also reverse hypotension, which results from β_2-adrenergic stimulation. Although β_2 receptor blockade can potentially cause bronchospasm in those with reactive or obstructive airway disease, this has not been reported when propranolol has been used in this setting. The selective beta$_1$ blocker esmolol can also be used for supraventricular tachycardias, and ventricular tachycardias can be treated with lidocaine or other antiarrhythmics. Volume expansion and an α agonist such as

norepinephrine can be given for hypotension. Repeated doses of charcoal shorten the serum half-life of theophylline by approximately 50% and are recommended for all patients. Hemodialysis and hemoperfusion are effective in removing theophylline and are indicated for patients with severe clinical toxicity or a serum drug level equal to or greater than that associated with such toxicity.

BIBLIOGRAPHY

GENERAL PRINCIPLES

HARDMAN JD et al (eds): *Goodman and Gilman's The Pharmacologic Basis of Therapeutics*, 9th ed. New York, McGraw-Hill, 1996

KLAASSEN CD (Ed): *Casarett and Doull's Toxicology: The Basic Science of Poisons*, 5th ed. New York, McGraw-Hill, 1996

EPIDEMIOLOGY

HENDERSON A et al: Experience with 732 acute overdose patients admitted to an intensive care unit over 6 years. Med J Austral 158:28, 1993

LITOVITZ TL et al: 1997 Annual Report of the American Association of Poison Control Centers Toxic Exposure Surveillance System. Am J Emerg Med 16:443, 1998

DIAGNOSIS

AABAKKEN et al: Osmolal and anion gaps in patients admitted to an emergency medical department. Hum Exp Toxicol 13:131, 1994

BRADBERRY SM, VALE JA: Disturbances of potassium homeostasis in poisoning. Clin Toxicol 33:295, 1995

CHAN TC et al: Drug-induced hyperthermia. Crit Care Clin 13:785, 1997

COUNCIL ON SCIENTIFIC AFFAIRS, AMERICAN MEDICAL ASSOCIATION: Scientific issues in drug testing. JAMA 257:3110, 1987

CURRY SC et al: Drug- and toxin-induced rhabdomyolysis. Ann Emerg Med 18:1068, 1989

HOFFMAN RS, GOLDFRANK LR: The poisoned patient with altered consciousness: Controversies in the use of the "coma cocktail." JAMA 274:562, 1995

OLSON KR et al: Physical assessment and differential diagnosis of the poisoned patient. Med Toxicol 2:52, 1987

ZACCARA G et al: Clinical features, pathogenesis, and management of drug-induced seizures. Drug Safety 5:109, 1990

TREATMENT

AMERICAN ACADEMY OF CLINICAL TOXICOLOGY/EUROPEAN ASSOCIATION OF POISONS CENTERS AND CLINICAL TOXICOLOGISTS: POSITION STATEMENTS ON GASTROINTESTINAL DECONTAMINATION: Introduction, ipecac syrup; gastric lavage; Single-dose activated charcoal; Cathartics; Whole bowel irrigation. Clin Toxicol 35: 695, 699, 711, 721, 743, 753, 1997

———: Multi-dose activated charcoal. Clin Toxicol 37:731, 1999

BRETT AS et al: Predicting the clinical course of intentional drug overdose: Implications for utilization of the intensive care unit. Arch Intern Med 147:133, 1987

BURGESS JL et al: Emergency department hazardous materials protocol for contaminated patients. Ann Emerg Med 34:205, 1999

COONEY DO: *Activated Charcoal in Medical Applications*. New York, Marcel Dekker, 1995

GARRETTSON LK, GELLER RJ: Acid and alkaline diuresis: When are they of value in the treatment of poisoning? Drug Safety 5:220, 1990

MANOGUERRA AS: Gastrointestinal decontamination after poisoning: Where is the science. Crit Care Clin 13:709, 1997

MINOCHA A, SPYKER DA: Acute overdose with sustained-release drug formulations: Perspectives in treatment. Med Toxicol 1:300, 1986

NEUVONEN PJ, OLKKOLA KT: Oral activated charcoal in the treatment of intoxications: Role of single and repeated doses. Med Toxicol 3:33, 1988

POND SM: Diuresis, dialysis and hemoperfusion: Indications and benefits. Emerg Med Clin North Am 2:29, 1984

STEAD AH, MOFFAT AC: A collection of therapeutic, toxic and fatal blood drug concentrations in man. Hum Toxicol 3:437, 1983

397 *Robert L. Norris, Paul S. Auerbach*

DISORDERS CAUSED BY REPTILE BITES AND MARINE ANIMAL EXPOSURES

Few topics in medicine are as controversial or as influenced by tradition as the management of bites and stings from venomous creatures. Because the incidence of serious bites and stings is relatively low in developed nations, there remains a paucity of relevant clinical research and literature, and therapeutic decision-making is often based on anecdotal information. Furthermore, the responses of different species to various toxins make it difficult to extrapolate data from animal studies to clinical application. This chapter outlines general principles for the evaluation and management of victims of venom poisoning or intoxication by certain reptiles and marine creatures and presents a clinical approach to these emergencies.

VENOMOUS SNAKEBITE

EPIDEMIOLOGY The venomous snakes of the world are grouped into the families Viperidae (subfamily Viperinae: the Old World vipers; subfamily Crotalinae: the New World and Asian pit vipers), Elapidae (including the cobras, coral snakes, and all Australian venomous snakes), Hydrophiidae (the sea snakes), Atractaspididae (the burrowing asps), and Colubridae (a large group of which only a few species are dangerously toxic to humans). The highest bite rates occur in temperate and tropical regions where people subsist by manual agriculture. Global estimates suggest that 30,000 to 40,000 persons die each year from venomous snakebite, but this range is likely an underestimate because of incomplete reporting.

SNAKE ANATOMY/IDENTIFICATION The typical snake-venom apparatus consists of bilateral venom glands—one on each side of the head, below and behind the eye—connected by ducts to hollow, anterior maxillary teeth. In viperids (vipers and pit vipers), these teeth are long, mobile fangs that retract against the roof of the mouth when the animal is at rest. In elapids and sea snakes, the fangs are less enlarged and are fixed in an erect position. Venomous snakes can bite without injecting venom. Approximately 20% of pit viper bites and an even higher percentage of bites inflicted by some other snake families (e.g., up to 75% for sea snakes) are "dry."

Differentiation of venomous from nonvenomous snake species can be difficult. Viperids are characterized by somewhat triangular heads (a feature shared with many harmless snakes); elliptical pupils (also seen in some nonvenomous snakes, such as boas and pythons); enlarged maxillary fangs; subcaudal scalation that involves a single scale running the full width of the ventral surface of the tail for several rows just distal to the anal plate (as opposed to two scales in each subcaudal row for most nonvenomous snakes); and, in the case of pit vipers, the heat-sensing pits (foveal organs located slightly inferior and anterior to the eyes on each side) for which they are named. Color pattern is notoriously misleading in identifying most venomous snakes except for the coral snakes, whose other body characteristics are similar to those of harmless colubrids. The American coral snakes can be identified by red, yellow (or white), and black bands completely encircling the body; a few species have red and black bands only. North of Mexico City, the immediate contiguity of red and yellow bands is fairly reliable for distinguishing a coral snake from its many harmless mimics. Further south, differentiation by color pattern is more problematic.

In many areas of the world, enzyme-linked immunoassay (ELISA) kits are available to aid in determining the specific snake species involved in a bite. These kits identify venom in the victim's blood, urine, or wound aspirate. No such kit is commercially available in the United States, however.

VENOMS AND CLINICAL MANIFESTATIONS Snake venoms are complex mixtures of enzymes, low-molecular-weight polypeptides, glycoproteins, and metal ions. Among the deleterious components are hemorrhagins that promote vascular leaking and cause both local and systemic bleeding. Various proteolytic enzymes cause local tissue necrosis, affect the coagulation pathway at various steps, and impair organ function. Myocardial depressant factors reduce cardiac output, and neurotoxins act either pre- or postsynaptically to inhibit peripheral nerve impulses. Most snake venoms have multisystem effects in their victims.

℞ **TREATMENT Field Management** Initial (prehospital) measures should focus on rapidly delivering the victim to definitive medical care while keeping him/her as inactive as possible to limit systemic spread of venom. Any other measures employed should at least do no further harm to the victim.

After viperid bites, local mechanical suction applied to the site within 3 to 5 min may remove a small percentage of deposited venom. A useful device is the Extractor (Sawyer Products, Safety Harbor, FL), which delivers one atmosphere of negative pressure to the wound. Suction should be continued for at least 30 min. Mouth suction should be avoided as it inoculates the wound with oral flora and theoretically can also result in the absorption of venom by the rescuer through lesions of the upper digestive tract. If the victim is >60 min from medical care, a proximal lympho-occlusive constriction band may limit the spread of venom when applied within 30 min. To avoid worsening tissue damage, however, the band should not interrupt arterial blood flow. The bitten extremity should be splinted if possible and kept at approximately heart level. Measures to be avoided include incising or cooling the bite site, giving the victim an alcoholic beverage, or applying electric shocks.

For elapid or sea snake bites, the Australian pressure-immobilization technique, in which the entire bitten extremity is wrapped with an elastic or crepe bandage and then splinted, is highly effective. The bandage is applied with the same snugness used for a sprained ankle. This technique greatly restricts absorption and circulation of venom. The utility of this method in viperid poisoning requires further research, as it theoretically could compound local tissue damage by restricting venom to the local tissues.

Hospital Management In the hospital, the victim should be closely monitored (vital signs, cardiac rhythm, and oxygen saturation) while a history is quickly obtained and a brief but thorough physical examination is performed. The level of erythema and/or swelling in a bitten extremity should be marked and limb circumferences measured in several locations every 15 min until swelling has stabilized. Large-bore intravenous access in unaffected extremities should be established. Early hypotension is due to pooling of blood in the pulmonary and splanchnic vascular beds. Hours later, hemolysis and loss of intravascular volume into soft tissues may play important roles. Fluid resuscitation with normal saline or Ringer's lactate should be initiated for clinical shock. If the blood pressure response is inadequate after administration of 20 to 40 mL/kg of body weight, then a trial of 5% albumin (10 to 20 mL/kg) is in order. If tissue perfusion fails to respond to volume resuscitation and antivenom infusion (see below), vasopressors (e.g., dopamine) should be administered. Invasive hemodynamic monitoring (central venous and/or pulmonary arterial pressures) can be helpful in such cases, although obtaining access is riskier if coagulopathy is present.

Blood should be drawn for laboratory evaluation as soon as possible. Blood typing and cross-matching procedures can be affected over time by circulating venom. Also important are a complete blood count to evaluate the degree of hemorrhage or hemolysis, studies of renal and hepatic function, coagulation studies to identify signs of consumptive coagulopathy, and testing of urine for blood or myoglobin. In severe cases or in the face of significant comorbidity, arterial blood gas studies, electrocardiography, and chest radiography are indicated.

Attempts to locate a source of appropriate antivenom should begin early in all cases of known venomous snakebite, regardless of symptoms. In the event that signs and symptoms progress rapidly, any delay in the administration of antivenom is dangerous. Antivenoms rarely offer cross-protection against snake species other than those used in their production unless the species are closely related. An example of good cross-protection is that of Australian tiger snake (*Notechis scutatus*) antivenom for sea snake bites (see below). The package insert accompanying a particular antivenom should be consulted for information regarding the spectrum of coverage. In the United States, assistance in finding antivenom can be obtained 24 hours a day from the University of Arizona Poison and Drug Information Center (telephone: 520-626-6016).

Rapidly progressive or severe local findings (soft tissue swelling, ecchymosis, petechiae, etc.) or manifestations of systemic toxicity (signs and symptoms or laboratory abnormalities) are indications for the administration of intravenous antivenom. The package insert outlines techniques for reconstitution of antivenom (when necessary), skin-testing procedures (for potential allergy), and appropriate starting doses. Most commercial antivenoms are of equine origin and carry a risk of anaphylactic, anaphylactoid, and delayed-hypersensitivity reactions. Skin testing does not reliably predict which patients will have an allergic reaction to equine antivenom; false-negative and false-positive results are common. Before antivenom infusion, the patient should receive appropriate loading doses of intravenous antihistamines (e.g., diphenhydramine, 1 mg/kg to a maximum of 100 mg; and cimetidine, 5 to 10 mg/kg to a maximum of 300 mg) in an effort to limit acute reactions. Modest expansion of the patient's intravascular volume with crystalloids may also be beneficial in this regard. Epinephrine should be immediately available, and the antivenom dose to be administered should be diluted (e.g., in 1000 mL of normal saline for adults or in 20 mL/kg for children). This volume can be decreased if necessary (e.g., if the victim has a history of congestive heart failure). The antivenom should be started slowly, with the physician at the bedside to intervene in the event of an acute reaction. The rate of infusion can be increased gradually in the absence of allergic phenomena until the total starting dose has been administered (over a total period of 1 to 4 h). Further antivenom may be necessary if the patient's clinical condition worsens. Laboratory values should be rechecked hourly, particularly if abnormal, until stability is apparent.

The management of a life-threatening envenomation in a victim with an apparent allergy to antivenom requires significant expertise. Consultation with a poison specialist, an intensive care specialist, and/or an allergist is recommended. Often antivenom can still be administered in these situations under closely controlled conditions and with intensive premedication (e.g., with epinephrine, antihistamines, and steroids).

Care of the bite wound should include application of a dry sterile dressing and splinting of the extremity with padding between the digits. Once the administration of an indicated antivenom has been initiated, the extremity should be elevated above heart level to relieve edema. Tetanus immunization should be updated as appropriate. The use of prophylactic antibiotics is controversial, as the incidence of secondary infection following venomous snakebite appears to be low. Many authorities, however, prescribe a broad-spectrum antibiotic (such as ampicillin or a cephalosporin) for the first few days.

If swelling in the bitten extremity raises concern that subfascial muscle edema may be impeding tissue perfusion (muscle-compartment syndrome), intracompartmental pressures should be checked by any minimally invasive technique (e.g., the wick catheter). If pressures are elevated and remain so despite antivenom administration, prompt surgical consultation for possible fasciotomy should be obtained. This complication, fortunately, is rare after snakebites.

Whether or not antivenom is given, any patient with signs of venom poisoning should be observed in the hospital for at least 24 h. A patient with an apparently "dry" bite should be watched for at least 6 to 8 h before discharge, as significant toxicity occasionally develops after a delay of several hours. The onset of systemic symptoms is commonly delayed for a number of hours after bites by several of the elapids (including the coral snakes) and sea snakes. Patients bitten by these reptiles should be observed in the hospital for 24 h.

Significant work is being done in several regions of the world to produce safer, more effective antivenoms. Much of this work involves production of ovine-based antivenoms that are further purified and enzymatically cleaved to yield functional F(ab) fragments of the immunoglobulin molecules. These antivenoms are currently in clinical use in many countries, and trials of one product are under way in the United States.

MORBIDITY AND MORTALITY The overall mortality rates for venomous snakebite are low in areas of the world with rapid access to medical care and appropriate antivenom. In the United States, for example, the mortality rate is <1% for victims who receive antivenom. Eastern and western diamondback rattlesnakes (*Crotalus adamanteus* and *C. atrox*, respectively) are responsible for most snakebite deaths in the United States. Snakes responsible for large numbers of deaths in other regions of the world include the cobras (*Naja* spp.) of Asia and Africa, the carpet and saw-scaled vipers (*Echis* spp.) of the Middle East and Africa, Russell's viper (*Daboia russelli*) of the Middle East and Asia, the large African vipers (*Bitis* spp.), and the lancehead pit vipers (*Bothrops* spp.) of Central and South America.

The incidence of morbidity in terms of permanent functional loss in a bitten extremity is difficult to estimate but is probably substantial. Such loss may be due to muscle, nerve, or vascular injury or to scar contracture. In the United States, such loss due to snakebite tends to be much more common and severe after rattlesnake bites than after bites by copperheads or water moccasins.

LIZARD BITES

Bites from the two species of venomous lizards (the gila monster, *Heloderma suspectum*, of the southwestern United States and the Mexican beaded lizard, *H. horridum*) are infrequent and usually follow attempts to capture or handle these creatures. The wounds are characterized by soft tissue trauma with surrounding local edema and occasionally local cyanosis and ecchymosis. Broken teeth may be embedded in the wounds. The venom contains proteases and phospholipases. Systemic effects may include hypotension, weakness, dizziness, and diaphoresis.

Prehospital care measures for these bites should follow the guidelines listed above for viperid bites. If the biting lizard is still attached to the victim, its jaws may need to be manually pried apart for removal.

The sparseness of data on the pathophysiologic effects of helodermatid venom precludes specific recommendations regarding laboratory evaluation, but routine studies (complete blood count, coagulation studies, electrolyte analysis, blood typing and cross-matching, urinalysis, and electrocardiography) are prudent in anything other than a trivial bite. Wounds should be cleansed thoroughly and irrigated when possible. Tetanus immunization should be updated as indicated. Soft tissue radiography of the bite site and sterile probing under local anesthesia may identify retained teeth. The extremity should be splinted and elevated, but antibiotic treatment is not usually required. Systemic care is supportive (e.g., crystalloid infusion for hypotension). No commercial antivenom exists. Pain due to local venom effects and mechanical trauma can be treated with opiates and regional nerve blocks. The mortality rate is extremely low.

MARINE ENVENOMATIONS

Management of venom poisoning by marine creatures is similar to that of venomous snakebite in that much of the treatment administered is supportive in nature. A few specific marine antivenoms can be used when appropriate.

INVERTEBRATES   *Hydroids, fire coral, jellyfish, Portuguese man-of-war,* and *sea anemones* possess specialized stinging cells called nematocysts. The venoms from these organisms are mixtures of proteins, carbohydrates, and other components. The clinical syndrome following envenomation by any of these species is similar but of variable severity. Victims usually report immediate prickling or burning, pruritus, paresthesia, and painful throbbing with radiation. A legion of neurologic, cardiovascular, respiratory, rheumatologic, gastrointestinal, renal, and ocular symptoms have been described. Victims in unstable condition with hypotension or respiratory distress should be treated supportively. During stabilization, the skin should be immediately decontaminated with a forceful jet of vinegar (5% acetic acid) or rubbing alcohol (40 to 70% isopropyl alcohol), which inactivates nematocysts. For the venomous *box-jellyfish* (*Chironex fleckeri;* **Plate**

vinegar should be used. Perfume, aftershave lotion, and high-proof ethanol are less efficacious and may be detrimental. Shaving the skin helps remove remaining nematocysts. Freshwater irrigation and rubbing lead to further stinging by adherent nematocysts and should be avoided. After decontamination, application of anesthetic ointments (lidocaine, benzocaine), antihistamine creams (diphenhydramine), or steroid lotions (hydrocortisone) may be helpful. Persistent pain following decontamination may be treated with morphine or meperidine. Muscle spasms may respond to 10% calcium gluconate (5 to 10 mL) or diazepam (2 to 5 mg, titrated upwards as necessary) given intravenously. An antivenom is available from Commonwealth Serum Laboratories (see section on antivenom sources, below) for stings from the box-jellyfish found in Australian waters.

Touching a *sea sponge* may result in dermatitis. If contact occurs, the skin should be gently dried and adhesive tape used to remove embedded spicules. Vinegar should be applied immediately and then for 10 to 30 min three or four times a day. Rubbing alcohol may be used if vinegar is unavailable. After spicule removal and skin decontamination, a steroid or antihistamine cream may be applied to the skin. Severe vesiculation should be treated with a 2-week course of systemic glucocorticoids.

Annelid worms (bristleworms) possess rows of soft, cactus-like spines capable of inflicting painful stings. Contact results in symptoms similar to those of nematocyst envenomation. Without treatment, pain usually subsides over several hours, but inflammation may persist for up to a week. Victims should resist the urge to scratch, since scratching may fracture retrievable spines. Visible bristles should be removed with forceps and adhesive tape, a commercial facial peel, or a thin layer of rubber cement. Use of vinegar, rubbing alcohol, or dilute ammonia or a brief application of unseasoned meat tenderizer (papain) may provide additional relief. Local inflammation should be treated with topical or systemic glucocorticoids.

Sea urchins possess either hollow, venom-filled, calcified spines or triple-jawed, globiferous pedicellariae with venom glands. Their venom contains several toxic components, including steroid glycosides, hemolysins, proteases, serotonin, and cholinergic substances. Contact with either venom apparatus produces immediate and intensely painful stings. The affected part should be immersed immediately in hot water (see below). Accessible embedded spines should be removed but may break off and remain lodged in the victim. Residual dye from the surface of a spine remaining after the spine's removal may mimic a retained spine but is otherwise of no consequence. Soft tissue radiography or magnetic resonance imaging can confirm the presence of retained spines; this finding may warrant referral for attempted surgical removal if the spines are located near vital structures (e.g., joints, neurovascular bundles). Retained spines may cause the formation of granulomas that are amenable to excision or to intralesional injection with triamcinolone hexacetonide (5 mg/mL).

Cone shells are predatory, carnivorous mollusks. The most dangerous of these creatures are found in the Indian and Pacific oceans. A neurotoxic venom comprising multiple peptides is delivered through harpoon-like darts propelled from an extensible proboscis. Clinically, the sting is like that of a bee. The victim may report wound, perioral, and generalized paresthesias. Bulbar dysfunction and systemic muscular paralysis indicate severe envenomation. The sting of the geographer cone (*Conus geographus*) can cause cerebral edema, coma, and death due to respiratory or cardiac failure. Immediately after envenomation, a circumferential pressure-immobilization dressing 15 cm wide should be applied over a gauze pad measuring approximately $7 \times 7 \times 2$ cm that has been placed directly over the sting. The dressing should be applied at venous-lymphatic pressure with the preservation of distal arterial pulses. Once the victim has been transported to the nearest medical facility, the bandage can be released. Provision should be made for cardiovascular and respiratory support.

Serious envenomations and deaths have followed bites of the *Australian blue-ringed octopuses* (*Octopus maculosus* and *O. lunulata*). Although these animals rarely exceed 20 cm in length, their venom contains a potent neurotoxin (maculotoxin) that inhibits peripheral nerve transmission by blocking sodium conductance. Within several minutes of a serious envenomation, oral and facial numbness develops and rapidly progresses to total flaccid paralysis, including failure of respiratory muscles. If respirations are assisted, the victim may remain awake although completely paralyzed. Since there is no antidote, treatment is supportive. Immediately after envenomation, attempts should be made to limit the dispersion of venom by application of a pressure-immobilization or venous-lymphatic pressure dressing. Hot-water immersion and cryotherapy are ineffective. Artificial respiration should be provided. Even with serious envenomations, significant recovery often takes place within 4 to 10 h. Sequelae are uncommon unless related to hypoxia.

VERTEBRATES A number of marine vertebrates, including stingrays, scorpionfish, catfish, surgeonfish, and weeverfish, can envenom humans. The management of most of these stings is similar.

A *stingray* injury is both an envenomation and a traumatic wound. The venom, which contains serotonin, 5'-nucleotidase, and phosphodiesterase, causes immediate and intense pain that may last up to 48 h. Systemic effects include weakness, diaphoresis, nausea, vomiting, diarrhea, dysrhythmias, syncope, hypotension, muscle cramps, fasciculations, paralysis, and (in rare cases) death.

The designation *scorpionfish* encompasses members of the family Scorpaenidae and includes not only scorpionfish but also lionfish and stonefish. A complex venom with neuromuscular toxicity is delivered through 12 or 13 dorsal, two pelvic, and three anal spines. Pectoral spines do not contain venom. The severity of envenomation depends on the species of fish, the number of stings, and the amount of venom released. In general, the sting of a stonefish is regarded as the most serious (severe to life-threatening); that of the scorpionfish is of intermediate seriousness; and that of the lionfish is the least serious. Like that of a stingray, the sting of a scorpionfish is immediately and intensely painful. Pain from a stonefish envenomation may last for days. The systemic manifestations are similar to those of stingray envenomations but may be more pronounced, particularly in the case of a stonefish sting. The rare deaths following stonefish envenomation usually occur within 6 to 8 h.

Two species of marine *catfish*, *Plotosus lineatus* (the oriental catfish) and *Galeichthys felis* (the common sea catfish), as well as several species of freshwater catfish are capable of stinging humans. Venom is delivered through a single dorsal spine and two pectoral spines. Clinically, a catfish sting is comparable to that of a stingray, although marine catfish envenomations are generally more severe than those of their freshwater counterparts. *Surgeonfish* (doctorfish, tang), *weeverfish*, and *horned venomous sharks* have also been implicated in human envenomations.

The stings of all these marine vertebrates are treated in a similar fashion. Except for stonefish and serious scorpionfish envenomations (see below), no antivenom is available. The affected part should be immersed immediately in nonscalding hot water (113°F/45°C) for 30 to 90 min or until there is significant relief of pain. This measure also helps inactivate the heat-labile components of the venoms. Recurrent pain may respond to repeated hot-water treatment. Cryotherapy is contraindicated. Opiates will help alleviate the pain, as will local wound infiltration or regional nerve block with 1% lidocaine, 0.5% bupivacaine, and sodium bicarbonate mixed in a 5:5:1 ratio. After soaking and anesthetic administration, the wound must be explored and debrided. Radiography may be helpful in the identification and location of foreign bodies. After exploration and debridement, the wound should be vigorously irrigated with warm sterile water, saline, or 1% povidone-iodine in solution. Bleeding can usually be controlled by sustained local pressure for 10 to 15 min. In general, wounds should be left open to heal by secondary intention or be treated by delayed primary closure. Tetanus immunization should be updated. Antibiotic treatment should be considered for serious wounds and for envenomation in immunocompromised hosts. The initial antibiotics should cover *Staphylococcus* and *Streptococcus* spp. If the victim is immunocompromised or an infection develops, antibiotic coverage should be broadened to include *Vibrio* spp.

Approach to the Patient

It is not uncommon for a physician to encounter a patient who has been envenomed by a marine creature that cannot be positively identified at the scene of the envenomation. Therefore, it is useful to be familiar with the local marine fauna and to recognize patterns of injury.

A large puncture wound or jagged laceration, particularly on the lower extremity, that is more painful than one would expect from the size and configuration of the wound is likely a stingray envenomation. Smaller punctures, as described above, represent the activity of a sea urchin or starfish. Stony corals cause rough abrasions and, in rare instances, lacerations or puncture wounds.

Coelenterate (marine invertebrate) stings sometimes create diagnostic skin patterns. A diffuse urticarial rash on exposed skin is often indicative of exposure to fragmented hydroids or larval anemones. A linear, whiplike print pattern appears where a jellyfish tentacle has contacted the skin. In the case of the dreaded box-jellyfish (**Plate IID-53**), a frosted cross-hatched appearance followed by dark purple coloration within a few hours of the sting heralds skin necrosis. An encounter with fire coral causes immediate pain and a red, swollen skin irritation in the pattern of contact, similar to but more severe than the imprint left by exposure to an intact feather hydroid. Seabather's eruption, caused by thimble jellyfishes and larval anemones, may cause a diffuse rash that consists of clusters of erythematous macules or raised papules, accompanied by intense itching. Toxic sponges (exposure to which usually occurs during handling) create a burning and painful red rash on exposed skin, which may blister and later desquamate. Virtually all marine stingers invoke the sequelae of inflammation, so that local erythema, swelling, and adenopathy are fairly nonspecific.

SOURCES OF ANTIVENOMS AND OTHER ASSISTANCE   An antivenom for stonefish (and severe scorpionfish) envenomation, made in Australia by the Commonwealth Serum Laboratories (CSL; 45 Poplar Road, Parkville, Victoria, Australia 3052; 61-3-389-1911; fax: 61-3-389-1434), is available in the United States through the pharmacies of Sharp Cabrillo Hospital Emergency Department, San Diego, CA, at (619) 221-3429, and Community Hospital of Monterey Peninsula (CHOMP) Emergency Department, Monterey, CA, at (408) 625-4900.

Polyvalent sea snake antivenom is available from CSL or CHOMP. If sea snake antivenom is unavailable, tiger snake (*N. scutatus*) antivenom should be used.

Divers Alert Network, a nonprofit organization designed to assist in the care of injured divers, may also help with the treatment of marine injuries. The network can be reached 24 h a day at (919) 684-8111 or on the Internet at www.dan.ycg.org.

MARINE POISONINGS

CIGUATERA   Ciguatera poisoning is the most common nonbacterial food poisoning associated with fish in the United States. The poisoning involves almost exclusively tropical and semitropical marine coral reef fish. Of reported cases, 75% (except in Hawaii) involve the barracuda, snapper, jack, or grouper. The ciguatera syndrome is associated with at least five toxins, all of which are unaffected by freeze-drying, heat, cold, and gastric acid and none of which affects the odor, color, or taste of fish.

The onset of symptoms may come within 15 to 30 min of ingestion and typically takes place within 1 to 3 h. Symptoms then increase in severity over the ensuing 4 to 6 h. Most victims develop symptoms within 12 h of ingestion, and virtually all are afflicted within 24 h. The more than 150 symptoms reported include abdominal pain, nausea,

vomiting, diarrhea, chills, paresthesias, pruritus, tongue and throat numbness or burning, sensation of "carbonation" during swallowing, odontalgia or dental dysesthesias, dysphagia, dysuria, dyspnea, weakness, fatigue, tremor, fasciculations, athetosis, meningismus, aphonia, ataxia, vertigo, pain and weakness in the lower extremities, visual blurring, transient blindness, hyporeflexia, seizures, nasal congestion and dryness, conjunctivitis, maculopapular rash, skin vesiculations, dermatographism, sialorrhea, diaphoresis, headache, arthralgias, myalgias, insomnia, bradycardia, hypotension, central respiratory failure, and coma. Death is rare.

Diarrhea, vomiting, and abdominal pain usually develop 3 to 6 h after ingestion of a ciguatoxic fish. Symptoms may persist for 48 h and then generally resolve (even without treatment). A pathognomonic symptom is the reversal of hot and cold tactile perception, which develops in some persons after 3 to 5 days and may last for months. Tachycardia and hypertension have been described, in some cases after potentially severe transient bradycardia and hypotension. More severe reactions tend to occur in persons previously stricken with the disease. Persons who have ingested parrotfish (scaritoxin) may suffer from classic ciguatera poisoning as well as a "second-phase" syndrome (after 5 to 10 days' delay) of disequilibrium with locomotor ataxia, dysmetria, and resting or kinetic tremor. This affliction may persist for 2 to 6 weeks.

The differential diagnosis of ciguatera includes paralytic shellfish poisoning, eosinophilic meningitis, type E botulism, organophosphate insecticide poisoning, tetrodotoxin poisoning, and psychogenic hyperventilation. At present, the diagnosis of ciguatera poisoning is made on clinical grounds because no routinely used laboratory test detects ciguatoxin in human blood. A ciguatoxin enzyme immunoassay or radioimmunoassay may be used to test small portions of the suspected fish.

Therapy is supportive and based on symptoms. Although not of proven efficacy, gastric lavage or syrup of ipecac–induced emesis followed by the administration of a slurry of activated charcoal (100 g) in sorbitol may be of limited value if performed within 3 h after ingestion. Nausea and vomiting may be controlled with an antiemetic, such as prochlorperazine (2.5 to 5 mg intravenously). Hypotension may require the administration of intravenous crystalloid and, in rare cases, a pressor drug. Bradyarrhythmias that lead to cardiac insufficiency and hypotension generally respond well to atropine (0.5 mg intravenously, up to 2 mg). Cool showers or the administration of hydroxyzine (25 mg orally every 6 to 8 h) may relieve pruritus. Amitriptyline (25 mg orally twice a day) reportedly ameliorates pruritus and dysesthesias. In three cases unresponsive to amitriptyline, tocainide appeared to be efficacious. Intravenous infusion of mannitol may be beneficial in moderate or severe cases, particularly for the relief of distressing neurologic or cardiovascular symptoms. The infusion is rendered initially as 1 g/kg per day over 45 to 60 min during the acute phase (days 1 to 5). The mechanism of the benefit against ciguatera intoxication is hyperosmotic water-drawing action, which reverses ciguatoxin-induced Schwann cell edema. Mannitol may also act in some fashion as a "hydroxyl scavenger."

During recovery from ciguatera poisoning, the victim should exclude the following from the diet: fish (fresh or preserved), fish sauces, shellfish, shellfish sauces, alcoholic beverages, and nuts and nut oils. Consumption of fish in ciguatera-endemic regions should be avoided. All oversized fish of any predacious reef species should be suspected of harboring ciguatoxin. Neither moray eels nor the viscera of tropical marine fish should ever be eaten.

PARALYTIC SHELLFISH POISONING   Paralytic shellfish poisoning (PSP) is induced by the ingestion of any of a variety of feral or aquacultured filter-feeding organisms, including clams, oysters, scallops, mussels, chitons, limpets, starfish, and sand crabs. The origin of their toxicity is the chemical toxin they accumulate and concentrate by feeding on various planktonic dinoflagellates and protozoan organisms. The unicellular phytoplanktonic organisms form the foundation of the food chain, and in warm summer months these organisms "bloom" in nutrient-rich coastal temperate and semitropical waters. A number of dinoflagellates produce a variety of toxins. These planktonic species can release massive amounts of toxic metabolites into the water and cause enormous mortality in bird and marine populations. The paralytic shellfish toxins are water-soluble as well as heat- and acid-stable; they cannot be destroyed by ordinary cooking. The best-characterized and most frequently identified paralytic shellfish toxin is saxitoxin, which takes its name from the Alaska butter clam *Saxidomus giganteus*. A toxin concentration of >75 $\mu g/100$ g of foodstuff is considered hazardous to humans. In the 1972 New England "red tide," the concentration of saxitoxin in blue mussels exceeded 9000 $\mu g/100$ g of foodstuff. Saxitoxin appears to block sodium conductance, inhibiting neuromuscular transmission at the axonal and muscle membrane levels.

Within minutes to a few hours after ingestion of contaminated shellfish, there is the onset of intraoral and perioral paresthesias, notably of the lips, tongue, and gums, that progress rapidly to involve the neck and distal extremities. The tingling or burning sensation later changes to numbness. Other symptoms rapidly develop and include lightheadedness, disequilibrium, incoordination, weakness, hyperreflexia, incoherence, dysarthria, sialorrhea, dysphagia, thirst, diarrhea, abdominal pain, nausea, vomiting, nystagmus, dysmetria, headache, diaphoresis, loss of vision, chest pain, and tachycardia. Flaccid paralysis and respiratory insufficiency may follow 2 to 12 h after ingestion. In the absence of hypoxia, the victim often remains alert but paralyzed.

Treatment is supportive and based on symptoms. If the victim comes to medical attention within the first few hours after poison ingestion, the stomach should be emptied by gastric lavage and then irrigated with 2 L (in 200-mL aliquots) of a solution of 2% sodium bicarbonate. The administration of activated charcoal (50 to 100 g) and a cathartic (sorbitol, 20 to 50 g) makes empirical sense but has not been proved effective. Some authors advise against administration of magnesium-based solutions, such as certain cathartics, cautioning that hypermagnesemia may contribute to suppression of nerve conduction.

The most serious problem is respiratory paralysis. The victim should be closely observed in a hospital for at least 24 h for respiratory distress. With prompt recognition of ventilatory failure, endotracheal intubation and assisted ventilation prevent anoxic myocardial and brain injury.

DOMOIC ACID INTOXICATION In late 1987 in eastern Canada, an outbreak of gastrointestinal and neurologic symptoms (amnestic shellfish poisoning) occurred after consumption of mussels found to be contaminated with domoic acid. A heat-stable neuroexcitatory amino acid whose biochemical analogs are kainic acid and glutamic acid, domoic acid binds to the kainate type of glutamate receptor with three times the affinity of kainic acid and is 20 times as powerful a toxin. Mussels can be tested for domoic acid by mouse bioassay and high-performance liquid chromatography. The regulatory limit for domoic acid in shellfish is 20 parts per million.

The abnormalities noted within 24 h of ingesting contaminated mussels (*Mytilus edulis*) include arousal, confusion, disorientation, and memory loss. The median time of onset is 5.5 h. Other prominent symptoms include severe headache, nausea, vomiting, diarrhea, abdominal cramps, hiccoughs, arrhythmias, hypotension, seizures, ophthalmoplegia, hemiparesis, mutism, grimacing, agitation, emotional lability, coma, copious bronchial secretions, and pulmonary edema. Histologic study of brain tissue taken at autopsy has shown neuronal necrosis or cell loss and astrocytosis, most prominently in the hippocampus and the amygdaloid nucleus—findings similar to those in animals poisoned with kainic acid. Several months after the primary intoxication, victims still demonstrate chronic residual memory deficits and motor neuronopathy or axonopathy. Nonneurologic illness does not persist.

Therapy is supportive and based on symptoms. Since kainic acid neuropathology seems to be nearly entirely seizure mediated, an emphasis should be placed on anticonvulsive therapy, for which diazepam appears to be as effective as any other drug.

SCOMBROID Scombroid (mackerel-like) fish include the albacore, bluefin, and yellowfin tuna; mackerel; saury; needlefish; wahoo; skipjack; and bonito. Nonscombroid fish that produce scombroid poisoning include the dolphinfish (mahimahi, *Coryphaena*), kahawai, sardine, black marlin, pilchard, anchovy, herring, amberjack, and Australian ocean salmon. In the northeastern and mid-Atlantic United States, bluefish has been linked to scombroid poisoning. Because greater numbers of nonscombroid fish are being recognized as scombrotoxic, the syndrome may more appropriately be called *pseudoallergic fish poisoning*.

Under conditions of inadequate preservation or refrigeration, the musculature of these dark- or red-fleshed fish undergoes bacterial decomposition, which includes the decarboxylation of the amino acid L-histidine to histamine, histamine phosphate, and histamine hydrochloride. Histamine levels of >20 to 50 mg/100 g are noted in toxic fish, with levels in excess of 400 mg/100 g on occasion. The toxin is heat stable and is not destroyed by domestic or commercial cooking. Affected fish typically have a sharply metallic or peppery taste; however, they may be normal in appearance, color, and flavor.

Symptoms occur within 15 to 90 min of ingestion and include flushing (sharply demarcated; exacerbated by ultraviolet exposure; particularly pronounced on the face, neck, or upper trunk), a sensation of warmth without elevated core temperature, conjunctival hyperemia, pruritus, urticaria, angioneurotic edema, bronchospasm, nausea, vomiting, diarrhea, epigastric pain, abdominal cramps, dysphagia, headache, thirst, pharyngitis, burning of the gingiva, palpitations, tachycardia, dizziness, and hypotension. Without treatment, the symptoms generally resolve within 8 to 12 h. The reaction may be more severe in a person who is concurrently ingesting isoniazid because of blockade of gastrointestinal tract histaminase.

Therapy is directed at reversing the histamine effect with antihistamines, either H-1 or H-2. If bronchospasm is severe, an inhaled bronchodilator—or in rare, extremely severe circumstances, injected epinephrine—may be used. Glucocorticoids are of no proven benefit. Protracted nausea and vomiting, which may empty the stomach of toxin, may be controlled with a specific antiemetic, such as prochlorperazine. The persistent headache of scombroid poisoning may respond to cimetidine or a similar antihistamine if standard analgesics are not effective.

PFIESTERIA In the summer of 1997, reports of adverse reactions after casual exposure to Maryland waters infested with the fish-eating dinoflagellate *Pfiesteria* prompted the Centers for Disease Control and Prevention (CDC) to undertake multistate surveillance and to establish a case definition. As defined by the CDC, the human disease syndrome associated with *Pfiesteria* is characterized by either of two groups of signs and symptoms: (1) memory loss, confusion, or acute skin burning on direct contact with infested water; or (2) at least three of the following: headache, rash (flat red sores), eye irritation, upper respiratory irritation, muscle cramps, and gastrointestinal symptoms. Since the initial reports from Maryland, many such cases have followed both casual exposure to infested water and laboratory work with *Pfiesteria* (which is currently conducted in biohazard III facilities).

Research on *Pfiesteria* has been complicated by a variety of factors, including the lack of a test for detection of its toxins, which have yet to be purified, and the organism's complex life cycle, which includes at least two dozen stages. In nature, the proximity of a school of fish elicits *Pfiesteria's* transformation into a flagellated zoospore that releases at least two toxins: a water-soluble, neuroactive toxin that kills fish within minutes, and a fat-soluble toxin that causes epidermal delamination. Polluted environments appear to favor *Pfiesteria*.

For the treatment of *Pfiesteria*-associated syndromes, one teaspoon of milk of magnesia followed by one scoop of cholestyramine in 8 ounces of water and 70% sorbitol solution is administered daily for 2 weeks.

BIBLIOGRAPHY

SNAKES AND LIZARDS

DART RC et al: Affinity-purified, mixed monoclonal specific crotalid antivenom ovine Fab for the treatment of crotalid venom poisoning. Ann Emerg Med 30:33, 1997

MEYER WP et al: First clinical experiences with a new ovine Fab *Echis ocellatus* snake bite antivenom in Nigeria: Randomized comparative trial with Institute Pasteur Serum (IPSER) Africa antivenom. Am J Trop Med Hyg 56:291, 1997

MINTON SA, NORRIS RL: Non-North American venomous reptile bites, in *Wilderness Medicine: Management of Wilderness and Environmental Emergencies*, 3d ed, PS Auerbach (ed). St. Louis, Mosby, 1995, pp 710–730

RUSSELL FE: *Snake Venom Poisoning*. New York, Scholium International, 1983

SULLIVAN JB et al: North American venomous reptile bites, in *Wilderness Medicine: Management of Wilderness and Environmental Emergencies*, 3d ed, PS Auerbach (ed). St. Louis, Mosby, 1995, pp 680–709

MARINE CREATURES

AUERBACH PS: Marine envenomation, in *Wilderness Medicine: Management of Wilderness and Environmental Emergencies*, 3d ed, PS Auerbach (ed). St. Louis, Mosby, 1995, pp 1327–1374

AUERBACH PS: Marine envenomations. N Engl J Med 325:486, 1991

BROWN CK, SHEPHERD SM: Marine trauma, envenomations, and intoxications. Emerg Med Clin North Am 10:385, 1992

BURNETT JW et al: Coelenterate venom research 1991–1995: Clinical, chemical and immunological aspects. Toxicon 34:1377, 1996

HALSTEAD BW, AUERBACH PS: *Dangerous Aquatic Animals of the World: A Color Atlas: With Prevention, First Aid, and Emergency Treatment Procedures*. Princeton, Darwin Press, 1992, pp 29–124, 241–252

MEIER J, WHITE J (eds): *Handbook of Clinical Toxicology of Animal Venoms and Poisons*. Boca Raton, FL, CRC Press, 1996, pp 89–176

MINES D et al: Poisonings: Food, fish, and shellfish. Emerg Med Clin North Am 15:157, 1997

STEWART MPM: Ciguatera fish poisoning: Treatment with intravenous mannitol. Trop Doct 21:54, 1991

TEITELBAUM JS et al: Neurologic sequelae of domoic acid intoxication due to the ingestion of contaminated mussels. N Engl J Med 322:1781, 1990

---

398 *James H. Maguire, Andrew Spielman*

ECTOPARASITE INFESTATIONS, ARTHROPOD BITES AND STINGS

Ectoparasites are arthropods or helminths that *infest* the skin of other animals from which they derive sustenance. They may penetrate beneath the surface of the host or attach superficially by their mouthparts. These organisms damage their hosts by inflicting direct injury, by eliciting a hypersensitivity reaction, or by inoculating toxins or pathogens. The main medically important ectoparasites are arachnids (including mites and ticks), insects (including lice, fleas, and flies), pentastomes (tongue worms), and leeches. Arthropods may also harm humans through brief encounters in which they take a blood meal or attempt to defend themselves by biting, stinging, or inoculating venoms. Various arachnids (spiders, scorpions), insects (including bees, hornets, wasps, ants, flies, bugs, caterpillars, and beetles), millipedes, and centipedes produce ill effects in this manner, as do certain ectoparasites of animals, including ticks, biting mites, and fleas (discussed in this chapter as biting arthropods). More people in the United States die each year as a consequence of arthropod stings than from poisonous snake bites.

ECTOPARASITE INFESTATIONS

SCABIES The human itch mite, *Sarcoptes scabiei*, which infests some 300 million persons each year, is one of the most common causes of itching dermatoses throughout the world. Gravid female mites measuring 0.3 to 0.4 mm in length burrow superficially beneath the stratum corneum for a month, depositing two or three eggs a day. Nymphs that hatch from these eggs mature in about 2 weeks through a series of molts and then emerge as adults to the surface of the skin, where they mate and subsequently reinvade the skin of the same or another host. Transfer of newly fertilized female mites from person to person occurs by intimate personal contact and is facilitated by crowding, uncleanliness, and multiple sexual partners. Medical practitioners are at particular risk of infestation. Transmission via sharing of contaminated bedding or clothing is infrequent because these mites cannot survive much more than a day without host contact. In the United States, scabies may account for 2 to 5% of visits to dermatologists; involved particularly often are children, immigrants from developing countries, and close household contacts. Outbreaks occur in nursing homes, mental institutions, and hospitals.

The itching and rash associated with scabies derive from a sensitization reaction directed against the excreta that the mite deposits in its burrow **(Plate IID-52)**. For this reason, an initial infestation remains asymptomatic for 4 to 6 weeks, and a reinfestation produces a hypersensitivity reaction without delay. Scratching generally destroys the burrowing mite, but symptoms remain even in its absence. Burrows become surrounded by infiltrates of eosinophils, lymphocytes, and histiocytes, and a generalized hypersensitivity rash later develops in remote sites. By destroying these pathogens, immunity and associated scratching limit most infestations to fewer than 15 mites per person. Hyperinfestation with thousands or millions of mites, a condition known as *crusted scabies* or *Norwegian scabies*, may result from glucocorticoid use, immunodeficiency diseases (including AIDS and infection with human T-lymphotropic virus type I), and neurologic and psychiatric illnesses that interfere with itching and scratching.

Patients with scabies report intense itching that worsens at night and after a hot shower. Typical burrows may be difficult to find because they are few in number and may be obscured by excoriations. Burrows appear as dark wavy lines in the epidermis, measure 3 to 15 mm, and end in a small pearly bleb that contains the female mite. Such lesions generally develop on the volar wrists, between the fingers, on the elbows, and on the penis. Small papules and vesicles, often accompanied by eczematous plaques, pustules, or nodules, are symmetrically distributed in these sites and in skin folds under the breasts and around the navel, axillae, belt line, buttocks, upper thighs, and scrotum. Except in infants, the face, scalp, neck, palms, and soles are spared. Burrows and other typical lesions may be sparse in persons who wash frequently, and topical glucocorticoid treatment and bacterial superinfection may alter the appearance of the rash. Atypical presentations of scabies include bullous lesions, which resemble those of bullous pemphigoid, and vesicular lesions, which resemble those of dermatitis herpetiformis. Superinfection with nephritogenic strains of streptococci has led to acute glomerulonephritis. Crusted scabies resembles psoriasis in its typical widespread erythema, thick keratotic crusts, scaling, and dystrophic nails. Characteristic burrows are not seen in crusted scabies, and patients usually do not itch, although their infestations are highly contagious and have been responsible for outbreaks of classic scabies in hospitals. Bacteremia occurs frequently in AIDS patients with crusted scabies and prominent fissures. Persons with massive infestations occasionally present with diffuse pruritus and generalized papules or with minimal or no cutaneous signs.

A diagnosis of scabies should be considered in patients with pruritus and symmetric polymorphic skin lesions in characteristic locations, particularly if there is a history of household contact with a case. Burrows should be sought and unroofed with a sterile needle or scalpel blade, and the scrapings should be examined microscopically for the mite, its eggs, and its fecal pellets. A drop of mineral oil facilitates removal of the sample. Biopsies or scrapings of papulovesicular lesions may also be diagnostic. In the absence of identifiable mites or mite products, the diagnosis is based on clinical presentation and history. The possibility of other sexually transmitted diseases should be excluded in adults with scabies.

℞ TREATMENT For the treatment of scabies, 5% permethrin cream is less toxic than the once commonly used 1% lindane preparations and is effective against lindane-tolerant infestations. Both scabicides are applied thinly but thoroughly behind the ears and from the neck down after bathing and are removed 8 h later with soap and water. Lindane is absorbed through the skin, and its overuse has led to seizures and aplastic anemia. It should not be applied to pregnant women or infants. Alternatives include topical crotamiton cream, benzyl benzoate, and sulfur ointments. Successful treatment of crusted scabies requires the application first of a keratolytic agent such as 6% salicylic acid (to improve the penetration of scabicides) and then of scabicides to the scalp, face, and ears (with care to avoid the eyes). Repeated treatments or the sequential use of several agents may be necessary. A single oral dose of ivermectin (200 μg/kg) effectively treats scabies in otherwise healthy persons. Patients with crusted scabies may require two or more doses of ivermectin. Although ivermectin may become the agent of choice for treating crusted scabies, it has not yet received approval by the U.S. Food and Drug Administration (FDA) for any form of scabies. Its use should be reserved for persons who fail to respond to topical scabicides, the elderly, persons with generalized eczema, and other persons who may not tolerate topical therapy.

Although effectively treated scabies infestations become noninfectious within a day, itching and rash due to hypersensitivity frequently persist for weeks or months. Unnecessary re-treatment of the affected patients may provoke contact dermatitis. Antihistamines, salicylates, and calamine lotion relieve itching during treatment, and topical glucocorticoids are useful for the pruritus that lingers after effective treatment. An oral antibiotic may be necessary for bacterial superinfections that fail to resolve with antiscabietic therapy. Relapses of scabies may be due to infestations of the scalp when topical therapy is applied only from the neck down. To prevent reinfestations, bedding and clothing should be washed in hot water, and close contacts, even if asymptomatic, should be treated simultaneously.

OTHER MITE INFESTATIONS Species of *Demodex*, the follicle mite, live in hair follicles and sebaceous glands of the face and ears. The wormlike mites measure up to 0.4 mm in length and, if carefully sought, can be found on almost all persons. They appear not to cause disease, although their density is high in persons with rosacea. House dust mites of the genus *Dermatophagoides* infest houses throughout the world, living on furniture and rugs and feeding on shed human dander. Exposure to their allergens causes asthma, rhinitis, conjunctivitis, and eczema in persons with house dust allergies. Management includes immunotherapy with mite extracts and environmental interventions such as frequent vacuuming and removal of rugs from bedrooms to reduce mite density.

PEDICULOSIS (LOUSE INFESTATIONS) All three species of human louse feed at least once a day on human blood. *Pediculus humanus* var. *capitis* infests the head, *P. humanus* var. *corporis* the clothing, and *Phthirus pubis* mainly the hair of the pubis. Females cement their eggs (nits) firmly to hair or clothing. The saliva of lice produces an intensely irritating maculopapular or urticarial rash in sensitized persons.

Head lice, which infest an estimated 6 to 12 million people in the United States, are transmitted directly from person to person and occasionally by shared headgear and grooming implements. The prevalence is highest among school-aged girls who wear long hair; in the United States, black children are less frequently infested than other children. Excoriations of pruritic lesions on the scalp, neck, and shoulders lead to oozing, crusting, matting of hair, bacterial infections, and regional lymphadenopathy. Adult lice are frequently seen crawling in the hair with a velocity that approaches 25 mm/min.

Body lice remain in clothing except when feeding and cannot survive more than a few hours away from the human host. It follows, therefore, that *P. humanus* var. *corporis* mainly infests disaster victims or indigent persons who do not change their clothes. Transmission by direct contact or by sharing of clothing and beds is enhanced under crowded conditions. The fact that the body louse leaves febrile persons or corpses as they become cold facilitates the transmission of typhus, louse-borne relapsing fever, and trench fever (Chap. 177). Trench fever

and endocarditis due to *Bartonella quintana* have emerged as diseases of homeless persons living in large cities of the United States and Europe. Pruritic lesions are particularly common around the neckline. Chronic infestations result in the postinflammatory hyperpigmentation and thickening of skin known as *vagabonds' disease.*

The cosmopolitan crab or pubic louse is transmitted mainly by sexual contact but can infest eyelashes, axillary hair, and hair in other sites as well as pubic hair. Children with pubic lice generally acquire their infestations from parents rather than via sexual transmission. Polymerase chain reaction (PCR) analysis of the blood meal of lice permits identification of host DNA in cases of child abuse or rape. Intensely pruritic lesions and 2- to 3-mm blue macules (maculae ceruleae) develop at the site of bites. Blepharitis commonly accompanies infestations of the eyelashes.

A suspected diagnosis of pediculosis is confirmed by the finding of nits or adult lice on hairs or in clothing. The dorsoventrally flattened adult lice measure 2 to 4 mm in length and have three pairs of legs ending in claws that enable them to grasp hair shafts or clothing. Oval nits measure 0.8 mm in length and are opaque white or cream-colored (body and head lice) or dark brown (pubic lice).

℞ TREATMENT The preferred treatment is a 10-min application of 1% permethrin creme rinse, which kills both lice and eggs and is available without prescription. An alternative, 0.5% malathion, requires a prescription and must be left in place for 8 to 12 h. Other agents, such as the more toxic 1% lindane and pyrethrins with piperonyl butoxide, are not ovicidal and require a second application 1 week after the first to kill hatching nymphs. Dead or hatched nits, which remain attached to hair sheaths and become translucent or opalescent, may falsely suggest an active infection. Resistance of head lice to permethrin, malathion, and lindane has been reported. When a properly applied treatment fails, a higher concentration (5%) of permethrin may be tried or the class of pediculicide changed (e.g., by switching from permethrin to malathion). Ivermectin may be useful in cases of resistance to both malathion and permethrin but has not been approved for this purpose by the FDA.

After louse infestations have been treated with insecticide, the hair should be combed with a fine-toothed nit comb to remove nits. Combs and brushes should be disinfected in hot water at 65°C for 5 min or soaked in insecticide for 1 h. Body lice can be eliminated by bathing and application of topical pediculicides from head to foot. Clothes and bedding are deloused by heat sterilization in a dryer at 65°C for 30 min or by fumigation. Infestations with pubic lice are treated with topical pediculicides except for eyelid infestations (*phthiriasis palpebrum*), which respond to a coating of petroleum applied for 3 to 4 days or 1% yellow oxide of mercury ointment applied four times daily for 2 weeks.

TUNGIASIS *Tunga penetrans*, like other fleas, is a wingless, laterally flattened insect measuring 2 to 4 mm in length that feeds on blood. Also known as the chigoe flea, sand flea, or jigger, it occurs in tropical regions of Africa and the Americas. Adults live in sandy soil and burrow under the skin between toes, under nails, or on the soles of bare feet. The fleas engorge on blood and grow from pinpoint to pea size over a 2-week period. The lesions resemble a white pustule with a central black depression and may be pruritic or painful. Occasional complications include tetanus, bacterial infections, and autoamputation of toes. Tungiasis is treated by removal of the intact flea with a sterile needle or scalpel, tetanus vaccination, and topical antibiotics.

MYIASIS *Myiasis* refers to infestations by maggots, mainly due to the larvae of metallic-colored screw-worm flies or botflies. Maggots invade living or necrotic tissue or body cavities and produce different clinical syndromes depending on the species of fly.

Furuncular Myiasis In forested parts of Central and South America, larvae of *Dermatobia hominis* (the human botfly) produce boil-like subcutaneous nodules 2 to 3 cm in diameter. The adult female captures a mosquito or other bloodsucking insect and deposits her eggs beneath its abdomen. When the carrier insect attacks a human or bovine host several days later, the warmth and moisture of the host's surface stimulate the larvae to hatch and penetrate the skin. After 6 to 12 weeks, the larvae mature and drop to the ground, where they pupate. The African tumbu fly, *Cordylobia anthropophaga*, produces similar lesions. Dozens of eggs are deposited on sand or drying laundry that is contaminated with urine or sweat. Larvae hatch on contact with the body, penetrate the skin, and produce boils from which they emerge 8 or 9 days later. A diagnosis of furuncular myiasis is suggested by uncomfortable lesions with a central breathing pore that emits bubbles when submerged in water. There is often a sensation of movement under the skin that may lead to severe emotional distress. Tumbu fly larvae can be removed by manual expression after the air pore is coated with petroleum to suffocate the larvae and induce them to emerge. Removal of *Dermatobia* larvae is facilitated by injection of a local anesthetic into the surrounding tissue, but surgical excision is often necessary because up-pointing spines hold the larva firmly in place.

Creeping Dermal Myiasis   Maggots of the horse botfly, *Gasterophilus intestinalis*, do not mature after penetrating human skin but migrate for weeks in the epidermis. The resulting pruritic and serpiginous eruption resembles cutaneous larva migrans caused by *Ancylostoma braziliense*. Horseback riders become infested when eggs deposited on the flank of the horse hatch against their bare legs. The black spines of the larvae can be identified after mineral oil is smeared over the lesion. Larva are removed with a needle. The larvae of the cattle botfly (*Hypoderma* species) invade more deeply and produce boil-like swellings.

Wound and Body Cavity Myiasis   Certain flies are attracted to blood and pus, and their newly hatched larvae enter wounds or diseased skin. Larvae of species such as *Phaenicia sericata*, the green-bottle fly, remain superficial and confined to necrotic tissue and were used in the past to debride purulent wounds. Other species, including the screw-worms (*Chrysomyia bezziana* in Asia and Africa and *Cochliomyia hominivorax* in Latin America) and the flesh fly (*Wohlfahrtia vigil* in northern North America), invade more deeply into viable tissue and produce large suppurating lesions. Larvae that infest wounds also may infest body cavities such as the mouth, nose, ears, sinuses, anus, vagina, and lower urinary tract, particularly in unconscious or otherwise debilitated patients. The consequences range from harmless colonization to destruction of the nose, meningitis, and deafness. Treatment involves removal of maggots and debridement of tissue.

Other Forms of Myiasis   The maggots responsible for furuncular and wound myiasis may also cause ophthalmomyiasis. Sequelae include nodules in the eyelid, retinal detachment, and destruction of the globe. In addition, the adult sheep botfly, *Oestrus ovis*, may deposit larvae in the eyes of persons tending sheep and goats, and the larvae may produce a conjunctival infestation and acute conjunctivitis. True intestinal myiasis occurs when eggs or larvae of the drone fly (*Eristalis tenax*) are ingested with contaminated food, mature in the gut, and cause enteritis. Most instances in which maggots are found in human feces are the result of larviposition by flesh flies on recently passed stools.

PENTASTOMIASIS   Pentastomids, or tongue worms, are parasites with characteristics of both helminths and arthropods and are classified in a separate phylum. The wormlike adults inhabit the respiratory passages of reptiles and carnivorous mammals. Human infestation with *Linguatula serrata* is common in the Middle East and occurs in the Sudan following ingestion of encysted larval stages in raw liver or lymph nodes of sheep and goats, the intermediate hosts. The larvae migrate to the nasopharynx and produce an acute self-limiting syndrome known as *halzoun* (*Marrara* in the Sudan), which is characterized by pain and itching of the throat and ears, coughing, hoarseness, dysphagia, and dyspnea. Severe edema may cause obstruction and necessitate tracheostomy, and ocular invasion has been described. Diagnostic larvae measuring 5 to 10 mm in length are found

in the copious nasal discharge or vomitus. Human beings become infected with *Armillifer armillatus* by ingesting eggs in contaminated food or drink or after handling the definitive host, the African python. Larvae encyst in various organs but rarely cause symptoms unless they compress vital structures or perforate an organ during migration. Cysts occasionally require surgical removal as they enlarge during molting, but they are usually encountered as an incidental finding at autopsy. There are reports of the cutaneous larva migrans syndrome due to other pentastomes (*Reighardia* and *Sebekia* species) in Southeast Asia and Central America.

LEECH INFESTATIONS   Medically important leeches are annelid worms that attach to their hosts with chitinous cutting jaws and draw blood with muscular suckers. The medicinal leech, *Hirudo medicinalis*, is still used occasionally to reduce venous congestion in surgical flaps or replanted body parts. This practice has been complicated by wound infections, myonecrosis, and sepsis due to *Aeromonas hydrophila*, which colonizes the gullets of commercially available leeches.

Ubiquitous aquatic leeches that parasitize fish, frogs, and turtles readily attach to the skin of human beings and avidly suck blood. More notorious are the land leeches (*Haemadipsa*) that live in moist vegetation of tropical rain forests. Attachment is usually painless. Hirudinin, a powerful anticoagulant secreted by the leech, causes continued bleeding after the leech has detached. Healing of the wound is slow, and bacterial infections are not uncommon. Several species of aquatic leeches in Africa, Asia, and southern Europe can enter through the mouth, nose, and genitourinary tract and attach to mucosal surfaces at sites as deep as the esophagus and trachea. Bleeding may be intense. Externally attached leeches are removed by steady gentle traction. Removal is hastened by application of alcohol, salt, vinegar, or a flame to the leech. Internally attached leeches may detach on exposure to gargled saline or may be removed by forceps.

DELUSIONAL INFESTATIONS   The groundless conviction that one is infested with arthropods or other parasites is an extremely difficult disorder to treat and unfortunately is not rare. Patients report infestations of their skin, clothing, or homes and describe sensations of something moving in or on their skin. Excoriations often accompany complaints of pruritus or insect bites. Patients bring in as evidence of infestation specimens that are identified microscopically as plant-feeding or peridomestic arthropods, pieces of skin, vegetable matter, or inanimate objects. In suspected cases, it is imperative to rule out true infestations and neuropathies, environmental irritants such as fragments of fiberglass, and other causes of tingling or prickling sensations. Pharmacotherapy with pimozide, which blocks dopamine receptors, has been more helpful than psychotherapy in treating this disorder.

ARTHROPOD BITES AND STINGS

SPIDER BITES   Of the >30,000 recognized species of spider, only about 100 defend themselves aggressively and have fangs sufficiently long to penetrate human skin. The venom that spiders use to immobilize and digest their prey can cause necrosis of skin and systemic toxicity. While the bites of most spiders are painful but not harmful, envenomations of the brown or fiddle spiders (*Loxosceles* species), widow spiders (*Latrodectus* species), and other species may be life-threatening. Identification of the offending spider should be attempted, since specific treatments exist for bites of widow and brown recluse spiders and since injuries attributed to spiders are frequently due to other causes.

Recluse Spider Bites and Necrotic Arachnidism   Severe necrosis of skin and subcutaneous tissue follows envenomation by *Loxosceles reclusa*, the brown recluse spider, and by at least four other species of *Loxosceles* in the southern and midwestern United States. Other spiders that produce necrotic ulceration include the hobo spider (*Tegenaria agrestis*) in the Pacific Northwest, the sac spiders (*Chiracanthium* species) throughout the United States and abroad, the South American brown spider *Loxosceles laeta* in Central and South Amerthese spiders measure 7 to 15 mm in body length and 2 to 4 cm in leg span. Recluse spiders are brown and have a dark violin-shaped spot on their dorsal surface; hobo spiders are brown with gray markings; and sac spiders may be pale yellow, green, or brown.

These spiders are not aggressive toward human beings and bite only if threatened or pressed against the skin. They hide under rocks and logs or in caves and animal burrows, and they emerge at night to hunt other spiders and insects. They invade homes, particularly in the fall, and seek dark and undisturbed hiding spots in closets, in folds of clothing, or under furniture and rubbish in storage rooms, garages, and attics. Bites often occur while the victim is dressing and are sustained primarily to the arms, neck, and lower abdomen.

The clear viscous venoms of these spiders contain an esterase, alkaline phosphatase, protease, and other enzymes that produce tissue necrosis and hemolysis. Sphingomyelinase B, the most important dermonecrotic factor, binds cell membranes and promotes chemotaxis of neutrophils, leading to vascular thrombosis and an Arthus-like reaction. Initially, the bite is painless or produces a stinging sensation. Within the next few hours, the site becomes painful and pruritic, with central induration surrounded by a pale zone of ischemia and a zone of erythema. In most cases, the lesion resolves without treatment over 2 to 3 days. In severe cases, the erythema spreads, and the center of the lesion becomes hemorrhagic and necrotic with an overlying bulla. A black eschar forms and sloughs several weeks later, leaving an ulcer that may be ≥25 cm in diameter and eventually a depressed scar. Healing usually takes place within 3 to 6 months but may take as long as 3 years if adipose tissue is involved. Local complications include injury to nerves and secondary infection. Fever, chills, weakness, headache, nausea, vomiting, myalgia, arthralgia, maculopapular rash, and leukocytosis may develop within 72 h of the bite. In rare instances, acute complications such as hemolytic anemia, hemoglobinuria, and renal failure are fatal.

TREATMENT Initial management includes local cleansing, application of sterile dressings and cold compresses, and elevation and loose immobilization of the affected limb. Analgesics, antihistamines, antibiotics, and tetanus prophylaxis should be administered if indicated. Within the first 48 to 72 h, the administration of dapsone, a leukocyte inhibitor, may halt the progression of lesions that are becoming necrotic. Dapsone is given in oral doses of 50 to 100 mg twice daily after glucose-6-phosphate dehydrogenase deficiency has been ruled out. The efficacy of locally or systemically administered glucocorticoids has not been demonstrated, and a potentially useful *Loxosceles*-specific antivenin has not been approved for use in the United States. Debridement and later skin grafting may be necessary after signs of acute inflammation have subsided, but immediate surgical excision of the wound is detrimental. Patients should be monitored closely for signs of hemolysis, renal failure, and other systemic complications.

Widow Spider Bites The bite of the female widow spider is notorious for the effect of its potent neurotoxin. *Latrodectus mactans*, the black widow, has been found in every state of the United States except Alaska and is most abundant in the southeast. It measures up to 1 cm in body length and 5 cm in leg span, is shiny black, and has a red hourglass marking on the ventral abdomen. Other dangerous North American *Latrodectus* species include *L. geometricus* (the brown widow), *L. bishopi* (the red widow), *L. variolus*, and *L. hesperus*, and there are related species in other temperate and subtropical parts of the world.

Widow spiders spin their webs under stones, logs, plants, or rock piles or in dark spaces in barns, garages, and outhouses. Bites are most common in the summer and early autumn and occur when the web is disturbed or when the spider is trapped or provoked. The buttocks or genitals are sites of bites incurred by humans while sitting in an outdoor privy.

The initial bite goes unnoticed or is perceived as a sharp pinprick.

Two small red marks, mild erythema, and edema develop at the fang entrance site. The oily yellow venom that is injected does not produce local necrosis, and some persons experience no other symptoms. However, α-latrotoxin, the most active component of the venom, binds irreversibly to nerves and causes release and eventual depletion of acetylcholine, norepinephrine, and other neurotransmitters from presynaptic terminals. Within 30 to 60 min, painful cramps spread from the bite site to large muscles of the extremities and the trunk. Extreme rigidity of the abdominal muscles and excruciating pain may suggest peritonitis, but the abdomen is not tender on palpation. Other features include salivation, diaphoresis, vomiting, hypertension, tachycardia, labored breathing, anxiety, headache, weakness, fasciculations, paresthesia, hyperreflexia, urinary retention, uterine contractions, and premature labor. Rhabdomyolysis and renal failure have been reported, and respiratory arrest, cerebral hemorrhage, or cardiac failure may end fatally, especially in very young, elderly, or debilitated persons. The pain begins to subside during the first 12 h but may recur during several days or weeks before resolving spontaneously.

TREATMENT Treatment consists of local cleansing, application of ice packs, and tetanus prophylaxis. Hypertension that does not respond to analgesics and antispasmodics, such as benzodiazepines or methocarbamol, requires specific antihypertensive medication. Intravenous administration of one or two vials of a widely available equine antivenin rapidly relieves pain and can be life-saving. Because of the risk of anaphylaxis and serum sickness, antivenin should be reserved for severe cases involving respiratory arrest, uncontrollable hypertension, seizures, or pregnancy.

Envenomations by Tarantulas and Other Spiders Tarantulas are long-lived, hairy spiders of which 30 species are found in the United States, primarily in the southwest. The tarantulas that have become popular household pets are usually imported species with bright colors and a leg span of up to 25 cm. Tarantulas bite only when threatened and cause no more harm than a bee sting, but the venom occasionally provokes deep pain and swelling. Several species are covered with urticating hairs that are launched in the thousands when a threatened spider rubs its hind legs across the dorsal abdomen. These hairs penetrate human skin and produce pruritic papules that last for weeks. Failure to wear gloves or to wash the hands after handling the Chilean Rose tarantula, the most popular pet spider, has resulted in transfer of hairs to the eye and devastating ocular inflammation. Treatment of bites includes local washing and elevation of the bitten area, tetanus prophylaxis, and analgesic administration. Antihistamines and topical or systemic glucocorticoids are given for exposure to urticating hairs.

Atrax robustus, the Sydney funnel-web spider of Australia, and *Phoneutria* species, the South American banana spiders, are among the most dangerous spiders in the world because of their aggressive behavior and potent neurotoxins. Envenomation by *A. robustus* causes a rapidly progressive neuromotor syndrome that can be fatal within 2 h. The bite of the banana spiders causes severe local pain followed by profound systemic symptoms and respiratory paralysis that can lead to death within 2 to 6 h. Specific antivenins for envenomation by each of these spiders are available. *Lycosa* species (wolf spiders) are found throughout the world and may produce painful bites and transient local inflammation.

SCORPION STINGS Scorpions are crablike arachnids that feed on ground-dwelling arthropods and small lizards, which they grasp with a pair of frontal pinchers and paralyze by injecting venom from a stinger on the tip of the tail. Painful but relatively harmless scorpion stings need to be distinguished from the potentially lethal envenomations that are produced by about 30 of the approximately 1000 known species and cause more than 5000 deaths worldwide each year. Scorpions feed at night and remain hidden during the day in crevices or burrows or under wood, loose bark, or rocks on the ground.

They seek cool spots under buildings and often enter houses, where they get into shoes, clothing, or bedding or enter bathtubs and sinks in search of water. Scorpions sting human beings only when disturbed.

Scorpions of the United States   Of the 40 or so scorpion species in the United States, only the bark scorpion (*Centruroides sculpturatus* or *C. exilicauda*) produces a venom that can be lethal. Stings of the other species, such as the common striped scorpion *C. vittatus* and the large *Hadrurus arizonensis*, cause immediate sharp local pain followed by edema, ecchymosis, and a burning sensation. Symptoms typically resolve within a few hours, and skin does not slough. Allergic reactions to the venom sometimes develop.

The deadly *C. sculpturatus* of the southwestern United States and northern Mexico measures about 7 cm in length and is yellow-brown in color. Its venom contains neurotoxins that cause sodium channels to remain open and neurons to fire repetitively. In contrast to the stings of nonlethal species, *C. sculpturatus* envenomations are usually associated with little swelling, but prominent pain, paresthesia, and hyperesthesia can be accentuated by tapping on the affected area (the tap test). These symptoms soon spread to other locations; dysfunction of cranial nerves and hyperexcitability of skeletal muscles develop within hours. Patients present with restlessness, blurred vision, abnormal eye movements, profuse salivation, lacrimation, rhinorrhea, slurred speech, difficulty in handling secretions, diaphoresis, nausea, and vomiting. Muscle twitching, jerking, and shaking may be mistaken for a seizure. Complications include tachycardia, arrhythmias, hypertension, hyperthermia, rhabdomyolysis, and acidosis. Symptoms progress to maximal severity in about 5 h and subside within a day or two, although pain and paresthesia can last for weeks. Fatal respiratory arrest is most common among young children and the elderly.

Other Dangerous Scorpions   Envenomations by *Leiurus quinquestriatus* in the Middle East and North Africa, by *Mesobuthus tamulus* in India, by *Androctonus* species along the Mediterranean littoral and in North Africa and the Middle East, and by *Tityus serrulatus* in Brazil cause massive release of endogenous catecholamines with hypertensive crises, arrhythmias, pulmonary edema, and myocardial damage. Acute pancreatitis occurs with stings of *Tityus trinitatis* in Trinidad, and central nervous toxicity complicates stings of *Parabuthus* and *Buthotus* scorpions of South Africa. Tissue necrosis and hemolysis may follow stings of the Iranian *Hemiscorpius lepturus*.

℞ **TREATMENT**   Identification of the offending scorpion aids in planning therapy. Stings of nonlethal species require at most ice packs, analgesics, or antihistamines. Because most victims of dangerous envenomations (such as those produced by *C. sculpturatus*) experience only local discomfort, they can be managed at home with instructions to return to the emergency department if signs of cranial-nerve or neuromuscular dysfunction develop. Aggressive supportive care and judicious use of antivenin can reduce or eliminate mortality from more severe envenomations. Keeping the patient calm and applying pressure dressings and cold packs to the sting site decrease the absorption of venom. A continuous intravenous infusion of midazolam controls the agitation, flailing, and involuntary muscle movements produced by scorpion stings. Close monitoring during treatment with this drug and other sedatives or narcotics is necessary for persons with neuromuscular symptoms because of the risk of respiratory arrest. Hypertension and pulmonary edema respond to nifedipine, nitroprusside, hydralazine, or prazosin, and bradyarrhythmias can be controlled with atropine.

Commercially prepared antivenins are available in several countries for some of the most dangerous species. A caprine *C. sculpturatus* antivenin (not yet FDA approved) is available as an investigational drug from the Arizona State University for use only in Arizona. Because of the risk of anaphylaxis or serum sickness following administration of goat serum, use of the antivenin is controversial. Intravenous administration of antivenin rapidly reverses cranial-nerve dysfunction and muscular symptoms but does not affect pain and paresthesia. The benefit of scorpion antivenin has not been established in controlled trials.

Prevention   In scorpion-infested areas, shoes, clothing, bedding, and towels should be shaken and inspected before being used. Removal of wood, stones, and debris from yards and campsites eliminates hiding places for scorpions, and household spraying of insecticides can deplete their source of food.

CHIGGERS AND OTHER BITING MITES   Chiggers are the larvae of trombiculid (harvest) mites that normally feed on mice in grassy or brush-covered sites in the tropics and subtropics and (less frequently) in temperate areas during warm months. They wait for hosts on low vegetation and attach themselves to passing animals or to people. The larva then pierces the skin of its host and deposits a tubelike structure in the dermis through which it imbibes lymph and tissue juices. This highly antigenic "stylostome" serves as the focus of an exceptionally pruritic papular, papulovesicular, or papulourticarial lesion that may be 2 cm in diameter and that develops within hours of attachment in persons previously sensitized to mite antigen. Feeding mites appear as tiny red vesicles in hair follicles. Scratching invariably destroys the body of a mite attached to a person. These lesions generally vesiculate and develop a hemorrhagic base. Itching and burning last for weeks. The rash is most common on the ankles or near tight-fitting clothes that obstruct the mites' movements. Chiggers are the vectors of scrub typhus in tropical and subtropical parts of Asia. Repellents are useful for preventing chigger bites.

Certain mesostigmatid mites that infest the nests of mice or birds feed on human beings when their usual hosts have been displaced. For example, intense episodes of itching dermatitis in humans may follow the removal of trash from a human residence or the departure of pigeons that have been nesting on a window air-conditioner. Other mites that infest grain, straw, cheese, or other animal products occasionally produce similar episodes. Persons who have close contact with dogs—and, to a lesser extent, cats—may develop a self-limited pruritic papulovesicular rash from bites of cheyletiellid mites that cause a mangelike condition in these animals. Mouse mites are the vectors of rickettsialpox in cities of the northeastern United States. Fowl and chicken mites transmit the viruses of St. Louis encephalitis and western equine encephalitis. Although sanitary measures effectively prevent rickettsialpox, removal of accumulated refuse may result in a transient period of elevated risk.

Diagnosis of mite-induced dermatitides (including those caused by chiggers) relies heavily on a history of exposure to the source of the mite, since the tiny mite may escape notice or may already have fallen off or been scratched off the lesions. Antihistamines or topical steroids effectively reduce mite-induced pruritus.

HYMENOPTERA STINGS   Insects that sting to defend their colonies or subdue their prey belong to the order Hymenoptera, which includes apids (bees and bumblebees), vespids (wasps, hornets, and yellow jackets), and ants. Their venoms contain a wide array of amines, peptides, and enzymes that are responsible for local and systemic reactions. Although the toxic effect of multiple stings can be fatal, nearly all of the 50 or more deaths due to hymenopteran stings in the United States each year are the result of allergic reactions.

Bee and Wasp Stings   Bees lose their venom apparatus in the act of stinging and subsequently die, while vespids can sting numerous times in succession. The familiar honeybees (*Apis mellifera*) and bumblebees (*Bombus* and other genera) attack when a colony is disturbed, but the extremely aggressive Africanized honeybees respond to minimal intrusions rapidly and in large numbers. Since their introduction into Brazil in 1957, these "killer bees" have spread through South and Central America to the southern and western United States.

The common vespids in the United States include the yellow jacket, notable for the yellow and black bands on its abdomen; the bald-faced hornet, with a black body and a white face; the brown hornet, measuring 2.5 to 3.5 cm in length; and the paper wasps, which have variously colored elongate bodies. Vespids sting in defense of their nests, which they often build near human dwellings and suspend from eaves or shubbery, plaster onto walls, or burrow into wood or soil. Yellow jackets feed on sugary substances and decaying meat and are annoyingly abundant at recreation sites and around garbage, particularly in the late summer and fall.

Venom is produced in glands at the posterior end of the abdomen and is expelled rapidly by contraction of muscles of the venom sac, which has a capacity of up to 0.1 mL in large insects. The venoms of different species of hymenopterans are biochemically and immunologically distinct. Direct toxic effects are mediated by mixtures of low-molecular-weight compounds such as serotonin, histamine, and acetylcholine and several kinins. Polypeptide toxins in honeybee venom include mellitin, which damages cell membranes; mast cell–degranulating protein, which causes histamine release; apamin, a neurotoxin; and adolapin, which has anti-inflammatory action. Enzymes in venom include hyaluronidase, which allows the spread of other venom components, and phospholipases, which may be among the major venom allergens. There appears to be little cross-sensitization between honeybee and wasp venoms.

Uncomplicated stings cause immediate pain, a wheal-and-flare reaction, and local edema and swelling that subside in a few hours. Stings from accidentally swallowed insects may induce life-threatening edema of the upper airways. Multiple stings can lead to vomiting, diarrhea, generalized edema, dyspnea, hypotension, and collapse. Rhabdomyolysis and intravascular hemolysis may cause renal failure. Death from the direct effects of venom has followed 300 to 500 honeybee stings.

Large local reactions that spread ≥10 cm around the sting site over 24 to 48 h are not uncommon. These reactions may resemble cellulitis but are caused by hypersensitivity rather than secondary infection. Such reactions tend to recur on subsequent exposure but are seldom accompanied by anaphylaxis and are not prevented by venom immunotherapy.

An estimated 0.4 to 4.0% of the U.S. population exhibits clinical immediate-type hypersensitivity to insect stings, and 15% may have asymptomatic sensitization manifested by positive skin tests. Persons who experience severe allergic reactions are likely to have similar reactions after subsequent stings; occasionally, adults who have had mild reactions later experience serious reactions. Mild anaphylactic reactions from insect stings, as from other causes, consist of nausea, abdominal cramping, generalized urticaria, flushing, and angioedema. Serious reactions, including upper airway edema, bronchospasm, hypotension, and shock, may be rapidly fatal. Severe reactions usually begin within 10 min of the sting and only rarely develop after 5 h. Unusual complications, including serum sickness, vasculitis, neuritis, and encephalitis, develop several days or weeks after a sting.

℞ TREATMENT Stingers embedded in the skin should be scraped or brushed off with a blade or a fingernail but not removed with forceps, which may squeeze more venom out of the venom sac. The site should be cleansed and disinfected and ice packs used to slow the spread of venom. Elevation of the affected site and administration of analgesics, oral antihistamines, and topical calamine lotion relieve symptoms; application of meat tenderizer containing papain is of no proven value. Large local reactions may require a short course of oral therapy with glucocorticoids. Patients with numerous stings should be monitored for 24 h for evidence of renal failure or coagulopathy.

Anaphylaxis is treated with subcutaneous injection of 0.3 to 0.5 mL of epinephrine hydrochloride in a 1:1000 dilution; treatment is repeated every 20 to 30 min if necessary. Intravenous epinephrine (2 to 5 mL of a 1:10,000 solution administered by slow push) is indicated for profound shock. A tourniquet may slow the spread of venom. Parenteral antihistamines, fluid resuscitation, bronchodilators, oxygen, intubation, and vasopressors may be required. Patients should be observed for 24 h for recurrent anaphylaxis.

Prevention Persons with a history of allergy to insect stings should carry a sting kit with a preloaded syringe containing epinephrine for self-administration in case of a sting. These patients should seek medical attention immediately after using the kit. To avoid stings when outdoors, individuals can wear shoes and protective clothing and avoid attracting insects with sweet foods, bright-colored clothes, perfumes, or cosmetics.

Venom Immunotherapy Repeated injections of purified venom produce a blocking IgG antibody response to venom and reduce the incidence of recurrent anaphylaxis from between 50 and 60% to <5%. Honeybee, wasp, yellow jacket, and mixed vespid venoms are commercially available for desensitization and for skin testing. Adults with a history of anaphylaxis should undergo desensitization. Results of skin tests and venom-specific radioallergosorbent tests aid in the selection of patients for immunotherapy and guide the design of such treatment. The risk of a systemic reaction to a sting is ~5 to 10% after discontinuation of a ≥5-year course of immunotherapy.

Stings of Fire Ants and Other Ants All ants that are large enough can bite human beings, and some can secrete repugnant substances when handled. Stinging fire ants are an important medical problem in the United States. The imported fire ants *Solenopsis richteri* and *S. invicta* were introduced from South America into Alabama in 1918 and now infest urban and rural areas of southern states from Texas to North Carolina, with colonies in California, New Mexico, Arizona, and Virginia. They excavate open fields and yards to build tall mounds that can harbor 200,000 worker ants. Slight disturbances of the mounds have provoked massive outpourings of ants and as many as 10,000 stings on a single person. Each year fire ants sting up to 60% of the inhabitants of some cities. Waterborne ants bite on contact during times of flooding. The elderly and immobile persons are at high risk for attacks when fire ants invade dwellings.

Red-brown or brown-black fire ants attach to human skin with powerful mandibles and rotate their bodies around their heads while repeatedly injecting venom with posteriorly situated stingers. The alkaloid venom consists of cytotoxic and hemolytic piperidines and several proteins with enzymatic activity. The initial wheal-and-flare reaction, burning, and itching resolve in about 30 min, and a sterile pustule develops within 24 h. The pustule ulcerates over the next 48 h and then heals a week or 10 days later unless it becomes secondarily infected. Large areas of erythema and edema lasting several days are not uncommon and in extreme cases may compress nerves and blood vessels. Anaphylaxis occurs in ~1 to 2% of persons, and seizures and mononeuritis have been reported. Stings are treated with ice packs, topical glucocorticoids, and oral antihistamines. Covering pustules with bandages and antibiotic ointment may prevent bacterial infection. Epinephrine and supportive measures are indicated for anaphylactic reactions. Whole-body extracts are available for skin testing and immunotherapy, which appears to lower the rate of anaphylactic reactions.

The western United States is home to harvester ants (*Pogonomyrmex* species) as well as to less aggressive fire ants not yet displaced by the introduced species. The painful local reaction following harvester ant stings often extends to lymph nodes and may be accompanied by anaphylaxis. Large Australian bulldog ants and the aggressive South American *Paranopera* ants deliver extremely painful stings and may cause systemic symptoms. Velvet ants that inhabit sandy beaches in the United States and sting the bare feet of bathers are actually wingless female wasps of the genus *Dasymutilla*.

TICK BITES AND TICK PARALYSIS In the United States, hard ticks (Ixodidae) have increased in abundance since the mid-1900s to become the most common carriers of vector-borne diseases. Deer ticks of the genus *Ixodes* transmit the pathogens of Lyme disease, babesiosis, and human granulocytic ehrlichiosis. Other ticks, such as *Dermacentor variabilis* (the dog tick), *D. andersoni* (the wood tick), and *Amblyomma americanum* (the Lone Star tick), are vectors of tularemia, Rocky Mountain spotted fever, Colorado tick fever, and human monocytic ehrlichiosis. Outside the United States, hard ticks transmit pathogenic rickettsiae and arboviruses as well. Soft ticks (Argasidae) of the genus *Ornithodoros* transmit tick-borne relapsing fever

(Chap. 175). Except in parts of Africa, soft ticks rarely attack human beings, and relapsing fever occurs only sporadically in the United States. Hard ticks differ from soft ticks by virtue of a dorsal scutum or plate and their preference for wooded, brushy, or weedy habitats. Soft ticks, which are nonscutate and leathery, are generally found in animal burrows and bird nests.

Ticks attach and feed painlessly; blood is their only food. Their secretions, however, produce local reactions, a febrile illness, or paralysis. Soft ticks attach for <1 h and produce erythematous macular lesions up to 2 to 3 cm in diameter. Some species in Africa, the western United States, and Mexico produce painful hemorrhagic lesions. At the site of hard-tick bites, small areas of induration with surrounding erythema and occasionally necrotic ulcers develop. Chronic nodules, or "tick granulomas," reach several centimeters in diameter and may require surgical excision. Tick-induced fever, associated with headache, nausea, and malaise, usually resolves within 24 to 36 h after the tick is removed. Tick paralysis is an ascending flaccid paralysis believed to be caused by a toxin in tick saliva that causes neuromuscular block and decreased nerve conduction. Throughout the world, this rare complication has followed the bites of more than 40 kinds of tick—most commonly, dog and wood ticks in the United States. Children, especially girls with long hair, are most often affected. Weakness begins in the lower extremities 5 to 6 days after the tick's attachment and ascends symmetrically over several days to result in complete paralysis of the extremities and cranial nerves. Deep tendon reflexes are diminished or lacking altogether, but sensory examination and findings on lumbar puncture are typically normal. Removal of the tick results in improvement within a few hours and usually in complete recovery after several days. Failure to remove the tick may lead to dysarthria, dysphagia, and ultimately death from aspiration or respiratory paralysis. Diagnosis depends on finding the tick, which often is hidden beneath hair and which, when engorged, may resemble a pedunculated nevus.

An antiserum to the saliva of *Ixodes holocyclus*, the usual cause of tick paralysis in Australia, effectively reverses paralysis caused by these ticks. Ticks should be removed by firm traction with a forceps placed near their point of attachment. The site of attachment should be disinfected (e.g., with tincture of iodine). Mouthparts remaining in the skin may cause persistent irritation or lead to secondary infection. Removal of ticks during the first 48 h of attachment nearly always prevents transmission of the agents of Lyme disease, babesiosis, and erhlichiosis. Gentle handling to avoid rupture of ticks and use of gloves may avert accidental contamination with tick fluids containing pathogens. Protective measures against ticks include avoidance of brushy vegetation, removal of ticks from pet dogs and cats, use of protective clothing sprayed with 0.5% permethrin, and application of a repellent containing *N,N*-diethyl-*m*-toluamide (DEET). The cuffs of trousers should be tucked inside the socks.

OTHER ARTHROPOD BITES AND ENVENOMATIONS
Dipteran (Fly and Mosquito) Bites In the process of feeding on vertebrate blood, adults of certain fly species inflict painful bites, produce local allergic reactions, or transmit infectious diseases. Unlike insect stings, insect bites rarely cause anaphylaxis. Mosquitoes are ubiquitous pests and are the vectors of malaria, filariasis, yellow fever, dengue, and viral encephalitides. Female mosquitoes require a blood meal to produce eggs and an environment of standing water in which to deposit them. Their bite typically produces a wheal and later a pruritic papule. In the United States, a similar reaction follows the bite of tiny but aggressive midges known as "no-see-ums," which attack in swarms during warm months, or of other *Culicoides* species that transmit "nonpathogenic" filariae in tropical climates. Nodular lesions at the site of midge bites may last for months. The bite of the small humpbacked blackfly of the genus *Simulium* leaves a large bleeding puncture and painful and pruritic sores that are slow to heal; regional lymphadenopathy, fever, or anaphylaxis occasionally ensues. Black-flies are common summertime nuisances in the United States and Canada and are vectors of onchocerciasis in Africa and Latin America. The widely distributed tabanids, including deerflies (*Chrysops* species) and horseflies (*Tabanus* species), are stout flies measuring 10 to 25 mm in length that attack during the day and produce large and painful bleeding punctures. Deerflies transmit loiasis in African equatorial rain forests and tularemia in the United States and elsewhere. Tsetse flies of the genus *Glossina* transmit African trypanosomiasis in sub-Saharan Africa. Tiny phlebotomine sandflies are the vectors of leishmaniasis, bartonellosis (Carrión's disease), sandfly fever, and other arboviral infections in warm climates. *Stomoxys calcitrans*, the stable fly, which resembles a large housefly, is a fierce biter of human beings and domestic animals and a major pest in seacoast areas. Houseflies do not bite.

℞ TREATMENT Treatment of fly bites is symptom-based. Topical application of antipruritic agents, glucocorticoids, or antiseptic lotions may relieve the itching and pain. Allergic reactions may require oral antihistamines. Antibiotics may be necessary for large bite wounds that become secondarily infected. Personal protection measures against biting flies include avoidance of infested areas, application of a DEET-containing repellent to exposed skin, and use of protective clothing and bed nets treated with permethrin. Higher concentrations of DEET provide longer-lasting protection, and 10 to 35% DEET provides adequate protection under most conditions. Repellents used on children should contain ≤10% DEET to avoid absorption of toxic levels that provoke encephalopathy and seizures. Permethrin applied to clothing maintains its potency for at least 2 weeks, even with laundering. It should not be applied to the skin.

Flea Bites Common human-biting fleas include the dog and cat fleas (*Ctenocephalides* species) and the rat flea (*Xenopsylla cheopis*), which inhabit the nests and resting sites of their hosts. Larval fleas feed on pellets of dried host blood that the adult fleas eject from their rectums while feeding. The high-jumping adults attack human beings or other available warm-bodied animals when the usual host abandons or is driven from its nest. The human flea (*Pulex irritans*) infests human bedding and furniture but mainly in relatively humid buildings that lack central heating. Sensitized persons develop erythematous pruritic papules, urticaria, and occasionally vesicles and bacterial superinfection at the site of the bite. Treatment consists of antihistamines and antipruritics.

Fleas transmit plague, murine typhus, a typhus-like illness due to *Rickettsia felis*, the rat and dog tapeworms, and *B. henselae*. Flea infestations are eliminated by frequent cleaning of the nesting sites and bedding of the host or judicious dusting or spraying of insecticides such as pyrethrin, DDT, or malathion.

Hemipteran (True Bug) Bites Several true bugs of the family Reduviidae inflict bites that produce allergic reactions and are sometimes painful. The cosmopolitan bedbug (*Cimex* species) hides in mattresses, behind bedboards, and under loose wallpaper during the day and takes its blood meal at night. The bite is painless, but sensitized persons develop erythema, itching, and wheals around a central hemorrhagic punctum. The cone-nose bugs, so called because of their elongated heads, include the assassin and wheel bugs, which feed on other insects and bite human beings only in self-defense, and the kissing bugs, which routinely feed on vertebrate blood. Assassin and wheel bugs inhabit many parts of the world, including the southwestern and southern United States, where they are notorious for their painful bites. The bites of the nocturnally feeding kissing bugs are painless and occur commonly in groups on the face and other exposed parts of the body. Reactions to such bites depend on prior sensitization and include tender and pruritic papules, vesicular or bullous lesions, giant urticaria, fever, lymphadenopathy, and anaphylaxis. *Triatoma infestans* and other species of kissing bug are the vectors of *Trypanosoma cruzi* in South and Central America and Mexico, but transmission of *T. cruzi* to human beings by species indigenous to the United States is exceedingly rare. Bug bites are treated with topical antipruritics or oral antihistamines. Persons with anaphylactic reactions to reduviid bites should keep an epinephrine kit available.

Centipede Bites and Millipede Dermatitis The fangs of centipedes of the genus *Scolopendra* can penetrate human skin and deliver a venom that produces intense burning pain, swelling, erythema, and lymphangitis. Dizziness, nausea, and anxiety are occasionally described, and rhabdomyolysis and renal failure have been reported. Treatment includes washing of the site, application of cold dressings, oral analgesic administration or local lidocaine infiltration, and tetanus prophylaxis. Species of *Scolopendra*, measuring up to 25 cm, occur widely in the southern United States and other areas with warm climates worldwide. The smaller house centipede *Scutigera coleopatrata*, which is common throughout the United States, is harmless.

Millipedes, unlike centipedes, do not bite but rather secrete and in some cases eject defensive fluids that burn and discolor human skin. Affected skin turns brown overnight and may blister and exfoliate. Secretions in the eye cause intense pain and inflammation that may lead to corneal ulceration and blindness. Management includes irrigation with copious amounts of water or saline, use of analgesics, and local care of denuded skin. Millipedes are found throughout the world in leaf litter and under rocks.

Caterpillar Stings and Dermatitis The surface of caterpillars of several moth species is covered with hairs or spines that produce mechanical irritation and may contain or be coated with venom. Contact with these caterpillars causes an immediate burning sensation followed by local swelling and erythema and occasionally by regional lymphadenopathy, nausea, vomiting, and headache; shock, seizures, and coagulopathy are rare complications. In the United States, stings are most often caused by io moth larvae and puss as well as saddleback and brown-tail moth caterpillars as they cling to leaves and branches. Contact with even detached hairs of other caterpillars, such as gypsy moth larvae (*Lymantria dispar*) in the northeastern United States, can produce a pruritic urticarial or papular rash hours later. Spines may be deposited on tree trunks and drying laundry or may be airborne and cause irritation of the eyes and upper airways. Treatment of caterpillar stings consists of repeated application of adhesive or cellophane tape to remove the hairs, which can then be identified microscopically. Local ice packs, topical steroids, and oral antihistamines relieve symptoms.

Beetle Vesication When disturbed, blister beetles extrude cantharidin, a low-molecular-weight toxin that produces thin-walled blisters measuring up to 5 cm in diameter 2 to 5 h after contact with the beetle. The blisters are not painful or pruritic unless broken, and they resolve without treatment in a week to 10 days. Nephritis may follow unusually heavy cantharidin exposure. In the southern United States, blister beetles of several *Epicauta* species are abundant in the summer months. Contact occurs when people sit on the ground, work in the garden, or deliberately handle the beetles. In other countries, different species of beetle produce different vesicants. No treatment is necessary, although ruptured blisters should be kept clean and bandaged until healing is complete.

BIBLIOGRAPHY

AUERBACH PS (ed): *Wilderness Medicine*, 3d ed. St. Louis, Mosby, 1995

DeSHAZO RD et al: Fire ant attacks on residents in health care facilities: A report of two cases. Ann Intern Med 131:424, 1999

DOWNS AM et al: Head lice: Prevalence in schoolchildren and insecticide resistance. Parasitol Today 15:1, 1999

FRADIN MS: Mosquitoes and mosquito repellents: A clinician's guide. Ann Intern Med 128:931, 1998

GODDARD J: *Infectious Diseases and Arthropods*. Totowa, NJ, Humana, 2000

HAWDON GM, WINKEL KD: Spider bite. A rational approach. Aust Fam Physician 26: 1380, 1997

KING MS: Pathogenesis of envenomation. Ann Emerg Med 34:411, 1999

LAVARDE V, FORNES P. Lethal infection due to *Armillifer armillatus* (*Porocephalida*): A snake-related parasitic disease. Clin Infect Dis 29:1346, 1999

MILLIKAN LE: Myiasis. Clin Dermatol 17:191, 1999

PETERS W: *A Colour Atlas of Arthropods in Clinical Medicine*. London, Wolfe, 1992

NOBEL PRIZE IN PHYSIOLOGY OR MEDICINE, 1977

Roger Guillemin was born on January 11, 1924, in Dijon, France. His early education was in the public schools in Dijon after which he received his B.A. and B.S. degrees there in college. In 1943 he pursued a medical degree in a joint program at the School of Medicine in Dijon and the University of Lyon. At the same time he also served in the French Resistance from 1940 to 1944. For his degree in medicine, Guillemin desired to write his thesis on hormonal adaptation to alarm reactions after meeting Dr. Hans Selye during his visit to Paris. Selye invited Guillemin to work at the new Institute of Experimental Medicine and Surgery at Montreal University in Canada. With this background in medicine and hormonal research, he began his search for the chemical structure of peptide hormones. Geoffrey W. Harris in England had provided anatomical evidence that the brain hypothalamus controlled the pituitary and suggested that this control was not by nerve impulses, but rather hormones that flowed through a capillary network connecting the hypothalamus and the pituitary.

Guillemin became a professor of physiology at the Baylor College of Medicine where in 1955 he demonstrated, in a co-culture experiment, the regulatory effect of the hypothalamus on the pituitary. Between 1960 and 1963 Guillemin held a temporary associate director position at the Laboratory of Experimental Endocrinology, Collège de France, where he collected from slaughterhouses, 5 million pieces of sheep hypothalamus weighing about 50 tons. From this material he and his collaborator, R. Burgus, isolated 1 mg of thyrotropin-releasing factor (TRF) from 300,000 sheep hypothalami. In 1969 he established the primary structure to be a tripeptide composed of three amino acids and demonstrated the hormone's stimulating effect on thyroid-stimulating hormone (TSH). In 1920 Guillemin, Burgus, and colleagues isolated luteinizing hormone–releasing factor (LHRF) from sheep hypothalami. LHRF was found to stimulate both luteinizing and follicle-stimulating hormones of the pituitary. The structure of LHRF was then determined in 1971. At the same time, Andrew Schally's group independently identified the structures of TRF and LHRF at Tulane University.

In 1970 Guillemin moved his neuroendocrinology laboratory from Baylor to the Salk Institute in La Jolla, California. After his identification of LHRF, Guillemin demonstrated an inhibitory effect of the hypothalamus on pituitary growth hormone and eventually identified the substance to be somatostatin or somatotrophin-release inhibiting factor. Guillemin did not stop there. In 1976, from 25,000 swine hypothalami, he isolated and purified a group of opiate-like substances called endorphins (endogenous morphine).

Andrew Victor Schally was born on November 30, 1926, in Wilno, Poland. His family fled Poland when Germany occupied it, and his father became a major general with the allied forces in World War II. After the war he moved to Scotland where he finished high school. Schally then became a research laboratory technician at the National Institute for Medical Research in London, but ultimately moved to Montreal where in 1957 he received his Ph.D. at McGill University. At McGill he worked with Murray Saffran, who was pursuing the possibility of hypothalamic hormones. In 1954 he joined Roger Guillemin's laboratory at Baylor University in Houston, but ultimately, they became scientific competitors rather than collaborators. In 1962 Schally became Chief of the Endocrine and Polypeptide Laboratory at the New Orleans Veterans Administration Hospital and a professor at Tulane University School of Medicine. Schally was successful in isolating TRF, but falsely concluded that the structure was not a peptide. He had worked a total of 11 years in his search of hypothalamic hormones and their structure. The National Institutes of Health Endocrine Study Section was considering terminating funding for the project. Both Schally and Guillemin had mistaken impurities for the TRF compound. However, Guillemin's colleague, Roger Burgus, finally purified the material and demonstrated that TRF was a tripeptide. There was, however, still another barrier since differing sequences of the amino acids demonstrated no biological activity until the cap at the end of the TRF molecule was found to curl back and create an internal loop in the molecule. The publisher received Schally's paper five weeks before Guillemin's paper, which arrived at a similar conclusion. Although the papers were published only a few days apart, Schally's was given credit for identifying the first hypothalamic hormone because of his earlier submission. Schally's team next turned to defining the structure of LHRF. From 160,000 pig brains, Schally extracted 250 μg of LHRF. Schally's colleague, Hisayuko Matsuo, knew that this amount of LHRF was not enough to determine the structure by standard means. Using the Yalow and Berson radioimmunoassay technique, he demonstrated that LHRF stimulated release of reproductive hormones, namely the luteinizing and follicle-stimulating hormones. The Schally team also isolated and identified somatostatin, an inhibitory hormone. Although rivals, Guillemin and Schally opened the era of hypothalamic hormones that was to have an enormous impact on the future of neuroendocrinology.

Rosalyn Sussman Yalow was born in the South Bronx, New York, the second child of Simon and Clara Sussman. Clara had emigrated from Germany at the age of four, and Simon ran a paper and twine business in the Bronx. Although neither parent finished high school, they instilled in their children the importance of education. Rosalyn Yalow graduated from Walton Public High School and attended Hunter College where she was the first ever to be graduated from that institution with a physics major. Her professors convinced her that as a woman she could never obtain a physics position in graduate school, but they were wrong. She was offered a teaching assistant position at the University of Illinois and she entered the College of Engineering as the only woman among 400 graduate students. She obtained her Ph.D. in nuclear physics in 1945. She met and married another physics graduate student, Aaron Yalow, and they had two children. During her graduate studies she learned laboratory techniques for measuring radioactivity, including constructing the necessary apparatus. This experience would become invaluable in her future work. During her free summer from teaching, however, she volunteered to work in Edith Quimby's laboratory at Columbia College of Physicians and Surgeons in order to obtain experience in using radioisotopes in medical research. This experience enabled her to obtain a part-time position at the Bronx Veterans Administration Hospital (VAH). She began to establish a radioisotope service and to conduct research out of a converted janitor's closet at the VAH. She then resigned her teaching position at Hunter College, accepted a full-time staff position at the Veterans Hospital, and was joined by a physician trained at New York University, Solomon Berson. Berson brought the clinical insights to this remarkable team, which spanned the disciplines of biochemistry, medicine, and nuclear physics. Their pivotal work began with an interest in adult-onset diabetes (type 2), where a hypothesis was proposed that insulin was being removed from the body too rapidly. Berson and Yalow, therefore, injected ^{131}I-labeled insulin into normal individuals and adult-onset diabetic patients and surprisingly found the opposite result. The insulin disappearance was slower in the diabetic patients. Further analysis of the data revealed that those diabetic patients who had been treated previously with insulin demonstrated the slowest disappearance of the hormone. Yalow and Berson then hypothesized that antibodies had developed against the bovine or pork insulin that the diabetic patients had received. They realized that the amount of injected labeled insulin that was bound by the antibody was dependent on the amount of endogenous insulin present in the body at the time of the injected radiolabeled insulin. This observation led to the development of the radioimmunoassay (RIA) that revolutionized medicine. This technique allowed the measurement of proteins in concentrations as small as 0.05 pmol, which was a million times smaller than any technique available at that time. The Yalow and Berson team extended their RIA technique from insulin to growth hormone, corticotropin, parathyroid hormone, and gastrin.

In 1977, Yalow was the second woman to receive the Nobel Prize in Physiology or Medicine, an award that would, no doubt, have been shared with Solomon Berson had it not been for his untimely death in 1972. In her Nobel lecture on receiving the award in Stockholm, Yalow concluded that, like the microscope, the RIA allowed for new avenues of biology to be explored. At the formal Nobel dinner she rose to speak on behalf of equal opportunities for women, stating that, "The world cannot afford the loss of talents of half of its people."

REFERENCES

1. Magill FN (ed): *Nobel Prize Winners: Physiology or Medicine*, vol 3. Pasadena, Salem Press, 1993
2. Schrier RW: *A Salute to Nobel Laureates in Physiology and Medicine*, Proceedings of the Association of American Physicians 108(1): Jan 1996

Robert W. Schrier, MD

A

LABORATORY VALUES OF CLINICAL IMPORTANCE

INTRODUCTORY COMMENTS

All laboratory appendices should be interpreted with caution since normal values differ widely among clinical laboratories. The values given in this Appendix are meant primarily for use with this text. In preparing the Appendix, the editors have taken into account the fact that the system of international units (SI, système international d'unités) is now used in most countries and in most medical and scientific journals.[1] However, clinical laboratories in many countries continue to report values in traditional units. Therefore, both systems are used in the Appendix. Values in SI units appear first and traditional units appear in parentheses after the SI units. The dual system is also used in the text except for (1) those instances in which the numbers remain the same but only the terminology is changed (mmol/L for meq/L or IU/L for mIU/mL), when only the SI units are given; and (2) most pressure measurements (e.g., blood and cerebrospinal fluid pressures), when the traditional units (mmHg, mmH$_2$O) are used. In all other instances in the text the SI unit is followed by the traditional unit in parentheses. The SI base units, SI derived units, other units of measure referred to in Appendix A, and SI prefixes are listed in Tables A-1 to A-3. Conversions from one system to another can be made as follows:

$$mmol/L = \frac{mg/dL \times 10}{\text{atomic weight}}$$

$$mg/dL = \frac{mmol/L \times \text{atomic weight}}{10}$$

TABLE A-1 RADIATION-DERIVED UNITS

Quantity	Old Unit	SI Unit	Name for SI Unit (and Abbreviation)	Conversion
Activity	curie (Ci)	Disintegrations per second (dps)	becquerel (Bq)	1 Ci = 3.7 × 10^{10} Bq 1 mCi = 37 mBq 1 μCi = 0.037 MBq or 37 GBq 1 Bq = 2.703 × 10^{-11} Ci
Absorbed dose	rad	joule per kilogram (J/kg)	gray (Gy)	1 Gy = 100 rad 1 rad = 0.01 Gy 1 mrad = 10^{-3} cGy
Exposure	roentgen (R)	coulomb per kilogram (C/kg)	—	1 C/kg = 3876 R 1 R = 2.58 × 10^{-4} C/kg 1 mR = 258 pC/kg
Dose equivalent	rem	joule per kilogram (J/kg)	sievert (Sv)	1 Sv = 100 rem 1 rem = 0.01 Sv 1 mrem = 10 μSv

[1]Young DS: Implementation of SI units for clinical laboratory data. Ann Intern Med 106:114, 1987

TABLE A-2 BODY FLUIDS AND OTHER MASS DATA

	Reference Range	
	SI Units	Conventional Units
Ascitic fluid: See Chap. 46		
Body fluid, total volume (lean) of body weight	50% (in obese) to 70%	
Intracellular	0.3–0.4 of body weight	
Extracellular	0.2–0.3 of body weight	
Blood		
Total volume		
Males	69 mL per kg body weight	
Females	65 mL per kg body weight	
Plasma volume		
Males	39 mL per kg body weight	
Females	40 mL per kg body weight	
Red blood cell volume		
Males	30 mL per kg body weight	1.15–1.21 L/m² of body surface area
Females	25 mL per kg body weight	0.95–1.00 L/m² of body surface area

TABLE A-3 CEREBROSPINAL FLUID[a]

	Reference Range	
Constituent	SI Units	Conventional Units
Osmolarity	292–297 mmol/kg water	292–297 mOsm/L
Electrolytes		
Sodium	137–145 mmol/L	137–145 meq/L
Potassium	2.7–3.9 mmol/L	2.7–3.9 meq/L
Calcium	1.0–1.5 mmol/L	2.1–3.0 meq/L
Magnesium	1.0–1.2 mmol/L	2.0–2.5 meq/L
Chloride	116–122 mmol/L	116–122 meq/L
CO$_2$ content	20–24 mmol/L	20–24 meq/L
P$_{CO_2}$	6–7 kPa	45–49 mmHg
pH	7.31–7.34	
Glucose	2.2–3.9 mmol/L	40–70 mg/dL
Lactate	1–2 mmol/L	10–20 mg/dL
Total protein	0.2–0.5 g/L	20–50 mg/dL
Albumin	0.066–0.442 g/L	6.6–44.2 mg/dL
IgG	0.009–0.057 g/L	0.9–5.7 mg/dL
IgG index[b]	0.29–0.59	
Oligoclonal bands (OGB)	<2 bands not present in matched serum sample	
Ammonia	15–47 μmol/L	25–80 μg/dL
Creatinine	44–168 μmol/L	0.5–1.9 mg/dL
Myelin basic protein	<4 μg/L	
CSF pressure		50–180 mmH$_2$O
CSF volume (adult)	~150 mL	
Leukocytes		
Total	<5 per μL	
Differential:		
Lymphocytes	60–70%	
Monocytes	30–50%	
Neutrophils	None	

[a] Since cerebrospinal fluid concentrations are equilibrium values, measurements of the same parameters in blood plasma obtained at the same time are recommended. However, there is a time lag in attainment of equilibrium, and cerebrospinal levels of plasma constituents that can fluctuate rapidly (such as plasma glucose) may not achieve stable values until after a significant lag phase.

[b] IgG index $= \dfrac{\text{CSF IgG(mg/dL)} \times \text{serum albumin(g/dL)}}{\text{Serum IgG(g/dL)} \times \text{CSF albumin(mg/dL)}}$

Constituent	Specimen	Reference Range	
		SI Units	Conventional Units
Acetoacetate	P	$<100\ \mu$mol/L	<1 mg/dL
Albumin	S	35–55 g/L	3.5–5.5 g/dL
Aldolase		0–100 nkat/L	0–6 U/L
Alpha$_1$ antitrypsin	S	0.8–2.1 g/L	85–213 mg/dL
Alpha fetoprotein (adult)	S	$<30\ \mu$g/L	<30 ng/mL
Aminotransferases	S		
Aspartate (AST, SGOT)		0–0.58 μkat/L	0–35 U/L
Alanine (ALT, SGPT)		0–0.58 μkat/L	0–35 U/L
Ammonia, as NH_3	P	6–47 μmol/L	10–80 μg/dL
Amylase	S	0.8–3.2 μkat/L	60–180 U/L
Angiotensin-converting enzyme (ACE)		<670 nkat/L	<40 U/L
Anticonvulsant drug levels: see Table 360-8			
Arterial blood gases			
[HCO_3^-]		21–28 mmol/L	21–30 meq/L
P_{CO_2}		4.7–5.9 kPa	35–45 mmHg
pH		7.38–7.44	
P_{O_2}		11–13 kPa	80–100 mmHg
β-Hydroxybutyrate	P	$<300\ \mu$mol/L	<3 mg/dL
Bilirubin, total	S (Malloy-Evelyn)	5.1–17 μmol/L	0.3–1.0 mg/dL
Direct	S	1.7–5.1 μmol/L	0.1–0.3 mg/dL
Indirect	S	3.4–12 μmol/L	0.2–0.7 mg/dL
Calcium, ionized		1.1–1.4 mmol/L	4.5–5.6 mg/dL
Calcium	P	2.2–2.6 mmol/L	9–10.5 mg/dL
Carbon dioxide content	P (sea level)	21–30 mmol/L	21–30 meq/L
Carbon dioxide tension (P_{CO_2})	Arterial blood (sea level)	4.7–5.9 kPa	35–45 mmHg
Carbon monoxide content	Blood	Symptoms with 20% saturation of hemoglobin	
Chloride	S (as Cl^-)	98–106 mmol/L	98–106 meq/L
Cholesterol: see Table A-9			
Complement	S		
C3		0.55–1.20 g/L	55–120 mg/dL
C4		0.20–0.50 g/L	20–50 mg/dL
Coproporphyrins (types I and III)	U	150–460 μmol/d	100–300 μg/d
Creatine kinase	S (total)		
Females		0.17–1.17 μkat/L	10–70 U/L
Males		0.42–1.50 μkat/L	25–90 U/L
Creatine kinase-MB		0–7 μg/L	
Creatinine	S	$<133\ \mu$mol/L	<1.5 mg/dL
Erythropoietin	S	5–36 U/L	
Fatty acids, free (nonesterified)	P	180 mg/L	<18 mg/dL
Ferritin	S		
Women		10–200 μg/L	10–200 ng/mL
Men		15–400 μg/L	15–400 ng/mL
Fibrinogen: See "Hematologic Evaluations: Platelets and Coagulation Parameters"			
Fibrinogen split products: See "Hematologic Evaluations: Platelets and Coagulation Parameters"			
Glucose (fasting)	P		
Normal		4.2–6.4 mmol/L	75–115 mg/dL
Diabetes mellitus		>7.8 mmol/L	>140 mg/dL
Glucose, 2 h postprandial	P		
Normal		<7.8 mmol/L	<140 mg/dL
Impaired glucose tolerance		7.8–11.1 mmol/L	140–200 mg/dL
Diabetes mellitus		>11.1 mmol/L	>200 mg/dL
Hemoglobin	B (sea level)		
Male		140–180 g/L	14–18 g/dL
Female		120–160 g/L	12–16 g/dL
Hemoglobin A_{1c} Up to 6% of total hemoglobin			
Iron	S	9–27 μmol/L	50–150 μg/dL
Iron-binding capacity	S	45–66 μmol/L	250–370 μg/dL
Saturation		0.2–0.45	20–45%
Lactate dehydrogenase	S	1.7–3.2 μkat/L	100–190 U/L
Lactate dehydrogenase isoenzymes	S (agarose)		
Fraction 1 (of total)		0.14–0.25	14–26%
Fraction 2		0.29–0.39	29–39%
Fraction 3		0.20–0.25	20–26%
Fraction 4		0.08–0.16	8–16%
Fraction 5		0.06–0.16	6–16%

(continued)

Constituent	Specimen	Reference Range	
		SI Units	**Conventional Units**
Lactate	P, venous	0.6–1.7 mmol/L	5–15 mg/dL
Lipase	S	0–2.66 μkat/L	0–160 U/L
Lipids: see Table A-9			
Lipids, triglyceride: S see "Triglycerides"			
Lipoprotein: see Table A-9			
Lipoprotein (a)	S	0–300 mg/L	0–3 mg/dL
Magnesium	S	0.8–1.2 mmol/L	1.8–3 mg/dL
Myoglobin	S		
Male		19–92 μg/L	
Female		12–76 μg/L	
Osmolality	P	285–295 mmol/kg serum water	285–295 mosmol/kg serum water
Oxygen content	B, arterial (sea level)		17–21 vol%
	B, venous arm (sea level)		10 to 16 vol%
Oxygen percent saturation (sea level)	B, arterial	0.97 mol/mol	97%
	B, venous, arm	0.60–0.85 mol/mol	60–85%
Oxygen tension (P_{O_2})	Blood	11–13 kPa	80–100 mmHg
pH	B	7.38–7.44	
Phosphatase, acid	S	0.90 nkat/L	0–5.5 U/L
Phosphatase, alkaline	S	0.5–2.0 nkat/L	30–120 U/L
Phosphorus, inorganic	S	1.0–1.4 mmol/L	3–4.5 mg/dL
Porphobilinogen	U	None	None
Potassium	S	3.5–5.0 mmol/L	3.5–5.0 meq/L
Prostate-specific antigen (PSA)	S		
Female		<0.5 μg/L	<0.5 ng/mL
Male: <40 years		0.0–2.0 μg/L	0.0–2.0 ng/mL
≥40 years		0.0–4.0 μg/L	0.0–4.0 ng/mL
PSA, free, in males 45–75 years, with PSA values between 4 and 20 μg/mL	S	>0.25 associated with benign prostatic hyperplasia	>25% associated with benign prostatic hyperplasia
Protein, total	S	55–80 g/L	5.5–8.0 g/dL
Protein fractions	S		
Albumin		35–55 g/L	3.5–5.5 g/dL (50–60%)
Globulin		20–35 g/L	2.0–3.5 g/dL (40–50%)
Alpha$_1$		2–4 g/L	0.2–0.4 g/dL (4.2–7.2%)
Alpha$_2$		5–9 g/L	0.5–0.9 g/dL (6.8–12%)
Beta		6–11 g/L	0.6–1.1 g/dL (9.3–15%)
Gamma		7–17 g/L	0.7–1.7 g/dL (13–23%)
Pyruvate	P, venous	60–170 μmol/L	0.5–1.5 mg/dL
Sodium	S	136–145 mmol/L	136–145 meq/L
Transferrin	S	2.3–3.9 g/L	230–390 mg/dL
Triglycerides	S	<1.8 mmol/L	<160 mg/dL
Troponin I	S	0–0.4 μg/L	0–0.4 ng/mL
Troponin T	S	0–0.1 μg/L	0–0.1 ng/mL
Urea nitrogen	S	3.6–7.1 mmol/L	10–20 mg/dL
Uric acid:	S		
Men		150–480 μmol/L	2.5–8.0 mg/dL
Women		90–360 μmol/L	1.5–6.0 mg/dL
Urobilinogen	U	1.7–5.9 μmol/d	1–3.5 mg/d

NOTE: B, blood; P, plasma; S, serum; U, urine.

TABLE A-5 DRUG LEVELS

Drug	Therapeutic Range		Toxic Level	
	Conventional Units	SI Units	Conventional Units	SI Units
Acetaminophen	10–30 μg/mL	66–199 μmol/L	>200 μg/mL	>1324 μmol/L
Amikacin				
Peak	25–35 μg/mL	43–60 μmol/L	>35 μg/mL	>60 μmol/L
Trough	4–8 μg/mL	6.8–13.7 μmol/L	>10 μg/mL	>17 μmol/L
Amitriptyline	120–250 ng/mL	433–903 nmol/L	>500 ng/mL	>1805 nmol/L
Amphetamine	20–30 ng/mL	148–222 nmol/L	>200 ng/mL	>1480 nmol/L
Barbiturates, most short-acting			>20 mg/L	>88 μmol/L
Bromide			>1250 μg/mL	>15.6 mmol/L
Carbamazepine	6–12 μg/mL	26–51 μmol/L	>15 μg/mL	>63 μmol/L
Chlordiazepoxide	700–1000 ng/mL	2.34–3.34 μmol/L	>5000 ng/mL	>16.7 μmol/L
Clonazepam	15–60 ng/mL	48–190 nmol/L	>80 ng/mL	>254 nmol/L
Clozapine	200–350 ng/mL	0.6–1 μmol/L		
Cocaine	100–500 ng/mL	330–1650 nmol/L	>1000 ng/mL	>3300 nmol/L
Desipramine	75–300 ng/mL	281–1125 nmol/L	>400 ng/mL	>1500 nmol/L
Diazepam	100–1000 ng/mL	0.35–351 μmol/L	>5000 ng/mL	>17.55 μmol/L
Digoxin	0.8–2.0 ng/mL	1.0–2.6 nmol/L	>2.5 ng/mL	>3.2 umol/L
Doxepin	30–150 ng/mL	107–537 nmol/L	>500 ng/mL	>1790 nmol/L
Ethanol			>300 mg/dL	>65 mmol/L
Behavioral changes	>20 mg/dL	>4.3 mmol/L		
Legal intoxication	>80 mg/dL	>17 mmol/L		
Ethosuximide	40–100 μg/mL	283–708 μmol/L	>150 μg/mL	>1062 μmol/L
Flecainide	0.2–1.0 μg/mL	0.5–2.4 μmol/L	>1.0 μg/mL	>2.4 μmol/L
Gentamicin				
Peak	8–10 μg/mL	16.7–20.9 μmol/L	>10 μg/mL	>21 μmol/L
Trough	<2–4 μg/mL	<4.2–8.4 μmol/L	>4 μg/mL	>8.4 μmol/L
Imipramine	125–250 ng/mL	446–893 nmol/L	>500 ng/mL	>1784 nmol/L
Lidocaine	1.5–6.0 μg/mL	6.4–26 μmol/L		
CNS or cardiovascular depression			6–8 μg/mL	26–34.2 μmol/L
Seizures, obtundation, decreased cardiac output			>8 μg/mL	>34.2 μmol/L
Lithium	0.6–1.2 meq/L	0.6–1.2 nmol/L	>2 meq/L	>2 mmol/L
Methadone	100–400 ng/mL	0.32–1.29 μmol/L	>2000 ng/mL	>6.46 μmol/L
Methotrexate	Variable	Variable		
Low-dose (1–2 weeks)			>9.1 ng/mL	>20 nmol/L
High-dose (48 h)			>227 ng/mL	>0.5 μmol/L
Morphine	10–80 ng/mL	35–280 μmol/L	>200 ng/mL	>700 nmol/L
Nitroprusside (as thiocyanate)	6–29 μg/mL	103–499 μmol/L		
Nortriptyline	50–170 ng/mL	190–646 nmol/L	>500 ng/mL	>1.9 μmol/L
Phenobarbital	10–40 μg/mL	43–170 μmol/L		
Slowness, ataxia, nystagmus			35–80 μg/mL	151–345 μmol/L
Coma with reflexes			65–117 μg/mL	280–504 μmol/L
Coma without reflexes			>100 μg/mL	>430 μmol/L
Phenytoin	10–20 μg/mL	40–79 μmol/L	>20 μg/mL	>79 μmol/L
Procainamide	4–10 μg/mL	17–42 μmol/L	>10–12 μg/mL	>42–51 μmol/L
Quinidine	2–5 μg/mL	6–15 μmol/L	>6 μg/mL	>18 μmol/L
Salicylates	150–300 μg/mL	1086–2172 μmol/L	>300 μg/mL	>2172 μmol/L
Theophylline	8–20 μg/mL	44–111 μmol/L	>20 μg/mL	>110 μmol/L
Thiocyanate				
After nitroprusside infusion	6–29 μg/mL	103–499 μmol/L		
Nonsmoker	1–4 μg/mL	17–69 μmol/L	>120 μg/mL	>2064 μmol/L
Smoker	3–12 μg/mL	52–206 μmol/L		
Tobramycin				
Peak	8–10 μg/mL	17–21 μmol/L	>10 μg/mL	>21 μmol/L
Trough	<4 μg/mL	<9 μmol/L	>4 μg/mL	>9 μmol/L
Valproic acid	50–150 μg/mL	347–1040 μmol/L	>150 μg/mL	>1040 μmol/L
Vancomycin				
Peak	18–26 μg/mL	12–18 μmol/L		
Trough	5–10 μg/mL	3–7 μmol/L	>80–100 μg/mL	>55–69 μmol/L

TABLE A-6 CIRCULATORY FUNCTION TESTS

Test	Results: Reference Range SI Units (Range)	Conventional Units (Range)
Arteriovenous oxygen difference	30–50 mL/L	30–50 mL/L
Cardiac output (Fick)	2.5–3.6 L/m² of body surface area per min	2.5–3.6 L/m² of body surface area per min
Contractility indexes		
Max. left ventricular dp/dt	220 kPa/s (176–250 kPa/s)	1650 mmHg/s (1320–1880 mmHg/s)
(dp/dt)/DP when DP = 5.3 kPa (40 mmHg)(DP, diastolic pressure)	(37.6 ± 12.2)/s	(37.6 ± 12.2)/s
Mean normalized systolic ejection rate (angiography)	3.32 ± 0.84 end-diastolic volumes per second	3.32 ± 0.84 end-diastolic volumes per second
Mean velocity of circumferential fiber shortening (angiography)	1.66 ± 0.42 circumferences per second	1.66 ± 0.42 circumferences per second
Ejection fraction: stroke volume/end-diastolic volume (SV/EDV)	0.67 (0.55–0.78)	0.67 (0.55–0.78)
End-diastolic volume	75 mL/m² (60–88 mL/m²)	75 mL/m² (60–88 mL/m²)
End-systolic volume	25 mL/m² (20–33 mL/m²)	25 mL/m² (20–33 mL/m²)
Left ventricular work		
Stroke work index	30–110 (g·m)/m²	30–110 (g·m)/m²
Left ventricular minute work index	1.8–6.6 [(kg·m)/m²]/min	1.8–6.6 [(kg·m)/m²]/min
Oxygen consumption index	110–150 mL	110–150 mL

Test	Results: Reference Range SI Units (Range)	Conventional Units (Range)
Maximum oxygen uptake	35 mL/min (20–60 mL/min)	35 mL/min (20–60 mL/min)
Pulmonary vascular resistance	2–12 (kPa·s)/L	20–120 (dyn·s)/cm⁵
Systemic vascular resistance	77–150 (kPa·s)/L	770–1500 (dyn·s)/cm⁵

TABLE A-7 NORMAL VALUES OF DOPPLER ECHOCARDIOGRAPHIC MEASUREMENTS IN ADULTS

	Range	Mean
RVD (cm)	0.9 to 2.6	1.7
LVID (cm)	3.5 to 5.7	4.7
Posterior LV wall thickness (cm)	0.6 to 1.1	0.9
IVS wall thickness (cm)	0.6 to 1.1	0.9
Left atrial dimension (cm)	1.9 to 4.0	2.9
Aortic root dimension (cm)	2.0 to 3.7	2.7
Aortic cusps separation (cm)	1.5 to 2.6	1.9
Percentage of fractional shortening	34 to 44%	36%
Mitral flow (m/s)	0.6 to 1.3	0.9
Tricuspid flow (m/s)	0.3 to 0.7	0.5
Pulmonary artery (m/s)	0.6 to 0.9	0.75
Aorta (m/s)	1.0 to 1.7	1.35

NOTE: RVD, right ventricular dimension; LVID, left ventricular internal dimension; LV, left ventricle; IVS, interventricular septum.
SOURCE: From H Feigenbaum, *Echocardiography,* 5th ed, Philadelphia. Lea & Febiger, 1994

TABLE A-8 GASTROINTESTINAL TESTS. SEE ALSO "STOOL ANALYSIS"

Test	Results SI Units	Conventional Units
Absorption tests		
D-Xylose: after overnight fast, 25 g xylose given in oral aqueous solution		
Urine, collected for following 5 h	33–53 mmol (or >20% of ingested dose)	5–8 g (or >20% of ingested dose
Serum, 1 h after dose	1.7–2.7 mmol/L	25–40 mg/dL
Vitamin A: a fasting blood specimen is obtained and 200,000 units of vitamin A in oil is given orally	Serum level should rise to twice fasting level in 3–5 h	Serum level should rise to fasting level in 3–5 h
Bentiromide test (pancreatic function): 500 mg bentiromide (chymex) orally; p-aminobenzoic acid (PABA) measured		
Plasma		>3.6 (±1.1) µg/mL at 90 min
Urine	>50% recovered in 6 h	>50% recovered in 6 h
Gastric juice		
Volume		
24 h	2–3 L	2–3 L
Nocturnal	600–700 mL	600–700 mL
Basal, fasting	30–70 mL/h	30–70 mL/h
Reaction		
pH	1.6–1.8	1.6–1.8
Titratable acidity of fasting juice	4–9 µmol/s	15–35 meq/h
Acid output		
Basal		
Females (mean ± 1 SD)	0.6 ± 0.5 µmol/s	2.0 ± 1.8 meq/h
Males (mean ± 1 SD)	0.8 ± 0.6 µmol/s	3.0 ± 2.0 meq/h
Maximal (after SC histamine acid phosphate, 0.004 mg/kg body weight, and preceded by 50 mg promethazine, or after betazole, 1.7 mg/kg body weight, or pentagastrin, 6 µg/kg body weight)		
Females (mean ± 1 SD)	4.4 ± 1.4 µmol/s	16 ± 5 meq/h
Males (mean ± 1 SD)	6.4 ± 1.4 µmol/s	23 ± 5 meq/h
Basal acid output/maximal acid output ratio	≤0.6	≤0.6
Gastrin, serum	40–200 µg/L	40–200 pg/mL
Secretin test (pancreatic exocrine function): 1 unit/kg body weight, IV		
Volume (pancreatic juice) in 80 min	>2.0 mL/kg	>2.0 mL/kg
Bicarbonate concentration	>80 mmol/L	>80 meq/L
Bicarbonate output in 30 min	>10 mmol	>10 meq

A-5

Substance	Specimen	Reference Range SI Units	Reference Range Conventional Units
Adrenocorticotropin (ACTH), 8 A.M.	P	1.3–16.7 pmol/L	6.0–76.0 pg/mL
Aldosterone, 8 A.M., (patient supine, 100 mmol/L Na and 60–100 mmol/L K intake)	P	<220 pmol/L	<8 ng/dL
Aldosterone	U	14–53 nmol/d	5–19 μg/d
Androstenedione	P		
Women		3.5–7.0 nmol/L	1–2 ng/mL
Men		3.0–5.0 nmol/L	0.8–1.3 ng/mL
Angiotensin II, 8 A.M.	P	10–30 nmol/L	10–30 pg/mL
Arginine vasopressin (AVP), random fluid intake	P	1.4–5.6 pmol/L	1.5–6.0 ng/L
Calciferols (vitamin D)	P		
1,25-dihydroxyvitamin D [1,25(OH)$_2$D]		40–160 pmol/L	16–65 pg/mL
25-hydroxyvitamin D [25(OH)D]		20–200 nmol/L	8–80 ng/mL
Calcitonin	P		
Women		≤8 ng/L	≤8 pg/mL
Men		≤4 ng/L	≤4 pg/mL
Catecholamines			
Epinephrine	U	<275 nmol/d	<50 μg/d
Free	U	<590 nmol/d	<100 μg/d
Metanephrine	U	<7 μmol/d	<1.3 mg/d
Norepinephrine	U	89–473 nmol/d	15–80 μg/d
Vanillylmandelic acid (VMA)	U	<40 μmol/d	<8 mg/d
Chorionic gonadotropin, β subunit (β-hCG), men and nonpregnant women	P	<3 IU/L	<3 mIU/mL
Cortisol			
Free	U	25–140 nmol/d	10–50 μg/d
8 A.M.	P	140–690 nmol/L	5–25 μg/dL
4 P.M.	P	80–330 nmol/L	3–12 μg/dL
Dehydroepiandrosterone (DHEA)	P	7–31 nmol/L	2–9 ng/dL
11-Deoxycortisol (compound S)	P	<30 nmol/L	<1 μg/dL
DHEA sulfate	P	1.3–6.8 μmol/L	500–2500 μg/dL
Estradiol	P		
Women (higher at ovulation)		70–220 pmol/L	20–60 pg/mL
Men		<180 pmol/L	<50 pg/mL
Gastrin	S	40–200 ng/L	40–200 pg/mL
Glucagon	P	50–100 ng/L	50–100 pg/mL
Gonadotropins			
Follicle-stimulating hormone (FSH)	P		
Women			
Mature, premenopausal, except at ovulation		1.4–9.6 IU/L	1.4–9.6 mIU/mL
Ovulatory surge		2.3–21 IU/L	2.3–21 mIU/mL
Postmenopausal		34–96 IU/L	34–96 mIU/mL
Men		0.9–15 IU/L	0.9–15 mIU/mL
Luteinizing hormone (LH)	P		
Children, prepubertal		1.0–5.9 IU/L	1.0–5.9 mIU/mL
Women			
Mature, premenopausal, except at ovulation		0.8–26 IU/L	0.8–26 mIU/mL
Ovulatory surge		25–57 IU/L	25–57 mIU/mL
Postmenopausal		40–104 IU/L	40–104 mIU/mL
Men		1.3–13 IU/L	1.3–13 mIU/mL
Growth hormone, after 100 g oral glucose		<2 μg/L	<2 ng/mL
Hemoglobin A$_{1c}$	WB	0.038–0.064	3.8–6.4%
17-Hydroxycorticosteroids	U	5.5–28 μmol/d	2–10 mg/d
5-Hydroxyindoleacetic acid (5-HIAA)	U	≤31.4 μmol/d	≤6 mg/d
17-Hydroxyprogesterone	P		
Women			
Follicular phase		0.6–3 nmol/L	0.2–1.0 μg/L
Luteal phase		1.5–10.6 nmol/L	0.5–3.5 μg/L
Men		0.2–9.0 nmol/L	0.06–3.0 μg/L
Insulin, fasting	S, P	43–186 pmol/L	6–26 μU/mL
Insulin-like growth factor (somatomedin C, IGF-1/SM C)	S		
16–24 years		182–780 μg/L	182–780 ng/mL
25–39 years		114–492 μg/L	114–492 ng/mL
40–54 years		90–360 μg/L	90–360 ng/mL
>54 years		71–290 μg/L	71–290 ng/mL
17-Ketosteroids	U		
Women		20–59 μmol/d	6–17 mg/d
Men		20–69 μmol/d	6–20 mg/d
Oxytocin			
Random		1–4 pmol/L	1.25–5 ng/L
Ovulatory peak in women		4–8 pmol/L	5–10 ng/L
Parathyroid hormone	S	10–60 ng/L	10–60 pg/mL
Parathyroid hormone–related protein	P	<1.3 pmol/L	<1.3 pmol/L
Progesterone	P		
Women, luteal, peak		6–60 nmol/L	2–20 ng/mL
Men, prepubertal girls, preovulatory women, postmenopausal women		<6 nmol/L	<2 ng/mL
Prolactin	S	2–15 μg/L	2–15 ng/mL
Radioactive iodine uptake, 24 h (range varies in different areas due to variations in iodine intake)			5–30%
Renin (adult, normal-Na diet)	P		
Supine		0.08–0.83 ng/(L·s)	0.3–3.0 ng/(mL/h)
Upright		0.28–2.5 ng/(L·s)	1.0–9.0 ng/(mL/h)
Resin triiodothyronine (T$_3$)		0.25–0.35	25–35%
Reverse T$_3$ (rT$_3$)	P	0.15–0.61 nmol/L	10–40 ng/dL
Semen analysis: see Chap. 335			
T$_3$	P	1.1–2.9 nmol/L	70–190 ng/dL
Testosterone	P		
Women		<3.5 nmol/L	<1 ng/mL
Men		10–35 nmol/L	3–10 ng/mL
Prepubertal boys and girls		0.17–0.7 nmol/L	0.05–0.2 ng/mL
Thyroglobulin	S	0–60 μg/L	0–60 ng/mL
Thyroid stimulating hormone (TSH)		0.4–5.0 mU/L	0.4–5.0 μU/mL
Thyroxine (T$_4$)	SR	64–154 nmol/L	5–12 μg/dL

NOTE: P, plasma; S, serum; SR; serum radioimmunoassay; U, urine; WB, whole blood.

TABLE A-10 CLASSIFICATION OF TOTAL CHOLESTEROL, LDL-CHOLESTEROL, AND HDL-CHOLESTEROL VALUES

	Total Plasma Cholesterol		LDL-Cholesterol		HDL-Cholesterol	
	SI, mmol/L	C, mg/dL	SI, mmol/L	C, mg/dL	SI, mmol/L	C, mg/dL
Desirable	<5.2	<200	<3.36	<130	>1.55	>60
Borderline	5.20–6.18	200–239	3.36–4.11	130–159	0.9–1.55	35–60
Undesirable	≥6.21	≥240	≥4.14	≥160	<0.9	<35

NOTE: LDL, low-density lipoprotein; HDL, high-density lipoprotein; SI, SI units; C, conventional units

SOURCE: Modified from the report of the Expert Panel on Detection, Evaluation, and Treatment of High Blood Cholesterol in Adults: Second Report of the National Cholesterol Education Program (NCEP) expert panel on detection, evaluation, and treatment of high blood cholesterol (Adult Treatment Panel II). Circulation 89:1329, 1994.

TABLE A-11 VITAMINS AND TRACE MINERALS

	Specimen	Reference Range SI Units	Reference Range Conventional Units
Carotenoids	S	0.9–5.6 μmol/L	50–300 μg/dL
Ceruloplasmin	S	270–370 mg/L	27–37 ng/dL
Copper	S	11–22 μmol/L	70–140 μg/dL
Folic acid	RC	340–1020 nmol/L cells	150–450 ng/mL cells
Folic acid	S	7–36 nmol/L cells	3–16 ng/mL cells
Lead	S	<1 μmol/L	<20 μg/dL
Vitamin A	S	0.7–3.5 μmol/L	20–100 μg/dL
Vitamin B_1 (thiamine)	S	0–75 nmol/L	0–2 μg/dL
Vitamin B_2 (riboflavin)	S	106–638 nmol/L	4–24 μg/dL
Vitamin B_6	P	20–121 nmol/L	5–30 ng/ml
Vitamin B_{12}	S	148–443 pmol/L	200–600 pg/mL
Vitamin C (ascorbic acid)	S	23–57 μmol/L	0.4–1.0 mg/dL
Vitamin D_3, 1,25-dihydroxy	S	60–108 pmol/L	25–45 pg/mL
Vitamin D_3, 25-hydroxy	P		
Summer		37.4–200 nmol/L	15–80 ng/mL
Winter		34.9–105 nmol/L	14–42 ng/mL
Vitamin E	S	12–42 μmol/L	5–18 μg/mL
Zinc	S	11.5–18.5 μmol/L	75–120 μg/dL

NOTE: P, plasma; RC, red cells; S, serum.

TABLE A-12 PULMONARY FUNCTION TESTS

See Table A-19: Summary of Values Useful in Pulmonary Physiology

TABLE A-13 RENAL FUNCTION TESTS

	Reference Range SI Units	Reference Range Conventional Units
Clearances (corrected to 1.72 m² body surface area):		
Measures of glomerular filtration rate:		
Inulin clearance (Cl)		
Males (mean ± 1 SD)	2.1 ± 0.4 mL/s	124 ± 25.8 mL/min
Females (mean ± 1 SD)	2.0 ± 0.2 mL/s	119 ± 12.8 mL/min
Endogenous creatinine clearance	1.5–2.2 mL/s	91–130 mL/min
Urea	1.0–1.7 mL/s	60–100 mL/min
Measures of effective renal plasma flow and tubular function:		
p-Aminohippuric acid clearance (Cl$_{PAH}$):		
Males (mean ± 1 SD)	10.9 ± 2.7 mL/s	654 ± 163 mL/min
Females (mean ± 1 SD)	9.9 ± 1.7 mL/s	594 ± 102 mL/min
Concentration and dilution test:		
Specific gravity of urine:		
After 12-h fluid restriction	≥1.025	≥1.025
After 12-h deliberate water intake	≤1.003	≤1.003
Protein excretion, urine	<0.15 g/d	<150 mg/d
Males	0–0.06 g/d	0–60 mg/d
Females	0–0.09 g/d	0–90 mg/d
Specific gravity, maximal range	1.002–1.028	1.002–1.028
Tubular reabsorption, phosphorus	0.79–0.94 of filtered load	79–94% of filtered load

TABLE A-14   HEMATOLOGIC EVALUATIONS. SEE ALSO "CHEMICAL CONSTITUENTS OF BLOOD"

	Reference Range			Reference Range	
	SI Units	Conventional Units		SI Units	Conventional Units
Bone marrow: see Table A-6			Platelets and coagulation parameters:		
Carboxyhemoglobin			Alpha$_2$ antiplasmin		70–130%
Nonsmoker	0–0.023	0–2.3%	Antithrombin III		80–120%
Smoker	0.021–0.042	2.1–4.2%	Bleeding time (Simplate)	<7 min	<7 min
Erythrocyte			Euglobulin lysis time	>2 h	>2 h
Count	4.15–4.90 × 10^{12}/L	4.15–4.90 × 10^6/mm^3	Factor II		60–100%
			Factor V		60–100%
Distribution width	0.13–0.15	13–15%	Factor VII		60–100%
Glucose-6-phosphate dehydrogenase	0.78 ± 0.13 MU/mol Hb	12.1 ± 2 IU/g Hb	Factor IX		60–100%
Life span			Factor X		60–100%
Normal survival	120 days	120 days	Factor XI		60–100%
Chromium-labeled, half-life ($t_{1/2}$)	28 days	28 days	Factor XII		60–100%
			Factor XIII		60–100%
Mean corpuscular hemoglobin (MCH)	28–33 pg/cell	28–33 pg/cell	Fibrinogen	2–4 g/L	200–400 mg/dL
Mean corpuscular hemoglobin concentration (MCHC)	320–360 g/L	32–36 g/dL	Plasminogen		2.4–4.4 CTA U/mL
			Protein C (antigenic assay)		58–148%
Mean corpuscular volume (MCV)	86–98 fl	86–98 μm^3	Protein S (antigenic assay)		58–148%
Ham's test (acid serum)	Negative	Negative	Partial thromboplastin time (activated PTT) comparable to control		
Haptoglobin (serum)	0.5–2.2 g/L	50–220 mg/dL	Prothrombin time (quick one-stage) control ± 1 s		
Hematocrit					
Males	0.42–0.52	42–52%	Platelets	130–400 × 10^9/L	130,000–400,000/mm^3
Females	0.37–0.48	37–48%			
Hemoglobin			Thrombin time control ± 3 s		
Plasma	0.01–0.05 g/L	1–5 mg/dL	von Willebrand's antigen		60–150%
Whole blood			Protoporphyrin, free erythrocyte (FEP)	0.28–0.64 μmol/L of red blood cells	16–36 μg/dL of red blood cells
Males	8.1–11.2 mmol/L	13–18 g/dL			
Females	7.4–9.9 mmol/L	12–16 g/dL			
Hemoglobin A$_2$ (HbA$_2$)	0.015–0.035	1.5–3.5%			
Hemoglobin, fetal (HbF)	<0.02	<2%	Red cells: see "Erythrocytes"		
Leukocytes			Schilling test, orally administered vitamin B$_{12}$ excreted in urine		7–40%
Alkaline phosphatase (LAP)	0.2–1.6 μkat/L	13–100 μ/L			
Count	4.3–10.8 × 10^9/L	4.3–10.8 × 10^3/mm^3	Sedimentation rate		
			Westergren, <50 years of age		
Differential			Males		0–15 mm/h
Neutrophils	0.45–0.74	45–74%	Females		0–20 mm/h
Bands	0–0.04	0–4%	Westergren, >50 years of age		
Lymphocytes	0.16–0.45	16–45%	Males		0–20 mm/h
Monocytes	0.04–0.10	4–10%	Females		0–30 mm/h
Eosinophils	0–0.07	0–7%	Sucrose hemolysis	Negative	Negative
Basophils	0–0.02	0–2%	Viscosity		
T cells: see Chap. 309			Plasma	1.7–2.1	1.7–2.1
Methemoglobin: <2 mg/L (<2 μg/mL)			Serum	1.4–1.8	1.4–1.8
Osmotic fragility			White blood cells: see "Leukocytes"		
Slight hemolysis		0.45–0.39%			
Complete hemolysis	0.33–0.30%				

TABLE A-15   DIFFERENTIAL NUCLEATED CELL COUNTS OF BONE MARROW

	Normal, Mean%[a]	Range, %[b]		Normal, Mean%[a]	Range, %[b]
Myeloid	56.7		Erythroid	25.6	
Neutrophilic series	53.6		Pronormoblasts	0.6	0.2–1.3
Myeloblast	0.9	0.2–1.5	Basophilic normoblasts	1.4	0.5–2.4
Promyelocyte	3.3	2.1–4.1	Polychromatophilic normoblasts	21.6	17.9–29.2
Myelocyte	12.7	8.2–15.7			
Metamyelocyte	15.9	9.6–24.6	Orthochromatic normoblasts	2.0	0.4–4.6
Band	12.4	9.5–15.3	Megakaryocytes	<0.1	
Segmented			Lymphoreticular	17.8	
Eosinophilic series	3.1	1.2–5.3	Lymphocytes	16.2	11.1–23.2
Basophilic series	<0.1	0–0.2	Plasma cells	2.3	0.4–3.9
			Reticulum cells	0.3	0–0.9

[a] From MM Wintrobe et al, *Clinical Hematology,* 8th ed. Philadelphia, Lea & Febiger, 1981.
[b] Range observed in 12 healthy men.

	Specimen	Reference Range	
		SI Units	Conventional Units
α_2 Antitrypsin (adult)	S	0.76–1.89 g/L	76–189 mg/dL
Antiglomerular basement membrane antibodies	S		
Qualitative		Negative	Negative
Quantitative		<5 kU/L	<5 U/mL
Antineutrophil cytoplasmic autoantibodies, cytoplasmic (C-ANCA)	S		
Qualitative		Negative	Negative
Quantitative (antibodies to proteinase 3)		<2.8 kU/L	<2.8 U/mL
Antineutrophil cytoplasmic autoantibodies, perinuclear (P-ANCA)	S		
Qualitative		Negative	Negative
Quantitative (antibodies to myeloperoxidase)		<1.4 kU/L	<1.4 U/mL
Autoantibodies			
Antiadrenal antibody	S	NA	Negative at 1:10 dilution
Anti-double-stranded (native) DNA	S	NA	Negative at 1:10 dilution
Antigranulocyte antibody	S	NA	Negative
Anti-Jo-1 antibody	S	NA	Negative
Anti-La antibody	S	NA	Negative
Antimitochondrial antibody	S	NA	Negative
Antinuclear antibody	S	NA	Negative at 1:40 dilution
Antiparietal cell antibody	S	NA	Negative at 1:20 dilution
Anti-Ro antibody	S	NA	Negative
Anti-RNP antibody	S	NA	Negative
Anti-Scl-70 antibody	S	NA	Negative
Anti-Smith antibody	S	NA	Negative
Anti-smooth-muscle antibody	S	NA	Negative at 1:20 dilution
Antithyroglobulin antibody	S	NA	Negative
Antithyroid antibody	S	<0.3 kIU/L	<0.3 IU/mL
Bence Jones protein	S	NA	None detected
Qualitative	U	NA	None detected in a 50-fold concentration
Quantitative	U		
Kappa		<0.03 g/L	<2.5 mg/dL
Lambda		<0.05 g/L	<5.0 mg/dL
C1 esterase-inhibitor protein	S		
Antigenic		0.12–0.25 g/L	12.4–24.5 mg/dL
Functional		Present	Present
Complement			
C3 (adult)	S	0.86–1.84 g/L	86–184 mg/dL
C4 (adult)	S	0.20–0.58 g/L	20–58 mg/dL
Total complement (adult)	S	63–145 kU/L	63–145 U/mL
Factor B	S	0.17–0.42 g/L	17–42 mg/dL
Cryoproteins	S	NA	None detected
CSF	CSF		
Agarose electrophoresis		NA	No banding seen in an 80-fold concentration
Quantitation of albumin (adult)		0.11–0.51 g/L	11.0–50.9 mg/dL
Quantitation of IgG (adult)		0.0–0.08 g/L	0.0–8.0 mg/dL
Immunoglobulins	S		
IgA		0.9–3.2 g/L	90–325 mg/dL
IgD		0–0.08 g/L	0–8 mg/dL
IgE		<0.00025 g/L	<0.025 mg/dL
IgG		8.0–15.0 g/L	800–1500 mg/dL
IgM		0.45–1.5 g/L	45–150 mg/dL
Rheumatoid factor	S, JF	<30 kIU/L	<30 IU/mL
Serum protein electrophoresis	S	NA	Normal pattern
T cells: see Chap. 309			
Viscosity	S	1.4–1.8 relative viscosity units, as compared with water	1.4–1.8 relative viscosity units, as compared with water

NOTE: CSF, cerebrospinal fluid; JF, joint fluid; S, serum; U, urine; NA, not applicable.   SOURCE: Adapted from A Kratz, KB Lewandrowski: N Engl J Med 339:1063, 1998.

TABLE A-17 STOOL ANALYSIS

	Reference Range	
	SI Units	Conventional Units
Bulk		
Wet weight	<197.5 (115 ± 41)g/d	<197.5 (115 ± 41) g/d
Dry weight	<66.4 (34 ± 15) g/d	<66.4 (34 ± 15) g/d
α_1 Antitrypsin	0.98 (±0.17) mg/g dry weight	0.98 (±0.17) mg/g dry weight
Coproporphyrin	600–1500 nmol/d	400–1000 µg/d
Fat (on diet containing at least 50 g fat), measured on a ≥ 3-day collection		
Fat		
Percent of dry weight	<0.30	<30.4%
Coefficient of fat absorption	>0.95	>95%
Fatty acid		
Free	0.01–0.10	1–10% of dry matter
Combined as soap	0.005–0.12	0.5–12% of dry matter
Nitrogen	<1.7 (1.4 ± 0.2) g/d	<1.7 (1.4 ± 0.2) g/d
Protein content	Minimal	Minimal
Urobilinogen	68–470 µmol/d	40–280 mg/d
Water	~0.65	~65%

TABLE A-18 URINE ANALYSIS

	Reference Range	
	SI Units	Conventional Units
Acidity, titratable	20–40 mmol/d	20–40 meq/d
Ammonia	30–50 mmol/d	30–50 meq/d
Amylase		4–400 U/L
Amylase/creatinine clearance ratio [(Cl$_{am}$/Cl$_{cr}$) × 100]	1–5	1–5
Calcium (10 meq/d or 200-mg/d dietary calcium)	<7.5 mmol/d	<300 mg/d
Creatine, as creatinine		
Women	<760 µmol/d	<100 mg/d
Men	<380 µmol/d	<50 mg/d
Creatinine	8.8–14 mmol/d	1.0–1.6 g/d
Glucose, true (oxidase method)	0.3–1.7 mmol/d	50–300 mg/d
5-Hydroxyindoleacetic acid (5-HIAA)	10–47 µmol/d	2–9 mg/d
Protein	<0.15 g/d	<150 mg/d
Potassium (varies with intake)	25–100 mmol/d	25–100 meq/d
Sodium (varies with intake)	100–260 mmol/d	100–260 meq/d

TABLE A-19 SUMMARY OF VALUES USEFUL IN PULMONARY PHYSIOLOGY

		Typical Values	
	Symbol	Man Aged 40, 75 kg, 175 cm Tall	Woman Aged 40, 60 kg, 160 cm Tall
PULMONARY MECHANICS			
Spirometry—volume-time curves			
Forced vital capacity	FVC	4.8 L	3.3 L
Forced expiratory volume in 1 s	FEV$_1$	3.8 L	2.8 L
FEV$_1$/FVC	FEV$_1$%	76%	77%
Maximal midexpiratory flow	MMF (FEF 25–27)	4.8 L/s	3.6 L/s
Maximal expiratory flow rate	MEFR (FEF 200–1200)	9.4 L/s	6.1 L/s
Spirometry—flow-volume curves			
Maximal expiratory flow at 50% of expired vital capacity	V$_{max}$ 50 (FEF 50%)	6.1 L/s	4.6 L/s
Maximal expiratory flow at 75% of expired vital capacity	V$_{max}$ 75 (FEF 75%)	3.1 L/s	2.5 L/s
Resistance to airflow:			
Pulmonary resistance	RL (R$_L$)	<3.0 (cmH$_2$O/s)/L	
Airway resistance	Raw	<2.5 (cmH$_2$O/s)/L	
Specific conductance	SGaw	>0.13 cmH$_2$O/s	
Pulmonary compliance			
Static recoil pressure at total lung capacity	Pst TLC	25 ± 5 cmH$_2$O	
Compliance of lungs (static)	CL	0.2 L cmH$_2$O	
Compliance of lungs and thorax	C(L + T)	0.1 L cmH$_2$O	
Dynamic compliance of 20 breaths per minute	C dyn 20	0.25 ± 0.05 L/cmH$_2$O	
Maximal static respiratory pressures:			
Maximal inspiratory pressure	MIP	>90 cmH$_2$O	>50 cmH$_2$O
Maximal expiratory pressure	MEP	>150 cmH$_2$O	>120 cmH$_2$O
LUNG VOLUMES			
Total lung capacity	TLC	6.4 L	4.9 L
Functional residual capacity	FRC	2.2 L	2.6 L
Residual volume	RV	1.5 L	1.2 L
Inspiratory capacity	IC	4.8 L	3.7 L
Expiratory reserve volume	ERV	3.2 L	2.3 L
Vital capacity	VC	1.7 L	1.4 L
GAS EXCHANGE (SEA LEVEL)			
Arterial O$_2$ tension	Pa$_{O_2}$	12.7 ± 0.7 kPa (95 ± 5 mmHg)	
Arterial CO$_2$ tension	Pa$_{CO_2}$	5.3 ± 0.3 kPa (40 ± 2 mmHg)	
Arterial O$_2$ saturation	Sa$_{O_2}$	0.97 ± 0.02 (97 ± 2%)	
Arterial blood pH	pH	7.40 ± 0.02	
Arterial bicarbonate	HCO$_3$$^-$	24 + 2 meq/L	
Base excess	BE	0 ± 2 meq/L	
Diffusing capacity for carbon monoxide (single breath)	DL$_{CO}$	0.42 mLCO/s/mmHg (25 mL CO/min/mmHg)	
Dead space volume	V$_D$	2 ml/kg body wt	
Physiologic dead space; dead space-tidal volume ratio	V$_D$/V$_T$		
Rest		≤35% V$_T$	
Exercise		≤20% V$_T$	
Alveolar-arterial difference for O$_2$	P(A − a)$_{O_2}$	≤2.7 kPa ≤20 kPa (≤20 mmHg)	

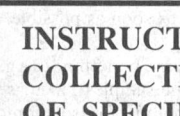

INSTRUCTIONS FOR COLLECTION AND TRANSPORT OF SPECIMENS FOR CULTURE

It is absolutely essential that the microbiology laboratory be informed of the site of origin of the sample to be cultured and of the infections that are suspected. This information determines the selection of culture media and the length of culture time.

Type of Culture (Synonyms)	Specimen	Minimum Volume	Container	Other Considerations
BLOOD				
Blood, routine (blood culture for aerobes, anaerobes, and yeasts)	Whole blood	10 mL in each of 2 bottles for adults and children; 5 mL, if possible, in each of 2 bottles for infants; less for neonates	See below.*a*	See below.*b*
Blood for fungi/*Mycobacterium* spp.	Whole blood	10 mL in each of 2 bottles, as for routine blood cultures, or in Isolator tube requested from laboratory	Same as for routine blood culture	Specify "hold for extended incubation," since fungal agents may require 4 weeks or more to grow.
Blood, Isolator (lysis centrifugation)	Whole blood	10 mL	Isolator tubes	Use mainly for isolation of fungi, *Mycobacterium*, or other fastidious aerobes and for elimination of antibiotics from cultured blood in which organisms are concentrated by centrifugation.
RESPIRATORY TRACT				
Nose	Swab from nares	1 swab	Sterile culturette or similar transport system containing holding medium	Swabs made of calcium alginate may be used.
Throat	Swab of posterior pharynx, ulcerations, or areas of suspected purulence	1 swab	Sterile culturette or similar swab specimen collection system containing holding medium	See below.*c*
Sputum	Fresh sputum (not saliva)	2 mL	Commercially available sputum collection system or similar sterile container with screw cap	*Cause for rejection:* Care must be taken to ensure that the specimen is sputum and not saliva. Examination of Gram's stain, with number of epithelial cells and PMNs noted, can be an important part of the evaluation process. Induced sputum specimens should not be rejected.
Bronchial aspirates	Transtracheal aspirate, bronchoscopy specimen, or bronchial aspirate	1 mL of aspirate or brush in transport medium	Sterile aspirate or bronchoscopy tube, bronchoscopy brush in a separate sterile container	Special precautions may be required, depending on diagnostic considerations (e.g., *Pneumocystis*).
STOOL				
Stool for routine culture; stool for *Salmonella, Shigella,* and *Campylobacter*	Rectal swab or (preferably) fresh, randomly collected stool	1 g of stool or 2 rectal swabs	Plastic-coated cardboard cup or plastic cup with tight-fitting lid. Other leak-proof containers are also acceptable.	If *Vibrio* spp. are suspected, the laboratory must be notified, and appropriate collection/transport methods should be used.
Stool for *Yersinia, E. coli* O157	Fresh, randomly collected stool	1 g	Plastic-coated cardboard cup or plastic cup with tight-fitting lid	*Limitations:* Procedure requires enrichment techniques.
Stool for *Aeromonas* and *Plesiomonas*	Fresh, randomly collected stool	1 g	Plastic-coated cardboard cup or plastic cup with tight-fitting lid	*Limitations:* Stool should not be cultured for these organisms unless also cultured for other enteric pathogens.
UROGENITAL TRACT				
Urine	Clean-voided urine specimen or urine collected by catheter	0.5 mL	Sterile, leak-proof container with screw cap or special urine transfer tube	See below.*d*
Urogenital secretions	Vaginal or urethral secretions, cervical swabs, uterine fluid, prostatic fluid, etc.	1 swab or 0.5 mL of fluid	Transwab containing Amies transport medium or similar system containing holding medium for *Neisseria gonorrhoeae;* modified Todd-Hewitt broth for group B *Streptococcus* surveillance cultures	Vaginal swab samples for "routine culture" should be discouraged whenever possible unless a particular pathogen is suspected. For detection of multiple organisms (e.g., group B *Streptococcus, Trichomonas, Chlamydia,* or *Candida* spp.), 1 swab per test should be obtained.

(continued)

Cerebrospinal fluid (lumbar puncture)	Spinal fluid	1 mL for routine cultures; ≥5 mL for *Mycobacterium*	Sterile tube with tight-fitting cap	Do not refrigerate; transfer to laboratory as soon as possible.
Body fluids	Aseptically aspirated body fluids	1 mL for routine cultures	Sterile tube with tight-fitting cap. Specimen may be left in syringe used for collection if the syringe is capped before transport.	For some body fluids (e.g., peritoneal lavage samples), increased volumes are helpful for isolation of small numbers of bacteria.
Biopsy and aspirated materials	Tissue removed at surgery, bone, anticoagulated bone marrow, biopsy samples, or other specimens from normally sterile areas	1 mL of fluid or a 1-g piece of tissue	Sterile "culturette"-type swab or similar transport system containing holding medium. Sterile bottle or jar should be used for tissue specimens.	Accurate identification of specimen and source is critical. Enough tissue should be collected for both microbiologic and histopathologic evaluations.
Wounds	Purulent material or abscess contents obtained from wound or abscess without contamination by normal microflora	2 swabs or 0.5 mL of aspirated pus	Culturette swab or similar transport system or sterile tube with tight-fitting screw cap. For simultaneous anaerobic cultures, send specimen in anaerobic transport device or closed syringe.	*Collection:* Abscess contents or other fluids should be collected in a syringe (see above) when possible to provide an adequate sample volume and an anaerobic environment.

SPECIAL RECOMMENDATIONS

Fungi	Specimen types listed above may be used. When urine or sputum is cultured for fungi, a first morning specimen is usually preferred.	1 mL or as specified above for individual listing of specimens. Large volumes may be useful for urinary fungi.	Sterile, leak-proof container with tight-fitting cap	*Collection:* Specimen should be transported to microbiology laboratory within 1 h of collection. Contamination with normal flora from skin, rectum, vaginal tract, or other body surfaces should be avoided.
Mycobacterium (acid-fast bacilli)	Sputum, tissue, urine, body fluids	10 mL of fluid or small piece of tissue. Swabs should not be used.	Sterile container with tight-fitting cap	Detection of *Mycobacterium* spp. is improved by use of concentration techniques. Smears and cultures of pleural, peritoneal, and pericardial fluids often have low yields. Multiple cultures from the same patient are encouraged. Culturing in liquid media shortens the time to detection.
Legionella	Pleural fluid, lung biopsy, bronchoalveolar lavage fluid, bronchial/transbronchial biopsy. Rapid transport to laboratory is critical.	1 mL of fluid; any size tissue sample, although a 0.5-g sample should be obtained when possible	—	
Anaerobic organisms	Aspirated specimens from abscesses or body fluids	1 mL of aspirated fluid or 2 swabs	An appropriate anaerobic transport device is required.[e]	Specimens cultured for obligate anaerobes should be cultured for facultative bacteria as well.
Viruses[f]	Respiratory secretions, wash aspirates from respiratory tract, nasal swabs, blood samples (including buffy coats), vaginal and rectal swabs, swab specimens from suspicious skin lesions, stool samples (in some cases)	1 mL of fluid, 1 swab, or 1 g of stool in each appropriate transport medium	Fluid or stool samples in sterile containers or swab samples in viral culturette devices (kept on ice but not frozen) are generally suitable. Plasma samples and buffy coats in sterile collection tubes should be kept at 4 to 8°C. If specimens are to be shipped or kept for a long time, freezing at −80°C is usually adequate.	Most samples for culture are transported in holding medium containing antibiotics to prevent bacterial overgrowth and viral inactivation. Many specimens should be kept cool but not frozen, provided they are transported promptly to the laboratory. Procedures and transport media vary with the agent to be cultured and the duration of transport.

[a] For samples from adults and children, two bottles (smaller for pediatric samples) should be used: one with dextrose phosphate, tryptic soy, or another appropriate broth and the other with thioglycollate or another broth containing reducing agents appropriate for isolation of obligate anaerobes. For special situations (e.g., suspected fungal infection, culture-negative endocarditis, or mycobacteremia), different blood collection systems may be used (Isolator systems; see table).

[b] *Collection:* An appropriate disinfecting technique should be used on both the bottle septum and the patient. Do not allow air bubbles to get into anaerobic broth bottles. *Special considerations:* There is no more important clinical microbiology test than the detection of blood-borne pathogens. The rapid identification of bacterial and fungal agents is a major determinant of patients' survival. Bacteria may be present in blood either continuously (as in endocarditis, overwhelming sepsis, and the early stages of salmonellosis and brucellosis) or intermittently (as in most other bacterial infections, in which bacteria are shed into the blood on a sporadic basis). Most blood culture systems employ two separate bottles containing broth medium: one that is vented in the laboratory for the growth of facultative and aerobic organisms and a second that is maintained under anaerobic conditions. In cases of suspected continuous bacteremia/fungemia, two or three samples should be drawn before the start of therapy, with additional sets obtained if fastidious organisms are thought to be involved. For intermittent bacteremia, two or three samples should be obtained at least 1 h apart during the first 24 h.

[c] Normal microflora includes alpha-hemolytic streptococci, saprophytic *Neisseria* spp., diphtheroids, and *Staphylococcus* spp. Aerobic culture of the throat ("routine") includes

screening for and identification of beta-hemolytic *Streptococcus* spp. and other potentially pathogenic organisms. Although considered components of the normal microflora, organisms such as *Staphylococcus aureus*, *Haemophilus influenzae*, and *Streptococcus pneumoniae* will be identified by most laboratories, if requested. When *Neisseria gonorrhoeae* or *Corynebacterium diphtheriae* is suspected, a special culture request is recommended.

[d] (1) Clean-voided specimens, midvoid specimens, and Foley or indwelling catheter specimens that yield ≥50,000 organisms/mL and from which no more than three species are isolated should have organisms identified. (2) Straight-catheterized, bladder-tap, and similar urine specimens should undergo a complete workup (identification and susceptibility testing) for all potentially pathogenic organisms, regardless of colony count. (3) Certain clinical problems (e.g., acute dysuria in women) may warrant identification and susceptibility testing of isolates present at concentrations of <50,000 organisms/mL.

[e] Aspirated specimens in capped syringes or other transport devices designed to limit oxygen exposure are suitable for the cultivation of obligate anaerobes. A variety of commercially available transport devices may be used. Contamination of specimens with normal microflora from the skin, rectum, vaginal vault, or another body site should be avoided. Collection containers for aerobic culture (such as dry swabs) and inappropriate specimens (such as refrigerated samples; expectorated sputum; stool; gastric aspirates; and vaginal, throat, nose, and rectal swabs) should be rejected as unsuitable.

[f] Laboratories generally use diverse methods to detect viral agents, and the specific requirements for each specimen should be checked before a sample is sent.

Bold number indicates the start of the main discussion of the topic; numbers with "f" and "t" refer to figure and table pages; italic roman numerals refer to the Color Atlas plates.

ISBN 0-07-007272-8
90000

9 780070 072725

BRAUNWALD/U.S.
SINGLE VOL.

TOPICAL CONTENTS